EDITED BY

LEE GOLDMAN, MD

Executive Vice President for Health and Biomedical Sciences
Columbia University
Dean, Faculties of Health Sciences and Medicine
Columbia University Medical Center
New York, New York

DENNIS AUSIELLO, MD

Jackson Professor of Medicine
Harvard Medical School
Physician-in-Chief
Massachusetts General Hospital
Boston, Massachusetts

SAUNDERS

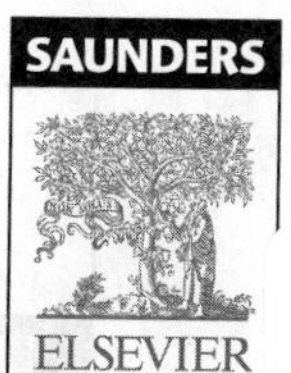

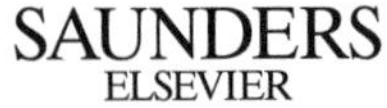

1600 John F. Kennedy Boulevard
Suite 1800
Philadelphia, PA 19103

CECIL MEDICINE, 23rd EDITION

ISBN: 978-1-4160-2805-5 (Expert Consult)
978-1-4160-4478-9 (Expert Consult Premium Ed.)
978-0-8089-2377-0 (International Ed.)

Notice

Knowledge and best practice in this field are constantly changing. As new research and experience broaden our knowledge, changes in practice, treatment, and drug therapy may become necessary or appropriate. Readers are advised to check the most current information provided (i) on procedures featured or (ii) by the manufacturer of each product to be administered to verify the recommended dose or formula, the method and duration of administration, and contraindications. It is the responsibility of practitioners, relying on their own experience and knowledge of their patients, to make diagnoses, to determine dosages and the best treatment for each individual patient, and to take all appropriate safety precautions. To the fullest extent of the law, neither the Publisher nor the Editors assume any liability for any injury and/or damage to persons or property arising out of or related to any use of the material contained in this book.

The Publisher

Library of Congress Cataloging-in-Publication Data

Cecil medicine / [edited by] Lee Goldman, Dennis Ausiello.—23rd ed.
p. ; cm.
Includes bibliographical references and index.
ISBN 987-1-4160-2805-5 [Expert Consult]; 978-1-4160-4478-9 [Expert Consult Premium Ed.]; 978-0-8089-2377-0 [International Ed.]
1. Internal medicine. I. Cecil, Russell L. (Russell La Fayette), 1881–1965. II. Goldman, Lee, MD. III. Ausiello, D. A. IV. Title: Textbook of medicine.
[DNLM: 1. Medicine. WB 100 C38888 2008]
RC46.C423 2007
616–dc22 2006047505

Publishing Director: Kimberly Murphy
Senior Acquisitions Editor: Rolla Couchman
Developmental Editor: Heather Krehling
Publishing Services Manager: Frank Polizzano
Project Manager: Lee Ann Draud
Design Direction: Steve Stave

Printed in the United States of America

Last digit is the print number: 9 8 7 6 5 4 3 2 1

Associate Editors

WILLIAM P. AREND, MD
Endowed Chair in Rheumatology
University of Colorado School of Medicine
Aurora, Colorado

Principles of Immunology and Inflammation
Diseases of Allergy and Clinical Immunology
Rheumatic Disease

JAMES O. ARMITAGE, MD
Professor, Internal Medicine, Section of Hematology & Oncology
University of Nebraska College of Medicine
Section of Hematology and Oncology
University of Nebraska Medical Center
Omaha, Nebraska

Hematologic Diseases
Oncology

DAVID R. CLEMMONS, MD
Chief, Division of Endocrinology and Metabolism
Sarah Graham Kenan Professor of Medicine
University of North Carolina at Chapel Hill School of Medicine
Chapel Hill, North Carolina

Metabolic Diseases
Nutritional Diseases
Endocrine Diseases
Women's Health
Diseases of Bone and Mineral Metabolism

JEFFREY M. DRAZEN, MD
Distinguished Parker B. Francis Professor of Medicine
Harvard Medical School
Senior Physician
Brigham and Women's Hospital
Editor-in-Chief
New England Journal of Medicine
Boston, Massachusetts

Respiratory Diseases
Critical Care Medicine

ROBERT C. GRIGGS, MD
Professor and Chair of Neurology, Professor of Medicine, Pediatrics, and Pathology and Laboratory Medicine
University of Rochester School of Medicine and Dentistry
Neurologist-in-Chief
Strong Memorial Hospital
Rochester, New York

Neurology

NICHOLAS LaRUSSO, MD
Chair, Department of Internal Medicine
Charles H. Weinman Endowed Professor of Medicine and Biochemistry/Molecular Biology
Distinguished Investigator of the Mayo Foundation
Division of Gastroenterology
Mayo Clinic College of Medicine
Rochester, Minnesota

Gastrointestinal Diseases
Diseases of the Liver, Gallbladder, and Bile Ducts

Coordinating Editors

ELIZABETH FOSTER, Ed.M
Massachusetts General Hospital
Boston, Massachusetts

JANE NEWMAN, MA
Teaching Associate
Harvard Medical School
Director of Special Projects
Department of Medicine
Massachusetts General Hospital
Boston, Massachusetts

Preface

The 23rd Edition of *Cecil Medicine* symbolizes a time of extraordinary advances in medicine and in technological innovations for the dissemination of information. This textbook and its associated electronic products incorporate the latest medical knowledge in formats that are designed to appeal to learners who prefer to access information in a variety of ways.

The contents of *Cecil* have remained true to the tradition of a comprehensive textbook of medicine that carefully explains the *why* (the underlying normal physiology and pathophysiology of disease, now at the cellular and molecular as well as the organ level) and the *how* (now frequently based on Grade A evidence from randomized controlled trials). Descriptions of physiology and pathophysiology include the latest genetic advances in a practical format that strives to be useful to the nonexpert. Medicine has entered an era when the acuity of illness and the limited time available to evaluate a patient have diminished the ability of physicians to satisfy their intellectual curiosity. As a result, the acquisition of information, quite easily achieved in this era, is often confused with knowledge. We have attempted to counteract this tendency with a textbook that not only informs but also stimulates new questions and gives a glimpse of the future path to new knowledge. Grade A evidence is specifically highlighted in the text and referenced at the end of each chapter. In addition to the information provided in the textbook, the Cecil website supplies expanded content and functionality. In many cases, the full articles referenced in each chapter can be accessed from the Cecil website. The website is also continuously updated to incorporate subsequent Grade A information, other evidence, and new discoveries.

The sections for each organ system begin with a chapter that summarizes an approach to patients with key symptoms, signs, or laboratory abnormalities associated with dysfunction of that organ system. As summarized in Table 1–1, the text specifically provides clear, concise information regarding how a physician should approach more than 100 common symptoms, signs, and laboratory abnormalities, usually with a flow diagram or a table, or both, for easy reference. In this way, *Cecil* remains a comprehensive text to guide diagnosis and therapy, not only for patients with suspected or known diseases but also for patients who may have undiagnosed abnormalities that require an initial evaluation.

Just as each edition brings new authors, it also reminds us of our gratitude to past editors and authors. Previous editors of *Cecil Medicine* include a short but remarkably distinguished group of leaders of American medicine: Russell Cecil, Paul Beeson, Walsh McDermott, James Wyngaarden, Lloyd H. Smith, Jr., Fred Plum, and J. Claude Bennett. As we welcome two new associate editors—David Clemmons and Nicholas LaRusso—we also express our appreciation to Don W. Powell, Gordon N. Gill, and W. Michael Scheld, editors from the previous edition on whose foundation we have built. We also would like to thank Steven Calderwood and Scott Hammer, who served as consulting editors for the Infectious Diseases and HIV/AIDS sections for this edition. Our returning associate editors—William P. Arend, James O. Armitage, Jeffrey M. Drazen, and Robert C. Griggs—continue to make critical contributions to the selection of authors and the review and approval of all manuscripts. The editors, however, are fully responsible for the book as well as the integration among chapters.

The tradition of *Cecil Medicine* is that all chapters are written by distinguished experts in each field. We are also most grateful for the editorial assistance in San Francisco of Deborah Airo and Vida Lynum. In addition to editorial support, Jane Newman and Elizabeth Foster in Boston brought us into the current century by developing a web-based manuscript submission system that consolidated workflow for both authors and editors, making our jobs much easier. These individuals have shown extraordinary dedication and equanimity in working with authors and editors to manage the unending flow of manuscripts, figures, and permissions. We thank Margaret Chesney, who helped update Chapter 36 during Dr. Stephen Straus's terminal illness. We also thank Benjamin Lebwohl, Kirsten O. Healy, Elizabeth C. Verna, and Shepard Weiner for their assistance with the Grade A references and Suggested Readings. At Elsevier, Rolla Couchman, Heather Krehling, Lee Ann Draud, and Frank Polizzano have been critical to the planning and production process under the direction of Kimberly Murphy. Many of the clinical photographs were supplied by Charles D. Forbes and William F. Jackson, authors of *Color Atlas and Text of Clinical Medicine*, Third Edition, published in 2003 by Elsevier Science Ltd. We thank them for graciously permitting us to include their pictures in our book. We have been exposed to remarkable physicians in our lifetimes and would like to acknowledge the mentorship and support of several of those who exemplify this paradigm—George DeVito, John Ausiello, Robert H. Gifford, and Lloyd H. Smith, Jr. Finally, we would like to thank our families—Jill, Jeff, Abigail, Daniel, and Robyn Goldman, and the Ausiello famiglia and its newest member, Mia—for their understanding of the time and focus required to edit a book that attempts to sustain the tradition of our predecessors and to meet the needs of today's physician.

LEE GOLDMAN, MD
DENNIS AUSIELLO, MD

Contents

Section XXIV: Human Immunodeficiency Virus and the Acquired Immunodeficiency Syndrome

Contributors

Nezam H. Afdhal, MD
Associate Professor of Medicine, Harvard Medical School; Chief of Hepatology, Beth Israel Deaconess Medical Center, Boston, Massachusetts
Diseases of the Gallbladder and Bile Ducts

Masood Akhtar, MD
Clinical Professor of Medicine, University of Wisconsin School of Medicine and Public Health; Section Head, Cardiovascular Disease Section, and Director, Clinical Cardiac Electrophysiology and Cardiovascular Disease Fellowship, Aurora Sinai Medical Center; Director, Arrhythmia Service, Milwaukee Heart Institute, Milwaukee, Wisconsin
Cardiac Arrhythmias with Supraventricular Origin

Cem Akin, MD, PhD
Assistant Professor of Medicine, Department of Internal Medicine, Division of Allergy and Immunology, University of Michigan Medical School, Ann Arbor, Michigan
Mastocytosis

Ban Mishu Allos, MD
Assistant Professor of Medicine and Preventive Medicine, Vanderbilt University School of Medicine, Nashville, Tennessee
Campylobacter *Infections*

David Altshuler, MD, PhD
Associate Professor of Genetics and of Medicine, Harvard Medical School; Department of Molecular Biology, Center of Human Genetic Research and Diabetes Unit, Massachusetts General Hospital; Director, Program in Medical and Population Genetics, Broad Institute of Harvard and Massachusetts Institute of Technology, Boston, Massachusetts
The Inherited Basis of Common Diseases

Michael J. Aminoff, MD, DSc
Professor of Neurology, University of California, San Francisco, School of Medicine; Attending Physician, University of California San Francisco Medical Center, San Francisco, California
Approach to the Patient with Neurologic Disease; Mechanical and Other Lesions of the Spine, Nerve Roots, and Spinal Cord

Jeffrey L. Anderson, MD
Professor of Internal Medicine, University of Utah School of Medicine; Associate Chief of Cardiology, LDS Hospital, Intermountain Healthcare, Salt Lake City, Utah
ST Segment Elevation Acute Myocardial Infarction and Complications of Myocardial Infarction

Karl E. Anderson, MD
Professor, Departments of Preventive Medicine and Community Health, Internal Medicine, and Pharmacology and Toxicology, University of Texas Medical Branch; Member, Medical Staff, University of Texas Medical Branch Hospital, Galveston, Texas
The Porphyrias

Larry J. Anderson, MD
Director, Division of Viral Diseases, National Center for Immunization and Respiratory Diseases, Centers for Disease Control and Prevention, Atlanta, Georgia
Coronaviruses

Nicholas Anthonisen, MD, PhD
Professor of Medicine and Dean Emeritus, University of Manitoba Faculty of Medicine; Respiratory Hospital, Winnipeg, Manitoba, Canada
Chronic Obstructive Pulmonary Disease

Karen Antman, MD
Provost, Boston University Medical Campus, and Dean, Boston University School of Medicine, Boston, Massachusetts
Sarcomas of Soft Tissue

Aśok C. Antony, MD, FACP
Professor of Medicine, Indiana University School of Medicine; Attending Physician, Indiana University Hospitals and The Richard Roudebush Veterans Affairs Medical Center, Indianapolis, Indiana
Megaloblastic Anemias

Michael A. Apicella, MD
Professor and Head, Department of Microbiology, University of Iowa Carver College of Medicine, Iowa City, Iowa
Meningococcal Infections

Gerald B. Appel, MD
Professor of Clinical Medicine, Columbia University College of Physicians and Surgeons; Director of Clinical Nephrology, New York–Presbyterian Hospital, New York, New York
Glomerular Disorders and Nephrotic Syndromes

Frederick R. Appelbaum, MD
Professor and Head, Division of Medical Oncology, University of Washington School of Medicine; Member and Director, Clinical Research Division, Fred Hutchinson Cancer Research Center, Seattle, Washington
The Acute Leukemias

Gordon L. Archer, MD
Associate Dean for Research and Professor of Medicine and Microbiology/Immunology, Medical College of Virginia Campus of Virginia Commonwealth University School of Medicine, Richmond, Virginia
Staphylococcal Infections

William P. Arend, MD
Endowed Chair in Rheumatology, University of Colorado School of Medicine, Aurora, Colorado
Approach to the Patient with Rheumatic Disease

Paul M. Arguin, MD
Commander and Medical Epidemiologist, U.S. Public Health Service Commissioned Corps, Atlanta, Georgia
Approach to the Patient before and after Travel

James O. Armitage, MD
Professor, Internal Medicine, Section of Hematology and Oncology, University of Nebraska College of Medicine; Section of Hematology and Oncology, University of Nebraska Medical Center, Omaha, Nebraska
Approach to the Patient with Lymphadenopathy and Splenomegaly; Non-Hodgkin's Lymphomas; Venomous Snake Bites

Cheryl A. Armstrong, MD
Associate Professor, Department of Dermatology, University of Colorado at Denver and Health Sciences Center, Denver, Colorado
Examination of the Skin and Approach to Diagnosing Skin Diseases

M. Amin Arnaout, MD
Professor of Medicine, Harvard Medical School; Chief, Nephrology Division, Massachusetts General Hospital, Boston, Massachusetts
Cystic Kidney Diseases

David Atkins, MD, MPH
Chief Medical Officer, Center for Outcomes and Evidence, Agency for Healthcare Research and Quality, Rockville, Maryland
The Periodic Health Examination

Dennis Ausiello, MD
Jackson Professor of Medicine, Harvard Medical School; Physician-in-Chief, Massachusetts General Hospital, Boston, Massachusetts
Approach to Medicine, the Patient, and the Medical Profession: Medicine as a Learned and Humane Profession; Disorders of Sodium and Water Homeostasis

Ricardo Azziz, MD, MPH, MBA
Professor of Obstetrics and Gynecology, David Geffen School of Medicine at UCLA; Chief, Division of Reproductive Endocrinology and Infertility, Cedars-Sinai Medical Center, Los Angeles, California
Hirsutism

Bruce R. Bacon, MD
James F. King, MD, Endowed Chair in Gastroenterology, Professor of Internal Medicine, and Director, Division of Gastroenterology and Hepatology, Saint Louis University School of Medicine, St. Louis, Missouri
Iron Overload (Hemochromatosis)

Grover C. Bagby, Jr., MD
Professor of Medicine, Oregon Health & Science University School of Medicine; Director, Oregon Health & Science University Cancer Center; Scientist, Portland Veterans Affairs Medical Center, Portland, Oregon
Leukopenia and Leukocytosis

Dean F. Bajorin, MD
Professor of Medicine, Weill Medical College of Cornell University; Attending Physician, Memorial Sloan-Kettering Cancer Center, New York, New York
Tumors of the Kidney, Bladder, Ureters, and Renal Pelvis

Laurence H. Baker, DO
Professor of Internal Medicine and Pharmacology, University of Michigan Medical School; Chairman, Southwest Oncology Group, Ann Arbor, Michigan
Bone Tumors: Primary and Metastatic Bone Lesions

Mark Ballow, MD
Professor of Pediatrics, School of Medicine and Biomedical Sciences, State University of New York at Buffalo; Chief, Division of Allergy and Clinical Immunology, Women and Children's Hospital of Buffalo, Buffalo, New York
Primary Immunodeficiency Diseases

Robert W. Baloh, MD
Professor of Neurology and Head and Neck Surgery, David Geffen School of Medicine at UCLA; Attending Physician, UCLA Medical Center, Los Angeles, California
Neuro-ophthalmology; Smell and Taste; Hearing and Equilibrium

Alan F. Barker, MD
Professor of Medicine, Oregon Health & Science University School of Medicine, Portland, Oregon
Bronchiectasis, Atelectasis, Cysts, and Localized Lung Disorders

Anna D. Barker, PhD
Deputy Director, National Cancer Institute, National Institutes of Health, Bethesda, Maryland
Cancer Biomarkers

A. James Barkovich, MD
Professor of Radiology, Neurology, Pediatrics, and Neurosurgery, University of California, San Francisco, School of Medicine, San Francisco, California
Congenital, Developmental, and Neurocutaneous Disorders

Richard J. Barohn, MD
Professor of Neurology, University of Kansas School of Medicine; Chairman, Department of Neurology, University of Kansas Medical Center, Kansas City, Kansas
Muscle Diseases

Murray G. Baron, MD
Professor of Radiology, Emory University School of Medicine; Attending Physician, Emory University Hospital, Atlanta, Georgia
Radiology of the Heart

Elizabeth Barrett-Connor, MD
Professor of Family and Preventive Medicine and Medicine and Chief, Division of Epidemiology, University of California, San Diego, School of Medicine, La Jolla, California
Menopause

Michael J. Barry, MD
Professor of Medicine, Harvard Medical School; Chief, General Medicine Unit, Massachusetts General Hospital, Boston, Massachusetts
Benign Prostate Disease and Prostatitis

Bruce A. Barshop, MD, PhD
Professor of Clinical Pediatrics and Benard L. Maas Chair in Inherited Metabolic Disease, University of California, San Diego, School of Medicine, La Jolla, California
Homocystinuria and Hyperhomocysteinemia

Robyn J. Barst, MD
Professor of Pediatrics in Medicine, Columbia University College of Physicians and Surgeons; Director, Pulmonary Hypertension Center, New York–Presbyterian Medical Center, New York, New York
Pulmonary Hypertension

John G. Bartlett, MD
Professor of Medicine, Johns Hopkins University School of Medicine; Chief, Division of Infectious Diseases, Johns Hopkins Hospital, Baltimore, Maryland
Bioterrorism; Clostridial Infections; Gastrointestinal Manifestations of Human Immunodeficiency Virus and Acquired Immunodeficiency Syndrome

Robert C. Basner, MD
Associate Professor of Clinical Medicine, Columbia University College of Physicians and Surgeons; Director, Cardiopulmonary Sleep and Ventilatory Disorders Center, and Director, Pulmonary Diagnostic Unit, Columbia University Medical Center, New York, New York
Obstructive Sleep Apnea-Hypopnea Syndrome

Stephen G. Baum, MD
Professor of Medicine, Microbiology, and Immunology, Albert Einstein College of Medicine, Bronx; Chairman, Department of Medicine, Beth Israel Medical Center, New York, New York
Mycoplasma *Infections*

Arnold S. Bayer, MD, FACP, FCCP
Professor of Medicine, David Geffen School of Medicine at UCLA, Los Angeles; Associate Chief, Infectious Disease, Los Angeles Biomedical Research Institute, Torrance, California
Infective Endocarditis

Hasan Bazari, MD
Assistant Professor of Medicine, Harvard Medical School; Attending Physician, Massachusetts General Hospital, Boston, Massachusetts
Approach to the Patient with Renal Disease

John H. Beigel, MD
Critical Care Medicine Department, National Institutes of Health, Bethesda, Maryland
Antiviral Therapy (Non-HIV)

Michael Bell, MD
Chief, Epidemiology Unit, Special Pathogens Branch, Division of Viral and Rickettsial Diseases, National Center for Infectious Diseases, Centers for Disease Control and Prevention, Atlanta, Georgia
Viral Hemorrhagic Fevers

George A. Beller, MD
Ruth C. Heede Professor of Cardiology and Professor of Internal Medicine, University of Virginia School of Medicine; University of Virginia Health System, Charlottesville, Virginia
Nuclear Cardiology and Computed Tomography

Robert M. Bennett, MD
Professor of Medicine and Nursing, Oregon Health & Science University School of Medicine, Portland, Oregon
Fibromyalgia and Chronic Fatigue Syndrome

Neal L. Benowitz, MD
Professor of Medicine, Psychiatry, and Biopharmaceutical Sciences, University of California, San Francisco, School of Medicine; Chief, Division of Clinical Pharmacology and Experimental Therapeutics, San Francisco General Hospital, San Francisco, California
Tobacco

Nora V. Bergasa, MD
Professor of Medicine, State University of New York at Downstate Medical Center; Vice Chair of Medicine, Woodhull Medical and Mental Health Center, Brooklyn, New York
Approach to the Patient with Liver Disease

Joseph R. Berger, MD
Ruth L. Works Professor and Chairman, Department of Neurology, and Professor, Department of Internal Medicine, University of Kentucky College of Medicine, Lexington, Kentucky
Cytomegalovirus, Epstein-Barr Virus, and Slow Virus Infections of the Central Nervous System; Neurologic Complications of Human Immunodeficiency Virus Infection; Acute Viral Encephalitis; Poliomyelitis; Rabies

Paul D. Berk, MD
Professor of Medicine, Columbia University College of Physicians and Surgeons; Attending Physician, New York–Presbyterian Hospital, New York, New York
Approach to the Patient with Jaundice or Abnormal Liver Test Results

Philip J. Bierman, MD
Associate Professor of Internal Medicine, University of Nebraska Medical Center, Omaha, Nebraska
Non-Hodgkin's Lymphomas

J. Andrew Billings, MD
Associate Professor of Medicine and Co-Director, Harvard Medical School Center for Palliative Care, Harvard Medical School; Director, Palliative Care Service, Massachusetts General Hospital, Boston, Massachusetts
Care of Dying Patients and Their Families

Alan L. Bisno, MD
Professor Emeritus, Department of Medicine, University of Miami Miller School of Medicine, Miami, Florida
Rheumatic Fever

Bruce R. Bistrian, MD, PhD, MPH
Professor of Medicine, Harvard Medical School; Chief, Clinical Nutrition, Beth Israel Deaconess Medical Center, Boston, Massachusetts
Nutritional Assessment

Joseph J. Biundo, MD
Clinical Professor of Medicine, Tulane University Health Sciences Center, New Orleans, Louisiana
Bursitis, Tendinitis, and Other Periarticular Disorders, and Sports Medicine

David J. Bjorkman, MD
Dean and Professor of Medicine, University of Utah School of Medicine, Salt Lake City, Utah
Gastrointestinal Hemorrhage and Occult Gastrointestinal Bleeding

Martin J. Blaser, MD
Frederick H. King Professor of Internal Medicine, Professor of Microbiology, and Chair, Department of Medicine, New York University School of Medicine, New York, New York
Acid Peptic Disease: Epidemiology and Pathobiology; Acid Peptic Disease: Clinical Manifestations, Diagnosis, Treatment, and Prognosis; Campylobacter *Infections*

William A. Blattner, MD
Professor of Medicine, University of Maryland School of Medicine; Director, Division of Epidemiology and Prevention, Institute of Human Virology, Baltimore, Maryland
Retroviruses Other than Human Immunodeficiency Virus

Thomas P. Bleck, MD
Vice Chair for Academic Affairs and Professor of Neurology, Neurological Surgery, and Medicine, Northwestern University Feinberg School of Medicine, Chicago; The Ruth Cain Ruggles Chairman of Neurology, Evanston Northwestern Healthcare, Evanston, Illinois
Arthropod-Borne Viruses Affecting the Central Nervous System

Linda K. Bockenstedt, MD
Professor of Medicine, Section of Rheumatology, Yale University School of Medicine, New Haven, Connecticut
Lyme Disease

Jean Bolognia, MD
Professor of Dermatology, Yale University School of Medicine, New Haven, Connecticut
Infections, Hyper- and Hypopigmentation, Regional Dermatology, and Distinctive Lesions in Black Skin

Larry Borish, MD
Professor of Medicine, University of Virginia School of Medicine; Staff Physician, University of Virginia Health Systems, Charlottesville, Virginia
Allergic Rhinitis and Sinusitis

Randall Brand, MD
Associate Professor of Medicine, Northwestern University Feinberg School of Medicine, Chicago; Evanston Northwestern Healthcare, Glenview, Illinois
Pancreatic Cancer

Itzhak Brook, MD, MSc
Professor of Pediatrics and Medicine, Georgetown University School of Medicine; Attending Physician, Georgetown University Medical Center, Washington, DC
Actinomycosis

Phillip A. Brunell, MD
Professor Emeritus of Pediatrics, David Geffen School of Medicine at UCLA, Los Angeles, California; Special Volunteer, Laboratory of Clinical Infectious Diseases, National Institute of Allergy and Infectious Diseases, National Institutes of Health, Bethesda, Maryland
Measles (Rubeola Virus Infection); Rubella (German Measles); Varicella (Chickenpox, Shingles)

Robert C. Brunham, MD, FRCP
Professor of Medicine, University of British Columbia Faculty of Medicine; Executive Director and Scientific Director, British Columbia Centre for Disease Control, Vancouver, British Columbia, Canada
Diseases Caused by Chlamydiae

John C. M. Brust, MD
Professor of Clinical Neurology, Columbia University College of Physicians and Surgeons; Director, Department of Neurology, Harlem Hospital Center, New York, New York
Nutrition- and Alcohol-Related Neurologic Disorders

David M. Buchner, MD, MPH
Chief, Physical Activity and Health Branch, Division of Nutrition and Physical Activity, Centers for Disease Control and Prevention, Atlanta, Georgia
Physical Activity

Daniel Burkhoff, MD, PhD
Adjunct Associate Professor of Medicine, Columbia University College of Physicians and Surgeons; Adjunct Associate Attending of Medicine, New York–Presbyterian Hospital, New York, New York
Cardiac Function and Circulatory Control

Joel N. Buxbaum, MD
Professor and Head, Division of Research Rheumatology, The Scripps Research Institute, La Jolla, California
The Amyloidoses

Peter A. Calabresi, MD
Associate Professor of Neurology, Johns Hopkins University School of Medicine; Director, Multiple Sclerosis Center, and Co-Director, Division of Neuroimmunology and Neuroinfectious Diseases, Johns Hopkins Hospital, Baltimore, Maryland
Multiple Sclerosis and Demyelinating Conditions of the Central Nervous System

Hugh Calkins, MD
Professor of Medicine, Johns Hopkins University School of Medicine; Director of Electrophysiology, Johns Hopkins Hospital, Baltimore, Maryland
Principles of Electrophysiology

Michael Camilleri, MD
Atherton and Winifred W. Bean Professor and Professor of Medicine and Physiology, Mayo Clinic College of Medicine; Consultant in Gastroenterology, Mayo Clinic, Rochester, Minnesota
Disorders of Gastrointestinal Motility

Grant W. Cannon, MD
Professor of Medicine, Division of Rheumatology, University of Utah School of Medicine; Associate Chief of Staff for Academic Affiliations, George E. Wahlen Veterans Administration Medical Center, Salt Lake City, Utah
Immunosuppressing Drugs Including Corticosteroids

Blase A. Carabello, MD
Professor of Medicine, Baylor College of Medicine; Medical Careline Executive, Michael E DeBakey Veterans Affairs Medical Center; Houston, Texas
Valvular Heart Disease

Edgar M. Carvalho, MD, PhD
Professor of Medicine, Universidade Federal da Bahia; Professor of Immunology, Escola Bahiana de Medicina e Saúde Pública; Head, Immunology Service, Hospital Universitário Prof. Edgard Santos, Salvador-Bahia, Brazil
Schistosomiasis (Bilharziasis)

Agustin Castellanos, MD
Professor of Medicine and Physiology and American Heart Association Chair in Cardiovascular Research, University of Miami Miller School of Medicine, Miami, Florida
Approach to Cardiac Arrest and Life-Threatening Arrhythmias

Hugo Castro-Malaspina, MD
Associate Professor, Weill Medical College of Cornell University; Associate Member, Memorial Sloan-Kettering Cancer Center, New York, New York
Aplastic Anemia and Related Disorders

Stephen D. Cederbaum, MD
Professor of Psychiatry, Pediatrics, and Human Genetics, David Geffen School of Medicine at UCLA; Attending Physician, UCLA Medical Center, Los Angeles, California
Disorders of Phenylalanine and Tyrosine Metabolism; Diseases of the Urea Cycle

Bartolome R. Celli, MD
Professor of Medicine, Tufts University School of Medicine; Chief, Pulmonary, Critical Care, and Sleep Medicine, Caritas–St. Elizabeth's Medical Center, Boston, Massachusetts
Diseases of the Diaphragm, Chest Wall, Pleura, and Mediastinum

Raju S. K. Chaganti, PhD
Professor of Cell Biology, Gerstner Graduate School, Sloan-Kettering Institute, Memorial Sloan-Kettering Cancer Center; Professor of Cell Biology and Genetics, Weill-Cornell Medical Center; Attending Geneticist and Cytogeneticist, Memorial Sloan-Kettering Cancer Center, New York, New York
Genetics of Cancer

David C. Christiani, MD, MPH
Professor of Medicine, Harvard Medical School, and Professor of Occupational Medicine and Epidemiology, Harvard School of Public Health; Physician, Pulmonary and Critical Care Unit, Massachusetts General Hospital, Boston, Massachusetts
Physical and Chemical Injuries of the Lung

David R. Clemmons, MD
Chief, Division of Endocrinology and Metabolism, and Sarah Graham Kenan Professor of Medicine, University of North Carolina at Chapel Hill School of Medicine, Chapel Hill, North Carolina
Principles of Endocrinology

Steven L. Cohn, MD, FACP
Clinical Professor of Medicine, State University of New York Downstate Medical Center College of Medicine; Chief, Division of General Internal Medicine, SUNY Downstate Medical Center, Brooklyn, New York
Preoperative Evaluation

Joseph M. Connors, MD
Clinical Professor, Department of Medicine, University of British Columbia Faculty of Medicine; Chair, Lymphoma Tumor Group, British Columbia Cancer Agency, Vancouver, British Columbia, Canada
Hodgkin's Lymphoma

Deborah J. Cook, MD, MSc (Epid), FRCPC
Professor of Medicine, Clinical Epidemiology, and Biostatistics, McMaster University Faculty of Medicine; Academic Chair, Critical Care Medicine, St. Joseph's Healthcare, Hamilton, Ontario, Canada
Approach to the Patient in a Critical Care Setting

G. Ralph Corey, MD
Professor of Medicine and Infectious Disease, Duke University School of Medicine; Gary Hock Distinguished Professor of Medicine and Director, Hubert/Yeargan Center for Global Health, Duke University Medical Center, Durham, North Carolina
Venomous Snake Bites

Kenneth H. Cowan, MD, PhD
Professor, Eppley Institute for Research in Cancer, and Professor, Section of Oncology/Hematology, University of Nebraska Medical Center; Director, UNMC Eppley Cancer Center; Director, Eppley Institute for Research in Cancer, Omaha, Nebraska
Biology of Cancer

William A. Craig, MD
Emeritus Professor of Medicine, University of Wisconsin School of Medicine and Public Health; Consultant, William S. Middleton Memorial Veterans Affairs Hospital, Madison, Wisconsin
Antibacterial Therapy

Michael H. Criqui, MD, MPH
Professor, Department of Family and Preventive Medicine and Department of Medicine, and Director, Preventive Cardiology Academic Award, University of California, San Diego, School of Medicine, La Jolla, California
Epidemiology of Cardiovascular Disease

Mary K. Crow, MD
Professor of Medicine, Weill Medical College of Cornell University; Benjamin M. Rosen Chair in Immunology and Inflammation Research, Hospital for Special Surgery, New York, New York
Systemic Lupus Erythematosus

Mark R. Cullen, MD
Professor of Medicine and Public Health, Yale University School of Medicine, New Haven, Connecticut
Principles of Occupational and Environmental Medicine

Gary C. Curhan, MD, DSc
Associate Professor of Medicine, Harvard Medical School; Associate Professor of Epidemiology, Harvard School of Public Health; Attending Physician, Brigham and Women's Hospital, Boston, Massachusetts
Nephrolithiasis

Edward Curtiss, MD*
Formerly Dean of Admissions and Professor of Medicine, University of Pittsburgh School of Medicine; Formerly Director, Central Heart Station, Cardiovascular Institute, University of Pittsburgh Medical Center, Pittsburgh, Pennsylvania
Electrocardiography
**deceased*

F. Michael Cutrer, MD
Assistant Professor, Mayo Clinic College of Medicine; Consultant, Mayo Clinic, Rochester, Minnesota
Headaches and Other Head Pain

Inger K. Damon, MD, PhD
Adjunct Clinical Faculty, Department of Medicine, Emory University School of Medicine; Chief (Acting) Poxvirus and Rabies Branch, Division of Viral and Rickettsial Disease, Centers for Disease Control and Prevention, Atlanta, Georgia
Smallpox, Monkeypox, and Other Poxvirus Infections

Troy E. Daniels, DDS, MS
Professor, University of California, San Francisco, Schools of Dentistry and Medicine, San Francisco, California
Diseases of the Mouth and Salivary Glands

Lisa M. DeAngelis, MD
Professor of Neurology, Weill Medical College of Cornell University; Chairman, Department of Neurology, and Attending Neurologist, Memorial Sloan-Kettering Cancer Center, New York, New York
Tumors of the Central Nervous System and Intracranial Hypertension and Hypotension

Leonard J. Deftos, MD, JD
Professor of Medicine, University of California, San Diego, School of Medicine, La Jolla; Physician, San Diego Veterans Affairs Medical Center, San Diego, California
Medullary Thyroid Carcinoma and Calcitonin

Carlos del Rio, MD
Professor of Medicine, Division of Infectious Diseases, Emory University School of Medicine; Chief of Medical Services, Grady Memorial Hospital, Atlanta, Georgia
Prevention of Human Immunodeficiency Virus Infection

Robert H. Demling, MD
Professor of Surgery, Harvard Medical School; Director of Education and Research, Department of Surgery, Brigham and Women's Hospital, Boston, Massachusetts
Medical Aspects of Trauma and Burn Care

Robert J. Desnick, MD, PhD
Professor and Chair, Department of Genetics and Genomic Science, Mount Sinai School of Medicine; Attending Physician, Department of Pediatrics, Mount Sinai Hospital, New York, New York
Lysosomal Storage Diseases

Patricia A. Deuster, PhD, MPH
Professor, Department of Military and Emergency Medicine, Uniformed Services University of the Health Sciences, F. Edward Hébert School of Medicine, Bethesda, Maryland
Rhabdomyolysis

Robert B. Diasio, MD
Professor of Molecular Pharmacology and Experimental Therapeutics and Professor of Oncology, Mayo Clinic College of Medicine; Director, Mayo Clinic Cancer Center, Mayo Clinic, Rochester, Minnesota
Principles of Drug Therapy

Anna Mae Diehl, MD
Professor, Department of Medicine, Division of Gastroenterology, Duke University School of Medicine; Chief, Division of Gastroenterology, Duke University Medical Center, Durham, North Carolina
Alcoholic and Nonalcoholic Steatohepatitis

John M. Douglas, Jr., MD
Director, Division of Sexually Transmitted Diseases Prevention, National Center for HIV, Hepatitis, Sexually Transmitted Diseases, and Tuberculosis Prevention, Centers for Disease Control and Prevention, Atlanta, Georgia
Papillomavirus

Jeffrey M. Drazen, MD
Distinguished Parker B. Francis Professor of Medicine, Harvard Medical School; Senior Physician, Brigham and Women's Hospital; Editor-in-Chief, *New England Journal of Medicine*, Boston, Massachusetts
Asthma

Stephen C. Dreskin, MD, PhD
Professor of Medicine and Immunology, University of Colorado School of Medicine; Practice Director, Allergy and Rheumatology, University of Colorado Hospital, Denver, Colorado
Urticaria and Angioedema

W. Lawrence Drew, MD, PhD
Professor of Laboratory Medicine and Medicine and Director, Clinical Virology Laboratory, University of California, San Francisco, School of Medicine; Chief, Infectious Diseases, UCSF Medical Center at Mount Zion, San Francisco, California
Cytomegalovirus

Mark K. Drezner, MD, PhD
Professor, University of Wisconsin School of Medicine and Public Health; Attending Physician, University of Wisconsin Hospital and Clinics, Madison, Wisconsin
Osteomalacia and Rickets

Raymond N. DuBois, MD, PhD
Professor of Cancer Medicine and Biology, The University of Texas M. D. Anderson Cancer Center, Houston, Texas
Neoplasms of the Large and Small Intestine

Thomas D. DuBose, Jr., MD
Tinsley R. Harrison Professor and Chair of Internal Medicine and Professor of Physiology and Pharmacology, Wake Forest University School of Medicine; Chief, Internal Medicine Service, North Carolina Baptist Hospital, Winston-Salem, North Carolina
Vascular Disorders of the Kidney

Herbert L. DuPont, MD
H. Irving Schweppe, Jr., Chair of Internal Medicine and Vice Chairman, Department of Medicine, Baylor College of Medicine; Chief Internal Medicine, St. Luke's Episcopal Hospital; Director, Center for Infectious Diseases, University of Texas–Houston School of Public Health, Houston, Texas
Approach to the Patient with Suspected Enteric Infection

Madeleine Duvic, MD
Professor of Internal Medicine and Dermatology, University of Texas Medical School—Houston; Chairman, Department of Dermatology, University of Texas M. D. Anderson Cancer Center, Houston, Texas
Urticaria, Drug Hypersensitivity Rashes, Nodules and Tumors, and Atrophic Diseases

Paul H. Edelstein, MD
Professor of Pathology and Laboratory Medicine, University of Pennsylvania School of Medicine; Director, Clinical Microbiology, Hospital of the University of Pennsylvania, Philadelphia, Pennsylvania
Legionella *Infections*

Lawrence H. Einhorn, MD
Distinguished Professor of Medicine, Indiana University School of Medicine, Indianapolis, Indiana
Testicular Cancer

Ronald J. Elin, MD, PhD
A. J. Miller Professor and Chair, Department of Pathology and Laboratory Medicine, University of Louisville School of Medicine; Medical Director, Pathology and Laboratory Medicine, University of Louisville Hospital, Louisville, Kentucky
Reference Intervals and Laboratory Values

George M. Eliopoulos, MD
Professor of Medicine, Harvard Medical School; Physician, Division of Infectious Diseases, Beth Israel Deaconess Medical Center, Boston, Massachusetts
Principles of Anti-infective Therapy

Diane L. Elliot, MD
Professor of Medicine, Division of Health Promotion and Sports Medicine, Oregon Health & Science University School of Medicine, Portland, Oregon
Pregnancy: Hypertension and Other Common Medical Problems

Louis J. Elsas II, MD
Professor of Pediatrics and Biochemistry and Director, Dr. John T. Macdonald Foundation Center for Medical Genetics, University of Miami Miller School of Medicine; Active Admitting Staff/Faculty, Jackson Memorial Hospital and Miami Children's Hospital, Miami, Florida
Approach to Inborn Errors of Metabolism; Galactosemia; Branched-Chain Aminoacidurias

Ezekiel J. Emanuel, MD, PhD
Chair, Department of Clinical Bioethics, National Institutes of Health, Bethesda, Maryland
Bioethics in the Practice of Medicine

Gregory F. Erickson, PhD
Professor Emeritus, Department of Reproductive Medicine, University of California, San Diego, School of Medicine, La Jolla California
Ovaries and Development; Menstrual Cycle and Fertility

Joel D. Ernst, MD
Director, Division of Infectious Diseases; Jeffrey Bergstein Professor of Medicine; and Professor of Medicine, Pathology, and Microbiology, New York University School of Medicine; Attending Physician, Bellevue Hospital Center, Tisch Hospital, and New York University Medical Center, New York, New York
Leprosy (Hansen's Disease)

Luis R. Espinoza, MD
Professor and Chief, Section of Rheumatology, Louisiana State University Health Sciences Center School of Medicine at New Orleans, New Orleans, Louisiana
Infections of Bursae, Joints, and Bones

David S. Ettinger, MD
Alex Grass Professor of Oncology, The Sidney Kimmel Comprehensive Cancer Center at Johns Hopkins, Johns Hopkins University School of Medicine, Baltimore, Maryland
Lung Cancer and Other Pulmonary Neoplasms

Murray J. Favus, MD
Professor of Medicine, Section of Endocrinology, Diabetes, and Metabolism, The University of Chicago Pritzker School of Medicine; Attending Physician and Director, Bone Program, University of Chicago Hospitals, Chicago, Illinois
Mineral and Bone Homeostasis

David P. Faxon, MD
Professor of Medicine, Harvard Medical School, Boston; Chief, Section of Cardiology, West Roxbury Veterans Affairs Health System, West Roxbury; Director, Strategic Planning, Brigham and Women's Hospital, Boston, Massachusetts
Catheterization and Angiography

Aaron Fay, MD
Assistant Professor of Ophthalmology, Harvard Medical School; Interim Director, Ophthalmic Plastic Surgery, Massachusetts Eye and Ear Infirmary, Boston, Massachusetts
Diseases of the Visual System

Judith E. Feinberg, MD
Professor of Medicine, University of Cincinnati College of Medicine; Attending Physician, University Hospital and Cincinnati Children's Hospital Medical Center, Cincinnati, Ohio
Pneumocystis *Pneumonia*

Eva L. Feldman, MD, PhD
Russell N. DeJong Professor, Department of Neurology, University of Michigan Medical School, Ann Arbor, Michigan
Amyotrophic Lateral Sclerosis and Other Motor Neuron Diseases

Stephan D. Fihn, MD, MPH
Head, Division of General Internal Medicine, and Professor, Departments of Medicine and Health Services, University of Washington School of Medicine; Director, Veterans Affairs Northwest Health Services Research and Development Center of Excellence, Veterans Affairs Puget Sound Health Care System, Seattle, Washington
Measuring Health and Health Care

Sydney M. Finegold, MD
Emeritus Professor of Medicine and of Microbiology, Immunology, and Molecular Genetics, David Geffen School of Medicine at UCLA; Staff Physician, Infectious Diseases Section, Veterans Affairs Medical Center West Los Angeles, Los Angeles, California
Lung Abscess

Gary S. Firestein, MD
Professor of Medicine and Chief, Division of Rheumatology, Allergy, and Immunology, University of California, San Diego, School of Medicine, La Jolla, California
Mechanisms of Inflammation and Tissue Repair

Neil Fishman, MD
Associate Professor of Medicine, University of Pennsylvania School of Medicine; Director, Department of Healthcare, Epidemiology, and Infection Control, University of Pennsylvania Medical Center, Philadelphia, Pennsylvania
Prevention and Control of Hospital-Acquired Infections

Garret A. FitzGerald, MD, DSc
Professor of Medicine and Elmer Bobst Professor of Pharmacology, University of Pennsylvania School of Medicine, Philadelphia, Pennsylvania
Prostaglandins, Aspirin, and Related Compounds

Marsha D. Ford, MD
Adjunct Professor of Emergency Medicine, University of North Carolina at Chapel Hill School of Medicine, Chapel Hill; Director, Carolinas Poison Center, and Director, Division of Medical Toxicology, Department of Emergency Medicine, Carolinas Medical Center, Charlotte, North Carolina
Acute Poisoning

Vance G. Fowler, Jr., MD, MHS
Associate Professor, Division of Infective Diseases, Department of Medicine, Duke University School of Medicine, Durham, North Carolina
Infective Endocarditis

Jay W. Fox, PhD
Professor, Department of Microbiology, and Assistant Dean for Research, University of Virginia School of Medicine, Charlottesville, Virginia
Venoms and Poisons from Marine Organisms

David O. Freedman, MD
Professor of Medicine and Epidemiology, William C. Gorgas Center for Geographic Medicine, Division of Infectious Diseases, University of Alabama School of Medicine, Birmingham, Alabama
Filariasis

Linda P. Fried, MD, MPH
Professor of Medicine and Epidemiology, Johns Hopkins University School of Medicine; Director, Division of Geriatric Medicine and Gerontology, and Director, Center on Aging and Health, Johns Hopkins Medical Institutions, Baltimore, Maryland
Epidemiology of Aging: Implications of the Aging of Society

Valentin Fuster, MD, PhD
Professor of Medicine, Department of Cardiology, Mount Sinai School of Medicine; Director, Wiener Cardiovascular Institute, and Director, Kravis Center for Cardiovascular Health, Mount Sinai Medical Center, New York, New York
Atherosclerosis, Thrombosis, and Vascular Biology

Kenneth L. Gage, PhD
Chief, Flea-Borne Diseases Activity, Division of Vector-Borne Infectious Diseases, Centers for Disease Control and Prevention, Fort Collins, Colorado
Plague and Other Yersinia *Infections*

Robert F. Gagel, MD
Professor of Medicine and Head, Division of Internal Medicine, University of Texas M. D. Anderson Cancer Center, Houston, Texas
Endocrine Manifestations of Tumors: "Ectopic" Hormone Production; Medullary Thyroid Carcinoma and Calcitonin

John N. Galgiani, MD
Professor and Director, Valley Fever Center for Excellence, University of Arizona College of Medicine; Program Director for Infectious Diseases, Southern Arizona Veterans Affairs Health Care System, Tucson, Arizona
Coccidioidomycosis

Eithan Galun, MD
Professor of Gene Therapy, Hebrew University Medical School; Director, Goldyne Savad Institute of Gene Therapy, Hadassah Hebrew University Hospital, Jerusalem, Israel
Cell and Gene Therapy

Leonard Ganz, MD
Associate Professor of Medicine, Temple University School of Medicine, Philadelphia; Staff Electrophysiologist, Western Pennsylvania Hospital, Pittsburgh, Pennsylvania
Electrocardiography

Guadalupe Garcia-Tsao, MD
Professor of Medicine, Yale University School of Medicine, New Haven; Chief, Digestive Diseases Section, VA Connecticut Healthcare System, West Haven, Connecticut
Cirrhosis and Its Sequelae

Jonathan D. Gates, MD
Assistant Professor of Surgery, Harvard Medical School; Director, Trauma Center, Brigham and Women's Hospital, Boston, Massachusetts
Medical Aspects of Trauma and Burn Care

M. Eric Gershwin, MD
Distinguished Professor of Medicine and Chief, Division of Rheumatology, Allergy, and Clinical Immunology, University of California, Davis, School of Medicine, Davis, California
Sjögren's Syndrome

Gordon N. Gill, MD
Professor of Medicine, Department of Endocrinology, University of California, San Diego, School of Medicine, La Jolla, California
Principles of Endocrinology

D. Gary Gilliland, MD, PhD
Professor of Medicine, Harvard Medical School; Senior Physician, Brigham and Women's Hospital and Dana-Farber Cancer Institute, Boston, Massachusetts
Myelodysplastic Syndrome

Gordon D. Ginder, MD
Professor of Internal Medicine, Division of Hematology-Oncology, Medical College of Virginia Campus of Virginia Commonwealth University School of Medicine; Director, Massey Cancer Center, and Lipman Chair in Oncology, Virginia Commonwealth University, Richmond, Virginia
Microcytic and Hypochromic Anemias

Jeffrey Ginsberg, MD
Professor, Department of Medicine, Faculty of Health Sciences at McMaster University, Hamilton, Ontario, Canada
Peripheral Venous Disease

Carol A. Glaser, MD
Chief, California Department of Health Services, Viral and Rickettsial Disease Laboratory, Richmond, California
Amebiasis

Michael Glogauer, DDS, PhD
Associate Professor, University of Toronto Faculty of Medicine and University of Toronto Faculty of Dentistry; Periodontist, Hospital for Sick Children, Toronto, Ontario, Canada
Disorders of Phagocyte Function

John W. Gnann, Jr., MD
Professor of Medicine, Pediatrics, and Microbiology, Division of Infectious Diseases, University of Alabama School of Medicine and Birmingham Veterans Affairs Medical Center, Birmingham, Alabama
Mumps

David E. Golan, MD, PhD
Professor of Medicine and Professor of Biological Chemistry and Molecular Pharmacology, Harvard Medical School; Attending Physician, Brigham and Women's Hospital and Dana-Farber Cancer Institute, Boston, Massachusetts
Hemolytic Anemias: Red Cell Membrane and Metabolic Defects

Marcia B. Goldberg, MD
Associate Professor of Medicine, Harvard Medical School; Attending Physician, Massachusetts General Hospital, Boston, Massachusetts
Shigellosis

Victor M. Goldberg, MD
Professor of Orthopaedics, Case Western Reserve University School of Medicine; Attending Physician, University Hospitals of Cleveland, Cleveland, Ohio
Surgical Treatment of Joint Diseases

Lee Goldman, MD, MPH
Executive Vice President for Health and Biomedical Sciences, Columbia University; Dean of the Faculties of Health Sciences and Medicine, Columbia University Medical Center, New York, New York
Approach to Medicine, the Patient, and the Medical Profession: Medicine as a Learned and Humane Profession; Approach to the Patient with Possible Cardiovascular Disease

Ellie J. C. Goldstein, MD
Clinical Professor of Medicine, David Geffen School of Medicine at UCLA, Los Angeles; Director, R. M. Alden Research Laboratory, Santa Monica, California
Diseases Caused by Non–Spore-Forming Anaerobic Bacteria

Lawrence T. Goodnough, MD
Professor of Pathology and Medicine, Stanford University School of Medicine; Director, Transfusion Service, Stanford University Medical Center, Stanford, California
Transfusion Medicine

Jörg J. Goronzy, MD, PhD
Mason I. Lowance, MD, Professor of Medicine, and Director, Kathleen B. and Mason I. Lowance Center for Human Immunology, Department of Medicine, Emory University School of Medicine, Atlanta, Georgia
The Innate and Adaptive Immune Systems

Eduardo Gotuzzo, MD
Professor, Universidad Peruana Cayetano Heredia; Chief, Department of Infectious, Tropical, and Dermatologic Diseases, Hospital Nacional Cayetano Heredia, Lima, Peru
Cholera and Other Vibrio *Infections*

Deborah Grady, MD, MPH
Associate Dean for Clinical and Translational Research, University of California, San Francisco, Schools of Medicine and Nursing; Professor of Epidemiology and Biostatistics and of Medicine, University of California, San Francisco, School of Medicine; Director, UCSF Women's Health Clinical Research Center, San Francisco, California
Menopause

Leslie C. Grammer, MD
Professor of Medicine, Northwestern University Feinberg School of Medicine; Clinical Chief, Allergy-Immunology Division, Northwestern Memorial Hospital, Chicago, Illinois
Drug Allergy

F. Anthony Greco, MD
Medical Director, Sarah Cannon Cancer Center, Nashville, Tennessee
Cancer of Unknown Primary Origin

Peter K. Gregersen, MD
Professor of Medicine and Pathology, New York University School of Medicine, New York; Investigator and Director, Robert S. Boas Center for Genomics and Human Genetics, Feinstein Institute for Medical Research, North Shore LIJ Institute for Medical Research, Manhasset, New York
The Major Histocompatibility Complex

Edward C. Grendys, Jr., MD
Associate Clinical Professor of Obstetrics and Gynecology, Northwestern University Feinberg School of Medicine, Chicago, Illinois; Florida Gynecologic Oncology, Bonita Springs, Florida
Management of Neoplastic Diseases during Pregnancy

Robert C. Griggs, MD
Professor and Chair of Neurology and Professor of Medicine, Pediatrics, and Pathology and Laboratory Medicine, University of Rochester School of Medicine and Dentistry; Neurologist-in-Chief, Strong Memorial Hospital, Rochester, New York
Approach to the Patient with Neurologic Disease

Lisa M. Guay-Woodford, MD
Professor of Medicine, University of Alabama School of Medicine, Birmingham, Alabama
Hereditary Nephropathies and Abnormalities of the Urinary Tract

Richard L. Guerrant, MD
Thomas H. Hunter Professor of International Medicine and Director, Center for Global Health, University of Virginia School of Medicine, Charlottesville, Virginia
Escherichia *Enteric Infections*

David Hackney, MD
Professor of Radiology, Harvard Medical School; Chief of Neuroradiology, Beth Israel Deaconess Medical Center, Boston, Massachusetts
Radiologic Imaging Procedures

Colleen Hadigan, MD, MPH
Staff Clinician, Laboratory of Immunoregulation, National Institute of Allergy and Infectious Diseases, National Institutes of Health, Bethesda, Maryland
Treatment of Human Immunodeficiency Virus Infection and Acquired Immunodeficiency Syndrome

John D. Hainsworth, MD
Chief Scientific Officer, Sarah Cannon Research Institute, Nashville, Tennessee
Cancer of Unknown Primary Origin

Judith G. Hall, MD, MS
Professor Emerita of Pediatrics and Medical Genetics, University of British Columbia Faculty of Medicine and British Columbia Children's Hospital, Vancouver, British Columbia, Canada
Single-Gene and Chromosomal Disorders

Kenneth R. Hande, MD
Professor of Medicine and Pharmacology, Vanderbilt University School of Medicine and Vanderbilt/Ingram Cancer Center, Nashville, Tennessee
Multiple-Organ Systems: Carcinoid Syndrome

H. Hunter Handsfield, MD
Clinical Professor of Medicine and Epidemiology, University of Washington Center for AIDS and STD; Senior Research Leader, Battelle Centers for Public Health Research and Evaluation, Seattle, Washington
Gonococcal Infections

Nancy Harris, MD
Department of Pathology, Massachusetts General Hospital, Boston, Massachusetts
Non-Hodgkin's Lymphomas

Raymond C. Harris, MD
Ann and Roscoe R. Robinson Professor of Medicine, and Chief, Division of Nephrology, Vanderbilt University School of Medicine, Nashville, Tennessee
Diabetes and the Kidney

Stephen Crane Hauser, MD
Assistant Professor of Medicine, Mayo Clinic College of Medicine; Consultant in Gastroenterology and Hepatology, Mayo Clinic, Rochester, Minnesota
Vascular Diseases of the Gastrointestinal Tract

Frederick G. Hayden, MD
Stuart S. Richardson Professor of Clinical Virology and Professor of Medicine and Pathology, University of Virginia School of Medicine; Staff Physician, University of Virginia Health System, Charlottesville, Virginia
Antiviral Therapy (Non-HIV); Influenza

Letha Healey, MD
Staff Clinician, Critical Care Medicine Department, Clinical Center, National Institutes of Health, Bethesda, Maryland
Treatment of Human Immunodeficiency Virus Infection and Acquired Immunodeficiency Syndrome

Douglas C. Heimburger, MD, MS
Professor of Nutrition Sciences and Professor of Medicine, University of Alabama School of Medicine; Director, Medical Nutrition Services, University of Alabama Hospital and Birmingham Veterans Affairs Medical Center, Birmingham, Alabama
Nutrition's Interface with Health and Disease

David K. Henderson, MD
Deputy Director for Clinical Care, Hospital Epidemiologist, and Senior Investigator, Clinical Center, National Institutes of Health, Bethesda, Maryland
Prevention and Control of Hospital-Acquired Infections

J. Owen Hendley, MD
Professor of Pediatrics, University of Virginia School of Medicine, Charlottesville, Virginia
The Common Cold

Janet B. Henrich, MD
Associate Professor of Medicine and of Obstetrics and Gynecology, Yale University School of Medicine, New Haven, Connecticut
Approach to Women's Health

Michael S. Hershfield, MD
Professor of Medicine and Biochemistry, Duke University Medical Center, Durham, North Carolina
Disorders of Purine and Pyrimidine Metabolism

Erik L. Hewlett, MD
Professor of Medicine and Pharmacology, University of Virginia School of Medicine, Charlottesville, Virginia
Whooping Cough and Other Bordetella *Infections*

William R. Hiatt, MD
Professor of Medicine, University of Colorado School of Medicine; President, Colorado Prevention Center, Denver, Colorado
Atherosclerotic Peripheral Arterial Disease

Richard E. Hillman, MD
Professor of Child Health, Biochemistry, and Pathology, University of Missouri School of Medicine and University of Missouri Hospital and Clinics, Columbia, Missouri
Primary Hyperoxaluria

Jack Hirsh, MD, FRCP, FRACP, FRSC, DSc
Professor Emeritus, McMaster University Faculty of Health Sciences; Consultant, Intellectual Property, Hamilton Health Sciences and McMaster University, Henderson Research Centre, Hamilton, Ontario, Canada
Antithrombotic Therapy

Craig J. Hoesley, MD
Associate Professor of Medicine, University of Alabama School of Medicine, Birmingham, Alabama
Disease Caused by Bartonella *Species*

V. Michael Holers, MD
Professor of Medicine and Immunology, Head, Division of Rheumatology, and Smyth Professor of Rheumatology, University of Colorado Health Sciences Center, Denver, Colorado
Complement in Health and Disease

Steven M. Holland, MD
Chief, Laboratory of Clinical Infectious Diseases, National Institute of Allergy and Infectious Diseases, National Institutes of Health, Bethesda, Maryland
The Nontuberculous Mycobacteria

David R. Holmes, Jr., MD
Professor of Medicine, Mayo Clinic College of Medicine; Consultant, Mayo Clinic, Rochester, Minnesota
Cardiogenic Shock

Waun Ki Hong, MD
American Cancer Society Professor; Samsung Distinguished University Chair in Cancer Medicine; Head, Division of Cancer Medicine; and Professor, Department of Thoracic/Head and Neck Medical Oncology, University of Texas M. D. Anderson Cancer Center, Houston, Texas
Cancer Prevention

Jay H. Hoofnagle, MD
Director, Liver Disease Research Branch, Division of Digestive Diseases and Nutrition, National Institute of Diabetes and Digestive and Kidney Diseases, National Institutes of Health, Bethesda, Maryland
Acute Viral Hepatitis; Chronic Hepatitis

Edward W. Hook III, MD
Professor of Medicine, Microbiology, and Epidemiology, University of Alabama School of Medicine; Medical Director, Sexually Transmitted Disease Program, Jefferson County Department of Health, Birmingham, Alabama
Chancroid; Granuloma Inguinale (Donovanosis); Syphilis; Nonsyphilitic Treponematoses

Keith A. Hruska, MD
Professor of Pediatrics, Medicine, and Cell Biology, Washington University in St. Louis School of Medicine; Director, Pediatric Nephrology, St. Louis Children's Hospital, St. Louis, Missouri
Renal Osteodystrophy

Laurence Huang, MD, MAS
Associate Professor of Medicine, University of California, San Francisco, School of Medicine; Chief, AIDS Chest Clinic, San Francisco General Hospital, San Francisco, California
Pulmonary Manifestations of Human Immunodeficiency Virus Infection and Acquired Immunodeficiency Syndrome

Leonard D. Hudson, MD
Professor of Medicine and Endowed Chair in Pulmonary Disease Research, University of Washington School of Medicine; Attending Physician, Harborview Medical Center, Seattle, Washington
Acute Respiratory Failure; Mechanical Ventilation

Steven E. Hyman, MD
Professor of Neurobiology, Harvard Medical School, and Provost, Harvard University, Cambridge, Massachusetts
Biology of Addiction

Robert D. Inman, MD
Professor of Medicine and Immunology, University of Toronto Faculty of Medicine; Consultant Rheumatologist, Toronto Western Hospital, Toronto, Ontario, Canada
The Spondyloarthropathies

Sharon K. Inouye, MD, MPH
Professor of Medicine, Beth Israel Deaconess Medical Center, Harvard Medical School; Director, Aging Brain Center, Institute for Aging Research, Hebrew Senior Life, Boston, Massachusetts
Neuropsychiatric Aspects of Aging; Delirium and Other Mental Status Problems in the Older Patient

Karl L. Insogna, MD
Professor of Medicine and Clinical Director, Yale University School of Medicine; Director, Yale Diabetes Center, Yale–New Haven Hospital, New Haven, Connecticut
The Parathyroid Glands, Hypercalcemia, and Hypocalcemia

Silvio E. Inzucchi, MD
Professor of Medicine, Department of Internal Medicine, and Clinical Director, Section of Endocrinology, Yale School of Medicine; Director, Yale Diabetes Center, Yale–New Haven Hospital, New Haven, Connecticut
Type 1 Diabetes Mellitus; Type 2 Diabetes Mellitus

Michael D. Iseman, MD
Professor of Medicine, University of Colorado Health Sciences Center, and Professor of Medicine, Mycobacterial and Respiratory Infections Section, National Jewish Medical and Research Center, Denver, Colorado
Tuberculosis

Eric M. Isselbacher, MD
Associate Professor of Medicine, Harvard Medical School; Associate Director, Massachusetts General Hospital Heart Center, and Co-Director, Thoracic Aortic Center, Massachusetts General Hospital, Boston, Massachusetts
Diseases of the Aorta

Michael D. Jensen, MD
Professor of Medicine, Mayo Clinic, Rochester, Minnesota
Obesity

Robert T. Jensen, MD
Chief, Cell Biology Section, Digestive Diseases Branch, National Institutes Of Health, Bethesda, Maryland
Pancreatic Endocrine Tumors

Selma M. B. Jeronimo, MD, PhD
Professor of Biochemistry, Department of Biochemistry, Universidade Federal do Rio Grande do Norte, Natal, Brazil
Leishmaniasis

Mariell Jessup, MD
Professor of Medicine, University of Pennsylvania School of Medicine; Medical Director, Heart Failure/Transplant Program, University of Pennsylvania Health System, Philadelphia, Pennsylvania
Cardiac Transplantation

Howard W. Jones III, MD
Professor, Department of Obstetrics and Gynecology, Vanderbilt University School of Medicine; Director of Gynecologic Oncology, Vanderbilt University Hospital, Nashville, Tennessee
Gynecologic Cancers

Ralph F. Józefowicz, MD
Professor of Neurology and Medicine, University of Rochester School of Medicine and Dentistry, Rochester, New York
Approach to the Patient with Neurologic Disease

Stephen G. Kaler, MD, MPH
Adjunct Associate Professor of Pediatrics and Pathology, George Washington University School of Medicine, Washington, DC; Clinical Director, National Institute of Child Health and Human Development, National Institutes of Health, Bethesda, Maryland
Wilson's Disease

Hagop Kantarjian, MD
Chairman, Department of Leukemia, The University of Texas M. D. Anderson Cancer Center, Houston, Texas
The Chronic Leukemias

Albert Z. Kapikian, MD
Head, Epidemiology Section, Laboratory of Infectious Diseases, National Institute of Allergy and Infectious Diseases, National Institutes of Health, Bethesda, Maryland
Rotaviruses, Noroviruses, and Other Gastrointestinal Viruses

David R. Karp, MD, PhD
Associate Professor of Internal Medicine, Chief, Rheumatic Diseases Division, and Harold C. Simmons Chair in Arthritis Research, University of Texas Southwestern Medical Center, Dallas, Texas
Complement in Health and Disease

Daniel L. Kastner, MD, PhD
Chief, Genetics and Genomics Branch, and Clinical Director and Director of Translational Research, National Institute of Arthritis and Musculoskeletal and Skin Diseases, National Institutes of Health, Bethesda, Maryland
The Systemic Autoinflammatory Diseases

Carol A. Kauffman, MD
Professor of Internal Medicine, University of Michigan Medical School; Chief, Infectious Diseases, Veterans Affairs Ann Arbor Healthcare System, Ann Arbor, Michigan
Histoplasmosis; Blastomycosis; Paracoccidioidomycosis; Cryptococcosis; Sporotrichosis; Candidiasis

Donald Kaye, MD
Professor of Medicine, Drexel University College of Medicine, Philadelphia, Pennsylvania
Salmonella *Infections (Including Typhoid Fever)*

Keith S. Kaye, MD, MPH
Associate Professor of Medicine, Duke University School of Medicine, Durham, North Carolina
Salmonella *Infections (Including Typhoid Fever)*

James W. Kazura, MD
Professor, Case Western Reserve University School of Medicine; Professor of Medicine, University Hospitals of Cleveland, Cleveland, Ohio
Nematode Infections

Emmet B. Keeffe, MD, MACP
Professor of Medicine and Chief of Hepatology, Stanford University School of Medicine; Co-Director, Liver Transplant Program, Stanford University Medical Center, Stanford, California
Hepatic Failure and Liver Transplantation

Craig M. Kessler, MD
Professor of Medicine and Pathology, Georgetown University School of Medicine; Director, Division of Coagulation, Lombardi Comprehensive Cancer Center, Georgetown University Hospital, Washington, DC
Hemorrhagic Disorders: Coagulation Factor Deficiencies

Matthew Kim, MD
Assistant Professor of Medicine, Division of Endocrinology and Metabolism, Johns Hopkins University School of Medicine, Baltimore, Maryland
Thyroid

Charles H. King, MD, MS
Professor of International Health, Center for Global Health and Diseases, Case Western Reserve University School of Medicine, Cleveland, Ohio
Cestode Infections

Beth D. Kirkpatrick, MD
Associate Professor of Medicine, Unit of Infectious Diseases, University of Vermont College of Medicine; Attending Physician, Fletcher Allen Health Care, Burlington, Vermont
Cryptosporidiosis

Samuel Klein, MD
William H. Danforth Professor of Medicine and Nutritional Science and Director, Center for Human Nutrition, Washington University School of Medicine, St. Louis, Missouri
Protein-Energy Malnutrition

David S. Knopman, MD
Professor of Neurology, Mayo Clinic College of Medicine; Consultant in Neurology, Mayo Clinic, Rochester, Minnesota
Regional Cerebral Dysfunction: Higher Mental Functions; Alzheimer's Disease and Other Dementias

Albert I. Ko, MD
Associate Professor of Medicine, Division of International Medicine and Infectious Disease, Weill Medical College of Cornell University, New York, New York; Visiting Researcher, Oswaldo Cruz Foundation, Brazilian Ministry of Health, Salvador, Brazil
Leptospirosis

Dimitrios P. Kontoyiannis, MD, MSc
Professor, University of Texas M. D. Anderson Cancer Center, Houston, Texas
Mycetoma

Kevin M. Korenblat, MD
Assistant Professor of Medicine, Washington University in St. Louis School of Medicine, St. Louis, Missouri
Approach to the Patient with Jaundice or Abnormal Liver Test Results

Bruce R. Korf, MD, PhD
Wayne H. and Sara Crews Finley Professor of Medical Genetics and Chair, Department of Genetics, University of Alabama School of Medicine, Birmingham, Alabama
Principles of Genetics: Overview of the Paradigm of Genetic Contribution to Health and Disease

Neil J. Korman, MD, PhD
Professor of Dermatology, Case Western Reserve University School of Medicine, Attending Physician, University Hospitals of Cleveland, Cleveland, Ohio
Macular, Papular, Vesiculobullous, and Pustular Diseases

Kris V. Kowdley, MD
Professor of Medicine, University of Washington School of Medicine, Seattle, Washington
Inherited and Metabolic Hepatic Disorders

Matthew J. Kraay, MS, MD
Professor of Orthopaedics, Case Western Reserve University School of Medicine; Director, Division of Joint Reconstruction and Arthritis Surgery, University Hospitals Case Medical Center, Cleveland, Ohio
Surgical Treatment of Joint Diseases

Monica Kraft, MD
Associate Professor of Medicine, Duke University School of Medicine; Director, Duke Asthma, Allergy, and Airway Center, Duke University Medical Center, Durham, North Carolina
Approach to the Patient with Respiratory Disease

Christopher M. Kramer, MD
Professor of Radiology and Medicine, University of Virginia School of Medicine; Director of Cardiac Magnetic Resonance Imaging, University of Virginia Health System, Charlottesville, Virginia
Nuclear Cardiology and Computed Tomography

Donald J. Krogstad, MD
William Henderson Professor and Chair of Tropical Medicine, Tulane University School of Public Health and Tropical Medicine; Professor of Medicine, Tulane University School of Medicine; Attending Physician, Tulane University Hospital and Clinic, Veterans Affairs Medical Center, and Charity Hospital of Louisiana, New Orleans, Louisiana
Malaria

Henry M. Kronenberg, MD
Professor of Medicine, Harvard Medical School; Chief, Endocrine Unit, Massachusetts General Hospital, Boston, Massachusetts
Polyglandular Disorders

Ernst J. Kuipers, MD, PhD
Chair, Departments of Gastroenterology and Hepatology and Internal Medicine, Erasmus MC University Medical Center, Rotterdam, The Netherlands
Acid Peptic Disease: Epidemiology and Pathobiology; Acid Peptic Disease: Clinical Manifestations, Diagnosis, Treatment, and Complications

Ruben I. Kuzniecky, MD
Professor of Neurology, New York University School of Medicine; Co-Director, New York University Epilepsy Center, New York, New York
Congenital, Developmental, and Neurocutaneous Disorders

Robert A. Kyle, MD
Professor of Medicine, Laboratory Medicine, and Pathology, Mayo Clinic College of Medicine; Consultant, Division of Hematology, Mayo Clinic, Rochester, Minnesota
Plasma Cell Disorders

Paul Ladenson, MD
John Eager Howard Professor of Endocrinology and Metabolism and Professor of Medicine, Pathology, Oncology, and Radiology, Johns Hopkins University School of Medicine; Director, Division of Endocrinology and Metabolism, Johns Hopkins Medical Institutions, Baltimore, Maryland
Thyroid

Nancy E. Lane, MD
Professor of Medicine and Rheumatology, University of California, Davis, School of Medicine; Director, Aging Center, University of California at Davis Medical Center, Davis, California
Osteoarthritis

Anthony E. Lang, MD, FRCPC
Professor, Department of Medicine (Neurology); Director, Division of Neurology; and Jack Clark Chair for Parkinson's Disease Research, University of Toronto Faculty of Medicine; Director, Movement Disorders Center, Toronto Western Hospital, Toronto, Ontario, Canada
Parkinsonism; Other Movement Disorders

George V. Lawry, MD
Professor of Medicine, University of Iowa Carver College of Medicine, Iowa City, Iowa
Approach to the Patient with Rheumatic Disease

Thomas H. Lee, MD, MSc
Professor of Medicine, Harvard Medical School; Network President, Partners Healthcare System, Boston, Massachusetts
Using Data for Clinical Decisions

William M. Lee, MD
Professor of Internal Medicine, Division of Digestive and Liver Diseases, University of Texas Southwestern Medical Center at Dallas, Dallas, Texas
Toxin- and Drug-Induced Liver Disease

James Leggett, MD
Associate Professor of Infectious Diseases, Oregon Health & Science University School of Medicine; Assistant Director, Medical Education, Providence Portland Medical Center, Portland, Oregon
Approach to Fever or Suspected Infection in the Normal Host

Bruce B. Lerman, MD
Hilda Altschul Master Professor of Medicine, Weill Medical College of Cornell University; Chief, Division of Cardiology, and Director, Cardiac Electrophysiology Laboratory, New York–Presbyterian Hospital, New York, New York
Ventricular Arrhythmias

Stuart Levin, MD
Professor of Medicine, Rush Medical College of Rush University; Chairman, Department of Internal Medicine, Rush University Medical Center, Chicago, Illinois
Zoonoses

Stephanie M. Levine, MD
Professor of Medicine, Division of Pulmonary and Critical Care Medicine, University of Texas Health Science Center at San Antonio; Audie L. Murphy Veterans Affairs Hospital, San Antonio, Texas
Alveolar Filling Disorders

Oliver Liesenfeld, MD
Professor of Medical Microbiology and Immunology of Infection and Head, Toxoplasmosis Counseling Laboratory, Charité Medical School, Berlin, Germany
Toxoplasmosis

Henry W. Lim, MD, DSc
Chairman and C. S. Livingood Chair, Department of Dermatology, Henry Ford Medical Center, Detroit, Michigan
Eczemas, Photodermatoses, Papulosquamous (Including Fungal) Diseases, and Figurate Erythemas

Aldo A. M. Lima, MD, PhD
Professor of Medicine, Department of Physiology and Pharmacology, Universidade Federal do Ceará; Coordinator, Unidade de Pesquisas Clínicas, Universidate Federal do Ceará, Fortaleza-Ceará, Brazil
Schistosomiasis (Bilharziasis)

Andrew H. Limper, MD
Professor of Medicine, Mayo Clinic College of Medicine; Consultant in Pulmonary and Critical Care, St. Mary's Hospital and Mayo Clinic, Rochester, Minnesota
Overview of Pneumonia

Geoffrey S. F. Ling, MD, PhD
Professor and Vice-Chair of Neurology, Uniformed Services University of the Health Sciences F. Edward Hébert School of Medicine, Bethesda, Maryland; Attending Physician in Neurology, Neurosurgery, and Critical Care Medicine and Director of Neurocritical Care, Walter Reed Army Medical Center, Washington, DC
Traumatic Brain Injury and Spinal Cord Injury

Scott M. Lippman, MD
Charles A. LeMaistre Distinguished Chair in Thoracic Oncology; Chair, Department of Thoracic/Head and Neck Medical Oncology; Professor, Divisions of Cancer Medicine and Cancer Prevention, The University of Texas M. D. Anderson Cancer Center, Houston, Texas
Cancer Prevention

Alan F. List, MD
Professor of Medicine, University of South Florida College of Medicine; Division Chief, Malignant Hematology, and Co-Director, Infusion Center, H. Lee Moffitt Cancer Center and Research Institute, Tampa, Florida
Myelodysplastic Syndrome

Richard F. Loeser, MD
Professor of Internal Medicine and Head, Section of Molecular Medicine, Wake Forest University School of Medicine, Winston-Salem, North Carolina
Connective Tissue Structure and Function

Bennett Lorber, MD
Thomas M. Durant Professor of Medicine and Professor of Microbiology and Immunology, Temple University School of Medicine; Chief, Section of Infectious Diseases, Temple University Hospital, Philadelphia, Pennsylvania
Listeriosis

John M. Luce, MD
Professor of Medicine and Anesthesia, University of California, San Francisco, School of Medicine; Chief Medical Officer, San Francisco General Hospital, San Francisco, California
Respiratory Monitoring in Critical Care

Daniel R. Lucey, MD, MPH
Co-Director, Master of Science Program in Biohazardous Threat Agents and Emerging Infectious Diseases, and Adjunct Professor, Department of Microbiology and Immunology, Georgetown University Medical Center; Director, Center for Biological Counterterrorism and Emerging Diseases, Washington Hospital Center, Washington, DC
Anthrax

Bruce W. Lytle, MD
Professor of Surgery, Cleveland Clinic Lerner College of Medicine of Case Western Reserve University; Chairman, Department of Thoracic and Cardiovascular Surgery, Cleveland Clinic, Cleveland, Ohio
Surgical Treatment of Coronary Artery Disease

Adel A. F. Mahmoud, MD, PhD
Professor, Department of Molecular Biology, Princeton University, Princeton, New Jersey; Adjunct Professor of Medicine, Case Western Reserve University School of Medicine, Cleveland, Ohio
Liver, Intestinal, and Lung Fluke Infections

Mark W. Mahowald, MD
Professor, Department of Neurology, University of Minnesota Medical School; Director, Minnesota Regional Sleep Disorders Center, Minneapolis, Minnesota
Disorders of Sleep

Juan-R. Malagelada, MD
Professor of Gastroenterology, Universitat Autònoma de Barcelona; Chief, Digestive Diseases, Hospital Universitari Vall d'Hebron, Barcelona, Spain
Acid Peptic Disease: Clinical Manifestations, Diagnosis, Treatment, and Prognosis

Stephen E. Malawista, MD
Professor of Medicine, Yale University School of Medicine, New Haven, Connecticut
Lyme Disease

Lionel A. Mandell, MD
Professor of Medicine, Faculty of Health Sciences at McMaster University: Department of Medicine, Attending Physician, Hamilton Health Sciences, Henderson Division, Hamilton, Ontario, Canada
Pneumococcal Pneumonia

Warren J. Manning, MD
Professor of Medicine and Radiology, Harvard Medical School; Section Chief, Non-invasive Cardiac Imaging, Beth Israel Deaconess Medical Center, Boston, Massachusetts
Cardiovascular Magnetic Resonance Imaging; Pericardial Disease

Peter Manu, MD
Professor of Clinical Medicine, Psychiatry, and Behavioral Sciences, Albert Einstein College of Medicine, Bronx; Director of Medical Services, Zucker Hillside Hospital, North Shore–Long Island Jewish Health System, Glen Oaks, New York
Medical Consultation in Psychiatry

Marsha D. Marcus, PhD
Professor of Psychiatry and Psychology, University of Pittsburgh School of Medicine; Chief, Eating Disorders Program, Western Psychiatric Institute and Clinic, University of Pittsburgh Medical Center, Pittsburgh, Pennsylvania
Eating Disorders

Ariane J. Marelli, MD
Associate Professor of Medicine, McGill University Faculty of Medicine; Director, McGill Adult Unit for Congenital Heart Disease (MAUDE), McGill University Health Centre, Montreal, Quebec, Canada
Congenital Heart Disease in Adults

George M. Martin, MD
Professor of Pathology Emeritus, University of Washington School of Medicine, Seattle, Washington
Biology of Aging

Joel B. Mason, MD
Associate Professor of Medicine and Nutrition, Tufts University School of Medicine; Attending Physician, Division of Clinical Nutrition and Gastroenterology, Tufts–New England Medical Center, Boston, Massachusetts
Vitamins, Trace Minerals, and Other Micronutrients

Barry M. Massie, MD
Professor of Medicine, University of California, San Francisco, School of Medicine; Chief, Cardiology Section, and Director, Heart Failure Program, San Francisco Veterans Affairs Medical Center, San Francisco, California
Heart Failure: Pathophysiology and Diagnosis

Henry Masur, MD
Clinical Professor of Medicine, George Washington University School of Medicine, Washington, DC; Chief, Critical Care Medicine Department, National Institutes of Health, Bethesda, Maryland
Treatment of Human Immunodeficiency Virus Infection and Acquired Immunodeficiency Syndrome

Toby Maurer, MD
Associate Professor, Department of Dermatology, University of California, San Francisco, School of Medicine; Chief of Dermatology, San Francisco General Hospital, San Francisco, California
Skin Manifestations in Patients with Human Immunodeficiency Virus Infection

Mitchell B. Max, MD
Chief, Clinical Pain Research Section, National Institute of Dental and Craniofacial Research, National Institutes of Health, Bethesda, Maryland
Pain

Charles E. McCulloch, PhD
Professor of Biostatistics, University of California, San Francisco, School of Medicine, San Francisco, California
Statistical Interpretation of Data

Margaret M. McGovern, MD, PhD
Professor of Genetics and Genomic Science and Pediatrics, Mount Sinai School of Medicine; Attending Physician, Mount Sinai Hospital, New York, New York
Lysosomal Storage Diseases

Michael A. McGuigan, MD, CM, MBA
Clinical Professor of Emergency Medicine, State University of New York, Stony Brook, School of Medicine, Stony Brook; Medical Director, Long Island Regional Poison & Drug Information Center, Winthrop-University Hospital, Mineola, New York
Chronic Poisoning: Trace Metals and Others

William McKenna, MD, DSc, FRCP
Professor of Cardiology, University College London; UCL Division of Medicine, Centre for Cardiology in the Young, Royal Free and University College Medical School; Clinical Director, The Heart Hospital, London, United Kingdom
Diseases of the Myocardium and Endocardium

Robert McMillan, MD
Professor Emeritus, The Scripps Research Institute, La Jolla, California
Hemorrhagic Disorders: Abnormalities of Platelet and Vascular Function

John J. V. McMurray, MD, FRCP
Professor of Medical Cardiology, University of Glasgow; Honorary Consultant Cardiologist, Western Infirmary, Glasgow, United Kingdom
Heart Failure: Management and Prognosis

Mary McNaughton-Collins, MD, MPH
Assistant Professor of Medicine, Harvard Medical School; Associate Physician, Massachusetts General Hospital, Boston, Massachusetts
Benign Prostate Disease and Prostatitis

Steven J. Mentzer, MD
Associate Professor of Surgery, Harvard Medical School; Director, Thoracic Intensive Care Unit, Brigham and Women's Hospital, Boston, Massachusetts
Surgical Approach to Lung Disease3

Frederick W. Miller, MD, PhD
Chief, Environmental Autoimmunity Group, Office of Clinical Research, National Institute of Environmental Health Sciences, National Institutes of Health, Bethesda, Maryland
Polymyositis and Dermatomyositis

Kenneth L. Minaker, MD, FRCP
Associate Professor of Medicine, Harvard Medical School; Chief, Geriatric Medicine Unit, Massachusetts General Hospital, Boston, Massachusetts
Common Clinical Sequelae of Aging

Michael Ming, MD, MSCE
Assistant Professor of Medicine, University of Pennsylvania School of Medicine; Director, Pigmented Lesion Clinic, Hospital of the University of Pennsylvania, Philadelphia, Pennsylvania
Melanoma and Nonmelanoma Skin Cancers

Daniel R. Mishell, Jr., MD
Lyle G. McNiele Professor, Department of Obstetrics and Gynecology, Keck School of Medicine of the University of Southern California; Chief, Division of Family Planning, Women's and Children's Hospital, Los Angeles, California
Contraception

William E. Mitch, MD
Gordon A. Cain Chair in Nephrology and Director, Division of Nephrology, Baylor College of Medicine, Houston, Texas
Chronic Kidney Disease

John F. Modlin, MD, MS
Professor of Pediatrics and Medicine, Dartmouth Medical School; Chairman, Department of Pediatrics, Dartmouth-Hitchcock Medical Center, Lebanon, New Hampshire
Enterovirus Infections

Mark E. Molitch, MD
Professor of Medicine, Northwestern University Feinberg School of Medicine; Attending Physician, Northwestern Memorial Hospital, Chicago, Illinois
Neuroendocrinology and the Neuroendocrine System; Anterior Pituitary

Bruce A. Molitoris, MD
Professor of Medicine, Indiana University School of Medicine, Indianapolis, Indiana
Acute Kidney Injury

Kelly L. Molpus, MD
Director of Gynecologic Oncology, Halifax Medical Center, Daytona Beach, Florida
Gynecologic Cancers

Fred Morady, MD
Professor, University of Michigan Medical School; Director, Clinical Electrophysiology Service, University of Michigan Medical Center, Ann Arbor, Michigan
Electrophysiologic Interventional Procedures and Surgery

Jeffrey A. Moscow, MD
Children's Miracle Network Professor of Pediatrics and Chief, Pediatric Hematology/Oncology, University of Kentucky College of Medicine; Director, Experimental Therapeutics Program, Markey Cancer Center, Lexington, Kentucky
Biology of Cancer

Michael A. Moskowitz, MD
Professor of Neurology and Faculty Member, Harvard-MIT Division of Health Sciences and Technology; Associate Neurologist and Associate Neurophysiologist, Massachusetts General Hospital, Boston, Massachusetts
Headaches and Other Head Pain

Andrew H. Murr, MD
Professor of Clinical Otolaryngology and Vice Chairman, Department of Otolaryngology/Head and Neck Surgery, University of California, San Francisco, School of Medicine; Chief of Service, San Francisco General Hospital, San Francisco, California
Approach to the Patient with Nose, Sinus, and Ear Disorders

Hyman B. Muss, MD
Professor of Medicine, University of Vermont College of Medicine and Vermont Cancer Center; Attending Physician, Fletcher Allen Health Care, Burlington, Vermont
Breast Cancer and Differential Diagnosis of Benign Lesions

Robert J. Myerburg, MD
Professor of Medicine, Division of Cardiology, University of Miami Miller School of Medicine, Miami, Florida
Approach to Cardiac Arrest and Life-Threatening Arrhythmias

Ronald L. Nagel, MD
Professor, Department of Physiology and Biophysics, and Irving D. Karpas Professor of Medicine, Albert Einstein College of Medicine of Yeshiva University; Head of Hematology, Montefiore Hospital, Bronx, New York
Methemoglobinemias and Unstable Hemoglobins

Stanley Naguwa, MD
Clinical Professor of Medicine, University of California, Davis, School of Medicine, Davis, California
Sjögren's Syndrome

Stanley J. Naides, MD
Medical Director, Immunology Research and Development, Quest Diagnostics Nichols Institute, San Juan Capistrano, California
Arthropod-Borne Viruses Causing Fever and Rash Syndromes

Avindra Nath, MBBS
Professor of Neurology and Neuroscience and Director of Neuroimmunology and Neurological Infections, Johns Hopkins University School of Medicine, Baltimore, Maryland
Cytomegalovirus, Epstein-Barr Virus, and Slow Virus Infections of the Central Nervous System; Neurologic Complications of Human Immunodeficiency Virus Infection; Brain Abscess and Parameningeal Infections; Acute Viral Encephalitis; Poliomyelitis; Rabies

Eric G. Neilson, MD
Chairman, Department of Medicine, and Hugh Jackson Morgan Professor of Medicine and Cell and Developmental Biology, Vanderbilt University School of Medicine; Physician-in-Chief, Vanderbilt University Hospital, Nashville, Tennessee
Tubulointerstitial Diseases

Heidi Nelson, MD
Professor of Surgery, Mayo Clinic College of Medicine; Consultant, Division of Colon and Rectal Surgery, and Fred C. Anderson Professor of Surgery, Mayo Foundation, Rochester, Minnesota
Diseases of the Rectum and Anus

Brent A. Neuschwander-Tetri, MD
Professor of Internal Medicine, Saint Louis University School of Medicine, St. Louis, Missouri
Bacterial, Parasitic, Fungal, and Granulomatous Liver Diseases

Franklin A. Neva, MD
National Institute of Allergy and Infectious Diseases, National Institutes of Health, Bethesda, Maryland
American Trypanosomiasis (Chagas' Disease)

James R. Newland, MD
Professor Emeritus of Pathology and Microbiology, University of Nebraska Medical Center; Courtesy Staff, University of Nebraska Hospital, Omaha, Nebraska
The Peripheral Blood Smear

Thomas B. Newman, MD, MPH
Professor of Epidemiology and Biostatistics and Pediatrics, University of California, San Francisco, School of Medicine; Attending Physician, University of California, San Francisco, Children's Medical Center and San Francisco General Hospital, San Francisco, California
Statistical Interpretation of Data

John Newsom-Davis, MD
Professor Emeritus, University of Oxford, Oxford, United Kingdom
Disorders of Neuromuscular Transmission

Lynnette K. Nieman, MD
Senior Investigator, Reproductive Biology and Medicine Branch, National Institute of Child Health and Human Development, National Institutes of Health, Bethesda, Maryland
Adrenal Cortex

S. Ragnar Norrby, MD, PhD
Director General, Swedish Institute for Infectious Disease Control, Solna, Sweden
Approach to the Patient with Urinary Tract Infection

David A. Norris, MD
Professor and Chairman, Department of Dermatology, University of Colorado at Denver and Health Sciences Center, Denver, Colorado
Structure and Function of the Skin

Susan O'Brien, MD
Professor of Medicine, Department of Leukemia, The University of Texas M. D. Anderson Cancer Center, Houston, Texas
The Chronic Leukemias

Francis G. O'Connor, MD, MPH
Associate Professor of Family Medicine, Uniformed Services University of the Health Sciences, F. Edward Hébert School of Medicine, Bethesda, Maryland
Rhabdomyolysis

Patrick G. O'Connor, MD, MPH
Professor of Medicine, Yale University School of Medicine; Chief, Section of General Internal Medicine, Yale–New Haven Hospital, New Haven, Connecticut
Alcohol Abuse and Dependence

James R. O'Dell, MD
Larson Professor of Medicine, University of Nebraska College of Medicine; Chief, Section of Rheumatology and Immunology and Vice-Chairman, Department of Internal Medicine, University of Nebraska Medical Center, Omaha, Nebraska
Rheumatoid Arthritis

Jeffrey E. Olgin, MD
Associate Professor and Melvin Scheinman Chair in Electrophysiology, University of California, San Francisco, School of Medicine, San Francisco, California
Approach to the Patient with Suspected Arrhythmia

Jeffrey W. Olin, DO
Professor of Medicine, Mount Sinai School of Medicine; Director, Vascular Medicine, Mount Sinai Medical Center, New York, New York
Other Peripheral Arterial Diseases

Richard J. O'Reilly, MD
Professor of Pediatrics, Weill Medical College of Cornell University; Chairman, Department of Pediatrics, Memorial Sloan-Kettering Cancer Center, New York, New York
Aplastic Anemia and Related Disorders

Walter A. Orenstein, MD
Professor of Medicine and Pediatrics, Emory University School of Medicine; Associate Director, Emory Vaccine Center, Atlanta, Georgia
Immunization

Roy C. Orlando, MD
Professor of Medicine and Adjunct Professor of Physiology, Tulane University School of Medicine; Chief, Gastroenterology and Hepatology, Tulane University Health Sciences Center, New Orleans, Louisiana
Diseases of the Esophagus

Catherine M. Otto, MD
J. Ward Kennedy-Hamilton Endowed Professor of Cardiology, Professor of Medicine, and Director, Cardiovascular Fellowship Training Program, University of Washington School of Medicine; Associate Director, Echocardiography Laboratory, University of Washington Medical Center, Seattle, Washington
Echocardiography

Joseph G. Ouslander, MD
Professor of Medicine and Director, Division of Geriatric Medicine and Gerontology, Emory University School of Medicine; Chief Medical Officer, Wesley Woods Center of Emory University, Atlanta, Georgia
Urinary Incontinence

Chung Owyang, MD
Professor of Internal Medicine, University of Michigan Medical School, Ann Arbor, Michigan
Pancreatitis

Stephen A. Paget, MD
Professor of Medicine, Weill Medical College of Cornell University; Physician-in-Chief and Chairman, Division of Rheumatology, Hospital for Special Surgery, New York, New York
Polymyalgia Rheumatica and Temporal Arteritis

Peter G. Pappas, MD, FACP
Professor of Medicine, Division of Infectious Diseases, University of Alabama School of Medicine, Birmingham, Alabama
Dematiaceous Fungal Infections

Joseph E. Parrillo, MD
Professor of Medicine, University of Medicine and Dentistry of New Jersey Robert Wood Johnson Medical School; Head, Division of Cardiovascular Disease and Critical Care Medicine; Director, Cooper Heart Institute; Director, Cardiovascular and Critical Care Service, Cooper University Hospital, Camden, New Jersey
Approach to the Patient with Shock

Pankaj Jay Pasricha, MD
Professor of Medicine and Chief, Division of Gastroenterology, University of Texas Medical Branch, Galveston, Texas
Gastrointestinal Endoscopy

Steven Z. Pavletic, MD
Head, Graft-versus-Host and Autoimmunity Unit, National Cancer Institute, National Institutes of Health, Bethesda, Maryland
Hematopoietic Stem Cell Transplantation

Richard D. Pearson, MD, FACP
Professor of Medicine and Pathology, University of Virginia School of Medicine; Professor of Medicine and Pathology, University of Virginia Health System, Charlottesville, Virginia
Antiparasitic Therapy; Leishmaniasis; Babesiosis and Other Protozoan Diseases

Eli N. Perencevich, MD, MS
Associate Professor, Department of Epidemiology and Preventive Medicine, University of Maryland School of Medicine; Attending Physician, Veterans Affairs Maryland Healthcare System, Baltimore, Maryland
Enterococcal Infections

Trish M. Perl, MD, MSc
Associate Professor of Medicine and Pathology Hospital Epidemiologist, Johns Hopkins Medical Institutions, Baltimore, Maryland
Enterococcal Infections

Michael C. Perry, MD, MS, FACP
Professor of Internal Medicine, Director of Division of Hematology/Medical Oncology, and Nellie B. Smith Chair of Oncology, University of Missouri School of Medicine; Deputy Director, Ellis Fischel Cancer Center, Columbia, Missouri
Principles of Cancer Therapy

William A. Petri, Jr., MD, PhD
Wade Hampton Frost Professor of Epidemiology; Professor of Medicine, Microbiology, and Pathology; and Chief, Division of Infectious Diseases and International Health, University of Virginia School of Medicine; Attending Physician, University of Virginia Hospitals, Charlottesville, Virginia
Relapsing Fever and Other Borrelia *Infections*

Marc A. Pfeffer, MD, PhD
Professor of Medicine, Harvard Medical School; Cardiovascular Division, Brigham and Women's Hospital, Boston, Massachusetts
Heart Failure: Management and Prognosis

James M. Phang, MD
Chief, Metabolism and Cancer Susceptibility Section, Laboratory of Comparative Carcinogenesis, National Cancer Institute at Frederick, National Institutes of Health, Frederick, Maryland
The Hyperprolinemias and Hydroxyprolinemia

Perry J. Pickhardt, MD
Associate Professor of Radiology, University of Wisconsin School of Medicine and Public Health, Madison, Wisconsin; Adjunct Assistant Professor of Radiology, Uniformed Services University of the Health Sciences, F. Edward Hébert School of Medicine, Bethesda, Maryland
Diagnostic Imaging Procedures in Gastroenterology

Gerald B. Pier, PhD
Professor of Medicine, Microbiology, and Molecular Genetics, Harvard Medical School; Microbiologist, Brigham and Women's Hospital, Boston, Massachusetts
Pseudomonas *and Related Gram-Negative Bacillary Infections*

Peter Piot, MD, PhD
Executive Director, UNAIDS, Geneva, Switzerland
Human Immunodeficiency Virus Infection and Acquired Immunodeficiency Syndrome: A Global Overview

David S. Pisetsky, MD, PhD
Professor of Medicine and Immunology and Chief of Rheumatology and Immunology, Duke University Medical Center; Chief of Rheumatology, Durham Veterans Affairs Medical Center, Durham, North Carolina
Laboratory Testing in the Rheumatic Diseases

Marshall Posner, MD
Associate Professor of Medicine, Harvard Medical School; Medical Director, Head and Neck Oncology Program, Dana-Farber Cancer Institute, Boston, Massachusetts
Head and Neck Cancer

Don W. Powell, MD
Professor of Neuroscience and Cell Biology, Department of Internal Medicine, and Program Director, General Clinical Research Center, University of Texas Medical Branch, Galveston, Texas
Approach to the Patient with Diarrhea and Malabsorption

Charlene Prather, MD
Associate Professor of Internal Medicine, Saint Louis University School of Medicine, St. Louis, Missouri
Inflammatory and Anatomic Diseases of the Intestine, Peritoneum, Mesentery, and Omentum

Deborah D. Proctor, MD
Associate Professor of Medicine, Section of Digestive Diseases, and Director, Gastroenterology Fellowship Training Program, Yale University School of Medicine; Attending Physician, Yale–New Haven Hospital, New Haven, Connecticut
Approach to the Patient with Gastrointestinal Disease

Basil A. Pruitt, Jr., MD
Professor of Surgery, Uniformed Services University of the Health Sciences, F. Edward Hébert School of Medicine; Bethesda, Maryland; Clinical Professor of Surgery, University of Texas Health Science Center at San Antonio; Staff Surgeon, University Hospital, San Antonio; Surgical Consultant, U.S. Army Institute of Surgical Research, Fort Sam Houston, Texas
Electric Injury

Reed E. Pyeritz, MD, PhD
Professor of Medicine and Genetics, University of Pennsylvania School of Medicine; Chief, Division of Medical Genetics, Hospital of the University of Pennsylvania, Philadelphia, Pennsylvania
Inherited Diseases of Connective Tissue

Anastacio de Queiroz Sousa, MD
Associate Professor, Department of Clinical Medicine, Federal University of Ceará; Physician, Hospital Saõ José for Infectious Disease, Ceará, Brazil
Leishmaniasis

Peter J. Quesenberry, MD
Professor of Medicine, Boston University School of Medicine, Boston, Massachusetts; Professor of Medicine, The Warren Alpert Medical School of Brown University; Director, Adele R. Decof Cancer Center and Blood and Marrow Transplant Program, Roger Williams Medical Center, Providence, Rhode Island
Hematopoiesis and Hematopoietic Growth Factors

Thomas C. Quinn, MD, MSc
Professor of Medicine, International Health, Epidemiology, and Molecular Microbiology and Immunology, Johns Hopkins University School of Medicine; Director, Johns Hopkins Center for Global Health, Baltimore; Senior Investigator, Laboratory of Immunoregulation, and Associate Director for International Research, National Institute of Allergy and Infectious Diseases, National Institutes of Health, Bethesda, Maryland
African Trypanosomiasis (Sleeping Sickness); Epidemiology of Human Immunodeficiency Virus Infection and Acquired Immunodeficiency Syndrome

Ganesh Raghu, MD, FACP, FCCP
Professor of Medicine and Laboratory Medicine (Adjunct), University of Washington School of Medicine; Chief, Chest Clinic, and Medical Director, Lung Transplant Program, University of Washington Medical Center, Seattle, Washington
Interstitial Lung Disease

S. Vincent Rajkumar, MD
Professor of Medicine, Mayo Clinic College of Medicine; Consultant, Division of Hematology, Mayo Clinic, Rochester, Minnesota
Plasma Cell Disorders

Didier Raoult, MD, PhD
Professor, Faculty of Medicine, Marseilles School of Medicine; Head Clinical Microbiology Department, Hôpital La Timone, Marseilles, France
Rickettsioses

Robert W. Rebar, MD
Volunteer Professor, Department of Obstetrics and Gynecology, University of Alabama School of Medicine, Birmingham, Alabama
Ovaries and Development; Menstrual Cycle and Fertility

Annette C. Reboli, MD
Professor of Medicine, University of Medicine and Dentistry of New Jersey Robert Wood Johnson Medical School; Head, Infectious Diseases Division, and Hospital Epidemiologist, Cooper University Hospital, Camden, New Jersey
Erysipelothrix *Infections*

Donald Redelmeier, MD, FRCP
Professor of Medicine and Canada Research Chair, University of Toronto Faculty of Medicine; Staff Physician, Division of General Internal Medicine, Sunnybrook Health Science Center; Director of Clinical Epidemiology, Sunnybrook Research Institute, Toronto, Ontario, Canada
Postoperative Care and Complications

John J. Reilly, Jr., MD
Associate Professor of Medicine, Harvard Medical School; Acting Chief, Division of Pulmonary and Critical Care Medicine, Brigham and Women's Hospital, Boston, Massachusetts
Surgical Approach to Lung Disease

Michael F. Rein, MD
Jordan Professor of Epidemiology in Medicine, University of Virginia School of Medicine, Charlottesville, Virginia
Approach to the Patient with a Sexually Transmitted Disease

David A. Relman, MD
Associate Professor of Medicine and Microbiology and Immunology, Stanford University School of Medicine, Stanford; Chief, Infectious Diseases, Veterans Affairs Palo Alto Health Care System, Palo Alto, California
Disease Caused by Bartonella *Species*

Herbert Y. Reynolds, MD
Professor Emeritus, Department of Medicine, Penn State College of Medicine, Hershey, Pennsylvania; Adjunct Professor of Medicine, Uniformed Services University of the Health Sciences, F. Edward Hébert School of Medicine, Bethesda; Medical Officer, Division of Lung Diseases, National Heart, Lung, and Blood Institute, National Institutes of Health, Bethesda, Maryland
Respiratory Structure and Function: Mechanisms and Testing

Robert A. Rizza, MD
Professor of Medicine, Mayo Clinic College of Medicine, Rochester, Minnesota
Hypoglycemia/Pancreatic Islet Cell Disorders

Lewis R. Roberts, MB ChB, PhD
Assistant Professor of Medicine, Mayo Clinic College of Medicine; Assistant Professor of Medicine and Consultant, Mayo Clinic, Rochester, Minnesota
Liver and Biliary Tract Tumors

Griffin P. Rodgers, MD, MSc
Chief, Molecular and Clinical Hematology Branch, National Institute of Diabetes and Digestive and Kidney Diseases, National Institutes of Health, Bethesda, Maryland
Hemoglobinopathies: The Thalassemias

John L. Rombeau, MD
Professor of Surgery, University of Pennsylvania School of Medicine; Attending Physician, Hospital of the University of Pennsylvania, Philadelphia, Pennsylvania
Enteral Nutrition

G. David Roodman, MD, PhD
Professor of Medicine, University of Pittsburgh School of Medicine; Director, Center for Bone Biology, University of Pittsburgh Medical Center; Vice Chair for Research, Veterans Affairs Pittsburgh Healthcare System, Pittsburgh, Pennsylvania
Paget's Disease of Bone

Clifford Rosen, MD
Professor of Nutrition, University of Maine, Orono; Senior Staff Scientist, The Jackson Laboratory, Bangor, Maine
Osteoporosis

Marc E. Rothenberg, MD, PhD
Professor of Pediatrics, University of Cincinnati College of Medicine; Director, Division of Allergy and Immunology, Cincinnati Children's Hospital Medical Center, Cincinnati, Ohio
Eosinophilic Syndromes

Hope S. Rugo, MD
Clinical Professor of Medicine and Director, Breast Oncology Clinical Trials Program, University of California, San Francisco, Comprehensive Cancer Center, San Francisco, California
Paraneoplastic Syndromes and Other Non-neoplastic Effects of Cancer

James A. Russell, MD, FRCPC
Professor, Department of Medicine and James Hugg Centre for Cardiovascular and Pulmonary Research, University of British Columbia Faculty of Medicine; Intensivist, Critical Care Medicine, St. Paul's Hospital, Vancouver, British Columbia, Canada
Shock Syndromes Related to Sepsis

Anil K. Rustgi, MD
T. Girier Miller Professor of Medicine and Genetics, University of Pennsylvania School of Medicine; Chief of Gastroenterology, Hospital of the University of Pennsylvania, Philadelphia, Pennsylvania
Neoplasms of the Stomach

Robert A. Salata, MD
Professor and Vice-Chair, Department of Medicine, and Chief, Division of Infectious Diseases and HIV Medicine, Case Western Reserve University School of Medicine; Attending Physician and Consultant, University Hospitals Case Medical Center, Cleveland, Ohio
Brucellosis

Jane E. Salmon, MD
Professor of Medicine, Weill Medical College of Cornell University; Attending Physician and Senior Scientist, Hospital for Special Surgery, New York, New York
Mechanisms of Immune-Mediated Tissue Injury

Jeffrey H. Samet, MD, MA, MPH
Professor of Medicine and Social and Behavioral Sciences, Boston University School of Medicine and School of Public Health; Chief, Section of General Internal Medicine, Boston Medical Center, Boston, Massachusetts
Drug Abuse and Dependence

Jonathan M. Samet, MD, MS
Professor and Chair, Department of Epidemiology; Director, Institute for Global Tobacco Control; and Co-Director, Risk Sciences and Public Policy Institute, Johns Hopkins Bloomberg School of Public Health, Baltimore, Maryland
Occupational Pulmonary Disorders

Renato M. Santos, MD
Assistant Professor of Internal Medicine and Associate Director, Cardiovascular Training Program, Wake Forest University School of Medicine, Winston-Salem, North Carolina
Vascular Disorders of the Kidney

Clifford B. Saper, MD, PhD
James Jackson Putnam Professor of Neurology and Neuroscience, Harvard Medical School; Chairman, Department of Neurology, and Neurologist-in-Chief, Beth Israel Deaconess Medical Center, Boston, Massachusetts
Autonomic Disorders and Their Management

Michael N. Sawka, PhD
Chief, Thermal & Mountain Medicine Division, U.S. Army Research Institute of Environmental Medicine, Natick, Massachusetts
Disorders Due to Heat and Cold

Paul E. Sax, MD
Associate Professor of Medicine, Harvard Medical School; Clinical Director, Division of Infectious Diseases, Brigham and Women's Hospital, Boston, Massachusetts
Immunopathogenesis of Human Immunodeficiency Virus Infection

Andrew I. Schafer, MD
The E. Hugh Luckey Distinguished Professor of Medicine and Chairman, Department of Medicine, Weill Medical College of Cornell University; Physician-in-Chief, New York–Presbyterian Hospital and Weill Cornell Medical Center, New York, New York
Approach to the Patient with Bleeding and Thrombosis; Hemorrhagic Disorders: Disseminated Intravascular Coagulation, Liver Failure, and Vitamin K Deficiency; Thrombotic Disorders: Hypercoagulable States

William Schaffner, MD
Professor and Chair, Department of Preventive Medicine, and Professor of Medicine (Infectious Diseases), Vanderbilt University School of Medicine, Nashville, Tennessee
Tularemia and Other Francisella *Infectious*

W. Michael Scheld, MD
Bayer–Gerald L. Mandell Professor of Infectious Diseases, Professor of Internal Medicine and Clinical Professor of Neurosurgery, University of Virginia Health System, Charlottesville, Virginia
Introduction to Microbial Disease: Host-Pathogen Interactions

Randolph B. Schiffer, MD
The Vernon and Elizabeth Haggerton Chair in Neurology and Chair, Department of Neuropsychiatry and Behavioral Science, Texas Tech University Health Sciences Center; Chief of Neurology and Psychiatry, University Medical Center, Lubbock, Texas
Psychiatric Disorders in Medical Practice

David Schlossberg, MD
Professor of Medicine, Temple University School of Medicine; Adjunct Professor of Medicine, University of Pennsylvania School of Medicine; Medical Director, Tuberculosis Control Program, Department of Public Health, Philadelphia, Pennsylvania
Arthropods and Leeches

Thomas J. Schnitzer, MD, PhD
Professor and Assistant Dean for Clinical Research, Northwestern University Feinberg School of Medicine, Chicago, Illinois
Osteoarthritis

Robert T. Schooley, MD
Professor of Medicine and Head, Division of Infectious Diseases, University of California, San Diego, School of Medicine, La Jolla, California
Epstein-Barr Virus Infection

David L. Schriger, MD, MPH
Professor, David Geffen School of Medicine at UCLA; Attending Physician, UCLA Emergency Medicine Center, Los Angeles, California
Approach to the Patient with Abnormal Vital Signs

Steven A. Schroeder, MD
Distinguished Professor of Health and Health Care, Department of Medicine, and Director, Smoking Cessation Leadership Center, University of California, San Francisco, School of Medicine, San Francisco, California
Socioeconomic Issues in Medicine

Lynn Schuchter, MD
Professor of Medicine, University of Pennsylvania School of Medicine; Hospital of the University of Pennsylvania, Philadelphia, Pennsylvania
Melanoma and Nonmelanoma Skin Cancers

Sam Schulman, MD, PhD
Thrombosis Service, McMaster Clinics, Hamilton Health Sciences General Hospital, Hamilton, Ontario, Canada
Antithrombotic Therapy

Frederick L. Schuster, PhD
Research Scientist, California Department of Health Services, Viral and Rickettsial Disease Laboratory, Richmond, California
Amebiasis

Lawrence B. Schwartz, MD, PhD
Professor of Medicine, Medical College of Virginia Campus of Virginia Commonwealth University School of Medicine, Richmond, Virginia
Systemic Anaphylaxis, Food Allergy, and Insect Sting Allergy

Robert S. Schwartz, MD
Distinguished Professor of Medicine, Tufts University School of Medicine; Deputy Editor, *New England Journal of Medicine*, Boston, Massachusetts
Autoimmune and Intravascular Hemolytic Anemias

Cynthia L. Sears, MD
Professor of Medicine, Divisions of Infectious Diseases and Gastroenterology, Johns Hopkins University School of Medicine; Attending Physician, Johns Hopkins Hospital, Baltimore, Maryland
Cryptosporidiosis; Giardiasis

Carlos Seas, MD
Associate Professor, Universidad Peruana Cayetano Heredia; Attending Physician, Department of Infectious, Tropical, and Dermatologic Diseases, Hospital Nacional Cayetano Heredia, Lima, Peru
Cholera and Other Vibrio *Infections*

Margretta R. Seashore, MD
Professor of Genetics and Pediatrics, Yale University School of Medicine; Attending Physician, Yale–New Haven Hospital, New Haven, Connecticut
Genetic Risk Assessment

Julian L. Seifter, MD
Associate Professor of Medicine, Harvard Medical School; Physician, Brigham and Women's Hospital, Boston, Massachusetts
Potassium Disorders; Acid-Base Disorders

Steven A. Seifert, MD
Professor, University of New Mexico School of Medicine; Director, New Mexico Poison and Drug Information Center, Albuquerque, New Mexico
Venomous Snake Bites

Clay F. Semenkovich, MD
Herbert S. Gasser Professor and Chief, Division of Endocrinology, Metabolism, and Lipid Research, Washington University in St. Louis School of Medicine, St. Louis, Missouri
Disorders of Lipid Metabolism

Carol E. Semrad, MD
Associate Professor of Medicine, The University of Chicago Pritzker School of Medicine; Attending Physician, The University of Chicago Hospitals, Chicago, Illinois
Approach to the Patient with Diarrhea and Malabsorption

F. John Service, MD, PhD
Professor of Medicine, Mayo Clinic College of Medicine; Consultant in Endocrinology and Metabolism, Mayo Clinic, Rochester, Minnesota
Hypoglycemia/Pancreatic Islet Cell Disorders

George M. Shaw, MD, PhD
Professor of Medicine and Microbiology, University of Alabama School of Medicine, Birmingham, Alabama
Biology of Human Immunodeficiency Viruses

Steven A. Shea, PhD
Associate Professor of Medicine, Harvard Medical School; Director, Sleep Disorders Research Program, Brigham and Women's Hospital, Boston, Massachusetts
Disorders of Ventilatory Control

Robert S. Sherwin, MD
C. N. H. Long Professor of Medicine; Director, Yale Center for Clinical Investigation; Director, Diabetes Endocrinology Research Center; and Interim Chief, Section of Endocrinology, Yale University School of Medicine; Attending Physician, Yale–New Haven Hospital, New Haven, Connecticut
Type 1 Diabetes Mellitus; Type 2 Diabetes Mellitus

Michael E. Shy, MD
Professor of Neurology and Professor of Molecular Medicine and Genetics, Wayne State University School of Medicine; Co-Director, Neuromuscular Division, Detroit Medical Center, Detroit, Michigan
Peripheral Neuropathies

Wilmer L. Sibbitt, Jr., MD
Professor, Internal Medicine, Rheumatology, and Neurology, University of New Mexico Health Sciences Center, Albuquerque, New Mexico
Multifocal Fibrosclerosis

Michael S. Simberkoff, MD
Professor of Medicine and Assistant Dean for Veterans Affairs, New York University School of Medicine; Chief of Staff, Veterans Affairs New York Harbor Healthcare System, New York, New York
Haemophilus *and* Moraxella *Infections*

David L. Simel, MD, MHS
Professor of Medicine, Duke University School of Medicine; Associate Chief of Staff for Ambulatory Care, Durham Veterans Affairs Medical Center, Durham, North Carolina
Approach to the Patient: History and Physical Examination

Roger P. Simon, MD
Adjunct Professor Neurology, Physiology, and Pharmacology, Oregon Health & Science University School of Medicine; Robert Stowe Dow Chair of Neurology and Director, Dow Neurobiology Laboratories, Legacy Research, Portland Oregon
Syncope; Coma and Disorders of Arousal

Karl Skorecki, MD
Annie Chutick Professor of Medicine, Rappaport Faculty of Medicine, Technion-Israel Institute of Technology; Director of Medical and Research Development, Rambam Health Care Campus, Haifa, Israel
Cell and Gene Therapy; Disorders of Sodium and Water Homeostasis

Arthur S. Slutsky, MD
Professor of Medicine, Surgery, and Biomedical Engineering and Director, Interdepartmental Division of Critical Care, University of Toronto Faculty of Medicine; Vice-President for Research, St. Michael's Hospital, Toronto, Ontario, Canada
Acute Respiratory Failure; Mechanical Ventilation

Eric J. Small, MD, PhD
Professor of Medicine and Urology, University of California, San Francisco, School of Medicine, San Francisco, California
Prostate Cancer

Gerald W. Smetana, MD
Associate Professor of Medicine, Harvard Medical School; Division of General Medicine and Primary Care, Beth Israel Deaconess Medical Center, Boston, Massachusetts
Principles of Medical Consultation

Susan B. Sorenson, PhD
Professor of Social Policy, School of Social Policy and Practice, University of Pennsylvania, Philadelphia, Pennsylvania
Violence and Injury

Frederick S. Southwick, MD
Professor of Medicine, University of Florida College of Medicine; Chief of Infectious Diseases, Shands Hospital at the University of Florida, Gainesville, Florida
Nocardiosis

P. Frederick Sparling, MD
Professor of Medicine, Division of Infectious Diseases, University of North Carolina at Chapel Hill School of Medicine; Director, North Carolina Sexually Transmitted Diseases Cooperative Research Center, Chapel Hill, North Carolina
Gonococcal Infections

Stephen A. Spector, MD
Professor of Pediatrics; Section Chief, Division of Infectious Diseases; and Director, Mother-Child-Adolescent HIV Program, University of California, San Diego, School of Medicine; Member, University of California, San Diego, Center for AIDS Research, La Jolla, California
Human Immunodeficiency Virus in Pregnancy

Susan S. Spencer, MD
Professor of Neurology, Yale University School of Medicine; Director, Clinical Epilepsy Service, Yale–New Haven Hospital, New Haven, Connecticut
Seizures and Epilepsy

Robert F. Spiera, MD
Associate Professor of Clinical Medicine, Weill Medical College of Cornell University; Director, Vasculitis and Scleroderma, Hospital for Special Surgery, New York, New York
Polymyalgia Rheumatica and Temporal Arteritis

Paul Stark, MD
Professor of Clinical Radiology, University of California, San Diego, School of Medicine; Chief of Cardiothoracic Radiology Section, Veterans Affairs San Diego Health Care System, La Jolla, California
Imaging in Pulmonary Disease

Lynne S. Steinbach, MD
Professor of Radiology and Orthopaedic Surgery and Chief, Musculoskeletal Imaging, University of California, San Francisco, School of Medicine, San Francisco, California
Imaging Studies in the Rheumatic Diseases

Martin H. Steinberg, MD
Professor of Medicine, Pediatrics, Pathology, and Laboratory Medicine, Boston University School of Medicine; Director, Center of Excellence in Sickle Cell Disease, Boston Medical Center, Boston, Massachusetts
Sickle Cell Disease and Associated Hemoglobinopathies

Beat Steinmann, MD
Professor in Pediatrics, Medical Faculty, University of Zurich; Division of Metabolism and Molecular Pediatrics, University Children's Hospital, Zurich, Switzerland
Disorders of Fructose Metabolism

William F. Stenson, MD
Professor of Medicine, Washington University in St. Louis School of Medicine; Attending Physician, Barnes-Jewish Hospital, St. Louis, Missouri
Inflammatory Bowel Disease

David A. Stevens, MD
Professor of Medicine, Stanford University School of Medicine, Stanford; Chief, Division of Infectious Diseases, Department of Medicine, Santa Clara Valley Medical Center; President, California Institute for Medical Research, San Jose, California
Systemic Antifungal Agents; Aspergillosis; Mucormycosis

Dennis L. Stevens, MD, PhD
Professor of Medicine, University of Washington School of Medicine, Seattle, Washington; Chief, Infectious Disease Section, Veterans Affairs Medical Center, Boise, Idaho
Streptococcal Infections

John H. Stone, MD, MPH
Instructor, Harvard Medical School; Associate in Medicine, Massachusetts General Hospital, Boston, Massachusetts
The Systemic Vasculitides

Stephen E. Straus, MD*
Director, National Center for Complementary and Alternative Medicine, National Institutes of Health, Bethesda, Maryland
Complementary and Alternative Medicine
**deceased*

Roland W. Sutter, MD, MPH&TM
Coordinator, Research and Product Development, Polio Eradication Initiative, World Health Organization, Geneva, Switzerland
Diphtheria and Other Corynebacteria Infections

Morton N. Swartz, MD
Professor of Medicine, Harvard Medical School; James Jackson Firm Chief, Medical Services, Massachusetts General Hospital, Boston, Massachusetts
Meningitis: Bacterial, Viral, and Other

Ronald S. Swerdloff, MD
Professor of Medicine, David Geffen School of Medicine at UCLA, Los Angeles; Chief, Division of Endocrinology, and Associate Chair of Medicine, Harbor–UCLA Medical Center, Torrance, California
The Testis and Male Sexual Function

Megan Sykes, MD
Harold and Ellen Danser Professor of Surgery and Professor of Medicine (Immunology), Harvard Medical School; Immunologist, Departments of Surgery and Medicine (Immunology), and Associate Director, Transplantation Biology Research Center, Massachusetts General Hospital, Boston, Massachusetts
Transplantation Immunology

Nicholas J. Talley, MD, PhD
Professor of Medicine, Division of Gastroenterology and Hepatology, Mayo Clinic College of Medicine, Rochester, Minnesota
Functional Gastrointestinal Disorders: Irritable Bowel Syndrome, Dyspepsia, and Noncardiac Chest Pain

Thomas A. Tami, MD, FACS
Director, Cincinnati Sinus Institute, Good Samaritan Hospital–Trihealth, Cincinnati, Ohio
Throat Disorders

Victor F. Tapson, MD
Professor of Medicine, Duke University School of Medicine; Director, Center for Pulmonary Vascular Disease, Duke University Medical Center, Durham, North Carolina
Pulmonary Embolism

Victoria M. Taylor, MD, MPH
Full Member, Fred Hutchinson Cancer Research Center, Seattle, Washington
Cultural Context of Medicine

Ayalew Tefferi, MD
Professor of Medicine and Hematology, Mayo Clinic College of Medicine; Consultant, Hematology and Internal Medicine, Mayo Clinic, Rochester, Minnesota
Nonhemolytic Normochromic, Normocytic Anemias; Polycythemias; Myeloproliferative Disorders: Essential Thrombocythemia and Primary Myelofibrosis

Paul S. Teirstein, MD, FRCP
Visiting Professor of Medicine, Columbia University College of Physicians and Surgeons, New York, New York; Chief of Cardiology and Director, Interventional Cardiology, Scripps Clinic, La Jolla, California
Percutaneous Coronary Interventions

Margaret Tempero, MD
Division of Hematology/Oncology, University of California, San Francisco, School of Medicine, San Francisco, California
Pancreatic Cancer

Robert Terkeltaub, MD
Professor of Medicine, University of California, San Diego, School of Medicine, La Jolla; Chief, Rheumatology Section, Veterans Affairs Medical Center, San Diego, California
Crystal Deposition Diseases

Pierre Théroux, MD, FACC, FRCPC, FAHA
Professor of Medicine, University of Montreal Faculty of Medicine; Cardiologist, Montreal Heart Institute, Montreal, Quebec, Canada
Angina Pectoris

Michael J. Thun, MD, MS
Rollins School of Public Health and Winship Cancer Institute, Emory University; Vice President of Epidemiology and Surveillance Research, American Cancer Society, Atlanta, Georgia
Epidemiology of Cancer

C. Craig Tisher, MD
Dean, College of Medicine; Folke H. Peterson/Dean's Distinguished Professor; and Professor of Medicine, Pathology, and Anatomy and Cell Biology, University of Florida College of Medicine; Attending Physician, Shands Hospital, Gainesville, Florida
Structure and Function of the Kidneys

Nina Tolkoff-Rubin, MD
Professor of Medicine, Harvard Medical School; Medical Director for Renal Transplantation, Massachusetts General Hospital, Boston, Massachusetts
Treatment of Irreversible Renal Failure

John J. Treanor, MD
Division of Infectious Diseases, Department of Medicine, University of Rochester School of Medicine and Dentistry; Attending Physician, Strong Memorial Hospital, Rochester, New York
Adenovirus Diseases

Arthur C. Upton, MD
Clinical Professor of Environmental and Community Medicine, University of Medicine and Dentistry of New Jersey, Robert Wood Johnson Medical School, Piscataway, New Jersey
Radiation Injury

Greet Van den Berghe, MD, PhD
Professor of Medicine, Catholic University of Leuven; Director, Department of Intensive Care Medicine, University Hospital Gasthuisberg, Leuven, Belgium
Parenteral Nutrition

Joseph G. Verbalis, MD
Professor of Medicine and Physiology, Georgetown University School of Medicine; Interim Chair, Department of Medicine, Georgetown University Medical Center, Washington, DC
Posterior Pituitary

Ronald G. Victor, MD
Professor of Medicine, Norman and Audrey Kaplan Chair in Hypertension, and Chief, Division of Hypertension, University of Texas Southwestern Medical Center, Dallas, Texas
Arterial Hypertension

Angela Vincent, MBBS
Professor of Neuroimmunology, University of Oxford; Professor of Neuroimmunology, Oxford Radcliffe Hospital Trust; Professor of Neuroimmunology, Weatherall Institute of Molecular Medicine, Oxford, United Kingdom
Disorders of Neuromuscular Transmission

Paul A. Volberding, MD, FACP
Professor of Medicine and Co-Director, Center for AIDS Research, University of California, San Francisco, School of Medicine; Chief, Medical Service, San Francisco Veterans Affairs Medical Center, San Francisco, California
Hematology and Oncology in Patients with Human Immunodeficiency Virus Infection

Julie M. Vose, MD
Professor of Medicine, University of Nebraska Medical Center, Omaha, Nebraska
Hematopoietic Stem Cell Transplantation

Robert M. Wachter, MD
Professor, Department of Medicine, University of California, San Francisco, School of Medicine; Chief of the Medical Service, University of California, San Francisco, Medical Center, San Francisco, California
Quality of Care and Safety of Patients

Bruce D. Walker, MD
Professor of Medicine and Director, Division of AIDS, Harvard Medical School; Director, Partners AIDS Research Center, Massachusetts General Hospital, Boston, Massachusetts
Immunopathogenesis of Human Immunodeficiency Virus Infection

Edward E. Walsh, MD
Professor of Medicine, University of Rochester School of Medicine and Dentistry; Physician, Rochester General Hospital, Rochester, New York
Respiratory Syncytial Virus; Parainflueneza Viral Disease

Christina Wang, MD
Professor of Medicine, David Geffen School of Medicine at UCLA, Los Angeles; Program Director, General Clinical Research Center, Harbor–UCLA Medical Center, Torrance, California
The Testis and Male Sexual Function

Stephen I. Wasserman, MD
Professor of Medicine, University of California, San Diego, School of Medicine, La Jolla, California
Approach to the Patient with Allergic or Immunologic Disease

David D. Waters, MD
Maurice Eliaser, Jr., Distinguished Professor of Medicine, University of California, San Francisco, School of Medicine; Chief of Cardiology, San Francisco General Hospital, San Francisco, California
Acute Coronary Syndrome: Unstable Angina and Non–ST Segment Elevation Myocardial Infarction

Steven E. Weinberger, MD
Adjunct Professor of Medicine, University of Pennsylvania School of Medicine; Senior Vice President for Medical Education and Publishing, American College of Physicians, Philadelphia, Pennsylvania
Sarcoidosis

Myron L. Weisfeldt, MD
William Osler Professor of Medicine, Johns Hopkins University School of Medicine; Director, Department of Medicine, Johns Hopkins Hospital, Baltimore, Maryland
Cardiac Function and Circulatory Control

Michael J. Welsh, MD
Professor of Internal Medicine and of Physiology and Biophysics, University of Iowa Carver College of Medicine, Iowa City, Iowa; Investigator, Howard Hughes Medical Institute, Chevy Chase, Maryland
Cystic Fibrosis

Richard P. Wenzel, MD
Professor and Chairman, Department of Internal Medicine, Medical College of Virginia Campus of Virginia Commonwealth University School of Medicine, Richmond, Virginia
Acute Bronchitis and Tracheitis

Victoria P. Werth, MD
Professor of Dermatology, University of Pennsylvania School of Medicine; Chief, Department of Dermatology, Philadelphia Veterans Affairs Medical Center, Philadelphia, Pennsylvania
Principles of Therapy

Sterling G. West, MD
Professor of Medicine and Rheumatology Fellowship Program Director, University of Colorado Health Sciences Center, Denver, Colorado
Systemic Diseases in Which Arthritis Is a Feature

Cornelia M. Weyand, MD, PhD
David Lowance Professor of Medicine and Director, Kathleen B. and Mason I. Lowance Center for Human Immunology, Department of Medicine, Emory University School of Medicine, Atlanta, Georgia
The Innate and Adaptive Immune Systems

David P. White, MD
Gerald E. McGinnis Professor of Medicine, Harvard Medical School, Boston, Massachusetts; Chief Medical Officer, Respironics, Inc., Pittsburgh, Pennsylvania
Disorders of Ventilatory Control

Perrin C. White, MD
Professor of Pediatrics, University of Texas Southwestern Medical Center; Chief of Endocrinology, Children's Medical Center Dallas, Dallas, Texas
Disorders of Sexual Differentiation

Richard J. Whitley, MD
Professor of Pediatrics, Microbiology, Medicine, and Neurosurgery and Loeb Eminent Scholar Chair in Pediatrics, University of Alabama School of Medicine, Birmingham, Alabama
Herpes Simplex Virus Infections

Michael P. Whyte, MD
Professor of Medicine, Pediatrics, and Genetics, Washington University School of Medicine; Medical Scientific Director, Center for Metabolic Bone Disease and Molecular Research, Shriners Hospitals for Children, St. Louis, Missouri
Osteonecrosis, Osteosclerosis/Hyperostosis, and Other Disorders of Bone

Jeanine P. Wiener-Kronish, MD
Professor of Anesthesia and Medicine and Vice-Chairman, Department of Anesthesia and Perioperative Care, University of California, San Francisco, School of Medicine, San Francisco, California
Overview of Anesthesia

Fredrick M. Wigley, MD
Professor of Medicine and Associate Director, Division of Rheumatology, Johns Hopkins University School of Medicine; Director, Johns Hopkins Scleroderma Center, Baltimore, Maryland
Scleroderma (Systemic Sclerosis)

Alexander Wilmer, MD, PhD
Professor of Medicine, Catholic University of Leuven, Chef de Clinic—Internal Medicine, University Hospital Gasthuisberg, Leuven, Belgium
Parenteral Nutrition

William Winkenwerder, MD, MBA
Washington, DC
Disorders Due to Heat and Cold

Joseph I. Wolfsdorf, MB, BCh
Professor of Pediatrics, Harvard Medical School; Clinical Director and Associate Chief, Division of Endocrinology, Children's Hospital Boston, Boston, Massachusetts
Glycogen Storage Diseases

Steven H. Woolf, MD, MPH
Professor of Family Medicine, Epidemiology, and Community Health, Medical College of Virginia Campus of Virginia Commonwealth University School of Medicine, Richmond, Virginia
Principles of Preventive Health Care

John J. Wysolmerski, MD
Associate Professor of Internal Medicine, Yale University School of Medicine; Attending Physician, Yale Bone Center, Yale–New Haven Hospital, New Haven, Connecticut
The Parathyroid Glands, Hypercalcemia, and Hypocalcemia

Lowell S. Young, MD
Clinical Professor of Medicine, University of California, San Francisco, School of Medicine; Director, Kuzell Institute for Arthritis and Infectious Diseases, California Pacific Medical Center Research Institute, San Francisco, California
Approach to Fever and Suspected Infection in the Compromised Host

Neal S. Young, MD
Chief, Hematology Branch, National Heart, Lung, and Blood Institute, National Institutes of Health, Bethesda, Maryland
B19 Parvovirus

William F. Young, Jr., MD, MSc
Professor of Medicine, Mayo Clinic College of Medicine; Consultant, Division of Endocrinology, Diabetes, Metabolism, and Nutrition, Mayo Clinic, Rochester, Minnesota
Adrenal Medulla, Catecholamines, and Pheochromocytoma

Alan S. L. Yu, MB, BChir
Associate Professor of Medicine, Keck School of Medicine of the University of Southern California, Los Angeles, California
Disorders of Magnesium and Phosphorus

Mark L. Zeidel, MD
Herrman L. Blumgart Professor of Medicine, Harvard Medical School; Chair, Department of Medicine, and Physician-in-Chief, Beth Israel Deaconess Medical Center, Boston, Massachusetts
Obstructive Uropathy

Martin Zeidler, MB, MRCP, DM, FRCP (Edinburgh)
Consultant Neurologist, Victoria Hospital, Kirkcaldy, United Kingdom
Prion Diseases

Justin A. Zivin, MD, PhD
Professor of Neurosciences, University of California, San Diego, School of Medicine, La Jolla; Staff Physician, San Diego Veterans Affairs Medical Center, San Diego, California
Approach to Cerebrovascular Diseases; Ischemic Cerebrovascular Disease; Hemorrhagic Cerebrovascular Disease

Kenneth S. Zuckerman, MD
Professor of Oncology, Internal Medicine, and Molecular Medicine, University of South Florida College of Medicine; Harold H. Davis Professor of Cancer Research, H. Lee Moffitt Cancer Center, Tampa, Florida
Approach to the Anemias

Global Advisory Board

FEATURES OF THE 23RD EDITION

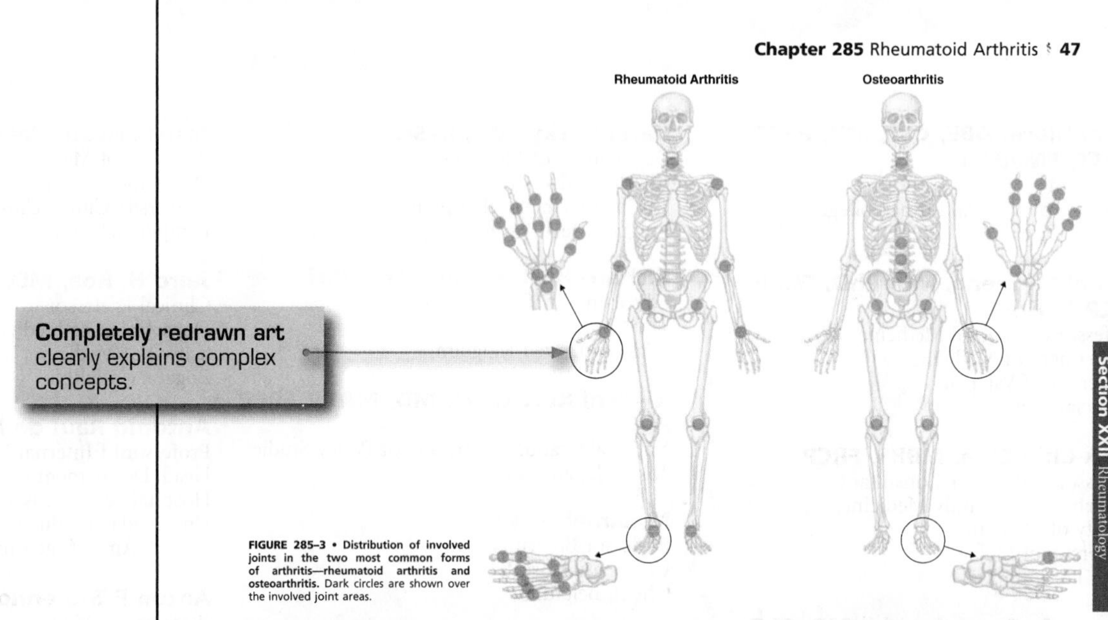

FIGURE 285–3 • Distribution of involved joints in the two most common forms of arthritis—rheumatoid arthritis and osteoarthritis. Dark circles are shown over the involved joint areas.

Summary tables present complicated information in an easily digestible form.

TABLE 285–3 DIFFERENTIAL DIAGNOSIS OF RHEUMATOID ARTHRITIS

Disorder	Subcutaneous Nodules	Rheumatoid Factor
Viral arthritis (hepatitis B and C, parvovirus, rubella, others)	–	±
Bacterial endocarditis	±	+
Rheumatic fever	+	–
Sarcoidosis	+	+
Reactive arthritis	–	–
Psoriatic arthritis	–	–
Systemic lupus erythematosus	±	+
Primary Sjögren's syndrome	–	+
Chronic tophus gout	+	–
Calcium pyrophosphate disease	–	–
Polymyalgia rheumatica	–	–
Osteoarthritis (erosive)	–	–

– = not present; + = frequently present; ± = occasionally present.

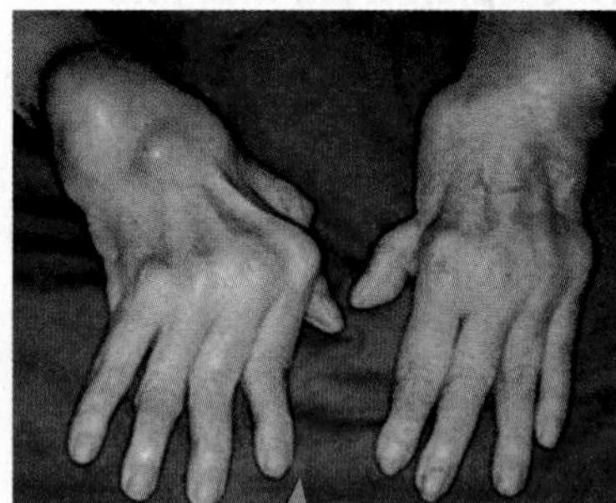

FIGURE 285–4 • Severe advanced rheumatoid arthritis of the hands. There is massive tendon swelling over the dorsal surface of both wrists, severe muscle wasting, ulnar deviation of the metacarpophalangeal joints, and swan-neck deformity of the fingers. (From Forbes CD, Jackson WF: Color Atlas and Text of Clinical Medicine, 3rd ed. London, Mosby, 2003.)

The DIP joints are rarely involved; significant involvement of the DIP joints should suggest the possibility of a different diagnosis. Figure 285–4 illustrates the classic ulnar deviation and swan-neck deformities (hyperextension of the PIP joints) that are commonly seen in late, more established disease. Boutonniere (or buttonhole) deformities also occur as a result of hyperextension of the MCP joints. If the clinical disease remains active, hand function deteriorates. Sudden loss of function of individual fingers may occur as a result of tendon rupture, which requires the expertise of a carefully selected hand surgeon to repair.

Feet

Feet, particularly the MTP joints, are involved early in most patients with RA. Radiographic erosions occur at least as early in the feet as in the hands. Subluxation of the toes is common and leads to the dual problem of breakdown of the skin with ulcers on the top of the toes and painful ambulation due to loss of the cushioning pads that usually protect the heads of the MTP joints.

Wrists

The wrist joints are involved in most patients with RA; radial deviation is the rule, and patients with severe involvement may progress to volar subluxation. Even early in the course of the disease, synovial proliferation in and around the wrists may compress the median nerve, causing carpal tunnel syndrome (Fig. 285–5). Later, this synovial proliferation may invade tendons and lead to rupture.

Color clinical photos show clinical manifestations as they are seen in real practice.

Main discussion of every disease in orange, as well as **consistent headings,** expedites access to the specific guidance you need.

Rx Treatment boxes summarize therapeutic options.

histamines. Agents that decrease the sensitivity of mast cells to degranulation, such as phosphodiesterase 4 inhibitors and syk kinase inhibitors, may also find a role in the treatment of this condition.

HEREDITARY ANGIOEDEMA AND RELATED DISEASES

Definition

Hereditary angioedema (HAE) and related illnesses are characterized by recurrent attacks of angioedema mediated by vasoactive peptides such as bradykinin.

Epidemiology

HAE affects approximately 1 in 50,000 people. It is an autosomal dominant disease and therefore affects 50% of offspring of both genders. Frequently, a history of several generations with this disease is obtained, but new mutations occur, and a negative family history is not uncommon. Acquired angioedema (AAE) is more rare and is not inherited; it affects older persons who often have paraproteinemia or malignancies such as lymphoma. Angioedema associated with ACE inhibitors occurs in 0.1 to 0.2% of treated patients.

Pathobiology

HAE and AAE are caused by either low levels or abnormal function of a regulatory protein in the plasma, C1 inhibitor (C1 INH), which exerts control of the complement, fibrinolytic, and kinin-generating pathways. Because there is one normal gene, levels of C1 INH are detectable but are not sufficient to control generation of kinins. The C1 esterase enzyme, when activated, cleaves two complement products, C4 and C2; without proper inhibition, this leads to low levels of circulating C4 and C2. C1 INH is also a critical modulator of the bradykinin pathway, and decreased C1 INH function leads to increased levels of bradykinin. Increased generation of bradykinin, and not mediators from mast cells or activation of complement, leads to capillary leakage and angioedema.

In HAE type I (85% of patients), the abnormal gene does not produce C1 INH. In HAE type II (15%), an antigenically detectable C1 INH protein is produced, but it is not functional. In HAE type III (very rare), C1 INH is present and functional, but there is a yet-to-be-defined abnormality in the generation of vasoactive compounds. In AAE, unknown factors activate C1 and deplete the C1 INH activity in plasma, or there is an autoantibody to C1 INH that interferes with its function. In ACE inhibitor–associated angioedema, the underlying problem is lack of catabolism of bradykinin; the complement pathway is unaffected.

Clinical Manifestations

Children with HAE can have attacks shortly after birth, but these tend to be mild. For most patients, the severity of the attacks worsens at puberty, with episodic attacks of swelling that can affect any external body surface, including the genitalia. Mucosal surfaces are also affected, and patients can have life-threatening swelling of the uvula and posterior pharynx leading to asphyxiation. Swelling of the submucosa of the gastrointestinal tract can cause symptoms of an "acute abdomen," leading to unnecessary exploratory laparotomy. About half of patients report that trauma, particularly that associated with local pressure, precipitates an attack, and about half of patients note an increased frequency of attacks during times of emotional stress. Attacks in patients with AAE are clinically similar to those in patients with HAE. Patients taking ACE inhibitors may have angioedema that manifests as severe swelling or simply as a chronic cough beginning days to months after ACE inhibitor therapy is initiated.

Diagnosis

pport the diagnosis of HAE or AAE are measure-
vel, C1 INH function, and C4 level, particularly

during an attack. The distinguishing features of AAE are lack of a family history, late onset, and the presence of a malignancy or paraproteinemia, as mentioned earlier. However, patients with AAE, in addition to having low C2 and C4, can have profound depressions in C1, a protein that is commonly normal in HAE. Patients with ACE inhibitor–associated angioedema can present within hours after initiation of therapy or after many months. The angioedema seen in urticaria/angioedema is distinctive in that it is usually associated with urticaria and is pruritic, responding to antihistamines, steroids, and epinephrine.

Section XXI Allergy

Treatment Rx

C1 INH concentrate (500 U) is available in Europe to treat acute attacks of HAE and is the treatment of choice, but this drug has not yet been approved by the FDA. In the United States, treatment of acute attacks of angioedema is currently suboptimal. Epinephrine is only modestly effective but is the safest agent available. Treatment should include nebulized racemic epinephrine delivered in the airway (1:1000 given by nebulization) and by intramuscular injections (0.2 to 0.3 mL of 1:1000 at intervals of 20 to 30 minutes). The addition of antihistamine for sedation may be helpful. Treating physicians must be prepared to perform nasotracheal intubation, preferably in the operating room under conditions in which tracheostomy can be performed if needed. Acute attacks can be terminated by administering 2 units of fresh-frozen plasma (FFP) to supply the missing C1 INH, but in rare instances patients become more edematous, presumably reflecting increased availability of the substrates for generation of kinins. Therefore, although FFP can be useful for treating non–life-threatening acute attacks, it is not recommended for treatment of life-threatening laryngeal edema.

Patients treated prophylactically with attenuated androgens, antifibrinolytic agents, FFP, or C1-INH concentrate have fewer attacks. Attenuated androgens, such as danazol (100 to 200 mg twice daily), increase the production of C1 INH and lead to marked amelioration of symptoms. Masculinizing side effects are usually mild but can be problematic. FFP (USA) or C1 INH concentrate (Europe) should be used before surgical or dental procedures to minimize edema attack due to trauma. Symptomatic treatment of AAE is similar to that for HAE, but definitive treatment requires amelioration of the underlying disease. Treatment of angioedema associated with the use of an ACE inhibitor includes antihistamines, epinephrine, or both, as appropriate, and discontinuation of the ACE inhibitor. Rare patients also will have angioedema when taking angiotension receptor blockers. An approach to the evaluation and treatment of patients with urticaria and angioedema is summarized in Figure 273–2.

Evidence-Based Treatments

Current therapy for HAE in the United States is directed toward prophylactic treatments, including attenuated androgens, antifibrinolytics, and FFP. Danazol was shown in a double-blind, placebo-controlled trial to significantly reduce the number of acute attacks. C1 INH has been used widely and successfully in Europe. In a study of 193 episodes of laryngeal edema treated with C1 INH concentrate, 192 responded within 60 minutes, and the remaining 1 case responded at 4 hours. [2]

Prognosis

The long-term outlook for patients with HAE depends greatly on the phenotype of the illness (more or fewer laryngeal attacks), the patient's willingness to take attenuated androgens, and how well the patient tolerates attenuated androgens. For most patients, life expectancy should be normal. AAE usually resolves with treatment of the underlying condition, but the ultimate prognosis for the patient depends on the nature of that illness. Angioedema associated with the use of an ACE inhibitor resolves after the medication is removed.

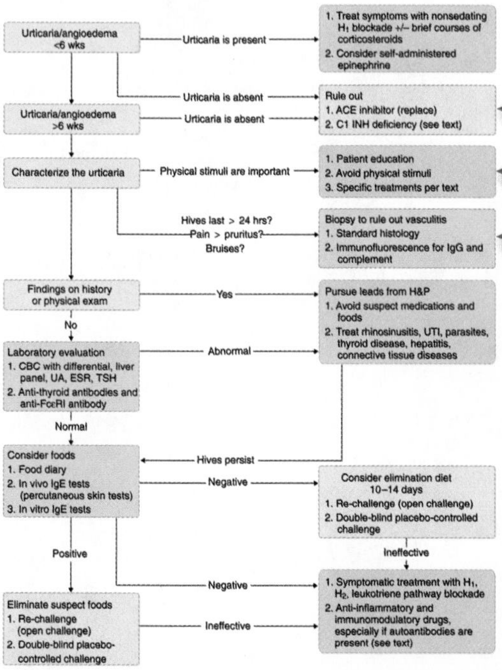

Section XXI Allergy

Urticaria/angioedema <6 wks — Urticaria is present → 1. Treat symptoms with nonsedating H_1 blockade +/– brief courses of corticosteroids 2. Consider self-administered epinephrine

Urticaria/angioedema <6 wks — Urticaria is absent → Rule out 1. ACE inhibitor (replace) 2. C1 INH deficiency (see text)

Urticaria/angioedema >6 wks — Urticaria is absent → Rule out 1. ACE inhibitor (replace) 2. C1 INH deficiency (see text)

Characterize the urticaria — Physical stimuli are important → 1. Patient education 2. Avoid physical stimuli 3. Specific treatments per text

Characterize the urticaria — Hives last > 24 hrs? Pain > pruritus? Bruises? → Biopsy to rule out vasculitis 1. Standard histology 2. Immunofluorescence for IgG and complement

Findings on history or physical exam — Yes → Pursue leads from H&P 1. Avoid suspect medications and foods 2. Treat rhinosinusitis, UTI, parasites, thyroid disease, hepatitis, connective tissue diseases

No ↓

Laboratory evaluation 1. CBC with differential, liver panel, UA, ESR, TSH 2. Anti-thyroid antibodies and anti-FcεRI antibody — Abnormal → Pursue leads from H&P

Normal ↓

Consider foods 1. Food diary 2. In vivo IgE tests (percutaneous skin tests) 3. In vitro IgE tests ← Hives persist — (from Pursue leads from H&P)

Consider foods — Negative → Consider elimination diet 10–14 days 1. Re-challenge (open challenge) 2. Double-blind placebo-controlled challenge

Consider elimination diet — Ineffective ↓ 1. Symptomatic treatment with H_1, H_2, leukotriene pathway blockade 2. Anti-inflammatory and immunomodulatory drugs, especially if autoantibodies are present (see text)

Consider foods — Negative → 1. Symptomatic treatment with H_1, H_2, leukotriene pathway blockade 2. Anti-inflammatory and immunomodulatory drugs, especially if autoantibodies are present (see text)

Consider foods — Positive ↓ Eliminate suspect foods 1. Re-challenge (open challenge) 2. Double-blind placebo-controlled challenge — Ineffective → 1. Symptomatic treatment with H_1, H_2, leukotriene pathway blockade 2. Anti-inflammatory and immunomodulatory drugs, especially if autoantibodies are present (see text)

FIGURE 273–2 • Evaluation and treatment of urticaria/angioedema. Treatment of urticaria with or without angioedema (AE) is similar. Treatment of AE without urticaria depends on the cause. If the AE is caused by an angiotensin-converting enzyme (ACE) inhibitor, discontinuation of the medication is required. Treatment of AE that is caused by a deficiency or dysfunction of C1 inhibitor (C1 INH) is discussed in the text. Idiopathic AE often responds to treatments described for urticaria/angioedema. ESR = erythrocyte sedimentation rate; FcεRI = high-affinity receptor for IgE; H_1 = histamine 1; H_2 = histamine 2; IgE = immunoglobulin E; TSH = thyroid-stimulating hormone; UA = urinalysis; UTI = urinary tract infection.

Color-coded algorithms outline strategies for diagnosing and treating common complaints and diseases.

- **Purple** boxes indicate diagnostic tests.
- **Green** boxes indicate treatments.
- **Orange** boxes are used for all other steps.

Future Directions

For treatment of HAE and related disorders, there is a strong effort to have the C1 INH concentrate approved for use in the United States. Finally, new therapies are being developed, including kallikrein inhibitors, bradykinin receptor antagonists, and recombinant C1 INH.

Grade A

1. Grattan CE, O'Donnell BF, Francis DM, et al: Randomized double-blind study of cyclosporin in chronic "idiopathic" urticaria. Br J Dermatol 2000;143:365–372.
2. Kunschak M, Engl W, Maritsch F, et al: A randomized, controlled trial to study the efficacy and safety of C1 inhibitor concentrate in treating hereditary angioedema. Transfusion 1998;38:540–549.

SUGGESTED READINGS

Bork K, Meng G, Staubach P, Hardt J: Hereditary angioedema: New findings concerning symptoms, affected organs, and course. Am J Med 2006;119:267–274. *A comprehensive review.*

Dibbern DA Jr, Dreskin SC: Urticaria and angioedema: An overview. Immunol Allergy Clin North Am 2004;24:141–162. *An overview of acute and chronic urticaria offering guidance to the evaluation of difficult patients.*

Joint Task Force on Practice Parameters: The diagnosis and management of urticaria: A practice parameter. I. Acute urticaria/angioedema. II. Chronic urticaria/angioedema. Ann Allergy Asthma Immunol 2000;85:S521–S544. *These guidelines are being updated in 2007 and will be available at* www.aaaai.org.

Kaplan AP: Chronic urticaria, pathogenesis and treatment. J Allergy Clin Immunol 2004;114:465. *A concise guide to the evaluation and treatment of chronic urticaria.*

Kozel MM, Sabroe RA: Chronic urticaria: Aetiology, management and current and future treatment options. Drugs 2004;64:2515–2536. *Contains references to many earlier double-blind, placebo-controlled studies of antihistamines as treatment for urticaria.*

Zuberbier T, Bindsley-Jensen C, Canonica W, et al: Management of urticaria. Allergy 2006;61:321–331. *A consensus guideline.*

Grade A **Highlighted Grade A evidence** references emphasize evidence-based treatments to foster cost-effective, best practice in clinical medicine.

Suggested readings expedite access to the articles that the experts recommend. Each includes a bottom-line expert commentary.

Section I

Social and Ethical Issues in Medicine

1 APPROACH TO MEDICINE, THE PATIENT, AND THE MEDICAL PROFESSION: MEDICINE AS A LEARNED AND HUMANE PROFESSION

Lee Goldman and Dennis Ausiello

APPROACH TO MEDICINE

Medicine is a profession that incorporates science and the scientific method with the art of being a physician. The art of tending to the sick is as old as humanity itself. Even in modern times, the art of caring and comforting, guided by millennia of common sense as well as a more recent, systematic approach to medical ethics (Chapter 2), remains the cornerstone of medicine. Without these humanistic qualities, application of the modern science of medicine is suboptimal, ineffective, or even detrimental.

The caregivers of ancient times and premodern cultures tried a variety of interventions to help the afflicted. Some of their potions contained what are now known to be active ingredients that form the basis for proven medications (Chapter 27). Others (Chapter 36) have persisted into the present era despite a lack of convincing evidence. Modern medicine should not dismiss the possibility that these unproven approaches may be helpful; instead, it should adopt a guiding principle that all interventions, whether traditional or newly developed, can be tested vigorously, with the expectation that any beneficial effects can be explored further to determine their scientific basis.

When compared with its long and generally distinguished history of caring and comforting, the scientific basis of medicine is remarkably recent. Other than an understanding of human anatomy and the later description, albeit widely contested at this time, of the normal physiology of the circulatory system, almost all of modern medicine is based on discoveries made within the last 150 years. Until the late 19th century, the paucity of medical knowledge was perhaps exemplified best by hospitals and hospital care. Although hospitals provided caring that all but well-to-do people might not be able to obtain elsewhere, there is little if any evidence that hospitals improved health outcomes. The term *hospitalism* referred not to expertise in hospital care but rather to the aggregate of iatrogenic afflictions that were induced by the hospital stay itself.

The essential humanistic qualities of caring and comforting can achieve full benefit only if they are coupled with an understanding of how medical science can and should be applied to patients with known or suspected diseases. Without this knowledge, comforting may be inappropriate or misleading, and caring may be ineffective or counterproductive if it inhibits a sick person from obtaining appropriate, scientific medical care. The *Cecil Textbook of Medicine* focuses on the discipline of *internal medicine,* from which neurology and dermatology, which are also covered in substantial detail in this text, are relatively recent evolutionary branches. The term *internal medicine,* which is often misunderstood by the lay public, was developed in 19th century Germany. *Inneren medizin* was to be distinguished from clinical medicine because it emphasized the physiology and chemistry of disease, not just the patterns or progression of clinical manifestations. The *Cecil Textbook of Medicine* follows this tradition by showing how pathophysiologic abnormalities cause symptoms and signs and by emphasizing how therapies can modify the underlying pathophysiology and improve the patient's well-being.

Modern medicine has moved rapidly past organ physiology to an increasingly detailed understanding of cellular, subcellular, and genetic mechanisms. For example, the understanding of microbial pathogenesis and many inflammatory diseases (Chapter 277) is now guided by a detailed understanding of the human immune system and its response to foreign antigens (Chapters 42 to 46).

Health, disease, and an individual's interaction with the environment are also substantially determined by genetics. In addition to many conditions that may be determined by a single gene (Chapter 39), medical science increasingly understands the complex interactions that underlie multigenic traits (Chapter 40). In the not-so-distant future, health care and medicine will probably be targeted according to an individual's genetic profile, and this approach will allow the development of robust presymptomatic disease management, as well as novel therapeutics for symptomatic disease. Currently, knowledge of the structure and physical forms of proteins helps explain abnormalities as diverse as sickle cell anemia (Chapter 167) and Creutzfeldt-Jakob disease (Chapter 442). Proteomics, which is the normal and abnormal protein expression of genes, also holds extraordinary promise for developing drug targets for more specific and effective therapies.

Concurrent with these advances in fundamental human biology has been a dramatic shift in methods for evaluating the application of scientific advances to the individual patient and to populations. The randomized controlled trial, sometimes with thousands of patients at multiple institutions, has replaced anecdote as the preferred method for measuring the benefits and optimal uses of diagnostic and therapeutic interventions (Chapter 9). As studies progress from those that show biologic effect, to those that elucidate dosing schedules and toxicity, and finally to those that assess true clinical benefit, the metrics of measuring outcome has also improved from subjective impressions of physicians or patients to reliable and valid measures of morbidity, quality of life, functional status, and other patient-oriented outcomes (Chapter 10). These marked improvements in the scientific methodology of clinical investigation have expedited extraordinary changes in clinical practice, such as recanalization therapy for acute myocardial infarction (Chapter 72), and have shown that reliance on intermediate outcomes, such as a reduction in asymptomatic ventricular arrhythmias with certain drugs, may unexpectedly increase rather than decrease mortality. Just as physicians in the 21st century must understand advances in fundamental biology, similar understanding of the fundamentals of clinical study design as it applies to diagnostic and therapeutic interventions is needed. An understanding of human genetics will also help stratify and refine the approach to clinical trials by helping researchers select fewer patients with a more homogeneous disease pattern to study the efficacy of an intervention.

This explosion in medical knowledge has led to increasing specialization and subspecialization, defined initially by organ system and more recently by locus of principal activity (inpatient vs. outpatient), reliance on manual skills (proceduralist vs. nonproceduralist), or participation in research. Nevertheless, it is becoming increasingly clear that the same fundamental molecular and genetic mechanisms are broadly applicable across all organ systems and that the scientific methodologies of randomized trials and careful clinical observation span all aspects of medicine.

APPROACH TO THE PATIENT

Patients commonly have complaints (symptoms). These symptoms may or may not be accompanied by abnormalities on examination (signs) or on laboratory testing. Conversely, asymptomatic patients may have signs or laboratory abnormalities, and laboratory abnormalities can occur in the absence of symptoms or signs.

Symptoms and signs commonly define *syndromes,* which may be the common final pathway of a wide range of pathophysiologic alterations. The fundamental basis of internal medicine is that diagnosis should elucidate the pathophysiologic explanation for symptoms and signs so that therapy may improve the underlying abnormality, not just attempt to suppress the abnormal symptoms or signs.

When patients seek care from physicians, they may have manifestations or exacerbations of known conditions, or they may have symptoms and signs that suggest malfunction of a particular organ system. Sometimes the pattern of symptoms and signs is highly suggestive or even pathognomonic for a particular disease process. In these situations, in which the physician is focusing on a particular disease, the *Cecil Textbook of Medicine* provides scholarly, yet practical approaches to the epidemiology, pathobiology, clinical manifestations, diagnosis, treatment, prevention, and prognosis of entities such as acute myocardial infarction (Chapter 72), chronic obstructive lung disease (Chapter 88), obstructive uropathy (Chapter 124), inflammatory bowel disease (Chapter 144), gallstones (Chapter 159), rheumatoid arthritis (Chapter 285), hypothyroidism (Chapter 244), tuberculosis (Chapter 345), and virtually any known medical condition in adults.

Many patients, however, have undiagnosed symptoms, signs, or laboratory abnormalities that cannot be immediately ascribed to a particular disease or cause. Whether the initial manifestation is chest pain (Chapter 48), diarrhea (Chapter 143), neck or back pain (Chapter 423), or a variety of more than 100 common symptoms, signs, or laboratory abnormalities, the *Cecil Textbook of Medicine* provides tables, figures, and entire chapters to guide the approach to diagnosis and therapy (Table 1–1). By

TABLE 1–1 GUIDE TO THE APPROACH TO COMMON SYMPTOMS, SIGNS, AND LABORATORY ABNORMALITIES

	Chapter	Specific Tables or Figures
SYMPTOMS		
CONSTITUTIONAL		
Fever	302	Tables 302–1 to 302–8
Fatigue	293	Table 293–3
Poor appetite	134	Table 134–1
Weight loss	134, 233, 238	Figure 134–3; Table 134–4
Obesity	233	Figure 233–2
Snoring, sleep disturbances	101, 429	Table 429–3
HEAD, EYES, EARS, NOSE, THROAT		
Headache	421	Table 421–1
Visual loss, transient	449	Tables 449–2, 450–1
Ear pain	452	Table 452–1
Hearing loss	454	Figure 454–1
Ringing in ears (tinnitus)	454	Figure 454–2
Vertigo	454	Figure 454–3
Nasal congestion	452	Figure 452–1
Rhinitis or sneezing	272	Figure 272–2
Loss of smell or taste	453	Table 453–1
Dry mouth	451	Table 451–7
Sore throat	455	Figure 455–2; Table 455–1
Hoarseness	455	
CARDIOPULMONARY		
Chest pain	48	Table 48–2
Bronchitis	96	
Shortness of breath	48, 83	Figures 48–1, 83–1
Palpitations	48, 61	Figure 61–1; Tables 48–3, 61–1
Dizziness	48, 61, 427	Figure 61–1; Table 427–1
Syncope	61, 427	Figures 61–1, 427–1; Tables 61–1, 427–1, 427–2
Cardiac arrest	62	Figures 62–2, 62–3
Cough	83	Figure 83–1; Tables 83–1, 83–2
Hemoptysis	83	Tables 83–5, 83–6
GASTROINTESTINAL		
Nausea and vomiting	134	Table 134–3
Dysphagia, odynophagia	134, 140	Table 134–1
Hematemesis	137, 157	Figure 137–3; Table 137–1
Heartburn/dyspepsia	139, 140	Figures 139–2, 140–3
Abdominal pain:		
Acute	134, 145	Figure 134–1; Table 134–2
Chronic	134, 139	Figure 134–2; Table 134–2
Diarrhea	139, 143	Figures 139–1, 143–2, 143–3, 143–8 to 143–10
Melena	137	Figure 137–4; Table 137–4
Constipation	138, 139	Figures 138–4, 139–1; Table 138–2
Fecal incontinence	148	Figure 148–4
Anal pain	148	Table 148–2
GENITOURINARY		
Dysuria	306, 307	
Frequency	130, 306	
Incontinence	24	Figure 24–1; Table 24–3
Urinary obstruction	124	Tables 124–1 to 124–3
Renal colic	127	Figure 127–3
Vaginal discharge	307	
Menstrual irregularities	256	Figure 256–9; Tables 256–3 to 256–5
Female infertility	256	Table 256–6
Hot flushes	262	Table 262–1
Erectile dysfunction	253	
Male infertility	253	Figures 253–11, 253–12
MUSCULOSKELETAL		
Neck or back pain	423	Figure 423–3; Tables 423–1 to 423–4
Painful joints	277	Table 277–2
EXTREMITIES		
Swollen feet, ankles, or legs		
bilateral	48	Figure 48–8
unilateral	81	Figure 81–2; Table 81–2
Claudication	79	Figure 79–2
NEUROLOGIC		
Weakness	418, 446, 447, 448	Tables 418–1, 446–2
Sensory loss	418, 446	Tables 446–1, 446–4 to 446–7
Memory loss	425	Figures 425–1, 425–2; Tables 425–1 to 425–6
Abnormal gait	418	Table 418–2
Seizures	426	Tables 426–1 to 426–4
INTEGUMENTARY		
Abnormal bleeding	178	Table 178–1
Rash	462	Figure 462–1; Tables 462–1 to 462–4
Hives	273, 466	Figure 273–2; Tables 273–1, 466–1
Abnormal pigmentation	467	Table 467–2
Hirsutism and alopecia	261, 467	Tables 261–1, 467–5
SIGNS		
VITAL SIGNS		
Fever	302, 303	Tables 302–1 to 302–8
Hypothermia	7, 110	Table 110–4
Tachycardia/bradycardia	7, 52, 61, 65	Figures 61–2, 61–3
Hypertension	66	Table 66–4
Hypotension/shock	7, 107	Figure 107–1
Altered respiration	7, 86, 105	Tables 86–1, 105–2
HEAD, EYES, EARS, NOSE, THROAT		
Red eye	449	Table 449–4
Dilated pupil	450	Figure 450–4
Nystagmus	450	Table 450–5
Papilledema	450	Table 450–2
Strabismus	450	Figure 450–6
Jaundice	150	Figure 150–3; Tables 150–1 to 150–3
Otitis	452	Figure 452–1
Sinusitis	272, 452	Figure 452–1
Oral ulcer	451	Tables 451–1, 451–3, 451–4
Salivary gland enlargement	451	Table 451–6
NECK		
Neck mass	200	Figure 200–3
Lymphadenopathy	174	Tables 174–1, 174–2, 174–5
Thyroid nodule	244	Figure 244–4
Thyromegaly/goiter	244	Figures 244–1, 244–3
BREAST		
Breast mass	208	
LUNGS		
Wheezes	83	Table 83–3
CARDIAC		
Heart murmur or extra sounds	48	Figure 48–4; Tables 48–6, 48–7
Jugular venous distention	48	Table 48–5
Carotid pulse abnormalities	48	Figure 48–5
ABDOMEN		
Hepatomegaly	149	Figure 149–4
Splenomegaly	174	Tables 174–6, 174–8
Acute abdomen	145	Tables 145–1 to 145–3
Abdominal swelling/ascites	146, 157	Table 157–3
Rectal bleeding/positive stool	137, 203	Figures 137–4, 137–5; Table 137–5
Hemorrhoids	148	Table 148–1

TABLE 1–1 GUIDE TO THE APPROACH TO COMMON SYMPTOMS, SIGNS, AND LABORATORY ABNORMALITIES—cont'd

	Chapter	Specific Tables or Figures
GENITOURINARY		
Scrotal mass	210	Figure 210–1
Vaginal discharge	307	
Genital ulcers or warts	307	
MUSCULOSKELETAL/EXTREMITIES		
Arthritis	277	
Edema	48	Figure 48–8
Cyanosis	48	
Clubbing	48	
NEUROLOGIC		
Delirium	26	Figure 26–1; Tables 26–1, 26–2
Psychiatric disturbances	420	Tables 420–1, 420–3 to 420–5, 420–7 to 420–9
Coma	428	Table 428–1
Stroke	431	Figure 431–4
Movement disorders	434	Tables 434–1 to 434–7
Neuropathy	446	Figure 446–1
SKIN AND NAILS		
Suspicious mole	214	Table 214–1
Nail diseases	467	Table 467–4
COMMON LABORATORY ABNORMALITIES		
HEMATOLOGY/URINALYSIS		
Anemia	162	Figure 162–2; Tables 162–4 to 162–6
Polycythemia	172	Figure 172–3; Table 172–2
Leukocytosis	173	Figure 173–7; Table 173–4
Lymphocytosis	173	Table 173–7
Monocytosis	173	Table 173–6
Eosinophilia	176	Figure 176–2; Table 176–1
Neutropenia	173	Figures 173–2, 173–5; Table 173–1
With fever	303	Figures 303–1, 303–2
Thrombocytosis	177	Figure 177–1; Table 177–2
Thrombocytopenia	179	Table 179–1
Prolonged PT or PTT	178	Figures 178–3, 178–4
Urinalysis	115	Table 115–1
CHEMISTRIES		
Abnormal liver enzymes	150	Figures 150–3 to 150–5
Elevated BUN/creatinine		
Acute	121	Figure 121–1; Tables 121–1 to 121–5
Chronic	131	Table 131–1
Hyperglycemia	247, 248	Table 248–2
Hypoglycemia	249	Table 249–1
Electrolyte abnormalities	117, 118	Tables 117–3, 117–4, 117–6, 118–2, 118–3
Acid–base disturbances	119	Tables 119–1 to 119–5
Hypercalcemia	266	Table 266–1
Hypocalcemia	266	Table 266–4
Hypo- and hyperphosphatemia	120	Tables 120–2, 120–3
Elevated Pco_2	86	Figure 86–3
CHEST RADIOGRAPH/ECG		
Solitary pulmonary nodule	201	Figure 201–5
Pleural effusion	100	Table 100–5
Suspected lung cancer	201	Figure 201–4
ECG abnormalities	52	Tables 52–2 to 52–5

BUN = blood urea nitrogen; ECG = electrocardiogram; PT = prothrombin time; PTT = partial thromboplastin time.

virtue of this dual approach to known disease as well as to undiagnosed abnormalities, this textbook, similar to the modern practice of medicine, applies directly to patients regardless of their mode of manifestation or degree of previous evaluation.

The patient-physician interaction proceeds through many phases of clinical reasoning and decision making. The interaction begins with an elucidation of complaints or concerns, followed by inquiries or evaluations to address these concerns in increasingly precise ways. The process commonly requires a careful history or physical examination, ordering of diagnostic tests, integration of clinical findings with test results, understanding of the risks and benefits of the possible courses of action, and careful consultation with the patient and family to develop future plans. Physicians can increasingly call on a growing literature of evidence-based medicine to guide the process so that benefit is maximized while respecting individual variations in different patients. Throughout the *Cecil Textbook of Medicine*, the best current evidence is highlighted with specific grade A references that can be accessed directly in the electronic version.

The increasing availability of evidence from randomized trials to guide the approach to diagnosis and therapy should not be equated with "cookbook" medicine. Evidence and the guidelines that are derived from it emphasize proven approaches for patients with specific characteristics. Substantial clinical judgment is required to determine whether the evidence and guidelines apply to individual patients and to recognize the occasional exceptions. Even more judgment is required in the many situations in which evidence is absent or inconclusive. Evidence must also be tempered by patients' preferences, although it is a physician's responsibility to emphasize evidence when presenting alternative options to the patient. The adherence of a patient to a specific regimen is likely to be enhanced if the patient also understands the rationale and evidence behind the recommended option.

To care for a patient as an individual, the physician must understand the patient as a person. This fundamental precept of doctoring includes an understanding of the patient's social situation, family issues, financial concerns, and preferences for different types of care and outcomes, ranging from maximum prolongation of life to the relief of pain and suffering (Chapters 2 and 3). If the physician does not appreciate and address these issues, the science of medicine cannot be applied appropriately, and even the most knowledgeable physician will fail to achieve the desired outcomes.

Even as physicians become increasingly aware of new discoveries, patients can obtain their own information from a variety of sources, some of which are of questionable reliability. The increasing use of alternative and complementary therapies (Chapter 36) is an example of patients' frequent dissatisfaction with prescribed medical therapy. Physicians should keep an open mind regarding unproven options but must advise their patients carefully if such options may carry any degree of potential risk, including the risk that they may be relied on to substitute for proven approaches. It is crucial for the physician to have an open dialogue with the patient and family regarding the full range of options that either may consider.

The physician does not exist in a vacuum, but rather as part of a complicated and extensive system of medical care and public health. In premodern times and even today in some developing countries, basic hygiene, clean water, and adequate nutrition have been the most important ways to promote health and reduce disease. In developed countries, adoption of healthy lifestyles, including better diet (Chapter 232) and appropriate exercise (Chapter 14), is the cornerstone to reducing the epidemics of obesity (Chapter 239), coronary disease (Chapter 69), and diabetes (Chapter 248). Public health interventions to provide immunizations (Chapter 16) and reduce injuries (Chapter 15) and the use of tobacco (Chapter 30), illicit drugs (Chapter 32), and excess alcohol (Chapter 31) can collectively produce more health benefits than nearly any other imaginable health intervention.

APPROACH TO THE MEDICAL PROFESSION

In a profession, practitioners puts the welfare of clients or patients above their own welfare. Professionals have a duty that may be thought of as a contract with society. The American Board of Internal Medicine and the European Federation of Internal Medicine have jointly proposed that medical professionalism should emphasize three fundamental principles: the primacy of patient welfare, patient autonomy, and social

TABLE 1–2 PROFESSIONAL RESPONSIBILITIES

Commitment to
- Professional competence
- Honesty with patients
- Patient confidentiality
- Maintaining appropriate relations with patients
- Improving the quality of care
- Improving access to care
- Just distribution of finite resources
- Scientific knowledge
- Maintaining trust by managing conflicts of interest
- Professional responsibilities

From Brennan T, Blank L, Cohen J, et al: Medical professionalism in the new millennium: A physician charter. Ann Intern Med 2002;1136:243–246.

justice. As modern medicine brings a plethora of diagnostic and therapeutic options, the interactions of the physician with the patient and society become more complex and potentially fraught with ethical dilemmas (Chapter 2). To help provide a moral compass that is not only grounded in tradition but also adaptable to modern times, the primacy of patient welfare emphasizes the fundamental principle of a profession. The physician's altruism, which begets the patient's trust, must be impervious to the economic, bureaucratic, and political challenges that are faced by the physician and the patient (Chapter 5).

The principle of patient autonomy asserts that physicians make recommendations but patients make the final decisions. The physician is an expert advisor who must inform and empower the patient to base decisions on scientific data and how these data can and should be integrated with a patient's preferences.

The importance of social justice symbolizes that the patient-physician interaction does not exist in a vacuum. The physician has a responsibility to the individual patient and to broader society to promote access and to eliminate disparities in health and health care.

To promote these fundamental principles, a series of professional responsibilities have been suggested (Table 1–2). These specific responsibilities represent practical, daily traits that benefit the physician's own patients and society as a whole. Physicians who use these and other attributes to improve their patients' satisfaction with care are not only promoting professionalism but also reducing their own risk for liability and malpractice.

An interesting new aspect of professionalism is the increasing reliance on team approaches to medical care, as exemplified by physicians whose roles are defined by the location of their practice—historically in the intensive care unit or emergency department and more recently on the inpatient general hospital floor. Quality care requires coordination and effective communication across inpatient and outpatient sites among physicians who themselves now typically work defined hours. This transition from reliance on a single, always available physician to a team, ideally with a designated coordinator, places new challenges on physicians, the medical care system, and the medical profession.

The changing medical care environment is placing increasing emphasis on standards, outcomes, and accountability. As purchasers of insurance become more cognizant of value rather than just cost (Chapter 11), outcomes ranging from rates of screening mammography (Chapter 208) to mortality rates with coronary artery bypass graft surgery (Chapter 74) become metrics by which rational choices can be made. Clinical guidelines and critical pathways derived from randomized controlled trials and evidence-based medicine can potentially lead to more cost-effective care and better outcomes.

These major changes in many Western health care systems bring with them many major risks and concerns. If the concept of limited choice among physicians and health care providers is based on objective measures of quality and outcome, channeling of patients to better providers is one reasonable definition of better selection and enlightened competition. If the limiting of options is based overwhelmingly on cost rather than measures of quality, outcomes, and patient satisfaction, it is likely that the historic relationship between the patient and the truly professional physician will be fundamentally compromised.

Another risk is that the same genetic information that could lead to more effective, personalized medicine will be used against the very people whom it is supposed to benefit—by creating a stigma, raising health insurance costs, or even making someone uninsurable. The ethical approach to medicine (Chapter 2), genetics, and genetic counseling (Chapter 38) provides means to protect against this adverse effect of scientific progress.

In this new environment the physician often has a dual responsibility: to the health care system as an expert who helps create standards, measures of outcome, clinical guidelines, and mechanisms to ensure high-quality, cost-effective care and to individual patients who entrust their well-being to that physician to promote their best interests within the reasonable limits of the system. A health insurance system that emphasizes cost-effective care, that gives physicians and health care providers responsibility for the health of a population and the resources required to achieve these goals, that must exist in a competitive environment in which patients can choose alternatives if they are not satisfied with their care, and that places increasing emphasis on health education and prevention can have many positive effects. In this environment, however, physicians must beware of overt and subtle pressures that could entice them to underserve patients and abrogate their professional responsibilities by putting personal financial reward ahead of their patients' welfare. The physician's responsibility to represent the patient's best interests and avoid financial conflicts by doing too little in the newer systems of capitated care provides different specific challenges but an analogous moral dilemma to the historic American system in which the physician could be rewarded financially for doing too much.

In the current health care environment, all physicians and trainees must redouble their commitment to professionalism. At the same time, the challenge to the individual physician to retain and expand the scientific knowledge base and process the vast array of new information is daunting. In this spirit of a profession based on science and caring, the *Cecil Textbook of Medicine* seeks to be a comprehensive approach to modern internal medicine.

SUGGESTED READINGS

Bowen JL: Educational strategies to promote clinical diagnostic reasoning. N Engl J Med 2006;355:2217–2225. *An educational review.*

Hafferty FW: Professionalism—the next wave. N Engl J Med 2006;355:2151–2152. *Redefining professionalism in medical education.*

Snyderman R, Yoediono Z: Prospective care: A personalized, preventative approach to medicine. Pharmacogenomics 2006;7:5–9. *How genetic information may allow targeting of preventive and therapeutic interventions.*

Stelfox HT, Gandhi TK, Orav EJ, et al: The relation of patient satisfaction with complaints against physicians and malpractice lawsuits. Am J Med 2005;118:1126–1133. *More satisfied patients are less likely to sue.*

Stern DT, Papadakis M: The developing physician—becoming a professional. N Engl J Med 2006;355:1794–1799. *Standards of professional behavior in new physicians.*

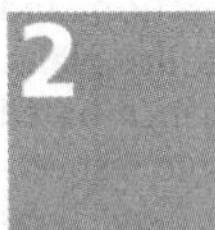

2 BIOETHICS IN THE PRACTICE OF MEDICINE

Ezekiel J. Emanuel

It commonly is argued that modern advances in medical technology, antibiotics, dialysis, transplantation, and intensive care units have created the bioethical dilemmas that confront physicians in the 21st century. In reality, however, concerns about ethical issues are as old as the practice of medicine itself. The Hippocratic Oath, composed sometime around 400 BC, attests to the need of ancient Greek physicians for advice on how to address the many bioethical dilemmas that they confronted. The Oath addresses issues of confidentiality, abortion, euthanasia, sexual relations between physician and patient, divided loyalties, and, at least implicitly, charity care and executions. Other Hippocratic works address issues such as termination of treatments to dying patients and telling the truth. Whether we agree with the advice dispensed or not, the important point is that many bioethical issues are not created by technology but are inherent in medical practice. Technology may make these issues more common and may change the context in which they arise, but there are underlying bioethical issues that seem timeless.

Many physicians have been educated that four main principles can be invoked to address bioethical dilemmas: autonomy, nonmaleficence, beneficence, and justice. Autonomy is the idea that people should have the right and freedom to choose, pursue, and revise their own life plans. Nonmaleficence is the idea that people should not be harmed or injured knowingly; this principle is encapsulated in the frequently repeated phrase that a physician has an obligation to "first do no harm"—*primum non nocere.* This phrase is not found either in the Hippocratic Oath or in other Hippocratic writing; the only related, but not identical, Hippocratic phrase is "at least, do not harm." Although nonmaleficence is about avoiding harm, beneficence is about the positive actions that the physician should undertake to promote the well-being of his or her patients. In clinical practice, this obligation usually arises from the implicit and explicit commitments and promises surrounding the physician-patient relationship. Finally, there is the principle of justice as the fair distribution of benefits and burdens.

Although helpful in providing an initial framework, these principles have limited value because they are broad and open to diverse and conflicting interpretations. In addition, as is clear with the principle of justice, they frequently are underdeveloped. In any difficult case, the principles are likely to conflict. Conflicting ethical principles are precisely why there are bioethical dilemmas. The principles themselves do not offer guidance on how they should be balanced or specified to resolve the dilemma. These principles are focused on the individual physician-patient context; they are not particularly helpful when the bioethical issues are institutional and systemic, such as setting priorities or establishing general policies. Finally, these four principles are not comprehensive. Other fundamental ethical principles and values, such as communal solidarity, duties to future generations, trust, and professional integrity, are important in bioethics but not encapsulated except by deformation in these four principles.

There is no formula or small set of ethical principles that mechanically or magically gives answers to bioethical dilemmas. Instead, medical practitioners should follow an orderly analytic process. First, practitioners need to obtain the facts relevant to the situation. Second, they must delineate the basic bioethical issue. Third, it is important to identify all the crucial principles and values that relate to the case and how they might conflict. Fourth, because many ethical dilemmas have been analyzed previously and subjected frequently to empirical study, practitioners should examine the relevant literature, whether it is commentaries or studies in medical journals, legal cases, or books. With these analyses, the particular dilemma should be reexamined; this process might lead to reformulation of the issue and identification of new values or new understandings of existing values. Fifth, with this information, it is important to distinguish clearly unethical practices from a range of ethically permissible actions. Finally, it is important not only to come to some resolution of the case but also to state clearly the reasons behind the decisions, that is, the interpretation of the principles used and how values were balanced. Although unanimity and consensus may be desirable ideals, reasonable people frequently disagree about how to resolve ethical dilemmas without being unethical or malevolent.

A multitude of bioethical dilemmas arise in medical practice, including issues of genetics, reproductive choices, and termination of care. In clinical practice, the most common issues revolve around informed consent, termination of life-sustaining treatments, euthanasia and physician-assisted suicide, and conflicts of interest.

PHYSICIAN-PATIENT RELATIONSHIP: INFORMED CONSENT

History

It commonly is thought that the requirement for informed consent is a relatively recent phenomenon. Suggestions about the need for a patient's informed consent can be found as far back as Plato, however. The first recorded legal case involving informed consent is the 1767 English case of *Slater v. Baker and Stapleton,* in which two surgeons refractured a patient's leg after it had healed improperly. The patient claimed they had not obtained consent. The court ruled:

> [I]t appears from the evidence of the surgeon that it was improper to disunite the callous without consent; this is the usage and law of surgeons: then it was ignorance and unskillfulness in that very particular, to do contrary to the rule of the profession, what no surgeon ought to have done.

Although there may be some skepticism about the extent of the information disclosed or the precise nature of the consent obtained, the notable fact is that an 18th century court declared that obtaining prior consent of the patient is not only the usual practice but also the ethical and legal obligation of surgeons. Failure to obtain consent is incompetence and inexcusable. In contemporary times, the 1957 case of *Salgo v. Leland Stanford Junior University Board of Trustees* constitutes a landmark by stating that physicians have a positive legal obligation to disclose information about risks, benefits, and alternatives to patients; this decision popularized the term *informed consent.*

Definition and Justification

Informed consent is a person's autonomous authorization of a physician to undertake diagnostic or therapeutic interventions for himself or herself. In this view, the patient understands that he or she is taking responsibility for the decision while empowering someone else, the physician, to implement it. Not any agreement to a course of medical treatment qualifies as informed consent, however.

There are four fundamental requirements for valid informed consent: mental capacity, disclosure, understanding, and voluntariness. Informed consent assumes that people have the mental capacity to make decisions; disease, development, or medications can compromise patients' mental capacity to provide informed consent. Adults are presumed to have the legal competence to make medical decisions, and whether an adult is incompetent to make medical decisions is a legal determination. Practically, physicians usually decide whether patients are competent on the basis of whether patients can understand the information disclosed, appreciate its significance for their own situation, and use logical and consistent thought processes in decision making. Incompetence in medical decision making does not mean a person is incompetent in all types of decision making and vice versa. Crucial information relevant to the decision must be disclosed, usually by the physician, to the patient. The patient should understand the information and its implications for his or her interests and life goals. Finally, the patient must make a voluntary decision (i.e., one without coercion or manipulation by the physician). It is a mistake to view informed consent as an event, such as the signing of a form. Informed consent is viewed more accurately as a process that evolves during the course of diagnosis and treatment.

Typically, the patient's autonomy is the value invoked to justify informed consent. Other values, such as bodily integrity and beneficence, have also been cited, especially in early legal rulings.

Empirical Data

Fairly extensive research has been done on informed consent. In general, studies show that in clinical situations, physicians frequently do not communicate all relevant information for informed decision making. In a study of audiotapes from 1057 outpatient encounters, physicians mentioned alternatives in only 11.3% of cases, provided pros and cons of interventions in only 7.8% of situations, and assessed the patient's understanding of the information in only 1.5% of decisions. The more complex the medical decisions, the more likely it was that the elements of informed consent would be fulfilled. Importantly, data suggest that disclosure is better in research settings, both in terms of the informed consent documents and in the discussions. For instance, in recorded interactions between researchers and prospective participants, the major elements of research, such as that the treatment was investigational and the risks and benefits, were disclosed in more than 80% of interactions. Greater disclosure in the research setting may be the consequence of requiring a written informed consent document.

Patients frequently fail to recall crucial information disclosed, although they usually think they have sufficient information for decision making. Whether patients fail to recall key information because they are overwhelmed by the information or because they do not find much of it salient to their decision is unclear. The issue is what patients understand at the point of decision making, not what they recall later.

Studies aimed at improving informed consent in the clinical setting suggest that interactive media, such as videos, can improve understanding by patients. Conversely, data from the research setting suggest that interactive media do not improve participants' understanding, whereas more personal interaction, whether as an additional telephone call by a research nurse or as an additional face-to-face meeting, does enhance understanding.

One of the most important results of empirical research on informed consent is the information–decision making gap. Many studies show that most patients want information, but far fewer prefer decision-making authority. One study showed that most patients wanted information, but only about one third desired decision-making authority, and patients' decision-making preferences were not correlated with their information-

TABLE 2–1 FUNDAMENTAL ELEMENTS FOR DISCLOSURE TO PATIENTS

Diagnosis and prognosis
Nature of proposed intervention
Reasonable alternative interventions
Risks associated with each alternative intervention
Benefits associated with each alternative intervention
Probable outcomes of each alternative intervention

seeking preferences. Several investigators found that patients' preference for decision-making authority increases with higher educational levels and declines with advancing age. Most important, the more serious the illness, the more likely patients are to prefer that physicians make the decisions. Several studies suggest that patients who have less of a desire to make their own decisions generally are more satisfied with how the decisions were made.

Practical Considerations

Implementing informed consent raises concerns about the extent of information to be disclosed and exceptions to the general requirement. A major area of ethical and legal disagreement has been what information to disclose and how to disclose it. As a practical matter, physicians should disclose at least six fundamental elements of information to patients: (1) diagnosis and prognosis, (2) nature of the proposed intervention, (3) alternative interventions, (4) risks associated with each alternative, (5) benefits of each alternative, and (6) likely outcomes of these alternatives (Table 2–1). Because risk is usually the key worry of physicians, it generally is recommended that physicians disclose (1) the nature of the risks, (2) their magnitude, (3) the probability that each risk will occur, and (4) when the consequence might occur. Some argue that minor risks need not be disclosed. In general, serious risks, even if rare, should be disclosed, as should common risks.

The central problem is that the physician should provide this detailed information within reasonable time constraints and yet not overwhelm patients with complex information in technical language. The result has been various legal standards defining how much information should be disclosed. The *physician* or *customary* standard, adapted from malpractice law, states that the physician should disclose information "which a reasonable medical practitioner would make under the same or similar circumstances." Conversely, the *reasonable person* or *lay-oriented* standard states that physicians should disclose all information that a "reasonable person in the patient's circumstances would find material to" the medical decision. The physician standard is factual and can be determined empirically, but the patient-oriented standard, which is meant to engage physicians with patients, is hypothetical. Currently, each standard is used by about half the states.

There are exceptions to the requirements of informed consent. In emergency situations, consent can be assumed because reasonable persons would want treatment. In some circumstances, physicians may believe the process of informed consent could harm the patient. In rare cases, the "therapeutic privilege" promoting a patient's well-being trumps autonomy, but physicians should be wary of invoking this exception too readily.

If patients are deemed incompetent, family members—beginning with spouse, children, parents, siblings, then more distant relatives—usually are selected as surrogates or proxies, although there may be concerns about conflicting interests or knowledge of the patient's wishes. In the relatively rare circumstance in which a patient formally designated a proxy, that person has decision-making authority.

The *substituted judgment* standard states that the proxy should choose what the patient would choose if he or she were competent. The *best interests* standard states that the proxy should choose what is best for the patient. Frequently, it is not clear how the patient would have decided because the situation was not discussed with the patient and he or she left no living will. Similarly, what is best for a patient is controversial because there are usually tradeoffs between quality of life and survival. These problems are exacerbated because a proxy's predictions about a patient's quality of life are poor; proxies tend to underestimate patients' functional status and satisfaction. Similarly, proxy predictions are inaccurate regarding life-sustaining preferences when the patient is mentally incapacitated; families tend to agree with patients less than 70% of the time in deciding whether to provide life-sustaining treatments if the patient became demented, when chance alone would generate agreement in 50% of the cases. Such confusion about how to decide for incapacitated patients can create conflicts among family members or between the family and medical providers. In such circumstances, an ethics consultation may be helpful.

TERMINATION OF MEDICAL INTERVENTIONS

History

Since the start of medicine, it has been viewed as ethical to withhold medical treatments from the terminally ill and "let nature take its course." Hippocrates argued that physicians should "refuse to treat those [patients] who are overmastered by their disease." In the 19th century, prominent American physicians advocated withholding of cathartic and emetic "treatments" from the terminally ill and use of ether to ease pain at the end of life. In 1900, editors of *The Lancet* argued that physicians should intervene to ease the pain of death but did not have an obligation to prolong a clearly terminal life. The contemporary debate on terminating care began in 1976 with the *Quinlan* case, in which the New Jersey Supreme Court ruled that patients had a right to refuse life-sustaining interventions on the basis of a right of privacy and that the family could exercise the right for a patient in a persistent vegetative state.

Definition and Justification

It generally is agreed that all patients have a right to refuse medical interventions. Ethically, this right is based on the patient's autonomy and is implied by the doctrine of informed consent. Legally, state courts have cited the right to privacy, right to bodily integrity, or common law to justify the right to refuse medical treatment. In the 1990 *Cruzan* case and in the subsequent physician-assisted suicide cases, the U.S. Supreme Court affirmed that there is a "constitutionally protected right to refuse lifesaving hydration and nutrition." The Court stated that "[A] liberty interest [based on the 14th Amendment] in refusing unwanted medical treatment may be inferred from our prior decisions." All patients have a constitutional and an ethical right to refuse medical interventions. These rulings were the basis of the consistent state and federal court rulings to permit the husband to terminate artificial nutrition and hydration in the *Schiavo* case.

Empirical Data

Data show that termination of medical treatments is now the norm. More than 85% of Americans die without cardiopulmonary resuscitation, and more than 90% of decedents in intensive care units do not receive cardiopulmonary resuscitation. Of decedents in intensive care units, 90% die after the withholding or withdrawal of medical treatments, with an average of 2.6 interventions being withheld or withdrawn per decedent. Since the 1990s, the trend has been to stop medical interventions more frequently.

Despite extensive public support for use of advance care directives and the passage of the Patient Self-Determination Act mandating that health care institutions inform patients of their right to complete such documents, only about 20% of Americans have completed one. Data suggest that attention generated by the *Schiavo* case appears to have increased completion of advanced directives by Americans to more than 30%. Efforts to improve completion of advance care directives have generated mixed results; even successful pilot efforts have not been adopted or reproduced widely. A persistent problem has been that even when patients complete advance care directives, the documents frequently are not available, physicians do not know they exist, or they tend to be too general or vague to guide decisions.

Just as proxies are poor at predicting patients' wishes, data show that physicians are probably even worse at determining patients' preferences for life-sustaining treatments. In many cases, life-sustaining treatments are continued even when patients or their proxies desire them to be stopped; conversely, many physicians discontinue or never begin interventions unilaterally without the knowledge or consent of patients or their surrogate decision makers. These discrepancies emphasize the importance of engaging patients early in their care about treatment preferences.

Practical Considerations

There are many practical considerations in enacting this right (Table 2–2). First, patients have a right to refuse any and all medical interventions, from blood transfusions and antibiotics to respirators, artificial hydration, and nutrition. Although initiation of cardiopulmonary resuscitation was the focus of the early court cases, this issue is viewed best as addressing just one of the many medical interventions that can be stopped or withheld. The attempt to distinguish ordinary from extraordinary or heroic treatments has been unhelpful in determining which treatments may be stopped.

Second, there is no ethical or legal difference between withholding an intervention and withdrawing it. If a respirator or other treatment is started because physicians are uncertain whether a patient would have wanted it, they always can stop it later when information clarifies the patient's wishes. Although physicians and nurses might find stopping a treatment to be more difficult psychologically, withdrawal is ethically and legally permitted—and required—when it is consonant with the patient's wishes.

Third, competent patients have the exclusive right to decide about terminating their own care. If there is a conflict between a competent patient and his or her family, the patient's wishes are to be followed. It is the patient's right to refuse treatment, not the family's right. For incompetent patients, the situation is more complex; if the patients left clear indications of their wishes, whether as explicit oral statements or as written advance care directives, these wishes should be followed. Physicians should not be overly concerned about the precise form patients use to express their wishes; because patients have a constitutional right to refuse treatment, the real concern is whether the wishes are clear and relevant to the situation. If an incompetent patient did not leave explicit indications of his or her wishes or designate a proxy decision maker, the physician should identify a surrogate decision maker and rely on the decision maker's wishes while being cognizant of the potential problems noted.

Fourth, the right to refuse medical treatment does not translate into a right to demand any treatment, especially treatments that have no pathophysiologic rationale, have already failed, or are known to be harmful. Attempts by physicians to invoke futility as a rationale for stopping treatments have been fraught with problems, however. Initially, some commentators advocated that an intervention was futile when the probability of success was 1% or lower. Although this threshold seems to be based on empirical data, it is a covert value judgment. Because the declaration of futility is meant to justify unilateral determinations by physicians, it generally has been viewed as an inappropriate assertion that undermines physician-patient communication and violates the principle of shared decision making. Similar to the distinction between ordinary and extraordinary, futility is viewed increasingly as more obfuscating than clarifying, and it is being invoked much less often.

ASSISTED SUICIDE AND EUTHANASIA

History

Since Hippocrates, euthanasia and physician-assisted suicide have been controversial issues. In 1905, a bill was introduced into the Ohio legislature to legalize euthanasia; it was defeated. In the mid-1930s, similar bills were introduced and defeated in the British Parliament and the Nebraska legislature. As of 2007, physician-assisted suicide is legal in Oregon, and euthanasia and physician-assisted suicide are legal in the Netherlands, Belgium, and Switzerland.

Definition and Justification

There has been much terminologic confusion about euthanasia and physician-assisted suicide. Table 2–3 provides accepted definitions. So-called passive and indirect euthanasia are misnomers and are not instances of euthanasia, and both are deemed ethical and legal.

There are four arguments against permitting euthanasia and physician-assisted suicide. First, Kant and Mill thought that autonomy did not permit the voluntary ending of the conditions necessary for autonomy, and as a result, both philosophers were against voluntary enslavement and suicide. Consequently, the exercise of autonomy cannot include the ending of life because that would mean ending the possibility of exercising autonomy. Second, many dying patients may have pain and suffering because they are not receiving appropriate care, and it is possible that adequate care would relieve much pain and suffering (Chapter 3). Although a few patients still may suffer uncontrolled pain and suffering despite optimal end-of-life care, it is unwise to use the condition of these few patients as a justification to permit euthanasia or physician-assisted suicide for any dying patient. Third, there is a clear distinction between intentional ending of a life and termination of life-sustaining treatments. The actual acts are different—injecting a life-ending medication, such as a muscle relaxant, or providing a prescription for one is not the same as removing or refraining from introducing an invasive medical intervention. Finally, adverse consequences of permitting euthanasia and physician-assisted suicide must be considered. There are disturbing reports of involuntary euthanasia in the Netherlands, and many worry about coercion of expensive or burdensome patients to accept euthanasia or physician-assisted suicide. Permitting euthanasia and physician-assisted suicide is likely to lead to further intrusions of lawyers, courts, and legislatures into the physician-patient relationship.

There are four parallel arguments for permitting euthanasia and physician-assisted suicide. First, it is argued that autonomy justifies euthanasia and physician-assisted suicide. To respect autonomy requires permitting individuals to decide when it is better to end their lives by euthanasia or physician-assisted suicide. Second, beneficence—furthering the well-being of individuals—supports permitting euthanasia and

TABLE 2–2 PRACTICAL CONSIDERATIONS IN TERMINATION OF MEDICAL TREATMENTS

Practical Question	Answer
Is there a legal right to refuse medical interventions?	Yes. The U.S. Supreme Court declared that competent people have a constitutionally protected right to refuse unwanted medical treatments based on the 14th Amendment.
What interventions can be legally and ethically terminated?	Any and all interventions (including respirators, antibiotics, intravenous or enteral nutrition, and hydration) can be legally and ethically terminated.
Is there a difference between withholding life-sustaining interventions and withdrawing them?	No. The consensus is that there is no important legal or ethical difference between withholding and withdrawing medical interventions. Stopping a treatment once begun is just as ethical as never having started it.
Whose view about terminating life-sustaining interventions prevails if there is a conflict between the patient and family?	The views of a competent adult patient prevail. It is the patient's body and life.
Who decides about terminating life-sustaining interventions if the patient is incompetent?	If the patient appointed a proxy or surrogate decision maker when competent, that person is legally empowered to make decisions about terminating care. If no proxy was appointed, there is a legally designated hierarchy, usually (1) spouse, (2) adult children, (3) parents, (4) siblings, and (5) available relatives.
Are advance care directives legally enforceable?	Yes. As a clear expression of the patient's wishes, they are a constitutionally protected method for patients to exercise their right to refuse medical treatments. In almost all states, clear and explicit oral statements are legally and ethically sufficient for decisions about withholding or withdrawing medical interventions.

TABLE 2–3 DEFINITIONS OF ASSISTED SUICIDE AND EUTHANASIA

Term	Definition
Voluntary active euthanasia	Intentional administration of medications or other interventions to cause the patient's death with the patient's informed consent
Involuntary active euthanasia	Intentional administration of medications or other interventions to cause the patient's death when the patient was competent to consent but did not (e.g., the patient may not have been asked)
Nonvoluntary active euthanasia	Intentional administration of medications or other interventions to cause the patient's death when the patient was incompetent and was mentally incapable of consenting (e.g., the patient might have been in a coma)
Passive euthanasia	Withholding or withdrawal of life-sustaining medical treatments from a patient to let him or her die (termination of life-sustaining treatments)
Indirect euthanasia	Administration of narcotics or other medications to relieve pain with the incidental consequence of causing sufficient respiratory depression to result in the patient's death
Physician-assisted suicide	A physician provides medications or other interventions to a patient with the understanding that the patient can use them to commit suicide

physician-assisted suicide. In some cases, living can create more pain and suffering than death; ending a painful life relieves more suffering and produces more good. Just the reassurance of having the option of euthanasia or physician-assisted suicide, even if people do not use it, can provide "psychological insurance" and be beneficial to people. Third, euthanasia and physician-assisted suicide are no different from termination of life-sustaining treatments that are recognized as ethically justified. In both cases, the patient consents to die; in both cases, the physician intends to end the patient's life and takes some action to end the patient's life; and in both cases, the final result is the same: the patient's death. With no difference in the patient's consent, the physician's intention, or the final result, there can be no difference in the ethical justification. Fourth, the supposed slippery slope that would result from permitting euthanasia and physician-assisted suicide is not likely. The idea that permitting euthanasia and physician-assisted suicide would undermine the physician-patient relationship or lead to forced euthanasia is completely speculative and not borne out by the available data.

In its 1997 decisions, the U.S. Supreme Court stated that there is no constitutional right to euthanasia and physician-assisted suicide but that there also is no constitutional prohibition against states legalizing these interventions. Consequently, Oregon's legalization of physician-assisted suicide was constitutional. In more recent years, however, voters consistently have defeated referenda to legalize physician-assisted suicide in other states, and bills have been defeated in state legislatures.

Empirical Data

Attitudes and practices related to euthanasia and physician-assisted suicide have been studied extensively. First, surveys indicate that 60 to 70% of Americans support euthanasia and physician-assisted suicide for terminally ill patients who suffer intractable pain, but public support declines significantly for euthanasia and physician-assisted suicide in other circumstances. American physicians are much less likely to support euthanasia and physician-assisted suicide, with oncologists being even more opposed than other types of physicians. Second, approximately 18 to 25% of American physicians have received requests for euthanasia or physician-assisted suicide; 43 to 63% of oncologists have received requests. Third, multiple studies indicate that less than 5% of American physicians have performed euthanasia or physician-assisted suicide. Among oncologists, 4% have performed euthanasia and 11% have performed physician-assisted suicide during their careers. Fourth, in many cases, the safeguards are violated. One study found that in 54% of euthanasia cases, it was the family who made the request; in 39% of euthanasia and 19% of physician-assisted suicide cases, the patient was depressed; in only half of the cases was the request repeated.

Counterintuitively, data indicate that it is not pain that motivates requests for euthanasia or physician-assisted suicide but rather psychological distress, especially depression and hopelessness. Interviews with physicians and with patients with amyotrophic lateral sclerosis, cancer, or infection with human immunodeficiency virus show that pain is not associated with interest in euthanasia or physician-assisted suicide; instead, depression and hopelessness are the strongest predictors of interest. Studies of patients in Australia and the Netherlands confirm the importance of depression in motivating requests for euthanasia.

Finally, data from the Netherlands and the United States suggest that there are significant problems in performing euthanasia and physician-assisted suicide. Dutch researchers reported that physician-assisted suicide causes complications in 7% of cases, and in 15% of cases, the patients did not die, awoke from coma, or vomited up the medication. Ultimately, in nearly 20% of physician-assisted suicide cases, the physician ended up injecting the patient with life-ending medication, converting physician-assisted suicide to euthanasia. These data raise serious questions about how to address complications of physician-assisted suicide when euthanasia is illegal or unacceptable.

Practical Considerations

There is widespread agreement that if euthanasia and physician-assisted suicide are used, they should be considered only after all attempts at physical and psychological palliation have failed. A series of safeguards have been developed and embodied in the Oregon and the Dutch procedures, as follows: (1) the patient must be competent and must request euthanasia or physician-assisted suicide repeatedly and voluntarily; (2) the patient must have pain and suffering that cannot be relieved by optimal palliative interventions; (3) there is a waiting period to ensure that the patient's desire for euthanasia or physician-assisted suicide is stable and sincere; and (4) the physician should obtain a second opinion from an independent physician. Oregon requires patients to be terminally ill, whereas the Netherlands, Belgium, and Switzerland have no such safeguard. Although there have been some prosecutions, there have been no convictions—except for Dr. Kevorkian—when physicians and others have participated in euthanasia and physician-assisted suicide.

FINANCIAL CONFLICTS OF INTEREST

History

Worrying about how payment and fees affect medical decisions is not new. In 1899, a physician reported that more than 60% of surgeons in Chicago were willing to provide a 50% commission to physicians for referring cases. He subsequently argued that in some cases, this fee splitting led to unnecessary surgical procedures. A 1912 study by the American Medical Association confirmed that fee splitting was a common practice. Selling patent medicines and patenting surgical instruments were other forms of financial conflicts of interest thought to discredit physicians a century ago. In the 1990s, the ethics of capitation for physician services and pharmaceutical prescriptions and payments by pharmaceutical and biotechnology companies to clinical researchers raised the issue of financial conflicts of interest.

Definition and Justification

It commonly is argued that physicians have certain primary interests: (1) to promote the well-being of their patients, (2) to advance biomedical research, (3) to educate future physicians, and more controversially, (4) to promote public health (Table 2–4). Physicians also have other, secondary interests, such as earning income, raising a family, and pursuing avocational interests. These secondary interests are not evil; typically, they are legitimate, even admirable. A conflict of interest occurs when one of these secondary interests compromises pursuit of a primary interest, especially the patient's well-being.

TABLE 2-4 PRIMARY INTERESTS OF PHYSICIANS

Promotion of the health and well-being of their patients
Advancement of biomedical knowledge through research
Education of future physicians and health care providers
Promotion of the public health

Conflicts of interest are problematic because they can or appear to compromise the integrity of physicians' judgment, compromising the patient's well-being or research integrity. Conflict of interest can induce a physician to do something—perform a procedure, fail to order a test, or distort data—that would not be in a patient's best interest. These conflicts can undermine the trust of patients and the public, not only in an individual physician but also in the entire medical profession. The appearance of conflicts of interest can be damaging because it is difficult for patients and the public "to determine what motives have influenced a professional decision." The focus on financial conflicts of interest is not because they are worse than other types of conflicts but because they are more pervasive and more easily identified and regulated compared with other conflicts. Since ancient times, the ethical norm on conflicts has been clear: the physician's primary obligation is to patients' well-being, and a physician's personal financial well-being should not compromise this duty.

Empirical Data

Financial conflicts are not rare. In Florida, it was estimated that nearly 40% of physicians were involved as owners of freestanding facilities to which they referred patients. Studies in the early 1990s consistently showed that self-referring physicians ordered more services, frequently charged more per service, and referred patients with less established indications. In one study, 4 to 4.5 times more imaging examinations were ordered by self-referring physicians than by physicians who referred patients to radiologists. Similarly, patients referred to joint-venture physical therapy facilities have an average of 16 visits compared with 11 at non–joint-venture facilities. Of greatest concern, licensed physical therapists at joint-venture facilities spent about 28 minutes per patient per visit compared with 48 minutes at non–joint-venture facilities. There are no comparable data on the influence of capitation on physicians' judgment.

Similarly, multiple studies have shown that interaction with pharmaceutical representatives can lead to prescribing of new drugs, nonrational prescribing, and decreased use of generic drugs by physicians. Industry funding for continuing medical education payment for travel to educational symposia increases prescribing of the sponsor's drug.

Regarding researcher conflicts of interest, the available data suggest that corporate funding does not compromise the design and methodology of clinical research; in fact, commercially funded research may be methodologically more rigorous than government- or foundation-supported research. Conversely, data suggest that financial interests do distort researchers' interpretation of data. The most important impact of financial interests, however, is on dissemination of research studies. Growing evidence suggests the suppression or selective publication of data unfavorable to corporate sponsors but the repeated publication of favorable results.

Practical Considerations

First, financial conflicts of interest are inherent in any profession when the professional earns income from rendering a service. Second, conflicts come in many different forms, from legitimate payment for services rendered to investments in medical laboratories and facilities, drug company dinners and payment for attendance at meetings, payment for enrolling patients in clinical research trials, and consultation with companies.

Third, in considering how to manage conflicts, it is important to note that people are poor judges of their own potential conflicts. Individuals often cannot distinguish the various influences that guide their judgments, do not think of themselves as bad, and do not imagine that payment shapes their judgments. Physicians tend to be defensive about charges of conflicts of interest. In addition, conflicts tend to act insidiously, subtly changing practice patterns so that they then become what appear to be justifiable norms.

Fourth, rules—whether laws, regulations, or professional standards—to regulate conflicts of interest are based on two considerations: (1) the likelihood that payment or other secondary interests would create a conflict and (2) the magnitude of the potential harm if there is compromised judgment. Rules tend to be of three types: (1) disclosure of conflicts, (2) management of conflicts, and (3) outright prohibition. Federal law bans certain types of self-referral of physicians in the Medicare program. The American Medical Association and the Pharmaceutical Research and Manufacturers of America have established joint rules that permit physicians to accept gifts of minimal value but "refuse substantial gifts from drug companies, such as the costs of travel, lodging, or other personal expenses . . . for attending conferences or meetings."

Fifth, although there is much emphasis on disclosure of conflicts, which may be useful in publications, it is unclear whether this is a suitable safeguard in the clinical setting. Disclosure just may make patients worry more. Patients may have no context in which to place the disclosure or to evaluate the physician's clinical recommendation, and patients may have few other options in selecting a physician or getting care, especially in an acute situation.

Finally, some conflicts can be avoided by a physician's own action. Physicians can refuse to engage in personal investments in medical facilities or to accept gifts from pharmaceutical companies at relatively little personal cost. In other circumstances, the conflicts may be institutionalized, and minimizing them can occur only by changing the way organizations structure reimbursement incentives. Capitation encourages physicians to limit medical services, and its potentially adverse effects are likely to be managed by institutional rules rather than by personal decisions.

FUTURE DIRECTIONS

In the near future, as genetics moves from the research to the clinical setting, practicing physicians are likely to encounter issues surrounding genetic testing, counseling, and treatment (Chapter 38). The use of genetic tests without the extensive counseling so common in research studies would alter the nature of the bioethical issues. Because these tests have serious implications for the patient and others, scrupulous attention to informed consent must occur. The bioethical issues raised by genetic tests for somatic cell changes, such as tests that occur commonly in cancer diagnosis and risk stratification, are no different from the issues raised with the use of any laboratory or radiographic test.

In some cases, ethics consultation services may be of assistance in resolving bioethical dilemmas, although current data suggest that consultation services are used mainly for problems that arise in individual cases and are not used for more institutional or policy problems.

SUGGESTED READINGS

Berg JW, Applebaum PS, Lidz CW, et al: Informed Consent: Legal Theory and Clinical Practice, 2nd ed. New York, Oxford University Press, 2001. *Principles and guidelines for obtaining informed consent.*

Curlin FA, Lawrence RE, Chin MH, et al: Religion, conscience, and controversial clinical practices. N Engl J Med 2007;356:593–600. *Explores interface of physicians' beliefs and their recommendations for medical procedures.*

Education in Palliative and End-of-life Care. Available at www.epec.net.

Partnership for Caring. Available at www.partnershipforcaring.org. *Frequently updated websites.*

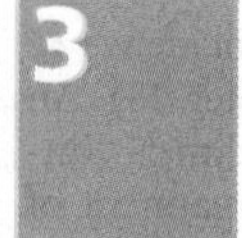

3 CARE OF DYING PATIENTS AND THEIR FAMILIES

J. Andrew Billings

What can a physician offer when a patient is dying? No procedure, no medicine, and no words can thwart death, and the physician is faced with a morass of difficult emotions in the patient, family, staff, and self. Death may be viewed as the physician's personal failure. The dying person may be an unwelcome reminder of the limitations of medicine, of the inevitability of loss and suffering in life, and of mortality. Few clinicians have been trained in providing good end-of-life care, and many feel uneasy, uncertain, or helpless about their role in these settings. Thus, physicians may tend to avoid terminally ill patients, thereby contributing to the isolation and loneliness regularly experienced by the dying.

Patients and families facing a terminal condition report hearing from clinicians, "There is nothing more we can do," a terrible dismissal that is never true. Physicians have a vital, active, and often satisfying role in the final stages of illness, ensuring safe passage for the patient and family and guiding them through an often complicated, frightening, unfamiliar, and difficult process. Good care for a person with an advanced, fatal condition means the physician, although recognizing the impossibility of cure, engages enthusiastically in the many opportunities to be helpful, primarily through preventing and treating physical, emotional, and spiritual suffering and by assisting in defining and achieving appropriate goals for the end of life. Such a transition from focusing primarily on cure and prolongation of life to attending primarily to comfort and quality of life—neither one nor the other exclusively, but whatever is the best for the patient—often proves difficult.

TALKING WITH DYING PATIENTS

How does one talk with a dying person? More important than anything that is said is the ability to listen carefully, to let patients express their understanding of the situation and their concerns and hopes. All the issues outlined in this chapter are likely to tumble out of the patient's mouth when the physician sits down with the dying person in a quiet, private setting; attends in a relaxed and unhurried manner; facilitates and encourages discussion and elaboration; tolerates occasional silences; pays close attention to verbal and nonverbal communication; discreetly encourages expression of emotion; provides empathic responses; tactfully probes difficult topics; and gently guides the discussion toward the common concerns of a person facing a fatal illness. Such a discussion often begins with the physician's asking some introductory questions (Table 3–1).

In the next sections of this chapter, four key issues in end-of-life care are addressed: pain and symptom control, shared decision making, psychosocial and spiritual support, and alternative sites of care.

Pain and Symptom Control: Is the Patient Comfortable?

A first step in good end-of-life care is meticulous attention to the management of a variety of disagreeable symptoms faced by the dying person—attending to "all that hurts," including physical distress, emotional suffering, functional limitations, and any other factors impairing quality of life. Comfort is a prerequisite for good coping. Assessment should precede treatment, although many symptoms in advanced disease do not require further diagnostic investigation to guide initial management, and sometimes the discomfort of such procedures outweighs their benefit. Treatment of pain in terminally ill patients does not need to await determination of the cause of pain (Chapter 28). Some symptoms are predictable and preventable (e.g., dyspnea from an enlarging cancer with lymphangitic spread), so the physician should anticipate and plan for alleviating such conditions before they cause serious distress, sometimes rehearsing next steps with the patient: "If the shortness of breath worsens, you can turn up the oxygen to 5 liters per minute and double the dosage of the morphine." In addition, patients and family members regularly harbor unrealistic fears about the future (e.g., of intractable pain or other severe suffering), so eliciting and addressing concerns about anticipated suffering can be as important as managing symptoms: "No, you don't have to worry about suffocating or choking with this sort of condition. We have excellent medication for breathlessness."

Numerous studies in a variety of settings show a high incidence of inadequately treated pain in many terminal illnesses (Chapter 28). An "epidemic of unnecessary pain" has been attributed to poor clinical education about pain management, a focus on diagnosis and treatment of underlying conditions rather than on patients' suffering, and inappropriate fears of opioids among laypersons and health professionals (Chapters 28 and 32). Relatively simple pharmacologic management can control about 75% of pain in advanced cancer, whereas more specialized interventions are successful for all but a small proportion of the remaining patients (see Fig. 28–5).

Disturbingly high rates of untreated nonpain symptoms, including dyspnea and anxiety, have been shown in adults and children with terminal illness (Table 3–2). Most patients report multiple disturbing symptoms. Depression (Chapter 420) and delirium (Chapter 26) often are underrecognized and inadequately managed.

Encouraging progress in the relief of many nonpain symptoms of advanced, terminal disease (e.g., nausea and vomiting) has occurred during the past few decades, and all of these symptoms can be alleviated although not necessarily eradicated. Common, underused interventions include opioids and benzodiazepines for dyspnea; antimuscarinics for excessive secretions and "death rattle"; glucocorticosteroids and progestational agents for anorexia; prokinetic agents for gastroparesis; glucocorticosteroids for fatigue, nausea, vomiting, pressure on nerves and other tissues with pain receptors, and obstruction of a viscus; neuroleptics (rather than benzodiazepines) for confusional states; oral naloxone for opioid-induced constipation; artificial saliva and good mouth care for xerostomia; and psychostimulants for depression, fatigue, and sedation. The physician, working closely with nurses and other allied health practitioners, should also become familiar with nonpharmacologic approaches to providing comfort (including careful skin and mouth care), adapting the home to the needs of a debilitated patient, and dealing with bowel and bladder management when a patient is bed bound.

Unnecessary and disagreeable treatments and diagnostic maneuvers that hold little promise of improving a patient's quality of life should be avoided. Many routines of hospital care, including venipunctures, endotracheal suction, noisy monitors, and vital sign monitoring or turning the patient in bed, especially when patients are trying to sleep, often can be discontinued, whereas heightened attention may be required for mouth comfort and regular bowel movements. The clinician may promote well-being and reduce suffering by choosing conservative management of selected conditions (e.g., managing partial small bowel obstruction without nasogastric suction); using simpler, less painful interventions in the place of complex, disagreeable approaches (e.g., sublingual administration of medications rather than starting an intravenous line); and forgoing inappropriate treatments (e.g., use of feeding tubes for advanced dementia).

Shared Decision Making: Is the Patient Well Informed, and Has an Individualized Plan of Care Been Developed?

What Is a "Good Death"?

There is no right way to die except for the way an informed patient desires, given the particular set of circumstances at hand. The patient's view of a "good death" is highly individualized and often different from the perspective held by physicians (Table 3–3). Psychosocial and spiritual goals regularly trump biomedical goals. Good end-of-life care requires eliciting a shared understanding of the patient's values and aspirations. Physicians tend to see their role as prolonging life at any reasonable cost, whereas patients may place higher priority on being at home, having meaningful time with their family, and avoiding unnecessary, expensive, or physically distressing prolongation of life. Family members, although hoping for a cure or prolonged survival, may recognize that communicating love and enjoying relationships are usually more important than having the patient live a few extra days, especially in discomfort.

Information Sharing and Hope

End-of-life care for a chronic, progressive illness inevitably places the physician in the role of repeatedly sharing bad news. No expertise in communication skills can make the conveying of distressing information painless for the patient and family or easy for the physician, but clinical guidelines promote a humane process (Table 3–4).

Patients cannot make good choices and intelligently set goals and participate in decisions unless they are reasonably well informed about their condition. Major gaps in terminally ill persons' understanding, especially about prognosis and alternatives to treatment, have been documented repeatedly. Although almost all dying patients report that they want general information about their medical condition, jargon-laden lectures about technical details are rarely appreciated. A few patients, reflecting their personal or cultural preferences (Chapter 4), do not want to be informed but instead favor delegating decisions to their family or physicians. Excess frankness or a presentation that is perceived as uncaring may be viewed as cruel or as taking away hope. In practice, patients and their health care professionals tend to collude in avoiding discussions of troubling topics or disagreeable news. Patients often seem to have unrealistically optimistic expectations about the value of treatments, regardless of what they have been told. The sharing of information and the making of decisions in the face of a life-threatening illness often are not totally rational processes, and neither the provision of better prognostic estimates

TABLE 3–1 SUGGESTED QUESTIONS FOR THE CLINICAL INTERVIEW WITH PATIENTS FACING THE END OF LIFE

Tell me the story of your illness. [the patient's perspective]

Tell me how you first found out about your illness. [hearing bad news]
- How were you told?
- What was it like? How did you feel then?

What is your understanding now about the illness? [patient's understanding or explanatory model]
- What have you been told? What do the doctors say? Your family?
- How did it begin? What caused it? Why did it happen?
- How has it been treated?
- What is happening with the illness now? What is likely to happen?
- What are your expectations and concerns about the future?

What do you want to be told about your illness? [shared decision making and information preferences]
- Part of my job is to assure that you have as much information as you wish about your health and that all your questions are answered in understandable terms. But people vary enormously in how much they want to know about their medical condition and their options for treatment—some want to hear as many of the details as possible, while others prefer to leave these matters to the doctors or their family.
- How much do you want to be told?
- If there is bad news, how do you want to be informed?
- How do you want us to communicate about these matters with your family?

How has the illness affected you? [patient's coping]
- What has it been like for you?
- How has it affected you physically?
  - Have you had pain?
  - Other disagreeable physical problems?
- How are you doing emotionally?
  - Have you been upset?
    - Nervous? Frightened? Worried?
    - Angry? Irritable?
    - Sad or depressed?
  - What has been most difficult about the illness?
  - What are your main worries now?
- Has there been any good side to what has happened?

How has your family (or close friends) been affected? [family's coping]
- What have you discussed with them?

How have you been helped? [supports]
- What gives you strength in facing these problems?
- How have you been helped by family and friends?
  - What do they say or do?
  - How are they not helpful or disappointing?
- How have you been helped by doctors and nurses?
  - Other health care workers?
  - How are they not helpful or disappointing?

Have there been other tough times you have had to face? [previous coping]
- Have there been other serious illnesses or losses?
- What was it like for you then?
- How did you manage? What helped?

Do you have a religious or spiritual practice or set of beliefs? [existential and spiritual concerns]
- Were you brought up in a religious tradition? Do you continue in this tradition? Are you connected to a minister (priest, rabbi)? To a church or congregation?
- How have your religious background and current religious or spiritual beliefs affected your experience of this illness?
- How have you made sense of this serious illness?
- How has your faith been important to you?
- Do you pray? What about? To whom?
- Do you believe in a life after death?

Have you been thinking about dying? [addressing death and dying]
- What kinds of thoughts have you had? What worries?
- Have you made plans because of it?

From Billings JA, Block SD: Program in palliative care education and practice, 2002. Available at http://www.hms.harvard.edu/cdi/pallcare/.

nor the encouragement to share information has been shown to affect outcomes. How much information a terminally ill patient wants to know or is able to appreciate about his or her medical condition varies enormously from person to person and from moment to moment for each individual. Requests for information may be requests for reassurance—pleas for offering hope. Especially when bad news is involved, patients may deal with matters with deep ambivalence or denial—at one moment, eager to absorb new information, and at a later moment, conducting themselves as if the conversation never occurred. Family members may behave similarly or differ from the patient in terms of preferences for information or ability to grasp distressing facts. The physician should not use the patient's reluctance to hear bad news as an excuse for avoiding difficult discussions.

Discussions about prognosis may be particularly treacherous because physicians usually can offer only an educated guess about the future. Nevertheless, laypersons may ascribe great certainty to the physician's

TABLE 3–2 COMMON SYMPTOMS IN SERIOUSLY ILL HOSPITALIZED PATIENTS (PERCENTAGE OF TOTAL PATIENTS)

	At Any Time	Severe and Frequent*
Pain	51%	23%
Dyspnea	49%	23%
Anxiety	47%	16%
Depression	45%	14%
Nausea	34%	6%

*Moderately or extremely severe symptoms occurring half to all the time.
After Desbiens NA, Mueller-Rizner N, Connors AF Jr, et al, for the SUPPORT Investigators: The symptom burden of seriously ill hospitalized patients. J Pain Symptom Manage 1999;17:248–255.

TABLE 3–3 PATIENTS' PERSPECTIVE ON A "GOOD DEATH"

Control pain and other symptoms
Avoid inappropriate prolongation of dying when life is no longer enjoyable
Relieve burden on the family
Achieve a sense of control
Strengthen relationships with loved ones

After Singer PA, Martin DK, Kelner M: Quality end-of-life care: Patients' perspective. JAMA 1999;218:163–168.

TABLE 3–4 SHARING BAD NEWS

Find an appropriate setting and adequate time. Ensure comfort, privacy, quiet, and absence of interruptions.

Prepare yourself. Rehearse key points. Monitor your personal reactions.

Consider involving the family (especially key decision makers) and other health professionals. Ask the patient who should be present. In the hospital, include the primary nurse. Unless the conversation occurs in the context of a well-established relationship, *begin by "aligning."* What does the patient and family know? What do they want to know? Let them ask questions and absorb information at their own pace. Understand their perspective and develop trust.

Listen. Attending to the patient is often more important than what you say. Listen for and respond to concerns and emotions. Tolerate silence. Encourage questions. Clarify. What is "hope" for this patient?

Be brief and simple, giving the key message in a few sentences. Give plain, clear explanations in jargon-free language. Beware of euphemisms. Repeat key points and write them down.

Set realistic goals for the initial discussion, avoiding information overload. Conveying bad news is a process, not an event. Tailor the information to the listener. Grade exposure to upsetting material. Keep in mind key objectives: What does the patient really need to know?

Be honest and exert a firm pressure for candor. Avoid false reassurance and false optimism but also excess bluntness. Respect cultural and personal preferences about sharing information. Avoid false certainty or precision, but give patients needed prognostic information.

Respond to affect. Actively elicit and encourage emotional reactions. Be supportive. Empathize. Acknowledge difficulty. Convey your caring. Identify current supports and offer additional resources.

Offer next steps that convey continued attention and, if reasonable, helpfulness (e.g., referral for treatment). Plan follow-up for sharing information, clarification, and support. Guarantee availability and continued attention.

Document the sharing of information, and communicate about it to the health care team.

estimates: "The doctor says he only has 3 months to live." Patients are entitled to a physician's best guesses, but speculations should be phrased in terms that reflect uncertainty and a wide range of possibilities: "The course of this cancer can be quite unpredictable, and physicians don't have a crystal ball. I think you should be aware of the possibility that your health may deteriorate quickly, and you should plan accordingly. We probably are dealing with a few months, while hoping that the disease stabilizes and allows us even longer. As time goes on, the course may become clearer, and if you wish, I might be able to be a little more precise about what we are facing."

The physician's duty is neither to protect the patient from bad news nor to confront denial head on but rather to tailor the sharing of information to a particular person at a particular time, guided by the patient's questions and reactions to disturbing information. The physician should convey realistic hopes while applying a firm but gentle pressure toward full appreciation of current facts. Honesty is a requisite for a relationship of trust, but truth can be shaded to meet the patient's needs of the moment. The challenge for most clinicians is turning conversations toward a recognition that death is likely without leaving the patient and family feeling hopeless or abandoned: "I see how you are striving to overcome this illness and to focus on the bright side of things, but I wonder if part of you doesn't also sometimes think about matters not working out so well?" The physician can help change the focus from exclusively curative or life-prolonging interventions to making the best of the remaining time while striving to reassure the patient and family that everything reasonable will be done, that comfort is a paramount concern, and that they will not be neglected. When a patient's expectations for cure or prolonged survival are unrealistic, the physician might reinforce more realistic optimism on such matters as hopes for acceptable physical well-being and level of function, enjoying the love of one's family or friends, and developing a sense of completing a meaningful life. A shift toward comfort as the goal of care does not mean helplessness, hopelessness, or loss of the physician's commitment to making the best of the situation. The physician's acceptance of the inevitability of death, combined with expectations for and enthusiastic engagement in achieving the best possible dying and death, can lead the patient and family toward better coping and can support their maintenance of hope.

Difficult Decisions

A common observation since the middle of the 20th century has been that advances in medical science lead to difficult new clinical and ethical decisions, such as whether to initiate cardiopulmonary resuscitation (CPR) or to withdraw ventilatory support in situations in which these technologic interventions seem to prolong or contribute to suffering without offering clear benefit (Chapter 103). Such decisions constitute some of the most difficult judgments in medical practice and can only become more frequent and complex in the future as the ability to forestall death improves. Interventions that at one time were considered routine and even morally required, such as the provision of intravenous fluids for patients unable to drink on their own, are increasingly seen as matters of choice. Even now, few patients with one of the chronic fatal illnesses that cause most deaths in the United States can die without some judgments being made about whether to prolong dying by providing cardiopulmonary support, hospitalization, intensive care, blood products, antibiotics, pressors, nutritional support, or fluids. The nostalgic notion of a "natural death," a death not involving difficult decisions about the use of technology or at least free of modern medical interventions, is limited to sudden deaths and patients who do not have access to good medical care. About a quarter of deaths now occur in intensive care units, and in one study of intensive care unit deaths, 90% involved the withholding and withdrawal of life support (Chapter 103). Death has been "medicalized."

Complicating matters further, studies of decision making in intensive care units reveal conflicts between staff and family in half of cases and among family members about a quarter of the time, with such conflicts centering primarily on decisions to limit life-sustaining treatment. Clinicians express high rates of dissatisfaction about burdensome treatments in end-of-life care. A frequently discussed intervention in this setting is CPR (Chapters 2 and 103). Without guidance from health care professionals, patients and families often have unrealistic notions of the utility of CPR and make ill-informed decisions to initiate it. Although CPR can be a life-saving measure in some settings, in most terminally ill patients, it is extremely unlikely to result in return of satisfactory cardiopulmonary function, survival to discharge from the hospital, or ability to live outside of an institution.

Advance Care Planning

Many terminally ill patients, especially patients hospitalized or facing the last few days of life, cannot participate meaningfully in health care decisions owing to confusion or other barriers to understanding and communication. In anticipation of difficult decisions when decisional capacity is lacking, patients have been encouraged to designate health care proxies and to create advance care planning documents, typified by the use of living wills (Chapter 2). These documents are meant to protect patients against unwanted treatments, and the courts, at times, have considered them essential if life-sustaining treatments are to be withheld or withdrawn. Discussions of such documents with health professionals and family members generally provoke important conversations about end-of-life care decisions and encourage patients to name a substitute decision maker, proxy, or surrogate who, should the patient become incapacitated, ideally can represent the patient's wishes and identify treatment preferences in specific situations.

The utility of a health care proxy seems incontrovertible. Advance care directives are prepared infrequently by patients, however, and rarely are documented in accessible medical records, even on hospital admission for a serious illness. Earlier decisions made by patients in a time of relative well-being may not reflect their true wishes in a later situation when they are faced by a serious illness, so documents must be reviewed regularly. When advance care directives, including do not resuscitate orders, are obtained, patients frequently have serious misunderstandings. Finally, physicians often do not understand or follow such directives. In one large multi-institutional study, physicians did no better than chance in identifying their seriously ill hospitalized patients' wishes to forgo CPR, and such wishes, even when known, rarely were respected when the physician believed that another course was appropriate. [1]

Psychosocial and Spiritual Support of the Patient and Family

Emotional, social, economic, and spiritual distresses among patients and their families near the end of life are even more complex phenomena than physical suffering. They challenge the clinician's ability to provide understanding, guidance, and support.

Emotional Suffering

Patients commonly face issues such as isolation and loneliness, fear and anxiety, feeling like a burden on loved ones, a heightened sense of vulnerability and loss of control, adaptation to disfigurement or disability, diminished self-esteem associated with inability to perform normal roles, worries about the future of loved ones, unrecognized or untreated depression, confusional states, wishes for a hastened death, economic pressures, and existential or spiritual predicaments. Despite strongly held beliefs about the nature of good psychosocial care, surprisingly little research has been conducted, and few interventions have been examined systematically. In general, successful psychosocial interventions appear to promote quality of life without influencing survival. [2] Social connectedness and a related concept—maintaining a sense of a valuable self despite the alterations in functioning attendant to the illness—have emerged as important factors in how patients cope with dying. For many families, a terminal illness allows greater cohesion, support, and expressions of affection; for others, it accentuates tensions and promotes distancing.

Dying patients experience considerable isolation, and they often harbor concerns that are not shared with family members. An attentive physician or other member of the health care team can counter this loneliness and provide valued support through careful listening and empathy. Key interventions include combating psychological isolation and identifying important goals by offering opportunities for open communication about all aspects of the illness. Common clinical tasks include conveying nonabandonment, facilitating life review, identifying and addressing fears and worries, providing appropriate reassurance, recognizing and treating depression and delirium (both of which cause significant, preventable morbidity), helping adults attend to the special needs of younger children affected by the illness, modeling equanimity and honesty in the face of frightening events, promoting reconciliation and forgiveness, and attending to the possibilities of personal growth in the face of dying. Consultation with a mental health clinician should be considered for selected patients, especially when there is a history of psychiatric illness or dysfunctional relationships, when there is evidence of major psychosocial dysfunction, or when patients simply seek more time and expertise in exploring their coping with the crisis of dying.

Spirituality

For patients and families facing the crisis of dying, existential or spiritual concerns are inevitable. Spirituality can provide a source of comfort and support—or provoke further distress. Taking a spiritual history allows clinicians to understand patients more fully, and most patients indicate an interest in sharing this important aspect of their lives with clinicians. The physician's role is not to answer profound questions about the meaning of life or to provide premature reassurance but rather to understand how spirituality influences the patient's coping and to help the dying person explore these issues and find supportive resources (e.g., the hospital chaplain).

Family Coping and the Burden of Care

Families and close friends of the person with a terminal illness suffer as surely as the patient does, and any rational health care system should address this suffering. Often neglected are the special needs for age-appropriate support for young children. Families also are regularly burdened with the physical care of the patient. Families may receive assistance from a variety of relatives, friends, formal caregivers, and volunteers, but the social and financial burden of a terminal illness—needing to quit work or to take off significant time, losing a major source of income, or using up savings—is often disastrous for families and underappreciated by health care professionals. Simply listening empathically to the family about their struggles is helpful, but arranging for a variety of concrete services and for more formal counseling should also be considered.

Bereavement

Bereavement care is a neglected field of medicine. Family grief may be associated with serious deterioration in psychological and social function and increased rates of substance abuse as well as premature death. At the same time, most bereaved persons adjust to loss during months and years without any formal help, albeit usually after considerable suffering.

The physician has an important role in assessing and assisting in bereavement through sensitive attention to the family before and at the time of death; attending funeral rituals; writing a letter of condolence; following up with the family; being available for later questions about the illness, the death, and the genetic basis of disease; and providing appropriate information and referral regarding bereavement. Individual counseling and support groups may improve outcomes for family and friends who are at high risk of complicated grief. Many other survivors benefit from opportunities to understand and to express their distress through the assistance of family, friends, clergy, other professional counselors, and support groups.

Alternatives to the Acute Care Hospital: Where Does the Patient Prefer to Receive Care?

An important theme in the hospice approach to death is that patients and families are generally happier when they are cared for in the home. In the United States, where about half of deaths occur in hospitals, the hospice movement has contributed to renewed attention to managing a terminal illness in the home when appropriate resources allow patients to feel well cared for and safe.

For about a quarter of patients in the United States, the site of death is a nursing home. High levels of pain and other symptoms, low support, excess use of tube feeding, and excess hospitalization have been shown in this setting, and access to palliative care is limited.

PALLIATIVE CARE AND HOSPICE

State-of-the-art end-of-life care and "best supportive care" are synonymous with *palliative care,* a term describing comprehensive (physical, psychosocial, and spiritual), interdisciplinary services that focus on alleviating suffering and promoting quality of life for patients and their families facing a life-threatening or terminal illness. The term *palliative* literally means "to cloak" and can be used derisively to describe measures that merely cover up a problem, but the term has become widely accepted as a description of approaches to providing comfort for dying persons without necessarily modifying the underlying medical condition (e.g., alleviating pain or dyspnea and improving quality of life without reducing the burden of tumor or enhancing cardiac function).

Palliative care will soon become a new specialty under the American Board of Internal Medicine. Palliative care programs, which are proliferating rapidly in the United States, typically include inpatient consultation, dedicated inpatient units, ambulatory care, and home care with or without hospice. Palliative care services may be provided at the earliest signs of a serious or complex illness, even in the intensive care unit, collaborating with general medical and specialty clinicians to offer care that concurrently optimizes survival as well as quality of life. These services not only assist the patient and family directly but also educate and support other involved clinicians.

Many aspects of palliative care, as with any specialty, are relevant to the general practice of medicine and to all clinicians who tend to dying persons. Palliative care has a role in the earliest phases of a life-threatening illness but assumes a more prominent or even dominant role in the final 3 to 6 months of common terminal conditions: advanced cancer, heart and lung failure, end-stage liver and renal disease, acquired immunodeficiency syndrome, and life-limiting neurologic diseases.

Hospice programs offer a widely recognized form of palliative care in the United States. In the United States, hospice refers to a specific, government-regulated form of end-of-life care, available under Medicare since 1982 but subsequently adopted by Medicaid and many other third-party insurers. Hospice care typically is given at home or in a nursing home (less commonly in an acute care hospital or specialized acute care unit) and is provided by an interdisciplinary team, which usually includes a physician, nurse, social worker, chaplain, volunteers, bereavement coordinator, and home health aides, all of whom collaborate with the primary care physician, patient, and family. Bereavement services are offered to the family for a year after the death.

Hospice regulations in the United States require that a patient agree to forgo measures with curative intent and to focus on comfort. Although hospice programs vary in their policies, many "aggressive," expensive interventions, such as surgery, radiation therapy, total parenteral nutrition, and transfusions, tend to be excluded. To many patients and families, hospice seems to signify "giving up," rather than being viewed as a model of compassionate care and of making the best of a situation with limited options. Also, to be eligible for a Medicare-certified hospice program, the primary physician must certify that the patient is likely to die within 6 months if the illness runs its usual course. No penalties exist, however, for referring a patient too early to hospice, and physicians generally use hospice care much later in the course of an illness than is appropriate.

A less regularly available option under hospice is palliative care in inpatient units, which tend to be furnished in a homelike fashion. They are quieter than the usual noisy hospital ward and are decorated with personally important objects from each patient; they typically lack, minimize, or obscure hospital paraphernalia. Patients are encouraged to wear their own clothes, and pets are allowed. Families (including children) have unlimited visiting privileges, use on-site cooking facilities or bring food, and are welcomed to stay overnight.

STRAINS AND REWARDS IN END-OF-LIFE CARE

No discussion of palliative care would be complete without touching on the importance of the inner life of clinicians and their personal relationships with the patient and family. Even with the best informed and most proactive consumers of health care, clinicians must shepherd the patient and family through an often terrifying, unfamiliar trajectory and attempt to provide safe passage, not only by applying technical skills to prevent and to reduce suffering but also by a reassuring presence—an intimate, individualized relationship that communicates concern, connectedness, equanimity in the face of death, realistic hope, nonabandonment, and an eagerness to address a broad range of physical, psychosocial, and spiritual concerns. Palliative care should involve a team of skilled professionals who can provide the patient and family with a variety of opportunities for supportive interactions.

Seriously ill and dying persons may evoke strong emotional reactions in clinicians, thrusting them into often intense, intimate relationships at a major crisis point in the lives of patients and their families. Clinicians may report a wearying sense of grief and depletion over recurrent losses as well as an exhilarating sense of privilege in witnessing how some patients and families cope with extraordinary dignity, acceptance, and love.

Staff support programs, which are routine aspects of most palliative care services, can help all clinicians develop and maintain a working environment that attends to emotional reactions, addresses staff conflict, and bolsters a personal capacity to deal with multiple losses without becoming hardened to suffering. The camaraderie and support that can accompany interdisciplinary teamwork is an important antidote to burnout of clinicians.

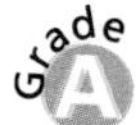

1. SUPPORT Principal Investigators: A controlled trial to improve care for seriously ill hospitalized patients. The study to understand prognoses and preferences for outcomes and risks of treatments (SUPPORT). JAMA 1995;274:1591–1598.
2. Goodwin PJ, Leszca M, Ennis M, et al: The effect of group psychosocial support on survival in metastatic breast cancer. N Engl J Med 2001;345:1719–1726.

SUGGESTED READINGS

Back AL, Arnold RM, Quill TE: Hope for the best, and prepare for the worst. Ann Intern Med 2003;138:439–443. *A practical approach to end-of-life care.*

Doyle D, Hanks GWC, Cherny NI, Calman K: Oxford Textbook of Palliative Medicine, 3rd ed. New York, Oxford Medical Publications, 2004. *An outstanding clinical resource that offers a comprehensive review of the scientific basis of palliative care.*

Ellershaw J, Ward C: Care of the dying patient: The last hours or days of life. BMJ 2003;326:30–34. *An overview of end-of-life care and of barriers to good care, focusing on the difficulties of "diagnosing dying" and its consequences.*

End of Life/Palliative Education Resource Center. Available at www.eperc.mcw.edu/. *Peer-reviewed instructional and evaluation materials on end-of-life care, core resources for educators, and opportunities for training and funding.*

Hanson LC, Ersek M: Meeting palliative care needs in post-acute care settings: "To help them live until they die." JAMA 2006;295:681–686. *A case-based review.*

National Consensus Project for Quality Palliative Care: Clinical Practice Guidelines for Quality Palliative Care, 2004. Available at www.nationalconsensusproject.org.

Truog RD, Cist AFM, Brackett SE, et al: Recommendations for end-of-life care in the intensive care unit: The Ethics Committee of the Society of Critical Care Medicine. Crit Care Med 2001;29:2332–2348. *Detailed guidelines on end-of-life care in the intensive care unit, including discontinuation of life supports.*

Wennberg J, Fisher E, Stukel TA, et al: Use of hospitals, physician visits, and hospice care during last six months of life among cohorts loyal to highly respected hospitals in the United States. BMJ 2004;328:607–611. *A contribution from the Dartmouth Atlas project reveals striking variations in the use of health care services near the end of life.*

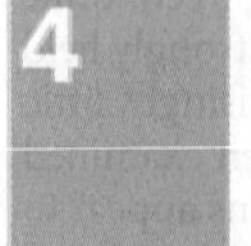

CULTURAL CONTEXT OF MEDICINE

Victoria M. Taylor

The 2000 United States Census counted more than 36 million Americans of African descent (13% of the population), nearly 12 million Asians (4% of the population), more than 4 million American Indians and Alaska Natives, and almost 1 million Native Hawaiians and other Pacific Islanders. In addition, more than 35 million Americans were of Hispanic or Latino descent (13% of the population). More than one tenth (11%) of the total population, 69% of Asians, and 40% of Latinos were foreign born. Residents of the United States now speak more than 300 languages, and 47 million speak a language other than English at home. In 2000, two fifths of Asians (40%) and Hispanics (41%) had limited English proficiency (i.e., did not speak English well or fluently), and the proportions were much higher among some Asian subgroups (Fig. 4–1).

During the last two decades, a large body of literature has documented significant disparities in health status, some of which are socioeconomic (Chapter 5) but many of which are not. Black men have a substantially higher age-adjusted prostate cancer incidence rate than do white men (272 per 100,000 versus 164 per 100,000). Mexican Americans and American Indians are more than twice as likely as non-Latino whites of a similar age to have diabetes. Compared with the general population, chronic hepatitis B infection is 25 to 75 times more common among Samoans and among immigrants from Cambodia, Laos, and Vietnam. Finally, numerous studies have documented high rates of suicidal behavior among gays and lesbians compared with heterosexuals. A major goal of Healthy People 2010 is to eliminate health differences among population subgroups for preventable and treatable conditions such as cancer, cardiovascular disease, diabetes, human immunodeficiency virus infection, and acquired immunodeficiency syndrome, among others.

Culture can be defined as a shared system of values, beliefs, and patterns of behavior, and it is not simply defined by race and ethnicity. Culture can also be shaped by factors such as country and region of origin, acculturation, language, religion, and sexual orientation. For instance, the black population of the northeastern United States includes individuals who moved from southern states decades ago as well as recent immigrants from Ethiopia. As the United States population becomes increasingly diverse and as pronounced differences in health status continue to be documented, consideration of the cultural context of medicine is becoming a national priority.

DISPARITIES IN HEALTH CARE ACCESS AND QUALITY

Components of health care access include the ability to get into the health care system as well as to obtain appropriate care once in the system. The availability of health care providers who meet an individual patient's needs is another key component of access to care. Quality care is based on scientific evidence (i.e., is effective), avoids injury to the patient (i.e., is safe), minimizes harmful delays (i.e., is timely), is responsive to the individual patient's needs (i.e., is patient centered), does not vary because of personal characteristics (i.e., is equitable), and avoids waste (i.e., is efficient) (Chapter 11).

Access to Health Care

Racial and ethnic minority groups, particularly Latinos, are disproportionally represented among those with health care access problems. The proportions of Latinos who lack health insurance and have no regular source of medical care are more than twice the proportions among non-Latino whites (Fig. 4–2). Latinos are significantly more likely to report problems in obtaining health care for illness or injury as well as referrals for specialist care than are non-Latino whites, even after differences in education, income, and insurance coverage are taken into account. Black heterosexual women have significantly higher levels of health insurance coverage than do black lesbian or bisexual women.

The Commonwealth Fund 2001 Health Care Quality Survey collected information on a cross section of adults representing people from diverse backgrounds. A series of questions were used to assess each respondent's interactions with the physician during his or her last office visit. Communication between patients and physicians was more of a problem among members of racial and ethnic minority groups than among whites (Table 4–1). In this survey, 33% of Latinos, 27% of Asians, 23% of blacks, and 16% of whites reported one or more of the following problems with communication: the doctor did not listen to everything they said, they did not fully understand the doctor, or they had questions that they did not ask during the visit. In addition, Latinos who spoke Spanish as their primary language (43%) were more likely to have one or more communication problems than were those who spoke English as their primary language (26%).

Blacks (23%) and Latinos (26%) are far less likely than whites (82%) to have regular physicians of their own race and ethnicity. Research has shown that racial concordance between physicians and patients can improve the processes and outcomes of care. For instance, patients in race-concordant relationships with their physician rate his or her decision-making style significantly more participatory and inclusive than do

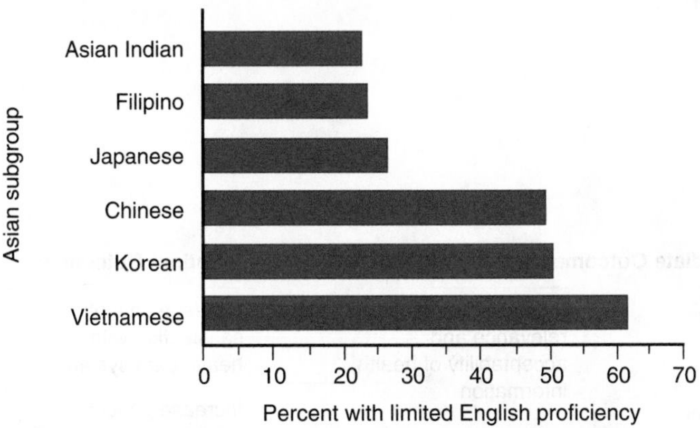

FIGURE 4–1 • Limited English proficiency among selected Asian subgroups: United States—2000. (U.S. Department of Commerce: We the People: Asians in the United States. Washington, DC, U.S. Department of Commerce, 2004.)

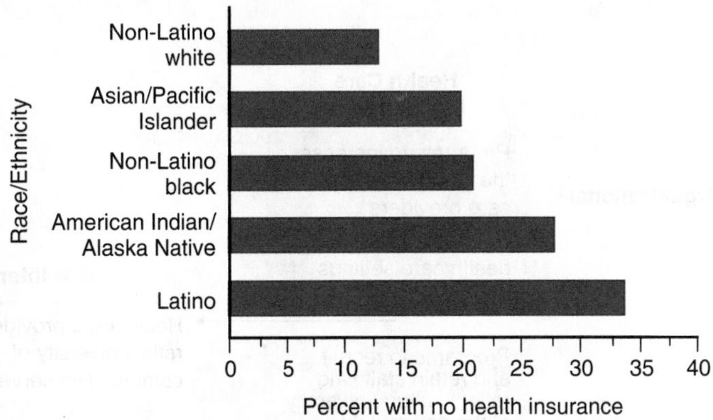

FIGURE 4–2 • Health insurance coverage by race/ethnicity: United States—2003. (Kaiser Commission on Medicaid and the Uninsured: The Uninsured: A Primer—Key Facts About Americans Without Health Insurance. Washington, DC, The Henry J. Kaiser Family Foundation, 2004.)

TABLE 4–1 PATIENT-PHYSICIAN INTERACTIONS DURING LAST VISIT BY RACE/ETHNICITY—2001

Patient Variable	White (%)	Black (%)	Asian (%)	Latino (%)
Doctor listened to everything they said	68	68	49	57
Understood everything doctor said	69	61	48	56
Had questions which they did not ask	10	13	14	19
Great deal of confidence in doctor	72	69	54	57
Treated with a great deal of dignity and respect	77	75	59	76
Involved in health care decisions as much as they wanted	78	73	56	65
Doctor spent as much time as they wanted	72	70	50	57

From Collins KS, Hughes DL, Doty MM, et al: Diverse Communities, Common Concerns: Assessing Health Care Quality for Minority Americans. New York, The Commonwealth Fund, 2002.

patients in race-discordant relationships. Furthermore, race-concordant office visits last significantly longer than do race-discordant visits.

Quality of Health Care

National surveys confirm population-level disparities in the quality of both preventive care and the management of chronic disease. Asian and American Indian/Alaska Native women are less likely to receive interval screening for breast cancer (Chapter 208) and cervical cancer (Chapter 209) than are women of other racial groups (Table 4–2). Compared with white diabetic adults, black and Latino adults with diabetes are more than 30% less likely to receive recommended preventive and screening services (Chapter 247) and are still less likely to receive them after adjustment for insurance coverage.

TABLE 4–2 BREAST AND CERVICAL CANCER SCREENING RATES BY RACE/ETHNICITY AND IMMIGRATION: UNITED STATES—2000

Characteristic	Mammogram within the Past 2 Years* (%)	Pap Test within the Past 3 Years† (%)
Race/ethnicity		
Non-Latino white	72	84
Non-Latino black	68	86
Latino	63	78
American Indian/ Alaska Native	52	78
Asian	57	68
Immigration		
Born in the United States	72	84
In the United States 10 years or more	65	79
In the United States less than 10 years	41	59

*Women aged 40 and older.
†Women aged 18 and older with uteri.
From American Cancer Society: Cancer Prevention and Early Detection Facts and Figures. Atlanta, American Cancer Society, 2004.

In a recent Institute of Medicine report, disparities were found in such specific clinical situations as the prescription of analgesia for pain control (blacks receive less pain medication than whites do for extremity fractures), the surgical treatment of cancer (blacks are less likely than whites to receive potentially curative surgery for stage I or stage II non–small cell lung cancer), and the management of end-stage renal disease (blacks are less likely to be entered on the transplant list than are whites). Moreover, disparities in the quality of care were consistently found even when variations in such factors as insurance status, income, age, and comorbid conditions were taken into account.

Disparities in health care quality exist even in systems that are generally believed to provide equal access. For example, in Veterans Health Administration facilities, black patients who were ideal candidates to receive thrombolytic therapy (Chapter 72) on arrival were less likely to receive it than comparable white patients. Black patients were also significantly less likely to have coronary artery bypass graft surgery during their index hospitalization or within 90 days after a myocardial infarction even after adjustment for clinical characteristics and differences in patients' preferences. Similarly, in Medicare-managed care plans, black patients were less likely than white patients to receive diabetic retinal examination, post-infarction β-blockers, and post-hospitalization follow-up for mental illness after adjustment for clinical characteristics and for clustering within health plans.

CULTURAL COMPETENCE IN HEALTH CARE

Health disparities can be reduced or perhaps even eliminated by maintaining culturally competent health care systems. Cultural competence may be defined as a set of congruent attitudes, behaviors, and policies that come together both among professionals and within systems to enable effective work in cross-cultural situations (Fig. 4–3). Ongoing efforts to improve cultural competence in the United States health care system target organizational, structural, and clinical barriers. These initiatives aim to close gaps in health status, to decrease differences in the quality of care, to enhance patients' satisfaction, and to increase patients' trust.

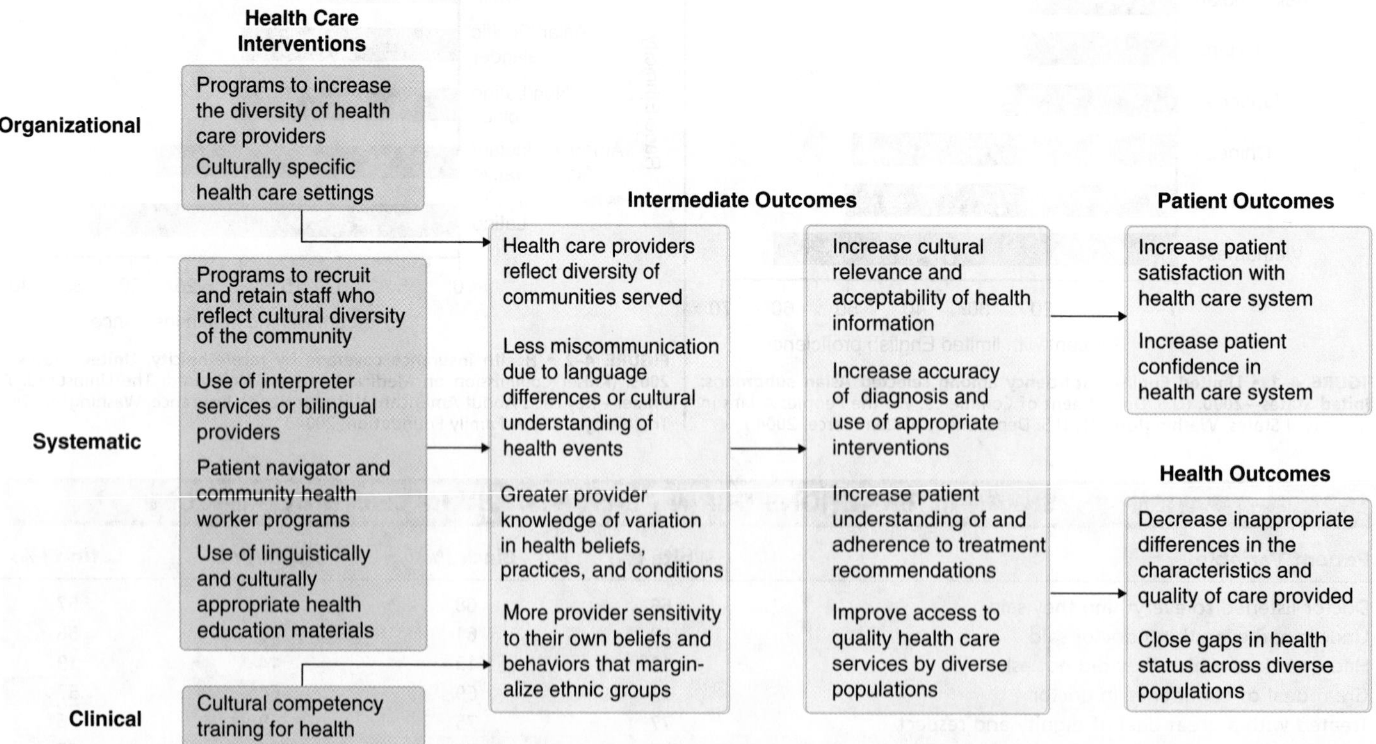

FIGURE 4–3 • Analytic framework for evaluating the effectiveness of health care interventions to increase cultural competence. (From Anderson LM, Scrimshaw SC, Fullilove MT, et al; Task Force on Community Preventive Services: Culturally competent healthcare systems: A systemic review. Am J Prev Med 2003;24 [Suppl]:68–79.)

Organizational Barriers and Interventions

Physicians of racial and ethnic minorities are more likely than their white colleagues to work in medically underserved communities. Moreover, they have a better understanding of barriers to health care (such as office hours that do not match community work patterns, bureaucratic intake processes that create fear of deportation among the undocumented, and long waiting times to get an appointment and, after arrival, to keep an appointment). Finally, minority physicians bring a nuanced awareness of the needs of diverse groups of patients and share it through the critical avenues of role-modeling and teaching. However, less than 15% of students enrolled in the 125 United States medical schools are black, American Indian/Alaska Native, or Latino. In addition, only 7% of medical school clinical faculty are members of one of these underrepresented minority groups.

The majority (approximately two thirds) of patients who receive care at federally funded community health centers in medically underserved areas are members of racial and ethnic minority groups. The community health center model has proved effective not only in increasing access to care but also in improving continuity of care and health outcomes. For example, one study found that medically underserved communities with federally qualifying community health centers had 5.8 fewer preventable hospitalizations per 1000 population over 3 years than did similar communities without health centers. Consequently, the Federal Health Center Growth Initiative, which aims to increase the capacity of community health centers by more than 50%, is likely to help reduce health disparities.

Structural Barriers and Interventions

Title VI of the Civil Rights Act protects against discrimination based on national origin by obligating medical care providers to offer interpreter services so that patients whose proficiency in English is limited can have access to medical services equal to that of English speakers. In addition, the Department of Health and Human Services has created standards on culturally and linguistically appropriate services to guide providers. However, interpreter services often remain ad hoc, with family members and untrained nonclinical employees acting as interpreters. Use of ad hoc services has potentially negative clinical consequences, including breach of the patient's confidentiality and inaccurate communication. One major obstacle to the implementation of professional interpreter programs is a lack of reimbursement; Medicare and most private insurers do not pay for interpretation and related services (such as translation or telephone language lines), and only a few states currently pay for interpretation under Medicaid.

Accumulating evidence suggests that trained professional interpreters and bilingual providers can have a positive impact on the satisfaction of patients and quality of care among individuals with limited English proficiency. For example, in a health maintenance organization, the introduction of professional interpreter services for Portuguese- and Spanish-speaking patients increased their use of recommended preventive services, office visits, and number of prescriptions written and filled.

Assistance with "navigation" represents one promising model to enable racial and ethnic minority patients to move through the health system effectively and to be actively involved in decision making about their medical care. Navigator programs rely on personal guides to shepherd disadvantaged patients with chronic diseases into standard care. Guides help patients and their families navigate the treatment process, steering them around obstacles that may limit their access to quality care. For example, guides (who may be nurses, social workers, or volunteers who are familiar with the health care system) help patients choose doctors and assess treatment options. A survey of more than 50 existing navigator programs for cancer patients in the United States found wide variations in the training of navigators, the services they provided, and the mixture of professional and lay navigators used. Most programs assessed needs and educated patients as well as assisted with transportation, appointment scheduling, and referrals. In addition, some programs developed action plans and coordinated interpretation services.

Community health workers are increasingly being used in attempts to close the gap in health care among various racial and ethnic minority populations. In general, community health workers live locally and share the language and culture of the population of patients served. Lay community health workers have several core functions; they provide cultural mediation between communities and the health care system, provide culturally appropriate and accessible health education and information, help people obtain the medical services they need, provide informal counseling and social support, and advocate for individuals within the health care system. The largest system formally to use the skills of community health workers is the Indian Health Service, which currently has about 1400 community health representatives who work with tribally managed or Indian Health Service programs in more than 550 American Indian/Alaska Native nations.

Evidence for the effectiveness of community health workers is provided by the breast and cervical cancer screening literature. For example, a randomized trial showed that a community health worker intervention (including a home visit as well as use of a video and print materials) was the best way to increase appropriate utilization of Pap smears among women of Chinese descent; a direct mail intervention (including a video and print materials) also was better than no intervention, but it was not nearly as good as the community health worker intervention. 1

Clinical Barriers and Interventions

Patients who are members of racial and ethnic minority groups often have an understanding of health and disease (i.e., explanatory model) that differs from that of the general population. For example, many Vietnamese people believe that disease is caused by an imbalance of the humoral forces of yin and yang. When ill, they commonly use Chinese herbal medicine as well as indigenous folk practices known as Southern medicine in an effort to restore the balance of humoral forces. In addition, Vietnamese patients may think that Western medicine is too strong and will upset the internal balance. Consequently, a hypertensive patient, for example, may use Chinese herbal medicines (Chapter 36) instead of prescribed antihypertensive medication. Alternatively, the patient may take a lower dose of medication than prescribed by his or her physician.

Standards for training in cultural diversity recently have become part of medical school curricula. Cultural competency training generally includes some balance of cross-cultural knowledge and communication skills, taught while avoiding stereotypes. Examples include the effect of prejudice on gays and lesbians and how this prejudice shapes their interactions with the health care system, and common spiritual practices that might interfere with prescribed therapies (such as Ramadan fasting practices, when observed by diabetic Muslim patients). Communication skills that can be addressed in cultural competence training include approaches to eliciting patients' explanatory models and use of traditional treatments as well as methods for negotiating different styles of communication and levels of family participation in decision making. Overall, there is excellent evidence that cultural competency training improves the attitudes and skills of health professionals and good evidence that cultural competence training improves patient satisfaction. 2 However, data are generally not available to document improved adherence by patients, better health outcomes, or cost-effectiveness.

SUMMARY

The average life expectancy of Americans increased by more than 30 years between 1900 and 2000. However, some groups have not fully benefited from the medical and public health achievements of the last century. Although there are demonstrated correlations between racial and ethnic background and socioeconomic status (Chapter 5), poverty alone cannot explain all the gaps in health and health care that exist between minorities and whites. Although the disparities were first documented in blacks in the United States, a growing body of evidence indicates that Latinos, who constitute the fastest growing minority population, and other minority groups as well as gays, lesbians, and bisexuals also experience significant problems with health care access and quality, especially when their English is not proficient.

Efforts to improve cultural competence in health care, whether they are used alone or in conjunction with socioeconomic initiatives (Chapter 5), are likely to play a significant role in reducing health disparities across population subgroups. The dissemination of successful interventions through linkages with payers, policymakers, provider groups, community organizations, and the media will be critical.

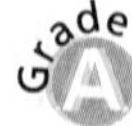

1. Taylor VM, Hislop TG, Jackson JC, et al: A randomized controlled trial of interventions to promote cervical cancer screening among Chinese women in North America. J Nat Cancer Inst 2002; 94:670–677.
2. Beach MC, Price EG, Gary TL, et al: Cultural competence—a systematic review of health care provider educational interventions. Med Care 2005;43:356–373.

SUGGESTED READINGS

Frist WH: Overcoming disparities in U.S. health care. Health Affairs 2005;24: 445–451. *Discusses approaches to reducing health care disparities.*

Kennedy EM: The role of the federal government in eliminating health disparities. Health Affairs 2005;24:452–457. *Discusses the role of government in eliminating health disparities.*

Minkler M, Fuller-Thomson E, Guralnik JM: Gradient of disability across the socioeconomic spectrum in the United States. N Engl J Med 2006;355:695–703. *A significant gradient was present up to, but not beyond, the age of 85 years.*

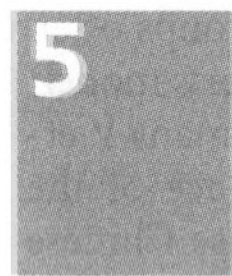

5 SOCIOECONOMIC ISSUES IN MEDICINE

Steven A. Schroeder

All nations—rich or poor—struggle with how to improve the health of the public, obtain the most value from medical services, and restrain rising health care expenditures. Most developed countries also wrestle with the paradox that their citizens have never been so healthy or so unhappy with their medical care. Despite the reality that only 10% of premature deaths result from inadequate medical care, the bulk of professional and political attention focuses on how to obtain and pay for state-of-the-art medical care. By comparison, 40% of premature deaths stem from unhealthy behaviors—smoking (Chapter 30), excessive or unwise drinking (Chapter 31), obesity (Chapter 239), insufficient physical activity (Chapter 14), illicit drug use (Chapter 32), and imprudent sexual behavior (Chapter 307) (Fig. 5–1). Genetics (Chapter 37) account for an additional 30%; social factors—discussed next—account for 15%, and environmental factors (Chapter 17) account for 5%.

SOCIAL STATUS INFLUENCES HEALTH

Socioeconomic status, or class, is a composite of many different factors, including income, education, occupation, and neighborhood. In general, people in lower classes are less healthy and die earlier than people at higher socioeconomic levels, a pattern that holds true in a stepwise fashion from the poorest to the richest. In the United States, the association between health and class is usually discussed in terms of racial and ethnic disparities; but in fact, race and class are independently associated with health status, and it can be argued that class is the more important factor. For example, income is a much stronger predictor of cardiovascular deaths than is race (Table 5–1). Yet, because class is less often captured in medical and death certificate data, race has become an imperfect proxy for class.

In part, the relationship between class and health is mediated by the higher rates of unhealthy behaviors among the poor, such as the inverse relationship between educational attainment and cigarette smoking (Fig. 5–2); but unhealthy behaviors do not fully explain the poor health of those in the lower socioeconomic classes. Even when behavior is held constant, people in lower socioeconomic classes are much more likely to die prematurely than are people of higher classes.

It currently is not clear which of the components of class—education, income (either absolute wealth or the extent of the gap between rich and poor), occupation, or neighborhood—makes the greatest impact on a person's health. Most likely, it is a combination of all of them. For example, the constant stress of a lower class existence—lack of control over one's life circumstances, social isolation, and the anxiety derived from the feeling of having low status—is linked to poor health. This stress may trigger a variety of neuroendocrinologic responses that are useful for short-term adaptation but bring long-term harm.

What can clinicians do with this knowledge? Clearly, it is difficult to write prescriptions for more income or for better schooling or neigh-

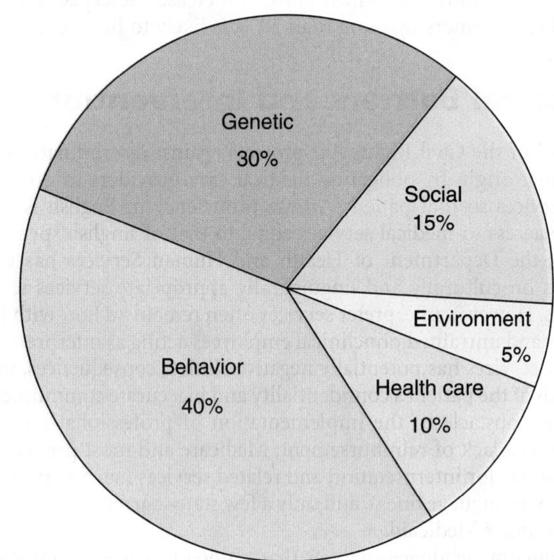

FIGURE 5–1 • Determinants of health. Health is influenced by genetic predisposition, behavioral patterns, environmental exposures, social circumstances, and health care. (Data from McGinnis MJ, Williams-Russo P, Knickman JR: The case for more active policy attention to health promotion. Health Affairs 2002;21:78–93.)

TABLE 5–1 AVERAGE ANNUAL, AGE-ADJUSTED RATES* OF DEATH FROM HEART DISEASE AMONG PERSONS 25 TO 64 YEARS OLD, 1979–1980

	Men			Women		
Annual Income	**White**	**Black**	**Ratio of Black Men to White Men**	**White**	**Black**	**Ratio of Black Women to White Women**
<$10,000	324.1	390.8	1.21	112.2	184.7	1.65
$10,000–$14,999	255.4	292.8	1.15	71.3	119.2	1.67
$15,000–$24,999	136.9	142.2	1.04	43.7	64.8	1.48
Ratio of lowest to highest income	2.4	2.7	—	2.6	2.9	—

*No. of deaths/100,000 person years.

From Isaacs SL, Schroeder SA: Class—the ignored determinant of a nation's health. N Engl J Med 2004;351:1137–1142. Data on income ranges (in 1980 dollars) and ratios of black men to white men and black women to white woman are from Williams DR: Race and health: Trends and policy implications. *In* Auerbach JA, Krimgold BK (eds): Income, socioeconomic status, and health: Exploring the relationships. Washington, DC, National Policy Association, 2001, p 69.

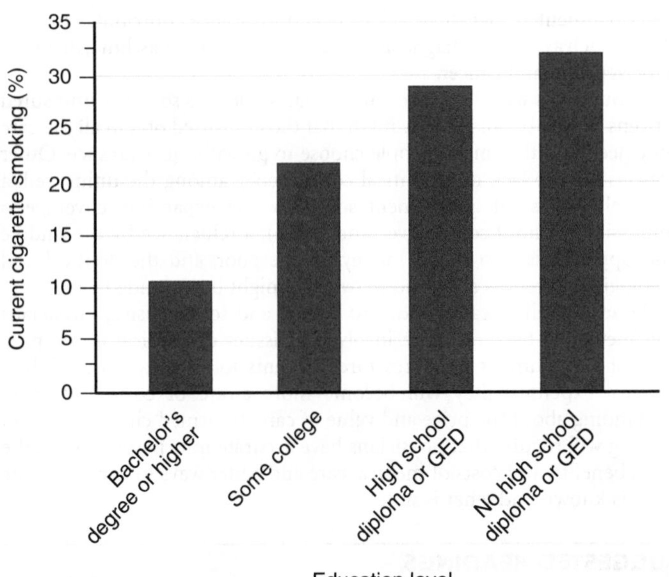

FIGURE 5–2 • Age-adjusted prevalence of cigarette smoking in 2000, among persons 25 years of age or older, according to educational level. GED, general equivalency diploma. (Data from Health, United States. Hyattsville, MD, National Center for Health Statistics, 2002, p 198. DHHS publication no. 2002–1232. Figure from Isaacs SL, Schroeder SA: Class—the ignored determinant of a nation's health. N Engl J Med 2004;351:1137–1142.)

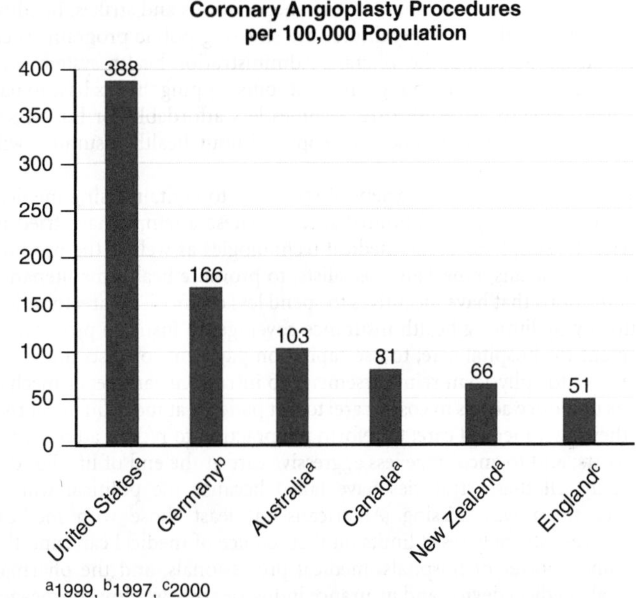

FIGURE 5–3 • Coronary angioplasty procedures per 100,000 population. (Data from OECD Health Data 2002. Organisation for Economic Co-operation and Development, U.K. Department of Health.)

borhoods or jobs, but physicians can encourage healthy behavior. At key times of transition, such as during discharge planning for hospitalized patients, physicians should be attentive to social circumstances. For patients who are likely to be socially isolated, clinicians should encourage or arrange interactions with family, neighbors, religious organizations, or community agencies to improve the likelihood of optimal outcomes. In addition, physicians should seek to identify and to eliminate any aspects of racism in health care institutions. Finally, in their role as social advocates, physicians can promote such goals as safe neighborhoods, improved schools, and equitable taxation policies.

ECONOMIC ISSUES IN MEDICAL CARE

Medical care today is on a collision course. On the one hand, an ever-expanding science continuously generates new technologies and drugs that promise a longer and healthier life. Add a public eager to obtain the latest breakthroughs touted in the media and over the Internet, plus a well-stocked medical industry eager to meet that demand, and it is easy to understand why expenditures continue to soar. On the other hand, payers for medical care—health insurance companies, government (federal, state, and local), and employers—increasingly bridle at the costs of medical care.

The United States continues to lead the world in health care expenditures. In 2003, it spent more than $1.7 trillion, amounting to 15.3% of its gross domestic product. It is projected that expenditures will continue to rise, reaching above 18% by 2014. Few other countries have double-digit health care expenditures, and none comes close to 15%. A potent combination of supply and demand factors explains why the United States spends so much for medical care. On the supply side, it far exceeds other countries in the availability and use of expensive diagnostic technologies, such as magnetic resonance imaging and computed tomography. For example, the United States has five times as many magnetic resonance imaging machines per capita as does Canada. Similar patterns exist for therapeutic technologies, whether coronary angioplasty (Fig. 5–3), cancer chemotherapy, or joint prostheses. The differences are especially dramatic in older patients. For example, in the 65- to 69-year age group, the United States performed 1.95 more carotid endarterectomy procedures per capita than did Canada; but above the age of 80 years, the ratio was 8.7.

Other supply factors that drive high medical expenditures in the United States include a fee-for-service payment system that compensates physicians much more for using expensive technologies than when they do not; a medical professional work force that earns much higher incomes relative to the population than in other nations and that emphasizes specialist rather than generalist practice; accelerated development of new and costly medications that are directly marketed to consumers; and a high rate of defensive medicine in response to pervasive fears about medical malpractice suits. Supply factors that do not seem to be unique in the United States are the number of physicians or hospitals. Many other developed countries have a much larger physician work force relative to their populations. The number of hospitals and hospital beds, the frequency of hospitalizations, and the length of hospital stay are relatively low in the United States, although it does have a much greater proportion of intensive care beds. Finally, recent analyses suggest that a principal driver of high expenditures on health care in the United States is the much greater price charged per unit of service compared with other developed countries.

Demand factors also drive medical expenditures. The extent to which the media and the medical profession feature medical "breakthroughs" is extensive and one-sided. New promising treatments merit front-page stories and commercial advertisements, whereas subsequent disappointing results are buried or ignored. The cumulative result is to whet patients' appetites for more and to leave the impression that good health depends only on finding the right treatment. This same quest explains the popularity of alternative medicine, for which patients are willing to spend more than $30 billion annually out of their own pockets (Chapter 36).

It could be argued that rising expenditures for medical care are not a bad thing, as what could be more important than ensuring maximal health? There are several rebuttals to that argument. First, it is not clear that money spent on medical care brings appropriate value in the United States, given that its health statistics are worse than those of virtually every other developed country. Second, there are substantial regional differences in the supply and use of medical care, such as a two-fold difference in the supply of acute hospital beds in metropolitan regions (even with adjustment for demographic variables) and a four-fold difference in the risk of being hospitalized in an intensive care unit at the end of life. Similar regional differences exist for procedures such as transurethral prostatectomy, hysterectomy, and coronary artery bypass surgery. Yet there is no evidence that "more is better" on a regional basis. In fact, geographic areas with higher consumption of medical services have been shown to have worse outcomes for some conditions, such as acute myocardial infarction.

Money spent on medical care means less to spend on other important social priorities—schools, the environment, job creation, and competition with overseas manufacturers that spend less on health care. Furthermore, many businesses are reducing their health insurance contributions to employees and retirees, passing those costs along to the beneficiaries. Consequently, health insurance coverage has emerged as the most important issue in labor contract negotiations and strikes. In addition, rising health care expenditures are stressing public programs such as Medicare, Medicaid, the Veterans Administration health system, and municipal hospitals, with budget requests outstripping the tax base to pay for them. Finally, as health care becomes less affordable for businesses and government, the number of people without health insurance will continue to increase.

Since the mid-1970s, a variety of strategies to contain rising medical expenditures have yielded limited success. These attempts have tried to restrict the supply of costly medical technologies as well as the production of physicians, especially specialists; to promote health maintenance organizations that have incentives to spend less on medical care; to ration indirectly by limiting health insurance coverage; to institute prospective payment for hospital care; to use capitation payments or discounted fee schedules for physician reimbursement; to introduce gatekeeper mechanisms to reduce access to costly care; to put patients at more financial risk for their own medical care; to reform malpractice; to reduce administrative costs; and to encourage less aggressive care at the end of life. Fundamentally, all these strategies have failed because the political will to enforce them was missing. Americans—at least those with medical insurance—strongly resist limits on their choice of medical care, and the combined power of hospitals, medical professionals, and the pharmaceutical, medical device, and insurance industries overwhelms the meager forces pushing cost containment. Add to that the continuous production of new technologies and drugs plus the public's avidity for the latest innovations, and it is not difficult to understand why medical costs are projected to keep rising. As a result, the costs of even modest health insurance plans are a challenge for most blue-collar and many middle-class families.

The payment for medical care varies by country. In the United States, health insurance coverage is an incomplete patchwork, consisting of government-sponsored programs for the elderly (Medicare), the poor (Medicaid), and veterans plus employer-based coverage for workers and their families. Medicare covers acute care services in the hospital and in physicians' offices but has limited coverage for prescription drugs and long-term care. More than half of all Medicare subscribers buy supplemental insurance. Medicaid covers more services than Medicare does, but Medicaid payments to physicians and hospitals are so low in many states that patients have restricted access to care. At any given time, more than 45 million Americans lack health insurance, and 70 million are without insurance at some point during the year. In addition, millions of immigrant workers are also uninsured. This large group must depend on charity care, often at community clinics and public hospitals, and it is well documented that their lack of health insurance contributes to poor health, such as delayed diagnosis and undertreatment of asthma, diabetes, hypertension, and cancer.

A country as wealthy as the United States tolerates so many uninsured citizens in part because of the myth that the uninsured obtain all the care they need and that many people choose to go without insurance. Other reasons are the lack of a political constituency among the uninsured, a cultural distrust of government solutions (yet expanding coverage is impossible without some government role), a reluctance by the middle and upper classes to spend money on the poor, and the political and ideologic differences about how coverage might be expanded.

Because medical care is both so valued and so expensive, physicians will inevitably become more involved in issues of medical economics. As cost-containment pressures force patients to assume more of their medical expenses, they will become more aware of costs and more demanding about the price and value of care. Informed clinical decision making will require that physicians have accurate information about the risks, benefits, and costs of medical care and better ways to communicate what is known and what is not.

SUGGESTED READINGS

Anderson GF, Reinhardt UE, Hussey PS, et al: It's the prices, stupid: Why the United States is so different from other countries. Health Affairs 2003;22:89–105. *Higher prices per unit of service account for a substantial proportion of the increased costs of U.S. health care.*

Bodenheimer T: Rising health care costs. Part 1: Seeking an explanation. Part 2: Technologic innovation. Part 3: The role of health care providers. Part 4: Can costs be controlled while preserving quality? Ann Intern Med 2005;142:847–854, 932–937, 996–1002; 143:26–31. *Comprehensive and excellent four-part summary of medical cost dilemma.*

Cutler DM, Rosen AB, Vijan S: The value of medical spending in the United States, 1960–2000. N Engl J Med 2006;355:920–927. *Increased spending over the 40-year period has been a good value.*

Fisher E, Wennbert D, Stukel T, et al: The implications of regional variations in Medicare spending. Part 2: Health outcomes and satisfaction with care. Ann Intern Med 2003;138:288–299. *Medicare enrollees in higher spending regions receive more medical care but do not have better outcomes.*

Institute of Medicine, National Academy of Sciences: Care without coverage: Too little, too late. Washington, DC, National Academy Press, 2002. Available at www.nap.edu. *Comprehensive review of how the health of the uninsured is worse than if they are insured, with particular impact on the health of the uninsured who are disadvantaged.*

Isaacs SL, Schroeder SA: Class—the ignored determinant of a nation's health. N Engl J Med 2004;351:1137–1142. *Reviews social class and health, including the potential impact of education, employment, and taxation policies on health.*

Section II

Principles of Evaluation and Management

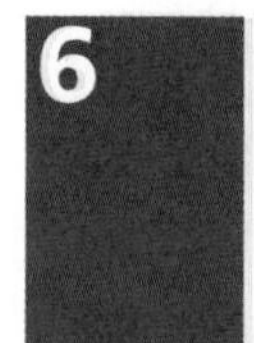

APPROACH TO THE PATIENT: HISTORY AND PHYSICAL EXAMINATION

David L. Simel

OVERVIEW

Physicians have several specific medical goals that assume varying degrees of importance in encounters with patients, depending on their individual characteristics and the care setting. These goals include but are not limited to the translation of symptoms and signs into diagnoses, assessment of stability or change in known conditions, provision of information and counseling for future prevention, and reaffirmation or alteration of therapeutic interventions.

In the context of these medical goals, the physician should also strive to address several related social goals whose achievement can synergistically improve medical outcomes, such as establishing a relationship and measure of trust. The interaction between the patient and physician represents not only a scientific encounter but also a social ritual centered on locus of control and meeting each other's expectations. Patients may not be able to express their needs fully and may fear loss of control in determining their own medical fate. Conversely, physicians also have expectations that they must consider and sometimes answer for themselves: a need to feel that they have not missed something important in addressing diagnostic challenges, a need to put limits on the time available for each interaction, and a need to maintain objectivity so that their evaluation and recommendations are not clouded by their emotional feelings about the patient. When the patient's needs are to establish the presence of health or the diagnosis for a symptom, the expertise of the physician is expressed through the performance and interpretation of a rational clinical examination.

Physical Examination Begins with the History

It is almost impossible to consider the history as distinct from the physical examination because the clinical examination begins as soon as the physician sees or hears the patient. Cynics contend that physical diagnostic skills have eroded because most diagnoses are made during the history and then confirmed by a more objective test, such as a laboratory value or a radiographic image. It is perhaps unfair to assume that clinical diagnostic skills have deteriorated because scientific principles were not applied to the clinical examination until the mid-1970s. Before then, the sparse literature that addressed the clinical examination was dominated by case reports and case series that provided anecdotal evidence in which the usefulness of the physical examination was often overstated. Even proponents of the clinical examination now demand proof of reasonable reproducibility and accuracy before they accept the value of specific components of the history and physical examination. No objective evidence supports the contention that physicians' diagnostic skills have deteriorated over time.

Quantitative Principles of the Clinical Examination

The clinical examination can be studied with the same principles as those applied to more traditional tests, such as laboratory results or diagnostic images. For each component of the history and physical examination, there is an associated sensitivity (the percentage of patients with a disorder who have an abnormal finding), specificity (the percentage of patients without a disorder who have a normal finding), and measure of precision (the agreement beyond chance between two observers) (Chapter 9). Current research on the clinical examination uses likelihood ratios (LRs) that inform clinicians how likely they are to observe a particular finding in a patient with a given condition as opposed to a patient without the condition. When it is estimated that an older patient who "shuffles her feet" when she walks has an LR of 3.0 for Parkinson's disease (Chapter 433), it means her risk of Parkinson's disease increases threefold compared with the baseline risk. Similarly, if a patient who insists that he does not have "shaking in his arms" has an LR of 0.25 for Parkinson's disease, he is one fourth as likely (a reduced chance) compared with the baseline risk. Evaluation of the precision of the examination uses the kappa (κ) statistic to describe the agreement beyond chance (0 = random agreement; +1 = perfect agreement).

How to Find Quantitative Information about the Clinical Examination

Finding data on the sensitivity, specificity, LRs, and observer variability of components of the clinical examination may require a MEDLINE search for evaluation of a disease-specific condition (e.g., melanoma) or a clinical finding (e.g., splenomegaly) (Table 6–1).

MEDICAL HISTORY

The basic approach to a complete medical history is outlined in Table 6–2. The history begins by asking patients to describe, in their own words, the reason for seeking medical care. Although patients may have many reasons for initiating a visit to the physician, they should be encouraged to select the single or two most important concerns they have. The patient should be reassured that the physician will not ignore other concerns but wants to understand what is most important to the patient. It is generally best to steer patients to describing a symptom or sign that prompted the visit rather than steering them to a diagnosis. For example, instead of accepting "I am here for my diabetes," the physician might preferentially elicit that "I am here because my blood sugar has been a little high."

History of the Present Illness

Initially, patients should be asked open-ended questions to permit a description of their problems in their own words. This initial process can be followed by a series of specific questions to fill in any gaps or to clarify important points. These questions should be asked in an order dictated by the story the patient tells and targeted to suit the individual problem. When the patient is acutely ill, the physician should limit the amount of time spent in open-ended discussion and move promptly to the most important features that allow quick evaluation and management. In general, the history of the problem under consideration includes the following:

- Description of onset and chronology
- Location of symptoms
- Character (quality) of symptoms
- Intensity
- Precipitating, aggravating, and relieving factors
- Inquiry into whether the problem or similar problems occurred before and, if so, whether a diagnosis was established at that time

Finally, it is often helpful to ask patients to express what they believe is the cause of the problem or what concerns them the most. This approach often uncovers other pertinent factors and helps establish that the physician is trying to meet the patient's needs.

Past Medical and Surgical History

Much of the past medical and surgical history is obtained when the patient relates the history of the problem in question. An astute clinician should not rely on patients to divulge all their prior problems, however, because they may forget, may assume that previous events are unrelated to their current problem, or simply may not want to discuss past events. An open-ended statement such as "Tell me about other medical illnesses you have had that we did not discuss" and "Tell me about any operations you have had" prompts the patient to consider other items. During the physical examination, the physician should ask the patient about unexplained surgical or traumatic scars.

A list of current medications should include prescriptions, over-the-counter medications, vitamins, and herbal preparations. When a patient is uncertain about the names of medications, the patient or family member should be asked to bring all medication bottles to the next visit. Patients may not consider topical medications (e.g., skin preparations or eye drops) as important, so they may need prompting.

Information about allergies (Chapter 275) is particularly important to collect but also challenging. Patients may attribute adverse reactions or intolerances to allergies, but many supposed allergic reactions are not

TABLE 6–1 MEDLINE SEARCH STRATEGY FOR IDENTIFYING QUANTITATIVE INFORMATION ON THE CLINICAL EXAMINATION USING THE OVID SEARCH SYSTEM*

1. exp physical examination/or physical exam$.mp
2. medical history taking.mp
3. professional competence.mp
4. (sensitivity and specificity).mp or (sensitivity and specificity).tw
5. (reproducibility of results or observer variation).mp
6. diagnostic tests, routine/
7. (decision support techniques or Bayes theorem).mp
8. 1 or 2 or 3 or 4 or 5 or 6 or 7
9. limit 8 to (Ovid full text available and human and English language)
10. exp knee injuries
11. 10 and 9
12. exp splenomegaly
13. 9 and 12

*OVID Technologies, Inc. A condition and a physical finding are given as examples. Abbreviations or search term abbreviations are as follows: "exp" indicates that the topic is "exploded" to include all subheadings for the topic. The "$" is a wildcard designator, so "exam$" would include the words *examination, examining,* and *examiner.* "mp" searches for the word or phrase in the title, abstract, registry number word, or mesh subject heading. Step 9 limits the search to studies that involve humans only and where the full manuscript is available online and is written in English. If the search yields too few topics, the limitation of full text available can be removed and the search repeated. If too many results are obtained, some of the items from step 8 can be eliminated.

truly drug allergies. Less than 20% of patients who claim a penicillin allergy are allergic on skin testing. Eliciting the patient's actual response to medications facilitates a determination of whether the response was a true allergic reaction.

Social and Occupational History and Risk Factors

The social history not only reveals important information but also improves understanding of the patient's unique values, support systems, and social situation. The social history should be tailored to the individual patient and allow for physician-centered questioning and patient-centered expression of values and concerns.

Data that may influence risk factors for disease should be gathered, including a nonjudgmental assessment of substance abuse. The tobacco history should include the use of snuff, chewing tobacco, and cigar and cigarette smoking (Chapter 30). Alcohol use should be determined quantitatively and by the effect that it has had on the patient's life (Chapter 31). Past or present use of illicit substances, prescription pain medications or sedatives, and intravenous drugs should be assessed (Chapter 32). The sexual history should include current sexual activity, including the number of partners and past history. The employment history should include the current and past employment history, military experience, and any significant hobbies. Information should be elicited from military veterans regarding their combat history, years of service, and areas of deployment.

The physician should also obtain information on socioeconomic status, insurance, the ability to afford or obtain medications, and past or current barriers to health care because of their impact on care of the patient (Chapter 5). Marital status and the living situation (i.e., whom the patient lives with, significant stressors for that patient) are important as risk factors for disease and to determine how best to care for the patient. A patient's culture (Chapter 4) and values should be known, including any prior advance directives or desire to overrule them (Chapter 3). The physician should explicitly elicit and record information regarding the next of kin; surrogate decision makers; emergency contacts; social support systems; and financial, emotional, and physical support available to the patient.

TABLE 6–2 PATIENT'S MEDICAL HISTORY

Description of the patient
- Age, gender, ethnic background, occupation

Chief reason for seeking medical care
- State the purpose of the evaluation (usually in the patient's words)

Other physicians involved in the patient's care
- Include the clinician that the patient identifies as his or her primary provider or the physician who referred the patient.
- Record contact information for all physicians who should receive information about the visit

History of the reason for seeking medical care
- In chronologic fashion, determine the evolution of the indication for the visit and then each major symptom. It is best to address the patient's reason for seeking care first rather than what the physician ultimately believes is most important
- Be careful to avoid "premature closure," in which a diagnosis is assumed before all the information is collected

Past medical and surgical history
- List other illnesses and previous surgeries not related to the current problem
- List all prescribed and over-the-counter medications with dose
- Remember to ask about vitamin and herbal supplements

Allergies and adverse reactions
- List allergic reactions to medications and food. Record the specific reaction (e.g., hives). Distinguish allergies from adverse reactions or intolerance to medication (e.g., dyspepsia from nonsteroidal anti-inflammatory agents)

Social and occupational history
- Describe the patient's current family and a typical day for patient. The occupational history should focus on current and past employment as it might relate to the current problem. For veterans, inquire about their military history, including combat exposure, years of service, and areas of deployment

Risk factors
- Include history of tobacco use, illegal drug use, and risk factors for sexually transmitted disease (including human immunodeficiency virus and hepatitis)

Family history
- History of any diseases in first-degree relatives and a listing of family members with any conditions that could be risk factors for the patient (e.g., cardiovascular disease at a young age, malignancy, known genetic disorders, longevity)

Review of systems (see Table 6–3)

The social history should be tailored to the individual patient and to the physician-patient encounter. An understanding of a patient's habits and social situation furthers understanding of risk factors, is crucial to developing an appropriate patient-physician relationship, and allows planning of optimal care.

Family History

The patient's family history is of increasing importance given the rapid expansion of knowledge about genetics in medicine. The family history is never diagnostic, but it allows risk stratification, which affects the pretest probability for an increasing number of disorders (e.g., heart disease, breast cancer, or Alzheimer's disease). For common diseases such as heart disease, additional inquiry into the age of onset in first-degree relatives and death attributed to the disease should be obtained (Chapter 49). When a patient reports that a first-degree relative had a myocardial infarction, the LR is 19 that the patient has a family history of myocardial infarction. Patients may lack appropriate information about the absence of disease, however, so a reported lack of a family history of myocardial infarction reduces the likelihood only by a third. In general, the specificity of the reported family history far exceeds its sensitivity; for example, only two thirds of patients with essential tremor (Chapter 434) report a family history, but 95% of such patients have first-degree relatives with tremor. The expansion of knowledge about genetic diseases (Chapter 37) requires clinicians not only to improve their skills in eliciting the family history but also to develop methods for confirming the information. For example, patients who report that a first-degree relative had carcinoma of the colon (LR 25), breast (LR 14), ovaries (LR 34), or prostate (LR 12) are usually providing accurate information.

Review of Systems

The review of systems, which is the structural assessment of each of the major organ systems, elicits symptoms or signs not covered, or overlooked, in the history of the present illness. In practice, the review of systems may be accomplished by direct questioning (Table 6–3) or by having the patient fill out a previsit questionnaire that constrains the answers to a specific time frame. When directly obtained, the best approach is not to use open-ended questions but rather to proceed efficiently and effectively by asking direct questions. The physician may ask the patient, "Has there been any recent change in your vision" or "Have you recently had shortness of breath, wheezing, or coughing?" The relative value of these approaches has not been investigated fully, but restricting the symptoms to a narrower time frame prevents a complete retelling of the history. One estimate is that the review of systems yields a new important diagnosis about 10% of the time. Nevertheless, the review of systems is an efficient mechanism for detecting issues and for obtaining a complete understanding of the patient's overall status.

PHYSICAL EXAMINATION

Chaperones

When asked in surveys, most patients of either sex and all ages report a lack of preference for a chaperone; it is not clear whether this response is their true feeling or a desire to give a "correct" response. Nevertheless, many adult women (29%) and adolescent girls (46%) do express a preference for a chaperone during a breast, pelvic, or rectal examination by a male physician (especially during their first examination). Examiners should offer patients the option of a chaperone, and a chaperone should be considered when the clinician and patient are of different genders. Many examiners prefer a chaperone to allay their own anxieties attributable to gender differences or to achieve a perceived need for protection should the patient become concerned during the procedure.

TABLE 6–3 REVIEW OF SYSTEMS*
FOCUS all questions on a specific time frame (e.g., within the past "month" or "now") and on items not already addressed during the clinical examination
Change in weight or appetite
Change in vision
Change in hearing
New or changing skin lesions
Chest discomfort or sensation of skipped beats
Shortness of breath, dyspnea on exertion
Abdominal discomfort, constipation, melena, hematochezia, diarrhea
Difficulty with urination
Change in menses
Joint or muscle discomfort not already mentioned
Problems with sleep
Difficulty with sexual function
Exposure to "street" drugs or medications not already mentioned
Depression (feeling "down, depressed, or hopeless"; loss of interest or pleasure in doing things)
A sensation of unsteadiness when walking, standing, or getting up from a chair

*Clinicians may start with this basic list and adapt the items to their specific patient population by considering factors such as age, gender, medications, and the problems identified during the examination. The process is facilitated by developing a routine personal approach to these questions, typically going through the systems from "head to toe."

Vital Signs

A nurse or assistant often obtains the vital signs. Vital signs include the pulse rate, blood pressure, respiratory rate, body temperature, and the patient's quantitative assessment of pain. Marked abnormalities require a rapid, focused evaluation that may take precedence over the typical structural approach to the remainder of the evaluation (Chapter 7).

The pulse should be recorded as not just the rate but also the rhythm. Physicians may prefer to initiate the examination by holding the patient's hand while palpating the pulse. This nonthreatening initial contact with the patient allows the physician to determine whether the patient has a regular or irregular rhythm.

When the blood pressure is abnormal, many physicians repeat the measurement. The instrument error that contributes to the greatest variability is the cuff size of the sphygmomanometer (Chapter 66). Many adults require a large adult cuff; using a narrow cuff can alter systolic/diastolic blood pressure by −8 to +10/+2 to +8 mm Hg. The appearance of repetitive sounds (Korotkoff sounds, phase 1) constitutes systolic pressure. After the cuff is inflated about 20 to 30 mm Hg above the palpated pressure, the Korotkoff sounds muffle and disappear as the pressure is released (phase 5). The level at which the sounds disappear is diastolic pressure. The American Heart Association recommends that each measure be rounded upward to the nearest 2 mm Hg.

The respiratory rate should be assessed at the same time that the patient is observed to determine whether there is any respiratory discomfort (dyspnea) (Chapter 83). The subjective sensation of dyspnea is caused by an increased work of breathing. The examiner should decide whether patients have tachypnea (a rapid rate of breathing) or hypopnea (a slow or shallow rate of breathing). Tachypnea is not always associated with hyperventilation, which is defined by increased alveolar ventilation resulting in a lower arterial carbon dioxide level (Chapter 104). In the evaluation of patients suspected of having pneumonia, examiners agree on the presence of tachypnea only 63% of the time.

The body temperature of adults is usually measured with an oral electric thermometer. These thermometers correlate well with the traditional mercury thermometer and are safer to use. Rectal thermometers reliably record temperatures 0.4° C higher than oral thermometers do. By comparison, newer tympanic thermometers may vary too much in comparison to oral thermometers (−1.2° C to +1.6° C vs. the oral temperature) to be reliable in hospitalized patients.

The Joint Commission on Accreditation of Healthcare Organizations has been a leading advocate of the systematic measurement of self-assessed pain in all patients, typically rated on a scale of 0 to 10 (no pain to worst pain ever) (Chapter 28). The validity, usefulness, and value of the adopted scales as a screening tool for clinical diagnosis are uncertain, however.

Head and Neck

Face

When looking at the face, the examiner can simplify the assessment by carefully judging for symmetry. Asymmetrical facial features should be noted and explained. Examples of asymmetry include skin lesions (Chapter 462), cranial nerve palsies (Chapter 418), parotid enlargement (Chapter 451), or the ptosis of Horner's syndrome (Chapter 445). A variety of disorders may cause symmetrical, abnormal facies; examples include acromegaly (Chapter 242), Cushing's syndrome (Chapter 245), and Parkinson's disease (Chapter 433).

Ears

Physicians may not recognize hearing loss unless they pay special attention (Chapter 454). When patients do not appreciate the whispered voice, the likelihood of hearing loss increases considerably (LR 6.0). Cerumen impaction is an easily treated cause of diminished hearing. Otoscopic evaluation of the tympanic membranes should reveal a translucent membrane and an obvious cone of light reflected where the eardrum meets the malleolus (see Fig. 452–6). Few data exist to determine observer variability in otoscopic examination of adult patients.

Nose

Patients frequently have nasal symptoms, such as a self-diagnosis of sinusitis (Chapter 452) or snoring (Chapter 429). The nares should be examined for the presence of polyps, which can be seen as obstructing, glistening mucosal masses. Transillumination performed in a dark room is useful for diagnosing sinusitis, especially when combined with visualization of a purulent discharge, a patient's report of a poor response to decongestants or antihistamines, a maxillary toothache, and the presence of discolored rhinorrhea (Chapter 452). These patients have an LR greater than 6 for bacterial sinusitis.

Mouth

The quality of the patient's dentition directly affects nutrition. Generalist physicians can be confident that the patient requires dental care if periodontal disease or dental caries is detected (LR > 4.0). The need for dental care cannot be excluded even in the absence of such findings (LR 0.7), however, and all patients should be encouraged to seek regular dental evaluations. Premalignant oral lesions (e.g., leukoplakia [see Fig. 200–1], nodules, ulcerations) found by generalist physicians are usually verified by dentists (LR > 6.5) (Chapter 451). Patients who use smokeless tobacco products are at significantly increased risk for premalignant and malignant oral lesions (Chapter 30). Bimanual palpation of the cheeks and floor of the mouth facilitates identification of potentially malignant lesions (Chapter 451).

Eyes

The eye examination begins with simple visual inspection to look for symmetry in the lids, extraocular movements, pupil size and reaction, and the presence of redness (Chapters 449 and 450). Abnormalities in extraocular movements should be grouped into nonparalytic (usually chronic with onset in childhood) or paralytic (third, fourth, or sixth cranial nerve palsy) causes. Pupillary abnormalities may be symmetrical or asymmetrical (anisocoria). Red eyes should be categorized by the pattern of ciliary injection, presence of pain, effect on vision, and papillary abnormalities. When the eye examination is approached systematically, the generalist physician can evaluate the likelihood of conjunctivitis, episcleritis or scleritis, iritis, and acute glaucoma.

Routine determination of visual acuity can help confirm or refute a patient's report of diminished vision but does not replace the need for formal ophthalmologic evaluation in patients with visual complaints (Chapter 449). Cataracts can be detected with direct ophthalmoscopy, but the generalist's proficiency in this evaluation is uncertain.

After identifying the optic disc by ophthalmoscopy, the examiner should note the border of the disc for clarity, color, and the size of the central cup in relation to the total diameter (usually less than half the diameter of the disc). A careful observer sees spontaneous venous pulsations that indicate normal intracranial pressure. Abnormalities of the optic disc include optic atrophy (a white disc), papilledema (see Fig. 449–18) (blurry margins with a pink, hyperemic disc), and glaucoma (a large, pale cup with retinal vessels that dive underneath and that may be displaced toward the nasal side). The generalist's examination inadequately detects early glaucomatous changes, so high-risk patients should undergo routine ophthalmologic examination for glaucoma.

After inspecting the disc, the examiner should examine the upper and lower nasal quadrants for the appearance of vessels and the presence of any retinal hemorrhages (see Fig. 449–17) or lesions. Proceeding from the nasal quadrants to the temporal quadrants decreases the risk of papillary constriction from the bright light focused on the fovea. Dilating the pupils leads to an improved examination. Despite the improved results in direct ophthalmoscopy after dilation, patients with diabetes (Chapter 247) should undergo routine examination by ophthalmologists to detect diabetic retinopathy because the sensitivity of a generalist's examination is not adequate to exclude diabetic retinopathy or monitor it over time.

Neck

Carotid Pulses

The carotid pulses should be palpated for contour and timing in relation to the cardiac impulse. Abnormalities in the carotid pulse contour reflect underlying cardiac abnormalities (e.g., aortic stenosis) but are generally appreciated only after detecting an abnormal cardiac impulse or murmur (Chapter 48).

Many physicians listen for bruits over the carotid arteries because asymptomatic carotid bruits are associated with an increased incidence of cerebrovascular and cardiac events in older patients (Chapters 430 and 431). In asymptomatic patients, the presence of a carotid bruit increases the likelihood of a 70 to 90% stenotic lesion (LR 4 to 10), but the absence of a bruit is of uncertain value. Unfortunately, clinical data do not provide adequate data for judging the importance of detecting bruits in asymptomatic patients.

Thyroid

The thyroid gland is felt best when standing behind the patient and using both hands to palpate the thyroid gland gently (Chapter 244). The palpatory examination is enhanced by asking the patient to swallow sips of water, which allows the thyroid to glide underneath the fingers, but the quantitative improvement achieved by this maneuver in detecting thyroid enlargement or nodules has not been evaluated rigorously. Inspection of the gland from the side is useful because lateral prominence of the thyroid between the cricoid cartilage and the suprasternal notch indicates thyromegaly. The generalist physician should estimate the size of the thyroid gland as normal or enlarged; the impression of an enlarged thyroid gland by a generalist physician has an LR of almost 4.0, whereas assessment that the gland is of normal size makes thyromegaly less likely (LR 0.4).

Lymphatic System

While palpating the thyroid, the examiner may also identify enlarged cervical lymph nodes (Chapter 174). In addition, lymph nodes can be palpated in the supraclavicular area, axilla, epitrochlear area, and inguinofemoral region. Simple lymph node enlargement confined to one region is common and as a single finding does not usually represent an important underlying disorder. Unexpected gross lymph node enlargement in a single area or diffuse lymph node enlargement is more important. Patients with febrile illnesses, underlying malignancy, or inflammatory diseases should routinely undergo an examination of each of the aforementioned areas for lymph node enlargement.

Chest

Inspection of the patient's posture may reveal lateral curves in the back (scoliosis) or kyphosis that may be associated with loss of vertebral height from osteoporosis (Chapter 264). When patients have back pain, the spine and paravertebral muscles should be palpated in a search for spasm and tenderness (Chapter 423). The patient may be placed through maneuvers to assess loss of mobility associated with ankylosing spondylitis (Chapter 286), but a history of loss of lateral mobility may be just as efficient in the early stages of spondylitis.

Lungs

Examination of the lungs begins with inspection of the shape of the chest, although a barrel chest, thought to be typical of obstructive airways disease, is present only in severely affected patients (Chapters 83 and 88). The incremental value of palpation and percussion of the chest to supplement the history, auscultation, and eventual chest radiograph is unknown. Medical students show more consistency than pulmonary specialists do in recording auscultatory abnormalities. The presence or absence of adventitial sounds (wheezes, crackles, or rubs) has good interobserver reliability ($\kappa = 0.30$ to 0.70). The best piece of information for increasing the likelihood of chronic obstructive pulmonary disease is a history of more than 40 pack years of smoking (LR 19). The presence of wheezing or downward displacement of the larynx to within 4 cm of the sternum (distance between the top of the thyroid cartilage and the suprasternal notch) increases the likelihood of obstructive pulmonary disease (LR 4 for either).

Heart

The patient should be examined in the sitting and lying positions (Chapter 48). Typically, the examination begins with auscultation of the precordium while the patient is sitting. Most examiners progress as follows: aortic area, pulmonic area, left sternal border, and apex. For auscultation over the aortic area, having the patient lean forward may increase the intensity of aortic murmurs. Palpation of the apical impulse when the patient lies down in the left lateral decubitus position helps detect a displaced apical impulse and can reveal a palpable S_3. When the apical impulse is lateral to the midclavicular line, the likelihood of radiographic cardiomegaly and an ejection fraction less than 50% increases appreciably (LR about 3.5 and 6.0).

A systematic approach to auscultation helps organize the examination. First, the physician should listen to the heart sounds and concentrate on their timing, intensity, and splitting with respiration. The first and second heart sounds are heard best with the diaphragm, as are pericardial rubs. Gallops (S_3 and S_4) are heard best with the stethoscope bell. Murmurs, depending on their origin, vary in pitch and may require switching from the diaphragm to the bell to assess their characteristics (see Table 48–6). The location, timing, intensity, radiation patterns, and respiratory variation of murmurs should be noted. Special maneuvers during auscultation (e.g., Valsalva, auscultation during sudden squatting/standing) do not usually need to be performed if the results of routine precordial examination are entirely normal.

There is considerable concern about the reliability and accuracy of the cardiac examination. When performed on patients (as opposed to cardiac simulators), the reliability of perceiving an S_3 or S_4 is no better than chance, and agreement on the finding among examiners does not seem to improve with the examiner's experience. Nevertheless, the presence of an S_3 on any examination is useful for detecting left ventricular systolic dysfunction (LR > 4.0 for identifying patients with an ejection fraction <30%). The presence of a systolic thrill (palpable murmur, LR 12) or a holosystolic murmur increases the likelihood of moderate to severe aortic stenosis or mitral regurgitation. Quiet systolic murmurs (LR 0.08) are much less likely to herald important cardiac abnormalities. A loud, early diastolic murmur (LR 4) or a diastolic murmur associated with an S_3 suggests severe aortic regurgitation.

Breast

The most important determinants of the accuracy of the breast examination are the duration of the examination; the patient's position; careful evaluation of the breast boundaries; the pattern of the examination; and the position, movement, and pressure of the examiner's fingers (Chapter 208). Interobserver variability is substantial (κ about 0.3 to 0.6) because these aspects of the examination vary among physicians. To obtain the best sensitivity, the duration of the breast examination needs to be 5 to 10 minutes total time, but few generalist physicians perform such a lengthy examination. Clinicians should recognize that the examination may make them (or their patient) feel uncomfortable—the presence of a chaperone may give the clinician the confidence to perform an intensive examination.

The patient should be examined with the pads of the fingers while she is supine, holding her hand first on her forehead (to flatten the lateral border of the breast) and then on her shoulder (to flatten the medial border). The examiner should make small circular motions with the fingers, moving up and down in parallel rows to span the entire breast-clavicle to the bra line. Cancerous breast lumps are difficult to distinguish from benign breast lumps on examination, but the presence of a fixed mass or a mass 2 cm in diameter has an LR of about 2 to 2.5 for cancer.

Abdomen

Palpation and percussion of the abdomen of patients with no symptoms or risk factors for an abdominal disorder rarely reveals important abnormalities (Chapter 134). The only caveat would be palpation of an older patient for asymptomatic widening of the abdominal aorta, which is useful when found (LR of 16 for detecting aneurysms >4 cm in diameter) but misses a substantial proportion of small to medium aneurysms (Chapter 78). After specific training in palpation techniques, general internists have good agreement on the presence or absence of an aortic aneurysm (κ = 0.53).

When patients have potential abdominal symptoms, the examination should be guided by the symptoms. If the history suggests an acute problem, the examination should focus initially on identifying patients who may require surgical evaluation.

Auscultation of the abdomen in patients with acute symptoms is directed toward listening for bowel sounds to evaluate possible intestinal obstruction. For patients without gastrointestinal symptoms or abnormalities on palpation, auscultation for bruits is important primarily to detect renal bruits in patients with hypertension (Chapters 66 and 126). The presence of an abdominal bruit in a hypertensive patient, if heard in systole and diastole, strongly suggests renovascular hypertension (LR ≈ 40).

Liver

Detection of liver disease depends mostly on the history and laboratory evaluations (Chapter 149). By the time that signs are present on physical examination, the patient usually has advanced liver disease. The first abnormalities on physical examination associated with liver disease are extrahepatic. The clinician should assess the patient for ascites, peripheral edema, jaundice, or splenomegaly as signs of liver disease. In patients with an enlarged liver, palpation should begin at the liver edge, but palpation of the edge below the costal margin increases the likelihood of hepatomegaly only slightly (LR 1.7). The upper border of the liver may be detected by percussion, and a span of less than 12 cm reduces the likelihood of hepatomegaly. In the absence of a known diagnosis (e.g., a hepatoma, which may cause a hepatic bruit), auscultation of the liver rarely is helpful.

Spleen

Examination for splenomegaly in patients without findings suggestive of a disorder associated with splenomegaly almost always reveals nothing (Chapter 174). Approximately 3% of healthy teenagers may have a palpable spleen. The examination for an enlarged spleen begins first with percussion in the left upper quadrant to detect dullness. Percussion is performed over the lowest left anterior axillary line during inspiration and expiration while the patient is supine. In the absence of dullness, the results of palpation do not establish or exclude splenomegaly, so a radiographic image (ultrasound or nuclear scintigraphy) is required. The presence of a palpable splenic edge in patients with dullness to percussion and clinical suspicion of splenomegaly confirms enlargement. Palpation can be performed by any of the following three approaches (κ about 0.2 to 0.4): palpating with the right hand while providing counterpressure with the left hand behind the spleen, palpating with one hand without counterpressure (with the patient in the right lateral decubitus position for both techniques), or placing the patient supine with the left fist under the left costovertebral angle while the examiner tries to hook the spleen with the hands.

Musculoskeletal System

The musculoskeletal examination in adult patients is almost always driven by symptoms (Chapters 277 and 284). Regional musculoskeletal complaints are ubiquitous, and the limited formal clinical training that most physicians receive on the evaluation and management of such disorders belies their impact on the generalist's daily professional activities.

Most patients have back pain at some point during their lives (Chapter 423). Back pain is second only to upper respiratory illness as a reason for seeking outpatient care. The goal is to be sure that the back pain is not representative of systemic disease and to exclude neurosurgical emergencies. The patient's history helps assess the likelihood of an underlying systemic disease (age, history of systemic malignancy, unexplained weight loss, duration of pain, responsiveness to previous therapy, intravenous drug use, urinary infection, or fever). The most important physical examination findings for lumbar disc herniation in patients with sciatica all have excellent reliability, including ipsilateral straight leg raising causing pain, contralateral straight leg raising causing pain, and ankle or great toe dorsiflexion weakness (all with κ > 0.6).

The generalist physician should evaluate an adult patient with knee discomfort for torn menisci or ligaments. The best maneuvers for demonstrating a tear in the anterior cruciate ligament is the anterior drawer or Lachman maneuver, in which the examiner detects the lack of a discrete end point as the tibia is pulled toward the examiner while the femur is stabilized. A variety of maneuvers that assess for pain, popping, or grinding along the joint line between the femur and tibia are used to evaluate for meniscal tears. As with many musculoskeletal disorders, no single finding has the accuracy of the orthopedist's examination, which factors in the history and a variety of clinical findings.

The shoulder examination is directed toward determining range of motion, maneuvers that cause discomfort, and assessment of functional disability. Hip osteoarthritis is detected by evidence of restriction of internal rotation and abduction of the affected hip. Generalist physicians often rely on radiographs to determine the need for referral to orthopedic physicians, but routine radiographs are not needed early in the course of shoulder or hip disorders. The degree of pain and disability experienced by the patient may prompt confirmation of the diagnosis and referral to evaluate for surgery.

The hands and feet may show evidence of osteoarthritis (local or as part of a systemic process) (Chapter 283), rheumatoid arthritis (Chapter 285), gout (Chapter 294), or other connective tissue diseases. In addition to regional musculoskeletal disorders, such as carpal tunnel syndrome, a variety of medical and neurologic conditions should prompt routine examination of the distal ends of the extremities to prevent complications (e.g., diabetes [neuropathy or ulcers] or hereditary sensorimotor neuropathy [claw toe deformity]).

Skin

The skin should be examined systematically under good lighting (Chapter 462). It is best to ask the patient to point out any spots on the skin that concern them. Examiner agreement on some of the most important features of melanoma (asymmetry, haphazard color, border irregularity) is fair to moderate (Chapter 466). A lesion that is symmetrical, has regular borders, is only one color, is 6 mm or smaller, or has not enlarged in size is unlikely to represent a melanoma (LR 0.07). However, an increasing number of findings greatly enhances the likelihood of melanoma (LR 2.6 for two or more findings and LR 98 for the presence of all five findings) (Chapter 214).

Basal cell carcinoma and squamous cell carcinoma occur even more frequently than melanoma (Chapter 214). These lesions can be detected during routine examination by paying careful attention to sun-exposed areas of the nose, face, forearms, and hands.

Neurologic Examination

Full details of the neurologic examination are given in Chapter 418.

Psychiatric Evaluation

During the general examination, much of the psychiatric assessment (including cognition) is accomplished while eliciting the routine history and performing the review of systems (Chapter 420). Observation of the patient's mannerisms, affect, facial expression, and behavior may suggest underlying psychiatric disturbances. When a screening survey and review of systems are obtained by a questionnaire completed by the patient, the clinician should review the responses carefully to determine whether the patient exhibits symptoms of depression. Specific questioning for symptoms of depression is appropriate for all adult patients.

Genitalia and Rectum

Pelvic Examination

A complete examination should result in a description of the external genitalia, appearance of the vagina and cervix as seen through a speculum, and bimanual palpation of the uterus and ovaries (Chapters 209 and 254). The precision of the pelvic examination is uncertain. In the emergency setting there is poor agreement between resident physicians and emergency physicians on the presence of cervical motion tenderness, uterine tenderness, adnexal tenderness, and adnexal masses (κ 0.2 to 0.25) (Chapter 307). Among gynecologists, assessment of uterine size by examination correlates reasonably well with measurement by pelvic ultrasound. In asymptomatic women, 10 to 15% have some abnormality on examination, and 1.5% have abnormal ovaries. Screening for ovarian cancer is limited by the low sensitivity of the physical examination for detecting early-stage ovarian carcinoma (Chapter 209).

Male Genitalia

Examination of the male genitalia should begin with a description of whether the penis is circumcised and whether there are any visible skin lesions (e.g., ulcers or warts). Palpation should confirm the presence of bilateral testes in the scrotum. The epididymis and testes should be palpated for nodules. The low incidence of testicular carcinoma means than most nodules are benign (Chapter 210).

The prostate should be examined in all quadrants with attention focused on surface irregularities or differences in consistency throughout the prostate (Chapter 211). An estimate of prostate size may be confounded by the size of the examiner's fingers. It may be best to estimate the size of the prostate in centimeters of width and height.

Rectum

Patients can be examined while lying on their side, although this approach may place the examiner in an awkward stance (Chapters 134 and 148). The rectal examination in women can be performed as part of a bimanual examination, with the index finger in the vagina and the third finger in the rectum to permit palpation of the rectovaginal vault. Men may be asked to stand and lean over the examining table; alternatively, they may be examined while on their back with their hips and knees flexed. This latter maneuver is not used often, although it may facilitate examination of the prostate, which falls into the finger in this position.

The rectal examination begins with inspection of the perianal area for skin lesions. A well-lubricated, gloved finger is placed on the anus, and while applying gentle pressure, the examiner asks that the patient bear down as though having a bowel movement. This maneuver facilitates entry of the finger into the rectum. A normal rectal response includes tightening of the anal sphincter around the finger. The examiner should palpate circumferentially around the length of the fully inserted finger for masses. On withdrawing the gloved finger, the finger should be wiped on a stool guaiac card for fecal blood testing to assess for acute blood loss. As a screening test for colorectal carcinoma (Chapter 203), digital examination does not replace the need for testing stool samples collected by the patient (or using alternative screening strategies, such as flexible sigmoidoscopy or colonoscopy).

SUMMARIZING THE FINDINGS FOR THE PATIENT

The physician should summarize the pertinent positive and negative findings for the patient and be willing to express uncertainty to the patient, provided that it is accompanied by a plan of action (e.g., "I will reexamine you on your next visit"). The rationale for subsequent laboratory, imaging, or other tests should be explained. A plan should be established for providing further feedback and results to the patient, especially when there is a possibility that bad news may need to be delivered. Some physicians ask the patient if there is "anything else" to be covered. Patients who express additional new concerns at the end of the visit may have been fearful to address them earlier (e.g., "by the way, doctor, I'm getting a lot of chest pain"), although this does not make them any less important. When the problems seem inconsequential, however, it is acceptable to reassure the patient and offer the promise of evaluating them further in a follow-up phone call or at the next visit.

FUTURE DIRECTIONS

The common assumption that physicians' diagnostic skills are deteriorating is not supported by evidence. There is considerable evidence that the scientific approach to understanding what is worthwhile and what is not worthwhile during the clinical examination identifies a core set of skills for clinical diagnosticians. Because good patient outcomes at good value are driven primarily by the quality of the information obtained during the clinical examination, continued application of scientific principles to the history and physical examination should improve diagnostic skills.

SUGGESTED READINGS

Boulware L, Marinopoulos S, Phillips K, et al: Systematic review: The value of the periodic health evaluation. Ann Intern Med 2007;146:289–300. *Improves delivery of some recommended preventive services and may lessen patient worry.*

Society of General Internal Medicine: Website for Clinical Examination Research Groups. Available at http://www.sgim.org/clinexam.cfm. *Facilitates personal literature searches for topics on the clinical examination and a bibliography of the "Rational Clinical Examination Series" published in the* Journal of the American Medical Association.

7 APPROACH TO THE PATIENT WITH ABNORMAL VITAL SIGNS

David L. Schriger

Care of the patient is guided by integration of the chief complaint, history, vital signs, and physical examination findings (Chapter 6). Physicians should be keenly aware of a patient's vital signs but should seldom make them the centerpiece of the evaluation.

THE IMPORTANCE OF VITAL SIGNS

The importance of vital signs in medical care is a conundrum for proponents of an evidence-based approach to care of patients. No experienced physician would be willing to care for patients without them, yet a formal evaluation of the utility of vital signs for making specific diagnoses would conclude that they are not particularly useful because their likelihood ratios are too low to differentiate those who have a condition from those who do not (Chapter 6). For uncommon conditions, their predictive value is even worse. For example, the probability of tachycardia in a patient in thyroid storm is high, yet the probability of thyroid storm in a patient with isolated tachycardia is low. This application of Bayes' theorem (Chapter 9) demonstrates why there is no justification for ordering thyroid tests for every tachycardic patient and why attempts to say "When vital sign *x* is high [low], do *y*" fail. Each vital sign can be normal or abnormal in almost every acute condition (Table 7–1), and vital signs can be transiently abnormal in healthy individuals. An algorithmic approach to testing and treatment in response to abnormal vital signs would be too vague and too complex to be of use.

Predictive Value

How can it be that vital signs are poor predictors of diagnoses but central to the practice of medicine? First, although vital signs are insufficiently predictive to be of use in rigid algorithms, these algorithms are but one of several heuristics used by physicians to diagnose and to treat patients. Pattern recognition and the hypothetico-deductive model are heuristics that are based not on average tendencies of a single factor (e.g., hypotension is present in *x*% of cases of septic shock) or a small number of factors (hypotension and tachycardia are present in *y*% of cases of septic shock) but on the complex interaction of multiple factors (e.g., because this patient is an ill-appearing elderly man with an enlarged prostate and a history of urinary tract infections, is tachycardic and hypotensive, has clear lungs and an enlarged but nontender prostate, and has an oxygen saturation of 97%, he should be treated for urosepsis [Chapter 306] while awaiting results of urinalysis and urine culture).

TABLE 7–1 NORMAL AND PANIC RANGES FOR KEY VITAL SIGNS IN ADULTS*

	Normal	Panic
Temperature	36–38° C (96.8–100.4° F)	40° C (104° F)
Pulse	60 to 100 per minute	<45 per minute, >130 per minute
Respirations	12 to 20 per minute	<10 per minute, >26 per minute
Oxygen saturation	95–100%	<90%
Systolic blood pressure	90–130 mm Hg	<80 mm Hg, >200 mm Hg
Diastolic blood pressure	60–90 mm Hg	<55 mm Hg, >120 mm Hg

*Normal values are for healthy adults. Values outside these ranges are common in patients who are ill or are anxious about their health care encounter. Panic values demand the health care provider's attention in any adult patient. These values are specific (rarely present in healthy patients) but not sensitive (most ill patients' vital signs will not include panic values). All vital signs must be interpreted in the context of the patient's presentation (see text).

Thus, vital signs can play an important function in medical decision making even though their likelihood ratios are unimpressive.

Vital Signs as Symptoms

Abnormal vital signs are seldom the fundamental pathophysiologic problem. In shock (Chapter 107), hypotension and tachycardia are manifestations of pathophysiologic processes occurring at cellular and molecular levels. Given the circuitous links from clinical disease to fundamental pathophysiology to abnormal vital signs, it is not surprising that the relationships between the ends of the chain are not strong. Until new technologies enable direct measurement of primary pathologic processes, vital signs remain an important, albeit imperfect, proxy.

The five key vital signs are temperature, pulse, blood pressure, respiratory rate, and oxygen saturation (pulse oximetry). Pulse oximetry is included because it has become widely available in acute care settings, is noninvasive and relatively inexpensive, and provides information unique from the respiratory rate. Advocates have suggested that pain, smoking status, and weight be considered routine vital signs; although a case can be made for each, they are not considered here. Clinicians should never forget that the most important vital sign is what the patient looks like; general appearance is a sign that guides the intensity and urgency of the evaluation.

MEASURING VITAL SIGNS

Although obtaining vital signs is generally straightforward, the validity and reliability of measurement depend on proper technique and, for blood pressure and pulse oximetry, well-maintained equipment. Rectal and oral temperatures are generally accurate (Chapter 302), although oral temperatures can be falsely depressed in patients who breathe through their mouths. Axillary temperature is unreliable and should not be used. There is wide variability in the validity and reliability of measurements performed with tympanic membrane thermometers. A hypothermia thermometer is preferred in patients with suspected hypothermia, and core temperature should be measured with an esophageal, bladder, or rectal temperature sensor in patients with severe hypothermia or hyperthermia (Chapter 110).

Blood pressure must be measured with an appropriately sized cuff (Chapter 66). Automated blood pressure machines occasionally provide spurious results, and questionable values should be confirmed by manual auscultation and by checking other limbs. Pulse is best obtained by palpation because this technique provides the opportunity to assess regularity and contour; the pulse should be counted for sufficient time for an accurate rate to be obtained (at least 15 seconds). High heart rates on the readout of a cardiac monitor must be confirmed by palpation because these monitors can spuriously count large P waves, T waves, or pacemaker spikes as R waves, thereby reporting a heart rate double the actual rate. Orthostatic vital signs—the comparison of blood pressure and pulse in the supine, sitting, and standing positions—are advocated by some but have proved to be insensitive and nonspecific for hypovolemia.

Because the typical respiratory rate is between 12 and 20 and because there is considerable breath to breath variation, the respiratory rate should be assessed for at least 30 seconds and preferably 1 minute. Oxygen saturation is dependent on technology, so an understanding of the idiosyncrasies of the device being used is critical; valid measurements are unlikely unless there is good correlation of the machine's pulse reading and the patient's pulse. The probe should be placed on a part of the body that is warm and well perfused. Pulse oximeters compare the absorption of light at two wavelengths, so readings may be spuriously high under conditions that change the color of oxygenated or deoxygenated hemoglobin, including carbon monoxide poisoning (Chapter 94), methemoglobinemia (Chapter 168), and some of the less common hemoglobinopathies.

THE ROLE OF VITAL SIGNS IN MANAGEMENT OF THE PATIENT

Abnormal vital signs should be remeasured. Certain abnormalities require prompt evaluation (Table 7–2). Other vital sign abnormalities should be rechecked in the future unless they have been previously noted, in which case a work-up can be initiated, guided by the patient's past history and physical examination findings. It is critical that the physician always "treat the patient, not the vital signs."

TABLE 7–2 ABNORMALITIES REQUIRING RAPID EVALUATION IN THE ASYMPTOMATIC PATIENT

An irregularly irregular rapid pulse (if it is not known to be chronic) should trigger an evaluation of the patient's rhythm so that atrial fibrillation can be identified, evaluated, and treated (Chapter 63), thereby decreasing the patient's risk of stroke.

A heart rate above 130 warrants an electrocardiogram to determine the patient's rhythm and a consideration of the differential diagnosis of tachycardia (anemia and thyroid disease in particular).

A markedly elevated diastolic blood pressure (e.g., >115 mm Hg) should stimulate an evaluation for hypertensive urgencies (Chapter 66). Note that hypertension in the absence of signs of acute end-organ damage does not require acute treatment, which can reduce intracranial perfusion pressure and cause stroke. Patients with elevated blood pressure should be offered the standard evaluation and treatment for chronic hypertension (Chapter 66).

Markedly low pulse or blood pressure in patients receiving cardioactive medications should lead to a confirmation that the patient is truly asymptomatic, an inquiry into the dosing of these medications, and a reconsideration of the regimen. Markedly low pulse in elderly patients who are not receiving rate-controlling drugs should trigger an evaluation of the patient's cardiac conduction system.

Oxygen saturation below 93% in the absence of known pulmonary problems should prompt an evaluation of the patient's pulmonary status.

Patients without Systemic Complaints

In patients presenting for a routine evaluation or nonsystemic complaint (e.g., knee pain), an abnormal vital sign will seldom be the harbinger of acute illness. Most commonly, it will be a false reading or a transient finding due to random variation or anxiety that requires no evaluation or treatment and can be rechecked in the future. On occasion, it will be the only or most apparent manifestation of a chronic condition or risk factor. The measurement of an elevated blood pressure leading to a diagnosis of hypertension is the classic example of the value of vital signs in such patients.

Patients Who Complain of Systemic Illness but Do Not Appear To Be Ill

Vital signs serve two additional roles in symptomatic patients who do not appear particularly ill. First, abnormalities in vital signs provide information that may suggest or support a diagnosis. The presence of elevated temperature in a patient with productive cough, shortness of breath, and localized rales and egophony supports a diagnosis of infectious pneumonia. Vital signs may also play a role in defining therapy and triage. For example, guidelines for patients with community-acquired pneumonia (Chapter 97) formally incorporate vital signs.

The second role of vital signs in the stable symptomatic patient is to provide warning that the patient is sicker than he or she appears. For example, the presence of hypotension in a well-appearing patient thought to have pyelonephritis may be an indication of sepsis or hypovolemia. However, for vital signs to be of use, the physician must be aware of them and must incorporate them explicitly into a thought process that considers the dangerous diagnoses associated with the abnormal vital sign. The physician then must decide whether the likelihood of each potentially dangerous diagnosis is high enough to warrant specific evaluation. Unfortunately, no quick or easy rules differentiate spurious abnormalities that can be ignored from those that should trigger additional testing or treatment. What can be said is that the well-trained physician who is aware of abnormal vital signs and is willing to contemplate a change in treatment or disposition in response to them is less likely to make mistakes.

A few specific points bear mention. First, for most vital signs, "normal" is relative. Blood pressure must be interpreted in the context of the patient. For example, a blood pressure of 88/64 mm Hg may be reasonable for an otherwise healthy, young 50-kg woman but should cause concern in a 90-kg middle-aged man. Similarly, a blood pressure of 128/80 mm Hg would be fine in a 60-year-old man but worrisome in a 34-week pregnant woman. Second, because vital signs are insensitive measures of disease, normal vital signs should not dissuade the physician from pursuing potentially critical diagnoses. For example, young, well-conditioned adults may maintain normal vital signs well into the course of shock.

Use of Vital Signs in Patients Who Appear To Be Ill

For some patients, abnormal vital signs are expected on the basis of their appearance and their symptoms. For patients in extremis, care should proceed according to established guidelines such as Advanced Cardiac Life Support (Chapter 62), Advanced Trauma Life Support, and algorithms for the treatment of shock (Chapters 108 and 109). For other ill-appearing patients, two processes must occur. In one, the physician, armed with knowledge of the differential diagnosis of each abnormal vital sign and the ability to take a thorough history and to perform an appropriate physical examination, narrows the list of potential diagnoses and decides which are of sufficient probability to warrant evaluation. Simultaneously, the physician considers the list of treatment options for all diagnoses associated with the abnormal vital sign and, before establishing a diagnosis, initiates those treatments for which the potential benefit of prompt administration exceeds potential harms. For example, antibiotics for febrile patients at risk for bacterial infection, hydrocortisone for hypotensive patients at risk for hypoadrenalism, and thiamine for hypothermic patients at risk for Wernicke's encephalopathy may improve outcome and are unlikely to cause harm even if the patient does not have the suspected condition. Although early presumptive treatment can be life-saving in selected patients, it should not be abused; physicians must avoid knee-jerk responses that can cause harm.

Differential Diagnosis and Treatment Options

Single Abnormal Vital Signs

Because vital signs can be abnormal in virtually any disease process, no differential diagnosis can be encyclopedic. The physician should focus initially on common diseases and diseases that require specific treatment. The thought process should begin with the chief complaint and history and then incorporate information about the vital signs and the remainder of the physical examination.

Multiple Abnormal Vital Signs

Patients who are acutely ill are likely to have several abnormal vital signs. Although certain patterns of abnormal vital signs predominate in specific conditions (e.g., hypotension, tachycardia, and hypothermia in profound sepsis), no pattern can be considered pathognomonic. The physician's goal is to work toward a diagnosis while simultaneously providing treatments whose benefits outweigh potential harms.

Fever is generally accompanied by tachycardia, with the general rule of thumb that the heart rate will increase by 10 beats per minute for every 1° C increase in temperature. The absence of tachycardia with fever is known as pulse-temperature dissociation and has been reported in typhoid fever (Chapter 329), legionnaires' disease (Chapter 335), babesiosis (Chapter 374), Q fever (Chapter 348), infection with *Rickettsia* sp (Chapter 348), malaria (Chapter 366), leptospirosis (Chapter 344), pneumonia caused by *Chlamydia* sp (Chapter 97), and viral infections such as dengue fever (Chapter 404), yellow fever (Chapter 404), and viral hemorrhagic fevers (Chapter 404), although the predictive value of this finding is unknown.

Much can be learned by comparing the respiratory rate with pulse oximetry. Hyperventilation in the presence of high oxygen saturation suggests a central nervous system process or metabolic acidosis rather than a cardiopulmonary process. Low respiratory rates in the presence of low levels of oxygen saturation suggest central hypoventilation, which may respond to narcotic antagonists.

Hypertension and bradycardia in the obtunded or comatose patient is known as the Cushing reflex, a relatively late sign of elevated intracranial pressure. The goal is diagnosis and treatment of the patient before the Cushing reflex develops.

Approach to Abnormalities of Specific Vital Signs

Elevated Temperature

Normal temperature is often cited as 37°C (98.6°F), but there is considerable diurnal variation and variation among individuals, so 38°C is the most commonly cited threshold for fever. Fever thought to be due to infection should be treated with antipyretics and appropriate antimicrobials (Chapter 302). The importance of early administration of antibiotics to potentially septic patients cannot be overstated (Chapters 109 and 302). Hyperthermia (temperature above 40°C) should be treated with cooling measures such as ice packs, cool misting in front of fans, cold gastric lavage, and, for medication-related syndromes, medications such as dantrolene (Chapter 110). Most hospital anesthesia departments will have a designated kit for the treatment of malignant hyperthermia (Chapters 458 and 460).

Low Temperature

The treatment of hypothermia is guided by its cause (Chapter 110). The body's temperature decreases when heat loss exceeds heat production. Every logically possible mechanism for this phenomenon has been observed. Decreased heat production can result from endocrine hypofunction (e.g., Addison's disease [Chapter 245], hypopituitarism [Chapter 242], hypothyroidism [Chapter 244]) and loss of the ability to shiver (e.g., drug-induced or neurologic paralysis or neuromuscular disorders). Malfunction of the hypothalamic regulatory system can be due to hypoglycemia (Chapter 247) and a variety of central nervous system disorders (Wernicke's encephalopathy [Chapter 443], stroke [Chapter 431], tumor [Chapter 199], and trauma [Chapter 422]). Resetting of the temperature set point can occur with sepsis. Increased heat loss can be due to exposure, behavioral and physical disorders that prevent the patient from sensing or responding to cold, skin disorders that decrease its ability to retain heat, and vasodilators (including ethanol). A careful history and physical examination should illuminate which of these possibilities is most likely.

Several considerations are worthy of emphasis. The spine of an obtunded hypothermic patient who is "found down" must be protected and evaluated because paralysis from a fall may have prevented the patient from seeking shelter and may have diminished the ability to produce heat. The physician should not forget to administer antibiotics to patients who may be septic (Chapter 109), thiamine to those who may have Wernicke's encephalopathy (Chapter 443), hydrocortisone to those who may be hypoadrenal (Chapter 245), and thyroid hormone to those who may have myxedema coma (Chapter 244). Severely hypothermic patients should be treated gently because any stimulation may trigger ventricular dysrhythmias; even in the absence of pulses, cardiopulmonary resuscitation should be used only in patients with ventricular fibrillation or asystole (Chapter 110).

Elevated Heart Rate

The rate, rhythm, and electrocardiogram differentiate sinus tachycardia from tachyarrhythmias (Chapters 61 to 64). Tachyarrhythmias can be instigated by conditions that may require specific treatment (e.g., sepsis [Chapter 109], electrolyte disorders [Chapters 117, 118, and 119], endocrine disorders [Chapters 240 and 241], and poisonings [Chapters 20 and 111]) before the arrhythmia is likely to resolve. For sinus tachycardia, treatment of the underlying cause is always paramount. Treatments may include antipyretics (for fever); anxiolytics; oral or intravenous fluids (for hypovolemia); nitrates, angiotensin-converting enzyme inhibitors, and diuretics (for heart failure and fluid overload [Chapter 58]); oxygen (for hypoxemia); α-blockers (for stimulant overdose); β-blockers (for acute coronary syndromes [Chapters 71 and 72] or thyroid storm [Chapter 244]); and anticoagulation (for pulmonary embolism [Chapter 99]). Tachycardia is often an appropriate response to a clinical condition and should not be treated routinely unless it is causing or is likely to cause secondary problems.

Low Pulse

Bradycardia can be physiologic (athletes and others with increased vagal tone), due to prescribed cardiac medications (e.g., β-blockers, calcium-channel blockers, digoxin), overdoses (e.g., cholinergics, negative inotropes), disease of the cardiac conducting system, electrolyte abnormalities (severe hyperkalemia), and inferior wall myocardial infarction (Chapters 63 and 72). Asymptomatic patients do not require immediate treatment. The goal of therapy is to produce a heart rate sufficient to perfuse the tissues and alleviate the symptoms (Chapter 62). Overdoses should be treated with specific antidotes (Chapter 111). Endocrine disorders should be treated with replacement therapy. In patients with acute coronary syndrome (Chapter 71), the goal is to restore perfusion and alleviate the ischemia. Patients with profound bradycardia or hypotension may require chronotropic drugs to increase perfusion even if they may increase myocardial oxygen demand. In normotensive patients with milder bradycardia, chronotropic agents should be used only if symptoms and ischemia cannot be resolved by other means. Atropine is the primary therapy for bradycardia; isoproterenol and cardiac pacing are reserved for those who do not respond (Chapter 62).

Elevated Blood Pressure

Elevated blood pressure does not require acute treatment in the absence of symptoms or signs of end-organ damage (Chapter 66). In patients whose blood pressure is markedly above their baseline, the history and physical examination should assess for the conditions that define "hypertensive emergency": evidence of encephalopathy, intracranial hemorrhage, ischemic stroke, heart failure, pulmonary edema, acute coronary syndrome, aortic dissection, renal failure, and preeclampsia. In the absence of these conditions, treatment should consist of restarting or adjusting the medications of patients with known hypertension and initiating a program of blood pressure checks and appropriate evaluation for those with no prior history of hypertension (Chapter 66).

The patient with a true hypertensive emergency should be treated with agents appropriate for the specific condition. Because rapid decreases in blood pressure can be as deleterious as the hypertensive state itself, intravenous agents with short half-lives, such as nitroprusside, labetalol, nitroglycerin, and esmolol, are preferred (Chapter 66).

Low Blood Pressure

Low blood pressure must be evaluated in the context of the patient's symptoms, general appearance, and physical examination findings. Treatment depends on context. The same blood pressure value may necessitate intravenous inotropic agents in one patient and no treatment in another.

In tachycardic hypotensive patients, the physician must rapidly integrate all available evidence to determine the patient's volume state, cardiac function, vascular capacitance, and primary etiology (Chapter 107). Not all patients with hypotension and tachycardia are in shock, and not all patients in shock will have hypotension and tachycardia. Patients in shock should be treated on the basis of the cause (Chapters 107 to 109).

Symptomatic hypotensive patients thought to be intravascularly volume depleted should receive intravenous fluid resuscitation with crystalloid or blood, depending on their hemoglobin level (Chapter 107). In patients with known heart disease, patients who are frail or elderly, and patients whose volume status is uncertain, small boluses of fluid (e.g., 250 mL of normal saline), each followed by reassessment, are critical to avoid precipitating heart failure. Inotropic support should be reserved for patients who do not respond to fluid resuscitation. High-output heart failure should be kept in mind in patients with possible thyroid storm or stimulant overdose.

Increased Respiratory Rate

Tachypnea is a normal response to hypoxemia (see later). Treatment of tachypnea in the absence of hypoxemia is directed at the underlying cause, which often is pain (Chapter 28). Anxiolytics (e.g., diazepam, 5 to 10 mg PO or IV; lorazepam, 1 to 2 mg PO, IM, or IV) or reassurance can calm patients with behavioral causes of hyperventilation. Breathing into a paper bag has been shown to be an ineffective treatment. Pulmonary embolism (Chapter 99) does not necessarily reduce the oxygen saturation or cause a low Po_2 and should always be considered in at-risk patients with unexplained tachypnea.

Decreased Respiratory Rate

Any perturbation of the respiratory center in the central nervous system can slow the respiratory drive (Chapter 86). Narcotics and other sedatives and neurologic conditions are common causes of a decreased respiratory rate. The primary treatment of apnea is mechanical ventilation (Chapter 106), but narcotic antagonists can be tried in patients with a history or physical examination findings (miosis, track marks, opiate patch) suggestive of narcotic use or abuse (Chapter 32). In nonapneic patients, mechanical ventilation is indicated for patients who are breathing too slowly to maintain an acceptable oxygen saturation and for patients who are retaining carbon dioxide in quantities sufficient to depress mental function. Patients who are unable to protect their airway should be intubated. Oxygen should be administered to all hypopneic patients who are hypoxemic (see earlier). Patients with chronic hypoventilation (Chapter 85) may have retained HCO_3^- to compensate for an elevated Pco_2 and so may depend on hypoxia to maintain respiratory drive; in these patients, overaggressive administration of oxygen can decrease the respiratory rate, increase the Pco_2, and increase obtundation (Chapter 105).

Decreased Oxygen Saturation

In hypopneic patients, initial efforts should try to increase the respiratory rate (see earlier) and tidal volume. Regardless of etiology, oxygen, in amounts adequate to restore adequate oxygen saturation ($Po_2 > 60$ mm Hg, oxygen saturation >90%), is the mainstay of therapy. When oxygen alone fails, noninvasive methods for improving ventilation or tracheal intubation are required (Chapter 105). Oxygen should increase the Po_2 in all patients except those who have severe right-to-left shunting (Chapter 68). Treatment of conditions that cause hypoxemia includes antibiotics (pneumonia), bronchodilators (asthma, chronic obstructive pulmonary disease), diuretics and vasodilators (pulmonary edema), anticoagulants (pulmonary embolism), hyperbaric oxygen (carbon monoxide poisoning), methylene blue (methemoglobinemia, sulfhemoglobinemia), and transfusion (anemia).

SUGGESTED READINGS

Cooper RJ, Schriger DL, Flaherty HL, et al: Effect of vital signs on triage decisions. Ann Emerg Med 2002;39:223–232. *How vital signs modified nurse triage decisions in 14,285 emergency department patients.*

Nurmi J, Harjola VP, Nolan J, et al: Observations and warning signs prior to cardiac arrest. Should a medical emergency team intervene earlier? Acta Anesthesiol Scand 2005;49:702–706. *Significant deterioration typically precedes arrest by an average of 3.8 hours and provides a window of therapeutic opportunity.*

8 STATISTICAL INTERPRETATION OF DATA

Thomas B. Newman and Charles E. McCulloch

ROLE AND LIMITATIONS OF STATISTICS

Much of medicine is inherently probabilistic. Not everyone with hypercholesterolemia who is treated with a statin is prevented from having a myocardial infarction, and not everyone not treated does have one, but statins reduce the *probability* of a myocardial infarction in such patients. Because so much of medicine is based on probabilities, studies must be performed on *groups* of people to estimate these probabilities. Three component tasks of statistics are (1) selecting a sample of subjects for study, (2) describing the data from that sample, and (3) drawing inferences from that sample to a larger population of interest.

SAMPLING: SELECTING SUBJECTS FOR A STUDY

The goal of research is to produce generalizable knowledge, so that measurements made by researchers on samples of individuals will eventually help draw inferences to a larger group of people than were studied. The ability to draw such inferences depends on how the subjects for the study (the sample) were selected. To understand the process of selection, it is helpful to begin by identifying the group to which the results are to be generalized and then work backward to the sample of subjects to be studied.

Target Population

The *target population* is the population to which it is hoped the results of the study will be generalizable. For example, to study the efficacy of a new drug to treat obesity, the target population might be all people with a certain level of obesity (e.g., body mass index [BMI] of ≥30 kg/m^2) who might be candidates for the drug.

Sampling

The *intended sample* is the group of people who are eligible to be in the study based on meeting *inclusion criteria,* which specify the demographic, clinical, and temporal characteristics of the intended subjects, and the group of people not meeting *exclusion criteria,* which specify the characteristics of subjects whom the investigator does not wish to study. For example, for a study of obesity, the intended sample (inclusion criteria) might be men and women 18 years or older who live in one of four metropolitan areas, who have a BMI of 30 kg/m^2 or higher, and who have failed an attempt at weight loss with a standard diet. Exclusion criteria might include an inability to speak English or Spanish, known alcohol abuse, plans to leave the area in the next 6 months, and women who are pregnant or planning to become pregnant in the next 6 months.

In some cases, particularly large population health surveys such as the National Health and Nutrition Examination Survey (NHANES), the intended sample is a *random* sample of the target population. A *simple random sample* is a sample in which every member of the target population has a known and equal chance of being selected. Simple random samples are the easiest to handle statistically but are often impractical. For example, if the target population is the entire population of the United States (as is the case for NHANES), a simple random sample would include subjects from all over the country. Getting subjects from thousands of distinct geographic areas to examination sites would be logistically difficult. An alternative, which is used in NHANES, is *cluster* sampling, in which investigators take a random sample of "clusters" (e.g., specific census tracts or geographic areas) and then try to study all or a simple random sample of the subjects in each cluster. Knowledge of the cluster sampling process is then used during analysis of the study (see later) to draw inferences correctly back to the target population.

Regardless of the method used to select the intended sample, the *actual sample* will almost always differ in important ways because not all intended subjects will be willing to enroll in the study and not all who begin a study will complete it. In a study on treatment of obesity, for example, those who consent to be in the study probably differ in important, but difficult-to-quantify ways from those who do not (and may be more likely to do well with treatment). Furthermore, subjects who respond poorly to treatment may drop out, thus making the group that completes the study even less representative.

Statistical methods address only some of the issues involved in making inferences from a sample to a target population. Specifically, the vast majority of *statistical methods address only the effect of random variation on the inference from the intended sample to the target population.* Estimating the effects of differences between the intended sample and the actual sample depends on the quantities being estimated and content knowledge about whether factors associated with being in the actual sample are related to those quantities. One rule of thumb about generalizability is that *associations between variables* are more often generalizable than measurements of single variables are. For instance, subjects who consent to be in a study of obesity may be more motivated than average, but this motivation would be expected to have less effect on the *difference* in weight loss between groups than on the average weight loss in either group.

DESCRIBING THE SAMPLE

Types of Variables

A key use of statistics is to describe sample data. Methods of description depend on the *type of variable* (Table 8–1). *Categorical* variables consist of named characteristics, whereas *numerical* variables describe the data with numbers. Categorical variables can be further divided into *dichotomous* variables, which can take on only two possible values (e.g., alive/dead); *nominal* variables, which can take on more than two values but have no intrinsic ordering (e.g., race); and *ordinal* variables, which have more than two values and an intrinsic ordering of the values (e.g., tumor stage). *Numerical* variables include *count* variables (e.g., the number of times a woman has been pregnant), *continuous* variables (those that have a wide range of possible values), and *time-to-event* variables (e.g., the time from initial treatment to recurrence of breast cancer). Numerical variables are also ordinal by nature and can be made binary by breaking the values into two disjointed categories (e.g., systolic blood

TABLE 8–1 TYPES OF VARIABLES AND COMMONLY USED STATISTICAL METHODS

		Associated Statistical Methods	
Type of Variable	**Examples**	**Bivariate**	**Multivariate**
Categorical (dichotomous)	Alive; readmission to the hospital within 30 days	2 × 2 table, chi-square analysis	Logistic regression
Categorical (nominal)	Race; cancer, tumor type	Chi-square analysis	Nominal logistic regression
Categorical (ordinal)	Glasgow Coma Scale	Mann-Whitney-Wilcoxon, Kruskal-Wallis	Ordinal logistic regression
Numerical (continuous)	Cholesterol; SF-36 scales*	*t* test, analysis of variance	Linear regression
Numerical (count)	Number of times pregnant; number of mental health visits in a year	Mann-Whitney-Wilcoxon, Kruskal-Wallis	Poisson regression, generalized linear models
Time to event	Time to breast cancer; time to viral rebound in HIV-positive subjects	Log-rank	Cox proportional hazards regression

*Numerical scores with many values are often treated as though they were continuous. HIV = human immunodeficiency virus; SF-36 = short form 36-item health survey.

pressure >140 mm Hg or not), and thus sometimes methods designed for ordinal or binary data are used with numerical variable types, either for freedom from restrictive assumptions or for ease of interpretation.

Univariate Statistics for Continuous Variables: The "Normal" Distribution

When describing data in a sample, it is a good idea to begin with *univariate* (one variable at a time) statistics. For continuous variables, univariate statistics typically measure *central tendency* and *variability.* The most common measures of central tendency are the *mean* (or average, i.e., the sum of the observations divided by the number of observations) and the *median* (the 50th percentile, i.e., the value that has equal numbers of observations above and below it).

One of the most commonly used measures of variability is the *standard deviation* (SD). SD is defined as the square root of the *variance,* which is calculated by subtracting each value in the sample from the mean, squaring that difference, totaling all of the squared differences, and dividing by the number of observations minus 1. Although this definition is far from intuitive, the SD has some useful mathematical properties, namely, that if the distribution of the variable is the familiar bell-shaped, "normal," or "gaussian" distribution, about 68% of the observations will be within 1 SD of the mean, about 95% within 2 SD, and about 99.7% within 3 SD. Even when the distribution is not normal, these rules are often approximately true.

For variables that are not normally distributed, the mean and SD are not as useful for summarizing the data. In that case, the median may be a better measure of central tendency because it is not influenced by observations far below or far above the center. Similarly, the range and pairs of percentiles, such as the 25th and 75th percentiles or the 15th and 85th percentiles, will provide a better description of the spread of the data than the SD will. The 15th and 85th percentiles are particularly attractive because they correspond, in the gaussian distribution, to about −1 and +1 SD from the mean, thus making reporting of the 50th, 15th, and 85th percentiles roughly equivalent to reporting the mean and SD.

Univariate Statistics for Categorical Variables: Proportions, Rates, and Ratios

For categorical variables, the main univariate statistic is the *proportion* of subjects with each value of the variable, a calculation that captures both central tendency and variability. For dichotomous variables, only one proportion is needed (e.g., the proportion female); for nominal variables and ordinal variables with few categories, the proportion in each group can be provided. Ordinal variables with many categories can be summarized by using proportions or by using medians and percentiles, as with continuous data that are not normally distributed.

It is worth distinguishing between *proportions, rates,* and *ratios* because these terms are often confused. *Proportions* are unitless, always between 0 and 1 inclusive, and express what fraction of the subjects have or develop a particular characteristic or outcome. Strictly speaking, *rates* have units of inverse time; they express the proportion of subjects in whom a particular characteristic or outcome develops over a specific time period. The term is frequently misused, however. For example, the term "false-positive rate" is widely used for the proportion of subjects without a disease who test positive, even though it is a proportion, not a rate. *Ratios* are the quotients of two numbers; they can range between zero and infinity. For example, the male-to-female ratio of people with a disease might be 3 : 1. As a rule, if a ratio can be expressed as a proportion instead (e.g., 75% male), it is more concise and easier to understand.

Incidence and Prevalence

Two terms commonly used (and misused) in medicine and public health are *incidence* and *prevalence. Incidence* is the number of subjects who *contract* a disease *over time* divided by the population at risk. Incidence is usually expressed as a rate (e.g., 7 per 1000 per year), but it may sometimes be a proportion if the time variable is otherwise understood or clear, as in the lifetime incidence of breast cancer or the incidence of diabetes during pregnancy. *Prevalence* is the number who *have* a disease at *one point in time* divided by the population at risk; it is always a proportion. At any point in time, the prevalence of disease depends on how many people contract it and how long it lasts: prevalence = incidence × duration.

Bivariate Statistics

Bivariate statistics summarize the relationship between two variables. In clinical research, it is often desirable to distinguish between *predictor* and *outcome variables.* Predictor variables include treatments received, demographic variables, and test results that are thought possibly to predict or cause the *outcome variable,* which is the disease or (generally bad) event or outcome that the test should predict or treatment prevent. For example, to see whether a bone mineral density measurement (the predictor) predicts time to vertebral fracture (the outcome), the choice of bivariate statistic to assess the association of outcome with predictor depends on the types of predictor and outcome variables being compared.

Dichotomous Predictor and Outcome Variables

A common and straightforward case is when both predictor and outcome variables are dichotomous and the results can thus be summarized in a 2 × 2 table. Bivariate statistics are also called "measures of association" (Table 8–2).

TABLE 8–2 COMMONLY USED MEASURES OF ASSOCIATION FOR DICHOTOMOUS PREDICTOR AND OUTCOME VARIABLES*

	Outcome		
Predictor	**Yes**	**No**	**Total**
Yes	a	b	a + b
No	c	d	c + d
Total	a + c	b + d	N
Risk ratio or relative risk (RR)	$\frac{a/(a+b)}{c/(c+d)}$		
Relative risk reduction (RRR)	1 − RR		
Risk difference or absolute risk reduction (ARR)	a/(a + b) − c/(c + d)		
Number needed to treat (NNT)	1/ARR		
Odds ratio (OR)	ad/bc		

*The numbers of subjects in each of the cells are represented by a, b, c, and d. Case-control studies allow calculation of only the odds ratio.

Relative Risk

The *relative risk* or *risk ratio* (RR) is the ratio of the proportion of subjects in one group in whom the outcome develops divided by the proportion in the other group in whom it develops. It is a general (but not universal) convention to have the outcome be something bad and to have the numerator be the risk for those who have a particular factor or were exposed to an intervention. When this convention is followed, an RR greater than 1 means that exposure to the factor was bad for the patient (with respect to the outcome being studied), whereas an RR less than 1 means that it was good. That is, risk factors that cause diseases will have RR values greater than 1, and effective treatments will have an RR less than 1. For example, in the Women's Health Initiative (WHI) randomized trial, conjugated equine estrogen use was associated with an increased risk for stroke (RR = 1.37) and decreased risk for hip fracture (RR = 0.61). 1

Relative Risk Reduction

The *relative risk reduction* (RRR) is 1 − RR. The RRR is generally used only for effective interventions, that is, interventions in which the RR is less than 1, so the RRR is generally greater than 0. In the aforementioned WHI example, estrogen had an RR of 0.61 for hip fracture, so the RRR would be 1 − 0.61 = 0.39, or 39%. The RRR is commonly expressed as a percentage.

Absolute Risk Reduction

The *risk difference* or *absolute risk reduction* (ARR) is the difference in risk between the groups, defined as earlier. In the WHI, the risk for hip fracture was 0.11% per year with estrogen and 0.17% per year with placebo. Again, conventionally the risk is for something bad and the risk in the group of interest is subtracted from the risk in a comparison group, so the ARR will be positive for effective interventions. In this case, the ARR = 0.06% per year, or 6 in 10,000 per year.

Number Needed to Treat

The *number needed to treat* (NNT) is 1/ARR. To see why this is the case, consider the WHI placebo group and imagine treating 10,000 patients for a year. All but 17 would not have had a hip fracture anyway because the fracture rate was 0.17% per year, and 11 subjects would sustain a fracture despite treatment because the fracture rate in the estrogen group was 0.11% per year. Thus, with treatment of 10,000 patients for a year, 17 − 11 = 6 fractures are prevented, or 1 fracture is prevented for each 1667 patients treated. This calculation is equivalent to 1/0.06% per year.

Risk Difference

When the treatment *increases* the risk for a bad outcome, the difference in risk between treated and untreated patients should still be calculated, but it is usually just called the risk difference rather than an ARR (because the "reduction" would be negative). In that case, the NNT is sometimes called the number needed to harm. This term is a bit of a misnomer. The reciprocal of the risk difference is still a number needed to treat; it is just a number needed to treat per person harmed rather than a number needed to treat per person who benefits. In the WHI, treatment with estrogens was estimated to cause about 12 additional strokes per 10,000 women per year, so the number needed to be treated for 1 year to cause a stroke was about 10,000/12, or 833.

Odds Ratio

Another commonly used measure of association is the *odds ratio* (OR). The OR is the ratio of the *odds* of the outcome in the two groups, where the definition of the odds of an outcome is $p/(1 - p)$, with p being the probability of the outcome. From this definition it is apparent that when p is very small, $1 - p$ will be close to 1, so $p/(1 - p)$ will be close to p and the OR will closely approximate the RR. In the WHI, the ORs for stroke (1.37) and fracture (0.61) were virtually identical to the RRs because both stroke and fracture were rare. When p is not small, however, the odds and probability will be quite different, and ORs and RRs will not be interchangeable.

Absolute Versus Relative Measures

RRRs are usually more generalizable than ARRs. For example, the use of statin drugs is associated with about a 30% decrease in coronary events in a wide variety of patient populations (Chapter 217). The ARR, however, will usually vary with the baseline risk, that is, the risk for a coronary event in the absence of treatment. For high-risk men who have already had a myocardial infarction, the baseline 5-year risk might be 20%, which could be reduced to 14% with treatment, an ARR of 6% and an NNT of about 17 for approximately 5 years. Conversely, for a 45-year-old woman with a high low-density lipoprotein cholesterol level but no history of heart disease, in whom the 5-year risk might be closer to 1%, the same RRR would give a 0.7% risk with treatment, a risk difference of 0.3% and an NNT of 333 for 5 years.

The choice of *absolute* versus *relative measures* of association depends on the use of the measure. As noted earlier, RRs are more useful as summary measures of effect because they are more often generalizable across a wide variety of populations. RRs are also more helpful for understanding causality. However, absolute risks are more important for questions about clinical decision making because they relate directly to the tradeoffs between risks and benefits—specifically, the NNT, as well as the costs and side effects that need to be balanced against potential benefits. RRRs are often used in advertising because they are generally more impressive than ARRs. Unfortunately, the distinction between relative and absolute risks may not be appreciated by clinicians, thereby leading to higher estimates of the potential benefits of treatments when RRs or RRRs are used.

Risk Ratios Versus Odds Ratios

The choice between RRs and ORs is easier: RRs are to be preferred because they are easier to understand. Because ORs that are not equal to 1 are always farther from 1 than the corresponding RR, they may falsely inflate the perceived importance of a factor. ORs are, however, typically used in two circumstances. First, in case-control studies (Chapter 10), in which subjects with and without the disease are sampled separately, the RR cannot be calculated directly. This situation does not usually cause a problem, however, because case-control studies are generally performed to assess rare outcomes, for which the OR will closely approximate the RR. Second, in observational studies that use a type of multivariate analysis called *logistic regression* (see later), use of the OR is convenient because it is the parameter that is modeled in the analysis.

Dichotomous Predictor Variable, Continuous Outcome Variable

Many outcome variables are naturally continuous rather than dichotomous. For example, in a study of a new treatment of obesity, the outcome might be change in weight or BMI. For a new diuretic, the outcome might be change in blood pressure. For a palliative treatment, the outcome might be a quality-of-life score calculated from a multi-item questionnaire. Because of the many possible values for the score, it may be analyzed as a continuous variable. In these cases, dichotomizing the outcome leads to loss of information. Instead, the *mean difference* between the two groups is an appropriate measure of the effect size.

Most measurements have units (e.g., kg, mm Hg), so differences between groups will have the same units and be meaningless without them. If the units of measurement are familiar (e.g., kg or mm Hg), the difference between groups will be meaningful without further manipulation. For measurements in unfamiliar units, such as a score on a new quality-of-life instrument, some benchmark is useful to help judge whether the difference in groups is large or small. What is typically done in that case is to express the difference in relation to the spread of values in the study, as measured by the SD. In this case, the *standardized mean difference* (SMD) is the difference between the two means divided by the SD of the measurement. It is thus expressed as the number of SDs by which the two groups are apart. To help provide a rough feel for this difference, a 1-SD difference between means (SMD = 1) would be a 15-point difference in IQ scores, a 600-g difference in birthweight, or a 40-mg/dL difference in total cholesterol levels.

Continuous Predictor Variable

When predictor variables are continuous, the investigator can either group the values into two or more categories and calculate mean differences or SMDs between the groups as discussed earlier or use a *model* to summarize the degree to which changes in the predictor variable are associated with changes in the outcome variable. Use of a model may more compactly describe the effects of interest but involves assumptions about the way the predictor and outcome variables are related. Perhaps the simplest model is to assume a linear relationship between the outcome and predictor. For example, one could assume that the relationship between systolic blood pressure (mm Hg) and salt intake (g/day) was linear over the range studied:

$$SBP_i = a + (b \times SALT_i) + \varepsilon_i$$

where SBP_i is the systolic blood pressure for study subject *i*, $SALT_i$ is that subject's salt intake, and ε_i is an error term that the model specifies must average out to zero across all of the subjects in the study. In this model, *a* is a constant, the *intercept,* and the strength of the relationship between the outcome and predictor can be summarized by the slope *b,* which has units equal to the units of SBP divided by the units of SALT, or mm Hg per gram of salt per day in this case.

Note that without the units, such a number is meaningless. For example, if salt intake were measured in grams per week instead of grams per day, the slope would only be one seventh as large. Thus, when reading an article in which the association between two variables is summarized, it is critical to note the units of the variables. As discussed earlier, when units are unfamiliar, they are sometimes standardized by dividing by the SDs of one or both variables.

It is important to keep in mind that use of a model to summarize a relationship between two variables may not be appropriate if the model does not fit. In the preceding example, the assumption is that salt intake and blood pressure have a linear relationship, with the slope equal to 1 mm Hg/g salt/day (the approximate value for hypertensives [2]). In that case, if the range of salt intake of interest is from 1 to 10 g/day, the predicted increase in blood pressure will be 1 mm Hg as a result of a 1-g/day increase in salt intake whether that increase is from 1 to 2 g/day or from 9 to 10 g/day. If the effect of a 1-g/day change in salt intake differed in subjects ingesting low- and high-salt diets, the model would not fit and misleading conclusions could result.

When the outcome variable is dichotomous, the relationship with the continuous predictor variable is often modeled with a *logistic* model:

$$\Pr\{Y_i = 1\} = \frac{1}{1+e^{-(a+bx_i)}}$$

where the outcome Y_i is coded 0 or 1 for study subject *i*, and x_i is that subject's value of the predictor variable. Once again, *a* is a constant, in this case related to the probability of the disease when the predictor is equal to zero, and *b* summarizes the strength of the association; in this case, it is the natural logarithm of the OR rather than the slope. The OR is the OR *per unit change* in the predictor variable. For example, in a study of lung cancer, an OR of 1.06 for pack years of smoking would indicate that the odds of lung cancer increase by 6% for each pack year increase in smoking.

Because the outcome variable is dichotomous, it has no units, and "standardizing" it by dividing by its SD is unnecessary and counterproductive. On the other hand, continuous predictor variables do have units, and the OR for the logistic model will be per unit change in the predictor variable or, if standardized, per SD change in the predictor variable. Re-expressing predictors in standardized or at least more sensible units is often necessary. For example, suppose 10-year mortality risk decreases by 0.8 for each increase in gross income of $10,000. The RR associated with an increase in gross income of $1 (which is what a computer program would report if the predictor were entered in dollars) would be 0.99998, apparently no effect at all because a change of $1 in gross income is negligible and associated with a negligible change in risk. To derive the coefficient associated with a $1 change, the coefficient for a $10,000 change is raised to the $^1/_{10,000}$ power: $0.8^{(1/10,000)} = 0.99998$.

Multivariable Statistics

In many cases, researchers are interested in the effects of multiple predictor variables on an outcome. Particularly in observational studies, in which investigators cannot assign values of a predictor variable experimentally, it will be of interest to estimate the effects of a predictor variable of interest *independent* of the effects of other variables. For example, in studying whether regular exercise decreases the risk for heart disease, investigators would realize that those who exercise may be different in many ways from those who do not and try to take differences in race, sex, age, cigarette smoking, blood pressure, and cholesterol into account. Trying to subdivide the data by race, sex, cigarette smoking status, blood pressure, and cholesterol would require a massive data set and raise issue of multiple testing (see later). Once again, models are generally used because they enable the information about individual predictors to be summarized by using the full data set. In this way, the estimated coefficients from the model are powerful descriptive statistics that allow a sense of the data in situations where simpler methods fail. These models are similar to those described earlier but include terms for the additional variables.

Multiple Linear Regression

The multiple linear regression model is

$$Y_i = a + (b_1 \times x_{1i}) + (b_2 \times x_{2i}) + \ldots + (b_k \times x_{ki}) + \varepsilon_i,$$

where the subscripts *1, 2, . . . , k* are for the first, second, . . . *kth* variables of the model and the *i* subscripts are for each individual. As before, the relationships between each of these predictor variables and the outcome variable are summarized by coefficients, or slopes, which have units of the units of *Y* divided by the units of the associated predictor. In addition, the linear combination of predictor variables adds a major simplifying constraint (and assumption) to the model: it specifies that the effects of each variable on the outcome variable are the same regardless of the values of other variables in the model. Thus, for example, if x_1 is the variable for salt intake and x_2 is a variable for sex (e.g., 0 for females and 1 for males), this model assumes that the average effect of a 1-g increase in daily salt intake on blood pressure is the same in men and women. If such is not believed to be the case, either based on previous information or from examining the data, the model should include *interaction* terms, or separate models should be used for men and women.

Multiple Logistic Regression

The logistic model expands to include multiple variables in much the same way as the linear model:

$$\Pr\{Y_i = 1\} = \frac{1}{1+e^{-(a+b_1x_{1i}+b_2x_{2i}+\ldots+b_{k1}x_{ki})}}$$

Again, the additional assumption when more than one predictor is included in the model is that in the absence of included interaction terms, the effect of each variable on the odds of the outcome is the same regardless of the values of other variables in the model. Because the logistic model is multiplicative, however, the effects of different predictors on the odds of the outcome are multiplied, not added. Thus, for example, if male sex is associated with a doubling of the odds for heart disease, this doubling will occur in both smokers and nonsmokers; if smoking triples the odds, this tripling will be true in both men and women, so smoking men would be predicted to have 2 × 3 = 6 times higher odds of heart disease than nonsmoking women.

Recursive Partitioning

Recursive partitioning, or "*classification and regression trees,*" which is a prediction method often used with dichotomous outcomes, avoids the use of linear combinations of the predictors and the assumptions of linearity. This technique creates prediction rules by repeatedly dividing the sample into subgroups, with each subdivision being formed by separating the sample on the value of one of the predictor variables. The optimal choice of variables and cut points may depend on the relative costs of false-positive and false-negative predictions, as set by the investigator. The end result is a treelike structure in which each final branch provides a yes/no prediction of the outcome. The methods of fitting the tree to data (e.g., cross-validation) help reduce overfitting (inclusion of unnecessary predictor variables), especially in cases with many potential predictors.

Proportional Hazards (Cox) Model

A multivariate model often used in studies in which subjects are monitored over time for development of the outcome is the *Cox* or *proportional hazards* model. Like the logistic model, the Cox model is used for continuous or dichotomous predictor variables, but in this case with a time-to-event outcome (e.g., time to a stroke). This approach models the *rate* at which the outcome occurs over time by taking into account the number of people still at risk at any given time. The coefficients in the Cox model are logarithms of *hazard ratios* rather than ORs, interpretable (when exponentiated) as the effect of a unit change in predictors on the *hazard* (risk in the next short time period) of the outcome developing. Like the logistic model, the Cox model is multiplicative; that is, it assumes that changes in risk factors multiply the hazard by a fixed amount regardless of the levels of other risk factors. A key feature of the Cox model and other *survival analysis* techniques is that they accommodate censored data (when the time to event is known only to exceed a certain value). For example, if the outcome is time to stroke, the study will end with many subjects who have not had a stroke, so their time to stroke is known only to exceed the time to their last follow-up visit.

INFERRING POPULATION VALUES FROM A SAMPLE

The next step after describing the data is drawing inferences from a sample to the population from which the sample was drawn. Statistics mainly quantify random error, which arises by chance because even a sample randomly selected from a population may not be exactly like the population from which it was drawn. Samples that were not randomly selected from populations may be unrepresentative because of *bias,* and statistics cannot help with this type of systematic (nonrandom) error.

Inferences from Sample Means: Standard Deviation versus Standard Error

The simplest case of inference from a sample to a population involves estimating a population mean from a sample mean. Intuitively, the larger the sample, the more likely that the sample mean will be close to the population mean, that is, close to the mean that would be calculated if every member of the population were studied. The more variability there is within the sample, the less accurate the estimate of the population mean is likely to be. Thus, the precision with which a population mean can be estimated is related to both the size of the sample and the SD of the sample. To make inferences about a population mean from a sample mean, the *standard error of the mean* (SEM), which equals the sample SD divided by the square root of the sample size, N, is calculated as:

$$\mathrm{SEM} = \frac{\mathrm{SD}}{\sqrt{N}}$$

To understand the meaning of the SEM, imagine that instead of taking a single sample of *N* subjects from the population, many such samples were taken. The mean of each sample could be calculated, as could the mean of those sample means and the SD of these means. The SEM is the best estimate from a single sample of what that SD of sample means would be.

Confidence Intervals

The SEM has an interpretation pertaining to means that is parallel to the SD for individual observations. Just as about 95% of *observations* in a population are expected to be within ±1.96 SD of the mean, 95% of *sample means* are expected to be within 1.96 SEM of the population mean, thereby providing the 95% confidence interval (CI), which is the range of values for the population mean consistent with what was observed from the sample.

CIs can similarly be calculated for other quantities estimated from samples, including proportions, ORs, RRs, regression coefficients, and hazard ratios. In each case, they provide a range of values for the parameter in the population consistent with what was observed in the study.

Significance Testing and *P* Values

Many papers in the medical literature include *P* values, but the meaning of *P* values is widely misunderstood and mistaught. *P* values start with calculation of a *test statistic* from the sample that has a known distribution under certain assumptions, most commonly the *null hypothesis,* which states that there is no association between variables. *P* values provide the answer to the question, "If the null hypothesis were true, what would be the probability of obtaining, by chance alone, a value of the test statistic this large or larger (suggesting an association between groups of this strength or stronger)?"

There are a number of common pitfalls in interpreting *P* values. The first is that because *P* values less than .05 are customarily described as being "statistically significant," the description of results with *P* values less than .05 sometimes gets shortened to "significant" when in fact the results may not be clinically significant (i.e., important) at all. This situation most commonly arises when studies have a large sample size and the measurement is of a continuous or frequently occurring outcome.

A second pitfall is concluding that no association exists simply because the *P* value is greater than .05. However, it is possible that a real association exists, but that it simply was not found in the study. This problem is particularly likely if the sample size is small because small studies have low *power,* defined as the probability of obtaining statistically significant results if there really is a given magnitude of difference between groups in the population. One approach to interpreting a study with a nonsignificant *P* value is to examine the power that the study had to find a difference. A better approach is to look at the 95% CI. If the 95% CI excludes all clinically significant levels of the strength of an association, the study probably had an adequate sample size to find an association if there had been one. If not, a clinically significant effect may have been missed. In "negative" studies, the use of CIs is more helpful than power analyses because CIs incorporate information from the study's results.

Finally, a common misconception about *P* values is that they indicate the probability that the null hypothesis is true (e.g., that there is no association between variables). Thus, it is not uncommon to hear or read that a *P* value less than .05 implies at least a 95% probability that the observed association is not due to chance. This statement represents a fundamental misunderstanding of *P* values. Calculation of *P* values is *based on the assumption* that the null hypothesis is true. The probability that an association is real depends not just on the probability of its occurrence under the null hypothesis but also on the probability of another basis for the association (see later)—an assessment that depends on information from outside the study, sometimes called the *prior probability* of an association (of a certain magnitude) estimated before the study results were known and requiring a different approach to statistical inference. Similarly, CIs do not take into account previous information on the probable range of the parameter being estimated.

Appropriate test statistics and methods for calculating *P* values depend on the type of variable, just as with descriptive statistics (see Table 8–1). For example, to test the hypothesis that the mean values of a continuous variable are equal in two groups, a *t* test would be used; to compare the mean values across multiple groups, analysis of variance would be used. Because there are many different ways for the null hypothesis to be false (i.e., many different ways that two variables might be associated) and many test statistics that could be calculated, there are many different ways of calculating a *P* value for the association of the same two variables in a data set, and they may not all give the same answer.

Meta-analysis

Statistical techniques for inferring population values from a sample are not restricted to samples of individuals. *Meta-analysis* is a statistical method for drawing inferences from a sample of *studies* to derive a single estimate of a treatment effect. Meta-analysis allows the formal combination of results while estimating and accommodating both the within-study and between-study variations. Meta-analysis is particularly useful when raw data from the studies are not available, as is typically the case in synthesizing information from multiple published results. For example, the previously cited estimate that a 1-g/day change in salt intake is associated with a 1–mm Hg change in blood pressure was obtained from a meta-analysis of randomized trials of low-salt diets in adults. 2

INFERRING CAUSALITY

In many cases, a goal of clinical research is not just to identify associations but to determine whether they are *causal,* that is, whether the predictor causes the outcome. Thus, if people who take vitamin E live longer than those who do not, it is important to know whether it is *because* they took the vitamin or for some other reason.

Determination of causality is based on considering alternative explanations for an association between two variables and trying to exclude or confirm these alternative explanations. The alternatives to a causal relationship between predictor and outcome variables are *chance, bias, effect-cause,* and *confounding. P* values and CIs help assess the likelihood of *chance* as the basis for an association. *Bias* occurs when systematic errors in sampling or measurements can lead to distorted estimates of an association. For example, if those making measurements of the outcome variable are not blinded to values of the predictor variable, they may measure the outcome variable differently in subjects with different values of the predictor variable.

Effect-cause is a particular problem in cross-sectional studies, in which (in contrast to longitudinal studies) all measurements are made at a single point in time, thereby precluding demonstration that the predictor variable preceded the outcome—an important part of demonstrating causality. Sometimes biology provides clear guidance about the direction of causality. For example, in a cross-sectional study relating levels of urinary cotinine (a measure of exposure to tobacco smoke) to decreases in pulmonary function, it is hard to imagine that poor pulmonary function caused people to be exposed to smoke. Conversely, sometimes inferring causality is more difficult: are people overweight because they exercise less, or do they exercise less because they are overweight (or both)?

Confounding

Confounding occurs when a third variable is associated with the predictor and is a cause of the outcome. For example, observational studies suggested that high doses of vitamin E might decrease the risk for heart disease. However, this association seems to have been largely due to confounding: people who took vitamin E were different in other ways from those who did not, including differences in factors causally related to coronary heart disease. If such factors are known and can be measured accurately, one way to reduce confounding is to *stratify* or *match* on these variables. The idea is to assemble groups of people who did and did not take vitamin E but who were similar in other ways. Multivariate analysis can accomplish the same goal—other measured variables are held constant statistically, and the effect of the variable of interest (in this case the use of vitamin E) can be examined. Multivariate analysis has the advantage that it can control simultaneously for more potentially confounding variables than can be considered with stratification or matching, but it has the disadvantage that a model must be created (see earlier) and this model may not fit the data well.

A new technique that is less dependent on model fit but still requires accurate measurements of confounding variables is the use of *propensity scores.* Propensity scores are used to assemble comparable groups in the same way as stratification or matching, but in this case the comparability is achieved on the basis of the *propensity* to be exposed to or be treated with the predictor variable of primary interest.

A major limitation of these methods of controlling for confounding is that the confounders must be known to the investigators and accurately measured. In the case of vitamin E, apparent favorable effects persisted after controlling for known confounding variables. It is for this reason that randomized trials provide the strongest evidence for causality. If the predictor variable of interest can be randomly assigned, confounding variables, both known and unknown, should be approximately equally distributed between the subjects who are and are not exposed to the predictor variable, and it is reasonable to infer that any significant differences in outcome that remain in these now comparable groups would be due to differences in the predictor variable of interest. In the case of vitamin E, a recent meta-analysis of randomized trials found no benefit whatsoever and in fact suggested harm from high doses. 3

OTHER COMMON STATISTICAL PITFALLS

Missing Data

Research on human subjects is challenging. People drop out of studies, refuse to answer questions, miss study visits, and die of diseases that are not being studied directly in the protocol. Consequently, missing or incomplete data are a fact of medical research. When the fact that data are missing is unrelated to the outcome being studied (which might be true, for example, if the files storing the data got partially corrupted), analyses using only the data present (sometimes called a complete case analysis) are unlikely to be misleading. Unfortunately, such is rarely the case. Subjects refusing to divulge family income probably have atypical values, patients not coming for scheduled visits in a study of depression may be more or less depressed, and patients in an osteoporosis study who die of heart disease probably differ in many ways from those who do not.

Whenever a sizable fraction of the data is missing (certainly if it is above 10 or 15%), there is the danger of substantial bias from an analysis that uses only the complete data. This is the gap noted earlier before between the intended and actual samples. Any study with substantial missing data should be clear about how many missing data there were and what was done to assess or alleviate the impact; otherwise, the critical consumer of such information should be suspicious. In a randomized trial, the general rule is that the primary analysis must include all subjects who were enrolled, regardless of whether they followed the study protocol, in an *intention-to-treat* analysis.

Clustered or Hierarchical Data

Data are often collected in a clustered (also called hierarchical) manner; for example, NHANES used a cluster sample survey, and a study of patient outcomes might be conducted at five hospitals, each with multiple admission teams. The cluster sample or the clustering of patients within teams within hospitals leads to correlated data. Said another way, and other things being equal, data collected on the same patient, by the same admission team, or in the same cluster are likely to be more similar than data from different patients, teams, or clusters. Failure to use statistical methods that accommodate correlated data can seriously misstate standard errors, widths of CIs, and *P* values. Unfortunately, standard errors, CIs, and *P* values can be estimated to be too small or too large when using a naïve analysis. Statistical methods for dealing with correlated data include *generalized estimating equations* and the use of *robust standard errors* and *frailty models* (for time-to-event data). Studies with obvious hierarchical structure that fail to use such methods may be in serious error.

Multiple Testing

The "multiple testing" or "multiple comparisons" issue refers to the idea that if multiple hypothesis tests are conducted, each at a significance level of .05, the chance that at least one of them will achieve a *P* value of less than .05 is considerably larger than .05, even when all the null hypotheses are true. For example, when comparing the mean value of a continuous variable across many different groups, analysis of variance is a time-tested method of performing an overall test of equality and avoiding making a large number of pairwise comparisons.

Because most medical studies collect data on a large number of variables, performing a test on each one may generate a number of false-positive results. The risk for falsely positive results is especially high with genomic studies, where a researcher may test 10,000 single-nucleotide polymorphisms for association with a disease.

A typical method for dealing with the problem of multiple testing is the *Bonferroni correction,* which requires a *P* value to be less than .05 *divided by the number of tests performed* (or even the number of tests considered). Although simple to use, a problem with this approach is that it is often difficult to decide how many tests make up the "universe" of tests. Some newer methods for genomic studies involve controlling the *false discovery rate.*

Studies with many listed or apparent outcomes or predictors (or both) are subject to inflation of the error rate to well above the nominal .05. Automated stepwise regression methods for choosing predictors in regression models typically *do not* alleviate and may exacerbate this problem. If no adjustment or method for dealing with multiple comparisons is used, the chance for a false-positive result in a study should be kept in mind.

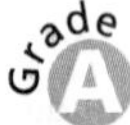

1. Anderson GL, Limacher M, Assaf AR, et al: Effects of conjugated equine estrogen in postmenopausal women with hysterectomy: The Women's Health Initiative randomized controlled trial. JAMA 2004;291:1701–1712.
2. He FJ, MacGregor GA: Effect of longer-term modest salt reduction on blood pressure. Cochrane Database Syst Rev 2004;3:CD004937.
3. Miller ER 3rd, Pastor-Barriuso R, Dalal D, et al: Meta-analysis: High-dosage vitamin E supplementation may increase all-cause mortality. Ann Intern Med 2005;142:37–46.

SUGGESTED READINGS

Hulley SB, Cummings SR, Browner WS, et al: Designing Clinical Research: An Epidemiologic Approach, 3rd ed. Philadelphia, Lippincott Williams & Wilkins, 2007. *A helpful text in which many of the epidemiologic concepts mentioned here are discussed in greater depth.*

Rothwell PM: External validity of randomised controlled trials: "To whom do the results of this trial apply?" Lancet 2005;365:82–93. *Practical issues in extrapolating results from randomized controlled trials to patients.*

Rothwell PM: Subgroup analysis in randomised controlled trials: Importance, indications, and interpretation. Lancet 2005;365:176–186. *Advantages and pitfalls of subgroup analyses.*

Thompson SG, Higgins JPT: Can meta-analysis help target interventions at individuals most likely to benefit? Lancet 2005;365:341–346. *A primer on how to interpret meta-analyses, remembering that they show only relative risk reductions whereas absolute risk reductions are more meaningful clinically.*

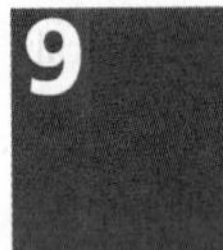

9 USING DATA FOR CLINICAL DECISIONS

Thomas H. Lee

Key functions in the professional lives of all physicians are the collection and analysis of clinical data. Decisions must be made on the basis of these data, including which therapeutic strategy is most appropriate for the patient and whether further information should be gathered before the best strategy can be chosen. This decision-making process is a blend of science and art in which the physician must synthesize a variety of concerns, including the patient's most likely outcome with various management strategies, the patient's worst possible outcome, and the patient's preferences among these strategies.

Only rarely does the physician enjoy true certainty regarding any of these issues, so a natural inclination for physicians is to seek as much information as possible before making a decision. This approach ignores the dangers inherent in the collection of information. Some of these dangers are direct, such as the risk of cerebrovascular accident associated with coronary angiography. Other dangers are indirect, such as the possibility that performance of a blood culture might lead to a contaminant result that might lead in turn to further blood cultures, unnecessary antibiotic therapy, and prolongation of hospitalization.

An additional concern is the cost of information gathering, including the direct costs of the tests themselves and the indirect costs that flow from decisions made on the basis of the test results. Standards of medical professionalism endorse the need for physicians to exert their influence to minimize inefficiency, but this challenge grows increasingly complex as medical progress leads to proliferation of alternative testing strategies.

For the physician, there are three key questions in this sequence: Should I order a test to improve my assessment of diagnosis or prognosis? Which test is best? Which therapeutic strategy is most appropriate for this patient?

SHOULD I ORDER A TEST?

The decision of whether to order a test depends on the physician's and the patient's willingness to pursue a management strategy with the current degree of uncertainty. This decision is influenced by several factors, including the patient's attitudes toward diagnostic and therapeutic interventions (e.g., a patient with claustrophobia might prefer an angiogram to magnetic resonance imaging) and the information provided by the test itself. The personal tolerance of the patient and physician for uncertainty also frequently influences test-ordering approaches. A decision to watch and wait rather than to obtain a specific test also should be considered an information-gathering alternative because the information obtained while a patient is being observed often reduces uncertainty about the diagnosis and outcome. In other words, the "test of time" should be recognized as one of the most useful tests available when this tactic does not seem inappropriately risky.

Most tests do not provide a definitive answer about diagnosis or prognosis but instead reduce uncertainty. Accordingly, the impact of information from tests often is expressed as *probabilities* (Table 9–1). A probability of 1.0 implies that an event is certain to occur, whereas a probability of 0 implies that the event is impossible. When all the possible events for a patient are assigned probabilities, these estimates should sum to 1.0.

It is often useful to use *odds* to quantify uncertainty instead of probability. Odds of 1 : 2 suggest that the likelihood of an event is only half the likelihood that the event will not occur. The relationship between odds and probability is expressed in the following formula:

$$\text{Odds} = P/(1 - P)$$

where P is the probability of an event.

Performance Characteristics

Sensitivity and *specificity* are key terms for the description of test performance. These parameters describe the test and are in theory true regardless of the population of patients to which the test is applied. Research studies that describe test performance often are based, however, on highly selected populations of patients; test performance may deteriorate when tests are applied in clinical practice. The result of a test for coronary artery disease, such as an electron beam computed tomography scan, rarely may be abnormal if it is evaluated in a low-risk population, such as high-school students. False-positive abnormal results secondary

TABLE 9–1 KEY DEFINITIONS*

Probability	A number between 0 and 1 that expresses an estimate of the likelihood of an event
Odds	The ratio of [the probability of an event] to [the probability of the event not occurring]
TEST PERFORMANCE CHARACTERISTICS	
Sensitivity	Percentage of patients with disease who have an abnormal test result
Specificity	Percentage of patients without disease who have a normal test result
Positive predictive value	Percentage of patients with an abnormal test result who have disease
Negative predictive value	Percentage of patients with a normal test result who do not have disease
BAYESIAN ANALYSIS	
Pretest (or prior) probability	The probability of a disease before the information is acquired
Post-test (or posterior) probability	The probability of a disease after new information is acquired
Pretest (or prior) odds	(Pretest probability of disease)/(1 – pretest probability of disease)
Likelihood ratio	(Probability of result in diseased persons)/(Probability of result in nondiseased persons)

**Disease* can mean a condition, such as coronary artery disease, or an outcome, such as postoperative cardiac complications.

to coronary calcification in the absence of obstructive coronary disease are common when the test is performed in middle-aged and elderly people.

Although researchers are interested in the performance of tests, the true focus of medical decision making is the patient. Physicians are more interested in the implications of a test result on the probability that a patient has a specific disease or outcome, that is, the predictive values of abnormal or normal test results. These predictive values are extremely sensitive to the population from which they are derived (Table 9–2; see also Table 9–1). An abnormal lung scan result in an asymptomatic patient has a much lower positive predictive value than that same test result in a patient with dyspnea and a diminished oxygen saturation. Bayes' theorem (see later) provides a framework for analyzing the interaction between test results and a patient's pretest probability of a disease.

As useful as the performance characteristics may be, they are limited by the fact that few tests truly provide dichotomous (i.e., positive or negative) test results. Tests such as exercise tests have several parameters (e.g., ST segment deviation, exercise duration, hemodynamic response) that provide insight into the patient's condition, and the normal range for many blood tests (e.g., prostate-specific antigen) varies markedly according to the age of the tested population and one's willingness to "miss" patients with disease. Tests that require human interpretation (e.g., radiologic studies) are particularly subject to variability in the reported results.

Bayes' Theorem

The impact of a test result on a patient's probability of disease was first quantified by Bayes, an 18th century English clergyman who developed a formula for the probability of disease in the presence of an abnormal test result. The classic presentation of Bayes' theorem is complex and difficult to use. A more simple form of this theorem is known as the *odds ratio* form, which describes the impact of a test result on the pretest odds (see Table 9–1) of a diagnosis or outcome for a specific patient.

To calculate the post-test odds of disease, the pretest odds are multiplied by the *likelihood ratio* (LR) for a specific test result. The mathematical presentation of this form of Bayes' theorem is as follows:

$$\text{Post-test odds} = (\text{Pretest odds}) \times (\text{LR})$$

The LR is the probability of a particular test result in patients with the disease divided by the probability of that same test result in patients without disease. In other words, the LR is the test result's sensitivity divided by the false-positive rate. A test of no value (e.g., flipping a coin and calling "heads" an abnormal result) would have an LR of 1.0 because half of patients with disease would have abnormal test results, as would half of patients without disease. This test would have no impact on a patient's odds of disease. The further an LR is above 1.0, the more that test result raises a patient's probability of disease. For LRs less than 1.0, the closer the LR is to 0, the more it lowers a patient's probability of disease.

When it is displayed graphically (Fig. 9–1), a test of no value (dotted line) does not change the pretest probability, whereas an abnormal or normal result from a useful test moves the probability up or down. For a patient with a high pretest probability of disease, an abnormal test result changes the patient's probability only slightly, but a normal test result leads to a marked reduction in the probability of disease. Similarly, for a patient with a low pretest probability of disease, a normal test result has

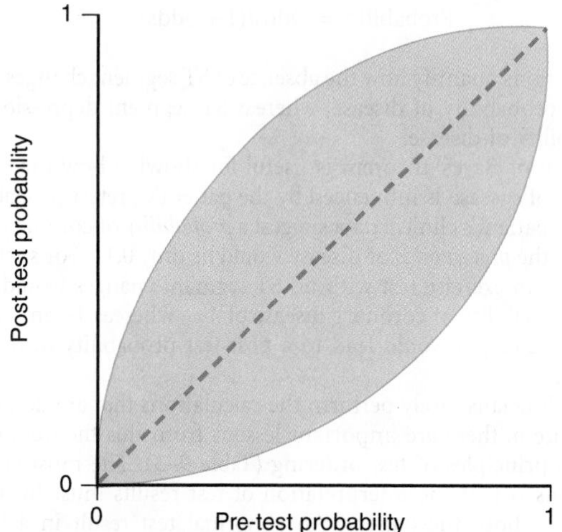

FIGURE 9–1 • Impact of various test results on the patient's probability of disease. The x axis depicts a patient's probability of disease before a test. If the test is of no value, the post-test probability (dotted line) is no different from the pretest probability. An abnormal test result raises the post-test probability of disease, as depicted by the concave downward arc, whereas a normal test result lowers the probability.

TABLE 9–2 EXAMPLE OF ODDS RATIO FORM OF BAYES' THEOREM

Question: What is the probability of coronary disease for a patient with a 50% pretest probability of coronary disease who undergoes an exercise test if that patient develops (a) no ST segment changes, (b) 1 mm of ST segment depression, or (c) 2 mm of ST segment depression?

Step 1. Calculate the pretest odds of disease:

$$P/(1 - P) = 0.5/(1 - 0.5) = 0.5/0.5 = 1$$

Step 2. Calculate the likelihood ratios for the various test results, using the formula LR = sensitivity/(1 − specificity). (Data from pooled literature.)

Test Result	Sensitivity	Specificity	Likelihood Ratio
No ST segment changes	0.34	0.15	0.4
1-mm ST segment depression	0.66	0.85	4.4
2-mm ST segment depression	0.33	0.97	11

Step 3. Calculate the post-test odds of disease and convert those odds to post-test probabilities:

Test Result	Pretest Odds	Likelihood Ratio	Post-test Odds	Post-test Probability
No ST segment changes	1	0.4	0.4	0.29
1-mm ST segment depression	1	4.4	4.4	0.81
2-mm ST segment depression	1	11	11	0.92

little impact, but an abnormal test result markedly raises the probability of disease.

Consider how various exercise test results influence a patient's probability of coronary disease (see Table 9–2). For a patient whose clinical history, physical examination, and electrocardiographic findings suggest a 50% probability of disease, the pretest odds of disease are 1.0. LRs for various test results are developed by pooling data from published literature. The sensitivity of an exercise test with any amount of ST segment changes is the rate of such test results in patients with coronary disease, and the specificity is the percentage of patients without coronary disease who do *not* have this test result. The LR for no ST change is less than 1, whereas the LRs for patients with ST changes are greater than 1 (see Table 9–2). Therefore, when the LRs for various test results are multiplied by the pretest odds to calculate post-test odds, the odds decrease for patients without ST segment changes but increase for patients with 1 or 2 mm of ST segment change. Post-test odds can be converted to post-test probabilities according to the following formula:

$$\text{Probability} = \text{Odds}/(1 + \text{odds})$$

The calculations quantify how the absence of ST segment changes reduces a patient's probability of disease, whereas ST segment depression raises the probability of disease.

This form of Bayes' theorem is useful for showing how the post-test probability of disease is influenced by the patient's pretest probability of disease. If a patient's clinical data suggest a *probability* of coronary disease of only 0.1, the *pretest odds* of disease would be only 0.11. For such a low-risk patient, an exercise test with no ST segment changes would lead to post-test probability of coronary disease of 4%, whereas 1-mm or 2-mm ST segment changes would lead to a post-test probability of disease of 33 or 55%.

Even if clinicians rarely perform the calculations that are described in Bayes' theorem, there are important lessons from this theorem that are relevant to principles of test ordering (Table 9–3). The most crucial of these lessons is that the interpretation of test results must incorporate information about the patient. An abnormal test result in a low-risk patient may not be a true indicator of disease. Similarly, a normal test result in a high-risk patient should not be taken as evidence that disease is not present.

Figure 9–2 provides an example of the post-test probabilities for positive and negative results for a test with a sensitivity of 85% and a specificity of 90% (e.g., radionuclide scintigraphy for diagnosis of coronary artery disease). In a high-risk population with a 90% prevalence of disease, the positive predictive value of an abnormal result is 0.99 compared with 0.31 for the same test result obtained in a low-risk population with a 5% prevalence of disease. Similarly, the negative predictive value of a normal test result is greater in the low-risk population than in the high-risk population.

Multiple Testing

Clinicians frequently obtain more than one test aimed at addressing the same issue and at times are confronted with conflicting results. If

TABLE 9–3 PRINCIPLES OF TEST ORDERING AND INTERPRETATION

The interpretation of test results depends on what is already known about the patient.
No test is perfect; clinicians should be familiar with their diagnostic performance (see Table 9–1) and never believe that a test "forces" them to pursue a specific management strategy.
Tests should be ordered if they may provide *additional* information beyond that already available.
Tests should be ordered if there is a reasonable chance that the data will influence the patient's care.
Two tests that provide similar information should not be ordered.
In choosing between two tests that provide similar data, use the test that has lower costs and/or causes less discomfort and inconvenience to the patient.
Clinicians should seek all of the information provided by a test, not just an abnormal or normal result.
The cost-effectiveness of strategies using noninvasive tests should be considered in a manner similar to that of therapeutic strategies.

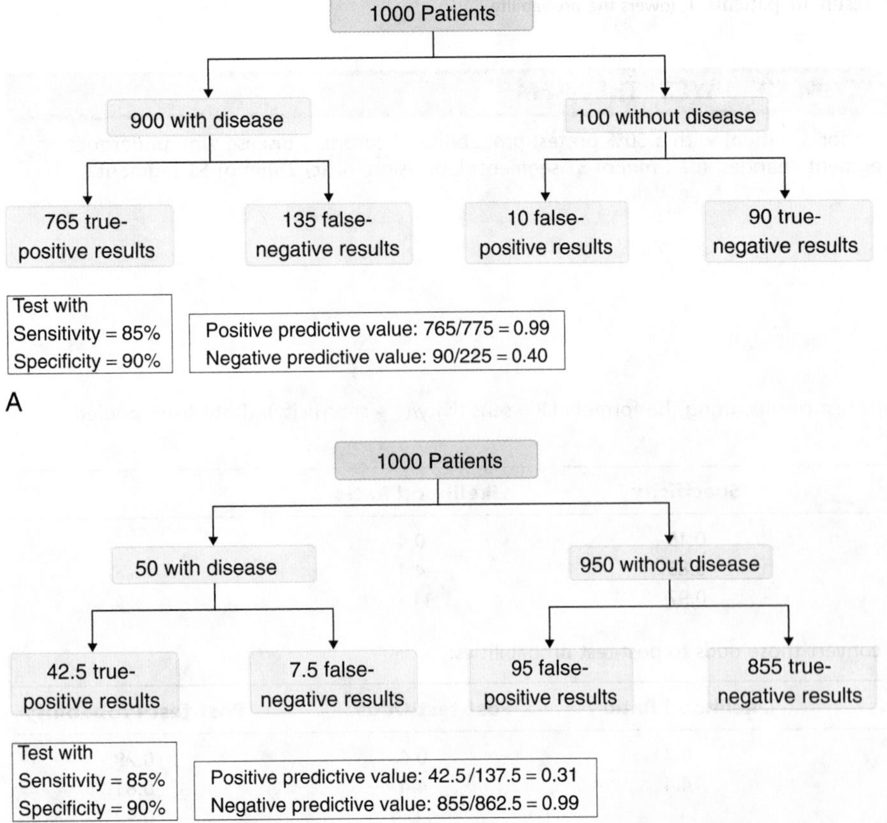

FIGURE 9–2 • Interpretation of test results in high-risk and low-risk patients. A, High-risk population (90% prevalence of disease). **B,** Low-risk population (5% prevalence of disease).

these tests are truly independent (i.e., the tests do not have the same basis in pathophysiology), it may be appropriate to use the post-test probability obtained through performance of one test as the pretest probability for the analysis of the impact of the second test result.

If the tests are not independent, this strategy for interpretation of serial test results can be misleading. Suppose a patient with chronic obstructive pulmonary disease and a history vaguely suggestive of pulmonary embolism is found to have an abnormal lung ventilation-perfusion scan. Obtaining that same test result over and over would not raise that patient's probability of coronary disease further and further. In this extreme case, the tests are identical; serial testing adds no information. More commonly, clinicians are faced with results from tests with related but not identical bases in pathophysiology, such as ventilation-perfusion scintigraphy and pulmonary angiography.

Regardless of whether tests are independent, the performance of multiple tests increases the likelihood that an abnormal test result will be obtained in a patient without disease. If a chemistry battery includes 20 tests and the normal range for each test has been developed to include 95% of healthy individuals, the chance that a healthy patient will have a normal result for any specific test is 0.95. However, the probability that all 20 tests will be normal is $(0.95)^{20}$, or 0.36. Most healthy people can be expected to have at least one abnormal result. Unless screening test profiles are used thoughtfully, false-positive results can subject patients to unnecessary tests and procedures.

Threshold Approach to Decision Making

Even if a test provides information, that information may not change management for an individual patient. Lumbar spine radiographs of a patient who is not willing to undergo surgery may reveal the severity of disease but expose the patient to needless radiation. Similarly, a test that merely confirms a diagnosis that already is recognized is a waste of resources (see Table 9–3).

Before ordering a test, clinicians should consider whether that test result could change the choice of management strategies. This approach is called the *threshold approach to medical decision making,* and it requires the physician to be able to estimate the threshold probability at which one strategy will be chosen over another. The management of a clinically stable patient with a high probability of coronary disease might not be changed by any of the post-test probabilities shown in Table 9–2. If that patient had no ST segment changes, the post-test probability of 0.29 still would be too high for a clinician to consider that patient free of disease. An abnormal test result that strengthened the diagnosis of coronary disease might not change management unless it suggested a greater severity of disease that might warrant another management strategy.

Testing for Peace of Mind

Physicians frequently order tests even when there is little chance that the outcomes will provide qualitatively new insights into a patient's diagnosis or prognosis or alter a patient's management. In such cases, the cited goal for testing may be to improve a patient's peace of mind. Although a decrease in uncertainty can improve quality of life for many patients, individuals with hypochondriasis and somatization disorders rarely obtain comfort from normal test results; instead, their complaints shift to a new organ system, and their demands focus on other tests. For such patients, management strategies using cognitive tactics are recommended.

WHICH TEST IS BEST?

If the clinician decided that more information is needed to reduce uncertainty, and if it appears possible that tests might lead to a change in management strategies, the question arises as to which test is most appropriate. Several factors influence this decision, including the patients' preferences, the risk associated with the tests, and the diagnostic performance of alternative tests.

Diagnostic performance of a test often is summarized in terms of sensitivity and specificity, but as shown in the example in Table 9–2, these parameters depend on which threshold (e.g., 1 mm vs. 2 mm of ST segment change) is used. A low threshold for calling a test result abnormal might lead to excellent sensitivity for detecting disease, but at the expense of a high false-positive rate. Conversely, a threshold that led to few false-positive results might cause a clinician to miss many cases of true disease.

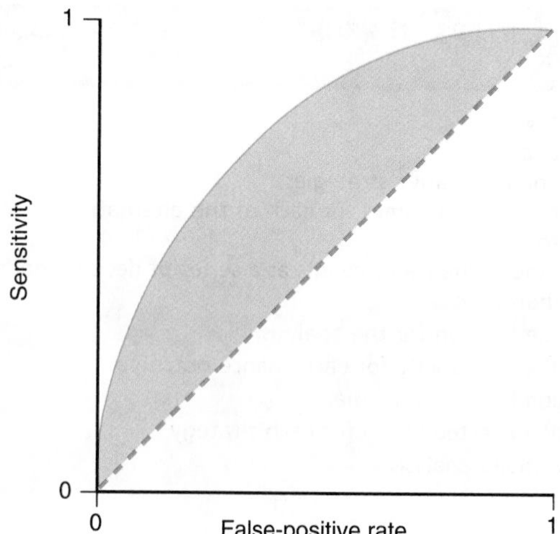

FIGURE 9–3 • Receiver operating characteristic curve. The points on the curve reflect the sensitivity and false-positive (1 – specificity) rates of a test at various thresholds. As the threshold is changed to yield greater sensitivity for detecting the outcome of interest, the false-positive rate rises. The better the test, the closer the curve comes to the upper left corner. A test of no value (e.g., flipping a coin) would lead to a curve with the course of the dotted line. The area under the curve is used often to compare alternative testing strategies.

The receiver operating characteristic (ROC) curve is a graphic form of describing this tradeoff and providing a method for comparing test performance (Fig. 9–3). Each point on the ROC curve describes the sensitivity and the false-positive rate for a different threshold for abnormality for a test. A test of no value would lead to an ROC curve with the course of the dotted line, whereas a misleading test would be described by a curve that was concave upward (not shown).

The more accurate the test, the closer its ROC curve comes to the upper left corner of the graph, which would indicate a test threshold that has excellent sensitivity and a low false-positive rate. The closer an ROC curve comes to the upper left corner, the greater the area under the curve. The area under ROC curves can be used to compare the information provided by two tests.

Even if one test is superior to another as shown by a greater area under its ROC curve, the question still remains as to what value of that test should be considered abnormal. The choice of threshold depends on the purpose of testing and on the consequences of a false-positive or false-negative diagnosis. If the goal is to screen the population for a disease that is potentially fatal and potentially curable, a threshold with excellent sensitivity is appropriate even if it leads to frequent false-positive results. In contrast, if a test is used to confirm a diagnosis that is likely to be treated with an invasive procedure, a threshold with high specificity is preferred. Only 1 mm of ST segment depression might be the appropriate threshold when exercise electrocardiography is used to evaluate the possibility of coronary disease in a patient with chest pain. If the question is whether to perform coronary angiography in a patient with stable angina in search of severe coronary disease that might benefit from revascularization, a threshold of 2 mm or more would be more appropriate.

CHOOSING A STRATEGY

Physicians and patients ultimately must use clinical information to make decisions. These choices usually are made after consideration of a variety of factors, including information from the clinical evaluation, patients' preferences, and expected outcomes with various management strategies. Insight into the impact of these considerations can be improved through the performance of decision analysis (Table 9–4).

The first step in a decision analysis is to define the problem clearly; this step often requires writing out a statement of the issue so that it can be scrutinized for any ambiguity. After the problem is defined, the next step is to define the alternative strategies.

Consider the question of which test is most appropriate to screen patients for breast cancer: mammography with or without breast magnetic resonance imaging—a newer technology that is highly sensitive for detecting breast cancer but is more costly and less specific. The expected outcomes for these strategies depend on each test's sensitivity and specificity for detecting breast cancer, which is influenced in turn by other

TABLE 9–4 STEPS IN PERFORMANCE OF DECISION ANALYSIS

Frame the question.
Create the decision tree.
Identify the alternative strategies.
List the possible outcomes for each of the alternative strategies.
Describe the sequence of events as a series of decision nodes and chance nodes.
Choose a time horizon for the analysis.
Determine the probability for each chance outcome.
Assign a value to each outcome.
Calculate the expected utility for each strategy.
Perform sensitivity analysis.

factors, such as the frequency with which the test is performed. Patients' outcomes also are influenced by their underlying risk for breast cancer and the likelihood that earlier detection of tumors reduces the risk for death.

Each of these variables must be known or estimated for calculations to be made of each strategy's predicted life expectancy and direct medical costs. These outcomes differ for patients according to age, medical history, family history, and presence or absence of genetic markers such as *BRCA* mutations. Optimal strategies for an elderly patient with a short life expectancy and low clinical risk of cancer are unlikely to be the same as for a younger patient with inherited mutations of the *BRCA1* or *BRCA2* gene, indicating a cumulative lifetime risk of breast cancer of 50 to 85% (Chapter 208).

The credibility of the decision analysis depends on the credibility of these estimates. Published reports often do not provide information on the outcomes of interest for specific subsets of patients, or there may not have been sufficient statistical power within subsets of patients for the

TABLE 9–5 ESTIMATED COST-EFFECTIVENESS OF COMMON HEALTH INTERVENTIONS

Disease Category	Intervention versus Comparator in Target Population	Cost per Quality-Adjusted Life Year*
Circulatory system	Stress echocardiography versus exercise electrocardiography in 55-year-old women with chest pain and risk factors that put them at intermediate pretest probability (25–75%) of coronary artery disease	$3,400
	Statin therapy versus usual care in patients aged 75–84 with a history of myocardial infarction	$21,000
	Exercise electrocardiography versus no testing in patients with no history of myocardial infarction presenting with typical angina	$35,000
	Exercise single-photon emission computed tomography versus exercise electrocardiography in patients with no history of myocardial infarction presenting with typical angina	$44,000
	Transesophageal echocardiography versus transthoracic echocardiography in 45-year-old patients with bacteremia and native heart valves and a pretest probability of endocarditis of 4–60%	$57,000
	Prophylactic implantable cardioverter defibrillator versus amiodarone therapy in patients who have had a prior myocardial infarction with an ejection fraction of 30% or less but who did not have sustained ventricular tachycardia	$76,000
	Prophylactic implantable cardioverter defibrillator versus no antiarrhythmic therapy in patients who have had a prior myocardial infarction and an ejection fraction of 31–40% but who did not have sustained ventricular tachycardia	$210,000
Endocrine	TSH screening versus no TSH screening in women undergoing 5-year periodic health examinations, beginning at age 35 years	$11,000
	Retinopathy screening every 5 years versus no screening in patients older than 40 years recently diagnosed with type 2 diabetes	$19,000
	Retinopathy screening every 3 years versus every 5 years in patients older than 40 years with recently diagnosed type 2 diabetes	$33,000
Digestive system	Surveillance every 1–5 years versus no surveillance in patients with Barrett's esophagus	$120,000
Infectious	HIV antibody testing versus no testing in blood donations	$440
	Treatment with interferon alfa for 6 months versus no treatment (conventional management only) in 40-year-old patients with chronic hepatitis C infection	$5,000
	Outreach initiative for pneumococcal and influenza vaccination versus usual vaccine availability in patients 65 years and older	$13,000
	Varicella vaccination without testing versus varicella antibody testing followed by vaccination if negative in 20- to 29-year-old adults with no history of chickenpox	$2,300,000
	Examination and culture for herpesvirus versus examination only in pregnant women with a history of genital herpes, active disease during pregnancy, or sexual partners with a proven history of genital herpes	$57 million
Injury	Driver-side air bags versus no air bags	$30,000
	Dual air bag versus driver air bags only	$76,000
Obstetrics	Elective cesarean section versus vaginal delivery in 25-year-old HIV-infected women with detectable HIV RNA	Cost savings
Oncology	Magnetic resonance imaging versus core-needle biopsy in women with suspicious breast lesions	$84,000
	Excisional biopsy versus core-needle biopsy in women with suspicious breast lesions	$310,000

*In 2002 U.S. dollars.
HIV = human immunodeficiency virus; TSH = thyroid-stimulating hormone.
Modified from CEA Registry: Comprehensive table of cost-utility ratios 1976–2001. Available at http://www.tufts-nemc.org/cearegistry/index.html. Accessed August 22, 2006.

findings to be statistically significant. Randomized trial data are relevant to the populations included in the trial; the extension of the findings to other genders, races, and age groups requires assumptions by individuals performing the analysis. For many issues, expert opinion must be used to derive a reasonable estimate of the outcome.

For many diseases, the potential outcomes are more complex than perfect health or death. With chronic diseases, patients may live many years in a condition somewhere between these two, and the goal of medical interventions may be to improve quality of life rather than to extend survival. The value of life in imperfect health must be reflected in decision analyses. These values by convention are expressed on a scale of 0 to 100, where 0 indicates the worst outcome and 100 indicates the best outcome.

Life-expectancy and quality-of-life estimates are combined in many decision analyses to calculate *quality-adjusted life years.* A strategy that leads to a 10-year life expectancy with such severe disability that utility of the state of health is only half that of perfect health would have a quality-adjusted life expectancy of 5 years. With such adjustments to life-expectancy data, the impact of interventions that improve quality of life but do not extend life can be compared with interventions that extend life but do not improve its quality or perhaps even worsen it.

After the value and the probability of the various outcomes have been estimated, the expected utility of each strategy can be calculated. In comparing the different strategies available at a decision node, the analysis generally selects the option with the highest expected utility. At chance nodes, the expected utility is the weighted average of the utility of the various possible branches.

After the analysis has been performed with the baseline assumptions, *sensitivity analyses* should be performed in which these assumptions are varied over a reasonable range. These analyses can reveal which assumptions have the most influence over the conclusions and identify threshold probabilities at which the conclusions would change. For example, the threshold at which breast magnetic resonance imaging should be added to mammography is likely to be influenced by the cost of the magnetic resonance imaging and the accuracy of the radiologists who interpret the images.

Cost-Benefit and Cost-Effectiveness Analyses

For clinicians and health care policymakers, the choices that must be addressed go beyond the choices within any single decision analysis. Because resources available for health care are limited, policymakers may have to choose among many competing "investments" in health. Although such decisions frequently are made on the basis of political considerations, cost-benefit and cost-effectiveness analyses can be informative in making the choices.

The methodology of these techniques is similar to that of decision analysis except that costs for the various possible outcomes and strategies also are calculated. *Discounting* is used to adjust the value of future benefits and costs because resources saved or spent currently are worth more than resources saved or expended in the future. In *cost-benefit* analyses, all benefits are expressed in terms of economic impact. Extensions in life expectancy are translated into dollars by estimating societal worth or economic productivity.

Because of the ethical discomfort associated with expressing health benefits in financial terms, *cost-effectiveness* analyses are used more commonly than cost-benefit analyses. In these analyses, the ratio of costs to health benefits is calculated; one frequently used method for evaluating a strategy is calculation of cost per quality-adjusted life year. These estimates can be used to compare strategies and to identify settings in which strategies that may be more expensive (e.g., coronary angiography) may "purchase" quality-adjusted life years at a lower cost than less aggressive strategies (e.g., observation).

Cost-effectiveness analyses can provide important insights into the relative attractiveness of different management strategies and can help guide policymakers in decisions about which technologies to make available on a routine basis. No medical intervention can have an attractive cost-effectiveness if its effectiveness has not been proved. The cost-effectiveness of an intervention depends heavily on the population of patients in which it is applied. An inexpensive intervention would have a poor cost-effectiveness ratio if it were used in a low-risk population unlikely to benefit from it. In contrast, an expensive technology can have an attractive cost-effectiveness ratio if it is used in patients with a high probability of benefiting from it. Table 9–5 shows cost-effectiveness estimates from published literature for some common medical and nonmedical interventions. Such estimates should be used only with understanding of the population for which they are relevant.

SUGGESTED READINGS

Akobeng AK: Understanding diagnostic tests 2: Likelihood ratios, pre- and post-test probabilities and their use in clinical practice. Acta Paediatr 2007;96: 487–491. *A practical overview for clinicians.*

CEA Registry: Comprehensive table of cost-utility ratios 1976–2001 and cost-utility ratios 2002–2003. Available at http://www.tufts-nemc.org/cearegistry/. Accessed April 8, 2007. *Through this website, the Harvard Center for Risk Analysis provides all published cost-effectiveness ratios, sorted by disease area and standardized according to 2002 dollars.*

Deeks JJ, Altman DG: Diagnostic tests 4: Likelihood ratios. BMJ 2004; 329:168–169. *Part of an excellent occasional series aimed at helping clinicians interpret published literature on diagnostic tests and use the information appropriately.*

Mulherin SA, Miller WC: Spectrum bias or spectrum effect? Subgroup variation in diagnostic test evaluation. Ann Intern Med 2002;137:598–602. *Describes hazards of interpreting test performance data without a full understanding of the population of patients from which the data were derived and provides guidance for minimizing that risk.*

10 MEASURING HEALTH AND HEALTH CARE

Stephan D. Fihn

The increasing emphasis on measuring and improving the quality of health care in the United States and elsewhere is based on several fundamental concerns. First is clear evidence that the health care system in the United States does not provide the highest quality of care possible. In one study, approximately 4600 randomly selected adults from 12 U.S. cities received recommended preventive, acute, or chronic care only slightly more than half the time. Second, substantial disparities in health care and outcomes persist, with women (Chapter 254), the poor (Chapter 5), and ethnic minorities (Chapter 4) typically faring less well than others. Third, there is growing concern that health care sometimes causes harm, as reflected by statistics indicating that 1 in 6.5 hospitalizations is complicated by a mistake in administering or prescribing medication, that 1 in 20 outpatient prescriptions is wrong, or that inpatient errors may cause as many as 44,000 to 98,000 deaths annually (Chapter 11). Fourth, health care is extraordinarily expensive, consuming nearly 15% of the U.S. gross domestic product in 2002 and projected to grow to more than 18% in 2013, with an annual expenditure of $3.4 trillion (Chapter 5). Moreover, there is substantial evidence that the delivery system is inefficient and wasteful, as illustrated by the fact that one in seven hospital admissions is prompted by lack of access to previous medical records, 12% of physicians' orders are not executed as written, and 20% of laboratory tests are requested because previous results are not readily available.

Findings such as these have fueled demands from the public, especially corporations that fund employee health care benefits, and from consumer groups for greater accountability and improved quality. In response, the information collected to measure health and health care has increased dramatically. Physicians and other health care providers are frequently confronted with these data in nearly every sphere of activity, including clinical care, education, and research. To interpret and apply this information correctly, health care providers should understand the basic principles of measuring the process and outcomes of health care.

MEASUREMENT OF HEALTH CARE

The basic paradigm that guides assessment of quality includes three fundamental domains: structure, process, and outcome. *Structure* refers to the stable elements that make up the health care system, such as the physical plant, administrative organizations, and qualifications of the staff. Because structural characteristics, such as whether floors are clean or doctors are board-certified, are often the easiest aspects of health care to observe and measure, they were the main focus of early efforts to improve quality. Over time, however, it became clear that a clean environment and qualified providers are essential but insufficient to guarantee high quality unless the process of care is effective.

Process refers to how care is delivered, including medical interventions and interpersonal interactions. Thus, it is important to understand, for instance, whether the right physician performs the right procedure on the right patient in the right way at the right time. Documenting these findings for the multitude of patients, however, can be expensive, difficult, and sometimes subjective because there may be a variety of acceptable approaches to a given clinical problem. Moreover, patients tend to be more concerned about achieving the best possible outcomes of care, such as curing disease, reducing symptoms, or improving function, than about the details of how these outcomes are achieved.

Outcomes represent the presumptive results of care that is delivered. The concept of health outcomes encompasses a broad array of clinical indicators that include death, adverse clinical events, persistence or recurrence of disease, disability, discomfort, and pain. Outcomes from the patient's perspective include self-reported health, ability to function, burden imposed by disease, or satisfaction with care. In addition, there may also be societal perspectives, such as cost-effectiveness and the cost-benefit ratio (Chapter 9). Judging care on the basis of outcomes, however, is handicapped because it may be difficult to measure outcomes reliably and because one-to-one linkage between optimal process and optimal outcome (and vice versa) is often lacking. Indeed, recent studies of the quality of health care demonstrate that it is important to select measures that are adequately specified to provide a "tight" linkage between process and outcome.

STANDARDS OF MEASUREMENT

Irrespective of what aspect of health care is being evaluated, the measures used should satisfy standards that help ensure that the data generated are trustworthy. These standards include reliability, validity, responsiveness, and interpretability. A *reliable* measure yields consistent results when repeated under similar circumstances. Although random error can never be eliminated, one would expect, for example, that two reviewers examining the same medical records would classify the outcomes in the same fashion in all but a small minority of cases. The level of reliability can be compared with common diagnostic procedures in medicine, many of which demonstrate only moderate reliability. For example, common methods of echocardiographic determination of ejection fraction vary up to 24% (Chapter 53), the intraclass coefficient for exercise treadmill tests performed a day apart is only 0.70, and the interobserver correlation for ascertaining the presence of coronary stenosis by highly trained experts is approximately 0.75 (Chapter 56).

Validity refers to accurate measurement of an intended effect or outcome. In the case of physiologic measures, such as diagnosis of coronary artery disease with electron beam computed tomography (Chapter 54), validity would be indicated by the likelihood of coronary stenoses demonstrated angiographically. In actuality, demonstrable coronary stenoses are present in only 55% to 84% of patients who have a positive result on electron beam computed tomography, which makes it a relatively invalid outcome measure. Validity for measures of subjective outcomes, such as pain, is typically documented through correlation with other related measures, such as the use of analgesic medications or limitation of activities.

Responsiveness reflects the sensitivity of a measure to clinically meaningful changes in status. Whereas a patient with worsening osteoarthritis might record no change on an instrument assessing activities such as bathing or dressing, this patient might exhibit declining scores on a measure that addresses more vigorous activities.

Interpretability is the degree to which the results of a measure can be understood and applied in clinical settings. Although most internists understand the clinical implications of a change in arterial pH from 7.42 to 7.30, they might not have the same appreciation for a change of 20 points on a 100-point physical function score.

These principles of measurement apply to both quality improvement studies and research, although the standards used in research are generally more rigorous. Measures are typically developed initially for use in research studies and, when shown to possess acceptable performance, are applied to routine quality improvement activities.

TYPES OF MEASURES

Driven largely by efforts to compare the performance of providers and different health care systems, considerable effort has been expended in standardizing measures at a national level. One example is the Health Employer Data and Information Set (HEDIS), which is a set of standardized performance measures designed to assist purchasers and consumers in comparing the performance of managed health care plans (Table 10–1). Most of these are process measures, although some structural measures and intermediate outcome measures (see later) are included.

Linkage between Process and Outcome Measures

Process measures are of greatest value when there is a close association, or tight linkage, between a process or action and an outcome. Numerous clinical trials, for example, have shown a substantial reduction in mortality when patients with hypercholesterolemia and ischemic heart disease are given a hydroxymethylglutaryl-coenzyme A (HMG-CoA) reductase inhibitor (statin) to lower low-density lipoprotein cholesterol (LDL-C) levels (Chapter 217). Accordingly, the use of statins in appropriate patients is a common indicator used to measure quality in many health care organizations. There are, however, limitations to using LDL-C measured at a single point in time because there may be a legitimate reason for it being over the target range in as many as half of patients who would otherwise appear to have received poor-quality care. Such reasons include having only recently started taking statins when the dosage is being titrated, having refused therapy, having a high LDL-C level despite maximal therapy, or having experienced an adverse effect of statins.

Intermediate and Combined Outcomes

Because many outcomes of interest, such as death or the occurrence of serious adverse events, may be relatively infrequent, *intermediate outcomes* are sometimes measured in lieu of the true outcome of interest. Intermediate outcomes are often physiologic variables such as blood pressure, cholesterol level, or hemoglobin A_{1c} concentration. For example, the primary rationale for treating diabetes is to prevent complications such as blindness, amputation, or renal failure, and the efficacy of treatment should ultimately be determined by a reduction in risk for these complications. Though important in the pathophysiology of diabetes, a change in the measured hemoglobin A_{1c} level is meaningful as an outcome measure (particularly to the patient) only in so far as it reflects a reduction in risk afforded by treatment. As opposed to standard physiologic measures, other intermediate outcomes reflect subclinical disease, for example, microalbuminuria, which indicates subclinical renal disease in diabetes (Chapter 247). Intermediate outcomes are attractive because they are often familiar to clinicians and can readily be measured repeatedly in most or all patients, whereas the outcome of interest (e.g., amputation) is a relatively infrequent event in patients treated for diabetes. Using intermediate outcomes, however, may be deceptive, particularly when the linkage to the true outcome of interest is loose. The presence of microalbuminuria in a patient with type 2 diabetes (Chapter 248), for instance, is associated with a $2^1/_2$-fold increase in the relative odds for death over a period of 6 years when compared with diabetic patients who have no protein in their urine. This sizable increase in relative risk, however, translates into a relatively small increase in absolute risk for any individual in any given year. Thus, changes in quality as measured by rates of microalbuminuria would not probably be reflected in outcome measures such as the incidence of cardiovascular events or renal failure except in extremely large populations. Moreover, it is also possible for a treatment to have a salutary effect on a surrogate outcome but a deleterious effect overall. Such was the case for short-acting dihydropyridines, such as nifedipine, which effectively lowered blood pressure in hypertensive patients but doubled the incidence of myocardial infarction.

Another strategy adopted when outcome events are infrequent is the use of combined end points. An example would be the incidence of cardiovascular events, including stroke, myocardial infarction, unstable angina, and sudden cardiac death. This approach can improve the statistical power of a study, but it tends to exaggerate the perceived efficacy of a particular intervention and may obscure specific effects, for example, if an intervention reduces the frequency of stroke more than it does myocardial infarction.

Patient-Oriented Measures

Although physiologic and standard clinical measures are important, assessment of outcomes from the patient's perspective has increasingly

TABLE 10–1 PARTIAL LISTING OF HEALTH EMPLOYER DATA AND INFORMATION MEASURES FOR ADULTS*

EFFECTIVENESS OF CARE

Inappropriate antibiotic treatment of adults with acute bronchitis
Screening for colorectal, breast, and cervical cancer
Chlamydia screening in women
Osteoporosis management in women who had a fracture
Controlling high blood pressure
Initial and ongoing β-blocker treatment after a heart attack
Comprehensive diabetes care
Use of appropriate medications for people with asthma
Use of spirometry in the diagnosis of chronic obstructive pulmonary disease
Follow-up after hospitalization for mental illness
Antidepressant medication management
Glaucoma screening in older adults
Use of imaging studies for low back pain
Disease-modifying antirheumatic drug therapy in patients with rheumatoid arthritis
Drugs to be avoided in the elderly
Medical assistance with smoking cessation
Flu shots and pneumonia vaccination for older adults
Management of urinary incontinence in older adults
Physical activity in older adults

ACCESS/AVAILABILITY OF CARE

Access to preventive/ambulatory health services
Initiation and engagement of alcohol and other drug dependence treatment
Call answer timeliness and abandonment

SATISFACTION WITH THE EXPERIENCE OF CARE
HEALTH PLAN STABILITY

Practitioner turnover
Years in business/total membership

USE OF SERVICES

Frequency of selected procedures
Inpatient utilization—general hospital/acute care
Ambulatory care
Inpatient utilization—nonacute care
Mental health utilization—inpatient discharges and average length of stay
Mental health utilization—percentage of members receiving inpatient and intermediate care and ambulatory services
Chemical dependency utilization—inpatient discharges and average length of stay
Identification of alcohol and other drug services
Outpatient drug utilization
Antibiotic utilization

COST OF CARE
INFORMED HEALTH CARE CHOICES
HEALTH PLAN DESCRIPTIVE INFORMATION

Board certification
Enrollment by product line
Race/ethnic diversity of membership
Language diversity of Medicaid membership

*For a complete and up-to-date listing, visit *http://www.ncqa.org/Programs/HEDIS/.*

been recognized as being of equal or even greater importance, especially when evaluating treatments that are intended to lessen symptoms or improve function rather than improve survival. Approaches that depend on a physician's perception of a patient's condition, such as the Canadian Cardiovascular Society Classification for cardiac symptoms (Chapter 48), are limited because physicians often tend to underestimate a patient's symptoms or disability and such assessments are difficult to standardize. Self-reporting of health and function by patients themselves via standardized questionnaires overcomes these problems. The terminology used to describe the hundreds of questionnaires now available is evolving and, at times, confusing, but the resulting scales generally address various aspects of health-related quality of life, which is a complex, multidimensional concept. Facets or subscales of quality of life may include the severity of symptoms, pain, physical functioning, social functioning, general perceptions of health, overall burden of disease, emotional well-being, and coping, among others.

General measures of health status or health-related quality of life, such as the Short-Form 36 (SF-36), do not focus on a specific disease or condition but seek to assess overall health and functioning. General measures may, however, be insensitive to a specific, yet clinically meaningful change in symptoms related to a particular condition. For this reason, *condition-specific measures* have been developed and there are now more than 1000 such measures reported. Whereas a patient's score on a questionnaire dealing with overall health might not change in response to successful treatment of gastroesophageal reflux, the score on a more specific questionnaire addressing symptoms of heartburn would demonstrate a substantial change.

In the past, measures of self-reported health were criticized as being "soft" and overly subjective. In fact, many general and condition-specific measures demonstrate reliability and validity that equal or exceed that of many physiologic or clinical measures commonly used in research or clinical settings. For example, in patients undergoing coronary artery bypass grafting (Chapter 74), a 10-point reduction in self-reported physical functioning (on a 100-point scale) increases the risk for death by the same magnitude that the presence of diabetes or chronic obstructive pulmonary disease does.

A shortcoming of nearly all outcome measures other than death is that it is difficult or impossible to use such measures to compare alternative treatments unless they are applied in precisely the same fashion. In the case of hypertension (Chapter 66), for example, different drugs might exhibit differential effects on the risk for stroke or heart failure and also on the risk for adverse events such as fatigue, hepatotoxicity or renal insufficiency. *Utility measures,* which are derived from economic and decision theory, seek to provide a standard method of comparing such disparate outcomes. *Utility* is the value or preference that an individual places on a given state of health or condition. Utility is scored from 0 (generally equivalent to death) to 1.0 (ideal health). Multiplication of individual utilities for different health states by their probabilities of occurrence permits computation of the overall utility of a treatment or intervention and enables comparison with therapeutic alternatives through the technique of decision analysis. When combined with probabilities of survival, utility can be used to calculate quality-adjusted life years, yet another way of comparing outcomes of different treatment strategies (Chapter 9). Outside the research setting, however, utilities have not been widely used because they are difficult to elicit from patients.

Satisfaction with health care is another patient-oriented measure that is often evaluated. Like health-related quality of life, satisfaction is a broad concept that can incorporate a number of different dimensions, including satisfaction with overall health care, systems of care, hospital care, outpatient care, specific types of treatments, individual health care providers, amenities, and other aspects. Because patients' satisfaction with their care may not correlate with other aspects of the process and outcomes of cares, results should be interpreted in the context of these other measures.

Measures of Cost and Resource Use

Given the dramatically rising expense of health care, costs are frequently measured. Because of the complexity of the health care market, including contractual arrangements and complicated formulas for reimbursement, charges (prices) rarely represent the true underlying cost of services. Therefore, careful accounting methods are necessary to accurately ascertain cost. Because these methods can be laborious and expensive, *utilization* of health care services, such as average length of stay or number of days in intensive care units, is often measured as a proxy for cost. When actually measured, the costs evaluated are generally those characterized as *direct,* or the actual fixed and variable expenses for labor, materials, and equipment necessary to provide a given clinical service. Because these costs are typically the responsibility of insurers and health systems, analyses that use direct costs assume their viewpoint. When more global perspectives are incorporated, including those of patients, it is also necessary to measure *indirect costs,* such as the loss of time and inconveniences incurred by patients or the societal burdens of disability or loss of productivity. Naturally, indirect costs are even more difficult and expensive to measure than direct costs.

From a policy or decision-making perspective, information about cost is most useful when it permits comparisons of alternatives such as different drugs to treat hypertension. *Cost-benefit* analysis attempts to summarize all costs of treatment and all potential benefits solely in monetary terms. This approach is controversial and not frequently applied because it necessitates assigning dollar costs to outcomes such as death or disability. *Cost-effectiveness* analysis is performed more frequently because the results are expressed in more comprehensible clinical terms, such cost per life saved or per quality-adjusted life year (using the utilities described earlier). When a new treatment is evaluated, it is desirable to calculate its *marginal cost-effectiveness,* which describes its costs and benefits in relation to an existing standard treatment.

SOURCES OF DATA FOR MEASUREMENT OF HEALTH AND HEALTH CARE

In ideal circumstances, data for measuring health care would be collected prospectively with techniques and instruments specifically designed for the patient population and problem being assessed. In reality, the time and expense required to develop or identify measures and collect primary data are often prohibitive for many important questions. In these situations, it may be advantageous to use information that is collected for administrative or billing purposes and that reflects the process of health care. Such secondary sources of data have increasingly been applied to a broad range of topics, including the use and outcomes of all types of health service.

Governmental Sources of Data

Historically, federal and state governments have collected data related to public health such as the occurrence of communicable diseases or causes of death. With the expansion of publicly funded health programs such as Medicare and Medicaid and the rise in chronic illnesses as the major cause of morbidity and mortality, governmental agencies now maintain a much broader range of databases, many of which can be accessed via the Internet (Table 10–2). These databases make available vast amounts of information about the incidence and prevalence of various medical conditions, characteristics of patients and health care providers, types of health care services used, burdens and cost of illness, and other health outcomes.

Clinical and Quality Data

Whereas up until the latter part of the 20th century most statistics on health care delivery and on the health of groups of patients, excluding individual medical records, were maintained by government agencies, there are now hundreds of public and private entities that collect, process, analyze, or disseminate this information. The consolidation of health care delivery systems within markets and the wide use of electronic health records have led to the creation of very large and rich clinical databases that can be an excellent substrate for monitoring and improving quality of care. These data sources can furnish clinical details about the severity and clinical course of illnesses not obtainable from administrative databases.

Another emerging source of data is quality measurement systems developed by peer review organizations, medical care organizations, health plans, professional organizations, consumer organizations, and bodies that perform accreditation. To a greater or lesser extent, all these groups have developed systems to measure and evaluate the performance of health care providers and systems. These data may be collected through extraction of data from secondary sources, manual abstraction of physical or electronic medical records, or primary data collection by clinical or administrative personnel. Despite the relatively low expense, ready availability, and large size of secondary data sources, there are serious potential limitations to their use (Table 10–3).

TABLE 10–2 EXAMPLES OF PUBLICLY AVAILABLE SOURCES OF SECONDARY DATA

FEDERAL AGENCIES

- Centers for Disease Control and Prevention, CDC Wonder: *http://wonder.cdc.gov*
- Centers for Disease Control and Prevention, AIDS Public Use Data by major metropolitan area: *http://wonder.cdc.gov/AIDSPublic.htm*
- Centers for Disease Control and Prevention, National Center for Injury Prevention and Control WISQARS Database (Web-based Injury Statistics Query and Reporting System): *http://www.cdc.gov/ncipc/wisqars**
- Centers for Disease Control and Prevention, Sexually Transmitted Disease Morbidity Data Request Screen (by state): *http://wonder.cdc.gov/sexu00.htm*
- Healthy People 2010 Database (DATA 2010)—state-level data queries that can provide some benchmarks: *http://wonder.cdc.gov/data2010/focus.htm*
- Indian Health Service: *http://www.ihs.gov*
- U.S. Census Bureau: *http://factfinder.census.gov/home/saff/main.html?_lang=en*
- Cancer data from the National Cancer Institute SEER program: *http://seer.cancer.gov*
- Department of Veteran Affairs: *http://www.virec.research.med.va.gov*

FEDERAL SURVEYS THROUGH THE NATIONAL CENTER FOR HEALTH STATISTICS: *http://www.cdc.gov/nchs/*

- National Health Interview Survey (NHIS): *http://www.cdc.gov/nchs/products/elec_prods/subject/nhis.htm*
- National Health and Nutrition Examination Survey (NHANES): *http://www.cdc.gov/nchs/nhanes.htm*
- Behavioral Risk Factor Surveillance System (BRFSS): *http://www.cdc.gov/brfss*
- Youth Risk Behavior Surveillance System (YRBSS): *http://www.cdc.gov/nccdphp/dash/yrbs/index.htm*
- National Immunization Study public use data files: *http://www.cdc.gov/nis/datafiles.htm*
- Ambulatory Health Care Data: *http://www.cdc.gov/nchs/about/major/ahcd/ahcd1.htm#Micro-data*
- National Hospital Discharge and Ambulatory Surgery data: *http://www.cdc.gov/nchs/about/major/hdasd/nhds.htm*
- National Nursing Home Survey data: *http://www.cdc.gov/nchs/about/major/nnhsd/nnhsd.htm*
- National Home and Hospice Care Survey data: *http://www.cdc.gov/nchs/about/major/nhhcsd/nhhcsd.htm*
- National Employer Health Insurance Survey data: *http://www.cdc.gov/nchs/about/major/nehis/nehis.htm*
- National Health Provider Inventory data: *http://www.cdc.gov/nchs/products/elec_prods/subject/nhpi.htm*
- National Survey of Family Growth data: *http://www.cdc.gov/nchs/nsfg.htm*
- State and Local Area Integrated Telephone Survey: *http://www.cdc.gov/nchs/slaits.htm*
- National Vital Statistics System: *http://www.cdc.gov/nchs/nvss.htm*

*WISQARS is an interactive database that provides customized reports of national injury data (fatal and nonfatal).

DESIGN OF MEASUREMENT STUDIES

Data used to measure the structure, process, and outcomes of health care can be obtained in a variety of ways. Investigators engaged in hypothesis-driven research generally use more rigorous methods of measurement and research designs, whereas those evaluating the quality of care provided within and among health care organizations tend to rely on observational studies or secondary sources of data (i.e., data that were initially collected for a different purpose, such as clinical care or claims processing). However, progressive overlap in the methods used and the proliferation of computerized data sources have begun to blur the boundaries between certain types of research and quality improvement studies.

TABLE 10–3 POTENTIAL LIMITATIONS OF SECONDARY DATA

Feature	Potential Limitations
Accuracy and precision of data	Basic information on patient characteristics, diagnoses, and procedures may be miscoded Data generally available only for people who use services or access the health care system during the period of interest Patients may be miscounted if they have multiple sites of residence or have undergone procedures in more than one system of care
Sample size	Large sample sizes may produce statistical significance without clinical or policy significance
Characterization of patients	Patients are incompletely characterized; key clinical data on processes and outcomes may be missing
Characterization of providers	Characteristics of providers may be missing, miscoded, or inconsistently recorded
Characterization of interventions	Services or procedures may be coded imprecisely or inaccurately
Ascertainment of outcomes	Outcomes of greatest relevance may not be captured (e.g., symptom relief, quality of life, out-of-hospital events, level of satisfaction)
Completeness of follow-up	Only data about discrete episodes of care may be coded. Longitudinal follow-up requires data linkage, which may not be possible

Adapted from Huston P, Naylor CD: Health services research: Reporting on studies using secondary data sources. Can Med Assoc J 1996;155:1697–1702.

Experimental Studies

Evaluation of the effects of treatments on clinical outcomes should generally be performed in randomized, controlled trials in which the intervention is randomly assigned to ensure that patients who do (subjects) and do not (controls) receive it are as similar as possible. Except for the experimental intervention, subjects and controls should be treated in an identical fashion to the greatest extent possible. In the case of drug studies, this method usually requires giving an identical placebo to control patients. In "double-blind" studies, not only is the patient kept uninformed about the treatment assignment, but the patient's physician and certain members of the investigative team are kept uninformed as well. Maintenance of blinding is more difficult in studies of interventions other than drugs, but even studies of surgery or acupuncture, for example, can have control patients undergo sham procedures. In studies evaluating more complex interventions, such as a team to manage diabetes or heart failure, blinding may be impractical. To help maintain equivalence in such cases, patients serving as controls may receive a less intensive educational program to help ensure that any observed difference in health outcomes between the intervention and control groups is the result of genuine treatment effects rather than nonspecific effects of increased attention.

In trials of interventions that are applied directly to patients, such as medications or procedures, allocation of the experimental treatment is generally random by patient, and results are analyzed at the level of the patient. Conversely, in trials of interventions that are designed to improve how care is delivered, the unit of randomization and analysis may be the health care provider or even the entire system of care, depending on the level at which the intervention is administered. In studying the clinical effects of an educational program for physicians, for example, participating physicians should be randomized along with their patient panels because the effects on patients within a panel would not be independent. Similarly, in a study of a new way to organize personnel within a practice to treat depression, entire practices might be the correct unit of randomization and analysis.

Although the randomized control trial is the most rigorous method of assessing treatment effects, this approach has several shortcomings. To achieve equivalence between treatment and control groups with respect to key demographic and clinical characteristics, eligibility is often restricted to a narrow range of individuals who fulfill strict criteria. Although this approach enhances the internal validity of a trial's results, applicability of the results to groups of patients who would have been deemed ineligible for the trial (often elderly or chronically ill patients) remains uncertain. Moreover, to help ensure that patients fully comply with the treatment being tested, study personnel frequently provide substantially more support and assistance to participants in randomized trials than similar patients would receive in ordinary clinical settings. This difference often raises additional concern about the generalizability of results. For this reason, tightly controlled randomized trials are often considered to establish the *efficacy* of an intervention, specifically, the potential benefit of an intervention under ideal conditions. To establish whether an intervention is successful in patients more typically seen in routine practice, investigators may conduct an *effectiveness trial,* also known as a *management* or *pragmatic trial.*

Other potential drawbacks of randomized trials are the long time required for planning and execution, high expense, and low statistical power to assess infrequent outcomes, especially for studies in which health care providers or systems of care are randomized. To compensate in part for these drawbacks, *cluster randomized trials* are designed to permit randomization at the level of the provider or system but use sophisticated statistical techniques to perform analyses at the level of the patient so that statistical power is preserved. This approach is particularly well suited to effectiveness trials, which often involved testing of clinical strategies or programs. Other novel approaches are sequential methods, such as the *group sequential response* and *adaptive clinical trial designs,* which provide an opportunity to terminate a study, adjust the expected sample size, or modify the intervention as the trial progresses on the basis of interim analysis at predetermined points in time. These approaches, which are especially attractive when preliminary data are limited, can enhance efficiency by terminating positive or negative trials earlier than might be the case when using only initial sample size estimates.

Nonexperimental Designs

Although randomized trials remain the best approach to assess the efficacy of therapeutic interventions, for the reasons enumerated, other study designs, such as *observational* or *case-control* studies, may be preferable under certain circumstances. *Cohort* studies are a type of observational study in which one or more groups of patients are selected because they have or have not been exposed to a particular condition or intervention. Exposures can be broadly defined and range from the presence of a particular disease or condition (e.g., pneumonia or heart failure), to receipt of a type of medication, to provision of a given medical service (e.g., a surgical procedure) or set of services (e.g., care received from a specialist physician or enrollment in a type of health plan), to exposure to a set of conditions (e.g., having health insurance). Cohort studies have numerous attractive features, including the ability to provide a direct estimate of the absolute risk for an outcome in exposed patients. The foremost liability common to these approaches is the possibility that any observed difference in outcomes is due to inherent differences between patients who do and do not receive the intervention because it is not randomly allocated. This dilemma can often be addressed by using statistical methods for *case mix adjustment* (described in the next section). In some circumstances, however, even extensive adjustment is inadequate, such as when there is *bias by indication.* This problem occurs in the study of a relationship between an exposure (e.g., a medication such as a short-acting calcium-channel blocker) and an outcome (e.g., myocardial infarction) when one indication for the medication is treatment that is directly related to the outcome (i.e., angina pectoris). One solution to this problem is to eliminate patients for whom this bias is likely to be present.

In the illustrative case, for example, a heightened risk for myocardial infarction in patients taking short-acting calcium-channel blockers was initially demonstrated in a study restricted to persons with hypertension but no known cardiovascular disease.

In a *prospective cohort study,* participants are identified at the time of exposure and followed forward in time according to a predefined protocol and with standard measures. Prospective cohort studies often permit enrollment of a broader cross section of patients than is possible in randomized trials and can be conducted under circumstances in which randomization is not feasible for ethical or logistic reasons. Like randomized trials, prospective cohort studies provide a means to be certain that the exposure under study truly precedes the outcome of interest. Limitations of prospective cohort studies include the need to enroll large numbers of patients (especially when evaluating rare outcomes), the frequent loss of participants during follow-up, and the high expense, often related to the duration of follow-up.

In a *retrospective cohort study,* exposure is typically defined by using secondary data (e.g., an admitting diagnosis of acute myocardial infarction or a procedure code for spinal fusion on a hospital discharge abstract) at some point in the past, and patients are followed forward in time by using previously collected data for outcomes (e.g., death, reoperation, or readmission). Formerly, retrospective cohort studies were limited in time and scope because they relied on often tedious manual abstraction of medical charts. With the proliferation of secondary electronic data sources, this approach has become extremely popular because of several advantages, chief among these the opportunity to study vast numbers of patients inexpensively, including patients with relatively rare conditions. Standardized coding for many variables, such as diagnoses and procedures, helps reduce the variability introduced by human chart abstractors. Moreover, electronic records are far less apt to be unavailable or incomplete than paper records are. On the other hand, retrospective cohort studies are subject to a number of potentially serious flaws. Hypotheses are usually generated and studies designed well after collection of the data, which were generally gathered for a wholly different purpose. Thus, the reliability and validity of the data are often unknown and beyond control of the investigator. This problem, in turn, can lead to misclassification of both exposures and outcomes. For example, a diagnosis of pneumonia coded for billing purposes may not satisfy the rigorous criteria used in research. Although a patient's complete electronic record is rarely lost, missing data within records is common. Unlike prospective studies, it may be difficult to be certain that an exposure preceded an outcome. A patient might, for example, have had a subclinical form of a disease at the time of a given exposure, thereby leading to an erroneous impression of a temporal sequence when the disease was recognized clinically. Apart from methodologic limitations, the sheer volume of data available encourages investigators to conduct numerous analyses, often without pre-stated hypotheses. Multiple comparisons performed with very large sample sizes readily lead to erroneous conclusions that random associations are clinically meaningful because they are of marginal statistical significance.

Case-control studies differ from cohort studies in that the case and control groups are defined on the basis of whether they have experienced an outcome rather than on the basis of exposure. Data from existing records or gathered by interview (or both) are then used to ascertain the proportion of case and control patients who experienced the exposure of interest. As in cohort studies, exposures can be defined broadly, including a medication, a type of clinical event, or receipt of a service. Case-control studies are attractive in many settings because they require fewer patients than prospective studies do to achieve a similar level of statistical power. This attribute makes them especially useful for investigating uncommon outcomes. For example, pharmacoepidemiologists often use case-control studies to identify serious adverse effects of medications when the events are too rare to study with clinical trials or cohort studies. Case-control studies are nonetheless subject to a number of potential biases. As with cohort studies, limitations of data from secondary sources can lead to misclassification of exposure or outcome. When exposure is determined by interview, differential recall by cases and controls can introduce bias. It may be even more difficult to be certain that an exposure truly occurred before the outcome than in retrospective cohort studies. Furthermore, the results of case-control studies do not yield estimates of absolute risk, as do randomized trials and cohort studies, but are expressed as the odds of an outcome in cases relative to controls. *Relative odds* only approximate the ratio of risk in cases to risk in controls.

Cross-sectional studies are performed when data on one or more groups of patients are collected at a single point in time. Although, this approach is inexpensive and can provide estimates of the prevalence of a condition or outcome, it is highly subject to nearly all the biases mentioned and is the weakest method in terms of making inferences about whether a particular exposure directly causes a given outcome.

Case Mix Adjustment

Only in prospective, randomized trials is it possible to control which patients do and do not receive a specific treatment, and even then, it may not be possible to ensure equivalence of all of the characteristics that affect outcomes between those in the control and experimental groups. In all nonexperimental research designs, allocation of the experimental intervention is not random but is a function of a patient's personal and clinical characteristics and those of the system care. Without consideration of such differences, it is impossible to differentiate the genuine effects of an intervention from bias related to allocation of the intervention to certain types of patients. Modern statistical techniques that can adjust for such differences are effective when many of the patient characteristics that exert an important influence on outcomes have been elucidated and are available. For example, the major factors that predict mortality after acute myocardial infarction include prolonged chest pain, tachycardia, hypotension, ST segment elevation on the admission electrocardiogram, poor left ventricular function, and initial laboratory measures that indicate a large infarct, such as a high troponin level. Thus, when comparing the outcomes of patients who are treated in different systems of care, it is essential to use multivariate statistical methods to adjust for these factors. Otherwise, differences observed between systems that are actually due to differing patient populations might erroneously be attributed to differences in quality of care. A related method is propensity scoring, which applies the results of modeling equations that predict how likely a person was to have received one intervention or the other based on personal and clinical characteristics. Even with sophisticated adjustments, however, studies of treatments that rely heavily on the judgment of physicians or the preference of patients, such as postmenopausal estrogen therapy, are likely to have biases that cannot be addressed by statistical modeling but rather require randomized trials.

TRENDS IN OUTCOME MEASUREMENT

In recent years, the topics of studies evaluating outcomes have expanded greatly. In addition to evaluating specific treatments, such as drugs or procedures, evaluations have extended to comparing various types of clinical programs, systems of care, types of providers, mechanisms of financing, patient safety, disparities among ethnic groups, and geographic variations in patterns of care (Table 10–4). It is safe to predict that studies on the processes and outcomes of health care will become

TABLE 10–4 EXPANDING AREAS OF STUDY FOR HEALTH CARE QUALITY AND OUTCOMES

General Area of Study	Example of Intervention or Outcome Evaluated
Effectiveness of clinical programs	Disease management programs, specialized clinics, consultative services
Organization of care	Health maintenance organizations vs. private practice
Effects of different mechanisms of financing	Capitation vs. fee-for-service; different levels of pharmacy copayments
Outcomes of different types of providers	Generalists vs. specialists
Disparities among ethnic groups	Receipt of preventive services or sophisticated procedures
Patient safety	Occurrence of adverse drug effects or medical errors
Geographic variations in patterns of care	Use of expensive procedures

even more ubiquitous with the expanding availability of electronic data, increasingly sophisticated statistical techniques, and growing public demand for accountability.

SUGGESTED READINGS

Higashi T, Shekelle PG, Adams JL, et al: Quality of care is associated with survival in vulnerable older patients. Ann Intern Med 2005;143:4:274–281. *Higher scores on 207 criteria for improved quality of care were associated with better 3-year survival.*

Landon BE, Hicks LS, O'Malley AJ, et al: Improving the management of chronic disease at community health centers. N Engl J Med 2007;356:921–934. *Shows it is easier to improve processes than to improve measurable outcomes in vulnerable populations.*

Trivedi AN, Zaslavsky AM, Schneider EC, et al: Trends in the quality of care and racial disparities in Medicare managed care. N Engl J Med 2005;353:692–700. *Over a 3- to 7-year period, performance related to mammography, diabetes, and ischemic heart disease improved, but disparities between white and black patients persisted.*

Williams SC, Schmaltz SP, Morton DJ, et al: Quality of care in U.S. hospitals as reflected by standardized measures, 2002–04. N Engl J Med 2005;353:255–264. *There was a 3 to 33% improvement on 15 measures over a 2-year period.*

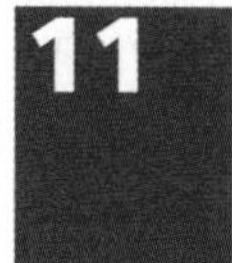

11 QUALITY OF CARE AND SAFETY OF PATIENTS

Robert M. Wachter

During the past two decades, scores of studies have demonstrated that the quality and safety of modern health care leave much to be desired, despite the fact that most physicians are well trained and work very hard. Yet the evidence is undeniable, with clear documentation of stunning variations in patterns of care that are neither supported by evidence nor justified by outcomes, major gaps between evidence-based best practices and current practice, and staggering numbers of serious medical errors. The recognition of these quality and safety problems has catalyzed a major transformation in thinking and practice, with new technologies, regulations, training models, incentive systems, and more.

To appreciate the problem and how to address it requires an understanding of quality measurement and improvement, safety of patients, and finally value, which is the confluence of safety, quality, and cost.

QUALITY

Definition

Quality of care, which has been defined by the Institute of Medicine as "the degree to which health services for individuals and populations increase the likelihood of desired health outcomes and are consistent with current professional knowledge," includes six aims for a quality health care system, emphasizing that quality involves more than the delivery of evidence-based care (Table 11–1). Nevertheless, evidence-based medicine (Chapter 9) provides much of the scientific underpinning for quality measurement and improvement. Previously, the lack of clinical evidence and the apprenticeship model of medical training promoted an idiosyncratic practice style by which a senior clinician or a marquee medical center determined the standard of care—a tradition now sometimes termed eminence-based medicine. Without discounting the value of experience and mature clinical judgment, the modern paradigm for determining optimal practice has changed, driven by the explosion in clinical research during the past 30 years; for example, the number of randomized clinical trials grew from 350 per year in 1970 to 14,000 per year in 2004. This research has helped define "best practices" in many areas of medicine, from preventive strategies for a healthy 62-year-old outpatient (Chapters 12 and 13) to the treatment of the patient with acute myocardial infarction and cardiogenic shock (Chapters 72 and 108).

Donabedian's triad, which divides quality measures into *structure* (how care is organized), *process* (what is done), and *outcomes* (what happens to the patient), represents the most popular construct for quality measurement. Each element of the triad has important advantages and disadvantages as a quality measure (Table 11–2). Most of the widely used quality measures are process measures, primarily in situations in which clinical research has established the link between such processes and improved outcomes. An example is the rate at which aspirin or a β-blocker is given to survivors of a myocardial infarction before hospital discharge (Chapter 72). However, when processes are less relevant and the science of case-mix adjustment is suitably advanced (e.g., cardiac bypass surgery; Chapter 74), outcome measurement is often used. In other areas in which the processes are complex, structural measures are used as proxies for quality; examples here include the presence of inten-

TABLE 11–1 THE INSTITUTE OF MEDICINE'S SIX QUALITY AIMS

Patient safety
Patient-centeredness
Effectiveness
Efficiency
Timeliness
Equity

From Committee on Quality of Health Care in America, Institute of Medicine: Crossing the Quality Chasm: A New Health System for the 21st Century. Washington, DC, National Academy Press, 2001.

TABLE 11–2 A COMPARISON OF THE THREE TYPES OF CLINICAL QUALITY MEASURES (THE DONABEDIAN TRIAD)

Measure	Simple Definition	Advantages	Disadvantages
Structure	How was care organized?	May be highly relevant in a complex health system	May fail to capture the quality of care by individual physicians Difficult to determine the "gold standard"
Process	What was done?	More easily measured and acted on than outcomes May not require case-mix adjustment No time lag—can be measured when care is provided May directly reflect quality (if carefully chosen)	A proxy for outcomes Not all may agree on "gold standard" processes May promote "cookbook" medicine, especially if physicians and health systems try to "game" their performance
Outcomes	What happened to the patient?	What we really care about	May take years to occur May not reflect quality of care Requires case-mix and other adjustment to prevent "apples-to-oranges" comparisons

Modified from Donabedian A: The quality of care. How can it be assessed? JAMA 1988;270:1743–1748; and Shojania KG, Showstack J, Wachter R: Assessing hospital quality: A review for clinicians. Eff Clin Pract 2001;4:82–90.

sivists to staff critical care units, a dedicated stroke service, and computerized physician order entry (CPOE) systems.

The Epidemiology of Quality Problems

It is now well established that there are large and clinically indefensible variations in care from one city to another. Furthermore, U.S. practice adheres with the best evidence only slightly more than 50% of the time, even when adherence is known to correlate with ultimate clinical outcomes.

Levers for Change

For physicians, policymakers, administrators, and patients, this evidence of major quality problems has led to a recognition of structural problems that prevent the highest quality of care from being delivered. These problems include the lack of information regarding the performance of a provider or institution, the absence of incentives for quality improvement, the difficulty for practicing physicians to stay abreast of modern evidence-based medicine, and the absence of an information technology support system for quality.

The first step in quality improvement begins with the creation of practice standards against which to measure quality. Literally scores of such measures have been promulgated by a variety of organizations, including payers (such as the Centers for Medicare and Medicaid Services), accreditors (such as the Joint Commission on Accreditation of Healthcare Organizations), and medical societies. These measures have identified many opportunities for improvement for individual physicians, practices, and hospitals.

Given the volume of new literature published each year, no individual physician can possibly remain abreast of all the evidence-based advances in his or her field. *Practice guidelines,* such as those for the care of community-acquired pneumonia (Chapter 97) or prophylaxis for deep venous thrombosis (Chapter 81), aim to synthesize evidence-based best practices into a set of summary recommendations. Although concerns about "cookbook medicine" linger, there is increasing consensus that best practices should be "hard-wired" if possible. The major challenges are to update guidelines as new knowledge accumulates and to recognize the complexity of guidelines when patients have multiple, potentially overlapping illnesses. *Clinical pathways* are similar to guidelines but attempt to codify a series of steps, usually temporal (on day 1, do the following; on day 2, . . .), and thus are more useful for stereotypical processes such as the postoperative management of patients after hip replacement.

Although professionalism (Chapter 1) should be a sufficient incentive for physicians to provide high-quality care, reaching this goal typically depends on a system organized to translate research into practice and to deliver the right care every time. Such a system requires significant investments (i.e., in education of physicians, hiring of case managers or clinical pharmacists, building of information systems, and development of guidelines). The historic payment system, which compensates physicians and hospitals equally whether quality is terrific or terrible, provides no incentive to make the requisite investments.

The Changing Environment for Quality

The recent recognition of major gaps in quality and of the need for systemic change to improve quality has led to a variety of initiatives to catalyze quality improvement. Virtually all involve several steps: defining reasonable quality measures (evidence-based measures; capturing appropriate structure, process, or outcomes), measuring the performance of providers or systems, and using these results to promote change. This final imperative creates the greatest degree of uncertainty and experimentation.

Although one might hope that simply giving a physician information about prior performance will generate meaningful improvement, this strategy yields only modest change at best. Increasingly, a more aggressive and transparent strategy, such as disseminating the results of quality measurement to key stakeholders, is being adopted. In some cases, simple transparency is the main strategy, in the hope that providers will find exposition of their gaps in quality to be sufficiently concerning or embarrassing to motivate improvement. Although there is little evidence that patients use such data to choose among physicians or hospitals, transparency itself has frequently resulted in impressive improvements in some publicly reported quality measures.

The newest strategy in the United States is to tie payments for service to quality performance (pay for performance, or P4P). A number of ongoing P4P experiments are testing whether differential payment will lead to significantly more improvement than that achieved by simple transparency. P4P also raises a host of concerns, including whether presently captured quality data are accurate, whether payments should go to best performers or those with the greatest improvements, whether existing measures adequately measure quality in patients with complex diseases, and whether P4P will create undue focus on certain measurable practices and relative inattention to other important processes that are not being compensated.

Quality Improvement Strategies

Whether the motivation is professionalism, embarrassment, or economics, the next question is how actually to improve the quality of care. There is no simple answer; successful institutions and physicians have used a variety of strategies. In general, most use a variation of a "Plan, Do, Study, Act" (PDSA) cycle, recognizing that quality improvement activities must be carefully planned and implemented, that their impact needs to be measured, and that the results of these activities will often be imperfect and require retooling.

In addition to the PDSA cycle, several other types of activities are useful. For quality improvement practices that require predictable repetition, efforts to "hardwire" the practice or to use alternative providers who focus on the activity are often beneficial. For example, the best strategy to increase the rate of pneumococcal vaccination (Chapter 16) of hospitalized patients with pneumonia is to embed it in a standard order set, either paper based or computerized. Another example is that having a nurse remove the patient's shoes before the physician's entry can increase rates of diabetic foot examinations in an outpatient practice (Chapter 247).

In some areas, though, quality improvement involves much more complex and interdependent activities. In these circumstances, bringing teams together to examine their practices and to participate in a PDSA cycle is the most likely path to success. For example, a group of cardiac surgeons in the northeastern United States participated in such an experiment, in which they observed each other's practices, agreed on best practices, and measured each other's outcomes; the result was a 24% reduction in mortality with cardiac surgery.

SAFETY OF PATIENTS

Epidemiology

The concept of "first, do no harm" began more than 2 millennia ago, and many hospitals have long hosted periodic forums (e.g., morbidity and mortality conferences) to discuss errors. Until recently, however, there has been little teaching about the nature of medical mistakes, investment in safety research, regulation of safety standards, or emphasis on safety improvements despite that an estimated 44,000 to 98,000 Americans die each year of medical mistakes—the equivalent of a jumbo jet crashing each day. These deaths are related to medication errors, gaps in the discharge process, communication problems in intensive care units, retained sponges in surgical patients—in short, virtually every aspect of modern medical care. Moreover, detailed clinical and statistical evidence of suboptimal safety has been reinforced by several high-profile and disquieting errors, sometimes apparently related to inadequate supervision and prolonged duty-hours of trainees, the wrong patient getting a major procedure, the wrong limb being operated on, chemotherapy overdoses, mistaken mastectomies, and more.

Because patients may be harmed despite receiving perfect care (i.e., from an accepted complication of surgery or a side effect of a medication), it is important to separate *adverse events* from *errors.* The patient safety literature commonly defines an error as "an act or omission that leads to an unanticipated, undesirable outcome or to substantial potential for such an outcome." Adverse events, on the other hand, are injuries due to medical management rather than the patient's underlying illness. This distinction is crucial—when a patient who was appropriately prescribed warfarin for chronic atrial fibrillation (Chapter 63) develops a gastrointestinal bleed despite a therapeutic international normalized ratio (INR), an adverse event but not a medical error has occurred. Conversely, if the INR was supratherapeutic because the physician prescribed a new medication without checking for possible drug interactions, a medical error would have occurred.

The Modern Approach to Safety of Patients

The historical approach to medical errors often has been to blame the provider who was most proximate: whoever performed the surgery, hung the intravenous medication, or mixed the chemotherapy. It is now recognized that this approach fails to appreciate that most errors are committed by hard-working, well-trained individuals, and such errors are unlikely to be prevented by admonishing people to be more careful or by shaming and suing them. Instead, the modern approach, known as systems thinking, holds that humans will inevitably err and that safety depends on creating systems that anticipate errors and either prevent or catch them before they cause harm. Such an approach has been the cornerstone of safety improvements in other high-risk industries for some time.

The "Swiss cheese model" of accidents, drawn from innumerable investigations of accidents in, for example, commercial aviation and nuclear power, emphasizes that single errors by one individual working in an otherwise safety-conscious system rarely cause harm. Instead, such errors must penetrate multiple incomplete layers of protection ("layers of Swiss cheese") to cause terrible harm. The lesson is to focus not on the futile goal of trying to perfect human behavior but rather on creating multiple overlapping layers of protection to decrease the probability that the holes in the Swiss cheese will ever align and let an error slip through.

How to Improve Safety of Patients

Drawing on these models, modern thinking emphasizes efforts to design and implement systems to prevent or catch errors. For example, errors in routine behaviors can best be prevented by building in redundancies and crosschecks in the form of checklists, read-backs, and other standardized safety procedures, such as sponge counts in the operating room, signing a surgical site before an operation, or asking patients their name before administering a medication. One way to decrease errors at the person-machine interface is by use of "forcing functions," engineering solutions that decrease the probability of human error. The classic example outside of medicine is the modification of automobile braking systems to make it impossible to place a car in reverse when the driver's foot is off the brake. In health care, forcing functions include changing the gas nozzles and connectors so that anesthesiologists cannot mistakenly hook up the wrong gas, such as nitrogen instead of oxygen, to a patient. Given the ever-increasing complexity of modern medicine, building in such forcing functions in intravenous pumps, defibrillators, mechanical ventilators, and computerized order entry systems will be crucial to safety.

In addition to better systems, communication and teamwork must be improved. All commercial pilots must take "crew resource management" courses, in which they train for emergencies with other crewmembers, learn to flatten hierarchies that might stifle open communication, communicate clearly with standard language, and use checklists and other systemic approaches. Although evidence that such interventions in medical care will improve the safety of patients is preliminary, the goal is a "culture of safety"—an environment in which teamwork, clear communication, and openness about errors, both with other health care professionals and with patients, is the norm.

Another key principle in the safety of patients is to learn from one's mistakes. Safe systems have a culture in which errors are openly discussed, often in "morbidity and mortality" conferences. To be useful, these discussions should involve nursing, identify when errors occurred, emphasize systems thinking and solutions, and not be punitive. In addition to the open discussion during conferences, safe organizations build in mechanisms to hear about errors from front-line staff, often through "incident reporting systems," and to perform detailed "root cause" analyses of major errors or "sentinel events" in an effort to define all the layers of Swiss cheese that need improvement.

Finally, there is increasing appreciation of the importance of a well-trained, well-staffed, and well-rested work force for delivery of safe care. Lower nurse-to-patient ratios, long resident work hours, and lack of board certification are all linked to poor outcomes for patients. Safer systems cannot be created if the providers are overextended or poorly trained or supervised.

In the absence of comparative evidence and in light of the high cost of interventions, such as improved staffing, computerized order entry, and teamwork training, even institutions committed to safety must oftentimes make difficult changes. Given the natural tendency to focus on practices that are measured, publicly reported, and compensated, institutions and physicians will tend to focus first on areas subject to regulation or on initiatives, such as computerization, with multiple potential benefits. Since improving culture is difficult to measure and to regulate, there is concern that it will not be as high a priority as it should be.

VALUE: CONNECTING SAFETY AND QUALITY TO COST

Outside of health care, most purchasing decisions are based on perceived value: (quality + safety) ÷ cost. Health care decisions historically have not been made this way, in part because of the limited ability of patients and payers to make rational judgments about the quality and safety of a given provider or system, and in part because health care insurance insulates patients from the full cost of care. Much of the recent push to measure and to improve quality and safety should be seen as part of a broader effort to allow patients and payers to make rational judgments about value and to choose their providers on the basis of such judgments. Given the stakes, it will be vitally important for physicians and other health care providers to participate in efforts to measure and to improve the quality and safety of care and to do so while being mindful of the price tag.

SUGGESTED READINGS

Aiken LH, Clarke SP, Sloane DM, et al: Hospital nurse staffing and patient mortality, nurse burnout, and job dissatisfaction. JAMA 2002;288:1987–1993. *An influential article that linked nurse-to-patient ratios to both clinical outcomes and nurse satisfaction.*

Boyd CM, Darer J, Boult C, et al: Clinical practice guidelines and quality of care for older patients with multiple comorbid diseases: Implications for pay for performance. JAMA 2005;294:716–724. *Adhering to evidence-based guidelines for a hypothetical 79-year-old woman with multiple common illnesses would result in polypharmacy and other negative effects.*

Brennan TA, Horwitz RI, Duffy FD, et al: The role of physician specialty board certification status in the quality movement. JAMA 2004;292:1038–1043. *Argues that board certification should be included among publicly reported quality measures.*

Landrigan CP, Rothschild JM, Cronin JW, et al: Effect of reducing interns' work hours on serious medical errors in intensive care units. N Engl J Med 2004;351:1838–1848. *ICU interns working traditional shifts of 24 hours or more made significantly more errors than those working shorter shifts.*

Leape LL, Berwick DM: Five years after To Err Is Human: What have we learned? JAMA 2005;293–2384–2390. *A thoughtful review of progress in safety and quality 5 years after the blockbuster Institute of Medicine report.*

Wachter RM: Expected and unanticipated consequences of the quality and information technology revolutions. JAMA 2006;295:2780–2783. *Describes the benefits and potential risks.*

Section III

Preventive and Environmental Issues

12 PRINCIPLES OF PREVENTIVE HEALTH CARE

Steven H. Woolf

Heart disease, cancer, diabetes, and other diseases that occupy the attention of physicians and claim the lives of patients can be ameliorated, if not averted entirely, by preventive measures such as early detection, immunizations (Chapter 16), and health behavior change. Fully 35% of the deaths that occur annually in the United States are attributable to tobacco use (Chapter 30), physical inactivity (Chapter 14), and poor diet (Chapter 232). Tobacco use alone accounts for 420,000 deaths annually in the United States.

It is intuitive that patients benefit more from upstream efforts to prevent diseases than from their treatment after symptoms emerge. Paradoxically, the latter consumes the vast resources of the health care system—trillions of dollars per year (Chapter 5)—in an enterprise that is often powerless to alter the course of disease, prolong survival, or forestall the pain and suffering of complications.

The inherent logic behind prevention has been advocated since ancient Greece but assumes heightened urgency in modern times, when an aging population is facing an increase both in the prevalence of chronic diseases and in treatment costs for these conditions. Employers, insurers, government, and patients are struggling with spiraling health care budgets. The impending convergence of these trends on both population health and the economy underscores the strategic leverage of prevention in stemming the rising incidence, severity, and cost of chronic diseases.

The most effective venues for prevention are the settings of daily life—home, work, and school—where people make choices about health habits (e.g., physical activity, diet) and obtaining medical care. Support in pursuing healthy lifestyles can come from various community sectors: employers, schools, public health departments, manufacturers, retailers, government agencies, health advocacy organizations, advertisers, community centers, and the media. The health care community often plays a peripheral role. For example, the most effective measures to prevent injuries involve legislation and product redesign more so than clinical intervention (Chapter 15). The Centers for Disease Control and Prevention's *Guide to Community Preventive Services* outlines a variety of strategies outside the clinical setting that are effective in preventing diseases.

Preventive health care involves primary and secondary prevention more so than tertiary prevention. *Primary prevention* refers to efforts among asymptomatic persons (individuals without signs or symptoms of the target condition) to prevent the occurrence of disease. Examples include smoking cessation and immunizations. *Secondary prevention* refers to screening asymptomatic persons for the early detection of preclinical disease or risk factors. Examples include Papanicolaou smears and measurement of serum lipids. *Tertiary prevention* refers to efforts in patients with known disease to avert related complications. An example is screening for retinopathy in persons with diabetes. Most of the nonpalliative care that is delivered to patients with disease is, by this definition, tertiary prevention.

Although the context for prevention is community-wide, clinicians maintain a prominent role in its implementation. First, physicians have cachet: studies consistently cite the advice of physicians among the most important factors that motivate patients to change health habits and obtain screening tests. Second, clinicians are essential to deliver *clinical preventive services,* or interventions that require a health professional (e.g., immunizations, colonoscopy). This chapter focuses on clinical preventive services, which include counseling about health behavior, immunizations, and screening tests.

BENEFIT, HARM, AND COST OF PREVENTIVE HEALTH CARE

Benefit

Evidence is growing that each form of prevention can be effective, but primary prevention offers the greatest promise. Because three types of health behavior—tobacco use (Chapter 30), unhealthy diet (Chapter 232), and physical inactivity (Chapter 14)—account for one in three deaths in the United States, reducing the prevalence of such behavior and stemming the rising prevalence of obesity would have a major impact on the health of the population and the incidence of related diseases (e.g., coronary artery disease, stroke, cancer, diabetes, chronic obstructive pulmonary disease). The number of lives that could be saved through primary prevention far exceeds the number of deaths averted by secondary or tertiary prevention (Table 12–1).

Individuals, however, find it difficult to sustain changes in health behavior, and there is only limited evidence that clinicians, offering advice during an office visit, can improve success rates. Such evidence exists for counseling about smoking cessation; even a few minutes of brief advice increases abstinence rates. [1] Counseling by clinicians also appears to influence the eating habits of individuals at high risk for cardiovascular disease and diabetes, [2] but evidence is insufficient to determine whether routine counseling about diet or physical activity is (or is not) effective in modifying the lifestyle of average-risk, asymptomatic individuals.

Another form of primary prevention—immunizations—is much easier to implement and is among the most clinically efficacious and cost-effective interventions available in health care (Chapter 16). Pneumococcal vaccine, which can be administered within seconds, can lower the incidence of invasive pneumococcal disease by 50%. [3] Pneumonia and influenza, which are also preventable through vaccination, together constitute the seventh leading cause of death in the United States.

Secondary prevention (screening) is effective for certain diseases. For example, randomized trials have demonstrated that mammography screening for breast cancer (Chapter 208) and fecal occult blood testing for colorectal cancer (Chapter 203) can reduce death rates by 15 to 20%. [4,5] Other cancer screening tests (e.g., Papanicolaou smears, sigmoidoscopy/colonoscopy), measurement of serum lipids, bone mineral testing, and screening for depression are among the list of evidence-based secondary prevention (early detection) maneuvers.

Finally, a robust literature supports the value of tertiary prevention in reducing the complications of certain diseases. Examples include highly effective preventive cardiology regimens in patients with coronary artery disease (Chapters 70 to 72) or heart failure (Chapter 58), physical activity to delay the progression of diabetes (Chapter 248), and smoking cessation by patients with chronic obstructive pulmonary disease (Chapters 30 and 88).

Harm

Most Americans, and many physicians as well, assume that early detection of diseases must be beneficial and that cost is the only conceivable counterargument to screening. Few appreciate that screening can harm the health of patients or that such harm could occur with sufficient frequency or severity to outweigh the benefits. The risk is not so much testing itself, which is usually trivial, but the downstream consequences generated by the test results. A seemingly innocuous blood test can trigger a cascade of follow-up tests that are invasive and induce greater risk for a potentially large portion of the screened population. For example, many women screened for ovarian cancer will have suspicious masses that require surgical exploration. Screening also induces psychological harm: patients awaiting evaluations for alarming diseases (e.g., cancer, human immunodeficiency virus infection) experience anxiety and worry. Physical and psychological harm occurs with little benefit if the screening test results are falsely positive.

The chances that a test's results will be falsely positive is less a function of *sensitivity* (the proportion of persons with the condition who test positive) than of *specificity* (the proportion of persons without the condition who test negative) and is compounded by a low pretest probability (prevalence) of the target condition (Chapter 9). That is, high specificity does not guarantee that a screening test will have a high *positive predictive value* (PPV, the probability that an abnormal test result is a true positive). As shown in Table 12–2, if the prevalence of a cancer is 1%, a screening test with a sensitivity and specificity of 95% will generate five false-positive results for every true cancer detected. If the prevalence is lowered to 0.1%, as might occur in a primary care setting, the same screening test will have a much lower PPV and generate 53 false-positive results for every true cancer detected (Table 12–3).

The difficult tradeoff between benefit and harm explains the policy of many agencies and health organizations to recommend screening only for select conditions rather than for all diseases that might potentially benefit from early detection. A group known for its close examination of such tradeoffs is the U.S. Preventive Services Task Force (USPSTF), an independent nonfederal panel that uses evidence-based methods to develop practice guidelines on clinical preventive services. The USPSTF recommends routine screening only if a systematic review of the evidence demonstrates that the test can accurately detect the condition, that early detection improves health outcomes, and that the benefit outweighs the harm of screening and treatment (see Table 13–3).

Cost

Preventive services that result in more good than harm are generally recommended, but not if the ratio between the cost of the service and its health benefits *(cost-effectiveness)* is exorbitant (Chapter 9). An expensive screening program that benefits only a few members of the screened population may be cost-effective if targeted to high-risk groups, but not if administered to individuals at lower risk.

TABLE 12–1 POTENTIALLY AVERTABLE DEATHS PER YEAR IN THE UNITED STATES THROUGH:

PRIMARY PREVENTION	
Smoking cessation	328,044
Physical activity	177,940
Lowering total cholesterol by 10%	132,777
Control of hypertension	68,382
Pneumococcal vaccination of elderly	9,922
SECONDARY PREVENTION	
Mammography	4,475
Fetal occult blood testing (FOBT)	9,632
Pap smears	3,644
TERTIARY PREVENTION	
Angiotensin-converting enzyme inhibitors for heart failure	11,000
β-blockers after acute myocardial infarction	17,023
Aspirin after acute myocardial infarction	10,365
Warfarin after atrial fibrillation	3,418
Total	776,622

Adapted from Woolf SH: The need for perspective in evidence-based medicine. JAMA 1999;282:2358–2365.

IMPLEMENTING PREVENTIVE HEALTH CARE IN PRACTICE

Establishing a Practice's Prevention Policies

Clinicians should establish guidelines regarding the preventive services that their practice will offer, the patients who will be eligible, and optimal starting/stopping ages and intervals. National guidelines provide a good starting point, and a recent report from the National Commission on Prevention Priorities has identified which services offer the greatest benefit and value. Individual practices, however, should customize generic guidelines to achieve "buy-in" from the practice and to ensure applicability to the health needs and circumstances of the patient population being served (Chapter 4).

Some preventive services require further individualization. For example, it may be necessary to calculate a patient's 5-year risk for stroke or cancer to determine whether the benefit of a screening test or preventive medication outweighs its harm. For some preventive services, the scientific uncertainty or the "close call" between benefit and harm may create the need for *shared decision making* to enable patients to consider personal preferences in deciding which option is best.

Clinicians and practices must decide which preventive services to deliver opportunistically (during acute and chronic care visits) or during wellness visits (i.e., periodic health/health maintenance examinations) so that clinicians can focus attention on the prevention agenda and spend more time, be free of competing demands, and receive more reimbursement than possible at routine visits (Chapter 13). The downsides of addressing prevention only at well-person visits are that problems (e.g., overdue screening, smoking relapse) may escape attention in the interim and many patients do not schedule wellness visits; often, they are the high-risk individuals most in need of preventive care.

Reminder Systems and Prompts

Preventive care is improved when practices adopt an electronic or paper-based system to remind clinicians when patients are due for tests, immunizations, or health behavior counseling. 6 Prompts generated

TABLE 12–2 ACCURACY OF A SCREENING TEST (SCENARIO A: PREVALENCE = 1%)

Population = 100,000, prevalence of cancer = 1%, test sensitivity = 95%, test specificity = 95%

Test Result	Cancer Present	Cancer Absent	Total	Positive Predictive Value	Ratio of False Positives to True Positives
Positive	950	4,950	5,900	0.16	5.2 (4,950/950)
Negative	50	94,050	94,100		
Total	1,000	99,000	100,000		

Administering a seemingly accurate cancer screening test to a hypothetical population of 100,000 persons can generate a large proportion of false-positive results if the prevalence of the target condition is low. The prevalence of cancer (pretest probability) in scenario A is assumed to be 1% (1000 individuals have the cancer). Of the 5900 persons who would test positive, only 950 (16%) would have cancer; 5 individuals would receive false-positive results for every true cancer case detected. The *positive predictive value* is the proportion of positive test results that are true positives, *prevalence* is the proportion of the population with disease, *sensitivity* is the proportion of persons with disease who test positive, and *specificity* is the proportion of persons without disease who test negative.

TABLE 12–3 ACCURACY OF A SCREENING TEST (SCENARIO B: PREVALENCE = 0.1%)

Population = 100,000, prevalence of cancer = 0.1%, test sensitivity = 95%, test specificity = 95%

Test Result	Cancer Present	Cancer Absent	Total	Positive Predictive Value	Ratio of False Positives to True Positives
Positive	95	4,995	5,090	0.02	52.6 (4,995/95)
Negative	5	94,905	94,910		
Total	100	99,900	100,000		

The positive predictive value of a test deteriorates as the prevalence of the target condition decreases. In this table, the assumptions used in Table 12–1 are retained but the prevalence of cancer (pretest probability) is lowered to 0.1% (100 individuals have the cancer). Of the 5090 persons who would test positive, only 95 (2%) would have cancer; 53 individuals would receive false-positive results for every true cancer case detected. The *positive predictive value* is the proportion of positive test results that are true positives, *prevalence* is the proportion of the population with disease, *sensitivity* is the proportion of persons with disease who test positive, and *specificity* is the proportion of persons without disease who test negative.

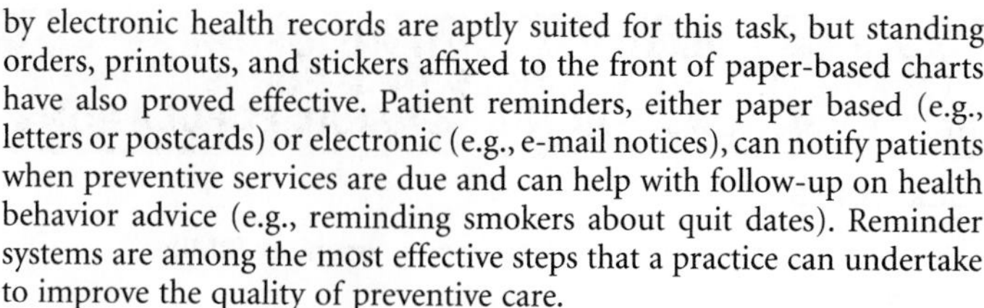

by electronic health records are aptly suited for this task, but standing orders, printouts, and stickers affixed to the front of paper-based charts have also proved effective. Patient reminders, either paper based (e.g., letters or postcards) or electronic (e.g., e-mail notices), can notify patients when preventive services are due and can help with follow-up on health behavior advice (e.g., reminding smokers about quit dates). Reminder systems are among the most effective steps that a practice can undertake to improve the quality of preventive care.

Teamwork

Physicians need not be the only members of the practice who deliver preventive services; indeed, they often lack the time, reimbursement, and skills. In a team model, the front desk, rooming staff, medical assistants, and nurses can play coordinated roles in identifying patients in need of preventive services; providing education, motivation, and links to community resources; and administering preventive procedures (e.g., immunizations). Staff can perform these roles in real time at the index office visit or offline by conducting group visits, classes, telephone counseling, and e-mail consultations.

Capitalizing on Continuity

Clinicians with continuity relationships (e.g., primary care clinicians and specialists who monitor patients over time) can deliver recommended preventive services longitudinally rather than compressing the entire prevention agenda into one office visit or hospitalization. Clinicians and patients should reach agreement on a health maintenance plan, identify the preventive issues to address first, and schedule one or more follow-up visits to address outstanding tests, immunizations, and lifestyle issues.

Practice Redesign

For preventive care and other services, practices should adopt modern models of care delivery to improve the quality and timeliness of service to patients, increase efficiency, and better monitor performance. Initiatives launched by specialty societies and quality improvement organizations, epitomized by the Institute for Healthcare Improvement (www.ihi.org), provide valuable resources and guidance in implementing practice redesign.

Reaching Out Beyond the Practice

Limited resources, time, and reimbursement make it difficult for even the most well designed practice to offer the full spectrum of assistance that patients need. For example, patients with unhealthy behavior are expected to receive the "5 A's": *Assess* (ask about the behavior), *Advise* (a clear, personal message of encouragement to change), *Agree* (set goals based on readiness to change), *Assist* (build the skills, confidence, and environmental support for change, supplemented by medical treatment when appropriate), and *Arrange* (establish follow-up). Busy clinicians usually lack the time, skills, and counseling staff to offer this level of assistance systematically.

A more realistic model is for clinicians to focus on the first two A's—identifying patients who need assistance *(Assess)* and conveying the importance of making a change *(Advise)*—and then refer patients to resources outside the practice for more intensive assistance (e.g., community programs, Internet resources). For example, smokers can be invited to receive free, high-quality telephone counseling from established quit line programs, which are more effective than brief physician advice. [1] The *Assess-Advise-Refer* model requires an upfront effort by the practice to establish a competent system to identify eligible patients, offer brief advice, streamline the referral process, and ensure a feedback loop to coordinate the off-site program with ongoing primary care.

FUTURE DIRECTIONS

Policy, technologic, and cultural forces will shape the content and direction of preventive care in the future. For example, advances in genetic technology are likely to enhance lead time and precision in identifying individuals at risk for disease and to introduce complicated ethical dilemmas. New models of community partnership will be necessary to help citizens adopt and maintain healthy lifestyles. The ability of clinicians to function effectively in this effort will depend on successes in addressing larger defects in the health care system. Society's actions to address the uninsured, fragmentation between health care institutions, spiraling cost, and inadequate information technology will affect preventive services, along with all aspects of medical care.

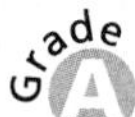

1. Lancaster T, Stead LF: Physician advice for smoking cessation. Cochrane Database Syst Rev 2004;2:CD000165.
2. Pignone MP, Ammerman A, Fernandez L, et al: Counseling to promote a healthy diet in adults: A systematic review for the U.S. Preventive Services Task Force. Am J Prev Med 2003;24:75–92.
3. Dear K, Holden J, Andrews R, et al: Vaccines for preventing pneumococcal infection in adults. Cochrane Database Syst Rev 2003;4:CD000422.
4. Humphrey LL, Helfand M, Chan BK, et al: Breast cancer screening: A summary of the evidence for the U.S. Preventive Services Task Force. Ann Intern Med 2002;137:347–360.
5. Pignone M, Rich M, Teutsch SM, et al: Screening for colorectal cancer in adults at average risk: A summary of the evidence for the U.S. Preventive Services Task Force. Ann Intern Med 2002;137:132–141.
6. Stone EG, Morton SC, Hulscher ME, et al: Interventions that increase use of adult immunization and cancer screening services: A meta-analysis. Ann Intern Med 2002;136:641–651.

SUGGESTED READINGS

Maciosek MV, Coffield AB, Edwards NM, et al: Priorities among effective clinical preventive services: Results of a systematic review and analysis. Am J Prev Med 2006;31:52–61. *Ranks more than 30 clinical preventive services based on their effectiveness and cost-effectiveness.*

Sheridan SL, Harris RP, Woolf SH, Shared Decision-Making Workgroup of the U.S. Preventive Services Task Force: Shared decision making about screening and chemoprevention: A suggested approach from the U.S. Preventive Services Task Force. Am J Prev Med 2004;26:56–66. *Outlines the rationale and principles for incorporating shared decision-making into the offering of preventive services.*

Smith RA, Cokkinides V, Eyre HJ: American Cancer Society guidelines for the early detection of cancer, 2006. CA Cancer J Clin 2006;56:11–25. *Recommendations for cancer of the breast, cervix, colon, rectum, and prostate.*

U.S. Preventive Services Task Force: Guide to Clinical Preventive Services, 2005. AHRQ Publication No. 05–0570, June 2005. Agency for Healthcare Research and Quality, Rockville, MD. Available at http://www.ahrq.gov/clinic/pocketgd.htm. *Recommendations for screening tests, counseling, and preventive medication.*

Woolf SH, Glasgow RE, Krist A, et al: Putting it together: Finding success in behavior change through integration of services. Ann Fam Med 2005;3 (Suppl. 2):S20–S27. *How primary care practices can partner with other resources to help patients receive preventive care.*

THE PERIODIC HEALTH EXAMINATION

David Atkins

An increasingly important part of adult primary health care is primary and secondary prevention (Chapter 12). The traditional concept of an annual visit structured around a physical examination and a standard battery of screening tests, however, has given way to an emphasis on a set of preventive services targeted to each individual. The appropriate services and their frequency vary with the age, gender, and individual risk factors of each patient. Although these services can be delivered in the context of ongoing care, a periodic health examination focusing on prevention increases the delivery of appropriate screening and lifestyle counseling. In the United States, Medicare has recently added coverage for a one-time preventive visit for new enrollees.

The most comprehensive prevention recommendations are produced by the U.S. Preventive Services Task Force (USPSTF), an ongoing panel of experts supported by the federal Agency for Healthcare Research and Quality *(http://preventiveservices.ahrq.gov)*. USPSTF recommendations are used by major primary care subspecialty groups (the American College of Physicians and the American Academy of Family Physicians), many health plans, and quality organizations. The USPSTF recommendations require evidence that a service can reduce disease-specific mortality or morbidity. Grade A recommendations generally require direct evidence from high-quality studies (e.g., large screening trials) and benefits that substantially exceed harms. USPSTF recommendations are thus more conservative than those of some subspecialty organizations that may be based on less direct evidence, such as earlier detection of disease without a proven effect on long-term outcomes. General recommendations of the USPSTF include the following: clinicians should be selective in their use of screening tests; clinicians and patients should share decision making about specific services, especially where benefits must be balanced against harms; and clinicians need to take advantage of opportunities to deliver services outside of the specifically scheduled prevention visit.

Specific components of the periodic health examination include history and risk assessment, screening for early disease or modifiable risk factors, counseling and behavioral interventions to promote healthy behaviors, immunizations, and discussions about chemoprevention.

HISTORY AND RISK ASSESSMENT

The history and risk assessment are important tools to guide decisions about other preventive interventions. Risk assessment can identify individuals who may need additional screening tests or immunizations not generally recommended for their age group or who may benefit from specific counseling to address unhealthy behaviors. Formal health risk appraisals can improve preventive care, but only when they are linked to a system to provide specific feedback and targeted interventions. Risk assessment should address the following:

- use of tobacco, alcohol, and other drugs (especially injection drugs) (Chapters 30, 31, and 32);
- diet (Chapter 232);
- physical activity (Chapter 14);
- sexual behavior that may increase risk of sexually transmitted diseases, including human immunodeficiency virus (HIV) infection, or unintended pregnancy (Chapters 307, 410, and 411);
- family history of cancer and heart disease;
- residence (community risk of infectious diseases); and
- presence of chronic diseases and cardiovascular risk factors (Chapter 49).

SCREENING FOR EARLY DISEASE OR ASYMPTOMATIC RISK FACTORS

Every year, new screening tests are introduced and marketed on the basis of their ability to detect unrecognized diseases or risk factors for disease. Other conditions need to be fulfilled for a screening test to be worthwhile for routine use, however (Table 13–1). Benefits of screening must also be balanced against the potential harms, including false-positive and false-negative results and the risks and costs of follow-up procedures or treatments. Even when tests have high specificity, the majority of positive results will be false-positives if the test is used to screen healthy populations for uncommon conditions such as cancer (Chapter 9). The number of screening tests proven to be beneficial for the general population is relatively small (Table 13–2), but additional tests may be indicated for specific populations at increased risk (Table 13–3). Finally, some commonly used tests are not recommended for routine screening (Table 13–4). For most other potential screening tests, current data are not adequate for a convincing case to be made for or against screening.

Depression

Depression is common and frequently undetected in primary care (Chapter 420). Simple screening instruments can increase the detection of patients with major depression. Two questions—During the past 2

TABLE 13–1 REQUIREMENTS OF AN EFFECTIVE SCREENING TEST

Disease is an important cause of morbidity and mortality
Screening can detect disease in early, presymptomatic phase
Screening and treatment of patients with early disease or risk factors produce better health outcomes than does treatment of patients when they present with symptoms
Screening test is acceptable to patients and clinicians—safe, convenient, acceptable false-positive rate, acceptable costs
Benefits of early detection and treatment are sufficient to justify potential harms and costs of screening

TABLE 13–2 RECOMMENDATIONS OF THE U.S. PREVENTIVE SERVICES TASK FORCE INTERVENTIONS FOR THE GENERAL POPULATION

SCREENING

Height and weight and calculate body mass index (BMI): periodically
Blood pressure: at least every 2 years
Screen for problem drinking
Brief screen for depression*
Total blood cholesterol and HDL cholesterol: men ≥35 yr, women ≥45 yr, and others with CVD risk factors; every 5 years
Colorectal cancer screening: age ≥50 yr (see above for options)
Mammogram every 1–2 years (± clinical breast examination): women ≥40 yr
Papanicolaou (Pap) test: sexually active women, at least every 3 years, ages 21 to 65 yr
Chlamydia: sexually active women ≤25 yr and older women at risk
Bone mineral density test: women ≥65 yr and at-risk women ages 60–64 yr
Vision screening: age ≥65 yr
Assess for hearing impairment: age ≥65 yr

COUNSELING

Substance use
  Tobacco cessation
  Reduce risky or harmful alcohol use
  Avoid alcohol and drug use while driving, swimming, boating†
Diet and exercise
  Limit saturated fat; maintain calorie balance; emphasize grains, fruits, and vegetables‡
  Adequate calcium intake (women)
  Regular physical activity†
Sexual behavior
  Unintended pregnancy: contraception
  STD prevention: avoid high-risk behavior,† use condoms or female barrier with spermicide†
Injury prevention
  Lap and shoulder belts
  Motorcycle, bicycle, and ATV helmets†
  Smoke detector†
  Safe storage and removal of firearms†
Dental health
  Regular visits to dental care provider†
  Floss, brush with fluoride toothpaste daily†

IMMUNIZATIONS

Pneumococcal vaccine (once, age ≥65 yr)
Influenza vaccine (annual, age ≥50 yr)
Tetanus-diphtheria (Td) boosters (every 10 yr)
Measles, mumps, rubella (MMR) vaccine (susceptible adults ages 19 to 49 yr)§
Varicella (2 doses, susceptible adults ages 19 to 49 yr)§
Human papilloma virus (HPV) vaccine (3 doses, women age ≤26 yr)

CHEMOPREVENTION

Multivitamin with folic acid (women planning or capable of pregnancy)
Discuss benefits and harms of aspirin to prevent myocardial infarction in middle-aged adults and others at increased risk of heart disease

*Depression screening is most effective where systems exist to improve management of depression.
†The ability of clinician counseling to influence this behavior is uncertain.
‡Diet counseling is most effective when it is targeted to at-risk groups.
§Immunity can be verified by serologic testing, documented history of illness, or vaccination.
HDL = high-density lipoprotein; CVD = cardiovascular disease; STD = sexually transmitted disease; ATV = all-terrain vehicle.

TABLE 13–3 RECOMMENDED SCREENING AND INTERVENTIONS FOR HIGH-RISK POPULATIONS

Potential Interventions	Population
Ultrasound examination for abdominal aortic aneurysm	Current or former smokers, ages 65 to 75 yr
HIV test	High-risk sexual behavior or IV drug use; consider local epidemiology*
Syphilis (RPR/VDRL)	High-risk sexual behavior; consider local epidemiology*
Gonorrhea screen	High-risk sexual behavior; consider local epidemiology*
PPD	Immigrants, tuberculosis contacts, alcoholics; consider local epidemiology*
Hepatitis B vaccine	Exposure to blood products; IV drug use; high-risk sexual behavior; travelers to specific countries
Hepatitis A vaccine	Persons living in or traveling to high-risk areas; institutionalized persons and workers in these institutions; certain chronic medical conditions
Meningococcal vaccine	First-year college students in dormitories; military recruits; asplenia; travelers to high-risk areas
Varicella vaccine	Adults born after 1980 without evidence of immunity
Discuss breast cancer chemoprevention	Women at increased risk for breast cancer and low risk of thromboembolic complications
Diabetes screen	Persons with elevated blood pressure or high cholesterol

*Routine screening may be indicated in communities or settings where infection is prevalent.
HIV = human immunodeficiency virus; IV = intravenous; RPR = rapid plasma reagin; VDRL = Venereal Disease Research Laboratory; PPD = purified protein derivative.

TABLE 13–4 INTERVENTIONS NOT RECOMMENDED FOR ROUTINE USE IN ASYMPTOMATIC AVERAGE-RISK ADULTS*

Resting or exercise electrocardiography or helical CT for asymptomatic coronary disease
Ultrasound examination for asymptomatic carotid artery disease
Chest radiograph or helical CT for early detection of lung cancer
Routine blood tests for anemia
Routine urine tests
Blood tests or ultrasound examination for ovarian cancer
Whole body CT
Brief tests of mental status
Vitamin supplements
Blood test for hepatitis C infection
Blood level of C-reactive protein to predict coronary risk

*These tests are not recommended for routine use because they are not supported by evidence that they improve clinical outcomes. Any of the tests may be appropriate for selected patients on the basis of clinical judgment, and some are under investigation for more widespread use.
CT = computed tomography.

weeks, have you felt down, depressed, or hopeless? and During the past 2 weeks, have you felt little interest or pleasure in doing things?—may be as sensitive as longer instruments. To improve outcomes, however, screening for depression must be linked to an organized system of follow-up and treatment.

High Blood Pressure

Blood pressure should be measured periodically (Chapter 66). As with lipid guidelines, intensity of treatment should be tailored to cardiovascular risk status rather than to blood pressure alone. [1]

Abnormal Lipids

The USPSTF recommends measuring total and high-density lipoprotein (HDL) cholesterol, which can be done on nonfasting samples, beginning in middle age. The National Cholesterol Education Program guidelines recommend fasting lipoprotein analysis beginning at the age of 20 years (Chapter 217). Either strategy will detect the high-risk patients who need lipid-lowering therapy, which can reduce coronary events by an estimated 25 to 30%. [2] Treatment decisions should be based on estimates of coronary heart disease risk, considering the presence and severity of other risk factors such as age, tobacco use, diabetes, and high blood pressure *(www.nhlbi.nih.gov/guidelines/cholesterol/index.htm)* (Chapter 49).

Abdominal Aortic Aneurysm

Between 5 and 9% of men older than 65 years have an abdominal aortic aneurysm (Chapter 78). The risk is higher in smokers and substantially lower in women. On the basis of four large trials in which screening reduced deaths from ruptured aneurysms in older men by up to 40%, the USPSTF recommends one-time screening for abdominal aortic aneurysms with ultrasound examination in men aged 65 to 75 years who are current or former smokers. [3]

Colorectal Cancer

Screening for colorectal cancer can reduce both incidence of and mortality from colorectal cancer. [4] Options for screening men and women older than 50 years include an annual fecal occult blood test, flexible sigmoidoscopy every 5 to 10 years; colonoscopy every 10 years, or barium enema every 5 to 10 years (Chapter 203). The choice should consider local resources and patients' preferences. Colonoscopy is the most sensitive test but carries higher costs and risks, and no single strategy has been proved to be more effective or cost-effective than the other alternatives. Evidence is not yet sufficient to support newer technologies such as computed tomographic colography or stool tests for DNA markers of neoplasia.

Breast Cancer

In large trials, mammography screening (with or without clinical breast examination) reduces breast cancer mortality by 20 to 30% (Chapter 208). [5] The decision of when to begin and when to discontinue screening should be a shared decision between a woman and her physician. Most but not all trials suggest benefits extend to women screened in their 40s, but the benefits are smaller and risks of false-positive results higher than in women aged 50 to 70 years. The marginal benefits of annual (versus biennial) mammography and of the clinical breast examination are uncertain; they increase the detection rate for cancer but at the expense of more false-positive results. Although many cancers are discovered by the patient, teaching of breast self-examination has not been proved to improve outcomes. Widespread screening for *BRCA1* or *BRCA2*, inherited mutations that increase the risk for breast cancer, is not recommended, but women with a suggestive family history (multiple first-degree relatives with breast or ovarian cancer) should be referred for genetic counseling.

Cervical Cancer

Papanicolaou (Pap) screening is highly effective in preventing invasive cervical cancer, but consensus has grown that prevailing practices in the United States excessively screen many low-risk women. Recent changes endorse less frequent screening (every 2 to 3 years) in women with previous normal test results (Chapter 209); delay of screening until the age of 21 years or 3 years after onset of sexual activity; offering low-risk women the option of discontinuation of screening after 65 years of age; and discontinuation of screening in women after total hysterectomy. Liquid-based cytology specimens have not been proved to improve clinical outcomes significantly, but they allow testing for human papillomavirus (Chapter 203), which may help in managing borderline Pap smear results, such as atypical squamous cells. Primary screening for human papillomavirus, although sensitive for cervical neoplasia, is not recommended for routine use because it identifies many younger women with transient infection. The availability of human papillomavirus vaccine (Chapter 16) may substantially alter appropriate screening practices.

Prostate Cancer

Screening with prostate-specific antigen (PSA) can increase the detection of organ-confined prostate cancer, but proof that regular prostate cancer screening can lower morbidity or mortality from prostate cancer is still lacking (Chapter 211). The prognosis of untreated prostate cancer varies with the grade of the tumor. For early prostate cancer, prostatectomy can reduce progression of cancer and deaths from prostate cancer, but the benefits of prostatectomy or irradiation may not apply to all cancers detected by PSA screening. Screening may increase morbidity in some men by leading to treatment of indolent cancers, especially in men older than 70 years. The USPSTF concluded that current evidence is not adequate for a recommendation to be made for or against regular screening. If early detection is effective, men who are between the ages of 50 and 70 years and in good health are most likely to benefit. The American Cancer Society and some specialty groups recommend offering PSA screening to men who have a life expectancy of at least 10 years, after potential benefits and harms have been discussed.

Osteoporosis

Tests of bone mineral density, by use of central or peripheral tests, can identify women who are at high risk of fracture and who may benefit from medications proven to lower the risk of fractures in women with osteoporosis (Chapter 264). Other risk factors, such as age, low body weight, and fracture history, can be incorporated along with bone mineral density to calculate more specific estimates of fracture risk *(http://courses.washington.edu/bonephys)*. The benefits of screening and treatment are clearest for women older than 65 years and for postmenopausal women with specific risk factors for fracture.

Thyroid Disease

Routine thyroid testing can identify patients with symptomatic but undiagnosed hypothyroidism (Chapter 244), but screening of healthy people primarily detects subclinical hypothyroidism, a disorder marked by elevations in thyroid-stimulating hormone with normal levels of free thyroxine. Because the benefits of treating subclinical hypothyroidism remain uncertain, the USPSTF does not recommend routine thyroid testing in the absence of symptoms. Clinicians should be alert to subtle signs of thyroid disease and have a low threshold for testing patients in high-risk groups, including postpartum and postmenopausal women.

Diabetes

Routine screening for diabetes beginning at the age of 45 years is recommended by some groups but not by the USPSTF (Chapter 248). Although tight glucose control can reduce the incidence of microvascular disease, the benefit of early detection on retinopathy, neuropathy, and nephropathy is likely to be small. More substantial benefits are achieved by screening for diabetes among patients who have hypertension or elevated lipid levels because more aggressive treatment of cardiovascular risk factors in patients with diabetes produces significant benefits during a relatively short period.

HIV Infection

The USPSTF recommends screening for HIV infection in all pregnant women and in adolescents and adults at increased risk. In an effort to reduce the estimated 25% of infected patients who have not yet been diagnosed, however, the Centers for Disease Control and Prevention now recommends that all adolescents and adults aged 13 to 64 years have at least one HIV test and annual tests if at high risk.

Sexually Transmitted Disease

Screening for chlamydia is recommended for all sexually active women younger than 25 years and for older women at risk. Early detection can reduce pelvic inflammatory disease, a risk factor for infertility and ectopic pregnancy (Chapter 307). [6] Similar benefits are likely from screening women for gonorrhea, but the risk of gonorrhea infection is more concentrated in high-risk urban and southeastern rural populations. New DNA-based tests, which can be performed on urine or cervical specimens, have largely supplanted culture techniques.

Vision and Hearing

Undetected but correctable vision and hearing problems are common in older adults and can be detected by asking about problems and performing simple tests of visual acuity and hearing.

BEHAVIORAL INTERVENTIONS

Lifestyle factors such as tobacco use, alcohol abuse, diet, lack of physical activity, and other risky behaviors contribute to a large proportion of preventable deaths in the United States. There is good evidence that brief interventions can have measurable effects on some behaviors such as smoking and problem drinking, but changing other behaviors usually requires more intensive interventions. The *5 As* framework—ask, assess, advise, assist, and arrange—that developed from smoking cessation research provides a useful framework for other behavioral interventions.

Tobacco Use

Brief interventions can produce small but clinically important increases in quit rates among smokers. Effects increase with more intensive counseling and support, including use of medication (Chapter 30).

Problem Drinking

A variety of screening instruments can detect patients with problems due to alcohol and those with risky patterns of alcohol consumption. Brief interventions can successfully reduce alcohol consumption in at-risk drinkers (Chapter 31).

Diet

Diet counseling can reduce intake of saturated fat and increase consumption of fruits and vegetables. Effects are most consistent with more intensive counseling (multiple sessions with trained counselors) and in higher risk patients, such as patients with elevated lipid levels (Chapter 232).

Physical Activity

Moderate physical activity reduces the risk of obesity, diabetes, and coronary heart disease, among other benefits. Studies of counseling in the primary care setting, however, have reported inconsistent effects on long-term levels of physical activity (Chapter 14).

Injury Prevention

Motor vehicle injuries are the leading cause of years of potential life lost before the age of 65 years (Chapter 15). In older persons, falls are a leading cause of unintentional injury and can be reduced with targeted interventions (Chapter 23).

IMMUNIZATIONS

Recommendations regarding immunization are regularly updated by the Advisory Committee on Immunization Practices of the Centers for Disease Control and Prevention *(www.cdc.gov/nip)* (Chapter 16). The most severe complications of influenza occur in adults older than 50 years and others at high risk because of chronic conditions or immunodeficiency, but annual immunization is also effective in healthy adults and can reduce transmission and lost work time. Pneumococcal immunization is recommended at least once at the age of 65 years or after for all adults and for younger adults with asplenia, chronic heart or lung disease, and other immune disorders. Revaccination is not generally recommended unless initial immunization was before 65 years of age or patients have immune-related risk factors.

Tetanus is rare in persons who have received a complete series of primary vaccinations. Revaccination every 10 years, however, incorporating diphtheria and acellular pertussis vaccine at least once, can reduce risk of pertussis and maintain levels of immunity against diphtheria.

DISCUSSIONS ABOUT CHEMOPREVENTION

Aspirin, postmenopausal hormone replacement therapy, and breast cancer chemopreventive drugs carry both benefits and risks. Decisions need to consider the likely benefits (which increase with the underlying risk of the disease being prevented), the probability of harm, and the individual preferences of each patient.

Aspirin

Aspirin reduces the risk of myocardial infarction by up to 30% in men and ischemic stroke by 25% in women, but it also increases risk of serious gastrointestinal bleeding and hemorrhagic stroke. [7] Benefits exceed risks as the 10-year risk of heart disease (for men) or stroke (for women) approaches 10%, but individual preferences should be considered (Chapters 49, 70, 72, 430, and 431).

Chemoprevention of Breast Cancer

Tamoxifen and raloxifene can reduce the incidence of invasive breast cancer by nearly 50% in women at increased risk, but both agents increase risk of thromboembolic events (including stroke) and worsen menopausal symptoms; tamoxifen also increases risk of endometrial cancer (Chapter 208). The balance of benefits and harm is most favorable in women younger than 60 years who have an increased risk of breast cancer due to family history. Tools are available to calculate risk of breast cancer based on age and individual risk factors (*http://cancer.gov/bcrisktool*).

Postmenopausal Hormone Therapy

Estrogen therapy reduces the risk of fracture, but it does increase the risk of thromboembolism and gallbladder disease (Chapter 262). When it is given with progestin, postmenopausal estrogen modestly increases the risk of heart disease, stroke, breast cancer, and dementia. [8] Risk is most pronounced in women older than 60 years. Use of hormone replacement should be limited to women with troublesome menopausal symptoms and should aim for the lowest effective dose for the shortest period.

Vitamin Supplementation

The USPSTF does not recommend routine vitamin supplementation because multiple large trials have failed to demonstrate benefits of vitamin A, C, or E against heart disease or cancer. Two studies suggested that β-carotene may increase risk of lung cancer in smokers. Ongoing studies are examining whether folic acid supplementation can reduce the risk of heart disease.

QUALITY MEASUREMENT AND IMPROVEMENT

Clinicians are increasingly accountable for delivering recommended preventive care. Health plans collect and report data on the delivery rates of a number of preventive services, including smoking cessation, immunizations, and cancer screening. These data are being extended to groups and individual clinicians in "pay for performance" strategies that link reimbursement rates to performance targets (Chapter 11). Improving regular delivery of preventive care requires a systems approach. Among the most effective interventions for increasing the delivery of preventive care are reminders aimed at patients and physicians, standing orders (especially for immunizations), and feedback on performance, all of which are facilitated by having an electronic medical record. Educational material alone does not have a consistent effect on patients or clinicians. A ranking of preventive services based on health gains, cost-effectiveness, and current delivery rates indicates that the highest priorities for improving clinical preventive services are tobacco cessation counseling, colorectal cancer screening, chlamydia screening, and pneumococcal immunization. [9]

FUTURE ISSUES

As the understanding of genetic factors that modify the risk of disease grows, clinicians may eventually be able to target screening, preventive treatments, or lifestyle interventions to those at greatest risk. Although the number of mutations associated with specific diseases is growing steadily, their value for routine use in primary care is limited by incomplete understanding of the predictive value of specific genotypes in the general population, the uncertain role of the information on clinical decisions, and concerns about the possible adverse effects of screening (anxiety or "labeling," false reassurance, or discrimination). A number of genetic screens for cancer risk are now commercially available, but their primary role is to assist in the counseling of individuals from high-risk families rather than to screen the general population (Chapter 38).

Important information on benefits and harms of new screening tests is expected from large ongoing trials of PSA screening, helical computed tomography for early detection of lung cancer, serum tumor markers and ultrasound examination for the detection of ovarian cancer, and alternative methods for screening for colorectal cancer (see *clinicaltrials.gov*).

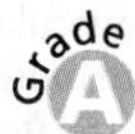

1. Chobanian AV, Bakris GL, Black HR, et al: The Seventh Report of the Joint National Committee on Prevention, Detection, Evaluation, and Treatment of High Blood Pressure. The JNC 7 report. JAMA 2003;289:2560–2572.
2. Grundy SM, Cleeman JI, Bairey CN, et al: Implications of recent clinical trials for the National Cholesterol Education Program Adult Treatment Panel III Guidelines. Circulation 2004;110:227–239.
3. Fleming C, Whitlock EP, Beil TL, Lederle FA: Screening for abdominal aortic aneurysm: A best-evidence systematic review. Ann Intern Med 2005;142:203–211.
4. Pignone M, Rich M, Teutsch SM, et al: Screening for colorectal cancer in adults at average risk: Summary of the evidence for the U.S. Preventive Services Task Force. Ann Intern Med 2002;137:132–141.
5. Humphrey LL, Helfand M, Chan BKS, Woolf SH: Breast cancer screening: Summary of the evidence. Ann Intern Med 2002;137:344–346.
6. Nelson HD, Helfand M: Screening for chlamydial infection. Am J Prev Med 2001;20:95–107. Available at http://www.elsevier.com/locate/ajpmonline.
7. Berger JS, Roncaglioni MC, Avanzini F, et al: Aspirin for the primary prevention of cardiovascular events in women and men: A sex-specific meta-analysis of randomized controlled trials. JAMA 2006;295:306–313.
8. Writing Group for the Women's Health Initiative Investigators: Risks and benefits of estrogen plus progestin in healthy postmenopausal women: Principal results from the Women's Health Initiative randomized controlled trial. JAMA 2002;288:321–333.
9. Maciosek MV, Coffield AB, Edwards NM, et al: Priorities among effective clinical preventive services: Results of a systematic review and analysis. Am J Prev Med 2006;31:52–61.

SUGGESTED READINGS

Boulware LE, Marinopoulos S, Phillips KA, et al: Systematic review: Value of the periodic health evaluation. Ann Intern Med 2007;146:289–300. *May improve preventive services and lessen worry.*

Canadian Task Force on Preventive Health Care. Available at http://www.ctfphc.org. *A practical guide to preventive health interventions.*

National Guideline Clearinghouse. Available at http://www.guidelines.gov. *Standardized descriptions of more than 1700 guidelines, with full text access to many of them. Guidelines can be searched by condition, intervention, or organization, and the site will construct a comparison of different guidelines on a given topic.*

PDQ—NCI's Comprehensive Cancer Database. Available at http://nci.nih.gov/cancertopics/pdq/cancerdatabase. *Up-to-date reviews of cancer prevention and screening topics.*

Task Force on Community Preventive Services; Zaza S, Priss PA, Harris KW (eds): The Guide to Community Preventive Services: What Works to Promote Health? New York, Oxford University Press, 2005. Available at http://www.thecommunityguide.org. *This guide, sponsored by the Centers for Disease Control and*

Prevention and available online, provides updated reviews and recommendations on a wide array of community-based preventive interventions.

U.S. Preventive Services Task Force. Available at http://preventiveservices.ahrq.gov. *This site includes all the recommendations and the supporting reviews of the USPSTF.*

14 PHYSICAL ACTIVITY

David M. Buchner

Regular physical activity has numerous health benefits and is an essential component of a healthy lifestyle. Characteristics of the individual, social environment, and physical environment influence levels of physical activity in ways that vary from person to person. Clinical interventions affect many behavioral determinants, and medical care plays a key role in promoting physical activity.

Definitions

Physical activity is defined as body movement that is produced by skeletal muscles and expends energy. *Exercise,* which is a subset of physical activity, involves a structured program designed to improve one or more components of physical fitness. *Physical fitness* refers to an individual's ability to perform physical activity. *Health-related physical fitness* refers to components of fitness that influence the risk for disease or produce functional limitations (or both): aerobic (or endurance) capacity, muscular strength and endurance, body composition, and flexibility. Attributes such as balance and bone strength may also be regarded as health-related measures of fitness.

The primary attributes of physical activity are *type* (mode), *frequency, duration,* and *intensity.* Types of physical activity (e.g., walking, swimming, lifting, stretching) are grouped according to their main physiologic effects into well-known categories: *aerobic* (or "cardio"), *muscle strengthening, flexibility,* and *balance.*

Evidence for the health benefits of aerobic activity is much more extensive than for the benefits of other types of activity. As a result, public health recommendations and clinical practice guidelines focus mainly on aerobic activity. The *absolute intensity* of aerobic activity is measured in metabolic equivalents (METs), with 1 MET being the resting metabolic rate, or an oxygen consumption of about 3.5 mL/kg/min. Moderate-intensity aerobic activity is in the range 3.0 to 6.0 METs; a brisk walk at 3 to 4 mph is a common example. Vigorous activity is greater than 6.0 METs, and light activity is less than 3.0 METs. The *volume* of aerobic activity (frequency × duration × intensity) is measured in units such as MET-hours per week—a sum across all activities of the MET intensity of an activity multiplied by time spent on that activity. When body weight is taken into account, volume is measured as activity-related caloric expenditure.

The *relative intensity* of aerobic activity is also of interest inasmuch as improvement in fitness depends on the intensity of aerobic activity relative to fitness. Relative intensity is measured on a scale of 0 to 100% as the percentage of oxygen uptake (aerobic capacity) reserve. In practice, the heart rate is used to monitor relative intensity because of the generally linear relationship between heart rate and percent oxygen uptake.

Epidemiology

The health benefits of physical activity do not depend on whether its purpose is recreation, work, transportation, or domestic tasks. National U.S. and state-based surveys initially tracked only leisure-time (recreational) physical activity, These surveys showed that the physical activity levels of American adults are low: about 30% of Americans are inactive (sedentary) in their leisure time, about 45% are insufficiently active, and only about 25% are active at recommended levels (defined later). Trends in leisure activity over time have been flat, with the exception of a gradual decline in the percentage of individuals who are inactive and a greater decline in older age groups, which have the highest rates of inactivity. For example, in 1990 about 50% of women 70 years and older were inactive as compared with about 40% in 2002. In more recent national surveys that track domestic, leisure-time, and transportation physical activity, about 45% of American adults are active at recommended levels.

Physical activity levels decline with age, and men report more activity than women. Higher levels of income and education are associated with greater physical activity. White Americans report higher levels of physical activity than other racial and ethnic groups do.

Prevention

Preventive Health Benefits

Regular physical activity reduces the risk for premature mortality and cardiovascular disease (Chapter 49), stroke, high blood pressure (Chapter 66), some lipid disorders (Chapter 217), type 2 diabetes mellitus (Chapter 248), osteoporosis (Chapter 264), colon cancer (Chapter 203), breast cancer (Chapter 208), and obesity (Chapter 239). There is substantial evidence that physical activity also reduces the risk for falls, age-related muscle loss, depression, and anxiety disorders (Chapters 23 and 420). Some evidence suggests that physical activity reduces the risk for sleep problems, cognitive impairment, osteoarthritis, and back pain. Observational studies consistently report that physical activity delays age-related functional limitations and loss of independence (disability).

The benefits of physical activity are independent of other risk factors. For example, a sedentary obese smoker achieves health benefits from exercise, even if smoking and obesity persist.

Epidemiologic studies report that low levels of activity are associated with an increase in risk for adverse health outcomes, including as large as a 52% increase in overall mortality, a doubling of mortality from cardiovascular disease, and a 29% increase in mortality from cancer. When a healthy diet, regular activity, and abstinence from smoking are simultaneously considered, the effect of lifestyle is dramatic. For example, one study attributed 82% of coronary events in women to lack of adherence to a healthy lifestyle.

The health benefits of physical activity are proportional to the amount, although the dose-response relationship is probably curvilinear such that the marginal benefit of activity at lower levels is large and the benefit decreases with higher activity levels. For example, in data from more than 70,000 women, the risk for cardiovascular disease, when compared with the least active women, was 11% less in women who averaged 4.2 MET-hr/wk but only 28% less in women who were five to six times more active (average of 23.4 MET-hr/wk). A randomized trial of two doses of exercise (doses equivalent to jogging 12 and 20 miles/wk) found that even a lower volume of exercise significantly improved plasma lipoproteins but the higher volume of exercise had greater beneficial effects. [1] The dose-response relationship also varies by disease. For example, the risks for premature mortality and cardiovascular disease are related to the volume of aerobic activity over a wide range of volume, whereas the dose-response relationship of activity with blood pressure is fairly flat, with most benefit occurring at lower levels of activity. Resistance training and high-impact activities have greater influence on bone density than the dose of aerobic activity does.

Treatment

Therapeutic Benefits

Clinical practice guidelines assign a substantial therapeutic role to physical activity in patients with coronary heart disease (Chapter 48), high blood pressure (Chapter 66), type 2 diabetes (Chapter 248), obesity (Chapter 239), osteoporosis (Chapter 264), osteoarthritis (Chapter 283), claudication (Chapter 79), and chronic obstructive pulmonary disease (Chapter 88). Physical activity also plays a role in the management of depression and anxiety disorders, elevated cholesterol levels, pain, heart failure, syncope, stroke, prophylaxis of venous thromboembolism, back pain, dementia, and constipation.

Physical activity effectively opposes age-related loss of fitness and functional limitations. Randomized controlled trials demonstrate that exercise by sedentary older adults improves health-related physical fitness (e.g., aerobic exercise improves aerobic capacity) and has beneficial effects on functional limitations, such as a slow gait speed. [2] Generally, the benefits are most demonstrable in older

Rx

adults with clinically significant functional limitations. Physical activity, especially balance training, prevents falls in older adults at increased risk for falls, such as those with frequent falls or impaired gait and balance. 3 It is probable that physical activity improves the ability to live independently, but evidence from randomized trials is incomplete.

Health Risks of Physical Activity

Physical activity and exercise have risks, and risk management strategies are important when recommending regular physical activity. Musculoskeletal overuse injuries, which are the most common adverse effect of physical activity, vary widely by setting. Research studies of exercise programs rarely report major injuries, possibly because such studies exclude participants with a high risk for injury or implement effective risk management strategies. By comparison, the incidence of injuries was reported to be greater than 50% in women undergoing 8 weeks of U.S. Army basic training. In a cohort study of community adults with above-average levels of activity, about 25% reported a musculoskeletal injury in a year.

Overall, regular physical activity decreases the risk for sudden cardiac death and myocardial infarction. However, vigorous physical activity acutely increases the risk for these events in both active and inactive adults. About 5 to 10% of myocardial infarctions are associated with vigorous activity. Sudden death is a rare event during exercise, with published rates in the range of one death per year in 18,000 ostensibly health men and one death per 2.6 million workouts in fitness facilities.

Recommended Amounts of Aerobic Activity for Prevention

The fundamental scientific basis for recommending aerobic physical activity was summarized in the 1996 Surgeon General's report *Physical Activity and Health:* a person achieves meaningful, significant health benefits from a moderate amount of physical activity. Additional health benefits can be gained from greater amounts of activity.

An adult can achieve the recommended levels of aerobic activity by engaging in either moderate-intensity or vigorous-intensity activity. To meet the vigorous recommendation developed in the 1980s, adults should perform at least 20 minutes of continuous vigorous aerobic activity on 3 or more days each week.

Alternatively, adults can engage in moderate-intensity aerobic activity according to a recommendation originally issued in 1995 by the Centers for Disease Control and Prevention and the American College of Sports Medicine. Adults should accumulate at least 30 minutes of moderate-intensity physical activity on 5 or more days each week. Bouts of moderate-intensity activity that count toward meeting the 30-minute minimum must be at least 10 minutes in duration. It is inappropriate to cite the recommendation as "a person needs only 30 minutes a day." Many people should exceed the minimal recommended amounts so that they obtain additional health benefits.

Recommended Amounts of Muscle-Strengthening Activity for Prevention

Adults should perform activities that strengthen the major muscle groups of the body at least 2 days each week. Historically, people engaged in muscle-strengthening activities as part of manual labor. Today, most people prefer weightlifting or other forms of resistance exercise. A typical resistance exercise program involves one to three sets of 6 to 10 exercises on 2 or 3 days each week, with at least 1 day off between exercise involving the same muscle group.

Flexibility Activity

There is insufficient evidence that flexibility activities have health benefit. Stretching exercises have been recommended to prevent injuries, but evidence for this benefit is inconclusive. Flexibility training does increase flexibility, and it is commonly recommended as part of exercise programs, in part because flexibility training may permit and facilitate the type of physical activity that has health

Rx

benefits. If so, flexibility training is more important for people with reduced flexibility, such as older adults who have experienced age- and disease-related changes in range of motion.

Balance Activity

Balance training is currently recommended only for adults at increased risk for falls, generally adults older than 65 years with impaired gait or balance or frequent falls. Randomized trials have demonstrated that multicomponent fall prevention programs that include physical activity are effective. Meta-analyses, which seek to identify the effective components in fall prevention programs, indicate that balance training is effective. The optimal frequency, duration, and type of balance training are unknown, but training three times a week was effective in several studies.

Recommending Physical Activity in Clinical Settings

Efforts to promote physical activity in clinical settings have used essentially the same steps as the five A's of smoking cessation: Ask, Advise, Assess, Assist, Arrange. (1) Ask about the amount of physical activity that a patient typically achieves each week by questionnaire or interview. (2) Advise all patients to get at least a moderate amount of physical activity each week. Advise patients who do not meet the recommendations to increase their physical activity gradually to a specified minimal level, and tailor the recommendations according to medical conditions. (3) Assess the next step or steps that a patient needs to take to become more active. (4) Assist the patient in taking these steps. (5) Arrange an appointment to follow up on efforts to increase activity.

Health care providers should ask and advise patients about physical activity regularly. A recent quality-of-care measure assesses whether asking and advising are done at least once a year in older adults. Asking at least once a year is reasonable, given the importance of physical activity and the fact that adults (especially older adults) identify their health care provider as an important source of advice on physical activity.

The evidence on the effectiveness of primary care–based counseling (i.e., assessing and assisting) with respect to physical activity is rated as inconclusive by the most recent U.S. Preventive Services Task Force review. A reasonable approach is to counsel selected patients, with selection partly based on patients' preferences. Some patients may prefer help from a health care provider or benefit from brief clinical counseling. Other patients may prefer help in increasing their activity levels from other sources, such as community exercise classes, self-help materials, and walking groups.

Exercise Prescription

For patients who prefer exercise, a clinician can provide an exercise prescription. The prescription includes (1) the type, frequency, duration, and intensity of aerobic exercise; (2) the exercise movements (e.g., bench press), repetitions, and sets for resistance exercise; (3) other exercises such as stretching, balance exercises, warm-up, and cool-down; and (4) risk management strategies, such as increasing levels of activity gradually over time.

For aerobic exercise, the American College of Sports Medicine recommends a minimum frequency of at least 3 days per week, a minimum duration of 20 minutes, and an intensity of 70 to 85% of the maximal heart rate (HR_{max}). When HR_{max} is measured, there is good confidence that the target heart range is appropriate. When HR_{max} is estimated, there is error in estimating the target range. Ratings of perceived exertion are useful in monitoring and adjusting exercise intensity in this situation. The aerobic exercise session should include warm-up and cool-down activities (Fig. 14–1). Moderate-intensity training (40 to 60% of oxygen uptake reserve or 50 to 69% of HR_{max}) is an option, although it typically requires more than 3 days per week to reach an adequate volume of exercise. Training at the upper limits of vigorous intensity (85 to 89% of HR_{max}) is discouraged because of concern about injury and adherence (higher exercise intensities are commonly regarded as less pleasant).

For resistance training, the recommendation is 8 to 10 separate exercises that train the major muscle groups. Adults should perform

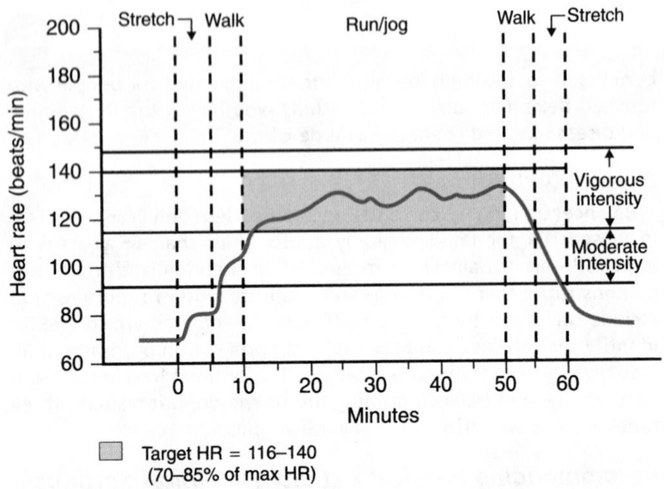

FIGURE 14–1 • Illustration of an aerobic exercise program. The figure illustrates a program for an adult with a maximal heart rate (HR_{max}) of 165 beats per minute and fitness sufficient for running and jogging. Moderate-intensity exercise is in the range of 91 to 115 beats per minute (55 to 69% of HR_{max}) and vigorous intensity in the range of 116 to 148 beats per minute (70 to 89% of HR_{max}). The target heart rate is in the range of 116 to 140 (70 to 85% of HR_{max}) because this range represents a good compromise in health benefits, fitness benefits, risk for injury, enjoyment, and time required to obtain the recommended amounts of physical activity in the average person. Walking precedes run/jog as a warm-up and follows run/jog as a cool-down. It is preferable to begin and end the exercise sessions with stretching exercises, although other approaches are acceptable given the lack of information on how stretching influences the risk for injury. The program would be performed on 3 or more days each week. Moderate-intensity training is acceptable for adults who prefer it or to reduce the risk for injury, in which case exercise typically occurs on more than 3 days per week to meet health and fitness goals.

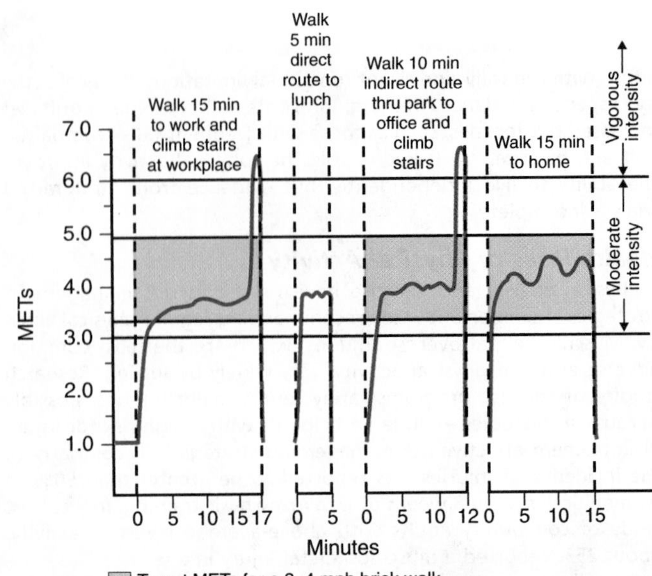

FIGURE 14–2 • Illustration of a walking program integrated into daily activities. A person obtains moderate-intensity aerobic activity (3.0 to 6.0 METs) at a target level of effort during a brisk walk (3.0 to 4.0 mph). Because moderate-intensity bouts of less than 10 minutes do not count toward the recommendations, the person obtains 40 min/day of moderate-intensity activity that counts toward recommendations: 15 minutes walking to work, 15 minutes walking home from work, and 10 minutes walking an indirect route from lunch to work. Although the 5-minute walk to lunch does not count toward the recommendations, it and the climbing of stairs at work expend calories and thereby assist in weight management. This program would be performed 5 days a week, preferably supplemented by leisure physical activity on other days.

Rx

at least one set of 8 to 12 repetitions of each exercise on 2 or 3 nonconsecutive days each week, except that older adults should do 10 to 15 repetitions in a set. Although more than one set is associated with larger gains in strength, these gains are usually modest in previously sedentary adults.

Lifestyle Prescription

The term "lifestyle intervention" broadly refers to approaches that integrate physical activity into daily life. Physical activity recommendations are met by activities such as domestic chores, walking for transportation, or gardening (Fig. 14–2). Moderate-intensity activities are in the range of 3.0 to 6.0 METs, and vigorous activities are above this range.

Tailoring the Recommendation

Recommendations need to be tailored according to individual abilities, individual preferences, medical conditions, and behavior techniques that improve adherence. Randomized trials show that home-based programs are superior to center-based programs in terms of long-term adherence. 4 Although center-based programs are preferred by some, in most cases they serve a short-term purpose, such as assisting adults to initiate regular exercise. Adults with chronic conditions should perform physical activity according to therapeutic recommendations and clinical practice guidelines. If able, adults should also meet preventive recommendations for aerobic and muscle-strengthening activity to prevent new chronic conditions. For example, 3 days per week of aerobic exercise is recommended as effective treatment of arthritis, but individuals with arthritis would still benefit from 5 or more days per week (if they are capable) so that other chronic diseases might be prevented.

A target level of physical activity below that of preventive recommendations is appropriate for adults with very low fitness, a large burden of chronic disease (such as severe chronic obstructive lung disease), or major functional limitations. An assessment of the nature of the activity limitation and the capability and preferences of the person will determine the target activity level and other details of the activity recommendation. Often, promoting physical

Rx

activity in such adults relies on health care and community resources designed for people with preexisting limitations, such as cardiac rehabilitation, pulmonary rehabilitation, and exercise classes for adults with arthritis.

Risk Management

A lack of research on effective strategies for reducing the risks associated with activity means that risk management strategies rely mainly on expert opinion, clinical experience, and legal liability concerns. Risk for activity-related injury is regarded as higher with (1) higher volumes of exercise, (2) participation in vigorous exercise, (3) rapid increases in activity, and (4) obesity. Risk for injury is regarded as lower with (5) higher levels of fitness, (6) supervision, (7) protective equipment such as bike helmets, and (8) well-designed environments that eliminate hazards. Each of these eight risk factors implies strategies for risk management. The type of activity also influences the risk for injury. Evidence supports the clinical experience that walking has a low risk for injury and is popular. Despite the lack of evidence that stretching prevents injury, it is reasonable to recommend stretching based on clinical experience and the lack of evidence that stretching has adverse effects. Arguably, the most importance risk management strategy is to increase physical activity gradually over time. Although exercise stress testing has been recommended by some to reduce the risk for sudden death with exercise, the U.S. Preventive Services Task Force does not recommend exercise testing or any other forms of mass screening for heart disease.

Coordination between Medical Care and Community

Many factors affecting physical activity levels are difficult to influence in medical care settings, such as the characteristics of the communal environment (e.g., parks and recreation facilities) and the social environment (e.g., crime and social support). Community-level interventions that address such characteristics are essential to promoting physical activity. Effective community-based interventions include school physical education, social support interventions, community-wide campaigns, enhancement of access to places for physical activity, and interventions that involve community design, such as improving the connectivity of streets and the walkability of neighborhoods. Medical care and community efforts should be synergistic and mutually supportive. For example, health plans should be advocates for evidence-based community interventions. Community programs should serve as resources for evidence-based therapeutic activity for selected chronically ill adults, such as exercise classes designed to reduce the risk of falls.

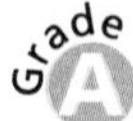

1. Kraus WE, Houmard JA, Duscha BD, et al: Effects of the amount and intensity of exercise on plasma lipoproteins. N Engl J Med 2002;347:1483–1492.
2. Latham NK, Bennett DA, Stretton CM, et al: Systematic review of progressive resistance strength training in older adults. J Gerontol A Biol Sci Med Sci 2004;59:48–61.
3. Robertson MC, Campbell AJ, Gardner MM, et al: Preventing injuries in older people by preventing falls: A meta-analysis of individual-level data. J Am Geriatr Soc 2002;50:905–911.
4. Ashworth NL, Chad KE, Harrison EL, et al: Home versus center based physical activity programs in older adults. Cochrane Database Syst Rev 2005;1:CD004017.

SUGGESTED READINGS

Gulati M, Black HR, Shaw LJ, et al: The prognostic value of a nomogram for exercise capacity in women. N Engl J Med 2005;353;468–475. *Exercise capacity is a strong predictor of mortality.*

Holmes MD, Chen WY, Feskanich D, et al: Physical activity and survival after breast cancer diagnosis. JAMA 2005;293:2479–2486. *Physical activity decreases the risk for development of breast cancer and may improve survival in women with breast cancer.*

Jeon CY, Lokken RP, Hu FB, et al: Physical activity of moderate intensity and risk of type 2 diabetes: A systematic review. Diabetes Care 2007;30:744–752. *Moderate exercise can reduce the risk of type 2 diabetes.*

Thompson PD, Buchner D, Pina IL, et al: Exercise and physical activity in the prevention and treatment of atherosclerotic cardiovascular disease: A statement from the Council on Clinical Cardiology (Subcommittee on Exercise, Rehabilitation, and Prevention) and the Council on Nutrition, Physical Activity, and Metabolism (Subcommittee on Physical Activity). Circulation 2003; 107:3109–3116. *A broad yet concise review of the role of physical activity in prevention and treatment of cardiovascular disease.*

U.S. Preventive Services Task Force: Screening for coronary heart disease: Recommendation statement. Ann Intern Med 2004;140:569–572. *The U.S. Preventive Services Task Force recommends against routine screening, such as by exercise treadmill testing, in adults at low risk for coronary heart disease.*

VIOLENCE AND INJURY

Susan B. Sorenson

Definition

Injuries are damage to the body by an energy exchange (due to mechanical, thermal, and other energies) that exceeds the body's capacities to withstand that energy. Injuries occur in identifiable patterns with associated risk factors. Injuries, therefore, usually are not accidents, a term that implies an event due to circumstances out of the control of humans.

Epidemiology

Injuries are the leading cause of death of all persons younger than 45 years in the United States. Among men, injuries account for 35% of the years of potential life lost before the age of 65 years, which is more years of potential life lost than are attributable to heart disease, malignant neoplasms, human immunodeficiency virus infection, liver disease, and diabetes combined. Injuries are not limited to the young, however. Falls and their attendant complications are common among the elderly (Chapter 23).

Motor vehicle crashes are the leading cause of death of 15- to 24-year-olds, accounting for more than one third of all deaths in this age group. Firearms, which also are a substantial problem in some populations, are the leading cause of death of 15- to 24-year old African American men. Motor vehicles and guns also account for a majority of the serious traumatic injuries (Chapter 113) treated in emergency departments across the nation. Other nonfatal injuries commonly seen in emergency departments include suicide attempts (Chapter 420) and injuries due to intimate partner violence.

A small fraction of all injuries result in fatalities. Most injuries are acute events with a relatively brief recovery period. Some injuries, however, are more severe and result in temporary and sometimes permanent disability (e.g., spinal cord injury and brain injury; Chapter 422). Injury is a common condition for which acute care and rehabilitation are sought.

Ethnicity, Nativity, and Gender

The risk of injury differs across ethnic and age groups. Injury rates are highest among American Indians for all ages below 75 years. In fact, the rate of unintentional injury alone is, with one exception, higher among American Indians than the rate of unintentional injury, homicide, and suicide combined for all other ethnic groups among 15- to 74-year olds (Fig. 15–1). Among 15- to 34-year olds, injuries account for a majority of the deaths due to all causes. These same trends are seen in women, but the absolute rates of fatal and nonfatal injury are much lower among women than among men.

Unintentional death rates due to injuries, previously on a declining pattern, have been increasing since 1992. However, the gap in life expectancy between African Americans and whites in the United States is narrowing, and part of the decrease in the gap is attributable to greater reductions in mortality due to unintentional injury among African Americans.

The rate of suicide is lower among African Americans, average age 34 years, than among whites, average age 44 years, in the United States. The risk of suicide differs by age and ethnicity, and suicide rates are highest among elderly white men (Chapter 420). Clinicians should be aware of suicide risk as it relates to the population of patients they serve.

By contrast, African Americans, Hispanics, and American Indians are at substantially greater risk than are whites of becoming a homicide victim. Homicide rates for young African American men are down from their peak of 140 per 100,000 in 1991, but homicide rates remain extraordinarily high—86.7 per 100,000—for 15- to 34-year-old African American men.

Ethnicity and immigration are linked in the United States. About one in nine U.S. residents is an immigrant, and the fraction is substantially higher in some parts of the country. For example, in California, home to nearly one of every eight U.S. residents, more than one fourth of the population was born outside the United States. Among young immigrants (15- to 34-year-olds), non-Hispanic white, Hispanic, and Asian immigrants are at increased risk of homicide; non-Hispanic white immigrants are at increased risk and Hispanic immigrants are at decreased risk of suicide; and non-Hispanic white immigrants are at increased risk of unintentional injury.

These demographic patterns relate to the pathogenesis of injury. In the United States, an increasing number of motor vehicle crashes occur at intersections, owing in part to noncompliance with traffic signals. Noncompliance with traffic laws and regulations is considered a major cause of motor vehicle crashes in Mexico. Are Hispanics in the United States less likely to comply with traffic laws? A study using 7 years of data from the national Fatality Analysis Report System found no differences among African American, white, and Hispanic drivers in rates of fatal crashes caused by running through red lights. One Hispanic group, however, was associated with running red lights—Hispanics who do not have a valid driver's license or a record of previous driver's license suspension, presumably because they are recent immigrants to the United States. Drinking and driving, by contrast, was strongly related to red light running. Nationally, representative data indicate that compared with whites of European origins, Hispanics are less likely to drink but consume more alcohol on the days that they drink. Clinicians whose practices include many immigrants would be wise to recognize that given the general pattern of similar or higher risk, the "healthy immigrant" phenomenon, by which immigrants generally are healthier than their U.S.-born counterparts, appears not to extend to fatal injuries.

Boys and men have much higher rates of both fatal and nonfatal injuries than do women. Less widely recognized, however, is the similarity of the relative risk of injuries as a cause of death for men and women: the rank of unintentional injuries, suicide, and homicide is nearly identical for men and women (Table 15–1). Another similarity among men's

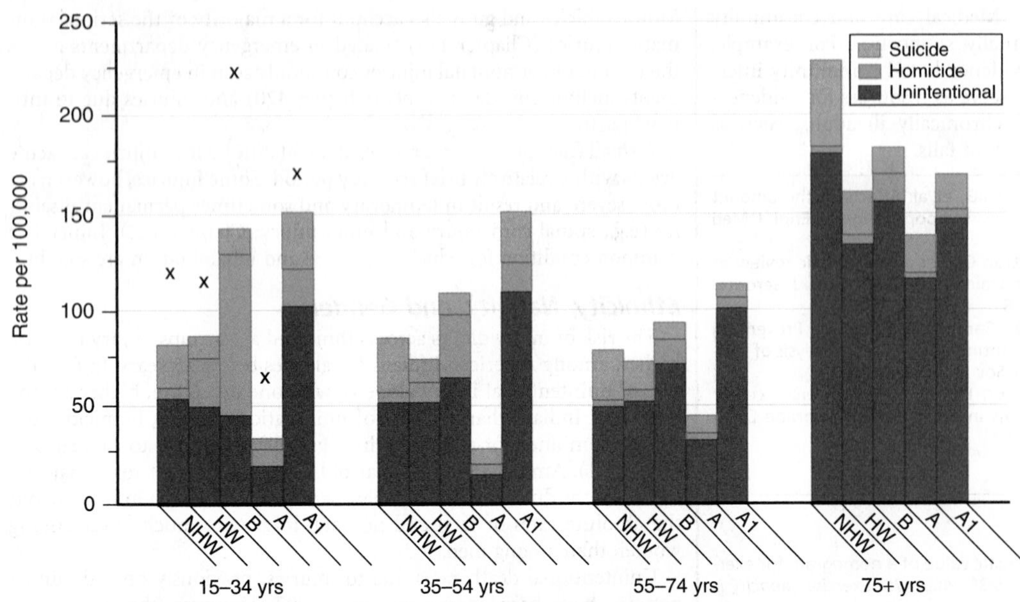

FIGURE 15–1 • Injury rates, U.S. men by age and ethnicity, 2002. A = Asian; AI = American Indian; B = black; HW = Hispanic white; NHW = non-Hispanic white. The X above each ethnic group for 15- to 34-year-olds indicates the death rate from all causes for that age group. Data accessed September 24, 2005, at *http://www.cdc.gov/hcipc/wisquars/*.

TABLE 15–1 RANK OF INJURIES AS A CAUSE OF DEATH, UNITED STATES, 2002, BY AGE AND SEX

	Age (years)										
Rank	**<1**	**1–4**	**5–9**	**10–14**	**15–24**	**25–34**	**35–44**	**45–54**	**55–64**	**65+**	**All ages**
1		MUI, FUI	MUI, FUI	MUI, FUI	MUI, FUI	MUI, FUI	MUI				
2					MH, FH	MS	FUI				
3		MH, FH		MS	MS	MH		MUI, FUI			
4			MH, FH	MH, FH	FS	FS	MS, FS		MUI		MUI
5				FS		FH		MS			
6	MUI								FUI		
7	FUI						MH				FUI
8							FH	FS	MS	MUI	MS
9										FUI	
10											

FS = female, suicide; FUI = female, unintentional injury; MH = male, homicide; MS = male, suicide; MUI = male, unintentional injury; SH = female, homicide.
Source: Data accessed September 26, 2005 at http://www.cdc.gov/hcipc/wisquars/

and women's injury deaths is the mechanism of injury. Motor vehicle crashes are the most common type of unintentional injury death for both men and women, and firearms, specifically handguns, are the most common mechanism of intentional injury (both suicide and homicide) for both men and women. Therefore, injuries are relevant to women's health as well (Chapter 254), especially when they are considered in the context of intimate partner violence.

Treatment

Rx

Prevention and Risk Reduction

Whereas efforts to reduce injuries in factories and other workplaces began in the late 1800s, the beginning of injury prevention as a science often is credited to Hugh DeHaven, an airplane pilot who incurred multiple injuries in a 1917 practice flight crash from which the other pilot walked away. The field of injury prevention grew to cover a wide range of unintentional injuries—motor vehicle crashes, burns (Chapter 113), acute poisonings (Chapter 111), submersions, suffocations, and the like. In the late 1980s, the field expanded to include intentional injuries—assaults, homicides, suicide, and other injuries—in its framework.

The unique contribution of injury prevention is its focus on the mechanism of injury—the motor vehicle, the firearm—rather than on characteristics or behaviors of the injured individual or the individual who might become injured. Having relatively little to show after decades of focusing on behavior, injury prevention turned to engineering and policy. Characteristics and behaviors of individuals (e.g., impulsivity, alcohol consumption) are acknowledged as important, but the mechanism of injury typically is given priority in interventions.

Diverging from traditional approaches, a primary focus of injury prevention is to reduce the *injury* rather than to eliminate the event that has the potential of producing an injury. One example of such attempts is the biomechanics researcher who drops helmeted cadaver heads from varying heights onto flat anvil surfaces. The goal of this work is not to prevent a motorcycle crash but to protect the skull and its contents in the event of a crash. This approach has gained widespread acceptance such that consumers can access online reports from the National Highway Traffic Safety Administration (NHTSA) and the Insurance Institute for Highway Safety to learn about the crashworthiness of motor vehicles and the ability of a given make and model of vehicle to protect its occupants in the event of a crash.

The importance of a multifaceted approach to reduce and to prevent injuries is illustrated well in an injury matrix developed by William Haddon, a physician with public health training who was

	Host	Vehicle	Environment	
			Social	Physical
Pre-event	Driver's education	Improved braking systems	Media campaigns to reduce drunk driving	Roadways that allow good visibility
Event	Maintaining good physical health	Rounded, padded interior surfaces Air bags	"Good Samaritan" norms and laws	Sand-filled barrels at freeway exit ramps
Post-event	Emergency and rehabilitative medical care	Vehicle repair services	Mandated emergency care regardless of insurance status	Physical proximity of trauma centers

FIGURE 15–2 • Preventing injuries from motor vehicle crashes. (From Haddon W Jr: A logical framework for categorizing highway safety phenomena and activity. J Trauma 1972;12:197.)

Rx

the first director of NHTSA, a U.S. federal agency established in 1970 to reduce deaths, injuries, and economic losses resulting from motor vehicle crashes. Two key concepts underlie the matrix: time—before the crash or other event that has the potential to produce an injury, the event itself, and after the event; and the target of the intervention—the person who could be injured, the mechanism that delivers the force or other energy that can produce an injury, the social environment, and the physical environment.

The example of motor vehicle injuries illustrates actions that would derive from the cross section of the concepts of time and target (Fig. 15–2). Each of these possible interventions could reasonably be expected to reduce motor vehicle crashes. Because interventions aimed at individual behavior change (e.g., drivers' education) have been met with limited success, the injury field has come to focus primarily on potential solutions based on engineering and policy (e.g., design of roadways and motor vehicles, laws mandating helmet use and reduced speed limits). By identifying multiple intervention points, the Haddon matrix emphasizes the interdependence of efforts to reduce death and disability due to injury.

Haddon's injury matrix for motor vehicles has been modified, with some success, to address intentional injuries. With assault and other injuries caused by another person, the matrix can be adapted to include a column for the other individual (the suspect, in criminal justice parlance). The focus on the external mechanism is useful, in no small part because only a few mechanisms are responsible for a substantial portion of deaths. In the United States, motor vehicle traffic-related injuries, gunshot wounds, poisons (Chapter 111), and falls (Chapter 113) account for about one in every four, one in every five, one in every six, and one in every ten injury deaths, respectively.

Intimate Partner Violence

Intimate partner violence includes physical, sexual, and psychological maltreatment at the hands of a current or former spouse or boyfriend or girlfriend. The inclusion of nonmarital relationships is important because such violence also occurs in relationships that are not legally sanctioned, relationships that are legally over, and relationships that involve same-sex partners.

Like homicides in general, the number of intimate partner homicides has dropped substantially during the past 25 years, especially homicides of men by intimate partners. Homicides remain highest for girlfriends. The most common weapon used in all intimate partner homicides is a firearm. Despite a general emphasis on "stranger danger," women are at higher risk of homicide by an intimate; women are 2.2 times as likely to be shot by a current or former intimate partner as to be shot, stabbed, strangled, bludgeoned, or killed in any other way by a stranger. The elevated risk is due largely to handguns; women are 1.6 times as likely to be killed by an intimate partner with a handgun than to be murdered in any other way by a stranger.

Health care providers, especially emergency department personnel, have tried to identify and more fully treat women who are victims of intimate partner violence. Although this identification and treatment is far from complete, the general trend has moved away from treat-the-injury-and-release and embraced an approach in which the underlying issues are addressed to reduce recurrent injury.

Attempts to "lay out the facts" and instruct a woman who has been battered to leave an abusive partner are generally ineffective. Economic, familial, psychological, and other considerations often influence a woman's decision about whether to stay with or to leave an abusive partner. The decision to stay, which often appears inconsistent with external logic, is consistent with theories of traumatic bonding and learned helplessness. A colloquial description that sometimes is useful is that of a frog in a pot of hot water. If a frog is placed in hot water, it will quickly try to escape, but if a frog is placed in cool water and the heat under the pot is gradually increased, the likely outcome is a cooked frog. A healthy woman facing a violent partner will seek to escape quickly; a healthy woman who has been exposed to ongoing and gradually increasing forms of psychological, sexual, and physical violence is less able to realize when that same point of danger has been passed.

Data suggest that on average, a woman makes seven attempts to leave an abusive relationship before finally leaving. Battered women are much like "healthy" women who are willing to give a relationship one more try for the sake of the children, because he has changed, because she really loves him, or myriad other reasons. Many, like the spouses of alcoholics (Chapter 31) who want the drinking but not the relationship to end, want the violence but not the relationship to stop. Furthermore, the risk of homicide at the hands of the intimate partner increases substantially as the woman attempts to end the relationship. As a result, when the woman does what the clinician and others tell her (i.e., leave the abusive partner), she increases her risk of being murdered. Thus, exhortations by medical personnel to leave the relationship are not likely to be acted on and actually increase risk to the woman, unless they incorporate safety planning to reduce the risk of harm.

Not surprisingly, an abused woman's risk of being killed by an intimate partner is higher if the partner has access to a firearm and if the partner has used a gun as part of the abuse. All 50 states have restraining orders, although they may be called by various names (e.g., orders of protection). U.S. federal law has added persons under a domestic violence restraining order and those convicted of a domestic violence misdemeanor to the list of persons who are prohibited from purchasing and possessing a firearm. Obtaining a civil order of protection is associated with fewer subsequent injuries and reduced abuse-related medical care. Clinicians can assess if a woman who has been abused is in extreme danger by asking whether the abuser has been arrested for domestic violence, has ever threatened the victim with a weapon, or has ever threatened to kill her and whether the partner has access to a firearm.

SUGGESTED READINGS

Evans L: Traffic Safety. Bloomfield Hills, MI, Science Service Society, 2004. *Covers important topics in traffic safety.*

Mitchell C, Anglin D (eds): Intimate Partner Violence: A Health-Based Perspecture. New York, Oxford University Press, 2007. *Medical textbook that reviews health issues related to intimate partner violence.*

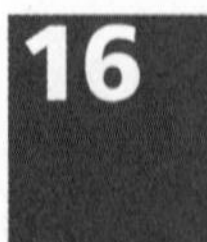

16 IMMUNIZATION

Walter A. Orenstein

Immunization is one of the most cost-effective means of preventing morbidity and mortality from infectious diseases. Routine immunization, particularly of children, has resulted in decreases of 90% or more in reported cases of measles, mumps, rubella, congenital rubella syndrome, poliomyelitis, tetanus, and diphtheria. In many circumstances, immunization not only prevents morbidity and mortality but also, in the long run, reduces health care costs.

GENERAL CHARACTERISTICS OF IMMUNIZATIONS

Immunization protects against disease or the sequelae of disease through the administration of an immunobiologic—vaccines, toxoids, immune globulin preparations, and antitoxins. Protection induced by immunization can be active or passive.

Active Immunization

Administration of a vaccine or toxoid causes the body to produce an immune response against the infectious agent or its toxins. Vaccines consist of suspensions of live (usually attenuated) or inactivated microorganisms or fractions thereof. Toxoids are modified bacterial toxins that retain immunogenic properties but lack toxicity. Active immunization generally results in long-term immunity, although the onset of protection may be delayed because it takes time for the body to respond. With live attenuated vaccines, small quantities of living organisms multiply within the recipient until an immune response cuts off replication. In contrast, inactivated vaccines and toxoids contain large quantities of antigen. In most recipients, a single dose of a live vaccine generally induces an immune response that closely parallels natural infection and induces long-term immunity. Killed vaccines, in contrast, often require multiple doses.

Passive Immunization

Passive immunization with use of immune globulins or antitoxins delivers preformed antibodies to provide temporary immunity. Immune globulins obtained from human blood may contain antibodies to a variety of agents, depending on the pool of human plasma from which they are prepared. Specific immune globulins are made from the plasma of donors with high levels of antibodies to specific antigens, such as tetanus immune globulin. Most immune globulins must be injected intramuscularly, although an intravenous preparation is also available. Antitoxins are solutions of antibodies derived from animals immunized with specific antigens (e.g., diphtheria antitoxin). Passive immunization usually is indicated to protect individuals immediately before anticipated exposure or shortly after known or suspected exposure to an infectious agent (Table 16–1), when active immunization either is not possible or has not been adequate.

TABLE 16–1 PASSIVE IMMUNIZATIONS FOR ADULTS

Disease	Name of Material	Comments and Use
Tetanus	Tetanus immune globulin, human	Management of tetanus-prone wounds in persons without adequate prior active immunization and treatment of tetanus
Cytomegalovirus	Cytomegalovirus immune globulin, intravenous	Prophylaxis for bone marrow and kidney transplant recipients
Diphtheria	Diphtheria antitoxin, equine	Treatment of established disease, high frequency of reactions to serum of nonhuman origin; in the United States, available only from CDC
Rabies	Rabies immune globulin, human	Postexposure prophylaxis of animal bites
Measles	Immune globulin, human	Prevention or modification of disease in contacts of cases, not for control of epidemics
Hepatitis A	Immune globulin, human	Protection of household contacts, pre-exposure prophylaxis for travelers who need protection before immunity can be achieved with hepatitis A vaccine
Hepatitis B	Hepatitis B immune globulin, human	Prophylaxis for needlestick or mucous membrane contact with HBsAg-positive persons, for sexual partners with acute hepatitis B or hepatitis B carriers, for infants born to mothers who are carriers of HBsAg, for infants whose mother or primary caregiver has acute hepatitis B
Varicella	Varicella-zoster immune globulin (varizig)	Persons with underlying disease and at risk of complications from chickenpox who have not had varicella or varicella vaccine and who are exposed to varicella; may be given after exposure to known susceptible adults, particularly if antibody negative.
Vaccinia	Vaccinia immune globulin	Treatment of eczema vaccinatum, vaccinia necrosum, and severe inadvertent inoculations such as ocular vaccinia after vaccinia (smallpox) vaccination
Erythroblastosis fetalis	Rh immune globulin	Rh-negative women who give birth to Rh-positive infants or who abort
Hypogammaglobulinemia	Immune globulin, intravenous	Maintenance therapy
Idiopathic thrombocytopenic purpura	Immune globulin, intravenous	Therapy for acute episodes
Botulism	Trivalent A, B, and E antitoxin, equine	Treatment of botulism; available through CDC
Snakebite	Antivenin, equine (North American coral snake antivenin)	Specific for North American coral snake, *Micrurus fulvius*
	Crotalidae, polyvalent	Effective for viper and pit viper bites, including rattlesnakes, copperheads, moccasins
Spider bite	Antivenin, equine	Specific for black widow spider, *Latrodectus mactans,* and other members of the genus

CDC = Centers for Disease Control and Prevention; HBsAg = hepatitis B surface antigen.

Route and Timing of Vaccination

Each immunobiologic has a preferred site and route of administration. In adults, vaccines containing adjuvants should be injected intramuscularly, preferably in the deltoid muscle. For most adults, intramuscular injections should be administered with a 1- to 1½-inch, 22- to 25-gauge needle. Use of the buttocks is discouraged except when large volumes are required because of the potential for damage to the sciatic nerve and because of diminished immune response to some vaccines, such as hepatitis B, probably because of injection into fat rather than into muscle. Subcutaneous vaccines also are usually administered in the deltoid area. In general, inactivated vaccines and toxoids can be given at the same visit at different sites. Live and inactivated vaccines usually can be administered at the same time. Measles, mumps, and rubella (MMR) vaccine can be administered at the same time as inactivated poliovirus vaccine and live attenuated varicella vaccine. With the exception of injected or intranasal vaccines, such as MMR and live attenuated influenza vaccine, live vaccines not delivered on the same day should be separated by at least 1 month to avoid interference. Orally administered live vaccines, such as oral typhoid vaccine, can be administered at any interval before or after live injected or intranasal vaccines. Immune globulin also may interfere with the replication of injected live vaccine viruses; ideally, most live vaccines should be administered at least 2 weeks before or 3 to 11 months after immune globulin. Immune globulin does not interfere with the response to yellow fever vaccine and is not believed to interfere with orally or intranasally administered live virus vaccines.

Adverse Reactions

No vaccine is completely safe or completely effective. Hypersensitivity to vaccine components, such as animal proteins, antibiotics, preservatives, and stabilizers, can lead to local and systemic reactions ranging from mild to severe. The egg protein contained in vaccines grown in chicken eggs (influenza and yellow fever vaccines) may cause reactions in persons severely allergic to eggs. In general, persons without anaphylactic-type allergies to eggs can be given these vaccines safely, but persons with anaphylactic reactions to eggs generally should not receive these vaccines except when it is absolutely necessary and then only under established protocols by physicians who are expert in such situations. Although measles and mumps vaccines are grown in chick embryo tissue culture, the risk of anaphylaxis even in persons with severe hypersensitivity to eggs is low, so they can be vaccinated without prior testing. Suspected adverse events temporally related to vaccinations should be reported to the Vaccine Adverse Events Reporting System (1-800-822-7967 or *www.vaers.hhs.gov*).

General Considerations

The major group that makes comprehensive, detailed recommendations regarding immunization of adults is the Advisory Committee on Immunization Practices of the U.S. Public Health Service, which publishes its information in *Morbidity and Mortality Weekly Report* (also available at *www.cdc.gov/nip/acip*). Immunizations for adults depend on age, lifestyle, occupation, and medical conditions. Two adult immunization schedules are available, one based on age group (Fig. 16–1A) and one based on underlying risk (Fig. 16–1B and Table 16–2). All adults should have a primary series of tetanus and diphtheria toxoids with boosters of combined toxoids (Td) every 10 years. Adults younger than 65 years of age should have a one-ime dose of combined tetanus and diphtheria toxoids and acellular pertussis vaccine (TdaP) followed by Td every 10 years. Persons born in or after 1957 should have evidence of immunity to measles, mumps, and rubella (e.g., documentation of vaccination or presence of antigen-specific immunoglobulin G). Vaccination of susceptible adolescents and adults against varicella is desirable. Pneumococcal polysaccharide vaccine (PPSV23) and annual vaccination against influenza are indicated for all adults 65 years old and older and younger adults with certain medical conditions that place them at high risk of complications. Influenza vaccine also is recommended for all adults 50 to 64 years of age. Household contacts of and people caring for patients at high risk of complications from influenza, including children younger than 5 years of age, should receive annual vaccination to decrease exposure of the high-risk patient to the virus. Health care workers exposed to blood or blood products should receive hepatitis

Recommended Adult Immunization Schedule, by Vaccine and Age Group
UNITED STATES, OCTOBER 2006–SEPTEMBER 2007

Vaccine	Age group (yrs) 19–49 years	50–64 years	≥ 65 years
Tetanus, diphtheria pertussis (Td/Tdap)[1]*		1 dose Td booster every 10 yrs Substitute 1 dose of Tdap for Td	
Human papillomavirus (HPV)[2]*	3 doses (females)		
Measles, mumps, rubella (MMR)[3]*	1 or 2 doses	1 dose	
Varicella[4]*	2 doses (0, 4–8 wks)	2 doses (0, 4–8 wks)	
Influenza[5]*	1 dose annually	1 dose annually	
Pneumococcal (polysaccharide)[6,7]	1–2 doses		1 dose
Hepatitis A[8]*		2 doses (0, 6–12 mos, or 0, 6–18 mos)	
Hepatitis B[9]*		3 doses (0, 1–2, 4–6 mos)	
Meningococcal[10]		1 or more doses	

NOTE: These recommendations must be read along with the footnotes, which can be found at MMWR 2006;55:1–4 and at http://www.cdc.gov/mmwr/PDF/wk/mm5540-Immunization.pdf.

*Covered by the Vaccine Injury Compensation Program.

For all persons in this category who meet the age requirements and who lack evidence of immunity (e.g., lack documentation of vaccination or have no evidence of prior infection)

Recommended if some other risk factor is present (e.g., based on medical, occupational, lifestyle, or other indications)

A

FIGURE 16–1 • Recommended immunization schedules for adults. A, Recommended adult immunization schedule by vaccine and age group.

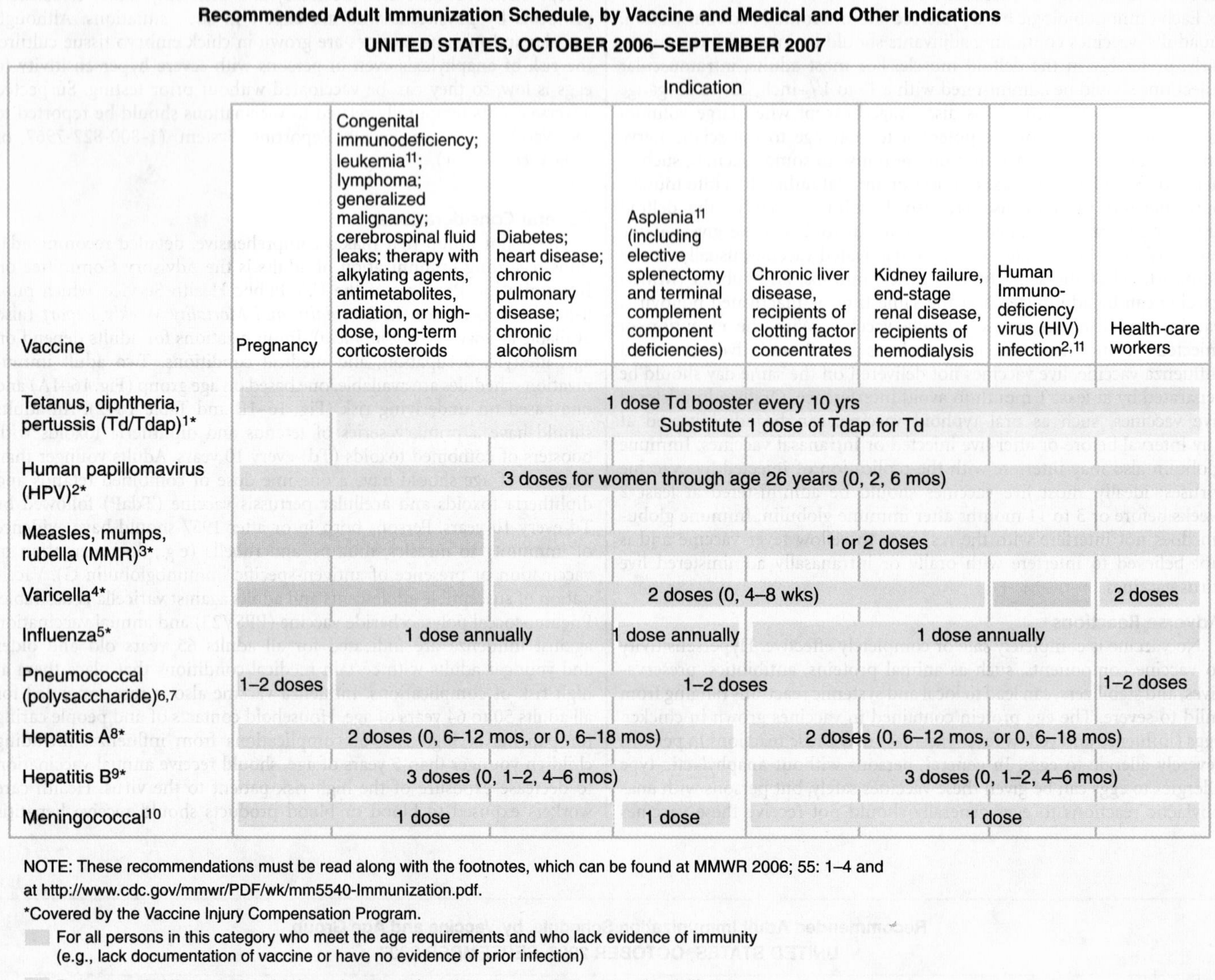

Recommended Adult Immunization Schedule, by Vaccine and Medical and Other Indications

UNITED STATES, OCTOBER 2006–SEPTEMBER 2007

	Indication							
Vaccine	Pregnancy	Congenital immunodeficiency; leukemia[11]; lymphoma; generalized malignancy; cerebrospinal fluid leaks; therapy with alkylating agents, antimetabolites, radiation, or high-dose, long-term corticosteroids	Diabetes; heart disease; chronic pulmonary disease; chronic alcoholism	Asplenia[11] (including elective splenectomy and terminal complement component deficiencies)	Chronic liver disease, recipients of clotting factor concentrates	Kidney failure, end-stage renal disease, recipients of hemodialysis	Human Immuno-deficiency virus (HIV) infection[2,11]	Health-care workers
Tetanus, diphtheria, pertussis (Td/Tdap)[1]*	1 dose Td booster every 10 yrs Substitute 1 dose of Tdap for Td							
Human papillomavirus (HPV)[2]*	3 doses for women through age 26 years (0, 2, 6 mos)							
Measles, mumps, rubella (MMR)[3]*			1 or 2 doses					
Varicella[4]*			2 doses (0, 4–8 wks)					2 doses
Influenza[5]*	1 dose annually			1 dose annually	1 dose annually			
Pneumococcal (polysaccharide)[6,7]	1-2 doses	1–2 doses						1-2 doses
Hepatitis A[8]*	2 doses (0, 6–12 mos, or 0, 6–18 mos)				2 doses (0, 6–12 mos, or 0, 6–18 mos)			
Hepatitis B[9]*	3 doses (0, 1–2, 4–6 mos)				3 doses (0, 1–2, 4–6 mos)			
Meningococcal[10]	1 dose			1 dose	1 dose			

NOTE: These recommendations must be read along with the footnotes, which can be found at MMWR 2006; 55: 1–4 and at http://www.cdc.gov/mmwr/PDF/wk/mm5540-Immunization.pdf.

*Covered by the Vaccine Injury Compensation Program.

For all persons in this category who meet the age requirements and who lack evidence of immunity (e.g., lack documentation of vaccine or have no evidence of prior infection)

Recommended if some other risk factor is present (e.g., based on medical, occupational, lifestyle or other indications)

Contraindicated

B

FIGURE 16–1, cont'd • B, Recommended adult immunization schedule by vaccine and medical and other indications. (The footnotes are available at *http://www.cdc.gov/nip/recs/adult-schedule-pss.pdf.*)

B vaccine. Health care workers likely to come in contact with persons transmitting measles, mumps, rubella, or varicella should be immune to those diseases.

Immunocompromise

Patients with conditions that compromise their immune systems should not receive live attenuated vaccines. Such patients include those with immunodeficiency diseases, leukemia, lymphoma, and generalized malignant disease and those who are immunosuppressed from therapy with corticosteroids, alkylating agents, antimetabolites, and radiation. An exception is infection with human immunodeficiency virus (HIV). Asymptomatic patients should receive MMR vaccine. MMR should be considered for symptomatic patients with HIV infection; however, severely immunocompromised persons should not be vaccinated. Patients with leukemia in remission who have not been receiving any chemotherapy for at least 3 months may receive live virus vaccines. Short-course therapy (<2 weeks) with corticosteroids, alternate-day regimens with low to moderate doses of short-acting corticosteroids, and topical applications or tendon injections are not ordinarily contraindications to the administration of live vaccines.

Immunocompromised patients can receive inactivated vaccines and toxoids, although the efficacy of such preparations may be diminished. Patients with known HIV infection should receive pneumococcal vaccine and annual influenza vaccination.

Pregnancy

In general, live vaccines should not be given to pregnant women because of the theoretical concern that the vaccines could adversely affect the fetus. No significant adverse events attributable to vaccination of pregnant women with MMR or varicella have been documented; nevertheless, pregnant women should not receive MMR or varicella vaccine, and women who do receive these vaccines should wait 1 month before becoming pregnant. Poliomyelitis and yellow fever vaccines usually should not be given to pregnant women unless the risk of disease is substantial. Td vaccination is especially indicated for pregnant women who are not appropriately vaccinated to prevent neonatal tetanus in their infants. Vaccination is done best after the first trimester to avoid attribution to a vaccine of an adverse outcome of pregnancy that was only coincidental. Most pregnant women should not receive TdaP. In such cases, however, TdaP should be administered postpartum provided at least 2 years have lapsed since the last dose of Td. All pregnant women should be screened for hepatitis B surface antigen (HBsAg). Offspring of HBsAg carrier mothers should receive hepatitis B vaccine and hepatitis B

Text continued on p. 80.

TABLE 16–2 SELECTED IMMUNIZING AGENTS INDICATED FOR ADULTS*

Disease	Immunizing Agent	Indications	Schedule	Major Contraindications and Precautions	Comments
Anthrax	Anthrax vaccine, adsorbed, an inactivated vaccine	Pre-exposure prophylaxis of persons at high risk of exposure (e.g., military, certain laboratory workers) Consider with antibiotics for postexposure prophylaxis	0.5-mL dose SC at 0, 2, and 4 wk and 6, 12, and 18 mo Manufacturer recommends booster annually thereafter If used after exposure, 3 doses at 0, 2, and 4 wk with antibiotics for at least 7–14 days after third dose	Severe allergic reaction to a vaccine component or after a prior dose Moderate or severe acute illness is a precaution to vaccination.	Effectiveness against aerosol exposure inferred primarily from animal data Limited data on the benefits of postexposure use
Diphtheria	Tetanus and diphtheria toxoids combined	All adults	Two doses IM 4 wk apart, third dose 6–12 mo after second dose for primary series Booster every 10 yr No need to repeat if schedule is interrupted	History of neurologic reaction after a previous dose Severe allergic reaction to a vaccine component or after a prior dose Moderate or severe acute illness is a precaution but not a contraindication.	Tetanus and diphtheria toxoids combined with acellular pertussis vaccine preferred for booster at age 11–12 yr
Hepatitis A	Inactivated hepatitis A vaccine	Travelers to highly or intermediately endemic countries Men who have sex with men Illegal drug users (injectors and noninjectors) Persons who work with hepatitis A virus–infected primates or who do research with the virus Persons with chronic liver disease Recipients of clotting factors	Two doses at least 6 mo apart for persons aged ≥1 yr	Severe allergic reaction to a vaccine component or after a prior dose Moderate or severe acute illness is a precaution to vaccination.	Recommended for all children Should be considered for outbreak control
Hepatitis B	Inactivated hepatitis B virus subunit vaccine containing HBsAg	Adolescents Health care and public safety workers potentially exposed to blood Clients and staff of institutions for the developmentally disabled Hemodialysis patients Men who have sex with men Users of illicit injectable drugs Recipients of clotting factors Household and sexual contacts of HBV carriers Inmates of long-term correctional facilities Heterosexuals treated for sexually transmitted diseases or with multiple sexual partners Travelers with close contact for ≥6 mo with populations with high prevalence of HBV carriage	IM; three doses at 0, 1, and 6 mo	Severe allergic reaction to a vaccine component or after a prior dose Moderate or severe acute illness is a precaution to vaccination.	Pregnancy is not a contraindication. Health care workers who have contact with patients or blood, sexual contacts of persons with chronic HBV infection, hemodialysis patients and other immunosuppressed persons, and recipients of clotting factor concentrates should be tested 1–2 mo after vaccination to determine serologic response.

Continued

TABLE 16–2 SELECTED IMMUNIZING AGENTS INDICATED FOR ADULTS*—cont'd

Disease	Immunizing Agent	Indications	Schedule	Major Contraindications and Precautions	Comments
Human papilloma virus	Inactivated L1 capsid proteins of types 6, 11, 16, and 18	Females at 11–12 yr; catch-up vaccination of females up through 26 yr	Three 0.5 mL doses IM at 0, 2, and 6 mo	Hypersensitivity to vaccine components. Vaccine is not recommended for pregnant women or for males.	The vaccine will not protect against types with associated existing infections. Because the types in the vaccine are not responsible for about 30% of infections associated with cervical cancer, screening for cancer should occur as for unvaccinated women.
Influenza	Inactivated influenza virus vaccine	All adults ≥50 yr, with greatest priority for those ≥65 yr Other adults with high-risk conditions Adults caring for persons with high-risk conditions, including medical personnel (see text) Women who will be pregnant during influenza season Household contacts of persons at high risk for complications of influenza, including children <5 years of age	Annual vaccination; see annual ACIP recommendation	Severe allergic reaction to a vaccine component (including eggs) or after a prior dose Moderate or severe acute illness is a precaution to vaccination.	Optimum timing for vaccination is October and November. However, vaccination can occur in December and later, particularly for health care workers and persons at high risk for complications who were not vaccinated earlier. Only one dose of influenza vaccine per season is recommended for adults.
Live attenuated influenza vaccine		Persons 5–49 yr without underlying conditions that place them at high risk of complications from influenza	Annual vaccination; see annual ACIP statement Administered intranasally	Persons <5 yr or ≥50 yr Underlying disorders that place them at high risk of influenza complications History of GBS Pregnant women Hypersensitivity to eggs or components of vaccine	Can be used for household contacts and health care workers caring for patients without severe immunocompromise
Japanese encephalitis	Inactivated Japanese encephalitis virus vaccine	Travelers to Asia spending at least 1 mo in endemic areas during transmission season	Three 1-mL doses SC on days 0, 7, 30; shortened schedule of 0, 7, 14 days may be used when necessary Booster doses may be given after 2 yr	Persons with a history of urticaria are at greater risk of adverse reactions to vaccine Pregnancy	No data exist on concurrent administration with vaccines other than DTP, drugs (e.g., chloroquine, mefloquine), or other biologics

Measles	Live virus vaccine (combined MMR vaccine preferred if one or more components are indicated)	All adults born after 1956 without history of live vaccine on or after first birthday, physician-diagnosed measles, or detectable measles antibody Persons born before 1957 generally can be considered immune.	One dose sufficient for most adults; 2 doses at least 1 mo apart indicated for persons entering college or medical facility employment, traveling abroad, or at risk of measles during outbreaks	Altered immunity (e.g., leukemia, lymphoma, generalized malignant disease, congenital immunodeficiency, immunosuppressive therapy) Immune globulin or other blood products within prior 3–11 mo, depending on dose of immune globulin or blood product received Untreated tuberculosis Anaphylactic hypersensitivity to neomycin or gelatin Pregnancy Thrombocytopenia	Persons with anaphylactic allergies to eggs may be vaccinated (see text). Vaccine should be administered to persons with asymptomatic HIV infection and should be considered for patients except those with severe immunocompromise.
Meningococcal disease (2 vaccines)	1. Meningococcal conjugate vaccine containing polysaccharide of serogroups A, C, W135, and Y conjugated to diphtheria toxoid 2. Polysaccharide vaccine containing tetravalent A, C, W135, and Y Polysaccharide vaccine is an acceptable alternative especially for college freshmen living in dormitories and persons with high-risk medical conditions. It is the only vaccine available for persons aged 2–10 yr.	1. All 11- to 12-year-olds, unvaccinated students entering high school (~age 15 yr), college freshmen living in dormitories Licensed for 11- to 55-year-old persons Persons with terminal complement component deficiencies, anatomic or functional asplenia, travelers who will live in areas with hyperendemic or epidemic diseases; may be useful during localized outbreaks 2. An acceptable alternative to MCV4 for persons aged 11–55 yr with the above conditions College freshmen living in dormitories Persons aged 2–10 yr or >55 yr with terminal complement component deficiencies, anatomic or functional asplenia, travelers who will live in areas with hyperendemic or epidemic diseases; may be useful during localized outbreaks	1. One dose 2. One dose	1. Allergic reactions to a component of the vaccine including diphtheria toxoid and latex	1. Conjugate vaccine is preferred to polysaccharide alone for persons aged 11–55 yr with indications. 2. An excess risk of Guillain-Barré syndrome on the order of 1.25 cases per million doses has been reported within 6 weeks of vaccination in 11–19 year olds. 3. Consider revaccination after 5 yr for adults at increased risk of disease.

Continued

TABLE 16–2 SELECTED IMMUNIZING AGENTS INDICATED FOR ADULTS*—cont'd

Disease	Immunizing Agent	Indications	Schedule	Major Contraindications and Precautions	Comments
Mumps	Live virus vaccine (combined MMR vaccine preferred if one or more components are indicated)	All adults born after 1956 without history of live vaccine on or after first birthday, physician-diagnosed mumps, or detectable mumps antibody Persons born before 1957 generally can be considered immune.	One dose sufficient for most adults; 2 doses at least 1 mo apart indicated for persons entering college or medical facility employment, or traveling abroad.	Altered immunity (e.g., leukemia, lymphoma, generalized malignant disease, congenital immunodeficiency, immunosuppressive therapy) Immune globulin or other blood products within prior 3–11 mo Anaphylactic hypersensitivity to neomycin or gelatin Pregnancy Thrombocytopenia if administered with measles vaccine	Although persons born after 1957 are generally immune, vaccine can be given to adults of all ages and may be particularly indicated for postpubertal males who are thought to be susceptible. Persons with anaphylactic allergies to eggs may be vaccinated.
Pertussis	Adult preparation of pertussis antigens combined with tetanus and diphtheria toxoids (Tdap)	All 11–12 yr Catch-up vaccination for all persons 13–64 years of age Preferred interval of 5 yr from prior dose of Td but may be given at shorter intervals if risk of pertussis is high	One dose	Severe allergic reaction to a vaccine component or after a prior dose Moderate or severe acute illness is a precaution to vaccination.	Two preparations are available, one licensed for 10- to 18-year-olds, one for 11-to 64-year-olds
Pneumococcal disease	23-Valent polysaccharide vaccine	Adults with cardiovascular disease, pulmonary disease, diabetes mellitus, alcoholism, cirrhosis, cerebrospinal fluid leaks, splenic dysfunction or anatomic asplenia, Hodgkin's disease, lymphoma, multiple myeloma, chronic renal failure, nephrotic syndrome, immunosuppression, HIV infection High-risk populations such as certain Native Americans and *all* adults ≥65 yr	One dose IM or SC. A second dose should be considered ≥5 yr later for adults at high risk of disease (e.g., asplenic patients) and those who lose antibody rapidly (e.g., nephrotic syndrome, renal failure, transplant recipients). Revaccinate adults who received a first dose when <65 yr who are now ≥65 yr and who received their vaccine at least 5 yr earlier.	Severe allergic reaction to a vaccine component or after a prior dose Moderate or severe acute illness is a precaution to vaccination.	A 7-valent conjugate pneumococcal vaccine is not indicated for adults.

Poliomyelitis	Inactivated poliovirus vaccine	Certain adults who are at greater risk of exposure to wild poliovirus than the general population, including travelers to countries where poliomyelitis is epidemic or endemic, members of community or specific populations with disease caused by wild poliovirus, laboratory workers handling specimens that may contain poliovirus, health care workers in close contact with wild poliovirus	For unvaccinated adults, two doses SC 4 wk apart and a third dose 6–12 mo after the second; if <4 wk available before protection is needed, a single dose of IPV For incompletely immunized adults, complete primary series that consists of three doses of IPV or prior OPV; no need to restart interrupted series A single dose of IPV can be given to adults who previously received a primary series but now are at high risk, such as travel to an endemic area.	On theoretical grounds, pregnant women should not receive IPV. If immediate protection is needed, IPV can be used. Severe allergic reaction to a vaccine component or after a prior dose Moderate or severe acute illness is a precaution to vaccination.	
Rabies	Inactivated vaccine, HDCV, PCEC, or RVA	High-risk persons, including animal handlers, selected laboratory and field workers, and persons traveling for ≥1 mo to areas with high risk of rabies	Pre-exposure prophylaxis: three doses of 1 mL IM for HDCV, PCEC, or RVA on days 0, 7, and 21 or 28	History of severe hypersensitivity reaction	Further doses needed after exposure
Rubella	Live virus vaccine (combined MMR vaccine preferred if one or more components are indicated)	Adults, particularly women of childbearing age, who lack history of rubella vaccine and detectable rubella-specific antibodies in serum Males and females in institutions where rubella outbreaks may occur, such as hospitals, the military, and colleges Persons born before 1957, except women who can become pregnant, generally can be considered immune.	One dose SC	Pregnancy, altered immunity (e.g., leukemia, lymphoma, generalized malignant disease, congenital immunodeficiency, immunosuppressive therapy) Immune globulin or other blood products within the 3–11 mo before vaccination Anaphylactic hypersensitivity to neomycin Administration of blood products should not contraindicate postpartum vaccination Thrombocytopenia if administered with measles vaccine	Women should be counseled to avoid pregnancy for 1 mo

Continued

TABLE 16–2 SELECTED IMMUNIZING AGENTS INDICATED FOR ADULTS*—cont'd

Disease	Immunizing Agent	Indications	Schedule	Major Contraindications and Precautions	Comments
Smallpox	Live vaccinia virus	Persons working with orthopox viruses Members of public health and health care response teams	One dose intracutaneously with a bifurcated needle Boosters every 10 yr and perhaps every 3 yr for persons working with virulent orthopox viruses	History or presence of eczema or other acute, chronic, or exfoliative skin condition Immunosuppression or pregnancy in patient or a close household or personal contact History of heart disease Breast-feeding Age <1 yr Allergy to a vaccine component No contraindications if exposed to smallpox	Some complications of vaccination are treatable with vaccinia immune globulin. Vaccine is effective 3–4 days after exposure to variola and perhaps longer to prevent or to modify the illness. Serious adverse events are rare but significant, including eczema vaccinatum, progressive vaccinia, myopericarditis, autoinoculation, and encephalitis. Vaccinia is transmissible.
Tetanus	Tetanus and diphtheria toxoids combined	All adults	Three doses IM needed for primary series: two doses 4 wk apart, third dose 6–12 mo after second dose Booster every 10 yr No need to repeat if schedule is interrupted	History of neurologic or severe hypersensitivity reaction after a previous dose	Special recommendations for wound treatment (see text) Persons with GBS within the first 6 wk after immunization, particularly adults who received a prior primary series, probably should not be revaccinated in most circumstances. Tetanus and diphtheria toxoids combined with acellular pertussis vaccine preferred for boosters at age 11–12 yr

Typhoid fever	Vi capsular polysaccharide vaccine Live attenuated Ty21a oral vaccine	Travelers to areas where the risk of prolonged exposure to contaminated food and water is high May be considered for family and intimate contacts of carriers and laboratory workers who work with *Salmonella typhi*	Vi polysaccharide vaccine: one dose IM 0.5 mL, boosters every 2 yr Oral vaccine: four doses on alternate days, boosters every 5 yr	Severe local or systemic reaction to a prior dose Ty21a vaccine should not be administered to persons with altered immunity or those receiving antimicrobial agents.	Efficacy only 50–77% Food and water precautions essential
Varicella: chickenpox	Attenuated varicella vaccine, Oka strain	Persons, including health care workers, who have contact with patients at high risk of complications from varicella Persons who work with children (e.g., teachers) Persons in institutions that may have outbreaks (e.g., colleges) Nonpregnant women of childbearing age International travelers Desirable for other susceptible adolescents and adults	Two 0.5-mL SC doses 4–8 wk apart for persons ≥13 yr A second dose is recommended for all persons who previously received one dose	Immunocompromise Pregnancy Allergy to vaccine components Manufacturer recommends avoidance of salicylate use for 6 wk after vaccination.	Adults with a history of prior varicella should be considered immune. Vaccine virus has rarely been transmitted to contacts from healthy vaccinees in whom rash developed. Women who receive vaccine should not become pregnant for 1 month.
Yellow fever	Live attenuated virus (17D strain)	Persons living or traveling in areas where yellow fever exists	One dose, booster every 10 yr	Immunocompromised persons History of anaphylactic allergies to eggs Pregnancy on theoretical grounds, although may be given if risk is high	Fever, jaundice, and multiple-organ system failure (viscerotropic disease) have been rarely reported in first-time recipients of 17D-derived yellow fever vaccinations. Vaccinate only persons traveling to areas endemic to yellow fever.
Varicella: zoster	Attenuated Ok a strain of varicella, approximately 14 times more potent than varicella vaccine	Persons ≥60 years of age	One 0.65 mL dose SC	Immunocompromise Allergy to vaccine components	

*See the text and package inserts for further details, particularly regarding indications, dosage, mode of administration, side effects, and adverse reactions and contraindications.
ACIP = Advisory Committee on Immunization Practices; DTP = diphtheria-tetanus-pertussis; GBS = Guillain-Barré syndrome; HBsAg = hepatitis B surface antigen; HBV = hepatitis B virus; HDCV = human diploid cell vaccine for rabies; HIV = human immunodeficiency virus; IM = intramuscularly; IPV = inactivated poliovirus vaccine; MMR = measles, mumps, and rubella vaccine; OPV = live trivalent oral poliovirus vaccine; PCEC = purified chick embryo cell culture rabies vaccine; RVA = rabies vaccine absorbed; SC = subcutaneously.

immune globulin within 12 hours of birth. Women who will be pregnant during the influenza season should receive influenza vaccine.

INDIVIDUAL IMMUNOBIOLOGICS

Hepatitis A

Two inactivated hepatitis A (Chapter 151) vaccines are available in the United States. Seroconversion rates after a single dose of either vaccine in persons older than 1 year exceed 95%. Antibody levels shown to be protective in animals develop in almost all persons.

Indications

The vaccine is indicated primarily for persons traveling to countries, generally the developing world, with high or intermediate endemicity for hepatitis A, but it is also recommended for other groups at high risk for infection or for development of severe hepatitis. In addition, children living in communities with high rates of endemic hepatitis A (anti–hepatitis A prevalence of 30 to 40% by 5 years of age) should be vaccinated. Health care workers have not been shown to be at higher risk than the general population for hepatitis A and do not need routine immunization. Although food handlers are not at increased risk of hepatitis A compared with the general population, the consequences of infection or suspected infection in this group, which can lead to extensive public health investigations, may make vaccination cost-effective in some settings. Hepatitis A vaccine can be given to children 1 year of age or older to control outbreaks in communities with high rates of prior infection and be considered for communities with intermediate levels of prior infection (anti–hepatitis A seroprevalence of 10 to 25% by 5 years of age). In 2006, the Advisory Committee on Immunization Practices recommended universal vaccination of children. Doses vary by age and product. All schedules call for a second dose at least 6 months after the first dose, with a permissible range for one of the products 18 months after the initial dose. Vaccines are not indicated for children younger than 1 year because adequate data on safety and efficacy are lacking.

Side Effects

The most common side effect has been tenderness and soreness at the injection site. Although rare and more serious adverse events have been reported in temporal association with vaccination, a causal relationship has not been established.

Hepatitis B

Hepatitis B (Chapter 151) vaccine is the first vaccine that can prevent cancer (an estimated 800 persons per year in the United States die of hepatitis B–related liver cancer; many times more die in the developing world). It also can prevent acute and chronic complications of hepatitis B, including an estimated 4000 deaths annually from cirrhosis and 250 deaths annually from fulminant hepatic disease in the United States. The original hepatitis B vaccine in the United States consisted of purified, inactivated, alum-adsorbed, 22-nm HBsAg particles obtained from human plasma. Currently produced vaccines are derived from insertion of the gene for HBsAg into *Saccharomyces cerevisiae.* Hepatitis B vaccine, the first licensed vaccine made by use of recombinant techniques, produces adequate antibody responses in more than 90% of normal adults and more than 95% of normal infants, children, and adolescents when it is administered in a three-dose series. The dosage depends on the product, the age group, and the underlying clinical condition and can be determined by consulting the package insert. The duration of vaccine-conferred immunity is not known, although follow-up of vaccinees for more than 16 years indicates persistence of protection against clinically significant infections (i.e., detectable viremia and clinical disease). Booster doses are not currently recommended. Vaccine must be injected intramuscularly, preferably in the deltoid.

Indications

Hepatitis B vaccine is indicated for adults at high risk of infection (see Fig. 16–1B). Because strategies targeting hepatitis B vaccine use only to high-risk populations have not had a significant impact on hepatitis B incidence, universal vaccination is now recommended for infants and for all adolescents who have not been previously vaccinated. Universal screening for HBsAg is recommended for all pregnant women; administration of three doses of vaccine and one dose of hepatitis B immune globulin is recommended for infants of acutely or chronically infected mothers.

Side Effects

The major side effect is soreness at the injection site. Alopecia, which is usually reversible, has been reported rarely. Hepatitis B vaccine has not been shown to induce multiple sclerosis in controlled studies and has not been shown to exacerbate illness in patients with multiple sclerosis who are vaccinated. There is no risk of acquiring HIV infection from either the recombinant or the plasma-derived vaccine.

Human Papillomavirus

In 2006, a quadrivalent human papillomavirus (HPV) vaccine was licensed. The vaccine consists of the L1 capsid protein of types 16 and 18, which account for about 70% of cases of cervical cancer, and types 6 and 11, which are the most common causes of anogenital warts. An additional bivalent vaccine consisting of types 16 and 18 is in clinical trials.

Routine vaccination of 11- to 12-year-old girls is recommended in a three-dose schedule at 0, 2, and 6 months. Catch-up vaccination should be undertaken for females up through 26 years of age. Recipients of HPV vaccine should follow the same recommendations for Pap smear screening as unvaccinated females. Persons with prior abnormal Pap smears or genital warts may be vaccinated to prevent persistent infection with types of HPV that are in the vaccine and have not yet been acquired.

Side Effects

The most common reactions are local pain, swelling, and erythema, which may, in part, be explained by the aluminum adjuvant rather than the L1 capsid protein. There is a slightly higher incidence of fever within 15 days of vaccination in vaccine recipients compared with that in placebo recipients.

Influenza

The two available influenza vaccines are the inactivated trivalent influenza vaccine (TIV) and the live attenuated influenza vaccine (LAIV). TIV, which contains split viruses of three major antigenic types, A (H3N2), A (H1N1), and B, is administered intramuscularly. LAIV, which consists of three cold-adapted, temperature-sensitive attenuated viruses, one for each of the expected circulating strains, is administered intranasally. LAIV is prepared by use of attenuated parent viruses that have been reassorted with circulating strains to contain six internal genes from the parent virus and genes for the surface hemagglutinin and neuraminidase of an A (H3N2), A (H1N1), or B strain.

Indications

Annual influenza (Chapter 387) vaccination with TIV is indicated for adults at high risk of complications from the disease: persons with chronic cardiopulmonary disorders, residents of nursing homes or other long-term care facilities, persons 65 years of age or older, patients with other chronic diseases (e.g., diabetes mellitus, kidney dysfunction, hemoglobinopathies, and immunosuppression) who have required regular medical follow-up or hospitalization in the prior year, adults and children who have any condition (e.g., cognitive dysfunction, spinal cord injuries, seizure disorders, or other neuromuscular disorders) that can compromise respiratory function or the handling of respiratory secretions or that can increase the risk for aspiration, and children receiving long-term aspirin therapy. Women who will be pregnant during the influenza season (usually late December through mid-March) also should be vaccinated. Vaccination also has been recommended for all adults 50 to 64 years old to reduce influenza. Influenza vaccine can be considered for providers of essential community services and anyone who wants to avoid disease. To reduce transmission of influenza to high-risk patients, health care workers and household contacts of high-risk patients should also be vaccinated annually, including contacts of children younger than 5 years of age.

LAIV is licensed only for patients 5 to 49 years of age without underlying conditions that place them at high risk of complications from influenza. LAIV can be used for contacts of high-risk patients, if the contacts are of the appropriate age. LAIV, for theoretical concerns about live virus transmission, is not recommended for contacts of severely immunosuppressed patients such as patients with bone marrow transplants but can be given to contacts of persons with mild to moderate immunologic impairment.

The efficacy of TIV varies with the host's condition and the degree to which antigens in the vaccine match viruses in circulation the following season. Provided the match is good, the vaccine's efficacy is usually 70 to 90% in normal healthy young adults. Efficacy is substantially lower, often between 30 and 40%, in the institutionalized elderly; nevertheless, it seems to be 60 to 80% protective against pneumonia and death. LAIV has been found to be more than 85% effective in young children, even in a year when the circulating strain had antigenically drifted from the vaccine strain. Similar effects were seen in challenge studies in adults.

Ideally, vaccines should be administered between October and November of each year, although earlier in the autumn suffices if circumstances require. If vaccine is available in December and January, vaccination should continue because it still can offer protection for many individuals. A review of 29 consecutive influenza seasons documented that peak activity did not occur until January or later in 24 seasons and until February or later in 18 seasons.

Side Effects

Persons with anaphylactic allergy to eggs should not be immunized. The most common side effect of TIV is soreness at the injection site. Fever, malaise, and myalgia may begin 6 to 12 hours after vaccination and persist for 1 to 2 days, although such reactions are most common in children exposed to vaccine for the first time. Severe allergic reactions are rare. If current influenza vaccines cause Guillain-Barré syndrome, it is likely to be rare, on the order of 1 case per 1 million doses. The most common adverse events after LAIV in adults are runny nose, headache, and sore throat.

Measles

Indications

Measles (Chapter 390) immunization is recommended for all persons born in or after 1957 who lack evidence of prior physician-diagnosed measles or laboratory evidence of immunity or appropriate vaccination. Before 1989, appropriate vaccination consisted of a single dose of live vaccine administered on or after the first birthday. Since then, a routine two-dose schedule has been recommended: the first dose, which is 93 to 98% effective, at 12 to 15 months of age and the second dose at entry to primary school. All children from kindergarten through the 12th grade should have a second dose. Most adults are considered to have been appropriately vaccinated if they received one dose of vaccine administered on or after their first birthday. Some adults who are at increased risk of measles (health care workers with direct contact with patients, students in college, international travelers) should receive a second dose of vaccine, however, unless they have documentation of prior physician-diagnosed measles or serologic evidence of immunity. Persons embarking on foreign travel ideally should have received two doses or have other evidence of measles immunity. Persons born before 1957 are usually immune as a result of natural infection and do not require vaccination, although vaccination is not contraindicated if they are believed to be susceptible.

During outbreaks of measles in institutions, all persons at risk who have not received two doses or who lack other evidence of measles immunity should be vaccinated. Measles vaccine is usually administered along with mumps and rubella vaccines as MMR to ensure immunity against all three diseases. Individuals already immune to one or more of the components may receive MMR without harm.

Measles vaccine is contraindicated for pregnant women on theoretical grounds, for persons with moderate to severe acute febrile illnesses, and for persons with altered immunocompetence except persons with HIV infection who are not severely immunocompromised. Patients with anaphylactic reactions to eggs can be vaccinated without prior skin testing.

Side Effects

In approximately 5 to 15% of susceptible recipients of measles vaccine, temperatures of 39.4° C or higher develop 5 to 12 days after vaccination and last 1 to 2 days. Transient rashes develop in about 5%. Thrombocytopenic purpura has been reported rarely after MMR. The overall rate of reactions after the second dose of a measles-containing vaccine is substantially lower than after the first dose. Encephalopathy or encephalitis after measles vaccination has been reported at a rate lower than the background or expected rate.

Meningococcal Vaccines

Two quadrivalent meningococcal polysaccharide vaccines against disease caused by serogroups A, C, Y, and W135 are available: meningococcal polysaccharide vaccine (MPSV4), which consists of 50 μg of polysaccharide of each of the four serogroups and is licensed for persons 2 years of age and older; and meningococcal conjugate vaccine (MCV4), which consists of 4 μg of each polysaccharide covalently linked to 48 μg of diphtheria toxoid and licensed for persons 11 to 55 years of age. The four serogroups in each vaccine account for approximately two thirds of meningococcal disease in the United States and about 75% of the disease in persons 11 years of age or older (Chapter 437). Serogroup A and C polysaccharide vaccines have had 85 to 100% efficacy in epidemic settings, whereas polysaccharide vaccines for the other groups have documented good immunogenicity in adults. Meningococcal conjugate vaccine type C (MCV-C) has been associated with an estimated effectiveness of 88 to 98% in the year following vaccination in the United Kingdom, where it has been used widely. In addition, MCV-C has reduced colonization by 66% and decreased disease among unvaccinated persons by 67% in 1- to 17-year-olds and by 35% among those older than 25 years. In contrast to polysaccharide vaccines, conjugate vaccines induce immunologic memory, result in higher and more durable levels of high-avidity antibodies, and have been documented to induce herd immunity. The duration of immunity for both MPSV4 and MCV4 is unknown, although protection in older children and adults probably persists for at least 3 years for both vaccines. Protection after MPSV4 in preschool children may be shorter.

Indications

Routine vaccination with a single dose of MCV4 is recommended for all adolescents at 11 to 12 years of age, all persons at high school entry (approximately age 15 years) who have not been previously vaccinated, and college freshman who will live in dormitories. Vaccination is also recommended for persons with terminal complement component deficiencies, asplenia or splenic dysfunction, and travelers and persons who will live in areas with hyperendemic or epidemic disease (e.g., the "meningitis belt" of sub-Saharan Africa, stretching from Mauritania to Ethiopia). MPSV4 should be used for persons 2 to 10 years and older than 55 years with an indication for vaccine. MPSV4 is an acceptable alternative for college freshman living in dormitories, travelers, and patients with high-risk medical conditions. Meningococcal vaccination may be useful during localized epidemics of serogroups in the vaccine.

Revaccination should be considered 2 to 3 years after primary immunization with MPSV4 for children younger than 4 years at the initial vaccination. Revaccination 5 years after the initial dose also may be considered for older adolescents and adults at continued risk. At present, there are no recommendations for booster doses for persons vaccinated with MCV4.

Side Effects

The major side effects of MPSV4 are local reactions lasting 1 to 2 days. The incidence of local reactions and low-grade fever is slightly higher after MCV4 than with MPSV4. An excess risk of 1.25 cases of Guillain-Barré syndrome per million doses has been noted with the vaccination.

Mumps

Indications

Mumps (Chapter 392) vaccine is indicated for all persons, especially susceptible males, without evidence of immunity. For most adults, such evidence consists of a prior history of vaccination on or after the first birthday, physician-diagnosed mumps, or laboratory evidence of immunity. For adults at high risk, including health care workers, international travelers, and students at post–high school educational institutions, two doses of mumps vaccine constitute acceptable evidence of immunity. Most persons born before 1957 can be considered immune as a result of natural infection, although vaccination is not contraindicated if such persons are thought to be susceptible.

Side Effects

Adverse events after the Jeryl Lynn strain of mumps vaccine, the strain used in the United States, are uncommon—fever, parotitis, and allergic manifestations. Thrombocytopenic purpura has been reported rarely in persons administered MMR. Mumps vaccine is contraindicated for pregnant women on theoretical grounds, for persons with moderate to severe acute febrile illnesses, and for persons with altered immunocompetence. When combined with measles vaccine, it may be given to persons with asymptomatic HIV infection and considered for persons with symptomatic infection if they are not severely immunocompromised. Patients with anaphylactic reactions to eggs can be vaccinated without skin testing (see Measles earlier).

Pertussis Vaccine

In 2005, two vaccines were licensed for boosting immunity to pertussis. Both vaccines are combined with the adult preparation of tetanus and diphtheria toxoids and have a reduced content of pertussis antigens compared with the childhood pertussis-containing vaccines (Tdap). Boostrix (GlaxoSmithKline), which is licensed for adolescents 10 to 18 years of age, contains three pertussis antigens—toxoid (PT), filamentous hemagglutinin (FHA), and pertactin (PRN). Adacel (Sanofi Pasteur, Inc.), which is licensed for 11- to 64-year-olds, contains five pertussis antigens, PT, FHA, PRN, and two fimbriae. Both vaccines, when administered to previously vaccinated adolescents and adults, induce serologic responses that are comparable to those induced during childhood vaccination with vaccines that have been proved to be effective. Adverse events, usually local reactions, are similar with the adult preparation of tetanus and diphtheria toxoids (Td) alone. Tdap is indicated for all adolescents at 11 to 12 years of age. Older adolescents should receive Tdap instead of Td if they have not received an adolescent Td booster. For patients who have received a Td booster, an interval of 5 years is encouraged before Tdap is received. However, Tdap can be given at any interval after Td when the risk of pertussis is judged to be high. All adults younger than 65 years of age should receive a single dose of TdaP to replace a Td booster.

Pneumococcal Vaccine

Pneumococcal polysaccharide vaccine consists of purified polysaccharide capsular antigens from the 23 types of *Streptococcus pneumoniae* that are responsible for 85 to 90% of the bacteremic disease in the United States (Chapter 311). Most adults, including the elderly and patients with alcoholic cirrhosis and diabetes mellitus, have a two-fold or greater rise in type-specific antibodies within 2 to 3 weeks of vaccination. Although the serologic response is generally acceptable, estimates of vaccine efficacy in preventing disease vary widely. Efficacy may be lower in some patients, such as patients with alcoholic cirrhosis or Hodgkin's disease. There is good evidence that vaccination is approximately 60% effective against bacteremic pneumococcal disease, which accounts for an estimated 50,000 cases annually. Evidence regarding efficacy against pneumonia in high-risk populations is not clear, however.

Indications

Regardless, the preponderance of information supports the use of pneumococcal vaccine in high-risk populations, including all persons older than 65 years. Special efforts should target hospitalized patients. Approximately two thirds of patients who are admitted later with pneumococcal disease had been hospitalized for other reasons within the preceding 5 years.

Immunity may decrease 5 years or more after initial vaccination; a single booster dose should be considered at that time for adults at highest risk of disease, such as asplenic patients, and for adults who lose antibody rapidly, such as patients with nephrotic syndrome or renal failure. Persons older than 65 years who received a dose more than 5 years earlier when they were younger than 65 years should be revaccinated.

Side Effects

Local reactions are frequent. Less than 1% of vaccinees experience severe local reactions or systemic illness, such as fever and malaise. Severe events such as anaphylaxis are rare. Because of the rarity of severe reactions in revaccinated patients, persons with indications for vaccination but with unknown histories of prior vaccination should be vaccinated.

A pneumococcal conjugate vaccine in which the polysaccharides of seven types are covalently linked to a protein carrier was licensed and recommended for universal use in children in 2000. This vaccine, which covers substantially fewer types than the 23-valent polysaccharide vaccine, is not indicated for persons 9 years of age or older. Widespread vaccination of children in the United States has led to substantial reductions of invasive pneumococcal disease in adults, suggesting that children are the source for many adult infections.

Poliomyelitis

The last documented cases of indigenously acquired poliomyelitis (Chapters 402 and 440) caused by wild polioviruses in the United States were reported in 1979. In 2000, an all inactivated poliovirus vaccine (IPV) schedule was recommended in the United States; this vaccine replaced the live attenuated oral poliovirus vaccine (OPV), which, although it had eliminated wild poliovirus in the United States, caused about eight cases per year on average among OPV recipients or their contacts. IPV is the only vaccine available in the United States. OPV is still the vaccine used in most countries around the world, however. Between 1988, when the goal was announced to eradicate wild poliovirus from the world, and 2003, cases of poliomyelitis worldwide decreased by an estimated 99%. Polio was limited to six countries in South Asia and Africa, but a resurgence in Nigeria in 2004 led to transmission in several African countries that had been polio free. Four endemic countries remain, and efforts to eradicate polio globally continue.

Indications

Routine vaccination of persons 18 years of age or older is not warranted given the small risk of exposure to wild virus in the United States. The major indication for adult vaccination is travel to areas where wild poliovirus is endemic or epidemic. Previously unvaccinated adults should receive IPV. Adult travelers who have histories of partial vaccination should complete a primary series of three doses with IPV. Adults who formerly received three doses of OPV or IPV should receive a single booster of IPV. Health care personnel who come in contact with wild viruses should be immune to polio.

A primary series of IPV consists of three doses. A fourth dose is administered to children at school entry.

Side Effects

No serious side effects of IPV have been reported.

Rabies

Indications

Rabies (Chapter 441) vaccine is indicated for pre-exposure prophylaxis of high-risk persons, including animal handlers, selected laboratory and field workers, and persons traveling for more than 1 month to areas where rabies is a constant threat. The pre-exposure regimen consists of three 1-mL intramuscular injections on days 0, 7, and 21 or 28 for all rabies vaccines. Testing for serum antibody or a booster every 2 years is indicated for persons with continuing risk. Postexposure treatment depends on prior exposure to vaccine (Chapter 441). Human rabies immune globulin is indicated for previously unvaccinated persons who are exposed.

Rubella

Indications

Rubella (Chapter 391) vaccine is indicated for susceptible adults born in 1957 or later and for susceptible women of any age who are considering becoming pregnant. Persons without a prior history of vaccination on or after the first birthday or laboratory evidence of immunity should be considered susceptible. A single dose of vaccine is 95% or more effective. Many persons receive two doses of rubella vaccine by the two-dose schedule of MMR.

Side Effects

Follow-up of susceptible pregnant women who received rubella vaccines within 3 months of the estimated date of conception has failed to reveal any evidence of defects compatible with congenital rubella syndrome in their offspring. Nevertheless, vaccine is contraindicated in pregnant women on theoretical grounds, and conception should be delayed for 1 month after rubella vaccination.

Adverse reactions occur only in susceptible persons. Arthralgia, usually of the small peripheral joints, develops in 40% of susceptible adults, and frank arthritis develops in 10 to 20%. Joint symptoms usually begin 1 to 3 weeks after vaccination and persist for 1 day to 3 weeks. Chronic recurrent or persistent joint symptoms have developed rarely after vaccination, but controlled studies have shown that the incidence of these events in vaccinees is similar to that in nonvaccinees. Other infrequent adverse events include transient peripheral neuritis and pain in the arms and legs. Thrombocytopenic purpura has been reported rarely when rubella vaccine is administered as MMR. Rubella vaccine is contraindicated for persons with moderate to severe acute febrile illnesses and for persons with reduced immunocompetence. When given with measles vaccine, it may be administered to persons with asymptomatic HIV infection and considered for persons with symptomatic infection without severe immunocompromise. Rubella vaccine is grown in human diploid cells and can be administered without problems to persons with allergy to eggs.

Tetanus and Diphtheria

Tetanus (Chapter 319) toxoid is one of the most effective immunizations, with more than 95% protection after a primary series. The adsorbed preparation is preferred to the fluid preparation because it induces protective levels of antitoxin that persist longer after fewer doses. A primary series consists of three doses. In persons aged 7 years or older, it should always be used in combination with diphtheria (Chapter 315) toxoid (Td), which is more than 85% effective in preventing disease. Combinations also including pertussis antigens (Tdap) are preferred to Td for routine immunization of adolescents. Doses need not be repeated if the schedule is interrupted. Boosters of Td are recommended every 10 years. An easy way to remember is to schedule immunization at the middle of each decade (e.g., 25 years, 35 years).

Indications

After a wound, persons of unknown immunization status or persons who have received fewer than three doses of tetanus toxoid should receive a dose of Td regardless of the severity of the wound. Td also is indicated for persons who have previously received three or more doses if more than 10 years has elapsed since the last dose, in the case of clean and minor wounds, and if more than 5 years has elapsed for all other wounds. Persons who have never received a dose of TdaP should receive it in place of Td for wound management. Tetanus immune globulin should be administered simultaneously at a separate site to persons who have not received at least three doses of toxoid and who have wounds that are not clean and minor.

Side Effects

Most reactions to Td consist of local inflammation and low-grade fever. Guillain-Barré syndrome and brachial neuritis rarely have been associated with tetanus toxoid.

Varicella: Chickenpox

A live attenuated varicella vaccine (Oka strain) was licensed in March 1995. A combination measles-mumps-rubella-varicella vaccine was licensed in September 2005. The vaccine protects 70 to 90% of recipients against any disease and more than 95% of recipients against severe disease. Vaccine effectiveness of at least 84% has been demonstrated up to 8 years after vaccination. Breakthrough infections in persons who have previously seroconverted have been reported. Such breakthroughs are typically mild and average fewer than 50 lesions compared with several hundred lesions in unvaccinated persons with varicella. Breakthrough illnesses do not seem to increase in incidence or severity with increasing time since vaccination, a finding compatible with long-term protection after initial vaccination. Persons 13 years or older require two doses at least 4 weeks apart to achieve seroconversion rates of approximately 99%, a rate comparable to that in younger children after one dose.

Indications

Varicella vaccine is indicated routinely for all children without a contraindication. A two-dose schedule is recommended, generally at 12 to 15 months of age and 4 to 6 years of age. For persons who previously received a single dose, catch-up vaccination with a second dose is recommended, provided at least 3 months have elapsed since the first dose. Persons who received a second dose at least 28 days after the first dose do not need a third dose. Persons with a prior history of varicella disease can be considered immune and do not need vaccination. Although a negative or unknown history of disease is predictive of susceptibility in children, many adults with such histories are immune. Serologic screening of adults in some situations may be cost-effective, provided that identified susceptible adults are vaccinated. The vaccine is contraindicated in the immunocompromised, persons with anaphylactic allergies to vaccine components, and pregnant women. Varicella vaccine is more temperature sensitive than other vaccines used in the United States. It must be stored frozen at −15° C or colder to retain potency, and it should be discarded if it is not used within 30 minutes of reconstitution.

Side Effects

The most common side effect is soreness at the injection site, which is reported in 25 to 35% of recipients 13 years or older. Varicella-like rashes at the injection site (median of two lesions) have been reported in 3% of recipients in this age group after the first dose and in 1% after the second dose. Nonlocalized rashes with a median of five lesions have been reported in 5.5% of recipients after the first dose and in 0.9% after the second dose. Although the vaccine can cause herpes zoster (shingles), the incidence is substantially lower than would be expected after natural varicella (Chapter 398). More severe events occurring in temporal relation to the vaccine have been reported rarely, although a causal relationship has not been established. Transmission of vaccine virus to a contact is extremely rare and seems to take place only with vaccinees in whom a varicella-like rash has developed.

Varicella: Zoster

Clinical trials of a varicella vaccine, approximately 14 times more potent than the varicella vaccine used routinely, among persons 60 years of age or older reported a 51% reduction in the incidence of zoster and a 67% decrease in postherpetic neuralgia. The efficacy against zoster declined with increasing age from 60 to 80 years or older, but there was evidence of continuing protection against postherpetic neuralgia. The vaccine requires special freezer storage.

Indications

Zoster vaccine is recommended as a single dose for persons 60 years of age or older. Persons with a prior history of zoster may be vaccinated. The vaccine is not recommended for immunocompromised persons.

Side Effects

The major side effect attributed to the vaccine is local reactions.

VACCINES INTENDED PRIMARILY FOR INTERNATIONAL TRAVELERS

Japanese Encephalitis Vaccine

Indications

Japanese encephalitis (Chapter 439) vaccine is indicated primarily for travelers to Asia who will spend a month or longer in endemic areas during the transmission season, especially if travel will include rural areas. In all instances, travelers should be advised to take personal precautions to reduce exposure to mosquito bites. The vaccine seems to be 80 to 91% effective in preventing clinical disease. The primary series consists of three subcutaneous 1-mL doses given on days 0, 7, and 30 (see Table 16–2). A shortened schedule given on days 0, 7, and 14 may be used when necessary. Booster doses may be given after 2 years.

Side Effects

The vaccine is contraindicated for pregnant women on theoretical grounds, but if such women travel to an endemic, high-risk area, they may be vaccinated. Local reactions are common and occur in about 20% of vaccinated persons, and systemic symptoms of fever, headache, chills, nausea, and abdominal pain have been noted in about 10%. A delayed urticaria-angioedema syndrome may occur a median of 12 hours after the first dose of vaccine and 2 weeks after the second dose. Vaccinees should be observed for at least 30 minutes after inoculation and, during the subsequent 10 days, should remain in areas with ready access to medical care.

Typhoid Vaccine

Indications

Two types of vaccines, a live attenuated Ty21a oral vaccine and a capsular polysaccharide vaccine (ViCPS), seem to be of comparable efficacy (50 to 77%). Typhoid (Chapter 329) vaccine is indicated primarily for travelers to areas where the risk of prolonged exposure to contaminated food and water is high. The vaccine is not optimally effective; food and water precautions are still essential. The vaccine also may be considered for family or other intimate contacts of typhoid carriers and laboratory workers who work with *Salmonella typhi.* For adults and children 6 years and older, either of the vaccines may be used. For Ty21a, one enteric-coated capsule is taken every other day for four doses. Alternatively, a single dose of the ViCPS vaccine may be given. The duration of protection with Ty21a is not known; repetition of the primary series is recommended every 5 years for persons at risk. Boosters are recommended every 2 years for the ViCPS vaccine if persons continue to be at risk. The ViCPS vaccine can be given to children 2 years of age.

Side Effects

Adverse reactions are rare.

Yellow Fever Vaccine

Indications

Yellow fever (Chapter 404) now occurs only in areas of South America and Africa. Vaccination with a single dose of the live attenuated 17D strain of virus confers protection to almost all recipients for at least 10 years. Boosters are recommended every 10 years for persons at risk.

Side Effects

Side effects are uncommon. A rare syndrome of yellow fever vaccine, febrile multiple organ system failure or viscerotropic disease, has been reported, with high rates of mortality, primarily among older adults and persons who have undergone thymectomy or have severe thymic dysfunction. Yellow fever vaccine should be administered with caution and only after careful counseling to elderly patients who are going to spend time in yellow fever endemic zones. Yellow fever vaccine should not be given to immunocompromised persons or persons with anaphylactic allergies to eggs. The vaccine is contraindicated in pregnant women on theoretical grounds, although if pregnant women must travel to a high-risk area, they may be vaccinated.

VACCINES FOR POSSIBLE BIOTERRORISM AGENTS

Anthrax Vaccine

Anthrax vaccine adsorbed (AVA) is prepared from a cell-free filtrate of a nonencapsulated strain of anthrax and contains many cell products including protective antigen. Protective antigen is responsible for binding to cells, allowing transport of lethal factor and edema factor into host cells.

Indications

Pre-exposure prophylaxis consists of six doses subcutaneously at 0, 2, and 4 weeks and 6, 12, and 18 months followed by annual boosters. Protective efficacy of an earlier form of the vaccine against cutaneous anthrax was 92.5%. Animal models suggest efficacy against inhalation anthrax. Pre-exposure vaccination is recommended for persons engaged in work involving exposure to high concentrations of *Bacillus anthracis* or in activities with high potential for aerosol production. Vaccine may be given with antibiotics for postexposure prophylaxis (Chapters 19 and 317); the antibiotics should be continued for 7 to 14 days after the third dose of vaccine is given.

Side Effects

The most common adverse events are local reactions, including subcutaneous nodules, which are thought to be due to the deposition of the aluminum-containing adjuvant in subcutaneous tissue. Studies are under way to determine if the number of doses can be reduced and whether switching to the intramuscular route results in fewer local reactions. In addition, a recombinant protective antigen (rPA) vaccine is in clinical trials.

Smallpox Vaccine

Smallpox vaccine uses vaccinia virus, an orthopox virus that is distinct from variola and cowpox viruses and that provides cross-protection from smallpox. With successful eradication of natural transmission and laboratory containment, variola virus is known to be in only two sites, the Centers for Disease Control and Prevention in Atlanta, Georgia, and the Russian State Research Center for Virology and Biotechnology, Koltsovo, Novosibirsk. Allegations that the former Soviet Union was engaged in use of variola virus in weapons and concerns that some scientists, with the break-up of the Soviet Union, may have given the virus to other countries or terrorist groups have raised the potential of a bioterrorist event with variola.

Smallpox vaccine is close to 100% effective when it is administered properly, with a bifurcated needle. Vaccination also prevents or modifies disease when it is administered within 3 to 4 days of exposure and perhaps even after greater delays. The skin usually does not need any special preparation. If alcohol is used for cleaning, the skin should be allowed to dry before vaccination to avoid inactivation of the vaccine. The needle is held perpendicular to the skin; 3 punctures for primary vaccination and 15 punctures for revaccination are made rapidly with enough vigor to ensure that a trace of blood appears within 15 to 20 seconds. With a primary take, the vaccination site should become reddened and pruritic by 3 or 4 days after vaccination; a large vesicle with a red areola forms and becomes pustular by 7 to 11 days. The lesion scabs by the third week. Fever is the most common adverse event. Other more serious complications include eczema vaccinatum, a local or disseminated vaccinia infection in persons with a history of eczema or other exfoliative dermatitis; vaccinia necrosum, which occurs in immunocompromised persons; autoinoculation, especially of the eye, which can cause keratitis and scarring; generalized vaccinia; myopericarditis; and encephalitis. The risk of death from vaccinia has been estimated to be approximately 1 per 1 million primary vaccinations.

The vaccine is indicated for persons who work with orthopox viruses. To increase preparedness for a smallpox attack, vaccination is often recommended for persons who will serve on public health or health care response teams. The duration of immunity is unclear. Revaccination is recommended at least every 10 years for persons who continue to be at risk. Contraindications include history or presence of eczema, other chronic or exfoliative skin conditions, and immunosuppression or pregnancy in the patient or a close household or other contact. Persons who are younger than 1 year, are breast-feeding, or have allergies to vaccine components should not be vaccinated. Because of reports of postvaccination cardiac events, vaccination should be deferred in persons with ischemia or other severe heart diseases or at high risk for ischemic heart disease events *(www.cdc.gov/smallpox).* In the event of exposure to variola, there are no contraindications. Should variola be introduced into a community, vaccination would be indicated for all exposed persons and their close contacts to prevent further spread, and recommendations for more widespread vaccination would have to be evaluated on a case-by-case basis.

Other Agents

Other organisms or products that have been considered potential bioterrorism threats include plague (Chapter 333) and botulinum toxin (Chapter 319). An inactivated whole cell plague vaccine had been available in the United States for persons whose occupation places them at risk; it is no longer being produced. Although the vaccine seemed to be effective against bubonic plague, animal studies suggest poor efficacy against pneumonic disease. At present, vaccine is not considered a major part of the response to a bioterrorist attack with *Yersinia pestis.*

Poisoning with botulinum toxin can be treated with a trivalent antitoxin, available from the Centers for Disease Control (see MMWR 2003;52:774). An experimental pentavalent botulinum toxoid can be obtained from the Centers for Disease Control and Prevention for laboratory workers at high risk of exposure to toxin. Pre-exposure vaccination is not warranted or feasible for the general population.

OTHER VACCINES

Many other vaccines are used in selected circumstances, including BCG (bacille Calmette-Guérin) vaccine, which has limited use in the United States, to prevent tuberculosis (Chapter 345). BCG vaccination of health care workers should be considered on an individual basis in settings in which (1) a high percentage of tuberculosis patients are infected with *Mycobacterium tuberculosis* strains resistant to isoniazid and rifampin, (2) transmission of drug-resistant *M. tuberculosis* strains to health care workers and subsequent infection are likely, and (3) comprehensive tuberculosis infection control has been implemented but has not been successful.

FUTURE DIRECTIONS

Although not available today, many vaccines are under development and may be licensed in the future. Example include combination vaccines, improved influenza vaccines, and vaccines to prevent or treat selected chronic diseases and many other infectious diseases.

SUGGESTED READINGS

Centers for Disease Control and Prevention: Recommendations of the Advisory Committee on Immunization Practices. *Comprehensive coverage on vaccine-preventable diseases, vaccines, indications, schedules, and adverse events. Published as available in the* Morbidity and Mortality Weekly Report *as "Recommendations and Reports" supplements and available at www.cdc.gov/nip/acip.*

Centers for Disease Control and Prevention: Traveler's Health. *A complete guide for the international traveler, including required and recommended vaccinations. Revised every 1 to 2 years. Available online at www.cdc.gov/travel.*

Centers for Disease Control and Prevention: Notice to Readers: Recommended Adult Immunization Schedule—United States, October 2006–September 2007. Available at www.cdc.gov/nip/recs/adult-schedule.htm#print. *The schedule is divided in two parts: (1) vaccines recommended by age group and (2) vaccines recommended by underlying medical condition.*

Committee on Infectious Diseases, American Academy of Pediatrics: Report of the Committee on Infectious Diseases, 27th ed. Elk Grove Village, IL, American Academy of Pediatrics, 2006. *The* Red Book *is published every 2 to 3 years and addresses in a comprehensive manner vaccination of children and adolescents and other issues relating to prevention, control, and treatment of infectious diseases.*

National Immunization Program (NIP), Centers for Disease Control and Prevention. *The NIP has established toll-free numbers for answering questions from the general public and physicians: 1–800–232–2522 (English), 1–800–232–0233 (Spanish). Inquiries can be made to the NIP by e-mail: nipinfo@cdc.gov or the NIP website at www.cdc.gov/nip.*

17 PRINCIPLES OF OCCUPATIONAL AND ENVIRONMENTAL MEDICINE

Mark R. Cullen

In the first several decades after World War II, when many American workers came to enjoy coverage by health insurance—for everything but workplace injuries and illnesses—the myth grew that modern work was largely free of the risks of the industrial horrors of past eras. Starting in the 1970s, however, resurgence of societal and medical interest in these consequences of work found that diseases related to work were not truly extinct, just not well observed or studied. Occupational physicians, largely cut off from mainstream medical practice, had difficulty changing the perception, and most practicing internists were largely oblivious. It is now recognized that a substantial burden of ill health and disability is due to work-associated physical, chemical, and biologic hazards. Another intriguing possibility, recognized by social epidemiologists, is that work may be injurious to health in ways beyond these tangible risks.

Although tens of thousands of toxic chemicals and other hazards can potentially cause or exacerbate a wide range of acute and chronic conditions, certain basic principles and clinical approaches apply broadly to general and specialty medical practice. This chapter outlines these basics, then briefly summarizes the most common occupational disorders seen by internists in developed countries, and finally reviews the effects of the environmental exposures most likely to be encountered.

PRINCIPLES OF OCCUPATIONAL AND ENVIRONMENTAL DISEASE

It is widely imagined that the major health effects of environmental and occupational exposures are unique disorders best recognized by their failure to fit easily into other diagnostic categories (e.g., arsenic poisoning). In reality, *the major consequences of chemical and physical exposures are, without further exploration of an environmental connection, indistinguishable in clinical presentations from disorders that make up the bulk of outpatient and inpatient medical practice:* rashes, abnormal liver function studies (Chapter 150), wheezing and irritative symptoms of the upper and lower respiratory tract (Chapter 87), various cancers (Chapter 185), peripheral neuropathies (Chapter 446), dysphoria (Chapter 420), and nonspecific cognitive dysfunction (Chapter 425). Although a handful of pathologically distinct disorders still occur, such as silicosis (Chapter 93) and lead poisoning (Chapter 20), when an environmental or workplace agent causes overt disease, physiologic and radiographic studies typically reveal manifestations completely consistent with common diagnoses such as asthma (Chapter 87), contact dermatitis (Chapter 464), fatty liver (Chapter 156), and lung cancer (Chapter 201). The underlying cause—whose recognition and modification could affect treatment and prognosis as well as appropriate apportionment of health and disability costs—may remain obscure unless the clinician adheres to a disciplined approach designed to investigate and exclude occupational or environmental causes whenever it is appropriate. The best approach is consistent use of the occupational and environmental history, a short series of questions that can be expanded on the basis of the replies (see later). The point is that the internist cannot "wait" to consider occupational or environmental issues until other diseases have been ruled out without running the risk of missing almost every occupational and environmental effect that he or she will encounter.

Each toxic material acts through one or more specific pathways to cause injury—effects tend to follow one of several well-defined temporal patterns. Put another way, easily searchable information about occupational and environmental hazards, although often incomplete or limited to only a few published studies in animals, can be used to evaluate the likelihood that a particular exposure might cause a specific health effect in an individual case. This approach provides the basis for narrowing down which organs might be affected by a particular material at what exposure dose (see later) and whether this effect would be expected soon after exposure begins (typical of solvents and metals) or after some biologic "latency" of years to decades after exposure began and possibly already ended (typical of dusts causing pneumoconioses or most physical and chemical hazards that cause cancer). These time sequences, in turn, inform the history-taking process.

Whatever the pathway or time course, exposure dose is the major determinant of the risk for development of disease. As in pharmacology (Chapter 27), it is impossible to make any meaningful statement about cause and effect without appreciation of dose. Consider, for example, the difference in health effects among aspirin at 65 mg, 650 mg, and 6500 mg (Chapter 34). Over this two-order magnitude of change, the chemical goes from having one therapeutic target organ to having many and to being potentially lethal. It is no different with lead or organophosphate pesticides or solvents, except that there is rarely as simple a way to determine dose as in the drug situation, where pill bottles are labeled and drug prescriptions are recorded. This limitation is exacerbated because, unlike with drugs, the range of toxic exposures may vary far more widely. For example, water in a contaminated drinking well or poor indoor air in an office could have toxins at a level that is two, three, or even four orders of magnitude (i.e., 10,000 times) lower than the level that may have been evaluated in an epidemiologic study of workers or tested in animals. Fortunately, it is much easier to "range find" than one might presuppose (see later discussion of history), and eagerness for precision—often unattainable—should not interfere with obtaining the great amount of information that *can* be readily gleaned and is often sufficient to act on. The key point is that no attempt to apply clinical information in relation to work or environment can be useful without some effort to characterize exposure dose.

Environmental hazards may affect preferentially vulnerable populations—those with underlying disease, those at the extremes of life, those with atopy, and those with other serious health risks such as smoking or diabetes. Genetic differences may underlie some differences, but few relevant genes have been sufficiently characterized for use in practice. Clinical studies of a host of common occupational diseases have identified behavioral and constitutional cofactors; for example, smoking dramatically increases the risk of lung cancer in asbestos-exposed workers (Chapter 201). This interaction creates a double demand on the clinician—the presence of smoking or atopy in a young woman with cough does not preclude the possibility of an occupational cause of her asthma but rather actually increases the likelihood that such a consideration may be important.

The Occupational and Environmental History and Exposure Assessment

Key to determining whether work and other environmental exposures may be causing or contributing to adverse health is the history. The approach to obtaining this information and to the use of available resources to corroborate and complement it depends on the clinical context. In primary and much specialty medical care, where it is anticipated that a patient will be observed during a long period into the future, the most important step is to establish the hazards to which the patient may be exposed at work presently, the activities that may have resulted in past harmful exposures potentially relevant to future health (because of latency), and whether the present residential environment, including air and water and food sources, is thought to be contaminated by harmful materials. The recommended approach is to use a simple questionnaire, which can be self-administered or supervised by a medical extender (Fig. 17–1, which is one among many published). These instruments can then be reviewed together by the patient and physician as time permits and updated over time. When jobs or materials are noted but the actual generic exposures are unknown, the patient and available reference sources can be enlisted to "translate" the history into specifics, such as which metals are being welded or what is actually contained in a cleaning agent or plastic. This information is obligatorily maintained and supplied on request by employers in most developed countries in the form of fact sheets termed Material Safety Data Sheets, many of which can be easily found online as well. In this way, the ongoing and former exposures, which may have an impact on health, can be noted and, where important, incorporated into routine preventive care or clinical surveillance for sequelae.

For patients with new clinical complaints or recently diagnosed conditions, the question of an environmental cause looms more urgently, so the approach must be more focused. If symptoms or signs of acute or subacute illness are suggested, the *timing* of recent or unusual environmental exposures in relation to the symptoms is key—more important than specific chemical detail. For example, if the patient develops shortness of breath shortly after the introduction of a new chemical or process at work or after a leak or spill, that fact should drive further questions, such as, Did others get sick as well? For recurrent symptoms, such as cough or rash, cyclic changes are most often the strongest clue: Do symptoms get worse on workdays and improve on days off or holidays? For more insidious symptoms, such as weakness or numbness of the extremities or new-onset hepatic dysfunction, the appropriate question would be whether the onset of the abnormality has followed by weeks or months some demonstrable change in the work or home environment. Again, the coincidence of others similarly affected may be more valuable than detailed knowledge of the constituents of that environment. When such a temporal pattern is suggested, further efforts to establish what exposure has actually occurred are warranted, often with specialty consultation when it is available.

In the elucidation of evidently more chronic conditions, such as pulmonary fibrosis, chronic renal insufficiency, or a malignant neoplasm, an alternative approach is suggested because the exposure, if relevant, is usually remote. In this situation, a detailed query about current work or ambient environments is not likely to be helpful in differential diagnosis, although knowledge of a past exposure to an important hazard (such as silica, asbestos, or cadmium) might, on the basis of the knowledge of its effects, influence the sequence of the evaluation. However, it is generally more efficient to explore past exposures *after* the pathophysiologic disturbance has been characterized, focusing inquiry exclusively on factors known to cause or suspected of causing that disorder—as is easily found in suggested texts or literature searches.

In acute or chronic cases, information about *what* the exposure has been (generically) must be augmented by an estimation of exposure dose. A brief exposure to a fume containing a small percentage of lead will not, in general, cause acute lead poisoning (although hosts may differ in their responses), nor will trace contamination of a drinking well with benzene typically cause blood dyscrasias. The patient will rarely be able to supply detailed information about past or even current "dose" but often can provide valuable clues: Did the exposure continue during many years? Were fumes or fibers grossly visible in the air? Were respirators or other protective gear necessary or offered? Have episodes of unprotected exposure ever resulted in irritation or acute discomfort? A positive reply to any of these questions would suggest "high" exposure, where the reference point is the level at which the risk for development of a health effect becomes substantial. Conversely, if exposure has occurred in an otherwise typical office or around a home renovation, the levels of exposure are more likely "low." Nevertheless, such low-level exposure does not exclude a health effect, especially one caused by idiosyncratic mechanisms or occurring in hosts who are more "sensitive" to chemical exposures, a health characteristic found in 2 to 10% of the population. Although not to be condoned because of broader public health consequences, exposures in food and drinking water are uncommon causes of perceptible clinical problems. When concern about the exposure is high, information from patients can be readily supplemented by information from employers (with the patient's consent!) and regulatory or health authorities or by consultation with specialists who should know the levels of most workplace hazards in the community. Finally, with an appropriate understanding of the limits of testing and awareness of "timing" issues in relation to exposure (as with measuring drug levels), an increasing number of hazardous chemicals can be biologically measured in blood or urine. Metals and some pesticides can be reliably tested now, and a broad array of organic chemicals should be amenable for testing in the near future.

OCCUPATIONAL AND ENVIRONMENTAL HEALTH DISORDERS COMMON IN PRACTICE

Although almost any medical complaint or condition may have an occupational or environmental cause or contribution, certain conditions encountered in medical practice *commonly* do (Table 17–1). For these conditions, attention to the history is most important and most often rewarding.

Asthma (Chapter 87)

Men and women with preexisting airways disease tolerate irritants in the workplace poorly and may experience exacerbations in temporal relation to one or more exposures. More important, numerous antigens are extant in the workplace, from large proteins, such as latex and animal danders, to small molecules, such as isocyanates needed to set polyurethane. More than 250 agents have been well characterized, and many others are suspect. Virtually no profession or work is immune. Presentation is often nonspecific; timing of symptoms during or slightly staggered from exposure is the clue to diagnosis. The reward for early recognition of such causes is the likelihood that airway inflammation will abate when the noxious exposure is eliminated; otherwise lifelong, often generalized asthma is the rule.

Chronic Interstitial and Parenchymal Lung Disorders

The rounded opacities of silicosis (Chapter 93) and coal workers' pneumoconiosis (Chapter 93) radiographically resemble sarcoid (Chapter 95); chronic beryllium disease (Chapter 93), a granulomatous disorder caused by sensitization to this widely used light metal, is clinically identical to sarcoid in almost all respects, but a reasonably specific test for blood and bronchoalveolar lavage fluid is now available to distinguish them. Asbestosis (Chapter 93) in every way is identical to idiopathic pulmonary fibrosis (Chapter 92) except that benign pleural changes often accompany asbestosis, which, unlike idiopathic pulmonary fibrosis, tends to run a far more indolent course and usually stops progressing when exposure ceases or within a few years thereafter. Hypersensitivity pneumonitis (Chapter 93) is rarely suspected outside of agricultural settings but is occurring far more often; the causes are likely to be microbial contaminants of work materials, but some chemicals, such as the isocyanates, may also be causal.

Cancers of the Respiratory Tract (Chapter 201)

Although most carcinomas of the lung and upper airway occur in smokers, occupational exposures to asbestos, silica, and the polyaromatic hydrocarbons in particulate air pollution, diesel exhaust, pitch, and asphalt contribute to the burden, as do radon and carcinogenic metals such as chromium and nickel found in most alloys. Some organic materials, such as formaldehyde, are also likely culprits. Until there is an

Occupational and Environmental Exposure History

Current employment (if not currently employed, fill out for last job held)

1. Job title ______
2. Name and address of employer______
3. Nature of work ______
4. How many hours a week do you usually work?______
5. Start date?______ If ended, last day worked ______
   If ended, why did you leave?______
6. Do you have to wear personal protective equipment (like a respirator or gloves or hearing protection) at your job? If yes, what kind(s)______
7. Exposures at this job. For each record whether "none", "a little" or "a lot"

	None	A little	A lot
Dust or fumes	______	______	______
Organic solvents or thinners	______	______	______
Other chemicals	______	______	______
Noise	______	______	______
Excessive heat			
Physical strain			
Mental stress			

Conflict between work and family

Any hazard at this job that you think might be making you sick? ______

Past employment

Please list all the jobs you had before this last one, working backwards towards school. For each list the title, years you held job, and whether there was any exposure you are worried about from that job.

Job Title	Years held	Exposure of concern?
______	______	______
______	______	______
______	______	______
______	______	______

Were you ever in the military service?

If yes, what years? ______ Were you in an active war zone?

Where?

Did hazardous exposures in any of these jobs make you sick?______

If so, explain

Environmental exposures

Are there any specific exposures in your home or neighborhood you are worried about?

If so, what?______

Please tell us about your home environment:

1. Is your drinking water from a city or town source? Private well? Any health problems with the water?______
2. Is your heating system oil? Gas? Electric? Any health problems with the heat?______
3. Are there sources of pollution near your home? ______ What?______
4. Does anyone smoke inside your home? ______ Who?______
5. Does anyone have hobbies at home involving chemicals or industrial materials? If so describe.
   ______
6. Does anyone bring dust or other materials home on clothes from work? If yes, what? ______

FIGURE 17–1 • A questionnaire for use during the "intake" of new patients for ongoing primary or specialty care. The instrument may be self-administered or supervised by a medical extender; it should then be reviewed by the patient and physician and periodically updated.

TABLE 17–1 COMMON OCCUPATIONAL AND ENVIRONMENTAL HEALTH CONDITIONS IN GENERAL PRACTICE

Condition	Exposure Settings	Comment
Asthma	Virtually any indoor or outdoor workplace	New-onset, recrudescent, or exacerbated asthma
Interstitial and parenchymal lung disorders	Dusts, metals, and organic materials	All parenchymal disorders have one or more environmental causes
Cancers of the respiratory tract	Asbestos, radon, silica, mineral oils, tars, and other carcinogens	Smokers are more likely to be affected
Sensorineural hearing loss	Noise, metals, and solvents	High-frequency loss, especially in younger workers
Musculoskeletal disorders of trunk and limbs	Heavy or stereotyped activities	Cold, vibration, and work stress contribute
Upper airway irritation	Dust and fumes	More common in smokers and atopic persons
Nonspecific building-related illness	Office work	Must exclude *specific* causes
Dermatitis, allergic or irritant	Repeated exposure to unprotected skin	Work and environmental exposures should be considered in every case
Multiple chemical sensitivities	Any	Complication of adverse environmental exposure

established strategy for secondary prevention, patients with these exposures should be observed expectantly; at a minimum, extraordinary efforts should be made to control smoking in these exposed individuals. Asbestos-exposed workers—smokers or otherwise—are additionally at risk for malignant mesothelioma (Chapters 100 and 201); but other than primary prevention, the only clinical implication is awareness for early diagnosis and compassionate care for this still largely incurable industrial disease.

Fatty Liver (Chapter 156)

With the widespread use of abdominal imaging, fatty liver has been recognized as more common than previously thought. This disorder is common among individuals exposed regularly to organic solvents, a possibility that should be considered at the same time that infectious, metabolic, and pharmaceutical causes are considered. Once it is suspected, whether or not other factors are also present, exposure should be reduced. Improvement tends to be slow, but the risk of progression is likely to have been averted or at least diminished.

Sensorineural Hearing Loss (Chapter 454)

Aside from aging, noise is the most important cause of high-frequency sensorineural hearing loss, recognizable as early as in adolescence. Hobbies such as shooting and loud music may combine with industrial and agricultural noise to accelerate hearing loss. Although it is the responsibility of employers to conduct routine audiograms and to control exposure, clinicians should test noise-exposed patients periodically and reinforce whatever control strategies may be in place at work. Exposure to metals such as lead and organic solvents may compound the risk further.

Musculoskeletal Disorders of the Upper Extremity and Trunk

The most common cause of work disability, including permanent disability, is injury to the back (Chapter 423) and wrist. Repetitive, heavy, awkward, and time-pressured activities are notorious contributors, as are cold and vibration. Although an anatomically localized lesion may be identified and specifically treated in a small fraction of cases, as in carpal tunnel syndrome (Chapter 446) or thoracic outlet obstruction, the most important modalities of care in the majority of cases are early recognition and avoidance of further insult. Physical therapy and medications may hasten recovery but cannot prevent recurrences and even progression unless the causal work and avocational activities are modified.

Upper Airway Irritation (Chapter 93)

Virtually any smoke, fume, dust, or chemical has potential to irritate the upper respiratory tract, causing acute or chronic symptoms indistinguishable from common allergic manifestations (Chapter 270) or upper respiratory infections (Chapter 96). Although the mucosae of the eyes, nose, sinuses, and throat tend to be forgiving, recurrent episodes are extremely nettlesome and cause substantial disability. Atopic patients and patients with frequent infections are often the most sensitive to these ubiquitous environmental insults, which must ultimately be addressed along with the symptoms themselves and secondary infections.

Dermatitis

Erythematous rashes are a common consequence of topical exposures to workplace, avocational, and household materials, including latex, plastics, and many foods (Chapter 464). Although the keys to recognition are timing and the anatomic relation to clothing, allergenic and irritating chemicals can find their way into unlikely places, such as the groin and belt lines. Specialty consultation and patch testing are warranted in intractable cases but should not supplant careful observation and history taking in most situations.

Sick Building Syndrome and Nonspecific Building-Related Illness

The effort to reduce the influx of "fresh" air into buildings to save heating and air-conditioning costs has resulted in upper airway and dermal irritation as well as vague central nervous system symptoms such as headache and fatigue, occurring shortly after beginning work and clearing minutes to hours after leaving the affected building. Many occupants are typically affected, especially those who spend the most time in one place. The cause is unknown, but recent evidence suggests that microbial materials may be the most common culprits. In every instance, a search for a specific allergen or irritant is worth undertaking (Chapter 270), but the most remedial sources are poor overall ventilation and dampness in which molds fester. When the cause is remedied, most building occupants typically experience symptomatic improvement. From a clinical perspective, the major consideration is whether any more serious problem, such as asthma, may have also developed.

Multiple Chemical Sensitivities

An environmental illness as transient as a single noxious inhalation or as persistent as a protracted course of nonspecific building-related illness can initiate a cycle of similar symptoms after exposures to odors or irritants at very low levels so that even everyday tasks such as shopping or driving become problematic. A patient typically complains of being "allergic" to everything, although there is no evidence for allergic mechanisms (Chapter 270); the cause of this vexing complication, most prevalent in women, is unknown and may involve psychological as well as physiologic factors. Despite the severity of complaints, which often include fatigue, muscle pain, stridor, chest tightness, and palpitations, laboratory test results are normal. Coexistent anxiety and depression

TABLE 17–2 COMMON HAZARDS IN THE WORKPLACE AND AMBIENT ENVIRONMENT

Hazard	Health Effects of Greatest Concern	Comments
Metals	Neurotoxicity, cancer	Most can be measured in blood or urine to assess dose
Organic solvents	Respiratory and dermal irritation, neurotoxicity, hepatotoxicity	Benzene and a few others have unique effects
Organohalides (e.g., DDT, PCBs)	Cancer population concern	Ubiquitous suspect carcinogens of high
Herbicides and pesticides	Rare acute neurotoxicity, unknown long-term effects	Widespread hazards of high population concern
Electromagnetic radiation	Leukemia, glioblastoma	Ubiquitous exposures with unproven effects
Mold	Allergy	High population concern regarding putative chronic effects
Mineral dusts (e.g., asbestos, silica)	Cancer	Old hazards still of high concern

DDT = dichlorodiphenyltrichloroethane; PCBs = polychlorinated biphenyls.

often prompt psychiatric referral (Chapter 420), but the disorder has proved relatively refractory to all treatment modalities. Sympathetic support, environmental modification as needed to provide some symptomatic relief, and candor regarding the unknown nature of the disorder are appropriate; extensive clinical investigations often serve only to reinforce the patient's "sick" role and are best avoided. Despite all efforts, the most severely affected individuals will often seek the care of alternative practitioners (Chapter 36) with compelling if unproved theories and expensive, potentially harmful remedies.

COMMON HAZARDOUS EXPOSURES IN THE WORKPLACE AND AMBIENT ENVIRONMENT

Tens of thousands of chemicals in the workplace as well as important physical and biologic hazards may be encountered in the general environment (Table 17–2). Several of these hazards are of major current concern in industrialized countries.

Metals

Exposures to lead and arsenic (Chapter 20), once commonplace in industry, are now generally controlled; concern remains highest for environmental settings, especially for children. There is now greater concern for mercury—entrained in large ocean fish worldwide—and manganese (Chapter 20), a potent neurotoxin in welding fumes and various alloys. For most metals—manganese being a notorious exception—blood or urine tests are available to quantify a patient's burden, but these tests must be mindful of timing, the form of metal, and possible "confounders" such as the largely benign form of arsenic excreted in urine for several days after even a single shellfish meal.

Organic Solvents (Chapter 111)

These petroleum derivatives remain ubiquitous in workplace and household products. All are irritating, potentially neurotoxic, and, to varying degrees, hepatotoxic. A few, such as trichloroethylene and *n*-hexane, are more potent but no longer are widely used. Benzene and the ethers of ethylene glycol are bone marrow toxins (Chapter 171).

Organohalides

Although these complex organic pesticides and industrial materials are no longer made and sold in developed countries, their remarkable biopersistence has resulted in entrainment into everyone's fat. Worse, the dread byproduct dioxin, once associated with herbicide manufacture, has now been recognized as a predictable consequence of combustion of any chlorine-containing materials. All are suspect carcinogens, although debate remains whether this effect is limited to soft tissue sarcomas (Chapter 213)—a relationship established for dioxin—or promotes cancers more globally.

Herbicides and Pesticides (Chapter 111)

The acute neurotoxicity and irritant properties of most herbicides and pesticides have been well studied. These agents are generally well controlled, although both occupational and residential overexposures occasionally occur.

Electromagnetic Radiation (Chapter 18)

Electric wires, appliances, and, notoriously, cell phones emit low-frequency electromagnetic radiation at levels far below those that cause local thermal injuries. These radiations are nonionizing, but there is some epidemiologic evidence of an increased risk of childhood leukemia with high-level exposure from household wiring and of excess brain tumors in adult workers with regular exposures. Moreover, recent reports from Europe suggest excess brain cancer in cell phone users. These data are difficult to interpret because study results differ according to how exposure is assessed; the only conclusion is that there is basis for concern and need for further study but not cause for widespread alarm or action other than precaution in the placement of new heavy power lines near schools and residences.

Mold

Molds are ubiquitous and long known for their unpleasant odors and potential for inducing allergic responses (Chapter 270), including asthma. Recently, concern has arisen over potential for serious effects from various mycotoxins, long problems in veterinary medicine when domestic animals consume contaminated feed; however, a consensus panel concluded that there is no evidence of human risks beyond those well established from living or working in a moldy environment. Mold formation should be prevented wherever possible, especially in schools and offices, where molds contribute to problems with indoor air quality. Identification, with eradication of leaks and other sources of water accumulation, is key.

Mineral Dusts

Although asbestos has been largely abated, silica and man-made mineral fibers remain widely distributed in the environment. Silica (Chapter 93), present in virtually every form of "rock," is a potent cause of lung injury and cancer, so respiratory exposure should be carefully controlled in every setting. The evidence of serious risk from fibrous glass, mineral wool, and other man-made mineral fibers is less clear; probably only the finest fibers, such as slag wool, have cancer-causing potential, but many are potent dermal and upper respiratory irritants and should be well controlled for that reason alone.

SUMMARY

Occupational and environmental health problems remain prevalent, although their spectrum and nature have changed as rapidly as any in medicine and are likely to change even faster as technology, work, and knowledge continue to evolve. Physicians need not necessarily develop a large base of "facts"—themselves subject to revision frequently—but rather an approach that incorporates key elements and provides a foundation for efficient recognition and management of current and future clinical syndromes.

SUGGESTED READINGS

Frank AL: Approach to the patient with an occupational or environmental illness. Prim Care 2000;27:877–894. *A practical overview.*

Nawrot TS, Nemmar A, Nemery B: Update in environmental and occupational medicine 2006. Am J Resp Crit Care Med 2007;175:758–762. *Update of recent advances.*

Rosenstock LR, Cullen MR, Brodkin CA, et al (eds): Textbook of Clinical Occupational and Environmental Medicine, 2nd ed. Philadelphia, Elsevier, 2005. *A comprehensive text.*

RADIATION INJURY

Arthur C. Upton

Definition

The term *radiation injury* denotes any abnormality of form or function caused by electromagnetic waves or accelerated atomic particles. The term is also often applied to the harmful effects of high-intensity ultrasound and electromagnetic fields. The different types of radiation differ markedly in their biologic effects, so that each must be dealt with separately in considering the injuries that it can cause.

Ionizing Radiation Injury

The ionizing radiations occur as electromagnetic waves of extremely short wavelength (Fig. 18–1) and as accelerated atomic particles (e.g., electrons, protons, neutrons, α-particles). The injuries they cause include mutagenic, carcinogenic, and teratogenic effects and various acute and chronic tissue reactions, such as erythema, cataract of the lens, sterility, and depression of hematopoiesis.

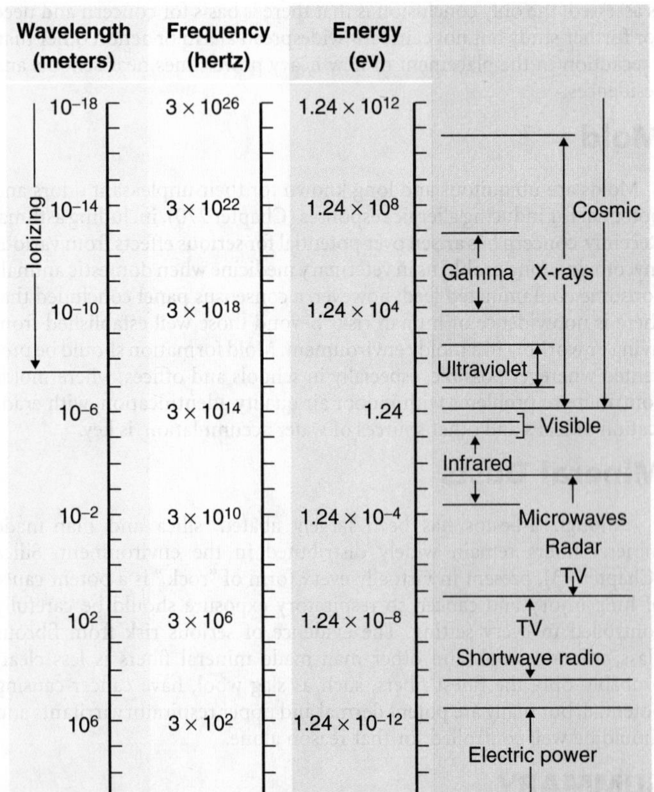

FIGURE 18–1 • The electromagnetic spectrum. (From Mettler FA, Upton AC: Effects of Ionizing Radiation, 2nd ed. Philadelphia, WB Saunders, 1995.)

Epidemiology

Precise data on the frequency of injuries caused by ionizing radiation are not available. Injuries attributable to excessive occupational exposure were prevalent among radiation workers in the era preceding modern safety standards but are seldom encountered in the United States today. The Chernobyl accident, however, caused radiation sickness in more than 200 emergency workers, injured 28 fatally, released enough radioactivity to require tens of thousands of inhabitants to be evacuated from the surrounding area, and resulted in a collective dose equivalent commitment of 600,000 person-Sv for the population of the Northern Hemisphere. Less catastrophic but more numerous than reactor accidents have been accidents with medical and industrial γ-ray sources, which are occasionally serious enough to be fatal. Noteworthy in this context is the potential for terrorist attacks (Chapter 19) in which nuclear weapons, conventional explosives ("dirty bombs"), or other means may be used to disperse hazardous amounts of radioactivity.

Also of ongoing public health concern is the risk of cancer incurred by the general population from current levels of exposure to ionizing radiation. Although no more than 3% of all cancers in the general population are thought to result from natural background ionizing irradiation, a substantially larger percentage of lung cancers are generally attributed to indoor radon. Another concern is the risk of heritable abnormalities resulting from the mutagenic and clastogenic effects of radiation, which have yet to be observed in humans but are well documented in other organisms.

Prenatal irradiation can also cause death, malformations, cataracts, mental retardation, impairment of growth, and behavioral disorders, depending on the dose and the developmental stage of the embryo at the time of exposure. Hence, special precautions now are taken to avoid exposure of the embryo to irradiation for prevention of such complications.

Pathobiology

The biologic effects of ionizing radiation result from damage to DNA and other vital molecules by locally deposited energy. Doses of ionizing radiation are therefore measured in terms of energy deposition (Table 18–1).

All humans are exposed continuously to natural background ionizing radiation from (1) cosmic rays; (2) radium and other radioactive elements in the earth's crust; (3) potassium 40, carbon 14, and other radionuclides normally present in human tissues; and (4) inhaled radon and its daughter elements (Table 18–2). In people residing at mile-high elevations, as in Denver, Colorado, the contribution from cosmic rays may be increased 2-fold; at jet aircraft altitudes, it may be increased more than 100-fold, exceeding 0.005 mSv (1 Sv = 100 rem) per hour. Likewise, in regions where the earth's crust is rich in radium, the contribution from this radionuclide may be increased correspondingly.

Among man-made sources of radiation, the largest is the use of x-rays in medical diagnosis. Smaller amounts of radiation are also received from radioactive minerals in building materials, phosphate fertilizers, and crushed rock; radiation-emitting components of television sets, smoke detectors, and other consumer products; radioactive fallout from atomic weapons; and nuclear power.

Workers in various occupations are exposed to additional doses of ionizing radiation, depending on their job assignments and working conditions. The average annual effective dose received by monitored radiation workers in the United States is less than 1 mSv, and less than 1% approach the maximum permissible dose limit (50 mSv) in any given year.

Pathogenesis

Ionizing radiation, colliding randomly with atoms and molecules in its path, gives rise to ions and free radicals, which break chemical bonds, cause other molecular alterations, and can ultimately injure the absorbing cell and its neighbors. Any molecule may thus be altered, but DNA is the critical biologic target because of the limited redundancy of its genetic information. A dose of radiation large enough to kill the average dividing cell (2 Sv) causes hundreds of lesions in its DNA molecules. Most such

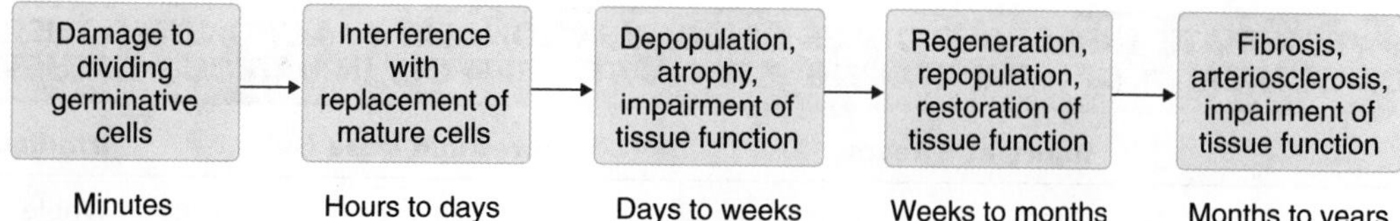

FIGURE 18–2 • Characteristic sequence of events in the pathogenesis of the nonstochastic effects of ionizing radiation. (From Upton AC: Radiological science. *In* Detels R, Holland W, McEwen J, Omenn GS [eds]: Oxford Textbook of Public Health, 3rd ed. New York, Oxford University Press, 2002, by permission of Oxford University Press.)

TABLE 18–1 RADIATION QUANTITIES AND DOSE UNITS

Quantity	Dose Unit*	Definition
Radioactivity	Becquerel (Bq)	One disintegration per second
Absorbed dose	Gray (Gy)	Energy deposited in tissue (1 J/kg)
Equivalent dose	Sievert (Sv)	Absorbed dose weighted for quality (potency) of the radiation
Effective dose	Sievert (Sv)	Equivalent dose weighted for sensitivity of the exposed organs
Collective effective dose	Person-Sv	Effective dose applied to a population
Committed effective dose	Sievert (Sv)	Effective dose from a given intake of radioactivity to be received during a period extending into the future

*The units of measurement listed are those of the International System, which have replaced earlier units such as the rad (1 rad = 0.01 Gy), the rem (1 rem = 0.01 Sv), and the curie (1 Ci = 3.7×10^{10} Bq).
Modified from Phillips TL: Radiation injury. *In* Wyngaarden JB, Smith LH Jr, Bennett JC (eds): Cecil Textbook of Medicine, 19th ed. Philadelphia, WB Saunders, 1992, p 2351.

TABLE 18–2 AVERAGE AMOUNTS OF IONIZING RADIATION RECEIVED ANNUALLY FROM DIFFERENT SOURCES BY A RESIDENT OF THE UNITED STATES

	Dose*	
Source	**mSv**	**%**
Natural		
Radon†	2.0	55
Cosmic	0.27	8
Terrestrial	0.28	8
Internal	0.39	11
Total natural	2.94	82
Artificial		
X-ray diagnosis	0.39	11
Nuclear medicine	0.14	4
Consumer products	0.10	<0.3
Occupational	<0.1	<0.3
Nuclear fuel cycle	<0.1	<0.3
Nuclear fallout	<0.1	<0.3
Miscellaneous‡	<0.1	<0.3
Total artificial	0.63	18
Total natural and artificial	~3.6	100

*Average effective dose.
†Average effective dose to bronchial epithelium.
‡Department of Energy facilities, smelters, and transportation.
Modified from National Research Council, National Academy of Sciences: Health Effects of Exposure to Low Levels of Ionizing Radiation: BEIR V. Washington, DC, National Academy Press, 1990.

lesions are reparable, but those produced by a densely ionizing radiation (e.g., proton or α-particle) are generally less reparable than those produced by a sparsely ionizing radiation (e.g., x-ray or γ-ray).

Unrepaired or misrepaired damage to DNA may be expressed in the form of mutations, the frequency of which approximates 10^{-5} to 10^{-6} per locus per sievert. Because the mutation rate tends to increase in proportion to the dose, it is inferred that a single ionizing particle traversing a genetic target may suffice to cause a mutation. Radiation damage also can cause changes in chromosome number and structure, the yields of which are characterized well enough that their frequency in lymphocytes can serve as a biologic dosimeter.

Radiation damage to genes, chromosomes, and other vital organelles may kill cells, especially dividing cells, which are radiosensitive as a class. Measured in terms of proliferative capacity, the survival of dividing cells tends to decrease exponentially with increasing dose; rapid exposure to 1 to 2 Sv generally reduces the surviving population of such cells by about 50%. Except for lymphocytes and oocytes, which tend to die in interphase, most cells killed by irradiation die in mitosis.

Although the killing of cells is a stochastic process, too few cells are killed by a dose less than 0.5 Sv to cause clinically detectable injury in most organs other than the testis and organs of the embryo. The killing of dividing progenitor cells, if sufficiently extensive, can interfere with the orderly replacement of senescent cells, especially in tissues such as the epidermis, bone marrow, and intestinal epithelium, which normally are characterized by high rates of cell turnover. The timing of the resulting atrophy (Fig. 18–2) varies, depending on the cell population dynamics within the tissue in question; in organs such as the liver and vascular endothelium, which are characterized by slow cell turnover, expression of the injury is delayed. Also, if the volume of tissue exposed is small or if the dose is accumulated slowly enough, the effects of irradiation may be counteracted in part by adaptive responses and by compensatory regenerative hyperplasia of surviving cells.

Clinical Manifestations

Ionizing radiation injuries encompass a diversity of tissue reactions that vary markedly in their dose-response relationships, manifestations, timing, and prognosis (Table 18–3). Except for mutagenic and carcinogenic effects, the reactions generally result from the killing of sizable numbers of cells in the exposed tissues and are not detectable unless the dose of radiation exceeds a substantial threshold. For this reason, the reactions are called *nonstochastic* (or *deterministic*) effects. In contrast, the mutagenic and carcinogenic effects of radiation are presumed to have no thresholds and are considered to be *stochastic* in nature. The existing data do not exclude the possibility, however, that the latter effects may have thresholds in the millisievert dose range, and the existence of adaptive responses to radiation (e.g., DNA repair processes) has been interpreted by some observers to support the hypothesis that the net effects of small doses may be beneficial ("radiation hormesis").

Tissues in which cells proliferate rapidly are generally the first to exhibit radiation injury. In such tissues, mitotic inhibition and cytologic abnormalities may be detectable immediately after irradiation, whereas ulceration, fibrosis, and other degenerative changes may not appear until months or years later (see Fig. 18–2).

TABLE 18–3 APPROXIMATE THRESHOLD DOSES OF CONVENTIONALLY FRACTIONATED THERAPEUTIC RADIATION FOR CLINICALLY DETRIMENTAL NONSTOCHASTIC EFFECTS IN VARIOUS TISSUES

Organ	Injury at 5 Years	Threshold Dose (sv)*	Irradiation Field (Area)
Fetus	Death	2	Whole
Bone marrow	Hypoplasia	2	Whole
Ovary	Permanent sterility	2–3	Whole
Lens	Cataract	5	Whole
Testes	Permanent sterility	5–15	Whole
Cartilage, child	Arrested growth	10	Whole
Breast, child	Hypoplasia	10	5 cm^2
Bone, child	Arrested growth	20	10 cm^2
Bone marrow	Hypoplasia, fibrosis	20	Localized
Muscle, child	Hypoplasia	20–30	Whole
Kidney	Nephrosclerosis	23	Whole
Lymph nodes	Atrophy	33–45	—
Liver	Liver failure, ascites	35	Whole
Lung	Pneumonitis, fibrosis	40	Lobe
Heart	Pericarditis, pancarditis	40	Whole
Stomach, small intestine, colon	Ulcer, perforation	45	100 cm^2
Thyroid	Hypothyroidism	45	Whole
Pituitary	Hypopituitarism	45	Whole
Lymphatics	Sclerosis	50	—
Central nervous system (brain)	Necrosis	50	Whole
Spinal cord	Necrosis, transection	50	5 cm^2
Salivary glands	Xerostomia	50	50 cm^2
Cornea	Keratitis	50	Whole
Capillaries	Telangiectasis, fibrosis	50–60	—
Breast, adult	Atrophy, necrosis	>50	Whole
Rectum	Ulcer, stricture	55	100 cm^2
Skin	Ulcer, severe fibrosis	55	100 cm^2
Eye	Panophthalmitis, hemorrhage	55	Whole
Oral mucosa	Ulcer, severe fibrosis	60	50 cm^2
Esophagus	Ulcer, stricture	60	75 cm^2
Cartilage, adult	Necrosis	60	Whole
Urinary bladder	Ulcer, contracture	60	Whole
Bone, adult	Necrosis, fracture	60	10 cm^2
Ear (inner)	Deafness	>60	Whole
Adrenal	Hypoadrenalism	>60	Whole
Vagina	Ulcer, fistula	90	5 cm
Muscle, adult	Atrophy	>100	Whole
Uterus	Necrosis, perforation	>100	Whole

*Dose causing effect in 1 to 5% of exposed persons.
Modified from Rubin P, Casarett GW: A direction for clinical radiation pathology: The tolerance dose. *In* Vaeth JM (ed): Frontiers of Radiation Therapy and Oncology. Basel, Karger, 1972; and Nonstochastic effects of ionizing radiation. ICRP publication 41. Ann ICRP 1984;14:1, with permission from Elsevier Science Ltd.

Skin

After rapid exposure to a dose of 6 Sv or more, erythema typically appears within 1 day, lasts a few hours, and is followed 2 to 4 weeks later by one or more waves of deeper and more prolonged erythema and epilation. Brief exposure to a dose greater than 10 to 20 Sv may cause transepithelial injury, with moist desquamation, necrosis, and ulceration within 2 to 4 weeks. The ensuing fibrosis of the underlying dermis and vasculature may lead to atrophy and a second wave of ulceration months or years later.

Bone Marrow and Lymphoid Tissue

A dose of 2 to 3 Sv delivered rapidly to the whole body destroys enough lymphocytes to depress the lymphocyte count and immune response within hours. Such a dose also can damage enough hematopoietic cells to cause profound leukopenia and thrombocytopenia within 3 to 5 weeks. If the dose exceeds 5 Sv, fatal infection and hemorrhage are likely to result (Table 18–4).

Intestine

The killing of epithelial stem cells is sufficiently extensive after an acute dose of 10 Sv to cause rapid denudation of the overlying intestinal villi. If the area affected is large, death from a fatal dysentery-like syndrome may ensue within days.

Respiratory Tract

Rapid exposure of the lung to a dose of 6 to 10 Sv damages alveolar cells and the pulmonary vasculature sufficiently to result in acute pneumonitis within 1 to 3 months. If extensive, the process may lead to fatal respiratory failure within 6 months or pulmonary fibrosis and cor pulmonale months or years later.

Gonads

Spermatozoa are relatively radioresistant, but spermatogonia are highly radiosensitive; a dose of 0.15 Sv delivered rapidly to both testes causes oligospermia after a latent period of about 6 weeks, and a dose of 2 to 4 Sv may cause permanent sterility. Oocytes also are radiosensitive; a dose of 1.5 to 2.0 Sv delivered to both ovaries causes temporary sterility, and a larger dose causes permanent sterility, depending on the woman's age at the time of exposure.

Lens of the Eye

Acute exposure of the lens to more than 0.5 Sv may lead within months to a microscopic posterior polar opacity, and 2 to 3 Sv received in a single

TABLE 18–4 SYMPTOMS, THERAPY, AND PROGNOSIS OF WHOLE BODY IONIZING RADIATION INJURY

	0–1 Sv	1–2 Sv	2–6 Sv	6–10 Sv	10–20 Sv	>50 Sv
Therapeutic needs	None	Observation	Specific treatment	Possible treatment	Palliative	Palliative
Vomiting	None	5–50%	>3 Gy, 100%	100%	100%	100%
Time to nausea, vomiting	—	3 hr	2 hr	1 hr	30 min	<30 min
Main locus of injury	None	Lymphocytes	Bone marrow	Bone marrow	Small bowel	Brain
Symptoms and signs	—	Moderate leukopenia, epilation	Leukopenia, hemorrhage, epilation	Leukopenia, hemorrhage, epilation	Diarrhea, fever, electrolyte imbalance	Ataxia, coma, convulsions
Critical period	—	—	4–6 wk	4–6 wk	5–14 days	1–4 hr
Therapy	Reassurance	Observation	Transfusion of granulocytes, platelets	Transfusion, antibiotics, bone marrow transplantation	Fluids and salts, possible bone marrow transplantation	Palliative
Prognosis	Excellent	Excellent	Guarded	Guarded	Poor	Hopeless
Lethality	None	None	0–80%	80–100%	100%	100%
Time of death	—	—	2 mo	1–2 mo	2 wk	1–2 days
Cause of death	—	—	Infection, hemorrhage	Hemorrhage, infection, pneumonitis	Enteritis, infection	Cerebral edema

Modified from Phillips TL: Radiation injury. *In* Wyngaarden JB, Smith LH Jr, Bennett JC (eds): Cecil Textbook of Medicine, 19th ed. Philadelphia, WB Saunders, 1992, p 2354.

brief exposure or 5.5 to 14 Sv accumulated during months may result in a vision-impairing cataract.

Other Tissues and Organs

Other tissues and organs, except in the embryo, are relatively less radiosensitive. All tissues, however, are more radiosensitive when they are rapidly growing.

Whole Body Radiation Injury

Brief exposure of a major part of the body to more than 1 Sv may cause the acute radiation syndrome, which is characterized by (1) an initial prodromal stage of malaise, anorexia, nausea, and vomiting; (2) an ensuing latent period; (3) a second (main) phase of illness; and (4) either recovery or death (see Table 18–4). The main phase of the illness usually takes one of four primary forms: (1) hematologic, (2) gastrointestinal, (3) neurovascular, or (4) pulmonary, depending on the size and anatomic distribution of the dose.

Localized or Regional Radiation Injury

In contrast to the acute radiation syndrome, manifestations of which are dramatic and relatively prompt, reactions to localized irradiation in most tissues tend to evolve more slowly and not to produce symptoms or signs unless the volume of tissue irradiated or the dose is large. Injury produced by a radionuclide follows the anatomic distribution of the radionuclide and its emitted radiation, which may be influenced by the physicochemical state in which the radionuclide is encountered and its portal of entry into the body.

Heritable (Genetic) Effects of Radiation

Radiation-induced heritable mutations and chromosome abnormalities are well documented in other organisms but have yet to be observed in humans. Intensive study of more than 76,000 children of Japanese atomic bomb survivors has failed to reveal definite evidence of heritable radiation effects detectable in terms of untoward outcomes of pregnancy, neonatal deaths, malignant neoplasms, balanced chromosome rearrangements, sex chromosome aneuploidy, alterations in serum or erythrocyte protein phenotypes, changes in gender ratio, or disturbances in growth and development. On the basis of the existing evidence, it is inferred that a dose of at least 1 Sv is required to double the rate of heritable mutations in human germ cells and that, consequently, less than 1% of all genetically determined disease is attributable to natural background irradiation.

TABLE 18–5 ESTIMATED LIFETIME RISK OF CANCER OF VARIOUS ORGANS ATTRIBUTABLE TO 0.1-SV RAPID IRRADIATION

	Excess Cancer Deaths Per 100,000	
Type or Site of Cancer	**No.**	**%***
Lung	205	3
Leukemia	86	14
Breast	73	2
Colon	61	3
Urinary bladder	25	5
Ovary	24	2
Stomach	22	4
Thyroid	8	16
Other	109	2
Total	613	3

*Percentage increase (values rounded) in the expected risk of death from cancer of the same organ in a nonirradiated population.

Modified from National Research Council, National Academy of Sciences: Health Risks from Exposure to Low Levels of Ionizing Radiation. Washington, DC, National Academy Press, 2005.

Carcinogenic Effects of Radiation

Many but not all types of benign and malignant growths have been observed to be inducible by irradiation; however, the induced growths have characteristically taken years or decades to appear and have possessed no features distinguishing them from growths resulting from other causes. With few exceptions, moreover, such growths have been detectable only after relatively large doses (>0.5 Sv) and have varied in frequency with the type of neoplasm and the age and gender of the exposed population. Because the existing data do not suffice to describe the dose-incidence relationship precisely or to define how long after irradiation the risk of cancer may remain elevated in an exposed population, assessment of the risks of low-level irradiation must be based on models incorporating assumptions about these parameters. Assessments (Table 18–5) have depended heavily on findings in atomic bomb survivors, whose overall incidence of cancer can be inferred to have increased as a linear nonthreshold function of their radiation dose. These estimates cannot be assumed to predict the risk of cancer attributable to a dose accumulated during weeks, months, or years, however, because experiments with laboratory animals have shown the carcinogenic potency of x-rays or γ-rays to decrease by a factor of 2 to 10 if the exposure is sufficiently prolonged. Furthermore, the estimates tabulated represent averages for a nominal population of males and females of all ages, whereas the estimates for breast cancer in women and for thyroid cancer in persons irradiated during childhood are substantially higher than those shown.

Effects on Lifespan

Mortality from cardiovascular, respiratory, and other non-neoplastic diseases as well as from various forms of cancer is increased in heavily irradiated populations. In lightly irradiated populations, however, these effects have not been evident, and survival has appeared to be enhanced in some instances. This finding has prompted some to infer that the effects of small doses may be beneficial on balance (radiation hormesis), but this hypothesis is highly controversial and remains to be validated.

Effects of Prenatal Irradiation

The embryo is especially vulnerable to death if it is exposed before implantation; it is susceptible to malformations and other developmental disturbances if it is exposed during subsequent stages in organogenesis, and it is sensitive throughout intrauterine life to the carcinogenic effects of radiation. Among various disturbances in growth and development, the dose-dependent increase in frequency of severe mental retardation and the dose-dependent decrease in IQ test scores in atomic bomb survivors who were irradiated between the 8th and the 15th week and, to a lesser extent, the 16th and the 25th week after conception are particularly noteworthy.

Diagnosis

Any facility likely to deal with radiation injuries should be able to cope with these injuries and should have personnel on call who are trained and equipped appropriately for the purpose. At the outset, to evaluate the dose and to determine whether the patient has been contaminated with radionuclides, the nature of the exposure and any measurements by film badges or other detectors should be reviewed in detail. If exposure to radionuclides is known or suspected, radioactivity measurements of the whole body, skin, other tissue, blood, urine, and body fluid may be indicated to identify the isotope and to evaluate the dose. Malaise, anorexia, nausea, and vomiting suggest a total body dose larger than 1 Sv, as do signs of erythema, hemorrhage, or infection in the skin, conjunctivae, or mucous membranes. The depth of lymphopenia within the first 24 hours also varies with the size of the total body dose. Although the granulocyte count may be elevated temporarily during the first 24 to 48 hours, the rapidity with which it and the platelet count fall in the ensuing 2 to 4 weeks also varies with the total body dose. Cytogenetic analysis of cultured lymphocytes for chromosome aberrations can provide another useful index of exposure.

Treatment

Rx

In managing radiation injury, good medical judgment and first aid are the priorities. Even if the patient has been heavily irradiated, the patient should be evaluated for other forms of injury, such as burns, mechanical trauma, and smoke inhalation. If radioactive contamination is known or suspected, rescue and medical personnel who handle the patient should wear gloves and other protective clothing and take precautions to isolate all contaminated objects.

Apart from symptomatic treatment, management of the hematologic form of acute radiation syndrome is similar to that of pancytopenic leukemia, including reverse isolation, antibiotics to combat infection, granulocyte and platelet transfusions as needed, and intravenous fluids as required to combat dehydration and electrolyte loss (Chapter 194). Colony-stimulating factors and interleukin may be beneficial in patients exposed to 6 to 10 Sv. Bone marrow transplantation (Chapter 184) may be life-saving after a dose of 7 to 10 Sv if a suitably matched donor is available; specimens of marrow and peripheral blood should be obtained for tissue typing as early as possible.

For localized injuries, treatment depends on the anatomic location and severity. Dry and moist desquamations of the skin, which are the most common injuries requiring treatment, usually are managed adequately by simple cleansing. Large or ulcerated lesions should be covered with lanolin and closed dressings that are changed regularly. Severe injuries may require resection of necrotic tissue and skin grafting.

In the event of radioactive contamination, steps should be taken to minimize the uptake and retention of isotope. Contaminated areas should be rinsed; the mouth, nose, and bronchial tree should be lavaged; and the gastrointestinal tract should be purged, if necessary. Additional measures to inhibit the uptake and retention of specific radionuclides may be indicated. Radioactive iodine may be released in a radiation accident or nuclear detonation and can pose a significant risk of thyroid cancer, especially in children. Stable potassium iodide should be administered to potentially exposed persons, except persons who are sensitive to iodine, to inhibit the uptake of radioactive iodine by the thyroid. The protective effect of a given dose persists for about 24 hours, and the optimal effect is achieved when potassium iodide can be given before exposure or concurrently with exposure. The recommended dose varies, depending on the recipient's age, expected level of thyroid exposure to radioactivity, and pregnancy or lactation status; recommendations range from 130 mg for adults to 16 mg for neonates.

Prevention

Because the mutagenic and carcinogenic effects of ionizing radiation may have no thresholds, unnecessary exposure should be avoided, and any doses to radiation workers and patients should be kept as low as reasonably achievable, with particular care that they not exceed the relevant maximum permissible doses (e.g., 50 mSv/year occupational whole body radiation). Facilities using radiation or radiation sources should be designed and equipped appropriately and should provide specialized training and supervision for all workers who may be occupationally exposed. Because indoor radon accounts for the bulk of the public's exposure to ionizing radiation, measures to limit excessive doses from this source also are warranted.

Prognosis

After a total body dose of 2 Sv or less, survival is probable with little or no treatment; in the 2- to 10-Sv range, appropriate treatment can afford a high rate of survival. If the injury is localized, the prognosis depends on the nature and severity of the reaction. Although recovery is the rule after minor, acute reactions, delayed reactions tend to be irreversible and progressive.

Nonionizing Radiation Injury

Ultraviolet Radiation

The ultraviolet (UV) radiation spectrum (see Fig. 18–1) is subdivided, for convenience, into three bands: UVA, or "black light," 315 to 400 nm; UVB, 280 to 315 nm; and UVC, which is germicidal, 200 to 280 nm. UV radiation does not penetrate deeply into human tissues, so the injuries it causes are confined chiefly to the skin and eyes.

Epidemiology

The largest source of UV radiation for the public is sunlight, which varies in intensity with latitude, elevation, and season. Important man-made sources include sun and tanning lamps, welding arcs, plasma torches, germicidal and black-light lamps, electric arc furnaces, hot-metal operations, mercury-vapor lamps, and some lasers. Low-intensity sources include fluorescent lamps and certain laboratory equipment.

Reactions of the skin to UV radiation, common among fair-skinned people, include sunburn, skin cancers (basal cell and squamous cell carcinomas and, to a lesser extent, melanomas), aging of the skin, solar elastosis, and solar keratosis. Injuries of the eye include photokeratitis, which may result from brief exposure to a high-intensity UV radiation source ("welder's flash") or more prolonged exposure to intense sunlight ("snow blindness"); cortical cataract; and pterygium.

Pathobiology

The effects of UV radiation are primarily attributable to its absorption in DNA; pyrimidine dimers are produced and cause mutational changes in exposed cells. Sensitivity to UV radiation may be increased by DNA repair defects (as in xeroderma pigmentosum), by agents (e.g., caffeine) that inhibit repair enzymes, and by photosensitizing agents (e.g., psoralens, sulfonamides, tetracyclines, nalidixic acid, sulfonylureas, thiazides, phenothiazines, furocoumarins, and coal tar) that produce UV radiation-absorbing DNA photoproducts. The carcinogenic action of UV radiation is mediated through direct effects on the exposed cells and depression of local immunity.

Clinical Manifestations

UVB in sunlight, although far less intense than UVA, plays a more important role in sunburn and skin carcinogenesis, but UVA also contributes to skin carcinogenesis, tanning, some photosensitivity reactions, and aging of the skin.

Treatment and Prevention

Rx

Excessive exposure to sunlight or other sources of UV radiation should be avoided, especially in fair-skinned individuals. Protective clothing, UV radiation–screening lotions or creams, and UV radiation–blocking sunglasses should be used. To protect occupationally exposed workers, the American Conference of Governmental Industrial Hygienists has recommended 8-hour exposure limits for the unprotected eye that range from 3 mJ/cm^2 to 10^6 mJ/cm^2, depending on the wavelength of the radiation (note: 1 J/s = 1 W). The protective layer of ozone in the stratosphere is being depleted globally by chlorofluorocarbons and other air pollutants, and every 1% decrease in ozone is expected to increase the UV radiation reaching the earth by 1 to 2% and thus to increase the rates of nonmelanotic skin cancer by 2 to 6%.

Visible Light

Visible light consists of electromagnetic waves varying in wavelength from 380 nm (violet) to 760 nm (red) (see Fig. 18–1).

Pathobiology

Bright, continuously visible light normally elicits an aversion response to protect the eye against injury, so few sources of light other than a laser or the sun in a solar eclipse are large or bright enough to cause a retinal burn under normal viewing conditions.

Pathogenesis

Photochemical reactions in the retina from sustained exposure to intensities exceeding 0.1 mW/cm^2, such as can result from fixing on a bright source of light, may suffice to produce photochemical blue-light injury. Brief exposure of the retina to intensities exceeding 10 W/cm^2, depending on image size, may cause a retinal burn.

Clinical Manifestations

Too little illumination can cause eyestrain or seasonal affective disorder, whereas too bright a light can injure the retina (Chapter 449).

Treatment and Prevention

Common sense usually suffices to prevent excessive exposure of the retina to light. However, in situations involving potential exposure to high-intensity sources, such as carbon arcs or lasers, appropriate training, proper design of equipment, and protective eye shields are important.

Infrared Radiation

Infrared radiation consists of electromagnetic waves ranging in wavelength from 7×10^{-5} m to 3×10^{-2} m. The injuries caused by infrared radiation are chiefly burns of the skin and cataracts of the lens of the eye.

Epidemiology

Potentially hazardous sources include furnaces, ovens, welding arcs, molten glass, molten metal, and heating lamps. The warning sensation of heat usually prompts aversion in time to prevent burning of the skin by infrared radiation; however, the lens of the eye is vulnerable because it lacks the ability to sense or dissipate heat.

Clinical Manifestations

Glass blowers, blacksmiths, oven operators, and people working around heating and drying lamps are at increased risk of infrared radiation–induced cataracts (Chapter 449).

Treatment and Prevention

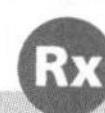

Control of infrared radiation hazards requires appropriate shielding of its sources, training of potentially exposed persons, and use of protective clothing and goggles.

Microwave Radiation

Microwave and radio frequency radiation consists of electromagnetic waves ranging in frequency from about 3 kHz to 300 GHz.

Epidemiology

Sources of microwave and radio frequency radiation are used widely in radar, televisions, cellular phones, radios, other telecommunications systems, various industrial operations (e.g., heating, welding, and melting of metals; processing of wood and plastic; high-temperature plasma), household appliances (e.g., microwave ovens), and medical applications (e.g., diathermy and hyperthermia).

Pathobiology

The biologic effects of microwave and radio frequency radiation are primarily thermal in nature. Because of the deep penetration of these types of radiation, the cutaneous burns they cause tend to involve dermal and subcutaneous tissues and heal slowly.

Clinical Manifestations

Isolated cases of skin burns, thermal injury to deeper tissues, and death from hyperthermia have been caused by industrial microwave and radio frequency radiation sources. Burns also have resulted from faulty or improperly used household microwave ovens and from the overexposure of patients with impaired cutaneous pain and temperature senses that usually warn of impending injury. Other effects reported in the literature but not as yet conclusively documented include cataract of the lens, impairment of fertility, developmental disturbances, neurobehavioral abnormalities, depression of immunity, and increased risk of cancer. Microwave and radio frequency radiation also can interfere with cardiac pacemakers (Chapter 65) and other medical devices.

Treatment and Prevention

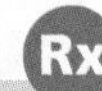

Microwave and radio frequency radiation sources must be designed and shielded properly, and potentially exposed persons, especially persons with cardiac pacemakers or other sensitive devices, must be trained and supervised properly. In general, detectable heating of tissue requires microwave and radio frequency radiation power densities greater than 10 W/cm^2; avoidance of such exposure, as prescribed by existing federal standards, suffices to prevent injury.

Extremely Low Frequency Electromagnetic Fields

Extremely low frequency electromagnetic fields range in frequency from 1 to 3000 Hz, including the 50- to 60-Hz fields associated with alternating currents in electric power distribution systems and appliances. Exposure to such fields is not known to be hazardous, but data suggesting that it may cause reproductive abnormalities and carcinogenic effects have aroused public health concern.

Epidemiology

The earth is surrounded by a naturally occurring electromagnetic field ranging in frequency from the low end of the extremely low frequency region to radio frequencies that exist briefly as a result of lightning discharges. Localized electromagnetic fields also are generated by electric power lines, transformers, motors, household appliances, video display tubes, and various medical devices, notably nuclear magnetic resonance imaging systems. These localized fields are generally stronger than naturally existing ones; electromagnetic field flux densities near common household appliances may range up to 270 mG compared with the average value of 0.6 mG for the earth's magnetic field.

Pathobiology

Evaluation of epidemiologic data is complicated by the lack of any known biologic basis for the effects of extremely low frequency electromagnetic fields on tissue, especially because the currents emanating from normal nerve and muscle activity are far stronger than the currents attributable to 1- to 10-mG external 60-Hz fields. Such fields nevertheless have been reported to influence ion transport, melatonin secretion, and tumor promotion in some model systems.

Clinical Manifestations

Exceptionally strong fields may affect electrically active tissues (nerves, neuromusculature, heart) and cardiac pacemakers and may raise body temperature. Conflicting epidemiologic studies have evaluated the possibility that (1) residential exposure of children to weaker electromagnetic fields may increase their risk of leukemia, (2) occupational exposure of male utility workers may increase their risk of brain cancer and leukemia, and (3) chronic exposure of pregnant women to video display tubes may increase their risk of miscarriage and of bearing children with birth defects; none of these links has been established.

Treatment and Prevention

Persons with pacemakers should avoid electromagnetic fields stronger than 0.5 mT, such as exist around transformers, accelerators, nuclear magnetic resonance systems, and other electrical devices; areas containing such fields should be posted with warning signs. Exposure of workers also should be limited, in accordance with national guidelines.

Ultrasound

Although frequently classified with nonionizing radiation, ultrasound consists of mechanical vibrations at inaudibly high frequencies (i.e., >16 kHz) and is not a component of the electromagnetic spectrum.

Epidemiology

High-power, low-frequency ultrasound is used widely in science and industry for cleaning, degreasing, plastic welding, liquid-extracting, atomizing, homogenizing, and emulsifying operations and in medicine for lithotripsy. Low-power, high-frequency ultrasound is used widely in analytic work and in medical diagnosis (e.g., ultrasonography).

Pathobiology

The biologic effects of high-power ultrasound are similar in mechanism to those of mechanical vibration-localized heating, agitation, and fragmentation of tissues.

Clinical Manifestations

Deleterious effects from prolonged exposure to high-power ultrasound include headache, malaise, tinnitus, vertigo, hypersensitivity to light and sound, and peripheral neuritis. Similar complaints may result from excessive exposure to high-frequency ultrasound through body contact with the source. However, adverse effects have not been shown to result from exposure to high-frequency ultrasound at the low power levels used in medical ultrasonography.

Treatment and Prevention

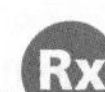

Protection against ultrasound injury requires appropriate isolation and insulation of generating sources and proper training and ear protective devices for persons working around such sources. Yearly audiometric and neurologic examinations of workers are advisable.

SUGGESTED READINGS

American Conference of Governmental Industrial Hygienists: 2005 Threshold Limit Values and Biological Exposure Indices. Cincinnati, OH, American Conference of Governmental Industrial Hygienists, 2005. *An authoritative listing of recommended maximum permissible occupational exposure limits of radiation of all types.*

Berrington de Gonzalez A, Darby S: Risk of cancer from diagnostic x-rays: Estimates for the UK and 14 other countries. Lancet 2004;363:345–351. *About 0.6% could be attributable to diagnostic x-rays.*

Huda W, Vance A: Patient radiation doses from adult and pediatric CT. Am J Roentgenol 2007;188:540–546. *The effective dose of one scan is about the same as 1 year of natural background radiation.*

Mettler FA, Voelz GL: Major radiation exposure—what to expect and how to respond. N Engl J Med 2002;346:1554–1561. *Overview of the consequences of and responses to a possible terrorist attack.*

National Research Council, National Academy of Sciences: Health Risks from Exposure to Low Levels of Ionizing Radiation. Washington, DC, National Academy Press, 2005. *A comprehensive review of the risks of genetic and carcinogenic effects that may result from exposure to low-level ionizing radiation.*

Wakeford R: The cancer epidemiology of radiation. Oncogene 2004;23:6404–6428. *A comprehensive review of the carcinogenic effects of ionizing and nonionizing radiations on human populations.*

Waselenko JK, MacVittie TJ, Blakely WF, et al: Medical management of the acute radiation syndrome: Recommendations of the Strategic National Stockpile Radiation Working Group. Ann Intern Med 2004;140:1037–1051. *A comprehensive review.*

19 BIOTERRORISM

John G. Bartlett

BIOLOGIC WEAPONS

Definition

Weapons of mass destruction are classified as biologic, chemical, or nuclear. Biologic weapons are microbes or microbial products that are used for bioterrorism. The potential for mass destruction is evident from a report from the U.S. Office of Technology, which predicted that release of 100 kg of anthrax spores upwind of Washington, DC, would cause 130,000 to 3,000,000 deaths, thus matching the lethal potential of a hydrogen bomb.

Epidemiology

Despite the enormous potential for mass destruction, the reality is that the actual application of bioterrorism has been quite limited. During World War II, there were major bioweapon programs in the United States, the Soviet Union, Japan, and Germany, but only Japan used it in any well-established way. The largest bioweapon program was by the Soviet Union, which had approximately 50 facilities and 60,000 employees. In 1972, the Biologic and Toxin Weapons Convention, which was established to eliminate the threat of bioterrorism, was signed by 140 nations, including the United States and the Soviet Union. The subsequent destiny of the enormous volume of products (smallpox virus, botulinum toxin, anthrax spores, etc.) and most of the scientists who were highly skilled in this area is largely unknown. Current estimates are that many nations continue to harbor bioweapon programs.

In addition to these large-scale national programs, there is also the potential for use of bioweapons by individuals or dissident groups. For example, in 1984 a religious cult in Oregon attempted to influence an election by contaminating restaurant salad bars with *Salmonella* to reduce voter turnout; the effort resulted in 751 cases of salmonellosis, but the election was not affected. Aum Shinrykio, a Japanese cult, was responsible for the release of sarin nerve gas in Tokyo, which resulted in 6000 casualties and 10 deaths.

More recently, there were 22 cases of anthrax in the United States during a 2-month period in 2001 as a result of contaminated letters sent to four sites. Of the 22 cases, 20 were traced directly to contaminated mail, all with the same molecular type of *Bacillus anthracis*. Some cases were cutaneous because the contaminated material in letters was milled to a relatively large particle size that contaminated surfaces via gravity. By contrast, letters with anthrax that was milled to nearly the size of a single spore resulted in particles that were aerosolized at release and inhaled, thereby causing inhalational anthrax. Exposed persons were advised to receive prophylactic doxycycline or ciprofloxacin, and in none of more than 10,000 persons who received even a single dose of either antibiotic did anthrax subsequently develop. For this terrorist act, the U.S. Centers for Disease Control and Prevention (CDC) assigned more than 1000 personnel to the epidemic and still needed more. In a 1-month period, the New York City Health Department managed over 15,000 telephone inquiries. During the outbreak, more than 200 mailed or telephoned threats of bioterrorism were recorded. Thus, despite a relatively small incident with just 22 cases over a 2-month period, the impact on society and health care resources was enormous.

Classification

The agents of bioterrorism are classified as A (greatest potential; Tables 19–1 and 19–2), B (less likely or important), or C (not believed to be a high bioterrorism risk). This classification is based on the following criteria:

1. Impact on public health in terms of illness and death
2. Ease of delivery based on stability of the agent and ability to mass produce and distribute
3. Potential for person-to-person transmission
4. Public perception in terms of potential for civil disruption
5. Requirements for a special public health response

TABLE 19–1 CLASSIFICATION OF BIOTERRORISM AGENTS

	Public Health Impact		Dissemination*			
Agent	Disease	Death	Delivery Potential	Person to Person	Public Perception†	Special Preparation‡
Smallpox (A)	+	++	+	+++	+++	+++
Anthrax (A)	++	+++	+++	0	+++	+++
Plague (A)	++	+++	++	+	++	+++
Botulism (A)	++	+++	++	0	++	+++
Tularemia (A)	++	++	+	0	+	+++
Viral hemorrhagic fever (A)	++	+++	+	++	+++	++
Viral encephalitis (B)	++	+	+	0	++	++
Q fever (B)	+	+	++	0	+	++
Brucellosis (B)	+	+	++	0	+	++
Glanders (B)	++	+++	++	0	0	++
Melioidosis (B)	+	+	++	0	0	++
Psittacosis (B)	+	+	++	0	0	+
Ricin toxin (B)	++	++	++	0	0	++
Typhus (B)	+	+	++	0	0	+
Cholera (B)	+	+	++	+/–	+++	+
Shigellosis (B)	+	+	++	+	+	+

*Potential for rapid large-scale dissemination.
†Media reports with +++ include more than 45 titles in surveying 233 newspapers and 70 TV/radio sources.
‡Needs therapeutics, surveillance, laboratory demands.
+++, Death in more than 50%; ++, 21 to 49%; +, less than 20%.
A = Greatest potential for bioterrorism; B = less likely or important for bioterrorism.

TABLE 19–2 CLINICAL FEATURES OF CATEGORY A AGENTS

	Anthrax (Inhalation)	Smallpox	Plague (Pneumonia)	Tularemia	Botulism	Viral Hemorrhagic Fever
Cases in U.S. per year	0	0	8–10	100–200	100–200	0
Clinical features	Flulike, then shock	Fever, then characteristic rash	Pneumonia, hemoptysis	Pneumonia	Descending paralysis and involvement of cranial nerves	Hemorrhage and fever
Diagnosis	Blood culture, CT of the chest	BSL-4 laboratory for virus	Blood and sputum culture	Sputum culture and radiograph	Toxin assay of blood, GI specimens; EMG	BSL-4 laboratory for virus
Mortality	40–50%	30%	10–20%	1–2%	60%	Variable
Treatment*	Cipro, Doxy, or Levo + 2nd agent,† 60–100 days	None	Gent/Strep (Cipro/Doxy), 10 days	Gent/Strep (Cipro/Doxy), 10 days	Antitoxin, ventilator	Ribavirin (some), 7 days
Prevention*	Cipro/Doxy	Vaccine	Cipro/Doxy	Cipro/Doxy	None	None
Infection control	Not transmitted	Contact and airborne precautions	Masks	Not transmitted	Not transmitted	Contact precautions

*Doses: Ciprofloxacin, 400 mg IV q8–12h or 500–750 mg PO bid; levofloxacin, 500–750 mg IV qd or 500 mg PO qd; doxycycline, 100 mg PO or IV bid; gentamicin, 5 mg/kg/day IM or IV; streptomycin, 1 g IM bid; ribavirin, 16 mg/kg/day IV × 4 days, then 8 mg/kg/day × 3 days or 1000–1200 mg/day PO × 7.
†Imipenem (500 mg IV q6h), rifampin (600 mg IV or PO qd), chloramphenicol (1 g IV q6h), clarithromycin (500 mg PO bid), vancomycin (1 g IV bid), or clindamycin (600 mg IV q8h).
BSL = Biologic Safety Level; Cipro = ciprofloxacin; CT = computed tomography; EMG = electromyography; GI = gastrointestinal; Levo = levofloxacin; Doxy = doxycycline; Gent = gentamicin; Strep = streptomycin; ( ) = alternative to preferred.

Anthrax

Definition

Infection is caused by *B. anthracis* (Chapter 317). The three recognized forms that reflect the portal of entry are inhalation, cutaneous exposure, and ingestion.

Epidemiology

The greatest concern for bioterrorism is the inhaled form, which results from the inhalation of *B. anthracis* spores and results in a devastating disease with a mortality rate of about 50% even with optimal management. The last naturally occurring case of inhalational anthrax in the United States was in 1976. The largest epidemic followed an accidental release of anthrax in Sverdlovsk, Russia, in 1979 and resulted in an estimated 80 to 250 cases. Cutaneous anthrax is the usual naturally occurring zoonotic form. An average of less than 1 case per year now occurs in the United States, with about 2000 naturally occurring cases in the world per year.

Pathobiology

With inhalational anthrax associated with bioterrorism, spores must be milled to less than 5 μm to permit both aerosolization and inhalation. The spores are taken up by alveolar macrophages and migrate to the mediastinal lymph nodes, where they revert to vegetative forms and produce toxins. The protective antigen combines with lethal toxin and edema toxin; these toxins are thought to account for the clinical features.

Clinical Manifestations

The incubation period is usually 4 to 5 days, but the range is from 2 to 43 days after exposure. Inhalational anthrax is a two-stage disease. The initial symptoms are nonspecific and flulike. Features that distinguish this stage from influenza are the lack of coryza and the anticipated exposure history. The second stage is profound sepsis with chest pain, chest compression from large pleural effusions and mediastinal expansion, multiple organ failure, obtundation, cyanosis, hypotension, and death, which may occur within hours. Cutaneous anthrax is characterized by a vesicle that progress to an eschar associated with substantial surrounding edema, often with regional adenopathy and systemic signs of infection.

Diagnosis

The diagnosis is established by recovery of *B. anthracis* from blood or the infected site. Virtually all patients with inhalational anthrax have positive blood cultures, frequently within 12 to 16 hours if cultures were obtained before therapy. Other highly characteristic features of the disease are a chest radiograph that shows a wide mediastinum and a computed tomography scan that shows hyperdense hilar and mediastinal lymph nodes, often with large pleural effusions. A highly characteristic feature of the disease is large bloody pleural collections. There may or may not be a pulmonary infiltrate.

Treatment

The most important facets of treatment of inhalational anthrax are supportive care, drainage of pleural effusions, and rapid administration of antibiotics. The drugs approved by the Food and Drug Administration (FDA) for *B. anthracis* are intravenous penicillin, doxycycline, ciprofloxacin, and levofloxacin (Table 19–2). Because no therapeutic trials have been conducted, these drugs are approved on the basis of efficacy shown in a primate model of inhalational anthrax. In reality, a bioterrorism event with inhaled anthrax will result in specific recommendations from the CDC. In 2001, the preferred agents were doxycycline or ciprofloxacin combined with a second agent such as penicillin, imipenem, rifampin, chloramphenicol, clarithromycin, vancomycin, or clindamycin based on sensitivity tests of the epidemic strain. After clinical improvement, the intravenous administration may be changed to oral agents such as

Rx

ciprofloxacin, levofloxacin, or doxycycline; the total recommended duration of treatment is 60 to 100 days. The prolonged course is suggested because studies in primates show persistence of spores after drugs were given for up to 30 days. For cutaneous anthrax, the recommendation is ciprofloxacin or doxycycline for a total of 60 to 100 days because of the assumption that a patient with cutaneous anthrax as a result of bioterrorism may have inhaled organisms as well.

Prevention

In the event of bioterrorism, prophylaxis appears to be critical because it is nearly 100% effective, whereas patients in whom the disease develops have substantial morbidity and mortality despite optimal management. During the 2001 epidemic, the recommendation was oral doxycycline or ciprofloxacin for 60 to 100 days; despite variable compliance, anthrax did not develop in any individual. An FDA-approved anthrax vaccine given in six administrations to wool sorters and other workers in high-risk occupations is highly effective, but other forms of anthrax vaccine are now being developed in the hope that they will require fewer administrations and have less adverse reactions.

Prognosis

Available data from the Sverdlovsk outbreak in Russia suggest a mortality rate of 60 to 87% despite appropriate antibiotics. In the 2001 epidemic in the United States there were five deaths (45%) in 11 patients despite aggressive management. In fatal cases, the interval between the onset of symptoms and death averaged 3 to 4 days.

Smallpox

Definition

Smallpox is a systemic infection caused by the virus Variola major or Variola minor (Chapter 395). The assumption is that any attempt at bioterrorism with smallpox would use V. major, which is associated with a substantially higher mortality rate. The virus is viewed as ideal for bioterrorism because it is easy to culture, survives well in aerosols, and is lethal in of 30% of cases. Furthermore, most humans are now susceptible because immunization was stopped in the United States and most of the world by 1973.

Epidemiology

The global campaign to eradicate smallpox was initiated in 1966, and the last naturally occurring case was reported in 1977. In 1980 the World Health Organization (WHO) declared smallpox eradicated and recommended that all laboratories destroy stocks of variola or transfer them to one of two WHO reference laboratories, one in Moscow and the other at the CDC in Atlanta. These remaining isolates were to be destroyed in 1999, but the WHO agreed to retain the supplies in an effort to develop an attenuated vaccine and antiviral drugs. The number of countries that have this virus other than Russia and the United States is not known.

Smallpox is spread from person to person in droplets from the oral pharynx. The greatest risk is to persons within 6 to 8 feet of an infected individual, and prior epidemics have consistently shown that most cases occur in household members and hospital contacts. The secondary attack rate in unvaccinated household members is 37 to 88%. Because the disease has been eradicated, any confirmed case of smallpox implies bioterrorism.

Clinical Manifestations

The incubation period is usually 12 to 14 days. Initial symptoms are high fever, malaise, prostration, headache, and backache. These symptoms are severe, and most patients are bedridden. The rash usually appears on day 3 as a maculopapular eruption that subsequently evolves through the vesicular and then pustular stages; at 2 to 3 weeks it forms scabs that separate and leave a characteristic pitted scar. The rash begins on the face and forearms and then spreads to the trunk and legs. Pustules have a characteristic firm, round, deep-seated appearance and measure 7 to 10 mm in diameter. Lesions are more dense on the face and extremities, all are in the same stage, and there may be involvement of the palms and soles. An important issue in terms of disease control is that transmission takes place during the rash phase and not during the early prerash period of illness.

Diagnosis

Laboratory diagnosis requires fluid collected from a typical vesicular or pustular lesion, preferably by a vaccinated person with appropriate protection. Laboratory testing must be done in a maximum containment facility (Biologic Safety Level 4 [BSL-4] laboratory); tissue culture is used to recover the virus, and polymerase chain reaction and restriction fragment length polymorphism are used to characterize the viral strain. For the clinician, the major issue is the distinction of smallpox from chickenpox or other illnesses that are also characterized by a vesicular rash (Table 19–3). With chickenpox (Chapter 398), the lesions are more superficial, have a centripetal distribution with more involvement of the trunk and face, and are not all at the same stage of evolution. Patients are also less seriously ill.

Other conditions in the differential diagnosis for a vesicular or pustular rash include disseminated herpes zoster or herpes simplex (Chapter 397), drug eruptions (Chapter 466), erythema multiforme (Chapter 464), enteroviral infection (Chapter 402), secondary syphilis (Chapter 340), monkeypox (Chapter 395), molluscum contagiosum (Chapter 464), and generalized vaccinia. With a generalized maculopapular rash, the differential diagnosis includes measles (Chapter 390), rubella (Chapter 391), drug rash, erythema multiforme, and scarlet fever (Chapter 311).

Treatment

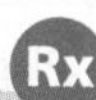

There is no therapy with established merit.

TABLE 19–3 MAJOR AND MINOR CRITERIA FOR SMALLPOX AND PRIORITY FOR REPORTING TO THE CENTERS FOR DISEASE CONTROL AND PREVENTION

MAJOR CRITERIA:

Fever (>38.3° C) 1–4 days before the onset of rash plus one of the following: headache, prostration, chills, vomiting, and abdominal pain
Typical smallpox lesions: firm, round, deep-seated vesicles or pustules with evolution to become umbilicated or confluent
Lesions same stage in development

MINOR CRITERIA:

Centrifugal distribution of the rash (face and extremities)
First lesions on oral mucosa, palate, face, and arms
Patient appears toxic or moribund
Slow evolution of lesions—each stage lasts at least 1–2 days
Lesions on palms and soles

REPORTING PRIORITY:

Report immediately: (1) febrile prodrome, (2) classic smallpox lesions, and (3) lesions in the same stage of development (need all 3)
Urgent assessment: (1) febrile prodrome and one other major smallpox criterion *or* (2) febrile prodrome plus ≥4 minor criteria
Manage as clinically indicated: febrile prodrome and ≥4 minor criteria

Prevention

Vaccination with vaccinia (cowpox) virus before exposure provides significant protection against smallpox. Persons in whom a vesicle or pustule develops or who have a pitted scar at a previous vaccination site have "a take" indicating an immune response. The duration of protection is not well known. Vaccination also provides some protection when given within 4 days after exposure because the immune response to vaccinia is faster than it is to smallpox. The major goal in the event of anticipated bioterrorism is to vaccinate persons with anticipated risks, such as military personnel or hospital-based smallpox response teams. In an outbreak, the highest priority will be first responders, household contacts, and others who have face-to-face contact with patients after the onset of fever.

Vaccination was associated with substantial risk when it was given routinely before 1973. The major currently recognized vaccine-associated complications (Chapter 16) include (1) postvaccinal encephalitis, which is probably a immune reaction; (2) progressive vaccinia, which is a progressive and rapidly lethal complication of disseminated vaccinia seen primarily in patients with defective cell-mediated immunity; (3) generalized vaccinia caused by dissemination of vaccinia; (4) accidental inoculation of other anatomic sites or other persons, usually bedmates; and (5) eczema vaccinatum in patients with a current or past history of eczema or atopic dermatitis. Complications that result from uncontrolled growth of vaccinia can be treated with vaccinia immune globulin. During the recent experience with smallpox vaccination in more than 500,000 U.S. military personnel and health care workers, the frequency of these adverse reactions was modest and no deaths were recorded; however, another major complication was recognized: myopericarditis, which was most common with primary vaccination, self-limited, and probably immune mediated.

Plague

Definition

Plague refers to infection by *Yersinia pestis* (Chapter 333).

Epidemiology

Approximately 10 cases of plague occur in the United States annually, but the pneumonic form of disease that would be anticipated in the event of bioterrorism is rare, with only about 7 cases in the past 50 years. Thus, any case of pneumonic plague, particularly if acquired in urban areas and outside endemic areas, should arouse suspicion of bioterrorism. An important clinical clue to the diagnosis is severe pneumonia associated with hemoptysis. It is known that *Y. pestis* was produced in large quantities by Soviet scientists for bioterrorism before abandoning this program in 1992. The WHO has estimated that a 50-kg release of *Y. pestis* over an urban area of 5 million people would result in 150,000 cases of plague pneumonia and 36,000 deaths.

Clinical Manifestations

The incubation period is 1 to 6 days. The pneumonic form is associated with bloody sputum, fever, dyspnea, and frequently gastrointestinal symptoms, including nausea, vomiting, abdominal pain, and diarrhea. The course is rapidly progressive with a sepsis syndrome at 2 to 6 days. Chest radiographs usually show consolidated infiltrates, and about 50% of patients have pleural effusions.

Diagnosis

Y. pestis is a gram-negative coccobacillus that demonstrates bipolar staining and resembles a safety pin. Although the organism may be recognized by Gram stain of sputum, most laboratories require extended periods to identify it with standard methods. If this diagnosis is suspected, the laboratory should be warned so that one culture can be incubated at 28° C for rapid growth and a second at 37° C to permit identification of the capsular antigen. Rapid diagnostic tests are available in some state health departments, the CDC, and some military facilities.

The differential diagnosis includes other severe forms of pneumonia or epidemic pneumonia, such as legionnaires' disease (Chapter 335), histoplasmosis (Chapter 353), anthrax (Chapter 317), tularemia (Chapter 332), and influenza (Chapter 387).

Treatment

The preferred drugs are streptomycin or gentamicin; doxycycline and fluoroquinolones such as ciprofloxacin or levofloxacin are alternative agents. The duration of treatment is 10 days.

Prevention

Limited data define the efficiency of person-to-person transmission. Current recommendations are for contact and droplet precautions with the use of masks, gowns, gloves, and eye protection. Isolation may be discontinued after 48 hours of antibiotic treatment and clinical improvement. Prophylactic doxycycline or ciprofloxacin is recommended for 7 days for household members, health care workers, and other close contacts of patients. Prophylactic antibiotics are also advocated for other persons with a common-source exposure. Like anthrax, prophylaxis is virtually 100% effective, whereas treatment after the onset of symptoms is much less successful.

Prognosis

The fatality rate of pneumonic plague approaches 100% without therapy. Mortality has been reduced to 5 to 14% with aminoglycoside treatment, but this experience is based largely on syndromes that are generally less severe than plague pneumonia.

Botulism

See Chapter 319.

Tularemia

Definition

Tularemia is an infection caused by *Francisella tularensis* (Chapter 332).

Epidemiology

About 100 to 200 cases of tularemia are diagnosed per year in the United States, primarily in rural areas, especially in Oklahoma, Arkansas, Missouri, South Dakota, and Montana. Since 2000, there have been more than 15 cases in Martha's Vineyard in Massachusetts. With bioterrorism, the expectation would be a large number of cases of acute nonspecific febrile illness with pneumonitis. However, aerosol delivery could result in multiple other forms, depending on the anatomic site of inoculation, including ulceroglandular (from contaminated wounds), ocular, and oropharyngeal tularemia.

Clinical Manifestations

The incubation period is 3 to 5 days. The illness is characterized by fever, sometimes with a temperature-pulse disassociation, and progresses to pharyngitis, bronchitis, and pneumonitis with pleurisy and hilar adenopathy. When compared with plague or anthrax, inhalational tularemia progresses much more slowly and has a low fatality rate. Other manifestations include pharyngeal (exudative pharyngitis with fever and cervical adenopathy) and typhoidal (fever prostration and septic shock) tularemia.

Diagnosis

The chest radiograph typically shows hilar adenopathy. Respiratory secretions contain small gram-negative coccobacilli but not the "safety pin" form of plague. The diagnosis is established by direct immunofluo-

TABLE 19–4 VIRAL HEMORRHAGIC FEVERS

Agent	Source	Vector	Clinical Features	P-P Tx	Treatment	Mortality
Ebola	Africa	Not known	Fever, rash, DIC	+	Supportive	50–90%
Marburg	Africa	Not known	Fever, rash	+	Supportive	20–70%
Lassa fever	Africa	Rodent	Fever, conjunctivitis	+	Ribavirin	15–20%
New World Arenaviridae	South America	Rodent	GI symptoms, conjunctivitis, adenopathy	+	Ribavirin	15–30%
Rift Valley fever	Africa, Saudi Arabia	Mosquito	Fever, jaundice, photophobia	No	Ribavirin	<1%
Yellow fever	Africa, Americas	Mosquito	Fever, jaundice, conjunctivitis	No	Supportive	20%
Omsk hemorrhagic fever	Central Asia	Tick	Fever, cough, conjunctivitis, adenopathy	No	Supportive	1–10%
Kyasanur	India	Tick	Biphasic encephalitis	No	Supportive	3–10%

DIC = disseminated intravascular coagulation; GI = gastrointestinal; P-P Tx = Person-to-person transmission; + = yes.

rescent antibody staining, but the reagents are available only from specialized laboratories in the Laboratory Response Network. The organism may be used, but the laboratory must be warned for two reasons: to use specialized media and to take special precautions to avoid exposure. Growth is slow, with 2 to 5 days generally required.

Treatment

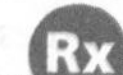

The preferred drugs are streptomycin or gentamicin given for 10 days; doxycycline and ciprofloxacin are alternatives. Exposed persons in whom fever develops within 14 days of exposure should be treated expectantly.

Prevention

The preferred antibiotic for postexposure prophylaxis is doxycycline or ciprofloxacin given for 14 days. There is no person-to-person spread, so health care workers, family members, and other close contacts with cases are at no risk.

Viral Hemorrhagic Fever

Definition

The hemorrhagic fever viruses include diverse organisms that cause a clinical illness characterized by fever and bleeding. These agents are grouped in four families: Filoviridae, Arenaviridae, Bunyaviridae, and Flaviviridae (Table 19–4). These viruses are attractive for bioweapons because the minimum infecting dose may be as low as 10 virions, they can be distributed by aerosols, mortality rates are virus dependent but often high, they generate great fear, many are transmitted person to person, and no good treatment is available.

Epidemiology

The hemorrhagic fever viruses are not normally found in the United States, Europe, or Australia. They are transmitted by contact with infected animals or arthropod vectors, although the natural reservoir for Ebola and Marburg viruses is not known. Any case of viral hemorrhagic fever in a patient in a nonendemic area who has not visited an endemic area within the previous 22 days is presumed to represent bioterrorism.

Clinical Manifestations

The onset of illness is generally nonspecific and consists of fever and myalgias. Additional symptoms are "virus dependent" (Table 19–4) and include rash, encephalitis, pharyngitis, adenopathy, and gastrointestinal symptoms. The syndrome progresses to thrombocytopenia with petechiae, hematuria, hematemesis, hemoptysis, and melena. Disseminated intravascular coagulation with shock, delirium, convulsions, and coma may then develop.

Diagnosis

Laboratory features include thrombocytopenia, as well as leukopenia, anemia, or hemoconcentration. All specimens from patients with suspected viral hemorrhagic fever should be referred to the CDC for testing in a BSL-4 laboratory. Personnel in the referring laboratory must be warned, and only designated technicians should be assigned to processing.

Treatment

Ribavirin has activity in vitro against Lassa fever virus, New World arenaviruses, and bunyaviruses, but clinical experience is limited. It is assumed that a limited number of cases involving these viruses would permit the use of intravenous ribavirin, but a mass casualty setting would require oral administration. Treatment of other hemorrhagic fever viruses would largely be limited to supportive care.

Prevention

The major concern is nosocomial and household transmission by contact with blood and other body fluids. Patients should be in a single-occupant negative-pressure room, and health care personnel should use N95 respirators or powered air purifying respirators (PAPRs), double gloves, impermeable gowns, goggles or face shields, and leg and shoe coverings. Nonessential staff and visitors should be excluded. Dedicated medical equipment such as stethoscopes and point-of-care analyzers should be available. Laboratory specimens should not be sent in pneumonic systems, contaminated objects should be cleaned with 1:100 household bleach or a similar disinfectant, and contaminated cloth items should be double-bagged and incinerated or autoclaved. Particular care needs to be exercised in managing corpses.

SUGGESTED READINGS

Arnon SS, Schecter R, Inglesby TV, et al: Botulinum toxin as a biological weapon: Medical and public health management. JAMA 2001;285:1059–1070. *Overview of botulism as a bioterrorism event.*

Blank S, Moskin LC, Zucker JR: An ounce of prevention is a ton of work: Mass antibiotic prophylaxis for anthrax, New York City 2001. Emerg Infect Dis 2003;9:615–622. *A review of the exemplary methods used to serve up to 10,000 persons exposed to anthrax.*

Borio L, Inglesby T, Peters CJ, et al: Hemorrhagic fever viruses as biological weapons: Medical and public health management. JAMA 2002;287:2391–405. *Overview of hemorrhagic fever viruses as agents of bioterrorism.*

Dennis DT, Inglesby TV, Henderson DA, et al: Tularemia as a biological weapon: Medical and public health management. JAMA 2001;285:2763–2773. *Overview of tularemia as a bioterrorism event.*

Inglesby TV, O'Toole T, Henderson DA, et al: Anthrax as a biological weapon, 2002: Updated recommendations for management. JAMA 2002;287: 2236–2252. *Overview of anthrax as a bioterrorism event.*

Moore ZS, Seward JF, Lane JM: Smallpox. Lancet 2006;367:425–435. *Review of smallpox, including recommendations for public health authorities.*

Prentice MB, Rahalison L: Plague. Lancet 2007;369:1196–1207. *A review, including plague as a bioterrorism event.*

Relman DA: Bioterrorism—preparing to fight the next war. N Engl J Med 2006;354:113–115. *Reviews the state of preparedness for bioterrorism.*

Smith BT, Inglesby TV, Brimmer E, et al: Navigating the storm: Report and recommendations from the Atlantic Storm exercise. Biosecur Bioterror 2005;3:256–267. *A bioterrorism simulation emphasizing that public health and diplomatic responses must be in place before any attack.*

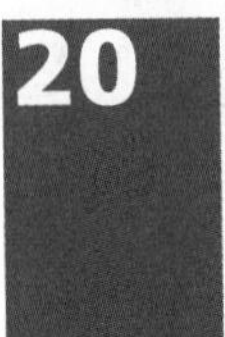

20 CHRONIC POISONING: TRACE METALS AND OTHERS

Michael A. McGuigan

Definition

The term *chronic poisoning* refers to toxicity that develops during repeated or continuous exposure to a substance during many months or years. A *trace metal,* which by definition is present in minute quantities, usually refers to metals that are essential to an organism's function, but this chapter includes a number of metals that are not physiologically required and does not discuss acute poisoning (Chapter 111).

Epidemiology

The source of most metals and the two other substances discussed in this chapter is the environment—the home, the workplace, or the outdoors—and most of the exposures are unintentional. Because many of these metals are essential to normal physiologic functions, another source may be dietary supplements (Chapter 237). The most common site of absorption is the gastrointestinal tract.

The medical literature on chronic low-level exposures is uneven. Although the clinical toxicology of each metal is presented individually, most if not all exposures involve a number of different metals, and the clinical impact of metal-metal interactions is poorly understood.

Lead

Epidemiology

Lead poisoning was recognized more than 2000 years ago. Although lead poisoning is often considered a problem primarily in the children of lower socioeconomic status families living in dilapidated housing with peeling lead-based paint, lead poisoning also occurs in adults exposed in occupational or nonoccupational activities (Table 20–1).

Pathobiology

Inhaled fine particulates (<5 μm in diameter) of inorganic lead reach the alveoli and are readily absorbed; larger particles come in contact with airway mucus and eventually are swallowed. Only 20 to 30% of orally ingested lead is absorbed. Organic lead compounds can also be absorbed through the skin. Absorbed lead distributes first into blood and soft tissue and then into bone, where more than 90% of total body lead is found. Factors contributing to bone demineralization (e.g., prolonged bedrest, pregnancy, menopause) promote the release of lead from bone. Lead is excreted primarily through the kidneys at a rate of about 30 μg/day, which may increase to 200 μg/day with higher body burdens.

Clinical Manifestations

Lead binds to sulfhydryl groups and adversely affects zinc- and calcium-dependent enzyme systems. This binding interferes with heme synthesis, DNA transcription, and calcium-dependent release of neurotransmitters and of protein kinase C, which regulate cell growth, learning, and memory. In addition, lead affects membrane integrity, steroid metabolism, and vitamin D synthesis in renal tubular cells, and it produces motor axon degeneration and segmental demyelination. The clinical manifestations of lead toxicity are roughly related to the blood lead level (Table 20–2).

Cardiovascular System

A cross-sectional study of 2165 women aged 40 to 59 years found that a change in blood lead levels from the lowest quartile (mean, 1.0 μg/dL; range, 0.5 to 1.6 μg/dL) to the highest quartile (mean, 6.3 μg/dL; range, 4.0 to 31.1 μg/dL) was associated with a significant increase in systolic (by 1.7 mm Hg) and diastolic (by 1.4 mm Hg) blood pressures. At blood lead levels between 10 and 40 μg/dL, lead increases systolic blood pressure by 1 to 2 mm Hg and diastolic pressure by 1.4 mm Hg for every doubling of the blood lead level. Workers with mean blood lead levels between 40 and 70 μg/dL have an increased risk of death from renal and

TABLE 20–1 COMMON SOURCES OF ADULT LEAD EXPOSURES

Occupational	Nonoccupational
Manufacturing	Shooting firearms
Manufacture of storage batteries	Remodeling or renovation activities
Secondary smelting	Hobbies (e.g., casting, ceramics, stained glass)
Manufacture of primary batteries	Retained bullets or gunshot wounds
Primary smelting	Pica
Welding and cutting operations	Contaminated food, liquid, or nontraditional medications
Construction	
Special trade contractors	
Painting, paperhanging, decorating	
Lead abatement workers	
Mining	
Mining of lead and zinc ores	
Wholesale trades	
Wholesale distribution of electrical apparatus and equipment, wiring supplies, and construction materials	
Retail trades	
Automobile repair shops	
Transportation, communication, electric, gas, and sanitary services	

TABLE 20–2 SUMMARY OF CLINICAL LEAD TOXICITY

Blood Lead Level (μg/dL)	Effects
<10	Aminolevulinic acid dehydrase inhibition
15–30	Elevation of erythrocyte protoporphyrin
30–39	Mild elevations in blood pressure Altered testicular function
40–49	Increased coproporphyrins and urinary aminolevulinic acid Slowed peripheral nerve conduction
50–59	Reduced hemoglobin synthesis Neurologic symptoms
60–69	Reproductive effects in women
80–90	Anemia Encephalopathy symptoms Nephropathy
100+	Encephalopathy signs

hypertensive cardiovascular disease. The progression, mechanisms, and effects of therapeutic interventions are unclear in lead-associated hypertension.

Reproductive System

Workplace exposure to lead is associated with decreased fertility, spontaneous abortions, stillbirths, low birthweights, and increased infant mortality. At mean blood lead levels above 23 μg/dL, lead has a direct toxic effect on spermatogenesis, resulting in decreased sperm counts and abnormal sperm morphology and function.

Renal System

Lead accumulates in proximal tubule cells. Reported clinical findings include Fanconi's syndrome, increased urate excretion, chronic interstitial nephritis, and interference in the renin-aldosterone system. In a population with a mean blood lead level of 8.1 μg/dL, an increase in blood lead level of 10 μg/dL was associated with a decrease in creatinine clearance of 10.4 mL/min.

Nervous System

Chronic encephalopathy (Chapter 439) is more common than acute encephalopathy. Early encephalopathic manifestations include changes in cognitive function and mood: early morning sleep disturbances, headache, irritability, lassitude, and loss of libido. Abnormalities in cognition or visual-motor function may be evident on psychometric testing. These findings may be found in workers with blood levels as low as 30 μg/dL but are more common with blood lead levels in the range of 40 to 60 μg/dL. The decrease in neuropsychological performance may be comparable to what would be expected during aging of up to 20 years, although debate continues about the predictability of the effects of blood lead levels below 70 μg/dL. Many of these manifestations respond at least partially to a reduction in the blood lead level.

Lead-induced peripheral axonal neuropathy (Chapter 446) most commonly involves the motor nerves, tending to be more severe in the upper extremities and on the dominant side. A subclinical decrease in ulnar nerve motor conduction velocity has been demonstrated at blood lead levels as low as 30 μg/dL. Lead poisoning also predisposes to the development of carpal tunnel and tarsal tunnel syndromes (Chapter 446).

Hematologic System

Lead affects the red cell membrane and interferes with enzymes involved in the synthesis of hemoglobin. The traditional findings in severe poisoning include a hypochromic microcytic anemia and basophilic stippling (Chapter 163).

Diagnosis

The initial steps in diagnosis of lead poisoning are to identify people involved in high-risk activities (see Table 20–1) and to determine the levels of lead in the venous (not capillary) blood. The diagnosis of lead poisoning should not rely on clinical symptoms and signs because these develop late and generally correlate poorly with blood lead levels. The blood lead level that triggers an intervention is not well established for adults, and no national guidelines exist for managing adults with lead poisoning. It is in the best interest of the patient to follow the most conservative standards: a confirmed venous blood lead level of 40 μg/dL or more should trigger an intervention, including improved industrial hygiene, better dust control, and increased ventilation.

Treatment

Treatment is designed to prevent further exposure, to reduce the blood lead level to an acceptable range, and to repair any existing damage. Removal of an individual from a lead environment is recommended if a blood lead level is 50 μg/dL or higher on two tests separated by 2 weeks or if a medical condition consistent with lead poisoning has been identified. Removal from the lead source often is associated with a gradual reduction in blood lead levels. Chelation therapy is generally recommended if symptoms or signs are present or if the blood lead level is above 60 μg/dL (Table 20–3).

Calcium disodium ethylenediaminetetraacetic acid ($CaNa_2EDTA$) is the first-line drug for treating asymptomatic adults with high blood lead levels. In the treatment of symptomatic lead poisoning (with or without encephalopathy), $CaNa_2EDTA$ is used in conjunction with dimercaprol (2,3-dimercaptopropanol or BAL). Larger doses of $CaNa_2EDTA$ (50 to 75 mg/kg/day) are used for more severely poisoned patients. A third chelator, succimer (meso-2,3-dimercaptosuccinic acid, DMSA), is approved for the treatment of children with blood lead levels above 45 μg/dL; although succimer has not been approved by the Food and Drug Administration (FDA) for the treatment of adult lead poisoning, adults have been successfully treated with succimer and it should be considered in place of $CaNa_2EDTA$ monotherapy. D-Penicillamine (3-mercapto-D-valine or penicillamine) is not recommended for the treatment of adult lead poisoning because of the high incidence of adverse drug reactions.

Chelation removes lead from the blood and soft tissues, but little is removed from bone. Redistribution of lead from deep stores after chelation may result in a rebound of blood lead levels and the redevelopment of clinical toxicity. For this reason, individuals who have been chelated should have blood lead levels measured 2 weeks after the course of chelation has been completed. In general, the clinical response to chelation therapy is variable and the data demonstrating improved outcomes are not robust. After chelation, blood lead levels tend to rise because of redistribution of lead. If the blood lead level rises into the toxic range or if symptoms recur, another course of chelation is indicated with the same dose and duration as in the original course.

Mercury

Definition

There are three chemical forms of mercury. Elemental or metallic mercury (Hg^0, quicksilver) is a silver liquid at room temperature. Inorganic mercury is in either a mercurous (Hg^+) or a mercuric (Hg^{++}) state. Organic mercurials are attached to short (ethyl or methyl) or long (alkyl or aryl) carbon chains. Each form of mercury may be found in a variety of occupations and products.

Epidemiology

The different chemical forms represent different delivery systems by which mercury enters and is distributed throughout the body. From a clinical perspective, the most important target organ is the central nervous system even though the kidney accumulates the most mercury regardless of the chemical type. Chronic poisoning with any of the chemical forms of mercury results in central nervous system toxicity. Ingestion of organic mercury is the most efficient way to get mercury into the brain, inhalation of elemental mercury vapor is second, and ingestion of inorganic mercury is the least efficient.

TABLE 20–3 GENERAL GUIDELINES FOR CHELATION THERAPY

Drug	Adult Dose	Indications	Cautions and Contraindications
Dimercaprol, British antilewisite (BAL)	3 to 5 mg/kg (75 mg/m²) IM every 4 hours for 2 days; then 3 mg/kg IM every 12 hours for 1 day; then 3 mg/kg one or two times daily	Lead: Symptomatic poisoning	Administration is by deep IM injection; injections are painful. The vehicle is peanut oil—do *not* use intravenously. Use is contraindicated if peanut allergy exists.
$CaNa_2EDTA$	20 to 30 mg/kg/day (1000 to 1500 mg/m²/day) as a continuous IV infusion for 5 days	Lead: Symptomatic poisoning or asymptomatic patients with high blood lead levels Manganese: Symptomatic patients with blood, serum, or urine manganese levels above reference values	Do *not* use Na_2EDTA. It can be given IM in two or three divided doses. High doses of $CaNa_2EDTA$ increase zinc excretion and may be toxic to the renal glomerulus and proximal tubule.
Dimercaptopropanesulfonate (DMPS)	100 mg orally four times per day for 7 days May repeat therapeutic course after 7 days of no therapy if levels still elevated	Arsenic: Symptomatic patients with urine arsenic levels ≥50 μg/L Asymptomatic patients with urine arsenic levels >200 μg/L Manganese: Symptomatic patients with blood, serum, or urine manganese levels above reference values Bismuth: Symptomatic patients with bismuth blood levels >50 μg/L or urine levels >150 μg/L	
Deferoxamine	6 g as a continuous IV infusion given in 24 hours May repeat if serum levels are still elevated	Aluminum: Symptomatic patients with serum aluminum levels >100 μg/L	
Succimer	10 mg/kg (350 mg/m²) orally every 8 hours for 5 days; then 10 mg/kg every 12 hours for 14 days	Lead: Symptomatic poisoning or asymptomatic patients with high blood lead levels Mercury: Symptomatic patients with mercury blood levels >10 μg/L or urine levels >20 μg/L	Succimer has a sulfur-like odor

Pathobiology

Mercury produces toxicity by binding to sulfhydryl groups, thereby inhibiting enzyme systems and disrupting cell membrane integrity. Mercury also binds to amide, amine, carboxyl, and phosphoryl groups. Methyl mercury inhibits choline acetyltransferase, a critical enzyme in the formation of acetylcholine.

Elemental mercury is or has been used in dental amalgams, calibration instruments, electroplating, gold extraction, manometers, and thermometers. Elemental mercury pooled under carpets or floorboards in homes has resulted in clinical toxicity. Ingested elemental mercury is poorly absorbed from the gastrointestinal tract and causes virtually no toxicity. Conversely, nearly 75% of inhaled elemental mercury vapor is absorbed through the lungs. Once it is absorbed, elemental mercury is distributed to the tissues and red blood cells, where it is oxidized to the mercuric form. Some elemental mercury crosses the blood-brain barrier, and oxidation within the central nervous system leads to accumulation of divalent mercury in the brain because ionized mercury does not readily cross the blood-brain barrier.

Inorganic mercury may be a component of disinfectants, fireworks, preservatives, and photograph developing chemicals. Inorganic mercury solutions are corrosive to the gastrointestinal tract, but up to 15% of ingested inorganic mercury is absorbed through the gastrointestinal mucosa. After absorption, the inorganic mercury salt is ionized and penetrates the blood-brain barrier poorly. However, absorbed divalent mercury can be reduced to the metallic form that will cross the blood-brain barrier.

Organic mercurials are used as pesticides, preservatives, and disinfectants. Coal-fired power plants are a major source of mercury in the environment. Elemental and inorganic mercurials deposited in the environment are bioconverted into organic mercury compounds that are a recognized contaminant of the food chain, particularly in fish. Consumption of fish is the source of nearly all of the methyl mercury in the general population. The FDA and the Environmental Protection Agency recommend avoidance of fish with the highest mercury concentrations—king mackerel, shark, swordfish, and tilefish from the Gulf of Mexico. Women of childbearing age and pregnant women should limit their consumption of medium-mercury fish: fresh tuna steaks, canned white or albacore tuna, grouper, orange roughy, saltwater trout, bluefish, lobster, halibut, haddock, snapper, and crabs. In addition, caution is urged regarding the consumption of fish from local lakes and ponds that may be more polluted than commercial fish sources.

Organic mercury is highly lipid soluble, well absorbed through the gastrointestinal tract, and widely distributed throughout the body. Organic mercury compounds are metabolized in the body; longer chain mercury compounds are rapidly metabolized to inorganic mercury, whereas short-chain mercury compounds (e.g., methyl mercury) are slowly metabolized to inorganic mercury. Organic mercury readily crosses the blood-brain barrier, and oxidation within the central nervous system leads to accumulation of mercuric ion in the brain.

Clinical Manifestations

The chronic inhalation of elemental mercury vapor results in two syndromes. The first syndrome consists of neuropsychiatric manifestations, gingivostomatitis, and tremor. The tremor (Chapter 434) is evident at rest or with motion and may be aggravated with purposeful movement. The second syndrome is erythism, a neuropsychiatric constellation of findings that includes fatigue, insomnia, memory impairment, nervousness, irritability, shyness, social withdrawal, loss of confidence, timidity, and depression.

Chronic occupational exposure to inorganic mercury may cause subclinical psychomotor and neuromuscular abnormalities as well as long-term behavioral impairment. Neuropsychiatric abnormalities (in attention, memory, construction, and motor performance) appear to be dose related (Chapter 425).

Methyl mercury poisoning is cumulative and develops during several years. Based on epidemics of methyl mercury poisoning in Japan and Iraq in which large quantities of organic mercury were consumed, the initial symptoms are fatigue and perioral and extremity paresthesia, followed by difficulty with hand movements and disturbances of vision. The classic picture of methyl mercury poisoning is the gradual onset of ataxia, constricted visual fields, and dysarthria. Other findings are paresthesia, deafness, incoordination, loss of voluntary movement, and mental retardation. The full picture of toxicity is that of psychological, cerebellar, sensory, and motor abnormalities. However, moderate amounts of methyl mercury in the diet have not been implicated as causing adverse effects in adults; most concern relates to potential toxic effects on the fetus and its developing central nervous system.

Diagnosis

The diagnosis of mercury poisoning requires a history of exposure, compatible clinical findings, and elevated mercury levels in blood or urine.

Mercury Levels

The mean total mercury levels in whole blood and urine in the general population are 1 to 8 μg/L and 4 to 5 μg/L, respectively. Although elevated blood or urine mercury levels are consistent with clinical toxicity, the correlation of clinical signs or symptoms with blood or urine mercury levels is poor because of substantial intra-individual and inter-individual variations. For example, data in urban adults (mean age, 59 years) found no significant association between blood mercury levels (mean, 2.1 μg/L; range, 0 to 16 μg/L) and neurobehavioral performance.

A ratio of red blood cell to plasma mercury of 1:1 suggests inorganic mercury poisoning, whereas a ratio of 10:1 suggests organic mercury toxicity. Red blood cell and plasma mercury levels could be requested if the source and type of the mercury exposure are unknown. Methyl mercury blood levels of 3 to 5 μg/dL may be found in patients with symptoms. Determination of a methyl mercury level is recommended if the exposure is to a contaminated environmental source.

Treatment

Rx

Asymptomatic patients with elevated urine mercury levels should have the analyses repeated after a 4-week period without fish consumption.

A patient with mercury poisoning should be immediately removed from the contaminated environment; the source of the mercury must then be identified and removed. Treatment is primarily symptomatic and supportive.

Chelation therapy (see Table 20–3) is used to increase the excretion of mercury even though improved clinical outcomes have not been demonstrated; increased urine excretion of mercury alone has become an accepted if empirical clinical goal. There is little agreement on the indications for initiation or cessation of chelation therapy. The presence of clinical toxicity combined with elevated mercury levels is an accepted indication for chelation therapy. The role of chelation therapy for asymptomatic individuals with mercury levels above background values is controversial. A reasonable end point for chelation is the achievement of background levels of mercury in urine or blood (<20 μg/L or 10 μg/L, respectively). Fish eaters with elevated mercury levels should avoid eating any fish or shellfish for 1 month, after which analysis of mercury levels in blood or urine should be repeated. If mercury levels have come down to reference values, low-mercury fish (shrimp, canned light tuna, salmon, pollock, catfish) can be reintroduced into the diet at a frequency of no more than two meals per week.

Succimer (see Table 20–3) is the chelator of choice because it can be given orally and has been effective in reducing brain levels of methyl mercury in animal studies. D-Penicillamine is less effective than succimer and has a higher adverse drug reaction rate. Dimercaprol is not recommended because of its potential to shift mercury from peripheral tissues into the brain. *N*-Acetylcysteine has been proposed as a chelator of methyl mercury, and repeated oral administration may interrupt the enterohepatic recirculation of methyl mercury; however, use of this drug for this purpose has not undergone clinical trials and is not approved by the FDA.

Arsenic

Definition

Arsenic is a naturally occurring omnipresent element that exists in three valence states: elemental or metallic arsenic (As^0), trivalent (arsenite, As^{3+}), and pentavalent (arsenate, As^{5+}). The trivalent form of arsenic (arsenite) is the most toxic and is responsible for the worldwide public health concern about chronic arsenic poisoning. Organic alkane arsenicals are of low toxicity, and elemental arsenic is virtually nontoxic.

Epidemiology

The major sources of human exposure to arsenic are the environment (mining, seafood, groundwater) and industry (pesticides, pigments, wood preservatives, glass or metal manufacturing, electronics, folk remedies). The arsenic content in the average North American adult diet is less than 1 μg/kg/day. Arsenic in seafood is primarily in the form of organic arsenicals, and the content is variable; freshwater fish may have up to 2 mg/kg, whereas lobster may have up to 22 mg/kg. The Environmental Protection Agency drinking water standard is 10 μg/L.

Pathobiology

Nearly 90% of ingested or inhaled arsenic is absorbed; little arsenic is absorbed through intact skin. Absorbed arsenic is widely distributed throughout the body, but no form of arsenic readily crosses the blood-brain barrier. Pentavalent arsenic and trivalent arsenic undergo oxidation-reduction reactions, converting one form to the other. Pentavalent arsenic is reduced by glutathione to the more toxic trivalent form. Methylation of trivalent arsenic produces the less toxic monomethylarsenate and dimethylarsenate metabolites that are excreted in the urine. Organic arsenicals, such as those found in seafood, are not toxic, are not metabolized to toxic forms of arsenic, and are rapidly excreted in the urine with an elimination half-life of 4 to 6 hours.

Arsenite (As^{3+}) binds to sulfhydryl groups, resulting in inhibition of many enzyme systems (glycolysis, pyruvate dehydrogenase, Krebs cycle) and decreased production of adenosine triphosphate. Arsenate (As^{5+}) replaces phosphate in microsomal enzyme systems, resulting in uncoupling of oxidative phosphorylation and decreased production of adenosine triphosphate. The pentavalent arsenate does not bind to sulfhydryl groups. Inorganic arsenic is a human carcinogen.

Clinical Manifestations

Chronic poisoning develops after ingestion or inhalation of arsenic during weeks to months, depending on the daily dose. Clinical manifestations develop gradually and are highly variable among exposed individuals. Typical initial manifestations include nonspecific complaints such as a metallic taste in the mouth, anorexia, weight loss, malaise, and weakness.

Skin lesions are some of the most common and earliest nonmalignant identifiable toxic effects. Typical dermal findings include melanosis (trunk and extremities), hyperpigmentation (tongue, oral mucosa, axillae), hyperkeratosis (palms, soles), and brittle nails. Less common or late findings include alopecia and white transverse bands (Mees' lines) (Chapter 467).

Later findings involve the nervous system and carcinogenesis. Neurologic effects are both central and peripheral. Central effects include mild dementia (Chapter 425) and headache; cranial nerves are normal. Peripheral sensory and motor neuropathies (Chapter 435) develop in a stocking-and-glove distribution and cause muscle weakness, muscle atrophy, and ataxia.

Malignant neoplasms include Bowen's disease, basal cell carcinoma, and squamous cell carcinomas (Chapter 214). Lung cancer (Chapter 201) may result from the inhalation of dust containing high levels of arsenic. Arsenic in drinking water has been associated with leukemias, bladder cancer, renal cancer, hepatic cancer, and uterine cancer (Chapter 185). The cancer risk from arsenic in drinking water may be dose related. Studies of populations outside the United States exposed to arsenic in drinking water show increases in cancer only at drinking water arsenic concentrations of more than several hundred micrograms per liter. Studies of United States populations exposed to average drinking water arsenic concentrations of about 190 µg/L have not demonstrated evidence of increased cancer.

Cardiovascular disease includes atherosclerosis, coronary artery disease, and hypertension. Blackfoot disease, peculiar to the southwest coast of Taiwan, is a form of peripheral vascular disease that results in gangrene of the lower extremities. Other manifestations of exposure to arsenic in drinking water include chronic cough, type 2 diabetes, and reproductive abnormalities such as congenital malformations, miscarriage, and low birthweight.

Diagnosis

The diagnosis of chronic arsenic poisoning depends on an appropriate history of exposure (including a source), compatible clinical manifestations, and documentation of an elevated body burden of arsenic. Principal sources of arsenic are environmental (contaminated water, air, soil) and occupational or industrial. Although seafood may be a source of organic arsenic, it is not associated with clinical toxicity.

Arsenic can be measured in the hair, blood, or urine. Hair analysis is a suboptimal method of determining chronic toxicity. Environmental arsenic is adsorbed to the external surface of the hair and is difficult to remove by washing, arsenic levels vary within a single hair and among hairs, and there is a significant inter-individual variability in adsorption of arsenic to hair. Nonetheless, the normal arsenic hair levels are less than 1 µg/g dry weight, and arsenic levels in hair from people with chronic toxicity range from 1 to 5 µg/g or more.

Blood levels of arsenic reflect only very recent exposures and are not reliable indicators of chronic exposure to low levels of arsenic. For example, there is no correlation between arsenic blood levels and arsenic drinking water levels of 6 to 125 µg/L.

Normal urine arsenic levels are 50 µg/L or 25 µg/24 hours in the absence of seafood consumption. Urine arsenic levels above 200 µg/L are abnormal. The average urine arsenic levels among people with chronic toxicity are 207 µg of inorganic arsenic per gram of creatinine. Because urine analysis measures total arsenic, elevated levels should be speciated to determine the fractions of inorganic arsenic and organic arsenic. If this analysis is not possible, seafood should be eliminated from the patient's diet for 1 week and the urine analysis then repeated.

A nerve conduction study is not a reliable tool for diagnosis of chronic arsenic toxicity. Among patients with elevated urine arsenic levels, the results of nerve conduction tests do not correlate well with the presence or absence of clinical neuropathy.

Treatment

Treatment approaches can be stratified according to symptoms and inorganic arsenic urine levels (Table 20–4). All patients who are symptomatic or who have inorganic arsenic urine levels of 50 µg/L or above should be removed from the source of the arsenic.

Dimercaptopropanesulfonate (DMPS) is the most widely studied chelating agent for chronic arsenic poisoning and the drug of choice, although it is not approved by the U.S. FDA. DMPS forms a water-soluble complex with monomethylarsenic that is excreted in the urine. In a randomized trial, DMPS therapy (100 mg orally four times per day on alternate weeks for 7 weeks) increased urine arsenic excretion and improved weakness, pigmentation, and lung disease, but it did not improve hematologic and blood chemistry abnormalities, neuropathy, hepatomegaly, keratosis, or skin histology. [1] Chelation should continue until the urine arsenic level is below 50 µg/L. Succimer has not been successful for treating chronic arsenic toxicity, and dimercaprol is not recommended because the lipid-soluble dimercaprol-arsenic complex penetrates the blood-brain barrier.

Cadmium

Epidemiology

Cadmium may be found as the metal and in a number of industrial chemicals. Cadmium may enter the environment through contamination, fuel combustion, or fertilizers. The majority of cadmium is used occupationally in nickel-cadmium batteries and to protect polyvinyl chloride against heat and light. Cadmium is used as a pigment in coloring "red bags" used for infectious hospital waste. When they are incinerated, these bags release cadmium into the environment, so medical waste incinerators are an important environmental source of cadmium. The largest source of most human exposure to cadmium is dietary, with an average daily intake of 10 to 30 µg. Cadmium exposure is doubled in people who smoke tobacco.

Pathobiology

Approximately 25% of inhaled cadmium is absorbed. Although only 5% of ingested cadmium is normally absorbed, gastrointestinal absorption is increased in the presence of calcium or iron deficiency or high dietary fat. Cadmium concentrates in the liver and kidneys. Cadmium is poorly excreted from the body; the half-life for elimination from kidney parenchyma is estimated to be more than 6 years. The kidney is the primary target organ in chronic toxicity.

Clinical Manifestations

The clinical picture of chronic cadmium toxicity is one of irreversible renal toxicity (Chapter 123). Proximal tubule damage results in high urine concentrations of low-molecular-weight proteins, amino acids, glucose, phosphate, and calcium. Decreased glomerular filtration rate and nephrolithiasis may occur. Renal failure is common.

TABLE 20–4 ARSENIC TREATMENT STRATIFICATION

Inorganic Arsenic Urine Levels	Symptomatic	Asymptomatic
<50 µg/L	Supportive care	No treatment
50–200 µg/L	Chelation*	Monitor 24-hour urine levels monthly
>200 µg/L	Chelation*	Chelation*

*Using DMPS (see Table 20–3).

The renal pathophysiologic process may result in calcium deficiency, osteoporosis, osteomalacia, and bone fractures. Other clinical manifestations of chronic cadmium poisoning include male infertility, slowing of visual-motor functioning, and peripheral neuropathies.

The Environmental Protection Agency and the International Agency for Research on Cancer have designated cadmium a probable human carcinogen. However, this designation is controversial, and chronic exposure to cadmium may not increase cancer rates. For example, residents of a cadmium-polluted village in England had no increase in cancer rates; a study of residents of a cadmium-polluted area in Belgium found no increase in prostate, kidney, or urinary tract cancers; a retrospective comparison of Japanese residents in high, low, and no cadmium-polluted areas found no differences in cancer mortality; and a study of copper-cadmium alloy workers found no increased risk of lung cancer.

Diagnosis

A tentative diagnosis of chronic cadmium poisoning can be confirmed by measuring elevated urinary cadmium levels (>5 μg/L) and elevated urinary microprotein levels, particularly α_1-microglobulin.

Treatment

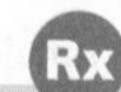

Treatment of the toxic effects of cadmium is symptomatic and supportive. There is no accepted way to reduce the body burden of cadmium. The use of $CaNa_2EDTA$ or dimercaprol may increase nephrotoxicity. Succimer and *N*-acetylcysteine have shown favorable results in animal studies, but neither has been adequately evaluated in human studies.

Manganese

Definition

Manganese is an increasingly important toxin, both environmentally and occupationally. Manganese exists as a metal (metallic manganese, ferromanganese), as inorganic manganese (e.g., chloride or sulfate salts), or as organic manganese.

Epidemiology

Metallic manganese is used in steel production. Inorganic manganese (Mn^{2+}, Mn^{3+}, and Mn^{4+}) is most commonly found in industry and in the environment. Various inorganic manganese compounds are involved in the manufacture of animal feed, batteries, fertilizers, fireworks, fungicides, matches, and potassium permanganate. Organic manganese compounds are used as a fuel oil additive, as fungicides, and as a gasoline additive (methylcyclopentadienyl manganese tricarbonyl, MMT).

Manganese is an essential nutrient, acting as a cofactor in enzymatic reactions involving bone mineralization as well as protein and carbohydrate metabolism. As such, it is often a component of parenteral nutrition preparations, and chronic infusion has resulted in manganese toxicity. Substantial exposure to manganese occurs in people who work in welding, mining, and foundry occupations. People who work with gasoline or as automobile mechanics may be exposed to MMT.

Pathobiology

Manganese is absorbed through the gastrointestinal and respiratory tracts and is distributed widely throughout the body. Manganese accumulates in the globus pallidus of the basal ganglia. Bile is the principal route of excretion. The elimination half-life is approximately 40 days but is longer for manganese in the central nervous system.

The primary target organ is the central nervous system, but the exact mechanisms of toxicity are unclear despite the fact that manganese adversely affects enzymes, receptors, and transport systems. A characteristic finding in chronic manganese poisoning is the selective destruction of dopaminergic neurons. The pathophysiologic mechanism is uncertain, but one hypothesis is that Mn^{2+} causes oxidation, production of free radicals or reactive oxygen species, or depletion of antioxidants.

Clinical Manifestations

People who work with manganese have developed a syndrome similar to but not identical with Parkinson's disease (Chapter 433). Findings include an extrapyramidal syndrome (masklike facies, tremor of the extremities at rest or on extension, bradykinesia, stooped posture, shuffling gait, propulsion abnormalities).

Parkinson's disease and manganese-induced parkinsonism are similar, but several clinical characteristics may help distinguish between the two. Manganese-poisoned patients have a "cock walk" and have a propensity to fall backward when they are pushed. Manganese-poisoned patients often exhibit psychological disturbances early in the disease process. The so-called manganese madness includes aggression, irritability, nervousness, and destructive behavior. Uncontrollable spasmodic crying or laughter, singing or dancing, or unfocussed running around have been described.

Diagnosis

The initial diagnosis of chronic manganese poisoning relies on a history of exposure and consistent clinical findings. In patients with significant central nervous system findings, a T1-weighted magnetic resonance imaging examination showing bilateral, symmetrical hyperdensities in the globus pallidus lends strong support to the diagnosis of chronic manganese poisoning.

Manganese levels in body fluids are helpful in establishing a diagnosis. Reference ranges have been established: blood, 40 to 140 μg/L; serum, 1.5 to 26.5 μg/L; and urine, 9.7 to 10.7 μg/L.

Treatment

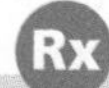

Treatment of chronic manganese toxicity starts with removing the source of the manganese and providing supportive care. The results of chelation with $CaNa_2EDTA$ or DMPS (see Table 20–3) have been equivocal. Although levodopa responsiveness is a hallmark of Parkinson's disease, welders with manganese-induced parkinsonism treated with levodopa showed no improvement over placebo-treated control subjects. 2

Nickel

Epidemiology

Nickel is absorbed through the lungs, gastrointestinal tract, and skin. Water-soluble nickel compounds (e.g., nickel chloride or sulfate) are absorbed better than insoluble nickel is. Approximately 25% of the nickel in drinking water is absorbed. Nickel applied to the skin is absorbed into the skin but may not reach the circulation. The urine is the primary means of excretion of nickel from the body.

Pathobiology

Nickel is used in a large number of metal alloys and in batteries, electroplating (e.g., table cutlery and some jewelry), coins, surgical staples, and some joint prostheses. Nickel also is present in drinking water; the Environmental Protection Agency standard is 0.02 mg/kg/day.

Nickel appears to be an essential element in the body, but the physiologic role of nickel in the body is unclear. Nickel crosses the cell membrane through calcium channels and competes with calcium for some receptors.

Clinical Manifestations

Contact dermatitis (Chapter 464) is the most common manifestation of nickel toxicity. Exposure to consumer products containing nickel, particularly jewelry, causes sensitization and contact dermatitis in as many as 30% of people. Once sensitization has occurred, the severity of subsequent reactions is related to the dose of nickel.

Chronic occupational exposures to nickel dusts and fumes have been associated with respiratory tract disease, including nasal, laryngeal, and lung cancers (Chapter 185). The Environmental Protection Agency identifies nickel dust and nickel subsulfide as class A human carcinogens. Exposures to nickel in nonindustrial settings, from ingestion of nickel in water or food or from dermal contact, have not been associated with an increased risk of cancer.

Diagnosis

Nickel levels in blood or urine are not useful in establishing either excessive exposure or risk of disease.

Treatment

There is no specific treatment of nickel-induced dermal sensitivity.

Other Toxic Metals

Aluminum

Epidemiology

Aluminum is the most abundant metal. It is widely available in consumer products such as food, water, cookware, food wraps, cans, antiperspirants, medications (especially antacids and phosphate binders), and dialysate fluids. North Americans consume 7 to 9 mg of aluminum in their diets each day. Industrial exposures to aluminum may result in significant toxicity.

Pathobiology

Gastrointestinal tract absorption of aluminum ranges from 0.1 to 1.0%. Once it is absorbed, aluminum is bound to transferrin and distributed throughout the body, concentrating in bone and lung. The kidneys are the primary route of aluminum excretion, and a compromised ability to excrete aluminum is an important factor in development of aluminum toxicity outside of the occupational setting. Rare individuals may accumulate significant amounts of aluminum from antiperspirants.

Aluminum blocks the incorporation of calcium into bones and inhibits osteoblastic and osteoclastic activity. In patients with renal failure, aluminum has been identified as a potential contributor to anemia, dialysis encephalopathy, and renal osteodystrophy.

Clinical Manifestations

The central nervous system is a target organ for aluminum toxicity. The findings in dialysis encephalopathy (Chapters 157, 236, and 443), which develops during months, include stuttering or stammering speech, directional disorientation, personality changes, myoclonus, motor apraxia, convulsions, and hallucinations. Industrial aluminum workers have developed cognitive defects, depression, incoordination, poor memory, and tremor. The relationship between aluminum exposure and Alzheimer's disease is controversial.

Chronic exposure to excessive aluminum may cause osteomalacia (Chapter 265), spontaneous fractures, and bone pain. Hypochromic, microcytic anemia (Chapter 163) unresponsive to iron therapy correlates with aluminum levels in the plasma or erythrocytes. Aluminum workers have increased risks for development of lung or bladder cancer (Chapter 185).

Diagnosis

The background serum aluminum levels in normal individuals are less than 10 μg/L. Patients undergoing chronic dialysis may have serum aluminum levels up to 50 μg/L. Levels above 60 μg/L indicate increased absorption; serum levels above 100 μg/L are potentially toxic; and serum levels above 200 μg/L are usually associated with clinical symptoms and signs of toxicity.

Treatment

Elevated serum aluminum levels can be brought down with extracorporeal clearance techniques, such as hemodialysis and hemofiltration. Deferoxamine chelates aluminum, and its use (see Table 20–3) is indicated when serum aluminum levels exceed 100 μg/L.

Beryllium

Epidemiology

Beryllium occurs naturally in rocks, coal, oil, soil, and volcanic dust. Commercially, beryllium is used in metal alloys for aerospace, aircraft, sports equipment (golf clubs, bicycle frames), and automotive manufacturing; in electronics and computers; in ceramics; and in defense weapons. Beryllium is naturally present in tobacco and may be inhaled during smoking.

Pathobiology

Inhaled beryllium is cleared from the respiratory tract by the mucociliary action and alveolar macrophages. Once it is absorbed, beryllium is distributed to the bone, liver, kidneys, lung parenchyma, and lymphatic system. The kidney is the primary route of beryllium excretion.

Repeated exposure to beryllium causes a cell-mediated immune response involving T lymphocytes and release of T_H1 cytokines in genetically susceptible persons (Chapter 93). The cell-mediated response is persistent and results in the accumulation of immune effector cells (sensitized T lymphocytes, macrophages) that form granulomas and mononuclear cell infiltrations. Dermal exposure to beryllium may cause irritative or atopic dermatitis as well as beryllium-containing foreign bodies and granulomas. The Environmental Protection Agency considers beryllium to be a probable human carcinogen.

Clinical Manifestations

Chronic beryllium disease is a progressive systemic hypersensitivity disease affecting the lungs and lymphatic system (Chapter 93). Clinical effects include progressive dyspnea, chest pain, weight loss, fatigue, anorexia, and fevers. Skin lesions, lymphadenopathy, and hepatosplenomegaly may occur. The pulmonary disease is progressive and may lead to respiratory failure within several years.

One third of patients will have a predominantly obstructive pattern, one fourth will have a predominantly restrictive pattern on pulmonary function testing, one third will have reduced carbon monoxide diffusion capacity with normal air flow and lung volumes, and some will have a mix of obstruction and restriction (Chapter 85). A chest radiograph will be normal early in the course but later will show diffuse bilateral infiltrates and hilar lymphadenopathy. Confirmation of beryllium sensitivity is made by the blood beryllium lymphocyte proliferation test. Tissue for histologic analysis from transbronchial or open lung biopsy may confirm the diagnosis.

Treatment

Treatment involves removing the patient from exposure to beryllium, slowing or halting the progression of the disease with corticosteroids, and providing symptomatic and supportive care.

Bismuth

Epidemiology

Bismuth has been used in the treatment of gastrointestinal disorders such as ulcers, diarrhea, and *Helicobacter pylori* infection. Two forms of bismuth are toxic; lipid-soluble organic compounds (e.g., bismuth subgallate) are neurotoxic, and some water-soluble organic compounds (e.g., bismuth triglycollamate) are nephrotoxic.

Pathobiology

Parenterally administered bismuth is distributed throughout the body but concentrates in the kidneys and liver. Elimination is through the kidneys with a terminal elimination half-life of 3 to 10 weeks.

In the blood, bismuth binds to macroglobulins, immunoglobulins, lipoproteins, and haptoglobin. In the kidney, bismuth concentrates in the proximal tubule and causes necrosis. The mechanism of the neurologic effects is unclear.

Clinical Manifestations

Chronic exposure to bismuth causes gastrointestinal, dermatologic, renal, and neurologic effects. Gastrointestinal effects include increased salivation, discoloration of the oral mucosa and gums, ulcerative stomatitis, nausea and vomiting, and diarrhea. Dermatologic effects are primarily a generalized rash after parental administration. Renal effects include nephritis, tubular necrosis, and renal failure.

The primary neurologic effect is an encephalopathy developing in two distinct phases. The prodrome lasts up to several months and consists of asthenia, somnolence, depression, anxiety, and sometimes hallucinations. This prodrome is followed by the rapid onset (1 to 2 days) of encephalopathy characterized by confusion progressing to coma or dementia, dysarthria, disturbances of walking and standing, and tremor with myoclonic jerks. Chronic bismuth poisoning is associated with a distinctive electroencephalographic pattern: bilateral low-voltage diffuse beta frequencies that are maximal in the frontal and central regions and that are accentuated during hyperventilation.

The diagnosis of chronic bismuth toxicity is based on the history of exposure and a consistent clinical picture. Blood and urine levels of bismuth may be helpful. In chronic toxicity, the blood bismuth level range is 50 to 1600 μg/L, and the urine level range is 150 to 1250 μg/L. The median blood bismuth levels in patients with bismuth encephalopathy are in the range of 680 to 700 μg/L. In patients taking a bismuth product therapeutically, a blood bismuth level above 50 μg/L is a concern; blood bismuth levels above 100 μg/L are an indication to discontinue bismuth therapy.

Treatment

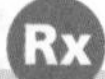

Treatment of bismuth toxicity starts with stopping exposure to bismuth. DMPS administration (see Table 20–3) has resulted in increased renal excretion of bismuth, but such therapy has not been shown to improve clinical outcomes.

Chromium

The most common forms of chromium in the environment are metallic chromium, trivalent chromium, and hexavalent chromium. Hexavalent chromium is the most toxic form. Trivalent chromium is essential for normal glucose tolerance; chromium picolinate is an alternative dietary supplement.

The trivalent and hexavalent chromiums are the most commonly used forms in industry. Chronic chromium toxicity is essentially an occupational disease related to tanning, metal alloys and electroplating (including surgical metals), photography, dyes, and cement.

Hexavalent chromium is absorbed through the gastrointestinal and respiratory tracts. The other valences are poorly absorbed. Hexavalent chromium is a skin and mucous membrane irritant. In dichromate compounds, hexavalent chromium binds to cellular and nuclear proteins and accumulates in red blood cells and platelets. Reduction of hexavalent to trivalent chromium creates intermediates that cause oxidative damage to DNA. Hexavalent chromium is a human carcinogen (lung cancer), but chromium and trivalent chromium are not classifiable. The Environmental Protection Agency standard for chromium in drinking water is 100 μg/L.

Chronic occupational exposure to high levels of airborne hexavalent chromium has been associated with upper airway irritation (including nasal septum ulceration), bronchospasm, and increased incidence of lung cancer. Repeated exposure to dichromate dust causes conjunctivitis and lacrimation. Dermal effects include irritation and chronic full-thickness ulcers. Chronic ingestion of high doses of chromium picolinate may cause renal impairment. Reference levels of serum chromium are 0.05 to 0.16 μg/L. Treatment of chromium toxicity is symptomatic and supportive.

Cobalt

Cobalt is a naturally occurring element that exists as a metal, as a stable isotope, and as radioactive isotopes. The general public is rarely exposed to the radioactive isotopes (^{60}Co is used in radiation therapy). The metal is in paints, enamels, and alloys used for household appliances, cutting tools, and joint replacements and surgical implants. Cobalt is a normal part of vitamin B_{12}. The average daily North American diet contains 5 to 40 μg of cobalt. Cobalt is absorbed through the gastrointestinal and respiratory tracts, distributed throughout the body, and excreted in the urine. Inhalation of cobalt is associated with obstructive and interstitial pulmonary disease. The interstitial pneumonitis is a fibrosing alveolitis with leukocyte and multinucleated giant cell infiltration (Chapter 92). The process may be an immunoglobulin E–mediated response to cobalt reactivity. Chronic ingestion of or industrial exposure to cobalt produces a cardiomyopathy with pericardial effusions and biventricular heart failure (the beer-drinkers' cardiomyopathy of the 1960s). Cobalt levels are not useful in the diagnosis or management of chronic cobalt poisoning. The diagnosis is based on a history of exposure and compatible pulmonary findings. Medical evaluation should use standard methods for assessing pulmonary and cardiac function. Treatment consists of removal of the patient from the source of the cobalt and symptomatic supportive care; both *N*-acetylcysteine and $CaNa_2EDTA$ have been used, but there is no definitive clinical evidence of benefit.

Selenium

Selenium is used in the vulcanization of rubber, the manufacture of some red glass, the electronics and semiconductor industry, and in some pharmaceutical products and dandruff shampoos. Selenium is absorbed through the gastrointestinal and respiratory tracts and accumulates primarily in the liver and kidneys. Selenium is cleared from the body in the urine and feces. The mechanism of toxicity of selenium is not clear, but one hypothesis is that it inhibits sulfhydryl enzymes and subsequent reduction in intracellular oxidative reactions.

Chronic exposure to selenium compounds in animals results in hepatotoxicity and decreased growth. In humans, dermal effects include alopecia, abnormal nail formation, and discoloration and decay of the teeth. Chronic high-dose dietary selenium has caused neurologic effects such as paresthesia and paresis. Elevated selenium levels in body fluids have been associated with clinical toxicity. The diagnosis of selenium toxicity relies on identification of a source, compatible clinical findings, and elevated whole blood selenium levels. Whole blood selenium levels vary with dietary intake; people with normal selenium intake (90 to 168 μg/day) have whole-blood selenium levels ranging from 0.143 to 0.211 μg/L. Treatment of a patient with chronic selenium toxicity consists of removing the patient from the selenium source and providing symptomatic and supportive care. Chelating agents are not useful.

Silver

Silver is used widely in photography, electronics, electrical equipment, metal alloys, and antibacterial agents. Silver is ingested in water and foods. Silver toxicity develops after ingestion of at least 25 g of silver during 6 months.

Silver is absorbed through the gastrointestinal tract, the lungs, and the skin. Ingested silver undergoes a significant hepatic first-pass effect. Silver has a high affinity for sulfhydryl groups and other proteins. Inorganic silver salts precipitate intracellularly and in turn are complexed with DNA, RNA, and other proteins; alternatively, ascorbic acid or catecholamines can reduce silver salts to the metallic form. Silver is not carcinogenic. Silver is eliminated primarily in the feces; little is excreted in the urine.

The dermal picture of chronic silver poisoning is argyria, an irreversible blue-gray pigmentation of the skin (Fig. 20–1). In the kidneys, silver is deposited in the basement membrane of the glomerulus; altered renal function is expected but has not been documented clinically. Silver levels in body fluids have not been useful in establishing the diagnosis of chronic silver intoxication. Diagnosis is based on a history of exposure and a compatible clinical picture. Reference levels of serum silver are less than 0.5 μg/L. Treatment of chronic silver intoxication consists of

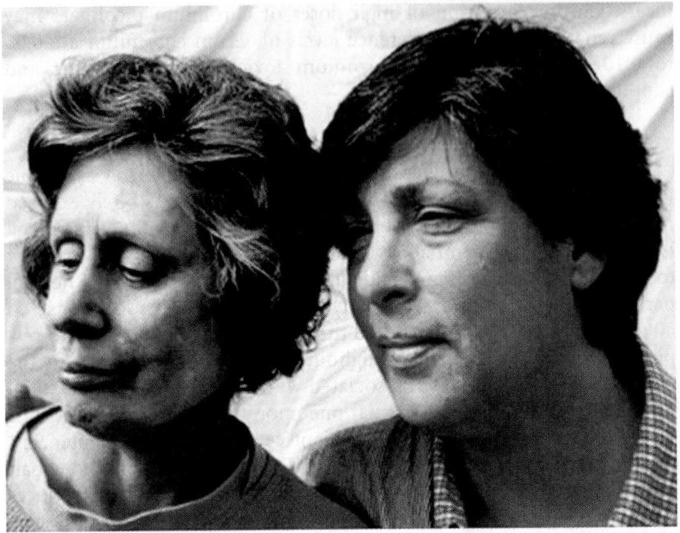

FIGURE 20–1 • A 56-year-old woman (on the left, with a normal person on the right) has had discolored skin since the age of 14 years. At the age of 11 years, the patient was given nose drops of unknown composition for "allergies," and 3 years later her skin turned gray. She has argyria, and a skin biopsy confirmed silver deposition. (From Bouts BA: Images in clinical medicine. Argyria. N Engl J Med 1999;340:1554.)

removing the patient from the silver source and providing symptomatic and supportive care. Chelating agents are not useful.

Uranium

Uranium causes toxicity because of its chemical effects or its radiation effects (Chapter 18). Uranium compounds are used in photography and as dyes or fixitives; depleted uranium is used in military equipment. Uranium is poorly absorbed from all exposed sites. Two percent of uranium in drinking water and food is absorbed into the body. Two thirds of the uranium in the body is in the bones, and about 15% is in the liver.

Uranium decays into radium and then into radon, a radioactive gas that seeps into building foundations in particular geographic areas. Although radon is a respiratory carcinogen (Chapter 201), uranium itself is not carcinogenic. The chemical toxicity of uranium affects the kidneys and lungs. Uranium is nephrotoxic but has not led to increased mortality from renal disease in uranium workers. The injury to the lungs is a nonmalignant damage to type II alveolar cells but does not increase mortality from respiratory disease in uranium workers. Treatment of uranium toxicity consists of removing the patient from the uranium source and providing symptomatic and supportive care. Chelators are not recommended.

Although alkalinization of the urine with sodium bicarbonate enhances removal of the uranium molecule from the body, no interventions reduce the effects of chronic uranium toxicity.

Zinc

Zinc is a common element found in air, soil, water, and food. It is widely used in metal alloys, cosmetics, and medications and as an alternative dietary supplement. The oral bioavailability of zinc is variable and depends on the formulation and amount ingested. After ingestion, zinc is concentrated in the liver before being distributed throughout the body. Muscle and bone contain 90% of the total body burden of zinc. High levels of zinc stimulate synthesis of metallothionein in the liver and in the gastrointestinal mucosal cells. Zinc is eliminated from the body primarily through the gastrointestinal tract. Chronic ingestion of zinc in doses as low as 2 mg/kg/day may lead to microcytic anemia secondary to zinc-induced copper deficiency (a result of increased gastrointestinal mucosal cell metallothionein). Other effects of chronic ingestion of high doses of zinc include nausea, vomiting, and abdominal cramping; variable increases in low-density lipoprotein levels and decreases in high-density lipoprotein levels; and impaired white blood cell function. Treatment of chronic zinc toxicity consists of removing the patient from the zinc source and providing symptomatic and supportive care. The use of chelating agents is not recommended.

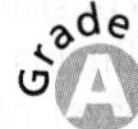

1. Mazumder DNG, De KB, Santra A, et al: Randomized placebo-controlled trial of 2,3-dimercapto-1-propanesulfonate (DMPS) in therapy of chronic arsenicosis due to drinking arsenic-contaminated water. J Toxicol Clin Toxicol 2001;39:665–674.
2. Koller WC, Lyons KE, Truly W: Effect of levodopa treatment for parkinsonism in welders: A double-blind study. Neurology 2004;62:730–733.

SUGGESTED READINGS

Clarkson TW, Magos L, Myers GJ: The toxicology of mercury—current exposures and clinical manifestations. N Engl J Med 2003;349:1731–1737. *Excellent review of the consequences of exposure to methyl mercury in fish, mercury vapor from dental amalgam, and ethyl mercury (in thimerosal).*

Department of Health and Human Services, Public Health Service, Agency for Toxic Substances and Disease Registry: Toxicological Profiles. Available at: http://www.atsdr.cdc.gov/toxpro2.html. *The most comprehensive review of environmental toxins available; each profile includes a Public Health Statement for consumers.*

Gidlow DA: Lead toxicity. Occup Med 2004;54:76–81. *Review of the current issues regarding lead toxicity.*

Kazantzis G: Cadmium, osteoporosis and calcium metabolism. Biometals 2004;17:493–498. *Excellent review of the characteristic toxicologic effect of cadmium.*

Kosnett MJ, Wedeen RP, Rothenberg SJ, et al: Recommendations for medical management of adult lead exposure. Environ Health Perspect 2007; 115:463–471. *Practical overview, cautions restraint in the use of chelation therapy.*

Krantz A, Dorevitch S: Metal exposure and common chronic diseases: A guide for the clinician. Dis Mon 2004;50:220–262. *Brief review of the clinical picture of poisoning from five metals.*

Mukherjee A, Sengupta MK, Hossain MA, et al: Arsenic contamination in ground water: A global perspective with emphasis on the Asian scenario. J Health Popul Nutr 2006;24:142–163. *Overview of the problem, especially in Bangladesh, India, and China.*

Section IV

Aging and Geriatric Medicine

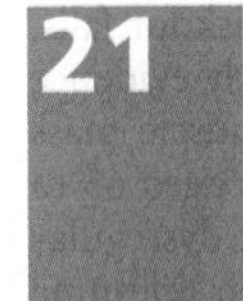

EPIDEMIOLOGY OF AGING: IMPLICATIONS OF THE AGING OF SOCIETY

Linda P. Fried

DEMOGRAPHIC REVOLUTION: TRANSITION TO AN AGING SOCIETY

There are now more than 35 million persons 65 years and older in the United States, or more than 12% of the population; in contrast, in 1900 there were 3 million persons 65 years and older, or just 4% of the population. By 2030, about 20% of the U.S. population will be older than 65. These increases represent similarly dramatic increases in life expectancy over the last century: in 1900, at birth, men could expect to live to 48 years and women could expect to live to 51 years on average; by 2002, life expectancy had increased to 75 and 80 years, respectively. Substantial years are now lived after the age of 65 by a large proportion of the population.

With this significant demographic shift, older adults have become the majority users of health care. One index of this statement is that a substantial proportion of persons with most chronic diseases are older than 65 years (Table 21–1). As a result of this burden of disease, people 65 years and older account for about 27% of U.S. health care expenditures. Older adults make, on average, 11 outpatient visits per year. People 75 and older make almost twice as many emergency department visits as people of all ages combined. Overall, older adults are the majority users of health services, including outpatient visits, hospital care, home care, and nursing home care.

HEALTH OF OLDER ADULTS

Changes in Health Status of Older Adults

By many measures, overall well-being is improving for the current generation of older adults as compared with previous birth cohorts. In 2002, 37% of persons 65 years and older reported being in excellent or very good health. Educational status, a strong predictor of health behavior and health outcome, is also increasing. In 1950, 70% of persons 65 years or older had attended eighth grade or less and 3% had 4 or more years of college; by 2004 these percentages had changed to 14% and 19%, respectively. In 1950, 17.7% of persons 65 years and older had a high-school diploma or higher and 3.6% had a bachelor's degree or higher; by 1998, these percentages had increased to 67% and 14.8%. Physical disability, which is an adverse outcome of chronic diseases and aging, is reported by 40% of older adults; however, the remaining 60% are not disabled, and disability rates appear to have declined in the last 10 years.

In 1900, pneumonia and influenza, tuberculosis, diarrhea, and enteritis were the leading causes of death and accounted for 30% of all deaths in persons older than 65 years. In 2002, heart disease was the leading cause of death in persons 65 and older, followed by cancer, stroke, chronic obstructive pulmonary diseases, pneumonia and influenza, and Alzheimer's disease (Table 21–2); the first three diseases accounted for 60% of all deaths. Among persons 85 years and older, heart disease alone is responsible for 40% of all deaths. Alzheimer's disease is the sixth leading cause of death in white women 85 and older, but it is a less common cause in black women and men of either race.

From 1981 through 2002, actual death rates declined by 38% for heart disease and by 37% for stroke. Both these declines are due to a combination of improved medical care, risk factor reductions, and changes in lifestyle. Conversely, mortality resulting from cancer, pneumonia, and influenza increased slightly, and death rates for chronic lower respiratory disease and diabetes increased 61% and 44%, respectively. Such evidence of improvements in health status and declines in mortality rates indicates that either many of the outcomes associated with aging are not inevitable or their onset can potentially be delayed until later in life by means of effective prevention or treatment.

Multiple Causes of Death in Older Adults

Mortality in older adults results from multiple contributing causes, even if one cause can be considered primary. One study of the predictors of 5-year mortality in older adults found that numerous types of health indices contribute: sociodemographic characteristics, health habits, cardiovascular risk factors, clinical and subclinical diseases, physical disability, and cognitive impairment (Table 21–3). After taking these risk factors and conditions into account, age itself becomes substantially less important as a predictor of mortality, up until the age of 85 years.

Disease Frequencies Rise with Increasing Age

Given the substantial number of years that are lived after the age of 65, patients and clinicians must focus on the conditions with which people live. After 65 years of age, 80% of persons report one or more chronic diseases, with the frequency of almost all chronic diseases increasing with age. For example, arthritis was reported by 8% of adults aged 18 to 44 years, by 30% of adults aged 45 to 64 years, and by 48% of adults 65 years and older in 2002 (Table 21–4). For conditions such as severe memory impairment, prevalence also rises rapidly with aging (Fig. 21–1). In the oldest age groups, arthritis, diabetes, hypertension, and possibly cerebrovascular disease are substantially more frequent in African Americans than in whites. Overall, the proportion who report very good or excellent health decreases with increasing age, from 72% of persons aged 25 to 44, to 60% of persons aged 45 to 54, to 52% of persons aged 55 to 64, and to 37% of persons 65 and older in 2002.

In addition to prevalent clinical disease, subclinical disease is common in older adults. Among the 6000 men and women aged 65 and older who participated in the Cardiovascular Health Study, 31% had evidence of clinical cardiovascular disease, whereas another 37% had subclinical disease by a variety of noninvasive measures. This subclinical disease in some circumstances may actually have clinical manifestations that are not yet diagnosed or diagnosable. For example, infarct-like lesions were found on magnetic resonance imaging in 28% of Cardiovascular Health Study participants without a known history of stroke. These imaging findings were associated with falling, balance problems, and cognitive decline, but not with clinically diagnosed stroke. Overall, subclinical cardiovascular disease is a stronger predictor of the older adults in whom clinical cardiovascular disease will develop than other classic risk factors are. These epidemiologic data suggest that detection of subclinical disease should become a focus of diagnostic attention and preventive interventions.

Onset of Geriatric Conditions

Health status in aging is a result of many factors, including the chronic diseases of aging and many other prevalent "geriatric" conditions that cannot be defined as classic "diseases" because they do not result from a single pathologic cause. Falls, which occur in a third of older adults, result in injuries, fractures, and high risk for disability and mortality (Chapter 23). Severe cognitive impairment (Chapters 25 and 26) and urinary incontinence (Chapter 24) have a substantial adverse impact on an older person, as does the sensory isolation resulting from hearing and visual impairment; all these conditions are frequent with aging.

Why Geriatric Patients Are Different

Comorbid Conditions

Older patients differ from young or middle-aged adults who have the same disease in many ways, one of which is the frequent occurrence of comorbid and subclinical disease. As a function of the high prevalence of disease, comorbidity (or the co-occurrence of two or more diseases in the same individual) is also common. Of people aged 65 and older, 50% have two or more chronic diseases, and these diseases can confer an additive risk for adverse outcomes, such as mortality. In some patients, cognitive impairment may mask the symptoms of important conditions. Treatment of one disease may affect another adversely, as in the use of aspirin to prevent stroke in individuals with a history of peptic ulcer disease. The risk for becoming disabled or dependent also increases with the number of diseases present. Specific pairs of diseases can synergistically increase the risk for disability. For example, arthritis and heart disease coexist in 18% of older adults; although the odds of disability developing are increased by 3-fold to 4-fold with either disease alone, the risk for disability increases 14-fold if both are present.

Nonspecific Signs and Symptoms

A second way in which older adults differ from younger adults is the greater likelihood that their diseases will have nonspecific symptoms and signs. Pneumonia and stroke may be associated with nonspecific changes in mentation as the primary symptom. Similarly, the frequency of silent myocardial infarction increases with increasing age, as does the proportion of patients who have a change in mental status, dizziness, or weakness rather than typical chest pain (Chapter 48). As a result, diagnostic evaluation of geriatric patients must consider a wider spectrum of diseases than would generally be considered in middle-aged adults.

Frailty

A third condition that is found primarily in older adults is frailty. Frailty is thought to be a wasting syndrome consisting of multiple symptoms and signs, including reduced muscle mass, weakness, poor exercise tolerance, slowed motor performance, low physical activity, and weight loss. Some estimates indicate that the full syndrome is found in 7% of community-dwelling people aged 65 and older and in 25% of community-dwelling people 85 and older. Many institutionalized older adults are also frail. Frailty is a state of decreased reserves and increased vulnerability to all kinds of stress, from acute infection or injury to hospitalization, and may identify individuals who cannot tolerate invasive therapies. The syndrome of frailty is associated with a high risk for falls, need for hospitalization, disability, and mortality. There is early evidence that a core component of frailty is sarcopenia, or loss of muscle mass associated with aging, which occurs in 13 to 24% of persons aged 65 to 70 and in 60% of persons aged 80 and older. It is likely that dysregulation of multiple physiologic systems, including inflammation, immune function, hormonal status, and glucose metabolism, underlies the syndrome, with resulting decreased ability to maintain homeostasis in the face of stress. Subclinical disease (e.g., atherosclerosis), end-stage chronic disease (e.g., heart failure), or a combination of comorbid diseases may precipitate the clinically apparent syndrome. Evidence from randomized, controlled trials shows that resistance exercise, with or without nutritional supplements, and home-based physical therapy can increase lean body mass and strength in even the frailest older adults. [1, 2] This evidence suggests that earlier stages of frailty may be remediable, although end-stage frailty probably presages death.

Cognitive Impairment

Fourth, cognitive impairment increases in prominence as people age (Chapters 25 and 26). Cognitive impairment is a risk factor for a wide

TABLE 21–1 PREVALENCE OF SELECTED CHRONIC CONDITIONS REPORTED BY PERSONS 65 YEARS AND OLDER (COMMUNITY DWELLING), UNITED STATES, 2002

	Number of Persons 65 Years and Older with the Disease (in Thousands)	Percentage Reporting the Disease Who Are 65 Years and Older, among All Individuals 18 Years and Older Reporting the Disease
Hypertension	17,509	38.1
Arthritis	16,621	36.3
Heart disease	10,729	45.6
Diabetes	5,671	40.5
Emphysema and chronic bronchitis	3,695	31.6
Stroke	2,816	60.2
Kidney disease	1,237	41.0
Malignant neoplasm	7,145	49.6
Hearing impairment	12,281	39.8
Visual impairment	5,783	30.3
Sinusitis	4,315	14.8
Liver disease	368	15.2
Ulcers	4,184	26.8
Obesity	6,980	15.2
Underweight	805	20.1

From Lethbridge-Çejku M, Vickerie J: Summary health statistics for U.S. adults: National Health Interview Survey, 2003. National Center for Health Statistics. Vital Health Stat 2005;10(225):16–63.

TABLE 21–3 PREDICTORS OF 5-YEAR MORTALITY IN MEN AND WOMEN 65 YEARS AND OLDER IN THE CARDIOVASCULAR HEALTH STUDY*

Sociodemographic	Age (older) Gender (male) Income (<$50,000/yr)
Anthropometric	Weight (lower)
Health habits	Physical activity (low) Smoking (pack years)
Cardiovascular risk factors	Brachial systolic blood pressure (elevated) Posterior tibial artery blood pressure (reduced) Diuretic use (in persons with severe CHF or liver disease) Fasting blood glucose (higher)
Serum measures	Albumin (lower) Creatinine (higher)
Clinically manifested disease	CHF
Subclinical disease, measured noninvasively	Forced vital capacity, mL (lower) Ejection fraction abnormal Aortic stenosis (moderate–severe) Major ECG abnormality Stenosis (maximal) of the internal carotid artery (greater)
Consequences of disease	Difficulty with instrumental activities of daily living (≥2) Cognitive impairment (greater) Poor self-assessed health

*Persons without cancer at the time of enrollment.
CHF = congestive heart failure; ECG = electrocardiographic.
Data from Fried LP, Kronmal RA, Newman AB, et al: Risk factors for 5-year mortality in older adults: The Cardiovascular Health Study. JAMA 1998;279:585–592.

TABLE 21–2 DEATH RATES (PER 100,000) FOR THE LEADING CAUSES OF DEATH IN PERSONS 65 YEARS OR OLDER, 1981–2002

	Heart Disease	Stroke	Cancer	COPD	Pneumonia and Influenza	Alzheimer's Disease
1981	2547	624	1056	186	207	6
2002	1585	393	1091	301	161	159
Percent change from 1981 to 2002	−38.5	−37.0	3.3	61.8	−22.2	2550

COPD = chronic obstructive pulmonary disease.
From National Vital Statistics System.

TABLE 21–4 MOST PREVALENT CONDITIONS AMONG COMMUNITY-DWELLING PERSONS 65 YEARS AND OLDER

Disease or Condition	Prevalence (per 1000)
Arthritis*	48.3
Disability†	40.0
Hypertension*	36.4
Falls†	30.0
Hearing impairment†	30.3
Heart disease*	26.9
Influenza*	21.4
Disabled in IADL and/or ADL†	21.0
Cataracts*	17.2
Orthopedic impairment†	15.8
Depression*	14.7
Malignant neoplasms*	14.5
Chronic sinusitis*	11.7
Diabetes mellitus*	10.0
Urinary incontinence†	8.8
Visual impairment†	8.4
Asthma, emphysema*	7.7
Alzheimer's disease*	7.0
Frailty†	6.9
Cerebrovascular disease*	6.5

*Clinical diseases.
†Geriatric conditions not associated with specific diseases.
ADL = activities of daily living; IADL = instrumental activities of daily living.

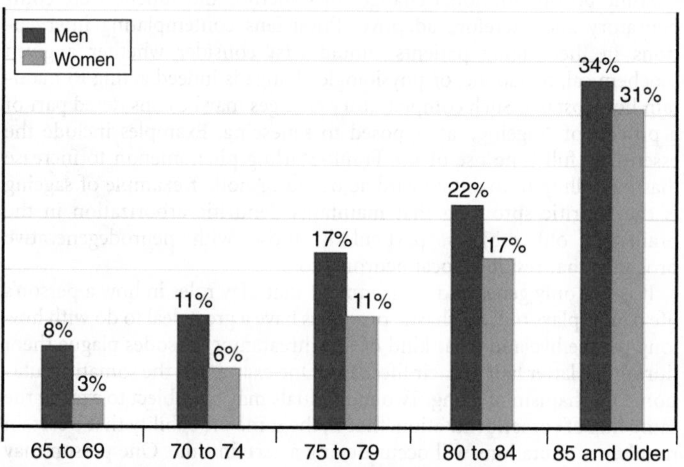

FIGURE 21–1 • Percentage of persons 65 years or older with moderate or severe memory impairment (defined as ≤4 words recalled out of 20 on combined immediate and delayed recall tests). (Data from Lethbridge-Cejku M, Vickerie J: Summary health statistics for U.S. adults: National Health Interview Survey, 2003. National Center for Health Statistics. Vital Health Stat 10; 2005. Data also from Annual Estimates of the Population by Sex and Five-Year Age Groups for the United States: April 1, 2000 to July 1, 2004 [NC-EST2004-01]. Source: Population Division, U.S. Census Bureau.)

range of adverse outcomes, including falls, immobilization, dependency, institutionalization, and mortality. Cognitive impairment complicates diagnosis, compromises independence, and requires additional caregiving to ensure safety.

Physical Disability

Finally, a serious and common outcome of chronic diseases of aging is physical disability, defined as having difficulty or being dependent on others for the conduct of essential or personally meaningful activities of life from basic self-care (e.g., bathing or toileting) to tasks required to live independently (e.g., shopping, preparing meals, or paying bills) to a full range of activities considered to be productive or personally meaningful. Of older adults, 40% report difficulty with tasks requiring mobility, and difficulty with mobility predicts the future development of difficulty in instrumental activities of daily living (IADL; household management tasks) and activities of daily living (ADL; basic self-care tasks) (Table 21–5). In community-dwelling persons aged 65 and older, difficulty with IADL is reported by 20%, and difficulty with ADL is reported by 11%; for both, the prevalence increases with age. People who have difficulty with tasks of IADL and ADL are at high risk of becoming dependent. Of persons older than 65 years, 5% reside in nursing homes, largely as a result of dependency in IADL or ADL (or both) secondary to severe disease. Generally, women live more years with disability, whereas men who become similarly disabled are more likely to die at a younger age. Although physical disability is primarily a result of chronic diseases and geriatric conditions, its onset and severity are modified by other factors, including treatments that control the underlying diseases, physical activity, nutrition, and smoking. Many intervention trials indicate that disability can be prevented or its severity decreased; 1-3 one trial showed improvements in functioning with resistance and aerobic exercise in older adults with osteoarthritis of the knee.

TABLE 21–5 ASSESSMENT OF PHYSICAL DISABILITY IN OLDER ADULTS

Disability Type	Descriptor
Ambulation	Difficulty in walking
Instrumental activities of daily living	Difficulty in
	Preparing meals
	Doing housework
	Using the telephone
	Shopping
	Medication management
	Financial management
Basic activities of daily living	Difficulty in
	Bathing
	Dressing
	Grooming
	Toileting
	Transfers
	Eating

For the full assessment instrument, see Reuben DB, Herr KA, Pacala JT, et al: Geriatrics at Your Fingertips. Maiden, MA, Blackwell, Inc, for the American Geriatrics Society, 2002.

Relationships Among Factors

Comorbidity, frailty, and disability are recognized as distinct clinical entities (Fig. 21–2), although they are related in the same causal pathway. Comorbidity may be a risk factor for frailty, and both are risk factors for disability. A vicious cycle may exist whereby inactivity resulting from disability precipitates or worsens frailty.

The health status of older adults includes a broader spectrum of issues than is found in middle-aged or younger patients, including prevalent chronic disease, recurrent disease, comorbidity, and geriatric conditions, each of which can be an independent problem or interact with other problems to cause disability, dependency, or death. There is also, however, great heterogeneity in health status among older adults, with robust, independent individuals even in the oldest age ranges. Because of this heterogeneity, older patients may require primary, secondary, or tertiary preventive health care (Table 21–6) tailored to their individual health status and inherent risk. Overall, preventive health care is effective in older adults (Chapter 12), and attention to clinical practices and health habits, from immunization to physical activity, can prevent adverse outcomes into the oldest ages. Preventive measures should also be targeted to situations of acute stress (e.g., hospitalization or immobilization), when the risk of decline in function is high. Health status can change rapidly as people age, so clinical care and services must evolve in concert with the health and function of the patient.

FUTURE DIRECTIONS

Clinical care of older adults will become more effective in improving health outcomes as clinical principles of geriatrics are broadly adopted and as new evidence emerges regarding how best to identify the subsets of older individuals who are at risk for adverse outcomes. The range of

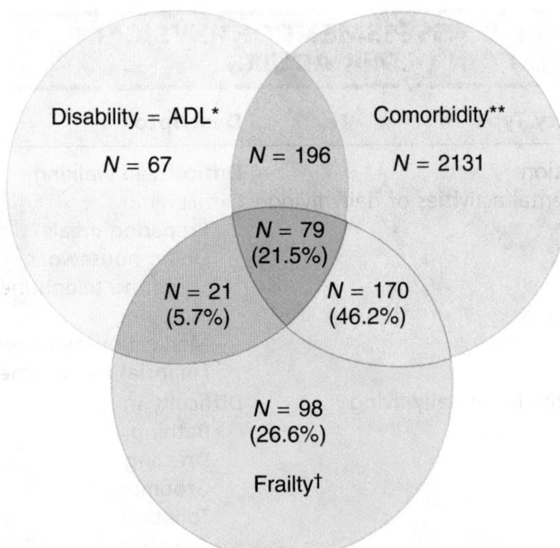

FIGURE 21–2 • Overlap of frailty, disability, and comorbidity in community-dwelling older adults participating in the Cardiovascular Health Study. The total represented was 2762 subjects who had comorbidity, disability, or frailty, or any combination of these conditions. **N* = 363 with a disability in activities of daily living (ADL); of these, 100 were frail. ***N* = 2576 with comorbidity, defined as two or more of the following nine diseases: myocardial infarction, angina, heart failure, claudication, arthritis, cancer, diabetes, hypertension, and chronic obstructive pulmonary disease. Of these, 249 were also frail. †*N* = 368 frail subjects. (Adapted from Fried LP, Tangen CM, Walston J, et al: Frailty in older adults: Evidence for a phenotype. J Gerontol A Biol Sci Med Sci 2001;56:M146–M156.)

TABLE 21–6 SPECTRUM OF HEALTH CARE AND PREVENTIVE CARE NEEDS AMONG OLDER ADULTS

Level of Prevention	Targeted Health Issues
Primary	Incident disease, geriatric conditions
Secondary	Screening, early detection of prevalent disease and geriatric conditions
	Treatment of morbidity
	Prevention of recurrent disease
Tertiary	Impact of disease and geriatric conditions
	Disability and dependency
	Hospitalization
	Institutionalization
	Death

outcomes for which more effective screening methods are being developed includes cardiovascular disease, hip fractures, frailty, disability, and susceptibility to medical procedures or polypharmacy.

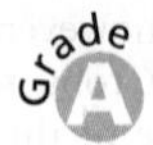

1. Gill TM, Baker DI, Gottschalk M, et al: A program to prevent functional decline in physically frail, elderly persons who live at home. N Engl J Med 2002;347:1068–1074.
2. Binder EF, Yarasheski KE, Steger-May K, et al: Effects of progressive resistance training on body composition in frail older adults: Results of a randomized, controlled trial. J Gerontol A Biol Sci Med Sci 2005;60:1425–1431.
3. Gill TM, Baker DI, Gottschalk M, et al: A prehabilitation program for the prevention of functional decline: Effect on higher-level physical function. Arch Phys Med Rehabil 2004;85:1043–1049.

SUGGESTED READINGS

Fried LP, Ferrucci L, Darer J, et al: Untangling the concepts of disability, frailty, and comorbidity: Implications for improved targeting and care. J Gerontol A Biol Sci Med Sci 2004;59:M255–M263. *Differentiating frailty, comorbidity, and disability in older patients is critical to effective diagnosis, prevention, and treatment, as well as outcomes research.*

Nummela OP, Sulander TT, Heinonen HS, et al: Self-rated health and indicators of SEC among the ageing in three types of communities. Scand J Public Health 2007;35:39–47. *Emphasizes that an adequate income is a key correlate of health, especially in urban areas.*

22 BIOLOGY OF AGING

George M. Martin

THE LIFE COURSE APPROACH TO UNDERSTANDING AGING

It is useful to think of organisms as protein-synthesizing factories. If that factory is to function at high levels of efficiency and stability for long periods, the builder should start with an excellent set of blueprints (hence the importance of understanding the constitutional genomes of individual patients), hire engineers and supervisors to oversee its construction and maturation (hence the relevance of understanding how development affects the adult phenotypes of our patients), ensure that the factory functions in a safe environment (hence the importance of protecting patients from teratogens, mutagens, carcinogens, and candidate "gerontogens," such as tobacco smoke), and finally initiate rigorous regimens of quality control throughout the lifespan of the factory (hence the importance of such biologic processes as DNA repair and the detection, reconstitution, and turnover of aberrant proteins). This rationale underlies the view of many biologists that aging begins at conception. Operationally, however, gerontologists typically use the terms *aging* and *senescing* interchangeably to refer to the slow, insidious declines in structure and function that unfold after the achievement of sexual maturation and the young adult phenotype. Given large populations of individuals, this process eventually translates into exponential increases in age-specific death rates, although those rates of increase have been shown to decline in exceedingly old organisms. The mechanisms underlying this paradoxical terminal slowing of mortality rates are not fully understood; because it can be observed even in genetically homogeneous experimental animals, it cannot be attributed solely to genetic differences.

Some postmaturational changes in structure and function are compensatory and therefore adaptive. Physicians contemplating interventions in their aging patients should first consider whether a given biochemical, metabolic, or physiologic change is indeed acting to maintain homeostasis. Such compensatory changes may be considered part of a process of "sageing," as opposed to senescing. Examples include the essentially full-time use of the Frank-Starling phenomenon to increase diastolic filling to maintain cardiac output. Another example of sageing is the neuritic sprouting that maintains dendritic arborization in the brains of old subjects, particularly those with neurodegenerative processes that result in focal neuronal loss.

It is not only genes and environment that play roles in how a person's life course plays out. Stochastic processes have a great deal to do with how long people live and what kind of life-threatening episodes plague them during the latter half of their lifespans. One example is the somatic mutational mechanism of aging. Two individuals may be subject to exactly the same flux of somatic mutation, that is, the same probability that a certain number of mutations will occur during a certain time. One person may be lucky, with all or most of the "hits" occurring in pseudogenes—dead, nonfunctional relics of genes; mutations here would have absolutely no functional consequences. Another person might be unlucky, however, with the hits preferentially involving tumor suppressor genes like *p53* or activating oncogenes like *ras*. Consider also two individuals who suffer from a comparable degree of coronary artery atherosclerosis or amyloid deposits in cerebral blood vessels. Physicians are not surprised by the fact that such individuals may differ substantially in the age at which some fatal precipitating event may take place (coronary artery thrombosis or cerebral hemorrhage). Although future discoveries may elucidate all of the interacting variables that determine the probability of such events, chance juxtapositions of sets of such variables are likely to be responsible for much of the variance. These considerations provide great difficulties for investigators who are interested in performing a genetic analysis of longevity—for example, the genetic issues contributing to achieving centenarian celebrity.

THE EVOLUTIONARY BIOLOGIC THEORY OF AGING PROVIDES A SATISFACTORY EXPLANATION FOR WHY HUMANS AGE

Why do animal species evolve such striking differences in their life history strategies? The answer appears to lie in an understanding of the different ecologies in which they have evolved. Consider, for example, an exceptionally hazardous environment—one with unreliable sources of food and water and a rich supply of predators, infectious agents, and dangerous terrains conducive to fatal accidents. In such ecologies, there is strong selective pressure to "get the job over with quickly." That "job," of course, is reproduction. Natural selection sculpts the genome to provide the maximum opportunity for enhancing reproductive fitness in a given ecologic niche. For a hazardous niche, natural selection will favor a life history characterized by rapid development, large numbers of progeny during a relatively short course of reproductively active adult life, and an abbreviated longevity. There is no need for nature to have designed energetically expensive quality control systems to maintain the soma for long periods. Such gene variations might well appear spontaneously and potentially benefit a rare long-lived individual within an age-structured population; but the chances of that individual's passing on that allelic variant to the gene pool of the next generation is negligible, as the bulk of the alleles would be derived from the much larger cohort of younger animals. Older animals would be much less frequent even in the absence of senescence, as they would have been eliminated with high probabilities because of disease, predators, and starvation. Thus, limited lifespans occur because the alleles that have the potential to provide enhanced lifespans escape the force of natural selection. Both laboratory and field experiments have proved, however, that when animals are provided with a much more benign ecology with low hazard functions, a different life history strategy can emerge, characterized by a slower rate of development, fewer progeny per gestation, but longer periods of fecundity and longer lifespans.

Various classes of gene actions conspire to modulate lifespans, including some that escape the force of natural selection.

Classes of Gene Action That Escape the Force of Natural Selection

Several classes of gene action escape the force of natural selection (Table 22–1). The term *good allele* refers to a variety of a gene that functions well and is adaptive, that is to say, contributes to organismal viability and durability. Some good alleles may be better than others, of course.

Longevity Assurance Genes

The first category involves alleles that are often referred to as longevity assurance genes and are good to have both early and late in the life course. Examples could include alleles at an array of DNA repair loci, alleles that function efficiently to scavenge reactive oxygen species, and alleles that reduce methionine sulfoxides.

TABLE 22–1 CLASSES OF GENE ACTION THAT CAN ESCAPE THE FORCE OF NATURAL SELECTION AND THUS HAVE THE POTENTIAL TO MODULATE THE RATES OF DEVELOPMENT OF SENESCENT PHENOTYPES AND THE DURATION OF THE LIFESPAN

Good alleles with good effects early and late ("longevity assurance genes")
Good alleles that are downregulated for good reasons
Good alleles that are inappropriately upregulated in late life (loss of "silencing")
Good alleles that have bad late effects ("antagonistic pleiotropy")
Good alleles that go bad by somatic mutation or epimutation
Bad alleles that do not reach a phenotypic level of expression until late in the life course (constitutional "mutation accumulation")

After Martin GM: The evolutionary substrate of aging. Arch Neurol 2002;59:1702.

Downregulation of Genes

The second category involves genes that function at high levels early in the life course but whose expressions are decreased during certain developmental epochs, presumably to enhance reproductive fitness. There is evidence in murine models, for example, that there is downregulation of sets of ribosomal DNA genes at about the time animals reach sexual maturity and the fully adult phenotype, after which there is no requirement for rapid somatic growth. Another example that may function adaptively to modulate rates of somatic growth is the gradual downregulation of the paternal *IGF2* allele; this downregulation ensures markedly decreased function of that gene product because the maternal allele is imprinted. In humans, there is evidence that this process may well begin at around puberty or shortly thereafter. Once such a process is initiated, it "has a life of its own." In both of these examples, there is continuing downregulation, eventually reaching very low levels late in the lifespan, when it may well have deleterious effects but when such phenotypic expression will have escaped the force of natural selection.

Genes Inappropriately Upregulated

A number of genetic loci may become upregulated during the process of sageing mentioned before, but genetic loci may also become inappropriately upregulated late in the lifespan. This process, which has been referred to as a loss of gene silencing, occurs, for example, when the inactive X chromosome becomes activated in aging mice. The molecular mechanisms for such loss of silencing have not been fully elucidated but may sometimes involve changes in the regulation of enzymes such as the NAD^+-dependent histone deacetylase, an enzyme required for chromatin-dependent gene silencing in yeast. Homologues of the responsible gene, *Sir2,* occur in mammals. Increased dosages of a *Sir2* gene have been shown to extend the lifespan of *Caenorhabditis elegans.*

Antagonistic Pleiotropy

The fourth class in Table 22–1 is one of two classic examples of gene action that escape the force of natural selection. It is often referred to as antagonistic pleiotropy, in that the alleles are associated with adaptive effects early in the lifespan but deleterious effects late in the lifespan. This class of gene action has received much recent attention in connection with evidence that levels of the tumor suppressor gene *p53* have been "fine-tuned" by evolution to decrease both the risk of cancer and the rate of aging. In mouse models, putative excessive functioning of *p53* protects from cancer but is associated with decreased lifespans and such conditions as osteopenia, multiple organ atrophy, and poor wound healing.

Somatic Mutation or Epimutation

Stochastic alterations in the primary nucleotide sequences or copy numbers of gene loci, termed somatic mutations, clearly occur during the aging of mammals. These changes accumulate exponentially with age and are proven causes of various age-related cancers. Less is known about what has been referred to as epimutations, which involve stochastic alterations in such epinucleic chemical changes as methylation and acetylation. Given that somatic mutations make their greatest impact late in the lifespan, they largely escape the force of natural selection. Experimental data provide support for stochastic variations in gene expression that are associated with intraspecific variations in longevity. It has been known for some time that despite all efforts to control genetic and environmental aspects in model organisms, such as fruit flies, roundworms, and mice, substantial variation in lifespans is regularly observed nevertheless. What might be called epigenetic drifts in gene expression have also been demonstrated in aging human identical twins.

Mutation Accumulation

A sixth class of gene action also escapes the force of natural selection. It involves inborn, constitutional mutations that have neutral or nearly neutral effects early in the life course but deleterious effects late in the life course. The prototypic example is Huntington's disease, which typically does not reach a level of expression until after the peak of reproduction. Although individually rare, there are potentially thousands of such examples. All patients are likely to have one or more such "private" modulations that can have an impact on patterns of aging. Moreover, even for constitutional mutations that may not have fully escaped the force of natural selection, there likely evolved a variety of suppressor mutations at other loci that act to postpone the age of phenotypic expression. Thus,

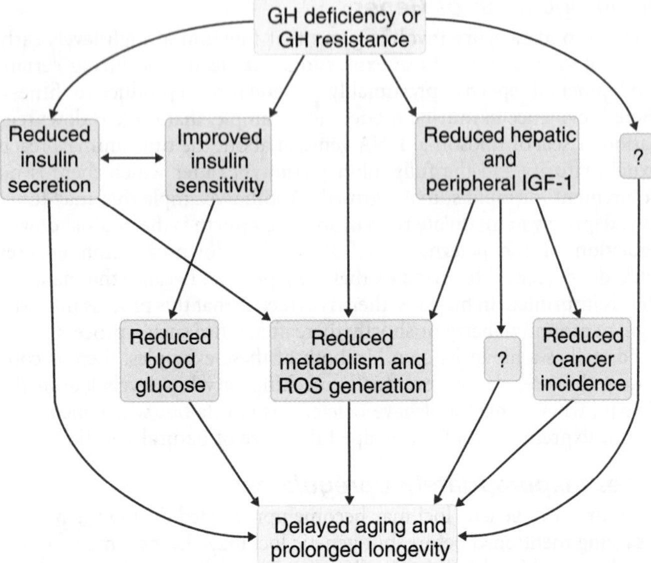

FIGURE 22–1 • Suggested mechanisms for the enhancement of longevity of hypopituitary, growth hormone–deficient and growth hormone–resistant mice. GH = growth hormone; IGF-1 = insulin-like growth factor 1; ROS = reactive oxygen species. (From Bartke A: Minireview: Role of the growth hormone/insulin-like growth factor system in mammalian aging. Endocrinology 2005;146:3718.)

individuals also are likely to carry their private arrays of suppressor mutations.

ARE THERE "PUBLIC" MODULATORS OF LONGEVITY AND AGING?

Most genetic research in biogerontology deals with an investigator's favorite experimental organism. It might be asked, however, if there is evidence of a specific pattern of gene action that makes a major difference in the longevities of a wide range of species. Such a pathway would be a "public" modulator of aging and longevity. A strong candidate for such a pathway, which is the signal transduction involving insulin-like growth factors and their receptors (Fig. 22–1), has indeed been observed in *Caenorhabditis elegans, Drosophila melanogaster,* and Monarch butterflies, and it may also operate in unusually long-lived dwarf mice. A human counterpart to one of these dwarf mutations involves the growth hormone receptor and is known in humans as a variant of the Laron syndrome, but there is insufficient information to know whether this syndrome is also associated with enhanced longevity. The pathway appears to have evolved to implement a mechanism for what might be called a "time out" in the usual progression of the life history or, to use the proper zoologic terminology, a diapause. Some investigators believe that this pathway may also be playing a role in what is arguably the most robust methodology for enhancing lifespan in the widest range of organisms, namely, calorie restriction.

HUMAN PROGEROID MUTATIONS

Progress in understanding the nature of gene action associated with differential rates of aging and longevity in experimental organisms did not come from a study of genes that shortened lifespan because it has been difficult to be certain that the associated phenotypes were valid models of accelerated normative aging. Real progress came only with the isolation and characterization of long-lived mutants, although in many cases, such mutations may merely have complemented some special vulnerability of a clonal strain. Research in humans on the discovery of gene mutations and polymorphic alleles that may lead to unusually robust structure and function during the latter half of the lifespan is in its infancy. Possible examples include loci that influence the size of lipoprotein particles, with large sizes being associated with unusual longevity in some studies. There have been several confirmations in different populations of associations of an unusual polymorphic allele (*APOE ε2*) in centenarians. In contrast, there is a relatively poor representation among centenarians of the *APOE ε4* allele, which is known to be a risk factor for dementia of the Alzheimer type as well as for various fatal cardiovascular disorders, so it can be presumed that there has been a winnowing of carriers for this more deleterious allele. That deleterious allele, however, may have evolved among groups of ancestors of some extant populations because it provided enhanced reproductive fitness in particular environments. If that were indeed the case, one can view this type of gene action as an example of antagonistic pleiotropy (fourth class of Table 22–1).

In contrast to the difficulties of determining the significance, for the biology of aging, of short-lived experimental animals like worms and fruit flies, gene action responsible for the abbreviated lifespans of at least a subset of human subjects can indeed be informative because phenotypic information on geriatric patients supports the consideration of two classes of "progeroid" syndromes.

Segmental Progeroid Mutations

One class, segmental progeroid mutations, involves gene actions that appear to lead to premature onsets and accelerated rates of development of numerous senescent phenotypes. The prototypic example is the Werner syndrome, sometimes known as progeria of the adult. It is caused by homozygosity for null mutations at a member of the RecQ family of DNA helicases. It is an unusual member of that family in that it has exonuclease as well as helicase functions. Its definitive role in pathophysiology remains to be defined, but the wild-type function probably acts to recognize and resolve unusual DNA structures during DNA replication and recombination, such as nucleotide mismatch "bubbles" and Holliday junctions. Deficient function results in high frequencies of somatic mutations, especially deletions and chromosome rearrangements. Deficient function also leads to marked limitations of the replicative potentials of somatic cells. These cellular and molecular phenotypes may explain the striking progeroid features, which include bilateral ocular cataracts, atherosclerosis, medial calcinosis, calcification of heart valves, type 2 diabetes mellitus, osteoporosis, gonadal atrophy, atrophy of skin and subcutaneous tissues, and premature thinning and graying of hair. These patients also suffer from a variety of benign and malignant neoplasms. There are a number of discordances, however, with usual aging, including a disproportionate number of mesenchymal neoplasms and an unusual distribution of osteoporosis. It therefore seems prudent to continue to refer to this syndrome as a progeroid syndrome rather than a "premature aging" syndrome. Nevertheless, research on the Werner syndrome has drawn attention to a potentially key role of somatic mutations and of replicative senescence in the pathogenesis of a wide array of geriatric disorders.

Unimodal Progeroid Syndromes

A second class of progeroid syndromes can be termed unimodal because they appear to involve only a single tissue or organ. Prototypic examples include the several forms of early-onset familial dementias of the Alzheimer type (Chapter 425), such as the autosomal dominant mutations at the presenilin 1 and 2 loci at chromosomes 14 and 1, respectively, and the β-amyloid precursor locus on chromosome 21. A strong argument can be made that Alzheimer pathology is part of normative aging because varying degrees of plaques and tangles and amyloid deposits are seen in the central nervous systems of virtually all very old human subjects. In any case, since the age-specific incidence of this form of dementia increases exponentially after the age of 65 years and the clinical diagnosis of probable Alzheimer's disease has been made in about 50% of all human subjects older than 85 years in a community-based population of Americans, it might be concluded that Alzheimer pathology goes hand in hand with aging in a large proportion of humanity. The advantage of studying unimodal progeroid syndromes is that it can potentially define biochemical pathways that operate to produce an array of specific geriatric disorders, thus opening the door to the development of interventions tailored to the needs of each geriatric patient.

SUMMARY

A genetic and evolutionary biologic approach to aging emphasizes that in age-structured populations (such as humans), genes that are very slow in reaching some phenotypic level of expression escape the force of natural selection because under the conditions in which humans have evolved, most reproducing individuals were young. Six classes of gene action can escape the force of natural selection, including the two "classic" types—antagonistic pleiotropy and the accumulation of constitutional mutations. Research in diverse species points to an important role for signal transduction pathways involving insulin-like growth factors and their receptors in the modulation of lifespan. There is also increasing evidence for stochastic variations in gene expression as the major explanation for intraspecific variations in longevity. Finally, research on genetic causes of progeroid syndromes may elucidate generalizable mechanisms of aging, with the hope that such research may eventually lead to rational interventions tailored to the specific vulnerabilities of geriatric patients.

SUGGESTED READINGS

Arking R: Biology of Aging: Observations and Principles, 3rd ed. New York, Oxford University Press, 2006. *This is one of very few textbooks that cover theoretical and experimental research on a wide range of organisms.*

Fraga MF, Ballestar E, Paz MF, et al: Epigenetic differences arise during the lifetime of monozygotic twins. Proc Natl Acad Sci USA 2005;102:10604–10609. *Epigenetic "drift" in aging identical twins.*

Fuster JJ, Andres V: Telomere biology and cardiovascular disease. Circ Res 2006;99:1167–1180. *Review of telomerase and telomere biology.*

Kenyon C: The plasticity of aging: Insights from long-lived mutants. Cell 2005;120:449–460. *An authoritative review of exciting recent research on the genetics of longevity.*

Martin GM: Genetic modulation of senescent phenotypes in *Homo sapiens.* Cell 2005;120:523–532. *A review of a subset of human progeroid syndromes.*

Science of Aging Knowledge Environment, sponsored by *Science* magazine and the American Association for the Advancement of Science. Available at http://sageke.sciencemag.org. *An intellectual home for scientists interested in research and teaching on the biology of aging; will increasingly embrace relevant clinical issues; includes links to other sites of interest to biogerontologists and geriatricians.*

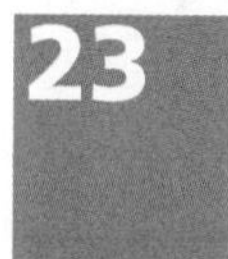

23 COMMON CLINICAL SEQUELAE OF AGING

Kenneth L. Minaker

Epidemiology

Increased longevity throughout the world is influencing medical care dramatically as more and more older individuals survive with more complex medical conditions. Although some elderly individuals present classically with single-system disease, others have presentations and responses to treatments that are different from those in younger patients. This variation in presentation and behavior of illnesses, which is due to the combined effect of aging and comorbid disease, must be understood if elderly patients are to receive successful care.

Pathobiology

Age-associated changes in health and disease are the result of (1) variations in the underlying physiologic changes that occur with age; (2) the presence of other diseases and medical conditions that have developed over time; (3) genetic predispositions for certain diseases; (4) lifestyle factors, including health-seeking behavior, diet, exercise, and exposure to medications and toxins; and (5) the variability intrinsic to diseases and medical conditions in general. Although no single hypothesis fully explains the process of aging at this time (Chapter 22), two major groupings have emerged (Table 23–1). The first concerns programmed causes, which are dominated by genetic theories. The second concerns stochastic causes, so-called process-of-living theories, in which genetic or environmental influences limit viability.

Spectrum of Changes Produced by Aging Processes

Perhaps the most important observation regarding normal aging is how much does not change. Most hormone levels, liver enzyme activities, electrolyte levels, body temperature, and basal glucose concentration remain constant throughout the lifespan. Long-term studies have indicated that there is no age-related anemia (Chapter 162), although the hematocrit declines slightly in men presumably because of the age-related decline in testosterone.

The passage of time results in changes that are not due to aging per se but rather may be considered "dose-time" related. For example, prolonged exposure results in the emergence of abnormalities and illnesses, such as skin cancer due to cumulative actinic injury (Chapter 214). Much of the lifetime exposure to sun is received before the age of 20 years, yet the resulting cancers follow decades later. Another example is polycystic kidney disease, which is an inheritable condition that does not appear until well into adulthood (Chapter 128); the passage of time allows the "full expression" of the genetic phenotype, but aging itself is not the key factor.

Some conditions become less likely with advancing age because of changes in the immune system. Immune disorders such as systemic lupus erythematosus (Chapter 287) and multiple sclerosis (Chapter 436) rarely appear in late life, presumably because changes in the immune system lead to less aggressive autoimmune activity. Similarly, although many cancers are more common in the elderly, many of the most aggressive tumors occur at a young age, suggesting that immune tolerance develops with advancing age.

Physiologic aging modulates the ways in which illnesses cause signs and symptoms. The elderly individual with hyperthyroidism often presents not with the systemic findings of agitation, irritability, hyperactivity, hyperphagia, and increased bowel movements but rather with apathy, anorexia, and atrial fibrillation (Chapter 244). The underlying pathophysiologic process may be no different, but age-related changes in physiology alter the body's sensitivity to dysfunction and influence the clinical presentation.

The most important physiologic change of aging is the predisposition to more generalized clinical syndromes and more severe disease. The lung function of a healthy 70-year-old is about 50% that of a 30-year-old (Chapters 83 and 85). Renal function commonly declines by 50% or more by the age of 70 years (Chapter 116). The resultant lack of physiologic reserve capacity does not affect day-to-day function but can affect the ability to recover from an extreme illness that exhausts the body's reserve capacity.

Geriatric syndromes emerge from these age-related changes. Many systems that maintain our upright posture are compromised by age, leading to increased postural sway. An older individual is much more likely to fall after a slip or a push. The consequences of that fall are more serious because of the age-related loss of bone mass (Chapter 264), resulting in fall-related fractures and spinal cord injuries.

Some physiologic changes imitate illness when they may be a normal part of aging. Diabetes mellitus may "appear" and "disappear" in the elderly (Chapters 247 and 248). The ability of insulin to stimulate glucose uptake declines with age and usually is manifested as postprandial hyperglycemia, but with normal fasting insulin and glucose levels. Under stress situations, older individuals can appear to be diabetic, but when the stressful situation is relieved, they no longer have chemical evidence of diabetes. Nevertheless, this loss of physiologic reserve understandably contributes to the increasing prevalence of diabetes with advancing age.

The age-related changes that make the elderly more vulnerable in daily life are often subtle. Older individuals are more likely to develop hypothermia or hyperthermia (Chapter 110) during extreme environmental exposure because of neurologic and thermoregulatory changes. The loss of brain stem neurotransmitters in older persons not only may cause a senile gait pattern but also predisposes to genetically determined conditions such as Parkinson's disease (Chapter 433). Decreases in the function of the frontal lobe inhibitory center predispose to urgency of urination.

Some age-related changes cause specific medical sequelae. Menopause (Chapter 262) is a normal aging process that produces symptoms and predisposes to future bone loss, urogenital atrophy, and atherosclerosis. Senile cataracts are caused by post-translational modifications in lens proteins combined with the inability of the lens to dispose of breakdown products associated with these processes; as a result, the lens becomes stiffer, thicker, and more opaque with age (Chapter 449).

EFFECTS OF AGING ON SPECIFIC ORGANS AND SYSTEMS

Cardiovascular System

Aging and Its Clinical Sequelae

Many important physiologic changes occur in the aging heart and help explain common age-associated cardiac disorders. Perhaps the most

TABLE 23–1 PATHOBIOLOGY OF AGING

Theory	Definition	Cause	Genetic (G) or Environmental (E)
PROGRAMMED THEORIES			
Programmed senescence	Aging results from gene interference with the ability of the cells to reproduce	Master clock	G
Hormonal	Biologic clock alters hormone secretion, resulting in tissue changes	Decrease in levels of insulin-like growth factor 1 and the hormones estrogen, testosterone, DHEA, and melatonin	G
Immunologic	T-cell function declines, increasing the chances for development of infections and cancer	Alteration in the cytokines that are responsible for communication between immune cells	G
Telomere shortening	Shortening of telomeres in somatic cells lessens the ability of cells to divide	Cells cannot divide	G, E
STOCHASTIC THEORIES			
Metabolic rate	The higher the basal metabolic rate (the rate at which the body, at rest, uses energy), the shorter the lifespan	Energy demands to maintain basal metabolism	G
Glycation	Glycation (browning) causes proteins to be joined, resulting in rigidity and decreased function	Elevated glucose	G, E
Somatic mutation	Mutations in genes occur with aging, eventually causing cells to stop functioning	Errors in the transmission of genetic messages over time	G
Wear and tear	Parts of cells wear out over time	Accumulated debris mechanically disrupts cell function	E
Oxygen free radicals	Tissue damage is caused by free radicals, such as superoxide or hydroxyl radicals; this is a specific form of the wear-and-tear theory	Oxygen free radicals are unstable chemical compounds that can oxidize cell components such as DNA and proteins	E

DHEA = dehydroepiandrosterone.

important physiologic change is the delay in left ventricular filling, which declines 50% between the ages of 20 and 80 years. Cardiac filling becomes more dependent on active filling late in diastole during atrial contraction (Chapter 50). This phenomenon commonly is related to thickening and stiffening of the left ventricular wall. Under normal conditions, systolic function remains unchanged, but the thickened ventricle will not produce normal output when volumes are low or be able to avoid elevated filling pressures and the resulting pulmonary congestion when volume is high. As a result, atrial natriuretic and brain natriuretic peptide levels increase with age as myocardial sensors detect greater pressures in the heart.

The resting heart rate slows slightly with advancing age, and maximum and submaximum exercise-induced heart rates show an age-related decline. The loss of sinus node pacemaker cells—up to 90% at 80 years—contributes to these changes. There also are changes in central and baroreflex-mediated heart rate control (Chapter 60). Heart valves thicken and stiffen, particularly in the mitral and aortic locations (Chapter 75). The functional significance of heart valve stiffening is minimal, but 25% of older individuals have flow murmurs (Chapter 48). The aorta dilates and its walls thicken as medial walls calcify; with this loss of elasticity, there is a secondary increase in systolic blood pressure (Chapter 66). The arteriosclerosis that is due to intimal disease further causes arterial walls to thicken, calcify, and lose their elasticity, thereby predisposing aging vessels to occlude or rupture (Chapter 69).

In most industrialized countries, there is a progressive increase in blood pressure with advancing age (Chapter 66). In general, systolic blood pressure increases after the age of 30 years, continues to rise until the mid-70s, then tends to fall slightly through the 80s and 90s. Diastolic blood pressure tends to parallel the usual increase in body weight that peaks in the early 50s in men and the early 60s in women; diastolic pressures subsequently fall slightly in older age. These changes in blood pressure are not universal, suggesting varied genetic and environmental causes, such as stress, sodium and potassium intake, and obesity.

Age-Related Cardiovascular Syndromes

Although atherosclerosis is the most important cause of symptomatic cardiac disease in the elderly, age-associated vascular stiffness predisposes to left ventricular stiffness, impaired diastolic filling, and the clinical syndrome of diastolic heart failure (Chapter 57). The most common arrhythmia in older individuals is atrial fibrillation (Chapter 63), which may occur in one third of older individuals undergoing surgery and may affect 4% of community-dwelling elderly individuals. Although thyroid disease, coronary artery disease, valvar heart disease, and intrinsic conduction system disease are common causes, atrial fibrillation in the elderly is often "lone" atrial fibrillation without a detectable underlying illness.

The combination of sensitivity to filling volumes and impaired heart rate response to stress may explain the increasingly prevalent syndrome of postural hypotension that is present in 20% of older individuals (Chapter 427). Postural hypotension is also common in the elderly after large meals; during infections severe enough to depress salt and water intake; and during volume-depleting stresses, such as diarrhea, diuretic therapy, and bowel preparation for colonoscopy. Stiffening of vessels in which baroreceptors reside also reduces the ability to modulate blood pressure with advancing age.

Perhaps the most important principle in the approach to cardiovascular signs and symptoms with advancing age is to recognize the narrowed homeostatic capacity of the elderly. Volume status must be managed carefully, attention should be paid to standing as opposed to sitting blood pressure in patients predisposed to postural hypotension, side effects of medications must be anticipated and monitored, and cardiovascular instability must be expected during almost any major illness that an older person may experience.

Respiratory System

The most characteristic change in the chest wall with advancing age is stiffening (Chapter 85). Cartilages thicken and calcify, and spinal ligaments and joints become stiffer. The primary internal change in the lungs is the loss of the elastic recoil. The result is a modest expansion of the chest wall with the appearance of a mild barrel chest. Although resting lung mechanics do not seem to change in any major way, the loss of maximum breathing capacity declines by approximately 40%. At the alveolar level, the capacity to exchange oxygen and carbon monoxide decreases by approximately 50% between the ages of 30 and 65 years, in part as a result of ventilation-perfusion mismatching (Chapter 85). Although these changes are not noticeable at rest, individuals experience fatigue or shortness of breath when the respiratory system is under stress (e.g., during exercise or major illness). Pulmonary reflexes such as coughing and ciliary function decrease, predisposing elderly individuals to the pooling of secretions.

These changes do not produce substantial abnormalities in resting oxygen saturation, but they produce a steady decline in arterial Po_2. The arterial Po_2 of many individuals older than 80 years is about 70 to 75 mm Hg. As with other age-related physiologic findings, these changes do not interfere with function under resting conditions but dramatically affect survival during severe respiratory illness.

Age-Related Respiratory Syndromes

The major clinical impact of normal physiologic aging in the lungs is an earlier appearance of shortness of breath as a warning signal of underlying disease. Myocardial infarction and heart failure can present primarily with shortness of breath, mainly due to age-related mechanical changes, an inability to clear blood from the lungs, and a decline in resting pulmonary function to near the threshold for clinical hypoxia. Aspiration pneumonia is caused by impaired swallowing and reduced clearance of lung secretions.

Gastrointestinal System

A broad series of changes occur in gastroenterologic tissues, but the redundancy of overall gastrointestinal function usually prevents clinical symptoms. Age-related changes in the mouth include slower production of dentine, shrinkage of the root pulp, and decreasing bone density of the jaw. Taste and smell decline progressively with advancing age, with rising thresholds for tasting salt, sweetness, and certain proteins (Chapter 453). The overall net effect is that food may taste more bitter, and more sugar is required before something tastes sweet. Salivary gland function normally does not change with age (Chapter 451). The loss of bone and tongue musculature makes the tongue appear to be enlarged.

The esophagus seems to function relatively normally. The strength of muscle contraction declines, however, and peristaltic waves slow with advancing age. There is also a tendency for the lower esophageal sphincter to become lax (Chapter 140).

The gastric mucosa secretes less acid with advancing age. Although these changes do not seem to affect digestion in most individuals, associated conditions, such as atrophic gastritis, may further decrease the absorption of nutrients to the point of producing illness. Most studies suggest that delayed gastric emptying is a feature of aging, leading to a sense of false or early satiety, which can impair subsequent food ingestion (Chapter 138).

Liver weight declines by one third between the ages of 30 and 90 years, primarily because of the loss of hepatocytes. The result is a decreased ability to process medications such as benzodiazepines and vitamin K–blocking agents. Doses of drugs often must be adjusted, and their blood levels should be monitored when possible.

Aging is associated with a significant reduction in small intestinal surface area with the consequence of reduced absorption of some dietary components, such as calcium. Colonic function declines with advancing age. Motility up to the rectosigmoid area, measured by passage of markers, does not seem to decline with advancing age (Chapter 138). Distal to this point, however, evacuation is characteristically slower with advancing age. Stool frequency tends to decline, and hardness of stools seems to increase with advancing age. Diverticula are present in approximately 50% of people older than 80 years and are likely to be related to reduced dietary fiber and the resulting greater intracolonic pressure (Chapter 145).

Age-Related Gastroenterologic Syndromes

The most important age-related symptom is constipation, which may affect 60% of individuals in late life. Obstipation can present atypically with confusion, nausea, and vomiting or as obscure fever resulting from stercoral ulcerations. Perhaps the most common abnormality related to declining hepatic function is increased sensitivity to medications that require hepatic metabolism.

Renal and Urinary Excretory System

Overall kidney size declines by approximately one third, and blood flow through the kidney declines by about 1% per year. Beginning in the late 30s, cortical nephrons appear to drop out and sclerose at a much higher rate than medullary nephrons, creating a hyperfiltration syndrome that limits maximum concentrating capacity (Chapter 116). Resulting functional changes include decreased ability to excrete a salt load, declining glomerular filtration rate, delayed ability to regain sodium and potassium balance during deprivation states, and difficulty in conserving water under situations of dehydration. Excretion of water loads is not strikingly impaired with age, but modest and perhaps clinically significant reductions in acid secretion have been shown in older individuals.

The bladder tends to become more irritable with advancing age and may generate less power during contraction. Because of the delay in sodium excretion and orthostatic changes, nocturia is common; older individuals seem to produce more urine at night than during the day. The most important bladder change may be the slight increase in residual bladder urine volume. Atrophy of vaginal and urethral tissues due to postmenopausal estrogen deprivation predisposes women to urinary tract infections (Chapter 262).

Age-Related Renal and Urinary Tract Syndromes

The age-related increases in asymptomatic bacteriuria and urinary tract infections are almost certainly due to increased residual bladder volume and loss of protective factors in the normal anatomic structures. As the prostate gland grows with advancing age, benign prostatic hypertrophy causes urinary retention in men (Chapter 130). Urinary incontinence (Chapter 24) is more prevalent in women. The kidney is more susceptible to the effects of medications, particularly nonsteroidal anti-inflammatory drugs, which can result in sodium and fluid retention and subsequent hypertension. In the elderly, a slight acidemia results from impaired acid excretion and may contribute to the development of osteoporosis.

Dehydration or volume depletion, which is increasingly more prevalent with advancing age, often accompanies acute infections and increases the morbidity and mortality of pneumonia or urinary tract infections. Dehydration is the most common fluid and electrolyte disorder in the frail elderly because of decreased fluid intake and increased fluid losses. Vomiting and diarrhea are the most common causes of isotonic dehydration. Fever associated with delirium is the leading cause of hypertonic dehydration. Hypotonic dehydration is seen most commonly with overuse of diuretics. Signs and symptoms of dehydration are notoriously vague or absent. Orthostatic tachycardia and hypotension are important clinical findings, and an acute decline in weight may be documented. Perhaps the most useful clinical parameter is a history of having missed one or more meals. Laboratory tests should measure the electrolytes, osmolality, creatinine, and blood urea nitrogen; a blood urea nitrogen–to–creatinine ratio greater than or equal to 25 is suggestive of dehydration.

Anticipation and prevention of dehydration are crucial. Adequate food intake should be maintained; 30 mL of daily fluid intake per kilogram of body weight is recommended. For an acute event, it is important to review any long-term medications, particularly diuretics, that may have contributed to dehydration and to define the ethically appropriate approach to future episodes. In terminally ill patients, death from dehydration becomes a natural event in which symptom-focused care relieves discomfort from dry mucous membranes (Chapter 3).

Endocrine System

Growth hormone levels fall with advancing age, with initial loss of nocturnal growth hormone spikes (Chapter 242). These declines contribute to the decreased muscle strength, thinning of bones and skin, and increased central fat associated with aging. It is currently unclear whether replacement of growth factors can induce a permanent reversal of muscle, bone, and skin changes with advancing age.

The production rates and clearance rates of thyroxine, triiodothyronine, and calcitonin seem to be constant with advancing age despite the increased prevalence of thyroid disease in late life (Chapter 244). There is an increase in parathyroid hormone levels, particularly in women, with advancing age, perhaps in compensation for the age-related decline of the kidney's ability to maintain normal levels of phosphorus and calcium in the blood (Chapter 266).

The adrenal glands maintain their ability to secrete cortisone with advancing age (Chapter 245). Dehydroepiandrosterone declines 85 to 90% by the age of 70 years, however, perhaps contributing to impaired immune or cardiovascular function with advancing age. Renin and aldosterone secretion rates decline progressively with advancing age and do not contribute to the increased rates of hypertension with advancing age.

The insulin content of the elderly pancreas is increased, but the release of insulin in response to stimulation may be blunted with advancing age (Chapters 247 and 248). There is also a concomitant decline in insulin clearance with advancing age, with the net result that plasma insulin levels in response to glucose seem to be relatively preserved. Insulin resistance may increase with advancing age, but glucagon secretion seems to be well preserved.

The ovaries show dramatic declines in estrogen and progesterone as fibrosis and scarring occur. Menopause occurs at an average age of 51 years with subsequent hot flashes, accelerated bone loss, and atrophy of estrogen-sensitive tissues (Chapter 262). Levels of testosterone decrease in some men beginning around 50 years, but declines do not seem to affect the potency of semen. Sexual function is relatively well preserved, albeit with an increase in the refractory period and time to arousal and a loss of tissue turgor (Chapter 253).

Age-Related Endocrine Syndromes

The most important age-related endocrine syndrome occurring with advancing age is menopause (Chapter 262). Most other endocrine changes with age may enhance the prevalence of common disorders seen with aging, especially diabetes.

Immune System

Normal aging produces an obvious decrease in the size of the thymus gland between puberty and 50 or 60 years of age, at which time the gland becomes difficult to identify anatomically. This decrease in size is accompanied by a corresponding drop in thymosin levels, which are related directly to the number of functional T cells found in older adults. T cells also seem to be less active in responding to the presence of foreign proteins, and they tend to reproduce more slowly than those in younger adults. Functional studies of immune responsiveness suggest that although antibody responses are produced by older individuals, they tend to be less robust and less long lasting than in younger individuals (Chapters 42 and 270).

Clinical Syndromes of Aging

There are increased morbidity and mortality associated with influenza and pneumonia with advancing age and reactivation of infections such as tuberculosis and herpes zoster. The decline in immune function also may make it less likely that older adults will develop autoimmune diseases, such as systemic lupus erythematosus.

Vaccine therapy for the prevention of herpes zoster is now recommended (Chapters 16 and 398). It is even more critical to maintain annual immunization against influenza (Chapter 16). Pneumovax and tetanus vaccination are also important in the elderly (Chapter 16).

Hematopoietic System

The pluripotent stem cell and the erythroid and myeloid progenitor cells show no age-related reduction, indicating that there is minimal or no change in basal hematopoiesis during aging (Chapter 160). The aging hematopoietic system is less able to respond to increased demands, however, as evidenced by a slower recovery from anemia and less of a rise of hemoglobin during hypoxia. The older marrow also seems to respond less well to erythropoietin.

Neutrophils from elderly individuals show less prekilling activity and lower levels of lysozyme (Chapter 175), with a significant reduction in signal transduction and less release of inositol 1,4,5-trisphosphate and diacylglycerol during stimulation. During nutritional deprivation, there seems to be impairment in the reserve capacity to kill phagocytosed bacteria, a change that may contribute to the high prevalence of serious bacterial infections among the nutritionally compromised elderly.

Age-Related Hematopoietic Syndromes

There are no specific syndromes of impaired hematopoiesis, aside from the clinical observation that during a comparable illness stress, hematologic abnormalities are more likely in the elderly.

Musculoskeletal System

Bone mass and density decrease with age after reaching maximum in the 20s. In women, this loss may be about 1% per year until menopause, when it can increase to 2 to 3% per year (Chapters 262 and 264). After 5 to 10 years post menopause, bone loss returns to a rate of loss of 1% per year, but it may accelerate again in the late 80s. Because men have more bone mass than women do and lose bone mass at a similar rate of about 1% per year, the clinical effects in men are not seen until advanced age.

Tendons and ligaments become less elastic with advancing age, contributing to a higher incidence of rupture, especially of the Achilles tendon, in older individuals. Cartilage and ligaments of the ribs and spine are more likely to become calcified and less elastic.

Muscles reach their ultimate size and strength in the 20s and 30s. By 70 years of age, muscle mass declines by approximately 25% for men and women unless it is offset by exercise. By the age of 80 years, muscle size and strength in most sedentary adults decrease by 30 to 40% from the mid-30s peak. Muscle mass in late life depends on exercise earlier in life to reach a higher early mass and exercise late in life to stimulate muscle preservation.

Age-Related Musculoskeletal Syndromes

The most important age-related clinical syndrome associated with advancing age is osteoporosis (Chapter 264). Sarcopenia, or diminished muscle mass, is a clear predisposing factor for falls, which is the leading cause of accidental death at home in older individuals. Bone and muscle mass respond well to gravitational stress and resistance exercises, respectively, even in the oldest age ranges.

Falls are a major age-related syndrome involving neural, musculoskeletal, and cardiovascular systems. Most falls in older adults are due to a combination of several factors rather than a single event. Internal contributors to falls include sensory impairment from poor eyesight, hearing loss, and balance disturbances; diseases of the brain, including motor and sensory disorders, cognitive impairment that produces poor judgment or apraxia, and depression; cardiovascular, respiratory, and metabolic diseases; and musculoskeletal conditions, such as lower limb weakness, poor grip strength, osteoporosis, rheumatoid arthritis, osteoarthritis, and foot disorders. External causes of falls include medications. The risk of falling increases in patients who receive four or more prescription medications; drugs specifically shown to increase the risk of falling include hypnotics, muscle relaxants, antihypertensives, diuretics, and antidepressants. Environmental problems increase the risk of falls. Inside the home, risks include stairs (coming down is more hazardous than climbing up, as the first and last steps often have no railing or an unusable one); loose objects, such as furniture, cords, and rugs; poor lighting, particularly in areas with dark and light variability; poorly fitting shoes; surfaces with glare or patterning; and lack of bathroom safety equipment. Outdoor risks include uneven pavements and surface roads made slippery from ice, water, or fallen leaves.

For a person who has fallen, the evaluation should include a detailed history of the circumstances surrounding the fall, medications, medical problems, and mobility; an examination of vision, gait, balance, and lower extremity joint function; an examination of neurologic function, including muscle strength; and an examination of the cardiovascular system. The investigations for falls and syncope (Chapters 61 and 427) are similar. Tests are needed only if the history and physical examination do not reveal the cause of falling or if they point to a particular abnormality that requires laboratory evaluation. These tests may include the following:

- blood tests to exclude anemia, infection, and metabolic problems such as diabetes and thyroid disease;
- an electrocardiogram to evaluate heart disease;
- a 24-hour electrocardiogram recording or loop monitor to evaluate arrhythmias (Chapter 65);
- an echocardiogram for patients with significant heart murmurs (Chapter 53);
- drug levels to check if a patient is being undertreated or overtreated with a particular drug;

- if focal neurologic signs or symptoms are present, a computed tomographic scan of the brain;
- if suggestive symptoms are present, a radiograph of the neck or spine to look for spinal stenosis (Chapter 423).

Prevention of Fractures

The prevention of fractures has three components. First, persons with lower bone densities are more likely to fracture a bone, given the same amount of trauma, than are persons with higher bone densities. Women should be assessed for osteoporosis and treated accordingly (Chapter 264). Osteoporosis often is underdiagnosed in men, and men with fractures or repeated falls should be evaluated for possible osteoporosis; however, screening strategies for elderly men have not been defined.

Fractures can be prevented if falls can be prevented. Older people who have recurrent falls should have regular exercise and balance training after their risk factors for falling are fully addressed. The optimal type, duration, and intensity of exercise are unclear, but balance training for 10 weeks or more has the best-proven benefit. Exercise must be sustained for continued benefit.

When someone falls, the damage may be reduced by the intrinsic padding of fat or by devices such as mechanical hip protectors. Randomized controlled trials of hip protectors to reduce fractures in nursing home patients and in ambulatory older individuals in Europe have shown mixed results in the United States. Compliance with these cumbersome devices is only 25 to 70%.

Nervous System

Brain size decreases with advancing age; after the age of 60 years, its size declines by 5 to 10%. The decrease in size is caused primarily by a decrease in the cerebral cortex. Novel adjustments to cell loss include the formation of new connections between remaining neurons. Aging is associated with a progressive decline in the synthesis of neurotransmitters and a decline in their corresponding receptors. A major functional change is slower reaction times, which may be the result of a slower nerve conduction or transsynaptic speed.

The farsightedness of aging is caused by the diminished ability of the lens to focus on nearby objects because of its thickening and stiffening (Chapter 449). There is reduced ability to distinguish colors, particularly blue, because of yellowing of the lens. Overall transmission of light through the lens may decline by 50 to 65% between the ages of 25 and 60 years; as a result, individuals require more ambient light. Older individuals experience more glare because light scatters through the thickened lens. Older individuals also notice more floaters as the vitreous jelly becomes slightly more liquefied and mobile with advancing age. Tear production is decreased, leading to a sense of grittiness in the older eye. Overall visual acuity tends to decrease with age, and by 65 years, 40% of men and 60% of women have a visual acuity of 20/70 or worse.

Approximately 25% of individuals older than 65 years experience hearing loss with age (Chapter 454), with men affected more than women. The degeneration of neural transmission from the ear to the brain results in difficulty in identifying a voice or understanding a spoken message when there is background noise. Presbycusis results in high-frequency sound loss and more difficulty in distinguishing high-pitched consonants and voices compared with lower pitched vowels and sounds.

Sleep patterns change with advancing age (Chapter 429). Functionally, older adults are more wakeful during the night and spend much more time in bed. The pattern of sleep characteristically changes from the fairly regular stepwise patterns of childhood and young adulthood to a more fragmented pattern, with frequent awakenings in late life.

Age-Related Neurologic Syndromes

Age-associated memory dysfunction is common (Chapters 25 and 425), and delirium (Chapter 26) may occur, especially during illnesses. Prevention of delirium is possible with a proactive consultation intervention, which can reduce the incidence of hospital delirium by about 40 to 50%. [1]

Sleep cycle disturbances are increasingly important with advancing age, and sleep-disordered breathing associated with sleep apnea seems to rise in prevalence with advancing age (Chapter 101). Anatomic changes, such as tissue laxity and diseases of the nose and sinuses, may contribute to sleep-disordered breathing. Sleep apnea may have a neurologic basis either in the sleep cycling center, leading to central sleep apnea, or in neurologic control of pharyngeal tissues.

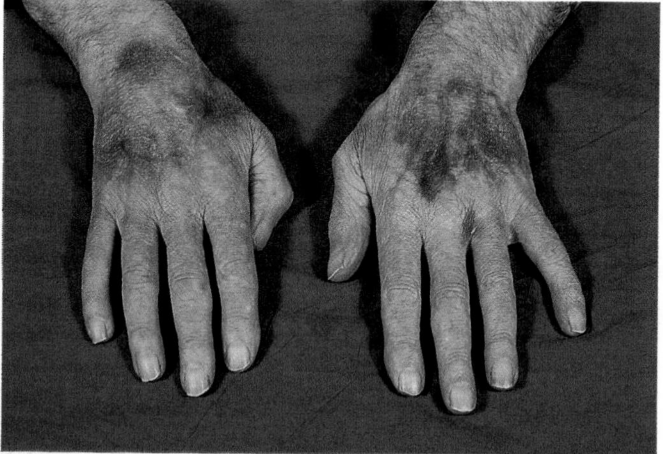

FIGURE 23–1 • Senile purpura is a common and benign condition that results from impaired collagen production and capillary fragility in the elderly. In the absence of other signs of disease, no investigation is necessary. (From Forbes CD, Jackson WF: Color Atlas and Text of Clinical Medicine, 3rd ed. London, Mosby, 2003, with permission.)

Integumentary System

Thinning of the subcutaneous tissue begins in most people in their mid-40s independent of the degree of sun exposure or protection from injury. The epidermis and dermis adhere less tightly, making the skin feel looser and increasing its tendency to blister and to be subject to friction burns or pressure ulceration (Chapter 461). This phenomenon also leads to senile purpura (Fig. 23–1) that results from tears in small venules when the skin is bumped or abraded (Chapter 466).

Environmental exposures, including ultraviolet sunlight, wind, and smoking, help promote the development of wrinkles by damaging the subcutaneous tissues and the epidermis, especially the elastin fibers. The process of photo injury (Chapter 464) leads to slow repair, particularly of tissues of the distal forearm and lower leg. Ultraviolet light exposure also predisposes to the development of skin cancer, the most common of which is basal cell cancer, but squamous cell cancer and melanoma are also age dependent (Chapter 214). Approximately two thirds of aging individuals experience at least one skin problem, and about 40% have two underlying skin disorders.

The most profound consequence of environmental exposure and age-related changes is that wound repair rates are significantly prolonged. In individuals older than 65 years, healing takes about 50% longer compared with individuals in their 30s; complete skin healing can take 5.5 weeks instead of 3.5 weeks.

Rates of epithelial cell regeneration decrease by about 50% from maturity to 70 years of age. A similar pattern is seen in hair, which grows more slowly. With advancing age, graying is variable but universal because the number of melanocytes within hair bulbs declines with age (Chapter 467). Changes in skin cell size and shape cause irregular patterning and may predispose to water-induced or environment-induced cracking.

Age-Related Integumentary Syndromes

Specific illnesses affecting the skin include basal cell cancer and rosacea (Chapters 464 to 467). Aging skin syndromes also include xerosis, thermoregulatory changes, skin thinning, and hair loss. The primary therapy for xerosis is the external application of treatments to protect and moisturize the skin (Chapter 463).

Diminished sweating poses a threat during times of high ambient and environmental temperatures or in the context of fever (Chapters 110 and 303). The absence of sweating lessens heat loss by conduction and evaporation, and it diminishes the urge to move to a more protected environment. As few elderly experience thirst, dehydration may occur quickly in these settings. Environmental protection from temperature extremes is crucial (Chapter 110).

Pressure sores are necrotic areas of muscle, subcutaneous fat, and skin as a result of compression and subsequent ischemia (Fig. 23–2). Pressure sores usually occur between underlying bone and a hard surface or a soft surface during a prolonged time. Among elderly patients in acute care hospitals, the incidence rate is 8% and the prevalence rate is 16%. Rates

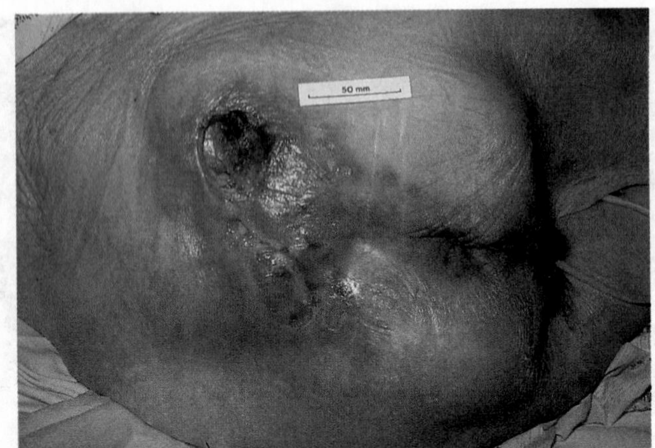

FIGURE 23–2 • Severe sacral pressure sore, one of the serious but preventable complications of immobility. (From Forbes CD, Jackson WF: Color Atlas and Text of Clinical Medicine, 3rd ed. London, Mosby, 2003, with permission.)

are even higher in patients who are in intensive care units or who have hip fractures.

A standard mattress can generate pressures as high as 150 mm Hg, well above the 30 to 35 mm Hg continuous pressure threshold needed to cause pressure sores. In addition to pressure injury, shear injury is important. Shear injury, which occurs when local blood vessels are stretched and separated from underlying perforating vessels, is more likely when the patient is in a sloped position or is rubbing constantly against underlying surfaces. Burning injury also can result from friction of the superficial skin layers. A complicating feature of all pressure ulcers is moisture, which leads to softening of the skin, sticking to underlying surfaces, and easy access for infection.

Individuals at higher risk include those who are immobile; those who are incontinent of bowel or bladder; and those who have compromised circulation due to hypotension, dehydration, or vascular disease. Neurologic disease, particularly peripheral neuropathy that impairs sensation, can predispose to pressure ulcers, as can any neurologic condition that causes spasticity, contractures, or poor mobility.

Preventive strategies encourage safe positioning, regular turning, and avoidance of direct pressure. Judicious use of pressure-reducing beds may lower the incidence of pressure ulcers after hip fractures. Deep foam mattresses and air suspension beds are even more effective.

When pressure sores appear, they should be photographed to establish a baseline. Nutrition should be improved, all pressure on the wound should be removed, and active vigilance should be focused to prevent additional pressure ulcers. Débridement of necrotic tissue should be considered; wet to dry dressings and surgical or chemical débridement are often used. Infections may require topical or systemic antibiotics. Semi-occlusive and occlusive dressings also can be helpful. Most pressure ulcers heal within 6 months, but operative repair is sometimes necessary.

Clinical Pharmacology

Of all prescription medications (Chapter 27), about 30% are taken by the elderly even though they compose only 14% of the population. Nonprescription medications are disproportionately consumed by older individuals and are increasingly implicated in drug-drug interactions.

The gastrointestinal absorption of medications generally does not change with advancing age, despite the theoretical possibility that medications requiring acidification in the stomach may be absorbed less well because of the higher frequency of atrophic gastritis and reduced gastric acid. Drug distribution changes significantly with advancing age because medications distribute to fat or muscle. As muscle mass declines with advancing age, fat increases as a proportion of total body weight. As a result, older individuals are more sensitive to the effects of water-soluble drugs (heart) and have prolonged effects from lipophilic drugs (brain).

The decline in renal function with normal aging reduces the clearance of many drugs, especially digoxin, aminoglycosides, and cimetidine. Hepatic metabolism also may decline with age. Oxidative reactions, so-called phase 1 reactions, become impaired with normal aging, whereas phase 2 reactions (conjugation and glucuronidization) are relatively spared. A clinical example is that diazepam, which requires phase 1 and phase 2 metabolism, has a prolonged half-life with advancing age, but oxazepam, which requires only phase 2 reactions to be metabolized, does not.

The overall impact of these pharmacokinetic changes is that the half-life, which is proportional to the volume of distribution divided by drug clearance, increases for many lipophilic drugs. Poorly nourished or frail elderly persons may have a low serum albumin level. The normal age-related decline in the serum albumin level is clinically insignificant. When the albumin level is less than 3 g/dL, however, drug levels have to be interpreted on the basis of their binding to albumin; albumin levels this low are associated with an increased risk of in-hospital death and longer lengths of hospital stay.

Independent of pharmacokinetic issues, the elderly are more sensitive to many medications. The brain appears to be increasingly sensitive to many compounds, including opiates, benzodiazepines, and neuroleptics. As a result, lower doses cause effects equivalent to those seen with higher doses in younger individuals. Warfarin, which acts primarily on the liver, will maintain therapeutic anticoagulation profiles at lower doses in the elderly because the aging liver is increasingly sensitive to blockage of vitamin K–dependent systems.

The elderly are at higher risk for nonadherence to prescribed regimens. Factors influencing nonadherence include the number of medications and their cost, inadequate education of the patient, unacceptable side effects, and complexity of the medical regimen. Individuals who take more than three prescription drugs have lower adherence. Below three medications per day, the elderly in general have high adherence rates. Unfortunately, no intervention has reliably improved adherence rates in the elderly. 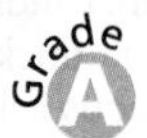

Perhaps the most important phenomenon in multiple drug regimens in older individuals is the progressive accumulation of anticholinergic effects, including dry mouth, constipation, poor vision, urinary retention, balance disorders, and cognitive difficulties. Anticholinergic drugs include neuroleptics, antispasmodics, antianxiety agents, antihistamines, and medications used for urinary incontinence.

Grade A

1. Marcantonio ER, Flacker JM, Wright JR, Resnick NM: Reducing delirium after hip fracture: A randomized trial. J Am Geriatr Soc 2001;49:516–522.
2. Higgins N, Regan C: A systematic review of the effectiveness of interventions to help older people adhere to medication regimes. Age Ageing 2004;33:224–229.

SUGGESTED READINGS

Cohen HJ, Feussner JR, Weinberger M, et al: A controlled trial of inpatient and outpatient geriatric evaluation and management. N Engl J Med 2002;346:905–912. *Significant reductions in functional decline and improvements in mental health were achieved at no increase in costs.*

Juurlink DN, Mamdani M, Kopp A, et al: Drug-drug interactions among elderly patients hospitalized for drug toxicity. JAMA 2003;289:1652–1658. *Many admissions for drug toxicity occur after administration of a drug known to cause drug-drug interactions.*

Kamel NS, Gammack JK: Insomnia in the elderly: Cause, approach, and treatment. Am J Med 2006;119:463–469. *A comprehensive review.*

Kannus P, Sievänen H, Palvanen M, et al: Prevention of falls and consequent injuries in elderly people. Lancet 2005;366:1885–1893. *A comprehensive review.*

Lachs MS, Pillemer K: Elder abuse. Lancet 2004;364:1263–1272. *A practical overview.*

Nair KS, Rizza RA, O'Brien P, et al: DHEA in elderly women and DHEA or testosterone in elderly men. N Engl J Med 2006;355:1647–1659. *Neither DHEA nor testosterone has physiologically relevant beneficial effects.*

Zakai NA, Katz R, Hirsch C, et al: A prospective study of anemia status, hemoglobin concentration, and mortality in an elderly cohort: The Cardiovascular Health Study. Arch Intern Med 2005;165:2214–2220. *Lower and higher hemoglobin concentrations and anemia were independently associated with increased mortality.*

24 URINARY INCONTINENCE

Joseph G. Ouslander

Definition

Urinary incontinence is defined as involuntary loss of urine of sufficient severity to be a health or social problem. Although it is commonly hidden and not discussed with health professionals, urinary incontinence is a prevalent, morbid, and expensive condition.

Epidemiology

Half of young and middle-aged women experience urinary incontinence, often in association with childbirth. Urinary incontinence is a common manifestation of benign and malignant prostate enlargement in middle-aged and older men. The prevalence and incidence of urinary incontinence are higher in women and increase with age. Among relatively healthy community-dwelling adults aged 60 years and older, about one third of women and nearly 20% of men have some degree of urinary incontinence. About 10% of both sexes have frequent (at least weekly) episodes or use protective padding. The prevalence is nearly 40% in hospitalized older adults and 70 to 80% in adults in long-term care institutions.

A recently defined syndrome, overactive bladder, includes urinary frequency (more than eight voids per 24 hours), nocturia (awakening at night from sleep to void), and urgency (the acute need to void), with or without incontinence. The prevalence of overactive bladder is about 16% in the adult population older than 40 years, but the prevalence rises to 31% in women 75 years and older and 42% in men 75 years and older.

Urinary incontinence causes considerable physical and psychosocial morbidity and health care costs. The condition is uncomfortable and predisposes to skin problems and falls in older patients rushing to the bathroom. It is a social stigma and can lead to embarrassment, isolation, and depression. Urinary incontinence is commonly an important precipitating factor in the decision to enter a long-term care facility. The annual health care costs of managing urinary incontinence and its complications have been estimated to be more than $20 billion.

Pathogenesis

Continence requires effective lower urinary tract functioning; adequate mobility, dexterity, cognition, and motivation to be continent; and absence of environmental and iatrogenic barriers (Table 24–1). From a lower urinary tract standpoint, incontinence results from (1) failure to store urine because of bladder overactivity or low urethral resistance, (2) failure to empty the bladder because of anatomic or physiologic obstruction or inadequate bladder contractility, or (3) a combination of these factors.

Aging does not cause urinary incontinence, but age-related changes can predispose to it. Among women, urethral resistance declines because of diminished estrogen effects and weakened periurethral and pelvic muscles. Among men, urethral resistance increases, and the urine flow rate decreases in association with prostatic enlargement. In both sexes, the bladder tends to become overactive and is affected by involuntary detrusor contractions (more so in men than in women). In many older individuals, impaired bladder contractility develops and can result in a condition termed detrusor hyperactivity with impaired contractility. Finally, age-related declines in renal concentrating mechanisms, loss of the normal diurnal rhythm of arginine vasopressin, and increases in atrial natriuretic peptide can predispose older patients to nocturnal polyuria and nighttime incontinence.

Several potentially reversible factors may cause or contribute to urinary incontinence, especially in geriatric patients (Table 24–2). The common reversible factors can be remembered by the mnemonic DRIP (delirium; restricted mobility, retention; infection, inflammation [atrophic vaginitis], impaction of stool; polyuria, pharmaceuticals).

TABLE 24–1 REQUIREMENTS FOR CONTINENCE

Effective lower urinary tract function
Storage
Accommodation by bladder of increasing volumes of urine under low pressure
Closed bladder outlet
Appropriate sensation of bladder fullness
Absence of involuntary bladder contractions
Emptying
Bladder capable of contraction
Lack of anatomic obstruction to urine flow
Coordinated lowering of outlet resistance with bladder contractions
Adequate mobility and dexterity to use toilet or toilet substitute and to manage clothing
Adequate cognitive function to recognize toileting needs and to find a toilet or toilet substitute
Motivation to be continent
Absence of environmental and iatrogenic barriers, such as inaccessible toilets or toilet substitutes, unavailable caregivers, or drug side effects

From Kane RL, Ouslander JG, Abrass IB: Essentials of Clinical Geriatrics, 5th ed. New York, McGraw-Hill, 2004. Copyright © by McGraw-Hill, Inc. Used by permission of McGraw-Hill Book Company.

Clinical Manifestations

Urinary incontinence may be of sudden onset. In geriatric patients, a sudden onset commonly is associated with an acute medical illness or one or more potentially reversible factors (see Table 24–2). More commonly, urinary incontinence is a chronic problem, and patients often delay for years after its onset before discussing it with a health professional. For this reason, the physician periodically should ask screening questions specifically about bladder control problems.

Persistent types of urinary incontinence can be categorized into four basic types (Table 24–3). *Stress* incontinence is far more common in women than in men, among whom it occurs only after sphincter damage from surgery or irradiation. *Urge* incontinence is the most common and bothersome symptomatic type of incontinence in the geriatric population and usually is associated with other symptoms of overactive bladder. The symptoms and signs of *overflow* incontinence are nonspecific and may mimic symptoms and signs of the stress and urge types. Men, patients with diabetes mellitus, and patients with neurologic disorders are at highest risk for overflow urinary incontinence. *Functional* incontinence refers to patients whose involuntary urine loss is related predominantly to impaired mobility or cognition. These basic types of urinary incontinence commonly coexist. A substantial proportion of women have symptoms of urge *and* stress incontinence (generally referred to as a *mixed* type). Frail geriatric patients commonly have urge incontinence with bladder overactivity and functional impairments that contribute to the incontinence problem.

Diagnosis

The basic evaluation of incontinent patients includes a focused history (which can be enhanced by a voiding diary), targeted physical examination, urinalysis, and postvoid residual determination (Fig. 24–1). Postvoid residual determination is essential in almost all patients because the symptoms of overflow incontinence are nonspecific, and the physical examination alone is not sensitive in detecting significant urinary retention (i.e., postvoid residual of more than 200 mL). A portable ultrasound device is available and can provide noninvasively an accurate estimate of bladder volume. The objectives of this basic evaluation are (1) to identify potentially reversible factors (see Table 24–1); (2) to determine, if possible, the most likely types and underlying causes (see Table 24–2); and (3) to identify patients who may require further evaluation.

Selected patients may benefit from further urologic, gynecologic, and urodynamic evaluation. Patients with sterile hematuria should be

TABLE 24–2 REVERSIBLE CONDITIONS THAT CAUSE OR CONTRIBUTE TO URINARY INCONTINENCE

Condition	Management
CONDITIONS AFFECTING THE LOWER URINARY TRACT	
Urinary tract infection (symptomatic with frequency, urgency, dysuria)	Antimicrobial therapy
Atrophic vaginitis, urethritis	Topical estrogen
Postprostatectomy, postpartum	Behavioral interventions; further evaluation if condition does not resolve over a few months
Stool impaction	Disimpaction; appropriate use of stool softeners, bulk-forming agents, and laxatives if necessary; high fiber intake; adequate exercise and fluid intake
DRUG SIDE EFFECTS	
Diuretics Anticholinergics α-Adrenergic agents Psychotropics Narcotics	Discontinue or change therapy if clinically appropriate; dosage reduction or modification (e.g., flexible scheduling of rapid-acting diuretics) also may help
INCREASED URINE PRODUCTION	
Metabolic (hyperglycemia, hypercalcemia)	Better control of diabetes mellitus; therapy for hypercalcemia depends on the underlying cause
Excess fluid intake	Reduction in intake of caffeinated beverages
Volume overload	
Venous insufficiency with edema	Support stockings, leg elevation, sodium restriction, diuretic therapy
Congestive heart failure	Medical therapy
IMPAIRED ABILITY OR WILLINGNESS TO REACH A TOILET	
Delirium	Diagnosis and treatment of underlying cause of acute confusional state
Chronic illness, injury, or restraint that interferes with mobility	Regular toileting; environmental alterations (e.g., bedside commode, urinal)
Psychological	Pharmacologic or nonpharmacologic treatment

From Kane RL, Ouslander JG, Abrass IB: Essentials of Clinical Geriatrics, 5th ed. New York, McGraw-Hill, 2004. Copyright © by McGraw-Hill, Inc. Used by permission of McGraw-Hill Book Company.

considered for urine cytology and cystoscopy. Women with severe pelvic prolapse should be referred to a gynecologist for consideration of pessary placement or surgery. Women or men with severe stress incontinence should be considered for referral for surgical intervention. Patients with significant urinary retention, patients with a neurologic disorder such as multiple sclerosis or spinal cord injury, and patients who fail initial treatment interventions should be considered for urodynamic evaluation. Complex urodynamic tests (multichannel cystometry, pressure-flow studies, leak point pressure) can assist in determining the precise underlying lower urinary tract pathophysiologic process and in targeting specific treatment on the basis of the findings.

Treatment

Rx

The most common method of managing urinary incontinence is adult diapers and pads. Although many of these products are well designed and helpful, they are nonspecific and expensive. Many patients cannot afford these products and instead design their own, often poorly hygienic substitutes. Use of adult diapers and pads may serve simply to hide a curable or potentially serious problem or foster dependency in frail geriatric patients. These products generally should be used as adjuncts to more specific interventions, and patients should be encouraged to undergo at least a basic evaluation of their condition.

Reversible factors identified by the basic evaluation outlined here should be treated (see Table 24–2). In some patients, the urinary incontinence resolves after treatment of one or more of these factors. Primary therapies for persistent types of urinary incontinence are listed in Table 24–3. A variety of behavioral therapies have been shown in randomized, controlled clinical trials to be highly effective for targeted patients. Functional, motivated patients with stress, urge, and mixed incontinence generally respond well to behavioral interventions. These interventions include education, self-monitoring with a voiding diary, modifications of fluid intake, various bladder training techniques (e.g., timed voiding and strategies to manage urgency), and pelvic muscle exercises. Many patients have difficulty isolating the appropriate pelvic muscles and benefit from adjunctive techniques, such as biofeedback (using surface electromyography of sphincteric and abdominal muscles), vaginal weights, and electrical stimulation (which can help identify and exercise pelvic muscles and help inhibit bladder activity, depending on the frequency of the stimulus). For some mobility-impaired or cognitively impaired patients in long-term care institutions and at home, reminders to void (or some other form of systematic toileting assistance) can be highly effective in managing urinary incontinence during the daytime.

Pharmacologic treatment is effective and may be combined with behavioral interventions (see Table 24–3 for specific drugs and dosages). For stress incontinence in women, α-adrenergic medications can enhance the contraction of periurethral smooth muscle. Pseudoephedrine may be helpful in some patients, but it must be used carefully in women with underlying cardiovascular disease. Duloxetine, a selective serotonin reuptake inhibitor that is approved in the United States for the treatment of depression, may also be effective for stress incontinence because it increases α-adrenergic tone to the urethra through a spinal cord mechanism; it is not, however, approved by the Food and Drug Administration for this indication. Topical estrogen may be useful in women who have stress and urge incontinence or overactive bladder symptoms and

TABLE 24–3 BASIC TYPES, CAUSES, AND TREATMENT OF PERSISTENT URINARY INCONTINENCE

Type	Clinical Manifestations	Common Causes	Primary Treatments
Stress	Involuntary loss of urine (usually small amounts) with increases in intra-abdominal pressure (e.g., cough, laugh, exercise) With sphincter weakness, symptoms may be constant wetting	Weakness of pelvic floor musculature and urethral hypermobility Bladder outlet or urethral sphincter weakness	Pelvic muscle exercises and other behavioral interventions Topical estrogen α-Adrenergic agonists (pseudoephedrine, 30–60 mg tid, or 120–240 mg sustained release daily; duloxetine, 40–60 mg daily*) Periurethral injections Surgical bladder neck suspension or sling
Urge	Leakage of urine (variable but often larger volumes) because of inability to delay voiding after sensation of bladder fullness is perceived	Detrusor overactivity, isolated or associated with one or more of the following: Local genitourinary condition such as tumors, stones, diverticula, or outflow obstruction CNS disorders such as stroke, dementia, parkinsonism, or spinal cord injury	Bladder training, pelvic muscle exercises, and other behavioral interventions Women: Topical estrogen Men: α-blockers (alfuzosin, 10 mg daily; tamsulosin, 0.4 mg daily; terazosin, 1–5 mg nightly) Bladder relaxants (darifenacin, 7.5–15 mg daily; oxybutynin short-acting, 2.5–5 mg 1–3 times daily; oxybutynin extended release, 5–30 mg daily; oxybutynin transdermal patch, one 3.9-mg patch every 3 days; solifenacin, 5–10 mg daily; tolterodine, 4 mg daily; trospium, 20 mg twice daily; start with once per day in the elderly with decreased renal function)
Overflow	Leakage of urine (usually small amounts without warning) resulting from mechanical forces on an overdistended bladder or from other effects of urinary retention on bladder and sphincter function	Anatomic obstruction by prostate, stricture, or cystocele Acontractile bladder associated with diabetes mellitus or spinal cord injury Neurogenic (detrusor-sphincter dyssynergy), associated with multiple sclerosis and other suprasacral spinal cord lesions	Surgical removal of obstruction Intermittent or chronic catheterization
Functional	Urinary accidents associated with inability to toilet because of impairment of cognitive or physical functioning, psychological unwillingness, or environmental barriers	Severe dementia and other neurologic disorders Psychological factors such as depression and hostility	Prompted voiding and other behavioral intervention Absorbent padding Drug treatment for bladder overactivity (selected patients)

*Not approved by the Food and Drug Administration for this indication.
CNS = central nervous system.

Rx

who have signs of severe vaginal atrophy or atrophic vaginitis on pelvic examination. Although data from large clinical trials suggest that oral estrogen with progestin may actually increase the risk for development of incontinence and worsen its severity, [1] topical estrogen should be considered for older postmenopausal women with bothersome symptoms of overactive bladder or incontinence.

Bladder relaxant medications can be effective in managing urge incontinence, but they often are limited by their anticholinergic side effects (especially dry mouth). Five drugs are approved for the management of urge incontinence and overactive bladder (see Table 24–3), and clinical trials suggest that all are equally efficacious. [2] These medications generally result in a 60 to 70% reduction in urge incontinence episodes and cause a 20 to 25% incidence of dry mouth, most of which is tolerable. Efficacy appears to be similar in older and younger patients. Short-acting oxybutynin has the highest incidence of side effects, but it is much less expensive and shorter acting than the other drugs, so it may be useful in selected patients for these reasons. Other side effects of concern in older patients include onset or exacerbation of constipation and gastroesophageal reflux, increased intraocular pressure in patients receiving therapy for glaucoma (which is not an absolute contraindication, but consultation with the patient's ophthalmologist is advisable), and cognitive impairment, especially in patients with preexisting mild cognitive impairment or dementia. In these last patients, careful questioning about any changes in cognition, mood, and behavior should guide therapy. α-Adrenergic blockers have been shown to improve irritative voiding symptoms, including frequency and urgency, in men with prostatic enlargement. Tamsulosin and alfuzosin appear to have

Rx

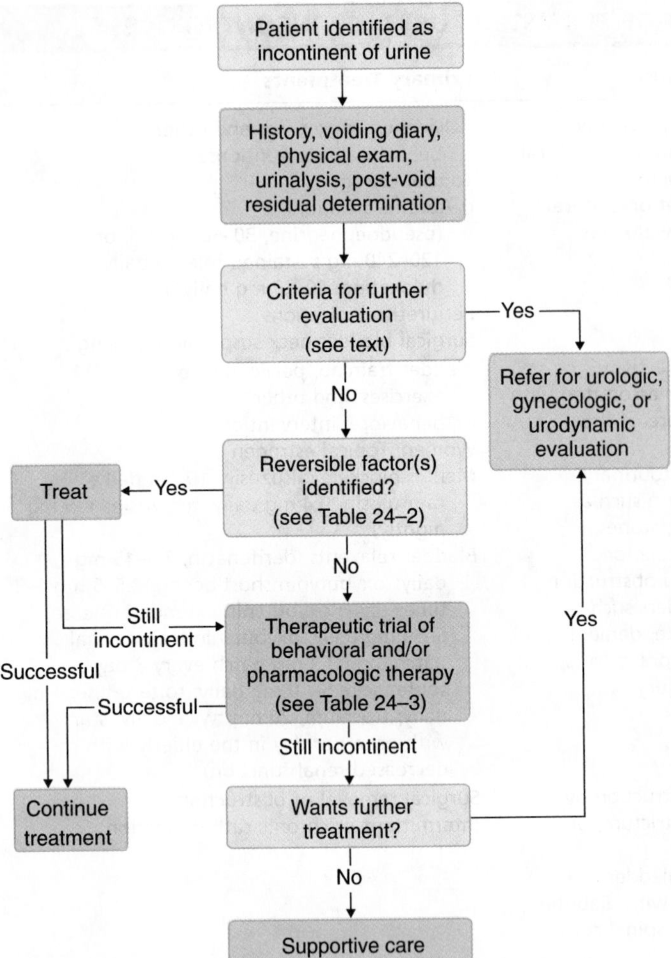

FIGURE 24–1 • Flow diagram for the evaluation and treatment of urinary incontinence in primary care practice. Criteria for further evaluation are outlined in the text.

Rx

fewer effects on blood pressure and may be safer in older men, especially those who have underlying cardiovascular disease and are taking other hypotensive agents. Pharmacologic treatment of an underactive bladder associated with chronic urinary retention and overflow incontinence is not generally effective.

Surgical treatment can be highly effective in women with stress incontinence, at least during a 1- to 5-year period. [3] Women with intrinsic sphincter weakness (as opposed to urethral hypermobility) may benefit from periurethral injections of collagen.

Future Directions

Defining the basic abnormalities that cause detrusor hyperactivity, including the role of sensory afferent innervation, is a crucial goal. New drugs and drug delivery systems to treat detrusor hyperactivity but minimize bothersome anticholinergic side effects will have a major impact on the treatment of urinary incontinence in the geriatric population.

Prevention

No strategies have proved effective in preventing urinary incontinence. Two approaches may be of some benefit, however, and are worthy of brief consideration. First, general education about bladder health and the behavioral and dietary factors that can affect it can help people understand that urinary incontinence and related urinary problems are not normal and that when such symptoms do occur, patients should seek evaluation and treatment. Second, pelvic muscle exercises may be an effective preventive measure. The long-term effectiveness of this intervention and the ability of patients to comply with an exercise program are currently under investigation.

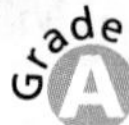

1. Hendrix SL, Cochrane BB, Nygaard IE, et al: Effects of estrogen with and without progestin on urinary incontinence. JAMA 2005; 293:935–948.
2. Herbison P, Hay-Smith J, Ellis G, et al: Effectiveness of anticholinergic drugs compared with placebo in the treatment of overactive bladder: Systematic review. BMJ 2003;326:1–7.
3. Brubaker L, Cundiff GW, Fine P, et al: Abdominal sacrocolpopexy with Burch colposuspension to reduce urinary stress incontinence. N Engl J Med 2006;354:1557–1566.

SUGGESTED READINGS

Brown JS, Bradley CS, Subak LL, et al: The sensitivity and specificity of a simple test to distinguish between urge and stress urinary incontinence. Ann Intern Med 2006;144:712–723. *The 31Q questionnaire is appropriate for use in primary care settings.*

Ouslander JG: Management of overactive bladder. N Engl J Med 2004; 350:786–799. *A comprehensive review.*

Teunissen TA, de Jonge A, van Weel C, et al: Treating urinary incontinence in the elderly—conservative therapies that work: A systematic review. J Fam Pract 2004;53:25–32. *A systematic review.*

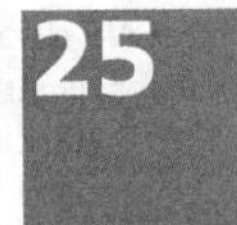

25 NEUROPSYCHIATRIC ASPECTS OF AGING

Sharon K. Inouye

Definition

The process of aging produces important physiologic changes in the central nervous system (Table 25–1), including neuroanatomic, neurotransmitter, and neurophysiologic changes. These processes result in age-related symptoms and manifestations (Table 25–2) for many older persons. These physiologic changes develop at dramatically variable rates in different older persons, however, the decline being modified by factors such as diet, environment, lifestyle, genetic predisposition, disability, disease, and side effects of drugs. These changes can result in the common age-related symptoms of benign senescence, slowed reaction time, postural hypotension, vertigo or giddiness, presbyopia, presbycusis, stiffened gait, and sleep difficulties. In the absence of disease, these physiologic changes usually result in relatively modest symptoms and little restriction in activities of daily living. These changes decrease physiologic reserve, however, and increase the susceptibility to challenges posed by disease-related, pharmacologic, and environmental stressors.

Epidemiology

Neuropsychiatric disorders, the leading cause of disability in older persons, account for nearly 50% of functional incapacity. Severe neuropsychiatric conditions have been estimated to occur in 15 to 25% of older adults worldwide. These conditions are due to diseases that increase with age but are not part of the normal aging process. Alzheimer's disease

TABLE 25–1 AGE-RELATED PHYSIOLOGIC CHANGES IN THE CENTRAL NERVOUS SYSTEM

Neuroanatomic changes
Brain atrophy
Decreased neuron counts
Increased neuritic plaques
Increased lipofuscin and melanin
Neurotransmitter changes
Decline in cholinergic transmission
Decreased dopaminergic synthesis
Decreased catecholamine synthesis
Neurophysiologic changes
Decreased cerebral blood flow
Electrophysiologic changes (slowing of alpha rhythm, increased latencies in evoked responses)

TABLE 25–2 NEUROPSYCHIATRIC MANIFESTATIONS OF AGE-RELATED PHYSIOLOGIC CHANGES

System	Manifestation
Cognition	Forgetfulness Processing speed declines throughout adult life Neuropsychological declines: selective attention, verbal fluency, retrieval, complex visual perception, logical analysis
Reflexes	Stretch reflexes lose sensitivity Decreased or absent ankle reflexes Decreased autonomic and righting reflexes, postural instability
Sensory	Presbycusis (high-frequency hearing loss), tinnitus Deterioration of vestibular system, vertigo Presbyopia (decreased lens elasticity) Slowed pupil reactivity, decreased upgaze Olfactory system deterioration Decreased vibratory sensation
Gait and balance	Gait stiffer, slowed, forward flexed Increased body sway and mild unsteadiness
Sleep	Decreased sleep efficiency, fatigue Increased awakenings, insomnia Decrease in sleep stages 3 and 4 Sleep duration more variable, more naps

TABLE 25–3 GERIATRIC DEPRESSION SCALE—SHORT FORM

1. Are you basically satisfied with your life?	yes/**NO**
2. Have you dropped many of your activities and interests?	**YES**/no
3. Do you feel that your life is empty?	**YES**/no
4. Do you often get bored?	**YES**/no
5. Are you in good spirits most of the time?	yes/**NO**
6. Are you afraid that something bad is going to happen to you?	**YES**/no
7. Do you feel happy most of the time?	yes/**NO**
8. Do you feel helpless?	**YES**/no
9. Do you prefer to stay home rather than going out and doing new things?	**YES**/no
10. Do you feel you have more problems with memory than most?	**YES**/no
11. Do you think it is wonderful to be alive now?	yes/**NO**
12. Do you feel pretty worthless the way you are now?	**YES**/no
13. Do you feel full of energy?	yes/**NO**
14. Do you feel that your situation is hopeless?	**YES**/no
15. Do you think that most people are better off than you are?	**YES**/no

Scoring: Answers indicating depression are **highlighted;** six or more highlighted answers indicate depressive symptoms.
Modified from Yesavage J, Brink T, Rowe T, et al: Development and validation of a geriatric depression screening scale: A preliminary report. J Psychiatr Res 1983;17:37–49.

and related dementias occur in approximately 10% of adults aged 65 years and older and 40% of adults older than 85 years (Chapter 425). Delirium occurs in 5 to 10% of all persons older than 65 years and in up to 80% of older persons, predominantly during hospitalizations for acute illnesses (Chapter 26). Severe depression (Chapter 420) occurs in approximately 5% of older adults, with 15% having significant depressive symptoms. Anxiety disorders occur in 10% of older adults. Older individuals also are subject to substantial morbidity and functional disability from cerebrovascular disease (Chapters 430 to 432), Parkinson's disease (Chapter 433), peripheral neuropathies (Chapter 446), degenerative myelopathies (Chapters 423 and 448), spinal stenosis and disc disease (Chapter 423), seizure disorders (Chapter 426 Epilepsies), sleep apnea (Chapter 101), falls (Chapter 23), incontinence (Chapter 24), and impotence (Chapter 253).

Diagnosis

To diagnose these conditions, physicians must understand and perform a mental status examination and an assessment of functional capacity and know the uses and side effects of psychoactive drugs in geriatric patients.

Mental Status Examination

In addition to a detailed neurologic examination, evaluation of neuropsychiatric disturbances in older persons requires a careful mental status examination, including an assessment of mood, affect, and cognition. Brief screening tests are available to evaluate these domains and to assist in the detection of potential problems requiring further evaluation and treatment. For depression screening, scores of 6 or more on the 15-item short-form Geriatric Depression Scale (Table 25–3) indicate substantial depressive symptoms requiring further evaluation. Alternative depression screening instruments include the Center for Epidemiologic Studies Depression scale (CES-D). For cognitively impaired patients, observer-rated depression scales, such as the Hamilton Depression Scale or Cornell Scale, are recommended.

Early cognitive deficits can be missed easily during conversation because intellectual impairment can be masked with intact social skills. Given the high frequency of cognitive impairment, formal cognitive screening is recommended for all older persons. Ideally, cognitive testing should evaluate at least the general domains of attention, orientation, language, memory, visuospatial ability, and conceptualization. To exclude delirium, attention should be assessed first by asking the patient to perform a task such as repeating five digits or reciting the months backward; the remainder of cognitive testing would not be useful in an inattentive patient. For further cognitive testing, many brief, practical screening instruments are available. The most widely used instrument is the Mini-Mental State Examination, a 19-item, 30-point scale that can be completed in 10 minutes (Table 25–4). A score of 25 or more generally indicates intact cognitive function, whereas a score of 24 or less requires further evaluation for potential dementia. Further bedside testing can include asking the patient to draw a clock with the hands at a set time to assess visuospatial ability and higher cortical functions. Questions to evaluate judgment and problem-solving ability in hypothetical situations, such as in a fire or when driving, can provide crucial insight into the patient's ability to function safely and independently.

Functional Assessment

Functional impairment, defined as difficulty in performing daily activities, is common among elderly persons. Although it is not routinely evaluated in the standard medical assessment, determination of the patient's degree of functional incapacity based on medical and neuropsychiatric conditions is crucial to understanding the burden of disease and its impact on the individual's daily life. The important relationship of functional status with health in older persons is reflected in the finding that functional measures are stronger predictors of mortality after hospitalization than are admitting diagnoses. Functional measures strongly predict other important hospital outcomes in the elderly, such as length of stay, functional status at discharge, future care needs, caregiver burden, risk for institutionalization, and long-term prognosis.

The functional assessment should include an assessment of the patient's ability to perform basic self-care activities of daily living and instrumental activities of daily living, the higher level activities needed for independent living. Performance of activities of daily living reflects the ability of the patient to perform basic self-care skills, such as feeding, grooming, bathing, dressing, toileting, transferring, and walking. Performance of instrumental activities of daily living reflects the ability of the patient to perform more complex tasks, including shopping, preparing meals, managing finances, housekeeping, using the telephone, taking medications, and driving or using public transportation. The functional assessment is conducted with the patient or the family, and the questions ascertain whether the patient can perform these activities independently. Other related domains that should be assessed include vision, hearing,

TABLE 25–4 MINI-MENTAL STATE EXAMINATION

Cognitive Domain	Maximum Score
ORIENTATION	
What is the (year) (season) (date) (day) (month)?	5
Where are we (city) (state) (county) (hospital) (floor)?	5
REGISTRATION	
Name 3 objects: 1 second to say each. Ask the patient for all 3 after you have said them. Give 1 point for each correct answer. Repeat them until all 3 are learned. Count the trials and record the number.	3
ATTENTION AND CALCULATION	
Serial 7s backward from 100 (stop after 5 answers). Alternatively, spell WORLD backward.	5
RECALL	
Ask for the 3 objects repeated above. Give 1 point for each correct answer.	3
LANGUAGE AND PRAXIS	
Show a pencil and watch, and ask the patient to name them.	2
Ask the patient to repeat the following: "No ifs, ands, or buts."	1
Three-stage command: "Take this paper in your right hand, fold it in half, and put it on the floor."	3
"Read and obey the following: Close your eyes."	1
"Write a sentence."	1
"Copy this design" (interlocking pentagons).	1

A score of 25 or more signifies intact cognitive function.
Modified from Folstein MF, Folstein SE, McHugh PR: "The Mini-Mental State": A practical method for grading the cognitive state of patients for the clinician. J Psychiatr Res 1975;12:189–198.

TABLE 25–5 DRUGS WITH PSYCHOACTIVE EFFECTS

- Sedative-hypnotics
  - Benzodiazepines (especially flurazepam, diazepam)
  - Barbiturates
  - Sleeping medications (chloral hydrate)
- Narcotics (especially meperidine)
- Anticholinergics
  - Antihistamines (diphenhydramine, hydroxyzine)
  - Antispasmodics (belladonna, Lomotil)
  - Heterocyclic antidepressants (amitriptyline, imipramine, doxepin)
  - Neuroleptics (chlorpromazine, haloperidol, thioridazine)
  - Antiparkinsonian (benztropine, trihexyphenidyl)
  - Atropine, scopolamine
- Cardiac
  - Digitalis glycosides
  - Antiarrhythmics (quinidine, procainamide, lidocaine)
  - Antihypertensives (β-blockers, methyldopa)
- Gastrointestinal
  - H_2-antagonists (cimetidine, ranitidine, famotidine, nizatidine)
  - Metoclopramide (Reglan)
- Miscellaneous
  - Nonsteroidal anti-inflammatory drugs
  - Corticosteroids
  - Anticonvulsants
  - Levodopa
  - Lithium
- Over-the-counter drugs
  - Cold and sinus preparations (antihistamines, pseudoephedrine)
  - Sleep aids (diphenhydramine, alcohol-containing elixirs)
  - Stay Awake (caffeine)
  - Nausea, gastrointestinal (Donnagel, meclizine, H_2-antagonists, loperamide)

continence, nutritional status, safety, falls, living situation, social supports, and socioeconomic status.

The onset of acute cognitive or functional decline is often the first and sometimes the only sign of serious acute illness in older persons and warrants immediate medical attention. Similarly, the onset or worsening of related conditions, such as delirium, falls, incontinence, depression, or failure to thrive, heralds the need for prompt medical evaluation.

Treatment

Psychoactive Effects of Drugs in Older Patients

Adverse Drug Events in the Elderly

Iatrogenic complications occur in 29 to 38% of older hospitalized patients, with a three-fold to five-fold increased risk in older compared with younger patients. Adverse drug events, the most common type of iatrogenic complication, account for 20 to 40% of all complications. The elderly are particularly vulnerable to adverse drug reactions because of multiple-drug regimens, multiple chronic diseases, relative renal and hepatic insufficiency, decreased physiologic reserve, and altered drug metabolism with aging. Inappropriate drug use has been reported in about 40% of hospitalized older patients, with more than one quarter of these patients having absolute contraindications to the drug and the others being given a drug that was unnecessary. Because 50% of adverse drug events occur in patients receiving inappropriate drugs, the potential for reducing these adverse events is substantial.

Rx

Drugs with Psychoactive Effects

Nearly every class of drugs has the potential to cause delirium in a vulnerable patient, but specific drugs have been most commonly implicated (Table 25–5) and should be used with caution in older patients. Many cases of delirium or cognitive decline in older patients may be preventable through avoidance, substitution, or dose reduction of these psychoactive drugs. Long-acting benzodiazepines (e.g., flurazepam and diazepam) are particularly problematic medications for the elderly and should be avoided whenever possible. If nonpharmacologic approaches to the management of insomnia are unsuccessful, short-term use of an intermediate-acting benzodiazepine without active metabolites (e.g., lorazepam, 0.5 mg, half-life of 10 to 15 hours) is recommended. Drugs with anticholinergic effects (e.g., antihistamines, antidepressants, neuroleptics, antispasmodics) produce a panoply of poorly tolerated side effects in older patients, including delirium, postural hypotension, urinary retention, constipation, and dry mouth. Of the narcotics, meperidine causes delirium more frequently than other agents because of an active metabolite, normeperidine. Cardiac drugs, such as digitalis and antiarrhythmic agents, have prolonged half-lives, narrowed therapeutic windows, and decreased protein binding in older patients. The clinician should be aware that toxicity with these agents (e.g., digoxin) can occur even at therapeutic drug levels. The H_2-receptor antagonists (e.g., cimetidine, ranitidine, famotidine, nizatidine) are among the most common causes of drug-induced delirium in the elderly because of their frequent use; clinicians should strongly consider the use of less toxic alternatives (e.g., sucralfate or antacids) or dosage reduction for older patients, especially when the medication is being used for prophylaxis rather than treatment of active disease. Proton pump inhibitors have been asso-

Rx

ciated with delirium in case reports; however, the overall rate of this adverse effect has not been systematically determined.

Psychoactive drugs account for nearly 50% of preventable adverse drug events, often in patients in whom three or more psychoactive drugs are prescribed, frequently at inappropriately high doses in the elderly. Delirium and cognitive impairment are the most frequent adverse outcomes of psychoactive drugs. The use of any psychoactive drug is associated with a four-fold increased risk of delirium or cognitive decline, but the outcomes of delirium and cognitive decline depend on the type or class of drug administered and total number of drugs received. Sedative-hypnotic drugs are associated with a 3-fold to 12-fold increased risk for delirium or cognitive decline, narcotics are associated with a 2-fold to 3-fold increased risk, and anticholinergic drugs are associated with a 5-fold to 12-fold increased risk. When more drugs are used, not only does each carry its own individual risk for adverse outcomes, but also the overall risk is compounded by the heightened potential for drug-drug interactions. If more than three drugs are added in a 24-hour period, the risk of delirium increases four-fold. Similarly, the risk of cognitive decline increases directly with the number of drugs prescribed, from a 3-fold increased risk with two or three drugs to a 14-fold increased risk with six or more drugs.

Principles of Drug Therapy in the Elderly

Physicians always should consider whether nonpharmacologic approaches (Chapter 36) may be used as alternatives to medications in older persons. Relaxation techniques, massage, and music are highly effective for the treatment of insomnia and anxiety; localized pain often can be managed effectively with local measures, such as injection, heat, ultrasound, and transcutaneous electrical stimulation.

When drug therapy is required in the elderly, physicians should choose the drug with the least toxic potential and emphasize drugs that have been well tested in older populations (Table 25–6). When the drug is chosen, it is often wise to start with 25 to 50% of the standard adult dosage for psychoactive drugs and increase the dose slowly. Drug regimens should be kept as simple as possible, with the fewest drugs and the fewest number of pills possible. Most important, the medication list should be reassessed frequently. Systematic interventions involving geriatricians and clinical pharmacists can significantly reduce the frequency of adverse drug reactions in older persons. 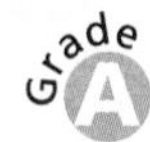

Even long-standing medications should be re-evaluated because the host is changing with age and illness. Long-term use does not justify continued use. The physician should review with the patient all prescribed and over-the-counter medications on a regular basis, preferably by having the patient bring in all medication bottles and indicate how each is being taken. Patients frequently underestimate the toxic potential of over-the-counter medications and herbal remedies, and they may be using a variety of such agents that could potentiate the side effects or directly counteract the desired effects of prescription medications (Chapter 27). For example, gingko biloba may interact with warfarin to cause bleeding, and many herbal remedies (such as kava kava and Chinese herbal preparations) are associated with the risk of hepatotoxicity.

TABLE 25–6 GUIDELINES FOR DRUG THERAPY IN THE ELDERLY

GENERAL PRINCIPLES

Remember that the elderly are highly sensitive to the psychoactive effects of all drugs.

Know the pharmacology of the drugs you prescribe. Know a few drugs well.

RECOMMENDED APPROACH

Use nonpharmacologic approaches whenever possible.

Avoid *routine* use of "as needed" drugs for sleep, anxiety, pain.

Choose the drug with the least toxic potential.

Substitute less toxic alternatives whenever possible (antacid or sucralfate for an H_2-blocker or proton pump inhibitors, Metamucil or Kaopectate for Imodium, scheduled acetaminophen regimen for pain management).

Reduce the dosage.

"Start low and go slow."

- Start with 25–50% of the standard dose of psychoactive drugs in the elderly.
- Titrate the drug slowly.
- Set realistic end points: titrate to improvement, not elimination of symptoms.

Keep the regimen simple.

Regularly reassess the medication list. Have the patient bring in all bottles and review what is being taken.

Re-evaluate long-time drug use because the patient is changing.

Review over-the-counter medication use.

Future Directions

Screening methods for cognitive and functional decline in older persons will continue to be refined and simplified. An important future direction will be to incorporate these screening and intervention measures into the routine care of all older persons in physicians' offices, clinics, hospitals, nursing homes, and other settings.

Grade A

1. Schmader KE, Hanlon JT, Pieper CF, et al: Effects of geriatric evaluation and management on adverse drug reactions and suboptimal prescribing in the frail elderly. Am J Med 2004;116:394–401.
2. Rollason V, Vogt N: Reduction of polypharmacy in the elderly: A systematic review of the role of the pharmacist. Drugs Aging 2003;20:817–832.

SUGGESTED READINGS

Juurlink DN, Mamdani M, Kopp A, et al: Drug-drug interactions among elderly patients hospitalized for drug toxicity. JAMA 2003;289:1652–1658. *Study of 909 older persons demonstrated that many admissions for drug toxicity were due to well-known and readily avoidable drug-drug interactions.*

Karlawish JHT, Clark CM: Diagnostic evaluation of elderly patients with mild memory problems. Ann Intern Med 2003;138:411–419. *Case-based discussion emphasizing a stepwise approach.*

Monastero R, Palmer K, Qui C, et al: Heterogeneity in risk factors for cognitive impairment, no dementia: Population-based longitudinal study from the Kungsholmen Project. Am J Geriatr Psychiatry 2007;15:60–69. *Shows that cognitive dysfunction without dementia, which is increased by polypharmacy, psychoses, and hip fracture, is then a risk factor for subsequent dementia.*

26 DELIRIUM AND OTHER MENTAL STATUS PROBLEMS IN THE OLDER PATIENT

Sharon K. Inouye

Mental status change, one of the most common presenting symptoms in acutely ill elders, is estimated to account for 30% of emergency evaluations for older patients. Mental status often serves as a barometer of the underlying health of an elderly patient and is commonly the only symptom of serious underlying disease. A broad range of medical, neurologic, and psychiatric conditions can lead to mental status changes (Chapters 420 and 425). A systematic approach aids in the evaluation of suspected mental status change in an older patient (see Fig. 26–1).

The first step in evaluating suspected altered mental status in an older patient is to obtain a detailed history from a reliable informant to establish the patient's baseline level of cognitive function and the clinical course of any cognitive changes. Chronic changes (i.e., changes occurring over months to years) most likely represent an underlying dementing illness, which should be evaluated accordingly (Chapter 425). Acute changes (i.e., changes occurring over days to weeks)—even if superimposed on an underlying dementia—should be evaluated further by detailed cognitive assessment to determine whether delirium is present. If features of delirium (e.g., inattention, disorganized thinking, altered level of consciousness, fluctuating symptoms) are not present, further evaluation for depression, acute nonorganic psychotic disorders, or other psychiatric conditions is indicated.

DELIRIUM

Delirium, a clinical syndrome characterized as an acute disorder of attention and cognitive function, is the most frequent complication of hospitalization for elders and a potentially devastating problem. Delirium often is unrecognized despite sensitive methods for its detection, and its complications may be preventable.

Definition

The definition and diagnostic criteria for delirium are evolving. The *Diagnostic and Statistical Manual of Mental Disorders,* fourth edition, has been used widely (Table 26–1), but development of the criteria in this manual was based on expert consensus, and their diagnostic sensitivity and specificity have not been determined. The Confusion Assessment Method provides a simple, operationalized diagnostic algorithm with a sensitivity of 94 to 100%, a specificity of 90 to 95%, and a high interrater reliability.

TABLE 26–1 DIAGNOSTIC CRITERIA FOR DELIRIUM

DSM-IV DIAGNOSTIC CRITERIA

A. Disturbance of consciousness (i.e., reduced clarity of awareness of the environment) with reduced ability to focus, sustain, or shift attention

B. A change in cognition (e.g., memory deficit, disorientation, language disturbance) or the development of a perceptual disturbance that is not better accounted for by a preexisting, established, or evolving dementia

C. The disturbance develops over a short period (usually hours to days) and tends to fluctuate during the course of the day

D. Evidence from the history, physical examination, or laboratory findings indicates that the disturbance is caused by the direct physiologic consequences of a general medical condition

CAM DIAGNOSTIC ALGORITHM*

Feature 1. Acute onset and fluctuating course

This feature is usually obtained from a family member or nurse and is shown by positive responses to the following questions: Is there evidence of an acute change in mental status from the patient's baseline? Did the (abnormal) behavior fluctuate during the day, that is, tend to come and go, or increase and decrease in severity?

Feature 2. Inattention

This feature is shown by a positive response to the following question: Did the patient have difficulty focusing attention, for example, being easily distractible or having difficulty keeping track of what was being said?

Feature 3. Disorganized thinking

This feature is shown by a positive response to the following question: Was the patient's thinking disorganized or incoherent such as rambling or irrelevant conversation, unclear or illogical flow of ideas, or unpredictable and switching from subject to subject?

Feature 4. Altered level of consciousness

This feature is shown by any answer other than "alert" to the following question: Overall, how would you rate this patient's level of consciousness (alert [normal], vigilant [hyperalert], lethargic [drowsy, easily aroused], stupor [difficult to arouse], or coma [unarousable])?

*The diagnosis of delirium by CAM requires the presence of features 1 and 2 and either 3 or 4.

DSM-IV = American Psychiatric Association: *Diagnostic and Statistical Manual of Mental Disorders,* fourth edition. Washington, DC, American Psychiatric Association, 1994; CAM = Confusion Assessment Method.

From Inouye SK, van Dyck CH, Alessi CA, et al: Clarifying confusion: The Confusion Assessment Method. A new method for detection of delirium. Ann Intern Med 1990;113:941–948.

Epidemiology

In the elderly, the prevalence of delirium at hospital admission is 13 to 60%. Delirium develops anew in 6 to 56% of patients during hospitalization. Higher rates are found when frequent surveillance is performed in older, surgical, and intensive care populations. Delirium occurs in 15 to 74% of postoperative patients and 60 to 80% of patients in medical intensive care units.

The associated hospital mortality rates for delirium are 25 to 33%, rates as high as those associated with acute myocardial infarction and sepsis. The problem of delirium in hospitalized elderly patients has assumed particular prominence because patients aged 65 years and older currently account for about 50% of all inpatient days of hospital care. Based on U.S. vital health statistics, delirium complicates hospital stays for at least 20% of the 12.5 million older persons hospitalized each year and increases hospital costs by more than $2500 per patient, amounting to more than $6.9 billion (2004 U.S. dollars) of Medicare expenditures yearly. Substantial additional costs are incurred after hospital discharge because of the increased need for rehabilitation services, nursing home placement, and home care. These extrapolations highlight the extensive economic and health policy implications of delirium.

Pathogenesis

Similar to other common geriatric syndromes (Chapter 23), delirium usually has multifactorial causes. A search for the innumerable potential underlying contributors requires clinical astuteness and a thorough medical evaluation, especially because many of these factors are treatable but, if untreated, may result in substantial morbidity and mortality. The process is made more challenging by the frequently nonspecific, atypical, or muted features of the underlying illness in older persons. Delirium is commonly the only initial sign of underlying life-threatening illness, such as pneumonia (Chapter 97), urosepsis (Chapter 306), or myocardial infarction (Chapter 72), in the older population.

The development of delirium usually involves a complex interrelationship between a vulnerable patient with pertinent predisposing factors and exposure to noxious insults or precipitating factors. Delirium may develop in vulnerable patients, such as cognitively impaired or severely ill patients, after a relatively benign insult, such as a single dose of sleeping medication. Conversely, in patients who are not vulnerable, delirium would develop only after exposure to multiple noxious insults. Previous studies have shown that the effects of these risk factors may be cumulative. The importance of this multifactorial causation to the clinician is that removal or treatment of one factor in isolation usually is not sufficient to resolve the delirium. The full spectrum of vulnerability and precipitating factors should be addressed.

Predisposing, or vulnerability, factors include preexisting cognitive impairment or dementia, severe underlying illness, high levels of comorbidity, functional impairment, advanced age, chronic renal insufficiency, dehydration, malnutrition, and vision or hearing impairment. Dementia is an important and consistent risk factor for delirium; demented patients have a two-fold to five-fold increased risk for delirium. Of delirious patients, 30 to 50% have underlying dementia. Delirious patients commonly have evidence of underlying chronic brain disease, particularly conditions associated with cognitive impairment, such as Alzheimer's disease, Parkinson's disease, cerebrovascular disease, and space-occupying lesions.

Medications, the most common remediable cause of delirium, contribute to delirium in 40% of cases (Chapter 25). Insufficiency or failure of any major organ system, particularly renal or hepatic failure, can precipitate delirium. Hypoxemia and hypercarbia have been associated with delirium. Clinicians must be attuned to occult respiratory failure, which in the elderly often lacks the usual signs and symptoms of dyspnea and tachypnea and can be missed by measurement of oxygen saturation alone. Acute myocardial infarction or heart failure can be manifested as delirium in an elderly patient without the usual symptoms of chest pain or dyspnea. Occult infection is a particularly notable cause of delirium. Older patients frequently fail to mount the febrile or leukocytotic response to infection, and clinicians must assess carefully for signs of pneumonia, urinary tract infection, endocarditis, abdominal abscess, or infected joints. A variety of metabolic disorders may contribute to delirium, including hypernatremia or hyponatremia, hypercalcemia, acid-base disorders, hypoglycemia and hyperglycemia, and thyroid or adrenal disorders. Immobilization and immobilizing devices (e.g., indwelling bladder catheters, physical restraints) have been shown to be important factors in precipitating delirium. Dehydration and volume depletion and nutritional decline during hospitalization (e.g., decline in weight, fall in serum albumin concentration) are well-documented factors contributing to delirium. Drug and alcohol withdrawal are important and often unsuspected causes of delirium in the elderly. Environmental factors, such as unfamiliar surroundings, sleep deprivation, deranged schedule, frequent room changes, sensory overload, and sensory deprivation, may aggravate delirium in the hospital. Psychosocial factors, such as depression, psychological stress, pain, and lack of social supports, also may precipitate delirium.

The basic pathogenesis of delirium is unclear. Most investigators agree that delirium seems to be a functional rather than structural lesion. Electroencephalographic studies show global functional derangements in patients with delirium, characterized by generalized slowing of cortical background activity with appearance of delta and theta activity. Neuroimaging studies coupled with cognitive testing demonstrate generalized disruption in higher cortical function, with dysfunction in prefrontal cortex, frontal and temporoparietal cortex, fusiform cortex, lingual gyri, subcortical structures, thalamus, and basal ganglia. The leading hypotheses for the pathogenesis of delirium focus on the roles of neurotransmission and inflammation. The most widely postulated mechanism for delirium is the failure of cholinergic transmission. Evidence supporting this hypothesis includes the frequent association of anticholinergic drugs with delirium, the reversal of delirium with pro-cholinergic drugs such as physostigmine, the increased levels of serum anticholinergic activity in some delirious patients, and the benefit of cholinesterase inhibitors for some delirium cases. Other neurotransmitter systems, such as dopamine, serotonin, tryptophan, norepinephrine, and γ-aminobutyric acid, may also play a role in delirium, but the evidence is less well developed. In special circumstances, such as infections or cancer, delirium may be mediated through cytokines, such as interleukin-2 and tumor necrosis factor. Although delirium has long been considered a transient syndrome, several of these basic mechanisms may not be completely reversible, particularly mechanisms resulting in hypoxic damage. The dose and duration of the noxious insults, along with the degree of vulnerability of the patient, also may exert great influence on the ultimate reversibility of the delirium.

Clinical Manifestations

The cardinal features of delirium include acute onset and inattention. Establishing the acuity of onset requires accurate knowledge of the patient's baseline cognitive function. Patients are inattentive; that is, they have difficulty focusing, maintaining, and shifting attention. They appear easily distracted and have difficulty maintaining conversation and following commands. Objectively, patients may have difficulty with simple repetitive tasks, digit spans, and recitation of months backward. Other key features include disorganization of thought processes, which is usually a manifestation of underlying cognitive or perceptual disturbances; altered level of consciousness, which typically is lethargy with reduced clarity of awareness of the environment; and fluctuation of cognitive symptoms. Although not cardinal elements, other features frequently occurring during delirium include disorientation, cognitive deficits, psychomotor agitation or retardation, perceptual disturbances such as hallucinations and illusions, paranoid delusions, and sleep-wake cycle reversal.

TABLE 26–2 EVALUATION OF DELIRIUM IN ELDERLY PATIENTS

Cognitive testing and determination of baseline cognitive functioning: establish the diagnosis of delirium.
Obtain a comprehensive history and perform physical examination, including careful neurologic examination for focal deficits and a search for occult infection.
Review the medication list: discontinue or minimize all psychoactive medications. Check the side effects of all medications.
Laboratory evaluation (tailored to the individual): complete blood count, electrolytes, blood urea nitrogen, creatinine, glucose, calcium, phosphate, liver enzymes, oxygen saturation.
Search for occult infection: physical examination, urinalysis, chest radiography, selected cultures (as indicated).
When no obvious cause is revealed from these steps, further targeted evaluation is considered in selected patients:
Laboratory tests: magnesium, thyroid function tests, B_{12} level, drug levels, toxicology screen, ammonia level
Arterial blood gas analysis: indicated in patients with dyspnea, tachypnea, any acute pulmonary process, or history of significant respiratory disease
Electrocardiography: indicated in patients with chest or abdominal discomfort, shortness of breath, or cardiac history
Cerebrospinal fluid examination: indicated when meningitis or encephalitis is suspected
Brain imaging: indicated in patients with new focal neurologic signs or with a history or signs of head trauma
Electroencephalography: useful in diagnosis of occult seizure disorder and in differentiation of delirium from nonorganic psychiatric disorders

Diagnosis

The cornerstone of evaluation of delirium is a comprehensive history and physical examination. The first step in evaluation (Table 26–2) is to establish the diagnosis of delirium through cognitive assessment and to determine whether the present condition represents an acute change from the patient's baseline cognitive function. Because cognitive impairment may not be apparent during conversation, brief cognitive screening tests, such as the Mini-Mental Status Examination and the Confusion Assessment Method (CAM), should be used. Attention should be assessed further with simple tests, such as a forward digit span (inattention indicated by an inability to repeat five digits forward) or recitation of the months backward. A delirium assessment for nonverbal (e.g., intubated) patients, called the CAM-ICU, has been developed. The history, which should be obtained from a reliable informant, is targeted to establish the patient's baseline cognitive function and the time course of any mental status change and to obtain clues about potential precipitating factors, such as recent medication changes, intercurrent infections, or medical illness. Physical examination should include a detailed neurologic examination for focal deficits and a careful search for signs of occult infection or an acute abdominal process.

Review of the medication list, including over-the-counter medications, is crucial, and use of medications with psychoactive effects should be discontinued or minimized whenever possible. In the elderly, these medications may cause psychoactive effects even at doses and measured drug levels that are within the "therapeutic range." Consideration should be given to the possibility that withdrawal from alcohol or other medications is a contributor to delirium.

Laboratory Findings

Laboratory evaluation must be tailored to the individual situation (see Table 26–2). In patients with preexisting cardiac or respiratory diseases or related symptoms, electrocardiography or arterial blood gas determination may be indicated. The need for cerebrospinal fluid examination is controversial except when it is clearly indicated, such as in a febrile delirious patient. Brain imaging should be reserved for patients with new focal neurologic signs, for patients with a history or signs of head trauma, and for patients without another identifiable cause of the delirium. Electroencephalography, with a false-negative rate of 17% and a false-positive rate of 22% for distinguishing delirious from nondelirious patients, has a limited role and is most useful for detection of an occult seizure disorder and in differentiation of delirium from psychiatric disorders.

Differential Diagnosis

A crucial difficulty in the differential diagnosis of delirium is distinguishing a long-standing confusional state (dementia) from delirium alone or delirium superimposed on dementia (Fig. 26–1). These two conditions are differentiated by the acute onset of symptoms in delirium (dementia is much more insidious) and the impaired attention and altered level of consciousness associated with delirium. The differential diagnosis also includes depression and nonorganic psychotic disorders. Although paranoia, hallucinations, and affective changes can occur with delirium, the key features of acute onset, inattention, altered level of consciousness, and global cognitive impairment assist in the recognition of delirium. At times, the differential diagnosis can be difficult, particularly with an uncooperative patient or when an accurate history is unavailable. Because of the potentially life-threatening nature of delirium, it is prudent to manage the patient as having delirium and to search for underlying precipitants (e.g., intercurrent illness, metabolic derangements, drug toxicity) until further information can be obtained.

TABLE 26–3 DELIRIUM RISK FACTORS AND POTENTIAL INTERVENTIONS

Risk Factor	Interventions
Cognitive impairment	Reality orientation program (reorienting techniques, communication) Therapeutic activities program
Sleep deprivation	Noise reduction strategies Scheduling of nighttime medications, procedures, and nursing activities to allow uninterrupted period of sleep
Immobilization	Early mobilization (e.g., ambulation or bedside exercises) Minimizing immobilizing equipment (e.g., bladder catheters)
Psychoactive medications	Restricted use of "as needed" sleep and psychoactive medications (e.g., sedative-hypnotics, narcotics, anticholinergic medications) Nonpharmacologic protocols for management of sleep and anxiety
Vision impairment	Provision of vision aids (e.g., magnifiers, special lighting) Provision of adaptive equipment (e.g., illuminated phone dials, large-print books)
Hearing impairment	Provision of amplifying devices Repair of hearing aids
Dehydration	Early recognition and volume repletion

Treatment

Rx

Prevention

The most effective strategy to reduce delirium and its associated complications is primary prevention of delirium before it occurs. Preventive strategies should address important delirium risk factors and target patients at a moderate to high risk for delirium at baseline (Table 26–3). Randomized trials have shown that a geriatrics consultation [1] or a multidisciplinary intervention [2,3] aimed at the risk factors for delirium can reduce the incidence of delirium by 40%. On a larger scale, preventive efforts for delirium require system-wide changes to educate physicians and nurses to improve recognition and heighten awareness of the clinical implications, to provide incentives to change practice patterns that lead to delirium (e.g., immobilization, use of sleep medications, bladder catheters, and physical restraints), and to create systems that enhance high-quality geriatric care (e.g., geriatric expertise, case management, clinical pathways, and quality monitoring).

Medical Therapy

In general, nonpharmacologic approaches should be used in all delirious patients and usually are successful for symptom management. Pharmacologic approaches should be reserved for patients in whom the delirium symptoms may result in interruption of needed medical therapies (e.g., intubation, intravenous lines) or may endanger the safety of the patient or other persons. No drug is ideal for the treatment of delirium symptoms, however; any choice may cloud the patient's mental status further and obscure efforts to monitor the course of the mental status change. Any drug chosen should be given in the lowest dose for the shortest time possible. Neuroleptics are the preferred agents of treatment. Haloperidol, the most widely used agent, causes less orthostatic hypotension and fewer anticholinergic side effects than thioridazine does and is available in parenteral form; however, it has a higher rate of extrapyramidal side effects and acute dystonias. If parenteral administration is required, intravenous use results in rapid onset of action with a short duration of effect, whereas intramuscular use has a more optimal duration of action and is preferred. The recommended starting dose is 0.5 to 1 mg of haloperidol orally or parenterally, repeated every 30 minutes after the vital signs have been rechecked until sedation has been achieved. The end point should be an awake but manageable patient. The average elderly patient who has not been treated previously with neuroleptics should require a total loading dose of no more than 3 to 5 mg of haloperidol. Subsequently, a maintenance dose consisting of half of the loading dose should be administered in divided doses during the next 24 hours, with doses tapered in the next few days as the agitation resolves.

Benzodiazepines are not recommended for the first-line treatment of delirium because of their tendency to cause oversedation and exacerbate the confusional state. They remain the drugs of choice, however, for treatment of withdrawal syndromes from alcohol and sedative drugs (Chapters 31 and 32).

Nonpharmacologic management techniques recommended for every delirious patient include encouraging the presence of family members, use of "sitters" to be orienting influences, and transfer of a disruptive patient to a private room or closer to the nurse's station for increased supervision. Interpersonal contact and communication, including verbal reorientation strategies, simple instructions and explanations, and frequent eye contact, are vital. Patients should be involved in their own care and allowed to participate in decision making as much as possible. Eyeglasses and hearing aids may reduce sensory deficits. Mobility, self-care, and independence should be encouraged, and physical restraints should be avoided, if possible, because of their tendency to increase agitation, their questionable efficacy, and their potential to cause injury. Attention must be focused on minimizing the disruptive influences of the hospital environment. Clocks and calendars should be provided to assist with orientation. Room and staff changes should be kept to a minimum. A quiet environment with low-level lighting is optimal for delirious patients. Perhaps the most important intervention is to schedule checking of vital signs, administration of medications, and procedures to allow an uninterrupted period for sleep at night. Nonpharmacologic approaches to relaxation, including music, relaxation tapes, and massage, can be highly effective.

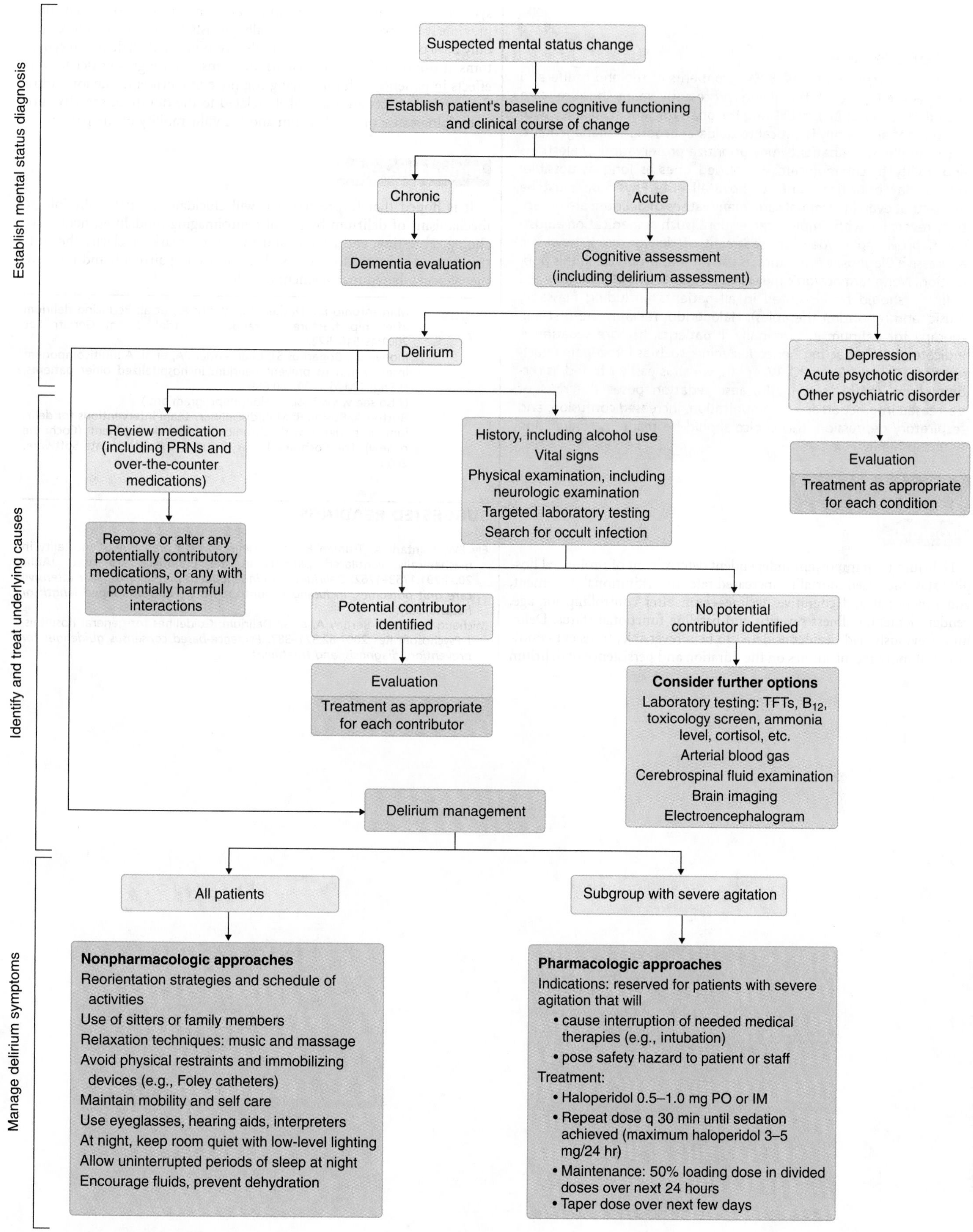

Establish mental status diagnosis

Suspected mental status change

↓

Establish patient's baseline cognitive functioning and clinical course of change

→ Chronic → Dementia evaluation

→ Acute → Cognitive assessment (including delirium assessment)

- → Depression / Acute psychotic disorder / Other psychiatric disorder → Evaluation; Treatment as appropriate for each condition
- → Delirium

Identify and treat underlying causes

Delirium →

- Review medication (including PRNs and over-the-counter medications) → Remove or alter any potentially contributory medications, or any with potentially harmful interactions
- History, including alcohol use; Vital signs; Physical examination, including neurologic examination; Targeted laboratory testing; Search for occult infection
  - → Potential contributor identified → Evaluation; Treatment as appropriate for each contributor
  - → No potential contributor identified → **Consider further options**: Laboratory testing: TFTs, B_{12}, toxicology screen, ammonia level, cortisol, etc.; Arterial blood gas; Cerebrospinal fluid examination; Brain imaging; Electroencephalogram
- → Delirium management

Manage delirium symptoms

Delirium management →

All patients →

Nonpharmacologic approaches

- Reorientation strategies and schedule of activities
- Use of sitters or family members
- Relaxation techniques: music and massage
- Avoid physical restraints and immobilizing devices (e.g., Foley catheters)
- Maintain mobility and self care
- Use eyeglasses, hearing aids, interpreters
- At night, keep room quiet with low-level lighting
- Allow uninterrupted periods of sleep at night
- Encourage fluids, prevent dehydration

Subgroup with severe agitation →

Pharmacologic approaches

Indications: reserved for patients with severe agitation that will

- cause interruption of needed medical therapies (e.g., intubation)
- pose safety hazard to patient or staff

Treatment:

- Haloperidol 0.5–1.0 mg PO or IM
- Repeat dose q 30 min until sedation achieved (maximum haloperidol 3–5 mg/24 hr)
- Maintenance: 50% loading dose in divided doses over next 24 hours
- Taper dose over next few days

FIGURE 26–1 • Algorithm for evaluation of suspected mental status change in an older patient. PRN = as needed; TFTs = thyroid function tests.

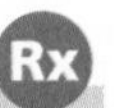

End-of-Life Care

Delirium occurs in at least 80% of patients at the end of life and is considered part of the dying process by many hospice care providers (Chapter 3). Establishing the goals for care in advance with the patient and family is critical to guide appropriate management. For example, some patients may prioritize preservation of alertness and ability to communicate with loved ones as long as possible; others may prioritize comfort above all else. Physicians must be aware that even in terminal care, many causes of delirium are potentially reversible with simple interventions (such as medication adjustment, providing oxygen, or treatment of dehydration); however, aggressive diagnostic evaluation is usually inappropriate in this population. Nonpharmacologic measures for treatment of agitation and delirium should be instituted in all patients (including massage, music, and relaxation therapies). Haloperidol remains the first-line therapy for delirium in terminally ill patients. If more sedation is indicated, a short-acting benzodiazepine, such as lorazepam (starting dose, 0.5 to 1.0 mg PO, IV, or SC), which is easily titrated, is recommended in this setting. Because sedation poses the risks of decreased interaction and communication, increased confusion, and respiratory depression, this choice should be made in conjunction with the family.

Prognosis

Delirium is an important independent determinant of prolonged hospital stay, increased mortality, increased rates of institutional placement, and functional and cognitive decline—even after controlling for age, gender, dementia, illness severity, and baseline functional status. Delirium previously had been considered to be a reversible, transient condition, but more recent studies on the duration and persistence of delirium symptoms document that delirium may be much more persistent than previously believed. Delirium typically persists for 30 days or more, and only 20% of patients may have complete resolution of all delirium symptoms at 6-month follow-up. Delirium seems to have greater deleterious effects in patients with underlying cognitive impairment. The long-term detrimental effects are most likely related to the duration, severity, and underlying cause of the delirium and the vulnerability of the patient.

Future Directions

It is hoped that future research will elucidate the pathophysiologic mechanisms of delirium by use of neuroimaging modalities, neuropsychological testing, and genetic and laboratory markers; clarify the contribution of delirium to irreversible cognitive impairment; and improve the evidence-based management of delirium.

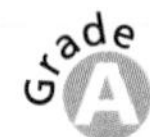

1. Marcantonio ER, Flacker JM, Wright RJ, et al: Reducing delirium after hip fracture: A randomized trial. J Am Geriatr Soc 2001;49:516–522.
2. Inouye SK, Bogardus ST, Charpentier PA, et al: A multicomponent intervention to prevent delirium in hospitalized older patients. N Engl J Med 1999;340:669–676. (Also see www.hospitalelderlifeprogram.org.)
3. Britton A, Russell R: Multidisciplinary team interventions for delirium in patients with chronic cognitive impairment (Cochrane review). The Cochrane Library, Issue 4. Oxford, Update Software, 2003.

SUGGESTED READINGS

Ely EW, Shintani A, Truman B, et al: Delirium as a predictor of mortality in mechanically ventilated patients in the intensive care unit. JAMA 2004;291:1753–1762. *Delirium is an independent predictor of poor intensive care unit outcomes, including 6-month mortality and prolonged length of hospital stay.*

Michaud L, Bula C, Berney A, et al: Delirium: Guidelines for general hospitals. J Psychosom Res 2007;62:371–383. *Evidence-based consensus guidelines for prevention, diagnosis, and treatment.*

Section V

Clinical Pharmacology

27 PRINCIPLES OF DRUG THERAPY

Robert B. Diasio

Under different conditions, a drug may produce diverse effects ranging from no effect to a desirable effect or, in other cases, an undesirable, toxic effect. Physicians must learn how to individualize the drug dosage under different conditions to ensure effective and safe therapy. This necessitates understanding the pharmacokinetics—the movement of a drug over time through the body—and the pharmacodynamics—the relationship between drug concentration and drug effect (Fig. 27–1). This chapter presents a review of the basic concepts of pharmacokinetics and pharmacodynamics, followed by guidelines on how to use this information to optimize therapeutic applications. Drug interactions and adverse drug responses are discussed with advice on how both can be recognized and minimized in clinical practice.

PHARMACOKINETIC PRINCIPLES

Administration

The most efficient and straightforward means of administering a drug into the systemic circulation is by intravenous injection of the drug as a bolus. With this route, the full amount of a drug is delivered to the systemic circulation almost immediately. The same dose also may be administered as an intravenous infusion during a longer time, resulting in a decrease in the peak plasma concentration with an accompanying increase in the time the drug is present in the circulation. Many other routes of administration can be used, including sublingual, oral, transdermal, rectal, inhalation, subcutaneous, and intramuscular; each of these routes carries not only a potential delay in the time it takes the drug to enter the circulation but also the possibility that a large fraction of it will never reach the circulation.

Absorption

Absorption refers to the transfer of a drug from the site where it was administered to the systemic circulation. Many drugs cross a membrane barrier by passive diffusion and enter the systemic circulation. Because passive diffusion in this setting depends on the concentration of the solute at the membrane surface, the rate of drug absorption is affected by the concentration of free drug at the absorbing surface. Factors that influence the availability of free drug affect drug absorption from the administration site; this effect can be exploited to design medications that provide a slow release of drug into the circulation by prolonging drug absorption. With certain sustained-released oral preparations, the rate of dissolution of the drug in the gastrointestinal tract determines the rate at which the drug is absorbed (e.g., timed-release antihistamines). Similarly, a prolonged drug effect can be obtained by use of transdermal medications (e.g., nitroglycerin) or intramuscular depot preparations (e.g., benzathine penicillin G).

First-Pass Effect

Some drugs that are administered orally are absorbed relatively well into the portal circulation but are metabolized by the liver before they reach the systemic circulation. Because of this "first-pass" or "presystemic" effect, the oral route may be less suitable than other routes of administration for such drugs. A good example is nitroglycerin, which is well absorbed but efficiently metabolized during the first pass through the liver. The same drug can achieve adequate systemic levels when it is given sublingually or transdermally.

Bioavailability

The extent of absorption of drug into the systemic circulation may be incomplete. The bioavailability of a particular drug is the fraction (F) of the total drug dose that ultimately reaches the systemic circulation from the site of administration. This fraction is calculated by dividing the amount of the drug dose that reaches the circulation from the administration site by the amount of the drug dose that would enter the systemic circulation after direct intravenous injection into the circulation (essentially the total dose). Bioavailability, or F, can range from 0, in which no drug reaches the systemic circulation, to 1.0, in which essentially all of the drug is absorbed. The bioavailability of a drug may change in different formulations because the overall absorption may differ. This variability has become a concern with the increasing use of generic preparations.

Distribution

After delivery of a drug into the systemic circulation either directly by intravenous injection or after absorption, the drug is transported throughout the body, initially to the well-perfused tissues and later to areas that are less perfused. The distribution phase can be assessed best by plotting the drug's plasma concentration on a log scale versus time on a linear scale (Fig. 27–2). For an intravenously administered drug, when absorption is not a factor, the initial phase, from immediately after administration through the rapid fall in concentration, represents the distribution phase, during which a drug rapidly disappears from the circulation and enters the tissues. This is followed by the elimination phase (see later), when drug in the plasma is in equilibrium with drug in the tissues. During this latter phase, the drug's plasma concentration is thought to be related to drug effect.

Volume of Distribution

The volume of distribution (VD) is a term used to relate the amount of drug in the body to the concentration of drug in the plasma. It is calculated by dividing the dose that ultimately gets into the systemic circulation by the plasma concentration at time zero (C_{p0}):

$$VD = \frac{\text{dose}}{C_{p0}} \tag{1}$$

The C_{p0} can be calculated by extrapolating the elimination phase back to time zero (see Fig. 27–2). The VD is best considered the "apparent VD" because it represents the apparent volume needed to contain the entire amount of the drug, assuming that the drug is distributed throughout the body at the same concentration as in the plasma. Table 27–1 lists pharmacokinetic data for commonly used drugs from several drug classes, showing the wide variation in VD. Digoxin can be seen to have a large VD (>5 L), whereas valproic acid has a relatively small VD (0.15 L). As discussed later, the VD is a useful pharmacokinetic term for calculating the loading dose and appreciating how various changes can affect a drug's half-life.

Elimination

Drugs are removed from the body by two major mechanisms: hepatic elimination, in which drugs are metabolized in the liver and excreted through the biliary tract; and renal elimination, in which drugs are removed from the circulation by either glomerular filtration or tubular secretion. For most drugs, the rates of hepatic and renal elimination are proportional to the plasma concentration of the drug. This relationship often is described as a "first-order" process. Two measurements, clearance and half-life, are used to evaluate elimination.

Clearance

The efficiency of elimination can be assessed from a quantification of how fast the drug is cleared from the circulation. Drug clearance is a measure of the volume of plasma cleared of drug per unit of time. It is similar to the measurement used clinically to assess renal function—creatinine clearance, which is the volume of plasma from which creatinine is removed per minute. Total drug clearance (Cl_{tot}) is the rate of elimination by all processes (El_{tot}) divided by the plasma concentration of the drug (C_p):

$$Cl_{tot} = \frac{El_{tot}}{C_p} \tag{2}$$

Drugs may be cleared by several organs; renal clearance and hepatic clearance are the two major mechanisms. Total drug clearance (Cl_{tot}) can be described best as the sum of clearances by each organ. For most drugs, this is essentially the sum of renal clearance and hepatic clearance:

$$Cl_{tot} = Cl_{Ren} + Cl_{Hep} \tag{3}$$

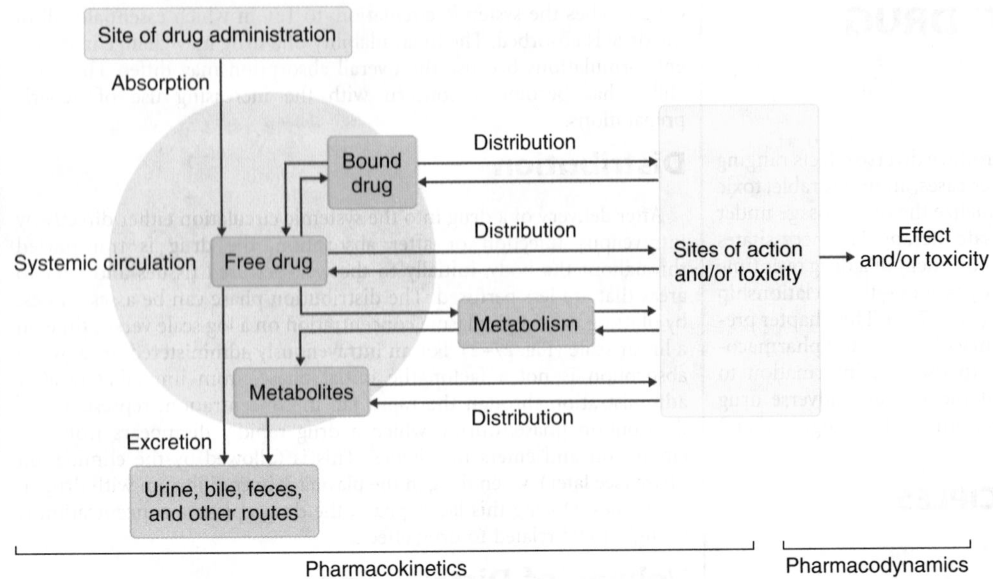

FIGURE 27–1 • Schematic of drug movement through the body, from site of administration to production of drug effect. The relationship between pharmacokinetics and pharmacodynamics is shown.

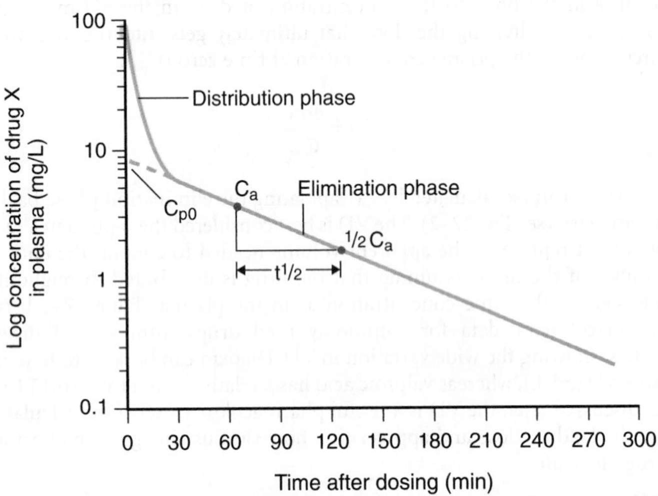

FIGURE 27–2 • Representative concentration versus time plot used in pharmacokinetic studies. Concentration of drug is plotted with a logarithmic scale on the ordinate, and time is plotted with a linear scale on the abscissa. The resultant curve is seen to have two phases: the distribution phase, the initial portion of the plotted line when the concentrations of drug decrease rapidly; and the elimination phase, the later phase when there is exponential disappearance of drug from the plasma with time. The dotted line extrapolated from the elimination phase back to time zero is used to calculate C_{p0}. During the elimination phase, the half-life can be calculated as the time it takes to decrease the concentration by half (shown here as the time needed to decrease from concentration C_a to $\frac{1}{2}C_a$).

Table 27–1 shows the wide variation in clearance values among commonly used medications; some drugs (e.g., phenobarbital) have relatively low clearances (<5 mL/min), and other drugs (e.g., aspirin) have relatively high clearances (>500 mL/min). Amikacin, gentamicin, and tobramycin are cleared almost entirely by the kidneys, whereas aspirin, carbamazepine, and phenytoin are cleared less than 5% by the kidneys.

Drug clearance is affected by several factors, including blood flow through the organ of clearance, protein binding to the drug, and activity of the clearance processes in the organs of elimination (e.g., glomerular filtration rate and tubular secretion in the kidney or enzyme activity in the liver). Drug clearance is not affected by distribution of drug throughout the body (VD) because clearance mechanisms act only on drug in the circulation.

Half-life

The amount of time needed to eliminate a drug from the body depends on the clearance and the VD. The first-order elimination constant (K_e) represents the proportion of the apparent VD that is cleared of drug per unit of time during the exponential disappearance of drug from the plasma over time (elimination phase):

$$K_e = \frac{Cl}{VD} \tag{4}$$

The value of this constant for a particular drug can be determined by plotting drug concentration versus time on a log-linear plot (see Fig. 27–2) and measuring the slope of the straight line obtained during the exponential (elimination) phase.

The time needed to eliminate the drug is described best by the drug half-life ($t_{1/2}$), which is the time required during the elimination phase (see Fig. 27–2) for the plasma concentration of the drug to be decreased by half. Mathematically, the half-life is equal to the natural logarithm of 2 (representing a reduction of drug concentration to half) divided by K_e. Substituting for K_e from Equation 4 and calculating the natural logarithm of 2, the half-life can be represented by the following equation:

$$t_{1/2} = \frac{0.693\ VD}{Cl} \tag{5}$$

From this equation, one can predict that at a given clearance, as the VD increases, the half-life increases. Similarly, at a given VD, as the clearance increases, the half-life decreases. Clinically, many disease states (see later) can affect VD and clearance. Because disease affects the VD and clearance differently, the half-life may increase, decrease, or not change much. Therefore, the half-life by itself is not a good indicator of the extent of abnormality in elimination.

The half-life is useful to predict how long it takes for a drug to be eliminated from the body. For any drug that has a first-order elimination, one would expect that by the end of the first half-life, the drug would be reduced to 50%; by the end of the second half-life, to 25%; by the end of the third half-life, to 12.5%; by the end of the fourth half-life, to 6.25%; and by the end of the fifth half-life, to 3.125%. In general, a drug can be considered essentially eliminated after three to five half-lives, when less than 10% of the effective concentration remains. Table 27–1 shows the wide variation in half-life for several commonly used drugs.

APPLYING PHARMACOKINETIC PRINCIPLES

Using a Loading Dose

To attain a desired therapeutic concentration rapidly, a loading dose often is used. In determining the amount of drug to be given, the physician must consider the "volume" within the body into which the drug may be distributed. This volume is best described by the apparent VD. The loading dose can be calculated by multiplying the desired concentration by the VD:

TABLE 27–1 PHARMACOKINETIC PARAMETERS FOR SOME COMMONLY USED DRUGS

	VD (L/kg)	Protein Binding (%)	Total Clearance (mL/min)	% of Total Clearance as Renal Clearance	Half-life (hr)	Therapeutic Range (mg/L)
Amikacin	0.25	<10	100	94–98	2–3	5–20 (TR) 20–30 (PK)
Aspirin (acetylsalicylic acid)	0.14–0.18	80–90	575–725	<2	0.2–0.3	20–250
Carbamazepine	1.2	75–90	50–125	1–3	12–17	4–12
Digoxin	5–7.3	20–30	75	50–70	34–44	0.5–2
Gentamicin sulfate	0.22–0.3	<10	60	>95	1.5–4	0.5–2 (TR) 4–8 (PK)
Lidocaine	3	60–80	700	<10	1.5–2	1–5
Lithium carbonate	0.7–1	0	20–40	95–99	20–270	0.4–1.4*
Penicillin G	0.5–0.7	45–68	—	20	0.4–0.9	Variable
Phenobarbital	0.6–0.7	20–45	4	25	2–6 days	<10–40*
Phenytoin	0.4–0.8	88–93	—	<5	7–26	10–20
Procainamide	2.2	14–23	470–600	40–70	2.5–4.7	4–8
Quinidine sulfate	2	80	180–300	10–20	6–8	0.3–6
Theophylline	0.3–0.7	60	36–50	<10	4–16	5–20
Tobramycin	0.25–0.30	<10	70	>95	2–4	0.5–2 (TR) 4–8 (PK)
Valproic acid	0.15	80–95	7	<10	5–20	50–100
Vancomycin	0.4–1	52–60	65	85	4–6	5–10 (TR) 25–35 (PK)

*Therapeutic range varies according to the indication for the drug. For example, lithium carbonate in the range of 0.4–1.3 mg/L is appropriate for affective schizophrenia disorder; a whole range of 1.0–1.4 mg/L is appropriate for mania. Phenobarbital concentration below 10 mg/mL is appropriate for anticonvulsant therapy; 40 mg/L is appropriate as a hypnotic.
PK = peak value; TR = trough value; VD = volume of distribution.

$$\text{Loading dose} = \text{desired concentration} \times \text{VD} \quad (6)$$

Administration of the entire loading dose rapidly may produce an initially high peak concentration that results in toxicity. This problem can be avoided either by administering the loading dose as a divided dose or by varying the rate of access to the circulation, such as by administering the drug as an infusion (with intravenous drug) or by taking advantage of the slower access to the circulation from various other routes (oral dose). This approach is illustrated by phenytoin (see Table 27–1), which may need to be administered with a loading dose to achieve a therapeutic level (10 to 20 mg/L) rapidly. Because the VD for phenytoin is approximately 0.6 L/kg, the loading dose calculated from Equation 6 is 420 mg/L to attain a minimally therapeutic level of 10 mg/L in a 70-kg adult. Administration of 420 mg of phenytoin by intravenous bolus carries the risk of cardiac arrest and death. By taking advantage of the reduced bioavailability (F = 0.8) and slow absorption of oral phenytoin, the loading dose can be administered safely as an oral dose of 500 mg.

The equation for the loading dose also can be used to calculate the dose needed to "boost" an inadequate blood level of drug to a desired therapeutic range. If the phenytoin level is observed on therapeutic monitoring to be 5 mg/L and the desired level is 15 mg/L, it is necessary to multiply the difference needed to achieve the desired concentration (10 mg/L) by the VD (0.6 L/kg) to determine the dose (in milligrams per kilogram) necessary to achieve this drug level after distribution. In a 70-kg individual, 0.6 mg/kg is multiplied by 70 kg to obtain the calculated loading dose (420 mg) that can be administered safely. A 500-mg oral dose with a bioavailability of less than 1 (e.g., F = 0.8) would deliver to the systemic circulation the approximate amount needed and avoid the risks associated with rapid intravenous administration.

Determining Drug Accumulation

Continuing to administer a drug, either as a prolonged infusion or as repeated doses, results in accumulation until a steady state occurs. Steady state is the point at which the amount of drug being administered equals the amount being eliminated so that the plasma and tissue levels remain constant. The elimination half-life determines not only the time course of drug elimination but also the time course of drug accumulation. This

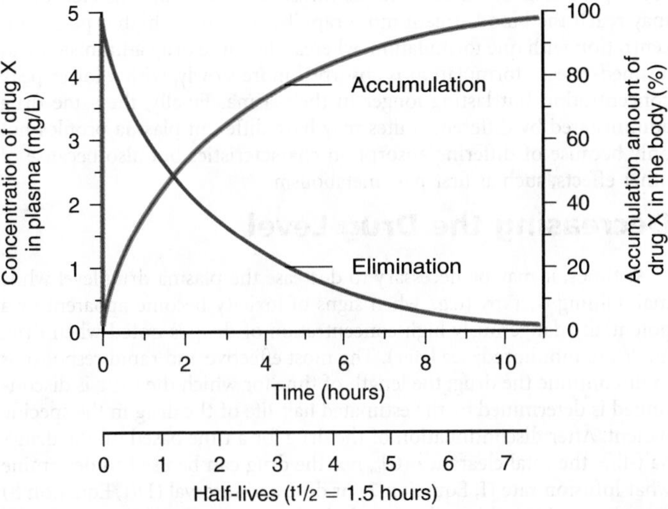

FIGURE 27–3 • Representative plot of the "mirror image" relationship between elimination of drug (after drug is discontinued) and accumulation of drug (during infusion). The plot shows the concentration on the left y-axis and time on the upper x-axis. The lower x-axis shows the time in half-lives, and the y-axis on the right shows the percentage of drug in the body. After three to five half-lives, elimination is essentially complete, and accumulation is essentially at a steady state.

"mirror image" pattern of drug accumulation and elimination is illustrated in Figure 27–3. As with drug elimination, three to five half-lives determine the time it takes to reach steady state during drug accumulation. Although drugs with short half-lives accumulate rapidly, drugs with long half-lives require a longer time to accumulate, with a potential delay in achieving therapeutic drug levels. For drugs with long half-lives, a loading dose may be needed to achieve drug accumulation rapidly and a more rapid therapeutic effect.

With each change in drug dose or rate of infusion, a change in steady state occurs. Although it is not obvious for drugs with short half-lives, the effects of dose adjustments for drugs with longer half-lives are delayed, and the time varies directly with the drug's half-life.

Using a Maintenance Dose

After steady state is reached in three to five half-lives with either a continuous infusion or intermittent doses, the rate of drug administered equals the rate of drug eliminated. For an intravenous drug, the administration rate is the infusion rate (I); for a drug administered by another route (e.g., oral dose), the administration rate is the dose per unit time (D/t). From Equation 3, the rate of elimination (total) can be seen to equal the $Cl_{tot} \times C_p$. It follows with an intravenously administered drug, because the infusion rate equals the elimination rate at steady state, that

$$I = Cl_{tot} \times C_p \qquad (7)$$

Similarly, with an orally administered drug, the dose administered per unit time equals the elimination rate at steady state, with the result that

$$D/t = Cl_{tot} \times C_p \qquad (8)$$

These equations show the direct relationship between the dose and the resultant plasma concentration at steady state. This relationship is independent of the distribution of the drug. By use of these equations, it is possible to determine the infusion rate or the interval and dose needed to achieve and to maintain a specified drug concentration in the plasma.

When it is administered intermittently, a drug approaches steady-state concentration over time with a pattern similar to that observed with continuous infusion (Fig. 27–4). With intermittent drug administration, such as with an oral dose, the drug concentration fluctuates; the magnitude of fluctuation between the peak and trough concentrations depends on the interval of administration, drug half-life, absorption characteristics, and site of administration. The effect of a change in the interval of administration for an oral drug is shown in Figure 27–4. As the intervals decrease below the half-life, the fluctuation decreases and approaches the curve produced by an intravenous infusion. Orally administered drugs may reach the blood stream more rapidly, attaining a higher peak concentration with one formulation, whereas the same drug administered as a timed-release formulation is absorbed more slowly, with a lower peak concentration but lasting longer in the plasma. Finally, the same drug administered by different routes may have different plasma profiles not only because of differing absorption characteristics but also because of other effects, such as first-pass metabolism.

Decreasing the Drug Level

At times, it may be necessary to decrease the plasma drug level while maintaining therapy (e.g., when signs of toxicity become apparent or a potentially dangerously high concentration of drug is noted when drug levels are monitored; see later). The most effective and rapid response is to discontinue the drug; the length of time for which the drug is discontinued is determined by the estimated half-life of the drug in the specific patient. After discontinuation of the drug for a time based on the drug's half-life, the total clearance (Cl_{tot}) of the drug can be used to determine what infusion rate (I, Equation 7) or dose and interval (D/t, Equation 8) must be used to achieve the new desired concentration (C_p).

DOSE-DEPENDENT PHARMACOKINETICS

Although the previously discussed pharmacokinetic principles can be a guide to the dose of most drugs, not all drugs behave the same when the dose is increased. The elimination of most drugs follows first-order or linear kinetics; the amount of drug eliminated is directly proportional to the concentration of drug in the plasma (Fig. 27–5A). A few drugs have a different pattern of elimination. Three of the most commonly used drugs that exhibit this different pharmacokinetic pattern are ethanol, phenytoin, and salicylate. These drugs have dose-dependent, nonlinear, saturation kinetics. As the dose of drug increases and the concentration of drug in the plasma rises, the relative amount of drug being eliminated falls (i.e., the clearance decreases) until the rate of drug metabolism is at its maximum. At this point, drug elimination is said to be zero order, and the drug concentration in plasma starts to increase much more (no longer a linear relationship) with each subsequent increase in dose (see Fig. 27–5B).

MONITORING OF DRUG CONCENTRATION AS A GUIDE TO THERAPY

Although published pharmacokinetic data (usually population averages) such as those listed in Table 27–1 are useful to determine initial drug dosing, modification of the dose still may be needed in the individual patient. For some drugs (e.g., certain antihypertensives or anticoagulants), the therapeutic effects (e.g., blood pressure or coagulation) can be quantified easily over a range of concentrations, permitting adequate

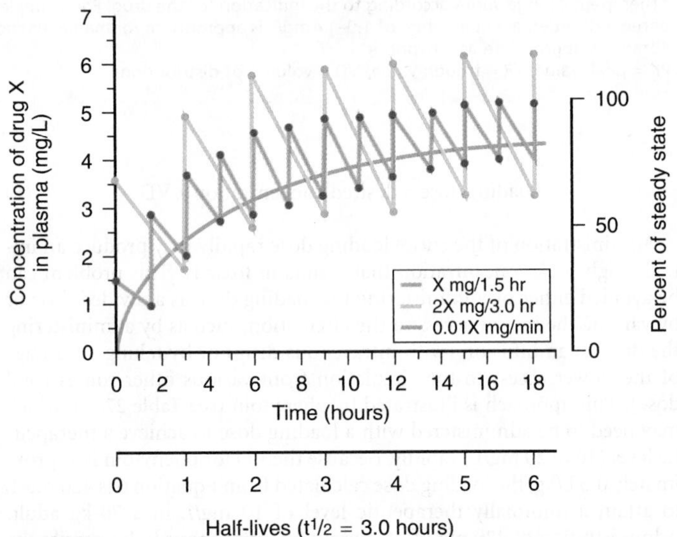

FIGURE 27–4 • The accumulation of drug over time approaching a steady state is shown. Time is depicted in hours (upper x-axis) and half-lives (lower x-axis, showing that steady state is reached in three to five half-lives). The green line depicts the pattern produced by an infusion of a hypothetical drug at a dose of 0.01X. The orange line shows the pattern resulting from oral administration of a 2X dose every 3 hours, and the blue line represents the pattern produced by oral administration of a dose X every 1.5 hours.

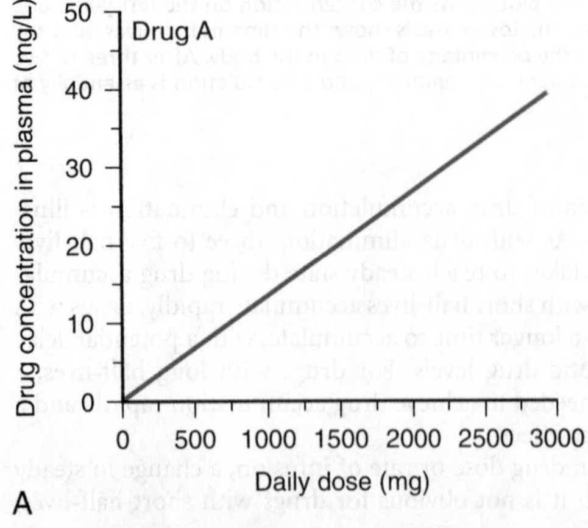

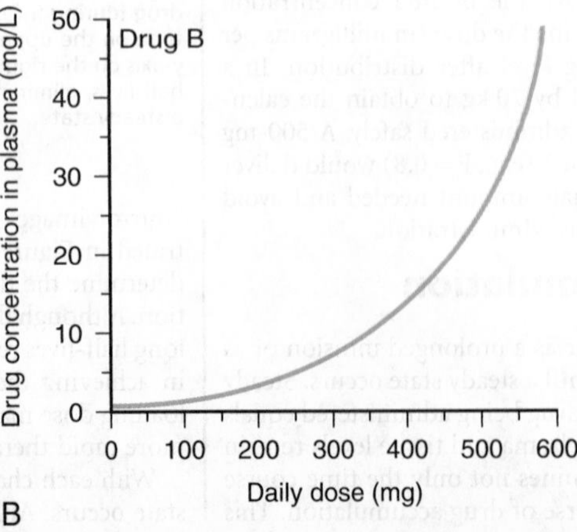

FIGURE 27–5 • The effect of increasing dose on serum concentration for drug A, which follows first-order or linear kinetics, and drug B, which follows zero-order or nonlinear (or saturable) kinetics.

drug adjustment. For many other drugs (e.g., some antiarrhythmics or antiseizure medications), therapeutic effects over a range of concentrations are not readily detectable. With these drugs, the plasma concentration of the drug may be used to provide further guidance in optimizing therapy if the plasma drug concentration is a reflection of the concentration at the site of action and the drug effects are reversible. A third, much smaller group of drugs produces irreversible effects (e.g., aspirin inhibition of platelet aggregation). With these drugs, plasma drug concentration does not correlate with drug effect, and drug monitoring is not useful.

To use drug concentrations as a guide to therapy, it is necessary to establish a range of concentrations from minimally to maximally efficacious with tolerable toxicity. This range of concentrations, or *therapeutic window,* usually is determined from a dose-response curve generated from a population of patients who have been examined closely for therapeutic and toxic effects (Fig. 27–6). This graph also may be used to determine the *therapeutic index,* a useful measure of drug toxicity calculated by dividing the 50% value from the toxicity curve by the 50% value of the efficacy curve. Because these curves are generated from population data, the values may not be applicable to all individuals.

Table 27–1, in addition to providing useful pharmacokinetic data, lists therapeutic ranges of several common drugs for which measuring the concentration and knowing the therapeutic range may be useful in clinical management. Many of these drugs are used to treat serious or life-threatening diseases. It is essential to avoid inadequate doses because therapeutic effect is needed. Excessive doses also must be avoided because of the risk of toxicity with many of these drugs that have a small therapeutic index. In contrast, it is not necessary to assay drug levels for other drugs used in noncritical diseases (no problem if inadequately treated) or for which the therapeutic index is large (overtreatment is not likely to produce toxicity).

Problems with Interpreting Drug Concentration

The time of blood collection, perhaps more than any other factor, contributes to the misinterpretation of drug levels. As can be seen from Figure 27–2, if sampling is performed too early, while the drug is still in the distribution phase, the drug level may be high and not reflect drug concentration at the site of action. It is therefore important to sample after the distribution phase.

For many drugs administered intermittently, a trough level, obtained immediately before the next dose is administered, is most useful for making decisions about dose adjustments (see Table 27–1). For drugs that are administered by infusion or intermittently at short intervals (see Fig. 27–4), the best time to draw blood is during steady state.

Protein binding is another major factor that contributes to the misinterpretation of drug levels. Free drug (not bound to protein and able to equilibrate with tissues and to interact with the site of action) is the critically important drug concentration when therapeutic decisions are being made. Many drugs are tightly bound to plasma protein, however. Table 27–1 shows that many commonly used drugs, such as aspirin, carbamazepine, phenytoin, and valproic acid, have protein binding of more than 75%. Because many of the commonly used drug assays determine total drug concentration (which includes protein-bound drug and free drug), assessment of the "true" free drug concentration may be inaccurate, particularly if the fraction of drug bound to protein varies. In addition, the drug's binding may be decreased by disease or other drugs, leading to increased unbound drug levels that alter the interpretation of the measured drug concentrations. Kidney and liver disease can change the binding of certain drugs (e.g., phenytoin) to protein because of a decrease in protein (e.g., decreased albumin as in nephrotic syndrome or liver disease) or as a result of competition for protein binding by endogenously produced substances (e.g., uremia in kidney disease or hyperbilirubinemia in liver disease). Similarly, other drugs may compete for binding to protein. A major problem that occurs secondary to the just-discussed changes in protein binding is that free drug is not typically measured in many of the common drug assays used by most clinical laboratories. Last, changes in drug binding to protein also can affect the pharmacokinetics of the drug, the main effect being on the VD, which increases as protein binding decreases.

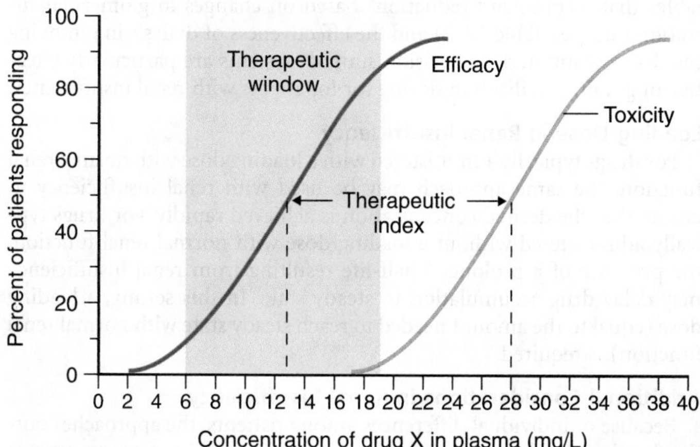

FIGURE 27–6 • The pattern produced in a dose-response population study in which both effect and toxicity are measured. The therapeutic window is shown as the range of therapeutically effective concentrations, which includes most of the efficacy curve and less than 10% of the toxicity curve. The therapeutic index is calculated by dividing the 50% value on the toxicity curve by the 50% value on the efficacy curve.

The usefulness of a drug assay also is limited by physiologic changes that may alter the response at a particular drug concentration. An example of this pharmacodynamic change is the response produced at a certain digoxin level in the presence of altered electrolyte concentration (e.g., potassium, calcium, or magnesium). Tolerance, a reduced response to a given concentration of drug with continued use, is another pharmacodynamic change that may alter how a drug concentration is interpreted. Tolerance commonly is observed with the continued use of narcotics (e.g., in terminal cancer patients); initially, adequate pain control is noted at a given drug concentration, but after long-term administration, the same drug concentration no longer is associated with pain relief.

ADJUSTING DRUG DOSE WITH DISEASE

Kidney Disease

The major questions to be answered in determining whether drug dosage needs to be adjusted in the setting of kidney disease are the following: Is the drug primarily excreted through the kidneys? Are increased drug levels likely to be associated with toxicity? If the answer to both is yes, it is likely that with decreased renal clearance, a drug will accumulate and become toxic. With renal failure, it is necessary to adjust the dosing regimen of such drugs, particularly for a drug with a long half-life and small therapeutic index (e.g., digoxin).

To obtain the desired concentration over time in the presence of decreased clearance, adjustments can be made by decreasing the dose while maintaining the dose interval (DD), maintaining the dose but increasing the interval between doses (II), or a combination of both (DD and II). Table 27–2 shows how these three different methods are used for several common drugs (previously characterized in Table 27–1 as to their pharmacokinetic properties with normal renal function) that require dosage adjustment with renal dysfunction. Although it may be possible with these adjustments to achieve an average concentration similar to that with normal renal function, there may be concomitant marked changes in the magnitude of peak and trough values. In choosing the type of drug adjustment, the physician should consider not only the therapeutic index of the drug but also (1) whether an effective concentration needs to be achieved quickly and maintained within a narrow range (i.e., there is a need to maintain an average drug concentration and to avoid trough levels when the drug is ineffective) and (2) whether toxicity is associated with elevated drug concentrations (i.e., toxicity with peak drug concentration).

Renal drug clearance has been shown to correlate with creatinine clearance (whether the drug uses glomerular filtration or tubular secretion); any adjustment of drug dose in kidney disease can use the creatinine clearance to calculate the dose needed because the renal drug clearance is proportional to the creatinine clearance. The creatinine clearance (Cl_{Cr}), which is used as an estimate of glomerular filtration rate, may be calculated directly from the serum creatinine concentration by the following equation:

Section V Pharmacology

TABLE 27–2 ADJUSTMENT OF DRUG DOSAGE IN RENAL FAILURE

Drug	Type of Elimination	Half-life (hr) Normal	Half-life (hr) End-stage Renal	Method*	Adjustment for Renal Failure GFR (mL/min) >50	10–50	<10	Removed by Dialysis†
Amikacin	Renal	2–3	30	DD II	60–90% 12 hr	30–70% 12–18 hr	20–30% 24 hr	Yes
Aspirin	Hepatic (renal)	2–19	Unchanged	II	4 hr	4–6 hr	Avoid	Yes
Carbamazepine	Hepatic (renal)	35	?	DD	Unchanged	Unchanged	75%	No
Digoxin	Renal (nonrenal 15–40%)	36–44	80–120	DD II	Unchanged 24 hr	25–75% 36 hr	10–25% 48 hr	No
Gentamicin sulfate	Renal	2	24–48	DD II	60–90% 8–12 hr	30–70% 12 hr	20–30% 24 hr	Yes
Lidocaine	Hepatic (renal <20%)	1.2–2.2	1.3–3	DD	Unchanged	Unchanged	Unchanged	No
Lithium carbonate	Renal	14–28	Prolonged	DD	Unchanged	50–75%	25–50%	Yes
Penicillin G	Renal (hepatic)	0.5	6–20	DD II	Unchanged 6–8 hr	75% 8–12 hr	25–50% 12–16 hr	Yes
Phenobarbital	Hepatic (renal 30%)	60–150	117–160	II	Unchanged	Unchanged	12–16 hr	Yes
Phenytoin	Hepatic (renal)	24	8	DD	Unchanged	Unchanged	Unchanged	No
Procainamide	Renal (hepatic 7–24%)	2.5–4.9	5.3–5.9	II	4 hr	6–12 hr	8–24 hr	Yes
Quinidine sulfate	Hepatic (renal 10–50%)	5–7.2	4–14	II	Unchanged	Unchanged	Unchanged	Yes
Theophylline	Hepatic	3–12	?	DD	Unchanged	Unchanged	Unchanged	Yes
Tobramycin	Renal	2.5	56	DD II	60–90% 8–12 hr	30–70% 12 hr	20–30% 24 hr	Yes
Valproic acid	Hepatic	Biphasic 1 and 12	10	DD	Unchanged	Unchanged	Unchanged	No
Vancomycin	Renal	6–8	200–250	II	24–72 hr	72–240 hr	240 hr	No

*Method: DD (alone)—decrease dose (maintain same interval). II (alone)—increase interval between doses (maintain dose). DD and II (together)—combination of both approaches.
†Dialysis refers to hemodialysis.
GFR = glomerular filtration rate.

$$Cl_{Cr} = \frac{(140 - \text{age}) \times \text{weight (kg)}}{72 \times \text{serum creatinine (mg/dL)}} \quad (9)$$

The calculated creatinine clearance should be multiplied by 0.85 for females. (*Note:* This calculation applies only when the serum creatinine concentration is less than 5 mg/dL and renal function is not rapidly changing.)

Using Clearance for Dose Adjustment

The dose of a drug used in renal insufficiency ($dose_{D-RI}$) can be shown to be proportional to the dose used with normal renal function ($dose_D$) in the same ratio as the clearance of the drug in renal insufficiency (Cl_{D-RI}) to the clearance with normal renal function (Cl_D). By rearranging, $dose_{D-RI}$ is defined as:

$$Dose_{D-RI} = dose_D \times \frac{Cl_{D-RI}}{Cl_D} \quad (10)$$

One can estimate the Cl_{D-RI} by multiplying the Cl_D by the ratio of the creatinine clearance in renal insufficiency (Cl_{Cr-RI}) over the Cl_{Cr} with normal renal function:

$$Cl_{D-RI} = Cl_D \times \frac{Cl_{Cr-RI}}{Cl_{Cr}} \quad (11)$$

As shown in Equation 3, total clearance is the sum of clearance by renal and nonrenal (typically hepatic) mechanisms. Any nonrenal clearance is assumed to remain normal, and only the renal clearance is adjusted, with total clearance being reduced only to the extent that renal clearance is reduced. The dose may be calculated from the total (adjusted) clearance and the desired plasma concentration by either Equation 7 or Equation 8. The calculated dose is only an initial guide to the dose needed, however. By monitoring of the drug response or the plasma drug concentration at various times after initial dosing, further dose adjustments can be made as necessary. From a practical perspective, most clinical dose adjustment of drugs in the presence of renal dysfunction can be guided by published tables that recommend reductions based on changes in glomerular filtration rate (see Table 27–2) and the effectiveness of dialysis in removing the drug. Computerized decision support systems are particularly effective in guiding medication dosing for inpatients with renal insufficiency.

Loading Dose in Renal Insufficiency

For drugs typically administered with a loading dose with normal renal function, the same approach may be used with renal insufficiency to ensure that the desired concentration is achieved rapidly. For drugs typically administered without a loading dose with normal renal function, the presence of a prolonged half-life resulting from renal insufficiency may delay drug accumulation to steady state. In this setting, a loading dose (equal to the amount needed to reach steady state with normal renal function) is required.

Additional Considerations in Renal Insufficiency

Because of individual differences among patients, the approaches outlined earlier should be considered only initial approximations to prevent ineffective (too low) or toxic (too high) doses. In planning further maintenance therapy, it is desirable to monitor blood levels to guide further dosing.

If a metabolite of the drug is responsible for effect or toxicity and accumulates in renal failure, the drug level alone may not provide sufficient guidance for planning therapy in the setting of renal insufficiency. The major metabolite of procainamide is *N*-acetylprocainamide, which has toxicity similar to that of the parent drug but only modest antiarrhythmic activity. In the setting of renal failure, *N*-acetylprocainamide may accumulate dramatically because it is more dependent on renal elimination. Measurement of procainamide levels alone does not assess accurately either the levels needed for antiarrhythmic effect or the risk of toxicity.

Liver Disease

Although many drugs are biotransformed in the liver, it is not possible to make any general recommendations for drug dose adjustments in liver disease. In contrast to renal disease, no useful laboratory test is available on which to base dose adjustments. It has been suggested that if the liver's capacity to produce protein (reflected by albumin concentration and the prothrombin time) is reduced significantly, the clearance of drugs metabolized by the cytochrome P-450 enzymes probably also is reduced.

One special situation that can develop with chronic liver disease and may require dose adjustment is the portacaval shunt. This condition produces not only a potential hemodynamic alteration, leading to decreased hepatic blood flow with accompanying decreased clearance, but also possible bypassing of a first-pass effect, resulting in higher concentrations of drug reaching the systemic circulation. Drugs with a large hepatic extraction that typically are administered orally (e.g., propranolol) may appear in the systemic circulation with higher, potentially toxic concentrations.

Hemodynamic Diseases

Decreased cardiac output and hypotensive conditions lead to decreased perfusion of the organs, including those responsible for eliminating drugs. As noted earlier with primary kidney disease, the dose can be adjusted for decreased renal perfusion by use of the creatinine clearance. The effect of decreased hepatic blood flow on pharmacokinetics is more difficult to assess. For drugs that have a high hepatic extraction (e.g., lidocaine), decreased hepatic blood flow suggests a need to reduce doses.

Altered hemodynamics also may affect the distribution of selected drugs. Drugs that have a relatively large VD (e.g., lidocaine, procainamide, and quinidine) may be affected by conditions leading to hypotension, such as shock, resulting in a decrease in the apparent VD. With a reduced VD, the loading dose of a drug should be reduced to avoid potentially toxic drug levels.

In general, in the setting of severely compromised hemodynamics, it is advisable to be conservative, avoiding potentially toxic loading and maintenance doses of drugs. Drug levels and the clinical status should be monitored closely, and drug doses should be adjusted as necessary.

APPROACH TO DRUG OVERDOSE

The pharmacokinetic principles discussed earlier can be used to determine the best approach to drug removal in the setting of a drug overdose, particularly if hemodialysis or hemoperfusion is contemplated. The major goal is to increase the overall clearance of drug, removing a substantial fraction of the total body load of drug. Examination of the VD and clearance values can provide some guidance. For drugs with a large VD (e.g., digoxin in Table 27–1), only a small amount of drug can be removed because clearance affects only the amount of drug present in the plasma, and a large portion of the drug in the body is outside the plasma compartment. Similarly, for drugs with high clearance values, hemoperfusion may increase the overall clearance only minimally and is not indicated. Table 27–2 provides data for determining whether hemodialysis is likely to be useful to remove several commonly prescribed drugs.

USING DRUGS IN THE ELDERLY

Administering drugs to the elderly is perhaps the most challenging area in adult therapeutics because of several factors: the increasing likelihood of multiple illnesses, often with multisystemic involvement; the need for these patients to take multiple drugs (often prescribed by different physicians); and the increasing probability of altered pharmacokinetics and pharmacodynamics. These factors together contribute to significantly increased frequency of drug interactions and adverse drug responses in this group of patients.

Pharmacokinetic Changes with Age

These changes can be secondary to the effects of general physiologic changes of aging, such as the change in body composition, or to specific changes in pharmacokinetically important organs (e.g., kidneys or liver). The distribution of drugs tends to change dramatically with age, mainly because of changes in body composition. Most typical is the increase in total body fat with the accompanying decrease in lean body mass and total body water. Changes also may occur in the concentration of plasma proteins, particularly albumin, which decreases as the liver ages. The changes in distribution are manifested as a change in the apparent VD. For water-soluble drugs that are not bound to plasma proteins, the apparent VD is reduced, in contrast to lipid-soluble drugs, for which the VD is increased. Minimal changes in metabolism accompany aging, but these alone cannot account for altered pharmacokinetics.

Excretion can be altered in the elderly. The clearance of many drugs is decreased. Cardiac output and blood flow to the kidneys and liver also may be decreased. Glomerular filtration rate may be reduced by 50%. Hepatic elimination of drugs is less affected except for drugs with a high hepatic clearance (e.g., lidocaine). The elimination half-life of many drugs is increased with aging as a consequence of a larger apparent VD and a decreased hepatic or renal clearance (see Equation 5).

Pharmacodynamic Changes with Age

These changes are a result of changes in the responsiveness of the target organ. They require use of smaller drug doses in the elderly, even if the pharmacokinetics are unchanged. Many examples exist of such changes with drugs commonly used in the elderly; for example, antianxiety drugs and drugs from the sedative-hypnotic class may produce increased central nervous system depression in the elderly at concentrations that are well tolerated in younger adults. Similarly, anticoagulants (e.g., warfarin) may produce hemorrhage in the elderly at concentrations that are well tolerated in younger adults.

General Recommendations

Several general principles apply to drug use in the elderly.

- The clearance of drugs eliminated by the kidneys may be reduced by 50%.
- Drugs that are eliminated primarily by the liver typically do not require adjustment for age except for drugs with high hepatic clearances, which may be affected by age-related decrease in hepatic blood flow.
- Because of potential for increased target organ sensitivity in the elderly, only the lowest effective dose should be used.
- Frequent reviews of the patient's drug history should be conducted, including not only prescription medications but also over-the-counter medications, keeping in mind the increased potential risk for drug interactions and adverse drug responses.

INTERACTIONS BETWEEN DRUGS

Because patients typically are treated today with multiple agents even for a single disease, the possibilities for drug interactions are great. In general, most clinically important drug interactions typically involve a drug with a low therapeutic index (e.g., warfarin) and an easily detectable pharmacologic effect (e.g., bleeding), such that a small increase in the amount of drug produces a significant effect (toxicity).

Epidemiology

It is difficult to assess accurately the prevalence of drug interactions in either the inpatient or ambulatory settings, particularly because no formal and comprehensive surveillance mechanism is available currently. The risk for drug interactions seems to be increasing, particularly for critically ill, hospitalized patients, who frequently are taking more than 10 medications.

Etiology

There are basically two types of drug interaction: pharmacokinetic drug interactions, caused by a change in the amount of drug or active metabolite at the site of action; and pharmacodynamic drug interactions (without a change in pharmacokinetics), caused by a change in drug effect.

Pharmacokinetic Drug Interactions

Less Drug at the Site of Action

Decreased Absorption

The gastrointestinal lumen is perhaps the best example of an area where drug interactions can result in decreased drug absorption. Examples of some commonly used drugs illustrate this type of interaction. For many drugs, a physicochemical interaction prevents the drug from being absorbed. Drugs such as colestipol and cholestyramine (resins used to lower cholesterol and bind bile acids) also can bind other drugs simultaneously present in the gastrointestinal lumen. Among the drugs that can be bound are digoxin and warfarin. Because of the potential for many other drugs also to be bound, it generally is recommended that other drugs not be administered within 2 hours of colestipol or cholestyramine. Another type of interaction occurs when metal ions (e.g., aluminum, calcium, and magnesium in antacids and iron in supplements to treat iron deficiency) form insoluble complexes with tetracyclines, which can act as chelating agents. Other commonly used medications that decrease absorption include kaolin-pectin suspensions to treat diarrhea. These medications can inhibit significantly the absorption of coadministered drugs (e.g., digoxin).

Drugs that are particularly susceptible to pH changes may have decreased absorption when they are coadministered with drugs that either affect gastric acidity or alter the extent of exposure to low pH. H_2-receptor antagonists, such as cimetidine, ranitidine, and famotidine, may elevate gastric pH, which can inhibit the dissolution and subsequent absorption of drugs that are weak bases (e.g., ketoconazole). Medications that delay gastric emptying (e.g., belladonna alkaloids) can increase the degradation of a coadministered acid-labile drug (e.g., levodopa), resulting in decreased absorption.

Altered Distribution

Drugs that use the same active transport process to reach their site of action can compete at the level of transport, resulting in lower levels of drug reaching the site of action. The classic example of this type of interaction is the coadministration of guanidinium-type antihypertensives with tricyclic antidepressants, phenothiazines, and certain sympathomimetic amines (e.g., ephedrine), which block the effects of the antihypertensive drug.

Increased Metabolism

Many drugs (e.g., barbiturates, such as phenobarbital, phenytoin, ethanol, glutethimide, griseofulvin, rifampin, and toxic compounds such as cigarette smoke and certain chlorinated hydrocarbons) can increase hepatic metabolism of other drugs (e.g., corticosteroids, cyclophosphamide, cyclosporine, certain β-adrenergic blockers, theophylline, and warfarin) by inducing the activity of the cytochrome P-450 mixed function oxidase (CYP) system.

More Drug at the Site of Action

Increased Absorption

Any drug that increases the rate of gastric emptying (e.g., metoclopramide) potentially can increase the absorption of acid-unstable drugs. Also, drugs that decrease intestinal motility (e.g., anticholinergics) may increase the absorption of drugs that are relatively poorly absorbed (e.g., digoxin tablets) by increasing the contact time of the drug with the absorbing surface.

Altered Distribution

Drugs bound to protein are limited in their distribution (particularly to the site of action) and are not available for metabolism or excretion. Drugs can compete with each other for binding to plasma proteins, resulting in drug interactions. Sulfonamides can displace barbiturates bound to serum albumin, leading to increased levels of free barbiturates with possible toxicity.

Decreased Metabolism

One of the most impressive drug interactions is produced when one drug inhibits the metabolism of another drug, leading to the second drug's accumulation and a significant risk of toxicity. This type of interaction results from use of 6-mercaptopurine, an antileukemic drug with a low therapeutic index, with allopurinol, often administered in this setting to control hyperuricemia. The interaction may result in potentially life-threatening toxicity.

Some drugs can inhibit the metabolism of many other drugs. For example, cimetidine can inhibit the metabolism of diazepam, imipramine, lidocaine, propranolol, quinidine, theophylline, and warfarin. Amiodarone inhibits the metabolism of calcium-channel blockers, phenytoin, quinidine, and warfarin. Of particular importance with amiodarone is its half-life of 1 to 2 months; it continues to inhibit drug metabolism for several months after it has been discontinued.

Other drugs are notable in that their metabolism is inhibited by a variety of different drugs. The metabolism of the commonly used anticoagulant warfarin is inhibited not only by cimetidine and amiodarone but also by many other drugs, including alcohol, allopurinol, disulfiram, metronidazole, phenylbutazone, sulfinpyrazone, and trimethoprim-sulfamethoxazole. Similarly, the metabolism of phenytoin also is inhibited by additional drugs, including chloramphenicol, clofibrate, dicumarol, disulfiram, isoniazid (slow acetylators), phenylbutazone, and valproic acid.

Although most of the examples just noted involve enzymes that metabolize the drug in the liver, drug-metabolizing enzymes outside the liver also may be affected by certain drugs. The best-known example is monoamine oxidase, which can be affected by nonspecific monoamine oxidase inhibitors, resulting in the accumulation of catecholamines at multiple sites after their release in response to eating of tyramine-containing foods such as aged cheese, aged or cured meats, and any potentially spoiled meat, poultry, or fish.

Decreased Excretion

Drugs can compete for the active transporters present in the kidney. Most of these interactions involve the acid transporters. The best-known interaction is the probenecid inhibition of penicillin transport, leading to decreased penicillin clearance with resultant increased plasma levels, an interaction that was used in the past to maximize penicillin therapy. A similar inhibitory effect on renal excretion of methotrexate can be produced by salicylates, phenylbutazone, and probenecid. The active transport of basic drugs (e.g., procainamide) also can be inhibited by other drugs (e.g., cimetidine or amiodarone).

Pharmacodynamic Drug Interactions

With pharmacodynamic interactions, drugs interact at the level of the receptor (target) or may produce additive effects by acting at separate sites on cells. An example of the first is the interaction of propranolol and epinephrine, which blocks β-adrenergic receptors with the result that the α-adrenergic effects of epinephrine are unopposed. This undesirable interaction can result in severe hypertension.

Many examples exist of additive effects between drugs. Aspirin, which can produce increased bleeding time by acting on platelets, can interact with warfarin, which affects clotting. The result is an increased risk of hemorrhage. Similarly, cardiac drugs, such as β-adrenergic blockers and calcium-channel blockers, have additive negative inotropic effects when they are coadministered, resulting in an increased risk of cardiac failure.

Diagnosis and Prevention of Drug Interactions

For a drug interaction to be recognized, the index of suspicion must be high whenever multiple drugs are used together. Because of the ever-increasing list of known and suspected drug interactions, it is impossible for a clinician to remember all or even many of the possible interactions.

Several clinical settings should raise concern about the possibility of drug interactions:

- The use of any drug with a low therapeutic index (Table 27–3) should be suspect.
- As the number of drugs being used concurrently increases, there is a disproportionately greater risk of drug interactions, particularly with more than 10 drugs.
- Critically ill patients who have multisystemic disease with compromised renal, hepatic, cardiac, or pulmonary function have an increased risk of drug interactions. This risk may be higher for patients with acquired immunodeficiency syndrome, who have an immunocompromised state as well as take a great number of drugs.

- Patients with various behavioral and psychiatric disorders (e.g., drug abusers taking not only a large number of prescription drugs but also illicit drugs and alcohol) are at risk for development of drug interactions.

Another type of drug interaction that is becoming increasingly important is the interaction of components of food (e.g., grapefruit juice) or natural products (e.g., herbs) with drugs. Concomitant use of grapefruit juice, through its inhibition of the intestinal cytochrome P-450 3A4 enzyme system, can raise levels of drugs (e.g., saquinavir, cyclosporine, or verapamil) metabolized by this pathway and result in toxicity or adverse drug effects.

Several steps can be taken to prevent drug interactions:

- In taking the medical history, it is important to document all the drugs the patient is taking (and has recently taken), including prescription, over-the-counter, and other addictive drugs.
- It is desirable to minimize the number of drugs the patient is taking by frequently reviewing the patient's drug list to ensure that each drug continues to be needed.
- There should be a high degree of suspicion when medications with a low therapeutic index known to have a high risk of drug interactions (see Table 27–3) are used.
- High-risk clinical settings, such as occur with critically ill patients, should raise suspicion of adverse drug interactions.
- Adverse drug interactions should be considered in the differential diagnosis whenever any change occurs in a patient's course.

ADVERSE REACTIONS TO DRUGS

An adverse drug response is an undesired effect produced by a drug at standard doses, which typically necessitates reducing or stopping the suspected agent and may require treatment of the noxious effect produced. Further harm may occur with continued or future therapy with the drug.

TABLE 27–3 DRUGS WITH LOW THERAPEUTIC INDICES AT HIGH-RISK FOR ADVERSE DRUG RESPONSE AND DRUG INTERACTIONS

Anticoagulants
Antiarrhythmics
Anticonvulsants
Digoxin
Lithium carbonate
Oral hypoglycemics
Theophylline

Epidemiology

The actual incidence of adverse drug responses is difficult to quantify because many cases are either not recognized or not reported. Several large studies have shown that the incidence may approach 20% for outpatients (even higher for patients taking more than 15 drugs) and 2 to 7% for inpatients. Meta-analyses of several prospective studies suggest that adverse drug reactions may be the fourth to sixth leading cause of death in hospitalized patients. It is clear from more recent surveys that a relatively small group of drugs (see Table 27–3) continues to be implicated in most of the reported adverse drug responses. Current trends suggest that the incidence of adverse drug responses is likely to increase as a result of more and more prescribed and over-the-counter medications being used.

Etiology

Most adverse drug responses are caused by an exaggerated (but predictable) pharmacologic effect of the drug or by a toxic or immunologic effect of the drug or a metabolite (not typically expected).

Exaggerated (Predictable) Response to a Drug

Exaggerated drug responses that cause adverse drug effects may be due to any condition that causes altered pharmacokinetics or pharmacodynamics (discussed earlier). There has been interest in the role of genetic factors as a cause of increased susceptibility to adverse drug responses, primarily through an effect on drug metabolism. Molecular changes in the genes coding for drug-metabolizing enzymes can account for variability in pharmacokinetics and drug effect observed in population studies. Three of the best-studied examples are the debrisoquine-sparteine, *N*-acetylation, and mephenytoin genetic polymorphisms. These are each associated with an autosomal recessive inheritance and together are responsible for the metabolism of approximately 40 drugs (Table 27–4). Individuals with autosomal recessive genes are "poor metabolizers" with potentially altered pharmacokinetics that result in elevated plasma drug concentrations and can lead to toxicity. A particularly impressive example occurs with certain cancer chemotherapy agents that have a relatively narrow therapeutic window and the potential to produce severe cytotoxicity (e.g., deficiency in dihydropyrimidine dehydrogenase activity can result in life-threatening toxicity after administration of 5-fluorouracil). These defects typically are not recognized until the patient is given the drug. They often are described as being "pharmacogenetic" syndromes.

Other genetic alterations do not affect metabolism specifically and do not produce a range of quantitative changes. These defects can produce "qualitative" defects and often are associated with structural defects. The classic example is glucose-6-phosphate dehydrogenase. Individuals who are deficient in this enzyme cannot tolerate oxidative stress that is

TABLE 27–4 GENETIC POLYMORPHISMS OF DRUG-METABOLIZING ENZYMES

Type	Primary Drug Examples	Other Drugs that Are Substrates	Incidence of "Poor Metabolizers" in Whites (%)	Enzyme Involved
Debrisoquine-sparteine polymorphism	Debrisoquine, sparteine, bufuralol	Antidepressants, antiarrhythmics, β-adrenergic receptor–blocking drugs, codeine, dextromethorphan, neuroleptics	5–10	Cytochrome P-450 IID6 (CYP2D6)
Mephenytoin polymorphism	Mephenytoin	Mephobarbital, hexobarbital, diazepam, omeprazole	4 (Japanese, Chinese, 15–20)	Cytochrome P-450 IIC (CYP2C)
N-acetylation polymorphism	Isoniazid, sulfadiazine	Isoniazid, hydralazine, phenelzine, procainamide, dapsone, sulfamethazine, sulfapyridine, aminoglutethimide, aminosalicylic acid, sulfadiazine, sulfasalazine	40–70 (Japanese, 10–20)	*N*-acetyltransferase (NAT2)
Methyl conjugation polymorphism	Catecholamines	L-Dopa, methyldopa	25–30	Catechol-*O*-methyltransferase (COMT)

produced by some drugs, leading to hemolysis (Chapter 165). Drugs that can produce this clinical picture include aspirin, nitrofurantoin, primaquine, probenecid, quinidine, quinine, sulfonamides, sulfones, and vitamin K. Another similar defect is deficiency of methemoglobin reductase, which results in an inability to maintain iron in hemoglobin in the ferrous state, causing methemoglobinemia after exposure to oxidizing drugs, such as nitrites, sulfonamide, and sulfones.

Unpredictable Toxic Responses to Drug

There are other toxic or immunologic adverse drug responses that are not predictable and not obviously due to an increase in drug concentration (pharmacokinetic) or drug effect (pharmacodynamic). Unpredictable toxic responses include direct reactions between drug and a specific organ (e.g., platinum-containing drugs, such as cisplatin, can produce direct toxicity in the kidney and the eighth cranial nerve). With other drugs, metabolism of the drug to an active intermediate must occur first. With a standard dose of acetaminophen, no untoward effects occur because the relatively small amount of reactive metabolite formed by oxidative metabolism is detoxified rapidly by reduced glutathione. In the presence of an overdose, the glutathione is depleted, and the remaining reactive metabolite can damage the liver. Understanding the mechanism of this toxicity has provided a rationale for treatment of acetaminophen overdose. Sulfhydryl-containing compounds (e.g., *N*-acetylcysteine), which can complex with the reactive metabolite, can be administered to reduce the amount of free toxic metabolite present, protecting the liver.

Immunologic reactions to drugs (Table 27–5) in general are not produced by the drug alone. Similar to other low-molecular-weight compounds (<1000 D), they are typically not antigenic themselves. When a drug or reactive metabolite combines with a protein to form a drug-protein complex, it can become antigenic, capable of eliciting an immune response.

Perhaps the most impressive form of drug allergy is anaphylaxis, which is due to an immunoglobulin E–mediated hypersensitivity. Many drugs from different classes have been shown to produce this type of drug allergy (see Table 27–5). The best-known example is the anaphylactic response produced by penicillin, which can occur after the

TABLE 27–5 SOME NOTABLE ADVERSE DRUG REACTIONS

MULTISYSTEMIC MANIFESTATIONS

ANAPHYLAXIS

Macromolecules
- Allergenic extracts
- Antisera
- Dextrans (including iron dextran)
- Enzymes
  - Asparaginase
  - Chymopapain
  - Trypsin
- Heparin
- Hormones (e.g., ACTH, insulin)
- Human gamma globulin
- Monoclonal antibodies
- Protamine
- Vaccines

Diagnostic agents
- Fluorescein
- Iodinated contrast media

Antimicrobials
- Aminosalicylic acid
- Amphotericin B
- Cephalosporins
- Cinoxacin
- Clindamycin
- Demeclocycline
- Ethambutol
- Kanamycin
- Lincomycin
- Nalidixic acid
- Penicillins
- Streptomycin
- Sulfonamides
- Tetracyclines
- Vancomycin

OTHER DRUGS, including nonsteroidal anti-inflammatory drugs (NSAIDs)
- Aspirin
- Benzyl alcohol
- Bleomycin
- Cisplatin
- Colchicine
- Cromolyn
- Cytarabine
- Dantrolene
- Ethylenediamine
- Etoposide
- Flucytosine
- Glucocorticoids
- Indomethacin
- Lidocaine
- Local anesthetics
- Mephyton
- Meprobamate
- Niacin
- Opiates
- Pentamidine
- Probenecid
- Procainamide
- Sulfite
- Thiopental
- Tolmetin
- Triamterene
- Tubocurarine and other muscle-relaxing agents
- Vitamin B_{12}

SERUM SICKNESS

Macromolecules
- Dextrans
- Heparin
- Hormones (e.g., insulin, ACTH)
- Vaccines
- Antisera

Antimicrobials
- Cephalosporins
- Griseofulvin
- Lincomycin
- Minocycline
- Penicillins
- Streptomycin
- Sulfonamides

Other drugs
- Barbiturates
- Hydralazine
- Phenylbutazone
- Phenytoin
- Procarbazine
- Propylthiouracil

DRUG FEVER

Antimicrobials
- 5-Aminosalicylic acid
- Amphotericin B
- Cephalosporins
- Erythromycin
- Isoniazid
- Kanamycin
- Nitrofurantoin
- Norfloxacin
- Penicillins
- Pyrazinamide
- Quinine
- Streptomycin
- Sulfonamides
- Tetracyclines

Other drugs
- Allopurinol
- Captopril
- Heparin
- Hydantoins
- Hydralazine
- Hydrochlorothiazide
- Methyldopa
- Penicillamine
- Phenobarbital
- Pneumococcal vaccine
- Procainamide
- Propylthiouracil
- Quinine

VASCULITIS
- Allopurinol
- Atenolol
- Busulfan
- Carbamazepine
- Colchicine
- Diphenhydramine
- Ethionamide
- Furosemide
- Hydantoins
- Hydroxyurea
- Ibuprofen
- Indomethacin
- Isoniazid
- Meprobamate
- Methamphetamine
- Naproxen
- Penicillins
- Phenothiazines
- Phenylbutazone
- Propranolol
- Propylthiouracil
- Streptokinase
- Sulfonamides
- Tetracyclines
- Thiazide diuretics
- Vaccines

TABLE 27–5 SOME NOTABLE ADVERSE DRUG REACTIONS—cont'd

SYSTEMIC LUPUS ERYTHEMATOSUS SYNDROME
5-Aminosalicylic acid
Chloroquine
Chlorpromazine
Ethosuximide
Griseofulvin
Hydralazine
Isoniazid
Methyldopa
Nitrofurantoin
Penicillamine
Penicillins
Phenytoin
Procainamide
Propylthiouracil
Quinidine
Tetracycline
Tocainide
Trimethadione

SKIN

URTICARIA AND ANGIOEDEMA
Antimicrobials
- Aminoglycosides
- 5-Aminosalicylic acid
- Cephalosporins
- Isoniazid
- Metronidazole
- Miconazole
- Nalidixic acid
- Penicillins
- Quinine
- Rifampin
- Spectinomycin
- Sulfonamides

Other drugs
- Asparaginase
- Aspirin and other NSAIDs
- Calcitonin
- Chloral hydrate
- Chlorambucil
- Cimetidine
- Cyclophosphamide
- Daunorubicin
- Doxorubicin
- Ergotamine
- Ethchlorvynol
- Ethosuximide
- Ethylenediamine
- Glucocorticoids
- Melphalan
- Penicillamine
- Phenothiazines
- Procainamide
- Procarbazine
- Quinidine
- Tartrazine
- Thiazide diuretics
- Thiotepa

MORBILLIFORM-MACULOPAPULAR RASH
Antimicrobials
- 5-Aminosalicylic acid
- Cephalosporins
- Erythromycin
- Gentamicin
- Penicillins
- Streptomycin
- Sulfonamides

Other drugs
- Allopurinol
- Barbiturates
- Captopril
- Coumarin
- Gold salts
- Hydantoins
- Thiazide diuretics

TOXIC EPIDERMAL NECROLYSIS, ERYTHRODERMA, AND EXFOLIATIVE DERMATITIS
Allopurinol
Amikacin
Captopril
Carbamazepine
Chloral hydrate
Chlorambucil
Chloroquine
Chlorpromazine
Cyclosporine
Diltiazem
Ethambutol
Ethylenediamine
Glutethimide
Gold salts
Griseofulvin
Hydantoins
Hydroxychloroquine
Minoxidil
Nifedipine
NSAIDs
Penicillin
Phenobarbital
Rifampin
Spironolactone
Streptomycin
Sulfonamides
Trimethadione
Trimethoprim
Tocainide
Vancomycin
Verapamil

ERYTHEMA MULTIFORME
Acetaminophen
Barbiturates
Carbamazepine
Chloroquine
Chlorpropamide
Clindamycin
Ethambutol
Ethosuximide
Gold salts
Hydantoins
Hydralazine
Hydroxyurea
Mechlorethamine
Meclofenamate
Penicillins
Phenolphthalein
Phenylbutazone
Rifampin
Streptomycin
Sulfonylureas
Sulindac
Vaccines

PHOTOSENSITIVE
Topical
- *p*-Aminobenzoic acid esters
- Fluorouracil
- Hexachlorophene
- Promethazine
- Sulfanilamide

Systemic
- Carbamazepine
- Chlorpromazine
- Griseofulvin
- Imipramine
- Lincomycin
- Nalidixic acid
- Naproxen
- Norfloxacin
- Phenothiazines
- Piroxicam
- Quinethazone
- Sulfonamides
- Sulfonylureas
- Thiazide diuretics
- Triamterene

FIXED DRUG ERUPTIONS
Acetaminophen
5-Aminosalicylic acid
Aspirin
Barbiturates
Benzodiazepines
Chloroquine
Dapsone
Dimenhydrinate
Diphenhydramine
Gold salts
Hydralazine
Hyoscine
Ibuprofen
Iodides
Meprobamate
Methenamine
Metronidazole
Penicillins
Phenobarbital
Phenolphthalein
Phenothiazines
Phenylbutazone
Procarbazine
Pseudoephedrine
Quinine
Saccharin
Streptomycin
Sulfonamides
Tetracyclines

ERYTHEMA NODOSUM
Bromides
Oral contraceptives
Penicillin
Sulfonamides

CONTACT DERMATITIS
Ambroxol
Amikacin
p-Aminobenzoic acid
Antihistamines
Bacitracin
Benzalkonium chloride
Benzocaine
Benzyl alcohol

Continued

TABLE 27–5 SOME NOTABLE ADVERSE DRUG REACTIONS—cont'd

Cetyl alcohol
Chloramphenicol
Chlorpromazine
Clioquinol
Colophony
Ethylenediamine
Fluorouracil
Formaldehyde
Gentamicin
Glucocorticoids
Glutaraldehyde
Heparin
Hexachlorophene
Iodochlorhydroxyquin
Lanolin
Local anesthetics
Minoxidil
Naftin
Neomycin
Nitrofurazone
Opiates
Parabens
Penicillins
Phenothiazines
Proflavine
Propylene glycol
Streptomycin
Sulfonamides
Thimerosal
Timolol

LUNGS

ASTHMA

Aspirin and other NSAIDs
Cromolyn
Occupational exposures to
- Cephalosporins
- Glutaraldehyde
- Pancreatic enzymes
- Papain
- Penicillins
- Psyllium
- Thimerosal

Sulfite
Tartrazine

EOSINOPHILIC PNEUMONITIS

5-Aminosalicylic acid
Azathioprine
Captopril
Carbamazepine
Chlorpropamide
Cromolyn
Desipramine
Gold salts
Imipramine
Nitrofurantoin
Penicillins
Phenytoin
Sulfonamides
L-Tryptophan

FIBROTIC AND PLEURAL REACTIONS

Bleomycin
Busulfan
Cyclophosphamide
Gold salts
Hydralazine
Hydrochlorothiazide
Melphalan
Methotrexate
Methysergide
Mitomycin
Nitrofurantoin
Procarbazine

LIVER

CHOLESTATIC

Chlorzoxazone
Erythromycin estolate
Ethchlorvynol
Imipramine
Nalidixic acid
Nitrofurantoin
Phenothiazines
Sulfamethoxazole
Sulfonylureas
Troleandomycin

HEPATOCELLULAR

5-Aminosalicylic acid
Amphotericin B
Azapropazone
Ethacrynic acid
Furosemide
Gold salts
Griseofulvin
Halothane
Hydantoins
Isoniazid
Methyldopa
Monoamine oxidase inhibitors
Nitrofurantoin
Propylthiouracil
Pyrazinamide
Quinidine
Rifampin
Sulfonamides
Trimethadione

CHRONIC ACTIVE HEPATITIS

Methyldopa
Nitrofurantoin

KIDNEY

GLOMERULITIS

Allopurinol
Captopril
Gold salts
NSAIDs
Penicillamine
Penicillins
Phenytoin
Probenecid
Sulfonamides
Thiazide diuretics

INTERSTITIAL NEPHRITIS

Allopurinol
Aztreonam
Captopril
Carbamazepine
Cephalosporins
Chloramphenicol
Cimetidine
Ciprofloxacin
Colistin
Furosemide
Minocycline
NSAIDs
Penicillins, especially methicillin
Phenytoin
Polymyxin B
Rifampin
Sulfonamides
Tetracycline
Thiazide diuretics

BONE MARROW AND BLOOD CELLS

BONE MARROW APLASIA

Chloramphenicol
Gold salts
Mephenytoin
Penicillamine
Phenylbutazone
Trimethadione

ANEMIA

Acetaminophen
5-Aminosalicylic acid
Captopril
Cephalosporins
Chlorpromazine
Cisplatin
Hydantoins
Ibuprofen
Insulin
Isoniazid
Levodopa
Mefenamic acid
Melphalan
Methyldopa
Methysergide
Penicillins
Quinidine
Quinine
Rifampin
Sulfonamides
Sulfonylureas

THROMBOCYTOPENIA

Acetaminophen
Acetazolamide
Acetylsalicylic acid
5-Aminosalicylic acid
Carbamazepine
Chloramphenicol
Chlorpheniramine
Cimetidine
Digitoxin
Diltiazem
Ethchlorvynol
Gold salts
Heparin
Hydantoins
Isoniazid
Levodopa
Meprobamate
Methyldopa
Penicillamine
Phenylbutazone
Procainamide
Quinidine
Quinine
Ranitidine
Rauwolfia alkaloids
Rifampin
Sulfonamides
Sulfonylureas
Thiazide diuretics

TABLE 27–5 SOME NOTABLE ADVERSE DRUG REACTIONS—cont'd

GRANULOCYTOPENIA	Phenothiazines	**LYMPHOID HYPERPLASIA**
Captopril	Phenylbutazone	Phenytoin
Cephalosporins	Phenytoin	Mephenytoin
Chloral hydrate	Procainamide	
Chlorpropamide	Propranolol	
Penicillins (semisynthetic)	Tolbutamide	

ACTH = adrenocorticotropic hormone; NSAIDs = nonsteroidal anti-inflammatory drug.
Modified from Reed CE: Drug allergy. *In* Wyngaarden JB, Smith LH Jr, Bennett JC (eds): Cecil Textbook of Medicine, 19th ed. Philadelphia, WB Saunders, 1992, pp 1480–1481.

administration of penicillin by any route. Skin testing with penicillin G, penicilloic acid, or penicilloyl polylysine can identify patients at risk and should be performed in patients with suspected penicillin allergy who need to be treated with penicillin. If the skin test result is positive, the patient must undergo desensitization before receiving penicillin. If the skin test result is negative, penicillin can be administered with caution.

Diagnosis of Adverse Drug Responses

Although many of the well-known adverse drug effects are due to a relatively small group of drugs, every drug potentially can cause an adverse drug response. The physician always should consider the possibility of an adverse drug response in the differential diagnosis even if none has been reported previously for the particular drug. Table 27–5 lists many diverse clinical presentations associated with adverse drug responses. In many instances, it is readily apparent that a specific drug has produced an adverse drug response, such as the appearance of a rash in an otherwise healthy patient who recently has been prescribed a single drug (e.g., penicillin). In other cases, the effect produced by the drug may be difficult to discern from other disease states. In still other cases, the adverse effect may mimic the illness being treated (e.g., development of an arrhythmia in a patient being treated with an antiarrhythmic drug).

From a public health perspective, it is highly desirable to have a mechanism available to detect, catalog, and track the incidence and severity of adverse drug responses not only for drugs at various stages of development but also for drugs that were approved earlier. The Food and Drug Administration tries to track adverse drug events through a voluntary reporting program, MedWatch. Health care professionals are encouraged to report any adverse events or product problems on a one-page form that can be sent by mail, fax, or electronically to the Food and Drug Administration. Although various methods for surveying adverse drug responses have been proposed, ultimately the cooperation of alert clinicians and health care professionals must be encouraged.

SUGGESTED READINGS

Cusack BJ: Pharmacokinetics in older persons. Am J Geriatr Pharmacother 2004;2:274–302. *Reviews the changes in pharmacokinetics due to age-related physiologic perturbations that can lead to altered dose requirements.*

Evans WE, McLeod HL: Pharmacogenomics—drug disposition, drug targets, and side effects. N Engl J Med 2003;348:538–549. *Describes how genetic differences affect drug metabolism.*

Gabardi S, Abramson S: Drug dosing in chronic kidney disease. Med Clin North Am 2005;89:649–687. *Specific recommendations are available for dosing of medications in chronic kidney disease.*

Greenblatt DL, von Moltke LL: Interaction of warfarin with drugs, natural substances, and foods. J Clin Pharmacol 2005;45:127–132. *This review documents the variability in the anticoagulant response to warfarin, one of the drugs most often associated with interactions with other drugs, natural substances, and foods.*

Mertens-Talcott SU, Zadezensky I, De Castro WV, et al: Grapefruit-drug interactions: Can interactions with drugs be avoided? J Clin Pharmacol 2006;46:1390–1416. *Review of clinically important drug interactions.*

Obach RS, Walsky RL, Venkatakrishnan K, et al: In vitro cytochrome P450 inhibition data and the prediction of drug-drug interactions: Qualitative relationships, quantitative predictions, and the rank-order approach. Clin Pharmacol Ther 2005;78:582–592. *In vitro inhibition data can be used in the prediction of in vivo drug-drug interactions.*

Relling MV, Hoffman JM: Should pharmacogenomic studies be required for new drug approval? Clin Pharmacol Ther 2007;81:425–428. *Makes the case for basic testing.*

Williamson EM: Interactions between herbal and conventional medicines. Expert Opin Drug Saf 2005;4:355–378. *Review of clinically important drug interactions that occur with commonly used herbal medicines and prescribed drugs.*

Wysowski DK, Swartz L: Adverse drug event surveillance and drug withdrawals in the United States, 1969–2002: The importance of reporting suspected reactions. Arch Intern Med 2005;165:1363–1369. *Despite limitations of underreporting and incomplete reporting, reports submitted to the Food and Drug Administration and pharmaceutical manufacturers often permit identification of serious adverse effects that can then be added to the product labeling.*

28 PAIN

Mitchell B. Max

Pain is the main symptom for which patients seek relief and is often a key clue for diagnosis. Only recently, however, have the mechanisms involved in the generation of pain been elucidated. Previously, the study of pain and its treatment were of relatively marginal interest to medical science and limited to anesthesiology, neurology, and a few other specialties. Now, basic neuroscientists are rapidly expanding the understanding of pain processing, making it possible for any interested clinician to translate these mechanistic insights into better diagnosis and treatment.

PAIN MECHANISMS AND THEIR IMPLICATIONS FOR PRACTICE

Pain Pathways and Mechanisms

Transmission

A conscious experience of pain generally requires signaling by two neurons in sequence (Fig. 28–1, left panel). The peripheral nociceptor has specialized tissue endings that transduce strong mechanical, thermal, or chemical stimuli into action potentials. This nerve fiber, which is nourished by a cell body in the dorsal root ganglion in the spinal canal, sends its central process into the dorsal horn of the spinal cord to synapse on a secondary neuron. The peripheral neuron releases excitatory neurotransmitters, such as glutamate and substance P, which cause the secondary neuron to discharge, sending impulses into its projections to the brain stem and thalamus. Projection of nociception to this level is sufficient to evoke pain experience and behavior, but additional processing by projections to the cerebral cortex contributes to the distinct sensory qualities, mood, and motor responses associated with the pain experience.

Modulation

Comparison of a crying child with a minor scrape of the knee, a college football hero running full speed on a broken ankle, and a depressed adult with multiple pain complaints and negative evaluations makes it clear that there is not a one-to-one correspondence between a peripheral lesion and the experience of pain. Such reflections led to the hypothesis that higher brain centers could modulate incoming pain signals. Decades of animal studies have elucidated systems that descend to the spinal dorsal horn (see Fig. 28–1, right panel) and either can inhibit or can amplify

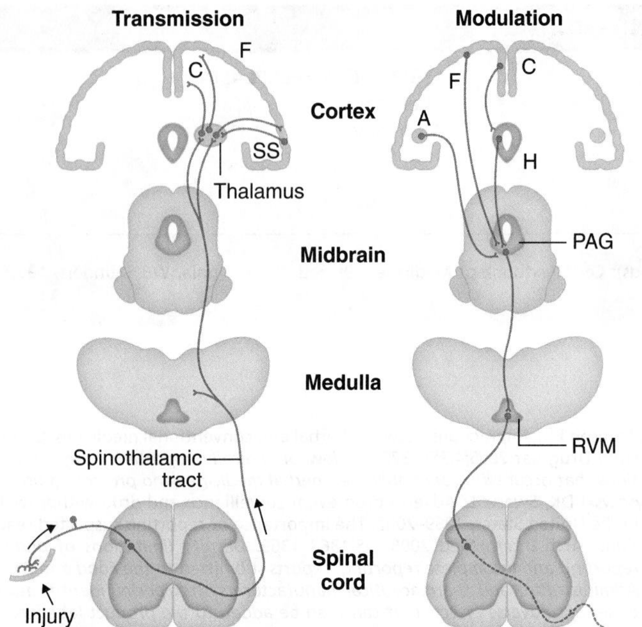

FIGURE 28–1 • Pain transmission and modulation pathways. Left, A noxious stimulus applied to the skin (lower left) elicits a train of impulses beginning in peripheral nociceptors and propagated to the dorsal horn of the spinal cord, where they activate the nerve cells of origin of the spinothalamic tract. The spinothalamic tract activates thalamic neurons, which project to and activate neurons in the cingulate cortex (C), frontal cortex (F), and somatosensory cortex (SS). Right, A variety of stimuli can activate pain modulation circuits. Frontal and cingulate cortex projections and afferents from the amygdala (A) and hypothalamus (H) converge on midbrain periaqueductal gray (PAG) neurons, which, through a relay in the rostral ventromedial medulla (RVM), control spinothalamic pain transmission neurons. (Redrawn from Fields HL: Pain modulation: Expectation, opioid analgesia and virtual pain. Progr Brain Res 2000;122:245–253. © 2000, with permission from Elsevier Science.)

pain signals, depending on the importance of pain to the organism in that situation. Neurophysiologic studies in nonhuman primates whose state of attention is modified during painful stimulation suggest mechanisms by which a variety of clinical interventions, such as reassurance, cognitive-behavioral therapy, and placebo effects associated with drug treatments, may not only change patients' interpretation of incoming pain messages but also markedly decrease the number of pain impulses arising at the spinal dorsal horn projection neuron.

Plasticity of Pain-Processing Circuits

Injuries to peripheral tissues or nerve and the resulting painful input alter subsequent pain processing. In the uninjured state (Fig. 28–2), noxious and innocuous stimuli trigger modest numbers of impulses in nociceptors and Aβ mechanoreceptors. Only the noxious stimuli result in pain. After injury to any kind of tissue, release of inflammatory mediators, such as prostaglandins, cytokines, bradykinin, and protons, sensitizes nociceptors (see Fig. 28–2) so that light touch can trigger impulses in these fibers, and noxious stimuli cause higher rates of firing than before. If nerve is injured, new sodium channels at sites of repair or regeneration give rise to spontaneous discharges, which can lead to steady or episodic pain in the absence of peripheral stimulation. In some cases, adrenoreceptors at the injury site trigger pain when activated by norepinephrine released by local sympathetic nerves or by circulating catecholamines (see Fig. 28–2). A barrage of painful impulses from injured nerve or tissue can sensitize the central neuron (see Fig. 28–2) so that light touch signals carried by Aβ fibers can trigger a central discharge sufficient to generate pain.

Additional mechanisms have been described in animals to explain the development of pain with light touch. One day or more after tissue injury, Aβ mechanoreceptors may begin to make a neurotransmitter, substance P, that is otherwise confined to pain-signaling fibers and excites central pain projection neurons. After nerve injury, Aβ mechanoreceptors, which normally synapse in a deep layer of the spinal cord that processes light touch, may grow new sprouts that synapse on pain projection neurons in the superficial dorsal spinal cord.

Implications for Diagnosis of Painful Complaints

Proximal Limbs, Trunk, and Viscera have Heavily Overlapping Input on a few Spinal Neurons

Patients' description of pain arising from many of these structures may be similar. Figure 28–3 shows that nociceptors from heart, esophagus, and deep tissues in the left shoulder and chest wall may synapse on the same spinal dorsal horn neuron. Noxious chemical stimulation of the heart (by ischemia) or esophagus (acid) may be described as pain in the left shoulder and proximal arm and the chest, whereas inflammation of the left chest wall may be perceived as deep visceral and local musculoskeletal pain. Commonly, patients with chest wall or esophageal inflammation present with sudden overwhelming chest pain indistinguishable from that described by patients with myocardial infarction and require hospitalization until stable electrocardiograms, cardiac biomarkers, and other test results exclude cardiac ischemia (Chapters 48 and 71). Current evidence suggests that some individuals have an increased tendency to develop central sensitivity to widely distributed thoracic visceral pain inputs after stimulation of a small area of the lower esophagus with acid. This physiologic trait appeared to be common in patients who had been hospitalized for chest pain with subsequent normal findings on cardiac evaluation. Similar interactions among noxious stimuli may occur in pelvic disease. In women with chronic renal stones, attacks of colic severe enough to require hospitalization tend to occur near the times of painful menses. Sensory studies show sensitization to stimulation of muscle fibers whose afferents feed into the same spinal segment as the uterine and renal pain.

Another example is the well-known phenomenon that disease in proximal body parts may refer to other parts of a limb. Bone and soft tissue disease in the spine often refers pain to the buttock or hip, and disease in the hip often refers pain to the knee. Figure 28–4 illustrates the timing and location of pain after the experimental infusion of hypertonic saline into the upper anterior tibialis muscle of normal volunteers. Local pain is described near the upper tibial injection site, but pain also is referred to an area just above the ankle (see Fig. 28–4A). The local muscle pain begins immediately (see Fig. 28–4B), whereas the referred pain is not reported for another 20 seconds. This sequence argues against the simple "converging input" model of referred pain illustrated in Figure 28–3. With the former model, one would expect the referred pain to be felt as soon as the local pain begins. The delay suggests that an additional process intervenes (e.g., that it takes 20 seconds for the pain input from the saline infusion to sensitize central neurons, after which they can be activated by low-level innocuous input from the ankle area).

Implications for Pain Treatment

The application of these physiologic principles to treatment may be illustrated by considering pain related to herpes zoster, one of the best-studied pain disorders. In the prodrome, zoster virus is produced by spinal dorsal root ganglion cells, where the zoster DNA has been dormant in neuronal nuclei for decades after a childhood chickenpox attack. Acute hemorrhagic inflammation first occurs in the ganglion, most commonly a thoracic ganglion. The patient may perceive severe pain in any of the structures innervated by that thoracic nerve, which may cause a misdiagnosis of biliary colic or myocardial ischemia. After several days, the virus is transported to the periphery, causing the pathognomonic belt of skin vesicles, and to the spinal cord. Depending on the severity of the inflammatory reactions, a few or almost all of the peripheral and central sensory nerve fibers may die.

In the acute phase, antiviral and anti-inflammatory medications are most effective in relieving pain and minimizing nerve fiber death. Nonsteroidal anti-inflammatory drugs (NSAIDs) reduce the amount of sensitization of primary afferents and contribute as well to reducing spinal cord excitation. Opioids may complement this analgesic effect by activating opioid receptors on peripheral pain nerve endings, reducing their excitability; on presynaptic spinal terminals of these fibers, reducing the amount of excitatory transmitter release; or on spinal or higher central nervous system neurons, directly inhibiting firing.

In herpes zoster cases with extensive neural damage, most common in elderly and immunosuppressed patients, pain may persist for months or years and is termed postherpetic neuralgia. The efficacy of various treatments may depend on the pattern of neural loss and activity. When

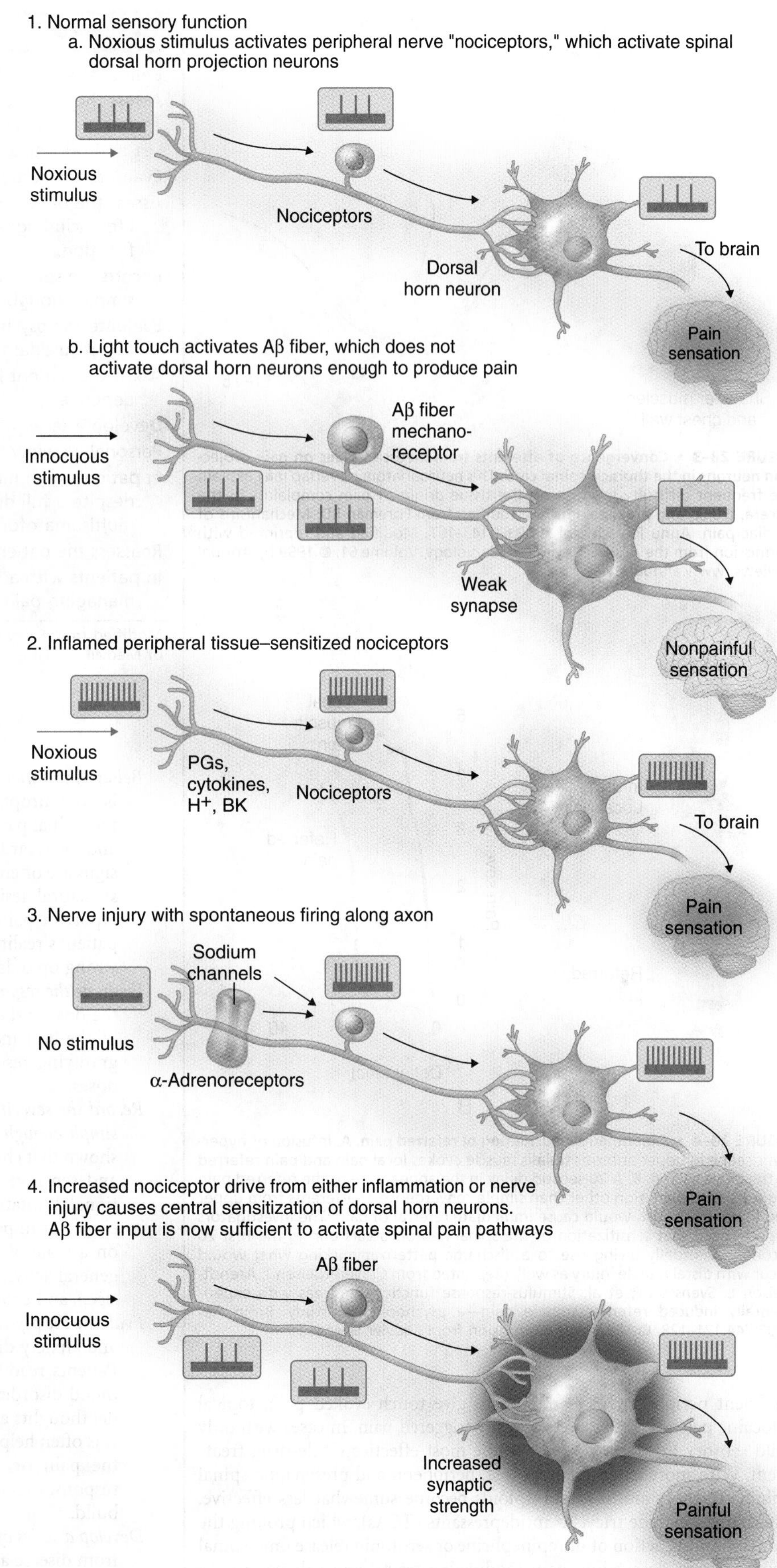

FIGURE 28–2 • Plasticity of pain-processing circuits. See text for explanation. Aβ = amyloid-beta; BK = bradykinin; PG = prostaglandins. (Modified from Woolf CJ, Mannion RJ: Neuropathic pain: Etiology, symptoms, mechanisms, and management. Lancet 1999;353:1959–1964.)

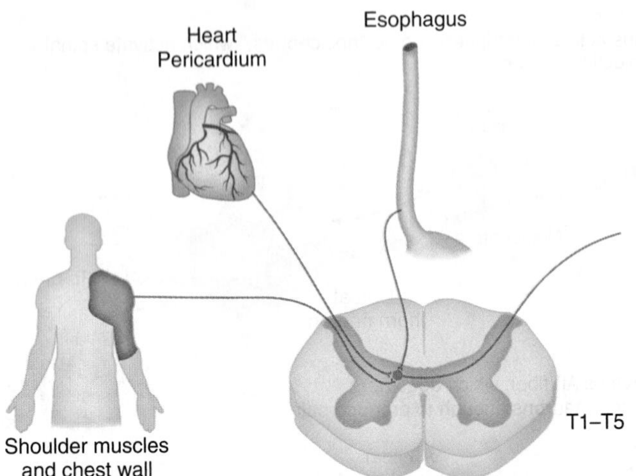

FIGURE 28–3 • Convergence of afferents from diverse tissues on pain projection neurons in the thoracic spinal cord. This neuroanatomic overlap may explain the frequent difficulty in inferring the tissue origin of pain complaints in the viscera, trunk, and proximal limbs. (Modified from Foreman RD: Mechanisms of cardiac pain. Annu Rev Physiol 1999;61:143–167. Modified and reprinted with permission from the Annual Review of Physiology, Volume 61. © 1999 by Annual Reviews, *www.annualreviews.org*.)

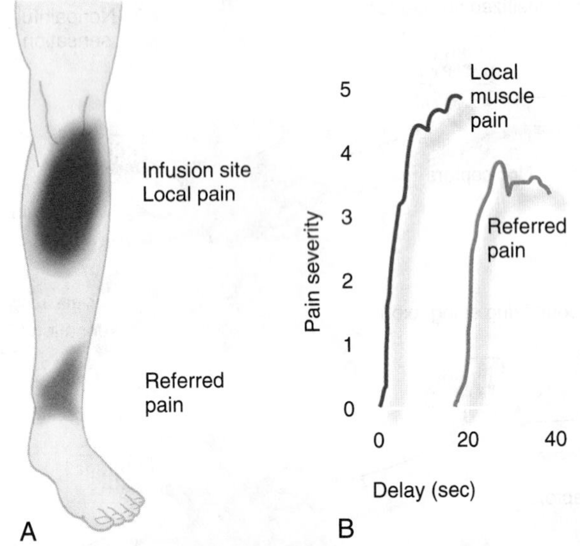

FIGURE 28–4 • Experimental elucidation of referred pain. A, Infusion of hypertonic saline in upper anterior tibialis muscle evokes local pain and pain referred to the ankle region. **B,** A 20-second delay in the appearance of the referred pain suggests an explanation other than simple convergence of afferents from upper and lower leg, which would cause immediate referral of pain. The investigators hypothesized that sensitization of the spinal neuron occurs during the first 20 seconds, eventually giving rise to a discharge pattern mimicking what would occur with distal muscle injury as well. (Reprinted from Graven-Nielsen T, Arendt-Nelson L, Svensson P, et al: Stimulus-response functions in areas with experimentally induced referred muscle pain—a psychophysical study. Brain Res 1997;744:121–128. © 1997, with permission from Elsevier Science.)

sufficient peripheral fibers remain to give touch-evoked pain, topical lidocaine patches reduce mechanically triggered pain. In cases with only mild sensory loss, opioids may be the most effective single-drug treatment. With more extensive fiber loss, peripheral and presynaptic spinal opioid receptors are lost, and opioids become somewhat less effective. Alternatives include tricyclic antidepressants (TCAs), which prolong the pain-inhibiting action of norepinephrine or serotonin release onto spinal neurons from descending pain-modulating tracts, and gabapentin, an anticonvulsant that blocks processes leading to sensitization of spinal cord sensory neurons.

APPROACH TO THE PATIENT WITH PAIN

Table 28–1 lists some of the principles of assessing and treating the patient with pain.

TABLE 28–1 CLINICAL ASSESSMENT OF PAIN

Believe the patient's complaint of pain.
Assess the characteristics of each pain, including site, referral pattern, and aggravating and relieving factors.
List and prioritize each pain complaint.
Evaluate the response to previous and current analgesic therapies.
Assess the patient's current level of functioning in work and family life, including what his or her priorities are for increasing function.
Record the severity of pain and functional impairment with a scale simple enough for repeated use.
Evaluate the psychological state of the patient, asking specifically about suicidal thoughts.
Ask if the patient has a past history of alcohol or drug dependence.
Develop a series of diagnosis-related hypotheses.
Personally review the dignostic procedures.
In patients with multiple chronic symptoms that are unexplained despite a full diagnostic evaluation, consider the possibility of multisomatoform disorder.
Reassess the patient's response to pain therapy.
In patients with advanced illness, discuss advance directives for managing pain and other symptoms.

Modified from Foley KM: Pain. *In* Goldman L, Bennett C (eds): Cecil Textbook of Medicine, 21st ed. Philadelphia, WB Saunders, 2000, p 104.

Believe the patient's complaint of pain. Despite decades of effort, there is no neurophysiologic or chemical test that can measure pain in individual patients. Objective observations of grimacing, limping, and tachycardia may be useful in assessing the patient, but these signs are often absent in patients with chronic pain caused by large structural lesions. The clinician can acknowledge the patient's report of pain before understanding its cause. Acceptance of the patient's reality of pain does not obligate the physician to provide strong opioids or other particular types of treatments.

Evaluate the response to previous and current analgesic therapies. Record the dose and duration of each previous treatment. Optimal doses of the best medication for a particular syndrome often produce gratifying results in patients who failed a brief trial with lower doses.

Record the severity of pain and functional impairment with a measure simple enough for repeated use. Extensive work in many diseases has shown that changes on a scale of 0 to 10 for pain intensity are valid and sensitive for detecting meaningful relief. Pain-related functional limitations can be assessed either by using the patient's choice of important activities or by asking the patient how much, on a scale of 0 to 10, pain has interfered with domains such as general activity, mood, walking, work, relations with other people, sleep, and enjoyment of life.

Evaluate the psychological state of the patient. Unrecognized depression and anxiety disorders are common in patients with chronic pain. Patients readily tell the clinician about these if asked, and these mood disorders are readily treatable. Assess the presence of suicidal thoughts and the pain's effect on the patient's sexual activities. It is often helpful to ask patients how they are coping in the face of the pain or what keeps them from giving up because these responses identify sources of strength on which the clinician can build.

Develop a series of diagnosis-based hypotheses. Because pain may result from disease at the pain site or be referred from other parts of the body, it may be helpful to list all the possibilities for the site of origin, particularly when the pain has been resistant to therapy. Persistent rib pain in a patient with metastatic cancer despite radiation therapy to the lesion in that rib would raise the possibility of referred pain from thoracic epidural tumor, which can be imaged and treated. For each potential site of the lesion, the list of the common disease processes in that area can be considered.

Personally review the diagnostic procedures. In the re-evaluation of difficult pain diagnoses, it is remarkable how often lesions had been missed previously on imaging procedures, particularly when the radiologist was not given a specific diagnostic hypothesis.

In patients with multiple chronic symptoms that are unexplained despite a full diagnostic evaluation, consider the possibility of multisomatoform disorder. This more recently proposed diagnosis, which applies to one tenth of primary care visits, is defined by the presence of three bothersome and unexplained complaints, some of which have troubled the patient on most days in the previous 2 years. Depending on the presenting complaint or the clinician's specialty, many of these patients are said to have fibromyalgia, chronic fatigue, irritable bowel syndrome, idiopathic low back pain, or chronic tension-type headaches, but most of these patients have multisystem complaints. Laboratory studies suggest that generalized amplification of symptoms by the central nervous system is common in these patients. Recognition of multisomatoform disorder alerts the clinician to look closely for depressive or panic disorders, whose prevalence is high in these patients; to treat with antidepressants or cognitive-behavioral treatment, shown to reduce symptoms; and to limit elaborate diagnostic testing or potentially hazardous medical treatments.

Reassess the patient's response to pain therapy. The principles of analgesic treatment are simple, but dose requirements and adverse effects vary widely. A daily phone call until the patient's treatment has been optimized is often the key to successful treatment. 

Treatment

Rx

Mastery of the principles of analgesic drug prescribing yields gratifying results (Fig. 28–5). Three key classes of analgesic drugs are traditional nonopioid analgesics, including acetaminophen, NSAIDs, and selective cyclooxygenase-2 (COX-2) inhibitors (of limited use because of cardiovascular side effects); opioid analgesics; and miscellaneous analgesics, including some antidepressant and anticonvulsant drugs.

Many novel analgesics are in early clinical development, and ongoing studies will define better the benefit-to-risk ratio of long-term opioid treatment in subsets of patients with nonmalignant pain. The greatest opportunity for advance may rest with medical and surgical specialists outside of the traditional pain research community who test current theories about pain physiology and treatment.

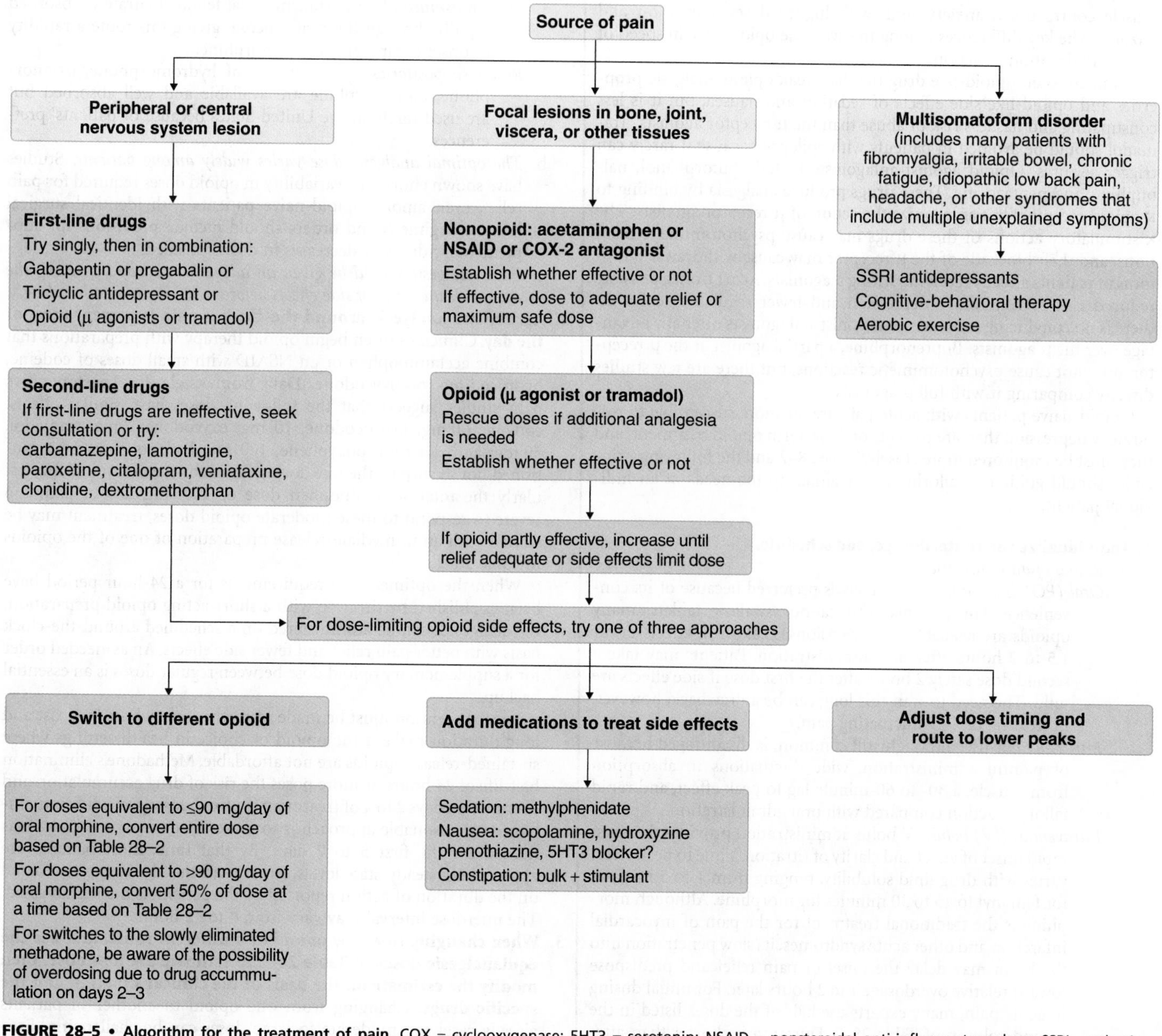

Source of pain

Peripheral or central nervous system lesion
→ **First-line drugs**: Try singly, then in combination: Gabapentin or pregabalin or Tricyclic antidepressant or Opioid (μ agonists or tramadol)
→ **Second-line drugs**: If first-line drugs are ineffective, seek consultation or try: carbamazepine, lamotrigine, paroxetine, citalopram, veniafaxine, clonidine, dextromethorphan

Focal lesions in bone, joint, viscera, or other tissues
→ **Nonopioid: acetaminophen or NSAID or COX-2 antagonist**: Establish whether effective or not. If effective, dose to adequate relief or maximum safe dose
→ **Opioid (μ agonist or tramadol)**: Rescue doses if additional analgesia is needed. Establish whether effective or not
→ If opioid partly effective, increase until relief adequate or side effects limit dose

Multisomatoform disorder (includes many patients with fibromyalgia, irritable bowel, chronic fatigue, idiopathic low back pain, headache, or other syndromes that include multiple unexplained symptoms)
→ SSRI antidepressants; Cognitive-behavioral therapy; Aerobic exercise

For dose-limiting opioid side effects, try one of three approaches:

Switch to different opioid
→ For doses equivalent to ≤90 mg/day of oral morphine, convert entire dose based on Table 28–2. For doses equivalent to >90 mg/day of oral morphine, convert 50% of dose at a time based on Table 28–2. For switches to the slowly eliminated methadone, be aware of the possibility of overdosing due to drug accummulation on days 2–3

Add medications to treat side effects
→ Sedation: methylphenidate. Nausea: scopolamine, hydroxyzine phenothiazine, 5HT3 blocker? Constipation: bulk + stimulant

Adjust dose timing and route to lower peaks

FIGURE 28–5 • Algorithm for the treatment of pain. COX = cyclooxygenase; 5HT3 = serotonin; NSAID = nonsteroidal anti-inflammatory drug; SSRI = selective serotonin reuptake inhibitor.

Nonopioid Analgesics

The chief advantage of nonopioid analgesics is that they do not cause sedation or other central nervous system side effects. Unless the patient has contraindications to these drugs or has been shown not to respond to several of them, any analgesic regimen should include a nonopioid drug even if pain is severe enough to require the addition of an opioid. Acetaminophen optimally is prescribed in doses approaching 4000 mg/day. Higher doses, or standard doses in patients who are fasting or who drink alcohol heavily, may cause hepatic necrosis. Acetaminophen lacks the antiplatelet or gastric erosive effects of the NSAIDs. NSAIDs and COX-2 inhibitors often provide better analgesia than acetaminophen (Chapter 34), although the possible cardiovascular risks of COX-2 inhibitors must be considered.

Opioid Analgesics

The μ receptor opioid agonists include morphine, codeine, oxycodone, hydrocodone, fentanyl, hydromorphone, methadone, and meperidine. More than a century of research has failed to reveal significant differences in the relative ratios of analgesia to side effects offered by different members of this class, although clinical anecdote suggests that individual patients may respond to one drug better than to another. The one exception is meperidine, which has a toxic metabolite that accumulates after several days of treatment and causes myoclonus (a brief, sudden muscle contraction), anxiety, and, with higher doses, confusion and seizures. The key differences among the available opioids are in speed of onset and duration of action.

Tramadol is an opioid-like drug that has weak opioid analgesic properties and opioid-like side effects of sedation and nausea, but it is less constipating and has less risk of abuse than the μ receptor agonists. Tramadol should be avoided in patients with epilepsy because it rarely can trigger seizures. Opioid agonist-antagonists include butorphanol, nalbuphine, and pentazocine. These drugs produce analgesia by binding to κ opioid receptors but antagonize the action of μ receptor agonists. The κ stimulatory actions of these drugs may cause psychotomimetic reactions, and their blockade of the μ receptor may cause withdrawal symptoms in patients already receiving strong μ agonists. Apart from a possibly reduced risk of respiratory depression and fewer regulatory controls, there is no convincing evidence that agonist-antagonists offer any advantage over the μ agonists. Buprenorphine, a partial agonist at the μ receptor, does not cause psychotomimetic reactions, but there are few studies directly comparing it with full μ agonists.

Opioid-naive patients with acute pain are far more susceptible to respiratory depression than are patients on long-term opioid treatment, and they must be monitored more closely. Table 28–2 and the following principles should guide the tailoring of a regimen to the needs of an individual patient.

1. **Individualize the route, dosage, and schedule.**
   a. *Routes of administration*
   Oral (PO). The oral route usually is preferred because of its convenience. For patients who cannot swallow tablets, many opioids are available in suspensions. Peak drug effects occur 1.5 to 2 hours after oral administration. Patients may take a second dose safely 2 hours after the first dose if side effects are mild. The need to wait this long can be a drawback, however, in treating rapidly fluctuating pain.
   Intramuscular use, although still common, is discouraged because of painful administration, wide fluctuations in absorption from muscle, a 30- to 60-minute lag to peak effect, and rapid falloff of action compared with oral administration.
   Intravenous (IV) bolus. IV bolus administration provides the most rapid onset of effect and clarity of titration. Time to peak effect varies with drug lipid solubility, ranging from 1 to 5 minutes for fentanyl to 15 to 30 minutes for morphine. Although morphine is the traditional treatment for the pain of myocardial infarction and other acute syndromes, its slow penetration into the brain may delay the onset of pain relief and predispose toward relative overdosage 1 to 2 hours later. For initial dosing in acute pain, many experts use half of the doses listed in the second column of Table 28–2. Duration is shorter than after intramuscular administration. If severe pain persists but side effects are minimal at the time of expected peak effect, another bolus may be given. Opioids with long elimination half-lives, such as methadone and levorphanol, are not recommended for rapid opioid titration because drug levels remain elevated for many hours if too high a dose is given.
   IV infusion. Continuous IV infusions provide steady blood levels, which should provide the most effective analgesia with the fewest side effects. Subcutaneous infusion is an alternative to IV infusion and produces equivalent blood levels at steady state. Subcutaneous boluses have slower onset and offset, however, and a lower peak effect than IV boluses.
   IV, patient-controlled analgesia. A popular and effective method for treating severe acute pain is to titrate the patient to temporary comfort with IV boluses, then start a patient-controlled analgesia machine. Usual patient-triggered bolus doses of morphine are 0.5 to 2 mg every 5 to 10 minutes.
   Transdermal. Fentanyl is available in a transdermal drug delivery system, providing a steady opioid infusion without pumps or needles. Several clinical trials suggest that constipation is reduced by use of the transdermal route, which avoids the local slowing effects of opioids in the gut. There is a 12- to 24-hour lag to analgesia after initial application of the patch as opioid is transferred to subcutaneous fat and a 24-hour offset after the patch is removed. Temperature higher than 39° F or a local heating pad accelerates absorption and may cause overdose.
   Oral transmucosal. Oral transmucosal fentanyl citrate is absorbed rapidly through the oral mucosa, giving this route a rapidity of onset comparable to IV morphine.
   Rectal suppositories. Suppositories of hydromorphone, oxymorphone, and morphine are available and well absorbed but are used rarely in the United States because of patients' preferences.
   b. *The optimal analgesic dose varies widely among patients.* Studies have shown enormous variability in opioid doses required for pain relief, even among opioid-naive patients with identical surgical lesions. Regimens and orders should include provisions for supplementary doses or decreases in dose if needed.
   c. *Each analgesic should be given an adequate trial by increasing the dose with the onset of side effects before switching to another drug.*
2. **Administer analgesic around-the-clock if pain is present most of the day.** Clinicians often begin opioid therapy with preparations that combine acetaminophen or an NSAID with small doses of codeine, hydrocodone, or oxycodone. Data from single-dose postoperative pain studies suggest that the following doses have similar effects: codeine, 60 mg; hydrocodone, 10 mg; oxycodone, 7 mg; tramadol, 50 mg; and dextropropoxyphene, 100 mg. Patients should be cautioned not to surpass the safe dosing limits for the nonopioid, particularly the total acetaminophen dose of 4000 mg/day. In pain too severe to respond to these moderate opioid doses, treatment may be started with an immediate-release preparation of one of the opioids in Table 28–2.

   When the optimal dose requirements for a 24-hour period have been established by titrating with a short-acting opioid preparation, the analgesics can be administered on a scheduled around-the-clock basis with better pain relief and fewer side effects. An as-needed order for a supplementary opioid dose between regular doses is an essential backup.

   Special mention must be made of methadone, whose low cost and long duration make it the opioid of choice in health settings where sustained-release opioids are not affordable. Methadone's elimination half-life of 24 hours or more poses the risk of drug accumulation and overdose on days 2 to 4 of treatment if a fixed dosing schedule is maintained. A reasonable approach is to prescribe doses of methadone as needed for the first 3 to 7 days. By that time, most patients are approaching steady-state levels. An around-the-clock regimen, based on the duration of action reported by the patient, is then established. The interdose interval may vary from 4 to 12 hours.
3. **When changing to a new opioid or a different route, first use the equianalgesic doses in Table 28–2 to estimate the new dose, then modify the estimate on the basis of the clinical situation and the specific drugs.** Changing from one opioid to another in patients already receiving moderate to large doses can be challenging. Estimates must take into account the wide interindividual variability, any

TABLE 28–2 OPIOID ANALGESICS COMMONLY USED FOR SEVERE PAIN

Name	Equianalgesic Dose (mg) Oral	Parenteral*	Comments	Precautions and Contraindications
MORPHINE-LIKE AGONISTS				
Morphine	30	10	Standard of comparison for opioid analgesics Sustained-release preparations (MS Contin, Oramorph SR, or generic morphine sulfate ER) release drug during 8–12 hr Recent addition of once-a-day sustained-release formulation (Kadian)†	For all opioids, caution in patients with impaired ventilation, bronchial asthma, increased intracranial pressure, liver failure
Hydromorphone (Dilaudid)	7.5	1.5	Slightly shorter duration than morphine	
Oxycodone	20	—	Sustained-release 8–12 hr preparation (OxyContin)	
Methadone (Dolophine)	20, acute 2–4, long term	10, acute 2–4, long term	Good oral potency, long plasma half-life (24–36 hr)	Accumulates with repeated dosing, requiring decreases in dose size and frequency, especially on days 2–5
Levorphanol (Levo-Dromoran)	4, acute 1, long term	2, acute 1, long term	Long plasma half-life (12–16 hr)	Accumulates on days 2–3
Fentanyl	—	0.1	Transdermal fentanyl (Duragesic), 25 μg/hr, roughly equivalent to sustained-release morphine, 45 mg/day Oral transmucosal fentanyl citrate now available for treatment of breakthrough pain in patients with chronic cancer pain already taking around-the-clock opioids	Because of skin reservoir of drug, 12-hr delay in onset and offset of transdermal patch Fever increases dose rate
Oxymorphone (Numorphan)	—	1	5 mg rectal suppository = 5 mg morphine IM	Same as IM morphine
Meperidine (Demerol)	300	75	Slightly shorter acting than morphine	Normeperidine (toxic metabolite) accumulates with repetitive dosing, causing central nervous system excitation Avoid in children and in all patients who have impaired renal function or who are receiving monoamine oxidase uneven inhibitors‡
MIXED AGONIST-ANTAGONISTS				
Nalbuphine (Nubain)	—	10	Not available orally Not scheduled under Controlled Substances Act	Incidence of psychotomimetic effects lower than with pentazocine May precipitate withdrawal in narcotic-dependent patients
Butorphanol (Stadol)	—	2	Same as nalbuphine	Same as nalbuphine
PARTIAL AGONISTS				
Buprenorphine (Buprenex)	—	0.4	Sublingual preparation (0.6 mg) now available in United States to treat addiction Lower abuse liability than with morphine Does not produce psychotomimetic effects	May precipitate withdrawal in narcotic-dependent patients Not readily reversed by naloxone Avoid in labor

*These are standard intramuscular (IM) doses for acute pain in adults and can be used to convert doses for intravenous (IV) infusions and repeated small IV boluses. For single IV boluses, use half the IM dose. For total 24-hour dose, IV and IM doses are similar.
†A once-a-day formulation (Kadian) is available as 20-, 50-, or 100-mg capsules. The sustained-release formulation is not destroyed by breaking the capsule and sprinkling it over food, such as applesauce.
‡Irritating to tissues with repeated IM injection.
Modified from Max MB, Payne R, Edwards WT, et al: Principles of Analgesic Use in the Treatment of Acute Pain and Cancer Pain, 4th ed. Glenview, IL, American Pain Society, 1999.

differences in the time course of absorption and metabolism, the expected course of the pain condition, and the possibility of incomplete cross-tolerance between opioids. For this reason, the general recommendation (see Fig. 28–5) is to convert only half of the dose of the old opioid to the new opioid at one time, in case the estimate in Table 28-2 is too high or too low for that patient.

4. **Anticipate and treat opioid side effects.** Sedation, constipation, nausea, itching, and respiratory depression are the most common side effects, and they may be treated by changing the dosing regimen to provide lower or more steady blood concentrations, by switching to a different opioid, or by adding a treatment that counteracts the adverse effect. Sedation may be counteracted partly by adding a stimulant such as caffeine, dextroamphetamine (2.5 to 10 mg PO), or methylphenidate (5 to 10 mg PO). To prevent constipation, patients should be given stool softeners and agents to increase bowel motility. A useful regimen includes dioctyl sodium sulfosuccinate, 100 to 300 mg/day, combined with senna, 2 to 6 tablets twice a day; laxative suppositories; or lactulose. Opioid-related nausea and vomiting often abate after the first few days of treatment but may be treated with transdermal scopolamine, hydroxyzine, or a phenothiazine antiemetic.

   Although respiratory depression is rare in patients receiving opioid treatment long term, even when doses are increased, it is a risk in the treatment of opioid-naive patients who require high opioid doses for severe pain. When pain is relieved, the patient may fall asleep, which considerably augments the opioid depressant effect and predisposes to closure of the airway by the tongue. In such situations, patients should be stimulated to keep them awake. If an opioid antagonist is required to reverse respiratory depression or coma in a patient on long-term opioids, the physician must be aware that these patients are exquisitely sensitive to antagonists. Experts often start with small doses of naloxone (e.g., one twentieth of a 0.4-mg ampule IV every 2 minutes).

5. **Carefully consider the risk-benefit balance and treatment alternatives before starting long-term opioid treatment for nonmalignant pain.** Large case series suggest that many patients with chronic malignant pain benefit from long-term opioid treatment. Patients often develop tolerance to opioid side effects (except constipation) without losing analgesia. In typical series of patients observed by pain specialists for 10 years or more, behaviors raising concerns about abuse have arisen in only 5 to 10% of patients—most commonly unauthorized dose increases—and usually responded to renegotiation of treatment between clinician and patient. Compared with most other drug classes, opioids are remarkably free of major organ toxicity, with the possible exception of decreased gonadotropic function, which may require estrogen or testosterone replacement (Chapter 32). Surgical pain specialists have reported that the use of opioids has reduced the need for surgical procedures in some chronic pain conditions. Many medical specialty societies and federal and state drug regulators have emphasized that the long-term prescription of opioids in nonmalignant pain is a legitimate medical option.

   There are no controlled trials of opioid therapy in nonmalignant pain beyond 2 months, and the increase in prescribing for nonmalignant pain may create new problems, including opioid abuse and diversion. Table 28–3 summarizes guidelines for appropriate prescribing that have been adopted by the Federation of State Medical Boards of the United States.

   Medication therapy alone rarely provides complete relief of pain. Most pain clinicians agree that the best results may be obtained from combinations of analgesic treatments with psychological and physical approaches to rehabilitation.

TABLE 28–3 GUIDELINES FOR USING CONTROLLED SUBSTANCES FOR THE TREATMENT OF CHRONIC NONMALIGNANT PAIN*

1. Conduct and record a complete history and physical examination, including nature and intensity of pain, current and past pain treatments, effect of pain on physical and psychological function, and whether there is a history of substance abuse. Document one or more recognized medical indications for use of a controlled substance.
2. Record objectives that will determine treatment success, such as pain relief and improved physical and psychosocial function, and indicate if further diagnostic evaluations or treatments are planned.
3. Discuss the risks and benefits of the prescribing of controlled substances with the patient or persons designated by the patient. The patient should receive prescriptions from one physician and one pharmacy whenever possible. If the patient is assessed to be at high risk for medication abuse, consider a written agreement outlining the patient's responsibilities, including urine/blood level screening when requested, the number and frequency of prescription refills, and circumstances, such as violation of the agreement, in which drug therapy may be stopped.
4. Review the course of treatment and reconsider the cause of the pain at reasonable intervals depending on the individual patient. If treatment goals are not being met despite medication adjustments, reconsider the appropriateness of the treatment. Monitor the patient's compliance with medication and other treatment plans.
5. Make referrals as indicated for additional evaluation or treatment. Consider consultation with a psychiatrist or substance abuse expert for patients with a history of substance abuse or a comorbid psychiatric disorder.
6. Keep records current and accessible, and document through the course of treatment how points 1–5 have been addressed.
7. Comply with state and federal controlled substance regulations.

*Abridged from Federation of State Medical Boards, 1998. The unabridged version of these guidelines and a wealth of other information about state and U.S. federal opioid regulatory policies are available at the website of the University of Wisconsin Pain and Policy Group, *http://www.painpolicy.wisc.edu.*

Miscellaneous Analgesics

First-Line Drugs for Pain from Nerve Lesions

Systematic reviews have suggested that three classes of medication have similar effectiveness in 1- to 2-month clinical trials in a variety of neuropathic pain syndromes: opioids (μ agonists and tramadol), TCAs, and gabapentin or its analog, pregabalin. 2 Each of these approaches provides clinically significant relief, defined as a 50% reduction in pain beyond that seen with placebo treatment, for one of every two or three patients. For refractory pain, higher doses of oral opioids provide incremental benefit. Of the TCAs, nortriptyline and imipramine probably have the best efficacy–to–side effect ratio. Amitriptyline is equally effective but sedating, and it should be reserved for bedtime dosing in patients with poor sleep. Desipramine may be less effective but has the least sedation. Specific serotonin reuptake inhibitors seem less effective than the first-generation TCAs. For treatment of pain, TCAs should be initiated at low dosages (10 to 25 mg in a single dose at bedtime) and increased weekly by the same amount as tolerated. Limited dose-response information suggests that an average dose of 125 to 150 mg/day is optimal, but because of interindividual variability in the cytochrome P-450 2D6 isoenzymes that metabolize TCAs, some patients need much lower or higher doses. Side effects include sedation; postural hypotension; weight gain; and anticholinergic effects, such as dry mouth, constipation, and urinary hesitancy. Because TCAs have a quinidine-like proarrhythmic effect in the presence of cardiac ischemia, they are contraindicated in patients with suspected coronary disease.

Gabapentin has efficacy similar to that of TCAs and opioids in neuropathic pain, but it is safer than TCAs because it has no cardiovascular effects or drug interactions. Treatment is started at 100 to 300 mg in a single dose at bedtime, then three times daily, and then titrated to 1800 to 3600 mg/day, which are the doses shown to be effective in randomized trials. Side effects include somnolence, dizziness, and peripheral edema. Dosage must be reduced in patients with renal impairment. Each drug alone usually produces no more than partial relief at maximally tolerated doses. There is preliminary evidence that combinations of drugs with different analgesic mechanisms, such as opioids plus gabapentin, may produce greater pain relief at similar levels of side effects than larger doses of a single agent. 3

Second-Line Drugs for Pain from Nerve Lesions

Second-line drugs include lamotrigine (which must be used with caution because of the uncommon complication of Stevens-Johnson syndrome), carbamazepine, selective serotonin reuptake blockers and venlafaxine, epidural or systemic clonidine, and high-dose dextromethor-phan.

Second-Line Drugs for Cancer Pain

High-dose steroids temporarily shrink many tumors and may be helpful in intractable pain secondary to malignant infiltration of nerves or the spinal cord. Rapid withdrawal of steroids may exacerbate pain. Pamidronate and other bisphosphonates and strontium 89 reduce pain caused by bone metastases.

Physical Therapy

Restoration of physical function is crucial in treating patients with pain. When pain limits physical activities, nerve blocks or coverage with extra analgesic doses may be especially valuable. Injection of painful soft tissue "trigger points" with local anesthetic or saline may be helpful, although controlled studies are lacking.

Cognitive and Behavioral Therapies

Cognitive-behavioral interventions (including training in coping skills and modification of thoughts, feelings, and behaviors) can increase function and reduce distress caused by pain. Some patients may be able to use relaxation techniques, biofeedback, meditation, imagery, or self-hypnosis to reduce muscle tension and emotional arousal or to enhance pain tolerance (Chapter 36). Experienced clinicians sometimes work with family members to encourage the patient to increase function, overriding the natural inclination to relieve the loved one of pain-provoking activities.

Nerve Blocks, Spinal Infusions, and Neurosurgical Interventions

Anesthetic and neurosurgical procedures are occasionally helpful in intractable pain. Nerve blocks are limited because motor, light touch, and position sense fibers accompany pain fibers in most nerves. Local anesthetics and permanent neurolytic treatments with alcohol or phenol usually cause unacceptable motor loss along with pain blockade. Temporary nerve blocks sometimes provide a window for physical therapy, however, which itself may give sustained relief. Selective blockade of sympathetic nerves may be helpful in pain conditions such as reflex sympathetic dystrophy or complex regional pain syndrome types I and II. Injection of the celiac plexus may provide selective analgesia of the pancreas and transverse colon by interrupting the afferent fibers that run through the ganglion.

Epidural or intrathecal infusion of opioids or local anesthetics may relieve pain below the midthorax with fewer cerebrally mediated side effects than with systemic opioids. Electrical spinal cord stimulators, which may activate endogenous pain-modulating systems, can be implanted as an outpatient procedure and have been shown to be moderately effective in complex regional pain syndrome. 4

Destructive neurosurgical procedures, such as anterolateral cordotomy, dorsal root entry zone destruction, midline myelotomies, and destruction of nerve roots with alcohol, have become uncommon since the more widespread use of systemic and epidural opioids. The exception is trigeminal neuralgia, in which neurosurgery remains an important option (Chapter 421). As with any major surgical procedure, benefits are greatest and complications minimized when these procedures are performed by experts who do them frequently.

Management of Pain in Terminal Illness

Pain may become severe in the final weeks of cancer and other illnesses (Chapters 2 and 3). Expert consultation should be sought early to prepare for possible worsening. Clinicians should not be reluctant to give as much opioid analgesic as needed, even though there is a possibility that major increases in dose may slow respiration and hasten death by hours or, rarely, days (Chapter 3). Regulatory authorities, medical societies, and ethicists are unanimous in their written policies stating that in this situation, pain relief is the prime concern, and clinicians should not be criticized or disciplined if death is hastened as a byproduct of this effort. On occasion, opioid tolerance develops to the point where opioids are unhelpful. At doses above several hundred milligrams per hour, morphine infusions may cause neuroexcitation or seizures, necessitating a switch to a different opioid. If opioids, NSAIDs, local anesthetics, and other measures are insufficient, sedation with barbiturates, benzodiazepines, propofol, or other anesthetic agents may provide comfort for the remaining hours of life.

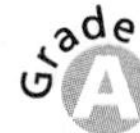

1. Miaskowski C, Dodd M, West C, et al: Randomized clinical trial of the effectiveness of a self-care intervention to improve cancer pain management. J Clin Oncol 2004;22:1713–1720.
2. Finnerup NB, Otto M, McQuay HJ, et al: Algorithm for neuropathic pain treatment: An evidence-based proposal. Pain 2005;118:289–305.
3. Gilron I, Bailey JM, Tu D, et al: Morphine, gabapentin, or their combination for neuropathic pain. N Engl J Med 2005;352:1324–1334.
4. Johnson M, Martinson M: Efficacy of electrical nerve stimulation for chronic musculoskeletal pain: A meta-analysis of randomized controlled trials. Pain 2007. Epub ahead of print.

SUGGESTED READINGS

Bradshaw DH, Nakamura Y, Chapman CR: National Institutes of Health grant awards for pain, nausea, and dyspnea research: An assessment of funding patterns in 2003. J Pain 2005;6:277–293. *An analysis of current U.S. academic pain research, whose major finding is that the extraordinary advances in understanding the molecular principles of pain have received little application yet in clinical areas such as cardiology, urology, gynecology, and gastroenterology.*

Federation of State Medical Boards of the United States, Inc: Model Guidelines for the Use of Controlled Substances for the Treatment of Pain. Available at www.painpolicy.wisc.edu/domestic/model04.pdf. *The most commonly used standards by which state medical boards judge whether prescription of opioids for chronic nonmalignant pain is within the standard of care.*

Koltzenburg M, McMahon SB (eds): Wall and Melzack's Textbook of Pain, 5th ed. London, Elsevier, 2006. *The leading pain textbook, particularly noteworthy for the fine reviews about basic pain mechanisms.*

Martell BA, O'Connor PG, Kerns RD, et al: Systematic review: Opioid treatment for chronic back pain: Prevalence, efficacy, and association with addiction. Ann Intern Med 2007;146:116–127. *Good short-term efficacy, but long-term efficacy unclear with a 6 to 24% risk of addictive behavior.*

Max MB, Lynn J (eds): Symptom Research: Methods and Opportunities. Available at http://symptomresearch.nih.gov. *A web-based interactive textbook that uses real data sets and research scenarios to teach clinical research approaches to pain, nausea, fatigue, constipation, anorexia, dyspnea, and other common symptoms.*

29 BIOLOGY OF ADDICTION

Steven E. Hyman

Addiction is a significant contributor to medical morbidity and mortality, both directly as a result of the toxic effects of abused drugs and indirectly through accidents, suicide, nonsterile needle use, and violence. By far the greatest contributors to illness and death are the widely used legal drugs tobacco and alcohol, although illegal addictive drugs and abuse of prescription drugs also contribute. Outside of medical statistics, addiction exacts an enormous toll on society by impairing the function of the addicted person in multiple life roles, disrupting families and neighborhoods, blighting productivity, and producing enormous costs for the criminal justice system.

Addiction is often remarkably frustrating to treat. The acts of obtaining and using drugs involve a series of voluntary behavior that an otherwise sentient patient seems unable or unwilling to control. What is worse, after enormous effort has been exerted to get a patient into treatment, relapse is all too common, even months and years after apparently successful detoxification and rehabilitation. The cardinal feature of addiction is compulsive substance use despite serious negative consequences. "Compulsive use" means that the addicted person cannot control substance use effectively despite powerful reasons to do so, such as drug-induced medical illness, arrest, or the threat of losing one's job or children; addicted individuals often fail to control use over time even when they strongly desire to do so. A result of this compulsion is a significant narrowing of life focus to seeking and using drugs. Tolerance, dependence, and withdrawal may occur but are neither necessary nor sufficient for addiction. Tolerance, dependence, "rebound," and withdrawal symptoms occur with a wide variety of drugs used in the practice of medicine, such as antidepressants, without producing compulsive use. The unfortunate selection of the term "dependence" to signify "addiction" in the fourth edition of the *Diagnostic and Statistical Manual of Mental Disorders* (DSM-IV) of the American Psychiatric Association has led to the confusion of physiologic dependence with addiction by physicians and patients alike, thus complicating the treatment of anxiety disorders, severe pain, and other conditions. Most importantly, addicted individuals remain at high risk for relapse long after detoxification and the cessation of withdrawal symptoms. If dependence and withdrawal were necessary factors in addiction, the phenomenon of late relapse would not be the major clinical problem that it is.

In recent years there has been progress in understanding both the risk factors and the pathophysiology of addiction. The most important goals of current research include elucidation of the disordered neural processes that contribute to compulsion and persistence of relapse risk. When compared with other neuropsychiatric disorders, the study of addiction has the advantage that the critical causative factors (the drugs themselves) are known, even though significant genetic and nongenetic risk factors remain unknown. This has permitted the development of a large number of useful animal models based on drug administration. However, even the most sophisticated models do not quite recapitulate the behavior of free-living addicted human beings, which makes such approaches as neuroimaging of clinical populations critically important.

RISK FACTORS

The best-established risk factors for drug addiction are male sex and a family history. The familial transmission of risk appears to be preponderantly, but not entirely explained by genes; this conclusion is based on evidence from twin studies that consistently show higher rates of concordance in monozygotic twin pairs than in dizygotic twin pairs for both heavy drug use and DSM-IV substance dependence. Adoption studies that have been performed for alcoholism show that adoptees resemble their biologic rather than their adoptive parents in this regard.

Although genes play a significant role in vulnerability to addiction and other substance use disorders, specific genes that confer risk have not yet been identified with certainty. Like all common neuropsychiatric disorders, the risk for addiction is genetically complex; there is strong evidence that multiple genetic and nongenetic risk factors interact to produce the disorder. Moreover, experience with genetically complex disorders suggests that no single gene is likely to prove necessary for a given disorder (Chapter 40). As a result, discovery of risk genes has proved challenging despite significant ongoing effort. As with other chronic medical disorders, genetic risk factors are being sought to find clues to pathophysiology and ultimately to aid in the discovery of new treatments.

Complicating the task of gene discovery, substance use disorders present substantial challenges for phenotype definition. There may be independent genetic and nongenetic risk factors for different stages of substance use disorders, such as drug experimentation, becoming addicted on experimentation, and treatment responsiveness once addicted. In addition, some evidence suggests that there are both shared risk factors for the abuse of any addictive drug and drug-specific risk factors.

NEUROBIOLOGY OF ADDICTIVE DRUG ACTION

Survival and perpetuation of the species require that humans, like other species, learn the circumstances under which they can reliably obtain food, water, and shelter, as well as opportunities for procreation. These survival-related goals function as rewards; their consumption or consummation produces a hedonic response—in humans this is typically reported as subjective pleasure. Such hedonic responses automatically activate associative learning mechanisms in the brain that imbue rewarding goals and the circumstances that predict their availability ("cues") with "incentive salience." This means that cues predictive of reward come to elicit "wanting" and activate behavioral repertoires aimed at obtaining the particular reward. The power of incentive stimuli is enhanced by the presence of motivational states, such as hunger, but conversely, cues (e.g., the smell of freshly baking bread) can elicit wanting and goal-directed behavior in the absence of prior hunger.

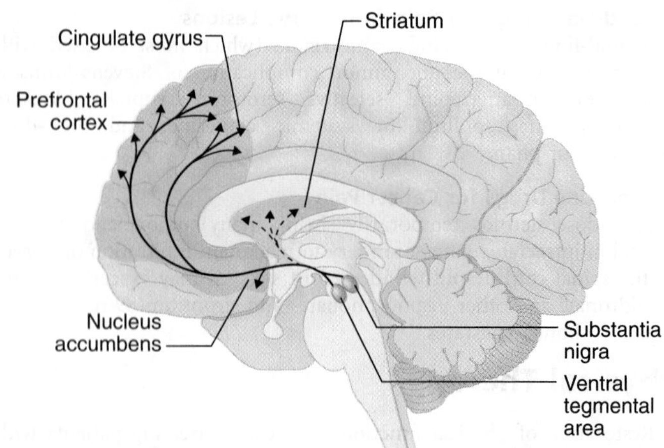

FIGURE 29–1 • Brain reward circuits. The major dopaminergic projections to the forebrain that underlie brain reward are shown superimposed on a diagram of the human brain: projections from the ventral tegmental area to the nucleus accumbens, and prefrontal cerebral cortex. Also shown are projections from the substantia nigra to the dorsal striatum (caudate and putamen and related structures) that play a role in habit formation and in well-rehearsed motor behavior, such as drug seeking and drug administration. (Reprinted from Hyman SE, Malenka RC, Nestler EJ: Neural mechanisms of addiction: The role of reward-related learning and memory. Annu Rev Neurosci 2006;29:565–598.)

A complex neural circuitry underlies the valuation and pursuit of rewards. At its center is a dopaminergic neural projection system that communicates information about the motivational state of the organism to the forebrain structures involved in valuation, learning of behavioral responses, and response selection. This projection extends from the ventral tegmental area (VTA) of the midbrain to multiple forebrain structures (Fig. 29–1). Dopamine is not required for hedonic responses themselves but rather acts to bind hedonic responses to valuation and action so that an organism can maximize the likelihood of obtaining such necessities as food, water, and shelter. In this regard it is noteworthy that nicotine produces little subjective pleasure as compared with cocaine, but it is very highly addicting.

Both natural rewards and addictive drugs increase dopamine in synapses made by neurons in the VTA, thus consolidating their incentive value and their ability to motivate behavior. Despite their lack of homeostatic or survival value (indeed, often quite the opposite), addictive drugs mimic and often exceed the dopamine-releasing effects of survival-relevant natural rewards because of their direct pharmacologic actions (Table 29–1). Cocaine blocks the dopamine uptake transporter (DAT) on the presynaptic terminals of dopamine-releasing neurons, thus blocking clearance of the neurotransmitter from synapses. Amphetamines enter dopamine neurons via the DAT and act within the presynaptic terminal on the vesicular monoamine transporter (VMAT) to cause leakage of dopamine out of vesicles into the cytoplasm, followed by "reverse transport" of dopamine out of the cell into the synapse via the DAT. Other addictive drugs (see Table 29–1) act indirectly. Opiates, nicotine, and cannabinoids act on receptors that relieve inhibitory influences on VTA dopamine neurons, thus disinhibiting them. Alcohol influences multiple receptors but ultimately produces dopamine release. In fact, opiates have some actions on reward systems that are dopamine independent, but as a general rule, dopamine plays a central role in connecting rewards to behavior.

Among the targets of the VTA dopamine projection, the nucleus accumbens (NAc) within the ventral striatum (see Fig. 29–1) has been shown to be required for both natural rewards and drugs such as cocaine to motivate behavior. Thus, for example, in rats, the NAc is required for the acquisition of cocaine self-administration. Once drug self-administration becomes established, however, the behavior becomes independent of the NAc and is supported by the dorsal striatum, the brain structure that underlies automatic behavior and habits. If such observations made in rats can be extended to addicted humans, the role of the striatal habit system would help explain the power of cues to elicit drug seeking that persists despite obstacles and seems to override conscious desires to resist. The VTA also supplies dopamine to the amygdala

TABLE 29–1 PROPERTIES OF ADDICTIVE DRUGS

Drug	Neurotransmitter	Drug Target	Effect after Binding
Opiates (morphine, heroin, oxycodone)	Endorphins	μ and δ opioid (agonist)	Activate G_i/G_o Activate K^+ channels
Psychostimulants (cocaine, amphetamines)	Dopamine (DA)	Dopamine transporter (DAT)* (antagonist)	Increase synaptic DA; stimulate presynaptic and postsynaptic DA receptors
Nicotine	Acetylcholine	Nicotinic acetylcholine receptors (nAChRs) (agonist)	Stimulate cation channel (may desensitize)
Alcohol	γ-Aminobutyric acid (GABA)	$GABA_A$ receptor (agonist)	Activate Cl^- channel
	Glutamate	*N*-methyl-D-aspartate (NMDA) receptor (antagonist)	Inhibit Ca^{2+} entry
Marijuana (D-9-tetrahydrocannabinol)	Anandamide	Cannabinoid CB_1 (agonist)	Activate G_i/G_o
Phencyclidine, ketamine	Glutamate	NMDA receptor channel (antagonist)	Inhibit Ca^{2+} entry

*The psychostimulants also interact with the norepinephrine and serotonin transporters, but under normal conditions, it is the DAT that is critical for rewarding and addictive properties. Unlike cocaine, amphetamines enter dopamine via the DAT and interact with a second target, the vesicular monoamine transporter (VMAT), to release DA into the cytoplasm and thence, via the DAT, to release it into the synapse.

Adapted from Hyman SE, Malenka RC, Nestler EJ: Neural mechanisms of addiction: The role of reward-related learning and memory. Annu Rev Neurosci 2006;29:565–598.

and the orbitofrontal cortex, which play roles in the valuation of rewards and in decision making.

The initial molecular targets in the nervous system have been cloned and characterized for all of the addictive drugs. Given the diversity of targets and their locations in the nervous system, these drugs produce many different effects (e.g., opiates are analgesic and sedating; cocaine is a potent stimulant). Their rewarding and addicting properties, however, are based on their shared ability to increase synaptic dopamine in the reward circuitry just described.

Effects of Repeated Drug Taking

Because they are rewarding, drugs that release dopamine may be taken repeatedly by vulnerable individuals and may thus produce long-term changes in brain function: tolerance, dependence, and addiction. Tolerance and dependence result from homeostatic adaptations in diverse neural cells and circuits. Depending on the locations of drug receptors and the effects of drugs on signaling, different drugs produce distinct adaptations and thus differ in the presence and nature of withdrawal symptoms. Alcohol and opiates may produce adaptations that when unmasked by drug cessation, produce serious physical withdrawal symptoms. The highly addictive drugs cocaine and amphetamine do not produce physical dependence and withdrawal. As discussed, however, tolerance and dependence are neither necessary nor sufficient for addiction. The compulsion that is the cardinal feature of addiction and long-term risk for relapse are thought to arise from long-term associative memory processes that occur in neural circuits that receive input from VTA dopamine neurons. Long-term memories are perhaps the most persistent changes in brain function that may occur in adult life; some may last for a lifetime. The neural substrates of memory include alterations in synaptic weights such as long-term potentiation (LTP) or long-term depression (LTD) and physical remodeling of synaptic connections.

The centrality of associative learning mechanisms for addiction was first recognized from clinical observation: much drug taking and, most notably, late relapses follow exposure to cues previously associated with drug use. Cues that can reinitiate drug use include environmental stimuli (e.g., persons with whom drugs have been used, drug paraphernalia) and bodily feelings. Based on current neurobiologic models, when drugs are taken, they further consolidate the association of "wanting" and drug-seeking behavior with drug cues. Because addictive drugs reliably increase synaptic dopamine as a result of their direct pharmacologic actions—indeed, they produce an excessive and grossly distorted dopamine signal—the brain receives a powerful impetus to connect the circumstances in which the drugs have been used with the motivation to take drugs again. Even if the drug is no longer pleasurable—often the case in late stages of alcoholism—the release of dopamine continues to reinforce drug wanting and seeking. The reliability and quantity of dopamine release give drugs a marked advantage over natural rewards.

It is increasingly possible to study the effects of drug cues on neural circuits, physiology, and subjective responses in humans based on functional neuroimaging. For example, drug-associated cues have been shown to elicit drug urges and physiologic responses, as well as activate identifiable neural circuits in addicted human subjects. Cocaine-related cues have also been shown to elicit dopamine release in the dorsal striatum in addicted subjects.

Investigations at the cellular and molecular levels have begun to examine the physiologic and molecular changes that might underlie the effects of addictive drugs on reward-related memory processes. There is now very strong evidence that addictive drugs produce LTP and LTD in brain reward circuits. There is also strong evidence that addictive drugs lead to marked changes in the phosphorylation of critical proteins, including the transcription factor CREB—a factor that has been implicated in multiple forms of learning and memory in several animal models. Dopamine and cocaine have been shown to regulate many genes downstream of CREB, including other transcription factors. For example, drugs such as cocaine alter the composition of activator protein 1 (AP-1) complexes in brain reward circuits. Overall, much current research is focused on the nature and function of gene expression and synaptic connections regulated by addictive drugs. Although there is a long way to go before the biology of this important clinical disorder is fully understood, research at the molecular, cellular, behavioral, and clinical levels is beginning to converge on the key issues of compulsion and the persistence of risk for relapse.

SUGGESTED READINGS

Berke JD, Hyman SE: Addiction, dopamine, and the molecular mechanisms of memory. Neuron 2000;25:515–532. *Reviews the actions of dopamine and argues that associative learning mechanisms underlie mechanisms of relapse.*

Chao J, Nestler EJ: Molecular neurobiology of drug addiction. Annu Rev Med 2004;55:113–132. *Reviews the molecular mechanisms underlying the long-term actions of addictive drugs with a major emphasis on gene expression.*

Childress AR, Mozley PD, McElgin W, et al: Limbic activation during cue-induced cocaine craving. Am J Psychiatry 1999;156:11–18. *One of the pioneering studies of cue-induced brain activation demonstrating craving-specific activation of emotion processing circuits.*

Everitt BJ, Robbins TW: Neural systems of reinforcement for drug addiction: from actions to habits to compulsion. Nat Neurosci 2005;8:1481–1489. *Describes mechanisms by which drug seeking becomes a deeply ingrained prepotent response to drug cues.*

Goldman D, Oroszi G, Ducci F: The genetics of addictions: uncovering the genes. Nat Rev Genet 2005;6:521–532. *Reviews the progress and challenge of finding genes that predispose to addiction, a genetically complex chronic disorder.*

Hyman SE: Addiction: a disease of learning and memory. Am J Psychiatry 2005;162(8):1414–1422. *Discusses limitations of older formulations which saw dependence and withdrawal as central to addiction with a central focus on the phenomenon of late relapse.*

Hyman SE, Malenka RC, Nestler EJ: Neural mechanisms of addiction: the role of reward-related learning and memory. Annu Rev Neuosci 2006;29:565–598. *Reviews mechanisms of neural plasticity that might underlie addiction.*

Hyman SE: The neurobiology of addiction: Implications for voluntary control of behavior. Am J Bioeth 2007;7:8–11. *Addicted individuals have complex impairments in the cognitive control of behavior.*

Kalivas PW, Volkow ND: The neural basis of addiction: a pathology of motivation and choice. Am J Psychiatry 2005;162:1403–1413. *Reviews human imaging data that implicate abnormal function of prefrontal cortex in choices made by addicted individuals.*

O'Brien CP, Childress AR, Ehrman R, et al: Conditioning factors in drug abuse: can they explain compulsion? Psychopharmacol 1998;12:15–22. *Describes clinical observations that point to the central role of drug-associated cues in maintaining drug taking and relapse.*

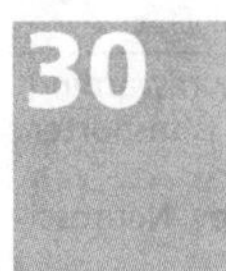

30 TOBACCO

Neal L. Benowitz

Definition

Harmful Constituents of Tobacco

Tobacco smoke is an aerosol of droplets (particulates) containing water, nicotine and other alkaloids, and tar. Tobacco smoke contains several thousand different chemicals, many of which may contribute to human disease. Major toxic chemicals in the particulate phase of tobacco include nicotine, benzo(a)pyrene and other polycyclic hydrocarbons, N′-nitrosonornicotine, β-naphthylamine, polonium 210, nickel, cadmium, arsenic, and lead. The gaseous phase contains carbon monoxide, acetaldehyde, acetone, methanol, nitrogen oxides, hydrogen cyanide, acrolein, ammonia, benzene, formaldehyde, nitrosamines, and vinyl chloride. Tobacco smoke may produce illness by way of systemic absorption of toxins or cause local pulmonary injury by oxidant gases.

Tobacco Addiction

Tobacco use is motivated primarily by the desire for nicotine. Drug addiction is defined as compulsive use of a psychoactive substance, the consequences of which are detrimental to the individual or society. Understanding addiction is useful in providing effective smoking cessation therapy. Nicotine is absorbed rapidly from tobacco smoke into the pulmonary circulation; it then moves quickly to the brain, where it acts on nicotinic cholinergic receptors to produce its gratifying effects, which occur within 10 to 15 seconds after a puff. Smokeless tobacco is absorbed more slowly and results in less intense pharmacologic effects. With long-term use of tobacco, physical dependence develops in association with an increased number of nicotinic cholinergic receptors in the brain. When tobacco is unavailable, even for only a few hours, withdrawal symptoms often occur, including anxiety, irritability, difficulty concentrating, restlessness, hunger, craving for tobacco, disturbed sleep, and, in some people, depression.

Epidemiology

Currently, about 46 million individuals in the United States are cigarette smokers, including 26% of men and 21% of women. People who are less well educated or have unskilled occupations are more likely to smoke. Smoking is responsible for about 430,000 preventable U.S. deaths annually. A lifelong smoker has about a one in three chance of dying prematurely of a complication of smoking. Smoking is the major preventable cause of death in developed countries.

Other forms of tobacco use include pipes and cigars (used by 8.7% of men and 0.3% of women) and smokeless tobacco (5.5% of men and 1% of women). Smokeless tobacco use in the United States is primarily oral snuff and chewing tobacco, whereas nasal snuff is used to a greater extent in the United Kingdom. Oral snuff (snus) is widely used by men in Sweden.

Addiction to tobacco is multifactorial, including a desire for the direct pharmacologic actions of nicotine, relief of withdrawal symptoms, and learned associations. Smokers report a variety of reasons for smoking, including pleasure, arousal, enhanced vigilance, improved performance, relief of anxiety or depression, reduced hunger, and control of body weight. Environmental cues, such as a meal, a cup of coffee, talking on the phone, an alcoholic beverage, or friends who smoke, often trigger an urge to smoke. Smoking and depression are strongly linked. Smokers are more likely to have a history of major depression than are nonsmokers. Smokers with a history of depression are also likely to be more highly dependent on nicotine and to have a lower likelihood of quitting. When they do quit, depression is more likely to be a prominent withdrawal symptom. Cigarette smoking is also more common in alcoholics and other substance abusers and in people with schizophrenia and attention-deficit disorder.

Most tobacco use begins in childhood or adolescence. Risk factors for youth smoking include peer and parental influences; behavioral problems (e.g., poor school performance); personality characteristics, such as rebelliousness or risk taking, depression, and anxiety; and genetic influences. Adolescent desire to appear older and more sophisticated, such as emulating more mature role models, is another strong motivator. Environmental influences such as advertising also are thought to contribute. Approaches to prevention of tobacco addiction in youth include educational activities in schools, aggressive anti-tobacco media campaigns, taxation, changing the social and environmental norms, and deglamorizing smoking (restricting indoor smoking, educating parents not to smoke around children).

Pathobiology

Health Hazards of Tobacco

Tobacco use is a major cause of death from cancer, cardiovascular disease, and pulmonary disease (Table 30–1). Smoking is also a major risk factor for osteoporosis, reproductive disorders, and fire-related and trauma-related injuries.

Cancer

Although it is the largest preventable cause of cancer (Table 30–2), smoking is responsible for about 30% of cancer deaths. Many chemicals in tobacco smoke may contribute to carcinogenesis as tumor initiators, cocarcinogens, tumor promoters, or complete carcinogens. Cigarette smoking induces specific patterns of *p53* mutations that are associated with squamous cell carcinomas of the lung, head, and neck. Lung cancer (Chapter 201) is the leading cause of cancer deaths in the United States and is predominantly attributable to cigarette smoking. The risk of lung and other cancers is proportional to how many cigarettes are smoked per day and the duration of smoking. Exposure in the workplace to asbestos or of uranium miners to α-radiation (Chapter 18) synergistically increases the risk of lung cancer in cigarette smokers. Alcohol use interacts synergistically with tobacco in causing oral, laryngeal, and esophageal cancer (Chapters 140, 200, and 451). The mechanism of interaction may involve alcohol-solubilizing tobacco carcinogens or alcohol-related induction of liver or gastrointestinal enzymes that metabolize and activate tobacco carcinogens. The tobacco-related risks of bladder and kidney cancer (Chapter 207) are enhanced by occupational exposure to aromatic amines, such as in the dye industry. Cervical cancer (Chapter 209) is more common in women who smoke, presumably the result of exposure to carcinogens in cervical secretions. Smoking seems to be involved in 20 to 30% of leukemia cases in adults (Chapters 194 and 195), including lymphoid and myeloid leukemia, and in 20% of colorectal cancers (Chapter 203).

Cardiovascular Disease

Cigarette smoking accounts for about 20% of cardiovascular deaths in the United States (Chapter 49). Risks are increased for coronary heart disease (Chapters 70 to 72), sudden death (Chapter 64), cerebrovascular disease (Chapters 430 and 431), and peripheral vascular disease (Chapter 81), including aortic aneurysm (Chapter 75). Cigarette smoking accelerates atherosclerosis (Chapter 69) and promotes acute ischemic events. The mechanisms of the effects of smoking are not fully elucidated but are believed to include (1) hemodynamic stress (nicotine increases the heart rate and transiently increases blood pressure; Chapter 66), (2) endothelial injury and dysfunction (nitric oxide release and resultant

TABLE 30–1 HEALTH HAZARDS OF TOBACCO USE (RISKS INCREASED BY SMOKING)

CANCER

See Table 30–2

CARDIOVASCULAR DISEASE

Sudden death
Acute myocardial infarction
Unstable angina
Stroke
Peripheral arterial occlusive disease (including thromboangiitis obliterans)
Aortic aneurysm

PULMONARY DISEASE

Lung cancer
Chronic bronchitis
Emphysema
Asthma
Increased susceptibility to pneumonia
Increased susceptibility to pulmonary tuberculosis and desquamative interstitial pneumonitis
Increased morbidity from viral respiratory infection

GASTROINTESTINAL DISEASE

Peptic ulcer
Gastroesophageal reflux
Crohn's disease

REPRODUCTIVE DISTURBANCES

Reduced fertility
Premature birth
Lower birth weight
Spontaneous abortion
Abruptio placentae
Premature rupture of membranes
Increased perinatal mortality

ORAL DISEASE

Oral cancer
Leukoplakia
Gingivitis
Gingival recession
Tooth staining

OTHER

Non–insulin-dependent diabetes mellitus
Earlier menopause
Osteoporosis
Cataract
Tobacco amblyopia
Age-related macular degeneration
Premature skin wrinkling
Graves' disease, including ophthalmopathy
Aggravation of hypothyroidism
Altered drug metabolism or effects

vasodilation are impaired), (3) development of an atherogenic lipid profile (smokers have on average higher low-density lipoprotein, more oxidized low-density lipoprotein, and lower high-density lipoprotein cholesterol than nonsmokers do; see Chapter 217), (4) enhanced coagulability (Chapter 178), (5) arrhythmogenesis (Chapter 60), and (6) relative hypoxemia because of the effects of carbon monoxide (Chapter 83). Carbon monoxide reduces the capacity of hemoglobin to carry oxygen and impairs the release of oxygen from hemoglobin to body tissues, both

TABLE 30–2 SMOKING AND CANCER MORTALITY

	Relative Risk among Smokers		Mortality Attributable to Smoking	
Type of Cancer	**Current**	**Former**	**Percentage**	**Number**
Lung				
Male	22.4	9.4	90	82,800
Female	11.9	4.7	79	40,300
Larynx				
Male	10.5	5.2	81	2400
Female	17.8	11.9	87	700
Oral cavity				
Male	27.5	8.8	92	4900
Female	5.6	2.9	61	1800
Esophagus				
Male	7.6	5.8	78	5700
Female	10.3	3.2	75	1900
Pancreas				
Male	2.1	1.1	29	3500
Female	2.3	1.8	34	4500
Bladder				
Male	2.9	1.9	47	3000
Female	2.6	1.9	37	1200
Kidney				
Male	3.0	2.0	48	3000
Female	1.4	1.2	12	500
Stomach				
Male	1.5	?	17	1400
Female	1.5	?	25	1300
Leukemia				
Male	2.0	?	20	2000
Female	2.0	?	20	1600
Cervix				
Female	2.1	1.9	31	1400

Modified from Newcomb PA, Carbone PP: The health consequences of smoking: Cancer. Med Clin North Am 1992;76:305–331.

of which combine to result in a state of relative hypoxemia. To compensate for this hypoxemic state, polycythemia develops in smokers, with hematocrits often 50% or more (Chapter 172). The polycythemia and the increased fibrinogen levels that are found in cigarette smokers also increase blood viscosity, which adds to the risk of thrombotic events. Cigarette smoking also induces a chronic inflammatory state, as evidenced by increased levels of C-reactive protein and other inflammatory markers in the blood of smokers. Chronic inflammation is thought to contribute to atherogenesis.

Cigarette smoking acts synergistically with other cardiac risk factors to increase the risk of ischemic heart disease. Although the risk of cardiovascular disease is roughly proportional to cigarette consumption, the risk persists even at low levels of smoking (e.g., one or two cigarettes per day). Cigarette smoking reduces exercise tolerance in patients with angina pectoris (Chapter 70) and intermittent claudication (Chapter 79). Vasospastic angina is more common, and the response to vasodilator medication is impaired in patients who smoke. The number of episodes and total duration of ischemic episodes as assessed by ambulatory electrocardiographic monitoring in patients with coronary heart disease are substantially increased by cigarette smoking. The increase in relative risk of coronary heart disease because of cigarette smoking is greatest in young adults, who in the absence of cigarette smoking would have a relatively low risk. Women who use oral contraceptives and smoke have a synergistically increased risk of myocardial infarction and stroke.

After acute myocardial infarction (Chapters 71 and 72), the risk of recurrent myocardial infarction is higher and survival is half during the next 12 years in persistent smokers compared with quitters. Smoking also interferes with revascularization therapy for acute myocardial infarction. After thrombolysis, the reocclusion rate is four-fold higher in smokers who continue than in quitters. The risk of reocclusion of a coronary artery after angioplasty or occlusion of a bypass graft is increased in smokers. Cigarette smoking is not a risk factor for hypertension but does increase the risk of complications, including the development of nephrosclerosis and progression to malignant hypertension. Cigarette smoking has been shown to be a substantial contributor to morbidity and mortality in patients with left ventricular dysfunction (Chapter 58). The mortality benefit of stopping smoking in such patients is equal to or greater than the benefit of therapy with angiotensin-converting enzyme inhibitors, β-blockers, or spironolactone.

Pulmonary Disease

More than 80% of chronic obstructive lung disease in the United States is attributable to cigarette smoking (Chapter 88). Pulmonary disease from smoking includes the overlapping syndromes of chronic bronchitis (cough and mucus hypersecretion), emphysema, and airway obstruction. The pathologic changes produced in the lung by cigarette smoking include loss of cilia, mucous gland hyperplasia, increased number of goblet cells in the central airways, inflammation, goblet cell metaplasia, squamous metaplasia, mucus plugging of small airways, destruction of alveoli, and reduced number of small arteries. The mechanism of injury is complex and seems to include direct injury by oxidant gases, increased elastase activity (a protein that breaks down elastin and other connective tissue), and decreased antiprotease activity. A genetic deficiency of α_1-antiprotease activity produces a similar imbalance between pulmonary protease and antiprotease activity and is a risk factor for early and severe smoking-induced pulmonary disease. Cigarette smoking is associated with an increased risk of desquamative interstitial pneumonitis (Chapter 92).

Cigarette smoking also increases the risk of respiratory infection, including pneumonia, and results in greater disability from viral respiratory tract infections. Smoking is a substantial risk factor for pneumococcal pneumonia and in particular with invasive pneumococcal disease. Cigarette smoking increases the risk for development of and the severity of viral infections including the common cold, influenza, and varicella. Tuberculosis is perhaps the most important smoking-associated infection. Smoking is a substantial risk factor for tuberculin skin test reactivity, skin test conversion, and development of active tuberculosis. A case-control study from India found a prevalence risk ratio of 2.9 and a mortality risk ratio of 4.2 to 4.5 (for rural and urban residents, respectively) for ever-smokers compared with never-smokers. 1 Thus, smoking contributes substantially to the worldwide disease burden of tuberculosis.

Other Complications

Ulcer

Cigarette smoking increases the risk of duodenal and gastric ulcers, delays the rate of ulcer healing, and increases the risk of relapse after ulcer treatment (Chapter 141). Smoking also is associated with esophageal reflux symptoms (Chapter 140). Smoking produces ulcer disease by increasing acid and pepsinogen secretion, reducing pancreatic bicarbonate secretion, impairing the gastric mucosal barrier (related to decreased gastric mucosal blood flow and inhibition of prostaglandin synthesis), and reducing pyloric sphincter tone.

Diabetes Mellitus

Cigarette smoking is an independent risk factor for the development of non–insulin-dependent diabetes mellitus (Chapter 248), which is a consequence of development of resistance to the effects of insulin. The effects of nicotine seem to contribute at least in part to insulin resistance, and insulin resistance has been described in users of smokeless tobacco, who are not exposed to tobacco combustion products.

Osteoporosis

Cigarette smoking is a risk factor for osteoporosis in that it reduces the peak bone mass attained in early adulthood and increases the rate of bone loss in later adulthood (Chapter 264). Smoking antagonizes the protective effect of estrogen replacement therapy on the risk of osteoporosis in postmenopausal women.

Reproductive Problems

Cigarette smoking is a major cause of reproductive problems and results in approximately 4600 U.S. infant deaths annually. Growth retardation from cigarette smoking has been termed the fetal tobacco syndrome. Cigarette smoking causes reproductive complications by causing placental ischemia mediated by the vasoconstricting effects of nicotine, the hypoxic effects of chronic carbon monoxide exposure, and the general increase in coagulability produced by smoking.

Other Adverse Effects

Other adverse effects of cigarette smoking include premature facial wrinkling, increased risk of cataracts (Chapter 449), olfactory dysfunction (Chapter 453), and fire-related injuries (Chapters 15 and 113); the last-mentioned contribute significantly to the economic costs of tobacco use. Smoking is associated with Graves' disease and especially increases the risk of more severe ophthalmopathy. Smoking also reduces the secretion of thyroid hormone in women with subclinical hypothyroidism and increases the severity of clinical symptoms of hypothyroidism in women with subclinical or overt hypothyroidism, the latter effect reflecting antagonism of thyroid hormone action (Chapter 244). Cigarette smoking also potentially interacts with a variety of drugs by accelerating drug metabolism or by the antagonistic pharmacologic actions that nicotine and other constituents of tobacco have with other drugs (Table 30–3).

Health Hazards of Smokeless Tobacco

Smokeless tobacco refers to snuff and chewing tobacco. Oral snuff is placed (as a "pinch") between the lip and gum or under the tongue; chewing tobacco is actively chewed and generates saliva that is spit out ("spit tobacco"). Smokeless tobacco products are usually flavored, many with licorice, and also contain sodium bicarbonate to keep the local pH alkaline to facilitate buccal absorption of nicotine. Nicotine absorption from smokeless tobacco is similar in magnitude to that from cigarette smoking. Other chemicals, including sodium, glycyrrhizinic acid (from licorice), and potentially carcinogenic chemicals such as nitrosamines also are absorbed systemically.

Smokeless tobacco is addictive and is associated with an increased risk of oral cancer at the site where the tobacco is usually placed (inside the lip, under the cheek or tongue) or nasal cancer in nasal snuff users (Chapter 200). Other oral diseases also associated with smokeless tobacco include leukoplakia, gingivitis, gingival recession, and staining of the teeth. Cardiovascular effects of smokeless tobacco include acute aggravation of hypertension or angina pectoris as a result of the sympathomimetic effects of nicotine, hypokalemia and hypertension secondary to the effects of glycyrrhizinic acid (a potent mineralocorticoid; Chapter 66), and excessive sodium absorption resulting in aggravated hypertension or sodium-retaining disorders.

Health Hazards of Secondhand Smoke

Considerable evidence indicates that exposure to secondhand smoke is harmful to the health of nonsmokers (Table 30–4). The U.S. Environmental Protection Agency classifies secondhand smoke as a class A carcinogen, which means that it has been shown to cause cancer in humans.

Secondhand smoke consists of smoke that is generated while the cigarette is smoldering and mainstream smoke that has been exhaled by the smoker. Of the total combustion product from a cigarette, 75% or more enters the air. The constituents of environmental tobacco smoke are qualitatively similar to those of mainstream smoke. However, some toxins, such as ammonia, formaldehyde, and nitrosamines, are present in much higher concentrations in secondhand smoke than in mainstream smoke. The Environmental Protection Agency has estimated that secondhand smoke is responsible for approximately 3000 lung cancer deaths annually in nonsmokers in the United States, is causally associated with 150,000 to 300,000 cases of lower respiratory tract infection in infants and young children up to 18 months of age, and is causally associated with the aggravation of asthma in 200,000 to 1 million children. Secondhand smoke exposure is also responsible for about 40,000 cardiovascular deaths per year. An appreciation of the hazards of secondhand smoke is important to the physician because it provides a basis for advising parents not to smoke when children are in the home, for insisting that child care facilities be smoke free, and for recommending smoking restrictions in work sites and other public places.

Treatment

Cessation Intervention

Of cigarette smokers, 70% would like to quit, and 46% try to quit each year. Spontaneous quit rates are about 1% per year. Simple advice from the physician to quit increases the quit rate to 3%. Minimal-intervention programs increase quit rates to 5 to 10%,

TABLE 30–3 INTERACTION BETWEEN CIGARETTE SMOKING AND DRUGS

Drug		Interaction (Effects Compared with Nonsmokers)	Significance
Antipyrine Caffeine Chlorpromazine Clozapine Desmethyldiazepam Estradiol Estrone Flecainide Fluvoxamine Haloperidol	Imipramine Lidocaine Olanzapine Oxazepam Pentazocine Phenacetin Phenylbutazone Propranolol Tacrine Theophylline	Accelerated metabolism	May require higher doses in smokers, reduced doses after quitting
Oral contraceptives		Enhanced thrombosis, increased risk of stroke and myocardial infarction	Do not prescribe to smokers, especially if older than 35 years
Cimetidine and other H_2-blockers		Lower rate of ulcer healing, higher ulcer recurrence rates	Consider the use of proton pump inhibitors
Propranolol		Less antihypertensive effect, less antianginal efficacy; more effective in reducing mortality after myocardial infarction	Consider the use of cardioselective β-blockers
Nifedipine (and probably other calcium blockers)		Less antianginal effect	May require higher doses or multiple-drug antianginal therapy
Diazepam, chlordiazepoxide (and possibly other sedative-hypnotics)		Less sedation	Smokers may need higher doses
Chlorpromazine (and possibly other neuroleptics)		Less sedation, possibly reduced efficacy	Smokers may need higher doses
Propoxyphene		Reduced analgesia	Smokers may need higher doses

TABLE 30–4 HEALTH HAZARDS OF ENVIRONMENTAL TOBACCO SMOKE IN NONSMOKERS

Children	Adults
Hospitalization for respiratory tract infection in first year of life	Lung cancer Myocardial infarction Reduced pulmonary function
Wheezing Middle ear effusion Asthma Sudden infant death syndrome	Aggravation of asthma and chronic obstructive pulmonary disease Irritation of eyes, nasal congestion, headache Cough

Rx

whereas more intensive treatments, including smoking cessation clinics, can yield quit rates of 25 to 30%. A practical office smoking cessation program developed by the U.S. Public Health Service consists of *5 As*: (1) *ask* about smoking at every opportunity, (2) *advise* all smokers to stop, (3) *assess* willingness to make a quit attempt, (4) *assist* the patient in stopping and maintaining abstinence, and (5) *arrange* follow-up to reinforce nonsmoking. Assistance in quitting should include providing self-help material or quit kits, which are widely available from governmental health agencies, professional societies, and local organizations such as cancer, heart, and lung associations. The physician may offer additional education and counseling through the office (most efficiently provided by office staff and by teaching aids such as videotapes) or through referral to community smoking cessation programs. Telephone counseling is effective in promoting smoking cessation. [2] Telephone quitlines are available at no cost in most states in the United States. Thus, the busiest physician can easily refer patients to telephone quitlines for counseling if personal counseling time is not available. Smokers who are interested should be offered nicotine replacement or other pharmacologic therapy.

Medical Therapy

Currently, three medications have been approved for smoking cessation: nicotine, bupropion, and varenicline. All types of smoking cessation medications, if used properly, double smoking cessation rates compared with placebo treatments.

Nicotine Replacement

Nicotine replacement medications include 2- and 4-mg nicotine polacrilex gum, 2- and 4-mg nicotine buccal lozenges, transdermal nicotine patches, nicotine nasal spray, and nicotine inhalers. All seem to have comparable efficacy, but in a randomized study, compliance was greatest for the patch, lower for gum, and very low for the spray and the inhaler. A smoker should be instructed to quit smoking entirely before beginning nicotine replacement therapies. Optimal use of nicotine gum includes instructions not to chew too rapidly, to chew 8 to 10 pieces per day for 20 to 30 minutes each, and to use it for an adequate period for the smoker to learn a lifestyle without cigarettes, usually 3 months or longer. Side effects of nicotine gum are primarily local and include jaw fatigue, sore mouth and throat, upset stomach, and hiccups. Nicotine lozenges have recently been marketed over-the-counter. The lozenges are placed in the buccal cavity where they are slowly absorbed for 30 minutes. Smokers are instructed to choose their dose according to how long after awakening in the morning they smoke their first cigarette (a measure of the level of nicotine dependence). Those who smoke within 30 minutes are advised to use the 4-mg lozenge, whereas

Rx

those who smoke their first cigarette at 30 minutes or more are advised to use 2-mg lozenges. Use is recommended every 1 to 2 hours.

Several different transdermal nicotine preparations are marketed; three deliver 21 or 22 mg during a 24-hour period, and one delivers 15 mg during 16 hours. Most have lower dose patches for tapering. Patches are applied in the morning and removed either the next morning or at bedtime, depending on the patch. Full-dose patches are recommended for most smokers for the first 1 to 3 months, followed by one or two tapering doses for 2 to 4 weeks each. Nicotine nasal spray, one spray into each nostril, delivers about 0.5 mg of nicotine systemically and can be used every 30 to 60 minutes. Local irritation of the nose commonly produces burning, sneezing, and watery eyes during initial treatment, but tolerance develops to these effects in 1 or 2 days. The nicotine inhaler delivers nicotine to the throat and upper airway, from where it is absorbed similarly to nicotine from gum. It is marketed as a cigarette-like plastic device and can be used ad libitum.

Nicotine medications seem to be safe in patients with cardiovascular disease and should be offered to cardiovascular patients. Although smoking cessation medications are recommended by the manufacturer for relatively short-term use (generally 3 to 6 months), the use of these medications for 6 months or longer is safe and may be helpful in smokers who fear relapse without medications. Combination therapy—combining bupropion and nicotine or combining slow-release nicotine patches with preparations with more rapid release, such as gum, inhaler, or nasal spray—increases the likelihood of cessation compared with single-drug therapy.

Bupropion

Bupropion, also marketed as an antidepressant drug, is dosed at 150 to 300 mg/day (150 mg BID) for 7 days before stopping smoking, then at 300 mg/day (150 mg BID) for the next 6 to 12 weeks; the sustained-release preparation should be used. Bupropion also can be used in combination with a nicotine patch. [3] Bupropion in excessive doses can cause seizures and should not be used in individuals with a history of seizures or with eating disorders (bulimia or anorexia). On average, nicotine medications or bupropion treatment doubles the cessation rates found with placebo treatment, and absolute rates of smoking cessation have increased from 12% (placebo) to 24% (active medication) in clinical trials.

Varenicline

Varenicline is an α4 β2 nicotinic acetylcholine receptor partial agonist. Thus, varenicline both stimulates the receptor and blocks actions of nicotine on the receptor. The α4 β2 receptor subtype is believed to mediate the rewarding properties of nicotine. Varenicline appears both to reduce craving and other withdrawal symptoms after stopping smoking and to block the nicotine satisfaction if a person lapses to smoking. Clinical trials find cessation rates for varenicline treatment to be greater than either placebo (odds ratio 2.82) or bupropion (odds ratio 1.56). [4] The main side effects are nausea and abnormal dreams. Treatment is started 1 week before the target quit date. Dose escalation is recommended to reduce the risk of nausea: 0.5 mg per day for 3 days; 0.5 mg twice daily for 4 days; then 1 mg twice daily for 12 weeks. For those who have quit successfully at 12 weeks but would like futher pharmacologic support, treatment for an additional 12 weeks has been shown to sustain higher quit rates.

Follow-up

Follow-up office visits or telephone calls during and after active treatment increase long-term smoking cessation rates. Even in the best treatment circumstances, 70% or more of smokers relapse. Most smokers go through a quitting process three or four times before they finally succeed. When a quit attempt fails, the health care provider should encourage patients to try again as soon as they are ready. Cost-effectiveness studies find average costs per year of life saved of $400 to $900 for brief counseling by a physician alone and an incremental cost for adding a course of nicotine patch therapy of $2000 to $4000, depending on the individual's gender and age, to aid cessation. Smoking cessation treatment is much less costly per year of life saved than are other widely accepted preventive therapies, including treatment of mild to moderate hypertension or hypercholesterolemia.

Primary Prevention

Benefits of Quitting Smoking

The benefits of quitting smoking are substantial for smokers of any age. A person who quits smoking before the age of 50 years has half the risk of dying in the next 15 years compared with a continuing smoker. Smoking cessation reduces the risks for development of lung cancer, with the risk falling to half that of a continuing smoker by 10 years and one sixth that of a smoker after 15 years' cessation. Quitting smoking in middle age substantially reduces lung cancer risk, with a 50% reduction in risk if a lifelong smoker quits at 55 years of age compared with 75 years. The risk of acute myocardial infarction falls rapidly after quitting smoking and approaches nonsmoking levels within a few years of abstinence. Cigarette smoking produces a progressive loss of airway function over time that is characterized by an accelerated loss of forced expiratory volume in 1 second (FEV_1) with increasing age. FEV_1 loss to cigarette smoking cannot be regained by cessation, but the rate of decline slows after smoking cessation and returns to that of nonsmokers. Women who stop smoking during the first 3 to 4 months of pregnancy reduce the risk of having a low-birth-weight infant to that of a woman who has never smoked.

After quitting, smokers gain an average of 5 to 7 pounds, which is perceived as undesirable and a reason not to quit by some smokers. Smokers tend to be thinner because of the effects of nicotine to increase energy expenditure and reduce compensatory increases in food consumption. After they quit smoking, ex-smokers tend to reach the weight expected had they never smoked. On balance, the benefits of quitting far outweigh the risks associated with weight gain, and patients should be counseled accordingly.

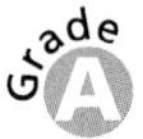

1. Gajalakshmi V, Peto R, Kanaka TS, et al: Smoking and mortality from tuberculosis and other diseases in India: Retrospective study of 43,000 adult male deaths and 35,000 controls. Lancet 2003;362:507–515.
2. Zhu SH, Anderson CM, Tedeschi GJ, et al: Evidence of real-world effectiveness of a telephone quitline for smokers. N Engl J Med 2002;347:1087–1093.
3. Jorenby DE, Leischow SJ, Nides MA, et al: A controlled trial of sustained-release bupropion, a nicotine patch, or both for smoking cessation. N Engl J Med 1999;340:685–691.
4. Gonzalez D, Rennard SI, Nides M, et al: Varenicline, and α4 β2 nicotinic acetylcholine receptor partial agonist, vs sustained-release bupropion and placebo for smoking cessation. JAMA 2006;296:47–55.

SUGGESTED READINGS

Arcavi L, Benowitz NL: Cigarette smoking and infection. Arch Intern Med 2004;164:2206–2216. *A review of mechanisms and epidemiology of infectious diseases caused by smoking.*

Ranney L, Melvin C, Lux L: Smoking cessation intervention strategies for adults and adults in special populations. Ann Intern Med 2006;145:845–856. *A systematic review.*

Rigotti NA: Treatment of tobacco use and dependence. N Engl J Med 2002;346:506–512. *A review of interventions includes behavioral and pharmacologic approaches to promote tobacco use cessation.*

Schroeder SA: What to do with a patient who smokes. JAMA 2005;294:482–487. *A clinician's approach to smoking cessation.*

Schnoll RA, Rukstalis M, Wileyto EP, et al: Smoking cessation treatment by primary care physicians: An update and call for training. Am J Prev Med 2006;31:233–239. *Shows suboptimal practices and makes suggestions for improvement.*

US Public Health Service: Treating tobacco use and dependence: Clinician's packet. *http://www.ahrq.gov/clinic/tobacco/. Consensus recommendations on implementing smoking cessation.*

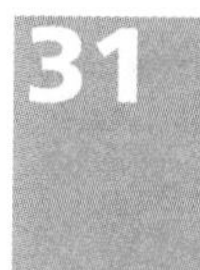

ALCOHOL ABUSE AND DEPENDENCE

Patrick G. O'Connor

Definition

A variety of terms have been used to describe the spectrum of medical, psychological, behavioral, and social problems associated with excessive consumption of alcohol (*alcohol problems*). *Alcoholism* is perhaps the most widely used term to describe patients with alcohol problems. In an attempt to define *alcoholism* more precisely, a panel of 23 experts convened by the National Council on Alcoholism and Drug Dependence and the American Society of Addiction Medicine developed a definition of alcoholism that included "a primary chronic disease with genetic psychosocial and environmental factors . . . often progressive and fatal . . . characterized by impaired control over drinking, preoccupation with the drug alcohol, use of alcohol despite future consequences, and distortions of thinking most notably denial." Because the term *alcoholism* is so broad, it also can be imprecise in defining the entire spectrum of alcohol problems.

Abstainers are individuals who consume no alcohol. *Moderate drinking* is defined by the National Institute on Alcohol Abuse and Alcoholism as the average number of drinks consumed daily that places an adult at low risk for alcohol problems. There is some epidemiologic evidence to suggest that moderate drinking may have some health benefits by reducing the risk of cardiovascular disease (Chapter 49). The scope of alcohol consumption that imparts this benefit may be low, however (e.g., less than one drink per day).

At-risk drinking is a level of alcohol consumption that imparts health risks (Table 31–1). This category of drinking behavior has been identified on the basis of epidemiologic evidence that certain threshold levels of alcohol consumption are associated with increased risk of specific health problems. At-risk drinking is defined differently for men younger than 65 years than for women of all ages because of generally lower body weights and lower rates of metabolism of alcohol in women; the definition in men older than 65 years is the same as in women because of the age-related increased risk of alcohol problems, in part due to changes in alcohol metabolism in older individuals. *Binge drinking* or *heavy drinking* is the episodic consumption of large amounts of alcohol, usually five or more drinks per occasion for men and four or more drinks per occasion for women. One standard drink contains 12 g of pure alcohol, an amount equivalent to that contained in 5 ounces of wine, 12 ounces of beer, or 1.5 ounces of 90-proof spirits. *Problem drinking* refers to a level of alcohol consumption that causes any problems for the patient (medical, psychiatric, behavioral, or social—*alcohol problems*).

Alcohol abuse and *alcohol dependence*, which are alcohol use disorders defined in the *Diagnostic and Statistical Manual of Mental Disorders*, 4th edition, require the presence of specific social or clinical phenomena (see Table 31–1). *Alcohol abuse* includes criteria that indicate social dysfunction or use in high-risk situations (e.g., driving). *Alcohol dependence* includes social consequences along with criteria related to physiologic aspects of dependence (e.g., tolerance, loss of control) and use despite physical or psychological problems. The distinction between *alcohol abuse* and *alcohol dependence* is important given the general need for more intensive treatment services for patients who are alcohol dependent.

TABLE 31–1 TERMS AND CRITERIA FOR PATTERNS OF ALCOHOL USE

AT-RISK DRINKING
Men: ≥15/week or ≥5 drinks/day
Women: ≥8/week or ≥4 drinks/day
ALCOHOL ABUSE
Maladaptive pattern of alcohol use leading to clinically significant impairment or distress, manifested within a 12-month period by one or more of the following:
Failure to fulfill role obligations at work, school, or home
Recurrent use in hazardous situations
Legal problems related to alcohol
Continued use despite alcohol-related social or interpersonal problems
Symptoms have never met criteria for alcohol dependence
ALCOHOL DEPENDENCE
Maladaptive pattern of alcohol use leading to clinically significant impairment or distress, manifested within a 12-month period by three or more of the following:
Tolerance (either increasing amounts used or diminished effects with the same amount)
Withdrawal (withdrawal symptoms or use to relieve or avoid symptoms)
Use of larger amounts for a longer period than intended
Persistent desire or unsuccessful attempts to cut down or control use
Great deal of time spent obtaining, using, or recovering from use
Important social relationships, occupations, or recreational activities given up or reduced
Use despite knowledge of alcohol-related physical or psychological problems

Epidemiology

In national surveys, 64% of American adults reported that they use alcoholic beverages (liquor, wine, or beer), whereas 36% reported that they were abstinent. Among individuals who use alcohol, many experience problems because of their drinking. It has been estimated that more than $100 billion is spent by American society each year to treat alcohol use disorders and to recover the costs of alcohol-related economic losses. Excessive alcohol consumption ranks as the third leading preventable cause of death in the United States after cigarette smoking and obesity. More than 100,000 deaths per year in the United States are attributed to alcohol use disorders.

Population-based epidemiologic studies have shown that alcohol use disorders are among the most prevalent medical behavioral or psychiatric disorders in the general population. An epidemiologic survey of the general population in the United States documented a prevalence of alcohol abuse and dependence estimated to be between 7.4 and 9.7%. The lifetime prevalence of abuse and dependence is estimated to be even higher. Despite higher thresholds and tolerance, men are at least twice as likely to meet criteria for alcohol abuse and dependence by standard diagnostic survey techniques. Although sociodemographic features, such as young age, low income, and low education level, have been associated with an increased risk for problem drinking, alcohol use disorders are prevalent throughout all sociodemographic groups, and all individuals should be screened carefully. The "skid row" stereotype of the alcohol-dependent patient is much more the exception than the rule.

The prevalence of alcohol use disorders is higher in most health care settings than it is in the general population because alcohol problems often result in treatment-seeking behaviors. The prevalence of problem drinking in general outpatient and inpatient medical settings has been estimated between 15 and 40%. These data strongly support the need for physicians to screen all patients for alcohol use disorders.

Pathobiology

Beverage alcohol contains ethanol, which acts as a sedative-hypnotic drug. Alcohol is absorbed rapidly into the blood stream from the stomach and intestinal tract. Because women have lower levels of gastric alcohol dehydrogenase, the enzyme primarily responsible for metabolizing alcohol, they experience higher blood alcohol concentrations than do men who consume similar amounts of ethanol per kilogram of body weight. The absorption of alcohol can be affected by other factors, including the presence of food in the stomach and the rate of alcohol consumption. By means of metabolism in the liver, alcohol is converted to acetaldehyde and acetate (Fig. 31–1). Metabolism is proportional to an

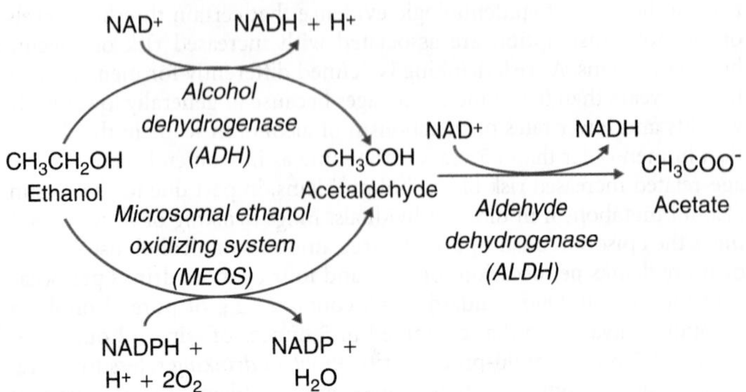

FIGURE 31–1 • Ethanol metabolism. Alcohol dehydrogenase (ADH) predominates at low to moderate ethanol doses. The microsomal ethanol-oxidizing system (MEOS) is induced at high ethanol levels of chronic exposure and by certain drugs. Aldehyde dehydrogenase (ALDH) inhibition (genetic or drug induced) leads to acetaldehyde accumulation.

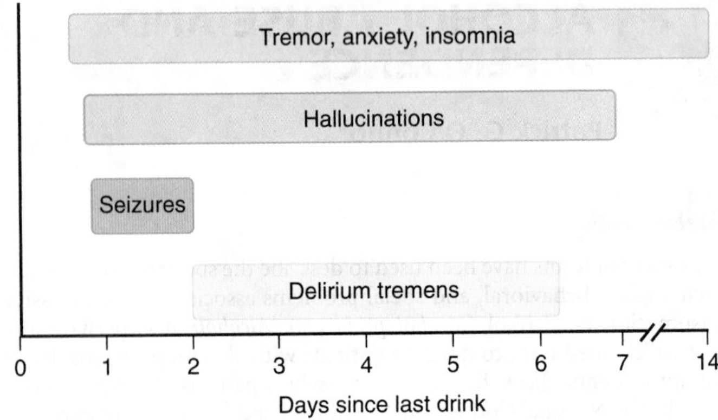

FIGURE 31–2 • Time course of alcohol withdrawal.

individual's body weight, but a variety of other factors can affect how alcohol is metabolized. A genetic variation in a significant proportion of the Asian population alters the structure of an acetaldehyde, aldehyde hydrogenase isoenzyme, resulting in the development of an alcohol flush reaction, which includes facial flushing, hot sensations, tachycardia, and hypotension.

In the brain, alcohol seems to affect a variety of receptors, including γ-aminobutyric acid (GABA), *N*-methyl-D-aspartate, and opioid receptors. Glycinuric and serotoninergic receptors also are thought to be involved in the interaction between alcohol and the brain. The phenomena of reinforcement and cellular adaptation are thought, at least in part, to influence alcohol-dependent behaviors. Alcohol is known to be reinforcing because withdrawal from ethanol and ingestion of ethanol itself are known to promote further alcohol consumption. After chronic exposure to alcohol, some brain neurons seem to adapt to this exposure by adjusting their response to normal stimuli. This adaptation is thought to be responsible for the phenomenon of tolerance, whereby increasing amounts of alcohol are needed over time to achieve desired effects. Although much has been learned about the variety of effects alcohol can have on various brain receptors, no single receptor site has been identified. A variety of neuropsychological disorders are seen in association with chronic ethanol use, including impaired short-term memory, cognitive dysfunction, and perceptual difficulties.

Although the brain is the primary target of alcohol's actions, a variety of other tissues have a major role in how alcohol affects the human body. Direct liver toxicity may be among the most important consequences of acute and chronic alcohol use (Chapter 156). A variety of histologic abnormalities ranging from inflammation to scarring and cirrhosis have been described. The pathophysiologic mechanism of these effects is thought to include the direct release of toxins and the formation of free radicals, which can interact negatively with liver proteins, lipids, and DNA. Alcohol also has substantial negative effects on the heart and cardiovascular system. Direct toxicity to myocardial cells frequently results in heart failure (Chapter 59), and chronic heavy alcohol consumption is considered to be a major contributor to hypertension (Chapter 66). Other organ systems that experience significant direct toxicity from alcohol include the gastrointestinal tract (esophagus, stomach), immune system (bone marrow, immune cell function), and endocrine system (pancreas, gonads).

Clinical Manifestations

Alcohol has a variety of specific acute and chronic effects. The acute effects seen most commonly are alcohol intoxication and alcohol withdrawal. Chronic clinical effects of alcohol include almost every organ system.

Acute Effects

Alcohol Intoxication

After entering the blood stream, alcohol rapidly passes through the blood-brain barrier. The clinical manifestations of alcohol intoxication are related directly to the blood level of alcohol. Because of tolerance, individuals chronically exposed to alcohol generally experience less severe effects at a given blood alcohol level than do individuals who are not chronically exposed to alcohol.

The symptoms of mild alcohol intoxication in nontolerant individuals typically occur at blood alcohol levels of 20 to 100 mg/dL and include euphoria, mild muscle incoordination, and mild cognitive impairment. At higher blood alcohol levels (100 to 200 mg/dL), more substantial neurologic dysfunction occurs, including more severe mental impairment, ataxia, and prolonged reaction time. Individuals with blood alcohol levels in these ranges can be obviously intoxicated with slurred speech and lack of coordination. These effects progress as the blood alcohol level rises to higher levels, to the point at which stupor, coma, and death can occur at levels equal to or greater than 300 to 400 mg/dL, especially in individuals who are nontolerant to the effects of alcohol. The usual cause of death in individuals with very high blood levels of alcohol is respiratory depression and hypotension.

Alcohol Withdrawal Syndrome

Alcohol withdrawal can occur when individuals decrease their alcohol use or stop using alcohol altogether. The severity of symptoms can vary greatly. Many individuals experience alcohol withdrawal without seeking medical attention, whereas others require hospitalization for severe illness. Because ethanol is a central nervous system depressant, the body's natural response to withdrawal of the substance is a hyperexcitable neurologic state. This state is thought to be the result of adaptive neurologic mechanisms being unrestrained by alcohol, with an ensuing release of a variety of neurohumoral substances, including norepinephrine. In addition, chronic exposure to alcohol results in a decrease in the number of GABA receptors and impairs their function.

The clinical manifestations of alcohol withdrawal include hyperactivity resulting in tachycardia and diaphoresis. Patients also experience tremulousness, anxiety, and insomnia. More severe alcohol withdrawal can result in nausea and vomiting, which can exacerbate metabolic disturbances. Perceptual abnormalities, including visual and auditory hallucinations and psychomotor agitation, are common manifestations of more moderate to severe alcohol withdrawal. Grand mal seizures commonly occur during alcohol withdrawal, although they do not generally require treatment beyond the acute withdrawal phase.

The time course of the alcohol withdrawal syndrome can vary within an individual and by symptom complex, and the overall duration of symptoms can be a few to several days (Fig. 31–2). Tremor is typically among the earliest symptoms and can occur within 8 hours of the last drink. Symptoms of tremulousness and motor hyperactivity typically peak within 24 to 48 hours. Although mild tremor typically involves the hands, more severe tremors can involve the entire body and greatly impair a variety of basic motor functions. Perceptual abnormalities typically begin within 24 to 36 hours after the last drink and resolve within a few days. When withdrawal seizures occur, they are typically generalized tonic-clonic seizures and most often occur within 12 to 24 hours after reduction of alcohol intake. Seizures can occur, however, at later time periods as well.

The most severe manifestation of the alcohol withdrawal syndrome is delirium tremens. This symptom complex includes disorientation, confusion, hallucination, diaphoresis, fever, and tachycardia. Delirium tremens typically begins after 2 to 4 days of abstinence, and the most severe form can result in death.

Chronic Effects

Acute manifestations, including intoxication and withdrawal, are generally stereotypical in their appearance and time course, but chronic manifestations tend to be more varied. Many patients with alcohol dependence may be without evidence of any chronic medical manifestations for many years. As time goes on, however, the likelihood that one or more of these manifestations will occur increases considerably. All major organ systems can be affected, but the primary organ systems involved are the nervous system, cardiovascular system, liver, gastrointestinal system, pancreas, hematopoietic system, and endocrine system (Table 31–2). Patients who drink are at risk for a variety of malignant neoplasms, such as head and neck, esophageal, and liver cancers (Chapters 140, 200, and 206). Excessive alcohol use often causes significant psychiatric and social morbidity that can be more common and more severe than the direct medical effects, especially earlier in the course of problem drinking.

Nervous System

In addition to the acute neurologic manifestations of intoxication and withdrawal, alcohol has major chronic neurologic effects. Approximately 10 million Americans have identifiable nervous system impairment from chronic alcohol use. Individual predisposition to these disorders is highly variable and is related to genetics, environment, sociodemographic features, and gender; the relative contribution of these factors is unclear.

In the central nervous system, the major effect is cognitive impairment. Patients may present with mild to moderate short-term or long-term memory problems or may have severe dementia resembling Alzheimer's disease (Chapter 425). The degree to which the direct toxic effect of alcohol is responsible for these problems or the impact of alcohol-related nutritional deficiencies is uncertain (Chapter 443). The deficiency of vitamins such as thiamine may have a major impact in terms of promoting alcoholic dementia and severe cognitive dysfunction, as is seen in Korsakoff's syndrome. Alcohol also causes a polyneuropathy that can present with paresthesias, numbness, weakness, and chronic pain (Chapters 443 and 446). As with the central nervous system, peripheral nervous system effects are thought to be caused by a combination of the direct toxicity of alcohol and nutritional deficiencies. A small proportion (<1%) of patients with alcohol dependence may develop midline cerebellar degeneration, which presents as an unsteady gait.

TABLE 31–2 ALCOHOL-RELATED COMPLICATIONS

System/Realm of Problem	Complications
Nervous system	Intoxication Withdrawal Cognitive impairment Cerebellar degeneration Peripheral neuropathy
Cardiovascular system	Cardiac arrhythmias Chronic cardiomyopathy Hypertension
Liver	Fatty liver Alcoholic hepatitis Cirrhosis
Gastrointestinal tract	
Esophagus	Chronic inflammation Malignant neoplasms Mallory-Weiss tears Esophageal varices
Stomach	Gastritis Peptic ulcer disease
Pancreas	Acute pancreatitis Chronic pancreatitis
Other medical problems	Cancers: mouth, oropharynx, esophagus Hepatoma Pneumonia Tuberculosis
Psychiatric	Depression Anxiety Suicide
Behavioral and psychosocial	Injuries Violence Crime Child or partner abuse Tobacco, other drug abuse Unemployment Legal problems

Cardiovascular System

The most common cardiovascular complications of chronic alcohol consumption are cardiomyopathy, hypertension, and supraventricular arrhythmias. Alcoholic cardiomyopathy (Chapter 59) can present clinically in a manner similar to other causes of heart failure (Chapter 57). It is the most common cause of nonischemic cardiomyopathy in Western countries, accounting for approximately 45% of cases. Like these other causes, alcoholic cardiomyopathy also responds to conventional treatments of heart failure (Chapter 58). Abstinence from alcohol can result in significant improvement in cardiomyopathy in some patients. Increasing levels of alcohol consumption also are associated with increasing levels of systolic and diastolic hypertension (Chapter 66).

The most common arrhythmias associated with chronic alcohol use include atrial fibrillation and supraventricular tachycardia; these are seen commonly in the setting of acute intoxication and withdrawal (Chapter 63). The prevalence of alcohol-induced arrhythmias is unclear. Alcoholic cardiomyopathy also is associated with arrhythmias, in particular, ventricular arrhythmias (Chapter 64).

Liver

Alcohol abuse is the major cause of morbidity and mortality from liver disease in the United States. It has been estimated that there are more than 2 million people with known alcoholic liver disease in the United States. Factors that predispose to early liver disease include the quantity and duration of alcohol exposure, female gender, and malnutrition. The range of clinical manifestations includes acute fatty liver, alcoholic hepatitis, and cirrhosis (Chapter 156). Fatty liver associated with alcohol ingestion can be asymptomatic or associated with nonspecific abdominal discomfort; it generally improves with abstinence from alcohol. Alcoholic hepatitis can present as an asymptomatic condition identified through abnormalities in liver enzymes or as an acute episode with abdominal pain, nausea, vomiting, and fever. Patients with alcoholic hepatitis have particularly high levels of aspartate aminotransferase in the blood and elevated levels of γ-glutamyltransferase. Alcoholic hepatitis typically improves with abstinence from alcohol.

Alcohol-related cirrhosis is a major cause of death in the United States (Chapter 157). Although patients are often asymptomatic, patients with more advanced cirrhosis may present with a variety of symptoms and signs, including jaundice, ascites, and coagulopathy. Cirrhosis also is associated with gastrointestinal bleeding from esophageal varices (Chapter 137). Although there is some controversy about the use of liver transplantation to treat patients with alcoholic cirrhosis, many believe that patients in established recovery are good candidates for liver transplantation (Chapter 158).

Gastrointestinal Disease

Chronic alcohol use is associated with a variety of esophageal problems, including esophageal varices, Mallory-Weiss tears, and squamous cell carcinoma of the esophagus. The risk of squamous cell carcinoma is increased further in patients who smoke tobacco and drink alcohol. Patients with these problems can present with difficulty swallowing, chest pain, gastrointestinal blood loss, and weight loss. Acute alcoholic gastritis typically presents with abdominal discomfort, nausea, and vomiting (Chapter 137).

Pancreas

The risk of pancreatitis in individuals with alcohol dependence is approximately four times that in the general population. Quantity and duration of alcohol exposure and a history of pancreatitis are predictive of future episodes. Acute alcoholic pancreatitis, which may present with severe abdominal pain, nausea, vomiting, fever, and hypotension, can be life-threatening (Chapter 147). Individuals who have recurrent acute pancreatitis may develop chronic pancreatitis, which typically presents with chronic abdominal pain, malabsorption, weight loss, and malnutrition.

Hematopoietic System

The anemia that commonly is seen in patients with chronic alcohol problems can be multifactorial (e.g., blood loss, nutrient deficiency, secondary to liver disease and hypersplenism). Studies of selected inpatients with alcohol dependence showed the prevalence of anemia to range from approximately 10 to 60%. Gastrointestinal blood loss due to Mallory-Weiss tears (Chapter 140), alcoholic gastritis (Chapter 137), or esophageal varices (Chapters 140 and 157) may be a key factor, and many patients develop subsequent iron deficiency. Dietary folate deficiency can be associated with megaloblastic anemias (Chapter 171). Alcohol also has a direct toxic effect on the bone marrow, which can lead to sideroblastic anemia that resolves after abstinence (Chapter 169).

Alcohol can suppress megakaryocyte production and cause thrombocytopenia, which may manifest as petechiae or bleeding (Chapter 178); the thrombocytopenia is particularly sensitive to abstinence, with platelet counts usually rebounding or returning to normal within 5 to 7 days after cessation of alcohol intake. Alcohol also appears to interfere directly with platelet function. Alcohol-related immune dysfunction, as evidenced by decreased production and function of white blood cells and derangement in humoral and cell-mediated immunity, explains why alcohol-dependent individuals are at higher risk for infectious diseases, such as pneumonia and tuberculosis. The hypersplenism that occurs in combination with cirrhosis also may contribute to the increased risk of serious infection in these patients (Chapters 157 and 174).

Malignant Neoplasms

Alcohol intake has been associated with upper digestive, respiratory, and liver malignant neoplasms. Alcohol use is associated with squamous cell carcinomas of the esophagus (Chapter 140) and of the head and neck (Chapter 200). The co-occurrence of alcohol and tobacco abuse seems to be synergistic. Either heavy alcohol use or smoking individually increases the rate of oropharyngeal cancer by about six or seven times that of the general population, whereas the rate for people with both risk factors is about 40 times that of the general population. Patients with alcohol-induced liver disease who also have a history of hepatitis B or C are at particularly increased risk for hepatocellular carcinoma (Chapter 206).

Chronic alcohol use also has been associated with malignant neoplasms of the breast (Chapter 208), prostate (Chapter 211), pancreas (Chapter 205), cervix (Chapter 209), lung (Chapter 201), and colon (Chapter 203). Women who have more than one or two alcoholic drinks per day may increase their breast cancer risk 1.5-fold or more. Hormonal mechanisms and direct carcinogenic effects of alcohol have been postulated as causes of this association. The association of cervical cancer with alcohol dependence may be due to alcohol-associated, high-risk sexual behaviors that are thought to increase the risk of cervical cancer.

Other Medical Issues

Gout has been associated with alcohol abuse, and flares can occur at lower serum urate levels than in nonalcoholic patients (Chapter 294). Alcoholic ketoacidosis (Chapter 119), which usually follows an alcoholic binge, presents as nausea, vomiting, abdominal pain, and volume depletion. Typically, ketoacidosis is seen with low or normal glucose readings. Mild or nonspecific abnormalities in thyroid function, especially in patients with underlying liver disease, may reflect abnormalities in the clearance of thyroid-stimulating hormone or the impact of elevated circulating estrogens (Chapter 244). Infertility and menstrual irregularities have been associated with chronic alcohol consumption, presumably due to alcohol-induced disruption in hypothalamic-pituitary dysfunction, gonadal toxicity, and impaired hepatic metabolism of circulating hormones (Chapter 256). Hypogonadism is highly prevalent in male alcoholics with cirrhosis (Chapter 253). Alcohol dependence also is associated with higher rates of dental and periodontal disease (Chapter 451) and with a variety of dermatologic problems including spider angiomas and, in patients with poor hygiene, skin infestations.

Psychiatric Issues

Psychiatric symptoms and illnesses (Chapter 420) are exceedingly common among individuals with alcohol problems. The prevalence of anxiety disorders is about 40%, and the prevalence of affective disorders is about 30%. Antisocial personality disorder is also more common in individuals with alcohol problems than in the general population. These psychiatric problems are more prevalent during periods of heavy drinking and withdrawal. All patients with alcohol use disorders require careful screening for psychiatric illnesses. Effective treatment of underlying psychiatric disorders may result in improved drinking behaviors.

Other Behavioral and Psychosocial Issues

Alcohol commonly is the underlying cause of domestic abuse injuries, trauma, motor vehicle accidents, and burns (Chapters 15 and 113). Patients presenting with injuries should be questioned carefully about their alcohol use. Tobacco (Chapter 30) and other drug abuse (Chapter 32) are more prevalent in people with alcohol problems than in the general population.

Diagnosis

Data from the history, physical examination, and laboratory generally are needed to provide a complete picture of the extent of alcohol problems in affected patients (Table 31–3).

Discussing the Diagnosis with Patients

In discussing alcohol problems, it is crucial that physicians be sensitive to the stigma and shame that may be felt by patients with alcohol problems and by their families. Alcohol-related diagnoses or problems should be discussed in a nonjudgmental manner, which forges a partnership and indicates commitment to helping with whatever problems the patients

TABLE 31–3 DIAGNOSIS OF ALCOHOL PROBLEMS

HISTORY

Step 1: Ask all patients about current and past use.
- Do you drink alcohol (ever or currently)?
- Do you have a family history of alcohol problems?

Step 2: Obtain detailed history regarding quantity and frequency of alcohol use.
- What types of alcohol do you consume?
- How often do you drink?
- How much do you usually drink?
- Do you ever drink more, and if so, how much?

Step 3: Standardized questionnaire
- CAGE questions:
- Have you ever felt that you should Cut down on your drinking?
- Have people Annoyed you by criticizing your drinking?
- Have you ever felt bad or Guilty about drinking?
- Have you ever taken a drink first thing in the morning (Eye opener) to steady your nerves or get rid of a hangover?

Step 4: Assess specific areas in suspected or known problem drinkers.
- Criteria for alcohol abuse and dependence
- Evidence of medical and psychiatric problems
- Evidence of behavioral or social problems
- Use of other substances
  - Tobacco
  - Mood-altering prescription drugs
  - Illicit drugs (e.g., heroin, cocaine)
- Prior alcohol or substance abuse treatment

PHYSICAL EXAMINATION

Thorough and complete examination important in all patients

Focus attention to system with identified problems

In all patients, carefully examine
- Central and peripheral nervous systems
- Cardiovascular system
- Liver
- Gastrointestinal tract

LABORATORY STUDIES (IN SELECTED PATIENTS)

Liver enzymes

Coagulation studies

Complete blood count

Carbohydrate-deficient transferrin

might have. Setting the stage for the discussion should include educating patients about the various levels of alcohol problems (e.g., at-risk drinking, alcohol abuse, alcohol dependence) so that patients have an understanding of the spectrum of alcohol problems. Many patients may have a skewed view of what qualifies as problem drinking and may believe that only individuals with severe alcohol problems are truly problem drinkers. The history, physical examination, and laboratory studies should be provided as "proof" that a problem may or does exist.

History

A four-step approach to the alcohol history includes comprehensive questions about alcohol use and a thorough evaluation for alcohol-related problems.

Step 1: Ask All Patients About Current and Past Alcohol Use

A single question—Do you currently or have you ever used alcohol?—can identify quickly patients who are not lifetime abstainers and require further screening. Patients who answer yes to this question should proceed through the subsequent three steps. Patients who answer no can be classified as lifetime abstainers from alcohol and require no further questioning unless their answer changes over time. It is crucial to ask about current and past alcohol use because many patients who meet lifetime criteria for alcohol dependence but who are currently in recovery answer no to the question about current use; unless it is specifically asked about, important past use information may be missed.

Step 2: Obtain Detailed History Regarding Quantity and Frequency of Alcohol Use

A question to be asked routinely is, What type or types of alcoholic drinks (beer, wine, spirits) do you consume? Many patients do not consider the use of beer or wine "drinking." Quantity should be determined for typical use—How much do you usually drink on a typical drinking day?—and for range of use—Do you ever drink more than your usual amount, and if so, how much? This second question can be particularly important for identifying binge drinking. Quantity questions offer easy identification of at-risk drinking. Asking about the frequency of alcohol consumption—How often do you drink?—helps distinguish daily from nondaily alcohol users. Binge drinkers who drink only on weekends tend to have significant alcohol problems yet not be daily drinkers. A major goal of step 2 is to acquire a complete characterization of current alcohol use behaviors and the pattern of quantity and frequency of alcohol use during the patient's lifetime.

Step 3: Use Standardized Screening Instruments

Many standardized questionnaires have been developed to detect alcohol abuse and dependence. The two questionnaires that have been evaluated most extensively in medical settings are the CAGE (Cut down, Annoyed, Guilty, and Eye opener) questionnaire (see Table 31–3) and the Alcohol Use Disorder Identification Test (AUDIT). The CAGE questionnaire includes four questions and is scored by giving 1 point for each positive response. Given that the word *ever* is used in the CAGE questions, by definition this instrument is designed to detect lifetime alcohol problems and does not distinguish between lifetime problems and current problems. To screen for alcohol abuse and dependence, the CAGE has a sensitivity of 43 to 94% and a specificity of 70 to 97% when a cutoff score of 2 is used to indicate a "positive" result.

The AUDIT's ten questions cover the quantity and frequency of alcohol use, drinking behaviors, adverse psychological symptoms, and alcohol-related problems. It was developed by the World Health Organization to identify hazardous (e.g., at-risk) drinking and harmful (e.g., alcohol use that results in physical or psychological harm) drinking. In contrast to the CAGE questionnaire, the AUDIT focuses on recent (current to past year) drinking behaviors. Each question is scored 0 to 4 (range for total score is 0 to 40), and a total score of 8 is considered to be a positive result.

Step 4: Assess Specific Areas in Suspected or Known Problem Drinkers

Questions asked in step 4 are based on the results of the questions asked in steps 2 and 3 to obtain more detailed information in patients with potential alcohol problems. Even patients who do not screen positive on the CAGE questionnaire may warrant detailed questioning about alcohol abuse and dependence (see Table 31–1), especially if they are drinking at or above at-risk levels or there is other evidence of possible alcohol problems. A detailed review for evidence of alcohol-related medical and psychiatric problems should occur, and the need for further medical and psychiatric evaluation should be determined. The physician should look for evidence of behavioral and social problems commonly associated with alcohol use and screen for family and occupational dysfunction and other problems, such as domestic violence. Patients should be asked about their use of tobacco, mood-altering prescription medications, and illicit drugs such as heroine and cocaine.

Finally, many patients with alcohol problems have prior treatment episodes that should be detailed. The inquiry should include questions not only about formal alcohol treatment (including number of episodes, duration of treatment, and inpatient versus outpatient treatment) but also about more informal treatments, such as attendance at self-help groups like Alcoholics Anonymous (AA). For patients who require a referral for treatment, knowledge of prior treatment experience is a crucial determinant of future referral recommendations.

The National Institute on Alcohol Abuse and Alcoholism has published *Helping Patients Who Drink Too Much: A Clinician's Guide,* which provides a similar approach to screening and evaluating patients for alcohol-related problems and includes an appendix of useful supporting materials.

Physical Examination

Patients with potential alcohol use disorders require a detailed physical examination to complement the history. In addition, attention should be focused to detect common alcohol-related problems, including the nervous system, cardiovascular system, liver, and gastrointestinal system (see Table 31–2).

Laboratory Findings

A variety of laboratory tests have been proposed to aid screening for alcoholic abuse and dependence. Aminotransferase levels, red blood cells, mean corpuscular volume, and carbohydrate-deficient transferrin, alone or in combination, are not as effective as screening questionnaires, such as the CAGE and the AUDIT.

Laboratory tests do have a role in diagnosis and assessment of patients with potential alcohol problems. Routine laboratory testing including liver enzymes (Chapter 150), bilirubin, complete blood count, and prothrombin time should be obtained in all patients with alcohol problems on a regular basis so that an appropriate and complete picture of the effects of alcohol on the individual can be obtained.

Prevention and Treatment

The relationship of change in alcohol use with prevention of subsequent problems has been well established. Treatment of alcohol use disorders should be based on the severity of potential or actual alcohol problems and tailored to meet the needs of individual patients. Separate advice and management approaches are suggested for nondependent at-risk or problem drinkers compared with individuals who are alcohol dependent (Table 31–4).

Treatment of At-Risk Drinkers

Evidence confirms that generalist physicians, in a cost-effective manner, can help patients reduce their alcohol intake and prevent subsequent alcohol-related problems by using brief (5 to 20 minutes), focused counseling techniques (brief interventions) that are well suited for primary care and other medical settings. The brief counseling strategy includes four main components: motivational techniques, feedback about the problems with alcohol use, discussion of the adverse effects of alcohol, and setting recommended drinking limits. Motivational techniques are designed to motivate patients to change their alcohol use behavior by identifying potential or actual problems with which their alcohol use is associated. Feedback about these problems can make it clear to the patient that the problems exist. For at-risk and problem drinkers who do not meet criteria for alcohol dependence, setting recommended drinking limits below at-risk levels (e.g., less than one drink per day for women and less than two drinks per day for men) is a realistic and suitable goal. Epidemiologic evidence suggests that drinking below these levels is less likely to be associated with problems. Several randomized clinical trials confirm that patients who receive brief interventions significantly decrease their alcohol intake, often to "safe" levels, and can decrease health care use as well. I

TABLE 31–4 ADVICE FOR PATIENTS WITH ALCOHOL PROBLEMS

State your medical concern:

Be specific about your patient's drinking patterns and related health risks.

Ask: How do you feel about your drinking?

Agree on a plan of action:

Ask: Are you ready to try to cut down or abstain?

Talk with patients who are ready to make a change in their drinking about a specific plan of action.

For patients who are not alcohol dependent:

Advise the patient to cut down if drinking is at or above at-risk drinking amounts (see Table 31–1) and there is no evidence of alcohol dependence.

Ask the patient to set a specific drinking goal: Are you ready to set a drinking goal? Some patients choose to abstain for a period of time or for good; others prefer to limit the amount they drink. What do you think will work best for you?

Provide patient education materials and tell the patient: It helps to think about your reasons for wanting to cut down and examine what situations trigger unhealthy drinking patterns. These materials will give you some useful tips on how to maintain your drinking goal.

For patients with evidence of alcohol dependence:

Advise to abstain if:
- Evidence of alcohol dependence
- History of repeated failed attempts to cut down
- Pregnant or trying to conceive
- Contraindicated medical condition or medication

Refer for additional diagnostic evaluation or treatment.
- Procedures for patient in making referral decisions:
- Involve your patient in making referral decisions.
- Discuss available alcohol treatment services.
- Schedule a referral appointment while the patient is in the office.

Rx

Treatment of Alcohol Dependence

Patients who meet criteria for alcohol dependence typically require more intensive services than do patients who meet criteria for at-risk drinking. Most patients can be managed in outpatient treatment settings, whereas patients with more severe alcohol dependence or comorbid problems initially may require inpatient management, specific counseling programs, and pharmacologic therapy. Before entering a formal program to maintain remission, many patients first require medical management of alcohol withdrawal. Professional organizations have published practice guidelines that provide useful recommendations for how to select among treatment options for patients with alcohol dependence.

Management of Alcohol Withdrawal

Many patients may not present for medical management of alcohol withdrawal and deal with it on their own. However, a substantial subset do present for alcohol withdrawal treatment. Patients with mild to moderate withdrawal generally can be managed safely as outpatients with close follow-up. Patients with moderate to severe withdrawal, as manifested by hypertension, tremor, and any mental status changes, especially patients with significant comorbid medical or psychiatric illnesses, generally are treated best as inpatients. Patients who have a history of severe withdrawal in the past (e.g., delirium tremens) or who have a history of alcohol withdrawal seizures also generally should be managed as inpatients. The three major goals of medical management of alcohol withdrawal are to minimize the severity of withdrawal-related symptoms; to prevent specific withdrawal-related complications, such as seizures and delirium tremens; and to provide referral to relapse prevention treatment.

A wide variety of medications have been evaluated for their effectiveness in managing the alcohol withdrawal syndrome (Table 31–5). Longer acting benzodiazepines are preferred because they provide a smoother withdrawal. Shorter acting benzodiazepines, such as oxazepam, may be indicated in individuals with severe liver disease. The most common approach is to administer a standing dose of a benzodiazepine, with additional medication being given "as

TABLE 31–5 MEDICATIONS FOR THE TREATMENT OF ALCOHOL DEPENDENCE*

Medication	Dose and Route	Frequency	Effects	Major Common Adverse Effects
ALCOHOL WITHDRAWAL				
Benzodiazepines‡				
Chlordiazepoxide*	25–100 mg, PO/IV/IM‡	Every 4–6 hr	Decreased severity of withdrawal; stabilization of vital signs; prevention of seizures and delirium tremens	Confusion, oversedation, respiratory depression
Diazepam†	5–10 mg, PO/IV/IM‡	Every 6–8 hr		
Oxazepam†	15–30 mg, PO‡	Every 6–8 hr		
Lorazepam†	1–4 mg, PO/IV/IM‡	Every 4–8 hr		
β-Blockers				
Atenolol	25–50 mg, PO	Once a day	Improvement in vital signs	Bradycardia, hypotension
Propranolol	10–40 mg, PO	Every 6–8 hr	Reduction in craving	
α-Agonists				
Clonidine	0.1–0.2 mg, PO	Every 6 hr	Decreased withdrawal symptoms	Hypotension, fatigue
Antiepileptics				
Carbamazepine	200 mg, PO	Every 6–8 hr	Decreased severity of withdrawal; prevention of seizures	Dizziness, fatigue, red blood cell abnormalities
PREVENTION OF RELAPSE				
Disulfiram†	125–500 mg, PO	Daily	Decreased alcohol use among those who relapse	Disulfiram-alcohol reaction, rash, drowsiness, peripheral neuropathy
Naltrexone†	50 mg, PO	Daily	Increased abstinence, decreased drinking days	Nausea, abdominal pain, myalgias-arthralgias
Acamprosate†	666 mg, PO	Three times a day	Increased abstinence	Diarrhea

*Most commonly used medications listed.
†Currently approved by Food and Drug Administration for the indication noted.
‡Dose and routes given for standard fixed-dose regimens, which indude dose tapers over time.

Rx

needed" on the basis of withdrawal symptoms. The specific benzodiazepine and dose often depend on the experience of the prescribing physician and the characteristics of the patient, including the severity of withdrawal (higher doses are used if withdrawal is more severe), the presence of liver disease (patients with severe liver disease should receive lower doses or shorter acting medications), and the response to prior doses of medication (higher doses are given if symptom control is inadequate; lower doses are given if adverse effects, such as oversedation, have occurred). In general, the amount of medication per dosing period is decreased gradually as the withdrawal syndrome abates. An individualized "symptom-triggered" dosing approach, in which benzodiazepines are administered on a dose-by-dose basis (e.g., 25 to 100 mg of chlordiazepoxide hourly) as guided by withdrawal symptoms, is safe and effective in certain patients and can reduce the total doses of benzodiazepines needed to treat withdrawal. [2] β-Blockers (atenolol and propranolol), α-agonists (clonidine), and antiepileptics (carbamazepine) improve signs and symptoms of alcohol withdrawal but are viewed best as adjunctive medications to be used in addition to benzodiazepines.

Prevention of Relapse

Counseling Strategies Used by Alcohol Treatment Programs

Three commonly used psychotherapeutic techniques are motivational enhancement therapy, 12-step facilitation, and cognitive-behavioral coping skills. Two of these techniques are designed to give patients specific tools to help them avoid relapse to alcohol use. In motivational enhancement therapy, patients identify reasons for staying away from alcohol. The 12-step facilitation therapy uses the principles of AA to help patients focus their attention on abstinence. In cognitive-behavioral coping skills therapy, the patient identifies triggers to alcohol use and develops strategies to help deal with the triggers when they are present.

Project MATCH (Matching Alcohol Treatments to Client Heterogenicity) showed equivalence among three counseling approaches (cognitive-behavioral coping skills therapy, motivational enhancement therapy, or 12-step facilitation therapy) to treat alcohol dependence. At 1-year follow-up, most enrolled patients either remained abstinent or significantly decreased their alcohol use.

Self-Help Groups

Self-help groups such as AA and Rational Recovery are an important source of support and treatment for many patients with alcohol dependence. AA has the advantage of being widely available throughout the United States and is free of charge. The overall approach to treatment is based on the 12 steps for maintaining abstinence and dealing with the various effects of alcohol. AA meetings can be either "open" to anybody in the community or "closed" for active members only. The meetings vary in format, size, location, and demographic makeup. In counseling patients about attending AA, it is important for physicians to make them aware that variations in the nature of specific meetings, especially location and demographics of participants, require patients to be willing to attend more than one meeting site on a trial basis so that they find a comfortable setting.

Research of the effectiveness of AA has been limited, and there are no large controlled studies. Indirect evidence suggests, however, a significant improvement in alcohol use behaviors.

Pharmacotherapy to Prevent Relapse to Alcohol Use

The addition of medication to enhance the effectiveness of counseling therapies has been the subject of research for the past 40 years. As the neurobiology of alcohol use disorders has become more clearly understood, the potential to develop medications that may promote abstinence or decreased alcohol use has grown. Three medications—disulfiram, naltrexone, and acamprosate—are approved for the treatment of alcohol dependence in the United States (see Table 31–5).

Disulfiram

Disulfiram is designed to prevent alcohol use by causing a severe adverse reaction when patients use alcohol. The disulfiram reaction, which includes flushing, nausea, vomiting, and diarrhea, is mediated by the inhibition of alcohol dehydrogenase and the resulting increase in serum levels of acetaldehyde and acetate after ingestion of alcohol. Disulfiram also affects monoamine metabolism, and the alcohol-disulfiram reaction may be related to changes in central monoamine functioning. Although disulfiram offers little benefit to most patients, it is effective in reducing alcohol intake in highly motivated patients who are supervised in an alcohol treatment program. [3]

Naltrexone

Naltrexone is thought to decrease alcohol use by diminishing the euphorigenic effects of alcohol and by decreasing craving in alcohol-dependent patients. Randomized, placebo-controlled trials generally have shown that alcohol-dependent patients who receive naltrexone (50 mg/day) are more likely to decrease their alcohol use or remain abstinent compared with patients who receive placebo, and the effects persist after discontinuation of treatment, although one randomized trial did not show benefit in male veterans with severe alcohol dependence. [4] Although most studies of naltrexone were performed in a specialty alcohol treatment setting and observed subjects for only 10 to 12 weeks, one study demonstrated that naltrexone can be effective in primary care settings in patients who were observed for up to 34 weeks. [5] Side effects of naltrexone are infrequent, most notably self-limited nausea in about 10% of patients. Dose-related hepatotoxicity has been reported in patients treated for obesity with high-dose naltrexone (300 mg/day). Mild liver enzyme abnormalities are not a contraindication to naltrexone, but patients should be followed up with repeated liver enzyme studies. Patients with acute hepatitis or liver failure should not use naltrexone.

Acamprosate

Approved by the Food and Drug Administration in 2004, acamprosate (calcium acetylhomotaurinate) has been identified as an effective agent for treatment of alcohol dependence. The precise mechanism of action of acamprosate is uncertain, but it may be related to its effects on neuroexcitatory amino acids and the inhibitory GABA system. In a randomized, placebo-controlled clinical trial, subjects who received acamprosate were more likely to remain abstinent compared with subjects who received placebo. [6] Side effects are minimal and typically include diarrhea. Like naltrexone, acamprosate is given as an adjunctive therapy to psychological treatments for alcohol dependence.

Other Pharmacologic Approaches to Prevent Relapse

There has been much interest in evaluation of the effectiveness of combinations of drug therapies to treat alcohol dependence. One study of 160 patients suggested that the combination of naltrexone and acamprosate was more effective than either medication alone. A larger federally funded study that enrolled 1383 subjects, Project COMBINE, examined naltrexone and acamprosate alone and in combination with two different psychological therapies to see which combination of pharmacologic and behavioral therapies is most effective. [7] The behavioral therapies were medical management, which was designed to approximate counseling that can be provided in primary care and other medical settings, and combined behavioral intervention, which incorporated counseling techniques that are provided in alcohol treatment specialty settings. Results from this study demonstrated that patients receiving medical management with naltrexone, combined behavioral intervention, or both fared best, lending further support to the idea that alcohol-dependent patients can be effectively treated in primary care and other medical settings. Interestingly, acamprosate was not shown to be effective in this study.

Topiramate, a fructopyranose derivative, has been shown to be an effective treatment of alcohol dependence in a randomized clinical trial at a dose of up to 300 mg/day. [8] A long-acting injectable formulation of naltrexone (up to 380 mg, administered monthly) has been shown to reduce heavy drinking in alcohol-dependent patients. [9] Other medications that have shown promise include

TABLE 31–6 OVERVIEW OF TREATMENT APPROACH FOR PATIENTS WITH ALCOHOL PROBLEMS

Evaluate all patients
For patterns of problem alcohol use (Table 31–1)
For alcohol-related complications, if indicated (Table 31–2)
With use of data collected from history, physical examination, and laboratory testing (Table 31–3)
For at-risk and nondependent problem drinkers
Advise to decrease alcohol use to below at-risk levels (Table 31–4)
Advise patients who cannot decrease use to below at-risk levels to abstain
For patients who are alcohol dependent
Assess for need for withdrawal management medications (Table 31–5)
Refer to an alcohol treatment program
Consider medication to prevent relapse (Table 31–5)

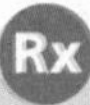

ondansetron, bromocriptine, and sodium valproate. Other drugs have shown possible benefits in patients with concurrent depression (e.g., fluoxetine) or anxiety (e.g., buspirone) or no effect (e.g., lithium).

Prognosis

Alcohol abuse and dependence are chronic disorders that are characterized by exacerbations and remissions. The prognosis is better for patients who seek treatment and receive it in a systematic way (Table 31–6), but it can be poor for patients with advanced liver disease and continued alcohol use. In addition, the use of combinations of medications (e.g., naltrexone plus acamprosate) is under investigation.

Future Directions

To date, most studies have focused on shorter term outcomes, from a few months to a year. It is important to understand more clearly what happens to these patients over time, especially the need for "booster sessions" to sustain improvements provided by brief interventions. Newer pharmacologic therapies may help many patients.

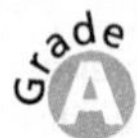

1. Fleming MF, Barry KL, Manwell LB, et al: Brief physician advice for problem alcohol drinkers: A randomized controlled trial in community-based primary care practices. JAMA 1997;277:1039–1045.
2. Saitz R, Mayo-Smith MF, Roberts MS, et al: Individualized treatment for alcohol withdrawal: A randomized double-blind controlled trial. JAMA 1994;272:519–523.
3. Fuller RK, Branchey L, Brightwell DR, et al: Disulfiram treatment of alcoholism: A Veterans Administration cooperative study. JAMA 1986;256:1449–1455.
4. Chick J, Anton R, Checinski K, et al: A multicentre, randomized, double-blind, placebo controlled trial of naltrexone in the treatment of alcohol dependence or abuse. Alcohol Alcohol 2000;35:587–593.
5. O'Malley SS, Rounsaville BJ, Farren C, et al: Initial and maintenance naltrexone treatment for alcohol dependence using primary care vs specialty care: A nested sequence of 3 randomized trials. Arch Intern Med 2003;163:1695–1704.
6. Tempesta E, Janiri L, Bignamini A, et al: Acamprosate and relapse prevention in the treatment of alcohol dependence: A placebo-controlled study. Alcohol Alcohol 2000;35:202–209.
7. Anton RF, O'Malley SS, Ciraulo, DA, et al: COMBINE Study Research Group: Combined pharmacotherapies and behavioral interventions for alcohol dependence. The COMBINE study: A randomized controlled trial. JAMA 2006;295:2003–2017.
8. Johnson BA, Ait-Daoud N, Akhtar FZ, et al: Use of oral topiramate to promote smoking abstinence among alcohol-dependent smokers: A randomized controlled trial. Arch Intern Med 2005;165:1600–1605.
9. Garbutt JC, Kranzler HR, O'Malley SS, et al: Vivitrex Study Group: Efficacy and tolerability of long-acting injectable naltrexone for alcohol dependence: A randomized controlled trial. JAMA 2005;293:1617–1625.

SUGGESTED READINGS

American Psychiatric Association Workgroup on Substance Use Disorders: Practice Guidelines for the Treatment of Patients with Substance Use Disorders. American Psychiatric Association, 2006. *Consensus guidelines.*

Kosten TR, O'Connor PG: Management of drug and alcohol withdrawal. N Engl J Med 2003;348:1786–1795. *Overview of inpatient and outpatient options.*

Moss M, Burnham EL: Alcohol abuse in the critically ill patient. Lancet 2006;368:2231–2242. *Review of how alcohol abuse can complicate up to 10% of admissions.*

National Institute on Alcohol Abuse and Alcoholism: Helping Patients Who Drink Too Much: A Clinician's Guide, 2005 edition. Available at http://pubs.niaaa.nih.gov/publications/Practitioner/CliniciansGuide2005/clinicians_guide.htm. *A useful overview of screening, assessing, and managing patients who drink too much.*

Saitz R, Horton NJ, Sullivan LM, et al: Addressing alcohol problems in primary care: A cluster randomized, controlled trial of a systems intervention. Ann Intern Med 2003;138:372–382. *When physicians are provided information and recommendations about their patients' alcohol habits, subsequent discussions may lead to decreased alcohol use.*

Saitz R, Palfai TP, Cheng DM, et al: Brief intervention for medical inpatients with unhealthy alcohol use: A randomized, controlled trial. Ann Intern Med 2007;146:167–176. *Brief intervention was unsuccessful.*

32 DRUG ABUSE AND DEPENDENCE

Jeffrey H. Samet

Definition

The terms *drug* (or substance) *dependence* and *drug abuse* have specific clinical meanings (Table 32–1). Dependence is the more severe disorder and frequently is associated with physiologic and psychological manifestations. *Tolerance* and *withdrawal* are the major physiologic manifestations of drug dependence. Tolerance is defined as either a need for increased amounts of the substance to achieve the desired effect or a diminished effect with continued use of the same amount of the substance. Withdrawal is manifested by a characteristic syndrome with sudden abstinence, but it may be relieved or avoided if the same or a closely related substance is taken. The other criteria for dependence relate to the pattern of drug use (i.e., taken in a larger amount or longer period than intended), the effects on life activities (i.e., great deal of time spent on activities to obtain, use, or recover from the substance; reduction in social, occupational, or recreational activities as a result of substance use), and the psychological need to use the substance (i.e., use despite awareness of adverse consequences, persistent desire for the substance, or inability to control its use).

A diagnosis of substance abuse requires the recurrent use of a substance during 12 months with subsequent adverse consequences (e.g., failure to fulfill a major role at work, school, or home; legal problems; persistent interpersonal problems) or placement of an individual in high-risk, physically hazardous situations. Addiction is a chronic, relapsing illness characterized by compulsive drug seeking and use.

The degree of harm associated with occasional drug use or "experimentation" is difficult to quantify, and no medical definition has been assigned formally to the use of illicit drugs with consequences less than those associated with abuse. The fear of progression to abuse or dependence, the potential morbidity of even isolated use of drugs such as cocaine, the criminality associated with drug use, and the high-risk behavior under the influence of a drug are the basis of recommendations to proscribe use of these substances.

Epidemiology

Drug abuse and dependence are important mainstream health problems as evidenced by consequences and costs. Injection drug use remains a major transmission risk for human immunodeficiency virus (HIV) infection; more than 1.5 million drug arrests occur in the United States each year and costs are enormous, estimated as more than $180 billion

TABLE 32–1 DIAGNOSTIC CRITERIA FOR DEPENDENCE AND DRUG ABUSE

Dependence (≥3 needed)	Abuse (≥1 for 12 months)
Tolerance Withdrawal The substance is often taken in larger amounts for a longer period than intended Any unsuccessful effort or a persistent desire to cut down or to control substance use A great deal of time is spent in activities necessary to obtain the substance or to recover from its effects Important social, occupational, or recreational activities given up or reduced because of substance use Continued substance use despite knowledge of having had persistent or recurrent physical or psychological problems that are likely to be caused or exacerbated by the substance	1) Recurrent substance use resulting in failure to fulfill major role obligations at work, school, or home 2) Recurrent substance use in situations in which it is physically hazardous 3) Recurrent substance-related legal problems 4) Continued substance use despite having persistent or recurrent social or interpersonal problems caused or exacerbated by the effects of the substance And: Never met criteria for dependence

in the United States in 2002. About 19.5 million people older than 12 years have used illicit drugs at least once during the past month, and about 4.4 million people are classified as drug dependent. Worldwide, 15.3 million persons have drug use disorders. The highest impact of illicit drugs on disease burden is among industrialized countries with otherwise low mortality. Medical complications of drug abuse are predominantly infectious but span organ systems and range from cocaine-related cardiac arrhythmia to neuropsychiatric effects of cannabis.

Etiology

A minority of people who ever experiment with an illicit drug progress to a clinical drug abuse diagnosis. The cofactors responsible for progression to dependence and abuse are only partially defined. Genetic susceptibility, social context of the drug use, and comorbid psychiatric conditions are considered important factors affecting an individual's potential for subsequent problems. Twin studies suggest that genetics plays a role in a person's positive or negative perception of a drug's effect. Despite the fact that an individual is required to be exposed to a drug to become addicted, the heritability of dependence to psychostimulants and opioids is high. This heritability seems to be directly related to addiction liability. The neurobiologic basis of this genetic association is likely to involve pathways that mediate reward, stress response, and compulsivity, among others. Knockout mouse strains have begun to identify specific gene products that may have a role in these mechanisms.

The social context in which drug abuse develops and is expressed is important. Returning Vietnam War veterans addicted to heroin were relatively easy to treat compared with addicts on the streets of the United States, in part because the veterans had become addicted in a setting different from the one they found on return home and were exposed to few enduring environmental cues. Psychiatric comorbidities, particularly depression and panic disorders, are high-risk conditions for the development of drug abuse and its consequences.

Treatment

Patients who use illicit drugs benefit from treatment if they recognize that their substance use is a problem. The transtheoretical model considers a patient on a continuum from precontemplation (denial) toward maintenance (abstinence/recovery) (Fig. 32–1). The clinical approach should be tailored to the patient's readiness to change behavior and enter treatment. For all abused drugs, medical follow-up after any acute toxic presentation is essential to address substance abuse issues and the very common coexisting medical and psychiatric problems.

The major goals of drug abuse treatment are detoxification, abstinence initiation, and relapse prevention. Treatment can be pharmacologic and nonpharmacologic. Pharmacologic approaches are offered by physicians specializing in addiction medicine and increasingly by other clinicians in the primary care setting.

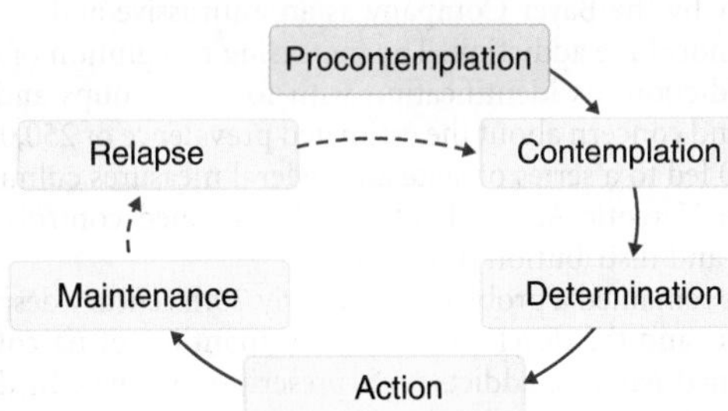

FIGURE 32–1 • Graphic depiction of the Prochaska and DiClemente model for readiness for behavioral change.

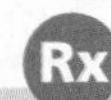

Some form of psychosocial treatment is the backbone of substance abuse treatment, be it psychotherapy, behavioral therapy, or counseling. Issues addressed in these encounters include teaching coping skills, changing reinforcement contingencies, fostering management of painful affective states, addressing motivation, improving interpersonal functioning, enhancing social supports, and encouraging compliance with and retention in pharmacotherapy. Much of this work is done by substance abuse care providers. Physicians are in an excellent position to detect drug abuse by asking about the use of specific drugs when they encounter a possible related clinical manifestation. Primary care physicians in particular can make significant contributions. Individuals with substance abuse–related medical conditions were more likely to remain abstinent when they were treated in an integrated medical care and substance abuse treatment program. 1

The active ingredients of a brief clinical intervention addressing substance use have been summarized by the acronym FRAMES: *feedback* of personal risk or impairment (e.g., sharing abnormal test results, discussing medical complications); emphasis on personal *responsibility* to change; clear *advice* to change; a *menu* of different options for change; provider *empathy;* and enhancement of the patient's *self-efficacy* or optimism. Physicians can refer to substance abuse treatment specialists; 12-step or mutual-help groups (e.g., Narcotics Anonymous) are often part of a successful abstinence maintenance program.

DRUGS OF ABUSE

Heroin and Other Opioids

Definition

Opioids, including naturally occurring alkaloids (opiates derived from the poppy plant *Papaver somniferum*), semisynthetic compounds (chemically altered alkaloids), and synthetic agents, are potent analgesics and produce an intense euphoria associated with nausea, drowsiness, miosis, and decreases in respiration, pulse, and blood pressure. Opioids also are valued for their calming, antitussive, and antidiarrheal properties. Depending on the particular effect on opioid cell membrane receptors, they may be classified as agonists (morphine, heroin, methadone), partial agonists-antagonists (buprenorphine), or antagonists (naloxone, naltrexone). These drugs have led to many medical complications because of their abuse potential and frequent parenteral route of administration.

History

In the 19th century, opioids were used commonly in many settings in the United States. The drug was supplied freely by physicians to treat symptoms of pain, anxiety, cough, and diarrhea. Opiates also were available without restriction in commercial medicinal remedies.

In 1806, a pure substance was isolated from opium and named morphine after the Greek god of dreams, Morpheus. By the middle of the 19th century, the advent of the hypodermic needle allowed this inexpensive, standard-strength agent to become a highly effective pain-killing and calming therapy. Smoking of opium, which has no medicinal value, also rose in the latter half of the 19th century. In 1898, heroin was introduced commercially by the Bayer Company as an antitussive and was used as therapy for morphine addiction. The increasing recognition of the perils of opiate addiction, its identification with foreign groups and internal minorities, and concern about the estimated prevalence of 250,000 opiate users in 1900 led to a series of state and federal measures culminating in the Harrison Narcotic Act in 1914, which legislated controls over the importation and distribution of opiates.

Opiate use remained a problem in the early 20th century despite interdiction efforts and the development and dismantling of narcotic clinics that maintained narcotic addicts with prescription drugs. In the 1920s, narcotic abuse became a predominantly underground activity. Efforts to treat narcotic addiction as a medical problem were limited until the advent of methadone maintenance therapy in the 1960s.

Epidemiology

In the United States, an estimated 3.7 million people have reported prior use of heroin. Globally, it is estimated that 9.2 million people use heroin. About 170,000 of the estimated 810,000 opioid-dependent persons in the United States are enrolled in opioid treatment programs. An estimated 150,000 individuals become new heroin users each year; 25% of these are younger than 19 years. Polysubstance abuse is increasingly common, with 50% of male and 25% of female narcotic addicts meeting the criteria for alcohol dependence. Nicotine is the most common substance used together with opiates.

The use of prescription opioids for nonmedical reasons (e.g., OxyContin) is currently one of the fastest growing dimensions of drug abuse in the United States, with a 225% increase from 1992 to 2000. This use far outpaced the relatively stable use of heroin (i.e., 1.5% increase) in this period. In 2003, an estimated 11.7 million Americans misused pain relievers. Opioid pill abuse can lead to injection opioid use.

Pathobiology

Opioids exert their effects on specific receptors for three distinct families of endogenous opioid peptides: enkephalins, endorphins, and dynorphins. In the central nervous system, three major classes of opioid receptors with unique selectivity and pharmacologic profiles have been identified: μ, κ, and δ. Subtypes of these major classes (μ_1, μ_2, κ_1, κ_2, κ_3, δ_1, δ_2) have been elucidated primarily by the use of selective receptor antagonists. The μ receptor activity is associated with the most prominent manifestations of morphine and heroin: respiratory depression, analgesia, euphoria, and development of dependence. It is thought that opioid peptides acting as neurotransmitters or neuromodulators exert their actions at neuronal synapses.

Heroin may be injected intravenously or subcutaneously, snorted, smoked, or ingested. The parenteral and inhaled routes of administration result in the most rapid delivery of drug to the brain and are the most potentially addicting. As the purity of street heroin has increased from less than 5% in the 1960s to 80% since the mid-1990s, its nonparenteral administration has risen. Heroin may be used intermittently or regularly. Intermittent users generally either quit or become regular users within 1 to 3 years. Given heroin's short half-life, regular users require two to four daily doses to avoid withdrawal symptoms.

Oral ingestion accounts for the majority of prescription opioid use, such as oxycodone (Percodan, Percocet), hydrocodone (Vicodin), hydromorphone (Dilaudid), and meperidine (Demerol). In particular, OxyContin, a long-acting opioid by virtue of its structural design giving delayed absorption of oxycodone, is abused by crushing the pill before ingestion, thus destroying its slow-release matrix. This medication, approved in 1995, provides a "rush" comparable to that of injectable heroin when it is taken in this manner. Despite this abuse potential, it is important for the physician to understand that it is uncommon for appropriate use of prescription opioids in the treatment of pain to lead to opioid dependence (Chapter 28).

Clinical Manifestations

Heroin's initial effect is an intense euphoria described as a rush or kick, compared in intensity and pleasure with an orgasm that lasts 45 seconds to several minutes. The initial effects may be perceived as a turning in the stomach with tingling and warmth. A user's first experience may be unpleasant because of nausea, vomiting, and anxiety, but these effects decrease or become less of a concern to the user over time. The intense euphoria is followed by an intoxicated pleasant feeling referred to as nodding, with decreased respiration and peristalsis. The depressant effect of heroin on the central nervous system is marked, particularly after parenteral administration. Sedation, mental clouding, decreased visual acuity, heavy feeling in the extremities, light sleep with vivid dreams, and reduction in anxiety are typical, at least until tolerance develops. Physical signs include miosis, decreased heart rate, and lowered blood pressure. In addition to these effects on opioid receptors, heroin causes the release of histamine, which may result in itching, scleral injection, and hypotension.

High levels of tolerance develop rapidly with regard to respiratory depression, analgesia, sedation, vomiting, and euphoric properties. Little tolerance develops for miosis or constipation, so a heroin addict with an acutely painful medical condition may complain of insufficient analgesia despite pinpoint pupils. Cross-tolerance is common among opioids.

From the patient's perspective, withdrawal from heroin or any chronic opioid is a dreaded clinical condition, a mix of emotional, behavioral, and physical signs and symptoms (Table 32–2). Although unpleasant, it is not life-threatening. Withdrawal symptoms, which are related directly to clearance of the drug, begin 4 to 8 hours after the last dose of heroin. The acute withdrawal syndrome peaks in intensity after 36 to 72 hours and resolves during 5 to 7 days.

TABLE 32–2 SIGNS AND SYMPTOMS OF WITHDRAWAL

OPIOID WITHDRAWAL	
Vital signs	Tachycardia, hypertension, fever
Central nervous system	Craving, restlessness, insomnia, muscle cramps, yawning, mydriasis
Eyes, nose	Lacrimation, rhinorrhea
Skin	Perspiration, piloerection
Gastrointestinal	Nausea, vomiting, diarrhea
COCAINE WITHDRAWAL	
Crash	Depression, fatigue
Withdrawal	Anxiety, high craving
Extinction	Normalization of mood, episodic craving
MARIJUANA WITHDRAWAL	
Central nervous system	Craving, irritability, insomnia, anxiety, increased aggression, tremors
Skin	Perspiration
Gastrointestinal	Nausea, decreased appetite

In addition to the acute abstinence syndrome, a protracted abstinence syndrome occurs and lasts 6 months or more. In contrast to the hyperadrenergic characteristics of the primary withdrawal syndrome (tachycardia, hypertension, elevated temperature, mydriasis, and diaphoresis), the period afterward can consist of sluggishness, sleep disturbance, and malaise. Craving can recur for years after cessation of drug use. An understanding of the nature of recovery from opioid use is important for setting appropriate expectations for the patient and the health care provider.

Complications

Most deaths and other opioid-related medical complications are a result of overdose and the spread of infectious agents by injection drug use among heroin addicts (Fig. 32–2). The manifestations of the infectious complications are protean but frequently nonspecific, such as fever, malaise, weight loss, pain, or dyspnea. The underlying causes include endocarditis, cellulitis, HIV infection, hepatitis, pneumonia, and a variety of abscesses.

Cardiac Complications

The major cardiac complication of opioid abuse is bacterial endocarditis (Chapter 76) caused by injection drug use. *Staphylococcus aureus* is the most frequently reported bacterial isolate, and the tricuspid valve is most commonly involved. Left-sided valvar infection is associated with a worse prognosis, as are the uncommon gram-negative and fungal infections.

Opioid abusers normally have acute rather than subacute endocarditis. The initial clinical finding can be fever alone in half the cases, or fever may be associated with pulmonary infiltrates from right-sided emboli or systemic embolic phenomena, such as arthritis, abscess, and osteomyelitis. The diagnosis of endocarditis in a febrile injection drug user is difficult because of the poor sensitivity and specificity of readily available clinical and laboratory data. Blood cultures are essential for these patients. If adequate outpatient follow-up is not possible, hospitalization generally is recommended until initial blood culture results are known. Other cardiac complications associated with opioid abuse include toxic cardiomyopathy, perivalvar abscess, abnormalities of the conduction system such as QT prolongation and ST-T wave changes, and cor pulmonale.

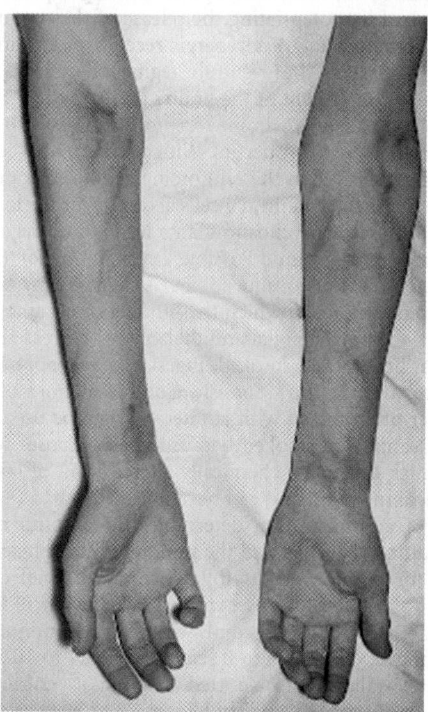

FIGURE 32–2 • Injection drug use typically leads to this appearance, which results from repeated superficial thrombophlebitis of accessible veins in the arm or elsewhere in the body. Sharing and reuse of syringes and needles puts these patients at risk of a wide range of infections, including bacterial septicemia, systemic fungal infection, hepatitis B, hepatitis C, and HIV infection. Right-sided endocarditis is a common complication. (From Forbes CD, Jackson WF: Color Atlas and Text of Clinical Medicine, 3rd ed. London, Mosby, 2003, with permission.)

Pulmonary Complications

The most common pulmonary complication is bacterial pneumonia, which is present in one third of injection drug users evaluated for fever. The risk for this infection probably results from a combination of factors, including hypoventilation, immune dysfunction, suppression of coughing, and aspiration during periods of clouded sensorium. Pulmonary hypertension can result from “talc granulomatosis,” the development of diffuse pulmonary granulomas caused by the intravenous injection of foreign substances, most notably talc. Other pulmonary complications associated with opioid abuse include acute pulmonary edema, bronchospasm, septic pulmonary emboli, and infectious or chemical mediastinitis.

Neurologic Complications

Neurologic complications of opioid abuse are infectious and noninfectious. Seizures, most often generalized, are the most common noninfectious neurologic complication. The cause of seizures includes overdose, with centrally mediated respiratory depression and hypoxia, and cerebral infarction. Meningitis, mycotic aneurysm, and abscesses (epidural, subdural, and brain) are well-described infectious conditions resulting from injection drug use. In HIV-infected patients, HIV-associated neurologic infectious and noninfectious diseases occur (Chapter 417).

Psychiatric Complications

Psychiatric conditions among opioid abusers are common and include alcohol abuse or dependence, major depression, phobic disorders, and antisocial personality; all have a greater than 15% lifetime prevalence. Men are four to seven times more likely to have an antisocial personality than are women; women more commonly have depression. Women are at high risk of being victims of violence.

Immunologic Complications

Immunologic abnormalities among heroin-dependent persons were described before the acquired immunodeficiency syndrome (AIDS) epidemic. In vitro, morphine decreases the number of T lymphocytes, and naloxone, an opiate antagonist, can reverse this decrease. Injection drug users' hypergammaglobulinemia, presumably resulting from repeated antigenic stimulation, is the explanation given for a high rate of false-positive indirect syphilis serologic test results. The long-term consequences of opioid-related immunologic effects are not clear. The most prominent clinical endocrine effect is amenorrhea.

The associated medical complications of HIV infection in drug users mirror those of noninjection drug users with HIV infection with a few caveats. HIV-infected drug users have an increased frequency of bacterial pneumonia and a decreased frequency of Kaposi's sarcoma. HIV testing with appropriate counseling should be recommended strongly for all opioid abusers. Behavioral changes to promote the use of condoms and the avoidance of sharing of needles can reduce HIV transmission. Needle exchange programs are efficacious in reducing the harm of heroin addiction.

Other Medical Complications

Renal complications of opioid abuse include acute diseases (myoglobinuria, necrotizing angiitis, glomerulonephritis associated with endocarditis or hepatitis) and chronic diseases (nephrotic syndrome, renal failure, renal amyloidosis). The pathologic process most commonly found in heroin-associated nephrotic syndrome is focal and diffuse glomerulosclerosis (Chapter 122). In HIV-infected patients, HIV-associated nephropathy also is found.

Of patients in methadone maintenance clinics, 50 to 90% have positive serologic studies for hepatitis B and C. Complications of these infections (Chapter 152) range from chronic asymptomatic antigenemia to cirrhosis and hepatocellular carcinoma.

Treatment

Pharmacologic treatment of opioid abuse includes agonist, antagonist, mixed agonist-antagonist, or symptomatic treatment. With detoxification, the goal is amelioration of the symptoms of heroin or other opioid withdrawal by agonist substitution (e.g., methadone, buprenorphine) or symptomatic treatment (e.g., clonidine). Buprenorphine has μ-receptor agonist and κ-receptor antagonist properties, which has yielded a better safety profile and less physical dependence. Hospitalized opioid-dependent patients can

TABLE 32–3 RELAPSE PREVENTION FOR OPIOID DEPENDENCE

Medication	Dose	Dosing Interval	Mechanism	Prescribing Regulations	Withdrawal
Methadone	60–100 mg orally	Daily	Agonist	Yes	++
Buprenorphine	8–32 mg sublingually	q1–2d	Partial agonist/antagonist	Yes	+
Naltrexone	50 mg orally	Daily	Antagonist	No	—

++ = moderate; + = mild; — = none.

Rx

be treated effectively with methadone for withdrawal symptoms by any physician. Methadone for the post-discharge treatment of opioid addiction is currently available only through specially licensed treatment facilities.

Pharmacologic treatment to prevent relapse to active opioid abuse is effective by substitution of a safer drug (i.e., methadone, buprenorphine) with similar pharmacologic properties to relieve the craving and withdrawal and to block some of the euphoric effects of heroin or other opioids (Table 32–3). These medications at effective doses (i.e., methadone, 60 to 100 mg; buprenorphine, 16 to 32 mg) substantially reduced use of illicit opioids compared with low-dose methadone (20 mg) in a randomized controlled trial. 2 The recent U.S. adoption of buprenorphine prescription for opioid dependence in primary care by physicians with limited additional training has expanded treatment opportunities for opioid-dependent persons. It has also facilitated engagement of younger patients with fewer of the medical complications that almost inevitably occur after years of opioid abuse. One pharmacologic option for a detoxified patient concerned about relapse is use of an opioid antagonist (i.e., naltrexone) that effectively blocks agonist stimulation. Brief weekly counseling and weekly medication is as good a maintenance therapy as more aggressive regimens, but only about 40 to 45% of patients comply with either approach. 3 Although an emphasis on the treatment and prevention of drug abuse is crucial, physicians also should promote measures to reduce harm for injection drug users who are not able or willing to cease drug use, including participation in needle exchange programs, avoidance of "shooting galleries" to obtain or to administer drugs, prescriptions for needles and syringes, and instructions never to share "works" (injection equipment).

Cocaine, Methamphetamine, and Other Psychostimulants

Definition

Cocaine (an alkaloid extracted from coca leaves), methamphetamine (a synthetic compound produced from over-the-counter medications), and other psychostimulants (e.g., amphetamine) rapidly increase the concentration of several neurotransmitters in synaptic junctions and stimulate the sympathetic and central nervous systems. Methamphetamine has no appropriate clinical role. Topical cocaine is used in otolaryngologic procedures, and psychostimulants are used either for their stimulant effects or for their paradoxical calming effect in some patients with attention-deficit/hyperactivity disorder.

History

The earliest recorded use of cocaine in the form of ingested coca leaf occurred around 3000 BC. In 1860, cocaine was isolated and incorporated into tonics, teas, and wines. In the 1880s, an Atlanta druggist patented a product that contained naturally occurring stimulants, cocaine and caffeine, which eventually became known as Coca-Cola; until 1903, it contained approximately 60 mg of cocaine per 8-ounce serving. In the late 19th century, reports of cocaine addiction surfaced, and its use was restricted after passage of the Harrison Narcotic Act of 1914. The abuse potential of amphetamines led to their being listed as schedule II drugs, which are defined as having a high potential for abuse with severe liability to cause psychic or physical dependence.

The advent of methamphetamine in the United States began with regional reports of its use in the Midwest and West in the 1990s, with more recent national use in specific groups (e.g., gay and bisexual men). It is currently described as one of the most socially destructive drugs of abuse.

Epidemiology

An estimated 1.5 million Americans, representing 0.8% of the population aged 12 years and older, have used cocaine in the past month. In 2002, 1.1 million Americans used cocaine for the first time, and 323,000 were methamphetamine initiates. Use of amphetamine-like stimulants appears to be growing in many countries; in fact, as of 1996, 20 countries reported greater use of these types of drugs than of heroin and cocaine combined (e.g., Japan, Korea). Although current cocaine use is highest in the unemployed (3.1%), 71% of adult users are employed full-time or part-time. Current cocaine use is similar for whites (0.9%), blacks (1.3%), and Hispanics (1.1%). Methamphetamine's local production in makeshift laboratories has facilitated its use and consequences in rural America, a setting with less reported drug abuse and fewer resources to address this scourge.

Pathobiology

Psychostimulants increase neurotransmitter concentrations at the synaptic terminal by blocking the reuptake of norepinephrine, dopamine, and serotonin and by potentiating the release of these monoamines. In the heart, α-adrenergic and β-adrenergic receptors are stimulated.

Dopamine activates the ventral tegmental–nucleus accumbens pathway, a major component of the brain's reward system. The system is complex, with at least five dopamine receptor subtypes with distinct molecular and pharmacologic properties. With cocaine, D_1, D_2, and D_3 receptors have been implicated in the reinforcing actions. Cocaine's ability to block sodium channels in neuronal cells accounts for the local anesthetic actions. Chronic use of psychostimulants leads to dysregulation of the brain's dopaminergic systems. Possible degeneration of dopaminergic terminals in the brains of cocaine addicts is suggested by positron emission tomographic studies in which the binding of cocaine to dopamine transporters in the basal ganglia and thalamus is decreased.

Cocaine can be snorted, smoked, ingested orally, applied to mucous membranes, or injected intravenously. Cocaine hydrochloride, a water-soluble powder often mixed with adulterants, can be used by all routes except that it cannot be smoked because it decomposes when burned. Freebase or crack cocaine, a chemically altered form of cocaine, vaporizes before decomposition and can be smoked.

The route of administration determines the amount of cocaine or methamphetamine absorbed and the rapidity of its uptake in the brain. The kinetics for cocaine are as follows: oral, peak effect in 1 hour; intranasal, 3 to 5 minutes for onset with a peak effect in 30 to 60 minutes; intravenous, onset in 12 to 16 seconds with 10- to 20-minute duration of effect; and smoked, onset in 6 to 8 seconds with 5- to 10-minute duration of effect. Swallowed or snorted (intranasal) cocaine penetrates biologic membranes poorly and undergoes 70 to 80% hepatic transformation. Similar absorption and onset of action are found with methamphetamine. Cocaine has an elimination half-life of 30 to 60 minutes. Less than 5% of cocaine appears unchanged in urine. Cocaine's major metabolites are benzoylecgonine and ecgonine methyl ester. Both are inactive, and benzoylecgonine is the main target in urine testing (Table 32–4). Methamphetamine's effects last 8 to 24 hours, and only 50% of

TABLE 32–4 URINE TESTING FOR ABUSED DRUGS

Drug	Compound Detected	Urine Detection Time
Heroin	Morphine, 6-acetylmorphine	1–3 days
Codeine	Codeine, morphine	1–3 days
Methadone	Methadone	2–4 days
Cocaine	Benzoylecgonine	1–3 days
Amphetamine	Amphetamine	2–4 days
Methamphetamine	Methamphetamine, amphetamine	2–4 days
Marijuana	Tetrahydrocannabinol	1–3 days for casual use, up to 30 days for chronic use
Phencyclidine	Phencyclidine	2–7 days for casual use, up to 30 days for chronic use
Benzodiazepines	Oxazepam, diazepam, other benzodiazepines	Up to 30 days
Barbiturates	Amobarbital, secobarbital, other barbiturates	2–4 days for short acting, up to 30 days for long acting

the drug is eliminated in 12 hours. With both of these drugs, casual users can progress to high-dose users with compulsive and uncontrollable bingeing. During a binge, cocaine is administered every 10 to 30 minutes, generally during 4 to 24 hours or more; methamphetamine can be taken every 2 to 3 hours for several days. Individuals on binges may forego food and sleep until exhaustion or the supply is depleted.

Clinical Manifestations

The acute effects of cocaine and methamphetamine include intense euphoria, increased energy and self-confidence, enhanced mental acuity and sensory awareness (including sexual), and decreased appetite. Sympathetic signs include tachycardia, mydriasis, and hyperthermia. Withdrawal symptoms are the inverse of the acute effects: depressed mood, lack of energy, limited interest in the environment, hyperphagia, hypersomnia, anxiety, and craving. The withdrawal syndromes are not as consistent as those of alcohol or opioid withdrawal. Chronic users become tolerant to its acute effects; symptoms of anxiety, agitation, inability to concentrate, and loss of sexual drive predominate. Beyond the initial withdrawal period, craving leading to relapse can be precipitated by conditioned cues in which the pleasurable effects of these drugs are associated with particular settings.

Cocaine

The most common medical complications of cocaine use involve the brain and the heart and include altered mental status, seizures, chest pain, palpitations, and syncope. Sudden death can occur by a variety of mechanisms, including arrhythmias, status epilepticus, intracerebral hemorrhage, and centrally mediated respiratory arrest.

Cocaine use leads to ischemia and myocardial infarction as a result of increased myocardial demand because of tachycardia and hypertension, diffuse and local coronary spasm in normal or atherosclerotic arteries, and a propensity to thrombus formation secondary to blood stasis in narrowed arteries and increased platelet aggregability. Myocardial infarction is unrelated to the dose of cocaine ingested, the frequency of use, or the route of administration; first-time, recreational, and habitual users are all at risk. Almost 90% of cocaine-associated myocardial infarctions occur in men. Most chest pain develops within minutes, but pain can be delayed 15 hours after use.

Other cardiac complications include supraventricular and ventricular arrhythmias, cardiomyopathy, and myocarditis. Arrhythmias are attributed to direct toxic effects and a cocaine-induced hyperadrenergic state. Myocardial damage may be similar to that seen in pheochromocytoma, in which norepinephrine excess results in a nonspecific pathologic finding, contraction band necrosis.

Cocaine addiction frequently is associated with psychiatric diseases, such as depression, anxiety, phobia, attention-deficit disorder, and antisocial personality disorder. High doses can result in transient psychosis, delirium, paranoid ideation, bizarre behavior, and suicide attempts.

Other complications of cocaine use include vascular headaches, rhabdomyolysis with acute renal failure, placental abruption, erosion of dental enamel, gingival ulceration, chronic rhinitis, perforated nasal septum, pulmonary edema, and sexual dysfunction. Sexually transmitted diseases, including HIV infection, have been associated strongly with cocaine use; HIV testing should be pursued in any patient with a cocaine abuse diagnosis. Ingested packets of cocaine can rupture and cause acute toxic reactions and cardiovascular collapse.

Methamphetamine

The synthetic psychostimulant methamphetamine, a particularly potent form of amphetamine, is highly addictive; it is cheaper and longer lasting than cocaine. Nicknames include speed, crank, and zip; the smokable form is called ice or crystal. Methamphetamine's neurotoxic effects can result in Parkinson's disease–like symptoms, a consequence of damage to cell endings causing reduced levels of dopamine. The range of central nervous system complications of methamphetamine use includes convulsions, tremors, aggression, paranoia, and hyperthermia. Cardiovascular damage can cause strokes, collapse, and death. Chronic users may exhibit psychotic symptoms (e.g., paranoia, hallucinations, uncontrollable rages, and delusions), which can lead to extremely violent behavior and suicidal ideation. Injection users of methamphetamine have an increased risk of acquiring infectious diseases such as hepatitis B and C and HIV infection. Although methamphetamine use can increase libido initially, chronic abuse may have the opposite effect. Damage to teeth characterized by rampant decay and caries has been termed meth mouth. This condition is caused by the drug's enamel-eroding hydrochloric acid as well as by the user's poor oral hygiene, tooth grinding, and consumption of sweet beverages due to dehydration and sugar cravings.

Treatment

Cocaine abuse is treated by psychotherapy, behavioral therapy, and 12-step programs. Acupuncture has been used for detoxification and for preventing relapse but has limited proven efficacy. As yet, no pharmacologic agent has been consistently effective in reducing cocaine use or craving. No antidote is known for acute cocaine overdose.

Physician referral to community-based programs (e.g., 12-step groups, rehabilitation programs) is appropriate treatment of methamphetamine abuse. Cognitive-behavioral therapy has been effective for cessation and the maintenance of abstinence from methamphetamine use.

Marijuana and Other Cannabinoids

Definition

Marijuana is the common name applied to the leaves, stems, and tops of the plant *Cannabis sativa,* which contains cannabinoids, the most active of which is Δ^9-*trans*-tetrahydrocannabinol (THC). It generally is smoked but can be ingested, mixed in food or tea. Although tolerance and physical dependence can occur, clinical presentation of these syndromes is not common. The changes in the brain, cardiovascular system, and lungs are typically acute and reversible. Marijuana or purified oral THC has been used as effective therapy for nausea in some patients.

Epidemiology

Cannabinoids are the most commonly used illicit drugs in the world. About 2.5% of the world population, 147 million people, consume cannabis each year. An estimated 25.2 million Americans, or about 10% of the population aged 12 years and older, have used cannabinoids within the past year, and more than 96 million have used marijuana in their lifetime.

Pathobiology

Cannabinoids bind to specific receptors for the endogenous ligand anandamide: CB1 in the brain and CB2 in the periphery. G protein activation is a result of receptor binding and has three effects: inhibition of adenylate cyclase, increased potassium ion conductance, and decreased calcium ion conductance. CB1 receptors are concentrated in the globus pallidus, hippocampus, cerebral cortex, cerebellum, and striatum.

Clinical Manifestations

Smoked marijuana results in a variety of acute changes within 3 minutes that peak within 20 to 30 minutes; when it is ingested, onset takes 30 to 60 minutes, and the peak effect occurs after 2 to 3 hours. An average cigarette contains 5 mg of THC, and 50 to 60% of it is absorbed. THC is lipophilic and distributed rapidly throughout the body. Because of slow release from adipose tissue, THC or its metabolites can be found in urine 1 to 3 days after use in nonchronic users and 30 days after use in chronic users (see Table 32–4).

Most effects last 2 to 3 hours after inhalation; psychomotor effects can last 11 hours. Effects include conjunctival injection, mild euphoria, impaired memory, dry mouth, motor incoordination, time-space distortion, increased visual and auditory awareness, increased hunger, sleepiness, and spontaneous laughter; some may experience nausea, headaches, tremors, decreased muscle strength, and increased anxiety. A withdrawal state occurs in approximately 9% of cannabis users and is similar to tobacco withdrawal (i.e., irritability, depressed mood, headaches, restlessness, trouble sleeping) except for its effect on appetite. Marijuana withdrawal results in decreased appetite. Its onset is usually 1 to 3 days after cessation of use and can last 4 to 14 days.

Treatment

Marijuana use rarely requires acute treatment in the medical setting. Reassurance generally is sufficient to manage the occasional dysphoric manifestations. On occasion, anxiety reactions require specific therapy with benzodiazepines; rarely, psychotic reactions are treated with haloperidol.

Hallucinogens

Definition

Hallucinogen use results predominantly in changes in thought, perception, and mood. Minimal impairment occurs in memory or intellect. This class of drugs is not generally associated with stupor, narcosis, or excessive stimulation. Users do not exhibit craving. The major categories of hallucinogens are indolamines (e.g., lysergic acid diethylamide [LSD], dimethyltryptamide, psilocybin) and phenylethylamines (e.g., methylenedioxyamphetamine, methylenedioxymethamphetamine [MDMA], mescaline). These drugs have no appropriate clinical role.

Epidemiology

In the United States, the lifetime prevalence of hallucinogen use is about 14% (34 million individuals). LSD was used widely on college campuses in the 1960s. After a decline in the 1970s and 1980s, use has increased. There were 1.1 million new users in 2002, with a modest recent decline.

Pathobiology

The classic hallucinogens are structurally similar to many major neurotransmitters, but serotonin (5-hydroxytryptamine [5-HT]) agonist or partial agonist properties have been associated most consistently with its actions. These drugs bind at $5\text{-}HT_{2A}$ and $5\text{-}HT_{2C}$ receptors with high affinity. These receptors are found in greatest density in brain cortical regions (cerebral cortex, claustrum, caudate putamen, globus pallidus, ventral pallidum, islands of Calleja, mammillary nuclei, and inferior olive) and may have a role in depression and suicide.

Clinical Manifestations

Hallucinogen use results in an altered perception of one's environment marked by a subjective feeling of enhanced mental activity, perceptual distortions, visual hallucinations, sharpened sense of hearing, and reduced ability to tell the difference between one's self and one's surroundings. These drugs can produce sympathomimetic effects, including mydriasis, flushed face, fine tremor, piloerection, high blood pressure, hyperthermia, and hyperglycemia. Panic attacks and psychosis are the major adverse effects. Clinically "desired" effects and adverse effects vary by specific hallucinogen. Altered perceptions can be associated with paranoid delusions, manic or depressed behavior, and confusion. Aggressive behavior has been described with psychosis; in particular, phencyclidine (PCP) has been implicated in violent crimes. The psychotic episodes can last hours or days, and flashbacks can occur. Precipitants for flashbacks are anxiety, stress, fatigue, emergence into a dark environment, and marijuana.

Diagnosis

Although tolerance can develop with hallucinogens, the clinical syndrome is unusual inasmuch as chronic use is uncommon. No clinically significant withdrawal symptoms are known. The use of hallucinogens may be detected in the acute setting when a patient with toxic manifestations is examined or may be noted when a history of drug use is obtained. After diagnosis, it is important to obtain a history of other substance abuse and psychiatric illness and a neurologic evaluation. No specific laboratory tests are required; a urine toxicologic screen for other drugs of abuse is recommended (see Table 32–4).

LSD often is sold as postage stamp–size papers impregnated with varying doses of LSD, from 50 µg to more than 300 µg. Doses of 20 µg can lead to psychological effects; doses of 100 µg cause hallucinogenic psychoactive manifestations within 1 to 2 hours. Clearing of symptoms begins in 10 to 12 hours, although symptoms of fatigue and tension can persist for an additional 24 hours.

Treatment

Specific therapy for the complications of hallucinogen use is nonpharmacologic and involves emotional reassurance and a calm supportive environment. No specific antagonists are clinically available for any of the hallucinogens. Medications are required only if the patient cannot be controlled adequately, in which case anxiolytic drugs are recommended.

Benzodiazepines and Other Sedatives

Benzodiazepines and the less commonly used barbiturates are legitimate therapeutic drugs with abuse potential. These drugs are designated schedule IV substances by the Drug Enforcement Agency and the Food and Drug Administration. Schedule IV drugs have a low potential for abuse and lead to limited physical or psychological dependence.

Nonmedical use of tranquilizers and sedatives occurs in less than 2% of U.S. adults annually; however, between 1992 and 2003, there was a 44% increase in abuse of prescription central nervous system depressants. The magnitude of the problem is substantially less than that of opioids, psychostimulants, and marijuana. This problem occurs largely in individuals who also abuse other substances. This finding is consistent with the experience in laboratory animals, which do not exhibit repeated self-administration, a standard measure of addictive potential, when they are exposed to benzodiazepines.

All benzodiazepines studied are capable of producing physiologic dependence even when they are used in low doses for prolonged periods as may be seen in clinical practice. The key to the diagnosis of benzodiazepine or other prescription drug abuse is evidence of inappropriate drug-taking behavior, including escalation in dose, obtaining prescriptions from multiple physicians, or taking the drug for reasons other than those for which it was prescribed. Before initiation of clinical use of benzodiazepines and other sedatives, a careful medical history must be obtained regarding current and prior substance abuse. Although benzodiazepines are not absolutely contraindicated in patients with such a history, particular caution and extra monitoring are appropriate with such individuals. Discontinuation of benzodiazepines can be accomplished in dependent patients by prescribing a regimen of gradual dose reduction. Alternatively, another long-acting sedative-hypnotic can be substituted for the drug of abuse and gradually withdrawn. It is important to attempt to verify that the patient has no alternative sources for these medications.

Other Drugs of Abuse

More recent drugs of abuse, such as 3,4-methylenedioxymethamphetamine (MDMA), γ-hydroxybutyrate (GHB), ketamine, phencyclidine (PCP), and anabolic steroids, are used in a variety of settings. The term *club drug* is inconsistently defined but may include any of the following substances: MDMA, GHB, ketamine, LSD, flunitrazepam (Rohypnol), and methamphetamine. When they are ingested in association with inadequate fluid intake, vigorous exercise, or a hot and humid environment, these drugs are particularly likely to cause complications. Inhalants, which are primarily used by children and teens, are found commonly in the household and can cause serious damage to major organs.

MDMA (Ecstasy)

MDMA, commonly referred to as ecstasy, is a synthetic analogue of amphetamine and shares properties with amphetamine and hallucinogenic drugs. It acts on the serotonin transporter, stimulating serotonin release and inhibiting its reuptake. Although it is usually taken in the pill form, MDMA can be snorted, injected, or administered per rectum. The purity of MDMA tablets may vary 70-fold, and tablets may include caffeine, heroin, or mescaline. Of high-school seniors, 7.5% report having used MDMA, 4% in the past year.

MDMA's clinical effects are predominantly sensory enhancement with distortion and decreased inhibitions. The onset of action is 30 to 60 minutes, the peak effects occur at 90 minutes, and the duration is 8 hours or more. Common adverse effects, which are similar to effects found with amphetamines and cocaine, include sweating, muscle spasms, involuntary teeth clenching, faintness, chills, and tachycardia. Psychological manifestations include confusion, depression, sleep problems, severe anxiety, and paranoia. High temperatures and muscle exertion from dancing seem to lower the threshold for serious MDMA-associated adverse effects, especially rhabdomyolysis; other reported adverse effects in the club setting include hyponatremia, dehydration, hypothermia, hypertensive crisis, and cardiac arrhythmias.

GHB

GHB, or liquid ecstasy, is a metabolite of the neurotransmitter γ-aminobutyric acid. It is thought to function as a neurotransmitter, producing a dopaminergic response and release of an endogenous opiate-like substance. Its half-life is approximately 30 minutes. GHB is used for its euphoric and anabolic effects. Behavioral changes include increased aggression, and neurologic changes range from mild ataxia to apnea. Withdrawal symptoms are similar to those of sedative abuse and persist for 3 to 7 days. There is no antidote for GHB overdoses, and treatment is limited to nonspecific supportive care.

Ketamine

Ketamine, commonly referred to as Special K, is a fast-acting intravenous or intramuscular anesthetic that delivers hypnotic, analgesic, and amnesic effects. Most of ketamine's activity is associated with *N*-methyl-D-aspartate receptors. Because it causes an intense dissociative state and loss of physical control, ketamine use is associated with a high risk of injuries. Ketamine usually is acquired from veterinary clinics.

PCP

PCP, also known as angel dust, originally was developed as an anesthetic in the 1950s but was abandoned because of frequent postoperative delirium and hallucinations. It can be obtained in various forms (powder, liquid, tablet, capsule, or sprayed on other drugs such as marijuana) and administered by several routes (smoked, ingested, snorted, or injected intravenously). The drug is water soluble and lipophilic, so it penetrates fat stores and has a long half-life, up to 3 days. A pronounced pharmacologic characteristic of PCP is its analgesia and amphetamine-like stimulation in addition to hallucination. Ataxia, slurred speech, nystagmus, and numbness commonly are observed at doses of 1 to 10 mg. Emotional withdrawal, catatonic posturing resembling schizophrenia, and physical violence can result from its use.

Methylphenidate

Methylphenidate (Ritalin), a central nervous system stimulant, is prescribed primarily for treatment of attention-deficit/hyperactivity disorder in children because of its paradoxical calming effect. About 5% of high-school seniors report using it in a nontherapeutic setting. Illicit users take the drug tablets orally, crush them for intranasal use, or dissolve and inject them.

Inhalants

Inhalants are toxic substances whose vapors create a psychoactive effect when inhaled. They are rarely if ever abused through any other route. Inhalants include volatile solvents (e.g., paint thinner), gases (e.g., butane, nitrous oxide), aerosols (e.g., hairspray), and nitrites (e.g., amyl, butyl), also known as poppers. Approximately 9% of eighth graders and 4% of high-school seniors abuse inhalants each year. These drugs are rapidly absorbed, producing a "quick high" lasting only a few minutes but that may be prolonged by repeated use during several hours. Inhalants, except nitrites, depress the central nervous system to produce short-term psychoactive alcohol-like effects. Nitrites increase the heartbeat and are often used to enhance sexual encounters. Chronic or prolonged exposure damages the brain, peripheral nervous system, heart, lungs, liver, and kidneys. Cognition, vision, and hearing can be affected. "Sudden sniffing death" can occur within minutes of repeated use, particularly with butane, propane, and aerosols.

Anabolic Steroids

Anabolic steroids are used to treat deficiencies in testosterone production and for body wasting due to AIDS and other diseases. These steroids enhance athletic performance or alter physical appearance. Approximately 2% of eighth graders and 3% of high-school seniors have used anabolic steroids in their lifetime. These drugs are taken orally or injected intravenously during a course of several weeks, then stopped and restarted at a later date (i.e., cycling). Side effects include liver damage, high blood pressure, increases in low-density lipoprotein cholesterol, decreases in high-density lipoprotein, kidney damage, acne, and aggression. Gender-specific side effects can also occur. Adolescents who abuse steroids may prematurely halt their growth.

Future Directions

With current understanding of the associated morbidities and costs of drug use and the increasing availability of medications for chronic treatment, increasing emphasis will be placed on the contributions that physicians can make in the care of patients with drug abuse and dependence. Opportunities exist to work with substance abuse providers to treat opioid-dependent patients in the primary medical care setting with pharmacologic therapy, including buprenorphine and methadone. Such future opportunities will increase the need for physicians to obtain skills to screen for drug abuse, to address use of illicit drugs, to treat related medical and mental health disorders, and to intervene to reduce the harm of these addictive behaviors.

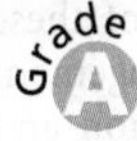

1. Weisner C, Mertens J, Parthasarathy S, et al: Integrating primary medical care with addiction treatment: A randomized controlled trial. JAMA 2001;286:1715–1723.
2. Johnson RE, Chutuape MA, Strain EC, et al: A comparison of levomethadyl acetate, buprenorphine, and methadone for opioid dependence. N Engl J Med 2000;343:1290–1297.

3. Fiellin DA, Pantalon MV, Chawarski MC, et al: Counseling plus buprenorphine-naloxone maintenance therapy for opioid dependence. N Engl J Med 2006;355:365–374.

SUGGESTED READINGS

Alford D, Compton P, Samet JH: Acute pain management for patients receiving maintenance methadone or buprenorphine therapy. Ann Intern Med 2006;144:127–134. *A perspective piece providing recommendations for treating acute pain in patients receiving methadone and buprenorphine.*

Cami J, Farre M: Drug addiction. N Engl J Med 2003;349:975–986. *A comprehensive review.*

Kosten TR, O'Connor PG: Management of drug and alcohol withdrawal. N Engl J Med 2003;348:1786–1795. *Overview of inpatient and outpatient options.*

Krantz MJ, Mehler PS: Treating opioid dependence: Growing implications for primary care. Arch Intern Med 2004;164:277–288. *An overview of two major approaches to treatment of opioid dependence—agonist maintenance and detoxification—and the role of the primary care provider.*

Volkow ND, Li TK: Drugs and alcohol: Treating and preventing abuse, addiction and their medical consequences. Pharmacol Ther 2005;108:3–17. *An overview of addiction research and the direction of future efforts by the Directors of the National Institute on Drug Abuse and the National Institute on Alcohol Abuse and Alcoholism.*

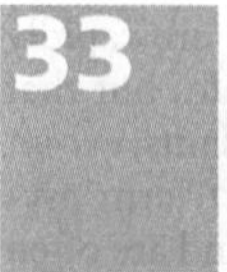

33 IMMUNOSUPPRESSING DRUGS INCLUDING CORTICOSTEROIDS

Grant W. Cannon

IMMUNOSUPPRESSIVE DRUGS

The immune response is an essential host defense mechanism to control and to fight infection. The ability to suppress immune reactions is a critical component in autoimmune disease treatment and transplantation management. During autoimmune diseases, the basic immune physiology is altered, and one or more components of this process do not function properly. Current challenges with the selection, dosing, monitoring, and development of immunosuppressing drugs involve identifying the component of the immune system to be altered by the immunosuppressive therapy while at the same time maintaining a competent immune response to fight infection. After organ transplantation, most patients have an immune response to reject the organ that has been implanted. Immunosuppression during transplantation management, in contrast to autoimmune disease, involves the suppression of normal immune reactions and not a pathologic process. Suppression of natural host immune responses must affect the ability of these protective mechanisms to fight infection. The general principles for selecting immunosuppressive therapy in transplantation patients involve specific monitoring of the organ rejection with subsequent selection of immunosuppressive therapy proportionate to the degree of rejection or for maintaining tolerance to the implanted organ. The selection of the most effective therapy requires an individualized treatment program. These decisions require an understanding of the underlying pathophysiologic process, prognosis, and potential adverse events for the agents selected.

This chapter describes the mechanism of action—including the components of the immune response affected by the therapy, indications, and adverse events associated with commonly used immunosuppressive agents in autoimmune diseases and transplantation. Whereas each of these agents has an individual discussion, these drugs are frequently used in combination as their complementary effects are employed. The understanding of the principles and adverse events associated with immunosuppressive therapy is important for all physicians as the use of these drugs becomes more widespread; however, their specific management and initiation, particularly in patients with organ transplantation and severe autoimmune diseases, should generally be limited to specialists with specific training in immunosuppressive therapies.

Corticosteroids

Corticosteroids are remarkable for their important action as anti-inflammatory and immunosuppressive agents. The development and understanding of corticosteroids throughout the 20th century and now into the new millennium have demonstrated the interplay of basic and clinical science in drug development. The lessons learned during this process have provided fundamental knowledge of the function of adrenal hormones, basic immunology, and clinical drug evaluations, particularly balancing risks with benefits in the selection and administration of immunosuppressive agents.

The adrenal extract cortisone was extracted in 1935, then synthesized in 1944 and named compound E. The initial enthusiasm for the marked clinical benefit of corticosteroids in the treatment of rheumatoid arthritis was dampened by the significant adverse events that developed after prolonged use. As opposed to many adverse events that may develop as allergic and idiosyncratic reactions to medications, the majority of adverse events with corticosteroid therapy are a direct action of the physiologic effects of the drug. This observation sparked a determined effort to understand the mechanisms of actions of corticosteroids at physiologic levels and therapeutic doses. The objectives of these investigations have been to develop modifications of the naturally occurring hormones to exploit the clinical benefits provided by corticosteroids while avoiding the associated adverse effects.

Mechanism of Action

Corticosteroids affect multiple physiologic functions at the molecular, cellular, and organ level. The final result of corticosteroid treatment represents the composite effects of the drug on these multiple functions, which vary with the particular agent, dose, route, and duration of treatment (Table 33–1).

Molecular Action

Genomic Effects

Corticosteroids are lipophilic and rapidly cross cell membranes into the cytosol, where they bind to the glucocorticoid receptor. The complex of glucocorticoid and its receptor then enters the nucleus and affects gene transcription by binding to glucocorticoid response elements. Depending on the specific gene, the complex may either stimulate or suppress gene transcription and subsequent protein production. This mechanism may have an impact on the function of 1% of all genes and suppresses the production of cytokines and other important inflammatory proteins. In addition to binding to glucocorticoid response elements, the glucocorticoid–glucocorticoid receptor complex also suppresses signal transduction pathways such as transcription factor activator protein 1 (AP-1), nuclear factor κB (NF-κB), and nuclear factor of activator of T cells (NF-AT). Corticosteroids may also act to affect post-transcription and post-translation steps of protein synthesis. Recent investigations have suggested that the anti-inflammatory actions of corticosteroids may be related to the action of these drugs on the NF-κB and AP-1 pathways; the adverse events produced are related more to the activation or suppression of gene transcription.

Nongenomic Effects

The genomic effects require the diffusion of the drug into the cell, binding to the receptor, entry into the nucleus, and alteration of transcription. The ultimate effect on protein synthesis is not immediate, and it generally takes at least 30 minutes before any response is seen. The observation that some actions of corticosteroids are seen immediately has directed a search for nongenomic effects of corticosteroids. The glucocorticoid–glucocorticoid receptor complex can inhibit arachidonic acid release. Recent data have suggested that in addition to the cytosol glucocorticoid receptor, a membrane-bound receptor may be present that may also mediate nongenomic functions.

Systemic Effects

Impact on Leukocytes

Corticosteroids have an impact on the activation, production, circulation, function, and survival of leukocytes. Whereas these impacts appear to be principally modulated by the genomic effects of corticosteroids on cytokines, corticosteroids also act on adhesion molecules and other mechanisms as well. The effects are seen on neutrophils, monocytes,

TABLE 33–1 CLASSIFICATION OF IMMUNOSUPPRESSIVE AGENTS

CORTICOSTEROIDS

Binding to cytosol glucocorticoid receptor: results in suppression of pro-inflammatory cytokines (genomic effects)
Inhibition of arachidonic acid release and binding to surface receptor (nongenomic effects)
Results of corticosteroid actions
- Leukocyte numbers
  - Increase in circulating neutrophils
  - Decrease in circulating lymphocytes, monocytes, eosinophils, and basophils
- Leukocyte function
  - Neutrophils: decrease in trafficking
  - Lymphocytes: decrease in cellular immune functions and immunoglobulin production
- Cytokines
  - Decrease in pro-inflammatory cytokines: IL-1, IL-2, IL-6, and tumor necrosis factor-α
  - Increase in anti-inflammatory cytokines: IL-4, IL-10, and IL-13
- Prostaglandins and leukotrienes: decreased production

PURINE PATHWAY INHIBITORS

Azathioprine: inhibition of DNA synthesis and purine synthesis
Mycophenolate mofetil: inhibition of purine synthesis

PYRIMIDINE PATHWAY INHIBITORS

Leflunomide: inhibits pyrimidine synthesis by inhibiting dihydroorotate dehydrogenase

IMMUNOPHILIN BINDING

Calcineurin inhibition
- Cyclosporine: binds with cyclophilin to inhibit calcineurin, resulting in decreased T-cell activation
- Tacrolimus: binds with FKBP12 to inhibit calcineurin, resulting in decreased T-cell activation

Mammalian target of rapamycin (mTOR) inhibition
- Sirolimus: binds to FKBP12 to inhibit mTOR, resulting in decreased T-cell activation

ALKYLATING AGENTS

Cyclophosphamide: alkylation of nucleic acids with cytotoxic action

FKBP12 = 12-kD FK-binding protein; IL = interleukin; mTOR = mammalian target of rapamycin.

macrophages, lymphocytes, eosinophils, and basophils. With corticosteroid therapy, neutrophils increase in the peripheral circulation, primarily because of demargination, in contrast to a decrease in monocytes, lymphocytes, eosinophils, and basophils. Although the number of circulating neutrophils may increase, trafficking appears to be impaired. The impact on T cells is more pronounced than the effects on B cells, with the induction of apoptosis particularly in immature and activated T cells. Although function of B cells and neutrophils is not affected as strongly as that of T cells, high-dose prolonged use of corticosteroids can lead to suppression of antibody production.

Changes in Inflammatory Mediators

Corticosteroids result in a decrease in multiple pro-inflammatory cytokines and interleukins (ILs). The cytokines affected include IL-1, IL-2, IL-6, and tumor necrosis factor-α at the same time that there is an increase in anti-inflammatory cytokines—IL-4, IL-10, and IL-13. Corticosteroids have been associated with a reduction in the production of prostaglandins, leukotrienes, and other arachidonic acid metabolites, probably related to the reduced production of cyclooxygenase-2 and phospholipase A_2–related pro-inflammatory compounds.

Treatment

Specific Issues with Corticosteroid Therapy

Multiple corticosteroid compounds and preparations are available. Many of the commonly employed compounds are listed in Table 33–2. These compounds have differences in potency, half-life, and sodium-retaining properties. In many conditions, the local administration of corticosteroids will provide clinical benefit without the systemic toxicity associated with oral therapy. Local therapies include topical, ophthalmic, inhaled, and local injection, such as soft tissue and intra-articular injections. Although the potential for adverse events is generally reduced with local therapy, local toxicities can develop as well as systemic effects if large doses of topical corticosteroids are used.

Whereas most conditions can be treated with local or oral corticosteroids, intravenous administration can provide pulse doses if desired. Pulse therapy is generally administered in high intravenous doses that are often given as divided treatments during 3 to 5 days. High-dose pulse therapy has particularly been advocated in acute organ transplantation rejection, severe systemic lupus erythematosus (SLE), aggressive vasculitis, and other acute and severe autoimmune disorders. The use of high-dose pulse corticosteroid therapy has been associated with the development of sudden cardiac arrhythmias and sudden death. Many of the patients described have had serious concurrent diseases that could in part be responsible for electrolyte abnormalities and other associated morbidities that could contribute to these observations. Despite the confusion about

TABLE 33–2 GLUCOCORTICOID PREPARATIONS

	Anti-inflammatory Potency	Equivalent Dose (mg)	Sodium-Retaining Potency	Plasma Half-life (min)	Biologic Half-life (hr)
Hydrocortisone	1	20	2+	90	8–12
Cortisone	0.8	25	2+	30	8–12
Prednisone	4	5	1+	60	12–36
Prednisolone	4	5	1+	200	12–36
Methylprednisolone	5	4	0	180	12–36
Triamcinolone	5	4	0	300	12–36
Betamethasone	20–30	0.6	0	100–300	36–54
Dexamethasone	20–30	0.75	0	100–300	36–54

From Garber EK, Targoff C, Paulus HE: Glucocorticoid preparations. *In* Paulus HE, Furst DE, Droomgoole SH (eds): Drugs for Rheumatic Diseases. New York, Churchill Livingstone, 1987, p 446.

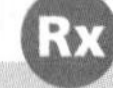

this association, close monitoring of patients receiving high-dose pulse corticosteroid therapy is warranted.

Indications

Corticosteroids are employed in a large range of autoimmune disorders and transplantation procedures. A listing of each indication for which corticosteroids have been employed and proven effective is beyond the scope of this chapter, but indications range from multiple rheumatologic disorders to transplantation and many other inflammatory conditions. For example, the demonstration that inflammation plays a significant role in reactive airway disease has dramatically increased the use of systemic and inhaled corticosteroids in asthma and chronic obstructive pulmonary disorders. The challenge is to determine the dose, route, and duration of therapy with these disorders. For severe autoimmune disorders, high doses of corticosteroids are employed. In many cases, oral administration of prednisone, 60 to 80 mg/day as single or divided doses, can be employed. If patients cannot take oral medication or high doses of corticosteroids are indicated, higher doses can be administered intravenously. Comparative data on the most appropriate doses and routes of administration are generally not available. Clinical judgment and empirical literature have formed the basis of these treatment regimens.

Adverse Effects

With most medications, adverse events are the results of allergic and frequently idiosyncratic reactions. The adverse events associated with corticosteroid use are generally caused by the physiologic action of these drugs. Investigations are ongoing to determine whether separate mechanisms might be more associated with the therapeutic benefits whereas other pathways are more involved in the adverse events of corticosteroids. Experimental compounds testing this hypothesis are in development with a hope to develop compounds with a higher benefit-to-risk ratio, but these agents are not yet available for therapeutic use. At the moment, currently available forms of corticosteroids do not selectively allow separation of the adverse events from the therapeutic effects. For example, the increase in infection associated with corticosteroids is the result of the impact of these drugs on leukocyte function and antibody production and is not an allergic reaction. The prevalence and severity of these adverse effects increase in proportion to the dose and duration of the therapy. The key to reducing adverse events with corticosteroids is to use the lowest needed dose and shortest possible duration for the required indication. Data also suggest that intermittent and every-other-day dosing may be associated with less toxicity than daily or divided daily doses.

Despite these limitations, corticosteroids are the only viable treatment option in many conditions, and efforts must be made to prevent, to detect development of, and to monitor for these adverse events. In most situations, education of the patient coupled with vigilant surveillance can detect these adverse events and often reduce their serious impact.

The following description of adverse events is not intended to be a comprehensive list of all reported adverse events associated with corticosteroids. The problems with infection, osteoporosis, metabolic abnormalities, and cardiovascular effects are highlighted because specific interventions can have an impact on these problems through proper education of the patient, monitoring, or prophylactic therapy. However, the most effective intervention is to limit the dose, duration, and frequency of administration of corticosteroids as much as possible.

Infections

Infections are increased in patients taking corticosteroids, particularly bacterial, fungal, and mycobacterial infections. These infections are representative of opportunistic infections that are seen much less frequently in healthy patients with normal immune function. The increased incidence and general severity of these infections are complicated by the anti-inflammatory actions of corticosteroids that can mask many of the cardinal signs of infection, such as fever, inflammation, and local discomfort. Patients taking corticosteroids should be alerted to the possibility of these "subclinical infections," and the provider must be vigilant in investigating signs and symptoms that may be less concerning in patients not taking corticosteroids. Management of infections in patients receiving corticosteroids requires close monitoring. Appropriate diagnostic procedures, antimicrobial therapy, and supportive measures are keys to successful management of infections in immunocompromised hosts. Patients with adrenal suppression may require "stress doses" of corticosteroids during the initial treatment. However, when possible, a reduction in corticosteroid dose may help restore a host immune response to the underlying infection, particularly with chronic infections.

Preventive measures that should be undertaken to reduce infections include proper immunizations. If possible, for example, in a patient being evaluated for future transplantation, immunizations should be given before the immunosuppressive therapy. In many cases, a delay of immunosuppressive therapy is not possible to allow immunizations to be updated. However, in patients receiving chronic immunosuppressive therapy, routine immunizations should be offered when the disease is stable. Prophylactic antibiotics are generally not recommended to prevent infections in patients receiving corticosteroid therapy. However, two notable exceptions are the use of antituberculosis therapy in purified protein derivative (PPD)-positive patients and trimethoprim-sulfamethoxazole therapy in patients receiving high-dose corticosteroid therapy for *Pneumocystis jirovecii* (previously named *Pneumocystis carinii*) prophylaxis.

Osteoporosis

Bone loss with corticosteroids affects multiple sites and has a greater impact on trabecular bone than on cortical bone. Common sites for involvement are the spine and femur with associated fracture rates that may be as high as 20%, depending on the duration and dose of therapy. On initiation of long-term corticosteroid therapy, all patients should be evaluated for osteoporosis prophylactic therapy. Unless it is contraindicated, patients should have adequate calcium and vitamin D through diet or supplements. In many patients, bisphosphonates will provide significant protection. Postmenopausal women should be evaluated for potential estrogen replacement therapy that may be helpful if benefits of therapy with corticosteroids are considered to outweigh the risks for cardiovascular disease and malignant disease. If osteoporosis develops in a patient receiving corticosteroids, efforts should be made to discontinue therapy or to reduce dose. Agents employed for treatment of osteoporosis should also be employed. An algorithm for prevention and treatment of glucocorticoid-induced osteoporosis is provided (Fig. 33–1).

Metabolic Effects

The metabolic effects of corticosteroids may affect glucose metabolism with results ranging from mild glucose intolerance to frank diabetes. Patients beginning corticosteroid therapy should be monitored for glucose intolerance and treated if significant hyperglycemia develops. The management of patients with existing diabetes is particularly challenging during corticosteroid therapy and requires close monitoring and adjustments of the diabetes management program.

Exogenous corticosteroids will suppress the hypothalamic-pituitary-adrenal (HPA) axis. The likelihood of adrenal suppression increases with dose and duration of therapy. HPA axis suppression should be considered in patients receiving doses of 20 mg/day or more for 3 weeks or longer, although suppression can occur with lower doses. Formal evaluations can be performed to test the integrity of the HPA axis, but in most cases a scheduled taper of corticosteroid dose during several weeks will allow the return of HPA axis function without signs of adrenal insufficiency. The ideal rate for tapering corticosteroids has not been evaluated by clinical trials. The rate in reduction in corticosteroid dose is often limited more by relapses of disease activity than by the development of adrenal insufficiency. In general, a rapid reduction in dose, as tolerated by the patient's clinical disease, can be undertaken until a dose reflecting the normal physiologic production of cortisol is achieved, about 10 mg prednisone-equivalent per day. After this point, reductions in dose of 1 to 2.5 mg/day every 1 to 2 weeks will generally be well tolerated and may be accomplished by decreasing the dose of alternate-day treatment during 6 to 8 weeks. However, with acute medical illness, patients who have received corticosteroid doses in the past sufficient to cause HPA suppression should receive stress doses of steroids for a period of up to 1 year after the steroid treatment. Other metabolic complications of corticosteroid treatment include weight gain with truncal obesity, electrolyte abnormalities including hypokalemia, and fluid retention.

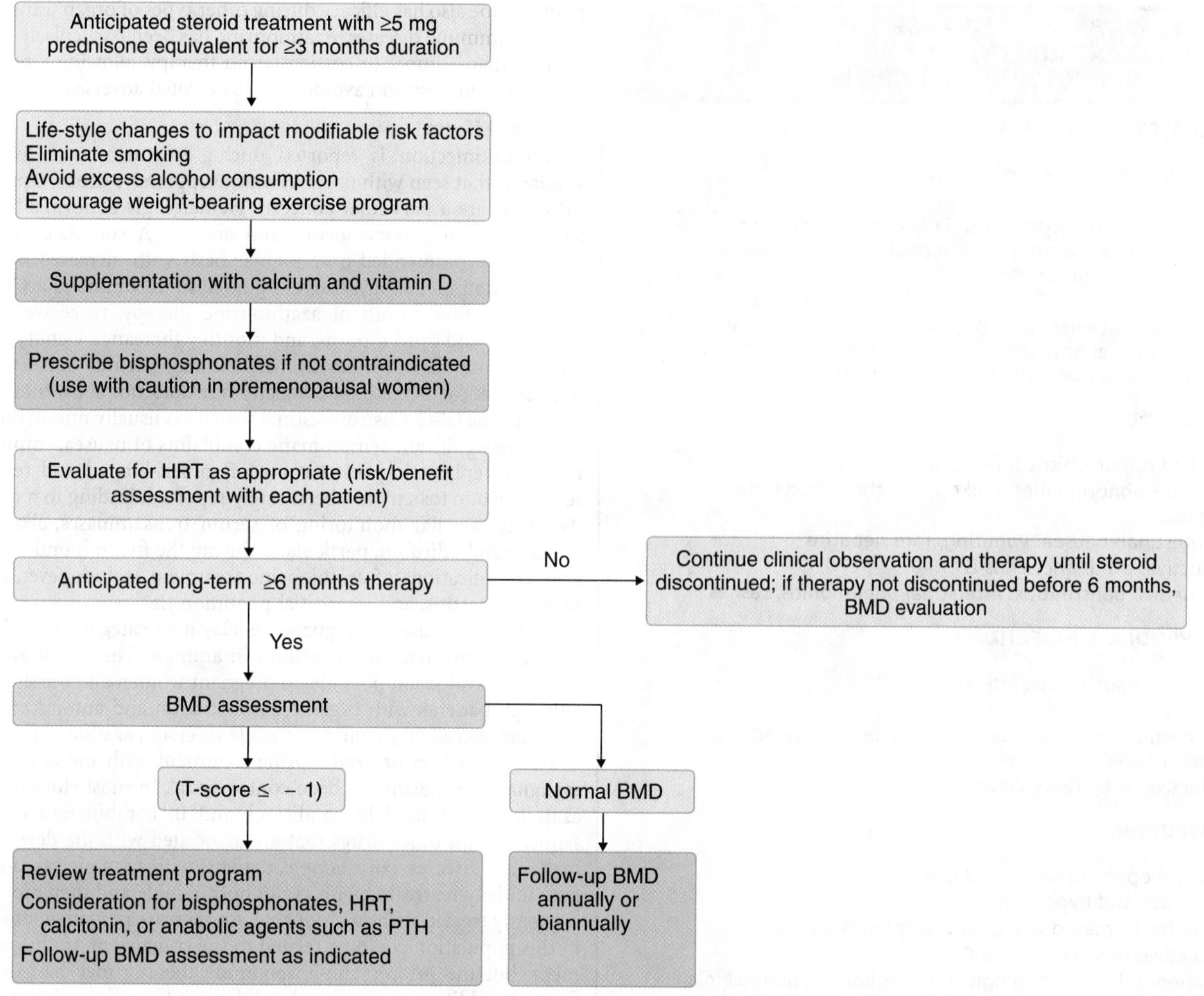

FIGURE 33–1 • Algorithm for prevention of steroid-induced osteoporosis on initiation of glucocorticoid therapy. BMD = bone mineral density; HRT = hormone replacement therapy; PTH = parathyroid hormone. (Modified from American College of Rheumatology Ad Hoc Committee on Glucocorticoid-Induced Osteoporosis: Recommendations for the prevention and treatment of glucocorticoid-induced osteoporosis. Arthritis Rheum 2001;44:1496–1503.)

Cardiovascular Effects

Corticosteroids may induce or exacerbate cardiovascular risk factors including hypertension, hyperlipidemia, and diabetes. Multiple mechanisms have been proposed for these effects, but the end result is that patients taking corticosteroids have an increased prevalence of atherosclerotic diseases and their associated complications. This problem is further complicated by the recent observation that many patients with inflammatory conditions including rheumatoid arthritis and SLE may have an increased risk for cardiovascular disease above that predicted by traditional risk factors. These observations have emphasized the need to monitor corticosteroid-treated patients closely for cardiovascular risk factors with aggressive treatment of detected abnormalities.

Other Adverse Effects

Many other adverse events have been noted with corticosteroid therapy and are listed in Table 33–3. Osteonecrosis (avascular necrosis) is common during corticosteroid therapy and particularly involves the femoral head. Peptic ulcer disease is increased independently of concurrent nonsteroidal anti-inflammatory therapy. Cataracts and a variety of dermatologic abnormalities are more common. Muscle weakness or steroid myopathy, alteration of mood and behavior, and psychosis may develop. This broad spectrum of clinical complications requires the prescriber of corticosteroids to be aware of and alert to the development of these adverse events.

Purine Inhibition

Purines are critical components of nucleic acids and are particularly important in proliferating cells as part of cell growth and division. The inhibition of purines by competitive inhibitors (azathioprine and 6-mercaptopurine) or blocking critical enzymes (mycophenolate mofetil) in the purine pathway is an effective method of immunosuppression.

Azathioprine and 6-Mercaptopurine

Mechanism of Action

Azathioprine is an inactive compound that is metabolized to the active compound 6-mercaptopurine (6-MP). The exact mechanisms of action of 6-MP and its metabolites have not been fully established. At high doses, 6-MP may be incorporated into RNA and DNA, resulting in a cytotoxic effect; however, this effect is probably not the major action of the drug at the doses generally employed. Most likely through feedback inhibition of de novo purine synthesis, 6-MP and its metabolites may reduce cell proliferation and thus produce immunosuppression. Genetically controlled differences in the activity of enzymes involved in the metabolism of 6-MP have been identified. The enzyme thiopurine *S*-methyltransferase is responsible for the metabolism of 6-MP to the metabolite methyl-6-MP. A rare homozygous (0.3%) and heterozygous (10%) defect in thiopurine *S*-methyltransferase is associated with increased toxicity with severe hematologic toxicity in the homozygous patients.

The drug is metabolized eventually by xanthine oxidase. Because xanthine oxidase is inhibited by allopurinol, the concurrent use of allopurinol and azathioprine or 6-MP can result in a significant reduction in the metabolism of the active compounds and a significant increase in drug toxicity. For this reason, the combination of allopurinol and azathioprine should be avoided.

Indications

Azathioprine is approved by the Food and Drug Administration (FDA) for prevention of rejection of renal transplantation and treatment of rheumatoid arthritis. Clinical trials and reports have suggested that

TABLE 33-3 MAJOR ADVERSE EVENTS ASSOCIATED WITH IMMUNOSUPPRESSIVE THERAPIES*

CORTICOSTEROIDS

Serious and opportunistic infections
Osteoporosis
Metabolic disorders: hyperglycemia, adrenal suppression, hyperlipidemia, electrolyte abnormalities, fluid retention, hypertension, truncal obesity
Cardiovascular
Miscellaneous: osteonecrosis, peptic ulcer disease, cataracts, dermatologic abnormalities, steroid myopathy, psychosis, growth retardation, altered mood and behavior

AZATHIOPRINE

Serious and opportunistic infections
Hematologic abnormalities: leukopenia, thrombocytopenia, anemia
Gastrointestinal: nausea, vomiting, rare hepatitis
Reproductive: pregnancy class D
Miscellaneous: pancreatitis, interstitial pneumonitis, rashes

MYCOPHENOLATE MOFETIL

Serious and opportunistic infections
Leukopenia
Gastrointestinal: diarrhea, nausea, dyspepsia, elevated transaminases
Reproductive: pregnancy class C

CYCLOSPORINE

Serious and opportunistic infections
Renal disease and hypertension
Potential for increased malignant neoplasms
Reproductive: pregnancy class C
Miscellaneous: hirsutism, gingival hyperplasia, hyperuricemia, electrolyte abnormalities

TACROLIMUS

Serious and opportunistic infections
Renal disease and hypertension, perhaps lower than with cyclosporine
Potential for increased malignant neoplasms
Post-transplantation diabetes mellitus
Neurotoxicity: tremor, headaches, motor function abnormalities, mental status alteration, sensory changes
Reproductive: pregnancy class C
Miscellaneous: hirsutism, gingival hyperplasia, myocardial hypertrophy

SIROLIMUS

Serious and opportunistic infections
Renal disease and hypertension
Potential for increased malignant neoplasms
Reproductive: pregnancy class C
Miscellaneous: hyperlipidemia, pneumonitis, interstitial lung disease

CYCLOPHOSPHAMIDE

Serious and opportunistic infections
Increased incidence of malignant neoplasms
Hematologic toxicity: leukopenia, thrombocytopenia, anemia
Reproductive: pregnancy class D, premature ovarian failure, oligospermia, fetal abnormalities
Urologic: hemorrhagic cystitis, bladder cancer
Miscellaneous: nausea, vomiting, diarrhea, pulmonary fibrosis

*This list is to highlight the most serious and common adverse events but does not include all reported adverse events with these agents.

azathioprine also has efficacy during other types of organ transplantation and autoimmune diseases. Azathioprine has been particularly effective at providing an adjunct to corticosteroid therapy, allowing a reduction in corticosteroid dose and avoiding the associated adverse events.

Adverse Effects

Serious infection is reported during treatment with azathioprine similar to that seen with other immunosuppressive drugs. Opportunistic infections are a particular concern. Hematologic abnormalities include leukopenia, thrombocytopenia, and anemia. A complete blood count (CBC) is recommended on a regular basis with increased frequency at the initiation of therapy. Current guidelines recommend a CBC weekly during the first month of azathioprine therapy, twice weekly during the second and third months, and monthly thereafter. Genotyping of the enzyme thiopurine *S*-methyltransferase may identify subjects with the highest risk for hematologic toxicity but does not substitute for monitoring of the CBC. Gastrointestinal toxicity is usually minor, but patients may have significant symptomatic complaints of nausea, vomiting, diarrhea, and epigastric pain that are often self-limited and reversible. A severe hepatic toxicity has been rarely reported, leading to a recommendation for regular monitoring of serum transaminases, alkaline phosphatase, and bilirubin, particularly during the first 6 months of therapy. Rare complications of azathioprine treatment include fever, arthralgia, rash, pancreatitis, and interstitial pneumonitis.

Azathioprine use in pregnancy is classified category D and has been associated with fetal abnormalities in animals. The use of azathioprine should be avoided, if possible, in pregnant women and nursing mothers, although patients with organ transplantation and autoimmune disease have had successful pregnancies while receiving azathioprine.

The association of azathioprine treatment with the development of malignant neoplasms has been controversial. In most clinical situations, azathioprine is used in conditions and in combination or temporal sequence with other drugs that are associated with the development of malignant diseases. For example, patients with systemic vasculitis or SLE may initially be treated with cyclophosphamide and then are often subsequently treated with azathioprine. An increase in malignant neoplasms in this population could be related to the concurrent azathioprine treatment, but the prior cyclophosphamide therapy may be a higher risk factor. In addition, patients with solid organ transplantation, another circumstance in which azathioprine is frequently employed, appear to have a higher rate of malignant neoplasms separate from the use of immunosuppressive drugs. Extensive efforts to identify an independent increased risk for malignant neoplasms with azathioprine have not produced consistent results. These results suggest that the risk for malignant transformation with azathioprine is very low if this risk exists at all.

Azathioprine is an important and effective therapy in organ transplantation and autoimmune disease. Often this drug is used in combination with other agents and as a corticosteroid-sparing drug. Surveillance for infection and monitoring for hematologic toxicity are important. Concurrent treatment with allopurinol should be avoided to prevent serious toxicity from an interaction of the two drugs.

Mycophenolate Mofetil

Mechanism of Action

Mycophenolate mofetil is a prodrug that is converted in vivo to the active compound mycophenolic acid. Mycophenolic acid acts through inhibition of the enzyme inosine monophosphate dehydrogenase, resulting in an increase in 6-thionosinic acid that is normally metabolized by this enzyme. The accumulation of 6-thionosinic acid works through a negative feedback loop to suppress the de novo synthesis of purines and associated DNA production. Although it is not a cytotoxic agent, the actions of mycophenolic acid are most pronounced on proliferating cells, such as lymphocytes, to reduce cell division and associated functions of these critical cells in the immune response.

Indications

Mycophenolate mofetil is approved by the FDA for the prevention of allograft rejection in renal, hepatic, and cardiac transplantation. In addition to these approved indications, mycophenolate mofetil has been evaluated in SLE, for which its principal use has been in patients with lupus nephritis, although the drug has been used for other manifestations. Current studies are seeking to determine whether this agent can replace cytotoxic agents, such as cyclophosphamide, in the treatment of SLE, particularly as initial and maintenance therapy for lupus nephritis. Limited use has been reported in other autoimmune diseases such as rheumatoid arthritis, vasculitis, and polymyositis.

Adverse Effects and Monitoring

Common adverse events with mycophenolate mofetil include hematologic and gastrointestinal complications. Leukopenia is reported in 20 to 35% of patients receiving this drug for organ transplantation; however, severe neutropenia is seen in only 2 to 3% of subjects. Patients receiving mycophenolate mofetil have a higher susceptibility to infections similar to that seen with other immunosuppressive agents but with a higher proportion of opportunistic infections. Diarrhea is a common symptom, as are nausea and dyspepsia. Abnormalities of liver enzymes are commonly noted and appear to be dose dependent. Rare complications include pulmonary fibrosis and malignant neoplasms. Mycophenolate mofetil is classified as category C by the FDA for use in pregnant women. Although the agent should be avoided in patients who are pregnant or not practicing adequate contraception, this drug appears to have less impact on the reproductive system than does cyclophosphamide. Patients with SLE having concerns with a potential severe impact of cyclophosphamide on reproductive organs might elect to use mycophenolate mofetil instead.

Monitoring of patients receiving mycophenolate mofetil should include a monthly CBC and hepatic enzyme activities. Clinical monitoring for gastrointestinal and infectious complications should be conducted during regular clinical follow-up.

Mycophenolate mofetil is an important and effective agent in the management of transplantation patients. Ongoing work is studying the role of this drug in other autoimmune diseases. It is hoped that mycophenolate mofetil can provide effective therapy for rheumatic and autoimmune disorders with less toxicity than is seen with currently available agents, with a particular potential for use in lupus nephritis.

Immunophilin-Binding Agents

The development of immunophilin inhibitors has significantly advanced organ transplantation. Each of these drugs, cyclosporine, tacrolimus (also known as FK506), and sirolimus (also known as rapamycin), has significant immunosuppressive activity on T cell–mediated functions. Whereas the mechanisms of action for each drug differ, they all have the common action of binding to a cytosolic protein specific to each agent. This binding results in a decrease in T-cell cytokine production and T-cell proliferation. These separate sites of action allow the use of these agents in combination in transplantation management. In addition, the differences in action and specific binding for each drug have resulted in unique profiles of adverse events.

Cyclosporine

Mechanism of Action

Cyclosporine acts by binding to the cytosolic protein cyclophilin to form a cyclosporine-cyclophilin complex. The cyclosporine-cyclophilin complex inhibits the enzyme calcineurin. Calcineurin is an enzyme involved in multiple T-cell functions and is of particular importance in enhancing the transcription of genes for pro-inflammatory cytokines. The use of cyclosporine inhibits the production of IL-2 with a resulting decrease in T-cell activation. Cyclosporine also inhibits the production of other cytokines including IL-3, IL-4, granulocyte-macrophage colony-simulating factor, tumor necrosis factor-α, and interferon-γ. The overall impact of these actions is to reduce immune function and inflammation.

Indications

The use of cyclosporine and other calcineurin inhibitors has revolutionized treatment after solid organ transplantation. The specific FDA-approved indications include renal, liver, and heart transplantation. Most often the drug is used in conjunction with other immunosuppressive agents including corticosteroids and azathioprine. The critical clinical challenge is to balance the potent immune suppressive effects of the drug against the adverse events produced by this agent, with particular attention to avoidance of infectious complications and monitoring for hypertension and renal toxicity. Because of these critical issues, prescribing information specifically limits this agent to physicians experienced with the use of immunosuppressive agents.

Oral cyclosporine is also approved for the treatment of rheumatoid arthritis as a disease-modifying anti-rheumatic drug (DMARD), either alone or in combination with methotrexate. Although it is effective in the treatment of rheumatoid arthritis and other rheumatic diseases, cyclosporine does not provide a substantially greater efficacy than the other DMARDs. Cyclosporine is also approved for the treatment of psoriasis. Because of the significant adverse event profile, cyclosporine is generally reserved for patients with autoimmune diseases whose therapy with more traditional and less toxic agents has failed.

Topical cyclosporine has been developed, proven effective, and approved for treatment to increase tear production presumed to be suppressed secondary to inflammation in patients with keratoconjunctivitis sicca syndrome. The topical treatment is associated with a much lower frequency of adverse drug events than is systemic cyclosporine therapy.

Adverse Effects

Close monitoring is required during cyclosporine therapy. Blood levels can be measured, which is useful in ensuring that the drug remains within a therapeutic range and below levels associated with increased toxicity. Because of multiple potential drug interactions that can both raise and lower cyclosporine levels as well as food interactions, particularly increased levels with grapefruit and grapefruit juices, patients should be constantly monitored and blood levels obtained when indicated. These evaluations should ensure that when medical therapy is added, changed, or deleted, these adjustments will not have an impact on the effects of the cyclosporine with its associated therapeutic and toxicity issues.

Infection

All infections have an increased potential for developing in patients receiving cyclosporine and other calcineurin inhibitors as with other immunosuppressive agents. Opportunistic infections associated with impaired cell-mediated immunity are particularly increased.

Renal Disease and Hypertension

Renal disease and hypertension are common adverse events during cyclosporine therapy and are increased in prevalence with increases in dose and duration of therapy. Close monitoring of blood pressure and serum creatinine concentration is critical during treatment with cyclosporine. In many cases, these conditions are reversible if they are detected early and appropriate dose adjustments are implemented. In many patients, a mild increase in serum creatinine concentration may be tolerated if the level remains stable. Although the mechanism of the renal disease and associated hypertension is not clearly defined, alteration in renal blood flow and thromboxane and endothelin levels has been suggested. Whereas renal abnormalities and hypertension are commonly identified during treatment of patients with cyclosporine, most patients will not require discontinuation of the drug if adjustments in dose or other interventions are undertaken to avoid these complications.

Malignant Neoplasia

Malignant neoplasms, particularly lymphomas, have been noted to be more common in patients receiving solid organ transplantation with associated immunosuppressive therapy. However, the exact cause of these malignant neoplasms has not been determined. In vitro mutagenesis assays with cyclosporine have been negative. In vivo animal studies have yielded equivocal results, with some data suggesting a possible increased rate of malignant neoplasms in rats and mice.

Issues with Reproduction

Cyclosporine is a pregnancy class C drug. Data in animals have demonstrated toxicity to both the embryo and fetus. Patients should practice effective contraception while receiving this drug. However, because some transplantation patients have become pregnant while taking cyclosporine and are also required to continue cyclosporine therapy throughout pregnancy, some data are available on the impact of cyclosporine in humans. However, these data are difficult to interpret because cyclosporine is generally not the only medical therapy received by these pregnant women and the impact of the disease associated with the organ transplantation is at times difficult to separate from the impact of therapy. Despite these limitations, normal pregnancies and early childhood development have been reported in many women receiving cyclosporine. Premature birth and low birthweight are more common in women receiving cyclosporine. These data suggest that although the use of cyclosporine during pregnancy and breast-feeding should be avoided if at all possible, in patients who become pregnant, an assessment should determine if the immunosuppressive therapy should be continued. In some cases, the risk of organ rejection with discontinuation of cyclosporine therapy may exceed the risk of exposure to the fetus during pregnancy.

Other Adverse Effects

Cyclosporine has also been associated with the development of hirsutism, gingival hyperplasia, hyperuricemia, and electrolyte abnormalities.

Tacrolimus

Mechanism of Action

Tacrolimus inhibits calcineurin through a mechanism different from that of cyclosporine. Whereas cyclosporine binds to cyclophilin, tacrolimus binds to a different protein, the 12-kD FK-binding protein (FKBP12). The binding of FKBP12 and tacrolimus forms a complex that inhibits calcineurin in a fashion similar to cyclosporine. Through this mechanism, tacrolimus has similar inhibitory effects on T-cell function and cytokine production.

Indications

Tacrolimus is approved for the prophylactic treatment of organ rejection after kidney and liver transplantation. Although there are data to support efficacy of this agent in other conditions, formal FDA approval has not been received. The efficacy and safety in rheumatoid arthritis is limited but encouraging. Experience with this agent is less extensive than the experience with cyclosporine.

Adverse Effects

The major adverse events with tacrolimus are similar to those of cyclosporine and include increased susceptibility to infection, renal disease, and hypertension. An increase in malignant neoplasia is also reported with a pattern similar to that reported in patients receiving cyclosporine.

Whereas many adverse events with tacrolimus are similar to those of other calcineurin inhibitors, some specific complications have been reported, including the development of post-transplantation diabetes mellitus. The development of post-transplantation diabetes mellitus was seen in 20% of subjects in phase III clinical trials of tacrolimus with an onset generally within the first 3 months of therapy. In many patients, post-transplantation diabetes mellitus will resolve after the drug is discontinued. Neurotoxicity is also reported; tremor, headache, motor function abnormalities, mental status alterations, and sensory changes are noted. Myocardial hypertrophy has been reported. Tacrolimus, like cyclosporine, is pregnancy class C. Patients receiving this drug should practice effective contraception.

Sirolimus

Mechanism of Action

Sirolimus (or rapamycin) in not a calcineurin inhibitor but has many actions and mechanisms similar to calcineurin inhibitors. The mechanism of action of sirolimus involves binding to FKBP12, the binding protein for tacrolimus, but the impact of this binding is different. Instead of acting on calcineurin, the sirolimus-FKBP12 complex binds to another protein, the mammalian target of rapamycin (mTOR), which is a key regulatory kinase. The inhibition of mTOR results in significant immunosuppression by decreasing T-cell proliferation and the progression from G_1 phase to S phase in the cell cycle. Because sirolimus works through a mechanism different from the mechanism of action for cyclosporine, the two drugs have been studied in combination. In renal transplantation patients, the use of these two agents in combination has a greater immunosuppressive effect than that of cyclosporine alone.

Indications

Sirolimus is approved for the prophylaxis of organ rejection in renal transplantation in combination with cyclosporine and corticosteroids for patients older than 12 years. The use in pediatric populations has not been sufficiently studied to allow extension of this drug to younger groups. Data with the use sirolimus in other populations, including subjects with autoimmune diseases, are limited and generally are derived only from animal models.

Adverse Effects

The adverse event profile for infection and malignant neoplasms with sirolimus is similar to that with calcineurin inhibitors. Renal disease with cyclosporine and sirolimus in combination has been reported more frequently than in patients receiving cyclosporine alone. Adverse reactions specific for sirolimus include hyperlipidemia, interstitial lung disease, and the syndrome of calcineurin-induced hemolytic-uremic syndrome, thrombotic thrombocytopenic purpura, and thrombotic microangiopathy.

Alkylating Agents

Alkylating agents are an important component of immunosuppressive therapy in autoimmune diseases. The use of these agents is limited by their associated toxicity, particularly the potential for development of malignant neoplasia, reproductive toxicity, and increased incidence of infection. Patients considered candidates for alkylating therapy should be fully informed of the potential risks and benefits of these drugs and concur with the decision for their use. Regular monitoring of the CBC and urinalysis are important in observing patients receiving these drugs.

Cyclophosphamide

Cyclophosphamide has been used primarily as a cytotoxic drug for the treatment of malignant neoplasms; it is currently approved for this indication as well as for biopsy-proven minimal change nephrotic disease in children. Several severe autoimmune diseases have also been shown to be responsive to cyclophosphamide often given in conjunction with initial high-dose corticosteroid therapy. Because of the significant toxicities associated with these drugs, a benefit-to-risk assessment and discussion should be undertaken with each patient as cyclophosphamide use is being considered. In most cases, the diseases warranting cyclophosphamide therapy will be life-threatening conditions with poor prognosis. In these cases, the severity of toxicity with cyclophosphamide may be justified.

Mechanism of Action

Cyclophosphamide is an inactive compound that can be administered either orally or intravenously and is metabolized to the active drug by the cytochrome P-450 mixed function oxidase system. This process produces the active compounds phosphoramide mustard and the toxic metabolite acrolein. The cytotoxic effect of this drug results from the alkylation of various cellular constituents, especially nucleic acids. In vitro and in vivo studies have demonstrated changes in immune function with cyclophosphamide. These changes include depletion of lymphoid tissues, with decreases in both B and T cells, suppression of cellular immune function, and decreased antibody production.

Indications

Treatment of lupus nephritis and severe systemic vasculitis is the most well studied and common use of cyclophosphamide in the rheumatic diseases. Controlled clinical trials have demonstrated improved outcomes in these conditions, particularly with reduced progression to end-stage renal disease in patients with SLE and improved survival with systemic vasculitis such as Wegener's granulomatosis. The evaluation of cyclophosphamide in patients with SLE has demonstrated the benefit of intermittent, usually monthly, intravenous pulse therapy as a method to avoid some of the most severe toxic side effects while maintaining therapeutic efficacy. However, pulse intravenous cyclophosphamide has not been found to be equally effective to continuous oral cyclophosphamide in all conditions, particularly Wegener's granulomatosis. With these favorable results, cyclophosphamide has been evaluated in multiple other conditions, such as polyarteritis nodosa, Takayasu's arteritis, and Churg-Strauss syndrome. These relatively rare conditions have been reported to benefit from cyclophosphamide; however, the low prevalence of these diseases has prohibited the conduct of controlled clinical trials to prove efficacy. Cyclophosphamide has also been demonstrated to be effective in the treatment of patients with rheumatoid arthritis, but it is generally not used in this condition because of the associated toxicity and availability of other effective agents.

Adverse Effects

Before the initiation of cyclophosphamide therapy, a frank discussion with the patient about potential serious and even life-threatening adverse events should be undertaken and documented. Patients should understand and be willing to accept these risks before therapy is initiated.

MALIGNANT NEOPLASIA. Malignant neoplasms may develop in patients receiving cyclophosphamide for the treatment of both malignant and nonmalignant diseases. The risk for malignant change appears to increase with the duration and dose of cyclophosphamide. The most common malignant neoplasms are bladder, myeloproliferative, and lymphoproliferative disorders. The use of intravenous pulse cyclophosphamide may reduce but not eliminate the risk of bladder malignant neoplasms. These malignant neoplasms may develop years after the discontinuation of the drug.

REPRODUCTIVE ISSUES. Cyclophosphamide can be teratogenic, affect female reproduction, and reduce male fertility. Cyclophosphamide is pregnancy category D and should not be used in pregnant women unless life-threatening disease is present that warrants this treatment. Whereas successful pregnancies have been reported in patients receiving cyclophosphamide during pregnancy, fetal abnormalities are well documented secondary to chromosome damage in patients receiving cyclophosphamide. The use of cyclophosphamide in premenopausal women can induce premature ovarian failure. The use of gonadotropin-releasing hormone analogues during intravenous pulse cyclophosphamide therapy may reduce premature ovarian failure in patients with SLE; however, the risk of this complication is still present. In males, temporary and permanent decrease in sperm count may occur with cyclophosphamide. Because the recovery of fertility after cyclophosphamide is variable, sperm banking should be considered before therapy is begun.

OTHER ADVERSE EFFECTS. As with other immunosuppressive agents, infections are more frequent and potentially more serious in patients receiving cyclophosphamide. Opportunistic infections are more likely to be seen in these subjects. Hematologic abnormalities can involve all cell lines and represent the directed cytotoxic activity of this drug. The CBC should be monitored regularly and cyclophosphamide discontinued or the dose reduced when cytopenias develop. Cyclophosphamide treatment may be complicated by hemorrhagic cystitis and bladder cancer, which are probably related to the toxic metabolite acrolein. Efforts to reduce the potential for hemorrhagic cystitis and bladder malignant neoplasms include the use of intravenous pulse therapy, hydration, frequent voiding, and treatment with agents containing sulfhydryl groups to scavenge acrolein. Regular urinalysis for blood is indicated to monitor for bladder toxicity. Patients may develop severe nausea, vomiting, and diarrhea with cyclophosphamide therapy.

Chlorambucil

Chlorambucil is another alkylating agent used in immunosuppressive therapy. Chlorambucil has not been evaluated as extensively as cyclophosphamide, but this agent appears to have properties and an adverse event profile similar to those of cyclophosphamide. Like cyclophosphamide, chlorambucil is associated with the development of malignant neoplasms and should be avoided during pregnancy.

Miscellaneous Agents

Other Small Molecules

Although principally prescribed for other indications, methotrexate and leflunomide have been evaluated and used for their potential immunosuppressive effects. Leflunomide blocks the enzyme dihydroorotate dehydrogenase, resulting in an inhibition of pyrimidine synthesis and a reduction in T-cell activation. Methotrexate has multiple mechanisms of action, but its major effect in autoimmune diseases is mediated by inhibition of the enzyme aminoimidazole-4-carboxamide ribonucleotide transformylase. This inhibition affects purine synthesis, increasing the intracellular concentration of aminoimidazole-4-carboxamide ribonucleotide, which stimulates the release of adenosine, a potent anti-inflammatory compound. Methotrexate has principally been advocated for its corticosteroid-sparing effects. Both methotrexate and leflunomide are effective DMARDs in the treatment of rheumatoid arthritis.

Biologic Agents

Biologic agents have been used to treat autoimmune diseases and to provide immunosuppression during transplantation. Initially, polyclonal antibodies have been used. These agents have included antithymocyte globulin in transplantation patients and intravenous immune globulin for immune thrombocytopenia. More recently, monoclonal antibodies and genetically designed molecules for targeted therapy have been employed. These agents include anti-CD3 and anti–IL-2 receptor antibodies (daclizumab and basiliximab) and costimulator molecule blockade (belatacept). The development of these agents has demonstrated that understanding of transplantation biology can direct the development of targeted therapy in these disorders. Inhibitors of tumor necrosis factor (etanercept, infliximab, and adalimumab) have been proved effective DMARDs in the treatment of rheumatoid arthritis. B cell–depleting antibody therapy (rituximab) is being evaluated in organ transplantation, rheumatoid arthritis, and other autoimmune diseases.

SUGGESTED READINGS

Buttgereit F, Burmester GR, Lipworth BJ: Optimised glucocorticoid therapy: The sharpening of an old spear. Lancet 2005;365:801–803. *A practical approach.*

Halloran PF: Immunosuppressive drugs for kidney transplantation. N Engl J Med 2004;351:2715–2729. *A detailed review.*

Rhen T, Cidlowski JA: Antiinflammatory action of glucocorticoids—new mechanisms for old drugs. N Engl J Med 2005;353:1711–1723. *A comprehensive overview.*

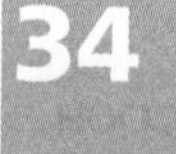

34 PROSTAGLANDINS, ASPIRIN, AND RELATED COMPOUNDS

Garret A. FitzGerald

Arachidonic acid is an unsaturated fatty acid that contains 20 carbon atoms and 4 double bonds ($\Delta^{5,8,11,14}$ $C_{20:4}$). It circulates in plasma in free and esterified forms and is a natural constituent of the phospholipid domain of cell membranes, bound to the glycerol backbone in the *sn*-2 position. Arachidonic acid is mobilized for release from the membrane by the action of various phospholipases A_2, particularly a type IV cytosolic phospholipase A_2 that has high affinity for arachidonic acid as a substrate. Diverse stimuli, including physical perturbation and hormones, mediate a calcium-dependent translocation of cytosolic phospholipase A_2 to the nuclear membrane and the endoplasmic reticulum, where it catalyzes the release of arachidonic acid. The lipid substrate is subject to metabolism by three major groups of enzymes: prostaglandin G/H synthase, which catalyzes the formation of prostaglandins; lipoxygenases, which result in the formation of leukotrienes; and cytochrome P-450 isozymes, which generate epoxyeicosatrienoic acids. Collectively, these products are known as eicosanoids, derived from the Greek εικφσι for the 20 carbons. Isoeicosanoids are free radical–catalyzed isomers of prostaglandins, leukotrienes, and epoxyeicosatrienoic acids formed by direct peroxidation of arachidonic acid in situ in cell membranes.

PROSTAGLANDINS AND THE CYCLOOXYGENASE PATHWAY

The best-known products of arachidonic acid are the prostaglandins, formed by the action of prostaglandin G/H synthase on arachidonic acid to form bisenoic products containing two double bonds, denoted by a subscript 2, such as prostaglandin E_2. Prostaglandin G/H synthase catalyzes the formation of monoenoic (Δ^{13}) prostaglandins (e.g., prostaglandin E_1) from eicosatrienoic acid ($C_{20:3}$; *n*-6) and of trienoic ($\Delta^{5,13,17}$) prostaglandins (e.g., prostaglandin E_3) from eicosapentaenoic acid ($C_{20:5}$; *n*-3), which is prevalent in fatty fish.

Prostaglandin G/H synthase is expressed as a dimer, homotypically inserted into the endoplasmic reticulum membrane. Prostaglandin G/H synthase contains cyclooxygenase (COX) and hydroperoxidase activities, sequentially catalyzing the transformation of arachidonic acid into the unstable cyclic endoperoxides prostaglandin G_2 and prostaglandin H_2 (Fig. 34–1). Prostaglandin H_2 is delivered to downstream isomerases and synthases that are expressed in a cell-specific manner and that generate evanescent products, the prostaglandins. It is presently not understood how arachidonic acid is delivered specifically to prostaglandin G/H synthase (colloquially known as COX) or how prostaglandin H_2 is presented to downstream enzymes. Prostaglandins activate G protein–coupled membrane receptors. Two COX genes have been identified: *COX1* is expressed constitutively in most cells; *COX2* is upregulated by cytokines, shear stress, and tumor promoters. These observations suggest that *COX1* accounts for prostaglandin formation that subserves housekeeping functions, such as gastric epithelial cytoprotection and hemostasis (see later), whereas *COX2* is the dominant source of prostaglandin formation in inflammation and cancer. Both isozymes are subject to developmental regulation, however, and both may contribute to prostaglandin forma-

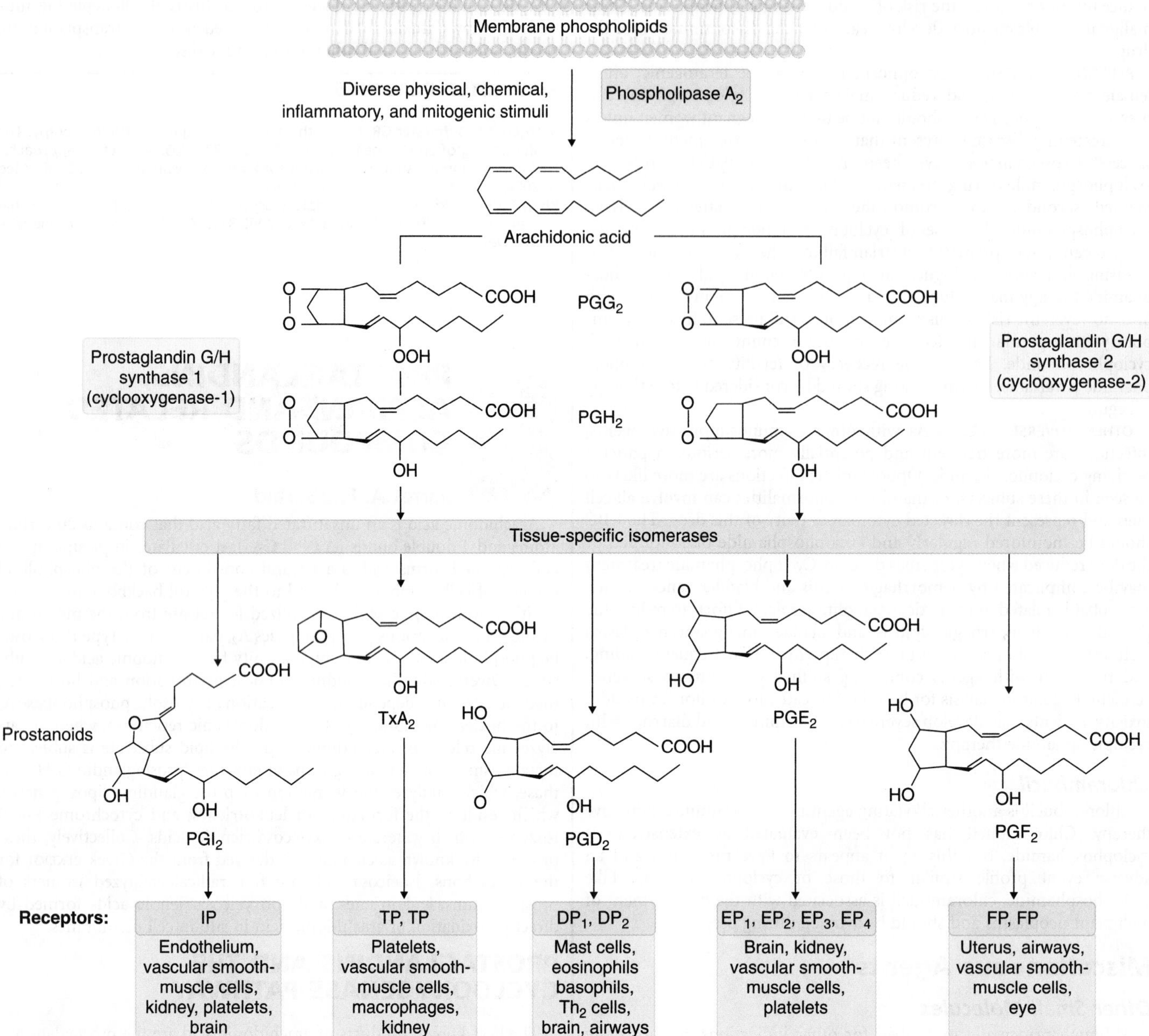

FIGURE 34–1 • Production and actions of prostaglandins and thromboxane. Arachidonic acid, a 20-carbon fatty acid containing four double bonds, is liberated from the *sn*-2 position in membrane phospholipids by phospholipase A_2, which is activated by diverse stimuli. Arachidonic acid is converted by cytosolic prostaglandin G/H synthases, which have cyclooxygenase and hydroperoxidase activities, to the unstable intermediate prostaglandin H_2 (PGH_2). The synthases are colloquially termed cyclooxygenases and exist in two forms, cyclooxygenase-1 and cyclooxygenase-2. Coxibs selectively inhibit cyclooxygenase-2. Prostaglandin H_2 is converted by tissue-specific isomerases to multiple prostanoids. These bioactive lipids activate specific cell membrane receptors of the superfamily of G protein–coupled receptors. Some of the tissues in which individual prostanoids exert prominent effects are indicated. DP = prostaglandin D_2 receptor; EP = prostaglandin E_2 receptor; FP = prostaglandin $F_{2\alpha}$ receptor; IP = prostacyclin receptor; TP = thromboxane receptor. (Modified from FitzGerald GA, Patrono C: The coxibs, selective inhibitors of cyclooxygenase-2. N Engl J Med 2001;345:433–442.)

tion in human inflammation; they are coexpressed in human atherosclerotic plaque and in synovial tissue in patients with rheumatoid arthritis. There is some evidence suggesting that *COX1* and *COX2* may heterodimerize with unknown consequences in terms of product formation or sensitivity to pharmacologic inhibitors. A splice variant of *COX1* termed *COX3* appears not to contribute significantly to prostaglandin formation in humans.

Deletion of *COX2* results in multiple defects of implantation and reproduction; it is difficult for these animals to breed. Offspring variably have had cardiac fibrosis, renal defects, and impairment of inflammatory responses. The expression of these phenotypes is modulated by genetic background. *COX1* deletion has been reported to impair certain inflammatory responses. Deletion of the *COX2* gene results in an increased frequency of patent ductus arteriosus. Although *COX1* deletion alone does not result in patent ductus arteriosus, coincidental deletion of *COX1* increases the frequency of the *COX2* knockout patent ductus arteriosus phenotype. Uses of COX knockouts and isozyme-specific inhibitors suggest that *COX1* and *COX2* are expressed in a spatially segregated manner at different times during thymic development and that they influence T-cell maturation. Deletion of one isozyme seems to have a variable, tissue-dependent impact on expression of the other.

COX-1 and COX-2 have been crystallized and bear a remarkable similarity at the atomic level (Fig. 34–2). One difference is a more accommodating hydrophobic tunnel for substrate access to the COX catalytic site in COX-2, reflected by a broader range of substrate specificity for this isozyme. Another is the existence of a side pocket in the hydrophobic channel of COX-2, which has afforded the structural basis for the development of selective inhibitors of this isozyme. Although immunogold studies suggest a similar subcellular distribution of both isoenzymes, each exhibits a preference for coupling with different downstream enzymes in heterologous expression systems and, apparently, in vivo. COX-1 preferentially couples with thromboxane synthase and prostaglandin F

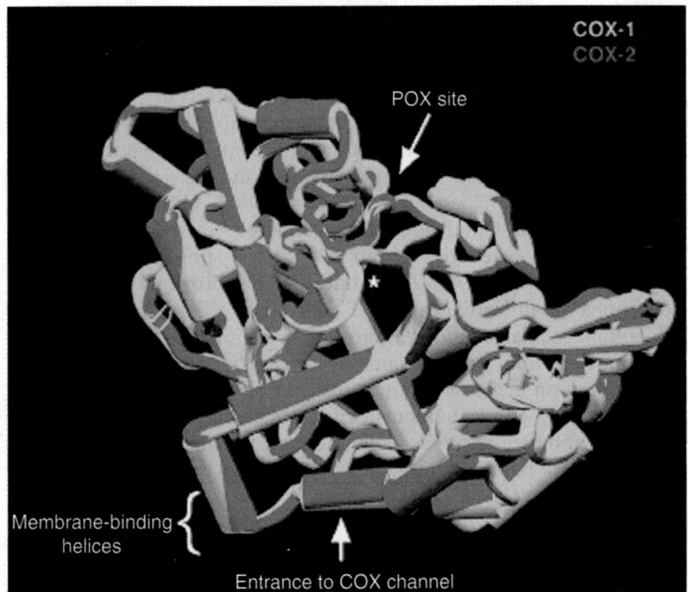

FIGURE 34–2 • The cyclooxygenase-1 (COX-1) and COX-2 backbones, overlaid. COX-1 is shown in yellow, and COX-2 is shown in red. The two structures are almost perfectly superimposable. The amphipathic helices that form the site of monotropic membrane attachment are indicated. The peroxidase (POX) active site lies on the side of the molecule opposite from the entrance to the COX active site channel. The actual position of the COX active center is marked by the asterisk, found near the center of the molecule. (From FitzGerald GA, Loll P: COX in a crystal ball: Current status and future promise of prostaglandin research. J Clin Invest 2001;107:1335–1337.)

synthase, whereas COX-2 prefers prostaglandin I synthase. Two classes of prostaglandin E synthases have been cloned. One is a family of microsomal prostaglandin E synthase (mPGES) isoenzymes that belong to the MAPEG (membrane-associated proteins in eicosanoid and glutathione metabolism) superfamily; these colocalize with COX-2 in several systems (but with both COXs in others) and are induced by cytokines and tumor promoters. A second is a family of cytosolic prostaglandin E synthase isozymes that colocalize with COX-1 and seem to favor this isozyme in heterologous coexpression systems. Deletion of mPGES-1 restrains the inflammatory response to a degree similar to traditional nonsteroidal anti-inflammatory drugs (NSAIDs) in mice and appears not to elevate blood pressure or to predispose to thrombosis in mice, at least on certain genetic backgrounds. This may reflect augmented prostaglandin I_2 formation due to prostaglandin H_2 substrate rediversion from biosynthesis of prostaglandin E_2. Deletion of mPGES-1 retards atherogenesis in hyperlipidemic mice. Two forms of prostaglandin D synthase and prostaglandin F synthase also have been identified. It seems likely that understanding of the diversity, function, and localization of the isomerases and synthases will expand dramatically in the near future.

Because of their short half-lives (seconds to minutes), prostaglandins act as autacoids rather than as circulating hormones. They activate membrane receptors at or close to the site of their formation, perhaps following their export by dodecahelical transporters. Specific heptahelical receptors have been cloned for all of the prostaglandins (see Fig. 34–1). Single receptors have been identified for prostacyclin/prostaglandin I_2 (the I prostanoid receptor), prostaglandin $F_{2\alpha}$ (the F prostanoid receptor), and thromboxane A_2 (the T prostanoid receptor). Four receptors have been cloned for prostaglandin E_2 (the E prostanoid receptors 1 through 4) and two for prostaglandin D_2 (D prostanoid receptor 1 and D prostanoid receptor 2). All except for D prostanoid receptor 2 seem to derive from an ancestral E prostanoid receptor and share high homology. The D prostanoid receptor 2, by contrast, is unrelated to the others and belongs to the *N*-formyl-Met-Leu-Phe receptor superfamily. It seems likely that other prostaglandin receptors will emerge. There is pharmacologic evidence for two functionally distinct forms of the T prostanoid receptor; however, this distinction is not attributable to the two carboxy-terminal variants of the cloned receptor (T prostanoid receptor α and T prostanoid receptor β) that presently have been identified. Receptor deletion studies in mice revealed the diversity of prostaglandin function in mammals.

Thromboxane A_2

Thromboxane A_2 is the major product of COX-1, the only isoform expressed in mature human platelets. Both COX isoforms have been identified in developing megakaryocytes. COX-2 is detectable in immature platelets released into the circulation in syndromes of accelerated platelet turnover. Its contribution to platelet thromboxane formation even under such circumstances seems trivial, however. Thromboxane A_2 is a potent vasoconstrictor and induces platelet activation in vitro. Deletion of the T prostanoid receptor reveals a mild hemostatic defect and resistance to arachidonic acid–induced platelet activation. Despite the diversity of platelet agonists, inhibition of platelet thromboxane formation is sufficient to account for cardioprotection from aspirin (see later). This finding may reflect the importance of thromboxane A_2 as an amplification signal for continuing the process of platelet aggregation induced by more potent agonists, such as thrombin and adenosine diphosphate. Thromboxane A_2 is also a major product of macrophage COX-2. Whereas platelet COX-1 is the major source, COX-2, probably in macrophages, also contributes to the increment in thromboxane A_2 biosynthesis in cigarette smokers. Elevated urinary thromboxane metabolites in chronic smokers fall rapidly on quitting. Deletion or antagonism of the T prostanoid receptor retards initiation and early development of atherogenesis and also modulates the proliferative response to vascular injury in mice. Overexpression of the T prostanoid receptor in vascular tissues results in a syndrome reminiscent of intrauterine growth retardation, probably secondary to placental ischemia.

Two forms of the T prostanoid receptor have been segregated pharmacologically: one mediating platelet shape change, the other mediating aggregation. The cloned splice variants do not seem to account for this distinction, however, and only T prostanoid receptor α is expressed in platelets. Activation of T prostanoid receptor β antagonizes the pro-angiogenic effects of fibroblast growth factor 2 by impairing ligand-induced internalization of its receptor. T prostanoid receptor activation also restrains angiogenesis induced by vascular endothelial cell growth factor. The only other differences that have emerged between the splice variants to date have related to affinity for coupling with downstream guanosine triphosphate–binding proteins (G proteins) and the rate of agonist-induced desensitization.

The cloned T prostanoid receptor isoforms couple via G_q, $G_{12/13}$, and G_h (which is also tissue transglutaminase II) to activate phospholipase C–dependent inositol phosphate generation and an elevation in intracellular calcium. Activation of the T prostanoid receptor also may inhibit adenylate cyclase via G_i and signal via G_q and related proteins to membrane-associated protein kinase signaling pathways. Analogous to its role in vascular proliferation, T prostanoid receptor activation also may mediate hypertrophy of myometrial cells and cardiomyocytes. The T prostanoid receptor is expressed abundantly in the thymus, but its role in lymphocyte development and function is presently unclear. A naturally occurring mutation in the first intracellular loop of the T prostanoid receptor has been associated with a mild bleeding diathesis and resistance to platelet aggregability by T prostanoid receptor agonists. Polymorphisms in the T prostanoid receptor have been linked to bronchodilator resistance in both allergic and aspirin-sensitive asthma.

Prostacyclin (Prostaglandin I_2)

Prostaglandin I_2 (PGI_2), the major product of COX-2 in healthy individuals and in mice, is a potent inhibitor of platelet aggregation induced by all recognized agonists and a vasodilator. Mice deficient in the I prostanoid receptor have an exaggerated response to hypertensive stimuli, such as dietary salt. Coincident deletion of the T prostanoid receptor protects these mice from the consequent myocardial injury without lowering blood pressure. Similarly, findings in I prostanoid receptor–deficient mice have implicated PGI_2 in the mediation of pain and inflammation. Both these effects and the hypertensive phenotype are conditioned by genetic background. Platelets of I prostanoid receptor knockout mice reveal resistance to disaggregation by I prostanoid receptor agonists. Deletion of this receptor augments the response to thrombogenic stimuli and fosters the initiation and early development of atherogenesis in genetically prone mice by increasing platelet and neutrophil interactions with the vasculature and the attendant oxidant stress. Estrogen acts through its ER-α receptor to upregulate COX-2–dependent PGI_2 formation, which in turn upregulates the antioxidant enzyme heme oxygenase 1. Deletion of the I prostanoid receptor undermines considerably the atheroprotection afforded by exogenous estrogen in ovariectomized hyperlipidemic mice. I prostanoid–deficient mice also exhibit an enhanced proliferative response to vascular injury and perturbed vascular remodeling in response to alterations in blood flow. Biosynthesis of PGI_2 is increased in syndromes of platelet activation, such as severe atherosclerosis and unstable angina (Chapters 69 and 71), perhaps as a homeostatic response to accelerated platelet vascular interactions.

Prostaglandin I synthase appears uniquely sensitive among the arachidonic acid biosynthetic enzymes to nitrative inactivation. Prostaglandin I synthase gene transfer diminishes the response to vascular injury in rodents and the response to thrombotic stimuli in dogs. Prostaglandin I synthase knockout mice have a phenotype—severe hypertension and renal lesions—that is distinct from that of I prostanoid receptor knockout mice. COX-2–dependent PGI_2 formation also limits oxidant injury in cardiomyocytes, reduces the pulmonary vasoconstriction induced by hypoxia, and blocks angiotensin II–induced renal vasoconstriction. Recent evidence suggests that PGI_2 may also accelerate viral clearance and modulate the phenotype evoked by infection with respiratory syncytial virus.

Prostaglandin D_2

Prostaglandin D_2 (PGD_2) is the major COX product formed by mast cells. It is released during allergic responses, including asthma and systemic mastocytosis. Infusion of PGD_2 in humans results in flushing, nasal stuffiness, and hypotension, although subsequent formation of F-ring metabolites may result in hypertension, presumably by activation of the F prostanoid receptor. PGD_2 activates a G protein–coupled receptor, the D prostanoid receptor 1, which is related closely to the other prostaglandin receptors. Deletion of the D prostanoid receptor 1 sharply reduces the infiltration of lymphocytes and eosinophils and decreases the airway's reactivity induced by ovalbumin in rodents, suggesting that PGD_2 may have a role in the mediation of asthma. Indeed, a selective inhibitor of D prostanoid receptor 1 affords relief from the symptoms of allergic rhinitis. High levels of D prostanoid receptor 1 are expressed in ileum where they appear important in regulation of blood flow. A chemoattractant receptor–homologous molecule (CRTH2) expressed on T helper type 2 cells has been recognized to function as a D prostanoid receptor 2. PGD_2 induces chemotaxis and migration of T helper type 2 cells through the D prostanoid receptor 2. D prostanoid receptor 2 and prostaglandin D synthase are expressed coordinately at the fetal-maternal interface in human deciduas, where they may participate in lymphocyte recruitment. Overexpression of prostaglandin D synthase increases the cellular and functional response to bronchial challenge with ovalbumin in mice.

PGD_2 is an abundant COX product in brain, where its functional significance is presently incompletely understood. Data from knockout mice suggest, however, that PGD_2 acts on arachnoid trabecular cells in the basal forebrain to mediate an increase in extracellular adenosine, which facilitates induction of sleep. Elevated levels of PGD_2 occur in African sleeping sickness (Chapter 367) and meningitis (Chapter 437). Localized infusions of PGE_2 into the third ventricle counter the effects of PGD_2 and induce wakefulness through E prostanoid receptor 1 and E prostanoid receptor 3. When it is infused into the subarachnoid space of the basal forebrain, PGE_2 also induces sleep, but through the E prostanoid 4 receptor. Prostaglandin D synthase is highly expressed in the leptomeninges and the choroid plexus, and it is a major protein in cerebrospinal fluid. Expression seems to be increased in meningiomas. Deletion of prostaglandin D synthase abolishes allodynia (sensitivity to pain) in mice. A second form of prostaglandin D synthase is found in blood cells, and abnormal levels have been described in the circulation in patients with coronary disease.

PGD_2 may be metabolized in vitro to prostaglandin J_2, from which the metabolite 15-deoxy-$\Delta^{12,14}$-prostaglandin J_2 is formed. Considerable interest has revolved around the possibility that the metabolite might function as a natural ligand for peroxisomal proliferator activator receptor γ and contribute to the resolution phase of inflammation. Although prostaglandin J_2 and its metabolite can activate the nuclear receptor in vitro, it seems unlikely that sufficient concentrations are formed to exert this effect in vivo. However, concentrations formed in vivo are sufficient to activate the D prostanoid receptor 2. COX-2–derived PGD_2 and its putative J_2 metabolite have been suggested to contribute to the resolution phase in inflammation in several animal models.

Prostaglandin E_2

Prostaglandin E_2 (PGE_2) is coupled to two receptors, the E prostanoid receptor 2 and the E prostanoid receptor 4, which activate adenylate cyclase through coupling to the guanosine triphosphate–binding (G) proteins. Mice deficient in the E prostanoid receptor 2 are normotensive, but have an increased sensitivity to salt and can develop pressor hormone–induced hypertension. PGE_2 and PGI_2 play crucial roles in maintaining renal blood flow under conditions of increased vasoconstrictor tone associated with activation of the sympathoadrenal and renin-angiotensin systems. COX-2 is induced in the proximal tubule under conditions of salt loading, and PGE_2 activates the E prostanoid receptor 2 to inhibit tubular sodium reabsorption. Inhibition of these prostanoids does not compromise renal blood flow under physiologic conditions, but COX inhibition may result in impairment of blood flow under renoprival conditions, with a consequent rise in systemic blood pressure, fluid retention, or deterioration in renal function. Experiments in mice suggest that COX-2 is the dominant source of these autoregulatory prostaglandins. It is unclear whether E prostanoid receptor 2 or E prostanoid receptor 4 plays a dominant role in mediating the vasodilator effects of PGE_2 in this setting and its ability to inhibit tubular sodium reabsorption.

Selective E prostanoid receptor 2 agonists inhibit myometrial contractility and are being investigated for use in the treatment of premature labor. COX-2–dependent PGE_2 activates the E prostanoid receptor 2 to enhance the development of intestinal polyposis in mice, apparently by inducing release of vascular endothelial growth factor and consequent angiogenesis. PGE_2 plays a complex role in the switch from the fetal to the adult circulation. Inactivation of the E prostanoid receptor 4, but not of the E prostanoid receptor 2, results in a patent ductus arteriosus and neonatal death, suggesting that PGE_2 is the major product mediating COX-2–dependent ductal remodeling and closure. An abrupt decline in the perinatal period results from induction of 15-PGE_2 dehydrogenase, the major inactivating enzyme of PGE_2. Low levels of PGE_2 signal through the E prostanoid 4 receptor to induce remodeling. Deletion of this enzyme sustains high levels of PGE_2 throughout the perinatal period. By contrast, these high levels of the prostaglandin mediate ductal patency through the E prostanoid 4 receptor. E prostanoid receptor 2 and E prostanoid receptor 4 also seem relevant to immune function; E prostanoid 2 receptors inhibit T-cell proliferation, and E prostanoid 2 and E prostanoid 4 receptors regulate antigen-presenting function in vivo. Both receptors mediate T-cell factor/lymphoid enhancer factor–mediated transcriptional activation. Finally, E prostanoid receptor 2 and E prostanoid receptor 4 interact in bone development and remodeling; E prostanoid receptor 4 antagonists limit osteoclastogenesis and bone resorption in vitro, whereas E prostanoid receptor 2 deletion reduces bone biomechanical strength in vivo. E prostanoid 4 receptor agonists limit bone loss and stimulate osteoblastogenesis in rodents, suggesting potential utility in osteoporosis.

E prostanoid receptor 1 and E prostanoid receptor 3 are coupled via G_q to phospholipase C activation and an inositol phosphate–mediated increase in intracellular calcium, similar to the T prostanoid and the F prostanoid receptors (see later). E prostanoid receptor 3 also inhibits adenylate cyclase via G_i. Activation of these receptor subtypes may result in a metalloproteinase-dependent transactivation of the epidermal growth factor receptor, also of potential relevance to proliferative effects of PGE_2 in cancer. Circulating levels of the cytokine interleukin-1β induce coordinate expression of COX-2 and microsomal prostaglandin E synthase at the blood-brain barrier, permitting activation of E prostanoid receptors in the brain and spine. The pyrexial response to a range of endogenous and exogenous pyrogens seems to be mediated by activation of the E prostanoid receptor 3 in neurons of the organum vasculosum of lamina terminalis, at the midline of the preoptic area. Spinal E prostanoid receptor 1 mediates allodynia, similar to the I prostanoid receptor and products of prostaglandin D synthase (see earlier), whereas E prostanoid receptor 3 seems to mediate hyperalgesia in mice. The implications of these findings in murine models for human syndromes of pain remain to be determined, however. E prostanoid 1 and 3 receptors seem to mediate the myometrial contractility caused by prostaglandin E analogues, such as misoprostol, used to induce labor. Myocardial overexpression of the E prostanoid receptor 3 attenuates reperfusion injury. The E prostanoid receptor 3 also mediates platelet aggregation, similar to the T prostanoid receptor. High concentrations of

PGE_2 can inhibit platelet function by activating the I prostanoid receptor. Such issues of functional redundancy and their implications for drug development are only beginning to be explored. Similarly, the role of E prostanoid subtypes may be conditioned by differential tissue expression. The cytoprotective effects of prostaglandin E analogues are mediated by E prostanoid receptor 1 in the murine stomach but by E prostanoid receptors 3 and 4 in the intestine and by E prostanoid receptor 4 in the colon. E prostanoid 3 receptor deletion attenuates chemically induced skin carcinogenesis in mice. Genetic studies have associated the E prostanoid receptor 3 with the phenotype of severe peripheral vascular disease. Whether this reflects a role for the receptor in pain or hemostatic activation is unknown, but an antagonist is currently under clinical evaluation in this condition.

Prostaglandin $F_{2\alpha}$

So far, one G protein–coupled receptor for prostaglandin $F_{2\alpha}$ ($PGF_{2\alpha}$), the F prostanoid receptor, has been cloned. It is coupled to G_q and can activate phospholipase C–dependent increases in intracellular calcium, culminating in activation of protein kinase C or a Rho-dependent kinase. Activation of the F prostanoid receptor is crucial to parturition. Mice deficient in the F prostanoid receptor do not deliver normal fetuses at term because of failure to induce the oxytocin receptor and absence of the normal decline in elevated progesterone levels. Ovariectomy restores responsiveness to oxytocin and permits successful parturition. COX-1–derived $PGF_{2\alpha}$ ligates the F prostanoid receptor to induce luteolysis. Both F and I prostanoid activation regulates expression of gonadotropin-releasing hormone receptors. COX-2 is upregulated subsequently, and its products, including $PGF_{2\alpha}$ and thromboxane A_2, play a role in the final stages of parturition. $PGF_{2\alpha}$ and its 15-hydroxy metabolite function as male pheromones in fish.

The F prostanoid receptor also is expressed in the ciliary body of the eye, and F prostanoid receptor agonists have shown clinical utility in the treatment of increased intraocular pressure in patients with glaucoma. The F prostanoid receptor is expressed abundantly in smooth muscle cells and its activation results in vasoconstriction, bronchoconstriction, vascular smooth muscle cell proliferation, and cardiomyocyte hypertrophy. The F and T prostanoids together mediate the tachycardiac response to administration of bacterial lipopolysaccharide. The role of $PGF_{2\alpha}$ in cardiopulmonary disease is poorly characterized, however. Similarly, activation of the F prostanoid receptor blocks preadipocyte differentiation in vitro, but the role of the F prostanoid receptor, if any, in obesity is poorly understood.

Prostaglandin F synthase is a member of the aldo-keto reductase family of enzymes. It catalyzes the reduction of prostaglandin H_2 to $PGF_{2\alpha}$ and of PGD_2 to $9\alpha11\beta$-prostaglandin F_2, and it has been shown to reduce retinal to retinol. Prostaglandin F synthase exists in at least two isoforms, identified initially in liver and lung. Prostaglandin F synthase is related closely to 20α-hydroxysteroid dehydrogenase, an aldo-keto reductase that inactivates progesterone to 20α-progesterone, is crucial to the maintenance of pregnancy, and is inhibited by NSAIDs. Prostaglandin F synthase is expressed in contractile tissues of the lung and in lymphocytes, the spinal cord, and the liver.

Isoeicosanoids

Isoeicosanoids are free radical–catalyzed isomers of the enzymatic products of arachidonic acid. Isoprostanes, isomers of the prostaglandins, are formed initially in situ in the membrane after peroxidation of arachidonic acid. Because they are inflexible molecules, they may contribute to membrane injury induced by oxidants. After formation, they are cleaved by phospholipases. The endogenous phospholipases that fulfill this function are unknown, but secretory type II phospholipases A_2 and the platelet-activating factor acetyl hydrolase exhibit this function in vitro. The isoprostanes are a much more complex family than the prostaglandins. Theoretically, 64 isomers, divided into four chemical classes (isoprostanes III, IV, V, and VI), may be formed for each prostaglandin by this mechanism.

Perhaps the most studied isoprostane is isoprostane $F_{2\alpha}$-III, a prostaglandin F isomer also known as 8-*iso* $PGF_{2\alpha}$. This compound acts as an incidental ligand at the T prostanoid receptor to modulate platelet function and to induce vascular smooth muscle cell contraction. Other isoprostanes exhibit diverse biologic actions by activating other eicosanoid G protein–coupled receptors or by acting as ligands for nuclear peroxisomal proliferator activator receptors in vitro. It is unknown, however, if the concentrations attained in vivo evoke these responses and contribute to the clinical manifestations of oxidant stress in human disease. Because isoprostanes are chemically stable, circulate, and are cleared into urine, they have attracted much attention as indices of lipid peroxidation in vivo. Urinary isoprostanes are elevated in syndromes of oxidant stress, such as during tissue reperfusion after ischemia. Elevated levels have been detected in atherosclerotic plaque, circulating low-density lipoprotein, and urine of hypercholesterolemic patients and in the senile plaques, cerebrospinal fluid, plasma, and urine of patients with Alzheimer's disease. Because isoprostane $F_{2\alpha}$-III is a minor urinary isoprostane and may be formed in a COX-dependent mechanism, attention has focused on members of the more abundant VI series, such as 8,12-*iso* isoprostane $F_{2\alpha}$-VI, as a preferable analyte. Quantification of urinary isoprostanes may facilitate a rational basis for selection of doses and patients for clinical trials of antioxidants.

INHIBITORS OF CYCLOOXYGENASE

Three classes of COX inhibitors include aspirin, traditional NSAIDs, and a subset of the NSAIDs developed specifically to target COX-2.

Aspirin

Aspirin irreversibly acetylates a serine (Ser529) residue close to, but not at, the COX catalytic site in prostaglandin G/H synthase. Interpolation of the bulky acetyl residue prevents access of the substrate to the catalytic site (Fig. 34–3). The anucleate platelet retains minimal capacity to generate new protein and is rendered a unique cellular target for aspirin action. This effect has two major clinical implications. First, doses of aspirin that incompletely block the capacity of platelet COX-1 to generate thromboxane A_2 have a cumulative effect until they produce maximal inhibition after repeated daily administration. This principle underlies the use of low doses of aspirin, such as 75 to 80 mg/day, for cardiac protection (Chapters 67 to 69). These doses take 3 to 4 days to reach a steady state and are expected to provide protection similar to that of high doses of aspirin while simultaneously reducing drug exposure and drug-related side effects. Complete inhibition of platelet COX-1 can be achieved with a single loading dose of 160 mg or more of aspirin. By comparison, nucleated cells, such as endothelial cells, generate PGI_2 and recover from aspirin exposure within hours owing to synthesis of new prostaglandin G/H synthase.

The second implication of aspirin's mechanism of action is that when platelet thromboxane A_2 is completely inhibited, new platelets must be generated to overcome aspirin's effects. Recovery of platelet function requires regeneration of only 10% of the normal platelet count, but there is a 1- to 2-day lag thought to reflect the impact of aspirin on marrow megakaryocytes. Platelet function begins to recover 4 to 5 days after inhibition by aspirin and is complete within 12 to 14 days, corresponding to platelet turnover time. This principle underlies the use of aspirin every other day, which is expected, under steady-state conditions, to be equally effective for cardiac protection.

So far, there are no large-scale prospective trials to assess the relative effectiveness of higher and lower doses of aspirin in cardiovascular disease. Doses of 81 mg/day, 324 mg/day, and 1300 mg/day all reduce myocardial infarction and death, however, each by 50%, in placebo-controlled trials in patients with unstable angina (Chapter 71). Meta-analyses suggest that doses greater than and less than 325 mg are similarly effective in the secondary prevention of myocardial infarction and stroke. No difference was seen in the effectiveness of daily doses of 30 mg versus 283 mg in the secondary prevention of these events in patients presenting with a transient ischemic attack or minor stroke. Insufficient data are available, however, to permit a rigorous analysis of the relative impact of lower dosing regimens on clinical outcomes. Because PGI_2 modulates the cardiovascular biology of thromboxane A_2 in vivo, one might speculate that lower doses may be more efficacious if PGI_2 were spared. Even low doses of conventionally formulated aspirin reduce biosynthesis of PGI_2 coincident with that of thromboxane A_2, however. Aspirin acetylates platelets as they circulate through the portal circulation. A slow-release, low-dose aspirin preparation takes advantage of the high first-pass metabolism of aspirin to its deacetylation product, salicylic acid, a weak reversible COX inhibitor, and confines aspirin's

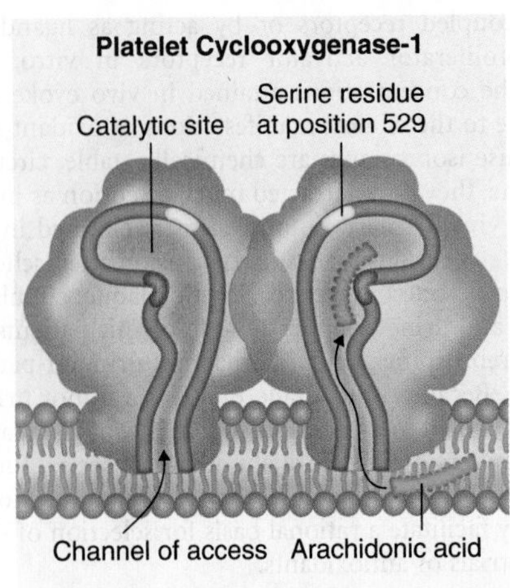

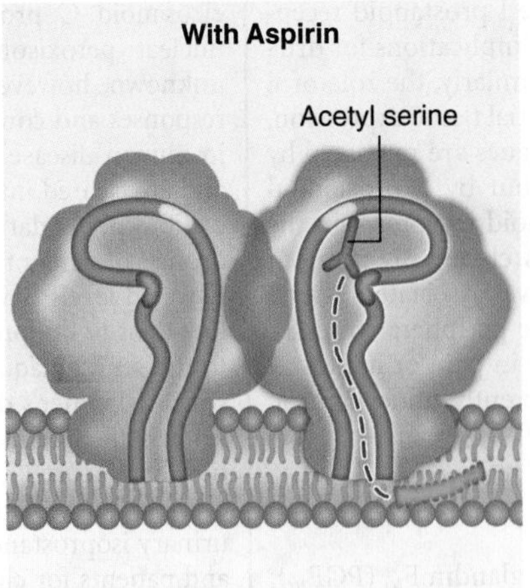

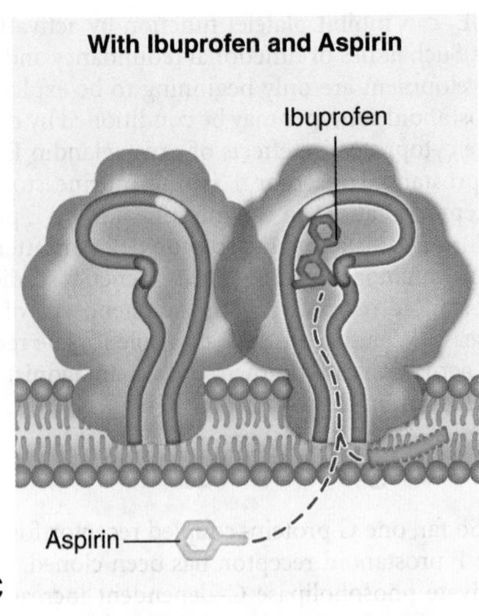

FIGURE 34–3 • The platelet prostaglandin G/H synthase-1 (cyclooxygenase-1) is depicted as a dimer. The arachidonic acid substrate gains access to the catalytic site (orange area) through a hydrophobic channel that leads into the core of the enzyme **(A)**. Aspirin blocks the access of arachidonic acid to the catalytic site by irreversibly acetylating a serine residue at position 529 in platelet cyclooxygenase-1, near but not within the catalytic site **(B)**. Interpolation of the bulky acetyl residue prevents metabolism of arachidonic acid into the cyclic endoperoxides prostaglandin G_2 and prostaglandin H_2 for the lifetime of the platelet. Because prostaglandin H_2 is metabolized by thromboxane synthase into thromboxane A_2, aspirin prevents the formation of thromboxane A_2 by the platelets until new platelets are generated. Nonsteroidal anti-inflammatory drugs, such as ibuprofen, are reversible, competitive inhibitors of the catalytic site **(C)** whose use results in the reversible inhibition of thromboxane A_2 formation during the dosing interval. Prior occupancy of the catalytic site by ibuprofen prevents aspirin from gaining access to its target serine. (From Catella-Lawson F, Reilly MP, Kapoor SC, et al: Cyclooxygenase inhibitors and the antiplatelet effects of aspirin. N Engl J Med 2001;345:1809–1837.)

action to the presystemic circulation. Because the systemic vasculature is protected from aspirin exposure, PGI_2 formation is not depressed coincident with thromboxane A_2 with this formulation; it is unknown if this confers a clinical advantage.

Overview analyses suggest that aspirin reduces the secondary incidence of important vascular events—nonfatal stroke, nonfatal myocardial infarction, and vascular death—by about 25%. Aspirin reduces the secondary incidence of myocardial infarction by about 30% and of stroke by about 15%. This disparity in aspirin action is explained partly by the reduction in thrombotic strokes being offset by an increase in the less common hemorrhagic strokes. Relatively short-term studies (follow-up of approximately 1 month) showed that aspirin reduces mortality in patients presenting with either acute stroke or acute myocardial infarction. [1] Benefit from aspirin is a function of the incidence of thrombotic events. The magnitude of the absolute benefit decreases as one moves from unstable angina to myocardial infarction to stroke to chronic stable angina, all conditions in which aspirin is more effective than placebo (Fig. 34–4). The place of aspirin in primary prevention is less clear. Controlled trials indicate that low-dose aspirin reduces the incidence of nonfatal myocardial infarction, but the number of myocardial infarctions prevented corresponds almost precisely to the number of serious upper gastrointestinal bleeds attributable to aspirin therapy. [2] Large trials are under way to address this issue more precisely.

Multiple epidemiologic studies have associated aspirin consumption with a reduced incidence of colon cancer (Chapter 203). Similar data have been obtained for NSAIDs. COX-2 expression is upregulated in many colonic cancers, and the intensity of protein expression has been related to tumor survival. COX-2 deletion and inhibition delay the development of intestinal polyps in mouse models of human familial polyposis coli, a precancerous condition. Deletion of COX-1 has a similar effect, however, and the interplay of the two enzymes in carcinogenesis is poorly understood. The inverse relationship between aspirin or NSAID consumption and tumor progression has been reported for tumors in sites other than the colon, including tumors of the breast, prostate, esophagus, and stomach. Overexpression of one or both COX isozymes has been reported in Alzheimer's disease plaques, but the direct contribution of COX activity, if any, to disease progression is poorly understood. Inhibition of inflammation might be expected to retard disease progression, and some NSAIDs decrease accumulation of a toxic $A\beta_{(1-42)}$ fragment in the amyloid plaques of Alzheimer's disease. This effect seems to be independent of COX inhibition and may result from inhibition of γ-secretase activity. There is some evidence from epidemiologic studies and small clinical trials that NSAIDs may delay the progression of Alzheimer's disease

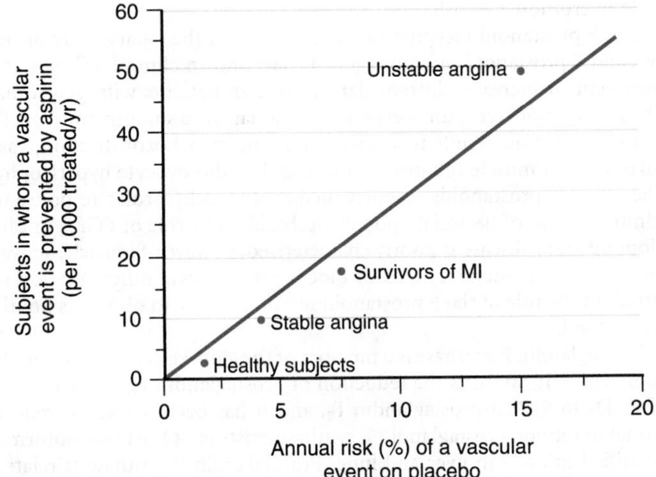

FIGURE 34–4 • The absolute risk of vascular complications is the major determinant of the absolute benefit of antiplatelet prophylaxis. Data are plotted from placebo-controlled aspirin trials in different clinical settings. For each category of patients, the abscissa denotes the absolute risk of experiencing a major vascular event as recorded in the placebo arms of the trials. The absolute benefit of antiplatelet treatment is reported on the ordinate axis as the number of subjects in whom an important vascular event (i.e., nonfatal myocardial infarction [MI], nonfatal stroke, or vascular death) is prevented by treatment of 1000 subjects with aspirin for 1 year. (From Patrono C, Coller B, Dalen JE, et al: Platelet-active drugs: The relationships among dose, effectiveness, and side effects. Chest 2001;119:39S–63S.)

(Chapter 425). On the other hand, some, but not all, COX inhibitors appear to activate in mice γ-secretase–catalyzed release of $A\beta_{42}$, suggesting a potential contribution to disease progression by these agents.

Multiple mechanisms of action have been proposed for aspirin beyond inhibition of COX, including modulation of signaling molecules of the NF-κB signaling pathway. The concentrations used in these studies are unlikely to be compatible with life, however. A possible exception is the interference with binding of the CCAAT/enhancer-binding protein β transcription factor to promoter elements in cytokine genes, which is observed in vitro at concentrations of salicylic acid that are attained after high doses of aspirin in vivo. This effect may explain in part the anti-inflammatory actions of salicylate, despite its weak reversible properties as a COX inhibitor.

Aspirin resistance is a term variably used for patients who have clinical thrombotic events or evidence of failed inhibition of COX activity or platelet function despite aspirin. Given the redundancy in the system, it is surprising that inhibition of just thromboxane A_2–dependent platelet activation should translate into a benefit detectable with as crude an instrument as a clinical trial. Aspirin resistance may reflect the relative importance of other pathways of platelet activation in some individuals, but it also may cover drug interactions, noncompliance, and pharmacokinetic or pharmacogenetic differences. The incidence of cardiovascular events is elevated in individuals who sustain high levels of urinary excretion of thromboxane metabolites despite being prescribed aspirin. All drugs are subject to such heterogeneous causes of "resistance" or "treatment failure." A molecular basis for this phenomenon and a reasonable estimate of its prevalence remain to be identified.

Nonsteroidal Anti-inflammatory Drugs

Traditional (t)NSAIDs are isoform nonselective, reversible active site inhibitors of COX. The class includes arylpropionic acids (ibuprofen, naproxen, flurbiprofen, ketoprofen), indole acetic acids (indomethacin, etodolac), heteroaryl acetic acids (diclofenac, ketorolac), enolic acids (piroxicam, phenylbutazone), and alkanones (nabumetone).

As a result of the reversible action of tNSAIDs, most attain maximal inhibition of platelet COX-1 only transiently during the dosing interval. Because of a nonlinear relationship between the inhibition of COX capacity to generate thromboxane A_2 and thromboxane A_2–dependent platelet function, the offset of their effects on platelet function is even more striking. Inhibition of more than 95% of platelet COX is thought to be necessary to provide cardiac protection. An exception to these generalities regarding tNSAIDs may be naproxen, which exhibits an extended pharmacodynamic half-life in some but not all treated patients. Epidemiologic analyses have yielded conflicting information as to the association of naproxen consumption with a reduced incidence of myocardial infarction. However, where benefit is detected (approximately 10% reduction in myocardial infarction), it is less than the 20 to 25% protection observed with aspirin, as might be expected from interindividual variation in its clinical pharmacology.

NSAIDs are anti-inflammatory, antipyretic, and analgesic. These effects are attributed largely to suppression of PGE_2 and PGI_2 formation. These same prostaglandins provide cytoprotection when they are made by gastric epithelial COX-1. Gastropathy, which is the most common adverse effect of tNSAIDs (Chapters 137 and 138), has two components: bleeding, due to inhibition of platelet COX-1; and impairment of gastric cytoprotection, which is attributed largely to epithelial COX-1. The recognition that COX-2 is readily induced by cytokines suggested that it might represent a discrete target for inhibition, bypassing inhibition of COX-1 and minimizing gastropathy. This conjecture is referred to as the COX-2 hypothesis.

tNSAIDs may prevent access of aspirin to its target in platelet COX-1. Predosing with ibuprofen, the most commonly consumed NSAID in the United States, 2 hours before aspirin administration provides a rapidly reversible inhibition of platelet thromboxane A_2 and aggregation, an effect not observed with a selective COX-2 inhibitor because mature human platelets express only COX-1. This interaction is evident in volunteers taking ibuprofen three times a day, even when the morning dose follows the daily low dose of aspirin. A similar interaction has been reported with naproxen, for which the implications, for reasons discussed before, may be different. Epidemiologic evidence for and against the clinical importance of these interactions has been acquired, and results compatible with but inconclusive of an aspirin-ibuprofen interaction have been obtained in one large randomized controlled trial, the Therapeutic Arthritis Research and Gastrointestinal Event Trial (TARGET). The FDA has issued a warning about these potential interactions.

Acetaminophen is also a nonspecific COX inhibitor. This effect is partial at 1000 mg, a dose commonly taken for mild pain and pyrexia. Epidemiologic studies suggest, however, that higher doses (≥2000 mg) trigger adverse gastrointestinal effects indistinguishable from those of traditional NSAIDs. The degree of COX inhibition would be expected to be dose related. It has been speculated that acetaminophen, which is a good reducing agent, might act to reduce COX from its active, oxidized form. If this were the basis for COX inhibition by acetaminophen, it would be expected to be most pronounced under conditions of low peroxide tone. Although other NSAIDs may be complicated by hepatotoxicity (e.g., diclofenac), this is a particular feature of overdose (usually >10 g) with acetaminophen (Chapter 150). Treatment is by gastric lavage, supportive therapy, and use of *N*-acetylcysteine, which is thought to restore hepatic glutathione.

NSAIDs, similar to aspirin, have had many actions attributed to them aside from inhibition of COX activity. High concentrations, unlikely ever to be attained in patients, have been reported to modify signaling molecules and to activate peroxisomal proliferator activator receptors. Little information exists on how genetic variation might modulate the response to any COX inhibitors. However, considerable interindividual and intraindividual differences in response to these agents have been documented. There is some suggestion of an impact of time of dosing on the pharmacokinetics of some NSAIDs.

Selective Inhibitors of COX-2 (The Coxibs)

The relative selectivity of NSAIDs is evaluated in whole blood assays based on the capacity of platelet COX-1 to generate thromboxane A_2 in serum and of bacterial lipopolysaccharide induction of monocyte COX-2–dependent PGE_2 formation in plasma, pretreated with aspirin to inhibit COX-1, which is expressed constitutively. Three coxibs have been approved initially as selective COX-2 inhibitors in the United States: celecoxib, rofecoxib, and valdecoxib (Table 34–1). All three drugs have established efficacy in inflammatory syndromes, such as the chronic arthritides, and are effective in the treatment of pain (Chapter 28). Overall, the coxibs seem to be as effective as the traditional NSAIDs, a finding compatible with the notion that COX-2 is the dominant source of prostaglandin formation in pain and inflammation. The development strategies that led to approval of these drugs were not designed to seek their superior efficacy over traditional NSAIDs. Furthermore, COX

TABLE 34–1 CLINICAL PHARMACOLOGY OF COXIBS

	Celecoxib	Rofecoxib	Valdecoxib
Formulation	Oral	Oral	Oral
Selectivity ratio	7.6×	35×	30×
Onset of action (min)	60	≤45*	60
T_{max} (hr)	3	2–3	2.25
Half-life (hr)	11	17	8.11
Bioavailability (%)	—	93	83
Protein binding (%)	97	87	98
Metabolism	P-450 2C9	Reduced by cytosolic enzymes	P-450 (3A4 and 2C9) and glucuronidation
Excretion	27% in urine; 57% in feces (changed)	72% in urine; 14% in feces (unchanged)	90% in urine (changed); 10% in feces

*In some studies, rofecoxib was shown to provide pain relief in 27 minutes.
T_{max} = time of maximum concentration.
Sources of data: Prescribing information for rofecoxib (Merck & Co, Inc); prescribing information for celecoxib and valdecoxib (Pharmacia); unpublished data.

Section V Pharmacology

isoenzymes are coexpressed in inflammatory tissues, such as the synovial lining of rheumatoid joints and in atherosclerotic plaque. Also, COX-1 contributes approximately 10 to 15% of the prostaglandin formation induced by bacterial lipopolysaccharide administered to volunteers, and both isoenzymes are expressed in circulating cells ex vivo.

Given these caveats, the trials that led to clinical approval of the COX-2 inhibitors were based on endoscopic evidence of less gastrointestinal ulceration at doses that were equally efficacious to doses of a traditional NSAID. Celecoxib, rofecoxib, and valdecoxib have fared well in these comparisons, compatible with the COX-2 hypothesis. Three randomized trials have sought to discriminate the incidence of real clinical events between purpose-built COX-2 inhibitors and traditional NSAIDs. In one of these trials, the Vioxx Gastrointestinal Outcome Research (VIGOR) study, [3] the incidence of complicated ulcers, mainly gastrointestinal bleeding and perforations, was reduced significantly with rofecoxib compared with naproxen, a traditional NSAID. In a second, the TARGET trial, which comprised two separate studies, the incidence of gastrointestinal events was reduced significantly by the COX-2 inhibitor lumiracoxib compared with either naproxen or ibuprofen. A third outcome study, the Celecoxib Long-term Arthritis Safety Study (CLASS), when published in full, failed to detect a difference between celecoxib and either ibuprofen or diclofenac in gastrointestinal events, despite celecoxib's becoming the best-selling COX-2 inhibitor on the U.S. market. [4]

Evidence has emerged from six placebo-controlled trials involving three purpose-built COX-2 inhibitors that they elevate the incidence of myocardial infarction, stroke, and heart failure. The most parsimonious explanation for this finding is that these drugs suppress COX-2–derived PGI_2 without concomitant inhibition of platelet COX-1–derived thromboxane A_2. Whereas these two COX products have opposite effects on platelet activation, vascular tone and proliferation, and atherogenesis, they are merely two of many endogenous mediators that exert contrasting effects on these cardiovascular parameters. Consequently, the concept of a "balance" or "ratio" is misleading when it is applied restrictively. As PGI_2 restrains the effects of any endogenous mediator of platelet activation, vasoconstriction, and vascular proliferation, suppression of thromboxane A_2 formation (e.g., by low-dose aspirin) would be expected to reduce rather than to abolish such a hazard. The biologic plausibility of such a mechanism has been established in vivo. Deletion, disruption, or inhibition of COX-2 and deletion of the I prostaglandin receptor elevate blood pressure and augment the response to thrombogenic stimuli in mice. These effects are attenuated in mice in which COX-1 has been knocked down to simulate treatment with low-dose aspirin. Selective deletion of COX-2 in cardiomyocytes impairs cardiac function in mice. Given that other factors (e.g., nitric oxide, ectoADPase) share many of the biologic properties of PGI_2, one might have expected them to have substituted for disruption of this pathway. However, just as the benefit from blocking one of the many pathways of platelet activation by low-dose aspirin (or of adenosine diphosphate–induced platelet activation by clopidogrel) can be detected in clinical trials, so also can the cardiovascular hazard of blocking COX-2–dependent PGI_2 be detected in mice and, apparently, in clinical trials.

Currently, the Food and Drug Administration in the United States [5] and the European Medicines Agency [6] both concluded that the selective COX-2 inhibitors under consideration—rofecoxib, celecoxib, and valdecoxib (together with etoricoxib and parecoxib, a prodrug of valdecoxib, in Europe)—confer a small but absolute cardiovascular hazard. Other regulatory bodies reached similar conclusions. Rofecoxib and valdecoxib are no longer available, and the remaining drugs are restricted by label warnings. Both agencies noted the absence of comparable information from placebo-controlled trials of the traditional NSAIDs. However, the Food and Drug Administration applied a "black box" warning to these drugs similar to that for celecoxib, whereas the European Medicines Agency decided not to alter guidance on the use of traditional NSAIDs on the basis of current information. Both agencies suggested use of any of the drugs in this class (COX-2 inhibitors and traditional NSAIDs all belong to the NSAID class) at as low a dose and for as short a time as possible.

The current situation is fluid, and it is likely that approval will be sought for lumiracoxib on the basis of the TARGET study (which was underpowered to address a cardiovascular hazard) and for etoricoxib on the basis of the Multinational Etoricoxib and Diclofenac Arthritis Long-term (MEDAL) study, a randomized comparison with diclofenac involving more than 30,000 patients. Serious thrombotic events and complicated ulcers did not differ between etoricoxib and diclofenac in MEDAL. However, congestive heart failure and hypertension was more common on etoricoxib, whereas uncomplicated ulcers and hepatic adverse effects were more common on diclofenac. If approved, these drugs are likely to be subject to caution concerning patients at recognized risk of cardiovascular events, such as currently applies to celecoxib.

Presently, there are important gaps in our information. Among the questions that need to be addressed are the following.

Do patients differ in their response to individual NSAIDs? Although patients often report anecdotally that a particular NSAID is the only one that affords them relief, there are no controlled trials to determine whether this indeed is the case and, if so, why.

Do patients who begin at low cardiovascular risk undergo risk transformation during long-term treatment with selective COX-2 inhibitors? Two of the placebo-controlled trials of COX-2 inhibitors were chemoprevention studies designed to determine whether intestinal polyp formation could be reduced by these drugs. In both the Adenomatous Polyp Prevention on Vioxx (APPROVe) study [7] of rofecoxib (which led to its withdrawal) and the Adenoma Prevention with Celecoxib (APC) study [8] of celecoxib, the data are compatible with (although not conclusive of) a time-dependent emergence of risk. Furthermore, this is biologically plausible. Disruption of COX-2–dependent PGI_2 formation results in a rise in blood pressure, modulation of the flow-dependent remodeling response, and acceleration of atherogenesis, with an exaggerated thrombotic and vasoconstrictor response on eventual plaque destabilization. We need to determine whether such risk transformation does indeed occur in humans and, if so, how to detect that minority of patients at rapidly emerging risk and to follow dissipation of risk on cessation of therapy.

Do drugs presently classed as traditional NSAIDs confer a cardiovascular hazard? Given the absence of randomized trials, information is restricted to basic and human pharmacology and observational studies. Presently, it seems plausible that heterogeneity with respect to cardiovascular risk exists among traditional NSAIDs. Several traditional NSAIDs—diclofenac, meloxicam (for which approval was sought and obtained as a COX-2 inhibitor in some countries), and nimesulide—resemble celecoxib in their selectivity for inhibition of COX-2. These drugs might be expected to confer a cardiovascular hazard similar to that of celecoxib and not to interact pharmacodynamically with low-dose aspirin. Others, such as ibuprofen, ketoprofen, and indomethacin, inhibit both enzymes to a similar degree reversibly during the dosing interval. They might be expected to be neutral in their own right (save for indomethacin, which is much the more potent and has documented "off-target" effects on the vasculature) but would interact to undermine cardioprotection from aspirin. Furthermore, a discordance in the nature of the relationship between inhibition of the COXs and the functional consequences of these effects might theoretically result in a small direct hazard from such drugs. However, this would be expected to require longer and larger trials to detect than was the case for those that detected hazard from the selective inhibitors of COX-2. Finally, naproxen might be expected to afford cardioprotection in some but not all individuals (a benefit further undermined by irregular compliance with drug intake). However, it also may undermine the benefit of cardioprotection from low-dose aspirin. Indeed, in retrospect, the five-fold divergence in cardiovascular events in VIGOR, in which aspirin was excluded, is most likely compatible with a cardiovascular hazard from rofecoxib *and* cardioprotection in some individuals from naproxen. Given the uncertainty about traditional NSAIDs, one can formulate therapeutic strategies such as those displayed in Table 34–2. However, these guidelines are likely to be refined by further controlled comparisons among the NSAIDs, by observational studies of sufficiently large, high-quality databases, and by the provision of data of individual patients by trial sponsors to permit overview analyses of all the randomized trials pertinent to this question.

Can variability in the response to NSAIDs be exploited to tailor efficacy and safety to individual needs? Unsurprisingly, there are considerable interindividual and intraindividual differences in the pharmacokinetic and pharmacodynamic response to administration of

TABLE 34–2 SUGGESTED CONSIDERATION FOR PREFERRED TREATMENT OPTIONS

PGHS inhibitors with proven cardioprotective efficacy
- Low-dose aspirin

PGHS inhibitors with potential cardioprotective efficacy, variable among individuals
- Naproxen

PGHS inhibitors with the potential to offset the cardioprotective effect of low-dose aspirin
- Ibuprofen, flurbiprofen, indomethacin
- Naproxen

PGHS-2 inhibitors with proven gastroprotective efficacy
- Rofecoxib (withdrawn)
- Lumiracoxib (FDA approval pending)

Treatment options for chronic treatment of patients with low cardiovascular and low gastrointestinal risk
- Naproxen
- Ibuprofen

Treatment options for chronic treatment of patients with low cardiovascular and high gastrointestinal risk
- Naproxen + proton pump inhibitor
- Ibuprofen + proton pump inhibitor
- Lumiracoxib
- Possibly celecoxib or, pending FDA approval, etoricoxib (although gastrointestinal protection superiority to tNSAIDS not proven)

Treatment options for chronic treatment of patients with high cardiovascular and low gastrointestinal risk
- Naproxen + clopidogrel
- Ibuprofen + clopidogrel

Treatment options for chronic treatment of patients with high cardiovascular and high gastrointestinal risk
- Naproxen + proton pump inhibitor + clopidogrel
- Ibuprofen + proton pump inhibitor + clopidogrel

FDA = food and drug administration; PGHS = prostaglandin G/H synthase.
Adapted from Grosser T, Fries S, FitzGerald GA: Biological basis for the cardiovascular consequences of COX-2 inhibition: Therapeutic challenges and opportunities. J Clin Invest 2006;116:4–15.

NSAIDs, including those specific for COX-2. Indeed, specificity at the individual level for COX-2 among these drugs is a continuous rather than a discrete variable. It is impossible presently to calculate the population risk from exposure to any of these drugs. The number of individual events within any of the placebo-controlled trials is too small and the observational studies are devoid of too many elements of information likely to condition the emergence of a hazard—underlying risk of cardiovascular or thrombotic disease, concomitant therapies (especially those acquired over-the-counter, like aspirin), evidence of compliance with prescribed dosing—to permit such extrapolation. However, it appears that for the duration of the trials, only a small percentage of patients exposed, perhaps 1 to 2%, culminate in clinical cardiovascular events. This raises the possibility of exploiting variability in genetic and other determinants of attained selectivity in vivo and intensity and duration of drug exposure to identify those at greatest risk.

Direct-to-consumer advertising fostered the rapid substitution of traditional NSAID use with purpose-designed prescription COX-2 inhibitors without any scientific evidence of superior efficacy. It has been estimated that less than 5% of patients taking such drugs had evidence of marked gastrointestinal intolerance of traditional NSAIDs. In the future, evidence of distinct efficacy might justify the use of these more expensive drugs beyond patients who have such traditional NSAID intolerance, now limited to those who are also at low risk of cardiovascular disease. This may emerge from studies of cancer chemoprevention or other novel indications. Celecoxib already has been approved for the treatment of patients with familial adenomatous polyposis, a precancerous condition of the colon (Chapter 203), on the basis of the outcome of a placebo-controlled trial, and rofecoxib reduced polyposis significantly in the APPROVe study. However, these studies, like most in chemoprevention, do not include a traditional NSAID control. Furthermore, a risk: benefit analysis of the celecoxib data does not support its selection for polyp prevention. Finally, although inflammation is a hallmark of atherosclerosis and trials to seek a cardiovascular *benefit* of COX-2 inhibitors have been suggested by some, the ethics of such an undertaking in the present context seems questionable.

NSAIDs remain among the most commonly consumed drugs, and aspirin has an established place in cardiovascular prophylaxis. Given the remarkably broad range of biologic effects mediated by prostaglandins, it seems likely that the development of more targeted, receptor-based therapeutics will be seen in the future. COX-2 inhibitors were developed for a niche safety indication yet marketed to attain rapidly blockbuster status. Perhaps the recent salutary experience involving these drugs will catalyze development of a more individualized approach to their use in the future. This might conserve their value for those in whom the likelihood of benefit exceeds drug-related risk.

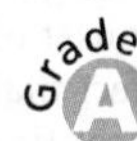

1. Antithrombotic Trialists' Collaboration: Collaborative meta-analysis of randomized trials of antiplatelet therapy for prevention of death, MI, and stroke in high risk patients. BMJ 2002;324:71–86.
2. Patrono C, Coller B, FitzGerald GA, et al: Platelet-active drugs: The relationships among dose, effectiveness, and side effects: The Seventh ACCP Conference on Antithrombotic and Thrombolytic Therapy. Chest 2004;126 (Suppl.):234S–264S.
3. Bombardier C, Laine L, Reicin A, et al: Comparison of upper gastrointestinal toxicity of rofecoxib and naproxen in patients with rheumatoid arthritis. N Engl J Med 2000;343:1521–1528.
4. Juni P, Rutjes MA, Dieppe PA: Are selective COX 2 inhibitors superior to traditional nonsteroidal anti-inflammatory drugs? BMJ 2002;324:1287–1288.
5. U.S. Food and Drug Administration, Center for Drug Evaluation and Research: Public Health Advisory: Non-Steroidal Anti-Inflammatory Drug Products (NSAIDS). Available at http://www.fda.gov/cder/drug/advisory/nsaids.htm.
6. European Medicines Agency, Committee on Medicinal Products for Human Use: EMEA Press Release. Available at http://www.emea.eu.int/pdfs/human/press/pr/24732305en.pdf.
7. Bresalier RS, Sandler RS, Quan H, et al: Cardiovascular events associated with rofecoxib in a colorectal adenoma chemoprevention trial. N Engl J Med 2005;352:1092–1102.
8. Solomon SD, McMurray JJ, Pfeffer MA, et al: Cardiovascular risk associated with celecoxib in a clinical trial for colorectal adenoma prevention. N Engl J Med 2005;352:1071–1080.

SUGGESTED READINGS

Brune K, Hintze B: Selective cyclooxygenase-2 inhibitors: Similarities and differences. Scand J Rheumatol 2004;33:1–6. *A comparative review of the inhibitors with an emphasis on pharmacokinetics.*

Grosser T, Fries S, FitzGerald GA: Biological basis for the cardiovascular consequences of COX-2 inhibition: Therapeutic challenges and opportunities. J Clin Invest 2006;116:4–15. *An overview of the evidence for a cardiovascular hazard from COX-2 inhibition and its mechanistic explanation.*

Hankey GJ, Eikelboom JW: Aspirin resistance. Lancet 2006;367:606–617. *A comprehensive review.*

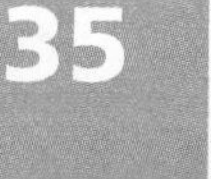

ANTITHROMBOTIC THERAPY

Jack Hirsh and Sam Schulman

Antithrombotic therapy suppresses the natural hemostatic mechanisms (Chapters 179 and 180) and is especially useful for patients with abnormalities of platelet or vascular function (Chapter 179) or with thrombotic disorders or a hypercoagulable state (Chapter 182). A variety of medications can interfere with various aspects of the coagulation system, sometimes with synergistic effects. In recent years, a remarkable number of randomized clinical trials have produced a substantial evidence-based literature to guide the use of antithrombotic therapy for a wide range of clinical conditions.

PHARMACOLOGIC AGENTS

Vitamin K Antagonists

For more than 50 years, vitamin K antagonists have been the only oral anticoagulants available for clinical use. However, with the development and clinical evaluation of novel oral agents that target single enzymes in the coagulation sequence, the situation is likely to change in the near future. Vitamin K antagonists are coumarin derivatives, of which warfarin is the most widely used. Coumarins produce their anticoagulant effect by inhibiting a vitamin K reductase that catalyzes the reduction of 2,3-epoxide (vitamin K epoxide), thereby leading to the depletion of vitamin KH_2. This reduced form of vitamin K is required for the production of functionally active (γ-carboxylated) coagulation proteins (factors II [prothrombin], VII, IX, and X) and anticoagulant proteins (protein C and protein S) (Chapter 180). Vitamin K_1 in food sources can reverse these effects of coumarins because it is reduced to vitamin KH_2 by a warfarin-insensitive vitamin K reductase (Fig. 35–1).

Warfarin is rapidly and almost completely absorbed from the gastrointestinal tract. It has a half-life of about 40 hours, a delayed onset of action (2 to 7 days, depending on dose), and an anticoagulant effect that is not completely reversed for up to 5 days after treatment is discontinued. The dose-response relationship of warfarin varies widely among individuals, and therefore the drug's effects must be monitored closely to prevent overdosing or underdosing. Laboratory monitoring is performed by measurement of the prothrombin time and is reported as an international normalized ratio (INR). The INR is prolonged in response to depression of three of the four vitamin K–dependent procoagulant clotting factors (prothrombin and factors VII and X). During initiation of warfarin therapy, the INR reflects primarily the depression of factor VII, which has a half-life of only approximately 6 hours, whereas during maintenance therapy, the INR is elevated by all three vitamin K–dependent factors. The dose response to warfarin is influenced by many factors, including age, body weight, liver disease, dietary vitamin K_1, genetic factors, concomitant drug use, compliance of the patient, and inappropriate dosage adjustments. Of these factors, inappropriate dosage adjustment and improved compliance through education of patients are the most readily correctable. Overanticoagulation during initiation of warfarin can be avoided by an average daily dose of 5 mg, with the expectation that a stable anticoagulant (and antithrombotic) effect will be achieved in 5 or 6 days. The starting dose should be reduced to 3 or 4 mg/day in the elderly because they are more sensitive to warfarin.

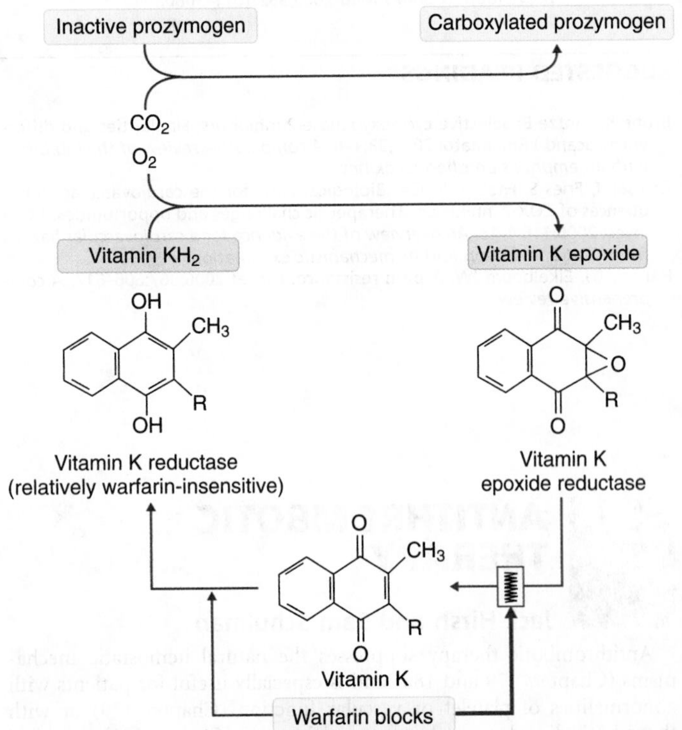

There is evidence that the reliability of warfarin monitoring is improved by having the dosage controlled by an anticoagulation management service and by using computer-assisted algorithms. The convenience of monitoring is increased, particularly in busy patients who travel frequently, by point-of-care testing with portable finger-prick monitors.

Inactive prozymogen

Carboxylated prozymogen

CO_2

O_2

Vitamin KH_2

Vitamin K epoxide

Vitamin K reductase (relatively warfarin-insensitive)

Vitamin K epoxide reductase

Vitamin K

Warfarin blocks

FIGURE 35–1 • Warfarin inhibits vitamin K epoxide reductase and leads to the intracellular depletion (in the hepatocyte) of vitamin KH_2. Vitamin KH_2 is required for the conversion (by γ-carboxylation) of functionally inactive to active coagulation proteins. The anticoagulant effect of warfarin can be reversed by vitamin K_1 in food because it is reduced to vitamin KH_2 by a warfarin-insensitive vitamin K reductase.

Warfarin

Indications for Warfarin

Warfarin is effective in the primary and secondary prevention of systemic embolism in patients with atrial fibrillation (Chapter 63); in the prevention of systemic arterial embolism in patients with valvular heart disease (bioprosthetic and mechanical heart valves; Chapter 75); in the primary and secondary prevention of venous thromboembolism (Chapters 81 and 99); in the prevention of acute myocardial infarction in high-risk patients (Chapter 72); and in the prevention of stroke, recurrent infarction, and death in patients with acute myocardial infarction (Chapter 72). A target INR of 2.5 (range, 2.0 to 3.0) is recommended for all indications except for patients with a mechanical prosthetic heart valve in the mitral position or in the aortic position in combination with other risk factors for systemic embolism and for patients with acute myocardial infarction, for whom an INR of 3.0 (range, 2.5 to 3.5) is recommended (Table 35–1).

Dosing and Monitoring

If a rapid anticoagulant effect is required, heparin and warfarin should be started at the same time and overlapped for at least 5 days. A loading dose of warfarin should not be used because it is safer to start with the estimated maintenance dose of about 5 mg/day; patients usually reach an INR of 2.0 in 4 or 5 days. If there is no increase of the INR after two or three doses, the daily dose should be progressively increased until an INR response is observed. The maintenance dose of warfarin varies among patients; in some, it can be as low as 1 mg/day, whereas doses up to 20 mg are required occasionally. Heparin treatment is discontinued when the INR has been in the therapeutic range for 2 days. If treatment is not urgent (e.g., chronic stable atrial fibrillation), warfarin treatment can be commenced out of the hospital at this same dose.

If treatment is started with a maintenance dose, the first INR measurement can be delayed until day 2 or 3 and then performed daily until the INR is in the therapeutic range. The INR is then performed two or three times weekly for 1 to 2 weeks and then less often, depending on the stability of INR results.

If the INR response remains stable, the frequency of testing can be reduced to intervals of every 4 weeks. If adjustments to the dose are

TABLE 35–1 RECOMMENDED THERAPEUTIC RANGE FOR ORAL ANTICOAGULANT THERAPY

Indication	INR
Prophylaxis of venous thrombosis (high-risk surgery)	2.0–3.0
Treatment of venous thrombosis	2.0–3.0
Treatment of pulmonary embolism	2.0–3.0
Prevention of systemic embolism	2.0–3.0
Tissue heart valves	
Aortic mechanical heart valves (low risk)	
Valvar heart disease	
Atrial fibrillation	
Recurrent systemic embolism	
Cardiomyopathy	
Mechanical prosthetic valves (high risk*)	2.5–3.5
Acute myocardial infarction†	2.5–3.5

*All mechanical prosthetic valves in the mitral position; caged-ball or caged-disc valves; presence of additional risk factors, such as atrial fibrillation, myocardial infarction, left atrial enlargement, endocardial damage, low ejection fraction, or systemic embolism in spite of a therapeutic INR.

†Aspirin is indicated in most patients, but an INR of 2.5 to 3.5 is recommended if warfarin is used.

INR = international normalized ratio.

required because the INR drifts out of the therapeutic range, the adjustments should be gradual and based on the weekly dose (e.g., a 10 to 20% change in weekly dose). Patients should be encouraged to keep a log of their dose and their INR response.

Adverse Effects

Warfarin-related bleeding is increased by the level of the INR; the risk of bleeding increases noticeably when the INR reaches 4.0 and even more sharply when the INR is higher than 5.0. For example, compared with an INR of 2.0 to 3.0, the risk of major bleeding is increased two- to three-fold at an INR of 4.5, about five-fold at an INR of 5.5, and eight- to ten-fold at an INR above 6.0. The risk of bleeding is also increased with concomitant aspirin use, in persons older than 65 years, in those with a history of stroke or gastrointestinal bleeding, and in those with serious comorbid conditions. Elderly patients are more sensitive to warfarin, requiring lower doses to reach the therapeutic range, and have an increased tendency to bleed, including intracranial bleeding, even when their INR is in the therapeutic range (Chapter 23). In addition, the elderly are more likely to be receiving one or more of the many drugs that interact with warfarin. When treatment with any new drug is indicated in any patient who is being treated with warfarin, the INR should be monitored more frequently during the initial stages of combined drug therapy.

Reversing the Effect of Warfarin

The anticoagulant effect of warfarin can be reversed in one of three ways: by discontinuation of therapy, with the expectation that the INR will return to baseline in about 5 days; by administration of vitamin K_1, with the expectation that the anticoagulant effect will be reduced in 6 hours and reversed in 24 hours; and by infusion of fresh-frozen plasma, prothrombin complex concentrate, or recombinant coagulation factor VIIa, which produces immediate reversal.

Patients whose INR is elevated up to 5.0 can be treated by appropriate dosage reduction. Patients with bleeding or whose INR is elevated above 5.0 may require more rapid reversal with vitamin K_1 treatment, whereas patients with serious bleeding commonly require fresh-frozen plasma in addition to vitamin K_1. When the INR is elevated to potentially dangerous levels and the patient is not bleeding, vitamin K_1 should be administered in a dose of 1 to 10 mg, depending on the level of the INR and if partial or complete reversal is needed. For an INR of 5.0 to 10.0, an oral dose of 1 to 2 mg of vitamin K_1 will usually bring the INR down to the range of 2.0 to 3.0 in less than 24 hours. Both the oral and intravenous (IV) routes give a predictable response, whereas the response to subcutaneous vitamin K_1 can be unpredictable. The oral route is recommended unless rapid reversal of warfarin is necessary, in which case vitamin K is administered by slow IV infusion.

Platelet-Active Drugs

The platelet-active drugs inhibit different steps in either platelet activation (aspirin, ticlopidine and clopidogrel, and dipyridamole) or platelet recruitment (the glycoprotein IIb/IIIa complex [GPIIb-IIIa] antagonists abciximab, tirofiban, and eptifibatide) (Fig. 35–2).

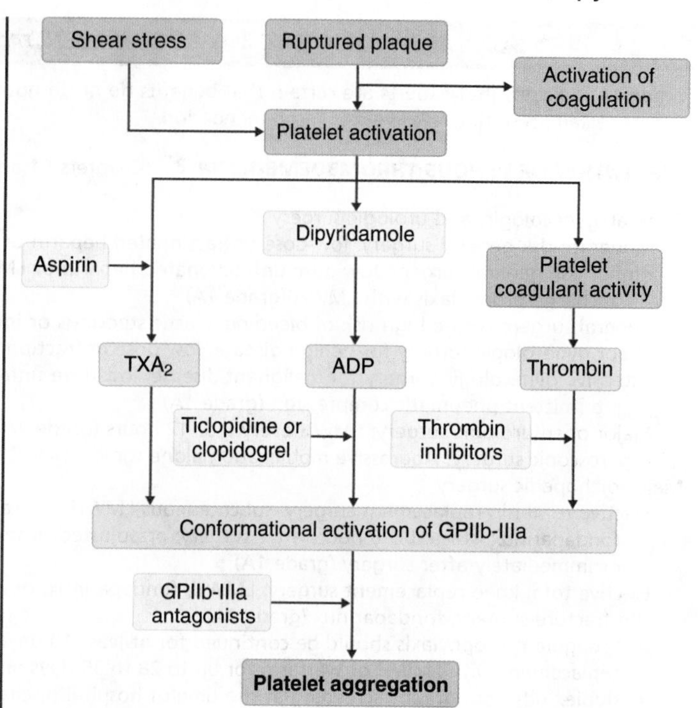

FIGURE 35–2 • Sites of action of platelet inhibitors. ADP = adenosine diphosphate; GPIIb-IIIa = glycoprotein IIb/IIIa complex; TXA_2 = thromboxane A_2.

Aspirin and Other Cyclooxygenase Inhibitors

Aspirin

On the basis of results of a meta-analysis of more than 50 secondary prevention cardiovascular trials, there is evidence that aspirin reduces vascular death by approximately 15% and nonfatal vascular events by about 30% in patients with cardiovascular disease [1] (Table 35–2). Aspirin is less effective than low-molecular-weight heparins (LMWHs) or warfarin for preventing venous thromboembolism and should not be used alone in hip fracture surgery. [1, 2]

Mechanism of Action

Aspirin permanently inactivates cyclooxygenase isoenzymes (COX-1 and COX-2) that catalyze the conversion of arachidonic acid to prostaglandin H_2, a precursor of a variety of prostaglandins including thromboxane A_2 and prostacyclin (prostaglandin I_2). Thromboxane A_2 is a potent inducer of platelet aggregation and vasoconstriction, whereas prostacyclin induces vasodilation. Aspirin is approximately 50- to 100-fold more potent at inhibiting platelet COX-1 than COX-2. Consequently, the COX-2–dependent anti-inflammatory effects of aspirin require larger doses of the drug (Chapter 34). The effect of aspirin on thromboxane A_2 production in platelets lasts for the lifespan of the platelet. In contrast to platelets, vascular endothelial cells process prostaglandin H_2 to produce prostacyclin. Low and even moderate doses of aspirin do not inhibit prostacyclin synthesis substantially because the effect of aspirin on endothelial cell–derived COX-1 is short-lived.

Pharmacology

Aspirin is rapidly absorbed in the stomach and upper intestine, attaining peak plasma levels at about 30 minutes after ingestion; it has a half-life of about 15 minutes. Inhibition of platelet function is evident by 1 hour with uncoated aspirin but can be delayed after administration of enteric-coated aspirin. Therefore, if only enteric-coated tablets are available when a rapid effect is required, the tablets should be chewed.

Aspirin potentiates the antithrombotic effects of warfarin (in high-risk subjects), dipyridamole (in those with ischemic stroke), clopidogrel (in those with coronary stents or acute myocardial ischemia), and heparin (in the prevention of recurrent miscarriages in pregnant women with antiphospholipid antibody syndrome and in patients with acute coronary ischemia). Aspirin produces a small increase in major bleeding and a very small increase in the risk of cerebral hemorrhage. It also potentiates bleeding when it is added to another antithrombotic agent.

Aspirin causes gastrointestinal side effects that are dose dependent and reduced by use of low doses (325 mg/day or less). Aspirin is contraindicated in individuals with peptic ulcer disease or aspirin-induced asthma or if gastrointestinal side effects are severe.

Clinical Uses

Aspirin reduces the incidence of myocardial infarction and death in patients with silent myocardial ischemia or stable angina, unstable angina, non–ST elevation myocardial infarction, ST elevation myocardial infarction, and ischemic cerebrovascular disease. [1, 3] Aspirin is also effective in patients after coronary angioplasty or coronary artery bypass surgery [1, 4, 5] and in preventing symptomatic coronary events in asymptomatic men and women older than 50 years. [1, 3] Aspirin has a favorable risk-to-benefit ratio for secondary prevention in patients with overt vascular disease, but the risk-to-benefit ratio is marginal when aspirin is used as primary prevention in asymptomatic individuals. Aspirin is less effective than oral anticoagulants in the prevention of recurrent stroke in atrial fibrillation and less effective than LMWH or warfarin in preventing venous thromboembolism. [2, 6]

Dipyridamole

Dipyridamole is a pyrimidopyrimidine derivative with vasodilator and antiplatelet properties. It inhibits platelet function by elevating platelet cyclic adenosine monophosphate levels. The absorption of conventional dipyridamole is variable but has been improved by a modified-release

TABLE 35–2 SUMMARY OF GRADE A RECOMMENDATIONS FOR ANTITHROMBOTIC THERAPY

Grade 1A indicates that experts are certain that benefits do or do not outweigh risks, burdens, and costs. Grade 2A indicates that they are less certain, resulting in a weaker recommendation.

PREVENTION OF VENOUS THROMBOEMBOLISM 2 (Chapters 81 and 99)

General, gynecologic, and urologic surgery
- Moderate-risk general surgery: low-dose unfractionated heparin or LMWH (grade 1A)
- Higher risk general surgery: low-dose unfractionated heparin or LMWH; in selected cases, including major cancer surgery: post-hospital discharge prophylaxis with LMWH (grade 1A)
- General surgery with a high risk of bleeding: elastic stockings or intermittent pneumatic compression (grade 1A)
- Major gynecologic surgery for benign disease: low-dose unfractionated heparin every 12 hours (grade 1A)
- Extensive gynecologic surgery for malignant disease: low-dose unfractionated heparin every 8 hours, higher doses of LMWH, or intermittent pneumatic compression (grade 1A)
- Major open urologic surgery: LMWH every 8 or 12 hours (grade 1A)
- Laparoscopic surgery: Aggressive mobilization alone (grade 1A)

Major orthopedic surgery
- Elective total hip replacement surgery: subcutaneous LMWH, started either 12 hours before or 12 to 24 hours after surgery; fondaparinux, started 6–8 hours after surgery; or adjusted-dose warfarin (INR target of 2.5; range, 2.0 to 3.0), started preoperatively or immediately after surgery (grade 1A)
- Elective total knee replacement surgery: LMWH, fondaparinux, or adjusted-dose warfarin (grade 1A)
- Hip fracture surgery: fondaparinux (grade 1A)
- Anticoagulant prophylaxis should be continued for at least 10 days (grade 1A). Extended prophylaxis should be given after total hip replacement with LMWH or warfarin for up to 28 to 35 days and after hip fracture surgery with fondaparinux (grade 1A). Routine duplex ultrasonography screening at the time of hospital discharge or during outpatient follow-up is not recommended in asymptomatic patients after total hip replacement or total knee replacement (grade 1A).

Neurosurgery, trauma, and acute spinal cord injury
- Neurosurgery: intermittent pneumatic compression with or without elastic stockings for intracranial neurosurgery (grade 1A)
- Trauma patients: all trauma patients with at least one risk factor for VTE and all patients with acute spinal cord injury should receive thromboprophylaxis, if it is not contraindicated (grade 1A). LMWH is started as soon as it is considered safe (grade 1A).

Medical conditions
- Acute myocardial infarction: anticoagulant therapy with subcutaneous low-dose unfractionated heparin or IV heparin in prophylactic or therapeutic doses
- Ischemic stroke with impaired mobility: low-dose unfractionated heparin or LMWH
- General medical patients with risk factors for VTE: low-dose unfractionated heparin or LMWH (grade 1A)

Critical care
- Most patients should, after appropriate assessment of the risk for VTE, receive thromboprophylaxis: if medically ill or postoperative—with unfractionated heparin or LMWH; with major trauma or orthopedic surgery—with LMWH (grade 1A).

TREATMENT OF VENOUS THROMBOEMBOLIC DISEASE 11 (Chapters 81 and 99)

Acute treatment
- Acute treatment: LMWH or unfractionated IV heparin or, for DVT, alternatively adjusted-dose subcutaneous heparin (grade 1A)
- Continue for at least 5 days. Start treatment with vitamin K antagonists on the first day and overlap with oral anticoagulation for at least 4 or 5 days and until INR is above 2.0 (grade 1A).

Long-term anticoagulation
- Patients with VTE and cancer: treat with LMWH for the first 3–6 months (grade 1A).
- Patients with a first episode of VTE and reversible or time-limited risk factors: treat with vitamin K antagonists for 3 months (grade 1A).
- Patients with a first episode of idiopathic VTE; or first episode of VTE with antithrombin deficiency, protein C or protein S deficiency, factor V Leiden or prothrombin 20210 gene mutation, homocystinemia, or high factor VIII levels: treat for at least 6–12 months and consider indefinite treatment (grade 1A).
- After two or more episodes: treat indefinitely (grade 2A).
- Adjust the dose of vitamin K antagonist to maintain a target INR of 2.5 with a range of 2.0 to 3.0 for all treatment durations (grade 1A).
- Prescribe an elastic compression stocking with an ankle pressure of 30 to 40 mm Hg for 2 years after an episode of DVT (grade 1A).

ATRIAL FIBRILLATION 6 (Chapter 63)

High-risk patients
- Standard approach: warfarin anticoagulation (INR of 2.5; range, 2.0 to 3.0) (grade 1A)
- Warfarin contraindicated or declined by patient: aspirin, 80 to 325 mg
- Aspirin plus low-, fixed-dose warfarin should not be used.

Moderate-risk patients
- Either oral anticoagulation or aspirin (grade 1A)

TABLE 35–2 SUMMARY OF GRADE A RECOMMENDATIONS FOR ANTITHROMBOTIC THERAPY—cont'd

VALVULAR HEART DISEASE [18] (Chapter 75)

Mitral valve prolapse
- Mitral valve prolapse with documented but unexplained TIA: long-term aspirin, 50 to 162 mg daily (grade 1A)

Mechanical prosthetic heart valves
- Vitamin K antagonists with a target INR of 2.5 (range, 2.0 to 3.0) for St. Jude bileaflet valve in the aortic position (grade 1A) and 3.0 (range, 2.5 to 3.5) in combination with aspirin, 75 to 100 mg, for caged-ball or caged-disc valves (grade 2A)

CORONARY THROMBOLYSIS AND ACUTE MYOCARDIAL INFARCTION [3, 12, 19-21] (Chapter 72)

Coronary thrombolysis
- All patients with acute myocardial infarction who receive fibrinolytic therapy should receive aspirin (160 to 325 mg), chewed and swallowed, on arrival to the hospital (grade 1A).
- Patients with ischemic symptoms for less than 12 hours who have ST segment elevation or left bundle branch block on the ECG should receive fibrinolytic therapy unless they undergo primary percutaneous intervention (grade 1A).
- Choice of fibrinolytic agent for patients with symptom duration <12 hours: streptokinase, anistreplase, reteplase, tenecteplase, or alteplase. Fibrinolytic therapy should be started within 30 minutes of arrival in the hospital (grade 1A).
- Choice of fibrinolytic agent for patients with symptom duration <6 hours: alteplase and tenecteplase are superior to streptokinase (grade 1A).

Acute myocardial infarction
- For patients receiving streptokinase: unfractionated heparin, 5000 U IV bolus, followed by 12,500 U every 12 hours for 48 hours (grade 2A)
- Aspirin: initial dose of 160 to 325 mg of non–enteric-coated aspirin to chew and swallow as soon as possible after the clinical impression of evolving acute myocardial infarction is formed (grade 1A)
- Maintenance dose of 75 to 162 mg daily should be continued indefinitely (grade 1A).
- Patients who have contraindications to aspirin should receive clopidogrel, 75 mg/day, indefinitely (grade 1A).
- High-risk patients should receive aspirin (<100 mg) in combination with vitamin K antagonists targeted at INR of 2.5 (2.0 to 3.0) (grade 2A).

UNSTABLE ANGINA [3] (Chapter 71)

Antiplatelet therapy
- Aspirin, non–enteric-coated, at an initial dose of 75 to 325 mg to chew and swallow as soon as possible after the clinical impression of unstable angina is formed (grade 1A). Aspirin by mouth, 75 to 162 mg, should be continued indefinitely (grade 1A).
- In cases of aspirin allergy or intolerance: clopidogrel at a bolus dose of 300 mg orally and then 75mg indefinitely (grade 1A), or triflusal in countries where it is available.

Thienopyridines
- Coronary angiography within 24 hours: start clopidogrel after the angiography (grade 2A).
- Delayed coronary angiography or coronary bypass until more than 5 days: start clopidogrel with a bolus dose of 300 mg, followed by 75 mg/day for 9 to 12 months in addition to aspirin (grade 1A).
- Clopidogrel should be discontinued for 5 days before scheduled surgery (grade 2A).

GPIIb-IIIa antagonists
- IV tirofiban or eptifibatide, in addition to aspirin and heparin, to patients with continuing ischemia or other high-risk features. The indication is strengthened by the detection of elevated troponin T or I. The infusion should continue for 48 to 72 hours or until PCI (grade 1A).
- Abciximab for 12 to 24 hours in patients who will undergo PCI within the following 24 hours, provided coronary angiography has been performed

Anticoagulants
- IV heparin (about 75 U/kg IV bolus, initial maintenance 1250 U/hr IV, aPTT 1.5 to 2 times control) in patients hospitalized with unstable angina for at least 48 hours or until the unstable pain pattern resolves (grade 1A)

CHRONIC CORONARY ARTERY DISEASE [3] (Chapter 70)

Aspirin for patients with stable angina, 75 to 162 mg daily (indefinitely) (grade 1A)

Primary prevention
- Moderate or high risk for a coronary event: aspirin, 75 to 162 mg daily (grade 2A)
- Very high risk with easily monitored INR: warfarin targeted at INR of approximately 1.5 (grade 2A)

CORONARY ARTERY BYPASS GRAFTS [5]

Aspirin, 75 to 162 mg, starting 6 hours after operation (grade 1A)
- In most patients, aspirin is indicated for life.

Patients with unstable angina: clopidogrel, 75 mg daily for 9 to 12 months in addition to aspirin (grade 1A)
- If it is started before surgery, discontinue clopidogrel 5 days before the operation (grade 2A).

Continued

TABLE 35–2 SUMMARY OF GRADE A RECOMMENDATIONS FOR ANTITHROMBOTIC THERAPY—cont'd

ANTITHROMBOTIC THERAPY IN PATIENTS UNDERGOING PERCUTANEOUS CORONARY INTERVENTION 4 (Chapter 73)

Oral antiplatelet agents
- Aspirin, 75 to 325 mg, should be administered before PCI (grade 1A).
- Aspirin, 75 to 162 mg daily, should be used for secondary prevention of cardiovascular events (grade 1A).

Thienopyridines
- Clopidogrel should be combined with aspirin for 9 to 12 months after stent placement (grade 1A). In patients with low atherosclerotic risk, clopidogrel should be given for 2 weeks after placement of a bare metal stent (grade 1A).

Platelet glycoprotein IIb/IIIa antagonists
- Abciximab (0.25 mg/kg bolus and 12-hour infusion at 10 μg/min) or eptifibatide (two bolus doses of 180 μg/kg 10 minutes apart and then 2 μg/kg/min for 18 hours) should be considered in all patients undergoing PCI, particularly patients with refractory unstable angina or with other high-risk features (grade 1A).

Direct thrombin inhibitors
- Bivalirudin
- When treatment with a glycoprotein IIb/IIIa antagonist is not used, bivalirudin should be given at an initial dose of 0.75 mg/kg, followed by 1.75 mg/kg/hr infusion for the duration of the coronary intervention (grade 1A).

ANTITHROMBOTIC THERAPY IN PERIPHERAL ARTERIAL OCCLUSIVE DISEASE 8 (Chapter 79)

Patients with clinical evidence of cerebrovascular disease or coronary artery disease should be treated indefinitely with aspirin, 75 to 325 mg daily (grade 1A).

Patients with carotid endarterectomy should be treated preoperatively and continued indefinitely with aspirin, 75 to 325 mg daily (grade 1A).

Peripheral vascular reconstructive surgery
- Reconstruction of low-flow arteries
- Patients having prosthetic, femoral-popliteal bypass operations: aspirin, 75 to 325 mg/day, begun preoperatively (grade 1A)

Intraoperative anticoagulation therapy
- Patients undergoing major vascular reconstructive operations should be systemically anticoagulated with heparin at the time of application of cross-clamps (grade 1A).

ANTITHROMBOTIC AND THROMBOLYTIC THERAPY FOR ISCHEMIC STROKE 7 (Chapter 431)

Acute ischemic stroke: treatment within 3 hours of onset of symptoms
- Thrombolytic therapy: in eligible patients, IV t-PA in a dose of 0.9 mg/kg (maximum of 90 mg), with 10% of the total dose given as an initial bolus and the remainder infused during 60 minutes (grade 1A).
- Streptokinase is not recommended except within the confines of a clinical trial (grade 1A).

Acute ischemic stroke: patients not receiving thrombolysis
- Aspirin, 160 to 325 mg/day, started early (grade 1A)
- Aspirin may be used safely in combination with low doses of subcutaneous heparin for DVT prophylaxis (grade 1A).

DVT or pulmonary embolism prophylaxis
- For acute stroke patients with restricted mobility: low-dose subcutaneous heparin or LMWHs or the heparinoid danaparoid, provided there are no contraindications to anticoagulation (grade 1A)

Stroke prevention
- Antiplatelet agents and anticoagulation
  - Noncardioembolic cerebral ischemic events (stroke or TIA; atherothrombotic, lacunar, or cryptogenic): aspirin, 50 to 325 mg/day (grade 1A). The combination of aspirin and extended-release dipyridamole (25/200 mg bid) and clopidogrel (75 mg qd) are acceptable options for initial therapy.
  - The combination of aspirin and extended-release dipyridamole (25/200 mg bid) is more effective than aspirin alone for the prevention of stroke (grade 2A).
  - Cardioembolic ischemic events: long-term vitamin K antagonists (target INR of 2.5; range, 2.0 to 3.0) for atrial fibrillation (grade 1A)
- Carotid endarterectomy: aspirin, 81 to 325 mg/day, before carotid endarterectomy and continued long term after the procedure

aPTT = activated partial thromboplastin time; DVT = deep venous thrombosis; ECG = electrocardiogram; INR = international normalized ratio; IV = intravenous; LMWH = low-molecular-weight heparin; PCI = percutaneous coronary intervention; TIA = transient ischemic attack; t-PA = tissue plasminogen activator; VTE = venous thromboembolism.

formulation. Dipyridamole has a terminal half-life of 10 hours and is eliminated primarily by biliary excretion. Results of clinical trials with conventional dipyridamole, used either alone or in combination with aspirin, have been disappointing. However, favorable results were obtained with the modified-release preparation in patients with prior stroke or transient ischemic attack, in whom the risk of stroke was reduced by 16% with dipyridamole alone and by 37% with aspirin and dipyridamole in combination, compared with placebo. 1, 7 Whether these favorable results reflect the use of a higher dose (400 vs. 225 mg daily) of dipyridamole than in prior trials or the improved systemic bioavailability of modified-release dipyridamole is uncertain.

Thienopyridines

Ticlopidine and clopidogrel are thienopyridines that inhibit adenosine diphosphate–induced platelet aggregation through the action of their active metabolites. Both drugs are administered orally, but their onset of action is delayed until their active metabolites are formed. Similarly, recovery of platelet function is delayed until the active thienopyridine metabolites are cleared and the circulating affected platelets replaced by newly formed, unaffected platelets.

Ticlopidine is more effective than aspirin in reducing stroke in patients with transient cerebral ischemia or minor stroke and more effective than placebo in patients with thromboembolic stroke, unstable angina, or peripheral vascular disease and after coronary bypass surgery. The combination of ticlopidine and aspirin is more effective than aspirin alone or aspirin plus warfarin in preventing thrombotic complications after coronary artery stent placement. However, ticlopidine has a number of important side effects, including hypercholesterolemia and neutropenia. Its use has also been associated with thrombocytopenia, aplastic anemia, and thrombotic thrombocytopenic purpura.

The better safety profile and equal efficacy of clopidogrel have resulted in its substitution for ticlopidine for essentially all indications. Clopidogrel is rapidly absorbed and metabolized, and the onset of the inhibition of platelet aggregation with clopidogrel is more rapid than with ticlopidine. Thus, inhibition of platelet aggregation is detectable as soon as 90 minutes after an oral loading dosing of 300 mg. With repeated daily administration of low doses (75 mg), there is cumulative inhibition of platelet function with a return to normal 7 days after the last dose of clopidogrel.

Clopidogrel is more effective than aspirin in patients who have experienced a recent stroke or recent myocardial infarction and in patients presenting with symptomatic peripheral arterial disease. [1, 3, 7, 8] The additional benefit over aspirin is modest and similar to that observed with ticlopidine (about 10% relative risk reduction). The combination of clopidogrel and aspirin is also more effective than aspirin alone in patients with unstable angina and non–ST elevation myocardial infarction (20% risk reduction), but at a cost of a modest increase in bleeding. The combination of clopidogrel and aspirin is also more effective than aspirin alone in patients who have percutaneous coronary intervention procedures. Clopidogrel appears to be as well tolerated as aspirin. [1]

Integrin $\alpha_{IIb}\beta_3$ (GpIIb-IIIa) Receptor Antagonists

The final common pathway of platelet aggregation is mediated by the binding of fibrinogen to the functionally active integrin $\alpha_{IIb}\beta_3$ (GPIIb-IIIa) on the platelet surface. Inhibitors of this process include monoclonal antibodies, synthetic peptides containing Arg-Gly-Asp (RGD) or Lys-Gly-Asp (KGD), and peptidomimetic and nonpeptide RGD mimetics. These compounds are administered intravenously and inhibit platelet function by competing with fibrinogen (and von Willebrand factor) for occupancy on the platelet integrin receptor. Severe but reversible thrombocytopenia occurs within a few hours in a small percentage of the patients.

Abciximab (ReoPro), a mouse-human chimeric 7E3 Fab antibody, inhibits platelet aggregation in a concentration-dependent manner. Abciximab is unique among the GPIIb-IIIa antagonists because it also blocks binding to the $\alpha_v\beta_3$ receptor on endothelial cells and to an activated form of the leukocyte $\alpha M\beta_2$ receptor. The role of these two unique actions in the antithrombotic effects of abciximab is unclear. Platelet function is impaired rapidly after an IV bolus of abciximab and gradually recovers during 24 to 48 hours. However, because of its tight binding to its integrin receptor, small amounts of abciximab can be detected on circulating platelets as late as 14 days after administration.

Tirofiban (MK-383, Aggrastat) is a nonpeptide derivative of tyrosine. It has a plasma half-life of 1.6 hours, and its effect on hemostasis is reversed within 4 hours of stopping treatment.

Eptifibatide (Integrilin) is a synthetic disulfide-linked cyclic heptapeptide. It has a rapid onset and offset of action, and its effect on platelet function is reduced by more than 50% after 4 hours.

All three GPIIb-IIIa receptor antagonists are effective IV agents in patients undergoing percutaneous coronary interventions, [4, 9] and tirofiban and eptifibatide are effective in patients with unstable angina or non–ST elevation myocardial infarction. [1, 4] The GPIIb-IIIa receptor antagonists are administered in combination with heparin and aspirin. Orally active nonpeptide GPIIb-IIIa inhibitors have been developed for long-term use, but the results of clinical trials have been disappointing.

Heparin and Low-Molecular-Weight Heparins

Heparin

Heparin acts as an anticoagulant by activating the plasma cofactor antithrombin, thereby increasing the rate at which the plasma cofactor inactivates thrombin, activated factor X (factor Xa), and other coagulation enzymes. Heparin accelerates the inactivation of thrombin by antithrombin by providing a template to which both the enzyme and the inhibitor bind to form a ternary complex (Fig. 35–3). In contrast, the inactivation of factor Xa by antithrombin-heparin complex does not require ternary complex formation and is achieved by binding of the activated antithrombin to factor Xa. Although effective clinically, heparin has biophysical limitations caused by the reduced ability of heparin to bind to and inactivate thrombin that is bound to fibrin and factor Xa that is bound to the platelet surface.

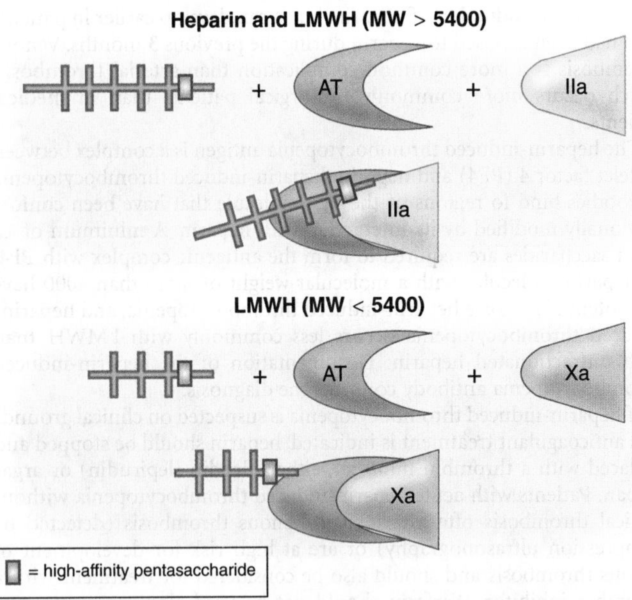

FIGURE 35–3 • Only one third of high-affinity pentasaccharide-containing heparin molecules and one fifth of pentasaccharide-containing low-molecular-weight heparin (LMWH) molecules activate antithrombin (AT). Virtually all of the high-affinity heparin molecules are large enough to bridge between AT and factor IIa (thrombin). In contrast, only 25 to 50% of LMWH molecules have a molecular weight of 5400 or more, and although these smaller molecules inactivate factor Xa, they do not inactivate factor IIa. Although heparin has equal anti–factor IIa and anti–factor Xa activities, LMWH has reduced anti–factor IIa activity.

Heparin binds to a number of plasma, platelet, and endothelial cell–derived proteins that compete with antithrombin for heparin binding. Binding of heparin to plasma proteins contributes to the variability of its anticoagulant response, whereas binding to hepatic macrophages is responsible for its dose-dependent clearance. Both properties contribute to the unpredictable anticoagulant effect of heparin and the need for laboratory monitoring.

Heparin is effective for the prevention and treatment of venous thromboembolism, [2, 10, 11] for the early treatment of patients with unstable angina and acute myocardial infarction, [3, 10] for patients who have cardiac surgery under cardiopulmonary bypass, [5] for patients undergoing vascular surgery, [8] and during and after coronary angioplasty and coronary stent placement. [4]

The anticoagulant effects of heparin are usually monitored by the activated partial thromboplastin time (aPTT). A therapeutic effect is achieved when the aPTT ratio is equivalent to a heparin level of 0.3 to 0.7 anti–factor Xa units, which for many reagents is an aPTT ratio of 1.5 to 2.5. The risk of bleeding complications is increased with increasing heparin dosage, which in turn is related to the anticoagulant response. However, other clinical factors, such as recent surgery, trauma, and invasive procedures, are also important as predictors of bleeding during heparin treatment.

For the treatment of venous thromboembolism, heparin is given in doses of 80 U/kg followed by 18 U/kg per hour by continuous infusion; the dose is adjusted according to the aPTT result at 6 hours by use of a validated nomogram. Lower doses (70 U/kg followed by 1000 U/hr) of heparin are used in patients with acute myocardial ischemia who also receive aspirin and GPIIb-IIIa antagonists or thrombolytic therapy.

The main complications of heparin are bleeding and heparin-induced thrombocytopenia. Less common complications are heparin-induced osteoporosis and hyperkalemia. Heparin-related bleeding is dose related, and the risk is increased in patients who undergo an invasive procedure and if heparin is used in combination with a GPIIb-IIIa antagonist or a thrombolytic agent.

Heparin-induced thrombocytopenia, which is an antibody-mediated adverse reaction to heparin, can be complicated by venous or arterial thrombosis. The diagnosis should be considered when a patient treated with heparin experiences an unexplained fall in the platelet count of 50% or more or develops skin lesions at sites of subcutaneous heparin injection. The fall in platelet count almost always occurs between days 5 and

15 after the introduction of heparin, but it can develop earlier in patients who had been exposed to heparin during the previous 3 months. Venous thrombosis is a more common complication than arterial thrombosis, which occurs more commonly in surgical patients than in medical patients.

The heparin-induced thrombocytopenia antigen is a complex between platelet factor 4 (PF4) and heparin; heparin-induced thrombocytopenia antibodies bind to regions of the PF4 molecule that have been conformationally modified by its interaction with heparin. A minimum of 12 to 14 saccharides are required to form the antigenic complex with PF4, so heparin molecules with a molecular weight of more than 4000 have the potential to cause heparin-induced thrombocytopenia, and heparin-induced thrombocytopenia occurs less commonly with LMWH than with unfractionated heparin. Documentation of the heparin-induced thrombocytopenia antibody confirms the diagnosis.

If heparin-induced thrombocytopenia is suspected on clinical grounds and anticoagulant treatment is indicated, heparin should be stopped and replaced with a thrombin inhibitor, either hirudin (lepirudin) or argatroban. Patients with acute heparin-induced thrombocytopenia without clinical thrombosis often have silent venous thrombosis (detected by compression ultrasonography) or are at high risk for development of venous thrombosis and should also be considered for treatment with a thrombin inhibitor. Warfarin should not be used alone to treat acute heparin-induced thrombocytopenia because it can aggravate the thrombotic process, but it is safe in combination with a thrombin inhibitor after the platelet count has risen above 100×10^9/L.

Low-Molecular-Weight Heparins

LMWHs are fragments produced by either chemical or enzymatic depolymerization of heparin. LMWHs are approximately one-third the size of heparin (Table 35–3). Depolymerization of heparin changes the anticoagulant profile. As a result, LMWHs have less protein and cellular binding and, as a consequence, have a more predictable dose response, better bioavailability, and a longer plasma half-life than regular heparin.

Compared with heparin, which has a ratio of anti–factor Xa to anti–factor IIa activity of approximately 1 : 1, the various commercial LMWHs have anti–factor Xa to anti–factor IIa ratios varying between 4 : 1 and 2 : 1, depending on their molecular size distribution. LMWHs bind much less avidly to heparin-binding proteins than does heparin, a property that contributes to superior bioavailability at low doses and to a more predictable anticoagulant response. LMWHs are cleared principally by the renal route. LMWHs are associated with a lower incidence of heparin-induced thrombocytopenia and heparin-induced osteoporosis than is heparin. LMWHs have a longer plasma half-life and a more predictable anticoagulant response than does heparin, thereby allowing LMWH to be administered once daily without laboratory monitoring, a property that facilitates out-of-hospital management of patients with venous thrombosis or unstable angina. LMWHs are administered subcutaneously.

LMWHs are effective in the prevention and treatment of venous thrombosis [2, 10, 11] (Chapter 81), in the treatment of patients with unstable angina and non–ST elevation myocardial infarction [3, 10] (Chapter 71), and as an adjunct to fibrinolytic therapy in patients with acute ST elevation myocardial infarction [12] (Chapter 72).

Pentasaccharides

On the basis of knowledge of the antithrombin-binding sequence on heparin, a pentasaccharide, fondaparinux, with high affinity for antithrombin has been synthesized. The structure of fondaparinux has been modified to increase its affinity to antithrombin. Fondaparinux inactivates factor Xa through an antithrombin-mediated mechanism. Because it is too short to bridge antithrombin to thrombin, fondaparinux has no activity against thrombin.

After subcutaneous injection, fondaparinux is rapidly and completely absorbed and exhibits a bioavailability of 100%. The volume of distribution is similar to the blood volume. The drug is mainly excreted unchanged in the urine with a terminal half-life of 17 hours in young volunteers and 21 hours in elderly volunteers.

Fondaparinux circulates extensively bound to antithrombin with minimal binding to other plasma proteins. Limited experimental and clinical studies suggest that fondaparinux has a lower risk of heparin-induced thrombocytopenia than that of heparin or LMWH as well as a lower risk of bone loss and of local skin reactions.

Fondaparinux is effective in the prevention of venous thrombosis after elective hip or knee arthroplasty, after hip fracture surgery, [13] after general surgery, and in high-risk medical patients. [14] Fondaparinux is also effective in the treatment of patients with venous thrombosis or pulmonary embolism.

Fibrinolytic Agents

Fibrinolytic agents convert plasminogen to the enzyme plasmin, which then degrades fibrin to soluble fragments, thereby lysing the thrombus. Of the available fibrinolytic agents, streptokinase and urokinase are not

TABLE 35–3 ANTICOAGULANT PROFILES, MOLECULAR WEIGHTS, PLASMA HALF-LIVES, AND RECOMMENDED DOSES OF COMMERCIAL LOW-MOLECULAR-WEIGHT HEPARINS

Agent	Anti-Xa/Anti-IIa Ratio	Molecular Weight	Plasma Half-life (min)	Recommended Dose (International anti-Xa Units): General Surgery Prophylaxis	Orthopedic Surgery Prophylaxis	Acute Treatment
Enoxaparin	2.7 : 1	4,500	129–180	4,000 U SC daily	4,000 U SC daily or 3,000 U SC bid	7,000 U SC bid*† or 10,500 U SC daily*
Dalteparin	2. : 1	5,000	119–139	2,500 U SC daily	2,500 U SC bid or 5,000 U SC daily	8,400 U SC bid*† or 14,000 U SC daily*
Nadroparin	3.2 : 1	4,500	132–162	2,850 U SC daily	2,700 U SC daily,* 4,000 U SC daily* from day 4	13,300 U SC daily*
Tinzaparin (Innohep)	1.9 : 1	4,500	111	3,500 U SC daily	3,500 U SC daily* or 4,500 U SC daily*	12,250 U daily*
Ardeparin	2. : 1	6,000	200		50 U/kg SC bid	
Danaparoid‡	20 : 1	6,500	1,100	750 U SC daily	750 U SC bid	2,500 U IV, then 4 hr each of 400 U/hr and 300 U/hr, then 200 U/hr; or 2,000 U SC bid

*Weight-adjusted dose; stated dose for 70-kg patient.
†The higher daily dose is for acute coronary syndromes; the lower dose is for deep venous thrombosis.
‡Danaparoid sodium is a heparinoid.
IV = intravenously; SC = subcutaneously.

fibrin specific; in contrast, recombinant tissue-type plasminogen activator (rt-PA, alteplase) and the rt-PA variant tenecteplase are relatively fibrin specific. In addition, the rt-PA variants tenecteplase and reteplase have been engineered to have a longer plasma half-life than rt-PA, allowing the variants to be administered as a bolus injection (see Table 72–5).

Streptokinase is an indirect fibrinolytic agent. It binds to plasminogen, converting it into a plasmin-like molecule that in turn converts plasminogen to plasmin. Streptokinase has a number of disadvantages. It is antigenic, rendering its repeated use problematic, and allergenic, producing chills, fever, and rigors in some patients and, in rare instances, anaphylaxis. Antistreplase (APSAC) is an acylated complex of streptokinase and Lys-plasminogen. Compared with streptokinase, it is more fibrin specific, has a longer plasma half-life, and is inactive until it is selectively activated by deacylation on the fibrin surface. Its side effect profile, antigenicity, and efficacy are similar to those of streptokinase.

Urokinase is a naturally occurring plasminogen activator that differs from streptokinase in that it directly activates plasminogen and is not antigenic. Urokinase was used extensively to treat peripheral vascular occlusions, but production problems have curtailed its availability.

In its natural state, tissue plasminogen activator is produced by vascular endothelium; rt-PA (alteplase) is produced by recombinant DNA technology. Alteplase is not antigenic or allergenic, and it has greater fibrin specificity than does streptokinase. It has a short half-life of about 3.5 minutes and therefore is given as a continuous IV infusion.

Truncated forms of rt-PA have been developed; the first was reteplase (r-PA), a single-chain deletion mutant that lacks certain domains. As a result, its half-life is about twice that of rt-PA, permitting double-bolus therapy 30 minutes apart. r-PA has lower affinity for fibrin than does rt-PA, but fibrinogen depletion with r-PA is less than that with streptokinase. No antigenicity has been reported with this compound.

Tenecteplase (TNK-tPA) is a mutant tissue plasminogen activator with amino acid substitution at three sites. Compared with rt-PA, it has a longer half-life, allowing single-bolus administration, increased fibrin specificity, and increased resistance to inhibition by plasminogen activator inhibitor 1.

New Anticoagulants

The limitations of established anticoagulants have prompted the development of a variety of new anticoagulant agents that target various specific steps in the coagulation mechanism.

Direct Thrombin Inhibitors

Direct thrombin inhibitors act independently of antithrombin to inactivate both free thrombin and thrombin bound to fibrin. The direct thrombin inhibitors include hirudin, synthetic hirudin fragments (hirugen and hirulog), and low-molecular-weight inhibitors that react with the active site of thrombin (melagatran and its oral prodrug ximelagatran, as well as dabigatran and argatroban). Although all of these inhibitors bind directly to thrombin, their sites of interaction are different. Hirulog is approved for use in coronary angioplasty (Chapter 73), and both argatroban and hirudin are approved in patients with heparin-induced thrombocytopenia (Chapter 179). Hirudin is more effective than heparin in the prevention of venous thrombosis (Chapter 81) and in patients with acute coronary syndromes (Chapter 71), but it causes more bleeding. [3, 15] Although the results of a meta-analysis suggested that bivalirudin is safer and possibly more effective than heparin in acute coronary syndromes (Chapter 71), this more favorable safety efficacy profile was not confirmed in a large study (HERO-2) of patients with acute myocardial infarction (Chapter 72). [15] Data comparing argatroban with hirudin in heparin-induced thrombocytopenia are too limited for conclusions to be drawn about their relative efficacy and safety at the current time.

Direct Factor Xa Inhibitors

A number of orally available, specific small-molecular-weight active site–directed factor Xa inhibitors have been designed and are in various stages of clinical development. Unlike heparins and pentasaccharides, direct inhibitors inactivate factor Xa without the need for antithrombin as a cofactor.

Activated Protein C and Soluble Thrombomodulin

Activated protein C, a naturally occurring anticoagulant, is available in plasma-derived and recombinant forms. Soluble thrombomodulin is available through recombinant DNA technology. Both are effective antithrombotic agents in a variety of experimental animal models, and they are administered by the parenteral route. Activated protein C is effective in reducing mortality in severe sepsis (Chapter 109). [16, 17] Soluble thrombomodulin is under evaluation for prophylaxis against venous thromboembolism in major orthopedic surgery.

Tissue Factor Pathway Inhibitor

Tissue factor pathway inhibitor is a naturally occurring inhibitor that blocks the generation of thrombin by inactivating factor Xa and factor VIIa. Tissue factor pathway inhibitor failed to show benefit in the treatment of disseminated intravascular coagulation that complicates severe sepsis (Chapter 109).

Another inhibitor of the tissue factor–factor VIIa complex is an 85–amino acid polypeptide, nematode anticoagulant protein c2 (NAPc2), from the canine hookworm *Ancylostoma caninum*. It is produced with recombinant DNA technique and binds to factor X-Xa to form an inhibitory complex. NAPc2 is being evaluated for prophylaxis against venous thromboembolism as well as in arterial thrombosis.

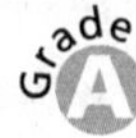

1. Patrono C, Coller B, FitzGerald GA, et al: Platelet-active drugs: The relationships among dose, effectiveness, and side effects. Chest 2004;126:234S–264S.
2. Geerts WH, Pineo GF, Heit JA, et al: Prevention of venous thromboembolism. Chest 2004;126:338S–400S.
3. Harrington RA, Becker RC, Ezekowitz M, et al: Antithrombotic therapy for coronary artery disease. Chest 2004;126:513S–548S.
4. Popma JJ, Berger P, Ohman EM, et al: Antithrombotic therapy during percutaneous coronary intervention. Chest 2004;126:576S–599S.
5. Stein PD, Schünemann HJ, Dalen JE, Gutterman D: Antithrombotic therapy in patients with saphenous vein and internal mammary artery bypass grafts. Chest 2004;126:600S–608S.
6. Singer DE, Albers GW, Dalen JE, et al: Antithrombotic therapy in atrial fibrillation. Chest 2004;126:429S–456S.
7. Albers GW, Amarenco P, Easton JD, et al: Antithrombotic and thrombolytic therapy for ischemic stroke. Chest 2004;126:483S–512S.
8. Clagett GP, Sobel M, Jackson MR, et al: Antithrombotic therapy in peripheral arterial occlusive disease. Chest 2004;126:609S–626S.
9. Bosch X, Marrugat J: Platelet glycoprotein IIb/IIIa blockers for percutaneous coronary revascularization, and unstable angina and non–ST-segment elevation myocardial infarction (Cochrane review). Cochrane Database Syst Rev 2001;4:CD002130.
10. Hirsh J, Raschke R: Heparin and low-molecular-weight heparin. Chest 2004;126:188S–203S.
11. Büller HR, Agnelli G, Hull RD, et al: Antithrombotic therapy for venous thromboembolic disease. Chest 2004;126:401S–428S.
12. Menon V, Harrington RA, Hochman JS, et al: Thrombolysis and adjunctive therapy in acute myocardial infarction. Chest 2004;126:549S–575S.
13. Turpie AGG, Bauer KA, Bengt I, et al: Fondaparinux versus enoxaparin for the prevention of venous thromboembolism in major orthopedic surgery. A meta-analysis of four randomized double-blind studies. Arch Intern Med 2002;162:1833–1840.
14. Cohen AT, Davidson BL, Gallus AS, et al: Efficacy and safety of fondaparinux for the prevention of venous thromboembolism in older acute medical patients: Randomised placebo controlled trial. BMJ 2006;332:335–339.
15. White H, Hirulog and Early Reperfusion or Occlusion (HERO)-2 Trial Investigators: Thrombin-specific anticoagulation with bivalirudin versus heparin in patients receiving fibrinolytic therapy for acute myocardial infarction: The HERO-2 randomised trial. Lancet 2001;358:1855–1863.
16. Weitz JI, Hirsh J, Samama MM: New anticoagulant drugs. Chest 2004;126:265S–286S.
17. Bernard GR, Vincet JL, Laterre PF, et al: Efficacy and safety of recombinant human activated protein C for severe sepsis. N Engl J Med 2001;344:699–709.
18. Salem DN, Stein PD, Al-Ahmad A, et al: Antithrombotic therapy in valvular heart disease—native and prosthetic. Chest 2004;126:457S–482S.
19. ISIS-2 (Second International Study of Infarct Survival) Collaborative Group: Randomised trial of intravenous streptokinase, oral aspirin, both, or neither among 17,187 cases of suspected acute myocardial infarction: ISIS-2. Lancet 1988;2:349–360.
20. van Es RF, Jonker JCJ, Verheugt FWA, et al: Aspirin and coumadin or both after acute coronary syndromes (the ASPECT-2 study): A randomised controlled trial. Lancet 2002;360:109–113.
21. Hurlen M, Abdelnoor M, Smith P, et al: Warfarin, aspirin, or both after myocardial infarction. N Engl J Med 2002;347:969–974.

SUGGESTED READING

Berger JS, Roncaglioni MC, Avanzini F, et al: Aspirin for the primary prevention of cardiovascular events in women and men: A sex-specific meta-analysis of randomized controlled trials. JAMA 2006;295:306–313. *Aspirin reduced ischemic stroke in women and MI in men; the risk of bleeding rose a similar degree among women and men.*

Bhatt DL, Fox KA, Hacke W, et al: Clopidogrel and aspirin versus aspirin alone for the prevention of atherothrombotic events. N Engl J Med 2006;354:1706–1717. *Clopidogrel plus aspirin was not significantly better than aspirin alone in reducing MI, stroke, or cardiovascular death.*

Heneghan C, Alonso-Coello P, Garcia-Alamino JM, et al: Self-monitoring of oral anticoagulation: A systematic review and meta-analysis. Lancet 2006;367: 404–411. *Patients capable of self-monitoring and self-adjusting therapy have fewer events and lower mortality than those who self-monitor alone.*

Hirsh J, Guyatt JH, Albers G, et al (eds): The Seventh ACCP Conference on Antithrombotic and Thrombolytic Therapy: Evidence-based guidelines. Chest 2004;126:163S–703S. *A comprehensive review of the pharmacology of antithrombotic agents with treatment recommendations based on the strength of evidence and on expert opinions.*

36 COMPLEMENTARY AND ALTERNATIVE MEDICINE

Stephen E. Straus

Despite dramatic advances in medical science and evidence-based practice, many people turn to other healing approaches, some derived from ancient medical traditions and others from new-age concepts. Although extraordinarily diverse in their nature and purpose, these approaches share enormous appeal, often despite the lack of compelling evidence that they are safe or effective. The term *alternative medicine* indicates practices that are used instead of mainstream approaches, whereas *complementary medicine* refers to practices that are used as adjuncts to conventional medicine. The most recent term for these approaches, *integrative medicine,* signals the hope that conventional medicine can embrace any modality that proves to be safe and effective, regardless of its origins, under a more inclusive health care umbrella. Complementary and alternative medicine commonly emphasizes therapies, many of which are based on unproven hypotheses regarding pathophysiology, and rarely focuses on specific diagnostic strategies.

Complementary and alternative medicine includes healing approaches that presently are not considered an integral part of conventional (allopathic) medicine as practiced in developed nations. Its many forms can be divided conveniently into four major categories: biologically based therapies, manipulative and body-based methods, mind-body interventions, and energy therapies. Whole alternative medical systems have been developed that employ many discrete practices from among these four categories.

ALTERNATIVE MEDICAL SYSTEMS

Alternative medical systems aim to prevent or to treat disease without relying on any elements of conventional Western medicine. Included are traditional Chinese medicine, Ayurveda (meaning "science of life") of India, and various Native American healing approaches. Each is a complex system that incorporates natural products, diet, spiritual elements, and other modalities. Of the various elements that are specific to some traditional medical systems, Americans are most familiar with herbal medicines and acupuncture, approaches that evolved during thousands of years through careful observation and empirical refinement. As practiced in traditional healing systems, herbs and acupuncture are but two of several tools commonly advised for relief of a particular condition, but in the United States, they typically are prescribed as stand-alone modalities. Many other alternative approaches similarly have been adapted to the tastes and interests of the broader American populace.

Newer, European-based or American-based alternative systems include homeopathic medicine and naturopathic medicine.

Homeopathic Medicine

Homeopathy was founded in the late 18th century as a reaction to the toxic and unsuccessful normative practices of the day, such as purging and leeching. The theory of homeopathy is that infinitesimal doses of a substance that causes particular symptoms in higher concentrations relieve similar symptoms, regardless of their cause. Previously a respected field that inspired some of the first placebo-controlled experiments and from which the original theory leading to allergen desensitization was derived, homeopathy is today a small and marginalized field in the United States. Only four states provide licenses for the practice of homeopathy. By contrast, homeopathy remains widely practiced in Germany and is well accepted within the National Health Service in the United Kingdom.

Naturopathic Medicine

Naturopathic medicine derived from the early 19th century German concept of natural healing (i.e., the body possesses an inherent ability to heal itself). The purpose of this approach is to guide the patient toward self-healing with gentle and nontoxic measures, proper diet, and a variety of other approaches. The emphasis is on outpatient-based primary care and family medicine. Training involves 4 years of postgraduate education leading to the Doctorate of Naturopathic Medicine (ND) degree. Practitioners are licensed for individual practice in 14 states in the United States.

Biologically Based Therapies

Because numerous drugs are of natural origin, it is presumed that nature harbors yet more medicinal gems awaiting discovery and characterization. Countless natural products and mixtures of products have been described in ancient medical texts, and contemporary versions of many of these products are sold to eager consumers as dietary supplements. The extraordinary popularity of these products, for which Americans spend billions of dollars each year, rests at least in part on the prevalent assumption that a natural product is healthy, whereas synthetic chemicals often are not. Under the Dietary Supplements Health and Education Act passed by the U.S. Congress in 1994, dietary supplements include vitamins, minerals, and all natural herbal and chemical products that are ingested for the maintenance of wellness or for the prevention and treatment of symptoms that arise from normal body processes, such as menopause, rather than from pathologic causes. These products are not deemed to be drugs and are not regulated as such; as a result, they do not require premarket review or approval by the Food and Drug Administration (FDA).

Manipulative and Body-Based Methods

Therapeutic massage and chiropractic and osteopathic manipulation are the best known of the manual therapies. Massage is widely practiced and licensed in 25 states. Manipulation procedures are practiced largely within chiropractic and osteopathic systems that emerged in the American heartland in the late 19th century. Both fields originally proposed that vertebral misalignments contribute to many diseases, each of which could be treated by appropriate manipulations. There were strong efforts by allopathic organizations to discredit chiropractic and osteopathic medicine. In part as reactions to these challenges, chiropractic medicine evolved as a discrete discipline that primarily uses spinal manipulation, most often to address musculoskeletal problems. Four years of postgraduate education lead to a Doctor of Chiropractic (DC) degree, and chiropractic physicians are licensed to practice in all states.

Osteopathic medicine also may use manipulative techniques, but historical differences between osteopathic medicine and allopathic medicine otherwise have disappeared. Other than teaching manipulation, undergraduate medical training for an osteopathic degree (DO) is now virtually indistinguishable from that which leads to the MD degree. Osteopathic physicians complete conventional residencies in osteopathic or allopathic hospitals and training programs, are licensed in all states, and have rights and responsibilities, such as military service, that are identical to those of allopathic physicians and surgeons.

Mind-Body Interventions

A major tenet of complementary and alternative medicine is that the mind influences body functions, and vice versa, and that the interactions between them can be affected for salutary purposes. This belief is both a remarkably ancient and a strikingly modern concept that conflicts with the Cartesian dissociation of mind from body that dominated Western philosophical thought for more than 300 years. Some uses for hypnosis, cognitive therapies, and biofeedback are well integrated within conventional medicine. Other approaches involving meditation, dance, music and art therapy, and prayer are considered complementary or alternative.

Energy Therapies

Ancient peoples postulated that health depends on the proper balance and flow of life energies, termed *qi* (pronounced "chee") in Chinese systems and the *doshas* in Ayurveda. Many strategies were developed with the goal of restoring the vitality and balance of a person's energies. In the aggregate, these approaches are controversial complementary and alternative medicine practices because neither these internal energy fields nor the activities they are assumed to possess have been shown convincingly. There are two general classes of energetic approaches. One involves the application of external electromagnetic fields, as with magnets inserted into clothing and mattresses. The other purports to manipulate a person's fields, such as by having a healer place hands in or through them. Therapeutic touch derives from the ancient practice of "laying on of hands" with the goal of allowing the therapist's healing force to restore that of the patient. Other related approaches include qigong and Reiki.

Acupuncture is a widely practiced energy healing art whose traditional justification may be less important than what contemporary science teaches about it. Acupuncture involves insertion of needles into empirically derived points on the body, or meridians, across which streams of energy are said to flow. Modern versions of acupuncture include attachment of electrodes to the needles and the application of small currents through them. Whatever the style of practice, acupuncture has moved progressively mainstream. Reports in the early 1970s of its use in China to substitute for general anesthetics excited the curiosity and fascination of Americans. Today, formal training leads to a license in acupuncture degree (LAc) that permits either independent practice or practice under the supervision of a physician in about 34 states.

Appeal and Use of Complementary and Alternative Medicine

A recent survey by the U.S. Centers for Disease Control and Prevention estimated that 36% of Americans employ complementary and alternative medicine therapies to help satisfy their personal health care needs. When one includes prayer specifically for health reasons, the estimated use of these practices rises to 62%. Americans spend billions of dollars on these therapies annually with little prospect of their reimbursement from insurance companies.

Surveys indicate that patients choose complementary and alternative medicine approaches to sustain or to restore their health and well-being, primarily to relieve symptoms of chronic or terminal illnesses that are not addressed adequately by conventional medical treatments. In general, it is not a reaction against or fundamental dissatisfaction with conventional medicine. Most use is as an adjunct to conventional treatment. Complementary and alternative medicine approaches are sought more frequently by women, people born after World War II, people with more years of formal education, people who think more about emotional stress and the environment, more affluent people, and people who are chronically ill.

Clinical Approach

A full inquiry into what ails patients includes an attempt to understand not only the clinical problems themselves but also what the patients believe the problems to represent and how they have attempted to address them. The physician must ask specifically about complementary and alternative medicine practices that patients may use. The broad range of complementary and alternative options available and the inundation of the public with unsubstantiated claims about them challenge physicians' abilities to guide their patients' choices. Merely to pontificate that none of these practices are meritorious may alienate a patient whose personal experience and firm convictions indicate otherwise. Yet a physician cannot accede to all preferences of all patients. Ultimately, a conscious decision must be made whether to prescribe a complementary and alternative treatment, to endorse a patient's choices for complementary and alternative medicine, to accept his or her choices (provided they do not interfere with the prescribed conventional approaches), or to advise against the complementary and alternative approach. First and foremost, the decision should be based on whether the approach could be harmful.

TABLE 36–1 SOME NATURAL MEDICINES THAT POTENTIATE OR INTERFERE WITH DRUGS

Natural Medicine	Known Drug Interactions
Ephedra	Theophylline (P)
Garlic	Anticoagulants (P), saquinavir (I)
Ginkgo leaf extract	Anticoagulants (P)
Glucosamine	Antidiabetic drugs (I)
Panax ginseng	Anticoagulants (P)
Saw palmetto	Hormone replacement therapies (P)
Soy	Estrogenic drugs (P)
St. John's wort	Antidepressants (P), HIV protease inhibitors (I), cyclosporine (I)
Valerian	Sedatives (P)
Yohimbe	Antihypertensives (I)

HIV = human immunodeficiency virus; I = interfere; P = potentiate.

Risks

That many complementary and alternative medicine practices are rooted in ancient health care systems and may involve natural products has been taken by many as ample proof of their safety if not also their effectiveness. This assumption is frequently incorrect. Few complementary and alternative medicine approaches have been studied rigorously, and some have not held up to scientific scrutiny at all. Despite millennia of empirically derived practices regarding which herbal medicines should be considered for a given condition (and in what form, quantity, and duration), Americans consume many such agents with impunity. It is common for individuals to self-medicate with dozens of different tablets, capsules, and liquid extracts daily. In the United States, there are no accepted standards for the manufacture, composition, or purity of herbal medicines. On occasion, products shown by the FDA to be inherently toxic, contaminated with toxic materials, or adulterated with proprietary drugs have been withdrawn. The Federal Trade Commission also has cited manufacturers for making unsubstantiated claims about their products. Many of the most popular dietary supplements have been shown to interact with conventional drugs and to affect their potential clinical effectiveness (Table 36–1).

A major concern regarding complementary and alternative medicine approaches is that an individual might choose them instead of mainstream practices that are known to be effective. Because few patients inform physicians about their consumption of dietary supplements and few physicians inquire about them, potential problems emerge in many clinical settings. Patients who consume medicinal herbs known to interfere with coagulation may be at increased risk of hemorrhage after surgery. With the increased awareness of the use and potential hazards of complementary and alternative medicine, more practitioners and institutions have begun to incorporate relevant questions into routine interactions with patients. By knowing what a patient is using and considering its potential hazards, the physician can begin to address the level of evidence supporting or negating a complementary and alternative medicine approach.

Evidence Base

If a modality were rigorously proven and widely accepted as such, it would no longer be considered complementary or alternative. The basis for claims regarding complementary and alternative medicine is frequently anecdotal, an aggregate of empirical observations, or a retrospective case series. Nonetheless, there have been hundreds of prospective controlled studies involving selected complementary and alternative medicine approaches. Thoughtful reviews of the data regarding some complementary and alternative medicine modalities have been conducted, including dozens by the members of the Cochrane Collaboration (*www3.Interscience.wiley.com/cgi-bin/mrwhome/106568753/HOME*). Many complementary and alternative medicine studies are flawed because of inadequate sample size, poor design, lack of blinding even when it is feasible, and failure to incorporate objective or standardized outcome instruments.

Credible information resources for the patient and the practitioner are accruing. Public databases such as PubMed of the National Library of Medicine highlight a complementary medicine subset with hundreds of thousands of articles. The National Cancer Institute and the National Center for Complementary and Alternative Medicine of the National Institutes of Health maintain active websites *(www.nih.gov)* that post relevant complementary and alternative medicine information. The database *ClinicalTrials.gov* lists all National Institutes of Health–supported clinical studies of complementary and alternative medical approaches that are actively accruing patients.

Failed Approaches

Desperation has long driven people to seek alternative and even radical therapies. A glimmer of hope, however faint, can be appealing; a mere anecdote can prove persuasive. Nonetheless, there is no justification for people to elect unconventional treatments when there is abundant evidence that such therapies are unsafe (Table 36–2) or ineffective.

An instructive example of a failed approach is that of laetrile, a cyanide-containing extract of apricot seeds. Through the 1970s, anecdotes and media reports that laetrile cured thousands of patients with inoperable cancers fanned public demand for the product. Finally, the National Cancer Institute funded two substantive prospective studies showing no clear evidence that laetrile could induce a partial or complete remission from cancer; these findings led to a dramatic reduction in requests for the product. Although laetrile remains available to determined and desperate patients, far fewer seek it today than in the 1970s. In the open-market environment in which alternative treatments are widely available, the fact that clear evidence affects consumers' demand may be as good a public health outcome as could be expected.

Acceptable Approaches

In considering complementary and alternative medicine approaches, patients and physicians must look to practices that at least make sense on the basis of clinical experience and what might be known of their mechanisms of action. Healthy skepticism must be balanced with thoughtful empiricism. Two categories of potentially acceptable complementary and alternative therapies exist: supportive approaches and specific therapies.

Supportive Approaches

Many complementary and alternative medicine practices are based on core elements that always have been a part of good medicine, what is known as the three T's—talk, touch, and time. It is unworthy of good medicine to have abandoned these core elements under the pressure of limited time or because of the emergence of more powerful technologies. Most current physicians cannot auscultate the chest or palpate a spleen as well as leading practitioners of prior generations, and modern imaging techniques are far better than physical diagnosis for detecting many pathologic changes. For reasons that might be cultural or even biologic, however, patients respond better to practitioners who listen well, care enough to touch them, and explain their findings and decisions. In the aggregate, these facets of the traditional physician-patient relationship may contribute to the placebo effect that facilitates healing. Rather than implying that a patient who recovers while receiving an inert substance was never really ill, placebos appear to operate through specific physiologic mechanisms. For example, imaging research indicates that placebos activate opioid receptor transmission, which may affect pain perception.

Anything that can relieve or distract a person suffering from severe pain can be a sensible approach (Chapter 28). Only in more recent years has pain management emerged as a distinct specialty, and its tools extend well beyond the wise and adequate use of narcotic analgesics. Increasingly, massage, yoga, and relaxation approaches have found their way into mainstream pain management. The evidence supporting acupuncture and hypnosis for some forms of pain is promising, but similar evidence is not available for many other complementary and alternative approaches to pain. Nonetheless, it is sensible to pursue some of these approaches in a logical and coherent sequence.

Contemporary medicine has acknowledged its historical shortcomings not only in pain management but also in the broader arena of palliative and end-of-life care (e.g., the success of the hospice movement) (Chapter 3). Dying patients need relief from pain or nausea; they also may seek spiritual guidance and a means to bring closure to their careers and their interactions with family and friends. Dying patients fear isolation, dependency, and the loss of intellectual and physical faculties. Hospitals have long housed chaplains, psychiatric social workers, and physical therapists. Increasingly, hospitals and hospice also are providing massage, art or music therapy, group counseling, meditation, and supportive services for the caregiver and the patient. These and other approaches to palliative care are increasingly being studied as strategies to enhance quality at the end of life.

Specific Therapies

Ubiquitous advertising might be all that some individuals need to be enticed to buy and use medicinal herbs. When published case series and pilot trials suggest that a product might be beneficial and there is little to indicate it is unsafe, the physician might be comfortable with the patient's wish to use it—especially if the patient is not neglecting more important health issues and proven effective therapies, if the patient can afford it, and if the complementary and alternative medicine seems to help and not cause side effects.

Valerian is an herb often consumed as a tea for improved sleep. Melatonin is a pineal hormone touted for the same purposes. Small studies suggest they might relieve insomnia, and there may be little harm in a trial course of either agent. Echinacea has long been taken to treat or to prevent colds, just as are zinc or high doses of vitamins. As yet, only moderate-sized studies have been conducted with echinacea or zinc, and their outcomes have been conflicting. Large trials of high doses of oral vitamin C showed little if any benefit in preventing or treating the common cold. Although there are not adequate data to recommend these agents, there also is no great urgency to demand they be abandoned. In talking with a patient, the physician instead might emphasize important health measures, such as avoidance of addictive substances, timely vaccination, and compliance with prescribed diet, exercise, and medications, rather than try to influence the patient's use of unproven but apparently safe complementary and alternative measures.

Encouraging Approaches

Physician and patients should be most comfortable in advising or accepting a complementary and alternative medicine approach when data from one or more fairly well designed, randomized controlled trials support it. Comparisons across trials are complicated by the absence of dosing guidelines for natural products or standardized protocols for practitioner-based intervention. Table 36–3 highlights some encouraging approaches that are now under increasingly rigorous scrutiny.

Herbal and Biochemical Medicine

Nature has long been the inspiration for and source of medicines, many of which are derived from plants, molds, or bacteria, including digoxin, morphine, aspirin, quinine, vincristine, taxol, the statins, penicillin, and cyclosporine. Although combinatorial chemistry provides more efficient ways to discover active agents, the screening of natural product repositories, especially if it is guided by claims of native practitioners, still yields promising compounds for drug development. One example is a new class of antimalarial drugs based on artemisinin, an extract of a plant used for treatment of fevers for more than 2000 years

TABLE 36–2 SOME NATURAL PRODUCTS WITH POTENTIALLY SERIOUS ADVERSE EFFECTS

Product	Adverse Effect
Aristolochia	Nephrotoxicity, carcinogenicity
Chaparral	Cholestatic hepatitis
Comfrey	Acute and chronic hepatitis
Digitalis leaf	Arrhythmias
Ephedra	Hypertension, stroke
Germander	Acute and chronic hepatitis
Khat	Tachycardia, psychosis
Kombucha	Hepatotoxicity, lactic acidosis
Mistletoe	Anaphylaxis
Skullcap	Seizures, acute and chronic hepatitis

TABLE 36-3 SOME COMPLEMENTARY AND ALTERNATIVE MEDICINE APPROACHES WITH ENCOURAGING CLINICAL RESULTS

Modality	Possible Indication
Artemisinin	Malaria
Acupuncture	Pain of osteoarthritis, nausea from chemotherapy
Chiropractic manipulation	Uncomplicated low back pain
Ginkgo biloba leaf extract	Dementia
Glucosamine, chondroitin sulfate	Osteoarthritis
Horse chestnut	Chronic venous insufficiency
Hypnosis	Pain
Omega-3 fish oils	Hyperlipidemia, depression
S-Adenosylmethionine	Osteoarthritis, depression
Saw palmetto	Benign prostatic hyperplasia
St. John's wort	Mild depressive illnesses

in southern China. Although plants serve as sources for discrete new chemical entities, it is also possible, as believed by herbal medicine advocates, that the aggregate of chemicals in an herb is superior to any of its constituents.

There are several medicinal herbs and natural substances for which existing data are encouraging. Extracts of *Ginkgo biloba* are well standardized and prescribed as drugs in Germany and most other European Union countries for prevention and treatment of dementia. This practice is supported by small but placebo-controlled, double-blind trials that in the aggregate show a significant improvement in cognitive performance in patients with Alzheimer's disease.

Glucosamine and chondroitin sulfate are found in the ground substance of cartilage. Crude extracts containing these agents are administered widely alone or in combination for the treatment and prevention of osteoarthritis, not only in humans but also in dogs and horses. Among 14 randomized controlled trials, 12 have found glucosamine to be superior to placebo for osteoarthritis. In one study of 1583 randomized subjects with painful knee osteoarthritis, followed for 24 weeks, glucosamine and chondroitin did not show overall benefit compared with placebo. However, for patients in the moderate-to-severe pain subgroup, glucosamine and chondroitin did provide statistically significant relief from pain, compared with placebo. [1]

St. John's wort, used for centuries to treat depression, was not found to be effective in treating moderate-to-severe major depression in a large, randomized trial. Smaller investigations continue to suggest that the herb may be beneficial for mild depression.

Acupuncture

Thousands of publications attest to the benefits of acupuncture, but few are scientific. Nonetheless, careful laboratory investigations have shown the induction of opioid-dependent brain pathways by which acupuncture might mediate an analgesic effect. In the aggregate, the research findings suggest its consideration in selected settings, although data are conflicting for well-studied indications, such as osteoarthritis of the knee and nausea associated with cancer drugs. A wristband that applies pressure to an "acupoint" associated with nausea was approved for management of seasickness by the FDA.

Spinal Manipulation

Manipulation is practiced most frequently by chiropractic and osteopathic physicians. Massage therapists practice their own specific forms of manipulation. Among all of the target indications for manipulation, its merits for treatment of back pain have been addressed the most. Although the conclusions from these studies are controversial, the aggregate data suggest that spinal manipulation for low back pain is superior to bedrest and at least equivalent to results with nonsteroidal drugs or back training exercises. [2]

PROSPECTS

Conventional medical practice may not evolve, as some have espoused, to a system in which patients are greeted routinely in a multimodality practice by a team of homeopaths, chiropractic and Ayurvedic physicians, herbalists, and spiritual counselors as well as by conventional physicians and nurses. There is no question, however, that patients increasingly are offered a menu of choices that is greater and more diverse than ever before. Witness the emergence of specialties and allied health professions that were unforeseen a generation ago. Today's patients interact with legions of medical technologists, therapists, counselors, dietitians, and hygienists, not to mention interventional radiologists, clinical psychopharmacologists, or cellular and molecular biologists in the guise of gene and stem cell therapists.

The question is, What elements of today's complementary and alternative medicine should become *integrated* into tomorrow's normative practice? The willingness of practitioners to commit adequate time, to listen carefully to patients, and to touch them physically and emotionally must remain part of conventional medicine. There are no longer any doubts that proper diet, exercise, intellectual and social engagement, and avoidance of stress and addictive substances are beneficial practices. Physicians must be trained to incorporate these messages into their routine interactions with patients. It also is appropriate that physicians acquaint themselves with other practices to which their patients might be drawn and negotiate thoughtfully and openly about their use to achieve the best outcome. It is unreasonable to expect physicians to master the rudiments of disciplines such as acupuncture, but they should understand how to access the evidence base and identify referrals as appropriate.

Complementary and alternative medicine, in some incarnation, is here to stay. It is important to appreciate the public interest and follow the scientific efforts that are under way to address its tenets as fairly and rigorously as possible.

The encouraging existing reports of several products, such as *Ginkgo biloba*, are under scrutiny in large, placebo-controlled, randomized multicenter trials involving thousands of patients. Studies such as these will help transform the question from does it work to should one recommend it?

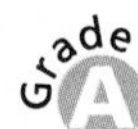

1. Clegg DO, Reda DJ, Harris CL, et al: Glucosamine, chondroitin sulfate, and the two in combination for painful knee osteoarthritis. N Engl J Med 2006;354:795–808.
2. Cherkin D, Deyo RA, Battie M, et al: A comparison of physical therapy, chiropractic manipulation, and provision of an educational booklet for the treatment of patients with low back pain. N Engl J Med 1998;339:1021–1029.

SUGGESTED READINGS

Bardia A, Barton DL, Prokop LJ, et al: Efficacy of complementary and alternative medicine therapies in relieving cancer pain: A systematic review. J Clin Oncol 2006;24:5457–5464. *None of these therapies has been proved to be effective.*

Barnes PM, Powell-Griner E, McFann K, Nahin RL: Complementary and alternative medicine use among adults: United States, 2002. Advance Data from Vital and Health Statistics; no. 343. Hyattsville, MD, National Center for Health Statistics, 2004, pp 1–20. *Reports national patterns of use.*

Berman BM, Lao L, Langenberg P, et al: Effectiveness of acupuncture as adjunctive therapy in osteoarthritis of the knee. Ann Intern Med 2004;141:901–910. *Showed benefit in a randomized trial of 570 patients.*

Ezzo JM, Richardson MA, Vickers A, et al: Acupuncture-point stimulation for chemotherapy-induced nausea or vomiting. Cochrane Database Systemic Rev 2006;(2)CD22285. *Meta-analysis suggesting a benefit.*

Goldberg RJ, Katz J: A meta-analysis of the analgesic effects of omega-3 polyunsaturated fatty acid supplementation for inflammatory joint pain. Pain 2007;129:210–223. *Patients reported benefits, but physician-assessed pain was not reduced.*

Nedrow A, Miller J, Walker M, et al: Complementary and alternative therapies for the management of menopause-related symptoms: A systematic evidence review. Arch Intern Med 2006;166:1453–1465. *Insufficient data to support efficacy of any complementary or alternative therapy.*

Niggemann B, Gruber C: Side-effects of complementary and alternative medicine. Allergy 2003;58:707–716. *Cautions about the many potential hazards.*

Scharf HP, Mansmann U, Streitberger K, et al: Acupuncture and knee osteoarthritis. Ann Intern Med 2006;145:12–20. *Randomized trial showing no significant benefit in 1007 patients.*

Section VI

Genetics

37 PRINCIPLES OF GENETICS: OVERVIEW OF THE PARADIGM OF GENETIC CONTRIBUTION TO HEALTH AND DISEASE

Bruce R. Korf

The elucidation of the structure and function of the genome is one of the great scientific triumphs of the 20th century. The relevance of inheritance to health and disease probably has been recognized throughout history, but it is only during the last century that the rules governing inheritance and the mechanisms whereby genetic information is stored and used have come to light. The application of this knowledge to medical practice so far has focused on relatively rare monogenic and chromosomal disorders. Major contributions have been made in these areas in the form of approaches to genetic counseling, genetic testing, prenatal diagnosis, newborn screening, carrier screening, and, to a limited extent, treatment. As important as these contributions are, however, their impact has been limited by the rarity of these disorders. New powerful tools resulting from the Human Genome Project are changing this situation. Genetic factors that contribute to common and rare disorders are being identified and will result in new approaches to diagnosis, prevention, and treatment. Genetics and genomics increasingly are going to occupy center stage in medical practice, guiding treatment decisions and preventive strategies. This chapter reviews the paradigm whereby genetics will be integrated into the routine practice of medicine.

GENETIC CONTRIBUTION TO DISEASE

It may be argued that no disorder is either completely determined genetically or completely determined by nongenetic factors. Even monogenic conditions, such as phenylketonuria, are modified by the environment, in this case by dietary intake of phenylalanine. Genetically determined host factors are known to modify susceptibility to infection or other environmental agents. Even individuals who are victims of trauma may find themselves at risk in part because of genetic traits that affect behavior or ability to perceive or escape from danger.

Multifactorial Inheritance

Complex traits that are important for both health and disease are the result of an interaction of multiple genes with one another and with the environment (Fig. 37–1). In some cases, individual genes or environmental factors contribute overwhelmingly to the cause of a disorder, as with a genetic condition, such as neurofibromatosis or Marfan syndrome, or an acquired disorder, such as bacterial infection or trauma. Other times, there may be interplay among many factors, making it difficult to dissect out the specific genes or environmental exposures.

From a medical perspective, it is helpful to divide the genetic contribution to disease into three categories: high-penetrance monogenic or chromosomal disorders, monogenic versions of common disorders, and complex, multifactorial disorders. Each of these has an impact on medical practice in distinctive ways.

High-Penetrance Monogenic or Chromosomal Disorders

High-penetrance monogenic or chromosomal disorders are the disorders that most clinicians think of as "genetic conditions." They include rare but familiar single-gene disorders, such as neurofibromatosis, Marfan syndrome, and cystic fibrosis, and chromosomal abnormalities, such as trisomy 21 (Down syndrome). At present, several thousand distinct human genetic disorders have been described and cataloged in *Mendelian Inheritance in Man* (available at *www.ncbi.nlm.nih.gov/Omim/*). These include mendelian dominant or recessive disorders, sex-linked disorders, and conditions that are due to mutations within the 16.6-kilobase mitochondrial genome. They also include major chromosomal aneuploidy syndromes and syndromes resulting from duplication or deletion of small regions of the genome that result in either reproducible syndromes, such as Williams syndrome (deletion of contiguous loci from a region of chromosome 7), or nonspecific mental retardation.

Role of the Nonspecialist

The internist or primary care physician plays a crucial role in the care of individuals with these disorders and faces significant challenges. Because of the rarity of many of these conditions, most practitioners have limited experience with a given disorder and are likely to need to refer the patient to an appropriate specialist for assistance with diagnosis and management. Nevertheless, the nonspecialist has many distinct roles in the care of these patients. These roles begin with the recognition of the fact that the patient may have a disorder and arrangement for appropriate diagnostic evaluation. Many genetic disorders produce obvious signs or symptoms that at least prompt referral even if they are not immediately suggestive of a diagnosis. Others can be more subtle, with nevertheless significant consequences if the diagnosis is missed. An example is Marfan syndrome (Chapter 281). The physician needs to be alert to the physical characteristics of patients with Marfan syndrome because life-threatening aortic dissection can be avoided with appropriate monitoring and treatment with β-blockers or surgery. Table 37–1 lists examples of some adult-onset monogenic conditions with which the internist should be familiar.

Treatment of Patients with Genetic Disorders

The treatment of patients with genetic disorders may require the assistance of a specialist, but the nonspecialist is likely to be the first contact when an affected individual is ill. The primary care physician needs to be familiar with the disorder and major potential complications. For example, the patient with neurofibromatosis who experiences chronic back pain may be presenting with a malignant peripheral nerve sheath tumor, requiring more aggressive evaluation than would be typical for an unaffected individual with back pain. Formation of a good working relationship between the specialist and nonspecialist is crucial to ensure effective care.

The nonspecialist also has a crucial role in supporting the patient and helping to explain the difficult choices that may be offered for management. This includes providing support for patients who have disorders that cannot be treated and for the emotional impact that accompanies knowledge that a disorder may be transmitted to one's offspring or shared with other relatives. Most patients have little understanding of the mechanisms of genetics and genetic disease. Although the responsibility to explain these issues may reside with specialists and counselors, the primary care provider has an important supportive role.

Advances in Genetics

Although many of the disorders in this group have been known for a long time, more recent advances in genetics have had a substantial impact on approaches to diagnosis and management. Genetic testing has been refined with the advent of molecular diagnostic tests that detect mutations within individual genes. Even rare disorders may be amenable to diagnostic testing; a database of testing laboratories can be found on the Internet (available at *www.genetests.org*). Population screening for carrier status of some disorders now is offered routinely. Some tests are targeted to particular ethnic groups, such as Ashkenazi Jews (Tay-Sachs disease, Canavan's disease, cystic fibrosis, Gaucher's disease) or individuals of African, Mediterranean, or Asian ancestry (hemoglobinopathies) (Table 37–2). Panethnic screening is now being made available for cystic fibrosis, although risks differ in different ethnic groups. Newborn screening is being expanded beyond inborn errors of metabolism such as phenylketonuria and galactosemia, particularly with the advent of tandem mass spectrometry. Efforts are now under way to standardize the screening panel from state to state. Finally, treatment of some monogenic disorders is becoming feasible. Life expectancy for patients with cystic fibrosis has been increasing gradually with better treatments for chronic lung disease; dietary therapy is available for many inborn errors of metabolism; novel therapies that use either pharmaceuticals or gene or enzyme replacement strategies are beginning to be tested for many conditions. The principles of management of genetic disorders are evolving rapidly so that care of patients increasingly requires active partnership of appropriate specialists and primary care providers.

Monogenic Versions of Common Disorders

Not all monogenic disorders produce obscure phenotypes, and not all common disorders are due to complex multifactorial causes. In more recent years, it has been recognized that some common disorders occur in some families as single-gene traits (Table 37–3). This is usually true for only a proportion of affected individuals; but in some cases, it is a significant proportion and represents an important group of patients to be recognized.

Breast Cancer

An example is breast cancer. About 7% of cases of this common form of cancer can be attributed to mutation in one of two genes, *BRCA1* or *BRCA2*. Women who inherit a mutation in one of these genes face a high risk of eventually developing breast or ovarian cancer—80% by age 70 years, depending in part on the specific mutation. Women at risk because of mutation do not look different from women with sporadic breast cancer but can be distinguished by many features, including family history of breast or ovarian cancer in multiple relatives, early age at onset of cancer, and multifocality of the cancer (e.g., bilateral breast cancer or breast and ovarian cancer).

Colon Cancer

Another example from cancer genetics is colon cancer. Two syndromes, familial adenomatous polyposis and hereditary nonpolyposis colon cancer, are autosomal dominantly inherited and convey a high risk of colon cancer. Other noncancer examples are hemochromatosis (Chapter 231), in which cirrhosis, cardiomyopathy, diabetes, joint disease, and other problems ensue from excessive iron absorption; 10% of whites carry an allele that predisposes to this recessive disorder. Mutations in the factor V gene or the prothrombin gene occur commonly and predispose to deep venous thrombosis. Rarer examples include inherited forms of cardiomyopathy, hypertension, and familial hypercholesterolemia.

Management

The physician may be called on to address these disorders in many ways. There is a compelling reason to make an early diagnosis of

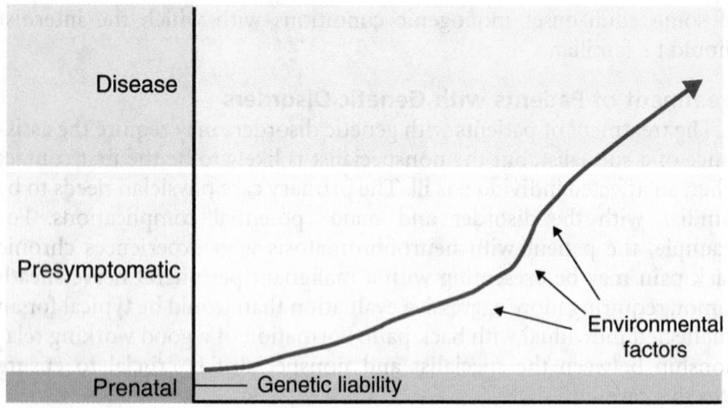

FIGURE 37–1 • Multifactorial etiology of disease. An individual is born with a genetic liability but remains in a presymptomatic state for some time until additional events occur, including exposure to environmental factors, that result in crossing a threshold that is identified as *disease*. In instances of high-penetrance monogenic disorders, the genetic liability may be overwhelming. In other instances, genetic factors may contribute only slightly to disease risk.

TABLE 37–2 MAJOR RECESSIVE DISORDERS FOR WHICH CARRIER SCREENING COMMONLY IS OFFERED IN THE UNITED STATES

Disorder	Major At-Risk Population	Carrier Frequency
Cystic fibrosis	White	1:25
	Ashkenazi Jewish	1:29
Sickle cell anemia	African American	1:10
β-Thalassemia	Mediterranean	1:60
α-Thalassemia	Southeast Asian, Chinese	1:50
Tay-Sachs disease	Ashkenazi Jewish	1:30
	French Canadian	1:30
Canavan's disease	Ashkenazi Jewish	1:40

TABLE 37–1 HIGH-PENETRANCE SINGLE-GENE DISORDERS THAT MAY PRESENT IN ADULTHOOD, WITH SOME MAJOR MEDICAL IMPLICATIONS*

Disorder	Inheritance	Major Medical Implications
CARDIOVASCULAR		
Marfan syndrome	AD	Risk of aortic dissection; lens dislocation
Long QT syndrome	AD, AR	Arrhythmia, sudden death
RENAL		
Adult polycystic kidney disease	AD	Renal failure
PULMONARY		
α_1-Antitrypsin deficiency	AR	Emphysema, cirrhosis
NEUROLOGIC		
NF1	AD	Benign and malignant nerve sheath tumors, gliomas
NF2	AD	Schwannomas (especially vestibular), meningiomas
von Hippel–Lindau	AD	Hemangioblastoma of cerebellum, brainstem, eye; pheochromocytoma; renal cell carcinoma
Huntington's disease	AD	Movement disorder, psychiatric disorder, dementia
HEMATOLOGIC		
Globin disorders	AR	Stroke, iron overload
ENDOCRINE		
MEN syndromes	AD	Tumors of thyroid and parathyroid, pheochromocytoma

*See Table 37–3 for examples of lower penetrance disorders.
AD = autosomal dominant; AR = autosomal recessive; MEN = multiple endocrine neoplasia; NF = neurofibromatosis.

Section VI Genetics

TABLE 37–3 SINGLE-GENE DISORDERS WITH INCOMPLETE PENETRANCE THAT MAY ACCOUNT FOR INHERITED FORMS OF SELECTED COMMON DISORDERS

Disorder	Inheritance: Genes	Major Medical Implications
Hemochromatosis	AR: *HFE*	Cirrhosis, cardiomyopathy, diabetes mellitus
Thrombophilia	AD, AR: multiple genes	Deep venous thrombosis
Breast and ovarian cancers	AD: *BRCA1, BRCA2*	Breast and ovarian cancers
Familial adenomatous polyposis	AD: *APC*	Multiple colonic polyps, colon cancer
Hereditary nonpolyposis colorectal cancer	AD: DNA mismatch repair genes	Colorectal cancer, endometrial cancer
Maturity-onset diabetes of the young	AD: multiple genes	Diabetes mellitus
Cardiomyopathy	AD: genes involved in cardiac contractile apparatus	Arrhythmia, heart failure

AD = autosomal dominant; AR = autosomal recessive.

hemochromatosis because the complications can be prevented, but not reversed, by phlebotomy and subsequent monitoring of iron stores. Individuals at risk of colon cancer can be offered surveillance with colonoscopy or surgical resection of the colon to reduce the risk of cancer. Individuals at risk of breast and ovarian cancer likewise can be offered surveillance or surgery. The benefits of knowledge of genetic risks are less clear in some instances. Carriers of the factor V Leiden mutation would not be treated with anticoagulation until after an event of thrombosis, and the treatment may not be different for a carrier versus a noncarrier. In some cases, knowledge of carrier status might help ensure prompt diagnosis, however.

Genetic Testing

As with other medical tests, the physician should carefully consider risks, benefits, and clinical utility in deciding to use a genetic test. Some distinct ethical and legal risks may apply to some genetic tests. These may include anxiety, stigmatization, guilt, and possibly discrimination for insurance or employment. Some of these risks may be addressed by legislation to maintain privacy of genetic information, but the risks of anxiety, guilt, and stigmatization cannot be legislated away. To some extent, further research may improve the basis for surveillance or lead to effective treatments. For now, many of these disorders present a double-edged sword of potentially useful knowledge and potentially harmful information.

Role of the Physician

The role of the physician in dealing with monogenic disorders includes recognition of individuals at risk and participation in formulation of a care plan. Individuals at risk cannot be identified by physical appearance and usually are not evident from medical history or physical examination findings. The most valuable screening tool is the family history. Directed questioning about a family history of major monogenic disorders, especially breast, ovarian, and colon cancer, as well as hypercholesterolemia, hypertension, deep venous thrombosis, cirrhosis, and diabetes can identify the relatively rare patient with mendelian segregation of these common disorders. Even if the information is of uncertain reliability, eliciting a family history can prompt referral for further evaluation, documentation of the family history, and consideration for genetic testing. The physician's job is not only to identify individuals at risk; some people believe they are at high risk even in the absence of well-documented risk factors. Addressing these misconceptions can bring peace of mind and usually does not require genetic testing.

In some instances, there may be a role for tests to screen for inherited disorders. The utility of screening for hemochromatosis has been considered on the basis of the argument that diagnosis before the onset of complications can avoid major morbidity and mortality. The utility of genetic testing is limited by incomplete penetrance of common *HFE* gene mutations, making it uncertain whether an individual with an at-risk genotype will develop iron overload. Screening for elevated iron stores and transferrin saturation may prove to be a better approach.

It is likely that the number of conditions in this category will increase in the coming years as genes that predispose to other common disorders are discovered. Although most affected individuals have only a small genetic contribution to their condition, a subset has a much more substantial genetic component. Discussions about the appropriateness of testing, surveillance, screening, and treatment are likely to increase in intensity in the near future.

Complex, Multifactorial Disorders

Understanding the genetics of common disorders is one of the great challenges of modern medicine, with the promise of major returns in terms of prevention, diagnosis, and treatment. The etiology of these disorders is complex in that they result from an interaction of multiple genes with one another and with environmental factors. The specific genes that are relevant may be different from one person to the next. Identification of these genes is difficult given this heterogeneity and the relatively small impact that any particular gene may have in a particular person.

Population Studies

Dissection of the genetic contribution to common disease cannot be accomplished by the standard genetic approaches involving study of rare variants or family-based linkage studies. Most recent efforts have focused on study of large groups of patients, comparing the prevalence of particular genetic markers in case patients and control subjects. The availability of markers has been boosted by the identification of single-nucleotide polymorphisms (SNPs). These are differences in single DNA bases between individuals that occur every several hundred bases. Some of these account for common genetic differences between people, including differences that may contribute to disease. The map of SNPs currently includes several million variants; it has been found that the genome has evolved as blocks of clusters of genes, making it possible to use only a limited number of SNPs within a given region to determine whether there is a gene in that region that is associated with a disease. The completion of the HapMap Project, which has provided a catalog of SNP blocks in humans, is expected to accelerate the identification of SNPs that are associated with common disorders.

The problem of establishing disease associations is made more difficult by differences between affected individuals and especially between large ethnic groups. This can result in spurious associations in case-control studies. To some extent, this problem is ameliorated by study of triads of an affected child and parents, but these studies are limited to instances in which nuclear families can be recruited for study.

It is likely that genetic risk factors for common disorders will come to light gradually during the next several years. The information derived from this effort probably will be used in a variety of ways but especially in risk assessment, disease stratification, and development of new approaches to treatment.

Genetic Testing

The goal of genetic risk assessment is the identification of individuals at risk of disease before the onset of signs or symptoms. In principle, the genetic factors could be identified at birth, or any time in life, by testing a DNA sample. Individuals found to be at risk might be offered treatment in advance of onset of the disease to avoid complications or might be advised to modify their lifestyle to avoid exposure to environmental factors that might increase their risk of disease.

Although this would appear to be an attractive paradigm, many questions may be raised about its practicality and implementation. First, predictive testing would be useful only insofar as it guides further management. This is likely to be a moving target because ability to test for risk can be developed more quickly than ability to modify that risk. The utility of interventions may be valued differently by different people. This already has been the case for testing of disorders such as breast cancer. Some women at risk choose not to know their *BRCA1* status because the options, including surveillance or prophylactic surgery, are unacceptable to them. If there were a low-cost, safe, and effective treatment that would neutralize any risk, the decision to test would be simple, but short of that, there are reasonable arguments on both sides of the issue of whether to test. For many disorders, it will take a long time to show the efficacy of any intervention because there may be a period of many years between the test and the onset of a disorder. Unless surrogate markers can be identified and followed, the task of proving a benefit to predictive testing may require years to decades in some instances.

Predictive value of Genetic Testing

A second issue surrounds the degree to which genetic testing would be predictive. Most genetic tests are likely to involve detection of relatively common polymorphic alleles that account for small increments of relative risk of disease. The predictive value of these tests would be modest, perhaps too low to induce an individual to modify behavior or to take medication. Here, again, much depends on the efficacy of any intervention that can be offered. There may be some disorders for which testing would have substantial predictive value and clinical utility and others for which testing would not be justified.

Social and Ethical Issues

A third concern relates to social and ethical issues. Will people use test results as an excuse to pursue self-destructive behaviors, having received what may be false reassurance of "immunity"? Will genetic testing further exacerbate the divide between individuals who can afford to pay for their care and those who cannot? Will individuals found to be at risk of disease on the basis of genetic testing become part of an underclass in terms of employability or insurability? Will people misinterpret results of testing in terms of a simplistic notion of genetic determinism, erroneously believing that their futures have been written, leaving them no recourse but to meet their fate? The rapid pace of technologic change is going to challenge the ability of the social and legal systems to keep pace.

Disease Stratification

A second application of genomics in medical practice entails stratification of disease. Even if genetic testing is not used to predict individuals at risk, it may well be used to determine the most appropriate treatment for a clinically diagnosed disorder. Probably most common disorders, such as hypertension and diabetes, are symptom complexes that result from a variety of causes. The particular combination of causes may differ in different individuals and may respond to different types of treatments. Choice of antihypertensive drug may depend at some point on genetic testing to determine the specific cause of hypertension in a patient. There are already examples of genotypes that predict response to commonly used drugs, for example, in asthma. Although they are not yet ready for routine clinical use, eventually it is possible that genetic tests will accompany many if not most treatment decisions.

Effects and Identification of Drugs

Aside from helping to choose the most efficacious drug, genetic testing may play a role in avoidance of side effects and in appropriate dosing. Many drugs are known to be associated with rare side effects, some of which are sufficiently severe as to lead the drug to be withdrawn from use. Some of these side effects may occur only in individuals who are susceptible on the basis of having a particular allele at a polymorphic locus. An example is the association of polymorphisms in certain sodium or potassium channel genes with risk of arrhythmia on exposure to specific drugs.

Absorption and metabolism of drugs is largely under genetic control. Several polymorphisms are known to lead to particularly rapid or slow metabolism, accounting for individuals who experience dose-related side effects or lack of efficacy at standard dosages (Table 37–4). Detection of these polymorphisms would allow customization of drug dosage to an individual's pattern of metabolism, increasing the likelihood of efficacy without a prolonged period of trial-and-error dosing.

The greatest gift of genetics and genomics to medicine may be in the ability to identify new drug targets and develop new approaches to treatment. Identification of genes that contribute to common disorders is revealing the cellular mechanisms that lead to disease. This knowledge offers the opportunity to develop new pharmaceutical agents that would target the physiologic mechanisms more precisely, leading to drugs that work better and cause fewer side effects. New approaches to gene replacement or insertion of genes into cells as localized drug delivery systems also may be developed. The treatment of common disorders likely would entail use of treatments developed as a result of genomics even in cases in which genetic testing is not used to predict individuals who are at risk.

TABLE 37–4 GENES IN WHICH COMMON POLYMORPHISMS AFFECT RATES OF DRUG METABOLISM

Gene	Medications (Examples)
CYP2C9	Phenytoin, warfarin
CYP2D6	Debrisoquin, β-blockers, antidepressants
Thiopurine methyltransferase	Mercaptopurine, azathioprine
N-Acetyltransferase	Isoniazid, hydralazine

CONCLUSION

The Human Genome Project began after most practicing physicians completed their medical training, and few are familiar with the methods and approaches of medical genetics and genomics. Nevertheless, physicians will be using the products of the genome project increasingly in their day-to-day practice during the coming years. Whether they are providing care for a patient with a rare genetic disorder or for a patient with a common condition not usually regarded as genetic, management choices increasingly will be informed by tests and treatments that in some way are based on information from the genome sequence.

The essence of the encounter between a physician and a patient can be distilled to two questions: Why this person? Why this time? A person who seeks medical care is doing so as the product of human evolution, as a member of an ethnic group with certain genetic vulnerabilities, because of inheritance of certain familial risk factors, because of exposure to some environmental factors, because of a particular physiologic process gone awry, because of behavioral traits that lead the person to seek medical care, because of prompting by family or friends to go to the doctor, because society makes medical services available, and because the person can afford to seek care. Genetics cannot answer all of these questions, but it is providing the key to addressing many of the biologic questions that underlie the medical mysteries that have puzzled humankind for generations.

SUGGESTED READINGS

Daly AK: Individualized drug therapy. Curr Opin Drug Discov Devel 2007; 10:29–36. *The promise of individualized treatments based on genetics and pharmacogenomics.*

Dervieux T, Bala MV: Overview of the pharmacoeconomics of pharmacogenetics. Pharmacogenomics 2006;7:1175–1184. *Practical examples of how pharmacogenomics can lead to cost-effective targeted treatment.*

Taylor MR, Edwards JG, Ku L: Lost in translation: Challenges in the expanding field of adult genetics. Am J Med Genet C Semin Med Genet 2006;142: 294–303. *Outlines an agenda for translating genetic advances into medical practice.*

GENETIC RISK ASSESSMENT

Margretta R. Seashore

UTILITY OF GENETIC RISK ASSESSMENT

Advances in genetics and genomics are making profound changes in medical practice. Using these advances, the physician can identify individuals at genetic risk and provide appropriate assessment and testing to aid in prevention and management of illness. The physician's response to questions and concerns about genetic risks depends on understanding how to identify these risks. Genetic factors confer an increased risk of developing a specific disorder compared with the prevalence of that disorder in the general population. Factors that result in increased genetic risk include genetic mutations that determine single-gene disorders, balanced chromosomal rearrangements, and genotypes that confer disease susceptibility. Multiple genes and environmental factors contribute to susceptibility to disease.

The challenge to the physician is to identify individuals and families who incur risks in time to provide information and interventions that may mitigate the risks or allow persons and families to make informed choices about them. Few well-controlled, prospective studies on genetic risk assessment exist. Current decision making depends on clinical observation and expert opinion. Nevertheless, a body of knowledge supports the utility of genetic assessment. Preventive therapy may enhance the medical care the physician can provide. Genetic risk information may offer the opportunity for reproductive decisions that enhance the chance for the birth of a healthy infant. Genetic testing can provide information that refines these risks. Ethnic background, medical history, and family history provide indicators of increased genetic risk and direct the kind of genetic testing to be done. When the physician and patient have decided that genetic testing will have a role in management of the patient, specific tests are selected and decisions about whom to test are made. This chapter addresses the use of genetic testing, ethnic background, and family history to refine the assessment of genetic risk in individuals and families.

Genetic Risk Assessment Using Genetic Testing

Genetic testing has been defined in the literature as the analysis of a specific gene, gene product or function, or other DNA or chromosome analysis to detect or exclude an alteration likely to be associated with a genetic disorder. This definition places the emphasis on the genetic test and correlation of the test result with the presence of, or predisposition to, a genetic disorder. The benefit of gene-based testing depends on many factors, including the characteristics of the test, the selection of whom to test and when to test, and an understanding of how to use the results of the test.

Characteristics of Genetic Tests

The development of gene-based diagnostic techniques for any disorder depends on understanding the disorder at the genetic level. The characteristics and the utility of the test are important factors in making the decision to use testing for assessment of genetic risk.

Validation

The precision and predictive value of gene-based testing determine whether a test is suitable. After investigators identify a new molecular or biochemical observation that correlates with disease, testing for the disease is developed on a research basis. Before research results can move into the clinical realm, tests for clinical use must undergo rigorous validation. The usual criteria to judge the validity of a medical test, including sensitivity, specificity, positive predictive value, and negative predictive value, must be determined. Technical standards and guidelines for performance and interpretation of genetic tests are in place. Laboratory testing in clinical use must conform to the requirements of the Clinical Laboratory Improvement Amendments of 1988 (CLIA). The Joint Test and Technology Transfer Committee Working Group of the American College of Medical Genetics (ACMG) and the College of American Pathologists have developed programs to help maintain quality assurance and proficiency standards for genetic testing. The ACMG provides position statements on the use of genetic testing in certain disorders.

After a test is known to provide reproducible results, the clinical utility of the test must be considered. Individual genetic testing may be helpful to confirm clinical findings when signs and symptoms suggest a genetic diagnosis. Genetic testing can provide assessment of increased risk for presymptomatic diagnosis. Finally, genetic testing can identify heterozygosity for genes that confer increased risk for adverse reproductive outcome when both members of the couple carry a mutation.

Selecting a Test

An understanding of the molecular pathology and the genetic heterogeneity of the disorder is crucial to the selection of an appropriate gene-based test. For some disorders, only a few mutations in a specific gene cause disease; these can be tested using DNA-based methods. DNA-based methods of gene testing include linkage studies of DNA haplotypes that are associated with disease (i.e., that segregate with the disorder) in a family, nucleic acid hybridization studies using DNA probes of normal and mutant sequences, polymerase chain reaction techniques that define specific DNA changes, and direct sequencing of DNA to identify mutations. Some DNA changes within a gene are normal polymorphisms and are not associated with increased disease risk. Some genetic alterations cannot be detected easily with today's technology. In conditions in which there are hundreds of different mutations or in which each affected family has a unique mutation, DNA-based methods may not be practical, and protein-based testing, such as enzymology and protein truncation studies, may provide more specific and more accurate information. In the future, expression testing based on microchip assays that show which proteins are being expressed may revolutionize genetic testing again. Gene expression profiling is under active study for use in cancer diagnosis and prediction of outcome of treatment. A recent example is the analysis of non–small cell lung cancers for selected mutations in the epidermal growth factor receptor, whose presence makes the tumor much more susceptible to a class of drugs that inhibit the kinase activity of the receptor. Microarray analysis in tissue samples may provide patterns that predict recurrence and survival in colorectal cancer. Clinical trials are underway to evaluate the utility of this approach in developing targeted therapy for breast and ovarian cancer.

Accuracy

In populations in which specific mutations and their frequencies are known, testing is highly accurate and predictive. For conditions in which a few specific mutations account for almost all the mutations within that population, gene-based testing can be straightforward, and detection of gene carriers may reach 90 to 95% or higher. If these correlations are not high, the utility of genetic testing is considerably less.

Predicting Clinical Outcome

Prediction of clinical outcome based on genetic testing depends on how well the genotype correlates with the phenotype. This correlation varies from one genetic disorder to another. Many single-gene disorders that manifest in childhood have a high correlation between genotype and phenotype. Examples include the four-base-pair insertion in exon 11 (4-bp ins, ex11) of the hexosaminidase A gene, which causes classic Tay-Sachs disease (TSD) in affected children of Ashkenazi Jewish ancestry. Another example is the glutamine-to-arginine substitution at protein position 188 (Q188R) in galactose-1-phosphate uridyltransferase, which is the classic severe galactosemia allele.

In selecting a genetic test, the physician must be aware of consequences of genetic locus heterogeneity, in which similar clinical disorders can result from mutations in different genes. This heterogeneity complicates genetic testing. For example, mutations in *BRCA1*, *BRCA2*, *TP53*, and *CHK2* can be associated with familial breast cancer. Before genetic testing can be of use to persons at risk for breast cancer in such a family, the associated mutation in an affected family member must be established. Even in the single-gene disorders that are inherited in a mendelian fashion, this kind of genetic heterogeneity adds to the complexity of testing. Genetic locus heterogeneity plays a role in such diverse conditions as Charcot-Marie-Tooth neuropathy, retinitis pigmentosa, and sensorineural deafness, each of which has multiple different genetic causes.

Defining the Purpose of the Test

The patient and the physician must consider the purpose of genetic testing when deciding whether to use a genetic test. They must have realistic expectations about the kind of information the test will provide and must determine whether multiple family members will need or wish to be tested. Integral to the process are communication of relevant information, obtaining consent, and providing results. For conditions in which there is a strong correlation between homozygosity or heterozygosity for specific mutations and clinical outcome, gene testing can provide clear guidance for selection of treatment options. To make the decision to use a genetic test, the patient and physician need to ask how well the test result predicts clinical outcome and what kind of action the physician or the patient can take based on the test result. Is there an effective treatment, a need for directed surveillance, or a reproductive option to select? Will a negative test result reduce the need for surveillance or invasive medical testing?

Deciding Whom and When to Test

Individuals and Families

Considerable ethical, legal, and social issues surround the use of genetic testing in individuals and families. Gene-based testing may uncover information about family members other than the individual who is being tested, and these persons frequently are not part of the decision to perform testing. If multiple family members are being tested, the results may reveal the fact that family biologic relationships are not what the family has believed. In families with multiple affected members, the results of testing may reveal who is and who is not at risk, and this information may cause grief or guilt in some tested members. Testing may not provide an answer in a particular family. Because these issues are complex, careful informed consent is an essential part of the process of obtaining genetic testing, and privacy of results must be assured. Communication of results requires sensitivity to all of these concerns.

Populations

Genetic testing can involve entire populations rather than single individuals or families. Population screening should identify treatable disease before symptoms occur, especially if the outcome may be improved by early identification. Such screening also can identify risk for adverse reproductive outcomes. Population-based screening includes public health measures, as in screening of newborns; community-based testing, as in TSD carrier screening; and practice-based testing, as in prenatal testing offered to all women.

Genetic Screening of Newborns

The experience gained in 40 years of screening of newborns shows a paradigm for widely based population genetic screening. Phenylketonuria (PKU), a disorder of phenylalanine metabolism that results in severe mental retardation, was the first disorder identified by newborn screening programs. The observation that early diagnosis of siblings of children with PKU and treatment of affected siblings with a phenylalanine-restricted diet resulted in normal cognitive development led, in 1962, to the establishment of newborn screening programs for PKU. These programs became the prototype for the development of newborn screening protocols for an increasing number of disorders. New methodology using tandem mass spectrometry has expanded the list of disorders that can be identified to more than 30. The success of newborn screening programs depends on the tracking and treatment programs that provide confirmatory testing, effective follow-up, and treatment for the disorders identified. Experience with PKU screening showed that what was thought to be a well-defined disorder also had variant, usually less severe forms not previously understood. Further outcome studies revealed that most of the disorders targeted in newborn screening programs show similar degrees of variation. Examples include the milder Duarte variant of galactosemia and the variability in age at onset of symptoms in medium-chain, acyl-coenzyme A dehydrogenase deficiency. Screening of newborns has enhanced understanding of long-term outcomes of the disorders screened and has identified surprising consequences, such as the teratogenic effects of high concentrations of blood phenylalanine in untreated maternal PKU. These programs have raised new considerations, such as the preservation of Guthrie cards for later use for other purposes, including identification in the event of kidnapping, diagnosis in the event of sudden death, and later research on genetic factors affecting health. The experience gained from screening of newborns also provides important guidance in the development of wider population-based genetic screening programs for adult-onset disorders.

Genetic Screening During Pregnancy

The adoption of screening panels for pregnant women or women contemplating pregnancy is another example of population-based genetic screening. This screening is offered to assess reproductive risk by identifying women who are heterozygous for genes that would be deleterious in the homozygous state. The tests offered are chosen based on population frequency of the disorder, ability to identify a substantial percentage of heterozygotes, severity of the disorder, and availability of reproductive options. Some tests are offered on the basis of increased risk based on ethnic background of the woman or her partner. Other tests are offered on the basis of maternal age, family history, or outcome of previous pregnancy. The American College of Obstetricians and Gynecologists (ACOG) and the ACMG have developed guidelines for prenatal screening. One recommendation is to offer testing for a panel of mutations in the *CFTR* gene that can identify at least 90% of heterozygotes for the alleles responsible for cystic fibrosis in a multiethnic population.

Genetic Screening of the General Population

Broad application of screening for genetic risks in the unselected general population is not yet practical. This screening would have the greatest value if it were inexpensive and could provide information about the risk of developing disease that could be mitigated by appropriate preventive action. Possible disorders amenable to screening include hemochromatosis and α_1-antitrypsin deficiency. Specific alleles in the apolipoprotein E locus may be associated with an increased risk of developing Alzheimer's disease. Pharmacogenomic traits that confer a high risk of adverse reaction to particular drugs, such as alterations in the cytochrome P-450 pathway, would be candidates. Before any of this new information could be of practical use, however, investigators would need to define the lifetime risk of disease or adverse outcome that such alleles confer.

So far, the identification of variant alleles that confer this kind of increased susceptibility is in its infancy, and such testing is not yet practical. New models must take genetic and environmental contributions to disease into account. Loci associated with an increased risk for common complex disorders, such as diabetes and hypertension, are not yet well defined; mutations in *MTHFR* that confer increased risk for neural tube defects are being investigated, but no practical test for increased risk for these conditions is available yet. In some disorders, such as hemochromatosis, mutations do not predict the clinical course well enough to warrant the use of population-based genetic testing. The lessons learned from screening of newborns and from prenatal genetic testing suggest, however, that when population screening on this level becomes available, attention to defining the genotype–phenotype correlations and the variability in phenotype within classes of genetic variations will play an important role in effective use of population testing. Testing of children for alleles that confer a risk for adult-onset disease if no intervention is available or necessary in childhood is controversial. New developments will increase its power, but genetic testing is already an effective tool; when properly used with appropriate expectations, it can guide clinical decisions and provide information that leads to action that can mitigate disease. Figure 38–1 is an algorithm for selecting genetic testing.

Genetic Risk Assessment Based on Ethnic Background

Race and Ethnicity

Genetic testing based on ethnic background is used commonly to assess susceptibility to disease and to provide information for reproductive choices. Ethnic background and race frequently are misconstrued to mean the same thing. The concept of "race" is a social construct, whereas facts about ethnic origin can convey genetic information. *Race,* as generally used, even by the U.S. Census Bureau, is a vague term without a scientific definition. There is more genetic variation among individuals within the races so construed than there is among the racial groups themselves. *Race* therefore is not helpful as a criterion for the use of genetic testing. However, founder effects, geographic isolation, social isolation, genetic drift, and similar factors can result in enrichment of particular disease-causing alleles within specific populations. Therefore, ethnic background, insofar as it represents these factors, may relate to an increased risk of having mutations that result in susceptibility to disease or increased risk of adverse reproductive outcome. When the full scope of human genomics and proteomics is understood and can be measured, identification of individual genetic risk based on gene expression or multiplex allelic testing may be possible. Until then, the use of ethnic background as a proxy for geographic origin or other isolating factors that imply an increased risk of specific mutations is advantageous. For this reason and within these limits, the physician can offer genetic testing based on self-reported ethnic origin.

All ethnic groups have mutations that increase disease frequency in that group compared with the rest of the population; no ethnic group is exempt from this liability. The frequencies of mutations that cause or predispose to disease vary among ethnic groups. Ethnic groups that should be considered in genetic risk assessment include northern European whites, southern European whites, sub-Saharan Africans, native indigenous peoples, Ashkenazi Jews, Jews of other geographic origin, Asians including Indians and Southeast Asians, Middle Eastern peoples, and Mediterranean peoples.

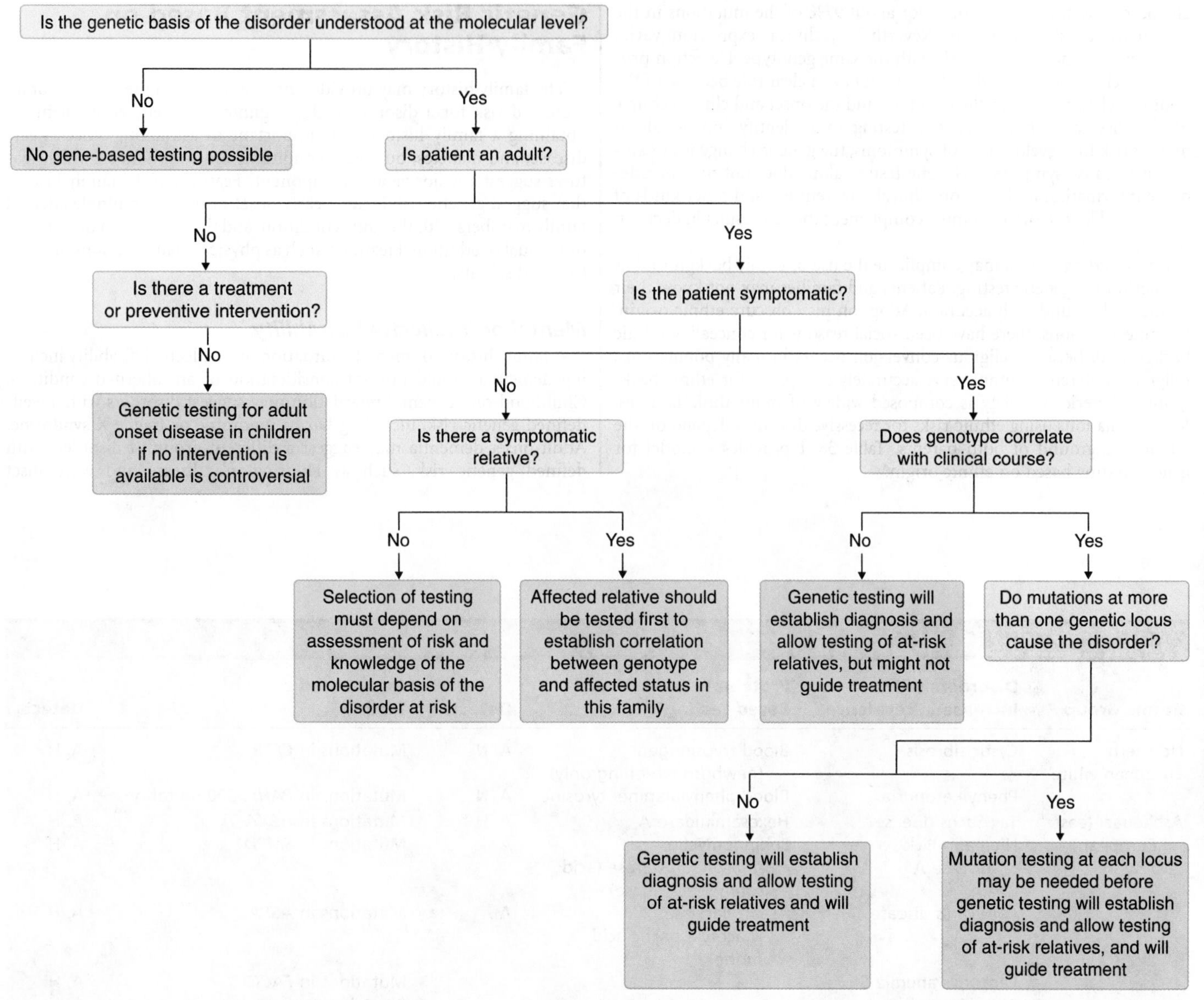

FIGURE 38–1 • Strategy for gene-based testing. The utility of gene-based testing depends on knowledge of the molecular pathology of the disorder. The correlation between genotype and clinical course guides the use of this testing. Testing may be able to confirm diagnosis, provide guidance for treatment, and offer assessment to family members at risk.

Goal of Genetic Testing of Ethnic Groups

The goal of genetic testing based on ethnic origin is to obtain information to guide medical interventions. Testing of prospective parents for heterozygosity for recessive alleles that cause serious disease in the homozygous state provides information for making reproductive decisions. Testing for mutations that cause or increase susceptibility to disease provides the basis for treatment or prevention of disease. In both cases, the utility of genetic testing depends on technical factors and on the correlation between mutation status and clinical outcome. Medical problems for which the genetic contribution has not yet been established also occur in certain ethnic groups, such as hypertension in people of African origin. Although specific genetic tests for these disorders are not yet available, clinical monitoring can be performed in an effort to identify disease in time to prevent serious complications.

Clear Role for Genetic Testing of Ethnic Groups: Tay-Sachs Disease

Testing for heterozygosity for TSD in individuals of Ashkenazi Jewish ancestry can serve as a model for the use of genetic testing in specific ethnic groups. TSD as it occurs in the Ashkenazi population is a recessively inherited neurologic condition that causes severe impairment and death in the early childhood years. The abnormality in the lysosomal enzyme hexosaminidase A that causes TSD was identified in the 1970s, and measurement of the activity of that enzyme was shown to distinguish heterozygotes from those who do not carry the mutation. This measurement is almost 100% sensitive in detecting heterozygotes. Educational programs for the population at risk, accurate testing, and sensitive prenatal testing provide reproductive options for couples in which both members carry a TSD mutation. Community-based heterozygote screening for TSD in the Ashkenazi Jewish community has been in use for about 30 years. These programs have decreased significantly the incidence of TSD in the Ashkenazi population. Now more than 80 TSD-causing mutations are known, and DNA-based testing can detect about 98% of TSD carriers in the Ashkenazi population. Enzyme testing combined with DNA testing to identify the specific mutations improves the detection rate of heterozygotes. DNA testing will facilitate prenatal diagnosis and testing of extended family members.

Unclear Role for Genetic Testing of Ethnic Groups: Gaucher's Disease

In contrast to TSD, Gaucher's disease provides an example of a disorder in which the role for genetic testing is not clear. Type I Gaucher's disease, the adult-onset form, occurs in about 1 in every 1000 Ashkenazi Jews, a higher risk than in other ethnic groups. Four mutations in the glucocerebrosidase gene account for about 97% of the mutations in the Ashkenazi Jewish population. Nevertheless, clinical expression varies considerably among individuals with the same genotype. Detection programs such as those used for TSD do not have a clear role because of the poor correlation between the genotype and the onset and clinical course of the disease. Although genetic testing may identify individuals at highest risk for development of symptoms, the genetic change is not sufficient to cause symptoms. Genetic testing alone does not provide adequate information to decide on clinical intervention, and other kinds of clinical and laboratory data must complement the test results in decision making.

Confounding factors may complicate the use of ethnic background as a criterion for genetic testing. Patients and families may not know their ethnic background with accuracy. Adoption may obscure ethnic origin. In some situations, there have been social reasons for concealing ethnic background. Because religious conversion occurs in many populations, religious preference cannot serve accurately as a proxy for ethnic background. American society is composed widely of multiethnic families. Risk calculations using ethnic risks for recessive disorders depend on the ethnic background of both parents. Table 38–1 provides a model for genetic testing based on ethnic origin.

Genetic Risk Assessment Based on Family History

The family history may provide important clues to the presence of an increased risk for a disorder with a significant genetic component. In obtaining a family history, it is important to ask about cancer, heart disease, and diabetes, but these conditions are common, so which features suggest a major genetic component? Features of the family history that suggest genetic risk include early onset of disease, multiple affected family members with the same condition, and the presence in the affected individual of additional features, such as physical malformations or intellectual disability.

Mental or Intellectual Disability

A family history of mental retardation or intellectual disability including dementia should prompt consideration of an inherited condition. Childhood-onset mental retardation may suggest disorders with a well-defined genetic risk, including Down syndrome or fragile X syndrome. Adult-onset dementia may suggest a different group of disorders with defined genetic risk, such as Huntington's disease and early-onset

TABLE 38–1 ETHNIC RISKS

Ethnic Group	Disorders with Increased Prevalence	Protein- or Biochemical-Based Testing	Detects	Gene-Based Testing	Detects
Northern European white	Cystic fibrosis	Blood trypsinogen (newborn screening only)	A, N	Mutations in *CFTR*	A, H
	Phenylketonuria	Blood phenylalanine, tyrosine	A, N	Mutations in *PAH:* >600 mutations	A, H
Ashkenazi (east European) Jewish	Tay-Sachs disease	Hexosaminidase A	A, H	Mutations in *HEXA*	A, H
	Niemann-Pick disease A	Sphingomyelin phosphodiesterase (acid sphingomyelinase)	A	Mutations in *SMPD1*	A, H
	Canavan's disease	Aspartylacylase; *N*-acetylaspartic acid (urine)	A	Mutations in *ASPA*	A, H
	Fanconi's anemia C			Mutations in *FACC*	A, H
	Bloom's syndrome			BlmAsh mutations in *BLM*	A, H
	Gaucher's disease	Glucocerebrosidase	A	Mutations in *GBA*	A, H
	Familial dysautonomia	IκB kinase complex–associated protein but not clinical testing		Mutations in *IKAP*	A, H
	Cystic fibrosis	Blood trypsinogen (newborn screening only)	A, N	Mutations in *CFTR*	A, H
African	Inherited anemias: sickle cell, thalassemias	Hematologic indices, hemoglobin electrophoresis	A, H	β-Globin gene mutations for prenatal diagnosis	A, H
Mediterranean	Inherited anemias: sickle cell, thalassemias	Hematologic indices, hemoglobin electrophoresis	A, H	β-Globin gene mutations for prenatal diagnosis	A, H
Hispanic	Inherited anemias: sickle cell	Hematologic indices, hemoglobin electrophoresis	A, H	β-Globin gene mutations for prenatal diagnosis	A, H
Asian	Inherited anemias: sickle cell, α-thalassemias	Hematologic indices, hemoglobin electrophoresis	A, H	β-Globin gene mutations for prenatal diagnosis; α-Globin deletion testing for prenatal diagnosis	A, H
Middle Eastern	Inherited anemias: sickle cell, thalassemias	Hematologic indices, hemoglobin electrophoresis	A, H	β-Globin gene mutations for prenatal diagnosis	A, H

A = testing for affected; H = testing for heterozygote; IκB = inhibitor of kappa light polypeptide gene enhancer in B-cells; N = newborn screening for affected infant.

Alzheimer's disease. A family history of mental retardation, neonatal death, or unexplained stillbirths, especially if associated with congenital malformations, may be the result of a chromosomal rearrangement in the family. Unexplained early or sudden death in children or adults may result from diverse genetic conditions such as Marfan syndrome, long QT syndrome, and disorders of fatty acid oxidation and transport.

Reaction to Medications

An unusual reaction to medications should raise the question of an inherited abnormality in the metabolism, transport, or activation of a drug. Polymorphisms in the *CYP* cytochrome P-450 genes alter the metabolism of a broad variety of medications, including coumarin anticoagulants, antihypertensives, and antiarrhythmic drugs. Although specific genetic tests are not yet widely available to confirm risk in an individual, a family history of an abnormal reaction to a specific medication should prompt concern and consideration of an alternative class of medications if possible. The alanine-to-glycine A1555G mutation in mitochondrial DNA alters metabolism of some aminoglycoside antibiotics. People carrying this mutation can be tested for sensorineural hearing loss after exposure to these antibiotics. DNA testing would need to provide very rapid results in order to use this testing to guide selection of an antibiotic in the face of acute infection.

Risks Associated with Consanguinity

The family history may reveal the presence of consanguinity. Genetic risks on the basis of consanguinity derive from the fact that, in a consanguineous couple, both individuals share a common ancestor, and both have inherited genes that are identical by descent from the common ancestor. If that ancestor passed on to them an abnormal allele for a recessively inherited condition, the consanguineous couple has a risk for having a child affected with that recessive disorder. The magnitude of this risk is significant if the members of the couple are first cousins or closer. If the couple belongs to an ethnic group with an increased chance of carrying abnormal alleles for recessive conditions, testing for those mutations is useful.

Clear Role for Genetic Testing Based on Family History: Colon Cancer

Colon cancer provides an example of how a family history of a genetic disorder can provide guidance for evaluation and management. The family history alerts the physician to the possibility of genetic risk. Properly defining that risk enhances the ability to target surveillance and to provide presymptomatic treatment (e.g., colectomy) in some patients. Genetic testing can help identify other family members at risk. Because many genes are involved in the development of colon cancer, testing must be targeted to the appropriate ones. Certain mutations are associated with cancer in other organs besides the colon, such as uterine cancer, thyroid cancer, or duodenal cancer, and the identification of these mutations suggests the need for wider surveillance. Still other mutations are associated with a predisposition to cancer but are not the only factors involved. The ACMG and the American Society of Human Genetics have developed a position statement on genetic testing for colon cancer that reviews the use of specific testing and counseling when there is a family history of colon cancer. Table 38–2 lists molecular testing used to identify risk for colon cancer.

When to Consider Genetic Factors

Family History with or without Mendelian Pattern

The taking of a family history should begin with obtaining a three-generation pedigree and learning about the health of each family

TABLE 38–2 GENETIC TESTS FOR SUSCEPTIBILITY TO COLON CANCER

Cancer Type	Test Name	Method (Reference)	Estimated Analytic Sensitivity/Specificity (%)	Sample	Indication
HNPCC	MSI, IHC	MSI analysis and immunohistochemical staining	85/85	Paraffin block (tumor)	Affected individuals with colon or uterine cancer in families with ≥3 cases of colon cancer or uterine cancer or early-onset colon cancer; if tumor manifests MSI, germline mutation analysis should be considered
HNPCC	MSH2, MLH1	DNA sequencing	70/99	Whole blood (14-mL lavender-top tube)	Affected individuals in families with ≥3 cases of colon or uterine cancer; if prior MSI tumor assay done, probability of germline mutation is low if tumor was microsatellite stable
HNPCC	MSH2	Protein truncation	50/99	Whole blood (7-mL lavender-top tube)	Affected individuals in families with ≥3 cases of colon cancer tested first; unaffected at-risk relatives tested only if mutation detected in affected patient
FAP	APC	Protein truncation	75/99	Whole blood (7-mL lavender-top tube)	Affected individuals tested first; unaffected at-risk relatives tested only if mutation detected in affected patient
Familial colon	APC11307K	ASO	99/99	Whole blood (7-mL lavender-top tube)	Affected and unaffected individual of Ashkenazi Jewish ethnicity with family history of colon cancer

APC = adenomatous polyposis coli; ASO = allele-specific oligonucleotide; FAP = familial adenomatous polyposis; HNPCC = hereditary nonpolyposis colorectal cancer; IHC = immunohistochemistry; MLH1 = test for the presence of the *MLH1* gene; MSH2 = test for the presence of the *MSH2* gene; MSI = microsatellite instability.
From Joint Test and Technology Transfer Committee Working Group, American College of Medical Genetics: Genetic testing for colon cancer: Joint statement of the American College of Medical Genetics and American Society of Human Genetics. Genet Med 2000;2:362–366.

member. Any time two or more people in the family have what seems to be the same condition, genetic factors should be considered, especially if the condition is relatively rare. If a clear mendelian pattern is seen or the disorder is a recognized mendelian condition, further assessment and testing can follow. If the family history fails to show a mendelian pattern, the diagnosis is reviewed and the medical literature is consulted to determine whether familial cases of the specific disorder have been reported. In autosomal recessive conditions, the birth of an affected child may be the first signal that both of the parents are heterozygous for a rare recessive condition. Here the genetic model depends on the correct diagnosis and the known inheritance pattern for that disorder.

X-Linked Conditions

For X-linked conditions, it must be determined whether the affected individual has a new mutation or has inherited a mutation from a heterozygous mother who by chance has no affected relatives. Twenty years ago, bayesian calculations based on the pedigree were the mainstay of this kind of analysis. Today, molecular diagnostic tools have refined the ability to determine heterozygosity in this situation.

Autosomal Dominant Conditions

For autosomal dominant conditions, the literature must be consulted to determine the proportion of patients who represent new mutations, a figure that can approach 50%. If a new mutation seems to be the explanation of the dominant condition, others in the family are not at risk, but each offspring of the affected individual has a 50% risk of inheriting the gene. Variable expression can confound the analysis in a family with an autosomal dominant condition. For example, gonadal mosaicism for the associated mutation accounts for rare recurrences of a dominant condition in families in which neither parent is affected, and no test can exclude this possibility. In general, however, the absence of the condition in any other family member makes it likely that the patient represents a new mutation.

Familial Aggregation

Frequently, no mendelian hypothesis can be sustained, yet there is familial aggregation of the disorder. Many conditions, such as neural tube defects, cleft lip and palate, pyloric stenosis, and multiple sclerosis, seem to be multifactorial in origin and have genetic and other, undefined components. Quantitative traits, such as hypertension, and common disorders, such as diabetes and heart disease, have familial aggregation. Genes governing these disorders are undergoing intense research. Genetic counseling for these conditions must rely on empirical figures for the specific condition until association with specific alleles is defined.

Using Information from Genetic Testing

Reproductive Planning

The use of information obtained from genetic testing, ethnic background, and family history depends on the interventions available for the condition under consideration. Actions can include informed reproductive decision making, presymptomatic surveillance or treatment to mitigate the risk or prevent the onset of disease, or prompt treatment of the newly diagnosed condition. Even if no further action is available, testing can result in a refined understanding of the cause of the disease. When the family has the genetic information, putting the risk in perspective is an important step. The perception of risk may be more important in family decision making than the actual numerical value of the risk. This perception depends on at least two factors: (1) risk compared with background risk and (2) overall burden, a combination of risk and severity. For example, in the case of PKU, the risk of recurrence in a second child, 1 in 4, is much greater than the risk in the general population, 1 in 10,000. Conversely, a risk of 1 in 10,000 may sound high to a couple who believe that the chances of something being wrong with an unborn child are 1 in a million. The presentation of such risk figures can change the perception of that risk. A 1 in 4 chance of recurrence of PKU is also a 3-to-1 chance against recurrence. The judgment of burden is a personal one. Physical handicap may be a severe burden for one family, whereas another family may find physical handicap tolerable but mental handicap unacceptable. Helping families to think about risks in these ways is an important component of genetic counseling. Families often are helped by being provided a description of the disorder that has been diagnosed or for which an increased risk has been determined. Many persons go to their local library in an attempt to find literature about the disorder or ask friends in the medical profession to do so. Often this results in misinformation or information that is out of date. Physicians can provide reliable, up-to-date written material and website information about the disorder. Medical genetics clinics have pamphlets, booklets, and other literature to provide. The family also should be furnished with a written report of the counseling, summarizing the important points. Thoughtful genetic counseling challenges the skills of the physician in diagnosis, analysis, communication, and support. From the initial evaluation, through development of the genetic model and identification of those at risk, to completion of the transfer of information, the use of these skills enables patients and their families to make intelligent, informed, and reasoned decisions for their future.

TABLE 38–3 REPRODUCTIVE OPTIONS FOR FAMILIES WITH GENETIC RISKS

Adoption
Reproductive assistance
In vitro fertilization with a donor egg
Artificial insemination by donor
Preimplantation genetic diagnosis
Prenatal diagnosis

Prenatal Diagnosis

If risk to future unborn children is at issue, the family at risk for a genetic disorder needs to know about the reproductive options that are available. Prenatal diagnosis and preconception diagnosis are important reproductive options that must be discussed, along with appropriate referral to experts in areas of assisted reproductive technologies. For the family at risk, these options can enhance the chances of having healthy children (Table 38–3).

The methods in prenatal diagnosis depend on imaging the fetus, examining DNA in cells of fetal origin, analyzing chromosomes in fetal cells, examining analytes, and measuring proteins and enzymes in cells of fetal origin. The major autosomal and sex chromosomal aneuploidies can be diagnosed in this way, along with chromosomal rearrangements, deletions, insertions, and the like. Prenatal DNA-based diagnosis uses fetal cells. Preimplantation genetic diagnosis uses embryo biopsy to examine one cell from a zygote obtained through in vitro fertilization, and is followed by implantation of an unaffected embryo. Testing depends on knowing the specific mutation or DNA change involved, and interpretation requires the assumption that one cell is representative of the entire fetus. For inherited single-gene disorders, this is a reasonable assumption, but it may be more difficult to exclude mosaicism in the case of chromosomal analysis. The range of single-gene disorders that have been identified using preimplantation genetic diagnosis includes autosomal recessive, autosomal dominant, and X-linked conditions. Multiplex testing for several disorders is a much bigger challenge, and efforts continue to develop fluorescence in situ hybridization (FISH) techniques for preimplantation chromosomal analysis.

In the past, the measurement of maternal serum α-fetoprotein (MSAFP), human chorionic gonadotropin (HCG), and unconjugated estriol (uE3) in maternal serum (triple screen) allowed detection of an estimated 70% of fetuses with Down syndrome regardless of maternal age. The addition of inhibin A (INH-A) to this panel identifies about 75 to 80% of fetuses with trisomy 21 (Down syndrome) and about 70% of fetuses with trisomy 18. Other aneuploidies are not detected. Measurement of MSAFP alone between 16 and 18 weeks of gestation detects 75 to 90% of open neural tube defects and at least 95% of anencephalic fetuses. Until recently, the standard recommendation was to offer multiple-marker maternal serum screening using these four markers in midtrimester. However, new studies have demonstrated that first-trimester screening using measurement of pregnancy-associated plasma protein A (PAPP-A) and ultrasound measurement of nuchal translucency in the fetus can provide a detection rate that is the same or better for trisomy 21 and trisomy 18 (Table 38–4). In addition, the results come in time for the woman to exercise the option of chorionic villus sampling (CVS) for earlier definitive testing. This approach has caveats. It will not detect open neural tube defects. In addition, the accuracy of the ultrasound measurement depends on special training and the specific skill of

TABLE 38–4 PRENATAL SCREENING USING MULTIPLE-MARKER SERUM SCREENING AND NUCHAL TRANSLUCENCY MEASUREMENT

Trimester	Test Recommended	Trisomy Detected	Open Neural Tube Detected
1	PAPP-A	18, 21	No
	Nuchal translucency	21	No
2	MSAFP, HCG, uE3, and INH-A	18, 21	Yes
	MSAFP	None	Yes

MSAFP = maternal serum α-fetoprotein; HCG = human chorionic gonadotropin; INH-A = inhibin A; PAPP-A = pregnancy-associated plasma protein A; uE3 = unconjugated estrogen (estriol).

TABLE 38–5 METHODS OF PRENATAL DIAGNOSIS

Method	Use	Risk
Preimplantation genetic diagnosis	Identify genetic abnormalities before implantation	Requires in vitro fertilization protocol
Ultrasonography	Estimate fetal age Assess growth Evaluate anatomy and organ function	None recognized
Amniocentesis or chorionic villus sampling (CVS)		
Amniocentesis (15–20 wk)	Amniotic fluid: analyze proteins, measure analytes of fetal origin	<0.5% risk of miscarriage
CVS (9–11 wk)	Fetal cells: analyze DNA, chromosomes, proteins	<2% risk of miscarriage
Periumbilical blood sampling	Fetal blood: analyze cells, measure serum analytes	<2% risk of miscarriage

the operator. The sequential use of maternal PAPP-A, HCG, and nuchal translucency measurement in the first trimester, followed by maternal serum measurements of MSAFP, HCG, uE3, and INH-A in the second trimester, offers the highest chance to identify an affected fetus with an open neural tube defect, trisomy 21, or trisomy 18 in the least invasive fashion. These modifications require the careful selection of cutoff values (to minimize false-positive results and maximize the detection rate). Special ultrasound skill is essential, and the woman must have access to an appropriate diagnostic test if the screening reveals an unacceptable risk. The ACMG recommends that women older than 35 years of age continue to be offered either CVS or amniocentesis for detection of trisomies 18 and 21, as well as other aneuploidies.

Indications, diagnostic uses, and risks of preimplantation diagnosis, midtrimester amniocentesis, CVS, and fetal blood sampling by cordocentesis are shown in Table 38–5. Studies of CVS suggest a small (1:3000 to 1:1000) risk of limb hypoplasia in infants born after that procedure. Fetoscopy is done only if other diagnostic avenues have failed; it is used to visualize fetal anatomy and to perform biopsy of fetal tissues, such as liver or skin.

It is crucial that the pregnant woman undergoing prenatal diagnosis have extremely clear counseling. Spelling out clearly the expectations and limitations of the testing before any procedures are performed is crucial. The diagnoses that are being sought must be explained, and it must be made clear that a normal result does not guarantee a normal infant. If the result of the test is not normal, the options for the woman are to terminate the pregnancy or to carry it to term. Rarely, surgical or medical treatment of the identified fetus can be offered, but this may be experimental, uncertain, and risky. The decision to terminate a pregnancy must be made in collaboration with the obstetrician who will perform the procedure, so that the process can be described and possible complications reviewed. Appropriate psychosocial support should be provided.

SUGGESTED READINGS

American College of Obstetricians and Gynecologists: ACOG Committee Opinion #296: First-trimester screening for fetal aneuploidy. Obstet Gynecol 2004;104:215–217.

Am PH: Newborn screening: Current status. Health Aff (Millwood) 2007;26: 559–566. *Advances in tandem mass spectometry make it possible to screen newborns for many rare inborn errors of metabolism, thereby raising issues about cost-effectiveness, ethics, quality, and oversight.*

Cunniff C, American Academy of Pediatrics Committee on Genetics: Prenatal screening and diagnosis for pediatricians. Pediatrics 2004;114:889–894. *Practice guidelines on prenatal diagnosis.*

Driscoll DA, Professional Practice and Guidelines Committee: Second trimester maternal serum screening for fetal open neural tube defects and aneuploidy. Genet Med 2004;6:540–541.

Ensenauer RE, Michels VV, Reinke SS: Genetic testing: Practical, ethical, and counseling considerations. Mayo Clin Proc 2005;80:63–73. *Case-based review of the use of genetic testing and counseling.*

Human Genome Project Information on Gene Testing: Available at www.ornl.gov/sci/techresources/Human_Genome/medicine/genetest.shtml (accessed June 2, 2006). *Website with reviews of genetic testing and links to sites providing testing information.*

Online Mendelian Inheritance in Man (OMIM): Available at http://www.ncbi.nlm.nih.gov/entrez/query.fcgi?db=OMIM. *Website of the catalog of known human mendelian traits with links to the genome database.*

van den Berg M, Timmermans DR, ten Kate LP, et al: Informed decision making in the context of prenatal screening. Patient Educ Couns 2006;63:110–117. *Prenatal screening decisions are often not informed decisions.*

Wade CH, Wilfond BS: Ethical and clinical practice considerations for genetic counselors related to direct-to-consumer marketing of genetic tests. Am J Med Genet C Semin Med Genet 2006;142:284–293. *Genetic counselors do not have an obligation to order DTC-advertised tests that have minimal clinical validity and utility.*

Wasson K, Cook ED, Helzlsouer K: Direct-to-consumer online genetic testing and the four principles: An analysis of the ethical issues. Ethics Med 2006;22:83–91. *The potential harms may outweigh the potential benefits.*

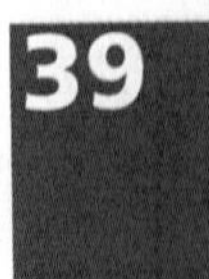

SINGLE-GENE AND CHROMOSOMAL DISORDERS

Judith G. Hall

SINGLE-GENE DISORDERS

Mendelian Inheritance

Single-gene or monogenic disorders are disorders in which inheritance results from a single mutant gene. Genes are "units of heredity," now known to be based in DNA. The concept of units of heredity first was described by Mendel in 1865. Consequently, this type of inheritance often is called *mendelian inheritance.* Mendel's work describing these invisible factors, which are passed from generation to generation and determine various traits or characteristics, was largely ignored until Bateson translated Mendel's work and reintroduced these concepts in the early 1900s.

Mendel's work was based on the characteristics he observed in his monastery's garden peas and led to four important conclusions:

1. Genes come in pairs, one from each parent.
2. The individual genes can have different forms (alleles) that can exert their effect on each other, being dominant or recessive. These various forms of the gene are transmitted entirely unchanged from generation to generation.
3. When germ cells are made, the two genes segregate/separate from each other so that the resultant gamete receives only one of the two alleles present in the parent.
4. The segregation/separation of a given gene (and the trait it produces) is independent of that for other traits.

What is remarkable about Mendel is that he was able to deduce these characteristics about the units of heredity from observing the transmission of characteristics that we now understand to have a basis in the physical nature of DNA. Although exceptions to each of Mendel's rules are now recognized, the concept of genes has been an extremely useful one. The idea that these units of heredity were arranged in linear sequence on each chromosome was anticipated long before the DNA basis of inheritance was defined.

The Human Genome Project

The Human Genome Project is in the process of defining the sequence, the normal position, and variations of all human genes. A great deal of additional work is needed to refine the variations and annotate unique areas. A major surprise of the project has been that there appear to be only about 20,000 to 30,000 genes. Because there are more than 100,000 human proteins, it was anticipated that there would be a gene for each protein. It is now recognized, however, that one gene may produce more than one protein by using different parts of the gene's sequence in what is called *alternative splicing.* In addition, many genes do not produce proteins but rather play a role in the regulation of gene expression. With a little more than 20,000 genes, it can be expected that the genes and their gene products will fall into approximately 1000 pathways, and that the pathways will interact in a variety of ways to form networks. It also can be anticipated that gene expression will occur in a time-specific and tissue-specific manner; however, the mechanisms of control of that orchestration are not yet understood. Clearly, gene expression is modified by environmental interactions.

Many single-gene disorders were recognized because of a change in the phenotype of affected individuals. In the case of diseases of adulthood, the phenotypic changes may not become obvious until long after puberty, even though the abnormal gene has been present since conception. Classically, genetic disorders were described on the basis of the presence of physical or functional abnormalities (phenotype). Only more recently has the DNA change (genotype) from "normal" and the molecular basis been understood. Consequently, the first descriptions of single-gene disorders came as a list of signs or symptoms that were inherited together, within a family, in recognizable patterns of inheritance (autosomal or X-linked, dominant or recessive).

In more recent years, the most useful listing of genes and genetic diseases for the clinician has been Online Mendelian Inheritance in Man (OMIM), available at *www.ncbi.nlm.nih.gov/entrez/query.fcgi?db=OMIM* (accessed June 2, 2006). Analysis of the mutations and the types of DNA changes that lead to the disease phenotypes has given much insight into (1) the mechanisms of disease, (2) the parts of the gene that lead to disease when changed, and (3) the complex biochemical pathways leading to disease.

Single-gene disorders are separated into autosomal and X-linked types. This classification is determined by whether the responsible gene is carried on one of the 22 autosomal chromosomes (chromosomes that are homologous in males and females) or on the X chromosome (females have two X chromosomes, whereas males have an X and a Y chromosome).

Patterns of Inheritance

Genes carried on the autosomes display different patterns of inheritance, which are reflected in the pedigree or family history (Table 39–1), compared with genes inherited on the X chromosome. *Dominant* and *recessive* refer to whether the disease phenotype produced by the mutant allele is manifested or observed when only a single copy of the abnormal allele is present (dominant) or whether expression requires, as in the case of recessively inherited traits, that no normal allele is present.

The terms *dominant* and *recessive* refer to the phenotypic expression. Now that the molecular basis of most genes is understood or at least clearer, it has become obvious that there are many mechanisms that can lead to the phenotypic expression. There are molecular mechanisms by which a mutant allele may exert an effect, such as by blocking a pathway or by overproduction or underproduction of a gene product. *Codominant* is the term used to describe the situation in which the products of both alleles exert an observable effect (e.g., hemoglobin S and hemoglobin C can be observed at the same time). Traditionally, recessive inheritance implied that both alleles must be mutant to produce a phenotypic effect, but today, using molecular techniques, most carriers of a recessive disorder can be identified and often have subtle or late-onset phenotypic features.

Most single-gene disorders are rare. If they are common, it reflects (1) that selection during evolution occurred (because of an advantage for survival); (2) that a population came from a few founders, one of whom carried the mutation; or (3) that the gene has a high mutation rate.

Because single-gene diseases have been described on a phenotypic basis, we refer to the abnormalities as *traits.* If the genes responsible for a given trait reside on one of the autosomes, it is called an *autosomally inherited trait.* There are normally two of each autosomal chromosome, one inherited from the father and one from the mother. The traits represent the expression of genes; the two different genes (alleles) on the two different chromosomes may express themselves in a manner such that one of the genes produces a trait that is dominant (i.e., is observed as the phenotype). This sometimes is called *dominant inheritance* of the trait. If the abnormal gene expresses itself in the phenotype only when it is present in a double dose, or homozygous state, this is called *recessive inheritance* of the trait. These terms, therefore, are used to describe the characteristics of the phenotype rather than the genotype.

Autosomal Dominant Inheritance Patterns

Autosomal dominant inheritance implies that the trait is observable and that the affected individual usually has an affected parent from whom the gene for the condition has been passed on (see Table 39–1). Occasionally, a mutation arises and is present in the germ cell that formed the affected individual. In this case, neither parent manifests the disorder, and the situation is described as a new (or de novo) mutation.

In autosomal dominant disorders, males and females are affected in equal numbers. An affected individual would be expected to have equal numbers of affected and unaffected offspring. Males and females can transmit the trait to males and females. The normal children of an affected individual have only normal offspring. If the trait does not impair reproductive capacity or viability, it is transmitted vertically through successive generations.

Many well-known autosomal dominant traits affect several organ systems. This is called a *pleiotropic* effect. There can be a great deal of variability from individual to individual, even within the same family, as to the age at onset of abnormalities and the degree of involvement. This is called *variable expressivity.* In other words, an abnormal gene is present, but it expresses in a variable way. *Penetrance* refers to whether or not there

TABLE 39–1 CHARACTERISTICS OF SINGLE-GENE INHERITANCE

Characteristic	Autosomal Dominant	Autosomal Recessive	X-Linked Dominant	X-Linked Recessive
Transmission	Vertical Successive generations	Usually horizontal Multiple sibs affected Usually only one generation	Daughters of affected males always inherit the disorder Sons of affected males never inherit the disorder Affected females can transmit the disorder to offspring of both sexes An excess of affected females exists in the pedigree	Mainly inherited by males through carrier women
Consanguinity	No increase	Parents often consanguineous	Consanguinity not increased	Affected males are at risk for transmission through their obligate carrier daughter
Risk of affected offspring	50% (both sexes)	25% affected, 50% carriers	50% affected	Males affected almost exclusively; females affected only with affected father and carrier mother (affected 50% of the time) or with skewed X-inactivation
Females affected	50%	Half of affected expected to be female	50% of daughters; however, twice as many affected women as affected men in family	Females are rarely affected; however, daughters of affected men are obligate carriers
Males affected	50% (expect male-to-male transmission)	Half of affected expected to be male	50% (no male-to-male transmission)	50% of sons of carrier females are affected; male-to-male transmission is not observed

is *any* expression of the gene. Some individuals carry an abnormal (usually dominant) gene but show no phenotypic features; this is called *nonpenetrance.*

In autosomal dominantly inherited traits, there is a 50% (1 in 2) chance that a child of either gender will inherit the trait. The normal individual in these families does not bear affected children unless it is a trait in which nonpenetrance occurs.

In classic autosomal dominant inheritance, the phenotype is said to be no worse in a homozygous state (i.e., when there are two abnormal genes) than when only one abnormal gene is present (heterozygous state). There are, however, only a few examples of this classic pattern. In almost all conditions of "double" dominance (homozygous mutant), the phenotype is more severe. There are many genes that are *sex-influenced* or *sex-limited* but inherited as autosomal traits. Baldness (which usually affects only males) and menstrual irregularities (only in females) are two such traits.

It is important to make a distinction between genotype and phenotype, because *genotype* refers to the actual gene and *phenotype* refers to the clinical expression of that gene in a functional or structural trait. Classically, genotypes are described as *homozygous* or *heterozygous,* implying that two genes are present and are, respectively, identical (both normal or both abnormal) or different (one normal and one abnormal). The term *allele* is often used for these two alternative genes inherited at the same position on the maternal and paternal chromosomes. Most of the time, each family has a unique mutation in the gene, and unless the parents are related, the actual mutations are not exactly the same. However, if an affected person has two abnormal alleles, they usually are still referred to as homozygous mutations if they produce the same abnormal trait.

Autosomal Recessive Inheritance Patterns

Autosomal recessive disorders are clinically apparent when the gene responsible is in the homozygous state (i.e., both alleles are mutant). Each parent of an affected offspring is a carrier for the mutant gene, but frequently the parents are phenotypically normal. As more is learned about gene function, carriers will be able to be identified on a biochemical or molecular basis.

Males and females are affected in equal proportions, and there is a 25% risk that each child of a male and a female carrier will be affected. Should the affected individuals (who have a homozygous mutant genotype) have children with individuals who are homozygous normal for that gene, none of their children will be affected, but all will be heterozygous carriers of the mutant gene. If two individuals who are homozygous for this gene mutation reproduce, all of their children will be homozygous and affected. Homozygous recessive traits are seen more commonly with consanguineous unions, because relatives are more likely to carry the same mutant genes. However, the mutant genes often differ slightly from each other. Such autosomal recessive inheritance is described as *heteroallelic* (i.e., with two different alleles, both of which are abnormal).

X-Linked Inheritance

X-linked inheritance refers to genes located on the X chromosome. Females have two X chromosomes; they may be heterozygous or homozygous for mutant X-linked genes. Males have only one X chromosome and thus one set of X-linked genes (called *hemizygous*); if the allele on the X chromosome of a male is abnormal, he is affected. Because males have only one X chromosome, they would be expected to express an X-linked trait whether it is recessive or dominant. X-linked dominant disorders also affect females who have only one copy of the abnormal gene. Most X-linked traits and diseases are recessive, and consequently females usually do not manifest these disorders or disease states. However, if a woman's father has the disorder and her mother is a carrier, she has a 50% chance of being affected.

Women carry two X chromosomes that are both active early in development; however, as tissue differentiation occurs, one of the X chromosomes becomes inactive. This process of X inactivation is thought to be random, and there is an equal chance that the paternal or the maternal X chromosome will be inactivated in a given cell. After one of the X chromosomes has been inactivated, it remains inactivated throughout all subsequent cell divisions. There are situations of skewed X inactivation, however, in which one or the other X chromosome is disproportionately inactivated. This can lead to females manifesting X-linked recessive disorders, such as hemophilia or color blindness.

X-linked dominant traits are traits in which the gene on the X chromosome is expressed in both males and females. Usually these are disorders that are dominant in females but lethal in males. X-linked recessive traits are traits that are fully expressed in the hemizygous affected male.

With X-linked recessive traits, heterozygote females are usually normal; however, because they can have skewed X inactivation, females occasionally are mildly affected, and in rare instances they may be as affected as a male. Females with X chromosome abnormalities such as deletions, translocations, and Turner's syndrome may also be affected by X-linked recessive disorders.

Gene Effects

Gene Function

Disorders typically have been described on a phenotypic basis, and when the mutations within the gene responsible have been found, in some cases a specific gene has turned out to be responsible for more than one disease. Sometimes these diseases are a part of a spectrum, as in the case of achondroplasia and thanatophoric dysplasia, both of which involve mutations in the fibroblast growth factor receptor 3 (*FGFR3*) gene. Other disorders caused by mutations in a single gene are apparently quite different, as in the case of Greig's cephalopolysyndactyly and polydactyly alone, both of which are mutations of the *GLI3* gene. Still more surprisingly, an abnormality of a gene may produce both dominant and recessive inheritance patterns, depending on the type and position of the DNA change. The differences in expression of specific genes are not entirely understood but seem to relate to the fact that genes are complex in their structures, so that different domains of the gene deal with different functions. A mutation in one domain may affect one biochemical pathway, whereas a mutation in another domain may affect a different process.

Gene Organization

As the structure of genes has become clearer, it is recognized that there are noncoding parts of genes that are important (i.e., the parts other than the *exons* whose sequence may or may not be transcribed into RNA). These include DNA sequences, distant from the gene, that enhance expression and determine whether the gene will be transcribed. There are also promoter elements close to the gene. Signal sequences are another part of the gene: one signals where transcription should begin, and another signals the point at which it should end. In addition, there are intervening sequences called *introns* that are transcribed into the RNA and then must be excised. The excision (splice) junctions are critical points. It is now clear that, in large genes, several different combinations of exons (sequences that express) can be transcribed. This is called *alternative splicing*, and it produces different proteins from the same gene. The DNA is copied to RNA in the nucleus of the cell, which is then transcribed into proteins using the genetic code in the cytoplasm of the cell.

When a protein is expressed, there are still modifications that need to be made to it so that it is folded properly and made functional. The mechanisms for control of the transcription process are not clear for most genes. There are many transcription factor genes that seem to be responsible for turning on other genes. These seem to be essential to the cascade of events that occur in differentiation, organ formation, and tissue-specific processes. Such transcription factor genes would be expected to have a major effect on many different pathways. For gene products to have an effect, not only do the proteins have to be made and properly processed, but also receptors for that protein need to be produced in a tissue-specific and time-specific way. In addition, the protein needs to "find" its proper place on the cell membrane, in the cytoplasm, or in an organelle. A great deal of work is needed to understand all of these processes and what controls their orderly, timely production.

Fundamental to determining single-gene disorders are the abilities to isolate DNA, to amplify it so that there is enough material with which to work, to recognize changes in the sequence, and to determine that a particular gene is in fact abnormal. (The molecular techniques for identifying abnormalities in genes are discussed elsewhere.) Newer technologies that recognize shortening (truncation) of a protein (which reflects mutations in the gene), alterations in triplet repeats, and other changes in gene structure will aid in the identification of the particular change in genetic information that has led to a disease. Most recently, the development of molecular microarray "chips" that can run thousands of tests simultaneously promises to change dramatically the approach to diagnosis of single-gene disorders.

Mutations

Until recently, mutations producing changes in a gene that lead to a disease phenotype were thought of as nucleotide changes or deletions. Several new classes of mutations, including expansion of genes through triple repeats and the presence of transposable elements that can disrupt a sequence but also can be removed, require the consideration of a new classification of the types of mutations that can lead to phenotypic changes in individuals.

Each time cell division occurs, it has been estimated that one or two errors occur during the replication of the total DNA of the cell. Because most of those errors occur in noncoding regions, they are not considered to be detrimental. However, if this type of error involves coding regions, it is the source of somatic mosaicism, in which an individual has some cells that are normal and some that have an abnormality. Somatic mosaicism may occur as patchy or streaky pigment or asymmetrical expression of abnormalities (as in segmented neurofibromatosis). It also may be expressed in milder manifestations, so mild that they may appear to be a different disorder (e.g., arthritis in the parent and severe spondyloepiphyseal dysplasia in the child).

There does seem to be a wide range of mutation rates. For some genes, such as the neurofibromatosis gene, mutations occur in approximately 1 of every 6000 individuals. In other genes, the rate of new mutations may be 1 in 50,000 individuals. It is not clear why these differences exist. Some of the variation may relate to the size of genes (i.e., large genes are likely to have more mutations). Some of it may relate to the type of mutation (i.e., deletions seem to occur when there are repeat segments within the gene, such that there is a slippage of one area of repeat sequences to another). Many mutations of a single nucleotide within a gene seem to occur during paternal meiosis. Mutations occur frequently at the site of a methylated CpG. The processes of mutation also seem to be specific for specific disorders—for example, somatic mutation in pseudoachondroplasia is relatively common, whereas somatic mutation in achondroplasia is rare. Mutations of the paternal germline gene in achondroplasia are extremely common (on the order of 1000 times the mutation rate of other genes).

Gene expression occurs in a time-specific, tissue-specific way. Some genes are used and reused in different tissues at different times in development and in normal physiology, so the control of expression is very important. Expression at one point in time can have a detrimental effect, whereas at another time or in another tissue there is no ill effect. The same gene product may be attracting other cells one day and a day later repelling cells, as in development of the nervous system. Abnormal time or place of expression of the gene product may be as detrimental as production of an abnormal gene product.

Mosaicism

Mosaicism is common in any multicellular organism (involving both single-gene mutations and chromosomal abnormalities). The question is whether its occurrence in a tissue will lead to a phenotype that will cause disease. Mutations that occur in stem cells give rise to many daughter cells with the same abnormality. Perhaps the most important consideration is whether the mutation has occurred in the germline. This would give the parent's germline more than one germ cell carrying the mutation, so that a phenotypically normal parent may have more than one affected child. This situation has been well documented in the case of osteogenesis imperfecta. Occasionally, a parent has some mild manifestation suggesting that he or she has some somatic cells that are affected, but germ cells that have the mutation produce a fully affected child. This situation is seen in individuals with pseudoachondroplasia, in which the parent has minimal expression (e.g., limitation of elbow extension) but the child has the full-blown disease.

In addition to mosaicism for mutations that occur during embryologic and fetal development of the individual, it is now clear that microchimerism also occurs. In microchimerism, an individual receives some cells (including stem cells) from the mother or from a dizygotic twin during pregnancy. A woman also may receive cells from her children, and those cells may find a niche where they become permanently housed and produce their own daughter cells, causing the woman to manifest chimerism.

Dominant Negative Mutations

Dominant negative mutations are mutations that interfere with the activity of the normal wild-type allele. These are particularly common in multimeric proteins, in which a mutation of one of the subunits interacts in a way that binds and alters the catalytic activity of the rest of the protein, so that it affects the entire multimeric structure. In these situations, most or all of the protein produced would be abnormal. Toxic protein alterations include those in which there is disruption of function or in which new functions are produced that involve totally new pathways. There are disorders that are inherited in what would appear to be an autosomal dominant pattern but should be considered recessive; examples include the changes seen in the retinoblastoma or *BRCA1* and *BRCA2* genes. These are situations in which both alleles must be abnormal to produce a cancer, but because the mutation rate of the second allele is high during the course of development, the production of a homozygous state somatically (including deletion or loss of the normal allele) is frequent. Therefore, inheritance of a single abnormal allele in these situations is likely to produce disease, because the second allele often becomes abnormal in the course of development.

Nontraditional, Epigenetic, and "Parent of Origin" Effects

Epigenetic refers to effects that are not part of a gene sequence but can be inherited. They include mechanisms that lead to differential control. There is a newly recognized class of genes, particularly related to growth, behavior, and placental function, in which, although two alleles are present, only the allele inherited from one parent is expressed. This is called *genomic imprinting.* It produces an unusual pattern of inheritance in the pedigree: expression of the abnormal phenotype occurs only when the gene is inherited from the parent of one gender.

Expression or exposure during development can have long-lasting effects. The growing understanding in developmental genetics reflects that there is an orderly hierarchy of processes in the course of development, including patterning information, tissue differentiation, organ development, and interdependent tissue function. If abnormalities occur during the process of formation, they are called *malformations.* If the structures have formed and are then lost because of some destructive mechanical force or loss of vascular supply, these are called *disruptions.* If an organ or tissue is formed and compression deforms that tissue, this type of abnormality is a *deformation. Dysplasias* are abnormalities of growth related to a specific tissue type. It is important in evaluating congenital anomalies to consider what type of process has led to the structural abnormalities. Different mechanisms underlie these different processes and reflect genetic versus environmental influences, recurrence risks, preventive strategies, and responses to therapy.

CHROMOSOMAL DISORDERS

Chromosomes are nuclear structures that become visible as cells divide. They represent the condensation of the cell's nuclear DNA together with histones and other proteins. They can be seen readily through special preparation and staining techniques. Disorders of single genes have been observed clinically because of a phenotypic change related to alterations in a protein or protein pathway that the gene normally would influence. Today, it is possible to define the exact change in the DNA (genotype) that leads to the change in phenotype. These changes are too small to see through a microscope and require a specialized molecular technique to define. By contrast, disorders of chromosomes almost always involve multiple genes and are a reflection of the absence or excess created by numerical or positional abnormalities of chromosome material.

Molecular techniques have enabled dramatic advances in the understanding of how genes and chromosomes function. These techniques allow amplification, sequencing, and even visualization of extremely small changes in genetic material. Most of what is inherited in humans resides along the 46 chromosomes; however, the mitochondria (inherited solely from the mother) also carry DNA. Other cell structures originally transferred from the egg and coming from the mother serve as templates for future cells, such as the cell wall and various organelles.

Characteristics of Chromosomes

The DNA of genes is packaged into chromosomes. Normally, humans have 46 chromosomes in the nucleus of every cell (44 autosomes and the X or Y sex chromosomes); for practical purposes, these carry the same (99.9%) genetic information (DNA) in one individual human being as in the next. The Y chromosome in males carries little genetic information but is important for determining the phenotypic sex of the individual. Extra chromosomes, missing chromosomes, missing parts of chromosomes, duplications, and rearrangements all can present a problem. There is an increased occurrence of chromosomal abnormalities among spontaneous abortions and stillbirths. Chromosomal abnormalities are a major cause of infertility in otherwise phenotypically normal individuals. Chromosomal rearrangements occur in most cancers. An obvious chromosomal anomaly is present in 0.5% of live-born infants, and at least half of these chromosomal abnormalities manifest clinically as recognizable syndromes. It is important to be aware of the problems related to the mechanisms that underlie chromosomal abnormalities, because they can have long-term effects on health in the adult.

Chromosomes are normally visible through the microscope only when they are in a contracted state going through cell division. However, a variety of new methods allow the visualization of chromosomes and chromosomal material at other times; these techniques include comparative genomic hybridization (CGH), representational oligonucleotide microarray analysis (ROMA), and florescence in situ hybridization (FISH) (see Figs. 39–3 to 39–5). Advances in molecular technology demonstrate submicroscopic deletions and duplications even during interphase. Microdeletions frequently are seen with many relatively common syndromes. In these deletions, more than one gene is lost, and usually affected individuals have multiple system involvement. However, small subtelomeric deletions are common (at least 10%) in persons with nonsyndromic mental retardation.

Nomenclature

Karyotype is the term used for the visual display of chromosomes (Figs. 39–1 and 39–2). This display is obtained by growing cells, usually fibroblast or lymphocytes, and arresting them during cell division at the specific cell cycle stage of metaphase. The cells are photographed, and the chromosomes are arranged in order according to size. This type of visual display also can be produced by computer.

In describing a karyotype, there are three elements to be defined:

1. The number of chromosomes
2. The sex chromosome constitution
3. Any abnormalities found

The normal karyotype for females is 46,XX, and for males it is 46,XY. Any abnormality observed is noted after the sex chromosome constitution. For example, in a male with Wolf-Hirschhorn syndrome, in which a piece of the short arm of chromosome 4 is missing, the karyotype is 46,XY,4p–. In a female with Down syndrome, in which there is an extra chromosome 21, the karyotype is 47,XX,+21.

Other types of abnormalities are noted by an abbreviation (e.g., *t* for translocation) and then the chromosomes that are involved. For instance, a male carrier with translocation between the long arms of 13 and 15 would be represented by 45,XY,t(13q15q). If a chromosome breaks along one of its arms, the band position in which the break occurs also is indicated within the brackets, such as 45,XY,t(13q2.3,15q3.2).

Types of Cell Division

Normally, there are two types of cell division: mitosis and meiosis.

Mitosis

In mitosis, two genetically identical daughter cells are produced from a single parent cell. Most cells in the body are produced by mitosis. During the first stage of mitosis, the chromosomes become condensed and are visible and easy to identify for karyotyping. Before the condensation and cell division, the DNA replicates so that there is already double the normal amount of DNA when the chromosomes condense. These chromosomes containing two identical copies of the DNA are called *sister chromatids.* The next phase of mitotic cell division is characterized by coiling of the chromosome threads to form recognizable chromosomes. The nuclear membrane and the nucleolus disappear, and a mitotic spindle forms. In the next stage, metaphase, the chromosomes condense and become clearly visible. The center structure of the chromosomes (centromere) attaches to microtubules of the mitotic spindle, and the chromosomes align in the middle of the cell along with the spindle.

In the next phase, called *anaphase,* the chromosomes separate along their longitudinal axis, and one of each pair of the sister chromatids is drawn into what will be the two daughter cells. The last phase, telophase, completes mitosis. During this stage, the nuclear membranes and the

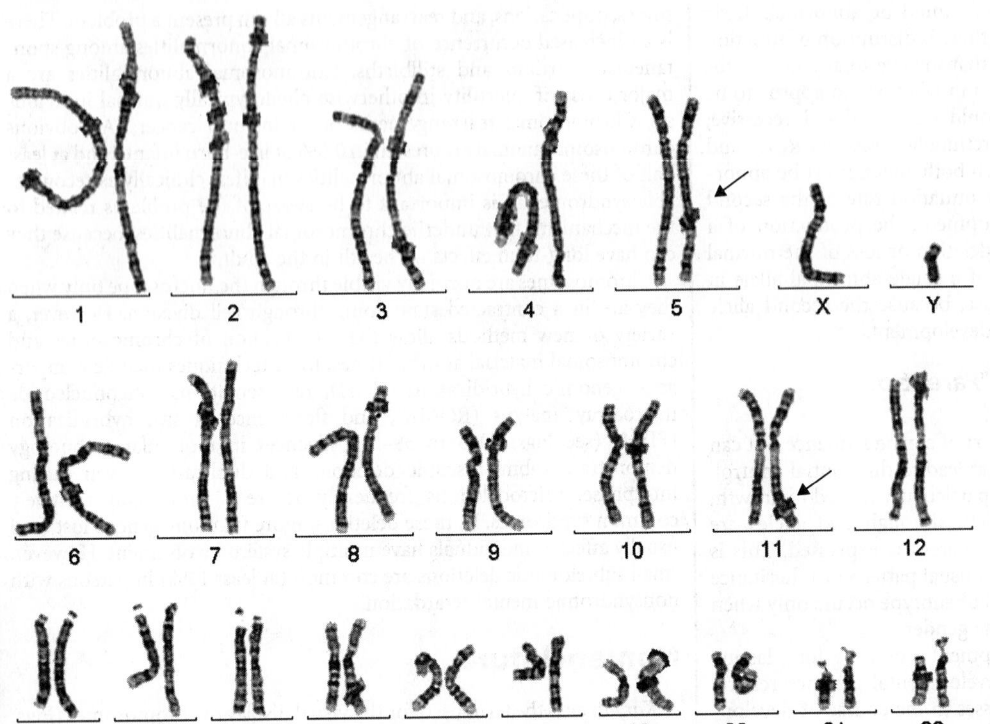

FIGURE 39–1 • Normal male karyotype (46,XY). G-banded chromosomes. Arrows indicate examples of areas where two chromosomes overlap. Resolution is greater than 550 bands.

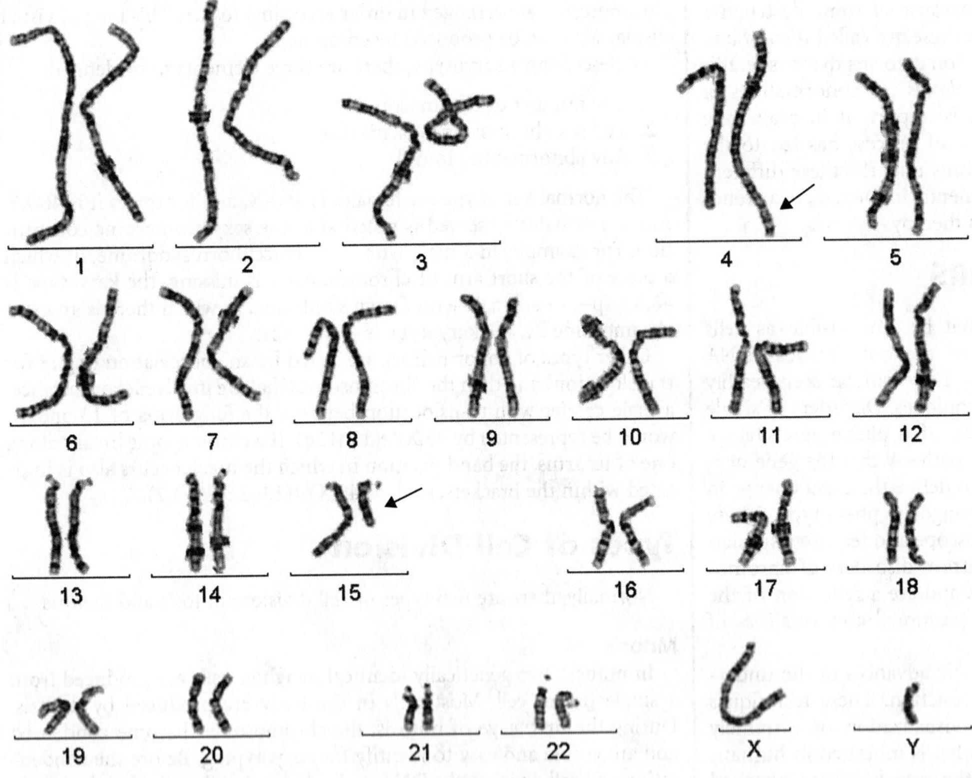

FIGURE 39–2 • Chromosome rearrangement in a normal male. Male karyotype shows a reciprocal translocation between the long arms of chromosome 4 and chromosome 15 (arrows). This translocation is balanced: no defect or excess of genetic material is apparent.

nucleoli reappear to form the two new daughter cells, each of which has 46 chromosomes (diploid).

Meiosis

The second form of cell division, meiosis, is involved in the formation of germ cells or gametes (sperm and egg). In this process, the normal set of 46 chromosomes is reduced to a half (haploid) set or 23 chromosomes, so that with fertilization the normal number of chromosomes can be reestablished. Meiosis is divided into two parts; the first is meiosis I, in which the DNA replicates. During the early stages of meiosis, the future germ cell replicates the DNA, resulting in two times the normal amount of DNA.

Male meiosis takes place after puberty. In male meiosis during this first cell division, each of these first daughter cells gets one of the duplicated chromosomes of a pair. In males, at the beginning of the second cell division of meiosis (meiosis II), each cell contains 23 chromosomes, the DNA of which has been duplicated; during meiosis II, the duplicated pairs separate, so that each of those daughter cells ends up with 23 chromosomes. Thus, there are four daughter cells (spermatids), each with half the normal number (haploid) set of chromosomes.

In females, meiosis begins during embryogenesis, and rather than going through cell divisions, the extra sets of duplicated chromosomes clump together on the side of the cell and form *polar bodies.* During meiosis I, one set of duplicated chromosomes condenses and forms the first polar body (which contains 46 chromosomes). Then, during meiosis II in females (which is not completed until after puberty), one of the other half sets of chromosomes forms the second polar body (which contains 23 chromosomes). The egg has two polar bodies and one set of half the normal number of chromosomes (i.e., 23 chromosomes, which is also the haploid number).

In the process of meiosis, there is exchange of segments of chromosomes (*crossing over* of chromosome segments). This leads to new alignments and new combinations of genes from both parents and their various allele states along the chromosomal DNA of the germ cells.

Two common errors in cell division that occur during meiosis and lead to abnormal numbers of chromosomes. The first is nondisjunction, in which the pair of chromosomes fails to separate, so that one of the new cells has two copies of that particular chromosome and one has no copy. The second type of error is anaphase lag, in which a chromatid is lost because it fails to move quickly enough during anaphase to become incorporated into one of the new daughter cells.

Chromosome Studies

Chromosome studies producing a karyotype can be obtained from any dividing nucleated cell. Because blood is readily accessible, cytogenetic studies usually are performed on lymphocytes, but studies of fibroblasts should be considered if there is a suspicion of mosaicism.

Chromosome studies for prenatal diagnosis are obtained from amniotic fluid, chorionic villus sampling, and fetal blood and by analysis of blastomeres when preimplantation diagnosis is performed. In cancer, chromosome studies are done to provide prognosis and identify the most appropriate therapy.

In routine karyotyping, the stains used allow 400 to 600 bands to become visible (see Fig. 39–1). Trypsin-Giemsa staining reveals G-bands, and quinacrine staining reveals Q-bands. Other special stains are used to show other chromosome structures, such as centromeres. If finer detail is necessary, prophase chromosomes may be examined. These are longer and have less condensation; they may show 600 to 1200 bands. Usually, chromosome studies done during prenatal diagnosis do not reveal as many as 1000 bands, and it may be necessary when looking for fine deletions or duplications to repeat the chromosome studies if the first set was done for prenatal diagnosis.

Comparative genomic hybridization is a molecular technique that allows simultaneous enumeration of every chromosome (Fig. 39–3). Test DNA is isolated from a single cell, then duplicated many times using polymerase chain reaction, and paired with reference DNA from a normal individual. The test DNA is labeled in a different way from the reference DNA using two different fluorescent dyes. Then the test and reference DNA are hybridized, and any excess of test DNA or excess of reference DNA can be identified, indicating duplications or deletions.

In situ hybridization can be employed using a probe for a particular chromosome, chromosome segment, or gene. It can be used on chromosome preparations or at interphase. It can be used on blood smears, fibroblasts, or buccal smears to identify the presence of numerical changes (i.e., trisomy or monosomy). Deletions, duplications, and translocations of specific chromosomes (as in the microdeletions associated with specific deletion syndromes) are most easily identified on metaphase chromosome spreads. Frequently, several fluorescent probes are used at the same time for FISH studies (Figs. 39–4 and 39–5). DNA microarrays using oligonucleotides are being developed which will identify duplications or deletions using only DNA.

Chromosomal Abnormalities

Chromosomal abnormalities occur in 0.5% of live births (Table 39–2). They are an important cause of mental retardation and congenital anomalies. Translocation carriers may be perfectly normal phenotypically, but they are at increased risk for having children with unbalanced chromosomal arrangements.

The phenotype associated with a particular chromosomal anomaly is often well established (see Fig. 39–2). Chromosomal anomalies include abnormalities of number and structure.

Abnormalities of Chromosome Number

The terminology for chromosome numbers relates first to whether there are a normal number of chromosome sets. *Haploid* means one set (in humans, 23 chromosomes—the number in a germ cell). *Diploid* means two sets (in humans, 46 chromosomes—the normal number of chromosomes in an organism). Any number of chromosomes that is an exact multiple of the haploid number (e.g., 23, 46, 69) is referred to as *euploid.* Euploid cells with more than the normal diploid number of 46 chromosomes are called *polyploid.* Polyploid conceptions are not viable. Polyploid cells are seen frequently in cancer. Polyploidy is occasionally present in mosaic form, which allows for survival of the individual (diploid/triploid/mixoploid). Cells with three sets of chromosomes are called *triploid* and are seen frequently in abortus material. Cells deviating from multiples of haploid numbers are called *aneuploid* (i.e., not euploid); this include all the variations of missing or extra chromosomes and deletions and duplications.

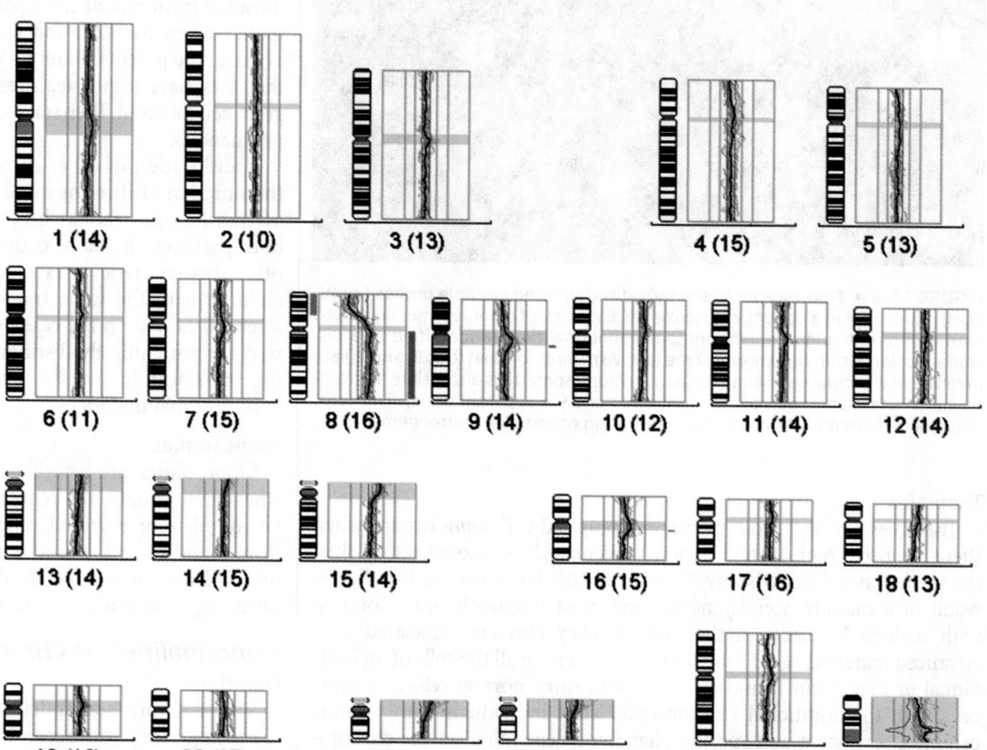

FIGURE 39–3 • Comparative genomic hybridization (CGH). CGH profile, showing a combined deletion of chromosome 8p (red, left shift) and duplication of chromosome 8q (green, right shift) on the same chromosome. This profile is consistent with a recombinant chromosome 8 resulting from a pericentric inversion in one parent.

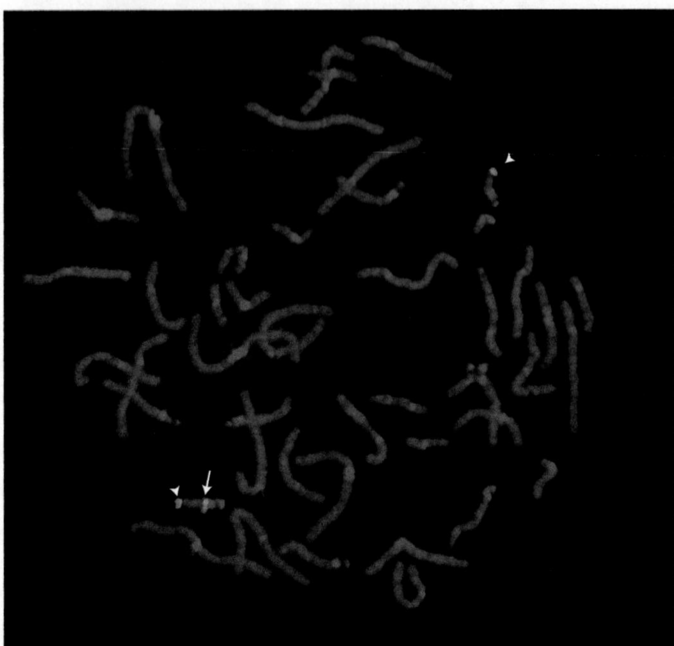

FIGURE 39–4 • Deletion 22q11.2. Dual-color fluorescence in situ hybridization (FISH), using a control probe mapping to the *ARSA* locus (green, arrowhead) at 22q13.3, and a test probe mapping to *TUPLE1* (red, arrow) at 22q11.2. One chromosome 22 is lacking the red signal.

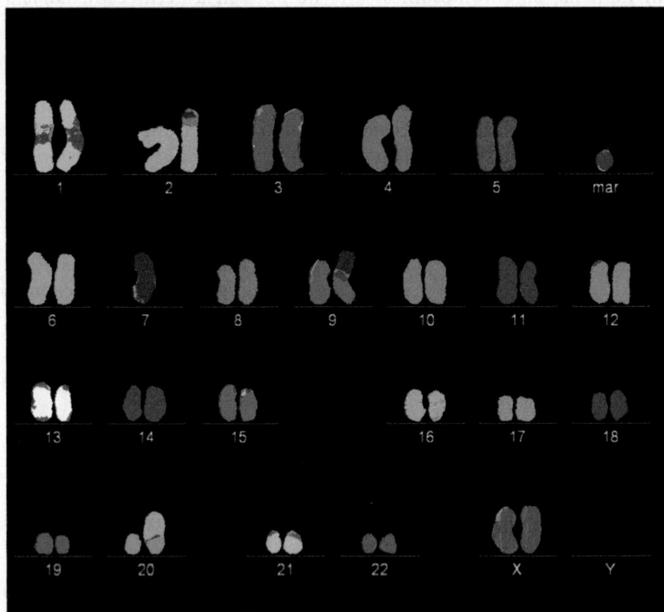

FIGURE 39–5 • Fluorescence in situ hybridization using multiple probes (multi-FISH). Multi-FISH in a patient with leukemia. Each pair of chromosomes is painted with a different color. Interchromosomal abnormalities are identified as a discrepant color within one chromosome (arrows). Chromosomes 2, 7, 9, and 20 are involved in a complex abnormality; a ring chromosome 18 is also visible. Pericentromeric heterochromatin of chromosomes 1 and 9 is apparent (blue). This technique allows identification and characterization of complex rearrangements.

Trisomies

Trisomies are the most common aneuploidy. *Trisomy* occurs when there are three representatives of a particular chromosome rather than the normal two (e.g., trisomy 21, trisomy 18). Trisomies are usually the result of a meiotic nondisjunction and most frequently are associated with meiosis I defects in the mother. They also are associated with advanced maternal age. Trisomy may be present in all the cells of an individual or may occur in mosaic form, with some normal cells and some cells with the additional chromosome. Most individuals with trisomy exhibit a consistent and specific phenotype depending on the chromosome involved. The most frequent and best known trisomy in humans is trisomy 21, or Down syndrome. Trisomies of chromosomes 18, 13, and X also occur relatively frequently. The incidence of trisomies among miscarriages is much higher than among live births. In the case of Down syndrome, at least twice as many conceptions of Down syndrome occur as there are live births. Conceptions with chromosomal abnormalities usually abort early in pregnancy.

TABLE 39–2 FREQUENCY OF CHROMOSOMAL DISORDERS AMONG NEWBORN INFANTS DETERMINED BEFORE AVAILABILITY OF PRENATAL DIAGNOSIS

Disorder	Frequency at Birth
AUTOSOMES	
Trisomy 21	1/600
Trisomy 18	1/5,000
Trisomy 13	1/15,000
SEX CHROMOSOMES	
Klinefelter's syndrome (47, XXY)	1/700 males
XYY syndrome	1/800 males
XXX syndrome	1/1,000 females
Turner's syndrome	1/4,000 females

The incidence of trisomies increases with advancing maternal age. The reason for this is not known. The incidence is sufficiently high by the age of 35 years, however, that prenatal diagnosis should be offered. Prenatal diagnosis usually involves amniocentesis or chorionic villus sampling to examine the fetal chromosomes. Most recently, maternal serum testing has been used for screening. In women younger than 35 years of age, maternal serum testing (triple screening) has been found to be efficacious in identifying those who are at risk for having a child with a chromosomal abnormality. Low maternal serum α-fetoprotein (MSAFP) concentration, low unconjugated estriol (uE3), and elevated human chorionic gonadotropin (HCG) are indicators of Down syndrome.

Among individuals with Down syndrome, most have three freestanding copies of chromosome 21; however, approximately 3% have a translocation involving chromosome 21. About one third of those with Down syndrome who have translocations have inherited the abnormal chromosome from one of their parents, who is usually completely asymptomatic. When translocation chromosomes are found, it is important to evaluate the parents. Rarely, a parent may have mosaic involvement such that they have minor features of Down syndrome and more than one germ cell involved. Prenatal diagnosis should be offered in all subsequent pregnancies.

Translocation of other chromosomes also may lead to aneuploidy. In the situation of three or more nonproductive pregnancies, the suspicion of translocation should be pursued by doing chromosome studies on both partners. In 5% of couples with multiple miscarriages, one or the other partner carries a translocation. Translocation carriers also can have children with the same translocations; all of their children should be screened as well. In the case of Down syndrome, those with a translocation are not clinically distinguishable from those with trisomy, because the translocation usually involves a complete extra set of functional chromosomal material.

Monosomies

Monosomies are another form of aneuploidy. Monosomies occur when there is only one representative of a chromosome pair. They may be complete or partial. Complete monosomies also are likely to result from nondisjunction and anaphase lag. Autosomal monosomies are usually lethal embryonically. Partial monosomies frequently occur in the offspring of individuals with translocations.

Abnormalities of Chromosome Structure

Deletions

Visible chromosomal deletions indicate that part of the chromosome is missing. They can occur as a simple deletion or as a deletion with a duplication (i.e., with a duplication of another segment). Deletions can

TABLE 39–3 MICRODELETIONS FOR SYNDROMES IN WHICH FLUORESCENCE IN SITU HYBRIDIZATION PROBES ARE AVAILABLE

Syndrome	Microdeletion
Alagille's syndrome	20p11.2
Angelman's syndrome	15.12q mat
Hemoglobin H-related mental retardation	16pter-p13.3
Miller-Dieker syndrome	17p13.12
Prader-Willi syndrome	15.12q pat
Rubinstein-Taybi syndrome	16p13.3
Smith-Magenis syndrome	17p11.2
Trichorhinophalangeal II (Langer-Giedion) syndrome	8q24.1
Velocardiofacial (DiGeorge) syndrome	22q11.2
WAGR	11p13
Williams syndrome	7q11.23

mat = maternal origin; pat = paternal origin; pter = short-arm terminal deletion; WAGR = Wilms' tumor, aniridia, genitourinary abnormalities, and mental retardation.

be located at the end of a chromosome or in an interstitial segment of the chromosome. Visible deletions usually are associated with mental retardation and/or malformations. Small telomeric deletions are relatively common in nonspecific mental retardation (10% of cases). The most commonly observed deletions in humans are 4p–, 5p–, 9p–, 11p–, 13q–, 18p–, and 18q–. These are associated with well-defined phenotypes.

Microdeletions

More recently, microdeletions have been found to be associated with specific syndromes, most of which also have been well described (Table 39–3). About half of these microdeletions are so small that they are not seen with microscopic studies and must be defined with the use of DNA probes. Microdeletions involve several genes, and the affected individuals can be expected to have a phenotype involving several organ systems. Known microdeletions identifiable with fluorescent probes include Williams syndrome, Langer-Giedion syndrome, Prader-Willi syndrome, Angelman's syndrome, Rubinstein-Taybi syndrome, Smith-Magenis syndrome, Miller-Dieker syndrome, Alagille's syndrome, and velocardiofacial (DiGeorge) syndrome.

Translocations

Translocations involve the transfer of chromosomal material from one chromosome to another and occur because of a break and reattachment of the chromosomes. They occur with a frequency of about 1 in 500 live births. They can be inherited from a parent or can occur de novo. When translocations are transmitted to children, there can be imbalances, with missing and/or extra chromosomal material. The two main types of translocation are robertsonian translocation and reciprocal translocation.

Robertsonian translocation involves acrocentric chromosomes (i.e., chromosomes in which the centromere is located near the end of the chromosome). This type of translocation involves fusion near the centromeric region, and consequently there is not loss of functional DNA. Robertsonian translocations comprise the fusion of the two long arms of two such chromosomes, and the individual carrying a robertsonian translocation has only 45 chromosomes. Individuals with robertsonian translocations are usually phenotypically normal; however, they are at increased risk of having offspring with translocation and trisomy.

Reciprocal translocations are the result of breaks of nonhomologous chromosomes with a reciprocal exchange of the broken segments. Carriers of various reciprocal translocations are usually phenotypically normal. Designation for reciprocal translocation includes the break points along the chromosome. For example, the designation 45,XY,t(13q2.1–14q1.3) indicates a male carrier of a translocation within the long arms of chromosomes 13 and 14.

Inversions

Inversions occur when the chromosome breaks at two points and the broken piece inverts and rejoins the chromosome. It can be *pericentric*, meaning that the breaks are in the two opposite arms of the chromosome, so that the inverted portion contains the centromere. *Paracentric* inversions occur within one arm of the chromosome.

Ring Chromosomes

Ring chromosomes are relatively rare and are frequently lost during mitosis, so individuals with a ring chromosome are often mosaic. The ring forms because there is a deletion at both ends of the chromosome, and the sticky ends join together to form a ring. The phenotype of a ring chromosome usually is similar to that of a deletion.

Duplications

Duplications occur when more than two copies of genetic material are present. Submicroscopic duplications also occur in some genetic disorders. Insertions occur when a piece of chromosome breaks and then is incorporated into part of another chromosome. Duplications and deletions frequently occur during crossing over in meiosis. Small deletions and duplications may not be obvious but have been found increasingly among children with moderate-to-severe mental retardation and no obvious phenotypic features. FISH and multitelomeric probes are becoming available to look for these small chromosomal changes.

Abnormalities of Sex Chromosomes

Turner's Syndrome

Turner's syndrome is the most common monosomy in live-born infants. The chromosome findings in Turner's syndrome involve loss of part or all of one of the sex chromosomes. Half of affected individuals have a 45,X karyotype in lymphocyte studies, suggesting that they do not have the other sex chromosome present in most cells. However, careful studies in fibroblasts and other tissues may reveal a Y chromosome in some cells in 2 to 3% of individuals with Turner's syndrome. The presence of Y-bearing cells is important, because these individuals have an increased risk of malignant degeneration of their gonads or masculinization at puberty. Half of individuals with Turner's syndrome have a variety of abnormalities of their other sex chromosome and may be mosaic. Turner's syndrome occurs in about 1 of every 4000 live-born females. The phenotype is almost always female, characterized by short stature and underdeveloped ovaries.

Klinefelter's Syndrome

Individuals with Klinefelter's syndrome are males with one or more extra X chromosomes, usually 47,XXY. The phenotype is male; they are usually relatively tall, they may have gynecomastia, and they almost always have azoospermia and small testes. Secondary sex characteristics may be late, and many men benefit from testosterone therapy.

Other Syndromes with Extra X Chromosomes

There are many syndromes described in which additional X chromosomes are observed. Males with an increasing number of X chromosomes are likely to be mentally retarded with radioulnar synostoses and genital anomalies. Women with 47,XXX are usually phenotypically normal and fertile.

47,XYY Male

The frequency of 47,XYY males is said to be about 1 in 1000 live-born males. Because XYY males do not have striking phenotype abnormalities, they often are not recognized, although they are said to be relatively tall and may have behavioral problems.

SUGGESTED READINGS

Iyengar SK: The quest for genes causing complex traits in ocular medicine: Successes, interpretations, and challenges. Arch Ophthalmol 2007;125:11–18. *Case study of the difficulty of finding a single disease-causing gene.*

Jalal SM, Harwood AR, Sekhon GS, et al: Utility of subtelomeric fluorescent DNA probes for detection of chromosome anomalies in 425 patients. Genet Med 2003;5:28–34. *These probes were instrumental in detecting anomalies.*

Jobanputra V, Sebat J, Troge J, et al: Application of ROMA (representational oligonucleotide microarray analysis) to patients with cytogenetic arrangements. Genet Med 2005;7:111–118. *Practical applications for a new technology.*

Malan V, Vekemans M, Turleau C: Chimera and other fertilization errors. Clin Genet 2006;70:363–373. *Overview with clinical examples.*

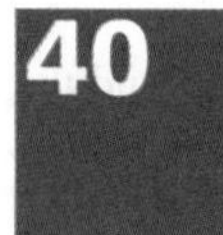

THE INHERITED BASIS OF COMMON DISEASES

David Altshuler

A central question in medicine is to understand why some people get sick and others do not. In some cases, a single environmental exposure plays a major role in disease risk (e.g., smoking and lung cancer or human immunodeficiency virus infection [HIV] and acquired immunodeficiency syndrome [AIDS]). In others, such as Huntington's disease or cystic fibrosis, mutation of a single gene is necessary and can be sufficient to cause illness. In most cases, however, disease is attributable neither to a single dominant environmental factor nor to mutation of a single gene. Rather, most cases of disease result from the combined action of inborn and somatically acquired alterations in gene sequence, environmental factors, and bad luck. Such disorders are termed complex traits.

Decades of careful epidemiologic research have documented that most common diseases are complex traits, with a significant fraction of interindividual variation in disease risk explained by inheritance. For this reason, studies of DNA sequence variation hold a key to unlocking information about the pathways that are causally responsible for human diseases as they exist in the general population. Because the sequence of the human genome is now known, it is possible for the first time to envision systematic and comprehensive surveys of common human genetic variation and its potential association to disease risk. This chapter reviews the paired concepts of heritability (the inherited contribution to disease risk) and heterozygosity (the inherited variation in genome sequence) and how they can be combined to illuminate the genetic architecture of common disease.

HERITABILITY: INHERITED VARIATION IN DISEASE RISK

Susceptibility to disease varies in the population. Studies of *familial aggregation* can determine the extent to which inheritance contributes to these patterns. These studies are simple in conception and ask whether members of the same family display more similar rates of disease than do individuals chosen at random from the population. When found, familial clustering can reflect not only shared genes but also shared environment. The contribution of shared genotype can be dissected further by comparing rates of disease within families as a function of the extent of genetic relatedness. The cleanest such design involves the comparison of disease concordance among dizygotic and monozygotic twin pairs. For common diseases such as types 1 and 2 diabetes mellitus, obesity, hypertension, coronary artery disease, autoimmune diseases, common cancers, schizophrenia, and bipolar disease, twin studies have documented that rates of concordance are significantly higher in monozygotic than in dizygotic twin pairs. For many other traits of clinical interest (e.g., most drug responses), formal tests of heritability have not yet been performed, and the role of inheritance in these characteristics is less clear.

Data about familial aggregation allow the calculation of *heritability,* or the fraction of interindividual variability in disease risk attributable to additive genetic influences. The remaining variability among individuals is due to all other contributions: environmental influences on disease, nonadditive (*epistatic*) genetic effects (e.g., gene-gene interactions or gene-environment interactions), error in the measurement of relatedness or disease, and random chance. For most clinically important traits (diseases and risk factors), empirical estimates of heritability range from 20 to 80% (see Online Mendelian Inheritance in Man, available at *http://www.ncbi.nlm.nih.gov:80/entrez/query.fcgi?db=OMIM,* for comprehensive information).

When interpreting estimates of heritability, it is important to consider two crucial factors: the effect of measurement errors and the environmental context. *Measurement errors* can decrease the estimate of the heritability of a trait. A single measurement of blood pressure is much less heritable than a composite score based on serial measures of blood pressure over time. That is, day-to-day variability and imprecision in clinical measures can obscure an underlying biologic susceptibility that is entrained by inheritance. For the patient and physician, this means that although the blood pressure on a given day may not be particularly heritable, the blood pressure over time (which is the risk factor for vascular disease) is heritable to a much greater extent.

Second, estimates of heritability have meaning only in the context of the environment in which the study was performed. In the case in which environmental triggers of disease are relatively constant across a study population, inherited factors may explain much of the variation in rates of disease. In contrast, in the case in which exposure to environmental causes of disease is highly varied across the study population, nongenetic factors may outweigh the contribution of inborn susceptibility. The rate and diversity of smoking histories have a major impact on how much of the variability in rates of lung cancer (in any given study or patient cohort) may be explained by inheritance. It is impossible to interpret or extrapolate measures of heritability without considering the environmental context in which the study was performed and that of the patient population of interest.

For these reasons, heritability is not a fixed characteristic of a disease, but an assessment of a given population, set of measurements, and the extent to which variability in genetic and environmental exposure explains disease risk. This sheds light on the apparent (but nonexistent) contradiction between rates of disease being highly heritable (in a given population) and yet varying dramatically across populations separated by time, geography, or socioeconomic status. In broad comparisons across groups, environmental exposure and methods of clinical ascertainment can vary substantially and contribute to secular changes in patterns of disease. Conversely, within a group exposed to a relatively uniform environment and studied in a standardized manner, genetic susceptibility may play a major role in determining individual risk. *Heritability* expresses the patterns of inherited variation in rates of disease; its doppelganger is *heterozygosity,* the pattern of inherited variation in genome sequence.

HETEROZYGOSITY: INHERITED VARIATION IN GENOME SEQUENCE

To what extent is there variation in the individual copies of the human genome sequence that we each inherit from our parents (Table 40–1)? A traditional measure of genetic variation is *heterozygosity,* defined as the proportion of sites on the chromosome at which two randomly chosen copies differ in DNA sequence. Because cells are *diploid* (carry two copies of the genome sequence) and because these two copies were selected in a semirandom manner from the population, heterozygosity is also equivalent to the fraction of base pairs that vary between the two copies in each

TABLE 40–1 CHARACTERISTICS OF HUMAN GENOME SEQUENCE VARIATION

Length of the human genome sequence (base pairs)	3,000,000,000
Number of human genes (estimated)	20,000
Fraction of base pairs that differ between the genome sequence of a human and a chimpanzee	1.3% (1 in 80)
Fraction of base pairs that vary between the genome sequence of any two humans	0.8% (1 in 1250)
Fraction of coding region base pairs that vary in a manner that alters the sequence of the encoded protein	0.2% (1 in 5000)
Number of sequence variants present in each individual as heterozygous sites	2,400,000
Number of amino acid–altering variants present in each individual as heterozygous sites	12,000
Number of sequence variants in the human population with a population frequency >1%	10,000,000
Number of amino acid polymorphisms present in the human genome with a population frequency >1%	75,000
Fraction of all human heterozygosity attributable to variants with a frequency >1%	90%

of our own cells. That is, heterozygosity is the rate of genetic variation in the individual.

There is limited heterozygosity in the human population. On average, less than 1 in 1200 positions in the human genome sequence varies between any two copies that are compared. In the coding regions of genes, rates of genetic variation are lower—less than 1 in every 2000 bases—secondary to darwinian selection against changes that alter the amino acid sequence of encoded proteins. These numbers are the same whether the two copies were sampled from a single geographic region or from groups whose ancestors lived in widely dispersed parts of the globe. The low rate of genetic diversity in the human population is quite unusual: chimpanzees, gorillas, and orangutans, primates closely related to humans, have 3 to 10 times as much genetic variation as humans do.

Much of the heterozygosity in the human population is due to single-nucleotide polymorphisms (SNPs)—sites at which a single letter in the DNA code has been swapped for a single alternate letter. The remaining variation is due to insertions and deletions of nucleotides, variation in the number of copies of repeat sequences, and larger-scale alterations. Until a short while ago, it was thought that larger-scale alterations (gains, losses, and inversions) were rare in the general population, but new technologies (with comprehensive scope, increased resolution, and falling cost) have revealed previously unappreciated variation in the content and structure of our genomes. Because both SNPs and larger-scale alterations presumably influence disease, both must be characterized to understand the inherited contribution to human health.

Among the limited fraction of sites that are heterozygous in any individual, approximately 90% are due to sequence variants that are *common* in the population (see Table 40–1). In cases in which the two copies in a single person differ, it is exceedingly likely that both versions would be found at an appreciable frequency in the population at large; only 10% of heterozygous sites in each individual are due to variants that exist at a frequency of less than 1% in the global human population. Because most human heterozygosity is due to common variants, it is possible to build catalogues that contain a substantial fraction of all human genetic diversity. A database containing all common (>1% frequency) sequence variants in the human population could be constructed that would sequence the genomes of only a few hundred individuals (drawn from all over the world) but would capture perhaps 90% of the heterozygous single-nucleotide changes present in any individual on the planet.

Sparked by the human genome project, efforts have sought to create such catalogues of common variants in the human genome sequence. At the time of this writing, the public database of SNPs contains more than 10 million candidate SNPs in the human genome (*http://www.ncbi.nlm.nih.gov:80/SNP/index.html*). Although not all of these SNPs are common (some are rare) and a small fraction may represent technical false positives, the existing collection represents the vast majority of the 10 million or so common SNPs thought to exist in the entire human population. Moreover, the frequencies of 3 million of these variants have been directly measured in human populations.

The major role of common variation in human sequence diversity is explained by the unique demographic history of the human population. Despite the global distribution of the current human population, it is now clear that all people on the planet are the descendants of a single population that lived in Africa only 10,000 to 40,000 years ago. The ancestral population was small (with an effective size of perhaps 10,000 individuals), lived a hunter-gatherer existence at low population densities (relative to other humans and later domesticated animals), and had evolved in Africa over millions of years. Most human genetic variation arose in this phase of human history, before the more recent migrations, expansions, and invention of technologies (e.g., farming) that resulted in widespread population of the globe. Most common human genetic variation predates the Diaspora and is shared by all populations on earth.

A second factor is that the rate of change in human DNA as a result of mutation and recombination is very slow when compared with the age of the human population. That is, any two people on the planet can trace their ancestry to a shared ancestor who lived at some point in the last million years since the emergence of modern humans. If we estimate the length of a human generation as being 20 years, the time to this shared ancestor is on the order of 10^3 to 10^4 generations. The rate of change in human DNA as a result of mutation, in contrast, is on the order of 10^{-8} per base pair per generation. In other words, considering the typical nucleotide in two unrelated humans, it is more likely that they trace back to a shared ancestor without any mutation having occurred than it is that a mutation has arisen in the intervening time. This explains why 99.9% of base pairs are identical when any two copies of the human genome are compared.

Another aspect of human variation is explained by these simple mathematical and population genetic relationships: the extent of human DNA sequence diversity attributable to rare and common variants. Each of us inherits from our parents some 3 million sites at which common polymorphisms exist. These common variants, which arose over hundreds of thousands of years, have the potential to influence traits in the population. We also inherit a set of less common variants that arose more recently, but these variants are fewer in number in each of us. Finally, given a genome that is 3,000,000,000 bases long and a mutation rate of 10^{-8} per base pair per generation, we inherit some 30 mutations that arose in the single generation from parent to child. The question of how these different classes of variants influence disease—the 3 million sites per person that are commonly varying and inherited from distant shared ancestors, the hundreds of thousands that are rare and arose in recent human history, and the 30 that arose in the last generation and are unique to the individual—is of central interest and importance to medical genetics.

The shared ancestry of human populations explains another aspect of human genetic variation: the correlations among nearby variants known as *linkage disequilibrium,* or *haplotypes.* Empirically, individuals who carry a particular variant at one site in the genome are much more likely than expected by chance to carry a particular set of variants at nearby positions along the chromosome. That is, not all combinations of nearby variants are observed in the population, but rather only a small subset of the possible combinations is observed. These correlations reflect the fact discussed earlier that most variants in our genomes arose once in human history (typically long ago) and did so on an arbitrary but unique copy carried by some individual in the population. The ancestral copy of the genome on which the mutation occurred can be recognized in the current population as a stretch of particular alleles (known as a *haplotype*) that track together in the population. That is, although most variations in our genome arose before written human history, the DNA sequence in each of us carries a record of the evolution and demographic history of the human population.

Studies have shown that these ancestral haplotypes, passed down from shared prehistoric ancestors in Africa, can be recognized in the current human population and explain the bulk of heterozygosity in each human. The relatively simple (modular) haplotype structure of the human genome offers a practical advantage in association studies of human disease. These haplotypes are typically long (spanning, on average, the size of a typical gene) and carry multiple variants always coinherited in the population. This can dramatically reduce the number of variants that need to be typed in patient samples to comprehensively assess common genetic variation across a region for contribution to disease risk. Developing a public database of human haplotypes is the goal of the recently completed International Haplotype Map Project.

MONOGENIC AND POLYGENIC FORMS OF DISEASE

With most diseases found to cluster in families and given increasingly powerful information and tools to investigate human genetic variation, there is great interest in identifying genetic risk factors that contribute to common human diseases. The design of studies to find these variations—and the probable implementation of any discoveries in clinical practice—depends on the underlying *genetic architecture* of each disease.

The genetic architecture of a disease refers to the number and magnitude of genetic risk factors that exist in each patient and in the population and their frequencies and interactions. Diseases can be due to a single gene *(monogenic)* in each family or to multiple genes *(polygenic).* It is easiest to identify genetic risk factors when only a single gene is involved and this gene has a major impact on disease. In cases in which a single gene is necessary and sufficient to cause disease, the condition is termed a *mendelian* disorder because the disease tracks perfectly with a mutation (in the family) that obeys Mendel's simple laws of inheritance.

Some single-gene disorders are caused by the same gene in all affected families; for example, cystic fibrosis is always caused by mutations in *CFTR.* Alternatively, a mendelian disorder can be due to a single genetic lesion in any given family, but in different families it can be due to mutations in a variety of genes. This phenomenon, termed *locus heterogeneity*, is illustrated by retinitis pigmentosa. Although mutation in a single gene is typically necessary and sufficient to cause retinitis pigmentosa, there are dozens of different genes in which retinitis pigmentosa mutations have been found (Online Mendelian Inheritance in Man #268000). In each family, however, only one such gene is mutated to cause disease.

Most single-gene disorders are rare (present in <1% of the population) and are manifested early in life. Many are severe and cause death before reproduction in the absence of modern medical care. The fact that most monogenic disorders are severe in childhood and rare in the population is probably not a coincidence but rather reflects the impact of *natural selection*. The deleterious effect of these mutations results in a decrease in reproductive fitness (in individuals unlucky enough to inherit them), and the mutations and the disease are unlikely to drift to high frequency in the population. There are exceptions to this general idea: cases in which the mutation causing a severe monogenic disease (such as *HbS*, the cause of sickle cell anemia, or the δ-508 mutation in *CFTR*) is common in the population at large. These cases appear as a result of a different kind of selection, known as *balancing selection:* situations in which a gene mutation is beneficial in one circumstance (a genotype or environment) but deleterious in another. It is believed that heterozygous carriers for *HbS* and δ-508 are relatively protected against infectious diseases and that this benefit balances the deleterious effect of the disease in homozygotes.

There has been spectacular success identifying the specific genetic mutations that cause mendelian disorders, with hundreds of genes identified for clinically important conditions (for comprehensive information, see *http://www.ncbi.nlm.nih.gov:80/entrez/query.fcgi?db=OMIM*). Progress was sparked by the development of a suite of powerful research techniques—*family-based linkage analysis* and *positional cloning*—in which the causal gene is first localized to a chromosomal region and then that chromosomal neighborhood is scoured for the genetic culprit. The power of these approaches was fuelled by the Human Genome Project, which provided the foundation of information on DNA structure, sequence, and genetic variation required to undertake such searches.

In most, but not all cases, the causal mutations found in mendelian disease are rare in the population, with each family carrying a different and novel mutation that severely alters the function of the encoded protein. The bias toward low-frequency mutations that are relatively unique to each family argues for the role of natural selection against the disease-causing mutations.

Similar to mendelian disorders, most common diseases are also influenced by inheritance. In contrast to mendelian disorders, the genetic contribution to common diseases seems to be due to the action of many genes rather than a single gene in each family and a limited number of genes in the population. Empirical evidence in favor of this model comes from efforts to use the same approach (positional cloning) for complex traits that was applied successfully to monogenic disorders. In the 1990s, the tools of family-based linkage analysis were applied to nearly all common disorders of the industrialized world. In many of these studies, dozens or hundreds of families were studied, and hundreds of genetic markers were typed in each individual. Despite this heroic effort and except for a few notable successes, these studies revealed few strong signals that localized the genes responsible for disease. In most of the dozens of such studies that have been published there are many weak statistical signals (few if any are statistically significant given the large number of hypotheses tested) and little agreement between different studies of the same disease.

In view of the well-understood statistical power of family-based linkage methods (based on their extensive use for monogenic disorders) and their relatively limited success despite extensive efforts in common diseases, it is reasonable to conclude that no single gene explains a large fraction of the risk for common diseases. If a single gene contained mutations that explained 30% of the inherited risk for type 2 diabetes, hypertension, or schizophrenia, it is extremely likely that its location would long since have been found. Supporting this idea is the exception to the general rule: HLA (human leukocyte antigen), which explains approximately 50% of the genetic risk for type 1 diabetes, has been strongly identified in every linkage study performed to date in that disease. The fact that few such findings (outside HLA) have been found for common diseases suggests that few single genetic risk factors (of this magnitude) are probably operative in complex traits. Rather, the typical situation seems to be a larger number of susceptibility factors, each of which more modestly contributes to disease.

MONOGENIC FORMS OF COMMON DISEASES

One potential shortcut to understanding the genetic determinants of common diseases is to identify and study rare, early-onset forms of diseases that demonstrate mendelian patterns of inheritance. Because these diseases display mendelian patterns of inheritance, the powerful tools of positional cloning can be and have been used successfully to identify the genes responsible. Important examples include the role of *BRCA1* and *BRCA2* in early-onset breast cancer, maturity-onset diabetes of the young as a form of type 2 diabetes, many monogenic disorders of blood pressure and electrolyte regulation, and early-onset Alzheimer's disease.

These successes are important because they provide diagnostic information for families burdened with severe, early-onset forms of disease and because they provide insight into the underlying pathways responsible for disease. More than a dozen genes have been identified that when mutated, cause rare mendelian disorders of blood pressure and electrolyte regulation. So far, every one of these genes is active in the kidney, and most are involved in the renin-angiotensin-aldosterone pathway. This result is a spectacular confirmation of the central importance of the kidney in human blood pressure regulation and has suggested new therapeutic targets of substantial promise.

It had long been hoped that the genes identified as being responsible for early-onset, monogenic forms of common diseases would contribute to the more common forms of disease in the population. In this scenario, severe mutations might cause early-onset forms, and more prevalent but subtle alterations in the same genes might contribute to common forms of disease. To date, convincing evidence in support of this hypothesis does not exist. Genes identified for the aforementioned, early-onset diseases have not yet been shown to contribute more generally to the population risk for disease. The hypothesis remains viable, however, because comprehensive evaluation of the genetic variation at any given gene is only now becoming possible as a result of developments in knowledge from the human genome and improved methods of genetic epidemiologic analysis.

MODELS FOR THE GENETIC ARCHITECTURE OF COMMON DISEASE

Although there is little specific knowledge about the genes and mutations responsible for most common diseases, two broad classes of models have been proposed to explain the genetic architecture of common disorders. In the first class of model, common diseases are not a single, homogeneous entity, but rather composites of many different rare disorders. Each of these disorders may be caused by mutations in different genes, with the mutations having characteristics (of low frequency and large magnitude of effect) similar to that in traditional mendelian disorders. In this model, which is reminiscent of retinitis pigmentosa, failure to achieve linkage (see earlier) occurs simply because the signal for any single gene is diluted by the large number of cases caused by mutations at other loci.

The second prominent model suggests that each case of disease is due to the combined influence of many different mutations and that disease ensues when the sum of susceptibility alleles outweighs the sum of alleles that are protective. In this scenario, many of these mutations must be common in the population because it is necessary for each affected person to inherit more than one such mutation and the diseases are common in the population. In this model, the relative risk attributable to any single mutation would be modest because disease would result only when each variant was inherited in concert with other such changes.

Two models are based on different precedents: the former from human genetics and the latter from epidemiology. Beyond argument by analogy, however, it is possible to base these arguments on the foundation of well-understood evolutionary principles and hypotheses about the evolutionary history of common diseases. Because most human genetic variation arose—and evolution took place—before the more recent expansions in the population and invention of modern society, it is likely that the relevant epoch of human history is that of the small, prehistoric ancestral population rather than the large, technologically advanced modern population.

If the disease (or other characteristic influenced by the genotype) had been neutral from the point of natural selection, the bulk of genetic variation contributing to the trait would be expected to be common. If the mutations led to traits that were evolutionarily disadvantageous (even mildly so), the bulk of disease-causing variants would be largely rare (as in most monogenic diseases). Finally, if the sum of the evolutionary effect of the disease-causing class of mutations was beneficial, the mutations would probably be more common than the genome-wide pattern.

One thing is certain: there will be no single answer, but rather examples of all such scenarios among the variety of common human diseases. It seems unlikely that mutations causing infertility would be found to be common in the population because the negative effect on reproduction is disadvantageous from an evolutionary perspective. In contrast, mutations that protect against infections or other major killers (e.g., famine or surviving the neonatal period) may well be common and could influence common diseases in the modern world. Mutations that cause a disease in the current environment may have had a different evolutionary impact in the environment in which humans evolved.

ASSOCIATION STUDIES

Despite this uncertainty, there has been significant progress identifying genes that contribute to the population risk for common diseases. Nearly all examples have been discovered through epidemiologic association studies of common genetic variation.

Genetic association studies are simple in conception. One or more putative causal variants are identified, and their frequency is compared between populations with the disease of interest and well-matched controls (drawn from the population at large or unaffected family members). Because association studies are a direct test of each allele, they offer the greatest sensitivity to detect the relationship between a variant and disease.

The *HLA* locus on chromosome 6 is probably the largest single determinant of susceptibility to common diseases because it plays a major (if complex) role in infectious and autoimmune diseases. Other robust and reproducible associations include the contribution of Apo-ε4 to Alzheimer's disease; factor V Leiden to deep venous thrombosis; a 32-base deletion in the chemokine receptor CCR5 to the risk for AIDS; common variants in the insulin gene, in PTPN22, and in CTLA4 to type 1 diabetes; SNPs in the peroxisome proliferator–activated receptor γ (PPAR-γ), the beta-cell potassium channel Kir6.2, and TCF7L2 to the risk for type 2 diabetes; and others (Table 40–2). A comprehensive survey of all published genetic association studies showed that although many published associations have been nonreproducible (probably because of inappropriate statistical thresholds for declaring or rejecting associations), true associations have been identified through this approach.

Perhaps the most spectacular recent results regarding the genetic basis of a common disease have come in the study of age-related macular degeneration (AMD). AMD appears to be a typical common, polygenic disease: there is evidence for heritability in that siblings of affected patients are perhaps three to six times as likely as unrelated individuals to become afflicted, and yet family-based linkage analysis revealed only modestly significant (and modestly reproducible) linkage results. Most importantly, the underlying pathophysiologic defects that explain why one person goes blind with AMD whereas another remains free of the disease were unknown.

TABLE 40–2 EXAMPLES OF GENES WITH COMMON INHERITED SEQUENCE VARIANTS THAT INFLUENCE COMMON, POLYGENIC HUMAN DISEASES

Gene	Disease
Apo-ε4	Alzheimer's disease
Factor V Leiden	Deep venous thrombosis
HLA (many)	Autoimmunity (many)
Insulin VNTR	Type 1 diabetes
PPAR-γ	Type 2 diabetes
Kir6.2	Type 2 diabetes
TCF7L2	Type 2 diabetes
CCR5 δ32	Protection against HIV infection
CTLA4 Thr17Ala	Graves' disease, type 1 diabetes
TPMT	Response to thiopurine
PTPN22	Rheumatoid arthritis, type 1 diabetes
CFH	Age-related macular degeneration
LOC387715	Age-related macular degeneration
IRF5	Systemic lupus erythematosus

In 2005, three groups simultaneously found that a common coding polymorphism in the gene for complement factor H is a major risk factor for AMD. The variant *(Y402H)* has a high population frequency (approximately 35% in European populations) and increases risk by 2.5- to 3.0-fold in heterozygotes and by 5- to 7-fold in homozygotes. Following on this work it was found that another factor, complement factor B (CFB), also carries common genetic variation that influences the risk for AMD in a highly reproducible manner (although the adjacent gene to CFB also shows association). Third, a common variant of high frequency and substantial effect was found in a previously unstudied gene on chromosome 10 *(LOC387715)* and shown by multiple groups to strongly influence risk.

The statistical association of genetic variants in these three genes explains perhaps half of the inherited risk for AMD and is able to stratify patients into risk groups with a quite different likelihood of disease. Such findings can, in principle, be used to design clinical trials with a much more precise estimate of risk in each patient. Perhaps most importantly, these findings unambiguously identify a previously unsuspected set of biologic actors as being causally involved in this common disease.

As in the examples presented, most of the known genetic influences on common disease are themselves common in the population. It is much too early, however, to conclude whether this will be a general feature of the genetic basis of common disease. On the one hand, it is possible that the high frequency of the common diseases is a byproduct of their evolutionary history. In this scenario, many common variants would be found, with many individually rare alleles that contribute a fraction to the overall genetic influence on the disease. On the other hand, the preponderance of common mutations identified thus far could reflect *ascertainment bias.* That is, it is possible that only a small subset of the mutations influencing common disease are common (with the rest being rare), but just those that are common could be found with the available information, tools, and methodologies. Only more data can resolve this question.

CHALLENGES TO THE IDENTIFICATION OF GENETIC FACTORS FOR COMMON DISEASES

The simple concepts of mutation and population history explain the relative contributions of rare and common variants to each individual's unique genome sequence. From one point of view, the human genome is 3,000,000,000 bases long, and with a mutation rate of 10^{-8} per base pair per generation, we each inherit some 30 mutations on each copy of the genome that arose in previous generation (from parent to child). Another perspective (which is equally true) is that each of us inherits some 3 million variants that are common and arose over the hundreds of thousands of years of human history. All of these variants, both common and rare, have the potential to influence traits in the population, so a key question for medicine is how these different classes of variants contribute to disease: the variants that are common and inherited from distant shared ancestors, the variants that arose in the thousand or so generations since humans left Africa (which tend to be lower in frequency and more population specific), and the few that arose in very recent history and are relatively unique to the individual.

The low likelihood of finding a gene and variant that play a role in disease requires that more stringent statistical thresholds be applied than is usually the case in epidemiologic research. This is often described as a problem of "multiple hypothesis testing," with the investigative community searching for associations between multiple genes, multiple variants in each gene, and multiple diseases. Given a large-scale and broad search, it becomes likely that a statistical fluctuation would be encountered (absent any true association) and lead to the false interpretation of a relationship between the exposure and disease of interest.

This problem is illuminated most clearly in a bayesian statistical framework. The human genome is now thought to contain approximately 20,000 genes. Each of these genes harbors dozens of common variants and many more changes that are rare. Absent any other knowledge of biology, each of these changes would have an equal (and exceedingly low) a priori likelihood of containing variation that confers risk for disease. Similar to the use of a screening test in a population that has a low rate of disease, the number of false-positive results is expected to outnumber true-positive results unless dramatically more stringent statistical thresholds are used. It is possible to increase the prior probability by guessing about candidate genes based on hypotheses about gene function, but these studies are by their nature limited and prone to bias. These concerns are supported by the published association literature, in which perhaps only 5 to 10% of the many hundreds of published genetic associations are found to be reproducible on repeated testing.

The statistical challenges increase exponentially when gene-gene or gene-environment interactions are considered. Although it is clear that gene-gene and gene-environment interactions exist, there is a huge potential universe of gene-gene or gene-environment pairs, and the prior probability of any given pair explaining a large degree of disease risk is correspondingly small. In the absence of a strong previous hypothesis (e.g., a known biochemical or physical interaction between proteins) or an extremely impressive statistical result, associations of this nature are more likely to represent a false-positive result arising from aggressive dredging of data rather than a biologically meaningful relationship to disease.

There is no simple, straightforward, or general answer to these challenges. As in most rapidly evolving fields of medical research, individual clinicians need to have access to reliable guidance on the interpretation of genetic studies and to extrapolate from the available literature to their own clinical practice.

FUTURE DIRECTIONS

Decades of epidemiology have shown that inherited factors contribute substantially to common human diseases. Progress in population genetics and genomics has revealed that most human heterozygosity is due to genetic variants that are common, old, and shared broadly across the planet. There is a narrow, but deep universe of less common variation that arose more recently in human history. Genome-wide catalogues of human genetic variation are becoming increasingly complete and offer an approach to testing the bulk of human heterozygosity for contribution to disease.

The exact path to apply these tools is uncertain because the evolutionary history and the genetic architecture of common diseases have not yet been defined. It is likely, however, that in the years and decades to come, the answers to these questions will come into much clearer focus. Over time, the tools of human genetics will help elucidate the pathways that cause common human diseases and, similar to the discovery of cholesterol and its association with vascular diseases, point toward the development of therapeutics of broad value to human health.

SUGGESTED READINGS

Daiger S: Was the Human Genome Project worth the effort? Science 2005;308:362–364. *Discusses strategies for gene discovery in the context of the novel finding of a common polymorphism in complement factor H that influences the risk for age-related macular degeneration.*

International Hapmap Consortium: A haplotype map of the human genome. Nature 2005;437:1299–320. *A genome-wide database of common human sequence variation as a resource for comprehensive genetic association studies of human disease.*

Kotowski IK, Pertsemlidis A, Luke A, et al: A spectrum of PCSK9 alleles contributes to plasma levels of low-density lipoprotein cholesterol. Am J Hum Genet 2006;78:410–422. *Common and rare variants in* PCSK9 *combine to influence low-density lipoprotein levels in the population.*

41 CELL AND GENE THERAPY

Karl Skorecki and Eithan Galun

CELL THERAPY

Cell therapy refers to the provision of living cells to patients for the prevention or treatment of human disease. The best established and most widely practiced form of cell therapy is the administration of blood and blood products in transfusion medicine, which provides therapeutic relief of a temporary deficit in formed blood elements such as erythrocytes, platelets, or white blood cells. Other emerging applications of cell therapy involve use of cells as vehicles for the delivery of genes or gene products, as discussed in the section on gene therapy.

Regenerative medicine is an emerging field wherein cells from various sources are administered to augment, repair, or replace tissue or organ system function damaged by disease, injury, or congenital anomaly. In this regard, solid organ transplantation can be considered a form of cell therapy. Like blood and blood product transfusion (Chapter 183), solid organ transplantation provides fully differentiated, functioning replacement cells of the transplanted organ (Chapters 82, 102, and 158).

One of the most important practical limitations of solid organ transplantation is the shortage of available organs relative to the growing demand. This situation is true to a greater or lesser extent for cardiac failure, end-stage renal disease, end-stage lung disease, diabetes mellitus, and advanced cirrhosis with hepatic failure. In certain forms of irreversible organ system failure, such as neurodegenerative disease, organ transplantation is not a therapeutic option. For these reasons, development of cell therapies is progressing.

Stem Cells of Human Origin

Stem cells are defined by their capacity for asymmetrical cell division (Fig. 41–1). In this process, a stem cell yields one daughter cell that is a replica of itself and has the capacity for further asymmetrical cell division. The second daughter cell loses this capacity and replaces it with other characteristics important for specialized cellular function. After asymmetrical cell division, non–stem cell derivatives may either generate a pool of organ system–restricted, transit-amplifying cells with enhanced proliferative capacity or differentiate by epigenetic and gene expression profile changes until reaching the terminally differentiated state. This framework was developed after the discovery of bone marrow cells that were capable of reconstituting the adult hematopoietic system. These hematopoietic stem cells constitute the basis for hematopoietic stem cell transplantation, the only form of stem cell therapy currently used in clinical practice (Chapter 184). More recent terminology has broadened use of the term "stem cells" to cover a wider array of cell types that contribute to organ development or have the capacity to repopulate tissues and organ systems. The term stem cell, together with the formulation noted earlier, has also recently been extrapolated to describe certain cellular subpopulations that may be principally responsible for the growth of malignant tumors. However, because cancer stem cells have no role in tissue regeneration, they are not considered further in this chapter.

Embryonic Stem Cells

Embryonic stem cells refer to stem cells derived during various stages of prenatal human development, beginning as a fertilized egg. The fertilized egg, or zygote, develops first into a blastocyst, then an embryo, and then a fetus. The blastocyst is evident on day 5 after fertilization and consists of 200 to 250 cells, 30 to 34 of which consist of the inner cell mass,

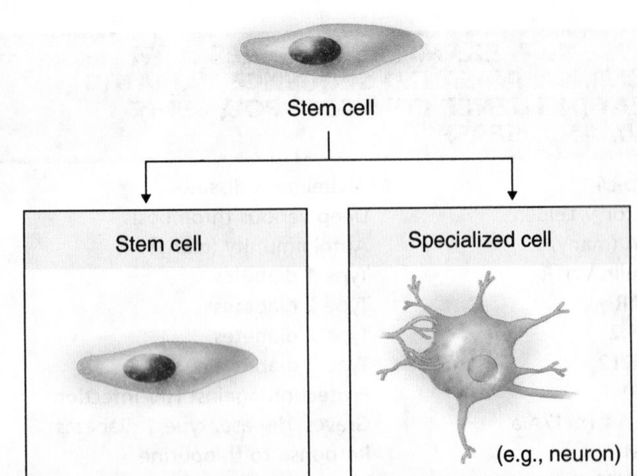

FIGURE 41–1 • Asymmetrical cell division. Although this first characteristic was considered a *required characteristic* for stem cells based on their original description in the adult hematopoietic system, not all cell types currently named as stem cells necessarily display this property. For instance, human embryonic stem cells divide by symmetrical cell division.

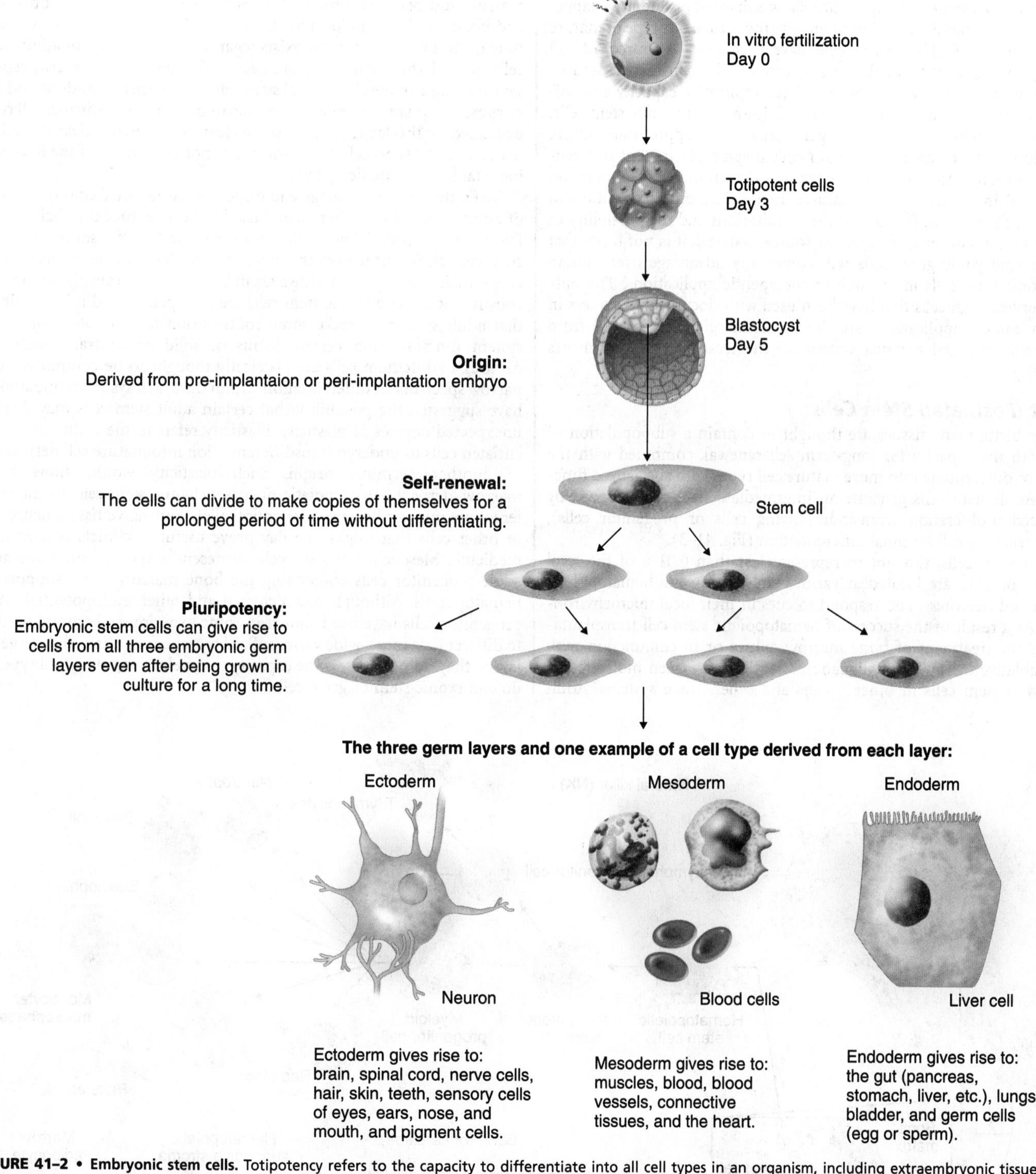

FIGURE 41–2 • Embryonic stem cells. Totipotency refers to the capacity to differentiate into all cell types in an organism, including extraembryonic tissues, placenta, and umbilical cord, a property confined to the fertilized egg itself, including the cells derived from the first few cell divisions after fertilization. Pluripotency refers to the capacity to differentiate into all the specialized cell types derived from the three germ layers (ectoderm, mesoderm, endoderm) of the developing embryo and is a hallmark feature of embryonic stem and germ cells.

or epiblast. The remaining cells are the outer cell mass (Fig. 41–2). After the entire blastocyst attaches to the lining of the uterus, embryonic and extraembryonic development begins. At the blastocyst stage, each cell in the inner cell mass has the capacity to differentiate into derivatives of all three germline layers (ectoderm, mesoderm, and endoderm). In normal development, these cells do not persist beyond the blastocyst stage. Unused preimplantation blastocysts created for in vitro fertilization can be used to generate human embryonic stem cells from the microdissected inner cell mass. Under appropriate culture conditions, these human embryonic stem cells exhibit unlimited or prolonged self-renewal in cell culture in the undifferentiated state without undergoing replicative senescence (i.e., losing the ability to divide). Embryonic stem cells exhibit high levels of expression of telomerase, an enzyme that maintains telomere integrity through multiple rounds of cell division. Under different culture conditions, human embryonic stem cells are pluripotent; they can differentiate into any of the known cell types of the body.

A major goal of embryonic stem cell research is to direct the differentiation process to enable enrichment to homogeneity of a replacement cell type by adding growth factors that activate cell signaling pathways used in normal embryonic development. This approach has yielded partial enrichment of cells with properties similar to those of authentic fetal pancreatic beta cells, vascular endothelial cells, and cardiomyocytes, as well as more mature cells with properties similar to those of bone, connective tissue, and retinal, neuronal, and hepatic cells.

During the later stages of prenatal human development, cells derived from fetal developmental origin often show enhanced proliferative capacity, as well as the ability to differentiate into more than one type of mature or specialized cell. Thus, these cells have been used as sources of cell therapy in regenerative medicine and can also be considered stem or progenitor cells—but with more restricted replicative capacity and differentiation potential than is the case with human embryonic stem cells. An exception is human embryonic germ cells. Under appropriate culture conditions, human embryonic germ cells display pluripotent differentiation, although they appear to have a limited number of population doublings, in contrast to the infinite replication capacity of human embryonic stem cells. Because of these limitations and the possibility of greater ethical concerns in terms of source material, it is not likely that human embryonic germ cells will confer any advantage over human embryonic stem cells in research or therapeutic applications. The only fetal-derived stem cells that have been used with documented success in human clinical applications are the dopaminergic cells derived from the developing fetal nervous system for the treatment of Parkinson's disease.

Adult (Postnatal) Stem Cells

After birth, many tissues are thought to contain a subpopulation of cells with the capacity for long-term self-renewal, combined with the ability to differentiate into more mature cell types with specialized functions. Adult stem cells generate an intermediate state characterized by enhanced proliferation (transit-amplifying cells or progenitor cells), before reaching full terminal differentiation (Fig. 41–3).

Adult stem cells, thought to represent less than 0.01% of the total number of cells, are located at various sites within the hematopoietic system and elsewhere, and respond to cues in their local microenvironment. As a result of the success of hematopoietic stem cell transplantation in the treatment of bone marrow failure or in conjunction with myeloablative therapy in malignancy, scientists have been motivated to find adult stem cells in other organs and other organ systems. Adult tissues and organ systems reported to contain stem cells include bone marrow and peripheral blood, the central nervous system, blood vessel endothelium, dental pulp, epithelia of the skin, digestive system, cornea, retina, and liver. Controversy exists regarding the existence of adult stem cells in the kidney, pancreas, and heart. Whether adult stem cells represent remnants of developmental stem cells that persist into adulthood for purposes of organ maintenance and repair or represent a distinct cell type dedicated for this latter purpose is not clear. However, it is clear that adult hematopoietic stem cells share some, but not all features of the developing fetal hematopoietic system.

Given their low percentage and dispersed tissue distribution, isolation of adult stem cells for therapeutic use has been technically challenging. Despite some promising results in animal models, the source of adult stem cells sufficient for cell therapy in the context of regenerative medicine remains to be proved. However, in bone marrow transplantation, the constituent hematopoietic stem cells are therapeutic, and it is also likely that adult stem cells make some contribution to restoration of organ system function after certain forms of solid organ transplantation. Although adult stem cells are classically thought to be committed to a narrow spectrum of differentiation within the organ system, some studies have suggested the possibility that certain adult stem cells may display unexpected degrees of plasticity. Plasticity refers to the ability of differentiated cells to undergo transdifferentiation into mature cell derivatives of another germline origin. Such plasticity would allow bone marrow–derived hematopoietic or mesenchymal stem cells to transdifferentiate into cardiac, vascular endothelial, connective tissue, neuronal, or other cells that might one day prove useful in clinical regenerative medicine. Mesenchymal stem cells represent a type of multipotential adult progenitor cells comprising the bone marrow niche supporting hematopoiesis. Although mesenchymal and other multipotential adult progenitor cells have been shown in some experimental animal models to differentiate into a wide variety of cell types representing all three germ layers, they do not possess the capacity to develop into every cell type, as do embryonic stem or germ cells.

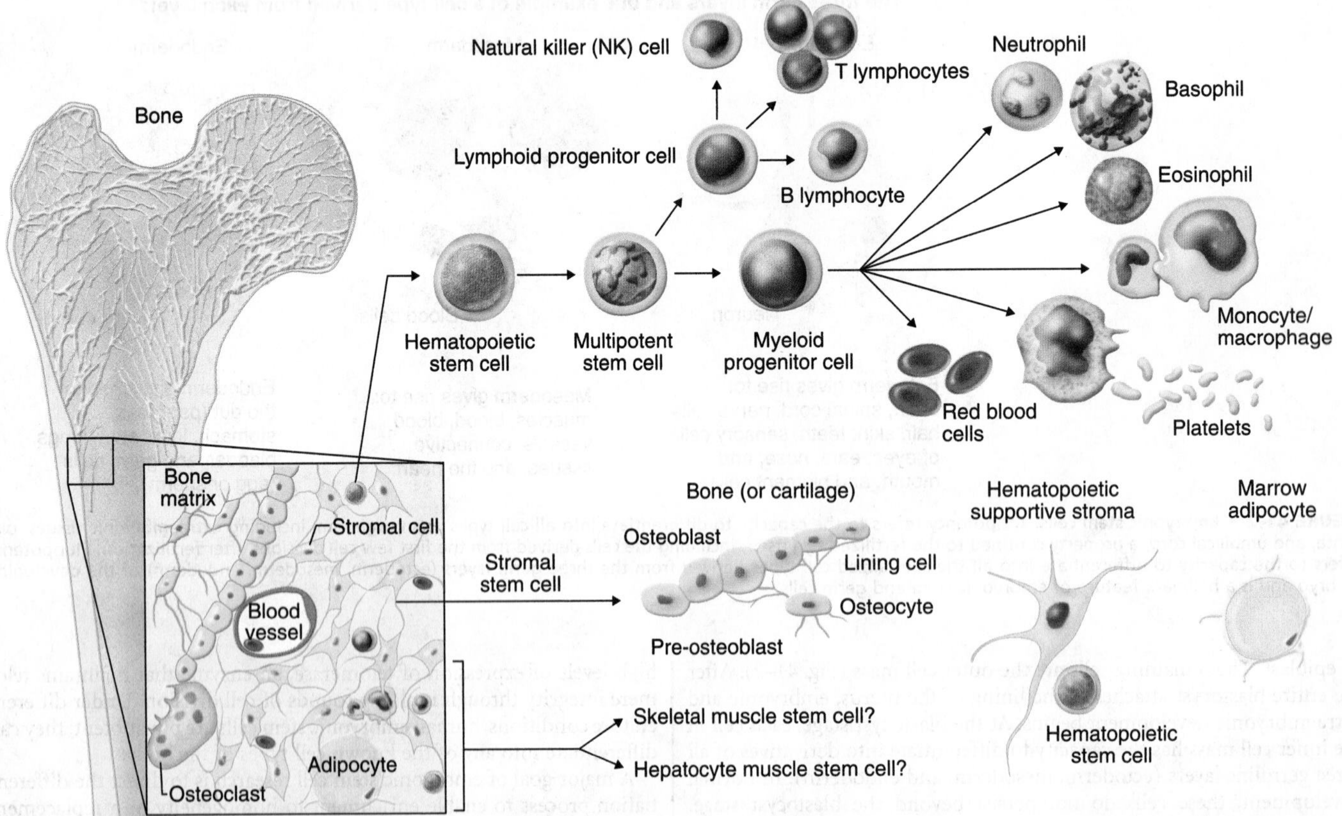

FIGURE 41–3 • Adult stem cells. Adult stem cells can be multipotent and have the capacity to differentiate into a limited number of different cell types, often restricted to a given tissue or organ system, as in the case of adult hematopoietic or epidermal stem cells. Two stem cell types have been isolated from adult bone marrow—the hematopoietic stem cell and the mesenchymal stem cell. Adult mesenchymal stem cells of bone marrow origin, although the range of differentiation has been shown to be broader than that of any other adult stem cell type, do not reach pluripotency. It is thought that in some organ systems, such as the gastrointestinal epithelium, a unipotent pool of progenitors exists for repopulating a rapid population turnover of only one type of cell—although it is difficult to be certain whether such progenitors can be distinguished from the overall population of fully differentiated cells in tissues with high cellular turnover.

TABLE 41–1 STRATEGIES FOR PREVENTING OR TREATING ALLOIMMUNOGENIC REJECTION IN STEM CELL THERAPY

Antirejection therapy, tolerance reduction, and chimerism
Adult stem cells from an autologous source
Banks for human embryonic stem cells corresponding to global major histocompatibility complex representation
Genetic manipulation of the major histocompatibility locus
Genetic engineering to introduce tolerogenic factors
Micro-encapsulation
Vaccination
Somatic nuclear transfer

Postnatal or adult stem cells have the potential to circumvent two of the obstacles in developmental stem cell therapy, including alloimmunologic rejection and ethical concerns regarding the use of cells of developmental origin. Embryonic stem cells and their derivatives generally emanate from a source not related to the potential recipient and can therefore be considered an allogeneic graft. Research studies have confirmed the immunogenicity of human embryonic stem cells despite their very early developmental origin. Although systemic antirejection immunosuppressive therapy can be used in a manner similar to that for allogeneic organ transplantation, several strategies have been investigated as a means of preempting such immunologic rejection in the first place. Adult stem cells of autologous origin should not elicit an alloimmunologic response and therefore offer a potential solution (see Table 41–1). On the other hand, when the underlying disease is an active autoimmune destructive process (e.g., type 1 diabetes mellitus), it can be expected that replacement cells of autologous origin might also be targets of the immune-mediated pathophysiologic process. Because their derivation is not associated with destruction of the organism, the other major advantage of using adult stem cells is avoidance of societal concerns regarding personhood status.

Specific Disease Applications in Cell Therapy

Except for hematopoietic stem cell and solid organ transplantation, experimental cell therapies have been implemented in a limited number of patient trials.

Parkinson's Disease

Parkinson's disease (Chapter 432) involves loss of melanin-containing dopaminergic neurons within the substantia nigra pars compacta of the midbrain, coupled with accompanying depletion of striatal dopamine. This cellular loss is responsible for the major motor features of the disease. Although pharmacologic dopaminergic replacement therapy is effective in the early stages of illness, prolonged treatment with pharmacologic agents alone is associated with refractoriness and complications and fails to halt the underlying neurodegeneration. In the search for more definitive therapy, cell replacement therapy and implantable electrical stimulation approaches, among others, have been suggested as candidate therapeutic tools. In the early 1970s, studies demonstrated that adrenal chromatin cells or embryonic dopaminergic neurons could be transplanted and followed into the rat anterior eye chamber. Neurite outgrowth and integration with the recipient nervous system were optimally achieved when the transplant source was of embryonic origin. These studies also underscored the importance of specificity of donor cells committed to a dopaminergic fate. As in the experimental animal systems, the first clinical trials began with the use of autografts of adrenal medullary origin. Improvements were modest and transient at best and were associated with unacceptable levels of morbidity and mortality. Subsequent work has focused on implantation of dopaminergic neuronal cells of fetal origin. Reports indicate significant and sustained improvement in motor function after intrastriatal implantation of human fetal mesencephalic tissue. The implanted cells in these trials were obtained from aborted human fetuses aged 6 to 9 weeks after conception. Long-term immunosuppressive treatment is essential to allow transplanted dopaminergic neurons to develop to their full functional potential despite the notion of an immunologic sanctuary within the brain. Clinical assessment standards have provided clear evidence of long-lived graft survival and clinical benefit after therapy with cells of fetal origin that has now lasted up to 10 years or longer. Further progress is limited by lack of sufficient source tissue to treat a large number of affected patients, prohibitive variability in functional outcome, and reports of serious dyskinesias in a subset of treated patients.

Research has have shown enrichment of dopaminergic neuronal derivatives in vitro, which has led to the hope that embryonic stem cell technologies may provide a potential source of dopaminergic neurons.

Investigations of stem cell–based approaches for the treatment of other neurodegenerative diseases, including Alzheimer's disease and spinal cord injury, are currently under way in animal models.

Muscular Dystrophies and Other Disorders of the Musculoskeletal System

The family of muscular dystrophies (Chapter 446) is characterized by progressive degeneration of skeletal muscle, with the various patterns depending on the underlying etiologic condition. In the major genetic forms of muscular dystrophy, a range of approaches have been developed that aim to correct the genetic defect, restore functional expression of the missing gene product (e.g., dystrophin), and thereby slow disease progression. These approaches can be divided into three categories: pharmacologic, genetic, and cell therapy. Maintenance plus regeneration of muscle fibers (myofibers) is necessary for normal muscle function. This process begins with activation of quiescent muscle precursor cells, which then form proliferating progenitors, which in turn fuse to generate differentiated myofibers. This has led to the proposal that implantation of myoblast muscle precursor cells might enable the improved repopulation of degenerating dystrophic muscles in these disease states. Although initial success in harvesting myoblasts was reported, clinical benefit did not ensue because of an inflammatory response that destroys the vast majority of injected myoblasts. Furthermore, failure of myoblasts to migrate meaningful distances from the injection site renders implantation by direct needle injection impractical in acute muscular dystrophy disorders.

A number of research groups have devised protocols for the development of mixed biomechanical substitutes for bone, tendon, cartilage, and other connective tissue that incorporate or produce relevant surrounding matrix. In these forms of cell therapy there may be an added advantage inasmuch as it is often an external source of matrix for scaffold that is the desired product. The connective tissue scaffold can be produced in vitro and then repopulated with endogenous recipient cells in the patient, thus potentially preempting immune rejection and other problems related to the presence of cells of allogeneic origin.

Heart Disease

Despite important advances in cardiovascular medicine, heart failure remains a major public health problem. Clinical limitations of therapy have motivated the search for cell-based therapies to restore or augment myocardial contractile function or reestablish functional cardiomyocytes in damaged cardiac regions.

Several sources of cells potentially suitable for restoring myocardial function have been considered and examined during experimental animal or human clinical trials. Skeletal myoblasts of autologous patient origin have been shown in clinical trials to grow in scarred cardiac tissue after direct intracardiac injection. However, histologic or functional evidence of electrical or mechanical coupling has not been seen. Moreover, the occurrence of severe ventricular dysrhythmias renders this approach unsafe and impractical at this time. The use of smooth rather than skeletal muscle as a source has been attempted in experimental animals with some success. In some cases, the apparent differentiation of cells of bone marrow origin into cardiac phenotypes has been subsequently refuted. For this reason, research continues to use embryonic stem cells because of their capacity for unlimited growth in the undifferentiated state, coupled with pluripotential differentiation capabilities. In cell culture, human embryonic stem cells are easily induced into a cardiomyocyte phenotype, including the following features: rhythmic contraction, gene and protein expression markers for cardiomyocyte differentiation, electrical coupling through gap junctions, responsiveness to chronotropic and inotropic agents, and electromechanical coupling with heterotypic cardiomyocytes derived from other sources. Cardiomyocytes of human embryonic stem cell origin have been shown to serve as a biologic pacemaker after conduction system ablation in experimental animals. They have also been shown to enhance cardiac contractility and performance parameters after myocardial infarction induced by coronary ligation in experimental animals.

Another potential application involving a combination of cell and gene therapy in heart disease entails the administration of genetically manipulated, autologously derived human fibroblasts for the treatment of refractory cardiac rhythm disturbances. This approach involves the stable expression of potassium conductance or other ion channels in skin fibroblasts derived from patients suffering from refractory rhythm disturbances, followed by their implantation into electrically unstable regions of the heart by endomyocardial injection guided by electrical mechanical navigation instrumentation.

Diabetes Mellitus

Successful pancreatic transplantation and improved glucocorticoid-free protocols for transplantation of islets of Langerhans have been shown not only to restore glucose control in patients with diabetes mellitus but also to prevent or even reverse some of the disease's complications (Chapter 247). However, whole organ or islet-based transplantation approaches are limited both by immunologic rejection and by limitation of an available source of transplantable tissues. This has motivated the search for cell types that can replace (type 1 diabetes mellitus) or augment (type 2 diabetes mellitus) deficient beta cell function. Although no clinical applications have been reported, significant progress has been made with cells of human origin tested in cell culture and in animal models. Strategies that have been pursued include the genetic manipulation of hepatic cells to provide them with the appropriate machinery for glucose-mediated insulin release. Protocols have also been established for differentiation of human embryonic stem cells to either a precursor or mature beta cell phenotype. These experiments mimic normal embryonic islet development by using growth factors that induce differentiation of definitive endoderm and derivative cell types relevant to differentiation of pancreatic islet cells. Exposure to growth factors such as activin led to the sequential appearance of markers of each of the stages involved in endocrine pancreas development and ultimately resulted in a differentiated population enriched in all the cell types of the endocrine pancreas. Because the pathogenesis of type 1 diabetes mellitus involves autoimmune destruction of pancreatic islet cells, the replacement beta cells might also become a target for autoimmune destructive processes unless measures are taken at the level of the cells or the recipient to preempt such an outcome. In addition, because glucose monitoring and insulin delivery systems are constantly improving, any cell therapy–based approach must provide a clear advantage over existing therapeutic modalities while meeting the most rigorous standards of patient safety.

Stem Cell–Derived Platforms in Gene and Drug Discovery

In addition to the generation of cells for regenerative applications, the ability to grow a wide variety of different specialized cell types of human origin in culture provides unparalleled opportunities for gene and drug discovery and testing. The ability to grow human cardiomyocytes in culture provides a preclinical human cellular-based experimental platform for screening newly developed drugs in terms of the potential for QT interval prolongation and hence the risk of inducing arrhythmia in the clinical setting. Other examples include the creation of an experimental tissue microenvironment of human origin for studying the stromal response to tumor growth and testing anticancer drugs that target tumorigenesis responses such as angiogenesis. By combining technologies such as RNA interference (RNAi) with human stem cell growth and technology (Fig. 41–4), it will also be possible to uncover the role of

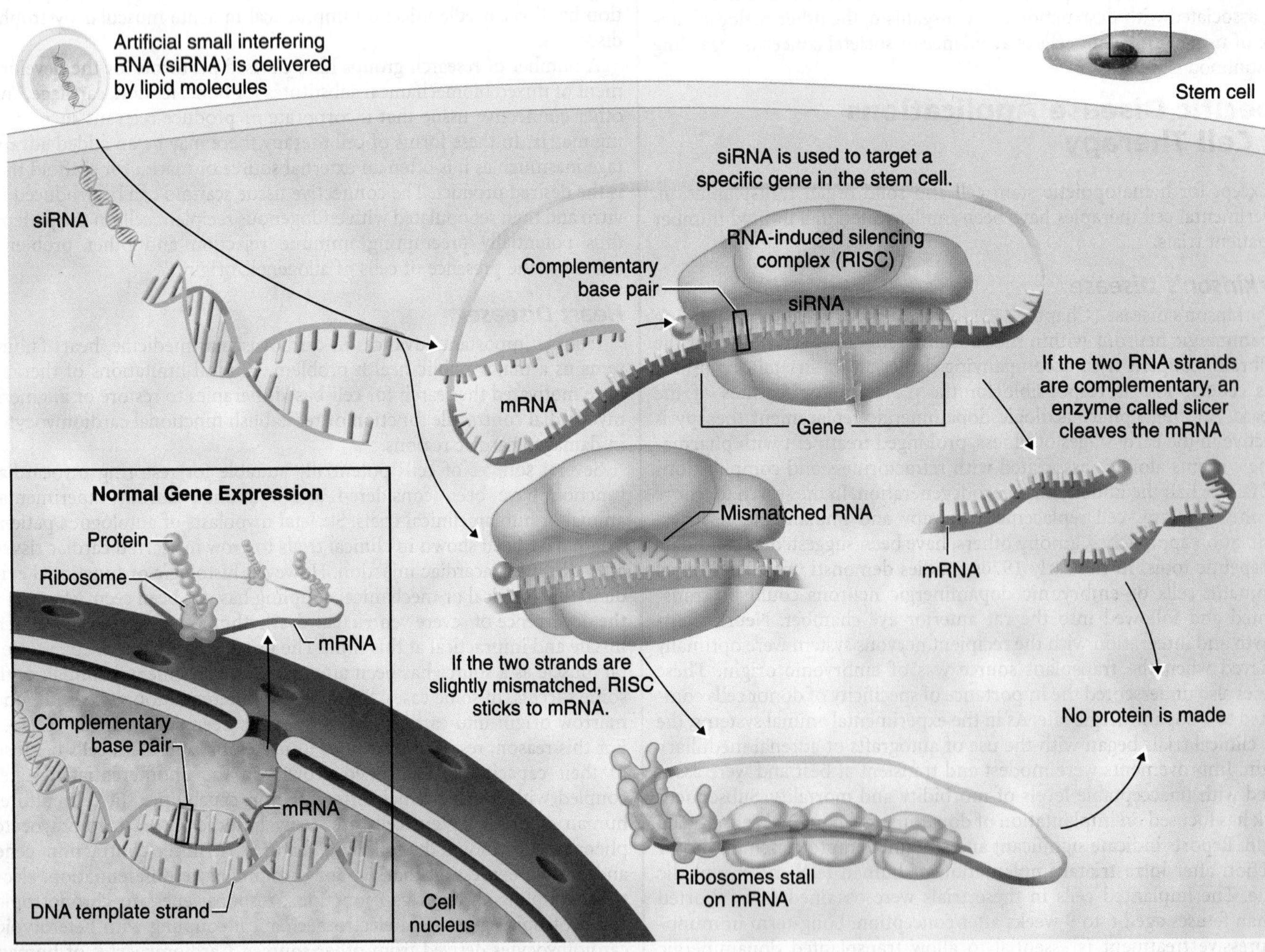

FIGURE 41–4 • RNA interference (RNAi). How RNAi can be used to modify stem cells.

certain gene products in the biochemical pathways and cellular responses in gene therapy.

Societal, Ethical, and Legal Considerations in Stem Cell Research and Therapy

Societal, ethical, and legal concerns about defining the concept of personhood status before birth have emerged among countries and political or religious constituencies in the field of stem cell research and therapy. Although there is a broad consensus that full personhood sanctity and associated rights should be accorded to each individual from at least the moment of birth, similar consensus does not apply to the status of an individual before birth. Various guidelines for research have been developed worldwide based on milestones in embryonic development. Bioethicists and legislators are often concerned about the possibility that research scientists and clinicians will move beyond allowable activities into prohibited domains. One area of concern relates to therapeutic cloning, in which the first step is somatic nuclear transfer, or replacement of the haploid nucleus of a harvested oocyte with the diploid nucleus derived from the somatic cell of a potential cell therapy recipient. The goal of this approach is to generate embryonic stem cells whose nuclear genome is identical to that of the potential recipient. This technique may provide a solution in circumventing alloimmunologic rejection in cell therapy with human embryonic stem cells. Because the initial step in therapeutic cloning is also the first step in reproductive cloning, certain constituencies have prohibited somatic cell nuclear transfer because of the fear of illegitimate extrapolation to reproductive cloning. However, there are key differences between therapeutic and reproductive cloning (highlighted in Table 41–2). Of particular note is that although the end product of therapeutic cloning is the generation of cells in culture, the end product of reproductive cloning is the generation of a cloned organism. Most bioethicists believe that appropriate legislation, regulation, and enforcement can preempt inappropriate research and clinical activities that might lead to reproductive cloning. Continued civil discourse will remain key to resolving the bioethical dilemmas raised by stem cell and related emerging biomedical technologies.

GENE THERAPY

The use of genes as therapeutic platforms emerged during the mid-20th century, and in the 1990s the first regulated registered studies were performed in the United States. Since then, over 7000 patients have been treated in more than 1000 studies in 15 countries across all continents with various modalities of gene therapy for a variety of diseases (see *http://www.wiley.co.uk/genmed/clinical/* and *http://www4.od.nih.gov/oba/rac/* for updated registries). About 40 studies have been performed for tracking gene delivery and more than 660 for therapeutic assessment. Sixty studies involved monogenic diseases and 470 involved cancer, which is also the most common disease category for gene therapy studies worldwide. Two gene therapy agents are currently available on the market. Fomivirsen (Vitravene) is used for the treatment of cytomegalovirus retinitis in patients with acquired immunodeficiency syndrome (AIDS). The p53 tumor suppressor coding sequence in an adenovirus vector is used for the treatment of head and neck cancer patients and is registered only in China. Most patients who participated in the first gene therapy clinical trials were administered marker or reporter genes rather than actual therapeutic genes. Of the thousands treated, two deaths have been attributed directly to gene therapy. The mortality statistics attributed to gene therapy are very low when compared with those associated with chemotherapy and transplantation, two therapeutic modalities frequently used today in clinical practice for disease targets of gene therapy.

Genetic Material

The therapeutic payload in most cases, the core of every gene therapy drug, is composed of an expression cassette (Fig. 41–5). Essential clinical objectives of gene therapy are based on controlling gene expression through regulation of a tissue-specific promoter for expression. Although a few systems have been developed in the experimental setting, none have yet received approval for clinical use by the Food and Drug Administration or any other regulatory authority.

Gene Therapy Delivery Methods

Gene therapy agents are often composed of two elements: the genetic material and the delivery system. The latter is usually the more complex and limiting component, and it is important to select the most efficient delivery method for any genetic therapy. Unfortunately, many gene therapy delivery methods are associated with potential adverse effects, thus necessitating tailoring of therapy to specific clinical considerations. The most commonly used delivery systems have used retrovirus- and adenovirus-based approaches. Viral-based approaches take advantage of the fact that viruses have been designed through evolution to serve as genetic material delivery systems. However, for each specific viral-based gene therapy vector there have been major disadvantages that should be balanced against potential therapeutic benefits. Nonviral methods have also been used in many studies. The most commonly used nonviral delivery methods involve the use of naked/plasmid DNA and liposome-mediated delivery. In cancer gene therapy, the immune response to the delivery vehicle carrying the anticancer genetic material can be used to advantage by serving as an adjuvant. However, the system for delivery of a gene to be expressed for a prolonged period to replace or supplement a missing gene product in monogenic disease states should preferably be ignored by the immune system.

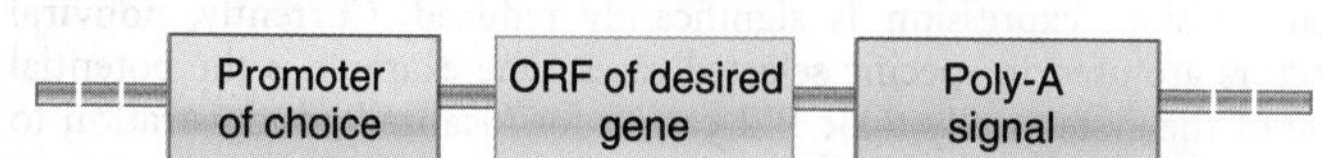

FIGURE 41–5 • Expression cassette. In gene therapy approaches an expression cassette is constructed to produce the desired protein. The three main components of an expression vector are depicted: **A,** the *promoter,* which determines binding of the enzyme RNA polymerase to initiate transcription for production of mRNA; **B,** the open reading frame (*ORF*), which is composed of a DNA sequence consisting of triplets of nucleic acids that can be translated into amino acids starting with an initiation codon and ending in a termination codon; and **C,** *poly(A) signal,* which is a stretch of approximately 200 bases of adenylic acid that is added to the 3′ end of mRNA after its synthesis for stabilization of the message.

TABLE 41–2 DIFFERENCES BETWEEN THERAPEUTIC AND REPRODUCTIVE CLONING

	Therapeutic Cloning	Reproductive Cloning
End product	Cells growing in a Petri dish	Human being
Purpose	To treat a specific disease of tissue degeneration	Replace or duplicate a human
Time frame	A few weeks (growth in culture)	9 months
Surrogate mother needed	No	Yes
Sentient human created	No	Yes
Ethical implications	Similar to all embryonic cell research	Highly complex issues
Medical implications	Similar to any cell-based therapy	Safety and long-term efficacy concerns

Modified from: Vogelstein B, Alberts B, Shine K: Please don't call it cloning. Science 2002;295:1237.

Naked/Plasmid DNA

In theory, the most straightforward approach to gene therapy would be the introduction of genetic material, such as an antisense molecule, short interfering RNA (siRNA), or an expression cassette, directly into the targeted cellular compartment (i.e., DNA into the nucleus or RNA into the cytoplasm). However, in clinical practice, this turns out not to be efficient. Systemic administration of naked DNA into the blood stream generally results in loss of the delivered genetic material, nonspecific interactions with serum proteins, and active degradation mediated by the innate immune system (e.g., tissue macrophages). Direct administration or application to target organs or tissues may circumvent some of these problems, but certain barriers must also be overcome. When the payload is a DNA expression cassette, it will need to interact with the cellular membrane and penetrate it, escape the endosomal compartment and cytosolic degradation by nucleases, and traverse the nuclear pores to reach the nucleus of the cell. This is a long process that is prone to failure unless supported by additional means that allow the DNA to pass the cellular barriers. Electroporation is an approach that has been applied to well-circumscribed body compartments or masses, such as muscle, skin, and tumors. Patients treated with electroporation have experienced tissue damage and associated pain. Additional methods have also been developed for the administration of naked DNA, including the different types of gene guns used for DNA vaccination and ultrasound energy for the transduction of endothelial cells, which could be used for cardiovascular applications and against tumor angiogenesis.

Naked DNA has also been formulated as part of DNA vaccination approaches to the treatment of cancer and immune and infectious diseases. Although preclinical studies have been promising, successful extrapolation to the clinic has not yet been achieved.

Nonviral Vectors

Nonviral vectors have been designed to overcome the cell membrane barrier and, in some cases, intracytoplasmic compartmentalization of the administered genetic material. These nonviral vectors are efficient at enhancing membrane penetration in vitro; however, their efficiency in vivo is significantly reduced. There are additional advantages to nonviral delivery systems: they are inexpensive and can carry large DNA molecules, and their structure can be modified to comply with specific needs, such as conjugation to short peptides for targeting. After systemic and, in some cases, local administration, these nonviral vectors stimulate the innate immune response by serving as adjuvants. They interact with serum proteins and undesirable nontargeted cells and extracellular matrix. Once the DNA reaches the nucleus, it is subject to silencing. After cell division, expression is significantly reduced. Currently, nonviral vectors are used in specific selected cases. One example is the potential use of the systemically toxic PEI carrier for localized administration to the bladder.

Adenovirus as a Viral Vector

Adenovirus is a nonenveloped DNA virus with the capacity to carry a large genetic payload. More than 50 adenovirus serotypes are recognized, but serotypes 2 and 5 have been the most commonly used in clinical gene therapy applications. Adenoviruses, as well as adenovectors (the virally based vector), transduce nondividing cells, a property that is important for gene therapy for many cell types, such as hepatocytes (<0.1% of hepatocytes are replicating in humans at any given time). These vectors have been modified to prevent their replication in healthy tissues. Replication-defective (RD) adenovectors are used for short-term expression. Additional modifications of the viral genome and the cellular system supporting production of the viral particles have enabled deletion of all the viral coding sequences, thereby converting it into a "gutted" vector (helper-dependent [HD] adenovector). It is possible to clone the therapeutic genes into the RD adenovirus and generate recombinant adenovectors in a relatively short time. An additional advantage of adenovectors is that the relatively simple production system enables the generation of a very high titer. High viral titers are essential when administration is parenteral or when production of a large amount of a given protein is needed, such as in disease states in which secretion of a protein is impaired and each cell needs to encode its own normal protein. The HD adenovectors, which do not harbor viral-encoded genes, are able to support the transgene expression for months and possibly for more than a year. RD adenovector–transduced cells express viral proteins and induce an immune response. They are thus used in clinical cases in which the therapeutic gene needs to be expressed at high levels for a short period.

Retroviral Vectors

Retroviral vectors are an RNA group of viruses that harbor two RNA genomic copies in each viral particle, which is composed of a capsid and surrounded by an envelope. For gene therapy applications, two groups of viruses have been modified for clinical assessment and use: the oncoretroviruses and the lentiviruses. Vectors generated from both groups have already entered clinical testing.

Gammaretroviral Vectors

Gammaretroviral vectors are derived from different gammaretroviruses, including the murine leukemia virus and the Moloney murine leukemia virus. RD viruses are produced in special packaging cells that supply all the essential components in *trans* for viral replication and structural proteins. The viral gene therapy vector is composed of (1) a genome without any encoded viral sequences that is responsible for the production of viral proteins, (2) the therapeutic genetic payload and the structural components, and (3) the capsid and envelope. These viral vectors can carry transgenic payloads up to 8 kilobases (kb) in length. Retroviral vectors are capable of transducing only dividing cells. If the DNA reaches the nucleus, integration of the viral genome into the host cell chromosome can occur and lead to stable, long-term transgene expression. At its peak, a multiplicity of infection (MOI) integration occurs at numerous sites. Therefore, if long-term correction of a genetic disorder is required, the target cells must first be induced to replicate. The integration is a random event, with preference within an approximately 5-kb nucleotide window around the transcription initiation site. Thus, there is concern that interference with normal cell function could occur, including the activation of oncogenes or the disruption of tumor suppressor genes. Such events have occurred and have led to the development of malignant transformation both in animal models (rodents and primates) and in humans. There is evidence that "young" cells of the hematopoietic system and hepatocytes are more susceptible to malignant transformation than are terminally differentiated cells. On the other hand, the selectivity for dividing cells is advantageous if one aims to deliver a toxin gene to a growing tumor surrounded by quiescent normal parenchyma. The production of retroviral vectors is less efficient than that of adenovectors. As a result, the application of retroviruses is, in most cases, not by systemic administration but by ex vivo or direct injection into normal or tumor tissue.

Lentiviral Vectors

This group of viruses has been developed more recently for gene therapy applications. Human immunodeficiency virus (HIV) and the feline, simian, and equine immunodeficiency virus (FIV, SIV, and EIV, respectively) lentivirus family members were converted to become lentivectors for gene therapy. These vectors are deprived of the structural and most nonstructural and accessory genomic sequences that are supplied in *trans* in the packaging cell line for vector production. In addition, the envelope glycoprotein is of nonlentivirus origin, and for safety measures, the origin of replication is inactivated to generate a self-inactivating vector. All these genomic manipulations have been introduced to improve the safety of the lentivector and to enable a large cloning capacity of up to 8 kb. The lentivectors have been applied in only a few gene therapy studies, mainly for the treatment of AIDS patients. However, additional studies using lentiviral-based delivery systems are under way in patients with hemoglobinopathies and other genetic diseases. The long-term risk of using retroviral vectors, including gammaretroviral and lentiviral vectors, is not known.

Adenovirus-Associated Virus

Adenovirus-associated virus (AAV) is a DNA nonenveloped, nonpathogenic human parvovirus. Currently, AAV serotype 2 is the best characterized and most commonly used delivery system for gene therapy vector preparations. The capacity of the AAV vector is 4.5 kb, which is a major limitation for AAV vector gene therapy approaches. Production of the vector involves the use of adenovirus or herpesvirus proteins expressed in the packaging line. The capacity for high titers (10^{13} transducing units per milliliter) of AAV serotypes enables systemic injections with reasonable MOI in targeted cells/tissues. An additional advantage of the AAV vector is that it transduces nondividing cells. After transduction, there is a slow rise in gene expression levels during the first 3 weeks, followed by a plateau. The innate immune system will detect the AAV and respond to it, and antibodies generated against the viral capsid after a single injection attenuate the effect of a second administration of AAV vector. However, there is almost no adaptive attack against the transduced cells. Several preclinical assessments indicate that long-term expression is detected with the use of AAV vectors. More than 20 phase I to III clinical studies have assessed the AAV vector for genetic, viral, inflammatory, degenerative, and malignant diseases.

Special Viral-Derived Vectors

In addition to the adenoviral, retroviral, and AAV vectors, numerous, more specialized viral-based vectors with interesting properties and clinical objectives have been developed during the past 10 years.

Herpes simplex virus type 1 (HSV-1) is a DNA virus that can be manipulated to become RD and accommodate a large amount of foreign DNA for gene delivery. Expression of the transgene payload is transient. The HSV-1 amplicon has been used in numerous clinical trials of gene therapy for neurologic diseases.

Viral-like particles (VLPs) were recently developed for vaccination or gene therapy. VLPs of human papillomavirus were recently used as empty particles for vaccination against cervical cancer with significant success. Viruses of the same group, including SV40, which is also a DNA virus, are used for the generation of VLPs to carry gene therapy payloads. One advantage of SV40 is the low immune response against the virus. Again, similar barriers will slow the development of these vehicles, such as limitation of titers and production capacity.

Recombinant vaccinia virus (rVV) was initially developed for the expression of proteins in transduced tissues. Clinical studies in this avenue have encountered limited success. However, recent development of rVV for the treatment of malignant diseases through the expression of antigens might yield clinical benefit.

Oncolytic Viruses

Oncolytic viruses replicate in tumor cells and induce a cytopathic effect or kill tumor cells through other means, such as induction of apoptosis. The major obstacle facing the current development of antitumor drugs is not their potency, but rather their low selectivity for tumor cells. High therapeutic selectivity is essential to enable a safe therapeutic window. Virotherapy has such properties, but these viruses are still waiting to be clinically proven. Tumor-targeted oncolytic viruses are composed of two groups. Genetically engineered viruses are designed to preferentially replicate in tumor cells. This group includes adenoviruses that can replicate only in the presence of a nonfunctioning tumor suppressor gene, such as p53 or Rb. The latter viruses will selectively replicate in tumor cells and induce their killing. However, the exact molecular mechanism of this effect is probably more complicated. The engineered HSV-1 and rVV viruses can also be included in this group. The second group consists of inherently antitumor-selective viruses found to possess antitumor effects through specific protein expression (reovirus) or viruses that activate the innate or adaptive immune response against the tumor, such as the Newcastle disease virus, measles virus strains, Sindbis virus, poliovirus, and vesicular stomatitis virus. The rationale for the use of reovirus as a virotherapeutic approach against cancer is based on the observation that reovirus infection activates host protein kinases to shut down protein production, an essential protection against the infection. Activated Ras signaling is known to interfere with protein kinase activation and with its signaling after reovirus infection. This allows the reovirus to continue to replicate in tumor cells and spare normal tissues. Such replication induces a specific cytopathic effect in malignant cells. Genetically engineered viruses and inherently antitumor-selective viruses have been tested in early clinical trials and are awaiting studies to determine their effectiveness in specific types of cancer.

Diseases Treated by Gene Therapy

Hematologic Conditions

Inherited Immunodeficiency

There have been 27 patients reported worldwide who have undergone treatment with different retroviral vectors for inherited immunodeficiencies. Patients with one of the following three diseases are included in this group: two types of severe combined immunodeficiency (SCID), both of which are characterized by dysregulation of T-cell development, and X-linked chronic granulomatous disease (X-CGD), an inherited immune deficiency with absent phagocyte reduced nicotinamide adenine diphosphate (NADPH) oxidase activity caused by mutations in the gp91 (*phox*) gene. Patients with adenosine deaminase (ADA) SCID suffer from premature death of T cells as a result of the accumulation of purine metabolites; patients with this condition have been treated with vectors expressing the ADA gene. In the first patients with ADA SCID, transduced T cells expressing transgenic ADA have been shown to persist for longer than 10 years; however, the therapeutic effect of gene therapy remained difficult to assess because of concomitant treatment with bovine polyethylene-glycol ADA (PEG-ADA). Discontinuation of PEG-ADA resulted in a strong selective advantage of gene-corrected T cells associated with restoration of T-cell function, but incomplete correction of the metabolic defect. Recently, an improved gene transfer protocol of bone marrow $CD34^+$ cells combined with low-dose busulfan resulted in multilineage, stable engraftment of transduced progenitors at substantial levels, restoration of immune function, correction of the ADA metabolic defect, and proven clinical benefit. Overall, no adverse effect or toxicity has been observed in patients treated with ADA gene transfer in mature lymphocytes or hematopoietic progenitors.

The X-linked type (X-SCID group), in which there is defective cytokine-dependent survival signaling in T and natural killer cells, was shown to be corrected by introduction of the wild-type sequence of the common γ (γ^c) chain, which is an essential component of five cytokine receptors. In one clinical study, hematologic malignancies developed in three patients. One of the three died of this complication. A group of patients treated with a different viral transduction protocol have been cured, with no reports of malignancy in 4 years of follow-up. Two adult X-CGD patients who suffered recurrent bacterial infections have been treated with $CD34^+$ cells transduced with a gammaretroviral vector expressing gp91 phox, with significant clinical improvement. However, in both these patients there was an expansion of gene-transduced cells caused by the transcriptional activation of growth-promoting genes without any clinical manifestations to date.

Additional inherited diseases have been treated in recent years with gene therapy. These diseases have included mostly hematologic conditions wherein a low amount of a secreted protein could reverse the clinical phenotype, and partial success has been achieved in various bleeding diathesis disorders. However, the response has not usually been sustained or has been accompanied by adverse reactions, such as increases in hepatic enzymes in the case of hepatic artery administration.

In the close to 30 patients worldwide treated with gene therapy for immunodeficiency disorders, significant clinical improvement has been observed in many. However, severe and even life-endangering adverse consequences have been encountered with certain viral vectors and protocols. Additional clinical information from long-term observation and new clinical studies will be important for clearer assessment of clinical benefit.

Cardiovascular and Pulmonary Conditions

Diverse approaches have been developed to treat cardiovascular-related syndromes with gene therapy. The most common cardiovascular-related syndromes are related to atherosclerotic arterial occlusive disease. To overcome arterial occlusions, especially when conventional therapies fail to improve blood supply to the ischemic organs, therapeutic angiogenesis has been advocated as a therapeutic option. Transfer of genes encoding angiogeneic growth factors (vascular endothelial growth factor and fibroblast growth factor) delivered by nonviral and viral vectors has been tested in phase II and III studies in patients with coronary and peripheral arterial disease.

Cystic Fibrosis

The molecular pathophysiology of cystic fibrosis (CF) (Chapter 89) is well understood, and experimental protocols for gene therapy for CF have been implemented since 1990. The cystic fibrosis transmembrane conductance regulator (CFTR) protein is mutated in patients with CF. Transducing the epithelium of the nasal and bronchial tree is potentially feasible through nonsystemic approaches. Nonviral gene therapy methods that deliver a copy of the CFTR gene to the airway of CF patients have been developed. Several placebo-controlled clinical trials of liposome-mediated CFTR gene transfer to the nasal epithelium have confirmed its safety and demonstrated variable degrees of functional correction. In addition, several clinical studies have assessed the potential of retrovectors, adenovectors, and AAV vectors for gene therapy for CF. With both nonviral and viral delivery systems there were only mild side effects. However, the long-term clinical benefit was marginal. Improved vectors are being assessed in preclinical studies.

Cancer

Cancer develops through selection of genetic mutations that abrogate the normal cellular balance between proliferation, differentiation, apoptosis, and senescence. Tumor cells derived from any of the more than 200 different cell types in humans develop after the accumulation of mutations in essential cellular regulators, such as tumor suppressor genes (loss of function) or the increased expression of oncogenes (gain of function). Gene therapy approaches to treatment of cancer have been based on perturbation of pathways in the tumorigenesis process, which has led to diverse anticancer gene therapy approaches.

Tumor-Specific Expression of Anticancer Proteins

Certain promoters are activated in many types of tumors (e.g., human telomerase or survivin), whereas others are activated in specific types of tumors (probasin in prostate cancer, ceruloplasmin in ovarian cancer, HER-2 in breast cancer, carcinoembryonic antigen in colon cancer). Targeting of tumor-specific promoters constitutes a rational basis for anticancer therapeutics, which may fall into different categories, including cellular proteins that are involved in apoptosis or antiproliferation, or both (i.e., p53, Fas, p202, E1A, and BAX). Their expression induces tumor-specific killing. The most clinically advanced gene therapy drug against cancer is the RD adenovector expressing the human p53 gene. This therapy (Gendicine) is approved in China for the treatment of patients with head and neck squamous cell carcinoma by direct administration into the tumor bed. According to the results emanating from China and clinical phase III studies in the United States, this treatment has therapeutic benefits. Additionally, the use of suicide genes is one of the most promising approaches for cancer gene therapy.

DNA Vaccines

Human clinical trials using DNA vaccines against cancer (as well as infectious diseases) have been conducted in the past several years. Although these studies have consistently demonstrated the safety of such DNA vaccines, the resultant immunologic responses have not been encouraging, including lack of or low antibody response detected in most cases and somewhat weak cellular response in some trials. Disappointing results were also reported with the use of DNA vaccines against HIV and other infectious agents. However, new methods are currently being assessed for DNA vaccination, such as electroporation and new generations of gene guns. Tumor gene knockdown has been used in many different clinical studies. This approach involves the use of antisense oligonucleotides (ASOs) to target genes involved in cancer progression. ASOs inhibit translation through a mechanism that involves the formation of an mRNA-ASO duplex, which leads to RNase-H–mediated cleavage of the target mRNA. The disappointing lack of clinical efficacy for some first-generation ASOs indicates that challenges remain to be confronted and overcome. These challenges are being addressed by advanced chemistry in the development of second-generation ASOs and by combining this approach as an adjunct to surgical tumor extirpation.

Gene Therapy Ethics and Regulation

There are major differences in the ethical issues pertaining to somatic as opposed to germline gene therapy. In most countries, germline gene therapy, because of its potential harmful effect on future generations, is appropriately outlawed. Our limited understanding of the complex interactions that have shaped human evolution, together with societal and cultural considerations, precludes the possibility of conceiving of responsible programs for germline genetic modifications in humans, as well as germline gene therapy approaches. However, somatic gene therapy is encouraged and performed worldwide under strict regulatory authority with remarkable congruency of guidelines in different countries and global constituencies (e.g., National Institutes of Health/Recombinant DNA Advisory Committee: *http://www4.od.nih.gov/oba/rac/guidelines/guidelines.html;* Food and Drug Administration/Center for Biologic Evaluation and Research: *http://www.fda.gov/cber/gdlns/gtindcmc.htm;* European Medicines Agency: *http://www.emea.eu.int/pdfs/human/bwp/308899en.pdf;* United Kingdom/Gene Therapy Advisory Committee: *http://www.advisorybodies.doh.gov.uk/genetics/gtac/publications.htm;* general: *www.clinigene.eu*). The concept that gene therapies constitute novel biologic drugs provides an appropriate framework for regulatory oversight.

Future Directions

In recent years, the genetic payload/transgene and delivery systems have experienced significant improvements. Rapid advances in understanding the molecular underpinnings of pathogenetic processes have facilitated translation to novel biologically based therapeutics, including gene therapy approaches. The major developments in recent years have been in the design of new types of transgenes. The discovery of RNAi (see Fig. 41–4) and the biogenesis and potential role of siRNA, including their apparent efficiency in the knockdown of gene expression, suggests that these developments will revolutionize gene therapy in the coming years. Preclinical applications involving localized and systemic administration are progressing. A clinical study targeting ocular neovascularization of patients suffering from adult macular degeneration with synthetic siRNA against vascular endothelial growth factor is in progress, with encouraging preliminary results. In addition, viral infections still pose a major threat to humanity. Because viruses are developing resistance to the current available therapies, there is an ongoing battle between the viruses and our ability to develop novel strategies to fight them. In vitro and in vivo experiments demonstrate the effectiveness of RNAi in inhibiting many viruses that cause severe health and economic problems, including respiratory syncytial, hepatitis C, and influenza viruses.

The tragic occurrence of tumors in three patients after retrovector-based treatment of X-SCID has motivated researchers to direct the integration of transgenes to specific human genomic sites. Assessment of these transgene insertion navigation tools will, it is hoped, help reduce the random occurrence of insertional mutagenic events. In addition to the development of novel transgenes, there is progress with viral and nonviral vectors. The AAV vector has experienced significant improvement as a delivery system in recent years because of its capacity for targeting with different capsid serotypes and more efficient production, and this has resulted in high-level AAV transgene expression early after transduction. The lentivectors are safer now than in earlier generations and will be the subject of newly planned clinical trials.

SUGGESTED READINGS

Cavazzana-Calvo M, Lagresle C, Hacein-Bey-Abina S, Fischer A: Gene therapy for severe combined immunodeficiency. Annu Rev Med 2005;56:585–602. *Unfolding the pathophysiologic basis of most SCID conditions enhanced the development of molecular therapy as an alternative to allogeneic hematopoietic stem cell transplantation.*

Collins SD, Baffour R, Waksman R: Cell therapy in myocardial infarction. Cardiovasc Revasc Med 2007;8:43–51. *The encouraging results of early clinical cell therapy studies have not been sustained by subsequent robust studies.*

Fischbach GD, Fishbach RL: Stem cells: Science, policy, and ethics. J Clin Invest 2004;114:1364–1370. *Issues in embryonic stem cell research ethics and public policy.*

Gleave ME, Monia BP: Antisense therapy for cancer. Nat Rev Cancer 2005;5:468–479. *Second-generation, chemically modified antisense oligonucleotides increase resistance to nuclease digestion, prolong tissue half-lives, and improve scheduling.*

Glover DJ, Lipps HJ, Jans JA: Towards safe, non-viral therapeutic gene expression in humans. Nat Rev Genet 2005;6:299–310. *Efficient, long-term gene expression can be achieved by nonviral vectors.*

Hacein-Bey-Abina S, Le Deist F, Carlier F, et al: Sustained correction of X-linked severe combined immunodeficiency by ex vivo gene therapy. N Engl J Med 2002;346:1185–1193. *Success was sustained.*

Ketzinel-Gilad M, Shaul Y, Galun E: RNA interference for antiviral therapy. J Gene Med 2006;8:933–950. *Antiviral applications for RNAi.*

Kimmelman J: Recent developments in gene transfer: Risk and ethics. BMJ 2005;330:79. *Gene therapy must be weighed carefully against the risks and efficacy of existing treatments, such as chemotherapy and transplantation.*

Manno CS, Pierce GF, Arruda VR: Successful transduction of liver in hemophilia by AAV–factor IX and limitations imposed by the host immune response. Nat Med 2006;12:342–347. *Only transient success could be achieved.*

Regenerative Medicine 2006. Department of Health and Human Services, August 2006. Available at http://stemcells.nih.gov/info/scireport/2006report.htm. *A comprehensive and well-illustrated overview of the application of stem cells to regenerative medicine.*

Rosenecker J, Huth S, Rudolph C: Gene therapy for cystic fibrosis lung disease: Current status and future perspectives. Curr Opin Mol Ther 2006;8:439–445. *Levels of CFTR expression are too low and only of limited duration.*

Sandel MJ: Embryo ethics—the moral logic of stem-cell research. N Engl J Med 2004;351:207–209. *A rigorous ethical analysis of human embryonic stem cell research.*

Schachinger V, Erbs S, Elsasser A, et al: REPAIR-AMI Investigators. Intracoronary bone marrow–derived progenitor cells in acute myocardial infarction. N Engl J Med 2006;355:1210–1221. *At 4 months, ejection fraction improved by 5.5% in treated patients versus 3.0% in controls.*

Verma IM, Weitzman MD: Gene therapy: Twenty-first century medicine. Annu Rev Biochem 2005;74:711–738. *A review of state-of-the art viral vectors used in gene therapy clinical trials.*

Tse HF, Yiu KH, Lau CP: Bone marrow stem cell therapy for myocardial angiogenesis. Curr Vasc Pharmacol 2007;5:103–112. *Issues to be addressed include development of a more efficient stem cell identification, purification, and expansion method.*

Section VII

Principles of Immunology and Inflammation

42 THE INNATE AND ADAPTIVE IMMUNE SYSTEMS

Jörg J. Goronzy and Cornelia M. Weyand

GENERAL PRINCIPLES OF THE IMMUNE SYSTEM

The immune system has evolved as a complex network of molecules, cells, and organs to defend against pathogenic microorganisms and noninfectious foreign substances. Beyond its role in host protection, it regulates tissue homeostasis and tissue repair by screening cell surfaces for the expression of specific molecules. Cells of the immune system identify and remove injured, dead, and malignant cells. Immune system cells derive from hematopoietic stem cells in the bone marrow, circulate in the blood and lymph, form complex microstructures in specialized lymphoid organs, and infiltrate virtually every tissue. These cells express characteristic profiles of surface molecules with which they sense other cells in their microenvironment. These cell surface molecules are collectively referred to as cluster of differentiation (CD) markers. Molecular structure, ligands, and main functions of more than 300 molecules have been defined; a selected list is given in Table 42–1. The anatomic organization of immune system cells in lymphoid organs and their ability to circulate throughout the body and to migrate between blood and lymphoid tissues are crucial components of host defense. On activation, these cells transcribe and release cytokines, small soluble proteins that serve to communicate between cells within the immune system or between immune system cells and cells in other tissues (Table 42–2).

Innate and Adaptive Immunity

Principally, host protection is accomplished by two types of immunity: innate and adaptive. These two arms of the immune system are not independent but are closely interlinked. The *innate immune system* is the older system; it is present in all vertebrates and is widely conserved among species. It provides the first line of defense and functions through immediate responses that use preformed proteins and preexisting cells. *Innate immunity,* broadly defined, includes physical barriers, such as epithelial layers, and chemical impediments, such as antimicrobial substances at these surfaces. Using a more narrow definition, the innate immune system mediates nonspecific protection through a diverse set of cells, including monocytes, macrophages, dendritic cells, natural killer (NK) cells, eosinophils, basophils, neutrophils, and mast cells. A variety of chemical mediators, such as members of the complement system, acute phase reactants, and cytokines, contribute to inflammatory responses that develop to prevent tissue invasion by pathogens. The need for immediacy is irreconcilable with selectivity and adaptivity. Response patterns of the innate immune system are broad, and collateral tissue damage is often unavoidable. Despite the lack of specificity, innate immunity is highly effective; microbial invasion frequently is controlled, and pathogens often are eliminated. The pathogenicity of microorganisms largely is related to their ability to resist and overcome the first line of defense mounted by the innate immune system.

If invading microorganisms succeed in escaping nonspecific host-defense mechanisms, a second line of defense, *adaptive immunity,* secures host survival. Adaptive immune responses depend on innate immunity for supplementation and augmentation and to provide crucial information on the nature of the attacker. The term *adaptive* relates to the ability of the system to adapt to the microbial challenge; it is also called *acquired* or *specific immunity*. The adaptive immune system is characteristic of higher vertebrates; it is evolutionarily younger than innate immunity and has unique attributes, such as specificity, diversity, memory, specialization, tolerance, and homeostasis.

Immune specificity relies on two major cell types: B cells and T cells. These cells possess receptors that specifically recognize antigenic determinants and that distinguish subtle differences on small protein structures. To contend with the gamut of possible antigens, the adaptive immune system requires an enormous spectrum of specific receptors. An extremely high degree of discriminatory specificity is achieved by clonal distribution of the recognition structures; each individual T cell and B cell expresses a unique receptor.

The diversity of the adaptive immune system is not inherited; it is acquired somatically and is called the *lymphocyte repertoire*. The lymphocyte repertoire is estimated to discriminate 10^9 to 10^{11} antigenic structures. The frequencies of T or B cells in the naïve repertoire specific for a particular antigenic determinant is less than 1 in 10^5 and therefore extremely low. On recognition of an antigen, the adaptive immune system reacts with clonal expansion of these infrequent antigen-responsive cells to build up a line of defense. Proliferating antigen-specific cells not only increase in frequency but also acquire new properties, including effector functions or the ability to function as memory cells. Because memory for the antigen is being generated, a second challenge from the same antigen elicits a faster and more efficient response. Specificity and memory are prerequisites for heightened reactivity to recurrent or persistent infections and also provide the basis for vaccination. Another example of the adaptive power of the specific immune system lies in specialized responses to different classes of microbes (e.g., parasites versus viral infections). Specialization is a consequence of differentiation during the evolution of the immune response; it results in selection of the most appropriate effector pathway for a particular microbial challenge.

Molding the responding lymphocyte population to the antigenic profile of the invading pathogen inevitably involves the risk of generating cells that respond to self-antigens. To prevent injury to the host, the adaptive immune system discriminates between self and non-self. Nonreactivity to self is actively acquired and is maintained by several mechanisms, collectively called *self-tolerance*. Distinguishing self and non-self is individualized for each host and requires the selection of an individual set of non-self–reactive receptors. Consequently, the outcome of self/non-self discrimination is not transferred from generation to generation and is devoid of evolutionary pressure. In contrast, innate immunity relies on genetically programmed recognition structures that respond to foreign antigens. Receptors that have been evolutionarily selected to recognize pathogens but not self should not carry the risk of autoimmunity. Therefore, autoimmune disease is generally considered as a failure in the adaptive immune system; however, the innate system contributes by setting the threshold for the induction of adaptive immune responses.

Together with the capability of generating tremendous diversity and specificity, the adaptive immune system has a built-in ability to self-limit responses and to regain homeostasis. This mechanism is crucial in preventing excessive immune responses and in providing space for emerging lymphocytes that are required for a new specific immune response.

The adaptive immune system is phylogenetically younger than the innate system. The subsequent and most recent evolutionary milestone in the development of the immune system has been the three-dimensional organization of its cellular components in lymphoid organs. In the highly specialized microenvironment of lymphoid tissues, both arms of the immune system interact intimately and collaborate efficiently to augment and optimize immune reactions. The earliest organized lymphoid structures developed during evolution were the gut-associated lymphoid tissues. More sophisticated secondary lymphoid organs, such as the spleen, thymus, and lymph nodes, are found only in higher vertebrates.

Leukocyte Migration and Homing

Mobility of the cellular constituents is fundamental to innate and adaptive immunity. To home to the site of tissue injury or to enter lymphoid organs, cells use a multistep process of adherence and activation. Initially, leukocytes roll on activated endothelial cells, activate chemokine receptors, increase adhesiveness, and eventually migrate through the endothelial layer across a chemokine gradient. The selectin family of proteins mediates the first steps of leukocyte migration. Selectins have a lectin domain and bind to carbohydrate ligands. L-selectin is present on virtually all leukocytes; P-selectin and E-selectin are expressed on activated endothelial cells; and P-selectins are also stored in platelets. Selectins capture floating leukocytes and initiate their attachment and rolling on activated endothelial cells. To transform attachment and rolling into firm adhesion, the concerted action of chemokines, chemokine receptors, and integrins is necessary. Integrins are heterodimers formed of many different α-chains and β-chains; different α/β combinations are expressed on different cell subsets. Only after

TABLE 42–1 CLUSTER OF DIFFERENTIATION (CD) MARKERS AND THEIR FUNCTIONS

CD Antigen	Main Cellular Expression	Ligand	Major Function
CD1a–e	Cortical thymocytes, dendritic cells, B cells, intestinal epithelium (CD1d)	T-cell receptor	MHC class I–like molecules, presentation of nonpeptide antigens to T cells
CD2	T cells, thymocytes, NK cells	CD48, CD58	T-cell activation, adhesion; also called LFA-2
CD3	Thymocytes, T cells		Associated with the T-cell antigen receptor, T-cell signaling complex
CD4	Helper T cells, monocytes, macrophages	MHC class II molecules	Coreceptor to T-cell receptor, signal transduction
CD8	Cytotoxic T cells, NK cells (α-chain)	MHC class I molecules	Coreceptor to T-cell receptor, signal transduction
CD11a	T cells, B cells, NK cells, monocyte/macrophage, neutrophils	ICAM-1 to -4	Pairs with CD18 to form LFA-1 (integrin), cell adhesion and migration
CD11b	Dendritic cells, monocytes/macrophages, NK cells, neutrophils	ICAM-1, complement component iC3b	Pairs with CD18, α-chain of complement receptor CR3, cell adhesion
CD11c	Dendritic cells, monocytes, neutrophils	ICAM-1, complement component iC3b	Pairs with CD18, α-chain of complement receptor CR4, cell adhesion
CD14	Monocytes/macrophages, neutrophils	LPS	Associates with TLR4, cell activation
CD16	NK cells, monocytes/macrophages, neutrophils	IgG Fc	Cell activation, phagocytosis, ATCC
CD18	T cells, B cells, NK cells, monocytes/macrophages, neutrophils	ICAM	Cell adhesion
CD19	B cells		Coreceptor for B-cell receptor, signal transduction
CD20	B cells		Regulates B-cell activation
CD21	B cells	Complement component C3d, EBV	Coreceptor for B-cell activation, complement receptor 2
CD23	Mature B cells, eosinophils, follicular dendritic cells	IgE	Low-affinity Fc receptor for IgE, B-cell activation
CD25	Activated T and B cells, NK cells	IL-2	Growth factor receptor
CD27	T cells, NK cells	CD70	Costimulation
CD28	T cells	CD80/CD86	Costimulation
CD31	Endothelial cells, naïve T cells, myeloid cells, B cells	CD38	Adhesion; also called PECAM-1
CD32	Myeloid cells, B cells	IgG	Low-affinity Fc receptor FcγRII, phagocytosis
CD34	Hematopoietic stem cells, endothelial cells	CD62 (L-selectin)	Adhesion
CD36	Monocytes/macrophages, platelets, endothelial cells	Thrombospondin, collagens, oxidized LDL	Scavenger receptor
CD40	B cells, monocytes, dendritic cells	CD154 (CD40 ligand)	B cell/dendritic cell costimulation
CD44	Lymphocytes, myeloid cells	Hyaluronic acid	Leukocyte homing
CD45	Leukocytes		Tyrosine phosphatase, augments signaling, alternative splicing produces multiple isoforms that correlate with cell differentiation
CD49a–f	B cells, memory T cells, monocytes	Matrix components	Also called VLA-1 through -6, associates with CD29 to form integrins, adhesion
CD54	T cells, B cells, monocytes/macrophages, endothelial cells	CD11a/CD18, rhinovirus	Adhesion molecule; also called ICAM-1
CD56	NK cells		Adhesion
CD58	Hematopoietic, endothelial and epithelial cells	CD2	LFA-3, adhesion
CD62E	Endothelial cells	Sialyl-Lewis X	E-selectin, adhesion, mediates leukocyte rolling
CD62L	B cells, T cells, NK cells, monocytes	CD34	L-selectin, adhesion, mediates rolling
CD62P	Platelets, endothelial cells	Sialyl-Lewis X	P-selectin, adhesion, mediates rolling of neutrophils
CD64	Monocytes/macrophages	IgG	High-affinity Fc receptor (FcγRI)
CD68	Monocytes/macrophages, neutrophils	LDL	Cytoplasmic localization, phagocytic activity
CD79a/b	B cells		Associated with the B-cell antigen receptor, signal transduction
CD80	Dendritic cells, macrophages, activated B cells	CD28, CD152 (CTLA-4)	Costimulatory ligand
CD85	T cells, B cells, NK cells, dendritic cells, monocytes/macrophages	MHC class I molecules	ILT family, modulates cell activation, mostly inhibition

TABLE 42–1 CLUSTER OF DIFFERENTIATION (CD) MARKERS AND THEIR FUNCTIONS—cont'd

CD Antigen	Main Cellular Expression	Ligand	Major Function
CD86	Dendritic cells, macrophages, activated B cells	CD28, CD152 (CTLA-4)	Costimulatory ligand
CD94	T cell subsets, NK cells	HLA-E	Inhibition of cell activation
CD95	Wide distribution	CD178 (Fas-ligand)	Induces apoptosis; also called Fas
CD102	Endothelial cells, T cells, B cells, monocytes	CD11a/CD18	Adhesion; also called ICAM-2
CD152	Activated T cells	CD80, CD86	Negative regulatory signal; also called CTLA-4
CD154	Activated T cells	CD40	Provides costimulatory signal
CD158a–k	T-cell subsets, NK cells	MHC class I molecules	Positive and negative regulatory signals; also called killer immunoglobulin-like receptor
CD159a/c	T cell subsets, NK cells	HLA-E	Associates with CD94, negative (a) and positive (c) regulatory signal
CD178	Activated T cells, various tissue cells	CD95	Induces apoptosis
CD195	Effector T cells, monocytes, neutrophils	RANTES, MIP-1α, MIP-1β	Chemokine receptor, induces migration to peripheral tissue, coreceptor for HIV; also called CCR5
CD197	Naïve and memory T cells, B cells, dendritic cells	Chemokines CCL19 and CCL21	Chemokine receptor, induces migration to secondary lymphoid tissue; also called CCR7
CD281–289	Dendritic cell, monocyte	Microbial products, PAMPs	Cell activation; also called TLR1–9

ADCC = antibody-dependent cellular cytotoxicity; CCL = CC chemokine ligand; CCR = CC chemokine receptor; CTLA = cytotoxic T-lymphocyte antigen; EBV = Epstein-Barr virus; Fc = crystallizable fragment of immunoglobulin; HIV = human immunodeficiency virus; HLA = human leukocyte antigen; ICAM = intercellular adhesion molecule; IgE = immunoglobulin E; IgG = immunoglobulin G; IL = interleukin; ILT = immunoglobin-like transcripts; LDL = low-density lipoprotein; LFA = leukocyte function–associated antigen; LPS = lipopolysaccharide; MHC = major histocompatibility complex; MIP = macrophage inflammatory protein; NK = natural killer; PAMPs = pathogen-associated molecular patterns; PECAM = platelet endothelial cell adhesion molecule; RANTES = regulated on activation, T-cell expressed and secreted; TLR = toll-like receptor; VLA = vascular leukocyte adhesion molecule.

activation can integrins interact with ligands on endothelial cells. Activation involves modification of the cytoplasmic domain of the β-chain, which leads to a structural change of the extracellular domains. This process is termed *inside-out signaling.* Integrin activation can be mediated by chemokines binding to leukocytes. The last step of homing is transendothelial migration. Here, the firmly attached leukocytes migrate through the endothelial cell monolayer and the basement membrane. Molecular components governing this process have not been identified.

INNATE IMMUNE SYSTEM

Activation of the Innate Immune System

Neutrophils, eosinophils, basophils, macrophages/monocytes, dendritic cells, and NK cells are the cellular constituents of the innate immune system. These cells depend on a variety of soluble factors, such as serum and tissue proteins, to generate nonspecific immune responses. Of particular importance is the complement system, a group of plasma enzymes and regulatory proteins that are converted from inactive proenzymes to active enzymes in a controlled and systematic cascade (Chapter 47). Cells of the innate immune system sense infection, cellular damage, and threat to tissue integrity by means of a variety of receptors and respond with an activation program. They possess surface receptors for complement factors. They are activated by binding antibody molecules through immunoglobulin crystallizable fragment (Fc) receptors. Finally, they express pattern recognition receptors (PRRs) that are instrumental in recognizing microbial invasion. Beyond its response to soluble factors, the innate immune system is able to screen cells for intactness by surveying cell surface molecules. In principle, recognition of membrane molecules provides inhibitory signals for constitutively activated cells of the innate immune system. Loss of these membrane molecules on the tissue abrogates inhibition and allows the generation of protective effector functions.

Activation by Pattern Recognition Receptors

The strategy of the innate immune system is to focus on the recognition of a few highly conserved structures that are preserved in large groups of microorganisms. It currently is estimated that the system uses a few hundred receptor structures to identify microbial invaders. This set of receptors is insufficient to cover the entire spectrum of antigens expressed on infectious agents. Innate responses are directed against structures that are shared by entire classes of pathogens and are essential for their survival and pathogenicity. Structures recognized by PRRs are collectively referred to as *pathogen-associated molecular patterns* (PAMPs). Examples of PAMPs are bacterial lipopolysaccharides, peptidoglycans, mannans, bacterial DNA, double-stranded RNA, and glucans.

PAMP-binding receptor families share structural characteristics, such as leucine-rich repeated domains, calcium-dependent lectin domains, and scavenger-receptor protein domains, and they use several different pathways to identify their microbial target. They can be secreted to act as opsonins; the best-characterized receptor of this class is the mannose-binding lectin that binds to microbial carbohydrates and activates the lectin pathway of complement activation. Another functional class of PRRs is expressed on the surface of phagocytes and facilitates endocytosis. The macrophage mannose receptor and the macrophage scavenger receptor are the best-known examples. These receptors are essential for the clearance of microbes from the circulation. A third class of PRRs controls cell activation (Fig. 42–1); the most important members are toll-like receptors (TLRs). Initially described in *Drosophila,* at least 10 TLRs have been identified in mammals. TLRs function by regulating the activity of nuclear factor-κB (NF-κB) signaling pathways and control the expression of many inflammatory cytokines and cell surface molecules. Prominent members of the TLR family are TLR4, which, in conjunction with other cell surface molecules, binds bacterial lipopolysaccharides; TLR2, which recognizes bacterial peptidoglycans and lipoproteins; and TLR9, which binds to bacterial DNA motifs.

PRRs used by the innate immune system are fundamentally different from the antigen-specific receptors generated in the adaptive immune system. The receptors of the innate immune system are encoded in the germline and are under evolutionary pressure. They are shared by many different effector cells, including macrophages and dendritic cells, and are not clonally distributed (i.e., different cell types display identical specificity). Finally, PRRs do not recognize self, so they do not carry the risk for autoimmune injury, although exceptions from this rule (e.g., recognition of heat shock proteins) have been described.

Regulation by Major Histocompatibility Complex Class I–Recognizing Receptors

PRRs dominate cell activation for some cell types and under certain conditions. Other cells of the innate immune system require reversal of

TABLE 42–2 CYTOKINES AND CYTOKINE FUNCTION

Cytokines	Major Producer Cells	Principal Action
HEMATOPOIETIN FAMILY		
IL-2	T cells	Proliferation of T cells, B cells, and NK cells
IL-3	T cells	Early hematopoiesis
IL-4	T cells, mast cells	B-cell activation, IgE switch, inhibition of T_H1 cells
IL-5	T cells, mast cells	Eosinophil growth and differentiation
IL-6	Macrophages, endothelial cells	T-cell and B-cell growth and differentiation, induction of acute phase proteins
IL-7	Bone marrow, thymic epithelium	Growth of pre-B cells and pre-T cells
IL-9	T cells	Stimulates mast cells and T_H2 cells
IL-11	Stromal fibroblasts	Hematopoiesis
IL-13	T cells	B-cell growth and differentiation, inhibition of T_H1 cells and macrophages
G-CSF	Fibroblasts and monocytes	Neutrophil development and differentiation
IL-15	Non-T cells	Growth of T cells and NK cells
GM-CSF	Macrophages, T cells	Growth and differentiation of myelomonocytic lineage cells
INTERFERON FAMILY		
IFN-α	Leukocytes	Antiviral, increases MHC class I expression
IFN-β	Fibroblasts	Antiviral, increases MHC class I expression
IFN-γ	T cells, NK cells	Macrophage activation, increases expression of MHC molecules, Ig class switching, inhibition of T_H2 cells
TNF FAMILY		
TNF-α	Macrophages, NK cells, T cells	Induction of proinflammatory cytokines, endothelial cell activation, apoptosis
TNF-β (LT-α)	T cells, B cells	Cell death, endothelial activation, lymphoid organ development
LT-β	T cells, B cells	Cell death, lymphoid organ development
OTHERS		
TGF-β	Monocytes, T cells	Anti-inflammatory, inhibits cell growth, induces IgA secretion
IL-1α, IL-1β	Macrophages, endothelial cells	Acute phase response, fever, macrophage activation, costimulation
IL-10, IL-1β	T cells, macrophages	Suppression of macrophage functions
IL-12	Macrophages, dendritic cells	NK cell activation, T_H1 cell differentiation
IL-16	T cells, mast cells, eosinophils	Chemoattractant for CD4 T cells, monocytes, and eosinophils
IL-17	CD4 memory cells	Cytokine production by epithelia, endothelia, and fibroblasts
IL-18	Macrophages	IFN-γ production by T cells and NK cells

CD = cluster of differentiation; G-CSF = granulocyte colony-stimulating factor; GM-CSF = granulocyte-macrophage colony-stimulating factor; IFN = interferon; Ig = immunoglobulin; IL = interleukin; LT = lymphotoxin; MHC = major histocompatibility complex; NK = natural killer; TGF = transforming growth factor; T_H = helper T lymphocyte; TNF = tumor necrosis factor.

inhibition to enter the activation cycle. Loss of inhibitory signals in constitutively activated cells is particularly important for NK cells. NK cells are poised constantly to attack, but they are held in check by inhibitory receptors that recognize major histocompatibility complex (MHC) class I or MHC class I–like molecules. The observation that NK cells kill target cells lacking MHC class I molecules led to the *missing-self hypothesis*. The principle that immune cells are kept in check by recognizing self-determinants is appreciated now as fundamental in the immune system. In addition to NK cells, other cells of the innate immune system and the adaptive immune system use this principle. Provision of negative signals is closely linked to the recognition of MHC class I molecules.

Currently, three types of MHC class I–recognizing receptors are known (see Table 42–1). C-type lectin receptors (CD159) (predominantly expressed on NK cells) recognize human leukocyte antigen E (HLA-E). Killer immunoglobulin-like receptors (CD158) are specific for HLA-C and, to a lesser extent, HLA-A and HLA-B. Immunoglobulin-like transcript receptors (CD85) are found preferentially on cells of the innate immune system other than NK cells. Immunoglobulin-like transcript receptor 2 is expressed on B cells, monocytes, dendritic cells, and macrophages. Immunoglobulin-like transcript receptors 3 and 4 have a more restrictive expression pattern and are encountered on monocytes, dendritic cells, and macrophages. By screening cell surfaces for the expression of MHC class I molecules, the innate immune system collects information about the intactness of tissues, emphasizing the crucial role of MHC class I molecules as markers of tissue integrity.

Recognition of MHC class I molecules provides a negative signal that suppresses cell activity. However, all receptor families also include stimulatory isoforms that mediate an activating signal. The balance between these opposing signals is finely tuned, ultimately determining whether innate immunity is initiated or not.

Activation by Fc Receptors

Most cells of the innate immune system possess Fc receptors (FcRs) and can bind antibodies attached to antigens (see Fig. 42–1 and Table 42–1). FcRs specifically interact with the constant region (Fc portion) of immunoglobulins. Each member of the FcR family displays specificity for one or a few immunoglobulin isotypes. The isotype of the antibody determines which cell type is activated in a given response. Triggering of most FcRs transmits activating signals; however, inhibitory FcRs do exist. Phagocytic cells, such as neutrophils and macrophages, are equipped with FcγRs that are activated by immunoglobulin G (IgG) antibodies, particularly IgG1. Ligation of an FcγR triggers phagocytosis of the antigen, activation of respiratory burst, and induction of cytotoxicity. On eosinophils, FcγRs mainly regulate granule release. On NK cells, FcγRs initiate

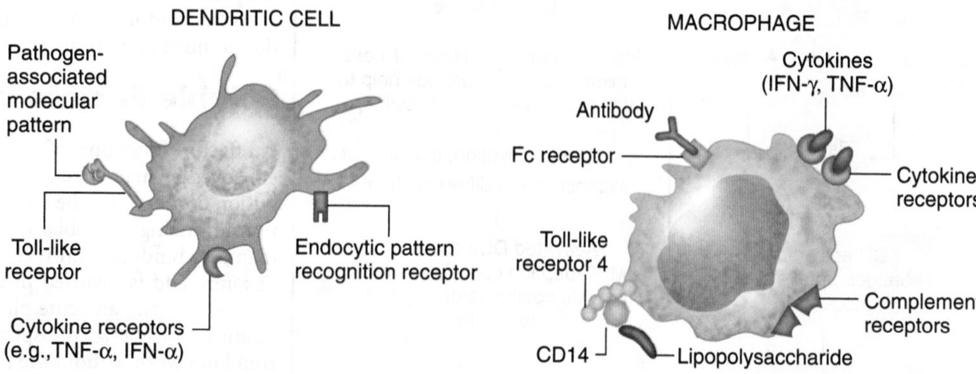

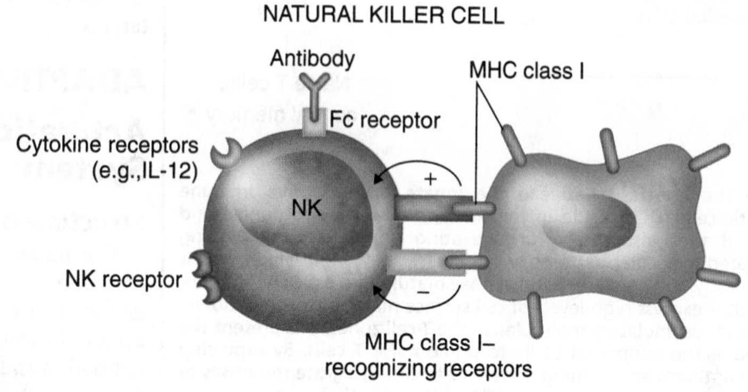

FIGURE 42–1 • Activation pathways in the innate immune system. Cells of the innate immune system recognize microorganisms and tissue damage caused by either infection or malignancy. Dendritic cells and monocytes/macrophages use a multitude of receptors to sense constituents of pathogens, often bacterial molecules common to many classes of microorganisms, and respond to cytokines and endogenous stimulators released from injured cells. Binding of complement factors also can trigger cell activation. Self-recognition of major histocompatibility complex (MHC) class I molecules by natural killer (NK) cells can deliver positive or negative signals. Lack of MHC class I molecules on the target cell surface activates NK cells to kill the target. IFN = interferon; IL = interleukin; TNF = tumor necrosis factor.

antibody-dependent, cell-mediated cytotoxicity. In this process, the cytolytic machinery of NK cells is triggered by the binding of IgG1-coated or IgG3-coated target cells. FcRs on mast cells, basophils, and activated eosinophils are specific for IgE. In contrast to other FcRs, they bind monomeric antibody molecules with extremely high affinity. Cross-linking of the constitutively cell surface–bound IgE induces cell activation and the release of cytoplasmic granules.

Activation by Cytokines

Generally, cells of the innate immune system are exquisitely sensitive to the action of cytokines. Cytokines are soluble, low-molecular-weight glycoproteins that derive from many tissue sources. They are chemical messengers that convey information between cells, regulate the differentiation of effector cells, and modulate immune responses. Important examples of cytokine-mediated signals in the innate immune system are interferon-γ (IFN-γ), produced by NK cells, which is the most potent activator of macrophages; interleukin-12 (IL-12) and IL-15, derived from macrophages and dendritic cells, which regulate the activity and proliferation of NK cells; and IFN-α, secreted by nonimmune cells at the time of injury, which activates NK cells and dendritic cells (see Fig. 42–1).

Cellular Elements of the Innate Immune System

Monocytes and Macrophages

Monocytes circulate in the peripheral blood with a half-life of 1 to 3 days. Macrophages arise from monocytes that have migrated out of the circulation and have proliferated and differentiated in tissue. Tissue macrophages are common in lymphoid organs, but they also are present in connective tissues, such as the perivascular space, and in the lining of serous cavities (pleura and peritoneum). Specialized macrophages include alveolar macrophages in the lung, Kupffer cells in the liver, osteoblasts in bone, microglia in the central nervous system, and type A synoviocytes in the synovial membrane. Macrophages are activated through triggering of PRRs or FcRs, and they respond vigorously to IFN-γ (see Fig. 42–1). They secrete a myriad of products, including hydrolytic enzymes, reactive oxygen species, cytokines (tumor necrosis factor-α [TNF-α], IL-1, IL-6, IL-10, IL-12, IL-15, and IL-18), and chemokines. They phagocytose and expose the engulfed microorganism to a wide range of toxic intracellular molecules, including reactive oxygen species, nitric oxide, antimicrobial cationic proteins and peptides, and lysosomal enzymes. In addition to attacking microbial organisms, macrophages remove dying and dead host cells. They recognize molecules expressed on apoptotic cells and eliminate them without initiating an inflammatory response. Finally, they play a crucial role in the recruitment of adaptive immune responses. After capturing antigen, they function as antigen-presenting cells for T lymphocytes. In this function, however, they are less important than dendritic cells. As a partner for IFN-γ–releasing T cells, macrophages mediate effector functions, contribute to tissue repair, and orchestrate immune responses through their release of cytokines, chemokines, and growth factors.

Dendritic Cells/Langerhans Cells

Dendritic cells represent the major cell type linking innate immunity to the adaptive immune system. Their primary function is the presentation of antigens to T cells. They are the only cell type that can activate naïve T cells and initiate adaptive immune responses. Dendritic cells are derived from lymphoid and myeloid lineages. When positioned in the skin and under the mucosal surface, dendritic cells are referred to as *Langerhans cells.* They constantly endocytose and digest extracellular molecules but usually do not display these molecules at a sufficient density to activate T cells. On receiving a stimulatory signal, they convert into highly efficient antigen-presenting cells. Activation signals can derive from PAMPs or from host cells that react to injury and secrete mediators such as TNF-α, IFN-α, or heat shock proteins (see Fig. 42–1). Activation causes dendritic cells to change their expression profile of chemokine receptors and to migrate from the local tissue to lymph nodes. In parallel, they begin expressing accessory molecules on their cell surface, a prerequisite for T-cell activation. When they arrive in the T-cell zone of the lymph node, they display MHC/peptide complexes with peptides derived from endocytosed and digested antigens. With high surface expression of MHC and accessory molecules, dendritic cells optimize the process of antigen presentation and T-cell priming (Fig. 42–2).

Natural Killer Cells

The current paradigm holds that NK cells provide the first line of defense against viral infections and other intracellular pathogens while adaptive responses are generated. NK cells are sensitized by cytokines released from macrophages and dendritic cells. They function by secreting cytokines, mainly IFN-γ, which activate macrophages and other cells.

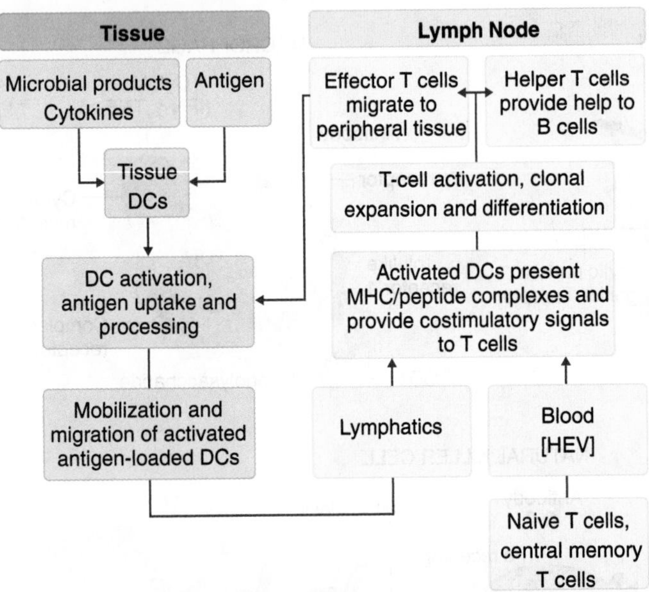

FIGURE 42–2 • The interface between the innate and adaptive immune systems. Dendritic cells (DCs) reside in the tissue, where they recognize and ingest antigens. If they also receive an activating signal (e.g., by binding pathogen-associated molecular patterns or cytokines), they enter lymph vessels to travel to regional lymph nodes. In parallel, they mature into efficient antigen-presenting cells that express high levels of cell surface major histocompatibility complex (MHC) and costimulatory molecules. In the T-cell zones, DCs present the antigen engulfed in the peripheral tissue to prime naïve T cells. By capturing and transporting antigens and priming naïve T cells, DCs integrate responses of the innate and adaptive immune systems. HEV = high endothelial venues.

They also are poised to kill virus-infected cells. NK cells induce apoptosis of the target cells by injecting pore-forming enzymes and granzymes. One of the interesting features of NK biology is the activation of these lymphocytes when MHC class I molecules on target cells are lost (see Fig. 42–1). NK cells are important in tumor surveillance because they are able to kill MHC class I–deficient tumor cells that no longer are susceptible to adaptive immune responses.

Neutrophils, Eosinophils, and Basophils

Neutrophils

Neutrophils are the most abundant circulating white blood cells. They are recruited rapidly to inflammatory sites and are capable of phagocytosing and digesting microbes. Activation of neutrophils and phagocytosis is facilitated through triggering of FcRs or complement receptors. During phagocytosis, the pathogen is first surrounded by the phagocyte membrane, then internalized in membrane-bound vesicles known as *phagosomes*. Phagosomes fuse with lysosomes, which contain enzymes, proteins, and peptides that inactivate and digest microbes. Beyond their phagocytic capability, neutrophils produce a variety of toxic products. Release of toxic products is known as *respiratory burst* because it is accompanied by an increase in oxygen consumption. During respiratory burst, oxygen radicals are generated by lysosomal reduced nicotinamide adenine dinucleotide phosphate (NADPH) oxidases. Neutrophils are short-lived cells, dying soon after they have been activated. Secretion of their granule products, in particular enzymes (myeloperoxidase, elastase, collagenase, and lysozyme), causes direct cellular injury and damages macromolecules at inflamed sites.

Eosinophils

In contrast to macrophages and neutrophils, eosinophils are only weakly phagocytic. They are potent cytotoxic effector cells against parasites. Their major effector mechanism is the secretion of various cationic proteins (major basic protein, eosinophil cationic protein, and eosinophil-derived neurotoxin). These proteins are released into the extracellular space, where they directly destroy the invading microorganism, but they also can damage host tissue.

Basophils

Basophils and tissue mast cells are important reservoirs of inflammatory mediators, such as histamines, prostaglandins, leukotrienes, and selected cytokines. Basophils and tissue mast cells have high-affinity receptors for monomeric IgE. They play a role in atopic allergies, in which allergens bind immunoglobulin (IgE) and cross-link FcεRs. Their function in normal immune responses is incompletely understood.

Soluble Factors in Innate Defenses

Effector functions of the cells of the innate immune system are enhanced by many circulating proteins. A particularly important contribution derives from the complement system, which holds a crucial position in linking microbial recognition to cellular effector functions. The mannose-binding lectin circulates in the plasma, functioning as an opsonin, and is involved in activation of the complement pathway. C-reactive protein, an acute phase protein, participates in opsonization by binding to bacterial phospholipids. Finally, the innate immune system could not work without the cytokines that regulate recruitment and activation of leukocytes (see Table 42–2). Cells of the innate immune system are not only the principal producers of such cytokines, but are also their targets.

ADAPTIVE IMMUNE SYSTEM

Activation of the Adaptive Immune System: Recognition of Antigen

Structure of Antigen-Specific Receptors

The innate immune system recognizes structural patterns that are common in the microbial world, whereas the adaptive immune system is designed to respond to the entire continuum of antigens. This goal is achieved through two principal types of antigen recognition receptors: antibodies and T-cell receptors (TCRs). These receptors distinguish antigens through subtle changes in shape. The antigen recognition structures are complementary to the shapes of the antigens and bind antigens noncovalently. Antibodies are expressed as cell surface receptors on B cells or are secreted. They recognize conformational structures, which are determinants formed by the tertiary configuration of proteins. In contrast, α/β TCRs fit specifically to epitopes formed by a small linear peptide embedded into MHC molecules on the surface of antigen-presenting cells.

Antibodies consist of two identical heavy chains and two identical light chains, which are covalently linked by disulfide bonds. The amino (N)-terminal domain of each chain is variable and represents the recognition structure that interacts with the antigen. Each antibody has two binding arms of identical specificity. The carboxy (C)-terminal ends of the heavy and the light chains form the constant region, which defines the subclass of the antibody (κ or λ for light chains and IgM, IgA, IgD, IgE, or IgG for heavy chains). Additional subclasses can be distinguished for IgG and IgA. The constant region of antibodies includes the Fc region. Fc regions can polymerize (IgA) or pentamerize in the presence of a J (joining) chain (IgM). Fc regions also are the ligand for the FcRs on cells of the innate immune system.

TCRs are dimers of α-chains and β-chains or of γ-chains and δ-chains, each of which contains three complementary-determining binding sites in the N-terminal domain. These complementary-determining sites define the specificity by contacting antigenic shapes. α/β TCRs exclusively recognize peptide fragments in the context of MHC molecules. γ/δ TCRs are more variable and can recognize certain glycolipid antigens in the context of MHC-like molecules or even unprocessed antigens, functioning similar to antibodies. The repertoires of antibodies and TCRs are extremely diverse and have been estimated in the human to account for 10^8 to 10^9 unique (of 10^{15} possible) combinations. This enormous diversity cannot be genetically encoded; it must be acquired. Its foundation consists of fewer than 400 genes that are recombined and modified. Immunoglobulin heavy chains are formed from four gene segments encoded on chromosome 14—the variable, diversity, joining, and constant region gene segments. Also, TCR β-chains and δ-chains are assembled by the recombination of variable, diversity, joining, and constant region segments of TCR genes. Immunoglobulin light chains and TCR α-chains and γ-chains lack the diversity segment and are composed of three gene segments. During antibody or TCR rearrangement, gene segments are cut out by nucleases and spliced together at the DNA level to form linear coding units for each receptor gene. Through the combination of several different mechanisms, an enormous diversity of receptors is generated. First, the genome contains multiple forms of gene segments; each receptor or antibody uses a different combination of these gene segments. Second, the splicing process is imprecise, introducing nucleotide variations at the variable/diversity, diversity/joining, or variable/joining junctions. These inaccuracies lead to frame shifts and result in completely different amino acid sequences. Finally, random nucleotides can be inserted at the junctional region by an enzyme, deoxyribonucleotidyl transferase.

When recombined, TCR sequences remain unchanged. This rule does not apply to immunoglobulins, which can undergo editing. Immunoglobulin editing includes replacement of an entire variable region (receptor editing); class switching during immune responses, in which the variable/diversity/joining unit combines with different constant region genes; or somatic hypermutation, in which the antigen contact areas of the antibody undergo mutations during an immune response.

Antigen Processing

T cells do not recognize native antigens but rather peptide fragments that are displayed in the context of MHC class I and class II molecules. The two classes of MHC molecules are used as restriction elements by two different subsets of T cells. $CD4^+$ T cells recognize antigen peptides embedded into MHC class II molecules, whereas $CD8^+$ T cells are directed against peptides complexed with MHC class I molecules. Generally, MHC class II molecules are expressed only on specialized antigen-presenting cells, such as dendritic cells, monocytes, macrophages, and B cells. Peptides bound to MHC class II molecules derive from extracellular antigens that are captured and internalized into endosomes to be digested by proteinases, notably cathepsin. Occasionally, intracellular proteins or membrane proteins also are funneled into this pathway. MHC class II molecules are assembled in the endoplasmic reticulum in association with a protein called the *invariant chain* (Fig. 42–3). The molecules are transported to the endosome, where the invariant chain is removed from

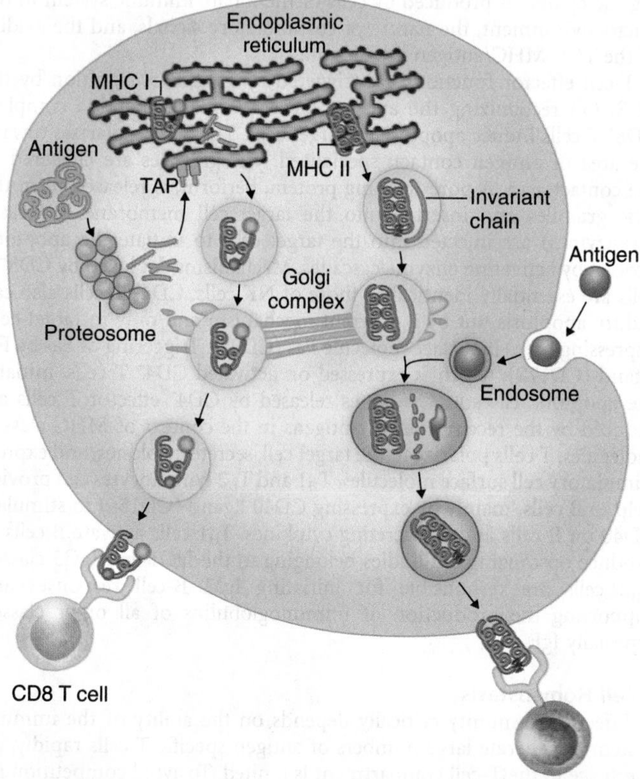

FIGURE 42–3 • Pathways of antigen processing and delivery to major histocompatibility complex (MHC) molecules. Cytosolic proteins are broken down by the proteosome to generate peptide fragments, which are transported into the endoplasmic reticulum by specialized peptide transporters (TAP). After peptides are bound to MHC class I molecules, MHC/peptide complexes are released from the endoplasmic reticulum and travel to the cell surface, where they are ligands for $CD8^+$ T-cell receptors (TCRs). Extracellular foreign antigens are taken into intracellular vesicles, endosomes. As the pH in the endosomes gradually decreases, proteases are activated that digest antigens into peptide fragments. After fusing with vesicles that contain MHC class II molecules, antigenic peptides are placed into the antigen-binding groove. Loaded MHC class II/peptide complexes are transported to the cell surface, where they are recognized by the TCRs of $CD4^+$ T cells.

the peptide-binding cleft, making the cleft accessible to peptides derived from extracellular proteins. MHC class II molecules, stabilized by peptides of 10 to 30 amino acids, are displayed on the cell surface, where they can be recognized by $CD4^+$ T cells.

MHC class I–associated peptides are produced in the cytosol by the proteosome, a large cytoplasmic multiprotein enzyme complex (see Fig. 42–3). Specialized transporter proteins, called *transporter in antigen processing,* facilitate translocation from the cytosol to the endoplasmic reticulum. Here, the peptides bind to newly formed MHC class I molecules and are transported to the cell surface, where they are recognized by antigen-specific $CD8^+$ T cells.

The nature of the antigen-processing pathway determines the sequence of events in immune responses. Extracellular antigens, in general, enter the endosomal pool and associate with MHC class II molecules to stimulate $CD4^+$ T cells. Cytosolic antigens, including antigens from intracellular infectious agents, are degraded and displayed in the context of MHC class I molecules to initiate $CD8^+$ T-cell responses.

Cellular Elements of the Adaptive Immune System

T Cells

T-Cell Development

T precursor cells derived from hematopoietic stem cells are seeded into the thymus, where all the subsequent stages of T-cell maturation occur (Fig. 42–4). Pre-T cells express two enzymes, recombinase and terminal deoxynucleotidyl transferase, enabling them to recombine TCR genes. The β-chain of the TCR is rearranged first and is expressed together with pre-TCR α-chain. Signals from the immature TCR complex inhibit rearrangement of the second β-chain allele and induce T-cell proliferation and expression of the CD4 and CD8 molecules. Subsequently, the TCR α-chain is recombined, and low levels of TCRs appear on the cell surface. From here, the T cell undergoes many differentiation and selection steps modulated by the thymic microenvironment, in particular by thymic epithelial cells, macrophages, and dendritic cells. Early stages of thymocytes reside in the thymic cortex, where they mostly interact with epithelial cells. They then migrate toward the medulla, encountering dendritic cells and macrophages at the corticomedullary junction. Thymic stromal cells regulate T-cell proliferation by secreting lymphopoietic growth factors, such as IL-7. Interactions of the TCR with MHC molecules expressed on epithelial cells and on dendritic cells/macrophages determine the fate of the thymocyte. Low-avidity recognition of peptide/MHC complexes on thymic epithelial cells by the TCR results in positive selection. This recognition event rescues cells from apoptotic cell death and ensures that only T cells with functional receptors survive. Thymocytes that express a receptor not fitting to any MHC antigen complex die by neglect. High-affinity interaction between the TCR and peptide/MHC complex induces apoptotic cell death of the recognizing T cell. This process of negative selection eliminates T cells with specificity for self-antigens and is responsible for central tolerance to many autoantigens. It has been estimated that approximately 1% of thymocytes survive the stringent selection process. While undergoing selection, T cells continue to differentiate with orderly expression of cell surface molecules. Thymocytes expressing CD4 and CD8 molecules develop into single-positive $CD4^+$ helper T cells that have been selected on MHC class II complexes or $CD8^+$ cytotoxic T cells that are restricted to MHC class I complexes.

T-Cell Stimulation and Accessory Molecules

T-cell activation is initiated when TCR complexes recognize antigenic peptides in the context of the appropriate MHC molecule on the surface of an antigen-presenting cell. Antigen recognition by T cells results in proliferation and differentiation and triggers various effector functions. Stimulation of the TCR is not sufficient and needs to be complemented by the interaction of accessory molecules on the T cell and their ligands on the antigen-presenting cell. A spectrum of accessory molecules is known (see Table 42–1). The coreceptors, CD4 and CD8, interact with MHC class II and class I molecules and support activation signals through the TCR. Adhesion molecules (integrins) stabilize the interactions between T cells and antigen-presenting cells. Finally, specialized costimulatory molecules provide a second signal in addition to the TCR signal. In the absence of such a second signal, T cells undergo apoptosis or are rendered nonresponsive and anergic.

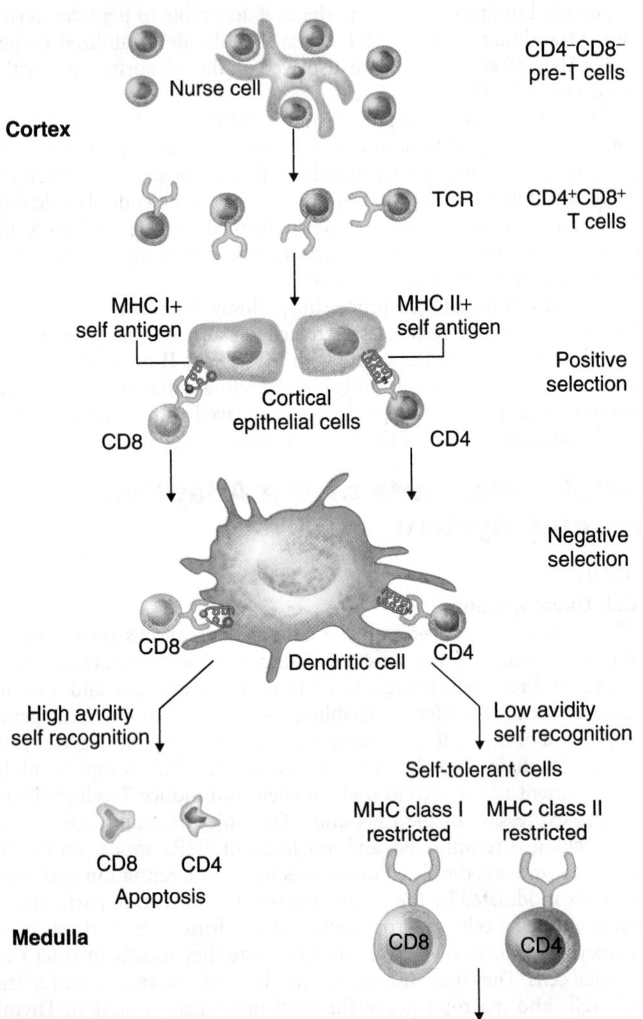

FIGURE 42–4 • Maturation of T cells in the thymus. Precursors committed to the T-cell lineage arrive in the thymus and begin to rearrange their T-cell receptor (TCR) genes. Immature T cells with receptors binding to self-major histocompatibility complex (MHC) on cortical epithelial cells receive signals for survival (positive selection). At the corticomedullary junction, surviving T cells probe self-antigens presented by dendritic cells and macrophages. T cells reacting strongly to self-antigens are deleted by apoptosis (negative selection). T cells released into the periphery are tolerant toward self and recognize foreign antigens in the context of self-MHC.

The best-known and best-studied costimulatory molecule expressed on T cells is the CD28 molecule, which binds to the CD80/CD86 ligands expressed on activated antigen-presenting cells. CD28-mediated signals are mandatory for the expression of many activation markers on the responding T cells, and in particular for the secretion of IL-2.

Signals from the TCR result in activation of many genes and entry of the T cell into the cell cycle. The signals are transmitted by a cascade of cytoplasmic events. Cross-linking of the TCR and associated CD3 molecules results in the recruitment and activation of phosphotyrosine kinases and the phosphorylation of molecular constituents of the TCR and various adapter molecules. Signals mediated through the TCR activate several biochemical pathways, such as the mitogen-activated protein (MAP) kinase, protein kinase C, and calcineurin pathways; the generation of phosphoinositol products; and the increase of intracellular calcium, which collectively lead to the activation of transcription factors that regulate gene expression.

Three major variables determine the outcome of TCR stimulation: the duration and affinity of the TCR/antigen interaction, the maturation stage of the responding T cell, and the nature of the antigen-presenting cell. Antigen-presenting cells are gatekeepers in the initiation of T-cell responses. They can upregulate the expression of accessory molecules that provide costimulatory signals. MHC/peptide complexes are particularly dense on dendritic cells, enabling them to activate naïve T cells. In contrast, memory and effector cells have a lower threshold for activation and can react to antigens presented on peripheral tissue cells.

T-Cell Differentiation and Effector Functions

T-cell activation induces T-cell proliferation with the goal of clonally selecting and expanding antigen-specific T cells. The extent of clonal proliferation is impressive. It has been estimated that the frequency of antigen-specific $CD8^+$ T cells increases by a factor of 50,000. $CD4^+$ T cells also are clonally selected but proliferate to a lesser extent. T-cell proliferation in response to antigen recognition is driven by autocrine mechanisms, predominantly by IL-2. During the phase of rapid growth, T cells differentiate from naïve T cells that are essentially devoid of effector functions into effector T cells. The transition into effector cells is associated with a fundamental shift in functional profile. First, effector T cells have a lower activation threshold; they do not require costimulation and can scan tissues that lack professional antigen-presenting cells. Second, they switch the expression of chemokine receptors and adhesion molecules to gain access to peripheral tissues. Finally, they gain effector functions. The principal effector function of $CD8^+$ T cells is to lyse antigen-bearing target cells. $CD4^+$ T cells produce many cytokines and express cell surface molecules that are important in the activation of phagocytes and other lymphocytes. $CD8^+$ T cells are committed to differentiating into cytotoxic T cells as they emerge from the thymus; the spectrum of options for $CD4^+$ T cells is larger. Different subsets of $CD4^+$ effector T cells can be distinguished based on the preferential production of certain cytokines (see Table 42–2). T_H1 T cells predominantly produce IFN-γ and TNF-α and are involved in cell-mediated immunity, such as delayed-type hypersensitivity reactions. T_H2 T cells preferentially produce IL-4, IL-5, and IL-13, cytokines that regulate B-cell responses and the activation of eosinophils. The decision as to which differentiation pathway to take is made during the early stages of T-cell activation and depends on many factors, including the cytokines produced by cells of the innate immune system in the microenvironment, the nature of costimulatory signals, and the avidity of the TCR-MHC/antigen interaction.

T-cell effector functions are triggered by antigen recognition by the TCR. On recognizing the appropriate MHC class I/peptide complex, $CD8^+$ T cells induce apoptosis in target cells. The T cell polarizes toward the area of antigen contact; specialized lytic granules are clustered in the contact area. A pore-forming protein, perforin, is released from the lytic granules and inserted into the target cell membrane. Proteases (granzymes) are injected into the target cells to initiate the apoptotic process by activating enzyme cascades. Mechanisms deployed by $CD8^+$ T cells are essentially identical to those of NK cells. $CD4^+$ T cells also can induce apoptosis but by a different mechanism and only in target cells expressing the cell-surface molecule Fas (CD95). Triggering of Fas by Fas ligand (CD178), which is expressed on activated $CD4^+$ T cells, initiates the apoptotic cascade. Cytokines released by $CD4^+$ effector T cells are induced by the recognition of antigens in the context of MHC class II molecules. T cells polarize to the target cell, secrete cytokines, and express stimulatory cell surface molecules. T_H1 and T_H2 lymphocytes can provide help to B cells, mainly by expressing CD40 ligand (CD154) to stimulate CD40 on B cells and by secreting cytokines. T_H1 cells activate B cells to produce opsonizing antibodies belonging to the IgG1 and IgG3 classes; T_H2 cells are responsible for initiating IgM B-cell responses and supporting the production of immunoglobulins of all other classes, especially IgE.

T-Cell Homeostasis

Effective immunity critically depends on the ability of the immune system to generate large numbers of antigen-specific T cells rapidly, yet the space in the T-cell compartment is limited. To avoid competition for space and resources and to prevent perturbation of T-cell diversity by life-long exposure to antigens, the adaptive immune system employs several counterbalancing mechanisms. In the later stages of the activation process, a strong negative signal derives from the interaction of the T-cell molecule cytotoxic T-lymphocyte antigen (CTLA)-4 (CD152) with CD80/CD86 on antigen-presenting cells. In addition, T cells undergo activation-induced cell death. Activated $CD4^+$ T cells begin to secrete Fas ligand and acquire sensitivity to Fas-mediated death, inducing apoptotic suicide and fratricide in neighboring T cells. These mechanisms impose constraints in the early stages of T-cell antigen responses. Other mechanisms control the rapid decline of expanded antigen-specific T cells when elimination of the antigen has been achieved. Removal of the driving antigen causes deprivation of cytokines and costimulatory molecules, and growth factor–deprived T cells die from apoptosis. It has been estimated that only 5% of the antigen-expanded population survives after antigen clearance.

B Lymphocytes

B-Cell Development

B cells are generated in the bone marrow. Supported by a specialized microenvironment of nonlymphoid stromal cells, lymphoid stem cells differentiate into distinctive B-lineage cells. Driven by chemokines (stromal cell–derived factor 1) and cytokines (IL-7), precursor B cells enter a process of tightly controlled sequential rearrangements of heavy-chain and light-chain immunoglobulin genes. On pre-B cells, the membrane μ-chain is associated with a surrogate light chain to form a pre-B-cell receptor (BCR). Signals provided through this receptor are believed to induce proliferation of a progeny that subsequently rearranges different light-chain gene segments.

It is estimated that only 10% of B cells generated in the bone marrow reach the recirculating pool. Losses are mostly due to negative selection and clonal deletion of immature B cells that express receptors directed against self-antigens. Cross-linking of surface IgM by multivalent self-antigens causes immature B cells to die. Such self-reactive B cells can be rescued from death by replacing the light chain with a newly rearranged light chain that is no longer self-reactive (receptor editing). On maturation, B cells begin to express surface IgD. B cells positive for IgD and IgM are exported from the bone marrow and seed peripheral lymphoid tissues (Fig. 42–5).

B-Cell Stimulation

Mature B cells are activated by soluble and cell-bound antigens to develop into antibody-secreting effector cells. B cells respond to a large variety of antigens, including proteins, polysaccharides, and lipids. Binding of antigen to cell surface IgM molecules induces BCR clustering. In addition to the antigen-binding immunoglobulin, the BCR comprises two proteins, Ig-α and Ig-β. The Ig-α/Ig-β heterodimer functions to transduce a signal and initiates the intracellular signaling cascade. The composition of the BCR, with a ligand-binding and a signal-transducing unit, and the signaling events that lead to gene induction are similar to those of the TCR. BCR triggering can be enhanced by coreceptors. The coreceptor complex is composed of CD81, CD19, and CD21; CD21 binds to complement fragments on opsonized antigens.

Naïve B cells require accessory signals in addition to the triggering of the immunoglobulin receptor. They receive second signals either from helper T cells or from microbial components. Microbial constituents, such as bacterial polysaccharides, can induce antibody production in the absence of helper T cells (thymus-independent antigens). In the case of protein antigens (thymus-dependent antigens), the initial BCR stimulation prepares the cell for subsequent interaction with helper T cells. These activated B cells start to enter the cell cycle; upregulate cell surface molecules, such as CD80 and CD86, that provide costimulatory signals to T cells; and upregulate certain cytokine receptors. These B cells are prepared to activate helper T cells and to respond to cytokines secreted by those T cells, but they cannot differentiate into antibody-producing cells in the absence of T-cell help.

B-Cell Differentiation

Subsequent differentiation of antigen-activated B cells depends on interaction with helper T cells. B cells use their antigen receptor, not only to recognize antigens, but also to internalize them. After processing endocytosed antigens, MHC class II/peptide complexes appear on the cell surface, where antigen-specific $CD4^+$ T cells detect them. Also, B cells express costimulatory molecules and provide optimal conditions for T-cell activation. On activation, $CD4^+$ T cells express CD154 on their surface and are able to stimulate the CD40 molecule on their B-cell partner. CD40/CD154 interaction is essential for subsequent B-cell proliferation and differentiation. Cytokines secreted by the helper T cells act in concert with CD154 to amplify B-cell differentiation and to determine the antibody type by controlling isotype switching. Isotypes greatly influence the versatility of antibodies as effector molecules, and cytokines drive switching by stimulating the transcriptional activation of heavy-chain constant region genes. The late events of T cell–dependent B-cell differentiation and maturation take place in germinal centers, specialized structures in secondary lymphoid tissues (see Fig. 42–5). Here, B cells undergo important modifications, finally leading to the production of large amounts of high-affinity antibodies. The variable regions of B cells are altered by somatic hypermutation. Subsequently, B cells that possess immunoglobulin receptors with high affinity for antigens in the germinal center are selected for survival (affinity maturation).

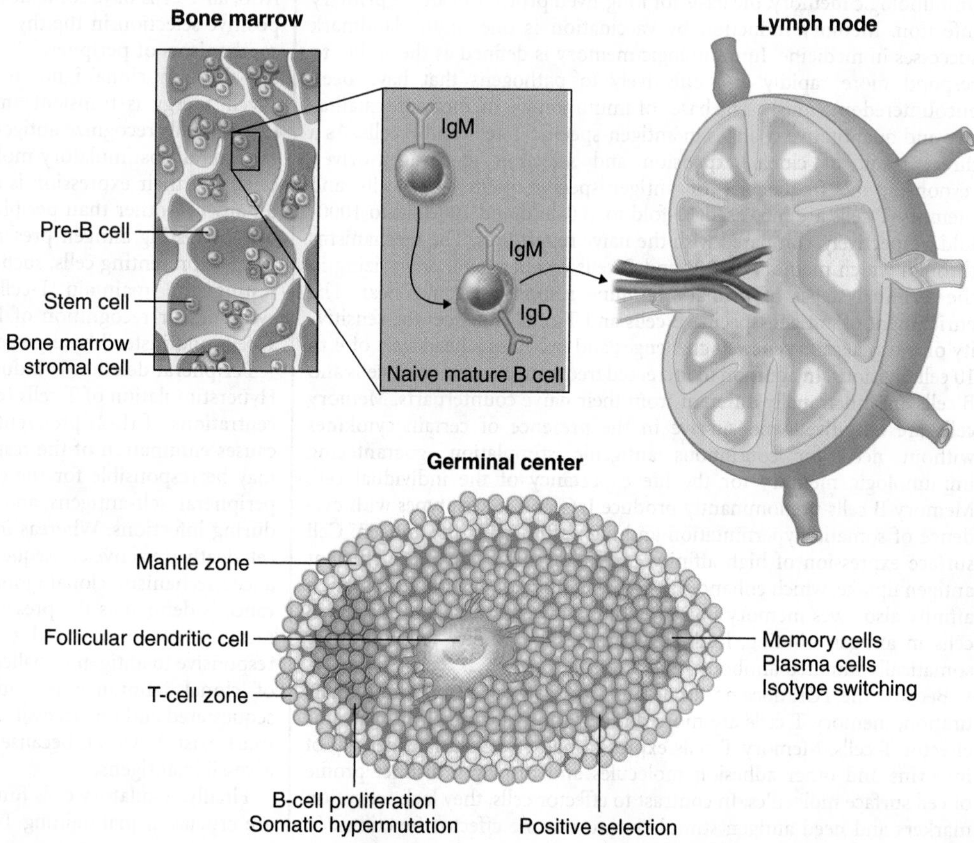

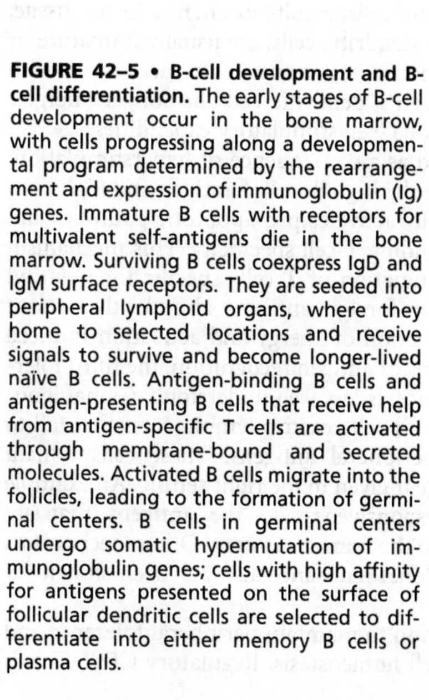

FIGURE 42–5 • B-cell development and B-cell differentiation. The early stages of B-cell development occur in the bone marrow, with cells progressing along a developmental program determined by the rearrangement and expression of immunoglobulin (Ig) genes. Immature B cells with receptors for multivalent self-antigens die in the bone marrow. Surviving B cells coexpress IgD and IgM surface receptors. They are seeded into peripheral lymphoid organs, where they home to selected locations and receive signals to survive and become longer-lived naïve B cells. Antigen-binding B cells and antigen-presenting B cells that receive help from antigen-specific T cells are activated through membrane-bound and secreted molecules. Activated B cells migrate into the follicles, leading to the formation of germinal centers. B cells in germinal centers undergo somatic hypermutation of immunoglobulin genes; cells with high affinity for antigens presented on the surface of follicular dendritic cells are selected to differentiate into either memory B cells or plasma cells.

Lymphocytes and Lymphoid Tissue

The initiation of adaptive immune responses depends on rare antigen-specific T cells and B cells meeting antigen-presenting cells and their relevant antigen. The recognition of a specific antigen in the tissue by uncommon T cells has a low probability, and it is unlikely that sufficient numbers of antigen-presenting cells and lymphocytes can be brought together to provide crucial momentum. The immune system uses specialized lymphoid microstructures to bring antigens to the site of lymphocyte traffic and accumulation. Secondary lymphoid organs include the spleen for blood-borne antigens, the lymph nodes for antigens that are encountered in peripheral tissues, the mucosa-associated lymphoid tissue, the bronchial-associated lymphoid tissue, and the gut-associated lymphoid tissue where antigens from epithelial surfaces are collected. Lymphocytes recirculate through secondary lymphoid organs, constantly searching for their antigen. Their homing to secondary lymphoid organs is facilitated by specialized microvessels, called high endothelial venules. Secondary lymphoid tissues have developed several strategies to sequester the relevant antigen. Antigens in peripheral tissue are encountered first by dendritic cells that, after activation, are mobilized to transport antigens into the local lymph nodes by the draining lymph. These antigen-bearing dendritic cells enter the lymph nodes through the afferent lymphatic vessel and settle in the T cell–rich zones to present processed antigens to T cells. The net result of this process is an accumulation and concentration of the antigen in an environment that can be readily screened by infrequent antigen-specific T cells (see Fig. 42–2).

B cells are segregated from T cells in the lymph nodes and are localized in follicles. If B cells find their cooperating T cells, they enter germinal centers. Germinal centers contain a network of follicular dendritic cells that capture particulate antigen or immune complexes on the cell surface. This unprocessed antigen is taken up by antigen-specific B cells, is processed and presented, and is recognized by antigen-specific T cells. These T cells provide cytokines and cell-cell contact signals to support the germinal center reaction, a process that leads to somatic hypermutation, affinity selection, and, eventually, isotype switching (see Fig. 42–5). Germinal centers are essential for generating antibody-secreting plasma cells and memory B cells.

Memory

An important consequence of adaptive immunity is the generation of immunologic memory, the basis for long-lived protection after a primary infection. Memory induction by vaccination is one of the landmark successes in medicine. Immunologic memory is defined as the ability to respond more rapidly and effectively to pathogens that have been encountered previously. The bases of immunologic memory are qualitative and quantitative changes in antigen-specific T cells and B cells. As a direct result of clonal expansion and selection in antigen-driven responses, the frequencies of antigen-specific memory B cells and memory T cells are increased 10-fold to 100-fold and 100-fold to 1000-fold, respectively, compared with the naïve repertoires. The mechanisms through which memory T cells and B cells escape clonal downsizing in the terminal stages of primary immune response are not clear. The enrichment of antigen-specific B cells and T cells enhances the sensitivity of the system to renewed challenges and provides a head start of 4 to 10 cell divisions. In addition to increased frequencies, memory T cells and B cells are functionally different from their naïve counterparts. Memory cells are long-lived and survive in the presence of certain cytokines without need for continuous antigenic stimulation, guaranteeing immunologic memory for the life expectancy of the individual cell. Memory B cells predominantly produce IgG and IgA isotypes with evidence of somatic hypermutation and high affinity for the antigen. Cell surface expression of high-affinity antibodies allows for more efficient antigen uptake, which enhances the crucial interaction with T cells. High affinity also gives memory B cells a competitive advantage over naïve B cells in antigen binding, leading to progressive affinity maturation of somatically mutated antibody molecules.

Because the TCR does not undergo isotype switching or affinity maturation, memory T cells are more difficult to distinguish from naïve or effector T cells. Memory T cells express a higher cell surface density of integrins and other adhesion molecules and display a distinct profile of cell surface molecules. In contrast to effector cells, they lack activation markers and need antigen stimulation to resume effector functions. In contrast to naïve T cells, memory T cells have a lower activation threshold toward antigen stimulation and are less dependent on costimulatory signals. In essence, their requirements for antigen stimulation are fewer, and their clonal size is larger, permitting fast, efficient responses to secondary antigen encounters. Also, memory T cells resume effector functions without having to undergo cell divisions.

Immunologic Tolerance and Autoimmunity

Unresponsiveness to self is a fundamental property of the immune system and is a condition, sine qua non, to maintain tissue integrity of the host. Self/non-self distinction is relatively straightforward for the innate immune system, in which receptors to non-self molecules are genetically encoded and evolutionarily selected. Self/non-self discrimination is much more complex for the adaptive immune system, in which antigen-specific receptors are generated randomly and the entire spectrum of antigens theoretically can be recognized. The adaptive immune system must acquire the ability to distinguish between self and non-self. Several different mechanisms are used, collectively called *tolerance*. Tolerance is antigen specific; its induction requires the recognition of antigen by lymphocytes in a defined setting. Failure of self-tolerance results in immune responses against self-antigens. Such reactions are called *autoimmunity* and may give rise to chronic inflammatory autoimmune disease.

Several tolerance mechanisms exist, some of which are shared between T cells and B cells. In central tolerance, self-reactive lymphocytes are deleted during development. Central tolerance implies that developing immature lymphocytes respond differently to antigen contact than do mature lymphocytes. This process of negative selection is particularly important for T cells. During thymic development, T cells that recognize antigen with high affinity are deleted. Negative selection ensures that T cells that recognize abundant antigens with high affinity, in particular antigens that are constitutively expressed on antigen-presenting cells, are deleted from the repertoire. Central tolerance for B cells follows the same principles. Recognition of antigen by developing B cells in the bone marrow induces apoptosis. Negative selection is particularly important for B cells that recognize multivalent antigens, because they do not depend on T-cell help and cannot be controlled peripherally.

Not all self-reactive T cells are centrally purged from the repertoire; certain antigens are not encountered at sufficient densities in the thymus. Also, all T cells have some degree of self-reactivity, which is necessary for positive selection in the thymus and for peripheral survival. Additional mechanisms of peripheral T-cell tolerance exist, such as anergy, peripheral deletion, clonal ignorance, and suppression of immune responses. T-cell anergy is transient and is actively maintained. It is induced if $CD4^+$ T cells recognize antigens without receiving costimulatory signals. In general, costimulatory molecules are restricted to antigen-presenting cells, and their expression is activation dependent. Antigen recognition on any cell other than peripheral antigen-presenting cells or on immature or resting antigen-presenting cells, results in anergy. In the tissue, antigen-presenting cells, such as dendritic cells, are usually immature or resting and maintain T-cell nonresponsiveness. On activation with cytokines or recognition of PAMPs, dendritic cells no longer anergize T cells and instead have powerful T-cell stimulatory capabilities.

Peripheral deletion is induced as a consequence of hyperstimulation. Hyperstimulation of T cells (e.g., by high doses of antigen and high concentrations of IL-2) preferentially activates pro-apoptotic pathways and causes elimination of the responding T-cell specificity. This mechanism may be responsible for the elimination of T cells specific for plentiful peripheral self-antigens and for foreign antigens abundantly present during infections. Whereas induction of anergy and activation-induced cell death are active consequences of antigen recognition, the third tolerance mechanism, clonal ignorance, is less well understood. Clonal ignorance is defined as the presence of self-reactive lymphocytes that fail to recognize or to respond to peripheral antigens. These cells remain responsive to antigenic challenge if given in the right setting. An example of clonal ignorance is nonresponsiveness to the antigens that are sequestered and not accessible to the immune system. Other mechanisms must exist, however, because clonal ignorance also has been shown for accessible antigens.

Finally, regulatory cells function to maintain peripheral tolerance and are crucial in maintaining T-cell homeostasis. Regulatory $CD4^+$ T cells are generated during T-cell differentiation in the thymus, recognize self-antigens, and are characterized by the constitutive expression of the IL-2 receptor and the transcription factor FoxP3. T cells with regulatory function are also generated during T-cell differentiation induced by antigen recognition. On antigen recognition, regulatory cells produce cytokines, such as transforming growth factor-β (TGF-β), IL-10, or IL-4, that dampen or suppress immune responses. Other subsets of regulatory cells maintain peripheral tolerance through contact-dependent mechanisms.

Peripheral tolerance of B cells is maintained through the absence of T-cell help. B cells require signals from T cells to differentiate into effector cells. B lymphocytes that recognize self-antigens in the periphery in the absence of T-cell help are rendered anergic or are not able to enter lymphoid follicles, where they could receive T-cell help, effectively excluding them from immune responses.

Generation and maintenance of self-tolerance for T cells and B cells is complex. This system can fail, in which case autoimmune responses are generated. Overall, chronic inflammatory diseases induced by tolerance failure occur in about 5% of the general population. Given the complexity of regulation, it is surprising that autoimmune diseases are not even more frequent. It currently is thought that most autoimmune diseases result from dysfunction of the adaptive immune system. Many models of autoimmunity rely on the hypothesis that peripheral anergy is broken. Aberrant expression of costimulatory molecules on nonprofessional antigen-presenting cells or inappropriate activation of tissue-residing dendritic cells would set the stage for the induction of "forbidden" T-cell responses. Also, autoreactive B cells that recognize self-antigen complexed with foreign antigen may engulf this complex and receive help from T cells specific for the foreign antigen. Autoimmunity also may emerge if antigen ignorance is broken. This could happen if tissue barriers break down and antigens that usually are sequestered from the immune system, such as antigens from the central nervous system or from the eye, become accessible. Tolerance mechanisms of anergy or clonal ignorance also can fail if a foreign antigen is sufficiently different from a self-antigen to initiate an immune response but sufficiently similar for activated T cells to elicit T-cell and B-cell effector functions (molecular mimicry).

Immunocompetence and Immunodeficiencies

Defects in any of the components of the immune system can compromise host protection and lead to increased susceptibility to infections. Patients with immune deficiencies also are prone to develop certain types of malignancies. Immunodeficiency can be inherited or acquired. Genetic defects have been instructive in defining the biologic relevance of various pathways in the immune system. Inherited defects that interfere with the development of the cellular components of the innate immune system have not been found, emphasizing that these deficiencies may not be compatible with survival. Few genetic defects exist that impair effector functions in innate immunity. Of these, complement deficiencies are most common. They increase susceptibility for certain infections and, in particular, predispose the host toward autoimmune disease (Chapter 47). Leukocyte adhesion deficiencies affect all cellular components of the innate and the adaptive immune systems and are associated with bacterial and fungal infections and impaired wound healing. Chédiak-Higashi syndrome is caused by the genetic defect of a protein involved in intracellular vesicle formation. Lysosomes cannot fuse properly, and intracellular killing is impaired. The clinical consequences are those of persistent bacterial infections. Another example of defective phagocytic cells is chronic granulomatous disease, in which phagocytes fail to produce reactive oxygen intermediates, and intracellular bacteria are inefficiently eliminated.

For the adaptive immune system, the underlying molecular defects for many types of inherited immunodeficiencies are now understood. As a common denominator, these immunodeficiencies severely impair the host's resistance to infection. Combined immunodeficiencies, affecting T cells and B cells, are rare and have been attributed to mutations in the cytokine receptor γ-chain or its proximal signaling molecules, defects in the recombination machinery of TCRs and BCRs, or a deficiency of the enzyme adenosine deaminase. Children born with severe combined immunodeficiencies often die from infections early in childhood (Chapter 271). Other primary immunodeficiency syndromes selectively target the T-cell or B-cell arm or interfere with T-cell and B-cell triggering. DiGeorge's syndrome (Chapter 271) is characterized by congenital malformation of the thymus. Congenital abnormalities in T-cell or B-cell activation and defects in MHC class I or II expression increasingly are understood at a molecular level. X-linked hyper-IgM syndrome results from mutations that disrupt T cell–mediated B-cell activation by CD40/CD154 interaction. The most frequent congenital immunodeficiencies are selective immunoglobulin isotype deficiencies, in which serum concentrations of one or more immunoglobulin subclasses are reduced. Affected individuals may not have any clinical manifestations or may present with recurrent bacterial infections.

More frequent than inherited immunodeficiency syndromes are acquired immunocompromised states. These conditions can be divided into infectious immunodeficiencies, iatrogenic immunodeficiencies, and immunoincompetence of the elderly. Infection with human immunodeficiency virus (HIV) causes the best-known acquired immunodeficiency. The virus paralyzes the immune system by targeting CD4-expressing helper T cells, macrophages, and dendritic cells (Chapter 408). More subtle strategies of subverting host immune responses are employed by other viruses. Cytomegalovirus is able to interfere with antigen processing and antigen presentation at several levels and compromises adaptive immune responses. Chemotherapy is regularly associated with acquired immunodeficiency, in particular in adult hosts. Although the innate immune system has a high degree of regenerative capacity, the adaptive immune system has limitations in its potential to repopulate. The ability to produce T cells progressively declines with age, and chemotherapy in adults frequently is associated with permanent defects in T-cell numbers and T-cell function. Other forms of iatrogenic immunodeficiencies are found in patients who require immunosuppressive therapy for transplant rejection (Chapter 46) or autoimmune disease. The acquired immunodeficiency associated with aging is termed *immunosenescence*. Age-related degeneration mostly affects functions of the adaptive immune system. The declines in T-cell diversity and function with advancing age lead to increased susceptibility for infections, reduced efficacy of vaccinations, increased risk of malignancies, and reactivation of viral infections. The dysfunction of the adaptive immune system in the elderly not only manifests as insufficient T-cell and B-cell responses but also impairs the maintenance of self-tolerance and predisposes these individuals to autoimmunity.

SUGGESTED READINGS

Abbas AK, Janeway CA Jr: Immunology: Improving on nature in the twenty-first century. Cell 2000;100:129–138. *A lucid review of immunologic concepts and landmark discoveries.*

Goodnow CC: Pathways for self-tolerance and the treatment of autoimmune diseases. Lancet 2001;357:2115–2121. *Discusses the premises and limitations of immunosuppressive treatments in the context of tolerance and autoimmunity models.*

Gregersen PK: Modern genetics, ancient defenses, and potential therapies. N Engl J Med 2007;356:1263–1266. *Links evolutionary immunity to modern medicine.*

Hoebe K, Janssen E, Beutler B: The interface between innate and adaptive immunity. Nat Immunol 2004;5:971–974. *Describes the key principles regarding how the innate immune system regulates adaptive immune responses.*

Krogsgaard M, Davis MM: How T cells "see" antigen. Nat Immunol 2005;6:239–245. *Summarizes the recent work on how T-cell receptors recognize peptide or lipid antigens in the context of major histocompatibility antigens and the implications for T-cell activation.*

Linton PJ, Dorshkind K: Age-related changes in lymphocyte development and function. Nat Immunol 2004;5:133–139. *Comprehensive review on the effect of age on the various different components of the immune system, from the hematopoietic stem cells to bone marrow and thymic function to mature lymphocytes.*

Medzhitov R, Janeway C Jr: Innate immunity. N Engl J Med 2000;343:338–344. *Excellent summary of the most recent concepts of how innate immunity is regulated.*

Sharpe AH, Abbas AK: T-cell costimulation-biology, therapeutic potential, and challenges. N Engl J Med 2006;355:973–975. *A concise overview.*

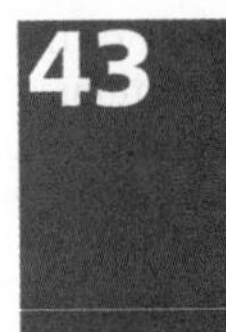

43 THE MAJOR HISTOCOMPATIBILITY COMPLEX

Peter K. Gregersen

HUMAN LEUKOCYTE ANTIGENS

The major histocompatibility complex (MHC) occupies a unique position in the nexus between clinical medicine, immunology, and genetics. Hundreds of diseases and clinical phenotypes have been associated with genes located within the MHC. The most important of these genes encode the human leukocyte antigens (HLAs), a family of cell surface proteins that are essential for normal immune function. HLA genes display a remarkably high degree of genetic variation between individuals in the population, and this variability is largely responsible for individual differences in immune responsiveness. These effects on immune responsiveness are in turn related to individual differences in susceptibility to a variety of autoimmune, inflammatory, and infectious disorders. Thus, the structural variability of the HLA molecules themselves underlies most, but not all, of the many HLA disease associations that have been reported over the last 3 decades.

The Structure of HLA Molecules

The x-ray crystallographic structure of an HLA molecule was first described in 1987. This discovery had a major impact on understanding the molecular basis of immune recognition by T cells. A ribbon diagram of the structure of an HLA class I molecule is shown in Figure 43–1. The "business end" of the molecule contains a peptide-binding cleft formed by the two membrane distal domains (α_1 and α_2) of the HLA class I heavy chain, as seen in the side view in panel A. A view from the top of this cleft is shown in panel B and illustrates that the base of the peptide-binding cleft is formed by β-pleated sheets, with two α-helical structures forming the sides of the cleft. Panel B can be thought of as the "T-cell view" of the HLA molecule.

It is now known that the T-cell receptor physically interacts with both the HLA molecule and the peptide bound within the cleft to form a "trimolecular complex" (Fig. 43–2). T-cell immune recognition (through α/β T-cell receptors) can be directly influenced by amino acid sequence variations that are present on the HLA molecule itself, as well as by the structure of the bound antigenic peptide. Thus, it is not surprising that structural differences in HLA molecules, particularly in amino acids surrounding the peptide-binding cleft, have a major role in many immunologically mediated diseases.

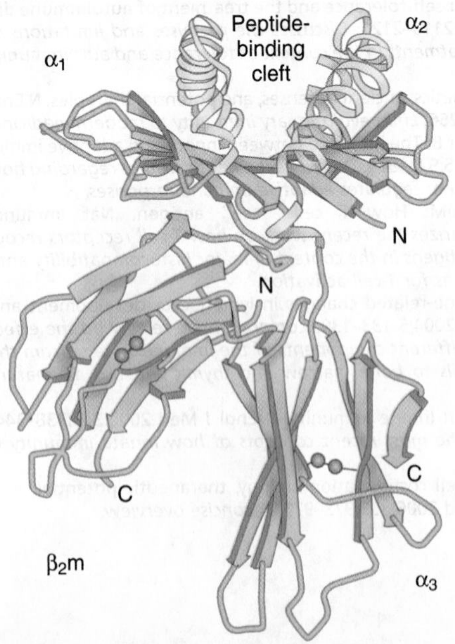

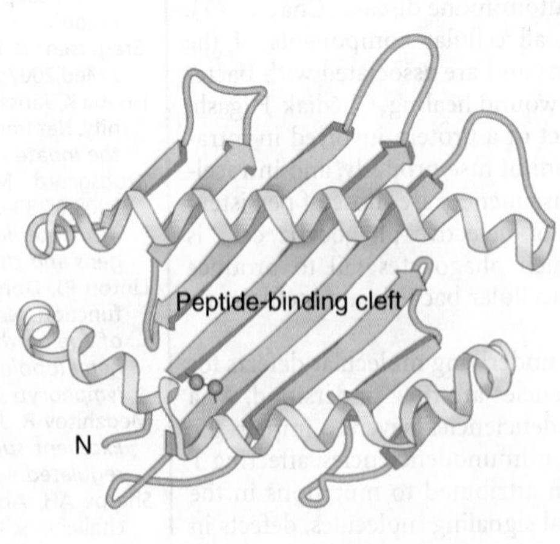

FIGURE 43–1 • Two views of an HLA class I molecule. A, Ribbon diagram showing the x-ray crystallographic structure of an HLA class I molecule (side view). The β-strand structures are indicated by the *thick green arrows* (oriented in an amino to carboxy direction), whereas connecting loops are indicated as *thin lines*. The α-helices are shown flanking a peptide-binding cleft at the top (membrane distal portion) of the molecule. The base (membrane proximal portion) of the molecule is formed by the noncovalent association between the α_3 domain of the class I α chain and β_2-microglobulin (β_2m). **B,** View from the top of the molecule emphasizing that the base of the peptide-binding cleft consists of β-pleated sheets flanked by α-helical structures. (Adapted from Bjorkman PJ, Saper MA, Samraoi B, et al: Structure of the class I histocompatibility antigen HLA-A2. Nature 1987;329:506–512.)

Properties of HLA Class I and Class II Isoforms

There are two major isoforms of HLA molecules, termed class I and class II. Both isoforms are anchored in the cell membrane and contain a peptide-binding cleft similar to that shown in Figure 43–1. However, their specific structural and functional features differ, as summarized in Figure 43–3 and Table 43–1. In the case of class I molecules, a highly variable α

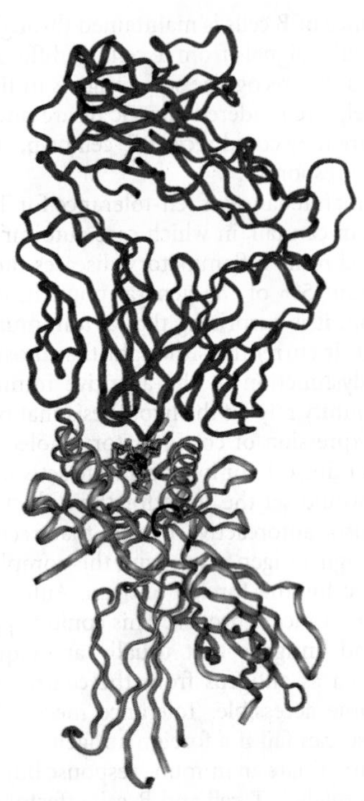

FIGURE 43–2 • HLA class II molecule. Ribbon diagram derived from the three-dimensional crystal structure of the trimolecular complex of a human α/β T-cell receptor (*top, blue*), influenza Ha antigen peptide (*green*), and the major histocompatibility complex class II molecule DRB1*0401 (*brown*). Note that the structure of this HLA class II molecule is highly similar to that of the HLA class I molecule shown in Figure 43-1. The structure shows that the peptide is bound within the binding cleft of the DR molecule and that the T-cell receptor directly interacts with both the bound peptide and the α-helical portions of the HLA-DR molecule. (Taken from Hennecke J, Wiley DC: Structure of a complex of the human alpha/beta T cell receptor [TCR] HAI.7, influenza hemagglutinin peptide, and major histocompatibility complex class II molecule, HLA-DR4 [DRA*0101 and DRB1*0401]: Insight into TCR cross-restriction and alloreactivity. J Exp Med 2002;195:571–581.)

TABLE 43–1 COMPARISON OF STRUCTURAL AND FUNCTIONAL FEATURES OF HLA CLASS I AND CLASS II ISOTYPES

	HLA Class I	HLA Class II
Chain structure of heterodimer	45-kD α chain 12-kD β_2-microglobulin	34-kD α chain 28-kD β chain
Tissue distribution	All nucleated cells	Antigen-presenting cells (monocytes, B cells, dendritic cells, Langerhans cells), thymic epithelium, and some T cells; inducible on other cell types by interferon-γ
Size of bound peptides	8–9 amino acids	10–20 amino acids
Source peptides	Cytosolic	Endosomal
Functions	Presentation of antigenic peptides to CD8⁺ T cells; ligands for natural killer cell receptors	Presentation of antigenic peptides to CD4⁺ T cells

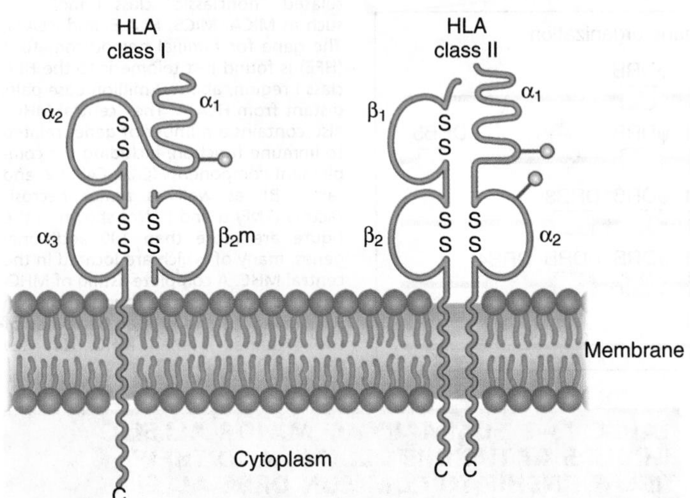

FIGURE 43–3 • Schematic comparison of the highly homologous heterodimeric structures of HLA class I and class II molecules. The peptide-binding cleft of each molecule is formed by the α_1 and α_2 domains in the case of class I, whereas the α_1 and β_1 domains form this structure in class II molecules.

chain (45 kD) forms a noncovalent heterodimer with an invariant β_2-microglobulin (12 kD) and is anchored to the cell by a single transmembrane segment on the α chain. In contrast, HLA class II molecules are formed by α (32 kD)- and β (28 kD)-chain heterodimers, and in many cases both chains exhibit structural variability among individuals. HLA class I molecules are expressed on nearly all nucleated cells. HLA class II molecules are found on more restricted cell populations, including B cells, monocytes, macrophages, dendritic cells, and other "professional" antigen-presenting cells such as Langerhans cells in the skin. Certain subsets of T cells also express class II molecules. In addition, HLA class II molecules are expressed on thymic epithelium, where they are involved in thymic selection of the T-cell receptor repertoire (see later). The size of the peptides bound to HLA class I molecules is circumscribed to 8 or 9 amino acids in length, whereas the peptides presented by HLA class II molecules are longer and more variable in size, with lengths usually ranging from 10 to 20 amino acids. HLA class I molecules generally present peptides for recognition by CD8⁺ T cells, such as in cytotoxic CD8⁺ T-cell responses against virally infected tissues. It has recently become apparent that class I molecules are also recognized by several types of receptors found on natural killer (NK) cells. In many cases, this recognition actually prevents killing of the cell by NK cells, a function of class I molecules that is largely independent of the particular antigenic peptide bound by the class I molecule. In contrast, HLA class II molecules are primarily involved in presenting antigenic peptides to CD4⁺ T cells.

Sources of the peptide antigens presented by class I and class II molecules are quite distinct. In the case of class I molecules, the bound peptides are derived from the cytosol and are loaded onto the class I molecules during their synthesis in the endoplasmic reticulum. Thus, either host or virally derived peptides may be present in the peptide cleft, and indeed, a peptide is required for proper folding and surface expression of class I molecules. In contrast, HLA class II molecules present peptides that are present in endosomes, and peptide loading onto class II molecules occurs in endocytic vesicles. These peptides are derived from sources exogenous to the cell, such as soluble proteins, particles, cell debris, or whole organisms. In the case of B cells, surface immunoglobulin can facilitate the internalization of highly specific antigens, whereas in macrophages and other antigen-presenting cells, endocytosis and phagocytosis mediate less specific cellular internalization of antigens. Mycobacteria and intracellular parasites such as *Leishmania* replicate inside vesicular compartments of the cell, and therefore peptides from these agents are generally presented on class II molecules.

Organization of HLA Molecules

Genetic Map of HLA Genes within the Major Histocompatibility Complex

The MHC is contained within a 3.6 million–base pair region located at chromosome 6p21 and encodes over 200 different genes, approximately 40% of which appear to have some role in immune function. Figure 43–4 shows a simplified map of the major HLA loci. The HLA class I and class II regions are separated by a gene-dense region often referred to as the "central" MHC. This central region encodes a number of genes of immunologic importance, including several complement components and tumor necrosis factor (TNF) α and β, to name only a few. The class I heavy chains for HLA-A, HLA-B, and HLA-C are encoded on the telomeric side of the MHC, along with a number of other class I–like molecules as shown in Figure 43-4. The HLA class II region is considerably more complicated, with multiple α and β chains encoded for each of the major HLA class II isotypes, HLA-DR, HLA-DQ, and HLA-DP. Of these, HLA-DR exhibits additional complexity in that a different gene organization of β chains is seen, depending on the particular DR haplotype.

HLA Typing Nomenclature and Patterns of Allelic Sequence Variation

In addition to the organizational complexity of the HLA region, the nomenclature for HLA typing of different alleles at each locus presents some challenges for the nonexpert. In the last decade, hundreds of HLA alleles have been sequenced, and each HLA allelic variant is defined by its locus and sequence. For example, B*2701 indicates allele 2701 at the HLA-B locus, and DRB1*0401 indicates allele 0401 at the DRB1 locus. This nomenclature is in principle quite straightforward. However, there are a very large number of different alleles at each of these loci; for example, more than 100 alleles have been identified at the HLA-B locus, and similar allelic diversity is seen at HLA-A and HLA-C, as well as in many of the HLA class II loci. The sequence relationships between alleles are both complex and informative for understanding HLA associations with disease, and to some degree this is reflected in the nomenclature. It is therefore worth understanding the origins of these naming conventions.

The current HLA nomenclature contains traces of the early history of HLA typing. Beginning in the 1960s, a serologic approach was initially

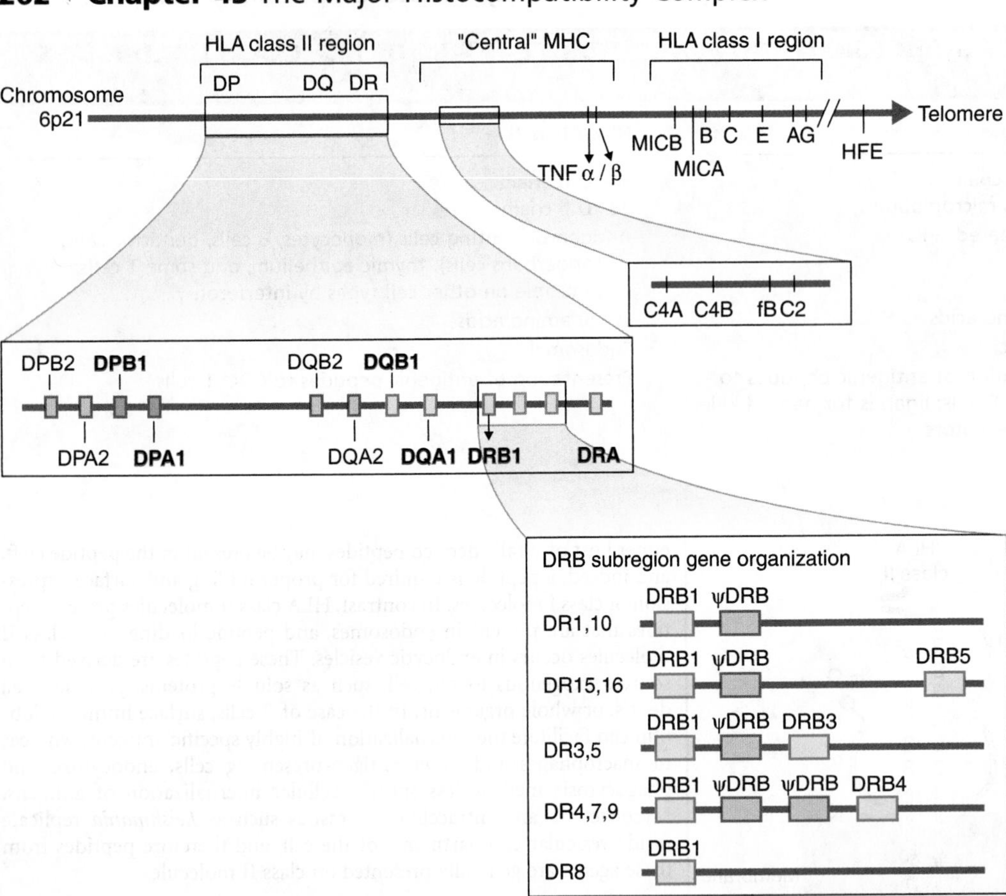

FIGURE 43–4 • Map of the human major histocompatibility complex (MHC) spanning approximately 3.5 million base pairs on the short arm of chromosome 6. The HLA class I and class II molecules are encoded in distinct regions of the MHC. The HLA class II region contains three subregions, DR, DQ, and DP. Each of these subregions contains a variable number of α- and β-chain genes. HLA class II loci with known functional protein products are labeled in bold. In the case of DR, different numbers of DRB genes are present in different haplotypes, some of which are nonfunctional pseudogenes (ψ). A summary of the most common of these are shown in the *box.* The DQ and DP subregions each contain one pair of functional α- and β-chain genes. The HLA class I region contains the three "classic" class I genes HLA-A, HLA-B, and HLA-C, as well as other related "nonclassic" class I molecules such as MICA, MICB, HLA-E, and HLA-G. The gene for familial hemochromatosis (HFE) is found just telomeric to the HLA class I region, about 3 million base pairs distant from HLA-A. The "central MHC" also contains a number of genes related to immune function, including the complement components (C4A, C4B, C2, and factor B), as well as tumor necrosis factors (TNF) α and β. Not shown in the figure are more than 100 additional genes, many of which are located in the central MHC. A complete listing of MHC-encoded genes can be found in Horton R, Wilming L, Rand V, et al: Gene map of the extended human MHC. Nat Rev Genet 2004;5:889–899.

used for HLA typing. HLA protein variation is highly immunogenic between individuals, and therefore typing alloantisera can be derived either from multiply transfused individuals (who make an antibody response to HLA molecules on the donor white cells) or from multiparous females (who commonly form antibodies to the paternal HLA antigens expressed by the fetus). Thus, by screening large numbers of individuals, panels of alloantisera were developed as the first HLA typing reagents and were shared by laboratories all over the world. Their names generally reflect their order of discovery, patterns of cross-reactivity, or "splits" of the original typing specificity. These original HLA typing sera did not distinguish all of the variation at a particular locus, and it is now apparent that serologic typing actually detects rather large groups of structurally related alleles. For example, the serologically defined allele "HLA-DR4" contains well over 30 different alleles at the DRB1 locus, although only a few of these alleles are common in the population. Table 43–2 summarizes the major allelic groups at the DRB1 locus and shows the relationship between the original serologic typing and the various groups of alleles defined at the sequence level. For some allelic groups, such as HLA-DR3, there is rather little sequence diversity within the group, depending on the population; thus, almost all white Europeans carry just one type of DR3 allele, DRB1*0301. As a result, the term "DR3" is often used in conversation to refer to the DRB1*0301 allele and is reasonably precise when talking about a white population. In contrast, the term "DR4" could refer to any one of several different alleles (see Table 43–2).

In addition to having large numbers of alleles at each locus, the frequency distribution of these alleles is also highly variable in human populations. As shown in Table 43–2, five DRB1 alleles predominate in the Northern European white population (shown in bold), with frequencies ranging from 10 to 30%. This frequency distribution will be quite different in a different population group, even among white subgroups, for example, comparing northern and southern European populations. In populations with a different major ancestry (such as African or Asian), many of these white alleles will not be present or are present at very different frequencies. These population differences emphasize the importance of matching controls to cases when comparing allele frequencies between them.

The overwhelming majority of amino acid sequence variations between different HLA alleles are clustered in and around the peptide-binding cleft. An example of the amino acid differences between five of the most common HLA-DRB1 alleles is shown in Figure 43–5. In this case, between 10 and 17 amino acid differences within the peptide-binding cleft distinguish these various alleles. These structural variations are found both at the base of the cleft and distributed along the α-helical

TABLE 43–2 SUMMARY OF MAJOR ALLELIC GROUPS AT THE DRB1 LOCUS AND THEIR RELATIONSHIP TO COMMON DRB1 ALLELES DEFINED AT THE SEQUENCE LEVEL

Allelic Groups (Serologic Typing)		Examples of Common Alleles (Northern European White Individuals) Defined by Sequence*†
MAJOR GROUPS	**SEROLOGIC "SPLITS"**	
DR1		DRB1***0101**, 0102, 0103
DR2	DR15	DRB1***1501**, 1502
	DR16	DRB1*1601
DR3		DRB1***0301**
DR4		DRB1***0401**, 0402, 0403, 0404, 0405, 0406, 0407, 0408
DR5	DR11	DRB1*1101, 1102, 1103, 1104
	DR12	DRB1*1201
DR6	DR13	DRB1*1301, 1302, 1303
	DR14	DRB1*1401
DR7		DRB1***0701**
DR8		DRB1*0801, 0802, 0803, 0804, 0806
DR9		DRB1*0901
DR10		DRB1*1001

*Alleles in bold are found in at least 10% of individuals in the population.
†From Williams F, Meenagh A, Single R, et al: High resolution HLA-DRB1 identification of a Caucasian population. Human Immunol 2004;65:66–77.

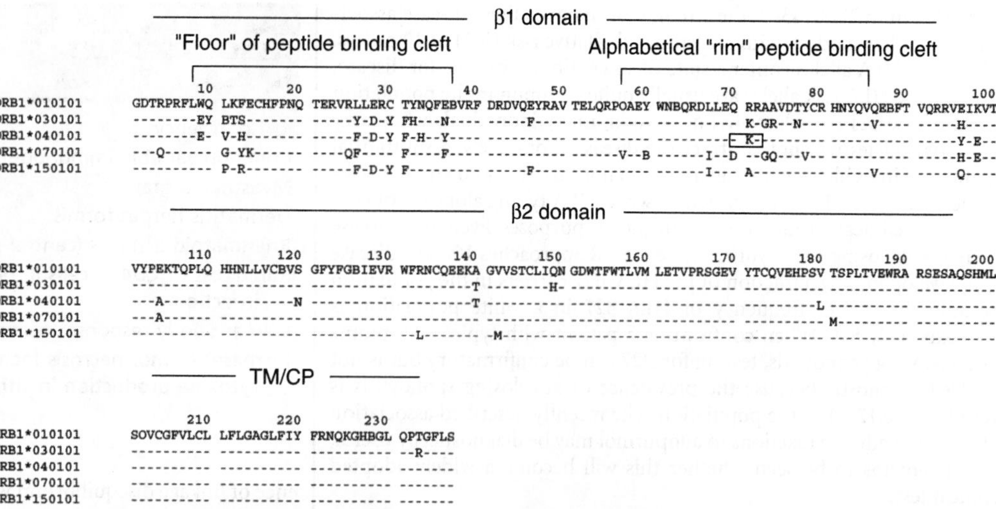

FIGURE 43–5 • Sequence comparisons of the five most common DRB1 alleles in a northern European white population (see Table 43–2). The membrane distal domain of the HLA class II molecule (β_1 domain, see Fig. 43–3) forms part of the peptide-binding cleft. Note that the majority of amino acid differences between these alleles occur in this domain and map either to the base of the peptide-binding cleft or to the α-helical rim of the cleft (see Figs. 43–1 and 43–2). In the case of HLA-DR, the α chain is invariant and does not contribute to structural variability between different HLA-DR molecules. The *boxed* region indicates the location of the five–amino acid "shared epitope" sequence on the DRB1*0401 allele that is associated with rheumatoid arthritis. TM/CP indicates transmembrane and cytoplasmic regions. A complete listing of alleles for all HLA loci can be found at *http://www.ebi.ac.uk/imgt/hla/*.

TABLE 43–3 SELECTED HLA ASSOCIATIONS WITH HUMAN DISEASES

Disease	Major HLA Association (Allelic Group or Haplotype)	Effect/Approximate Relative Risk/Relative Hazard	Probable Causative Loci/Alleles/Sequence
AUTOIMMUNE DISEASES			
Type 1 diabetes	DR3-DQ2 DR4-DQ3	10	DQB1*0201, 0302, and others with absence of Asp57 on the DQβ chain; DRB1 alleles also play a role
Multiple sclerosis	DR2-DQ1	3–5	DRB1*1501 and other related ?DQB alleles
Celiac disease	DR3-DQ2 DR4-DQ3	30	DQB1*0201 and DQB1*0302
Rheumatoid arthritis	DR1, DR4	2–5	DRB1*0101, 0401, 0404, and others; share the sequence QK/RRAA at positions 70–74 of the DRB1 chain
Systemic lupus erythematosus	DR2, DR3, DR8	2–10	?DQ locus, ?DRB1 locus, ?others
Ankylosing spondylitis	B27	100	Multiple B27 alleles
Psoriasis	Cw6	10	C*0601
INFECTIOUS DISEASES			
Progression to AIDS	B35	2–3	B*3502, B*3503, but *not* B*3501
Severe malaria	B53	0.5 (protective)	B*5301 and others
Transient vs. persistent	DR11-DQ3	5–10	?DRB1*1101, ?DQB1*0301
HEPATITIS C INFECTION			
OTHER			
Hemochromatosis	A3	10	HFE
Adverse drug reaction (allopurinol)	B58	>100	?B*5801
Cervical cancer	DR11-DQ3	2–3	?

AIDS = acquired immunodeficiency syndrome; HFE = hereditary hemochromatosis gene.

rim of the cleft. This rather large number of amino acid differences between HLA alleles is characteristic and emphasizes the very high degree of allelic diversity within the HLA system. In the case of the HLA-DR molecule, this diversity is restricted to the DRβ chain because the DRα chain is invariant at the HLA-DR locus. However, in the case of the DQ and DP loci, both the α_1- and β_1-chain domains show this general pattern of variation, and a similar degree of diversity is seen in the α_1 and α_2 domains of the HLA-A, HLA-B, and HLA-C class I molecules. From their location in the peptide-binding cleft, it is apparent that these amino acid differences can directly influence the structure of the peptides that can be bound to these alleles, as well as influence the specific T-cell receptor interactions with the peptide-HLA complex.

HLA Associations with Disease—The Concept of Disease Susceptibility

Table 43–3 provides a representative sample of some well-established HLA associations with human disease. The overwhelming majority of these studies have been conducted with a case-control design in which the frequency of alleles is compared in subjects with appropriately matched controls. Matching of controls is a critical part of the study design because HLA alleles can differ so greatly between different populations; as a result, many first reports in the literature turn out to be false positives. Nevertheless, hundreds of diseases and medically relevant phenotypes have confirmed associations with HLA alleles.

As shown in Table 43–3, the strength of many of these disease associations is rather modest, with an estimated relative risk (RR) of 10 or less. Therefore, HLA alleles confer a state of susceptibility, or risk, for disease. Because the HLA risk alleles are usually quite common in the population and the diseases are relatively uncommon, many individuals who carry these risk alleles will not contract the disease. Conversely, a substantial number of individuals with the disease do not carry the known HLA risk-conferring alleles. Thus, in a practical sense, HLA typing alone is not very useful in a clinical setting for most diagnostic purposes. Even for a disease such as ankylosing spondylitis, where the RR approaches 100, the disease will develop in only a fraction of the HLA-B27 carriers in the population because the carrier frequency of HLA-B27 in a white population is approximately 8%. When confronting a patient with typical symptoms of ankylosing spondylitis, testing for B27 can be confirmatory but is not in itself diagnostic because the prevalence of ankylosing spondylitis is very low (≈0.12%) in the population. The recently described association of B58 with adverse reactions to allopurinol may be diagnostically useful, but it remains to be seen whether this will become a widely adopted clinical test.

This pattern of association, in which HLA alleles confer a state of risk or susceptibility to disease, implies that other factors must be involved for disease to actually become manifested. In general, these other factors can include other genes, environmental factors, and nongenetic factors such as stochastic or "epigenetic" events that may occur at any time during development. Somatic rearrangements of T-cell and B-cell receptor genes are one example of such a stochastic process. These factors explain why concordance rates for many autoimmune disorders in monozygotic twins are only in the range of 30%, even though these diseases all exhibit significant genetic associations with particular HLA alleles and have a strong genetic component. The genetic predisposition conferred by the MHC is only part of the overall genetic contribution to most autoimmune disorders, and the MHC component varies in importance, depending on the particular disease.

Linkage Disequilibrium

An understanding of the concept of linkage disequilibrium is critical to proper interpretation of HLA associations or, indeed, any genetic associations with human diseases. The term *linkage disequilibrium* is used to describe the fact that alleles at adjacent loci are often found together on the same chromosomal segment, or haplotype, more frequently than predicted by chance. This phenomenon occurs throughout the genome, and the MHC is no exception. Indeed, because of the high degree of allelic diversity at HLA loci, the pattern of linkage disequilibrium between HLA alleles can be quite complicated and, like the alleles themselves, often varies among different population groups. For example, in most white populations, the DRB1*0301 allele is almost always found on the same haplotype with the DQB1*0201 allele at the DQB1 locus. (Note that the DQB1 locus is situated several hundred thousand base pairs away from the DRB1 locus—Fig. 43–4.) Likewise, DR4 alleles (at DRB1) are often found to be in linkage disequilibrium with DQB1*0302. These two haplotypes are both associated with type 1 diabetes (see Table 43–3).

Occasionally, linkage disequilibrium can extend to very long chromosomal segments. For example, a common haplotype in northern European white populations extends to several million base pairs and contains the HLA alleles A*0101-B*0801-DRB1*0301-DQB1*0201, often referred to as the "A1-B8-DR3" or "8.1" haplotype. This particular haplotype accounts for about a third of all DR3 haplotypes in a U.S. white population and is of particular interest because it is associated with a variety of diseases, some of which are listed in Table 43–4. Because haplotypes such as these are inherited as a unit, it can be difficult to determine which specific genes on the haplotype are actually responsible for the disease association in a population.

There are a number of possible explanations for linkage disequilibrium. In part it reflects the fact that meiotic recombination in the genome is discontinuous, and some loci have very low recombination rates between them—such as between the DRB1 and DQB1 loci. In addition, population migrations can introduce haplotypes into new population groups and thereby generate common "founder" haplotypes. Finally, some haplotypes may be kept intact because of selection. For example, it may be that the combination of genes found on the A1-B8-DR3 haplotype confers a survival advantage. Whatever the underlying reason, it is important to keep in mind that any HLA association may reflect the presence of linkage disequilibrium with another allele at another locus on the same haplotype.

TABLE 43–4 DISEASES AND PHENOTYPES ASSOCIATED WITH THE A1-B8-DR3 (8.1) HAPLOTYPE
IgA deficiency
Common variable immunodeficiency
Myasthenia gravis
Dermatitis herpetiformis
Rheumatoid arthritis (central portion of the 8.1 haplotype only)
Rapid loss of CD4$^+$ T cells in human immunodeficiency virus infection
Low antibody response to hepatitis B immunization
Increases (tumor necrosis factor) or decreases (interleukin-5) in cytokine production in vitro

HLA Associations with Autoimmune and Infectious Diseases

The majority of autoimmune disorders exhibit some association with HLA class II alleles, although because of linkage disequilibrium it is not always clear which locus is actually responsible for the association. In the case of type 1 diabetes, the bulk of evidence suggests that alleles at the HLA-DQ locus play a predominant role by virtue of specific amino acid substitutions that are present on multiple different DQB1 alleles. Thus, both associated haplotypes (DR3-DQ2 and DR4-DQ3) contain DQB1 alleles that lack an aspartic residue at position 57 of the DQβ chain (see Table 43–3). The arguments for the importance of amino acid residues at position 57 are statistical and result from an examination of all the various DQB1 alleles and their relationship to risk for type 1 diabetes in many different populations. It is supported by biochemical evidence that this residue plays an important role in the detailed structure of the peptide-binding cleft of the DQ molecule. However, it is not the entire explanation for the HLA association with type 1 diabetes. For example, certain DRB1 alleles, such as DRB1*0403, modify the degree of risk conferred by DQB1, and particular combinations of haplotypes, such as DR3/DR4, confer very high degrees of risk. These observations cannot be accounted for solely on the basis of amino acid substitutions at position 57 on DQB1 alleles.

Rheumatoid arthritis is another autoimmune disorder in which the molecular basis of HLA class II associations is partially worked out. In this case, a series of DRB1 alleles, including DRB1*0101, *0401, *0404, *0405, all share a common amino acid sequence (Q-K or R-R-A-A) at positions 70 to 74 of the DRβ1 chain, located on the rim of the peptide-binding cleft (see Fig. 43–5). This sequence is known as the "shared epitope" and provides an appealing unifying explanation for the complex patterns of HLA-DR associations with rheumatoid arthritis. However, as in type 1 diabetes, this single structure cannot fully account for all the data. For example, the DRB1*0101 allele has a weaker relative association (RR ≈2) than the DRB1*0401 or DRB1*0404 alleles (RR ≈4 to 5). Also similar to type 1 diabetes, certain heterozygous combinations of alleles, such as DRB1*0401/DRB1*0404, confer very high degrees of risk (RR ≈30).

For most of the HLA-associated diseases, the exact molecular basis of the association has not been definitively established, and in some cases even the causative locus is uncertain (see Table 43–3). For ankylosing spondylitis, it appears that most allelic variants of HLA-B27 are associated with disease. Recent genetic data provide support for the C*0601 allele being causative for psoriasis. However, in the case of systemic lupus erythematosus and multiple sclerosis, the relative importance of DRB1 versus DQB1 alleles is not clear.

For infectious disorders, such as the role of HLA-B35 in the progression of acquired immunodeficiency syndrome (AIDS), there is evidence again that particular amino acid residues on the HLA-B molecule are especially important. The amino acids that distinguish risk alleles (B*3502, B*3503) from nonrisk alleles (B*3501) alter the structure of a "pocket" within the peptide-binding cleft on the various HLA-B35 proteins and therefore can affect the kinds of human immunodeficiency virus (HIV) antigenic peptides that are bound by these alleles. Other

HLA-B alleles, such as B27 and B58, protect against progression of HIV, apparently by similar mechanisms. Aside from HLA-B associations with HIV outcome, specific structural explanations such as this have not yet been defined for most of the HLA associations with infectious disorders.

Mechanisms Explaining HLA Associations with Disease

It is fair to say that the mechanisms underlying HLA disease associations are still not fully explained for any disorder and the mechanisms clearly differ for different diseases. However, there are two general categories of mechanisms that are likely to be important. First, a pattern of immune responsiveness, or lack of immune responsiveness, can be related to the ability of an individual's HLA molecules to bind and present antigenic peptides (either foreign or self) to T cells. This mechanism is often referred to as "determinant selection," which means that HLA molecules are involved in selecting which antigenic determinants are selected for presentation to responding T cells. A mentioned earlier, this probably underlies the contrasting HLA-B allelic associations with AIDS progression.

An alternative mechanism invokes the role of HLA molecules in regulating thymic selection of the mature T-cell repertoire. During thymic development, thymocytes either survive or die of apoptosis, depending in large part on their ability to recognize "self" HLA molecules (and associated "self" peptides) on thymic epithelium or on other antigen-presenting cells in the thymus. This recognition is mediated through the α/β T-cell receptor. Thus, the structural repertoire of T-cell receptors in the mature circulating T-cell population is shaped by the structural variation of the selecting HLA molecules. This may lead to "holes" in the T-cell repertoire or, alternatively, enrichment for particular T-cell specificities. In this view, the presence of particular sets of potentially responding T cells provides a risk factor for response, or lack of response, to autoantigens or foreign antigens. It implies the need for an environmental trigger to actually make this risk manifest itself as overt clinical disease.

In addition to these two basic models, it has also been proposed that HLA molecules can themselves serve as a source of antigenic peptides and may predispose to disease by means of molecular mimicry or other more complex mechanisms. However, none of these proposed mechanisms have been definitively proved for any disorder.

HLA Associations with Disease Can Sometimes Reflect Linkage Disequilibrium with Non-HLA Genes

In most cases, HLA associations such as those given in Table 43–2 probably reflect the mechanistic involvement of the HLA molecules themselves in the disease or phenotype under study. However, the MHC is one of the most gene-dense segments in the human genome, and other genes in the region may in fact be responsible for the observed disease association. A good example of this is hemochromatosis. Early studies showed that certain HLA class I alleles, such as HLA-A3, were highly associated with this disorder. However, it is now clear that the causative gene, *HFE*, is actually over 3 million base pairs distant from the HLA-A locus (see Fig. 43–4). The HLA-A3 association is observed because the *HFE* C282Y allele (causative for hemochromatosis) is frequently found on the same haplotype as HLA-A3 in many white populations.

Some of the associations with the A1-B8-DR3 haplotype almost certainly reflect linkage disequilibrium with genes other than HLA class I and class II genes (see Table 43–4). Although the HLA genes may contribute to some of these disorders, it is likely that other genes on the 8.1 haplotype also contribute to risk. The central portion of the MHC in particular (see Fig. 43–4) is very gene dense with many genes of uncertain function, as well as important inflammatory cytokines such as TNF and complement components C2 and C4. Indeed, it may well be that the combination of several different genes explains why this haplotype is associated with so many different immunologic disorders.

HLA Typing and Bone Marrow Transplantation

As the term *histocompatibility* implies, the ability of the MHC to control graft rejection in experimental animals led to the realization that matching at HLA is important for transplant survival. For solid organ transplantation, treatment with immunosuppressive agents can often prevent the rejection of HLA-mismatched transplants. However, for bone marrow transplantation, careful matching of the major HLA class I and class II loci is important for a successful outcome, regardless of whether the donor is related or unrelated to the recipient. Because of the extensive sequence diversity of HLA alleles, very large numbers of unrelated donors are required to ensure a reasonable probability of a match for any given recipient who does not have a living related donor. This has led to the development of international bone marrow donor registries that now contain more than 10 million potential registered donors who have been screened for HLA type. If transplantation is performed in the presence of a significant mismatch at either class I or class II loci, T cells from the recipient may recognize the donor HLA molecules or their bound peptides as foreign and initiate an immune response and graft rejection. Interestingly, even when HLA molecules are completely matched, T cells still occasionally initiate rejection because of individual differences in "minor" histocompatibility antigens that are not encoded within the MHC but are processed and presented as antigenic peptides that appear foreign to the host.

HLA Class I—Alternative Forms and Functions

The HLA class I region of the MHC contains a number of genes that encode so-called nonclassic class I genes, including HLA-E, HLA-G, MICA, and MICB (see Fig. 43–4). These molecules do not present peptides to α/β T cells but rather interact with a variety of other ligands that are generally found on NK cells and some other types of T cells. In addition, certain allelic subsets of the "classic" class I molecules (e.g., HLA-A, -B, and -C) can also interact with some of these other ligands. Table 43–5 summarizes the various categories of interactions between these alternative ligands and class I molecules. Some of these ligands, such as the KIR (killer cell immunoglobulin-like receptor) family, display a large degree of genetic variation in both gene structure and gene number and have been associated with human disease. For example, certain combinations of HLA class I alleles and KIR alleles have been associated with risk for rheumatoid vasculitis, as well as outcome of HIV infection. These genetic relationships are complex and this aspect of HLA class I function in disease has been relatively understudied.

TABLE 43–5 ALTERNATIVE FORMS, LIGANDS, AND FUNCTIONS OF HLA CLASS I MOLECULES

HLA Class I Isoforms or Alleles	Ligands	Functions of Ligands
HLA-B (Bw4), HLA-C (S77/N80), HLA-A, HLA-G?	Killer cell immunoglobulin-like receptor (KIR) family (9 members)	Inhibitory (most often) or activating for NK and T cells
HLA-E	CD94/NKG2A	Inhibiting NK, γ/δ T cells, and subsets of $CD8^+$ T cells
HLA-E	CD94/NKG2C	Activating NK, γ/δ T cells, and subsets of $CD8^+$ T cells
MICA, MICB	NKG2D	Activation/increased cytotoxicity of NK cells, CD8 T cells
HLA-A, B, C, E, F	LILRB1	? Function; ligand expressed on all B cells and monocytes, some NK and T cells

LILRB1 = leukocyte immunoglobulin-like receptor, subfamily B, Member 1; NK = natural killer.

Section VII Immunology

HLA and Clinical Medicine

The identification of risk genes within the MHC potentially holds the key to understanding a large number of immunologically related disorders. However, we are far from identifying all of these genes, and in the few cases in which the actual risk alleles are known with confidence, their mechanism of action is not clear. Moreover, most HLA-associated disorders are complex, with additional genetic or environmental factors (or both) likely to be involved, most of which have not yet been identified. Therefore, in most cases, HLA typing alone has limited diagnostic utility. On the other hand, HLA typing may be very useful diagnostically in the future if used in combination with other genetic markers, and HLA typing remains critical to successful bone marrow transplantation. Thus, it is likely that future advances in immunology and genetics will lead to more active clinical use of genetic typing of HLA genes, as well as other genes, within the MHC.

SUGGESTED READINGS

Carrington M, Martin MP: The impact of variation at the KIR gene cluster on human disease. Curr Top Microbiol Immunol 2006;298:225–257. *A thorough review of the complex genetics of killer inhibitory receptors, an important group of ligands for HLA class I molecules with emerging disease associations.*

Cooke GS, Hill AV: Genetics of susceptibility to human infectious disease. Nat Rev Genet 2001;2:967–977. *A concise review of the genetics of infectious disease with an emphasis on HLA.*

Gao X, Bashirova A, Iversen AK, et al: AIDS restriction HLA allotypes target distinct intervals of HIV-1 pathogenesis. Nat Med 2005;11:1290–1292. *A detailed analysis of the role of HLA class I alleles in HIV pathogenesis.*

Kelly MA, Rayner ML, Mijovic CH, et al: Molecular aspects of type 1 diabetes. J Clin Pathol Mol Pathol 2003;56:1–10. *A discussion of the potential mechanisms involved in the association of HLA class II alleles with type 1 diabetes.*

Price P, Witt C, Allcock R, et al: The genetic basis for the association of the 8.1 ancestral haplotype (A1, B8, DR3) with multiple immunopathological diseases. Immunol Rev 1999;167:257–274. *A review of the unique role of the A1-B8-DR3 haplotype in human autoimmune diseases.*

44 MECHANISMS OF IMMUNE-MEDIATED TISSUE INJURY

Jane E. Salmon

THE ADAPTIVE IMMUNE RESPONSE

Definition

The adaptive immune response is a crucial component of host defense against infection. Its distinguishing and unique feature is the ability to recognize pathogens specifically, based on clonal selection of lymphocytes bearing antigen-specific receptors. Antigens unassociated with infectious agents also may elicit adaptive immune responses. Many clinically important diseases are characterized by normal immune responses directed against an inappropriate antigen, typically in the absence of infection. Immune responses directed at noninfectious antigens occur in allergy, in which the antigen is an innocuous foreign substance, and in autoimmunity, in which the response is to a self-antigen.

Effector mechanisms that eliminate pathogens in adaptive immune responses are essentially identical to those of innate immunity. The specific antigen recognition feature of the adaptive immune response seems to have been appended to the preexisting innate defense system. As a result, the inflammatory cells and molecules of the innate immune system are essential for the effector functions of B and T lymphocytes. In addition to initiating protective responses, they mediate tissue injury in allergy, hypersensitivity, and autoimmunity.

Effector Mechanisms

Effector actions of antibodies depend almost entirely on recruiting cells and molecules of the innate immune system. Antibodies are adapters that bind antigens to nonspecific inflammatory cells and direct their destructive effector responses. Antibodies also activate the complement system, which enhances opsonization of antigens, recruits phagocytic cells, and amplifies (or "complements") antibody-triggered damage. The isotype or class of antibodies produced determines which effector mechanisms are engaged.

Cell-bound receptors for immunoglobulin (Ig) constitute the link between humoral and cellular aspects of the immune cascade and play an integral part in the process by which foreign and endogenous opsonized material is identified and destroyed. These cell-based binding sites for antibodies, termed *Fc receptors,* interact with the constant region (Fc portion) of the immunoglobulin heavy chain of a particular antibody class or subclass regardless of its antigen specificity. Accessory cells that lack intrinsic specificity, such as neutrophils, macrophages, and mast cells, are recruited to participate in inflammatory responses through the interaction of their Fc receptors with antigen-specific antibodies. Distinct receptors for different immunoglobulin isotypes are expressed on different effector cells.

Receptors for IgG (FcγRs) are a diverse group of receptors expressed as hematopoietic cell surface molecules on phagocytes (macrophages, monocytes, neutrophils), platelets, mast cells, eosinophils, and natural killer (NK) cells. FcγRs often are expressed as stimulatory and inhibitory pairs. Triggering of stimulatory FcγRs initiates a series of events including phagocytosis; antibody-dependent, cell-mediated cytotoxicity; secretion of granules; and release of inflammatory mediators, such as cytokines, reactive oxidants, and proteases. Extensive structural diversity among FcγR family members leads to differences in binding capacity, signal transduction pathways, and cell type–specific expression patterns. This diversity allows IgG complexes to activate a broad program of cell functions relevant to inflammation, host defense, and autoimmunity. Phagocyte activation is triggered by stimulatory FcγRs, facilitating the recognition, uptake, and destruction of antibody-coated targets, whereas multivalent IgG binding to FcγRs on platelets leads to platelet aggregation and thrombosis, and binding to FcγRs on NK cells mediates cytotoxicity of antibody-coated targets.

IgE binds to high-affinity FcεRs on mast cells, basophils, and activated eosinophils. In contrast to FcγRs, which are low affinity and bind multivalent IgG to antigen rather than circulating individual IgG molecules, FcεRs can bind monomeric IgE. A single mast cell may be armed with IgE molecules specific for many different antigens, all bound to surface FcεRs. Mast cells, localized beneath the mucosa of the gastrointestinal and respiratory tracts and the dermis of the skin, await exposure to multivalent antigens, which cross-link surface IgE bound to FcεRs and cause release of histamine-containing granules and generation of cytokines and other inflammatory mediators. IgE-mediated activation of eosinophils, cells normally present in the connective tissue of underlying respiratory, urogenital, and gut epithelium, leads to the release of highly toxic granule proteins, free radicals, and chemical mediators such as prostaglandins, cytokines, and chemokines. These amplify local inflammatory responses by activating endothelial cells and recruiting and activating more eosinophils and leukocytes. Prepackaged granules and high-affinity FcεRs that bind to free monomeric IgE enable an immediate response to pathogens or allergens at the first site of entry, a location where FcεR-bearing cells reside.

Inhibitory FcγRs, which modulate activation thresholds and terminate stimulating signals, are key elements in the regulation of effector function. Given that inhibitory and stimulatory Fc receptors are often coexpressed on the same cells, the effector response to a specific stimulus in a particular cell represents the balance between stimulatory and inhibitory signals. Inhibitory FcγRs can dampen responses triggered by FcεRs on mast cells and FcγR-mediated inflammation at sites of immune complex deposition.

Effector activities targeted by IgG and IgM also may be mediated by components of the complement system (Chapter 47). Antigen-bound multimeric immunoglobulin can initiate activation of the classical pathway of complement, causing enhanced phagocytosis of antigen-antibody complexes, increased local vascular permeability, and recruitment and activation of inflammatory cells. The target of injury is specified by the antibody, and the extent of damage is determined by the synergistic activities of immunoglobulin and complement.

Antigen-specific effector T cells also may initiate tissue injury. On exposure to an appropriate antigen, memory T cells are stimulated to release cytokines and chemokines that activate local endothelial cells and recruit and activate macrophages and other inflammatory cells. The effector cells directed by T cell–derived cytokines, or cytolytic T cells themselves, mediate tissue damage. T_H1 cells produce interferon-γ (IFN-γ) and activate macrophages to cause injury, whereas T_H2 cells produce interleukin 4 (IL-4), IL-5, and eotaxin (an eosinophil-specific chemokine) and trigger inflammatory responses in which eosinophils predominate.

HYPERSENSITIVITY REACTIONS

In predisposed individuals, innocuous environmental antigens may stimulate an adaptive immune response, immunologic memory, and, on subsequent exposure to the antigen, inflammation. These "overreactions" of the immune system to harmless environmental antigens (allergens), called *hypersensitivity* or *allergic reactions,* produce tissue injury and can cause serious disease. Hypersensitivity reactions are grouped into four types according to the effector mechanisms by which they are produced (Table 44–1). The effectors for types I, II, and III hypersensitivity reactions are antibody molecules, whereas type IV reactions are mediated by antigen-specific effector T cells.

Autoimmune disease is characterized by the presence of antibodies and T cells specific for self-antigens expressed on target tissues. The mechanisms of antigen recognition and effector function that lead to tissue damage in autoimmune disease are similar to the mechanisms elicited in response to pathogens and environmental antigens. These mechanisms resemble certain hypersensitivity reactions and may be classified accordingly (Table 44–2). Autoimmune disease caused by antibodies directed against cell surface or extracellular matrix antigens corresponds to type II hypersensitivity reactions; disease caused by formation of soluble immune complexes that subsequently are deposited in tissue corresponds to type III hypersensitivity; and disease caused by effector T cells corresponds to type IV hypersensitivity. Typically, several of these pathogenic mechanisms are operative in autoimmune disease. However, IgE responses are not associated with damage in autoimmunity.

Type I Hypersensitivity Reactions

Type I hypersensitivity reactions (Fig. 44–1) are triggered by the interaction of antigen with antigen-specific IgE bound to FcεRs on mast cells, which causes mast cell activation. Proteolytic enzymes and toxic mediators, such as histamine, are released immediately from preformed granules, and chemokines, cytokines, and leukotrienes are synthesized after activation. Together, these mediators increase vascular permeability, break down tissue matrix proteins, promote eosinophil production and activation (interleukin [IL]-3, IL-5, and granulocyte-macrophage colony-stimulating factor [GM-CSF]), and cause influx of effector leukocytes (tumor necrosis factor-α [TNF-α], platelet-activating factor, and macrophage inflammatory protein [MIP-1]), constriction of smooth muscle, stimulation of mucus secretion, and amplification of T_H2 cell responses (IL-4 and IL-13). Eosinophils and basophils, activated through cell surface FcεRs, rapidly release highly toxic granular proteins (major basic protein, eosinophil peroxidase, and collagenase) and, over a longer period, produce cytokines (IL-3, IL-5, and GM-CSF), chemokines (IL-8), prostaglandins, and leukotrienes that activate epithelial cells, leukocytes, and eosinophils to augment local inflammation and tissue damage.

FcεR-bearing effectors act in a coordinated fashion. The immediate allergic inflammatory reaction initiated by mast cell products is followed by a late-phase response that involves recruitment and activation of eosinophils, basophils, and T_H2 lymphocytes. The manifestations of IgE-mediated reactions depend on the site of mast cell activation. Mast cells reside in vascular and epithelial tissue throughout the body. In a sensitized host (an individual with IgE responses to antigens), re-exposure to antigen leads to type I hypersensitivity responses only in the mast cells exposed to the antigen. Inhalation of antigens produces bronchoconstriction and increased mucus secretion (asthma and allergic rhinitis); ingestion of antigens causes increased peristalsis and secretion (diarrhea and vomiting); and the presence of subcutaneous antigens initiates increased vascular permeability and swelling (urticaria and angioedema). Blood-borne antigens cause systemic mast cell activation, increased capillary permeability, hypotension, tissue swelling, and smooth muscle contraction—the characteristics of systemic anaphylaxis.

Type II Hypersensitivity Reactions

Type II hypersensitivity reactions (Fig. 44–2) are caused by chemical modification of cell surface or matrix-associated antigens that generates "foreign" epitopes to which the immune system is not tolerant. B cells respond to this antigenic challenge by producing IgG that binds to these modified cells and renders them susceptible to destruction through complement activation, phagocytosis, and antibody-dependent cytotoxicity.

This phenomenon is seen clinically when drugs interact with blood constituents and alter their cellular antigens. Hemolytic anemia caused

TABLE 44–1 FOUR MAJOR TYPES OF IMMUNOLOGICALLY MEDIATED HYPERSENSITIVITY REACTIONS*

Immunologic Specificity	Type I (IgE Antibody)	Type II (IgG Antibody)	Type III (IgG Antibody)	Type IV (T Cells): T_H1 cells	Type IV (T Cells): T_H2 cells	Type IV (T Cells): T cells
Antigen	Soluble antigen allergen	Cell- or matrix-associated antigen	Soluble antigen	Soluble antigen	Soluble antigen	Cell-associated antigen
Effector mechanism	FcεRI- or FcγRIII-dependent mast cell activation, with release of mediators/cytokines	FcγR⁺ cells (phagocytes, NK cells), complement	FcγR⁺ cells, complement	Macrophage activation	Eosinophil activation	Direct cytotoxicity
Examples	Systemic anaphylaxis, asthma, allergic rhinitis, urticaria, angioedema	Certain drug reactions and reactions to incompatible blood transfusions	Arthus reaction and other immune complex–mediated reactions (e.g., serum sickness, subacute bacterial endocarditis)	Contact dermatitis, tuberculin reaction	Chronic allergic inflammation (e.g., chronic asthma, chronic allergic rhinitis)	Contact dermatitis (e.g., poison ivy), reactions to certain virus-infected cells, some instances of graft rejection

*Hypersensitivity reactions were classified into four types by Coombs and Gell (1963) and modified by Janeway and colleagues (2001). (Coombs RRA, Gell PGH: Classification of allergic reactions responsible for clinical hypersensitivity and disease. In Gell PGH, Coombs RA [eds]: Clinical Aspects of Immunology, Oxford, Blackwell, 1963; Janeway C, Travers P, Walport M, Shlomchick M: Immunobiology: The Immune System in Health and Disease, 5th ed. New York, Garland Publishing, 2001.)

FcγR, Fc receptor for immunoglobulin G; FcεR, Fc receptor for immunoglobulin E; NK, natural killer.

TABLE 44–2 CLASSIFICATION OF AUTOIMMUNE DISEASES ACCORDING TO MECHANISM OF TISSUE INJURY

Hypersensitivity Reaction	Autoimmune Disease	Autoantigen
TYPE II		
Antibody against cell-surface antigens	Autoimmune hemolytic anemia	Rh blood group antigens, I antigen
	Autoimmune thrombocytopenic purpura	Platelet integrin glycoprotein IIb:IIIa
Antibody against receptors	Graves' disease	Thyroid-stimulating hormone receptor (agonistic antibodies)
	Myasthenia gravis	Acetylcholine receptor (antagonistic antibodies)
Antibody against matrix antigens	Goodpasture's syndrome	Basement membrane collagen (α_3-chain of type IV collagen)
	Pemphigus vulgaris	Epidermal cadherin (desmoglein)
TYPE III		
Immune complex diseases	Mixed essential cryoglobulinemia	Rheumatoid factor IgG complexes (with or without hepatitis C antigens)
	Systemic lupus erythematosus	DNA, histones, ribosomes, ribonuclear proteins
TYPE IV		
T cell–mediated diseases	Insulin-dependent diabetes mellitus	Pancreatic beta-cell antigen
	Rheumatoid arthritis	Unknown synovial joint antigen
	Multiple sclerosis	Myelin basic protein, proteolipid protein

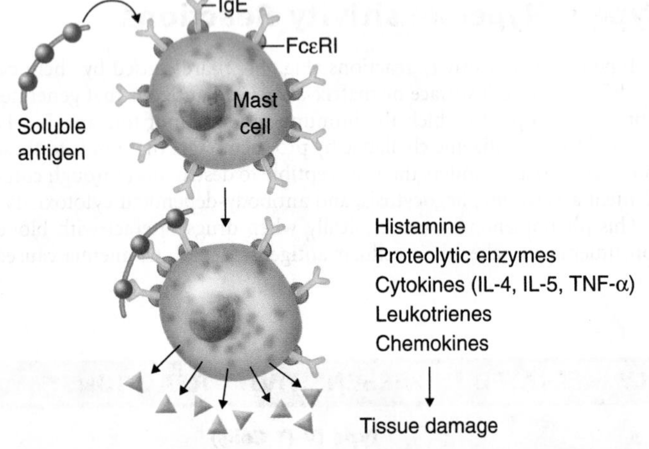

FIGURE 44–1 • Type I hypersensitivity. Type I responses are mediated by immunoglobulin E (IgE), which induces mast cell activation. Cross-linking of the Fc receptor for IgE (FcεR) on mast cells, triggered by the interaction of multivalent antigen with antigen-specific IgE bound to FcεR, causes the release of preformed granules containing histamine and proteases. Cytokines, chemokines, and lipid mediators are synthesized after cell activation. IL = interleukin; TNF = tumor necrosis factor.

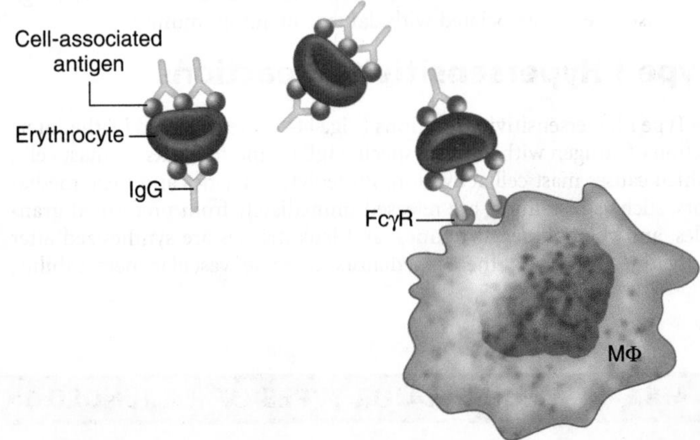

FIGURE 44–2 • Type II hypersensitivity. Type II responses are mediated by immunoglobulin G (IgG) directed against cell surface or matrix antigens, which initiates effector responses through the Fc receptor for IgG (FcγR) and complement. The relative contributions of these pathways vary with the IgG subclass and the nature of the antigen. Only FcγR-mediated phagocytosis by macrophages (MΦ) is depicted in this figure. Activation of complement components would result in binding of C3b to the red blood cell membrane, rendering red blood cells susceptible to phagocytosis and leading to formation of the membrane attack complex and cell lysis.

by immune-mediated destruction of erythrocytes and thrombocytopenia caused by destruction of platelets, both type II hypersensitivity reactions, are adverse effects of certain drugs. Chemically reactive drug molecules bind covalently to the surface of red blood cells or platelets. This modification of human proteins creates new epitopes that, in a small subset of individuals, are recognized as foreign antigens by the immune system and stimulate production of IgM and IgG antibodies reactive with the conjugate of drug and cell surface protein. Penicillin-specific IgG binds to penicillin-modified proteins on red blood cells. The binding of these antibodies to blood cells triggers activation of the complement cascade. Activation of complement components C1 through C3 results in covalent binding of C3b to the red blood cell membrane and renders circulating red blood cells susceptible to phagocytosis by FcγR-bearing and complement receptor–bearing macrophages in the spleen or liver. Activation of complement components C1 through C9 and formation of the membrane attack complex causes intravascular lysis of red blood cells. The factors that predispose only some people to drug-induced type II hypersensitivity reactions are unknown. Penicillin, quinidine, and methyldopa have been associated with hemolytic anemia and/or thrombocytopenia through this mechanism. Another example is heparin-induced thrombocytopenia/thrombosis, a severe, life-threatening complication that occurs in 1 to 3% of patients exposed to heparin. Interactions among heparin, human platelet factor 4, antibodies to the human platelet factor 4/heparin complex, platelet FcγRIIA, and splenic FcγRs (which remove opsonized platelets) are involved in the pathogenesis of this disease.

Autoantibodies directed at antigens on the cell surface or extracellular matrix cause tissue damage by mechanisms similar to type II hypersensitivity reactions. IgG or IgM antibodies against erythrocytes lead to cell destruction in autoimmune immune hemolytic anemia, because opsonized cells (coated with IgG or IgM and complement) are removed from the circulation by phagocytes in the liver and spleen or are lysed by formation of the membrane attack complex. Platelet destruction in autoimmune thrombocytopenic purpura occurs through a similar process. Because nucleated cells express membrane-bound complement regulatory proteins (Chapter 45), they are less sensitive to lysis through the membrane attack complex, but when coated with antibody they become targets for phagocytosis or antibody-dependent cytotoxicity. This mechanism is responsible for autoimmune and alloimmune neutropenia.

IgM and IgG antibodies recognizing antigens within tissue or binding to extracellular antigens cause local inflammatory damage through FcγR and complement mechanisms. Pemphigus vulgaris is a serious blistering disease that results from a loss of adhesion between keratinocytes caused by autoantibodies against the extracellular portions of desmoglein 3, an intercellular adhesion structure of epidermal keratinocytes. Another example of a type II hypersensitivity reaction is Goodpasture's disease, in which antibodies against the α_3-chain of type IV collagen (the collagen in basement membranes) are deposited in glomerular and lung basement membrane. Tissue-bound autoantibodies activate monocytes, neutrophils, and basophils through FcγRs, initiating release of proteases, reactive oxidants, cytokines, and prostaglandins. Local activation of complement, particularly C5a, recruits and activates inflammatory cells and amplifies tissue injury. Neighboring cells are lysed by assembly of the membrane attack complex or by FcγR-initiated, antibody-dependent cytotoxicity.

Autoantibodies against cell surface receptors produce disease by stimulating or blocking receptor function. In myasthenia gravis, autoantibodies against the acetylcholine receptors on skeletal muscle cells bind the receptor and induce its internalization and degradation in lysosomes, reducing the efficiency of neuromuscular transmission and causing progressive muscle weakness. In contrast, Graves' disease is characterized by autoantibodies that act as agonists. Autoantibodies to thyroid-stimulating hormone receptors bind the receptor, mimicking the natural ligand, inducing thyroid hormone overproduction, disrupting feedback regulation, and causing hyperthyroidism.

Type III Hypersensitivity Reactions

Type III hypersensitivity reactions (Fig. 44–3) are caused by tissue deposition of small soluble immune complexes that contain antigens and high-affinity IgG antibodies directed at these antigens. Localized deposition of immune complexes activates FcγR-bearing mast cells and phagocytes and initiates the complement cascade, all effectors of tissue damage.

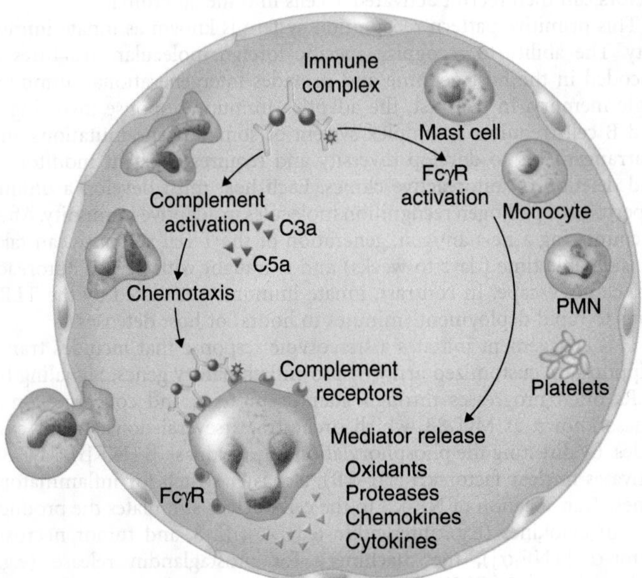

FIGURE 44–3 • Type III hypersensitivity. Type III responses are mediated by immunoglobulin G (IgG) directed against soluble antigens. Localized deposition of immune complexes activates mast cells, monocytes, neutrophils, and platelets bearing the Fc receptor for IgG (FcγR), and initiates the complement cascade, all effectors of tissue damage. Generation of complement components C3a and C5a recruits and stimulates inflammatory cells and amplifies effector functions. PMN, polymorphonuclear leukocyte (also called neutrophil).

Immune complexes are generated in all antibody responses. The formation and the fate of immune complexes depend on the biophysical and immunologic properties of the antigen and the antibody. These properties include the size, net charge, and valence of the antigen; the class and subclass of the antibody; the affinity of the antibody-antigen interaction; the net charge and concentration of antibody; the molar ratio of available antigen and antibody; and the ability of the immune complex to interact with the proteins of the complement system. The lattice size of the immune complex is influenced strongly by the physical size and valence of the antigen, the association constant of antibody for that antigen, the molar ratio of antigen and antibody, and the absolute concentrations of the reactants. Larger aggregates fix complement more efficiently, present a broader multivalent array of ligands for complement and FcγRs to bind, and are taken up more readily by mononuclear phagocytes in the liver and spleen and thereby removed from the circulation. Smaller immune complexes, which form in antigen excess, as occurs early in an immune response, circulate in the blood and are deposited in blood vessels, where they initiate inflammatory reactions and tissue damage through interactions with FcγRs and complement receptors.

The Arthus reaction is an example of a localized type III hypersensitivity reaction. It is induced by subcutaneous injection of a soluble protein antigen into the skin of an individual who has IgG antibodies against the sensitizing antigen. Local immune complexes form and bind to FcγRs on mast cells and phagocytes, causing release of inflammatory mediators that increase vascular permeability and induce influx and activation of leukocytes, further propagating injury. Complement also is activated and amplifies inflammation.

Serum sickness is a systemic type III hypersensitivity reaction, historically described in patients injected with therapeutic horse antiserum for the treatment of bacterial infections. In general, serum sickness occurs after the injection of large quantities of a soluble antigen. Clinical features include chills, fever, rash, urticaria, arthritis, and glomerulonephritis. Disease manifestations become evident 7 to 10 days after exposure to the antigen, when antibodies are generated against the foreign protein and form immune complexes with these circulating antigens. Immune complexes are deposited in blood vessels, where they activate phagocytes and complement, producing widespread tissue injury and clinical symptoms. The effects are transient, however, and resolve after the antigen is cleared.

A syndrome similar to serum sickness occurs in chronic infections in which pathogens persist in the face of continued immune response. In subacute bacterial endocarditis, antibody production continues but fails to eliminate the infecting microbes. As the pathogens multiply, generating new antigens, immune complexes form in the circulation and are deposited in small blood vessels, where they lead to inflammatory damage of skin, kidney, and nerve. Hepatitis B virus infection may be associated with immune complex deposition early in its course, during a period of antigen excess because antibody production in response to hepatitis B surface antigen is as yet relatively insufficient; some anicteric patients may present with acute arthritis. Mixed essential cryoglobulinemia, which may be associated with hepatitis C viral infection, is an immune complex–mediated vasculitis in which deposition of complexes containing IgG, IgM, and hepatitis C antigens causes inflammation in peripheral nerves, kidneys, and skin. Serum sickness also can develop in transplant recipients who are treated with mouse monoclonal antibodies specific for human T cells to prevent rejection, and in patients with myocardial infarction who are treated with the bacterial enzyme streptokinase to effect thrombolysis.

Systemic lupus erythematosus, the prototypical immune complex–mediated autoimmune disease, is characterized by circulating IgG directed against common cellular constituents, typically DNA and DNA-binding proteins. Small immune complexes are deposited in skin, joints, and glomeruli, with FcγRs playing a dominant role in initiating local tissue damage.

Type IV Hypersensitivity Reactions

Type IV hypersensitivity reactions (Fig. 44–4), also known as *delayed-type hypersensitivity reactions,* are mediated by antigen-specific effector T cells. They are distinguished from other hypersensitivity reactions by the lag time from exposure to the antigen until the response is evident (1 to 3 days). Antigen is taken up, processed, and presented by macrophages

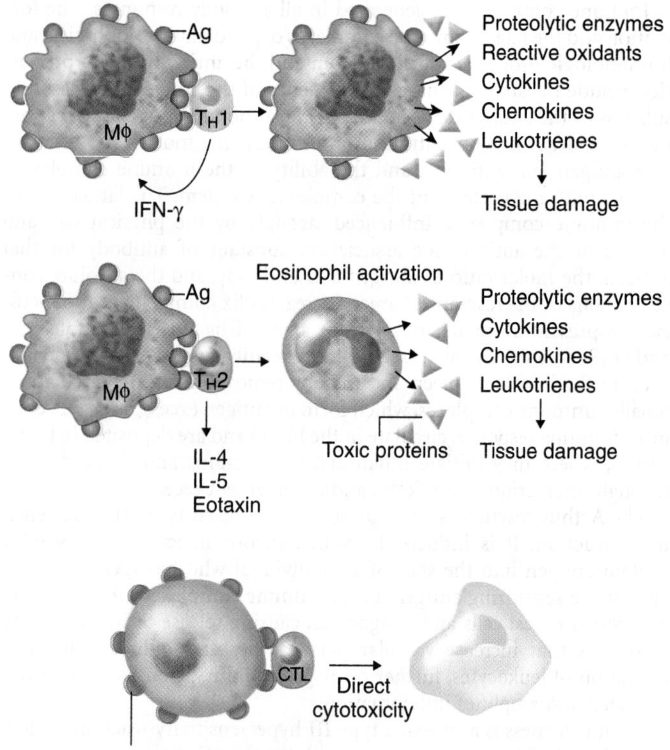

FIGURE 44–4 • Type IV hypersensitivity. Type IV responses are mediated by T cells through three different pathways. In the first, type 1 helper T (T_H1) cells recognize soluble antigens and release interferon-γ (IFN-γ) to activate effector cells, in this case macrophages (Mϕ), and cause tissue injury. In T_H2-mediated responses, eosinophils predominate. T_H2 cells produce cytokines to recruit and activate eosinophils, leading to their degranulation and tissue injury lymphocytes (CTLs). In the third pathway, damage is caused directly by cytolytic T. IL, interleukin.

or dendritic cells. Type 1 helper T (T_H1) effector cells that recognize the specific antigen (these are scarce and take time to arrive) are stimulated to release chemokines, which recruit macrophages to the site and release cytokines that mediate tissue injury. IFN-γ activates macrophages and enhances their release of inflammatory mediators, whereas TNF-α and TNF-β activate endothelial cells, enhance vascular permeability, and damage local tissue. The prototypical type IV hypersensitivity reaction is the tuberculin test, but similar reactions can occur after contact with sensitizing antigens (e.g., poison ivy, certain metals) and lead to epidermal reactions characterized by erythema, cellular infiltration, and vesicles. $CD8^+$ T cells also may mediate damage by direct toxicity.

In contrast to T_H1-mediated hypersensitivity reactions, in which the effectors are macrophages, eosinophils predominate in T_H2-mediated responses. T_H2 effector T cells are associated with tissue damage in chronic asthma. T_H2 cells produce cytokines to recruit and activate eosinophils (IL-5 and eotaxin), leading to degranulation, further tissue injury, and chronic, irreversible airway damage.

In some autoimmune diseases, effector T cells specifically recognize self-antigens to cause tissue damage, either by direct cytotoxicity or by inflammatory responses mediated by activated macrophages. In type I insulin-dependent diabetes mellitus, T cells mediate destruction of beta cells of the pancreatic islets. IFN-γ–producing T cells specific for myelin basic proteins have been implicated in multiple sclerosis. Rheumatoid arthritis is another autoimmune disease caused, at least in part, by activated T_H1 cells.

SUGGESTED READINGS

Kamradt T, Mitchison NA: Tolerance and autoimmunity. N Engl J Med 2001;344:655–664. *A basic review.*

Navratil JS, Liu CC, Ahearn JM: Apoptosis and autoimmunity. Immunol Res 2006;36:3–12. *Review of the mechanisms.*

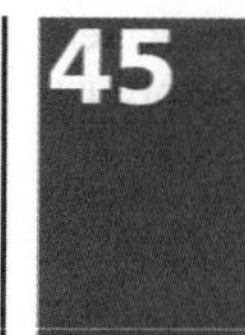

45 MECHANISMS OF INFLAMMATION AND TISSUE REPAIR

Gary S. Firestein

THE INFLAMMATORY RESPONSE

Host defense mechanisms have evolved to rapidly recognize pathogens, render them harmless, and repair the damaged tissue. This complex and highly regulated sequence of events can also be triggered by environmental stimuli such as noxious mechanical and chemical agents. The cascade is characterized clinically by the classically described signs and symptoms of "rubor et tumor cum calore et dolore," or redness and swelling with heat and pain. Under normal circumstances, tightly controlled responses protect against further injury and clear damaged tissue. In disease states, however, pathologic inflammation can lead to marked destruction of the extracellular matrix (ECM) and organ dysfunction.

Initiation of the Inflammatory Response

Toll-like Receptors and Innate Immunity

When normal tissue encounters a pathogen, resident cells are stimulated by engagement of pattern recognition receptors expressed on their cell membranes. These receptors include the toll-like receptor (TLR) family of proteins, which bind molecular structures on microbial pathogens that normally are not found in mammalian cells. Of the TLRs identified to date, perhaps the best studied is TLR2, which is activated primarily by bacterial peptidoglycan and lipoproteins, and TLR4, which is activated by lipopolysaccharide (LPS, or endotoxin) (Table 45–1). In addition, TLR9 is activated by unmethylated bacterial sequences that are enriched for CpG motifs, and TLR3 is important for antiviral defense because it binds double-stranded viral RNA. The range of recognized microbial stimulants is increased through the structural diversity of the TLR intracytoplasmic domains, their ability to heterodimerize, and their associations with tissue-specific accessory molecules. In addition to exogenous molecules, some endogenous structures can bind to TLRs, including heat shock proteins and oxidized low-density lipoproteins (oxLDLs). The latter might be especially important in the pathogenesis of atherosclerosis, where TLR4 is activated by LDL within vascular plaques. Local endothelial cell– and macrophage-derived chemotactic factors can then recruit activated T cells into the atheroma.

This primitive pattern recognition system is known as innate immunity. The ability to recognize specific foreign molecular structures is encoded in the host genome and provides intergenerational immunologic memory. In contrast, the adaptive immune response involving T and B cells requires a complex system of somatic gene mutations and rearrangements to develop diversity and requires constant monitoring and deletion of autoreactive clones. Each host must develop a unique repertoire of pathogen recognition molecules in adaptive immunity. After encountering a new antigen, generation of the T-cell response can take considerable time (days to weeks) and is fraught with peril if autoreactive clones escape. In contrast, innate immunity mediated by the TLRs leads to rapid deployment (minutes to hours) of host defenses.

TLR engagement initiates a stereotypic response that includes transcription of a customized array of pro-inflammatory genes. Signaling by TLRs often progresses through adaptor proteins and converges on a kinase known as MyD88, which orchestrates several downstream cascades. By directing the phosphorylation of IκB kinase-β (IKKβ), MyD88 activates nuclear factor-κB (NF-κB), a master switch for inflammatory genes. Translocation of NF-κB to the cell nucleus stimulates the production of cytokines (e.g., interleukin-6 [IL-6], IL-8, and tumor necrosis factor-α [TNF-α]), the machinery for prostaglandin release (e.g., cyclooxygenase 2 [COX2]), and genes that regulate the ECM (e.g., metalloproteinases). This rapid response is normally transient, although it can persist in pathogenic states. MyD88-indpendent pathways that stimulate innate immunity also exist. For instance, TLR3 stimulation by RNA viruses uses a separate pathway involving IKKε and interferon regulating factor-3 (IRF-3). IRF-3, in combination with several other transcription factors, induces the expression of genes such as interferon-β (IFN-β) to establish an antiviral state. The mitogen-activated protein (MAP) kinases,

TABLE 45–1 TOLL-LIKE RECEPTORS AND LIGANDS

Receptor	Ligands
TLR1/2	Human cytomegalovirus
TLR2/6	Peptidoglycan Lipoteichoic acid Zymosan Diacylated bacterial lipoprotein Modulin
TLR3	Double-stranded viral RNA
TLR4	Lipopolysaccharide β-Defensin 2 Oxidized low-density lipoprotein Hyaluronic acid fragments Heparan sulfate Fibronectin Fibrinogen
TLR5	Flagellin
TLR6	Macrophage-activating lipoprotein 2
TLR7	Resiquimod Single-stranded viral RNA
TLR8	Resiquimod
TLR9	CpG DNA motifs
TLR10	Unknown
TLR11	Uropathogenic bacteria

TABLE 45–2 EXAMPLES OF INFLAMMATION PATHWAYS IN DISEASE

Disease	Activated Pathways
Atherosclerosis	Toll-like receptor activation (e.g., oxLDL) Chemokine-mediated leukocyte recruitment (e.g., MCP-1)
Cancer	Reactive oxygen and nitrogen intermediate-induced mutations Cyclooxygenase 2–mediated neoplasia (e.g., colon, breast) NF-κB activation prolongs survival of damaged cells
Asthma	IgE-mediated mast cell activation T_H2 cytokine-mediated leukocyte activation Leukotriene-induced bronchospasm Protease-induced airway remodeling
Rheumatoid arthritis	Toll-like receptor activation (e.g., peptidoglycan) Macrophage/fibroblast cytokine production Cyclooxygenase 2 induction Protease-mediated cartilage destruction Synovial complement activation
Systemic lupus erythematosus	Complement activation in multiple organs α-Interferon production

IgE = immunoglobulin E; MCP-1 = monocyte chemoattractant protein 1; NF-κB = nuclear factor-κB; oxLDL = oxidized low-density lipoprotein; T_H2 = helper T lymphocytes type 2.

such as p38, extracellular signal–regulating kinase (ERK), and c-Jun N-terminal kinase (JNK), are also phosphorylated after ligation of many TLRs and can enhance production of cytokines and proteases.

Activation of transcription factors and signaling cascades has an element of peril for the host. The genes expressed primarily offer protection against pathogens by initiating key defense mechanisms. However, these same pathways can create a hazardous milieu that is toxic to normal cells through the production of oxygen radicals, nitric oxide, and other reactive intermediaries. These molecules can damage DNA and harm bystander cells, or even lead to neoplasia (Table 45–2). For instance, long-standing inflammation in the colon, as in ulcerative colitis, is associated with adenocarcinoma. Increased COX2 expression as a result of NF-κB translocation is another mechanism that also contributes to the development of tumors at inflammatory sites. An unanticipated finding is that NF-κB itself can also directly augment carcinogenesis by serving as a survival signal for damaged cells that would normally be deleted by apoptosis.

The TLR signal transduction mechanisms, initiated by broad categories of nonmammalian structures, integrate the environmental stimuli and generate a broadly antipathogen response. Fine-tuning of host defenses against unique pathogen structures to provide long-lived immunity requires the slower, more precise adaptive immune system. Although it is more cumbersome and primitive, innate immunity provides signals that activate adaptive responses. For instance, TLRs can stimulate dendritic cells (DCs), which have internalized and processed antigen, to migrate from peripheral tissues to central lymphoid organs. The dendritic cells can also produce cytokines and, after maturation, present antigens to T cells in the context of class II major histocompatibility molecules and surface costimulatory proteins. The activated T cells can then migrate to the tissue to enhance and amplify the host response. T cells also provide help to B cells, thereby stimulating antibody production and activating other components of innate immunity (e.g., the complement system).

Immune Complexes and Complement

The complement system is another ancient defense mechanism that links innate immunity and the humoral arm of adaptive immunity (see Chapter 47). Both the classical complement pathway, activated by immunoglobulin G (IgG)- and IgM-containing immune complexes, and the alternative pathway, activated by bacterial products, converge at the third component of complement, C3, with proteolytic release of fragments that amplify the inflammatory response and mediate tissue injury. The anaphylotoxins C3a and C5a directly increase vascular permeability and contraction of smooth muscle. C3a and C3a desArg also induce TNF-α and interleukin-1β (IL-1β) production by peripheral blood mononuclear cells. C5a induces mast cell release of histamine, thereby indirectly mediating increased vascular permeability. C5a also activates leukocytes and enhances their chemotaxis, adhesion, and degranulation, with release of proteases and toxic metabolites. C5b attaches to the surface of cells and microorganisms and is the first component in the assembly of the C5b–9 membrane attack complex.

Complement plays a critical role in immune regulation, and individuals with genetic or acquired deficiencies have increased susceptibility to many diseases. Individuals with abnormalities of the early complement components, especially C1q, C2, and C4, usually have a minimally increased incidence of infection but demonstrate an enhanced risk of developing autoimmune diseases such as systemic lupus erythematosus (SLE). The mechanism of increased disease susceptibility is probably related to inefficient clearance of immune complexes. Enhanced activation and consumption of complement proteins can also occur in SLE accompanied by low plasma C3 and C4 levels, especially in association with disease exacerbations. C3 or C5 deficiency causes increased susceptibility to bacterial infections, whereas defects in the late components that form the membrane attack complex result in an increase incidence of *Neisseria* bacteremia.

Environmental Stress and Tissue Damage

Tissue injury due to direct trauma or noxious stimulus also initiates an inflammatory response and is associated with microvascular damage, extravasation of leukocytes through vascular walls, and leakage of plasma and proteins into the tissue. Hemostasis at the site of damaged vessels quickly ensues to stem the flux. Platelets then release fibrinogen, fibronectin, thrombospondin, and von Willebrand's factor, which permit homotypic aggregation as well as adherence to collagen. The resulting thrombus not only serves as a mechanical plug but also begins the inflammatory cascade through the release of vasoactive amines (e.g., serotonin), release of lysosomal proteases, and formation of eicosanoid products. The platelets can also later regulate healing with release of growth factors such as platelet-derived growth factor (PDGF) and transforming growth factor-β (TGF-β).

Second Wave of the Inflammatory Response

Activation of innate immunity quickly leads to the robust influx of inflammatory cells. Resident cells, such as vascular endothelial cells (ECs), mast cells, dendritic cells, and interstitial fibroblasts, respond by releasing soluble mediators, including the eicosanoids and pro-inflammatory cytokines (Table 45–3). These mediators amplify the inflammatory response and recruit additional leukocytes. Locally stimulated cells, along with the newly arrived inflammatory cells, release toxic reactive intermediates of nitrogen and oxygen as well as a myriad of proteases, principally matrix metalloproteinases (MMPs), serine proteases, and cysteine proteases. These molecules are designed to help destroy infectious agents and remove damaged cells, thus clearing the injured site for tissue repair. Although these processes are carefully balanced and controlled under ordinary circumstances, prolonged stimulation of acute inflammatory mechanisms can cause severe tissue destruction. However, in the vast majority of situations, the normal physiologic response is an exquisitely coordinated program that utilizes proteolytic enzymes to remodel the ECM and promote a supportive environment for wound healing rather than tissue damage.

TABLE 45–3 SIGNALS FOR INDUCTION AND REPAIR OF INFLAMMATION

Inflammation	Resolution and Tissue Repair
CYTOKINES AND GROWTH FACTORS	
TNF-α	TGF-β
IL-1 family (IL-1, IL-18)	IL-10
IL-6 family (IL-6, IL-11, LIF, osteopontin)	FGF
IL-13	Osteoprotegerin
IL-15	IL-1RII
IL-17	IL-1Ra
IL-12 family (IL-12, IL-23)	Soluble TNF-R
VEGF	IL-18 binding protein
Chemokines	
PROTEASES	
Matrix metalloproteinases (MMPs)	TIMPs
Collagenases	SERPINs
Gelatinases	α_2-Macroglobulin
Stromelysins	
Matrilysins	
Serine proteases	
Trypsin	
Chymotrypsin	
Cysteine proteases	
Aggrecanases	
ADAM family	
SMALL MOLECULE MEDIATORS	
Prostaglandins (especially PGE_2)	Lipoxins
Leukotrienes (especially LTB4)	Cyclopentenone
C3a and C5a	Antioxidants
Histamine	
Bradykinin	
Reactive oxygen	
Reactive nitrogen	
APOPTOSIS REGULATORS	
Soluble Fas ligand	Fas
	TRAIL
	Reactive oxygen
	Reactive nitrogen

ADAM = a disintegrin and metalloproteinase family; FGF = fibroblast growth factor; IL = interleukin; LIF, leukemia inhibitory factor; R = receptor; Ra = receptor antagonist; SERPINs = serine protease inhibitors; TGF = transforming growth factor; TIMPs = tissue inhibitors of metalloproteinase; TNF = tumor necrosis factor; TRAIL, TNF-related apoptosis-inducing ligand; VEGF = vascular endothelial growth factor.

Cellular Response

Inflammatory cell infiltration at the site of initial tissue damage typically progresses in an orderly fashion. The process begins with release of chemokines and soluble mediators from resident cells, including interstitial fibroblasts, mast cells, and vascular endothelial cells. Signaling from these events alters the local adhesion molecule profile and creates a chemotactic gradient that recruits cells from the blood stream. Mast cells, in particular, play an important role by releasing vasoactive amines. In fact, some immune complex animal models of inflammation, such as the passive K/BxN arthritis model in mice, have an absolute requirement for mast cells. This model involves activation of complement by autoantibody complexes with glucose-6-phosphate isomerase and is dependent on the alternative complement pathway. Rapid mast cell activation by these autoantibodies increases vascular permeability, enhancing articular immune complex deposition and inflammatory cell ingress into the synovium. In most acute responses, polymorphonuclear leukocytes (PMNs) are the first inflammatory cells to extravasate from the circulation and arrive at the site of injury, followed later by mononuclear cells under the influence of separate signals.

Most resident tissue fibroblasts and vascular endothelial cells are quiescent before migration of PMNs into the tissue. However, these resident cells can be triggered to proliferate and migrate toward the site of injury as well as to synthesize cytokines, proteases, and ECM components. Growth factors are released, such as basic fibroblast growth factor (bFGF) and vascular endothelial growth factor (VEGF), stimulating new blood vessel formation. Together with granulocyte-macrophage colony-stimulating factor (GM-CSF), these locally released growth factors contribute to cellular proliferation and amplification of the inflammatory response and also induce maturation of dendritic cells that process antigens. In addition, fibroblasts and endothelial cells secrete new ECM proteins, MMPs, and other ECM-digesting enzymes. The balance of protease and ECM production varies as tissue is remodeled during the course of inflammation. Initially, the response favors proteolytic activity to clear damaged infrastructure. This is followed by a shift to increased production of new ECM to allow tissue repair and wound healing.

Coordinated with the changes induced in the ECM through proteolysis, alterations in endothelial morphology affect the barrier function of the ECM. Increased vascular permeability, caused by disruption of endothelial cell tight junctions, allows blood-borne proteins such as fibrinogen, fibronectin, and vitronectin to extravasate into the perivascular ECM. Interaction with preexisting ECM allows the assembly of new ligands for a subset of adhesion molecules (e.g., integrins α5β1 and αvβ3). This increased vascular permeability and change in the profiles of adhesion molecules and ligands, in conjunction with release of chemoattractant molecules, leads to the recruitment of leukocytes to sites of inflammation with subsequent retention. Some of the chemokines involved are IL-8 (for neutrophils), RANTES (regulated on activation, T-cell expressed and secreted; for monocytes and eosinophils), and IL-16 (for $CD4^+$ T cells).

The precise combination of chemokines and adhesion molecules present in an inflammatory lesion determines the specificity of time and event for the recruitment of subsets of inflammatory cells. For instance, in the synovial lining and microvasculature of patients with rheumatoid arthritis, induction of the adhesion molecule intercellular adhesion molecule 1 (ICAM-1) on endothelial cells and fibroblasts, in combination with chemokines such as IL-8 and monocyte chemoattractant protein 1 (MCP-1), serves to recruit neutrophils and monocytes using the β2 integrins. Similarly, vascular cell adhesion molecule 1 (VCAM-1) recruits T cells and monocytes that express α4β1 integrin. PMNs lack α4β1 and therefore are not recruited by expression of VCAM-1 by vascular endothelium. Thus, the selective expression of integrins and other adhesion molecules regulates the time course of migration of various cell lineages into inflamed tissue. Ligation of these integrins on leukocytes also prolongs cell survival once they have moved into the tissue, by preventing apoptosis. The central role of certain specific adhesion molecule–ligand pairs has been confirmed in human diseases. For instance, α4β1 plays a key role in the recruitment of lymphocytes to the central nervous system in multiple sclerosis, and blocking this interaction suppresses disease activity. Eosinophils also use the same adhesion receptors to migrate into the lung in allergen-induced asthma.

Increased expression of ICAM-1 and VCAM-1, as well as increased chemokine expression, is also evident in other cell types, such as the airway epithelium after allergen challenge in asthma. Rapid and transient influx of neutrophils occurs in allergic airway disease, along with activation of the local T cells and mast cells. These neutrophils produce lipid mediators, reactive oxygen intermediates, and proteases such as elastase, which may contribute to airflow obstruction, epithelial damage, and remodeling. Neutrophil elastase, together with chemokines released by both recruited and allergen-activated T cells and mast cells, serves to recruit eosinophils.

Soluble Mediators

In addition to the activation of local cells and the recruitment of leukocytes, the inflammatory response leads to the production of soluble mediators. In some cases, as with cytokines, these products serve as a primary communication system between cells, orchestrating subsequent infiltration and activation. Other molecules, such as reactive oxygen intermediates, act as effectors that directly kill pathogens. However, damage to normal tissues can be a byproduct of these events.

Pro-inflammatory Cytokines

Pro-inflammatory cytokines, often derived from macrophages and fibroblasts, are primary mediators that activate the immune system. Scores of factors have been identified, but IL-1 and TNF-α are among the most important. The pro-inflammatory members of the IL-1 family (IL-1α, IL-1β, and IL-18) and TNF-α have pleiotropic activities and can enhance adhesion molecule expression on endothelial cells, induce proliferation of endogenous cells, and stimulate antigen presentation. IL-1 and TNF-α also increase expression of matrix-degrading enzymes, such as collagenase and stromelysin. In addition, they stimulate synthesis of inflammatory mediators such as prostaglandin E_2 (PGE_2) from fibroblasts. Direct injection of these cytokines into animals induces local inflammatory responses, and IL-1 or TNF-α blockade abrogates tissue damage in many animal models of inflammation. Inhibitors of TNF-α are effective therapeutic agents in inflammatory diseases such as rheumatoid arthritis and inflammatory bowel disease, and IL-1 inhibitors are beneficial in genetic diseases such as Muckle-Wells syndrome and familial cold autoinflammatory syndrome.

IL-1 and TNF-α comprise only a small fraction of the acute cytokine response. Many other factors also participate, including IL-6 and its related cytokines (IL-11, osteopontin, and leukemia inhibitory factor), which can both induce acute phase reactants and bias an immune response toward a helper T type 1 (T_H1) or T_H2 phenotype (see Chapter 44). GM-CSF can regulate dendritic cell maturation, increase expression of human leukocyte antigen (HLA-DR) on these cells, and enhance antigen-specific responses, in addition to increasing bone marrow production of myeloid cells. Specialized chemoattractant cytokines called chemokines recruit specific cell types to the site of injury. Through G protein–coupled receptors, some of these molecules act to activate neutrophil effector functions directly. The T-cell lymphokine IFN-γ, although generally considered part of the secondary wave that ensues after T-cell activation, can also induce expression of HLA-DR, increase expression of endothelial cell adhesion molecules, and inhibit collagen production. IL-15, IL-17 (a T cell–derived pro-inflammatory factor that is stimulated by the production of macrophage-derived IL-23), and many other mediators participate in this complex cytokine network.

Cytokines play a key role in the establishment and perpetuation of inflammatory diseases. In rheumatoid arthritis, autocrine and paracrine cytokine networks play a critical role in the perpetuation of inflammation. Effects of IL-1 and TNF-α are often central to continued synovitis, and there is increasing evidence that IL-15 participates by enhancing TNF-α production. IL-17 contributes to synoviocyte activation, and IL-18 can trigger T-cell differentiation toward a T_H1 phenotype. Factors such as MCP-1 recruit and activate macrophages into atheromas containing oxLDLs and foam cells. In allergic asthma, IL-13 is emerging as a central inflammatory cytokine. IL-13 functions through binding to cell surface IL-4 receptors, and IL-4Rα–deficient mice are relatively resistant to the development of asthma. In addition, overexpression of IL-13 in the murine lung causes inflammation, mucus hypersecretion, subepithelial fibrosis, and production of chemokines for eosinophils. Administration of IL-13 directly into the airways of mice induces hyperreactivity, eosinophilia, and increased production of IgE. Finally, the administration of soluble IL-13 receptors leads to an antagonism of these responses, reducing bronchial hyperreactivity and mucus production in the mouse model of asthma.

Eicosanoids

In addition to cytokines and immune complexes, local inflammatory responses lead to the release of eicosanoids, which are lipid-derived molecules. Because lipids are present in the cell membrane, they are readily available substrates for the synthesis of mediators. These molecules are functional immediately adjacent to sites of synthesis, and their half-lives range from seconds to minutes. Eicosanoids are not stored but are produced de novo from membranes when cell activation by mechanical trauma, cytokines, growth factors, or other stimuli leads to release of arachidonic acid (AA). Cytosolic phospholipase A_2 ($cPLA_2$) is the key enzyme in eicosanoid production. Cell-specific and agonist-dependent events coordinate the translocation of $cPLA_2$ to the nuclear envelope, endoplasmic reticulum, and Golgi apparatus, where interaction with cyclooxygenase (in the case of prostaglandin synthesis) or 5-lipoxygenase (in the case of leukotriene synthesis) can occur. The temporal sequence of events in acute inflammation may be governed by eicosanoid profile switching. This shift can be mediated, in part, by the induction of COX2 in macrophages and fibroblasts after exposure to IL-1 or TNF-α.

Prostaglandins

Prostanoids are produced when AA is released from the plasma membrane of injured cells by phospholipases and metabolized by cyclooxygenases and specific isomerases. These molecules act both at peripheral sensory neurons and at central sites within the spinal cord and brain to evoke pain and hyperalgesia. Their production is increased in most acute inflammatory conditions, including arthritis and inflammatory bowel disease. In response to exogenous and endogenous pyrogens, PGE_2 derived from COX2 mediates a central febrile response. In addition, prostaglandins synergize with bradykinin (BK) and histamine to enhance vascular permeability and edema. The levels of prostaglandins are usually very low in normal tissues and increase rapidly with acute inflammation, well before leukocyte recruitment. Levels increase further with cellular infiltration and local cytokine production. COX2 induction with inflammatory stimuli most likely accounts for the high levels of prostanoids in chronic inflammation.

COX2 also plays a key role in platelet–endothelial cell interactions by increasing the production of prostacyclin (PGI_2) in endothelial cells. Increased risk of myocardial infarction associated with the use of selective COX2 inhibitors might be related to unopposed production of thromboxane A_2 by COX1 in platelets. Of interest, prostacyclin production also protects against atherosclerosis in female mice, and COX2 blockade abrogates this beneficial effect. Increased appreciation of the inflammatory nature of atherosclerosis and recent prospective studies evaluating cardiovascular events suggest that COX inhibitors might have a long-term stimulatory effect on thrombotic events and the progression of atherosclerosis.

Leukotrienes

In addition to prostaglandins, a distinct set of enzymes direct AA metabolites towards the synthesis of leukotrienes. Their relative importance depends on the specific target organ of an inflammatory response. For instance, leukotriene receptor antagonists have demonstrated efficacy in asthma, whereas similar approaches have been less impressive in rheumatoid arthritis. Unlike prostaglandins, leukotrienes are primarily produced by inflammatory cells such as neutrophils, macrophages, and mast cells. 5-Lipoxygenase (5-LO) is the key enzyme in this cascade, transforming released AA to the epoxide leukotriene A_4 (LTA_4) in concert with 5-lipoxygenase–activating protein (FLAP). LTA_4 can be hydrolyzed by cytosolic LTA_4 hydrolase to LTB_4, a potent neutrophil chemoattractant and stimulator of leukocyte adhesion to endothelial cells. LTA_4 can also conjugate with glutathione to form LTC_4 by LTC_4 synthase at the nuclear envelope. LTC_4 migrates out of the cell, using transporters such as the multidrug resistance–associated protein, and can be metabolized extracellularly to LTD_4 and LTE_4. These three cysteinyl leukotrienes comprise the "slow-reacting substance of anaphylaxis" for their slow and sustained smooth muscle–contracting abilities. They promote plasma leakage from postcapillary venules, upregulation of expression of cell surface adhesion molecules, and bronchoconstriction.

Histamine

One of the hallmarks of allergic inflammation is the activation of mast cells with release of histamine. This mediator is a vasoactive amine produced by basophils and mast cells that markedly increases capillary leakage. In basophils, histamine is released in response to bacterial formylmethionyl-leucyl-phenylalanine (f-MLP) sequences, complement fragments C3a and C5a, and IgE. The resultant edema can be readily observed clinically in urticaria and allergic rhinitis. Despite the production of histamine in asthma and in acute synovitis, histamine blockers have minimal therapeutic effect in these conditions. The stimulus for release of histamine from mast cell granules is the same as in basophils, except for the absence of f-MLP receptors in this cell type. Histamine can also synergize with locally produced LTB_4 and LTC_4. In addition, histamine enhances leukocyte rolling and firm adhesion, and induces gaps in the endothelial cell lining, enhancing leukocyte extravasation.

Kinins

Pain plays a key role in host responses as a mechanism to protect damaged sites from subsequent trauma by modulating behavior. Although these pathways are quite complex, the kinins are known to participate in vasodilation, edema, and smooth muscle contraction, as well as in pain and hyperalgesia through stimulation of C fibers. They are formed from high- and low-molecular-weight kininogens by the action of serine protease kallikreins in plasma and peripheral tissues. The primary products of kininogen digestion are bradykinin and lysylbradykinin. These products have high affinity for the B2 receptor, which is widely expressed and is responsible for the most common effects of kinins. The peptides desArg-BK and Lys-desArg-BK are generated by carboxypeptidases and bind the kinin B1 receptor subtype, which is not expressed in normal tissues but is rapidly upregulated by LPS and cytokines. The kinin B2 receptor is internalized rapidly and desensitized, whereas the B1 receptor remains highly responsive. Both receptors belong to the G protein–coupled receptor superfamily; they signal through phospholipase C with activation of protein kinase C and subsequent flux of intracellular calcium. Kinin actions are associated with the secondary production of other mediators of inflammation, including nitric oxide, mast cell–derived products, and the pro-inflammatory cytokines IL-6 and IL-8. In addition, kinins can increase IL-1α production through initial stimulation of TNF-α, and can increase prostanoid production through activation of phospholipase A_2 and release of AA.

Mechanisms of Tissue Damage in Inflammation

Reactive Oxygen and Nitrogen

Macrophages, neutrophils, and other phagocytic cells can generate large amounts of highly toxic reactive oxygen intermediates (ROIs) and reactive nitrogen intermediates (RNIs) that can directly kill pathogens. These molecules can damage DNA, oxidize membrane lipids, and nitrosylate proteins. Hence, their roles in inflammatory responses caused by infections are obvious. The ability of ROIs or RNIs to serve as critical signal transduction molecules that regulate expression of inflammatory genes is equally important.

Uncontrolled production of ROIs and RNIs can also lead to tissue damage. Release of reactive intermediates can be initiated by microbial products such as LPS and lipoproteins, by cytokines such as IFN-γ or IL-8, or by engagement of Fc receptors by IgG. These events cause translocation of several cytosolic proteins, including Rac2 and Rho-family guanosine triphosphatase (GTPase) to the membrane-bound complex carrying cytochrome *c*, with subsequent activation of reduced nicotinamide adenine dinucleotide phosphate (NADPH) oxidase. The reaction catalyzed by NADPH oxidase leads primarily to production of superoxide, which can be converted to hydrogen peroxide, hydroxyl radicals and anions, hypochlorous acid, and chloramines.

ROIs are critically important to the antimicrobial activity of neutrophils, but it is not clear to what extent other phagocytes utilize ROIs for control of intracellular bacteria in vivo. In some cases, ROIs can contribute directly to the initiation of chronic disease. Atherosclerosis is an especially important example. Lipid oxidation produces aldehydes that substitute lysine residues in apolipoprotein B-100. This altered moiety either binds to TLR2 to induce cytokine production or is internalized by macrophages, leading to the production of foam cells and fatty streaks, the primary lesions of atherosclerosis. Subsequently, altered epitopes in damaged host proteins can be presented to T cells to initiate an adaptive immune response that amplifies the inflammatory vascular lesion.

Nitric oxide synthases (NOS) convert L-arginine and molecular oxygen to L-citrulline and nitric oxide (NO). There are three known isoforms of NOS: neuronal NOS (ncNOS or NOS1) and endothelial cell NOS (ecNOS or NOS3) are both constitutively expressed, whereas macrophage NOS (macNOS, iNOS, or NOS2) is induced by inflammatory cytokines such as TNF-α and IFN-γ. The expression of NOS2 is suppressed by TGF-β. Products of viruses, bacteria, protozoa, and fungi, as well as low oxygen tension and low environmental pH, enhance NOS2 gene transcription.

Together with prostaglandins, the production of NO by NOS2 and ROIs by NADPH oxidase are key mechanisms by which macrophages paradoxically impair T-cell proliferation in response to mitogens or antigens. This may serve to control inflammatory processes or to delete autoreactive T cells, but it at least partially accounts for the immunosuppressed state seen in certain infections, malignancies, and graft-versus-host reactions. In addition, the intracellular balance of ROIs and RNIs may help to govern cell survival at a site of inflammation. For example, hydrogen peroxide promotes apoptosis in natural killer (NK) cells, but it contributes to macrophage resistance to NO-mediated apoptosis (presumably via scavenging of NO). Even within the lineage of a single cell, ROIs and RNIs may have both pro-apoptotic and anti-apoptotic effects. NO can prevent activity of caspases, a family of enzymes that can initiate apoptosis. Increased NADPH oxidase activity in neutrophils suppresses caspase activity but promotes externalization of phosphtidylserine, which signals the presence of an apoptotic cell to macrophages. Thus ROIs, like endogenous NO, may inhibit caspase function and simultaneously mediate neutrophil clearance through translocation of phosphotidlyserine and stimulation of cell death.

Proteases

Production of enzymes that degrade the ECM represents a key mechanism of tissue turnover in inflammation. This process is generally considered detrimental in diseases marked by overproduction of proteases (e.g., cartilage in osteoarthritis, synovium in rheumatoid arthritis, alveoli in chronic obstructive lung disease, and colonic epithelium in inflammatory bowel disease). However, reconfiguring of the matrix plays an important role in the host response by remodeling damaged tissue, releasing matrix-bound growth factors and cytokines, preparing the tissue for the ingrowth of new blood vessels, and altering the local milieu to permit adherence and retention of newly recruited cells.

The MMPs are a family of more than 20 extracellular endopeptidases that participate in degradation and remodeling of the ECM matrix (Table 45–4). They are produced as pro-enzymes and require limited proteolysis or partial denaturation to expose the catalytic site. Their name is derived from their dependence on metal ions (zinc/metzincin superfamily) for activity and from their potent ability to degrade structural ECM proteins. MMPs can also cleave cell surface molecules and other pericellular nonmatrix proteins, thereby regulating cell behavior. For instance, MMPs can alter cell growth by digesting matrix proteins associated with growth factors. FGF and TGF-β have high affinities for matrix molecules that serve as depots for storage of these cytokines in their activation state. Matrix proteolysis releases some growth factors and can make them available to cell surface receptors. In addition, MMPs can directly cleave and activate growth factors, as in the processing of latent TGF-β into its active form by MMP-2 and MMP-9. MMP-2, -3, and -9 also change IL-1β from its biologically inactive precursor into its active mature form. MMPs affect cell migration by altering cell–matrix or cell–cell receptor sites. For instance, the adhesion molecule β4 integrin is cleaved by MMP-7. MMP-3 and MMP-7 digest E-cadherin and not only disrupt endothelial cell junctions but also stimulate cell migration.

Degradation of the ECM is usually initiated by collagenases, which cleave native collagen. Denatured collagen is then recognized and further degraded by gelatinases and stromelysins. Unlike the collagenases, stromelysins demonstrate broad substrate specificity and act on many ECM proteins, such as proteoglycan, fibronectin, laminin, and many cartilage proteins. Stromelysins can also amplify the remodeling process by activating collagenase through limited proteolysis. MMP gene expression can be induced by many pro-inflammatory cytokines, including TNF-α, IL-1, IL-17, and IL-18, through MAP kinase signal transduction pathways. The MAP kinase pathway involving JNK is particularly important;

TABLE 45–4 COMMON MATRIX METALLOPROTEINASES (MMPs) AND THEIR SUBSTRATES

MMP Family	Matrix Substrates	Other Substrates
Collagenases	Collagen I, II, III, VII, and X	Pro-MMP-1, -2, -8, -9, and -13
	Aggrecan	Pro-TNF-α
Entactin	α1-proteinase inhibitors	
	Gelatin	
	Tenascin	
Gelatinases	Aggrecan	Pro-MMP-1, -2, and -13
	Denatured collagen	Pro-TNF-α
	Elastin	Pro-IL-1β
	Fibronectin	Latent TGF-β
	Laminin	
	Vitronectin	
Matrilysins	Proteoglycans	Pro-MMP-2 and -7
	Denatured collagens	Pro-TNF-α
	Entactin	Membrane-bound Fas ligand (FasL)
	Fibrin/fibrinogen	
	Fibronectin	Plasminogen
	Gelatin	β4 integrins
	Laminin	
	Tenascin	
	Vitronectin	
Stromelysins	Proteoglycans	Pro-MMP-1, -3, -7, -8, -9, -10, and -13
	Aggrecan	
	Collagen III, IV, V, IX, X, and XI	Pro-TNF-α
		Pro-IL-1β
	Entactin	Plasminogen
	Fibrin/fibrinogen	α1-proteinase inhibitors
	Fibronectin	
	Gelatin	
	Laminin	
	Tenascin	
	Vitronectin	

IL = interleukin; TNF = tumor necrosis factor.

it phosphorylates c-Jun, a component of the activator protein 1 (AP-1) transcription factor complex. The other two MAP kinase pathways, involving ERK and p38, can also activate MMP gene expression, depending on the specific cell type. NF-κB translocation can also enhance MMP production.

Several other classes of proteases contribute to matrix remodeling, including serine proteases and cysteine proteases. High levels of active serine proteases, such as trypsin, chymotrypsin, and elastase, are released by infiltrating PMNs at sites of inflammation and can directly digest the ECM or activate the pro-enzyme forms of secreted MMPs. The ADAM (a disintegrin and metalloproteinase) family can cleave the extracellular domain of cytokine receptors (e.g., ADAM-17 and cleavage of TNF-α). ADAM-related proteins and the ADAMT family and differ by the presence of multiple copies of thrombospondin 1–like repeats. These ECM proteases include two members of the aggrecanase family that are implicated in the degradation of cartilage in arthritis.

Tissue Repair and Resolution of Inflammation

Inflammation is a normal physiologic response, but it can cause serious host injury if it is allowed to persist. Hence, additional mechanisms are required to reestablish homeostasis once this response is initiated (Fig. 45–1). Suppression of acute inflammation by removal or deactivation of mediators and effector cells permits the host to repair damaged tissues through elaboration of appropriate growth factors and cytokines. The precise mechanisms controlling the switch from predominantly pro-inflammatory to anti-inflammatory pathways are not fully understood. However, as in the initial generation of an inflammatory response, components of resolution include a cellular response (apoptosis), formation of soluble mediators (such as anti-inflammatory cytokines and antioxidants), and production of direct effectors (such as protease inhibitors).

Deletion of Inflammatory Cells by Apoptosis

Apoptosis is a highly regulated process in eukaryotic cells that leads to cell death and marks the surface membrane for rapid removal by phagocytes. This clearance process does not elicit an inflammatory response, in contrast to cell death by necrosis, in which the release of intracellular contents into the microenvironment surrounding the dying cells promotes inflammation. Apoptosis is a normal process by which inflammatory cells are removed from healing sites, with the clearance of neutrophils

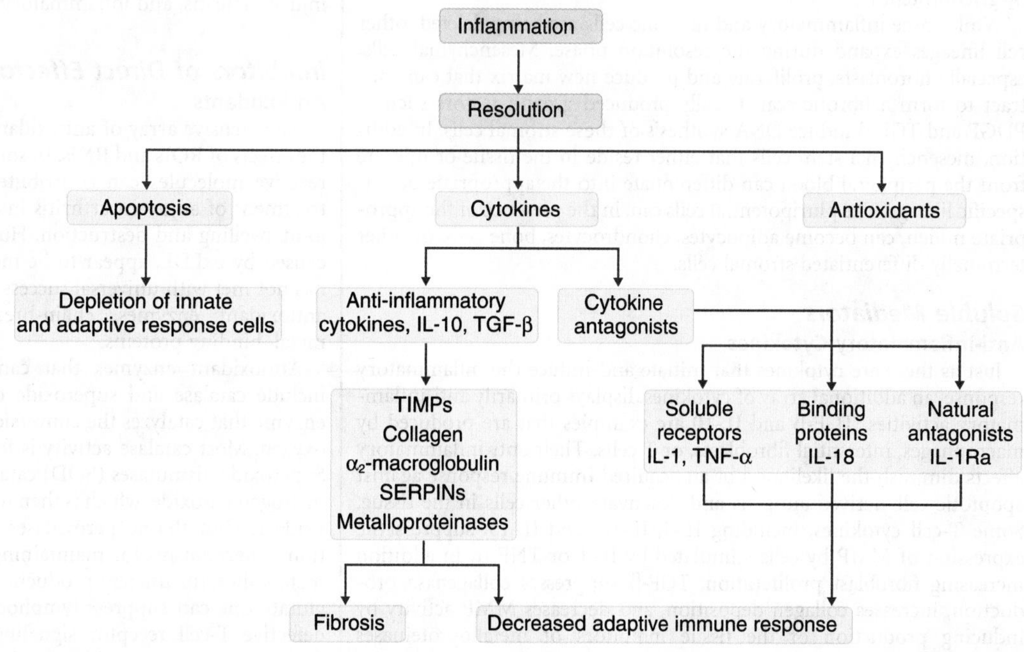

FIGURE 45–1 • Anti-inflammatory mechanisms that resolve inflammation and lead to repair of the extracellular matrix. IL = interleukin; SERPINs = serine protease inhibitors; TGF = transforming growth factor; TIMPs = tissue inhibitor of metalloproteinases; TNF = tumor necrosis factor.

representing a prominent example. PMN phagocytes have a very short half-life in the tissue, and the persistence or release of their contents into the microenvironment after death can be deleterious. In some pathologic conditions, such as leukocytoclastic vasculitis, abundant neutrophil apoptosis is readily apparent on histopathologic examination; in fact, it is one of the pathologic criteria for this diagnosis. Other cells, including T lymphocytes, undergo postactivation apoptosis to prevent their overwhelming of host responses. Defective apoptosis or even persistence of apoptotic cells that escape clearance may contribute to chronic inflammatory and autoimmune diseases. For instance, loss of tolerance to self-antigens might participate in autoimmune responses in SLE. Specific molecular defects in apoptosis pathways, such as the Fas–Fas ligand (FasL) system, induce lupus-like conditions in mice.

Commitment of a cell to apoptosis can be initiated by a number of factors, including the ROIs in the cellular microenvironment, as well as signaling through several death receptor pathways (e.g., FasL/Fas and TNF-related apoptosis-inducing ligand [TRAIL]). The former can damage DNA, which is a common sequela of the genotoxic environment created by inflammation. In this context, the p53 tumor suppressor protein is induced, leading to p21-dependent cell cycle arrest. If DNA damage is excessive, repair by tightly regulated mismatch repair mechanisms is terminated, and programmed cell death begins. The burden of mutations induced by ROIs or RNIs in chronic inflammation can potentially accumulate over time and eventually lead to amino acid substitutions in key regulatory proteins. Ultimately, as has been observed in ulcerative colitis, neoplastic disease can ensue.

Removal of apoptotic bodies, or the remnants of packaged apoptotic cells, is rapid and can be accomplished by macrophages, fibroblasts, epithelial and endothelial cells, muscle cells, and dendritic cells. The surface receptors used in recognition and engulfment of apoptotic cells include integrins (e.g., αvβ3), lectins, scavenger receptors, adenosine triphosphate (ATP)-binding cassette transporter 1, LPS receptor, CD14, and complement receptors CR3 and CR4. However, some of these membrane molecules can be utilized in both pro-inflammatory and apoptotic pathways, the divergence of which may be based on differing ligands and accessory molecules. For example, in macrophages, the CD14-dependent pro-inflammatory process in clearance of LPS depends on LPS-binding protein, whereas CD14-dependent apoptotic cell clearance does not.

Apoptotic cells display a series of membrane-associated molecular patterns that interact with receptors on phagocytes. The details of interactions between apoptotic cells and phagocytes are only partially understood. A general feature of apoptotic cells is loss of phospholipid asymmetry, with external presentation of phosphotidylserine. Externalized phosphatidylserine may be sufficient to trigger phagocytosis, but other apoptotic cell surface structures exist, including sugars (e.g., mannose), ICAM-3 (on leukocytes), oxidized surface structures (including phospholipids), thrombospondin, complement components, and β_2-glycoprotein I.

While some inflammatory and immune cells are being deleted, other cell lineages expand during the resolution phase. Mesenchymal cells, especially fibroblasts, proliferate and produce new matrix that can contract to form a fibrotic scar. Locally produced growth factors such as PDGF and TGF-β induce DNA synthesis of these stromal cells. In addition, mesenchymal stem cells that either reside in the tissue or migrate from the peripheral blood can differentiate into the appropriate organ-specific lineage. The pluripotential cells can, in the presence of the appropriate milieu, can become adipocytes, chondrocytes, bone cells, or other terminally differentiated stromal cells.

Soluble Mediators

Anti-Inflammatory Cytokines

Just as there are cytokines that initiate and induce the inflammatory response, an additional array of cytokines displays primarily anti-inflammatory activities. TGF-β and IL-10 are examples that are produced by macrophages, interstitial fibroblasts, or T cells. Their anti-inflammatory effects diminish the likelihood of an acquired immune response against apoptotic cell–derived antigens and deactivate other cells in the tissue. Some T-cell cytokines, including IL-4, IL-10, and IL-13, suppress the expression of MMP by cells stimulated by IL-1 or TNF-α. In addition increasing fibroblast proliferation, TGF-β suppresses collagenase production, increases collagen deposition, and decreases MMP activity by inducing production of the tissue inhibitors of metalloproteinases (TIMPs). Although resolution of inflammation clearly is necessary for normal wound healing, it is abnormal in diseases in which tissue fibrosis represents a major pathologic manifestation. For example, scleroderma is marked by diffuse fibrosis and is accompanied by high levels of TGF-β and increased production of ECM.

Cytokine decoy receptors can also downregulate the inflammatory response. These surface receptors recognize certain cytokines with high affinity and specificity but do not transduce intracellular signals. The receptors can also be shed from the cell surface after proteolytic cleavage and can absorb cytokines, thereby preventing them from ligating functional receptors on cell membranes. These cytokine inhibitors can be released as a coordinated attempt to prevent unregulated inflammation, as in septic shock, in which endotoxin induces production of soluble receptors after initial massive production of TNF-α and IL-1. Other types of cytokine-binding proteins are also produced as counter-regulatory mechanisms, including IL-18–binding protein (IL-18BP), which is an Ig superfamily-related receptor that captures IL-18. In bone remodeling, interactions of receptor activator of NF-κB (RANK) with RANK ligand are required for osteoclast-mediated resorption. The competitive antagonist osteoprotegerin (OPG) is a member of the TNF receptor family that binds to RANK ligand and inhibits osteoclast activation.

The need for tight control of the pro-inflammatory cytokine IL-1 is demonstrated by the existence of two separate mechanisms. An IL-1 decoy receptor, known as the type II IL-1R, has both cell membrane and soluble forms that neutralize IL-1 activity. In addition, a natural IL-1 antagonist, IL-1Ra, can bind to functional IL-1 receptors and compete with IL-1α or IL-1β. However, IL-1Ra does not transduce a signal to the cell and blocks the biologic functions of ambient IL-1. The balance of IL-1 and IL-1Ra production depends on many influences. For instance, monocytes produce more IL-1, whereas mature macrophages produce IL-1Ra, especially after engagement of Fc receptors by IgG.

Prostanoids/Cyclooxygenase

COX2 induced by pro-inflammatory mediators appears early and can contribute to inflammatory responses. However, COX2 expression late in the process has led to speculation that it also functions in the resolution of inflammation. This regulation might occur through formation of the cyclopentenone prostaglandins (CyPG). CyPG production is suppressed by COX inhibition and inhibits pro-inflammatory gene transcription. The prostanoids can serve as ligands for peroxisome proliferator-activated receptors (PPARs). There are three main classes PPAR receptors, PPARα, PPARβ/δ, and PPARγ, all of which bind to DNA as heterodimers in association with the retinoid X receptor. Activation of PPARγ by CyPG is associated with the suppression of AP-1 and signal transducer and activator of transcription (STAT) transcriptional pathways in macrophages. In addition, CyPG can directly inhibit IKKβ, thus preventing NF-κB activation. A variety of natural and synthetic PPAR agonists have demonstrated efficacy in models of ischemia-reperfusion injury, arthritis, and inflammatory airway disease.

Inhibitors of Direct Effectors

Antioxidants

An extensive array of antioxidant defenses exists to protect cells from the effects of ROIs and RNIs. In some cases, the damage induced by these reactive molecules can contribute to disease pathology. For instance, treatment of adjuvant arthritis in rats with antioxidants helps suppress joint swelling and destruction. Human diseases, such as atherosclerosis caused by oxLDL, appear to be more complex, and use of these agents has not met with universal success. Antioxidants can be divided into the antioxidant enzymes, chain-breaking antioxidants, and transition metal–binding proteins.

Antioxidant enzymes that can inactivate the toxic intermediates include catalase and superoxide dismutase. Catalase is a peroxisomal enzyme that catalyzes the conversion of hydrogen peroxide to water and oxygen. Most catalase activity is found in the liver and in erythrocytes. Superoxide dismutases (SOD) catalyze the dismutation of superoxide to hydrogen peroxide, which is then removed by catalase or glutathione peroxidase. Glutathione peroxidases and glutathione reductase are additional mechanisms for maintaining redox balance and removal of toxic metabolites. Insufficient production of intracellular antioxidants such as glutathione can suppress lymphocyte responses and could account for defective T-cell receptor signaling and blunted immunity in T cells derived from rheumatoid arthritis synovium.

Interactions of free radicals with surrounding molecules can generate secondary radical species in a self-propagating chain reaction. Chain-breaking antioxidants are small molecules that can receive or donate an electron and thereby form a stable byproduct with a radical. These antioxidant molecules are categorized as either aqueous phase (vitamin C, albumin, reduced glutathione) and lipid phase (vitamin E, ubiquinol-10, carotenoids, and flavonoids). In addition, transition metal–binding proteins (ceruloplasmin, ferritin, transferrin, and lactoferrin) can serve as antioxidants by sequestering cationic iron and copper and thereby inhibiting the propagation of hydroxyl radicals.

Protease Inhibitors

Mechanisms to protect the host and prevent tissue destruction using a complex system of protease inhibitors have evolved as part of the repair process. Protease inhibitors regulate the function of endogenous proteases and reduce the likelihood of collateral damage to tissues. These proteins form two functional classes, active site inhibitors and α_2-macroglobulin (α2M). The latter class of protease inhibitors acts by covalently linking the protease to the α2M chain and thereby blocking access to substrates. α2M binds to all classes of proteases and, after forming a covalent bond, conveys them to cells through receptor-mediated endocytosis with subsequent enzymatic inactivation. The family of inhibitors of serine proteases (SERPINs) are the most abundant members of the former class of protease inhibitors and play a major role in regulation of blood clot resolution and inflammation, as indicated by many of their names: anti-thrombin III, plasminogen activator inhibitors 1 and 2, α_2-antiplamsin, α_1-antitrypsin, and kallistatin. In addition to direct inactivation via protease inhibitors, serine proteases can be inactivated by oxidation. In contrast, MMPs are activated by partial denaturation in the toxic environment.

A specialized mechanism for inhibiting MMP function has also evolved and can be induced during the reparative phase of inflammation. A family of TIMPs inhibits most members of the MMP family. The TIMPs bind to activated MMPs and irreversibly block their catalytic sites. Examples of disease states with an unfavorable balance between TIMPs and MMPs include loss of cartilage in arthritis and regulation of tumor metastasis. TIMP-MMP imbalance in destructive forms of arthritis appears be caused by the limited production capacity for protease inhibitors, which is overwhelmed by the prodigious expression of MMPs. Whereas IL-1 and TNF-α induce MMPs, IL-6, TGF-β, and several other growth factors suppress production of MMPs and increase levels TIMPs. TGF-β also increases the production of matrix proteins such as collagen. Therefore, the cytokine profile has a pivotal influence on the status of remodeling. When pro-inflammatory cytokines predominate, the balance favors matrix destruction; in the presence of pro-inflammatory cytokine inhibitors and growth factors, matrix protein production increases and MMPs are inhibited by TIMPs.

SUGGESTED READINGS

Blank M, Shiloh Y: Programs for cell death: Apoptosis is only one way to go. Cell Cycle 2007;6:686–695. *Review of molecular basis of apoptotic and non-apoptotic cell death.*

Clevers H: At the crossroads of inflammation and cancer. Cell 2004;118:671–674. *Describes common mechanisms and processes.*

Parks WC, Wilson CL, Lopez-Boado YS: Matrix metalloproteinases as modulators of inflammation and innate immunity. Nat Rev Immunol 2004;4:617–629. *A comprehensive review.*

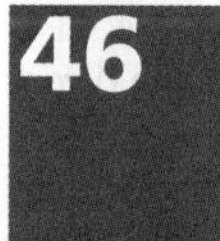

TRANSPLANTATION IMMUNOLOGY

Megan Sykes

DEFINITION

Clinical transplantation encompasses transplantation of organs and islet of Langerhans cells, in which it is necessary to overcome the host-versus-graft (HVG) immune response to avoid rejection, as well as hematopoietic cell transplantation (HCT), in which not only the HVG but also the graft-versus-host (GVH) immune response must be contended with. Because preparations of marrow or mobilized peripheral blood stem cells (mPBSCs) contain mature T cells, their administration to conditioned, and consequently immunoincompetent, recipients is associated with the risk of GVH disease. Organs transplanted include corneas, kidneys, livers, hearts, lungs, small intestines, pancreata, and even hands. The list of transplanted allogeneic cells is likely to expand in the future to include other cell types, such as hepatocytes, myoblasts, and stem cell–derived replacement cells. Transplants originating from a member of the same species are referred to as *allotransplants.* However, transplants from other species, termed *xenografts,* are believed by many to be a promising solution to the severely inadequate supply of allogeneic organs and tissues, and such grafts may be used in the future.

Antigens in Transplantation

The major antigens recognized during graft rejection and the cell types targeting them are summarized in Table 46–1.

Major Histocompatibility Antigens

The major histocompatibility complex (MHC; human leukocyte antigens [HLAs] in the human) presents the strongest immunologic obstacle to all types of allografts. Because of its uniquely extensive polymorphism, truly MHC-identical, unrelated donors are almost impossible to find in an outbred species such as humans. The reason for the strong immunogenicity of allogeneic MHC molecules relates to the manner in which T cells are selected in the thymus; developing thymocytes do not survive unless they can weakly recognize a self MHC/peptide complex on a thymic stromal cell. This process is termed "positive selection." Thymocytes whose receptors have high affinity for self/MHC complexes are deleted, however, so strongly autoreactive T cells rarely make it into the peripheral T-cell pool. Allogeneic antigens are not part of this "negative selection" process. Therefore, the net result of these two selection steps is that the human T-cell "repertoire" is strongly biased to have cross-reactivity to allogeneic MHC molecules, providing a barrier to organ and hematopoietic cell transplantation. In the case of organ transplantation, in which long-term pharmacotherapy with powerful immunosuppressive drugs is used in an effort to prevent graft rejection, this translates into improved results with matched organs in some situations. However, for unrelated, cadaveric donor transplantation, the benefits of HLA matching may be outweighed by the disadvantages associated with prolonged graft ischemia when attempts are made to transport organs to the most closely matched recipient. For hematopoietic cell transplantation, the risks of GVH disease and marrow graft failure are so greatly amplified in the presence of extensive HLA mismatches that such transplants are generally avoided; if a sufficiently matched, related donor cannot be found, a search is conducted through large registries containing millions of volunteer unrelated donors.

Minor Histocompatibility Antigens

MHC antigens do not present the only immunologic barrier to allografts. "Minor" histocompatibility antigens are peptides derived from polymorphic peptides presented by an MHC molecule. Even genotypically HLA-identical siblings have different minor histocompatibility antigens. These are sufficient to induce graft rejection if immunosuppressive pharmacotherapy is not used. In the case of HCT, significant GVH disease frequently (about 30 to 50% of the time) complicates transplantation between HLA-identical siblings, even with the use of pharmacologic immunoprophylaxis.

Other Antigens

Other antigens are also relevant for transplantation. The major blood group (ABO) antigens can be the target of a dramatic "hyperacute" rejection process that occurs when mismatched vascularized grafts are transplanted; recognition of blood group antigens on the endothelial surface of the graft vessels by recipient "natural" antibodies (antibodies that are present despite the lack of sensitization to the specific antigens) activates the complement and coagulation cascades, resulting in rapid graft thrombosis and ischemia. A similar outcome can occur after transplantation to an individual with preformed anti–donor HLA antibodies resulting from presensitization by prior transplantations, transfusions, or pregnancies. Consequently, until recently, transplantation could not be successfully performed in the presence of a positive anti-donor cross-match (see Chapter 133). Recently, however, considerable success has been achieved

TABLE 46–1 LYMPHOCYTES INVOLVED IN GRAFT REJECTION

Cell Type	Antigens Recognized	Function	Role in Transplantation
CD4⁺ T cells	Allogeneic class II MHC (± peptide) Self class II MHC + donor peptide	1. Assistance (cytokines and costimulation) in CD8⁺ T-cell activation, expansion, and CTL differentiation; B-cell Ig class switching, expansion, and effector differentiation 2. Cytotoxicity 3. Regulatory function	Organ allografts Cellular allografts Xenografts GVHD
CD8⁺ T cells	Allogeneic class I MHC (± peptide) Self class I MHC + donor peptide	1. Cytotoxicity 2. Cytokine production 3. Regulatory function	Organ allografts Cellular allografts Xenografts GVHD
NK cells	Class I MHC (activates or inhibits NK cell function) Other activating ligands	1. Cytotoxicity 2. Cytokine production	? Organ allografts Cellular allografts Xenografts
B cells	Class I and class II MHC Blood group antigens Xenogeneic carbohydrates	1. Antibody-mediated rejection (hyperacute, acute humoral, and chronic rejection)	Organ allografts Cellular allografts Xenografts

CTL = cytotoxic T lymphocyte; GVHD = graft-versus-host disease; Ig = immunoglobulin; MHC = major histocompatibility complex; NK = natural killer.

in the transplantation of ABO-mismatched kidneys and hearts (the latter in the neonatal period only), and in transplantation of kidneys to highly presensitized patients. In the case of kidney transplantation, initial removal of the antibody and sometimes of B cells, as well as the infusion of intravenous immunoglobulin (IVIG), has led to these successes. ABO-mismatched neonatal heart transplantation has succeeded because the transplants are performed before the recipient has developed high levels of anti–blood group antigen antibodies, and the B cells seem to be rendered tolerant to the donor blood group antigen by the grafting process. Recognition of blood group antigens can also be of significance in HCT, in which ABO barriers are routinely crossed in both directions. This can cause hemolysis of recipient erythrocytes if the mismatch is in the GVH direction, but this complication can be avoided by washing the cellular product before infusion. Mismatches in the HVG direction can cause more persistent problems due to ongoing destruction of donor erythropoietic cells, resulting in pure red cell aplasia. More often, however, donor erythropoiesis is successfully established and anti-donor isohemagglutinins disappear from the circulation.

A and B blood group antigens are the consequence of the presence or absence of specific glycosylation enzymes in different individuals. Likewise, an antigenic specificity of the utmost importance in xenotransplantation is a carbohydrate epitope, Galα1–3Galα1–4GlcNAc (αGal), which is produced by a specific galactosyl transferase. Humans and old world monkeys lack a functional αGal transferase and produce high levels of natural antibodies against the ubiquitous αGal epitope. Because animals of interest as xenograft sources (e.g., pigs) express αGal at high levels on their vascular endothelium, transplantation of vascularized organs from pigs results in hyperacute rejection unless something is done to absorb the antibodies or inactivate complement. The recent development of αGal-knockout pigs, therefore, is an important milestone, and encouraging results have been obtained in pig-to-primate transplantation in initial studies.

In another type of transplant reaction, recognition as foreign results not from the presence of an antigen, but paradoxically from the absence of a "self" MHC molecule. Natural killer (NK) cells express a series of surface inhibitory and activating receptors that, collectively, determine whether the NK cell does or does not kill a potential target cell. The ligands for the inhibitory receptors are MHC class I molecules, and the receptors recognize specific groups of alleles. An NK cell may kill an allogeneic target that lacks a "self" MHC inhibitory ligand. This phenomenon has been shown in animal models to result in rapid bone marrow rejection when the donor marrow cells are not given in excess numbers or when a fraction of them is destroyed by an incompletely suppressed T-cell response. A similar phenomenon has not been clearly demonstrated in clinical HCT. The possibility that NK cells play a role in organ allograft rejection has long been an area of controversy. NK cells may be of particular importance in xenotransplantation, where they appear early in infiltrates of organ xenografts undergoing acute vascular rejection. NK cells clearly play a strong role in rejection of xenogeneic bone marrow, an observation that is relevant in one approach to inducing tolerance (see later discussion).

Mechanisms of Rejection and Graft-versus-Host Disease

Cellular Mediators

Many different cell types participate in rejection responses, and there is considerable redundancy. T cells are key players in most forms of rejection, with the exception of rejection that can be induced by antibodies in the absence of T-cell help. These include hyperacute and acute vascular rejection processes that may be induced by natural antibodies, as described earlier, or by antibodies that are present due to presensitization. The possible role of NK cells has already been discussed.

Direct and Indirect Allorecognition

T-cell responses are induced by antigen-presenting cells (APCs) that present alloantigens. There are two forms of alloantigen recognition, termed "direct" and "indirect" (Fig. 46–1). Direct allorecognition denotes recognition of donor antigens on donor APCs provided by the graft. The extraordinarily high frequency of T cells with alloreactivity is caused by direct recognition of allogeneic MHC. Indirect recognition is the recognition of donor antigens that are picked up and presented on recipient MHC molecules on recipient APCs. The indirect response is more similar to "normal" T-cell responses, in which professional APCs presents peptide antigens to T cells that are present at relatively low frequency in the naïve repertoire.

In organ transplantation, direct alloreactivity is particularly important in the early post-transplantation period, when APCs within the transplanted organ are still present; many of these cells migrate to the lymphoid tissues, where they initiate the alloresponse. However, the APC supply that comes with the donor graft is not renewable, so, if the direct response is not maintained by recognition of donor antigens on endothelial cells or other cells in the graft, it recedes in importance. The indirect response, on the other hand, can be maintained by the constantly renewed pool of recipient APCs. The indirect response is of particular importance in inducing antibody responses.

Effector Mechanisms of Rejection

T cells can promote graft rejection through several effector mechanisms. One is the antibody-dependent processes that have already been discussed, which can be induced by CD4⁺ helper T cells that promote differentiation and immunoglobulin (Ig) class switching of B cells that

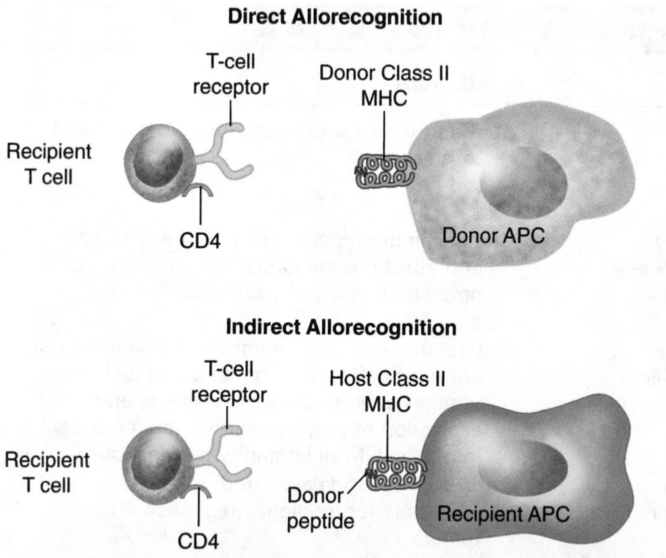

FIGURE 46–1 • Direct and indirect allorecognition. Direct allorecognition involves the recognition by a T-cell receptor of major histocompatibility complex (MHC) molecules (with or without a peptide) on a donor antigen-presenting cell (APC). Indirect allorecognition involves recognition by the T-cell receptor of a donor peptide presented on a recipient APC that has picked up and processed donor antigens.

recognize other specificities on the same alloantigens. T cells provide cognate help to B cells when they recognize complexes of self MHC with donor MHC-derived peptide antigens (produced by B cells whose surface Ig receptors recognize and pick up the donor MHC antigen). If anti-donor antibody is not present before transplantation but is induced afterward, the response can lead to the pathologic picture of acute humoral rejection. Antibodies may also participate in a slower, poorly understood process of chronic rejection, which, in the case of kidney and heart, is characterized by unique vascular lesions with intimal thickening and loss of the vessel space, and in the case of lung transplantation, by obliterative bronchiolitis. The mechanisms underlying these chronic rejection lesions are not well understood, and several different immune processes may in fact lead to similar lesions.

Another major effector pathway leading to graft rejection involves cytotoxic T lymphocytes (CTLs), which are predominantly members of the $CD8^+$ T-cell subset but also include $CD4^+$ T cells. Several effector mechanisms lead to killing of target cells by CTLs, and these include the granzyme/perforin–mediated pathway and the pathways involving Fas/Fas ligand (FasL) and other members of the tumor necrosis factor (TNF) receptor family and their ligands (see Chapter 42). Because $CD8^+$ cells recognize class I MHC molecules, which are widely expressed, it is not difficult to envision graft destruction by $CD8^+$ CTLs. $CD8^+$ CTLs may be activated via an APC that is stimulated initially through contact with an alloreactive $CD4^+$ cell. This is one form of CD4 "help" for $CD8^+$ cells. In addition, $CD8^+$ cells may be dependent on cytokines such as interleukin-2 (IL-2) from $CD4^+$ cells for their expansion and cytotoxic differentiation. However, there are also many examples of $CD8^+$ cell–mediated rejection that is independent of "help" from $CD4^+$ cells. Class II MHC, which is recognized by $CD4^+$ T cells, is less widely expressed on graft tissues than is class I MHC, although it may be induced on endothelial cells and graft parenchymal cells in the presence of inflammatory cytokines such as interferon-γ (IFN-γ).

In addition to cytotoxic mechanisms resulting from direct allorecognition, $CD4^+$ and $CD8^+$ T cells with indirect specificity seem to also be capable of causing graft destruction under some circumstances. Cytokines such as IFN-γ have been implicated in some instances, but in general the pathways of indirect graft destruction are not well understood. A $CD8^+$ cell–mediated form of skin graft rejection that is dependent on donor antigens cross-presented on recipient MHC molecules (a form of indirect allorecognition for $CD8^+$ cells) has been described in an animal model. This form of graft rejection may be directed at antigen presented on endothelial cells of recipient vessels that revascularize the graft. This mechanism would not apply to primarily vascularized organ allografts.

The Role of T-Cell Trafficking

All of the rejection processes described require trafficking of T cells into the graft. This process is made possible after the initial activation of naïve T cells in the lymphoid tissues. Naïve T cells can migrate into lymph nodes because of their expression of the CCR7 chemokine receptor and the adhesion molecule L-selectin. These T cells are activated by migratory graft APCs that also enter the lymph nodes. T-cell activation is associated with loss of CCR7 and L-selectin expression and acquisition of a new set of chemokine receptors and adhesion molecules that allow rolling and adhesion on the graft endothelium and entry into the graft parenchyma (see Chapter 44). Inflammation in the graft, such as that induced by ischemia/reperfusion injury and the transplantation procedure, as well as that induced by initially responding T cells, is associated with upregulation of chemokines and adhesion ligands that promote entry of lymphocytes into the graft. Nevertheless, well healed-in grafts can be slowly rejected by adoptively transferred memory T cells, demonstrating that acute graft injury and inflammation are not essential for rejection in the presence of an established memory T-cell response. Rejection of hematopoietic cell grafts may involve many of the same mechanisms as those discussed for solid organs, though less detailed work has been done in this area.

Mechanisms of Graft-versus-Host Disease

Initiation of GVH disease requires that donor T cells recognize host alloantigens. The disease involves attacks on a variety of recipient epithelial tissues, namely skin, the intestine, and liver. Animal models have demonstrated clear roles for both $CD4^+$ and $CD8^+$ cells in initiating GVH disease, and each subset is able to do so independently of the other. The mechanisms of GVH disease include activation of alloreactive donor T cells by recipient APCs, leading to the differentiation of effector cells with direct cytotoxic activity and cytokine production in response to host antigens. A prominent role is played by TNF-α, whose production is induced in part by the translocation of bacteria across the intestinal wall, and hence lipopolysaccharide production, which promotes innate immune system activation via a toll-like receptor (see Chapter 42).

T cell priming in the Peyer's patches plays a critical role in the induction of GVH disease. An intensely pro-inflammatory environment is produced by the combination of conditioning-induced tissue injury and disruption of mucosal barriers, bacterial activation of the innate immune system, and the GVH alloresponse. An important role is beginning to be appreciated for the inflamed microenvironment in target tissues in promoting the trafficking of GVH-reactive T cells into these tissues.

Strategies to Prevent Graft-versus-Host Disease

In view of the critical role of donor T cells in inducing GVH disease, an obvious strategy for preventing this complication is to remove mature T cells from the marrow graft. This approach has indeed been shown in both animal models and clinical studies to effectively prevent GVH disease. However, there are several disadvantages to this approach. One is that adult humans, particularly those who have undergone prior chemotherapy and radiotherapy, have little remaining thymic tissue and therefore demonstrate sluggish T-cell recovery, leading to serious opportunistic infections.

The second disadvantage applies to the most common indication for allogeneic HCT, namely the treatment of hematologic malignancies. In this setting, T-cell depletion is often associated with an increased relapse rate due to loss of a graft-versus-tumor (GVT) effect, which is in large part mediated by GVH alloreactivity. Separation of GVH disease from GVT effects is a major goal of research in HCT, and some promising strategies are being explored (Table 46–2). These include control of T-cell trafficking so that the GVH alloresponse is confined to the lymphohematopoietic tissues where the tumor resides and host conditioning with total lymphoid irradiation in combination with anti-thymocyte globulin in an attempt to enrich "NK/T" cells, which may inhibit GVH disease without impeding GVT effects.

The third disadvantage of donor T-cell depletion in HCT is that it increases the rate of engraftment failure. GVH alloreactivity and a "veto" effect of donor T cells helps to overcome host resistance to donor engraftment. A "veto" cell, which may be a T cell or an NK cell, kills a CTL that recognizes it. Although the phenomenon has been well established in

TABLE 46–2 EXPERIMENTAL STRATEGIES TO PREVENT GRAFT-VERSUS-HOST DISEASE

Strategy	Advantages	Limitations
T_H2 polarization of donor T cells (e.g., conditioning with ATG and TLI; in vitro stimulation with cytokine exposure)	May preserve GVL	May limit GVL; T_H2 can contribute to acute and chronic GVHD
Induction of tolerance in donor T cells (e.g., costimulatory blockade, regulatory cells)	Some strategies may selectively tolerize GVH-reactive T cells (e.g., in vitro antigen exposure with costimulatory blockade)	Global immunosuppression may limit GVL and anti-infectious immunity; tolerance (i.e., GVH protection) may be incomplete
Depletion of donor T cell plus infusion of NK cells with MHC class I–mismatched transplantation	NK cells do not cause GVHD but may mediate antitumor effects; donor NK cells may eliminate host APCs that trigger GVHD	May require very large numbers of donor NK cells; antitumor effect may not apply to all tumors; requires appropriate MHC disparity and expression of polymorphic NK cell receptors; insufficient T-cell immunity to infection
Depletion of donor T cells followed by delayed DLI	Preserves high level of GVL due to GVH reactivity; GVHD does not occur if host inflammation from conditioning has subsided and initial HCT was devoid of donor T cells	Antitumor effect delayed until time of DLI; most applicable for indolent lymphohematopoietic tumors
Depletion of donor T cells that recognize host alloantigens by in vitro activation/depletion (i.e., "allodepletion")	Preserves anti-infectious immunity and tumor antigen–specific responses	Loss of GVH reactivity limits GVL; highly efficient allodepletion methods are not yet available; residual T cells cause GVHD
Depletion of donor T cells with infusion of expanded infection-specific (e.g., CMV-specific, EBV-specific) T cells	Reduced GVHD potential while protecting against significant infectious organisms	Lack of GVL effect; lack of broad anti-infectious immunity; expense and inefficiency of in vitro T-cell expansion; loss of survival/homing potential of cultured T cells
Depletion of donor T cells with infusion of expanded tumor antigen–specific T cells	GVL without GVHD	Lack of anti-infectious immunity; expense and inefficiency of in vitro expansion of tumor-specific T cells; loss of survival/homing potential of cultured T cells
Insertion of suicide gene (e.g., thymidine kinase) into donor T cells	Drug targeting the inserted gene (e.g., ganciclovir) kills donor T cells to treat GVHD after GVL is initiated	Expense and inefficiency of in vitro transduction of T cells; loss of function and survival/homing potential of cultured T cells; risk of GVHD if transduction is incomplete; curtailment of GVL when donor T cells are killed in vivo

APC = antigen-presenting cell; ATG = anti-thymocyte globulin; CMV = cytomegalovirus; DLI = donor lymphocyte infusion; EBV = Epstein-Barr virus; GVHD = graft-versus-host disease; GVL = graft-versus-leukemia effects; HCT = hematopoietic cell transplantation; MHC = major histocompatibility complex; NK = natural killer; T_H2 = helper T lymphocytes type 2; TLI = total lymphoid irradiation.

animal models, its mechanisms are not clearly established, and its potential role in humans is uncertain. A recent report suggested that NK-cell recognition in the GVH direction resulting from the absence in the recipient of a class I MHC ligand (Fig. 46–2) that can trigger a donor NK-cell inhibitory receptor (KIR) may promote donor marrow engraftment and anti-tumor effects in the setting of T-cell–depleted, HLA-mismatched HCT.

Clinically, pharmacologic immunosuppressive prophylaxis is usually used in at least the first 6 months after HCT to minimize the complication of GVH disease. Additionally, HLA matched or closely matched donors are chosen whenever possible, because GVH disease increases in frequency and severity as increased HLA barriers are transgressed. These measures, nevertheless, are insufficient, and GVH disease remains a major complication of HCT. Therefore, many of the new strategies being explored in organ transplantation and other fields are also being examined for the prevention of GVH disease in experimental models. It should be borne in mind, however, that tolerance of donor T cells to recipient alloantigens (see later discussion) might not be entirely beneficial in the HCT setting for the treatment of malignant disease, because loss of GVH alloreactivity is likely to come with loss of anti-tumor effects.

Strategies to Prevent Allograft Rejection

Nonspecific Immunosuppression

Immunosuppressive drugs are the mainstay of clinical organ transplantation, and improvements in these drugs have brought the transplantation of hearts, lungs, pancreatic islets, and livers into clinical practice in the past 25 years. The mechanisms of action of these agents are discussed in Chapter 33 and will not be covered here. However, it is noteworthy that, despite these improvements and their enormous impact on early graft survival, these agents have been less effective in attenuating late graft loss. Because chronic immunologic rejection processes and side effects of the immunosuppressive drugs themselves are responsible for much of this late graft loss, improved immunosuppressive agents and induction of immune tolerance (see later discussion) are major research goals in transplantation.

Costimulatory Blockade

As understanding of immune responses has increased, recent years have seen the exploration of numerous biologic agents, including antibodies and small molecules targeting receptors of the immune system, as well as cell-based therapies, in efforts to improve allograft survival. Because of the central role played by T cells in the immune response, considerable attention has been focused on blockers of T-cell costimulation. When a naïve T cell recognizes antigen through its unique T-cell receptor, additional "costimulatory" signals are required to allow full activation, expansion, and differentiation to occur. These signals are often provided by APCs in the form of ligands (e.g., B7-1, B7-2) for costimulatory receptors (e.g., CD28) on the T cell. Cross-talk between the T cell and the APC (e.g., due to CD40 activation by CD154 upregulation on the activated T cell) further amplifies the costimulatory activity of the APC, allowing it to effectively activate other T cells as well. The CD154 (T

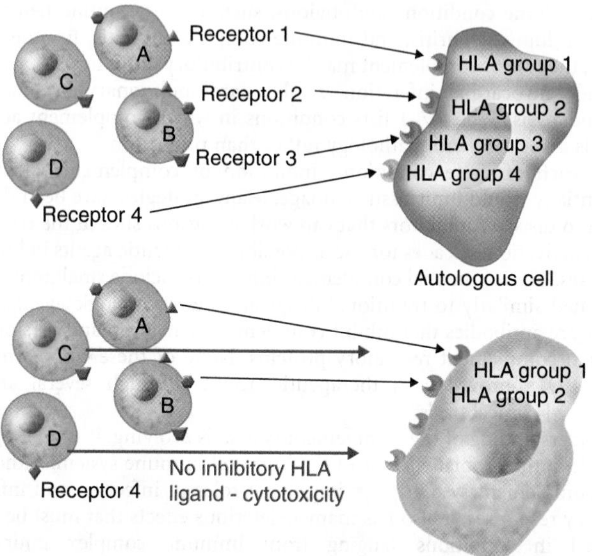

FIGURE 46–2 • Killing of allogeneic targets by natural killer (NK) cells due to "missing self." NK cells express clonally distributed inhibitory receptors (KIRs) with specificity for different groups of class I major histocompatibility complex (MHC) alleles, referred to in the figure as human leukocyte antigen (HLA) groups 1, 2, 3, and 4. Four different NK cells (A, B, C, and D) are shown, each with a different set of KIRs (referred to as receptors 1, 2, 3, and 4). Examples of HLA allele groups in the human are the HLA-Cw4, HLA-Cw3, and HLA-Bw4 groups; examples of KIRs are the ligands for these allele groups, namely KIR2DL1, KIR2DL2/3, and KIR3DL1, respectively. Each functional NK cell has one or more inhibitory receptors that recognize a "self" (autologous) HLA molecule. Although some of the NK cells (e.g., cells A and B in the example shown) will also find an HLA ligand to which its receptor binds on allogeneic cells, some (e.g., cells C and D) will not. The latter cells therefore will not receive inhibitory signals from the allogeneic cells and will kill them due to recognition by other (activating) receptors.

cell)–CD40 (B cell) interaction also promotes Ig class switching and functioning of B cells as APCs. Blockade of these processes (e.g., by CTLA4Ig and anti-CD154 monoclonal antibodies [mAbs]) has led to marked prolongation of allograft survival in stringent rodent and large-animal models. In bone marrow transplantation, robust, systemic tolerance has been achieved in rodents receiving costimulatory blockade. Some of these agents have been or are currently under evaluation as immunosuppressive agents in clinical trials in transplantation and autoimmune diseases. Anti-CD154 antibodies have been associated with thromboembolic complications, however, and their evaluation in transplantation trials is currently on hold. Numerous additional costimulatory and inhibitory pathways that affect T-cell responses have been described, and these all are potential targets for further manipulation of the alloresponse.

Immune Tolerance

Immune tolerance denotes a state in which the immune system is specifically unreactive to the donor graft (or recipient in the case of GVH reactivity), while remaining normally responsive to other antigens. Tolerance is distinct from the state produced by nonspecific immunosuppressive agents, which leads to increased risks of infection and malignancy due to their nonspecific immunosuppressive properties. Numerous approaches to tolerance induction have been described in rodent models, largely due to the strong tolerogenicity of primarily vascularized heart, liver, and kidney grafts in these animals. Because such grafts are less tolerogenic in humans, none of these strategies has been effectively applied clinically to date. Therefore, tolerance strategies that are appropriate for clinical evaluation must first be tested in "stringent" models, including relatively non-tolerogenic grafts such as MHC-mismatched skin in rodents and vascularized organ graft models in large animals. In most of the models, only a superficial understanding of the mechanisms leading to tolerance is currently available.

The three major mechanisms of T-cell tolerance are deletion, anergy, and suppression (often referred to as "regulation"). *Deletion* denotes the destruction of T cells with receptors that recognize donor antigens; it can be achieved during T-cell development in the thymus, for example by induction of mixed chimerism in T cell–depleted hosts. Deletion can also be applied to mature T cells in the periphery, for example, by transplantation of a tolerogenic organ or marrow graft in combination with blockade of costimulatory molecules. *Anergy* denotes the inability of T cells to respond fully to antigens they recognize, and it can be induced by antigen presentation without costimulation. *Suppression* has attracted considerable interest since the discovery that constitutively CD25$^+$ T cells of the CD4$^+$ subset have suppressive activity. These and other types of suppressive T cells (e.g., NK/T cells) have been implicated in many rodent transplantation tolerance models and in prevention of autoimmunity. However, it seems likely that large numbers of regulatory cells recognizing the relevant antigens would be needed to apply this type of cellular therapy clinically, and the ultimate practicality of the approach remains to be determined. Nevertheless, an improved understanding of this type of immune regulation may lead to effective strategies for favoring the suppressive immune response over destructive alloimmunity.

The developments in animal models and understanding of immune mechanisms described here have provided impetus for efforts to achieve immune tolerance in clinical transplantation. Every transplantation center has anecdotal cases of patients who have removed themselves from chronic immunosuppression without experiencing graft rejection. However, for every such patient, there are dozens more who have experienced rejection episodes on dose reduction or removal of immunosuppressive drugs. Although several centers are now undertaking efforts to minimize and even slowly withdraw nonspecific immunosuppressive therapy completely in organ transplant recipients, a major current limitation is the inability to identify predictors of success. Recent hopes have focused on the goal of identifying an "immune signature" that predicts tolerance. However, given the multiple immune mechanisms of tolerance and rejection, combined with genetic and environmental heterogeneity of transplant recipients, individual differences in underlying and intercurrent illnesses, donor–recipient immunologic disparity, and differing drug therapies, it seems unlikely that there will be a single "signature" indicating the ability to accept an organ without immunosuppression.

One approach developed in animal models has been successfully applied to the induction of immune tolerance in a small group of patients receiving renal allografts. This approach, involving bone marrow transplantation after nonmyeloablative conditioning, which is much less toxic than standard HCT conditioning, was shown to be effective in the most stringent rodent and large-animal models before being evaluated clinically. Initial success using combined kidney and bone marrow transplantation in patients with renal failure due to multiple myeloma has led to ongoing pilot studies sponsored by the Immune Tolerance Network in the United States, with encouraging preliminary results. This approach and others that have emerged from ongoing investigations provide hope that in the future transplantation might be routinely performed without the need for chronic immunosuppressive therapy, with its attendant complications and limited ability to control chronic rejection. Because autoimmune diseases are major contributors to end-stage renal disease, diabetes, and other types of organ failure, the potential of tolerance strategies to reverse autoimmunity while inducing allograft tolerance is also a source of hope. All of these approaches must, however, be undertaken with the caution that successful regimens could also lead to immune tolerance to active infectious organisms.

SUGGESTED READINGS

Bluestone JA: Regulatory T-cell therapy: Is it ready for the clinic? Nat Rev Immunol 2005;343–349. *A scholarly update.*

Brennan DC, Daller JA, Lake KD: Rabbit antithymocyte globulin versus basiliximab in renal transplantation. N Engl J Med 2006;355:1967–1977. *In a randomized trial, the two regimens were roughly equivalent.*

Chakraverty R, Cote D, Buchli J, et al: An inflammatory check point regulates recruitment of graft-versus-host reactive T cells to peripheral tissues. J Exp Med 2006;203:2021–2031. *A mechanistic review.*

Chalasani G, Li Q, Konieczny BT, et al: The allograft defines the type of rejection (acute versus chronic) in the face of an established effector immune response. J Immunol 2004;172:7813–7820. *Memory T cells are generally responsible for chronic rejection.*

Fan X, Ang A, Pollock-Barziv SM, et al: Donor-specific B-cell tolerance after ABO-incompatible infant heart transplantation. Nat Med 2004;10:1227–1233. *ABO mismatched heart transplants can succeed in infants before they develop high-level antibodies.*

Fudaba Y, Spitzer TR, Shaffer J, et al: Myeloma responses and tolerance following combined kidney and nonmyeloablative marrow transplantation: In vivo and in vitro analyses. Am J Transplant 2006;6:2121–2133. *This approach was successful in a small series.*

Hubscher SG: Transplantation pathology. Semin Diagn Pathol 2006;23:170–181. *A clinicopathologic overview.*

Lowsky R, Takahashi T, Liu YP, et al: Protective conditioning for acute graft-versus-host disease. N Engl J Med 2005;353:1321–1331. *Total lymphoid irradiation plus antithymocyte globulin decreased acute graft-versus-host disease in leukemia and lymphoma patients undergoing stem cell transplantation.*

Murai M, Yoneyama H, Ezaki T, et al: Peyer's patch is the essential site in initiating murine acute and lethal graft-versus-host reaction. Nat Immunol 2003;4:154–160. *The gut is a key regulator of immunity.*

Parham P: MHC class I molecules and KIRs in human history, health and survival. Nat Rev Immunol 2005;5:201–214. *An evolutionary approach to understanding modern immunology.*

Warren DS, Zachary AA, Sonnenday CJ, et al: Successful renal transplantation across simultaneous ABO incompatible and positive crossmatch barriers. Am J Transplant 2004;4:561–568. *Removal of ABO antibodies and sometimes B cells, combined with IVIG, can be successful.*

Watts TH: TNF/TNFR family members in costimulation of T cell responses. Annu Rev Immunol 2005;23:23–68. *A scholarly overview.*

47 COMPLEMENT IN HEALTH AND DISEASE

David R. Karp and V. Michael Holers

The term *complement* was coined by 19th century microbiologists who noted the fact that fresh immune serum could kill bacteria, whereas heated serum could not. They defined two activities in the serum: a heat stabile *antibody*, and a heat labile *complementary* factor. It is now known that the complement system consists of more than 30 serum and membrane proteins that participate in both host defense and a wide variety of pathologic states.

The complement system serves many protective functions ascribed to the innate immune system. As originally described, it helps to maintain blood sterility by depositing the membrane attack complex (MAC) in bacterial cell walls and lysing them. It also participates in the opsonization of pathogens for phagocytic removal. The peptide *anaphylatoxins* produced during complement activation promote inflammatory responses with microbicidal effects. The deposition of complement on immune complexes helps to keep them soluble and remove them from the circulation.

There also is increasing evidence that complement can shape the adaptive immune response. Antigens decorated by complement proteins are taken up by B cells and other antigen-presenting cells, resulting in T-cell activation. Studies from mice deficient in various complement proteins have shown that complement activation is needed for optimal antibody production by B cells. Lastly, it is well known that humans and experimental animals that are deficient in early complement components are often predisposed to autoimmune diseases, particularly systemic lupus erythematosus (SLE). This observation suggests that complement is required in some way to identify soluble self-antigens and eliminate self-reactive B cells.

Complement is activated immediately on exposure to immune complexes, but it lacks the immunologic memory of T or B cells with clonotypic receptors that discriminate between self and non-self. Activated complement can be deposited on host and pathogenic surfaces. This potentially dangerous situation is controlled by a series of genetically, structurally, and functionally similar proteins termed the *regulators of complement activation* (RCA). These proteins provide species-specific downregulation of complement activation on host tissues.

Inappropriate complement action occurs when the nondiscriminating activating proteins function in excess of the regulatory proteins that limit damage on self-tissues. This can be seen in almost any inflammatory disease. Some conditions are obvious, such as autoimmune hemolytic anemia, lupus nephritis, and immune complex vasculitis. In other diseases, the role of complement may be contributory but is less clear. These include myocardial infarction, stroke, cardiopulmonary bypass, and hemodialysis. Table 47–1 lists conditions in which complement activation is associated with pathology rather than protection.

In each of these conditions, inhibition of complement activation potentially would limit tissue damage. Many strategies have been developed to discover inhibitors that can work at various sites in the complement activation cascades for use as possible therapeutic agents in human diseases. These potential complement inhibitors include small molecules designed similarly to traditional drugs and newer, biologic agents. The latter are antibodies that inhibit complement activation and versions of human complement regulatory proteins. None of these compounds is currently approved as a therapeutic agent, although several are in advanced clinical trials.

Understanding of the complement system is evolving. It is no longer a simple antimicrobial effector of the humoral immune system. Although the complement system plays important roles in infection and inflammatory responses, it also has many deleterious effects that must be controlled in conditions ranging from immune complex injury to reproduction. The critical feature of complement-mediated pathology is the alternative pathway amplification loop. As shown in Figure 47–1, failure to control this response results in the generation of potent inflammatory signals and the recruitment of tissue-damaging neutrophils, monocytes, and mast cells. Because more than half of the proteins associated with the complement system are dedicated to the control of activation or effector functions, it is clear that discrimination between "self" and "non-self" must occur even in the innate immune system.

Knowledge of how complement is activated and how it can be controlled offers new opportunities for the development of therapeutic agents for human diseases. It is anticipated that within the next few years many of these drugs will be approved for clinical use. The most likely successful therapeutic target will be antibodies to factor B, C5, or C5a, and the diseases most likely to be improved by complement inhibition are ischemic injury to the heart and brain and autoimmune/inflammatory injury to joints and the kidney.

ACTIVATION OF COMPLEMENT

As an essential component of the innate immune system, complement is endowed with redundant, yet carefully controlled activation pathways. The molecular events that occur during activation not only are responsible for the pathology of complement-associated disease states, but also offer opportunities for the rational design of inhibitors. For simplicity, it is convenient to think of the different parts of the complement activation pathways as involving *recognition*, *convertase/amplification*, and *effector* mechanisms.

TABLE 47–1 PATHOLOGIC CONDITIONS PRIMARILY ASSOCIATED WITH COMPLEMENT ACTIVATION

Allotransplantation	Macular degeneration
Alzheimer's disease	Meconium pneumonitis
ARDS	Multiple sclerosis
Arthus reaction	Multisystem organ failure
Asthma	Myasthenia gravis
Bullous pemphigoid	Post-cardiopulmonary bypass
Burns	Psoriasis
Crohn's disease	Recurrent spontaneous abortion
Glomerulonephritis (many causes)	Rheumatoid arthritis
Hemodialysis	Septic shock
Hemolytic anemia	Stroke
Hereditary angioedema	Systemic lupus erythematosus
Immune complex vasculitis	Traumatic brain injury
Ischemia-reperfusion injury	Xenotransplantation

ARDS = adult respiratory distress syndrome.

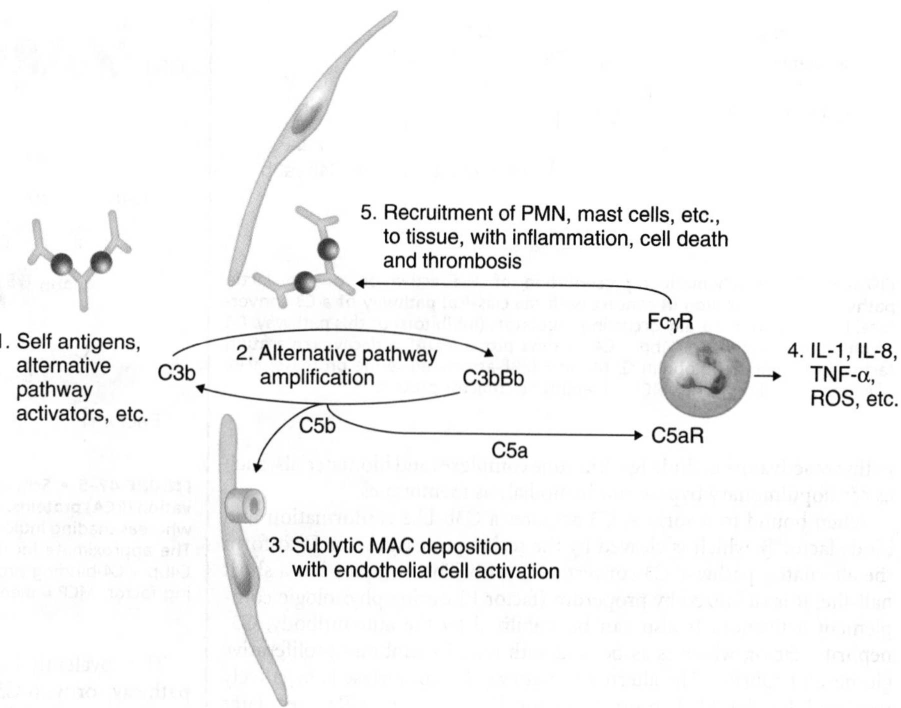

FIGURE 47–1 • Pathogenic effect of complement. 1, Complement is activated by immune complexes or the exposure of surfaces that lack regulatory proteins. **2,** In the absence of effective regulation, the alternative pathway activation loop produces large amounts of both C5a and C5b. **3,** C5b initiates the deposition of sublytic amounts of the membrane attack complex (MAC), leading to cellular activation and proliferation. **4,** C5a is a potent chemoattractant and activator of polymorphonuclear neutrophils (PMN), mast cells, and other leukocytes, resulting in production of inflammatory cytokines and chemokines. **5,** Leukocytes also express Fc receptors (e.g., FcγR) that interact with immunoglobulin G bound to damaged tissue, further amplifying the generation of inflammatory mediators and activating coagulation pathways. IL = interleukin; ROS = reactive oxygen species; TNF-α = tumor necrosis factor-α.

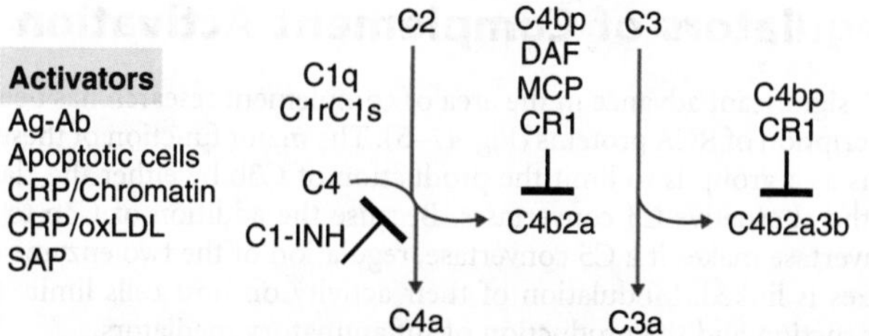

FIGURE 47–2 • Schematic representation of the activation of the classical pathway and generation of its C3 convertase. Included are naturally occurring regulators (inhibitors) of this pathway. Ag-Ab = antigen-antibody complex; C1-INH = C1 inhibitor; C4bp = C4 binding protein; CR = complement receptor; CRP = C-reactive protein; DAF = decay-accelerating factor; MCP = membrane cofactor protein; oxLDL = oxidized low-density lipoprotein; SAP = serum amyloid protein.

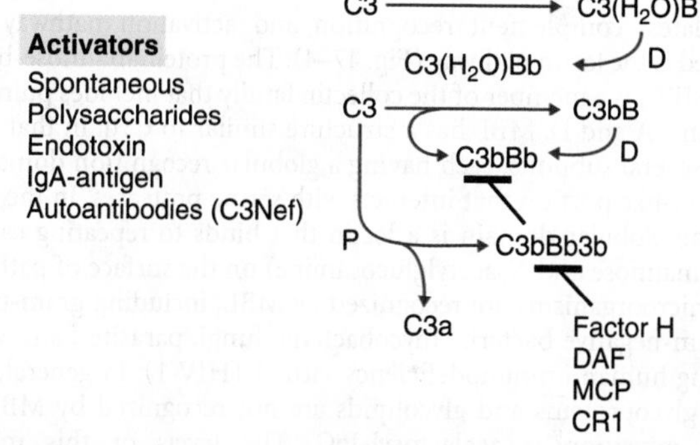

FIGURE 47–3 • Schematic representation of the activation of the alternative pathway and generation of its C3 convertase. Included are naturally occurring regulators (inhibitors) of this pathway. C3Nef = C3-nephritic factor; CR = complement receptor; DAF = decay-accelerating factor; IgA = immunoglobulin A; MCP = membrane cofactor protein.

Classical Pathway

Although traditionally thought of as activated only by immune complexes containing immunoglobulin M (IgM) or IgG, the classical pathway has been shown to be activated by targets other than immune complexes (Fig. 47–2). Notably, apoptotic cells bind C1q and activate the C1 proteases. C1 also is activated by the accumulated Aβ protein found in the neuritic plaques of patients with Alzheimer's disease. C-reactive protein (CRP) and serum amyloid protein bind to chromatin and other ribonucleoprotein complexes released from apoptotic cells. The CRP/nuclear antigen complexes bind and activate C1. C1q and the classical pathway seem to play a role in the opsonization and removal of nuclear materials that frequently contain autoantigens. The few patients with hereditary C1q deficiency all eventually develop SLE. Similarly, mice that have been engineered to lack C1q develop a lupus-like illness and have deposition of apoptotic bodies in their glomeruli. The addition of CRP and enzymatically modified low-density lipoprotein to human serum causes the activation of complement, as determined by the almost quantitative conversion of C3 to C3b. Finally, deposits of CRP and activated C1 have been shown in infarcted human myocardium. Together, these observations suggest that activation via the antibody-independent classical pathway is important in protective immune responses and in pathogenic inflammatory reactions.

Regulation of the classical pathway activation occurs at several levels. First is the serine protease inhibitor (serpin), C1-inhibitor (C1-INH). C1-INH blocks the activity of many proteases, including factor XIIa, kallikrein, and factor XIa of the clotting system and C1r and C1s of the complement system. The importance of C1-INH is seen in the disease hereditary angioedema. In this instance, the heterozygous deficiency of C1-INH allows uncontrolled proteolysis of C2 and C4 after minor trauma. A vasoactive peptide is released from C2 and leads to painless (but occasionally life-threatening) soft tissue swelling. Treatment of acute attacks of hereditary angioedema includes purified C1-INH and antifibrinolytic drugs such as ε-aminocaproic acid.

Classical pathway activation also is regulated by RCA proteins. These proteins form the basis for the ability of the complement system to discriminate self from non-self targets. They are discussed in depth later in this chapter. The RCA proteins C4-binding protein (C4-bp) and complement receptor 1 (CR1) are specific to classical pathway regulation.

Alternative Pathway

The alternative pathway is much less stringent in its recognition requirements. It takes advantage of the fact that C3 undergoes spontaneous low-grade activation in the fluid phase (Fig. 47–3). Based on estimates of the glomerular filtration of C3a and its steady-state serum concentration, it has been suggested that 1 to 2% of serum C3 is activated in serum each hour. This allows the covalent attachment of C3 to the polysaccharides of fungi and bacteria and to other appropriately charged targets, such as endotoxin and virally infected cells. Other alternative

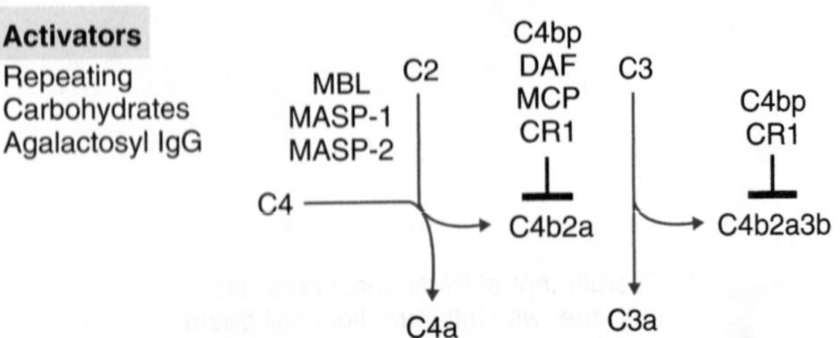

FIGURE 47–4 • Schematic representation of the activation of the lectin pathway and generation in concert with the classical pathway of a C3 convertase. Included are naturally occurring regulators (inhibitors) of this pathway. CR = complement receptor; C4bp = C4 binding protein; DAF = decay-accelerating factor; IgG = immunoglobulin G; MASP = MBL-associated serine protease; MBL = mannose-binding lectin; MCP = membrane cofactor protein.

pathway activators include IgA immune complexes and biomaterials, such as cardiopulmonary bypass and hemodialysis membranes.

When bound to a surface, C3 acquires a C3b-like conformation and binds factor B, which is cleaved by the serine protease factor D to form the alternative pathway C3 convertase C3bBb. This complex has a short half-life. It is stabilized by properdin (factor P) during physiologic complement activation. It also can be stabilized by the autoantibody, C3-nephritic factor, which is associated with type I membranoproliferative glomerulonephritis. The alternative pathway C3 convertase is negatively regulated by the RCA proteins factor H, DAF, and CR1 (see later discussion).

Lectin Pathway

The latest complement recognition and activation pathway to be described is the lectin pathway (Fig. 47–4). The protein mannose-binding lectin (MBL) is a member of the collectin family that includes pulmonary surfactants A and D. MBL has a structure similar to C1q, in that it consists of several subunits, each having a globular recognition domain and a collagen-like portion that interacts with serine proteases. In the case of MBL, the globular domain is a lectin that binds to repeating carbohydrates (mannose and *N*-acetylglucosamine) on the surface of pathogens. Many microorganisms are recognized by MBL, including gram-positive and gram-negative bacteria, mycobacteria, fungi, parasites, and viruses, including human immunodeficiency virus 1 (HIV-1). In general, mammalian glycoproteins and glycolipids are not recognized by MBL. One notable exception is agalactosyl-IgG. The levels of this modified immunoglobulin are increased in inflammatory conditions such as rheumatoid arthritis, raising the possibility that excessive activation of the lectin pathway is clinically relevant.

Two serine proteases, MASP-1 and MASP-2, associate with MBL, presumably through the collagen-like domain. Although not formally proven, this is analogous to the association of C1r and C1s with C1q. Activation of MASP-1 and MASP-2 results in cleavage of C2 and C4, with the subsequent formation of the classical pathway C3 convertase (C4b2a).

Variation in the structural and regulatory portions of the MBL gene leads to wide individual differences in serum levels. Low levels have been associated with recurrent infections in children and adults and have been shown to be a minor risk factor for the development of SLE. More striking is the association of low levels of MBL with infection in SLE. In a study of Danish lupus patients, heterozygous MBL deficiency was associated with a four-fold increase in the risk of bacterial pneumonia, and homozygous deficiency with a more than 100-fold increase.

C3 and C5 Convertases

The three activation pathways converge at C3. C3 (and C4) contains a reactive glutamic acid residue buried within the three-dimensional structure of the protein. Normally the γ-carboxy group of the reactive glutamic acid in C3 (and C4) is linked to a nearby cysteine in an "internal thioester." On activation, the thioester is exposed to the surface of the protein, where it can react with amino or hydroxyl groups. Most of the thioesters are hydrolyzed by water to form inactive C3 or C4. Some form amide or ester bonds to proteins or carbohydrates, covalently attaching C3b (and C4b) to target surfaces. This enables cells bearing CR1 to bind these targets and opsonize them, representing one of the effector mechanisms of complement.

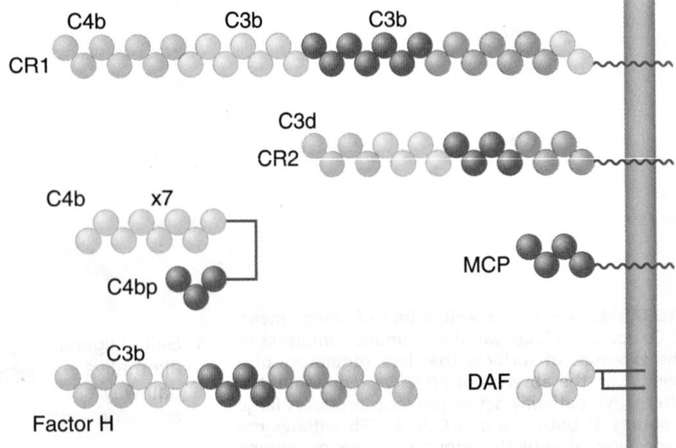

FIGURE 47–5 • Schematic representation of the regulators of complement activation (RCA) proteins. Circles represent individual short consensus repeats (SCRs), whereas shading indicates higher organizational units composed of several SCRs. The approximate locations for binding of C3 and C4 fragments are indicated. C4bp = C4-binding protein; CR = complement receptor; DAF = decay-accelerating factor; MCP = membrane cofactor protein.

The covalently bound C3b associates with C4b2a (classical or lectin pathway) or with C3bBb (alternative pathway) to form a convertase for C5. C3b is part of the alternative-pathway C3 convertase, and its product generates an amplification loop that can deposit thousands of C3b molecules on a target, regardless of the initial activation step.

Regulators of Complement Activation

A significant advance in the area of complement research has been the description of RCA proteins (Fig. 47–5). The major function of these proteins as a group is to limit the production of C3b by either the classical or the alternative C3 convertases. Because the addition of C3b to a C3 convertase makes it a C5 convertase, regulation of the two enzyme complexes is linked. Modulation of their activity on host cells limits tissue destruction and the production of inflammatory mediators.

There are six RCA proteins that control the C3/C5 convertases (Table 47–2). They are factor H, C4 binding protein (C4bp), membrane cofactor protein (MCP [CD46]), decay accelerating factor (DAF [CD55]), complement receptor 1 (CR1 [CD35]), and complement receptor 2 (CR2 [CD21]). The genes for all of these proteins are found in a cluster on human chromosome 1.q32. Structurally, they are composed of repeating subunits termed *short consensus repeats* (SCRs), sometimes referred to as *complement control protein* modules. Each SCR has approximately 60 amino acids with four invariant cysteine residues. The pairing of the disulfides leads to a four– to five–β pleated sheet structure, causing the SCRs to appear like beads on a string.

Although the SCRs are structurally related, the individual RCA proteins may recognize different parts of the C3 molecule. They do so using specific combinations of SCRs. The RCA proteins function to control complement activation by two processes. First is *decay acceleration.* This refers to the process whereby the RCA protein binds to C3b or C4b in the convertase and dissociates the other members of the complex, rendering it enzymatically inactive. The second effect is *cofactor* activity. Some of the RCA proteins facilitate the recognition of C3b or C4b by a serum protease, factor I. Cleavage of C3b or C4b by factor I also renders the convertase inactive.

Despite their relatedness, the RCA proteins exhibit differences in their overall structure, distribution, and function. All of the RCA proteins except MCP and CR2 have decay acceleration activity; it is the only function of DAF. This glycosyl phosphatidylinositol-linked protein is widely expressed and causes the removal of C2a or Bb from the C3 and C5 convertases. DAF lacks the cofactor activity seen with the other RCA proteins (except CR2). Factor H and C4bp are serum proteins. MCP and DAF are ubiquitously expressed membrane proteins. CR1 and CR2 are membrane proteins expressed primarily on hematopoietic cells.

RCA proteins have been linked to several disease states. DAF is missing from the abnormal erythrocytes of patients with paroxysmal nocturnal hemoglobinuria. Although the hemolysis of these cells is ultimately due to the fact that the cells also lack CD59 (see later discussion), the DAF

TABLE 47–2 DISTRIBUTION AND FUNCTION OF REGULATORS OF COMPLEMENT ACTIVATION (RCA) PROTEINS

RCA Protein	Distribution	Function
C4 binding protein	Serum	Cofactor for C4b; decay of classical C3/C5 convertases
Factor H	Serum	Cofactor for C3b; decay of alternative C3/C5 convertases
Decay-accelerating factor	Widely distributed on most cell types	Decay of classical and alternative C3/C5 convertases
Membrane cofactor protein	Widely distributed on most cell types (not RBCs)	Cofactor for C3b and C4b
Complement receptor 1	Most blood cells; mast cells	Cofactor for C3b and C4b; decay of C3/C5 convertases; receptor for C3b/C4b
Complement receptor 2	B cells; follicular dendritic cells	Receptor for C3b fragments; regulation of B cells

RBCs = red blood cells.

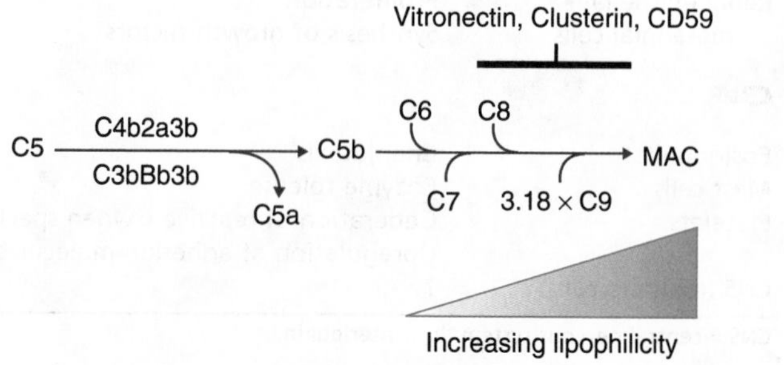

FIGURE 47–6 • Schematic representation of the assembly of the membrane attack complex (MAC) on a cell membrane.

deficiency promotes complement activation on these cells. Genetic factor H deficiency has been associated with type II membranoproliferative glomerulonephritis in humans and in a strain of Yorkshire pigs. Renal biopsy specimens in both cases showed evidence of robust alternative pathway activation. There is also evidence that mutations in factor H and MCP are responsible for some of the pathology seen in either sporadic or familial hemolytic-uremic syndrome. Lastly, low levels of CR1 and/or CR2 have been seen in patients with SLE. CR1 has cofactor and decay activity, and its major role is in the removal of immune complexes from the circulation. CR2 is necessary for optimal B-cell regulation, including the downmodulation of autoreactive B cells.

Membrane Attack Complex

The cleavage of C5 by either convertase generates C5a, the most potent of the complement anaphylatoxins, and C5b. C5b associates with C6 and C7 to create a lipophilic trimer as part of the MAC (Fig. 47–6). On the surface of a target cell, fewer than 1% of the C5b67 trimers that are formed insert into the lipid bilayer and serve as binding sites for C8. This attracts C9 to the membrane, and C9 has the capacity to self-polymerize. A total of 12 to 18 C9 molecules form a ring structure, completing the MAC. In its complete form, the MAC appears like a doughnut with a 10-nm pore running through the center. This pore can allow water and ions to enter the cells, ultimately leading to cell lysis. A MAC with only one or two C9 molecules also can cause lysis, however, suggesting that the MAC disrupts the lipid integrity in its general vicinity, rather than creating holes in the membrane.

The MAC itself appears to be largely redundant in terms of protection against infection. It seems to be essential only for efficient elimination of *Neisseria* species. Individuals who are homozygous deficient for C6, C7, C8, or C9 are at risk for meningococcal and gonococcal infection. C9 deficiency is the most common immunodeficiency in Japan, with a heterozygote frequency of 3 to 5%. Absence of an efficient MAC is not deleterious to the population in general and may have some selective advantage.

Extensive complement activation during an inflammatory response can result in sufficient MAC deposition to cause host cell lysis. Most nucleated cells have mechanisms to resist the osmotic changes caused by the MAC, however, and they may "disassemble" the MAC as it is formed. Rather, the nonlethal effects of sublytic MAC deposition are more likely

TABLE 47–3 RESPONSES TO SUBLYTIC MEMBRANE ATTACK COMPLEX ACTIVATION

Cell Type	Effects
Most cells	Increased intracellular calcium flux Activation of G protein Activation of protein kinases Activation of transcription factors Proliferation
Neutrophils and macrophages	Release of reactive oxygen species Activation of phospholipase A_2 Release of prostaglandins, thromboxane, and leukotrienes
Platelets	Release of ATP Increased P-selectin expression Procoagulant membrane changes
Endothelial cells	Increased synthesis of IL-1α Increased release of tissue factor Increased release of von Willebrand factor Increased synthesis of basic fibroblast and platelet-derived growth factors
Synoviocytes	Increased synthesis of prostaglandin Increased synthesis of IL-6 Increased production of matrix metalloproteinase
Glomerular epithelium	Activation of phospholipase A_2 Synthesis of prostaglandin Increased synthesis of collagen and fibronectin
Oligodendrocytes	Increased synthesis of myelin basic protein and proteolipid Increased proliferation

ATP = adenosine triphosphate; IL = interleukin.

to contribute to pathology. In most cells, this occurs through a general activation of multiple cell signaling pathways. Calcium enters the cell, activating protein kinases and phospholipase C, and upregulates the production of cyclic adenosine monophosphate (cAMP). G proteins and their associated factors are concentrated at the cell membrane, perhaps localized to C9 directly. The mitogen-activated protein kinase pathways (extracellular signal–regulated kinase [ERK], c-Jun N-terminal kinase [JNK], and p38) are activated, resulting in the induction of transcription factors such as c-jun and fos, cell proliferation, and inhibition of apoptosis.

The response to MAC deposition depends on the cell type (Table 47–3). In phagocytic cells, such as polymorphonuclear neutrophils or macrophages, sublytic MAC activation leads to the production of reactive oxygen species (e.g., superoxide, hydrogen peroxide), as well as prostaglandins and leukotrienes. Platelets undergo the exposure of phosphatidylserine on their outer membrane, resulting in greater formation of blood coagulation enzyme complexes. This has a potentially procoagulant effect. On endothelial cells, MAC deposition leads to many important events. It induces the synthesis of interleukin-1α (IL-1α), which leads to further autocrine and paracrine endothelial cell activation. It stimulates a procoagulant state by altering the phospholipid composition of the endothelial membrane, inducing the synthesis of tissue factor and upregulating the synthesis of plasminogen activator inhibitor. MAC treatment of endothelial cells causes an increase in the expression of adhesion molecules, including intercellular adhesion molecule 1 (ICAM)-1 and E-selectin. Finally, the MAC stimulates endothelial cells to proliferate through growth factor production. Despite the fact that cell death does not occur, deposition of the sublytic levels of MAC leads to a potentially more dangerous situation, with increased inflammation, coagulation, and cellular proliferation.

Regulation of MAC formation is important clinically and has become an area of therapeutic research. Two fluid-phase proteins, clusterin and S-protein (vitronectin), bind the C5b-7 complex and prevent its association with the lipid membrane. C8 and usually two to four C9 molecules bind to this soluble complex, termed *sC5b-9*, which is lytically inactive. CD59 is a membrane-bound inhibitor of MAC formation. This small glycoprotein is attached to the cell membrane through a glycosyl phosphatidylinositol tail. It binds tightly to C5b-8, preventing the binding and polymerization of C9. CD59 shows strong species restriction. That is, it is most effective in the inhibition of MAC formation by the same or closely related species. Lastly, the expression of CD59 is defective in patients with paroxysmal nocturnal hemoglobinuria, owing to the failure to synthesize the glycosyl phosphatidylinositol tail on this and many other cell surface proteins, including DAF. The clinical features of paroxysmal nocturnal hemoglobinuria are protean. The hemolysis is believed to be caused by low-grade complement activation on red blood cells, however; without CD59, MAC formation proceeds and allows hemolysis.

TABLE 47–4 DISTRIBUTION OF ANAPHYLATOXIN RECEPTORS AND THEIR CELLULAR RESPONSES

Cell Type	Responses
C5aR (CD88)	
Neutrophils Eosinophils Basophils Mast cells Monocytes	Chemotaxis Enzyme release Generation of reactive oxygen species Upregulation of adhesion molecules Increased synthesis of IL-1, IL-6, and IL-8 Prostaglandin/leukotriene synthesis
Hepatocytes	Increased synthesis of acute phase reactants
Pulmonary epithelium	Increased IL-8
Neuronal cells	?
Endothelial cells	Increased expression of P-selectin
Renal epithelial/ mesangial cells	Proliferation Synthesis of growth factors
C3aR	
Eosinophils Mast cells Platelets	Chemotaxis Enzyme release Generation of reactive oxygen species Upregulation of adhesion molecules
CNS (multiple cells)	?

CNS = central nervous system; IL = interleukin.

Anaphylatoxins

In addition to the MAC, the other major source of pathologic damage resulting from complement activation comes from the action of the anaphylatoxins. These are the peptides C3a, C4a, and C5a, which are cleaved from their respective proteins during activation. They were named by Friedberger in 1910 to describe toxic effects after the transfer of complement-activated serum into laboratory animals. They are 77 (C3a and C4a) or 74 (C5a) amino acids long and contain a carboxy (C)-terminal arginine. The structures of C3a and C5a have been determined by x-ray crystallography and nuclear magnetic resonance; they exhibit a compact amino (N)-terminal region that is held together by conserved disulfide bonds. This part of the molecule contains cationic amino acids that are believed to interact with the anaphylatoxin receptors. The C-terminal regions of the anaphylatoxins are extended sequences. Only the last five amino acids are required for activity. In plasma, the C-terminal arginine is removed rapidly by carboxypeptidase N from anaphylatoxins not bound to their receptors. Depending on the response studied, this removal totally inactivates the anaphylatoxin or reduces its potency by 1000-fold.

Understanding of anaphylatoxin effects has been aided greatly by the identification of their receptors, through a combination of molecular cloning and immunochemical techniques. The C5a receptor (C5aR [CD88]) was the first anaphylatoxin receptor to be characterized. It is a seven-transmembrane-spanning protein that couples ligand binding to G-protein signaling. Traditionally, it was thought to be expressed only on myeloid cells, particularly neutrophils and eosinophils. It mediates the potent chemoattractant property of C5a for both of these cell types. Signaling through CD88 leads to rapid secretion of all granule contents. These include proteases, peroxidases, and lactoferrin from neutrophils, and peroxidase, major basic protein, and eosinophil cationic protein from eosinophils. C5a also induces the release of cytokines, such as tumor necrosis factor (TNF), IL-1, IL-6, and IL-8, and adhesion molecules, promoting the inflammatory response.

The C5aR also has been found on numerous other tissues (Table 47–4). These include hepatocytes, bronchial and alveolar epithelium, vascular endothelium, renal mesangial and tubular epithelial cells, and brain astrocytes, microglia, and neurons. The function of C5a in these tissues is not clear. In vitro experiments have shown that these cells are activated by exposure to the anaphylatoxins, leading to production of cytokines, chemokines, and prostaglandins, and to cell proliferation.

The C3a receptor has been identified; it is also a seven-transmembrane-domain protein. Similar to the C5aR, the tissue distribution of the C3aR is much greater than previously thought. It is expressed on almost all myeloid cells, including mast cells, where it mediates the release of allergic mediators. The C3aR also has been detected on many tissues, including in the brain, by Northern blot analysis for RNA expression.

The anaphylatoxins have many biologic effects. In general, they cause smooth muscle contraction and recruitment of granulocytes, monocytes, and mast cells. In theory, they can contribute to the pathophysiology of any inflammatory condition. C3a and C5a have been shown to play a role in diseases such as adult respiratory distress syndrome, multisystem organ failure, septic shock, myocardial ischemia-reperfusion injury, asthma, rheumatoid arthritis, SLE, and inflammatory bowel disease. The anaphylatoxin peptides also are responsible for the "postpump" syndrome seen in patients undergoing cardiopulmonary bypass or hemodialysis. Exposure of blood to dialysis or perfusion membranes leads to complement activation. Within minutes of starting bypass, there is a sharp increase in the level of C3a and C5a in the extracorporeal circuit being returned to the patient. This increase can be associated with respiratory distress, pulmonary hypertension, and pulmonary edema. It has been shown that the length of time that patients stay on the ventilator after bypass surgery depends on the level of C3a generated during reperfusion.

C3a and C5a have been implicated in the initiation and prolongation of adult respiratory distress syndrome and multisystem organ failure. After severe trauma, levels of C3a have been measured that suggest activation of the entire circulating C3 pool. This activation leads to bronchoconstriction, increased vascular permeability, and vascular plugging with leukocytes. The activation of white blood cells continues the cycle of tissue damage with further complement activation. Continued elevation of C3a in shock or adult respiratory distress syndrome is a poor prognostic sign.

The role of C5a in pulmonary pathology has been shown using C5aR-knockout mice. A model of immune complex damage to the lung was studied. The wild-type mice had the expected increases in lung permeability and leukocyte infiltration after induction of intrapulmonary ovalbumin/anti-ovalbumin complexes. These effects were not seen in the

C5aR-deficient animals. In other animal models, antibodies to C5a have been shown to limit infarct size secondary to myocardial ischemia-reperfusion and to decrease tissue damage in experimental septic shock.

COMPLEMENT INHIBITORS

Given the many disease states in which complement is one of the central mediators of pathology, it is no surprise that several complement inhibitors are in preclinical or clinical development for treatment of human diseases. These inhibitors take several different forms. Some are variations of physiologic inhibitors, whereas others are the products of molecular biologic searches for novel compounds.

It is important to consider where in the complement pathway to design an inhibitor to act. Inhibition of the activation pathways limits the production of biologically active peptides. All three pathways need to be inhibited, however, for this approach to be effective. Inhibiting the activation of C3 not only prevents the generation of the C3a anaphylatoxin but also may leave the patient susceptible to infection by limiting the deposition of C3b on targets as an opsonin. Inhibition of C3b deposition also theoretically would decrease the patient's ability to clear immune complexes, resulting in renal, pulmonary, and vascular damage. It also might promote the development of antibodies to self-antigens.

Inhibition of the C5 convertases is an attractive goal because it would prevent the generation of the C5a anaphylatoxin and the MAC. This strategy would inhibit complement activation from any cause without the potentially immunosuppressive effects of limiting C3b deposition. Inhibitors based on this concept are the farthest along in clinical trials.

Other concerns about complement inhibition include the questions whether it is short-term or long-term and whether it is systemic or localized. Long-term inhibition of complement, particularly at early steps, is likely to predispose the patient to infection. Short-term (hours to days) inhibition at any step is unlikely to cause problems. Given that inflammation is usually a local phenomenon, there are several mechanisms being tested to target complement inhibitors to these sites. In this way, higher levels of inhibition can be achieved where needed with lower doses of inhibitor.

Natural Complement Inhibitors

There is a large literature on naturally occurring compounds that control complement activation. These include products or extracts of plants, fungi, insects, venoms, and cell lines. The mechanism of complement inhibition by some of these natural products is known and is of clinical and experimental importance. Cobra venom factor isolated from *Naja naja* is a 144,000-D glycoprotein that forms an alternative pathway convertase in association with Bb; this leads to massive activation of complement that causes pulmonary microvascular injury in experimental animals. This injury is usually not fatal, however, and the end result is a total depletion of complement that lasts 4 to 6 days. During this window, it has been possible to show the importance of the complement system in animal models of immune complex vasculitis, glomerulonephritis, multiple sclerosis, and graft rejection.

Perhaps the most widely used natural inhibitor of complement activation is heparin. Although heparin has been known to inhibit complement since 1929, the mechanism is not clear. It decreases activation of the classical and the alternative pathways. It has been reported to block association of C3b with Bb, inhibit binding of C4 to C1s and C2, and inactivate C1q. In clinical practice, the anticomplementary effect of heparin has been used to prevent complement activation during cardiopulmonary bypass. Measurement of complement activation products such as C3a or soluble C5b-9 after bypass showed decreases of 35 to 70% for adult and pediatric patients when heparin-coated extracorporeal circuits (e.g., Duraflo II) were used. Although numerous studies have looked at the decrease in complement activation by heparin-coated bypass circuits, there have been few attempts to correlate this with clinical outcome.

Soluble CR1

Soluble CR1 (sCR1) was the first rationally designed complement inhibitor to undergo extensive testing. The idea behind the use of this RCA protein was that it had multiple mechanisms of action. It has two separate binding sites for C3b and one for C4b. It not only serves as a cofactor for the enzymatic degradation of C3b and C4b but also can dissociate the classical (C3b4b) and the alternative (C3b2) C5 convertases. It is produced by recombinant methodology in animal cells. It consists of the entire extracellular portion of CR1 (30 SCRs). A modified version is produced in a manner that decorates the protein with the carbohydrate sialyl Lewis^x, the ligand for P-selectin and E-selectin. This modification targets sCR1 directly to activated (inflamed) endothelium. Another modified form of sCR1 has been developed that contains, rather than the entire 30-SCR protein, just the first three SCRs that retain complement-inactivating capacity in association with a cationic peptide at the C terminus followed by a myristyl group. This sCR1 targets the protein to the lipid membrane of cells. This technique has been shown to be effective in situations in which sCR1 can be delivered locally, such as intra-articular injections or the perfusion of donor organs before transplantation.

Similar to its membrane-bound counterpart, sCR1 binds C3b and C4b and blocks human classical and alternative pathway activation. It also blocks activation of complement in many experimental animals, leading to almost 100 publications describing its utility in a wide number of disease models.

The first disease model that was tested with sCR1 was myocardial ischemia-reperfusion injury in rats. These disease models include intestinal ischemia in mice and rats and middle cerebral artery ligation in mice. In each case, the administration of sCR1 was associated with decreased tissue injury, less neutrophil accumulation, and lower concentrations of inflammatory mediators, such as leukotriene B_4. In allograft transplantation, the donor organ undergoes significant ischemia-reperfusion injury. Animal models of allogeneic renal and lung transplantation have shown that sCR1 prolongs graft survival, which may prevent early rejection episodes. In pig-to-primate cardiac xenotransplantation, sCR1 prolonged graft survival remarkably. In one study of human lung transplantation, patients were randomly assigned to receive or not receive a single infusion of 10 mg/kg of sCR1 before restoration of blood flow in the graft. Complement activation was suppressed for 2 days after surgery. There were trends for all patients toward decreased time on the ventilator and in the intensive care unit that did not reach statistical significance. For patients who had been receiving cardiopulmonary bypass during surgery (and may have had more complement activation), however, there was a 56% decrease ($P = .035$) in time spent on the ventilator postoperatively if they were treated with sCR1.

sCR1 has been tested in models of autoimmune disease. Given intravenously, sCR1 delays the onset of collagen-induced arthritis in rats and inhibits the progression of established disease. In experimental autoimmune neuritis, a model for Guillain-Barré syndrome, daily sCR1 administration prevented the development of paresis and sciatic nerve damage. Similar beneficial results were seen in models of myasthenia gravis, multiple sclerosis, and glomerulonephritis.

CD55-CD46

Another soluble RCA protein under development as a therapeutic complement inhibitor is based on DAF and MCP. As stated earlier, DAF acts as only a decay accelerator of C3 and C5 convertases, whereas MCP acts as a cofactor for the degradation of C3. A recombinant fusion protein has been made that uses the four SCRs of MCP followed by the four SCRs of DAF. This protein now has decay-accelerating and cofactor activity, similar to sCR1.

Transgenic Animals

Xenotransplantation offers a solution to the chronic lack of solid organs for transplantation. The most studied donor animal is the pig, because swine have many desirable experimental and practical characteristics, such as size and ease of production. Although immunosuppression and other strategies may be able to overcome cellular immune barriers, the most pressing current problem facing xenotransplantation is hyperacute rejection. This is the immediate (within minutes) cessation of graft function owing to natural IgM antibodies that react with the vascular endothelium of the xenograft. The target of these antibodies is mainly the carbohydrate moiety galactose-(α1,3)-galactose present on the graft. These antibodies quickly activate complement, leading to intravascular coagulation, tissue edema, hemorrhage, and endothelial activation. Prevention of hyperacute rejection would require reducing the levels of antibodies or of their antigens, inhibiting complement activation, or a combination of all three.

Because complement regulatory proteins display species specificity, the approach to limit complement activation in xenografts has been to make transgenic pigs that express one or more membrane proteins of human origin. In one approach, pigs were generated that were transgenic for human CD55 (DAF), CD59, and the enzyme α1,3-fucosyltransferase. This enzyme modifies the carbohydrate antigen and has been shown to prolong the life of orthotopic heart transplants in mice. Kidneys from the triple-transgenic pigs were transplanted into bilaterally nephrectomized baboons. No immunosuppression or pretreatment of the recipients was given. Under these circumstances, the function of a nontransgenic pig kidney ceases within 3 minutes, and the graft rapidly becomes nonviable. The function of transgenic kidneys was maintained with good urine output for 3 to 5 days in the six baboons that received these grafts.

C3A and C5A Receptor Antagonists

The profound biologic effects of the anaphylatoxins and the many conditions in which C3a and/or C5a are believed to play a pathologic role make the development of specific inhibitors of these proteins attractive. Because the active portion of the anaphylatoxins is contained in the C-terminal part of the protein, it is possible that small-molecule antagonists could be developed that are orally available, easy to synthesize, and inexpensive. These are all advantages over the use of biologics such as monoclonal antibodies or recombinant RCA proteins.

To date, several synthetic C5a antagonists have been described. One is a cyclic analogue of C5a, acetyl-Phe[L-ornithine-Pro-D-cyclohexylalanine-Trp-Arg]. This compound inhibits C5a binding to CD88 with a 50% inhibitory concentration (IC_{50}) of 20 nmol/L. In vivo, it inhibits an Arthus-type reaction, completely blocking vascular permeability, cellular efflux, and systemic production of IL-6 and TNF. The other C5a antagonist that has been studied is a mutant version of C5a itself, which was selected using random phage methodology. This compond also was effective in inhibition of Arthus reactions in mice and prevention of ischemia-reperfusion injury. C5a inhibitors are in early human clinical trials. Finally, a potent small-molecule inhibitor of C3a has been reported. This compound is active in vitro as an inhibitor of C3a-mediated cellular activation, chemotaxis, and smooth muscle contraction.

Anti-Factor B

Inactivation of the factor B gene in mice prevents a number of autoimmune or inflammatory diseases. Presumably, this represents the necessity for an intact alternative pathway to amplify subclinical complement activation. Inhibition of the alternative pathway activation loop is an attractive target for therapy, because it would allow for protective immunity against pathogens through the classical pathway. The efficacy of this approach has been demonstrated using a monoclonal antibody to factor B that inhibits its function. This antibody blocks activation of the alternative pathway in the serum of a number of species, including mice, rats, nonhuman primates, and humans. In a mouse model of complement-mediated pregnancy loss, administration of the anti-factor B antibody resulted in a 50% decrease in fetal death. In models of asthma and renal ischemia-reperfusion injury, this antibody ameliorated disease. This strategy could have wide applicability in a number of disease states.

Anti-C5

The complement inhibitor that has achieved the widest attention as a potential therapeutic agent is a monoclonal antibody to C5. The advantage to this strategy is that it prevents the generation of C5a, the most potent of the anaphylatoxins, and of the MAC. The generation of C3b and C4b opsonins still would occur, allowing proper clearance of pathogens and immune complexes even if C5 conversion were inhibited chronically. Because there is evidence that activation of early complement components is important for the maintenance of tolerance to self-antigens, inhibition of C5 activation would be less worrisome than inhibition of C3 activation. Lastly, there seems to be little detrimental effect of genetic C5 deficiency. Certain inbred mouse strains are C5 deficient with no apparent increase in infections or decrease in lifespan. The only consequence of C5 deficiency in humans seems to be an increased risk of *Neisseria* infection.

Several groups have reported the use of an anti-C5 monoclonal antibody in either complement activation assays or animal model systems. All of these antibodies block the formation of the MAC, and a subset of them also block the generation of C5a. These are the anti-C5 monoclonal antibodies that have been selected for clinical development.

Arthritis

The availability of naturally C5-deficient mice has enabled the generation of monoclonal mouse anti–mouse C5 to test some of these therapies. Collagen-induced arthritis is a model for human rheumatoid arthritis. Mice are immunized with bovine type II collagen in complete Freund's adjuvant, resulting in an inflammatory peripheral arthritis with histopathology similar to rheumatoid arthritis. Treatment of the mice with anti-C5 for 3 weeks before the first immunization with collagen decreased the level of total hemolytic complement by about 60%. It totally prevented the appearance of arthritis in the mice. Histology of mice with arthritis that received a control antibody showed the typical proliferative synovitis with neutrophil and monocyte infiltration along with cartilage loss and bone erosion. In contrast, the anti-C5–treated mice had normal joints with smooth articular surfaces. The investigators then looked at the ability of anti-C5 to ameliorate established disease. Either anti-C5 or control antibody was given only after arthritis was evident clinically. The mice that received control antibody exhibited continued increases in paw thickness, clinical score, and number of joints involved. The mice treated with anti-C5 showed a halt in the progression of the arthritis and some indication of regression of disease, with a significant decrease in the number of joint erosions. These and other results have led to clinical trials of anti-C5 in human rheumatoid arthritis, paroxysmal nocturnal hemoglobinuria, membranoproliferative glomerulonephritis, and lupus nephritis.

Cardiopulmonary Bypass and Myocardial Ischemia

A smaller version of the anti-C5 antibody has been produced as a "single-chain Fv" that is a recombinant protein of approximately 30,000 molecular weight with characteristics of the Fab portion of the original monoclonal antibody. It binds to C5 and inhibits the C5 convertases with almost identical effectiveness as the intact antibody. This reagent is being developed for use in unstable angina, thrombolysis/angioplasty after myocardial infarction, and myocardial damage after cardiopulmonary bypass.

Graft Rejection

Similar to soluble CR1 and the other complement inhibitors described, anti-C5 treatment has been used to prolong xenograft survival. These results suggest that anti-C5 could play a role in managing acute graft rejection in humans.

Other Inflammatory Conditions

Anti-C5 has several other therapeutic uses. It has been shown to delay the onset of proteinuria and prolong survival in the (NZB × NZW)F_1 mouse model of SLE.

SUGGESTED READINGS

Girardi G, Bulla R, Salmon JE, Tedesco F: The complement system in the pathophysiology of pregnancy. Mol Immunol 2005;43:68–77. *A comprehensive discussion of the human and animal data on the essential role of complement in the antiphospholipid syndrome.*

Kemper C, Atkinson JP: T-cell regulation: With complements from innate immunity. Nat Rev Immunol 2007;7:9–18. *Reviews the role of complement in regulating T cells.*

Mastellos D, Germenis AE, Lambris JD: Complement: An inflammatory pathway fulfilling multiple roles at the interface of innate immunity and development. Curr Drug Targets Inflamm Allergy 2005;4:125–127. *An intriguing analysis of the data suggesting a critical role of complement in development and regeneration.*

Toapanta FR, Ross TM: Complement mediated activation of the adaptive immune responses: Role of C3d in linking the innate and adaptive immunity. Immunol Res 2006;36:197–210. *Overview of the importance of C3.*

Cecil Medicine 23

Section VIII

Cardiovascular Disease

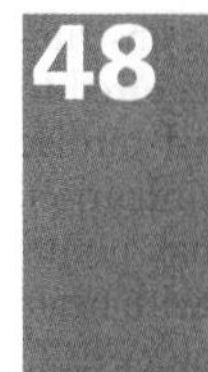

48 APPROACH TO THE PATIENT WITH POSSIBLE CARDIOVASCULAR DISEASE

Lee Goldman

Patients with cardiovascular disease may present with a wide range of symptoms and signs, each of which may be caused by noncardiovascular conditions. Conversely, patients with substantial cardiovascular disease may be asymptomatic. Because cardiovascular disease is a leading cause of death in the United States and other developed countries, it is crucial that patients be evaluated carefully to detect early cardiovascular disease, that symptoms or signs of cardiovascular disease be evaluated in detail, and that appropriate therapy be instituted. Improvements in diagnosis, therapy, and prevention have contributed to a 70% or so decline in age-adjusted cardiovascular death rates in the United States since the 1960s. However, the absolute number of deaths from cardiovascular disease in the United States has not declined proportionately because of the increase in the population older than 40 years as well as the aging of the population in general.

In evaluating a patient with known or suspected heart disease, the physician must determine quickly whether a potentially life-threatening condition exists. In these situations, the evaluation must focus on the specific issue at hand and be accompanied by the rapid performance of appropriately directed additional tests. Examples of potentially life-threatening conditions include acute myocardial infarction (Chapter 72), unstable angina (Chapter 71), suspected aortic dissection (Chapter 78), pulmonary edema (Chapter 58), and pulmonary embolism (Chapter 99).

USING THE HISTORY TO DETECT CARDIOVASCULAR SYMPTOMS

Patients may complain spontaneously of a variety of cardiovascular symptoms (Table 48–1), but sometimes these symptoms are elicited only by obtaining a careful, complete medical history. In patients with known or suspected cardiovascular disease, questions about cardiovascular symptoms are key components of the history of present illness; in other patients, these issues are a fundamental part of the review of systems.

Chest Pain

Chest discomfort or pain is the cardinal manifestation of myocardial ischemia resulting from coronary artery disease or any condition that causes myocardial ischemia by an imbalance of myocardial oxygen demand compared with myocardial oxygen supply (Chapter 70). New, acute, often ongoing pain may indicate an acute myocardial infarction, unstable angina, or aortic dissection; a pulmonary cause, such as acute pulmonary embolism or pleural irritation; a musculoskeletal condition of the chest wall, thorax, or shoulder; or a gastrointestinal abnormality, such as esophageal reflux or spasm, peptic ulcer disease, or cholecystitis (Table 48–2). The chest discomfort of myocardial infarction commonly occurs without an immediate or obvious precipitating clinical cause and builds in intensity for at least several minutes; the sensation can range from annoying discomfort to severe pain (Chapter 72). Although a variety of adjectives may be used by patients to describe the sensation, physicians must be suspicious of any discomfort, especially if it radiates to the neck, shoulder, or arms. The chest discomfort of unstable angina is clinically indistinguishable from that of myocardial infarction except that the former may be precipitated more clearly by activity and may be more rapidly responsive to antianginal therapy (Chapter 71). Aortic dissection (Chapter 78) classically presents with the sudden onset of severe pain in the chest and radiating to the back; the location of the pain often provides clues to the location of the dissection. Ascending aortic dissections commonly present with chest discomfort radiating to the back, whereas dissections of the descending aorta commonly present with back pain radiating to the abdomen. The presence of back pain or a history of hypertension or other predisposing factors, such as Marfan syndrome, should prompt a careful assessment of peripheral pulses to determine if the great vessels are affected by the dissection and of the chest radiograph to evaluate the size of the aorta. If this initial evaluation is suggestive, further testing with transesophageal echocardiography, computed tomography, or magnetic resonance imaging is indicated. The pain of pericarditis (Chapter 77) may simulate that of an acute myocardial infarction, may be primarily pleuritic, or may be continuous; a key physical finding is a pericardial rub. The pain of pulmonary embolism (Chapter 99) is commonly pleuritic in nature and is associated with dyspnea; hemoptysis also may be present. Pulmonary hypertension (Chapter 67) of any cause may be associated with chest discomfort with exertion; it commonly is associated with severe dyspnea and often is associated with cyanosis.

Recurrent, episodic chest discomfort may be noted with angina pectoris and with many cardiac and noncardiac causes (Chapter 70). A variety of stress tests can be used to provoke reversible myocardial ischemia in susceptible individuals and to help determine whether ischemia is the pathophysiologic explanation for the chest discomfort (Chapter 70).

Dyspnea

Dyspnea, which is an uncomfortable awareness of breathing, is commonly due to cardiovascular or pulmonary disease. A systematic approach (Fig. 48–1) with selected tests (see Table 83–4) nearly always reveals the cause. Acute dyspnea can be caused by myocardial ischemia, heart failure, severe hypertension, pericardial tamponade, pulmonary embolism, pneumothorax, upper airway obstruction, acute bronchitis or pneumonia, or some drug overdoses (e.g., salicylates). Subacute or chronic dyspnea is also a common presenting or accompanying symptom in patients with pulmonary disease (Chapter 83). Dyspnea also can be caused by severe anemia (Chapter 162) and can be confused with the fatigue that often is noted in patients with systemic and neurologic diseases (Chapters 277 and 418).

In heart failure, dyspnea typically is noted as a hunger for air and a need or an urge to breathe. The feeling that breathing requires increased work or effort is more typical of airway obstruction or neuromuscular disease. A feeling of chest tightness or constriction during breathing is typical of bronchoconstriction, which is commonly caused by obstructive airway disease (Chapters 87 and 88) but also may be seen in pulmonary edema. A feeling of heavy breathing, a feeling of rapid breathing, or a need to breathe more is classically associated with deconditioning.

In cardiovascular conditions, chronic dyspnea usually is caused by increases in pulmonary venous pressure as a result of left ventricular failure (Chapters 57 and 58) or valvular heart disease (Chapter 75). Orthopnea, which is an exacerbation of dyspnea when the patient is recumbent, is due to increased work of breathing because of either increased venous return to the pulmonary vasculature or loss of gravitational assistance in diaphragmatic effort. Paroxysmal nocturnal dyspnea is severe dyspnea that awakens a patient at night and forces the assumption of a sitting or standing position to achieve gravitational redistribution of fluid.

Palpitations

Palpitations (Chapter 61) describe a subjective sensation of an irregular or abnormal heartbeat. Palpitations may be caused by any arrhythmia (Chapters 63 and 64) with or without important underlying structural heart disease. Palpitations should be defined in terms of the duration and frequency of the episodes; the precipitating and related factors; and any associated symptoms of chest pain, dyspnea, lightheadedness, or syncope. It is crucial to use the history to determine whether the palpitations are caused by an irregular or a regular heartbeat. The feeling associated with a premature atrial or ventricular contraction, often described as a "skipped beat" or a "flip-flopping of the heart," must be distinguished from the irregularly irregular rhythm of atrial fibrillation and the rapid but regular rhythm of supraventricular tachycardia. Associated symptoms of chest pain, dyspnea, lightheadedness, dizziness, or diaphoresis suggest an important effect on cardiac output and mandate further evaluation. In general, evaluation begins with ambulatory electrocardiography (ECG) (Table 48–3), which is indicated in patients who have palpitations in the presence of structural heart disease or substantial accompanying symptoms. Depending on the series, 9 to 43% of patients have important underlying heart disease. In such patients, more detailed evaluation is warranted (see Fig. 61–1).

Lightheadedness or *syncope* (Chapters 61 and 427) can be caused by any condition that decreases cardiac output (e.g., bradyarrhythmia, tachyarrhythmia, obstruction of the left ventricular or right ventricular inflow or outflow, cardiac tamponade, aortic dissection, or severe pump failure), by reflex-mediated vasomotor instability (e.g., vasovagal, situational, or carotid sinus syncope), or by orthostatic hypotension (see Table 427–1). Neurologic diseases (e.g., migraine headaches, transient ischemic attacks, or seizures) also can cause transient loss of consciousness. The history, physical examination, and ECG are often diagnostic of the cause of syncope (see Table 427–2). Syncope caused by a cardiac arrhythmia usually occurs with little warning. Syncope with exertion or just after conclusion of exertion is typical of aortic stenosis and hypertrophic obstructive cardiomyopathy. In many patients, additional testing is required to document central nervous system disease, the cause of reduced cardiac output, or carotid sinus syncope. When the history, physical examination, and ECG do not provide helpful diagnostic information that points toward a specific cause of syncope, it is imperative that patients with heart disease or an abnormal ECG be tested with continuous ambulatory ECG monitoring to diagnose a possible arrhythmia (see Fig. 427–1); in selected patients, formal electrophysiologic testing may be indicated (Chapter 61). In patients with no evident heart disease, tilt testing (Chapters 61 and 427) can help detect reflex-mediated vasomotor instability.

TABLE 48–1 CARDINAL SYMPTOMS OF CARDIOVASCULAR DISEASE

Chest pain or discomfort
Dyspnea, orthopnea, paroxysmal nocturnal dyspnea, wheezing
Palpitations, dizziness, syncope
Cough, hemoptysis
Fatigue, weakness
Pain in extremities with exertion (claudication)

Other Symptoms

Nonproductive *cough* (Chapter 83), especially a persistent cough (see Fig. 83–1), can be an early manifestation of elevated pulmonary venous pressure and otherwise unsuspected heart failure. *Fatigue* and *weakness* are common accompaniments of advanced cardiac disease and reflect an inability to perform normal activities. A variety of approaches have been used to classify the severity of cardiac limitations, ranging from class I (little or no limitation) to class IV (severe limitation) (Table 48–4). *Hemoptysis* (Chapter 83) is a classic presenting finding in patients with

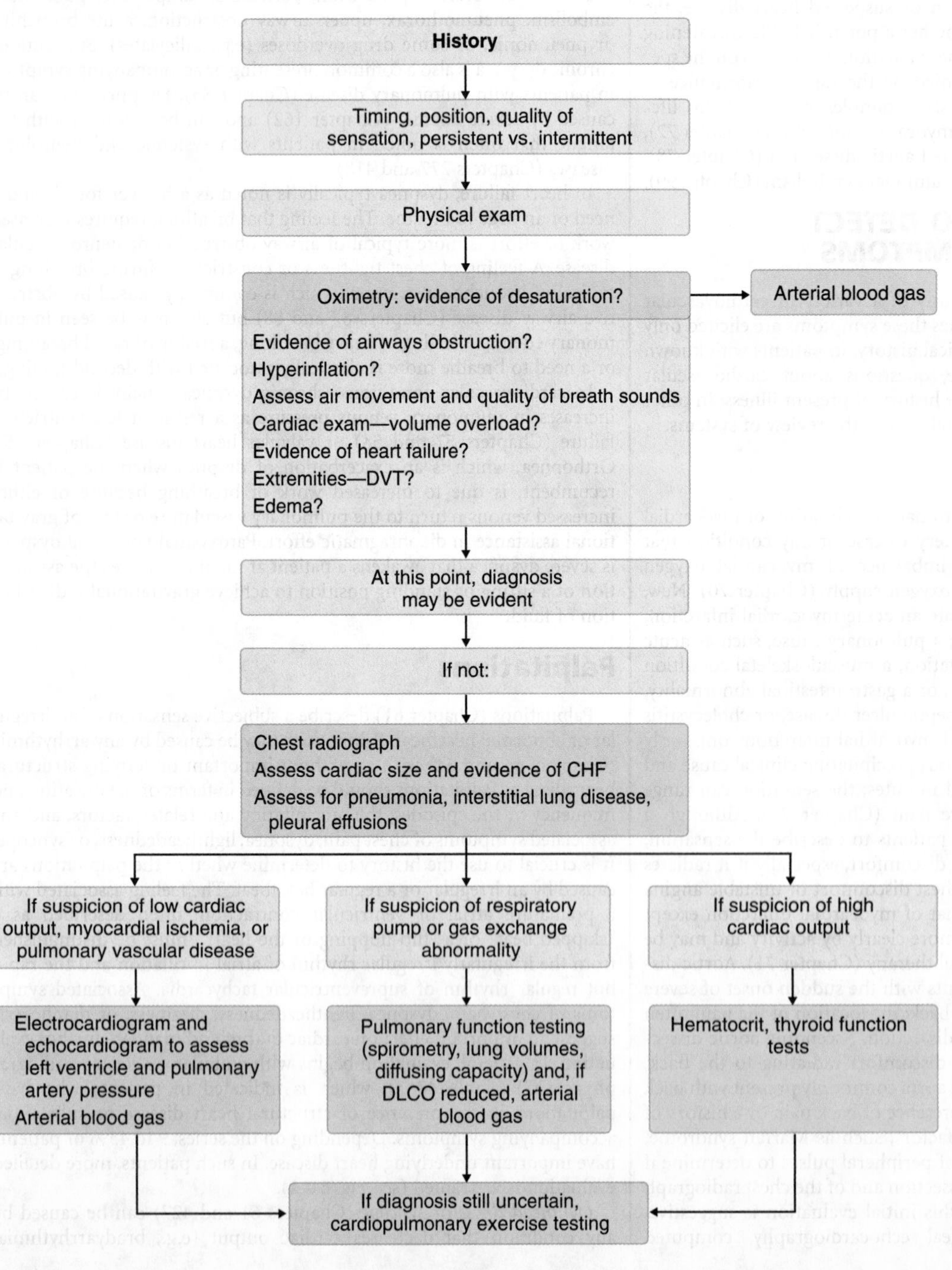

FIGURE 48–1 • Algorithm for the evaluation of a patient with dyspnea. The pace and completeness with which one approaches this framework depend on the intensity and acuity of the patient's symptoms. In a patient with severe, acute dyspnea, an arterial blood gas measurement may be one of the first laboratory evaluations, whereas it might not be obtained until much later in the work-up of a patient with chronic breathlessness of unclear cause. A therapeutic trial of a medication, such as a bronchodilator, may be instituted at any point if one is fairly confident of the diagnosis on the basis of data available at that time. CHF = congestive heart failure; DLCO = diffusing capacity of the lung for carbon monoxide; DVT = deep venous thrombosis. (From Schwartzstein RM, Feller-Kopman D: Approach to the patient with dyspnea. *In* Braunwald E, Goldman L [eds]: Primary Cardiology, 2nd ed. Philadelphia, WB Saunders, 2003.)

TABLE 48–2 CAUSES OF CHEST PAIN

Condition	Location	Quality	Duration	Aggravating or Relieving Factors	Associated Symptoms or Signs
CARDIOVASCULAR CAUSES					
Angina	Retrosternal region; radiates to or occasionally isolated to neck, jaw, epigastrium, shoulder, or arms (left common)	Pressure, burning, squeezing, heaviness, indigestion	<2–10 min	Precipitated by exercise, cold weather, or emotional stress; relieved by rest or nitroglycerin; atypical (Prinzmetal's) angina may be unrelated to activity, often early morning	S_3 or murmur of papillary muscle dysfunction during pain
Rest or unstable angina	Same as angina	Same as angina but may be more severe	Usually <20 min	Same as angina, with decreasing tolerance for exertion or at rest	Similar to stable angina, but may be pronounced; transient heart failure can occur
Myocardial infarction	Substernal and may radiate like angina	Heaviness, pressure, burning, constriction	≥30 min but variable	Unrelieved by rest or nitroglycerin	Shortness of breath, sweating, weakness, nausea, vomiting
Pericarditis	Usually begins over sternum or toward cardiac apex and may radiate to neck or left shoulder; often more localized than the pain of myocardial ischemia	Sharp, stabbing, knifelike	Lasts many hours to days; may wax and wane	Aggravated by deep breathing, rotating chest, or supine position; relieved by sitting up and leaning forward	Pericardial friction rub
Aortic dissection	Anterior chest; may radiate to back	Excruciating, tearing, knifelike	Sudden onset, unrelenting	Usually occurs in setting of hypertension or predisposition, such as Marfan syndrome	Murmur of aortic insufficiency, pulse or blood pressure asymmetry; neurologic deficit
Pulmonary embolism (chest pain often not present)	Substernal or over region of pulmonary infarction	Pleuritic (with pulmonary infarction) or angina-like	Sudden onset; minutes to <1 hr	May be aggravated by breathing	Dyspnea, tachypnea, tachycardia; hypotension, signs of acute right ventricular failure, and pulmonary hypertension with large emboli; rales, pleural rub, hemoptysis with pulmonary infarction
Pulmonary hypertension	Substernal	Pressure; oppressive	Similar to angina	Aggravated by effort	Pain usually associated with dyspnea; signs of pulmonary hypertension
NONCARDIAC CAUSES					
Pneumonia with pleurisy	Localized over involved area	Pleuritic, localized	Brief or prolonged	Painful breathing	Dyspnea, cough, fever, dull to percussion, bronchial breath sounds, rales, occasional pleural rub
Spontaneous pneumothorax	Unilateral	Sharp, well localized	Sudden onset, lasts many hours	Painful breathing	Dyspnea; hyperresonance and decreased breath and voice sounds over involved lung
Musculoskeletal disorders	Variable	Aching	Short or long duration	Aggravated by movement; history of muscle exertion or injury	Tender to pressure or movement
Herpes zoster	Dermatomal in distribution	Burning, itching	Prolonged	None	Vesicular rash appears in area of discomfort
Esophageal reflux	Substernal, epigastric	Burning, visceral discomfort	10–60 min	Aggravated by large meal, postprandial recumbency; relief with antacid	Water brash
Peptic ulcer	Epigastric, substernal	Visceral burning, aching	Prolonged	Relief with food, antacid	
Gallbladder disease	Epigastric, right upper quadrant	Visceral	Prolonged	May be unprovoked or follow meals	Right upper quadrant tenderness may be present
Anxiety states	Often localized over precordium	Variable; location often moves from place to place	Varies; often fleeting	Situational	Sighing respirations, often chest wall tenderness

Modified from Andreoli TE, Carpenter CCJ, Griggs RC, Loscalzo J: Evaluation of the patient with cardiovascular disease. *In* Cecil Essentials of Medicine, 6th ed. Philadelphia, WB Saunders, 2004, pp 34–35.

TABLE 48–3 AMERICAN HEART ASSOCIATION/AMERICAN COLLEGE OF CARDIOLOGY GUIDELINES FOR USE OF DIAGNOSTIC TESTS IN PATIENTS WITH PALPITATIONS*

AMBULATORY ELECTROCARDIOGRAPHY	
Class I	Palpitations, syncope, dizziness
Class II	Shortness of breath, chest pain, or fatigue (not otherwise explained, episodic, and strongly suggestive of an arrhythmia as the cause because of a relation of the symptom with palpitation)
Class III	Symptoms not reasonably expected to be due to arrhythmia
ELECTROPHYSIOLOGIC STUDY	
Class I	1. Patients with palpitations who have a pulse rate documented by medical personnel as inappropriately rapid and in whom electrocardiographic recordings fail to document the cause of the palpitations 2. Patients with palpitations preceding a syncopal episode
Class II	Patients with clinically significant palpitations, suspected to be of cardiac origin, in whom symptoms are sporadic and cannot be documented; studies are performed to determine the mechanisms of arrhythmias, to direct or provide therapy, or to assess prognosis
Class III	Patients with palpitations documented to be due to extracardiac causes (e.g., hyperthyroidism)
ECHOCARDIOGRAPHY	
Class I	Arrhythmias with evidence of heart disease Family history of genetic disorder associated with arrhythmias
Class II	Arrhythmias commonly associated with, but without evidence of, heart disease Atrial fibrillation or flutter
Class III	Palpitations without evidence of arrhythmias Minor arrhythmias without evidence of heart disease

*Class I, general agreement the test is useful and indicated; class II, frequently used, but there is a divergence of opinion with respect to its utility; class III, general agreement the test is not useful.
From Braunwald E, Goldman L (eds): Primary Cardiology, 2nd ed. Philadelphia, WB Saunders, 2003, p 132.

pulmonary embolism, but it is also common in patients with mitral stenosis, pulmonary edema, pulmonary infections, and malignant neoplasms (see Table 83–5). *Claudication*, which is pain in the extremities with exertion, should alert the physician to possible peripheral arterial disease (Chapters 79 and 80).

Complete Medical History

The complete medical history should include a thorough review of systems, family history, social history, and past medical history (Chapter 13). The review of systems may reveal other symptoms that suggest a systemic disease as the cause of any cardiovascular problems. The family history should focus on premature atherosclerosis or evidence of familial abnormalities, such as may be found with various causes of the long QT syndrome (Chapter 64) or hypertrophic cardiomyopathy (Chapter 59).

The social history should include specific questioning about cigarette smoking, alcohol intake, and use of illicit drugs. The past medical history may reveal prior conditions or medications that suggest systemic diseases, ranging from chronic obstructive pulmonary disease, which may explain a complaint of dyspnea, to hemochromatosis, which may be a cause of restrictive cardiomyopathy. A careful history to inquire about recent dental work or other procedures is crucial if bacterial endocarditis is part of the differential diagnosis.

PHYSICAL EXAMINATION FOR DETECTION OF SIGNS OF CARDIOVASCULAR DISEASE

The cardiovascular physical examination, which is a subset of the complete physical examination, provides important clues to the diagnosis of asymptomatic and symptomatic cardiac disease and may reveal cardiovascular manifestations of noncardiovascular diseases. The cardiovascular physical examination begins with careful measurement of the pulse and blood pressure (Chapter 7). If aortic dissection (Chapter 78) is a consideration, blood pressure should be measured in both arms and, preferably, in at least one leg. When coarctation of the aorta is suspected (Chapter 68), blood pressure must be measured in at least one leg and in the arms. Discrepancies in blood pressure between the two arms also can be caused by atherosclerotic disease of the great vessels. Pulsus paradoxus, which is more than the usual 10 mm Hg drop in systolic blood presure during inspiration, is typical of pericardial tamponade (Chapter 77).

General Appearance

The respiratory rate may be increased in patients with heart failure. Patients with pulmonary edema are usually markedly tachypneic and may have labored breathing. Patients with advanced heart failure may have Cheyne-Stokes respirations.

Systemic diseases, such as hyperthyroidism (Chapter 244), hypothyroidism (Chapter 244), rheumatoid arthritis (Chapter 285), scleroderma (Chapter 288), and hemochromatosis (Chapter 231), may be suspected from the patient's general appearance. Marfan syndrome (Chapter 281), Turner's syndrome (Chapter 255), Down syndrome (Chapter 39), and a variety of congenital anomalies also may be readily apparent.

Ophthalmologic Examination

Examination of the fundi may show diabetic (see Fig. 449–15) or hypertensive retinopathy (see Fig. 66–11) or Roth's spots (see Fig. 449–17) typical of infectious endocarditis. Beading of the retinal arteries is typical of severe hypercholesterolemia. Osteogenesis imperfecta, which is associated with blue sclerae, also is associated with aortic dilation and mitral valve prolapse. Retinal artery occlusion (see Fig. 449–20) may be caused by an embolus from clot in the left atrium or left ventricle, a left atrial myxoma, or atherosclerotic debris from the great vessels. Hyperthyroidism may present with exophthalmos and typical stare (see Fig. 449–14), whereas myotonic dystrophy, which is associated with atrioventricular block and arrhythmia, often is associated with ptosis and an expressionless face (see Fig. 447–2).

Jugular Veins

The external jugular veins help in assessment of mean right atrial pressure, which normally varies between 5 and 10 cm H_2O; the height (in centimeters) of the central venous pressure is measured by adding 5 cm to the height of the observed jugular venous distention above the sternal angle of Louis (Fig. 48–2). The normal jugular venous pulse, best seen in the internal jugular vein (and not seen in the external jugular vein unless

TABLE 48–4 A COMPARISON OF THREE METHODS OF ASSESSING CARDIOVASCULAR DISABILITY

Class	New York Heart Association Functional Classification	Canadian Cardiovascular Society Functional Classification	Specific Activity Scale
I	Patients with cardiac disease but without resulting limitations of physical activity Ordinary physical activity does not cause undue fatigue, palpitation, dyspnea, or anginal pain.	Ordinary physical activity, such as walking and climbing stairs, does not cause angina. Angina with strenuous or rapid or prolonged exertion at work or recreation	Patients can perform to completion any activity requiring ≥7 metabolic equivalents, e.g., can carry 24 lb up 8 steps; carry objects that weigh 80 lb; do outdoor work (shovel snow, spade soil); do recreational activities (skiing, basketball, squash, handball, jog or walk 5 mph)
II	Patients with cardiac disease resulting in slight limitation of physical activity They are comfortable at rest. Ordinary physical activity results in fatigue, palpitations, dyspnea, or anginal pain.	Slight limitation of ordinary activity Walking or climbing stairs rapidly, walking uphill, walking or stair climbing after meals, in cold, in wind, or when under emotional stress, or only during the few hours after awakening Walking >2 blocks on the level and climbing >1 flight of ordinary stairs at a normal pace and in normal conditions	Patient can perform to completion any activity requiring ≥5 metabolic equivalents but cannot and does not perform to completion activities requiring ≥7 metabolic equivalents, e.g., have sexual intercourse without stopping, garden, rake, weed, roller skate, dance fox trot, walk at 4 mph on level ground
III	Patients with cardiac disease resulting in marked limitation of physical activity They are comfortable at rest. Less than ordinary physical activity causes fatigue, palpitations, dyspnea, or anginal pain.	Marked limitation of ordinary physical activity Walking 1 or 2 blocks on the level and climbing >1 flight in normal conditions	Patient can perform to completion any activity requiring ≥2 metabolic equivalents but cannot and does not perform to completion any activities requiring ≥5 metabolic equivalents, e.g., shower without stopping, strip and make bed, clean windows, walk 2.5 mph, bowl, play golf, dress without stopping
IV	Patients with cardiac disease resulting in inability to carry on any physical activity without discomfort Symptoms of cardiac insufficiency or of the anginal syndrome may be present even at rest. If any physical activity is undertaken, discomfort is increased.	Inability to carry on any physical activity without discomfort—anginal syndrome *may be* present at rest	Patient cannot or does not perform to completion activities requiring ≥2 metabolic equivalents; *cannot* carry out activities listed above (Specific Activity Scale, class III)

From Goldman L, Hashimoto B, Cook EF, Loscalzo A: Comparative reproducibility and validity of systems for assessing cardiovascular functional class: Advantages of a new specific activity scale. Circulation 1981;64:1227–1234. Reproduced by permission of the American Heart Association.

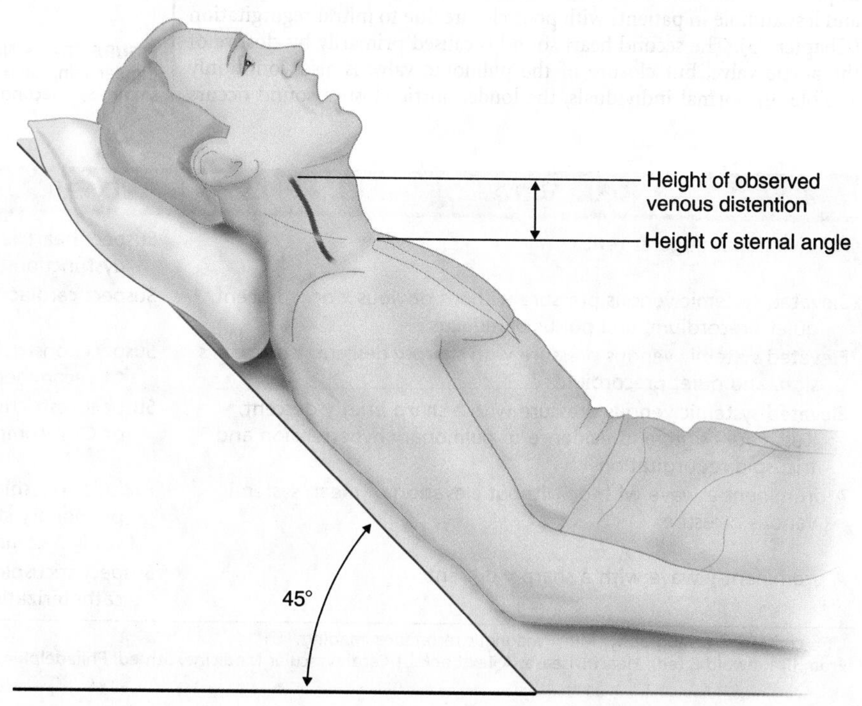

FIGURE 48–2 • Jugular venous distention is defined by engorgement of the internal jugular vein more than 5 cm above the sternal angle at 45%. The central venous pressure is the observed venous distention above the sternal angle plus 5 cm. (From American Academy of Family Physicians Online. *http://www.aafp.org/afp/20000301/1319.html.*)

insufficiency of the jugular venous valves is present), includes an *a* wave, caused by right atrial contraction; a *c* wave, reflecting carotid artery pulsation; an *x* descent; a *v* wave, which corresponds to isovolumetric right ventricular contraction and is more marked in the presence of tricuspid insufficiency; and a *y* descent, which occurs as the tricuspid valve opens and ventricular filling begins (Fig. 48–3). Abnormalities of the jugular venous pressure (Fig. 48–4) and pulse are useful in detecting conditions such as heart failure, pericardial disease, tricuspid valve disease, and pulmonary hypertension (Table 48–5).

Carotid Pulse

The carotid pulse should be examined in terms of its volume and contour. The carotid pulse (Fig. 48–5) may be increased in frequency and may be more intense than normal in patients with a higher stroke volume secondary to aortic regurgitation, arteriovenous fistula, hyperthyroidism, fever, or anemia. In aortic regurgitation or arteriovenous fistula, the pulse may have a bisferious quality. The carotid upstroke is delayed in patients with valvular aortic stenosis (Chapter 75) and has a normal contour but diminished amplitude in any cause of reduced stroke volume.

Cardiac Inspection and Palpation

Inspection of the precordium may reveal the hyperinflation of obstructive lung disease or unilateral asymmetry of the left side of the chest because of right ventricular hypertrophy before puberty. Palpation may be performed with the patient either supine or in the left lateral decubitus position; the latter position moves the left ventricular apex closer to the chest wall and increases the ability to palpate the point of maximal impulse and other phenomena. Low-frequency phenomena, such as systolic heaves or lifts from the left ventricle (at the cardiac apex) or right ventricle (parasternal in the third or fourth intercostal space), are felt best with the heel of the palm. With the patient in the left lateral decubitus position, this technique also may allow palpation of an S_3 gallop in cases of advanced heart failure or an S_4 gallop in cases of poor left ventricular distensibility during diastole. The left ventricular apex is more diffuse and sometimes may be frankly dyskinetic in patients with advanced heart disease. The distal palm is best for feeling thrills, which are the tactile equivalent of cardiac murmurs. By definition, a thrill denotes a murmur of grade 4/6 or louder. Higher frequency events may be felt best with the fingertips; examples include the opening snap of mitral stenosis or the loud pulmonic second sound of pulmonary hypertension.

Auscultation

The first heart sound (Fig. 48–6), which is largely produced by closure of the mitral and—to a lesser extent—the tricuspid valves, may be louder in patients with mitral valve stenosis and intact valve leaflet movement and less audible in patients with poor closure due to mitral regurgitation (Chapter 75). The second heart sound is caused primarily by closure of the aortic valve, but closure of the pulmonic valve is also commonly audible. In normal individuals, the louder aortic closure sound occurs

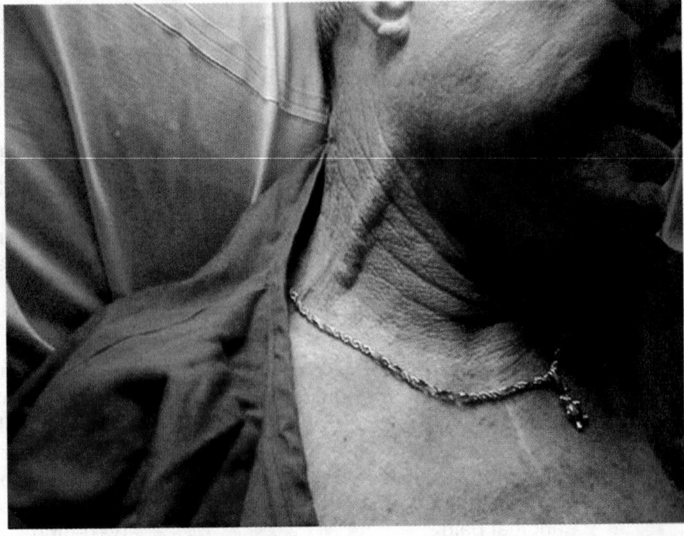

FIGURE 48–3 • Typical distention of the internal jugular vein. (From *http://courses.cvcc.vccs.edu/WisemanD/jugular_vein_distention.htm.*)

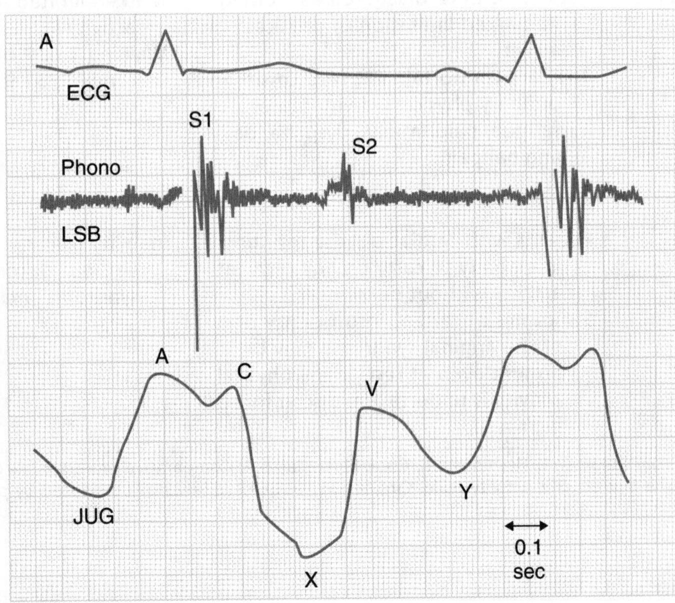

FIGURE 48–4 • Normal jugular venous pulse. ECG = electrocardiogram; JUG = jugular vein; LSB = left sternal border; phono = phonocardiogram; S_1 = first heart sound; S_2 = second heart sound.

TABLE 48–5 ABNORMALITIES OF VENOUS PRESSURE AND PULSE AND THEIR CLINICAL SIGNIFICANCE

Finding	Significance
Positive hepatojugular reflux	Suspect heart failure, particularly left ventricular systolic dysfunction (echocardiography recommended)
Elevated systemic venous pressure without obvious *x* or *y* descent, quiet precordium, and pulsus paradoxus	Suspect cardiac tamponade (echocardiography recommended)
Elevated systemic venous pressure with sharp *y* descent, Kussmaul's sign, and quiet precordium	Suspect constrictive pericarditis (cardiac catheterization and MRI or CT recommended)
Elevated systemic venous pressure with a sharp brief *y* descent, Kussmaul's sign, and evidence of pulmonary hypertension and tricuspid regurgitation	Suspect restrictive cardiomyopathy (cardiac catheterization and MRI or CT recommended)
A prominent *a* wave with or without elevation of mean systemic venous pressure	Exclude tricuspid stenosis, right ventricular hypertrophy due to pulmonary stenosis, and pulmonary hypertension (echo-Doppler study recommended)
A prominent *v* wave with a sharp *y* descent	Suspect tricuspid regurgitation (echo-Doppler or cardiac catheterization to determine etiology)

CT = computed tomography; MRI = magnetic resonance imaging.
From Braunwald E (ed): Heart Disease: A Textbook of Cardiovascular Medicine, 5th ed. Philadelphia, WB Saunders, 1997.

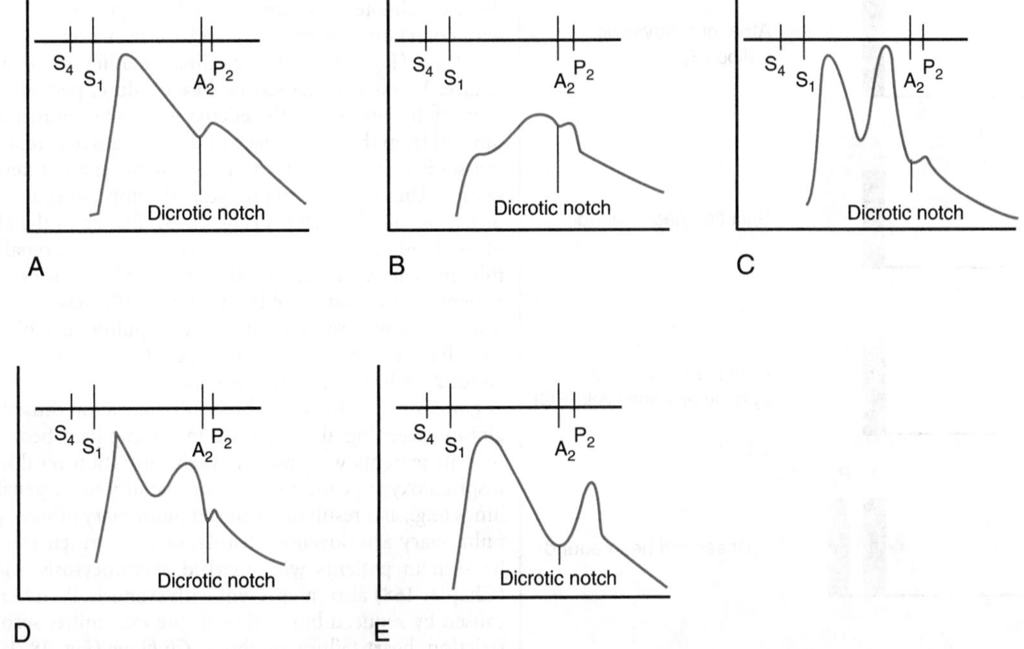

FIGURE 48–5 • Schematic diagrams of the configurational changes in the carotid pulse and their differential diagnosis. Heart sounds also are illustrated. **A,** Normal. **B,** Anacrotic pulse with slow initial upstroke. The peak is close to the second heart sound. These features suggest fixed left ventricular outflow obstruction, such as valvular aortic stenosis. **C,** Pulsus bisferiens, with percussion and tidal waves occurring during systole. This type of carotid pulse contour is observed most frequently in patients with hemodynamically significant aortic regurgitation or combined aortic stenosis and regurgitation with dominant regurgitation. It rarely is observed in patients with mitral valve prolapse or in normal individuals. **D,** Pulsus bisferiens in hypertrophic obstructive cardiomyopathy. This finding rarely is appreciated at the bedside by palpation. **E,** Dicrotic pulse results from an accentuated dicrotic wave and tends to occur in sepsis, severe heart failure, hypovolemic shock, and cardiac tamponade and after aortic valve replacement. A_2 = aortic component of the second heart sound; P_2 = pulmonary component of the second heart sound); S_1 = first heart sound; S_4 = atrial sounds. (From Chatterjee K: Bedside evaluation of the heart: The physical examination. *In* Chatterjee K, et al [eds]: Cardiology: An Illustrated Text/Reference. Philadelphia, JB Lippincott, 1991, pp 3.11–3.51.)

first, followed by pulmonic closure. With expiration, the two sounds are virtually superimposed. With inspiration, by comparison, the increased stroke volume of the right ventricle commonly leads to a discernible splitting of the second sound. This splitting may be fixed in patients with an atrial septal defect (Chapter 68) or a right bundle branch block. The split may be paradoxical in patients with left bundle branch block or other causes of delayed left ventricular emptying. The aortic component of the second sound is increased in intensity in the presence of systemic hypertension and decreased in intensity in patients with aortic stenosis. The pulmonic second sound is increased in the presence of pulmonary hypertension.

Early systolic ejection sounds are related to forceful opening of the aortic or pulmonic valve. These sounds are common in congenital aortic stenosis, with a mobile valve; in hypertension, with forceful opening of the aortic valve; and in healthy young individuals, especially when cardiac output is increased. Midsystolic or late systolic clicks are caused most commonly by mitral valve prolapse (Chapter 75). Clicks are relatively high frequency sounds that are heard best with the diaphragm of the stethoscope.

An S_3 corresponds to rapid ventricular filling during early diastole. It may occur in normal children and young adults, especially if stroke volume is increased. After about 40 years of age, however, an S_3 should be considered abnormal; it is caused by conditions that increase the volume of ventricular filling during early diastole (e.g., mitral regurgitation) or that increase pressure in early diastole (e.g., advanced heart failure). A left ventricular S_3 gallop is heard best at the apex, whereas the right ventricular S_3 gallop is heard best at the fourth intercostal space at the left parasternal border; both are heard best with the bell of the stethoscope. An S_4 is heard rarely in young individuals but is common in adults older than 40 or 50 years because of reduced ventricular compliance during atrial contraction; it is a nearly ubiquitous finding in patients with hypertension, heart failure, or ischemic heart disease.

The opening snap of mitral and, less commonly, tricuspid stenosis (Chapter 75) occurs at the beginning of mechanical diastole, before the onset of the rapid phase of ventricular filling. An opening snap is high pitched and is heard best with the diaphragm; this differential frequency should help distinguish an opening snap from an S_3 on physical examination. An opening snap commonly can be distinguished from a loud pulmonic component of the second heart sound by the differential location (mitral opening snap at the apex, tricuspid opening snap at the left third or fourth intercostal space, pulmonic second sound at the left second intercostal space) and by the longer interval between S_2 and the opening snap.

Heart murmurs may be classified as systolic, diastolic, or continuous (Table 48–6). Murmurs are graded by intensity on a scale of 1 to 6. Grade 1 is faint and appreciated only by careful auscultation; grade 2, readily audible; grade 3, moderately loud; grade 4, loud and associated with a palpable thrill; grade 5, loud and audible with the stethoscope only partially placed on the chest; and grade 6, loud enough to be heard without the stethoscope on the chest. Systolic ejection murmurs usually peak in early to mid systole when left ventricular ejection is maximal; examples include fixed valvular, supravalvular, or infravalvular aortic stenosis and pulmonic stenosis. The murmur of hypertrophic obstructive cardiomyopathy has a similar ejection quality, although its peak may be later in systole when dynamic obstruction is maximal (Chapter 59). Pansystolic murmurs are characteristic of mitral or tricuspid regurgitation or with a left-to-right shunt from conditions such as a ventricular septal defect (left ventricle to right ventricle). A late systolic murmur is characteristic of mitral valve prolapse (Chapter 75) or ischemic papillary muscle dysfunction. Ejection quality murmurs also may be heard in patients with normal valves but increased flow, such as occurs with marked anemia, fever, or bradycardia secondary to congenital complete heart block; they also may be heard across a valve that is downstream from increased flow because of an intracardiac shunt. Maneuvers such as inspiration, expiration, standing, squatting, and hand gripping can be especially useful in the differential diagnosis of a murmur; however, echocardiography commonly is required to make a definitive diagnosis of cause and severity (Table 48–7).

High-frequency, early diastolic murmurs are typical of aortic regurgitation and pulmonic regurgitation from a variety of causes. The murmurs of mitral and tricuspid stenosis begin in early to mid diastole and tend to diminish in intensity later in diastole in the absence of effective atrial contraction, but they tend to increase in intensity in later diastole if effective atrial contraction is present.

Continuous murmurs may be caused by any abnormality that is associated with a pressure gradient in systole and diastole. Examples include

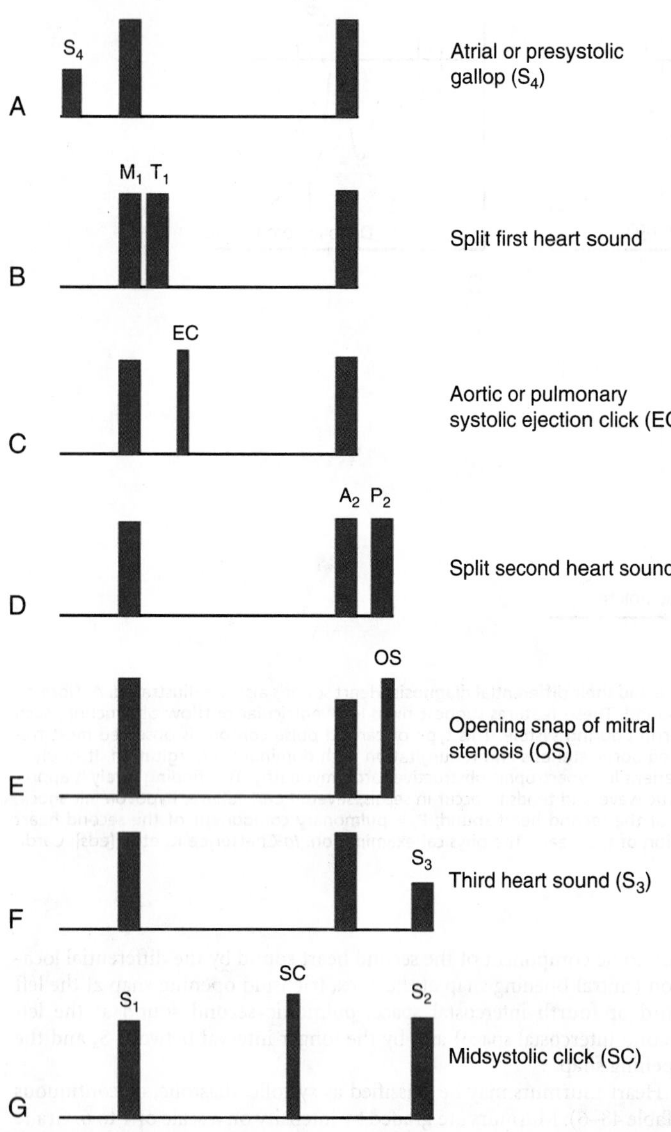

FIGURE 48–6 • Timing of the different heart sounds and added sounds. (Modified from Wood P: Diseases of the Heart and Circulation, 3rd ed. Philadelphia, JB Lippincott, 1968, with permission.)

a patent ductus arteriosus, ruptured sinus of Valsalva aneurysm, arteriovenous fistula (of the coronary artery, pulmonary artery, or thoracic artery), and a mammary soufflé. In some situations, murmurs of two coexistent conditions (e.g., aortic stenosis and regurgitation; atrial septal defect with a large shunt and resulting flow murmurs of relative mitral and pulmonic stenosis) may mimic a continuous murmur.

Abdomen

The most common cause of hepatomegaly in patients with heart disease is hepatic engorgement from elevated right-sided pressures associated with right ventricular failure of any cause. Hepatojugular reflux is elicited by pressing on the liver and showing an increase in the jugular venous pressure; it indicates advanced right ventricular failure or obstruction to right ventricular filling. Evaluation of the abdomen also may reveal an enlarged liver caused by a systemic disease, such as hemochromatosis (Chapter 231) or sarcoidosis (Chapter 95), which also may affect the heart. In more severe cases, splenomegaly and ascites also may be noted. Large, palpable, polycystic kidneys (Chapter 128) commonly are associated with hypertension. A systolic bruit suggestive of renal artery stenosis (Chapter 126) or an enlarged abdominal aorta (Chapter 78) is a clue of atherosclerosis.

Extremities

Extremities should be evaluated for peripheral pulses, edema, cyanosis, and clubbing. Diminished peripheral pulses suggest peripheral arterial disease (Chapters 79 and 80). Delayed pulses in the legs are consistent with coarctation of the aorta and are seen after aortic dissection.

Edema (Fig. 48–7) is a cardinal manifestation of right-sided heart failure. When it is caused by heart failure, pericardial disease, or pulmonary hypertension, the edema is usually symmetrical and progresses upward from the ankles; each of these causes of cardiac edema commonly is associated with jugular venous distention and often with hepatic congestion. Unilateral edema suggests thrombophlebitis or proximal venous or lymphatic obstruction (Fig. 48–8). Edema in the absence of evidence of right-sided or left-sided heart failure suggests renal disease, hypoalbuminemia, myxedema, or other noncardiac causes. Among unselected patients with bilateral edema, about 40% have an underlying cardiac disease, about 40% have an elevated pulmonary blood pressure, about 20% have bilateral venous disease, about 20% have renal disease, and about 25% have idiopathic edema.

Cyanosis (Fig. 48–9) is a bluish discoloration caused by reduced hemoglobin exceeding about 5 g/dL in the capillary bed. Central cyanosis is seen in patients with poor oxygen saturation resulting from a reduced inspired oxygen concentration or inability to oxygenate the blood in the lungs (e.g., as a result of advanced pulmonary disease, pulmonary edema, pulmonary arteriovenous fistula, or right-to-left shunting); it also may be seen in patients with marked erythrocytosis. Methemoglobinemia (Chapter 168) also can present with cyanosis. Peripheral cyanosis may be caused by reduced blood flow to the extremities secondary to vasoconstriction, heart failure, or shock. *Clubbing* (Fig. 48–10), which is loss of the normal concave configuration of the nail as it emerges from the distal phalanx, is seen in patients with pulmonary abnormalities such as lung cancer (Chapter 201) and in patients with cyanotic congenital heart disease (Chapter 68).

Examination of the Skin

Examination of the skin may reveal bronze pigmentation typical of hemochromatosis (Chapter 231); jaundice (see Fig. 150–2) characteristic of severe right-sided heart failure or hemochromatosis; or capillary hemangiomas typical of Osler-Weber-Rendu disease (see Fig. 179–2), which also is associated with pulmonary arteriovenous fistulas and cyanosis. Infectious endocarditis may be associated with Osler's nodes (see Fig. 76–2), Janeway's lesions, or splinter hemorrhages (Fig. 48–11) (Chapter 76). Xanthomas (Fig. 48–12) are subcutaneous deposits of cholesterol seen on the extensor surfaces of the extremities or on the palms and digital creases; they are found in patients with severe hypercholesterolemia.

Laboratory Studies

All patients with known or suspected cardiac disease should have an ECG and chest radiograph. The ECG (Chapter 52) helps identify rate, rhythm, conduction abnormalities, and possible myocardial ischemia. The chest radiograph (Chapter 51) yields important information on chamber enlargement, pulmonary vasculature, and the great vessels.

Blood testing in patients with known or suspected cardiac disease should be targeted to the conditions in question. In general, a complete blood cell count, thyroid indices, and lipid levels are part of the standard evaluation.

Echocardiography (Chapter 53) is the most useful test to analyze valvular and ventricular function. By use of Doppler flow methods, stenotic and regurgitant lesions can be quantified. Transesophageal echocardiography is the preferred method to evaluate possible aortic dissection and to identify clot in the cardiac chambers. Radionuclide studies (Chapter 54) can measure left ventricular function, assess myocardial ischemia, and determine whether ischemic myocardium is viable.

Stress testing by exercise or pharmacologic stress is useful to precipitate myocardial ischemia that may be detected by ECG abnormalities, perfusion abnormalities on radionuclide studies, or transient wall motion abnormalities on echocardiography. These tests are often crucial in diagnosis of possible myocardial ischemia (Chapter 70) and in establishment of prognosis in patients with known ischemic heart disease.

Cardiac catheterization (Chapter 56) can measure precise gradients across stenotic cardiac valves, judge the severity of intracardiac shunts, and determine intracardiac pressures. Coronary angiography provides a definitive diagnosis of coronary disease and is a necessary prelude to coronary revascularization with a percutaneous coronary intervention (Chapter 73) or coronary artery bypass graft surgery (Chapter 74).

TABLE 48–6 SOME COMMON CAUSES OF HEART MURMURS*

	Usual Location	Common Associated Findings
SYSTOLIC		
Holosystolic		
Mitral regurgitation	Apex → axilla	↑ with handgrip; S_3 if marked mitral regurgitation; left ventricular dilation common
Tricuspid regurgitation	LLSB	↑ with inspiration; right ventricular dilation common
Ventricular septal defect	LLSB → RLSB	Often with thrill
Early–mid systolic		
Aortic valvular stenosis	RUSB	
Fixed supravalvular or subvalvular	RUSB	Ejection click if mobile valve; soft or absent A_2 if valve immobile; later peak associated with more severe stenosis
Dynamic infravalvular	LLSB → apex + axilla	Hypertrophic obstructive cardiomyopathy; murmur louder if left ventricular volume lower or contractility increased, softer if left ventricular volume increased†; can be later in systole if obstruction delayed
Pulmonic valvular	LUSB	↑ with inspiration
stenosis Infravalvular (infundibular)	LUSB	↑ with inspiration
Supravalvular	LUSB	↑ with inspiration
"Flow murmurs"	LUSB	Anemia, fever, increased flow of any cause‡
Mid–late systolic		
Mitral valve prolapse	LLSB or apex → axilla	Preceded by click; murmur lengthens with maneuvers that decrease left ventricular volume†
Papillary muscle dysfunction	Apex → axilla	Ischemic heart disease
DIASTOLIC		
Early diastolic		
Aortic regurgitation	RUSB, LUSB	High pitched, blowing quality; endocarditis, diseases of the aorta, associated aortic valvular stenosis; signs of low peripheral vascular resistance
Pulmonic valve regurgitation	LUSB	Pulmonary hypertension as a causative factor
Mid–late diastolic		
Mitral stenosis, tricuspid stenosis	Apex, LLSB	Low pitched; in rheumatic heart disease, opening snap commonly precedes murmur; can be due to increased flow across normal valve‡
Atrial myxomas	Apex (L), LLSB (R)	"Tumor plop"
Continuous		
Venous hum	Over jugular or hepatic vein or breast	Disappears with compression of vein or pressure of stethoscope
Patent ductus arteriosus	LUSB	
Arteriovenous fistula		
Coronary	LUSB	
Pulmonary, bronchial, chest wall	Over fistula	
Ruptured sinus of Valsalva aneurysm	RUSB	Sudden onset

*See also Chapters 68 and 75.
†Left ventricular volume is decreased by standing or during prolonged, forced expiration against a closed glottis (Valsalva maneuver); it is increased by squatting or by elevation of the legs; contractility is increased by adrenergic stimulation or in the beat after an extrasystolic beat.
‡Including a left-to-right shunt through an atrial septal defect for tricuspid or pulmonic flow murmurs, and a ventricular septal defect for pulmonic or mitral flow murmurs.
LLSB = left lower sternal border (4th intercostal space); LUSB = left upper sternal border (2nd–3rd intercostal spaces); RLSB = right lower sternal border (4th intercostals space); RUSB = right upper sternal border (2nd–3rd intercostal spaces).

TABLE 48–7 SENSITIVITY AND SPECIFICITY OF BEDSIDE MANEUVERS IN THE IDENTIFICATION OF SYSTOLIC MURMURS

Maneuver	Response	Murmur	Sensitivity (%)	Specificity (%)
Inspiration	↑	RS	100	88
Expiration	↓	RS	100	88
Valsalva maneuver	↑	HC	65	96
Squat to stand	↑	HC	95	84
Stand to squat	↓	HC	95	85
Leg elevation	↓	HC	85	91
Handgrip	↓	HC	85	75
Handgrip	↑	MR and VSD	68	92
Transient arterial occlusion	↑	MR and VSD	78	100

HC = hypertrophic cardiomyopathy; MR = mitral regurgitation; RS = right sided; VSD = ventricular septal defect.
Modified with permission from Lembo NJ, Dell'Italia IJ, Crawford MH, et al: Bedside diagnosis of systolic murmurs. N Engl J Med 1988;318:1572–1578.

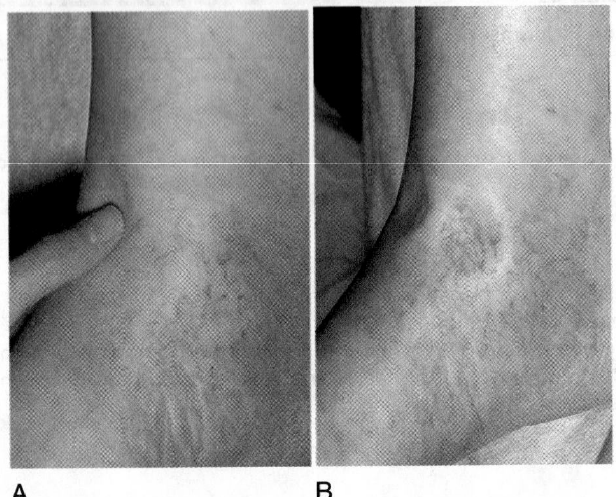

FIGURE 48–7 • Pitting edema in a patient with cardiac failure. A depression ("pit") remains in the edema for some minutes after firm fingertip pressure is applied. (From Forbes CD, Jackson WD: Color Atlas and Text of Clinical Medicine, 3rd ed. London, Mosby, 2003, with permission.)

Continuous ambulatory ECG monitoring can help diagnose arrhythmias. A variety of newer technologies allow longer term monitoring in patients with important but infrequently occurring symptoms (Chapter 61). Formal invasive electrophysiologic testing can be useful in the diagnosis of ventricular or supraventricular wide-complex tachycardia, and it is crucial for guiding a wide array of new invasive electrophysiologic therapies (Chapter 65).

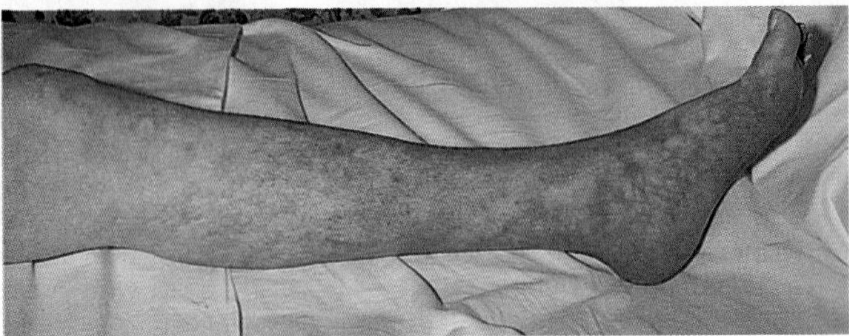

FIGURE 48–9 • Arterial embolism causing acute ischemia and cyanosis of the leg. Initial pallor of the leg and foot was followed by cyanosis. (From Forbes CD, Jackson WD: Color Atlas and Text of Clinical Medicine, 3rd ed. London, Mosby, 2003, with permission.)

Unilateral or bilateral?
- Unilateral → R/O DVT
  - Yes → Anticoagulation
  - No → Pain?
    - Yes → Fever or increased WBC?
      - Yes → Cellulitis or other infection? → Antibiotic treatment
      - No → Characteristic physical signs of popliteal cyst or gastrocnemius rupture
        - Yes → Initiate symptomatic therapy
        - No → Consider MRI
    - No → Postphlebitic syndrome?
      - Yes → Continue anticoagulation
      - No → R/O malignancy; Detailed history; Pelvic exam; Rectal exam
- Bilateral → Detailed history; Physical exam → Urine dipstick
  - – → Obvious findings of CHF?
    - Yes → Initiate appropriate therapy → Pursue further diagnostic work-up as appropriate
    - No → Creatinine; Electrolytes; Albumin; Cholesterol; Prothrombin time; Liver enzymes; TSH; Chest X-ray; Cardiac echo
      - → Renal disease; Occult CHF; Cirrhosis; Hypo-thyroidism; Other or idiopathic
      - Follow-up abnormalities; Initiate appropriate therapy
  - + → R/O concurrent cardiac and hepatic disease → Consider renal biopsy → Initiate appropriate therapy

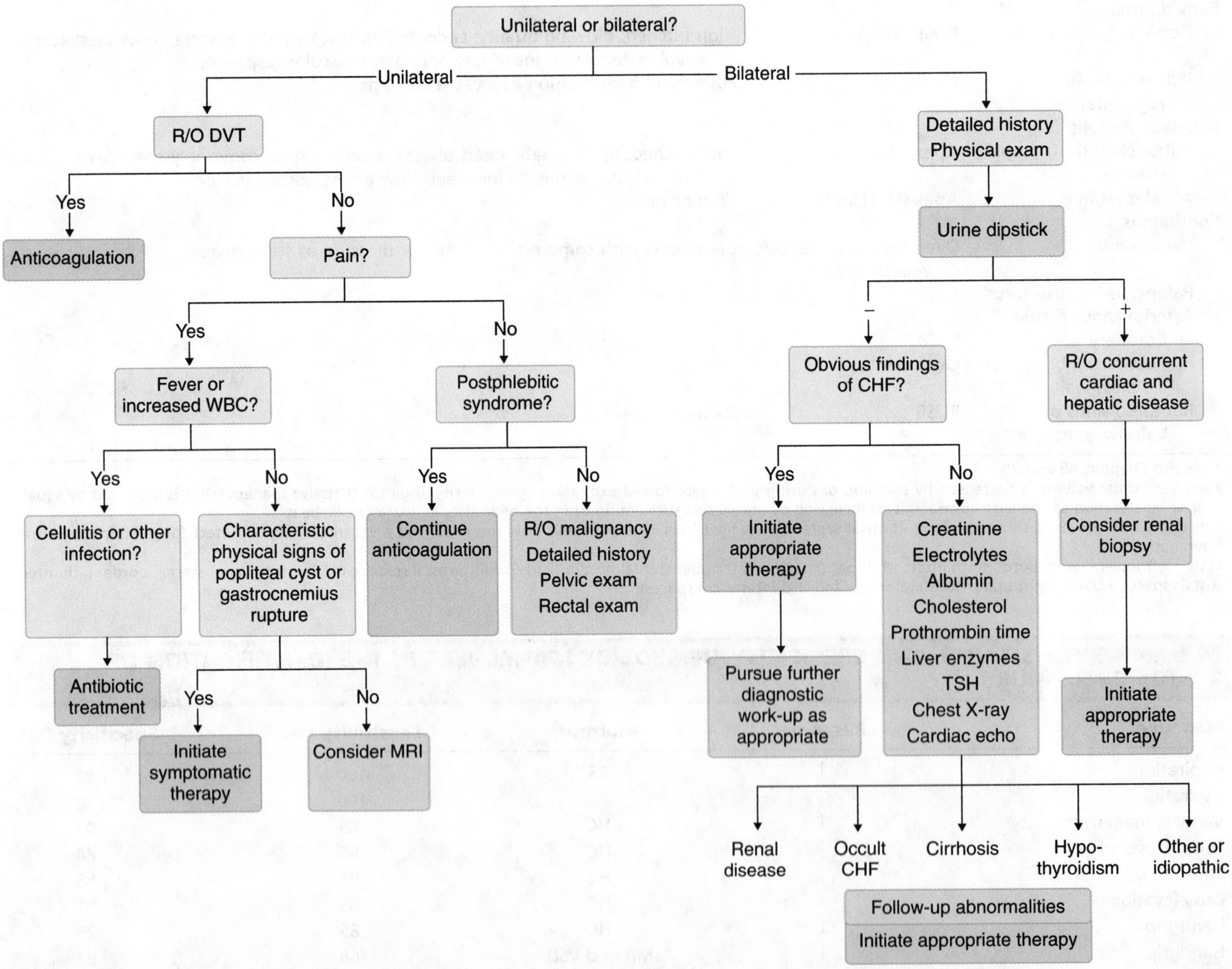

FIGURE 48–8 • Diagnostic approach to patients with edema. CHF = congestive heart failure; DVT = deep venous thrombosis; MRI = magnetic resonance imaging; R/O = rule out; TSH = thyroid-stimulating hormone; WBC = white blood cell count. (From Chertow G: Approach to the patient with edema. *In* Braunwald E, Goldman L [eds]: Primary Cardiology, 2nd ed. Philadelphia, WB Saunders, 2003, with permission.)

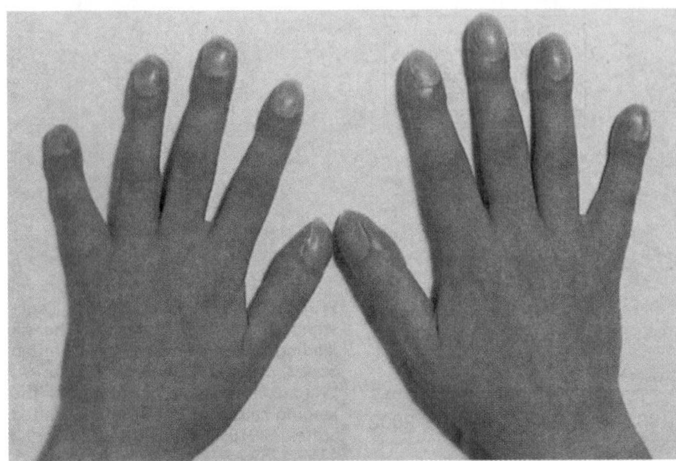

FIGURE 48–10 • Severe finger clubbing in a patient with cyanotic congenital heart disease. (From Forbes CD, Jackson WD: Color Atlas and Text of Clinical Medicine, 3rd ed. London, Mosby, 2003, with permission.)

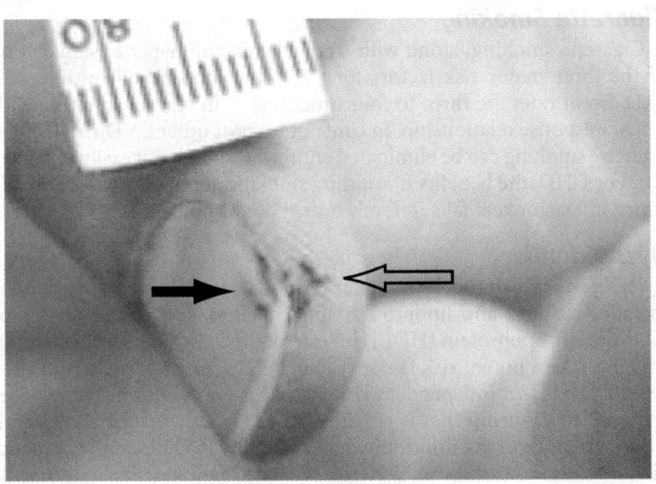

FIGURE 48–11 • Splinter hemorrhage (solid arrow) and Janeway's lesions (open arrow). These findings should stimulate a work-up for endocarditis. (From American Academy of Family Physicians Online. *http://www.aafp.org/afp/20040315/1417.html.*)

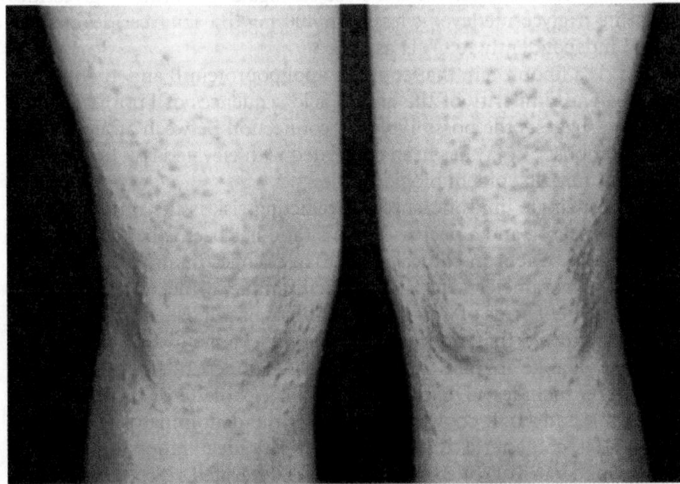

FIGURE 48–12 • Eruptive xanthomas of the extensor surfaces of the lower extremities. This patient had marked hypertriglyceridemia. (From Massengale WT, Nesbitt LT Jr: Xanthomas. *In* Bolognia JL, Jorizzo JL, Rapini RP [eds]: Dermatology. Philadelphia, Mosby, 2003, p 1449.)

SUMMARY

The history, physical examination, and laboratory evaluation should help the physician establish the cause of any cardiovascular problem; identify and quantify any anatomic abnormalities; determine the physiologic status of the valves, myocardium, and conduction system; determine functional capacity; estimate prognosis; and provide primary or secondary prevention. Key preventive strategies, including diet modification, recognition and treatment of hyperlipidemia, cessation of cigarette smoking, and adequate physical exercise, should be part of the approach to every patient, with or without heart disease.

SUGGESTED READINGS

Braunwald E: The clinical examination. *In* Braunwald E, Goldman L (eds): Primary Cardiology, 2nd ed. Philadelphia, WB Saunders, 2003, pp 29–46. *A practical approach.*

Marcus GM, Vessey J, Jordan MV, et al: Relationship between accurate auscultation of a clinically useful third heart sound and level of experience. Arch Intern Med 2006;166:617–622. *The S3 auscultated by more experienced physicians demonstrated fair agreement with phonocardiographic findings.*

Shah MG, Cho S, Atwood JE, et al: Peripheral edema due to heart disease: Diagnosis and outcome. Clin Cardiol 2006;29:31–35. *A case series showing that cardiac causes are difficult to diagnose but associated with high mortality.*

Treadway K: Heart sounds. N Engl J Med 2006;1112–1113. *Common heart sounds on audio.*

Vukanovic-Criley JM, Criley S, Warde CM, et al: Competency in cardiac examination skills in medical students, trainees, physicians, and faculty: A multicenter study. Arch Intern Med 2006;166:610–616. *Emphasizes the limitations of physical examination of training and cardiology experience, except cardiologists.*

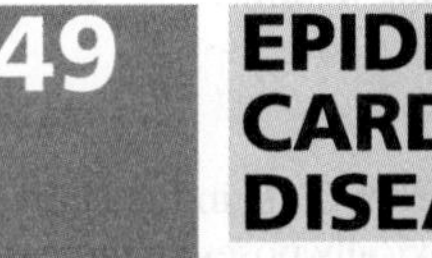

49 EPIDEMIOLOGY OF CARDIOVASCULAR DISEASE

Michael H. Criqui

CARDIOVASCULAR DISEASES

The three major clinical manifestations of atherosclerotic cardiovascular disease (CVD) are coronary heart disease (CHD) (Chapters 70 through 74), stroke (Chapters 430 to 432), and peripheral arterial disease (PAD) (Chapter 79). Atherosclerosis also can be found in other arterial beds, especially the renal arteries, where it causes about two thirds of cases of renal artery stenosis (Chapters 66 and 126).

The epidemiology of CVD has been evaluated in many study designs, including ecologic, case-control, cross-sectional survey, prospective cohort, and clinical trial designs (Chapters 9 and 10). In general, the strength of the causal inference one can draw from a study increases along this continuum, with policy changes typically appropriate only when supported by solid evidence from clinical trials.

IMPACT OF CARDIOVASCULAR DISEASE

More than 70 million Americans are estimated to have one or more types of CVD: 65 million have hypertension, 13 million have CHD, and 5.4 million have had a stroke. More than 8 million Americans have PAD, of whom about 40% do not report symptoms. Overall, about one in four Americans currently have some form of CVD.

CVD contributes to about 1.4 million deaths annually in the United States, or 40% of all deaths. Approximately 32% of CVD deaths occur prematurely (i.e., in persons <75 years old). Each year, about 1.2 million Americans have a new or recurrent myocardial infarction (MI), and more than 40% of these events are fatal. The annual incidence of new or recurrent stroke is about 700,000 per year, and about 275,000 Americans die from a stroke each year.

Secular Trends

Between 1970 and 2002, the death rate in the United States decreased 52% from heart disease and 63% from stroke (Fig. 49–1). The incidence of PAD has also declined somewhat. These observations have raised the

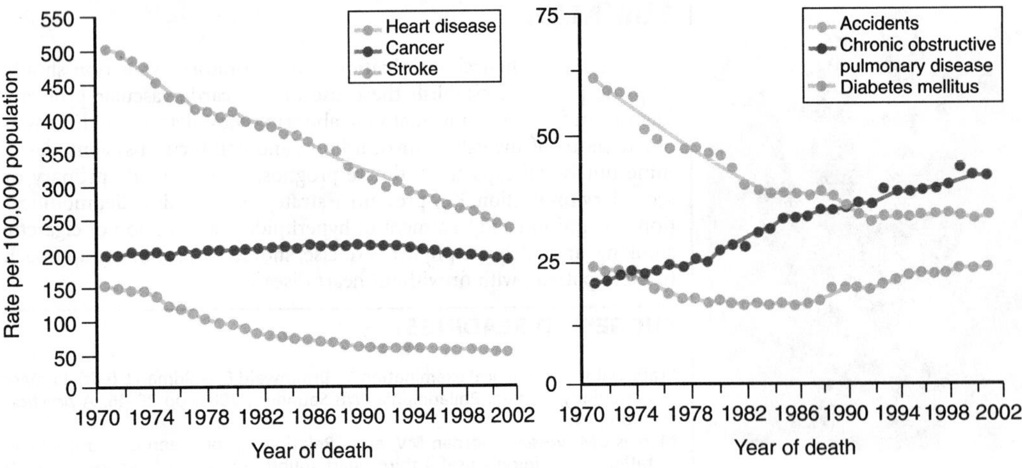

FIGURE 49–1 • Trends in age-standardized death rates for the six leading causes of death in the United States, 1970–2002. (From Jemal A, Ward E, Hao Y, et al: Trends in the leading causes of death in the United States, 1970–2002. JAMA 2005;294: 1255–1259.)

question of whether this decline in mortality is due to a true reduction in incidence at the population level, which logically could be attributed to improved prevention, or simply to a decline in case-fatality rates, which presumably would be attributable mostly to better treatment. Several studies have evaluated this question, and the consensus is that both prevention and therapy have contributed and that both population incidence rates and case-fatality rates have declined.

Despite this decline, CVD is still the leading cause of death in developed countries by a considerable margin. CHD and stroke are the second and third leading causes of mortality in developing nations.

Economic Impact

Despite the age-adjusted decline in mortality from CVD in the United States and many Western countries, CVD paradoxically poses an increasing economic burden, owing largely to two factors: (1) an aging population, which keeps the actual numbers of CVD cases relatively stable, and (2) technologic improvements, which allow more aggressive and extensive therapy. Hospital discharges and deaths from heart failure (Chapters 57 and 64), which is a frequent consequence of chronic CHD, increased substantially in the 1990s, as did the number of CVD operations and procedures (Chapters 73 and 74).

NATURAL HISTORY OF CARDIOVASCULAR DISEASE

Arterial lesions begin as fatty streaks, often early in life (Chapter 69). Autopsies of teenagers and young adults who were victims of accidental and other non-CVD causes of mortality show early fatty streaks, and these changes have correlated with traditional CVD risk factors. These fatty streaks can progress to raised lesions, which progressively can occlude the lumen of the artery.

Symptoms that typically occur in vascular beds well before the lesions completely occlude the lumen include angina pectoris from lesions in the coronary arteries (Chapters 70 and 71), transient ischemic attacks from lesions in the cerebrovascular arteries (Chapter 431), and intermittent claudication from lesions in the arteries in the lower extremities (Chapter 79). Although each of these pain syndromes has a classic prototype, patients can present with atypical symptoms despite significant disease. Many patients do not experience symptoms or ignore warning symptoms, and their first presentation may be a severe or fatal MI or stroke.

RISK FACTORS FOR CARDIOVASCULAR DISEASE

Unmodifiable Cardiovascular Disease Risk Factors

Several CVD risk factors are essentially immutable, including older age, male gender, and a family history of CVD. Nonetheless, these risk factors are important to consider in evaluating risk in an individual patient.

Modifiable Cardiovascular Disease Risk Factors

Cigarette Smoking

Cigarette smoking, along with dyslipidemia and hypertension, is one of the three major risk factors for CHD, thromboembolic stroke, and PAD. Event rates are three to four times higher in regular smokers, with a dose-response relationship. In contrast to most other CVD risk factors, cigarette smoking can be eliminated entirely, although not easily (Chapter 30). For CHD, the benefits of quitting smoking are dramatic: CHD incidence in ex-smokers falls to levels near those of nonsmokers in 2 years.

Dyslipidemia

Dyslipidemia is probably a better term than *hyperlipidemia* because it includes all lipid and lipoprotein abnormalities, such as low levels of high-density lipoprotein (HDL) cholesterol (hypoalphalipoproteinemia), which can be a potent risk factor (Chapter 225). An elevated serum cholesterol level is an independent risk factor for CVD, with a strong dose-response relationship that is exponential at higher levels of cholesterol. Although much of the interindividual variability in cholesterol is genetic, dietary consumption of cholesterol, saturated fat, and *trans*-fatty acids (typically formed by partial hydrogenation [saturation] of unsaturated vegetable fat) increases serum cholesterol.

Total cholesterol (TC) is carried on three lipoproteins in the blood, resulting in three separate cholesterol fractions with differing prognostic significance: very-low-density lipoprotein (VLDL) cholesterol, low-density lipoprotein (LDL) cholesterol, and HDL cholesterol. LDL cholesterol is positively related and HDL cholesterol is inversely related to CVD incidence. VLDL cholesterol is a close surrogate for serum triglycerides when the triglyceride level is less than 400 mg/dL. Triglycerides may be related independently to CVD as well.

Lp(a) is a lipoprotein that contains apolipoprotein B and apolipoprotein (a). The similarity of the amino acid sequences of Lp(a) and plasminogen suggests the possibility of a connection between atherogenesis and thrombosis. Lp(a) has been associated with elevated risk for CHD in most, but not all, epidemiologic studies.

The best single lipid measure in predicting risk is the ratio of TC to HDL cholesterol, and a decrease in this ratio has been a better predictor of treatment benefit in clinical trials than changes in any other lipid or lipoprotein parameter (Fig. 49–2). For example, a meta-analysis of 17 active treatment arms of lipid intervention trials published between 1987 and 2003 showed that, after considering the change in the TC-to-HDL ratio, the change in LDL itself was not an independent predictor of benefit. TC includes LDL cholesterol, VLDL cholesterol (a triglyceride surrogate), and HDL cholesterol, whereas the denominator is the protective HDL cholesterol. Ratios less than 3 are ideal, ratios of 3 to 5 are average, and ratios greater than 5 represent elevated risk, but risk continues to rise throughout the range of TC-to–HDL cholesterol values.

Hypertension

Elevated blood pressure is a potent risk factor for all forms of atherosclerotic CVD and is the dominant risk factor for stroke (Chapters 430

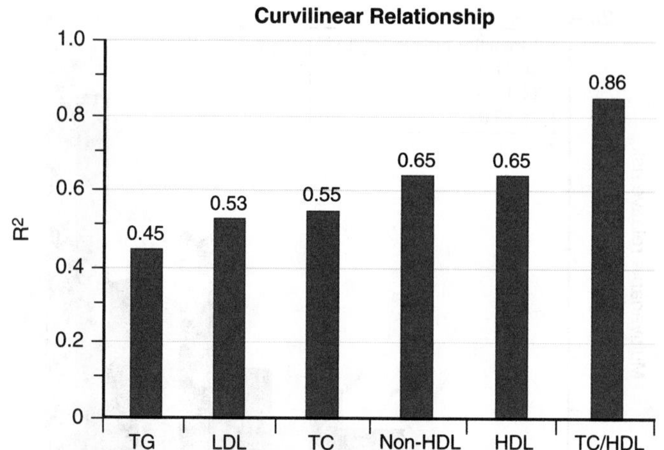

FIGURE 49–2 • Relationship between lipid parameters and relative risk reduction in coronary heart disease (univariate regression) in a meta-analysis of 17 lipid intervention trials. HDL = high-density lipoprotein; LDL = low-density lipoprotein; R^2 = coefficient of determination; TC = total cholesterol; TG = triglycerides.

to 432). In epidemiologic studies, there is a graded relationship between the level of blood pressure, even at the lowest levels, and CVD outcomes (Chapter 66). In general, systolic blood pressure is related more strongly to incident CVD than is diastolic blood pressure, particularly in the elderly. In some studies of older adults, pulse pressure (systolic blood pressure minus diastolic blood pressure) shows the strongest association. Early trials in severe hypertension unequivocally showed the benefits of reducing very high blood pressure levels, with a sharp reduction in morbidity and mortality from CVD. Meta-analyses of pharmacologic treatment of mild hypertension also showed benefit. Systolic pressure rises with age throughout life in Western populations, whereas diastolic pressure plateaus in late midlife and decreases thereafter. Trials of blood pressure lowering in isolated systolic hypertension in the elderly have shown dramatic benefits for reducing stroke and CHD, with the absolute benefit of treatment remaining stable or rising with increasing age. Multiple classes of antihypertensive drugs are now available, but a meta-analysis suggested that, for a given blood pressure reduction, low-dose diuretics were as effective or more effective than each of the other drug classes. [1] In most patients, blood pressure and other CVD risk factors can be improved to a greater or lesser degree by lifestyle changes, including weight loss, exercise, and a diet that is rich in fruits and vegetables and avoids excess sodium and alcohol (Chapters 14 and 232).

Physical Inactivity

Persons who exercise more or are better conditioned are at lower risk for CVD (Chapter 14). Evidence shows significant changes in multiple risk factors with exercise, including improved insulin resistance, blood pressure, HDL cholesterol, triglycerides, and fibrinolysis. Randomized trials of cardiac rehabilitation for secondary prevention also suggest benefit. Prior concerns about the possible acute risk for cardiac ischemia with exercise in susceptible persons are outweighed by the benefits for most people; nevertheless, high-risk individuals should be evaluated carefully before beginning an exercise program.

Diabetes Mellitus

Patients with either type 1 or type 2 diabetes mellitus are at increased risk for CVD (Chapters 247 and 248). In type 2 diabetes, CVD risk is approximately doubled in men and increased four-fold in women, sharply attenuating the typical relative CVD protection in women. In type 1 diabetes, the risks are higher, particularly in patients with proteinuria.

Patients with type 2 diabetes mellitus commonly exhibit evidence of insulin resistance well before the onset of chemical diabetes. Insulin resistance and type 2 diabetes usually are accompanied by one or more of many metabolic abnormalities, including increased levels of insulin, glucose, blood pressure, and triglycerides and lower HDL cholesterol levels. Evidence suggests that correction of the lipid abnormalities in type 2 diabetes substantially decreases the risk of CHD. Controversy persists, however, as to whether reduction of glucose levels improves macrovascular risk. New oral agents that lower glucose and insulin and improve insulin resistance may help resolve this issue. With weight loss and exercise, insulin resistance improves, triglyceride levels decrease, LDL particles become larger and less dense, HDL cholesterol increases, and hypertension tends to improve. Diet and exercise can reduce dramatically the likelihood of new-onset diabetes in high-risk patients. Angiotensin-converting enzyme inhibitors can reduce the risk of progressive renal disease and CHD events in patients with existing diabetes mellitus.

Obesity

Obesity (Chapter 239) has increased dramatically in recent years in the United States for unclear reasons. Suggested causes include the automobile, television, the Internet, a decrease in school-based physical activity programs, high-fat foods, low-fat foods, fast food, large portion sizes, homes in which both parents work, and neighborhoods unsuitable for walking. Obesity contributes to increased CVD risk by aggravating known CVD risk factors, including hypertension, insulin resistance, low HDL cholesterol, and hypertriglyceridemia. Clustering of these obesity-associated risk factors has been labeled the "metabolic syndrome" (Chapter 248), although the risk of the "metabolic syndrome" in a given patient varies as a function of the number and severity of these factors. Even adjusting for these risk factors, obesity seems to contribute independently to CVD risk. Although the body mass index, defined as weight divided by height, has been the traditional measure of obesity in epidemiologic studies, measures of central obesity or abdominal fat (e.g., waist circumference) may be better predictors of CVD risk. In theory, the obesity epidemic should result in both earlier and more CVD. However, the first available evidence suggests that CVD rates are stable, apparently because increased use of medications to treat hypertension and dyslipidemia is balancing the obesity and its associated risk factors.

Gonadal Hormones

Estrogen raises HDL cholesterol, lowers LDL cholesterol, and may have a beneficial effect on arterial flow. In randomized trials, however, both estrogen-progestin and unopposed estrogen resulted in an increase in total CVD events compared with placebo [2,3] (Chapter 262). New "designer estrogens," such as raloxifene, are now available and are being studied in long-term clinical trials.

Antioxidants

Intake of supplemental antioxidants, such as vitamin C or E, has been associated with a significant CVD risk reduction in observational studies, but clinical trials have repeatedly shown no benefit of antioxidants for reducing CVD. [4] As a result, there is currently no role for their prescription to reduce or prevent CVD.

Alcohol

Alcohol consumption (Chapter 31) up to three drinks per day is associated with protection against CHD in epidemiologic studies. Thrombotic stroke and PAD show similar associations. This protective effect seems to be mediated by increases in HDL cholesterol and by possible effects on coagulation and fibrinolytic factors and on insulin resistance. Some of the apparent benefit of moderate alcohol consumption could reflect selection bias. Clinical trials of alcohol for CVD end points have not and most likely will not be conducted, however, because of technical and ethical difficulties with study design. For nonatherosclerotic CVD, such as hemorrhagic stroke (Chapter 432) and cardiomyopathy (Chapter 59), risk is increased by alcohol consumption. At higher levels of alcohol consumption (three or more drinks per day), blood pressure increases, arrhythmias may be induced, rebound hypercoagulability may develop, direct myocardial damage can occur, and total CVD risk is increased. Maximum overall benefit for alcohol is reached at a single drink per day, and consumption of more than two drinks per day is associated with increases in morbidity and mortality from total cardiovascular causes, cirrhosis, accidents and violence, and certain cancers. Of particular concern is the consistent increase in breast cancer observed in women in epidemiologic studies, even with only modest levels of drinking. The benefit of alcohol for CHD is essentially limited to older persons who are at relatively high risk for CHD; younger persons and those at lower risk for CHD have minimal CHD benefit but easily could suffer alcohol-related harm. For these reasons and because of the high abuse potential of alcohol, it seems unwise to recommend alcohol for cardioprotection.

Thrombotic and Fibrinolytic Factors

Increasing attention has been paid to factors that influence thrombosis and fibrinolysis. The most consistent and reproducible risk factor in this group is fibrinogen, and epidemiologic studies have reported consistent and independent associations of fibrinogen with CHD, stroke, and PAD. Several other coagulation factors showed associations in some studies, including factor VII, factor VIII, and various measures of platelet aggregability. Aspirin therapy inhibits platelet aggregation and, as a result, reduces CVD risk. Low-dose aspirin generally seems to be as efficacious as a higher dose, but the lower dose shows fewer side effects, such as bleeding.

Plasminogen activator inhibitor 1 has been correlated with MI and carotid disease. Tissue-type plasminogen activator has shown positive and inverse associations with CVD, with the counterintuitive positive associations possibly explained by ongoing fibrinolysis, which similarly may explain the findings of an elevated D-dimer level in patients with CVD.

Homocysteine

Numerous studies have shown homocysteine to be a strong, independent risk factor for CVD, including CHD, stroke, and PAD. The potential for intervention is theoretically good, because folic acid supplementation alone or in combination with other B vitamins is known to lower total plasma homocysteine levels. Nevertheless, randomized trial results to date have shown that reducing homocysteine levels does not reduce CVD risk, suggesting that homocysteine may be a marker rather than a direct cause of CVD.

Infection

Research has given support to an old theory that infectious agents may be involved in the pathogenesis of atherosclerosis (Chapter 69). The evidence is strongest for *Chlamydia pneumoniae,* which has been isolated from atherosclerotic plaques. *C. pneumoniae* titer levels after MI may predict CVD events. In animals, herpesviruses can stimulate atherosclerosis, and cytomegalovirus titers have been reported to be increased in some studies of CVD patients. Evidence for other infectious agents, such as *Helicobacter pylori,* is weaker than for cytomegalovirus or *C. pneumoniae.* However, randomized trials of antibiotic therapy for the secondary prevention of CVD have not shown benefit. 6

Inflammation

Inflammatory markers, such as C-reactive protein, may reflect ongoing atherogenic inflammation at the level of the vessel wall. In this sense, such inflammatory markers can be thought of as measures of subclinical CVD. The level of C-reactive protein is a strong, independent predictor of future fatal and nonfatal CHD events and may be helpful in making treatment decisions in patients who are classified as being at intermediate risk by the Framingham risk score (Fig. 49–3). Data suggest that aspirin and statin therapy may reduce the CVD risk associated with elevated levels of C-reactive protein.

Psychosocial Factors

Psychosocial factors, such as anger, anxiety, depression, hostility, type A behavior, and various measures of social support, have been associated with the occurrence or recurrence of CVD. In addition, measures of cardiovascular physiologic reactivity have been correlated with CVD outcomes. Currently, data are inadequate to ascertain whether psychosocial interventions can reduce CVD risk.

Synergy of Risk Factors

CVD risk factors seem to interact synergistically in producing risk. The observed rate of CHD death among men who smoke, have serum cholesterol levels of 250 mg/dL or higher, and have diastolic blood pressure levels of 90 mm Hg or higher is almost twice as great as would be predicted by adding the risks attributable to each of these three factors to the baseline risk. Multivariate statistical models have confirmed the multiplicative effect of CVD risk factors acting in concert. These data also imply that control of one risk factor provides a substantial preventive benefit in persons with multiple risk factors.

RISK FACTORS IN PRIMARY AND SECONDARY PREVENTION

Primary prevention refers to preventing CVD in healthy persons. Secondary prevention refers to preventing recurrent CVD and death in

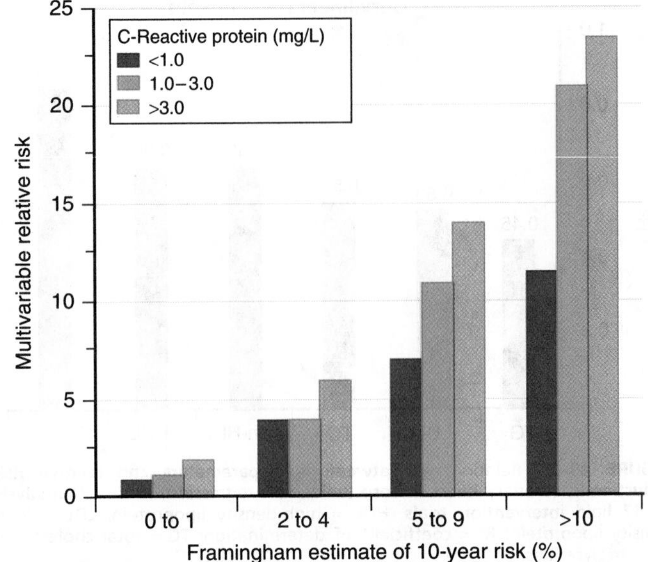

FIGURE 49–3 • Association of high sensitivity C-reactive protein with 8-year risk for cardiovascular disease in the Women's Health Study, stratified by Framingham risk score. $N = 27{,}939$. **(From Ridker PM, Rifai N, Rose L, et al: Comparison of C-reactive protein and low-density lipoprotein cholesterol levels in the prediction of first cardiovascular events. N Engl J Med 2002;347:1557–1565.)**

patients with extant CVD (Chapter 10). The major difference between primary and secondary CVD prevention is that event rates are much greater in secondary prevention, approximately five-fold higher, and the proportion of morbidity and mortality attributable to CVD is much higher. These simple facts have major clinical implications. First, the short-term benefit of intervention for a given patient is much greater in absolute terms in secondary prevention. Second, if a given intervention has any hazard (e.g., bleeding due to antiplatelet therapy), such a hazard is likely to be of greater importance in primary prevention, in which CVD event rates in the near term are relatively low.

In general, CVD risk factors and preventive interventions have similar effects on outcomes in primary and secondary prevention. Smoking cessation after MI cuts recurrent CHD risk in half, and cholesterol lowering after MI can reduce new CHD events by about 35% (Chapter 72).

Age-Related Effects of Risk Factors

The risk of CVD increases linearly with age. Older persons at any given level of risk factor burden have a higher risk for CVD than younger persons. Therefore, although the relative risks of essentially all CVD risk factors decrease with age, the absolute risks associated with them do not. As a result, the benefit for risk factor intervention does not appear to decrease with age and sometimes actually increases.

Gender Issues

The epidemiology of CVD in women and in men is similar. The major gender difference is the greater absolute age-specific risk for CVD among men, particularly at younger ages. Because absolute CVD risk is lower overall in women, the incremental risk produced by a given risk factor tends to be less. The exception is diabetes, in which the relative and the incremental risks for heart disease are greater among women.

Ethnic Issues

Minority ethnic groups are increasing as a proportion of the total U.S. population, with Hispanics being the fastest-growing group (Chapter 4). Considerable evidence exists for differences in CVD epidemiology among whites versus African Americans and Native Americans. African Americans have higher blood pressure levels and worse hypertensive outcomes than do whites, as well as a greater burden of PAD. Some Native American groups have a sharp excess of diabetes. Data also suggest excess obesity and diabetes among Hispanics and a high risk of insulin resistance and CHD among immigrants from the Indian subcontinent.

TABLE 49–1 RELATIVE STRENGTH OF ESTABLISHED AND NEWER CARDIOVASCULAR DISEASE RISK FACTORS FOR CORONARY HEART DISEASE, STROKE, AND PERIPHERAL ARTERIAL DISEASE

Risk Factors	CHD	Stroke	PAD
ESTABLISHED			
Advanced age	+++	++++	++++
Male gender	++	+	+
Cigarette smoking	+++	+	++++
Hypertension	++	++++	++
High LDL cholesterol	++	+	+
Low HDL cholesterol	+++	+	+++
Triglycerides	++	+	+++
Diabetes mellitus	+++	+	++++
NEWER			
Homocysteine	++	++	+++
Fibrinogen	++++	++	+++
C-reactive protein	++++	++	++
Lp(a)	++	++	+++
Chlamydia pneumoniae	++	+	++

CHD =coronary heart disease; HDL = high-density lipoprotein; Lp(a) = lipoprotein (a); LDL = low-density lipoprotein; PAD = peripheral arterial disease.

RISK FACTOR DIFFERENCES FOR CORONARY HEART DISEASE, STROKE, AND PERIPHERAL ARTERIAL DISEASE

Table 49–1 shows comparative associations of established and newer risk factors with CHD, stroke, and PAD. Important differences include the strength of inflammatory factors in CHD, the dominance of hypertension for stroke, and the importance of cigarette smoking and diabetes for PAD.

SUBCLINICAL CARDIOVASCULAR DISEASE

Tests for subclinical CVD include cerebral magnetic resonance imaging, retinal photography, and carotid duplex imaging in the cerebral circulation (Chapters 419 and 430); cardiac magnetic resonance imaging, echocardiography, ambulatory electrocardiography, and computed tomography (CT) for calcium in the coronary circulation (Chapters 53 to 55); CT for calcium in the aorta (Chapter 78); and reactive hyperemia, duplex imaging, and systolic blood pressure measurements at the ankle (ankle-brachial index) and at the toe, relative to the arm, in the lower-extremity arteries (Chapters 79 and 80). Current evidence for prognostic significance is strongest for carotid duplex imaging and the ankle-brachial index; significant carotid stenosis or an ankle-brachial index of 0.9 or less independently predicts a four-fold or greater increase in future CVD events. Coronary calcification on CT correlates well with anatomic coronary stenosis and predicts CVD events (Chapter 54).

FUTURE DIRECTIONS

It is unclear why some persons can tolerate higher levels of CVD risk factors, whereas others develop clinical CVD despite "normal" levels. Now that numerous traditional and newer CVD risk factors have been identified, research will focus on the transition from risk factors to subclinical and then clinical disease and on the key factors in this transition.

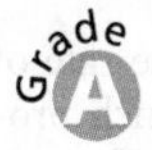

1. Psaty BM, Lumley T, Furberg CD, et al: Health outcomes associated with various antihypertensive therapies used as first-line agents: A network meta-analysis. JAMA 2003;289:2534–2544.
2. Rossouw JE, Anderson GL, Prentice RL, et al: Writing Group for the Women's Health Initiative Investigators: Risks and benefits of estrogen plus progestin in healthy postmenopausal women: Principal results from the Women's Health Initiative randomized controlled trial. JAMA 2002;288:321–333.
3. Anderson GL, Limacher M, Assaf AR, et al: Women's Health Initiative Steering Committee: Effects of conjugated equine estrogen in postmenopausal women with hysterectomy. JAMA 2004;291:1701–1712.
4. Heart Protection Study Collaborative Group: MRC/ BHF Heart Protection Study of antioxidant vitamin supplementation in 20,536 high-risk individuals: A randomized placebo-controlled trial. Lancet 2002;360:23–33.
5. Lonn E, Yusuf S, Arnold MJ, et al: Heart Outcomes Prevention Evaluation (HOPE) 2 Investigators. Homocysteine lowering with folic acid and B vitamins in vascular disease. N Engl J Med 2006;354:1567–1577.
6. Grayston JT, Kronmal RA, Jackson LA, et al: ACES Investigators: Azithromycin for the secondary prevention of coronary events. N Engl J Med 2005;352:1637–1645.

SUGGESTED READINGS

Howard BV, Van Hom L, Hsia J, et al: Low-fat dietary pattern and risk of cardiovascular disease: The Women's Health Initiative randomized controlled dietary modification trial. JAMA 2006;295:655–666. *The diet had no significant effects on incident CHD, stroke, or CVD.*

Ninomiya JK, L'Italien G, Criqui MH, et al: Association of the metabolic syndrome with history of myocardial infarction and stroke in the Third National Health and Nutrition Examination Survey. Circulation 2004;109:42–46. *Illustrates the relationship of the metabolic syndrome and its five components to myocardial infarction and stroke.*

Steg PG, Bhatt DL, Wilson PW, et al: One-year cardiovascular event rates in outpatients with atherothrombosis. JAMA 2007;297:1197–1206. *Outpatients with established atherosclerotic arterial disease experienced relatively high annual cardiovascular event rates.*

Yusuf S, Hawken S, Ounpuu S, et al: Effect of potentially modifiable risk factors associated with myocardial infarction in 52 countries (the INTERHEART study): Case-control study. Lancet 2004;364:937–952. *Lipid levels, smoking, blood pressure, diabetes, obesity, stress, lack of exercise, alcohol consumption, and daily consumption of fruit and vegetables explain 90% of the worldwide risk of MI.*

CARDIAC FUNCTION AND CIRCULATORY CONTROL

Daniel Burkhoff and Myron L. Weisfeldt

The heart is a muscular pump connected to the systemic and pulmonary vascular systems. Working together, the job of the heart and vasculature is to maintain adequate circulation of blood to the organs at rest and during periods of exercise. To understand perturbations that cause symptoms and disease, it is first necessary to understand the normal anatomy and physiology of the heart, its interaction with the vascular system, and its regulation by the autonomic nervous system.

ANATOMY OF THE HEART

The left ventricle, which is geometrically approximated by an axisymmetrical, truncated ellipsoid with approximately 1-cm-thick walls, consists of billions of cardiac muscle cells (myocytes) connected end to end at their *gap junctions* to form a network of branching muscle fibers that wrap around the chamber in an organized manner. The right ventricle is a roughly crescent-shaped structure formed by a 3- to 5-mm-thick sheet of myocardial fibers (the *right ventricular free wall*) that interdigitate at the anterior and posterior insertion points with the muscle fibers of the outer layer of the left ventricle. The right ventricular and left ventricular (LV) chambers share a common wall, the *interventricular septum*, that divides the chambers. Both the right and left atria are thin-walled muscular structures that receive blood from a low-pressure venous system. The *tricuspid valve* in the right heart and the *mitral valve* in the left heart separate each atrium from its associated ventricle, prohibit backward flow during forceful contraction of the ventricles, and are attached to fibrous rings that encircle each valve annulus. The central regions of these valves attach via *chordae tendineae* to *papillary muscles* that emerge from the ventricular walls. The predominant factor that determines valve opening and closure is the pressure gradient that exists between the ventricle and the atrium. However, the papillary muscles contract synchronously with the other heart muscles and aid in maintaining proper valve leaflet position, thus helping prevent regurgitant flow during contraction. A second set of tissue valves, the *aortic valve* and the *pulmonary valve*, separate each ventricle from its accompanying arterial connection and ensure unidirectional flow by preventing blood from flowing from the artery back into the ventricle. Pressure gradients across these valves are the major determinants of whether they are open or closed.

CARDIAC MUSCLE PHYSIOLOGY

The ability of the ventricles to generate blood flow and pressure derives from the ability of individual myocytes to shorten and generate force. Myocytes are tubular structures. During contraction, the muscles shorten and generate force along their long axis. Force production and shortening of cardiac muscle are created by regulated interactions among contractile proteins, which are assembled in an ordered and repeating structure called the *sarcomere* (Fig. 50–1). The lateral boundaries of each sarcomere are defined on both sides by a band of structural proteins at the Z lines to which the so-called *thin filaments* attach. The *thick filaments* are centered between adjacent Z lines and are held in register by a strand of proteins at the central M line. The alternating light and dark bands, as seen in cardiac muscle under light microscopy, result from the alignment of thick and thin filaments and give cardiac muscle its typical striated appearance.

The thin filaments are composed of linearly arranged globular actin molecules. The thick filaments are composed of bundles of myosin strands, with each strand having a tail, a hinge, and a head region. The tail regions bind to each other in the central portion of the filament, and the strands are aligned along a single axis. The head regions extend out from the center of the thick filament in both directions to create a central bare zone and head-rich zones on both ends of the thick filament. Each actin globule has a binding site for the myosin head. The hinge region allows the myosin head to protrude from the thick filament and make contact with the actin filament. In addition to the actin binding site, the myosin head contains an enzymatic site that cleaves the terminal phosphate molecule of adenosine triphosphate (ATP, myosin ATPase) to provide the energy used for repeatedly generating force. Force is produced when myosin binds to actin and, with hydrolysis of ATP, the head rotates and extends the hinge region. The force generated by a single sarcomere is proportional to the number of actin-myosin bonds. The state of actin-myosin binding after ATP hydrolysis is referred to as the *rigor state* because in the absence of additional ATP, the actin-myosin bond will persist and maintain high muscle tension. Relaxation, which requires uncoupling of the actin-myosin bond, occurs when a new ATP molecule binds to the ATPase site on the myosin head.

Actin-myosin interactions are regulated by troponin and tropomyosin. Tropomyosin is a thin protein strand that sits on the actin strand and, under normal resting conditions, covers the actin-myosin binding site, inhibits the interaction of actin and myosin, and prevents force production. Troponin, which is associated with tropomyosin, has calcium binding sites. When calcium binds to troponin, a conformational change causes the tropomyosin molecule to be pulled away from the actin-myosin binding site; as a result, inhibition of the actin-myosin interaction is eliminated, thus allowing force to be produced. This arrangement of proteins provides a means by which variations in intracellular calcium can readily modify instantaneous force production. The rise and fall in calcium levels during each beat is the basis for the cyclic rise and fall of muscle force. The greater the peak calcium, the greater the number of potential actin-myosin bonds and the greater the amount of force production.

In addition to the structural and regulatory proteins described, it is becoming increasingly clear that a multitude of other proteins are important for normal sarcomere structure, for the attachment of sarcomeres to the sarcolemma, and for proper transmission of force between sarcomeres and cells. These proteins include, among others, titin, desmin, dystrophin, α-actinin, talin, vinculin, and muscle LIM protein (MLP). Titin runs through the thick filaments, connects to adjacent Z lines, and helps maintain proper thick filament alignment within sarcomeres. Dystrophin links the sarcomere to the sarcolemma by binding sarcomeric and cytoskeletal actin to a glycoprotein complex on the sarcolemma. Desmin is a filamentous cytoskeletal protein found throughout the cell and at the Z lines; it appears to stabilize the sarcomeric actin via α-actinin, which in turn associates with the actin filament via talin, vinculin, and MLP. The physiologic roles of these structural proteins in maintaining normal contractile function has become clear recently by the use of murine models in which these genes are underexpressed and by the identification of specific inherited human cardiomyopathies that are due to point mutations of the genes encoding each of these proteins.

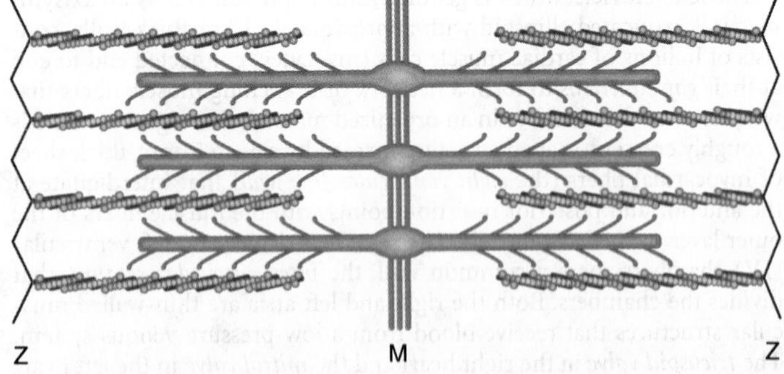

FIGURE 50–1 • Basic structure of the sarcomere. Thin filaments composed of actin with the associated regulatory proteins tropomyosin and troponin insert into structural proteins at the Z line, which defines the boundaries of the sarcomere. Thick filaments composed of myosin sit between the thin filaments and send their heads out in proximity to the actin molecules. During diastole (state of low intracellular calcium), tropomyosin strands block the interactions between actin and myosin. The thick filaments are kept in register at their centers by structural proteins at the M line. During systole (state of high calcium), calcium binds to troponin, which causes tropomyosin to shift away from the myosin binding site on actin, thus allowing the actin-myosin interactions that underlie force generation.

Excitation-Contraction Coupling

The sequence of events that lead to myocardial contraction is triggered by electrical depolarization of the cell; electrical depolarization increases the probability of sarcolemmal calcium channel opening, which in turn results in calcium influx into the cell (Fig. 50–2). An increase in calcium concentration then occurs in the subsarcolemmal space near the *lateral cisternae* of the sarcoplasmic reticulum. This increase in local calcium concentration causes the release of a larger pool of calcium stored in the sarcoplasmic reticulum through calcium release channels (originally known as *ryanodine receptors*), which are found in high concentration near the lateral cisternae. The mechanisms by which the subsarcolemmal increase in calcium concentration results in calcium release from the sarcoplasmic reticulum, a process referred to as *calcium-induced calcium release*, are not fully elucidated; the tight anatomic coupling between the sarcolemmal calcium channels and ryanodine receptors has suggested that conformational changes in calcium channel proteins can directly influence the properties of the ryanodine receptor. The calcium released from the sarcoplasmic reticulum diffuses through the myofilament lattice and is available for binding to troponin, which disinhibits actin and myosin interactions and results in force production.

Calcium release is rapid and does not require energy because of the large calcium concentration gradient between the sarcoplasmic reticulum and the cytosol during diastole. In contrast, removal of calcium from the cytosol and from troponin occurs up a concentration gradient and is an energy-requiring process. Calcium sequestration is primarily accomplished by pumps on the sarcoplasmic reticulum membrane that consume ATP (sarcoplasmic reticulum Ca^{2+}-ATPase pumps); these pumps are located in the central portions of the sarcoplasmic reticulum and are in close proximity to the myofilaments. Sarcoplasmic reticulum Ca^{2+}-ATPase activity is regulated by the phosphorylation status of another sarcoplasmic reticulum protein, phospholamban. To maintain calcium homeostasis, an amount of calcium equal to what entered the cell through the sarcolemmal calcium channels must also exit with each beat. This equilibrium is accomplished primarily by the sarcolemmal sodium-calcium exchanger, a transmembrane protein that translocates calcium across the membrane down its concentration gradient in exchange for sodium ions moved in the opposite direction. Sodium homeostasis is in turn regulated largely by the ATP-requiring sodium-potassium pump on the sarcolemma.

As suggested earlier, the amount of calcium released and the rate of calcium uptake are regulated by the β-adrenergic pathway, which provides a ready means of enhancing contractile force in settings of stress. β-Agonist (e.g., epinephrine or norepinephrine) binding to the β-receptor activates membrane-bound adenylyl cyclase, which results in the generation of cyclic adenosine monophosphate and then activation of

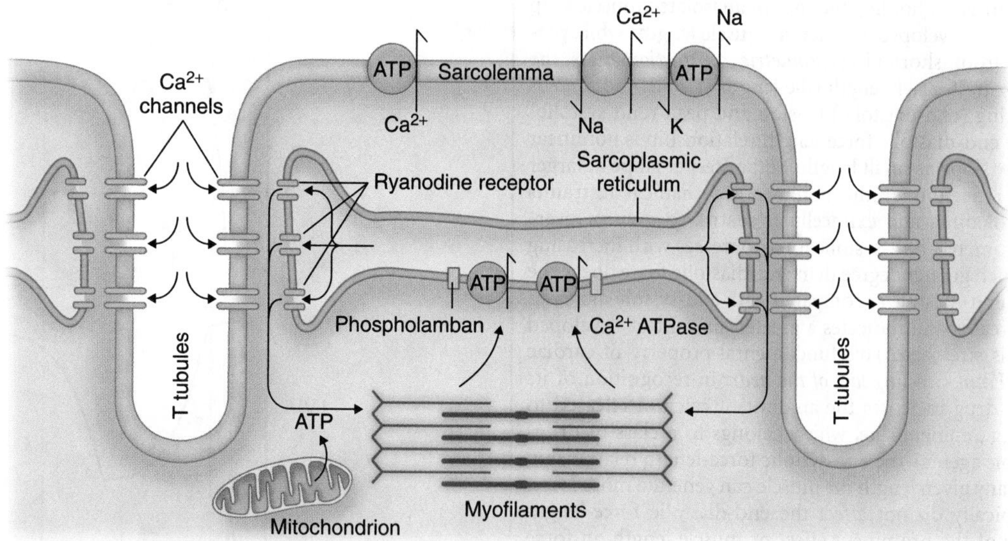

FIGURE 50–2 • Important features of the cardiac cell with an emphasis on aspects related to calcium metabolism. Arrows indicate calcium fluxes. The contraction cycle begins with calcium entering the cell via calcium channels and inducing the release of calcium from the lateral cisternae of the sarcoplasmic reticulum. This calcium binds to myofilaments and allows cross-bridge interactions that lead to force generation. A majority of the cytosolic systolic calcium is sequestered at the midportion of the sarcoplasmic reticulum by adenosine triphosphate (ATP)-dependent calcium pumps; the activity of these pumps is modified by the phosphorylation status of phospholamban. The sodium-calcium exchanger removes an amount of calcium during diastole equal to what entered through calcium channels to maintain calcium homeostasis. The sodium-potassium pump (an ATP-dependent pump) influences intracellular sodium concentrations, which in turn can influence the activity of the sodium-calcium exchanger and thus influence intracellular calcium and contractility.

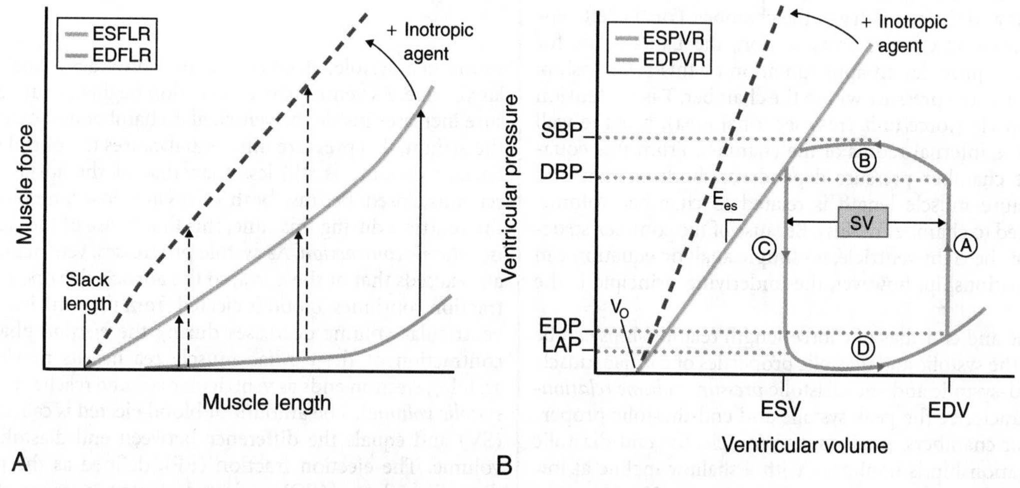

FIGURE 50–3 • The similar relationship between muscle length and force in isolated muscle and in the intact ventricle. A, Isolated muscle. When stretched from the slack length (the length at which no force is generated), both diastolic and systolic forces increase and result in the end-diastolic force-length relationship (EDFLR) and the end-systolic force-length relationship (ESFLR). The ESFLR increases much more steeply than the EDFLR does, so the force developed (difference between the two curves, indicated by the arrows) increases as the muscle is stretched. Pharmacologic agents that acutely increase contractile strength (contractility) have little effect on the EDFLR, but the ESFLR increases and consequently the force developed at any given length increases. **B,** The intact ventricle. Contractile properties are characterized by end-diastolic and end-systolic pressure-volume relationships (EDPVR and ESPVR). The slack length in muscle corresponds with V_0, the volume at which no pressure is generated. The ESPVR is nearly linear and characterized by a slope, E_{es}, that varies in relation to contractility. The pressure-volume loop sits within the boundaries defined by the EDPVR and ESPVR. The four phases of the cardiac cycle are indicated by isovolumic contraction (A), ejection (B), isovolumic relaxation (C), and filling (D). DBP = diastolic aortic blood pressure; EDP = end-diastolic pressure; EDV = end-diastolic volume; ESV = end-systolic volume; LAP = left atrial pressure; SBP = peak systolic blood pressure; SV = stroke volume.

phosphokinase A. Phosphokinase A activation results in phosphorylation of phospholamban, the calcium channel, the ryanodine receptor, and sarcomeric regulatory proteins. The modification in protein function caused by such phosphorylation results in a coordinated increase in calcium entry, uptake, and release, along with an associated increase in contractile strength.

Force-Length Relationships

In addition to calcium, cardiac muscle length exerts a major influence on production of force (Fig. 50–3). Because each muscle is composed of a linear array of sarcomere bundles from one end of the muscle to the other, muscle length is directly proportional to the average sarcomere length. Changes in sarcomere length alter the geometric relationship between thick and thin filaments. For myofilaments in general, maximal force is achieved when sarcomere length is about 2.2 to 2.3 μm, the length that provides optimal overlap of thick and thin filaments. As sarcomere length is decreased to less than about 2.0 μm, the tips of apposing thin filaments hit each other, the thick filaments approach the Z lines, and the lateral distance between thick and thin filaments increases. Each of these factors contributes to a reduction in force with decreasing sarcomere length. In skeletal muscle, when sarcomeres are stretched beyond 2.3 μm, force decreases because fewer myosin heads can reach and bind with actin; skeletal muscle can typically operate in this so-called *descending limb* of the sarcomere force-length relationship. In cardiac muscle, however, constraints imposed by the sarcolemma prevent myocardial sarcomeres from being stretched beyond 2.3 μm, even under conditions of severe heart failure when very high stretching pressures are imposed on the heart.

Force-length relationships are conveniently used to characterize the systolic and diastolic contractile properties of cardiac muscle. These relationships are measured by holding the ends of an isolated muscle strip and measuring the force developed at different muscle lengths while preventing the muscle from shortening *(isometric contractions)*. As the muscle is stretched from its slack length (the length at which no force is generated), both resting (end-diastolic) tension and peak (end-systolic) tension increase. The end-diastolic force-length relationship is nonlinear and exhibits a shallow slope at small lengths and a steeper slope at larger lengths, which is a reflection of the nonlinear mechanical restraints imposed by the sarcolemma and extracellular matrix to prevent overstretching of the sarcomeres. End-systolic force increases with increasing muscle length to a much greater degree than end-diastolic force does. The difference in force at end-diastole as compared with end-systole increases as muscle length increases and indicates a greater amount of developed force as the muscle is stretched. This fundamental property of cardiac muscle is called the *Frank-Starling law of the heart* in recognition of its two discoverers. If a drug increases the amount of calcium released to the myofilaments (e.g., epinephrine, which belongs to a class of drugs referred to as inotropic agents), the end-systolic force-length relationship shifts upward and at any given length the muscle can generate more force. Inotropic agents typically do not affect the end-diastolic force-length relationship. In view of the prominent effect of muscle length on force generation, the intrinsic strength of cardiac muscle, commonly referred to as muscle *contractility*, should be indexed by the end-systolic force-length relationship and not simply by peak force generation.

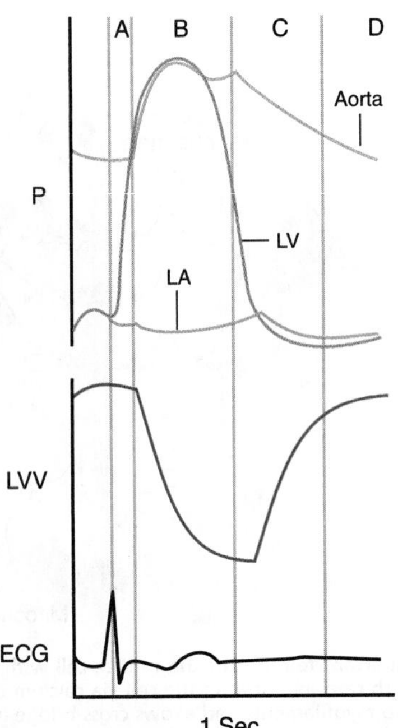

FIGURE 50–4 • Time sequence of events during a single cardiac cycle. Pressures (P) in the aorta, left ventricle (LV), and left atrium (LA) are shown. The four phases of the cardiac cycle are also illustrated: isovolumic contraction (A), ejection (B), isovolumic relaxation (C), and filling (D). ECG = electrocardiogram; LVV = left ventricular volume.

From Muscle to Chamber

Muscle length and the force generated by muscles in the walls of the ventricles are interrelated with the volume and pressure of the chambers. It is intuitively clear that as ventricular chamber volume varies, so too does muscle and sarcomere length. Ventricular pressure is related to the force within the walls and the geometry of the chamber. For the left ventricle, which has a roughly circular cross section, the Laplace law for thick-walled structures provides an approximation of this relationship: $P \approx 2 \cdot T \cdot h/R$, where P is the pressure within the chamber, T is the tension developed by the muscle (force/unit cross-sectional area), h is the wall thickness, and R is the internal radius of the chamber. From this equation, it follows that chamber pressure depends on both tension and muscle length (because muscle length is related to chamber volume, which in turn is related to chamber radius). Because of the complex structure and geometry of the right ventricle, no simple analytic equation can describe this interrelationship; however, the underlying principle is the same.

Just as end-systolic and end-diastolic force-length relationships can be used to characterize the systolic and diastolic properties of cardiac muscle fibers, so too can end-systolic and end-diastolic *pressure-volume relationships* be used to characterize the peak systolic and end-diastolic properties of the ventricular chambers. Analogous to muscle, the end-diastolic pressure-volume relationship is nonlinear, with a shallow incline at low pressures and a steep rise at pressures in excess of 20 mm Hg. However, the end-systolic pressure-volume relationship is typically linear, and as for muscle, ventricular pressure-generating capability is increased as ventricular volume is increased. Also analogous to muscle, the end-systolic pressure-volume relationship is used to index ventricular chamber *contractility*. Because the end-systolic pressure-volume relationship is roughly linear, it can be characterized by a slope and volume axis intercept. The slope of the line, which has units of myocardial stiffness or volume elastance (mm Hg/mL), is called E_{es} (*end-systolic elastance*), and the volume axis intercept (analogous to slack length of the muscle) is referred to as V_0. When muscle *contractility* is increased (e.g., by administration of an *inotropic agent*), the slope of the end-systolic pressure-volume relationship (E_{es}) increases, whereas little change occurs in V_0 (discussed later).

The Cardiac Cycle

The heart beats roughly once every second and repeatedly cycles through a sequence of hemodynamic events that can be divided into four phases. This cycle can be summarized by tracking the time course of change in ventricular pressure and volume along with atrial and aortic pressures in relation to events noted on the electrocardiogram (Fig. 50–4). At end-diastole, ventricular pressure is at its resting level *(end-diastolic pressure)* and ventricular volume is at its maximal value *(end-diastolic volume)*. Aortic pressure declines gradually during this period as the blood ejected into the aorta during the previous ventricular contraction is discharged to the peripheral circulation. Just before the onset of ventricular systole, atrial contraction provides a final boost to ventricular volume. As ventricular contraction begins about 120 msec later, pressure increases inside the ventricular chamber and exceeds the pressure in the atrium; this pressure differential causes the mitral valve to close. Ventricular pressure is still less than that of the aorta, so the aortic valve remains closed. Because both valves are closed, no blood enters or leaves the ventricle during this time; this first phase of the cardiac cycle is called *isovolumic contraction*. As systole progresses, ventricular pressure eventually exceeds that of the aorta, so the aortic valve opens. As muscular contraction continues, blood is ejected from the ventricle into the aorta, and ventricular volume decreases during the *ejection* phase of the cycle. As contraction of the cardiac muscle reaches its maximal effort (end of systole), ejection ends as ventricular volume reaches its lowest point (*end-systolic volume*). The amount of blood ejected is called the stroke volume (SV) and equals the difference between end-diastolic and end-systolic volume. The ejection fraction (EF), defined as the percentage of end-diastolic volume (EDV) ejected during a contraction ($EF = 100 \cdot SV/EDV$), provides a practical means of indexing heart strength in the clinical setting. As the muscles relax, ventricular pressure falls below that in the aorta, and the aortic valve closes. Muscular relaxation proceeds, and pressure continues to decrease. Ventricular volume is constant during this phase of *isovolumic relaxation* because both the mitral and aortic valves are closed. Eventually, ventricular pressure falls below the pressure in the left atrium, the mitral valve opens, and blood can flow from the atrium into the ventricle during the *filling* phase.

The four phases of the cardiac cycle are also illustrated by a *pressure-volume diagram* (see Fig. 50–3). The plot of instantaneous ventricular pressure versus volume for one cardiac cycle forms a loop called the *pressure-volume loop*, which sits within the boundaries defined by the end-diastolic and end-systolic pressure-volume relationships. The right ventricle, coupled with the right atrium and the pulmonary artery, undergoes a sequence of events nearly identical to that of the left ventricle except that the magnitudes of the peak pressures are approximately a sixth that of the left ventricle (Table 50–1).

Determinants of Cardiac Performance

Two primary measurements of overall cardiovascular performance are arterial blood pressure and cardiac output (mean arterial blood flow) because both adequate blood pressure and adequate cardiac output are necessary to maintain life. In general terms, these aspects of cardiac performance depend on four fundamental factors: *preload*, *afterload*, *ventricular contractility*, and *heart rate* (Chapter 57).

Preload, which refers to the degree to which sarcomeres are stretched just before the onset of systole, is generally defined for the ventricle as either end-diastolic pressure or end-diastolic volume—two parameters that are interrelated by the nonlinear end-diastolic pressure-volume relationship. As for myocytes, ventricular pressure and flow-generating capacity vary with preload (Frank-Starling law of the heart); a decrease in preload corresponds to a decrease in both end-diastolic volume and pressure, which are associated with decreases in peak pressure and stroke volume (Fig. 50–5). An increase in preload leads to an increase in ventricular pressure and generation of flow, but there are limits to how high preload pressures can be increased; LV end-diastolic pressures in excess of about 20 to 25 mm Hg typically cause exudation of fluid into the alveoli, and the resulting pulmonary edema limits blood oxygenation.

Afterload refers to the physical forces that must be overcome for myocytes to shorten and for the ventricle to eject blood. From the point of view of myocardium, peak arterial pressure provides a measure of the peak stress experienced by myocytes because stress is related to pressure according to Laplace's law. In the absence of LV outflow obstruction, arterial pressure is an appropriate index for quantifying myocyte afterload in vivo. Another parameter that characterizes the ventricular afterloading properties of the arterial system is *total peripheral resistance* (TPR), which predominantly relates to the vasomotor tone of the resistance vessels.

TPR is calculated as the ratio between the mean pressure decrease across the arterial system (mean arterial pressure [MAP] minus mean central venous pressure [CVP]) and cardiac output (CO): TPR = (MAP – CVP)/CO. When compared with the baseline pressure-volume loop, the loop obtained with increased TPR (but a similar preload volume) exhibits a higher peak pressure and a decrease in stroke volume and ejection fraction (see Fig. 50–5).

Contractility refers to the intrinsic strength of the cardiac muscle *(myocardial contractility)* or the ventricle *(ventricular contractility)*, independent of external conditions imposed by either preload or afterload. Inotropic agents such as epinephrine change muscle contractility and therefore induce shifts of the end-systolic pressure-volume relationship and changes in cardiac performance. When compared with the baseline pressure-volume loop, the loop obtained at increased contractility exhibits greater pressure, stroke volume, and ejection fraction despite a constant preload volume and arterial resistance. Although the end-systolic pressure-volume relationship fundamentally provides a load-independent index of ventricular contractility, it is difficult to measure in patients and is usually limited to the research setting. Even though the ejection fraction is influenced by afterload resistance, as well as by changes in contractility, the ejection fraction can help assess response to therapy and is a strong correlate of survival in patients with cardiac disease. Thus, despite theoretical limitations, the ejection fraction provides a simple and useful clinical indicator of overall LV contractile strength.

The importance of the *heart rate* in determining cardiac performance is appreciated by noting that cardiac output measured in liters per minute is equal to the amount of blood ejected at each heartbeat (stroke volume in liters per beat) multiplied by the number of beats per minute. Because blood pressure is related to cardiac output and TPR, heart rate variations also provide a means of influencing mean arterial pressure. Thus, the ability to vary the heart rate provides an effective means of influencing cardiovascular performance.

Cardiac output and mean arterial pressure can be related to the measures of preload, afterload, contractility, and heart rate (see Fig. 50–5B) by Frank-Starling curves. These curves plot end-diastolic pressure versus either cardiac output or mean arterial pressure to provide an overall characterization of LV pump function in practical terms and demonstrate the dependence of pump function on afterload resistance and contractility.

TABLE 50–1 RANGE OF NORMAL RESTING VALUES

PRESSURE
Central venous (mean): 0–5 mm Hg
Right atrial (mean): 0–5 mm Hg
Right ventricular (systolic/diastolic): 20–30/0–5 mm Hg
Pulmonary artery (systolic/diastolic): 20–30/8–12 mm Hg
Left atrial (mean): 8–12 mm Hg
Left ventricular (systolic/diastolic): 100–150/8–12 mm Hg
Aortic (systolic/diastolic): 100–150/70–90 mm Hg
VOLUME-RELATED MEASURES
Right ventricular end-diastolic volume: 70–100 mL
Left ventricular end-diastolic volume: 70–100 mL
Stroke volume: 40–70 mL
Cardiac index: 2.5–4. L/min/m^2
Ejection fraction: 55–70%
ARTERIAL RESISTANCE
Systemic vascular resistance: 10–20 mm Hg·min/L
Pulmonary vascular resistance: 0.5–1.5 mm Hg·min/L

Determination of Myocardial Oxygen Consumption and Energy Metabolism

The heart relies almost exclusively on oxidation of fatty acids and glucose as an immediate source of energy. The heart normally extracts

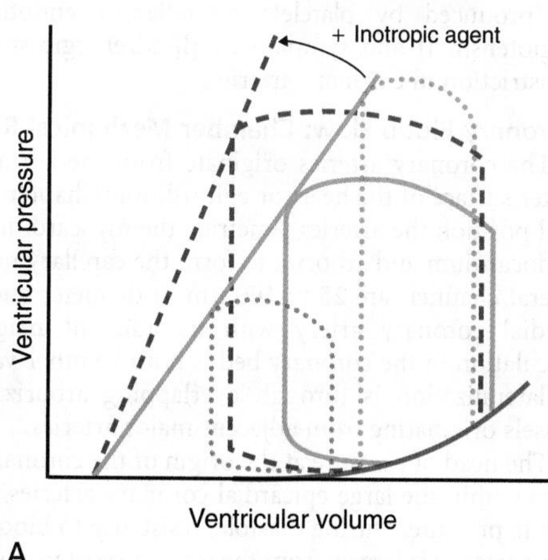

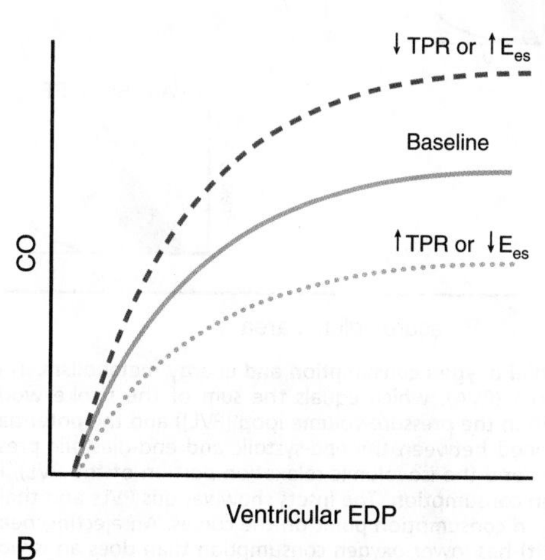

FIGURE 50–5 • Cardiac performance. A, Baseline end-systolic pressure-volume relationship (ESPVR) and pressure-volume loop shown by the solid green lines. The effect of a decrease in filling volume (but constant vascular resistance) on the loop is shown by the dotted purple line. The effect of increased afterload resistance (but nearly constant preload volume) on the loop is shown by the orange dotted-dashed line. The effect of a positive inotropic agent on the ESPVR and on the pressure-volume loop with constant afterload resistance and nearly constant preload is shown by the blue dashed line. With the exception of the inotropic agent, the changes in pressure and stroke volume do not reflect changes in intrinsic cardiac function. **B,** The dependence of cardiac output (CO) on contractility (E_{es}) and total peripheral resistance (TPR) is summarized by Frank Starling curves, which plot CO as a function of filling pressure (EDP). The nature of this interdependence is summarized by modern theories of ventricular vascular coupling according to the following equations: CO ≈ HR · [EDV – V_0]/[1 + TPR/(T · E_{es})], and mean arterial pressure (MAP) ≈ [EDV – V_0]/[T/TPR + 1/E_{es}], where T is the duration of the cardiac cycle (i.e., T = 60/HR), HR is heart rate, and EDV is end-diastolic volume.

free fatty acids preferentially from the coronary blood for oxidative energy production. Under conditions of limited oxygen supply, this preference is changed to glucose because glucose metabolism generates a greater amount of ATP for a given amount of oxygen consumed. In the heart, anaerobic metabolism (i.e., glycolysis) provides very limited energy, and muscular contraction cannot be supported under such conditions; as a result, the heart is dependent on the availability of oxygen to continue its function. Thus, when oxygen is unavailable (e.g., hypoxia, ischemia, carbon monoxide poisoning), heart function deteriorates remarkably rapidly, essentially on a beat-to-beat basis.

The oxygen and energy consumption of the heart is determined principally by four major independent factors: basal metabolism, total mechanical work performed by the heart, contractility, and heart rate. The latter three directly relate to contraction. Only 10 to 20% of the total oxygen consumption of the heart is used to maintain functions other than contraction, such as basal metabolism. As detailed earlier, the two processes that require energy during each contraction are breaking of the rigor complex of the myofilaments and sequestration of the calcium dump by the sarcoplasmic reticulum.

Myocardial oxygen consumption is tightly related to the total amount of mechanical work performed, which can be indexed by the total *pressure-volume area* (PVA; Fig. 50–6). PVA is the sum of external work performed by the heart in propelling the blood from the ventricle to the aorta (which is the area inside the pressure-volume loop) plus unliberated internal energy stored in the myocardium at the end of contraction. PVA is related to the number of cross-bridges formed (and therefore required to break) during the contraction.

With an increase in the contractile state, an additional obligatory increase in oxygen consumption is produced above what is related to the heart rate and PVA because with only a few important exceptions, changes in contractility are mediated by an increase in the amount of calcium released to the myofilaments. Thus, increased ATP and therefore increased oxygen consumption are needed for the increased sarcoplasmic reticular ATPase activity.

Finally, a more rapid heart rate requires a greater rate of oxygen consumption per unit time because of the greater number of contractions. Interestingly, at a given contractility and a given set of loading conditions, oxygen consumption *per beat* is roughly constant. The only determinant of oxygen consumption that does not change with heart rate is basal metabolism. Thus, if the heart rate increases from 60 to 180 beats per minute during exercise or stress, oxygen consumption increases almost three-fold over the basal value.

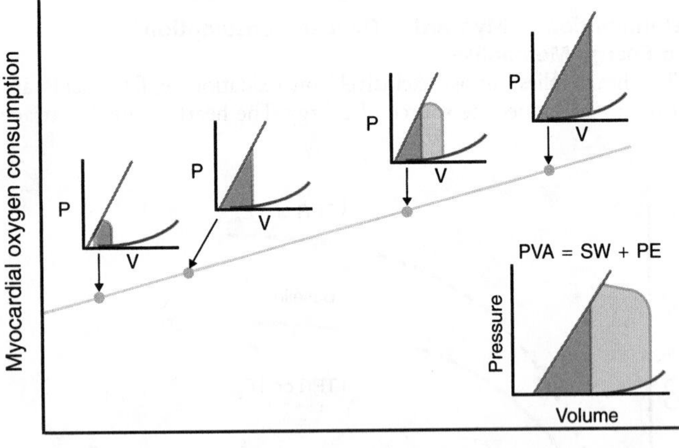

FIGURE 50–6 • Myocardial oxygen consumption and energy metabolism. The total pressure-volume area (PVA), which equals the sum of the stroke work ([SW]; area contained within the pressure-volume loop [PVL]) and the potential energy ([PE]; area contained between the end-systolic and end-diastolic pressure-volume relationships and the isovolumic relaxation portion of the PVL), is linearly related to oxygen consumption. The insets show various PVLs and their corresponding PVA–oxygen consumption point on the curves. An ejecting beat at low filling volume (left) has lower oxygen consumption than does an isovolumic beat at the same filling volume (second from the left). For isovolumic contractions, there is no external SW; all generated energy is PE. When filling is increased, PVA increases for both ejecting and isovolumic contractions in proportion to the increase in PVA. The nonzero y-axis intercept indicates the substantial energy requirements for basal metabolism and for calcium cycling, which are not directly related to energy for force generation. At increased contractility, the PVA–oxygen consumption curve shifts upward in a parallel manner, which is related largely to the fuel required for cycling the increased amount of calcium present at the increased contractility.

Coronary Blood Flow: Metabolic and Neurohormonal Regulation

The myocardium relies on a continuous supply of oxygen delivered via coronary perfusion. The myocardium extracts 80 to 90% or more of the oxygen delivered to it in blood, even under basal resting conditions. Thus, the striking increases in energy consumption that occur with the development of high tension, higher heart rates, or high contractility are met almost entirely by increases in coronary blood flow. High rates of myocardial oxygen consumption and coronary flow are characteristic of exercise.

The predominant mechanisms involved in this augmentation of coronary blood flow from normal values of 60 to 100 mL/100 g/min to values that are six-fold higher are metabolic factors, especially adenosine released in the setting of increased breakdown of ATP. Adenosine is the byproduct of the breakdown of ATP to adenosine monophosphate and then to adenosine. A second control of the magnitude of coronary blood flow under increased workload or demand conditions is nitric oxide, which is produced by coronary vascular endothelial cells and has a direct local vasodilating effect on coronary arteries and the more distal bed. Nitric oxide is a byproduct in a number of reactions that lead to an increase in the activity of nitric oxide synthase, an enzyme that produces nitric oxide from the amino acid L-arginine. In addition to adenosine and nitric oxide, other longer-acting coronary vasodilators such as bradykinin, prostaglandins, and CO_2 may have a direct effect in maintaining coronary artery blood flow.

Coronary artery mechanical changes also contribute to regulation of coronary flow. As coronary arteries are stretched by higher luminal pressure, they constrict; as pressure within the coronary artery is reduced, the artery dilates. These very potent changes, which help maintain coronary blood flow under circumstances of altered coronary flow hemodynamics but maintained oxygen demands, are termed *autoregulatory* mechanisms for coronary blood flow.

In addition to the metabolic and other factors that lead to coronary vasodilation, a series of factors can lead to coronary arterial vasoconstriction. The exact roles of these vasoconstricting factors in health are unclear, but in disease these factors may have a profoundly important effect. A local regulating factor is the endothelin system, which consists of peptides that are synthesized and controlled locally within small arteries or arterioles and have a profound vasoconstricting effect on resistance arteries within the coronary circulation. Constricting endothelins may be produced at the site of coronary artery atherosclerotic lesions and lead to vasoconstriction at these sites. In addition, at sites of coronary artery atherosclerosis where the endothelium is disrupted or abnormal, circulating vasoconstrictor substances gain access to smooth muscle receptors that are ordinarily covered by coronary arterial endothelium (Chapter 69). These substances include circulating serotonin, 5-hydroxytryptamine, and other serotonin-like substances, as well as thromboxane, which may be produced by platelets or adjacent endothelium. In addition, angiotensin II and sympathetic β_1-adrenergic stimulation cause vasoconstriction in coronary arteries.

Coronary Blood Flow: Chamber Mechanical Regulation

The coronary arteries originate from the aorta and spread over the outer surface of the heart or epicardium (Chapter 56). From this epicardial position the arteries penetrate the myocardium from epicardium to endocardium and arborize to form the capillary network. Coronary collateral channels are 25 to 100 μm in diameter and link one major epicardial coronary artery with its adjacent neighbor. The collateral circulation in the coronary bed is not like other vascular beds, in which collateralization is through overlapping arborization of small blood vessels originating from adjacent major arteries.

The head of pressure at the origin of the coronary artery and the pressure within the large epicardial coronary arteries directly reflect central aortic pressure. During diastole, resistance to blood flow from the coronary arteries is largely from the tone of resistance vessels. During systole, coronary perfusion pressure (which equals aortic pressure) is determined by LV intracavitary pressure. In turn, cavitary pressure equals the pressure within the inner myocardial wall. It is not surprising, then, that the endocardial coronary arteries are remarkably compressed during systole. The systolic pressure within the thick LV wall toward the epicardial surface is not nearly as high as that in the endocardial portion of the wall. Therefore, coronary blood flow during both systole and diastole is directed toward the epicardium but is essentially exclusively limited to diastole in the subendocardium.

In addition, if LV workload is increased or myocardial contractility or function is decreased, LV diastolic pressure will increase. This increase in diastolic pressure acts as a compressor force on the subendocardial vessels and limits myocardial blood flow during this critical period of diastole. Finally, the influence of heart rate on coronary blood flow, particularly to the subendocardium, is important and dramatic. As the heart rate increases, the period of diastole between beats becomes shorter and shorter. This limitation of coronary flow to the subendocardium during tachycardia can have profound effects in the setting of coronary artery disease and heart failure such that drugs that block tachycardia during exercise may be very useful therapeutically.

Neurohormonal Regulation of the Cardiovascular System

The major constituents of the neurohormonal systems that regulate cardiovascular function are the sympathetic and parasympathetic components of the autonomic nervous system and the renin-angiotensin system (Chapter 57). The major attributes of the sympathetic nervous system in responding rapidly to stress are the ability to increase the heart rate, to increase myocardial contractility, and to regulate vascular tone in the various organs. Most of these functions are performed by the sympathetic nervous system through release of norepinephrine at the nerve endings throughout the circulation. Under more profound stress, the sympathetic nervous system elaborates epinephrine from the adrenal gland. Norepinephrine and epinephrine act principally through the β-adrenergic vasoconstricting mechanisms in the periphery and by increasing contractility primarily by stimulating β-adrenergic receptors in the heart. Epinephrine has a more striking β-adrenergic effect than norepinephrine does, especially at low circulating levels. Through these β-adrenergic actions, epinephrine profoundly increases the heart rate and, at the same time, induces vasodilation of the central arterial bed, thereby reducing impedance to LV ejection. The coronary circulation operates in a mixed fashion, with evidence of coronary artery vasoconstriction occurring in response to β-adrenergic stimulation and vasodilation in response to lower doses of epinephrine.

The most important parasympathetic innervation is that of the sinoatrial and atrioventricular nodes, where these nerves slow the firing rate of pacemaker tissue and slow conduction in the atrioventricular node (Chapter 60). The neurotransmitter for the parasympathetic nervous system is acetylcholine. Ventricular muscle is poorly innervated by the parasympathetic nervous system and vagal tone has very little effect on contractility under normal resting conditions; however, increased vagal tone depresses myocardial contractility when sympathetic tone is high. At rest, the heart rate is under control of the parasympathetic nervous system rather than the sympathetic system. Thus, β-adrenergic blocking drugs have little effect on the heart rate at rest but markedly reduce augmentation of the heart rate particularly at high levels of exercise.

The sympathetic nervous system also has a profound vasoconstrictive effect on the venous system, especially the capacitance bed within the splanchnic or abdominal circulation. Thus, in forms of stress that are associated with rapid loss of blood or fluids, the venous constrictive effects of sympathetic stimulation can be life-saving.

The renin-angiotensin system is a second coordinated system that regulates blood pressure, peripheral vasoconstriction, and contractility in a fashion complementary to the sympathetic nervous system. Generally, action of the renin-angiotensin system is not nearly as immediate or profound as that of the sympathetic nervous system, but it operates principally as an intermediate- and long-term regulator. Under pathologic conditions such as heart failure, the system can remain chronically activated (Chapter 57). Renin is a hormone released by macula densa cells within the juxtaglomerular apparatus of the kidney under conditions of decreased perfusion to the kidney, decreased delivery of sodium to the macula densa, or increasing sympathetic activity (Chapter 116). Once renin is released, it acts exclusively through the production of angiotensin II, a potent peripheral vasoconstrictor and coronary artery constrictor, within the circulation and at individual organ sites. Angiotensin II induces release of the sodium-retaining hormone aldosterone from the adrenal gland (Chapter 246). All these actions tend to retain sodium in the circulation and increase arterial blood pressure. Angiotensin, which is also a potent stimulus to both myocardial and peripheral vessel hypertrophy, promotes the release of norepinephrine from peripheral sympathetic nervous system sites.

Cardiovascular Response to Exercise

High levels of exercise require truly remarkable augmentation of heart function and performance, as well as adaptation of the peripheral circulation. Enhanced blood flow is needed to the exercising muscles and restriction of blood flow away from parts of the body that are not essential during the period of exercise. Blood flow is also augmented to the skin and oral mucosa for dissipation of the heat produced by exercising muscles.

Oxygen consumption for the entire body during strenuous exercise increases approximately 18-fold. Two thirds of this increase in oxygen consumption results from greater cardiac output and the remaining third from an increase in oxygen extraction from arterial blood. Arterial oxygen saturation usually remains near 100%, whereas venous oxygen saturation decreases from approximately 75 to 25%. This increase in oxygen extraction is mostly related to the increase in blood flow to the exercising muscle, which essentially extracts most of the oxygen within the blood. The increase in blood flow to the exercising muscle occurs as a result of an increase in arterial pressure and perfusion of the exercising limbs and profound vasodilation of the arteries of the exercising muscle. Arterial dilation is a consequence of the release of potassium and other vasodilating substances from the exercising muscle. Whereas overall cardiac output may increase 6-fold, blood flow to the exercising muscle may increase 40- or 50-fold from rest to exercise.

This increase in blood flow to the exercising muscle and the increase in skin blood flow augment venous return to the heart. The heart accommodates this augmentation in venous return by increasing cardiac function remarkably. The major element in this increase in cardiac function in normal young individuals is an augmentation in sympathetic drive to the heart and a withdrawal of vagal tone. The heart rate is increased, contractility is increased (resulting in increased ventricular ejection and an increase in the ventricular ejection fraction), ejection and filling rates are increased, aortic impedance is decreased, and systolic blood pressure is increased.

In a young individual, withdrawal of vagal tone and greater sympathetic drive during maximal exercise increase the heart rate from 60 to 70 beats per minute at rest to 170 to 200 beats per minute. At this rapid heart rate, not only must ejection of blood be more rapid, but it is also essential to use mechanisms to augment the rate of filling the heart. These increases in contractility with associated increases in the velocity of ejection and filling occur as a result of augmented sympathetic drive to the heart, which increases the amount of calcium cycling within the cell and increases the rate of sarcoplasmic reticulum ATPase activity to hasten calcium sequestration.

Another sympathetic adaptation during exercise is arterial vasodilation of the aorta and central arteries. This β-sympathetic central arterial vasodilation decreases the impedance to LV ejection, but the augmentation in cardiac output is so great that even though impedance is lowered, systolic arterial blood pressure rises. The final mechanism available to the heart to augment cardiac function beyond that created by the withdrawal of vagal tone and the increase in sympathetic tone is an enhancement of preload (the Frank-Starling mechanism). A young individual at maximum exercise uses this mechanism very little, but when the sympathetic nervous system is blocked or when the sympathetic response is limited by aging or chronic heart failure, preload recruitment operates as a reserve mechanism to augment cardiac output during exercise. With increased preload, the left ventricle (and presumably the right ventricle) dilates acutely to a larger diastolic volume. This increase in diastolic volume results in stretching of myocardial fibers and augmentation of pump function.

Physiologic Principles Underlying Heart Failure

Heart failure is generally defined as an inability of the heart to provide sufficient blood flow to meet the metabolic demands of the body, which it can do only at a pathologically increased filling pressure (Chapter 57). When heart failure is due to systolic dysfunction and volume overload, the heart increases its size (rightward shift of the end-diastolic pressure-volume relationship) as a result of myocyte hypertrophy (increased cell length and width with concomitant molecular and extracellular matrix changes characteristic of hypertrophy) and fiber rearrangement.

Age Changes in the Cardiovascular System

In the cardiovascular system, intrinsic cardiac muscle function, the inotropic response to nonsympathetic mediators, and coronary perfusion are well maintained with age (Chapter 22). With age, however, cellular hypertrophy occurs because of both cell dropout and increased stiffening of the vascular tree; the result is increased afterload on the left ventricle. As a consequence of the hypertrophy, systole is prolonged.

Large arteries stiffen with age. Thus, even without hypertension, an age-related increase in impedance to ejection, a greater systolic load, and an increased pulse wave velocity occur. In addition, the *chronotropic* (i.e., heart rate response) and inotropic response to sympathetic mediation is diminished, so conditions that put sudden loads on the left ventricle, such as acute hypertension or myocardial infarction (Chapter 72), have more severe consequences in the elderly. Furthermore, disease and stress may produce less compensatory hypertrophy in the elderly and therefore place more stress on the left ventricle with age.

With exercise or other forms of stress, the effects of a decreased β-sympathetic response in the elderly are dominant. Older individuals have less of an increase in heart rate and contractility and a larger increase in impedance. Fortunately, the intrinsic cardiac muscle reserve is adequate to compensate for these limitations in exercise response if no cardiac disease is present. In the presence of disease, however, cardiac reserve is diminished. Therefore, older individuals or victims of acute myocardial infarction or heart failure have much greater difficulty during exercise because the heart rate increases less, load or impedance is greater, and preload recruitment may already be near the maximally tolerated level.

SUGGESTED READINGS

Burkhoff D, Mirsky I, Suga H: Assessment of systolic and diastolic ventricular properties via pressure-volume analysis: A guide for clinical, translational, and basic researchers. Am J Physiol Heart Circ Physiol 2005;289:H501–H512. *A comprehensive, practical overview.*

Burkhoff D, Dickstein ML, Ferber P: The Heart Simulator. Available at http://www.columbia.edu/itc/hs/medical/heartsim/. *A useful learning tool for cardiac physiology.*

Cingolani HE, Ennis IL: Sodium-hydrogen exchanger, cardiac overload, and myocardial hypertrophy. Circulation 2007;115:1090–1100. *Summary of the causative factors and pathophysiologic correlation of cardiac overload and the sodium-hydrogen exchanger.*

Knaapen P, Germans T, Knuuti J, et al: Myocardial energetics and efficiency: Current status of the noninvasive approach. Circulation 2007;115:918–927. *A review of the principle of mechanical efficiency and its invasive and noninvasive assessment.*

51 RADIOLOGY OF THE HEART

Murray G. Baron

The heart casts a homogeneous shadow on the chest film. No internal detail can be seen within its contours because the radiodensity of blood, myocardium, and other cardiac tissues is so similar that one cannot be distinguished from the others. Only two borders of the heart, where it contacts the radiolucent, air-containing lung, can be discerned in any one projection. Changes in the size or shape (or both) of the chambers of the heart and the great vessels usually alter the shape of the cardiac silhouette. However, because the heart is a three-dimensional structure, multiple views are required for complete radiographic evaluation. With the advent of echocardiography, the need for this "cardiac series" has disappeared. However, a remarkable amount of information regarding the heart is contained on standard frontal and lateral chest films, which remain a useful tool for detecting disease, evaluating the severity of known disease, documenting the progress of disease, and assessing the efficacy of treatment.

RADIOLOGIC ANATOMY

Except for the more complex cardiac anomalies, which are rare, especially in adults, the positions and spatial relationships of the cardiac chambers and the great vessels are the same from one patient to the next and are not significantly affected by disease. On a frontal chest film, the right cardiac border is composed of a straight vertical upper half formed by the superior vena cava and a gently convex lower half representing the lateral wall of the right atrium (Fig. 51–1). The break in the contour of this border of the heart indicates the caval-atrial junction. Some patients are able to inhale deeply enough to uncover a small, straight segment of the inferior vena cava between the diaphragm and the right atrium.

Abnormalities of the caval segment are usually due to dilation of the ascending aorta. A localized bulge in its midportion usually indicates post-stenotic dilation secondary to aortic valve stenosis, whereas aortic insufficiency is commonly associated with a more generalized dilation of the aorta. A bulge in the region of the caval-atrial junction may be due to an aneurysm of either the right coronary artery or the noncoronary sinus of Valsalva or to a markedly enlarged left atrium. Dilation of either atrium tends to extend the cardiac silhouette to the right, whereas dilation of either ventricle enlarges the silhouette to the left.

The left cardiac border is composed of four distinct segments. The uppermost bulge represents the aortic knob, the most distal portion of the aortic arch where it turns downward to become the descending aorta. The prominence below the knob is formed by the main pulmonary artery and the subvalvular portion of the outflow tract of the right ventricle. The lowermost third of this border represents the anterolateral wall of the left ventricle. Between this bulge and that of the pulmonary artery is a short, flat, or slightly concave segment where the left atrial appendage reaches the border of the heart.

Aneurysms of the descending thoracic aorta commonly involve its most proximal portion in the region of the ligamentum arteriosum and appear as a dilated aortic knob. Prominence of the pulmonary artery segment is common in younger individuals, but after the age of 35 to 40 years, such dilation is almost always an indicator of pulmonary arterial hypertension.

In the lateral view (see Fig. 51–1C), the anterior border of the cardiac silhouette is formed by the body and the outflow tract of the right ventricle. The heart lies in the anterior portion of the chest, and the right ventricle abuts the lower third of the sternum. Both the outflow tract and the pulmonary artery slope posteriorly. Air-containing lung interposed between this portion of the heart and the anterior chest wall forms the "retrosternal clear space." The posterior border of the heart extends from the level of the pulmonary carina to the diaphragm. Its upper half is formed by the back of the left atrium, and the lower half represents the posterior wall of the left ventricle. The shadow of the inferior vena cava is usually seen in the lateral projection extending obliquely upward and anteriorly from the diaphragm to enter the posterior aspect of the right atrium. The lowermost contour of the normal left ventricle curves anteriorly and crosses the inferior vena cava about 2 cm above the left side of the diaphragm.

Alterations in the contour of the heart usually reflect dilation or hypertrophy of the chambers, or both. Many times the pattern of these changes, together with the appearance of the pulmonary vasculature, points to a specific underlying cardiac abnormality. Chest films are most sensitive for detecting chamber dilation. Cardiac hypertrophy is more difficult to recognize because the thickened myocardium tends to encroach on the ventricular lumen more than extending outward and enlarging the cardiac silhouette. With severe hypertrophy, as in hypertrophic cardiomyopathy, the heart enlarges to the left and the apex becomes blunted, but this appearance is not pathognomonic.

HEART SIZE

A normal-sized heart does not guarantee the absence of cardiac disease. Angina, for example, no matter how severe, does not affect heart size until the left ventricle decompensates. Similarly, patients with restrictive cardiomyopathy may be in severe heart failure with a normal-appearing heart. Conversely, an enlarged heart always indicates the presence of cardiac or pericardial disease. Therefore, accurate evaluation of heart size is important.

Heart size, in the absence of disease, is directly related to the habitus of the patient. The cardiothoracic ratio, which compares the transverse diameter of the heart with the width of the chest, gives a readily obtainable, rough estimate of heart size. This ratio is measured by dropping a vertical line through the heart and summing the greatest distance to the right and left cardiac borders (Fig. 51–2) to give the transverse cardiac diameter. The transverse thoracic diameter, the greatest width of the chest, is measured from the inner surfaces of the ribs. Dividing the cardiac diameter by the chest diameter gives the cardiothoracic ratio. A value of less than 0.6 can be considered within the limits of normal. Setting this value at 0.5, as is often done, produces too many false-positive results.

In most cases, exact measurement of the cardiac silhouette is not necessary, and a reasonably experienced observer can achieve an acceptable degree of accuracy by visual estimation. With either method, several cau-

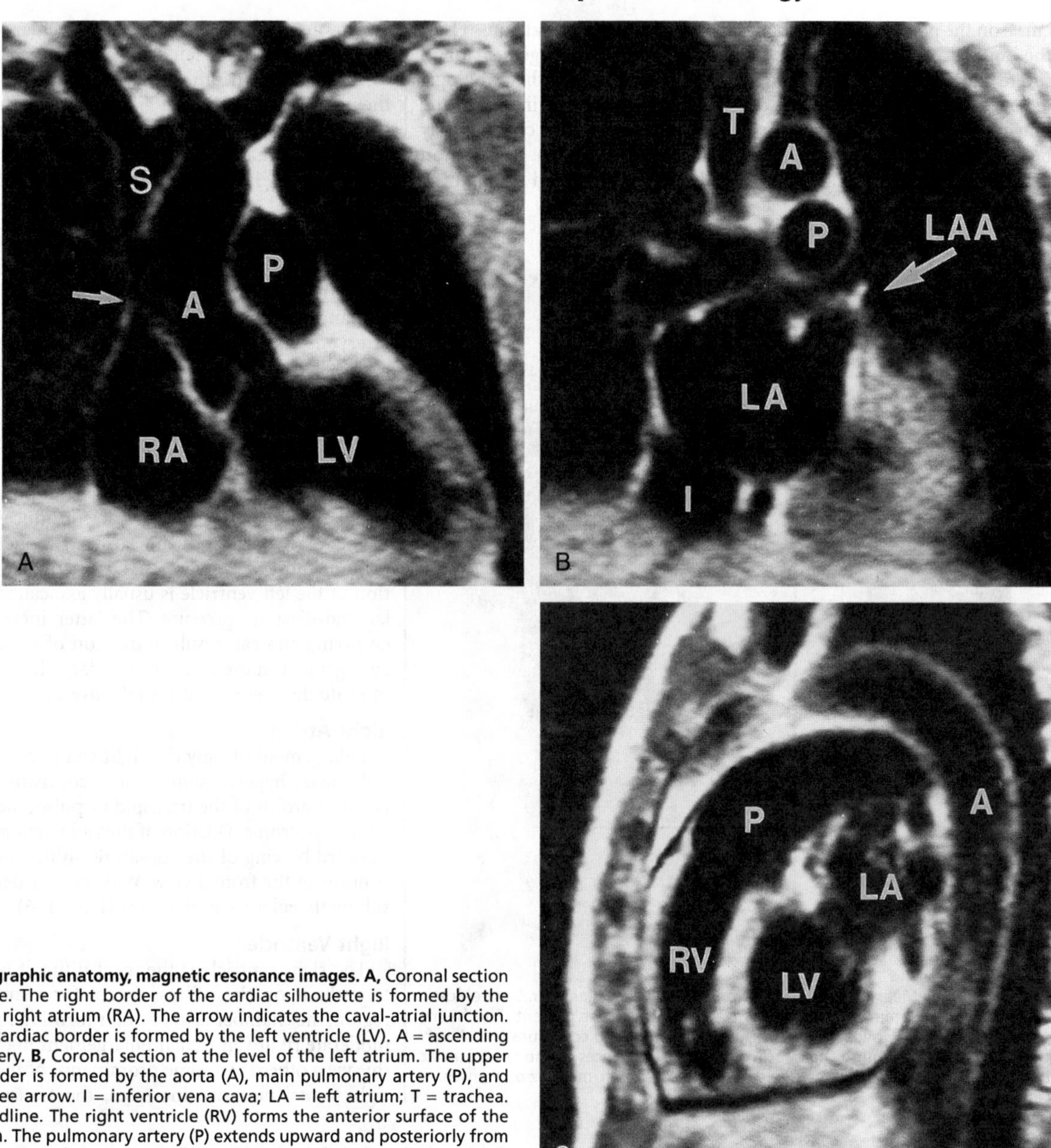

FIGURE 51–1 • Normal radiographic anatomy, magnetic resonance images. A, Coronal section at the level of the aortic valve. The right border of the cardiac silhouette is formed by the superior vena cava (S) and the right atrium (RA). The arrow indicates the caval-atrial junction. The lower portion of the left cardiac border is formed by the left ventricle (LV). A = ascending aorta; P = main pulmonary artery. **B,** Coronal section at the level of the left atrium. The upper portion of the left cardiac border is formed by the aorta (A), main pulmonary artery (P), and left atrial appendage (LAA), see arrow. I = inferior vena cava; LA = left atrium; T = trachea. **C,** Sagittal section near the midline. The right ventricle (RV) forms the anterior surface of the heart, which abuts the sternum. The pulmonary artery (P) extends upward and posteriorly from the ventricle. The posterior border of the heart is formed by the left atrium (LA) and left ventricle (LV). The aorta (A) is behind the heart.

tions must be observed. The single greatest effect on apparent cardiac size is the degree of inspiration. The volume of the heart is essentially constant throughout the cardiac cycle. As the diaphragm moves up with expiration, the vertical diameter of the heart is shortened and its transverse diameter increases. Because heart size is estimated primarily from its width, the heart appears larger on expiratory films. The degree of inspiration can be determined from the relationship of the diaphragm to the ribs. On a properly positioned frontal chest film, a reasonable degree of inspiration is indicated if the diaphragm is lowered to at least the level of the posterior portion of the ninth rib.

When the anteroposterior diameter of the chest is small, the heart may be compressed between the sternum and the spine so that it splays to one or both sides. For this reason, the heart often appears enlarged in patients with the straight back syndrome or with a pectus excavatum deformity of the sternum. An epicardial fat pad (actually it is extrapleural fat outside the pericardium) can occur in one or both cardiophrenic angles and make the heart appear larger than it actually is. The fat pad can be recognized because the cardiophrenic angle appears obtuse or the cardiac apex is indistinct. In addition, the slightly greater density of the heart can usually be distinguished from the more radiolucent image of the fat.

A change in size of the cardiac silhouette can also occur between systole and diastole. This point is important because chest films are exposed at random with reference to the cardiac cycle, so a change in heart size between two examinations may be solely due to the timing of filming. In the majority of cases, the difference in the transverse cardiac diameter between systole and diastole is small, no more than several millimeters. However, in younger patients, especially the more athletic with a slow heart rate and a large stroke volume, phasic change in the normal cardiac diameter can be as large as 2 cm.

CHAMBER ENLARGEMENT

Left Atrium

Dilation of the left atrium alone, in the absence of a left-to-right shunt, is most often due to disease of the mitral valve, although it can also result simply from atrial fibrillation. The two "popular" radiologic signs of left atrial enlargement—a double contour within the right cardiac border and elevation of the left main bronchus—are accurate when present, but they are insensitive and seen in only about half the cases of mitral valve disease. To produce a discernible margin within the cardiac silhouette in the frontal projection, the thickness of the heart must increase sharply at some point. This increase in thickness occurs in mitral disease when the left atrium enlarges and protrudes posteriorly from the back of the heart. The right border of the left atrium is then silhouetted where it abuts the right lung, and its contour is seen within the cardiac silhouette (Fig. 51–3A). This pattern is not apparent with lesser degrees of left atrial enlargement. Conversely, when the right atrium also enlarges, as is common in long-standing mitral valve disease, it forms a continuous curve on the posterior cardiac border with the enlarged left atrium. Thus, the double contour is not seen with mild left atrial enlargement or in severe cases of mitral valve disease. Furthermore, because the radiologic technique used for chest films is chosen to provide optimal images of the lungs, the enlarged heart is underexposed and the double contour may be hidden within its opaque silhouette. For the same reason, the position of the left main bronchus often cannot be clearly visualized through the mediastinal shadow.

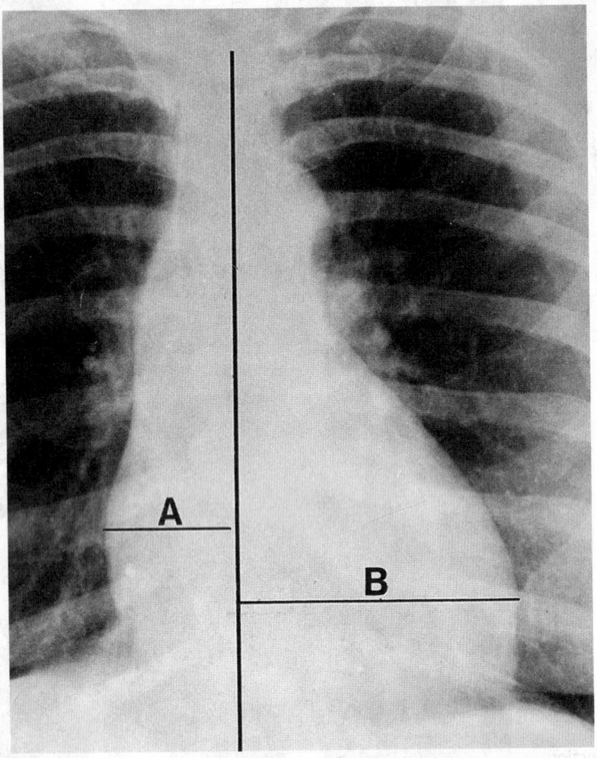

FIGURE 51–2 • Measurement of the transverse cardiac diameter. Severe aortic stenosis with a 95-mm systolic gradient across the valve is present. The heart, though considerably hypertrophied, is normal in size and configuration. A vertical line is drawn through the heart. The greatest distances to the right cardiac border (A) and to the left cardiac border (B) are then measured. Transverse cardiac diameter = A + B.

A more sensitive sign of left atrial enlargement in the frontal projection is dilation of the left atrial appendage. The appendage extends anteriorly from the atrium along the left side of the heart, below the level of the pulmonary artery (see Fig. 51–1B). It forms the part of the left heart border between the pulmonary artery segment and the left ventricular segment. Normally, the border of the appendage is flat or slightly concave. Any convexity is abnormal and usually indicates left atrial enlargement.

Left Ventricle

The shape of the dilated left ventricle depends to a large extent on the underlying cause. When it is due to insufficiency of the aortic or mitral valve, the ventricle elongates and its apex is displaced downward, to the left, and posteriorly (Fig. 51–4). When the dilation is due to coronary artery disease or primary myocardial disease, the ventricle tends to assume a more globular shape. In the lateral view, the downward extension of the enlarged left ventricle covers more of the vena cava shadow than normal, and the crossing point of their posterior borders occurs nearer to the diaphragm than normal. Unfortunately, the usefulness of this sign is limited because of the distortion produced by even slight rotation of the patient from the true lateral position.

Enlargement of the left ventricle produces a smoothly curved dilation of the lower portion of the cardiac silhouette. A localized bulge in this contour most often represents a ventricular aneurysm (Fig. 51–5). Dilation of the left ventricle is usually associated with elevated left ventricular end-diastolic pressure. The latter increases resistance to left atrial emptying and can result in dilation of the atrium. Therefore, left atrial enlargement in the presence of a large left ventricle does not necessarily indicate the presence of mitral valve disease.

Right Atrium

Enlargement of only the right chambers of the heart is seen in severe pulmonary hypertension without coexisting left heart failure, in bacterial endocarditis of the tricuspid or pulmonic valve (or both), and in carcinoid syndrome. Dilation of the right atrium causes an accentuation and outward bowing of the curvature on the lower half of the right cardiac contour in the frontal view. With greater degrees of dilation, the cardiac silhouette enlarges to the right (Fig. 51–6).

Right Ventricle

The right ventricle is the most difficult of the four cardiac chambers to evaluate on chest films. Except for a small area in the subpulmonic region, the chamber is not border forming in the frontal projection. Even moderate right ventricular enlargement may produce no abnormality in this view other than some prominence of the main pulmonary artery. As right ventricular size increases, the transverse diameter of the heart

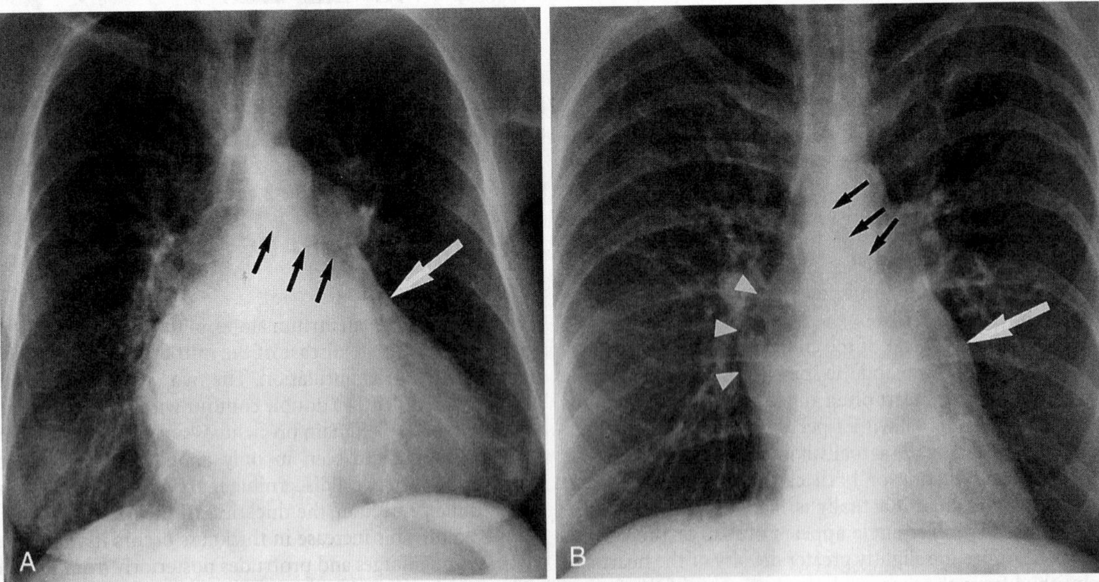

FIGURE 51–3 • Left atrial enlargement in mitral valve disease. A, Patient 1: The enlarged left atrium is causing the central portion of the cardiac silhouette to be abnormally dense. The right border of the atrium is seen within the right side of the cardiac silhouette. The left main bronchus (small arrows) is elevated. The region of the left atrial appendage (white arrow) is slightly concave because this structure was resected at a previous mitral commissurotomy. **B,** Patient 2: The enlarged left atrial appendage bulges from the left side of the heart (white arrow), whereas the body of the atrium (arrowheads) extends beyond the right atrium to form a part of the right heart border. No double density is seen within the heart, and the left main bronchus (small arrows) is not elevated.

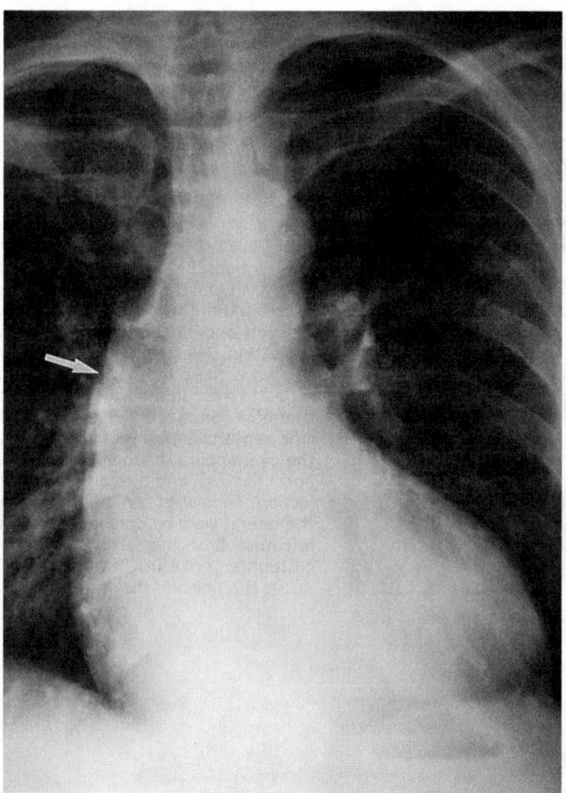

FIGURE 51–4 • Left ventricular dilation, aortic insufficiency. The apex of the heart is displaced downward and to the left. The ascending aorta (arrow) is diffusely dilated. The pulmonary vasculature is normal.

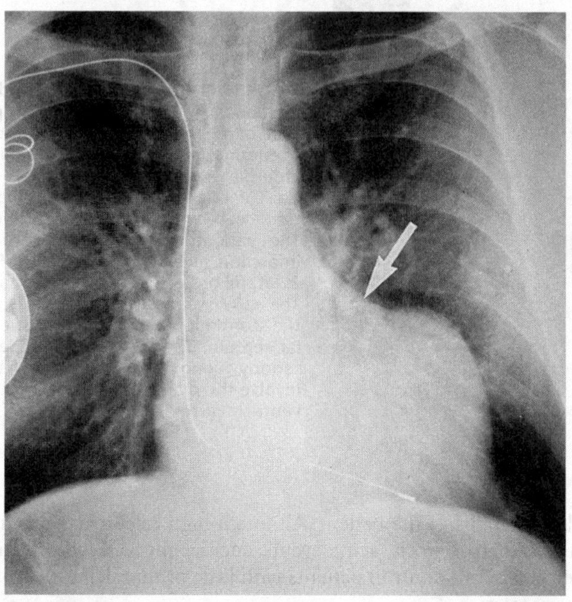

FIGURE 51–5 • Left ventricular aneurysm. A bulge on the lower portion of the left cardiac border, formed by the anterolateral wall of the left ventricle, represents a ventricular aneurysm. The patient had suffered a myocardial infarction 1 year previously. The left atrial appendage segment (arrow) is normal. A transvenous pacemaker has been inserted through the right subclavian vein. The electrode tip is situated in the apex of the right ventricle.

enlarges to the left, and the cardiac apex becomes blunted and elevated (see Fig. 51–6). Enlargement of either or both ventricles displaces the apex of the heart to the left. It is not often possible to distinguish between biventricular enlargement and dilation of one or the other ventricle.

As the right ventricle enlarges, its area of contact with the sternum increases and tends to obliterate the retrosternal clear space in the lateral view. This sign is nonspecific inasmuch as it also depends on the shape of the chest and the size of the left ventricle, as well as the size of the right ventricle.

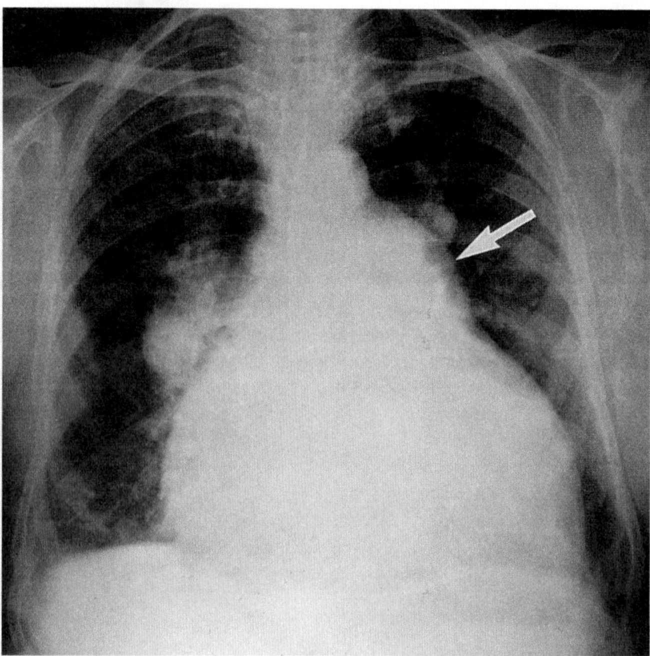

FIGURE 51–6 • Right ventricular enlargement seen in a patient with resistive pulmonary hypertension secondary to an atrial septal defect. The main pulmonary artery (arrow) and the right pulmonary artery are markedly dilated. The left pulmonary artery was also dilated but is hidden by the heart in this view. The sudden "cutoff" of the vascular shadows just beyond the hila is characteristic of resistive pulmonary hypertension. Enlargement of the right ventricle is elevating the cardiac apex and displacing it to the left. Accentuation of the curvature of the lower right cardiac border and enlargement of the cardiac silhouette to the right are caused by dilation of the right atrium.

CALCIFICATION

Most calcifications involving the heart occur in cardiac structures as a result of inflammatory or necrotic processes (or both) or degenerative disease. Because the calcific deposits have greater radiodensity than cardiac tissues do, they can often be seen within the cardiac silhouette.

The aortic and mitral valves abut each other, both inserting on the central fibrous tendon of the heart. On a frontal chest film, the two valves lie next to each other in the midportion of the cardiac silhouette, to the left of the spine (Fig. 51–7A), the aortic valve being slightly higher. It is often difficult to determine which valve is calcified in this view. They can be separated by fluoroscopy because the aortic valve tends to move in a vertical direction as the heart beats whereas the motion of the mitral valve approximates the horizontal. This distinction can also be made accurately from the lateral chest film. If a line is drawn from the left main bronchus, seen as a dark circular shadow over the lower end of the trachea, to the anterior costophrenic angle, the mitral valve lies below the line and the aortic valve is above it (Fig. 51–7B).

In the United States, calcification of only the aortic valve is most likely to represent degenerative disease of the cusps (a process in older patients akin to coronary artery calcification) or deterioration of a congenitally bicuspid valve (Chapter 75). In developing countries, calcification of the aortic or mitral valves, or both, is usually a late sequela of rheumatic fever. Calcification of the mitral annulus, which is seen in patients older than 70 years and is about four times more frequent in women than in men, is only rarely of clinical significance. The pattern of calcification is characteristic and should not be confused with that of the mitral valve. Calcium is deposited mainly between the base of the posterior mitral leaflet and the posterior wall of the left ventricle. It is seen as a broad, curvilinear band of calcium in a "C" shape, open superiorly and to the right on the frontal film and anteriorly on the lateral. In severe cases, the calcific deposits may also extend across the base of the anterior mitral leaflet and then form an "O" encircling the mitral orifice.

Calcification of the myocardium almost always indicates a previous transmural infarction and, frequently, a ventricular aneurysm. The calcified scar appears as a fine, curvilinear density, most commonly on the anterolateral aspect of the heart, best seen on the frontal view (Fig. 51–8A), or in the lower portion of the interventricular septum, best seen

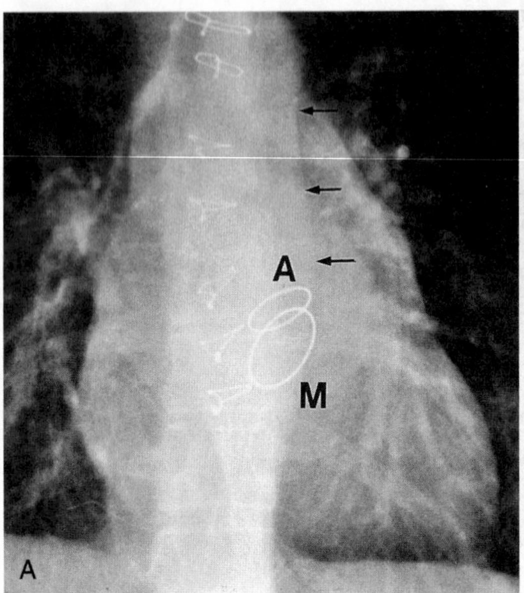

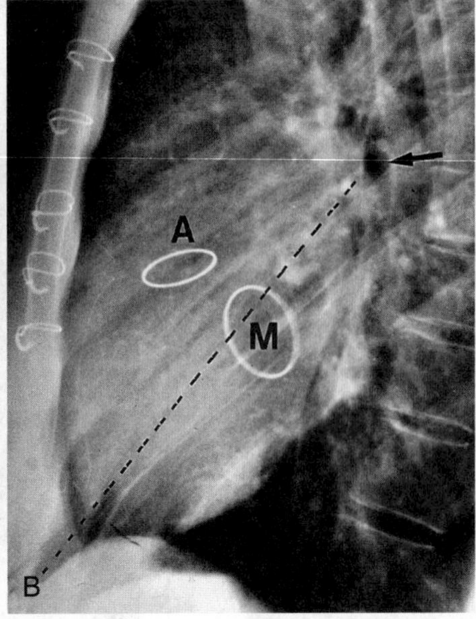

FIGURE 51–7 • Location of the mitral and aortic valves. Both the mitral (M) and aortic (A) valves have been replaced by porcine heterografts. The circular stents indicate the location and tilt of each valve. **A,** Frontal projection. The two valves are normally in contact with each other, and it is difficult to separate them in the frontal projection. Furthermore, on a routinely exposed film, calcific deposits are not easily seen because of the overlapping shadows of the descending aorta (arrows) and the spine. **B,** Lateral projection. The valves can be differentiated on the lateral view by drawing a line from the left main bronchus (arrow) to the anterior costophrenic sulcus. The aortic valve lies above this line and the mitral valve below it.

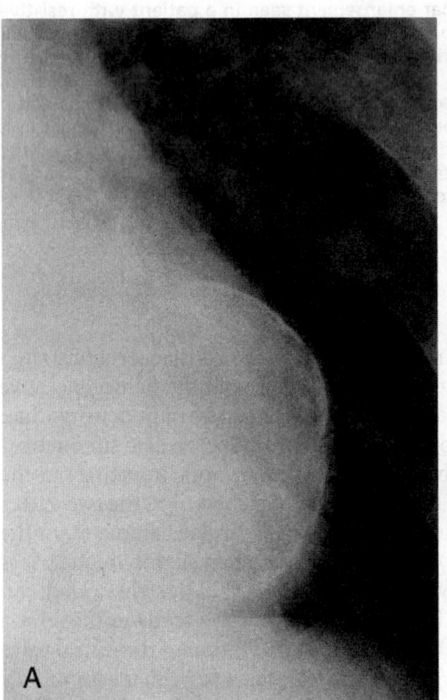

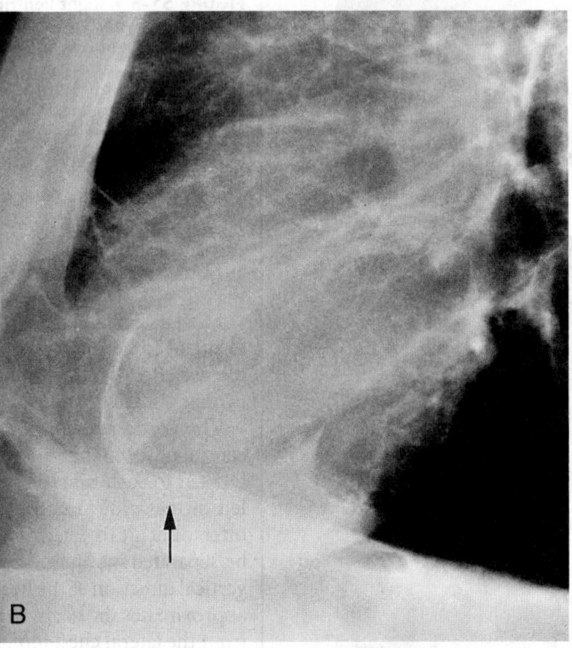

FIGURE 51–8 • Calcified myocardial infarctions. A, Patient 1: frontal projection of an anterolateral left ventricular aneurysm. The fine calcific line outlines an anterolateral aneurysm of the left ventricle. The calcific deposit is much finer than that seen with pericardial calcification. The patient had suffered a myocardial infarction several years earlier. **B,** Patient 2: lateral projection of a septal infarction. The curvilinear calcific deposit is within the scarred lower portion of the ventricular septum. The infarction extended posteriorly along the base of the heart to involve the diaphragmatic wall of the left ventricle (arrow).

on the lateral projection (see Fig. 51–8B). Calcification of the pericardium is usually coarser and tends to occur in clumps. Often, pericardial calcium is distributed primarily over the interventricular sulcus and the atrioventricular grooves, but when extensive, the deposits may coalesce and completely surround the heart (Fig. 51–9).

Calcification of the coronary arteries is a specific sign of complicated atheromatous plaques in which previous hemorrhage has occurred. Not uncommonly, this type of plaque, which may not produce significant narrowing of the vessel, is the site of acute thrombosis and vascular occlusion leading to myocardial infarction. There is no correlation between the sites of calcium deposition and the sites of greatest stenosis, but a strong correlation exists between the extent of coronary artery calcification and the extent of coronary arterial sclerosis.

Calcification of the coronary arteries is difficult to visualize on chest films because the deposits are thin and their shadows are blurred by the motion of the heart. Ultrafast computed tomography (CT) scanning using either electron beam or helical CT is very sensitive and accurate for detecting and quantifying the extent of coronary arterial calcification (Chapter 54). However, the data accumulated to date have not clearly shown a correlation between the volume of coronary calcification and the clinical status of the patient. Although high calcium scores indicate extensive atherosclerosis, acute events, such as myocardial infarction or sudden death, can occur in patients with little or no calcification of their coronary arteries.

PERICARDIAL EFFUSION

The pericardium completely invests the heart, except for a small area on its posterior surface between the entrances of the pulmonary veins and the superior and inferior venae cavae. When fluid accumulates in the pericardium, the sac distends smoothly to enlarge the cardiac silhouette and give it a flask-shaped appearance. A similar shape can occur with a dilated, failing heart.

The two conditions are readily differentiated by the appearance of the pulmonary hila on a frontal chest film. The pericardial sac extends onto the great vessels and up to or slightly above the level of the bifurcation of the main pulmonary artery (Fig. 51–10). As the sac distends with fluid, it tends to overlap and obscure the hilar vessels. Conversely, when the heart fails, the vessels become congested and appear more prominent than normal (Fig. 51–11).

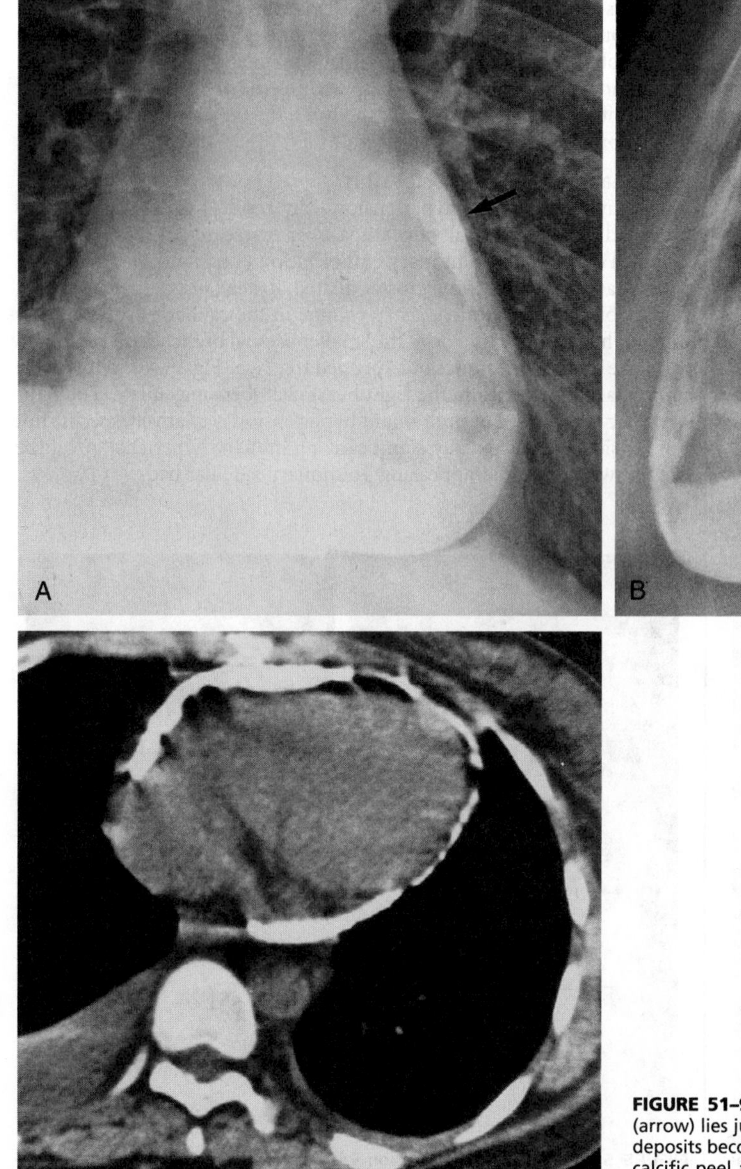

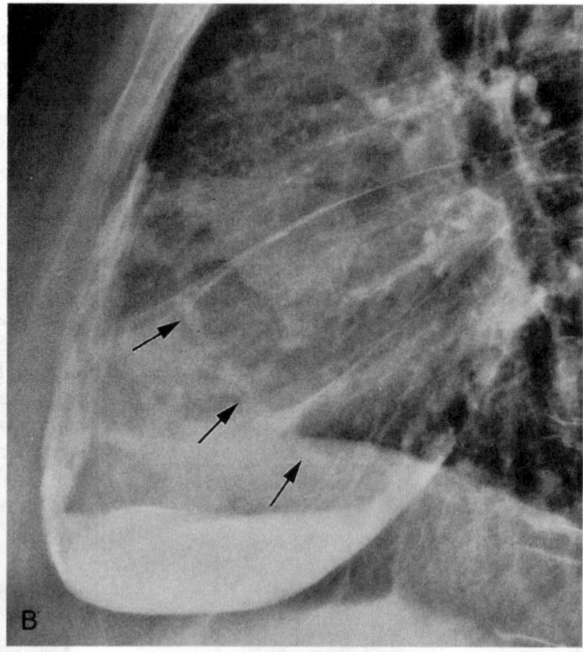

FIGURE 51–9 • Calcific pericarditis. A, Frontal projection. A large, thick, calcific plaque (arrow) lies just below the level of the left upper lobe bronchus. More caudad, the calcific deposits become confluent and cover the diaphragmatic surface of the heart. **B,** The dense calcific peel around the cardiac apex and the diaphragmatic aspect of the heart is better seen. Linear calcific deposits (arrows) lie within the atrioventricular sulcus. **C,** Nonenhanced computed tomography shows the irregular, thick, calcific peel almost encircling the heart.

Posterior displacement of the epicardial fat line is a second reliable sign of pericardial effusion (Chapter 77). In adults, fat is often insinuated between the myocardium and the visceral pericardium (the epicardium) and is sometimes seen on the lateral projection as a curvilinear, radiolucent shadow paralleling the anterior aspect of the heart. The anterior surface of the parietal pericardium borders the retrosternal mediastinal fat. The soft tissue density between these two fat lines therefore represents the pericardium, the epicardium, and the fluid between them. When normal, this stripe is no more than 2 to 4 mm thick. As fluid accumulates in the pericardial sac, the epicardial fat line is displaced posteriorly and the pericardial stripe widens (Fig. 51–12).

PULMONARY VASCULATURE

Almost all of the linear shadows in the lung represent large and medium-sized pulmonary arteries and veins. The terminal branches of the vessels are too small to be visualized as individual structures. The same is true of the interstitial tissues that support the alveoli and form the primary and secondary interlobular septa. However, summation of the minimal densities cast by these structures gives the pulmonary fields an overall grayish cast. The large vessels are seen because their soft tissue density is contrasted against the surrounding air-containing alveoli.

The caliber of the pulmonary vessels reflects the volume of blood flowing through the lungs. When this volume is diminished because of a right-to-left shunt, venous blood bypasses the pulmonary vessels and as a result these vessels are smaller in caliber and the lungs appear abnormally radiolucent. Increased size and prominence of the pulmonary vessels, both central and peripheral, usually indicate an increase in pulmonary blood flow secondary to a left-to-right shunt (Fig. 51–13A). The vessels in the lower as well as the upper lung fields are dilated. Although pulmonary arteries and veins also become abnormally prominent in patients with heart failure, the vessels are not usually sharply outlined, and additional signs of pulmonary venous hypertension or interstitial edema are present (Chapter 67).

The vessels to the lower lobes carry about 60 to 70% of the pulmonary blood flow and are normally of greater caliber than the vessels to the upper lobes. As pulmonary venous pressure increases, the lower lobe vessels become constricted, so more blood is distributed to the upper lobes, which makes their vessels more prominent. This redistribution of the pulmonary vasculature is a reliable sign of pulmonary venous hypertension (see Fig. 51–13B), although it is often difficult to recognize unless quite marked. With a sufficient further increase in venous pressure, pulmonary edema develops.

Pulmonary Edema

Normally, extravascular circulation of fluid in the lungs from the capillaries through the interstitium and back to the blood stream by way of the lymphatics is constant. When pulmonary venous pressure increases, more and more fluid leaks from the capillary bed, the capacity of the lymphatics to remove the fluid is exceeded, and the interstitium becomes waterlogged. Because the interlobular septa in the outer portions of the lung bases are oriented parallel to the x-ray beam on an erect film, when thickened, they are seen as parallel, short horizontal lines extending to the pleural surfaces (Kerley B lines). Kerley A lines also represent thickened interlobular septa, but they are longer and are seen in the upper lung fields. These lines are within the depth of the lung and do not usually reach the pleural surface. Most of the other septa, even when thickened, are too fine to be identified as individual structures. However, the summation pattern creates random "noise" on the film that obscures the shadows of the pulmonary vessels (Fig. 51–14). A ground-glass appearance of the lung fields without identifiable vascular markings within them is characteristic of interstitial pulmonary edema (Chapter 58). The patient is generally severely tachypneic at this stage, but rales may not be present. Interstitial edema also causes thickening of the bronchial walls and peribronchial connective tissue, best seen when they are projected on end. This "peribronchial cuffing" is best visualized in the superior portion of the pulmonary hila, where the anterior segmental bronchus of the upper lobes is viewed on end. When the interstitium can no longer accommodate the excess fluid, it spills into the alveoli (Fig. 51–15). At this point, as air bubbles through the fluid, the typical auscultatory findings of pulmonary edema appear.

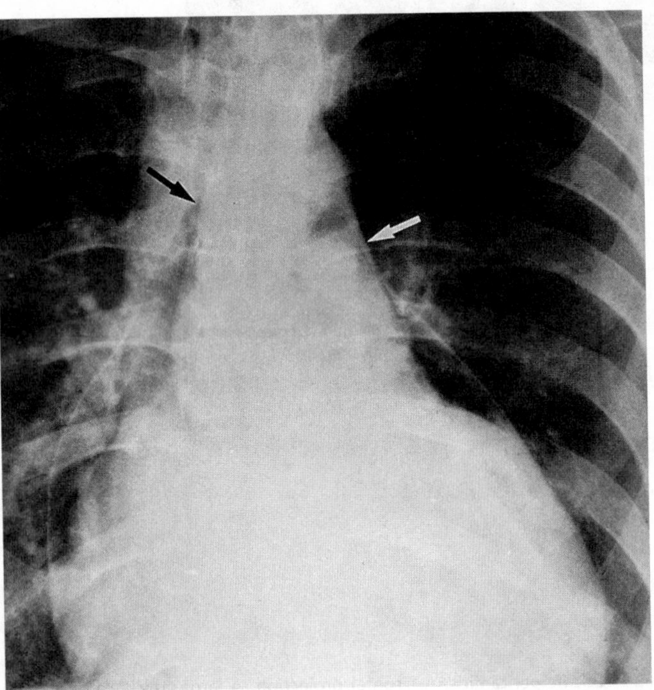

FIGURE 51–10 • Superior pericardial reflection with effusion after a tap. During pericardiocentesis, some of the fluid withdrawn was replaced with air. The normal pericardium is now outlined between the intrapericardial air and the air in the lungs and is seen as a thin linear shadow along the outer border of the cardiac silhouette. The film is made in the erect position and the air has risen to the highest point of the pericardial cavity (arrows), above the level of the pulmonary hila and almost reaching the aortic arch.

Pulmonary Arterial Hypertension

Resistive pulmonary hypertension can result from a left-to-right intracardiac shunt, mitral valve disease, or extracardiac disease, such as repeated episodes of pulmonary embolization (Chapter 67). The central pulmonary arteries become grossly dilated. Instead of gradually tapering as they bifurcate, a sudden, sharp change in the caliber of the vessels is noted. The size and number of the smaller arterial branches decrease, and they take on the appearance of a "pruned tree" (see Fig. 51–6). With severe pulmonary hypertension, the right heart chambers may dilate. The radiographic appearance of pulmonary hypertension is relatively specific but not sensitive, and clinically significant pulmonary hypertension can be present with a normal-appearing pulmonary vascular bed.

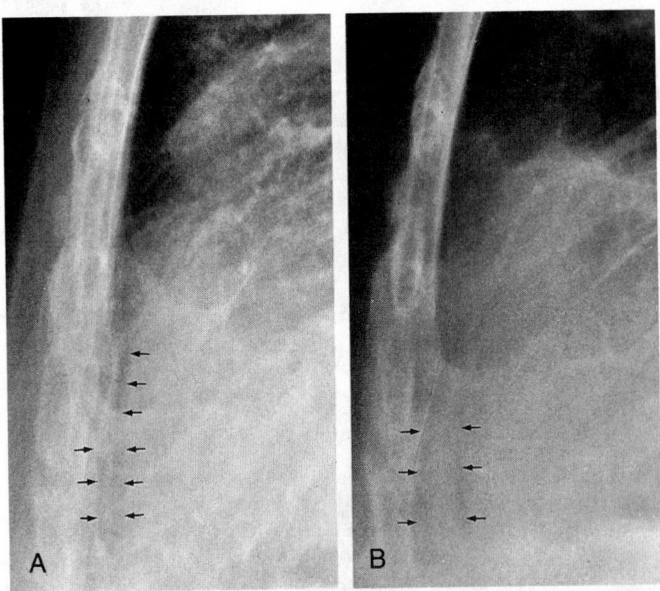

FIGURE 51–12 • Pericardial effusion with posterior displacement of the epicardial fat line. The two lines of arrows point to the substernal fat and the subepicardial fat layers. **A,** Normal. The fine line of soft tissue density between the fat layers represents the epicardium, the pericardium, and the fluid between them. **B,** Same patient with a pericardial effusion. The epicardial fat line is displaced posteriorly, and the pericardial stripe is abnormally wide.

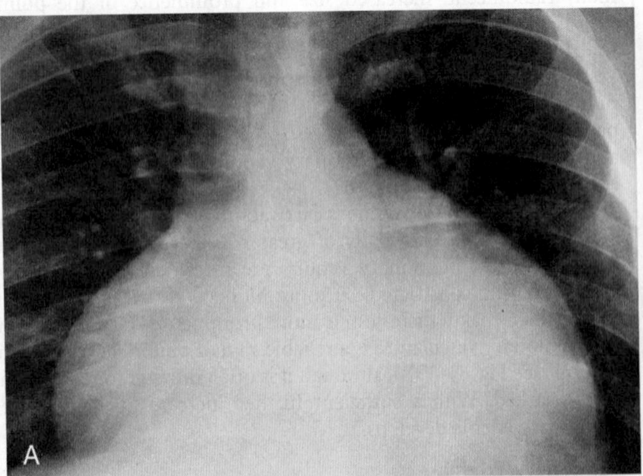

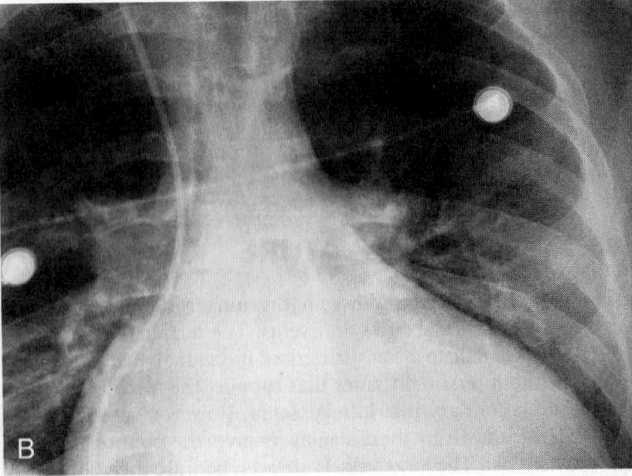

FIGURE 51–11 • Hilum overlay sign. A, Pericardial effusion. The heart is diffusely enlarged. Its silhouette extends outward and is obscuring the hilar shadows in each lung. **B,** Dilated cardiomyopathy. The heart is diffusely enlarged. The failing left ventricle has caused congestion of the hilar vessels, and they are more prominent than normal.

THE HEART AND PORTABLE FILMS

Not uncommonly, cardiac patients are too ill to be transported, so their studies must be performed with portable equipment at the bedside. The resulting images are less sharp and have less contrast, and the degree of magnification of the intrathoracic structures can vary considerably. Portable images can also vary from one to the next because the positioning of the patient and the film and the distance between the patient and the x-ray tube are all dependent, in practice, on visual estimation of the technologist. Despite these differences, the same principles of interpretation also apply to portable images, with a few important caveats:

1. The size of the heart, especially relative to the width of the chest, is magnified on a portable image, so the cardiothoracic ratio is not particularly useful. Furthermore, small changes in cardiac size from one portable film to the next have little significance because of the likelihood of variations in technique. Conversely, if the heart appears smaller on a portable than on an erect film, the decrease in size is almost certainly real.
2. If the technologist tilts the x-ray tube even slightly toward the patient's head, the heart will appear even larger and will be projected over the hilar vessels, thereby mimicking the "hilum overlay" sign of a pericardial effusion. Thus, this sign is not useful with portable images.
3. Free pleural fluid collects in the dependent portions of the pleural space, at first in the costophrenic sulci. With fixed equipment in which the x-ray beam is horizontal, the lateral costophrenic sulci are usually obliterated by the fluid, and the upper level of the fluid can be seen. When the patient is supine or slightly tilted, the fluid flows out of the costophrenic sulci and layers along the posterior chest wall. The x-ray beam, though still at right angles to the patient, is no longer horizontal, so the fluid, now viewed en face, appears as an ill-defined haze.
4. Portable films are frequently used to confirm the position of various inserted devices. Without any sense of depth, however, all that is really known is that the object is "projected over" the region of interest; it could actually be some distance away (Fig. 51–16).

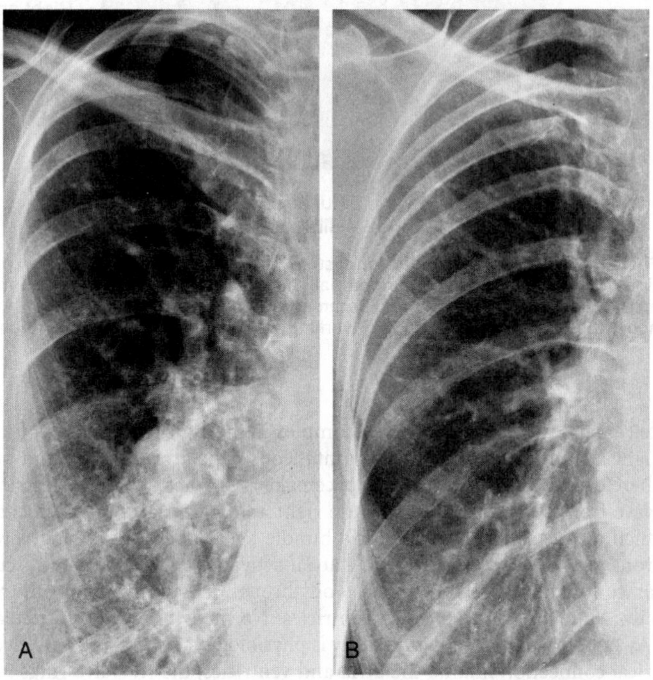

FIGURE 51–13 • Pulmonary vasculature. A, Atrial septal defect, left-to-right shunt. All pulmonary vessels, to the lower lobes as well as to the upper lobes, are dilated, which is indicative of increased blood flow. **B,** Mitral stenosis, pulmonary venous hypertension with redistribution of the pulmonary vasculature. The lower lobe vessels are constricted and the upper vessels, which now carry more blood, are of greater caliber.

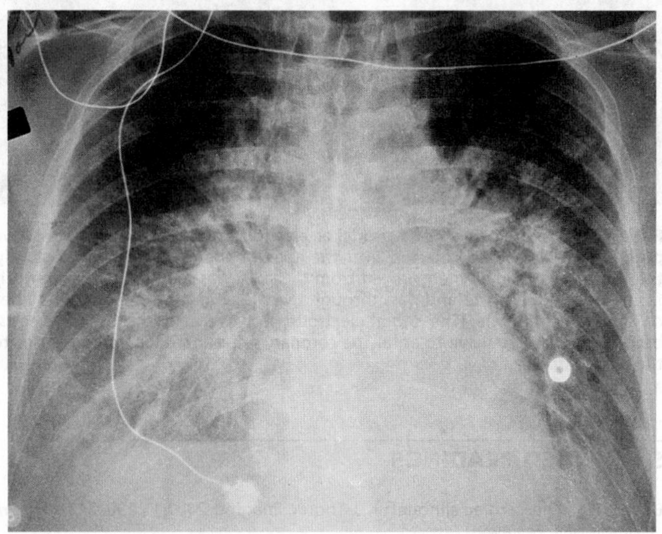

FIGURE 51–15 • Alveolar pulmonary edema, acute myocardial infarction. Patchy areas of consolidation can be seen in the perihilar regions of both lungs. Dilation of the heart after a massive myocardial infarction may not be seen for the first 24 to 48 hours.

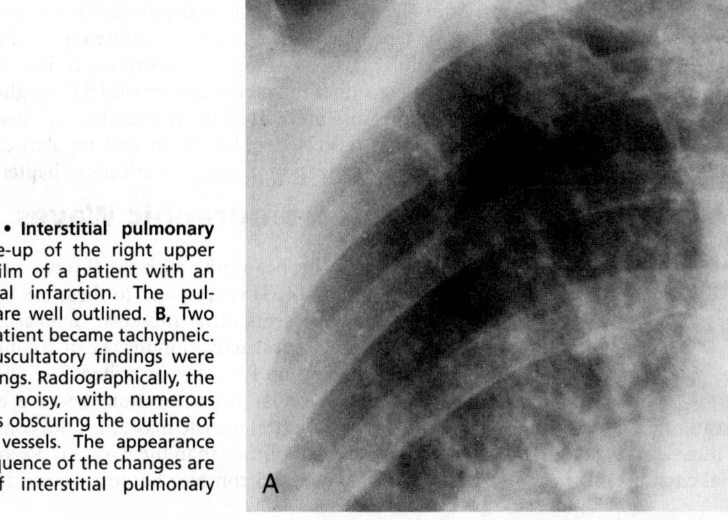

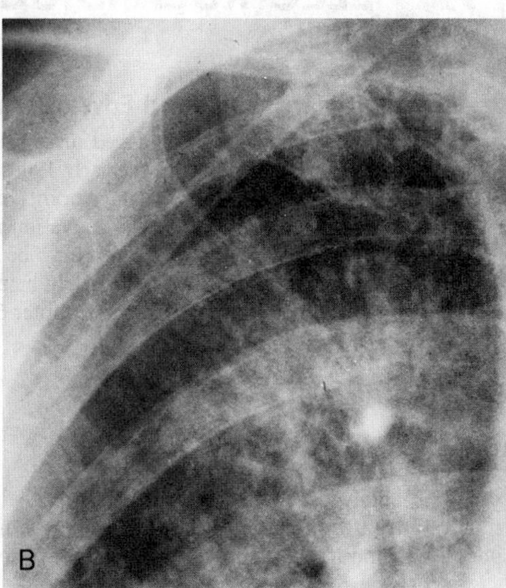

FIGURE 51–14 • Interstitial pulmonary edema. A, Close-up of the right upper lobe; portable film of a patient with an acute myocardial infarction. The pulmonary vessels are well outlined. **B,** Two days later, the patient became tachypneic. No abnormal auscultatory findings were present in the lungs. Radiographically, the lung fields are noisy, with numerous random shadows obscuring the outline of the pulmonary vessels. The appearance and the time sequence of the changes are characteristic of interstitial pulmonary edema.

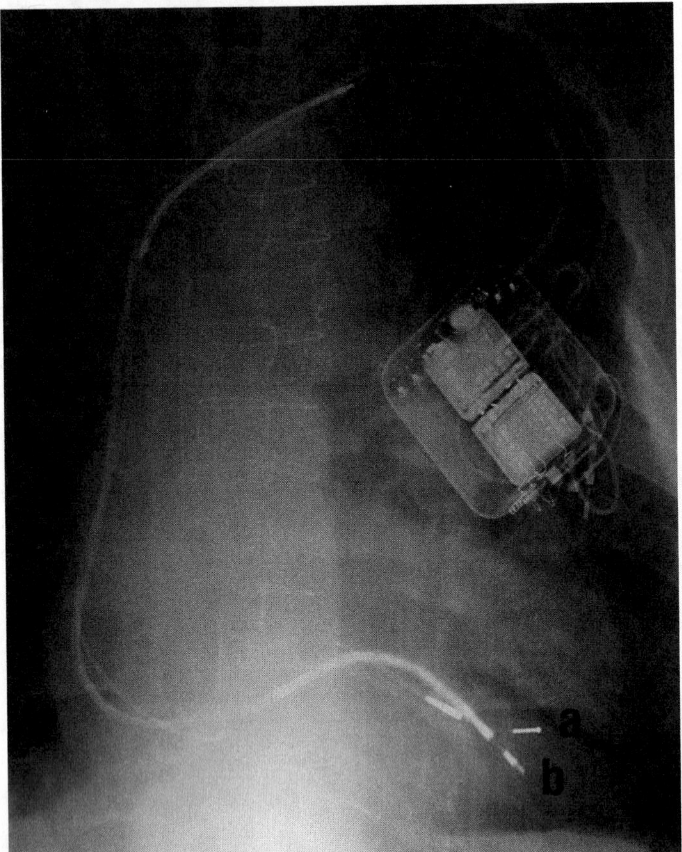

FIGURE 51–16 • Position of pacemaker electrodes. A frontal film shows two pacemaker electrodes projected over the apex of the right ventricle. Actually, the thicker electrode, when viewed from the side, was seen to curve anteriorly from the right ventricle and pass through the tricuspid valve and into the apex of the right ventricle. The other electrode, however, curved posteriorly just before the tricuspid valve to enter the coronary sinus and is located posterior to the left ventricle.

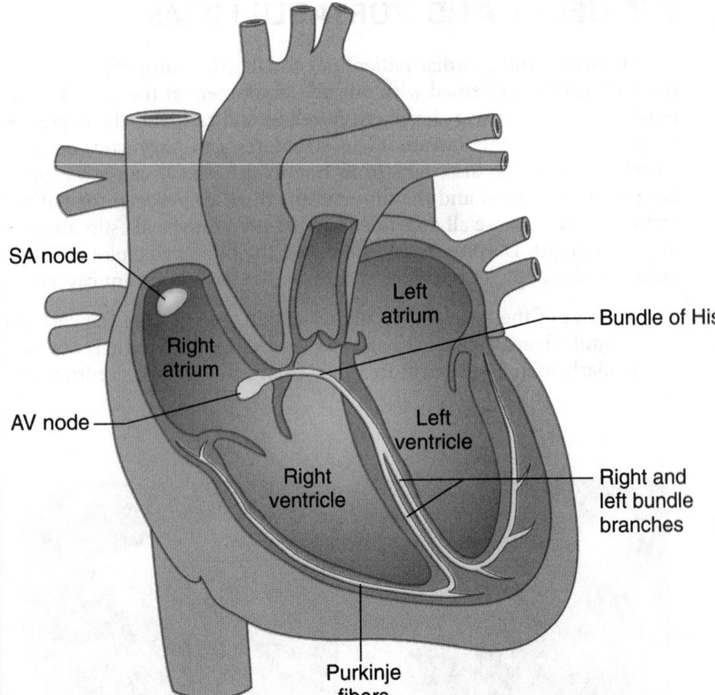

FIGURE 52–1 • Cardiac conduction system. The normal conducting system consists of pacemaker cells in the sinoatrial (SA) nodal complex, specialized intra-atrial conducting tracts (including Bachmann's bundle), the atrioventricular (AV) node, the His-Purkinje system, and working atrial and ventricular myocardium.

SUGGESTED READINGS

Baron MG: The cardiac silhouette. J Thorac Imaging 2000;15:230–242. *A comprehensive review.*

Miller RR, Ely EW: Radiographic measures of intravascular volume status: The role of vascular pedicle width. Curr Opin Crit Care 2006;12:255–262. *Assessment of the value of radiographic markers of volume status.*

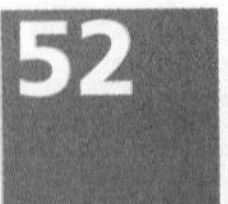

52 ELECTROCARDIOGRAPHY

Leonard Ganz and Edward Curtiss

Electrocardiography, which has changed surprisingly little since it was initially introduced by Einthoven in the early 1900s, allows recording of myocardial activation from several vantage points on the body's surface, thereby permitting analysis of electrical activation in different myocardial regions. Surface electrocardiography may be supplemented with intracardiac recordings, which are particularly helpful in the diagnosis and management of cardiac arrhythmias (Chapter 61).

NORMAL FUNCTION AND ELECTROCARDIOGRAM

Normal Cardiac Activation

Electrical activation of the heart depends on the spread of a depolarizing wave front from pacemaker cells through cardiac muscle, as well as specialized conducting tissues (Fig. 52–1). Under normal circumstances, cells in the sinoatrial (SA) nodal complex in the high lateral aspect of the right atrium have the highest spontaneous depolarization rate and are therefore the dominant cardiac pacemaker (Chapter 60). This electrical wave front spreads throughout the right and left atria; specialized conducting tracts called Bachmann's bundle speed the depolarizing wave front to the left atrium. Electrical atrial activation triggers atrial muscular contraction, which pumps blood through the tricuspid and mitral valves into the right and left ventricles. Normally, the atrioventricular (AV) node, where conduction delay is physiologic, serves as the only electrical connection linking the atria and ventricles; the AV valve rings are insulated. The depolarizing wave front exits the AV node into the bundle of His, a specialized conducting tissue capable of rapid conduction. The bundle of His bifurcates into right and left bundle branches; the left bundle branch divides into the left anterior and left posterior fascicles. The bundle branches, as well as their more distal ramifications of specialized conducting tissue, are called the Purkinje system. From these specialized conducting tissues, the depolarizing wave front enters into and then moves through ventricular muscle. As in the atria, ventricular electrical activation begets muscular contraction, which pumps blood through the semilunar valves into the pulmonary and systemic circulations. After electrical activation, or depolarization, a period of electrical recovery, or repolarization, is necessary before repeated activation.

At the cellular level, a complex orchestration of ion channels opening and closing determines the membrane potential throughout this process. The flow of ions into and out of the myocardial cells inscribes an action potential, which reflects depolarization and repolarization, as well as spontaneous depolarization of pacemaker cells (Chapter 60).

The Electrocardiographic Waves

Labeled alphabetically, beginning with the P wave, the basic waves of the electrocardiogram (ECG) correspond to these electrical events (Fig. 52–2). The P wave represents atrial muscular depolarization; in severe hyperkalemia, atrial electrical activation may be unaccompanied by atrial muscular activation, and no P wave is inscribed. The QRS complex represents ventricular muscular depolarization; because of the disparity between ventricular and atrial muscle mass, the QRS complex is typically much larger in voltage amplitude than the P wave is. Recorded from multiple vantage points, the QRS complex harbors tremendous information

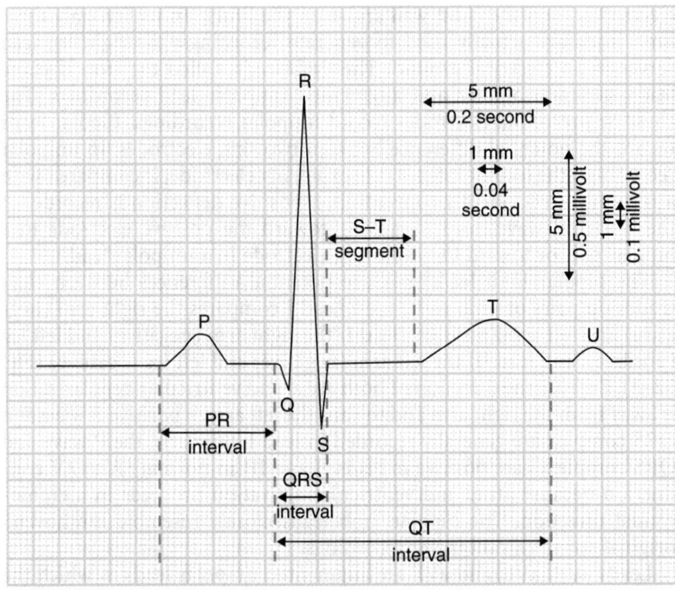

FIGURE 52–2 • Inscription of a normal electrocardiogram (ECG). Sinoatrial nodal depolarization is not visible on the surface ECG; the P wave corresponds to atrial mechanical contraction. The PR interval denotes conduction through the atrial muscle, atrioventricular node, and His-Purkinje system. The QRS complex reflects ventricular muscle depolarization. The ST segment and T wave correspond to ventricular repolarization. Atrial repolarization also occurs, but the signal is of low amplitude and buried underneath the QRS complex. Note the gridlines. On the horizontal axis, each 1-mm line ("small" box) denotes 0.04 second (40 msec); a "big" box denotes 0.2 second (200 msec). On the vertical axis, 1 mm ("small" box) corresponds to 0.1 mV; 10 mm (two "big" boxes) therefore denotes 1 mV.

about the structure and function of ventricular tissue. Under normal circumstances, the PR interval, which is the segment from the onset of the P wave to the onset of the QRS complex, represents the delay between atrial and ventricular depolarization. The ST segment and T wave (and occasionally the U wave) reflect ventricular repolarization, a process of electrical recovery that must take place before the ventricle can be depolarized again. Atrial muscle also requires repolarization before the next depolarizing wave front. Because ventricular mass far exceeds atrial muscular mass, the low-amplitude atrial repolarization wave is buried underneath the QRS complex and is rarely manifested on the ECG.

Electrocardiography Standards

A standard ECG is recorded on paper with 1-mm ("small" boxes) as well as 5-mm ("big" boxes) gridlines. Voltage amplitude is measured on the vertical axis (typically 10 mm equaling 1 mV) and time on the horizontal axis. Because the usual ECG recording speed is 25 mm/sec, each 1-mm gridline ("small" box) represents 0.04 second (40 msec), and each 5-mm gridline ("big" box) equals 0.2 second (200 msec). These parameters are the usual calibration or standardization. Necessary for proper interpretation, the standardization parameters are typically printed on the ECG.

A standard ECG is recorded over a 10-second period, although a rhythm or monitor strip can be recorded for substantially longer if necessary. Multiple leads are typically recorded simultaneously from the top to the bottom of the page. The usual groupings of leads include I, II, and III; aVR, aVL, and aVF; V_1, V_2, and V_3; and V_4, V_5, and V_6 (see later). Each group of leads is recorded for 2.5 seconds. A single lead (or multilead) rhythm strip is recorded below for the entire 10 seconds. Thus, as the ECG is scanned from left to right, one sees 10 seconds of cardiac activity, with each complex recorded simultaneously in multiple leads.

Normal Intervals

Each of the various ECG waves and intervals has normal ranges, defined from large numbers of electrocardiographic recordings in (presumably) healthy subjects (Table 52–1; see Fig. 52–2).

TABLE 52–1 NORMAL ELECTROCARDIOGRAPHIC INTERVALS

Heart rate	50–100 beats per minute
P wave duration	<0.12 sec (120 msec)
PR interval	0.09 (90 msec) to 0.20 sec (200 msec)
QRS duration	0.07 (70 msec) to 0.11 sec (110 msec)
QTc	0.44 sec (440 msec)
QRS axis	−30 to +100 degrees

The RR interval (or PP interval), which is the measurement from R wave to R wave (or P wave to P wave), allows calculation of the heart rate. Because there are 60,000 msec in a minute, the heart rate (HR) in beats per minute can be easily calculated from the RR or PP interval in milliseconds:

$$HR = \frac{60{,}000}{RR}$$

Although traditionally the normal resting heart rate has been defined as being from 60 to 100 beats per minute, a range of 50 to 90 at rest may actually be more reflective of normal physiology. When the heart rate is grossly irregular, as in atrial fibrillation (Chapter 63), the RR interval can be averaged over a number of cardiac cycles to estimate the heart rate. Because a standard ECG records 10 seconds in time, the heart rate (beats per minute) will equal the number of QRS complexes recorded on a standard ECG multiplied by 6.

P Wave Duration

The P wave duration, from the beginning to the end of a P wave, is typically less than 0.12 second (120 msec, three small boxes) in length. A broader P wave reflects an intra-atrial or interatrial conduction delay, or both. Abnormalities in P wave amplitude, morphology, and axis may reflect atrial enlargement.

PR Interval

The PR interval, which is measured from the onset of the P wave to the onset of the QRS complex, is normally between 0.09 and 0.2 second (90 to 200 msec). One-to-one AV conduction with a PR interval greater than 0.2 second has traditionally been called a *first-degree AV block,* but "delayed AV conduction" may be a more appropriate term. Conduction through the atrial tissue, the AV node, and the His-Purkinje system all contribute to the PR interval. When the PR interval is prolonged, delay is usually present in the AV node, although other sites of delay are possible. A short PR interval may reflect ventricular pre-excitation (Wolff-Parkinson-White syndrome), a junctional rhythm, or other conditions.

QRS Complex

The QRS complex, which reflects ventricular muscular electrical activation, carries important information in patients with coronary artery disease, cardiomyopathy, metabolic abnormalities, and other conditions. Capital letters (Q, R, S) denote large-amplitude deflections (>5 mm or 0.5 mV), whereas lowercase letters (q, r, s) signify low-amplitude deflections (<5 mm or 0.5 mV). Q, q, S, and s waves are negative excursions from the isoelectric baseline, whereas R and r waves are positive deflections. Q and q waves are initial negative deflections, and S and s waves are negative deflections that follow a positive deflection (R or r wave); a QS complex is an entirely negative deflection. An R′ or r′ wave refers to a second positive deflection after an S (or s) wave. The duration of the QRS complex reflects the time required for ventricular depolarization. Ventricular activation usually requires at least 0.07 second (70 msec, nearly two small boxes). There is some debate regarding the upper limit of the normal range for QRS duration; upper limits of 0.1 second (100 msec, 2.5 small boxes) or 0.11 second (110 msec, nearly 3 small boxes) are generally quoted. If the QRS duration is prolonged, an intraventricular or interventricular conduction delay (IVCD), or both, is present. Particular patterns of IVCD have been termed bundle branch block (see later).

QT Interval

The QT interval, which reflects ventricular repolarization, is measured from the onset of the QRS complex to the end of the T wave. Accurate assessment of the repolarization interval is important inasmuch as patients with prolonged repolarization, either congenital or acquired, may be at risk for a torsades de pointes ventricular tachycardia (Chapter 64). The QT interval must be corrected to allow comparison of this interval at differing heart rates. Bazett's formula defines a corrected QT interval (QTc):

$$QTc = \frac{QT}{\sqrt{RR}}$$

Bazett's formula works reasonably well at heart rates in the normal range but overcorrects at high rates and undercorrects at low rates. Although more complex regression formulas has been developed to correct the QT interval at different heart rates, none has achieved widespread clinical use. Irregular rhythms (notably atrial fibrillation) complicate calculation of the QTc. Calculating multiple QTc intervals and then taking the average is reasonable; alternatively, the QTc after the longest RR interval can be considered the "worst-case scenario" of the repolarization interval.

The presence of a U wave complicates measurement of the QT (and therefore QTc) interval because it is not always clear where the T wave ends and whether the U wave should be included in a QTU interval. If the isoelectric baseline is reached between the T and U waves, the U wave is not generally included in the QT interval. If the T wave "merges" into the U wave without reaching the isoelectric baseline, the U wave is included in the QT (or QTU) interval. Short QTc intervals are unusual. The upper limit of a normal QTc is somewhat debatable, but a cutoff of 0.44 second (440 msec) is frequently quoted. The QTc in a given patient may vary somewhat over the course of the day and tends to be slightly longer in women than in men. The QT interval is quite sensitive to drug effects, as well as to electrolyte and metabolic derangements.

Electrocardiographic Leads

Recording a single ECG lead allows calculation of the heart rate and, frequently, accurate diagnosis of the heart rhythm. When the ECG is recorded from multiple skin leads simultaneously, the direction (or vector) of activation as the electrical wave front moves through the heart can be inferred. Although a number of different lead systems are possible (and some are actually used in research settings), standard electrocardiography uses 12 leads from 12 vantage points, recorded with 10 electrodes, 6 on the chest wall and 4 on the limbs. In reality, only three limb leads are actually used to generate recordings; the right leg lead serves as an electrical ground. The limb leads, called the frontal plane leads, generate bipolar and augmented unipolar lead recordings. The chest or precordial electrodes record unipolar recordings. Bipolar leads record the potential difference between two skin electrodes. In unipolar recordings, the lead of interest, the exploring electrode, is compared with a reference electrode. By convention, a positive deflection is recorded if the electrical wave front is moving toward the positive electrode in a bipolar pair or toward the exploring electrode in a unipolar lead.

The bipolar limb leads measure potential differences between electrodes on pairs of limb electrodes. Lead I compares the right arm (negative) and left arm (positive), lead II the right arm (negative) and left leg (positive), and lead III the left arm (negative) and left leg (positive) (Fig. 52–3). Because the direction of both atrial and ventricular depolarization is away from the right arm and toward the left arm, a positive P wave and QRS complex are generally recorded in lead I. Similarly, the P wave and QRS complexes are positive in leads II and III in normal SA to AV conduction because atrial and ventricular activation proceeds in a craniocaudal direction. The bipolar limb leads closely resemble Einthoven's original string galvanometer recordings.

Leads aVR, aVL, and aVF are augmented unipolar leads in which the potential in each limb is compared with a reference electrode. For lead aVR, the potential of the right arm is compared with a reference composed of the left arm and left leg electrodes. Lead aVL compares the left arm potential with a reference combining the right arm and left leg; aVF compares the left leg with a right and left arm reference. Because atrial and ventricular activation normally moves from right to left and in a craniocaudal direction, the P wave and QRS complex are negative in lead aVR but positive in lead aVF. In lead aVL, P waves and QRS complexes are generally upright, although an rS complex may be recorded, particularly in young patients.

The precordial electrodes are positioned at specific points on the chest wall (Fig. 52–4A). These unipolar leads compare electrical potential between the chest electrode and a reference electrode called the Wilson central terminal. The Wilson central terminal combines the right arm, left arm, and left leg potentials through 5000-Ω resistors. The six precordial leads define atrial and ventricular activation with respect to a somewhat transverse plane through the chest wall (see Fig. 52–4B). In this plane, atrial activation moves from right to left. Initial ventricular activation involving the septum is directed from left to right; left ventricular depolarization, which dominates right ventricular depolarization because of the differential in myocardial mass, then moves apically and laterally. In lead V_1, to the right of the sternum, the P wave is biphasic

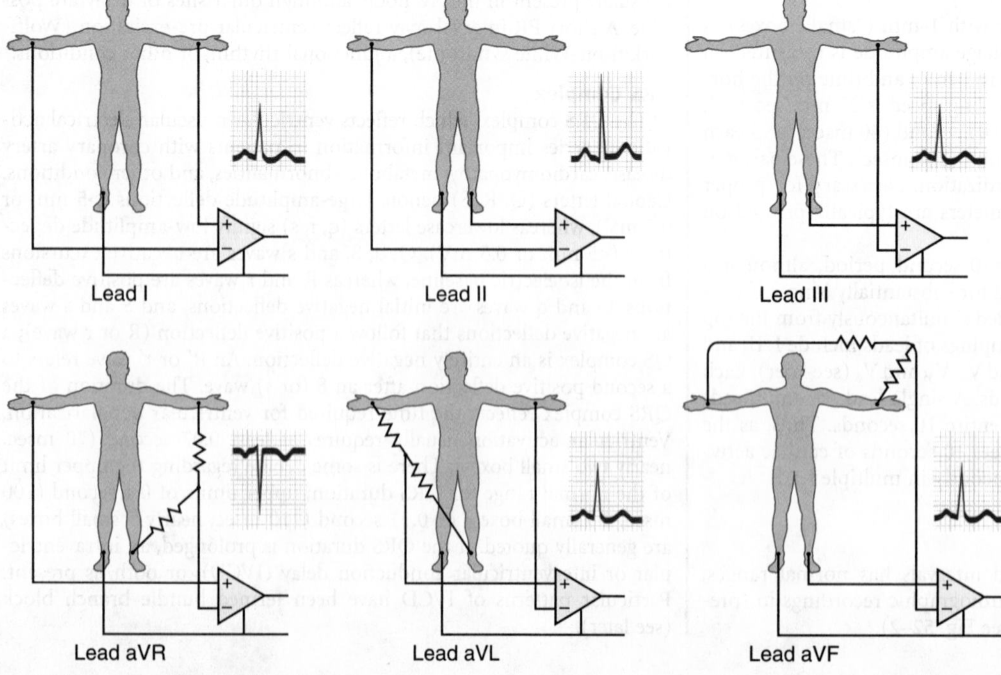

FIGURE 52–3 • Normal cardiac activation as manifested in the limb leads. Under normal circumstances, P waves and QRS complex are typically upright in leads I, II, III, and aVF and inverted in aVR. In lead aVL, P waves are usually upright, although QRS complexes may be either upright or inverted. The right leg electrode serves to ground the system.

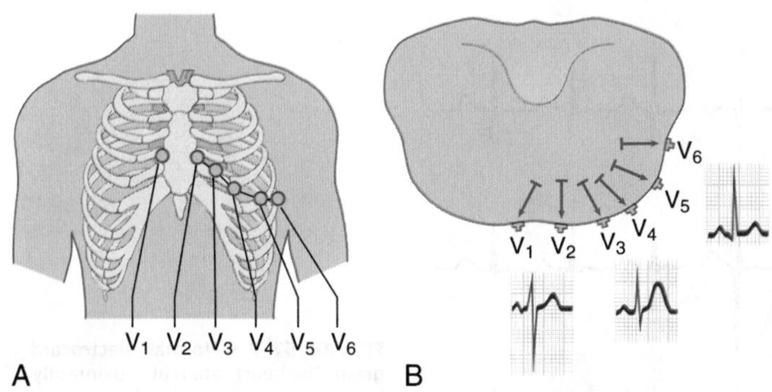

FIGURE 52–4 • Precordial leads. A, Positioning of the precordial leads on the chest wall. **B,** Normal cardiac activation as manifested in the precordial leads. Note the small r wave and deep S wave in lead V_1, the transition at around V_3 or V_4, and the "septal" q wave and large R wave in lead V_6.

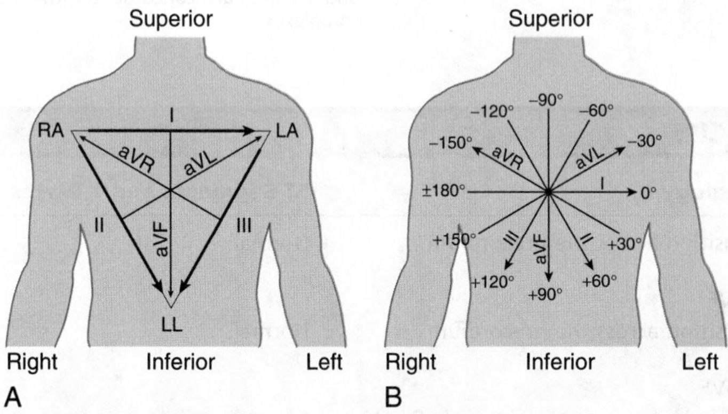

FIGURE 52–5 • Axis of electrical activation. A, Vectors for the limb leads in the frontal plane. **B,** Hexaxial reference for determining the frontal plane axis. Note that the vectors for leads I, II, and III are in the same direction as in **A,** but now, like the augmented limb leads, these standard limb lead vectors have been moved so that they emanate from the center of the figure.

(reflecting right and then left atrial activation). Initial ventricular activation of the septum inscribes an r wave, whereas subsequent activation away from lead V_1 records a dominant S wave. In lead V_6, the P wave is positive. Initial septal depolarization inscribes a tiny "septal" q wave (usually ≤0.02 second), and subsequent ventricular depolarization records a dominant R wave.

Right-sided chest leads should be recorded when right ventricular abnormalities are suspected. RV_3, the mirror image of lead V_3, is routinely recorded in pediatric patients because of the possibility of congenital heart disease. In adults, ST elevation in lead RV_3 is quite specific for acute right ventricular infarction in those being evaluated for an acute inferior wall myocardial infarction.

Axis

An axis of electrical activation can be defined in the frontal plane axis by combining the bipolar and augmented unipolar limb leads (Fig. 52–5A). By convention, the axis parallel to lead I, toward the left arm, is called 0 degrees. A frontal plane axis between −30 and +100 degrees is normal; other axes are abnormal (Fig. 52–6). Mild right axis deviation is a normal variant in children and young adults. The frontal plane axis can be estimated by identifying the limb lead in which the QRS complex is most nearly isoelectric (similar positive and negative deflections); the axis is perpendicular to this lead (see Fig. 52–5B). Because two lines pointing 180 degrees apart can be drawn perpendicular to any given line, examination of the other limb leads defines the direction in which the axis points. If the QRS complex is positive in any given limb lead, the axis will be oriented toward that limb lead, not away from it. Alternatively, the axis is in the normal range if the QRS complexes are primarily positive in both leads I and II.

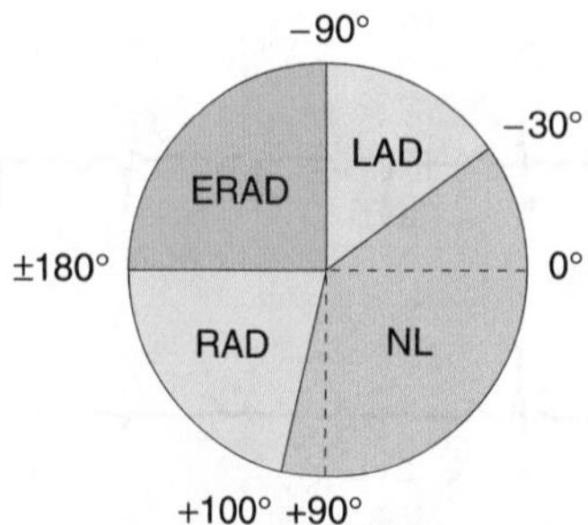

FIGURE 52–6 • Chart of frontal plane axes. Normal (NL) = −30 to +100 degrees; left axis deviation (LAD) = −30 to −90 degrees; right axis deviation (RAD) = +100 to +180 degrees; extreme right axis deviation (ERAD) = −90 to ±180 degrees. Mild RAD is considered normal in children, adolescents, and young adults.

TABLE 52–2 STEPWISE APPROACH TO INTERPRETING THE ELECTROCARDIOGRAM

Estimate the heart rate
Define the heart rhythm (regular vs. irregular; relationship of P waves to QRS complexes)
Measure intervals (PR, QRS duration, QT)
Calculate/estimate QTc
Estimate QRS axis
Examine P wave morphology, duration, and axis
Examine QRS progression and transition in precordial leads
Examine QRS complexes in regional groupings (septal leads [V_1,V_2], anterior leads [V_2, V_3, V_4], lateral leads [I, aVL, V_5, V_6], inferior and posterior leads [II, III, aVF, V_1,V_2])
Examine ST segments in regional groupings
Examine T waves in regional groupings

An axis per se is not defined in the precordial leads. Rather, because the typical progression from leads V_1 to V_6 is from a predominantly negative to a positive QRS complex, the transition point is usually defined as the point at which the amplitude of the R wave begins to exceed the amplitude of the S wave.

APPROACH TO INTERPRETING THE ELECTROCARDIOGRAM

A stepwise approach to interpreting the ECG ensures that no features of the tracing will be overlooked (Table 52–2).

Normal Electrocardiogram

Figure 52–7 is an example of a normal ECG. Sinus rhythm occurs at about 78 beats per minute, with minor variations in the RR intervals (sinus arrhythmia). The PR interval, QRS duration, and QTc are all normal. The QRS complex is most nearly isoelectric in lead aVL, so the QRS axis will be perpendicular to lead aVL. Because aVL points to −30 degrees, the QRS axis must be approximately −120 or +60 degrees. Because the QRS complex is positive in leads I and II (large R waves), the QRS axis is approximately +60 degrees. The transition in the precordial leads is between leads V_3 and V_4. The P wave is biphasic in lead V_1 and then positive in the other precordial leads. Septal q waves, reflecting not septal infarction but normal early septal depolarization, are present in leads V_5 and V_6. Tiny q waves, a normal variant, are seen in the inferior leads.

Abnormal Electrocardiogram

Electrocardiography in patients with coronary artery disease is reviewed in Chapters 70 to 72 and arrhythmias in Chapters 60 to 65.

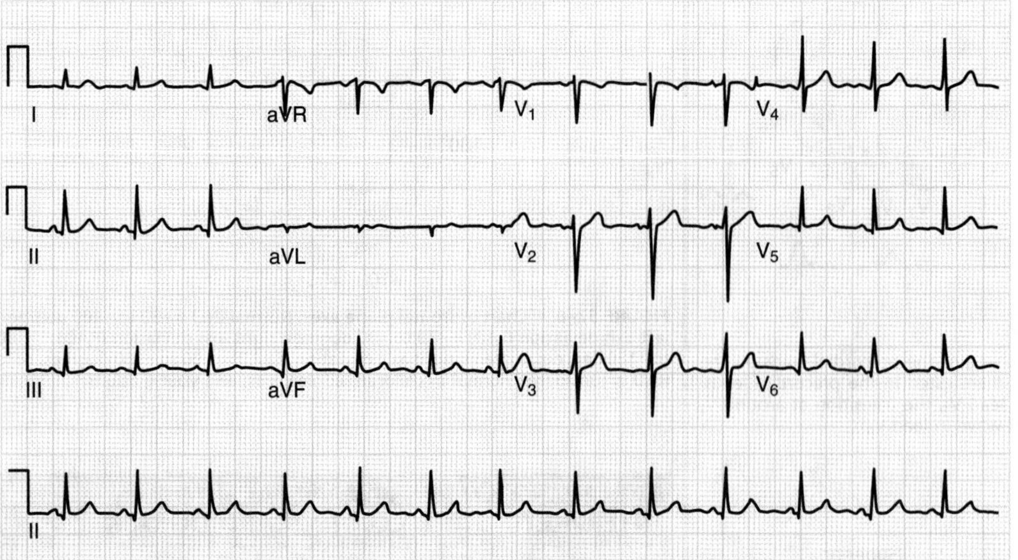

FIGURE 52–7 • Normal electrocardiogram. The heart rate is approximately 78 beats per minute, with minor irregularity. Sinus arrhythmia is present. The axis is approximately +60 degrees. The PR, QRS, and QT intervals are approximately 140, 90, and 360 msec, respectively. P wave morphology, duration, and axis are normal. The transition is between leads V_3 and V_4. No abnormal Q waves are present. ST segments are isoelectric, and T waves are concordant with QRS complexes.

TABLE 52–3 FASCICULAR AND BUNDLE BRANCH BLOCKS

	QRS Duration	Axis	QRS Morphology	ST Segments and T Waves
LAFB	<0.12 sec (120 msec)	<–45 degrees	Delayed transition across the precordium qR I, aVL rS in II, III, aVF	Normal
LPFB	<0.12 sec (120 msec)	>+120 degrees	Delayed transition across the precordium rS I, aVL qR in II, III, aVF	Normal
RBBB	≥0.12 sec (120 msec)	Normal	rsr′, rsR′, rSR′ in V_1 (and usually V_2); wide S in V_6 and I	Discordant in V_1 and V_2
RBBB with LAFB	≥0.12 sec (120 msec)	<–45 degrees	rsr′, rsR′, rSR′ in V_1 (and usually V_2); wide S in V_6 and I	Discordant in V_1 and V_2
RBBB with LPFB	≥0.12 sec (120 msec)	>+120 degrees	rsr′, rsR′, rSR′ in V_1 (and usually V_2); wide S in V_6 and I	Discordant in V_1 and V_2
LBBB	≥0.12 sec (120 msec)	Normal or LAD	rS or QS in V_1 (S wide and notched); wide notched R with q in V_6, I, aVL	Discordant in V_1 to V_6

LAD = left axis deviation; LAFB = left anterior fascicular block; LBBB = left bundle branch block; LPFB = left posterior fascicular block; RBBB = right bundle branch block.

Conduction Abnormalities and Axis Deviation

Abnormalities of the specialized conduction system (i.e., His-Purkinje system) reflect slow or absent conduction in a particular structure, but fascicular blocks do not prolong normal QRS duration (Table 52–3). An IVCD is generally defined as a QRS duration of more than 0.10 second (100 msec). When the QRS has a duration of at least 0.12 second (120 msec), it often has the configuration of a specific bundle branch block (Fig. 52–8).

Chamber Hypertrophy

A number of criteria for defining left ventricular hypertrophy (LVH; Fig. 52–9) and right ventricular hypertrophy (RVH) have been proposed. All of the LVH criteria suffer from poor sensitivity (ranging from 30 to 50%), although the specificity is good (85 to 95%). The Cornell voltage criteria, developed with an echocardiographic standard for LVH, simply add the S wave amplitude in V_3 and the R wave amplitude in aVL; a total greater than 2.0 mV in women and 2.8 mV in men implies LVH. In many clinical settings, the Cornell criteria have replaced the more complicated Romhilt-Estes criteria, which assign points for QRS amplitude, repolarization abnormalities ("strain" pattern), left axis deviation, and other electrocardiographic features. RVH is much less common than LVH. Electrocardiographic criteria for diagnosing RVH have even lower sensitivity (10 to 20%), although the specificity is similar to that for LVH. The Sokolow-Lyon criteria for RVH adds the R wave amplitude in V_1 to the S wave amplitude in lead V_5 or V_6; a sum of 1.1 mV or greater implies RVH.

Low Qrs Voltage

Low QRS voltage is defined as limb lead voltage less than 5 mm (0.5 mV) in all leads or precordial voltage less than 10 mm (1 mV) in all leads. The differential diagnosis is broad (Table 52–4), and no underlying explanation is defined in many cases.

Repolarization Abnormalities

Abnormalities of the ST segment or T waves, or both, are extremely common (Table 52–5). Electrolyte and other metabolic abnormalities, drug effects (particularly digoxin and antiarrhythmic drugs), and secondary effects caused by LVH or bundle branch block are all commonly encountered.

Pitfalls of Automated Computerized Electrocardiographic Readings

Automatic interpretations of ECG tracings are generally quite accurate for calculating heart rates, axes, and intervals. Interpretation of the significance of repolarization abnormalities may be less accurate, and diagnosis of rhythms is the striking weakness of these programs. Thus, over-reading of the computerized interpretation by the physician and comparison with previous tracings, when available, remain mandatory.

A

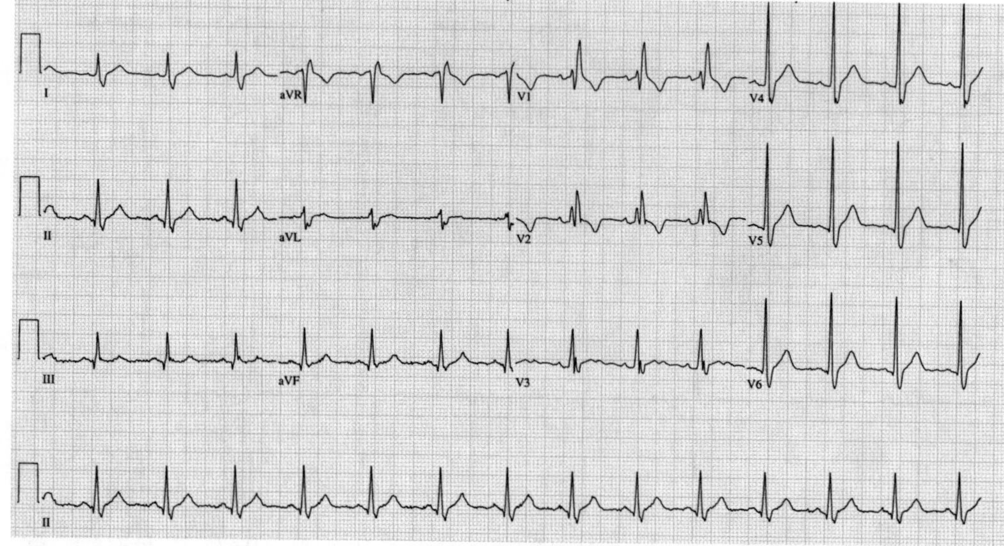

B

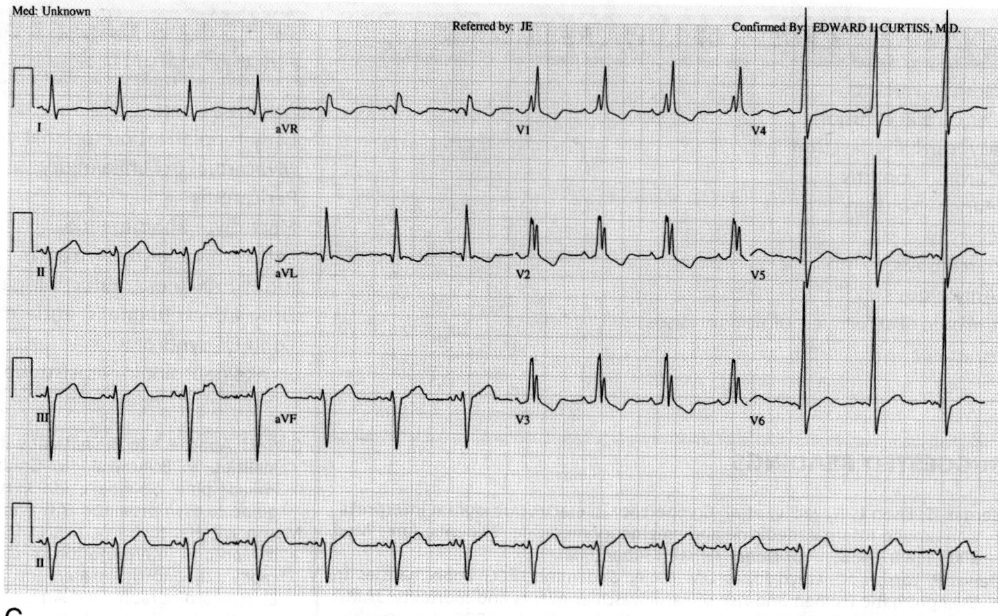

C

FIGURE 52–8 • Fascicular and bundle branch blocks. A, Left anterior fascicular block (LAFB). Left axis deviation is present; the axis is approximately –60 degrees. The QRS duration is normal, and there is a delay in R wave progression across the precordial leads (late transition). Small q waves are present in leads I and aVL and small r waves in leads II, III, and aVF. **B,** Right bundle branch block (RBBB). The QRS is widened, with an rsR′ pattern in lead V_1 and a wide terminal S wave in lead V_6. ST segments are downsloping, and T waves are discordant with the QRS complex in the right precordial leads. The axis is normal, and signs of normal septal activation (q waves in lead V_6) are present. **C,** RBBB and LAFB. In addition to features diagnostic of RBBB, an axis of –60 degrees is present.

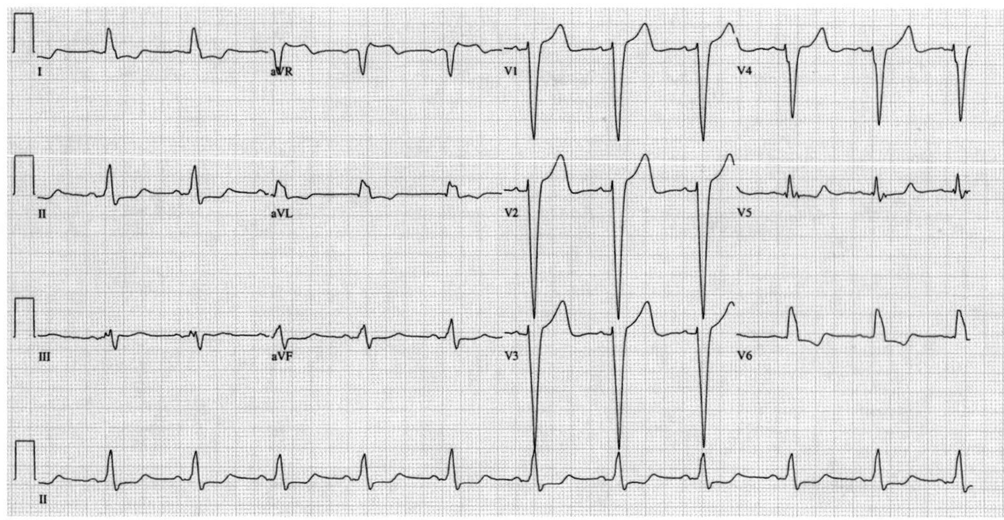

D

FIGURE 52–8, cont'd • D, Left bundle branch block (LBBB). The QRS is widened, with a broad, notched complex in leads I, aVL, and the left precordial leads. Small r waves and broad, deep S waves are present in the right precordial leads. With LBBB, the axis is usually normal or deviated to the left. ST segments and T waves are discordant with the QRS complex throughout the precordium.

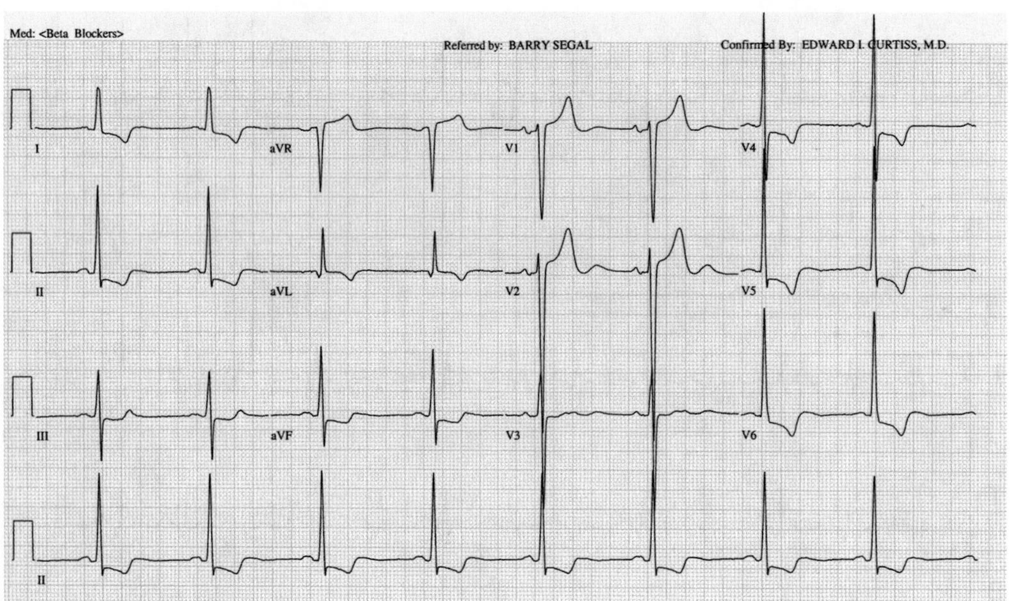

FIGURE 52–9 • **Left ventricular hypertrophy.** Note the striking S wave amplitude in the right precordial leads and R wave amplitude in the left precordial leads. Repolarization abnormalities are present in the left precordial leads, as well as the limb leads. The S wave amplitude in V_3 (2.4 mV) plus the R wave amplitude in aVL (1.0 mV) total 3.4 mV, easily satisfying the Cornell voltage criteria in this 76-year-old hypertensive man. Sinus bradycardia (50 beats per minute) is present as well.

TABLE 52–4 CAUSES OF LOW QRS VOLTAGE
Normal variant
Pericardial effusion
Myocardial infarction
Cardiomyopathy
Hypothyroidism
Obesity
Sarcoidosis
Amyloidosis
Chronic obstructive pulmonary disease
Anasarca

TABLE 52–5 CAUSES OF REPOLARIZATION ABNORMALITIES
Athlete's heart
Early repolarization (normal variant)
Myocardial ischemia/injury
Pericarditis
Electrolyte abnormalities
Left ventricular hypertrophy
Intraventricular conduction delay/bundle branch block
Drug effects (digitalis, antiarrhythmic drugs, etc.)
Long QT syndrome
Stroke/neurologic catastrophe

SUGGESTED READINGS

Berger JS, Eisen L, Nozad V, et al: Competency in electrocardiogram interpretation among internal medicine and emergency medicine residents. Am J Med 2005;118:873–880. *Proficiency remains suboptimal.*

Denes P, Larson JC, Lloyd-Jones DM: Major and minor ECG abnormalities in asymptomatic women and risk of cardiovascular events and mortality. JAMA 2007;297:978–985. *Clinically relevant baseline and incident ECG abnormalities are independently associated with increased risk of cardiovascular events among asymptomatic postmenopausal women.*

Elizari MV, Acunzo RS, Ferreiro M: Hemiblocks revisited. Circulation 2007;115:1154–1163. *A review of the criteria for the electrocardiographic and vectorcardiographic diagnosis of left anterior and posterior hemiblock.*

Ganz LI: Approach to the patient with asymptomatic electrocardiographic abnormalities. *In* Braunwald E, Goldman L (eds): Primary Cardiology, 2nd ed. Philadelphia, Saunders, 2003, pp 169–192. *A practical yet comprehensive guide to asymptomatic ECG findings.*

Mason JW, Hancock EW, Gettes LS, et al: Recommendations for the standardization and interpretation of the electrocardiogram: Part II: Electrocardiography diagnostic statement from the American Heart Association Electrocardiography and Arrhythmias Committee, Council on Clinical Cardiology; the American College of Cardiology Foundation; and the Heart Rhythm Society. J Am Coll Cardiol 2007;49:1128–1135. *A review of the diagnostic terms for ECG interpretation.*

53 ECHOCARDIOGRAPHY

Catherine M. Otto

Echocardiography is the clinical standard for evaluating cardiac function in patients with known or suspected heart disease. This chapter reviews the basic principles of echocardiography, echocardiographic approaches, quantitative measurements, and clinical indications. The specific use of echocardiography and additional images are shown in other chapters on individual types of cardiovascular disease.

ECHOCARDIOGRAPHIC IMAGING

Principles

Echocardiography is based on the use of a piezoelectric crystal that converts electrical to mechanical energy, and vice versa, allowing both transmission and reception of an ultrasound signal. The frequency of ultrasound waves used for diagnostic imaging ranges from 2 to 10 MHz, with lower frequencies having greater tissue penetration and higher frequencies providing better image resolution. Each transducer consists of a complex array of piezoelectric crystals arranged to provide images in a fanlike two-dimensional image with the narrow top of this sector scan indicating the origin of the ultrasound signal. Transducers also include an acoustic lens that determines the focal depth, height, and width of the ultrasound beam.

Images are generated based on the reflection of ultrasound from acoustic interfaces; for example, the boundary between the blood in the left ventricle and the myocardium. The time delay between transmission and reception is used to determine the depth of origin of the ultrasound reflection. A graph of the depth of the reflected signal along a single beam versus time is called motion (M)-mode echocardiography. When signals from multiple ultrasound beams are combined, a two-dimensional image is generated. The speed of signal analysis allows acquisition of two-dimensional ultrasound images at frame rates of 30 to 60 per second.

Ultrasound is strongly attenuated by bone and air, so echocardiography relies on acoustic "windows" where, for example, ultrasound can penetrate to the heart while avoiding the ribs and lungs. With transthoracic imaging, the patient is positioned to bring the cardiac structures close to the chest wall, usually in a left lateral decubitus position, and the transducer is placed on the chest, using gel to provide acoustic coupling between the transducer and skin. Standard acoustic windows are parasternal, apical, subcostal, and suprasternal notch.

Standard Image Planes

From the parasternal window, the image plane is adjusted manually by an experienced physician or sonographer to provide long- and short-axis views. Standard cardiac imaging planes are aligned relative to the axis of the heart, with the long axis defined as the plane that intersects the cardiac apex and the middle of the aortic valve. Short-axis views are perpendicular to this long axis, with standard image planes at the cardiac base (aortic valve level), mitral valve, and midventricular levels. From the apical window, the transducer is rotated to provide three views oriented 60 degrees from each other, producing a four-chamber, a two-chamber, and a long-axis view (Fig. 53–1).

Measurements

Echocardiography provides accurate cardiac dimensions from two-dimensional or two-dimensional-guided M-mode recordings. The measurements typically provided include left ventricular (LV) end-diastolic and end-systolic internal dimensions, LV wall thickness, left atrial anterior-posterior diameter, and aortic root dimension. LV ejection fraction (EF) is determined by visual estimation or, more accurately, by tracing the endocardial borders at end-diastole and end-systole in two orthogonal views. End-diastolic and end-systolic ventricular volumes (EDV and ESV, respectively) are calculated using validated formulas, and the EF is determined as follows:

$$EF = (EDV - ESV)/EDV$$

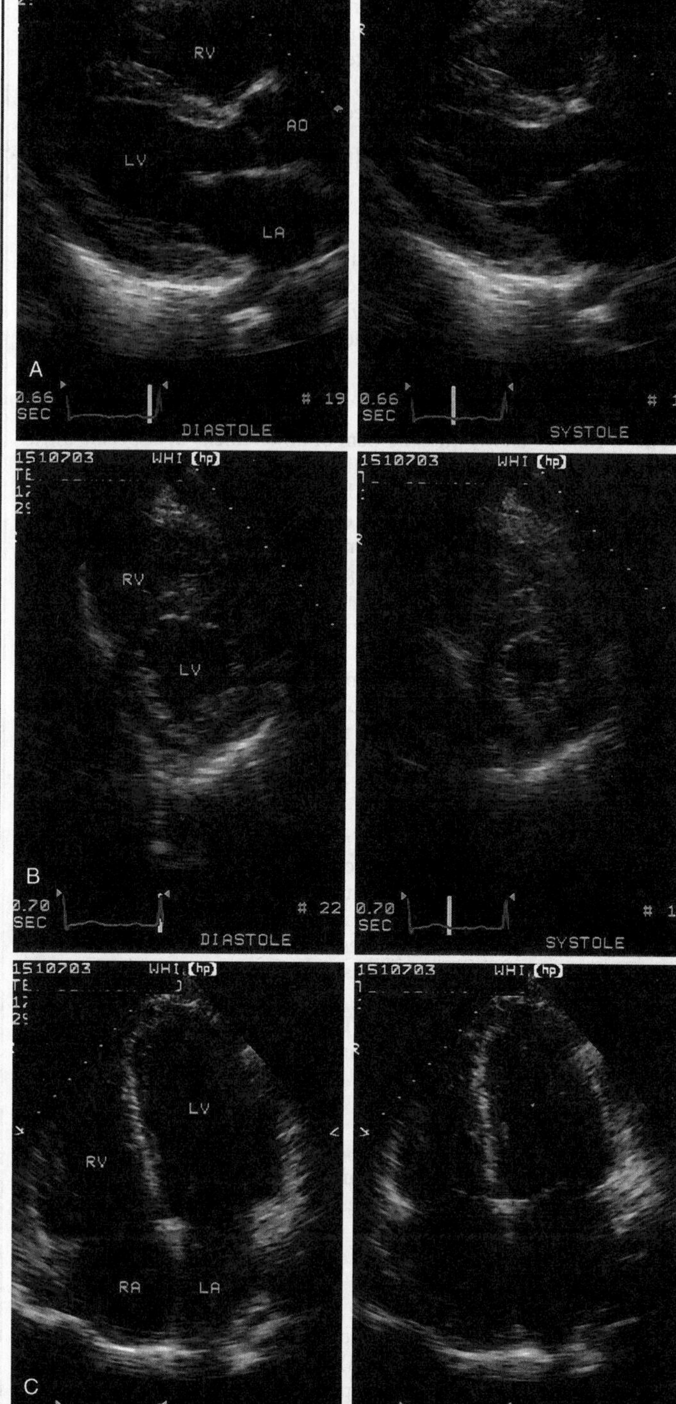

FIGURE 53–1 • Normal two-dimensional transthoracic echocardiogram in systole and diastole. A, With the transducer in the left parasternal location, images can be obtained parallel to the longitudinal axis of the left ventricle. This long-axis view depicts an elliptical left ventricle as visualized from the left shoulder, with the apex to the left and the base to the right. **B,** With the transducer in the left parasternal location, a perpendicular (short-axis) view of the left ventricle is obtained. The left ventricle appears as a circular cross section in the short-access view. **C,** Positioning the transducer at the apical impulse provides images of the perimeter of all four cardiac chambers and both the mitral and tricuspid valves (four-chamber view).

Limitations

Echocardiography is a very accurate, widely available, and widely used imaging approach. However, the quality of images can be suboptimal because of poor tissue penetration (e.g., excessive adipose tissue, position of the lungs relative to the heart), although images are nondiagnostic in fewer than 5% of patients with current instrumentation. Reflections are stronger when the interface is perpendicular to the ultrasound beam, so structures that are parallel to the beam may not be visible, an artifact called "echo dropout." This potential limitation may be avoided by the use of appropriate images planes and the integration of data from multiple transducer positions. Ultrasound artifacts, such as beam width, shadowing, and reverberations, may be misinterpreted by inexperienced observers.

DOPPLER ECHOCARDIOGRAPHY

Principles

Ultrasound energy that is backscattered from moving red blood cells is shifted to a higher frequency when the blood is moving toward the transducer and a lower frequency when it is moving away. The magnitude of this Doppler shift corresponds to the velocity of blood flow.

Modalities

Pulsed Doppler allows measurement of flow velocity at a specific intracardiac site with the advantages of high spatial and temporal resolution. However, spatial localization is based on intermittent sampling at a time interval corresponding to the depth of interest. The sampling frequency, which is depth dependent, limits the maximum detectable velocity because of a phenomenon called signal aliasing. Normal intracardiac flow velocities are about 1 m/second, which can usually be recorded with pulsed Doppler.

Continuous wave Doppler allows measurement of high velocities along the entire length of the ultrasound beam, but the origin of the high-velocity signal must be inferred from the two-dimensional images. With stenotic and regurgitant valves, blood flow velocities may be as high as 5 to 6 m/second, requiring the use of the continuous wave Doppler mode. Both pulsed and continuous wave Doppler velocities are displayed as a graph of velocity versus time, with the density of the spectral display corresponding to signal strength.

Color Doppler flow imaging is a modification of pulsed Doppler in which the flow velocity is displayed across a two-dimensional image using a color scale to indicate direction and velocity. The advantage is a visually appealing display of intracardiac flow patterns. Disadvantages are low temporal resolution (frame rates of 10 to 30 per second) and poor velocity resolution due to signal aliasing.

Tissue Doppler uses the Doppler principle to record the velocity of motion of the myocardial wall. Tissue Doppler recordings of the myocardium adjacent to the mitral annulus are used to evaluate diastolic ventricular function.

Measurements

A standard echocardiographic study includes pulsed Doppler measurement of antegrade flow velocities (transmitral and transaortic) and evaluation for valve regurgitation using continuous wave and color Doppler modalities. Other Doppler measurements depend on the specific clinical indication.

Quantitative measurements using Doppler data are derived from two basic concepts: volume flow rate and the pressure-velocity relationship. Stroke volume (in cubic centimeters) can be calculated as the volume of a cylinder, where the base is the spatial cross-sectional area (CSA, in square centimeters) of flow, determined as the area of a circle from a two-dimensional diameter measurement. The height of the cylinder is the distance the average blood cell travels in one cardiac cycle, which is the velocity time integral (VTI, in centimeters) of flow. Therefore,

$$\text{SV (cm}^3) = \text{CSA (cm}^2) \times \text{VTI (cm)}$$

This approach has been validated for measurement of transaortic, transmitral, and transpulmonic flow. Measurement of volume flow rate at two different intracardiac sites allows quantitation of intracardiac shunts and valvular regurgitation.

The relationship between the pressure gradient (ΔP) across a narrowing and the velocity (v) of blood flow is described by the simplified Bernoulli equation:

$$\Delta P = 4v^2$$

This equation allows calculation of maximum and mean gradients across stenotic valves, estimation of pulmonary systolic pressure, and detailed evaluation of intracardiac hemodynamics with regurgitant valves.

ECHOCARDIOGRAPHIC APPROACHES

Several echocardiographic modalities are in clinical use. If it is unclear which modality is optimal in a specific clinical setting, consultation with the echocardiographer is appropriate.

Transthoracic echocardiography (TTE) is the standard clinical approach in most patients with suspected or known cardiac disease. Advantages are that it is noninvasive, has no known adverse effects, and provides detailed data on cardiac anatomy and physiology. Limitations include poor image quality in some patients, limited visualization of structures distant from the transducer (e.g., atrial septum, left atrial appendage), and shadowing by prosthetic heart valves.

Transesophageal echocardiography (TEE) offers superior image quality because of a shorter distance between the transducer and the heart, the absence of interposed bone or lung, and the use of a higher-frequency transducer. TEE usually is well tolerated, but intubation of the esophagus entails some risk, and most clinicians do this procedure with the patient under conscious sedation. TEE is much more sensitive than TTE for detection of left atrial thrombus (95% vs. 50%), valvular vegetations (99% vs. 60%), and prosthetic mitral valve regurgitation.

Handheld echocardiography refers to the use of smaller, less expensive ultrasound systems that can be carried by the physician, who can perform quick, limited examinations in the office or at the bedside. These laptop-sized echocardiography units range from the very simple, with only two-dimensional imaging and limited controls, to systems with high-quality imaging and all Doppler modalities. The role of handheld echocardiography has not yet been fully defined, but it can serve as an adjunct to the physical examination, such as in distinguishing ventricular dilatation from a pericardial effusion.

Contrast echocardiography may be performed using intravenous injection of agitated saline to opacify the right-sided heart chambers. These microbubbles are relatively large and do not pass through pulmonary capillaries. Therefore, appearance of contrast in the left side of the heart within one or two beats after right heart opacification is consistent with an intracardiac shunt. Although most atrial-level shunts are predominantly left-to-right, a small amount of right-to-left shunting occurs, which is the basis of this approach (Fig. 53–2).

Contrast echocardiography also may be performed with commercially available microbubbles in the range of 1 to 5 μm. Because these microbubbles are smaller than the pulmonary capillaries, right heart opacification is followed by left heart opacification, which can enhance the evaluation of systolic function when image quality is suboptimal, especially during stress echocardiography (Fig. 53–3).

Three-dimensional echocardiography is commercially available but is not routinely used for clinical diagnosis (Fig. 53–4), although it can provide excellent images in patients with congenital heart diseases.

Stress echocardiography is a standard approach for evaluating patients with known or suspected coronary artery disease; it has a sensitivity (85 to 95%) and a specificity (80 to 90%) similar to those of radionuclide stress imaging (Chapters 54 and 70). Myocardial infarction results in thinning and akinesis of the affected wall. However, in the absence of infarction, resting myocardial function is normal, even when severe epicardial coronary disease is present. The increased myocardial demand associated with exercise or pharmacologic stress leads to myocardial ischemia, which results in a regional wall motion abnormality, often before the onset of chest pain or electrocardiographic changes.

In patients who can exercise, standard views of the left ventricle are recorded at baseline and immediately after maximal treadmill or bicycle exercise. If endocardial definition is suboptimal, left-sided contrast is used. The rest and exercise images are compared in a side-by-side cine loop format. Myocardial ischemia is present if resting wall motion is normal but hypokinesis or akinesis is seen after exercise. The pattern of regional wall motion accurately identifies the area of myocardium at risk and is reasonably reliable for identification of the affected coronary artery. With three-vessel coronary disease, rather than a regional wall motion abnormality, the only clue on imaging may be an absence of the expected decrease in chamber size at peak exercise, caused by diffuse ischemia. Interpretation of an exercise echocardiogram includes exercise duration, hemodynamic response, symptoms, and electrocardiographic changes, in addition to the echocardiographic images (Fig. 53–5).

In patients who are unable to exercise, stress testing is performed using a graded intravenous infusion of dobutamine, beginning at 5 to 10 μg/kg/minute and increasing every 3 minutes to a maximum dose of 40 to 50 μg/kg/minute. If needed, atropine is used to achieve 85% of the

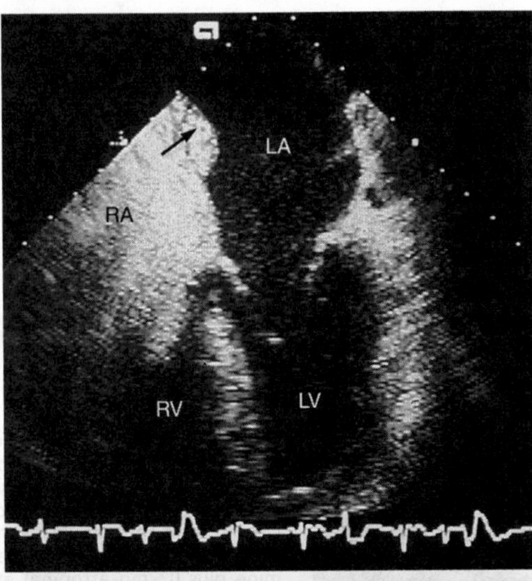

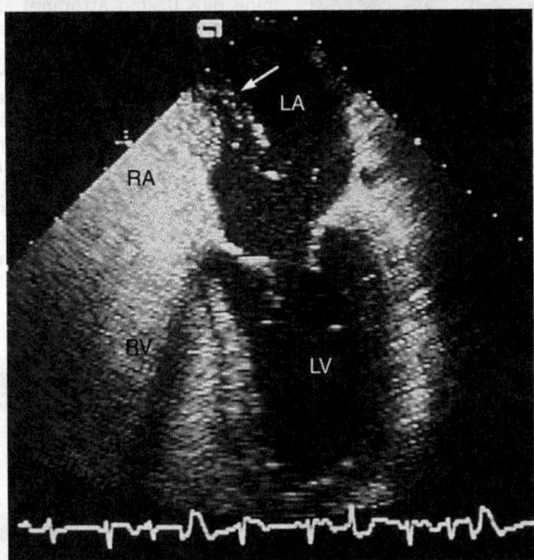

FIGURE 53–2 • Atrial septal aneurysm (top) with a patent foramen ovale (bottom) demonstrated on transesophageal echocardiography in a four-chamber view after injection of agitated saline solution in a peripheral vein. Small microbubbles (arrows) are seen traversing the defect from the opacified right atrium into the unopacified left atrium. LA = left atrium; LV = left ventricle; RA = right atrium; RV = right ventricle. (From Otto CM: Textbook of Clinical Echocardiography, 3rd ed. Philadelphia, Elsevier Saunders, 2004, p 424, Fig. 15–25.)

maximum predicted heart rate. In addition to evaluation for myocardial ischemia, dobutamine stress echocardiography can assess myocardial viability in areas of stunning or hibernation, based on an improvement in endocardial motion from baseline to low-dose dobutamine, with subsequent worsening of function at higher doses—the "biphasic" response.

Intracardiac echocardiography (ICE) is performed using an ultrasound probe on a catheter that is inserted into the right side of the heart via the femoral vein. ICE is used in the cardiac catheterization laboratory to guide percutaneous closure of a patent foramen ovale (PFO) and other procedures. In the electrophysiology laboratory, ICE helps guide catheter positioning and identify complications.

CARDIAC FUNCTION MEASUREMENTS

In addition to qualitative descriptions of cardiac anatomy and physiology, echocardiography provides precise and accurate quantitation of cardiac function including ventricular systolic and diastolic function, an estimate of the severity of valve stenosis and regurgitation, and a noninvasive estimate of pulmonary pressures.

Systolic Ventricular Function

Overall LV systolic function is graded by visual estimation, with an approximate correspondence to EF as follows: normal (EF >55%), mildly

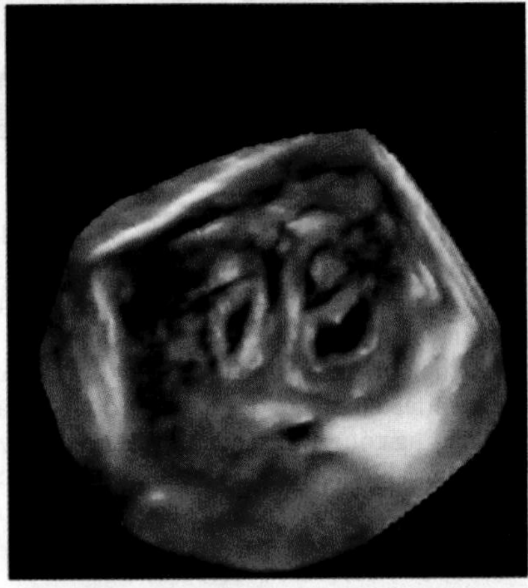

FIGURE 53–4 • Real-time three-dimensional image showing the tricuspid and mitral valves from the perspective of the left and right atrium. (Courtesy of Phillips Ultrasound, Andover, MA. From Otto CM: Textbook of Clinical Echocardiography, 3rd ed. Philadelphia, Elsevier Saunders, 2004, p 100, Fig. 4–6.)

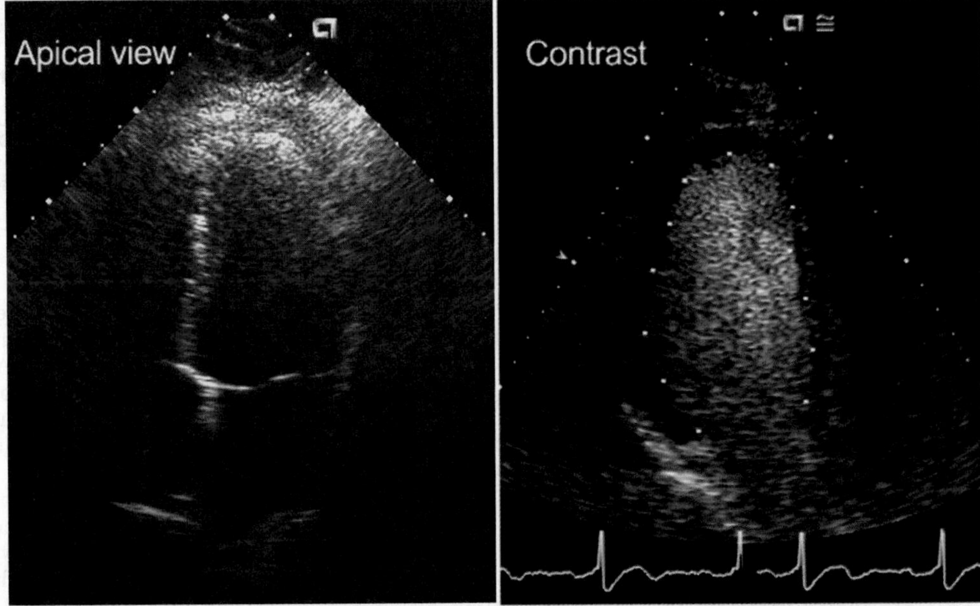

FIGURE 53–3 • Poor-quality apical view (A) with marked improvement in definition of the left ventricular cavity after opacification using contrast echocardiography (B). The dots indicate the left ventricular endocardial tracing for calculation of ejection fraction.

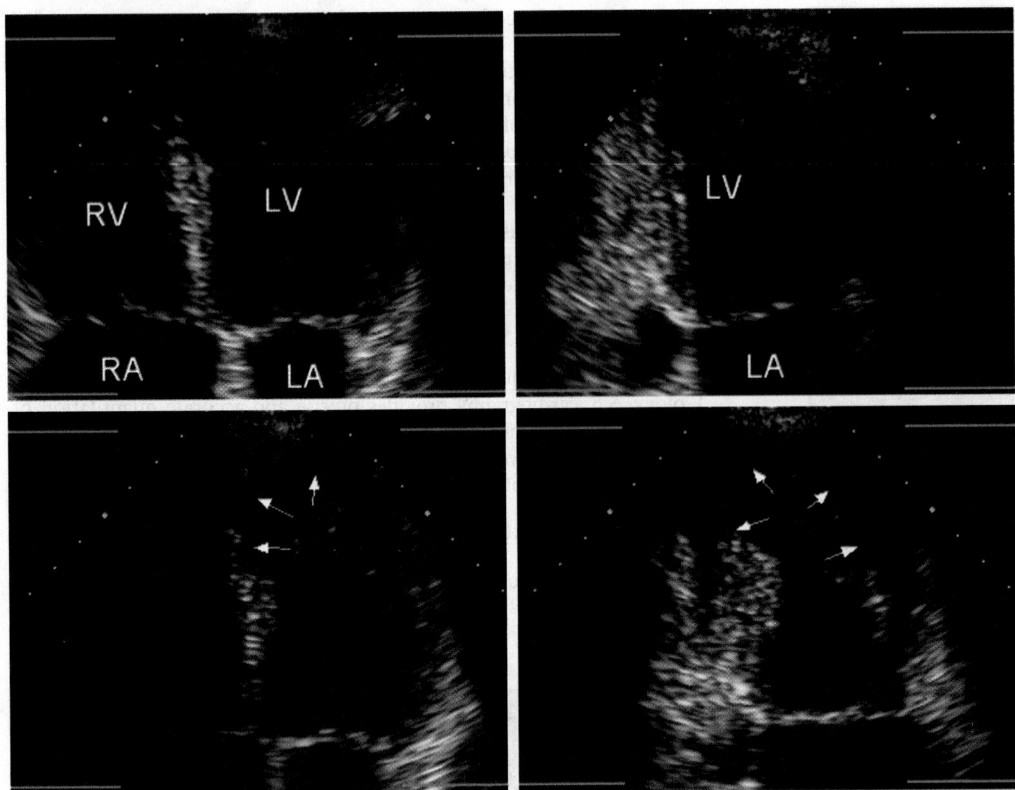

FIGURE 53–5 • Example of an abnormal dobutamine stress echocardiographic study. Baseline images at end-systole in an apical four-chamber view (top) and an apical two-chamber view (bottom) are shown on the left; the peak dose (40 mg/kg/minute dobutamine plus 0.5 mg atropine) end-systolic images are shown on the right. The apical segments of the septum and the anterior and inferior walls became akinetic at peak dobutamine dose (arrows), indicating significant coronary artery disease in the distribution of the left anterior descending artery. LA = left atrium; LV = left ventricle; RA = right atrium; RV = right ventricle. (From Otto CM: Textbook of Clinical Echocardiography, 3rd ed. Philadelphia, Elsevier Saunders, 2004, p 207, Fig. 8–13.)

reduced (EF 40 to 55%), moderately reduced (EF 20 to 40%), severely reduced (EF <20%). More precise quantitation is performed when clinically indicated by calculation of a biplane ejection fraction (see Fig. 53–4). Cardiac output calculations are not routine but may be helpful for noninvasive monitoring of therapy in patients with heart failure. Because EF measurements are affected by preload and afterload, measures that are less dependent on loading conditions, including the end-systolic dimension or volume, are generally preferred for clinical decision making in situations such as the timing of surgery for chronic valvular regurgitation.

Diastolic Ventricular Function

Evaluation of diastolic ventricular function is challenging because the patterns of ventricular filling are affected by preload, heart rate, and coexisting valvular regurgitation in addition to the diastolic properties of the ventricle. However, echocardiography can classify diastolic function based on the combination of LV inflow, pulmonary vein flow, tissue Doppler velocities, and the isovolumic relaxation time. An estimated of LV filling pressure (e.g., LV end-diastolic pressure) also can be inferred using these approaches.

Valvular Stenosis

Echocardiography is the clinical standard for evaluation of valvular heart disease (see Fig. 75–1). Cardiac catheterization can be reserved for cases in which echocardiography is nondiagnostic, clinical data are discrepant with echocardiographic findings, or coronary anatomy needs to be assessed (Chapter 75).

In patients with aortic stenosis, the most direct measure of stenosis severity is the antegrade velocity across the valve, indicating mild (<3 m/second), moderate (3 to 4 m/second), or severe (>4 m/second) valve obstruction. The maximum and mean transaortic pressure gradients also can be calculated using the Bernoulli equation (Fig. 53–6). Accurate evaluation depends on a careful examination by an experienced echocardiographer.

Aortic valve area (AVA) is calculated using the continuity equation, based on the concept that volume flow rates proximal to and within the narrowed orifice are equal:

$$AVA \times VTI_{AS} = CSA_{LVOT} \times VTI_{LVOT}$$

or

$$AVA = (CSA_{LVOT} \times VTI_{LVOT})/VTI_{AS}$$

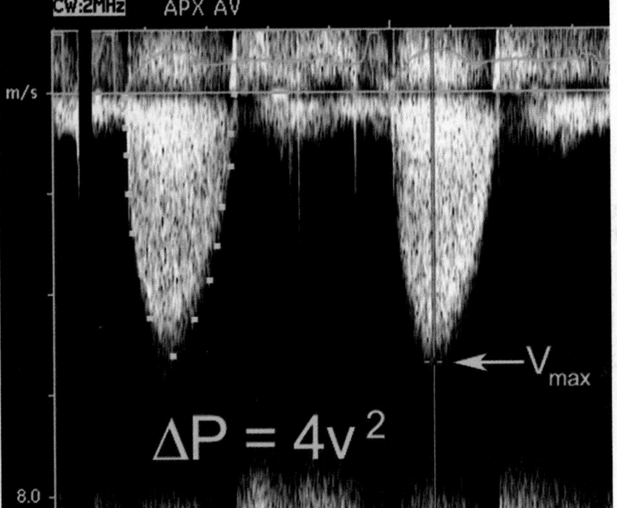

FIGURE 53–6 • In a patient with aortic stenosis, the aortic jet velocity is recorded with continuous wave Doppler from the window that yields the highest velocity signal. Maximum velocity (V_{max}) is used to calculate the maximum systolic gradient. The Doppler curve is traced, as shown, to calculate the mean systolic gradient, using the Bernoulli equation, by which the pressure gradient (ΔP) equals 4 times the square of the velocity.

where LVOT = left ventricular outflow tract, VTI = velocity time integral, CSA = cross-sectional area, and AS = aortic stenosis. It is especially important to calculate the AVA when LV systolic dysfunction accompanies aortic valve disease. In some patients, dobutamine stress echocardiography is helpful in distinguishing ventricular dysfunction caused by severe aortic stenosis from primary myocardial disease with concurrent moderate stenosis.

The evaluation of mitral stenosis (see Fig. 75–2) includes measurement of the mean transmitral gradient from the velocity curve and calculation of the valve area, both from two-dimensional planimetry of a short-axis image of the orifice and from the deceleration slope of the Doppler curve (pressure half-time method).

Valvular Regurgitation

The current approach to evaluating valvular regurgitation is based on the proximal geometry of the regurgitant jet and on calculation of regurgitant volume (RV), regurgitant fraction (RF), and regurgitant orifice area (ROA). Although color flow visualization of jets may be helpful for detection of regurgitation and for understanding the mechanism of valve dysfunction, this approach should no longer be used to evaluate severity.

The first step in evaluation of aortic regurgitant severity is measurement of the narrowest jet width (vena contracta) just beyond the regurgitant orifice (see Fig. 75–5). A narrow vena contracta (<3 mm) indicates mild regurgitation, whereas a wide vena contracta (>6 mm) indicates severe regurgitation. Additional evaluation of the severity of aortic regurgitation is based on the presence of holodiastolic flow reversal in the abdominal aorta and the density and slope of the continuous wave Doppler velocity curve. The approach to evaluating mitral regurgitation (see Fig. 75–4) is similar, beginning with measurement of the vena contracta. In addition to calculation based on transmitral vs. transaortic volume flow rates, the proximal acceleration of flow into the regurgitant orifice allows evaluation with central regurgitant jets. Color flow shows a proximal isovelocity surface area (PISA).

Pulmonary Pressures

Estimation of pulmonary artery systolic pressure (PAP) is a standard component of a complete examination. The systolic pressure difference between the right ventricle and right atrium is calculated from the peak velocity in the tricuspid regurgitant (V_{TR}) jet, using the Bernoulli equation. Then, the right atrial pressure (RAP) is estimated from the size and appearance of the inferior vena cava. Because right ventricular and pulmonary artery systolic pressures are equal (in the absence of pulmonic stenosis),

$$PAP = 4(V_{TR})^2 + RAP$$

A small amount of tricuspid regurgitation is present in most patients, so pulmonary pressures can be estimated with this approach in more than 90% of patients. Because this approach measures only pulmonary systolic pressure, not pulmonary vascular resistance, invasive evaluation may still be needed is some clinical situations (Chapter 67).

THE ECHOCARDIOGRAPHIC EXAMINATION

Clinical Indications

Echocardiography is an effective approach to the initial evaluation of many cardiac signs and symptoms (Table 53–1). Even when transesophageal imaging might be helpful, most clinicians begin with a transthoracic examination; exceptions are for the patient with a possible acute aortic dissection (Chapter 78), in whom TEE should be performed as quickly as possible, and in the evaluation of possible left atrial thrombosis before cardioversion without anticoagulation (Chapter 63). It is important to remember that resting echocardiography is not helpful for diagnosis of coronary artery disease; stress imaging is needed if this diagnosis is suspected (Chapter 70). In patients with known cardiac disease, echocardiography is used to evaluate severity, assess the results of medical and surgical interventions, and guide procedures (Table 53–2).

TABLE 53–1 COMMON SYMPTOMS AND SIGNS EVALUATED BY ECHOCARDIOGRAPHY

Reason for Echocardiography	Possible Echocardiographic Findings or Diagnosis
Chest pain	Coronary artery disease
	Acute myocardial infarction on resting echocardiography
	Stress echocardiography needed to detect coronary disease
	Aortic dissection
	Pericarditis
	Valvular aortic stenosis
	Hypertrophic cardiomyopathy
Heart failure	Left ventricular systolic dysfunction (global or segmental)
	Valvular heart disease
	Left ventricular diastolic dysfunction
	Pericardial disease
	Right ventricular dysfunction
Palpitations	Left ventricular systolic dysfunction
	Mitral valve disease
	Congenital heart disease (e.g., ASD, Ebstein's anomaly)
	Pericarditis
	No structural cardiac disease
Cardiac murmur	Flow murmur (no valve abnormality)
Systolic	Aortic stenosis, subaortic obstruction, hypertrophic obstructive cardiomyopathy
	Mitral regurgitation
	Ventricular septal defect
	Pulmonic stenosis
	Tricuspid regurgitation
Diastolic	Mitral stenosis
	Aortic regurgitation
	Pulmonic regurgitation
	Tricuspid stenosis
Cardiomegaly on chest radiography	Pericardial effusion
	Dilated cardiomyopathy
	Specific chamber enlargement (e.g., left ventricle in chronic aortic regurgitation)
Systemic embolic event	Left ventricular systolic function and segmental wall motion abnormalities (aneurysms)
	Left ventricular thrombus
	Aortic valve disease
	Mitral valve disease
	Left atrial thrombus (TTE has low sensitivity, TEE required)
	Patent foramen ovale

ASD = atrial septal defect; TEE = transesophageal echocardiography; TTE = transthoracic echocardiography.
From Otto CM: Textbook of Clinical Echocardiography, 3rd ed. Philadelphia, Elsevier Saunders, Philadelphia, 2004, pp 118–110, Tables 5–2 and 5–3.

TABLE 53–2 INDICATIONS FOR ECHOCARDIOGRAPHY BY KNOWN DIAGNOSIS

Clinical Diagnosis	Key Echocardiographic Findings	Limitations of Echocardiography	Alternative Approaches
Valvular heart disease			
Valve stenosis (Chapter 75)	Etiology of stenosis, valve anatomy Transvalvular ΔP, valve area Chamber enlargement and hypertrophy LV and RV systolic function Associated valvular regurgitation	Possible underestimation of severity of stenosis Possible coexisting coronary artery disease	Cardiac catheterization; MRI
Valve regurgitation	Mechanism and etiology of regurgitation Severity of regurgitation Chamber enlargement LV and RV systolic function PA pressure estimate	TEE may be needed to evaluate severity of mitral regurgitant and valve anatomy (especially before MV repair)	Cardiac catheterization; MRI
Prosthetic valve function	Evidence for stenosis Detection of regurgitation Chamber enlargement Ventricular function PA pressure estimate	Imaging of prosthetic valves is limited by shadowing and reverberations TEE is needed for suspected prosthetic MR due to "masking" of the LA on TTE	Cardiac catheterization
Endocarditis (Chapter 76)	Detection of vegetations (TTE sensitivity 70–85%) Presence and degree of valve dysfunction Chamber enlargement and function Detection of abscess Possible prognostic implications	TEE more sensitive for detection of vegetations (>90%) A definite diagnosis of endocarditis also depends on bacteriologic criteria TEE more sensitive for detecting an abscess	Blood cultures and clinical findings also are diagnostic criteria for endocarditis
Coronary artery disease			
Acute myocardial infarction (Chapters 71 and 72)	Segmental wall motion abnormality reflects "myocardium at risk" Global LV function (EF) Complications: Acute MR vs. VSD Pericarditis LV thrombus, aneurysm RV infarct	Coronary artery anatomy itself is not directly visualized	Coronary angiography Radionuclide LV angiography Cardiac catheterization
Angina (Chapter 70)	Global and segmental LV systolic function Exclude other causes of angina (e.g., AS, HOCM)	Resting wall motion may be normal despite significant CAD Stress echocardiography is needed to induce ischemia and wall motion abnormality	Coronary angiography Stress thallium ETT
Pre-revascularization/ post-revascularization	Assess wall thickening and endocardial motion at baseline Improvement in segmental function after procedure	Dobutamine stress and/or contrast echocardiography is needed to detect viable but nonfunctioning myocardium	MRI PET Thallium ETT Contrast echocardiography
End-stage ischemic disease	Overall LV systolic function (EF) PA pressures Associated MR LV thrombus RV systolic function	—	Coronary angiography Radionuclide EF

Cardiomyopathy (Chapters 57–59)			
Dilated	Chamber dilation (all four) LV and RV systolic function (qualitative and EF) Coexisting atrioventricular valve regurgitation PA systolic pressure LV thrombus	Indirect measures of LVEDP Accurate EF may be difficult if image quality is poor	Radionuclide EF LV and RV angiography
Restrictive	LV wall thickness LV systolic function LV diastolic function PA systolic pressure	Must be distinguished from constrictive pericarditis	Cardiac catheterization with direct, simultaneous RV and LV pressure measurement after volume loading
Hypertrophic	Pattern and extent of LV hypertrophy Dynamic LVOT obstruction (imaging and Doppler) Coexisting MR Diastolic LV dysfunction	—	—
Hypertension (Chapter 66)	LV wall thickness and chamber dimensions LV mass LV systolic function Aortic root dilation	—	—
Pericardial disease (Chapter 77)	Pericardial thickening Detection, size, and location of PE 2D signs of tamponade physiology Doppler signs of tamponade physiology	Diagnosis of tamponade is a hemodynamic and clinical diagnosis Constrictive pericarditis is a difficult diagnosis Not all patients with pericarditis have an effusion	Intracardiac pressure measurements for tamponade or constriction MRI or CT to detect pericardial thickening
Diseases of the aorta (Chapter 78)			
Aortic root dilation	Etiology of aortic dilation Accurate aortic root diameter measurements Anatomy of sinuses of Valsalva (especially Marfan syndrome) Associated aortic regurgitation	—	CT, MRI aortography
Aortic dissection	2D images of ascending aorta, aortic arch, descending thoracic and proximal abdominal aorta Imaging of dissection "flap" Associated aortic regurgitation Ventricular function	TEE more sensitive (97%) and more specific (100%) Cannot assess distal vascular beds	Aortography CT MRI TEE

Continued

TABLE 53–2 INDICATIONS FOR ECHOCARDIOGRAPHY BY KNOWN DIAGNOSIS—cont'd

Clinical Diagnosis	Key Echocardiographic Findings	Limitations of Echocardiography	Alternative Approaches
Cardiac masses (Chapter 59)			
LV thrombus	High sensitivity and specificity for diagnosis of LV thrombus Suspect with apical wall motion abnormality or diffuse LV systolic dysfunction	Technical artifacts can be misleading 5-MHz or higher frequency transducer and angulated apical views needed TEE is needed to detect LA thrombus reliably	LV thrombus may not be recognized on radionuclide or contrast angiography
LA thrombus	Low sensitivity for detection of LA thrombus, although specificity is high Suspect with LA enlargement, MV disease		TEE
Cardiac tumors	Size, location, and physiologic consequences of tumor mass	Extracardiac involvement is not well seen Cannot distinguish benign from malignant tumor, or tumor from thrombus	TEE CT MRI (with cardiac gating) Intracardiac echocardiography
Pulmonary hypertension (Chapter 67)	Estimate of PA pressure Evidence of left-sided heart disease to account for increased PA pressures RV size and systolic function (cor pulmonale) Associated TR	Indirect PA pressure measurement Cannot determine pulmonary vascular resistance accurately	Cardiac catheterization
Congenital heart disease (Chapter 68)	Detection and assessment of anatomic abnormalities Quantitation of physiologic abnormalities Chamber enlargement Ventricular function	No direct intracardiac pressure measurements Complicated anatomy may be difficult to evaluate if image quality is poor (TEE is helpful)	MRI with 3D reconstruction Cardiac catheterization TEE

2D = two-dimensional; 3D = three-dimensional; AS = aortic stenosis; CAD = coronary artery disease; CT = computed tomography; EF = ejection fraction; ETT = exercise treadmill test; HCM = hypertrophic obstructive cardiomyopathy; LA = left atrial; LV = left ventricular; LVEDP = left ventricular end-diastolic pressure; LVOT = left ventricular outflow tract; MR = mitral regurgitation; MRI = magnetic resonance imaging; MV = mitral valve; ΔP = pressure gradient; PA = pulmonary artery; PE = pericardial effusion; PET = position emission tomography; RV = right ventricular; TEE = transesophageal echocardiography; TR = tricuspid regurgitation; TTE = transthoracic echocardiography; VSD = ventricular septal defect.

From Otto CM: Textbook of Clinical Echocardiography, 3rd ed. Philadelphia, Elsevier Saunders, Philadelphia, 2004, pp 128–130.

Normal Findings

Trace to mild regurgitation is considered "physiologic" and is seen with 70 to 80% of mitral valves, 80 to 90% of tricuspid valves, and 70 to 80% of pulmonic valves in normal individuals. The prevalence of aortic regurgitation increases with age, but it is found in only 5% of young normal adults; the presence of aortic regurgitation raises the possibility of subtle aortic valve or root abnormalities. Prophylaxis of endocarditis (Chapter 76) is based on the presence of pathologic regurgitation and an underlying anatomic abnormality of the valve. Endocarditis prophylaxis is not needed for physiologic valvular regurgitation.

A PFO (Chapter 68) is present in 25 to 35% of normal individuals and may be identified by color Doppler or by contrast echocardiography. Use of the Valsalva maneuver enhances identification of a PFO, because the slight elevation in right atrial pressure may lead to a brief right-to-left shunt. The significance of a PFO in patients without clinical events is unclear. Other common anatomic variants seen on echocardiography include aberrant chords (or "webs") in the left ventricle; small, linear, mobile echoes associated with the valves (Lambl's excrescences); and normal ridges in the left and right atrium.

Unexpected abnormal findings also may be found on studies requested for other indications. A bicuspid aortic valve is present in 1 to 2% of the population; most of these patients are asymptomatic until late in life, so many are diagnosed "incidentally" by echocardiography. Aortic valve sclerosis, which is a frequent unexpected echocardiographic diagnosis, is a marker of cardiovascular disease and an increased risk of myocardial infarction even if valve function is normal.

INTEGRATING THE ECHOCARDIOGRAPHIC AND CLINICAL FINDINGS

The echocardiographic request should indicate the specific reason for the study and any relevant symptoms or signs. The echocardiographic examination then can be tailored to answer the clinical question. The echocardiographic results should be interpreted in conjunction with other clinical data. If the echocardiographic data seem discrepant with the clinical data, the requesting physician should review the images with the echocardiographer to identify areas of uncertainty and to determine the next best diagnostic step.

SUGGESTED READING

Cheitlin MD, Armstrong WF, Aurigemma GP, et al: ACC/AHA/ASE 2003 guideline update for the clinical application of echocardiography—Summary article: A report of the American College of Cardiology/American Heart Association Task Force on Practice Guidelines (ACC/AHA/ASE Committee to Update the 1997 Guidelines for the Clinical Application of Echocardiography). J Am Coll Cardiol 2003;42:954–970 and Circulation 2003;108:1146–1162. *Clinical guidelines for the use of echocardiography.*

Otto CM: Textbook of Clinical Echocardiography, 3rd ed. Philadelphia, Elsevier Saunders, 2004. *An introduction to echocardiography.*

Thomas JD, Popovic ZB: Assessment of ventricular function by cardiac ultrasound. J Am Coll Cardiol 2006;4:2012–2025. *The clinical impact of echocardiography and its future directions.*

Weyman AE: The year in echocardiography. J Am Coll Cardiol 2007;49: 1212–1219. *An overview of the developments in echocardiography.*

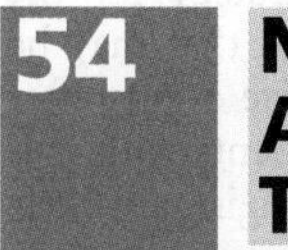

NUCLEAR CARDIOLOGY AND COMPUTED TOMOGRAPHY

George A. Beller and Christopher M. Kramer

NUCLEAR CARDIOLOGY

The techniques of nuclear cardiology permit the noninvasive imaging of myocardial perfusion under stress and resting conditions and of resting regional and global function by use of radionuclide imaging agents and gamma or positron cameras with associated computer processing. All these techniques are based on acquiring images of radioactivity emanating from tracers localized in heart muscle or in the blood pools of the left and right ventricles. Myocardial perfusion imaging is the most commonly performed nuclear cardiology technique, and it is employed most often in conjunction with either exercise or pharmacologic stress intended to produce flow heterogeneity between relatively hypoperfused and normally perfused myocardial regions. Radionuclide angiography, in which technetium-99m (^{99m}Tc)-labeled red blood cells or other ^{99m}Tc-labeled agents are injected intravenously, is used for measurement of left ventricular ejection fraction and assessment of regional wall motion. This technique is used most commonly to monitor changes in global left ventricular function in patients undergoing chemotherapy for cancer when drugs with the potential for cardiac toxicity are administered. Positron emission tomography (PET) can assess regional myocardial metabolism to estimate myocardial viability, most often with fluorine 18–labeled 2-deoxyglucose (FDG), as well as myocardial perfusion by use of rubidium (Rb) 82.

Myocardial Perfusion Imaging

Imaging Agents

Thallium-201 (^{201}Tl), a monovalent cation that is biologically similar to potassium, initially was the most commonly employed radionuclide agent for the assessment of myocardial perfusion. Now, however, ^{99m}Tc-labeled perfusion agents, which provide higher quality images more quickly, are used more commonly than ^{201}Tl for exercise or pharmacologic stress perfusion imaging to evaluate patients with suspected or known coronary heart disease (CHD). For clinical imaging, the major advantage of ^{99m}Tc perfusion imaging is the improved specificity for detecting coronary disease because its higher energy reduces attenuation artifacts and permits the images to be gated with the electrocardiogram (ECG) to assess regional systolic thickening on tomographic images throughout the cardiac cycle. Of the various ^{99m}Tc-labeled agents, ^{99m}Tc-sestamibi and ^{99m}Tc-tetrofosmin are the most common. ^{99m}Tc-sestamibi, an isonitrile, is superior in many ways to ^{201}Tl for myocardial perfusion imaging. ^{99m}Tc agents provide simultaneous assessment of regional and global left ventricular function with gated single-photon emission computed tomography (SPECT) technology. Left ventricular ejection fraction and end-diastolic and end-systolic volumes are measured accurately on gated SPECT images.

Some laboratories use dual-isotope rest ^{201}Tl/stress ^{99m}Tc-sestamibi imaging, in which patients undergo ^{201}Tl imaging at rest, then immediately afterward undergo ^{99m}Tc-sestamibi imaging during stress. Reversibility is identified by comparing the perfusion pattern on the stress ^{99m}Tc-sestamibi images with the pattern on the baseline resting ^{201}Tl images. The major advantage of this technique is the marked decrease in total imaging time.

Detection of Coronary Heart Disease

The major indications for stress and rest myocardial perfusion imaging are to diagnose CHD, to assess prognosis, and to detect myocardial viability. Exercise or pharmacologic stress ^{201}Tl or ^{99m}Tc-sestamibi SPECT imaging in patients with chest pain yields a sensitivity for detecting CHD in the 85 to 90% range. The specificity for excluding CHD is in the 85% range for ^{99m}Tc-sestamibi SPECT imaging and increases to 90% when gated images are used. Exercise or pharmacologic stress SPECT ^{201}Tl perfusion imaging and exercise or pharmacologic stress SPECT ^{99m}Tc perfusion imaging have sensitivities and specificities that are superior to those of exercise ECG testing alone. The specificity of gated SPECT for detecting CHD with use of one of the ^{99m}Tc-labeled perfusion agents is 20 to 30% higher than that of ^{201}Tl SPECT in women.

Radionuclide stress perfusion imaging is of particular value compared with exercise ECG testing alone in (1) patients with resting ECG abnormalities, such as those seen with left ventricular hypertrophy, digitalis effect, Wolff-Parkinson-White syndrome, and intraventricular conduction abnormalities, and (2) patients who fail to achieve more than 85% of maximum predicted heart rate. Approximately 40% of patients with a low to intermediate pretest likelihood of CHD who manifest 1.0 mm or more of horizontal or downsloping ST segment depression have no evidence of CHD (false-positive findings). The addition of stress perfusion imaging can assist in differentiating true-positive from false-positive ST depression. Detection of proximal left anterior descending stenoses and proximal multivessel CHD is enhanced by identifying regional systolic thickening or wall motion abnormalities on the gated SPECT images

TABLE 54–1 HIGH-RISK RESULTS IN EXERCISE MYOCARDIAL PERFUSION SCANNING

Abnormal regional perfusion in regions supplied by two or more coronary arteries (e.g., defects in the left anterior descending artery and left circumflex artery territories)
Extensive reversible defects, even if only in the region of one major coronary artery (e.g., defects in the anterior wall, septum, and apex corresponding to the left anterior descending coronary artery territory)
Large defect size (>20% of the left ventricular myocardium) on quantitative SPECT
Increased lung ^{201}Tl uptake, best assessed by quantitating the lung-to-heart ^{201}Tl ratio
Transient ischemic left ventricular cavity dilation in the stress compared with the resting state
Extensive regional systolic thickening or wall motion abnormalities on gated ^{99m}Tc SPECT images

compared with assessment based on perfusion alone. If possible, drugs such as long-acting nitrates, β-blockers, and rate-lowering calcium blockers should be discontinued for 24 hours before exercise stress testing that is performed to diagnose or to exclude CHD as the cause of chest pain.

Pharmacologic Stress Imaging

Certain patients are unable to exercise to adequate heart rates and workloads on exercise stress testing protocols. Pharmacologic stress testing with use of vasodilators, such as dipyridamole and adenosine, or inotropic agents, such as dobutamine, is an alternative to exercise for detecting physiologically significant coronary artery stenoses. Sensitivity and specificity for CHD detection are comparable for dipyridamole and adenosine. The addition of limited exercise to dipyridamole or adenosine imaging can prevent the vasodilator-induced hypotension, improve the ECG detection of ischemia, and enhance image quality by increasing the heart-to-liver ratio of tracer uptake. Dobutamine stress is preferred in patients who have bronchospasm or a history of asthma or who have consumed caffeine, which is an adenosine receptor antagonist, within 12 hours before testing. Patients who experience side effects such as hypotension and chest pain during dipyridamole or adenosine infusion should be treated with intravenous aminophylline, an adenosine antagonist that immediately reverses these side effects.

Assessment of Prognosis

One of the chief applications of stress myocardial perfusion imaging is the identification of patients at either high or low risk for future ischemic cardiac events. Numerous studies have shown that the extent of hypoperfusion on post-stress SPECT perfusion images provides important incremental prognostic information when it is added to clinical variables, the resting left ventricular ejection fraction, exercise ECG stress test variables, and even coronary artery anatomy. Nondiabetic patients with chest pain and a normal myocardial perfusion scan at peak exercise or under vasodilator stress have a subsequent cardiac death or infarction rate of less than 1% per year and are generally appropriate candidates for medical therapy or require further diagnostic evaluation for a noncardiac cause of chest pain (Chapters 48 and 139). Conversely, patients with high-risk imaging results (Table 54–1), may benefit from early referral for invasive strategies, including coronary revascularization (Chapters 73 and 74), even if symptoms are mild. Patients who show inducible ischemia involving more than 20% of the left ventricular myocardium appear to have a better outcome with coronary revascularization compared with medical therapy. Patients who have diabetes and who show inducible ischemia have a higher cardiac event rate than that of nondiabetics who have a similar extent and severity of perfusion abnormalities on exercise or pharmacologic stress SPECT images. Patients with a non–high-risk scan or mild perfusion defects (e.g., a single-vessel disease pattern) and a normal left ventricular ejection fraction generally can be treated medically without initially pursuing an invasive strategy.

Transient ischemic left ventricular cavity dilation, by which the left ventricular cavity appears more dilated on stress images compared with rest images, is a particularly high-risk finding on SPECT. This finding

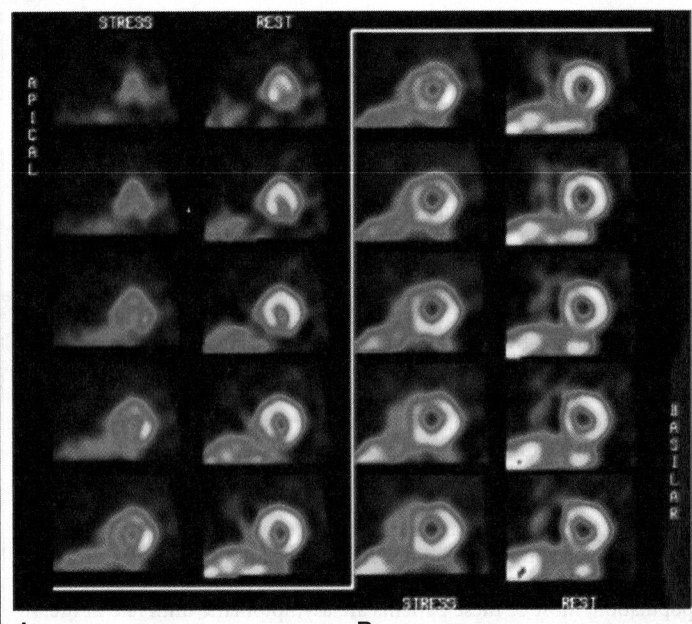

FIGURE 54–1 • Stress and rest short-axis ^{99m}Tc-sestamibi tomograms in a patient with chest pain and 3 mm of upsloping ST-segment depression on exercise electrocardiogram stress testing. Note a large defect involving the anterior wall, septum, and inferior wall; the defect is reversible on the resting study. These findings indicate significant inducible ischemia in the region of a proximal left anterior descending coronary artery stenosis. This patient was referred for further invasive evaluation.

occurs when subendocardial ischemia after stress causes a decrease in tracer uptake in the subendocardium, yielding what appears to be a larger left ventricular cavity than was observed on the resting images. Figure 54–1A shows adenosine stress and rest short-axis tomograms in a diabetic patient with reversible defects in the apex, anterior wall, septum, inferior wall, and posterolateral wall with transient ischemic left ventricular dilation. This finding is in contrast to the images of a normal patient with no coronary artery disease, in which tracer activity is uniformly distributed in all myocardial segments on stress and rest images.

Patients with abnormal pharmacologic stress studies have a worse prognosis than that of patients with comparable defect patterns seen on exercise scans, perhaps because their inability to exercise is also a prognostic factor. Assessment of regional left ventricular function on post-stress gated SPECT images enhances the detection of three-vessel CHD. Exercise or pharmacologic stress perfusion imaging also provides useful prognostic information for predischarge risk stratification in clinically low- to intermediate-risk patients who have experienced an uncomplicated myocardial infarction or unstable angina. Demonstration of defects remote from the zone of infarction (which indicate underlying multivessel disease), evidence for residual ischemia within the infarct zone, or both identify patients with an increased risk of reinfarction and subsequent cardiac death. Patients with only a nonreversible defect within the zone of infarction have a better long-term outcome unless the total defect size exceeds 15% of the left ventricular myocardium. Patients with peripheral vascular disease may be limited by claudication and not manifest exertional angina despite substantial CHD. Preoperative pharmacologic stress perfusion imaging offers a noninvasive strategy for the detection of physiologically important coronary stenoses that may be associated with an increased risk of early and late cardiac events after peripheral vascular or aortic surgery (Chapter 457). Patients with evidence for inducible ischemia on preoperative perfusion imaging are likely to benefit from preoperative β-blocker therapy.

Exercise or pharmacologic stress perfusion imaging is superior to exercise ECG testing alone for detection of coronary restenosis in patients presenting with recurrence of symptoms after a percutaneous coronary intervention (Chapter 73). Stress perfusion imaging also has proved useful for identifying high-risk patients who have undergone previous coronary artery bypass graft surgery but who are asymptomatic. Ischemia induced at a low workload, particularly in patients with depressed left ventricular function, merits an invasive evaluation in post-bypass patients (Chapter 74).

Determination of Myocardial Viability with Single-Photon Emission Computed Tomography or Positron Emission Tomography

SPECT perfusion imaging is performed in the resting state with ^{201}Tl- or ^{99m}Tc-labeled agents to identify residual myocardial viability in zones corresponding to severe regional wall motion abnormalities in patients with CHD and depressed left ventricular function. When severe left ventricular dysfunction is caused by "hibernation" (a state of chronic reduced contractility because of substantial ischemia) and not by irreversible myocardial necrosis, areas of resting hypoperfusion that are viable and contributing to hibernation show initial defects on early images and delayed redistribution or mild nonreversible defects on delayed images. If uptake ultimately exceeds 50% or 60% of peak uptake in these regions, there is a high probability (65 to 75%) that regional myocardial function will improve after successful revascularization. Myocardial zones of asynergy showing less than 50% on resting images have only a 10 to 20% probability of showing improved regional function after revascularization. Resting gated SPECT after nitroglycerin administration also can assess viability in a similar manner.

Regional myocardial metabolism can be assessed noninvasively by PET with FDG and a flow tracer such as [^{13}N]ammonia. FDG is a glucose analogue that is taken up initially in myocardial cells and is trapped by conversion to FDG-6-phosphate. FDG is cell membrane impermeable and remains within viable cells at high concentrations for more than 40 to 60 minutes. Increased FDG activity on clinical PET images in areas of diminished regional blood flow, as determined by [^{13}N]ammonia imaging, is characteristic of myocardial viability. These areas of blood flow/FDG mismatch usually show improved regional function after coronary revascularization. Regions of the heart that show diminished ^{13}N uptake and FDG uptake (a "match" pattern) represent predominantly nonviable myocardium, and these segments have only a 10 to 15% probability of showing improved systolic function after revascularization.

Patients with CHD with predominantly viable myocardium as the cause of left ventricular dysfunction have better survival and more improvement of heart failure symptoms after revascularization than with medical therapy. Patients who have an ischemic cardiomyopathy with poor viability on either resting SPECT or PET have a worse outcome after coronary revascularization compared with patients with predominantly viable myocardium.

Imaging of Ventricular Function

Global and segmental left and right ventricular function can be evaluated accurately by gated cardiac blood pool imaging with either the first-pass method or the equilibrium method to provide a radionuclide angiogram or ventriculogram. A uniform diminution of left ventricular systolic function without segmental wall motion abnormalities suggests nonischemic dilated cardiomyopathy, whereas depressed global left ventricular function associated with segmental wall motion abnormalities suggests ischemic heart disease.

First-Pass Method

First-pass radionuclide angiography analyzes rapidly acquired image frames to observe the fate of a bolus of ^{99m}Tc as it traverses the venous system to the right side of the heart, pulmonary artery, lungs, left atrium, and left ventricle. Time-activity curves are generated by measuring radioactive counts in the blood pools over time. Ejection fraction values are obtained by dividing the stroke counts (end-diastolic counts minus end-systolic counts) by the end-diastolic counts. It is also possible to estimate end-systolic and end-diastolic volumes.

Equilibrium Method

The equilibrium radionuclide angiographic approach is performed after thorough mixing of ^{99m}Tc-labeled blood cells within the intravascular compartment. Because ^{99m}Tc remains within the blood pool, serial imaging studies can be acquired during several hours. Acquisition of the images is synchronized with the QRS complex on the ECG through a multigated approach by which each cardiac cycle is divided into multiple frames. From the frame images accumulated during multiple cardiac cycles, regional wall motion and global left ventricular function can be evaluated in a cine mode.

CARDIAC COMPUTED TOMOGRAPHY

Technical Aspects

Computed tomography (CT) imaging is based on x-rays derived from a source that rotates around the body and emits a fan-shaped beam. The beam is focused by collimators and then detected sensitively. A cross-sectional image is derived from the detected x-rays obtained in multiple angles. Each pixel of the reconstructed image has a characteristic x-ray attenuation value or Hounsfield unit. Because of cardiac motion, high temporal resolution is required for cardiac imaging, which also must be gated to the ECG and obtained during a breath-hold to yield snapshots of the heart reconstructed from the same phase of the cardiac cycle.

Electron beam computed tomography (EBCT) uses a high-voltage electron beam that is deflected and focused by electromagnetic coils over a semicircular target, creating a fan of x-rays that pass through the patient and are subsequently detected. The strengths of the technique are its speed (33 to 100 msec temporal resolution) and its low radiation dose.

Multidetector computed tomography (MDCT) provides better temporal resolution and imaging. However, the radiation dose for coronary artery imaging is currently at least 8 to 11 mSv, equivalent to three or more times the background radiation in the United States per year for the average patient.

Coronary Artery Calcium Scoring

Coronary calcium is an indicator of the burden of atherosclerotic plaque, and very high levels confer an increased risk of future cardiac events (Fig. 54–2). Calcium scores are generally calculated as an Agatston score, which corresponds to each coronary lesion's calcium area multiplied by the maximum CT attenuation value of that lesion, and then summed for the entire coronary tree. In a large prospective, population-based study, the coronary calcium score predicted coronary events independently of either standard risk factors or C-reactive protein and was a better predictor than the Framingham risk score. Calcium scores above 100 were associated with a 9.2 times elevated risk of nonfatal myocardial infarction and death. The utility of calcium scoring may be highest in intermediate-risk patients on the basis of Framingham risk data. However, absolute event rates are low in asymptomatic persons, even in the highest risk group, and thus the utility of calcium scoring as a screening test has yet to be defined. Importantly, there is no correlation between coronary calcium and the physiologic or anatomic significance of a stenosis.

CT Coronary Angiography

CT is an excellent technique for diagnosis of anomalous coronary arterial anatomy in adults when equivocal findings are noted on echocardiography or x-ray angiography. The experience and accuracy for detecting stenoses in patients with coronary disease have progressed rapidly. Initially, EBCT was the technique of choice because of excellent temporal resolution, but 25% of coronary arteries could not be evaluated owing to low contrast-to-noise ratios or severe calcifications. By MDCT with as many as 64 detectors, fewer arteries (approximately 6 to 12%) cannot be evaluated. Studies with 16-detector scanners and 64-detector scanners compared with x-ray angiography as the "gold standard" have consistently demonstrated sensitivities on a per-segment basis in the 95% range, specificities of 85 to 98%, and positive and negative predictive values of 66 to 87% and about 98%, respectively. Thus, the technique appears to be an excellent way to exclude significant CHD (Fig. 54–3). The accuracy for detecting stenoses in bypass grafts is similar. However, MDCT tends to overestimate the percentage of stenosis, and the lumen of heavily calcified vessels still cannot be accurately assessed.

It remains unclear in which population of patients MDCT coronary angiography will be best applied. One possibility may include patients with atypical chest pain or patients with chest pain in emergency departments (Chapter 48) without overt evidence of myocardial damage by ECG or cardiac biomarkers.

Other Cardiac Applications

The same data acquired by MDCT for coronary artery imaging can be reformatted and used for functional cardiac imaging, including left ventricular volumes, ejection fraction, wall thickness, and global and

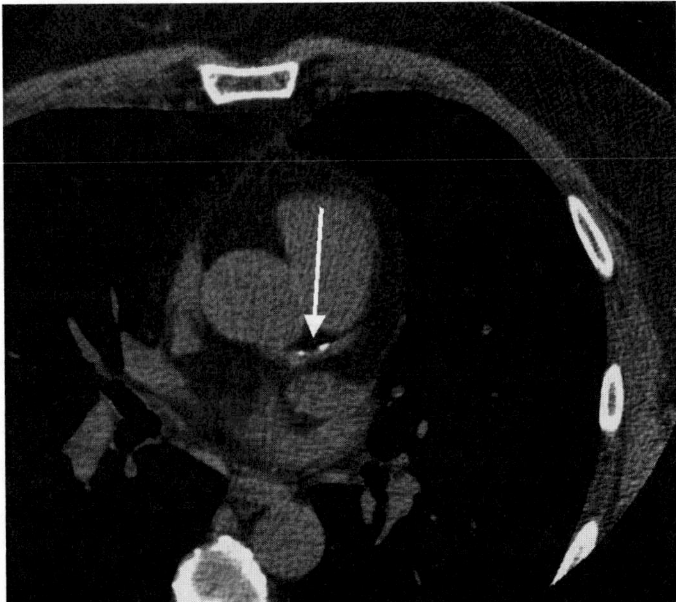

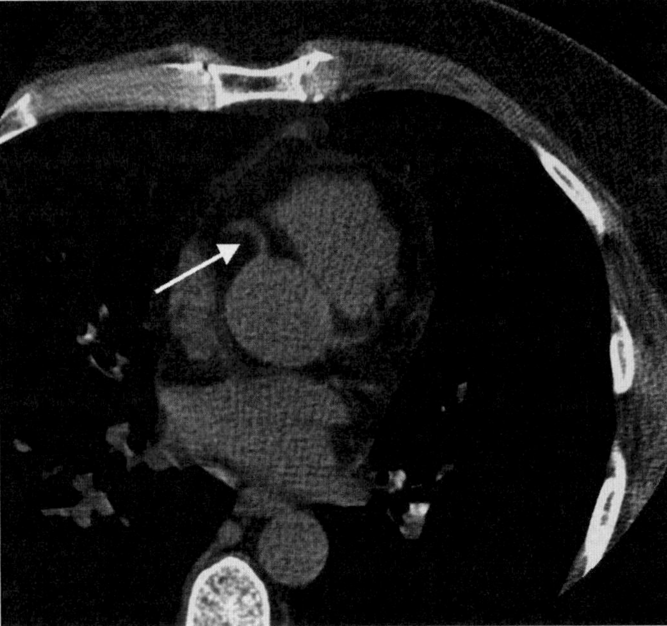

FIGURE 54–2 • Nonenhanced cardiac CT demonstrating focal calcification of the proximal left anterior descending artery (see arrow in top image) and lack of calcification in the proximal right coronary artery (see arrow in bottom image).

segmental wall motion. However, the measurement of end-diastolic volume, end-systolic volume, and left ventricular mass by MDCT is significantly different from that of cardiac magnetic resonance. Thus, MDCT provides only a rough estimate of left ventricular volumes and function and should not be used in a quantitative manner at present.

In acute myocardial infarction, areas of reduced perfusion can be seen both early and late after injection of contrast material on CT. Compared with late gadolinium-enhanced cardiac magnetic resonance, a more sensitive marker of infarct size than SPECT, MDCT fares well.

EBCT and MDCT can determine the degree of aortic valve calcification, with good agreement with surgical findings. An aortic valve calcium score of 1100 or higher is a strong marker of severe aortic stenosis.

Cardiac CT is increasingly used to image the left atrium and pulmonary venous anatomy for preprocedural planning for pulmonary vein ablations for atrial fibrillation (Chapter 65). Cardiac venous anatomy may be imaged to aid in the implantation of left ventricular pacemakers in the cardiac venous system for biventricular pacing for heart failure (Chapters 58 and 65).

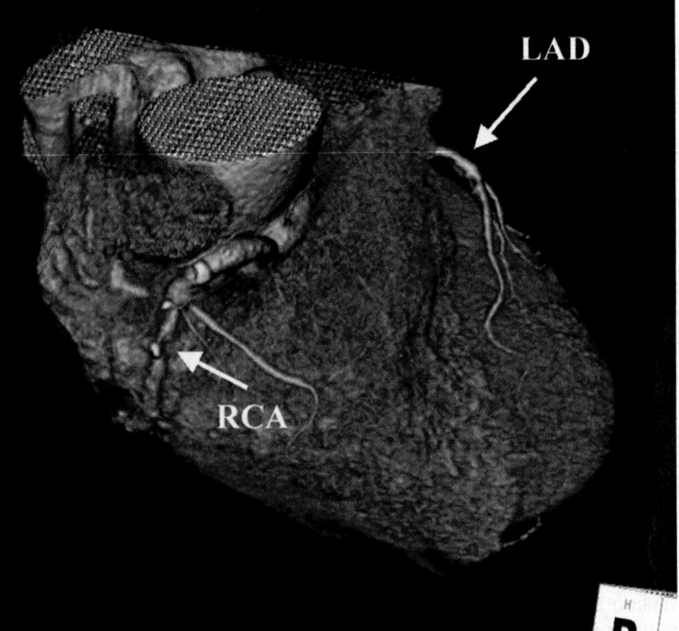

FIGURE 54–3 • Three-dimensional display of a contrast-enhanced CT coronary angiogram demonstrating multiple calcified lesions in the right coronary artery (RCA), with one focal obstructive lesion noted (see arrow). The left anterior descending artery (LAD) is also displayed and is without focal stenoses.

SUGGESTED READINGS

Abidov A, Germano G, Hachamovitch R, et al: Gated SPECT in assessment of regional and global left ventricular function: Major tool of modern nuclear imaging. J Nucl Cardiol 2006;13:261–279. *A comprehensive review.*

Greenland P, Bonow RO, Brundage BH, et al: ACCF/AHA 2007 clinical expert consensus document on coronary artery calcium scoring by computed tomography in global cardiovascular risk assessment and in evaluation of patients with chest pain: A report of the American College of Cardiology Foundation Clinical Expert Consensus Task Force (ACCF/AHA Writing Committee to Update the 2000 Expert Consensus Document on Electron Beam Computed Tomography). Circulation 2007;115:402–426. *A review of the guidelines for coronary artery calcium scoring by CT in CV risk assessment and the evaluation of chest pain.*

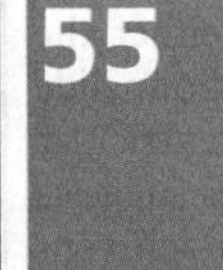

55 CARDIOVASCULAR MAGNETIC RESONANCE IMAGING

Warren J. Manning

UTILITY AND TYPES OF CARDIOVASCULAR MAGNETIC RESONANCE IMAGING

The combined attributes of superior image quality and flexibility for assessment of cardiac anatomy, ventricular function, great vessel and coronary anatomy and blood flow, myocardial viability, and myocardial perfusion, without the use of potentially harmful ionizing radiation or iodinated contrast agents, give cardiovascular magnetic resonance imaging (CMR) tremendous potential clinical utility for evaluation of the cardiovascular system. Current clinical applications of CMR are rapidly expanding (Table 55–1), and specialized CMR expertise is now available at most major institutions. Given the relative cost disadvantage of CMR in comparison with other noninvasive technologies such as ultrasound (echocardiography; Chapter 53), the ultimate clinical role of CMR is likely to depend on strategies that eliminate the need for other cardiovascular imaging tests such as nuclear imaging (Chapter 54), computed tomography (Chapter 54), or diagnostic x-ray coronary angiography (Chapter 56).

The most common CMR approaches are *spin-echo* ("black blood") imaging, which is used for mediastinal and cardiac anatomy; *gradient-echo* ("bright blood") and steady-state free precession techniques, which are used for cine imaging (e.g., ventricular function); and phase velocity

TABLE 55–1 CLINICAL APPLICATIONS FOR CARDIOVASCULAR MAGNETIC RESONANCE IMAGING (CMR)

Diagnosis and monitoring of evaluation of thoracic aorta
- Aneurysm
- Dissection
- Hematoma
- Coarctation
- Penetrating ulcer

Assessment of simple and complex congenital heart disease
- Spatial relationships of aorta, pulmonary arteries, cardiac chambers, venous system
- Identification of anomalous coronary arteries
- Quantification of intracardiac shunt

Quantitative left and right ventricle volumes, ejection fraction, mass
- Regional and global systolic function

Primary or secondary cardiac tumors, especially tumors that involve extracardiac structures

Pericardial disease
- Constriction
- Pericardial effusions, especially loculated effusions

Assessment of specific cardiomyopathies
- Hypertrophic cardiomyopathy, distribution of hypertrophy
- Sarcoidosis
- Hemochromatosis
- Right ventricular dysplasia
- Discrimination of ischemic vs. nonischemic etiology with coronary magnetic resonance angiography and/or delayed enhancement imaging

Coronary artery disease
- Regional myocardial viability
- Regional ischemia (dobutamine or vasodilator stress CMR)
- Multivessel proximal/middle coronary artery disease

Valvular heart disease
- Quantification of regurgitant volumes
- Assessment of severity of valvular stenosis

Pulmonary veins
- Assessment of anatomy before and after pulmonary vein ablation

Adapted from Pennell DJ, Sechtem UP, Higgins CB, et al: Clinical indications for cardiovascular magnetic resonance (CMR): Consensus Panel report. J Cardiovasc Magn Reson 2004;6:727–765.

methods (quantification of blood flow). Regions of local turbulence (e.g., valvular regurgitation or stenosis) are depicted as low-signal-intensity techniques on gradient echocardiography and, less so, on steady-state free precession methods. For most current CMR applications, electrocardiographic (ECG) gating is essential. Exogenous intravenous contrast material (gadolinium-diethylenetriamine pentaacetic acid [Gd-DTPA]) may be helpful in some situations, such as magnetic resonance angiography (MRA) of the aorta or assessment of myocardial viability, but it is not needed for most anatomic assessments of function and flow.

LIMITATIONS OF THE USE OF CMR IN CARDIAC PATIENTS

In addition to general restrictions regarding magnetic resonance (e.g., intracranial clips, transcutaneous electrical nerve stimulation units, intra-auricular implants), special considerations are required when considering CMR in cardiac patients. CMR is considered safe for all bioprosthetic and mechanical heart valves, but signal loss and image distortion occur in the region immediately surrounding the prosthesis and will obscure nearby pathology. Similarly, sternotomy wires and thoracic vascular clips are not a contraindication to CMR, but localized artifacts are common. CMR appears to be safe for patients with intracoronary stents.

In general, patients with cardiac pacemakers and implantable cardioverter-defibrillators should *not* undergo CMR because of concern regarding reprogramming of the device, direct stimulation of the heart during gradient switching, and/or localized heating in the lead system. Similarly, patients with retained permanent pacemaker leads and those with pulmonary artery catheters that include pacing or thermistor wires should not undergo magnetic resonance imaging (MRI). However, preliminary reports have demonstrated the safety of scanning in patients with modern (post-2000) pacemaker systems.

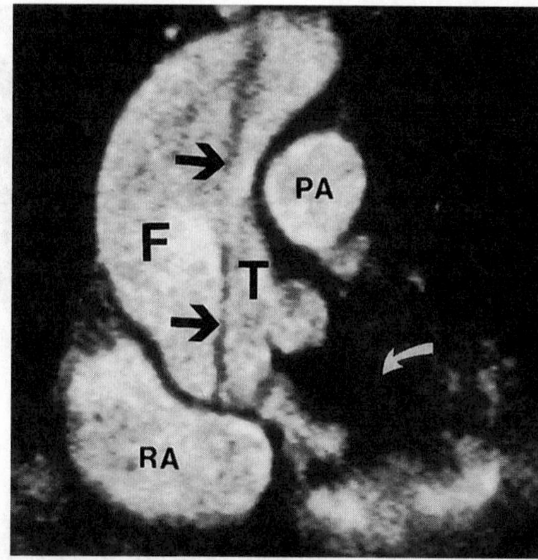

FIGURE 55–1 • Ascending aortic dissection: coronal orientation, gradient-echo sequence. Note that the dissection flap (black arrows) begins immediately superior to the aortic valve leaflet. Flow (white signal) is seen in both the true (T) and the false (F) lumen. Signal void (turbulence) is seen in the left ventricular cavity immediately below the aortic valve and is caused by associated aortic insufficiency (curved white arrow). PA = pulmonary artery; RA = right atrium.

CLINICAL APPLICATIONS OF CMR

Thoracic Aorta, Great Vessels, and Pulmonary Vein

CMR has a major clinical role in the assessment of the thoracic aorta in patients with known or suspected thoracic aortic aneurysm or aortic dissection (Chapter 78) (Fig. 55–1). ECG-gated spin-echo transverse, coronal, and sagittal images are typically acquired along with oblique three-dimensional contrast-enhanced MRA. The "sine qua non" of aortic dissection (Chapter 78) is the identification of an intimal "flap" separating the true and false lumens. Cine gradient-echo or steady-state free precession imaging often helps to define the flap's mobility as well as blood flow in both lumens. Eccentric aortic wall thickening may also be seen, representing an early dissection or intramural hematoma. In experienced hands, CMR, multidetector computed tomography (MDCT), and multiplane transesophageal echocardiography (TEE) all have similarly high sensitivity, specificity, and accuracy for the identification of thoracic aortic dissection. CMR and computed tomography have specific advantages (compared with TEE) for providing information on the full extent of the dissection with regard to involvement of the great vessels, entry and exit points, and the presence of a thrombosed lumen. Both TEE and CMR permit assessment of aortic valve involvement and aortic regurgitation, although valve morphology is better appreciated by TEE and quantification of aortic regurgitation by CMR. Both TEE and CMR can provide information regarding the involvement of the proximal coronary arteries. With current techniques, CMR assessment can be safely completed within 30 minutes. Both ECG rhythm monitoring and noninvasive blood pressure monitoring are strongly recommended during the examination.

CMR is also useful for delineation of aortic coarctation, patent ductus arteriosus, and more complex congenital abnormalities (conduits) involving the great vessels (Chapter 68). In general, patients with congenital lesions are referred for CMR to confirm or to better define an abnormality already identified or suspected on prior imaging by echocardiography or invasive x-ray angiography. Among patients undergoing pulmonary vein ablation for treatment of atrial fibrillation (Chapter 65), serial pulmonary vein CMR angiography is often used to monitor

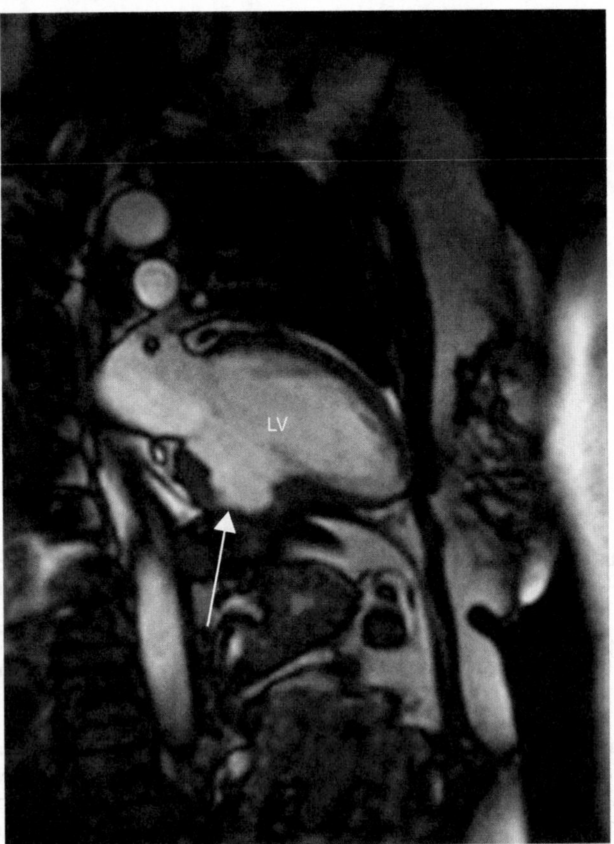

FIGURE 55–2 • Cine cardiovascular magnetic resonance image demonstrating a basal inferior aneurysm (arrow). LV = left ventricle.

complications (e.g., pulmonary vein stenosis), with the lack of ionizing radiation being a particular advantage (as compared with cardiac computed tomography).

Quantitative Assessment of Ventricular Volumes and Mass

Although less often used clinically because of its relative cost disadvantage in comparison with echocardiography, volumetric CMR methods are considered the "gold standard" for the *quantitative* assessment of left and right ventricular volumes and ejection fraction, as well as regional systolic function of both ventricles. When compared with two-dimensional echocardiography, which has suboptimal results in many patients, breath-hold cine-CMR can be readily performed in almost all patients in less than 10 minutes. Modern steady-state free precession cine methods provide superior definition of endocardial borders (Fig. 55–2). Semiautomated methods allow for delineation of the endocardial and epicardial borders with very high accuracy and reproducibility for determination of ventricular volumes, stroke volume, and ejection fraction. The superior accuracy and reproducibility of CMR methods may be especially valuable for monitoring quantitative ventricular volumetric data in patients with valvular regurgitation and for monitoring left ventricular mass and regression of hypertrophy in response to antihypertensive therapy or aortic valve replacement. The accurate evaluation of *right* ventricular volumes and ejection fraction is also relatively unique to CMR.

Cardiomyopathies

The ability of CMR to acquire images of the entire heart in true tomographic planes makes it ideal for the evaluation of patients with hypertrophic cardiomyopathies, especially those with asymmetrical hypertrophy (Chapter 59). Investigative CMR "tagging" methods may also be helpful in the further assessment of patients with hypertrophic cardiomyopathy, but this application remains to be more fully elucidated. Delayed-enhancement cardiovascular magnetic resonance (DE-CMR) can demonstrate interstitial myocardial fibrosis.

CMR is also useful in the assessment of patients with dilated cardiomyopathy. In addition to biventricular volumetric and mass data, CMR may confirm excess iron deposition as the cause of depressed systolic function in a patient with suspected hemochromatosis (Chapter 231). With spin-echo imaging, depressed T2* correlates with impaired systolic function and with the severity of iron deposition. DE-CMR methods using non-nephrotoxic agents may depict specific patterns of hyperenhancement that help discriminate ischemic from nonischemic cardiomyopathies, including sarcoidosis (Chapter 95), hypertrophic cardiomyopathy (Chapter 59), Fabry's disease (Chapter 223), or myocarditis (Chapter 59).

Spin-echo CMR can be used to identify transmural or focal fatty infiltration in the right ventricular free wall of patients with suspected arrhythmogenic right ventricular cardiomyopathy, a condition associated with ventricular arrhythmias and sudden death and in which the right ventricular free wall myocardium is diffusely or focally replaced with fatty or fibrous tissue (Chapters 59 and 64). Associated focal wall thinning, aneurysms, and systolic dysfunction with delayed hyperenhancement are also often present.

Coronary Artery Disease

In addition to the quantification of global ventricular volumes and the assessment of regional systolic function in patients with deformed ventricles after myocardial infarction, CMR can assess regional myocardial viability. With DE-CMR, the severity of transmural hyperenhancement is inversely linearly related to the likelihood of functional recovery after mechanical revascularization with percutaneous techniques or coronary bypass surgery. For patients with regional dysfunction and absent hyperenhancement, functional recovery is expected, whereas functional recovery is unlikely (<10%) if there is greater than 50% hyperenhancement. CMR of bypass grafts can determine their patency.

Cardiac Tumors and Masses

Although the high spatial resolution of CMR allows for depiction of intracavitary tumors or masses (e.g., myxoma; Chapter 59), these tumors are generally well appreciated by echocardiography. CMR adds information primarily in situations in which a mass extends into the myocardium and/or neighboring mediastinal structures (e.g., venae cavae, pulmonary veins, pericardial space) and a three-dimensional representation of the mass can help guide the surgical approach. The pathognomonic features of fat on CMR make it the ideal tool for characterizing benign lipomatous hypertrophy of the interatrial septum, which may sometimes be misdiagnosed as an atrial septal "tumor" on echocardiography.

Pericardium and Pericardial Effusions

The normal pericardium is seen as a thin black line between visceral and parietal pericardial fat on spin-echo CMR. Normal pericardial thickness is less than 3 mm. In patients with constrictive pericarditis (Chapter 77), the thickened (≥6 mm) pericardium is readily appreciated by CMR. Computed tomography is also valuable in this situation and is better than CMR for the assessment of pericardial *calcifications* (Chapters 54 and 77). However, although both CMR and computed tomography accurately quantify focal pericardial thickening, the isolated presence of global or focal pericardial thickening is not diagnostic of constrictive physiology, and constriction in the *absence* of pericardial thickening has also been described.

Congenital Heart Disease

CMR is useful for the assessment of both simple and complex congenital heart disease (Chapter 68). Although atrial septal defects and ventricular septal defects in adults are generally well appreciated by transthoracic echocardiography and/or TEE, phase velocity CMR readily allows for quantification of blood flow through the major blood vessels, thereby facilitating accurate quantification of the ratio of pulmonary to systemic blood flow. CMR is particularly valuable for assessing congenital heart disease outside the cardiac chambers, such as aortic coarctation (Fig. 55–3) or anomalous pulmonary venous drainage, and in patients with complex congenital heart disease who have undergone prior corrective or palliative shunt surgery.

CMR approaches can also readily identify anomalous coronary arteries (Fig. 55–4; Chapter 56). Although uncommon, with a prevalence of only 1 to 2%, an anomalous vessel that courses between the aorta and the

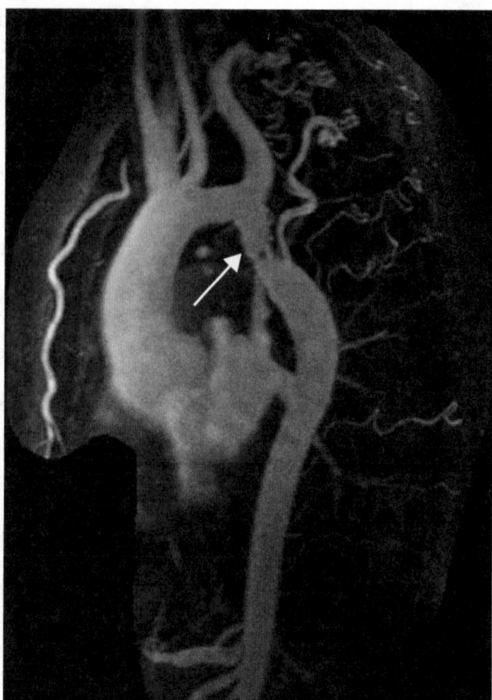

FIGURE 55–3 • Three-dimensional contrast-enhanced magnetic resonance angiogram in a patient with an aortic coarctation (arrow).

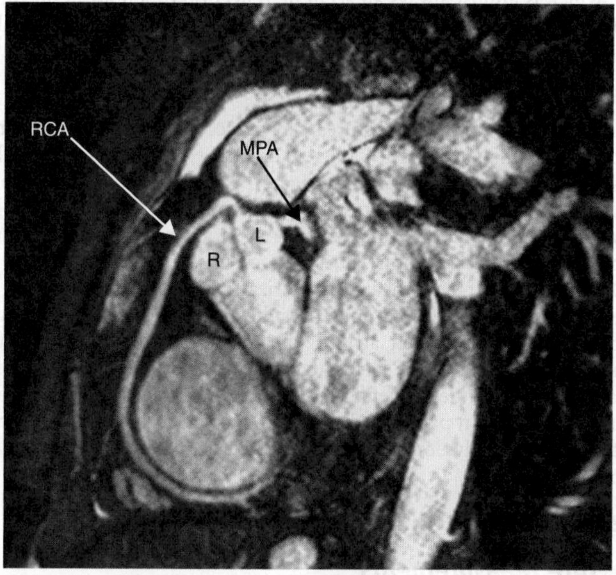

FIGURE 55–4 • Coronary cardiovascular magnetic resonance image in a patient with an anomalous right coronary artery (RCA) originating from the left (L) aortic sinus of Valsalva and traversing between the aorta and the main pulmonary artery (MPA). The left main coronary artery (black arrow) is also seen. R = right aortic sinus. (Courtesy of Franz Aepfelbacher, MD.)

pulmonary artery is associated with an increased risk of sudden death and myocardial infarction in young adults. Even among patients with anomalous coronary arteries identified by invasive x-ray angiography, the course of the anomalous vessel may be misinterpreted because of the projection method, making CMR a preferred technique.

SUGGESTED READINGS

Hendel RC, Patel MR, Kramer CM, et al: CF/ACR/SCCT/SCMR/ASNC/NASCI/SCAI/SIR 2006 appropriateness criteria for cardiac computed tomography and cardiac magnetic resonance imaging: A report of the American College of Cardiology Foundation Quality Strategic Directions Committee Appropriateness Criteria Working Group, American College of Radiology, Society of Cardiovascular Computed Tomography, and others. J Am Coll Cardiol 2006;48: 1475–1497. *Guidelines for the use of cardiac MRI.*

Pennell DJ, Sechtem UP, Higgins CB, et al: Clinical indications for cardiovascular magnetic resonance (CMR): Consensus Panel report. J Cardiovasc Magn Reson 2004;6:727–765. *Consensus guidelines.*

Shellock FG: Reference Manual for Magnetic Resonance Safety, Implants, and Devices—2005. Philadelphia, WB Saunders, 2005. *Excellent continuously updated reference for the safety of magnetic resonance; the related website is* www.mrisafety.com.

Sommer T, Naehle CP, Yang A, et al: Strategy for safe performance of extrathoracic magnetic resonance imaging at 1.5 tesla in the presence of cardiac pacemakers in non–pacemaker-dependent patients: A prospective study with 115 examinations. Circulation 2006;114:1285–1292. *Extrathoracic MRI of non–pacemaker-dependent patients can potentially be performed safely under controlled conditions.*

56 CATHETERIZATION AND ANGIOGRAPHY

David P. Faxon

Cardiac catheterization and angiography provide for detailed assessment of the anatomy and physiology of the heart and vasculature and represent the "gold standard" for assessment of cardiac disease. The technique first was applied to humans by Forssmann in 1929, but it was expanded into a diagnostic tool by Cournard and Richards; in 1956, all three physicians shared the Nobel Prize for their discovery. Selective coronary angiography was introduced by Sones in 1963 and modified further by Judkins. Cardiac catheterization is now the second most common operative procedure in the United States, with almost 2 million procedures performed annually.

CARDIAC CATHETERIZATION

Indications

Cardiac catheterization is performed most commonly to determine the nature and extent of a suspected cardiac problem in a symptomatic patient in whom surgical, electrophysiologic, or interventional therapy is anticipated (Table 56–1). It also is used to exclude the presence of significant disease when findings from other modalities, such as stress testing or echocardiography, are equivocal or when the patient continues to be severely symptomatic and a definitive diagnosis is important for management.

Because coronary angiography is the most accurate method to define the severity and extent of coronary disease, it is essential in the assessment of patients being considered for revascularization. If significant coronary disease is unlikely and noninvasive testing and/or imaging can define accurately the cardiac abnormality, cardiac catheterization is not necessary in young adults or children with simple congenital anomalies, such as atrial septal defect, or in young adults with valvular heart disease, such as aortic stenosis or mitral stenosis.

Contraindications and Risks

The risks of diagnostic cardiac catheterization and coronary angiography are low, with a 0.05% risk of myocardial infarction, a 0.07% risk of stroke, and a reported mortality rate of 0.1%. By comparison, interventional procedures carry a mortality rate of 1 to 1.5% and risk for myocardial infarction of 0.6%. However, these risks are increased substantially in certain subsets of patients, such as those undergoing an emergency procedure, those with an acute myocardial infarction, and those who are hemodynamically unstable. In patients who require catheterization as a prelude to a potentially life-saving intervention, there are no absolute contraindications, but relative contraindications include acute renal failure, pulmonary edema, bacteremia, acute stroke, active gastrointestinal bleeding, and documented anaphylactic reaction to contrast dye. The most common complication of cardiac catheterization, occurring in 1.5 to 2% of patients, is bleeding at the local vascular entry site.

Of all the potential complications, allergic reactions and renal failure induced by contrast media are particularly important, because they are common even in relatively healthy patients, and because precautions can reduce these risks. The frequency of allergic reactions is 5%, and life-threatening anaphylactic reactions occur in 0.1% of patients undergoing angiographies. Pretreatment of patients who have had prior allergic reactions with corticosteroids, antihistamines, and histamine 2 (H_2) antagonists can reduce substantially the risk of a subsequent reaction. Contrast medium–induced renal failure occurs in 3 to 7% of all patients but is

TABLE 56–1 INDICATIONS FOR CARDIAC CATHETERIZATION AND ANGIOGRAPHY

CORONARY ARTERY DISEASE
ASYMPTOMATIC OR SYMPTOMATIC
High risk for adverse outcome based on noninvasive testing
After resuscitation from cardiac arrest or sustained ventricular tachycardia
SYMPTOMATIC
Severe angina on medical therapy
Unstable angina (high or intermediate risk)
Acute myocardial infarction
Primary reperfusion with angioplasty
Recurrent ischemic episodes during hospitalization
Shock or hemodynamic instability
Mechanical complications such as mitral regurgitation or ventricular septal defect
Chest pain of uncertain origin and equivocal results on noninvasive testing
High-risk patients undergoing noncardiac surgery
VALVULAR HEART DISEASE
AORTIC STENOSIS
Symptomatic patients (angina, heart failure, syncope) with suspected severe aortic stenosis
Hypertrophic cardiomyopathy with angina
AORTIC REGURGITATION
Symptomatic patients (angina, heart failure, syncope) with suspected severe aortic regurgitation
Asymptomatic patients with progressive cardiac enlargement or reduction of ejection fraction
MITRAL STENOSIS
Symptomatic patients (dyspnea, heart failure, emboli) with suspected severe mitral stenosis
MITRAL REGURGITATION
Symptomatic patients (dyspnea, heart failure, emboli) with suspected severe mitral regurgitation
OTHER
CONGENITAL HEART DISEASE
Before cardiac surgery or percutaneous correction
PERICARDIAL DISEASE
Symptomatic patients with suspected constrictive pericarditis or tamponade
VASCULAR DISEASE
Aortic dissection or aneurysm with suspected concomitant coronary disease
CONGESTIVE HEART FAILURE
New onset
Suspected to be secondary to coronary artery disease
CARDIAC TRANSPLANTATION
Presurgical and postsurgical evaluation

Adapted from American College of Cardiology/American Heart Association Ad Hoc Task Force on Practice Guidelines: ACC/AHA guidelines for coronary angiography. Circulation 1999;99:2345–2357.

most common in patients with diabetes and/or preexisting renal failure, in whom the incidence is 12 to 30%. Preprocedural and postprocedural hydration for 12 hours with 5% normal saline at 50 mL/hour reduces the risk of subsequent renal failure. Pretreatment and post-treatment for 2 days with acetylcysteine appears to reduce the incidence of contrast-induced nephropathy in patients with moderate renal failure. In addition, pretreatment with sodium bicarbonate, use of low-osmolar contrast medium, and limiting contrast to less than 100 mL also may reduce the risk. Diabetic patients taking metformin should have the drug withdrawn 48 hours before the procedure to reduce the risk of contrast-induced lactic acidosis.

Technique

Patients should be fasting and sedated, but awake, for the procedure. Antibiotics are not necessary. Oral anticoagulation should be stopped before the procedure, but emergency cardiac catheterization can be performed despite full anticoagulation or even after the recent administration of thrombolytic agents.

Vascular Access

Most procedures are performed percutaneously through the femoral artery and vein. A brachial or radial (rarely, axillary) approach is used if peripheral vascular disease precludes access from the lower extremity. After the femoral approach, 4 to 6 hours of local compression and bed rest is desirable before the patient ambulates and is discharged. If percutaneous closure devices are used, earlier ambulation (2 to 4 hours) is possible.

Right-Sided Heart Catheterization

The most commonly used catheter is a balloon flotation catheter that is introduced into the femoral, brachial, subclavian, or internal jugular vein and then passed, with or without fluoroscopic guidance, into the right atrium, right ventricle, and pulmonary artery. If necessary, measurements of oxygen saturation can be obtained as the catheter is passed into the pulmonary artery. In the pulmonary artery, inflation of the balloon at the tip of the catheter occludes the smaller pulmonary arteries and allows for measurement of the pulmonary capillary wedge pressure, which is almost always an accurate reflection of left atrial pressure. With a thermistor-tipped balloon, thermal dilution cardiac output also can be measured.

Left-Sided Heart Catheterization

The left-sided cardiac structures can be accessed from the femoral, brachial, or radial artery. The catheters are passed retrograde under fluoroscopic guidance into the ascending aorta. Because embolization of a clot from a catheter in the arterial circulation could lead to a stroke, heparin is used if the procedure is prolonged. Hemodynamic measurements and oxygen saturation values also are usually obtained.

Occasionally, left-sided heart catheterization can be accomplished by a needle-tipped catheter that punctures the atrial septum from the right atrial side to enter the left atrium; the needle is withdrawn, and the catheter is advanced to the left ventricle. This technique is reserved for situations in which the left ventricle cannot be accessed by the retrograde approach, such as in patients who have aortic valve prostheses, or when aortic or mitral valvuloplasty or invasive electrophysiology studies are being done.

Hemodynamic Assessment

Pressure Measurements

The measurement of intracardiac pressure is an essential component of cardiac catheterization and is performed through fluid-filled catheters that are attached to an external pressure transducer (Table 56–2). The shape and magnitude of the waveforms provide important diagnostic information. An elevated mean right atrial pressure associated with a rapid descent and an early rise (square root sign), with equalization of right atrial, right ventricular diastolic, left atrial, and left ventricular diastolic pressures is characteristic of *constrictive pericarditis. Cardiac tamponade* (Chapter 77) results in equalization of diastolic chamber pressures but without a prominent descent. A large v wave (two times greater than the mean pressure) in the right atrium or left atrium suggests severe *tricuspid* or *mitral regurgitation.* Simultaneous recording of pressures in the proximal and distal cardiac chambers can allow for assessment of valvular stenosis. A pressure gradient in diastole between the pulmonary capillary wedge pressure or left atrial pressure and the left ventricle is found in patients with *mitral stenosis.* A gradient between the aorta and left ventricular systolic pressure is present when *aortic stenosis* (Chapter 75) occurs (Fig. 56–1). Simultaneous measurement of blood flow is important in the assessment of valvular disease. In the presence of regurgitation, an increasing gradient is evident because of an increase in blood flow across the valve. When a premature ventricular contraction

TABLE 56–2 NORMAL HEMODYNAMIC MEASUREMENTS

Parameter	Range
PRESSURES (mm Hg)	
RIGHT HEART	
Right atrium	
Mean	0–5
a wave	1–7
v wave	1–7
Right ventricle	
Peak systole	17–32
End-diastole	1–7
Pulmonary artery	
Peak systole	17–32
Diastole	4–13
Mean	9–19
Pulmonary capillary wedge (mean)	4–12
LEFT HEART	
Left atrium	
Mean	4–12
a wave	4–15
v wave	4–15
Left ventricle	
Peak systole	90–140
End-diastole	5–12
Aorta	
Peak systole	90–140
Diastole	60–90
Mean	70–105
CARDIAC OUTPUT AND RESISTANCES	
Cardiac index (L/min/m^2)	2.8–4.2
Arteriovenous oxygen difference (vol%)	3.5–4.8
Systemic vascular resistance (dyne-sec-cm^{-5})	900–1400
Pulmonary vascular resistance (dyne-sec-cm^{-5})	40–120
Oxygen consumption (mL/min)	115–140

induces a large pressure gradient between the aorta and left ventricle and a reduction in pulse pressure in the aorta (Brockenbrough's effect), *hypertrophic obstructive cardiomyopathy* (Chapter 73) is suggested. *Severe aortic regurgitation* (Chapter 75) causes an elevation in aortic systolic pressure, a fall in aortic diastolic pressure, and equalization of the end-diastolic pressures in the ventricle and aorta.

Cardiac Output

Cardiac output can be measured by the direct Fick method, by indicator dilution methods, or by angiographic techniques. The Fick method is the most accurate method in states with low cardiac output, and the indicator dilution method is most accurate in high-output conditions. When an accurate assessment of cardiac output is essential (e.g., in assessing the degree of valvular stenosis), the Fick and indicator dilution techniques are frequently used. The Fick principle states that the amount of a substance taken up or released by an organ is the product of its blood flow and the arterial-venous difference in concentration of the substance. Because oxygen can be measured reliably, the Fick method determines oxygen consumption by measuring inhaled and exhaled oxygen content and the arterial and venous blood oxygen content. Most commonly, oxygen consumption is estimated based on age and body surface area. The formula for calculating Fick cardiac output (in L/minute) is

$$\text{Cardiac output} = (\text{oxygen consumption})/(\text{arterial-venous oxygen difference})$$

where oxygen consumption is measured in mL O_2/minute and the arterial-venous oxygen difference (in vol% ×10) is equal to 1.39 (oxygen-carrying capacity of blood) × hemoglobin (g/dL) × (arterial-oxygen saturation difference).

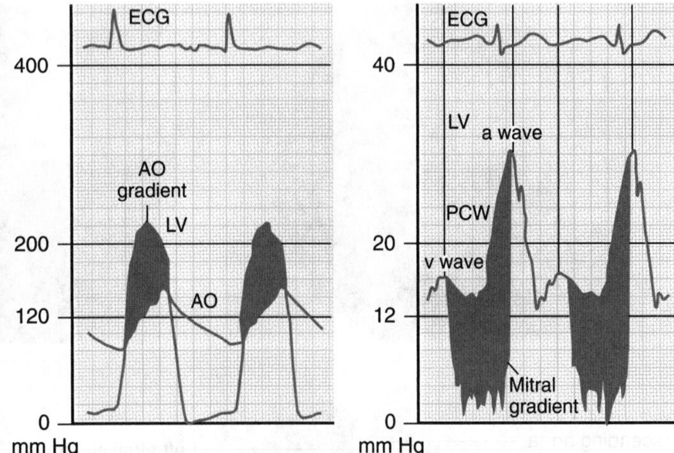

FIGURE 56–1 • Examples of the hemodynamic findings in aortic and mitral stenosis. Left panel, Simultaneous recording of aortic (AO) and left ventricular (LV) pressure shows a 50-mm Hg systolic pressure gradient. Right panel, There is a 15-mm Hg diastolic gradient between the pulmonary capillary wedge pressure (PCW) and the left ventricular pressure (LV). The a wave in the PCW tracing is larger than the v wave, indicating increased resistance to left ventricular filling in this patient. ECG = electrocardiogram.

The indicator dilution method is based on the Stewart-Hamilton equation, in which cardiac output is determined by the following formula:

$$\text{Cardiac output} = (I \times 60)/(mc \times t)$$

where *I* is amount of indicator injected, *60* is the number of seconds in 1 minute, *mc* is mean indicator concentration (mg/L), and *t* is total indicator circulatory time in seconds. The indicator dilution method involves injection of a substance that can be measured in blood. The indicator is injected at one site and sampled at another. Because the completeness of mixing of the indicator is crucial, injection and sampling optimally are done in cardiac chambers that are not adjacent (e.g., injection into the right atrium and sampling in the pulmonary artery). Thermodilution techniques are most common: Temperature is the indicator, and the mean change in temperature is the indicator concentration that is sampled distally. Because cardiac output varies with body size, it is customary to calculate the cardiac index (L/min/m^2) by dividing cardiac output by body surface area.

Valve Areas and Resistances

The resistance to blood flow can be calculated in a manner similar to Ohm's law of electrical resistance, as the ratio of the mean pressure gradient to the flow:

$$\text{Resistance} = (\text{mean pressure gradient})/(\text{mean flow})$$

The resistance through the systemic circulation is calculated as the mean aortic pressure minus the mean right atrial pressure, divided by cardiac output, multiplied by 80 to convert to dynes-seconds-cm^{-5}. Likewise, pulmonary vascular resistance is calculated as mean pulmonary artery pressure minus mean pulmonary capillary wedge pressure multiplied by 80 divided by cardiac output. The valve area in stenotic valves is the inverse of resistance. The most commonly used formula for calculation of valve stenosis is the Gorlin formula, where *K* is a constant (44.3 for aortic valve and 37.7 for mitral valve):

$$\text{Valve area} = (\text{flow across the valve})/(K \times \text{valvular gradient})$$

Severe aortic stenosis is considered to be present when the mean valvular gradient is greater than 50 mm Hg and the aortic valve area is less than or equal to 0.8 cm^2. For the mitral valve, a valve area of less than 1.0 cm^2 is considered severe.

Shunts

Patients with known or suspected congenital heart disease (Chapter 68) should have hemodynamic assessment and estimation of the location and degree of cardiac shunting if present. Estimation of the shunt can be made by changes in oxygen saturation and by angiography. Measurement

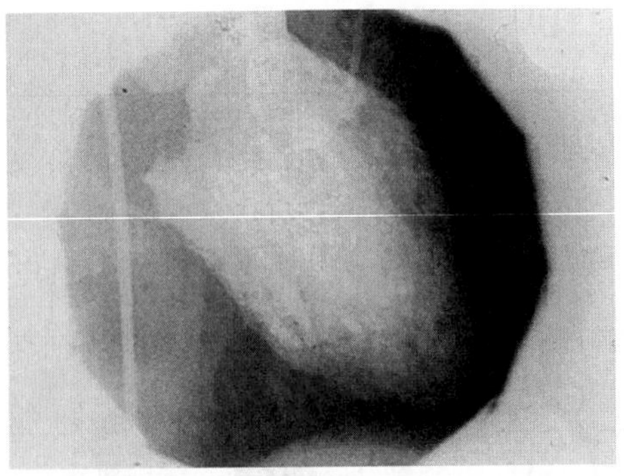
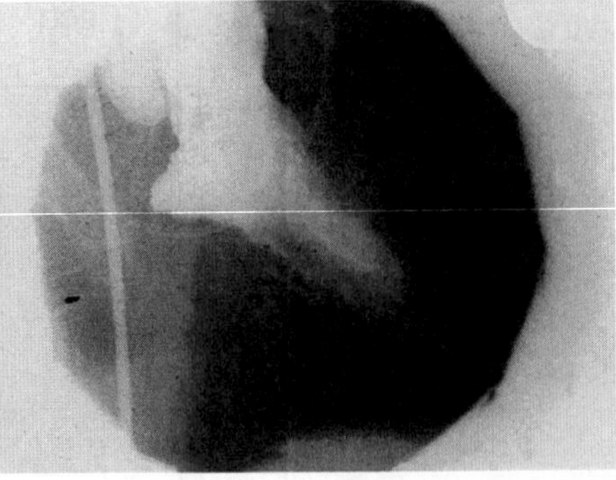

FIGURE 56–2 • An example of left ventriculography. The ventricular contour is seen in diastole (left panel) and in systole (right panel).

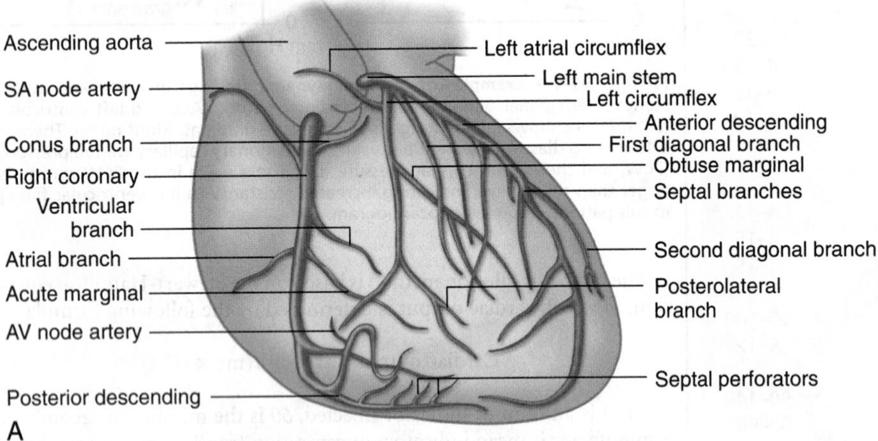

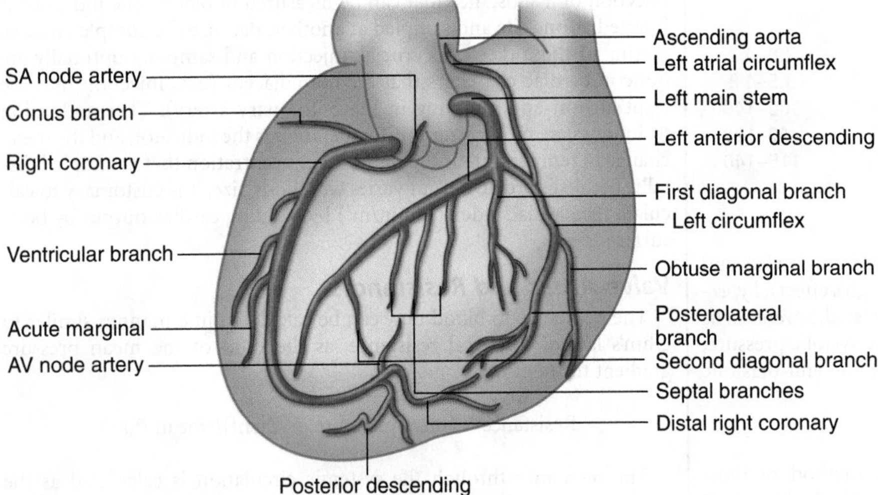

FIGURE 56–3 • The coronary vessels in the right anterior oblique (A) and left anterior oblique (B) view are shown. The major arteries are the left main, left anterior descending, circumflex, and right coronary arteries. SA, sinoatrial. (From Yang SS, Bentivoglio LG, Maranhao V, Goldberg H [eds]: From Cardiac Catheterization Data to Hemodynamic Parameters. Philadelphia, Oxford University Press, 1988. Used by permission of Oxford University Press, Inc.)

of oxygen saturation in each of the cardiac chambers and vessels can detect a "step up" in oxygen content in the right side of the heart when a left-to-right shunt is present or a "step down" in oxygen content in the left side of the heart when a right-to-left shunt is present. Systemic blood flow can be calculated from the Fick principle by obtaining oxygen saturations from the aorta and both venae cavae. Pulmonary blood flow is calculated using oxygen saturation measurements from the pulmonary artery and left atrium. The shunt ratio (ratio of pulmonary blood flow to systemic blood flow) measures the severity of a shunt; for an atrial or ventricular septal defect, a shunt ratio of greater than 1.5 : 1 is considered significant.

CARDIAC ANGIOGRAPHY

Angiography almost always is performed during cardiac catheterization by injection of an iodine-containing radiopaque contrast agent. These agents are highly viscous and can cause cardiac arrhythmias and adverse hemodynamic changes secondary to ionic changes, volume expansion, and negative inotropic effects. Use of more expensive, low-osmolar, nonionic agents reduces these adverse effects and may reduce the incidence of contrast-induced nephropathy.

Aortography

Aortography allows for the assessment of aortic size and structure, as well as the extent of aortic regurgitation. It also determines the location of coronary bypass grafts, if present.

Left Ventriculography

Left ventriculography frequently is performed with coronary angiography, because it allows for assessment of left ventricular size and function and the presence and extent of mitral regurgitation (Fig. 56–2). Left ventricular volume in end-diastole and end-systole can be calculated by the area-length method (normal = 70 ± 20 mL and 25 ± 10 mL, respectively). The difference between end-diastole and end-systole is the stroke volume. Cardiac output is calculated by multiplying the stroke volume by the heart rate. The ratio of angiographic stroke volume to end-

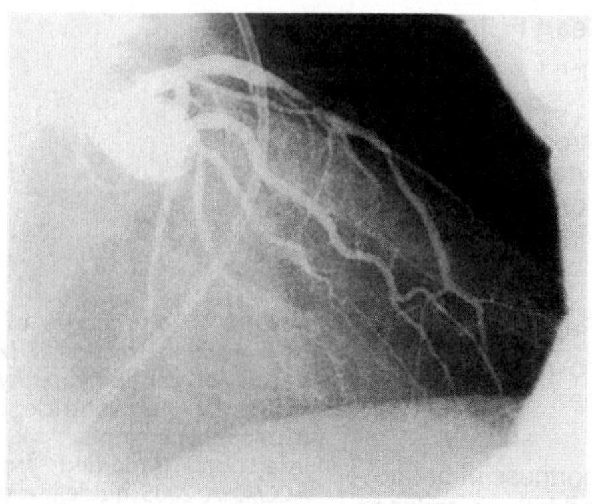

FIGURE 56–4 • An example of a significant stenosis in the left anterior descending coronary artery.

diastolic volume is the ejection fraction, which is an estimate of contractile function. Normal ejection fraction ranges from 0.5 to 0.7. Wall motion abnormalities, which are usually indicative of coronary artery disease, also can be assessed during angiography and classified as hypokinetic (reduced motion), akinetic (no motion), or dyskinetic (paradoxical motion). Estimation of mitral regurgitation by angiography uses a semiquantitative technique by which 1+ is minimal regurgitation into the left atrium in systole, 2+ is mild-to-moderate regurgitation of contrast material to outline the left atrium, 3+ is moderate-to-severe regurgitation from which the left atrium becomes as dense as the left ventricle, and 4+ is severe regurgitation from which the left atrium becomes more dense than the left ventricle. Usually 3+ to 4+ mitral regurgitation is considered to be hemodynamically significant and a relative indication for mitral valve surgery.

Coronary Angiography

Coronary angiography defines the coronary anatomy, the degree of obstruction of the coronary arteries, and the states of any coronary artery bypass grafts by means of injection of a contrast agent selectively into the ostium of the right or left coronary artery or bypass conduit (Figs. 56–3 and 56–4). The degree of obstruction is expressed as the percent stenosis, which is the ratio of the most severely narrowed segment in any view compared with the "normal" proximal and/or distal segment. A narrowing of greater than 50% of the diameter is considered significant. Visual assessments can overestimate the severity of the stenosis, but quantitative techniques reduce the variability of the measurement. The normal coronary vasculature can be highly variable but generally includes three major vessels—the left anterior descending, left circumflex, and right coronary arteries, with the first two emanating from the left main artery. A *right dominant* circulation occurs when the posterior wall of the left ventricle is served by the right coronary artery, and a *left dominant* circulation occurs when it is served by the left circumflex artery; the circulation is *codominant* when it is served by both vessels.

ADJUNCTIVE METHODS TO ASSESS CORONARY STENOSIS

Coronary angiography is limited to assessment of changes in the lumen diameter. Because atherosclerosis is a diffuse process and in the early stages results in compensatory dilation of the vessel, angiography can underestimate the severity of the stenosis; furthermore, angiography does not provide direct assessment of the physiologic significance of a stenosis. Intravascular ultrasound uses a small, flexible catheter with a 20- to 30-mHz transducer at its tip that can be passed over an angioplasty guidewire into the coronary artery. Accurate assessment of the degree of atherosclerosis and the percent stenosis can be obtained by this technique. Intracoronary Doppler flow measurements use a Doppler probe mounted on a small angioplasty-type guidewire. Measurement of the change in flow velocity before and after coronary vasodilation with agents such as adenosine can provide an estimate of coronary flow reserve and help assess the severity of the stenosis. A significant reduction in coronary flow reserve is present when the ratio of flow at rest to flow after vasodilation is less than 2 : 1. Measurement of the pressure gradient across a stenosis using a small wire transducer also can assess functional severity. Fractional flow reserve is the ratio of the distal pressure to the proximal pressure after maximum vasodilation. A fractional flow reserve of less than 0.75 indicates a significant stenosis. Measurement of blood flow velocity and coronary artery diameter before and after administration of acetylcholine can assess the possibility that coronary vasospasm or abnormalities in coronary endothelial function are present. Intravascular ultrasound, fractional flow reserve, and Doppler flow studies are used most commonly in conjunction with interventional procedures.

FUTURE DIRECTIONS

The cardiac catheterization laboratory of the future is likely to incorporate new methods of cardiac imaging, real-time magnetic resonance angiography, and the imaging of atherosclerotic plaques with magnetic resonance techniques.

SUGGESTED READING

Berry C, L'Allier PL, Gregoire J, et al: Comparison of intravascular ultrasound and quantitative coronary angiography for the assessment of coronary artery disease progression. Circulation 2007;115:1851–1857. *Disease progression on QCA is associated with significant increases in plaque volume on IVUS compared with no angiographic progression.*

Tobis J, Azarbal B, Slavin L: Assessment of intermediate severity coronary lesions in the catheterization laboratory. J Am Coll Cardiol 2007;49:839–848. *A review of the importance of IVUS and fractional flow reserve index in the management of patients with serial stenosis, bifurcation lesions, left main disease, saphenous vein graft disease, and acute coronary syndrome.*

57 HEART FAILURE: PATHOPHYSIOLOGY AND DIAGNOSIS

Barry M. Massie

HEART FAILURE

Definition

Heart failure is a heterogeneous syndrome in which abnormalities of cardiac function are responsible for the inability of the heart to pump blood at an output sufficient to meet the requirements of metabolizing tissues or the ability to do so only at abnormally elevated diastolic pressures or volumes. The heart failure syndrome is characterized by signs and symptoms of intravascular and interstitial volume overload (shortness of breath, rales, elevated jugular venous pressure, and edema) and/or manifestations of inadequate tissue perfusion (impaired exercise tolerance, fatigue, signs of hypoperfusion, renal dysfunction). Heart failure may occur as a result of (1) impaired myocardial contractility (systolic dysfunction, commonly characterized as reduced left ventricular [LV] ejection fraction [EF]); (2) increased ventricular stiffness or impaired myocardial relaxation (diastolic dysfunction, which is commonly associated with a relatively normal LVEF); (3) a variety of other cardiac abnormalities, including obstructive or regurgitant valvular disease, intracardiac shunting, or disorders of heart rate or rhythm; or (4) states in which the heart is unable to compensate for increased peripheral blood flow or metabolic requirements. In adults, LV involvement is almost always present even if the manifestations are primarily those of right ventricular (RV) dysfunction (fluid retention without dyspnea or rales). Heart failure may result from an acute insult to cardiac function, such as a large myocardial infarction (MI), or, more commonly, from a chronic process. The focus in this chapter is on the syndrome of *chronic* heart failure, including its presentation in an acutely decompensated state. The most common causes of de novo acute heart failure, such as MI (Chapter 72), valvular disease (Chapter 75), myocarditis (Chapter 59), and cardiogenic shock (Chapter 108), are discussed elsewhere.

Epidemiology

Both the incidence and the prevalence of heart failure are growing, as is the resulting burden of deaths and hospitalizations. Although these trends primarily reflect the strong association between heart failure and advancing age, they also are influenced by the rising prevalence of precursors such as hypertension, diabetes, dyslipidemia, and obesity in

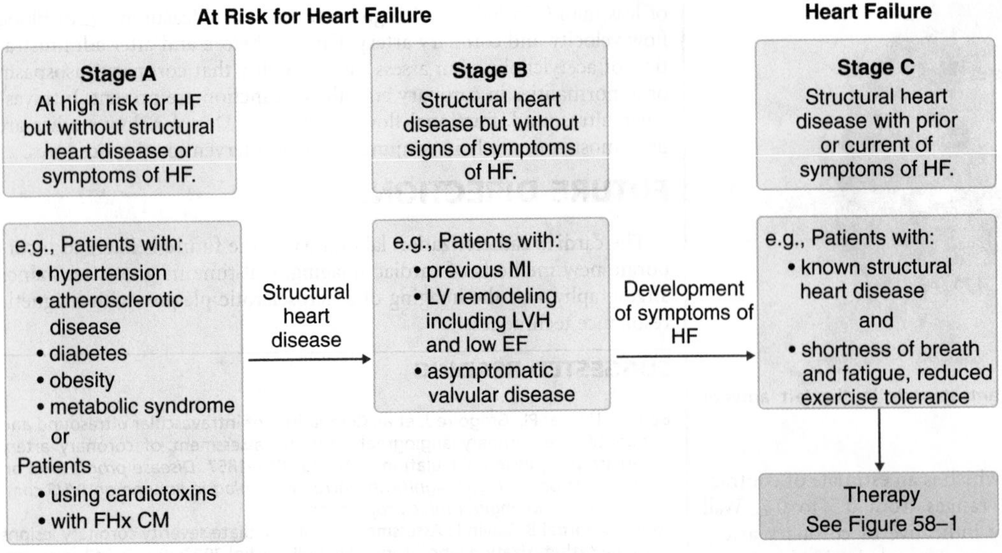

FIGURE 57–1 • Stages of heart failure. EF = ejection fraction; FHx CM = family history of cardiomyopathy; HF = heart failure; LV = left ventricle; LVH = left ventricular hypertrophy; MI = myocardial infarction. (Modified from Hunt SA: ACC/AHA 2005 guideline update for the diagnosis and management of chronic heart failure in the adult: A report of the American College of Cardiology/American Heart Association Task Force on Practice Guidelines [Writing Committee to Update the 2001 Guidelines for the Evaluation and Management of Heart Failure]. J Am Coll Cardiol 2005;46:e1–e82.)

industrialized societies and the improved long-term survival of patients with ischemic and other forms of heart disease. The annual incidence of new cases of heart failure rises from less than 1 per 1000 patient-years among those younger than 45 years of age, to 10 per 1000 patient-years for those older than 65 years, to 30 per 1000 patient-years (3%) for those older than 85 years. Prevalence figures follow a similar exponential pattern, increasing from 0.1% before 50 to 55 years of age to almost 10% after age 80 years. In the United States, there are an estimated 5.1 million patients with heart failure, of whom approximately 75% are 65 years of age or older. Although the relative incidence and prevalence of heart failure are lower in women than men, women constitute at least half of the cases because of their longer life expectancy.

Any condition that causes myocardial necrosis or produces chronic pressure or volume overload can induce myocardial dysfunction and heart failure. In developed countries, the causes of heart failure have changed greatly over several decades. Valvular heart disease, with the exception of calcific aortic stenosis, has declined markedly, whereas coronary heart disease has become the predominant cause in men and women, being responsible for 60 to 75% of cases. Hypertension, although less frequently the primary cause of heart failure than in the past, continues to be a major factor in 75%, including most of the patients with coronary disease.

Prevention of Heart Failure

Treatment of hypertension, with a focus on the systolic pressure, reduces the incidence of heart failure by 50%. This intervention remains effective even in patients older than 75 years of age (Chapter 66). Any intervention that reduces the risk of a first or recurrent MI (e.g., treatment of hypertension or dyslipidemia, antiplatelet therapy in high-risk individuals, and aggressive management of diabetes) will also reduce the incidence of heart failure (Chapter 49). In post-MI patients (Chapter 72), these measures plus β-blockers and angiotensin-converting enzyme (ACE) inhibitors, with coronary revascularization in selected individuals, can still prevent the development of heart failure. In patients with reduced LVEF, ACE inhibitors and β-blockers prevent or delay progressive LV dysfunction and dilation and the onset or worsening of heart failure. Well-timed intervention for progressive valvular disease affords another opportunity to prevent eventual heart failure (Chapter 75).

Stages of Heart Failure

The recognition that most patients who develop heart failure have underlying risk factors or predisposing clinical conditions that precede its development, usually by many years, has led to a greater emphasis on early detection and treatment of predisposing factors, on the staging of heart failure (Fig. 57–1), and on early intervention. *Stage A* heart failure includes patients who are at risk for development of heart failure but do not as yet have either symptoms or apparent structural abnormalities of the heart; this includes patients with hypertension, atherosclerotic disease, diabetes, obesity, or the metabolic syndrome and individuals with ongoing excessive alcohol intake, use of cardiotoxic drugs, a familial history of cardiomyopathy, or a known genetic abnormality associated with cardiomyopathy (Chapter 59). *Stage B* encompasses asymptomatic patients who have demonstrable structural abnormalities that predispose to heart failure, such as prior MI, LV hypertrophy by electrocardiography or echocardiography, reduced LVEF or LV dilatation, or asymptomatic but hemodynamically significant valvular heart disease. Stage C heart failure includes patients who have exhibited symptoms or signs of heart failure. These patients may have improved to the point of being relatively asymptomatic, but they still are classified as Stage C and usually continue to receive treatment with agents that are known to improve their natural history, such as β-blockers and inhibitors of the renin-angiotensin-aldosterone system.

Pathobiology

Differing Mechanisms of Heart Failure

Heart failure is a syndrome that may result from many cardiac and systemic disorders (Table 57–1). Some of these disorders, at least initially, do not involve the heart, and the term "heart failure" may be confusing. Even in high-output states, however, the patient may present with the classic findings of exertional dyspnea and edema *(high-output heart failure)* that resolve if the underlying disorder is eliminated. If they persist, these conditions may impair myocardial performance secondarily as a result of chronic volume overload or direct deleterious effects on the myocardium. Other conditions, including mechanical abnormalities, disorders of rate and rhythm, and pulmonary abnormalities, do not primarily affect myocardial function but are frequent causes of heart failure.

Abnormalities of Cardiac Function

Systolic Function

In the normal ventricle, stroke volume increases over a wide range of end-diastolic volumes (the Frank-Starling effect). If contractility (or the inotropic state of the myocardium) is enhanced, such as during exercise or catecholamine stimulation, this increase is correspondingly greater (Table 57–2). In the failing heart with depressed contractility, there is relatively little increment in systolic function with further increases in LV volume, and the ventricular function curve is shifted downward and flattened (Chapter 50). In the clinical setting, systolic dysfunction is characterized by depressed stroke volume despite elevated ventricular filling pressures. The resulting symptoms are those of pulmonary or systemic congestion, activity intolerance, and organ dysfunction.

Assessment of systolic function clinically is more problematic. The most useful measure is the LVEF (stroke volume/end-diastolic volume, usually expressed as a percentage), which reflects a single point on the ventricular function curve. The EF is "load dependent," however, meaning that alterations in afterload (see later discussion) can affect it independently of contractility. In addition, mitral regurgitation, which facilitates ejection into the low-pressure left atrium, may lead to an overestimation of systolic function by the EF. Nonetheless, with the excep-

TABLE 57–1 PATHOGENESIS OF HEART FAILURE

IMPAIRED SYSTOLIC (CONTRACTILE) FUNCTION
Ischemic damage or dysfunction
Myocardial infarction
Persistent or intermittent myocardial ischemia
Hypoperfusion (shock)
Chronic pressure overloading
Hypertension
Obstructive valvular disease
Chronic volume overload
Regurgitant valvular disease
Intracardiac left-to-right shunting
Extracardiac shunting
Nonischemic dilated cardiomyopathy
Familial/genetic disorders
Toxic/drug-induced damage
Immunologically mediated necrosis
Infectious agents
Metabolic disorders
Infiltrative processes
Idiopathic conditions
IMPAIRED DIASTOLIC FUNCTION (RESTRICTED FILLING, INCREASED STIFFNESS)
Pathologic myocardial hypertrophy
Primary (hypertrophic cardiomyopathies)
Secondary (hypertension)
Aging
Ischemic fibrosis
Restrictive cardiomyopathy
Infiltrative disorders (amyloidosis, sarcoidosis)
Storage diseases (hemochromatosis, genetic abnormalities)
Endomyocardial disorders
MECHANICAL ABNORMALITIES
Intracardiac
Obstructive valvular disease
Regurgitant valvular disease
Intracardiac shunts
Other congenital abnormalities
Extracardiac
Obstructive (coarctation, supravalvular aortic stenosis)
Left-to-right shunting (patent ductus)
DISORDERS OF RATE AND RHYTHM
Bradyarrhythmias (sinus node dysfunction, conduction abnormalities)
Tachyarrhythmias (ineffective rhythms, chronic tachycardia)
PULMONARY HEART DISEASE
Cor pulmonale
Pulmonary vascular disorders
HIGH-OUTPUT STATES
Metabolic disorders
Thyrotoxicosis
Nutritional disorders (beriberi)
Excessive blood flow requirements
Chronic anemia
Systemic arteriovenous shunting

tions indicated earlier, when the EF is normal (>50 to 55% in most laboratories), systolic function is usually adequate. LVEFs that are mildly (40 to 50%), moderately (30 to 40%), or severely (<30%) depressed are associated with reduced survival and, in the severe range, with reduced functional reserve, if not overt symptoms of heart failure. Cardiac output, in

TABLE 57–2 MAJOR DETERMINANTS OF CARDIAC PERFORMANCE

Ventricular systolic function (contractility)
Ventricular diastolic function
Relaxation
Stiffness
Ventricular preload
Ventricular afterload
Cardiac rate and conduction
Myocardial blood flow

contrast, is a poor measure of systolic function because it can be affected markedly by heart rate, systemic vascular resistance, and the degree of LV dilation.

Diastolic Function

Diastole is the portion of the cardiac cycle between aortic valve closure and mitral valve closure. Diastole consists of three phases: (1) active relaxation, (2) the conduit phase, and (3) atrial contraction. If relaxation is delayed or if the myocardium is abnormally stiff (e.g., an excessively steep relationship between change in pressure and change in volume [$\Delta P/\Delta V$]), passive filling may be impaired and atrial pressures are abnormally elevated. In this setting of a noncompliant ventricle (compliance is the inverse of stiffness—the change in volume for a given change in pressure), atrial contraction is responsible for a disproportionately large amount of diastolic filling.

The importance of abnormalities of diastolic function in the pathogenesis of heart failure is increasingly appreciated. Because relaxation is energy dependent, it frequently is impaired in the presence of ischemia or hypoxemia. Recurring myocardial ischemia, pathologic myocardial hypertrophy, chronic volume overload, and aging all are associated with increased interstitial fibrosis and poor relaxation.

In the left ventricle with diastolic dysfunction, LV filling pressures rise because of the compliance changes, with resulting left atrial hypertension and pulmonary congestion. Cardiac output may be reduced if ventricular filling is sufficiently impaired. With activity, these abnormalities are exaggerated, resulting in exertional dyspnea and exercise intolerance.

Ventricular Preload

In the intact heart, preload is best characterized by the end-diastolic volume or pressure, which are indirect indicators of end-diastolic fiber length (Chapter 50). The performance of the normal left ventricle is highly preload dependent, but the failing heart operates at high preloads and on the flat part of the LV function curve (see Fig. 50-3 in Chapter 50). In contrast to the normal ventricle, a modest decrease in preload has little effect on LV filling pressures, whereas an increase in preload does not improve systolic function but worsens pulmonary congestion further. Preload reduction by diuresis or by reduction of venous return with venodilating agents generally has a beneficial effect on symptoms of heart failure.

Ventricular Afterload

LV afterload frequently is equated with arterial pressure or systemic vascular resistance, but a more accurate measurement of afterload is systolic wall stress (Chapter 50), defined as follows:

$$\text{Systolic wall stress} = (\text{Pressure} \times \text{radius of left ventricle}) \div (2 \times \text{thickness of left ventricle})$$

At any given arterial pressure, afterload is increased with a dilated, thin-walled ventricle and decreased with a smaller or thicker ventricle. Increased afterload has an effect similar to that of depressed contractility, so afterload reduction can improve cardiac performance.

Heart Rate and Rhythm

Heart rate affects cardiac performance by two mechanisms. First, increasing the heart rate enhances the inotropic state by upregulating cytosolic calcium concentrations. Second, heart rate is an important determinant of cardiac output and is the primary mechanism by which cardiac output is matched to demand in situations such as exercise.

Because stroke volume is relatively fixed in the failing heart, heart rate becomes the major determinant of cardiac output. Chronic tachycardia impairs ventricular performance, however, and cardiac function often improves with control of tachyarrhythmias such as atrial fibrillation.

Optimal cardiac performance depends on a well-coordinated sequence of contraction. Normal atrioventricular conduction times (0.16 to 0.20 second) enhance the contribution of atrial contraction to LV filling, which is particularly important in the noncompliant ventricle. Patients with heart failure frequently have intraventricular conduction abnormalities, which result in dyssynchronous contractions, such that the septum and parts of the anterior wall begin contracting only after systole has ended in other regions.

Myocardial Blood Flow and Oxygen Requirements

In the normal heart, myocardial blood flow is closely coupled to oxygen requirements, and it is not ordinarily considered a determinant of cardiac performance. However, myocardial ischemia is associated with a rapid decline in contractile function that may persist long beyond the episode (myocardial stunning). Chronically inadequate blood flow may lead to a reduction in contractility, which reestablishes the balance between oxygen delivery and demands (hibernation). Low arterial diastolic pressures may interfere with the autoregulatory reserve of the coronary circulation, which is limited at diastolic pressures of less than 60 mm Hg. Endothelial dysfunction, which is common in patients with heart failure, also may limit blood flow. At the same time, tachycardia, increased afterload, and substantial LV hypertrophy increase myocardial oxygen requirements. Inadequate myocardial blood flow plays an important role in the pathogenesis of cardiac dysfunction, sometimes even in patients without obstructive coronary disease.

Genetic Causes of Dilated Cardiomyopathy

Although much less is known about the genetics of dilated cardiomyopathy than that of hypertrophic cardiomyopathy (Chapter 59), several forms of familial cardiomyopathy have been recognized, most of which are inherited in an autosomal dominant pattern. Mutations of genes encoding for nuclear membrane proteins (emerin, lamin) or for contractile or cytoskeletal proteins (desmin, a cardiac myosin, vinculin) have been identified. Cardiomyopathy also is associated with muscular dystrophies (Duchenne's, Becker's, and limb-girdle dystrophies; Chapter 447) and other forms of myopathy. As research in this area burgeons, it is estimated that genetic abnormalities may be involved in 20 to 30% of cases of idiopathic dilated cardiomyopathy.

Heart Failure Syndrome

Chronic heart failure is a multifaceted syndrome with diverse presentations (Fig. 57–2). The initial manifestations of hemodynamic dysfunction are a reduction in stroke volume and a rise in ventricular filling pressures, perhaps in the basal state but consistently under conditions of increased systemic demand for blood flow. These changes have downstream effects on cardiovascular reflexes and systemic organ perfusion and function, which in turn stimulate a variety of interdependent compensatory responses involving the cardiovascular system, neurohormonal systems, and alterations in renal physiology. It is this constellation of responses that leads to the characteristic pathophysiology of the heart failure syndrome. Recognition of the role of neurohormonal activation in heart failure has grown with the increasing understanding of its pathophysiology and with evidence that blockade of some of these responses can have a profound effect on the natural history of the disease (Table 57–3). The number of hormonal systems that are known to be activated in heart failure continues to grow.

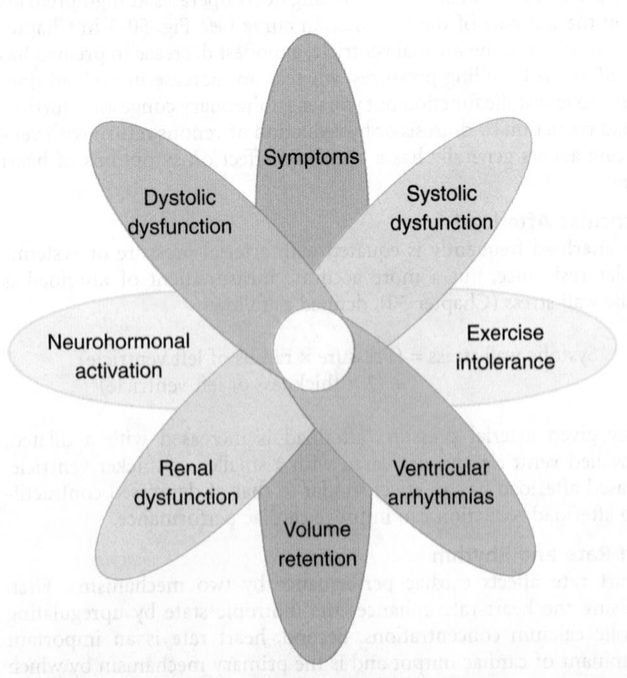

FIGURE 57–2 • Pathophysiology of heart failure, illustrated by Venn diagram.

Neurohormonal Responses

Sympathetic Nervous System

Initial activation of the sympathetic nervous system probably results from reduced pulse pressures, which activate arterial baroreceptors, and renal hypoperfusion. Evidence for its activation comes from elevated levels of circulating norepinephrine, direct sympathetic nerve recordings showing increased activity, and increased release of norepinephrine by several organs, including the heart. As cardiac function deteriorates, responsivity to norepinephrine diminishes, as evidenced by baroreceptor desensitization and downregulation of cardiac adrenergic receptors and signal transduction. This densensitization may further stimulate sympathetic responses.

The adaptive role of norepinephrine is to stimulate heart rate and myocardial contractility and to produce vasoconstriction. All of these actions reverse the depression of cardiac output and blood pressure. Increased levels of plasma norepinephrine are associated with a worse prognosis, although it is unclear whether this is a cause-and-effect relationship. There is also convincing, albeit circumstantial, evidence that norepinephrine has adverse effects on the myocardium. In this regard, β-adrenoceptor blockade, which once was considered dangerous in heart failure because it would interfere with important compensatory mechanisms, consistently improves LV function and prognosis. The roles of other catecholamines in heart failure remain undefined.

Renin-Angiotensin-Aldosterone System

Elements of the renin-angiotensin-aldosterone system are activated relatively early in heart failure. The presumptive mechanisms of induction include renal hypoperfusion, β-adrenergic system stimulation, and hyponatremia. All may be activated further by diuretic therapy. Angiotensin II increases blood pressure by vasoconstriction; it enhances glomerular filtration by increasing renal pressure and maintaining glomerular flow through its intrarenal hemodynamic effects. Aldosterone

TABLE 57–3 NEUROHORMONES THAT MAY BE INCREASED IN CHRONIC HEART FAILURE
Norepinephrine
Epinephrine
Plasma renin activity
Angiotensin II
Aldosterone
Prostaglandins
Vasopressin
Neuropeptide Y
Vasoactive intestinal peptides
Natriuretic peptides
Endothelin
Endorphins
Calcitonin gene-related peptide
Growth hormone
Cortisol
Proinflammatory cytokines
Neurokinin A
Substance P

causes sodium retention, which restores normal cardiac output by enhancing intravascular volume. These adaptations have deleterious consequences, however. Excessive vasoconstriction can depress LV function, and sodium retention worsens the already elevated ventricular filling pressures. There also is experimental evidence indicating that angiotensin II may have pathologic effects on the myocardium and may induce vascular hypertrophy, whereas aldosterone induces myocardial fibrosis. The striking success of ACE inhibitors and, more recently, of spironolactone in improving the natural history of heart failure suggests that the adverse effects of renin-angiotensin-aldosterone activation may outweigh their benefit.

Other Neurohormonal Systems

Levels of several natriuretic peptides are elevated consistently in heart failure, and they may counterbalance the vasoconstricting and sodium-retaining actions of the renin-angiotensin-aldosterone and sympathetic nervous systems. However, the renal responses to these natriuretic hormones are downregulated, so that they do not have the same natriuretic effects in patients with chronic heart failure that they manifest in normal individuals. Elevated circulating and tissue levels of vasodilating prostaglandins may improve glomerular hemodynamics, and inhibitors of prostaglandin synthesis (including aspirin and other nonsteroidal anti-inflammatory agents) interfere with the hemodynamic and renal actions of ACE inhibitors.

Endothelin and arginine vasopressin are elevated in many patients with heart failure, and interference with their actions may promote vasodilation and aquaresis. Arginine vasopressin induces vasoconstriction through a vascular (V-1) receptor and reduces free water clearance through a renal tubular (V-2) receptor. Endothelin causes prolonged vasoconstriction, reductions in glomerular filtration, mesangial hypertrophy, bronchoconstriction, and pulmonary arteriolar constriction. Although endothelin is a theoretically attractive target for therapy, clinical trials with endothelin antagonists have yielded unimpressive results, indicating that interdiction of neurohormonal activation is not uniformly beneficial.

Cytokine Activation

Circulating levels of many proinflammatory cytokines, including tumor necrosis factor-α (TNF-α), interleukin-1β, and interleukin-6, are elevated in patients with relatively severe heart failure and may be involved in the syndrome of cardiac cachexia. These cytokines also may induce contractile dysfunction, myocardial fibrosis, and myocyte necrosis, perhaps by mediating some of the deleterious responses to catecholamines and angiotensin II. Nonetheless, trials using antagonists of TNF-α have not shown clinical benefit.

Altered Renal Physiology

In most patients with chronic heart failure, the kidneys are anatomically and structurally normal. Reduced blood pressure, diminished stroke volume, and reduced renal perfusion pressure and flow are sensed as reduced blood volume by the high-pressure baroreceptors and the juxtaglomerular apparatus, which maintain cardiovascular homeostasis. In chronic heart failure, these receptors become desensitized, generating reduced afferent responses. The low-pressure intracardiac pressure and volume receptors also are desensitized. Thirst and fluid intake may be increased as a result of activation of the cerebral thirst center. Although heart failure usually is associated with a normal or increased blood volume, it paradoxically is characterized by activation of the same homeostatic responses as those that act in hemorrhage and shock; the result is abnormal retention of sodium and water. In advanced heart failure, which is usually characterized by low cardiac output and/or hypotension (or coexisting renal vascular disease), the glomerular filtration rate may become so severely reduced that sodium and fluid retention becomes refractory to diuretic therapy.

Left Ventricular Remodeling and Progression of Heart Failure

After an initial insult precipitates heart failure, progressive alterations occur in myocardial structure and function owing to continuing damage by the underlying process and responses to hemodynamic stresses and neurohormonal activation. The left ventricle progressively dilates and changes from the normal ellipsoid shape to a more spherical geometry. This "remodeling" is accompanied by changes in the cardiac interstitium that lead to altered orientation of the myofibrils and progressive fibrosis. The result is more discoordinate and less effective contraction. ACE inhibitors and β-blockers slow, halt, or reverse this remodeling process, preventing LV dilation, geometric distortion, and deterioration in contractile function.

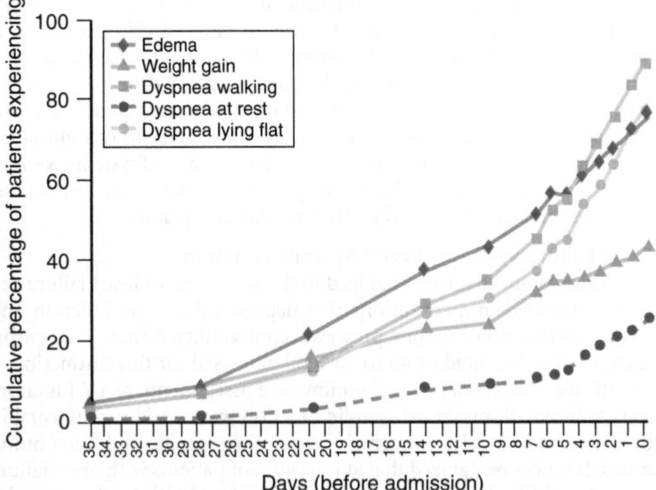

FIGURE 57–3 • Number of days from onset of worsening of selected symptoms of heart failure to admission to hospital: cumulative percentage of patients. (Reprinted with permission from Schiff GD, Fung S, Speroff T, et al: Decompensated heart failure: Symptoms, patterns of onset, and contributing factors. Am J Med 2003;114:625–630.)

Clinical Manifestations

Heart failure may manifest acutely in a de novo manner, chronically, or as an acute exacerbation of chronic heart failure.

Acute Decompensation of Heart Failure

Most episodes of acute worsening of heart failure occur in patients with previously recognized symptoms of chronic heart failure. Patients with such decompensations usually present with shortness of breath, generally after a period of fluid retention or signs of congestion, as manifested by worsening edema and some degree of worsening dyspnea (Fig. 57–3). Occasionally, the presentation may be more acute, with rapid progression to resting dyspnea and/or pulmonary edema. The latter presentation is often associated with hypertension and is particularly characteristic of patients who have diastolic dysfunction and whose stiff left ventricle tolerates fluid retention poorly. In patients without a preceding history of heart failure, other precipitating factors, such as acute MI (Chapter 72), tachyarrhythmias (Chapters 63 and 64), previously unrecognized or new valvular abnormalities (Chapter 75), toxic damage (including alcohol excess), or acute myocarditis (Chapter 59), should be considered. Rapid diagnosis by noninvasive testing, early cardiac catheterization, and, in selected cases, endomyocardial biopsy is essential. Treatment is cause specific and may include early coronary revascularization, valve repair or replacement, or supportive care (e.g., inotropic support, intra-aortic balloon pumping, ventricular assist devices). If the condition is not reversed, cardiac transplantation (Chapter 82) may be the best option for appropriate candidates.

Chronic Heart Failure

Left-Sided and Right-Sided Heart Failure

Most adult patients with heart failure have abnormalities of the left ventricle as the underlying cause. Nonetheless, the clinical presentation may be variable, sometimes suggesting predominantly or even exclusively RV dysfunction. The manifestations of LV dysfunction are related to elevated filling (diastolic) pressures, which are transmitted backward to the left atrium and pulmonary veins, or inadequate cardiac output. The former results in dyspnea (sometimes at rest but usually with activity) and, when severe, pulmonary edema (classically associated with rales and possibly pleural effusions). The cardiac output may be insufficient to support peripheral organ function, causing exertional muscle fatigue, impaired renal function and salt excretion, or depressed mentation.

Right-sided heart failure results from either chronic RV pressure overload (e.g., pulmonary hypertension resulting from cor pulmonale or pulmonary vascular disease) or intrinsic dysfunction of the right ventricle or its valves. However, the most common cause of RV pressure overload is left-sided heart dysfunction, which results in pulmonary hypertension. If the symptoms and signs of left-sided heart failure are absent or difficult to elicit, the physician inappropriately may seek a primarily right-sided pathology. The primary manifestations of right-sided failure are related to chronically elevated right atrial and systemic venous pressures: jugular venous distention, peripheral edema, ascites, hepatic and bowel edema, and varied gastrointestinal complaints.

Heart Failure with Preserved Systolic Function

Myocardial mechanisms that lead to the syndrome of heart failure can be differentiated into conditions that depress LV systolic function and conditions that occur despite preserved contractility. Although it is arbitrary, a LVEF threshold of 45 to 50% often is used for this distinction.

Until the widespread use of noninvasive assessments of LV function, heart failure with preserved systolic function was considered unusual in the absence of valvular abnormalities or other specific and uncommon causes. It is now recognized that at least 40% of patients with heart failure have normal EFs. In the ongoing Cardiovascular Health Study, a population-based study of more than 5000 patients aged 65 years and older, more than 70% of the patients developing heart failure had normal or only mildly impaired systolic function. It is likely that more elderly patients with heart failure have diastolic dysfunction as the primary cause of their symptoms.

Although there are many potential causes of heart failure with preserved systolic function, most patients have current hypertension or a history of treated hypertension; the resulting LV hypertrophy and fibrosis are probably responsible for increased chamber stiffness. Ischemic heart disease also may contribute to heart failure with preserved systolic function, probably by virtue of subendocardial fibrosis or as a result of acute, intermittent ischemic dysfunction. Diabetes mellitus is often present, especially in women. Age itself is a crucial predisposing factor, because it causes loss of myocytes (apoptosis), increased fibrosis with shifts to more rigid forms of collagen, and loss of vascular compliance.

The mortality rate of patients with preserved systolic function is lower than the rate for those with low EFs but remains higher than in the general population, even among similarly older-aged individuals. Hospitalization and rehospitalization rates for these patients are comparable to the rates for patients with reduced EFs, and there are few data on treatment to guide physicians.

Although patients who have heart failure with preserved systolic function often are considered to have *diastolic dysfunction,* other explanations for this presentation must be considered, some of which are reversible or warrant specific therapy (Table 57–4). The first two questions to consider are whether the patient's symptoms are caused by heart failure of any type and whether important valvular abnormalities are present. LVEF measurements may be inaccurate, particularly if their technical quality is suboptimal. Regurgitant valve disease may lead to a dissociation between the LVEF and underlying myocardial dysfunction, because afterload may be low in this setting. There also are many conditions in which LV function is impaired transiently, but subsequently measured EFs may be normal. Intermittent ischemia, presenting as episodic heart failure ("flash pulmonary edema"), is the most important of these conditions, because revascularization may be indicated. Severe hypertension with subsequent treatment and transient arrhythmias also may have temporary effects on EF. Some patients with alcoholic cardiomyopathy exhibit rapid recovery in EF when they cease drinking.

The remaining patients most likely have diastolic dysfunction as the underlying disorder. The noninvasive measurement of diastolic function remains problematic. The most commonly used test, Doppler echocardiography, is neither sensitive nor specific for diastolic dysfunction. Particularly in the elderly, Doppler mitral valve filling patterns show impaired early diastolic filling in most subjects, whether or not they have evidence of heart failure. Diastolic dysfunction is basically a diagnosis of exclusion based on accompanying conditions and circumstantial evidence.

Factors Precipitating Acute Decompensation of Chronic Heart Failure

Many patients with chronic heart failure maintain a stable course, then abruptly present with acutely or subacutely worsening symptoms. Although this decompensation may reflect unrecognized gradual progression of the underlying disorder, many precipitating events must be considered and, if present, addressed (Table 57–5). An important focus is on changes in medications (by patient or physician), diet, or activity. Superimposed new or altered cardiovascular conditions, such as arrhythmias, ischemic events, hypertension, or valvular abnormalities, should be considered. Systemic processes, such as fever, infection, or anemia, also can cause cardiac decompensation.

TABLE 57–4 CAUSES OF (AND ALTERNATIVE EXPLANATIONS FOR) HEART FAILURE WITH PRESERVED SYSTOLIC FUNCTION (LEFT VENTRICULAR EJECTION FRACTION >45–50%)

Inaccurate diagnosis of heart failure (e.g., pulmonary disease, obesity)
Inaccurate measurements of ejection fraction
Systolic function overestimated by ejection fraction (e.g., mitral regurgitation)
Episodic, unrecognized systolic dysfunction
Intermittent ischemia
Arrhythmia
Severe hypertension
Alcohol abuse
Diastolic dysfunction
Abnormalities of myocardial relaxation
Ischemia
Hypertrophy
Abnormalities of myocardial compliance
Hypertrophy
Aging
Fibrosis
Diabetes
Infiltrative disease (amyloidosis, sarcoidosis)
Storage disease (hemochromatosis)
Endomyocardial disease (endomyocardial fibrosis, radiation, anthracyclines)
Pericardial disease (constriction, tamponade)

TABLE 57–5 FACTORS THAT MAY PRECIPITATE ACUTE DECOMPENSATION OF CHRONIC HEART FAILURE

Discontinuation of therapy (patient noncompliance or physician initiated)
Initiation of medications that worsen heart failure (calcium antagonists, β-blockers, nonsteroidal anti-inflammatory drugs, antiarrhythmic agents)
Iatrogenic volume overload (transfusion, fluid administration)
Dietary indiscretion
Alcohol consumption
Increased activity
Pregnancy
Exposure to high altitude
Arrhythmias
Myocardial ischemia or infarction
Worsening hypertension
Worsening mitral or tricuspid regurgitation
Fever or infection
Anemia

Diagnosis

The diagnosis of heart failure is straightforward when a patient presents with classic symptoms and accompanying physical findings. In patients with chronic heart failure, however, the diagnosis is often delayed or missed entirely because no single sign or symptom is diagnostic.

Clinical Evaluation

The most frequent symptoms, dyspnea and fatigue, are not specific for heart failure, especially in the older population, but their presence always should lead to a more complete evaluation. The more specific symptoms of orthopnea, paroxysmal nocturnal dyspnea, and edema are much less common. Although the physical examination may be helpful, characteristic physical findings may be absent. The chest radiograph (Chapter 51), on which many physicians rely, adds relatively little to the clinical evaluation.

The key to making the timely diagnosis of chronic heart failure is to maintain a high degree of suspicion, particularly in high-risk patients with coronary artery disease, chronic hypertension, diabetes, a history of heavy alcohol use, and/or advanced age. If such patients present with any of the symptoms or physical findings suggestive of heart failure, additional testing (see later discussion) should be undertaken, typically beginning with echocardiography (Chapter 53).

The common symptoms of heart failure are well known but are frequently absent and variably specific for this condition. The symptoms generally reflect, but may be dissociated from, the hemodynamic derangements of elevated left-sided and right-sided pressures and impaired cardiac output or cardiac output reserve.

Dyspnea

Dyspnea (Chapter 83), or perceived shortness of breath, is the most common symptom of heart failure. In most patients, dyspnea is present only with activity or exertion. The underlying mechanisms are multifactorial. The most important is pulmonary congestion with increased interstitial or intra-alveolar fluid, which activates juxtacapillary J receptors, stimulating a rapid and shallow pattern of breathing. Increased lung stiffness may enhance the work of breathing, leading to a perception of dyspnea. Central regulation of respiration may be disturbed in those with more severe heart failure, resulting in disordered sleep patterns and sleep apnea. Cheyne-Stokes respiration, or periodic breathing, is common in advanced heart failure, is usually associated with low-output states, and may be perceived by the patient (and the patient's family) as either severe dyspnea or transient cessation of breathing. Hypoxia, which is uncommon in heart failure unless there is accompanying pulmonary disease, suggests the presence of pulmonary edema. Dyspnea is a relatively sensitive symptom of heart failure, provided that a careful history is taken of the patient's level of activity, but dyspnea may become less prominent with the onset of RV failure and tricuspid regurgitation, which may lead to lower pulmonary venous pressures. Dyspnea is a common symptom of patients with pulmonary disease (Chapter 83), obesity, or anemia and of sedentary individuals.

Orthopnea and Paroxysmal Nocturnal Dyspnea

Orthopnea is dyspnea that is positional, occurring in the recumbent or semirecumbent position. It occurs as a result of the increase in venous return from the extremities and splanchnic circulation to the central circulation with changes in posture, with resultant increases in pulmonary venous pressures and pulmonary capillary hydrostatic pressure. Nocturnal cough may be a manifestation of this process and is an under-recognized symptom of heart failure. Orthopnea is a relatively specific symptom of heart failure, although it may occur in patients with pulmonary disease who breathe more effectively in an upright posture and in individuals with significant abdominal obesity or ascites. Most patients with mild or moderate heart failure do not experience orthopnea if they are treated adequately.

Paroxysmal nocturnal dyspnea is an attack of acute, severe shortness of breath that awakens the patient from sleep, usually 1 to 3 hours after the patient retires. Symptoms usually resolve over 10 to 30 minutes after the patient arises, often gasping for fresh air from an open window. Paroxysmal nocturnal dyspnea results from increased venous return and mobilization of interstitial fluid from the extremities and elsewhere, with accumulation of alveolar edema. Paroxysmal nocturnal dyspnea almost always represents heart failure, but it is a relatively uncommon finding.

Acute Pulmonary Edema

Pulmonary edema results from transudation of fluid into the alveolar spaces due to acute rises in capillary hydrostatic pressures caused by an acute depression of cardiac function or an acute rise in intravascular volume. The initial symptoms may be cough or progressive dyspnea. Because alveolar edema may precipitate bronchospasm, wheezing is common. If the edema is not treated, the patient may begin coughing up pink (or blood-tinged), frothy fluid and become cyanotic and acidotic.

Exercise Intolerance

Activity or exercise intolerance is, together with dyspnea, the most characteristic symptom of chronic heart failure. Intuitively, it might be assumed that exercise would be limited by shortness of breath because of rising pulmonary venous pressures and pulmonary congestion. Although this mechanism may contribute, it is only one of many operating. Blood flow to exercising muscles is impaired as a result of reduced cardiac output reserve and impaired peripheral vasodilation; oxygen delivery is limited, and early fatigue ensues. Heart failure is associated with additional abnormalities of skeletal muscle itself, including biochemical changes and alterations in fiber types, which increase muscle fatigue and impair muscle function. Finally, heart failure may affect adversely respiratory muscle function and ventilatory control.

Fatigue

Fatigue is a common, if nonspecific, complaint of patients with heart failure. Perhaps the most common origin of this complaint is muscle fatigue. Fatigue also may be a nonspecific response to the systemic manifestations of heart failure, such as chronic increases in catecholamines and circulating levels of cytokines, sleep disorders, and anxiety.

Edema and Fluid Retention (Ascites, Pleural Effusion, Pericardial Effusion)

Elevated right atrial pressures increase the capillary hydrostatic pressures in the systemic circulation, with resultant transudation. The location of edema fluid is determined by position (e.g., dependent) and by the accompanying pathology. Most commonly, edema accumulates in the extremities and resolves at night, when the legs are not dependent. Edema may occur only in the feet and ankles, but if it is more severe, it may accumulate in the thighs, scrotum, and abdominal wall. Edema is more likely and more severe in patients with accompanying venous disease, in those who have had veins harvested for coronary bypass surgery, and in patients taking calcium channel blockers, which themselves cause edema. Fluid retention precipitated by the thiazolidinediones (Chapter 248) may precipitate heart failure or mimic it.

Fluid also may accumulate in the peritoneal cavity and in the pleural or pericardial space. Ascites occurs as a result of elevated pressures in the hepatic, portal, and systemic veins draining the peritoneum. Ascites is unusual in heart failure and almost always is associated with peripheral edema. Most commonly, there is severe tricuspid regurgitation, with potential damage to the liver. Otherwise, significant primary liver disease should be suspected as an exacerbating factor or cause of ascites. Pleural effusions are fairly common in chronic heart failure, especially when they are accompanied by left-sided and right-sided manifestations. The effusions result from an increase in transudation of fluid into the pleural space and from impaired lymphatic drainage caused by elevated systemic venous pressures. Pericardial effusions are far less frequent but may occur.

Abdominal and Gastrointestinal Symptoms

Passive congestion of the liver may lead to right upper quadrant pain and tenderness and mild jaundice. Usually only mild elevations of transaminase levels and modest increases in bilirubin levels are observed. With severe, acute rises in central venous pressures, especially if associated with systemic hypotension, a severe congestive and ischemic hepatopathy may occur, with striking elevations in liver function markers and hypoglycemia. Recovery is usually rapid and complete if the hemodynamic abnormalities are corrected.

Bowel wall edema may lead to early satiety (a common symptom in heart failure), nausea, diffuse abdominal discomfort, malabsorption, and a rare form of protein-losing enteropathy. The potential role of heart failure in producing these nonspecific gastrointestinal symptoms is often overlooked, leading to extensive diagnostic testing or unnecessary discontinuation of medications.

Sleep Disorders and Central Nervous System Manifestations

Periods of nocturnal oxygen desaturation to less than 80 to 85% are relatively common in patients with heart failure; they coincide with episodes of apnea (Chapter 101), and often are preceded or followed by episodes of hyperventilation. These are similar to, and may represent truncated forms of, Cheyne-Stokes respiration. These episodes reflect altered central nervous system ventilatory control and have been associated with diminished heart rate variability. Supplemental oxygen seems to reverse some of the ventilatory disorders, and the apneic spells respond to nasal positive-pressure ventilation. In some patients, these interventions have a striking beneficial effect on fatigue and other symptoms of heart failure.

Aside from the common complaint of fatigue, which originates in part in the central nervous system, brain function is not affected in most patients with heart failure. In advanced heart failure, cerebral hypoperfusion can cause impairment of memory, irritability, limited attention span, and altered mentation.

Cardiac Cachexia

In chronic, severe heart failure, unintentional chronic weight loss may occur, leading to a syndrome of cardiac cachexia. The cause of this syndrome is unclear, but it may result from many factors, including increased levels of pro-inflammatory cytokines (e.g., TNF), elevated metabolic rates, loss of appetite, and malabsorption. Cardiac cachexia carries a poor prognosis.

Physical Examination

The physical findings associated with heart failure generally reflect elevated ventricular filling pressures and, to a lesser extent, reduced cardiac output. In chronic heart failure, many of these findings are absent, often obscuring the correct diagnosis.

Appearance and Vital Signs

Compensated patients may be comfortable, but patients with more severe symptoms are often restless, dyspneic, and pale or diaphoretic. Although the heart rate is usually at the high end of the normal range or higher (>80 beats per minute), it may be lower in patients with chronic, stable heart failure. Premature beats and arrhythmias are common. Pulsus alternans (alternating amplitude of successive beats) is a sign of advanced heart failure (or of a large pericardial effusion). The blood pressure may be normal or high, but in advanced heart failure it is usually on the low end of normal or lower.

Jugular Veins and Neck Examination

Examination of the jugular veins is one of the most useful aspects of the evaluation of patients with heart failure. The jugular venous pressure should be quantified in centimeters of water (normal = 8 cm H_2O) (Chapter 48), estimating the level of pulsations above the sternal angle (and arbitrarily adding 5 cm H_2O in any posture). The presence of abdominal-jugular reflux should be assessed by putting pressure on the right upper quadrant of the abdomen for 30 seconds and avoiding an induced Valsalva maneuver; a positive finding is a rise in the jugular pressure of at least 1cm. Either an elevated jugular venous pressure or an abnormal abdominal-jugular reflux has been reported in 80% of patients with advanced heart failure. No other simple sign is nearly as sensitive.

An additional important finding in the neck is evidence of tricuspid regurgitation—a large "cv" wave, usually associated with a high jugular venous pressure. This finding is confirmed by hepatic pulsations, which can be detected during the abdominal-jugular reflux determination. The carotid pulses should be evaluated for evidence of aortic stenosis, and thyroid abnormalities should be sought.

Pulmonary Examination

Although dyspnea is the most common symptom of patients with heart failure, the pulmonary examination is usually unremarkable. Rales, representing alveolar fluid, are a hallmark of heart failure; when they are present in patients without accompanying pulmonary disease, they are highly specific for the diagnosis. In chronic heart failure, they are usually absent, however, even in patients known to have pulmonary capillary wedge pressures greater than 20 mm Hg (normal, <12 mmHg). LV failure cannot be excluded by the absence of rales. Pleural effusions, which are indicative of bilateral heart failure in patients with appropriate symptoms, are relatively rare.

Cardiac Examination

The cardiac examination is a crucial part of the evaluation of the patient with heart failure, but it is more useful for identification of associated cardiac abnormalities than for assessment of the severity of the heart failure (Chapter 48). Assessment of the point of maximal impulse may provide information concerning the size of the heart (enlarged if displaced below the fifth intercostal space or lateral to the midclavicular line) and its function (if sustained beyond one third of systole or palpable over two interspaces). Additional precordial pulsations may indicate an LV aneurysm. A parasternal lift is valuable evidence of pulmonary hypertension.

The first heart sound (S_1) may be diminished in amplitude when LV function is poor, and the pulmonic component of the second heart sound (P_2) may be accentuated when pulmonary hypertension is present. An apical third heart sound (S_3) is a strong indicator of significant LV dysfunction, but it is present only in a few patients with low EFs and elevated LV filling pressures. A fourth heart sound (S_4) is not a specific indicator of heart failure, but it is usually present in patients with diastolic dysfunction. An S_3 at the lower left or right sternal border or below the xiphoid indicates RV dysfunction. Murmurs may indicate the presence of significant valvular disease as the cause of heart failure, but mitral and tricuspid regurgitation also are common secondary manifestations of severe ventricular dilation and dysfunction.

Examination of the Abdomen and Extremities

The size, pulsatility, and tenderness of the liver should be evaluated as evidence of passive congestion and tricuspid regurgitation. Ascites and edema should be sought and quantified.

Characterization: Essential and Contingent Tests

Essential Tests

Chest Radiography

Although the standard posteroanterior and lateral chest radiographs provide limited information about chamber size, the presence of overall cardiomegaly (a cardiothoracic ratio >0.50, especially if >0.60) is a strong indicator of heart failure or another cause of cardiomegaly (especially valvular insufficiency) (Chapter 51). However, almost 50% of patients with heart failure do not have this high a cardiothoracic ratio.

Most patients with acute heart failure, but only a few of those with chronic heart failure, have evidence of pulmonary venous hypertension (upper lobe redistribution, enlarged pulmonary veins), interstitial edema (haziness of the central vascular shadows or increased central interstitial lung markings), or pulmonary edema (perihilar or patchy peripheral infiltrates). The absence of these findings reflects the subjectivity of interpretation and the increased capacity of the lymphatics to remove interstitial and alveolar fluid in chronic heart failure. This absence of radiographic findings is consistent with the absence of rales in most patients with chronic heart failure despite markedly elevated pulmonary venous pressures. Pleural effusions are important adjunctive evidence of heart failure. Characteristically, these are more common and larger on the right than on the left side, reflecting the greater pleural surface area of the right lung.

Electrocardiography

The major importance of the electrocardiogram is to evaluate cardiac rhythm, identify prior MI, and detect evidence of LV hypertrophy (Chapter 52). Prior MI suggests that the cause is ischemic cardiomyopathy with systolic dysfunction. LV hypertrophy is a nonspecific finding but may point toward LV diastolic dysfunction if the EF is not depressed.

Echocardiography

Noninvasive cardiac imaging is a crucial part of the diagnosis and evaluation of heart failure. The most useful procedure is the transthoracic echocardiogram (Chapter 53), which provides a quantitative assessment of LV function; in the presence of appropriate symptoms and signs, it can confirm the presence of heart failure resulting from systolic dysfunction, or indicate whether the patient has heart failure with preserved systolic function. The echocardiogram also provides a wealth of additional valuable information, including assessment of LV and RV size and regional wall motion (as an indicator of prior MI), evaluation of the heart valves, and diagnosis of LV hypertrophy. The echocardiogram generally has replaced the chest radiograph in the diagnostic assessment of heart failure.

Measurements of Natriuretic Peptides

Serum levels of natriuretic peptides can be measured quickly and accurately, including point-of-care testing at the bedside. B-type natriuretic peptide (BNP) and amino (N)-terminal pro-BNP are relatively sensitive and specific markers for clinically confirmed heart failure These peptides have been found to be useful adjuncts in the diagnosis of patients presenting in the acute care setting with possible heart failure, particularly when the diagnosis remains uncertain. [1] However, levels of both BNP and N-terminal pro-BNP increase with age in the absence of clinical heart failure, especially in women, probably reflecting increased ventricular stiffness associated with aging and hypertension. BNP levels may also be increased slightly in patients with chronic obstructive pulmonary disease, in whom elevations may reflect diastolic dysfunction or RV dysfunction but nonetheless may lead to a false-positive clinical diagnosis of heart failure. Elevated natriuretic peptide measurements are associated with a worse prognosis and may be helpful in assessing the response to therapy. However, the clinical value of serial measurements in guiding therapy, and whether they can facilitate improved outcomes, have not been assessed.

Contingent Tests

After the diagnosis of heart failure is made, the goal of additional testing is to identify potentially correctable or specifically treatable causes and to obtain further information that is necessary for future management.

Laboratory Testing

An extensive battery of laboratory tests is not required for most patients with heart failure. Routine testing should include a complete blood cell count (to detect anemia and systemic diseases with hematologic manifestations); measurement of renal function and electrolytes, including magnesium (to exclude renal failure and to provide a baseline for subsequent therapy); liver function tests (to exclude accompanying liver pathology and provide a baseline); and blood glucose and lipid testing (to diagnose diabetes and dyslipidemia, both of which should be managed aggressively in patients with heart failure).

A few additional tests may be indicated. Thyrotoxicosis, and to a lesser extent hypothyroidism, may cause heart failure and may be difficult to diagnose clinically, especially in older patients (Chapter 244). Many guidelines recommend thyroid function tests for all patients, or at least all elderly patients and those with atrial fibrillation. Hemochromatosis (Chapter 231) is a potentially treatable cause of heart failure; particularly if there is accompanying diabetes or hepatic disease, measurement of serum ferritin levels is indicated. Sarcoidosis (Chapter 95) is another potentially treatable cause, although it would be unusual not to have evidence of accompanying lung disease. Amyloidosis (Chapter 296) should be considered in patients with other manifestations, but treatment of the cardiac manifestations is rarely successful except with heart transplantation.

Assessment of Left Ventricular Function

Although heart failure is a syndrome with many pathogenic mechanisms, the most common are LV systolic dysfunction and LV diastolic dysfunction. In some patients, it is almost impossible to distinguish between these two forms of heart failure by clinical evaluation, because both may present with the same symptoms and with only subtle differences on physical examination. However, it is essential to distinguish between these two entities, because they may require different diagnostic evaluations and different therapeutic approaches (Chapter 58). The most useful and practical test is the echocardiogram (Chapter 53); alternative approaches include radionuclide measurements of LVEF (Chapter 54) and left ventriculography if cardiac catheterization (Chapter 56) is being performed. All of these tests allow the detection of significant systolic dysfunction; diastolic dysfunction sometimes can be documented (Chapter 53) but often is identified primarily as a process of exclusion in patients with preserved systolic function. Randomized trials have found no benefit, in terms of days alive and out of hospital or in a number of other relevant end points, among patients who were monitored with pulmonary artery catheterization compared with those who were not. [2]

Diagnostic Evaluation

Assessment for Coronary Artery Disease

Coronary artery disease is the most common cause of heart failure in industrialized societies. Often it is known that a patient has coronary disease based on a prior history of MI or positive results on an angiogram or noninvasive test, but in some patients MI can be silent. There are two reasons to identify the coexistence of heart failure and coronary disease: first, to treat symptoms that may be caused by ischemia and, second, to improve prognosis (Chapters 70, 71, and 72). A prudent approach is to divide patients with heart failure into three groups: (1) those with clinical evidence of ongoing ischemia (active angina or a possible ischemic equivalent), (2) those who have had a prior MI but do not currently have angina, and (3) those who may or may not have underlying coronary disease. The first group of patients may be evaluated most expeditiously by coronary angiography, because they stand to benefit in terms of symptoms and probably have more extensive ischemia. In the second group are patients with heart failure and prior MI who by other criteria (age, absence of other major comorbid conditions) are good candidates for coronary revascularization; they generally should undergo noninvasive stress testing in conjunction with nuclear myocardial perfusion imaging or echocardiography. These procedures identify individuals with extensive ischemic but viable myocardium, whose prognosis and symptoms also may be improved with revascularization. The third group, patients without either angina or prior MI, are much less likely to benefit from an evaluation for asymptomatic coronary disease.

Myocardial Biopsy

There is no rationale for routine myocardial biopsy in patients with heart failure, even in the subgroup without apparent coronary disease. Few entities that might be detected are amenable to specific therapy, and those that are (hemochromatosis, sarcoidosis) usually can be detected by their other manifestations or other procedures. A possible exception is acute fulminant myocarditis (Chapter 82), particularly eosinophilic and giant cell myocarditis, which may respond to immunosuppressive therapy. Another potential exception is in the patient being evaluated for cardiac transplantation (Chapter 82), because the presence of some entities may preclude this procedure.

Assessment of Exercise Capacity

Quantitative assessment of exercise capacity provides additional insight into prognosis beyond the clinical evaluation and measurements of cardiac function, particularly when a detailed history of activity tolerance cannot be obtained. Exercise testing with measurements of peak oxygen uptake by respiratory gas exchange has become a routine part of the evaluation for transplantation (Chapter 82) because it provides an indication of need for early intervention and an additional method for follow-up. In most patients, testing is not necessary, however. Emphasis should be placed on eliciting each patient's maximum tolerated activity and the minimum activity associated with symptoms; both can be monitored from visit to visit as a guide to management.

Assessment of Arrhythmias

Ventricular arrhythmias are extremely common in patients with chronic heart failure, with 50 to 80% of patients exhibiting nonsustained ventricular tachycardia during 24-hour monitoring. Because approximately 50% of cardiac deaths in these patients are sudden, these arrhythmias have been viewed with concern. In multivariate analyses, asymptomatic ventricular arrhythmias carry little independent prognostic significance when the severity of symptoms, EF, and presence of concurrent coronary disease are taken into account. Arrhythmias are no more predictive of sudden death than of total mortality. Further evaluation of asymptomatic arrhythmias is not warranted. In contrast, ventricular arrhythmias associated with syncope or hemodynamic compromise must be taken seriously and require further evaluation and treatment (Chapter 64).

Differential Diagnosis

Although it is not difficult to make the definitive diagnosis of heart failure in a patient who presents with the classic symptoms and signs, several alternative diagnoses need to be considered in less clear-cut situations, such as in the patient with normal LV function and less definitive clinical evidence. The most important alternative is possible pulmonary disease, for which pulmonary function testing is usually helpful (Chapter 85). If LV systolic function is normal, it may be difficult to make a conclusive determination of the relative role of diastolic heart failure compared with other concomitant conditions, such as severe obesity, chronic anemia, or other systemic illnesses; in some patients, a therapeutic trial of treatment for heart failure (Chapter 58) may be diagnostic.

Follow-Up Testing

After the diagnosis of heart failure is confirmed and the initial evaluation is complete, there is little need for further testing beyond the laboratory tests necessary to monitor therapy (primarily renal function and electrolytes). If the status of ventricular function is known, there are few indications for retesting. Exceptions are monitoring for transplantation and important changes in clinical status, such as marked deterioration in a patient previously known to have preserved LV function or the occurrence of new murmurs in conjunction with declining status.

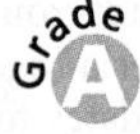

1. Doust JA, Glasziu PP, Pietrzak E, et al: A systematic review of the diagnostic accuracy of natriuretic peptides for heart failure. Arch Intern Med 2004;164:1978–1984.
2. The ESCAPE Investigators: Evaluation study of congestive heart failure and pulmonary artery catheterization effectiveness. The ESCAPE trial. JAMA 2005;294:1625–1633.

SUGGESTED READINGS

Hunt SA: ACC/AHA 2005 guideline update for the diagnosis and management of chronic heart failure in the adult: A report of the American College of Cardiology/American Heart Association Task Force on Practice Guidelines (Writing Committee to Update the 2001 Guidelines for the Evaluation and Management of Heart Failure). J Am Coll Cardiol 2005;46:e1–e82. *Consensus guidelines.*

Lee DS, Pencina MJ, Benjamin EJ, et al: Association of parental heart failure with risk of heart failure in offspring. N Engl J Med 2006;355:138–147. *Data emphasize the contribution of familial factors to the heart failure burden in the community.*

Le Jemtel TH, Padeletti M, Jelic S, et al: Diagnostic and therapeutic challenges in patients with coexistent chronic obstructive pulmonary disease and chronic heart failure. J Am Coll Cardiol 2007;49:171–180. *A review of the diagnostic challenges.*

Morita H, Seidman J, Seidman CE: Genetic causes of human heart failure. J Clin Invest 2005;115:518–526. *Review of the genetic abnormalities underlying both dilated and hypertrophic cardiomyopathy.*

Swedberg K (chairperson): The Task Force for the Diagnosis and Treatment of Chronic Heart Failure of the European Society of Cardiology. Guidelines for the diagnosis and treatment of chronic heart failure: Executive summary (update 2005). Eur Heart J 2005;26:1115–1140. *Consensus guidelines.*

Wang CS, FitzGerald JM, Schulzer M, et al: Does this dyspneic patient in the emergency department have congestive heart failure? JAMA 2005;294:1944–1956. *Practical discussion of the assessment of patients presenting with shortness of breath.*

58 HEART FAILURE: MANAGEMENT AND PROGNOSIS

John J. V. McMurray and Marc A. Pfeffer

EVALUATION AND MANAGEMENT OF HEART FAILURE

Heart failure is an overarching term for a syndrome (i.e., a constellation of signs and symptoms) that encompasses a vast spectrum of cardiovascular disorders and is associated with a greatly heightened risk of death and nonfatal adverse cardiovascular events (Chapter 57). Treatment is initially directed toward prevention of cardiac injury (e.g., due to hypertension or myocardial infarction) or toward limiting structural progression if cardiac damage has already occurred (e.g., left ventricular remodeling with declining left ventricular ejection fraction) and delaying the development of symptomatic heart failure. Once symptoms develop, treatments are also directed at improving functional status as well as prognosis.

Approximately one in five adults will develop heart failure. In the United States, the nearly 1 million annual hospitalizations with a primary diagnosis of heart failure account for 5 million hospital days. The estimated cost of heart failure management ranges from $15 billion to $40 billion annually, depending on the formula used.

Randomized controlled clinical trials (RCTs) supply the framework for quantifying what different therapeutic approaches can offer. Even when they are definitive, RCTs only generate data about average risks and benefits of the tested therapeutic option in a selected cohort. Because an individual patient's responses can only be implied from the overall estimated group responses, RCTs cannot definitively direct the approach of every patient or answer the myriad questions that confront the practitioner regarding the specific circumstances of the patient. Another major limitation of RCTs is the relatively narrow time frame of observation, generally only months to several years, compared with epidemiologic experiences during decades. Despite these limitations, RCTs are the premier tool of evidence-based medicine, and the field of heart failure has fortunately been the focus of relatively high quality RCTs that have provided robust evidence to improve clinical care and prognosis (Table 58–1). Indeed, the implementation of evidence from RCTs into clinical practice has resulted in impressive temporal improvements in survival after discharge from a first hospital admission for heart failure. Moreover, the age at which symptomatic heart failure first becomes evident has increased. Despite these tangible advances, heart failure continues to be a leading cause of morbidity and mortality in the elderly.

STAGES OF HEART FAILURE

The 2005 American Heart Association/American College of Cardiology Guidelines for the Evaluation and Management of Chronic Heart Failure in the Adult use a staging classification to underscore the evolution and progression of heart failure severity (Fig. 58–1). This classification emphasizes the use of different strategies and therapeutic options across the full spectrum of the syndrome, from prevention of heart failure to palliation of patients with end-stage disease.

Stage A: Individuals at Risk for Development of Heart Failure

Stage A designates patients at risk for development of heart failure based on concomitant cardiovascular diseases such as hypertension, coronary artery disease, and diabetes mellitus. Also included in stage A are individuals with prior exposure to cardiotoxic agents such as doxorubicin (Chapter 192) and those with a family history of a cardiomyopathy (Chapter 59). Although these predisposing factors do not by themselves technically constitute the syndrome of heart failure, the guidelines stress the importance of identifying individuals with modifiable factors because this represents an important opportunity to reduce the reservoir of patients at risk.

Population-based preventive approaches can reduce the incidence of heart failure. For example, public health programs targeting the eradication of the insect vector for *Trypanosoma cruzi* (Chapter 368) have reduced the incidence of Chagas' cardiomyopathy (Chapter 59) in endemic regions of South and Central America.

Other population-based approaches to reduce the incidence of heart failure require specific screening efforts to identify individuals with modifiable risk factors. The most important although unfortunately nonmodifiable risk factor for the development of heart failure is advanced age; the incidence of heart failure rises sharply per decade after the age of 45 years (Chapter 57). For each decade of age after 45 years, the incidence of heart failure doubles, and heart failure is the leading hospital diagnosis for patients older than 65 years in the United States.

Hypertension

Of the modifiable factors, hypertension (Chapter 66) undoubtedly contributes the greatest population attributable risk for heart failure. In other words, even though the increased risk of heart failure in an individual with hypertension is modest, the high prevalence of hypertension in the general population means that at a population level, hypertension is the major cause of heart failure.

The contribution of hypertension to the risk of heart failure was a consistent finding from all major cardiovascular epidemiologic studies, and the earliest RCTs of antihypertensive therapy showed unambiguous reductions in the risk of heart failure. Of the components of blood pressure, elevated systolic pressure has a greater influence on the incidence of heart failure than does diastolic pressure. In fact, aging is associated with

TABLE 58–1 CONTROLLED TRIALS* IN SYMPTOMATIC HEART FAILURE WITH REDUCED SYSTOLIC FUNCTION

Trial, Treatment, and Year Published	N	Severity of Heart Failure	Estimated First-Year Placebo/Control Group Mortality	Background Treatment†	Treatment Added	Trial Duration (years)	Primary End Point	Relative Risk Reduction (%)‡	Events Prevented per 1000 Patients Treated¶¶		
									DEATH	HF HOSP.	DEATH OR HF HOSP.
ACE INHIBITORS											
CONSENSUS, 1987[a]	253	End stage	52	Spironolactone	Enalapril, 20 mg bid	0.54‡	Death	40	146	—	—
SOLVD-T, 1991[b]	2569	Mild-severe	15.7	—	Enalapril, 20 mg bid	3.5	Death	16	45	96	108
β-BLOCKERS											
CIBIS-2, 1999[c]	2647	Moderate-severe	13.2	ACE-I	Bisoprolol, 10 mg qd	1.3‡	Death	34	55	56	—
MERIT-HF, 1999[d]	3991	Mild-severe	11.0	ACE-I	Metoprolol CR/XL, 200 mg qd	1.0‡	Death	34	36	46	63
COPERNICUS, 2001[e]	2289	Severe	19.7	ACE-I	Carvedilol, 25 mg bid	0.87‡	Death	35	55	65	81
ANGIOTENSIN RECEPTOR BLOCKERS											
Val-HeFT, 2001[8]	5010	Mild-severe	~8.0	ACE-I	Valsartan, 160 mg bid	1.9	CV death or morbidity	13	0	35	33¶
CHARM-Alternative, 2003[7]	2028	Mild-severe	12.6	BB	Candesartan, 32 mg qd	2.8	CV death or HF hosp.	23	30	31	60
CHARM-Added, 2003[9]	2548	Moderate-severe	10.6	ACE-I + BB	Candesartan, 32 mg qd	3.4	CV death or HF hosp.	15	28	47	39
ALDOSTERONE BLOCKADE											
RALES, 1999[11]	1663	Severe	~25	ACE-I	Spirolactone, 25–50 mg qd	2.0[‡]	Death	30	113	95	—
HYDRALAZINE-ISDN											
V-HeFT-1, 1986[f]	459	Mild-severe	26.4	—	Hydralazine, 75 mg tid-qid ISDN, 40 mg qid	2.3	Death	34	52	0	—
A-HeFT, 2004[14]	1050	Moderate-severe	~9.0	ACE-I + BB + spironolactone	Hydralazine, 75 mg tid ISDN, 40 mg tid	0.83‡	Composite	—	40	80	—
DIGITALIS GLYCOSIDES											
DIG, 1997[13]	6800	Mild-severe	~11.0	ACE-I	Digoxin	3.1	Death	0	0	79	73

Continued

TABLE 58–1 CONTROLLED TRIALS* IN SYMPTOMATIC HEART FAILURE WITH REDUCED SYSTOLIC FUNCTION—cont'd

Trial, Treatment, and Year Published	N	Severity of Heart Failure	Estimated First-Year Placebo/ Control Group Mortality	Background Treatment†	Treatment Added	Trial Duration (years)	Primary End Point	Relative Risk Reduction (%)‡	Events Prevented per 1000 Patients Treated¶¶		
									DEATH	HF HOSP.	DEATH OR HF HOSP.
CRT											
COMPANION, 2004[17]	925	Moderate-severe	19.0	ACE-I + BB + spironolactone	CRT	1.35[‡]	Death or any hospital admission	19	38	—	87
CARE-HF, 2005[g]	813	Moderate-severe	12.6	ACE-I + BB + spironolactone	CRT	2.45	Death or CV hospital admission	37	97	151	184
CRT-D											
COMPANION, 2004[17]	903	Moderate-severe	19.0	ACE-I + BB + spironolactone	CRT-ICD	1.35[‡]	Death or any hospital admission	20	74	—	114
IMPLANTABLE CARDIOVERTER DEFIBRILLATOR											
SCD-HeFT, 2005[16]	1676	Mild-severe	~7.0	ACE-I + BB	ICD	3.8	Death	23	—	—	—
VENTRICULAR ASSIST DEVICE											
REMATCH, 2001[h]	129	End stage	75	ACE-I + spironolactone	LVAD	1.8	Death	48	282	—	—

*Excluding active-controlled trials.
†In more than one third of patients, ACE-I + BB means that ACE inhibitors were used in almost all patients and BB in the majority; most patients were also taking diuretics, and many digoxin (except in DIG). Spironolactone was used at baseline in 5% Val-HeFT, 8% MERIT-HF, 17% CHARM-Added, 19% SCD-HeFT, 20% COPERNICUS, and 24% CHARM-Alternative.
‡Relative risk reduction in primary end point.
§Stopped early for benefit.
¶¶Individual trials may not have been designed or powered to evaluate effect of treatment on these outcomes.
¶Primary end point that also included treatment of heart failure with intravenous drugs for 4 hours or more without admission and resuscitated cardiac arrest (both added small numbers).
[a]The CONSENSUS Trial Study Group: Effects of enalapril on mortality in severe congestive heart failure. Results of the Cooperative North Scandinavian Enalapril Survival Study (CONSENSUS). N Engl J Med 1987;316:1429–1435.
[b]The SOLVD Investigators: Effect of enalapril on survival in patients with reduced left ventricular ejection fractions and congestive heart failure. N Engl J Med 1991;325:293–302.
[c]The Cardiac Insufficiency Bisoprolol Study II (CIBIS-II): A randomised trial. Lancet 1999;353:9–13.
[d]Effect of metoprolol CR/XL in chronic heart failure: Metoprolol CR/XL Randomised Intervention Trial in Congestive Heart Failure (MERIT-HF). Lancet 1999;353:2001–2007.
[e]Packer M, Coats AJ, Fowler MB, et al: Effect of carvedilol on survival in severe chronic heart failure. N Engl J Med 2001;344:1651–1658.
[f]Cohn JN, Archibald DG, Ziesche S, et al: Effect of vasodilator therapy on mortality in chronic congestive heart failure. Results of a Veterans Administration Cooperative Study. N Engl J Med 1986;314:1547–1552.
[g]Cleland JG, Daubert JC, Erdmann E, et al: The effect of cardiac resynchronization on morbidity and mortality in heart failure. N Engl J Med 2005;352:1539–1549.
[h]Rose EA, Gelijns AC, Moskowitz AJ, et al: Long-term mechanical left ventricular assistance for end-stage heart failure. N Engl J Med 2001;345:1435–1443.
ACE-I = ACE inhibitor; BB = β-blocker; CRT = cardiac resynchronization therapy (biventricular pacing); CRT-D = CRT device that also defibrillates; CV = cardiovascular; HF hosp. = patients with at least one hospital admission for worsening heart failure—some patients had multiple admissions; ICD = implantable cardioverter defibrillator; ISDN = isosorbide dinitrate; LVAD = left ventricular assist device.
Modified from McMurray JJ, Pfeffer MA: Heart failure. Lancet 2005;365:1877–1889.

a progressive rise in systolic blood pressure and fall in diastolic pressure as the compliance of the arterial tree diminishes (Chapter 66). In community-based studies, isolated systolic hypertension and elevated pulse pressure have been the most predictive blood pressure measurements for development of heart failure. In the Systolic Hypertension in the Elderly Program, one of the last placebo-controlled antihypertensive trials, antihypertensive treatment with chlorthalidone followed by atenolol reduced the incidence of new heart failure by about 50%. In general, the actual extent of blood pressure lowering achieved, not the agent used, is the most important factor in reducing overall rates of major cardiovascular events. However, the greatest reduction in risk of heart failure seems to be seen when initial therapy is based on a diuretic and angiotensin-converting enzyme (ACE) inhibitor. By comparison, treatment with α-blockers increases the risk of heart failure compared with other antihypertensive drugs. Most important, it is estimated that effective treatment of hypertension (Chapter 66) will substantially reduce the age-adjusted incidence of heart failure by approximately 60% in women and 50% in men.

Other Risk Factors

Treatment of atherosclerotic risk factors, such as hypercholesterolemia (Chapter 217), and promotion of measures that encourage healthier lifestyles, such as smoking cessation (Chapter 30), weight control (Chapter 239), and aerobic exercise (Chapter 14), should also reduce the number of individuals who progress from stage A to stage B (structural heart disease but without symptoms of heart failure). ACE inhibitors protect against the development of heart failure in patients with diabetes mellitus or with evidence of atherosclerosis. Although obesity is correlated with hypertension, lipid abnormalities, and glucose intolerance, an elevated body mass index is also an independent risk factor for the development of heart failure.

Stage B: Asymptomatic Structural or Functional Heart Disease

Stage B identifies asymptomatic (class I; Chapter 48) patients who have a structural or functional cardiac disorder (e.g., left ventricular hypertrophy, enlargement, or dysfunction and valvar abnormalities) but do not have the signs and symptoms, such as dyspnea and fatigue, of the heart failure syndrome. In addition to history, physical examination, and electrocardiography (Chapter 52), more extensive screening with echocardiography (Chapter 53) or other imaging modalities (Chapter 54) is often required to detect patients with asymptomatic cardiac structural abnormalities.

A patient who has an acute myocardial infarction is an obvious example of someone who transitions from stage A to stage B. Rapid pharmacologic or mechanical coronary reperfusion is one of the immediate goals of therapy, with the aim of limiting the extent of myocardial injury and reducing the risk of death and future development of heart failure (Chapters 71 and 72). Survivors of the acute phase of myocardial infarction, a well-studied stage B cohort, are at particularly high risk for the future development of heart failure, with an overall annual incidence of 2% per year—but higher in patients who are older, have a lower left ventricular ejection fraction (LVEF), do not routinely perform at least moderate exercise, or have concomitant hypertension or diabetes mellitus. For example, a clinically stable asymptomatic patient who has recovered from a myocardial infarction but who is older than 60 years with an LVEF of less than 50% and a history of diabetes and hypertension has an estimated 30% 5-year likelihood of experiencing death or heart failure; without diabetes or hypertension, the 5-year estimated rate becomes 12%. By comparison, a younger myocardial infarction survivor who has an LVEF over 50% and does not have hypertension or diabetes would be anticipated to have a 5-year rate for heart failure or death of only 3%. Recent data also suggest that an assessment of right ventricular function provides further independent incremental prediction for the risk of developing heart failure. With the continued improvements in care of patients with acute myocardial infarction (Chapters 71 and 72) and the use of implantable cardioverter defibrillators after myocardial infarction in patients with reduced LVEF, this pool of stage B patients, who represent a reservoir for new-onset heart failure, has been expanding.

The impaired left ventricle, often due to a prior myocardial infarction, can undergo progressive chamber enlargement. This process, also termed left ventricular remodeling, describes the time-dependent and often insidious structural alterations of the impaired left ventricle, whereby the relationship of the left ventricular cavity volume increases out of proportion to mass, so the overall ventricular geometry becomes more distorted, usually more spherical. These structural changes produce regional and global increases in myocardial wall stress, which can promote further remodeling and contribute to the progressive deterioration of cardiac function and structure often associated with the later stages of symptomatic heart failure.

Treatment

ACE Inhibitors and Angiotensin Receptor Blockers

Mechanistic studies confirm that ACE inhibitors inhibit progressive left ventricular enlargement by reducing wall stress during the entire cardiac cycle as well as by more direct inhibition of the intracellular signaling pathways involved in myocardial hypertrophy and interstitial fibrosis. This attenuation of ventricular remodeling by ACE inhibitors reduces the development of symptomatic heart failure and death in stage B asymptomatic patients with left ventricular dysfunction by about 20%. [1,2] In addition, deaths, often sudden and unexpected, attributed to cardiovascular causes, are reduced in stage B patients by ACE inhibitor therapy.

Several ACE inhibitors are effective as prophylactic therapy for high-risk stage B patients (see Fig. 58–1), and the target dose of each agent is established (Table 58–2). The angiotensin receptor blocker (ARB) valsartan (Table 58–3) is as effective as captopril in reducing risk of cardiovascular death and other nonfatal cardiovascular outcomes, [3] thereby providing an alternative pharmacologic class of agents. Importantly, in patients with left ventricular dysfunction or acute heart failure in the context of a myocardial infarction, the combination of an ACE inhibitor and ARB is not better than either alone, so combination therapy is not recommended in this setting.

β-Blockers

β-Adrenergic receptor blockers (β-blockers) have long been known to reduce death and recurrent myocardial infarction when they are administered during the acute phase of myocardial infarction in patients without pulmonary congestion (Chapter 72). However, carvedilol (Table 58–4) also improves survival, reduces subsequent nonfatal myocardial infarctions, and has a favorable trend for reduced hospitalizations for heart failure in patients with a recent myocardial infarction and reduced LVEF (≤40%) when it is added to an ACE inhibitor. [4] For stage B patients whose left ventricular dysfunction does not have an ischemic etiology, the evidence for β-blockers is less firm.

Treatment of Arrhythmias

Functional as well as structural problems may lead to the development of heart failure. For example, a persistently rapid ventricular rate in patients with atrial fibrillation can cause a rate-related (tachycardia-induced) cardiomyopathy (Chapter 63). Adequate pharmacologic control of the ventricular rate or interventions to restore sinus rhythm or to ablate re-entry pathways (Chapter 65) may reduce the risk of heart failure.

Other Therapies

Any treatments that control hypertension or reduce the risk of myocardial infarction will benefit stage B patients. Examples include statins, antiplatelet agents, and smoking cessation.

Stages C and D: Symptomatic Heart Failure

The development of symptoms and signs of the heart failure syndrome defines the transition from patients in the asymptomatic “at-risk” stages (A and B) to those who fulfill the clinical diagnosis of symptomatic heart failure (Chapter 57). This transition to the symptomatic phase underscores the progressive nature of heart failure and heralds a marked decline in prognosis. In one study, for example, the 2-year mortality rate was 27% in symptomatic patients compared with 10% in asymptomatic patients despite similarly reduced LVEFs and comorbidities.

Trials

Stage A	Stage B	Stage C	Stage D
High risk for HF without structural heart disease or symptoms of HF	**Structural heart disease but without signs or symptoms of HF**	**Structural heart disease with prior or current symptoms of HF**	**Refractory HF requiring specialized interventions**
Patients with • Hypertension • Artherosclerotic disease • Diabetes • Obesity • Metabolic syndrome or Patients using • Cardiotoxins with family history of cardiomyopathy (FHx CM)	Patients with • Previous MI • LV remodeling including LVH and low EF • Asymptomatic valvular disease	Patients with • Known structural heart disease • Shortness of breath and fatigue, reduced exercise tolerance	Patients with marked symptoms at rest despite maximal medical therapy (e.g., those who are recurrently hospitalized or cannot be safely discharged from the hospital without specialized interventions)
↓	↓	↓	↓
THERAPY	**THERAPY**	**THERAPY**	**THERAPY**

Goals
• Treat hypertension
• Encourage smoking cessation
• Treat lipid disorders
• Encourage regular exercise
• Discourage alcohol intake, illicit drug use
• Control metabolic syndrome
Drugs
• ACEI or ARB asappropriate patients for vascular or diabetes
	Goals
	• Treat hypertension
	• Encourage smoking cessation
	• Treat lipid disorders
	• Encourage regular exercise
	• Discourage alcohol intake, illicit drug use
	• Control metabolic syndrome
	Drugs
	• ACEI or ARB as appropriate patients for vascular or diabetes
	• Beta-blockers in appropriate patients
		Goals
		• Treat hypertension
		• Encourage smoking cessation
		• Treat lipid disorders
		• Encourage regular exercise
		• Discourage alcohol intake, illicit drug use
		• Control metabolic syndrome
		• Dietary salt restriction
		Drugs for routine use
		• ACEI
		• Beta-blockers in appropriate patients
		Drugs in selected patients
		• Aldosterone antagonist
		• ARBs
		• Digitalis
		• Hydralazine/nitrates
		Devices in selected patients
		• Biventricular pacing
		• Implantable defibrillators
			Goals
			• Appropriate measures under Stages A, B, C
			• Decision re: appropriate level of care
			Options
			• Compassionate end-of-life care/hospice
			• Extraordinary measures
			  • Heart transplant
			  • Chronic inotropes
			  • Permanent mechanical support
			  • Experimental surgery or drugs

Therapy	Stage A	Stage B	Stage C	Stage D
Antihypertensives	VA Study I and II SHEP HOT ALLHAT			
Statins	HPS WOSCOPS ASCOT-LLA AFCAPS-Texcaps	HPS 4S CARE →	→	→
Beta-blockers		BHAT Norwegian beta-blocker trial CAPRICORN	COPERNICUS CIBIS II MERIT HF COMET →	→
ACE inhibitors	HOPE EUROPA (PEACE)	SAVE AIRE TRACE SOLVD-P	SOLVD-T CONSENSUS →	→
Angiotensin II receptor blockers (ARBs)		VALIANT	CHARM alternative CHARM added Val-HeFT →	→
Hydralazine/ nitrates			V-HeFT I and II A-HeFT	
Digoxin			DIG	
Aldosterone antagonists		EPHESUS →	→ RALES →	→
Implantable cardioverter-defibrillator (ICD)		MADIT II	SCD-HeFT →	→
Cardiac resynchronization therapy (CRT)			COMPANION CARE HF →	→
Left ventricle assist device (LVAD)				REMATCH

TABLE 58–2 PRACTICAL GUIDANCE ON THE USE OF ANGIOTENSIN-CONVERTING ENZYME INHIBITORS IN PATIENTS WITH HEART FAILURE DUE TO LEFT VENTRICULAR SYSTOLIC DYSFUNCTION

WHY?

Two major randomized trials (CONSENSUS I and SOLVD-T) and a meta-analysis of smaller trials have conclusively shown that angiotensin-converting enzyme (ACE) inhibitors increase survival, reduce hospital admissions, and improve NYHA class and quality of life in patients with *all* grades of symptomatic heart failure. Other major randomized trials in patients with systolic dysfunction after acute myocardial infarction (SAVE, AIRE, TRACE) have shown that ACE inhibitors increase survival. In patients with heart failure (ATLAS), the composite end point of death or hospital admission was reduced by higher doses of ACE inhibitor compared with lower doses. ACE inhibitors have also been shown to delay or to prevent the development of symptomatic heart failure in patients with *asymptomatic* left ventricular systolic dysfunction.

IN WHOM AND WHEN?

Indications
- Potentially *all* patients with heart failure and a low ejection fraction
- First-line treatment (along with β-blockers) in patients with NYHA class II–IV heart failure; start as early as possible in course of disease. ACE inhibitors are also of benefit in patients with asymptomatic left ventricular systolic dysfunction (NYHA class I).

Contraindications:
- History of angioedema
- Known bilateral renal artery stenosis

Cautions/seek specialist advice
- Significant hyperkalemia ($K^+ > 5.0$ mmol/L)
- Significant renal dysfunction (creatinine 221 μmol/L or >2.5 mg/dL)
- Symptomatic or severe asymptomatic hypotension (systolic blood pressure <90 mm Hg)

Drug interactions to look out for
- K^+ supplements/K^+-sparing diuretics, e.g., amiloride and triamterene (beware combination preparations with furosemide)
- Aldosterone antagonists (spironolactone, eplerenone), angiotensin receptor blockers, NSAIDs*
- "Low-salt" substitutes with a high K^+ content

WHERE?

In the community for most patients
Exceptions—see Cautions/seek specialist advice

WHICH ACE INHIBITOR AND WHAT DOSE?

	Starting dose	*Target dose*
Captopril	6.25 mg thrice daily	50 mg thrice daily
Enalapril	2.5 mg twice daily	10–20 mg twice daily
Lisinopril	2.5–5.0 mg once daily	20–35 mg once daily
Ramipril	2.5 mg once daily	5 mg twice daily or 10 mg once daily
Trandolapril	0.5 mg once daily	4 mg once daily

HOW TO USE?

Start with a low dose (see above).
Double dose at *not less than* 2-week intervals.
Aim for target dose (see above) or, failing that, the highest tolerated dose.
Remember: *some* ACE inhibitor is better than no ACE inhibitor.
Monitor blood pressure and blood chemistry (urea/blood urea nitrogen, creatinine, K^+).
Check blood chemistry 1–2 weeks after initiation and 1–2 weeks after final dose titration.
When to stop up-titration, reduce dose, stop treatment—see PROBLEM SOLVING.
A specialist heart failure nurse may assist with education of the patient, follow-up (in person or by telephone), biochemical monitoring, and dose up-titration.

Continued

FIGURE 58–1 • Stages of heart failure (HF). 4S = Scandinavian Simvastatin Survival Study; AFCAPS-Texcaps = Air Force/Texas Coronary Atherosclerosis Prevention Study; A-HeFT = African American Heart Failure Trial; AIRE = Acute Infarction Ramipril Efficacy study; ALLHAT = Antihypertensive and Lipid Lowering to Prevent Heart Attack Trial; ASCOT-LLA = Anglo-Scandinavian Cardiac Outcomes Trial – Lipid Lowering Arm; BHAT = The Beta-Blocker Heart Attack Trial; CAPRICORN = Carvedilol Post-Infarct Survival Control in LV Dysfunction; CARE = Cardiac Resynchronization in Heart Failure; CARE HF = Cardiac Resynchronization in Heart Failure; CHARM added = Candesartan in Heart Failure—Added Trial; CHARM alternative = Candesartan in Heart Failure—Alternative Trial; CIBIS II = Cardiac Insufficiency Bisoprolol Study II; COMET = Carvedilol Or Metoprolol European Trial; COMPANION = Comparison of Medical Therapy, Pacing, and Defibrillation in Heart Failure; CONSENSUS = Cooperative North Scandinavian Enalapril Survival Study; COPERNICUS = Carvedilol Prospective Randomized Cumulative Survival Trial; DIG = Digitalis Investigation Group; EPHESUS = Eplerenone Post-Acute Myocardial Infarction Heart Failure Efficacy and Survival Study; EUROPA = European Trial on Reduction of Cardiac Events With Perindopril in Stable Coronary Artery Disease; HOPE = Heart Outcomes Prevention Evaluation; HOT = Hypertension Optimal Treatment; HPS = Heart Protection Study; MADIT II = Multicenter Automatic Defibrillator Implantation Trial II; MERIT-HF = Metoprolol CR/XL Randomized Intervention Trial in Congestive Heart Failure; PEACE = Prevention of Events with ACE inhibition; RALES = Randomised Aldactone Evaluation Study; REMATCH = Randomized Evaluation of Mechanical Assistance for the Treatment of Congestive Heart Failure; SAVE = Survival and Ventricular Enlargement trial; SCD-HeFT = Sudden Cardiac Death in Heart Failure Trial; SHEP = Systolic Hypertension in the Elderly Program; SOLVD-P = Studies of Left Ventricular Dysfunction-Prevention; SOLVD-T = Studies of Left Ventricular Dysfunction-Treatment; TRACE = Trandolapril Cardiac Evaluation; VALIANT = Valsartan in Acute Myocardial Infarction Trial; VHeFT = Vasodilator–Heart Failure Trials; WOSCOPS = West of Scotland Coronary Prevention Study.

TABLE 58–2 PRACTICAL GUIDANCE ON THE USE OF ANGIOTENSIN-CONVERTING ENZYME INHIBITORS IN PATIENTS WITH HEART FAILURE DUE TO LEFT VENTRICULAR SYSTOLIC DYSFUNCTION—cont'd

ADVICE TO PATIENT

Explain expected benefits (see WHY?).
Treatment is given to improve symptoms, to prevent worsening of heart failure leading to hospital admission, and to increase survival.
Symptoms improve within a few weeks to a few months of starting treatment.
Advise patients to report principal adverse effects, (i.e., dizziness/symptomatic hypotension, cough)—see PROBLEM SOLVING.
Advise patients to avoid NSAIDs* not prescribed by a physician (self-purchased over-the-counter) and salt substitutes high in K^+—see PROBLEM SOLVING.

PROBLEM SOLVING

Asymptomatic low blood pressure
- Does not usually require any change in therapy

Symptomatic hypotension
- If dizziness, lightheadedness, or confusion and a low blood pressure, reconsider need for nitrates, calcium-channel blockers,† and other vasodilators
- If no signs or symptoms of congestion, consider reducing diuretic dose
- If these measures do not solve problem, seek specialist advice.

Cough
- Cough is common in patients with heart failure, many of whom have smoking-related lung disease.
- Cough is also a symptom of pulmonary edema, which should be excluded when a new or worsening cough develops.
- ACE inhibitor–induced cough rarely requires treatment discontinuation.
- When a troublesome cough does develop (e.g., one stopping the patient from sleeping) and can be proved to be due to ACE inhibition (i.e., recurs after ACE inhibitor withdrawal and rechallenge), substitution of an angiotensin receptor blocker can be considered (see Table 58–3).

Worsening renal function
- Some rise in urea (blood urea nitrogen), creatinine, and potassium is to be expected after initiation of an ACE inhibitor; if an increase is small and asymptomatic, no action is necessary.
- An increase in creatinine of up to 50% above baseline, or 266 μmol/L (3 mg/dL), whichever is the smaller, is acceptable.
- An increase in potassium to ≤5.5 mmol/L is acceptable.
- If urea, creatinine, or potassium does rise excessively, consider stopping concomitant nephrotoxic drugs (e.g., NSAIDs*) and other potassium supplements or retaining agents (triamterene, amiloride, spironolactone-eplerenone‡) and, if no signs of congestion, reducing the dose of diuretic.
- If greater rises in creatinine or potassium than those outlined above persist despite adjustment of concomitant medications, the dose of the ACE inhibitor should be halved and blood chemistry rechecked within 1–2 weeks; if there is still an unsatisfactory response, specialist advice should be sought.
- If potassium rises to >5.5 mmol/L or creatinine increases by >100% or to above 310 μmol/L (3.5 mg/dL), the ACE inhibitor should be stopped and specialist advice sought.
- Blood chemistry should be monitored frequently and serially until potassium and creatinine have plateaued.

Note: It is very rarely necessary to stop an ACE inhibitor, and clinical deterioration is likely if treatment is withdrawn. Ideally, specialist advice should be sought before treatment discontinuation.
*Avoid nonsteroidal anti-inflammatory drugs (NSAIDs) unless essential.
†Calcium-channel blockers should be discontinued unless absolutely essential (e.g., for angina or hypertension).
‡The safety and efficacy of an ACE inhibitor used with an angiotensin receptor blocker *and* spironolactone (as well as β-blocker) are uncertain, and the use of all three inhibitors of the renin-angiotensin-aldosterone system together is not recommended.
Modified from McMurray J, Cohen-Solal A, Dietz R, et al: Practical recommendations for the use of ACE inhibitors, β-blockers, aldosterone antagonists and angiotensin receptor blockers in heart failure: Putting guidelines into practice. Eur J Heart Fail 2005;7:710–721.

Treatment

The goals of treatment for patients with stage C and stage D heart failure are relief of symptoms, avoidance of hospital admission, and prevention of premature death. In general, the preventive measures that are of value during stages A and B should be sustained in patients with stages C and D heart failure.

Heart Failure with Reduced Left Ventricular Ejection Fraction

Pharmacologic Treatment

Drugs are the mainstay of the treatment of patients with symptomatic heart failure on the basis of the cumulative experiences from RCTs (see Table 58–1), particularly for patients with reduced LVEF. However, devices and surgery have an important and increasing role in patients with advanced symptomatic heart failure (stages C and D; see Fig. 58–1). How care is structured and delivered is also important. Although lifestyle measures are also considered important, the evidence base for these interventions is less robust.

Rx

Diuretics

MECHANISM OF ACTION. Diuretics act by blocking sodium reabsorption at specific sites in the renal tubule, thereby enhancing urinary excretion of sodium and water.

CLINICAL BENEFITS. Although not proven to improve mortality and morbidity in large trials, diuretics are required in nearly all patients with symptomatic heart failure (stages C and D) to relieve dyspnea and the signs of sodium and water retention ("congestion"), that is, peripheral and pulmonary edema. No other treatment relieves symptoms and the signs of sodium and water overload as rapidly and effectively. Once a patient needs a diuretic, treatment is usually necessary for the rest of the patient's life, although the dose and type of diuretic may vary.

PRACTICAL USE. The key principle is to prescribe the minimum dose of diuretic needed to maintain an edema-free state ("dry weight"). Excessive use can lead to electrolyte imbalances, such as hyponatremia, hypokalemia (and risk of digitalis toxicity), hyperuricemia

TABLE 58–3 PRACTICAL GUIDANCE ON THE USE OF ANGIOTENSIN RECEPTOR BLOCKERS IN PATIENTS WITH HEART FAILURE DUE TO LEFT VENTRICULAR SYSTOLIC DYSFUNCTION

WHY?

Added to standard therapy, including an angiotensin-converting enzyme (ACE) inhibitor, in patients with all grades of symptomatic heart failure, the angiotensin receptor blockers (ARBs) valsartan and candesartan have been shown, in two major randomized trials (Val-HeFT and CHARM), to reduce heart failure hospital admissions, to improve NYHA class, and to maintain quality of life. The two CHARM low–left ventricular ejection fraction trials (CHARM-Alternative and CHARM-Added) also showed that candesartan reduced all-cause mortality. In patients previously intolerant of an ACE inhibitor, candesartan has been shown to reduce the risk of the composite outcome of cardiovascular death or heart failure hospitalization, to reduce the risk of heart failure hospital admission, and to improve NYHA class. These findings in heart failure are supported by another randomized trial in patients with left ventricular systolic dysfunction, heart failure, or both complicating acute myocardial infarction (VALIANT) in which valsartan was as effective as the ACE inhibitor captopril in reducing mortality and cardiovascular morbidity.

IN WHOM AND WHEN?

Indications
- Potentially *all* patients with heart failure
- First-line treatment (along with β-blockers) in patients with NYHA class II–IV heart failure intolerant of an ACE inhibitor
- Second-line treatment (after optimization of ACE inhibitor and β-blocker*) in patients with NYHA class II–IV heart failure

Contraindications
- Known bilateral renal artery stenosis

Cautions/seek specialist advice
- Significant hyperkalemia ($K^+ > 5.0$ mmol/L)
- Significant renal dysfunction (creatinine 221 μmol/L or >2.5 mg/dL)
- Symptomatic or severe asymptomatic hypotension (systolic blood pressure < 90 mm Hg)

Drug interactions to look out for
- K^+ supplements/K^+-sparing diuretics, e.g., amiloride and triamterene (beware combination preparations with furosemide)
- Aldosterone antagonists (spironolactone, eplerenone), ACE inhibitors, NSAIDs†
- "Low-salt" substitutes with a high K^+ content

WHERE?

In the community for most patients
Exceptions—see Cautions/seek specialist advice

WHICH ARB AND WHAT DOSE?

	Starting dose	*Target dose*
Candesartan	4 or 8 mg once daily	32 mg once daily
Valsartan	40 mg twice daily	160 mg twice daily

HOW TO USE?

Start with a low dose (see above).
Double dose at *not less than* 2-week intervals.
Aim for target dose (see above) or, failing that, the highest tolerated dose.
Remember: *some* ARB is better than no ARB.
Monitor blood pressure and blood chemistry (urea/blood urea nitrogen, creatinine, K^+).
Check blood chemistry 1–2 weeks after initiation and 1–2 weeks after final dose titration.
When to stop up-titration, reduce dose, stop treatment—see PROBLEM SOLVING.
A specialist heart failure nurse may assist with education of the patient, follow-up (in person or by telephone), biochemical monitoring, and dose up-titration.

ADVICE TO PATIENT

Explain expected benefits (see WHY?).
Treatment is given to improve symptoms, to prevent worsening of heart failure leading to hospital admission, and to increase survival.
Symptoms improve within a few weeks to a few months of starting treatment.
Advise patients to report principal adverse effect (i.e., report dizziness/symptomatic hypotension)—see PROBLEM SOLVING.
Advise patients to avoid NSAIDs† not prescribed by a physician (self-purchased over-the-counter) and salt substitutes high in K^+—see PROBLEM SOLVING.

PROBLEM SOLVING

Asymptomatic low blood pressure
- Does not usually require any change in therapy

Symptomatic hypotension
- If dizziness, lightheadedness, or confusion and a low blood pressure, reconsider need for nitrates, calcium-channel blockers,‡ and other vasodilators
- If no signs or symptoms of congestion, consider reducing diuretic dose
- If these measures do not solve problem, seek specialist advice.

Continued

TABLE 58–3 PRACTICAL GUIDANCE ON THE USE OF ANGIOTENSIN RECEPTOR BLOCKERS IN PATIENTS WITH HEART FAILURE DUE TO LEFT VENTRICULAR SYSTOLIC DYSFUNCTION—cont'd

Worsening renal function

Some rise in urea (blood urea nitrogen), creatinine, and potassium is to be expected after initiation of an ARB; if the increase is small and asymptomatic, no action is necessary.

An increase in creatinine of up to 50% above baseline, or 266 μmol/L (3 mg/dL), whichever is the smaller, is acceptable.

An increase in potassium to ≤5.5 mmol/L is acceptable.

If urea, creatinine, or potassium does rise excessively, consider stopping concomitant nephrotoxic drugs (e.g., NSAIDs†) and potassium supplements or retaining agents (triamterene, amiloride, spironolactone-eplerenone*) and, if no signs of congestion, reducing the dose of diuretic.

If greater rises in creatinine or potassium than those outlined above persist despite adjustment of concomitant medications, the dose of the ARB should be halved and blood chemistry rechecked within 1–2 weeks; if there is still an unsatisfactory response, specialist advice should be sought.

If potassium rises to >5.5 mmol/L or creatinine increases by >100% or to above 310 μmol/L (3.5 mg/dL), the ARB should be stopped and specialist advice sought.

Blood chemistry should be monitored frequently and serially until potassium and creatinine have plateaued.

Note: It is very rarely necessary to stop an ARB, and clinical deterioration is likely if treatment is withdrawn. Ideally, specialist advice should be sought before treatment discontinuation.

*The safety and efficacy of an ARB used with an ACE inhibitor *and* spironolactone (as well as a β-blocker) are uncertain, and the use of all three inhibitors of the renin-angiotensin-aldosterone system together is not recommended.

†Avoid nonsteroidal anti-inflammatory drugs (NSAIDs) unless essential.

‡Calcium-channel blockers should be discontinued unless absolutely essential (e.g., for angina or hypertension).

Modified from McMurray J, Cohen-Solal A, Dietz R, et al: Practical recommendations for the use of ACE inhibitors, β-blockers, aldosterone antagonists and angiotensin receptor blockers in heart failure: Putting guidelines into practice. Eur J Heart Fail 2005;7:710–721.

(and risk of gout), and uremia. The risk of renal dysfunction is increased by concomitant use of nonsteroidal anti-inflammatory drugs (NSAIDs). Diuretic-induced hypovolemia may also cause symptomatic hypotension and prerenal azotemia. Restriction of dietary sodium intake may help reduce but does not eliminate the requirement for diuretics. Diuretic dosing should be flexible, with temporary increases for evidence of fluid retention (e.g., increasing symptoms, weight gain, edema) and decreases for evidence of hypovolemia (e.g., as a consequence of increased electrolyte loss due to gastroenteritis, decreased fluid intake, or both).

In some patients with milder symptoms of heart failure (stage C), a thiazide diuretic such as chlorthalidone may suffice. In more advanced heart failure (stage D) or in patients with concomitant renal dysfunction, a loop diuretic such as furosemide is often needed. Loop diuretics cause a rapid onset of an intense but relatively short-lived diuresis compared with the longer lasting but gentler effect of a thiazide diuretic. The timing of administration of a loop diuretic, which need not be taken first thing every morning, can be adjusted according to the patient's social activities. The dose may be postponed or even temporarily omitted if the patient has to travel or has another activity that might be compromised by the prompt action of the diuretic. In severe heart failure (stage D), the effects of long-term administration of a loop diuretic may be diminished by increased sodium reabsorption at the distal tubule. This problem can be offset by use of the combination of a loop diuretic and a thiazide or thiazide-like diuretic (e.g., hydrochlorothiazide or metolazone), which act in synergy with a loop diuretic by blocking sodium reabsorption in different segments of the nephron. This combination requires more frequent monitoring of electrolytes and renal function for diuretic-induced hyponatremia, abnormalities of the serum potassium level, and prerenal azotemia.

A period of intravenous loop diuretic, given either as bolus injections or by continuous infusion, may be required in patients who become resistant to the action of oral diuretics. Why this resistance develops is uncertain, but factors thought to be important include impaired absorption of oral diuretics due to gut edema, hypotension, reduced renal blood flow, and adaptive changes in the nephron.

Patients with advanced heart failure (stage D) should usually also be treated with an aldosterone antagonist, such as spironolactone, which increases excretion of sodium but not of potassium. Patients receiving a combination of diuretics require careful monitoring of blood chemistry and clinical status. The use of a potassium-sparing diuretic or aldosterone antagonist along with an ACE inhibitor or ARB (treatment with all three is not recommended) requires particular care and surveillance for hyperkalemia.

Although they are highly effective in relieving symptoms and signs, diuretics alone are not sufficient for treatment of heart failure. In cases of severe resistant volume overload, mechanical removal of fluid by ultrafiltration may be considered. The addition of other treatments will better maintain clinical stability, slow structural progression, and reduce the risk of hospital admission and premature death.

ACE Inhibitors

MECHANISM OF ACTION. These drugs act by inhibiting the enzyme that converts the inactive decapeptide angiotensin I to the active octapeptide angiotensin II. In patients with heart failure, excessive angiotensin II is thought to exert myriad harmful actions mediated through stimulation of the angiotensin II type 1 receptor subtype (AT_1R), including vasoconstriction (which increases ventricular afterload), excessive growth of myocytes and the extracellular matrix (contributing to maladaptive left ventricular remodeling), activation of the sympathetic nervous system, prothrombotic actions, and augmentation of the release of arginine vasopressin and the retention of sodium (both directly and through stimulation of aldosterone secretion).

ACE inhibitors also reduce the breakdown of bradykinin (as ACE is identical to kininase II), and the resultant accumulation of bradykinin is directly or indirectly responsible for two of the specific adverse effects of ACE inhibitors, cough and angioedema. Bradykinin may, however, also have beneficial effects (vasodilation, inhibition of adverse cardiovascular remodeling, and antithrombotic actions), although the importance of these bradykinin-mediated actions to the clinical benefits of ACE inhibition is uncertain.

CLINICAL BENEFITS. Clinical trials have shown that treatment with an ACE inhibitor, when it is used alone or added to diuretics and digoxin, decreases left ventricular size, improves systolic function, reduces symptoms and hospital admissions, and prolongs survival 5,6 (see Table 58–1). These agents also reduce the risk for development of myocardial infarction, diabetes, and atrial fibrillation. Consequently, treatment with an ACE inhibitor is recommended for all patients with systolic dysfunction, irrespective of symptoms or etiology. ACE inhibitors are not a substitute for a diuretic but mitigate diuretic-induced hypokalemia.

PRACTICAL USE. ACE inhibitors should be introduced as early as possible in a patient's treatment. The only contraindications are current

TABLE 58–4 PRACTICAL GUIDANCE ON THE USE OF β-BLOCKERS IN PATIENTS WITH HEART FAILURE DUE TO LEFT VENTRICULAR SYSTOLIC DYSFUNCTION

WHY?

Several major randomized controlled trials (i.e., USCP, CIBIS II, MERIT-HF, COPERNICUS) have shown, conclusively, that certain β-blockers increase survival, reduce hospital admissions, and improve NYHA class and quality of life when added to standard therapy (diuretics, digoxin, and angiotensin-converting enzyme [ACE] inhibitors) in patients with *stable* mild and moderate heart failure and in some patients with severe heart failure. In the SENIORS trial, which differed substantially in design from the aforementioned studies (older patients, some patients with preserved left ventricular systolic function, longer follow-up), nebivolol appeared to have a smaller treatment effect, although direct comparison is difficult. One other trial (BEST) did not show a reduction in all-cause mortality but did report a reduction in cardiovascular mortality and is otherwise broadly consistent with the aforementioned studies. The COMET trial showed that carvedilol was substantially more effective than a low dose of short-acting metoprolol tartrate* (long-acting metoprolol succinate was used in MERIT-HF).

IN WHOM AND WHEN?

Indications
- Potentially *all* patients with *stable* mild and moderate heart failure; patients with severe heart failure should be referred for specialist advice
- First-line treatment (along with ACE inhibitors) in patients with *stable* NYHA class II–III heart failure; start as early as possible in course of disease

Contraindications
- Asthma
- Second- or thrid-degree atrioventricular block

Cautions/seek specialist advice
- Severe (NYHA class IV) heart failure
- Current or recent (<4 weeks) exacerbation of heart failure (e.g., hospital admission with worsening heart failure, heart block, or heart rate <60/minute).
- Persisting signs of congestion, hypotension/low blood pressure (systolic < 90 mm Hg), raised jugular venous pressure, ascites, marked peripheral edema

Drug interactions to look out for
- Verapamil, diltiazem (should be discontinued)†
- Digoxin, amiodarone

WHERE?

In the community in stable patients (NYHA class IV/severe heart failure patients should be referred for specialist advice)
Not in unstable patients hospitalized with worsening heart failure
Other exceptions—see Cautions/seek specialist advice

WHICH β-BLOCKER AND WHAT DOSE?

	Starting dose	*Target dose*
Bisoprolol	1.25 mg once daily	10 mg once daily
Carvedilol	3.125 mg twice daily	25–50 mg twice daily
Metoprolol CR/XL	12.5–25 mg once daily	200 mg once daily*
Nebivolol	1.25 mg once daily	10 mg once daily

HOW TO USE?

Start with a low dose (see above).
Double dose at *not less than* 2-week intervals.
Aim for target dose (see above) or, failing that, the highest tolerated dose.
Remember: *some* β-blocker is better than no β-blocker.
Monitor heart rate, blood pressure, and clinical status (symptoms, signs—especially signs of congestion, body weight).
Check blood chemistry 1–2 weeks after initiation and 1–2 weeks after final dose titration.
When to stop up-titration, reduce dose, stop treatment—see PROBLEM SOLVING.
A specialist heart failure nurse may assist with education of the patient, follow-up (in person or by telephone), and dose up-titration.

ADVICE TO PATIENT

Explain expected benefits (see WHY?).
Treatment is given to improve symptoms, to prevent worsening of heart failure leading to hospital admission, and to increase survival.
Symptomatic improvement may develop slowly after starting treatment, taking 3–6 months or longer.
Temporary symptomatic deterioration *may* occur during initiation or up-titration phase; in the long term, β-blockers improve well-being.
Advise patient to report deterioration (see PROBLEM SOLVING) and that deterioration (tiredness, fatigue, breathlessness) can usually be easily managed by adjustment of other medication; patients should be advised not to stop β-blocker therapy without consulting the physician.
To detect and to treat deterioration early, patients should be encouraged to weigh themselves daily (after waking, before dressing, after voiding, before eating) and to increase their diuretic dose should their weight increase, persistently (>2 days), by >1.5–2.0 kg.‡

Continued

Section VIII Cardiovascular

TABLE 58–4 PRACTICAL GUIDANCE ON THE USE OF β-BLOCKERS IN PATIENTS WITH HEART FAILURE DUE TO LEFT VENTRICULAR SYSTOLIC DYSFUNCTION—cont'd

PROBLEM SOLVING

Worsening symptoms or signs (e.g., increasing dyspnea, fatigue, edema, weight gain)
- If increasing congestion, increase dose of diuretic or halve dose of β-blocker (if increasing diuretic does not work)
- If marked fatigue (or bradycardia—see below), halve dose of β-blocker (rarely necessary); review patient in 1–2 weeks; if not improved, seek specialist advice
- If serious deterioration, halve dose of β-blocker or stop this treatment (rarely necessary); seek specialist advice

Low heart rate
- If <50 beats/minute and worsening symptoms, halve dose of β-blocker or, if severe deterioration, stop β-blocker (rarely necessary)
- Review need for other heart rate–slowing drugs (e.g., digoxin, amiodarone, diltiazem, or verapamil†)
- Arrange electrocardiogram to exclude heart block
- Seek specialist advice

Asymptomatic low blood pressure
- Does not usually require any change in therapy

Symptomatic hypotension
- If dizziness, lightheadedness, or confusion and a low blood pressure, reconsider need for nitrates, calcium-channel blockers,† and other vasodilators
- If no signs or symptoms of congestion, consider reducing diuretic dose or ACE inhibitor
- If these measures do not solve problem, seek specialist advice.

Note: β-Blockers should not be stopped suddenly unless absolutely necessary (there is a risk of a "rebound" increase in myocardial ischemia or infarction and arrhythmias). Ideally, specialist advice should be sought before treatment discontinuation.
*Metoprolol tartrate should not be used in preference to an evidence-based β-blocker in heart failure.
†Calcium-channel blockers should be discontinued unless absolutely necessary, and diltiazem and verapamil are generally contraindicated in heart failure.
‡This is generally good advice for all patients with heart failure.
Modified from McMurray J, Cohen-Solal A, Dietz R, et al: Practical recommendations for the use of ACE inhibitors, β-blockers, aldosterone antagonists and angiotensin receptor blockers in heart failure: Putting guidelines into practice. Eur J Heart Fail 2005;7:710–721.

Rx

symptomatic hypotension and bilateral renal artery stenosis (Chapter 126); the latter is often associated with a prompt and marked increase in serum levels of blood urea nitrogen and creatinine when renal perfusion is reduced precipitously by inhibiting the production and actions of angiotensin. Treatment should be started in a low dose (see Table 58–2), with the dose gradually increased toward a target dose proven of benefit in a clinical trial. The patient should be evaluated for symptomatic hypotension, uremia, and hyperkalemia after each dose increment; these adverse effects are uncommon and can usually be resolved by reduction in the dose of diuretic (if the patient is edema free) or concomitant hypotensive or nephrotoxic medications (e.g., nitrates, calcium-channel blockers, or NSAIDs). A dry, nonproductive cough occurs in approximately 15% of patients treated with an ACE inhibitor, and if it is troublesome, substitution of an ARB is recommended. In the rare cases of angioedema (Chapter 273), the ACE inhibitor should be stopped and not used again; an ARB can be cautiously substituted.

Angiotensin Receptor Blockers

MECHANISM OF ACTION. Instead of inhibiting the production of angiotensin II through ACE, ARBs block the binding of angiotensin II to the AT_1R. This pharmacologically distinct mechanism of action may be important because angiotensin II is also believed to be produced by other enzymes, such as chymase. ARBs do not inhibit kininase II or the breakdown of bradykinin, so they do not cause cough and cause less angioedema than do ACE inhibitors.

CLINICAL BENEFITS. When they are used as the sole agent in heart failure, ARBs produce benefits similar to those of ACE inhibitors and can be substituted for them in patients who have cough or angioedema with ACE inhibitors. [7,8] When they are used in clinically effective doses, other adverse effects such as hypotension, renal dysfunction, and hyperkalemia are encountered as frequently as with an ACE inhibitor. As with an ACE inhibitor, the specific agents, dosing regimens, and target doses that were of demonstrable benefit in clinical trials are recommended (see Table 58–1).

In the broader population of patients with symptomatic (stage C or stage D, functional class II–IV) heart failure that can be treated with an ACE inhibitor, an ARB *in combination* with an ACE inhibitor (and β-blocker) further improves LVEF, relieves symptoms, reduces the risk of hospital admission for worsening heart failure, and can also reduce the risk of cardiovascular death (see Table 58–3). [8,9] Consequently, the addition of an ARB to both an ACE inhibitor and a β-blocker should be considered in any patient with persisting symptoms (stages C and D). There is, however, also strong evidence that addition of an aldosterone antagonist to an ACE inhibitor is of benefit in patients with advanced (class III–IV) heart failure (see later), but the efficacy and safety of the four-drug combination of an ACE inhibitor, β-blocker, ARB, and aldosterone antagonist are uncertain. Consequently, either an ARB or an aldosterone antagonist, but not both, should be added to an ACE inhibitor and a β-blocker in such patients.

The approach to initiation, titration, and monitoring of an ARB is similar to that of an ACE inhibitor (see Table 58–3). The adverse effects, with the exception of cough and angioedema, are similar. Use of multiple inhibitors of the renin-angiotensin-aldosterone system requires even more diligent monitoring, especially in patients at higher risk of uremia, hypotension, or hyperkalemia (i.e., patients 75 years of age and older or with a systolic blood pressure below 100 mm Hg, diabetes, or renal impairment).

As with ACE inhibitors, β-blockers, and aldosterone antagonists, treatment with ARBs should be indefinite unless there is intolerance.

β-Blockers

MECHANISM OF ACTION. Heart failure is characterized by excessive activation of the sympathetic nervous system, which causes vasoconstriction and sodium retention, thereby increasing cardiac preload and afterload and often inducing myocardial ischemia or arrhythmias. In addition, norepinephrine can cause hypertrophy of myocytes and augment their apoptosis. β-Blockers counteract many of these harmful effects of the hyperactivity of the sympathetic nervous system.

CLINICAL BENEFITS. The long-term addition of a β-blocker to an ACE inhibitor (and diuretic and digoxin) further improves left ventricular function and symptoms, reduces hospital admissions, and strikingly improves survival. [10] Consequently, a β-blocker is recommended for all patients with symptomatic systolic dysfunction, irrespective of etiology and severity, and the combination of a β-blocker with an ACE inhibitor is now the cornerstone of the treatment of symptomatic heart failure (see Fig. 58–1).

Rx

PRACTICAL USE. The major contraindications to use of a β-blocker in heart failure are asthma (although it is important to note that the dyspnea caused by pulmonary congestion can be confused with reactive airway disease) and second- or third-degree atrioventricular block. Initiation of treatment during an episode of acute decompensated heart failure should also generally be avoided. In addition, caution is advised in patients with a heart rate below 60 beats per minute or a systolic blood pressure below 90 mm Hg. It is recommended that a β-blocker shown to produce benefits in a randomized trial be used (see Table 58–1).

Like ACE inhibitors, β-blockers should be introduced as early as possible in a patient's treatment, started in a low dose (see Table 58–4), and increased gradually toward a target dose used in a clinical trial (the "start low–go slow" approach). The patient should be checked for symptomatic hypotension and excessive bradycardia after each dose increment, but both of these side effects are uncommon, and hypotension can often be resolved by reduction in the dose of other nonessential blood pressure–lowering medications (e.g., nitrates and calcium-channel blockers). Bradycardia is more likely in patients who are also taking digoxin or amiodarone, and the simultaneous use of these agents should be reviewed if excessive bradycardia occurs. On occasion, symptomatic worsening and fluid retention (e.g., weight gain or edema) may occur after initiation of a β-blocker or during dose up-titration; these side effects usually can be resolved by a temporary increase in the diuretic dose without necessitating discontinuation of the β-blocker.

Treatment with a β-blocker should be given for life, although the dose may need to be decreased or discontinued during episodes of acute decompensation if the patient shows signs of circulatory underperfusion or refractory congestion.

Aldosterone Antagonists

MECHANISM OF ACTION. Aldosterone, which is the second effector hormone in the renin-angiotensin-aldosterone cascade, has detrimental vascular, renal, autonomic, and cardiac actions when it is produced in excess in patients with heart failure. Excessive aldosterone promotes sodium retention and hypokalemia, and it is believed to contribute to myocardial fibrosis, all of which predispose to arrhythmias. Aldosterone antagonists block these undesirable actions and act as potassium-sparing diuretics.

CLINICAL BENEFITS. The aldosterone antagonist spironolactone (Table 58–5) improves symptoms, reduces hospital admissions, and increases survival when it is added to an ACE inhibitor (and diuretics and digoxin) in patients with a reduced LVEF and severely symptomatic heart failure. [11] Eplerenone, another aldosterone antagonist, reduces mortality and morbidity when it is added to both an ACE inhibitor and β-blocker in patients with a reduced LVEF and heart failure or diabetes after a recent myocardial infarction [12] (see Table 58–5). Consequently, an aldosterone antagonist should be considered in patients who remain in severe heart failure (class III or IV) despite treatment with a diuretic, ACE inhibitor (or ARB), and β-blocker. When begun, it should be given indefinitely. The value of an aldosterone antagonist in patients with milder heart failure is uncertain, and at present, the combination of an ACE inhibitor, an ARB, and an aldosterone antagonist has not been adequately evaluated and is not recommended.

Treatment with an aldosterone antagonist should be initiated with a low dose (see Table 58–5) with careful monitoring of serum electrolytes and renal function. Hyperkalemia and uremia are the adverse effects of greatest concern (as with ACE inhibitors and ARBs), and an aldosterone antagonist should not be given to patients with a serum potassium concentration of more than 5.0 mmol/L, serum creatinine concentration above 2.5 mg/dL (>221 μmol/L), or other evidence of markedly impaired renal function. The importance of selection of patients and dose is underscored by reports of a worrisome incidence of serious hyperkalemia in community practice settings. Spironolactone can have antiandrogenic effects, especially painful gynecomastia, in men; because eplerenone does not block the androgen receptor, it is a reasonable substitute in patients who experience this adverse effect.

Rx

Digoxin

MECHANISM OF ACTION. Digitalis glycosides inhibit the cell membrane Na^+,K^+-ATPase pump, thereby increasing intracellular calcium and myocardial contractility. In addition, digoxin is thought to enhance parasympathetic and reduce sympathetic nervous activity as well as to inhibit renin release.

CLINICAL BENEFITS. Only one large RCT has examined the effects of starting (as opposed to withdrawing) digoxin on mortality and morbidity in patients with heart failure in sinus rhythm. In that trial, digoxin did not reduce mortality but did decrease the risk of admission to hospital for worsening heart failure when it was added to a diuretic and an ACE inhibitor. [13] In patients in sinus rhythm, addition of digoxin is recommended only for those whose heart failure remains symptomatic despite standard three-drug treatment with a diuretic, ACE inhibitor, and β-blocker plus an ARB or aldosterone antagonist. In patients with atrial fibrillation, digoxin may be used at an earlier stage if a β-blocker fails to control the ventricular rate (ideally less than 70/minute at rest and less than 100/minute during exercise; Chapter 63). Digoxin can also be used to control the ventricular rate when β-blocker treatment is being initiated or up-titrated.

If the effect of digoxin is needed urgently, loading with 10 to 15 μg/kg *lean* body weight, given in three divided doses 6 hours apart, may be used. The maintenance dose should be one third of the loading dose. Smaller maintenance doses (e.g., one quarter of the loading dose and not more than 62.5 μg/day) should be used in the elderly and in patients with reduced renal function as well as in patients with a low body mass. Monitoring of the serum digoxin concentration is recommended because of the narrow therapeutic window. A steady state is reached 7 to 10 days after treatment is started; blood should be collected at least 6 hours (and ideally 8 to 24 hours) after the last dose. The currently recommended therapeutic range is 0.5 to 1.0 ng/mL).

Digoxin can cause anorexia, nausea, arrhythmias, confusion, and visual disturbances, especially if the serum concentration is above 2.0 ng/mL. Hypokalemia increases susceptibility to the adverse effects. The dose of digoxin should be reduced in the elderly and patients with renal dysfunction. Certain drugs increase serum digoxin concentration, including amiodarone.

Hydralazine and Isosorbide Dinitrate

MECHANISM OF ACTION. Hydralazine is a powerful direct-acting arterial vasodilator. Its mechanism of action is not understood, although it may inhibit enzymatic production of superoxide, which neutralizes nitric oxide and may induce nitrate tolerance. Nitrates dilate both veins and arteries, thereby reducing preload and afterload by stimulating the nitric oxide pathway and increasing cyclic guanosine monophosphate in vascular smooth muscle. Neither drug on its own nor any other direct-acting vasodilator has been demonstrated to be beneficial in heart failure.

CLINICAL BENEFITS. Although this combination has been known for some time to improve systolic function and to reduce death in class II–IV heart failure compared with placebo, head-to-head comparisons showed that an ACE inhibitor is superior for improving survival. Nevertheless, on the basis of subgroup analyses suggesting that African Americans responded better to hydralazine and isosorbide dinitrate, a subsequent RCT showed that the addition of hydralazine and isosorbide dinitrate in African Americans, most of whom were receiving an ACE inhibitor and β-blocker and many of whom were taking spironolactone, further reduced mortality and hospital admissions for heart failure and improved quality of life. [14] A fixed combination of 37.5 mg of hydralazine and 20 mg of isosorbide dinitrate was used in the trial; one tablet was given and if tolerated, a second was given 12 hours later. One tablet was then prescribed three times daily for 3 to 5 days, at which point the dose was increased to the target maintenance of two tablets three times daily, that is, a daily dose of 225 mg hydralazine and 120 mg isosorbide dinitrate. Because of the limited inclusion criteria of this RCT, however, it is uncertain whether this combination of vasodilators is an effective addition in other populations of patients.

PRACTICAL USE. Other than for African Americans, the main indication for hydralazine and isosorbide dinitrate is as a substitute in

TABLE 58–5 PRACTICAL GUIDANCE ON THE USE OF SPIRONOLACTONE IN PATIENTS WITH HEART FAILURE DUE TO LEFT VENTRICULAR SYSTOLIC DYSFUNCTION

WHY?

The RALES study showed that low-dose spironolactone increased survival, reduced hospital admissions, and improved NYHA class when added to standard therapy (diuretic, digoxin, angiotensin-converting enzyme [ACE] inhibitor, and, in a minority of cases, β-blocker) in patients with severe (NYHA class III or IV) heart failure. These findings in heart failure are supported by another randomized trial in patients with left ventricular systolic dysfunction and heart failure (or diabetes) complicating *acute* myocardial infarction (EPHESUS), in which another aldosterone antagonist, eplerenone, increased survival and reduced hospital admissions for cardiac causes.

IN WHOM AND WHEN?

Indications
- Potentially all patients with symptomatically moderately severe or severe heart failure (class III–IV NYHA)
- Second-line therapy (after ACE inhibitors and β-blockers*) in patients with NYHA class III–IV heart failure; there is no evidence of benefit in patients with milder heart failure

Cautions/seek specialist advice
- Significant hyperkalemia ($K^+ > 5.0$ mmol/L)†
- Significant renal dysfunction (creatinine > 221 μmol/L or 2.5 mg/dL)†

Drug interactions to look out for
- K^+ supplements/K^+-sparing diuretics, (e.g., amiloride and triamterene; beware combination preparations with furosemide)
- ACE inhibitors, angiotensin receptor blockers, NSAIDs‡

"Low-salt" substitutes with a high K^+ content

WHERE?

In the community or in the hospital
Exceptions—see Cautions/seek specialist advice

WHICH DOSE?†

	Starting dose	*Target dose*
Spironolactone	25 mg once daily or on alternate days	25–50 mg once daily
Eplerenone	25 mg once daily	50 mg once daily

HOW TO USE?

Start with a low dose (see above).
Check blood chemistry at 1, 4, 8, and 12 weeks; 6, 9, and 12 months; 6-monthly thereafter.
If K^+ rises above 5.5 mmol/L or creatinine rises to 221 μmol/L (2.5 mg/dL), reduce dose to 25 mg on alternate days and monitor blood chemistry closely.
If K^+ rises to >6.0 mmol/L or creatinine to >310 μmol/L (3.5 mg/dL), stop spironolactone immediately and seek specialist advice.
A specialist heart failure nurse may assist with education of the patient, follow-up (in person or by telephone), biochemical monitoring, and dose up-titration.

ADVICE TO PATIENT

Explain expected benefits (see WHY?).
Treatment is given to improve symptoms, to prevent worsening of heart failure leading to hospital admission, and to increase survival.
Symptom improvement occurs within a few weeks to a few months of starting treatment.
Avoid NSAIDs‡ not prescribed by a physician (self-purchased over-the-counter) and salt substitutes high in K^+.
If diarrhea or vomiting occurs, patients should stop spironolactone and contact the physician.

PROBLEM SOLVING

Worsening renal function/hyperkalemia
- See HOW TO USE? section.

Major concern is hyperkalemia (>6.0 mmol/L); although this was uncommon in RALES, it has been seen more commonly in clinical practice. Conversely, a high-normal potassium level may be desirable in patients with heart failure, especially if they are taking digoxin.
It is important to avoid other K^+-retaining drugs (e.g., K^+-sparing diuretics such as amiloride and triamterene) and nephrotoxic agents (e.g., NSAIDs‡)
The risk of hyperkalemia and renal dysfunction when an aldosterone antagonist is given to patients already taking an ACE inhibitor *and* angiotensin receptor blocker is higher than when an aldosterone antagonist is added to just an ACE inhibitor or angiotensin receptor blocker given singly; close and careful monitoring is mandatory.*
Some "low-salt" substitutes have a high K^+ content.
Male patients treated with spironolactone may develop breast discomfort or gynecomastia (these problems are significantly less common with eplerenone).

*The safety and efficacy of spironolactone used with an ACE inhibitor *and* an angiotensin receptor blocker (as well as a β-blocker) are uncertain, and the use of all three inhibitors of the renin-angiotensin-aldosterone system together is not recommended.
†It is extremely important to adhere to these cautions and doses in light of recent evidence of serious hyperkalemia with spironolactone in usual clinical practice in Ontario.
‡Avoid nonsteroidal anti-inflammatory drugs (NSAIDs) unless essential.
Modified from McMurray J, Cohen-Solal A, Dietz R, et al: Practical recommendations for the use of ACE inhibitors, β-blockers, aldosterone antagonists and angiotensin receptor blockers in heart failure: Putting guidelines into practice. Eur J Heart Fail 2005;7:710–721.

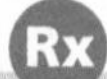

patients with intolerance to an ACE inhibitor and an ARB. Hydralazine and isosorbide dinitrate should be used as additional treatment in African Americans and considered for other patients who remain symptomatic with other proven therapies. The main dose-limiting adverse effects with hydralazine and isosorbide dinitrate are headache and dizziness. A rare adverse effect of higher doses of hydralazine, especially in slow acetylators, is a systemic lupus erythematosus–like syndrome (Chapter 287).

Other Pharmacologic Issues

Other therapies of proven value for cardiovascular conditions underlying or associated with heart failure, but not specifically tested in heart failure, include statins (Chapter 217) and antiplatelet treatment in patients with coronary heart disease (Chapter 35). Warfarin is indicated in patients with atrial fibrillation, provided there is no contraindication to its use (Chapter 63). Warfarin may also be used in patients with evidence of intracardiac thrombus (e.g., detected during echocardiographic examination) or systemic thromboembolism. The many interactions of warfarin with other drugs, including some statins and amiodarone (Chapter 35), must always be considered when warfarin or another drug in a patient taking warfarin is initiated. Heparin prophylaxis (Chapter 35) against deep venous thrombosis is indicated when patients with heart failure are bed bound, for example, during hospital admission.

Vaccination against influenza and pneumococcal infection is advised (Chapter 16) in all patients with heart failure. The stress of even mild infection can lead to clinical deterioration.

The aforementioned treatments are the only pharmacologic therapies shown to be of benefit in patients with heart failure and a reduced LVEF. Other treatments have been tested in randomized trials and shown to have a neutral (e.g., amlodipine) or uncertain (e.g., bosentan and etanercept) effect on mortality and morbidity or to increase mortality (e.g., milrinone, flosequinan, vesnarinone, and moxonidine).

Drugs to Use with Caution in Heart Failure

Patients with heart failure, especially if it is severe, often have renal and hepatic dysfunction, so any drug excreted predominantly by the kidneys or metabolized by the liver may accumulate (Chapter 27). Similarly, because of their extensive comorbidity, patients with heart failure are inevitably treated with multiple drugs, thereby increasing the risk of drug interactions.

Drugs that should be avoided, if possible, in heart failure include most antiarrhythmic drugs (with the exception of amiodarone and dofetilide), most calcium-channel blockers (with the exception of amlodipine), corticosteroids, NSAIDs, and many antipsychotics and antihistamines. Metformin (because of the risk of lactic acidosis) and thiazolidinediones (because of the risk of fluid retention) should be used with caution. Some salt substitutes contain substantial amounts of potassium and must be used cautiously. Other dietary constituents (e.g., grapefruit and cranberry juice) and supplements such as St. John's wort can interact with drugs taken by patients with heart failure, especially warfarin and digoxin.

Organization of Care

Several studies have shown that organized, nurse-led, multidisciplinary care can improve outcomes in patients with heart failure, particularly by reducing recurrent hospital admissions. The most successful approach seems to involve education of the patients, their families, and caregivers about heart failure and its treatment (including flexible diuretic dosing and reinforcing the importance of adherence), recognizing (and acting on) early deterioration (dyspnea, weight gain, edema), and optimizing proven pharmacologic treatments. [15] A home-based rather than clinic-based approach may be best, although trials are needed to compare these types of interventions directly. Even telephone follow-up is of value. New technology enabling noninvasive home telemonitoring of physiologic measures (e.g., heart rate and rhythm, blood pressure, temperature, respiratory rate, weight, and estimated body water content) and implanted devices, which collect similar data and may be interrogated remotely, are also being tested as aids to monitoring and management.

TABLE 58–6 TOPICS THAT SHOULD BE DISCUSSED WITH A PATIENT WITH HEART FAILURE AND WITH HIS OR HER FAMILY AND CAREGIVERS

- General advice
  - Explain what heart failure is and why symptoms occur
    - Causes of heart failure
    - How to recognize symptoms
    - What to do if symptoms occur
    - Self-weighing (to identify fluid retention)
  - Rationale for treatments
  - Importance of adhering to pharmacologic and nonpharmacologic (e.g., dietary) treatments
  - Smoking advice
  - Prognosis
- Drug counseling
  - Rationale (i.e., benefits of individual drugs)
  - Dose and time of administration
  - Potential adverse affects (and what, if any, action to take)
  - What to do in case of missed or skipped doses
  - Self-management (e.g., flexible diuretic dosing)
- Rest and exercise
  - Rest
  - Exercise and activities related to work
  - Daily physical activity
  - Sexual activity
  - Rehabilitation
- Vaccinations and immunizations
- Travel
- Driving
- Dietary and social habits
  - Control sodium intake when necessary (e.g., some patients with severe heart failure)
  - Avoid excessive fluids in severe heart failure
  - Avoid excessive alcohol intake

Modified from Swedberg K, Cleland J, Dargie H, et al; Task Force for the Diagnosis and Treatment of Chronic Heart Failure of the European Society of Cardiology: Guidelines for the diagnosis and treatment of chronic heart failure: Executive summary (update 2005). Eur Heart J 2005;26:1115–1140.

Education

Education of the patient, family, and caregivers is invaluable (Table 58–6). Detection of early signs and symptoms of deterioration provides for earlier intervention. Counseling on the proper use of therapies, with an emphasis on adherence, is critical.

Useful patient-oriented material is available from the Heart Failure Society of America (*http://www.hfsa.org/hf_modules.asp*), American Heart Association (*http://www.americanheart.org/presenter.jhtml?identifier=1486*), National Heart, Lung and Blood Institute (*http://www.nhlbi.nih.gov/*), and other organizations.

MEDICATION USE COUNSELING. When appropriate, a patient should be taught how to adjust the dose of diuretic within individualized limits. The dose should be increased (or a supplementary diuretic added) if there is evidence of fluid retention (symptoms of congestion) and decreased if there is evidence of hypovolemia (e.g., increased thirst associated with weight loss or postural dizziness, especially during hot weather or an illness causing decreased fluid intake or sodium and water loss). If hypovolemia is more marked, the doses of other medications also will have to be reduced.

The expected effects, beneficial and adverse, of other drugs should also be explained in detail (e.g., possible association of cough with ACE inhibitor). It is useful to inform patients that improvement with many drugs is gradual and may become fully apparent only after several weeks or even months of treatment. It is also important to explain the need for gradual titration with ACE inhibitors, ARBs, and β-blocking drugs to a desired dose level, which again may take weeks or even months to achieve. Patients should be advised not to use NSAIDs without consultation and to be cautious about using herbal or other nonproprietary preparations (Chapter 36).

Rx

ADHERENCE. Education and counseling of the patient, caregiver, and family promotes adherence, which is associated with better outcomes. Drug adherence can also be helped by certain pharmacy aids, such as dose allocation (dosette) boxes.

EXERCISE. Exercise helps avoid physical deconditioning and improves symptoms and functional capacity. Exercise should be tailored according to the individual patient's clinical status, and the optimal regimen in heart failure is uncertain. Aerobic exercise, such as walking at a rate and distance that do not cause undue symptoms, is thought to be safe and beneficial.

DIET, NUTRITION, ALCOHOL. Most guidelines advocate avoidance of foods containing relatively high salt content in the belief that doing so may reduce the need for diuretic therapy. Although there is little evidence from clinical trials to support this recommendation, clinical experience suggests that excess sodium intake can be a precipitant of clinical decompensation. Some salt substitutes have a high potassium content, which can lead to hyperkalemia.

Restriction of fluid intake is indicated only during episodes of decompensation associated with peripheral edema or hyponatremia. In these situations, daily intake should be restricted to 1.5 to 2.0 L to help facilitate reduction in extracellular fluid volume and to avoid hyponatremia.

Reducing excessive weight will reduce the work of the heart and may lower blood pressure (Chapter 66). Conversely, malnutrition is common in severe heart failure, and the development of cardiac cachexia is an ominous sign. Reduced food intake is sometimes caused by nausea (e.g., related to digoxin use or hepatosplenic congestion) or abdominal bloating (e.g., due to ascites). In these cases, small frequent meals and high-protein and high-calorie liquids may be helpful. In severe decompensated heart failure, eating may be difficult because of dyspnea.

Moderate alcohol intake is not thought to be harmful in heart failure, although excessive intake can cause cardiomyopathy and atrial arrhythmias in susceptible individuals. In patients with suspected alcoholic cardiomyopathy, abstinence from alcohol may improve cardiac function.

SMOKING. Smoking causes peripheral vasoconstriction, which is detrimental in heart failure. Nicotine replacement therapy (Chapter 30) is believed to be safe in heart failure. The safety of bupropion in heart failure is uncertain, especially as it is known to increase blood pressure.

SEXUAL ACTIVITY. Sexual activity need not be restricted in patients with compensated heart failure, although dyspnea may be limiting. In men with erectile dysfunction (Chapter 253), treatment with a cyclic guanine monophosphate phosphodiesterase type 5 inhibitor can be useful, but these drugs must not be taken within 24 hours of prior nitrate use, and nitrates must not be restarted for at least 24 hours afterwards.

DRIVING. Patients with heart failure can continue to drive, provided their condition does not induce undue dyspnea, fatigue, or other incapacitating symptoms. Patients with recent syncope, cardiac surgery, percutaneous coronary intervention, or device placement may be restricted from driving, at least temporarily, according to local regulations. Patients holding an occupational or commercial license may also be subject to additional restrictions.

TRAVELING. Short flights are unlikely to cause problems for a patient with compensated heart failure. Cabin pressure is generally maintained to provide an oxygen level no lower than equivalent to 6000 feet above sea level, which should be well tolerated in patients without severe pulmonary disease or pulmonary hypertension. Longer journeys may cause limb edema and dehydration, thereby predisposing to venous thrombosis. Adjustment of the dose of diuretics and other treatments should be discussed with the patient wishing to travel to a warm climate or a country where the risk of gastroenteritis is high. It is also advisable for heart failure patients to carry a list of medications and contact information for their health care provider.

Comorbidity

Comorbid conditions, which are common and important in patients with heart failure, may be due to the underlying cardiovascular disease that caused or contributed to heart failure (e.g., hypertension, coronary artery disease, diabetes mellitus), may arise as a complication of heart failure (e.g., arrhythmias), or can result from an adverse effect of treatment given for heart failure (e.g., gout). The exact causes of other comorbidities in heart failure, such as renal dysfunction and anemia, are complex and uncertain. These and other comorbid conditions, such as chronic obstructive pulmonary disease and asthma, are important because they are a major determinant of prognosis and may limit the use of certain treatments for heart failure (e.g., renal dysfunction limiting use of ACE inhibitors or asthma limiting β-blockers) and because treatment of comorbidities may affect the stability of heart failure (e.g., NSAIDs needed for rheumatic conditions can cause salt and water retention and renal dysfunction). Both prevention (e.g., diabetes mellitus) and treatment (e.g., anemia) of comorbidities are being evaluated as a potential new therapeutic goal in heart failure.

ANGINA. β-Blockers are of benefit in both angina (Chapter 70) and heart failure. Nitrates relieve angina but on their own are not of proven value in chronic heart failure. Calcium-channel blockers should generally be avoided in heart failure as they have a negative inotropic action and cause peripheral edema; only amlodipine has been shown to have no adverse effect on survival. Percutaneous (Chapter 73) and surgical (Chapter 74) revascularization is also of value in relieving angina in selected patients with heart failure.

ATRIAL FIBRILLATION. Atrial fibrillation (Chapter 63) may be the cause of or a consequence of heart failure in a patient presenting with atrial fibrillation and a rapid ventricular rate, and the distinction can be difficult, especially as prolonged atrial fibrillation may lead to a rate-related cardiomyopathy. Thyrotoxicosis (Chapter 244) and mitral valve disease (Chapter 75), especially stenosis, must be excluded. Alcohol abuse should also be considered. β-Blockers and digoxin are given to control the ventricular rate. The patient should be supervised closely after the initiation of these treatments because underlying sinus node dysfunction may raise the risk of bradycardia. Unless the patient presents emergently with symptoms or signs of heart failure, myocardial ischemia, or hypertension, there is little or no evidence to support a strategy of restoring sinus rhythm rather than controlling the ventricular rate in most patients with heart failure (Chapter 63). Atrioventricular node ablation and pacing may be required to control ventricular rate (Chapter 65). There is current interest in catheter ablation to cure atrial fibrillation in patients with heart failure, although this approach remains experimental (Chapter 65). There is a strong indication for thromboembolism prophylaxis with warfarin in patients with heart failure and atrial fibrillation (Chapter 63).

ASTHMA AND REVERSIBLE AIRWAYS OBSTRUCTION. Asthma is a contraindication for use of a β-blocker, but most patients with chronic obstructive pulmonary disease (Chapter 88) can tolerate a β-blocker. Pulmonary congestion can mimic chronic obstructive pulmonary disease. Systemic administration of a corticosteroid to treat reversible airways obstruction may cause sodium and water retention and exacerbate heart failure, whereas inhalation therapy is better tolerated.

DIABETES MELLITUS. Diabetes mellitus is discussed in detail elsewhere (Chapters 247 and 248). The prevalence and incidence of diabetes mellitus are high in heart failure, and the risk for development of type 2 diabetes may be reduced by ACE inhibitors and ARBs. β-Blocker treatment is not contraindicated and is of benefit in patients with diabetes and heart failure. Thiazolidinediones cause sodium and water retention and may lead to decompensation. Metformin may cause lactic acidosis. As a result, neither drug is recommended in patients with severe heart failure.

ABNORMAL THYROID FUNCTION. Both thyrotoxicosis and hypothyroidism can cause heart failure (and thyrotoxicosis can cause atrial fibrillation, which may precipitate heart failure). Amiodarone can also induce both hypothyroidism and hyperthyroidism, the latter being particularly difficult to diagnose.

GOUT. Hyperuricemia and gout (Chapter 294) are common in heart failure and, in part, are caused by diuretic treatment. Allopurinol may prevent gout, and acute attacks are better treated with colchicine, oral steroids, or intra-articular steroids rather than by an NSAID.

RENAL DYSFUNCTION. Most patients with heart failure have a reduced glomerular filtration rate. ACE inhibitors, ARBs, and aldosterone antagonists often cause a further small reduction in glomerular filtration rate and rise in serum blood urea nitrogen and creatinine levels, which, if limited, should not lead to discontinuation of treatment. Marked increases in blood urea nitrogen and creatinine, however, should prompt consideration of underlying renal artery stenosis (Chapter 126). Renal dysfunction may also be caused by sodium and water depletion, leading to relative hypovolemia (e.g., due to excessive diuresis, diarrhea, and vomiting) or hypotension. Nephrotoxic agents such as NSAIDs are also a common cause of renal dysfunction in heart failure.

PROSTATIC OBSTRUCTION. For prostatic disease (Chapter 130), a 5α-reductase inhibitor may be preferable to an α-adrenoceptor antagonist, which can cause hypotension and salt and water retention. Prostatic obstruction should also be considered in male patients with deteriorating renal function.

ANEMIA. A normocytic, normochromic anemia (Chapter 169) is also common in heart failure, in part because of the high prevalence of renal dysfunction. Malnutrition and blood loss may also contribute. The role of erythropoietic stimulating substances in treatment of the anemia of heart failure is under investigation.

DEPRESSION. Depression (Chapter 420) is common in patients with heart failure, perhaps partly owing to disturbance of the hypothalamic-pituitary axis and other neurochemical pathways but also as a result of social isolation and the adjustment to chronic disease. Depression is associated with worse functional status, reduced adherence to treatment, and poor clinical outcomes. Both psychosocial interventions and pharmacologic treatment are helpful. Selective serotonin reuptake inhibitors are believed to be the best tolerated pharmacologic agents, whereas tricyclic antidepressants should be avoided because of their anticholinergic actions and potential to cause arrhythmias.

CANCER. Many anticancer drugs, particularly anthracyclines, cyclophosphamide, and trastuzumab (Herceptin), can cause myocardial damage and heart failure, as can mediastinal radiotherapy. Pericardial constriction can be a result of previous radiotherapy, and malignant pericardial involvement can cause effusion and tamponade (Chapter 77).

Devices and Surgery

Implantable Cardioverter Defibrillators

About half of patients with heart failure die suddenly, mainly as the result of a ventricular arrhythmia. The relative risk of sudden death, as opposed to death from progressive heart failure, is greatest in patients with milder heart failure. In patients with more advanced heart failure, progressive pump failure deaths are relatively more common. Antiarrhythmic drugs have not been shown to improve survival in heart failure, but implantable cardioverter defibrillators (Chapter 65) reduce the risk of death in selected patients after myocardial infarction (Chapter 72) and improve survival in patients with class II–III heart failure and systolic dysfunction who were otherwise treated with optimal medical therapy. [16,17] There is still no consensus about exactly which patients with heart failure should receive an implantable cardioverter defibrillator, but patients with class II and class III heart failure and LVEF below 30% without other conditions greatly limiting life expectancy or the quality of life should be considered.

Cardiac Resynchronization Therapy

About 25% of patients with heart failure have substantial prolongation of the QRS duration on the surface electrocardiogram, which is a marker of abnormal electrical activation of the left ventricle causing dyssynchronous contraction, less efficient ventricular emptying, and, often, mitral regurgitation. Atrioventricular coupling may also be abnormal, as reflected by a prolonged PR interval, as may interventricular synchrony. Cardiac resynchronization therapy (CRT) with atrial-biventricular or multisite pacing optimizes atrioventricular timing and improves synchronization of cardiac contraction. In selected patients with severe heart failure, CRT improves pump function, reduces mitral regurgitation, relieves symptoms, and significantly prolongs exercise capacity. In two major trials, CRT reduced the composite of death or hospital admission in patients with severe heart failure (see Table 58–1) by more than 35%, [17,18] and in one trial it also reduced the risk of death from any cause by 36%. [18] Many other outcome measures, including quality of life, were also improved.

The current debate focuses on how best to select patients who will benefit from CRT. The key trials to date selected patients on the basis of a markedly prolonged QRS duration, usually manifested as left bundle branch block and a QRS duration of more than 120 msec. Tissue Doppler echocardiography and other imaging techniques may become alterna-tives for identifying patients likely to benefit from CRT, although such approaches remain to be proved. Whether patients with right bundle branch block, atrial fibrillation, dyssynchrony without marked QRS prolongation, and milder heart failure are helped by CRT is uncertain. There is no consensus yet about whether (or in whom) CRT alone or a CRT with implantable cardioverter defibrillator capabilities should be used.

Surgery

With the exception of cardiac transplantation and ventricular assist devices, there are no generally accepted criteria for surgical intervention. Use of operative procedures is therefore variable among centers and greatly dependent on local experience and expertise. Expert imaging and detailed hemodynamic and functional assessments are usually required when any patient with heart failure is considered for surgery, and close liaison between the relevant experts in these fields is essential. The collective expertise in surgical centers is often used to make highly individualized decisions about whether to operate and what procedures will be attempted. "Established" operative treatments for patients with heart failure include coronary artery bypass grafting, surgery for mitral valve incompetence, left ventricular remodeling surgery (including aneurysmectomy), implantation of ventricular assist devices, and heart transplantation. "Experimental" approaches include ventricular constraint devices and intramyocardial cell transplantation.

PERCUTANEOUS CORONARY INTERVENTION OR CORONARY ARTERY BYPASS GRAFTING. Percutaneous coronary intervention (Chapter 73) or coronary artery bypass grafting (Chapter 74), as appropriate, is indicated for relief of angina. The extent of ischemia and residual myocardial viability can be determined by noninvasive assessments such as dobutamine echocardiography (Chapter 53), magnetic resonance imaging (Chapter 55), and positron emission tomographic scanning (Chapter 54) in patients with impaired LVEF. Whether coronary artery bypass grafting is beneficial in patients with coronary artery disease but without angina is uncertain, but it is postulated that improvement of coronary blood flow to viable but noncontracting ("hibernating") myocardium may improve ventricular function and clinical outcomes even in patients without provokable ischemia.

LEFT VENTRICULAR ASSIST DEVICES. One RCT showed that a left ventricular assist device led to a short but significant prolongation of survival in patients who had end-stage heart failure and were ineligible for transplantation. However, the rates of infective and thrombotic complications as well as mechanical dysfunction are high with these devices, and the technology is evolving rapidly because of the limited availability of donor organs. These devices are increasingly used both as a "bridge to transplantation" and even as a final "destination therapy," that is, as the permanent, definitive procedure for some patients with advanced heart failure.

CARDIAC TRANSPLANTATION. Cardiac transplantation (Chapter 82) remains the most accepted surgical intervention in heart failure. Selection criteria usually focus on patients with refractory heart failure, that is, those with severe symptoms and functional limitations (peak oxygen consumption of less than 10 mL/kg/min), as well as a particularly worrisome clinical course and prognosis. These patients are often dependent on intravenous inotropic agents.

The role of surgical ventricular remodeling and surgery for mitral valve incompetence is currently under evaluation. Cardiomyoplasty and partial left ventriculectomy are recently developed operations for heart failure now thought to be without benefit.

Heart Failure with Preserved Left Ventricular Ejection Fraction (Diastolic Dysfunction)

Although all patients with symptomatic heart failure share a constellation of signs and symptoms, impaired physical capacity, and

Rx

reduced quality of life, some have a preserved LVEF (generally above 40 or 50%) and are classified as having diastolic heart failure (Chapter 57). Diastolic heart failure often has a cause different from that of systolic heart failure and a better survival rate (Chapters 50, 57, and 59), but sometimes it is simply the early manifestation of what will evolve into heart failure with a reduced LVEF. The distinction is important, however, because most of the RCTs that generated the evidence for treatment of heart failure included only patients with reduced LVEFs (see Table 58–1). Treatment of the underlying cardiovascular and other disorders that contribute to symptomatic stage C and stage D of heart failure with preserved LVEF, such as hypertension, myocardial ischemia, and diabetes, is critical and is as for stages A and B (see earlier). In patients with atrial fibrillation, control of the ventricular rate with a β-blocker or a rate-limiting calcium-channel blocker (or restoration of sinus rhythm) is particularly important (Chapter 63). Diuretics are used empirically to treat sodium and water retention, according to the same principles as in heart failure with reduced LVEF. Treatment with an ARB decreases the risk of hospital admission for heart failure but not the composite outcome of cardiovascular death or hospital admission for worsening heart failure. [19] Smaller studies in patients in sinus rhythm have shown that the calcium-channel blocker verapamil or the nonselective β-adrenergic blocker propranolol can improve symptoms and exercise capacity in patients with heart failure and preserved LVEF, possibly by reducing heart rate and thereby increasing the duration of diastolic left ventricular filling as well as by directly enhancing myocardial relaxation. There are, however, no RCTs in which these drugs decisively reduced mortality or morbidity in patients with heart failure and preserved LVEF, so treatment currently is aimed to relieve symptoms.

Heart Failure Due to Valvular Heart Disease

Heart failure also can arise as a result of regurgitant and stenotic valve disease (Chapter 75). It can sometimes be difficult to determine whether mitral regurgitation is primary or secondary in a patient with heart failure and left ventricular dilation, although a prior history of known valve disease or rheumatic fever may suggest a primary valve problem. The objective of treatment of primary valve disease is the prevention of heart failure by surgical repair or replacement of the diseased valve or valves (Chapter 75). The development of overt heart failure is an ominous sign, sometimes requiring emergent valve replacement (e.g., aortic stenosis) but sometimes indicating that valve replacement may not be possible (e.g., because of severe pulmonary hypertension). Surgery sometimes will result in clinical improvement (e.g., mitral valve surgery in a patient with severe mitral regurgitation), but some patients will have such advanced left ventricular dysfunction that they will not achieve substantial benefit. Valve repair or annuloplasty may, however, have a role in the treatment of some carefully selected patients with secondary mitral regurgitation caused or exacerbated by left ventricular dilation.

Heart Failure Due to Nonischemic Cardiomyopathy

Patients with heart failure and normal coronary arteries should be evaluated for possible reversible causes. Untreated hypertension is now an unusual cause of dilated cardiomyopathy in the United States, but hypertension was once a leading cause in the United States and still remains a major consideration in many parts of the world. Infiltrative cardiomyopathies (e.g., hemochromatosis, amyloid, sarcoid) sometimes have specific recommended therapies (Chapters 59, 95, 231, and 296). Chagas' disease (Chapter 368) must be considered in patients from endemic areas. However, most cases of nonischemic cardiomyopathy will be "idiopathic" (i.e., no specific etiology can be determined), and these patients should be treated in the same way as are patients whose dilated, poorly contracting left ventricle is a result of coronary artery disease.

Heart failure can arise in patients with hypertrophic cardiomyopathy because of predominant diastolic dysfunction, associated mitral incompetence, or the development of systolic dysfunction. The management of hypertrophic cardiomyopathy and its complications is oftentimes very different from the management of dilated

TABLE 58–7 SOME COMMON PRECIPITATING CAUSES OF HEART FAILURE

Myocardial ischemia or infarction
Atrial fibrillation or other supraventricular tachycardias
Uncontrolled hypertension
Valvar disease
Ventricular tachycardia
Pulmonary embolism
Pericardial disease
Sepsis
Anemia
Nutritional and medical noncompliance
Adverse drug effects
Hyperthyroidism or hypothyroidism

From Kimmelstiel CD, DeNofrio D, Konstam MA: Heart failure. *In* Wachter RM, Goldman L, Hollander H (eds): Hospital Medicine, 2nd ed. Philadelphia, Lippincott Williams & Wilkins, 2005, p 360.

Rx

cardiomyopathy (Chapter 59), thereby underscoring the value of echocardiography in the evaluation of the patient with heart failure.

Acute Decompensated Heart Failure and Pulmonary Edema

Patients presenting with acute heart failure include those who develop heart failure "de novo" as a consequence of another cardiac event, usually a myocardial infarction, and those who present for the first time with decompensation of previously asymptomatic and often unrecognized cardiac dysfunction (patients previously in stage B). However, because of frequent recurrences, most episodes of acute decompensation occur in patients with established, chronic heart failure that has worsened as a result of the unavoidable natural progression of the syndrome, with an intercurrent cardiac (e.g., arrhythmia) or noncardiac (e.g., pneumonia) event, or as a consequence of an avoidable reason, such as nonadherence with treatment or use of an agent that can alter renal function. Although it is not always identified, searching for a reversible precipitant is an important aspect of the initial therapy plan (Table 58–7).

Most patients with acute heart failure require admission to the hospital, especially if pulmonary edema is present. In contrast to chronic heart failure, data from RCTs generally are not available to guide effective therapy for patients with acute decompensated heart failure. The principal goals of management of this heterogeneous group of patients are to relieve symptoms, the most important of which is extreme dyspnea, and to maintain or to restore vital organ perfusion. An intravenous bolus or infusion of a loop diuretic, an intravenous opiate, and, in hypoxemic patients, oxygen are the key first-line treatments. Intravenous infusion of a nitrate is also valuable in patients with a systolic blood pressure of 100 mm Hg or higher (Fig. 58–2). Intravenous nesiritide (human B-type natriuretic peptide) can reduce the pulmonary capillary wedge pressure more promptly than intravenous nitroglycerin, but the effect of this short-term therapy on other clinical outcomes is controversial. In volume overloaded patients with severe heart failure unresponsive to diuretics, ultrafiltration is an option at specialized centers.

In patients with marked hypotension or other evidence of organ hypoperfusion, an inotropic agent such as dobutamine or a phosphodiesterase inhibitor (e.g., milrinone) should be considered, although neither treatment has ever been shown to reduce in-hospital deaths. In some countries, the calcium sensitizer levosimendan is also available for use in these patients. In general, potent inotropic agents should be used in a cardiac monitored setting at the lowest clinically effective dose and for the shortest duration possible (Chapter 108). Although there are limited data supporting a benefit, low-dose dopamine may be administered in an attempt to improve renal function.

In more critically ill patients, mechanical support (e.g., with an intra-aortic balloon pump) may also be considered (Chapter 108).

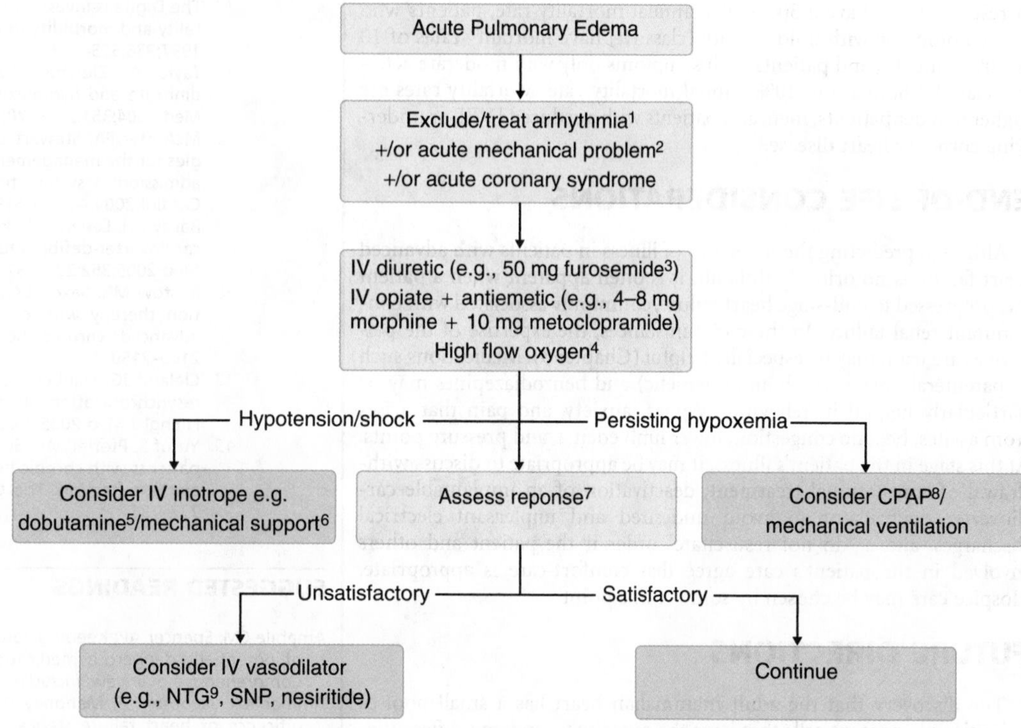

[1] Causal arrhythmia (e.g., ventricular tachycardia). It can be difficult to determine whether atrial fibrillation is a primary cause of acute pulmonary edema or secondary to it. An ECG is an essential investigation.

[2] Acute mechanical problems include ventricular septal rupture and mitral valve papillary muscle rupture. Mechanical support (e.g., an intra-aortic balloon pump) and urgent surgery should be considered. An echocardiogram should be performed as soon as possible, especially in a patient without a prior diagnosis of heart failure/other relevant heart disease (e.g., prior myocardial infarction or valve disease).

[3] Dose of diuretic depends on prior diuretic use and renal function—a lower dose may suffice if preserved renal function and no prior diuretic use.

[4] Oxygen causes an increase in systemic vascular resistance and a reduction in heart rate and cardiac output and should only be administered to patients with hypoxemia.

[5] e.g., an intra-aortic balloon pump

[6] An intravenous infusion of dobutamine may be started at a dose of 2.5 μg/kg/min, doubling every 15 minutes according to response and tolerability (dose titration usually limited by excessive tachycardia, arrhythmias or ischemia). A dose above 20 μg/kg/min is rarely needed.

[7] Improvement in symptoms and peripheral perfusion and adequate urine output—patient should be monitored closely and usually a response will occur within 30 minutes. Bladder catheterization may help in monitoring urine output.

[8] Continuous Positive Airways Pressure (CPAP) is valuable in severe pulmonary edema, especially if associated with hypoxemia. Endotracheal intubation and mechanical ventilation should be considered in patients with persisting hypoxemia and physical ventilatory exhaustion.

[9] An intravenous infusion of nitroglycerin (NTG) should be started at a dose of 10 μg/min and doubled every 10 minutes according to response and tolerability (usually dose up-titration is limited by hypotension). A dose of more than 100 μg/min is rarely needed.

FIGURE 58–2 • Approach to the patient with acute pulmonary edema.

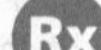

The aim of treatment is to support the patient's circulation and vital organ function until either the patient's own heart recovers or a definitive operative procedure can be performed (e.g., transplantation or permanent implantation of a ventricular assist device).

In patients admitted to the hospital, discharge planning and subsequent management to reduce the risk of readmission are important. Ideally, an effective oral diuretic regimen should have been identified, and fluid-volume and biochemical stability should have been achieved. This optimization of volume status and development of a stable oral regimen before discharge is thought to reduce the risk of early readmission. Treatment with an ACE inhibitor, β-blocker, and ARB or aldosterone antagonist, as appropriate, should also be started and titrated in the stabilized patient before discharge. Outpatient follow-up should be arranged to ensure that any of those treatments that have not been started before discharge are initiated after discharge and that the dose of each drug is increased, as tolerated, to the appropriate target.

Outpatient Follow-up

The key to successful follow-up is the careful tracking of clinical symptoms and the patient's weight, which often involves interviewing not only the patient but also family members, who may be more aware of changes in status than the patient is. Continuity of care and seamless transitions from the inpatient to the outpatient setting are crucial aspects of optimal management. Patients with advanced heart failure and patients requiring frequent hospitalization require special handling. Programs that provide telephone-based tracking of daily weights and symptoms can detect deterioration in time to intervene before the need for hospitalization. Although these programs may be costly, several evaluations have found them to be cost-effective. Because the management of these patients requires considerable experience and expertise, specialized heart failure programs and clinics have been developed and may provide additional benefit compared with traditional care.

Prognosis

The prognosis of patients with heart failure is poor despite advances in therapy. Of patients who survive the acute onset of heart failure, only 35% of men and 50% of women are alive after 5 years. Although it is difficult to predict prognosis in individual patients, patients with symptoms at rest (class IV) have a 30 to 50% annual mortality rate, patients who are symptomatic with mild activity (class III) have mortality rates of 10 to 20% annually, and patients with symptoms only with moderate activity (class II) have a 5 to 10% annual mortality rate. Mortality rates are higher in older patients, men, and patients with a reduced LVEF or underlying coronary heart disease.

END-OF-LIFE CONSIDERATIONS

Although predicting the trajectory of illness in patients with advanced heart failure is notoriously difficult, it is often apparent when a patient has progressed to end-stage heart failure, commonly associated with concomitant renal failure. In these circumstances, the expertise of the palliative care team may be especially helpful (Chapter 3). Medications such as parenteral opiates (with an antiemetic) and benzodiazepines may be particularly helpful in relieving dyspnea, anxiety, and pain that arises from ascites, hepatic congestion, lower limb edema, and pressure points. At this stage in the patient's illness, it may be appropriate to discuss withdrawal of conventional treatment, deactivation of an implantable cardioverter defibrillator to avoid undesired and unpleasant electrical discharges, and a "do not resuscitate" order if the patient and others involved in the patient's care agree that comfort-care is appropriate. Hospice care may be chosen by some at this point.

FUTURE DIRECTIONS

The discovery that the adult mammalian heart has a small pool of primitive pluripotent cells that have the capacity to undergo differentiation and to restore contractile tissue has generated considerable optimism about novel clinical approaches for the treatment of patients with impaired systolic function. Although animal studies have shown that stem cells can be isolated from the myocardium and can differentiate into contractile tissue to populate damaged areas, data in humans with use of progenitor cells from the bone marrow are suggestive but too preliminary.

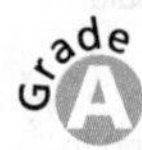

1. Pfeffer MA, Braunwald E, Moyé LA, et al: Effect of captopril on mortality and morbidity in patients with left ventricular dysfunction after myocardial infarction. Results of the survival and ventricular enlargement trial. The SAVE Investigators. N Engl J Med 1992;327:669–677.
2. Effect of enalapril on mortality and the development of heart failure in asymptomatic patients with reduced left ventricular ejection fractions. N Engl J Med 1992;327:685–691.
3. Pfeffer MA, McMurray JJ, Velazquez EJ, et al: Valsartan, captopril, or both in myocardial infarction complicated by heart failure, left ventricular dysfunction, or both. N Engl J Med 2003;349:1893–1906.
4. Dargie HJ: Effect of carvedilol on outcome after myocardial infarction in patients with left-ventricular dysfunction: The CAPRICORN randomised trial. Lancet 2001;357:1385–1390.
5. Effects of enalapril on mortality in severe congestive heart failure. Results of the Cooperative North Scandinavian Enalapril Survival Study (CONSENSUS). The CONSENSUS Trial Study Group. N Engl J Med 1987;316:1429–1435.
6. Effect of enalapril on survival in patients with reduced left ventricular ejection fractions and congestive heart failure. The SOLVD Investigators. N Engl J Med 1991;325:293–302.
7. Granger CB, McMurray JJ, Yusuf S, et al: Effects of candesartan in patients with chronic heart failure and reduced left-ventricular systolic function intolerant to angiotensin-converting-enzyme inhibitors: The CHARM-Alternative trial. Lancet 2003;362:772–776.
8. Cohn JN, Tognoni G: A randomized trial of the angiotensin-receptor blocker valsartan in chronic heart failure. N Engl J Med 2001;345:1667–1675.
9. McMurray JJ, Östergren J, Swedberg K, et al: Effects of candesartan in patients with chronic heart failure and reduced left-ventricular systolic function taking angiotensin-converting-enzyme inhibitors: The CHARM-Added trial. Lancet 2003;362:767–771.
10. Packer M, Coats AJ, Fowler MB, et al: Effect of carvedilol on survival in severe chronic heart failure. N Engl J Med 2001;344:1651–1658.
11. Pitt B, Zannad F, Remme WJ, et al: The effect of spironolactone on morbidity and mortality in patients with severe heart failure. Randomized Aldactone Evaluation Study Investigators. N Engl J Med 1999;341:709–717.
12. Pitt B, Remme W, Zannad F, et al: Eplerenone, a selective aldosterone blocker, in patients with left ventricular dysfunction after myocardial infarction. N Engl J Med 2003;348:1309–1321.
13. The Digitalis Investigation Group: The effects of digoxin on mortality and morbidity in patients with heart failure. N Engl J Med 1997;336:525–533.
14. Taylor AL, Ziesche S, Yancy C, et al: Combination of isosorbide dinitrate and hydralazine in blacks with heart failure. N Engl J Med 2004;351:2049–2057.
15. McAlister FA, Stewart S, Ferrua S, et al: Multidisciplinary strategies for the management of heart failure patients at high risk for admission: A systematic review of randomized trials. J Am Coll Cardiol 2004;44:810–819.
16. Bardy GH, Lee KL, Mark DB, et al: Amiodarone or an implantable cardioverter-defibrillator for congestive heart failure. N Engl J Med 2005;352:225–237.
17. Bristow MR, Saxon LA, Boehmer J, et al: Cardiac-resynchronization therapy with or without an implantable defibrillator in advanced chronic heart failure. N Engl J Med 2004;350:2140–2150.
18. Cleland JG, Daubert JC, Erdmann E, et al: The effect of cardiac resynchronization on morbidity and mortality in heart failure. N Engl J Med 2005;352:1539–1549.
19. Yusuf S, Pfeffer MA, Swedberg K, et al: Effects of candesartan in patients with chronic heart failure and preserved left-ventricular ejection fraction: The CHARM-Preserved Trial. Lancet 2003;362:777–781.

SUGGESTED READINGS

Amabile CM, Spencer AP: Keeping your patient with heart failure safe: A review of potentially dangerous medications. Arch Intern Med 2004;164:709–720. *Comprehensive overview, including NSAIDs.*

Ammar KA, Jacobsen SJ, Mahoney DW, et al: Prevalence and prognostic significance of heart failure stages: Application of the American College of Cardiology/American Heart Association heart failure staging criteria in the community. Circulation 2007;115:1563–1570. *An assessment of the prevalence of HF stages and their associated mortality.*

Heart Failure Society of America. Executive Summary: HFSA 2006 Comprehensive heart failure practice guideline. J Card Failure 2006;12:10–38. *Consensus guidelines.*

Hunt SA, Abraham WT, Chin MH, et al: ACC/AHA 2005 Guideline Update for the Diagnosis and Management of Chronic Heart Failure in the Adult—Summary Article: A report of the American College of Cardiology/American Heart Association Task Force on Practice Guidelines (Writing Committee to Update the 2001 Guidelines for the Evaluation and Management of Heart Failure): developed in collaboration with the American College of Chest Physicians and the International Society for Heart and Lung Transplantation: endorsed by the Heart Rhythm Society. Circulation 2005;112:1825–1852. *Detailed consensus guidelines.*

Jarcho JA: Biventricular pacing. N Engl J Med 2006;355:288–294. *A careful overview.*

McMurray J, Cohen-Solal A, Dietz R, et al: Practical recommendations for the use of ACE inhibitors, β-blockers, aldosterone antagonists and angiotensin receptor blockers in heart failure: Putting guidelines into practice. Eur J Heart Fail 2005;7:710–721. *A clear guide to clinical prescription.*

McMurray JJ, Pfeffer MA: Heart failure. Lancet 2005;365:1877–1889. *A concise review.*

Owan TE, Hodge DO, Herges RM, et al: Trends in prevalence and outcome of heart failure with preserved ejection fraction. N Engl J Med 2006;355:251–259. *The prevalence of heart failure with preserved ejection fraction increased over a 15-year period, while the rate of death from this disorder remained unchanged.*

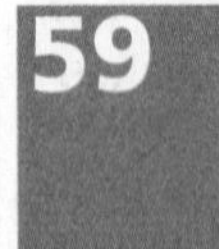

DISEASES OF THE MYOCARDIUM AND ENDOCARDIUM

William McKenna

MYOCARDIAL DISEASE

Although descriptive rather than etiologic, the usual designation of *cardiomyopathy* as hypertrophic, dilated, or restrictive has provided a useful clinical and prognostic framework for diagnosis and management (Table 59–1). Many infectious, metabolic, toxic, inflammatory, and other causes have been implicated, but most patients who present with symptoms or incidental abnormalities on routine cardiac evaluation in the absence of significant systemic hypertension, valvular heart disease, or atherosclerotic coronary artery disease have cardiomyopathies that have historically been considered idiopathic (Fig. 59–1). However, most of

TABLE 59–1 HEMODYNAMIC TYPES OF MYOCARDIAL DISEASE

	Hypertrophic	Dilated	Restrictive
Causes	Genetic (see Table 59–2) Secondary to pressure overload (e.g., hypertension, aortic stenosis)	Myocarditis (see Table 59–5) Chronic (see Table 59–7) Genetic (see Table 59–3) Arrhythmogenic right ventricular dysplasia (see Table 59–9)	Infiltrative or storage diseases (see Table 59–12) Endomyocardial (e.g., Löffler's, carcinoid)
Ejection fraction (normal >55%)	>60%	<30%	25–50%
Left ventricular diastolic dimension (normal <55 mm)	Often decreased	≥60 mm	<60 mm
Left ventricular wall thickness	Increased	Decreased	Normal or increased
Atrial size	Increased	Increased	Increased; may be massive
Valvular regurgitation	Mitral regurgitation	Mitral first during decompensation; tricuspid regurgitation in late stages	Frequent mitral and tricuspid regurgitation, rarely severe
Common first symptoms*	Exertional intolerance; may have chest pain	Exertional intolerance	Exertional intolerance, fluid retention
Congestive symptoms*	Primary exertional dyspnea	Left before right, except right prominent in young adults	Right often exceeds left
Risk for arrhythmia	Ventricular tachyarrhythmias, atrial fibrillation	Ventricular tachyarrhythmias; atrial fibrillation; conduction block in Chagas' disease, giant cell myocarditis, and some families	Atrial fibrillation; ventricular tachyarrhythmias uncommon except in sarcoidosis; conduction block in sarcoidosis and amyloidosis

*Left-sided symptoms of pulmonary congestion: dyspnea on exertion, orthopnea, paroxysmal nocturnal dyspnea. Right-sided symptoms of systemic venous congestion: discomfort on bending, hepatic and abdominal distention, peripheral edema.

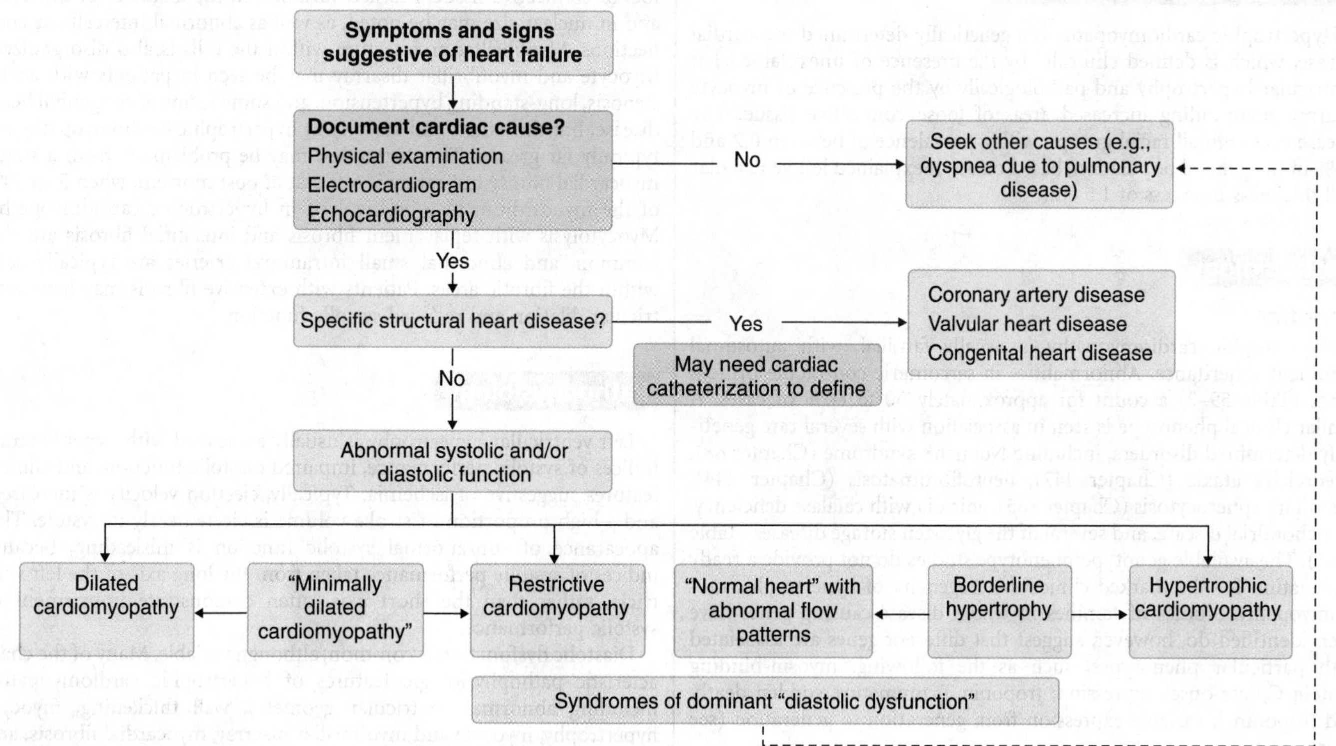

FIGURE 59–1 • Initial approach to classification of cardiomyopathy. The evaluation of symptoms or signs consistent with heart failure first includes confirmation that they can be attributed to a cardiac cause. Although this conclusion is often apparent from routine physical examination and electrocardiography, echocardiography serves to confirm cardiac disease and provides clues to the presence of other cardiac disease, such as focal abnormalities, suggesting primary valve disease or congenital heart disease. Having excluded these conditions, cardiomyopathy is generally considered to be dilated, restrictive, or hypertrophic, as shown in Table 59–1. Patients with apparently normal cardiac structure and contraction are occasionally found to demonstrate abnormal intracardiac flow patterns consistent with diastolic dysfunction but should also be evaluated carefully for other causes of their symptoms. Most patients with so-called diastolic dysfunction also demonstrate at least borderline criteria for left ventricular hypertrophy, frequently in the setting of chronic hypertension and diabetes. A moderately decreased ejection fraction without marked dilation or a pattern of restrictive cardiomyopathy is sometimes referred to as "minimally dilated cardiomyopathy," which may represent either a distinct entity or a transition between acute and chronic disease.

TABLE 59–2 FAMILIAL HYPERTROPHIC CARDIOMYOPATHY GENES, PROTEINS, AND ESTIMATED FREQUENCY OF MUTATIONS IN PATIENTS WITH THE PHENOTYPE

Gene	Protein	Frequency
MYH7	β-Myosin heavy chain	25–35%
MYBPC3	Cardiac myosin binding protein C	20–30%
TNNT2	Cardiac troponin T	3–5%
TNNI3	Cardiac troponin I	<5%
TPM1	α-Tropomyosin	<5%
MYL2	Regulatory myosin light chain	<5%
MYL3	Essential myosin light chain	Rare
ACTC	α-Cardiac actin	Rare
TTN	Titin	Rare
TNNC1	Cardiac troponin C	Rare
MYH6	α-Myosin heavy chain	Single study
CRP3	Muscle LIM protein	Rare

TABLE 59–3 GENETIC CONDITIONS ASSOCIATED WITH PHENOTYPIC LEFT VENTRICULAR HYPERTROPHY

Disorder	Disease Gene
METABOLIC DISEASE	
Glycogen storage diseases	
Pompe's disease	*GAA*
Forbes' disease	*AGL*
Danon's disease	*LAMP2*
Wolff-Parkinson-White syndrome, conduction disease	*PRKAG2*
Fabry's disease	*GLA*
Mitochondrial cytopathy (MELAS, MERRF, LHON)	Various mitochondrial genes
SYNDROMIC HYPERTROPHIC CARDIOMYOPATHY	
Noonan's syndrome	*PTPN11*
LEOPARD syndrome	*PTPN11*
Friedreich's ataxia	*FRDA*

these patients actually have familial disease involving the sarcomere (hypertrophic cardiomyopathy), the cytoskeleton (dilated cardiomyopathy), or cell adhesion (arrhythmogenic right ventricular cardiomyopathy), although most family members have incomplete gene expression and do not fulfill conventional clinical diagnostic criteria.

Hypertrophic Cardiomyopathy

Definition and Epidemiology

Hypertrophic cardiomyopathy is a genetically determined myocardial disease, which is defined clinically by the presence of unexplained left ventricular hypertrophy and pathologically by the presence of myocyte disarray surrounding increased areas of loose connective tissue. The disease occurs in all racial groups, with a prevalence of between 0.2 and 0.5% in the general population, based on an unexplained left ventricular wall thickness in excess of 1.5 cm.

Pathobiology

Genetics

Hypertrophic cardiomyopathy is usually familial, with autosomal dominant inheritance. Abnormalities in sarcomeric contractile protein genes (Table 59–2) account for approximately 50 to 60% of cases. A similar clinical phenotype is seen in association with several rare genetically determined disorders, including Noonan's syndrome (Chapter 68), Friedreich's ataxia (Chapter 447), neurofibromatosis (Chapter 444), hereditary spherocytosis (Chapter 165), aniridia with catalase deficiency, mitochondrial disease, and several of the glycogen storage diseases (Table 59–3). The available genotype/phenotype studies do not provide a ready explanation for the marked clinical heterogeneity of hypertrophic cardiomyopathy. Studies of families in whom disease-causing genes have been identified do, however, suggest that different genes are associated with particular phenotypes, such as the following: myosin-binding protein C, late-onset expression; troponin T, premature sudden death; and troponin I, variable expression from generation to generation (see later).

Pathology

Typically, heart weight is increased and the interventricular septum is hypertrophic, although virtually any pattern of thickening may occur. In the normal heart, the true apex is often relatively thinner than other segments. Apical variants characterized by relative or absolute thickening are rare, although hypertrophy commonly is predominantly in the distal ventricle below the papillary muscles. Macroscopically, one often sees a characteristic patch of endocardial thickening on the septum as a consequence of contact with the anterior leaflet of the mitral valve, which is correspondingly thickened.

Histologically, the hallmark of hypertrophic cardiomyopathy is myocyte disarray. This appearance results from the loss of the normal parallel arrangement of myocytes, with cells forming in whorls around foci of connective tissue. Marked variation in the diameter of myocytes and in nuclear size may be noted, as well as abnormal intercellular connections. Myofibrillar architecture within the cells is also disorganized. Myocyte and myofibrillar disarray may be seen in patients with aortic stenosis, long-standing hypertension, and some forms of congenital heart disease, but the extent and severity in hypertrophic cardiomyopathy are typically far greater. The distinction may be problematic from a single myocardial biopsy but rarely is difficult at post mortem, when 5 to 40% of the myocardium may be involved in hypertrophic cardiomyopathy. Myocytolysis with replacement fibrosis and interstitial fibrosis are also common, and abnormal small intramural arteries are typically seen within the fibrotic areas. Patients with extensive fibrosis may have ventricular dilation and reduced systolic function.

Pathophysiology

Left ventricular hypertrophy is usually associated with hyperdynamic indices of systolic performance, impaired diastolic function, and clinical features suggestive of ischemia. Typically, ejection velocity is increased, and a high proportion of stroke volume is ejected early in systole. This appearance of supranormal systolic function is misleading, because indices of systolic performance taken from the long axis of the left ventricle, rather than the short axis, often demonstrate impairment of systolic performance.

Diastolic dysfunction is common, although variable. Many of the characteristic pathophysiologic features of hypertrophic cardiomyopathy, including abnormal ventricular geometry, wall thickening, myocyte hypertrophy, myocyte and myofibrillar disarray, myocardial fibrosis, and ischemia would be expected to impair diastolic function. In most cases, relaxation is slow and prolonged, with elevation of diastolic pressures. A few patients have rapid early filling with restrictive hemodynamic physiology, markedly elevated filling pressures, and atrial dilation, with evidence of right-sided congestion, which may occur in the absence of significant myocardial hypertrophy or impairment of systolic performance. How the recognized genetic mutations cause these histologic and pathophysiologic changes is poorly understood, but inefficient utilization of adenosine triphosphatase by the sarcomere may be the final common pathway, because many of the mitochondrial and metabolic disorders and congenital syndromes that may mimic hypertrophic cardiomyopathy are associated with changes in adenosine triphosphatase synthesis and/or regulation.

Clinical Manifestations

The clinical expression of left ventricular hypertrophy usually occurs during periods of rapid somatic growth, which may be during the first year of life or childhood but more typically during adolescence and, occasionally, in the early 20s. The de novo development of myocardial hypertrophy later in life is uncommon but typically is associated with the development of mild to moderate systolic hypertension in patients with mutations in myosin-binding protein C.

Most patients are asymptomatic or have only mild or intermittent symptoms. Symptomatic progression is usually slow, age related, and associated with a gradual deterioration in left ventricular function over decades. Fewer than 5% of patients may have rapid, symptomatic deterioration in association with progressive myocardial wall thinning, increased left ventricular end-systolic dimensions, and an overall reduction in systolic performance. Such a rapid course is not associated with any particular genetic abnormality.

Symptoms and Signs

Symptoms may develop at any age, even many years after the appearance of electrocardiographic (ECG) or echocardiographic manifestations of left ventricular hypertrophy. Occasionally, sudden death may be the initial presentation. Experience from evaluating families suggests, however, that most affected individuals have few or only paroxysmal symptoms. Approximately 30% of adults develop exertional chest pain (Chapters 48 and 70), which may be atypical, prolonged, and noted at rest or nocturnally. Postprandial angina associated with mild exertion is typical. Mild to moderate dyspnea is common in adults and may relate to left ventricular outflow tract obstruction and/or mitral regurgitation; it probably develops as a consequence of ventricular diastolic dysfunction and raised pulmonary venous pressures.

Occasionally, patients without significant symptoms present with or develop paroxysmal nocturnal dyspnea. Such episodes suggest transient myocardial ischemia or arrhythmias, although evaluations often fail to identify the mechanism.

Approximately 20% of patients experience syncope (Chapter 427), and a similar proportion complain of presyncope. Such symptoms are often attributed to arrhythmias, but documentation may require prolonged ECG monitoring or implantation of an ECG recorder (Chapter 61); in many cases, no underlying cause is identified. Exertion-related syncope or presyncope raises the suspicion of labile left ventricular outflow tract obstruction, exertion-related mitral regurgitation, or ischemia.

Palpitations are a frequent complaint and are usually attributable to supraventricular or ventricular ectopy or to forceful cardiac contractions. Sustained palpitations are usually caused by supraventricular tachyarrhythmias. Initial presentation with a symptomatic arrhythmia, usually atrial fibrillation, is uncommon.

Patients with distal or apical hypertrophy have fewer symptoms, better exercise capacity, no arrhythmias, and good prognosis. Occasionally, however, patients with distal or apical hypertrophy may have severe refractory chest pain or may present with troublesome supraventricular arrhythmias.

Diagnosis

The initial diagnostic evaluation includes a family history focusing on premature cardiac disease or death, a comprehensive medical history focusing on cardiovascular symptoms, a careful physical examination, a 12-lead ECG study, and a two-dimensional echocardiogram. In patients with resting left ventricular outflow tract obstruction (~20%), the physical examination may demonstrate a rapid upstroke of the arterial pulse, often followed by a second late systolic peak (spike and dome). The left ventricular impulse is forceful, and the typical murmur is heard in late systole, loudest at the left sternal edge, and radiating to the aortic and mitral areas but not into the neck or axilla (Chapter 48). Physiologic and pharmacologic maneuvers that decrease afterload or venous return (e.g., standing, Valsalva maneuver, inhalation of amyl nitrite) or contractility (e.g., a post-extrasystole beat) will increase the intensity of the murmur, whereas interventions that increase afterload and venous return (e.g., squatting or handgrip) will reduce it (see Table 48–2). In contrast, in the majority of patients who do not have left ventricular outflow tract obstruction, the physical signs are subtle and are limited to features reflecting the hyperdynamic contraction (rapid upstroke pulse) and poorly compliant right (prominent a wave in jugular venous pressure) and left (S_4 gallop, double-apex beat) ventricles (Chapter 48).

More than 90% of patients have abnormal ECG findings, but no changes are disease specific. The most common abnormalities are left axis deviation (15 to 20%), abnormal Q waves (25 to 30%, most commonly in inferolateral leads), and ST segment or T wave changes (>50%). An isolated increase in the QRS voltage without ST segment changes or T wave inversion is rare in hypertrophic cardiomyopathy. The presence of predominantly distal or apical thickening is associated with giant negative T wave inversion on the ECG tracing.

Two-dimensional echocardiography (Chapter 53) is the mainstay of diagnostic imaging, although magnetic resonance imaging (Chapter 55) and computed tomography (Chapter 54) provide alternatives if the echocardiogram is of poor quality. A wall thickness of more than two standard deviations above the mean, corrected for age, gender, and height, is generally accepted as diagnostic: in adults, this value is typically 1.5 cm or greater in men and 1.3 cm or greater in women. In most patients, the hypertrophy is asymmetrical and involves the anterior and posterior intraventricular septum (Fig. 59–2). The hypertrophy, however, may be more generalized and may involve the free wall of the left ventricle, or it may be localized and confined to areas other than the septum, such as the free wall or posterior wall of the left ventricle.

The echocardiogram can measure left ventricular outflow tract obstruction, both at rest and after maneuvers (e.g., amyl nitrite, Valsalva) that may worsen or provoke obstruction. Patients with 30 mm Hg or more of left ventricular outflow tract obstruction typically have systolic anterior motion of the mitral valve, with contact of either the anterior (or less commonly) the posterior mitral leaflet with the intraventricular septum during systole, in association with a posteriorly directed jet of mitral regurgitation, the severity of which is usually proportionate to the severity of the obstruction. Most patients with hypertrophic cardiomyopathy have mild to moderate left atrial enlargement as well as echocardiographic evidence of diastolic dysfunction.

Diagnostic Criteria in Patients and First-Degree Relatives

Because genetic analysis is not routinely available outside of research centers, the diagnosis in first-degree relatives relies on the echocardiographic features of unexplained left ventricular hypertrophy. When genetic testing is available, it is at best confirmatory in individuals who meet echocardiographic criteria because the recognized sarcomeric contractile protein gene abnormalities account for only 60% of the cases of hypertrophic cardiomyopathy. Genetic testing is most helpful in first-degree relatives who do not meet conventional echocardiographic criteria but who may, nonetheless, be at risk of the complications of hypertrophic cardiomyopathy. Given the 50% probability of disease in a first-degree relative of a patient with hypertrophic cardiomyopathy, modified diagnostic criteria (Table 59–4) consider the high probability that their otherwise unexplained ECG and echocardiographic findings reflect incomplete disease expression, with the corresponding risks of complications and of passing the gene to their children.

When available, cardiopulmonary exercise testing with metabolic gas exchange measurements provides an accurate and reproducible assessment of exercise capacity, which can be followed serially. Cardiac catheterization is rarely required for diagnosis or management, but it may be indicated when measurement of intracardiac pressures is required to guide therapeutic decisions (e.g., in patients with severe mitral regurgitation) and for the exclusion of coexistent coronary artery disease in patients with chest pain.

Differential Diagnosis

In the presence of other causes of left ventricular hypertrophy, such as long-standing systemic hypertension or aortic stenosis, the diagnosis of hypertrophic cardiomyopathy may be problematic. However, secondary

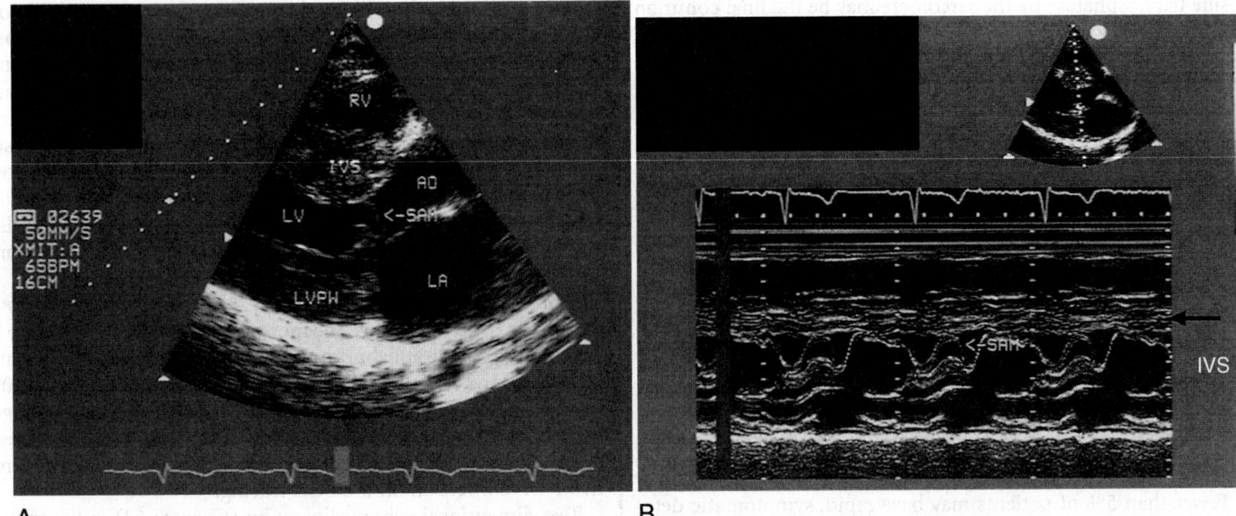

FIGURE 59–2 • Hypertrophic obstructive cardiomyopathy. A, The two-dimensional long-axis parasternal view shows the chambers of the heart. The left ventricle posterior wall (LVPW) is thickened, and the most striking abnormality is the hypertrophy of the interventricular septum (IVS). Another characteristic feature is a Venturi effect: as blood leaves the left ventricle (LV), it sucks the anterior leaflet of the mitral valve forward, a phenomenon called systolic anterior motion (SAM). This phenomenon is more clearly shown in the parasternal long-axis M-mode echocardiogram (**B**). The massive thickening of the septum is also obvious in the M-mode image (IVS). AO = aorta; LA = left atrium; RV = right ventricle. (From Forbes CD, Jackson WF: Color Atlas and Text of Clinical Medicine, 3rd ed. London, Mosby, 2003.)

TABLE 59–4 DIAGNOSTIC CRITERIA FOR HYPERTROPHIC CARDIOMYOPATHY IN FIRST-DEGREE RELATIVES OF AFFECTED PATIENTS*

Major Criteria	Minor Criteria
ECHOCARDIOGRAPHY	
Left ventricular wall thickness ≥13 mm in the anterior septum or posterior wall or ≥15 mm in the posterior septum or free wall	Left ventricular wall thickness of 12 mm in the anterior septum or posterior wall or of 14 mm in the posterior septum or free wall
Severe SAM of the mitral valve (septal-leaflet contact)	Moderate SAM of the mitral valve (no mitral leaflet-septal contact)
	Redundant mitral valve leaflets
ELECTROCARDIOGRAPHY	
Left ventricular hypertrophy with repolarization changes (Romhilt and Estes)	Complete bundle branch block or (minor) interventricular conduction defects (in left ventricular leads)
T wave inversion in leads I and aVL (≥3 mm) (with QRS-T wave axis difference ≥30 degrees), V_3–V_6 (≥3 mm) or II and III and aVF (≥5 mm)	Minor repolarization changes in left ventricular leads
	Deep S wave in lead V_2 (>25 mm)
Abnormal Q waves (>40 msec or >25% R wave) in at least two leads from II, III, aVF (in absence of left anterior hemiblock), and V_1–V_4; or I, aVL, V_5–V_6	Unexplained chest pain, dyspnea, or syncope

*The diagnosis of hypertrophic cardiomyopathy in first-degree relatives of patients with the disease is based on the presence of one major criterion or two minor echocardiographic criteria or one minor echocardiographic and two minor electrocardiographic criteria.
aVF = augmented voltage unipolar left foot lead; aVL = augmented voltage unipolar left arm lead; SAM = systolic anterior motion.
Adapted from McKenna WJ, Spirito P, Desnos M, et al: Heart 1997;77:130–132.

hypertrophy from other causes rarely exceeds 1.8 cm. Hypertrophy in the highly trained athlete is usually less than 1.6 cm and typically occurs in association with an increased left ventricular end-diastolic dimension and stroke volume, rather than at the expense of the size of the left ventricular cavity. An ECG tracing showing Q waves or inferolateral repolarization changes favors the diagnosis of hypertrophic cardiomyopathy.

Treatment

Rx

The aims of management are to improve symptoms and prevent disease-related complications (Fig. 59–3).

Medical Therapy

Symptomatic therapy is influenced by left ventricular morphology and hemodynamics. Patients with left ventricular outflow tract gradients and those with mitral regurgitation have higher rates of

endocarditis and should undergo antibiotic prophylaxis whenever the risk of bacteremia exists (Chapter 76).

Therapeutic options in patients *without left ventricular outflow gradients* are limited predominantly to pharmacologic therapy. β-Blockade (starting at a dose equivalent to propranolol, 120 mg/day) may improve chest pain and dyspnea, but patients' responses are variable. The dose should be titrated to achieve a target heart rate of 50 to 70 beats per minute at rest and 130 to 140 beats per minute at peak exercise. The calcium antagonists, verapamil (starting at a dose of 120 mg/day) and diltiazem (starting at a dose of 180 mg/day), provide useful alternatives, particularly in patients with refractory chest pain, but high doses (e.g., verapamil ≥480 mg/day, diltiazem ≥360 mg/day) may be required. In patients with paroxysmal nocturnal dyspnea despite no evidence of ventricular

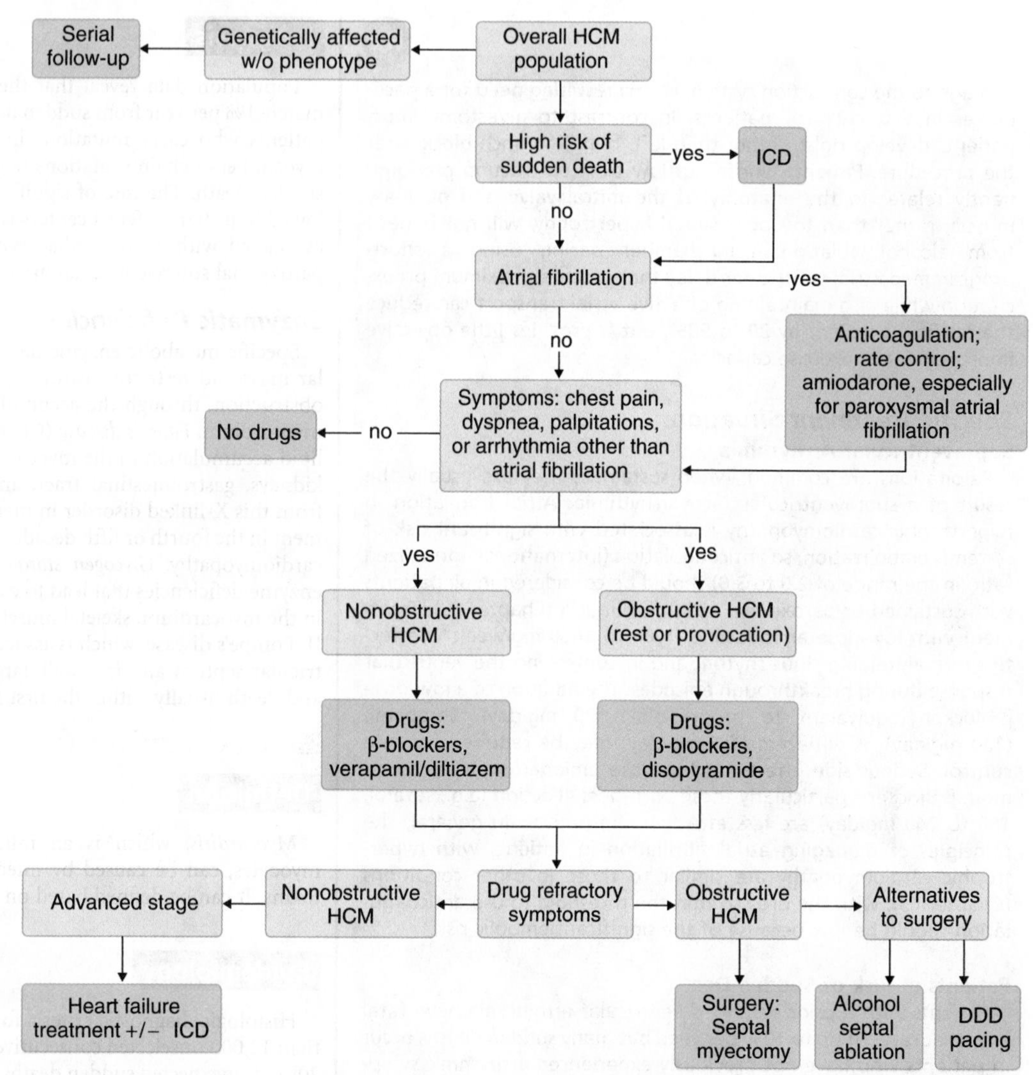

FIGURE 59–3 • Approach to the management of hypertrophic cardiomyopathy (HCM). ICD = implantable cardioverter-defibrillator. (Adapted from Maron BJ, McKenna WJ, Danielson GK, et al: American College of Cardiology/European Society of Cardiology Clinical Expert Consensus Document on Hypertrophic Cardiomyopathy. J Am Coll Cardiol 2003;42:1687–1713.)

Rx

outflow obstruction, a transient mechanism such as myocardial ischemia or arrhythmia may be the cause, although investigations usually fail to identify the precise mechanism. Such patients, as well as those with chronically raised pulmonary pressures, may require diuretics. The dose (typically starting with furosemide, 20 to 40 mg orally as needed, followed by 20 mg/day if required) and duration of diuretic therapy should be minimized because injudicious use of these drugs can be dangerous, particularly in patients with severe diastolic impairment or labile obstruction.

In patients *with symptoms associated with significant left ventricular outflow tract obstruction,* the main aim of treatment is to reduce the gradient. Options include negative inotropic drugs, surgery, atrioventricular sequential pacing, and percutaneous alcohol ablation. Approximately 60 to 70% of patients improve with β-blockers, although high doses (equivalent to propranolol at 480 mg/day) are frequently required, and side effects are often limiting. When β-blockade alone is ineffective, disopyramide, titrated to the maximum tolerated dose (usually between 400 and 600 mg/day), may be effective in up to two thirds of patients, but side effects, principally related to the anticholinergic effects (e.g., dry eyes and mouth) limit this drug's use. Disopyramide should be given concomitantly with a small to medium dose of a β-blocker (e.g., propranolol, 120 to 240 mg/day), which will slow the heart rate and also blunt rapid atrioventricular nodal conduction should supraventricular arrhythmias develop. In patients who have left ventricular outflow tract obstruction and who are receiving a β-blocker and disopyramide, other antiarrhythmic drugs that alter repolarization (e.g., sotalol or amiodarone) must be avoided because of the potential pro-arrhythmic effect. In patients with outflow tract gradients, verapamil's effects are unpredictable, and acute hemodynamic collapse has been described, particularly in patients with substantial gradients or elevated pulmonary pressures.

Invasive Treatments

Surgery should be considered for significant outflow obstruction (gradient >50 mm Hg) in patients who have symptoms refractory to medical therapy or an exercise capacity less than 70% of predicted. The most commonly performed surgical procedure, ventricular septal myectomy, either abolishes or significantly reduces the gradient in 95% of cases, reduces mitral regurgitation, and improves exercise capacity and symptoms; benefits are maintained long term in 70 to 80% of patients. Surgery should be performed in an experienced center, where mortality rates should be less than 2%. The main complications (atrioventricular block, ventricular septal defects) are rare with intraoperative transesophageal echocardiography and current surgical techniques. In some patients, concomitant mitral valve repair or replacement may be required.

In experienced centers, the selective injection of alcohol into a targeted septal perforator branch of the left anterior descending coronary artery to create a localized septal scar yields outcomes similar to surgery in terms of reducing the outflow gradient and improving symptoms and exercise capacity. The main complication is

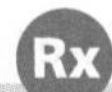

damage to the conduction system, with a resulting need for a pacemaker in 5 to 10% of patients. In contrast to myectomy, most patients develop right, rather than left, bundle branch block after the procedure. Patients whose outflow tract obstruction predominantly relates to the anatomy of the mitral valve and papillary muscle, rather than to upper septal hypertrophy, will not benefit from alcohol ablation. Dual-chamber pacing using a short-programmed atrial ventricular delay that provides maximum preexcitation while also maintaining effective atrial transport can reduce the outflow gradient by 30 to 50%, but it provides little objective improvement in exercise capacity.

Specific Treatment Situations

Supraventricular Arrhythmia

Palpitations are common; when sustained, they are usually the result of a supraventricular tachyarrhythmia. Atrial fibrillation in hypertrophic cardiomyopathy is associated with significant risk of systemic embolization, so anticoagulation (international normalized ratio in the range of 2.0 to 3.0) should be considered in all patients with sustained or paroxysmal atrial fibrillation (Chapter 63). Treatment with low-dose amiodarone, 1000 to 1400 mg/week, is effective in maintaining sinus rhythm and in controlling the ventricular response during breakthrough episodes. The addition of a low-dose β-blocker (equivalent to propranolol, 120 mg/day), verapamil (120 mg/day) or diltiazem (180 mg/day) may be required for rate control. Serious side effects on low-dose amiodarone are uncommon. β-Blockers, particularly those with class III action (e.g., sotalol, 160 to 240 mg/day) are less effective alternatives. In general, the principles of managing atrial fibrillation in patients with hypertrophic cardiomyopathy are similar to those in other conditions (Chapter 63), with the proviso that the threshold to use anticoagulation should be low because of the significant embolic risk.

Patients at Risk of Sudden Death

Patients with a prior sustained ventricular arrhythmia have fatal events at rates of up to 10% per year, but many sudden deaths occur in patients who have not previously experienced arrhythmic symptoms. Clinical features associated with an increased risk of sudden death include a family history of premature sudden death from hypertrophic cardiomyopathy, unexplained syncope, the presence of nonsustained ventricular tachycardia during ambulatory ECG monitoring, the finding of an abnormal blood pressure response during upright exercise, and severe left ventricular hypertrophy (≥3.0 cm). The presence of two or more of these risk markers is associated with annual sudden death rates of 3 to 6%, and the consensus is that such individuals, as well as those who have experienced symptomatic sustained ventricular arrhythmias, should receive an implantable cardioverter-defibrillator (ICD; Chapter 65). In such patients, the subsequent primary and secondary prevention discharge rates of 5 and 11%, respectively, support the benefit of the approach. Current clinical practice also supports consideration of an ICD in adolescents and young adults with any one of these risk factors. Patients with hypertrophic cardiomyopathy should be advised to avoid competitive sports and intense physical exertion. However, this advice arises from consensus guidelines, although no data prove that abstention from vigorous physical activity modifies risk or prevents sudden death.

Family Screening

First-degree relatives should undergo 12-lead ECG and two-dimensional echocardiographic studies annually during puberty and adolescence and then every 5 years as adults. Family evaluation should include genetic counseling regarding the risk of developing hypertrophic cardiomyopathy and its complications. Efforts to identify early markers of disease expression in adolescents who are known to carry disease-causing genes have focused on echocardiographic Doppler indices of impaired relaxation, which may be abnormal in the absence of left ventricular hypertrophy. The earliest changes are usually seen in the 12-lead ECG tracing: pathologic Q waves, left axis deviation, and inferolateral T wave inversion.

Prognosis

Population data reveal that the mortality rate in adults is approximately 1% per year from sudden death, and preliminary data suggest that patients who carry mutations in cardiac troponin T or in certain β-myosin heavy chain mutations (e.g., Arg403Glu) are at increased risk of sudden death. The rate of significant embolic events in individuals followed in tertiary referral centers is 1 to 4% per year. Embolic strokes are associated with more cardiac symptoms, left atrial enlargement, and paroxysmal supraventricular arrhythmias.

Enzymatic Deficiencies

Specific metabolic enzyme deficiencies also cause increased ventricular mass and restrictive cardiomyopathy, usually without outflow tract obstruction, through the accumulation of abnormal metabolites in the myocardium. *Fabry's disease* (Chapter 223) results in intracellular glycolipid accumulation in the myocardium, valves, vessel walls, skin, cornea, kidneys, gastrointestinal tract, and central nervous system. Mortality from this X-linked disorder in men results from multiple organ involvement in the fourth or fifth decade. Heterozygous women also can develop cardiomyopathy. *Glycogen storage disease* (Chapter 219) results from enzyme deficiencies that lead to excessive deposition of normal glycogen in the myocardium, skeletal muscle, and liver. The most common is type II, Pompe's disease, which is associated with dramatic thickening of ventricular septum and free wall, large QRS amplitude, short PR interval, and death usually within the first few years of life.

Myocarditis

Definition

Myocarditis, which is an inflammatory process involving cardiac myocytes, can be caused by infections, immune-mediated damage, or toxins. It can be defined based on histopathologic or clinical criteria.

Epidemiology

Histologic diagnostic criteria for myocarditis were met in 1% of more than 12,000 unselected consecutive autopsies in a Swedish study, in up to 20% of unexpected sudden deaths in young persons, and in 40% of cases of new-onset heart failure in children. Approximately 5% of a virus-infected population have clinical evidence of cardiac involvement.

A wide range of infectious, immune-mediated, toxic, and genetic causes has been implicated (Table 59–5). Viral genome studies of myocardium obtained by endomyocardial biopsy reveal evidence of adenovirus, enterovirus, or cytomegalovirus in 35 to 40% of patients with an acute presentation and histologic features of myocarditis. *Trypanosoma cruzi* infection (Chagas' disease; Chapter 368) is prevalent in South America, hepatitis C (Chapter 152) myocarditis is more common in Japan, and the parvovirus (Chapter 394) genome is increasingly recognized in Europe and North America. Cardiac involvement in human immunodeficiency virus (HIV) infection (Chapter 407) is associated with a lymphocytic myocarditis and is a strong predictor of poor prognosis. Recently, smallpox vaccination (Chapter 16) has been documented to cause myopericarditis, with a reported incidence of 7.8 cases per 100,000 vaccine administrations.

Pathobiology

Current knowledge of viral pathogenesis arises predominantly from inoculation of enterovirus (often coxsackievirus B3; Chapter 402) into various strains of mice. Direct myocardial invasion by cardiotropic virus progresses quickly (<5 to 7 days) to immunologic activation, initially with an inflammatory cellular infiltration, and later to activation of cell-mediated immunity, as well as development of autoantibodies directed against contractile (antimyosin), structural (antisarcolemmal), mitochondrial (adenine nucleotide translocator), and receptor (anti–β-adrenergic and anti-M2) proteins. In genetically predisposed mouse strains, immune-mediated myocarditis with production of serum autoantibodies develops following immunization with the relevant organ-specific autoantigens (e.g., cardiac myosin) in the absence of viral inoculation, similar to other autoimmune diseases. In humans, the detection of viral

TABLE 59–5 CAUSES OF MYOCARDITIS

INFECTIONS

Viral
- Coxsackievirus, human immunodeficiency virus, echovirus, adenovirus, influenza, measles, mumps, parvovirus, poliovirus, rubella, varicella-zoster virus, herpes simplex virus, cytomegalovirus, hepatitis C virus, rabies virus, respiratory syncytial virus, vaccine virus, dengue virus, yellow fever virus

Protozoal
- *Trypanosoma cruzi, Toxoplasma gondii*

Bacterial
- *Brucella, Corynebacterium diphtheriae, Salmonella, Haemophilus influenzae, Mycoplasma pneumoniae, Neisseria meningitidis* (meningococcus), *Streptococcus pneumoniae, Staphylococcus, Mycobacterium, Neisseria gonorrhoeae* (gonococcus), *Vibrio cholerae*

Spirochetal
- *Treponema pallidium, Borrelia, Leptospira*

Fungal
- *Aspergillus, Candida, Cryptococcus, Actinomyces, Blastomyces, Histoplasma, Coccidioides*

Rickettsial
- *Coxiella burnetii, Rickettsia rickettsii, Rickettsia tsutsugamushi*

Parasitic
- *Trichinella spiralis, Echinococcus granulosus, Taenia solium*

IMMUNE-MEDIATED DISORDERS

Alloantigens
- Heart transplant rejection

Autoantigens
- Churg-Strauss syndrome, celiac disease, Whipple's disease, giant cell myocarditis, Kawasaki's disease, systemic lupus erythematosus, systemic sclerosis, sarcoidosis, scleroderma, polymyositis, thrombocytopenic purpura

Allergens (drugs)
- Penicillin, sulfonamides, tetracycline, methyldopa, streptomycin, tricyclic antidepressants, thiazide diuretics, dobutamine, indomethacin

TOXIC CAUSES

Drugs
- Anthracyclines, catecholamines, amphetamines, cocaine, cyclophosphamide, 5-fluorouracil, herceptin, interferon, interleukin-2

Physical agents
- Electric shock, radiation, hyperpyrexia

Heavy metals
- Copper, iron, lead

Others
- Arsenic, snake bites, scorpion bites, wasp and spider stings, phosphorus, carbon monoxide

GENETIC DISORDERS

Inherited cardiomyopathies with immune-mediated pathogenesis (dilated and right ventricular cardiomyopathy)

TABLE 59–6 LABORATORY EVALUATION OF CARDIOMYOPATHY

CLINICAL EVALUATION

Thorough history and physical examination to identify cardiac and noncardiac disorders*
Assessment of ability to perform routine and desired activities*
Assessment of volume status*

LABORATORY EVALUATION

Electrocardiogram*
Chest radiograph*
Two-dimensional and Doppler echocardiogram*
Chemistry
- Serum sodium,* potassium,* glucose, creatinine,* blood urea nitrogen,* calcium,* magnesium*
- Albumin,* total protein,* liver function tests,* serum iron, ferritin
- Urinalysis
- Creatine kinase
- Thyroid-stimulating hormone*

Hematology
- Hemoglobin/hematocrit*
- White blood cell count with differential,* including eosinophils
- Erythrocyte sedimentation rate

INITIAL EVALUATION IN SELECTED PATIENTS ONLY

Titers for suspected infection
- Acute viral (coxsackievirus, echovirus, influenza virus)
- Human immunodeficiency virus, Epstein-Barr virus
- Lyme disease, toxoplasmosis
- Chagas' disease

Catheterization with coronary angiography in patients with angina who are candidates for intervention*
Serologic studies for active rheumatologic disease
Endomyocardial biopsy

*Level I recommendations from ACC/AHA 2005 Guideline Update for the Diagnosis and Management of Chronic Heart Failure in the Adult. (Hunt SA, Abraham WT, Chin MH, et al: Circulation 2005;112:e154–e235.)

genome following presumed myocardial infection suggests that viral persistence may contribute to ongoing myocardial damage as a component of the immunologic response to infection.

Immune-mediated myocarditis is seen in association with certain systemic inflammatory disorders but is probably more common when no infectious or associated disorder is identified. So-called autoimmune myocarditis may reflect progression of undiagnosed early dilated cardiomyopathy or a response to unrecognized triggers. Antibiotics, antidepressants, anti-inflammatory agents, and diuretics may cause hypersensitivity myocarditis that is associated with peripheral eosinophilia and a myocardial infiltrate with lymphocytes and eosinophils.

Clinical Manifestations

The clinical presentation is variable, ranging from asymptomatic ECG changes, symptoms of arrhythmia, or acute coronary syndromes to the new onset of heart failure. Acute fulminant myocarditis may develop rapidly, with fever, leukocytosis, severe heart failure, and cardiogenic shock. A viral prodrome is reported in 10 to 80% of patients who fulfill histologic diagnostic criteria.

Diagnosis

Evaluation of new-onset features of possible myocarditis should include a history of cardiac symptoms or premature (<40 years of age) familial cardiac disease. A careful history and physical examination should be supplemented by both routine and targeted laboratory testing (Table 59–6). Serum biomarkers of myocardial damage (troponin I or T) have high (>80%) positive predictive value if performed within 1 month of the onset of symptoms, whereas markers of inflammation appear to have low sensitivity and specificity. Noninvasive tests including 12-lead and exercise ECG and two-dimensional echocardiographic studies are recommended. Other studies of possible value include the following: gallium-67 scintigraphy, which detects the extent of myocardial inflammation; antimyosin imaging with indium-111, which detects the extent of myocyte necrosis; and early and late gadolinium-enhanced magnetic resonance imaging, which reflects both inflammation and necrosis.

Histologic evaluation based on endomyocardial biopsy tissue in patients with new-onset heart failure does not correlate with symptoms or prognosis, nor does it guide therapy. In addition, biopsy yields diagnostic information in only 10 to 20% of patients who present with clinical features of myocarditis. The low yield of biopsy may relate to sampling error (myocarditis is patchy), the timing of biopsy (acute versus chronic disease), interobserver variability in interpretation, and the overall low sensitivity of histologic evaluation in isolation. Biopsy is generally reserved for patients with heart failure (subacute or acute) refractory to standard management, features suggestive of associated cardiac (e.g., conduction defects, arrhythmia) or systemic disease (e.g., connective tissue disease, amyloidosis, hemochromatosis, sarcoidosis), or suspicion of giant cell myocarditis because of new-onset heart failure associated with tachyarrhythmias or conduction disease.

Treatment

Rx

Treatment of most patients with myocarditis is supportive. The severity of heart failure determines the level of pharmacologic intervention (Chapter 58) and hemodynamic support. In patients with fulminant myocarditis and severe left ventricular dysfunction, an aggressive short-term approach (e.g., left ventricular assist device, extracorporeal membrane oxygenation) is warranted because of the probability of spontaneous complete recovery. For giant cell myocarditis, which is a usually fatal disease of relatively young healthy adults, heart transplantation is the treatment of choice for most patients.

Recognition that pathogenesis involves immune-mediated damage has led to trials of immunosuppression, but data regarding benefit are unconvincing. [1] In general, immunosuppression using high-dose prednisolone (tapered over 3 to 6 months from 60 mg/day down to 5 mg/day) plus azathioprine (1 mg/kg twice daily for ≤6 months) is reserved for patients who have virus-negative myocarditis and whose disease progresses despite maximal supportive therapy, for patients with systemic autoimmune disease or progressive sarcoidosis, or for patients who have idiopathic giant cell myocarditis and are not able to undergo heart transplantation.

Prognosis

Patients with acute myocarditis with mild heart failure or symptoms suggestive of myocardial ischemia/infarction typically improve within weeks without sequelae. An acute presentation of myocarditis with advanced heart failure (ejection fraction <35%) may resolve (25%) but typically (50%) leads to chronic left ventricular dysfunction (dilated cardiomyopathy) or progresses to death or cardiac transplantation (25%). Patients who present with acute fulminant myocarditis, however, have an excellent prognosis, with survival rates of more than 90%. Giant cell myocarditis is usually fatal without heart transplantation.

Myocarditis Syndromes

Viral Myocarditis

Viral myocarditis may be suspected from the clinical picture of recent febrile illness, often with prominent myalgias, followed by angina-like chest pain, dyspnea, or arrhythmias. Elevated troponin levels support the diagnosis, and increasing viral titers (to coxsackievirus, echovirus, adenovirus, or influenza virus) confirm recent infection. The general prognosis of truly "new-onset" heart failure attributed to recent viral infection is major improvement in left ventricular function in up to 50% of patients. If deterioration continues during the months after diagnosis, the prognosis for recovery becomes poor.

Giant Cell Myocarditis

Patients with giant cell myocarditis, which accounts for 10 to 20% of biopsy-positive cases of myocarditis, present with the rapid onset of chest pain, fever, and hemodynamic compromise, often with ventricular tachycardia and/or atrioventricular block. When ventricular tachyarrhythmias are a major feature of myocarditis, particularly in a young person, endomyocardial biopsy is generally recommended to determine whether giant cell myocarditis is present, even though the diagnosis is statistically unlikely. Immunosuppression, although frequently used, does not appear to improve the clinical course, which is usually characterized by rapid deterioration and death from heart failure and refractory ventricular tachyarrhythmias unless cardiac transplantation can be performed.

Human Immunodeficiency Virus Cardiomyopathy

Clinical cardiomyopathy occurs in 10 to 40% of patients infected with HIV (Chapter 407), owing to HIV itself or to coinfection with cytomegalovirus. Treatment is of the underlying HIV infection.

Chagas' Disease

Chagas' disease (Chapter 368), which is caused by infection with *Trypanosoma cruzi*, affects up to 15% of rural populations in South America, is common in Central America, and is seen elsewhere in immigrants from these endemic areas. The acute tissue-invasive phase can present as myocarditis but is usually silent. Progressive myocardial disease and heart failure are manifested by apical aneurysms, right bundle branch block, and arrhythmias. Serologic diagnosis is made by the complement-fixation (Machado-Guerreiro) test and by immunofluorescent and immunosorbent assays. Antiparasitic agents such as nifurtimox and benzimidazole reduce parasitemia, but benefit in late-phase disease is not established. ICDs may decrease the risk of sudden death from conduction block or tachyarrhythmias. After the development of symptomatic heart failure, the 5-year survival rate is 20%.

Toxoplasmosis

Toxoplasmosis (Chapter 370) myocarditis, owing to intermittent rupture of cysts in the myocardium, can cause atypical chest pain, arrhythmias, pericarditis, and symptomatic heart failure. Diagnosis is made from antibody titers. Therapy is with pyrimethamine and sulfadiazine, but relapses are common.

Lyme Disease

Lyme carditis (Chapter 342) classically presents with conduction system abnormalities resulting from infection with *Borrelia burgdorferi*, which is diagnosed serologically. However, isolated cases of heart failure occur.

Immune-Mediated Myocarditis

Myocardial inflammation can be associated with polymyositis (Chapter 290) or systemic lupus erythematosus (Chapter 287), although pericarditis and coronary artery vasculitis are more common. Hypersensitivity reactions, especially to drugs (Chapter 275), can cause myocarditis that often is associated with peripheral eosinophilia and can be confirmed by endomyocardial biopsy. Treatment includes discontinuation of the offending agent and corticosteroid therapy.

Peripartum Cardiomyopathy

Peripartum cardiomyopathy appears in the last month of pregnancy or in the first 5 months after delivery in the absence of preexisting cardiac disease (Chapter 259). The incidence is between 1 in 3000 to 15,000 deliveries, with increased risk in older mothers or in the setting of twins, malnutrition, tocolytic therapy, toxemia, or hypertension. Lymphocytic myocarditis, found in 30 to 50% of biopsy specimens, suggests an immune component, perhaps cross-reactivity between uterine and cardiac myocyte proteins or an enhanced susceptibility to viral myocarditis. Presentation is usually with orthopnea and dyspnea on minimal exertion, most often within the first weeks after delivery when the excess volume of pregnancy would normally be mobilized. Preexisting cardiac disease must be excluded. Diuretics facilitate postpartum diuresis, and angiotensin-converting enzyme inhibitors improve symptoms. The prognosis is improvement to normal or near-normal ejection fraction during the next 6 months in more than 50% of patients.

Dilated Cardiomyopathy

Definition and Epidemiology

Dilated cardiomyopathy is characterized by ventricular dilation and impaired contractile performance, which may involve the left or both ventricles. It may develop as a consequence of prior myocarditis or as a result of a recognized toxin, infection, predisposing cardiovascular

TABLE 59–7 CAUSES OF DILATED CARDIOMYOPATHY

CARDIOVASCULAR DISORDERS
Systemic hypertension
Ischemic heart disease
Valvular heart disease
Myocarditis
Peripartum cardiomyopathy
TOXINS
Alcohol
Catecholamines
Anthracyclines
Radiation
Cocaine
ASSOCIATED SYSTEMIC DISEASES
Systemic lupus erythematosus
Polyarteritis nodosa
Rheumatoid arthritis
Scleroderma
Dermatomyositis
MUSCULAR DISORDERS
Duchenne's muscular dystrophy
Becker-type muscular dystrophy
Myotonic dystrophy
Mitochondrial disorders
HIGH-OUTPUT STATES
Thiamine deficiency
Thyrotoxicosis
Severe anemia
Arteriovenous fistulas/shunts
Incessant tachycardia

disease (e.g., hypertension, ischemic or valvular heart disease), or systemic metabolic, neuromuscular, or inflammatory disorder (Table 59–7). For some patients, identification of the specific cause and associated disease will strongly influence diagnosis, management, and prognosis, even though the principles related to the management of heart failure are generic (Chapter 58).

In the population, about 36 persons per 100,000 have unexplained left ventricular dysfunction with an ejection fraction of less than 40%—a finding that is indicative of advanced disease. Evidence from population data and family studies, however, indicates a higher frequency of asymptomatic left ventricular dysfunction. When no cause or associated disease is identified, dilated cardiomyopathy has been termed idiopathic, although pedigree studies revealed that 50 to 60% of such patients have familial disease, and disease-causing mutations currently can be identified in 10 to 20% of such families.

Pathobiology

In dilated cardiomyopathy, systolic dysfunction may result from a variety of causes (e.g., toxins, infection, ischemia) and pathologic states (e.g., inflammation, high output, genetic abnormalities). The altered hemodynamic parameters of decreased stroke volume and increased chamber pressures trigger the recognized neurohumoral changes of heart failure (Chapter 57) and produce ventricular remodeling with eccentric hypertrophy and cavity dilation, which is distinct from the remodeling seen in hypertrophic and restrictive cardiomyopathy but is similar for all other causes of dilated cardiomyopathy. The insult to myocyte integrity may be relatively acute and may trigger programmed cell death (apoptosis); however, insidious progression is the rule in inherited dilated cardiomyopathy and is also seen with viral persistence, anthracycline toxicity, and autoimmune dilated cardiomyopathy. The systolic dysfunction may reflect a combination of irreversible cell death and reversible dysfunction from inflammatory mediators. Current conventional treatment aims to minimize myocardial stress and triggers of ongoing inflammatory damage. Examples of significant improvement in systolic function raise the possibility of myocardial regenerative capacity, which is being investigated in the context of stem cell and myoblast therapies.

Dilated cardiomyopathy that develops in the absence of significant valvular, hypertensive, or ischemic heart disease is usually familial. Endomyocardial biopsy and long-term follow-up of asymptomatic relatives suggest a natural history of slowly progressive, immune-mediated myocardial damage, with age-related disease expression reaching 90% by the fifth decade. Symptomatic clinical presentation may be triggered by a respiratory tract infection, pregnancy, alcohol, or a salt and water load.

The concept of a trigger with immune-mediated pathogenesis in genetically predisposed individuals is supported by the finding of mutations in genes encoding important structural proteins in 20 to 30% of families with dilated cardiomyopathy; sarcomeric genes (10%) and lamin A/C (5%) are the most common (Table 59–8). One third of probands and family members develop low-titer, organ-specific autoantibodies to cardiac α-myosin, antibodies that are rare in other cardiac diseases or in physiologically normal individuals. The presence of autoantibodies is associated with markers of early disease and may reflect exposure of the immune system to the normally unseen intracytoplasmic antigens from the structurally damaged myocytes. Viral persistence has also been implicated as an ongoing trigger of immune-mediated damage. Preliminary studies do not suggest major phenotypic differences among families with mutations that affect various structural elements in the Z band (i.e., actin), in intermediate filaments (i.e., actinin), or in binding to the extracellular matrix (i.e., dystrophin). Lamin A/C mutations in the nuclear envelope, however, are associated with several distinct phenotypes, including premature conduction disease with late-onset dilated cardiomyopathy, severe early dilated cardiomyopathy with sudden death, and dilated cardiomyopathy in association with Emery-Dreifuss muscular dystrophy (Chapter 447).

Clinical Manifestations

The classic presentation with a gradual decrease in exercise capacity may be appreciated only in retrospect. The initial presentation is often with acute decompensation triggered by an unrelated problem, such as anemia, thyrotoxicosis, or infection (Chapter 57). Atypical chest pain may be prominent, perhaps reflecting myopericarditis. Presentation with an embolic event from the left ventricle or left atrium or with a sustained arrhythmia is less common. Symptoms relating to raised filling pressures (e.g., orthopnea, nocturnal cough, paroxysmal nocturnal dyspnea, peripheral edema) often precede symptoms of low cardiac output (e.g., dyspnea on exertion). An obvious family history of dilated cardiomyopathy is present in 5 to 10% of patients, although pedigree evaluation elicits suggestive evidence of unexplained premature cardiac disease or embolic events in up to 30% of patients.

Diagnosis

The diagnosis of dilated cardiomyopathy historically has relied on signs or symptoms of heart failure accompanied by indices of advanced left ventricular impairment and dilation. Unexplained less severe abnormalities on physical examination, 12-lead ECG tracings, or two-dimensional echocardiographic study, however, may reflect an early stage of disease with the opportunity to intervene and attenuate or prevent disease progression.

An early diagnosis of dilated cardiomyopathy requires consideration of the common recognized causes: systemic hypertension, valvular heart disease, associated systemic disorders, high-output states, and the muscular dystrophies, each of which is often suggested by the history, physical examination, 12-lead ECG study, and two-dimensional echocardiogram. Coronary angiography may be required, however, to exclude ischemic heart disease in patients with chest pain, risk factors for

TABLE 59–8 FAMILIAL DILATED CARDIOMYOPATHY: GENES, PROTEINS, AND PHENOTYPES

Gene	Protein Sarcomeric	Phenotype	Comment
MYH7	β-Myosin heavy chain	DCM	
MYBPC3	Cardiac myosin binding protein C	DCM	
TNNT2	Cardiac troponin T	DCM	
TNNI3	Cardiac troponin I	DCM	
TPM1	α-Tropomyosin	DCM	
ACTC	α-Cardiac actin	DCM	
TNNC1	Cardiac troponin C	DCM	
MYH6	α-Myosin heavy chain	DCM	Single study
SARCOMERE AND Z-DISC RELATED			
TTN	Titin	DCM	
CRP3	Muscle LIM protein	DCM	
VCL	Metavinculin	DCM	
LDB3	Cypher/ZASP	DCM, noncompaction	
INTERMEDIATE FILAMENTS			
DES	Desmin	DCM	
LMNA	Lamin A/C	DCM, conduction defect, muscular dystrophy	
CYTOSKELETAL			
DMD	Dystrophin	DCM	X-linked
SGCD	δ-Sarcoglycan	DCM	
ION CHANNEL AND ION-CHANNEL RELATED			
SCN5A	Cardiac sodium channel	DCM, conduction defect, arrhythmia	Single study
SUR2A/ABCC9	ATP-sensitive potassium channel	DCM, rhythm disturbances	Single study
PLN	Phospholamban	DCM	
MITOCHONDRIAL			
G4.5	Tafazzin	DCM, myopathy (Barth's syndrome)	X-linked

ATP = adenosine triphosphate; DCM = dilated cardiomyopathy; ZASP = z-band alternatively spliced; PDF = motif protein.

coronary disease, or age greater than 40 years. Recommended tests (see Table 59–6) include the following: a complete blood count; tests of renal, thyroid, and hepatic function; a chest radiograph to exclude infection; iron and transferrin levels to exclude hemochromatosis; and creatine kinase levels to exclude subclinical skeletal myopathy. Specific viral titers may be required if evidence suggests myocarditis (see Table 59–8).

The ECG changes of early disease are not specific and may include left axis deviation and T wave abnormalities. With progressive and advanced disease, conduction abnormalities develop: PR prolongation, QRS widening, and left bundle branch block. The rapid development of conduction disease in association with left ventricular dysfunction may suggest giant cell myocarditis, whereas progressive conduction disease in the absence of significant left ventricular dysfunction should raise suspicion of sarcoidosis (Chapter 95), myotonic dystrophy (Chapter 447), or disease caused by a mutation in lamin A/C.

As a baseline and for serial assessment to monitor disease progression and the effect of treatment, patients should have a two-dimensional echocardiogram (with measurement of chamber dimensions and calculated indices of systolic function) and a maximal exercise test (ideally with metabolic gas exchange measurements) to provide structural and functional characterization of their disease. Cardiac magnetic resonance imaging (Chapter 55) may provide more accurate measurements of ventricular volume but is generally less practical for serial evaluation. Gadolinium-enhanced magnetic resonance imaging, however, may be very helpful in differentiating segmental wall motion abnormalities in dilated cardiomyopathy from previous myocardial infarction. A myocardial biopsy occasionally should be considered in patients with potential unexplained myocarditis.

Treatment

Rx

In the absence of a specific underlying cause or aggravating factor, treatment is as described for the various stages of heart failure (Chapter 58). Supportive therapy includes sodium and fluid restriction, avoidance of alcohol and other toxins, and use of established heart failure medications. Although older recommendations emphasized rest and avoidance of exercise, this advice should be limited to patients with myocarditis or peripartum cardiomyopathy; for other patients, a submaximal exercise regimen is desirable to sustain mobility, to avoid deconditioning, and to maintain physical and psychological well-being. Patients with atrial fibrillation or with echocardiographic evidence of a left atrial or left ventricular mural thrombosis should be anticoagulated to an international normalized ratio of 2.0 to 3.0. An ICD is preferred over medication for ventricular arrhythmias, 2 and some patients require management for advanced heart failure (Chapter 58) with biventricular pacing, inotropic medications, ventricular assist devices, and cardiac transplantation (Chapter 82).

Prevention

Familial evaluation of first-degree relatives by history, by physical examination, and with 12-lead ECG and two-dimensional echocardiographic studies is warranted at the time of diagnosis and serially thereafter. Precise algorithms to determine the interval of evaluation remain to be determined; in the absence of acute myocarditis, disease progression is usually slow, and evaluation about every 5 years until age 50 years appears appropriate. The detection of early disease in a family member offers an opportunity to initiate treatment, usually with an angiotensin-converting enzyme inhibitor or β-blocker, but the efficacy of such therapy remains to be proven.

Prognosis

Prognosis relates to specific treatable causes (e.g., valvular heart disease) and to the overall prognosis of any associated disease (e.g., scleroderma). The prognosis of idiopathic and genetically determined dilated cardiomyopathy is related to the severity of disease at the time of presentation and the response to initial treatment. Most patients improve with treatment, but 5-year survival is less than 50% in patients who present with severe disease (e.g., ejection fraction <25%, left ventricular end-diastolic dimension >65 mm, peak oxygen consumption <12 mL/kg/minute).

Specific Causes of Dilated Cardiomyopathy

Alcoholic Cardiomyopathy

In the United States, excess alcohol consumption (Chapter 31) contributes to more than 10% of cases of heart failure. Alcohol and its metabolite, acetaldehyde, are cardiotoxins acutely and chronically. Myocardial depression is initially reversible but, if sustained, can lead to irreversible vacuolization, mitochondrial abnormalities, and fibrosis. Even in chronic stages, however, the heart failure represents a sum of both reversible and irreversible depression. The amount of alcohol necessary to produce symptomatic cardiomyopathy in susceptible individuals is not known but has been estimated to be six drinks (~4 oz of pure ethanol) a day for 5 to 10 years. Frequent binging without heavy daily consumption may also be sufficient. Alcoholic cardiomyopathy can develop in patients without social evidence of an alcohol problem. Abstinence leads to improvement in at least 50% of patients with severe symptoms, some of whom normalize their left ventricular ejection fractions. Patients with other causes of heart failure should also limit alcohol consumption.

Chemotherapy

Doxorubicin (Adriamycin) cardiotoxicity (Chapter 192) causes characteristic histologic changes on endomyocardial biopsy, with overt heart failure in 5 to 10% of patients who receive doses greater than or equal to 450 mg/m^2 of body surface area. Patients who have received anthracyclines in the prepubertal period without apparent cardiotoxicity may develop cardiac failure in young adulthood. The risk is higher in patients who have lower baseline ejection fractions, concomitant radiation therapy, or higher doses of doxorubicin. Cyclophosphamide and ifosfamide can cause acute severe heart failure and malignant ventricular arrhythmias. Imatinib (Chapter 195) therapy has recently been associated with decreased left ventricular function. 5-Fluorouracil can cause coronary artery spasm and depressed left ventricular contractility. Trastuzumab has been associated with an increased incidence of heart failure, particularly in patients who have received previous chemotherapy for breast cancer (Chapter 208). Interferon-α may be associated with hypotension and arrhythmias in up to 10% of patients, and interleukin-2 rarely has been associated with cardiotoxicity. Treatment consists of discontinuation of chemotherapy and, usually, standard therapy for heart failure (Chapter 58).

Metabolic Causes

Excess catecholamines, as in *pheochromocytoma* (Chapter 246), may injure the heart by compromising the coronary microcirculation or by direct toxic effects on myocytes. *Cocaine* (Chapter 32) increases synaptic concentrations of catecholamines by inhibiting reuptake at nerve terminals; the result may be an acute coronary syndrome or chronic cardiomyopathy.

Thiamine deficiency from poor nutrition or alcoholism (Chapter 237) can cause beriberi heart disease, with vasodilation and high cardiac output followed by low output. *Calcium deficiency* resulting from hypoparathyroidism, gastrointestinal abnormalities, or chelation directly compromises myocardial contractility. *Hypophosphatemia* (Chapter 120), which may occur in alcoholism, during recovery from malnutrition, and in hyperalimentation, also reduces myocardial contractility. Patients with *magnesium depletion* owing to impaired absorption or increased renal excretion (Chapter 120) also may present with left ventricular dysfunction.

Hypothyroidism (Chapter 244) depresses contractility and conduction and may cause pericardial effusions, whereas *hyperthyroidism* increases cardiac output, can worsen underlying heart failure, and may rarely be the sole cause of heart failure. The presenting sign of *diabetes* (Chapter 247) can be cardiomyopathy, especially with diastolic dysfunction, independent of epicardial coronary atherosclerosis, for which it is a major risk factor. *Obesity* (Chapter 239) can cause cardiomyopathy with increased ventricular mass and decreased contractility, which improve after weight loss, or it can aggravate underlying heart failure from other causes.

Skeletal Myopathies

Duchenne's muscular dystrophy and Becker's X-linked skeletal muscle dystrophy (Chapter 447) typically include cardiac dysfunction. Emery-Dreifuss muscular dystrophy with abnormalities of the anchoring protein emerin occurs in an X-linked pattern, whereas the same phenotype in an autosomal dominant pattern results from abnormalities of nuclear laminar proteins. Maternally transmitted mitochondrial myopathies such as Kearns-Sayre syndrome (Chapter 447) frequently cause cardiac myopathic changes that can be rapidly progressive in young adulthood.

Overlap with Restrictive Cardiomyopathy

Diseases causing primarily restrictive cardiomyopathies (see later) can occasionally overlap to cause a picture consistent with dilated cardiomyopathy. For example, *hemochromatosis* (Chapter 231) and *sarcoidosis* (Chapter 95) should be considered when evaluating any patient with a cardiomyopathy, although these conditions are more often considered with the restrictive diseases. *Amyloidosis* (Chapter 296) is less commonly confused with dilated than with hypertrophic cardiomyopathy but should be considered in a patient with a thick-walled ventricle with moderately depressed contractile function.

Arrhythmogenic Right Ventricular Cardiomyopathy

Definition and Epidemiology

Arrhythmogenic right ventricular cardiomyopathy (Chapter 64) is a genetically determined heart muscle disorder characterized by fibrofatty replacement of right ventricular myocardium. It is associated with arrhythmia, heart failure, and premature sudden death. The disease is seen in patients of European, African, and Asian descent, with an estimated prevalence in adults of between 1 in 1000 and 1 in 5000.

Pathobiology

Genetics

Arrhythmogenic right ventricular cardiomyopathy is inherited as an autosomal dominant disease, usually with incomplete penetrance, although recessive forms with cutaneous manifestations are recognized (Table 59–9). To date, recognized mutations account for approximately 40% of cases. Mutations in the cardiac ryanodine receptor produce a clinical picture with a closer resemblance to familial catecholaminergic polymorphic ventricular tachycardia (Chapter 64).

Pathology

The main pathologic feature is progressive loss of right ventricular myocardium, which is replaced by adipose and fibrous tissue. These changes, which are localized, begin in the inflow, outflow, and apical regions of the right ventricle. Aneurysm formation in these areas is typical. Progressive myocardial involvement may lead to global right ventricular dilation. Severe right ventricular disease is usually associated with fibrofatty substitution of the left ventricular myocardium, with the posterolateral wall preferentially affected.

The impairment of desmosomal function under conditions of mechanical stress is hypothesized to cause myocyte detachment and cell death. The acute phase of myocardial injury may be accompanied by inflammation; repair by fibrofatty replacement occurs because regeneration in cardiomyocytes is limited. The increased distensibility of the thin-walled right ventricle appears to confer vulnerability to cell adhesion defects. Early disease shows predilection for the thinnest portions of the right ventricle, whereas left ventricular involvement is often initially in

TABLE 59–9 FAMILIAL ARRHYTHMOGENIC RIGHT VENTRICULAR CARDIOMYOPATHY: GENES, PROTEINS, AND PHENOTYPES

Gene	Protein	Phenotype	Comment
DSP	Desmoplakin	ARVC with or without cutaneous abnormalities	Autosomal dominant or recessive
		ARVC, palmoplantar keratoderma, woolly hair (Carvajal's syndrome)	Autosomal recessive
JUP	Plakoglobin	ARVC, palmoplantar keratoderma, woolly hair (Naxos disease)	Autosomal recessive
PKP-2	Plakophilin-2	ARVC	Autosomal dominant
DSG2	Desmoglein-2	ARVC	Autosomal dominant
DSC2	Desmoglein-2	ARVC	Autosomal dominant
TGF-β3	Transforming growth factor-β3	ARVC	ARVD1 type
RyR2	Cardiac ryanodine receptor	Catecholamine-induced ventricular tachycardia	ARVD2 type

ARVC = arrhythmogenic right ventricular cardiomyopathy; ARVD = arrhythmogenic right ventricular dysplasia.

the relatively thin posterolateral wall with sparing of the thicker septum and free wall.

Clinical Manifestations

In general, four phases of disease relate to age. In the early phase, patients are usually asymptomatic, but resuscitated cardiac arrest and sudden death may be the initial manifestations, particularly in children, adolescents, and young adults. The overt arrhythmic phase most often first occurs in adolescents and young adults, when patients note palpitations or syncope. Symptomatic sustained arrhythmias are usually accompanied by morphologic and functional abnormalities of the right ventricle. The third phase, characterized by diffuse right ventricular disease, usually is recognized in the middle and later decades; patients may present with right-sided heart failure despite relatively preserved left ventricular function. In the advanced stage, obvious left ventricular involvement and biventricular heart failure are seen. More than 75% of deaths occur in patients with prior arrhythmic events and/or clinical heart failure.

Diagnosis

Clinical evaluation includes inquiry for symptoms of arrhythmia (syncope, presyncope, sustained palpitation), a family history of premature cardiac symptoms and/or sudden death, 12-lead, 24-hour, and maximal exercise ECG testing, and two-dimensional echocardiography with specific right ventricular views. Contrast echocardiography may be required to obtain better endocardial definition of the right ventricular myocardium and apex of the left ventricle. Magnetic resonance imaging may provide accurate assessment of ventricular volumes as well as noninvasive characterization of fibrous tissue and fat.

Ventricular arrhythmias with a left bundle branch block morphology, consistent with a right ventricular origin, are characteristic. Presentation during the arrhythmic phase may be with an arrhythmia of right ventricular outflow tract origin (left bundle branch block with inferior axis). However, the ECG and arrhythmic manifestations are not specific to arrhythmogenic right ventricular cardiomyopathy and overlap with many other disease states, so standard criteria are recommended for diagnosis (Table 59–10). Because these criteria are highly specific but lack sensitivity for detecting early disease, more sensitive criteria are recommended for first-degree relatives of known cases (Table 59–11). The diagnosis of arrhythmogenic right ventricular cardiomyopathy in a proband also raises the possibility of mutation analysis throughout the family to identify those at risk and in need of serial evaluation, as well as those who need no specific follow-up.

Differential Diagnosis

The differential diagnosis includes other inherited cardiomyopathies (e.g., hypertrophic, dilated), the inherited arrhythmias (long QT syndrome, Brugada syndrome, and catecholaminergic polymorphic ventricular tachycardia; Chapter 64) as well as anomalous coronary arteries (Chapter 56). The differentiation from so-called benign right ventricular outflow tract tachycardia may be problematic, although in the latter the 12-lead ECG and right ventricular imaging studies are typically normal, and no familial disease is present.

Treatment

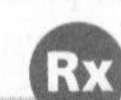

Treatment of patients with symptomatic ventricular arrhythmias is with an ICD, with supplemental metoprolol (50 to 200 mg/day), sotalol (160 to 240 mg/day), or even amiodarone (maintenance dose of 200 mg/day) if needed because of atrial fibrillation or frequent shocks.

Restrictive Cardiomyopathy

Definition and Epidemiology

Restrictive cardiomyopathies are characterized by impaired filling and reduced diastolic volume of the left and/or right ventricle despite normal or near-normal systolic function and wall thickness. Primary forms are uncommon, whereas secondary forms, in which the heart is affected as part of a multisystem disorder, usually present at the advanced stage of an infiltrative disease (e.g., amyloidosis or sarcoidosis) or a systemic storage disease (e.g., hemochromatosis). Idiopathic restrictive cardiomyopathy affects both male and female patients and may manifest in children and young adults.

Pathobiology

Genetics

Restrictive cardiomyopathy may be familial. Of the secondary forms, transthyretin amyloidosis (Chapter 296), hemochromatosis, several of the glycogen storage diseases (Chapter 219), and Fabry's disease (Chapter 223) all have a genetic basis (Table 59–12). Familial idiopathic restrictive cardiomyopathy also is part of the genetic and phenotypic expression of hypertrophic cardiomyopathy caused by sarcomeric contractile protein gene abnormalities. Restrictive cardiomyopathy has also been reported in association with skeletal myopathy and conduction system disease as part of the phenotypic spectrum caused by mutations in lamin A or C.

Pathophysiology

The characteristic dip and plateau (or square root) hemodynamic pattern (Fig. 59–4) during diastole, which is caused by an increased stiffness of the endocardium or myocardium, induces ventricular pressures to rise disproportionately to small changes in volume until a maximum

Section VIII Cardiovascular

TABLE 59–10 ARRHYTHMOGENIC RIGHT VENTRICULAR CARDIOMYOPATHY: CRITERIA FOR DIAGNOSIS IN PROBANDS*

Major	Minor
FAMILY HISTORY	
Familial disease confirmed at necropsy or surgery	Family history of premature sudden death (<35 yr) from suspected ARVC; family history (clinical diagnosis based on present criteria)
ECG DEPOLARIZATION/CONDUCTION ABNORMALITIES	
ε waves or localized prolongation (>110 msec) of QRS complex in right precordial leads (V_1–V_3)	Late potentials on signal-averaged ECG
ECG REPOLARIZATION ABNORMALITIES	
	Inverted T waves in right precordial leads (V_2 and V_3) in persons >12 years of age and in the absence of right bundle branch block
ARRHYTHMIAS	
	Sustained or nonsustained left bundle branch block–type ventricular tachycardia documented on ECG or Holter monitoring or during exercise testing; frequent ventricular extrasystoles (>1000/24 hr on Holter monitoring)
GLOBAL OR REGIONAL DYSFUNCTION AND STRUCTURAL ALTERATIONS	
Severe dilation and reduction of right ventricular ejection fraction with no or mild left ventricular involvement; localized right ventricular aneurysms (akinetic or dyskinetic areas with diastolic bulgings); severe segmental dilation of right ventricle	Mild global right ventricular dilation or ejection fraction reduction with normal left ventricle; mild segmental dilation of right ventricle; regional right ventricular hypokinesia
TISSUE CHARACTERISTICS OF WALLS	
Fibrofatty replacement of myocardium on endomyocardial biopsy	

*Diagnosis requires two major, one major and two minor, or four minor criteria.
ARVC = arrhythmogenic right ventricular cardiomyopathy; ECG = electrocardiogram.
From McKenna WJ, Thiene G, Nava A, et al: Diagnosis of arrhythmogenic right ventricular dysplasia/cardiomyopathy. Br Heart J 1994;71:215–218.

TABLE 59–11 ARRHYTHMOGENIC RIGHT VENTRICULAR CARDIOMYOPATHY: CRITERIA FOR DIAGNOSIS OF FIRST-DEGREE RELATIVES WHO DO NOT FULFILL CRITERIA AS PROBANDS*

ARVC in a first-degree relative plus one of the following:	
ECG	T wave inversion in right precordial leads (V_2 and V_3)
Signal-averaged ECG	Late potentials seen on signal-averaged ECG
Arrhythmia	Left bundle branch block–type ventricular tachycardia on ECG, Holter monitoring, or during exercise testing; >200 extrasystoles over a 24-hour period
Structural or functional abnormality of the right ventricle	Mild global right ventricular dilation or reduction in ejection fraction with normal left ventricle; mild segmental dilation of the right ventricle; regional right ventricular hypokinesia

*Any one criterion is adequate for the diagnosis.
ARVC = arrhythmogenic right ventricular cardiomyopathy; ECG = electrocardiogram.
From Hamid MS, Norman M, Quraishi A, et al: Prospective evaluation of relatives for familial arrhythmogenic right ventricular cardiomyopathy reveals a need to broaden diagnostic criteria. J Am Coll Cardiol 2002;40:1445–1450.

is reached. In infiltrative diseases such as amyloidosis or sarcoidosis, the increased stiffness results from infiltrates within the interstitium between myocardial cells. In the storage disorders, the deposits are within the cells.

Clinical Manifestations

The presenting clinical features develop as a consequence of raised ventricular filling pressures and are generally not distinguishable from those of heart failure resulting from systolic impairment. In the early stages, the patient may have a decrease in exercise capacity, whereas advanced disease is typically associated with extreme fatigue and dyspnea at rest as part of a low cardiac output state. Atrial dilation and atrial fibrillation are common. Pulmonary congestion, hepatic engorgement, ascites, and peripheral edema develop with advanced disease.

Diagnosis

Diagnosis is based on the demonstration of the abnormal filling pattern and can most usefully be achieved by Doppler echocardiographic evaluation (Chapter 53). Contrast echocardiography or magnetic resonance imaging is useful to delineate the distribution of disease and the extent of mitral and tricuspid valve involvement.

The diagnostic evaluation aims to exclude potentially reversible conditions (e.g., most of the secondary causes of restrictive cardiomyopathy). In such cases, the cardiac manifestations may provide the clues, but definitive diagnosis relies on the demonstration of disease-specific features, such as the following: the presence of abnormal amyloid protein in amyloidosis (Chapter 296), a noncaseating granuloma in sarcoidosis (Chapter 95), abnormal iron studies in hemochromatosis (Chapter 231),

TABLE 59–12 CAUSES OF RESTRICTIVE CARDIOMYOPATHIES

INFILTRATIVE DISORDERS
Amyloidosis
Sarcoidosis
STORAGE DISORDERS
Hemochromatosis
Fabry's disease
Glycogen storage diseases
FIBROTIC DISORDERS
Radiation
Scleroderma
Drugs (e.g., doxorubicin, serotonin, ergotamine)
METABOLIC DISORDERS
Carnitine deficiency
Defects in fatty acid metabolism
ENDOMYOCARDIAL DISORDERS
Endomyocardial fibrosis
Hypereosinophilic syndrome (Löffler's endocarditis)
MISCELLANEOUS CAUSES
Carcinoid syndrome

and reduced α_1-galactosidase levels in Fabry's disease (Chapter 223). Endomyocardial biopsy, although potentially definitive, is rarely required to make these diagnoses. It is often important to exclude constrictive pericarditis (Chapter 77), which is also characterized by rapid early diastolic filling.

Differential Diagnosis

In pericardial constriction, the capacity of the heart to expand is limited by the rigid pericardium, so increases in filling pressures will not result in an increased cardiac volume (Chapter 77). In restrictive cardiomyopathy, by comparison, increases in volume will increase filling pressures and, as a result, increase systemic blood pressure; by the same principle, patients with restrictive cardiomyopathy may be very sensitive to volume depletion.

Although the strictest definition of a restrictive cardiomyopathy requires normal or near-normal left ventricular systolic function and wall thickness with the dip and plateau hemodynamic pattern, diastolic impairment with or without restrictive physiology is also part of the spectrum of the clinical presentation of both hypertrophic and dilated cardiomyopathies. Patients with hypertension (Chapter 66) also may first present with diastolic dysfunction and mild left ventricular hypertrophy before progressing to more marked left ventricular hypertrophy or dilation.

Treatment Rx

In patients with secondary restrictive cardiomyopathies, treatment must address both the underlying systemic disease and the heart failure itself (Chapter 58; Tables 58–2 through 58–5). Diuresis is key but must be undertaken carefully so as not to reduce left ventricular filling pressures to the point of causing hypotension. Angiotensin-converting enzyme inhibitors and β-blockers are commonly recommended despite fewer data on their benefit than in dilated cardiomyopathy. For idiopathic restrictive cardiomyopathy, treatment of heart failure is the only option.

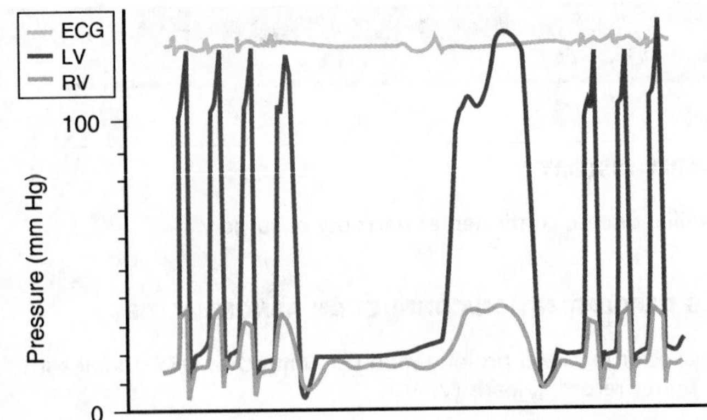

FIGURE 59–4 • Idiopathic restrictive cardiomyopathy. Right ventricular (RV) and left ventricular (LV) pressure electrocardiographic (ECG) tracings in a patient with idiopathic restrictive cardiomyopathy. A dip-and-plateau pattern is seen in both ventricles, and diastolic filling pressures are elevated. The plateaus occur at different pressures, approximately 16 mm Hg for the RV tracing compared with 20 mm Hg for the LV tracing. The diagnosis of restrictive disease was confirmed by thoracotomy. (Redrawn from Benofti JR, Grossman W, Cohn PF: The clinical profile of restrictive cardiomyopathy. Circulation 1980;61:1206.)

Prognosis

In restrictive cardiomyopathy, the clinical course is usually slow and protracted with an antecedent history that, in retrospect, may go back 5 years or more. Survival from the time of diagnosis is often 10 years or more, except for amyloidosis, which progresses much more rapidly. Symptoms of heart failure with mitral and tricuspid regurgitation are generally progressive and respond poorly to treatments for heart failure. Referral for transplant assessment should be considered early because pulmonary hypertension may develop and necessitate heart and lung transplantation.

Specific Clinical Syndromes

Sarcoidosis

Although cardiac involvement is found in up to 50% of patients with sarcoidosis (Chapter 95) at autopsy, clinical cardiac involvement occurs in fewer than 10% of patients. The presentation is often with conduction defects or ventricular tachyarrhythmias, although granulomas can also compromise the coronary circulation and cause ischemia or infarction. On echocardiogram, the cardiomyopathy may be dilated or restrictive. Biopsy of extracardiac sites is usually adequate for the diagnosis, but a gallium scan often demonstrates cardiac inflammation. A myocardial biopsy may show granulomas or, because of the focal distribution of the lesions, may be nondiagnostic. Corticosteroid therapy may improve arrhythmias, but heart failure may worsen despite such therapy. An ICD is generally indicated for ventricular arrhythmias.

Amyloidosis

Amyloidosis (Chapter 296), which is the most common cause of restrictive cardiomyopathy, can result from either primary amyloidosis in patients with multiple myeloma (Chapter 215) or familial amyloidosis in patients in whom an abnormal transthyretin is deposited in the kidney, liver, and sometimes the heart (Chapter 296). By comparison, secondary amyloidosis rarely involves the heart. Senile amyloidosis, involving normal transthyretin, occasionally causes clinical heart failure in elderly patients but progresses quite slowly compared with primary amyloidosis. Amyloid fibrils infiltrate into the interstitium, stiffen the ventricles, replace some contractile elements, and frequently affect the conduction system, thereby leading to bradyarrhythmias. When amyloid also surrounds the arterioles, it may lead to anginal chest pain and even myocardial infarction. Some patients may present with orthostatic hypotension resulting from amyloid autonomic neuropathy. Macroglossia, carpal tunnel syndrome with hypothenar wasting, skin friability, nephrotic syndrome, or multiple myeloma may also suggest the diagnosis of amyloidosis.

The ECG tracing characteristically shows markedly decreased voltage despite increased wall thickness on echocardiography. Specific diagnosis in some cases can be made from a characteristic sparkling refractile pattern on echocardiography (Fig. 59–5). Up to 80% of patients have a

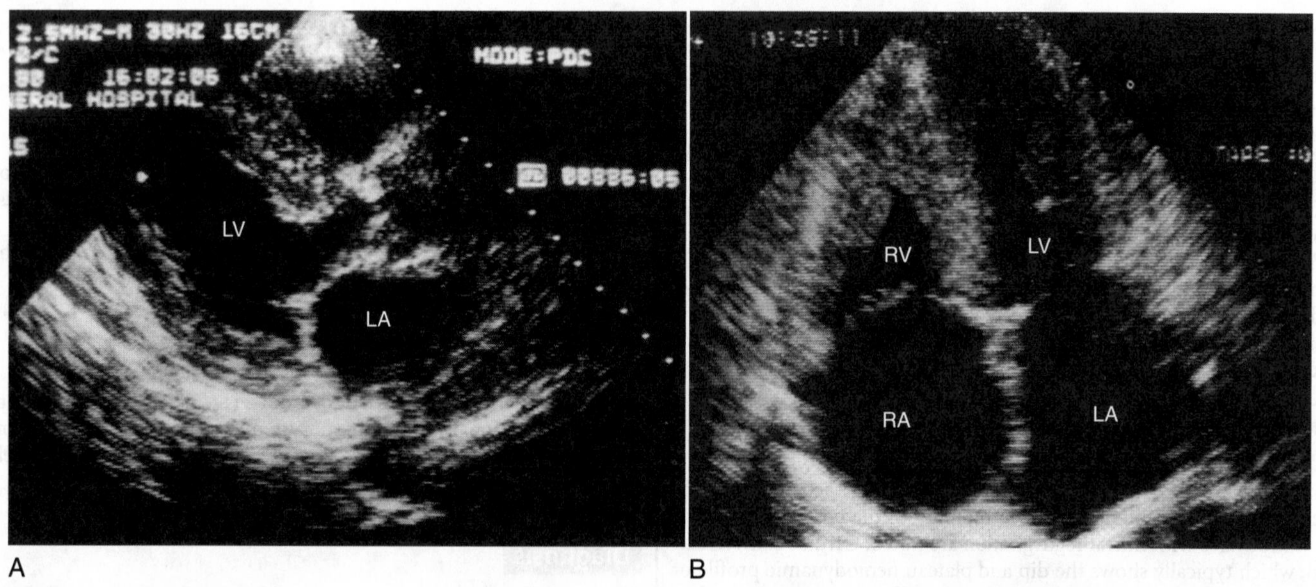

FIGURE 59–5 • Amyloidosis. A, Parasternal long-axis echocardiographic image shows a "sparkling" granular myocardial texture in the interventricular septum in a patient with biopsy-proved amyloidosis. LA = left atrium; LV = left ventricle. **B,** An apical four-chamber echocardiographic image demonstrates biventricular hypertrophy in a patient with biopsy-proved amyloidosis. RA = right atrium; RV = right ventricle. (From Levine RA: Echocardiographic assessment of the cardiomyopathies. *In* Weyman AE [ed]: Principles and Practice of Echocardiography, 2nd ed. Philadelphia: Lea & Febiger, 1994, p 810.)

monoclonal protein identified from either serum or urine. Biopsy of subcutaneous fat or the rectum frequently reveals amyloidosis, so endomyocardial biopsy is rarely required.

Therapy with colchicine or with combined melphalan and prednisone provides a 20 to 30% response rate in patients with monoclonal gammopathy. Vasodilator therapy is less effective than in dilated cardiomyopathy, owing to less pronounced systolic dysfunction, greater reliance on high filling pressures, and the frequently accompanying autonomic neuropathy, which predisposes to postural hypotension. Amyloidosis is usually a contraindication to cardiac transplantation because it recurs in the donor heart and can progress rapidly in other organs.

Patients with amyloidosis with heart failure have a median survival of less than 1 year and a 5-year survival of less than 5%. Most deaths occur suddenly. Patients with familial amyloidosis have a slower course than do patients with a monoclonal gammopathy.

Hemochromatosis

In hemochromatosis (Chapter 231), which can result from a genetic defect in iron regulation or from iron overload related to hemolytic anemia and transfusions, iron in the perinuclear areas of myocytes disrupts cellular architecture and mitochondrial function, thereby leading to cell death and replacement fibrosis. The atrioventricular node may be involved. Restrictive physiologic features dominate earlier in the course, followed by dilation generally to a left ventricular diastolic dimension less than 60 mm; ejection fractions in severe cases are often less than 30%. The diagnosis is generally made from the clinical picture, an elevated serum iron level, and high transferrin saturation (>50%). Genetic testing may be helpful, and the diagnosis can be confirmed by endomyocardial biopsy. Phlebotomy and iron chelation therapy with deferoxamine (Chapter 231) may improve cardiac function before cell injury becomes irreversible. Standard heart failure treatment (Chapter 58) is generally recommended. Deaths from hemochromatosis result more often from cirrhosis and liver carcinoma than from cardiac disease.

Fabry's Disease

In Fabry's disease and glycogen storage diseases, restrictive physiology is associated with increases in left ventricular mass (see Hypertrophic Cardiomyopathy). Treatment is for the underlying systemic disease, with careful treatment of the heart failure caused by the restrictive myopathy (Chapter 58).

Fibrotic Restrictive Cardiomyopathies

Radiation therapy for thoracic malignant disease (Chapters 18 and 201) can produce restrictive cardiomyopathy, usually within several years, although occasionally up to 15 years later, and sometimes with constrictive pericarditis (Chapter 77). In the scleroderma-affected heart (Chapter 288), interstitial fibrosis is common, perhaps related to small vessel ischemia with microinfarction; left ventricular dilation is uncommon, and the congestive symptoms may be refractory to therapy.

Unclassified Cardiomyopathies

Left Ventricular Noncompaction

Failure of the trabecular or spongiform layer of the myocardium to compact may occur with congenital heart disease, including atrial and ventricular septal defects and coarctation of the aorta (Chapter 68), and with the rare X-linked multisystem disorder, Barth's syndrome. With recent improvements in imaging technology, it has also been recognized in patients with hypertrophic and dilated cardiomyopathy. The prevalence of localized areas of noncompaction is unknown, but clinically significant, isolated left ventricular noncompaction in the absence of other cardiac abnormalities is uncommon.

Areas of noncompacted myocardium may be best delineated from normal myocardium by the demonstration of flow within the myocardium by Doppler or contrast echocardiography. When extensive areas are involved, systolic performance may be impaired, and there is a risk of ventricular arrhythmias and systemic emboli. Treatment, when necessary, is for associated heart failure (Chapter 58), arrhythmias (Chapter 61), and the risk of emboli (Chapter 99. Natural history and prognosis are not well established.

Tako-Tsubo Cardiomyopathy

Tako-Tsubo cardiomyopathy is a syndrome of transient apical left ventricular dysfunction that mimics myocardial infarction. Postulated mechanisms include coronary artery spasm, myocarditis, and dynamic midcavity obstruction. Analogous permanent apical outpouchings develop in patients with hypertrophic cardiomyopathy and midventricular obstruction.

The clinical syndrome classically includes chest pain, ST segment elevation, and raised cardiac biomarkers in association with emotional or physical stress. Coronary arteriography reveals normal epicardial vessels. Conservative treatment with rehydration and removal of the determinants of stress usually results in rapid resolution within hours of the symptoms, ECG changes, and wall motion abnormalities.

DISEASES OF THE ENDOCARDIUM

Löffler's Endocarditis and Endocardial Fibroelastosis

In equatorial Africa, endomyocardial fibrosis accounts for 15 to 25% of cardiac deaths. It can cause dense thickening of the ventricular inflow tracts and atrioventricular valves and of one or more commonly both ventricles. However, the underlying myocardium is usually spared, and systolic function is normal. The atria may be very large, and pericardial effusions may be present. Endocardial disease can also cause a clinical syndrome similar to restrictive cardiomyopathy.

In Löffler's endocarditis, which is seen as part of hypereosinophilic syndrome (Chapter 176), degranulated eosinophils are involved in an inflammatory endocardial process that predominantly involves the left ventricle. The mechanism of the fibrotic response, which develops in either or both ventricles, is unknown. Löffler's endocarditis occurs in temperate climates and is characterized by older age, male predominance, and a more aggressive course than endomyocardial fibrosis. Persistent eosinophilia of more than 1500 eosinophils/mm^3 without other causes leads to dysfunction of the heart, lungs, and other organs.

Diagnosis

In Löffler's endocarditis and endocardial fibrosis, the apices of the ventricle typically are obliterated, and immobility of the posterior leaflet of the mitral valve with mitral regurgitation are noted. Cardiac catheterization, which typically shows the dip and plateau hemodynamic profile of restrictive cardiomyopathy (see Fig. 59–4), usually is not necessary unless the quality of noninvasive studies is suboptimal. Endomyocardial biopsy in Löffler's endocarditis and endocardial fibrosis is important for diagnosis, although it may be difficult to obtain adequate tissue.

Treatment

Rx

In Löffler's endocarditis, treatment depends on the stage of disease and the activity of degranulating lymphocytes; anecdotal success has been reported with corticosteroids, hydroxyurea, and interferon. For both endomyocardial fibrosis and Löffler's endocarditis, diuretics and anticoagulation are important adjuncts to therapy. Surgical débridement of the fibrous plague with repair or replacement of the mitral or tricuspid valves may dramatically improve symptoms, albeit with significant perioperative mortality of 10 to 20%. In endomyocardial fibrosis, the prognosis is poor because progressive disease leads to death from heart failure, embolism, or ventricular arrhythmia.

Carcinoid Syndrome

Epidemiology and Pathobiology

Once a carcinoid tumor (Chapter 251) has metastasized to the liver, up to two thirds of patients will have endocardial involvement, usually with thickening and scarring of the right atrial and right ventricular endocardium as well as of the tricuspid and/or pulmonary valves. Valvular involvement may result in both stenosis and regurgitation, with tricuspid regurgitation oftentimes predominating. In patients with a patent foramen ovale, left-sided valvular involvement is common. Occasional patients may have concomitant myocardial metastases and pericardial effusions from direct tumor invasion, but the endocardial changes are typically related to the vasoactive substances produced by the tumor in the liver, rather than by actual tumor involvement.

Clinical Manifestations

The most common presentation is with dyspnea and signs and symptoms of right-sided heart failure. Cardiac involvement may be a major contributor to death in many patients.

Treatment

Treatment of the underlying carcinoid with a somatostatin analogue can improve systemic symptoms (Chapter 251). Valve replacement has occasionally been performed, but the operative mortality rate is markedly higher than is typical for valve replacement, and the advisability of such surgery must be weighed against the natural history of the noncardiac extent of disease (Chapter 251).

Endocardial Manifestations of Cancer

Nonbacterial Thrombotic (Marantic) Endocarditis

Epidemiology and Pathobiology

Platelet-fiber masses that are adherent to the mitral and/or aortic valves are seen in about 20% of patients with malignant tumors, especially mucin-producing adenocarcinomas, melanomas, leukemias, and lymphomas. The lesions are sterile, commonly verruciform, and without accompanying inflammation.

Clinical Manifestations

Nonbacterial thrombotic endocarditis is virtually always asymptomatic but occasionally is a source of systemic emboli. Because of the small size of many of the emboli, the first presentation is often with cerebral symptoms.

Diagnosis

Larger lesions are detectable by echocardiography, but even transesophageal echocardiography is not sufficiently sensitive to identify lesions that may be found at autopsy and that may have been the source of systemic emboli.

Treatment

No treatment has proven efficacious. However, systemic anticoagulation similar to that used in patients with tumor-associated deep venous thrombosis is often tried (Chapters 81 and 189).

CARDIAC TUMORS

Myocardial Tumors

Most primary cardiac tumors are benign. However, all tumors that extend from other tissues into the heart are malignant, as are metastatic lesions.

Epidemiology and Pathobiology

Primary tumors of the heart are unusual, with a prevalence of 1 in 2000 to 1 in 4000 in autopsy series. Nearly all these primary tumors are benign myxomas, although fibromas, lipomas, and fibroelastomas also occur. Rhabdomyomas are seen in children, especially with tuberous sclerosis (Chapter 444). The rare primary malignant tumors include sarcomas, especially angiosarcomas (Table 59–13). Rarely, a primary mesothelioma or lymphoma may originate in the heart.

TABLE 59–13 CARDIAC TUMORS

PRIMARY	SECONDARY
Benign	**Direct Extension**
Myxoma	Lung cancer
Lipoma	Breast cancer
Fibroma	Mediastinal tumors
Rhabdomyoma	
Fibroelastoma	**Metastatic Tumors**
Malignant	Malignant melanoma
Sarcoma	Leukemia
Mesothelioma	Lymphoma
Lymphoma	
	Venous Extension
	Renal cell cancer
	Adrenal cancer
	Liver cancer

Up to 20% of advanced cancers may involve the pericardium, epicardium, or cardiac chambers either by direct extension of the primary tumor or by metastatic disease. Direct extension occurs principally from cancers of the lung, breast, esophagus, and mediastinum. Extension through the inferior vena cava to the right atrium and even to the right ventricle occurs with cancers of the kidney, adrenal gland, and liver. Metastatic spread is most common with melanomas or lymphomas.

Pericardial Tumors

Clinical Manifestations

Pericardial tumors almost always result from direct extension of tumors, principally lung and breast, which produce a pericardial effusion that can progress to cardiac tamponade (Chapter 77). Patients typically are asymptomatic or minimally symptomatic in terms of the cardiac involvement until the effusion is very large, although they often may be very ill owing to progressive tumor elsewhere.

Diagnosis

The diagnosis is often suspected in a patient with advanced malignant disease based on evidence of heart failure, hypertension, or arrhythmia and is confirmed by echocardiography. The differentiation between pericardial involvement by tumor as compared with postradiation pericarditis depends on pericardiocentesis, often guided by echocardiography, and cytologic examination.

Treatment

Rx

Cardiac tamponade must be treated with urgent pericardiocentesis, preferably under echocardiographic or radiologic guidance (Chapter 77). Although such a procedure can be life-saving and provide short-term to immediate-term palliation, control of the effusion often requires prolonged drainage, administration of intrapericardial chemotherapeutic agents, or limited or full pericardiectomy (Chapter 77). Some patients with pericardial tumors may respond to aggressive systemic chemotherapy, but recurrent accumulation of fluid is sufficiently likely that creation of a pericardial window should be considered before hospital discharge.

Prognosis

In many cases, a tumor that is causing pericarditis has extended or will eventually extend through the pericardial space and into the myocardium, so no therapy is likely to be successful. The prognosis is very poor, except in unusual cases when the tumor responds dramatically to systemic therapy.

Intracavitary Tumors

Myxoma

Definition and Epidemiology

A *myxoma* is a benign polypoid neoplasm that originates from endocardial cells and is attached to the interatrial septum, usually protruding into the left atrium but occasionally into the right atrium and rarely into the ventricles. Myxomas are more common in women, especially between the ages of 30 and 60 years, than in men. These tumors can be familial and are rarely associated with other systemic abnormalities.

Clinical Manifestations

Myxomas are slow growing and usually do not produce symptoms or signs until they enlarge. The typical presentation is with a tumor embolus, whereby usually small portions of the myxoma break loose and cause a single embolism or a shower of emboli. However, a large embolism from a myxoma can be of sufficient size to obstruct a medium-size artery. Some patients have systemic symptoms including fever, malaise, and arthralgias as part of a clinical syndrome that may be confused with bacterial endocarditis (Chapter 76) or a collagen vascular disease. Large myxomas can prolapse into the mitral valve orifice during diastole, or they may obstruct blood flow from the left atrium to the left ventricle and mimic rheumatic mitral stenosis.

Diagnosis

A myxoma large enough to obstruct the mitral orifice can produce an audible "tumor plop" when the myxoma prolapses and obstructs blood flow during diastole, at the same time that the opening snap of mitral stenosis would typically be heard. If obstruction is incomplete, the tumor plop may be followed by a diastolic rumble. As obstruction becomes more severe, cardiac output may fall precipitously. Echocardiography (Chapter 53) is usually definitive; transesophageal echocardiography provides a higher sensitivity than does transthoracic echocardiography.

Treatment

Surgical removal is generally curative, although myxomas can be multiple or recur in about 5% of cases. Follow-up postoperative echocardiography is generally recommended. However, the optimal frequency and duration for follow-up screening are uncertain.

Other Primary Intracavitary Tumors

Papillary fibroelastomas are rare, typically frondlike tumors that may arise from a cardiac valve, often the mitral valve, and are generally detected incidentally by echocardiography. However, like myxomas, they can manifest with systemic or even coronary emboli. Surgical excision is usually successful.

Angiosarcomas, which are more frequent in men than in women, typically involve the pericardium and right atrium. They cause obstruction with clinical signs and symptoms of right-sided heart failure. These sarcomas are generally not amenable to therapy.

Extension of Tumor into the Cardiac Cavities

Direct extension of tumor up the inferior vena cava into the right atrium can be seen with renal cell carcinomas and less commonly with liver and adrenal cancers. In some cases, tumor extension will be accompanied by adherent clot, and either the tumor or the clot may cause obstruction or pulmonary emboli (Chapter 99). No treatments are generally successful, and the prognosis is grim.

Intramyocardial Tumors

Benign tumors in the myocardium include lipomas, fibromas, and rhabdomyomas. Primary malignant tumors include sarcomas, lymphomas, and mesotheliomas. Metastatic tumors include melanomas, lymphomas, and leukemias. The tumors may be clinically silent, or they may produce arrhythmias or even impinge on coronary arteries, thereby causing ischemic syndromes. Large tumors may protrude into the cardiac chamber and cause obstruction. Therapies are not successful, except for occasional patients whose metastatic tumors may respond to systemic chemotherapy or whose primary tumors have been cured by heart transplantation.

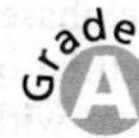

1. Mason JW, O'Connell JB, Herskowitz A, et al: A clinical trial of immunosuppressive therapy for myocarditis: The Myocarditis Treatment Trial Investigators. N Engl J Med 1995;333:269–275.
2. Kadish A, Dyer A, Daubert JP, et al: Prophylactic defibrillator implantation in patients with nonischemic dilated cardiomyopathy. N Engl J Med 2004;350:2151–2158.

SUGGESTED READINGS

Arad M, Maron BJ, Gorham JM, et al: Glycogen storage disease presenting as hypertrophic cardiomyopathy. N Engl J Med 2005;352:362–372. *A detailed analysis.*

Burkett EL, Hershberger RE: Clinical and genetic issues in familial dilated cardiomyopathy. J Am Coll Cardiol 2005;45:969–981. *Echocardiographic and ECG screening of first-degree relatives is indicated.*

Section VIII Cardiovascular

Doughan AR, Williams BR: Cardiac sarcoidosis. Heart 2006;92:282–288. *A comprehensive review.*
Elliott P, McKenna WJ: Hypertrophic cardiomyopathy. Lancet 2004;363: 1881–1891. *A practical review.*
Falk RH: Diagnosis and management of the cardiac amyloidoses. Circulation 2005;112:2047–2060. *A detailed review.*
Kirkpatrick JN, Wong T, Bednarz JE, et al: Differential diagnosis of cardiac masses using contrast echocardiographic perfusion imaging. J Am Coll Cardiol 2004;43;1412–1419. *Compared with adjacent myocardium, malignant and vascular tumors hyperenhanced, whereas stromal tumors and thrombi hypoenhanced.*
Magnani JW, Dec GW: Myocarditis: Current trends in diagnosis and treatment. Circulation 2006;113:876–890. *An excellent comprehensive review.*
Moller JE, Connolly HM, Ruin J, et al: Factors associated with progression of carcinoid heart disease. N Engl J Med 2003;348:1005–1015. *Details the relationship among serotonin levels, the progression of cardiac disease, and the effect of therapy on patients with carcinoid heart disease.*
Pinede L, Duhaut P, Loire R: Clinical presentation of left atrial cardiac myxoma: A series of 112 consecutive cases. Medicine (Baltimore) 2001;80:159–172. *Clinical and surgical data from a consecutive series of 112 patients seen over a 40-year period.*
Rassi A Jr, Rassi A, Little WC, et al: Development and validation of a risk score for predicting death in Chagas' heart disease. N Engl J Med 2006;355:799–808. *Functional class, cardiomegaly, systolic dysfunction, ventricular tachycardia, and low voltage were key prognostic factors.*
Sen-Chowdhry S, Syrris P, McKenna WJ: Genetics of right ventricular cardiomyopathy. J Cardiovasc Electrophysiol 2005;16:927–935. *Review of genetics and pathogenesis.*
Sliwa K, Fett J, Elkayam U: Peripartum cardiomyopathy. Lancet 2006;368:687–693. *A careful overview.*

60 PRINCIPLES OF ELECTROPHYSIOLOGY

Hugh Calkins

The function of the human heart requires rhythmic beating on the average of 70 times a minute, 24 hours a day, for 80 years or more. The close to 3 billion contractions of the cardiac musculature that must occur without fail are coordinated by an intricate network of specialized, electrically active cells that are integrated with the myocytes that compose the predominant mass of the heart. Any loss of electrical activity, even for a few seconds, results in syncope (Chapters 61 and 427); loss of electrical activity for a few minutes may end in death.

CARDIAC ELECTROPHYSIOLOGY

Ion channels are integral membrane-spanning proteins that allow the rapid movement of specific ions, most importantly Na^+, K^+, Cl^-, and Ca^{2+}, across the cell membrane at rates of 10^8 ions per second. The opening and closing of the channels occur through a process of gating, whereby changes in the voltage, ligand, or receptor associated with the channel lead to alterations in the conformation of the proteins that activate or inactivate the channel pore. Voltage gating is the predominant method of regulating ion channels in the heart and is found in sodium and various potassium channels. Ligand-gated ion channels use ligands such as neurotransmitters, ions such as intracellular calcium, and metabolic products such as adenosine triphosphate to activate a variety of channels, including those for potassium. Receptor-gated channels use changes in the physical environment, such as stretch, to activate channels, including those for chloride, that regulate intracellular volume.

The coordinated activity of numerous ion channels contributes to the creation of the cardiac action potential (Fig. 60–1). There are five phases to the cardiac action potential. At rest, the transmembrane potential of the cell exists close to −90 mV (the inside of the cell is positive with respect to the outside). With depolarization of the cell either from depolarization of adjacent cells or from an external change in voltage, sodium channels change from a closed to an open state and rapidly move sodium ions down a gradient into the interior of the cell, creating the sodium current I_{Na} and the rapid upstroke of phase 0 of the action potential. At the peak of depolarization, approximately +40 mV, the sodium current is inactivated, and the transient outward current I_{to} is activated with the opening of various voltage-gated potassium channels, resulting in the rapid decrease in voltage and phase 1 of the action potential. The plateau of the action potential, phase 2, follows and is an amalgamation of multiple currents representing inward and outward movement of ions. Contributors to this phase include the rapid component of the delayed rectifier potassium current I_{Kr}, the slow component of the delayed rectifier potassium current I_{Ks}, the L-type calcium channel, and the Na^+-Ca^{2+} exchanger. As the outward potassium currents increase and the calcium current decreases at the end of phase 2, the action potential progresses to phase 3, the phase of rapid repolarization. The inward rectifier potassium current I_{K1} contributes significantly to this final phase of repolarization and brings the action potential to its resting membrane potential. During phase 4, the heart is in diastole, with most cells at −85 to −90 mV. Specialized cells in the sinoatrial (SA) and atrioventricular (AV) nodes repolarize to approximately −60 mV and contain currents that contribute to spontaneous depolarization during phase 4. These pacemaker cells contain the inward activation or funny current I_f activated by hyperpolarization and carried by sodium and the background sodium current I_{Na-B}. The calcium currents $I_{Ca,L}$ and $I_{Ca,T}$, the Na^+-K^+ pump $I_{Na,K}$, and the Na^+-Ca^{2+} exchanger $I_{Na,Ca}$ additionally may contribute to diastolic depolarization.

Variations in the duration and shape of the cardiac action potential exist, depending on its location in the heart (Fig. 60–2). Likewise, alterations of ion channel expression and activity in disease states contribute to prolongation of the action potential. The atrial action potential has a typical duration of 100 to 200 msec; the ventricular action potential typically lasts 250 to 300 msec. Different layers of the ventricle exhibit marked changes in the action potential. Epicardial cells have a prominent phase 1 compared with endocardial cells, in which phase 1 is blunted. The phase 2 plateau is decreased in epicardial cells, leading to less activation of the delayed rectifier currents and a prolonged action potential in epicardial cells. M cells found in the midmyocardium have the longest action potential duration and may contribute to the U wave seen on the surface electrocardiogram (ECG). The J (Osborne) wave seen on the ECG in cases of hypothermia (see Fig. 110–1) may be due to the increased prominence of I_{to} in the epicardial cells. Prolongation of the action potential is seen in cardiac hypertrophy or failure. At the molecular level, downregulation of the transient outward current I_{to} plays a prominent role in these disease states.

In a normal heart, the source of initial depolarizations occurs in the pacemaker cells of the sinus node (see Fig. 60-2). The SA node is found at the lateral border of the superior vena cava and right atrial junction in the sulcus terminalis. It is an ovoid structure measuring up to 2 cm long × 0.5 cm wide. The sinus node artery, branching from either the right coronary artery (55 to 60%) or the left coronary artery (40 to 45%), runs through the middle of the sinus node. Pacemaker cells, seen as spider-shaped and spindle-shaped cells in the node, spontaneously depolarize during diastole. The wave of depolarization spreads through the sinus node and into the surrounding myocardium. The sympathetic and parasympathetic nervous systems affect the sinus rate. Adrenergic stimulation increases the rate by increasing $I_{Ca,L}$ and I_f activities. Cholinergic stimulation by the parasympathetic nervous system decreases the rate by decreasing $I_{Ca,L}$ and I_f activities. Stretch mediators found in the node and coupled to chloride channels also may increase the atrial rate with increasing atrial pressure. The SA node is the predominant pacemaker in the heart because of its rapid rates of depolarization and overdrive suppression of secondary pacemakers.

Depolarization occurs through the atria to the AV node and from the right atrium to the left atrium. Three intra-atrial pathways—anterior, middle, and posterior—connect the right and left atria. Three intranodal pathways—superior, middle, and inferior tracts—also may connect the SA node to the AV node, although various investigators have disputed their presence. The P wave on the ECG is formed by atrial depolarization. The AV node is found at the apex of the triangle of Koch, formed by the tendon of Todaro on one side and the tricuspid annulus on the other, on the right side of the heart and anterior to the os of the coronary sinus. The arterial supply of the AV node arises from the right coronary artery in 85 to 90% of cases. The AV node itself is complex and can be divided into three general regions, with further subdivisions possible. A transitional zone contains multiple atrial inputs that extend to the compact AV node, which penetrates the central fibrous body and becomes the bundle of His. The compact AV node ranges from 5 to 7 mm by 2 to 5 mm. At least two distinct populations of AV node cells, rod shaped and ovoid, have been described. These cells spontaneously depolarize because of a strong I_f current. Most ovoid cells lack I_{Na} and I_{to}, leading to slower depolarization. Conduction is relatively slow through the AV node compared with atrial and ventricular tissue, in part because

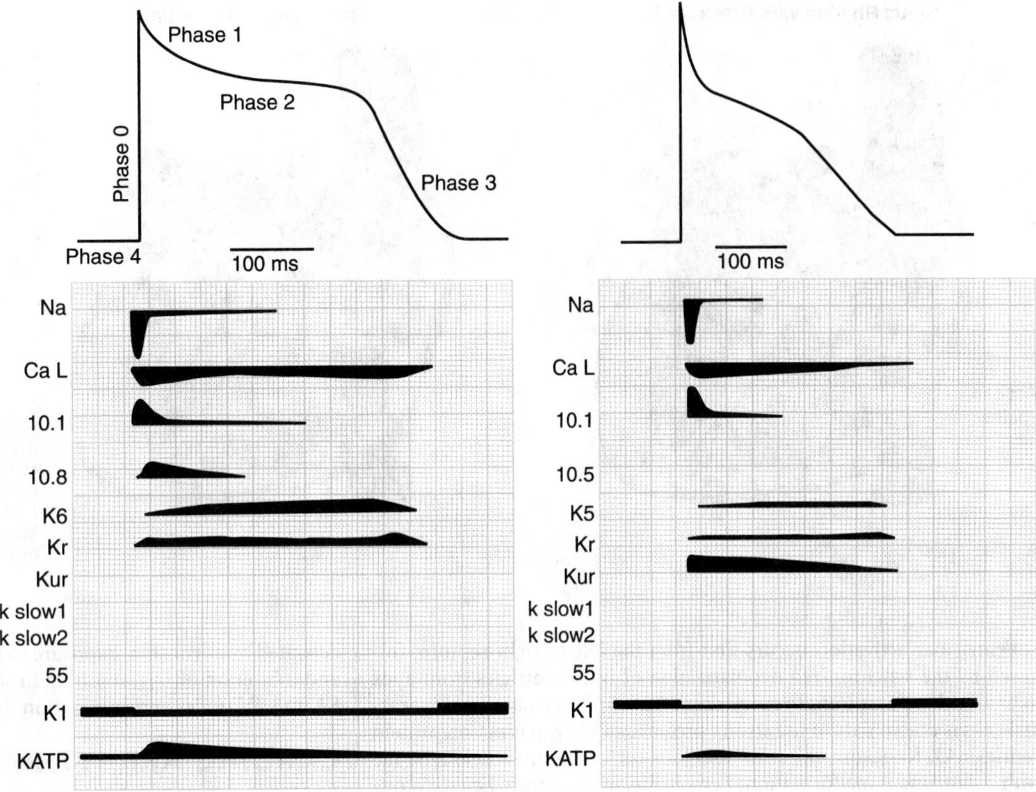

FIGURE 60–1 • The cardiac action potential waveforms and underlying ionic currents in adult human ventricular (left) and atrial (right) myocytes. The time- and voltage-dependent properties of the voltage-gated inward Na^+ (Nav) and Ca^{2+} (Cav) currents expressed in human atrial and ventricular myocytes are similar. In contrast, there are multiple types of K^+ currents, particularly Kv currents, contributing to atrial and ventricular action potential repolarization. The properties of the various Kv currents are distinct, and in contrast to the inward currents, there are multiple Kv currents expressed in individual myocytes throughout the myocardium. (From Nerbonne JM, Kass RS: Molecular physiology of cardiac repolarization. Physiol Rev 2005;85:1207.)

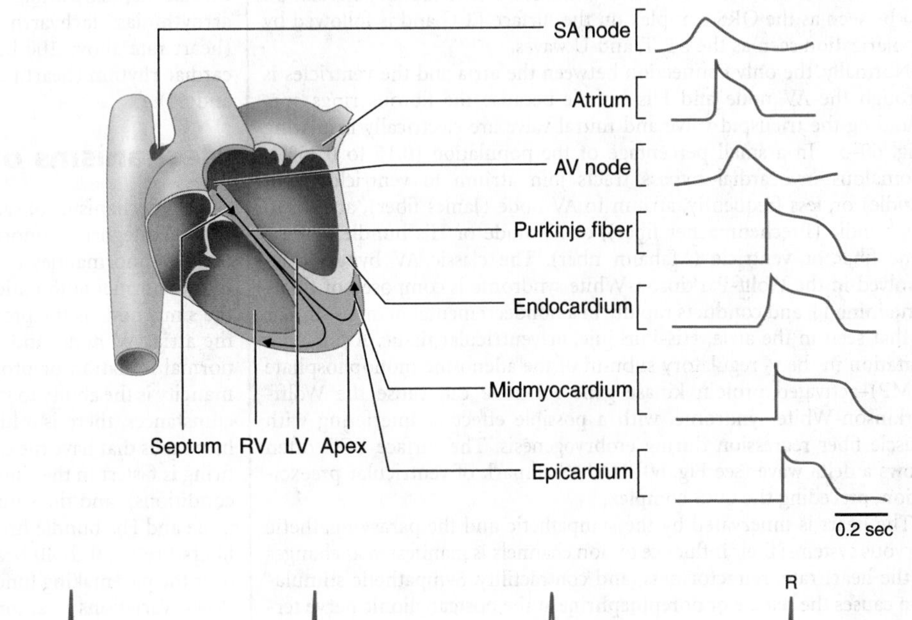

FIGURE 60–2 • Electrical activity in the myocardium. Top, schematic of a human heart with illustration of typical action potential waveforms recorded in different regions. Bottom, schematic of a surface electrocardiogram; three sequential beats are displayed. (From Nerbonne J, Kass R: Molecular physiology of cardiac repolarization. Physiol Rev 2005;85:1206.)

of the decreased density of gap junction proteins, such as connexin43, which is 33 times less prevalent in the AV node compared with ventricular cells. This reduction in gap junctions and intercalated discs leads to slower depolarization of neighboring cells. On the surface ECG, most of the PR interval depends on this slow AV node conduction.

The bundle of His arises from the compact AV node as it enters the central fibrous body. Conduction through the His bundle is rapid, on the order of 35 to 55 msec to the ventricles, because of the presence of rapidly acting sodium channels. The arterial supply of the bundle of His originates from the left anterior descending artery in 90% of cases; 10% emanate from the right coronary artery. The right and left bundle branches originate from the bundle of His. The left bundle branch further subdivides into the left anterior fascicle and left posterior fascicle before supplying the ventricular endocardium with Purkinje fibers. The right bundle branch trifurcates distally into a network that supplies the anterolateral papillary muscle, the low right septum, and the parietal band. Activation of the His-Purkinje system can be seen as the later portion of the PR interval on the surface ECG.

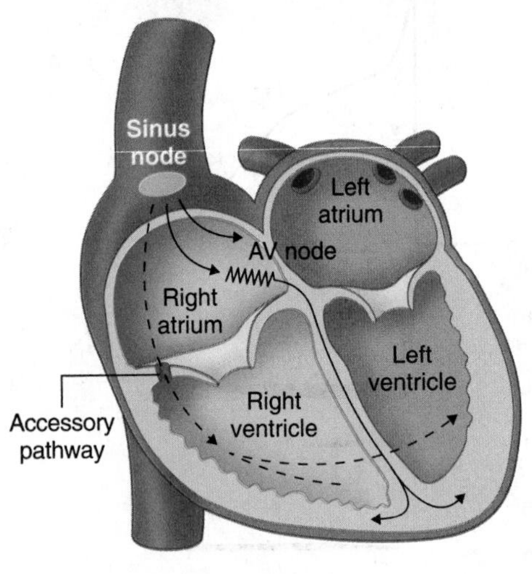

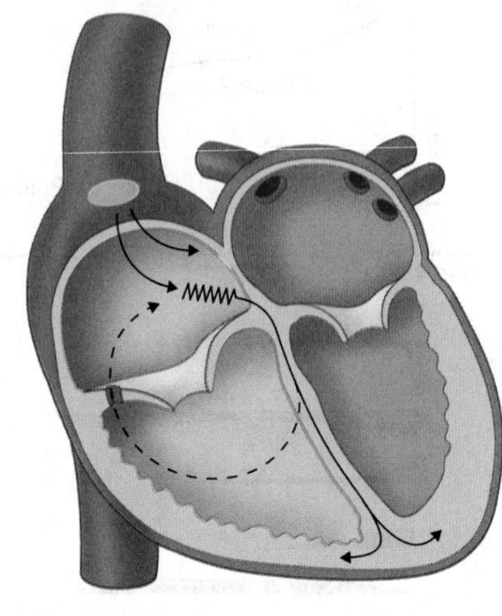

FIGURE 60–3 • Accessory pathway in sinus rhythm and in orthodromic re-entrant tachycardia. (From Basson CT: A molecular basis for Wolff-Parkinson-White syndrome. N Engl J Med 2001;344:1861. Copyright © 2001 Massachusetts Medical Society. All rights reserved.)

Ventricular activation occurs first from the left to right septum, followed by the synchronized depolarization of both ventricles from apex to base and endocardium to epicardium. The rapid activation of myocardial cells is due in part to the strong presence of the gap junction protein connexin43. Knockout mice homozygous for connexin43 deletions die with conotruncus malformations early in life, whereas mice heterozygous for connexin43 deletion ($Cx43^{+/-}$) have significant decreases in ventricular conduction in otherwise normal ventricles. Ventricular depolarization can be seen as the QRS complex on the surface ECG and is followed by repolarization seen as the ST, T, and U waves.

Normally, the only connection between the atria and the ventricles is through the AV node and His bundle because the fibrous rings surrounding the tricuspid valve and mitral valve are electrically insulating (Fig. 60–3). In a small percentage of the population (0.15 to 0.25%), anomalous myocardial bypass tracts join atrium to ventricle (Kent bundle) or, less frequently, atrium to AV node (James fiber), atrium to His bundle (Brechenmacher fiber), or AV node or His bundle to Purkinje fiber or ventricle (Mahaim fiber). The classic AV bypass tract involved in the Wolff-Parkinson-White syndrome is composed of fibers containing I_{Na} and conducts rapidly in a nondecremental manner similar to that seen in the atria, His-Purkinje, or ventricular tissue. A missense mutation in the γ_2 regulatory subunit of the adenosine monophosphate (AMP)–activated protein kinase gene *PRKAG2* can cause the Wolff-Parkinson-White syndrome, with a possible effect of interfering with muscle fiber regression during embryogenesis. The surface ECG often shows a delta wave (see Fig. 60–4), the hallmark of ventricular preexcitation, preceding the QRS complex.

The heart is innervated by the sympathetic and the parasympathetic nervous systems; their influence on ion channels is manifested as changes in the heart rate, refractoriness, and contractility. Sympathetic stimulation causes the release of norepinephrine at the postganglionic nerve terminal, leading to β_1-adrenergic and β_2-adrenergic receptor activation, followed by G protein–mediated adenylate cyclase production, which increases production of cAMP, which leads to the activation of protein kinase A, ultimately resulting in the phosphorylation of ion channels, which alter their gating and function. Parasympathetic activity leads to release of acetylcholine at the nerve terminal, which stimulates muscarinic cholinergic receptors, followed by direct G protein–mediated activation of channels or indirect G protein–mediated secondary messenger activation with use of cAMP. Multiple membrane currents are influenced by sympathetic or parasympathetic activity. The L-type calcium channel current $I_{Ca,L}$ is increased four times with β-adrenergic stimulation, leading to increased conduction of the SA and AV nodes. β-Adrenergic stimulation also leads to a cAMP-mediated change in the activation of I_f, with the result being increased activity of cardiac pacemaker cells and higher heart rates. Parasympathetic stimulation leads to activation of the acetylcholine-activated potassium current I_{KACh}, which results in decreased pacemaker activity and slowing of conduction over the AV node. Purinergic receptors are a third family of G protein–coupled receptors that are activated by adenosine. Exposure to adenosine leads to activation of I_{KACh} and inhibition of $I_{Ca,L}$, resulting in slowing of the pacemaker activity for SA and AV nodes and conduction delay through the AV node.

CARDIAC ARRHYTHMIA

A cardiac arrhythmia is an abnormality in the timing or sequence of cardiac depolarization. There are two predominant types of cardiac arrhythmias: tachyarrhythmia, an abnormally rapid cardiac rhythm (heart rate above 100 beats per minute); and bradyarrhythmia, a slow cardiac rhythm (heart rate below 60 beats per minute) (Chapters 61, 63, and 64).

Mechanisms of Tachyarrhythmias

The mechanisms of cardiac tachyarrhythmias can be grouped into two general categories, abnormalities of impulse formation and re-entry (Fig. 60–4). Abnormalities of impulse formation can be subdivided further into abnormal automaticity and triggered activity. In the normal heart, the sinus node is the predominant pacemaker; secondary pacemakers in the atria, AV node, and His-Purkinje system function in the event that normal initiation or propagation is affected by disease or drugs. Automaticity is the ability to initiate spontaneous impulses. Under normal circumstances, there is a hierarchical sequence in the rate of firing of the heart cells that have the capacity for automaticity. Normally, spontaneous firing is fastest in the sinus node (70 to 80 beats per minute under resting conditions), and the sinus node is the predominant pacemaker. The AV node and His bundle fire at 50 to 60 beats per minute, and the Purkinje fibers fire at 30 to 40 beats per minute. The lower pacemaker may take over the pacemaking function of the heart if the faster pacemaker fails or slows. Variations in autonomic tone may have a major effect on normal automaticity. In general, activation of the sympathetic nervous system increases automaticity, whereas activation of the parasympathetic nervous system decreases automaticity. Under pathologic conditions that depolarize cells, myocardial cells outside the specialized conduction system also may acquire automaticity, a phenomenon termed abnormal automaticity.

Triggered activity is an uncommon mechanism of cardiac arrhythmias. Triggered activity occurs when a preceding depolarization does not repolarize completely before depolarizing again. Early afterdepolarizations occur during phase 2 and phase 3 of the action potential. The basis for early afterdepolarizations seems to involve the L-type calcium channel. Early afterdepolarizations are facilitated by increased repolarization times, as seen in either congenital or acquired long QT syndromes. With drugs that prolong the QT interval, such as erythromycin, quinidine, sotalol, and procainamide, the block of potassium channels involved in repolarization leads to prolongation of the action potential. The ultimate effect of early afterdepolarizations may be in initiating polymorphic ventricular tachycardia or torsades de pointes (Chapter 64). Delayed after-

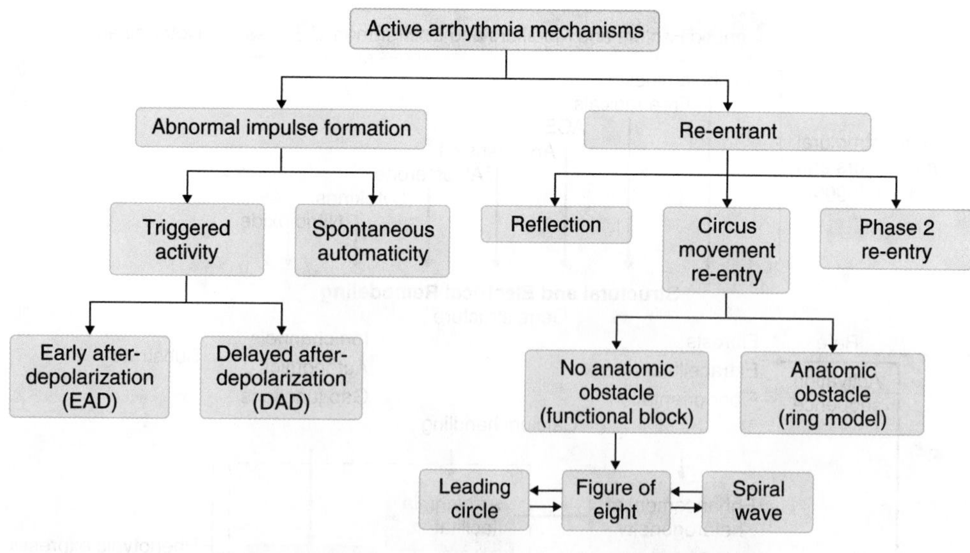

FIGURE 60–4 • Classification of cardiac arrhythmia mechanisms. (From Antzelevitch C: Basic mechanisms of reentrant arrhythmias. Curr Opin Cardiol 2001;16:1–7.)

depolarizations arise during phase 4 of the action potential, when the cell membrane is completely repolarized. Transient inward currents, which are not normally present, may be initiated by the action of elevated intracellular calcium on the Na^+-Ca^{2+} exchanger or by release of calcium from the sarcoplasmic reticulum, and they may form the basis for delayed afterdepolarizations. Rapid heart rates, increased extracellular calcium, and adrenergic stimulation may contribute to delayed afterdepolarizations. Delayed afterdepolarizations are thought to form the basis of arrhythmias resulting from digitalis, idiopathic ventricular tachyarrhythmias, and idioventricular rhythms, and they may be reduced by drugs that block the uptake of calcium by the sarcoplasmic reticulum. Multifocal atrial tachycardia is another example of an arrhythmia that results from delayed afterdepolarization–mediated triggered activity. The third type of automaticity, depolarization-induced automaticity, has been reproduced in cardiac tissues but may not lead to clinically relevant arrhythmias. Depolarization-induced automaticity arises from the constant application of current to muscle, a process that leads to spontaneous firing of the muscle.

Reentry is the most common mechanism of cardiac arrhythmias. Reentry generally occurs in the setting of abnormalities in impulse conduction. The abnormalities in impulse conduction may result from an anomalous electrical connection in the heart (i.e., an accessory pathway) or from poor impulse propagation. The basis for poor propagation of the depolarizing wave front in the heart may be attributed to disease, drugs, or hormonal modulation of the conduction system. Fibrosis or calcification of the AV node, His bundle, or right and left bundle branches may lead to AV block or right and left bundle branch blocks. AV nodal block may be a result of high vagal tone, as seen during sleep or in a well-conditioned athlete, or it may be due to agents that act on the AV node, such as digitalis, β-adrenergic blockers, or calcium-channel blockers. Slowing of conduction in the atrium and ventricles also may be affected directly by hyperkalemia or ischemia.

Poor propagation of the depolarizing wave front in the heart usually results from pathologic changes in patients with structural heart disease, including coronary artery disease, left ventricular hypertrophy, and heart failure. Fibrotic changes in the heart, with increases in collagen and intracellular matrix as seen in hypertrophy or infarction, can lead to areas of slow conduction and provide portals for reentry. Changes in the gap junction proteins have been noted in hypertrophy with increases of connexin43. These changes typically result from advanced age or the presence of structural heart disease, such as a prior myocardial infarction or a cardiomyopathy. In ischemia, the action potential is abbreviated because of activation of I_{KACh}; in hypertrophy and failure, action potential prolongation from loss of I_{to} is found. Other influences on remodeling include catecholamines, free radicals, angiotensin-converting enzyme, angiotensin II, aldosterone, cytokines, and nitric oxide. Re-entry occurs when there is continuation of a propagating wave front, which reactivates areas of the heart that previously have depolarized and are not refractory. The refractory period, which is the time interval in which the cells are unable to depolarize after a second stimulus, often persists until the transmembrane voltage is +60 mV at the activation threshold of I_{Na}.

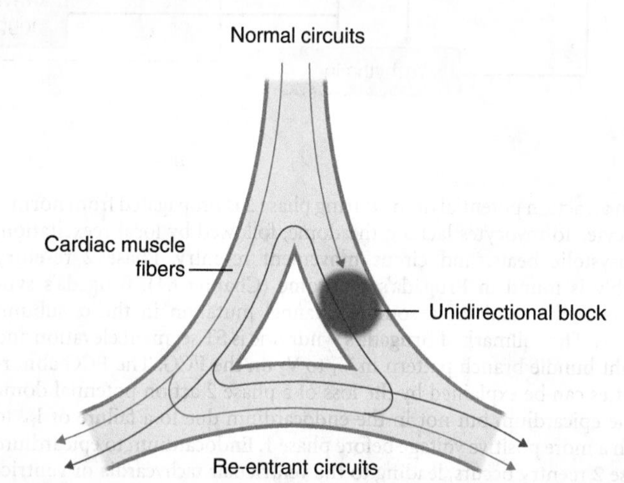

FIGURE 60–5 • Unidirectional block as a result of abnormal repolarization, conduction, or intracellular calcium homeostasis. Red arrows show normal conduction, and blue arrows show reentry through previously refractory tissue. (From Keating MT, Sanguinetti MC: Molecular and cellular mechanisms of cardiac arrhythmias. Cell 2001;104:569.)

Three types of re-entry have been described: circus movement re-entry, reflection, and phase 2 reentry. The simplest model of circus movement tachycardia, the ring model, requires the presence of unidirectional block, in which the wave front can travel only in one direction, and a long enough circuit, in which recovery from refractoriness occurs before the approach of the leading edge of depolarization (Fig. 60–5). The length of the circuit must be equal to or greater than the wavelength (conduction velocity × refractory period) of the tachycardia. Three criteria for circus movement tachycardia include the presence of unidirectional block, the presence of a distinct path of recurrent propagation, and the fact that disrupting the circuit at any point along the path terminates the tachycardia. AV reciprocating tachycardia is an example of a re-entrant tachycardia (see Fig. 60–3). During sinus rhythm, the cardiac impulse activates the ventricle through the AV node and the accessory pathway. The tachycardia is initiated when a premature atrial impulse blocks the accessory pathway and conducts down the AV node (owing to differences in refractoriness). The impulse then returns to the atria by conduction through the accessory pathway, resulting in a re-entrant or circus movement tachycardia. Atrial fibrillation is the most common type of arrhythmia that results from reentry. In contrast to arrhythmias with an accessory pathway in which there is only a single fixed re-entrant circuit, however, atrial fibrillation results from the presence of many functional re-entrant wavelets that propagate throughout the atria simultaneously. It has been estimated that at least three re-entrant wavelets must coexist for atrial fibrillation to be sustained. Re-entry resulting from reflection occurs when an impulse proceeds back and forth over a functionally unexcitable pathway, depolarizing proximal tissue on each return cycle. Phase 2 re-entry occurs

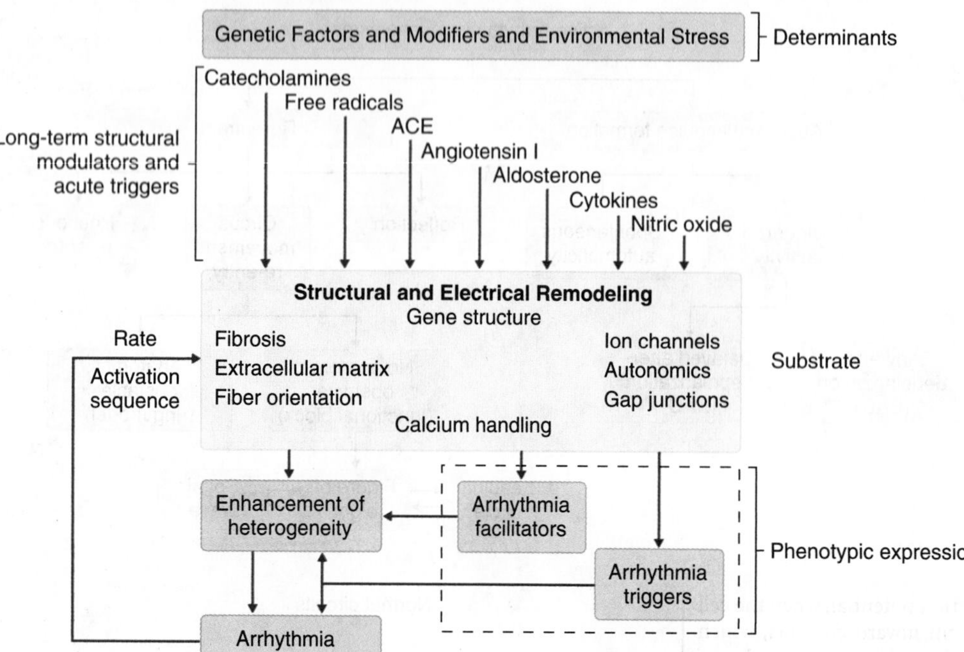

FIGURE 60–6 • Determinants of cardiac arrhythmias. (From Members of the Sicilian Gambit: New approaches to antiarrhythmic therapy: Emerging therapeutic applications of the cell biology of cardiac arrhythmias. Cardiovasc Res 2001;52:345, with permission.)

when an action potential dome during phase 2 is propagated from normal myocytes to myocytes lacking the dome, followed by local reexcitation, extrasystolic beats, and circus movement re-entry. Phase 2 re-entry notably is found in Brugada's syndrome (Chapter 64). Brugada's syndrome is the result of a sodium channel mutation in the α subunit SCN5A. The hallmark of Brugada's syndrome is ST segment elevation and a right bundle branch pattern in V_1 to V_3 on the ECG. The ECG abnormalities can be explained by the loss of a phase 2 action potential dome in the epicardium but not in the endocardium due to a failure of I_{Na} to reach a more positive voltage before phase 1. Endocardium to epicardium phase 2 reentry occurs, leading to the ventricular tachycardia or ventricular fibrillation that is seen in Brugada's syndrome.

Multiple intrinsic and extrinsic factors can affect the initiation and propagation of cardiac arrhythmias (Fig. 60–6). At the molecular level, multiple mutations contribute to the inherited long QT syndrome and to idiopathic ventricular fibrillation (Brugada's syndrome). At least eight different genes can cause the long QT syndrome, but 50% or so of phenotypic cases have not yet been linked to these genes (Chapter 64). These mutations affect the sodium channel and potassium channels involved in repolarization with either gain of function for the sodium channel or loss of function for the potassium channels, resulting in a prolonged phase 2. For example, the most common subtype, LQT1, is a disorder of the potassium channel α subunit KVLQT1 responsible in part for I_{Ks}. LQT2 is due to mutations in HERG, a component of I_{Kr}. LQT3 affects the sodium channel SCN5A at a site leading to incomplete inactivation and a continuing inward current. LQT4 is due to mutations in MiRP, the α subunit that associates with HERG to form I_{Kr}. LQT5 results from mutations in minK that associates with KVLQT1 to form I_{Ks}. Brugada's syndrome has been shown to be due to mutations in SCN5A, which causes faster inactivation of the sodium channel. Familial polymorphic ventricular tachycardia has been linked to mutations in the cardiac ryanodine receptor (RyR2) gene of the cardiac sarcoplasmic reticulum, mutations that may lead to changes in calcium-induced activation.

Mechanism of Bradyarrhythmias

Cardiac bradyarrhythmias may result from either abnormalities in impulse formation or abnormalities in impulse conduction. Sinus bradycardia is the most common type of bradyarrhythmia. Sinus bradycardia results from a decreased rate of firing of the sinus node, which may be physiologic and result from increased parasympathetic tone (i.e., during sleep) or pathologic and result from a fibrosis of the sinus node, such as occurs with aging. Bradyarrhythmias also occur when abnormalities of conduction interrupt the normal sequence of cardiac depolarization. Depending on the site of block, subsidiary pacemakers begin to fire, creating an "escape" rhythm. Conduction block usually is due to fibrosis or calcification of the AV node, His bundle, or right and left bundle branches. Conduction block also may result from increased parasympathetic tone, however, as seen during sleep or in a well-conditioned athlete, or it may be due to agents that act on the AV node, such as digitalis, β-adrenergic blockers, and calcium-channel blockers.

SUGGESTED READINGS

Nerbonne J, Kass R: Molecular physiology of cardiac repolarization. Physiol Rev 2005;85:1205–1253. *Excellent review of cardiac electrophysiology.*

Roberts R: Genomics and cardiac arrhythmias. J Am Coll Cardiol 2006;47:9–21. *Considers the genetics of supraventricular and ventricular arrhythmias.*

Sipido KR: Calcium overload, spontaneous calcium release, and ventricular arrhythmias. Heart Rhythm 2006;3:977–979. *Discusses calcium ion channels and their relation to arrhythmogenesis.*

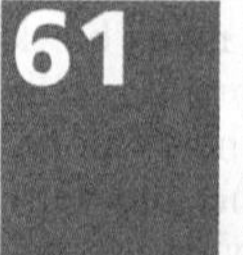

61 APPROACH TO THE PATIENT WITH SUSPECTED ARRHYTHMIA

Jeffrey E. Olgin

Clinical Manifestations

Patients with suspected arrhythmias can present in a variety of ways. Typical symptoms include palpitations, syncope, and presyncope (dizziness). On occasion, arrhythmias can manifest more subtly as exercise intolerance, lethargy, and vague complaints of malaise or without any symptoms at all. Conversely, arrhythmias occasionally manifest as aborted sudden cardiac death (cardiac arrest) (Chapter 62). The specific differential diagnosis, prognosis, and treatment of these symptoms are determined by the severity of the symptom (i.e., whether it results in syncope) and whether the patient has underlying structural heart disease. In general, the likelihood of a life-threatening arrhythmia, such as ventricular tachycardia or ventricular fibrillation, in a patient with symptoms of palpitations or syncope is significantly greater in a patient who has structural heart disease. Therefore, determination of whether a patient has structural heart disease is a key step in the diagnosis and prognosis of patients with suspected arrhythmias.

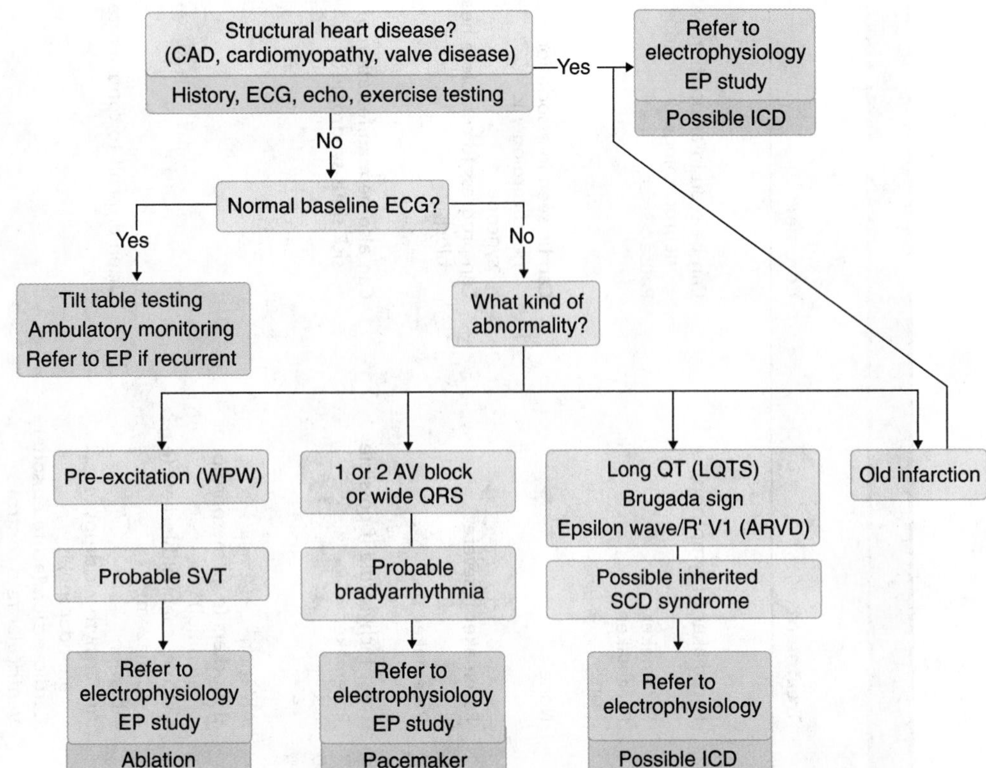

FIGURE 61–1 • Algorithm for evaluation of patients with symptoms of palpitation, dizziness, or syncope. ARVD = arrhythmogenic right ventricular dysplasia; AV = atrioventricular; CAD = coronary artery disease; ECG = electrocardiography; Echo = echocardiography; EP = electrophysiology; ICD = implantable cardioverter-defibrillator; LQTS = long QT syndrome; SCD = sudden cardiac death; WPW = Wolff-Parkinson-White syndrome.

Palpitations

Palpitations, defined as an awareness of an irregular or rapid heartbeat, are most commonly due to ectopic beats, namely, premature atrial contractions (PACs; Chapter 63) and premature ventricular contractions (PVCs; Chapter 64), or to tachyarrhythmias. A careful history can often distinguish benign palpitations from those that need further evaluation. It can be useful to have the patient tap out with a finger what the palpitations feel like. An irregularly irregular pattern suggests atrial fibrillation, whereas a more regular, rapid pattern suggests a sustained tachycardia. Conversely, most patients who complain of symptoms from PACs or PVCs are often more aware of the post-extrasystolic pause or the accentuated output of the post-extrasystolic beat than of the actual premature beat itself. The majority of patients who have symptoms suggestive of premature beats but not of sustained tachycardia do not require further evaluation if they have no other symptoms and no evidence of structural heart disease, that is, an otherwise normal cardiac history, physical examination, and electrocardiogram (ECG). If, however, the symptoms are not due to a single occasional extrasystole or are accompanied by presyncope or syncope, further evaluation is required (Fig. 61–1). Antiarrhythmic therapy is usually not necessary for treatment of PACs or PVCs unless the symptoms are frequent or severe. β-Blockers (metoprolol, 25 mg/day, or atenolol, 25 mg/day) are first-line therapy in those highly symptomatic patients with documented PACs or PVCs.

Palpitations are the most common presentation of tachyarrhythmias. The majority of tachyarrhythmias in patients without structural heart disease are due to supraventricular tachycardias (Chapter 63) that resolve spontaneously within several seconds. When the tachyarrhythmia is more prolonged, however, it often will resolve with simple interventions. Patients themselves can cough several times, perform the Valsalva maneuver, exhale forcefully against a closed glottis for several seconds, or even rub gently on their eyeballs. A physician can use carotid sinus massage, performed by pressing and rubbing the carotid pulse just below the angle of the mandible for 5 to 15 seconds. This maneuver should be avoided in elderly patients and in patients who have a history of a previous cerebrovascular accident, known carotid artery stenosis, or a carotid bruit on auscultation. In patients with structural heart disease, palpitations may signify ventricular tachycardia (Chapter 62), particularly if they occur with syncope (Chapter 427) or presyncope. Rarely do bradyarrhythmias manifest as palpitations.

Syncope and Presyncope

Syncope and presyncope, defined as a sudden loss of consciousness (syncope) or lightheadedness (presyncope), can be a manifestation of tachyarrhythmias, bradyarrhythmias, or neurocardiogenic syncope or can be unrelated to any arrhythmia (Chapter 427). A careful history and physical examination are necessary to exclude other cardiac causes (such as acute ischemia, aortic stenosis) or neurologic causes. Important historical features that suggest an arrhythmic cause are association with palpitations and lack of any neurologic deficits preceding or following the event. Important differential diagnoses include conditions other than lightheadedness that may be termed dizziness by the patient. Vertigo (Chapter 454), a sense of imbalance or of the "room spinning," and ataxia (Chapter 434) can usually be distinguished by the history and physical examination. The possibility of seizures (Chapter 426) must also be evaluated because syncope from an arrhythmia or neurocardiogenic syncope occasionally results in seizure-like activity and because seizures can sometimes be confused with syncope. The most important distinguishing feature is that postictal symptoms, a key feature of seizure disorders, are absent when syncope is a result of an arrhythmia. Patients with syncope from an arrhythmia will usually awaken without any neurologic residual, unless the patient had a cardiac arrest with prolonged hypoxia and required resuscitation.

Diagnosis

Arrhythmias are generally categorized as bradyarrhythmias (slow heart rates), tachyarrhythmias (fast heart rates), or premature beats (single extrasystoles from the atria or the ventricle, PACs [see Fig. 63–1] or PVCs [see Fig. 64–1], respectively) (Table 61–1). Although not a primary arrhythmia, neurocardiogenic syncope, also known as vasovagal syncope, is a related diagnostic and management issue because its symptoms are frequently similar to those of arrhythmias and because neurocardiogenic syncope secondarily results in bradycardia (see later).

Bradyarrhythmias

Bradyarrhythmias (Chapter 63) can be due to dysfunction in the sinoatrial node, atrioventricular (AV) node, or His-Purkinje system (below

TABLE 61–1 ARRHYTHMIC CAUSES OF PALPITATIONS AND SYNCOPE

Etiology	Specific Arrhythmia	Symptoms: Palpitations	Symptoms: Dizziness	Symptoms: Syncope	Treatment	Comment
BRADYARRHYTHMIAS						
Sinus node dysfunction	Sinus bradycardia	No	Occasional	Rare	Pacemaker (if symptoms)	Can be seen in association with neurocardiogenic syncope
	Sinus arrest	Occasional	Yes	Occasional	Pacemaker	Pause >3 sec
	Sick sinus syndrome	Occasional	Yes	Occasional	Pacemaker	
AV nodal disease	First-degree AV block	No	No	No	None	
	Type I second-degree AV block	Occasional	No	No	None	Can be seen in association with neurocardiogenic syncope
	Type II second-degree AV block	Occasional	Rare	No	Pacemaker if severe	Can progress to complete heart block
	Third-degree AV block	Yes	Yes	Yes	Pacemaker	
Tachy-brady syndrome		Yes	Yes	Occasional	Treat tachycardia if possible Pacemaker	Can also be manifestation of sick sinus syndrome
TACHYARRHYTHMIAS						
SVT	Atrial tachycardia	Yes	Occasional	Rare	Ablation β-Blockers (e.g., metoprolol or atenolol)* Calcium-channel blockers (e.g., diltiazem)*	
	Atrial flutter	Yes	Occasional	Rare	Ablation Antiarrhythmic drugs (e.g., amiodarone)* Cardioversion (acute episode)	Often difficult to control rate
	Atrial fibrillation	Yes	Occasional	Rare	Ventricular rate control Warfarin Antiarrhythmic drugs (e.g., amiodarone)* Cardioversion (acute episode) Ablation	
	AV nodal re-entrant tachycardia	Yes	Yes	Rare	Ablation β-Blockers (e.g., metoprolol or atenolol)* Calcium-channel blockers (e.g., diltiazem)	
	AV re-entrant tachycardia (WPW)	Yes	Yes	Rare	Ablation Antiarrhythmic drugs*	

VT	Idiopathic (RV outflow tract, fascicular)	Yes	Yes	Occasional	Ablation	Absence of structural heart disease Low risk of sudden death
	VT secondary to CAD, cardiomyopathy	Yes	Yes	Yes	ICD Amiodarone (400 mg qd)* Ablation	Increased incidence of sudden death
	Bundle branch re-entry	Yes	Yes	Yes	Ablation	Usually in the setting of LV dysfunction and baseline intraventricular conduction delay
	Genetic syndromes (e.g., long QT syndrome, Brugada's, arrhythmic right ventricular dysplasia)	Occasional	Yes	Yes	ICD	Not always a clear family history Increased incidence of sudden death
ECTOPY	PACs	Occasional	No	No	None β-Blockers (e.g., atenolol or metoprolol) if symptomatic*	
	PVCs	Occasional	No	No	None β-Blockers (e.g., atenolol or metoprolol) if symptomatic*	Benign in absence of structural heart disease
NEUROCARDIOGENIC SYNCOPE		No	Yes	Yes	Behavioral (hydration, avoid triggers, abort episodes) β-Blockers (e.g., atenolol or metoprolol)* Fludrocortisone (0.1 mg qd) Midodrine (10 mg tid) Paroxetine (10–20 mg qd)	

*See Table 63–3 for drug doses.

AV = atrioventricular; CAD = coronary artery disease; ICD = implantable cardioverter-defibrillator; LV = left ventricle; PACs = premature atrial contractions; PVCs = premature ventricular contractions; RV = right ventricle; SVT = supraventricular tachycardia; VT = ventricular tachycardia; WPW = Wolff-Parkinson-White syndrome.

the AV node). Sinus bradycardia is manifested as a slow atrial (sinus) rate and can occur at rest or as an inappropriately slow rate during exercise (chronotropic incompetence). Sinus arrest can be intermittent when transient loss of sinus activity (loss of the P wave on the ECG) causes brief sinus pauses or persistent with prolonged loss of atrial activation. The sinus rate and even the presence of sinus pauses are influenced by autonomic tone. Therefore, healthy individuals—particularly younger patients and well-trained athletes (with high vagal tone)—will have occasional sinus slowing, often during sleep. A sinus pause of more than 3 seconds is considered pathologic when it is associated with symptoms. Sinus bradycardia and sinus arrest can also be the result of medications, typically β-blockers and calcium-channel blockers. When not "physiologic" or due to medications, sinus bradycardia and sinus arrest are the result of intrinsic conduction system disease. Sinus bradycardia, especially if it is intermittent, can also signify coronary disease of the right coronary artery.

Bradyarrhythmias from AV nodal disease are a result of failure of impulse conduction from the atrium to the ventricle. Like the sinus node, the AV node is also dramatically affected by autonomic tone. Mobitz type I second-degree AV block (Wenckebach; see Fig. 63–7B) can be seen during periods of high vagal tone and is not necessarily pathologic; for example, it does not progress to complete heart block and is not associated with a widened QRS. Many drugs, such as β-blockers and calcium-channel blockers, commonly cause first-degree AV block and should be considered a potential cause for any degree of AV block. Mobitz type II block (see Fig. 63–7C) signifies that the level of AV block is below the AV node in the His-Purkinje system, which is not sensitive to autonomic tone; the resulting QRS is widened, and there is a high likelihood of progression to complete heart block (third-degree AV block; see Fig. 63–8B and C). Intermittent complete heart block, which can result in drop attacks or Stokes-Adams attacks, is usually preceded by abnormal baseline findings on the ECG, such as a bundle branch block or second-degree AV block. The treatment of choice for symptomatic bradyarrhythmias or those likely to progress to complete heart block is implantation of a permanent pacemaker (Chapter 65).

Tachyarrhythmias

Tachyarrhythmias can arise from the atrium or AV node (supraventricular tachycardia) or from the ventricle (ventricular tachycardia). Supraventricular tachyarrhythmias that may be associated with palpitations, presyncope, or syncope include atrial tachycardia (see Fig. 63–2C), AV nodal re-entrant tachycardia (see Fig. 63–2E), AV junctional tachycardia (see Fig. 63–2F), atrial flutter (see Fig. 63–3A and B), and atrial fibrillation (see Fig. 63–3D), sometimes in association with accessory conduction pathways that facilitate the re-entry needed to sustain the arrhythmia. Ventricular tachyarrhythmias include the various forms of ventricular tachycardia (see Fig. 64–3). Treatments are guided by the specific tachyarrhythmia and its underlying cause (see Tables 61–1 and 63–3) (Chapters 62 to 65).

Neurocardiogenic Syncope

Neurocardiogenic syncope (Chapter 427) is the sudden onset of lightheadedness or loss of consciousness as a result of autonomic reflexes and is more common in younger patients (teenage to third decade of life). It is sometimes called a vasovagal episode or a common faint. In this form of neurocardiogenic syncope, heightened parasympathetic output, either due to direct stimulation (e.g., coughing, micturition, gastrointestinal conditions) or as a reflex in response to sympathetic stimulation (e.g., seeing blood, abrupt cessation of exercise), results in arterial dilation (called the vasodilatory response) and an inhibition of sinus and AV node activity (the cardioinhibitory response). The result is a transient decrease in blood pressure, often manifested as lightheadedness or syncope. Because they are associated with parasympathetic (vagal) output, episodes are frequently associated with nausea, diaphoresis, and salivation.

Treatment of this form of syncope can be challenging. The most effective therapies are behavioral (avoidance of triggers), wearing of compression stockings, and maintenance of adequate hydration and salt intake. Lying down with the feet elevated and performing isometric hand exercises may abort an acute episode. Medical therapy, including β-blockers (pindolol, 5 to 15 mg twice daily), mineralocorticoids (fludrocortisone, 0.1 mg/day), paroxetine (10 to 20 mg/day), and midodrine (an α-adrenergic agonist and vasoconstrictor; 2.5 to 5 mg three times daily), has shown some efficacy in reducing recurrence rates (Chapter 427), although the efficacy of ß-blockers for reducing syncopal episodes has been inconsistent. Even though bradycardia is a dominant feature of neurocardiogenic syncope, a pacemaker is not an effective therapy for prevention of episodes because most patients also have a major vasodilatory component. 1

A related cause of syncope is carotid body hypersensitivity, in which vagal tone is increased by direct stimulation of the carotid body. This condition is frequently seen in older patients, in whom episodes are associated with mechanical stimulation of the neck (e.g., turning the head, shaving, wearing a tight collar or necktie). This form of syncope is diagnosed by documenting pauses longer than 3 seconds in response to carotid sinus massage and is curable with a pacemaker because carotid body stimulation does not cause significant vasodilation.

Diagnostic Tests

Electrocardiography

The baseline ECG is critical in the evaluation of the patient with palpitations or syncope. The presence of ventricular pre-excitation, as manifested by a short PR interval and a delta wave (see Fig. 63–4A), not only establishes the diagnosis of Wolff-Parkinson-White syndrome in a patient with palpitations and AV reciprocating tachycardia (Chapter 63) as the likely cause of the symptoms but also can be used to determine the location of the responsible accessory pathway. The baseline ECG also provides useful predictive information about the likelihood of conduction system abnormalities as a possible explanation for bradyarrhythmias (e.g., sinus bradycardia suggests sinus node dysfunction, a prolonged PR interval suggests the possibility of AV nodal disease, and a widened QRS suggests disease below the AV node) and in diagnosis of prior myocardial infarction (i.e., pathologic Q waves), which raises the likelihood of ventricular tachycardia as a potential cause of syncope or palpitations. Abnormalities such as a prolonged QT interval in a patient with syncope and a family history of syncope or sudden death suggest one of the congenital long QT syndromes (Chapter 64). An incomplete right bundle branch block with coved ST segment elevation in ECG lead V_1 or V_2 in a patient with syncope or palpitations suggests Brugada's syndrome (Chapter 64). An epsilon wave, incomplete right bundle branch block, and inverted T waves in V_1 are ECG findings suggestive of right ventricular dysplasia (Chapter 64). All of these syndromes carry an increased risk of recurrent syncope and sudden death if untreated (Chapters 62, 63, and 64).

An ECG during an episode of palpitations is extremely useful in making a definitive diagnosis. For narrow–QRS complex tachycardias, the specific supraventricular tachycardia can often be surmised from the 12-lead ECG obtained during symptoms (Fig. 61–2). Moreover, for wide–QRS complex tachycardias, the 12-lead ECG is useful in distinguishing a supraventricular tachycardia (with aberrancy) from a ventricular tachycardia (Fig. 61–3). The presence of fusion beats or AV dissociation during a wide–QRS complex tachycardia makes the diagnosis of ventricular tachycardia. For ventricular tachycardias, the morphology of the QRS complex is useful in determining the location of the ventricular tachycardia focus and in identifying idiopathic ventricular tachycardia (right ventricular outflow tract or fascicular), which has a much more benign course than ventricular tachycardia in the setting of coronary disease (Chapter 64).

The effect on tachycardia of carotid sinus massage or intravenous bolus administration of adenosine (given as a rapid IV bolus of 6 mg and repeated at a dose of 12 mg if the initial dose is ineffective) is also useful in narrowing the differential diagnosis of a tachycardia. Both maneuvers slow conduction through the AV node. Therefore, tachycardias that terminate with either maneuver are likely to involve the AV node as a critical component of the re-entrant circuit (AV nodal re-entrant tachycardia or AV re-entrant tachycardia). If the maneuver induces AV block but does not terminate the arrhythmia, likely causes of tachycardias that persist are atrial fibrillation, atrial flutter, and atrial tachycardias (or occasionally ventricular tachycardia if the QRS is wide). On rare occasion, atrial tachycardias and some idiopathic ventricular tachycardias are "adenosine responsive" and can terminate in response to adenosine. Important clues to the specific mechanism can be obtained at the onset or at the termination of tachycardia, so obtaining a continuous 12-lead ECG during carotid sinus massage or the administration of adenosine is useful.

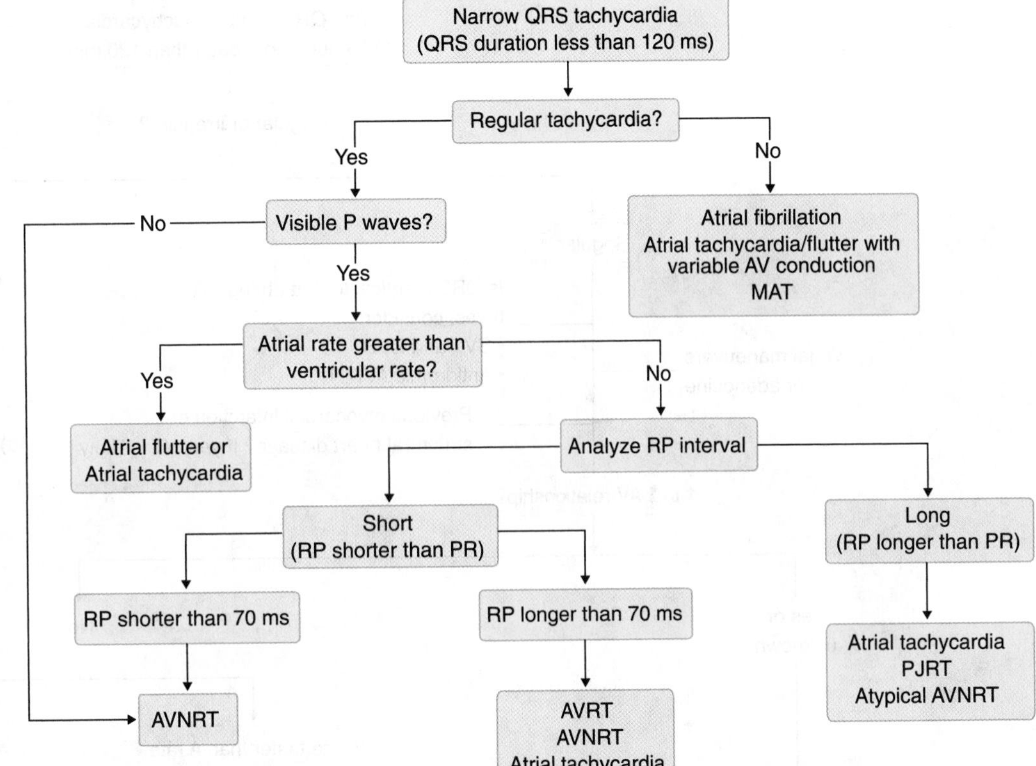

FIGURE 61–2 • ECG algorithm for diagnosis of narrow-complex tachycardias. AVRT = atrioventricular reciprocating tachycardia; AVNRT = atrioventricular nodal reciprocating tachycardia; MAT = multifocal atrial tachycardia; PJRT = permanent form of junctional reciprocating tachycardia. (From Blomstrom-Lundqvist C, Scheinman MM, Aliot EM, et al: ACC/AHA/ESC guidelines for the management of patients with supraventricular arrhythmias—executive summary. Circulation 2003;108:1871–1909.)

During bradycardias, the ECG is useful in determining the level of the conduction system (sinus node, AV node, or His bundle) responsible for the bradycardia. Sinus bradycardia is diagnosed when a slow (<50 per minute at rest) atrial rate (P wave) conducts to the ventricle. Sinus arrest or sinus pauses (see Fig. 63–6) are diagnosed by absent or dropped P waves. First-degree AV block (see Fig. 63–7A) is defined as a prolonged PR interval (>200 msec), and second-degree AV block is defined by P waves that occasionally do not conduct to the ventricle (P wave without an ensuing QRS); Mobitz type I second-degree AV block (also known as Wenckebach block; see Fig. 63–7B) is characterized by progressive lengthening of the PR interval until one P wave does not conduct to the ventricle. This form of AV block is often seen in younger patients, is usually benign, and rarely progresses to complete AV block (third-degree AV block). Mobitz type II second-degree AV block (see Fig. 63–7C), which is characterized by sudden unexpected loss of conduction of a P wave to the ventricle (dropped QRS), signifies disease of the His-Purkinje system and often progresses to complete heart block. Complete heart block or third-degree AV block (see Fig. 63-8C) is diagnosed by dissociation of P waves from QRS complexes, with an atrial rate faster than the ventricular rate.

Ambulatory Monitoring

For intermittent symptoms such as palpitations, dizziness, or syncope, it is often difficult to obtain a 12-lead ECG during the symptoms. Therefore, ambulatory monitoring, which allows ECG monitoring during long periods, is a vital tool in the diagnosis of these symptoms. There are currently three types of ambulatory monitors: Holter monitors, which continuously record the ECG for 24 to 48 hours; event recorders, which are wearable loop recorders that record only during specific events (at times when the patient activates the recorder because of symptoms or the recorder detects a heart rate above or below a specified threshold) but can be worn for 1 month or more; and implantable loop recorders, which function similarly to event recorders but can be used for up to 14 months. 2 More recently, home telemetry units have been developed, by which patients undergo prolonged continuous remote monitoring by wireless or Internet connections. The choice among ambulatory monitoring options is largely determined by the frequency of the symptoms and the likelihood of capturing an episode in a given monitoring period.

Ambulatory monitoring is diagnostic only if there are abnormalities during symptoms or if the patient has typical symptoms without any concurrent abnormalities. A "normal" monitoring record is nondiagnostic if the patient does not have symptoms during the period.

Holter Monitors

Holter monitors use a tape or digital media to record either a three- or five-lead surface ECG continuously for 24 to 48 hours. Processing, printing, and analysis of the recordings are performed offline with commercial systems. In addition to recording of the rhythm, analyses such as heart rate variability, ST segment changes, and accurate counts of PACs and PVCs can be automated. Some systems allow extrapolation to produce a "virtual 12-lead" recording at any time during the monitoring period. Holter monitoring is useful for detection of symptoms that are frequent (multiple times daily) and for diagnosis of sinus node dysfunction (sinus node arrest, sick sinus syndrome) or intermittent AV block. It can also be useful to assess the adequacy of the control of the ventricular rate in a patient with atrial fibrillation.

Event Monitors

Event monitors, also known as loop recorders, are designed to record intermittent episodes during long periods (weeks to months) and are thus useful for patients with less frequent symptoms. The system records the ECG into a loop buffer that is continuously updated and overwritten. The duration of memory varies from a few seconds to a few minutes and is usually programmable. When activated, the information is "locked" into memory and continues to record forward for a preprogrammed amount of time. Newer systems allow both patient-activated (when symptoms occur) and event-triggered (when the heart rate is above or below a preset threshold) recording. Some recorders have algorithms to detect and record atrial fibrillation automatically, regardless of the heart rate. After episodes have been recorded, the patient then transmits the recording over the telephone to centralized receivers. Some event monitors require leads similar to Holter monitors, whereas others are worn on the wrist or are put into small credit card–sized devices that are placed on the chest during symptoms. The latter type is useful only in patients whose symptoms last for several minutes and who do not have syncope.

Implantable Loop Recorders

Implantable loop recorders are small devices with integrated leads that are implanted in a small subcutaneous pocket during a simple surgery, usually in the electrophysiology laboratory. They function similarly to the event recorders in terms of recording ECGs. Patients can activate the device with a small transmitter, or the device can autotrigger on the basis of preprogrammed heart rates. The device can be interrogated by a

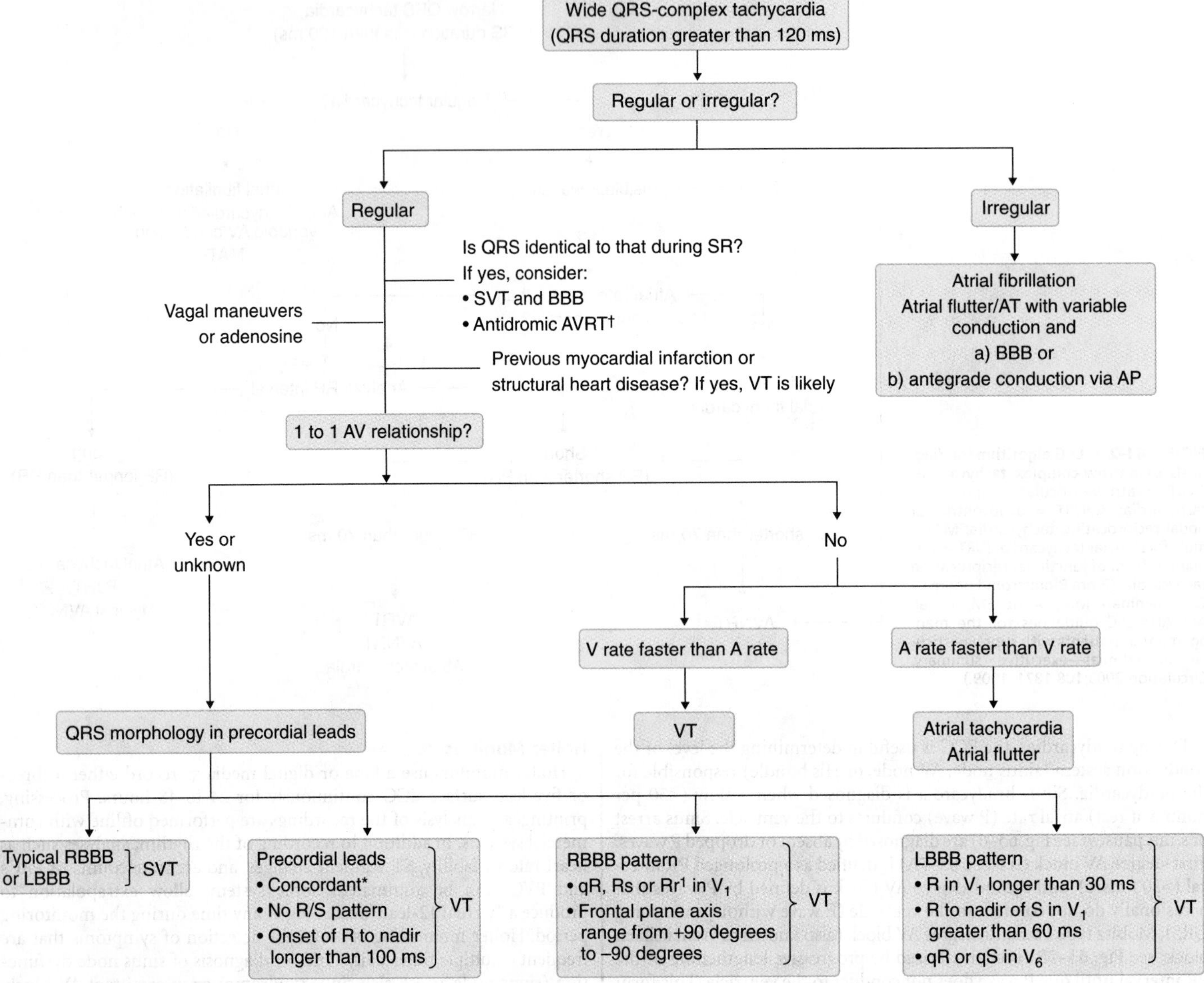

FIGURE 61–3 • ECG algorithm for diagnosis of wide-complex tachycardias. A = atrial; AP = accessory pathway; AT = atrial tachycardia; AV = atrioventricular; AVRT = atrioventricular reciprocating tachycardia; BBB = bundle branch block; LBBB = left bundle branch block; RBBB = right bundle branch block; SR = sinus rhythm; SVT = supraventricular tachycardia; V = ventricular; VF = ventricular fibrillation; VT = ventricular tachycardia. (From Blomstrom-Lundqvist C, Scheinman MM, Aliot EM, et al: ACC/AHA/ESC guidelines for the management of patients with supraventricular arrhythmias—executive summary. Circulation 2003;108:1871–1909.)

computer, similar to the way pacemakers are interrogated, to program the device's parameters and to retrieve ECGs that have been recorded. Implantable loop recorders are useful in patients with infrequent episodes, elderly patients who have difficulty using wearable recorders, or patients who cannot otherwise wear an event recorder (e.g., someone who is symptomatic during swimming).

Tilt Table Testing

Tilt table testing is used to confirm the diagnosis of neurocardiogenic syncope. The test involves continuous heart rate and blood pressure monitoring during head-up tilting. After baseline measurements in the supine position, the patient is tilted (head-up to 60 to 80 degrees) for 60 minutes. Some laboratories use isoproterenol or nitroglycerin as additional provocation. A positive result is a sudden and precipitous fall in blood pressure and heart rate, with concurrent reproducibility of symptoms (syncope). Because there is an appreciable false-positive rate, the test is best used as a confirmatory test in patients with a history suggestive of neurocardiogenic syncope or in patients with syncope in whom structural heart disease and other causes of syncope have been excluded.

Electrophysiologic Studies

Electrophysiologic studies involve placement of several transvenous catheters in the heart to perform temporary measurements of intracardiac electrograms and to perform pacing. Electrophysiologic studies are useful to identify the precise mechanism of tachyarrhythmias and are a necessary prelude to a curative ablation (Chapter 65). Most arrhythmias, especially those with re-entrant mechanisms, can be readily induced during electrophysiologic studies. In addition, the existence and characteristics of accessory AV pathways (i.e., those responsible for the Wolff-Parkinson-White syndrome or other re-entrant tachyarrhythmia) can be readily assessed by an electrophysiologic study. In patients with a previous myocardial infarction, electrophysiologic studies are useful in determining the existence of the substrate for ventricular arrhythmias (Chapter 64), which may be treated with ablation or implantable defibrillators (Chapter 65). Electrophysiologic studies are also useful to determine the integrity of the conduction system and the precise mechanism of bradyarrhythmias that may be causing syncope. Therefore, electrophysiologic studies are indicated in patients with documented or suspected tachyarrhythmias as a prelude to curative ablation; in patients with a previous myocardial infarction and syncope, presyncope, or palpitations to exclude ventricular tachycardia; and in patients with severe or prolonged symptoms and no apparent diagnosis by history or ambulatory monitoring, especially in the setting of an abnormal ECG.

Other Tests

Echocardiography

Echocardiography (Chapter 53) can be useful to ensure that a patient does not have underlying structural heart disease, which can be an important prognostic factor in patients with ventricular tachycardia or syncope.

Echocardiography should be performed in patients who present with syncope that is not obviously neurocardiogenic to ensure that there is no valvar or myocardial cause.

Exercise Testing

Exercise testing (Chapter 48) can be useful to assess arrhythmias, particularly in patients in whom symptoms are exercise related. Exercise testing can also be useful in the evaluation of patients with bradyarrhythmias to diagnose chronotropic incompetence and can be useful in differentiating AV block due to autonomic tone (improves with exercise) from intrinsic conduction disease (generally worsens with increasing rate).

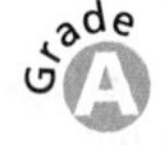

1. Connolly SJ, Sheldon R, Thorpe KE, et al: Pacemaker therapy for prevention of syncope in patients with recurrent severe vasovagal syncope: Second Vasovagal Pacemaker Study (VPS II): A randomized trial. JAMA 2003;289:2224–2229.
2. Krahn AD, Klein GJ, Yee R, et al: Randomized assessment of syncope trial: Conventional diagnostic testing versus a prolonged monitoring strategy. Circulation 2001;104:46–51.

SUGGESTED READINGS

Blomstrom-Lundqvist C, Scheinman MM, Aliot EM, et al: ACC/AHA/ESC guidelines for the management of patients with supraventricular arrhythmias—executive summary: A report of the American College of Cardiology/American Heart Association Task Force on Practice Guidelines and the European Society of Cardiology Committee for Practice Guidelines (Writing Committee to Develop Guidelines for the Management of Patients With Supraventricular Arrhythmias). Circulation 2003;108:1871–1909. *Guidelines for management of patients with supraventricular arrhythmias, including algorithms for the evaluation of patients with palpitations and syncope.*

Gregoratos G, Abrams J, Epstein AE, et al: ACC/AHA/NASPE 2002 guideline update for implantation of cardiac pacemakers and antiarrhythmia devices: Summary article: A report of the American College of Cardiology/American Heart Association Task Force on Practice Guidelines (ACC/AHA/NASPE Committee to Update the 1998 Pacemaker Guidelines). Circulation 2002;106: 2145–2161. *Guidelines for and comprehensive review of bradyarrhythmias and pacemaker indications.*

Grubb BP: Clinical practice. Neurocardiogenic syncope. N Engl J Med 2005;352:1004–1010. *A comprehensive review.*

Scheinman MM, Keung E: The year in clinical electrophysiology. J Am Coll Cardiol 2006;47:1207–1213. *A review on updates in the field.*

Sud S, Massel D, Klein GJ, et al: The expectation effect and cardiac pacing for refractory vasovagal syncope. Am J Med 2007;120:54–62. *The apparent response of pacemaker therapy may be due to a strong expectation response.*

Wever EF, Robles de Medina EO: Sudden death in patients without structural heart disease. J Am Coll Cardiol 2004;43:1137–1144. *A comprehensive review.*

62 APPROACH TO CARDIAC ARREST AND LIFE-THREATENING ARRHYTHMIAS

Robert J. Myerburg and Agustin Castellanos

Cardiac arrest is characterized by an abrupt loss of consciousness because of loss of effective blood flow. If not treated promptly, it will lead to central nervous system injury or death within minutes. Cardiac arrest is often forewarned by a change in symptoms related to the occurrence of transient arrhythmias or other clinical disturbances such as chest pain, dyspnea, lightheadedness, near-syncope, or weakness. Cardiac arrest may occur suddenly in an apparently previously healthy individual, in a patient with known previous cardiac disease, or as the end-stage final common pathway of any systemic disease.

The most common electrical mechanisms for cardiac arrest are the ventricular tachyarrhythmias—ventricular fibrillation (VF) or rapid (pulseless) ventricular tachycardia (VT). In a substantial minority of cardiac arrests, severe bradyarrhythmia, asystole, or pulseless electrical activity is the first rhythm abnormality noted; these rhythms may be the actual initiating mechanism of the cardiac arrest or a result of deterioration of untreated VT/VF to asystole or pulseless electrical activity.

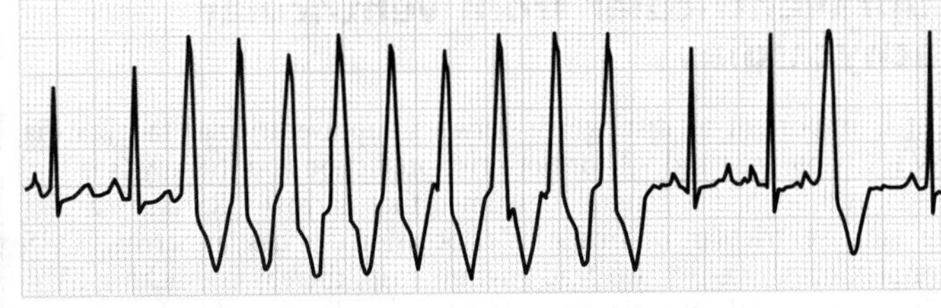

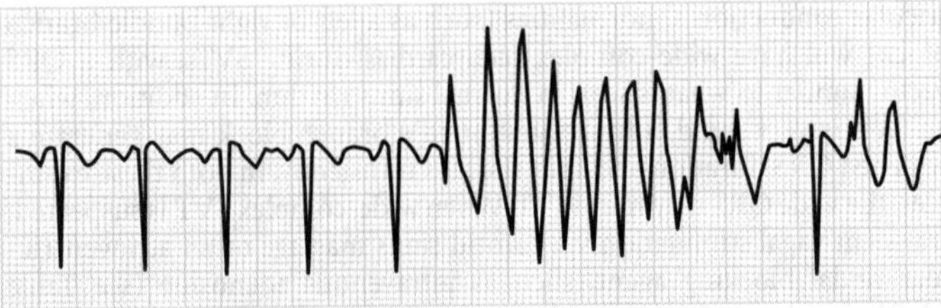

FIGURE 62–1 • Nonsustained ventricular tachycardia. Monomorphic patterns **(A)** are characterized by a slower and more stable electrical pattern than polymorphic patterns are **(B)**. Both have long-term prognostic implications in patients with advanced structural heart disease, but monomorphic patterns tend to be more stable over the short term.

Pulseless electrical activity may also be seen after termination of VT/VF by electrical cardioversion. Pulseless electrical activity is defined as secondary when it occurs in the setting of predisposing factors, such as hypoxia or other metabolic disorders, and primary when it is the initial rhythm noted in patients with predisposing cardiac disorders. The probability of survival after intervention is far better for ventricular tachyarrhythmias than for bradyarrhythmic or asystolic mechanisms. The interval between cardiac arrest and the initiation of resuscitation and cardioversion is the major determinant of survival.

PREDISPOSING WIDE–QRS COMPLEX TACHYCARDIAS

Sustained tachycardias with wide QRS complexes should be considered to be of ventricular origin and high risk until determined otherwise. Most wide-QRS tachycardias are initially approached as a medical urgency or emergency, whereas most narrow-QRS tachycardias of supraventricular origin can be managed with less urgency (Chapters 63 and 64).

Management of Sustained Ventricular Tachycardia

Sustained VT occurs most commonly in the presence of structural heart disease and must be interpreted as a forewarning of fatal arrhythmia in that setting. It is characterized by QRS complexes that are usually greater than 0.12 second, with a mean vector that is markedly different from the QRS vector of conducted impulses. The rate of most VTs is between 140 and 200 impulses per minute, but rates may be slower or faster. Sustained VTs may be electrically stable (such as monomorphic VT patterns at relatively slow rates; Fig. 62–1A) or unstable (such as polymorphic VTs or monomorphic VTs at rates exceeding 190 to 200 per minute; Fig. 62–1B) (Chapter 64). Slower monomorphic VT may be well tolerated, whereas rapid VT is typically associated with hypotension and hypoperfusion. In the latter circumstance, VT must be managed as a life-threatening or imminently fatal event, analogous to a VT/VF cardiac arrest (see later). Well-tolerated, slow monomorphic VT, especially in the absence of structural heart disease, may be treated with less urgency, usually with antiarrhythmic drugs or β-adrenergic blocking agents (see Table 63–3). Long-term management strategies, often involving consideration of implantable cardioverter-defibrillator therapy, are based on consideration of the likelihood of recurrent tachycardias and the extent of underlying disease (Chapter 64).

Dilemmas in Distinguishing Supraventricular from Ventricular Tachycardias

It is important to distinguish between supraventricular tachycardia (SVT; Chapter 63) and VT for both risk prediction and therapy (see Fig. 61–3). Although it is generally assumed that narrow-QRS tachycardias are supraventricular in origin, VT occasionally has a narrow QRS complex on a one- or two-lead rhythm strip, thereby mimicking SVT. Whenever possible, the diagnosis of a tachycardia should be based on a 12-lead electrocardiogram, although hemodynamically stable patients may occasionally be sent urgently for electrophysiologic testing to clarify an uncertain diagnosis (Chapter 61). Conversely, patients with intraventricular conduction abnormalities (such as a left or right bundle branch block) will have wide-complex tachycardias during SVTs, with a QRS vector similar to what is seen in normal sinus rhythm. In addition, when an SVT is very rapid, a functional bundle branch block may generate a widened QRS duration and shift the axis transiently. In both these examples, the wide QRS may mimic VT. When wide-complex SVT is suspected, transient vagal stimulation via carotid sinus massage or an atrioventricular nodal blocking agent, such as intravenous adenosine (see Table 63–3), may be useful for slowing the rate or terminating an SVT. Intravenous calcium-blocking agents should not be used for the diagnosis or treatment of wide-QRS tachycardias, especially in the presence of structural heart disease because of their myocardial depressant effects, except when it is known with certainty that the tachycardia is an SVT in a patient with normal or near-normal left ventricular function.

SVTs can result in a risk for life-threatening arrhythmias that require prompt therapy in two circumstances. One is in patients with high-grade coronary artery stenoses, in whom rapid heart rates can cause myocardial ischemia because of the dependence of coronary blood flow on the diastolic interval; the arrhythmia should be treated urgently, usually by electrical direct current (DC) cardioversion (Chapter 65), unless specific medical therapy is available and controls the rate promptly (Chapter 63). The second is in patients with Wolff-Parkinson-White syndrome, who may have ventricular rates greater than 300 beats per minute during atrial fibrillation when the accessory pathway has a short refractory period (see Fig. 63–5). This arrhythmia, which can cause hypotensive VT or VF, requires prompt therapy (Chapter 63).

GENERAL MANAGEMENT OF CARDIAC ARREST

Basic life-support (BLS) and advanced cardiac life support (ACLS) strategies for initial and definitive responses to cardiac arrest have improved survival in victims of cardiac arrest. The principles of BLS and ACLS apply to both in-hospital and out-of-hospital cardiac arrest, but their applications and outcomes depend on the setting. In the hospital, the probability of survival is determined by the specific patient category (acute syndromes better than end-stage diseases), the mechanism of cardiac arrest (better for tachyarrhythmias than for bradyarrhythmias, asystole, or pulseless electrical activity), and the hospital site (better in intensive care units or other monitored settings than on an unmonitored general care unit). In many acute care settings, including patients with acute coronary syndromes (Chapters 71 and 72), outcomes can be excellent. For other in-hospital settings and most out-of-hospital settings, the absolute number and proportion of survivors remain low, except in unique out-of-hospital settings that can provide an extraordinarily rapid response time to victims in VF or VT. When immediate defibrillation in highly protected environments is available, such as monitored intensive care units and electrophysiology laboratories, where response times of less than 60 seconds are the norm, the survival rate after VF is greater than 90% in the absence of pathophysiologic conditions that favor persistence of the potentially fatal arrhythmia. A newly emerging strategy is in-hospital monitoring linked to automated defibrillation.

Once 2 to 3 minutes has elapsed from the onset of cardiac arrest to defibrillation, the survival probability falls below 50% in most in-hospital and out-of-hospital circumstances. Survival rates also fall rapidly thereafter such that they are 25% or less by 4 to 6 minutes and less than 10% by 10 minutes. Although immediate defibrillation is the preferred method within the first few minutes after the onset of cardiac arrest, a brief period of cardiopulmonary resuscitation (CPR) to provide oxygenation of the victim improves survivability when the time to defibrillation exceeds 4 to 5 minutes. [1]

Basic Life Support

The activities included within BLS encompass the initial responses for diagnostic evaluation, followed by a seamless flow into establishing ventilation and perfusion via the techniques of CPR. The first action is to confirm that the collapse is the result of a cardiac arrest. After an initial evaluation for response to voice or tactile stimulation, observation for respiratory movements and skin color, and simultaneous palpation of major arteries for the presence of a pulse, the determination that a life-threatening incident is in progress should immediately prompt a call to an emergency medical rescue system (911).

Although the absence of a carotid or femoral pulse is a primary diagnostic criterion for the health care professional, palpation for a pulse is no longer recommended for lay responders. Instead, the absence of respiratory efforts or the presence of only agonal respirations, in conjunction with an absent pulse, is diagnostic of cardiac arrest. In contrast, absence of respiratory efforts or severe stridor with persistence of a pulse suggests a primary respiratory arrest that will lead to cardiac arrest in a short time; skin color may be pale or intensely cyanotic. In the latter circumstance, initial efforts should include oropharyngeal exploration in search of a foreign body and the Heimlich maneuver, which entails wrapping the arms around the victim from the back and delivering a sharp thrust to the upper part of the abdomen with a closed fist, particularly in a setting in which aspiration is likely (e.g., collapse in a restaurant).

Once a pulseless collapse is established, a blow to the chest (precordial thump) may be attempted by a properly trained rescuer as part of ACLS in response to a *pulseless* cardiac arrest when monitoring and a defibrillator are not immediately available. A precordial thump should not be used in an unmonitored patient with a perceptible rapid tachycardia or without complete loss of consciousness because of concern about converting organized electrical activity into VF. The technique involves one or two blows delivered firmly to the junction of the middle and lower thirds of the sternum from a height of 8 to 10 inches, but the effort should be abandoned if a spontaneous pulse does not immediately occur or if the patient begins to breathe.

As soon as the diagnosis of cardiac arrest is established, CPR is begun to maintain viability of the central nervous system, heart, and other vital organs until a definitive intervention can be carried out. CPR can be performed by professional and paraprofessional personnel, by experienced emergency medical technicians, and by trained laypersons. Time is the key element for success, and there should be minimal delay between the diagnosis and preparatory efforts in the initial response and institution of CPR. If only one witness is present, the only activity that should precede BLS is telephone contact (911) of emergency personnel.

Clearing the airway, which is a critical step in preparing for successful resuscitation, includes tilting the head backward and lifting the chin, in addition to exploring the airway for foreign bodies—including dentures—and removing them. The Heimlich maneuver should be performed if there is reason to suspect a foreign body lodged in the oropharynx. When the person at the scene has insufficient physical strength to perform the maneuver, mechanical dislodgment of a foreign body can sometimes be achieved by abdominal thrusts with the unconscious patient in a supine position. If there is suspicion that respiratory arrest precipitated the cardiac arrest, particularly in the presence of a mechanical airway obstruction, a second precordial thump should be delivered after the airway has been cleared.

With the head properly placed and the oropharynx clear, mouth-to-mouth respiration can be initiated if no specific rescue equipment is available. To a large extent, the procedure used for establishing ventilation depends on the site at which the cardiac arrest occurs. A variety of devices are available, including plastic oropharyngeal airways, esophageal obturators, a masked Ambu bag, and endotracheal tubes. Intubation is the preferred procedure, but time should not be sacrificed, even in the in-hospital setting, while awaiting an endotracheal tube or a person trained to insert it quickly and properly. Temporary support with Ambu bag ventilation is the usual method in the hospital until endotracheal intubation can be accomplished; in the out-of-hospital setting, mouth-to-mouth resuscitation is performed while awaiting emergency rescue personnel. The lungs should be inflated twice in succession after every 30 chest compressions.

TABLE 62–1 AUTOMATED EXTERNAL DEFIBRILLATOR STRATEGIES FOR RAPID RESPONSE TO CARDIAC ARRESTS CAUSED BY VENTRICULAR FIBRILLATION

Deployment	Examples	Rescuers	Advantages	Limitations
Emergency vehicles	Police cars Fire engines Ambulances	Trained emergency personnel	Experienced users Broad deployment Objectivity	Deployment time Arrival delays Community variations
Public access sites	Public buildings Stadiums, malls Airports Airliners	Security personnel Designated rescuers Random laypersons	Population density Shorter delays Lay and emergency personnel access	Low event rates Inexperienced users Panic and confusion
Multifamily dwellings	Apartments Condominiums Hotels	Security personnel Designated rescuers Family members	Familiar locations Defined personnel Shorter delays	Infrequent use Low event rates Geographic factors
Single-family dwellings	Private homes Apartments Neighborhood "Heart Watch"	Family members	Immediate access Familiar setting	Acceptance Victim may be alone One-time user; panic

The third element of BLS, circulation, is intended to maintain blood flow until definitive steps can be taken. The rationale is based on the hypothesis that chest compression maintains an externally driven pump function by sequential emptying and filling of its chambers, with competent valves favoring the forward direction of flow. The palm of one hand is placed over the lower part of the sternum while the heel of the other rests on the dorsum of the lower hand. The sternum is then depressed with the resuscitator's arms straight at the elbows to provide a less tiring and more forceful fulcrum at the junction of the shoulders and back. With this technique, sufficient force is applied to depress the sternum about 4 to 5 cm, with abrupt relaxation. The cycle is carried out at a rate of about 100 compressions per minute.

Automated External Defibrillators—Intermediate Life Support

Because time to defibrillation is the major determinant of survival, despite any temporizing benefit of BLS, and because ACLS strategies are generally implemented by in-hospital personnel or out-of-hospital emergency medical rescue system responders, an intermediate strategy has emerged that is based on the availability of automated external defibrillators (AEDs) for use by nonconventional first responders. Referred to as public access defibrillation or lay first-responder systems, the strategy relies on devices that prompt the user to deliver a defibrillation shock when deemed appropriate by a computerized rhythm detection system in the device. The operators can be trained police officers, security guards, airline personnel, or trained (or even untrained) lay responders (Table 62–1). A number of studies have suggested improved survival rates when such strategies are deployed. AED programs are not a replacement for ACLS (see later), but rather an intermediate supplement to the BLS-ACLS sequence that is intended to achieve earlier defibrillation while awaiting the arrival of ACLS personnel.

Advanced Cardiac Life Support

ACLS methods, other than those directly related to control of tachyarrhythmias, have led to the generation of comprehensive protocols to guide responders over a broad expanse of clinical circumstances and mechanisms of cardiac arrest ranging from transient clinical events to end-stage multisystem disease. The general goals of ACLS are to restore a hemodynamically effective cardiac rhythm, optimize ventilation, and maintain and support the restored circulation. Thus, during ACLS, the patient's cardiac rhythm is promptly cardioverted or defibrillated as the first priority, if appropriate equipment is immediately available, although a short period of closed-chest cardiac compression immediately before defibrillation enhances the probability of survival if the cardiac arrest has lasted for 4 to 5 minutes before the availability of a defibrillator. [1] After the initial attempt to restore a hemodynamically effective rhythm, the patient is intubated and oxygenated, if needed, and the heart is paced if a bradyarrhythmia or asystole occurs. An intravenous line is established to deliver medications. After intubation, the goal of ventilation is to reverse hypoxemia and not merely to achieve a high alveolar Po_2. When available, oxygen rather than room air should be used to ventilate the patient, and arterial O_2 saturation should be monitored, if possible. In the out-of-hospital setting, a facemask or an Ambu bag by means of an endotracheal tube is generally used; in the hospital, respiratory support is typical.

MANAGEMENT OF TACHYARRHYTHMIC CARDIAC ARRESTS

DC Cardioversion

When VF or a rapid VT is recognized on a monitor or by telemetry, defibrillation should be carried out immediately (Fig. 62–2). A normal rhythm can be successfully restored in up to 90% of VF victims weighing up to 90 kg with a DC shock of up to 360 J. Failure of the initial shock to cardiovert the patient to an effective rhythm is a poor prognostic sign. Although some algorithms suggest a succession of shock energies from 200 to 360 J during a sequence of attempts to defibrillate, there is little to be gained from beginning with energies less than 300 J during a cardiac arrest.

After a single shock at 300 or 360 J of energy, the patient should be checked for restoration of a spontaneous pulse; CPR should be continued for 5 cycles if a pulse remains absent. Subsequently, a second shock should be delivered, followed by epinephrine, 1 mg intravenously (IV). If a pulse is still absent, CPR is repeated for 5 cycles before the next shock. Epinephrine may be repeated at 3- to 5-minute intervals with defibrillator shocks in between, but high-dose epinephrine does not appear to provide added benefit. Vasopressin, 40 U given IV once, is an equally good alternative to epinephrine. [2]

Pharmacotherapy for Resistant Arrhythmias

For a patient who continues in VF or pulseless VT despite multiple attempts at DC cardioversion after epinephrine or who has recurrent episodes of VF or VT after cardioversion, electrical stability may be achieved by intravenous antiarrhythmic agents while continuing resuscitative efforts (see Fig. 62–2). Amiodarone (150 mg IV over a 10-minute period, followed by 1 mg/min for up to 6 hours and 0.5 mg/min thereafter) is the initial treatment of choice. [3] Additional bolus dosing, to a maximum of 500 mg, can be tried if the initial bolus is unsuccessful. Amiodarone need not be given as a routine to individuals who respond to initial defibrillation with a persistently stable rhythm, but it is preferred for those who have recurrent episodes of VT or VF after initial defibrillation and oxygenation.

If there is sufficient clinical evidence that the cardiac arrest was heralded by the onset of an acute coronary syndrome, lidocaine, (1.0- to 1.5-mg/kg bolus given IV, with the dose repeated in 2 minutes) is

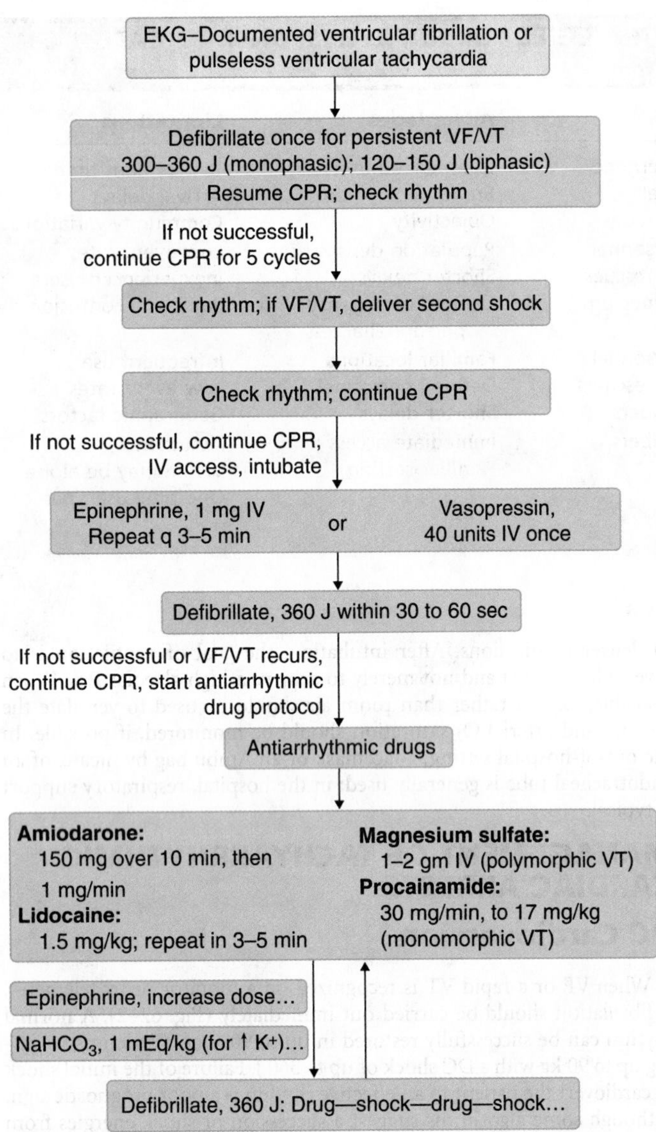

FIGURE 62–2 • General algorithm for advanced cardiac life support (ACLS) response to ventricular fibrillation (VF) or pulseless ventricular tachycardia (VT). For more detail, see the ACLS guidelines in Suggested Readings. CPR = cardiopulmonary resuscitation; EKG = electrocardiogram.

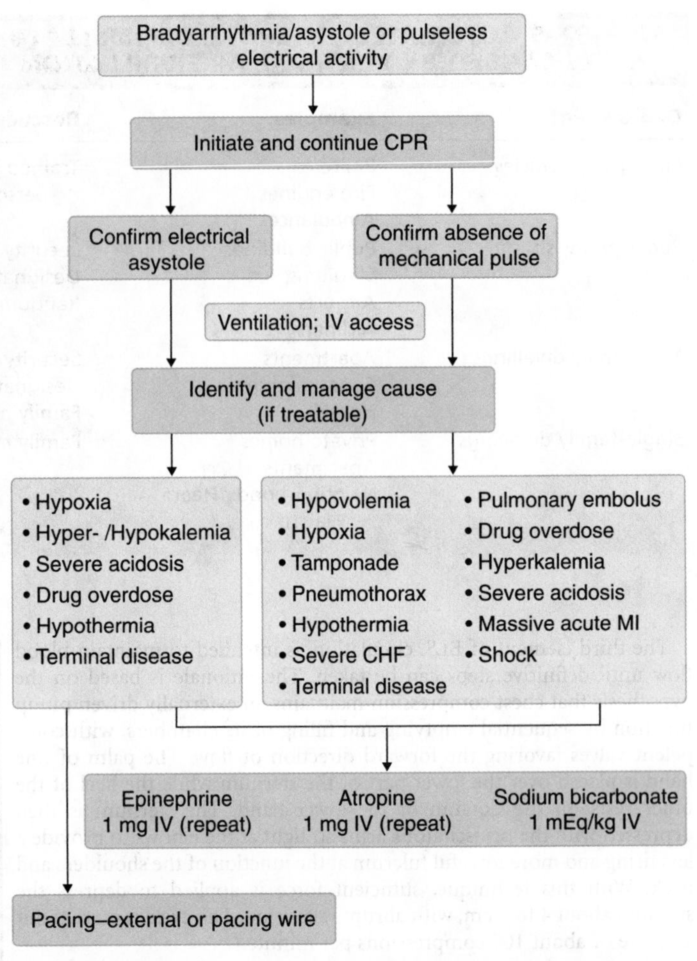

FIGURE 62–3 • General algorithm for advanced cardiac life support response to bradycardic or asystolic cardiac arrest or pulseless electrical activity. For more detail, see Suggested Readings. CHF = congestive heart failure; CPR = cardiopulmonary resuscitation; MI = myocardial infarction.

preferred over amiodarone. When acute ischemia or resistant or recurrent arrhythmias are not thought to be the mechanism, intravenous amiodarone should be used. Intravenous procainamide (loading infusion of 100 mg/5 min to a total dose of 500 to 800 mg, followed by a continuous infusion at 2 to 5 mg/min) is now rarely used but may be tried in those with persisting, hemodynamically unstable arrhythmias. In patients with acute hyperkalemia as the triggering event for resistant VF, hypocalcemia, or arrest potentially caused by excess doses of calcium-blocking drugs, 10% calcium gluconate (5 to 20 mL infused at a rate of 2 to 4 mL/min) may be helpful. Otherwise, calcium should not be used routinely during resuscitation, even though ionized Ca^{2+} levels may be low during resuscitation from cardiac arrest. Some resistant forms of polymorphic VT (*torsades de pointes*), rapid monomorphic VT, ventricular flutter (rate >260/min), or resistant VF may respond to $MgSO_4$ (1 to 2 g IV given over a 1- to 2-minute period) or to β-blocker therapy (propranolol, 1-mg boluses IV to a total dose of up to 15 to 20 mg; or metoprolol, 5 mg IV, up to 20 mg).

Adjunctive Therapeutic Actions

During or after therapy targeted to restoration of an electrically stable cardiac rhythm, the patient's general metabolic state should be addressed by improving oxygenation and reversing acidosis. Intravenous sodium bicarbonate (1 mEq/kg), with up to 50% of this dose repeated every 10 to 15 minutes during the course of CPR, is recommended for patients with known or suspected preexisting bicarbonate-responsive causes of acidosis, for certain drug overdoses (Chapter 111), and after prolonged and unsuccessful attempts at resuscitation. Caution must be exercised, however, because excessive quantities of sodium bicarbonate can be deleterious by causing alkalosis, hypernatremia, and hyperosmolality. When possible, arterial pH, Po_2, and Pco_2 should be monitored during the resuscitation.

MANAGEMENT OF CARDIAC ARREST CAUSED BY ASYSTOLE, BRADYARRHYTHMIAS, OR PULSELESS ELECTRICAL ACTIVITY

The approach to a patient with bradyarrhythmic or asystolic arrest, or pulseless electrical activity, differs from the approach to patients with tachyarrhythmic events (VT/VF). Once this form of cardiac arrest is recognized, efforts should focus on first establishing control of the patient's cardiorespiratory status (i.e., continue CPR, intubate, and establish intravenous access), then reconfirming the rhythm (in two leads if possible), and finally taking actions that favor the emergence of a stable spontaneous rhythm or attempt to pace the heart. Possible reversible causes, particularly for bradyarrhythmia and asystole, should be considered and excluded (or treated) promptly (Fig. 62–3), including hypovolemia, hypoxia, cardiac tamponade, tension pneumothorax, preexisting acidosis, drug overdose, hypothermia, and hyperkalemia. Epinephrine (1.0 mg IV every 3 to 5 minutes) and atropine (1.0 to 2.0 mg IV) or isoproterenol (up to 15 to 20 μg/min IV), which are commonly used in an attempt to elicit spontaneous electrical activity or increase the rate of a bradycardia, have only limited success. In the absence of an intravenous line, epinephrine (1 mg, i.e., 10 mL of a 1 : 10,000 solution) may be given by the intracardiac route, but there is danger of coronary or myocardial laceration. Sodium bicarbonate, 1 mEq/kg, may be tried for known or strongly suspected preexisting hyperkalemia or bicarbonate-responsive acidosis.

Pacing of a bradyarrhythmic or asystolic heart has been limited in the past by the unavailability of personnel capable of performing such procedures at the scene of cardiac arrests. With the development of more effective external pacing systems (Chapter 65), emergency pacing should be used for out-of hospital bradycardic or asystolic arrest, although its influence on outcome is not well documented. In the hospital setting, external pacing is generally used during the initial response to a bradycardic or asystolic arrest, but it should be superseded by transvenous pacing if the arrest is prolonged, if continuous pacing is needed, or if the external device fails to pace. Unfortunately, an *asystolic* patient continues to have a very poor prognosis despite available techniques.

LONG-TERM MANAGEMENT

Survivors of a cardiac arrest that is not due to transient factors remain at high risk for recurrent cardiac arrest and sudden cardiac death. A number of clinical trials have demonstrated improved survival rates in those who receive implantable cardioverter-defibrillators (Chapter 64).

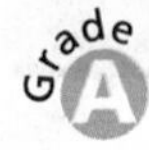

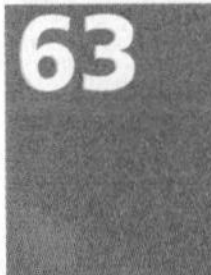

1. Wik L, Hansen TB, Fylling F, et al: Delaying defibrillation to give basic cardiopulmonary resuscitation to patients with out-of-hospital ventricular fibrillation: A randomized trial. JAMA 2003;289:1389–1395.
2. Aung K, Htay T: Vasopressin for cardiac arrest: A systematic review and meta-analysis. Arch Intern Med 2005;165:17–24.
3. Dorian P, Cass D, Schwartz B, et al: Amiodarone as compared with lidocaine for shock-resistant ventricular fibrillation. N Engl J Med 2002;346:884–890.
4. Huikuri HV, Castellanos A, Myerburg RJ: Sudden death due to cardiac arrhythmias. N Engl J Med 2001;345:1473–1482.

SUGGESTED READINGS

Cooper JA, Cooper JD, Cooper JM: Cardiopulmonary resuscitation: History, current practice, and future direction. Circulation 2006;114:2839–2849. *A comprehensive review.*

International Liaison Committee on Resuscitation: 2005 International Consensus on Cardiopulmonary Resuscitation and Emergency Cardiovascular Care Science with Treatment Recommendations. Circulation 2005;112:IV-1–IV-196. *Consensus guidelines.*

Wik L, Kramer-Johansen J, Myklebust H, et al: Quality of cardiopulmonary resuscitation during out-of-hospital cardiac arrest. JAMA 2005;293:299–304. *Emphasizes how frequently CPR is not done properly.*

63 CARDIAC ARRHYTHMIAS WITH SUPRAVENTRICULAR ORIGIN

Masood Akhtar

Definition and Pathobiology

Both of the atria and corresponding ventricles are electrically insulated from each other by fibrous tissue that is the anatomic atrioventricular (AV) junction. The fibrous structures in the AV junction are the annuli of the mitral and tricuspid valves and the fibrous portion of the interventricular septum. In the absence of an electrical bridge, the atrial impulses cannot cross this fibrous gap. Normally, the AV node and the connected His-Purkinje system (HPS) provide the only electrical conduit. Some individuals, however, have additional electrical bridges, which bypass the AV node–HPS to connect the atria directly with ventricles or fascicles. These pathways, often referred to as accessory pathways, include AV connections (Kent bundle), which form the anatomic basis for Wolff-Parkinson-White (WPW) syndrome, and atriofascicular fibers (previously called Mahaim fibers).

Any arrhythmia that arises above the bifurcation of the His bundle into the right and left bundle branches or activates the ventricles through an accessory pathway is classified as supraventricular. The resultant QRS complex morphology either can be normal or may be wide owing to bundle branch or fascicular block (aberrant conduction) or conduction over an accessory pathway (anomalous conduction or preexcitation). Supraventricular cardiac arrhythmias can be categorized broadly into tachyarrhythmias or bradyarrhythmias.

TACHYARRHYTHMIAS

Definition

Supraventricular tachyarrhythmias can occur either as single or consecutive premature complexes or in the form of nonsustained or sustained tachycardias. The most frequent definition of nonsustained tachycardias is an arrhythmia with a rate of more than 100 beats per minute lasting 3 beats or more but less than 30 seconds. Sustained tachycardia is a prolonged episode of tachycardia lasting at least 30 seconds or terminated earlier with an intervention, such as intravenous medication, overdrive pacing, or direct current electrical cardioversion because of the urgency of the situation.

Premature Atrial Complexes

Premature atrial complexes (PACs) can arise from any part of the right or left atrium or any adjacent tissue where a sleeve of atrial muscle extends, such as the pulmonary veins. The P wave morphology depends on the origin but differs from sinus rhythm unless PACs arise near the upper right atrial junction with the superior vena cava, that is, close to the location of sinus node. The P wave always precedes the QRS complex (Fig. 63–1A); if it encounters the absolute refractory period of the AV node or the HPS, the P wave is blocked and is not followed by a QRS complex. A blocked PAC may be confused with second-degree AV block unless its prematurity is recognized or with sinus node dysfunction (SND) if it is inconspicuous. Altered appearance of the ST-T segment is often a clue to the presence of a P wave. When a premature QRS complex has the morphology of the underlying sinus rhythm but is not preceded by a P wave, it is labeled *AV junctional* (see Fig. 63–1B). When two or more morphologically distinct P waves result in a rate less than 100 beats per minute, the rhythm is termed *wandering atrial pacemaker.*

Premature complexes from the atria or AV junction usually lead to the same intraventricular conduction pattern seen during sinus complexes; that is, if the sinus rhythm shows a normal QRS complex or bundle branch block pattern, the same configuration would be expected during the premature complexes (see Fig. 63–1B). If the premature complexes are relatively early (i.e., closely coupled), however, they can encroach on the refractory period of the right or left bundle branches, resulting in aberrant conduction and producing a right or left bundle branch or fascicular block pattern (see Fig. 63–1A) despite normal intraventricular conduction during sinus rhythm. Closely coupled PACs also frequently initiate sustained or nonsustained supraventricular tachycardias.

Sustained Supraventricular Tachycardias

Supraventricular tachycardias can be categorized broadly into atrial and AV junctional (Table 63–1). Atrial tachycardias are independent of AV nodal conduction, so that effective vagal maneuvers (e.g., carotid sinus massage, Valsalva) or medications that slow AV nodal conduction cause AV block, but the atrial process continues (Fig. 63–2A). Conversely, most AV junctional tachycardias require propagation through the AV node to continue, and AV junctional tachycardias generally terminate if vagal maneuvers induce AV nodal block (see Fig. 63–2B).

Atrial Tachycardias

Sinus Tachycardia

Sinus tachycardia is usually due to an enhancement of normal automaticity seen in the settings of increased adrenergic drive. Because sympathetic stimulation and vagal withdrawal also enhance AV nodal conduction, the PR interval is not prolonged despite acceleration of the sinus rate. The P wave configuration is the same as with sinus rhythm—upright in leads II, III, and aVF (see Fig. 63–2A and B) and biphasic in V_1—because of the normal sequence with which the sinus node depolarizes the two atria. The atrial rate during sinus tachycardia seldom exceeds 200 beats per minute and is generally less than 150 beats per minute.

Sinus Node Re-Entry

The P wave morphology is similar to sinus rhythm, but the underlying mechanism is re-entry in the region of the sinus node. In contrast to

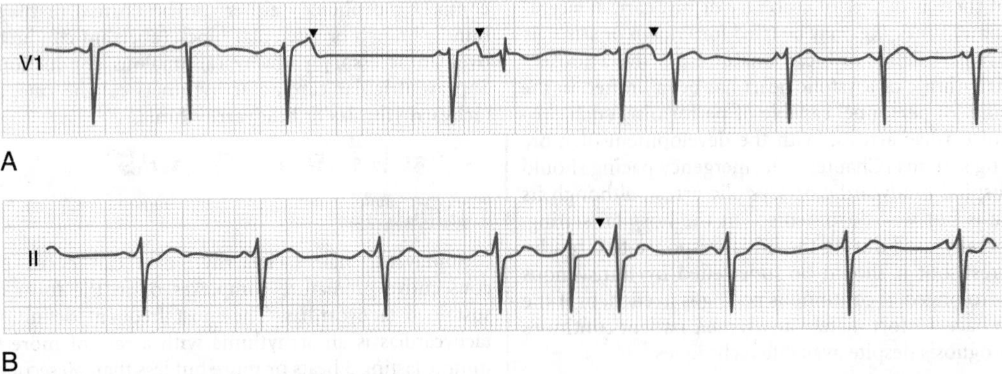

FIGURE 63–1 • Isolated premature complexes. A, Three premature atrial complexes (arrows). The first one is blocked, whereas the remaining two conduct to the ventricles with QRS morphology different from that of sinus complexes owing to encroachment of premature impulses on the refractory period of the His-Purkinje system (aberrant conduction). **B,** Premature junctional complex (fifth complex). Note the similarity of the QRS complex between the sinus and premature beat that is not preceded by a P wave. The next sinus P wave (arrow), which is superimposed on the T wave of the premature beat, occurs on time and conducts to the ventricles. Electrocardiographic leads are labeled. (Modified from Akhtar M: Examination of the heart: Part V. The electrocardiogram, 1990. With permission from the American Heart Association, Dallas, TX.)

TABLE 63–1 SUPRAVENTRICULAR TACHYCARDIAS

	R-R Regularity	P Wave Morphology
Atrial tachycardias		
Sinus tachycardia	Regular	Positive in II, III, aVF
Sinus node re-entry	Regular	Positive in II, III, aVF
Atrial tachycardia, unifocal	Regular	P different from sinus
Atrial tachycardia, multifocal	Irregular	≥3 different P wave morphologies
Atrial flutter, common, counterclockwise	Regular, irregular if variable AV block	Sawtooth flutter waves; regular waveform; negative in II, III, aVF
Atrial flutter, uncommon, clockwise	Regular, irregular if variable AV block	Upright flutter waves; positive waveform II, III, aVF
Atrial fibrillation	Irregularly irregular	Irregular fibrillation waves
AV junctional tachycardias		
AV re-entry (using accessory pathways)		
Orthodromic	Regular	Retrograde P in ST-T wave
Antidromic	Regular preexcited	Retrograde P, short RP
Slow conducting	Regular	Retrograde P at end of T wave or later (long RP)
Atriofascicular (antidromic)	Regular preexcited	Retrograde P, short RP
AV nodal re-entry		
Common (slow-fast)	Regular	Retrograde P obscured by QRS or alters the end of QRS (short RP)
Uncommon (fast-slow)	Regular	Retrograde P at end of T wave or later (long RP)
Others (slow-slow)	Regular	PR-RP approximately equal
Nonparoxysmal junctional tachycardia*	Regular, slow rate	AV dissociation
Automatic junctional tachycardia*	Regular	AV dissociation

*Site of origin usually infranodal.
AV = atrioventricular.

the physiologic form of sinus tachycardia, which has a gradual onset and termination, sinus node re-entry starts and ends abruptly. As with many other atrial re-entrant tachycardias, sinus node re-entry is generally triggered by a PAC. Sudden acceleration of the atrial rate prolongs the PR interval or may lead to AV nodal block owing to the expected physiologic delay in AV nodal conduction unless subsequent sympathetic stimulation facilitates AV nodal conduction. The atrial rates range between 150 and 250 beats per minute. Depending on the state of AV conduction, 1:1 AV conduction or a variable degree of AV block may be noted.

Atrial Tachycardia

Any tachycardia arising above the AV junction that has a P wave configuration different from sinus rhythm is called *atrial tachycardia* (see Fig. 63–2C). In general, impulses arising in the superior portion of the right or left atrium produce a positive P wave in the inferior leads (i.e., leads II, III, and aVF), whereas impulses arising in the lower or inferior portions result in negative P waves in the same leads. Atrial tachycardias can result from enhanced normal automaticity, abnormal automaticity, triggered activity, and re-entry (Chapter 60). The re-entrant forms can be reproduced easily in the electrophysiology laboratory with electrical stimulation of the atria (Chapter 61). When the P wave configuration is uniform from beat to beat, the tachycardia is unifocal; the term *multifocal atrial tachycardia* implies several different P wave morphologies. Atrial rates range between 100 and 250 beats per minute, and the ventricular response depends on the status of AV conduction; a 1:1 ratio of P wave to QRS complex is common with rates less than 200 beats per minute, whereas at higher rates various degrees of block (e.g., 3:2, 2:1, 3:1) are common (see Fig. 63–2C). Atrial rates and AV conduction can be altered markedly by cardioactive drugs, particularly antiarrhythmic agents.

Atrial Flutter

Atrial flutter causes regular atrial rates ranging from 250 to 350 beats per minute (300 being the most common). Common atrial flutter, with a "sawtooth" appearance in leads II, III, and aVF, has a fairly uniform route of impulse propagation localized to the right atrium. The re-entrant impulse travels over the anterolateral right atrium, through a

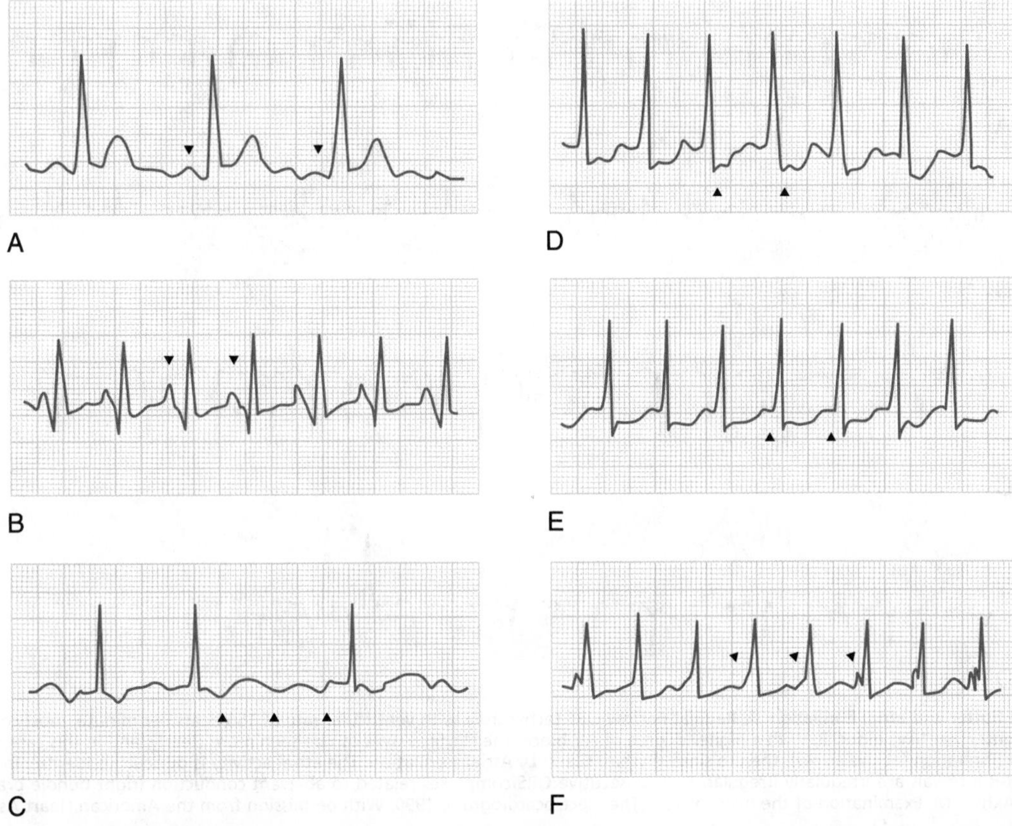

FIGURE 63–2 • P-QRS relationship in supraventricular tachycardia. Sinus rhythm (**A**), usual type of sinus tachycardia (**B**), and unifocal atrial tachycardia (**C**) are shown. Note the positive P wave and normal PR interval during sinus tachycardia. Atrial tachycardia (**C**) originates in the low atrium (negative P wave) and is accompanied by a variable degree of atrioventricular (AV) block. Among the AV junctional tachycardias, the P wave follows the QRS and is in the ST segment during AV re-entry (**D**) and buried in the QRS complex during common AV nodal re-entry (**E**). Nonparoxysmal junctional tachycardia in which the atria and ventricles are stimulated independently is shown (**F**). Resultant AV dissociation occurs because the junctional rate accelerates and competes with the sinus mechanism. Note the gradual march of P waves in and out of the QRS. Electrocardiogram lead II in all panels.

narrow isthmus in the posteroseptal area, then along the atrial septum toward the superior portion of the right atrium (counterclockwise). Incidental left atrial activation produces a negative sawtooth flutter wave in the inferior leads. A reverse of this direction in the circuit could cause a positive flutter wave in the same leads (uncommon or clockwise); both clockwise and counterclockwise atrial flutters are also referred to as isthmus dependent. Flutter waves with other configurations may have different origins, including the left atrium. At atrial rates of 300 beats per minute, the ventricular response is usually 2:1 (Fig. 63–3A) or 4:1, representing ventricular rates of 150 and 75 beats per minute, respectively. A 3:1 AV ratio is uncommon and fairly well tolerated. A 1:1 AV response is rare and can cause serious hemodynamic consequences.

Atrial Fibrillation

Atrial fibrillation (AF) is the most common sustained arrhythmia in adults. More than 2 million individuals in the United States have AF, with at least 160,000 new cases diagnosed every year. The incidence of AF increases with advancing age, affecting more than 6% of the population older than 75. A rapidly firing focus in one or more of the pulmonary veins is the usual trigger, with subsequent disorganized and asymmetrical conduction through the atria resulting in multiple wavelets of re-entry to sustain the AF. During AF, the atria have disorganized, rapid, irregular electrical activity exceeding 400 beats per minute (see Fig. 63–3B and 3C). The ventricular response is also irregular and variable (irregularly irregular). The atria do not contract effectively so that intra-atrial clot formation is promoted. With subsequent resumption of atrial contraction, embolism can occur with devastating consequences. On the surface electrocardiogram (ECG), the AF waves may be coarse, fine, or difficult to discern, but the irregularity of the RR wave makes the diagnosis of AF relatively easy. Aberrant conduction may be noted if the impulses reach the bundle branches during their refractory period (see Fig. 63–3D). In the absence of accessory pathways, the average ventricular response by the AV node–HPS is seldom more than 200 beats per minute and is generally less than 150 beats per minute. With a rapidly conducting accessory pathway, ventricular rates can exceed 300 beats per minute, however, and precipitate ventricular fibrillation.

Atrioventricular Junctional Tachycardia

Most AV junctional tachycardias (see Table 63–1) requiring long-term management are re-entrant. AV re-entry in the WPW syndrome is the classic example and is usually (>90%) initiated by atrial or ventricular premature complexes, or both.

Wolff-Parkinson-White Syndrome and Associated Tachycardias

A combination of a short PR interval and initial slurring of the QRS (Fig. 63–4A) is termed *ventricular preexcitation*, which in association with a history of tachycardia constitutes the WPW syndrome. Normally, the sinus impulse must travel through the AV node–HPS to reach the ventricles, resulting in a PR interval of 120 to 200 msec. When an accessory pathway (often called the *Kent bundle*) directly connects the atrium with the ventricle, it bypasses the AV nodal conduction delay and the impulse reaches the ventricles sooner than expected, hence the term *preexcitation* (Chapter 60). The length of the PR interval is a function of proximity of the accessory pathway to the origin of impulse and conduction time through it. When location or relatively slow conduction delays the accessory impulse, ventricular depolarization may occur through the normal pathway. In a typical case of WPW, however, the impulse reaches the ventricle first through the accessory pathway and starts the QRS earlier, resulting in a shorter PR interval.

Because the initial QRS activation is due to muscle-to-muscle conduction, as opposed to Purkinje-to-muscle activation during normal QRS, the beginning of the QRS is slurred and produces a so-called delta wave. Soon after, ventricular activation also starts through the normal pathway and is spread more rapidly through the ventricular myocardium, resulting in a fusion QRS activation with a rapid inscription after the delta wave. If the atrial or sinus impulse never reaches the ventricle through the accessory pathway because of either delayed arrival at or lack of anterograde conduction over the accessory pathway, the term *concealed*

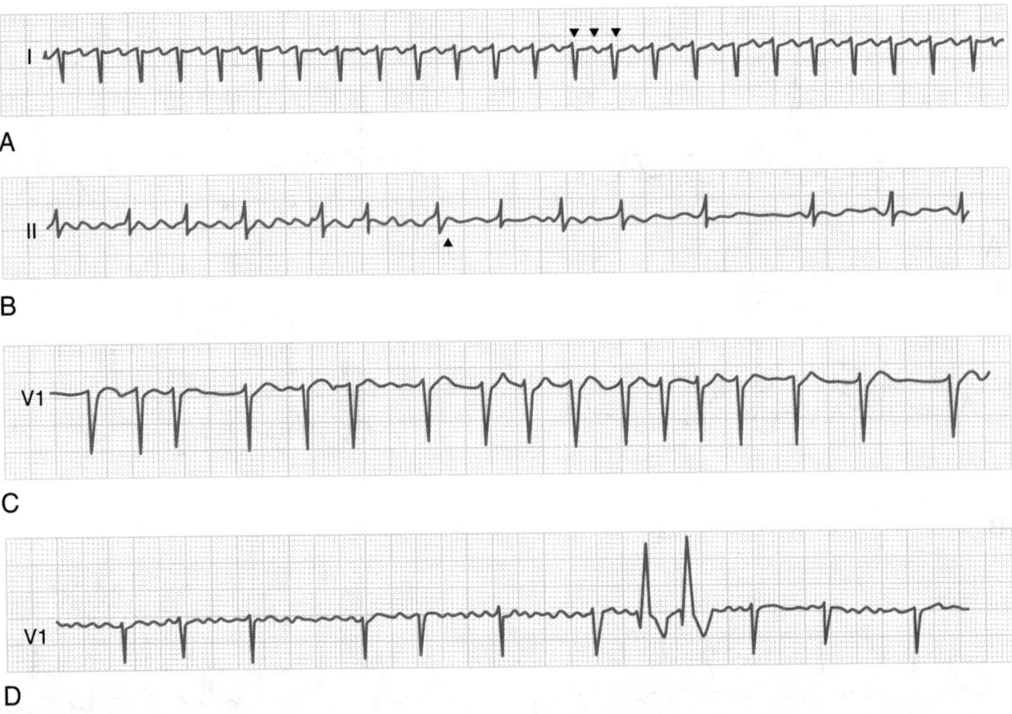

FIGURE 63–3 • Atrial flutter and atrial fibrillation. A, Regular narrow QRS tachycardia with ventricular rate of 150 beats per minute, most commonly seen in atrial flutter with 2:1 atrioventricular (AV) block. **B,** With a higher degree of AV block, the flutter waves can be seen more clearly, and in this case, the atrial flutter converted briefly to atrial fibrillation (at the arrow), then to sinus rhythm. **C and D,** Atrial fibrillation. The atrial activity is difficult to identify in C, but it is clear in D; in both tracings, the R-R intervals are irregularly irregular. Two consecutive QRS complexes related to aberrant conduction (right bundle branch block) are noted in D. (Modified from Akhtar M: Examination of the heart: Part V. The electrocardiogram, 1990. With permission from the American Heart Association, Dallas, TX.)

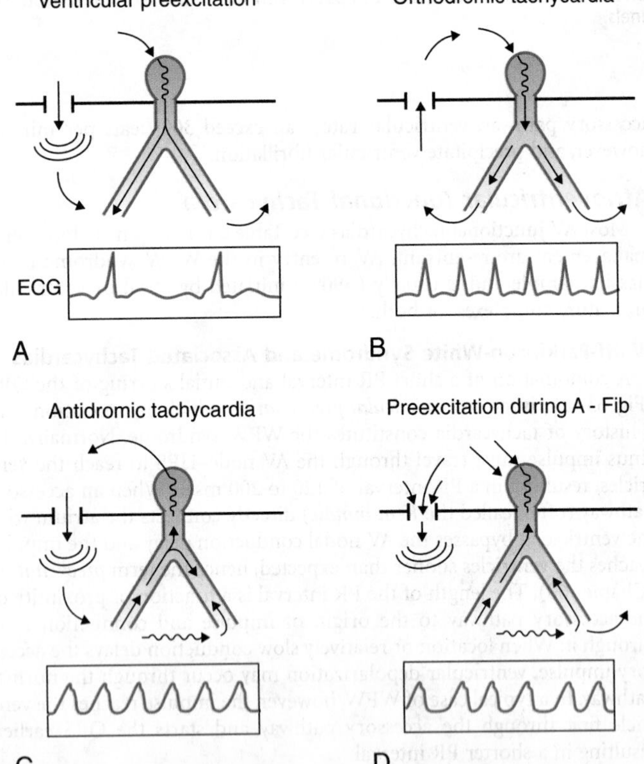

FIGURE 63–4 • Wolff-Parkinson-White syndrome. A, Ventricular preexcitation (short PR and delta wave) owing to earlier ventricular activation through the accessory pathway. **B,** Narrow QRS tachycardia with anterograde conduction over the atrioventricular node–His-Purkinje system and retrograde propagation through the accessory pathway (orthodromic tachycardia). **C,** The reversal of this re-entrant circuit produces antidromic tachycardia with regular and preexcited complexes. **D,** During atrial fibrillation, preferential conduction over the accessory pathway produces rapid irregular preexcited complexes. (Modified from Akhtar M: Examination of the heart: Part V. The electrocardiogram, 1990. With permission from the American Heart Association, Dallas, TX.)

WPW syndrome is used because retrograde conduction through the accessory pathway may be intact and able to cause orthodromic tachycardia. The most common accessory pathway (>50%) is in the left ventricle free wall, that is, left atrium–to–left ventricle connection. Posteroseptal pathways (connecting the right atrium with the left ventricle) are the next most common (30%). Right free wall and anteroseptal accessory pathways, both of which are right atrium–to–right ventricle connections, account for the remaining pathways.

The most common sustained arrhythmia in patients with WPW syndrome is orthodromic AV re-entry (see Fig. 63–2D and 4B), in which the impulse propagates to the ventricles by means of the normal pathway and in retrograde fashion to the atria through the accessory pathway; there is no evidence of ventricular preexcitation during the tachycardia. In rare instances, the circuit of re-entry may be reversed (antidromic) so that the impulse reaches the ventricle through the accessory pathway and in retrograde conducts to the atria through the normal pathway and produces a preexcited QRS complex (see Fig. 63–4C). The second most common arrhythmia and frequently the most serious is AF (see Fig. 63–4D), which is experienced by 40% of patients with WPW syndrome. If the accessory pathway conducts rapidly during AF, a relatively fast ventricular rate may occur and cause severe hypotension or syncope, or both, and even precipitate ventricular fibrillation. Other accessory pathways implicated in clinical tachycardias are the atriofascicular fibers (previously referred to as Mahaim fibers) and slowly conducting retrograde pathways.

Atrioventricular Nodal Re-entry

In the absence of ventricular preexcitation, the most common AV junctional tachycardia is AV nodal re-entry (AVNR). The entire re-entry circuit is localized to the region of the AV node and results from differences of conduction and refractory periods in various portions of the AV node. Faster conducting fibers (fast pathway) are situated more anteriorly and have longer refractory periods, whereas slower conducting fibers are posterior and have a shorter refractory period. In the common type of AVNR, anterograde conduction is over the slow pathway and retrograde conduction is through the fast pathway such that the conduction times of the impulse anterograde to the ventricles and retrograde to the atria are similar (see Fig. 63–2E), resulting in near-simultaneous P and QRS complexes. The retrograde P wave either is obscured by the QRS complex or alters the appearance of the terminal portion of the QRS and

TABLE 63-2 SELECTION OF MEDICATIONS FOR SPECIFIC SUPRAVENTRICULAR ARRHYTHMIAS

Arrhythmia	Acute Intravenous Management	Long-Term Oral Therapy*	Long-Term Anticoagulation
Atrial fibrillation	Verapamil, diltiazem, metoprolol, or digoxin for rate control Ibutilide for cardioversion	No organic cardiac disease—classes IA IC, class III, amiodarone Heart failure—amiodarone or dofetilide Hypertension—sotalol or class IC	Not necessary Yes Yes Yes
Atrial fibrillation with rapid rate owing to Wolff-Parkinson-White syndrome	Ibutilide or procainamide; avoid verapamil or digoxin	Amiodarone, sotalol, or class IA or IC	No
Atrial flutter	Verapamil, diltiazem, metoprolol, esmolol, or digoxin	Amiodarone, sotalol, class IA or IC	Yes
Paroxysmal supraventricular tachycardia	Adenosine, verapamil, propranolol, esmolol, or metoprolol	β-Blockers, calcium-channel blockers, class IA or IC, or sotalol	No

*Class IA = procainamide, quinidine, disopyramide; class IC = flecainide, propafenone; class III = sotalol, dofetilide.
Adapted in part from Scheinman MM, Kaushik V: Recognition and management of patients with tachyarrhythmias. *In* Braunwald E, Goldman L (eds): Primary Care Cardiology, 2nd ed. Philadelphia, WB Saunders, 2003, pp 503–528.

may be recognized in the early part of the ST segment. This type of AVNR is also referred to as slow-fast AVN re-entry. Less frequently, the direction of conduction through the re-entry circuit is reversed, with anterograde conduction to the ventricle over the fast pathway and retrograde conduction to the atria through the slow pathway; the result is a shorter PR interval (fast-slow). If the P wave follows the T wave, its retrograde morphology (i.e., negative in leads II, III, and aVF) is clearly recognizable. Sustained AVNR and AV re-entry together account for more than 75% of cases, frequently but incorrectly labeled as *paroxysmal atrial tachycardia.*

Nonparoxysmal Junctional Tachycardia

Nonparoxysmal junctional tachycardia arises within the region of the His bundle and activates the ventricles with a QRS morphology similar to that of sinus beats (see Fig. 63–2F). Retrograde conduction through the AV node may or may not take place. If there is retrograde block, sinus rhythm remains uninterrupted, and the sinus P wave also blocks when the AV node is refractory because of retrograde AV nodal penetration of the junctional impulse; AV dissociation may result. A 1:1 P wave–QRS complex relationship may also occur in some situations, and if the P wave is negative, junctional origin is suggested. Ventricular rates seldom exceed 150 beats per minute, and when the rate is less than 100 beats per minute, the term *accelerated junctional rhythm* is applied. The underlying mechanism is enhanced normal automaticity.

Automatic Junctional Tachycardia

The main difference between automatic junctional tachycardia and nonparoxysmal junctional tachycardia on the surface ECG is the rate. In the automatic variety, rates are faster (range, 130 to 200 beats per minute). This arrhythmia can be episodic or persistent. Because the rates are fairly comparable to those of paroxysmal AV junctional re-entrant tachycardia and the QRS complex morphology is similar to that of sinus beats, the presence of AV dissociation is the main distinction from re-entrant arrhythmias on the ECG. The underlying cause is abnormal automaticity in the AV junction.

Clinical Manifestations

The usual type of sinus tachycardia is caused by increased metabolic demands from high adrenergic states, such as fever, physical exertion, hypovolemia, heart failure (Chapter 57), sympathomimetic or parasympatholytic medications, thyrotoxicosis (Chapter 244), and pheochromocytoma (Chapter 246). Sinus tachycardia is an appropriate response to the need for an increase in cardiac output, and the accelerated rate is seldom the major symptom. All other supraventricular tachycardias represent abnormalities of rhythm and commonly produce tachycardia-related symptoms, including palpitation, racing of the heart, dizziness, shortness of breath, chest discomfort, presyncope, and sometimes frank syncope. Incessant supraventricular tachycardia and uncontrolled ventricular rates in AF can cause tachycardia-related cardiomyopathy, which is reversible with control of these arrhythmias.

Atrial dilation, fibrosis, and acute or chronic inflammatory states involving atrial myocardium or pericardium may cause atrial tachycardias. Multifocal atrial tachycardia is relatively frequent in the presence of chronic pulmonary disease. AF is often associated with aging, hypertension, valvular and pulmonary diseases, acute and chronic coronary disease, hyperadrenergic states, and metabolic abnormalities such as diabetes and thyrotoxicosis. AF may also be noted in the absence of any detectable cardiac pathology, in which case it is termed *lone AF.* The risk of thromboembolism in AF increases with age, diabetes mellitus, hypertension, previous embolic episodes, valvular disease, and heart failure. The lowest incidence (<1% annually) is in patients younger than 65 years with lone AF.

Re-entrant tachycardias have an abrupt onset and an abrupt ending, particularly when terminated with vagal maneuvers or intravenous medications. Although a functioning accessory pathway is a congenital abnormality, its clinical manifestation can occur at any age. If no ECG is obtained, asymptomatic ventricular preexcitation can go undetected for many years. When discovered, ventricular preexcitation can mimic inferior or anteroseptal myocardial infarction, right ventricular hypertrophy, and right and left bundle branch block. WPW syndrome is not clearly associated with mitral valve prolapse or hypertrophic cardiomyopathy, but single and multiple right-sided accessory pathways are more common with Ebstein's anomaly.

Nonparoxysmal AV junctional tachycardia is seen frequently with high adrenergic drive, that is, after myocardial infarction or cardiac surgery, with sympathomimetic and parasympatholytic agents, or with digitalis toxicity. Automatic junctional tachycardia is not known to be associated with any particular cardiovascular pathology.

Treatment

Rx

See Tables 63–2 and 63–3. See also Chapter 65.

Acute Therapy

Isolated premature beats seldom pose significant risk, do not cause severe arrhythmic symptoms, and do not warrant aggressive therapy. Conversely, sustained or prolonged repeated episodes of nonsustained supraventricular tachycardias generally require effective therapy. Whenever rapid control of supraventricular tachycardia is desired (e.g., in patients with myocardial ischemia or hypotension), cardioversion is the best solution (Chapter 65). Atrial tachycardias, including atrial flutter or AF, may also convert spontaneously or convert after treatment of an underlying cause, such as

TABLE 63–3 DRUGS AND DOSES USED TO TREAT SUPRAVENTRICULAR TACHYCARDIAS

Drug	Intravenous Bolus	Intravenous Infusion	Oral Dose
Digoxin	0.5–1 mg		0.125–0.5 mg/day
Adenosine	6–12 mg		
β-Blockers			
Esmolol	5 μg/kg/min	3 μg/kg/min	
Propranolol	1–3 mg		10–40 mg tid
Metoprolol	5 mg (can repeat ×2)		25–200 mg/day (or 12.5–100 mg bid)
Calcium-channel blockers			
Verapamil	5–15 mg		120–480 mg/day (3–4 times per day in divided doses or use long-acting form)
Diltiazem	15–25 mg	15 mg/kg	120–360 mg/day (2–3 times per day in divided doses or use long-acting form)
Class IA			
Procainamide	10–15 mg/kg	5 mg/kg	750–1500 mg qid
Quinidine			300–600 mg qid
Disopyramide			100–200 mg tid
Class IC			
Flecainide			50–200 mg bid
Propafenone			150–300 mg tid
Class III			
Ibutilide	1–2 mg		
Sotalol			80–160 mg bid
Dofetilide			125–500 mg bid
Amiodarone	2–3 mg/kg	0.5–1 mg/min	600–1200 mg/day for 7- to 10-day loading dose, then 100–400 mg/day, aiming for 100–200 mg/day maintenance dose by 3 months

hypoxia or heart failure, or after cessation of precipitating medications.

An acute episode of junctional tachycardia from either AVNR or AV re-entry can usually be terminated with vagal maneuvers, such as carotid massage, which produce sinus slowing and AV nodal block. In most atrial tachycardias, adenosine (see Table 63–3) or vagal stimulation, or both, produce enough AV block to unmask the atrial origin of the tachycardia. However, some atrial tachycardias, particularly those arising near the sinus node, may also terminate after administration of adenosine. Intravenous β-blockers and calcium-channel blockers (see Table 63–3) can be used for the same purpose. For sustained control of the ventricular rate during atrial tachycardia, intravenous esmolol and diltiazem are effective.

For acute AF without hypotension, rate control is crucial and can be accomplished with esmolol, metoprolol, verapamil, or diltiazem (see Table 63–3); digoxin is usually a third-line agent (Fig. 63–5). All patients with new-onset AF should receive anticoagulation acutely with heparin (Chapter 35). If the patient is seen within 8 hours of the onset of AF, transesophageal echocardiography should be performed (Chapter 53); if no clot is detected in the left atrium, it is safe to proceed to cardioversion followed by warfarin anticoagulation for 4 weeks. If transesophageal echocardiography detects clot, however, the patient should receive at least 3 weeks of oral anticoagulation before elective cardioversion. A variety of medications can be used to sustain sinus rhythm in patients with AF. Amiodarone (see Table 63–3) is the most effective but should be used selectively because of its potential side effects. If ventricular response during AF is through a rapidly conducting accessory pathway, intravenous digitalis and calcium-channel blockers are contraindicated, and procainamide is a better choice.

Long-Term Management

For symptomatic patients with sustained AV junctional re-entry, control sometimes can be achieved with digitalis, β-blockers, and calcium-channel blockers or with class I and class III drugs (see Table 63–3). In patients with atrial tachycardia or atrial flutter, ventricular rate control is possible through AV nodal block with digitalis, β-blockers, and calcium-channel blockers. Radio frequency ablation, which is curative, is now the preferred choice for most symptomatic sustained regular re-entrant supraventricular tachycardias, including atrial tachycardia and atrial flutter (Chapter 65).

For prevention of recurrent AF, oral amiodarone is significantly more effective than propafenone or sotalol, which are usually the recommended alternatives (see Table 63–2). For most patients with AF, however, control of the ventricular rate, usually to less than about 80 beats per minute at rest and no more than 100 to 110 per minute with exercise (typically with diltiazem, verapamil, metoprolol, or digoxin), combined with chronic warfarin anticoagulation is as good as attempts to restore and maintain sinus rhythm with medication or cardioversion, or both, in terms of longevity and quality of life. [1-3] In occasional patients with chronic AF, however, the loss of the atrial contraction may be sufficient to exacerbate symptoms of heart failure or low cardiac output despite rate control and medications for heart failure. In these situations, radio frequency ablation of the AF focus, usually in a pulmonary vein, can be curative. [4] Whether this approach or other catheter-based treatments will become first-line treatment is still unproved

In patients with recurrent paroxysmal AF, another alternative is oral, out-of-hospital, self-administration ("pill in the pocket") of either propafenone (600 mg for patients who weigh >70 kg, 450 mg otherwise) or flecainide (300 mg for patients who weigh >70 kg, 200 mg otherwise) after first demonstrating the safety and efficacy of either drug in the hospital setting. In this subgroup of patients, outpatient self-treatment is 84% successful and can reduce emergency department visits and hospitalizations.

Long-term anticoagulation therapy with warfarin is generally recommended in all patients who are older than 65 years, who have persistent or paroxysmal AF, and who have no contraindications to anticoagulation. [5] Warfarin alone is superior to the combination of clopidogrel and aspirin. [6] The international normalized ratio (INR) goal is 2.0 to 3.0 unless mitral stenosis is present, in which case the target is an INR of 2.5 to 3.5. Aspirin may be better than no

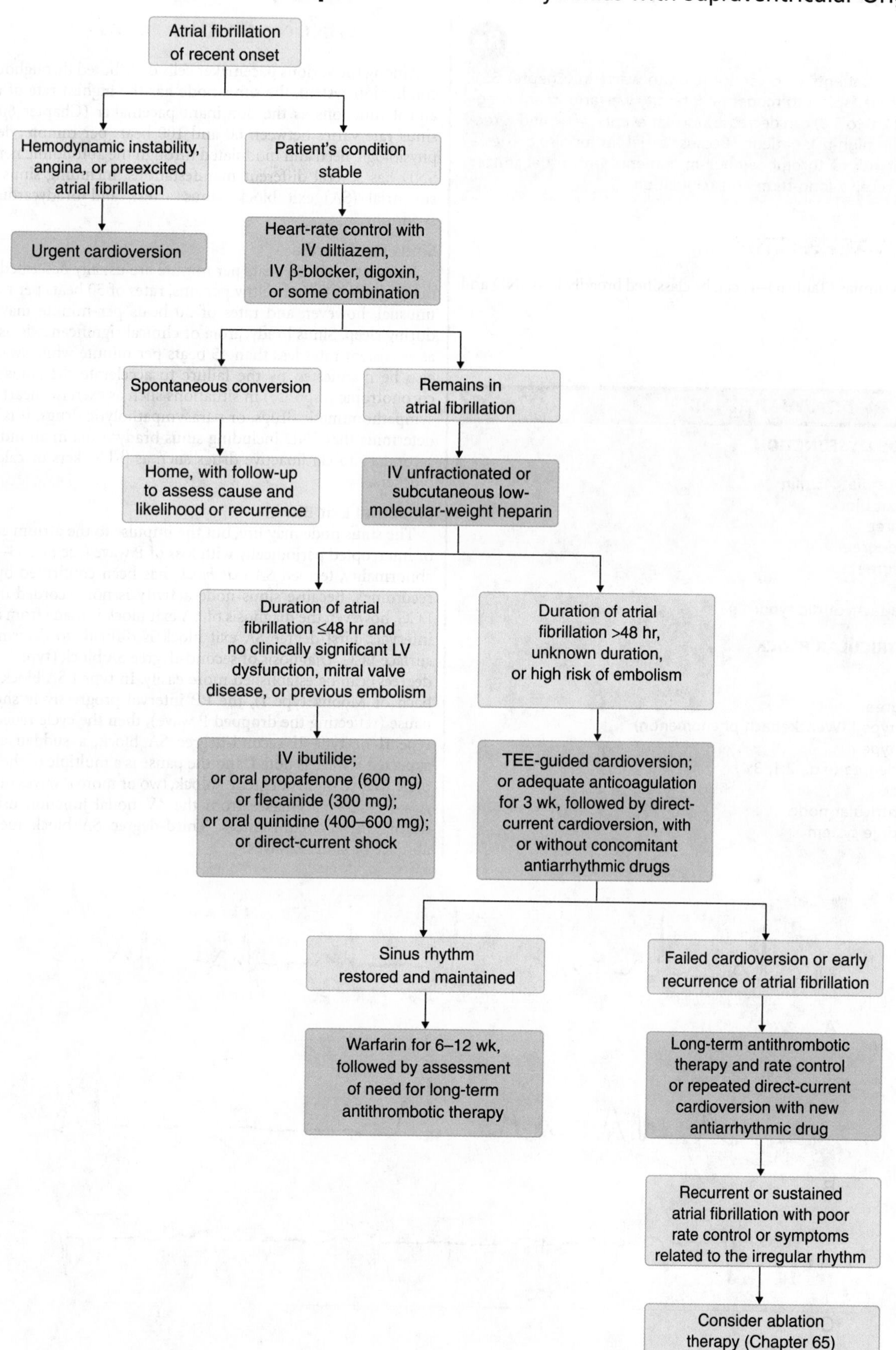

FIGURE 63–5 • Management of recent-onset atrial fibrillation. IV, intravenous; LV, left ventricular, TEE, transesophageal echocardiography. (From Scheinman MM, Kaushik V: Recognition and management of patients with tachyarrhythmias. *In* Braunwald E, Goldman L [eds]: Primary Cardiology, 2nd ed. Philadelphia, WB Saunders, 2003, p 510. Reprinted, by permission, from Falk RH: Atrial fibrillation. N Engl J Med 2001;344:1067–1078.)

Rx

treatment for patients who cannot tolerate warfarin (Chapter 35). The addition of aspirin to moderate-intensity warfarin in anticoagulation (INR 2.0 to 3.0) can decrease vascular events [5, 7] and is recommended in high-risk patients. Because atrial flutter also carries a 3% per year risk of thromboembolism, patients with atrial flutter should also receive long-term anticoagulation.

BRADYARRHYTHMIAS

Bradyarrhythmias (Table 63–4) can be classified broadly into SND and AV blocks.

TABLE 63–4 BRADYCARDIAS

SINUS NODE DYSFUNCTION
Sinus bradycardia <45/min
Sinoatrial exit block
First degree
Second degree
Third degree
Sinus arrest
Bradycardia-tachycardia syndrome
ATRIOVENTRICULAR BLOCK
First degree
Second degree
Mobitz type I (Wenckebach phenomenon)
Mobitz type II
Higher degree (e.g., 2:1, 3:1)
Third degree
Atrioventricular node
His-Purkinje system

Sinus Node Dysfunction

Among the various pacemaker cells distributed throughout the cardiac conduction system, the sinus node has the highest rate of automaticity, and it functions as the dominant pacemaker (Chapter 60). The usual sinus rate varies between 60 and 100 beats per minute, determined by physiologic need and modulated through the autonomic nervous system. SND has several different manifestations, including sinus bradycardia, sinoatrial (SA) exit block, sinus arrest, and bradycardia-tachycardia syndrome.

Sinus Bradycardia

Rates less than 60 beats per minute are usually described as bradycardia (Fig. 63–6A). In healthy persons, rates of 50 beats per minute are not unusual, however, and rates of 30 beats per minute may be recorded during sleep. Sinus bradycardia of clinical significance is usually defined as persistent rates less than 45 beats per minute while awake. SND may also be manifested by the failure to accelerate the sinus rate (lack of chronotropic response) in situations such as exercise, heart failure, fever, sympathomimetic drugs, or parasympatholytic drugs. It is important to determine that SND including sinus bradycardia in an individual is not secondary to cardioactive drugs such as β-blockers or calcium-channel blockers.

Sinoatrial Exit Block

The sinus node may fire, but the impulse to the atrium can be delayed or interrupted periodically with loss of P wave (see Fig. 63–6A to C); this abnormality, termed *SA exit block*, has been confirmed by intracardiac recordings. Because sinus node activity is not recorded on the surface ECG, however, the diagnosis of SA exit block is made from analysis of PP intervals. First-degree SA exit block is difficult to determine from the surface ECG. Diagnosis of second-degree SA block (type I, II, and higher degrees) can be established more easily. In type I SA block (SA Wenckebach or Mobitz type I), the PP interval progressively shortens after a pause (reflecting the dropped P wave), then the cycle repeats. In Mobitz type II or type II second-degree SA block, a sudden absence of an expected P wave is noted, and the pause is a multiple of the dominant PP cycle. With a higher degree of block, two or more P waves may be missing. A subsidiary pacemaker from the AV nodal junction usually emerges during these circumstances. Third-degree SA block means complete absence of sinus P waves.

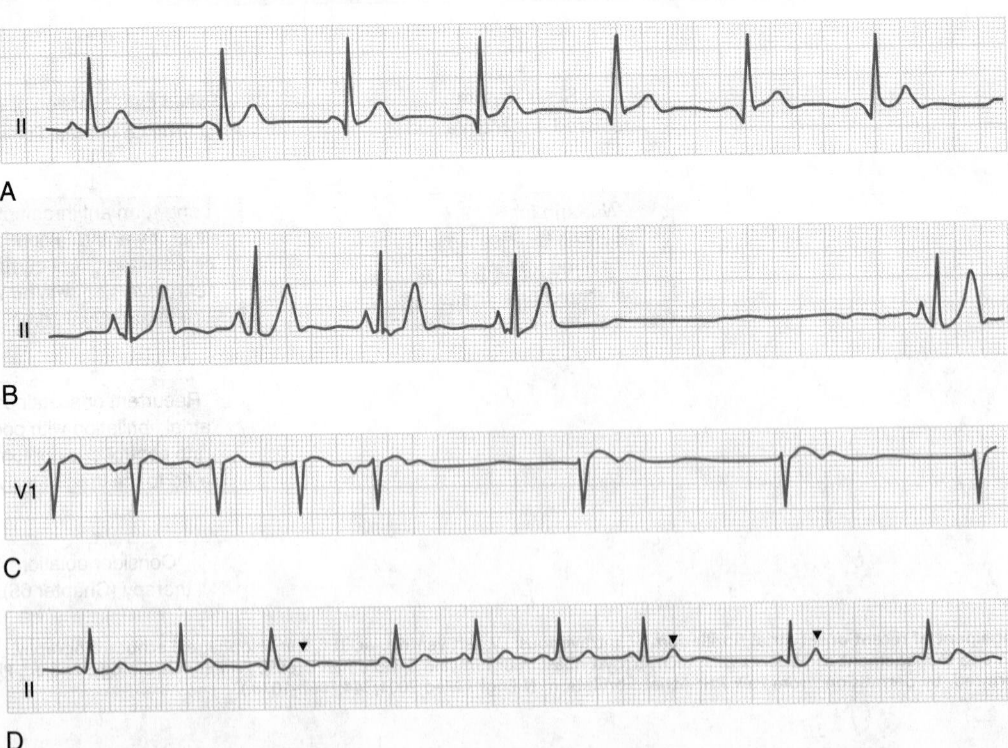

FIGURE 63–6 • Sinus node dysfunction. A, Sinus bradycardia. Sudden loss of sinus activity (no P waves). Sinus rhythm resumes after a 4.5-second pause **(B)**, whereas junctional rhythm emerges as a subsidiary mechanism in **C.** The exact cause (i.e., sinoatrial exit block versus sinus arrest) cannot be determined from the surface electrocardiogram in these examples. **D,** Blocked premature atrial complexes (note distortion of the T wave at arrows compared with sinus cycles) mimic sinus node dysfunction.

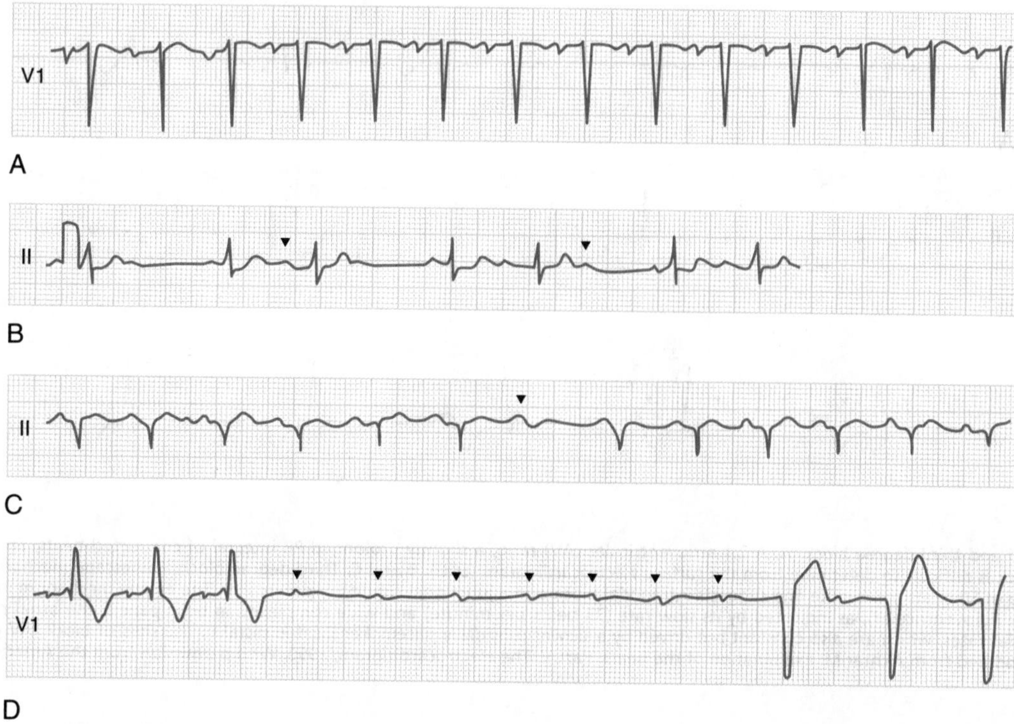

FIGURE 63–7 • Atrioventricular (AV) block. A, First-degree AV block (long PR interval). A 3:2 Wenckebach (Mobitz type I) second-degree AV block is seen in **B** and Mobitz type II second-degree block in **C.** Note the PR interval prolongation before the block in **B** but no PR increase in **C. D,** A sudden block of consecutive P waves. No AV conduction following 1:1 AV conduction with a normal PR interval and right bundle branch block suggests infra-His block. After a long escape interval, a stable subsidiary pacemaker from the peripheral Purkinje network emerges (idioventricular rhythm). (Modified from Akhtar M: Examination of the heart: Part V. The electrocardiogram, 1990. With permission from the American Heart Association, Dallas, TX.)

Sinus Arrest

Sudden disappearance of P waves could be due to either SA exit block or cessation of sinus node pacemaker function. The two are difficult to distinguish unless the resultant PP interval has a predictable periodicity or is a multiple of sinus PP cycle. SA exit block and sinus arrest must be distinguished from blocked PACs (see Fig. 63–6D) and sinus arrhythmia. Blocked PACs are likely to distort the ST-T segment and reset the sinus node so that the PP cycle with a blocked atrial premature contraction is less than two PP intervals. Sinus arrhythmia, which is a physiologic variation of PP change, usually follows the respiratory cycle (phasic sinus arrhythmia). The nonphasic variety may result in an abrupt sinus pause and may be confused with SND.

Bradycardia-Tachycardia Syndrome

Because SND often represents atrial disease processes (e.g., fibrosis, degeneration, inflammation), coexistence of atrial tachyarrhythmias with bradycardia is not surprising. When an atrial tachycardia such as AF is terminated, the underlying rhythm may reveal sinus bradycardia, SA exit block, or even complete atrial standstill with an escape rhythm from a lower pacemaker in the AV junction or the HPS.

Atrioventricular Blocks

In a resting state, the normal AV node is capable of conducting 200 impulses per minute. With facilitation of AV nodal conduction owing to adrenergic stimulation or vagal withdrawal, this rate can reach 250 impulses per minute and even 300 impulses per minute in exceptional cases. With rapid atrial tachycardia, atrial flutter, and AF, some degree of AV block (in the AV node) is expected. Abnormal AV block is defined when some impulses are delayed or do not reach the ventricle during sinus rhythm or sinus tachycardia.

Electrophysiologic and Electrocardiographic Features

First-Degree Atrioventricular Block (Prolonged Atrioventricular Conduction or PR Interval with 1:1 P-QRS Relationship)

The normal PR interval is 120 to 200 msec. Because the PR interval incorporates intra-atrial, AV nodal, and HPS conduction, it could be prolonged because of conduction delay in any of these areas. The intra-atrial conduction time, which contributes to the PR interval, can be estimated from the onset of the P wave on the surface ECG to the onset of atrial deflection on the His bundle electrogram. The AH interval (from the onset of the atrial deflection to the His bundle potential) represents conduction through the AV node and is normally 60 to 140 msec; the HPS time estimated by the HV interval (from the onset of the His bundle potential to the earliest venticular deflection) is 35 to 55 msec. When the PR interval is prolonged, delay is usually in the AV node (Fig. 63–7A); intra-atrial conduction delays and abnormal HPS conduction time seldom prolong the PR interval to more than 200 msec and are highly unlikely to prolong it to more than 300 msec. Block in the AV node or within the His bundle does not alter the QRS complex morphology compared with sinus rhythm; if a concomitant fascicular or bundle branch block is noted, infra-His block is likely.

Second-Degree Atrioventricular Block (Intermittent Atrioventricular Conduction)

With second-degree AV block, some P waves fail to produce a QRS complex. In type I, also called *Mobitz type I* or *Wenckebach phenomenon,* there is a progressive increase in the PR interval, despite a constant PP rate, until a P wave blocks and the cycle is repeated (see Fig. 63–7B). Any P-to-QRS ratio can be seen (e.g., 3:2, 4:3, 5:4). In a typical Wenckebach phenomenon, the PR interval after the block is the shortest. The largest increase in PR interval occurs after the second conducted beat; the R-R interval after the pause, which contains the blocked P wave, progressively shortens until the next pause. The Wenckebach phenomenon can be found in all cardiac conducting tissues, but the magnitude of PR prolongation or shortening from beat to beat is maximum in the AV node and therefore most noticeable. The AV node is the likely site of block when the PR interval increment with any subsequent PP cycle exceeds 100 msec, PR shortening is more than 100 msec after the block, or the absolute value of PR interval with any of the conducted beats is greater than or equal to 300 msec. Most but not all type I second-degree AV blocks are localized to the AV node.

Type II AV, or Mobitz type II, block causes a sudden, unexpected block of a P wave without a discernible change in the PR interval before the AV block (see Fig. 63–7C). AV block associated with marked prolongation of PR interval (i.e., >300 msec) is usually within the AV node, but type II AV block typically suggests disease in the HPS. When the QRS complex of the conducted beat is normal or narrow, the block is within the His bundle; an associated bundle branch block or fascicular block suggests

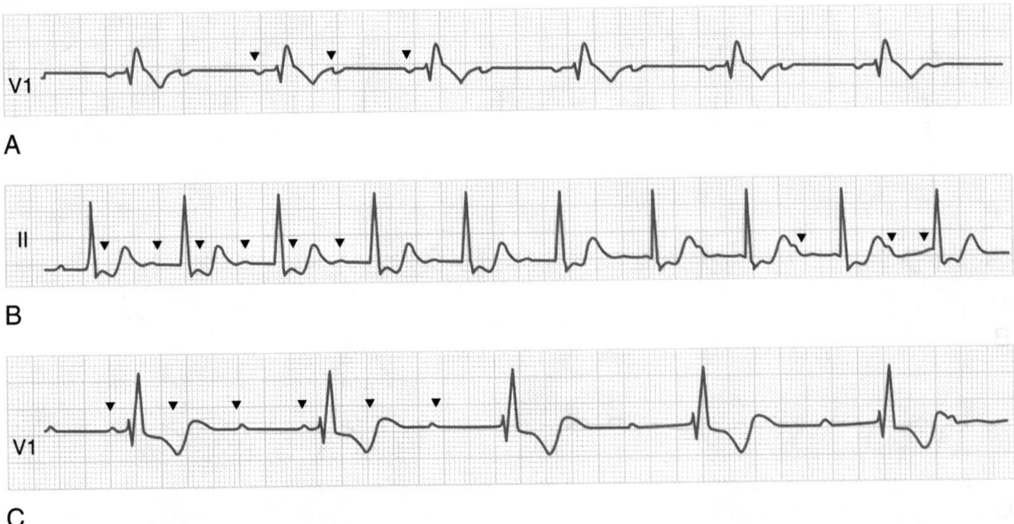

FIGURE 63–8 • A 2:1 and third-degree block. A, A 2:1 atrioventricular (AV) ratio, a slightly prolonged PR interval of conducted beats, and right bundle branch block. The site of block is difficult to determine from the surface electrocardiogram (ECG). **B** and **C,** Third-degree block. The escape mechanism has a narrow QRS complex in **B** at a rate of 50 beats per minute and suggests intranodal block and a junctional subsidiary pacemaker. The escape mechanism in **C** is from the peripheral Purkinje network (idioventricular), as indicated by its slow rate (33 beats per minute) and wide complexes. In both panels, the atrial rates are constant and unrelated to ventricular rates, which are also constant but driven by a slower subsidiary pacemaker located distal to the sites of block (AV dissociation). The ECG leads are labeled. (Modified from Akhtar M: Examination of the heart: Part V. The electrocardiogram, 1990. With permission from the American Heart Association, Dallas, TX.)

an infra-His site (see Fig. 63–7D). With a normal or only slightly prolonged PR interval, HPS is a more likely location of block.

A 2:1, 3:1, or higher AV ratio of AV block (Fig. 63–8A) may be noted with progression of Mobitz I or II to third-degree AV block. The site of block is more difficult to decipher with a 2:1 conduction ratio when the PR and the R wave of the conducted beat are normal. Documentation of progression from Mobitz type I or II is helpful in determining the site of block. In the presence of bundle branch block and a normal PR interval, HPS block should be suspected. Conversely the AV node is the more likely site of block when the PR of the conducted beat is 300 msec or more because a junctional escape rhythm emerges from a relatively normal HPS. When the HPS is the site of block, subsidiary pacemakers from a diseased HPS tend to have a slower escape rate and permit several blocked P waves before an escape mechanism emerges. In the absence of marked vagal influences, a 3:1 or 4:1 ratio is seldom noted with AV nodal block during sinus rhythm so that HPS is the more likely site of block. Vagally mediated AV block is accompanied by concomitant slowing of sinus rate.

Third-Degree (Complete) Atrioventricular Block (No Atrioventricular Conduction)

Complete failure of impulse propagation along the AV conduction system necessitates emergence of a subsidiary pacemaker distal to the site of block. Normally, the rate of resting pacemaker activity is highest in the sinus node (60 to 100 beats per minute), followed by the AV junction (40 to 60 beats per minute) and the bundle branch–Purkinje system (20 to 40 beats per minute). When the tissues expected to function as subsidiary pacemakers are abnormal, the rates may be even slower. During intact AV conduction, all of the subsidiary pacemakers remain suppressed (overdrive suppression). With abrupt cessation of AV conduction, the first subsidiary pacemaker response (often referred to as escape beat) is almost always slower than the subsequent rate from the same subsidiary foci; the rate of the emergent pacemaker below the site of block gradually accelerates (warm-up phenomenon) to its usual anticipated rate.

When the AV node is the site of third-degree AV block, the AV junctional pacemakers drive the ventricular rates. The QRS complex morphology is similar to that of sinus beats and normally warms up to 40 to 60 beats per minute. With infra-His block, the escape rhythm shows a wide QRS complex, originates distally in the HPS (idioventricular), and has a relatively slow rate. When the block is within the His bundle and the escape rhythm is also in the His bundle distal to the block, a narrow QRS complex appears at a slower than expected escape rate because of the disease process involving the junctional pacemakers.

AV dissociation occurs when the atria and ventricles are driven by different pacemakers. AV dissociation is generally due to AV or ventriculoatrial block. Complete AV block requires a subsidiary pacemaker to depolarize the ventricles; in this situation, the P wave is faster than the QRS complexes, and the two are unrelated (see Fig. 63–8B and C). AV dissociation also occurs when the rate of subsidiary pacemakers is faster than a normal sinus, such as nonparoxysmal junctional tachycardia (see Fig. 63–2F) or ventricular tachycardia; if there is retrograde (ventriculoatrial) block, the atria are driven by the SA node or other atrial pacemakers. *Isorhythmic AV dissociation* is the term used when atria and ventricles are driven independently but have a similar rate.

Clinical Manifestations

Aside from vagal influences and medications such as digitalis and antiarrhythmic drugs, the exact cause for SND is frequently difficult to determine. The most common causes for SND are atrial muscle degeneration, fibrosis with advanced age, and cardiac pathology such as coronary artery disease. Acute inferior wall myocardial ischemia or infarction associated with disease of the proximal right coronary artery may cause transient SND. Other, less common causes include acute or chronic inflammation from myocarditis or pericarditis and prior cardiac surgery with trauma to the sinus node. Congenital SND and complete atrial standstill with no detectable sinus node activity are seen rarely.

AV nodal blocks can be caused by digitalis, antiarrhythmic drugs, and vagal influences. Involvement of the AV junctional area with any inflammatory or other disease process can result in AV nodal block of varying degrees. The most common cause of chronic AV block in the HPS is progressive fibrosis or calcification in the HPS, or both, with aging or myocardial fibrosis of any cause. Because of the proximity of aortic and mitral valves to the distal His bundle and proximal bundle branches, annular calcification or valve surgery can cause acute or chronic intra-His and infra-His block. Myocardial infiltration by an infectious agent (i.e., Chagas' disease; Chapter 368) is an important cause of chronic heart block in Latin American countries. Acute inferior wall ischemia or infarction, or both, can cause various degrees of AV nodal block because of ischemia in the nodal artery distributions. Involvement of HPS during acute anterior myocardial infarction can lead to bundle branch block or AV block, or both.

Sinus bradycardia and various degrees of AV nodal blocks are also noted during sleep even in otherwise healthy people. Asymptomatic first- and second-degree AV block, particularly when partially or completely reversed by exercise, points toward a benign condition. Persistent second-degree and third-degree AV nodal block during the waking hours and during activity is abnormal and is often associated with symptoms of bradycardia, including dizziness, fatigue, exertional dyspnea, worsening of heart failure, near-syncope, or syncope. Third-degree AV block with a good junctional escape mechanism that accelerates during exercise, as often noted in patients with congenital AV block, may remain asymptomatic. Patients with congenital heart block may not appreciate their potential for a more active lifestyle because of the lack of a reference point but often feel much better when an appropriate heart rate acceleration can be achieved after pacemaker therapy.

Bradycardias of all types may be secondary to profound vagal influences, as seen with neurally mediated syndromes such as vasovagal episodes, vomiting, abdominal surgery, and upper and lower gastrointestinal invasive procedures. Periods of prolonged sinus arrest and AV nodal block with marked suppression of subsidiary pacemaker can occur and lead to symptomatic asystole. Vasovagal (neurocardiogenic) syndromes are a common cause of syncope in relatively healthy populations (Chapters 61 and 427); in most cases, vasodepression (hypotension) is the primary cause of syncope, and rate control alone does not relieve symptoms.

Treatment

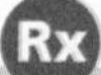

Asymptomatic SND or AV nodal block requires no therapy. Acute management of symptomatic SND and second- and third-degree AV block includes administration of intravenous atropine (1 mg) or isoproterenol (usually 1 to 2 µg/min infusion) to increase the heart rate. Temporary cardiac pacing may be needed. When SND or AV block is due to transient abnormalities, such as drug-induced or acute ischemic syndromes, temporary pacing is usually sufficient; however, when infra-His or intra-His block is suspected (e.g., exercise-induced AV block or asymptomatic Mobitz type II block) and the site can be documented with His bundle recording, permanent pacing (Chapter 65) is indicated. For all forms of persistent symptomatic SND or second-degree or third-degree AV block, permanent pacing is the therapy of choice (Chapter 65). Nevertheless, even prolonged paroxysmal asystole resulting from a neurocardiogenic mechanism is not an indication for permanent pacing; instead, pharmacologic therapy that relieves hypotension controls bradycardiac symptoms as well. As a general rule, bradycardia in individuals younger than 55 is vagal in origin and does not require permanent pacing unless proved otherwise.

Future Directions

Ablation of atrial tissue in or outside the pulmonary veins and atrial defibrillation therapy are likely to be used more frequently because of technologic advances and patients' preferences, although it is also conceivable that pharmacologic agents with more targeted effects and fewer side effects will be developed. Pulmonary vein isolation and ablation to cure AF may become a first-line therapy.

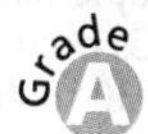

1. Hohnloser SH, Kuck K-H, Lilienthal J: Rhythm or rate control in atrial fibrillation—Pharmacological Intervention in Atrial Fibrillation (PIAF): A randomized trial. Lancet 2000;356:1789–1794.
2. Wyse DG, Waldo AL, DiMarco JP, et al: A comparison of rate control and rhythm control in patients with atrial fibrillation. N Engl J Med 2002;347:1825–1833.
3. Van Gelder IC, Hagens VE, Bosker HA, et al: A comparison of rate control and rhythm control in patients with recurrent persistent atrial fibrillation. N Engl J Med 2002;347:1834–1840.
4. Wazni O, Marrouche N, Martin D: Radiofrequency ablation vs. antiarrhythmic drugs as first-line treatment of symptomatic atrial fibrillation: A randomized trial. JAMA 2005;293:2634–2640.
5. Perez-Gomez F, Alegria E, Berjon J, et al: Comparative effects of antiplatelet, anticoagulant, or combined therapy in patients with valvular and nonvalvular atrial fibrillation: A randomized multicenter study. J Am Coll Cardiol 2004;44:1557–1566.
6. The ACTIVE Writing Group on behalf of the ACTIVE investigators. Clopidogrel plus aspirin versus oral anticoagulation for atrial fibrillation in the atrial fibrillation clopidogrel trial with irbesartan for prevention of vascular events (ACTIVE W): A randomised controlled trial. Lancet 2006;367:1903–1912.
7. Taylor FC, Cohen H, Ebrahim S: Systematic review of long term anticoagulation or antiplatelet treatment in patients with nonrheumatic atrial fibrillation. BMJ 2001;322:321–326.

SUGGESTED READINGS

Alboni P, Botto GL, Baldi N, et al: Outpatient treatment of recent-onset atrial fibrillation with the "pill-in-the-pocket" approach. N Engl J Med 2004;351:2384–2391. *In selected patients with recurrent atrial fibrillation, pill-in-the-pocket treatment is feasible and safe.*

Delacretaz E: Supraventricular tachycardia. N Engl J Med 2006;354:1039–1051. *A scholarly review.*

Fuster V, Ryder LE, Cannom DS, et al. ACC/AHA/ESC 2006 guidelines for the management of patients with atrial fibrillation—Executive summary. Circulation 2006;114:700–752. *A consensus review.*

Gage BF, Birman-Deych E, Kerzner R, et al: Incidence of intracranial hemorrhage in patients with atrial fibrillation who are prone to fall. Am J Med 2005;118:612–617. *Patients with AF at high risk for falls were at substantially increased risk of intracranial hemorrhage but still did better with anticoagulation.*

Ghali WA, Wasil BI, Brant R, et al: Atrial flutter and the risk of thromboembolism: A systematic review and meta-analysis. Am J Med 2005;118:101–107. *The risk is increased and appears to be about 3% per year.*

Page RL: Newly diagnosed atrial fibrillation. N Engl J Med 2004;351:2408–2416. *A case-based review.*

Pappone C, Augello G, Sala S, et al: A randomized trial of circumferential pulmonary vein ablation versus antiarrhythmic drug therapy in paroxysmal atrial fibrillation: The APAF study. J Am Coll Cardiol 2006;48:2340–2347. *Ablation was more successful than drugs to prevent AF, with few complications.*

Zimetbaum P: Amiodarone for atrial fibrillation. N Engl J Med 2007;356:935–941. *A review of mechanism of action, indications, and side effects.*

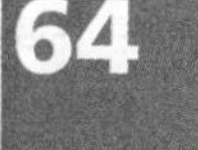

64 VENTRICULAR ARRHYTHMIAS

Bruce B. Lerman

PREMATURE VENTRICULAR COMPLEXES

Definition and Electrocardiographic Features

Premature ventricular complexes (PVCs) are ubiquitous arrhythmias that are recognized on the surface electrocardiogram (ECG) by their wide (generally >120 msec) and bizarre QRS morphology, which occurs independently of atrial activation (P waves). Late-cycle PVCs may follow a P wave that occurs on time and are identified by a shorter than normal PR interval. PVCs may be due to enhanced automaticity, triggered activity, or re-entry.

Most PVCs are followed by a "compensatory pause" because the PVC fails to conduct retrogradely to the atria and cannot affect or reset the electrical activity of the sinus node. The interval between the first sinus beat and the PVC plus the interval between the PVC and the next sinus beat equals two normal sinus intervals (Fig. 64–1). Occasionally, PVCs may be interpolated between two sinus beats (i.e., produce no pause), and rarely, PVCs may penetrate and reset the sinus node.

PVCs may be isolated or occur in groups. Two consecutive PVCs are termed a *couplet.* Three or more consecutive PVCs at a rate of 100 beats per minute or higher are termed *ventricular tachycardia* (VT). Single PVCs may occur sporadically or as bigeminy (every other beat is a PVC), trigeminy (every third beat is a PVC), or higher-order periodicities. A patient may manifest PVCs with two or more different morphologies, in which case the ectopy is termed *multiform.* Single PVCs, regardless of whether they occur sporadically or in a periodic pattern, are sometimes referred to as "simple" ventricular ectopy, whereas multiform PVCs, closely coupled PVCs (so-called R-on-T phenomenon), ventricular couplets, and nonsustained VT are referred to as "complex" ventricular ectopy. Fusion beats result from simultaneous activation of the ventricle by a normally conducted supraventricular beat and a concurrent PVC and have a morphology with some similarities to the supraventricular and ventricular beats.

Epidemiology

Ventricular ectopy is exceedingly rare in infants but increases in frequency with age. PVCs occur in patients with and without structural heart disease. Holter monitoring (Chapter 61) reveals at least one PVC in 40 to 75% and complex ventricular ectopy in 5 to 10% of normal

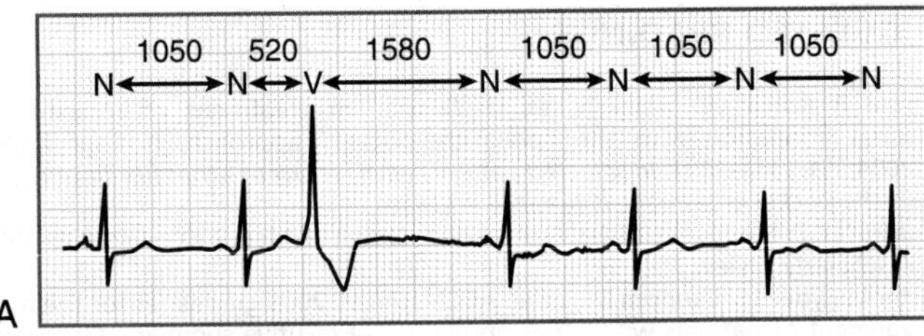

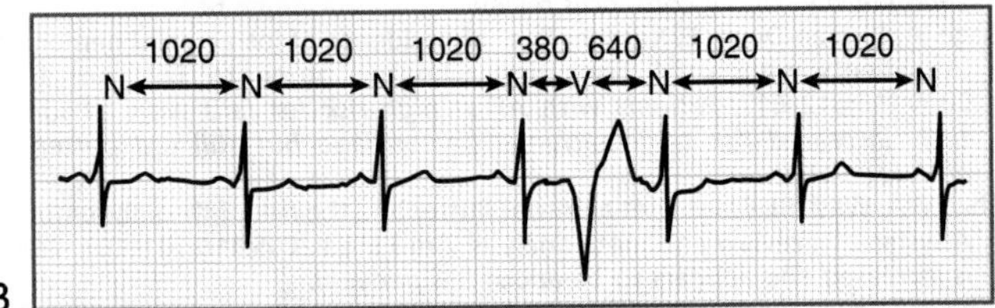

FIGURE 64–1 • Multiform premature ventricular complexes (PVCs). A, PVC followed by a compensatory pause. **B,** A recording from the same individual shows an interpolated PVC of a different morphology. Tracings are from lead I. N = normal sinus beat; V = premature ventricular beat. Intervals are given in milliseconds.

adults. PVCs occur with greater frequency and complexity in patients with structural heart disease, especially ischemic and valvar heart disease and idiopathic cardiomyopathy. PVCs may also occur in the setting of drug toxicity (e.g., digitalis intoxication) or electrolyte disturbances (e.g., hypokalemia).

Prognosis

In general, the frequency and complexity of PVCs are not associated with an adverse outcome in patients without structural heart disease. Rare exceptions do exist, however. In very occasional patients without structural heart disease, single but repetitive PVCs originating from the Purkinje network or right ventricular outflow tract can initiate ventricular fibrillation (VF). In some patients with frequent PVCs originating from the right ventricular outflow tract (10 to 40% of all ventricular beats), a secondary cardiomyopathy may develop that can be reversed by ablating the arrhythmogenic focus.

Among patients with a previous myocardial infarction (MI; Chapter 72), frequent (>10 PVCs per hour) and complex ventricular ectopy is associated with an increased risk for death. This risk is concentrated in patients with depressed left ventricular function, however. Likewise, in patients with valvar heart disease, sudden death is rare when ventricular function is normal (e.g., uncomplicated mitral valve prolapse), but risk increases when complex ventricular ectopy is observed in patients with depressed left ventricular function. R-on-T PVCs may be more likely than later coupled PVCs to result in VF or polymorphic VT. This relationship is weak, however, and has limited prognostic utility.

Sustained re-entrant ventricular arrhythmias probably result from the interaction of a critically timed triggering event (PVC) with an appropriate substrate (myocardial scarring resulting in mechanical and electrical ventricular dysfunction). Because of the high prevalence of ventricular ectopy in patients with structural heart disease, however, the predictive value for future events is low. Even among patients for whom PVCs indicate a poor prognosis, antiarrhythmic drug therapy aimed specifically at suppressing PVCs does not provide benefit. Suppression of PVCs with encainide, flecainide, or moricizine results in a significant increase in mortality in patients with frequent PVCs after MI.

Treatment

Because there is no evidence that treatment directed at suppressing PVCs improves overall mortality, the primary indication for treatment is to relieve symptoms. Although most PVCs are asymptomatic, in some patients they may result in troubling palpitations. Frequent PVCs can also cause a pounding sensation in the neck secondary to cannon *a* waves from atrioventricular dissociation. Because PVCs result in reduced stroke volume, patients with frequent PVCs may occasionally have fatigue, exertional intolerance, dyspnea, and lightheadedness.

Most patients with symptomatic PVCs in the absence of structural heart disease can be managed with a β-blocker such as atenolol (25 to 100 mg/day) or metoprolol (50 to 200 mg/day). Class I or class III antiarrhythmic drugs may be considered, but the potential for proarrhythmia and organ toxicity must be weighed. An alternative to antiarrhythmic drug therapy for highly symptomatic patients, particularly those without structural heart disease whose PVCs originate from the right ventricular outflow tract, is radiofrequency catheter ablation of the arrhythmogenic focus (Chapter 65).

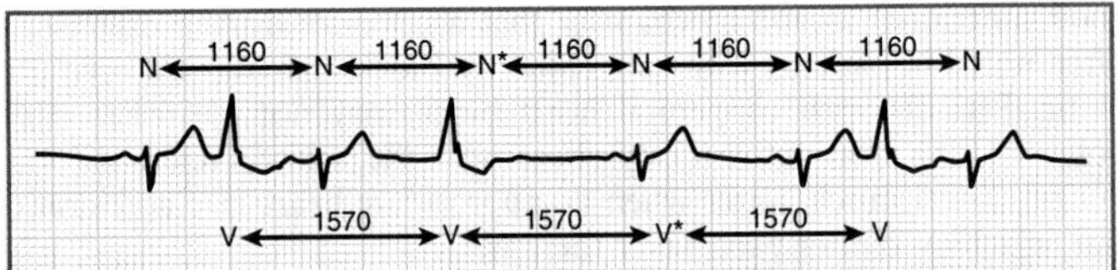

FIGURE 64–2 • Parasystole: sinus rhythm with a competing ventricular parasystolic focus. N = normal sinus beat; N* = timing of normal sinus discharge (occurring during the ventricular refractory period); V = ventricular parasystolic beat; V* = timing of ventricular parasystolic discharge (occurring during the ventricular refractory period). Intervals are given in milliseconds.

PARASYSTOLE

Ventricular parasystole results when an automatic focus arises from the ventricles and fires independently of supraventricular impulses conducted through the atrioventricular node. Classically, a surrounding region of depressed conductivity protects the focus by creating a complete entrance block that prevents supraventricular beats from resetting the focus. Independence of the parasystolic focus from the underlying rhythm is shown by variable coupling intervals between the ectopic beats and the preceding sinus beats and a fixed minimum time interval between PVCs, with any longer interectopic intervals being integral multiples of this minimum interval (reflecting an exit block from the parasystolic focus) (Fig. 64–2).

The entrance block surrounding the parasystolic focus can be partial rather than complete, so conducted supraventricular beats may influence depolarization of the parasystolic focus and either delay or accelerate its next discharge. Clinically, parasystole may be manifested as sporadic PVCs or as bigeminy or trigeminy.

ACCELERATED IDIOVENTRICULAR RHYTHM

Definition and Electrocardiographic Features

An accelerated idioventricular rhythm (AIVR) refers to an ectopic ventricular rhythm characterized by three or more consecutive PVCs occurring at a rate faster than the normal ventricular escape rate of 30 to 40 beats per minute but slower than VT. No single rate differentiates "fast" AIVR from "slow" VT, however. In general, the upper rate limit for AIVR is 100 to 120 beats per minute. Because AIVR has different prognostic and therapeutic implications than VT does, it is important to recognize AIVR's gradual onset, acceleration ("warm-up"), and deceleration before termination (consistent with an automatic mechanism) as compared with the paroxysmal initiation and abrupt termination characteristic of re-entrant VT. AIVR is generally brief (<1 minute) and is suppressed when the sinus rate exceeds its rate.

Clinical Manifestations

AIVR occurs most often in patients with acute MI, particularly after reperfusion, and usually resolves spontaneously. AIVR is also observed in patients with rheumatic heart disease, dilated cardiomyopathy, acute myocarditis, hypertensive heart disease, digitalis toxicity, and cocaine intoxication and in those without structural heart disease. It is generally

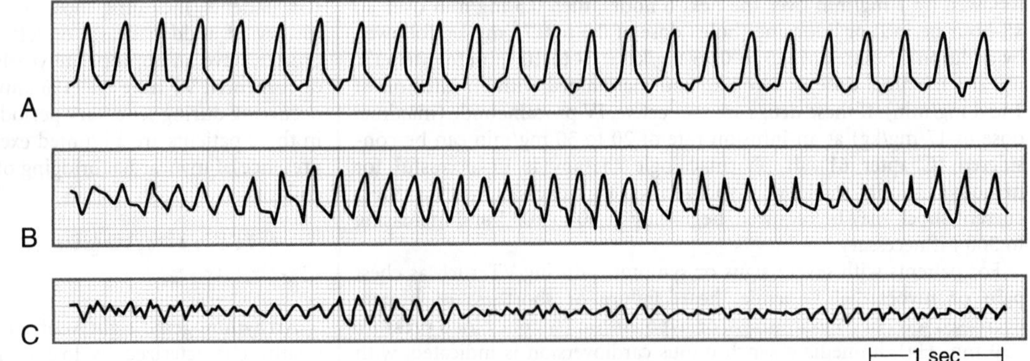

FIGURE 64–3 • Ventricular tachyarrhythmias. A, Rhythm strip showing monomorphic ventricular tachycardia. **B,** Example of polymorphic ventricular tachycardia. **C,** Example of ventricular fibrillation. All tracings are from lead V_1.

benign, and because most runs of AIVR are brief and asymptomatic, it requires no specific treatment. If patients with left ventricular dysfunction do not tolerate AIVR because of the loss of atrioventricular synchrony, increasing the atrial rate with intravenous (IV) atropine (1 mg) or by pacing suppresses AIVR.

VENTRICULAR TACHYCARDIA

Definition

VT, which originates below the bundle of His at a rate greater than 100 beats per minute, is a wide-complex rhythm that may be monomorphic (uniform) or polymorphic with beat-to-beat changes in the QRS configuration (Fig. 64–3). Sustained VT persists for 30 seconds or longer or requires termination because of hemodynamic instability. Sustained polymorphic VT is generally unstable and often degenerates into VF. Sustained monomorphic VT may be stable for long periods or, with faster rates or myocardial ischemia, may degenerate into polymorphic VT or VF. Torsades de pointes (TdP), a particular form of polymorphic VT, has a characteristic morphology ("twisting around a point") and is associated with prolongation of the QT interval on the surface ECG.

Electrocardiographic Features

It is important to distinguish monomorphic VT from supraventricular tachycardia with aberrant conduction because both are manifested as wide-complex tachycardias (Table 64–1). Features on the surface ECG permit differentiation of VT from supraventricular tachycardia with an overall accuracy that approaches 90%. Atrioventricular dissociation, which can be identified on the surface ECG in 25% of VTs, strongly suggests a ventricular origin. The presence of a one-to-one atrioventricular relationship does not imply a supraventricular origin, however, because some patients with VT have one-to-one retrograde conduction from the ventricles to the atria during tachycardia. Capture and fusion beats also suggest VT but are generally seen only during slow VT. A capture beat represents activation of the ventricles by a supraventricular impulse that conducts via the His-Purkinje system. This beat prematurely "captures" both ventricles during VT and results in a single narrow QRS interposed between wide tachycardia complexes. Other features of the surface ECG that permit differentiation of VT from supraventricular tachycardia include QRS width, axis, and morphology. Though helpful in most situations, these morphologic criteria are not 100% specific. An irregular wide-complex rhythm with essentially a single QRS morphology raises the possibility of atrial fibrillation with ventricular pre-excitation (Chapter 63), particularly in patients without structural heart disease.

Other diagnostic measures include the response of the tachycardia to vagal maneuvers and adenosine. Most VT is insensitive to vagal maneuvers, such as carotid sinus massage and the Valsalva maneuver, and to adenosine, whereas most forms of supraventricular tachycardia terminate or persist with a transient high-grade atrioventricular block in response to these measures. Idiopathic right ventricular outflow tract tachycardia in patients with normal hearts may also terminate with vagal maneuvers and adenosine, however.

Clinical Manifestations and Acute Treatment

Patients with monomorphic VT may initially be seen in sudden cardiac death (SCD) or with symptoms of impaired consciousness, such as syncope or near-syncope. Associated symptoms may include chest pain, dyspnea, and palpitations. Occasionally, patients with VT and slow rates may be asymptomatic, and hemodynamic stability is unreliable in distinguishing VT from supraventricular tachycardia.

Physical examination during VT may reveal signs of cardiogenic shock, including pulselessness, apnea, cool extremities, and cyanosis, as well as hypotension or signs of heart failure, such as pulmonary rales or jugular venous distention. Characteristic features during VT include cannon a waves and variable intensity of S_1, both of which result from atrioventricular dissociation.

Acute therapy for VT depends on the degree of hemodynamic instability that accompanies the arrhythmia. For stable VT in patients with left ventricular dysfunction, pharmacologic therapy should be initiated with either IV amiodarone (150 mg administered over a period of 10 minutes,

TABLE 64–1 ELECTROCARDIOGRAPHIC CHARACTERISTICS OF VENTRICULAR TACHYCARDIA

ATRIOVENTRICULAR RELATIONSHIP
Atrioventricular dissociation
Sinus capture beats
Fusion beats
QRS WIDTH
Left bundle branch block >160 msec
Right bundle branch block >140 msec
QRS AXIS
Extreme left axis (−90 to −180 degrees)
Right axis deviation in the presence of a left bundle branch block (+90 to +180 degrees)
QRS MORPHOLOGY
Right bundle branch block
Morphology in V_1
Monophasic R wave
Biphasic (qR or RS)
Triphasic with R > R′
Morphology in V_6
R/S ratio <1
Left bundle branch block
Morphology in V_1
Broad R wave (>30 msec)
Onset of R wave to nadir of S wave >60 msec
Notched downstroke in lead V_1
Morphology in V_6
QR or QS complex
Onset of R wave to nadir of S wave >100 msec in any precordial lead
Absence of RS wave in any precordial lead
Positive or negative precordial concordance

followed by 1 mg/min over the next 6 hours, then 0.5 mg/min over an 18-hour period) or lidocaine (bolus dose of 0.5 to 0.75 mg/kg, followed by additional boluses of 0.5 to 0.75 mg/kg at 5- to 10-minute intervals, up to a maximal dose of 3 mg/kg and maintained with an infusion of 1 to 4 mg/min). If these drugs are ineffective, IV procainamide (maximal dose of 17 mg/kg) at an infusion rate of 20 to 30 mg/min can be considered (Chapter 61). If pharmacologic therapy is unsuccessful for hemodynamically stable VT, synchronized cardioversion with a direct current shock may be required, beginning at 50 to 100 J and increasing to 360 J if necessary.

For patients with severe signs or symptoms during VT, such as chest pain or myocardial ischemia, heart failure or shortness of breath, decreased level of consciousness, or hypotension (systolic blood pressure <90 mm Hg), immediate synchronous cardioversion is indicated, with subsequent IV antiarrhythmic therapy to maintain sinus rhythm. After resuscitation from VT, the patient must be evaluated for a possible primary cause, such as electrolyte imbalance, acid-base disturbance, hypoxemia, drug toxicity, and myocardial ischemia.

Diagnosis and Treatment

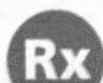

Invasive electrophysiologic testing (Chapter 65) can guide pharmacologic or device-based therapy (Chapter 65) in patients with sustained monomorphic VT and previous MI. In these patients, a sustained ventricular tachyarrhythmia can be induced with programmed stimulation in approximately 90%. When compared with antiarrhythmic therapy, an implantable cardioverter-defibrillator (ICD) improves outcome in patients who are hypotensive with their VT.

Ischemic Heart Disease

VT during acute MI (Chapter 72) may be monomorphic or polymorphic. Sustained ventricular arrhythmias within the first 48 hours of an acute MI do not convey an increased risk for future spontaneous arrhythmias. Coronary revascularization or antianginal medical therapy may be sufficient to control arrhythmias resulting from acute ischemia. Antiarrhythmic medications, such as lidocaine, are likewise useful to control recurrent sustained arrhythmias in this setting. Polymorphic VT and VF can also result from coronary vasospasm, which may occur in diseased or normal coronary arteries.

Sustained monomorphic VT occurs most frequently in patients with previous MI and depressed left ventricular function. VT arises from the border zone of the MI, where viable myocytes scattered within areas of fibrosis form a chronic substrate for re-entry. VT can occur days to decades after the MI, with an incidence that declines with time. The strongest risk factors for sustained ventricular arrhythmias late after MI are depressed left ventricular function and increased frequency and complexity of ventricular ectopy. Patients with a left ventricular ejection fraction less than 30% after MI have a nearly threefold increased risk for mortality or arrhythmic events.

Patients with VT beyond the first 48 hours after MI have a high recurrence rate, with an annual risk that approaches 30% in the absence of treatment. In general, coronary revascularization does not reduce the risk for recurrent VT arising from a chronic substrate after a remote MI, and therefore definitive antiarrhythmic therapy is required. Randomized trials have shown the superiority of ICDs over antiarrhythmic medications in patients with sustained monomorphic VT (Chapter 65). Catheter ablation may have an adjunctive role in controlling frequent ventricular arrhythmias in selected patients.

Cardiomyopathy

Monomorphic VT and polymorphic VT occur in patients with nonischemic dilated cardiomyopathy (Chapter 59). The signal-averaged ECG and invasive programmed stimulation (Chapter 65) have limited sensitivity and specificity for predicting future risk in these patients. VF, polymorphic VT, and to a lesser extent, monomorphic VT occur in patients with hypertrophic cardiomyopathy as a result of myocyte disarray, fibrosis, or ischemia. ICDs are effective for primary and secondary prevention in patients with hypertrophic cardiomyopathy. ICDs implanted in high-risk patients, including those with syncope, nonsustained VT, a family history of sudden death, or left ventricular wall thickness 30 mm or greater, have an appropriate yearly discharge rate of 5% (patients with documented VF have an 11% annual discharge rate), with most shocks occurring during sedentary periods. Other potential risk factors for SCD in these patients are a blunted exercise blood pressure response and the presence of myocardial bridging of the left anterior descending artery in children.

Arrhythmogenic Right Ventricular Dysplasia

Arrhythmogenic right ventricular dysplasia (ARVD) is a cardiomyopathy characterized by loss of myocytes in the right ventricle with replacement by fibroadipose tissue. ARVD causes SCD in adolescents and young adults, most commonly while the patient is sedentary, with a peak occurrence between 30 and 40 years of age. Patients have a propensity for re-entry ventricular arrhythmias involving diseased portions of the right ventricle, although dysplasia confined primarily to the left ventricle may occur.

The condition may be sporadic or familial. In most families, inheritance shows an autosomal dominant pattern with incomplete penetrance. ARVD has been linked to mutations in at least four desmosomal genes: plakophilin-2 *(PKP2)*, which is observed in 25% of unrelated probands; plakoglobin, which is responsible for Naxos disease (ARVD, palmoplantar keratoderma, and wooly hair); desmoplakin; and desmoglein-2. Desmosomes are protein complexes that mediate mechanical coupling between cardiac cells; mutations in desmosomal proteins cause cell death with subsequent fibrofatty replacement. The surface ECG of patients with ARVD may show a terminal notch on the QRS complex (e wave) in lead V_1, T wave inversions in the anterior precordial leads, and an S wave duration of 55 msec or longer in V_1 to V_3. A right bundle branch block is present in approximately 25% of patients. Echocardiography (Chapter 53) and right ventriculography show abnormalities of the right ventricle, including enlargement, wall motion abnormalities, decreased systolic function, and aneurysmal dilation. Magnetic resonance imaging (Chapter 55) reveals fatty replacement of the right ventricle, thinning of the right ventricular wall, and wall motion abnormalities. Endomyocardial biopsy may show characteristic fatty replacement and fibrosis, particularly in the so-called triangle of dysplasia—the right ventricular inflow tract, apex, and infundibulum. During invasive electrophysiologic testing, multiple morphologies of monomorphic VT may be inducible, usually with a left bundle branch block configuration.

Treatment of ARVD is an ICD, sometimes with the addition of an antiarrhythmic medication such as metoprolol (50 to 200 mg/day) or sotalol (160 to 320 mg/day). Catheter ablation, though not always curative, may ameliorate frequent ventricular arrhythmias.

Idiopathic Ventricular Tachycardia/Ventricular Fibrillation

Idiopathic monomorphic VT may be manifested as a sustained arrhythmia facilitated by exercise or as repetitive nonsustained VT that occurs at rest. The most common form of idiopathic monomorphic VT typically arises from the right ventricular outflow tract and has a left bundle branch block morphology and inferior axis. A somatic mutation in the inhibitory G protein ($G_{\alpha i2}$) is responsible for the right ventricular outflow tract tachycardia in some patients. Right ventricular outflow tract tachycardia is due to cyclic adenosine monophosphate–mediated, triggered activity resulting from intracellular calcium overload. Right ventricular outflow tract tachycardia can be cured by radio frequency catheter ablation (Chapter 65). In 10% of patients, tachycardia may originate from the left ventricular outflow tract. Identifying features of this form of VT are its responsiveness to adenosine and its sensitivity to vagal maneuvers and IV verapamil (10 mg). For patients reluctant to proceed with ablative therapy, consideration can be given to treatment with β-blockers (e.g., metoprolol, 50 to 200 mg/day, or atenolol, 25 to 100 mg/day) or class IC antiarrhythmic medications (e.g., flecainide, 100 to 300 mg/day), provided that there is no evidence of ischemic heart disease.

A less common form of monomorphic VT that also occurs in patients without structural heart disease is *fascicular re-entrant tachycardia.* This arrhythmia usually originates in the left ventricular region of the left posterior fascicle and has a right bundle branch block, left superior axis morphology. The tachycardia terminates in response to verapamil (10 mg) but not adenosine, vagal maneuvers, or β-blockers, and it is readily treated by radio frequency catheter ablation.

Idiopathic VF is initiated or triggered by extrasystoles that originate from the Purkinje system or right ventricular outflow tract myocardium. The coupling interval of the extrasystole with the preceding sinus beat may be short, intermediate, or long. Preliminary findings suggest that successful mapping and ablation of the initiating extrasystole can eliminate the VF. Until these data can be confirmed in a large number of patients, however, this approach should be considered palliative and definitive therapy should include an ICD.

Long QT Syndrome

Congenital Long QT Syndrome

The *congenital* long QT syndromes (LQTS) are related to cardiac ion channel defects that affect cardiac repolarization and result in prolongation of the QT interval and TdP. In the United States, the estimated prevalence of LQTS is 1 in 7000. Traditionally, congenital LQTS was classified into two forms: the Romano-Ward syndrome (more common; autosomal dominant and associated with normal hearing) and the Jervell and Lange-Nielsen syndrome (autosomal recessive and associated with congenital sensorineural deafness).

Molecular genetics has identified at least eight genes that account for genotypic designations (representing 50% of patients with LQTS). LQT1 accounts for approximately 45% of genotyped patients. The responsible gene, *KvLQT1* (also known as *KCNQ1*), is found on chromosome 11 and encodes a potassium channel pore-forming α subunit. Coexpression of *KvLQT1* with *KCNE1*, which encodes the non–pore-forming minK β subunit, forms I_{Ks}, the slowly activating component of the delayed rectifier potassium current. LQT2 (45% of genotyped patients) is due to mutations in the *HERG* (or *KCNH2*) gene located on chromosome 7. *HERG* encodes a potassium channel α subunit, and four *HERG* subunits assemble with *MiRP1* (*minK*-related protein; β subunit), which is encoded by *KCNE2*, to form I_{Kr}, the rapidly activating component of the delayed rectifier potassium current. Failure of these potassium channels to activate normally ("loss of function") prolongs the action potential duration and provokes early afterdepolarizations. LQT3 (5%) is due to a mutation in the gene *SCN5A*, which encodes the cardiac sodium channel and is located on chromosome 3. Failure of this channel to inactivate prolongs the action potential duration. Mutations in *MinK* and *MiRP1* are also linked to compromised potassium flux and inherited LQT5 and LQT6. The mutation responsible for LQT4 (chromosome 4) is found in *ANKB*, which encodes ankyrin-B, an adapter protein thought to anchor ion channels to the cell membrane. Mutations in one allele (heterozygous condition) of any one of the six known genes responsible for LQTS cause the Romano-Ward syndrome, whereas homozygous mutations in *KvLQT1* or *minK* or the compound heterozygous condition (simultaneous heterozygous mutations in the two genes) results in the Jervell and Lange-Nielsen syndrome, thus suggesting that mutation of a single allele is sufficient to produce QT prolongation whereas mutation of both alleles is necessary to produce congenital deafness.

Two other ion channelopathies have been identified that result in multisystem diseases and LQTS. Andersen-Twail syndrome (LQT7), which is associated with periodic paralysis, skeletal abnormalities, and a prolonged QT interval, is due to mutations in *KCNJ2*, which encodes the α subunit (Kir2.1) of the inward rectifier potassium channel. Timothy's syndrome (LQT8), which in addition to being associated with a long QT interval can also be manifested as cognitive impairment, autism, and webbing of the fingers and toes, is due to a splice variant of the gene *CACNA1*, which encodes the α subunit (Cav1.2) of the L-type calcium channel.

The corrected QT interval (QTc) in LQTS is usually greater than 0.46 in men and 0.47 in women (each associated with 100% specificity), although a third of affected individuals may have QTc intervals that fall within the normal or nondiagnostic range. A QTc interval of 0.40 or less in men and 0.42 or less in women virtually excludes LQTS. The QT interval fails to shorten normally or may be prolonged with exercise in patients with LQT1 and to a lesser extent in patients with LQT2. Other diagnostic features on the surface ECG include ST-T wave patterns. In LQT1, the T wave may be broad based or normal with a late onset. Very young patients may have a juvenile ST-T wave pattern. LQT2 patients generally have low-amplitude, bifid or notched T waves, whereas LQT3 patients have either late-onset peaked/biphasic T waves or asymmetrical peaked T waves. T wave alternans can also be observed in LQTS.

The genetic locus, QTc, and gender affect the prognosis. The most common trigger for a cardiac event in patients with LQT1 is exercise (particularly swimming). In LQT2 patients, the most frequent precipitant is emotional stress (auditory stimuli). Most events in patients with LQT3 occur during sleep or rest, thus suggesting that they are at higher risk at slow heart rates. Syncope and sudden death are more of a risk in individuals with mutations at the LQT1 locus than in those with LQT2 and LQT3. Events are more frequent in women than men with LQT2 but are more frequent in men than women with LQT3. In general, a QTc interval of 500 msec or longer is associated with a worse prognosis.

A genotype-specific approach to therapy may potentially improve the long-term outcome in patients with congenital LQTS. Patients with LQT1 respond well to β-blockers (e.g., propranolol, 80 to 240 mg/day) and should refrain from strenuous physical activity. β-Blockers may also have a role in patients with LQT2 because of their risk associated with auditory stimuli, but they are less effective than in patients with LQT1. An ICD should be considered in high-risk patients, including survivors of sudden death, those with recurrent syncope despite therapy with β-blockers, and those with marked prolongation of the QTc interval or a family history of sudden death from LQTS. Because of the unpredictable nature of the disease, it is not unreasonable to broaden the indications for an ICD in selected cases. Although patients with LQT1 and LQT2 have higher rates of syncope, patients with LQT3 have the highest mortality rate, and ICDs should be strongly considered, particularly in male patients and those with a QTc of 500 msec or longer. β-Blockers may cause potential harm and should not be used in these patients.

Acquired Long QT Syndrome

Acquired LQTS, which predisposes to TdP, occurs more frequently in women, is usually related to drugs that block the potassium channel I_{Kr}, and is potentiated by subclinical LQTS, hypokalemia, hypomagnesemia, bradycardia, heart block, and heart failure. Evidence suggests that there may be a genetic predisposition to these types of arrhythmias because sporadic mutations and single-nucleotide polymorphisms in ion channel genes have been identified in some patients. Offending agents may include antidepressants (most commonly tricyclics), neuroleptics, antibiotics (macrolides and quinolones), antifungal agents, tamoxifen, methadone, prokinetic agents, and class IA (quinidine, procainamide, and disopyramide) and class III (sotalol, dofetilide, and ibutilide) antiarrhythmic medications. A liquid protein diet, starvation, grapefruit juice, and central nervous system disease may also predispose to QT prolongation and TdP. Drugs that interfere with the hepatic metabolism of agents that directly prolong the QT interval by inhibiting one or more cytochrome P-450 isoenzymes (most commonly CYP3A4) can be a particularly hazardous combination; such drugs include calcium-channel blockers, macrolide antibiotics (e.g., erythromycin), antiretroviral agents, antifungal agents, selective serotonin reuptake inhibitors, and cyclosporine. A polymorphism in the CYP2D6 isoenzyme, found in approximately 7% of white and African American individuals, causes loss of function and therefore impairs the elimination of drugs that prolong the QT interval and are metabolized by CYP2D6, such as the antipsychotic drug thioridazine. Therapy for acquired LQTS is directed at reversing the metabolic abnormalities or withholding the offending medication. Infusion of magnesium and temporary pacing decrease the QT interval and prevent pause-dependent arrhythmias, whereas isoproterenol is a temporizing measure used to increase the sinus rate. Lidocaine (IV bolus, 1 to 2 mg/kg × 2, then an IV infusion at 2 to 4 mg/min), which tends to shorten the action potential duration and decrease the QT interval, may also be used.

Brugada's Syndrome

Brugada's syndrome is typically seen in individuals without known structural heart disease. It is thought to be responsible for the sudden and unexplained nocturnal death syndrome in Southeast Asian men and may account for 20% of sudden deaths in patients with normal hearts. The syndrome is associated with malignant ventricular arrhythmias, most commonly polymorphic VT occurring during rest or sleep.

Brugada's syndrome is associated with an autosomal dominant mode of inheritance with variable penetrance. In 20 to 30% of patients, mutations in the *SCN5A* gene (encodes the α subunit of the sodium channel) result in a diminished inward sodium current, which leads to heterogeneous loss of the action potential dome in the right ventricular epicardium, and ST segment elevation.

The characteristic finding on the ECG is a coved right precordial ST segment elevation (at least 0.2 mV) followed by a negative T wave. However, right precordial ST segment elevation can also be observed in normal subjects and in patients with other clinical conditions. The ECG findings in Brugada's syndrome may be transient and can be provoked by sodium-channel blockers such as procainamide and flecainide (approximate positive predictive value of 35%), as well as by vagotonic agents and β-adrenergic blockade. Magnetic resonance imaging, cardiac catheterization, and myocardial biopsy findings are normal. The diagnosis is supported by ST segment elevation in two or more right precordial leads, a spontaneous episode of VF or polymorphic VT, inducibility of VT on electrophysiologic testing, a family history of sudden death before 45 years of age, or a history of syncope.

An ICD is the most effective treatment for symptomatic patients. Preliminary data suggest that quinidine (1200 to 1500 mg/day) may have some therapeutic effect because of its inhibitory effects on the transient inward current I_{to}, the current responsible for loss of the action potential dome in these patients. Although asymptomatic patients with a spontaneous Brugada ECG pattern have a more favorable prognosis than symptomatic patients do, they are still at increased risk for sudden death as compared with the general population. Therefore, the general recommendation for asymptomatic patients is to undergo an electrophysiologic study and, for patients with an inducible ventricular arrhythmia, to receive an ICD.

Catecholaminergic Polymorphic Ventricular Tachycardia

Sporadic and familial forms of catecholaminergic polymorphic VT have been identified in children and adults with normal hearts. Autosomal dominant missense mutations in the myocardial ryanodine receptor gene, which encodes the ryanodine receptor (RyR2) that controls calcium release from the sarcoplasmic reticulum during excitation-contraction coupling, have been identified in patients with this arrhythmia. Mutant RyR2 has diminished binding affinity for the binding protein (FKBP12.6), which stabilizes interactions between RyR2s by coordinating opening and closing of the channels. Catecholamine activation of protein kinase A and phosphorylation of RyR2 cause dissociation of FKBP12.6 from the channel; however, in the presence of mutated channels, protein kinase A markedly augments calcium release (leak) during diastole and thereby potentiates ventricular arrhythmias. An autosomal recessive form of catecholaminergic polymorphic VT is due to mutations in the calsequestrin gene *(CASQ2)*.

Patients can have bidirectional VT, polymorphic VT, or idiopathic VF. The arrhythmias are precipitated by exercise, catecholamines, or emotional stress and are usually associated with syncope or SCD. In children, the condition may be misdiagnosed as a seizure disorder. Provocative testing with adrenaline (starting at 0.05 μg/kg/min and increasing to 0.10, 0.20, 0.30, and 0.40 μg/kg/min at 5-minute intervals) may unmask polymorphic ventricular ectopy or nonsustained VT. Patients often respond to β-blockers (e.g., metoprolol, 50 to 200 mg/day; propranolol, 120 to 240 mg/day), and strong consideration should be given to use of an ICD because the disease is highly lethal and β-blockers are not fully protective.

Short QT Syndrome

A consistently short QTc interval (<320 msec), termed short QT syndrome (SQTS), is associated with syncope and sudden death in people without structural heart disease. Three forms of SQTS have been identified, all associated with gain-of-function mutations in three different potassium currents, each of which results in accelerated repolarization and abbreviation of the action potential, thereby shortening the QT interval. SQT1 is caused by a mutation in the *KCNH2* gene, which encodes the α subunit of I_{Kr}; SQT2 is caused by a mutation in *KCNQ1*, which encodes the α subunit of I_{Ks}; and SQT3 is due to a mutation in the *KCNJ2* gene, which encodes for the inward rectifier I_{K1}. The ST segment may be abbreviated or absent. The QT interval does not shorten with exercise and may even paradoxically shorten at slow heart rates. Young patients may initially be seen with atrial fibrillation. SQTS occurs over the entire spectrum of age. Secondary causes of a short QT interval should be considered, including hyperkalemia, hypercalcemia, and acidosis.

Patients in whom SQTS is diagnosed should be treated with an ICD. Preliminary data suggest that quinidine (800 mg/day) may have an adjunctive role in patients with mutations in *KCNH2*.

Postoperative Tetralogy of Fallot

Patients who have undergone surgical repair of the tetralogy of Fallot through a right ventriculotomy are at an increased risk for sudden death and VT (Chapter 68). The tachycardia is due to re-entry around the right ventriculotomy scar in the infundibulum. Catheter or surgical ablation or resection is effective in preventing recurrent VT.

Bundle Branch Re-entry

Patients with dilated cardiomyopathy and disease in the His-Purkinje system are prone to the development of a specific form of VT known as bundle branch re-entry, in which the right and left bundle branches participate in a macro re-entrant tachycardia circuit, with one branch involved in the antegrade limb and the other in the retrograde limb. The tachycardia typically has a left bundle branch block morphology and is often associated with presyncope or syncope. The diagnosis is made by invasive electrophysiologic testing, and the tachycardia may be cured by catheter ablation of one of the bundle branches.

Digitalis Toxicity

Ventricular arrhythmias seen in patients with digitalis toxicity include single PVCs, nonsustained VT, and sustained polymorphic or monomorphic VT. Some digitalis toxic rhythms are due to triggered activity from the intracellular calcium overload that results from inhibition of Na^+, K^+-ATPase. A characteristic digitalis toxic rhythm is bidirectional VT, characterized by a right bundle branch block configuration and alternating right and left axis deviation. Therapy for severe digitalis toxic arrhythmias includes infusion of digoxin immune Fab fragments, which may be life-saving. Alternatives are class IB antiarrhythmic medications such as lidocaine (IV bolus, 1 to 2 mg/kg × 2, then an IV infusion, 2 to 4 mg/min) or phenytoin (3.5 to 5 mg/kg intravenously).

VENTRICULAR FLUTTER AND FIBRILLATION

Definition

VF is a malignant arrhythmia characterized by disorganized electrical activity resulting in failure of sequential cardiac contraction and an inability to maintain cardiac output (see Fig. 64–3). If not promptly terminated (Chapter 62), VF results in hypoxemia and eventually SCD. Ventricular flutter is an extremely rapid, hemodynamically unstable VT that typically progresses to VF. The evaluation and management of ventricular flutter should parallel that for VF.

Epidemiology and Pathobiology

With rare exceptions, VF occurs in patients with underlying structural heart disease, especially ischemic heart disease with left ventricular systolic dysfunction. In patients resuscitated from an episode of VF, it is imperative to identify the cause of the arrhythmia and to search for evidence of an acute ischemic event. Patients who survive an episode of VF within 48 hours of acute MI generally have a good prognosis, with a 2% recurrence rate at 1 year.

De novo VF can be caused by myocardial ischemia, which results in complex changes in the electrophysiologic properties of the ventricle, including delays in conduction and changes in refractoriness, that potentiate the multiple re-entrant wave fronts that characterize VF. Alternatively, PVCs during the vulnerable period of ventricular repolarization (R-on-T phenomenon) may initiate VF. Prolonged VT can result in hypotension and myocardial ischemia and cause degeneration of VT to VF.

Electrocardiographic Features

The ECG during ventricular flutter is characterized by a sinusoidal QRS complex, without a distinct ST segment or T wave, at a rate of 240

TABLE 64–2 CAUSES OF SUDDEN CARDIAC DEATH

STRUCTURAL HEART DISEASE

Coronary artery disease
Myocarditis
Cardiomyopathy
  Hypertrophic
  Infiltrative (e.g., amyloidosis, hemochromatosis, sarcoidosis)
Cardiac tumors
Valvular heart disease
Congenital heart disease
Anomalous origin of coronary arteries
Arrhythmogenic right ventricular dysplasia

WITHOUT STRUCTURAL HEART DISEASE

Long QT syndrome
  Congenital
  Acquired (e.g., drugs, electrolyte abnormalities)
Short QT syndrome
Brugada's syndrome
Catecholaminergic polymorphic ventricular tachycardia
Chest wall trauma (commotio cordis)
Wolff-Parkinson-White syndrome
Idiopathic ventricular fibrillation

to 280 beats per minute. In contrast, VF is an irregular rhythm with an undulating low-amplitude baseline without organized QRS complexes or T waves.

SUDDEN CARDIAC DEATH

Definition and Epidemiology

Half of all cardiac deaths are sudden, and they account for approximately 300,000 deaths per year in the United States. SCD is death from instantaneous, unanticipated circulatory collapse within 1 hour of initial symptoms and is often, but not always, due to a cardiac arrhythmia. More than 70% of all sudden natural deaths have a cardiac cause, and 80% of them are attributable to coronary artery disease (Table 64–2). Approximately 70% of SCDs occur in men. As compared with routine activities, vigorous exercise increases the immediate risk for SCD 17-fold. In more recent years, the incidence of SCD has declined in parallel with the decrease in coronary artery disease, probably secondary to a reduction in cardiac risk factors, more effective secondary preventive measures, improved resuscitative efforts, and expansion of emergency medical services. SCD has a diurnal pattern, with a primary peak in the morning hours after awakening, from 8 to 11 AM, and a secondary peak from 4 to 7 PM. β-Blockers attenuate the morning peak pattern. SCD also shows a seasonal predilection, with a higher incidence in December and January than in the summer months (in the Northern Hemisphere), a trend that is attributed to colder temperatures, holiday stress, and shorter daylight hours. Prodromal symptoms in the 2 weeks preceding collapse may include fatigue, dyspnea, and chest pain. Risk factors for SCD are identical to those for coronary artery disease and include age, male gender, hypertension, tobacco use, hypercholesterolemia, and left ventricular hypertrophy.

Holter monitor data indicate that approximately 85% of the rhythms leading to SCD are ventricular tachyarrhythmias, with the remaining 15% being bradyarrhythmias. Among tachyarrhythmias, 75% are due to VT, either monomorphic (two thirds) or polymorphic (one third), and 25% are due to TdP and primary VF. When VT precedes VF, it usually persists for 30 seconds to 3 minutes before degenerating into VF. By 4 minutes after collapse, VF is identified in nearly 90% of SCD cases, whereas asystole is identified in 10%. As more time elapses, asystole and pulseless electrical activity are identified in more than 40% of victims, which suggests that these rhythms reflect prolonged hypoxemia. This prolonged hypoxemia probably explains the lower long-term survival rates (1 to 4%) in SCD patients with these arrhythmias, in contrast to an approximate 30% rate of survival to hospital discharge in patients found to be in VF after a witnessed arrest (Chapter 62).

Pathobiology

Most cardiac arrest survivors have structural heart disease, with nearly 75% having coronary artery disease. VF may be the first manifestation of coronary artery disease in 25 to 50% of patients with ischemic heart disease. Only 20% of patients have evidence of a new Q wave MI at the time of cardiac arrest, whereas a remote MI is present in 40 to 80% of victims. Acute coronary occlusion is found in 50% of survivors of out-of-hospital cardiac arrest.

Of SCD survivors, 10 to 15% have a dilated cardiomyopathy that may be idiopathic or due to viral myocarditis, sarcoidosis, hemochromatosis, or amyloidosis (Chapter 296). In patients with dilated cardiomyopathy, the risk for SCD is related to symptomatic status. The annual mortality in patients who are New York Heart Association functional class II is estimated to be 5 to 15%, of which 50 to 80% is due to SCD. In patients who are functional class IV, the annual mortality is 30 to 70%, of which 5 to 30% is arrhythmogenic. Another cause of SCD is valvar heart disease. In younger patients, particularly those who sustain arrests during physical activity, causes such as hypertrophic cardiomyopathy (with or without outflow obstruction), ARVD, LQTS, anomalous origin of the coronary arteries, and Wolff-Parkinson-White syndrome should be considered in those who can conduct rapidly over the accessory pathway during atrial fibrillation. Other causes include acute myocarditis, cardiac tumors, and repair of congenital anomalies such as transposition of the great arteries and tetralogy of Fallot (Chapter 68). In a small subset of patients, including those with Brugada's syndrome, exercise-related polymorphic VT, LQTS (congenital and acquired), SQTS, drug toxicity (including cocaine use), and electrolyte disturbances, no structural heart disease is detected. More recently, it has been appreciated that a nonpenetrating blow to the chest caused by bodily collision or a projectile, such as a baseball or a hockey puck (commotio cordis; Chapter 113), can precipitate VF, presumably by occurring during the vulnerable phase of the T wave.

Although SCD is not usually associated with an acute Q wave MI, transient ischemia often precedes SCD. In patients with stable high-grade atherosclerotic plaques (>75% occlusion) but no previous MI or unstable ischemia, VF may be due to coronary vasospasm. The true prevalence and significance of ischemia in precipitating VF are unknown, especially in view of the fact that ischemic ST segment changes are rarely present at the time of SCD. An acute coronary thrombus may be observed in 50% of patients with preexisting coronary artery disease, however. The electrophysiologic consequences of acute ischemia that ultimately result in VF are mediated through acidosis, potassium efflux from the cell with membrane depolarization, increased intracellular calcium, and an increase in adrenergic tone.

Diagnosis

See Chapter 62.

Treatment

Rx

A key element for success is bystander initiation of cardiopulmonary resuscitation (see Fig. 62–2), but the most important factor that determines the outcome of cardiac arrest secondary to VF or pulseless VT is the time until defibrillation (Chapter 62).

Prognosis

Despite public education in bystander cardiopulmonary resuscitation and efforts to train emergency medical technicians, early in-hospital mortality is 50 to 60%, and only 4 to 40% of patients with out-of-hospital SCD survive to discharge from the hospital, thus underscoring the importance of primary and secondary prevention. A third of deaths are attributable to heart failure or cardiogenic shock; 90% of patients who recover from coma with meaningful function do so by the third hospital

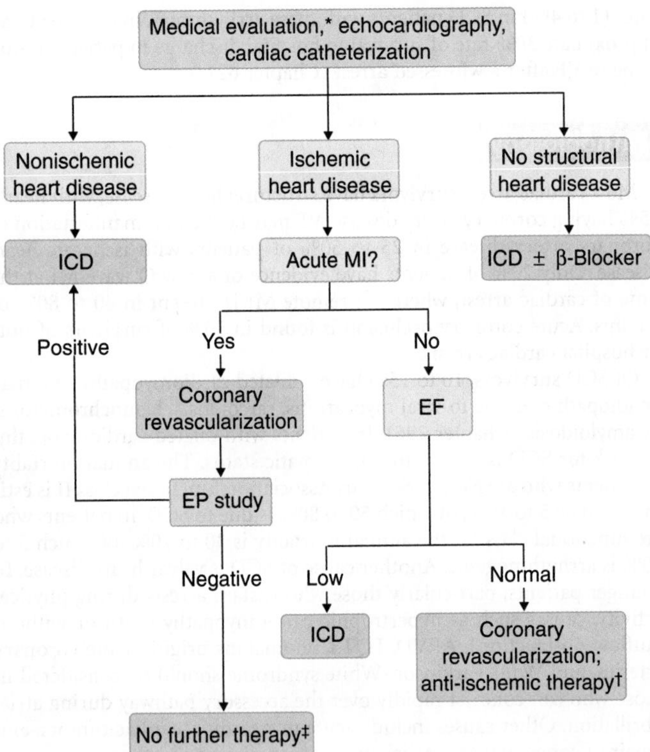

FIGURE 64–4 • Approach to a patient resuscitated from ventricular fibrillation. EF = ejection fraction; EP = electrophysiology; ICD = implantable cardioverter-defibrillator; MI = myocardial infarction. *Diagnose and treat reversible causes of ventricular fibrillation, such as drug toxicity and electrolyte imbalance. †Consider an electrophysiologic study. ‡If the EF is low, consider an ICD.

day. Public access defibrillation with the automatic external defibrillator, which recognizes VF and delivers high-energy shocks, allows laypersons and nonmedical personnel to function as first responders and has the potential to have a positive impact on survival.

A primary episode of SCD has a 10 to 30% 1-year recurrence rate. Identifiable reversible precipitants of secondary VF include transient ischemia, possibly related to vasospasm; hypokalemia resulting from diuretics; hyperkalemia secondary to renal failure, angiotensin-converting enzyme inhibitors, prostaglandin inhibitors, or potassium-sparing diuretics; proarrhythmia secondary to antiarrhythmic medications, tricyclic antidepressants, and antihistamines; or substance abuse with drugs such as cocaine and amphetamines. SCD related to acute ischemia in the absence of a previous MI is often associated with severe proximal coronary artery disease, normal left ventricular function, and noninducibility (absence of VT) during electrophysiologic study. In patients who undergo early defibrillation after an MI and survive to discharge from the hospital, the 5-year survival rate is equivalent to that of age-, sex-, and disease-matched controls.

Prevention

Primary Prevention of Sudden Cardiac Death

Primary preventive approaches to SCD involve the prophylactic treatment of patients identified as being at high risk and generally include reduction or elimination of myocardial ischemia with antianginal agents or coronary revascularization, or both (Fig. 64–4). Regardless of whether residual ischemia is present, initial therapy in all patients without contraindications should include a β-blocker, which reduces SCD and total mortality (25%) in survivors of MI. Results are similarly persuasive in patients with heart failure who can tolerate β-blockers. The beneficial effects of β-blockers in prevention of SCD occur independently of their limited effect on suppression of PVCs. Angiotensin-converting enzyme inhibitors also reduce SCD and overall mortality in survivors of MI with a left ventricular ejection fraction of 35% or less (Chapter 72). Fish oil, tested in two randomized trials, does not appear to be beneficial.

Antiarrhythmic drugs have proved to be proarrhythmic and often decrease survival (Table 64–3). In contrast, amiodarone reduces arrhythmic deaths in MI survivors who have an ejection fraction of 40% or less and either frequent PVCs or nonsustained VT, but it does not seem to improve overall mortality.

Most data regarding risk stratification have been derived from post-MI patients, in whom left ventricular dysfunction (particularly an ejection fraction <35%) is the strongest independent predictor of SCD. The combination of an ejection fraction less than 30% and 10 or more PVCs per hour carries a greater risk for SCD than either risk factor does alone, but drug suppression of ventricular ectopy does not improve the prognosis. However, electrophysiologic testing in post-MI patients without sustained ventricular arrhythmias helps identify those who will benefit from an ICD (Fig. 64–5).

ICDs offer no mortality benefit in acute survivors of MI with left ventricular dysfunction when implanted between 6 and 40 days after the event. [1] However, ICDs reduce mortality in MI survivors who have a low ejection fraction, nonsustained VT, and inducible sustained VT. ICDs also reduce total mortality in patients who are risk-stratified solely on the basis of severely impaired left ventricular function (ejection fraction ≤30%). [2, 3] This effect is more pronounced as the time from MI increases and remains apparent for at least 15 years after MI. In contrast, ICDs do not decrease mortality in patients undergoing elective coronary revascularization who have reduced left ventricular function and a positive signal-averaged ECG. These discrepant results may be due to several factors, including the positive effects of revascularization on outcome, the relative limitations of the signal-averaged ECG to stratify risk (vs. an electrophysiologic study), and the high incidence of nonarrhythmic deaths (70%), which overwhelms the 45% reduction in arrhythmic deaths by ICDs.

An ejection fraction of 35% or less in patients with heart failure is considered sufficient justification to proceed directly to an ICD. [2, 4] Patients with syncope and left ventricular dysfunction are known to have rates of SCD and total mortality similar to those who survive cardiac arrest. Sustained VT is induced in more than 40% of patients with syncope and impaired left ventricular function secondary to coronary artery disease. Despite receiving ICDs and having a high incidence of appropriate therapy, these patients have a considerably worse prognosis than do those who are not inducible. Likewise, syncope in patients with nonischemic dilated cardiomyopathy carries a poor prognosis.

Identification of polymorphisms linked to SCD will probably play a more prominent role in risk stratification in the future. For example, a polymorphism in the *SCN5A* gene that results in a substitution of tyrosine for serine (S1102Y) is found in 13% of African Americans and is associated with SCD.

Prevention of Recurrent Sudden Cardiac Death

Most patients who have survived SCD should undergo a comprehensive evaluation of myocardial function and coronary anatomy (see Fig. 64–4). Echocardiography is useful for excluding hypertrophic cardiomyopathy and valvar heart disease (Chapter 53), magnetic resonance imaging for diagnosing ARVD (Chapter 55), and myocardial biopsy for identifying infiltrative diseases such as myocarditis, amyloidosis, hemochromatosis, and sarcoidosis (Chapter 59). Coronary angiography should be performed to assess for the presence of coronary occlusive disease and to exclude coronary artery anomalies (Chapters 56 and 68). Myocardial perfusion scintigraphy provides complementary data for assessing ischemic burden (Chapter 54). Left ventricular function can be assessed by contrast ventriculography, radionuclide ventriculography, or echocardiography.

Sustained monomorphic VT is inducible by electrophysiologic testing (Chapter 61) in 40 to 50% and polymorphic VT in 10 to 20%; in 30 to 50%, no sustained arrhythmia is induced. In patients with ischemic heart disease and left ventricular dysfunction, inducibility of sustained VT carries a poor prognosis. A low ejection fraction is associated with a poor prognosis, however, regardless of whether sustained VT is inducible; patients who have an ejection fraction of 30% or less and who are noninducible have a 25% arrhythmia recurrence rate at 1 year, whereas noninducible patients with an ejection fraction greater than 30% have a 10 to 15% recurrence rate. An ICD is routinely recommended in such patients unless electrophysiologic testing shows a specific problem that can be cured by catheter ablation.

Coronary revascularization is the principal mode of secondary prevention in patients with significant coronary disease and those in whom VT cannot be induced during electrophysiologic study (Chapter 74).

TABLE 64–3 CLINICAL TRIALS FOR PREVENTION OF SUDDEN CARDIAC DEATH

Study	Background/Premise	Purpose	Entry Criteria	Design	Outcome
PRIMARY PREVENTION AFTER MYOCARDIAL INFARCTION: DRUGS					
CAST	PVCs in survivors of MI are a risk factor for SCD	Assess whether suppression of PVCs with antiarrhythmic drugs reduces risk for SCD	Asymptomatic/mildly symptomatic PVCs (≥6/hr) after MI	1. Primary prevention 2. Titration: encainide, flecainide, or moricizine 3. Randomized: suppressive drug vs. placebo 4. End point: SCD	Antiarrhythmic drugs: 1. Increase overall mortality 2. Increase risk for SCD
SWORD	Post-MI patients with decreased EF have increased mortality	Assess whether D-sotalol vs. placebo reduces mortality	1. Recent MI 2. EF ≤40%	1. Primary prevention 2. Randomized: D-sotalol vs. placebo 3. End point: mortality	1. D-Sotalol associated with increased mortality 2. Increased mortality presumed to be secondary to proarrhythmia
CAMIAT	Frequent or repetitive PVCs after MI increase mortality 1–2 yr after event	Assess effect of amiodarone on risk for VF	1. Post-MI status 2. ≥10 PVCs/hr or ≥one 3-beat run	1. Primary prevention 2. Randomized: amiodarone vs. placebo 3. End point: resuscitated VF or arrhythmic death	1. Amiodarone reduces VF and arrhythmic death (relative risk reduction: 38%) 2. No difference between groups in overall mortality
EMIAT	Post-MI patients with decreased EF are at increased risk for SCD	Assess whether amiodarone reduces mortality in post-MI patients with decreased EF	1. Post-MI status 2. EF ≤40%	1. Primary prevention 2. Randomized: amiodarone vs. placebo	1. 35% risk reduction in arrhythmic deaths with amiodarone 2. No difference in mortality between amiodarone and placebo
PRIMARY PREVENTION AFTER MYOCARDIAL INFARCTION/CORONARY ARTERY DISEASE: IMPLANTABLE CARDIOVERTER-DEFIBRILLATOR					
CABG patch	Patients with CAD, decreased EF, and (+) SAECG are at increased risk for SCD	Assess effect of prophylactic ICD at time of elective CABG surgery on survival	1. CAD 2. EF ≤35% 3. (+) SAECG	1. Primary prevention 2. Randomized: ICD vs. control 3. End point: mortality	1. No difference in mortality between ICD and control patients
MADIT	Post-MI patients with NSVT and decreased EF have 30% 2-yr mortality	Assess whether prophylactic ICD vs. conventional medical therapy improves survival	1. Previous MI 2. EF ≤35% 3. NSVT 4. Inducible but nonsuppressible VT with antiarrhythmic drug during EPS	1. Primary prevention 2. Randomized: ICD vs. conventional medical therapy 3. End point: mortality	1. Prophylactic ICD reduces mortality by 54% at 27 mo
MUSTT	Post-MI patients with decreased EF are at high risk for SCD	Assess whether EPS-guided antiarrhythmic therapy decreases risk for SCD	1. Previous MI/CAD 2. EF ≤40% 3. NSVT 4. Induced sustained VT	1. Primary prevention 2. Antiarrhythmic drugs or ICD vs. no antiarrhythmic therapy 3. End point: SCD	1. ICD results in a 27% reduction in risk for SCD at 5 yr

Continued

TABLE 64–3 CLINICAL TRIALS FOR PREVENTION OF SUDDEN CARDIAC DEATH—cont'd

Study	Background/Premise	Purpose	Entry Criteria	Design	Outcome
MADIT-II	Post-MI patients with decreased EF are at high risk for SCD	Assess effect of ICD on survival	1. Previous MI 2. EF ≤30%	1. Primary prevention 2. Randomized ICD vs. conventional therapy 3. End point: mortality	1. ICD associated with a 29% reduction in mortality at 20 mo
SCD-HeFT	SCD is a major cause of death in CHF	Assess relative efficacy of amiodarone or ICD vs. conventional therapy	1. NYHA class II/III CHF 2. EF ≤35%	1. Primary prevention 2. Randomized conventional CHF therapy vs. amiodarone vs. ICD 3. End point: mortality	1. ICD decreased risk for death (hazard ratio = .77; *P* = .007) 2. Amiodarone was associated with similar risk for death as conventional therapy 3. ICD benefits were similar in ischemic and nonischemic patients
DEFINITE	Patients with nonischemic dilated cardiomyopathy are at increased risk for SCD	Assess effect of ICD on survival	1. Nonischemic cardiomyopathy 2. EF ≤35% 3. PVCs/NSVT	1. Primary prevention 2. Randomized conventional therapy vs. ICD 3. End point: mortality	1. ICD did not reduce mortality (hazard ratio = .65, *P* = .08) 2. ICD reduced risk for SCD (hazard ratio = .20; *P* = .006)
DINAMIT	ICDs improve survival of high-risk cardiac patients	Assess benefit of ICD early after MI	1. Recent MI (6–40 days) 2. EF ≤35% 3. Impaired autonomic function	1. Primary prevention 2. Randomized ICD vs. control 3. End point: mortality	1. No mortality benefit from ICD 2. Arrhythmic death was reduced by ICD (hazard ratio = .42; *P* = .009)
SECONDARY PREVENTION OF SUDDEN CARDIAC DEATH/HYPOTENSIVE VENTRICULAR TACHYCARDIA: IMPLANTABLE CARDIOVERTER-DEFIBRILLATOR					
AVID	Patients who survive VF or hypotensive VT are at increased risk for recurrence	Assess relative efficacy of ICD vs. amiodarone (majority) or sotalol on mortality	1. VF 2. VT and syncope/presyncope (EF ≤40%)	1. Secondary prevention 2. Randomized: ICD vs. antiarrhythmic drugs 3. End point: mortality	1. ICD reduces mortality when compared with amiodarone 2. Relative risk reduction of 39 and 31% at 1 and 3 yr
CIDS	Patients who survive VF or hypotensive VT are at increased risk for recurrence	Assess relative efficacy of ICD vs. amiodarone on mortality	1. VF 2. VT and syncope/presyncope 3. Syncope and spontaneous/induced VT	1. Secondary prevention 2. Randomized: ICD vs. amiodarone 3. End point: mortality	1. ICD therapy results in a 20% relative risk reduction in mortality (*P* = .14)
CASH	Survivors of SCD are at high risk for recurrent event	Assess relative efficacy of class I, II, and III antiarrhythmic drugs and ICD	1. Survivor of SCD caused by VF/VT	1. Secondary prevention 2. Randomized: propafenone vs. metoprolol vs. amiodarone vs. ICD 3. End point: mortality	1. ICD reduces mortality 42 and 28% (1 and 3 yr) when compared with amiodarone/metoprolol (*P* = .8) 2. Propafenone arm aborted because of increased mortality vs. ICD

AVID = Antiarrhythmics Versus Implantable Defibrillators; CABG = coronary artery bypass graft; CAD = coronary artery disease; CAMIAT = Canadian Amiodarone Myocardial Infarction Arrhythmia Trial; CASH = Cardiac Arrest Study Hamburg; CAST = Cardiac Arrhythmia Suppression Trial; CHF = congestive heart failure; CIDS = Canadian Implantable Defibrillator Study; DEFINITE = Defibrillators in Non-Ischemic Cardiomyopathy Treatment Evaluation; DINAMIT = Defibrillator in Acute Myocardial Infarction Trial; EF = ejection fraction; EMIAT = European Myocardial Infarct Amiodarone Trial; EPS = electrophysiology study; ICD = implantable cardioverter-defibrillator; MADIT = Multicenter Automatic Defibrillator Implantation Trial; MI = myocardial infarction; MUSTT = Multicenter Unsustained Tachycardia Trial; NSVT = nonsustained ventricular tachycardia; NYHA = New York Heart Association; PVCs = premature ventricular complexes; SCD = sudden cardiac death; SAECG = signal-averaged electrocardiogram; SCD-HeFT = Sudden Cardiac Death in Heart Failure Trial; SWORD = Survival With Oral D-Sotalol; VF = ventricular fibrillation; VT = ventricular tachycardia.

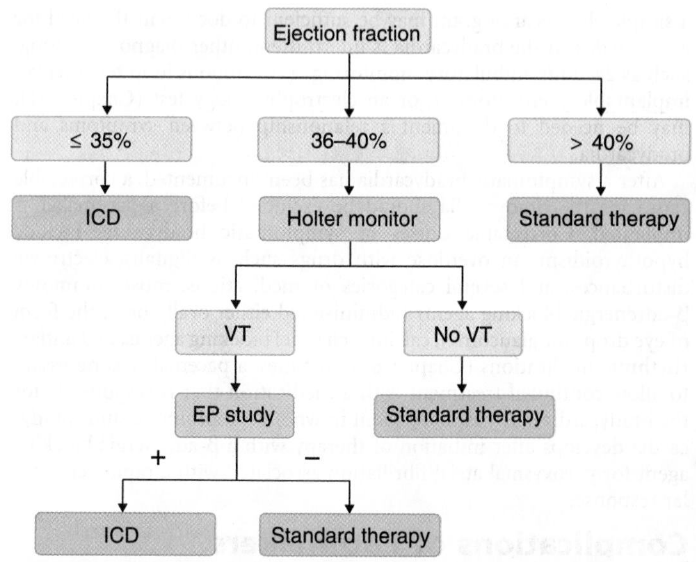

FIGURE 64–5 • Risk stratification for primary prevention of death in patients with ischemic and nonischemic cardiomyopathy. Standard therapy may include aspirin, anti-ischemic therapy, lipid-lowering therapy, a β-blocker, or an angiotensin-converting enzyme inhibitor (Chapter 72). EP = electrophysiology; ICD = implantable cardioverter-defibrillator; VT = ventricular tachycardia.

Revascularization is not effective, however, in preventing VT in patients with sustained monomorphic VT secondary to scars from a previous MI; treatment with catheter ablation may be effective in patients with hemodynamically tolerated VT. However, data suggest that 3-year mortality rates in patients with stable VT are equivalent to rates in patients with unstable VT. An ICD should be strongly considered in these patients.

Secondary prevention trials for sudden death survivors secondary to VF/VT or patients with hemodynamically unstable VT in the aggregate show a 20 to 30% reduction in mortality at 3 years with ICD therapy versus amiodarone, which is the best antiarrhythmic therapy. Thus, an ICD is the most effective therapy for primary and secondary prevention of SCD.

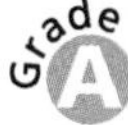

1. Hohnloser SH, Kuck KH, Dorian P, et al: Prophylactic use of an implantable cardioverter-defibrillator after acute myocardial infarction. N Engl J Med 2004;351:2481–2488.
2. Bardy GH, Lee KL, Mark DB, et al: Amiodarone or an implantable cardioverter-defibrillator for congestive heart failure. N Engl J Med 2005;352:225–237.
3. Moss AJ, Zareba W, Hall WJ, et al: Prophylactic implantation of a defibrillator in patients with myocardial infarction and reduced ejection fraction. N Engl J Med 2002;346:877–883.
4. Kadish A, Dyer A, Daubert JP, et al: Prophylactic defibrillator implantation in patients with nonischemic dilated cardiomyopathy. N Engl J Med 2004;350:2151–2158.

SUGGESTED READINGS

Antzelevitch C, Brugada P, Borggrefe M, et al: Brugada syndrome: Report of the second consensus conference. Circulation 2005;111:659–670. *Comprehensive review of Brugada's syndrome.*

Buxton AE: Not everyone with an ejection fraction ≤30% should receive an implantable cardioverter-defibrillator. Circulation 2005;111:2537–2542. *Review of data that support the view that the decision to implant a prophylactic defibrillator should not be based on a low ejection fraction alone.*

Josephson M, Wellens HJJ: Implantable defibrillators and sudden cardiac death. Circulation 2004;109:2685–2691. *Review of the pathophysiology and treatment of sudden cardiac death.*

Moss AJ: Everyone with an ejection fraction less than or equal to 30% should receive an implantable cardioverter-defibrillator. Circulation 2005;111:2542–2548. *Summary of data that support prophylactic implantation of defibrillators in patients risk- stratified according to ejection fraction alone.*

Priori SG, Schwartz PJ, Napolitano C, et al: Risk stratification in the long QT syndrome. N Engl J Med 2003;348:1866–1874. *Risk stratification of LQTS based on genotype.*

Zipes DP, Camm AJ, Borggrefe M, et al: ACC/AHA/ESC Guidelines for management of patients with ventricular arrhythmias and the prevention of sudden cardiac death. J Am Coll Cardiol 2006;48:247–346. *Consensus guidelines with a comprehensive review of the literature.*

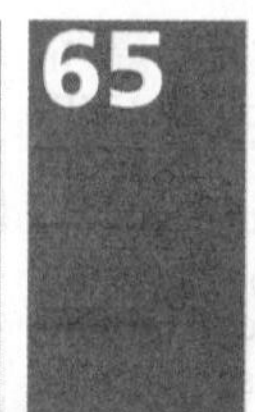

65 ELECTROPHYSIOLOGIC INTERVENTIONAL PROCEDURES AND SURGERY

Fred Morady

PACEMAKERS

Pacemaker Generators and Leads

Pacemaker batteries, which are lithium iodide cells that typically have a lifespan of 7 to 8 years, now often weigh less than 30 g. They are usually implanted subcutaneously in the infraclavicular area (Fig. 65–1). The programmability of many different variables has become standard, as has the ability of the pacemaker to provide diagnostic and telemetric data.

Pacemaker leads are generally bipolar, with the distal electrode serving as the cathode. Unipolar leads are less commonly used because of the potential for pacing chest wall muscles and for inhibition of pacing by skeletal muscle myopotentials. The leads are inserted into the heart either percutaneously through a subclavian vein or by cutdown into a cephalic vein. Atrial leads are usually positioned in the right atrial appendage, and ventricular leads are placed in the right ventricular apex. Fixation to the myocardium is achieved either passively with tines or actively with a screw mechanism. Newer electrode designs, such as porous carbon or steroid-eluting electrodes, have resulted in lower acute and chronic pacing thresholds.

Pacing Modes

The mode of pacing is described in shorthand fashion by a three- to five-letter code. The first letter designates the chamber being paced (A for atrium, V for ventricle, D for dual chamber); the second letter designates the chamber being sensed (A, V, D, or O for no sensing); the third letter designates whether the pacemaker functions in an inhibited (I) or tracking mode (T), in both modes (D), or asynchronously (O); and the fourth letter indicates whether the pacemaker is capable of rate modulation independent of atrial activity. An additional fifth letter may be used to designate the capability for antitachycardia pacing (P), delivery of shocks (S), or both (D). The most commonly used pacing modes are VVI (pacing and sensing within the ventricle in inhibited fashion), VVIR (VVI plus rate responsiveness), and DDD (pacing and sensing of the atrium and ventricle in both inhibited and tracking fashion).

The most appropriate pacing mode must always be determined on an individual basis, the goal being to meet the patient's physiologic needs with the simplest system possible. For example, in a patient with chronic atrial fibrillation who has symptomatic pauses but not chronotropic incompetence, a VVI pacemaker is sufficient. However, if the patient also has chronotropic incompetence, a VVIR pacemaker is necessary to restore a normal rate response to exercise. In a patient with a high-degree atrioventricular (AV) block and normal sinus node function, DDD pacing is optimal. However, if a patient with a high-degree AV block also has sinus node dysfunction, the ideal pacing mode is DDDR.

In patients who have paroxysmal atrial fibrillation and a high-degree AV block, no single pacing mode is optimal. DDD pacing is ideal when the patient is in sinus rhythm, but during atrial fibrillation, DDD pacing may result in tracking of the atrium at the upper rate limit of the pacemaker. Conversely, VVIR pacing, which is ideal during atrial fibrillation, will not provide AV synchrony during periods of sinus rhythm. The development of mode-switching pacemakers has solved this dilemma. Mode-switching pacemakers are capable of pacing in the DDD mode during sinus rhythm and automatically switching to rate-responsive ventricular pacing during atrial fibrillation or other supraventricular arrhythmias (Fig. 65–2).

The choice between ventricular (VVIR) and atrial (AAIR) or dual-chamber (DDDR) pacing remains controversial. Although a randomized trial of 225 patients with sinus node dysfunction reported a significant reduction in cardiovascular death at 8 years with AAIR versus VVIR pacing, 1 studies of nearly 5000 patients have shown no survival differences when patients were randomized to DDDR or VVIR pacing. Dual-chamber pacing, like atrial pacing, reduces the incidence of atrial fibrillation and appears to result in slightly better quality of life. [2] In these randomized trials, 5 to 25% of patients who initially received VVIR pacemakers "crossed over" to DDDR pacing because of physician-diagnosed pacemaker syndrome (see Complications of Pacemakers).

Several studies have demonstrated that the ventricular dyssynchrony induced by right ventricular pacing may have deleterious effects on ventricular function and functional capacity and may also predispose to the development of atrial fibrillation. Therefore, pacemakers should always be programmed to minimize the amount of ventricular pacing.

Indications for a Permanent Pacemaker

In general, pacemakers are implanted either to alleviate symptoms caused by bradycardia or to prevent severe symptoms in patients in whom symptomatic bradycardia is likely to develop (Tables 65–1 and 65–2). The most common bradycardia-induced symptoms are dizziness or lightheadedness, syncope or near-syncope (Chapters 61 and 427), exercise intolerance, or symptoms of heart failure. Because these symptoms are nonspecific, documentation of an association between symptoms and bradycardia should be obtained before pacemaker implantation. If the bradycardia is persistent, such as in a patient with a complete AV block, a simple electrocardiogram may be sufficient to document the need for a pacemaker. If the bradycardia is intermittent, other diagnostic testing, such as 24-hour ambulatory monitoring, a continuous loop recorder, an implantable event monitor, or an electrophysiology test (Chapter 61), may be needed to document a relationship between symptoms and bradycardia.

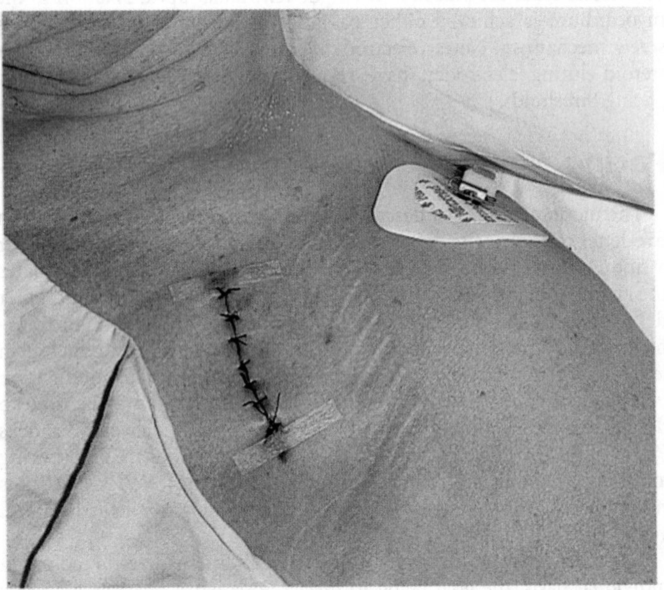

FIGURE 65–1 • Site of implantation of a permanent pacemaker or automatic implantable cardioverter-defibrillator. The pacemaker is usually implanted in the left pectoral region, but it may be placed elsewhere if necessary. (From Forbes CD, Jackson WF: Color Atlas and Text of Clinical Medicine, 3rd ed. London, Mosby, 2003.)

After a symptomatic bradycardia has been documented, a correctable cause for the bradycardia should be excluded before a pacemaker is implanted. Correctable causes of symptomatic bradycardia include hypothyroidism, an overdose with drugs such as digitalis, electrolyte disturbances, and several categories of medications, most commonly β-adrenergic blocking agents (administered either orally or in the form of eye drops for glaucoma), calcium-channel blocking agents, and antiarrhythmic medications (Chapter 63). At times, a pacemaker is necessary to allow continued treatment with a medication that is responsible for the bradycardia, such as in a patient in whom symptomatic sinus bradycardia develops after initiation of therapy with a β-adrenergic blocking agent for paroxysmal atrial fibrillation associated with a rapid ventricular response.

Complications of Pacemakers

Complications related to the implantation procedure occur in less than 2% of patients and include pneumothorax, perforation of the atrium or ventricle, lead dislodgement, infection, and erosion of the pacemaker pocket. Thrombosis of the subclavian vein occurs in 10 to 20% of patients and is more likely in the presence of multiple leads; it rarely causes symptoms.

Pacemaker-mediated tachycardia is a possible complication of DDD pacing when the atrial lead senses retrograde depolarizations because of ventriculoatrial conduction. The resulting tachycardia often has a rate equal to the upper rate limit of the pacemaker. Pacemaker-mediated tachycardia can be eliminated by various reprogramming maneuvers, such as lengthening of the postventriculoatrial refractory period.

The pacemaker syndrome consists of symptoms of weakness, lightheadedness, exercise intolerance, or palpitations caused by the absence of AV synchrony during ventricular pacing. It is treated by restoring AV synchrony with DDD pacing or, if AV conduction is intact, with AAI pacing. During long-term follow-up after pacemaker implantation, potential problems include failure to pace, failure to capture, and changes in the pacing rate. These problems may be a manifestation of suboptimal programming, fracture of a lead or a break in the insulation, generator malfunction, or battery depletion.

Temporary Pacemakers

Temporary pacemaker leads are generally inserted percutaneously into an internal jugular or subclavian vein or by cutdown into a brachial vein and then positioned under fluoroscopic guidance in the right ventricular apex and attached to an external generator. Temporary pacing is used to stabilize patients awaiting permanent pacemaker implantation, to correct a transient symptomatic bradycardia caused by drug toxicity or a

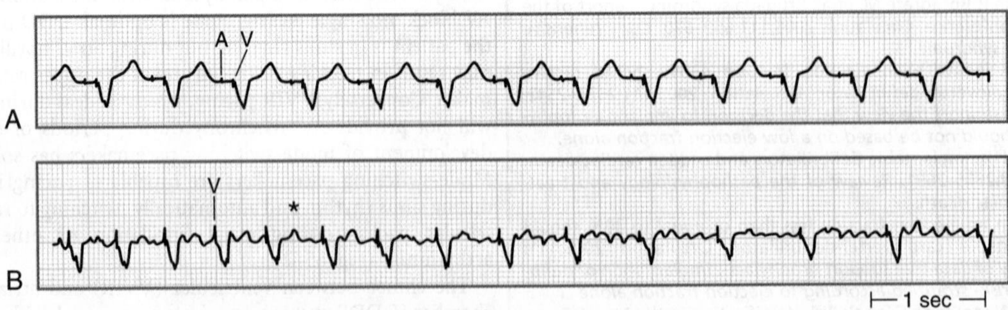

FIGURE 65–2 • Rhythm strips from a Holter monitor in a patient with complete atrioventricular block, sinus bradycardia, paroxysmal atrial fibrillation, and a rate-responsive dual-chamber pacemaker with mode-switching capability. A, When the patient is in sinus rhythm, the pacemaker functions in a DDDR mode, with synchronized atrial and ventricular pacing at 105 beats per minute while the patient is walking. **B,** At the onset of an episode of atrial fibrillation, there is tracking of the atrium that results in ventricular pacing at 140 beats per minute, which is the upper rate limit of the pacemaker. Within 2 seconds (asterisk), the mode-switch feature results in VVIR pacing, and the ventricular pacing rate gradually falls to 70 beats per minute, which is the lower rate limit of the pacemaker. A = atrial stimulus; V = ventricular stimulus.

TABLE 65–1 CLASS I INDICATIONS* FOR IMPLANTATION OF A PERMANENT PACEMAKER

I. Atrioventricular block
   A. Third-degree atrioventricular block associated with symptoms
   B. Third-degree atrioventricular block with pauses >3 seconds or with an escape rate <40 beats per minute in awake patients
   C. Postoperative atrioventricular block that is not expected to resolve
   D. Second-degree atrioventricular block associated with symptoms
   E. Chronic bifascicular or trifascicular block with an intermittent third-degree atrioventricular block or type II second-degree atrioventricular block or alternating bundle branch block
II. Atrioventricular block associated with myocardial infarction
   A. Second- or third-degree atrioventricular block in the His-Purkinje system
   B. Transient second- or third-degree infranodal atrioventricular block and associated bundle branch block
   C. Persistent, symptomatic second- or third-degree atrioventricular block
III. Sinus node dysfunction
   A. Symptomatic sinus bradycardia or sinus pauses
   B. Symptomatic chronotropic incompetence
IV. Carotid sinus syndrome: recurrent syncope or near-syncope as a result of carotid sinus syndrome

*Class I indications are conditions for which there is general agreement that a pacemaker is indicated.
Adapted from Gregoratos G, Abrams J, Epstein AE, et al: ACC/AHA/NASPE guideline update for implantation of cardiac pacemakers and antiarrhythmia devices—summary article. J Am Coll Cardiol 2002;40:1703–1719.

TABLE 65–2 CLASS II INDICATIONS* FOR IMPLANTATION OF A PERMANENT PACEMAKER

I. Atrioventricular block
   A. Asymptomatic third-degree atrioventricular block with an escape rate >40 beats per minute
   B. Asymptomatic Mobitz II second-degree atrioventricular block with a narrow QRS
   C. Asymptomatic Mobitz I second-degree atrioventricular block in the His-Purkinje system
   D. Bifascicular or trifascicular block and syncope without an identifiable cause
   E. His-ventricular interval >100 msec
   F. Pacing-induced block in the His-Purkinje system
II. Atrioventricular block associated with myocardial infarction: persistent second- or third-degree atrioventricular block at the level of the atrioventricular node
III. Sinus node dysfunction
   A. Heart rate <40 beats per minute, without a clear association between symptoms and bradycardia
   B. Unexplained syncope and sinus node dysfunction demonstrated in an electrophysiologic study
IV. Neurocardiogenic syncope: recurrent neurocardiogenic syncope associated with significant bradycardia during spontaneous syncope or during tilt-table testing

*Class II indications are conditions for which pacemakers are often used, but without unanimous agreement among experts that a pacemaker is necessary.
Adapted from Gregoratos G, Abrams J, Epstein AE, et al: ACC/AHA/NASPE guideline update for implantation of cardiac pacemakers and antiarrhythmia devices—summary article. J Am Coll Cardiol 2002;40:1703–1719.

metabolic defect, or to suppress torsades de pointes by maintaining a rate of 85 to 100 beats per minute until the causative factor has been eliminated. Temporary pacing may also be used in prophylactic fashion in patients at risk for symptomatic bradycardia during a surgical procedure or high-degree AV block in the setting of an acute myocardial infarction. The most common complication of temporary pacemakers is infection; this risk is minimized by limiting the use of a pacemaker lead to 48 hours. In emergency situations, ventricular pacing can be instituted immediately by transcutaneous pacing with electrode pads applied to the chest wall.

TRANSTHORACIC CARDIOVERSION AND DEFIBRILLATION

Mechanism of Action

Direct current defibrillators store an electrical charge and discharge it across two paddle electrodes in a damped, sinusoidal waveform. The shock terminates arrhythmias caused by re-entry by simultaneously depolarizing large portions of the atria or ventricles, thereby causing the re-entry circuits to extinguish (Chapters 60, 63, and 64).

A nonsynchronized shock that is delivered coincident with the T wave during supraventricular tachycardia (SVT) or ventricular tachycardia (VT) may precipitate ventricular fibrillation (VF). Cardioversion refers to the termination of SVT or VT by delivery of a shock in synchrony with the QRS complex. When shocks are delivered to terminate VF, synchronization to the QRS complex is not necessary, and this process is referred to as defibrillation.

Technique

Whenever cardioversion or defibrillation is performed on an elective basis, the patient should be in a fasting state. Intravenous access to a peripheral vein should be established, and oxygen, suction, and equipment needed for airway management should be readily available. Transthoracic shocks are painful, and drugs commonly used for anesthesia or amnesia include short-acting barbiturates such as methohexital or a short-acting amnestic agent such as midazolam. In the anteroapical configuration, one electrode is positioned to the right of the sternum at the level of the second intercostal space, and the second electrode is positioned at the midaxillary line, lateral to the apical impulse. In the anteroposterior configuration, an electrode is placed to the left of the sternum at the fourth intercostal space, and the second electrode is positioned posteriorly, to the left of the spine, at the same level as the anterior electrode. These two electrode configurations result in similar success rates of cardioversion and defibrillation.

Important variables affecting the success of cardioversion or defibrillation are the shock waveform and shock strength. Defibrillators that deliver biphasic shocks are now clinically available and have a significantly higher success rate than conventional defibrillators do. Other technique-dependent variables that maximize delivery of energy to the heart include firm paddle pressure, delivery of the shock during expiration, and repetitive shocks. Patient-related variables that may decrease the probability of successful cardioversion/defibrillation include metabolic disturbances, long arrhythmia duration, some antiarrhythmic drugs such as amiodarone, and body weight in excess of 80 kg.

Because cardioversion of atrial fibrillation (Chapter 63) may be complicated by thromboembolism, anticoagulation with warfarin is generally necessary for 3 weeks before cardioversion and for 1 month after cardioversion whenever atrial fibrillation has been present for 48 hours or longer. The 3-week period of anticoagulation before cardioversion can be eliminated if no atrial thrombi are seen on a transesophageal echocardiogram, but anticoagulation for 1 month after cardioversion is still necessary to prevent thrombus formation secondary to transient, postconversion atrial stunning.

Indications

The most common arrhythmias treated by cardioversion/defibrillation are VF, VT, atrial fibrillation, and atrial flutter (Chapters 62, 63, and 64). Treatment of VF is always an emergency, and a 200-J shock should be delivered as quickly as possible, followed by one or more 360-J shocks if necessary. Depending on the patient's hemodynamic status, cardioversion of VT may be performed electively or on an emergency basis; if elective, an initial shock strength of 50 J is appropriate, followed by higher energy levels if additional shocks are needed. An initial energy level of 50 J is appropriate for cardioversion of atrial flutter. In atrial fibrillation, in which cardioversion is generally performed on an elective basis, an initial shock of 100 to 200 J is appropriate, depending on the patient's body weight. Shocks of 300 to 360 J are then used if necessary. If atrial fibrillation must be treated on an urgent basis, for example, in a patient with Wolff-Parkinson-White syndrome who has a very rapid ventricular rate and hemodynamic compromise, an initial shock of 200 J should be followed by 360-J shocks, as needed. Because the defibrillation energy requirement is a probability function and not a discrete value, subsequent shocks may be effective for cardioversion/defibrillation even when the first 360-J shock is ineffective.

Complications

Asynchronous shocks may precipitate VF. Rarely, VF may occur even when shocks are synchronized to the QRS complex. The risk for post-shock ventricular arrhythmias is increased in the presence of a supratherapeutic plasma concentration of digitalis, so cardioversion in patients with digitalis toxicity should be avoided.

Transient ST segment elevation may occur after cardioversion and is usually of no clinical consequence. Mild myocardial necrosis may occasionally occur if a total energy exceeding 425 J is delivered in a short period. Another rare complication of cardioversion is pulmonary edema, which may be due to transient left ventricular dysfunction.

Post-shock bradycardia or asystole may occur because of vagal discharge or an underlying sick sinus syndrome. At times, atropine or emergency transcutaneous pacing may be necessary. In patients who have a pacemaker or implantable cardioverter-defibrillator (ICD), the shocking electrodes should be positioned as far away from the generator as possible, and the generator and pacing threshold should be checked afterward.

IMPLANTABLE CARDIOVERTER-DEFIBRILLATORS

ICD Pulse Generators and Leads

ICDs now weigh as little as 60 g, are multiprogrammable, have improved detection algorithms, are capable of antitachycardia and antibradycardia (including dual-chamber) pacing, can deliver biphasic shocks at strengths of less than 1 to 42 J, and provide a record of the electrograms recorded during arrhythmic episodes. An ICD that delivers shocks to terminate atrial fibrillation, as well as VT and VF, is now clinically available. Biventricular ICDs are available for patients who need an ICD and have advanced (class III or IV) heart failure and a bundle branch block.

With the development of pulse generators small enough to implant in the infraclavicular area and endocardial leads that are inserted transvenously, the implantation procedure has been greatly simplified and is now very similar to that for permanent pacemakers.

A single lead that contains a pacing-sensing electrode and two defibrillating coils can be used. If adequate defibrillation is not achieved with a single-lead configuration, a subcutaneous patch electrode or subcutaneous array can be added. In another commonly used configuration, the pulse generator itself functions as an electrode, and a lead that has a pacing-sensing electrode at its tip and a distal defibrillating coil electrode is positioned at the right ventricular apex. Multiple other combinations of a chest wall patch electrode and defibrillating electrodes in the right ventricular apex, superior vena cava, or coronary sinus can also be used. When a biventricular ICD is implanted, a lead is inserted into a branch of the coronary sinus for left ventricular pacing.

Indications

ICDs have become first-line therapy in patients who have survived an episode of VF not associated with acute myocardial infarction or who have had an episode of hemodynamically significant, sustained VT (Chapter 64). [3] ICDs are also implanted in individuals at high risk for cardiac arrest, including patients with idiopathic, dilated cardiomyopathy and unexplained syncope or patients with coronary artery disease (CAD), an ejection fraction less than 35%, spontaneous episodes of nonsustained VT, and inducible sustained VT in the electrophysiology laboratory (Chapter 64). [4] Based on the results of large-scale clinical trials, the indications for implantation of an ICD were recently expanded to include patients with a previous myocardial infarction and an ejection fraction of 30% or less, as well as patients with dilated cardiomyopathy (ischemic or nonischemic), an ejection fraction of 35% or less, and class II or III heart failure. [5-7]

Programming of ICDs

Testing is performed at the time of implantation to determine the energy requirement for defibrillation. A safety margin of at least 10 J should be present; for example, if the maximum output of the pulse generator is 32 J, successful defibrillation should be achieved with shocks of 22 J or less in strength. If the patient has had episodes of VT, antitachycardia pacing can be evaluated and programmed as needed to terminate the VT. Appropriate programming of the device is performed during predischarge testing.

With ICDs that are tiered-therapy devices, as many as two VT zones and one VF zone are available to provide individualized therapy for ventricular arrhythmias that have different rates. The rate threshold and various sequences of antitachycardia pacing and low- or high-energy shocks can be programmed for each of the two VT zones. The VF zone is a high-rate zone in which high-energy shocks are delivered. Optimal programming is important for many reasons, including minimizing patient discomfort, reducing the chance of syncope with an arrhythmia episode, maximizing the battery life of the pulse generator, and preventing inappropriate shocks.

Complications

Complications related to the implantation procedure include pneumothorax, myocardial perforation, and infection, all of which should have an incidence less than 1%. Complications associated with the subcutaneous or submuscular pocket into which the device is placed include hematoma formation and erosion of the pocket. The endocardial leads that are used in the ICD system occasionally become dislodged shortly after implantation, thus necessitating a second procedure to reposition the leads. Other lead complications include fracture or breakdown of the insulation, either of which may result in failure to defibrillate. Fracture of a lead may also result in an artifact that mimics VF and triggers inappropriate shocks.

Patients who have an ICD do not require evaluation every time that they experience a device discharge. However, urgent evaluation is necessary if the patient experiences flurries of discharges. Analysis of stored electrograms often reveals the underlying problem (Fig. 65–3). The frequent shocks may be appropriate shocks triggered by flurries of VT or VF; if a correctable cause such as a metabolic defect or proarrhythmic drug cannot be identified, antiarrhythmic drug therapy or catheter ablation, or both, should be used to eliminate these arrhythmia flurries. Flurries of shocks may be triggered by atrial fibrillation with a rapid ventricular response, in which case aggressive management of the atrial fibrillation is indicated. In addition, flurries of shocks may be a manifestation of a lead fracture, in which case lead replacement is necessary.

RADIO FREQUENCY CATHETER ABLATION

Tissue Effects of Radio Frequency Energy

Radio frequency ablation is a percutaneous catheter technique that can permanently eliminate a variety of SVTs and VTs that previously required either chronic pharmacologic treatment for suppression or surgery for cure. Radio frequency energy is delivered through an electrode catheter whose tip is in contact with tissue that is critical to maintenance of the tachycardia. The radio frequency energy results in resistive heating of the tissue and irreversible tissue destruction when the tissue temperature exceeds 50° C. The lesions that are created are 5 to 6 mm in diameter and 2 to 3 mm deep. Chronic lesions demonstrate coagulation necrosis and are well demarcated.

Procedural Aspects

Diagnostic electrophysiologic testing (Chapter 61) and radio frequency ablation are often performed during the same procedure, commonly on an outpatient basis. Various pacing techniques or infusions of isoproterenol (or both) are used to induce the patient's arrhythmia and

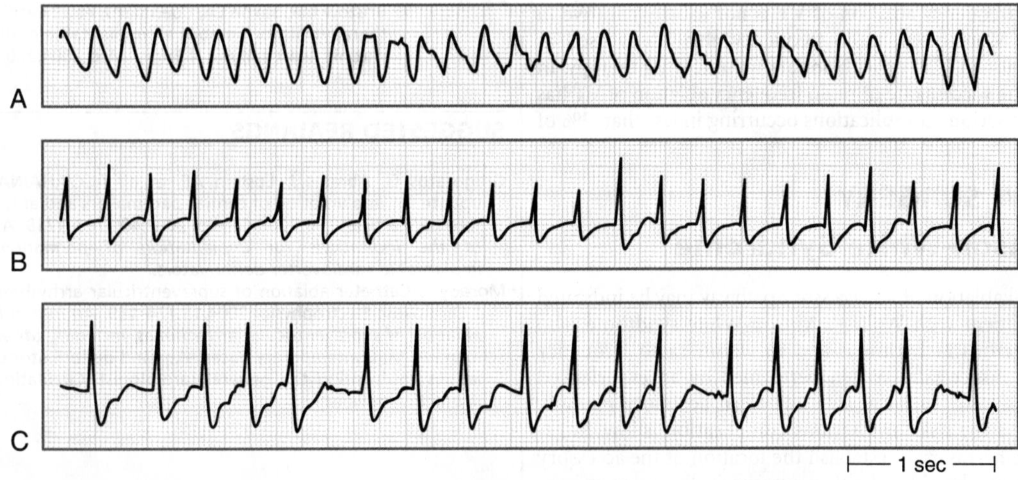

FIGURE 65–3 • Examples of stored electrograms obtained several hours after three different patients had experienced a flurry of shocks from an implantable cardioverter-defibrillator and showing the rhythm recorded by the device immediately before a shock was delivered. A, In this patient, the stored electrogram demonstrates ventricular tachycardia at a rate of 300 beats per minute, thus indicating that the shock was appropriate. He was treated with amiodarone to reduce the frequency of episodes of ventricular tachycardia. **B,** This patient received shocks because of paroxysmal supraventricular tachycardia at a rate of 206 beats per minute, which exceeded the programmed rate cutoff of 170 beats per minute. He underwent radio frequency ablation of the paroxysmal supraventricular tachycardia and received no further inappropriate shocks. **C,** The stored electrograms in this patient indicate that the patient received inappropriate shocks that were triggered by atrial fibrillation at a rate of 180 beats per minute. The rate cutoff of the device in this patient was 150 beats per minute. This patient was treated with a β-blocker to keep the ventricular rate less than 150 beats per minute during atrial fibrillation.

allow the specific mechanism of the tachycardia to be determined. Depending on the type of tachycardia, the sites in the heart targeted for ablation are determined by the results of mapping or as guided by specific anatomic landmarks. Radio frequency energy is delivered, typically in applications of 1 minute, at a power setting sufficient to result in adequate tissue heating of 60 to 70° C.

Radio Frequency Ablation of Supraventricular Arrhythmias

AV nodal re-entrant tachycardia (Chapter 63), the most common type of paroxysmal SVT, is eliminated by radio frequency ablation of either the "fast" or "slow" limb of the re-entry circuit. For slow-pathway ablation, which is the preferred technique, target sites for ablation are located in the posteroseptal aspect of the right atrium, near the ostium of the coronary sinus. Slow-pathway ablation has a success rate of 98 to 100% and is associated with a 0 to 1.3% risk for high-degree AV block.

Left-sided accessory pathways are ablated by using either a retrograde aortic or a transseptal approach, and those that are right sided or septal are ablated with a venous approach. Detailed mapping of the accessory pathway is essential for identification of an appropriate ablation site, and the ablation catheter is positioned on either the atrial or the ventricular aspect of the mitral or tricuspid annulus. The success rate of accessory pathway ablation is 90 to 98%, and the complication rate is 2 to 3%. A fatal complication occurs in less than 0.1% of patients. The most common nonfatal but serious complications are cardiac tamponade as a result of mechanical perforation of the heart by an electrode catheter and high-degree AV block in patients with a septal accessory pathway. Cryoablation is associated with a lower risk for AV block and is useful for ablation of accessory pathways located near the AV node.

Detailed mapping is also needed to identify sites for ablation of atrial tachycardias (Chapter 63). Most atrial tachycardias arise in the right atrium and are mapped by using a venous approach, but left atrial tachycardias are mapped via a transseptal approach. Assuming that the atrial tachycardia is arising only at one site, the success rate of ablation is approximately 90%, and complications are rare.

Type I atrial flutter (Chapter 63) arises in the right atrium and can be eliminated by radio frequency ablation directed at a critical isthmus in the low right atrium, between the tricuspid annulus and the inferior vena cava. The success rate of this type of ablation is greater than 90%, and the risk for a serious complication is less than 1%.

In patients with drug-refractory atrial fibrillation (Chapter 63) associated with an uncontrolled ventricular rate, either radio frequency ablation or modification of the AV node can improve symptoms, functional capacity, and left ventricular function. In AV node ablation, a third-degree AV block is intentionally induced; the success rate is 100%, and all patients require a permanent pacemaker. In the AV node modification procedure, the intent is to slow the ventricular rate without creating the need for a pacemaker. The success rate of the modification procedure is 75%, and the remaining 25% of patients require a pacemaker because of intentional or unintentional ablation of the AV node.

Catheter ablation aimed at the elimination of atrial fibrillation has been demonstrated to be useful in patients with symptomatic, drug-refractory atrial fibrillation. The 1-year efficacy of catheter ablation appears to be in the range of 75 to 85% for paroxysmal atrial fibrillation and 65 to 75% for chronic atrial fibrillation. The most serious complications are myocardial perforation, thromboembolism, and atrio-esophageal fistula, with an overall risk of 1 to 2%. Pulmonary vein stenosis is a potentially serious complication that can be avoided by not delivering radio frequency energy applications within the tubular portion of the pulmonary veins. Ablation techniques for atrial fibrillation are still evolving, and although early data are encouraging, their long-term efficacy is not yet established.

Inappropriate sinus tachycardia can also be managed with radio frequency ablation, but this approach should be recommended only as a last resort. The sinus node, located in the high lateral portion of the right atrium, is targeted for ablation. The success rate is 80%, and 10% of patients require a pacemaker because of an inadequate atrial escape rate.

Because of a very favorable risk-benefit ratio, radio frequency ablation is appropriate first-line therapy for any patient with paroxysmal SVT, Wolff-Parkinson-White syndrome, or type I atrial flutter that is symptomatic enough to warrant therapy (Chapter 63). In the case of atrial flutter other than type I, atrial fibrillation, and inappropriate sinus tachycardia, an ablation procedure is appropriate only in patients with severe symptoms who are refractory to medication.

Radio Frequency Ablation of Ventricular Tachycardia

Radio frequency ablation has been used as first-line treatment of idiopathic VT. The most common type of idiopathic VT arises in the outflow tract of the right ventricle and has a left bundle branch block configuration and superior axis. Another type of idiopathic VT has a right bundle branch block configuration and a superior axis and arises in the inferoapical aspect of the left ventricle (Chapter 64). The success rate of radio frequency ablation of these types of VT has been 85 to 100%, and complications have been rare.

In patients with CAD, VT usually arises in diseased tissue adjacent to an area of previous infarction in the left ventricle. Because the disease process is diffuse instead of focal and because VT may originate at multiple sites, radio frequency ablation of VT is not usually curative in patients with CAD. More often, radio frequency ablation is used as adjunctive therapy with an ICD or with antiarrhythmic drug therapy. In the setting of CAD, the success rate of radio frequency ablation of VT has been 65 to 95%, with serious complications occurring in less than 2% of patients.

ARRHYTHMIA SURGERY

Wolff-Parkinson-White Syndrome

At present, surgical ablation of an accessory pathway may be indicated for the occasional patient with Wolff-Parkinson-White syndrome who has potentially dangerous arrhythmias and in whom radio frequency catheter ablation is unsuccessful. When performed by an experienced surgeon, the success rate of surgical ablation of an accessory pathway approaches 100%, and the risk for a serious complication is low. Intraoperative mapping is necessary to establish the location of the accessory pathway, which then can be ablated either cryosurgically via an epicardial approach or by direct dissection via an endocardial approach.

Ventricular Tachycardia in Patients with Coronary Artery Disease

Subendocardial resection may be appropriate at the time of another surgical cardiac procedure in patients with CAD and recurrent, sustained, monomorphic VT. The substrate for monomorphic VT in patients with CAD usually lies within visually apparent scar tissue surrounding an area of previous myocardial infarction (Chapter 64). Subendocardial resection has been successful in eliminating VT when performed either on a visual basis, with resection or cryoablation of all visually apparent scar tissue, or on a map-guided basis, with resection or cryoablation limited to the areas found to be participating in generation of the VT. At centers experienced in this type of surgery, the success rate of subendocardial resection has been 85 to 90%, and the operative mortality rate has been in the range of 5 to 10%. Although subendocardial resection has the potential advantage of preventing recurrences of VT, the relatively high operative mortality rate and the widespread availability of ICDs have discouraged its use.

Atrial Fibrillation

In the Maze procedure, a series of incisions or linear lesions or both (created by cryoablation or radio frequency ablation) are made in specific regions of the left and right atria to subdivide the atria into parts too small to sustain atrial fibrillation. The operative mortality rate associated with the Maze procedure is less than 2%, and more than 90% of patients have had no recurrences of atrial fibrillation during long-term follow-up. However, because it requires extensive surgery, the Maze procedure is performed by only a small number of surgeons.

A variety of simpler operative procedures for atrial fibrillation have been developed, some of which can be performed with minimally invasive surgery. The long-term efficacy of these simpler procedures is lower than that of the Maze procedure, but because of their ease and low risk, their use has become widespread, mostly as an adjunct to valve or coronary bypass surgery.

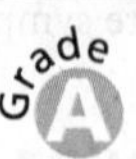

1. Connelly SJ, Kerr CR, Gent M, et al: Effects of physiological pacing versus ventricular pacing on the risk of stroke and death due to cardiovascular causes. N Engl J Med 2000;342:1385–1391.
2. Lamas GA, Lee KL, Sweeney MO, et al: Ventricular pacing or dual-chamber pacing for sinus-node dysfunction. N Engl J Med 2002;346:1854–1862.
3. The Antiarrhythmics versus Implantable Defibrillators (AVID) Investigators: A comparison of antiarrhythmic-drug therapy with implantable defibrillators in patients resuscitated from near-fatal ventricular arrhythmias. N Engl J Med 1997;337:1576–1583.
4. Buxton AE, Lee KL, Fisher JD, et al: A randomized study of the prevention of sudden death in patients with coronary artery disease. Multicenter Unsustained Tachycardia Trial Investigators. N Engl J Med 1999;341:1882–1890.
5. Moss AJ, Zareba W, Hall WJ, et al: Prophylactic implantation of a defibrillator in patients with myocardial infarction and reduced ejection fraction. N Engl J Med 2002;346:877–883.
6. Bardy GH, Lee KL, Mark DB, et al: Amiodarone or an implantable cardioverter-defibrillator for congestive heart failure. N Engl J Med 2005;352:225–237.
7. Bristow MR, Saxon LA, Boehmer J, et al: Cardiac-resynchronization therapy with or without an implantable defibrillator in advanced chronic heart failure. N Engl J Med 2004;350:2140–2150.

SUGGESTED READINGS

Gregoratos G, Abrams J, Epstein AE, et al: ACC/AHA/NASPE 2002 guideline update for implantation of cardiac pacemakers and antiarrhythmia devices—summary article. J Am Coll Cardiol 2002;40:1703–1719. *A detailed description of the indications for implantation of permanent pacemakers and implantable cardioverter-defibrillators.*

Morady F: Catheter ablation of supraventricular arrhythmias: State of the art. J Cardiovasc Electrophysiol 2004;15:124–139. *An in-depth review of catheter ablation of supraventricular arrhythmias, including atrial fibrillation.*

Schoenfeld M: Contemporary pacemaker and defibrillator device therapy: Challenges confronting the general cardiologist. Circulation 2007;115:638–653. *A practical review.*

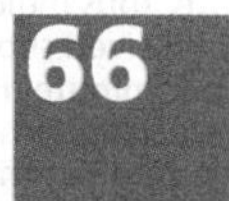

66 ARTERIAL HYPERTENSION

Ronald G. Victor

Definition

Across populations, the risks of heart disease and stroke increase continuously and logarithmically with increasing levels of systolic and diastolic blood pressure at or above 115/75 mm Hg (Fig. 66–1). Thus, the dichotomous separation of "normal" from "high" blood pressure is artificial, and the definition of arterial hypertension (i.e., high blood pressure) has been a moving target. On the basis of results of randomized clinical drug trials, *hypertension* currently is defined as a usual blood pressure of 140/90 mm Hg or higher (Table 66–1), the value above which the benefits of treatment appear to outweigh the risks. *Prehypertension* is a new designation for mildly elevated blood pressures between 120/80 and 139/89 mm Hg, a level at which progression to hypertension is twice as likely as with a blood pressure below 120/80 mm Hg, and cardiovascular risk retains its continuous log-linear function compared with lower blood pressures. The cardiovascular mortality rate is only half as great at 120/80 mm Hg as at 140/90 mm Hg, but it is unknown whether the benefits of treating prehypertension outweigh the risks.

Epidemiology

Affecting one quarter of the adult population (60 million in the United States and 1 billion people worldwide), arterial hypertension is the leading cause of death in the world and the most common cause for an outpatient visit to a physician; it is the most easily recognized treatable risk factor for stroke (Chapters 430, 431, and 432), myocardial infarction (Chapters 71 and 72), heart failure (Chapters 57 and 58), peripheral vascular disease (Chapter 79), aortic dissection (Chapter 78), atrial fibrillation (Chapter 63), and end-stage kidney disease (Chapter 131). Despite this knowledge and unequivocal scientific proof that treatment of hypertension can prevent many of its life-altering complications, hypertension remains untreated or undertreated in the majority of affected individuals in all countries, including those with the most advanced systems of medical care (Fig. 66–2). Inadequate treatment of hypertension is a major factor contributing to some of the adverse secular trends since the early 1990s, including an increased incidence of stroke, heart failure, and kidney failure plus a leveling off of the decline in coronary heart disease mortality.

The asymptomatic nature of the condition impedes early detection, which requires regular blood pressure measurement. Because most cases of hypertension cannot be cured, blood pressure control requires lifelong treatment with prescription medication, which is costly and often causes more symptoms than the underlying disease process. Effective management requires continuity of care by a regular and knowledgeable physician as well as sustained active involvement by an educated patient.

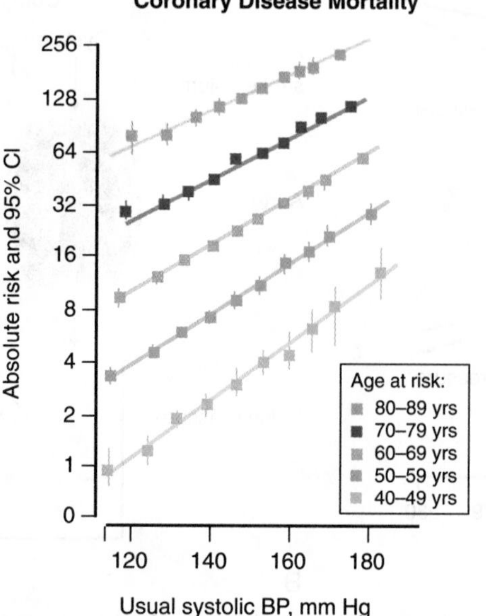

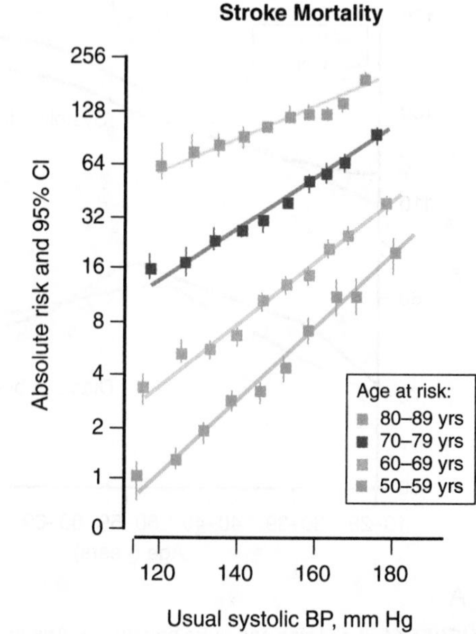

FIGURE 66–1 • Absolute risk of coronary artery disease and stroke mortality by usual systolic blood pressure (BP) levels. (From Lewington S, Clarke R, Qizilbash N, et al; Prospective Studies Collaboration: Age-specific relevance of usual blood pressure to vascular mortality: A meta-analysis of individual data for one million adults in 61 prospective studies. Lancet 2002;360:1903–1913.)

TABLE 66–1 STAGING OF OFFICE BLOOD PRESSURE*

Blood Pressure Stage	Systolic Blood Pressure (mm Hg)	Diastolic Blood Pressure (mm Hg)
Normal	<120	<80
Prehypertension	120–139	80–89
Stage 1 hypertension	140–159	90–99
Stage 2 hypertension	≥160	≥100

*Calculation of seated blood pressure is based on the mean of two or more readings on two separate office visits.
From Chobanian A, Bakris G, Black H, et al: The Seventh Report of the Joint National Committee on the Prevention, Evaluation, and Treatment of High Blood Pressure. The JNC 7 report. JAMA 2003;289:2560–2572.

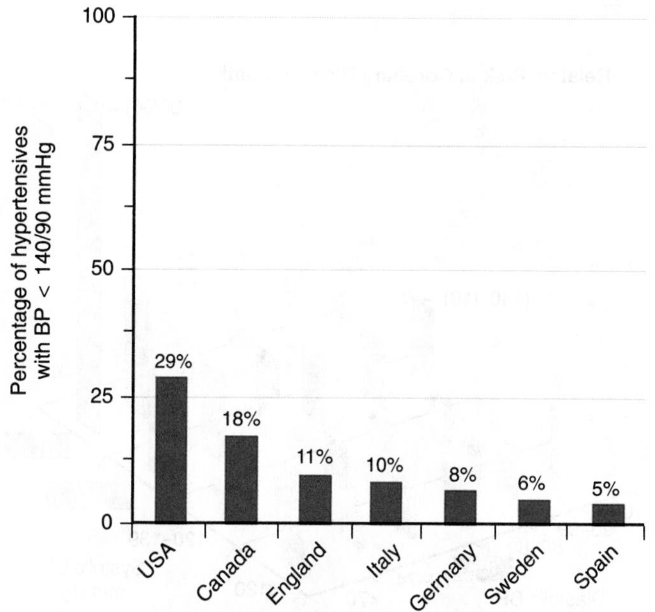

FIGURE 66–2 • Hypertension control rates in North America and Europe. (From Wolf-Maier K, Cooper RS, Kramer H, et al: Hypertension treatment and control in five European countries, Canada, and the United States. Hypertension 2004;43:10–17.)

Aging and Pulse Pressure

Patients often ask which is more important, systolic or diastolic blood pressure. The answer depends on the age of the patient. In industrialized societies, systolic pressure rises progressively with age; if individuals live long enough, almost all (>90%) develop hypertension. This age-dependent rise in blood pressure is not an essential part of human biology. In less industrialized societies where consumption of calories and salt is low, blood pressures remain low and do not rise with age. In industrialized societies, diastolic pressure rises until the age of 50 years and decreases thereafter, producing a progressive rise in pulse pressure (systolic pressure minus diastolic pressure) (Fig. 66–3).

Different hemodynamic faults underlie hypertension in younger and older individuals. Patients who develop hypertension before the age of 50 years typically have *combined systolic and diastolic hypertension:* systolic pressure above 140 mm Hg *and* diastolic pressure above 90 mm Hg. The main hemodynamic fault is vasoconstriction at the level of the resistance arterioles. In contrast, the majority of patients who develop hypertension after the age of 50 years have *isolated systolic hypertension:* systolic pressure above 140 mm Hg but diastolic pressure below 90 mm Hg (often below 80 mm Hg). In isolated systolic hypertension, the primary hemodynamic fault is decreased distensibility of the large conduit arteries. Collagen replaces elastin in the elastic lamina of the aorta, a process that is accelerated by both aging and hypertension. When pulse wave velocity increases sufficiently, the rapid return of the arterial pulse wave from the periphery augments central systolic (rather than diastolic) pressure. The augmented systolic load on the left ventricle increases myocardial oxygen demands, whereas the rapid diastolic runoff compromises myocardial perfusion. For these reasons, a blood pressure of 160/60 mm Hg (pulse pressure of 100 mm Hg) carries twice the risk of fatal coronary heart disease as 150/110 mm Hg (pulse pressure of 40 mm Hg) (Fig. 66–4). In the United States and Europe, the majority of uncontrolled hypertension occurs in older patients with isolated systolic hypertension.

Gender and Ethnicity

Before the age of 50 years, the prevalence of hypertension is somewhat lower in women than in men, suggesting a protective effect of estrogen. After menopause, the prevalence of hypertension increases rapidly in women and exceeds that in men.

In the United States, one in three African Americans has hypertension compared with one in four or five whites and Mexican Americans. In African Americans, hypertension also starts at a younger age, is more severe, and causes greater target organ damage, leading to premature disability and death. In the Bogalusa Heart Study, higher blood pressures in African American than in white children were already evident by grade school. Nevertheless, hypertension is more prevalent in the white populations of several European countries (Finland, Germany, Spain) than in African Americans and is rare among Africans living in Africa (Fig. 66–5).

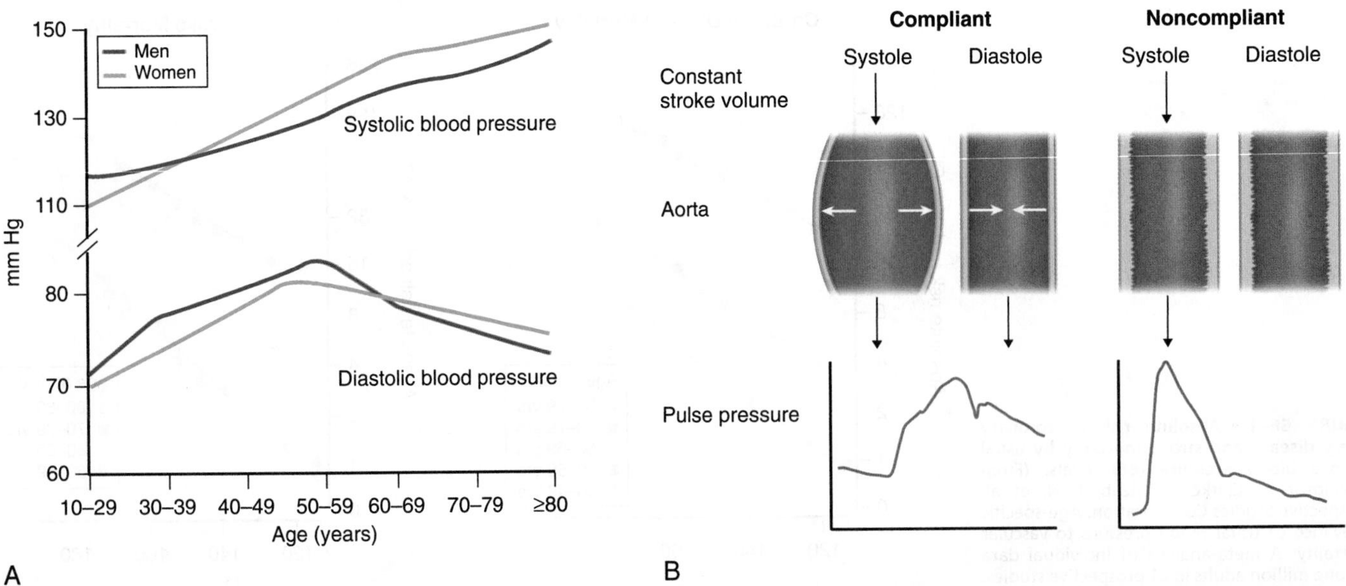

FIGURE 66–3 • Aging and pulse pressure. A, Age-dependent changes in systolic and diastolic blood pressure in the United States. (From Burt V, Whelton P, Rocella EJ, et al: Prevalence of hypertension in the U.S. adult population. Results from the Third National Health and Nutrition Examination Survey, 1988–1991. Hypertension 1995;25:305–313.) **B,** Schematic diagram showing the relation between aortic compliance and pulse pressure. (Courtesy of Dr. Stanley Franklin, University of California at Irvine, with permission.)

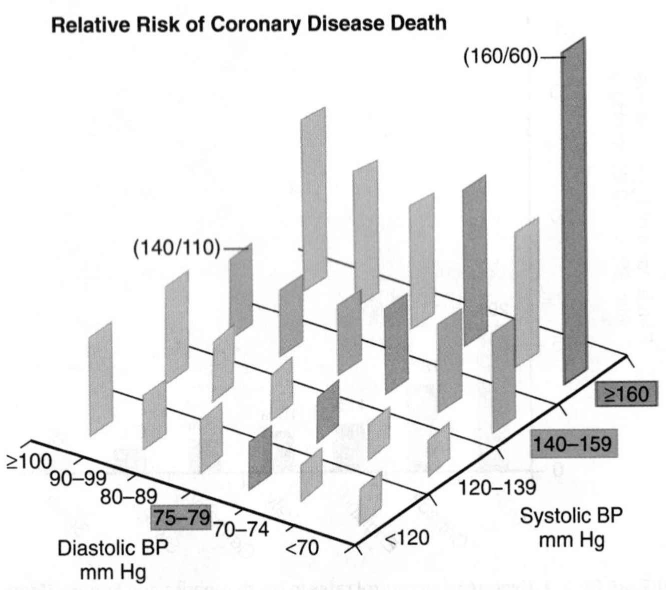

FIGURE 66–4 • Joint influences of systolic blood pressure and diastolic blood pressure on coronary heart disease risk in the Multiple Risk Factor Intervention Trial. (From Neaton JD, Wentworth D: Serum cholesterol, blood pressure, cigarette smoking, and death from coronary heart disease. Overall findings and differences by age for 316,099 white men. Arch Intern Med 1992;152:56–64.)

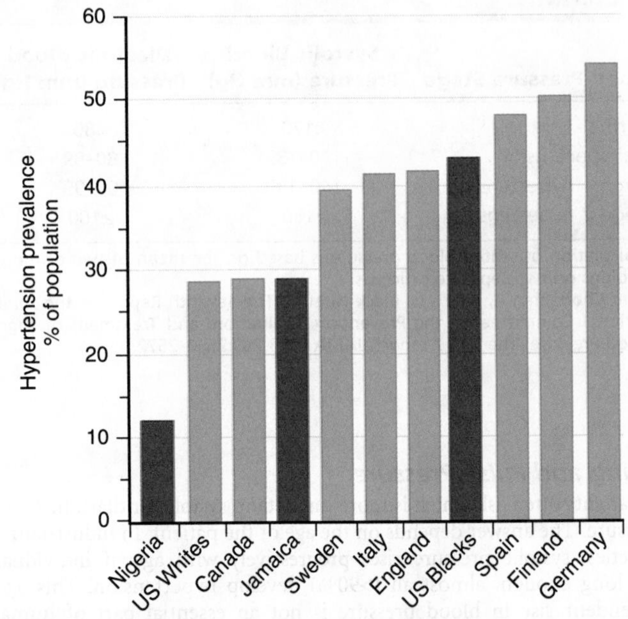

FIGURE 66–5 • Geographic variation in hypertension prevalence in populations of African and European ancestries. (From Cooper RS, Wolf-Maier K, Luke A, et al: An international comparative study of blood pressure in populations of European vs. African descent. BMC Med 2005;3:1–8.)

Pathobiology

In 90 to 95% of hypertensive patients, a single reversible cause of the elevated blood pressure cannot be identified, hence the term *primary hypertension.* However, in most patients with primary hypertension, readily identifiable behaviors—habitually excessive consumption of calories, salt, or alcohol—contribute to the elevated blood pressure. In the remaining 5 to 10%, a more discrete mechanism can be identified, and the condition is termed *secondary or identifiable hypertension.* At the organ-system level, hypertension results from a gain in function of pathways that promote vasoconstriction and renal sodium retention or a loss in function of pathways that promote vasodilation and renal sodium excretion. Neural, hormonal, and vascular mechanisms are involved. There is increasing evidence that neurohormonal activation contributes to the early pathogenesis by compromising vascular function (e.g., endothelium-dependent vasodilation) and structure (e.g., inward remodeling) that precede hypertension.

Behavioral Determinants of Human Blood Pressure Variation

The most important behavioral determinants of blood pressure are related to dietary consumption of calories and salt. Across populations, the prevalence of hypertension increases linearly with average body mass index. With the unrelenting obesity epidemic in both developed and developing societies, increasing attention is being paid to the *metabolic syndrome* (Chapter 248) that often accompanies hypertension. The metabolic syndrome refers to the frequent clustering of elevated blood pressure with abdominal ("male pattern") adiposity, insulin resistance with glucose intolerance, and a dyslipidemic pattern consisting typically of elevated plasma triglyceride and low high-density lipoprotein cholesterol levels. In the Framingham Heart Study, obesity has been estimated to account for as much as 60% of the new cases of hypertension. The underlying mechanisms by which weight gain leads to hypertension are incompletely understood, but there is mounting evidence for an expanded plasma volume plus sympathetic overactivity. The sympathetic overactivity is thought to be a compensatory attempt to burn fat but at the expense of peripheral vasoconstriction, renal salt and water retention, and hypertension. In some obese individuals, sleep apnea (Chapter 101) is an important cause of hypertension. Repeated arterial desaturation sensitizes the carotid body chemoreceptors, causing sustained sympathetic overactivity even during waking hours.

Dietary sodium intake is another key behavioral determinant of human hypertension. In the INTERSALT study of 52 locations around the world, the risk for development of hypertension during three decades of adult life was linearly and tightly related to dietary sodium intake. However, interindividual variability in blood pressure responses to dietary sodium loading and sodium restriction indicates an important genetic underpinning.

Genetic Determinants of Human Blood Pressure Variation

Concordance of blood pressures is greater within families than in unrelated individuals, greater between monozygotic twins than between dizygotic twins, and greater between biologic siblings than between adoptive siblings living in the same household. As much as 70% of the familial aggregation of blood pressure is attributed to shared genes rather than to shared environment. Despite the mapping of the human genome, as yet little is known about the genetic determinants of blood pressure variation in the general population.

In contrast, genetic research has identified 14 genes that cause mendelian forms of hypertension and 9 genes that cause mendelian forms of hypotension. In every case, the mechanism involves the renal handling of salt and water, thereby emphasizing the pivotal importance of the renin-angiotensin-aldosterone system in human blood pressure regulation. However, the identified mendelian forms of hypertension altogether are responsible for a tiny fraction of the 60 million cases of hypertension in the United States, and thus far there is little evidence that milder mutations in any of these 23 genes, alone or in combination, confer resistance against or sensitivity to the hypertensive effects of the common environmental exposures in the general population.

Clinical Manifestations

Hypertension has been termed the silent killer, an asymptomatic chronic disorder that silently damages the blood vessels, heart, brain, and kidneys if it is undetected and untreated. Although headaches (Chapter 421) are common in patients with mild to moderate hypertension, episodes of headaches do not correlate with fluctuations in ambulatory blood pressure. Rather, they correlate with a person's awareness of his or her diagnosis.

Diagnosis

Initial Evaluation for Hypertension

The initial evaluation for hypertension should accomplish three goals: (1) stage the blood pressure, (2) assess the patient's overall cardiovascular risk, and (3) detect clues of secondary hypertension that require further evaluation. *The initial clinical data needed to accomplish these goals are obtained by a thorough history and physical examination, routine blood tests, spot (preferably first morning) urine specimen, and resting 12-lead electrocardiogram.* In some patients, ambulatory blood pressure monitoring and echocardiography provide helpful additional data about the time-integral burden of blood pressure on the cardiovascular system.

Goal 1: Accurate Assessment of Blood Pressure

Office Blood Pressure

Because blood pressure normally varies widely throughout a 24-hour period, multiple readings on more than one occasion are required to obtain a clear picture of a person's "usual" blood pressure. For this reason, *hypertension should not be diagnosed on the basis of a single elevated reading.*

To minimize variability in office readings, blood pressure should be measured at least twice after 5 minutes of rest with the patient seated, the back supported, and the arm bare and at heart level. The most common mistake in measuring blood pressure is use of a standard-issue cuff that is too small for a large arm, thereby producing spuriously elevated readings. Most overweight adults will require a "large-adult" cuff. Tobacco and caffeine should be avoided for at least 30 minutes. To avoid underestimation of systolic pressure in older persons who may have an "auscultatory gap" due to arteriosclerosis, radial artery palpation should be performed to estimate systolic pressure; then the cuff should be inflated to a value 20 mm Hg higher than the level that obliterates the radial pulse and deflated at a rate of 3 to 5 mm Hg/sec. Blood pressure should be measured in both arms and after 5 minutes of standing to exclude a significant postural fall in blood pressure, particularly in older persons and in those with diabetes or other conditions (e.g., Parkinson's disease) that predispose to autonomic insufficiency.

Blood pressure currently is staged as normal, prehypertension, or hypertension on the basis of the average of two or more readings taken at two or more office visits. When a person's average systolic and diastolic pressures fall into different stages, the higher stage applies (see Table 66–1).

Home and Ambulatory Blood Pressure Monitoring

Cuff inflation and visits to the physician's office often evoke transient adrenergic responses that vary in magnitude from one patient to the next. In most patients, blood pressures are higher in the physician's office than when they are measured at home or during normal daily life outside the home. Self-monitoring of blood pressure outside of the physician's office actively engages a patient in his or her own health care and provides a better estimate of a person's usual blood pressure for medical decision making. Many electronic home monitors are manufactured, but only a handful of recommended models have been rigorously validated against mercury sphygmomanometry (see *www.dableducational.com*). Even then, each patient's monitor needs to be checked in the office for accuracy. To reduce reporting bias, patients should be instructed to record their pressures at fixed intervals, to keep all the readings, and if possible to use a monitor that is equipped with a printer.

Ambulatory monitoring provides automated measurements of blood pressure during a 24-hour period while patients are engaging in their usual activities, including sleep. Prospective outcome studies in both treated and untreated patients have proved that ambulatory blood pressure measurement is superior to standard office measurement in predicting fatal and nonfatal myocardial infarction and stroke. With ambulatory monitoring, current recommendations for *upper limits of normal* are a mean daytime blood pressure of 135/85 mm Hg, a mean nighttime blood pressure of 120/70 mm Hg, and a mean 24-hour blood pressure of 130/80 mm Hg. However, an *optimal* mean daytime ambulatory blood pressure is less than 130/80 mm Hg. With self-monitoring of blood pressure at home, an average value of 130/80 mm Hg should be considered the upper limit of normal; blood pressure should be lower in one's own home than with daily activities outside the home.

Up to one third of patients with elevated office blood pressures have normal home or ambulatory blood pressures. If the 24-hour blood pressure profile is completely normal (including a mean daytime ambulatory blood pressure below 130/80 mm Hg) and there is no target organ damage despite consistently elevated office readings, the patient has "office only" or "white coat" hypertension, presumably due to a transient adrenergic response to the measurement of blood pressure in the physician's office. In such rigorously defined white coat hypertension, the 5-year mortality rate in multiple large studies has been indistinguishable from that of patients with normal office blood pressures. However, many patients do not have pure white coat hypertension; rather, they have "white coat aggravation," a white coat reaction superimposed on persistent ambulatory or nocturnal hypertension that needs treatment. Currently, the only Medicare-approved indication for ambulatory monitoring is elevated office blood pressure with repeatedly normal home readings in the absence of demonstrable target organ damage (ICD 796.2).

Recent data argue that the indications for ambulatory monitoring should be expanded (Table 66–2). In up to 30% of treated patients with persistently elevated office blood pressures, ambulatory monitoring documents adequate or excessive control of hypertension, eliminating overtreatment (Fig. 66–6). In other patients, office readings underestimate ambulatory blood pressures, presumably because of sympathetic overactivity in daily life due to job or home stress, tobacco abuse, or other adrenergic stimulation that dissipates when the patient comes to the office. Such documentation prevents underdiagnosis and undertreatment of this "masked hypertension," which is present in up to 10% of patients and clearly increases cardiovascular risk (despite normal office blood pressure readings).

Ambulatory monitoring is the only way to detect nocturnal hypertension. Blood pressure normally dips during sleep at night and increases sharply when a person awakens and becomes active in the morning (see Fig. 66–6). Persistent nocturnal hypertension increases the aggregate blood pressure burden on the cardiovascular system and is a much stronger predictor of cardiovascular outcomes than daytime ambulatory blood pressure or standard office measurements are. Nocturnal hypertension is particularly common in patients with chronic kidney disease (Chapter 131), presumably because of their sustained sympathetic overactivity, which does not shut down during sleep, and centralization of blood volume with nocturnal recumbence. The morning surge in blood pressure is strongly associated with the peak incidence of stroke, myocardial infarction, and sudden cardiac death. Thus, medication ideally should be finely tuned to normalize the entire 24-hour blood pressure profile, particularly in high-risk patients (see Table 66–2).

Goal 2: Cardiovascular Risk Stratification

Most patients with blood pressures in the prehypertensive or hypertensive range will have one or more additional risk factors for atherosclerosis. The gradient between increasing levels of systolic blood pressure and cardiovascular risk becomes progressively steeper as additional risk factors are added (Fig. 66–7). For example, in a 50-year-old woman with no other cardiovascular risk factors, her 5-year risk of a cardiovascular complication is 1% if her systolic pressure is 110 mm Hg and only 3% if her systolic pressure is as high as 180 mm Hg. If the same woman were a smoker with a total cholesterol value of 240 mg/dL and a high-density lipoprotein cholesterol value of 40 mg/dL, her 5-year risk of a cardiovascular complication would increase from 5% if her systolic pressure is 110 mm Hg to 18% if her systolic pressure is 180 mm Hg. As the overall risks multiply, blood pressure control becomes more important.

The latest U.S. treatment guidelines recommend a usual blood pressure of 140/90 mm Hg as the threshold for initiation of a lifetime of antihypertensive medication in most patients, with a lower threshold of 130/80 mm Hg for high-risk patients with diabetes or chronic kidney disease. On the basis of subsequent data, it is reasonable to expand the definition of "high risk" to include diabetes mellitus, chronic kidney disease (estimated glomerular filtration rate below 60 mL/min/1.73 m^2 or estimated urinary albumin excretion above 300 mg per 24 hours), clinically evident cardiovascular disease (coronary disease, stroke, or heart failure), and left ventricular hypertrophy by electrocardiography or echocardiography (Table 66–3).

TABLE 66–2 RECOMMENDED INDICATIONS FOR AMBULATORY BLOOD PRESSURE MONITORING

Suspected "white coat hypertension"*
Suspected "white coat aggravation" in a patient with medically refractory hypertension
Suspected masked hypertension or suspected nocturnal hypertension
Hypertension of pregnancy
Suspected orthostatic hypotension or autonomic failure

*Medicare currently reimburses for ambulatory monitoring only to confirm the diagnosis of white coat hypertension that is suspected on the basis of three normal home readings in patients with no evidence of target organ damage despite repeatedly elevated office blood pressure readings (ICD 796.2).
Modified from O'Brien E, Asmar R, Beilin L, et al: Practice guidelines of the European Society of Hypertension for clinic, ambulatory and self blood pressure measurement. J Hypertens 2005;23:697–701.

Goal 3: Identification and Treatment of Secondary (Identifiable) Causes of Hypertension

A thorough search for secondary causes (Table 66–4) is not cost-effective in most patients with hypertension but becomes critically important in two circumstances: (1) when there is a compelling finding on the initial evaluation and (2) when the hypertensive process is so severe that it either is refractory to intensive multiple-drug therapy or requires hospitalization.

Renal Parenchymal Hypertension

Chronic kidney disease (Chapter 131) is the most common cause of secondary hypertension. Hypertension is present in more than 85% of patients with chronic kidney disease and is a major factor causing their increased cardiovascular morbidity and mortality. The mechanisms causing the hypertension include an expanded plasma volume and peripheral vasoconstriction; the peripheral vasoconstriction is caused by both activation of vasoconstrictor pathways (renin-angiotensin and sympathetic nervous systems) and inhibition of vasodilator pathways (nitric oxide).

Renal insufficiency should be considered when there is proteinuria by dipstick or when the serum creatinine level is greater than 1.2 mg/dL in hypertensive women or greater than 1.4 mg/dL in hypertensive men. The diagnosis and staging of chronic kidney disease are done by a simple spot urine collection and standard blood chemistries revealing an estimated glomerular filtration rate below 60 mL/min/1.73 m^2 or albuminuria, defined as a urine albumin–to–urine creatinine ratio of 30 mg/g (equivalent to excretion of 30 mg of albumin per 24 hours) or higher. Several calculators of glomerular filtration rate are readily available on the Internet (*www.nephron.com; www.newtech.kidney.org*).

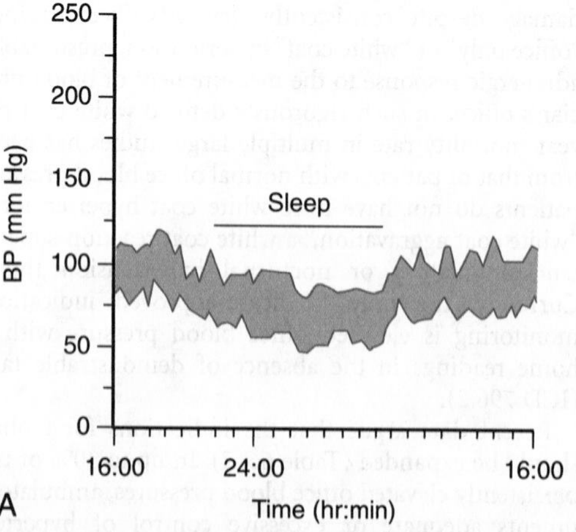

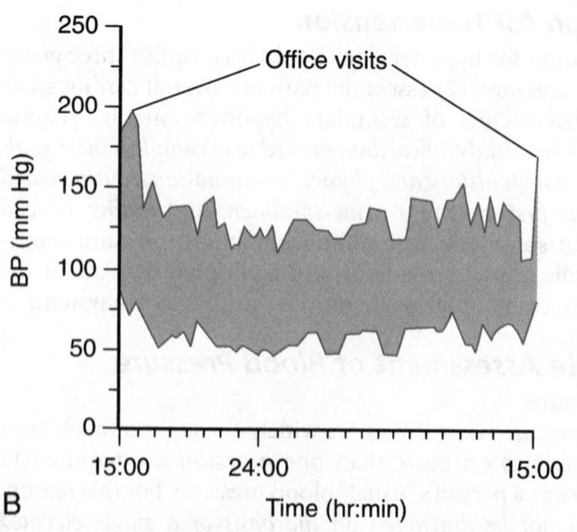

FIGURE 66–6 • The 24-hour ambulatory blood pressure (BP) monitor tracings of two different patients. A, Optimal blood pressure in a healthy 37-year-old woman. Note the normal variability in blood pressure, the nocturnal dip in blood pressure during sleep, and the sharp increase in blood pressure on awakening. (Tracing courtesy of Ronald G. Victor, MD, Hypertension Division, Department of Internal Medicine, University of Texas Southwestern Medical Center, Dallas, Texas.) **B,** Pronounced white coat effect in an 80-year-old woman referred for evaluation of medically refractory hypertension. Documentation of the white coat effect prevented overtreatment of the patient's isolated systolic hypertension. (Tracing provided by Wanpen Vongpatanasin, MD, Hypertension Division, Department of Internal Medicine, University of Texas Southwestern Medical Center, Dallas, Texas.)

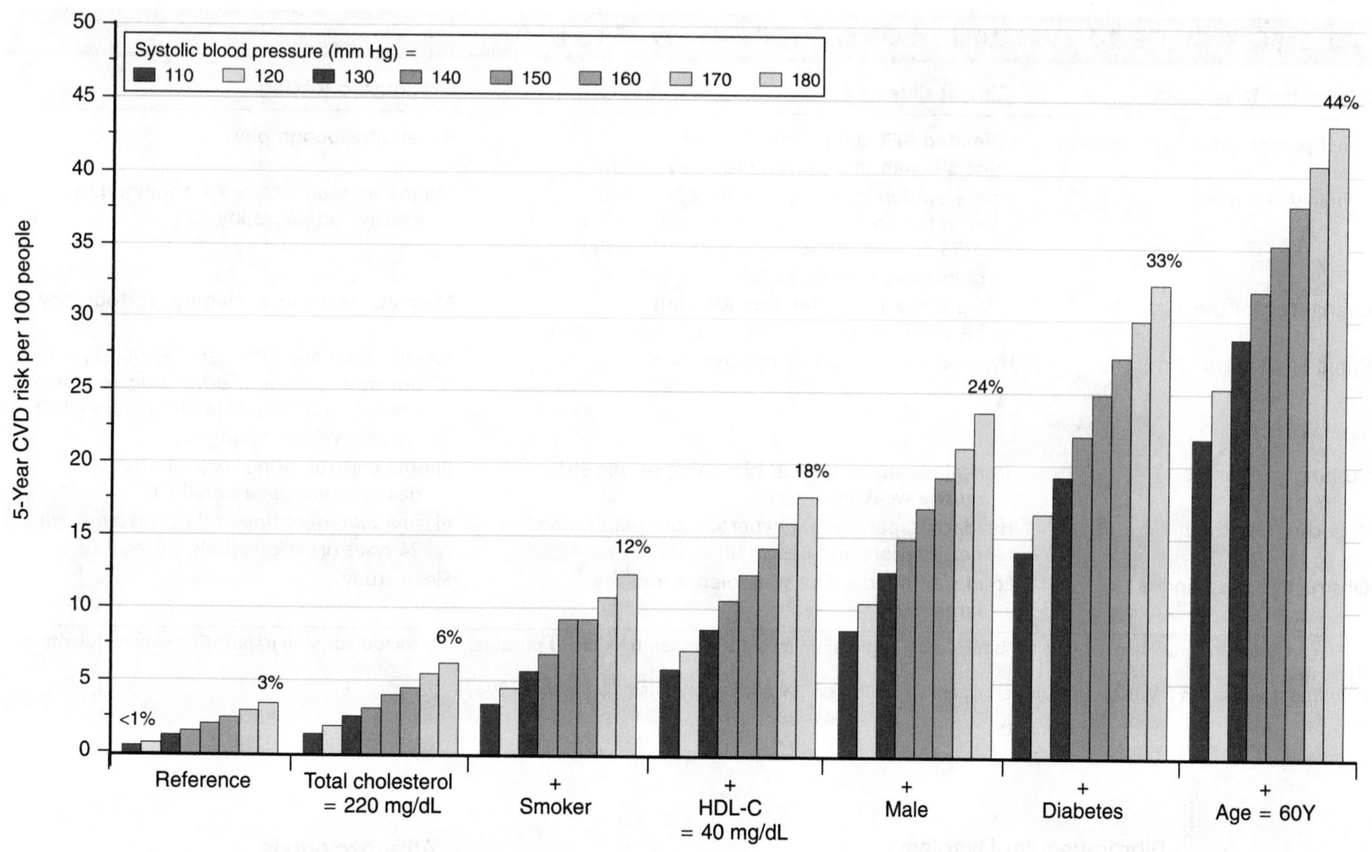

FIGURE 66–7 • Absolute risk of cardiovascular disease (CVD) during 5 years in patients by systolic blood pressure at specified levels of other risk factors. The reference category is a nondiabetic, nonsmoking woman aged 50 years with a total cholesterol value of 190 mg/dL and a high-density lipoprotein cholesterol (HDL-C) value of 60 mg/dL. Risks are given for systolic pressures of 110, 120, 130, 140, 150, 160, 170, and 180 mm Hg. In the other categories, additional risk factors are added consecutively. (From Jackson R, Lawes CMM, Benett DA, et al: Treatment with drugs to lower blood pressure and blood cholesterol based on an individual's absolute cardiovascular risk. Lancet 2005;365:434–441.)

TABLE 66–3 RECOMMENDED (TARGET) BLOOD PRESSURE VALUES

Uncomplicated hypertension: target BP <140/90 mm Hg
Accepted indications for target BP <130/80 mm Hg
Diabetes mellitus
Chronic kidney disease
GFR <60 mL/min/1.73 m²
Urine albumin-to-creatinine ratio ≥30 mg/g
Additional considerations for target BP <130/80 mm Hg
Stable coronary artery disease
Secondary prevention of stroke or TIA
Left ventricular hypertrophy

BP = blood pressure; GFR = glomerular filtration rate; TIA = transient ischemic attack.

In patients with mild (stage 2: glomerular filtration rate of 60 to 90 mL/min/1.73 m^2) or moderate (stage 3: glomerular filtration rate of 30 to 60 mL/min/1.73 m^2) chronic kidney disease, stringent blood pressure control is imperative both to slow the progression to end-stage renal disease and to reduce the excessive cardiovascular risk. In patients with severe chronic kidney disease, hypertension often becomes difficult to treat and may require either (1) intensive medical treatment with loop diuretics, potent vasodilators (e.g., minoxidil), high-dose β-adrenergic blockers, and central sympatholytics or (2) initiation of chronic hemodialysis as the only effective way to reduce plasma volume. In chronic hemodialysis patients, the challenge is to control interdialytic hypertension without exacerbating dialysis-induced hypotension. The gross annual mortality rate in the hemodialysis population is 25%; half of this excessive mortality is caused by cardiovascular events that are related, at least in part, to hypertension.

Renovascular Hypertension

Unilateral or bilateral renal artery stenosis is present in less than 2% of hypertensive patients in a general medical practice but up to 30% of patients referred to a hypertension specialist for refractory hypertension. The main causes of renal artery stenosis are atherosclerosis (85% of cases), typically in older persons with other clinical manifestations of systemic atherosclerosis, and fibromuscular dysplasia (15% of cases; Chapter 126), typically in women between the ages of 15 and 50 years. Unilateral renal artery stenosis leads to underperfusion of the juxtaglomerular cells, thereby producing renin-dependent hypertension even though the contralateral kidney is able to maintain normal blood volume. In contrast, bilateral renal artery stenosis (or unilateral stenosis with a solitary kidney) constitutes a potentially reversible cause of progressive renal failure and volume-dependent hypertension. The following clinical clues increase the suspicion of renovascular hypertension: any hospitalization for urgent or emergent hypertension; recurrent "flash" pulmonary edema; recent worsening of long-standing, previously well controlled hypertension; severe hypertension in a young adult or after the age of 50 years; precipitous and progressive worsening of renal function in response to angiotensin-converting enzyme (ACE) inhibition or angiotensin II receptor blockade; unilateral small kidney by any radiographic study; extensive peripheral arteriosclerosis; and a flank bruit.

The diagnosis of fibromuscular dysplasia (Chapter 126) in a young woman with recent-onset hypertension is readily supported by noninvasive testing with magnetic resonance or spiral computed tomographic angiography showing the classic "string of beads" appearance of a renal artery (Fig. 66–8A). Once the diagnosis is confirmed with invasive angiography, balloon angioplasty is the treatment of choice, with complete cure of hypertension in 40% of patients, improved blood pressure control in almost all patients, and a restenosis rate of only 10%. Medical therapy with an ACE inhibitor also may be effective, but the risks of teratogenicity must be considered in women of childbearing age.

In contrast, the approach to the older patient with generalized atherosclerosis and renal artery stenosis (see Fig. 66-8B) is not straightforward

TABLE 66–4 GUIDE TO EVALUATION OF SECONDARY HYPERTENSION

Suspected Diagnosis	Clinical Clues	Diagnostic Testing
Renal parenchymal hypertension	Estimated GFR <60 mL/min/1.73 m^2 Urine albumin-to-creatinine ratio ≥30 mg/g	Renal ultrasonography
Renovascular disease	New elevation in serum creatinine, marked elevation in serum creatinine with initiation of ACEI or ARB, refractory hypertension, flash pulmonary edema, abdominal bruit	Magnetic resonance or CT angiography, invasive angiography
Coarctation of the aorta	Arm pulses > leg pulses, arm BP > leg BP, chest bruits, rib notching on chest radiography	Magnetic resonance imaging, aortography
Primary aldosteronism	Hypokalemia, refractory hypertension	Plasma renin and aldosterone, 24-hour urine potassium, 24-hour urine aldosterone and potassium after salt loading, adrenal CT, adrenal vein sampling
Cushing's syndrome	Truncal obesity, wide and blanching purple striae, muscle weakness	Plasma cortisol, urine cortisol after dexamethasone, adrenal CT
Pheochromocytoma	Headaches, paroxysmal hypertension, palpitations, perspiration, and pallor; diabetes	Plasma metanephrine and normetanephrine, 24-hour urine catechols, adrenal CT
Obstructive sleep apnea	Loud snoring, daytime somnolence, obesity, large neck	Sleep study

ACEI = angiotensin-converting enzyme inhibitor; ARB = angiotensin receptor blocker; BP = blood pressure; CT = computed tomography; GFR = glomerular filtration rate.
Modified from Kaplan NM: Kaplan's Clinical Hypertension, 8th ed. Philadelphia, Williams & Wilkins, 2002.

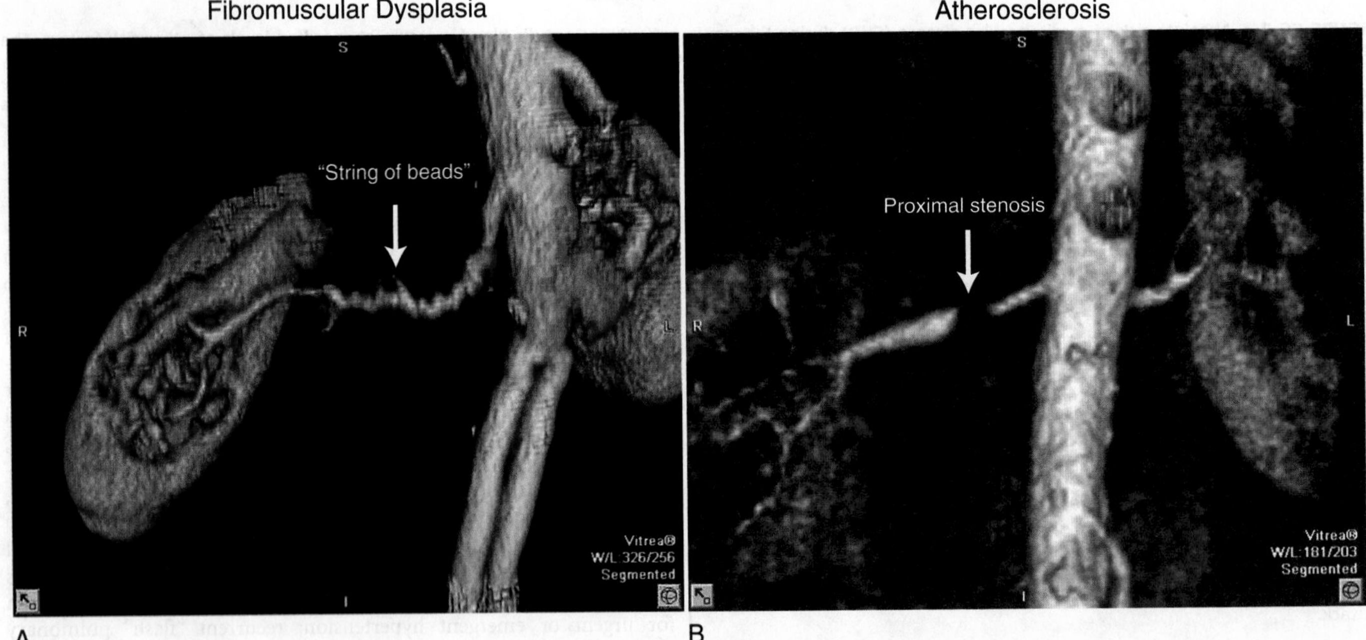

FIGURE 66–8 • Computed tomographic angiogram with three-dimensional reconstruction. A, The classic "string of beads" lesion of fibromuscular dysplasia (bilateral in this patient). **B,** A severe proximal atherosclerotic stenosis of the right renal artery and mild stenosis of the left renal artery. (Images courtesy of Bart Domatch, MD, Radiology Department, University of Texas Southwestern Medical Center, Dallas, Texas.)

and must be highly individualized. Primary hypertension and renovascular hypertension frequently coexist in older persons, and angiographic documentation of renal artery stenosis does not prove that the lesion is an important and reversible cause of the hypertension. For this reason, angioplasty improves hypertension in less than 30% of patients, and complete cures are rare; surgical revascularization is often reserved for patients undergoing simultaneous aortic reconstruction. In the absence of definitive data from randomized trials, revascularization should be considered for medically refractory hypertension, progressive renal failure with medical therapy, and bilateral renal artery stenosis or stenosis of a solitary functioning kidney.

Mineralocorticoid-Induced Hypertension Due to Primary Aldosteronism

The most common causes of primary aldosteronism (Chapter 245) are a unilateral aldosterone-producing adenoma and bilateral adrenal hyperplasia. Because aldosterone is the principal ligand for the mineralocorticoid receptor in the distal nephron, excessive aldosterone production causes excessive renal Na^+-K^+ exchange, often resulting in hypokalemia. The diagnosis should always be suspected when hypertension is accompanied by either unprovoked hypokalemia (serum potassium concentration below 3.5 mmol/L in the absence of diuretic therapy) or a tendency to develop excessive hypokalemia during diuretic therapy (serum potas-

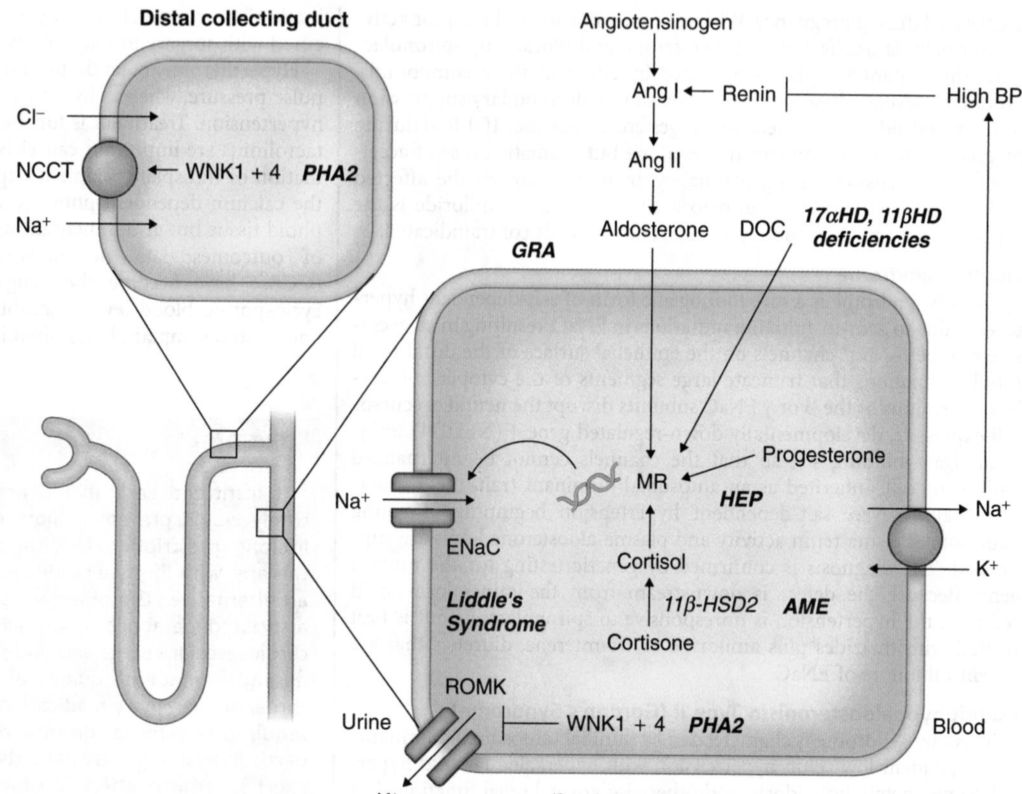

FIGURE 66–9 • Mendelian forms of hypertension that cause mineralocorticoid-induced hypertension. AME = apparent mineralocorticoid excess; Ang = angiotensin; BP = blood pressure; GRA = glucocorticoid-remediable aldosteronism; 17αHD and 11βHD = 17α- and 11β- hydroxylase deficiency; 11β-HSD2 = 11β-hydroxysteroid dehydrogenase type 2; DOC = deoxycorticosterone; ENaC = epithelial Na^+ channel; HEP = hypertension exacerbated by pregnancy; MR = mineralocorticoid receptor; NCCT = sodium-chloride cotransporter; PHA2 = pseudohypoaldosteronism type 2; ROMK = rectifying outer medullary K^+ channel; WNK = with no lysine kinases. See text for explanation. (Modified from Lifton RP, Gharavi AG, Geller DS: Molecular mechanisms of human hypertension. Cell 2001;104:545–556.)

sium concentration below 3.0 mmol/L). However, more than one third of patients do not have hypokalemia on initial presentation, and the diagnosis should also be considered in any patient with resistant hypertension. Laparoscopic surgery and mineralocorticoid receptor blockade with eplerenone constitute highly effective therapeutic options that target the disease-causing mechanism with a favorable risk-to-benefit ratio.

Mendelian Forms of Mineralocorticoid-Induced Hypertension

Almost all the rare mendelian forms of hypertension are mineralocorticoid induced and involve excessive activation of the epithelial Na^+ channel (ENaC), the final common pathway for reabsorption of sodium from the distal nephron (Fig. 66–9). Thus, salt-dependent hypertension can be caused both by gain-of-function mutations of ENaC or the mineralocorticoid receptor and by increased production or decreased clearance of mineralocorticoid receptor ligands, which are aldosterone, deoxycorticosterone, and cortisol.

Glucocorticoid-Remediable Aldosteronism

Fewer than 100 cases of glucocorticoid-remediable aldosteronism have been reported, but many additional cases probably go unreported or are undetected or misdiagnosed as bilateral adrenal hyperplasia. Inherited as an autosomal dominant mutation, glucocorticoid-remediable aldosteronism mimics an aldosterone-producing adenoma by causing severe mineralocorticoid-induced hypertension with hypokalemia, elevated plasma aldosterone, and suppressed plasma renin activity.

In the normal adrenal gland, angiotensin II acts on the enzyme aldosterone synthase in the zona glomerulosa to drive production of aldosterone; adrenocorticotropic hormone (ACTH) causes transcriptional activation of the enzyme 11β-hydroxylase in the zona fasciculata to drive production of cortisol. Glucocorticoid-remediable aldosteronism is caused by a gene duplication arising by unequal crossing over between the genes encoding aldosterone synthase and 11β-hydroxylase. The resulting chimeric gene encodes a hybrid protein that has aldosterone synthase activity, is expressed "ectopically" in the zona fasciculata, and is regulated entirely by ACTH rather than by angiotensin II. Thus, aldosterone production becomes inappropriately linked to cortisol production. In the attempt to maintain the appropriate production of normal levels of cortisol, aldosterone is constantly produced, resulting in volume-dependent hypertension. Although the expanded plasma volume suppresses plasma renin activity and thus angiotensin II, the reduced angiotensin II cannot downregulate aldosterone production.

The clinical clue to the diagnosis is that the hypertension is familial and discovered before the age of 20 years. In contrast, primary aldosteronism is sporadic and usually discovered between the ages of 30 and 60 years. The diagnosis of glucocorticoid-remediable aldosteronism is confirmed by Southern blot analysis for the chimeric gene, a test available at no cost through the International Registry for Glucocorticoid-Remediable Aldosteronism *(www.bwh.partners.org/gra)*. By suppressing ACTH and thus aldosterone secretion from the zona fasciculata, low-dose dexamethasone completely reverses the biochemical abnormalities in glucocorticoid-remediable aldosteronism and is the recommended therapy.

Hypertension Caused by Deoxycorticosterone

The rare but distinctive hypertensive syndromes caused by deoxycorticosterone include those due to congenital deficiency of either 11β-hydroxylase or 17α-hydroxylase. In both cases, decreased production of cortisol reduces feedback inhibition on ACTH, which drives overproduction of deoxycorticosterone (a potent mineralocorticoid). These patients typically present to the pediatrician with hypertension plus abnormal sexual development.

Hypertension Caused by Cortisol

Cortisol is a mineralocorticoid as well as a glucocorticoid, so both excessive production of cortisol (Cushing's syndrome; Chapter 245) and defective cortisol metabolism cause hypertension plus hypokalemia. Normally, the enzyme 11β-hydroxysteroid dehydrogenase type 2 converts cortisol to cortisone, which cannot bind the mineralocorticoid receptor. The *syndrome of apparent mineralocorticoid excess,* which is an autosomal recessive disease due to a loss-of-function mutation of this protective enzyme, results in early-onset hypertension with hypokalemia accompanied by suppressed plasma renin activity and undetectable plasma aldosterone. Glycerrhetinic acid, a metabolite found in licorice (and often used as a flavoring in chewing tobacco and an increasing number of herbal supplements) is a potent inhibitor of 11β-hydroxysteroid dehydrogenase type 2. Thus, habitual ingestion of these substances causes a phenocopy of apparent mineralocorticoid excess. Biochemical confirmation consists of elevations in urinary free cortisol. The congenital syndrome is treated with spironolactone, whereas the phenocopy is treated with diet.

Hypertension Caused by Progesterone

A gain-in-function mutation in the mineralocorticoid receptor is a rare cause of autosomal dominant, early-onset hypertension that is markedly accelerated during pregnancy. Whereas mineralocorticoid receptor activity normally is unaffected by progesterone and blocked by spironolactone, the mutant receptor is activated by either of these compounds, producing severe salt-sensitive hypertension with secondary suppression of renin and aldosterone. Because progesterone increases 100-fold during pregnancy, this mutation constitutes a rare but dramatic cause of accelerated hypertension during pregnancy. In one family, all the affected males developed hypertension before 20 years of age. Amiloride is the suggested treatment of choice, and spironolactone is contraindicated.

Liddle's Syndrome

Liddle's syndrome is a rare monogenic form of salt-dependent hypertension due to gain-in-function mutations in ENaC, resulting in an excessive number of Na^+ channels on the epithelial surface of the distal renal tubule. Mutations that truncate large segments of the cytoplasmic carboxyl terminus of the β or γ ENaC subunits disrupt the neural precursor cell expressed, developmentally down-regulated gene 4 (NEDD4) ubiquitin ligase–binding site so that the channels cannot be internalized within the cell. Inherited as an autosomal dominant trait, these mutations cause severe salt-dependent hypertension beginning in young adulthood. Plasma renin activity and plasma aldosterone levels are suppressed. The diagnosis is confirmed by genetic testing for the mutant gene. Because the defect is downstream from the mineralocorticoid receptor, the hypertension is unresponsive to spironolactone but is best treated with thiazides plus amiloride or triamterene, diuretics that are potent inhibitors of ENaC.

Pseudohypoaldosteronism Type II (Gordon's Syndrome)

This rare syndrome is characterized by familial (autosomal dominant) salt-dependent low-renin hypertension with hyperkalemia, mild hyperchloremic metabolic acidosis, and otherwise normal renal function. The disease-causing genes encode WNK1 and WNK4, members of a novel family of serine-threonine kinases that normally regulate the thiazide-sensitive Na^+-Cl^- cotransporter, which is overactive in affected individuals. Both the hypertension and all its associated metabolic abnormalities are exquisitely sensitive to treatment with thiazide diuretics.

Familial Brachydactyly and Hypertension

Severe autosomal dominant hypertension can be associated with brachydactyly and short stature. The gene has been mapped to the short arm of chromosome 12, but the mechanism of the hypertension is unknown. Unlike the other mendelian forms of hypertension, plasma renin and aldosterone levels are normal, and the hypertension is not salt sensitive.

Pheochromocytomas

Pheochromocytomas are rare catecholamine-producing tumors of the adrenal (or sometimes extra-adrenal) chromaffin cells (Chapter 246). The diagnosis should be suspected when hypertension is accompanied by frequent or refractory headaches or by paroxysms of headache, palpitations, pallor, or diaphoresis. In some patients, pheochromocytoma is misdiagnosed as panic disorder. A family history of early-onset hypertension may suggest pheochromocytoma as part of the multiple endocrine neoplasia syndromes (Chapter 250). If the diagnosis is missed, outpouring of catecholamines from the tumor can cause unsuspected hypertensive crisis during unrelated surgical or diagnostic procedures, such as the intravenous administration of contrast material; in such cases, mortality exceeds 80%.

Other Neurogenic Causes

Other causes of neurogenic hypertension that can be confused with pheochromocytoma include sympathomimetic agents (cocaine, methamphetamine; Chapter 32), baroreflex failure, and obstructive sleep apnea. A history of surgery and radiation therapy for head and neck tumors (Chapter 200) raises suspicion of baroreceptor damage. Snoring and somnolence suggest sleep apnea; continuous positive airway pressure or corrective surgery can improve blood pressure control in some patients with sleep apnea (Chapter 101).

Other Causes of Secondary Hypertension

Coarctation of the aorta typically occurs just distal to the origin of the left subclavian artery, so the blood pressure is lower in the legs than in the arms (opposite of the normal situation) (Chapter 68; see Fig. 55–3). The clue is that the pulses are weaker in the lower than in the upper extremities, indicating the need to measure blood pressure in the legs as well as in both arms. Intercostal collaterals can produce bruits on examination and rib notching on the chest radiograph. Coarctations can be cured with surgery or angioplasty.

Hyperthyroidism tends to cause systolic hypertension with a wide pulse pressure, whereas hypothyroidism tends to cause mainly diastolic hypertension. Treatment is for the underlying disease. Cyclosporine and tacrolimus are important causes of secondary hypertension in the population of transplant recipients, apparently by inhibition of calcineurin, the calcium-dependent phosphatase that is expressed not only in lymphoid tissue but also in neural, vascular, and renal tissue. In the absence of outcomes data, non-dihydropyridine calcium-channel blockers (CCBs) have become the drugs of first choice, but they increase cyclosporine blood levels. Combination therapy with diuretics, CCBs, and central sympatholytics often is required.

Prevention and Treatment of Hypertension

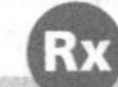

If instituted early in life and sustained, lifestyle modifications surely would prevent millions of cases of hypertension. However, lifelong prescription medication is the cornerstone of effective therapy, with lifestyle modification serving as an adjunct but not as an alternative. The objective is to reduce the blood pressure and associated metabolic abnormalities sufficiently to reduce the risk of cardiovascular events and end-stage renal disease without compromising the patient's quality of life. Multidrug regimens with two, three, or even more medications of different drug classes often are required to achieve currently recommended blood pressure goals, particularly in high-risk patients. Low-dose fixed-drug combinations exert synergistic effects on blood pressure, minimize side effects, and reduce pill burden as well as cost. For a large proportion of patients with hypertension, low-dose aspirin and lipid-lowering therapy are indicated as part of a comprehensive cardiovascular risk reduction strategy.

Lifestyle Modification

Every antihypertensive regimen should include lifestyle modification. The Seventh Report of the Joint National Committee on Prevention, Detection, Evaluation, and Treatment of High Blood Pressure (JNC 7) recommended a trial of lifestyle modification alone for an unspecified time (6 to 12 months in prior guidelines) before antihypertensive medication is prescribed, even for high-risk patients. More recent data suggest greater urgency in achieving rapid pharmacologic control of high blood pressure to minimize cardiovascular risk, especially because nonpharmacologic reductions in blood pressure often are small and recidivism is high. Nevertheless, in sufficiently motivated individuals, lifestyle modification can decrease medication requirements, have a favorable impact on associated cardiovascular risk factors, and emphasize the active role patients can play in controlling their blood pressure.

Moderate dietary sodium reduction (Chapter 232) reduces renal potassium wasting during diuretic therapy and lowers blood pressure by 2/2 mm Hg on average. Most dietary sodium comes from processed foods rather than from the salt shaker. Without draconian measures, daily salt consumption can be reduced from 10 to 6 g by teaching patients to read food labels (6 g of NaCl = 2.4 g of sodium = 100 mmol of sodium). The Dietary Approaches to Stop Hypertension (DASH) study showed that individuals with prehypertension or stage 1 hypertension can lower their blood pressures by as much as 11/6 mm Hg even without restricting calorie or sodium intake if they adhere to a diet rich in fresh fruits and vegetables (for high potassium content) and low-fat dairy products. This diet (*www.nhlbi.nih.gov/health/public/heart/hbp/dash/*) is strongly recommended because the blood pressure–lowering effects can approach the magnitude of drug monotherapy, can be enhanced by an additional 2/1 mm Hg by dietary sodium restriction, and are seen in all ethnic groups, especially African Americans.

Smokers should be counseled to quit because tobacco (Chapter 30) is such a potent risk factor for coronary heart disease, stroke, and progression of hypertensive nephrosclerosis to end-stage renal disease. Because blood pressure increases transiently by 10 to 15 mm Hg after each cigarette, smokers of more than 20 cigarettes per day

Rx

often have higher blood pressures out of the office. Blood pressure increases similarly with the first morning cup of coffee, but the pressor response to caffeine usually (but not always) habituates throughout the day. Thus, caffeine consumption need not be eliminated.

Moderate alcohol (Chapter 31) consumption (one or two drinks per day) seems to decrease cardiovascular risk and does not increase the risk of hypertension. However, heavy drinking (three or more standard-sized drinks per day, 5 days or more per week) activates the sympathetic nervous system and is associated with an increased incidence and severity of hypertension, which is reversible if alcohol consumption decreases.

After a bout of aerobic exercise (Chapter 14), a small reduction in blood pressure can persist for several hours. Relaxation techniques (e.g., meditation, biofeedback, breathing exercises) can decrease blood pressure transiently but generally produce little effect on ambulatory blood pressure (Chapter 36). However, in some individuals in whom overwhelming home or job strain is a major determinant of high blood pressure, stress management techniques and anxiolytics may be beneficial. Patients often associate hypertension directly with life stress and should be counseled that stress management alone without medication rarely is sufficient to control their hypertension.

Pharmacologic Therapy

More than 100 antihypertensive medications are marketed (Table 66–5). Randomized controlled trials have provided unequivocal proof that lowering blood pressure with medication dramatically reduces cardiovascular disability and death and slows the progression of chronic kidney disease.

Classes of Oral Antihypertensive Drugs

The various classes of oral antihypertensive drugs have different mechanisms of actions, which explain the therapeutic principles of their use as well as their major contraindications and side effects (Table 66–6).

Diuretics

MECHANISM OF ACTION. With initiation of diuretic therapy, contraction of blood volume causes the initial fall in blood pressure. With continued therapy, blood volume is partially restored, and vasodilator mechanisms (e.g., opening of ATP-sensitive K^+ channels) sustain the antihypertensive action. Loop diuretics block Na^+-K^+-$2Cl^-$ transport in the thick ascending loop of Henle, where a large portion of the filtered sodium is reabsorbed. Thiazide diuretics and the indoline derivative indapamide block Na^+-Cl^- cotransporter in the distal convoluted tubule, where a smaller portion of the filtered sodium is reabsorbed. Spironolactone and eplerenone prevent aldosterone from activating the mineralocorticoid receptor, thereby inhibiting the downstream activation of ENaC, whereas triamterene and amiloride block ENaC directly; because less sodium is presented to the Na^+,K^+-ATPase on the vascular side of the collecting duct cells, less potassium is excreted in the urine.

THERAPEUTIC PRINCIPLES. Diuretics are the oldest, least expensive, and still among the best antihypertensive medications. In the Antihypertensive and Lipid-Lowering Treatment to Prevent Heart Attack Trial (ALLHAT), the thiazide-type diuretic chlorthalidone was at least as effective as (and in some instances more effective than) newer, more expensive agents (the ACE inhibitor lisinopril or the dihydropyridine CCB amlodipine) in lowering blood pressure and preventing the attendant cardiovascular complications in all subgroups of patients. [1] Combined with other classes of antihypertensive medications, diuretics exert a synergistic effect on blood pressure. The most common cause of apparent drug-resistant hypertension is the failure to include a diuretic in the therapeutic regimen or to dose it correctly.

Because of their long half-lives, thiazides are much more effective than the short-acting loop diuretics for most patients with hypertension. Chlorthalidone, the thiazide-type diuretic used in the ALLHAT and many other trials, is more potent and has a much longer duration of action than hydrochlorothiazide, which for decades has replaced chlorthalidone as the main thiazide-type diuretic in clinical practice. Low-dose hydrochlorothiazide (12.5 mg/day), often in fixed-dose combination with an ACE inhibitor or angiotensin II receptor blocker, is recommended for uncomplicated hypertension, whereas chlorthalidone (typically 25 mg/day, which has a potency equivalent to about 40 mg of hydrochlorothiazide) is recommended for resistant hypertension.

When the glomerular filtration rate falls below 50 mL/min/1.73 m^2, standard doses of hydrochlorothiazide become ineffective, although metolazone or much higher doses of thiazides can be effective. Loop diuretics are the diuretics of choice for treating hypertension in patients with chronic kidney disease or heart failure. Because the duration of action of furosemide is less than 6 hours, torsemide is a better choice owing to its longer half-life. The addition of low-dose metolazone to a loop diuretic can sometimes restore blood pressure responsiveness in patients with resistant hypertension due to severe volume expansion in the setting of advanced chronic kidney disease.

Eplerenone (100 mg/day) has replaced spironolactone as the drug of choice for primary aldosteronism. Low-dose eplerenone (6.25 to 25 mg/day) or spironolactone (6.25 to 12.5 mg/day) can be effective in treatment of primary hypertension, particularly low-renin hypertension in African Americans.

Angiotensin-Converting Enzyme Inhibitors and Angiotensin Receptor Blockers

MECHANISM OF ACTION. The renin-angiotensin-aldosterone system is one of the most important targets for antihypertensive drugs. The interaction of angiotensin II with G protein–coupled receptors, termed AT_1 receptors, accelerates numerous cellular processes that contribute not only to hypertension but also to its end-organ damage. ACE inhibitors block the conversion of angiotensin I to angiotensin II, initially leading to a dramatic fall in plasma angiotensin II levels; with continued treatment, however, plasma angiotensin II levels return to normal (the phenomenon of "ACE escape"), because ACE inhibitors do not block alternative pathways that generate angiotensin II. The sustained antihypertensive action of ACE inhibitors is explained in part by their ability to block the metabolism of bradykinin, a potent endothelium-dependent vasodilator. These agents slow the deterioration of renal function in patients with chronic kidney disease by causing greater dilation of the efferent renal arteriole, thereby reducing intraglomerular pressure.

By comparison, angiotensin II receptor blockers (ARBs) lower blood pressure specifically by blocking the interaction of angiotensin II on the AT_1 receptors. Thus, ARBs do not increase bradykinin, which has been implicated in both the therapeutic benefits and the side effects of ACE inhibitors (i.e., cough, angioedema).

THERAPEUTIC PRINCIPLES. Because of their low side effect profiles and putative ancillary benefits on vascular health, ACE inhibitors and ARBs have been gaining popularity for the general treatment of hypertension. As monotherapy, they generally are less potent than diuretics or CCBs, particularly in African Americans, but they amplify the effects of these other drug classes when they are used in combination. Randomized trials have dispelled the fear that ACE inhibitors and ARBs are contraindicated for patients with mild or moderate degrees of renal impairment by showing that the incidence of hyperkalemia or acute renal failure is low and that renoprotection is provided. Serum creatinine and potassium concentrations need to be monitored in all patients receiving an ACE inhibitor or ARB. In patients with chronic kidney disease, initiation of an ACE inhibitor or ARB often causes small and transient increases in serum creatinine concentration that do not necessitate discontinuation. ACE inhibitors and ARBs can precipitate acute renal failure in patients with bilateral renal artery stenosis or hypovolemia. After correction of hypovolemia, the ACE inhibitor or ARB usually can be restarted safely at a lower dose.

The most common side effect of ACE inhibitors is a dry cough. Patients may complain not of a cough but rather of having to clear the throat or loss of voice later in the day. These symptoms occur in

TABLE 66–5 ORAL ANTIHYPERTENSIVE AGENTS

Drug	Dose Range, Total, mg/day (doses per day)	Usual Starting Dose, mg/day (doses per day)
DIURETICS		
Thiazide diuretics		
Chlorthalidone	6.25–50 (1)	12.5 (1)
HCTZ	6.25–50 (1)	12.5 (1)
Indapamide	1.25–5 (1)	1.25 (1)
Metolazone	2.5–5 (1)	2.5 (1)
Loop diuretics		
Bumetanide	0.5–2 (2)	1 (2)
Ethacrynic acid	25–100 (2)	25 (2)
Furosemide	20–160 (2)	20 (2)
Torsemide	2.5–20 (1–2)	5 (2)
Potassium sparing		
Amiloride	5–20 (1)	10 (2)
Eplerenone	25–100 (1–2)	25 (1)
Spironolactone	6.25–400 (1–2)	6.25 (1)
Triamterene	25–100 (1)	37.5 (1)
β-BLOCKERS		
Acebutolol	200–800 (2)	200 (2)
Atenolol	25–100 (1)	25 (1)
Betaxolol	5–20 (1)	5 (1)
Bisoprolol	2.5–20 (1)	2.5 (1)
Carteolol	2.5–10 (1)	2.5 (1)
Metoprolol	50–450 (2)	50 (2)
Metoprolol XL	50–200 (1–2)	50 (1)
Nadolol	20–320 (1)	40 (1)
Penbutolol	10–80 (1)	10 (1)
Pindolol	10–60 (2)	10 (1)
Propranolol	40–180 (2)	40 (2)
Propranolol LA	60–180 (1–2)	60 (1)
Timolol	20–60 (2)	20 (2)
β-/α-BLOCKERS		
Carvedilol	6.25–50 (2)	6.25 (2)
Labetalol	200–2400 (2)	200 (2)
CALCIUM-CHANNEL BLOCKERS		
Dihydropyridines		
Amlodipine	2.5–10 (1)	2.5 (1)
Felodipine	2.5–20 (1–2)	2.5 (2)
Isradipine CR	2.5–20 (2)	2.5 (2)
Nicardipine SR	30–120 (2)	30 (2)
Nifedipine XL	30–120 (1)	30 (1)
Nisoldipine	10–40 (1–2)	10 (2)
Non-dihydropyridines		
Diltiazem CD	120–540 (1)	180 (1)
Verapamil HS	120–480 (1)	180 (1)
ANGIOTENSIN-CONVERTING ENZYME INHIBITORS		
Benazepril	10–80 (1–2)	20 (1)
Captopril	25–150 (2)	25 (2)
Enalapril	2.5–40 (2)	5 (2)
Fosinopril	10–80 (1–2)	20 (2)
Lisinopril	5–80 (1–2)	40 (2)
Moexipril	7.5–30 (1)	7.5 (1)
Perindopril	4–16 (1)	4 (1)
Quinapril	5–80 (1–2)	40 (2)
Ramipril	2.5–20 (1)	2.5 (1)
Trandolapril	1–8 (1)	2 (1)

Continued

TABLE 66–5 ORAL ANTIHYPERTENSIVE AGENTS—cont'd

Drug	Dose Range, Total, mg/day (doses per day)	Usual Starting Dose, mg/day (doses per day)
ANGIOTENSIN RECEPTOR BLOCKERS		
Candesartan	8–32 (1)	16 (1)
Eprosartan	400–800 (1–2)	400 (1)
Irbesartan	150–300 (1)	150 (1)
Losartan	25–100 (2)	50 (1)
Olmesartan	5–40 (1)	20 (1)
Telmisartan	20–80 (1)	40 (1)
Valsartan	80–320 (1–2)	160 (2)
α-BLOCKERS		
Doxazosin	1–16 (1)	1 (1)
Prazosin	1–40 (2–3)	1 (2)
Terazosin	1–20 (1)	1 (1)
Phenoxybenzamine	20–120 (2) for pheochromocytoma	20 (2)
CENTRAL SYMPATHOLYTICS		
Clonidine	0.2–1.2 (2–3)	0.2 (2)
Clonidine patch	0.1–0.6 (weekly)	0.1 (weekly)
Guanabenz	2–32 (2)	2 (2)
Guanfacine	1–3 (1) (qhs)	1 (1)
Methyldopa	250–1000 (2)	250 (2)
Reserpine	0.05–0.25 (1)	0.05 (1)
DIRECT VASODILATORS		
Hydralazine	10–200 (2)	20 (2)
Minoxidil	2.5–100 (1)	2.5 (1)
FIXED-DOSE COMBINATIONS		
Amiloride/HCTZ	5/50 (1)	5/50 (1)
Amlodipine/benazepril	2.5–5/10–20 (1)	2.5/10 (1)
Atenolol/chlorthalidone	50–100/25 (1)	50/25 (1)
Benazepril/HCTZ	5–20/6.25–25 (1)	20/6.25 (1)
Bisoprolol/HCTZ	2.5–10/6.25 (1)	2.5/6.25 (1)
Candesartan/HCTZ	16–32/12.5–25 (1)	16/12.5 (1)
Enalapril/HCTZ	5–10/25 (1–2)	5/25 (1)
Eprosartan/HCTZ	600/12.5–25 (1)	600/12.5 (1)
Fosinopril/HCTZ	10–20/12.5 (1)	10/12.5 (1)
Irbesartan/HCTZ	150–300/12.5–25 (1)	150/12.5 (1)
Losartan/HCTZ	50–100/12.5–25 (1)	50/12.5 (1)
Olmesartan/HCTZ	20–40/12.5 (1)	20/12.5 (1)
Spironolactone/HCTZ	25/25 (½–1)	25/25 (1/2)
Telmisartan/HCTZ	40–80/12.5–25 (1)	40/12.5 (1)
Trandolapril/verapamil	2–4/180–240 (1)	2/180 (1)
Triamterene/HCTZ	37.5/25 (½–1)	37.5/25 (1/2)
Valsartan/HCTZ	80–160/12.5–25 (1)	160/12.5 (1)

HCTZ = hydrochlorothiazide.

Rx

3 to 39% of patients, resolve in a few days after the drug is discontinued, and can be eliminated by switching the patient to an ARB. The incidence is higher in African Americans than in whites and is highest in Asians.

The ARBs seem to be less effective than dihydropyridine CCBs in controlling hypertension but are increasingly popular because they have a more favorable side effect profile than ACE inhibitors. Their efficacy is enhanced considerably by addition of low-dose hydrochlorothiazide, and numerous fixed-dose combinations are available (see Table 66–5). Losartan, the prototype, differs from the other ARBs in two ways: a shorter duration of action, requiring twice-daily dosing if it is used as monotherapy, and a uricosuric effect, which may be beneficial in patients with hyperuricemia. Newer ARBs vary in potency and duration of action.

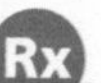

Direct Renin Inhibitors

Aliskerin is the first in a new class of orally effective, nonpeptide, low-molecular-weight renin inhibitors. Direct renin inhibitors block

TABLE 66–6 MAJOR CONTRAINDICATIONS AND SIDE EFFECTS OF ANTIHYPERTENSIVE DRUGS

Drug Class	Major Contraindications	Side Effects
Diuretics		
Thiazides	Gout	Insulin resistance, new-onset type 2 diabetes (especially in combination with β-blockers) Hypokalemia, hyponatremia Hypertriglyceridemia Hyperuricemia, precipitation of gout Erectile dysfunction (more than other drug classes) Potentiate nondepolarizing muscle relaxants Photosensitivity dermatitis Interstitial nephritis
Loop diuretics	Hepatic coma	Hypokalemia Potentiate succinylcholine Potentiate aminoglycoside ototoxicity
Potassium-sparing diuretics	Serum potassium concentration >5.5 mEq/L GFR <30 mg/mL 1.73 m^2	Fatal hyperkalemia if used with salt substitutes, ACE inhibitors, ARBs, high-potassium food, NSAIDs
ACE inhibitors	Pregnancy Bilateral renal artery stenosis Hyperkalemia	Cough Hyperkalemia Angioedema Leukopenia Fetal toxicity Cholestatic jaundice (rare fulminant hepatic necrosis if the drug is not discontinued)
Dihydropyridine CCBs	As monotherapy in chronic kidney disease with proteinuria	Headaches Flushing Ankle edema CHF Gingival hyperplasia Esophageal reflux
Non-dihydropyridine CCBs	Heart block Systolic heart failure	Bradycardia, AV block (especially with verapamil) Constipation (often severe with verapamil) Worsening of systolic function, CHF Gingival edema or hypertrophy Increase cyclosporine blood levels Esophageal reflux
ARBs	Pregnancy Bilateral renal artery stenosis Hyperkalemia	Hyperkalemia Angioedema (very rare) Fetal toxicity
β-Adrenergic blockers	Heart block Asthma Depression Cocaine and methamphetamine abuse	Insulin resistance, new-onset type 2 diabetes (especially in combination with thiazides) Heart block, acute decompensated CHF Bronchospasm Depression, nightmares, fatigue Cold extremities, claudication (β_2 effect) Stevens-Johnson syndrome Agranulocytosis
α-Adrenergic blockers	Orthostatic hypotension Systolic heart failure Left ventricular dysfunction	Orthostatic hypotension Drug tolerance (in the absence of diuretic therapy) Ankle edema CHF First-dose effect (acute hypotension) Potentiate hypotension with PDE-5 inhibitors (e.g., sildenafil)
Central sympatholytics	Orthostatic hypotension	Depression, dry mouth, lethargy Erectile dysfunction (dose dependent) Rebound hypertension with clonidine withdrawal Coombs-positive hemolytic anemia and elevated liver enzymes with α-methyldopa
Direct vasodilators	Orthostatic hypotension	Reflex tachycardia Fluid retention Hirsutism, pericardial effusion with minoxidil Lupus with hydralazine

ACE = angiotensin-converting enzyme; ARBs = angiotensin receptor blockers; AV = atrioventricular; CCBs = calcium-channel blockers; CHF = congestive heart failure; GFR = glomerular filtration rate; NSAIDs = nonsteroidal anti-inflammatory drugs; PDE-5 = phosphodiesterase-5.

Rx

the renin-angiotensin-aldosterone system at its origin without increasing bradykinin. Short-term studies in patients with mild or moderate hypertension suggest that once-daily low-dose (150 mg) or high-dose (300 mg) aliskerin is at least equivalent to an ARB in terms of its blood pressure–lowering effect, and it has an almost placebo-like side effect profile. By eliminating the reactive rise in plasma renin activity seen with ACE inhibitors and ARBs, direct renin inhibition may represent a significant advance over ARBs in the treatment of hypertension, and prevention of its cardiovascular sequelae is currently unknown.

Calcium-Channel Blockers

MECHANISM OF ACTION. The CCBs are antiarrhythmic, antianginal, and antihypertensive because they block the opening of voltage-gated (L-type) Ca^{2+} channels in cardiac myocytes and vascular smooth muscle cells. The resultant decrease in the cytosolic Ca^{2+} signal decreases heart rate and ventricular contractility and relaxes vascular smooth muscle. Blood pressure lowering is related mainly to peripheral arterial vasodilation, with the rank order of potency being dihydropyridines > diltiazem >> verapamil. In contrast, for negative chronotropic and inotropic effects, the rank order of potency is verapamil >> diltiazem > dihydropyridines.

THERAPEUTIC PRINCIPLES. *Short-acting dihydropyridines should not be used to treat hypertension.* By triggering an abrupt fall in blood pressure with reflex sympathetic activation, these rapidly acting arterial vasodilators can precipitate myocardial ischemia, infarction, stroke, and death. By comparison, the safety and efficacy of long-acting dihydropyridine CCBs was confirmed by ALLHAT and the VALUE (Valsartan Antihypertensive Long-term Use Evaluation) trial. 2 For most hypertensive patients, these are among the most potent, best tolerated, and safest antihypertensive medications available, but there are some caveats. For comparable degrees of blood pressure lowering, dihydropyridine CCBs exert protection against myocardial infarction and stroke equivalent to that of diuretics, but their use is associated with a greater risk of heart failure. For patients with renal insufficiency and proteinuria, dihydropyridine CCB–based therapy is less renoprotective than ARB- or ACE inhibitor–based therapy. However, in most patients with renal disease, multiple classes of medications, including dihydropyridines, are required to achieve blood pressure goals. Thus, dihydropyridine CCBs should not be used as first-line therapy for hypertension in patients with proteinuria, but they may be used as adjunctive therapy once the dose of the ACE inhibitor or ARB has been maximized in combination with an appropriate diuretic.

Verapamil is a weak antihypertensive and of limited utility because of dose-dependent constipation. Diltiazem is intermediate in potency between verapamil and the dihydropyridines; it is usually well tolerated.

Adrenergic Receptor Blockers and Central Sympatholytics

Sympathetic drive to the sinus node increases heart rate and cardiac output through β-adrenergic receptors, whereas sympathetic drive to the peripheral vasculature causes neurogenic vasoconstriction through α-adrenergic receptors. Sustained activation of the sympathetic nervous system is thought to contribute to chronic hypertension by vascular remodeling, renin release, and attenuation of renal sodium excretion by an action on the distal tubules.

β-Adrenergic Blockers

MECHANISM OF ACTION. Interaction of epinephrine or norepinephrine with β_1-adrenoreceptors in the heart causes G protein–linked activation of adenylate cyclase, resulting in positive chronotropic and inotropic effects. Interaction of catecholamines with β_2-adrenoreceptors relaxes bronchiolar and arteriolar smooth muscle. With the initiation of β-blocker therapy, blood pressure at first is little affected because the fall in cardiac output is offset by a compensatory increase in peripheral resistance. Over time, blood pressure falls progressively as the peripheral vasculature relaxes. Thus, the antihypertensive effect of β-blockade involves decreases in cardiac output (β_1-receptors), renin release (β_1-receptors), and norepinephrine release (prejunctional β_2-receptors).

Rx

First-generation agents (e.g., propranolol) nonselectively block both β_1- and β_2-receptors. *Second-generation* agents (e.g., metoprolol, atenolol, acebutolol, bisoprolol) are *relatively* cardioselective. In low doses, they exert a greater inhibitory effect on β_1- than on β_2-receptors, but selectivity is lost at high doses. Combined α- and β-blockers (labetalol, carvedilol) cause vasodilation by blocking α_1-adrenoreceptors on vascular smooth muscle.

THERAPEUTIC PRINCIPLES. β-Blockers, which are effective in reducing myocardial oxygen demands, are first-line therapy for hypertensive patients with coronary artery disease. Unless contraindicated, they should be prescribed in all patients who also have sustained a myocardial infarction (Chapters 71 and 72) and in those with compensated heart failure (Chapter 57).

However, ever-increasing evidence of their diabetogenic potential suggests that standard β-blockers may not be the best choice for uncomplicated hypertension in younger patients or those with the metabolic syndrome (Chapter 248). In addition, recent meta-analyses suggested that atenolol, one of the most popular drugs of this class, is less effective than other classes of antihypertensive agents (and often no better than placebo) in protecting against cardiovascular events and that β-blockers as a class are not as good as other medications for protecting against stroke. 3 In older patients with isolated systolic hypertension, β-blockers generally are less effective than other drug classes in reducing central aortic pressure and pulse pressure. In contrast, combined α- and β-blockers are powerful antihypertensive agents that appear to have a metabolic profile more favorable than that of standard β-blockers; as part of combination regimens, they can be effective in controlling otherwise difficult hypertension.

α-Adrenergic Blockers

MECHANISM OF ACTION. By blocking the interaction of norepinephrine on vascular α-adrenergic receptors, these drugs cause peripheral vasodilation, thereby lowering blood pressure. By increasing skeletal muscle blood flow, they increase insulin sensitivity. By dilating urethral smooth muscle, they improve symptoms of prostatism. Prazosin, doxazosin, terazosin, and intravenous phentolamine selectively block α_1-adrenoreceptors; phenoxybenzamine blocks both α_1- and α_2-receptors.

THERAPEUTIC PRINCIPLES. Phenoxybenzamine remains the drug of choice for preoperative management of pheochromocytoma (Chapter 246); after α-blockade is achieved, a β-blocker should be added to block an otherwise excessive reflex tachycardia. The selective α_1-blockers are not first-line agents and should not be used as monotherapy because their propensity to cause fluid retention can lead to tachyphylaxis and unmask or exacerbate heart failure. However, when they are prescribed as part of a combination regimen that includes a diuretic, they are effective third- or fourth-line therapy for difficult hypertension and are particularly useful in older men with prostatism. Although marketed specifically for prostatism and not as an antihypertensive agent, the selective α_{1A}-blocker tamsulosin lowers blood pressure in some men.

Central Sympatholytics

MECHANISM OF ACTION. Stimulation of postsynaptic α_2-adrenergic receptors and imidazoline receptors in the central nervous system lowers central sympathetic outflow, whereas stimulation of presynaptic α_2-receptors causes feedback inhibition of norepinephrine release from peripheral sympathetic nerve terminals. The combined effect is reduced sympathetic drive to the heart and peripheral circulation, thereby leading to decreased heart rate, cardiac output, and peripheral vascular resistance.

THERAPEUTIC PRINCIPLES. The central sympatholytics are best reserved for short-term oral treatment of severe uncontrolled hypertension. They are potent antihypertensive agents that may be needed as fourth- or fifth-line therapy for very difficult hypertension, but their troublesome central nervous system side effects greatly limit the adherence of patients in uncomplicated hypertension. The serious rebound hypertension seen with rapid discontinuation of clonidine is less of a problem with longer acting preparations (guanfacine, clonidine patch). α-Methyldopa remains the drug of choice for chronic hypertension in pregnancy (Chapter 259).

TABLE 66–7 "COMPELLING" INDICATIONS AND PUBLISHED EVIDENCE

Compelling Indication	Primary Outcome	Drug Class (Relevant Clinical Trials*)
Systolic heart failure	CV events	ACEI (CONSENSUS, SAVE) ARB (Val-HeFT, CHARM) β-Blocker (MERIT-HF, COMET) Aldosterone antagonist (RALES)
Recent MI	Recurrent MI or death	β-Blockers (ISIS)
Reduced left ventricular function after MI	Recurrent MI, CHF hospitalization	ACEI (SAVE, TRACE) Aldosterone antagonist (EPHESUS) β-Blocker (CAPRICORN)
Type 1 diabetes	Deterioration in renal function	ACEI (CCSG)
Type 2 diabetes	CV events	ACEI (MICRO-HOPE)
Type 2 diabetic nephropathy	Deterioration in renal function Progression of microalbuminuria	ARB (IDNT, RENAAL, IRMA-2, MOSES)
Nondiabetic chronic kidney disease	Deterioration in renal function	ACEI (REIN, AIPRI, AASK) ACEI + ARB (COOPERATE)
CV disease	CV events	ACEI (HOPE, EUROPA)
Prior stroke or TIA	Stroke and CV events	ACE + thiazide (PROGRESS)
Isolated systolic hypertension in older persons	CV events	DHP-CCB (Syst-Eur, Syst-China, STOP-2) Thiazide (SHEP) ACEI (STOP-2) ARB (SCOPE, second-line)
Left ventricular hypertrophy by electrocardiography	Stroke	ARB (LIFE)

*CONSENSUS, Cooperative North Scandinavian Enalapril Survival Study (N Engl J Med 1987;316:1429–1435); SAVE, Survival and Ventricular Enlargement study (N Engl J Med 1992;327:669–677); Val-HeFT, Valsartan Heart Failure Trial (N Engl J Med 2001;345:1667–1675); CHARM, Candesartan in Heart Failure: Assessment of Reduction in Morbidity and Mortality (Lancet 2003;362:759–766); MERIT-HF, Metoprolol Randomized Intervention Trial in Congestive Heart Failure (JAMA 2000;283:1295–1302); COMET, comparison of carvedilol and metoprolol on clinical outcomes in patients with chronic heart failure in the Carvedilol Or Metoprolol European Trial (Lancet 2003;362:7–13); RALES, Randomized Aldactone Evaluation Study (N Engl J Med 1999;341:709–717); ISIS, International Study of Infarct Survival (Lancet 1986;2:57–66); TRACE, Trandolapril Cardiac Evaluation (N Engl J Med 1995;333:1670–1676); EPHESUS, Eplerenone Post–Myocardial Infarction Heart Failure Efficacy and Survival Study (N Engl J Med 2003;348:1309–1321); CAPRICORN, effect of carvedilol on outcome after myocardial infarction in patients with left-ventricular dysfunction (Lancet 2001;357:1385–1390); CCSG, Captopril Cooperative Study Group (N Engl J Med 1993;323:1456–1462); MICRO-HOPE, Microalbuminuria, Cardiovascular and Renal Outcomes substudy of the Heart Outcomes Prevention Evaluation (Lancet 2000;355:253–259); IDNT, Irbesartan Diabetic Nephropathy Trial (N Engl J Med 2001;345:841–860); RENAAL, Reduction of Endpoints in NIDDM with the Angiotensin II Antagonist Losartan (N Engl J Med 2001;345:861–869); IRMA-2, Irbesartan Microalbuminuria study 2 (N Engl J Med 2001;345:870–878); REIN, Ramipril Evaluation in Nephropathy trial (Lancet 1998;352:1252–1256); AIPRI, ACE Inhibition in Progressive Renal Insufficiency (Kidney Int 1997;63 [Suppl.]:S63–S67); AASK, African American Study of Kidney Disease and Hypertension (JAMA 2002;288:2421–2431); COOPERATE, Combination treatment of angiotensin-II receptor blocker and angiotensin-converting-enzyme inhibitor in non-diabetic renal disease (Lancet 2003;361:117–124); HOPE, Heart Outcomes Prevention Evaluation (N Engl J Med 2000;342:145–153); EUROPA, European Reduction of Cardiac Events with Perindopril in Stable Coronary Artery Disease (Lancet 2003;362:782–788); PROGRESS, Perindopril Protection Against Recurrent Stroke Study (Lancet 2001;358:1033–1041); Syst-Eur, Systolic Hypertension in Europe trial (Lancet 1997;360:757–764); Syst-China, Systolic Hypertension in China trial (J Hypertens 1998;16:1823–1829); STOP-2, Swedish Trial in Old Patients with Hypertension 2 (Lancet 1999;354:1751–1756); SHEP, Systolic Hypertension in the Elderly Program (JAMA 1991;265:3255–3264); SCOPE, Study on Cognition and Prognosis in the Elderly (J Hypertens 2003;21:875–886); LIFE, Losartan Intervention for Endpoint Reduction (Lancet 2002;359:995–1003).

ACE = angiotensin-converting enzyme; ACEI = angiotensin-converting enzyme inhibitor; ARB = angiotensin receptor blocker; CHF = congestive heart failure; CV = cardiovascular; DHP-CCB = dihydropyridine calcium-channel blocker; MI = myocardial infarction; TIA = transient ischemic attack.

Modified from Elliott WJ: Compelling indications for antihypertensive drugs. ASH Clinical Hypertension Review Course. New York, American Society of Hypertension, 2005, pp 333–351.

Rx

Direct Vasodilators

MECHANISM OF ACTION. Minoxidil and hydralazine are potent hyperpolarizing arterial vasodilators that work by opening vascular ATP-sensitive K^+ channels.

THERAPEUTIC PRINCIPLES. By causing selective and rapid arterial dilation, both drugs cause profound reflex sympathetic activation and tachycardia as well as ankle edema. For this reason, hydralazine has largely been replaced by the longer acting dihydropyridine CCBs. However, hydralazine remains the treatment of choice for acute severe hypertension in pregnancy (Chapter 259). A combination of hydralazine plus nitroglycerin now is recommended for the treatment of heart failure specifically in African Americans, in whom hypertensive heart disease is the most common cause of heart failure  (Chapter 58). Difficult-to-control hypertension in advanced chronic kidney disease (Chapter 131) is the main indication for minoxidil, which must be combined with a β-blocker to prevent excessive reflex tachycardia and with a loop diuretic to prevent excessive fluid retention.

Drug Interactions That Affect Blood Pressure Control

Grapefruit juice (even a single glass) increases the bioavailability of dihydropyridine CCBs by inhibiting the intestinal cytochrome P-450 3A4 system, which is responsible for the first-pass metabolism of many oral medications. This effect is marked with felodipine, which has the least bioavailability of the dihydropyridines, and less with amlodipine and nifedipine, which have greater bioavailability.

By inhibiting renal sodium excretion, nonsteroidal anti-inflammatory drugs, including the cyclooxygenase-2 inhibitors, can markedly impair the antihypertensive action of diuretics as well as drugs that block the renin-angiotensin system, especially ACE inhibitors. Similar problems may occur with daily doses of aspirin in excess of 325 mg but do not seem to occur with 81 mg/day.

Rx

Which Drugs for Which Patients?

Choosing the best drugs to treat hypertension in a given patient is based on two considerations: (1) effective lowering of blood pressure and prevention of hypertensive complications with minimal side effects and cost and (2) concomitant treatment of comorbid cardiovascular diseases (e.g., angina, heart failure). According to a strict evidence-based approach, a "compelling indication" is defined as a comorbid condition for which the use of a specific antihypertensive drug has been shown to improve disease outcomes in a randomized controlled trial (Table 66–7).

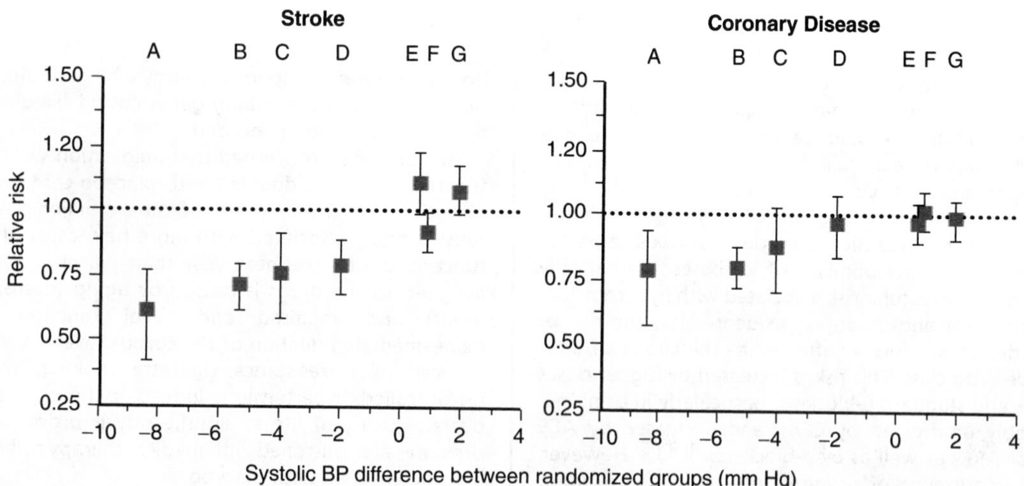

FIGURE 66–10 • Meta-meta-analysis of randomized controlled intervention trials. Meta-analysis of 29 randomized trials (n = 162,341 hypertensive patients). Regardless of drug classes being compared, the reduction in risk of stroke or coronary heart disease is mainly a function of the difference in achieved blood pressure in the treatment arms. A = CCB versus placebo; B = ACE inhibitor versus placebo; C = more intensive versus less intensive blood pressure lowering; D = ARB versus control; E = ACE inhibitor versus CCB; F = CCB versus diuretic or β-blocker; G = ACE inhibitor versus diuretic and β-blocker. (From Blood Pressure Lowering Treatment Trialists' Collaboration: Effects of different blood-pressure-lowering regimens on major cardiovascular events: Results of prospectively-designed overviews of randomised trials. Lancet 2003;362:1527–1535.)

Rx

Choice of Therapy for the Patient with "Uncomplicated" Hypertension

To date, a few DNA sequence variations have been proposed to identify individual patients whose blood pressure is particularly sensitive to a specific drug class. However, none of the reported effects has been sufficiently robust to have an impact on clinical decision making.

In the absence of such ideal scientific information, JNC 7 recommends a thiazide-type diuretic as cost-effective first-line therapy for most patients with hypertension. It also recommends initiation of therapy with two drugs (one being a thiazide) for stage 2 hypertension. In contrast, the European Society of Hypertension makes no specific drug class recommendation, arguing that the most effective drugs are those that the patient will tolerate and take. The British Hypertension Society advocates initiation of therapy with an ACE inhibitor, ARB, or β-blocker ("A" or "B" drug) for young white patients (younger than 55 years), who often have high-renin hypertension, but a CCB or diuretic ("C" or "D" drug) for older and black patients, who often have low-renin hypertension. A related approach that has not gained widespread endorsement is to use measured renin levels to guide therapy.

In contrast, an impressive body of evidence from clinical trials emphasizes the overriding importance of lowering blood pressure with combinations of drugs with different mechanisms of action (see Table 66–5), rather than belaboring the choice of the single best initial agent, to reach currently recommended blood pressure levels (<140/90 mm Hg for most patients, <130/80 mm Hg for high-risk patients). Unfortunately, systolic blood pressure goals are achieved in only 50 to 60% of subjects even in the idealized setting of a randomized trial (Fig. 66–10).

Low-dose combination drug therapy is not only the best way to control blood pressure but also the best way to minimize side effects because the dose-response relationship for blood pressure is rather flat, occurring at the lower end of the dose range for most medications, whereas many of the side effects are steeply dose dependent. Synergistic combinations achieve blood pressure control at lower doses. Fixed-dose combinations reduce pill burden and cost.

For these reasons, one simplified approach is to prescribe triple therapy consisting of (1) a low-dose thiazide diuretic, (2) an ACE inhibitor or ARB, and (3) a low-dose CCB (a dihydropyridine or diltiazem). The ARB dose typically can be maximized rapidly with minimal side effects. Treatment can be initiated with any two drug classes or all three, depending on the severity of the hypertension. As a rule of thumb, each agent added will lower systolic pressure by an additional 10 mm Hg. All the ACE inhibitors and ARBs are available as fixed-dose combinations with a low dose of hydrochlorothiazide; ACE inhibitor–CCB combinations are available as well (see Table 66–5). The triple combination regimen has synergistic effects on blood pressure because the ACE inhibitor or ARB counteracts the neurohormonal activation produced by the diuretic and CCB. Dihydropyridine CCBs cause dose-dependent ankle edema because they preferentially dilate arteries rather than veins, thereby elevating hydrostatic pressure; the resulting ankle edema often can be relieved by the addition of a thiazide diuretic or an ACE inhibitor or ARB, which dilates the veins as well as the arteries. In difficult or high-risk hypertension, the addition of an α- and β-blocker, selective α_1-blocker, or central sympatholytic may be needed as fourth-line therapy to block the reflex sympathetic activation caused by the diuretic and CCB. Pure β-blockers are no longer recommended as first-line therapy for uncomplicated hypertension because of their comparatively weak antihypertensive efficacy and clear-cut diabetogenic potential.

1. *Cardiovascular benefits of lowering blood pressure versus ancillary benefits of antihypertensive drug class beyond blood pressure lowering.* Despite much compelling basic research on ancillary benefits of ACE inhibitors and ARBs to block the adverse pleiotropic effects of angiotensin II on vascular health, there is increasing evidence and consensus that most of the cardiovascular benefit derived from these and all other classes of antihypertensive agents comes directly from lowering blood pressure. [1, 2, 5-8] Nevertheless, the participants in clinical trials typically are older than 60 years and have established hypertension or coronary artery disease, so the possibility remains that renin system blockers will more effectively block the vasculopathic effects of angiotensin II if they are introduced earlier in life before hypertension is fully established and vascular damage is far advanced. Regardless of the drug classes being compared or demographics of the patients, there are consistently fewer heart attacks, strokes, and cardiovascular deaths in the patients randomized to treatment with the drug that lowered blood pressure better than its comparator (see Fig. 66–10). Across clinical trials, systolic blood pressure is such a powerful and quantitative cardiovascular risk factor that a reduction of even 5 mm Hg during 5 years leads to a 20% average reduction in the risk of myocardial infarction and a 30% average reduction in the risk of stroke. An important caveat is that compared with all other

Rx

classes of antihypertensive drugs, the α_1-adrenergic antagonists and the CCBs have a greater propensity to precipitate heart failure and thus should be avoided in hypertensive patients with known heart failure and those with asymptomatic left ventricular systolic dysfunction.

2. *Antihypertensive drug class and risk of new-onset diabetes.* Both obesity and hypertension are powerful risk factors for diabetes, and the development of diabetes dramatically increases the cardiovascular risk associated with hypertension. There is consistent and mounting evidence that the risk of new-onset diabetes is further affected by the choice of antihypertensive drug class. This risk is increased by higher doses of thiazides and standard β-blockers, particularly in combination; probably unaffected by CCBs; and decreased by ACE inhibitors or ARBs as well as by α-blockers. [1, 2, 5] However, the clinical importance of drug-related changes in incident diabetes on cardiovascular outcomes is the subject of ongoing controversy. In the ALLHAT, the absolute differences in blood glucose concentrations between treatment groups were small and did not seem to negate the cardiovascular protection afforded by lowering blood pressure with a thiazide-type diuretic. [1] On the other hand, the 5-year duration of most clinical trials may be too short to observe the cardiovascular complications of newly developed diabetes, which typically take two or more decades to become manifest. For now, there are better choices than the traditional β-blocker–thiazide combination for treating hypertension in prediabetic individuals or younger persons who will require a lifetime of exposure to antihypertensive medication.
3. *Benefits of a more rapid approach to blood pressure reduction.* Many more strokes and other cardiovascular events are prevented by early rather than delayed treatment of isolated systolic hypertension in older patients. Early rapid control of hypertension may also explain why cardiovascular protection in high-risk hypertensive patients was greater with dihydropyridine CCB (amlodipine)–based treatment than with ARB (valsartan)–based treatment in one trial [2] and with a dihydropyridine plus ACE inhibitor (amlodipine plus perindopril) regimen compared with a β-blocker plus thiazide diuretic (atenolol plus bendroflumethiazide) regimen in another trial. [5] Thus, for many high-risk hypertensive patients, failure to control blood pressure within the first few months after diagnosis may be a cause of preventable cardiovascular complications. [2, 9]
4. *Expanded role for lipid-lowering therapy in patients with hypertension* (ASCOT-LLA [10]). Along with antihypertensive medication and lifestyle modification, additional cardiovascular risk reduction with low-dose aspirin (81 mg) (Chapter 35) and lipid-lowering medication (Chapter 217) should be strongly considered as an integral part of cardiovascular risk reduction. In treated hypertensive patients, low-dose aspirin reduces the risk of myocardial infarction by 36% without increasing the risk of intracerebral hemorrhage. [11] In patients with moderate hypertension, additional cardiovascular risk factors, and an average low-density lipoprotein cholesterol level of 130 mg/dL, the addition of 10 mg of atorvastatin to the antihypertensive regimen resulted in a 36% reduction in fatal and nonfatal myocardial infarction and a 27% reduction in fatal and nonfatal stroke. [10] Thus, statin therapy should be used in such patients with the goal of reducing the low-density lipoprotein cholesterol level to below 100 mg/dL or even lower (Chapter 217).

Medication Adherence

Medication adherence and costs are major barriers to control of hypertension. Several principles have been shown to facilitate adherence of patients: engaging the patients by teaching them to know their own goal blood pressure values and to monitor the effectiveness of therapy at home; prescribing long-acting preparations with once-daily dosing; prescribing low-dose drug combinations to achieve therapeutic synergy while avoiding dose-dependent side effects; and prescribing generics and fixed-dose combinations to reduce cost and pill burden.

Men are often concerned that medication will cause erectile dysfunction, but in a double-blind, placebo-controlled trial, thiazide diuretics were the only one of the six major classes of antihypertensive drugs associated with more new cases of male sexual dysfunction during the next year than placebo. Some of the blame assigned to the drugs is caused by aging (decreased testosterone levels) and impaired endothelial function (impaired nitric oxide–mediated dilation of the corpus cavernosum) due to obesity-induced insulin resistance, cigarette smoking, hyperlipidemia, and uncontrolled hypertension. Indeed, patients generally rate their overall quality of life as significantly improved when their blood pressures are controlled with medical therapy rather than when they are uncontrolled with placebo.

Hypertension in African Americans

The lower plasma renin levels common in hypertensive African Americans may suggest volume-dependent hypertension requiring diuretic therapy. Alternatively, lower plasma renin levels may be caused by a longer duration and greater severity of hypertension or by concomitant nephrosclerosis, which is a compelling indication for ACE inhibitor–based therapy. As monotherapy, an ACE inhibitor or ARB or a β-blocker generally yields a smaller decrease in blood pressure in African American than in white hypertensive patients. However, when high doses of an ACE inhibitor or ARB are used in combination with a diuretic, antihypertensive efficacy is amplified and ethnic differences seem to disappear. Among African American participants in the ALLHAT, the risk of fatal stroke was 40% greater in patients randomized to the ACE inhibitor lisinopril than to the diuretic chlorthalidone, probably because blood pressure control was also much poorer. [10] As part of an appropriate multidrug regimen, ACE inhibitor–based treatment can achieve excellent control of hypertension in African American patients.

Hypertensive Nephrosclerosis

Hypertension is the second most common cause of chronic kidney disease (Chapter 131), accounting for more than 25% of cases. Hypertensive nephrosclerosis, which is thought to be caused by severe constriction of the afferent renal arteriole, results in chronic glomerular ischemia. Typically, proteinuria is mild (<0.5 g/24 hr), and the diagnosis should be questioned in the presence of heavier degrees of proteinuria or in the absence of additional target organ damage (retinopathy, left ventricular hypertrophy). Mild to moderate nondiabetic renal insufficiency is now considered to be a compelling indication for ACE inhibitor–based antihypertensive therapy (or an ARB for ACE-intolerant patients). ACE inhibitors cause greater dilation of the efferent renal arterioles, thereby minimizing intraglomerular hypertension. In contrast, arterial vasodilators such as dihydropyridine CCBs, when used without an ACE inhibitor or ARB, preferentially dilate the afferent arteriole and impair renal autoregulation; glomerular hypertension can result if systemic blood pressure is not lowered sufficiently. In African Americans with moderate hypertensive nephrosclerosis and baseline proteinuria, an ACE inhibitor (ramipril)–based regimen has been shown to be superior to a dihydropyridine CCB (amlodipine)–based regimen in slowing the deterioration of renal function. [12] The ACE inhibitor should be withdrawn only if the rise in serum creatinine concentration exceeds 30% of the baseline value or the serum potassium concentration increases to more than 5.6 mmol/L.

Hypertension in Patients with Diabetes

Compared with its 25% prevalence in the general adult population, hypertension is present in 75% of diabetic patients and is a major factor contributing to an excessive risk of myocardial infarction, stroke, heart failure, microvascular complications, and diabetic nephropathy progressing to end-stage renal disease (Chapter 247). Compared with less intensive treatment, more intensive reduction of blood pressure has been proved repeatedly to reduce cardiovascular and microvascular end points dramatically in patients with dia-

Section VIII Cardiovascular

betes. To reduce these risks, blood pressures should be lowered to less than 130/80 mm Hg, a goal that typically requires three to five drugs. On the basis of data from randomized trials, type 1 diabetes (Chapter 247) with renal insufficiency is a compelling indication for ACE inhibitor–based antihypertensive therapy, whereas type 2 diabetes (Chapter 248) with renal insufficiency is now considered to be a compelling indication for ARB-based antihypertensive therapy because similar data do not yet exist for ACE inhibitor–based regimens in type 2 diabetics. However, an ACE inhibitor or ARB alone rarely achieves the stringent blood pressure goals; a loop diuretic is usually needed to shrink the expanded plasma volume, and a dihydropyridine CCB is usually needed for antihypertensive synergy. To optimize renal protection, the CCB should not be started until antihypertensive therapy has been initiated with an ACE inhibitor or ARB. A β-blocker should be added if the patient has coronary disease, which is prevalent in diabetes or heart failure. The α- and β-blocker carvedilol has a better metabolic profile than that of the pure β-blockers.

Hypertension in Patients with Coronary Artery Disease

To lower myocardial oxygen demands in patients with coronary disease, the antihypertensive regimen should reduce blood pressure without causing reflex tachycardia. For this reason, a β-blocker is often prescribed in conjunction with a dihydropyridine CCB or diltiazem. In patients with stable coronary disease and blood pressure in the prehypertensive range, the progression of coronary disease may be slowed more by lowering blood pressure with the dihydropyridine CCB amlodipine (which also is antianginal) than with the ACE inhibitor enalapril. β-Blockers are indicated for hypertensive patients who have sustained a myocardial infarction (Chapters 71 and 72) and for most patients with chronic heart failure (Chapter 58), and they are typically first-line therapy in patients with angina (Chapter 70). ACE inhibitors are indicated for almost all patients with left ventricular systolic dysfunction (Chapters 58 and 59) and may be considered for post–myocardial infarction patients even in the absence of ventricular dysfunction (Chapters 71 and 72). In patients with very high cardiovascular risk profiles but without known left ventricular dysfunction, the ACE inhibitor ramipril (10 mg/day) reduces cardiovascular events, an effect that may or may not be beyond what can be explained by blood pressure reduction alone. [13] In normotensive patients with stable coronary artery disease, there are conflicting data as to whether the addition of an ACE inhibitor reduces the risk of subsequent cardiovascular events.

Isolated Systolic Hypertension in Older Persons

In older persons with isolated systolic hypertension, lowering systolic pressure from above 160 to below 150 mm Hg has been shown unequivocally to reduce the risk of stroke by 30%, myocardial infarction by 23%, and overall cardiovascular mortality by 18%; it also reduces heart failure admissions and slows the progression of dementia. Trial data do not yet exist in older persons to determine whether the treatment of isolated elevations in systolic pressure between 140 and 160 mm Hg is beneficial; however, in the absence of such data, most authorities recommend treatment. As yet, studies have specifically tested for a mortality benefit of treating systolic hypertension in patients older than 80 years; however, post hoc analyses strongly suggest a large reduction in strokes and heart failure admissions.

Physicians often are overly conservative when it comes to treatment of isolated systolic hypertension, largely because of fears about precipitating acute myocardial ischemia if a low diastolic blood pressure is further reduced. Although this fear is certainly relevant in hospitalized patients with acute coronary syndromes, the risk associated with persistently undertreated systolic hypertension in the outpatient setting outweighs the risk of additional reduction of diastolic pressure.

On the basis of data from several large randomized trials, low-dose thiazide diuretics and dihydropyridine CCBs are the most effective drugs and should be the drugs of choice for isolated systolic hypertension. For many older hypertensive patients, especially those with diabetes, the addition of an ACE inhibitor or an ARB will be necessary to achieve recommended blood pressure goals.

Because of slower drug metabolism and slower postural autonomic reflexes in older persons, it is particularly important to start with low doses of antihypertensive medication. If orthostatic hypotension is present, medication must be titrated to standing blood pressure. In some older patients, even low-dose thiazides cause unacceptable degrees of hyponatremia; β-blockers should be restricted to those with coronary disease or heart failure and should be used with caution because they are more likely to precipitate heart block, to impair exercise tolerance, and to cause depression.

Blood Pressure Lowering for Secondary Prevention of Stroke

Most neurologists recommend minimal or no blood pressure reduction during an acute ischemic stroke unless the patient is a candidate for thrombolytic therapy (Chapters 431 and 432). Once the patient's condition has stabilized, however, lowering blood pressure by 12/5 mm Hg with a combination of the thiazide diuretic indapamide plus the ACE inhibitor perindopril reduces the risk of recurrent stroke by 43%. [14]

Hypertension Associated with Oral Contraceptives and Estrogen Replacement

Oral contraceptives, particularly current low-dose estrogen preparations, cause a small increase in blood pressure in most women but rarely cause a large increase into the hypertensive range. The mechanism is unknown, but women older than 35 years and those who smoke or are overweight appear to be at increased risk. If hypertension develops, oral contraceptive therapy should be discontinued in favor of other methods of contraception. Oral estrogen replacement therapy after menopause seems to cause a small increase in blood pressure, whereas transdermal estrogen (which bypasses first-pass hepatic metabolism) seems to cause a small decrease in blood pressure.

Hypertension in Pregnancy

Hypertension, the most common nonobstetric complication of pregnancy, is present in about 10% of all pregnancies (Chapter 259). About one third is caused by chronic hypertension and two thirds by preeclampsia, defined as an increase in blood pressure to 140/90 mm Hg or more after the 20th week of gestation, accompanied by proteinuria (>300 mg/24 hr) and pathologic edema. Preeclampsia sometimes also is accompanied by seizures (eclampsia) and the multisystem HELLP syndrome (Chapter 154) of hemolysis, elevated liver enzymes, and low platelets. Preeclampsia is the most common cause of maternal mortality and perinatal mortality. Given the current trend of childbearing in women older than 35 years, the prevalence of chronic hypertension in pregnancy is rising. In the absence of randomized trials, α-methyldopa remains the drug of choice for chronic hypertension in pregnancy, and hydralazine (plus bedrest) for preeclampsia. In preeclampsia, magnesium sulfate is predictably effective in preventing seizures but, despite being a vasodilator, has inconsistent effects on blood pressure.

Resistant Hypertension

Defined as persistence of usual blood pressure above 140/90 mm Hg despite treatment with full doses of three or more different classes of medications including a diuretic in rational combination, resistant hypertension is the most common reason for referral to a hypertension specialist. In practice, the problem usually falls into one of four categories: (1) pseudoresistance, (2) an inadequate medical regimen, (3) nonadherence or ingestion of pressor substances, or (4) secondary hypertension. Pseudoresistant hypertension is caused by white coat aggravation, a white coat effect superimposed on chronic hypertension that is well controlled with medication outside the physician's office. As many as half of patients referred to hypertension specialists have pseudoresistance, which is readily documented with ambulatory monitoring. Increasing evidence indicates that even when a patient's office blood pressure remains elevated despite multidrug treatment, a mean daytime ambulatory blood pressure below 135/85 mm Hg is a reassuring indicator of a favorable prognosis and adequate therapy.

Rx

The most common cause of apparent drug resistance is the absence of appropriate diuretic therapy: no diuretic, inappropriate use of a loop diuretic in a patient with normal renal function, infrequent dosing with a short-acting loop diuretic (e.g., once-a-day furosemide), or a low-dose thiazide in a patient with impaired renal function. Significant impairment in renal function can be present with serum creatinine concentrations in the range of 1.2 to 1.4 mg/dL or even lower, particularly in older patients with little muscle mass. For avoidance of this pitfall, calculation of glomerular filtration rate by equations based on serum creatinine concentration, age, and weight as well as measurement of the urinary albumin-to-creatinine ratio from a spot urine specimen should be an essential part of the routine evaluation of every patient with hypertension. Other common shortcomings of the medical regimen include reliance on monotherapy and inadequate dosing.

Several common causes of apparently resistant hypertension are related to the patient's behavior: nonadherence with medication; recidivism with lifestyle modification (obesity, a high-salt diet, excessive alcohol intake); or habitual use of pressor substances such as sympathomimetics (tobacco, cocaine, methamphetamine, phenylephrine-containing cold or herbal remedies) or nonsteroidal anti-inflammatory drugs, which cause renal sodium retention.

If the three other causes of apparent resistance have been excluded, the search should begin for secondary hypertension (see earlier). The most common causes are unrecognized chronic kidney disease and primary aldosteronism.

Acute Severe Hypertension

Twenty-five percent of all emergency department patients present with an elevated blood pressure (Chapter 7). *Hypertensive emergencies* are acute, often severe, elevations in blood pressure, accompanied by acute (or rapidly progressive) target organ dysfunction, such as myocardial or cerebral ischemia or infarction, pulmonary edema, or renal failure. *Hypertensive urgencies* are severe elevations in blood pressure without severe symptoms and without evidence of acute or progressive target organ dysfunction. The key distinction depends on the state of the patient and the assessment of target organ damage, not just the absolute level of blood pressure.

The full-blown clinical picture of a hypertensive emergency is a critically ill patient who presents with a blood pressure above 220/140 mm Hg, headaches, confusion, blurred vision, nausea and vomiting, seizures, pulmonary edema, oliguria, and grade 3 or grade 4 hypertensive retinopathy (Fig. 66–11). Hypertensive emergencies require immediate intensive care unit (ICU) admission for intravenous therapy and continuous blood pressure monitoring; hypertensive urgencies often can be managed with oral medications and appropriate outpatient follow-up in 24 to 72 hours. The most common hypertensive cardiac emergencies include acute aortic dissection (Chapter 78), hypertension after coronary artery bypass graft surgery (Chapter 74), acute myocardial infarction (Chapter 72), and unstable angina (Chapter 71). Other hypertensive emergencies include eclampsia (Chapter 259), head trauma (Chapter 422), severe body burns (Chapter 113), postoperative bleeding from vascular suture lines, and epistaxis that cannot be controlled with anterior and posterior nasal packing. Neurologic emergencies—acute ischemic stroke, hemorrhagic stroke, subarachnoid hemorrhage, and hypertensive encephalopathy—can be difficult to distinguish from one another (Chapters 430 to 432). Hypertensive encephalopathy (Chapter 432) is characterized by severe hypertensive retinopathy (retinal hemorrhages and exudates, with or without papilledema) and a posterior leukoencephalopathy (affecting mainly the white matter of the parieto-occipital regions) seen on cerebral magnetic resonance imaging or computed tomographic scanning. A new focal neurologic deficit suggests a stroke in evolution, which demands a much more conservative approach to the elevated blood pressure (Chapter 431).

In most other hypertensive emergencies, the goal of parenteral therapy is to achieve a controlled and gradual lowering of blood pressure. A good rule of thumb is to lower the initially elevated arterial pressure by 10% in the first hour and by an additional 15% during the next 3 to 12 hours to a blood pressure of no less than 160/110 mm Hg. Blood pressure can be reduced further during the next 48 hours. The principal exceptions to this rule are aortic dissection (Chapter 78) and postoperative bleeding from vascular suture lines, two situations that demand much more rapid normalization of blood pressure. In most other cases, unnecessarily rapid correction of the elevated blood pressure to completely normal values places the patient at high risk for worsening cerebral, cardiac, and renal ischemia. In chronic hypertension, cerebral autoregulation is reset to higher than normal blood pressures. This compensatory adjustment prevents tissue overperfusion (increased intracranial pressure) at very high blood pressures, but it also predisposes to tissue underperfusion (cerebral ischemia) when an elevated blood pressure is lowered too quickly (Chapter 431). In patients with coronary disease, overly rapid or excessive reduction in diastolic blood pressure in the ICU can precipitate an acute myocardial ischemia or infarction.

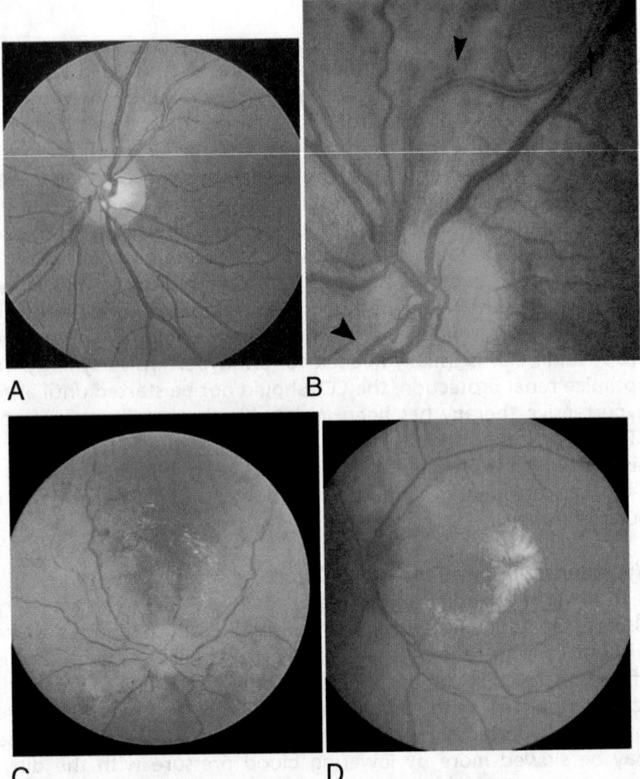

FIGURE 66–11 • Hypertensive retinopathy is traditionally divided into four grades. A, Grade 1 shows early and minor changes in a young patient. Increased tortuosity of a retinal vessel and increased reflectiveness (silver wiring) of a retinal artery are seen at 1 o'clock in this view. Otherwise, the fundus is completely normal. **B,** Grade 2 also shows increased tortuosity and silver wiring (arrowheads). In addition, there is "nipping" of the venules at arteriovenous crossings (arrow). **C,** Grade 3 shows the same changes as grade 2 plus flame-shaped retinal hemorrhages and soft "cotton wool" exudates. **D,** In grade 4, there is swelling of the optic disc (papilledema), retinal edema is present, and hard exudates may collect around the fovea, producing a typical "macular star." (From Forbes CD, Jackson WF: Color Atlas and Text of Clinical Medicine, 3rd ed. London, Mosby, 2003, with permission.)

Rx

Hypertensive Emergencies

Sodium nitroprusside, which is a nitric oxide donor that causes both venous and arterial dilation, is the most widely used agent for hypertensive emergencies because it can be titrated rapidly to control blood pressure (Table 66–8). Intravenous nitroglycerin, another nitric oxide donor, is a potent coronary vasodilator and therefore the drug of choice for hypertension in the setting of acute coronary syndromes, when it typically is combined with intravenous β-blockade (metoprolol) to reduce the double product (systolic blood pressure times heart rate) and thus myocardial oxygen

TABLE 66–8 PARENTERAL AGENTS FOR MANAGEMENT OF HYPERTENSIVE EMERGENCIES

Agent	Dose	Onset of Action	Precautions
PARENTERAL VASODILATORS			
Sodium nitroprusside	0.25–10 μg/kg/min IV infusion	Immediate	Thiocyanate toxicity with prolonged use
Nitroglycerin	5–100 μg/min IV infusion	2–5 min	Headache, tachycardia, tolerance
Nicardipine	5–15 mg/hr IV infusion	1–5 min	Protracted hypotension after prolonged use
Fenoldopam mesylate	0.1–0.3 μg/kg/min IV infusion	1–5 min	Headache, tachycardia, increased intraocular pressure
Hydralazine	5–10 mg as IV bolus or 10–40 mg IM; repeat q4–6h	10 min IV 20 min IM	Unpredictable and excessive falls in pressure; tachycardia; angina exacerbation
Enalaprilat	0.625–1.25 mg q6h IV bolus	15–60 min	Unpredictable and excessive falls in pressure; acute renal failure in patients with bilateral renal artery stenosis
PARENTERAL ADRENERGIC INHIBITORS			
Labetalol	20–80 mg as slow IV injection q10min, or 0.5–2 mg/min IV as infusion	5–10 min	Bronchospasm, heart block, orthostatic hypotension
Metoprolol	5 mg IV q10min × 3 doses	5–10 min	Bronchospasm, heart block, heart failure, exacerbation of cocaine-induced myocardial ischemia
Esmolol	500 μg/kg IV during 3 min, then 25–100 mg/kg/min as IV infusion	1–5 min	Bronchospasm, heart block, heart failure
Phentolamine	5–10 mg IV bolus q5–15 min	1–2 min	Tachycardia, orthostatic hypotension

Rx

demands. Nitroglycerin also is a potent venodilator and therefore lowers preload in patients with hypertension in the setting of exacerbated heart failure. However, nitroprusside (balanced arterial and venous dilation) may be necessary if pulmonary edema results from severe hypertension (increased afterload). Compared with nitroprusside, the fall in blood pressure is less predictable with nitroglycerin. Intravenous labetalol is an effective treatment of hypertensive crisis, particularly in the setting of myocardial ischemia with preserved ventricular function. Nicardipine is a parenteral dihydropyridine CCB that is particularly useful in the postoperative cardiac patient as well as in renal failure (to avoid thiocyanate toxicity with nitroprusside). Fenoldopam mesylate is a selective dopamine-1 receptor agonist that causes both systemic and renal vasodilation as well as increased glomerular filtration, natriuresis, and diuresis; it is a good choice for hypertensive emergencies in the setting of acute renal failure except for its high cost ($598 per patient versus $2.70 per patient with nitroprusside).

After the blood pressure has been brought under acute control, oral labetalol and dihydropyridine CCBs are particularly useful agents in weaning patients from parenteral therapy so they can be transferred from the ICU. A few doses of intravenous furosemide are often needed to overcome drug resistance due to secondary volume expansion resulting from parenteral vasodilator therapy.

Secondary hypertension should be suspected in every patient admitted to the ICU with hypertensive crisis. Normal 24-hour urinary catecholamine values or normal plasma normetanephrine and metanephrine values collected when the blood pressure is the highest (first 24 hours in ICU) effectively rule out pheochromocytoma (Chapter 246). Renal artery stenosis (Chapter 126) and other secondary causes should be excluded after the patient has been transferred out of the ICU but before discharge from the hospital.

Oral Medications for Hypertensive Urgencies

Most patients who present to the emergency department with hypertensive urgencies either are nonadherent with their medical regimen or are being treated with an inadequate regimen. To expedite the necessary changes in medications, outpatient follow-up should be arranged within 72 hours. For management of the patient during the short interim period, labetalol is effective in a dose of 200 to 300 mg, which can be repeated in 2 to 3 hours and then prescribed in twice-daily dosing. If a β-blocker is contraindicated, clonidine is effective in an initial dose of 0.1 or 0.2 mg followed by additional hourly doses of 0.1 mg. Patients can be prescribed 0.1 to 0.2 mg twice daily on discharge. Captopril, a short-acting ACE inhibitor, lowers blood pressure within 15 to 30 minutes of oral dosing. A small test dose of 6.25 mg should be used to avoid an excessive fall in blood pressure in hypovolemic patients; then, the full oral dose is 25 mg, which can be repeated in 1 to 2 hours and prescribed as 25 to 75 mg twice daily.

Incidental Blood Pressure Elevation in the Emergency Department

Blood pressures above 160/110 mm Hg are a common incidental finding among patients who present to emergency departments and other acute care settings for urgent medical or surgical care of symptoms that are unrelated to blood pressure (e.g., musculoskeletal pain, orthopedic injury). In these settings, the elevated blood pressure more often is the first indication of chronic hypertension than a simple physiologic stress reaction, so there is an important opportunity to initiate primary care referral for formal evaluation of possible chronic hypertension. Home and ambulatory blood pressure monitoring is indicated to determine whether the patient's blood pressure normalizes completely once the acute illness has resolved.

Prognosis

One of the most important prognostic factors in hypertension is electrocardiographic or echocardiographic left ventricular hypertrophy, with the latter already present in as many as 25% of patients with newly diagnosed hypertension. In a multicenter observational study of hypertensive patients with no prior history of cardiovascular or renal disease, echocardiographic left ventricular hypertrophy at baseline was accompanied by a three-fold increase in the cumulative 4-year incidence of cardiovascular events.

Because of the firmly established prognostic significance of left ventricular hypertrophy, numerous studies have examined the ability of antihypertensive therapy to cause regression of left ventricular hypertrophy. Meta-analyses estimate that left ventricular mass can be reduced by 11 to 12% with an ACE inhibitor, ARB, or CCB; 8% with a thiazide diuretic; but only 5% with a β-blocker. In contrast, in patients undergoing valve replacement for aortic stenosis, nearly complete surgical normalization of systolic load results in a rapid and dramatic 35% reduction in left ventricular mass. The comparatively disappointing effects of the antihypertensive drug trials are likely to be related to the incomplete normalization of systolic load in monotherapy trials.

Despite the impressive body of randomized clinical trial data, it remains to be determined whether even intensive antihypertensive therapy can completely normalize the excessive risks of cardiovascular and renal disease associated with untreated hypertension. In a large hypertensive referral clinic in Gothenburg, Sweden, treatment of hypertension in initially middle-aged men to a goal of 160/90 to 95 mm Hg with diuretics and β-blockers for 20 years did not completely normalize the risk of myocardial infarction. The persistently elevated risks in the treated patients were related to the existence of associated risk factors, such as cigarette smoking and elevated blood lipid levels, and emphasize the need for global risk reduction and larger reductions in blood pressure. Randomized trials have not yet established whether even lower blood pressure goals than those presently endorsed would produce further reductions in cardiovascular morbidity and mortality and in the risk of end-stage renal disease. *Because of their relatively short duration (typically less than 5 years), randomized trials underestimate the life-time protection against premature disability and death afforded by several decades of antihypertensive therapy in clinical practice.* In the Framingham Heart Study, treatment of hypertension for 20 years in middle-aged adults reduced total cardiovascular mortality by 60%, which is considerably greater than the results of most randomized trials despite the less intense treatment guidelines when therapy was initiated in the 1950s to 1970s.

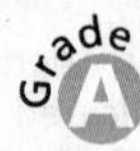

1. The ALLHAT Officers and Coordinators for the ALLHAT Collaborative Research Group: The major outcomes in high-risk hypertensive patients randomized to angiotensin-converting enzyme inhibitor or calcium channel blocker vs. diuretic: The Antihypertensive and Lipid-Lowering Treatment to Prevent Heart Attack Trial (ALLHAT). JAMA 2002;288:2981–2997.
2. Julius S, Kjeldsen SE, Weber M, et al: Outcomes in hypertensive patients at high cardiovascular risk treated with regimens based on valsartan or amlodipine: The VALUE randomised trial. Lancet 2004;363:2022–2031.
3. Lindholm LH, Carlberg B, Samuelsson O: Should beta blockers remain first choice in the treatment of primary hypertension? A meta-analysis. Lancet 2005;366:1545–1553.
4. Taylor AL, Ziesche S, Yancy C, et al: Combination of isosorbide dinitrate and hydralazine in blacks with heart failure. N Engl J Med 2004;351:2049–2057.
5. Dahlof B, Sever PS, Poulter NR, et al: Prevention of cardiovascular events with antihypertensive regimen of amlodipine adding perindopril as required versus atenolol adding bendroflumethiazide as required, in the Anglo-Scandinavian Cardiac Outcomes Trial—Blood Pressure Lowering Arm (ASCOT-BPLA): A multicentre randomised controlled trial. Lancet 2005;366:895–906.
6. Braunwald E, Domanski MJ, Fowler SE, et al; PEACE Trial Investigators: Angiotensin-converting-enzyme inhibition in stable coronary artery disease. N Engl J Med 2004;351:2058–2068.
7. Staessen JA, Wang JG, Thijs L: Cardiovascular protection and blood pressure reduction: A quantitative overview updated until 1 March 2003. J Hypertens 2003;21:1055–1076.
8. Blood Pressure Lowering Treatment Trialists' Collaboration: Effects of different blood-pressure-lowering regimens on major cardiovascular events: Results of prospectively-designed overviews of randomised trials. Lancet 2003;362:1527–1535.
9. Staessen JA, Thijs L, Fagard R, et al: Effects of immediate versus delayed antihypertensive therapy on outcome in the Systolic Hypertension in Europe Trial. J Hypertens 2004;22:847–857.
10. Sever PS, Dahlof B, Poulter NR, et al: Prevention of coronary and stroke events with atorvastatin in hypertension patients who have average or lower-than-average cholesterol concentrations, in the Anglo-Scandinavian Cardiac Outcomes Trial—Lipid Lowering Arm (ASCOT-LLA): A multicentre randomized controlled trial. Lancet 2003;361:1149–1158.
11. Hansson L, Zanchetti A, Carruthers SG, et al: Effects of intensive blood-pressure lowering and low-dose aspirin in patients with hypertension: Principal results of the Hypertension Optimal Treatment (HOT) randomised trial. Lancet 1998;351:1755–1762.
12. Agodoa LY, Appel L, Bakris GL, et al: Effect of ramipril vs amlodipine on renal outcomes in hypertensive nephrosclerosis: A randomized controlled trial. JAMA 2001;285:2719–2728.
13. Yusuf S, Sleight P, Pogue J, et al: Effects of an angiotensin-converting-enzyme inhibitor, ramipril, on cardiovascular events in high-risk patients. The Heart Outcomes Prevention Evaluation Study Investigators. N Engl J Med 2000;342:145–153.
14. PROGRESS Collaborative Group: Randomised trial of a perindopril-based blood-pressure-lowering regimen among 6,105 individuals with previous stroke or transient ischaemic attack. Lancet 2001;358:1033–1041.

SUGGESTED READINGS

Chobanian A, Bakris G, Black H, et al: The Seventh Report of the Joint National Committee on Prevention, Detection, Evaluation, and Treatment of High Blood Pressure. The JNC 7 report. JAMA 2003;289:2560–2572. *The latest U.S. consensus guidelines.*

Dieterle T, Schuurmans MM, Strobel W, et al: Moderate-to-severe blood pressure elevation at ED entry: Hypertension or normotension? Am J Emerg Med 2005;23:474–479. *A 24-hour ambulatory blood pressure monitoring confirmed that an incidental blood pressure elevation of 165/105 or higher is likely to indicate chronic hypertension.*

Dolan E, Stanton A, Thijs L, et al: Superiority of ambulatory over clinic blood pressure measurement in predicting mortality: The Dublin outcome study. Hypertension 2005;46:156–161. *Ambulatory blood pressure measurement predicted total and cardiovascular mortality over and beyond clinic blood pressure measurement and other cardiovascular risk factors.*

Julius S, Nesbitt SD, Egan BM, et al: Feasibility of treating prehypertension with an angiotensin-receptor blocker. N Engl J Med 2006;354:1685–1697. *After 4 years, hypertension developed more often in the placebo group (relative risk reduction, 16%; $P < 0.01$).*

Moser M, Setaro JF: Resistant or difficult-to-control hypertension. N Engl J Med 2006;355:385–392. *Overview of treatment guidelines.*

Pickering TG, Shimbo D, Haas D: Ambulatory blood-pressure monitoring. N Engl J Med 2006;354:2368–2374. *Review of techniques developed to improve the estimate of true blood pressure.*

Victor RG (ed): Clinical Hypertension Review Course Syllabus. The American Society of Hypertension, Inc, 2005. Available at: www.ash-us.org. *A comprehensive update and review for hypertension specialists.*

Wang JG, Staessen JA, Franklin SS, et al: Systolic and diastolic blood pressure lowering as determinants of cardiovascular outcome. Hypertension 2005;45:907–913. *Meta-analysis indicating the safety and benefit of lowering systolic blood pressure even when diastolic blood pressure falls below 70 mm Hg.*

Williams B, Poulter NR, Brown MJ, et al: British Hypertension Society guidelines for hypertension management 2004 (BHS-IV): Summary. BMJ 2004;328:634–640. *The latest British consensus guidelines.*

Wong T, Mitchell P: The eye in hypertension. Lancet 2007;369:425–435. *Discusses the ocular effects of blood pressure.*

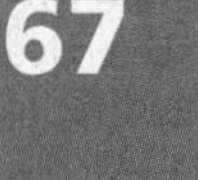

67 PULMONARY HYPERTENSION

Robyn J. Barst

Definition

Pulmonary hypertension is a common accompaniment of many cardiac and pulmonary disorders, for which the status of the pulmonary vascular bed is oftentimes the principal determinant of the clinical manifestations, course, and feasibility of surgical treatment. The prognosis varies greatly, depending on the cause of the pulmonary hypertension and its severity at the time of diagnosis. Although knowledge about the pulmonary circulation has advanced substantially, why one patient behaves differently from another with what appears to be the same degree of pulmonary hypertension remains unclear.

The pulmonary circulation is a low-resistance, highly distensible circulation. In normal individuals lying supine, systolic pressures are of the order of 15 to 25 mm Hg; the corresponding diastolic pressures are 5 to 10 mm Hg (Table 67–1). The mean driving pressure, or the difference between mean blood pressure in the pulmonary artery and in the left atrium, is about 10 to 12 mm Hg, one eighth of that in the systemic circulation. Because blood flow (cardiac output) is the same in both circulations in the absence of any systemic-to-pulmonary communications, pulmonary vascular resistance is about one eighth of systemic vascular resistance. The large aggregate cross-sectional area of the pulmonary circulation is responsible for this low resistance, which is reflected in the

TABLE 67–1 ADULT VALUES FOR NORMAL PULMONARY HEMODYNAMICS AT SEA LEVEL (REST AND MILD EXERCISE) AND AT ELEVATED ALTITUDE (REST)

	Sea Level: Rest	Sea Level: Mild Exercise	Altitude (≈15,000 ft): Rest
Pulmonary arterial pressure (mean), mm Hg	20/10 (15)	30/13 (20)	38/14 (26)
Cardiac output, L/min	6.0	12.0	6.0
Left atrial pressure (mean), mm Hg	5.0	9.0	5.0
Pulmonary vascular resistance, units	1.7	0.9	3.3

sparsity of muscle in the pulmonary resistance vessels, the large runoff of blood from the pulmonary arterial tree during each systole, the large capacity and expansibility of the pulmonary arterial tree, and the large number of minute vessels that are held in reserve. During exercise, pulmonary blood flow increases. Accompanying this increase in blood flow is a decrease in pulmonary vascular resistance brought about by recruitment of new parts of the pulmonary vascular bed, as well as by widening of the calibers of vessels that were already open. As a result of these accommodations, a considerable increase in pulmonary blood flow elicits only a moderate increase in pulmonary arterial pressure. For an adult at sea level, pulmonary hypertension is said to exist when the mean pulmonary arterial pressure is greater than 25 mm Hg at rest or greater than 30 mm Hg during exercise. However, this level, which would represent a modest increase for adults at sea level, is normal for adults at high altitude.

Classification

In 2003, the Third World Symposium on Pulmonary Arterial Classification identified five categories of pulmonary hypertension (Table 67–2): (1) pulmonary arterial hypertension, (2) pulmonary venous hypertension, (3) pulmonary hypertension associated with disorders of the respiratory system or hypoxia, (4) pulmonary hypertension secondary to thrombotic or embolic disease, and (5) pulmonary hypertension caused by diseases directly affecting the pulmonary vasculature. This classification is now widely accepted and used in clinical practice.

Epidemiology

In adults, the most common cause of pulmonary hypertension is lung disease, especially chronic obstructive pulmonary disease (COPD). An estimated 30,000 persons die each year of COPD, many of whom have pulmonary hypertension and resulting right ventricular failure as a contributing cause of death (Chapter 88). Patients with interstitial lung disease (Chapter 92), cystic fibrosis (Chapter 89), sleep apnea syndrome (Chapter 101), and lung disorders caused by occupational and other exposures (Chapters 93 and 94) also commonly exhibit secondary pulmonary hypertension when they become chronically hypoxic. In the United States, about 200,000 patients die annually of acute pulmonary embolism (Chapter 99), often with acute right ventricular failure secondary to acute and severe pulmonary hypertension. Pulmonary hypertension is also seen in patients with chronic or recurrent pulmonary embolism, regardless of the source of the embolic material.

Estimates of the incidence of idiopathic pulmonary arterial hypertension (formerly termed primary pulmonary hypertension) range from one to two newly diagnosed cases per million people per year in the general population. The prevalence of pulmonary vascular disease in patients with other illnesses is not known, but it appears that 1 to 2% of patients with portal hypertension (Chapter 157) or human immunodeficiency virus (HIV) infection (Chapter 413) have pulmonary arterial hypertension. The incidence of pulmonary arterial hypertension in patients with collagen vascular disease ranges from 2 to 35% in patients with scleroderma (Chapter 288) and may reach 50% in patients with limited scleroderma (formerly termed the CREST variant [calcinosis cutis, Raynaud's phenomenon, esophageal dysfunction, sclerodactyly, and telangiectasia]). Pulmonary arterial hypertension has been reported to occur in 23 to 53% of patients with mixed connective tissue diseases (Chapter 280) and in 1 to 14% of cases of systemic lupus erythematosus (Chapter 287), but it is rare in patients with rheumatoid arthritis (Chapter 285), Sjögren's syndrome (Chapter 289), or dermatomyositis

TABLE 67–2 CLASSIFICATION OF PULMONARY HYPERTENSION

- Pulmonary arterial hypertension
  - Idiopathic
  - Familial
  - Associated with
    - Collagen vascular disease
    - Congenital systemic-to-pulmonary shunts
    - Portal hypertension
    - HIV infection
    - Drugs and toxins
    - Other (thyroid disorders, glycogen storage disease, Gaucher's disease, hereditary hemorrhagic telangiectasia, hemoglobinopathies, myeloproliferative disorders, splenectomy)
  - Associated with significant venous or capillary involvement
    - Pulmonary veno-occlusive disease
    - Pulmonary capillary hemangiomatosis
  - Persistent pulmonary hypertension of the newborn
- Pulmonary hypertension with left heart disease
  - Left-sided atrial or ventricular heart disease
  - Left-sided valvular heart disease
- Pulmonary hypertension associated with lung diseases and/or hypoxemia
  - Chronic obstructive pulmonary disease
  - Interstitial lung disease
  - Sleep-disordered breathing
  - Alveolar hypoventilation disorders
  - Chronic exposure to high altitude
  - Developmental abnormalities
- Pulmonary hypertension caused by chronic thrombotic and/or embolic disease
  - Thromboembolic obstruction of proximal pulmonary arteries
  - Thromboembolic obstruction of distal pulmonary arteries
  - Nonthrombotic pulmonary embolism (tumor, parasites, foreign material)
- Miscellaneous
  - Sarcoidosis, histiocytosis X, lymphangiomatosis, compression of pulmonary vessels (adenopathy, tumor, fibrosing mediastinitis)

(Chapter 290). In addition, idiopathic pulmonary arterial hypertension has been associated with autoimmune phenomena, including Raynaud's syndrome (Chapter 288), positive antinuclear antibodies, and autoimmune thyroid disorders (Chapter 244). It is also estimated that the approximately 5% rate of increased pulmonary arterial reactivity in patients with mitral stenosis (Chapter 75) or left ventricular dysfunction (Chapter 57) may represent a genetic predisposition to pulmonary arterial hypertension.

Pulmonary vascular obstructive disease related to congenital systemic-to-pulmonary shunts, or the Eisenmenger syndrome (Chapter 68), develops after a period of decreased pulmonary vascular resistance and increased pulmonary flow. The high rates of pulmonary vascular obstructive disease in patients with uncorrected congenital heart disease (Table 67–3) demonstrate that even if all other causes of death could be

TABLE 67–3 RISK FOR PULMONARY VASCULAR DISEASE IN PERSONS WITH CONGENITAL HEART DISEASE*

Lesion	%	Total No.	No. at Risk
Ventricular septal defect	30	9,000	3,000
Patent ductus arteriosus	9	2,700	900
Atrial septal defect	7	2,100	700
Atrioventricular septal defect	3	900	800
Aortic stenosis	5	1,500	0
Pulmonic stenosis	7	2,100	0
Coarctation	6	1,800	0
Tetralogy of Fallot	5	1,500	200
Transposition of the great arteries	5	1,500	500
Truncus arteriosus	1	300	300
Hypoplastic right heart	2	600	50
Hypoplastic left heart	1	300	0
Double-outlet right ventricle	0.2	60	60
Total anomalous pulmonary venous connection	1	300	300
Univentricular heart	0.3	90	90
Miscellaneous	17.5	5,250	2,625
Total	100.0	30,000	9,525 (32%)

*Assumptions: 3 million live births per year; 1% incidence of congenital heart disease.

eliminated, approximately a third of these patients would eventually die of pulmonary vascular disease. Why irreversible pulmonary vascular obstructive disease develops in some patients in the first year of life and other patients remain "operable" from a pulmonary vascular disease standpoint into the second or third decade of life or later with the same congenital cardiac defect remains unknown. For example, the prevalence of the Eisenmenger syndrome in patients with a secundum atrial septal defect (Chapter 68) is 6 to 9% and is unrelated to the size of the defect. In contrast, a large ventricular septal defect or a large patent ductus arteriosus invariably leads to the Eisenmenger syndrome. Although secundum atrial septal defects are twice as common in females as in males, the Eisenmenger syndrome is still more prevalent in female patients with a secundum atrial septal defect (5:1 ratio in some series), a pattern reminiscent of what is observed with idiopathic pulmonary arterial hypertension (2:1). For other congenital heart defects, the risk for development of the Eisenmenger syndrome is not sex related, which raises the question of whether some patients with Eisenmenger's syndrome and an atrial septal defect do, in fact, have idiopathic pulmonary arterial hypertension.

Risk Factors

Pulmonary arterial hypertension probably reflects an interaction between a genetic predisposition and exposure. Risk factors can be categorized according to the strength of the association with pulmonary arterial hypertension and a possible causal role (Table 67–4).

TABLE 67–4 RISK FACTORS AND ASSOCIATED CONDITIONS FOR PULMONARY ARTERIAL HYPERTENSION IDENTIFIED DURING THE EVIAN MEETING (1998) AND CLASSIFIED ACCORDING TO THE STRENGTH OF EVIDENCE

A. Drugs and toxins
1. Definite
   - Aminorex
   - Fenfluramine
   - Dexfenfluramine
   - Toxic rapeseed oil
2. Very likely
   - Amphetamines
   - L-Tryptophan
3. Possible
   - Meta-amphetamines
   - Cocaine
   - Chemotherapeutic agents
4. Unlikely
   - Antidepressants
   - Oral contraceptives
   - Estrogen therapy
   - Cigarette smoking

B. Demographic and medical conditions
1. Definite
   - Gender
2. Possible
   - Pregnancy
   - Systemic hypertension
3. Unlikely
   - Obesity

C. Diseases
1. Definite
   - HIV infection
2. Very likely
   - Portal hypertension/liver disease
   - Collagen vascular diseases
   - Congenital systemic-pulmonary-cardiac shunts
3. Possible
   - Thyroid disorders

Pathobiology

Genetics

Familial pulmonary arterial hypertension, which represents at least 6% of all cases and perhaps considerably more, is inherited as an autosomal dominant disorder with reduced or incomplete penetrance. It is estimated that individuals in an affected family have a 5 to 10% lifetime risk for the development of pulmonary arterial hypertension.

Mutations in two receptors of the transforming growth factor-β family, bone morphogenetic protein receptor type II (BMPR-II) and activin receptor–like kinase type 1 (ALK-1), have been identified in patients with familial pulmonary arterial hypertension and indicate the critical role of this superfamily in vascular homeostasis and in embryologic development (Fig. 67–1). Mutations in *BMPR2* are found in approximately 50% of patients with familial pulmonary arterial hypertension and in approximately 10% of patients with idiopathic pulmonary arterial hypertension, whereas ALK-1 mutations are seen in a minority of patients who have hereditary hemorrhagic telangiectasia with coexistent pulmonary arterial hypertension. *BMPR2* mutations have also been identified in patients whose pulmonary arterial hypertension is related to the use of appetite suppressants and congenital systemic-to-pulmonary arterial shunts, but not to date in cases related to connective tissue disease, HIV infection, or portal hypertension. Mutations in *BMPR2* confer a 15 to 20% lifetime chance for development of pulmonary arterial hypertension. Hence, gene-gene or gene-environmental interactions must either promote or prevent the disease in individuals who carry a mutation.

Pathology

The vascular endothelium is an important source of locally active mediators that contribute to the control of vasomotor tone. Imbalances in the production or metabolism of vasoactive mediators of pulmonary vascular tone include increased thromboxane and endothelin and decreased prostacyclin and nitric oxide. Thromboxane and endothelin are vasoconstrictors as well as mitogens; in contrast, prostacyclin and nitric oxide are vasodilators with antiproliferative effects. Vasoconstrictors may also serve as factors or cofactors that stimulate the growth of smooth muscle or elaboration of matrix. It appears likely that endothelial injury results in the release of chemotactic agents, thereby leading to

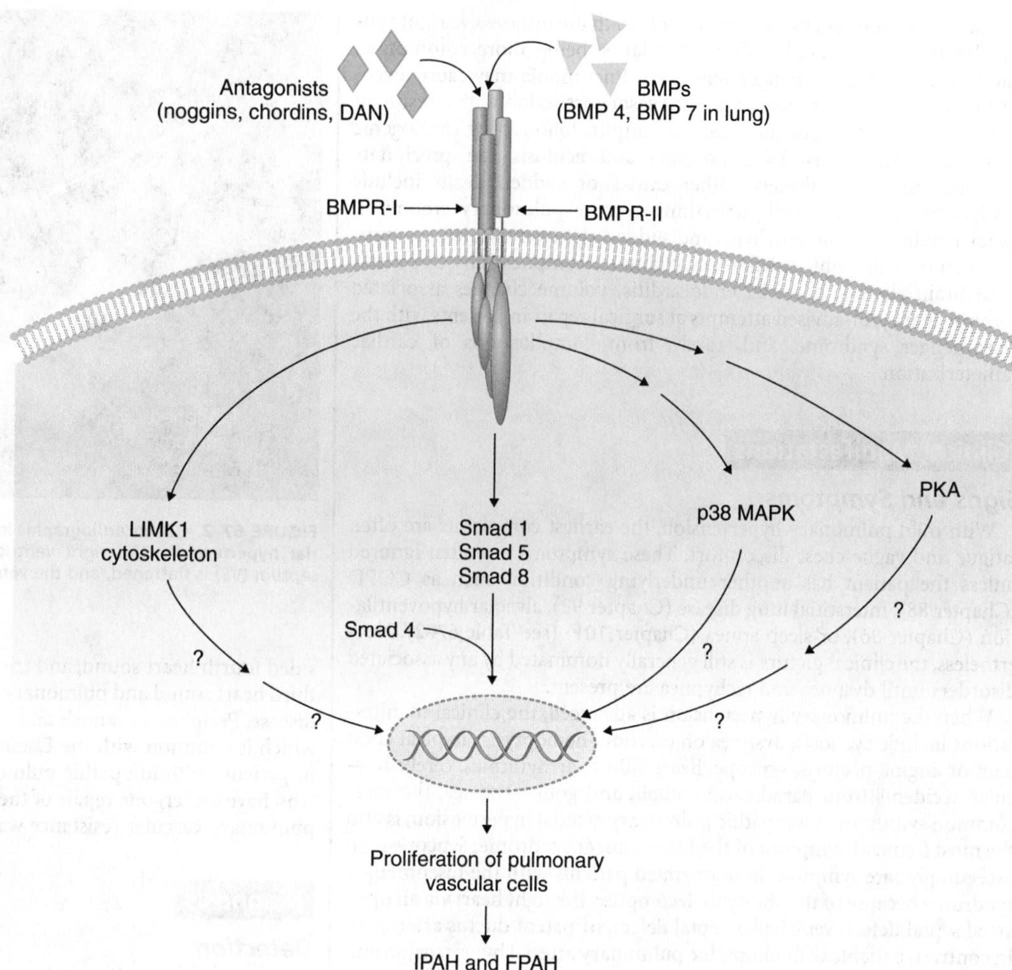

FIGURE 67–1 • Signaling pathways of the bone morphogenetic protein receptor type II (BMPR-II). In the extracellular space, the BMP receptor ligands bind directly to BMPR-II on the cell membrane. The bioavailability of BMPs is regulated by the presence of BMPR-II receptor antagonists such as noggins, chordins and DAN (differential screening–selected gene aberrative in neuroblastoma). Binding of ligands to BMPR-II leads to the recruitment of BMPR-I to form a heteromeric receptor complex at the cell surface. This complex results in phosphorylation and activation of the kinase domain of BMPR-I. Activated BMPR-I subsequently phosphorylates and activates the cytoplasmic signaling proteins Smad 1, 5, and 8. Phosphorylated Smads bind to the common mediator Smad 4, and the resulting Smad complex moves from the cytoplasm into the nucleus and regulates gene transcription. Other downstream signaling pathways that can be activated after the engagement of BMPR-I and BMPR-II by BMPs include cell-type dependent activation of p38 mitogen-activated protein kinase (p38 MAPK) and protein kinase A (PKA). In addition, the cytoplasmic tail of BMPR-II has been shown to interact with the LIM motif–containing protein kinase 1 (LIMK1) that is localized in the cytoskeleton. Germline mutations of the gene encoding BMPR-II underlie idiopathic and familial pulmonary arterial hypertension, which is characterized by the abnormal proliferation of pulmonary vascular cells. However, the specific cytoplasmic proteins and nuclear transcription factors that are involved in the development of idiopathic and familial pulmonary arterial hypertension have not been identified.

migration of smooth muscle cells into the vascular wall. This endothelial injury, coupled with excessive release of vasoactive mediators locally, promotes a procoagulant state that leads to further vascular obstruction. The process is therefore characterized by an inexorable cycle of endothelial dysfunction leading to the release of vasoconstrictive and vasoproliferative substances and ultimately progressing to vascular remodeling and progressive vascular obstruction and obliteration.

Pathophysiology

Pulmonary artery wedge pressure is elevated in patients with pulmonary venous hypertension but normal in other patients with pulmonary hypertension unless there is incidental, coexisting left heart disease. In patients with pulmonary venous hypertension (e.g., mitral stenosis or left ventricular dysfunction), the same elevation in pulmonary venous pressure may result in very different pulmonary artery pressures because of individual differences in pulmonary arterial vasoreactivity.

Pulmonary hypertension can be classified according to the site of increased pulmonary vascular resistance. In patients with precapillary pulmonary hypertension, the abnormalities occur in the pulmonary arteries or arterioles. In passive pulmonary hypertension, the increase in pulmonary artery pressure is caused by an increase in pulmonary venous pressure as a result of disease of the pulmonary veins or, more commonly, increased left atrial pressure secondary to diseases of the mitral valve, left ventricle (systolic or diastolic), or aortic valve. In passive pulmonary hypertension, the increase in pulmonary arterial blood pressure is a direct reflection of the increase in pulmonary venous pressure.

In reactive pulmonary hypertension, increased pulmonary venous pressure leads to reactive precapillary pulmonary artery abnormalities that raise pulmonary arterial pressure more than would be expected based on the pulmonary venous hypertension alone. This mixed picture, which was commonly seen with long-standing mitral valve disease during the rheumatic fever era, is less often seen today. The pulmonary hypertension related to idiopathic and familial pulmonary arterial hypertension, as well as to connective tissue disease, drugs, and toxins, is precapillary. Similarly, in the Eisenmenger syndrome, high pulmonary blood flow causes precapillary pulmonary hypertension, which then progresses independent of flow via a reactive phase.

The normal pulmonary vascular bed has a remarkable capacity to dilate and recruit unused vasculature to accommodate increases in blood flow. In pulmonary hypertension, however, this capacity is lost, and pulmonary artery pressure is increased at rest and further elevated during exercise. In response to this increased afterload, the right ventricle hypertrophies. Initially, the right ventricle is capable of sustaining normal cardiac output at rest, but the ability to increase cardiac output with exercise is impaired. As pulmonary vascular disease progresses, the right ventricle fails, and resting cardiac output decreases. As right ventricular dysfunction progresses, right ventricular diastolic pressure increases, and evidence of right ventricular failure, the most ominous sign of pulmonary hypertension, becomes manifest. Although the left ventricle is not directly affected by pulmonary vascular disease, progressive right ventricular dilation can impair left ventricular filling and lead to modestly increased left ventricular end-diastolic and pulmonary capillary wedge pressure. Dyspnea, the most frequent initial complaint in patients with pulmonary hypertension, is due to impaired oxygen delivery during physical activity as a result of an inability to increase cardiac output in the presence of increased oxygen demands. Chest pain (Chapter 48) most often results from right ventricular ischemia as coronary blood flow is impaired in the setting of increased right ventricular mass and elevated systolic and diastolic pressure; however, the left main coronary artery can become compressed by an enlarged main pulmonary artery, thereby causing left ventricular ischemia. Syncope (Chapters 48, 61, and 427), which is often exertional or postexertional, implies severely restricted cardiac output and diminished cerebral blood flow, which may be exacerbated by peripheral vasodilation during physical exertion.

The two most frequent mechanisms of death are progressive right ventricular failure and sudden death, the latter being more common in patients with the Eisenmenger syndrome. Pneumonia may cause alveolar hypoxia, which worsens pulmonary vasoconstriction with a resultant inability to maintain adequate cardiac output, followed by cardiogenic shock and death. Arterial hypoxemia and acidosis can precipitate life-threatening arrhythmias. Other causes of sudden death include bradyarrhythmias and tachyarrhythmias, acute pulmonary embolism, massive pulmonary hemorrhage, and sudden right ventricular ischemia. In patients with right-to-left cardiac shunts, complications can result from brain abscess, bacterial endocarditis, volume changes associated with pregnancy, ill-advised attempts at surgical repair in patients with the Eisenmenger syndrome, and, rarely, from complications of cardiac catheterization.

Clinical Manifestations

Signs and Symptoms

With mild pulmonary hypertension, the earliest complaints are often fatigue and vague chest discomfort. These symptoms are often ignored unless the patient has another underlying condition such as COPD (Chapter 88), interstitial lung disease (Chapter 92), alveolar hypoventilation (Chapter 86), or sleep apnea (Chapter 101) (see Table 67–2). Nevertheless, the clinical picture is still generally dominated by any associated disorders until dyspnea and tachypnea are present.

When the pulmonary hypertension is advanced, the clinical manifestations include cyanosis, dyspnea on exertion, hemoptysis, atypical chest pain or angina pectoris, syncope, heart failure, arrhythmias, cerebrovascular accidents from paradoxical emboli, and gout. Dyspnea, the most common symptom of idiopathic pulmonary arterial hypertension, is also the most frequent symptom of the Eisenmenger syndrome. Syncope is an exceedingly rare symptom in unoperated patients with the Eisenmenger syndrome because of the ability to decompress the right heart via an open atrial septal defect, ventricular septal defect, or patent ductus arteriosus. In contrast, patients with idiopathic pulmonary arterial hypertension and an intact atrial septum (i.e., without a patent foramen ovale) and patients with elevated pulmonary vascular resistance after complete surgical repair of congenital shunts may have syncope. Angina, a common symptom that is often underappreciated, most often results from right ventricular ischemia (but can result from left ventricular ischemia secondary to compression of the left main coronary artery by an enlarged main pulmonary artery). Edema is generally a reflection of right ventricular failure and is more likely to be associated with advanced pulmonary vascular disease.

Physical Examination

Each underlying or associated condition (see Table 67–2) affects the clinical findings. For example, COPD is usually associated with hyperinflation of the lungs, and this hyperinflation often shifts the position of the heart so that heart sounds are more difficult to hear. With interstitial lung disease, tachypnea invariably occurs. Nevertheless, certain physical findings (e.g., an increased intensity of P_2, a palpable P_2, a right-sided third heart sound, and as the pulmonary hypertension progresses, murmurs of pulmonary and tricuspid insufficiency) typically develop. Ultimately, the neck veins are distended and the liver is pulsatile, and peripheral edema, pleural effusions, and ascites may develop. In patients with pulmonary venous hypertension (e.g., mitral stenosis, systemic hypertension, or heart failure), the findings are frequently overshadowed by signs of left-sided heart disease (Chapters 57, 66, and 75). In idiopathic pulmonary arterial hypertension, there is no evidence of underlying pulmonary or cardiac disease.

Physical examination in a patient with the Eisenmenger syndrome demonstrates central cyanosis, clubbing of the digits, right ventricular lift, a palpable P_2, increased intensity of P_2 (frequently with a single loud second heart sound), a pulmonic ejection sound associated with a dilated pulmonary trunk, and a diastolic murmur of pulmonary insufficiency (Chapter 68). In the presence of heart failure, edema, ascites, and hepatosplenomegaly develop. In patients who have undergone corrective surgery for congenital heart disease when pulmonary vascular resistance was already elevated, the physical examination is similar to that in patients with idiopathic pulmonary arterial hypertension, specifically, an increase in the pulmonic component of the second heart sound, a right-sided fourth heart sound, and tricuspid regurgitation; a right ventricular third heart sound and pulmonary insufficiency generally reflect advanced disease. Peripheral cyanosis and edema are frequently present. Clubbing, which is common with the Eisenmenger syndrome, is typically not seen in patients with idiopathic pulmonary arterial hypertension or in those who have undergone repair of the congenital heart defect or defects after pulmonary vascular resistance was already increased.

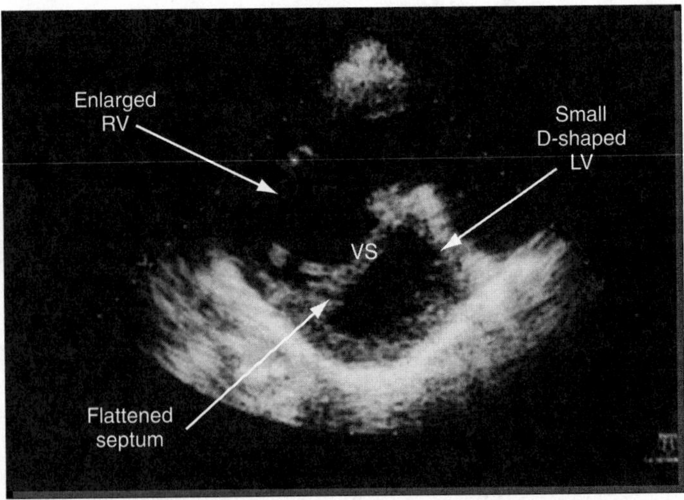

FIGURE 67–2 • Echocardiographic image from a patient with pulmonary arterial hypertension. The right ventricle (RV) is enlarged, the interventricular septum (VS) is flattened, and the ventricular cavity is small. LV = left ventricle.

Diagnosis

Detection

With current medical technology, a correct diagnosis and assessment of the severity of the pulmonary hypertension in a given individual can be made with a high level of confidence. Once pulmonary hypertension is suspected, an electrocardiogram (ECG) and chest radiograph should be performed. Although the ECG may be unremarkable, it more frequently shows right axis deviation and right ventricular hypertrophy with secondary T wave changes; however, the ECG changes often do not parallel the severity of the pulmonary hypertension (see Fig. 42–6). The chest radiograph demonstrates a large right ventricle, dilated hilar pulmonary arteries, and variably oligemic peripheral lung fields, depending on the amount of pulmonary blood flow (see Fig. 49–6).

If the ECG and chest radiograph are either nondiagnostic or consistent with pulmonary hypertension, the evaluation continues with an echocardiogram to exclude congenital heart disease, myocardial dysfunction, and valvar disease. The classic echocardiographic appearance of a patient with idiopathic pulmonary arterial hypertension shows right ventricular and right atrial enlargement with normal or reduced left ventricular size (Fig. 67–2). Pulmonic and tricuspid insufficiency is also often easily detected by Doppler interrogation (Chapter 53). The right ventricular pressure overload in advanced disease reverses the normal interventricular septal curvature. Underfilling of the left ventricle, manifested by reduced dimensions, is a reflection of the severity of the pulmonary vascular disease. Doppler ultrasound is useful for estimating pulmonary artery systolic pressure noninvasively as the sum of systemic venous pressure plus four times the tricuspid regurgitation velocity squared (Chapter 53). Transesophageal echocardiography can provide a more precise assessment of intracardiac defects, including detection of a patent foramen ovale. Saline contrast echocardiography can also be used to assess the integrity of the atrial septum.

Characterization of the Cause of Pulmonary Hypertension

The echocardiogram is the key to detecting congenital or acquired heart disease as the cause of pulmonary hypertension. Pulmonary function tests and cardiopulmonary exercise tests help evaluate patients with uncertain causes of dyspnea. When a cardiac cause is not found, the evaluation should follow a systematic approach (Fig. 67–3). Based on the

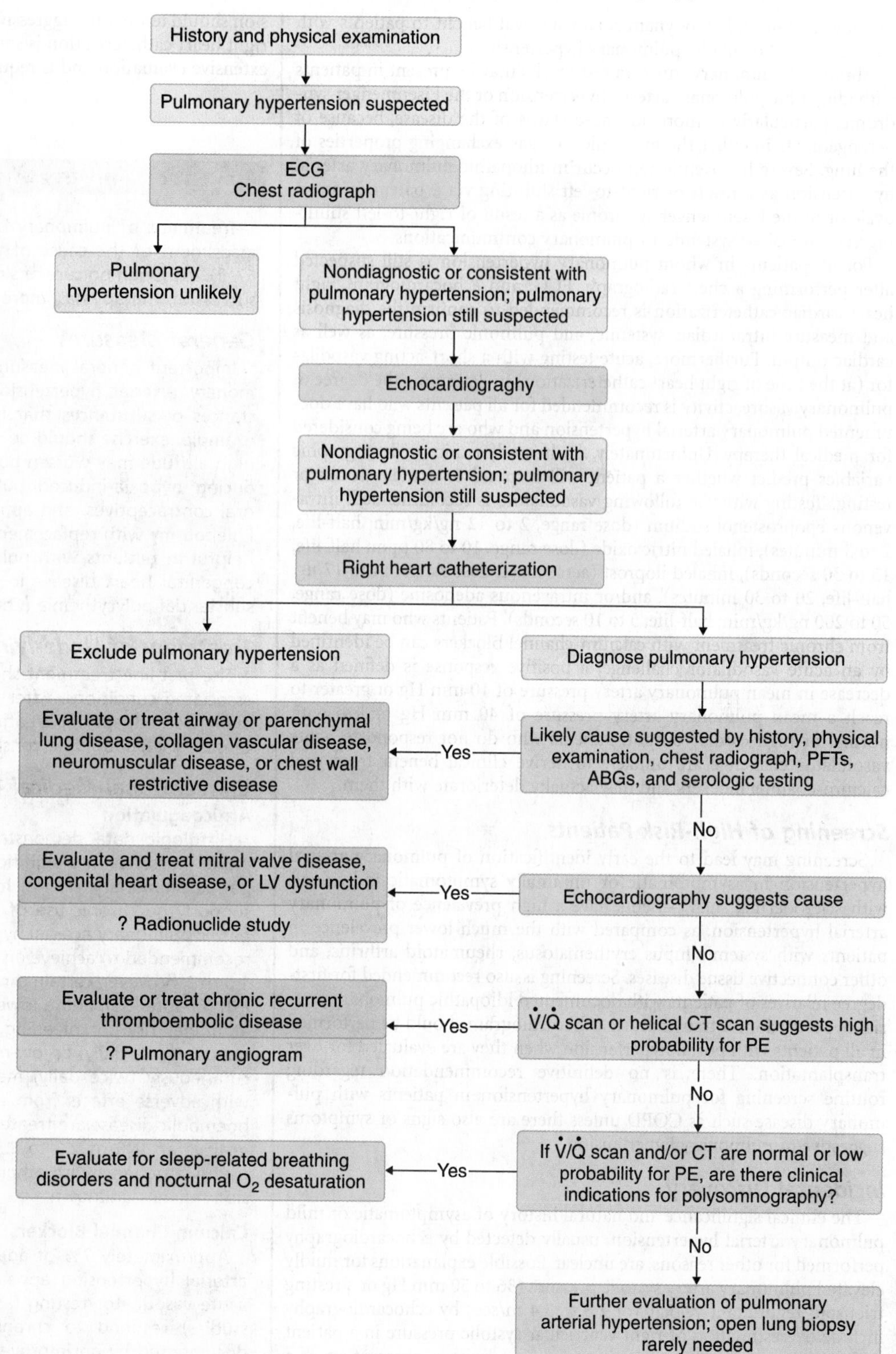

FIGURE 67–3 • An approach to determining the cause of pulmonary hypertension. ABG = arterial blood gas; CT = computed tomography; ECG = electrocardiogram; PFTs = pulmonary function tests. (From Widlitz A, Barst RJ: Pulmonary arterial hypertension in children. Eur Respir J 2003;21:155–176.)

results of the sequentially performed tests, underlying causes or related conditions, or both, can be diagnosed (see Table 67–2).

Magnetic resonance imaging (MRI; Chapter 55) and computed tomography (CT; Chapter 54) can help assess the anatomy in patients with cardiac defects, and high-resolution CT is very useful for the evaluation of patients with suspected interstitial lung disease. Exercise testing is useful for the initial assessment of functional capacity before initiating treatment, as well as serially to assess the response to therapy.

An assessment for sleep-disordered breathing (Chapter 101) is recommended in the evaluation of patients with pulmonary arterial hypertension, even though the prevalence of pulmonary arterial hypertension in the setting of sleep-disordered breathing is quite low and the severity of the pulmonary hypertension is most often mild. Pulmonary hypertension in patients with sleep-disordered breathing is most strongly associated with other risk factors such as left-sided heart disease, parenchymal lung disease, nocturnal desaturation, and obesity. For patients with documented obstructive sleep apnea and pulmonary arterial hypertension, treatment of the obstructive sleep apnea with positive airway pressure therapy will decrease but rarely normalize pulmonary pressure.

Ventilation-perfusion lung scanning and spiral CT are useful screening tests for chronic thromboembolic disease, although pulmonary angiography remains the "gold standard" for this assessment (Chapter 99). In chronic thromboembolic pulmonary hypertension, the clots are incorporated into the wall of the pulmonary arteries and become endothelialized; therefore, pulmonary angiography may underestimate the extent of the obstruction or be difficult to interpret. Angioscopy or MRI may be useful in selected cases. It is extremely important to diagnose chronic thromboembolic disease because thromboendarterectomy provides a clinical, hemodynamic, and survival benefit to patients with chronic thromboembolic pulmonary hypertension.

Abnormal pulmonary function test results may be present in patients with idiopathic pulmonary arterial hypertension or the Eisenmenger syndrome, particularly in more advanced stages of the disease, because of derangements in either the mechanical or gas-exchanging properties of the lung. Severe hypoxemia can occur in idiopathic pulmonary arterial hypertension as a result of right-to-left shunting via a patent foramen ovale or in the Eisenmenger syndrome as a result of right-to-left shunting via unrepaired systemic-to-pulmonary communications.

For all patients in whom pulmonary hypertension is still suspected after performing a chest radiograph, ECG, and echocardiogram, right heart cardiac catheterization is recommended to confirm the diagnosis and measure intracardiac, systemic, and pulmonic pressure, as well as cardiac output. Furthermore, acute testing with a short-acting vasodilator (at the time of right heart catheterization) to determine the degree of pulmonary vasoreactivity is recommended for all patients who have documented pulmonary arterial hypertension and who are being considered for medical therapy. Unfortunately, no hemodynamic or demographic variables predict whether a patient will respond to acute vasodilator testing. Testing with the following vasodilators is recommended: intravenous epoprostenol sodium (dose range, 2 to 12 ng/kg/min; half-life, 2 to 3 minutes), inhaled nitric oxide (dose range, 10 to 80 ppm; half-life, 15 to 30 seconds), inhaled iloprost (aerosolized dose range, 14 to 17 μg; half-life, 20 to 30 minutes), and/or intravenous adenosine (dose range, 50 to 200 ng/kg/min; half-life, 5 to 10 seconds). Patients who may benefit from chronic treatment with calcium-channel blockers can be identified by an acute vasodilator challenge; a positive response is defined as a decrease in mean pulmonary artery pressure of 10 mm Hg or greater to reach a mean pulmonary artery pressure of 40 mm Hg or less with normal or high cardiac output. Patients who do not respond to acute vasodilator challenge are unlikely to derive clinical benefit from oral calcium-channel blockers and may actually deteriorate with them.

Screening of High-Risk Patients

Screening may lead to the early identification of pulmonary arterial hypertension in asymptomatic or minimally symptomatic individuals with scleroderma; such patients have a high prevalence of pulmonary arterial hypertension, as compared with the much lower prevalence in patients with systemic lupus erythematosus, rheumatoid arthritis, and other connective tissue diseases. Screening is also recommended for first-degree relatives of patients with documented idiopathic pulmonary arterial hypertension. A transthoracic echocardiogram should be performed in all patients with portal hypertension when they are evaluated for liver transplantation. There is no definitive recommendation regarding routine screening for pulmonary hypertension in patients with pulmonary disease such as COPD unless there are also signs or symptoms suggestive of pulmonary hypertension.

Incidental Discovery

The clinical significance and natural history of asymptomatic or mild pulmonary arterial hypertension, usually detected by echocardiography performed for other reasons, are unclear. Possible explanations for mildly elevated pulmonary artery systolic pressure (36 to 50 mm Hg or a resting tricuspid regurgitant velocity of 2.8 to 3.4 m/sec) by echocardiography include overestimation of right ventricular systolic pressure in a patient with truly normal pulmonary pressure; serendipitous observation of a rare transient pressure elevation in an otherwise healthy individual; discovery of stable mild pulmonary hypertension, possibly of long duration; or discovery of early progressive pulmonary hypertension in an individual with pulmonary arterial hypertension.

There is a high correlation between measurements of pulmonary artery systolic pressure by transthoracic echocardiography and right heart catheterization, with a reported sensitivity of transthoracic echocardiography for detection of pulmonary hypertension ranging from 79 to 100% with a specificity of 60 to 98%. However, right ventricular systolic pressure increases with age, body mass index, and greater athletic conditioning. For example, pulmonary artery systolic pressure higher than 40 mm Hg is present in 6% of otherwise normal individuals older than 50 years and in 5% of healthy individuals with a body mass index greater than 30 kg/m^2. In general, any degree of pulmonary hypertension by echocardiography should prompt an attempt to define or exclude possible causes. However, the severity of pulmonary hypertension should temper the aggressiveness of the evaluation. Confirmation by right heart catheterization is sometimes warranted before embarking on extensive evaluation and is required before considering treatment.

Prevention and Treatment

Treatment of pulmonary hypertension depends on an accurate assessment of the cause of the pulmonary hypertension (see Fig. 67–3). Although no cure or single therapeutic approach is uniformly successful, therapy has improved substantially (Fig. 67–4).

General Measures

Important general measures for patients with all forms of pulmonary arterial hypertension include the avoidance of circumstances or substances that may aggravate the disease state. For example, exercise should be guided by symptoms, and exposure to high altitude may worsen pulmonary arterial hypertension by producing hypoxia-induced pulmonary vasoconstriction. Pregnancy, oral contraceptives, and appetite suppressants should be avoided. Phlebotomy with replacement of fluids (e.g., plasma or albumin) is helpful in patients with pulmonary vascular disease and cyanotic congenital heart disease in whom severe hypoxemia has evoked substantial polycythemia (Chapter 68).

Treatment of Underlying Conditions

The first-line treatment should be directed at any underlying or associated conditions. After these other disorders have been optimally treated, specific treatment of the pulmonary arterial hypertension itself should be considered.

Conventional Medical Therapy

Anticoagulation

Histologic data demonstrate thrombotic lesions in small pulmonary arteries in a significant percentage of patients with idiopathic pulmonary arterial hypertension, and limited clinical data support the chronic use of anticoagulation in patients with idiopathic pulmonary arterial hypertension. Warfarin anticoagulation is recommended to achieve an international normalized ratio (INR) of 1.5 to 2; however, certain clinical circumstances may require a higher INR (Chapter 35), and a lower INR is often appropriate for patients at higher risk for bleeding. Heparin (5000 to 10,000 U subcutaneously twice daily) or low-molecular-weight heparin (1 mg/kg subcutaneously twice daily) may be suitable alternatives in patients with adverse effects from warfarin. Patients with chronic thromboembolic disease are treated with higher doses of warfarin (i.e., to achieve an INR of 2.5 to 3.5). Whether chronic anticoagulation is useful in patients with other forms of pulmonary arterial hypertension remains unknown.

Calcium-Channel Blockers

Approximately 7% of adult patients with idiopathic pulmonary arterial hypertension appear to have a favorable response with acute vasodilator testing (as defined earlier) and (in uncontrolled studies) respond to chronic oral calcium-channel blockade, as documented by an improvement in symptoms, exercise tolerance, hemodynamics, and survival. Although most studies have used calcium-channel blockers at relatively high doses, such as long-acting nifedipine, 120 to 240 mg daily, or amlodipine, 20 to 40 mg daily, the optimal dosing for patients with idiopathic pulmonary arterial hypertension is uncertain. Patients with no evidence of an acute hemodynamic response to these drugs are unlikely to benefit from chronic therapy and should not be exposed to its frequent adverse effects.

Inotropic Agents/Diuretics

The efficacy and toxicity of cardiac glycosides in patients with pulmonary arterial hypertension remain unknown. Diuretics can reduce the increased intravascular volume and hepatic congestion that occur in patients with right heart failure, although great care should be taken to avoid the excessive diuresis that can decrease cardiac output in patients who are highly dependent on preload.

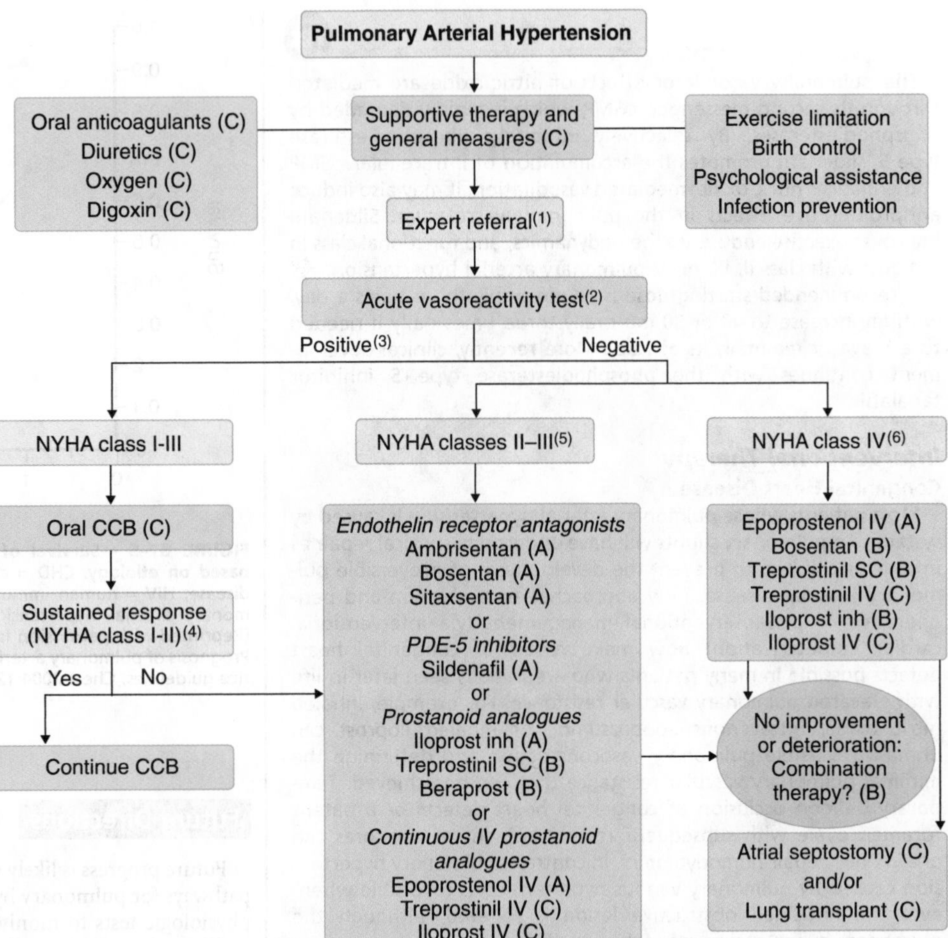

FIGURE 67–4 • Evidence-based treatment algorithm, including clinical trials published through 2005. A, B, and C are levels of evidence, defined as level of evidence A—data derived from multiple randomized clinical trials or meta-analyses; level of evidence B—data derived from a single randomized clinical trial or from multiple randomized clinical trials with heterogeneous results; level of evidence C—data derived from small nonrandomized studies and/or consensus opinion of experts; inh = inhaled; IV = continuous intravenous. (1) Because of the complexity and dangers associated with acute vasoreactivity tests and the treatment options available, it is strongly recommended that consideration be given to referral of patients with pulmonary arterial hypertension to a specialized center. (2) An acute vasoreactivity test should be performed in all patients. (3) A positive acute response to vasodilators is defined as a drop in mean pulmonary artery pressure of at least 10 mm Hg to 40 mm Hg or less, with an increase or unchanged cardiac output during acute challenge with inhaled nitric oxide, IV epoprostenol, or IV adenosine. (4) Sustained response to calcium-channel blockers (CCBs) is defined as patients being in functional New York Heart Association (NYHA) class I or II with near-normal hemodynamics after several months of treatment. (5) In patients in functional class III, first-line therapy may include oral endothelin receptor antagonists, phosphodiesterase type 5 (PDE-5) inhibitors, or prostanoid analogues. (6) Most experts believe that unstable functional class IV patients should be treated with long-term intravenous prostanoid analogues.

Supplemental Oxygen

Supplemental low-flow oxygen alleviates the arterial hypoxemia and attenuates the pulmonary hypertension in patients with chronic pulmonary parenchymal disease. In contrast, most patients with the Eisenmenger syndrome derive little hemodynamic benefit from supplemental oxygen, although all patients may benefit from supplemental ambulatory oxygen if they experience oxygen desaturation with activity.

Targeted Medical Therapy

Prostaglandins

Prostacyclin (epoprostenol) or prostacyclin analogue treatment is supported by the imbalance of thromboxane to prostacyclin and the demonstration of a reduction in prostacyclin synthase in the pulmonary arteries of patients with idiopathic pulmonary arterial hypertension. Continuous intravenous epoprostenol improves exercise endurance and hemodynamics in patients with functional class III or IV idiopathic pulmonary arterial hypertension [1] or pulmonary arterial hypertension related to connective tissue disease [2]; in addition, survival is improved with continuous intravenous epoprostenol in patients with functional class III or IV idiopathic pulmonary arterial hypertension. [1] The starting dose is 1 to 2 ng/kg/min with incremental increases, especially during the first several months of initiation. A mean dose after 1 year is 20 to 40 ng/kg/min for most patients, although there appears to be significant variability in the optimal dose. Continuous intravenous epoprostenol has also been used to treat patients with pulmonary arterial hypertension related to congenital systemic-to-pulmonary shunts, portal hypertension, HIV infection, or drugs and toxins, with reported improvement in exercise capacity, hemodynamics, and possibly survival in uncontrolled studies.

In an attempt to avoid intravenous therapy, prostacyclin analogues administered by continuous subcutaneous infusion (treprostinil) or by inhalation (iloprost; six to nine inhalations per day; 2.5 to 5 µg per dose) are alternatives. [3, 4] Treprostinil is started at 1 ng/kg/min and increased to achieve an optimal dose; treprostinil is approximately 30 to 40% as potent as epoprostenol. Treprostinil and iloprost can also be administered by continuous intravenous infusion; stability at room temperature and longer 4.5-hour half-life are advantages over continuous intravenous epoprostenol. Treprostinil administered by inhalation (four inhalations per day) is in clinical development.

Endothelin Receptor Antagonists

Endothelin-1 (ET-1), one of the most potent vasoconstrictors identified to date, has been implicated in the pathobiology of pulmonary arterial hypertension. The ET_A/ET_B antagonist bosentan was the first approved oral therapy for pulmonary arterial hypertension. [5] Bosentan is initiated at 62.5 mg twice daily for 4 weeks, then increased to 125 mg twice daily. The orally active, selective ET_A receptor antagonists sitaxsentan (100 mg once daily) [6] and ambrisentan (5 or 10 mg once daily) are approved in the European Union and United States, respectively. Adverse effects of endothelin receptor antagonists include acute liver toxicity with an increase in hepatic aminotransferase levels. Sitaxsentan also reduces the metabolism of warfarin.

Nitric Oxide and Phosphodiesterase Inhibitors

In pulmonary vascular smooth muscle cells, nitric oxide activates guanylate cyclase, which increases cyclic guanosine monophosphate (cGMP) and decreases intracellular calcium concentrations, thereby leading to smooth muscle relaxation. When inhaled, the rapid combination of nitric oxide with hemoglobin inactivates any nitric oxide diffusing into the blood, thereby preventing systemic vasodilation. Nitric oxide is therefore a potent and selective pulmonary vasodilator when administered by inhalation, thus making it a useful short-term treatment of pulmonary hypertension; chronic administration of nitric oxide, however, is cumbersome.

The pulmonary vasodilator effects of nitric oxide are mediated through its second messenger, cGMP, which is rapidly degraded by phosphodiesterases. By selectively inhibiting phosphodiesterase type 5, sildenafil promotes the accumulation of intracellular cGMP and enhances nitric oxide–mediated vasodilation; it may also induce antiproliferative effects in the pulmonary vasculature. Sildenafil improves exercise endurance, hemodynamics, and functional class in patients with class II, III, or IV pulmonary arterial hypertension. 7 The recommended starting dose is 20 mg orally three times a day, with an increase to 40 or 80 mg orally three times daily if needed to achieve or maintain its efficacy. More recently, clinical development continues with the phosphodiesterase type 5 inhibitor tadalafil.

Interventional Therapy

Congenital Heart Disease

Most patients whose pulmonary arterial hypertension is caused by systemic-to-pulmonary shunts will have undergone surgical repair as infants or children to prevent the development of irreversible pulmonary vascular disease. New approaches to evaluation and perioperative or peri-interventional management (via interventional cardiac catheterization) now make repair of congenital heart defects possible in many patients who are initially seen later in life with elevated pulmonary vascular resistance. For example, inhaled nitric oxide, intravenous epoprostenol, or inhaled iloprost can unmask reversible pulmonary vasoconstriction and determine the minimal pulmonary vascular resistance that can be achieved. Temporary balloon occlusion of congenital heart defects or a patent foramen ovale with subsequent remeasurement of pressures can predict postrepair hemodynamics. In contrast, pulmonary hypertension caused by pulmonary venous hypertension is reversible whenever the left-sided obstructive lesion is relieved, although the pulmonary hypertension may take months to resolve.

These newer approaches to the evaluation of surgical operability or repair via interventional cardiac catheterization in patients with congenital heart disease are also being applied to treating perioperative and postoperative acute pulmonary hypertensive crises in patients with pulmonary arterial hypertension who are undergoing noncardiac operations (Chapter 457). If a patient with elevated pulmonary resistance is being considered for surgery, there is an increased risk for postoperative pulmonary hypertensive crises. Knowing whether the pulmonary circulation will respond favorably to inhaled nitric oxide, intravenous epoprostenol, inhaled iloprost, or sildenafil will help in the management of this potential life-threatening perioperative complication.

Atrial Septostomy

The rationale for the creation of an atrial septostomy in patients with pulmonary arterial hypertension is based on experimental and clinical observations suggesting that an interatrial defect allowing right-to-left shunting may be beneficial in the setting of severe pulmonary arterial hypertension. This procedure, though still investigational, may help patients who have severe pulmonary arterial hypertension, recurrent syncope, or right ventricular failure despite maximal medical therapy and who have an intact atrial septum or a restrictive patent foramen ovale. It is also used for temporary palliation as a bridge to transplantation, in which case the atrial septostomy can be closed at the time of transplantation.

Heart-Lung or Lung Transplantation

Since 1981, more than 1800 patients have undergone either single-lung, double-lung, or heart-lung transplantation for progressive pulmonary hypertension worldwide (Chapters 82 and 102). The operative mortality ranges between 15 and 30% and is affected by the primary diagnosis. The 1-year survival rate is 65 to 75%, the 3-year survival rate is 45 to 55%, the 5-year survival rate is 40 to 45%, and the 10-year survival rate is 20 to 25%. The timing of referral for transplantation depends on the patient's prognosis with optimal medical therapy, the anticipated waiting time for transplantation in the region, and the expected survival after transplantation.

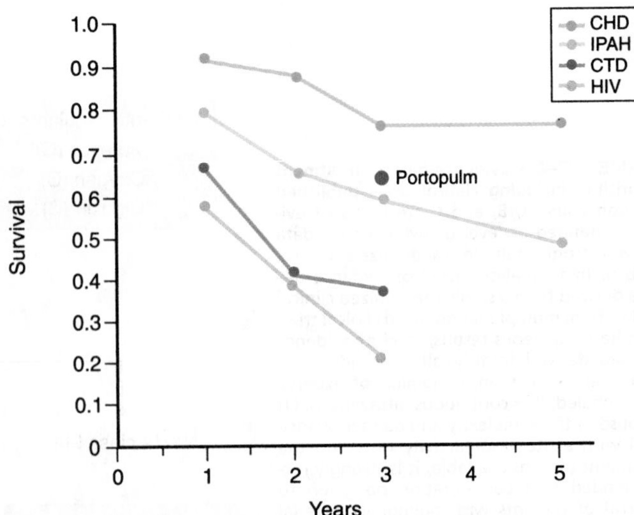

FIGURE 67–5 • Survival of patients with pulmonary arterial hypertension based on etiology. CHD = congenital heart disease; CTD = connective tissue disease; HIV = human immunodeficiency virus related; IPAH = idiopathic pulmonary arterial hypertension; Portopulm = portopulmonary hypertension. (Reprinted with permission from McLaughlin VV, Presberg KW, Doyle RW, et al: Prognosis of pulmonary arterial hypertension: ACCP evidence-based clinical practice guidelines. Chest 2004;126(Suppl.):78S–92S.)

Future Directions

Future progress is likely to focus on attempts to discover final common pathways for pulmonary hypertensive diseases, to develop molecular and physiologic tests to monitor and diagnose pulmonary vascular disease, and to test currently available therapies and develop new ones based on established pathobiologic mechanisms. Investigations are needed to further elucidate the genetic basis of pulmonary arterial hypertension, including candidate genes likely to modify risk.

Prognosis

The prognosis depends on the underlying cause (Fig. 67–5), as well as the severity. The prognosis in patients who have only mild pulmonary hypertension as a result of underlying pulmonary diseases such as COPD is generally much better than for idiopathic pulmonary arterial hypertension. In most cases, it is the natural history of the COPD that determines the patient's ultimate prognosis. In patients with pulmonary venous hypertension, the prognosis depends on the degree of hypertension and the prognosis of the heart failure itself. Patients with pulmonary arterial hypertension related to connective tissue disorders have a worse prognosis than do those with idiopathic pulmonary arterial hypertension, whereas patients with pulmonary arterial hypertension related to congenital systemic-to-pulmonary shunts have a much more slowly progressive course than do patients with idiopathic pulmonary arterial hypertension.

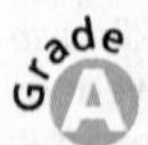

1. Barst RJ, Rubin LJ, Long WA, et al: A comparison of continuous intravenous epoprostenol (prostacyclin) with conventional therapy in primary pulmonary hypertension. N Engl J Med 1996;334:296–301.
2. Badesch DB, Tapson VF, McGoon MD, et al: A comparison of continuous intravenous epoprostenol with conventional therapy for pulmonary hypertension secondary to the scleroderma spectrum of disease. Ann Intern Med 2000;132:425–434.
3. Simonneau G, Barst RJ, Galie N, et al: Continuous subcutaneous infusion of treprostinil, a prostacyclin analogue, in patients with pulmonary arterial hypertension: A double-blind randomized controlled trial. Am J Respir Crit Care Med 2002;165:800–804.
4. Olschewski H, Simonneau G, Galie N, et al: Inhaled iloprost for severe pulmonary hypertension. N Engl J Med 2002;347:322–329.
5. Rubin LJ, Badesch DB, Barst RJ, et al: Bosentan in patients with pulmonary arterial hypertension. N Engl J Med 2002;346:896–903.
6. Barst RJ, Langleben D, Badesch D, et al: Sitaxsentan therapy for pulmonary arterial hypertension. J Am Coll Cardiol 2006;47:2049–2056.

7. Galie N, Ghofrani HA, Torbick A, et al: Sildenafil citrate therapy for pulmonary arterial hypertension. N Engl J Med 2005;353: 2148–2157.

SUGGESTED READINGS

Hoeper MM, Mayer E, Simonneau G, et al: Chronic thromboembolic pulmonary hypertension. Circulation 2006;113:2011–2020. *A practical review.*

McLaughlin W, McGoon MD: Pulmonary arterial hypertension. Circulation 2006;114:1417–1431. *A comprehensive review.*

Rubin LJ, Badesch DB: Evaluation and management of the patient with pulmonary arterial hypertension. Ann Intern Med 2005;143:282–292. *A comprehensive overview.*

Sitbon O, Humbert M, Jaïs X, et al: Long-term response to calcium channel blockers in idiopathic pulmonary arterial hypertension. Circulation 2005;111:3105–3111. *Less than 10% of 557 patients were long-term responders.*

68 CONGENITAL HEART DISEASE IN ADULTS

Ariane J. Marelli

The convergence of major progress in medicine, pediatrics, and cardiovascular surgery has resulted in the survival to adulthood of an increasingly large number of patients with complex structural heart lesions. Adult physicians are becoming increasingly responsible for these patients, commonly in concert with a cardiologist and a tertiary care facility.

Definitions

Patients can be subdivided into three categories according to the surgical status: not operated on, surgically palliated, or physiologically repaired. Congenital heart lesions can be classified as *acyanotic* or *cyanotic*. *Cyanosis* refers to a blue discoloration of the mucous membranes resulting from an increased amount of reduced hemoglobin. Central cyanosis occurs when the circulation is mixed because of a right-to-left shunt.

A *native lesion* refers to an anatomic lesion present at birth. Acquired lesions, naturally occurring or as a result of surgery, are superimposed on the native anatomy. *Palliative* interventions are performed in patients with cyanotic lesions and are defined as operations that serve either to increase or to decrease pulmonary blood flow while allowing a mixed circulation and cyanosis to persist (Table 68–1). *Physiologic* repair applies to procedures that provide total or nearly total anatomic and physiologic separation of the pulmonary and systemic circulations in complex cyanotic lesions and result in patients who are acyanotic.

Eisenmenger's complex refers to flow reversal across a ventricular septal defect (VSD) when pulmonary vascular resistance exceeds systemic levels. *Eisenmenger's physiology* designates the physiologic response in a broader category of shunt lesions in which a right-to-left shunt occurs in response to an elevation in pulmonary vascular resistance. *Eisenmenger's syndrome* is a term applied to common clinical features shared by patients with Eisenmenger's physiology.

Each congenital lesion can influence the course of another. For example, the physiologic consequences of a VSD are different if it occurs in isolation or in combination with pulmonary stenosis. A *simple lesion* is defined as either a shunt lesion or an obstructive lesion of the right or left heart occurring in isolation. A *complex lesion* is a combination of two or more abnormalities.

Epidemiology

In 90% of patients, congenital heart disease is attributable to multifactorial inheritance; only 5 to 10% of malformations are due to primary genetic factors, either chromosomal or related to a single mutant gene. The most common defect observed in patients with chromosomal aberrations is a VSD, which occurs in 90% of patients with trisomy 13 and trisomy 18. Defects of the endocardial cushions and the ventricular septum are found in 50% of patients with Down syndrome (trisomy 21). The most frequently observed defects in patients with Turner's syndrome (45,X) are aortic coarctation, aortic stenosis, and atrial septal defect (ASD). About 15% of patients with tetralogy of Fallot have a deletion on chromosome 22q11; prevalence is higher in those with a right aortic arch. Abnormalities involving the chromosomal band 22q11 can also result in a group of syndromes, the most common of which is DiGeorge syndrome. The shared phenotypic features are designated CATCH-22 syndromes, that is, a combination of cardiac defects, *a*bnormal facies, *t*hymic hypoplasia, *c*left palate, and *h*ypocalcemia. The recurrence risk for families with a child who carries a congenital cardiac malformation due to a chromosomal anomaly is related to the recurrence risk of the chromosomal anomaly itself.

TABLE 68–1 PALLIATIVE SURGICAL SHUNTS FOR CONGENITAL HEART LESIONS

Palliative Shunt	Anastomosis
SYSTEMIC ARTERIAL TO PULMONARY ARTERY SHUNTS	
Classic Blalock-Taussig	Subclavian artery to PA
Modified Blalock-Taussig	Subclavian artery to PA (prosthetic graft)
Potts anastomosis	Descending aorta to left PA
Waterston shunt	Ascending aorta to right PA
SYSTEMIC VENOUS TO PULMONARY ARTERY SHUNTS	
Classic Glenn	SVC to right PA
Bidirectional Glenn	SVC to right and left PA
Bilateral Glenn	Right and left SVC to right and left PA

PA = pulmonary artery; SVC = superior vena cava.
From Marelli A, Mullen M: Palliative surgical shunts for congenital heart lesions. Clin Paediatr 1996;4:189.

Typically, single mutant genes are also associated with syndromes of cardiovascular malformations, although not every patient with the syndrome has the characteristic cardiac anomaly. Examples include osteogenesis imperfecta (autosomal recessive), associated with aortic valve disease; Jervell and Lange-Nielsen syndrome (autosomal recessive) and Romano-Ward syndrome (autosomal dominant), associated with a prolonged QT interval and sudden death; and Holt-Oram syndrome (autosomal dominant), in which an ASD occurs with a range of other skeletal anomalies. Osler-Weber-Rendu telangiectasias are associated with pulmonary arteriovenous fistulas. Williams syndrome occurs with supravalvular aortic stenosis in most cases. Noonan's syndrome is associated with pulmonary stenosis, ASD, and hypertrophic cardiomyopathy. Although autosomal dominant inheritance has been implicated for both, most cases are sporadic. Deletion at chromosome 7q11.23 has been identified in patients with Williams syndrome, and a gene defect has been mapped to 12q22-qter in patients with Noonan's syndrome.

The risk of recurrence when the mother carries a sporadically occurring congenital lesion varies from 2.5 to 18%, depending on the lesion. Obstructive lesions of the left ventricular outflow tract have the highest recurrence rates in offspring. When the father carries the lesion, 1.5 to 3% of the offspring are affected. When a sibling has a congenital cardiac anomaly, the risk of recurrence in another sibling varies from 1 to 3%.

Incidence and Prevalence

Cardiac malformations occur at a rate of 8 per 1000 live births, or 32,000 infants with new diagnoses yearly in the United States. The prevalence of congenital heart disease has increased in the general population, with the steepest rise observed in adults with severe or complex lesions. An estimated 20% die in the first year of life—a substantial decrease from the late 1960s. An overall prevalence of 4 per 1000 adults has been documented. The median age of patients with severe lesions has increased from childhood to late adolescence. Currently, about 900,000 patients are thought to be alive in the United States with congenital heart disease.

Bicuspid aortic valve occurs in about 2% of the general population, is the most common congenital cardiac anomaly encountered in adult populations, and accounts for up to half of surgical cases of aortic stenosis in adults (Chapter 75). ASDs constitute 30 to 40% of cases of congenital heart disease in adults, with ostium secundum ASD accounting for 7% of all congenital lesions. A solitary VSD accounts for 15 to 20% of all congenital lesions and is the most common congenital cardiac lesion observed in the pediatric population; its high spontaneous closure rates explain the lesser prevalence in adults. Patent ductus arteriosus (PDA) accounts for 5 to 10% of all congenital cardiac lesions in infants with a normal birthweight. Pulmonary stenosis and coarctation of the aorta account for 3 to 10% of all congenital lesions.

Tetralogy of Fallot is the most common cyanotic congenital anomaly observed in adults. Together with complete transposition of the great arteries, these lesions account for 5 to 12% of congenital heart disease in infants. More complex lesions such as tricuspid atresia, univentricular heart, congenitally corrected transposition of the great arteries, Ebstein's anomaly, and double-outlet right ventricle account for 2.5% or less of all congenital heart disease.

Clinical Manifestations

Congenital heart disease is a lifelong condition during which the patient and the lesion evolve concurrently. A patient may have been monitored for many years because of an erroneous diagnosis made in infancy or childhood when diagnostic techniques were more limited. The differential diagnosis of native and surgical anatomy in the adult with an unknown diagnosis depends on whether the patient is cyanotic or acyanotic. On completion of the evaluation, the following questions should be answered (Fig. 68–1): What is the native anatomy? Has this patient undergone surgery for the condition? What is the physiology? What can and should be done for this patient both medically and surgically, and importantly, who should do it?

If the patient has not undergone surgery, the question is, Why not? If the patient is palliated, has the degree of cyanosis progressed as evidenced by a drop in systemic saturation or a rise in hemoglobin? If the patient has undergone a physiologic repair, what procedure was performed? Are residual lesions present and have new lesions developed as a consequence of surgery? The patient's physiology is determined by the presence or absence of cyanosis, pulmonary hypertension, adequate filling of the cardiac chambers, and any resulting medical complications.

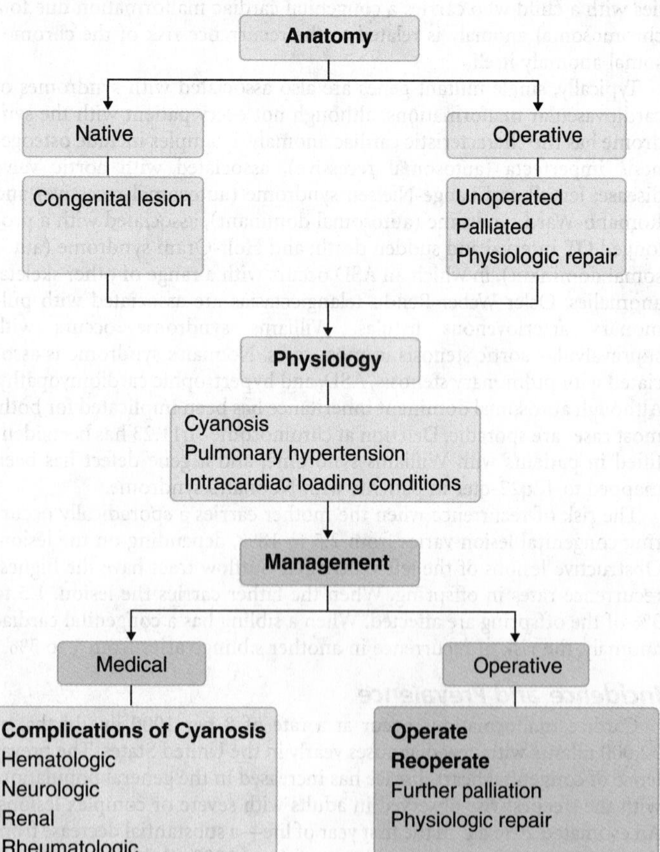

FIGURE 68–1 • The goals of complete clinical assessment in congenital heart disease are to define the anatomy and physiology to determine appropriate management.

A clinical assessment, 12-lead electrocardiogram (ECG), chest radiograph, and baseline oxygen saturation should be part of every initial assessment. Two-dimensional transthoracic echocardiography (Chapter 53) and Doppler and color flow imaging are used to establish the diagnosis and to monitor the evolution of documented hemodynamic complications. Transesophageal echocardiographic examination is particularly useful in adults and is increasingly important during interventional catheter-guided therapy and surgery. Magnetic resonance imaging (Chapter 55) and computed tomography (Chapter 54) are useful adjuncts. Cardiac catheterization for congenital heart disease has shifted from pure diagnosis to include intervention. Coronary arteriography is recommended for adults older than 40 years in whom surgical intervention is contemplated.

Pulmonary Hypertension

Pulmonary hypertension secondary to structural disease of the heart or circulation can occur with or without an increase in pulmonary vascular resistance. Pulmonary vascular obstructive disease occurs when pulmonary vascular resistance rises and becomes fixed and irreversible. In the most common congenital anomalies, pulmonary hypertension is a result of increased pulmonary blood flow because of a native left-to-right shunt. Examples include ASD, a moderately sized VSD, PDA, and a variety of complex lesions. The rate at which pulmonary hypertension progresses to become pulmonary vascular obstructive disease varies from one lesion to another and depends at least in part on the source of pulmonary blood flow. Pulmonary hypertension typically develops in patients with an ASD after the fourth decade; Eisenmenger's syndrome is a late complication seen in only 5 to 10% of cases. In contrast, in patients with a large VSD or persistent PDA, progressive elevation in pulmonary vascular resistance occurs rapidly because the pulmonary vascular bed is exposed not only to the excess volume of the left-to-right shunt but also to systemic arterial pressures. As a result, Eisenmenger's complex develops in approximately 10% of patients with a large VSD during the first decade. Surgical pulmonary artery banding is a palliative measure aimed at decreasing pulmonary blood flow and protecting the pulmonary vascular bed against the development of early pulmonary vascular obstructive disease.

If forward flow from the right side of the heart is insufficient, native collaterals or surgical shunts provide an alternative source of pulmonary blood flow (see Table 68–1). With large surgical shunts, however, direct exposure of the pulmonary vascular bed to the high pressures of the systemic circulation causes pulmonary vascular obstructive disease. As a result, systemic to pulmonary arterial shunts are currently less favored in neonates and infants, in whom systemic venous to pulmonary arterial shunts are now preferred.

Eisenmenger's Syndrome

The term *Eisenmenger's syndrome* should be reserved for patients in whom pulmonary vascular obstructive disease is present and pulmonary vascular resistance is fixed and irreversible. These findings in combination with the absence of left-to-right shunting render the patient inoperable.

The clinical manifestations of Eisenmenger's syndrome include dyspnea on exertion, syncope, chest pain, congestive heart failure, and symptoms related to erythrocytosis and hyperviscosity. On physical examination, central cyanosis and digital clubbing are hallmark findings. Systemic oxygen saturations typically vary between 75 and 85%. The pulse pressure narrows as the cardiac output falls. Examination of jugular venous pressure can reveal a dominant *a* wave reflecting a noncompliant right ventricle until tricuspid insufficiency is severe enough to generate a large *v* wave. A prominent right ventricular impulse is felt in the left parasternal border in end-expiration or in the subcostal area in end-inspiration. A palpable pulmonary artery is commonly felt. The pulmonary component of the second heart sound is increased and can be felt in most cases. Pulmonary ejection sounds are common when the pulmonary artery is dilated with a structurally normal valve. Right atrial gallop is heard more frequently when the *a* wave is dominant. A murmur

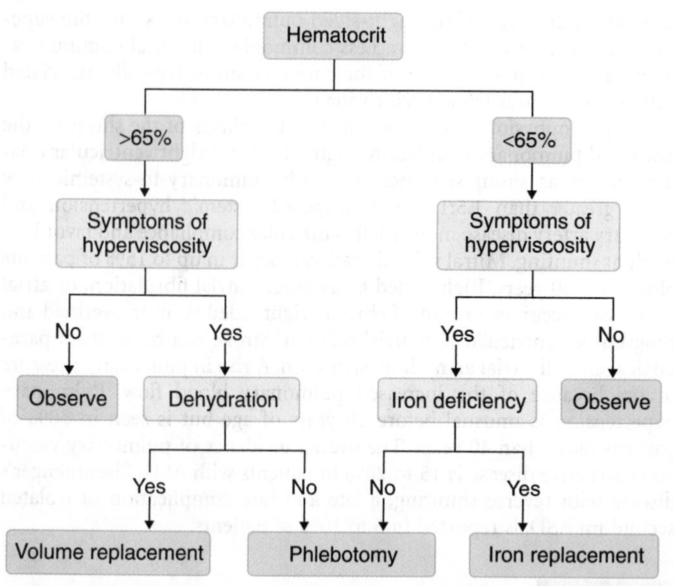

FIGURE 68–2 • Treatment algorithm for erythrocytosis of cyanotic congenital heart disease.

of tricuspid insufficiency is common, but the inspiratory increase in the murmur (Carvallo's sign) disappears when right ventricular failure occurs. In diastole, a pulmonary insufficiency murmur is often heard. The 12-lead ECG shows evidence of right atrial enlargement, right ventricular hypertrophy, and right axis deviation. Chest radiographic findings include a dilated pulmonary artery segment, cardiac enlargement, and diminished pulmonary vascular markings. Echocardiography confirms the right-sided pressure overload and pulmonary artery enlargement as well as the tricuspid and pulmonary insufficiency. Cardiac catheterization is indicated if doubt exists about the potential reversibility of the elevated pulmonary vascular resistance in a patient who might otherwise benefit from surgery.

Systemic Complications of Cyanosis

Cyanosis occurs when persistent venous to arterial mixing results in hypoxemia. Adaptive mechanisms to increase oxygen delivery include an increase in oxygen content, a rightward shift in the oxyhemoglobin dissociation curve, a higher hematocrit, and an increase in cardiac output. When cyanosis is not relieved, chronic hypoxemia and erythrocytosis result in hematologic, neurologic, renal, and rheumatic complications.

Hematologic complications of chronic hypoxemia include erythrocytosis, iron deficiency, and bleeding diathesis. Hemoglobin and hematocrit levels as well as red blood cell indices should be checked regularly and correlated with systemic oxygen saturation levels. Symptoms of hyperviscosity include headaches, faintness, dizziness, fatigue, altered mentation, visual disturbances, paresthesias, tinnitus, and myalgia. Symptoms are classified as mild to moderate when they interfere with only some activities, or they can be marked to severe and interfere with most or all activities. Patients with compensated erythrocytosis establish an equilibrium hematocrit at higher levels in an iron-replete state with minimal symptoms. Patients with decompensated erythrocytosis manifest unstable, rising hematocrit levels and experience severe hyperviscosity symptoms.

In the iron-replete state, moderate to severe hyperviscosity symptoms typically occur when hematocrit levels exceed 65%. If no evidence of dehydration is present, removal of 500 mL of blood during a 30- to 45-minute period should be followed by quantitative volume replacement with normal saline or dextran (Fig. 68–2). The procedure may be repeated every 24 hours until symptomatic improvement occurs.

Hemostatic abnormalities can occur in up to 20% of cyanotic patients with erythrocytosis. Bleeding is usually mild and superficial and leads to easy bruising, skin petechiae, or mucosal bleeding, but epistaxis, hemoptysis, or even life-threatening postoperative bleeding can occur. A variety of clotting factor deficiencies and qualitative and quantitative platelet disorders have been described.

Treatment for spontaneous bleeding is dictated by its severity and the abnormal hemostatic parameters (Fig. 68–3). For severe bleeding, platelet transfusions, fresh-frozen plasma, vitamin K, cryoprecipitate, and desmopressin have been used. Reduction in erythrocyte mass also improves hemostasis, so cyanotic patients undergoing surgery should have prophylactic phlebotomy if the hematocrit is greater than 65%.

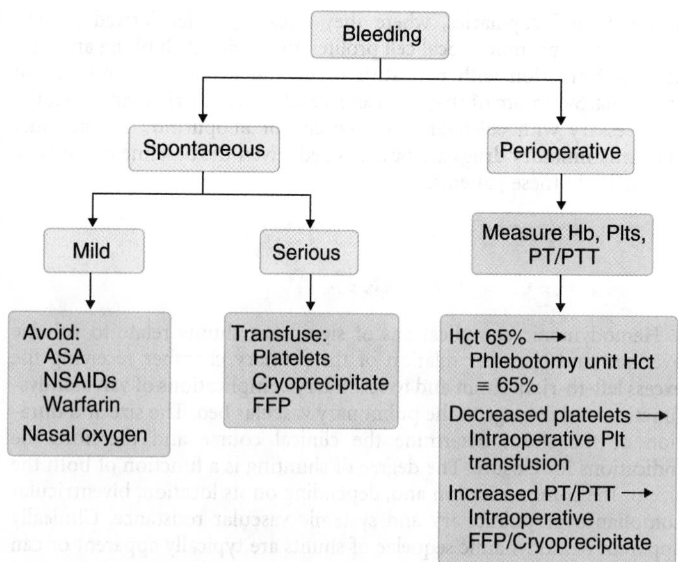

FIGURE 68–3 • Treatment algorithm for bleeding diathesis of cyanotic congenital heart disease. ASA = acetylsalicylic acid; FFP = fresh-frozen plasma; Hb = hemoglobin; Hct = hematocrit; NSAIDs = nonsteroidal anti-inflammatory drugs; Plts = platelets; PT = prothrombin time; PTT = partial thromboplastin time.

Iron deficiency is common in cyanotic adult patients because of excessive bleeding or phlebotomy. In contrast to normocytic erythrocytosis, which is rarely symptomatic at hematocrit levels less than 65%, iron deficiency may be manifested by hyperviscosity symptoms at hematocrit levels well below 65%. The treatment of choice is not phlebotomy but oral iron repletion until a rise in hematocrit is detected, typically within 1 week.

Neurologic complications, including cerebral hemorrhage, can be caused by hemostatic defects and are most often seen after inappropriate use of anticoagulant therapy. Patients with right-to-left shunts may be at risk for paradoxical cerebral emboli. Focal brain injury may provide a nidus for brain abscess if bacteremia supervenes. Attention should be paid to the use of air filters in peripheral intravenous lines to avoid paradoxical emboli through a right-to-left shunt.

Prophylactic phlebotomy has no place in the prevention of cerebral arterial thrombosis. Indications for phlebotomy are the occurrence of symptomatic hyperviscosity in an iron-repleted patient and prevention of excessive bleeding perioperatively.

Pulmonary complications include massive pulmonary hemorrhage and in situ arterial thrombosis. A rapid clinical deterioration associated with progressive hypoxemia often marks the terminal stage of disease. No clear benefits are observed with the use of anticoagulants (systemic or intrapulmonary) because of the risk of prolonged bleeding due to the underlying coagulopathy. The chronic disease process and high mortality prohibit pulmonary endarterectomy.

Chronic oxygen therapy is unlikely to benefit hypoxemia secondary to right-to-left shunting in the setting of a fixed pulmonary vascular resistance. Chronic oxygen therapy results in mucosal dehydration with an increased incidence of epistaxis and is therefore not recommended.

Renal dysfunction can be manifested as proteinuria, hyperuricemia, or renal failure. Focal interstitial fibrosis, tubular atrophy, and hyalinization of afferent and efferent arterioles can be seen on renal biopsy. Increased blood viscosity and arteriolar vasoconstriction can lead to renal hypoperfusion with progressive glomerulosclerosis. Hyperuricemia is commonly seen in patients with cyanotic congenital heart disease and is thought to be due mainly to the decreased reabsorption of uric acid rather than overproduction from erythrocytosis. Asymptomatic hyperuricemia need not be treated because lowering of uric acid levels has not been shown to prevent renal disease or gout.

Rheumatologic complications include gout and hypertrophic osteoarthropathy, which is thought to be responsible for the arthralgias affecting up to one third of patients with cyanotic congenital heart disease. In patients with right-to-left shunting, megakaryocytes released from the bone marrow bypass the lung and are entrapped in systemic arterioles and capillaries, where they release platelet-derived growth factor, which promotes local cell proliferation. Digital clubbing and new osseous formation with periostitis occur and cause the symptoms of arthralgia. Symptomatic hyperuricemia and gouty arthritis can be treated as necessary with colchicine, probenecid, or allopurinol; nonsteroidal anti-inflammatory drugs are best avoided, given the baseline hemostatic anomalies in these patients.

SPECIFIC SIMPLE LESIONS

Isolated Shunt Lesions

Hemodynamic complications of significant shunts relate to volume overload and chamber dilation of the primary chamber receiving the excess left-to-right shunt and to secondary complications of valvular dysfunction and damage to the pulmonary vascular bed. The size and duration of the shunt determine the clinical course and therefore the indications for closure. The degree of shunting is a function of both the size of the communication and, depending on its location, biventricular compliance or pulmonary and systemic vascular resistance. Clinically apparent hemodynamic sequelae of shunts are typically apparent or can be expected to occur when pulmonary-to-systemic flow ratios exceed 1.5 to 1.

Shunt size can be inferred and measured with cardiac ultrasonography. Secondary enlargement of the cardiac chambers receiving excess shunt flow in diastole occurs as the shunt size becomes hemodynamically significant; in addition, the pulmonary artery becomes enlarged as pulmonary pressure rises. When tricuspid insufficiency occurs primarily from right ventricular dilation or secondary to pulmonary hypertension, the regurgitant jet can be used to estimate the pulmonary pressure as another indicator of shunt significance. When the pulmonary-to-systemic flow ($\dot{Q}p:\dot{Q}s$) exceeds 2:1, the volume of blood in both circulations can be estimated by comparing the stroke volume at the pulmonary and aortic valves. Shunt detection and quantification can also be obtained by a first-pass radionuclide study. As a bolus of radioactive substance is injected into the systemic circulation, the rise and fall of radionuclide activity can be measured in the lungs. When a shunt is significant, the rate of persistent activity in the lungs over time can be used to calculate the shunt fraction. For both echocardiographic and radionuclide quantification of shunt size, sources of error are multiple. The most predictable results are obtained only in experienced laboratories. Uncertainty about the physiologic significance of a borderline shunt can be minimized by integrating serial determinations from multiple clinical and relevant diagnostic sources rather than basing management decisions on a single calculated shunt value.

Atrial Septal Defect

Classification of ASDs is based on anatomic location. Most commonly, an ostium secundum ASD occurs in the central portion of the interatrial septum as a result of an enlarged foramen ovale or excessive resorption of the septum primum. The combination of a secundum ASD and acquired mitral stenosis is known as Lutembacher's syndrome, the pathophysiology of which is determined by the relative severity of each. Abnormal development of the embryologic endocardial cushions results in a variety of atrioventricular canal defects, the most common of which consists of a defect in the lower part of the atrial septum in the ostium primum location, typically accompanied by a cleft mitral valve and mitral regurgitation. The sinus venosus defect, which accounts for 2 to 3% of all interatrial communications, is located superiorly at the junction of the superior vena cava and right atrium and is generally associated with anomalous drainage of the right-sided pulmonary veins into the superior vena cava or right atrium. Less commonly, interatrial communications can be seen at the site of the coronary sinus, typically associated with an anomalous left superior vena cava.

The pathophysiology is determined by the effects of the shunt on the heart and pulmonary circulation. Right atrial and right ventricular dilation occurs as shunt size increases with pulmonary-to-systemic flow ratios greater than 1.5:1.0. Superimposed systemic hypertension and coronary artery disease modify left ventricular compliance and favor left-to-right shunting. Mitral valve disease can occur in up to 15% of patients older than 50 years. Right-sided heart failure, atrial fibrillation, or atrial flutter can occur as a result of chronic right-sided volume overload and progressive ventricular and atrial dilation. Stroke can result from paradoxical emboli, atrial arrhythmias, or both. A rise in pulmonary pressure occurs because of the increased pulmonary blood flow. Pulmonary hypertension is unusual before 20 years of age but is seen in 50% of patients older than 40 years. The overall incidence of pulmonary vascular obstructive disease is 15 to 20% in patients with ASD. Eisenmenger's disease with reverse shunting, a late and rare complication of isolated secundum ASD, is reported in 5 to 10% of patients.

Diagnosis

Although most patients are minimally symptomatic in the first three decades, more than 70% become impaired by the fifth decade. Initial symptoms include exercise intolerance, dyspnea on exertion, and fatigue caused most commonly by right-sided heart failure and pulmonary hypertension. Palpitations, syncope, and stroke can occur with the development of atrial arrhythmias.

On physical examination, most adults have a normal general physical appearance. When Holt-Oram syndrome is present, the thumb may have a third phalanx or may be rudimentary or absent. With an uncomplicated nonrestrictive communication between both atria, the *a* and *v* waves are equal in amplitude. Precordial palpation typically discloses a normal left ventricular impulse unless mitral valve disease occurs. Characteristically, if the shunt is significant, a right ventricular impulse can be felt in the left parasternal area in end-expiration or in the subxiphoid area in end-inspiration. A dilated pulmonary artery can sometimes be felt in the second left intercostal space. On auscultation, the hallmark of an ASD is the wide and fixed splitting of the second heart sound. Pulmonary valve closure, as reflected by P_2, is delayed because of right ventricular overload and the increased capacitance of the pulmonary vascular bed. The A_2-P_2 interval is fixed because the increase in venous return elevates the right atrial pressure during inspiration, thereby decreasing the degree of left-to-right shunting and offsetting the usual phasic respiratory changes. In addition, compliance of the pulmonary circulation is reduced from the high flow, thus making the vascular compartment less susceptible to any further increase in blood flow. A soft midsystolic murmur generated by the increased flow across the pulmonary valve is usually heard in the second left interspace. In the presence of a high left-to-right shunt volume, increased flow across the tricuspid valve is heard as a mid-diastolic murmur at the lower left sternal border. With advanced right-sided heart failure, evidence of systemic venous congestion is present.

The ECG characteristically shows an incomplete right bundle branch block pattern (Fig. 68–4). Right axis deviation and atrial abnormalities, including a prolonged PR interval, atrial fibrillation, and flutter, are also seen. Typically, the chest radiograph shows pulmonary vascular plethora with increased markings in both lung fields consistent with increased pulmonary blood flow (see Fig. 51–13). The main pulmonary artery and both its branches are dilated. Right atrial and right ventricular dilation

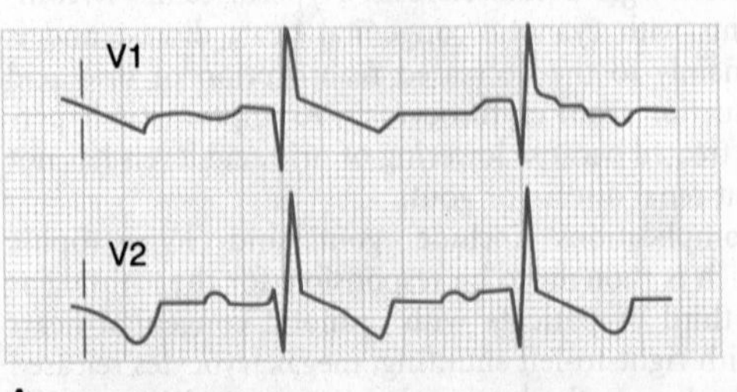

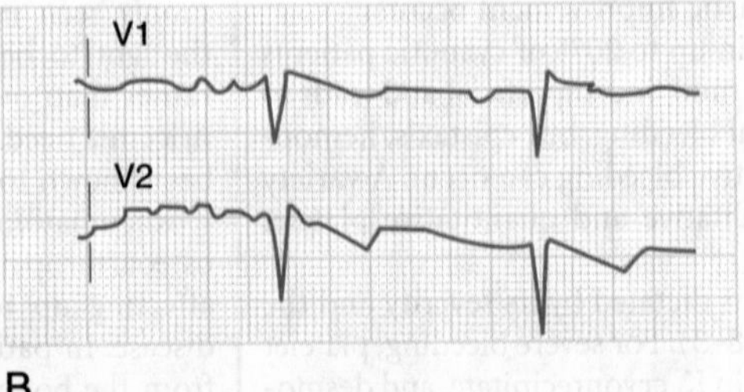

FIGURE 68–4 • Electrocardiographic hallmark in atrial septal defect. Right precordial leads V_1 and V_2 illustrate two variants of an incomplete right bundle branch block pattern, the rSrT pattern (A) and the rsR′ pattern (B).

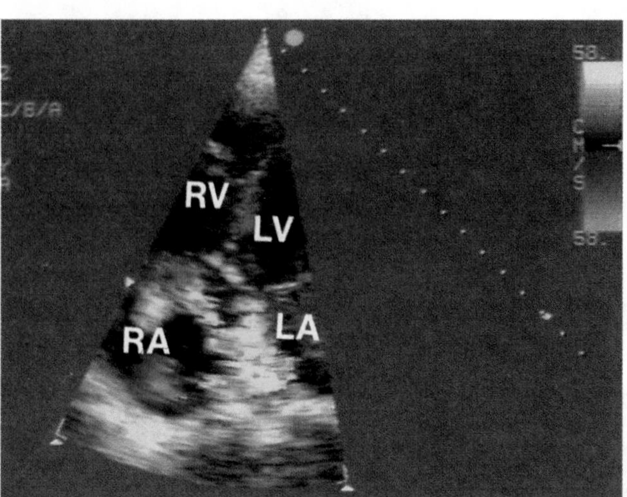

FIGURE 68–5 • Color flow Doppler apical four-chamber view showing blood flow from the left atrium (LA) to the right atrium (RA) through a moderately sized atrial septal defect. LV = left ventricle; RV = right ventricle. (From Forbes CD, Jackson WF: Color Atlas and Text of Clinical Medicine, 3rd ed. London, Mosby, 2003.)

can be seen. Cardiac ultrasonography is diagnostic and provides important prognostic information (Fig. 68–5). Ostium primum and secundum ASDs are easily identifiable with transthoracic imaging, but a sinus venosus ASD can be missed unless it is specifically sought. For more accurate visualization of the superior interatrial septum and localization of the pulmonary veins, transesophageal echocardiography is useful. With Doppler study, pulmonary artery pressures can be quantified, and the Q̇p:Q̇s can be measured.

Treatment

Rx

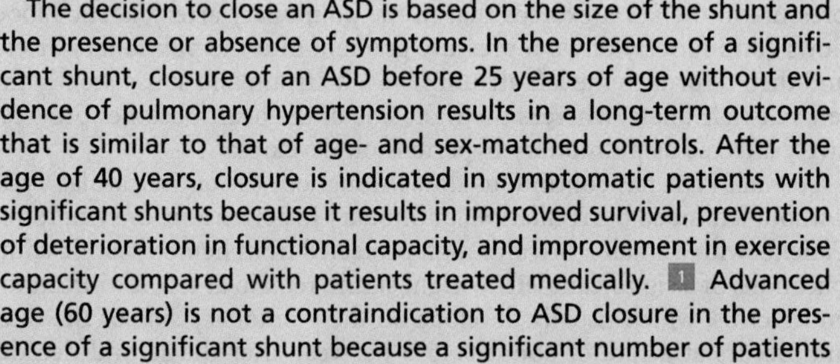

The decision to close an ASD is based on the size of the shunt and the presence or absence of symptoms. In the presence of a significant shunt, closure of an ASD before 25 years of age without evidence of pulmonary hypertension results in a long-term outcome that is similar to that of age- and sex-matched controls. After the age of 40 years, closure is indicated in symptomatic patients with significant shunts because it results in improved survival, prevention of deterioration in functional capacity, and improvement in exercise capacity compared with patients treated medically. 1 Advanced age (60 years) is not a contraindication to ASD closure in the presence of a significant shunt because a significant number of patients will show evidence of symptomatic improvement. Closure is also indicated in patients with systemic embolization in the presence of patent foramen ovale.

Uncomplicated secundum ASDs may be closed surgically in children and adults with minimal operative mortality, in the range of 1 to 3% or less. Preoperative pulmonary artery pressure and the presence or absence of pulmonary vascular disease are important predictors of successful surgical outcome.

Centrally located defects measuring up to 3.5 cm can be occluded by transcatheter techniques in a cardiac catheterization laboratory. Advantages of this approach include the avoidance of sternotomy and cardiopulmonary bypass. Complications, including device fracture with embolization and residual shunts, should decrease as newer devices are used.

Patent Foramen Ovale

Integrity of the fetal circulation depends on the patency of the foramen ovale. In the majority of cases, the fall in pulmonary vascular resistance at birth induces the foramen to become sealed. Necropsy studies have revealed that the foramen ovale remains patent beyond the first year of life in about 30% of individuals, and clinical studies have demonstrated that the prevalence of patent foramen ovale is three times greater in patients with cryptogenic stroke (Chapter 431), particularly before the age of 55 years, because of right-to-left shunting and paradoxical embolization of material from the venous circulation. Cardiac investigation of the patient with cryptogenic stroke includes transesophageal echocardiography with agitated saline injection to visualize the presence of a right-to-left shunt (Chapter 53). Patent foramen ovale most likely to result in future paradoxical embolization is found in patients younger than 55 years with a prior cryptogenic stroke, in association with a hypermobile septum with aneurysm formation, and when a significant amount of right-to-left shunting is present at rest without provocative maneuvers. Some data suggest that a patent foramen ovale also may be associated with migraine headaches.

Treatment

Rx

There are no indications for primary stroke prevention in a patient in whom a patent foramen ovale is fortuitously diagnosed on routine echocardiography. Warfarin to an international normalized ratio of 2.0 to 3.0 is usually preferred to aspirin for secondary stroke prevention in high-risk patients. Primary closure of a patent foramen ovale is indicated when a patient has contraindications to medical therapy, if medical therapy has failed, or in the presence of a hypercoagulable state not treatable by medical therapy. Device closure in experienced centers is usually preferred to surgical closure, although surgical closure is performed if the patient undergoes cardiac surgery for other reasons. Device closure appears to be associated with a low incidence of yearly recurrence rates.

Ventricular Septal Defect

For anatomic classification of VSDs, the interventricular septum can be divided into four regions. Defects of the membranous septum, or infracristal VSDs, are located in a small translucent area beneath the aortic valve and account for up to 80% of VSDs. These VSDs typically show a variable degree of extension into the inlet or outlet septum, hence their designation as perimembranous. Infundibular defects or supracristal outlet VSDs occur in the conal septum above the crista supraventricularis and below the pulmonary valve. Inlet defects are identified at the crux of the heart between the tricuspid and mitral valves and are usually associated with other anomalies of the atrioventricular canal. Defects of the trabecular or muscular septum can be multiple and occur distal to the septal attachment of the tricuspid valve and toward the apex.

The pathophysiology and clinical course of VSDs depend on the size of the defect, the status of the pulmonary vascular bed, and the effects of shunt size on intracardiac hemodynamics. Unlike ASDs, a VSD may decrease in size with time. Approximately half of all native VSDs are small, and more than half of them close spontaneously; moderate or even large VSDs may also close in 10% or less of cases. The highest closure rates are observed in the first decade of life; spontaneous closure in adult life is unusual.

Patients who have a small defect with trivial or mild shunts are defined as those with a Q̇p:Q̇s of less than 1.5 and normal pulmonary artery pressure and vascular resistance. Patients with moderate defects have a Q̇p:Q̇s ratio of greater than 1.2 and elevated pulmonary artery pressure but not elevated pulmonary vascular resistance. Patients with a large and severe defect have an elevated Q̇p:Q̇s ratio with high pulmonary pressure and elevated pulmonary vascular resistance. Eisenmenger's complex develops in about 10% of patients with VSDs, usually when there is no resistance to flow at the level of the defect, which can be as large as the aorta. When a systolic pressure gradient is present between the ventricles, the physiologic severity may be trivial or mild but can also be moderate or severe.

Minimal or mild defects usually cause no significant hemodynamic or physiologic abnormality. A moderate or severe defect causes left atrial and ventricular dilation consistent with the degree of left-to-right shunting. Shunting across the ventricular septum occurs predominantly during systole when left ventricular pressure exceeds that on the right; diastolic filling abnormalities occur in the left atrium. With moderate or severe defects, the right side of the heart becomes affected as a function of the rise in pulmonary pressure and pulmonary blood flow.

Diagnosis

An adult with a VSD most commonly has a small restrictive lesion that either was small at birth or has undergone some degree of spontaneous closure. A second group of patients consists of those with large, nonrestrictive VSDs that have not been operated on; these patients have had Eisenmenger's complex for most of their lives. Patients with a moderately sized defect are typically symptomatic as children and are therefore more likely to have repair at a young age.

Patients with a trivial or mild shunt across a small, restrictive VSD are usually asymptomatic. Physical examination discloses no evidence of systemic or pulmonary venous congestion, and jugular venous pressure is normal. A thrill may be palpable at the left sternal border. Auscultation reveals a normal S_1 and S_2 without gallops. A grade 4 or louder, widely radiating, high-frequency, pansystolic murmur is heard maximally in the third or fourth intercostal space and reflects the high-pressure gradient between the left and right ventricles throughout systole. The striking contrast between a loud murmur and an otherwise normal cardiac examination is an important diagnostic clue. The ECG and chest radiograph are also normal in patients with small VSDs.

At the other end of the spectrum are patients with Eisenmenger's complex (see earlier). Between these two extremes are patients with a moderate defect, whose pathology reflects a combination of pulmonary hypertension and left-sided volume overload resulting from a significant left-to-right shunt. In adults, shortness of breath on exertion can be the result of both pulmonary venous congestion and elevated pulmonary pressure. On physical examination, a diffuse palpable left ventricular impulse occurs with a variable degree of right ventricular hypertrophy and an accentuated second heart sound. A systolic murmur persists as long as pulmonary vascular resistance is below systemic resistance. The ECG commonly shows left atrial enlargement and left ventricular hypertrophy. The chest radiograph shows shunt vascularity with an enlarged left atrium and ventricle. The degree of pulmonary hypertension determines the size of the pulmonary artery trunk.

Echocardiography can identify the defect and determine the significance of the shunt by assessing left atrial and ventricular size, pulmonary artery pressure, and the presence or absence of right ventricular hypertrophy. Cardiac catheterization is reserved for those in whom surgery is considered. Adults with a small defect of no physiologic significance need not be studied invasively. Those with Eisenmenger's complex have severe pulmonary vascular disease and are not surgical candidates. Patients who have a moderately sized shunt that appears hemodynamically significant and in whom pulmonary pressures are elevated are most likely to benefit from direct measurements of pulmonary vascular resistance and reactivity.

Treatment

All patients with a VSD of any size require endocarditis prophylaxis (Chapter 76). Patients with Eisenmenger's complex have pulmonary vascular resistance that is prohibitive to surgery. For this group of patients, management centers on the medical complications of cyanosis (see earlier). In a few patients with small defects, complications can relate to progressive tricuspid insufficiency caused by septal aneurysm formation or to acquired aortic insufficiency when an aortic cusp becomes engaged in the high-velocity jet flow generated by the defect. The intermediate group of patients with a defect of moderate physiologic significance should have surgical closure unless it is contraindicated by high pulmonary vascular resistance.

Late results after operative closure of isolated VSDs include residual patency in up to 20% of patients, only about 5% of whom need a reoperation. Rhythm disturbances after surgical closure of VSDs include tachyarrhythmias and conduction disturbances. Right bundle branch block occurs in one third to two thirds of patients, whereas first-degree atrioventricular block and complete heart block occur in less than 10%. Sudden cardiac death after surgical repair of VSD occurs in 2% of patients.

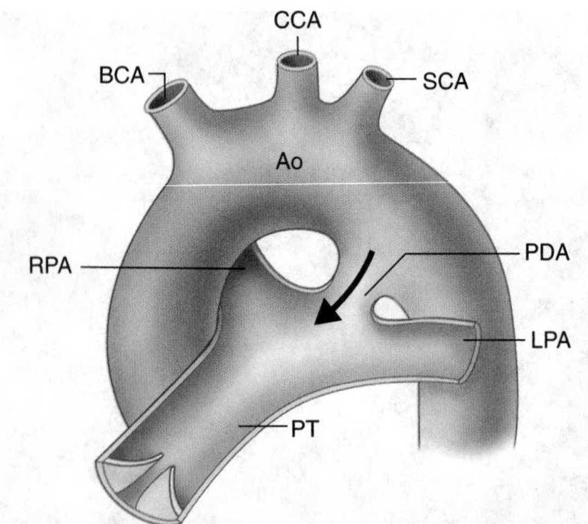

FIGURE 68–6 • The anatomy of a patent ductus arteriosus is shown. Note the relation between the position of the ductus, the left subclavian artery, and the pulmonary artery bifurcation. Ao = aorta; BCA = brachiocephalic; CCA = common carotid artery; L = left; PDA = patent ductus arteriosus; PT = pulmonary trunk; RPA = right pulmonary artery; SCA = subclavian artery. (From Perloff JK [ed]: Clinical Recognition of Congenital Heart Disease, 4th ed. Philadelphia, WB Saunders, 1994, p 510.)

Patent Ductus Arteriosus

The ductus arteriosus connects the descending aorta to the main pulmonary trunk near the origin of the left subclavian artery (Fig. 68–6). Normal postnatal closure results in fibrosis and degenerative changes in the ductal lumen, leaving in its place the residual ligamentum arteriosum, which rarely can become part of an abnormal vascular ring. When the duct persists, significant calcification of the aortic ductal end is observed.

The physiologic consequences of a PDA are determined by its size and length as well as by the ratio of pressure and resistance of the pulmonary and aortic circulations on either end of the duct. If systolic and diastolic pressure in the aorta exceeds that in the pulmonary artery, aortic blood flows continuously down a pressure gradient into the pulmonary artery and then returns to the left atrium. The left atrium and subsequently the left ventricle dilate, whereas the right side of the heart becomes progressively affected as pulmonary hypertension develops.

A small PDA has continuous flow throughout the entire cardiac cycle without left-sided heart dilation, pulmonary hypertension, or symptoms. Patients with a small PDA, although protected from hemodynamic complications of a significant left-to-right shunt, remain at risk for infectious endarteritis, which usually develops on the pulmonary side of the duct and occurs at a rate of about 0.45% per year after the second decade. Because endarteritis accounts for up to one third of the total mortality in patients with PDA, ductal closure should be considered even when the PDA is small.

A PDA is of moderate or large size but still restrictive when a left-to-right shunt occurs throughout systole and diastole is of variable duration. Left atrial or ventricular dilation and pulmonary hypertension will vary with the quantity of left-to-right shunting as well as with the secondary effects on the pulmonary vascular bed. Symptoms generally increase by the second and third decades and include dyspnea, palpitations, and exercise intolerance. As heart failure, pulmonary hypertension, or endarteritis develops, mortality rises to 3 to 4% per year by the fourth decade, and two thirds of patients die by 60 years of age. Eisenmenger's physiology with systemic or suprasystemic pulmonary pressure and a right-to-left shunt develops in 5% of patients with an isolated PDA.

Diagnosis

In patients with Eisenmenger's physiology, a right-to-left shunt from the pulmonary artery to the descending aorta results in decreased oxygen saturation in the lower extremities compared with the upper extremities. This difference in cyanosis and clubbing are most prominent in the toes; the left arm is variably affected through the left subclavian artery, and the right arm is typically spared. With a large left-to-right shunt, the pulse pressure widens as diastolic flow into the pulmonary artery lowers systemic diastolic pressure. The arterial pulse becomes bounding as a result of increased stroke volume. Precordial palpation discloses variable left and right ventricular impulses as determined by the relative degree of left-sided volume overload and pulmonary hypertension. In the presence of a continuous aortopulmonary gradient, the classic "machinery" murmur of a PDA can be heard at the first or second left intercostal space below the left clavicle. As the pulmonary pressure rises, the diastolic component of the murmur becomes progressively shorter. With the development of Eisenmenger's physiology and equalization of aortic and pulmonary pressure, the entire murmur may disappear and the clinical findings are dominated by pulmonary hypertension.

In adult patients with a significant left-to-right shunt, the ECG shows a bifid P wave in at least one limb lead consistent with left atrial enlargement and a variable degree of left ventricular hypertrophy. The PR interval is prolonged in about 20% of patients. In older patients, the chest radiograph shows calcification at the location of the PDA. Characteristically, the ascending aorta and pulmonary artery are dilated, and the left-sided chambers are enlarged. Echocardiography may not directly visualize the PDA but can accurately identify it by a Doppler signal that often parallels the length of the murmur. Left-sided heart dilation and pulmonary hypertension can be quantified and monitored. Cardiac catheterization to assess pulmonary vascular resistance is commonly indicated before closure.

Treatment Rx

After ligation of a PDA in infancy or early childhood, bacterial endocarditis prophylaxis is not required, cardiac function is commonly normal, and no special follow-up is required. In patients with an audible PDA by auscultation but without Eisenmenger's disease, the combined risk of endarteritis, heart failure, and late mortality provides the rationale for shunt closure. If pulmonary artery pressure and pulmonary vascular resistance are substantially elevated, preoperative evaluation should assess the degree of reversibility. With Eisenmenger's disease, closure is contraindicated.

The PDA can be closed surgically or by transcatheter methods. Reported operative mortality rates vary from less than 1 to 8%, depending on the presence of calcification and the degree of pulmonary hypertension. Transcatheter or coil occlusion is an accepted procedure in adults. Residual shunt rates vary from 0.5 to 8%, depending on the device used. Small residual defects that are detected by echocardiography but are not associated with an audible murmur or hemodynamic findings do not appear to carry a significant risk for endarteritis.

Aortopulmonary Window

An aortopulmonary window is typically a large defect across the adjacent segments of both great vessels above their respective valves and below the pulmonary artery bifurcation. The pathophysiology is similar to that of a PDA. The shunt is usually large, so pulmonary vascular resistance rises rapidly and abolishes the aortopulmonary gradient in diastole. The murmur is usually best heard at the third left intercostal space. With a right-to-left shunt, differential cyanosis never occurs because the shunt is proximal to the brachiocephalic vessels. Differentiation of an aortopulmonary window from a PDA can usually be confirmed with echocardiography; the left-to-right shunt is seen in the main pulmonary artery in the aortopulmonary window compared with the left pulmonary artery bifurcation in PDA. Cardiac catheterization confirms the diagnosis and hemodynamics. Surgical repair is necessary unless pulmonary vascular obstructive disease precludes closure.

Pulmonary Arteriovenous Fistulas

Pulmonary arteriovenous fistulas can occur as isolated congenital disorders or as part of generalized hereditary hemorrhagic telangiectasia (Osler-Weber-Rendu syndrome). These fistulas typically occur in the lower lobes or the right middle lobe and can be small or large, single or multiple. The arterial supply usually comes from a dilated, tortuous branch of the pulmonary artery.

The most common finding is that of abnormal opacity on a chest radiograph in a patient with buccal ruby patches or in an otherwise healthy adult who has mild cyanosis. Shunting between deoxygenated pulmonary arterial blood and the oxygenated pulmonary venous blood results in a physiologic right-to-left shunt. The degree of shunting is typically small and not significant enough to result in dilation of the left atrium and ventricle. Heart failure is unusual. Hemoptysis can result if a fistula ruptures into a bronchus. In patients with hereditary hemorrhagic telangiectasia, angiomas occur on the lips and mouth as well as in the gastrointestinal tract and on pleural, liver, and vaginal surfaces. Epistaxis is most common, but cerebrovascular accidents can also occur. Patients with hereditary hemorrhagic telangiectasia can have symptoms that resemble those of a transient ischemic attack even in the absence of right-to-left shunting. On physical examination, cyanosis and clubbing can be notable or barely detectable. Auscultation can disclose soft systolic or continuous noncardiac murmurs on the chest wall adjacent to the fistula. The murmur typically increases with inspiration. The ECG is usually normal. The chest radiograph shows one or more densities, typically in the lower lobes or in the right middle lobe. An echocardiogram can confirm the presence of the fistula by showing early opacification of the left atrium in the absence of any other intracardiac communication when saline is injected into a peripheral vein. The absence of a hemodynamically significant shunt can be confirmed by documenting normal cardiac chamber size.

If the hypoxemia is progressive or if a neurologic complication is documented to have occurred because of paradoxical emboli, fistula closure should be considered. Options include percutaneous catheter techniques if the fistula is small and accessible or a pulmonary wedge resection or lobectomy if the fistula is large. Multiple or recurrent fistulas create a major therapeutic challenge.

Isolated Obstructive Lesions of the Right and Left Ventricular Outflow Tract

Complications of obstructive lesions of the outflow tract relate to the secondary effects of exposure to pressure overload in the chamber proximal to the obstruction. The inability to increase systemic or pulmonary blood flow in the face of a fixed obstruction can cause exercise intolerance, inadequate myocardial perfusion, ventricular arrhythmias, and sudden death.

Right Ventricular Outflow Tract Obstruction

Obstruction of the right ventricular outflow tract can occur at the level of the pulmonary valve (see later), above it in the main pulmonary artery or its branches, or below it in the right ventricle itself. Supravalvular and branch pulmonary artery stenoses are important and common complications of patients with the tetralogy of Fallot (see later). Residual supravalvar pulmonary stenosis is sometimes seen after palliative pulmonary artery banding to decrease pulmonary blood flow in patients with large left-to-right shunts. Congenital branch pulmonary artery stenosis can occur in isolation or with valvar pulmonary stenosis, shunt lesions, or a variety of syndromes. Patients with Noonan's syndrome have a characteristic phenotypic facial appearance, short stature, and webbed neck; cardiac lesions may include a dysplastic pulmonary valve, left ventricular hypertrophic cardiomyopathy, and peripheral pulmonary artery stenosis. Supravalvular pulmonary stenosis can be seen with supravalvular aortic stenosis in Williams (elfin facies) syndrome.

Pulmonary atresia refers to an absent, imperforate, or closed pulmonary valve, which typically occurs in conjunction with other malformations. Pulmonary atresia with a nonrestrictive VSD is a complex cyanotic malformation that is discussed later.

Primary infundibular stenosis with an intact ventricular septum can result from a fibrous band just below the infundibulum. In a double-chambered right ventricle, obstruction is caused by anomalous muscle bundles that divide the right ventricle into a high-pressure chamber below the hypertrophied muscle bundles and a low-pressure chamber above the bundles and below the valve. The clinical features vary according to the presence or absence of other lesions, such as pulmonary valvular stenosis or VSD.

Valvular Pulmonary Stenosis

Isolated congenital valvular pulmonary stenosis (Chapter 75) is a common lesion due to a bicuspid valve in 20% of cases, a dysplastic valve caused by myxomatous changes and severe thickening in 10% of cases, and an abnormal trileaflet valve in most of the remaining cases. Fusion of the leaflets results in a variable degree of thickening and calcification in older patients.

The 25-year survival of patients with valvular pulmonary stenosis is greater than 95% but is worse in those with severe stenosis and peak systolic gradients greater than 80 mm Hg. For patients with mild (<50 mm Hg gradients) and moderate (50 to 80 mm Hg gradients) pulmonary stenosis, bacterial endocarditis, complex ventricular arrhythmias, and progression of the stenosis are uncommon.

Diagnosis

A patient with moderate or even severe pulmonary stenosis may be asymptomatic. With severe stenosis, exercise intolerance can be associated with presyncope and ventricular arrhythmias. Progressive right-sided heart failure is the most common cause of death. On physical examination of patients with significant pulmonary stenosis, jugular venous pressure has a dominant *a* wave, reflecting a noncompliant right ventricle. Palpation discloses a sustained parasternal lift of right ventricular hypertrophy. An expiratory systolic ejection click is characteristic if the leaflets are still mobile. In moderate or severe stenosis, a grade 3 or louder systolic murmur can be heard and felt in the second left interspace. The length of the murmur increases as it peaks progressively later in systole with an increasing degree of obstruction. If right-sided heart failure occurs, tricuspid insufficiency and systemic venous congestion develop. The ECG can show right axis deviation and tall, peaked right atrial P waves in lead II. With more than mild stenosis, the R wave exceeds the S wave in lead V_1. On chest radiography, the main pulmonary artery can be dilated even if the stenosis is mild. Characteristically, the left pulmonary artery is more dilated than the right because of the leftward direction of the high-velocity jet. A variable degree of right ventricular hypertrophy is manifested as right-sided chamber enlargement. Echocardiography can establish the diagnosis and determine the severity by Doppler ultrasound examination.

Treatment

Rx

For patients with valvular pulmonic stenosis and gradients less than 50 mm Hg, conservative management is usually indicated unless symptoms are present. For patients with gradients greater than 80 mm Hg by cardiac catheterization and for symptomatic patients with gradients greater than 50 mm Hg, intervention is recommended. Percutaneous pulmonary angioplasty is the procedure of choice for adults, who achieve persistently good results at 10-year follow-up. For patients with subvalvular stenosis (double-chambered right ventricle), surgical resection of right ventricular muscle bands can be performed.

Left Ventricular Outflow Tract Obstruction

Stenosis of the left ventricular outflow tract can occur at, below, or above the aortic valve. Discrete subaortic stenosis, most commonly caused by a fibromuscular ring just below the valve, accounts for 15 to 20% of all cases of congenital obstruction of the left ventricular outflow tract. Concomitant aortic insufficiency occurs in 50% of cases. Supravalvular aortic stenosis results from thickened media and intima above the aortic sinuses; early coronary atherosclerosis or even ostial coronary obstruction can occur.

Congenital Valvular Aortic Stenosis

The normal aortic valve has three cusps and commissures. A unicuspid aortic valve accounts for most cases of severe aortic stenosis in infants (Chapter 75). A bicuspid aortic valve, which is the most common congenital cardiac malformation, functions normally at birth but often becomes gradually obstructed as calcific and fibrous changes occur; prolapse of one or both cusps can cause aortic insufficiency.

The pathophysiology of aortic stenosis depends not only on its severity but also on the age at diagnosis. When a functionally normal bicuspid aortic valve becomes stenotic in adulthood because of degenerative changes, criteria for diagnosis and intervention parallel those for other forms of acquired aortic stenosis (Chapter 75). When the valve is congenitally stenotic, myocardium with a lifelong exposure to pressure overload behaves differently than if the hemodynamic burden occurred later in life.

The estimated overall 25-year survival rate for patients with congenital valvular aortic stenosis diagnosed in childhood is 85%. Children with initial peak cardiac catheterization gradients less than 50 mm Hg have long-term survival rates of higher than 90%, as opposed to survival rates of 80% in those with gradients of 50 mm Hg or greater.

Diagnosis

Symptoms include angina, exertional dyspnea, presyncope, and syncope and may progress to heart failure. The auscultatory hallmark of a bicuspid aortic valve is an audible systolic ejection click that is typically of a higher pitch than the first heart sound and is best heard not at the cardiac base but at the apex. The sound is caused by sudden movement of the stenotic valve as it moves superiorly in systole and is followed by the typical aortic stenosis murmur (Chapter 75). When significant calcification of the valve results in reduced mobility, the ejection sound is no longer heard. The diagnosis is easily confirmed by two-dimensional echocardiography, with which the number and orientation of aortic cusps can readily be identified.

Treatment

Rx

Conservative management is generally indicated for mild stenosis with a peak gradient of less than 25 mm Hg, but close supervision is required because 20% of these patients require an intervention during long-term follow-up. Unlimited athletic participation is allowed only for asymptomatic patients with peak gradients of less than 20 to 25 mm Hg, a normal ECG, and a normal exercise test. For children who are symptomatic or have gradients greater than 30 mm Hg but do not have significant aortic insufficiency, transcatheter aortic valvotomy is preferred. Aortic valvuloplasty can be considered in young adults, but calcification limits its success, and valve replacement is usually required (Chapter 75). For adults, treatment decisions are similar to those for aortic stenosis from other causes. For patients with subvalvular aortic stenosis, surgical intervention is indicated in the presence of peak gradients above 50 mm Hg, symptoms, or progressive aortic insufficiency.

Coarctation of the Aorta

Aortic coarctation typically occurs just distal to the left subclavian artery at the site of the aortic ductal attachment or its residual ligamentum arteriosum. Less commonly, the coarctation ridge lies proximal to the left subclavian. A bicuspid aortic valve is the most common coexisting anomaly, but VSDs and PDAs are also seen. Pseudocoarctation refers to buckling or kinking of the aortic arch without the presence of a significant gradient.

The most common complications of aortic coarctation are systemic hypertension (Chapter 66) and secondary left ventricular hypertrophy with heart failure. Systemic hypertension is caused by decreased vascular compliance in the proximal aorta and activation of the renin-angiotensin system in response to renal artery hypoperfusion below the obstruction. Left ventricular hypertrophy occurs in response to chronic pressure overload. Congestive heart failure occurs most commonly in infants and then after 40 years of age. The high pressure proximal to the obstruction stimulates the growth of collateral vessels from the internal mammary, scapular, and superior intercostal arteries to the intercostals of the descending aorta. Collateral circulation increases with age and contributes to perfusion of the lower extremities and the spinal cord. This mechanism, although adaptive in a patient who has not undergone surgery, accounts for significant morbidity during surgery when the motor impairment results from inadequate protection of spinal perfusion. Aneurysms occur most notably in the ascending aorta and in the circle of Willis. Premature coronary disease is thought to be related to the resulting hypertension. Complications, including bacterial endarteritis at the coarctation site or, more commonly, endocarditis at the site of a bicuspid aortic valve, cerebrovascular complications, myocardial infarction, heart failure, and aortic dissection, occur in 2 to 6% of patients, more frequently in those with advancing age who have not undergone surgery.

Diagnosis

Young adults may be asymptomatic with incidental systemic hypertension and decreased lower extremity pulses. Coarctation should always be considered in adolescents and young adult men with unexplained upper extremity hypertension. The pressure differential can cause epistaxis, headaches, leg fatigue, or claudication. Older patients have angina, symptoms of heart failure, and vascular complications.

On physical examination, the lower half of the body is typically slightly less developed than the upper half. The hips are narrow and the legs are short, in contrast to broad shoulders and long arms. Blood pressure measurements should be obtained in each arm and one leg; an abnormal measurement is an increase of less than 10 mm Hg in popliteal systolic blood pressure compared with arm systolic blood pressure. The diastolic pressure should be the same in the upper and lower extremities. A pressure differential of more than 30 mm Hg between the right and the left arms is consistent with compromised flow in the left subclavian artery. Right brachial palpation characteristically reveals a strong or even bounding pulse compared with a slowly rising or absent femoral, popliteal, or pedal pulse. Examination of the eyegrounds can reveal tortuous or corkscrew retinal arteries. Precordial palpation is consistent with left ventricular pressure overload. On auscultation, a systolic ejection sound reflecting the presence of a bicuspid aortic valve should be sought. The coarctation itself generates a systolic murmur heard posteriorly, in the midthoracic region, the length of which correlates with the severity of the coarctation. Over the anterior of the chest, systolic murmurs reflecting increased collateral flow can be heard in the infraclavicular areas and the sternal edge or in the axillae.

In adult coarctation, the most common finding on the ECG is left ventricular hypertrophy. Chest radiographic findings are diagnostic. Location of the coarctation segment between the dilated left subclavian artery above and the leftward convexity of the descending aorta below results in the "3 sign" (Fig. 68–7). Bilateral rib notching as a result of dilation of the posterior intercostal arteries is seen on the posterior of the third to eighth ribs when the coarctation is below the left subclavian. Unilateral rib notching sparing the left ribs is observed when the coarctation occurs proximal to the left subclavian artery. Transthoracic echocardiography documents the gradient in the descending aorta and determines the presence of left ventricular hypertrophy. Magnetic resonance imaging (Chapter 55) is the best modality for visualizing the anatomy of the descending aorta. Cardiac catheterization should measure pressures and assess collaterals when surgery is contemplated.

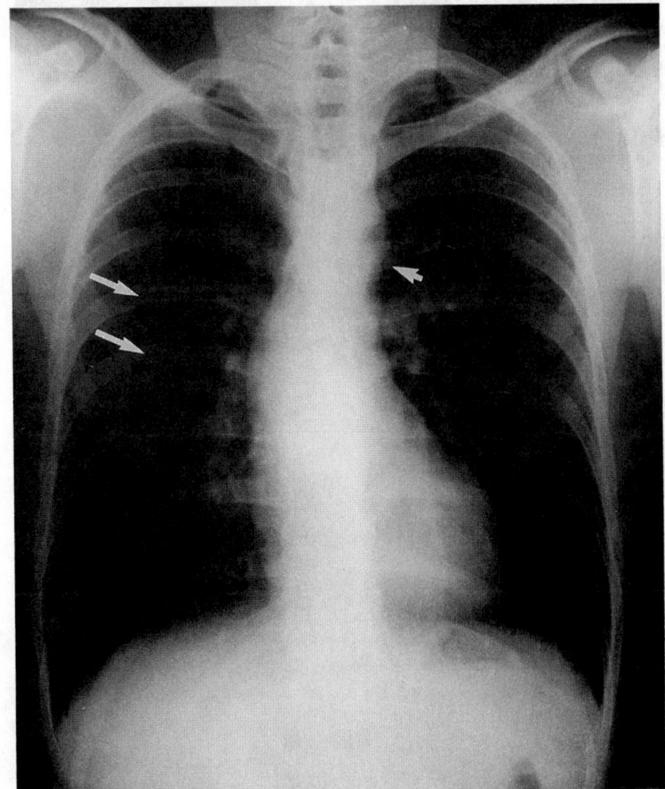

FIGURE 68–7 • Chest radiograph of a patient with coarctation of the aorta showing the radiographic "3" formed by the dilated subclavian artery above and the dilated aorta below (short arrow). Note the notching best seen at the level of the seventh and eighth ribs (long arrows). The dilated ascending aortic segment can also be seen.

Treatment

Rx

Intervention is considered in patients with gradients greater than 30 mm Hg on cardiac catheterization (Chapter 56). Fifty percent of patients repaired when they are older than 40 years have residual hypertension, whereas those who have undergone surgery between the ages of 1 and 5 years have a less than 10% prevalence of hypertension on long-term follow-up. Balloon angioplasty is the treatment of choice for focal recoarctation in patients who have previously been operated on. The incidence of incomplete relief and restenosis is decreased in adults by endovascular stent placement. Focal complications include aortic aneurysms and, rarely, aortic rupture.

Anomalies of the Sinuses of Valsalva and Coronary Arteries

Sinus of Valsalva Aneurysms

At the base of the aortic root, the aortic valve cusps are attached to the aortic wall, above which three small pouches, or sinuses, are seated. The right coronary artery originates from one sinus and the left main coronary artery from a second; the third is called the noncoronary sinus. A weakness in the wall of the sinus can result in aneurysm formation with or without rupture. In more than 90% of cases, the aneurysm involves the right or noncoronary cusp. Rupture typically occurs into the right side of the heart at the right atrial or ventricular level with a resulting large left-to-right shunt driven by the high aortic pressure.

A previously asymptomatic young man typically has chest pain and rapidly progressing shortness of breath sometimes after physical strain. The physical examination is consistent with significant heart failure. Even if the communication is between the aorta and the right side of the heart, biventricular failure is not unusual. The classic murmur is loud and continuous, often with a thrill. A murmur of aortic insufficiency secondary to damage to the adjacent aortic valve may be superimposed. The chest radiograph shows volume overload of both ventricles with evidence of shunt vascularity and pulmonary venous congestion. The echocardiogram is diagnostic. Cardiac catheterization can verify the integrity of the coronary artery adjacent to the ruptured aneurysm.

Even though symptoms may abate as the heart dilates, progressive cardiac decompensation typically results in death within 1 year of the rupture. A ruptured sinus of Valsalva aneurysm therefore requires urgent surgical repair.

Coronary Artery Fistulas

Fistulas arise from the right or left coronary arteries and in 90% of cases drain into the right ventricle, the right atrium, or the pulmonary artery in order of decreasing frequency. Typically, young patients are asymptomatic, but supraventricular arrhythmias are seen with progressive dilation of the intracardiac chambers. Angina can occur as the fistula creates a coronary steal by diverting blood away from the myocardium. Heart failure is seen with large fistulas. A continuous murmur heard in a young, otherwise normal acyanotic, asymptomatic patient should suggest the diagnosis. Most fistulas are associated with a small shunt, and hence the murmur is often less than grade 3 and is heard in the precordial area. Unless the shunt is large, the ECG is normal, as is the chest radiograph. The echocardiogram, especially the transesophageal echocardiogram, is diagnostic. Percutaneous transcatheter closure with coil embolization is preferred, but surgical ligation is also an alternative.

Anomalous Origin of the Coronary Arteries

The left main coronary artery normally arises from the left sinus of Valsalva and courses leftward, posterior to the right ventricular outflow tract. The right coronary artery arises from the right sinus of Valsalva and courses rightward to the right ventricle. Isolated ectopic or anomalous origins of the coronary arteries (see Fig. 55–4) are seen in 0.6 to 1.5% of patients undergoing coronary angiography.

The most common anomaly is ectopic origin of the left circumflex artery from the right sinus of Valsalva, followed by anomalous origin of the right coronary artery from the left sinus and anomalous origin of the left main coronary artery from the right sinus. If the anomalous coronary artery does not course between the pulmonary artery and aorta, the prognosis is favorable. Risks of ischemia, myocardial infarction, and death are greatest when the left main coronary artery courses between both great vessels.

Coronary arteries can also originate from the pulmonary trunk. If both the right and left arteries originate from the pulmonary trunk, death usually occurs in the neonatal period. If only the left anterior descending coronary artery originates from the pulmonary trunk, the rate of survival to adulthood is approximately 10%, depending on the development of collateral retrograde flow to the anomalous artery from a normal coronary artery. This collateral flow may cause a continuous murmur along the left sternal border, congestive heart failure from the large shunt, and a coronary steal syndrome as blood is diverted away from the normal artery.

A single coronary ostium can provide a single coronary artery that branches into right and left coronary arteries, the left then giving rise to the circumflex and the anterior descending arteries. The ostium can originate from the right or left aortic sinus. The coronary circulation is functionally normal unless one of the branches passes between the aorta and the pulmonary artery.

Diagnostic procedures include angiography, magnetic resonance imaging, and transesophageal echocardiography. For an anomalous coronary artery that originates from the pulmonary artery, surgical reimplantation into the aorta is preferred. For an anomalous artery that courses between the pulmonary artery and aorta, a bypass graft to the distal vessel is preferred.

SPECIFIC COMPLEX LESIONS

Tetralogy of Fallot

Tetralogy of Fallot, the most common cyanotic malformation, is characterized by superior and anterior displacement of the subpulmonary infundibular septum, which causes the tetrad of pulmonary stenosis, VSD, aortic override, and right ventricular hypertrophy. The VSD is perimembranous in 80% of cases. Additional cardiac anomalies include a right-sided aortic arch in up to 25% of patients. An anomalous left anterior descending artery originating from the right coronary cusp and crossing over the right ventricular outflow tract is seen in 10% of cases. Other associated anomalies include ASD, left superior vena cava, defects of the atrioventricular canal, and aortic insufficiency. With pulmonary atresia, pulmonary blood flow occurs through aortic to pulmonary collaterals. Life expectancy is limited unless staged reconstructive surgery is performed.

The physiology in unrepaired tetralogy of Fallot is determined by the severity and location of the pulmonic outflow obstruction and by the interaction of pulmonary and systemic vascular resistance across a nonrestrictive VSD. Because the pulmonary stenosis results in a relatively fixed pulmonary resistance, a drop in systemic vascular resistance as occurs with exercise is associated with increased right-to-left shunting and increasing cyanosis. A child who squats after running is attempting to reverse the process by increasing systemic vascular resistance by crouching with bent knees. Native pulmonary blood flow is typically insufficient. Unless a PDA has remained open, a cyanotic adult will typically have undergone a palliative procedure to increase pulmonary blood flow.

Examination of unrepaired patients reveals central cyanosis and clubbing. The right ventricular impulse is prominent. The second heart sound is single and represents the aortic closure sound with an absent or inconspicuous P_2. Typically, little or no systolic murmur is heard across the pulmonary valve because the more severe the obstruction, the more right-to-left shunting occurs and the less blood flows across a diminutive right ventricular outflow tract. A diastolic murmur of aortic insufficiency is often heard in adults. In the presence of a palliative systemic arterial to pulmonary artery shunt, the high-pressure gradient generates a loud continuous murmur. In a patient who has not undergone surgery, progressive infundibular stenosis and cyanosis occur. Before the advent of palliative surgery, mortality rates were 50% in the first few years of life and survival past the third decade was unusual.

Complete surgical repair consists of patch closure of the VSD and relief of the right ventricular outflow tract obstruction. Adequate pulmonary blood flow is ensured by reconstruction of the distal pulmonary artery bed. Previous palliative shunts are usually taken down. Complete repair in childhood yields a 90 to 95% 10-year survival rate with good functional results, and 30-year survival rates may be as high as 85%. Total correction with low mortality and a favorable long-term follow-up is possible even in adulthood.

After repair, residual pulmonary stenosis, proximal or distal, with a right ventricular pressure greater than 50% of systemic occurs in up to 25% of patients. Some degree of pulmonary insufficiency is common, particularly if a patch has been inserted at the level of the pulmonary valve or if a pulmonary valvotomy has been performed. Residual VSDs can be found in up to 20% of patients. Patients may be asymptomatic or may have symptoms related to long-term complications after surgical repair. Symptoms can reflect residual right ventricular pressure or volume overload or arrhythmias at rest or with exercise. Angina can occur in a young patient if surgical repair has damaged an anomalous left anterior descending artery as it courses across the right ventricular outflow tract. In acyanotic adults, clubbing commonly regresses. A right ventricular impulse is often felt as a result of residual pulmonary insufficiency or stenosis. Typically, no functioning pulmonary valve is present, and hence the second heart sound is still single. A systolic murmur can represent residual pulmonary stenosis, residual VSD, or tricuspid insufficiency. A diastolic murmur can reflect aortic or pulmonary insufficiency. Ventricular arrhythmias are common after repair, with an incidence of sudden death as high as 5%.

The ECG in unrepaired tetralogy of Fallot shows right axis deviation, right atrial enlargement, and dominant right ventricular forces over the precordial leads. The most common finding after repair is complete right bundle branch block, which is seen in 80 to 90% of patients. The chest radiograph typically shows an upturned apex with a concave pulmonary artery segment giving the classic appearance of a boot-shaped heart. Figure 68–8 demonstrates the findings in an adult after repair. The apex

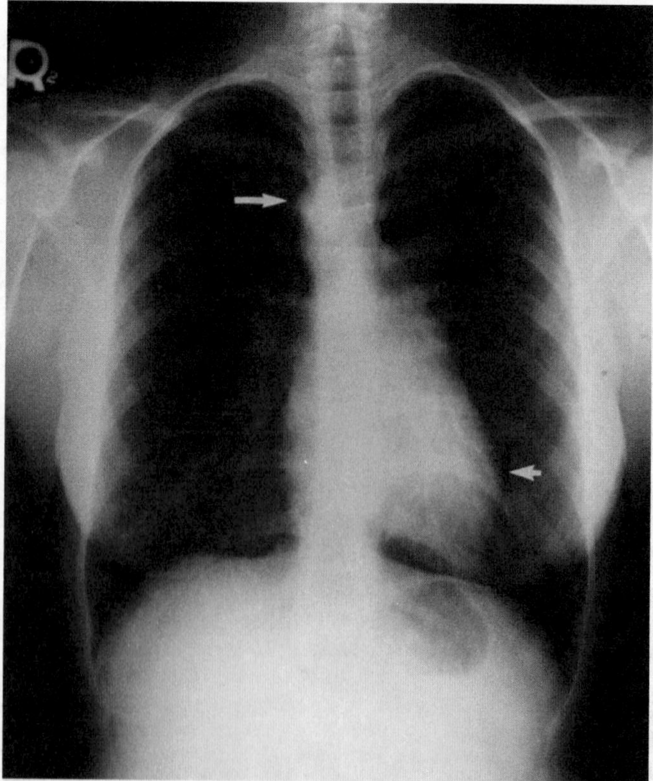

FIGURE 68–8 • Chest radiograph of an adult after tetralogy of Fallot repair. A right aortic arch with rightward indentation of the trachea (long arrow) can be seen. The right ventricular apex remains upturned (short arrow). Note the sternal wires consistent with intracardiac repair, thus clarifying the fullness of the pulmonary artery segment often seen after extensive enlargement of the right ventricular outflow tract.

is persistently upturned, although the pulmonary artery segment is no longer concave. Echocardiography can confirm the diagnosis and document intracardiac complications in repaired and unrepaired patients. Shunt patency can be determined by Doppler examination. Magnetic resonance imaging can accurately document stenosis in the distal pulmonary artery bed. Cardiac catheterization is reserved for patients in whom operative or reoperative treatment is contemplated or in whom the integrity of the coronary circulation needs to be verified.

Patients with a change in exercise tolerance, angina, or evidence of heart failure as well as those with symptomatic arrhythmias or syncope should be referred for complete evaluation. Surgical reintervention is generally considered when right ventricular pressure is more than two thirds as high as systemic pressure because of residual right ventricular outflow tract obstruction, free pulmonary regurgitation occurs with right ventricular dysfunction or sustained arrhythmias, or a residual VSD causes a significant shunt.

Complete Transposition of the Great Arteries

Complete transposition of the great arteries is the second most common cyanotic lesion, and surgically corrected adults are increasingly common. In simple transposition of the great arteries, the atria and ventricles are in their normal positions but the aorta arises from the right ventricle and the pulmonary artery arises from the left ventricle. When the aorta is anterior and rightward with respect to the pulmonary artery, as is most common, D-transposition is present. The native anatomy has the pulmonary and systemic circulations in parallel, with deoxygenated blood recirculating between the right side of the heart and the systemic circulation, whereas oxygenated blood recirculates from the left side of the heart to the lungs. The condition is incompatible with life unless a VSD, PDA, or ASD is present or an ASD is created; a hemodynamically significant VSD is present in 15% of cases. Subpulmonary obstruction of the left ventricular outflow tract occurs in 10 to 25% of cases.

The Senning or Mustard atrial baffle repairs, which were the first corrective procedures, redirect oxygenated blood from the left atrium to the right ventricle so that it may be ejected into the aorta while deoxygenated blood detours the right atrium and heads for the left ventricle and into the pulmonary artery. Although this operation results in acyanotic physiology, the right ventricle assumes a permanent position under the aorta and pumps against systemic pressures, a lifelong task for which it was not designed. When the subpulmonary obstruction is significant, the Rastelli procedure reroutes blood at the ventricular level by tunneling the left ventricle to the aorta inside the heart through a VSD. A conduit is then inserted outside the heart between the left ventricle and aorta. More recently, the arterial switch operation transects the aorta and pulmonary artery above their respective valves and switches them to become realigned with their physiologic outflow tracts and appropriate ventricles. The proximal coronary arteries are translocated from the sinuses of the native aorta to the neoaorta (native pulmonary artery). In this operation, each ventricle reassumes the role that it was embryologically destined to fulfill.

If an adult patient is cyanotic and has a native intracardiac shunt or a palliative shunt, referral to an appropriate facility should be undertaken to explore the possibility of intracardiac repair. At present, adults with transposition of the great arteries most commonly have undergone an atrial baffle repair, with an expected 15-year survival rate of 75% and a 20-year survival rate of 70%. For patients with an atrial baffle procedure, symptoms include exercise intolerance, palpitations caused by bradyarrhythmias or atrial flutter, and right ventricular failure. The patient is typically acyanotic unless a baffle leak exists. The clinical findings are determined by the presence or absence of systemic right ventricular failure. On auscultation, the second heart sound is classically single. The ECG reveals sinus bradycardia, but nodal rhythms and heart block occur as the patient ages. The chest radiograph shows a variable degree of right ventricular enlargement. Echocardiography can be used to confirm the diagnosis and to explore related abnormalities. Cardiac catheterization is performed when an operation or reoperation is contemplated. Reoperation is performed in approximately 20% of patients for baffle-related complications, progressive left ventricular outflow tract stenosis, or severe tricuspid regurgitation.

Congenitally Corrected Transposition of the Great Arteries

In congenitally corrected transposition of the great arteries, the great arteries are transposed, the ventricles are inverted, but the atria remain in their normal position. The systemic circulation (left atrium, morphologic right ventricle, and aorta) and pulmonary circulation (right atrium, morphologic left ventricle, and pulmonary artery) are in series. The patient is therefore acyanotic unless an intracardiac shunt is also present. The right ventricle is aligned with the aorta and performs lifelong systemic work, which accounts in part for its eventual failure. Associated lesions include a VSD, pulmonary stenosis, and Ebstein's malformation of the left-sided tricuspid valve. Complete heart block develops at a rate of 2% per year. Patients with congenitally corrected transposition of the great arteries and no other associated defects can remain free of symptoms until the sixth decade, at which time significant atrioventricular valve regurgitation, failure of the right (systemic) ventricle, supraventricular arrhythmias, and heart block occur.

Right-Sided Ebstein's Anomaly

The septal and posterior cusps of the tricuspid valve are largely derived from the right ventricle as it liberates a layer of muscle that skirts away from the cavity to become valve tissue. When this process occurs abnormally, the posterior and septal cusps of the tricuspid valve remain tethered to the muscle and adhere to the right ventricular surface—hence the diagnostic hallmark of Ebstein's anomaly, apical displacement of the septal tricuspid leaflet.

In right-sided Ebstein's anomaly of the tricuspid valve, the right side of the heart consists of three anatomic components: the right atrium proper, the true right ventricle, and the atrialized portion of the right ventricle between the two. The displaced septal and posterior tricuspid leaflets lie between the atrialized right ventricle and the true right ventricle. In mild Ebstein's anomaly, the degree of tricuspid leaflet tethering is only mild, the anterior leaflet retains mobility, and the size of the true right ventricle is only mildly reduced. Severe Ebstein's anomaly is associated with severe tethering of the tricuspid leaflet tissue and a diminutive, hypocontractile true right ventricle. Functionally, the valve is regurgitant because it is unable to appose its three leaflets during ventricular contraction. Valvular regurgitation and asynchronous, abnormal right ventricular function cause the dilation and right-sided heart failure observed in the more severe forms of the lesion. The wide spectrum of severity of the anomaly is based on the degree of tricuspid leaflet tethering and the relative proportion of atrialized and true right ventricle. The most common associated cardiac defect, a secundum ASD or patent foramen ovale, is reported in more than 50% of patients. On physical examination, a clicking "sail sound" is heard as the second component of S_1 when tricuspid valve closure becomes loud and delayed.

The 12-lead ECG typically shows highly peaked P waves with a wide, often bizarre-looking QRS complex. Preexcitation occurs in 20% of patients; supraventricular tachyarrhythmias, atrial fibrillation, and atrial flutter occur in 30 to 40% of patients and constitute the most common findings in adolescents and adults with right-sided Ebstein's anomaly.

When patients of all ages are taken together, the predicted mortality is approximately 50% by the fourth or fifth decade. Complications include atrial arrhythmias due to severe right atrial enlargement and cyanosis caused by a right-to-left atrial shunt as tricuspid insufficiency increases and the right ventricle fails. Atrial arrhythmias, cyanosis, and the presence of an intra-atrial communication also increase the risk of stroke.

Intervention is considered when functional status or cyanosis worsens, significant atrial arrhythmias are documented, or a cerebrovascular accident occurs. Surgical options include replacement or repair of the tricuspid valve and closure of the ASD. The feasibility of tricuspid valvuloplasty depends on the size and mobility of the anterior tricuspid leaflet, which is used to construct a unicuspid right-sided valve.

Atrioventricular Canal Defect

Embryologic septation of the atrioventricular canal results in closure of the inferior portion of the interatrial septum and the superior portion of the interventricular septum. Septation is achieved with the growth of endocardial cushions, which also contribute to development of the mitral and tricuspid valves. Hence, the nomenclature *atrioventricular canal defect* or *endocardial cushion defect* is used to designate this group of anomalies.

A partial atrioventricular canal defect refers to an ostium primum ASD with a cleft mitral valve. The anomaly is manifested as a hemodynamic combination of an ASD with a variable degree of mitral regurgitation. The 12-lead ECG shows the typical findings of left axis deviation with a Q wave in leads I and aVL and a prolonged PR interval. The echocardiogram shows a defect in the inferior portion of the interatrial septum and a cleft mitral valve.

A complete atrioventricular canal defect is an uncommon defect consisting of a primum ASD, an inlet VSD that usually extends to the membranous interventricular septum, and a common atrioventricular valve. Adults who have not been operated on usually have Eisenmenger's syndrome unless concomitant pulmonary stenosis has protected the pulmonary vascular bed or the VSD has undergone spontaneous closure, in which case the physiologic consequences are similar to those of a partial atrioventricular canal.

Surgical repair of an atrioventricular defect consists of closing the interatrial or interventricular communication with reconstruction of the common atrioventricular valve or closure of the cleft in the mitral valve. An adult who has undergone repair may have significant residual regurgitation of the mitral or tricuspid valve. Even after surgery, acquired subaortic obstruction can occur in the long left ventricular outflow tract, which has a classic gooseneck deformity on cardiac angiography.

Univentricular Heart and Tricuspid Atresia

The terms *single ventricle, common ventricle,* and *univentricular heart* have been used interchangeably to describe the double-inlet ventricle, in which one ventricular chamber receives flow from both the tricuspid and mitral valves. In 75 to 90% of cases, the single ventricle is a morphologic left ventricle. Obstruction of one of the great arteries is common, and life expectancy is short without an operation. The patients most likely to survive to adulthood palliated or, rarely, without surgery have a single ventricle of the left morphologic type, with pulmonary stenosis protecting the pulmonary vascular bed.

In tricuspid atresia, no orifice is found between the right atrium and right ventricle, and an underdeveloped or hypoplastic right ventricle is present. The morphologic left ventricle is consistently normally developed and therefore becomes the single functional ventricle. Typically, blood flows into the right atrium, then through an obligatory ASD and to the left atrium, where it then proceeds to the left ventricle. Variable features include a VSD, the abnormal position of the great arteries, and the relative degree of pulmonary stenosis, all of which are used to classify tricuspid atresia. Without surgery, 50% of patients die in the first 6 months and 90% in the first decade.

Adult patients rarely have not been operated on. They may be acyanotic after the Fontan operation; if cyanotic and palliated, the patient may benefit from further palliation or may be eligible for the Fontan operation. With the Glenn shunt or the Fontan operation, a direct anastomosis is created between the systemic venous and pulmonary circulations. Venous blood flows passively from the systemic veins to the pulmonary circulation and returns oxygenated to a left-sided atrium and into the single functional ventricle, which then pumps oxygenated blood into the systemic circulation. The Glenn anastomosis diverts part of the systemic venous return to the lungs, whereas the Fontan procedure makes the patient acyanotic by diverting the entire systemic venous circulation to the pulmonary vascular bed. For optimum results, a successful Fontan operation requires low pulmonary vascular resistance, preserved single ventricular function, and unobstructed anastomosis between the systemic veins and the pulmonary arteries. At 5-year follow-up, 80% or more of Fontan survivors are in New York Heart Association functional class I or II, with successful pregnancy reported in a small number of patients. When patients of all ages are considered together, 10-year survival rates vary from 60 to 70%. Late deaths are due to reoperation, arrhythmia, ventricular failure, and protein-losing enteropathy.

Vascular Malformations

Aortic Arch Anomalies

Vascular Rings and other Arch Anomalies

One of the most frequent developmental errors of the aortic arch is an aberrant right subclavian artery originating distal to the left subclavian and coursing rightward behind the esophagus at the level of the third thoracic vertebrae. Although the finding is frequent, symptoms are uncommon. When symptoms occur, the term *dysphagia lusoria* has been used in reference to swallowing difficulties that result from esophageal compression. Abnormal development of the brachial arches and dorsal aorta can result in a variety of anomalies that lead to the formation of vascular rings around the trachea and esophagus. The outcome is often benign, but symptoms of respiratory compromise or dysphagia warrant surgery. When the left pulmonary artery arises from the right and passes leftward between the trachea and esophagus, a pulmonary artery sling occurs. Symptoms of tracheal compression warrant correction.

A right aortic arch occurs when the aortic arch courses toward the right instead of the left. Mirror-image branching is the most common anatomic variant. In most cases, this anomaly coexists with other congenital lesions, notably tetralogy of Fallot.

Anomalous Venous Connections

Anomalies of Systemic Venous Return

A persistent left superior vena cava can be fortuitously diagnosed on chest radiography or on echocardiography. Its clinical relevance depends on development of the coronary sinus. If the coronary sinus is normally formed, typically the left superior vena cava drains into the right atrium through the coronary sinus. If the coronary sinus is not normally developed, the persistent left superior vena cava drains into the left atrium and cyanosis results from the obligatory right-to-left shunt. The latter commonly occurs with an ASD or a complex cardiac anomaly.

Venous return above the renal veins can be abnormal with inferior vena cava interruption and azygos or hemiazygos continuation. In the former, inferior vena cava flow above the renal veins continues into the azygos vein, which courses normally up the right of the spine to empty into the junction between the superior vena cava and right atrium. In a less common anatomic arrangement, the caval flow empties into a hemiazygos vein, which empties into a persistent left superior vena cava. The finding rarely occurs in isolation but can be seen in patients with associated simple or complex malformations.

Anomalies of Pulmonary Venous Return

In partial anomalous pulmonary venous return, one or more but not all four pulmonary veins are not connected to the left atrium. The most common pattern has the right pulmonary veins connected to the superior vena cava, usually with a sinus venosus ASD. Anomalous connection of the right pulmonary veins to the inferior vena cava results in a chest radiographic shadow that resembles a Turkish sword, hence the designation scimitar syndrome. Associated anomalies include hypoplasia of the right lung, anomalies of the bronchial system, hypoplasia of the right pulmonary artery, and dextroposition of the heart. Partial anomalous pulmonary venous return results in a left-to-right shunt physiology similar to that of an ASD.

In total anomalous pulmonary venous return, all the pulmonary veins connect abnormally to either the right atrium or one of the systemic veins above or below the diaphragm. Concurrent obstruction of the pulmonary veins is present when drainage occurs below the diaphragm and variable when drainage occurs above it. An ASD is essential to sustain life. One third of cases occur with major complex cardiac malformations.

In cor triatriatum, the pulmonary veins drain into an accessory chamber that is usually connected to the left atrium through an opening of variable size. The hemodynamic consequences are determined by the size of this opening and are similar to those of mitral stenosis. If symptoms of pulmonary venous hypertension occur, surgical treatment is indicated.

Cardiac Malpositions

The normal heart is left sided and hence the designation levocardia. Cardiac malpositions are defined in terms of the intrathoracic position of the heart in relation to the position of the viscera (visceral situs), which are usually concordant with the position of the atria. That is, when the liver is on the right and the stomach is on the left, the atrium receiving

TABLE 68–2 EXERCISE RECOMMENDATIONS IN ADULTS WITH CONGENITAL HEART DISEASE

Condition	Unrestricted	Low-Moderate Intensity*	Prohibited
ASD†	No PHT; no arrhythmia; normal ventricular function	PA pressure >40 mm Hg *with* normal ETT; no arrhythmia	Eisenmenger's
VSD†	Small; no PHT; no arrhythmia; normal ventricular function	Moderate VSD	Eisenmenger's
PDA†	Small; no PHT; no arrhythmia; normal ventricular function	PA pressure >40 mm Hg *with* normal ETT; no arrhythmia	Eisenmenger's
Coarctation‡	Gradient ≤20 mm Hg arm to leg; normal BP at rest and exercise	Gradient ≥20 mm Hg arm to leg *with* normal BP and normal ETT	Gradient ≥50 mm Hg arm to leg *or* aortic aneurysm
PS	Gradient <50 mm Hg; no arrhythmia; normal ventricular function	Gradient ≥50 mm Hg	Gradient ≥70 mm Hg *or* ventricular arrhythmia
AS	Gradient ≤20 mm Hg; normal ECG; normal ETT; asymptomatic	Gradient >20 mm Hg *with* normal ECG, normal ETT; asymptomatic	Gradient ≥50 mm Hg *or* ventricular arrhythmia
TOF after repair	Normal RV pressure; no shunt; no arrhythmia	Increased RV pressure *or* moderate PR *or* SVT	RV pressure ≥65% systemic *or* ventricular; arrhythmia on ETT *or* severe PR
Mustard or Senning		No cardiomegaly, arrhythmia, or syncope; normal ETT	Cardiomegaly *or* arrhythmia at rest or exercise
c-TGA unoperated	No cardiomegaly; mild TR; no arrhythmia; normal ETT	Moderate RV dysfunction, moderate TR; no arrhythmia	Severe TR *or* uncontrolled arrhythmia
Ebstein's	Mild Ebstein's; no arrhythmia; operated with mild TR	Moderate TR *with* no arrhythmia	Severe Ebstein's *or* uncontrolled arrhythmia
Fontan		Normal O_2 saturation *with* near-normal ETT and ventricular function	Moderate-severe MR or TR *or* uncontrolled arrhythmia

*Based on peak dynamic and static components of exercise during competition for individual sports (see credit line).
†Unoperated or 6 months after surgery.
‡Unoperated or 1 year after surgery.
AS = aortic stenosis; ASD = atrial septal defect; BP = blood pressure; c-TGA = corrected transposition of the great arteries; ECG = electrocardiogram; ETT = exercise tolerance test; MR = mitral regurgitation; PA = pulmonary artery; PDA = patent ductus arteriosus; PHT = pulmonary hypertension; PR = pulmonary regurgitation; PS = pulmonary stenosis; RV = right ventricle; SVT = supraventricular tachyarrhythmia; TOF = tetralogy of Fallot; TR = tricuspid regurgitation; VSD = ventricular septal defect.
Based on guidelines recommended in Graham TP, Bricker TJ, James FW, et al: 26th Bethesda conference: Recommendations for determining eligibility for competition in athletes with cardiovascular abnormalities. Task Force 1: Congenital heart disease. J Am Coll Cardiol 1994;24:867. Reprinted with permission of the American College of Cardiology.

systemic venous blood (right atrium) is right sided and the atrium receiving pulmonary venous blood (left atrium) is left sided. Asplenia and polysplenia syndromes are associated with a variety of complex cardiovascular malformations.

Dextrocardia and Mesocardia

In dextrocardia, the heart is on the right side of the thorax with or without situs inversus. When the heart is right sided with inverted atria, a right-sided stomach, and a left-sided liver, the combination is dextrocardia with situs inversus. In this arrangement, also called mirror-image dextrocardia, the ventricles are inverted, but so are the viscera and therefore the atria. The heart usually functions normally, and the diagnosis is often fortuitous. The heart sounds are louder on the right side of the chest and the liver is palpable on the left. The chest radiograph shows a right-sided cardiac apex with a lower left hemidiaphragm and a right-sided stomach bubble. The ECG shows an inverted P and T wave in lead I with a negative QRS deflection and a reverse pattern between aVR and aVL. A mirror-image progression is seen from V_1 to a right-sided V_6 lead. An echocardiogram should be performed to ensure that intracardiac anatomy is normal.

When dextrocardia with situs solitus occurs, the ventricles are inverted but not the viscera and therefore not the atria. Associated severe cardiac malformations are typical.

In mesocardia, the heart is centrally located in the chest with normal atrial and visceral anatomy. The apex is central or rightward displaced on the chest radiograph. Typically, no associated cardiac malformations are present.

Specialized Issues

Endocarditis Prophylaxis

Prolonged survival of patients with complex congenital heart disease has resulted in a population at increased risk for infective endocarditis (Chapter 76). Infection most commonly affects sites of turbulent blood flow on the low-pressure side of gradients. Such sites include restrictive VSDs, PDAs, cleft mitral valve, aortic coarctation (most often at the site of an associated bicuspid aortic valve), and prosthetic shunts, valves, and conduits in a postoperative patient. The risk of endocarditis associated with isolated low-pressure lesions in the right side of the heart is low.

Endocarditis should be suspected early and culture specimens obtained before antibiotic therapy is begun. Current recommendations for the prevention of bacterial endocarditis apply to most congenital heart lesions, with the exception of an isolated ASD and surgically repaired ASD, VSD, or PDA without residual shunting beyond 6 months after repair.

Exercise

The goal of exercise evaluation is to assess the functional results of therapeutic interventions and to provide guidelines for exercise prescriptions. Patients with residual hemodynamic lesions or unrepaired congenital cardiac anomalies should be evaluated on an annual basis with a physical examination, an ECG, and a cardiac ultrasonographic examination if indicated. Pertinent additional tests may include Holter monitoring and exercise testing. Attention should be directed to the detection of pulmonary hypertension, arrhythmias, myocardial dysfunction, and symptoms such as exercise-induced dizziness, syncope, dyspnea, or chest pain.

A series of exercise guidelines have been proposed for major groups of congenital heart defects (Table 68–2). Patients beyond 6 months after repair of a single shunt lesion without pulmonary hypertension, arrhythmias, or evidence of myocardial dysfunction can participate in all sports. With residual shunts, if the peak pulmonary artery pressure is less than 40 mm Hg in the absence of ventricular dysfunction or significant arrhythmias, patients can enjoy a free range of activity. Patients with elevated pulmonary vascular resistance are at risk of sudden death during intense exercise; although most self-limit their activity, participation in competitive sports is contraindicated. Patients with aortic and pulmonary stenosis should be counseled as recommended earlier, according to gradient severity. For patients with uncomplicated aortic coarctation, athletic participation is permitted if the arm-leg blood pressure gradient is 20 mm Hg or less at rest and the peak systolic blood pressure during exercise is normal. For patients after tetralogy of Fallot repair, repair of transposition of the great arteries, and the Fontan operation, exercise recommendations vary according to residual ventricular function and the presence or absence of arrhythmias.

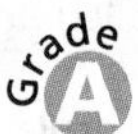

1. Attie F, Rosas M, Granados N, et al: Surgical treatment for secundum atrial septal defects in patients >40 years old. A randomized clinical trial. J Am Coll Cardiol 2001;38:2035–2042.

SUGGESTED READINGS

Chassot PG, Bettex DA: Anesthesia and adult congenital heart disease. J Cardiothorac Vasc Anesth 2006;20:414–437. *Overview with specific recommendations.*

Chessa M, Carrozza M, Butera G, et al: The impact of interventional cardiology for the management of adults with congenital heart defects. Catheter Cardiovasc Interv 2006;67:258–264. *Overview of percutaneous therapeutic procedures.*

Diller GP, Gatzoulis MA: Pulmonary vascular disease in adults with congenital heart disease. Circulation 2007;115:1039–1050. *A review of pulmonary arterial hypertension and Eisenmenger syndrome.*

Minette MS, Sahn DJ: Ventricular septal defects. Circulation 2006;114:2190–2197. *A review of this common congenital defect.*

Therrien J, Dore A, Gersony W, et al: Canadian Cardiovascular Society Consensus Conference 2001 update: Recommendations for the management of adults with congenital heart disease. Parts I and II. Can J Cardiol 2001; 17:940–959, 1029–1050. *Practical guidelines for the management of all the major congenital lesions seen in adults, with graded recommendations for intervention.*

Walsh EP, Cecchin F: Arrhythmias in adult patients with congenital heart disease. Circulation 2007;115:534–545. *A review of these clinical manifestations.*

Webb G, Gatzoulis MA: Atrial septal defects in the adult: Recent progress and overview. Circulation 2006;114:1645–1653. *A thoughtful review.*

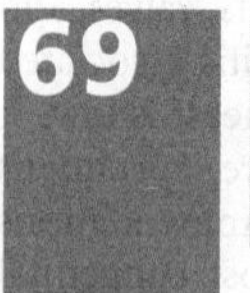

69 ATHEROSCLEROSIS, THROMBOSIS, AND VASCULAR BIOLOGY

Valentin Fuster

Definition

Atherothrombosis is a complex arterial disease in which cholesterol deposition, inflammation, extracellular matrix, and thrombus formation play major roles. Atherothrombotic cardiovascular disease refers to the diffuse condition of atherothrombosis, involving the heart (coronary arteries), brain (carotid, vertebral, cerebral arteries), aorta, and peripheral arteries. Most of the risk factors that apply to one arterial bed also apply to the others. The presence of atherothrombotic disease in one arterial bed increases the risk of developing disease in others.

Pathobiology

Morphology of Atherothrombosis

Normal Artery

The normal artery (Fig. 69–1A) consists essentially of a tube with an internal lining or *intima* covered by a continuous layer of endothelial cells that maintains the circulating blood flow (antithrombotic), acts as a barrier to keep circulating monocyte-macrophages from entering into the vessel wall (antiadhesion or migration), and regulates smooth muscle cell function (relaxation or antigrowth); the *media*, which consists of smooth muscle cells that contract and maintain the tone of the artery wall and of extracellular matrix or fibrils (elastin, collagen, and proteoglycans) that provide supportive structure; and the *adventitia*, which is composed of loose connective tissue (fibroblasts, extracellular matrix, and vasa vasorum).

Arteriosclerosis, Atherosclerosis-Thrombosis

Arteriosclerosis is the generic term for thickened and stiffened arteries of all sizes. By comparison, *atherosclerosis* (see Fig. 69–1B) is the descriptive term for thickened and hardened lesions of the medium and large muscular and elastic arteries. These lesions are lipid rich and occur within the intima, although the media and adventitia may also be involved. Lesions are generally eccentric and, if they become complicated by mural or occlusive thrombosis, may cause ischemia with onset of clinical angina or necrosis with the characteristic clinical sequelae of myocardial infarction (MI) (Chapter 72), cerebral infarction (Chapters 430 and 431), or gangrene of the extremities (Chapter 79); hence, the term *atherothrombosis* (see Fig. 69–1C).

Phases of the Lesions of Coronary Atherothrombosis

According to a simplified modification of the criteria previously set forth by the American Heart Association, progression of the atherosclerotic plaque in any arterial bed can be subdivided into six pathologic or clinically relevant phases (Fig. 69–2). *Phase 1* represents small lesions that are commonly found in persons younger than 30 and that may progress over several years. Type I lesions consist of macrophage-derived foam cells that contain lipid droplets, type II lesions contain macrophages and smooth muscle cells with mild extracellular lipid deposits, and type III lesions contain smooth muscle cells surrounded by extracellular connective tissue, fibrils, and lipid deposits.

Phase 2 includes the so-called vulnerable or high-risk plaques that, although not necessarily stenotic, may be susceptible to disruption because of their high lipid content, increased inflammation, and thin fibrous cap. These plaques are categorized morphologically as one of two variants. Type IV lesions consist of confluent cellular lesions with a great deal of extracellular lipid mixed with normal intima, which may predominate as an outer layer or cap. Type Va lesions possess an extracellular lipid core covered by a thin fibrous cap.

Phase 3 and *phase 4* include acutely complicated type VI lesions in the form of fixed or repetitive mural nonobstructive or obstructive thrombosis, respectively. Approximately two thirds of the acute coronary syndromes (Chapter 71) are related to phase 4 or "complicated" type VI occlusive thrombosis and are the result of mild disruption of nonseverely stenotic lipid-rich plaques of phase 2.

Phase 5 consists of phase 3 or phase 4 plaques that evolve, by a process of organized thrombus with extracellular matrix, into fibrotic type Vb or Vc lesions, respectively with or without predominant calcification. In the coronary arteries, such significantly stenotic or occlusive and fibrotic lesions may cause angina (Chapter 70); however, because the preceding stenosis or occlusion with associated ischemia can give rise to protective collateral circulation, these lesions may be silent clinically.

Phase 6: About one third of acute coronary syndromes are related to complicated type VI occlusive thrombus overlying a superficial erosion of a markedly stenotic and fibrotic plaque (see phase 5). Therefore, two different mechanisms, plaque disruption and erosion, can give rise to the occlusive arterial thrombosis of the acute coronary syndromes. The terms "high-risk plaques" and "vulnerable plaques" can be used as synonyms to describe plaques with an increased risk of thrombosis.

Early Atherosclerosis and the Intimal Layer

Endothelial Dysfunction

The endothelium is a dynamic autocrine and paracrine organ that regulates anti-inflammatory, mitogenic, and contractile activities of the vessel wall as well as the hemostatic process within the vessel lumen (see Fig. 69–1A). A single molecule, nitric oxide (NO), is responsible for these regulatory processes. A dysfunctional endothelium, characterized by decreased NO synthesis, facilitates vessel wall entry and oxidation of circulating lipoproteins, monocyte entry and internalization (inflammation), proliferation of smooth muscle cells, deposition of extracellular matrix, vasoconstriction, and a prothrombotic state within the vessel lumen (see Fig. 69–1B).

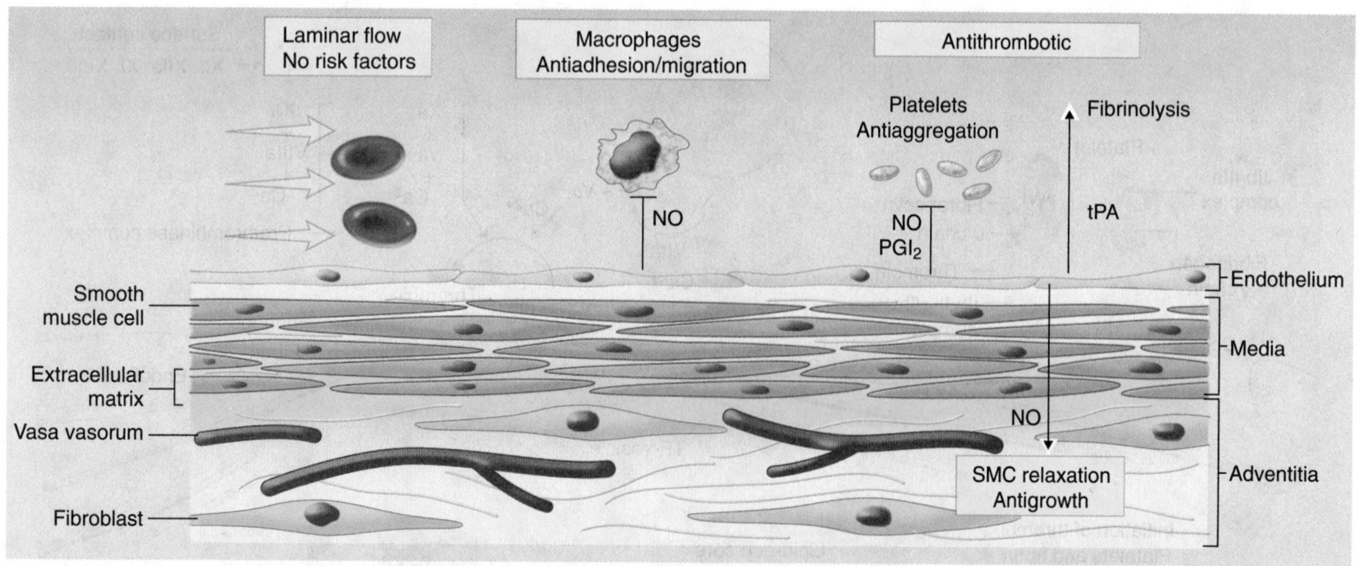

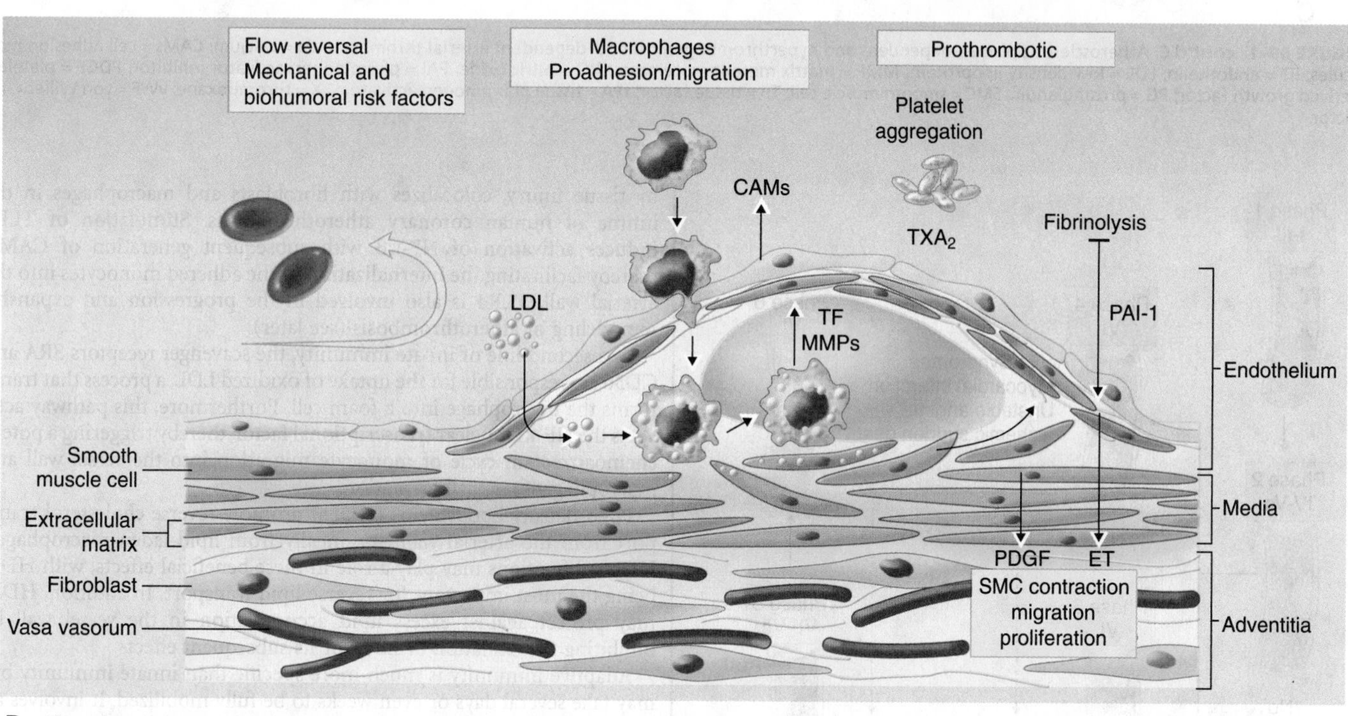

FIGURE 69–1 • Schematic representation of arterial wall biology and shear stress. A, Laminar shear stress and normal artery. **B,** Low shear stress/flow reversal and early events of atherosclerosis. CAMs = cell adhesion molecules; ET = endothelin; LDL = low-density lipoprotein; MMP = matrix metalloproteinases; NO = nitric oxide; PAI-1 = plasminogen activator inhibitor 1; PDGF = platelet-derived growth factor; PGI_2 = prostaglandin inhibitor 2; SMC = smooth muscle cell; TF = tissue factor; tPA = tissue plasminogen activator; TXA_2 = thromboxane A_2.

Endothelial dysfunction, traditionally the earliest manifestation of atherothrombosis, is often the result of a disturbance in the physiologic pattern of blood flow—flow reversal or oscillating shear stress—at bending points and near bifurcations. Endothelial cells respond to changes in local shear rates by modulating the induction or repression, or both, of several genes. A common mechanism of action of the gene modulation, in part, seems to be mediated by shear stress responding elements. Thus, as a response to reversal or oscillatory shear stress, endothelial cell activation is characterized by the expression of cell adhesion molecules (CAMs, such as intercellular adhesion molecule 1 and vascular cell adhesion molecule 1) (see Fig. 69–1B) from the selectin superfamily (E- and P-selectins), which attract monocytes to adhere to the vessel wall (see later). In addition to biomechanical shear forces enhanced by hypertension, the coexistence of other biohumoral risk factors such as hypercholesterolemia, advanced glycation end products in diabetes and in elderly persons, chemical irritants in tobacco smoke, circulating vasoactive amines, and immunocomplexes has been associated with endothelial activation and dysfunction.

Lipoprotein Entry and Infiltration

As a result of hypertension and biohumoral risk factors that induce endothelial dysfunction, low-density lipoproteins (LDLs) infiltrate through the arterial endothelium into the intima (see Fig. 69–1B). This binding appears to be related to an ionic interaction of apolipoprotein (apo) B with matrix proteins including proteoglycans, collagen, and

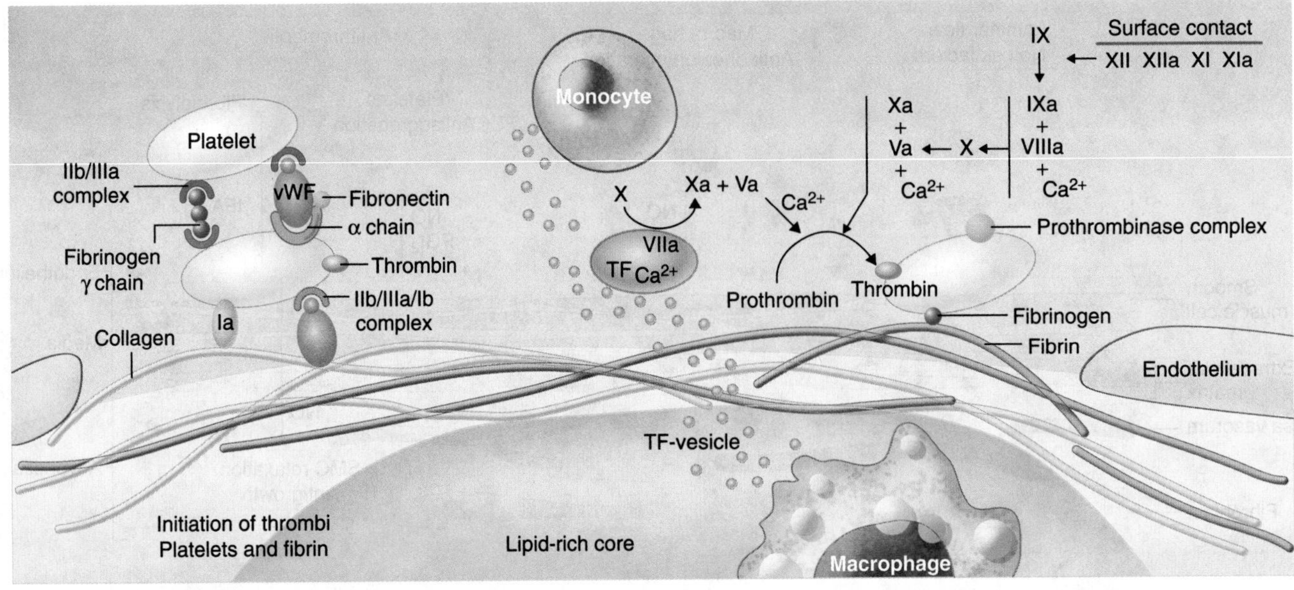

FIGURE 69–1, cont'd C, Atherosclerotic plaque–dependent and hyperthrombogenic blood–dependent arterial thrombosis. Ca = calcium; CAMs = cell adhesion molecules; ET = endothelin; LDL = low-density lipoprotein; MMP = matrix metalloproteinases; NO = nitric oxide; PAI = plasminogen activator inhibitor; PDGF = platelet-derived growth factor; PG = prostaglandin; SMC = smooth muscle cell; TF = tissue factor; tPA = tissue plasminogen activator; TX = thromboxane; vWF = von Willebrand factor.

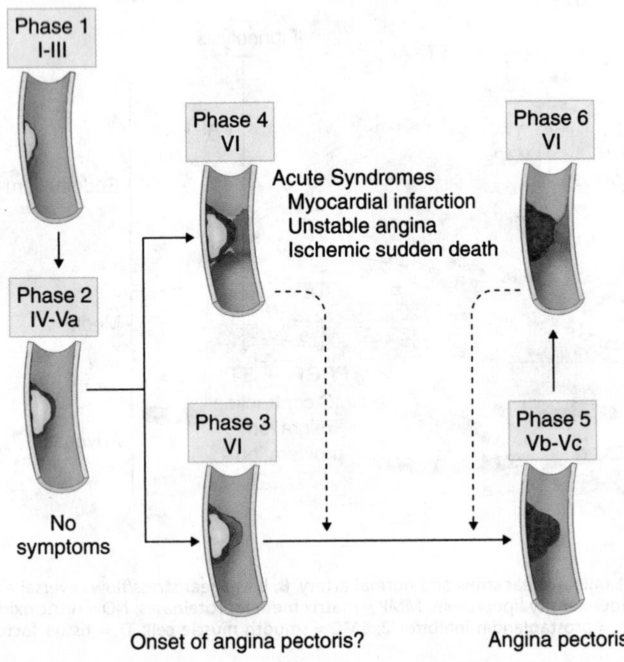

FIGURE 69–2 • Phases and morphology of the progression of coronary atherothrombosis according to clinical and gross pathology findings.

fibronectin. The interactions between oxidized LDLs and proteoglycans are crucial in early atherosclerosis, leading to lipoprotein chemical modification and retention as well as induction of inflammation. As a result of the lipoprotein entry and activation of the transcriptional nuclear factor NF-κB, subsequent expression of CAM peptides further facilitates the adherence and internalization of monocytes into the arterial wall. Such peptide-cellular interaction may be considered a defense mechanism but, if too intense, may become proatherogenic.

Inflammation and Reverse Cholesterol Transport

The development of atherosclerosis is influenced by innate and adaptive immune responses. The most important receptors for innate immunity in atherothrombosis are the Toll-like receptors (TLRs) and the macrophage scavenger receptors. For example, TLR4, which recognizes fibronectin and endogenous autoantigens produced by lipoprotein and by tissue injury, colocalizes with fibroblasts and macrophages in the intima of human coronary atherothrombosis. Stimulation of TLR4 induces activation of NF-κB with subsequent generation of CAMs, thereby facilitating the internalization of the adhered monocytes into the arterial wall. TLR4 is also involved in the progression and expansive remodeling of atherothrombosis (see later).

In a second line of innate immunity, the scavenger receptors SRA and CD36 are responsible for the uptake of oxidized LDL, a process that transforms the macrophage into a foam cell. Furthermore, this pathway activates the NF-κB nuclear transcriptional factor, thereby triggering a potent chemoattractant cycle of monocyte migration into the vessel wall and macrophage–foam cell formation.

High-density lipoproteins (HDLs) promote reverse cholesterol transport from the arterial wall, specifically from lipid-laden macrophages. HDL subfractions may play a role in these beneficial effects, with HDL_2 being the most important for reverse lipid transport. In addition, HDLs may protect against excess lipid accumulation in the vessel wall by inhibiting the oxidation of LDLs or its subsequent effects.

Adaptive immunity is much more specific than innate immunity but may take several days or even weeks to be fully mobilized. It involves an organized immune response leading to generation of T- and B-cell receptors and immunoglobulins, which can recognize antigens that are generated in atherogenesis. This type of immunity may provide the basis for future therapies, such as immunization and immunosuppressive drugs, that target adaptive immune responses.

Progression of Atherosclerosis and the Adventitia/Media

Eccentric Vascular Remodeling

Eccentric plaque growth, even without luminal compromise, is common in the early stages of atherogenesis (Fig. 69–3). Structural components involved in eccentric remodeling are vasa vasorum neovascularization, intraplaque hemorrhage, and inflammation generated in the adventitia and medial layers. Furthermore, atherosclerotic plaques that undergo remodeling, which is typical in atherosclerotic lesions that are responsible for unstable coronary syndromes, are characterized by a large lipid core.

Vasa Vasorum Neovascularization and Inflammation

Nourishment of normal blood vessels is accomplished by oxygen diffusion from the lumen of the vessel or from the adventitial vasa vasorum. When vessel wall thickness exceeds the effective diffusion distance of oxygen, vasa vasorum proliferate in the outer and inner layers of the vessel wall, where they are normally absent (see Fig. 69–1B). Vasa

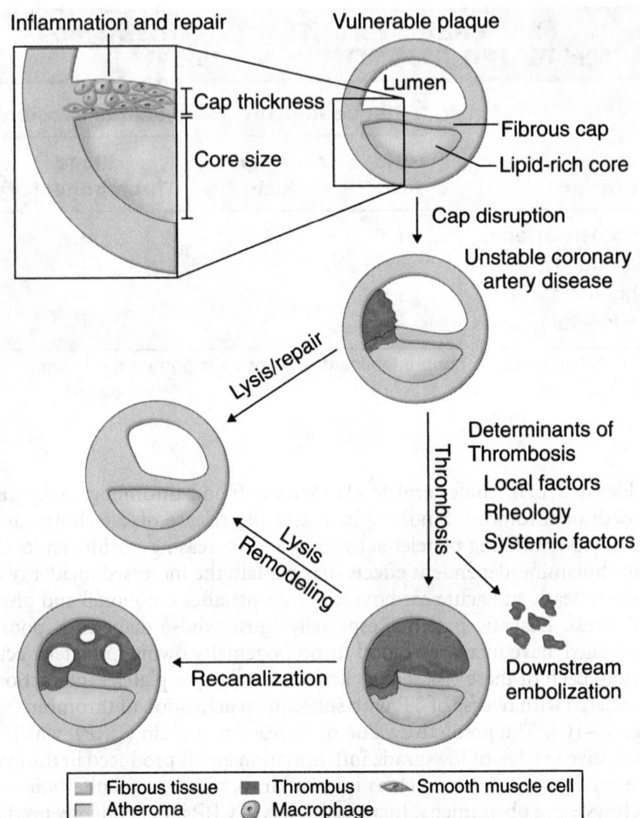

FIGURE 69–3 • Pathogenesis of a frequent type of unstable angina: anatomic changes (plaque disruption and thrombosis) leading to acute coronary syndromes and subsequent plaque remodeling. An element of vasoconstriction is usually present. (Modified from Théroux P, Fuster V: Acute coronary syndromes. Unstable angina and non-Q-wave myocardial infarction. Circulation 1998;97: 1195–1206.)

vasorum surround and penetrate the adventitia and outer media of large vessels including the aorta and the coronary, femoral, and carotid arteries. In the coronary arteries, vasa originate from bifurcation segments of epicardial vessels; in the ascending aorta, vasa originate from coronary and brachiocephalic arteries; in the descending thoracic aorta, vasa originate from intercostal arteries; and in the abdominal aorta, vasa arise from the lumbar and mesenteric arteries. First-order vasa run longitudinally to the lumen of the host vessel, whereas second-order vasa are arranged circumferentially around the host vessel. Normally, vasa remain constant in number throughout life, but atherosclerotic vasa can proliferate and lead to extensive neovascularization involving the tunica media and the intima of diseased vessels.

Vasa vasorum appear to proliferate toward regions of intimal lipoprotein infiltration, presumably to remove the excess of lipid accumulation. Therefore, intimal disease is considered a prerequisite for vessel wall and plaque neovascularization as a mechanism of defense. As cholesterol exits the plaque through the adventitia/media vasa vasorum, neovascularization and the atherosclerotic plaque may regress.

However, the neovessels are characterized by a complex morphology including sprouting, red blood cell extravasation or hemorrhage, and perivascular inflammation. Monocyte-macrophages, attracted by extravasation of red cells from the neovessels, are responsible for the cytokine production that supports neovessel growth as well as for metalloproteinase activation, which may predispose to plaque disruption. Thus, adventitia/media neovessel content and monocyte-macrophage infiltration appear to be significantly increased in ruptured plaques, with the neovessels being the source of such inflammatory components.

Vulnerable Lipid-Rich Plaque and Its Disruption

Independent predictors for plaque disruption include eccentric vascular remodeling, neovessel content in the adventitia and media, and inflammation. Type IV and Va lesions are commonly composed of an abundant crescentic mass of lipids, separated from the vessel lumen by a discrete component of extracellular matrix or cap (see Fig. 69–3). Coronary lesions that may appear relatively small on angiography as a result of remodeling may be associated with acute progression to severe thrombotic stenosis or total occlusion. In other words, the unpredictable and episodic progression of apparently small plaques is most likely caused by disruption of type IV and V lesions with subsequent thrombus formation, which changes the plaque's geometry and leads to acute or intermittent growth and acute occlusive coronary syndromes.

Two mechanisms independently or together trigger plaque rupture. The first is related to physical forces and occurs most frequently where the fibrous cap is thinnest, most heavily infiltrated by foam cells, and therefore weakest. Vulnerability to rupture depends on circumferential wall stress or cap fatigue; the location, size, and consistency of the atheromatous core; and blood flow characteristics, particularly the impact of flow on the proximal aspect of the plaque (i.e., the configuration and angulation of the plaque).

The second mechanism involves an active process within the plaque. Atherectomy specimens from patients with acute coronary syndrome reveal areas very rich in macrophages and T cells. These cells are capable of degrading extracellular matrix by phagocytosis or secretion of proteolytic enzymes, which lyse the extracellular matrix, weaken the fibrous cap, and predispose it to rupture. Destruction of the internal elastic lamina as a result of the adventitia/media infiltration by monocytes, which release matrix metalloproteinases mostly at areas of neovascularization, also appears to contribute significantly to plaque disruption.

The continuing entry, survival, and replication of monocyte-macrophages within plaques are partly dependent on factors such as CAMs, macrophage-monocyte chemoattractant protein 1, or macrophage-monocyte colony-stimulating factor. Cytokines regulate macrophage uptake of modified lipoprotein by scavenger receptors. Most important, interferon-γ, tumor necrosis factor-α, and interleukin-1 activate macrophage apoptosis. Thus, macrophages, following what appears to be a defensive mission to protect the vessel wall from lipoprotein accumulation, may eventually undergo apoptotic death. This phenomenon leads to the shedding of membrane microparticles, thereby exposing phosphatidylserine, a major contributor to arterial thrombosis after plaque rupture, on the cell surface (see Fig. 69–1C). There is an excellent correlation among macrophage density, markers of apoptosis, and the expression of tissue factor (TF) in atherosclerotic lesions.

Acute Thrombosis, Occlusive or Mural

Disruption of a vulnerable or unstable plaque with a subsequent change in plaque geometry and thrombosis results in a complicated lesion (see Figs. 69–2 and 69–3). This rapid change in geometry may result in acute occlusion or subocclusion, with clinical manifestations of unstable angina or other acute coronary syndromes (Chapter 71). More frequently, however, the rapid changes seem to result in nonocclusive mural thrombosis of the coronary arterial wall, with or without clinical angina. At the time of coronary plaque disruption, many factors—degree of disruption, local vessel wall substrate, rheology, and systemic circulation—may influence the magnitude and stability of the thrombus. Such a thrombus may be partially lysed or become replaced by collagen in the process of organization by the vascular repair response, increasing plaque size and contributing to disease progression.

Plaque-Dependent Thrombogenic Substrate

Exposure of a thrombogenic substrate is a key factor determining thrombogenicity at the local arterial site (Table 69–1). Heterogeneity of plaque composition varies even within the same subject. Lipid-rich plaques are by far the most thrombogenic, which explains why rupture of lipid-rich plaques is the most frequent cause of coronary thrombosis in the acute coronary syndrome (see Fig. 69–2, phases 3 and 4). Such thrombogenicity is modulated by the content of TF, mostly located in macrophage-rich areas (see Fig. 69–1C). TF, which is a low-molecular-weight glycoprotein, initiates the extrinsic clotting cascade and is believed to be a major regulator of coagulation, hemostasis, and thrombosis. TF forms a high-affinity complex with coagulation factors VII and VIIa; TF-VIIa complex activates factors IX and X, which in turn lead to thrombin generation.

Analysis of specimens of culprit lesions from patients with unstable angina shows a strong relationship between TF and macrophages. Thus, TF is often colocalized in LDL-overloaded macrophages that are undergoing apoptotic death and releasing microparticles, rather than in biologically active macrophages. This relationship suggests a cell-mediated thrombogenicity in patients with unstable angina and other acute coro-

TABLE 69–1 THE VIRCHOW TRIAD OF THROMBOGENICITY

LOCAL VESSEL WALL SUBSTRATES

Atherosclerosis
- Degree of plaque disruption (i.e., erosion, ulceration)

Vessel wall inflammation
- Components of plaque (i.e., lipid core)
- Macrophages and generation of microparticles (i.e., tissue factor content)

Postinterventional vessel wall injury
- Plaque disruption after percutaneous transluminal coronary angioplasty, atherectomy, or stenting
- Injury of smooth muscle cells (i.e., rich in thrombin)

RHEOLOGY

High shear stress
- Severe stenosis (i.e., change in geometry with plaque disruption, residual thrombus)
- Vasoconstriction (i.e., serotonin, thromboxane A_2, thrombin, dysfunctional endothelium)

Oscillatory shear stress
- Bifurcation of arteries, plaque irregularities

Postinterventional slow blood flow or local stasis (i.e., dissecting aneurysm)

SYSTEMIC FACTORS OF THE CIRCULATING BLOOD

Metabolic or hormonal factors
- Dyslipoproteinemia (triglycerides, increased low-density lipoprotein or oxidized low-density lipoprotein cholesterol, decreased high-density lipoprotein cholesterol, lipoprotein [a])
- Diabetes mellitus (i.e., glycosylation)
- Catecholamines (i.e., smoking, stress, cocaine use)
- Renin-angiotensin system (i.e., high-renin hypertension)

Plasma variables of hemostasis
- Tissue factor, factor VII, factor VII, fibrinogen, thrombin generation (fragments 1 and 2), thrombin activity (fibrinopeptide A), plasminogen activator inhibitor-1, tissue plasminogen activator
- Infectious (i.e., *Chlamydia pneumoniae*, cytomegalovirus, *Helicobacter pylori*) and cellular blood elements (i.e., monocytes and white blood cells)

nary syndromes. Residual mural thrombus in itself is also highly thrombogenic, presumably as a result of monocyte/TF-related activation with generation of thrombin.

Rheology and Thrombosis

The degree of stenosis caused by the ruptured plaque and the overlying mural thrombi are also key factors for determining thrombogenicity at the local arterial site (see Table 69–1). Specifically, shear rate is directly related to flow velocity and inversely related to the third power of the lumen diameter. Thus, acute platelet deposition after plaque rupture is highly modulated by the degree of narrowing after rupture. Changes in geometry may increase platelet deposition, whereas sudden growth of thrombus at the injury site may create further stenosis and thrombotic occlusion. Most platelets are deposited at the apex of a stenosis, where the highest shear rate develops. Furthermore, mural thrombus formation may contribute to vasoconstriction, which increases shear force–dependent platelet deposition.

Systemic Procoagulant Activity

About one third of coronary thromboses occur at sites of superficial erosion of a fibrotic plaque (see Fig. 62–2, phase 6). Complicated thrombi may be dependent on a hyperthrombotic state triggered by systemic factors. Two major pathways are deeply involved in systemic procoagulant activity: coronary risk factors and circulating TF (see Table 69–1).

TABLE 69–2 PREDOMINANT MECHANISMS IN COMPLICATED ATHEROTHROMBOSIS

	Plaque Rupture		Plaque Evosion
Location	**Lipid Rich**	**Non–Lipid Rich**	**Blood Thrombogenicity**
Coronary arteries	+	±	+
Carotid arteries	±	+	–
Thoracic aorta	+	–	–
Peripheral arteries	–	–	+

+ = Predominant; ± = nonpredominant; – = not an important mechanism.

Elevated LDL cholesterol levels increase blood thrombogenicity and growth of thrombus. Smoking increases the release of catecholamines, thereby potentiating platelet activation and increasing fibrinogen levels. Catecholamine-dependent effects may explain the increased incidence of sudden death and acute cardiovascular events after emotional and physical stress. Diabetic patients, especially those whose diabetes is poorly controlled, have increased blood thrombogenicity owing to platelet activation. Each of these risk factors activates leukocyte-platelet interactions associated with release of TF, with subsequent activation of thrombin (see Fig. 69–1C). The predictive value of C-reactive protein (CRP), which is a sensitive marker of low-grade inflammation and is produced in the liver as a result of mediators such as interleukin-6, may be a manifestation of such systemic phenomena. Increased levels of CRP independently predict acute coronary events even in persons whose blood lipid values fall below the median levels in the population. Whether CRP reflects the inflammatory component of atherosclerotic plaques or of the circulating blood and whether it is a surrogate marker or a biologically active element in the process of plaque development or thrombus formation are not known.

Noncoronary Atherothrombosis

Two different mechanisms, plaque rupture and erosion, can give rise to arterial thrombosis (Table 69–2). Thrombosis and thromboemboli originating in carotid plaques are frequently caused by rupture or dissection of a heterogeneous plaque, as is seen in about two thirds of coronary events, presumably as a result the impact of the systemic high-energy blood flow against the resistance offered by the plaque. Intraplaque hemorrhage caused by the rupture of vasa vasorum may play a significant role in the carotid arteries. Thrombosis and thromboemboli from the thoracic aorta also result from plaque rupture.

By comparison, thrombosis in the peripheral arteries is most frequently observed in the surface of stenotic and fibrotic plaques, as is seen in about one third of acute coronary events, predominantly as the consequence of thrombogenic blood associated with risk factors such as smoking, diabetes, and hyperlipidemia. Acute occlusion of the peripheral vasculature frequently results from thromboemboli from a cardiac or abdominal aortic source.

Clinical Manifestations

Atherothrombosis as a Systemic Disease

As previously mentioned, atherothrombotic cardiovascular disease is a diffuse condition involving the heart (coronary arteries), brain (carotid arteries), aorta, and peripheral arteries. At the time of clinical presentation, about 3 to 8% of patients have symptomatic atherosclerotic disease in three main arterial distributions and 23 to 32% of patients have clinical disease in two.

In patients with atherothrombotic disease, myocardial ischemia or MI (Chapters 70 to 72) causes 70% of deaths. Cerebrovascular disease (Chapter 430) causes approximately 10 to 17% of deaths, and another 10% are caused by ruptured thoracic or abdominal aortic aneurysms (Chapter 78). Peripheral arterial disease (Chapter 79) does not directly cause mortality, but it is an ominous manifestation of underlying disseminated atherosclerosis and portends an increased mortality related to coronary and cerebrovascular disease.

Coronary Atherothrombotic Disease

Coronary atherothrombotic disease includes a wide spectrum of conditions, ranging from silent ischemia and exertion-induced angina (Chapter 70) to the acute coronary syndromes (Chapter 71). Stable angina (usually exertional) or stable silent ischemia commonly results from increases in myocardial oxygen demand that outstrip the ability of stenosed coronary arteries to increase oxygen delivery. In contrast, acute coronary syndromes are characterized by an abrupt mismatch, with about one third caused by transient increases in myocardial oxygen demand and two thirds caused by a thrombotic occlusion related to local vessel wall substrates (i.e., plaque ulceration or erosion), rheology (i.e., high shear stress after plaque disruption or distortion, vasoconstriction), and systemic factors (i.e., blood hyperthrombogenicity). Such factors also contribute in various degrees to the completeness and duration of the occlusion and, as a consequence, to whether the acute coronary syndrome is manifested clinically as unstable angina, non–ST segment elevation acute MI, or ST segment elevation acute MI (Chapter 72).

A fairly small fissuring of a lipid-rich plaque may lead to an acute change in plaque structure and a reduction in coronary blood flow, resulting in exacerbation of angina. Transient episodes of thrombotic occlusion at the site of plaque damage, perhaps lasting only 10 to 20 minutes, may precipitate angina at rest. In addition, release of a vasoactive substance (serotonin, thromboxane A_2) by platelets, the vasoconstrictive effect of thrombin, and vasoconstriction secondary to neighboring endothelial vasodilator dysfunction may further contribute to a reduction in coronary flow.

In patients with non-ST segment elevation acute MI, a more persistent thrombosis may cause occlusion for up to 2 hours; in about 25% of patients, an infarct-related vessel occlusion may persist for longer if the distal myocardial territory is supplied by collaterals. Spontaneous thrombolysis, resolution of vasoconstriction, and presence of collateral circulation are important in preventing the development of ST segment elevation MI by limiting the duration of myocardial ischemia. In non-ST segment elevation infarction, the formation of a fixed and persistent thrombus, which leads to an abrupt cessation of myocardial perfusion for more than 2 hours, results in transmural necrosis of the involved myocardium. Some cases of sudden coronary death (Chapter 62) probably involve a rapidly progressive coronary lesion in which plaque disruption or superficial erosion, with resultant thrombosis, leads to ischemic and fatal ventricular arrhythmias in the absence of collateral flow. Platelet microemboli may also contribute to the development of sudden ischemic death.

Diagnosis

The diagnosis of disease in the various vascular beds is usually initiated by the presence of symptoms. Presymptomatic screening (Chapter 6) may identify subclinical disease, emphasizing the increased need for aggressive treatment of atherothrombotic risk factors. For coronary disease, screening options include exercise electrocardiography (Chapters 48 and 70), nuclear perfusion scanning (Chapter 54), computed tomography (CT; Chapter 54), and magnetic resonance imaging (MRI; Chapter 55). For the aorta, screening abdominal ultrasonography is appropriate in some situations (Chapter 78). Preclinical disease in the peripheral arteries can be diagnosed by an ankle-brachial index (Chapter 79). Screening for asymptomatic disease in the carotid circulation is controversial (Chapter 430).

Two of these modalities, CT and MRI, are particularly well suited for visualization of the vessel wall in both asymptomatic and symptomatic stages of atherothrombotic disease. CT can accurately quantify the coronary calcium burden (Chapter 54). Atherosclerotic coronary calcifications, mainly composed of hydroxyapatite and of a noncollagenous protein or osteopontin, are most frequently found in advanced collagen-rich lesions (plaque type Vb) rather than in vulnerable lipid-rich plaques, but they may also occur in earlier lesions. The presence of coronary calcification is a sensitive marker of obstructive disease, but only a significant extent of calcification offers reliable specificity. Individuals with no or low calcium scores are less likely to develop clinical events than those with high scores (Chapter 54). Noninvasive coronary angiography with contrast-enhanced CT also shows promise for the detection of coronary stenoses in high-risk patients.

Contrast-enhanced, whole body magnetic resonance angiography can potentially detect areas of luminal narrowing in the entire arterial system. Most important, high-resolution MRI allows noninvasive in vivo detection and characterization of atherosclerotic plaques and quantitative evaluation of the burden of atherosclerotic disease. Because of the lack of radiation and high reproducibility, the examination can be repeated over time to investigate the progression of disease or the response to therapy (i.e., statins) noninvasively. Plaque components are differentiated on the basis of biophysical and biochemical parameters, such as chemical composition, water content, physical state, molecular motion, or diffusion. These components include the lipid core, fibrous cap, fibrocellular tissue, adventitia, calcium, and thrombus or hemorrhage.

Future Directions

New targeted contrast agents may, in the future, provide information about the cellular and molecular activity of the plaque. CT and MRI also may, in the near future, provide unique information on subclinical disease, the progression of atherothrombosis, and its response to therapy. [1]

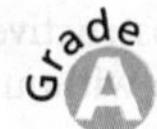

1. Corti R, Fuster V, Fayad ZA: Effects of aggressive versus conventional lipid-lowering therapy by simvastatin on human atherosclerotic lesions: A prospective, randomized, double-blind trial with high-resolution magnetic resonance imaging. J Am Coll Cardiol 2005;46:106–112.

SUGGESTED READINGS

Fenchel M, Scheule AM, Stauder NI, et al: Atherosclerotic disease: Whole-body cardiovascular imaging with MR system with 32 receiver channels and total-body surface coil technology—Initial clinical results. Radiology 2006; 238:280–291. *Whole-body arterial MRA is now feasible.*

Fuster V, Moreno PR, Fayad ZA, et al: Atherothrombosis and high-risk plaque. Part I, Evolving concepts and Part II, Approaches by noninvasive computed tomographic/magnetic resonance imaging. J Am Coll Cardiol 2005;46: 937–954; J Am Coll Cardiol 2005;46:1209–1218. *An overview of pathogenesis as well as the diagnostic and therapeutic role of noninvasive imaging.*

Hansson GK: Inflammation, atherosclerosis, and coronary artery disease. N Engl J Med 2005;352:1685–1695. *A pathophysiologic overview.*

Miller DT, Ridker PM, Libby P, et al: Atherosclerosis: The path from genomics to therapeutics. J Am Coll Cardiol 2007;49:1589–1599. *An overview of new technologies and their applications.*

Naghavi M, Falk E, Hecht HS, et al: From vulnerable plaque to vulnerable patient—Part III. Executive summary of the Screening for Hearth Attack Prevention and Education (SHAPE) Task Force report. Am J Cardiol 2006; 98:2H–15H. *An overview of screening to prevent major clinical events.*

Virmani R, Kolodgie FD, Burke AP, et al: Atherosclerotic plaque progression and vulnerability to rupture: Angiogenesis as a source of intraplaque hemorrhage. Arterioscler Thromb Vasc Biol 2005;25:2054–2061. *Neovascularization, cholesterol deposition in the monocyte membrane, and hemorrhage increase a plaque's vulnerability and risk of rupture.*

70 ANGINA PECTORIS

Pierre Théroux

Definition

Angina is the most frequent clinical expression of myocardial ischemia. Ischemia, which rapidly develops when a mismatch arises between myocardial oxygen needs and myocardial oxygen supply, can be manifested clinically in many different ways besides angina, from no symptoms (e.g., silent ischemia) to unstable angina (Chapter 71), myocardial infarction (MI; Chapters 69, 71, and 72), or sudden death (Chapter 62). It may remain stable for a long time or be rapidly progressive. Conversely, atherosclerosis, which is the most common cause of myocardial ischemia, may evolve for years without any manifestations of ischemia.

Chest pain (Chapter 48), which can be caused by various conditions that can originate from the heart or another source, may be ischemic or nonischemic and may or may not be related to coronary artery disease.

In almost all instances, the diagnosis of angina is first clinical and then subsequently supported by appropriate diagnostic testing.

Epidemiology

It has been estimated that at least half of the 13 million individuals with coronary artery disease in North America suffer from angina pectoris and that more than 400,000 new cases emerge every year (Chapter 49). An estimated 5.5 million patients come to emergency departments annually for chest pain, and about 1.5 million of them are hospitalized for unstable angina or non–ST segment elevation acute MI (Chapter 71). Half of the 1.2 million patients hospitalized for ST segment elevation MI had prior angina. The annual death rate in patients with stable angina ranges from 1 to 3.2%, depending on the population studied. Although women may have typical angina less frequently than men do, coronary artery disease is the most common cause of death in women, and more women than men die annually of coronary heart disease (CHD) or its complications in the United States. Perhaps because of delayed diagnosis or less optimal therapy, the steady decline in CHD mortality in the United States and other developed countries has been greater in men than in women. It is estimated that the risk of coronary artery disease, MI, and angina among the 10.3 million Americans suffering from obstructive sleep apnea (Chapter 101) is 4.5 times higher than in patients without sleep apnea.

Pathobiology

Atherosclerosis (Chapter 69) by far is the most common anatomic substrate of angina, although angina can also often be evident in the absence of documented atherosclerosis on the angiogram. Ischemia develops when fixed obstructions become severe enough to impede coronary blood flow or when a clot or a spasm is superimposed on a less severe obstruction. Ischemia can further be modulated by hemodynamic status, emotional status, and associated diseases such as anemia (Chapter 162) and hyperthyroidism (Chapter 244). The immediate triggers are consequences of an excessive myocardial oxygen demand or a reduced capacity of supply. In stable angina, the trigger typically is exercise in the presence of a stenosis that reduces the lumen of an epicardial coronary artery by 50% or more, corresponding to a 75% or more reduction in the artery's cross-sectional diameter.

Angina, which appears after only a few minutes of ischemia, is a complex phenomenon; its mechanisms are only partly explained. Primary angina is initiated by a reduction in oxygen supply, as found, for example, in Prinzmetal's variant angina and acute MI. In secondary angina, such as effort angina, an increase in demand is the precipitating event. Angina also can be of mixed nature, with elements of both supply and demand. Mental stress, emotions, nycthemeral variations, the postprandial state, exposure to cold, and other personal circumstances may simultaneously reduce coronary flow and increase myocardial oxygen consumption.

Mechanisms for Chest Pain

Ischemia promotes the release of active substances, such as adenosine, bradykinin, lipoxygenase byproducts, and protons, that activate chemosensitive and mechanosensitive receptors and the vanilloid receptor 1 (VR1) widely expressed on capsaicin-sensitive nerves in the cardiovascular system. The signals are transmitted to afferent nerves that connect in the upper fifth sympathetic ganglia and upper thoracic spinal cord to converge with other afferent somatic nerves and descending supraspinal signals to be transmitted to the thalamus and the cortex. These interconnections explain the various facets of the somatic presentation of the anginal pain.

Myocardial Energetics

Myocardial metabolism is essentially aerobic. Free fatty acids and protons accumulate within a few seconds after oxygen deprivation; ST segment changes ensue within minutes, followed by appearance of chest pain. The major determinants of myocardial oxygen consumption associated with heart contraction are, in decreasing order of importance, heart rate, wall tension generated during systole (afterload), inotropic state of the myocardial cell (contractility), and end-diastolic volume (preload) (Chapter 50).

Coronary Circulation

As myocardial oxygen extraction is already high in the basal state (75% at rest, 90% during ischemia), the adaptation of the heart to increasing demand is achieved mainly through vasodilation of coronary resistance vessels. During exercise, coronary blood flow can increase five-fold to six-fold from the resting value of 0.8 mL/g/min by means of the ability of the coronary circulation to autoregulate in response to changes in perfusion pressure and oxygen demand. This autoregulation is modulated by sympathetic and parasympathetic influences; by metabolic factors (primarily adenosine, a potent vasodilator resulting from oxidative phosphorylation of adenosine nucleotides that are produced when adenosine triphosphate use exceeds production); and by many other important vasoactive substances, such as nitric oxide and endothelin.

Coronary perfusion of the left ventricle is mainly during diastole, when wall tension and coronary resistance are lowest. As per Laplace's law, an intramural gradient in tension—highest in the subendocardium and lowest in the subepicardium—renders subendocardial areas more sensitive to ischemia. The ischemia with both increased demand and decreased supply will therefore be more promptly evident in the subendocardium. More severe ischemia progresses transmurally from the subendocardial to the subepicardial areas. Acute occlusion in the absence of a collateral circulation is directly manifested as ST elevation.

A gradient of pressure across the coronary obstruction builds up as the severity of luminal obstruction increases. The pressure drop through a stenosis is influenced mainly by the cross-sectional area of the stenosis (Δ pressure $\times$ 1/area^2 $\times$ length of stenosis $\times$ flow rate). The reduced distal pressure is associated with vasodilation, which limits the potential coronary reserve (i.e., the potential for any further increase in flow). Diagnostic tests such as the administration of adenosine and dipyridamole and the measure of the fractional flow reserve are based on this phenomenon (Chapter 54).

In the absence of adequate collateralization, stenoses of more than 75% of the cross-sectional area (corresponding to more than 50% lumen diameter by angiography) result in ischemia when the energy requirements are high, as during exercise in stable effort angina. The threshold for ischemia decreases as the severity of the obstruction increases. The extreme is chest pain at rest caused by severe stenoses with inadequate collateral circulation, by thrombus formation in acute coronary syndromes (Chapter 71), or by inappropriate spasm in Prinzmetal's variant angina. An important contributor to ischemia in acute coronary syndromes is the shedding and distal embolization of plaque and thrombus material, which may occlude the microvasculature and result in cell necrosis and release of troponin.

Endothelium

The endothelium is an extremely active surface that produces potent vasoactive, anticoagulant, procoagulant, and fibrinolytic substances and inflammatory mediators (Chapter 69). Nitric oxide, which is the most potent modulator of endothelial function, increases the intracellular content of cyclic guanosine monophosphate and mediates the vasodilator response to shear rate and a variety of vasoactive products, such as acetylcholine, adenosine diphosphate, bradykinin, and serotonin. The nitric oxide system, although important, is fragile and becomes ineffective in atherosclerotic vessels and when the endothelium is rendered dysfunctional by the presence of risk factors such as smoking, hypercholesterolemia, hypertension, and diabetes mellitus. Prostacyclin derived from the metabolism of arachidonic acid relaxes smooth muscle cells and inhibits platelet aggregation through an increase in the intracellular concentration of cyclic adenosine monophosphate. Endothelin produced by the endothelium is a potent vasoconstrictor with prolonged effect. The so-called syndrome X or microvascular angina relates to microvascular dysfunction in the absence of a detectable coronary occlusion or spasm in the large coronary vessels. It is a frequent and often disturbing cause of chest pain.

Inflammation and Active Plaque

Atherosclerosis is a degenerative process of the vessel wall associated with inflammation and autoimmune processes in response to injury such as oxidative stress and oxidized low-density lipoprotein cholesterol. The early endothelial dysfunction is accompanied by expression of cell adhesion molecules, monocyte-macrophage and lymphocyte infiltration, foam cell formation, cytokine production, and proliferation and migration of smooth muscle cells (Chapter 69). In acute coronary syndromes,

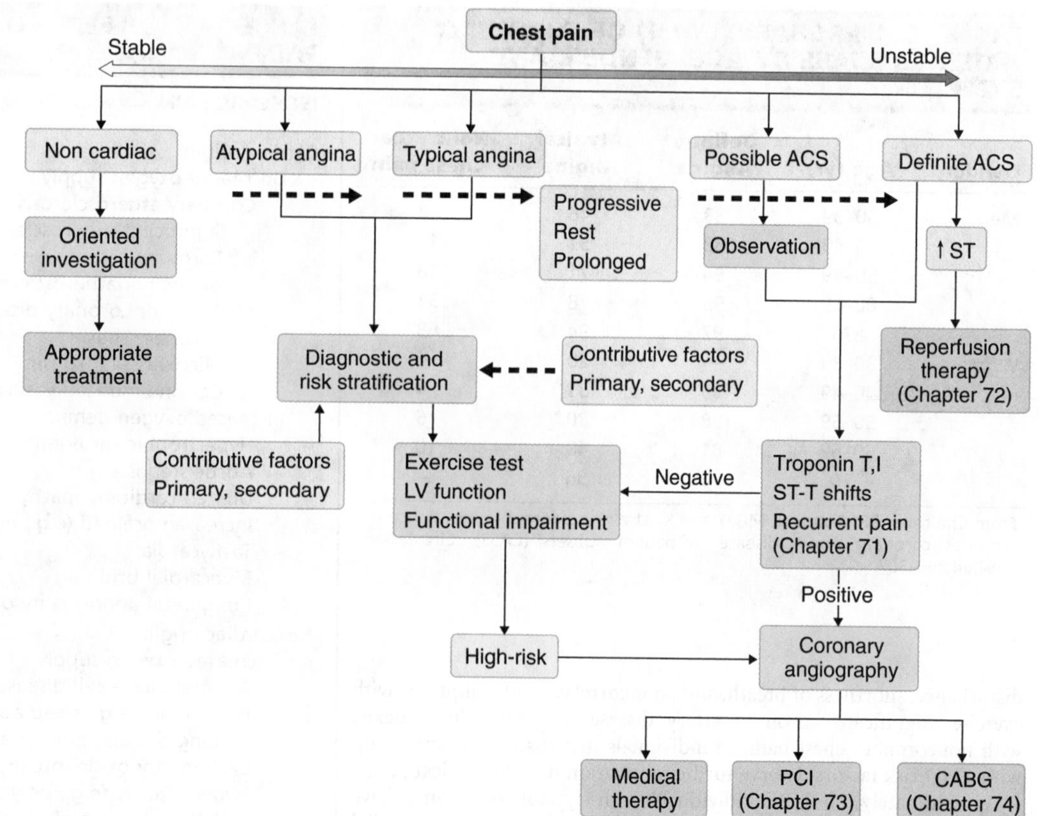

FIGURE 70–1 • Evaluation of chest pain. ACS = acute coronary syndrome; CABG = coronary artery bypass graft; LV = left ventricular; PCI = percutaneous coronary intervention.

the culprit lesion is the site of exaggerated inflammatory reaction accompanied by degeneration of the matrix, rendering the plaque friable and prone to rupture under hemodynamic stress. Rupture exposes tissue factor to the circulating blood, resulting in thrombus formation. Conversely, the plaques in stable angina contain more collagen and a thicker cap, and they are less inflammatory. The elevation of inflammatory markers, particularly C-reactive protein in patients with CHD, is believed to be related to this inflammatory component of atherosclerosis.

Clinical Manifestations

Angina is most often identified by the characteristics of the chest pain (see Table 48–2). The pain usually builds up rapidly within 30 seconds and disappears in decrescendo within 5 to 15 minutes, more promptly when nitroglycerin is used. The pain may have visceral, somatic, and cerebral components. It is variably described but typically presents as tightness, squeezing, or constriction; some patients describe an ache, a feeling of dull discomfort, indigestion, or burning pain. The discomfort is most commonly midsternal and classically radiates to the neck, left shoulder, and left arm. It also can be precordial, and it may radiate to the right arm or back, jaw, and teeth (but rarely higher) or to the epigastrium (but rarely lower). The intensity of pain ranges from mild to severe discomfort, and its characteristics and triggers, although variable among patients, are usually reproducible in any given patient. A clenching of the fist over the sternum while describing the pain (Levine's sign) is a classic representation of a patient with angina.

It is important to recognize angina equivalents in patients who deny pain or discomfort and instead report shortness of breath, dizziness, fatigue, sweating, or gastrointestinal complaints. When these symptoms occur in response to exercise or other stress, patients must be evaluated for possible myocardial ischemia.

Some patterns of angina are of particular interest. First-effort, warm-up, second-wind, or walk-through angina is manifested on first effort, often in the morning, and disappears with continued lighter exercise without reappearing on subsequent equivalent efforts. The mechanism probably is related to the phenomenon of ischemic preconditioning, which is reduced severity of ischemia after repeated short periods of occlusion and ischemia. Nocturnal angina may occur soon after lying down in patients with subclinical heart failure because of an increase in venous return; in the early morning hours, at the time the sympathetic tone is highest in patients with vasospastic disease; or any time in patients with sleep apnea.

Postprandial angina develops during or soon after meals because of an increased oxygen demand in the splanchnic vascular bed. New-onset or de novo angina and progressive angina imply a period of instability that may be defined as unstable angina, especially if the pain occurs at rest or the symptoms are progressive; these patients need close observation until the pattern stabilizes. Silent ischemia is diagnosed when no or minimal symptoms can be evoked despite objective documentation of myocardial ischemia, but in retrospect, subtle symptoms can often be elicited in these patients. At the other extreme, status anginosus is severe class IV angina that has reached a chronic phase and that is refractory to treatment; it is usually associated with extensive atherosclerosis not amenable to reperfusion.

Classifications of Angina

Various classifications have addressed the pathophysiology, diagnosis, severity, and prognosis of angina. The distinction between unstable and stable angina (Fig. 70–1) is based on the pattern of angina: its frequency, triggers, thresholds, severity, duration, accompanying manifestations, and responsiveness to rest or nitroglycerin. Angina is considered stable when symptoms have not been changing recently but rather are precipitated by a degree of effort that is reasonably predictable from day to day and are relieved by rest, more rapidly when nitroglycerin is used. Conversely, a lowering threshold to pain and progression in frequency, severity, or duration of symptoms evoke a diagnosis of unstable angina (Chapter 71).

Typical angina is defined by an affirmative answer to three simple questions: (1) Is the discomfort substernal? (2) Is it precipitated by exertion? and (3) Is it promptly relieved by rest or nitroglycerin? The interpretation of two affirmative answers is atypical angina, and none or one is noncardiac chest pain. Atypical angina is more frequent in women, who often have a more variable angina threshold as well as a pain that may have an atypical location or description. Elderly patients often complain of dyspnea, weakness, and sweating. Diabetic patients may feel no or subtle symptoms in association with myocardial ischemia. However, unstable angina by definition exhibits atypical features. The prodromal symptoms to an acute coronary syndrome can include fatigue, sleep

TABLE 70–1 PROBABILITY (%) OF CORONARY ARTERY DISEASE BY AGE, GENDER, AND SYMPTOMS

Gender	Age (yr)	Definite Angina	Atypical Angina	Noncardiac Chest pain
Men	30–39	83	46	3
	40–49	88	57	12
	50–59	94	71	18
	60–69	95	78	31
	≥70	97	94	63
Women	30–39	—	20	4
	40–49	56	31	4
	50–59	68	30	6
	60–69	81	48	10
	≥70	96	56	—

From Chaitman BR, Bourassa MG, Davis K, et al: Angiographic prevalence of high-risk coronary artery disease in patient subsets (CASS). Circulation 1981;64:360–367.

disturbance, shortness of breath, and poor correlation of symptoms with exercise. Significant coronary artery disease also can often coexist with noncoronary chest pain, so individuals in a susceptible age group with CHD risk factors deserve further evaluation despite atypical pain.

Approximately 80% of individuals with typical symptoms have demonstrable coronary artery disease and evidence of myocardial ischemia; 20% of patients, however, including a higher percentage of younger patients without risk factors, have no evidence of myocardial ischemia despite typical complaints (Table 70–1). In patients with atypical angina, the prevalence of underlying coronary artery disease and myocardial ischemia varies widely from 20% to more than 90%, depending on age and CHD. The Canadian Cardiovascular Society classification, which is the most widely used approach assessing disability due to angina (see Table 48–4), helps guide management, even though its predictive value for the extent and severity of coronary artery disease is poor and its prognostic value for subsequent events is weak.

Diagnosis

History

Chest pain can be due to a variety of extracardiac or cardiac causes, and cardiac pain can be ischemic or not (Table 70–2). Ischemic pain is generally related to obstructive coronary atherosclerosis, but it also can be caused by congenital anatomic abnormalities interfering with epicardial flow, such as a congenital abnormality of the coronary circulation, or focal systolic compression of a tunneled epicardial artery by an overlying band of cardiac muscle (termed a myocardial bridge).

Angina can also result from conditions that increase myocardial oxygen demand beyond supply, including tachyarrhythmias, aortic valve stenosis (Chapter 75), hypertrophic cardiomyopathy (Chapter 59), uncontrolled hypertension (Chapter 66), and cocaine intoxication (Chapter 32), or conditions that limit oxygen delivery, such as anemia and carbon monoxide intoxication. Angina or ischemia that is associated with normal epicardial coronary arteries is commonly related to endothelial dysfunction with failure of normal vasodilation in resistance vessels; a lowered threshold to pain may also contribute in some patients.

Nonischemic, noncardiac pain can be caused by pulmonary, gastrointestinal, chest wall, and psychogenic conditions (Chapter 48). In acute situations, aortic dissection (Chapter 78), acute pericarditis (Chapter 77), pulmonary embolism (Chapter 99), or pneumothorax (Chapter 100) must be considered. The clinical picture and differential diagnosis of chest pain can be blurred by the interactions that exist between the different mechanisms of chest pain and the locations of referred pain.

An accurate diagnosis of angina requires an objective documentation of myocardial ischemia associated with the chest pain. No historical evidence, physical examination findings, or other diagnostic tests are perfectly accurate for the diagnosis.

TABLE 70–2 DIFFERENTIAL DIAGNOSIS OF CHEST PAIN

ISCHEMIC PAIN

- Cardiac origin
  - Decreased oxygen supply
    - Coronary atherosclerosis
      - Significant atherosclerosis
      - Coronary thrombosis
    - Coronary, nonatherosclerotic causes
      - Aortic or coronary dissection
      - Coronary spasm
      - Microvascular spasm
      - Cocaine-induced vasoconstriction
  - Increased oxygen demand
    - Hypertrophic cardiomyopathy
    - Aortic stenosis
    - Dilated cardiomyopathy
    - Increased preload (e.g., aortic or mitral valve regurgitation)
    - Tachycardia
    - Myocardial bridging
    - Congenital abnormality of the coronary circulation
- Noncardiac origin
  - Decreased oxygen supply
    - Anemia, sickle cell disease
    - Hypoxemia (e.g., sleep apnea, pulmonary fibrosis, chronic lung disease, pulmonary embolism)
    - Carbon monoxide intoxication
    - Hyperviscosity (e.g., polycythemia, hypergammaglobulinemia)
  - Increased oxygen demand
    - Hyperthyroidism
    - Hyperthermia
    - High inotropic state (e.g., adrenergic stimulation)

NONISCHEMIC PAIN

- Cardiac origin
  - Pericarditis
  - Aortic dissection
- Noncardiac origin
  - Gastrointestinal: esophageal (esophagitis, spasm, reflux, rupture, ulcer); biliary (colic, cholecystitis); gastric (peptic ulcer); pancreatitis
  - Psychogenic: anxiety disorders (hyperventilation, panic); affective disorders (depression); somatization; cardiac psychosis
  - Pulmonary: pulmonary embolism, pneumothorax, pleuritis, pneumonia, pulmonary hypertension
  - Neuromuscular: costochondritis, fibrositis, Tietze's syndrome, rib fracture, herpes zoster, thoracic outlet syndrome, sternoclavicular arthritis

Physical Examination

The physical examination is of limited help in evaluating a patient with chest pain. The examination can occasionally identify cardiac or noncardiac causes of chest discomfort other than CHD, such as aortic stenosis, pericarditis, aortic dissection, costochondritis, and pulmonary disorders (see Tables 48–2 and 70–2). The physical examination may also increase the likelihood of CHD by detecting hypertension, xanthomas, xanthelasma, corneal arcus, obesity, diminished pulses, or vascular bruits. Indirect signs of transient myocardial ischemia on the physical examination include pulmonary rales, S_4 or S_3 gallop, sustained or dyskinetic left ventricular impulse, transient murmur of mitral regurgitation caused by papillary muscle dysfunction, and paradoxical splitting of S_2 due to transient left ventricular dysfunction or left bundle branch block.

Diagnostic Tests

Blood Tests

Routine blood tests are not diagnostic in angina but are important to assess risk factors and abnormalities that may precipitate or worsen

TABLE 70–3 OTHER LABORATORY TESTS SUGGESTED IN PATIENTS WITH STABLE ANGINA

LDL and HDL cholesterol levels (apolipoprotein B, apolipoprotein A-I)
Triglyceride level
Fasting glucose concentration
Creatinine levels
Homocysteine level in patients with strong family history, especially if not explained by other risk factors
Hemoglobin, hematocrit
Test of thyroid function (T_4 or TSH level)
Consider C-reactive protein levels*
Troponin T or troponin I, CK-MB†

*C-reactive protein levels are useful to assess prognosis and may help treatment selection, such as statin therapy.
†Should be obtained when a diagnosis of acute coronary syndrome is considered.
CK-MB = creatine kinase MB; HDL = high-density lipoprotein; LDL = low-density lipoprotein; T_4 = thyroxine; TSH = thyroid-stimulating hormone.
Modified from Braunwald E, Goldman L (eds): Primary Care Cardiology, 2nd ed. Philadelphia, WB Saunders, 2003.

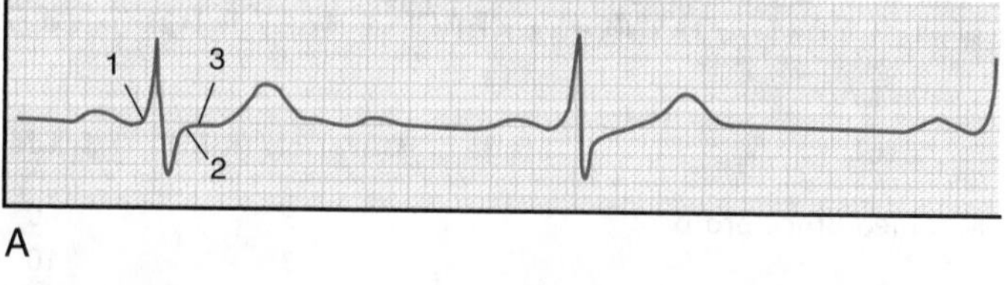

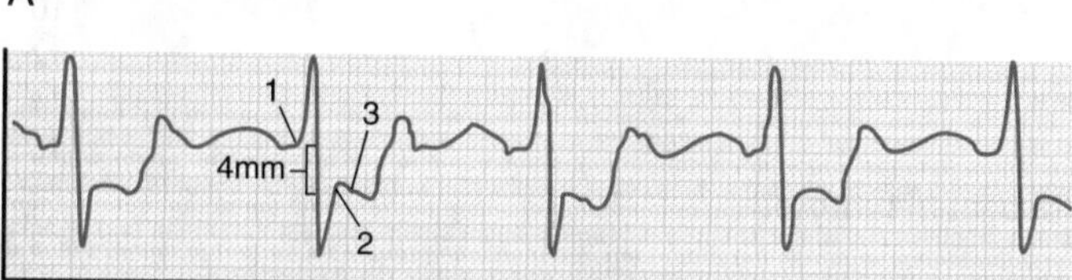

FIGURE 70–2 • Typical electrocardiographic ST segment depression associated with myocardial ischemia. A, Lead V_5 at rest. **B,** Lead V_5 at peak exercise. The PQ junction (1) that serves as the baseline reference, the J point (2), and the ST segment at 80 msec past the J point (3) are represented. In this case, the amount of ST segment depression measured 80 msec past the J point is 0.4 mV or 4 mm, and the slope between the J point and 80 msec past the J point is nonexistent since the ST segment is horizontal and not upsloping.

angina and to distinguish unstable angina from a non–ST elevation acute MI (Table 70–3). The laboratory evaluation should include a complete blood cell count to exclude anemia and thyroid function tests to exclude hyperthyroidism or hypothyroidism, which may precipitate or worsen angina. Creatinine and blood urea nitrogen levels assess the possibility of renal insufficiency as a precipitating or aggravating cause, may influence drug therapy, and help determine prognosis. Patients should also be routinely evaluated for CHD risk factors, including an evaluation for hyperlipidemia (Chapter 217) and diabetes mellitus (Chapter 247). Elevated levels of C-reactive protein identify patients at higher risk for an adverse outcome. Homocysteine levels can also be assessed, although the benefit of treatment has not yet been documented. Markers of myocyte damage (troponin T, troponin I, creatine kinase [CK]-MB) are not routinely indicated except to distinguish unstable angina from a non–ST segment elevation MI (Chapter 71).

Resting Electrocardiogram

A 12-lead electrocardiogram (ECG) recorded in a pain-free state may show arrhythmias, a previous MI, or left ventricular hypertrophy. Obtained during or shortly after an episode of chest pain, the ECG is extremely useful for the diagnosis of ischemia as well as its location, extent, and severity. ST segment shift, most often depression, is the most specific finding, followed by T wave inversion (Fig. 70–2). Pseudonormalization of these anomalies during pain is also a reliable indicator of ischemia. Transient ST segment elevation during pain is indicative of Prinzmetal's angina or of a severely obstructive lesion with impending MI. Deep T wave inversion in the anterior leads, sometimes more evident in the hours or days that follow an episode of angina, is a marker of significant stenosis of the left anterior descending coronary artery. Diffuse ST changes with an elevation in lead aVR suggest left main disease or multivessel disease.

Radiology

A chest radiograph (Chapter 51) is recommended when an intrathoracic disease such as lung disease, pulmonary embolism, or aortic aneurysm is a diagnostic possibility and in patients with suspected heart failure.

Electron beam computed tomography (Chapter 54) permits detection and quantification of coronary artery calcification with a high sensitivity, but calcification alone cannot predict the severity of stenoses. Computed tomography and magnetic resonance angiography are promising tests that are not yet recommended for routine use.

Echocardiography

Echocardiography (Chapter 53) is useful for the evaluation of left ventricular function and valve disease. An echocardiogram should be obtained in patients with a systolic murmur suggestive of aortic stenosis, hypertrophic cardiomyopathy, or mitral regurgitation and to evaluate the severity of ischemic wall motion abnormalities when the test can be obtained during pain or within 30 minutes after its resolution. In patients who have angina and a history of previous MI or symptoms of heart failure, left ventricular function should be assessed quantitatively by echocardiography (Chapter 53) or nuclear techniques (Chapter 54). The combination of significant coronary artery disease and left ventricular dysfunction is associated with a poor prognosis that can often be improved with revascularization (see later). Segmental dysfunction can relate to stunned myocardium (transient dysfunction secondary to acute ischemia) or hibernating myocardium (poorly functioning myocardium secondary to chronic hypoperfusion). These conditions are reversible with appropriate treatment.

Provocative Testing

Standard stressors for provocative testing are exercise on the treadmill or cycle ergometer and pharmacologic stimulation with dobutamine, dipyridamole, or adenosine. Dobutamine produces ischemia by increasing myocardial oxygen needs through chronotropic and inotropic stimulation; adenosine, by potent vasodilation that produces heterogeneous perfusion in the presence of flow-limiting stenoses while the vasodilation in nonobstructed arteries may steal blood away from vessels that already are maximally dilated distal to an occluded vessel; and dipyridamole, by adenosine release. Markers of ischemia during testing are ST segment shifts on the ECG (see Fig. 70–2), a perfusion defect on a planar or single-photon emission computed tomography nuclear scan (see Fig. 54-1) or on a positron emission tomography scan, and wall motion abnormalities and systolic thinning on an echocardiogram (see Fig. 53–6). Combined computed tomography and positron emission tomography allow concomitant studies of coronary anatomy, myocardial perfusion, and metabolism.

Exercise testing with ECG monitoring remains the provocative test recommended for routine use because it mimics physiology and is readily available, inexpensive, and safe. Death or MI occurs in less than one case per 2500 tests if the test is avoided in patients with severe aortic stenosis, severe hypertension, or uncontrolled heart failure. Other contraindications are acute MI, symptomatic arrhythmias, acute pulmonary embolism, pericarditis, and acute aortic dissection. Relative contraindications are hypertension greater than 200 mm Hg systolic or 110 mm Hg diastolic, hypertrophic cardiomyopathy, and high-degree atrioventricular block.

The exercise test protocol is usually adjusted to a patient's tolerance, aiming for 6 to 12 minutes of exercise time to achieve maximal oxygen consumption. Exercise that is too strenuous with rapid workload increments shortens the duration of the test and may lower the sensitivity for detecting ischemia and estimating exercise capacity; tests that are too easy become measures of endurance. In the commonly used and well-validated Bruce protocol (Table 70–4), the increase in workload between the various stages is relatively large. Less aggressive protocols, such as the Naughton, Weber, and Asymptomatic Cardiac Ischemia Pilot (ACIP) study or a ramp protocol, are preferred in patients with a reduced tolerance.

TABLE 70–4 COMMON EXERCISE TEST PROTOCOLS

Protocol	Stage	Duration (min)	Grade (%)	Rate (mph)	Metabolic Equivalents at Completion	Functional Class
Modified Bruce protocol*	1	3	0	1.7	2.5	III
	2	3	10	1.7	5	II
	3	3	12	2.5	7	I
	4	3	14	3.4	10	I
	5	3	16	4.2	13	I
Naughton protocol†	0	2	0	2	2	III
	1	2	3.5	2	3	III
	2	2	7	2	4	III
	3	2	10.5	2	5	II
	4	2	14	2	6	II
	5	2	17.5	2	7	I

Ramp protocols in which the workload is gradually increased on the basis of the patient's estimated functional capacity to achieve maximal effort in approximately 10 minutes are also useful.
*Commonly used in ambulatory patients.
†Commonly used in patients with recent myocardial infarction, unstable angina, or other conditions that are expected to limit exercise.
Modified from Braunwald E, Goldman L (eds): Primary Cardiology, 2nd ed. Philadelphia, WB Saunders, 2003.

An issue with exercise testing is its predictive value. On the basis of Bayes' theorem (Chapter 9), ST segment shifts on exercise testing in patients with a low probability of angina will most often be false-positives, whereas the same changes in patients with a higher clinical probability of the disease will almost always represent true-positives. It can be argued that a positive test result only confirms a diagnosis when the probability of CHD is high, whereas a negative test result is not discriminatory enough for diagnosis, and that a negative test result is only confirmatory when the probability is low, whereas a positive test result has little effect on the probability (Fig. 70–3). As a result, the strongest indication for diagnostic exercise testing is in patients with an intermediate (10% and 90%) pretest probability of CHD (see Table 70–1). The test is less useful for diagnosis in patients with a high or a low pretest probability, and it is not recommended for patients with an abnormal baseline ECG (e.g., left bundle branch block, resting ST segment elevation or depression, use of digitalis, Wolff-Parkinson-White syndrome, electrolyte abnormalities) that precludes the interpretation of ST segment change. However, exercise testing can be helpful for purposes other than the diagnosis of CHD, such as the evaluation of exercise tolerance and functional capacity, arrhythmias, and prognosis. An exercise test also may be appropriate in asymptomatic individuals with diabetes or other CHD risk factors before they undertake an exercise program or in individuals with calcifications on electron beam computed tomography (Chapter 54). A negative test result in asymptomatic persons or in individuals with noncardiac chest pain (probability of coronary artery disease less than 15%) virtually excludes ischemic heart disease.

In many patients, the standard exercise ECG can be complemented with perfusion imaging for more precise diagnosis (see Fig. 70-3) or should be replaced by an alternative diagnostic approach (Table 70–5). Exercise perfusion or echocardiography is preferred to an exercise ECG in patients with resting ST segment abnormalities secondary to left ventricular hypertrophy, intraventricular conduction defect, preexcitation, electrolyte abnormalities, or digitalis use. Imaging is also indicated in patients with an abnormal ECG after a previous MI or coronary artery bypass grafting.

Pharmacologic stress testing with dipyridamole or adenosine is preferred to exercise in patients who cannot exercise adequately; ischemia is then assessed by perfusion scintigraphy with thallium Tl-201 or technetium Tc-99m–sestamibi (Chapter 54) or by echocardiography (Chapter 53). Fixed perfusion deficits usually represent previous MI, whereas reversible deficits present only after exercise represent transient ischemia. Alternatively, reversible wall motion abnormalities and systolic wall thinning on echocardiography are indicators of reversible ischemia.

The overall sensitivity of exercise ECG for detecting coronary artery disease is about 70%, and its specificity for excluding coronary artery disease is about 75% (Table 70–6). ECG abnormalities most likely to indicate significant ischemia are horizontal or downsloping ST segment depression of more than 1 mV (see Fig. 70-2) and occurrence of symptoms consistent with angina. Many other specific and nonspecific features, such as dyspnea and a low tolerance, are of prognostic significance.

The sensitivity and specificity of imaging approaches are, in general, higher than those of the ECG, although they are also influenced by the pretest likelihood of the disease (see Table 70–6). False-negative perfusion scans occur in patients with three-vessel disease and global left ventricular ischemia because low flow is diffuse rather than focal. The positron emission tomography scan provides high-quality imaging corrected for soft tissue attenuation and is the "gold standard" for assessing viability in areas of dysfunction. The choice among stress perfusion imaging, stress echocardiography, and positron emission tomography is largely a matter of local expertise, although a patient's individual characteristics occasionally can be compelling (see Table 70–5).

Continuous ECG monitoring allows detection of otherwise clinically silent ischemia. Many patients with symptomatic angina also experience multiple additional episodes of asymptomatic ischemia with a total ischemic burden higher than clinically suspected. Control of asymptomatic ischemia by approaches that reduce ischemic burden rather than focus on symptoms may improve prognosis in some patients with episodes of silent ischemia.

Coronary Angiography

Coronary angiography (Chapter 56) remains the current standard for assessing the presence and severity of CHD and is required for guiding revascularization procedures (Table 70–7). Indeed, some patients may be incorrectly diagnosed with CHD for years until angiography shows no disease, whereas other patients may be treated symptomatically for noncardiac diseases until angiography documents CHD.

Fractional Flow Reserve Coronary Angiography

Fractional flow reserve (FFR) can be measured only in the catheterization laboratory. A pressure guidewire positioned distal to the stenosis provides the distal pressure (Pd); the aortic pressure (Pa) is measured through the guiding catheter. Maximal hyperemia is induced by the administration of a potent vasodilator such as adenosine, adenosine triphosphate, or papaverine and measured as the ratio of mean distal pressure to mean aortic pressure (FFR = Pd/Pa). A cutoff value of 0.75 permits accurate discrimination between coronary obstructive lesions that induce ischemia and those that do not. Although it is simple and helpful to evaluate the prognosis of patients and to establish the indication for revascularization of stenoses of doubtful significance, its application has been limited because of the hardware required.

Other Anginal Syndromes

Variant Angina or Prinzmetal's Angina

The diagnosis is based on the documentation of transient ST segment elevation during an episode of chest pain in the absence of a focal, severe,

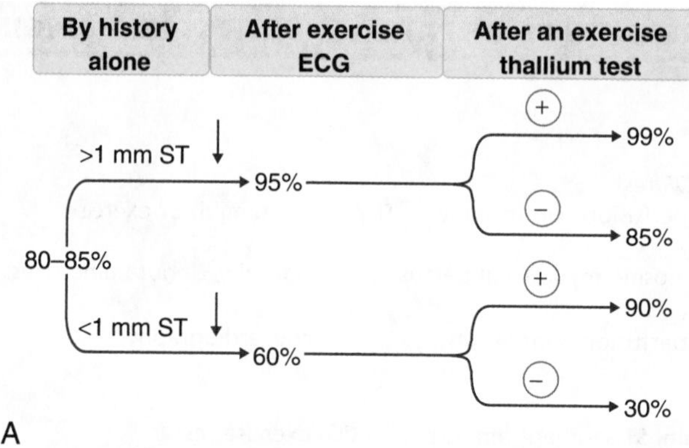

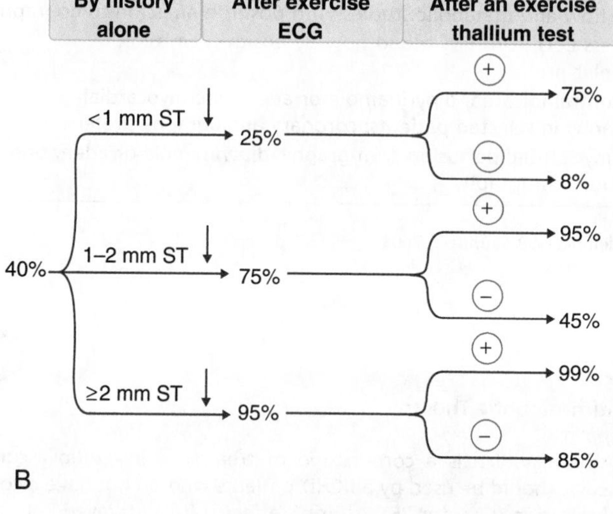

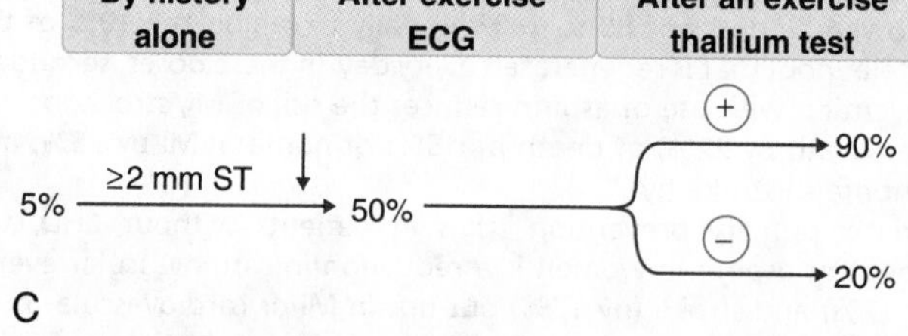

FIGURE 70–3 • A, Approximate probability of coronary artery disease before and after noninvasive testing in a patient with typical angina pectoris. These percentages demonstrate how the sequential use of an ECG and an exercise thallium test may affect the probability of coronary artery disease in a patient with typical angina pectoris. **B,** Approximate probability of coronary artery disease before and after noninvasive testing in a patient with atypical angina symptoms. **C,** Approximate probability of coronary artery disease before and after noninvasive testing in an asymptomatic subject in the coronary artery disease age range. (Redrawn from Branch WB Jr [ed]: Office Practice of Medicine, 3rd ed. Philadelphia, WB Saunders, 1994, p 45.)

fixed coronary stenosis. The chest pain occurs predominantly at rest, although approximately one third of patients may also experience the pain during exercise. There is a predilection for the pain to wake the patient in the early morning hours when sympathetic activity is increasing. The syndrome is often cyclical, with periods of exacerbation with repetitive episodes of chest pain that may persist only for seconds or be more prolonged and severe, alternating with periods with few or no symptoms. The pain is typically relieved by nitroglycerin. The ST segment elevation accompanying the pain signifies transmural ischemia due to total abrupt occlusion of a nonsignificant stenosis in the absence of a collateral circulation. The subsequent rapid reperfusion may explain the high prevalence of severe life-threatening arrhythmias.

Prinzmetal's variant angina typically is caused by an occlusive spasm superimposed on a nonsevere coronary artery stenosis; however, at times, no underlying stenoses are seen, or the underlying stenosis may be severe. Because of these uncertainties, it is mandatory to perform coronary angiography in all patients with vasospastic disease. Associated Raynaud's phenomenon and migraine headache have been described in some patients, suggesting that the syndrome may be part of a more generalized vasospastic disorder. A provocative test for spasm with acetylcholine or ergonovine is useful to establish the diagnosis and to assess the response to therapy in patients with normal or nearly normal coronary angiograms, in whom the diagnosis is otherwise unclear.

Angina with Normal Coronary Angiography

The chest pain in this syndrome occurs most frequently at rest, often in relation to emotional stress; periods of exacerbation commonly alternate with symptom-free periods. It is more frequent in women, and an important component is altered perception of pain or hypersensitivity to certain stimuli. The diagnosis requires objective documentation of ischemia with ST-T segment changes, of a metabolic abnormality, of transient regional perfusion defect, or of endothelial dysfunction that limits blood flow reserve. β-Blockers may be useful, particularly when a relative tachycardia, hypertension, or decreased heart rate variability on Holter monitoring is present. Nitroglycerin can relieve symptoms in approximately 50% of patients, and long-acting nitrates or calcium antagonists are sometimes helpful. Prognosis in general is favorable and not different from that of a general age-matched population in the absence of coronary artery disease.

Risk Stratification

Risk stratification incorporates demographic data (e.g., age, sex), risk factors, findings on physical examination, and diagnostic testing (Fig. 70–4). Abnormal blood lipids and cigarette smoking are the two most important risk factors, and these two plus high blood pressure, diabetes, abdominal obesity, stress, lack of daily consumption of fruits and vegetables, lack of daily exercise, and absence of regular consumption of small amounts of alcohol predict more than 90% of the risk of an MI worldwide.

High-risk findings on an exercise test include ST segment depression of 2 mm or more, ST segment depression of 1 mm or more in the first stage of the Bruce protocol, sustained ST segment depression of 5 minutes or more after cessation of exercise, blood pressure decrease of 10 mm Hg or more, severe ventricular arrhythmias during or after exercise at a heart rate of 120 beats per minute, and inability to complete the equivalent of 6 minutes of the Bruce protocol. Less specific symptoms, such as dyspnea, are also important for prognosis.

High-risk features on the nuclear scan are ischemia of more than 15% of the left ventricle, multiple perfusion defects in more than one vascular bed, large and severe perfusion defects, left ventricular dilation, uptake of the tracer in the lung with exercise, and postexercise left ventricular dilation. High-risk stress echocardiographic criteria are multiple reversible wall motion abnormalities and more severe and extensive abnormalities (see Table 70–8).

The extent of disease evaluated by the number of diseased vessels (>50% lumen diameter reduction) is the traditional angiographic marker of risk. In this assessment, left main disease is considered a separate high-risk entity or the equivalent of two-vessel disease, and specific attention is paid to proximal left anterior artery disease (Table 70–9).

Treatment

Rx

The management of angina pectoris aims to prevent death and MI, reducing ischemic episodes to improve quality of life and slowing or even reversing the process of atherosclerosis. Success requires physicians and often a team of health care professionals with programs that address individual patients' needs with information, counseling, lifestyle adjustments, medications, and judicious use of interventions (Table 70–10 and Fig. 70–5).

Cardiovascular Health

Control of Risk Factors and General Status

Control of risk factors is the cornerstone of primary and secondary prevention. Lifestyle interventions should address smoking cessation, weight reduction, physical fitness, and diet. Drugs that clearly improve outcomes (e.g., aspirin, statins, and medications to control blood pressure) are routinely indicated. Associated diseases that can

TABLE 70–5 SUGGESTED NONINVASIVE TESTS IN DIFFERENT TYPES OF PATIENTS WITH STABLE ANGINA

Exertional angina, mixed angina, walk-through angina, postprandial angina with or without prior myocardial infarction	
Normal resting ECG	Treadmill exercise ECG test
Abnormal, uninterpretable resting ECG	Exercise myocardial perfusion scintigraphy (^{201}Tl, ^{99m}Tc-sestamibi) or exercise echocardiography
Unsuitable for exercise	Dipyridamole or adenosine myocardial perfusion scintigraphy, dobutamine stress echocardiography
Atypical chest pain with normal or borderline abnormal resting ECG or with nondiagnostic stress ECG, particularly in women	Exercise myocardial perfusion scintigraphy, exercise echocardiography
Vasospastic angina	ECG during chest pain, ST segment ambulatory ECG, exercise test
Dilated ischemic cardiomyopathy with typical angina or for assessment of hibernating or stunned myocardium	Regional and global ejection fraction by radionuclide ventriculography or two-dimensional echocardiography, radionuclide myocardial perfusion scintigraphy; in selected patients, flow and metabolic studies with positron emission tomography
Syndrome X	Treadmill exercise stress ECG, coronary blood flow by positron emission tomography, Doppler probe
Known severe aortic stenosis or severe hypertrophic cardiomyopathy with stable angina	Exercise stress tests contraindicated; dipyridamole or adenosine myocardial perfusion scintigraphy in selected patients; coronary angiography preferred
Mild aortic valvar disease or hypertrophic cardiomyopathy with typical exertional angina	"Prudent" treadmill myocardial perfusion scintigraphy, dipyridamole or adenosine myocardial perfusion scintigraphy

ECG = 12-lead electrocardiogram.
Modified from Braunwald E, Goldman L (eds): Primary Care Cardiology, 2nd ed. Philadelphia, WB Saunders, 2003.

TABLE 70–6 APPROXIMATE SENSITIVITY AND SPECIFICITY OF COMMON TESTS TO DIAGNOSE CORONARY ARTERY DISEASE

	Sensitivity	Specificity
Exercise electrocardiography		
>1 mV ST depression	0.70	0.75
>2 mV ST depression	0.33	0.97
>3 mV ST depression	0.20	0.99
Perfusion scintigraphy		
Exercise SPECT	0.88	0.72
Pharmacologic SPECT	0.90	0.82
Echocardiography		
Exercise	0.85	0.81
Pharmacologic stress	0.81	0.79
PET	0.95	0.95

PET = positron emission tomography; SPECT = single-photon emission computed tomography.
From Gibbons RJ, Abrams J, Chatterjee K, et al: ACC/AHA 2002 guideline update for the management of patients with chronic stable angina—summary article: A report of the American College of Cardiology/American Heart Association Task Force on Practice Guidelines (Committee on Management of Patients with Chronic Stable Angina). Circulation 2003;107:149–158.

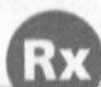

worsen CHD or precipitate ischemia, such as anemia, thyrotoxicosis, fever, infection, chronic lung disease, sleep apnea, diabetes, renal failure, and depression, must be recognized and addressed. The physician must also diagnose and treat associated cardiac conditions, such as valvar heart disease, bradyarrhythmias and tachyarrhythmias, and heart failure.

Prevention of Death and Myocardial Infarction

Death and MI can be prevented by antithrombotic and statin therapy and, in many patients, by β-blockers and angiotensin-converting enzyme inhibitors. Revascularization with coronary artery bypass graft (CABG) or percutaneous coronary intervention (PCI) can also prolong life and prevent MI in patients with critical coronary artery stenoses.

Antithrombotic Therapy

Aspirin

Aspirin, which is a cornerstone of treatment in cardiovascular disease, should be used by all CHD patients who do not have a contraindication (Chapter 35). Aspirin's effect is fully achieved with an initial dose of 300 mg, which inhibits the pretreatment platelet pool, followed by doses of 80 to 160 mg daily to inhibit the 10% of the platelet pool that is regenerated every day. In these doses, secondary prevention with use of aspirin reduces the risk of MI, stroke, or vascular death by 22%; of death by 15%; of nonfatal MI by 35%; and of nonfatal stroke by 25%. [1]

In six primary prevention trials in patients without CHD, the benefit of aspirin in women is a reduction in cardiovascular events (by 12%) and stroke (by 17%) but not in MI or cardiovascular mortality. By comparison, the benefit in men is a reduction in cardiovascular events (by 14%) and MI (by 32%) but not in stroke or cardiovascular mortality (Chapter 35). [2]

Clopidogrel

Clopidogrel is a thienopyridine that irreversibly inhibits the adenosine diphosphate PY12 receptor (Chapter 35). At a dose of 75 mg/day, it is slightly more effective than aspirin for the secondary prevention of cardiovascular events in patients with a recent stroke or MI or with symptomatic peripheral vascular disease, with no increase in adverse effects. The combination of aspirin plus clopidogrel (loading dose of 300 mg followed by 75 mg/day) reduces the risk of cardiovascular death, nonfatal MI, or stroke by 20% ($P < .0001$) during an average follow-up of 9 months. [3] However, clopidogrel plus aspirin was no better than aspirin alone in a large study of patients with clinical cardiovascular disease or multiple risk factors, with a suggestion of benefit in the former group and harm in the latter group. [4] The general recommendation is to use aspirin as a first-line agent for primary and secondary prevention, clopidogrel as an alternative in patients who are intolerant of aspirin or develop an ischemic event while taking aspirin, and the combination of aspirin and clopidogrel after stent implantation (Chapter 72) and for 9 to 12 months after an acute coronary syndrome (Chapter 71).

Anticoagulant Therapy

Warfarin is as effective as aspirin for secondary prevention but is associated with a higher risk of bleeding. Combination therapy with

TABLE 70–7 CORONARY ANGIOGRAPHY FOR DIAGNOSIS AND RISK STRATIFICATION IN PATIENTS WITH ANGINA

FOR DIAGNOSTIC PURPOSE

Recommended on the basis of evidence or general consensus

Patients with suspect angina or with a changing angina pattern surviving sudden cardiac death

Weight of evidence or opinion is in favor

Uncertain diagnosis after noninvasive testing, and the benefit of a more certain diagnosis outweighs the risk and cost of coronary angiography

Inability to undergo noninvasive testing because of disability, illness, or morbid obesity

Occupational requirement for a definitive diagnosis

Suspected nonatherosclerotic cause of myocardial ischemia

Suspicion of a coronary spasm

High pretest probability of left main or three-vessel disease

Recurrent hospitalization for chest pain in the absence of definitive diagnosis

Overriding desire for a definitive diagnosis and a greater than low probability of CAD

Not recommended

Significant comorbidity in patients in whom the risk of coronary arteriography outweighs the benefit of the procedure

Overriding personal desire for a definitive diagnosis and a low probability of CAD

FOR RISK STRATIFICATION OR TREATMENT

Recommended on the basis of evidence or general consensus

With disabling (CCS class III and class IV) chronic stable angina despite medical therapy

With high-risk criteria on noninvasive testing regardless of anginal severity

Patients with angina who have survived sudden cardiac death or serious ventricular arrhythmia

Angina and symptoms and signs of congestive heart failure

Clinical characteristics that indicate a high likelihood of severe CAD

Weight of evidence or opinion is in favor

Significant left ventricular dysfunction (EF <45%), CCS class I or class II angina, and demonstrable ischemia but less than high-risk criteria on noninvasive testing

High-risk criteria suggesting ischemia on noninvasive testing

Inadequate prognostic information after noninvasive testing

Clinical characteristics that indicate a high likelihood of severe CAD

CCS class I or class II angina, preserved left ventricular function (EF >45%), and less than high-risk criteria on noninvasive testing

CCS class III or class IV angina that improves to class I or class II with medical therapy

CCS class I or class II angina but intolerance (unacceptable side effects) to adequate medical therapy

Not recommended

CCS class I or class II angina in patients who respond to medical therapy and who have no evidence of ischemia on noninvasive testing

Patients who prefer to avoid revascularization after adequate explanation

CAD = coronary artery disease; CCS = Canadian Cardiovascular Society; CHD = coronary heart disease; EF = ejection fraction.

Modified from Gibbons RJ, Abrams J, Chatterjee K, et al: ACC/AHA 2002 guideline update for the management of patients with chronic stable angina—summary article: A report of the American College of Cardiology/American Heart Association Task Force on Practice Guidelines (Committee on Management of Patients with Chronic Stable Angina). Circulation 2003;107:149–158.

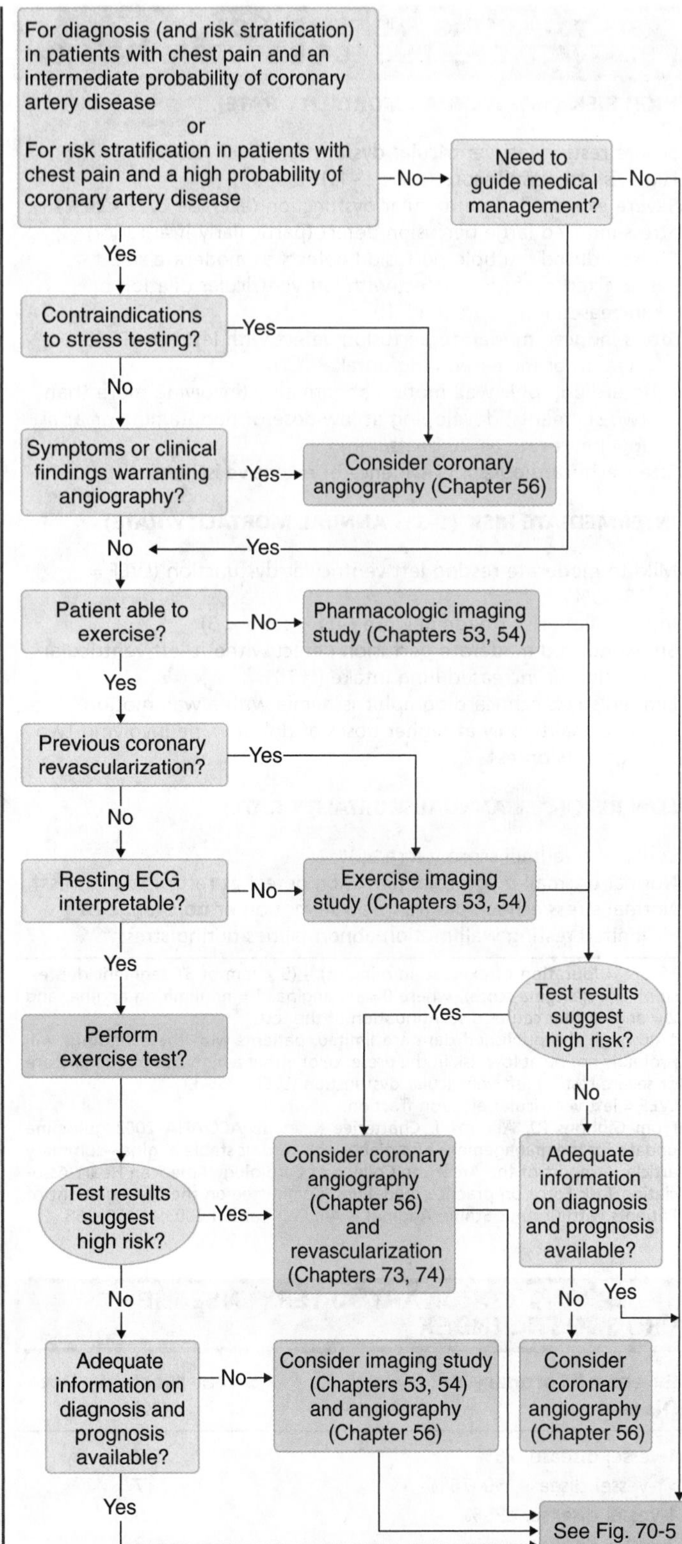

FIGURE 70–4 • Approach to the use of stress testing and angiography for the evaluation of chronic stable angina. ECG = electrocardiogram. (Modified from American College of Cardiology/American Heart Association Task Force on Practice Guidelines: Management of Patients with Chronic Stable Angina. ACC/AHA/ACP-ASIM Pocket Guidelines. Elsevier Science, 2000.)

TABLE 70-8 USING THE RESULTS OF NONINVASIVE TESTING FOR RISK STRATIFICATION

HIGH RISK (>3% ANNUAL MORTALITY RATE)

Severe resting left ventricular dysfunction (LVEF <35%)
High-risk treadmill score (score ≤–11)*
Severe exercise left ventricular dysfunction (exercise LVEF <35%)
Stress-induced large perfusion defect (particularly if anterior)
Stress-induced multiple perfusion defects of moderate size
Large, fixed perfusion defect with left ventricular dilation or increased lung uptake (^{201}Tl)
Stress-induced moderate perfusion defect with left ventricular dilation or increased lung uptake (^{201}Tl)
Echocardiographic wall motion abnormality (involving more than two segments) developing at low dose of dobutamine or at a low heart rate (<120 beats/min)
Stress echocardiographic evidence of extensive ischemia

INTERMEDIATE RISK (1–3% ANNUAL MORTALITY RATE)

Mild to moderate resting left ventricular dysfunction (LVEF = 35–49%)
Intermediate-risk treadmill score (–11 < score < 5)*
Stress-induced moderate perfusion defect without left ventricular dilation or increased lung intake (^{201}Tl)
Limited stress echocardiographic ischemia with a wall motion abnormality only at higher doses of dobutamine involving two segments or less

LOW RISK (<1% ANNUAL MORTALITY RATE)

Low-risk treadmill score (score ≥5)*
Normal or small myocardial perfusion defect at rest or with stress†
Normal stress echocardiographic wall motion or no change of limited resting wall motion abnormalities during stress†

*Score = (duration of exercise in minutes) – (5 × mm of ST segment depression) – (4 × angina score), where 0 = no angina, 1 = nonlimiting angina, and 2 = angina that causes discontinuation of the test.
†Although the published data are limited, patients with these findings will probably not be at low risk in the presence of either a high-risk treadmill score or severe resting left ventricular dysfunction (LVEF <35%).
LVEF = left ventricular ejection fraction.
From Gibbons RJ, Abrams J, Chatterjee K, et al: ACC/AHA 2002 guideline update for the management of patients with chronic stable angina—summary article: A report of the American College of Cardiology/American Heart Association Task Force on practice guidelines (Committee on the Management of Patients with Chronic Stable Angina). J Am Coll Cardiol 2003;41:159–168.

TABLE 70-9 CORONARY ARTERY DISEASE PROGNOSTIC INDEX

Extent of Coronary Artery Disease	5-Year Mortality Rate (%)*
1-vessel disease, 75%	7
>1-vessel disease, 50–74%	7
1-vessel disease, ≥95%	9
2-vessel disease	12
2-vessel disease, both ≥95%	14
1-vessel disease, ≥95% proximal LAD	17
2-vessel disease, ≥95% LAD	17
2-vessel disease, ≥95% proximal LAD	21
3-vessel disease	21
3-vessel disease, ≥95% in at least 1	27
3-vessel disease, 75% proximal LAD	33
3-vessel disease, ≥95% proximal LAD	41

*Assuming medical treatment only.
LAD = left anterior descending coronary artery.
From Califf RM, Armstrong PW, Carver JR, et al: Task Force 5: Stratification of patients into high, medium and low risk subgroups for purposes of risk factor management. J Am Coll Cardiol 1996;27:1007–1019.

TABLE 70-10 TREATMENT OF PATIENTS WITH STABLE ANGINA

GENERAL MEASURES

Rule out and control aggravating conditions
- Associated noncardiac diseases
- Associated cardiac disease
- Use of drugs aggravating angina

Smoking cessation
Dietary counseling for body weight and lipids control
Exercise prescription
Treat to targets
- Hypertension
- Blood lipids
- Diabetes

PHARMACOLOGIC THERAPY: RECOMMENDATIONS FOR PHARMACOTHERAPY TO PREVENT MI AND DEATH AND TO REDUCE SYMPTOMS

Recommended on the basis of evidence or general consensus
Aspirin in the absence of contraindications
β-Blockers as initial therapy in the absence of contraindications in patients with prior MI or without prior MI
Angiotensin-converting enzyme inhibitor in all patients with CAD who also have diabetes or left ventricular systolic dysfunction
Low-density lipoprotein–lowering therapy in patients with documented or suspected CAD and LDL cholesterol greater than 130 mg/dL, with a target LDL of less than 100 mg/dL
Sublingual nitroglycerin or nitroglycerin spray for the immediate relief of angina
Calcium-channel antagonists or long-acting nitrates as initial therapy for reduction of symptoms when β-blockers are contraindicated
Calcium-channel antagonists or long-acting nitrates in combination with β-blockers when initial treatment with β-blockers is not successful
Calcium-channel antagonists and long-acting nitrates as a substitute for β-blockers if initial treatment with β-blockers leads to unacceptable side effects
Weight of evidence or opinion is in favor
Clopidogrel when aspirin is contraindicated
Long-acting non-dihydropyridine calcium-channel antagonists instead of β-blockers as initial therapy
In patients with documented or suspected CAD and LDL cholesterol level of 100 to 129 mg/dL, several therapeutic options are available (Level of Evidence: B)
- Lifestyle and/or drug therapies to lower LDL to less than 100 mg/dL
- Weight reduction and increased physical activity in persons with the metabolic syndrome
- Institution of treatment of other lipid or nonlipid risk factors; consider use of nicotinic acid or fibric acid for elevated triglycerides or low HDL cholesterol
- Angiotensin-converting enzyme inhibitor in patients with CAD or other vascular disease

Usefulness unclear
Low-intensity anticoagulation with warfarin in addition to aspirin
Not recommended
Dipyridamole
Chelation therapy

CAD = coronary artery disease; HDL = high-density lipoprotein; LDL = low-density lipoprotein; MI = myocardial infarction.
From Gibbons RJ, Abrams J, Chatterjee K, et al: ACC/AHA 2002 guideline update for the management of patients with chronic stable angina—summary article: A report of the American College of Cardiology/American Heart Association Task Force on practice guidelines (Committee on the Management of Patients with Chronic Stable Angina). J Am Coll Cardiol 2003;41:159–168.

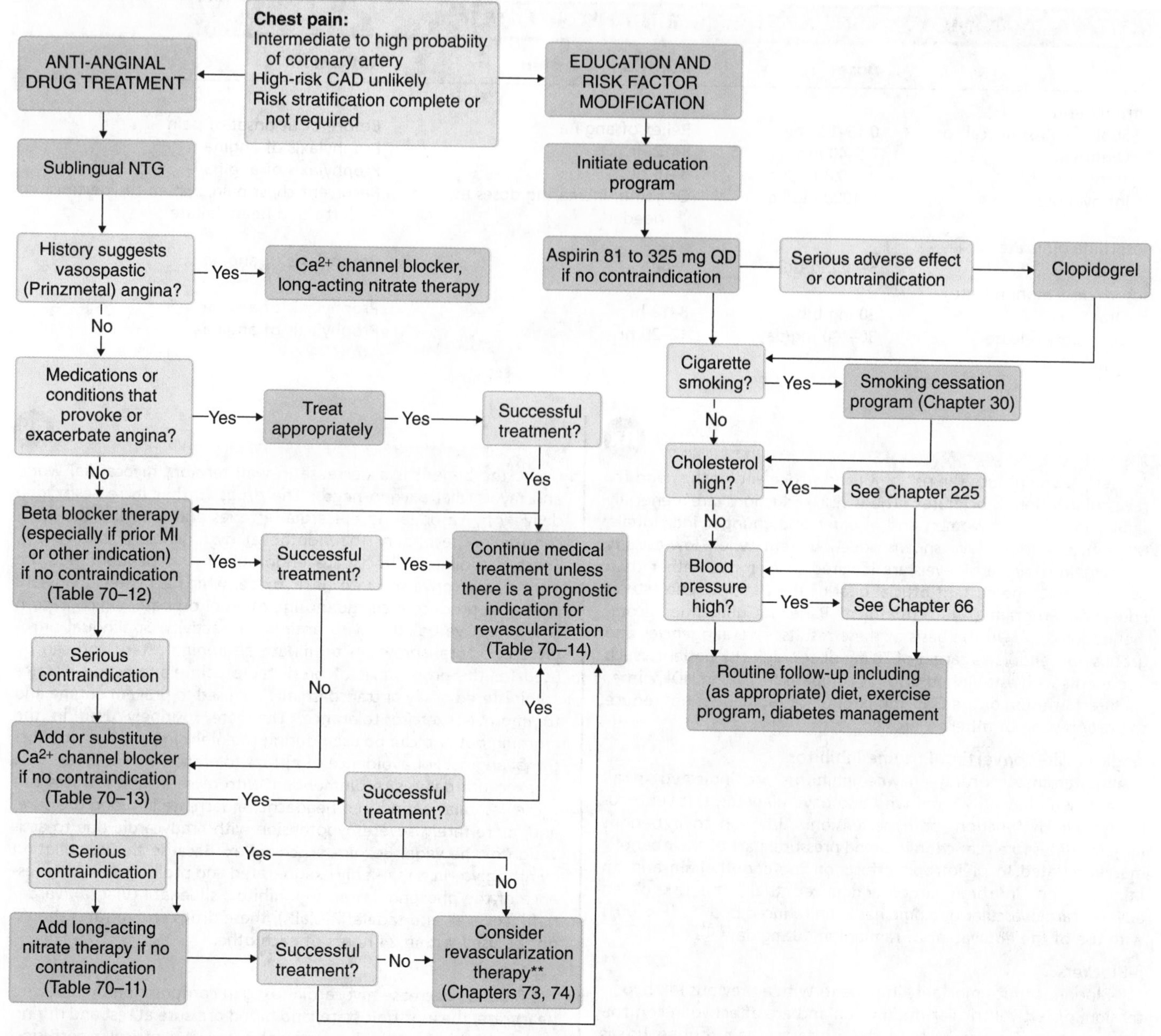

*Conditions that exacerbate or provoke angina:

Medications:
Vasodilators
Excessive thyroid replacement
Vasoconstrictors

Other medical problems:
Profound anemia
Uncontrolled hypertension
Hyperthyroidism
Hypoxemia

Other cardiac problems:
Tachyarrythmias
Bradyarrythmias
Valvular heart disease (espec. AS)
Hypertrophic cardiomyopathy

**At any point in this process, based on coronary anatomy, severity of anginal symptoms, and patient preferences, it is reasonable to consider evaluation for coronary revascularization. Unless a patient is documented to have left main, three-vessel, or two-vessel CAD with significant stenosis of the proximal left anterior descending coronary artery, there is no demonstrated survival advantage associated with revascularization in low risk patients with chronic stable angina; thus, medical therapy should be attempted in most patients before considering PTCA or CABG.

FIGURE 70–5 • Algorithm for the treatment of stable angina. AS = aortic stenosis; CABG = coronary artery bypass graft; CAD = coronary artery disease; MI = myocardial infarction; NTG = nitroglycerin; PTCA = percutaneous transluminal coronary angioplasty. (Modified from American College of Cardiology/American Heart Association Task Force on Practice Guidelines: Management of Patients with Chronic Stable Angina. ACC/AHA/ACP-ASIM Pocket Guidelines. Elsevier Science, 2000.)

Rx

warfarin plus aspirin is superior to aspirin alone, provided the international normalized ratio is maintained above 2.0, but the benefit of the combination needs to be weighed against a risk of bleeding in 1 of 100 patient years of treatment, mainly when the international normalized ratio is higher than 3. [5] Anticoagulants are used more liberally in Europe than in America. Atrial fibrillation (Chapter 63) is a strong indication for warfarin; aspirin should be added in patients with CHD unless a contraindication is present.

Rx

Statins

Statins inhibit 3-hydroxy-3-methylglutaryl–coenzyme A reductase in the liver, thereby leading to enhanced expression of the low-density lipoprotein receptors that capture blood cholesterol (Chapter 217). Clinical trials and meta-analyses of primary and secondary prevention trials with statins have consistently documented reductions of 30% in low-density lipoprotein cholesterol levels, 30% in the risk of a major coronary event, and 21% in the risk of death.

TABLE 70–11 CLINICAL USE OF NITROGLYCERIN AND NITRATES

	Dose	Duration of Action	Indication
Nitroglycerin			
Sublingual or buccal spray	0.15–1.5 mg	Relief of angina	Before or at onset of pain
Ointment	7.5–40 mg	8–12 hr	Prophylaxis of angina
Transdermal	0.2–0.8 mg/hr	8–16 hr	Prophylaxis of angina
Intravenous	5–1000 mg/hr	Ongoing; increasing doses as needed	Recurrent chest pain, systemic hypertension, left-sided heart failure
Isosorbide dinitrate			
Oral	5–40 mg tid	6–8 hr	Prophylaxis of angina
Isosorbide-5-mononitrate			
Oral	20 mg bid	8–12 hr	Prophylaxis of angina
Oral, slow release	30–240 mg/day	12–20 hr	Prophylaxis of angina

Rx

6 Statins also reduce the risk of MI and stroke and of the need for revascularization procedures. These risk reductions are generally similar in men and women and in older and younger individuals. More recent trials have shown added benefit when low-density lipoprotein cholesterol levels are lowered to 70 mg/dL rather than to 100 mg/dL, the current official goal of the National Cholesterol Education Program (Adult Treatment Panel III) guideline recommendations. 7 On the basis of these results, several agencies and groups now endorse a target of 70 mg/dL for high-risk patients, such as patients with established CHD. By comparison, raising HDL, either via direct infusion or the CTEP inhibitor torcetrapib, does not reduce the progression of atherosclerosis.

Angiotensin-Converting Enzyme Inhibitors

Angiotensin-converting enzyme inhibitors are indicated in all patients who have CHD and who also have diabetes, left ventricular systolic dysfunction, or hypertension. Although their benefit largely relates to a reduction in blood pressure, part of their benefit may be related to pleiotropic effects on the endothelium and on inflammation. In three large randomized trials, the risk of an adverse cardiovascular outcome has been reduced by 14% ($P < .001$) with use of the equivalent of ramipril at 10 mg/day. 8

β-Blockers

β-Blockers reduce mortality in patients with a previous MI, hypertension, or left ventricular dysfunction and are effective in controlling ischemia. On the basis of these effects, their routine use is recommended in patients with angina, although a benefit on survival has not been convincingly documented in patients who have angina alone without these other risk factors.

Revascularization Procedures

Revascularization with PCI or CABG is indicated to improve survival in patients with left main vessel disease, two- or three-vessel disease and moderate to severe left ventricular dysfunction, two-vessel disease with involvement of the proximal left anterior descending coronary artery independently of left ventricular function, left ventricular dysfunction regardless of symptoms, proximal left anterior disease when ischemia is documented, and class III or class IV angina with medical therapy (Chapters 73 and 74). The presence of a large ischemic zone on noninvasive testing is also an indicator of better survival with revascularization. In the absence of these criteria, coronary revascularization can still be useful for the control of angina, but medical therapy offers equivalent outcomes in terms of subsequent MI and death. 9,10

Control of Symptoms

Medical Management

β-Blockers, nitrates, and calcium antagonists reduce myocardial oxygen demand. Nitrates and calcium antagonists also increase coronary blood flow.

Nitroglycerin and nitrates produce immediate venous and arteriolar vasodilation, thereby reducing preload and afterload, respectively; the benefit is a decrease in wall tension, myocardial work, and myocardial oxygen needs. The drugs further increase oxygen delivery by vasodilating epicardial arteries and relieving the vasoconstriction secondary to endothelial dysfunction (Table 70–11). These vasodilator effects are endothelium independent because nitrates are converted into nitric oxide, which activates guanylate cyclase to produce cyclic guanosine monophosphate, which in turn is a potent vasodilator with antiplatelet activity. Sublingual nitroglycerin or oral spray can terminate an angina attack and can be used for the prophylaxis of predictable pain. Long-acting nitrates administered orally or transdermally are used to prevent angina and to improve exercise tolerance. They are routinely used in the morning but also can be used during the night in patients with nocturnal angina. For avoidance of nitrate tolerance, 8 to 12 hours free of exposure daily is recommended. Nitroglycerin and nitrates can cause vasodilation-induced headache, a decrease in blood pressure, and, more rarely, severe hypotension with bradycardia due to activation of the vagal Bezold-Jarisch reflex. Because the vasodilation by nitroglycerin is markedly exaggerated and prolonged in the presence of the phosphodiesterase inhibitors sildenafil (Viagra), vardenafil (Levitra), and tadalafil (Cialis), these drugs and nitrates should not be used within 24 hours of each other.

Rx

β-Blockers

β-Blockers decrease myocardial oxygen consumption by reducing heart rate, the inotropic state, and blood pressure at rest and during exercise (Table 70–12). They also enhance left ventricular perfusion by prolonging the diastolic filling time. An additional gain is a reduction of the degree of hemodynamic stress imposed on fragile coronary lesions, thereby preventing their rupture. Although different β-blockers have different pharmacokinetic and pharmacodynamic properties, they all are effective in delaying or avoiding the ischemic threshold by reducing the heart rate–blood pressure product during exercise. Doses are usually titrated to reduce the resting heart rate to 55 to 60 beats per minute, and even to less than 50 beats per minute if there are no associated symptoms or ECG abnormalities. It is sometimes useful to adjust the dose by monitoring the heart rate during exercise so that it goes no higher than approximately 75% of the heart rate that is associated with the onset of ischemia.

All β-blockers block β_1-receptors. Some agents, such as metoprolol, atenolol, and carvedilol, are more selective, at least at low doses, whereas others also act on the β_2-receptors that dilate bronchi and induce glycogenolysis in liver and muscles. A selective agent is therefore advantageous in bronchospastic disease. Some agents, such as acebutolol and pindolol, possess intrinsic sympathomimetic activity effects; others, such as labetalol and carvedilol, also have α-adrenergic blocking. The property of intrinsic sympathomimetic activity is useful in patients with significant bradycardia at rest, in whom such drugs mainly prevent the acceleration of heart during exercise, and in patients with peripheral vasospasm. Agents without intrinsic sympathetic activity may increase triglyceride levels and reduce high-density lipoprotein cholesterol levels. Sotalol also possesses class III

TABLE 70–12 CLINICAL USE OF β-BLOCKERS

Compound by Receptor Activity	Intrinsic Sympathomimetic Activity*	Membrane Stability Effect	Half-life (hr)	Excretion	Use
β_1 AND β_2					
Propranolol	–	++	1–6	Hepatic	20–80 mg bid-tid
Propranolol long-acting	–	++	8–11	Hepatic	80–360 mg od
Nadolol	–	–	40–80	Renal	40–80 mg od
Pindolol	+	+	3–4	Renal	2.5–7.5 mg tid
Sotalol	–	–	7–18	Renal	40–160 mg bid
Timolol	–	–	4–5	Hepatic-renal	10–15 mg bid
β_1 SELECTIVE					
Acebutolol	+	+	3–4	Hepatic	200–600 mg bid
Atenolol	–	–	6–9	Renal	50–200 mg od
Bisoprolol	–	–	9–12	50% renal	5–20 mg od
Metoprolol	–	–	3–7	Hepatic	50–200 mg bid
Metoprolol long-acting	–	–	14–25	Hepatic	100–400 mg
Esmolol	–	–	4.5 min	Esterases in red cells	Bolus 500 µg/kg 50–300 µg/kg/min IV
β_1, β_2, α_2					
Labetalol	+	–	6	Hepatic	200–600 mg bid
Carvedilol	–	+	6–10	Hepatic	200–600 mg bid

*Presence commonly associated with maintenance of or increase in heart rate; absence associated with decrease in heart rate.

TABLE 70–13 PROPERTIES OF CALCIUM-CHANNEL BLOCKING DRUGS IN CLINICAL USE

Drugs	Usual Dose	Elimination Half-life (hr)	Hemodynamic Effect HR	Hemodynamic Effect PVR	Side Effects
DIHYDROPYRIDINES					
Nifedipine PA*	10–40 mg bid	10	↑↑	↓↓↓	Hypotension, dizziness, flushing, edema, constipation
Nifedipine XL*	30–180 mg od	24	↑	↓↓	
Amlodipine	2.5–10 mg od	30–50	=	↓↓↓	Headache, edema
Felodipine	2.5–10 mg od	11–16	↑	↓↓↓	Headache, dizziness
Isradipine	2.5–10 mg bid	8	=	↓↓↓	Headache, fatigue
Nicardipine	20–40 mg tid	2–4	↑	↓↓↓	
Nicardipine SR*	30–60 mg bid	8–10	↑	↓↓	Headache, dizziness, flushing, edema
Nisoldipine	10–40 mg od	7–12	=	↓↓↓	As for nifedipine
Nitrendipine	20 mg od-bid	5–12	↑	↓↓↓	As for nifedipine
OTHERS					
Bepridil	200–400 mg od	24–40	↓	↓	Arrhythmias, dizziness, nausea
Diltiazem	30–90 mg tid	4–6	↓	↓	Hypotension, dizziness, bradycardia, edema
Diltiazem CD*	120–440 mg od	—	↓	↓	
Verapamil	80–160 mg tid	3–8	↓	↓↓	
Verapamil SR*	120–480 mg od	—	↓	↓↓	Hypotension, heart failure, edema, bradycardia

*PA, XL, SR, CD: long acting.
HR = heart rate; PVR = peripheral vascular resistance.

Rx

amiodarone-like antiarrhythmic activity, which makes it useful in patients with arrhythmias. Lipid solubility tends to be associated with more central nervous system side effects, more rapid absorption, and metabolism by the liver. Contraindications to β-blockers are significant bradyarrhythmias, acute but not chronic heart failure, and active asthma. Relative contraindications are Raynaud's phenomenon, severe claudication, severe depression, and diabetes with labile blood glucose levels. A few reports have described an exaggeration of angina in patients with Prinzmetal's angina. The most frequent side effects are fatigue, nightmares, asthma, and erectile

Rx

dysfunction, but the increased risk of these side effects is low in placebo-controlled trials.

Calcium-Channel Antagonists

These drugs reduce calcium flux through the voltage-sensitive L-type calcium channels. All calcium-channel antagonists are potent coronary vasodilators that can relieve coronary artery spasm. These drugs also decrease myocardial oxygen needs by slowing heart rate and by reducing blood pressure and contractility. Significant differences exist between drugs in the in vivo expression of these properties (Table 70–13). The dihydropyridines are more potent vasodilators, resulting in reflex adrenergic stimulation that masks the negative chronotropic effects. Short-acting nifedipine and other dihydropyridines may be associated with poorer outcomes in unstable angina and should be avoided unless the patient is also effectively treated with β-blockers. Verapamil has potent effects on cardiac conduction and contractility. The heart rate and vasodilator properties of diltiazem are intermediate between those of the dihydropyridines and verapamil, often resulting in a more favorable side effect profile. The dihydropyridines are advantageous when a bradyarrhythmia is present, and the new dihydropyridines are a better choice in heart failure. Verapamil and diltiazem are contraindicated in sinus node disease, in atrioventricular nodal block, and in patients with left ventricular dysfunction after MI; they are better choices in patients with atrial tachyarrhythmias. Calcium-channel antagonists are as effective as β-blockers for improving effort angina and are better in rest angina, particularly Prinzmetal's angina. Side effects related to vasodilation include hypotension, headache, and peripheral edema. Worsening of heart failure can occur with all drugs, whereas bradycardia and atrioventricular dissociation can occur with verapamil and diltiazem, particularly in combination with β-blockers. Constipation is common with verapamil.

Ranolazine was recently approved in the United States for the treatment of chronic angina in patients who do not respond to amlodipine, β-blockers, and sublingual nitrates. It improves exercise tolerance without decreasing blood pressure or heart rate, although its mechanism of action is not fully understood. The most frequent side effects are dizziness, headache, constipation, and nausea. The drug prolongs the QT interval and is contraindicated in patients with preexisting QT interval prolongation, in patients receiving drugs that prolong the QTc interval (such as class Ia or class III antiarrhythmic agents, macrolide antibiotics, and certain antipsychotics), and in patients taking medications that inhibit the metabolic enzyme cytochrome P-450 3A (CYP3A).

Revascularization

Successful PCI (Chapter 73) and CABG surgery (Chapter 74) immediately relieve the obstruction to blood flow and angina. The option of revascularization should be investigated by coronary angiography (Chapter 56) in patients with stable angina whenever symptoms are not satisfactorily controlled (Table 70–14). Angiography also should be performed in high-risk patients, including patients with left ventricular dysfunction, unless it is contraindicated.

Coronary Artery Bypass Graft versus Percutaneous Coronary Intervention

Factors to be weighed in selecting PCI compared with CABG include number of diseased vessels, location and characteristics of the obstructive lesions, left ventricular function, age, comorbidities, diabetes, local expertise, and preference of the patient. Symptomatic and angiographic improvement is expected in more than 90% of patients undergoing PCI, with a complication rate less than 5%. Elective CABG surgery is associated with a mortality rate of 0.2%. The risk of CABG surgery is affected by many factors, including age, comorbid diseases, left ventricular function, and extent of coronary artery disease. Internal thoracic artery grafts are associated with a better short-term and long-term outcome.

Observational studies and clinical trials have generally showed that PCI and CABG have a similar benefit for survival and for preventing MI. Patients with left ventricular dysfunction, proximal left

TABLE 70–14 CURRENT RECOMMENDATIONS FOR MYOCARDIAL REVASCULARIZATION IN PATIENTS WITH CHRONIC STABLE ANGINA

CABG SURGERY VERSUS MEDICAL THERAPY

Among patients with medically refractory angina pectoris, CABG surgery is indicated for symptom improvement. [9]
Among patients with medically stable angina pectoris, CABG surgery is indicated to prolong life in left main coronary artery disease or three-vessel disease (regardless of left ventricular function) and, possibly, help symptoms.
CABG surgery may be indicated for prolongation of life if the proximal left anterior descending coronary artery is involved (regardless of the number of diseased vessels).

PCI VERSUS MEDICAL THERAPY

Among patients with medically refractory angina pectoris, PCI is indicated for symptom improvement. [9, 10]
PCI may be indicated in the presence of severe myocardial ischemia, regardless of symptoms. PCI does not appear to improve survival compared with medical treatment among patients with one- or two-vessel disease. [10]
In the absence of symptoms or myocardial ischemia, PCI is not indicated (merely for the presence of an anatomic stenosis).

PCI VERSUS CABG SURGERY

For single-vessel disease, PCI and CABG surgery provide excellent symptom relief, but repeated revascularization procedures are required more frequently after PCI. Intracoronary stenting is preferred to regular PCI, but direct comparison with CABG surgery is limited. [9, 11–13]
For treated diabetics with two- or three-vessel disease, CABG surgery is the treatment of choice. [11]
For nondiabetics, multivessel PCI and CABG surgery are acceptable alternatives. The choice of PCI or CABG surgery for initial treatment depends primarily on local expertise and the patient's and physician's preferences. [9]
In general, PCI is preferred for patients at low risk and CABG surgery for patients at high risk.
Large differences in mortality are unlikely, but smaller, potentially important differences in mortality cannot be excluded by the available data.
CABG surgery is associated with more complete revascularization and superior early relief of angina, but these differences diminish after 3–5 years.
No significant differences in rates of myocardial infarction have been shown.
Repeated revascularization procedures are required significantly more often after PCI; this problem is reduced with drug-eluting stents.
Initial costs, quality of life, and return to work are initially more favorable with PCI than with CABG surgery, but these outcomes roughly equalize during 3–5 years.

CABG = coronary artery bypass graft; PCI = percutaneous coronary intervention.
Modified from Rihal CS, Gersh BJ, Yusuf S: Chronic coronary artery disease: Coronary artery bypass surgery vs. percutaneous transluminal coronary angioplasty vs. reduced therapy. Reproduced from Braunwald E, Goldman L (eds): Primary Care Cardiology, 2nd ed. Philadelphia, WB Saunders, 2003.

Rx

anterior descending coronary artery disease, and diabetes [11] usually fare better with CABG. PCI is generally preferred in patients with single-vessel disease. In patients with multivessel disease, PCI allows a more prompt return to normal life, but CABG often permits a more complete revascularization, with better long-term control of

Rx

angina and less need for subsequent revascularization procedures. 12, 13 To the extent to which the advantages of CABG are related to restenosis at the site of a PCI, drug-eluting stents may narrow the advantage; however, CABG retains the benefit of providing an alternative conduit as native disease progresses in segments of an artery that initially were not appropriate for PCI. PCI is preferred in patients who have associated valve disease that is not yet severe enough to require surgery, whereas CABG is preferred if concurrent valve surgery is indicated. Other considerations include coronary anatomy, local expertise, comorbid conditions, and preferences of the patient. PCI and CABG surgery are constantly evolving, so choices between the two are likely to continue to evolve.

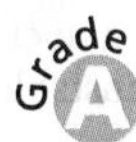

1. Antithrombotic Trialists' Collaboration: Collaborative meta-analysis of randomised trials of antiplatelet therapy for prevention of death, myocardial infarction, and stroke in high risk patients. BMJ 2002;324:71–86.
2. Berger JS, Roncaglioni MC, Avanzini F, et al: Aspirin for the primary prevention of cardiovascular events in women and men: A sex-specific meta-analysis of randomized controlled trials. JAMA 2006;295:306–313.
3. Yusuf S, Zhao F, Mehta SR, et al: Effects of clopidogrel in addition to aspirin in patients with acute coronary syndromes without ST-segment elevation. N Engl J Med 2001;345:494–502.
4. Bhatt DC, Fox KA, Hacke W, et al: Clopidogrel and aspirin versus aspirin alone for the prevention of atherothrombotic events. N Engl J Med 2006;354:1706–1717.
5. Anand SS, Yusuf S: Oral anticoagulants in patients with coronary artery disease. J Am Coll Cardiol 2003;41:62S–69S.
6. Baigent C, Keech A, Kearney PM, et al; Cholesterol Treatment Trialists' (CTT) Collaborators: Efficacy and safety of cholesterol-lowering treatment: Prospective meta-analysis of data from 90,056 participants in 14 randomised trials of statins. Lancet 2005; 366:1267–1278.
7. Cannon CP, Braunwald E, McCabe CH, et al: Intensive versus moderate lipid lowering with statins after acute coronary syndromes. N Engl J Med 2004;350:1495–1504.
8. Dagenais GR, Pogue J, Fox K, et al: Angiotensin-converting enzyme inhibitors in stable vascular disease without left ventricular systolic dysfunction or heart failure: A combined analysis of three trials. Lancet 2006;368:581–588.
9. Hueb W, Lopes NH, Gersh BJ, et al: Five-year follow-up of the Medicine, Angioplasty, or Surgery Study (MASS II): A randomized controlled clinical trial of 3 therapeutic strategies for multivessel coronary disease. Circulation 2007;115:1082–1089.
10. Boden WE, O'Rourke RA, Teo KK, et al: Optimal medical therapy with or without PCI for stable coronary disease. N Engl J Med 2007;356:1503–1516.
11. BARI Investigators: Comparison of coronary bypass surgery with angioplasty in patients with multivessel disease. N Engl J Med 1996;335:217–225.
12. Serruys PW, Ong ATL, van Herwerden LA, et al: Five-year outcomes after coronary stenting versus bypass surgery for the treatment of multivessel disease: The final analysis of the Arterial Revascularization Therapies Study (ARTS) randomized trial. J Am Coll Cardiol 2005;46:575–581.
13. Hannan EL, Racz MJ, Walford G, et al: Long-term outcomes of coronary-artery bypass grafting versus stent implantation. N Engl J Med 2005;352:2174–2183.

SUGGESTED READINGS

Gibbons RJ, Abrams J, Chatterjee K, et al: ACC/AHA 2002 guideline update for the management of patients with chronic stable angina—summary article: A report of the American College of Cardiology/American Heart Association Task Force on Practice Guidelines (Committee on Management of Patients with Chronic Stable Angina). Circulation 2003;107:149–158. *Executive guidelines and extensive review of diagnosis, risk stratification, and management of stable angina.*

Hemingway H, McCallum A, Shipley M, et al: Incidence and prognostic implications of stable angina pectoris among women and men. JAMA 2006; 295;1404–1411. *Women have a similarly high incidence of stable angina, with similarly high absolute rates of poor outcomes.*

Nissen SE, Tardif JC, Nicholls SJ, et al: Effect of torcetrapib on the progression of coronary atherosclerosis (ILLUSTRATE). N Engl J Med 2007;356:1304–1316. *This CETP inhibitor was associated with a 61% increase in HDL and a 20% decrease in LDL, but also with an increase in blood pressure; there was no decrease in the progression of atheroma.*

71 ACUTE CORONARY SYNDROME: UNSTABLE ANGINA AND NON–ST SEGMENT ELEVATION MYOCARDIAL INFARCTION

David D. Waters

Definition

Acute coronary syndrome (ACS) describes the continuum of myocardial ischemia that ranges from unstable angina at one end of the spectrum to non–ST segment elevation myocardial infarction (MI) at the other end. Unstable angina is distinguished from stable angina (Chapter 70) by the new onset or worsening of symptoms in the previous 60 days or by the development of post-MI angina 24 hours or more after the onset of MI. When the clinical picture of unstable angina is accompanied by elevated markers of myocardial injury, such as troponins or cardiac isoenzymes, non–ST segment elevation MI is diagnosed. The distinction between non–ST segment elevation MI and MI with ST segment elevation (Chapter 72) is clinically important because acute recanalization therapy is critical for improving the outcome in ST elevation MI but is less urgent in non–ST segment elevation MI.

Classification

Distinguishing *primary* from *secondary* unstable angina is of clinical value. Acute worsening of a coronary stenosis causes primary unstable angina by limiting coronary blood flow. Secondary unstable angina arises as a consequence of increased myocardial oxygen demand superimposed on severe underlying coronary disease. The conditions with the potential to provoke secondary unstable angina include tachyarrhythmia, fever, hypoxia, anemia, hypertensive crisis, and thyrotoxicosis. Secondary unstable angina should resolve with successful treatment of the precipitating condition. Patients with non–ST segment elevation ACS should be categorized according to their level of short-term risk because patients at higher risk benefit from earlier, more aggressive treatment, whereas low-risk patients do not.

Various classifications have been proposed for primary unstable angina on the basis of presenting symptoms. The most common approach (Table 71–1) includes three levels of severity and three clinical circumstances, to yield nine categories in all. This classification is used frequently to categorize patients for research purposes, but no system is used widely in clinical practice.

The recognition of three specific subtypes of primary unstable angina is worthwhile because their pathophysiologic processes, prognosis, and management are different from those of typical unstable angina. *Variant* or *Prinzmetal's angina* is caused by coronary spasm and usually can be controlled by calcium-channel blockers. *Unstable angina within 6 to 9 months after percutaneous coronary intervention* (Chapter 73) almost invariably is caused by restenosis or stent thrombosis. *Unstable angina in a patient with previous coronary artery bypass graft surgery* (Chapter 74) often involves advanced atherosclerosis of venous bypass grafts or progression of native vessel disease and portends a lower likelihood of long-term symptomatic relief compared with other patients with unstable angina. For each of these presentations, unstable angina may progress to non–ST segment elevation MI if adequate treatment is not instituted promptly.

Epidemiology

Whether ACS is defined clinically as unstable angina or non–ST segment elevation MI, the pathophysiologic mechanisms are the same. In most instances, ACS is caused by nonocclusive thrombosis in a native vessel, a vessel that has been the previous site of a coronary angioplasty (Chapter 73), or a coronary artery bypass graft (Chapter 74). In other situations, ACS may be precipitated by coronary spasm or by an increase in myocardial oxygen demand superimposed on preexisting fixed coronary stenoses. From a clinical perspective, the presentation of patients with ACS ranges from that of typical unstable angina to a presentation

TABLE 71–1 CLASSIFICATION OF UNSTABLE ANGINA

SEVERITY	
Class I	New-onset, severe or accelerated angina (angina <2 months in duration, severe or occurring >3 times/day, or angina that is distinctly more frequent and precipitated by distinctly less exertion; no rest pain within 2 months)
Class II	Angina at rest, subacute (angina at rest within the preceding month but not within the preceding 48 hours)
Class III	Angina at rest, acute (angina at rest within the preceding 48 hours)
CLINICAL CIRCUMSTANCES	
Class A	Secondary unstable angina (a clearly identified condition extrinsic to the coronary vascular bed that has intensified myocardial ischemia, e.g., anemia, hypotension, tachyarrhythmia)
Class B	Primary unstable angina
Class C	Post-infarction unstable angina (within 2 weeks of a documented myocardial infarction)
INTENSITY OF TREATMENT	
1.	Absence of treatment or minimal treatment
2.	Standard therapy for chronic stable angina (conventional doses of oral β-blockers, nitrates, and calcium-channel blockers)
3.	Maximal therapy (maximally tolerated doses of all three categories of oral therapy and intravenous nitroglycerin)

Modified from Braunwald E: Unstable angina: A classification. Circulation 1989;80:410–414.

indistinguishable from ST segment elevation MI. Regardless of the clinical presentation, however, the rapid clinical detection of ACS is key to the institution of appropriate therapy, which is different from that for stable angina, on the one hand, or ST segment elevation MI, on the other hand.

Approximately 1.5 million patients are hospitalized annually in the United States with unstable angina or non–ST segment elevation MI. These conditions are more common in older people, in people with a history of coronary disease, and in people with atherosclerosis known to be present in other vascular beds or with multiple coronary risk factors.

Pathobiology

With the exception of ACS caused by the systemic stresses listed previously, plaque rupture or erosion with overlying thrombosis is considered to be the initiating mechanism of ACS, including unstable angina and non–ST segment elevation MI (Chapter 69). Mechanical factors contribute to plaque disruption. A thin fibrous cap is more likely to rupture than a thick one is, and plaque rupture occurs commonly where the plaque joins the adjacent vessel wall. Plaque erosion and plaque rupture can initiate an ACS. Erosion usually occurs centrally through a thinning cap rather than at the lateral edge of the plaque.

Inflammation also seems to play a key role in plaque disruption. Macrophages and T lymphocytes accumulate in atherosclerotic plaques because of the expression of adhesion molecules on monocytes, endothelial cells, and leukocytes. These cells release growth factors and chemotactic factors, which lead to local oxidation of low-density lipoprotein cholesterol, proliferation of smooth muscle cells, and production of foam cells. Most patients with ACS have multiple inflamed coronary lesions.

Increased serum levels of C-reactive protein are found in most patients with unstable angina and MI, but not in stable angina, and elevated C-reactive protein levels are a strong predictor of subsequent coronary events in patients with coronary disease. The cytokine interleukin-6, which is the main producer of C-reactive protein in the liver, similarly is elevated in unstable angina but not in stable angina.

The stimulus that initiates the acute inflammatory process in ACS has not been identified. *Chlamydia pneumoniae*, cytomegalovirus, and *Helicobacter pylori* have been identified within human atherosclerotic lesions, and antibodies against *Chlamydia* heat shock proteins can cross-react against heat shock proteins produced by endothelium, resulting in endothelial damage and accelerated atherosclerosis. Antibodies to *Chlamydia*, cytomegalovirus, and *Helicobacter* are found more often in patients with atherosclerosis than in control subjects. These associations do not prove causality, however, and clinical trials of antibiotic therapy in patients with ACS have shown no benefit.

Platelet deposition onto the exposed, thrombogenic surface of the ruptured plaque is an important step in the pathogenesis of ACS, yet only a small fraction of disrupted plaques culminate in symptoms. Patients with coronary or peripheral vascular disease have increased platelet reactivity compared with normal controls. Healthy endothelium releases nitric oxide, which inhibits platelet aggregation. This protective mechanism is attenuated in atherosclerosis.

In ACS, platelets are activated and generate thromboxane and prostaglandin metabolites. Severe or persistent unstable angina is associated with the highest thromboxane output, and stabilization of unstable angina is accompanied by a return to normal levels.

Activated platelets and leukocytes interact to stimulate the coagulation system. Monocytes release tissue factor, a small glycoprotein that initiates the extrinsic clotting cascade, leading to an increase in thrombin generation. Transient increases in thrombin–antithrombin III and prothrombin fragment 1 + 2 can be shown in the hour after an ischemic attack in most patients with ACS.

Tissue factor is also present in the lipid-rich core of atherosclerotic plaque and may be one of the major determinants of the thrombogenicity of plaques when they rupture. When tissue factor specifically is inhibited, the deposition of platelets and fibrin onto the ruptured plaque is reduced. Patients with ACS and high circulating levels of tissue factor have unfavorable outcomes.

Overactivity of other components of the coagulation system has been reported in unstable angina, including levels of factor XII, bradykinin precursor, and fibrinogen. Lower levels of tissue-type plasminogen activator and plasminogen activator inhibitor 1 indicate that an impairment of the fibrinolytic system also is present.

Culprit lesions in unstable angina and non–ST segment elevation MI exhibit a heightened response to vasoconstrictor stimuli. This response is not present in other coronary segments and is not seen in culprit lesions of patients with stable angina. One explanation for this finding is that endothelin levels are higher in culprit lesions as a result of inflammation. Under experimental conditions, the degree of vasoconstriction varies, however, directly with the amount of platelet deposition. The process of platelet aggregation and thrombus formation releases potent vasoconstrictors, such as thromboxane A_2 and serotonin. Vasoconstriction, or the absence of appropriate vasodilation, probably contributes significantly to the development of ischemic episodes in ACS and is a potential target for therapy.

The angiographic aspects of the culprit lesion have been defined before, during, and after the episode of unstable angina or non–ST segment elevation MI. If a patient with ACS previously has had coronary angiography, the culprit lesion usually can be documented to have progressed markedly since that time. Lesions that progress to cause acute coronary events usually are not severely stenotic; two thirds cause less than a 50% reduction in diameter and would not be targets for revascularization. Angiographic features of a lesion predicting that it will precipitate an acute coronary event include greater asymmetry, greater length, and steeper outflow angle.

At the time of an episode of unstable angina or a non–ST segment elevation MI, the culprit lesion is more likely to be asymmetrical or eccentric, with a narrow base or neck, compared with control lesions. These angiographic features reflect the underlying plaque disruption with thrombus. Obvious thrombus is visible at angiography in a few patients with unstable angina. Coronary angioscopy reveals plaque rupture with overlying thrombus in most culprit lesions, however.

During the months after an episode of unstable angina or non–ST segment elevation MI, the initial culprit lesion is far more likely to progress and to precipitate another coronary event than are other lesions in the same patient or lesions in stable patients. Lesions with irregular borders, overhanging edges, or obvious thrombus at angiography are more likely to precipitate another event in the ensuing months than are smooth lesions.

Clinical Manifestations

Symptoms

The patient with unstable angina or non–ST segment elevation MI seeks medical attention because he or she has recognized either that new symptoms have appeared or that a previously stable pattern of symptoms has become unstable. Patients with non–ST segment elevation MI also may present with a pattern of increasing anginal episodes at rest or at lower levels of activity, but these patients are more likely to experience a prolonged episode of discomfort at rest. In many patients, the clinical presentation is indistinguishable from acute ST segment elevation MI (Chapter 72), whereas other patients may have nonspecific symptoms (Chapter 48).

The sensation of myocardial ischemia usually is located in the retrosternal area but may be felt only in the epigastrium, back, arms, or jaw. The description may include adjectives such as burning, squeezing, pressure-like, and heavy and, less often, sharp, jabbing, and knifelike. The physician should be cautioned that atypical features do not exclude unstable angina (Chapter 48).

Nausea, sweating, or shortness of breath may accompany episodes of acute myocardial ischemia. In elderly or diabetic patients, these symptoms may be the only indication that myocardial ischemia is present. Women who present with ACS are more likely to have diabetes, hypertension, hyperlipidemia, and heart failure and to be older than men; they are less likely to be smokers and to have had a previous MI or a previous coronary revascularization.

Physical Examination

On physical examination, transient signs of left ventricular dysfunction, such as basilar rales or a ventricular gallop, may accompany or follow shortly after an episode of unstable angina. More ominous signs of severe transient left ventricular dysfunction, such as hypotension or peripheral hypoperfusion, are not encountered commonly in the absence of myocardial necrosis. When ACS is manifested as a non–ST segment elevation MI, however, signs and symptoms may be similar to those of ST segment elevation MI (Chapter 72), depending on the size and location of the damage. Physical examination may reveal precipitating causes of or contributing factors to unstable angina, such as pneumonia or uncontrolled hypertension.

Diagnosis

Patients with suspected ACS must be evaluated rapidly and efficiently. A prompt and accurate diagnosis permits the timely initiation of appropriate therapy, which is important because complications are clustered in the early phases of ACS, and appropriate treatment reduces the rate of complications.

Patients with chest pain lasting longer than 20 minutes, hemodynamic instability, or recent syncope or presyncope should be referred to a hospital emergency department. Other patients with suspected unstable angina may be seen initially either in an emergency department or in an outpatient facility where 12-lead electrocardiography can be performed quickly.

The initial assessment should be directed toward determination of whether the symptoms are caused by myocardial ischemia and, if so, the level of risk. The probability of MI can be estimated from the history, physical examination, and electrocardiography (Fig. 71–1). This information and the assessment of the patient's clinical features should indicate whether the probability that symptoms are due to myocardial

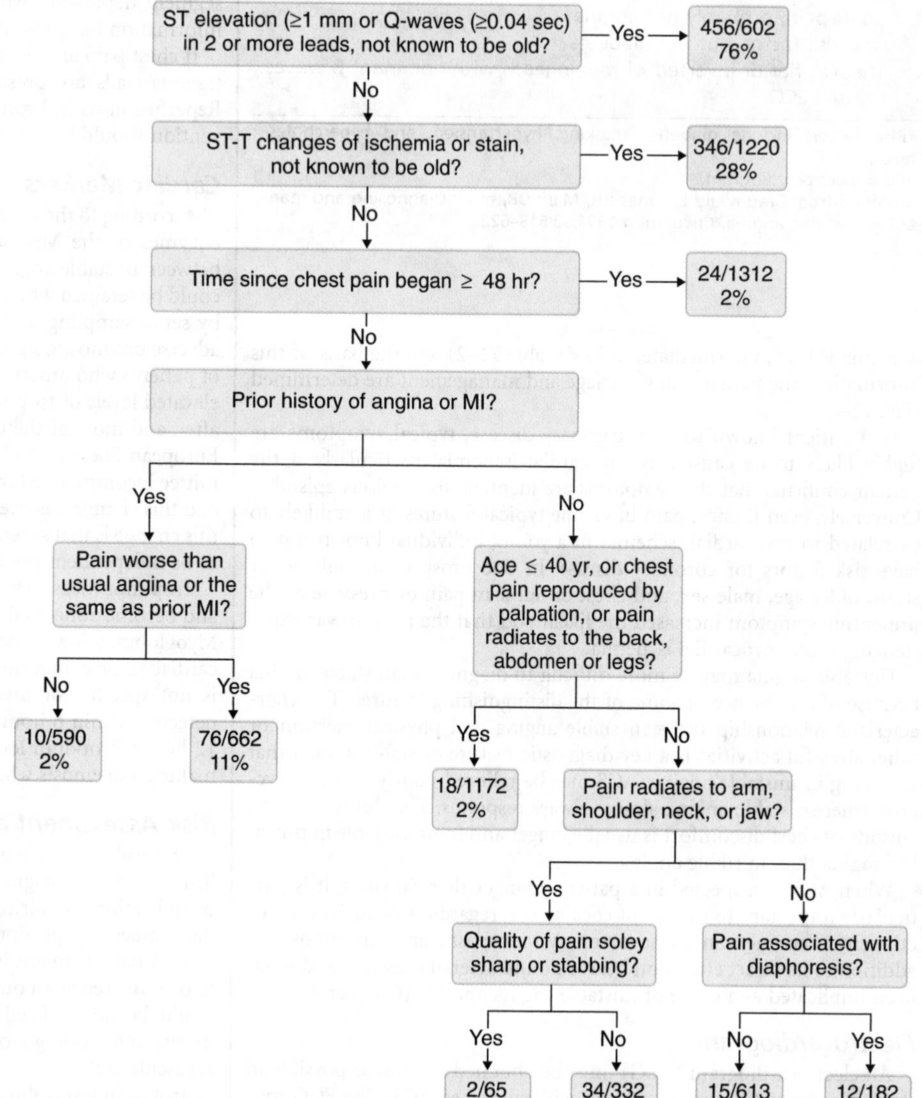

FIGURE 71–1 • Flow diagram to estimate the risk of acute myocardial infarction (MI) in emergency departments in patients with acute chest pain. For each clinical subset, the numerator is the number of patients with the set of presenting characteristics who had a myocardial infarction; the denominator is the total number of patients presenting with that characteristic or set of characteristics. (Modified from Pearson SD, Goldman L, Garcia TB, et al: Physician response to a prediction rule for the triage of emergency department patients with chest pain. J Gen Intern Med 1994;9:241–247.)

TABLE 71–2 LIKELIHOOD THAT UNSTABLE ANGINA SYMPTOMS ARE CAUSED BY MYOCARDIAL ISCHEMIA

HIGH LIKELIHOOD
Any of the following features:
Known coronary disease
Definite angina in men ≥60 years or women ≥70 years
Hemodynamic or ECG changes during pain
Variant angina
ST elevation or depression of at least 1 mm
Marked symmetrical T wave inversion in multiple precordial leads
INTERMEDIATE LIKELIHOOD
Absence of high-likelihood features and any of the following:
Definite angina in men <60 years or women <70 years
Probable angina in men ≥60 years or women ≥70 years
Probably not angina in diabetics, or in nondiabetics with ≥2 other risk factors*
Extracardiac vascular disease
ST depression 0.5–1 mm
T wave inversion of at least 1 mm in leads with dominant R waves
LOW LIKELIHOOD
Absence of high- or intermediate-likelihood features, but may have the following:
Chest pain, probably not angina
One risk factor, but not diabetes
T waves flat or inverted <1 mm in leads with dominant R waves
Normal ECG

*Risk factors include diabetes, smoking, hypertension, and hypercholesterolemia.
ECG = electrocardiogram.
Modified from Braunwald E, Jones RH, Mark DB, et al: Diagnosing and managing unstable angina. Circulation 1994;90:613–622.

ischemia is high, intermediate, or low (Table 71–2). On the basis of this information, the patient's initial triage and management are determined (Fig. 71–2).

In a patient known to have coronary disease, typical symptoms are highly likely to be caused by myocardial ischemia, particularly if the patient confirms that the symptoms are identical to previous episodes. Conversely, even if chest pain has some typical features, it is unlikely to be related to myocardial ischemia in a young individual known not to have risk factors for coronary disease. In one prospective multicenter study, older age, male sex, and chest or left arm pain or pressure as the presenting symptom increased the likelihood that the patient was experiencing acute myocardial ischemia.

Unstable angina may be more difficult to diagnose than stable angina because of an absence of some of the distinguishing features. The characteristic relationship between stable angina and physical exertion or other stressful activities is a key diagnostic feature of stable angina that is lacking in unstable angina. ACS may be relieved poorly by nitroglycerin, whereas stable angina almost always responds. The duration of an episode of chest discomfort is usually longer and more variable in unstable angina than in stable angina.

When ACS is suspected in a patient younger than 50 years, it is particularly important to ask about cocaine use, regardless of social class or ethnicity. Cocaine can cause coronary vasospasm and thrombosis in addition to its direct effects on heart rate and arterial pressure, and it has been implicated as a cause of unstable angina and MI (Chapter 32).

Electrocardiogram

An electrocardiogram (ECG) must be obtained as soon as possible in the initial evaluation of any patient with suspected ACS. The ECG may be entirely normal or show only nonspecific abnormalities in patients with unstable angina or non–ST segment elevation MI. The diagnostic yield is enhanced greatly if a tracing also can be recorded during an episode of chest pain. Transient ST segment depression of at least 1 mm that appears during chest pain and disappears with relief is objective evidence of transient myocardial ischemia. A normal ECG during chest pain does not exclude unstable angina; however, it does indicate that an ischemic area, if present, is not extensive or severe enough to induce ECG changes, and this finding is a favorable prognostic sign.

When ST segment depression is a persistent feature of ECGs recorded with or without chest pain, the finding commonly represents non–ST segment elevation MI. A common ECG pattern of patients with unstable angina or non–ST segment elevation MI is a persistently negative T wave, which usually indicates that a severe stenosis is present in the corresponding coronary artery. Deeply negative T waves occasionally are seen across all of the precordial leads, a pattern that suggests a severe, proximal stenosis of the left anterior descending coronary artery as the culprit lesion.

The ECG in ACS may show Q waves from an old MI or left bundle branch block due to extensive prior left ventricular damage. Patients with these findings are at increased risk because they are less likely than other patients to be able to tolerate an additional insult to the myocardium. ECG abnormalities may appear or evolve in the absence of new symptoms in patients with ACS. The development of significant Q waves may be the first indicator that the diagnosis is non–ST segment elevation MI, not unstable angina. T wave abnormalities may appear, worsen, or resolve. It is worthwhile to obtain serial ECGs during the first 48 hours and during episodes of chest pain.

Continuous 12-lead ECG monitoring can be performed with multiprocessor-controlled, programmable devices. The limited clinical experience with this technology suggests that it can detect episodes of ST segment depression when the presenting ECG is normal and that this information has prognostic and diagnostic value.

If chest pain and ST segment elevation greater than 1 mm in two contiguous leads are present, the diagnosis is ST segment elevation MI. Reperfusion with thrombolytic therapy or percutaneous coronary intervention should be considered without delay (Chapter 72).

Cardiac Markers

According to the traditional paradigm, elevated serum levels of cardiac enzymes or the MB isoenzyme of creatine kinase (CK) distinguished between unstable angina and acute MI. The diagnosis of unstable angina could be retained when minor elevations of CK or CK-MB were detected by serial sampling, but it was recognized that these elevations were an adverse prognostic sign. It now is recognized that one fifth to one quarter of patients who otherwise would be diagnosed with unstable angina have elevated levels of troponin T or troponin I on admission or soon thereafter, and most of them have normal levels of CK-MB. In 2000, a Joint European Society of Cardiology/American College of Cardiology committee recommended that these patients be classified as having acute MI, and this change has been widely adopted (Chapter 72). The rationale for this change is that several large studies have shown elevations of troponin to be independent predictors of adverse events.

Troponin measurements may be normal early after the onset of ACS and become abnormal later, usually by 6 and almost always by 12 hours. Myoglobin, a low-molecular-weight heme protein found in skeletal and cardiac muscle, may be detected 2 hours after the onset of symptoms but is not specific for myocardial damage. CK-MB subforms are usually detected within 6 hours, and troponin T or I is usually elevated within 12 hours. Troponin levels remain elevated for 1 week and are useful in making a diagnosis when the patient presents late after a coronary event.

Risk Assessment and Initial Triage

The evaluation of a patient with a possible ACS requires not only establishment of the diagnosis but also assessment of the short-term risk of complications requiring intensive care (Fig. 71–3). This risk assessment determines the appropriate intensity of therapy. At the low end of the risk scale, a patient might be discharged home with aspirin and a β-blocker, to be observed as an outpatient. At the opposite end of the scale, a patient might be hospitalized in a coronary care unit, treated with multiple drugs, and undergo coronary arteriography urgently as a prelude to revascularization.

Troponin levels should be measured when the patient first is seen and again 6 to 12 hours later (Chapter 72). Myocardial perfusion imaging

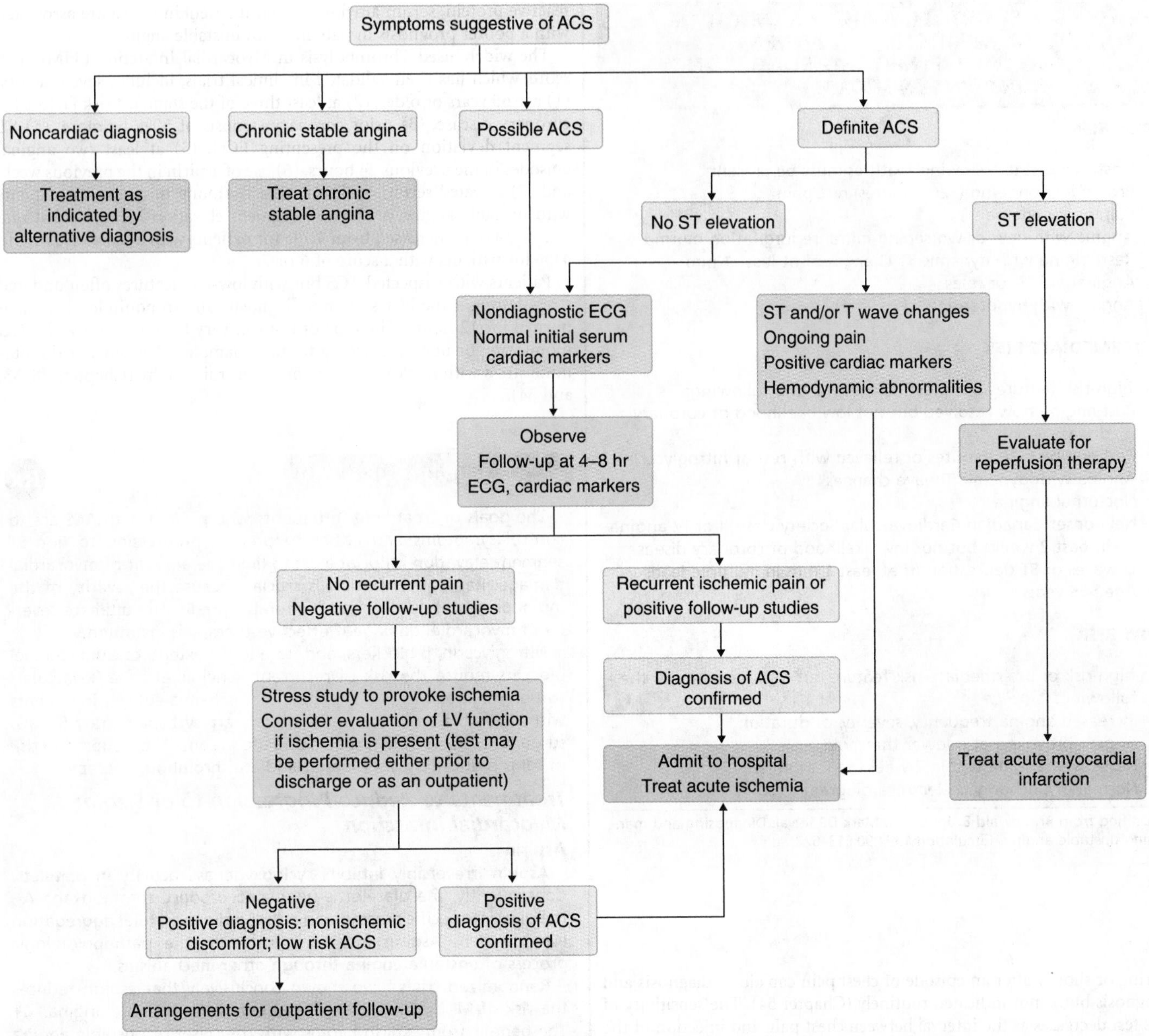

Symptoms suggestive of ACS

Noncardiac diagnosis → Treatment as indicated by alternative diagnosis

Chronic stable angina → Treat chronic stable angina

Possible ACS → Nondiagnostic ECG; Normal initial serum cardiac markers

Definite ACS → No ST elevation; ST elevation

No ST elevation → Nondiagnostic ECG; Normal initial serum cardiac markers

No ST elevation → ST and/or T wave changes; Ongoing pain; Positive cardiac markers; Hemodynamic abnormalities → Admit to hospital; Treat acute ischemia

ST elevation → Evaluate for reperfusion therapy → Treat acute myocardial infarction

Nondiagnostic ECG; Normal initial serum cardiac markers → Observe; Follow-up at 4–8 hr; ECG, cardiac markers

Observe → No recurrent pain; Negative follow-up studies → Stress study to provoke ischemia; Consider evaluation of LV function if ischemia is present (test may be performed either prior to discharge or as an outpatient)

Observe → Recurrent ischemic pain or positive follow-up studies → Diagnosis of ACS confirmed → Admit to hospital; Treat acute ischemia

Stress study → Negative; Positive diagnosis: nonischemic discomfort; low risk ACS → Arrangements for outpatient follow-up

Stress study → Positive diagnosis of ACS confirmed → Admit to hospital; Treat acute ischemia

FIGURE 71–2 • Initial triage for patients with symptoms suggestive of an acute coronary syndrome (ACS). ECG = electrocardiogram; LV = left ventricular. (Modified from Braunwald E, Antman EM, Beasley JW, et al: ACC/AHA guidelines for the management of patients with unstable angina and non–ST-segment elevation myocardial infarction. A report of the American College of Cardiology/American Heart Association Task Force on Practice Guidelines. J Am Coll Cardiol 2000;36:970–1062, with permission.)

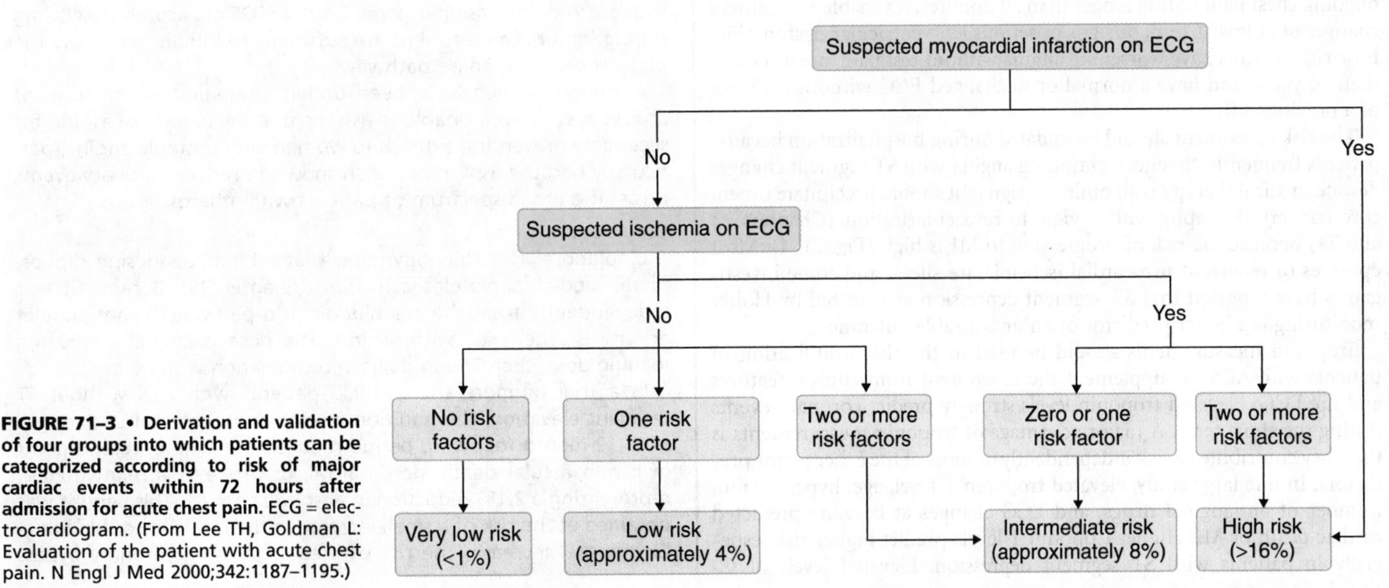

FIGURE 71–3 • Derivation and validation of four groups into which patients can be categorized according to risk of major cardiac events within 72 hours after admission for acute chest pain. ECG = electrocardiogram. (From Lee TH, Goldman L: Evaluation of the patient with acute chest pain. N Engl J Med 2000;342:1187–1195.)

TABLE 71–3 SHORT-TERM RISK OF DEATH OR MYOCARDIAL INFARCTION IN PATIENTS PRESENTING WITH SYMPTOMS SUGGESTING ACUTE CORONARY SYNDROME

HIGH RISK
At least one of the following features must be present:
Prolonged, ongoing (>20 minutes) rest pain
Pulmonary edema
Angina with new or worsening mitral regurgitation murmurs
Rest angina with dynamic ST changes of at least 1 mm
Angina with S_3 or rales
Angina with hypotension
INTERMEDIATE RISK
No high-risk features but must have any of the following:
Rest angina now resolved but not low likelihood of coronary disease
Rest angina (>20 minutes or relieved with rest or nitroglycerin)
Angina with dynamic T wave changes
Nocturnal angina
New-onset Canadian Cardiovascular Society class III or IV angina in past 2 weeks but not low likelihood of coronary disease
Q waves or ST depression of at least 1 mm in multiple leads
Age >65 years
LOW RISK
No high-risk or intermediate-risk feature but may have any of the following:
Increased angina frequency, severity, or duration
Angina provoked at a lower threshold
New-onset angina within 2 weeks to 2 months
Normal or unchanged electrocardiogram

Modified from Braunwald E, Jones RH, Mark DB, et al: Diagnosing and managing unstable angina. Circulation 1994;90:613–622.

during or shortly after an episode of chest pain can aid in diagnosis and prognosis but is not indicated routinely (Chapter 54). The sensitivity of this test decreases as the interval between chest pain and injection of the nuclear tracer lengthens. Large or multiple reversible perfusion defects indicate increased risk.

Patients with symptoms that suggest ACS can be categorized into low-risk, intermediate-risk, and high-risk groups on the basis of data available at the time of first assessment (Table 71–3). High-risk patients have ongoing chest pain lasting longer than 20 minutes, reversible ST segment changes of at least 1 mm, or signs of serious left ventricular dysfunction. Low-risk patients have worsening angina without rest pain, are not older than 65 years, and have a normal or unchanged ECG without evidence of a previous MI.

The risk assessment should be updated during hospitalization because patients frequently change. Continuing angina with ST segment changes despite medical therapy is an ominous sign that should precipitate urgent coronary arteriography with a view to revascularization (Chapters 73 and 74) because the risk of progression to MI is high (Fig. 71–4). Most episodes of recurrent myocardial ischemia are silent, and some investigators have reported that ST segment depression as detected by Holter monitoring is a better predictor of an unfavorable outcome.

Troponin measurements should be used in the risk stratification of patients with ACS to supplement the assessment from clinical features and the ECG. Elevated troponin levels strongly predict coronary events during the short term. A major advantage of troponin measurements is that they contribute to risk independently of most of the other major predictors. In one large study, elevated troponin T level, age, hypertension, number of antianginal drugs, and ECG changes at baseline predicted cardiac death or MI. Higher troponin T levels predict higher risk, especially in patients with ST segment depression. Elevated levels of C-reactive protein, serum amyloid A, and interleukin-6 also are associated with a poorer prognosis in patients with unstable angina.

The widely used Thrombolysis in Myocardial Infarction (TIMI) risk score, which has been validated in clinical trials, includes seven factors: (1) age 65 years or older, (2) at least three of the standard risk factors for coronary disease, (3) prior coronary stenosis of 50% or more, (4) ST segment deviation on the presenting ECG, (5) at least two anginal episodes in the previous 24 hours, (6) use of aspirin in the previous week, and (7) elevated serum cardiac markers. Among thousands of patients with unstable angina or non–ST segment elevation MI, the event rate during 14 days increased from 4.7% for patients with a score of 0 or 1 to 41% for patients with a score of 6 or 7.

Patients with suspected ACS but with low-risk features often undergo stress testing if the ECGs are nondiagnostic and troponin levels remain normal for 12 hours. The type of test can vary from exercise with ECG monitoring or nuclear imaging to dipyridamole, adenosine, or dobutamine stress with nuclear imaging or echocardiography (Chapters 48, 53, and 54).

Prevention and Treatment

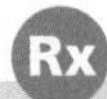

The goals of treatment in patients who present with ACS are to control symptoms and either to prevent progression to non–ST segment elevation MI or at least to limit the amount of myocardial damage. Rapid intervention is crucial because the severity of the initial presentation does not inalterably predict the ultimate severity of myocardial damage if effective therapy is instituted.

Nitroglycerin, β-blockers, and, to a lesser extent, calcium-channel blockers reduce the risk of recurrent ischemic attacks. Revascularization (Chapters 73 and 74) eliminates ischemia entirely in patients with favorable anatomy, and coronary artery bypass graft (CABG) surgery has been shown to prolong life in some subgroups. The risk of MI is reduced by antiplatelet and antithrombotic therapy.

Treatments to Reduce Progression to or Size of Myocardial Infarction

Aspirin

Aspirin irreversibly inhibits cyclooxygenase activity in platelets. Consequently, the platelet is unable to produce thromboxane A_2, the platelet-specific prostaglandin that induces platelet aggregation (Chapter 34). Aspirin also may influence the pathophysiologic process of unstable angina through other mechanisms.

Randomized trials have shown conclusively that aspirin reduces the risk of MI by 50 to 67% in patients with unstable angina. [1] The benefit from aspirin begins with the onset of unstable angina and extends for more than 1 year. Because aspirin reduces the risk of MI in patients with stable coronary disease (Chapter 70), the drug should be continued for life after an episode of unstable angina. The dose of aspirin in trials of patients with unstable angina has ranged from 75 to 1300 mg/day. Gastrointestinal side effects increase with increasing dosage. Doses of 325 mg acutely and 81 mg during long-term treatment are sufficient to inhibit maximally the platelet cyclooxygenase pathway.

Although women have been underrepresented in the trials of aspirin, it seems reasonable to assume that the benefit of aspirin for secondary prevention extends to women with unstable angina, particularly because aspirin has been shown to reduce coronary events across the broad spectrum of patients with atherosclerosis.

Clopidogrel

Clopidogrel is a thienopyridine that inhibits adenosine diphosphate–mediated platelet activation (Chapter 35). Because it acts independently from the arachidonic acid pathway, its antiplatelet activity is synergistic with aspirin. The dose is an initial 300 mg loading dose, then 75 mg daily, in combination with aspirin.

In a trial of more than 12,000 patients with ACS without ST segment elevation, the addition of clopidogrel to aspirin during a 3- to 12-month follow-up period reduced the composite end point of cardiovascular death, nonfatal MI, or stroke by a relative 20%, representing a 2.1% reduction in absolute risk. [2] This benefit was obtained at the risk of a small increase in the incidence of bleeding. Clopidogrel increases the risk of bleeding during coronary bypass

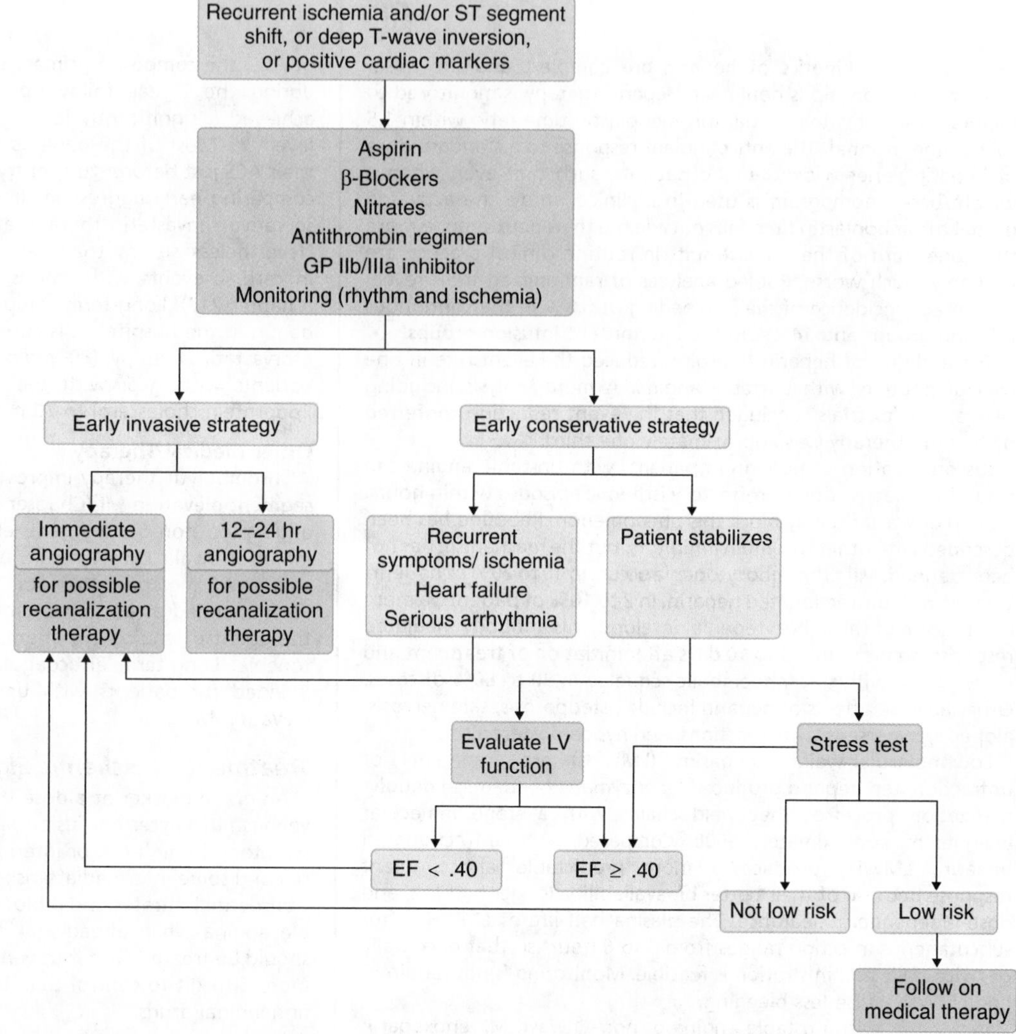

FIGURE 71–4 • Approach to the high-risk patient with an acute coronary syndrome. EF = ejection fraction; GP = glycoprotein; LV = left ventricular. (Modified from Braunwald E, Antman EM, Beasley JW, et al: ACC/AHA guidelines for the management of patients with unstable angina and non–ST-segment elevation myocardial infarction. A report of the American College of Cardiology/American Heart Association Task Force on Practice Guidelines. J Am Coll Cardiol 2000;36:970–1062, with permission.)

Rx

surgery, so this drug usually is not started if the patient may become a surgical candidate.

Platelet Glycoprotein IIB/IIIA Receptor Inhibitors

Platelet membranes contain glycoprotein (GP) receptors. The GPIIb-IIIa receptor changes from its resting to its active state when the platelet is activated by agonists or other platelets and serves as a receptor for fibrinogen and von Willebrand factor. Fibrinogen binding is central to platelet aggregation and thrombus formation in the arterial circulation. In contrast to aspirin and clopidogrel, which do not block thrombin-induced platelet aggregation, GPIIb-IIIa inhibitors block aggregation in response to all potential agonists.

Three GPIIb-IIIa blockers have been approved and are used widely clinically. Abciximab is the Fab fragment of a monoclonal antibody, eptifibatide is a peptide GPIIb-IIIa inhibitor, and tirofiban is a smaller molecule. These drugs must be administered by parenteral infusion; oral GPIIb-IIIa inhibitors failed to reduce events in large clinical trials and have not been approved for use.

Platelet GPIIb-IIIa inhibition at the time of percutaneous coronary intervention (PCI) reduces ischemic complications in patients with ACS. The benefit is less with eptifibatide and tirofiban (15 to 20%) than with abciximab (30 to 60%). In addition, five large trials have assessed the value of these drugs in the broader population of patients with unstable angina or non–Q wave MI. Although abciximab was the most successful drug in the PCI trials, eptifibatide and tirofiban predominate in the ACS trials.

The value of GPIIb-IIIa inhibitors in patients with unstable angina who are not undergoing intervention is not fully defined. GPIIb-IIIa inhibitors have not been compared with clopidogrel or with low-molecular-weight heparins or studied in patients taking these drugs as background therapy. The current high cost of these drugs makes it tempting to limit their use to high-risk patients. Patients with troponin elevations or other high-risk features benefit from GPIIb-IIIa blockade, but low-risk patients may not.

Current guidelines recommend that eptifibatide or tirofiban be added to aspirin and heparin in the treatment of patients with high-risk features or with refractory ischemia. 3 These drugs should be continued during PCI (Chapter 73) and for 12 to 24 hours after the procedure for tirofiban (0.4 μg/kg/min for 30 minutes, then 0.1 μg/kg/min) and for 24 to 72 hours after the procedure for eptifibatide (180 μg/kg IV bolus, then 2 μg/kg/min until discharge or CABG, up to 72 hours). Abciximab also can be used in patients with unstable angina in whom PCI is planned within the following 24 hours (0.25 g/kg followed by 18- to 24-hour infusion of 10 μg/min, ending 1 hour after the procedure). When abciximab is administered before diagnostic coronary angiography, however, the prolonged platelet inhibition it induces may force a delay in the urgent CABG surgery that is needed for some patients. When aspirin and unfractionated heparin are used with GPIIb-IIIa inhibitors, the dose of heparin should be conservative during coronary procedures, and heparin should be discontinued after the procedure if it is uncomplicated.

Heparin

The principal inhibitory effect of heparin on coagulation is probably through the inhibition of thrombin-induced activation of factor V and factor VIII (Chapter 35). Platelets inhibit the anticoagulant effect of heparin by binding factor Xa and protecting it from inactivation.

The pharmacokinetics of heparin are complex, and the dose-response relationship is nonlinear. Heparin therapy is monitored to maintain the activated partial thromboplastin time ratio within 1.5 to 2.5 times normal. The anticoagulant response to a standard dose of heparin varies widely among patients, such that even when a weight-based nomogram is used in a clinical study, the activated partial thromboplastin time falls outside the therapeutic range more than one third of the time. Results in routine clinical practice are probably much worse. Pooled analyses of randomized trials reveal an average incidence of major bleeding of 6.8% in the continuous infusion groups and 14.2% in the intermittent infusion groups.

The addition of heparin to aspirin reduced the event rate in one trial of patients with unstable angina. A meta-analysis including several smaller trials concluded that the event reduction conferred by heparin therapy was approximately one third. [4]

Discontinuation of heparin in patients with unstable angina can result in a reactivation of refractory ischemic episodes within hours. Aspirin or warfarin may block this phenomenon. Rebound has been described with other thrombin inhibitors, but the mechanism has not been defined. Mild thrombocytopenia occurs in 10 to 20% of patients treated with unfractionated heparin. In 2 to 10% of patients, a more severe form of thrombocytopenia develops. This antibody-mediated response occurs within 5 to 10 days after initiation of treatment and is associated with thromboembolic sequelae in 30 to 80% of cases. Other adverse effects of heparin include osteoporosis, skin necrosis, alopecia, hypersensitivity reactions, and hypoaldosteronism.

Low-molecular-weight heparins (LMWHs) are fragments of unfractionated heparin produced by enzymatic or chemical depolymerization processes that yield chains with average molecular weights of approximately 5000. Compared with unfractionated heparin, LMWHs produce a more predictable anticoagulant response because of their better bioavailability, longer half-life, and dose-independent clearance. The plasma half-life of LMWHs after subcutaneous injection ranges from 3 to 6 hours so that once-daily or twice-daily administration is feasible. Monitoring is not required, and LMWHs cause less bleeding.

In patients with unstable angina or non–Q wave MI, enoxaparin is superior to unfractionated heparin for the first few days of therapy. The early benefit of treatment with LMWHs seems to dissipate in the ensuing months, and continuing therapy was not beneficial in most trials. In one trial, treatment from 5 days to 3 months with dalteparin produced an impressive reduction in death or MI at 1 month, with gradual loss of this benefit thereafter.

Heparin is recommended for the acute treatment of all patients with unstable angina except patients determined to be at low risk. Unfractionated heparin should be started with an intravenous bolus of 60 to 70 U/kg followed by a constant infusion of approximately 16 U/kg/hr, adjusted to maintain the activated partial thromboplastin time at 1.5 to 2.5 times control, or 50 to 70 seconds. Subcutaneous administration of enoxaparin or dalteparin may be used instead of unfractionated heparin. [5] The dose of enoxaparin is 1 mg/kg twice daily, and the dose of dalteparin is 120 IU/kg (maximum, 10,000 IU) twice daily. Either standard heparin or LMWHs should be continued for 2 to 5 days or until the patient has been stabilized for 24 hours or revascularization is performed. The dose of unfractionated heparin should be reduced during coronary angioplasty when aspirin and GPIIb-IIIa inhibitors are being administered concomitantly, and heparin should be discontinued after an uncomplicated procedure. Information is accumulating on the combined use of LMWHs and GPIIb-IIIa inhibitors; in one large randomized trial, enoxaparin was at least equivalent to unfractionated heparin when it was used in combination with tirofiban in patients with unstable angina or non–Q wave MI. More recent data suggest that fondaparinux is superior to enoxaparin.

Statins

In one randomized trial of patients with unstable angina or non–Q wave MI for whom early revascularization was not planned, high-dose atorvastatin for 16 weeks reduced the composite primary end point. [6] In another randomized trial comparing atorvastatin (80 mg) with pravastatin (40 mg) begun within 10 days of an episode of ACS, the composite primary end point was significantly reduced during the 2-year follow-up in the atorvastatin group, which achieved a significantly lower low-density lipoprotein cholesterol level. [7] Most of the patients in this trial had undergone PCI for their ACS just before study entry. However, a third randomized trial comparing early aggressive simvastatin therapy with a more conservative simvastatin therapy after ACS showed no early benefit. Nevertheless, several trials have demonstrated long-term reduction in cardiac events with statins in patients with coronary disease (Chapter 217). Long-term compliance is improved if this therapy is begun in the hospital. It is currently recommended that high-dose atorvastatin therapy (80 mg/day) be initiated in the hospital in patients with ACS, with the goal of reducing the low-density lipoprotein cholesterol to 70 mg/dL or lower.

Other Medical Therapy

Thrombolytic therapy improves the outcome of patients with ST segment elevation MI (Chapter 72) but is of no benefit in unstable angina or non–ST segment elevation MI. The direct thrombin inhibitor bivalirudin (1 mg/kg IV bolus followed by 4-hour IV infusion at 2.5 mg/kg/hr, then for 20 hours at 0.2 mg/kg/hr) has been recommended as an improvement over heparin during PCI and is the agent of choice in patients with heparin-induced thrombocytopenia. Long-term anticoagulation with warfarin is not recommended for patients with unstable angina or non–ST segment elevation MI.

Treatment of Ischemic Signs and Symptoms

An oral β-blocker at a dose that reduces heart rate and an intravenous nitroglycerin infusion are reasonable treatments to control symptoms in high-risk or intermediate-risk patients with ACS. Low-risk and some intermediate-risk patients can be treated with oral or transdermal nitrates and β-blockers. A patient who develops unstable angina while already taking two or three antianginal drugs should be treated with intravenous nitroglycerin, but symptoms are more difficult to control than in a patient who previously took no antianginal drugs.

Nitroglycerin and Nitrate Therapy

In patients with unstable angina, sublingual nitroglycerin (0.4 mg every 5 minutes ≤3 doses/15 minutes) usually relieves attacks promptly, although it may be less efficacious than in stable angina. Nitroglycerin is a venodilator at low doses and an arteriolar dilator at higher doses; it reduces preload and afterload and myocardial oxygen consumption. The drug directly dilates coronary stenoses and increases oxygen delivery to the ischemic region. Nitroglycerin increases collateral flow and favorably redistributes regional coronary flow. Because of its preferential effect on capacitance as opposed to resistance vessels, it does not induce a coronary steal, in contrast to other vasodilators.

Nitroglycerin and longer acting nitrates act by releasing nitric oxide in vascular smooth muscle through an enzymatic process. Sulfhydryl-donating compounds are necessary for this activity, and their rapid depletion during long-term therapy with nitroglycerin or other nitrate preparations rapidly leads to tolerance to the hemodynamic effects of the drug. This phenomenon is a major problem when nitrates are used as long-term therapy but is less relevant to their use in ACS. Nitroglycerin inhibits platelet aggregation and, in experimental models, reduces platelet thrombus deposition. This effect seems to persist even after tolerance develops for the hemodynamic effects of the drug.

Patients with unstable angina often are treated with an infusion of intravenous nitroglycerin to prevent further attacks. A common starting dose is 10 μg/min. The dose can be increased by increments of 10 μg/min until symptoms are controlled or unwanted side effects develop. The most common adverse effects are headache, nausea, dizziness, hypotension, and reflex tachycardia.

The evidence that intravenous nitroglycerin prevents ischemic attacks in patients with unstable angina is based on small, uncontrolled studies. No studies of sufficient power have examined whether intravenous nitroglycerin or other nitrate preparations reduce the risk of MI in unstable angina.

Rx

Angina episodes usually disappear entirely when patients with unstable angina or non–ST segment elevation MI are hospitalized and given medical therapy. At that point, intravenous nitrates often are replaced with transdermal or oral nitrates.

β-Blockers

Although it is accepted widely that β-blockers are useful to control ischemic episodes in patients with unstable angina or non–ST segment elevation MI, the data to support this claim are mainly inferential or derived from small trials without placebo-treated controls from the early 1980s, an era when patients were not treated routinely with aspirin and heparin. Taken together, these trials indicate that β-blockers effectively reduce symptoms in patients with unstable angina who are not already taking one of these drugs on admission. Whether a β-blocker also reduces the risk of MI is uncertain because the trials in unstable angina are underpowered to answer this question.

During long-term therapy, a long-acting β-blocker is preferable to a short-acting one because it can be given once daily. In the context of ACS, it is reasonable to try to achieve β-blockade within hours, however, and not days. One approach is to begin metoprolol at an oral dose of 50 mg every 6 to 8 hours and to increase the dose as necessary to control heart rate, blood pressure, and symptoms. β-Blockade sometimes is initiated with intravenous boluses titrated to reduce heart rate. Early heart rate control is particularly important in high-risk patients and in patients with tachycardia or a high arterial pressure on admission. A reasonable target heart rate is 50 to 60 beats per minute at rest.

The main contraindications to β-blockers in unstable angina are reactive airway disease, sinus node dysfunction or atrioventricular block, and severe heart failure. Most patients with chronic obstructive pulmonary disease tolerate a β-blocker; a β_1-selective agent (e.g., metoprolol or atenolol) is theoretically less likely to provoke bronchoconstriction. In some patients with conduction system disease, permanent pacing may be indicated in part so that long-term β-blocker therapy can be given. Mild heart failure that is stable is not a contraindication to β-blockers in unstable angina. Diltiazem or verapamil should be considered when a β-blocker cannot be used.

Calcium-Channel Blockers

Calcium-channel blockers increase coronary blood flow globally and to the ischemic zone. Diltiazem and verapamil slow heart rate, reduce afterload, and reduce myocardial contractility; they reduce myocardial oxygen demand and are useful to control ischemic symptoms. Diltiazem and verapamil have been compared with placebo or a β-blocker in several small clinical trials in unstable angina, and they seem to be more effective than placebo and equivalent to a β-blocker in preventing recurrent angina episodes.

Most dihydropyridine calcium-channel blockers induce a reflex increase in heart rate in the absence of β-blockade, a feature that is likely to mitigate any benefit on myocardial ischemia. The rapid absorption and short half-life of the short-acting formulation of nifedipine (10 mg three times daily up to 30 mg four times daily) produce frequent abrupt changes in arterial pressure and heart rate. The calcium-channel blocker that has been used most often in the limited number of studies in unstable angina is this formulation of nifedipine. Taken together, these trials provide fairly strong evidence that nifedipine is harmful when it is used in patients with unstable angina not receiving β-blockers but that it may be helpful in controlling angina in patients with an adequate level of β-blockade. Whether the poor results seen with nifedipine in trials of unstable angina and post-MI patients would have been different with a long-acting formulation or newer dihydropyridines such as amlodipine is open to debate because these drugs have not been evaluated under these conditions.

Diltiazem (180 to 360 mg/day) and verapamil (240 to 480 mg/day) are reasonable choices for treatment of unstable angina when β-blockers are contraindicated. The scant evidence suggests that both drugs reduce the frequency of attacks in unstable angina, but there is no evidence that they prevent MI. The combination of either diltiazem or verapamil with a β-blocker is not generally used in patients with unstable angina because the effects of these calcium-channel blockers on heart rate and myocardial contractility are additive to the effects of β-blockers.

Rx

Diltiazem reduced the risk of reinfarction within 14 days in a placebo-controlled trial among patients with non–Q wave MI in the early 1980s. Diltiazem and β-blockers have not been compared in this situation, and the relevance of this old trial to the current management of non–ST segment elevation MI is uncertain.

Recurrent or Refractory Unstable Angina

In most patients hospitalized with unstable angina, symptoms do not recur after institution of antianginal therapy. Patients with refractory unstable angina have a high risk for development of MI. Patients whose angina is labeled refractory often become asymptomatic when medical therapy is intensified.

Intra-aortic balloon counterpulsation prevents myocardial ischemia effectively in patients whose unstable angina is truly refractory. This mechanical approach improves myocardial blood flow and reduces myocardial oxygen demand by collapsing the resistance to left ventricular ejection in early systole. Intra-aortic balloon counterpulsation is needed for control of symptoms in less than 1% of patients with unstable angina, but it also is used in high-risk cases at the time of PCI to provide a margin of safety. Intra-aortic balloon counterpulsation causes lower limb ischemia in approximately 10% of cases, but this complication almost always resolves with removal of the device.

Coronary Revascularization

CABG surgery (Chapter 74) and PCI (Chapter 73) are performed frequently in patients with unstable angina; however, the precise indications for revascularization, the choice of procedure, and its timing are controversial. CABG surgery relieves angina completely in approximately 90% of patients who undergo the procedure, and symptoms usually do not recur for many years.

In patients with lesions amenable to PCI, angina also almost always is relieved, but repeated procedures are more common during follow-up than in CABG patients. The introduction of drug-eluting stents has almost totally eliminated restenosis, and the incidence of stent thrombosis is low. Whether revascularization prolongs survival and prevents future coronary events in patients at different levels of risk has not been determined adequately from trials.

An overview of the 10-year results from the clinical trials comparing CABG surgery with medical treatment for stable angina indicates that patients with left main coronary artery stenosis or three-vessel disease obtain the most benefit from surgery. In low-risk groups, such as patients with single-vessel involvement, no survival advantage can be shown with CABG surgery. These conclusions also may be relevant to patients with unstable angina.

Trials of coronary revascularization in unstable angina have compared an "aggressive" approach with a "conservative" approach. The aggressive approach involves early coronary angiography with revascularization by either PCI or CABG surgery, depending on the coronary anatomy. Formerly, patients with one or two severe stenoses were treated with PCI, and patients with more extensive disease underwent CABG surgery. More recently, the near elimination of restenosis with drug-eluting stents has increased the use of PCI and decreased the use of CABG surgery in patients with multivessel disease. The conservative approach usually limits coronary arteriography to patients who require revascularization to control persistent symptoms and to patients with high-risk features.

Although early trials suggested that the conservative approach was as good as or better than the aggressive approach in patients with ACS, more recent studies of patients with either unstable angina or non–ST segment elevation MI tend to show that patients randomized to routine catheterization within 4 to 48 hours and revascularization "as appropriate" have a better outcome than do patients for whom catheterization is limited to objective evidence of recurrent ischemia or an abnormality on stress testing. In one study, for example, the composite end point of death, nonfatal MI, or rehospitalization for ACS within 6 months was reduced by about 20%, with the benefit restricted almost entirely to high-risk patients (e.g., patients with elevated troponin levels). 8

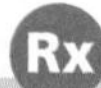

Complications

Patients with non–ST segment elevation MI can develop all of the complications associated with ST segment elevation MI, including arrhythmias, heart failure, and mechanical complications (Chapter 72). However, with the exception of recurrent ischemia, complications are less common in non–ST segment elevation MI because the amount of myocardial damage tends to be less.

Integrated Approach to Treatment

The treatment of unstable angina should be individualized to consider the specific features of the disease and the particular circumstances of the patient. Nevertheless, algorithms provide a useful framework (see Fig. 71–1).

Unstable angina is an acute episode related to one active culprit lesion, but the patient has diffuse atherosclerosis. Coronary disease is a chronic condition that usually causes recurrent events spread out during many years. Smoking cessation (Chapter 30), cholesterol lowering (Chapter 217), control of hypertension (Chapter 66) and diabetes (Chapter 248), and other risk factor reductions (Chapters 70 and 72) are more important long term than are the specific treatment decisions related to the acute event. Maintaining compliance long term with medical therapy appears to reduce the risk of a future coronary event by up to 80%. An episode of unstable angina may be viewed as an opportunity to improve the patient's profile with respect to secondary prevention.

Prognosis

Prognosis in unstable angina and non–ST segment elevation MI can be viewed as a composite of the expected prognosis based on the extent of coronary disease and left ventricular function, overlaid with the short-term risk associated with the culprit lesion and the unstable state. The short-term risk is related almost entirely to MI and its complications and to recurrences of unstable angina. Risk is highest in the hours, days, and first month after the onset of symptoms. The incremental risk associated with the unstable state dissipates completely by 1 year. Of unstable angina patients in one series, 11% experienced an MI between hospital discharge and 1 year, but the subsequent annual MI rate was less than 2%.

Published data on prognosis in unstable angina are influenced by selection of patients and treatment and can be misleading. The inclusion and exclusion criteria for clinical trials may bias the prognosis by eliminating either low-risk or high-risk patients. If large numbers of younger patients with atypical symptoms and no objective evidence of myocardial ischemia are included, the prognosis of the cohort tends to be better. Conversely, if ECG changes or elevated troponin levels are required, the prognosis tends to be worse.

Prognosis has improved dramatically since the 1980s with the introduction of increasingly more sophisticated medical therapy and revascularization techniques. In a compilation of 10 representative series with a total of nearly 2000 patients with unstable angina, excluding patients with new-onset or post-MI angina, the mortality was 4% in the hospital and 10% at 1 year. Survival without MI was 89% at 1 month and 79% at 1 year. Among 4488 patients with unstable angina in another large study, the mortality rate was 2.4% at 30 days, 5% at 6 months, and 7% at 1 year; the MI rate was 4.8% at 30 days and 6.2% at 6 months. Recurrent ischemia has a major impact on these rates; the 30-day MI rate increases from 2.3 to 7.2 to 21.7% in patients with no ischemia, ischemia, and refractory ischemia. These outcomes represent what can be expected now with modern therapy.

Grade A

1. Antithrombotic Trialists' Collaboration: Collaborative meta-analysis of randomised trials of antiplatelet therapy for prevention of death, myocardial infarction, and stroke in high risk patients. BMJ 2002;324:71–86.
2. Yusuf S, Mehta SR, Zhao F, et al, on behalf of the CURE (Clopidogrel in Unstable angina to prevent Recurrent Events) Trial Investigators: Early and late effects of clopidogrel in patients with acute coronary syndromes. Circulation 2003;107:966–972.
3. Boersma E, Harrington RA, Moliterno DJ, et al: Platelet glycoprotein IIb/IIIa inhibitors in acute coronary syndromes: A meta-analysis of all major randomised clinical trials. Lancet 2002;359:189–198.
4. Oler A, Whooley MA, Oler J, et al: Adding heparin to aspirin reduces the incidence of myocardial infarction and death in patients with unstable angina: A meta-analysis. JAMA 1996;276:811–815.
5. Wong GC, Giugliano RP, Antman EM: Use of low-molecular-weight heparins in the management of acute coronary artery syndromes and percutaneous coronary intervention. JAMA 2003;289:331–342.
6. Schwartz GG, Olsson AG, Ezekowitz MD, et al: Effects of atorvastatin on early recurrent ischemic events in acute coronary syndromes. The MIRACL study: A randomized controlled trial. JAMA 2001;265:1711–1718.
7. Cannon CP, Steinberg BA, Murphy SA, et al: Meta-analysis of cardiovascular outcomes trials comparing intensive versus moderate statin therapy. J Am Coll Cardiol 2006;48:438–445.
8. Mehta SR, Cannon CP, Fox KA, et al: Routine vs selective invasive strategies in patients with acute coronary syndromes: A collaborative meta-analysis of randomized trials. JAMA 2005;23:2908–2917.

SUGGESTED READINGS

Kastrati A, Mehilli J, Neumann FJ, et al: Abciximab in patients with acute coronary syndromes undergoing percutaneous coronary intervention after clopidogrel pretreatment: The ISAR-REACT 2 randomized trial. JAMA 2006;295:1531–1538. *In patients with an elevated troponin, adverse events were significantly lower in the abciximab group (13.1% versus 18.3%).*

Morrow DA, Cannon CP, Jesse RL, et al: National Academy of Clinical Biochemistry Laboratory Medicine Practice Guidelines: Clinical characteristics and utilization of biochemical markers in acute coronary syndromes. Circulation 2007;115:e356–375. *A consensus review.*

Peterson ED, Roe MT, Mulgund J, et al: Association between hospital process performance and outcomes among patients with acute coronary syndromes. JAMA 2006;295:1912–1920. *Every 10% increase in adherence was associated with a 10% decrease in mortality.*

Yusuf S, Mehta SR, Chrolavicius S, et al: Comparison of fondaparinux and enoxaparin in acute coronary syndromes. N Engl J Med 2006;354:1464–1476. *Fondaparinux substantially reduced major bleeding and improved long term mortality and morbidity.*

72 ST SEGMENT ELEVATION ACUTE MYOCARDIAL INFARCTION AND COMPLICATIONS OF MYOCARDIAL INFARCTION

Jeffrey L. Anderson

Definition

Conceptually, myocardial infarction (MI) is myocardial necrosis caused by ischemia. Practically, MI can be diagnosed and evaluated by clinical, electrocardiographic, biochemical, radiologic, and pathologic methods. Technologic advances in detecting much smaller amounts of myocardial necrosis than previously possible (e.g., by troponin determinations) have required a redefinition of MI. Given these developments, the term MI now should be qualified with regard to size, precipitating circumstance, and timing. This chapter focuses on acute MI associated with ST segment elevation on the electrocardiogram (ECG). This category of acute MI is characterized by profound ("transmural") acute myocardial ischemia affecting relatively large areas of myocardium. The underlying cause essentially always is *complete* interruption of regional myocardial blood flow (resulting from coronary occlusion, usually atherothrombotic) (Chapter 69). This clinical syndrome should be distinguished from non–ST segment elevation MI, in which the blockage of coronary flow is incomplete and for which different acute therapies are appropriate (Chapter 71).

Epidemiology

Cardiovascular disease is responsible for almost one half of all deaths in the United States and other developed countries and for one fourth of deaths in the developing world (Chapter 49). By 2020, cardiovascular disease will cause one of every three deaths worldwide. Cardiovascular

TABLE 72–1 CONDITIONS OTHER THAN CORONARY ATHEROSCLEROSIS THAT CAN CAUSE ACUTE MYOCARDIAL INFARCTION

Coronary emboli	Causes include aortic or mitral valve lesions, left atrial or ventricular thrombi, prosthetic valves, fat emboli, intracardiac neoplasms, infective endocarditis, and paradoxical emboli
Thrombotic coronary artery disease	Can occur with oral contraceptive use, sickle cell anemia and other hemoglobinopathies, polycythemia vera, thrombocytosis, thrombotic thrombocytopenic purpura, disseminated intravascular coagulation, antithrombin III deficiency and other hypercoagulable states, macroglobulinemia and other hyperviscosity states, multiple myeloma, leukemia, malaria, and fibrinolytic system shutdown secondary to impaired plasminogen activation or excessive inhibition
Coronary vasculitis	Seen with Takayasu's disease, Kawasaki's disease, polyarteritis nodosa, lupus erythematosus, scleroderma, rheumatoid arthritis, and immune-mediated vascular degeneration in cardiac allografts
Coronary vasospasm	Can be associated with variant angina, nitrate withdrawal, cocaine or amphetamine abuse, and angina with "normal" coronary arteries
Infiltrative and degenerative coronary vascular disease	Can result from amyloidosis, connective tissue disorders (e.g., pseudoxanthoma elasticum), lipid storage disorders and mucopolysaccharidoses, homocystinuria, diabetes mellitus, collagen vascular disease, muscular dystrophies, and Friedreich's ataxia
Coronary ostial occlusion	Associated with aortic dissection, luetic aortitis, aortic stenosis, and ankylosing spondylitis syndromes
Congenital coronary anomalies	Including Bland-White-Garland syndrome of anomalous origin of the left coronary artery from the pulmonary artery, left coronary artery origin from the anterior sinus of Valsalva, coronary arteriovenous fistula or aneurysms, and myocardial bridging with secondary vascular degeneration
Trauma	Associated with and responsible for coronary dissection, laceration, or thrombosis (with endothelial cell secondary to trauma such as angioplasty) and with radiation and cardiac contusion
Augmented myocardial oxygen requirements exceeding oxygen delivery	Encountered with aortic stenosis, aortic insufficiency, hypertension with severe left ventricular hypertrophy, pheochromocytoma, thyrotoxicosis, methemoglobinemia, carbon monoxide poisoning, shock, and hyperviscosity syndromes

disease causes almost 1 million deaths in the United States each year; it accounts for 37% of all deaths and contributes to 58% of deaths. Annually, an estimated 1.2 million U.S. residents suffer a fatal or nonfatal acute MI. Coronary heart disease, the leading cause of cardiovascular death, underlies or is a contributing cause of 650,000 deaths annually. Half of coronary heart disease deaths (250,000/year) are directly related to acute MI, and at least half of these acute MI–related deaths occur within 1 hour of onset of symptoms and before patients reach a hospital emergency department.

More than 5 million people visit emergency departments in the United States each year for evaluation of chest pain and related symptoms, and almost 1.5 million are hospitalized for an acute coronary syndrome (Chapter 48). The presence of ST segment elevation or new left bundle branch block (LBBB) on the ECG distinguishes patients with acute MI who require consideration of immediate recanalization therapy from other patients with an acute coronary syndrome (non–ST segment elevation MI/unstable angina; Chapter 71). Changing demographics, lifestyles, and medical therapies have led to a decrease in the ratio of ST segment elevation MI to non–ST segment elevation acute coronary syndromes over the past 10 to 15 years, so ST segment elevation MI now accounts for about 30% of all MIs. However, ST segment elevation MI is associated with greater in-hospital (but not post-hospital) mortality than non–ST segment elevation MI, and it remains an important contributor to total population mortality.

Pathobiology

Erosion, fissuring, or rupture of vulnerable atherosclerotic plaques has been determined to be the initiating mechanism of coronary thrombotic occlusion, thereby precipitating intraplaque hemorrhage, coronary spasm, and occlusive luminal thrombosis (Chapter 70). Plaque rupture most frequently occurs in lipid-laden plaques with an endothelial cap weakened by internal collagenase (metalloproteinase) activity derived primarily from macrophages. These macrophages are recruited to the plaque from blood monocytes responding to inflammatory mediators and adhesion molecules.

With plaque rupture, elements of the blood stream are exposed to the highly thrombogenic plaque core and matrix containing lipid, tissue factor, and collagen. Platelets adhere, become activated, and aggregate; vasoconstrictive and thrombogenic mediators are secreted; vasospasm occurs; thrombin is generated and fibrin formed; and a partially or totally occlusive platelet- and fibrin-rich thrombus is generated. When coronary flow is occluded, electrocardiographic ST segment elevation occurs (ST segment elevation acute MI). Partial occlusion, occlusion in the presence of collateral circulation, and distal coronary embolization result in unstable angina or non–ST segment elevation MI (Chapter 71). Ischemia from impaired myocardial perfusion causes myocardial cell injury or death, ventricular dysfunction, and cardiac arrhythmias.

Although most MIs are caused by atherosclerosis, occasional patients can develop complete coronary occlusions owing to coronary emboli, in situ thrombosis, vasculitis, primary vasospasm, infiltrative or degenerative diseases, diseases of the aorta, congenital anomalies of a coronary artery, or trauma (Table 72–1). In a canine model of coronary occlusion and recanalization, myocardial cell death begins within 15 minutes of occlusion and proceeds rapidly in a wave front from endocardium to epicardium. Partial myocardial salvage can be achieved by releasing the occlusion within 3 to 6 hours; the degree of salvage is inversely proportional to the duration of ischemia and occurs in a reverse wavefront from epicardium to endocardium. The extent of myocardial necrosis can also be altered by modification of metabolic demands and collateral blood supply. The temporal dynamic of infarction in human disease, although more complex, is generally similar.

Clinical Manifestations

Traditionally, the diagnosis of acute MI has rested on the triad of ischemic-type chest discomfort, ECG abnormalities, and elevated serum cardiac markers. Acute MI was considered present when at least two of the three were present. With their increasing sensitivity and specificity, serum cardiac markers (e.g., troponin I [TnI] or troponin T [TnT]) have assumed a dominant role in confirming the diagnosis of acute MI in patients with suggestive clinical and/or ECG features.

History

Ischemic-type chest discomfort is the most prominent clinical symptom in the majority of patients with acute MI (see Table 48–1). The discomfort is characterized by its quality, location, duration, radiation, and precipitating and relieving factors. The discomfort associated with acute MI is qualitatively similar to that of angina pectoris but more severe. It often is perceived as heavy, pressing, crushing, squeezing, bandlike, viselike, strangling, constricting, aching, or burning; it rarely is perceived as sharp pain and generally not as stabbing pain (Chapters 48 and 70).

The primary location of typical ischemic pain is most consistently retrosternal, but it also can present left parasternally, left precordially, or across the anterior chest (Chapter 48). Occasionally, discomfort is predominantly perceived in the anterior neck, jaw, arms, or epigastrium. It

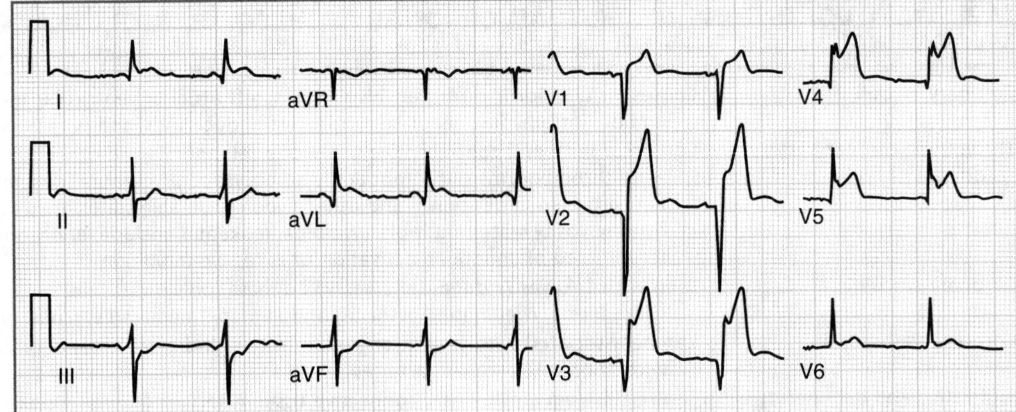

FIGURE 72–1 • Electrocardiographic tracing shows an acute anterolateral myocardial infarction. Note ST segment elevation in leads I, L, and V_1 to V_6 with Q waves in V_1 to V_4.

generally is somewhat diffuse; highly localized pain (finger point) is rarely angina or acute MI. The most characteristic pattern of radiation is to the left arm, but the right arm or both arms can be involved. The shoulders, neck, jaw, teeth, epigastrium, and interscapular areas also are sites of radiation. Discomfort above the jaws or below the umbilicus is not typical of acute MI. Associated symptoms often include nausea, vomiting, diaphoresis, weakness, dyspnea, restlessness, and apprehension.

The discomfort of acute MI is more severe and lasts longer (typically 20 minutes to several hours) than angina, and it is not reliably relieved by rest or nitroglycerin. The onset of acute MI usually is unrelated to exercise or other apparent precipitating factors. Nevertheless, acute MI begins during physical or emotional stress and within a few hours of arising more frequently than explained by chance.

It is estimated that at least 20% of acute MIs are painless ("silent") or atypical (unrecognized). Elderly patients and patients with diabetes are particularly prone to painless or atypical MI, which occurs in as many as one third to one half of such patients. Because the prognosis is worse in elderly patients and in those patients with diabetes, diagnostic vigilance is required. In these patients, acute MI can present as sudden dyspnea (which can progress to pulmonary edema), weakness, lightheadedness, nausea, and/or vomiting. Confusional states, sudden loss of consciousness, a new rhythm disorder, or an unexplained fall in blood pressure are other uncommon presentations. The differential diagnosis of ischemic chest discomfort also should include gastrointestinal disorders (e.g., reflux esophagitis; Chapter 140), musculoskeletal pain (e.g., costochondritis), anxiety or panic attacks, pleurisy or pulmonary embolism (Chapter 99), and acute aortic dissection (Chapter 78; see Table 48–2).

Physical Examination

No physical findings are diagnostic or pathognomonic of acute MI. The physical examination can be entirely normal or may reveal only nonspecific abnormalities. An S_4 gallop frequently is found if carefully sought. Blood pressure often is initially elevated, but it may be normal or low. Signs of sympathetic hyperactivity (tachycardia and/or hypertension) often accompany anterior wall MI, whereas parasympathetic hyperactivity (bradycardia and/or hypotension) is more common with inferior wall MI.

The examination is best focused on an overall assessment of cardiac function. Adequacy of vital signs and peripheral perfusion should be noted. Signs of cardiac failure, both left and right sided (e.g., S_3 gallop, pulmonary congestion, elevated neck veins) should be sought, and observation for arrhythmias and mechanical complications (e.g., new murmurs) is essential. If hypoperfusion is present, determination of its primary cause (e.g., hypovolemia, right heart failure, left heart failure) is critical to management.

Diagnosis

Electrocardiogram

In patients with a possible acute MI, an ECG must be obtained immediately. Although the initial ECG is neither perfectly specific nor perfectly sensitive in all patients who develop acute ST segment elevation MI, it plays a critical role in initial stratification, triage, and management (Chapter 48). In an appropriate clinical setting, a pattern of regional ECG ST segment elevation suggests coronary occlusion causing marked myocardial ischemia; hospital admission is indicated with triage to the coronary care unit (CCU). An emergency recanalization strategy (primary angioplasty or fibrinolysis) should be used unless it is contraindicated. Other ECG patterns (ST segment depression, T wave inversion, nonspecific changes, normal ECG) in association with ischemic chest discomfort are consistent with a non–ST segment elevation acute coronary syndrome (non–ST segment elevation MI or unstable angina) and are treated with different triage and initial management strategies (Chapter 71).

Electrocardiographic Evolution

Serial ECG tracings improve the sensitivity and specificity of the ECG for the diagnosis of acute MI and assist in assessing the outcomes of therapy. When typical ST segment elevation persists for hours and is followed within hours to days by T wave inversions and Q waves, the diagnosis of acute MI can be made with virtual certainty. The ECG changes in ST segment elevation acute MI evolve through three overlapping phases: (1) hyperacute or early acute, (2) evolved acute, and (3) chronic (stabilized).

Early Acute Phase

This earliest phase begins within minutes, persists, and evolves over hours. T waves increase in amplitude and widen over the area of injury (hyperacute pattern). ST segments evolve from concave to a straightened to a convex upward pattern (acute pattern). When prominent, the acute injury pattern of blended ST-T waves can take on a "tombstone" appearance (Fig. 72–1). ST segment depressions that occur in leads opposite those with ST segment elevation are known as "reciprocal changes" and are associated with larger areas of injury and a worse prognosis but also with greater benefits from recanalization therapy.

Other causes of ST segment elevation must be considered and excluded. These conditions include pericarditis (Chapter 77), left ventricular (LV) hypertrophy with J point elevation, and normal variant early repolarization (Chapter 52). Pericarditis (or perimyocarditis) is of particular concern because it can mimic acute MI clinically, but fibrinolytic therapy is *not* indicated and can be hazardous.

Evolved Acute Phase

During the second phase, ST segment elevation begins to regress, T waves in leads with ST segment elevation become inverted, and pathologic Q or QS waves become fully developed (>0.03-second duration and/or depth >30% of R wave amplitude).

Chronic Phase

Resolution of ST segment elevation is quite variable. It is usually complete within 2 weeks of inferior MI, but it can be delayed further after anterior MI. Persistent ST segment elevation, often seen with a large anterior MI, is indicative of a large area of akinesis, dyskinesis, or ventricular aneurysm. Symmetrical T wave inversions can resolve over weeks to months or can persist for an indefinite period; hence, the age of an MI in the presence of T wave inversions is often termed *indeterminate.* Q waves usually do not resolve after anterior MI but often disappear after inferior wall MI.

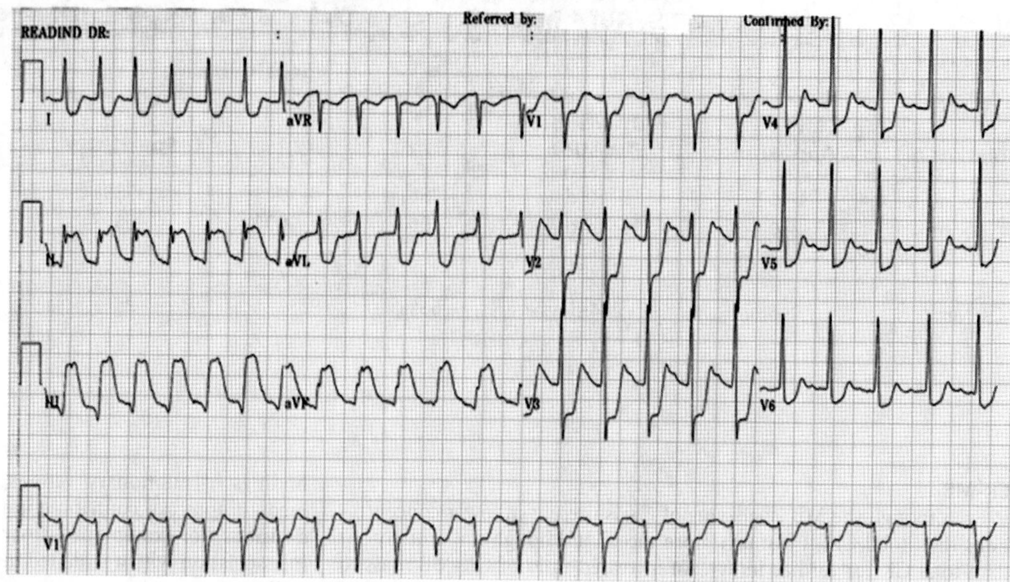

FIGURE 72–2 • Electrocardiographic tracing shows an acute inferoposterior myocardial infarction.

Early recanalization therapy accelerates the time course of ECG changes so that, on coronary recanalization, the pattern can evolve from acute to chronic over minutes to hours instead of days to weeks. ST segments recede rapidly, T wave inversions and losses of R wave occur earlier, and Q waves may not develop or progress and occasionally may regress. Indeed, failure of ST segment elevation to resolve by more than 50 to 70% within 1 to 2 hours suggests failure of fibrinolysis and should prompt urgent angiography for "rescue angioplasty."

True Posterior Myocardial Infarction and Left Circumflex Myocardial Infarction Patterns

"True posterior" MI presents a mirror-image pattern of ECG injury in leads V_1 to V_2 to V_4 (Fig. 72–2). The acute phase is characterized by ST segment depression, rather than ST segment elevation. The evolved and chronic phases show increased R wave amplitude and widening instead of Q waves. Recognition of a true posterior acute MI pattern should lead to an early recanalization strategy. Other causes of prominent upright anteroseptal forces include right ventricular (RV) hypertrophy, ventricular preexcitation variants (Wolff-Parkinson-White syndrome; Chapter 63), and normal variants with early R wave progression. New appearance of these changes or the association with an acute or evolving inferior MI usually allows the diagnosis to be made.

Occlusion of the left circumflex artery, especially when it is nondominant, often is not associated with diagnostic ST segment elevation and is therefore more difficult to recognize, to prioritize by triage appropriately, and to manage. Extending the ECG to measure left posterior leads V_7 to V_9 increases sensitivity for detecting left circumflex–related posterior wall injury patterns with excellent specificity (Chapter 52).

Right Ventricular Infarction

Proximal occlusion of the right coronary artery before the acute marginal branch can cause RV as well as inferior acute MI in about 30% of cases. Because the prognosis and treatment of inferior acute MI differ in the presence of RV infarction, it is important to make this diagnosis. The diagnosis is assisted by obtaining right precordial ECG leads, which are routinely indicated for inferior acute MI (Chapter 52). Acute ST segment elevation of at least 1 mm (0.1 mV) in one or more of leads V_{4R} to V_{6R} is both sensitive and specific (>90%) for identifying acute RV injury, and Q or QS waves effectively identify RV infarction.

Diagnosis in the Presence of Bundle Branch Block

The presence of LBBB often obscures ST segment analysis in patients with suspected acute MI. The presence of a new (or presumed new) LBBB in association with clinical (and laboratory) findings suggesting acute MI is associated with high mortality; patients with new-onset LBBB benefit substantially from recanalization therapy and should undergo triage and treatment in the same way as patients with ST segment elevation MI. Certain ECG patterns, although relatively insensitive, suggest acute MI if present in the setting of LBBB: Q waves in two of leads I, aVL, V_5, V_6; R wave regression from V_1 to V_4; ST segment elevation of 1 mm or more in leads with a positive QRS complex; ST segment depression of 1 mm or more in leads V_1, V_2, or V_3; and ST segment elevation of 5 mm or more associated with a negative QRS complex. The presence of right BBB (RBBB) usually does not mask typical ST-T wave or Q wave changes, except for rare cases of isolated true posterior acute MI, characterized by tall right precordial R waves and ST segment depressions.

Serum Cardiac Markers

The increasing sensitivity and specificity of serum cardiac markers have made them the "gold standard" for detection of myocardial necrosis. However, because of the 1- to 12-hour delay after the onset of symptoms before markers become detectable or diagnostic, and given laboratory delays even when markers are positive, the decision to proceed with an urgent recanalization strategy (primary angioplasty or fibrinolysis) must be based on the patient's clinical history and initial ECG (Chapter 48).

Serum cardiac markers of acute MI are macromolecules (proteins) released from myocytes undergoing necrosis. Ideal markers are not normally present in serum, become rapidly and markedly elevated during acute MI, and are not released from other injured tissues. In recent years, TnI and TnT have emerged as the best markers, although the MB isoenzyme of creatine kinase (CK) continues to be useful in selected settings (Table 72–2).

Troponins I and T

Cardiac-derived TnI (cTnI) and TnT (cTnT), proteins of the sarcomere, have amino acid sequences distinct from their skeletal muscle isoforms. These troponins are not normally present in the blood. With even small acute MIs, troponins increase to 20-fold or more above the lower limits of the assay, and elevations persist for several days. Troponins have replaced CK-MB because they are more specific in the setting of injuries to skeletal muscle or other organs that release CK and (to a lesser extent) CK-MB, and they also are more sensitive in the setting of minimal myocardial injury.

The troponins generally are first detectable 2 to 4 hours after the onset of acute MI, are maximally sensitive at 8 to 12 hours, peak at 10 to 24 hours, and persist for 5 to 14 days. Their long persistence has allowed them to replace lactate dehydrogenase and its isoenzymes for the diagnosis of acute MI in patients presenting late (>1 to 2 days) after symptoms. However, this persistence can obscure the diagnosis of recurrent MI, for which more rapidly cleared markers (i.e., CK-MB) are more useful. Clinically, cTnI and cTnT appear to be of approximately equivalent utility. However, renal failure is more likely to be associated with false-positive elevations of cTnT than of cTnI. Although qualitative point-of-service troponin tests can speed the diagnosis of acute MI in the emergency department, serum cardiac markers are often negative within the first few hours after the onset of symptoms.

TABLE 72–2 FEATURES OF SERUM MARKERS OF ACUTE MYOCARDIAL INFARCTION

Marker	Time to Appearance	Duration of Elevation	Sensitivity at: 6 hr	Sensitivity at: 12 hr	Specificity	Comments
Troponin I	2–6 hr	5–10 days	~75%	90–100%	~98%	Generally regarded as test of choice
Troponin T	2–6 hr	5–14 days	~80%	95–100%	~95%	Test of choice; less specific than troponin I (elevated in renal insufficiency)
CK-MB	3–6 hr	2–4 days	~65%	~95%	~95%	Test of choice for recurrent angina once troponin is elevated

CK-MB

Even though the MB isoenzyme of CK is present in lower concentrations than total CK, it is much more specific (although not entirely so) than total CK for cardiac injury. An increased ratio of CK-MB mass to total CK activity substantially improves the specificity of the diagnosis of acute MI with only a modest reduction in sensitivity. A problem in using the ratio occurs when total CK is markedly elevated (in the presence of skeletal muscle damage, including prolonged cardiac resuscitation) and CK-MB is elevated by units but not by ratio. Another clinical dilemma occurs when total CK is within the normal range but the ratio is elevated. Serial measurements of CK and CK-MB are more useful than single measurements in assessing diagnosis, timing, sizing, and success of therapy of acute MI. CK-MB increases within 3 to 4 hours after the onset of acute MI, is maximally sensitive within 8 to 12 hours, peaks at 12 to 24 hours, and returns to normal in 2 to 4 days.

The total quantity of CK/CK-MB protein released correlates with infarct size. Peak concentrations (e.g., for CK/CK-MB) correlate generally but less well with infarct size. Early reperfusion leads to higher and earlier peaks but similar or smaller integrated concentrations over time (consistent with myocardial salvage). The timing of the peak CK-MB can provide useful insight into the success (peak at 10 to 18 hours) or failure (peak at 18 to 30 hours) of recanalization therapy.

It does not appear to be cost-effective to measure both a cardiac-specific troponin and CK/CK-MB serially over time in every patient with suspected acute MI. However, CK/CK-MB still is useful for certain applications, such as to confirm the diagnosis when the troponin level is elevated in a confusing clinical setting, to evaluate possible reinfarction in patients with recurrent chest pain, and, in specific settings, to assess the success of recanalization noninvasively (using time to peak).

Other Laboratory Tests

On admission, routine assessment of complete blood count and platelet count, standard blood chemistry studies, a lipid panel, and coagulation tests (prothrombin time, partial thromboplastin time) are useful. Results assist in assessing comorbid conditions and prognosis and in guiding therapy. Hematologic tests provide a useful baseline before initiation of antiplatelet, antithrombin, and fibrinolytic therapy or coronary angiography or angioplasty. Myocardial injury precipitates polymorphonuclear leukocytosis, commonly resulting in an elevation of white blood cell count of up to 12,000 to 15,000/μL, which appears within a few hours and peaks at 2 to 4 days. The metabolic panel provides a useful check on electrolytes, glucose, and renal function. On hospital admission or the next morning, a fasting lipid panel is recommended to assist in decision making for inpatient lipid lowering (e.g., statin therapy if low-density lipoprotein is greater than 70 mg/dL; Chapter 217). Unless carbon dioxide retention is suspected, finger oximetry is adequate to titrate oxygen therapy. The C-reactive protein level increases with acute MI, but its incremental prognostic value in the acute setting is unknown. B-type natriuretic peptide, which increases with ventricular wall stress and relative circulatory fluid overload, may provide useful incremental prognostic information in the setting of acute MI.

Imaging

A chest radiograph is the only imaging test *routinely* obtained on admission for acute MI. Although the chest radiograph is often normal, findings of pulmonary venous congestion, cardiomegaly, or widened mediastinum can contribute importantly to diagnosis and management decisions. For example, a history of severe, "tearing" chest and back pain in association with a widened mediastinum should raise the question of a dissecting aortic aneurysm (Chapter 78). In such cases, fibrinolytic therapy must be withheld pending more definitive diagnostic imaging of the aorta. Other noninvasive imaging (e.g., echocardiography [Chapter 53], cardiac nuclear scanning [Chapter 54], and other testing) is performed for evaluation of specific clinical issues, including suspected complications of acute MI. Coronary angiography (Chapter 56) is performed urgently as part of an interventional strategy for acute MI or later for risk stratification in higher-risk patients who are managed medically.

Echocardiography

Two-dimensional transthoracic echocardiography with color-flow Doppler imaging is the most generally useful noninvasive test obtained on admission or early in the hospital course (Chapter 53). Echocardiography efficiently assesses global and regional cardiac function and enables the clinician to evaluate suspected complications of acute MI. The sensitivity and specificity of echocardiography for regional wall motion assessment are high (>90%), although the age of the abnormality (new versus old) must be distinguished clinically or by ECG. Echocardiography is helpful in determining the cause of circulatory failure with hypotension (relative hypovolemia, LV failure, RV failure, or mechanical complication of acute MI). Echocardiography also can assist in differentiating pericarditis and perimyocarditis from acute MI. Doppler echocardiography is indicated to evaluate a new murmur and other suspected mechanical complications of acute MI (papillary muscle dysfunction or rupture, acute ventricular septal defect, LV free wall rupture with tamponade or pseudoaneurysm). Later in the course of acute MI, echocardiography may be used to assess the degree of recovery of stunned myocardium after recanalization therapy, the degree of residual cardiac dysfunction and indications for angiotensin-converting enzyme (ACE) inhibitors and other therapies for heart failure, and the presence of LV aneurysm and mural thrombus (requiring oral anticoagulants).

Radionuclide, Magnetic Resonance, and Other Imaging Studies

Radionuclide techniques generally are too time consuming and cumbersome for routine use in the acute setting. More commonly, they are used in risk stratification before or after hospital discharge to augment exercise or pharmacologic stress testing (Chapter 54). Thallium-201 and technetium-99m-sestamibi alone or, more commonly, together (dual isotope imaging) are currently the most frequently used "cold spot" tracers to assess myocardial perfusion and viability, as well as infarct size. Infarct avid tracers to identify, locate, and size recent myocardial necrosis are available but are rarely required for ST segment elevation MI. Computed tomography (Chapter 54) and magnetic resonance imaging (Chapter 55) can be useful to evaluate patients with a suspected dissecting aortic aneurysm and, together with positron-emission tomography, for research purposes and in selected clinical applications such as for assessment of myocardial viability (infarct sizing). When the issue of a nonatherosclerotic cause of myocardial necrosis is raised (e.g., perimyocarditis simulating acute MI), contemporary multislice (e.g., 64-slice) coronary computed tomography (Chapter 54) can assess coronary artery disease qualitatively and semiquantitatively, and it can also distinguish other causes of chest pain syndromes.

Treatment

Rx

Assessment and Management

Prehospital Phase

More than one half of deaths related to acute MI occur within 1 hour of onset of symptoms and before the patient reaches a hospital emergency department. Most of these deaths are caused by ischemia-related ventricular fibrillation (VF) and can be reversed by defibrillation (Chapters 62 and 65). Rapid defibrillation allows resuscitation in 60% of patients when treatment is delivered by a bystander using an on-site automatic external defibrillator or by a first-responding medical rescuer (Chapter 62). Moreover, the first hour represents the best opportunity for myocardial salvage with recanalization therapy. Thus, the three goals of prehospital care are as follows: (1) to recognize symptoms promptly and seek medical attention; (2) to deploy an emergency medical system team capable of cardiac monitoring, defibrillation and resuscitation, and emergency medical therapy (e.g., nitroglycerin, lidocaine, atropine); and (3) to transport the patient expeditiously to a medical care facility staffed with personnel capable of providing expert coronary care, including recanalization therapy (primary angioplasty or fibrinolysis).

The greatest time lag to recanalization therapy is the patient's delay in calling for help. Public education efforts have yielded mixed results, and innovative approaches are needed. The feasibility of initiating fibrinolytic therapy by highly trained ambulance personnel in coordinated ambulance and emergency department systems has been shown. In coordinated systems and when transportation delays are substantial, initiation of fibrinolytic or other antithrombotic therapy in the field may be considered, thereby shortening the time to recanalization.

Hospital Phases

Emergency Department

The goals of emergency department care are to identify patients with acute myocardial ischemia rapidly, to stratify them into acute ST segment elevation MI as compared with other acute coronary syndromes (see Figs. 71–1 and 72–1), to initiate a recanalization strategy and other appropriate medical care in qualifying patients with acute ST segment elevation MI, and to prioritize by triage rapidly to inpatient (CCU, step-down unit, observation unit) or outpatient care (patients without suspected ischemia) (see Fig. 71–2).

The evaluation of patients with chest pain and other suspected acute coronary syndromes begins with a 12-lead ECG even as the physician is beginning a focused history, including contraindications to fibrinolysis, and a targeted physical examination. Continuous ECG monitoring should be started, an intravenous line should be established, and admission blood tests should be drawn (including cardiac markers such as cTnI or cTnT). As rapidly as possible, the patient should be stratified as having a probable ST segment elevation acute MI, a non–ST segment elevation acute MI, probable or possible unstable angina, or likely noncardiac chest pain.

In patients with ST segment elevation acute MI by clinical and ECG criteria, a recanalization strategy must be selected: alternative choices are primary percutaneous coronary intervention (primary PCI; the patient is transferred directly to the cardiac catheterization laboratory with a goal of door-to-balloon time of less than 90 minutes) or fibrinolysis (begun immediately in the emergency department with a goal of door-to-needle time of less than 30 minutes) (Fig. 72–3).

Aspirin (162 to 325 mg) should be given to all patients unless it is contraindicated (see Fig. 72–3). Intravenous heparin (initial bolus 60 IU/kg, maximum, 4000 IU, then 12 IU/kg/hour, maximum 1000 IU/hour, for patients >70 kg, adjusted to maintain activated partial thromboplastin time 1.5 to 2 times the control value) or low-molecular-weight heparin (LMWH; e.g., enoxaparin, 30 mg intravenous bolus, then 1 mg/kg subcutaneously twice daily, for patients <75 years old without renal insufficiency) is appropriate in most patients. Patients with chest pain should be given sublingual nitroglycerin (0.4 mg every 5 minutes for a total of three doses) after which an assessment should be made of the need for intravenous nitroglycerin. Persistent ischemic pain may be treated with titrated to intravenous doses of morphine (i.e., 2 to 4 mg intravenously [IV], repeated every 5 to 15 minutes to relieve pain). Initiation of β-blocker therapy is usually indicated, especially in patients with hypertension, tachycardia, and ongoing pain; however, decompensated heart failure is a contraindication to the acute initiation of β-blocker therapy, particularly by the intravenous route. Oxygen should be used in doses sufficient to avoid hypoxemia (e.g., initially at 4 L/minute by nasal cannula; fingertip oximetry may be used to monitor effect). The ideal systolic blood pressure is 100 to 140 mm Hg. Excessive hypertension usually responds to titrated nitroglycerin, β-blocker therapy, and morphine (also given for pain). Relative hypotension could require discontinuation of these medications, fluid administration, or other measures as appropriate to the hemodynamic subset (Table 72–3). Atropine (0.5 to 1.5 mg IV) should be available to treat symptomatic bradycardia and hypotension related to excessive vagotonia. Direct transfer to the catheterization laboratory or fibrinolysis followed by transfer to the CCU should occur as expeditiously as possible.

Early Hospital Phase: Coronary Care

Coronary care for early hospital management of acute MI has reduced in-hospital mortality by more than 50%. The goals of CCU care include (1) continuous ECG monitoring and antiarrhythmic therapy for serious arrhythmias (i.e., rapid defibrillation of VF), (2) initiation or continuation of a coronary recanalization strategy to achieve myocardial reperfusion, (3) initiation or continuation of other acute medical therapies, (4) hemodynamic monitoring and appropriate medical interventions for different hemodynamic subsets of patients, and (5) diagnosis and treatment of mechanical and physiologic complications of acute MI. General care and comfort measures also are instituted. A sample of CCU admission orders is given in Table 72–4.

General care measures include attention to activity, diet and bowels, education, reassurance, and sedation. Bedrest is encouraged for the first 12 hours. In the absence of complications, dangling and bed-chair and self-care activities can begin within 24 hours. When stabilization has occurred, usually within 1 to 3 days, patients may be transferred to a step-down unit where progressive reambulation occurs. The risk of emesis and aspiration or the anticipation of angiography or other procedures usually dictates nothing by mouth or clear liquids for the first 4 to 12 hours. Thereafter, a heart-healthy diet in small portions is recommended. In patients at high risk for bleeding gastric stress ulcers, a proton pump inhibitor or an H_2-antagonist is recommended for prophylaxis in patients receiving antithrombotic therapy. Many patients benefit from an analgesic (e.g., morphine sulfate, in 2- to 4-mg increments) to relieve ongoing pain and an anxiolytic or sedative during the CCU phase. A benzodiazepine is frequently selected. Sedatives should not be substituted for education and reassurance from concerned caregivers to relieve emotional distress and improve behavior; routine use of anxiolytics is neither necessary nor recommended. Constipation often occurs with bedrest and narcotics; stool softeners and a bedside commode are advised.

The ECG should be monitored continuously in the CCU (and usually in the step-down unit) to detect serious arrhythmias and to guide therapy. Measures to limit infarct size (i.e., coronary recanalization) and to optimize hemodynamics also stabilize the heart electrically. Routine antiarrhythmic prophylaxis (e.g., with lidocaine or amiodarone) is not indicated, but specific arrhythmias require treatment (see later text).

Hemodynamic evaluation is helpful in assessing prognosis and in guiding therapy (see Table 72–3). Clinical and noninvasive evaluation of vital signs is adequate for normotensive patients without pulmonary congestion. Patients with pulmonary venous congestion alone can usually be managed conservatively. Invasive monitoring is appropriate when the cause of circulatory failure is uncertain and when titration of intravenous therapies depends on hemodynamic measurements (e.g., pulmonary capillary wedge pressure and cardiac output). Similarly, an arterial line is not necessary in all patients and may be associated with local bleeding after fibrinolysis or potent antiplatelet and antithrombin therapy. Arterial

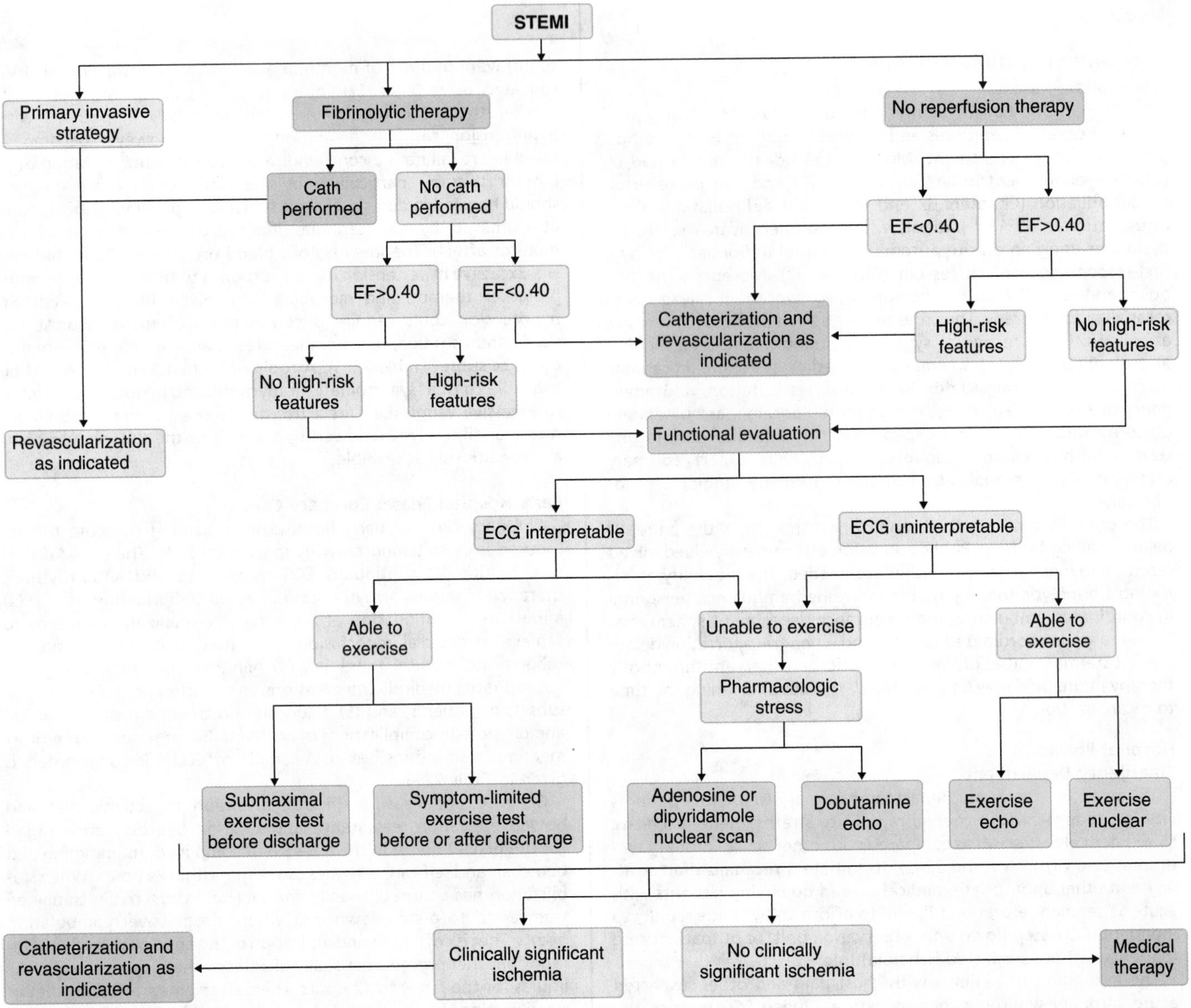

STEMI
Primary invasive strategy
Fibrinolytic therapy
No reperfusion therapy
Cath performed
No cath performed
EF<0.40
EF>0.40
EF>0.40
EF<0.40
Catheterization and revascularization as indicated
High-risk features
No high-risk features
No high-risk features
High-risk features
Revascularization as indicated
Functional evaluation
ECG interpretable
ECG uninterpretable
Able to exercise
Unable to exercise
Able to exercise
Pharmacologic stress
Submaximal exercise test before discharge
Symptom-limited exercise test before or after discharge
Adenosine or dipyridamole nuclear scan
Dobutamine echo
Exercise echo
Exercise nuclear
Catheterization and revascularization as indicated
Clinically significant ischemia
No clinically significant ischemia
Medical therapy

FIGURE 72–3 • Evidence-based approach to need for catheterization (cath) and revascularization after ST segment elevation myocardial infarction (STEMI). This algorithm shows treatment paths for patients who initially undergo a primary invasive strategy, receive fibrinolytic therapy, or do not undergo reperfusion therapy for STEMI. Patients who have not undergone a primary invasive strategy and have no high-risk features should undergo functional evaluation with one of the noninvasive tests shown. When clinically significant ischemia is detected, patients should undergo catheterization and revascularization as indicated; if no clinically significant ischemia is detected, medical therapy is prescribed after STEMI. (From Antman EM, Anbe DT, Armstrong PW, et al: 2004 Update: ACC/AHA Guidelines for the Managment of Patients with ST-Elevation Myocardial Infarction—Exective Summary. A Report of the American College of Cardiology/American Heart Association Task Force on Practice Guidelines. Circulation 2004;110:588–636.) ECG = electrocardiography; Echo = echocardiography; EF = ejection fraction.

catheters are appropriate and useful in clinically unstable, hypotensive patients who do not respond to intravenous fluids to replete or expand intravascular volume (see the later discussion of complications).

Later Hospital Phase

Transfer from the CCU to the step-down unit usually occurs within 1 to 3 days, when the cardiac rhythm and hemodynamics are stable. The duration of this late phase of hospital care is usually an additional 2 to 3 days in uncomplicated cases. Activity levels should be increased progressively under continuous ECG monitoring. Medical therapy should progress from parenteral and short-acting agents to oral medications appropriate and convenient for long-term outpatient use.

Risk stratification and functional evaluations are critical to assess prognosis and to guide therapy as the time for discharge approaches. Functional evaluation also can be extended to the early period after hospital discharge. Education must be provided about

diet, activity, smoking, and other risk factors (e.g., lipids, hypertension, diabetes).

Specific Therapeutic Measures

Recanalization Therapy

Early reperfusion of ischemic, infarcting myocardium represents the most important conceptual and practical advance for ST segment elevation acute MI and is the primary therapeutic goal. Coronary recanalization is accomplished by using primary PCI with angioplasty and, commonly, stenting or with fibrinolytic (thrombolytic) therapy. With broad application of recanalization therapy, 30-day mortality rates from ST segment elevation acute MI have progressively declined over the past 3 decades (from 20 to 30% to 5 to 10%).

Fibrinolytic Therapy

Various fibrinolytic agents (Table 72–5) are useful in patients with ST segment elevation or new or presumed-new LBBB who present for

TABLE 72–3 HEMODYNAMIC SUBSETS OF ACUTE MYOCARDIAL INFARCTION

	Blood Pressure (Relative)	Typical Physical Findings	Cardiac Index ($L/min/m^2$)	PA Wedge Pressure (mm Hg)	Suggested Interventions
Normal	Normal	$+/-S_4$	>2.5	≤12	None required
Hyperdynamic	Normal or high	Anxious	>3	<12	Control pain, anxiety; β-blocker; treat SBP to <140 mm Hg
Hypovolemia	Low	Dry	≤2.7	≤9	Add fluids to maintain normal pressure; can develop pulmonary edema if hypotension caused by unrecognized LV failure
Mild LV failure	Low to high	Rales, $+/-S_3$	2–2.5	>15	Diuresis; nitrates, ACE inhibitor; consider low-dose β-blocker
Severe LV failure	Low to normal	Above $+S_3$, +/– ↑ JVP, +/– edema	<2	>20	Diuresis; nitrates; low-dose ACE inhibitor; avoid β-blockers; consider inotropes, urgent revascularization
Cardiogenic shock	Very low	Above + cool, clammy; ↓ mental or renal function	≤1.5	>25	Avoid hypotensive agents; place intra-aortic balloon pump; urgent revascularization if possible
RV infarct	Very low	↑ JVP with clear lungs	<2.5	≤12	Give IV fluids; avoid nitrates and hypotensive agents; dobutamine if refractory to fluids

↑ = increased; ↓ = decreased; ACE = angiotensin-converting enzyme; IV = intravenous; JVP = jugular venous pressure; LV = left ventricle; PA = pulmonary artery; RV = right ventricle; SBP = systolic blood pressure.

Adapted from Forrester JS, Diamond G, Chatterjee K, Swan HJ: Medical therapy of acute myocardial infarction by application of hemodynamic subsets (second of two parts). N Engl J Med 1976;295:1404–1413.

TABLE 72–4 SAMPLE ADMISSION ORDERS FOR ST SEGMENT ELEVATION ACUTE MYOCARDIAL INFARCTION

Diagnosis:	Acute ST segment elevation myocardial infarction
Admit:	Coronary care unit with telemetry
Condition:	Serious
Vital signs:	q1/2h until stable, then q4h and prn; pulse oximetry ×24 hr; notify if heart rate <50 or >100; respiratory rate <8 or >20; SBP <90 or >150 mm Hg; O_2 saturation <90%
Activity:	Bedrest ×12 hr with bedside commode; thereafter, light activity if stable
Diet:	NPO except for sips of water until pain-free and stable; then 2 g sodium, heart-healthy diet as tolerated, unless on call for catheterization (or other test requiring NPO)
Laboratory tests*:	Troponin I or T and CK/CK-MB q8h ×3; comprehensive blood chemistry, magnesium, CBC with platelets; PT/INR, aPTT; BNP; lipid profile (fasting in morning); portable CXR
IV therapy:	D_5W or NS to keep vein open (increase fluids for relative hypovolemia); second IV if IV medication given
Recanalization therapy*:	Emergency primary coronary angioplasty, or fibrinolysis (if appropriate) 1. Primary angioplasty (preferred if available within 90 min) 2. Tenecteplase, alteplase, reteplase, or streptokinase (see Table 72–5 for doses)
Medications:	1. Nasal O_2 at 2 L/min ×6 hr, then by order (per O_2 saturation) 2. Aspirin 325 mg chewed on admission, then 162 mg PO qd (enteric coated) 3. IV heparin, 60 U/kg bolus (maximum, 4000 U) and 12 U/kg/hr (maximum, 1000 U/hr) or enoxaparin 30 mg IV then 1 mg/kg SQ q12h (maximum SQ doses, 100 mg on day 1) 4. Metoprolol, 12.5 PO q6h, incremented to 25–50 mg q6h as tolerated (hold for SBP <100, pulse <50, asthma, heart failure); may consider IV metoprolol if immediate effect required (tachyarrhythmia, severe hypertension, unrelieved pain) *in the absence of heart failure* 5. Consider IV nitroglycerin drip ×24–48 hr (titrated to SBP 100–140 mm Hg) 6. Morphine sulfate, 2–4 mg IV and increment at 5–15 min prn for unrelieved pain 7. Stool softener 8. Anxiolytic or hypnotic if needed 9. ACE inhibitor for hypertension, anterior acute MI, or LV dysfunction, in low oral dose (e.g., captopril 6.25 mg q8h), begun within 24 hours or when stable (SBP >100 mm Hg) and adjusted upward 10. Consider: lipid-lowering agent (i.e., statin if LDL >70–100 mg/dL or, optionally, for all with total cholesterol >135 mg/dL), GPIIb/IIIa inhibitor (e.g., eptifibatide or tirofiban) "upstream" from planned PCI, and clopidogrel, 300 mg PO, then 75 mg PO qd immediately after PCI (if CABG not planned) 11. Specific treatments for hemodynamic subgroups (see Table 72–3)

*If not ordered in the emergency department.

ACE = angiotensin-converting enzyme; aPTT = activated partial thromboplastin time; BNP = brain natriuretic peptide; CABG = coronary artery bypass graft surgery; CBC = complete blood count; CK = creatine kinase; CXR = chest radiograph; D_5W = 5% dextrose in water; GP = glycoprotein; INR = international normalized ratio; IV = intravenous; LDL = low density lipoprotein; LV = left ventricle; MI = myocardial infarction; NPO = nothing by mouth; NS = normal saline; PCI = percutaneous coronary intervention; PO = orally; prn = as needed; PT = prothrombin time; qd = once daily; SBP = systolic blood pressure; SQ = subcutaneous.

Adapted from Antman EM, Anbe DT, Armstrong PW, et al: 2004 Update: ACC/AHA guidelines for the management of patients with ST-elevation myocardial infarction—executive summary: A report of the American College of Cardiology/American Heart Association Task Force on Practice Guidelines. Circulation 2004;110:588–636.

TABLE 72–5 CHARACTERISTICS OF INTRAVENOUS FIBRINOLYTIC AGENTS APPROVED BY THE FOOD AND DRUG ADMINISTRATION

	Streptokinase (SK)	Alteplase (t-PA)	Reteplase (r-PA)	Tenecteplase (TNK–t-PA)
Dose	1.5 MU in 30–60 min	100 mg in 90 min*	10 U +10 U, 30 min apart	30–50 mg[†] over 5 sec
Circulating half-life (min)	≅20	≅4	≅18	≅20
Antigenic	Yes	No	No	No
Allergic reactions	Yes	No	No	No
Systemic fibrinogen depletion	Severe	Mild to moderate	Moderate	Minimal
Intracerebral hemorrhage	≅0.4%	≅0.7%	≅0.8%	≅0.7%
Patency (TIMI-2/3) rate, 90 min[‡]	≅51%	≅73–84%	≅83%	≅77–88%
Lives saved per 100 treated	≅3[§]	≅4[¶]	≅4	≅4
Cost per dose (approximate U.S. dollars)	300	1800	2200	2200

*Accelerated t-PA given as follows: 15-mg bolus, then 0.75 mg/kg over 30 min (maximum, 50 mg), then 0.50 mg/kg over 60 min (maximum, 35 mg).
[†]TNK–t-PA is dosed by weight (supplied in 5 mg/mL vials): <60 kg = 6 mL; 61–70 kg = 7 mL; 71–80 kg = 8 mL; 81–90 kg = 9 mL; >90 kg = 10 mL.
[‡]TIMI = Thrombolysis in Myocardial Infarction. Data from Granger CB, Califf RM, Topol EJ: Thrombolytic therapy for acute myocardial infarction: A review. Drugs 1992;44:293–325; and Bode C, Smalling RW, Berg G, et al: Randomized comparison of coronary thrombolysis achieved with double-bolus reteplase (recombinant plasminogen activator) and front-loaded, accelerated alteplase (recombinant tissue plasminogen activator) in patients with acute myocardial infarction: The RAPID ‖Investigators. Circulation 1996;94:891–898.
[§]Patients with ST segment elevation or bundle branch block, treated <6 hr.
[¶]Based on the finding from the GUSTO trial that t-PA saves one more additional life per 100 treated than does SK. Data from The GUSTO investigators: An international randomized trial comparing four thrombolytic strategies for acute myocardial infarction. N Engl J Med 1993;329:673–682; and Simes RJ, Topol EJ, Holmes DR Jr, et al: Link between the angiographic substudy and mortality outcomes in a large randomized trial of myocardial reperfusion: Importance of early and complete infarct artery reperfusion. GUSTO-I Investigators. Circulation 1995;91:1923–1928.

TABLE 72–6 INDICATIONS AND CONTRAINDICATIONS TO FIBRINOLYTIC THERAPY

INDICATIONS

Ischemic-type chest discomfort or equivalent for 30 min–12 hr with new or presumed new ST segment elevation in two contiguous leads of ≥2 mm (≥0.2 mV) in leads V_1, V_2, or V_3 or ≥1 mm in other leads
New or presumed-new left bundle branch block with symptoms consistent with myocardial infarction
Absence of contraindications

CONTRAINDICATIONS, ABSOLUTE

Active bleeding or bleeding diathesis (menses excluded)
Prior hemorrhagic stroke, other strokes within 1 year
Intracranial or spinal cord neoplasm or arteriovenous malformation
Suspected or known aortic dissection
Closed head or facial trauma within 3 months

CONTRAINDICATIONS, RELATIVE

Severe, uncontrolled hypertension by history or on presentation (>180/110 mmHg)
Anticoagulation with therapeutic or elevated international normalized ratio (>2–3)
Old ischemic stroke (>3 mo ago); intracerebral disease other than above
Recent (<3 wk) major trauma/surgery or prolonged (>10 min) cardiopulmonary resuscitation or internal bleeding
Active peptic ulcer
Recent noncompressible vascular punctures
Pregnancy
For streptokinase/anistreplase: prior exposure (especially if >5 day ago) or allergic reaction

Adapted from Antman EM, Anbe DT, Armstrong PW, et al: 2004 Update: **ACC/AHA guidelines for the management of patients with ST-elevation myocardial infarction—executive summary: A report of the American College of Cardiology/American Heart Association Task Force on Practice Guidelines.** Circulation 2004;110:588–636.

Rx

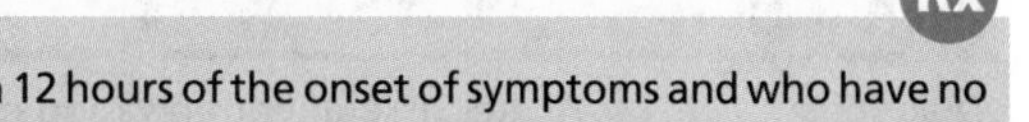

treatment within 12 hours of the onset of symptoms and who have no contraindications to the use of these agents (Table 72–6). Compared with no recanalization therapy, older fibrinolytics such as streptokinase reduced mortality by 18% (from 11.5% to 9.8%) at 5 weeks. [1] Patients with anterior ST segment elevation benefit more (37 lives saved per 1000) than those with inferior ST segment elevation only (8 lives saved per 1000), and younger patients benefit more than the elderly (>75 years). No benefit or a slight adverse effect is seen in patients presenting with normal ECGs or ST depression alone. Benefit is time dependent; it declines from about 40 lives or more saved per 1000 within the first hour, to 20 to 30 lives saved per 1000 for hours 2 to 12, to a nonsignificant 7 lives saved per 1000 for hours 13 to 24. An accelerated regimen of tissue plasminogen activator (t-PA plus intravenous heparin) further reduces mortality at 30 days (by 14%, from 7.3 to 6.3%), compared with streptokinase, [2] because the patency rate of the infarct-related artery at 90 minutes is higher with t-PA (81%) than with streptokinase (53 to 60%). Longer-acting variants of t-PA, given by single-bolus (tenecteplase) or double-bolus (reteplase) injections are now in widespread clinical use because they are more convenient to give, but they have not improved survival further.

The major risk of fibrinolytic therapy is bleeding. Intracerebral hemorrhage is the most serious and frequently fatal complication; its incidence rate is 0.5 to 1% with currently approved regimens. Older age (>70 to 75 years), female gender, hypertension, and higher relative doses of t-PA and heparin increase the risk of intracranial hemorrhage. The risk-to-benefit ratio should be assessed in each patient when fibrinolysis is considered and specific regimens are selected.

Primary Percutaneous Coronary Intervention

PCI has emerged as an alternative, and usually the preferred, recanalization strategy (Table 72–7). [3,4] PCI achieves mechanical recanalization by inflation of a catheter-based balloon centered within the thrombotic occlusion (Chapter 73). Percutaneous transluminal coronary angioplasty (PTCA) is generally augmented by placing a stent at the site of occlusion as a scaffold to enlarge the lumen and to retain optimal post-angioplasty expansion. Preference is often given to drug-eluting stents (e.g., sirolimus, paclitaxel), which markedly reduce the rates of restenosis but can increase the risk of late thrombosis.

TABLE 72–7 INDICATIONS FOR PRIMARY ANGIOPLASTY AND COMPARISON WITH FIBRINOLYTIC THERAPY

INDICATIONS

Alternative recanalization strategy for ST segment elevation or LBBB acute MI within 12 hr of symptom onset (or >12 hr if symptoms persist)
Cardiogenic shock developing within 36 hr of ST segment elevation/Q wave acute MI or LBBB acute MI in patients <75 yr old who can be revascularized within 18 hr of shock onset
Recommended only at centers performing >200 PCI/yr with backup cardiac surgery and for operators performing >75 PCI/yr

ADVANTAGES OF PRIMARY PCI

Higher initial recanalization rates
Reduced risk of intracerebral hemorrhage
Less residual stenosis; less recurrent ischemia or infarction
Usefulness when fibrinolysis contraindicated
Improvement in outcomes with cardiogenic shock

DISADVANTAGES OF PRIMARY PCI (COMPARED WITH FIBRINOLYTIC THERAPY)

Access, advantages restricted to high-volume centers, operators
Longer average time to treatment
Greater dependence on operators for results
Higher system complexity, costs

LBBB = left bundle branch block; MI = myocardial infarction; PCI = percutaneous coronary intervention (includes balloon angioplasty, stenting).

Rx

The relative benefits of primary PTCA or PCI over fibrinolysis are confirmed by a meta-analysis that found a significantly lower mortality rate (4.4% versus 6.5%; odds ratio, 0.66) and lower rates of nonfatal reinfarction (2.9% versus 5.3%; odds ratio, 0.53) and intracerebral hemorrhage with primary PTCA compared with fibrinolysis. [3] PCI yields better outcomes than fibrinolysis across all age groups when it is performed within 1 to 2 hours of presentation to a health care facility.

Currently, a primary PCI strategy may begin with initiation of a glycoprotein (GP) IIb/IIIa inhibitor in the emergency department, together with aspirin and heparin, followed by rapid application of coronary angioplasty with stenting. [5] Whether the addition of a reduced dose of a plasminogen activator to GPIIb/IIIa therapy in the field or emergency department could further improve outcomes in selected patients who undergo early PCI without compromising safety is not conclusively resolved but appears doubtful (except possibly in selected patient subgroups), and this approach is not generally recommended. [6, 7]

Operator and institutional experience is an issue more important to outcomes with primary PCI than fibrinolysis and has been incorporated into current recommendations (see Table 72–7). Primary PCI is feasible in community hospitals without surgical capability, but concerns about timing and safety remain. Current guidelines allow that primary PCI "might be considered" in hospitals without on-site cardiac surgery, provided (1) there is a proven plan for rapid and safe transport to a nearby hospital with cardiac surgery capability and availability, and (2) the PCI is done by a skilled operator (≥75 PCIs/year) in a hospital with adequate experience (≥36 primary PCIs/year).

Mechanical reperfusion, primarily with stenting and abciximab, for patients presenting more than 12 but less than 48 hours after the onset of symptoms, also can reduce infarct size and perhaps adverse events. [8] Extending PCI to ST segment elevation MI beyond 12 hours deserves further testing in larger studies.

An additional important indication is cardiogenic shock occurring within 36 hours of the onset of acute MI and treated within 18 hours of the onset of shock. [9] However, benefit was not established for patients older than 75 years of age, and benefit was greater with earlier PCI.

Rx

Selecting a Recanalization Regimen

Whether to use PCI or fibrinolytic therapy depends on local resources and experience, as well as on patient factors. Outcomes appear to be determined both by timing and by institutional and operator experience. In general, in experienced facilities (≥200 PCIs/center; surgical capability; ≥75 PCIs/operator annually; frequent primary PCI, e.g., ≥36/year/center; ≥four/operator/year) that are able to mobilize and treat patients quickly (<90 minutes to balloon inflation), primary PCI is considered the preferred strategy, with stenting preferred over balloon PTCA. PCI is particularly preferred for patients at higher risk for mortality (including shock), for later presentations (>3 hours), and for patients with greater risk of intracerebral hemorrhage (age >70 years, female gender, therapy with hypertensive agents). Ancillary antithrombotic therapy with primary PCI includes aspirin, unfractionated heparin or LMWH, and a GPIIb/IIIa inhibitor (preferably initiated on admission before catheterization). Clopidogrel is begun directly after PCI and is continued after discharge.

For other situations, fibrinolytic therapy becomes the recommended recanalization strategy. If time since the onset of symptoms is within 3 hours and the difference between expected time to PCI and fibrinolytic administration is more than 1 hour, fibrinolysis is often the preferred strategy. Fibrinolysis also is preferred in centers without sufficient PCI experience or capability. In hospitals with long ambulance transport times (>60 to 90 minutes), a strategy for initiating prehospital fibrinolysis may be considered. Very early or prehospital fibrinolysis (followed by an invasive strategy on hospital arrival, i.e., "pharmacoinvasive therapy"), although an appealing concept, appears to cause a *higher* rate of in-hospital mortality, cardiac ischemic events, and strokes compared with primary PCI alone, [10] and its use cannot be recommended as a primary recanalization strategy. Whether fibrinolysis before PCI will be beneficial in selected subgroups with MI, such as patients seen within the first hour of symptoms and with an expected delay to PCI of 2 hours or more, deserves further testing. Currently, however, efforts should be made to provide primary PCI to a larger percentage of patients with acute MI.

The selection of a specific fibrinolytic regimen is based on the risk of complications of the acute MI, the risk of intracerebral hemorrhage, and a consideration of economic constraints. Using these factors, longer-acting variants of t-PA (i.e., tenecteplase and reteplase) have become dominant in the United States and other affluent medical markets; in other countries, less costly streptokinase is still widely used. A nonimmunogenic fibrinolytic agent is preferred for patients with a history of prior streptokinase use. Streptokinase has a lower risk of intracerebral hemorrhage than other regimens if excessive heparin is avoided. Tenecteplase combined with enoxaparin was more effective than tenecteplase with standard heparin or with a GPIIb/IIIa inhibitor (abciximab) and heparin in one but not another trial. Reteplase with abciximab showed no mortality advantage when combined (in half-dose) with abciximab than with heparin alone; ischemic events decreased, but intracerebral hemorrhage increased, especially in elderly patients. Over the past decade, the application of recanalization therapy has remained relatively constant in the United States and other Western countries at 70 to 75% of "eligible" patients with acute MI. Primary PCI use has increased (31% of time-eligible patients in one recent international study), although fibrinolytic therapy continues to be more commonly applied (45% of eligible patients).

Ancillary and Other Therapies

Antiplatelet Therapy

Aspirin

Platelets form a critical component of coronary thrombi. Aspirin inhibits platelet aggregation by irreversibly blocking cyclooxygenase 1 activity by selective acetylation of serine at position 530. Cyclooxygenase 1 catalyzes the conversion of arachidonic acid to thromboxane-A_2, a potent platelet aggregator (Chapter 34).

Rx

Aspirin has been extensively tested to prevent coronary heart disease (Chapter 35). Aspirin trials in ST segment elevation acute MI have been more limited but positive. The most important trial of aspirin in ST segment elevation acute MI randomized more than 17,000 patients with "suspected acute MI" (representing mostly, but not entirely, ST segment elevation acute MI) to aspirin or control and to intravenous streptokinase or control. At 5 weeks, the relative risk of vascular death was reduced 21% by aspirin alone, 25% by streptokinase alone, and 40% by aspirin in combination with streptokinase. Since that time, aspirin has been included as standard therapy in most treatment regimens for ST segment elevation acute MI.

Current guidelines strongly recommend aspirin (class I indication) on admission in a dose of 162 to 325 mg, preferably chewed. Aspirin administration is continued throughout hospitalization and then indefinitely in a maintenance dose of 75 to 162 mg/day on an outpatient basis (enteric-coated forms are popular).

Adenosine Diphosphate Receptor Antagonists

The thienopyridine clopidogrel exerts potent antiplatelet effects by blocking the platelet membrane adenosine diphosphate receptor (Chapter 35). For patients allergic to aspirin, clopidogrel has become the alternative of choice for short- and long-term therapy of ST segment elevation acute MI. A single loading dose of 300 mg is given (600 mg has been successfully tested in recent trials to achieve earlier onset of platelet inhibition, i.e., within 1 to 2 hours, if needed). The maintenance dose is 75 mg/day.

In patients who can take aspirin, the addition of clopidogrel (300 mg followed by 75 mg/day) to aspirin and fibrinolytic therapy in patients 75 years of age or younger reduces predischarge occlusion rates of infarct-related arteries (by 41%) and reduces ischemic complications at 30 days (by 20%) without increasing rates of intracerebral hemorrhage. [11] When given without a loading dose but also without an upper age restriction, clopidogrel reduces 15-day ischemic complications by 9% and death from any cause by 7%. [12] Hence, clopidogrel appears to represent a beneficial initial adjunctive therapy in patients with ST segment elevation MI who are treated with fibrinolytic agents. However, clopidogrel increases the risk of bleeding with coronary artery bypass grafting (CABG), so it is commonly initiated only after coronary angiography has been performed and early surgery has been excluded as a therapeutic choice; if CABG is planned, clopidogrel should be withheld for 5 to 7 days unless the urgency of surgery outweighs the risk of excessive bleeding.

Clopidogrel added to aspirin on admission for patients with non–ST segment elevation acute MI or unstable angina (Chapter 71) or after a PCI reduces vascular events (by 22%) at 3 to 12 months compared with aspirin alone. Extrapolation of these findings led to the recommendations that clopidogrel be used for 3 to 12 months as an alternative antiplatelet agent in patients with ST segment elevation acute MI when aspirin is contraindicated and that it be considered routinely (in addition to aspirin) in patients after primary PCI.

Glycoprotein IIB/IIIA Inhibitors

Inhibitors of the platelet membrane GPIIb/IIIa receptor, a fibrinogen receptor, have been shown to benefit high-risk patients with non–ST segment elevation acute coronary syndrome (Chapters 35 and 71) on admission or after PCI. The benefit in ST segment elevation MI is smaller when routine stenting is used and when GPIIb/IIIa therapy is administered only in the catheterization laboratory. Earlier ("upstream") GP inhibition before hospital admission or in the emergency department (precatheterization) is effective in improving coronary patency by the time of emergency angiography and, possibly, clinical outcomes, although data from clinical trials are limited for ST segment elevation MI. [13] If early CABG is a possibility after angiography, a shorter-acting inhibitor (eptifibatide, tirofiban) may impart a lower perioperative risk of bleeding than abciximab. For patients with ST segment elevation acute MI who are treated with fibrinolysis, a GPIIb/IIIa inhibitor added to reduced-dose t-PA (e.g., half-dose t-PA) improves early coronary patency. However, improved survival has not been shown, and the risk of serious bleeding (including intracerebral hemorrhage) is increased. [6, 7]

Rx

Antithrombin Therapy

Unfractionated Heparin

On injection, heparin complexes with antithrombin III. The heparin–antithrombin III complex inactivates circulating thrombin and, less effectively, factor X. Clot-bound thrombin is resistant. Evidence for the contribution of heparin to antithrombotic regimens is mostly observational, indirect, or inferential (Chapter 35).

Heparin is recommended for patients undergoing primary PCI and for those receiving fibrin-specific lytic agents (i.e., alteplase, reteplase, or tenecteplase; see Fig. 72–3 and Table 72–4). It is also recommended with intravenous streptokinase or anistreplase for patients at high risk for systemic emboli (e.g., large or anterior acute MI with LV thrombus, atrial fibrillation [AF]). Low-dose subcutaneous heparin (7500 to 12,500 U twice daily) was recommended in the past for patients with acute MI, to prevent deep vein thrombosis in the absence of intravenous heparin; however, current early reambulation after acute MI and routine use of aspirin have made the utility of *routine* subcutaneous heparin uncertain.

Excessive bleeding when heparin is used in combination with antithrombotic regimens has led to reductions in heparin doses, with improved safety. When given with a fibrinolytic, intravenous heparin is begun concurrently and is given for 48 hours. Currently recommended doses include a 60 U/kg bolus (maximum, 4000 U), followed initially by a 12 U/kg/hour infusion (maximum, 1000 U/hour), with adjustment after 3 hours based on activated partial thromboplastin time (target of 50 to 70 seconds, 1.5 to 2 times control). Experimental regimens including a GPIIb/IIIa inhibitor and a fibrinolytic agent have used even lower heparin doses. During primary PCI, high-dose heparin is used (activated clotting time, 300 to 350 seconds). Given together with a GPIIb/IIIa inhibitor during PCI, the dose of heparin is adjusted to a lower activated clotting time range (150 to 300 seconds).

Low-Molecular-Weight Heparins and Factor Xa Inhibitors

LMWHs have enhanced inhibitory activity for factor Xa (Chapter 35). They also have more reliable bioavailability and longer durations of action, thus permitting subcutaneous administration once or twice daily in fixed (weight-adjusted) doses. LMWHs have been extensively tested for the non–ST segment elevation acute coronary syndromes and for prophylaxis of deep vein thrombosis. Evidence suggests that in patients with ST segment elevation acute MI who are treated with fibrinolytic therapy, LMWH can improve angiographic outcomes and can reduce reinfarction rates by 25% and mortality by about 10%. For example, in the largest trial of 20,506 patients, enoxaparin, given throughout the index hospitalization, reduced the composite outcome of death or nonfatal reinfarction at 30 days from 12.0 to 9.9%, compared with unfractionated heparin. [14] Enoxaparin may thus be preferred over unfractionated heparin as an antithrombotic agent for ST segment elevation acute MI in most patients treated with a fibrinolysis strategy. When used as ancillary therapy with a fibrinolytic agent, enoxaparin may be given to patients less than 75 years old who do not have renal insufficiency as a 30-mg intravenous bolus, followed by 1 mg/kg subcutaneously twice daily until hospital discharge, and to those 75 years and older as 0.75 mg/kg subcutaneously twice daily without a bolus.

Selective factor Xa inhibitors (e.g., fondaparinux, 2.5 mg once daily for up to 8 days during index hospitalization) reduce the end point of death or reinfarction at 30 days by 18 to 23% independent of heparin use in patients who receive fibrinolysis or no recanalization therapy but have no benefit in patients who have undergone PCI. [15] These results suggest that fondaparinux may be a preferred alternative to unfractionated heparin or no heparin (e.g., in patients who present later, in patients treated with streptokinase) in patients with ST segment elevation MI who are not undergoing a primary PCI strategy.

Direct Antithrombins

Direct-acting antithrombins, such as hirudin and its analogues (e.g., bivalirudin), do not require antithrombin III for activity; they inhibit clot-bound heparin and are not neutralized by plasma proteins (Chapter 35). Unlike heparin, hirudins do not induce thrombocytopenia. Early studies using surrogate end points were promising. However, bleeding and optimal dose administration were problematic, and major clinical trials did not show a survival advantage. Bivalirudin is clinically available and is considered a useful alternative to unfractionated heparin for patients with known heparin-induced thrombocytopenia who are receiving streptokinase. Bivalirudin has had limited experience as an adjunct to primary PCI.

Other Pharmacologic Therapies

Nitrates

Nitroglycerin and other organic nitrates (isosorbide dinitrate and isosorbide mononitrate) induce vascular smooth muscle relaxation by generating vascular endothelial nitric oxide. The resulting vasodilation of veins and peripheral and coronary arteries can beneficially reduce excessive cardiac preload and afterload, increase coronary caliber in responsive areas of stenosis, reverse distal small coronary arterial vasoconstriction, improve coronary collateral flow to ischemic myocardium, and inhibit platelet aggregation in acute MI (Chapter 70). The results are improved oxygen delivery and reduced oxygen consumption. Potential clinical benefits include relief of ischemia, limitation of infarct size, prevention of dilative remodeling, control of hypertension (afterload), and relief of congestion (preload).

In the era before reperfusion, nitrates appeared to confer a mortality benefit in acute MI. In the context of fibrinolytic therapy and aspirin, however, mortality benefits are modest, with a relative survival benefit of about four lives saved per 1000 treated. [16] Nitroglycerin is definitely recommended for the first 24 to 48 hours for patients with acute MI and pulmonary congestion, large anterior MI, persistent ischemia, or hypertension. For other patients without contraindications, nitrates are possibly useful.

When nitrates are clearly indicated early in acute MI, intravenous nitroglycerin is preferred. Intravenous nitroglycerin may begin with a bolus injection of 12.5 to 25 μg followed by an infusion of 10 to 20 μg/minute. The infusion dose is increased by 5 to 10 μg every 5 to 10 minutes up to about 200 μg/minute during hemodynamic monitoring until clinical symptoms are controlled or blood pressure targets are reached (blood pressure decreased by 10% in normotensive patients or by 30% in hypertensive patients but not less than 80 mm Hg mean or 90 mm Hg systolic).

β-Blockers

β-Adrenoceptor blockers reduce heart rate, blood pressure, and myocardial contractility, and they stabilize the heart electrically. These actions provide clinical benefit to most patients with acute MI by limiting myocardial oxygen consumption, relieving ischemia, reducing infarct size, and preventing serious arrhythmias.

In the era before fibrinolysis, a meta-analysis of 28 randomized trials involving 27,500 patients found a modest early benefit on mortality (14% odds reduction), cardiac arrest (16% reduction), and nonfatal reinfarction (19% reduction). In patients with acute MI who are receiving fibrinolytic therapy, immediate (intravenous then oral) metoprolol reduces recurrent ischemic events and reinfarction compared with deferred oral therapy. Further experience has shown that moderate to severe heart failure should preclude the early use of intravenous β-blockers, but not predischarge and outpatient oral therapy initiated in small doses and carefully adjusted once stability is achieved.

Early (first-day) initiation of oral β-blockade is generally recommended for patients with acute MI who have ongoing or recurrent ischemic pain or tachyarrhythmias if they do not have heart failure or other contraindications (asthma, hypotension, severe bradycardia), regardless of concomitant fibrinolysis or PCI. Intravenous initiation (e.g., metoprolol, 5 mg over 2 minutes to a total of 15 mg over 10 to 15 minutes, or atenolol, 2.5 to 5 mg over 2 minutes to a total of 10 mg over 10 to 15 minutes) is reasonable in the absence of contraindications if an indication for immediate therapy is present, such as a tachyarrhythmia or hypertension. However, the routine, short-term initiation of intravenous β-blockade should be avoided because it is not associated with benefit and, indeed, causes a small excess of early death from cardiogenic shock, primarily in patients with preexisting heart failure. [12] All patients without contraindications or intolerance to β-blocker therapy should receive oral doses, titrated to tolerance or goal (e.g., metoprolol, 25 to 100 mg twice daily, atenolol, 50 to 100 mg/day, or carvedilol, 6.25 to 25 mg twice daily). β-Blocker therapy should begin promptly, in the absence of heart failure and if not otherwise contraindicated, and should be continued during the in-hospital convalescent phase of ST segment elevation MI and beyond.

Renin-Angiotensin-Aldosterone System Inhibitors

The renin-angiotensin-aldosterone system is activated in acute MI and heart failure. Use of an ACE inhibitor has been shown to improve remodeling after acute MI (especially after large anterior MI). ACE inhibitors also have demonstrated efficacy in heart failure, wherein they prevent disease progression, hospitalization, and death (Chapter 58). A meta-analysis of three major trials and 11 smaller ones involving more than 100,000 patients showed an overall mortality reduction of 6.5%, representing about five lives saved per 1000 patients treated. Benefit is concentrated and greater in higher-risk patients with large or anterior MI and with LV dysfunction or heart failure, [16] although patients with lesser degrees of LV dysfunction and only moderate cardiovascular risk can also benefit in the long term. [17]

Oral *ACE inhibitor therapy* should begin within the first 24 hours in patients with anterior infarction, pulmonary congestion, or low ejection fraction (<0.40) in the absence of hypotension (systolic pressure <100 mm Hg or >30 mm Hg less than usual baseline) or known contraindications. An *angiotensin receptor blocker* (ARB) should be given to otherwise qualifying patients who are intolerant of ACE inhibitors. An ACE inhibitor or an ARB also should be considered for other patients with ST segment elevation MI, especially those with a relative indication (e.g., hypertension, diabetes, or mild renal insufficiency), with the expectation of a smaller but worthwhile benefit. All patients without contraindications or intolerance to initial ACE inhibitor or ARB therapy also should receive these drugs during the in-hospital convalescent phase. ACE inhibitor therapy should begin with low oral doses and should be progressively adjusted to full dose as tolerated. For example, the short-acting agent captopril may be started in a dose of 6.25 mg or less and adjusted over 1 to 2 days to 50 mg twice daily. Before discharge, a transition may be made in graded dose schedules to longer-acting agents such as ramipril (2.5 mg titrated to 10 mg/day), lisinopril (2.5 to 5 mg titrated to 10 mg/day), or enalapril (2.5 mg, titrated to up to 20 mg twice daily). In patients who cannot tolerate ACE inhibitors (e.g., because of cough), graded doses of an ARB may be substituted (e.g., valsartan, 80 to 160 mg twice daily, or losartan, 50 to 100 mg/day).

Selective *aldosterone receptor blockade* with eplerenone (25 to 50 mg/day) reduces total and cardiovascular mortality (including sudden death) as well as cardiovascular hospitalizations in post-MI who have an ejection fraction of 0.40 or less and heart failure or diabetes and who are already receiving other optimal therapies, including ACE inhibitors. [18] Spironolactone also benefits patients with advanced heart failure, including those in whom it is caused by a remote MI. Hence, aldosterone receptor blockade should be added to other standard therapies during convalescence in patients with these characteristics. Hyperkalemia, which is the most common side effect, requires monitoring (Chapter 58).

Antiarrhythmic Agents

Antiarrhythmic therapy is reserved for treatment of, or short-term prevention after, symptomatic or life-threatening ventricular arrhythmias, together with other appropriate measures (cardioversion, treatment of ischemia and metabolic disturbances). An implantable cardioverter-defibrillator (ICD) is indicated in patients with VF or hemodynamically significant sustained ventricular tachycardia (VT) occurring more than 2 days after ST segment elevation MI or in patients with inducible VT or VF at electrophysiologic study and a depressed ejection fraction (≤0.40) at least 1 month after ST segment elevation MI (Chapter 64). An ICD also may be considered for patients with severe LV dysfunction (ejection fraction ≤0.30) at least 1 month after ST segment elevation MI and 3 months after CABG without spontaneous or induced VT or VF [21] (Chapter 65).

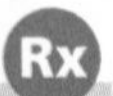

Inotropes

Digitalis and intravenous inotropes can increase oxygen demand, provoke serious arrhythmias, and extend infarction. Current recommendations support the use of digoxin in selected patients recovering from acute MI who develop supraventricular tachyarrhythmias (e.g., AF) or heart failure refractory to ACE inhibitors and diuretics. Intravenous inotropes (e.g., dobutamine, dopamine, milrinone, and norepinephrine) are reserved for temporary support of patients with hypotension and circulatory failure that is unresponsive to volume replacement (Chapters 58 and 108). Other treatment measures for these patients (e.g., intra-aortic balloon pump, early revascularization) are discussed herein.

Lipid-Lowering Therapy

Lipid lowering, particularly with hydroxymethylglutaryl-coenzyme A reductase inhibitors (statins), reduces event rates in patients with coronary disease, and a more aggressive approach appears to provide superior benefits [19] (Chapter 217). A fasting lipid profile should be obtained on admission, so a statin can be started promptly in the hospital with a low-density lipoprotein cholesterol goal of less than 70 mg/dL.

Other Medical Therapies

Calcium channel blockers, although anti-ischemic, also are negatively inotropic and have not been shown to reduce mortality after ST segment elevation acute MI. With certain agents and in specific groups of patient, harm has been suggested. For example, short-acting nifedipine has been reported to cause reflex sympathetic activation, tachycardia, hypotension, and increased mortality. Verapamil or diltiazem (heart rate–slowing drugs) may be given to patients in whom β-blockers are ineffective or contraindicated for control of rapid ventricular response with AF or relief of ongoing ischemia *in the absence of heart failure, LV dysfunction, or atrioventricular (AV) block.*

Magnesium is of no benefit in patients with acute MI who are treated with fibrinolysis. Supplementation is recommended if the magnesium level is lower than normal or in patients with torsades de pointes–type VT associated with a prolonged QT interval.

Glucose-insulin-potassium affords no benefit on mortality, cardiac arrest, or cardiogenic shock when this combination is added to usual care in patients with acute ST segment elevation MI. [20] However, *glucose control,* using an insulin infusion to normalize high blood glucose, is recommended for patients in the acute phase of ST segment elevation MI, especially for those with a complicated course. After the acute phase, individualized treatment is indicated using agents or combinations of agents that best achieve glycemic control and are well tolerated (Chapters 247 and 248).

Management of Complications

Recurrent Chest Pain

When chest pain recurs after acute MI, the diagnostic possibilities include post-infarction ischemia, pericarditis, infarct extension, and infarct expansion. Characterization of the pain, physical examination, ECG, echocardiography, and cardiac marker determinations assist in differential diagnosis. CK-MB often discriminates reinfarction better than cTnI or cTnT.

Post-infarction angina developing spontaneously during hospitalization for acute MI despite medical therapy usually merits coronary angiography. β-blockers (IV, then orally) and nitroglycerin (IV, then orally or topically) are recommended medical therapies. Pain with recurrent ST segment elevation or recurrent elevation of cardiac markers may be treated with (re)administration of t-PA or, possibly, a GPIIb/IIIa inhibitor, together with nitroglycerin, β-blockade, and heparin. Streptokinase, which induces neutralizing antibodies, generally should not be reutilized after the first few days. If facilities for angiography, PCI, and surgery are available, an invasive approach is recommended to relieve discomfort occurring hours to days after an acute MI that is associated with objective signs of ischemia. Radionuclide testing (e.g., adenosine thallium) can be helpful in patients with discomfort that is transient or of uncertain ischemic origin.

Infarct expansion implies circumferential slippage with thinning of the infarcted myocardium. Infarct expansion can be associated with chest pain but without recurrent elevation of cardiac markers. Expansive remodeling can lead to an LV aneurysm. The risk of remodeling is reduced with early recanalization therapy and administration of ACE inhibitors.

Acute pericarditis most commonly manifests on days 2 to 4 in association with large, "transmural" infarctions causing pericardial inflammation. Occasionally, hemorrhagic effusion with tamponade develops; thus, excessive anticoagulation should be avoided. Pericarditis developing later (2 to 10 weeks) after acute MI could represent Dressler's syndrome, which is believed to be immune mediated. The incidence of this post-MI syndrome has decreased dramatically in the modern reperfusion era. Pericardial pain is treated with aspirin (preferred, especially in the acute setting) or other nonsteroidal agents (e.g., indomethacin); patients with severe symptoms could require corticosteroids.

Rhythm Disturbances

Ventricular Arrhythmias

Acute MI is associated with a proarrhythmic environment that includes heterogeneous myocardial ischemia, heightened adrenergic tone, intracellular electrolyte disturbance, lipolysis and free fatty acid production, and oxygen free radical production on recanalization (Chapters 62 and 64). Arrhythmias thus are common early during acute MI. Micro-re-entry is likely the most common electrophysiologic mechanism of early phase arrhythmias, although enhanced automaticity and triggered activity also are observed in experimental models.

Primary VF, the most serious MI-related arrhythmia, contributes importantly to mortality within the first 24 hours. It occurs with an incidence of 3 to 5% during the first 4 hours and then declines rapidly over 24 to 48 hours. Polymorphic VT and, less commonly, monomorphic VT are associated life-threatening arrhythmias that can occur in this setting. Clinical features (including warning arrhythmias) are not adequately specific or sensitive to identify patients at risk for sustained ventricular tachyarrhythmias, so all patients should be continuously monitored. Prophylactic lidocaine, which reduces primary VF but does not decrease (and may increase) mortality, is not recommended. Primary VF is associated with a higher rate of in-hospital mortality, but long-term prognosis is unaffected in survivors.

Accelerated idioventricular rhythm (60 to 100 beats per minute) frequently occurs within the first 12 hours and is generally benign (i.e., is not a risk factor for VF). Indeed, accelerated idioventricular rhythm frequently heralds recanalization after fibrinolytic therapy. Antiarrhythmic therapy is not indicated except for sustained, hemodynamically compromising accelerated idioventricular rhythm.

Late VF, which is defined as VF developing more than 48 hours after the onset of acute MI, often occurs in patients with larger MIs or heart failure, portends a worse prognosis for survival, and is an indication for aggressive measures (e.g., consideration of an ICD). Monomorphic VT resulting from re-entry in the context of a recent or old MI also can appear late after MI, and patients may require long-term therapy (e.g., an ICD).

Electrical cardioversion is required for VF and sustained polymorphic VT (unsynchronized shock) and for sustained monomorphic VT that causes hemodynamic compromise (synchronized shock) (Chapters 62 and 65). Brief intravenous sedation is given to conscious, "stable" patients. For slower, stable VT and nonsustained VT requiring therapy, intravenous amiodarone or intravenous lidocaine is commonly recommended. After episodes of VT/VF, infusions of antiarrhythmic drugs may be given for 6 to 24 hours; the ongoing risk of arrhythmia then is reassessed. Electrolyte and acid-base imbalance and hypoxia should be corrected. β-Blockade is useful in patients with frequent polymorphic VT associated with adrenergic activation ("electrical storm"). Additional, aggressive measures should be considered to reduce cardiac ischemia (e.g., emergency PCI or CABG) and LV dysfunction (intra-aortic balloon pump) in

Rx

patients with recurrent polymorphic VT despite the use of β-blockers and/or amiodarone.

Patients with sustained VT or VF occurring late in the hospital course should be considered for long-term prevention and therapy. An ICD provides greater survival benefit than antiarrhythmic drugs in patients with ventricular arrhythmias and can improve survival after acute MI for patients with an ejection fraction of 30% or less, regardless of their rhythm status. 21

Atrial Fibrillation and other Supraventricular Tachyarrhythmias

AF occurs in up to 10 to 15% of patients after an acute MI, usually within the first 24 hours (Chapter 63). The incidence of atrial flutter or another supraventricular tachycardia is much lower. The risk of AF increases with age, larger MIs, heart failure, pericarditis, atrial infarction, hypokalemia, hypomagnesemia, hypoxia, pulmonary disease, and hyperadrenergic states. The incidence of AF is reduced by effective early recanalization. Hemodynamic compromise with rapid rates and systemic embolism (in ~2%) are adverse consequences of AF. Systemic embolism can occur on the first day, so prompt anticoagulation with heparin is indicated.

Recommendations for management of AF include the following: electrical cardioversion for patients with severe hemodynamic compromise or ischemia; rate control with intravenous digoxin for patients with ventricular dysfunction (i.e., give 1.0 mg, one half initially and one half in 4 hours), with an intravenous β-blocker (e.g., metoprolol, 5 mg over 2 minutes to a total of 15 mg over 10 to 15 minutes) in those without clinical ventricular dysfunction, or with intravenous diltiazem or verapamil in hemodynamically compensated patients with a contraindication to β-blockers; and anticoagulation with heparin (or LMWH). Amiodarone, which is generally reserved for patients with or at high risk for recurrence, may be continued for 6 weeks if sinus rhythm is restored and maintained.

Bradycardias, Conduction Delays, and Heart Block

Sinus and AV nodal dysfunction are common during acute MI. Sinus bradycardia, a result of increased parasympathetic tone often in association with inferior acute MI, occurs in 30 to 40% of patients. Sinus bradycardia is particularly common during the first hour of acute MI and with recanalization of the right coronary artery (Bezold-Jarisch reflex). Vagally mediated AV block also can occur in this setting. Anticholinergic therapy (atropine, 0.5 to 1.5 mg IV) is indicated for *symptomatic* sinus bradycardia (heart rate generally <50 beats per minute associated with hypotension, ischemia, or escape ventricular arrhythmia), including ventricular asystole, and *symptomatic* second-degree (Wenckebach) or third-degree block at the AV nodal level (narrow QRS complex escape rhythm). Atropine is not indicated and can worsen infranodal AV block (anterior MI, wide complex escape rhythm).

New-onset infranodal AV block and intraventricular conduction delays or BBBs predict substantially increased in-hospital mortality. Fortunately, their incidence has declined in the recanalization era (from 10 to 20% to ~4%). Mortality is related more to extensive myocardial damage than to heart block itself, so cardiac pacing only modestly improves survival. Prophylactic placement of multifunctional patch electrodes, which allow for immediate transcutaneous pacing (and defibrillation) if needed, is indicated for symptomatic sinus bradycardia refractory to drug therapy, infranodal second-degree (Mobitz II) or third-degree AV block, and new or indeterminate-age bifascicular (LBBB; RBBB with left anterior or left posterior fascicular block) or trifascicular block (bilateral or alternating BBB [any age], BBB with first-degree AV block). Transcutaneous pacing is uncomfortable and is intended for prophylactic and temporary use only. In patients who require a pacemaker to maintain a rhythm or who are at very high risk (>30%) of requiring pacing (including patients with alternating, bilateral BBB, with new or indeterminate-age bifascicular block with first-degree AV block, and with infranodal second-degree AV block) should have a transvenous pacing electrode inserted as soon as possible.

Indications for permanent pacing after acute MI depend on the prognosis of the AV block and not solely on symptoms. Class I indications include even transient second- or third-degree AV block in association with BBB and symptomatic AV block at any level. Advanced block at the AV nodal level (Wenckebach) rarely is persistent or symptomatic enough to warrant permanent pacing.

Heart Failure and Other Low-Output States

Cardiac pump failure is the leading cause of circulatory failure and in-hospital death from acute MI. Manifestations of circulatory failure can include a weak pulse, low blood pressure, cool extremities, a third heart sound, pulmonary congestion, oliguria, and obtundation. However, several distinct mechanisms, hemodynamic patterns, and clinical syndromes characterize the spectrum of circulatory failure in acute MI. Each requires a specific approach to diagnosis, monitoring, and therapy (see Table 72–3).

Left Ventricular Dysfunction

The degree of LV dysfunction correlates well with the extent of acute ischemia or infarction. Hemodynamic compromise becomes evident when impairment involves 20 to 25% of the left ventricle, and cardiogenic shock or death occurs with involvement of 40% or more (Chapter 108). Pulmonary congestion and S_3 and S_4 gallops are the most common physical findings. Early recanalization (with fibrinolytic agents, PCI, or CABG) is the most effective therapy to reduce infarct size, ventricular dysfunction, and associated heart failure. Medical treatment of heart failure related to the ventricular dysfunction of acute MI is otherwise generally similar to that of heart failure in other settings (Chapter 58) and includes adequate oxygenation and diuresis (begun early, blood pressure permitting, and continued on a long-term basis if needed). Morphine sulfate (i.e., 2 to 4 mg IV, with increments as needed after 5 to 15 minutes or more) is useful for patients with pulmonary congestion. Nitroglycerin also reduces preload and effectively relieves congestive symptoms. Titrated oral ACE inhibitor therapy (e.g., captopril, incremented from 3.125 to 6.25 mg three times daily to 50 mg twice daily as tolerated) also is indicated for heart failure and pulmonary edema unless excessive hypotension (systolic blood pressure <100 mm Hg) is present. Treatment can be begun sublingually (0.4 mg every 5 minutes three times), and then the transition can be made to intravenous therapy (initially 5 to 10 μg/minute, incrementing by 5 to 20 μg/minute until symptoms are relieved or until mean arterial pressure falls by 10% in normotensive or 30% in hypertensive patients but not <90 mm Hg or >30 mm Hg lower than baseline). Intravenous vasodilator therapy to reduce preload and afterload, inotropic support, and intra-aortic balloon counterpulsation (IABP), together with urgent recanalization, are indicated in cardiogenic shock (Chapter 108).

Volume Depletion

Relative or absolute hypovolemia is a frequent cause of hypotension and circulatory failure and is easily corrected if it is recognized and treated promptly. Poor hydration, vomiting, diuresis, and disease- or drug-induced peripheral vasodilation can contribute to this condition. Hypovolemia should be identified and corrected with intravenous fluids before more aggressive therapies are considered. An empirical fluid challenge may be tried in the appropriate clinical setting (e.g., for hypotension in the absence of congestion, for inferior or RV infarction, and for hypervagotonia). If filling pressures are measured, cautious fluid administration to a pulmonary capillary wedge pressure of up to about 18 mm Hg may optimize cardiac output and blood pressure without impairing oxygenation.

Right Ventricular Infarction

RV ischemia and infarction occur with proximal occlusion of the right coronary artery (before the take-off of the RV branches). Ten to 15% of inferior acute ST segment elevation MIs show classic hemodynamic features, and these patients form the highest risk subgroup for morbidity and mortality (25 to 30% versus <6% hospital mortality). Improvement in RV function commonly occurs over time, a finding suggesting reversal of ischemic stunning and other favorable accommodations, if short-term management is successful.

Hypotension in patients with clear lung fields and elevated jugular venous pressure in the setting of inferior or inferoposterior acute MI should raise the suspicion of RV infarction. Kussmaul's sign (dis-

Rx

tention of the jugular vein on inspiration) is relatively specific and sensitive in this setting. Right-sided ECG leads show ST segment elevation, particularly in V_{4R} (Chapter 52), in the first 24 hours of RV infarction. Echocardiography is helpful in confirming the diagnosis (RV dilation and dysfunction are observed). When right-sided heart pressures are measured, a right atrial pressure of 10 mm Hg or greater and 80% or more of the pulmonary capillary wedge pressure are relatively sensitive and specific for RV ischemic dysfunction.

Management of RV infarction consists of early maintenance of RV preload with intravenous fluids, reduction of RV afterload (i.e., afterload-only reducing drugs as for LV dysfunction; consider intra-aortic balloon pump), early recanalization, short-term inotropic support if needed, and avoidance of venodilators (e.g., nitrates) and diuretics used for LV failure (they may cause marked hypotension). Volume loading with normal saline solution alone is often effective. If the cardiac output fails to improve after 0.5 to 1 L fluid, inotropic support with intravenous dobutamine (starting at 2 μg/kg/minute and titrating to hemodynamic effect or tolerance, up to 20 μg/kg/minute) is recommended. High-grade AV block is common, and restoration of AV synchrony with temporary AV sequential pacing can lead to substantial improvement in cardiac output. The onset of AF (in up to one third of RV infarcts) can cause severe hemodynamic compromise requiring prompt cardioversion. Early coronary recanalization with fibrinolysis or PCI markedly improves outcomes.

Cardiogenic Shock

Cardiogenic shock (Chapter 108) is a form of severe LV failure characterized by marked hypotension (systolic pressures <80 mm Hg) and reductions in cardiac index (to <1.8 L/minute/m^2) despite high LV filling pressure (pulmonary capillary wedge pressure >18 mm Hg). The cause is loss of a critical functional mass (>40%) of the left ventricle. Cardiogenic shock is associated with mortality rates of more than 70 to 80% despite aggressive medical therapy. Risk factors include age, large (usually anterior) acute MI, previous MI, and diabetes. In patients with suspected shock, hemodynamic monitoring and IABP are indicated. Intubation often is necessary. Vasopressors are often needed. Early urgent mechanical revascularization (PCI or CABG), if feasible, affords the best chance for survival, especially in patients less than 75 years old [9] (Chapter 108).

IABP remains useful for patients with medically refractory unstable ischemic syndromes and for cardiogenic shock. The deflated balloon catheter is introduced into the femoral artery and is advanced into the aorta. The ECG triggers balloon inflation during early diastole, thereby augmenting coronary blood flow; deflation then occurs in early systole, thereby reducing LV afterload. Primary IABP therapy for cardiogenic shock associated with acute MI provides temporary stabilization but does not reduce mortality (>80%). IABP is currently recommended in the setting of acute MI as a stabilizing measure for patients undergoing angiography and subsequent PCI or surgery for (1) cardiogenic shock, (2) mechanical complications (acute mitral regurgitation, acute ventricular septal defect), (3) refractory post-MI ischemia, or (4) recurrent intractable VT or VF associated with hemodynamic instability. IABP is not useful in patients with significant aortic insufficiency or severe peripheral vascular disease.

Mechanical Complications

Mechanical complications usually occur within the first weeks and account for approximately 15% of MI-related deaths. Such complications include acute mitral valve regurgitation, ventricular septal defect, free wall rupture, and LV aneurysm. Suspicion and investigation of a mechanical defect should be prompted by a new murmur and/or sudden, progressive hemodynamic deterioration with pulmonary edema and/or a low output state. Transthoracic or transesophageal Doppler echocardiography usually establishes the diagnosis. A balloon flotation catheter can be helpful in confirming the diagnosis. Arteriography to identify correctable coronary artery disease is warranted in most cases. Surgical consultation should be requested promptly, and urgent repair is usually indicated.

Acute mitral valve regurgitation (Chapter 75) results from infarct-related rupture or dysfunction of a papillary muscle. Total rupture leads to death in 75% of patients within 24 hours. Medical therapy is initiated with nitroprusside (beginning with 0.1 μg/kg/minute and titrating upward every 3 to 5 minutes to the desired effect, as tolerated by blood pressure response, up to 5 μg/kg/minute), to lower preload and to improve peripheral perfusion, and inotropic support (e.g., dobutamine, titrated from 2 up to 20 μg/kg/minute in normotensive patients; dopamine, titrated from 2 up to 20 μg/kg/minute in hypotensive patients; or combined dobutamine and dopamine). An IABP is used to maintain hemodynamic stability. Emergency surgical repair (if possible) or replacement is then undertaken. Surgery is associated with high mortality (≥25 to 50%), but it leads to better functional and survival outcomes than medical therapy alone.

Post-infarction septal rupture with *ventricular septal defect,* which occurs with increased frequency in elderly patients, in patients with hypertension, and possibly after fibrinolysis, also warrants urgent surgical repair. Because a small post-MI ventricular septal defect can suddenly enlarge and cause rapid hemodynamic collapse, all septal perforations should be repaired. On diagnosis, invasive monitoring is recommended, together with vasodilators (e.g., nitroprusside, initially 0.1 μg/kg/minute, titrated upward every 3 to 5 minutes to desired effect, as tolerated by blood pressure response, up to 5 μg/kg/minute) and, if needed, judicious use of inotropic agents (e.g., dobutamine, titrated from 2 up to 20 μg/kg/minute in normotensive patients; dopamine, titrated from 2 up to 20 μg/kg/minute in hypotensive patients; or combined dobutamine and dopamine). An IABP should be inserted, a surgical consultation promptly obtained, and surgical repair undertaken as soon as feasible.

LV free wall rupture usually causes acute cardiac tamponade with sudden death. In a small percentage of cases, however, resealing or localized containment ("pseudoaneurysm") can allow medical stabilization, usually with inotropic support and/or an IABP, followed by emergency surgical repair.

An *LV aneurysm* can develop after a large, usually anterior, acute MI. If refractory heart failure, VT, or systemic embolization occurs despite medical therapy and PCI, aneurysmectomy with CABG is indicated.

Thromboembolic Complications

Thromboembolism has been described in approximately 10% of clinical series and 20% of autopsy series, a finding suggesting a high rate of undiagnosed events. Thromboembolism contributed to up to 25% of hospital deaths from acute MI in the past, but the incidence has declined in the recanalization era in association with greater use of antithrombotics, reductions of infarct size, and earlier ambulation. Systemic arterial emboli (including cerebrovascular emboli) typically arise from an LV mural thrombus, whereas pulmonary emboli commonly arise from thrombi in leg veins. Arterial embolism can cause dramatic clinical events, such as hemiparesis, loss of a pulse, ischemic bowel, or sudden hypertension, depending on the regional circulation involved.

Mural thrombosis with embolism typically occurs in the setting of a large (especially anterior) ST segment elevation acute MI and heart failure. The risk of embolism is particularly high when a mural thrombus is detected by echocardiography. Thus, in patients with anterior ST segment elevation acute MI and in other high-risk patients, echocardiography should be performed during hospitalization; if results are positive, anticoagulation should be started (with an antithrombin), if not already initiated, and continued (with warfarin) for 6 months.

Deep vein thrombosis can be prevented by lower extremity compression therapy, by limiting the duration of bedrest, and by the use of subcutaneous unfractionated heparin or LMWH (in patients at risk not receiving intravenous heparin) until patients are fully ambulatory (Chapter 81). Patients with pulmonary embolism are treated with intravenous heparin, then oral anticoagulation for 6 months (Chapter 99).

Risk Stratification after Myocardial Infarction

The goal of risk stratification before and early after discharge for acute MI is to assess ventricular and clinical function, latent ischemia,

and arrhythmic risk, to use this information for patient education and prognostic assessment, and to guide therapeutic strategies (see Fig. 72–3).

Cardiac Catheterization and Noninvasive Stress Testing

Risk stratification generally involves functional assessment by one of three strategies: cardiac catheterization, submaximal exercise stress ECG before discharge (at 4 to 6 days), or symptom-limited stress testing at 2 to 6 weeks after discharge. Many or most patients with ST segment elevation acute MI undergo invasive evaluation for primary PCI or after fibrinolytic therapy. Catheterization generally is performed during hospitalization for patients at high risk. In others, predischarge submaximal exercise testing (to peak heart rate of 120 to 130 beats per minute or 70% of the predicted maximum) appears safe when it is performed in patients who are ambulating without symptoms; it should be avoided within 2 to 3 days of acute MI and in patients with unstable post-MI angina, uncompensated heart failure, or serious cardiac arrhythmias. Alternatively or in addition, patients may undergo symptom-limited stress testing at 2 to 6 weeks before they return to work or resume other increased physical activities. Abnormal test results include not only ST segment depression but also low functional capacity, exertional hypotension, and serious arrhythmias. Patients with positive test results should be considered for coronary angiography.

The sensitivity of stress testing can be augmented with radionuclide perfusion imaging (thallium-201 and/or technetium-99m-sestamibi; Chapter 54) or echocardiography (Chapter 53). Supplemental imaging also can quantify the LV ejection fraction and size the area of infarction and/or ischemia (e.g., by cardiac magnetic resonance imaging; Chapter 55). For patients taking digoxin or for those with ST segment changes that preclude accurate ECG interpretation (e.g., baseline LBBB or LV hypertrophy), an imaging study is recommended with initial stress testing. In others, an imaging study may be performed selectively for those in whom the exercise ECG test result is positive or equivocal. For patients unable to exercise, pharmacologic stress testing can be performed using adenosine or dipyridamole scintigraphy or dobutamine echocardiography.

Electrocardiographic Monitoring

Modern telemetry systems capture complete rhythm information during hospital observations and allow for identification of patients with serious arrhythmias, so routine 24- to 48-hour ambulatory ECG (Holter) monitoring before or after hospital discharge is not recommended. Sustained VT or VF occurring late during hospitalization or provoked during electrophysiologic study in patients with nonsustained VT on monitoring are candidates for an ICD, especially if the ejection fraction is less than 40% (Fig. 72–4) (Chapters 64 and 65). Prophylactic ICD placement prevents sudden death after acute MI for patients with severely depressed function (ejection fraction ≤0.30) regardless of the rhythm status. 21

Secondary Prevention, Patient Education, and Rehabilitation

Secondary Prevention

Advances in secondary prevention have resulted in increasingly effective measures to reduce recurrent MI and cardiovascular death. Secondary prevention should be conscientiously applied after acute MI (Table 72–8).

A fasting *lipid profile* is recommended on admission, and *lipid-lowering therapy,* typically with a statin, is begun in the hospital, generally with an LDL cholesterol goal of less than 70 mg/dL (Chapter 217). Continued smoking doubles the subsequent mortality risk after acute MI, and *smoking cessation* reduces the risk of reinfarction and death within 1 year (Chapter 30). An individualized smoking cessation plan should be formulated, including pharmacologic aids (nicotine gum and patches, bupropion).

Antiplatelet therapy (Chapter 35; Fig. 72–5) should consist of aspirin, given on a long-term basis to all patients without contraindications (maintenance dose, 75 to 162 mg/day). Clopidogrel (75 mg/day) is given to patients who received PCI with stenting and

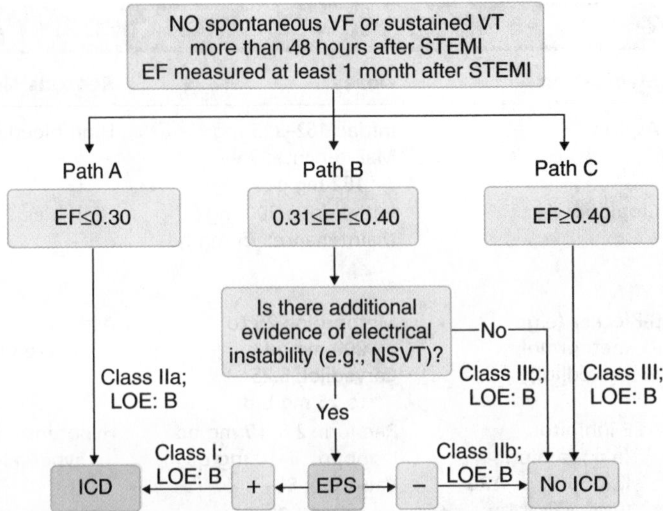

FIGURE 72–4 • Algorithm to aid in selection of implantable cardioverter-defibrillator (ICD) in patients with ST segment elevation myocardial infarction (STEMI) and diminished ejection fraction (EF). The appropriate management path is selected based on left ventricular EF measured at least 1 month after STEMI. All patients, whether an ICD is implanted or not, should receive medical therapy. (From Antman EM, Anbe DT, Armstrong PW, et al: 2004 Update: ACC/AHA Guidelines for the Managment of Patients with ST-Elevation Myocardial Infarction—Exective Summary. A Report of the American College of Cardiology/American Heart Association Task Force on Practice Guidelines. Circulation 2004;110:588–536.) EPS = electrophysiologic studies; LOE = level of evidence; NSVT = nonsustained ventricular tachycardia; VF = ventricular fibrillation; VT = ventricular tachycardia.

Rx

is also appropriate for others at higher risk for recurrent vascular events. Therapy is recommended for a minimum of 1 month after a bare metal stent, for at least 3 months for sirolimus-eluting stents, and for at least 6 months for paclitaxel-eluting stents. If patients are not at high risk of bleeding, therapy is continued for up to 1 year or more.

Anticoagulant therapy (i.e., warfarin, with an international normalized ratio goal of 2.0 to 3.0) is indicated after acute MI for patients unable to take antiplatelet therapy (aspirin or clopidogrel), for those with persistent or paroxysmal AF, for those with LV thrombus, and for those who have suffered a systemic or pulmonary embolism. Anticoagulants also may be considered for patients with extensive wall motion abnormalities and markedly depressed ejection fraction with or without heart failure. Data on the benefit of warfarin instead of or in addition to aspirin are inconclusive.

ACE inhibitor therapy can prevent adverse myocardial remodeling after acute MI and can reduce heart failure and death; it is clearly indicated for long-term use in patients with anterior acute MI or an LV ejection fraction less than 40%. ACE inhibitors also reduce recurrent MI in higher-risk patients with an ejection fraction greater than 40%. In contrast, ACE inhibition, when added to other contemporary therapies, provides little additional benefit in reducing cardiovascular events in patients who have stable coronary disease and a low risk (<5%/year) of a coronary event. These data suggest a rationale for the long-term use of ACE inhibitors (e.g., ramipril, 2.5 mg titrated to 10 mg/day, or lisinopril, 2.5 to 5 mg titrated to 10 mg/day) in all patients after MI, except perhaps those at lowest risk (i.e., without heart failure, hypertension, glucose intolerance, or reduced ejection fraction). An ARB (e.g., valsartan, 80 to 160 mg twice daily, or losartan, 50 to 100 mg/day) should be substituted in patients who cannot tolerate an ACE inhibitor; in patients with advanced heart failure, both an ACE inhibitor and an ARB may be complementary (Chapter 58). An aldosterone receptor blocker (e.g., eplerenone, 25 mg/day orally, increased to 50 mg/day after 4 weeks if tolerated, with monitoring of serum potassium levels) also should be added to the ACE inhibitor or ARB (but not both) regimen on a long-term

TABLE 72–8 DISCHARGE MEDICATION CHECKLIST AFTER MYOCARDIAL INFARCTION*

Medication	Doses	Reasons Not to Use	Comments
Aspirin	Initial: 162–325 mg Maintenance: 75–162 mg qd	High bleeding risk	Reduces mortality, reinfarction, and stroke
Clopidogrel	Initial dose: 300 mg Maintenance: 75 mg qd	High bleeding risk	Indicated after PCI for 3 mo–1 yr; also reduces vascular events when added to aspirin in non–ST segment elevation acute MI (also useful based on recent clinical trials after ST segment elevation acute MI)
β-Blocker (e.g., metoprolol, carvedilol)	Metoprolol: 25 to 200 mg qd Carvedilol: 6.25 to 25 mg bid	Asthma, bradycardia, severe CHF	Reduces mortality, reinfarction, sudden death, arrhythmia, hypertension, angina, atherosclerosis progression
ACE inhibitor (e.g., ramipril, lisinopril) or ARB (e.g., valsartan, losartan)	Ramipril: 2.5–10 mg qd Lisinopril: 5–10 mg qd Valsartan: 80–160 mg qd–bid Losartan: 50–100 mg qd	Hypotension, allergy, hyperkalemia	Reduces mortality, reinfarction, stroke, heart failure, diabetes, atherosclerosis progression
Lipid-lowering agent (e.g., a statin) (e.g., atorvastatin, simvastatin)	Atorvastatin: 10–80 mg qd Simvastatin: 20–40 mg qd	Myopathy, rhabdomyolysis, hepatitis	Goal = LDL <100 and preferably <70 (statins also can benefit patients with lower LDL[†]); consider addition of niacin or fibrate for high non-HDL cholesterol, low HDL
Nitroglycerin sublingual	0.4 mg SL prn for angina	Aortic stenosis; sildenafil (Viagra) use	Instruct on prn use and appropriate need for medical attention

*Medications given at hospital discharge improve long-term compliance. See also Antman EM, Anbe DT, Armstrong PW, et al: 2004 Update: ACC/AHA guidelines for the management of patients with ST-elevation myocardial infarction—executive summary: A report of the American College of Cardiology/American Heart Association Task Force on Practice Guidelines. Circulation 2004;110:588–636.
[†]Heart Protection Study (Lancet 2002;360:7); and PROVE-IT Study (N Engl J Med 2004;350:1495.)
ARB = angiotensin receptor blocker; bid = twice daily; CHF = congestive heart failure; HDL = high-density lipoprotein; LDL = low-density lipoprotein; MI = myocardial infarction; PCI = percutaneous coronary intervention; prn = as needed; qd = once daily, SL = sublingual.

Rx

basis in patients with depressed ejection fraction (≤0.40) and clinical heart failure or diabetes, unless this approach is contraindicated.

Long-term *β-blocker therapy* is strongly recommended for all MI survivors without uncompensated heart failure or other contraindications. Long-term therapy in patients at low risk (normal ventricular function, successful recanalization, absence of arrhythmias) is reasonable but not mandatory.

Nitroglycerin (0.4 mg) is prescribed routinely for sublingual or buccal administration for acute anginal attacks. Longer-acting oral therapy (isosorbide mononitrate, 30 to 60 mg orally every morning, or dinitrate, 10 to 40 mg orally two to three times daily) or topical nitroglycerin (e.g., start 0.5 inch, can titrate up to 2 inches, every 6 hours for 2 days) may be added to treatment regimens for angina or heart failure in selected patients.

Calcium-channel blockers are negatively inotropic and are *not* routinely given on a long-term basis; however, they may be given to selected patients without LV dysfunction (ejection fraction >0.40) who are intolerant of β-blockers and who require these drugs for antianginal therapy (e.g., amlodipine, 5 to 10 mg/day orally, or diltiazem, 120 to 480 mg/day orally as sustained release or divided doses) or for control of heart rate in AF (e.g., diltiazem, 120 to 480 mg/day orally, or verapamil, 180 to 480 mg/day orally, as sustained release or in divided doses). Short-acting nifedipine should be avoided.

Hormone therapy with estrogen with or without progestin is not begun after an acute MI because it increases thromboembolic risk and does not prevent reinfarction. For women already receiving hormone replacement, therapy should be discontinued unless it is being given for another compelling indication.

Hypertension (Chapter 66) and diabetes mellitus (Chapter 247) must be assessed and tightly controlled in patients after acute MI.

Rx

ACE inhibitors or β-blockers as described earlier are usually the first-choice therapies for hypertension, with ARBs indicated when ACE inhibitors are not tolerated. ACE inhibitors and ARBs also can reduce the long-term complications of diabetes.

Antioxidant supplementation (e.g., vitamin E, vitamin C) does not benefit patients after acute MI and is *not* recommended. Folate therapy reduces homocyst(e)ine levels, but it has not been effective in reducing clinical events in large secondary prevention trials. Evidence regarding fish oil supplements is insufficient to make recommendations for or against them.

Antiarrhythmic drugs are *not* generally recommended after acute MI, and class I antiarrhythmic agents can increase the risk of sudden death. Class III drugs (amiodarone, sotalol, dofetilide) may be used as part of the management strategy for specific arrhythmias (e.g., AF, VT) (Chapter 63 and 64).

Patient Education and Rehabilitation

The hospital stay provides an important opportunity to educate patients about their MI and its treatment, coronary risk factors, and behavioral modification. Education should begin on admission and should continue after discharge. However, the time before hospital discharge is particularly opportune. Many hospitals use case managers and prevention specialists to augment physicians and nurses, to provide educational materials, to review important concepts, to assist in formulating and actualizing individual risk-reduction plans, and to ensure proper and timely outpatient follow-up. This follow-up should include early return appointments with the patient's physician (within a few weeks). Instructions on activities also should be given before discharge. Many hospitals have cardiac rehabilitation programs that provide supervised, progressive exercise.

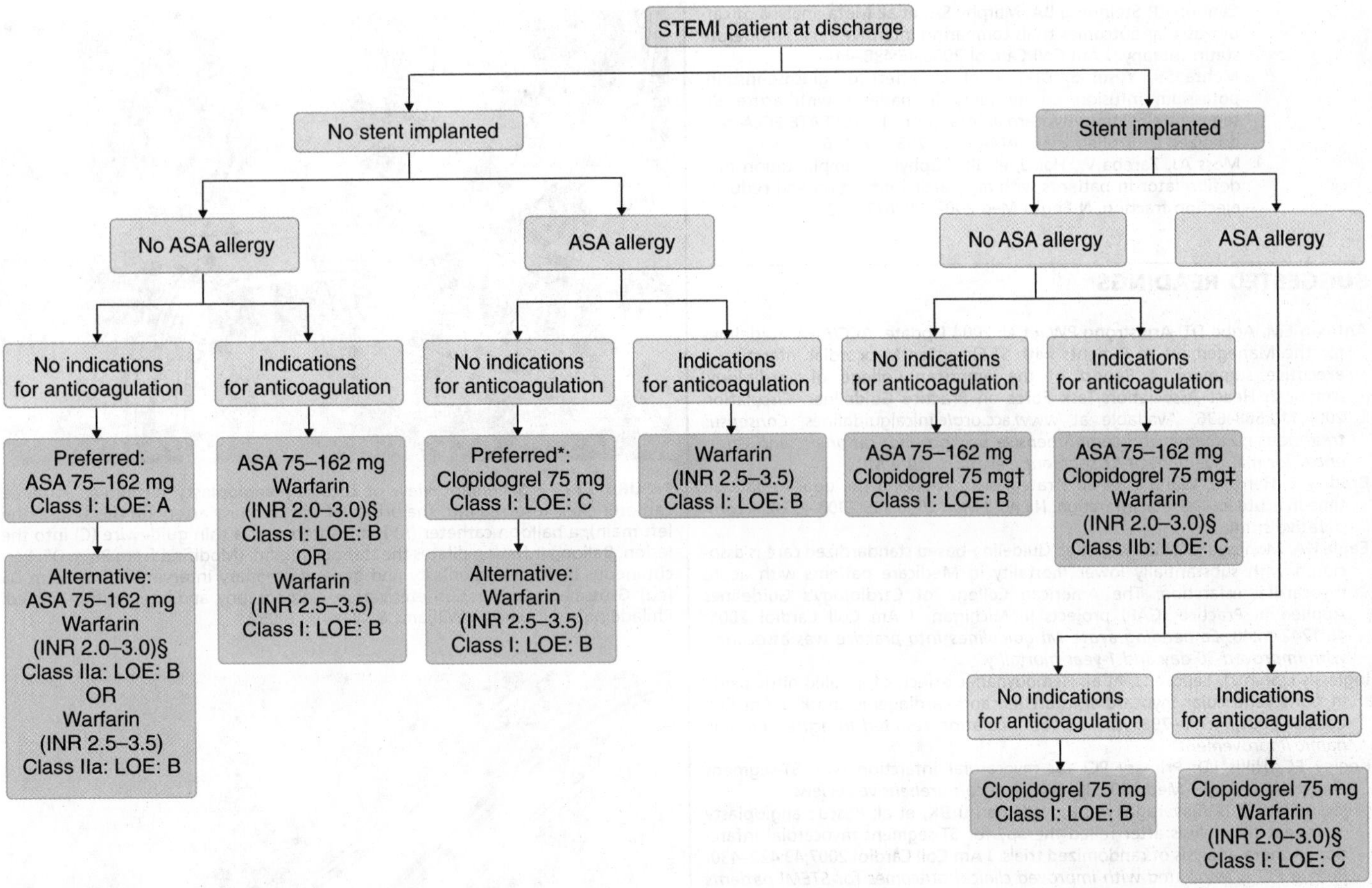

- STEMI patient at discharge
  - No stent implanted
    - No ASA allergy
      - No indications for anticoagulation
        - Preferred: ASA 75–162 mg Class I: LOE: A
        - Alternative: ASA 75–162 mg Warfarin (INR 2.0–3.0)§ Class IIa: LOE: B OR Warfarin (INR 2.5–3.5) Class IIa: LOE: B
      - Indications for anticoagulation
        - ASA 75–162 mg Warfarin (INR 2.0–3.0)§ Class I: LOE: B OR Warfarin (INR 2.5–3.5) Class I: LOE: B
    - ASA allergy
      - No indications for anticoagulation
        - Preferred*: Clopidogrel 75 mg Class I: LOE: C
        - Alternative: Warfarin (INR 2.5–3.5) Class I: LOE: B
      - Indications for anticoagulation
        - Warfarin (INR 2.5–3.5) Class I: LOE: B
  - Stent implanted
    - No ASA allergy
      - No indications for anticoagulation
        - ASA 75–162 mg Clopidogrel 75 mg† Class I: LOE: B
      - Indications for anticoagulation
        - ASA 75–162 mg Clopidogrel 75 mg‡ Warfarin (INR 2.0–3.0)§ Class IIb: LOE: C
    - ASA allergy
      - No indications for anticoagulation
        - Clopidogrel 75 mg Class I: LOE: B
      - Indications for anticoagulation
        - Clopidogrel 75 mg Warfarin (INR 2.0–3.0)§ Class I: LOE: C

FIGURE 72–5 • Long-term antithrombotic therapy at hospital discharge after ST segment elevation myocardial infarction (STEMI). *Clopidogrel is preferred over warfarin because of increased risk of bleeding and low patient compliance in warfarin trials. †For 12 months. ‡Discontinue clopidogrel 1 month after implantation of a bare metal stent or several months after implantation of a drug-eluting stent (3 months after sirolimus and 6 months after paclitaxel) because of the potentially increased risk of bleeding with warfarin and two antiplatelet agents. Continue aspirin (ASA) and warfarin on a long-term basis if warfarin is indicated for other reasons such as atrial fibrillation, left ventricular thrombus, cerebral emboli, or extensive regional wall motion abnormality. §An international normalized ratio (INR) of 2.0 to 3.0 is acceptable with tight control, but the lower end of this range is preferable. The combination of antiplatelet therapy and warfarin may be considered in patients less than 75 years old who have a low bleeding risk and who can be monitored reliably. LOE = level of evidence. (Redrawn from Antman EM, Anbe DT, Armstrong PW, et al: ACC/AHA guidelines for the management of patients with ST-elevation myocardial infarction—executive summary: A report of the American College of Cardiology/American Heart Association Task Force on Practice Guidelines (Writing Committee to Revise the 1999 Guidelines for the Management of Patients with Acute Myocardial Infarction). Circulation 2004;110:588–636.)

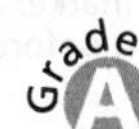

1. Fibrinolytic Therapy Trialists' (FTT) Collaborative Group: Indications for fibrinolytic therapy in suspected acute myocardial infarction: Collaborative overview of early mortality and major morbidity results from all randomised trials of more than 1000 patients. Lancet 1994;343:311–322.
2. GUSTO investigators: An international randomized trial comparing four thrombolytic strategies for acute myocardial infarction. N Engl J Med 1993;329:673–682.
3. Keeley EC, Boura JA, Grines CL: Primary angioplasty versus intravenous thrombolytic therapy for acute myocardial infarction: A quantitative review of 23 randomised trials. Lancet 2003;361:13–20.
4. Andersen HR, Nielsen TT, Rasmussen K, et al: A comparison of coronary angioplasty with fibrinolytic therapy in acute myocardial infarction. N Engl J Med 2003;349:733–742.
5. Stone GW, Grines CL, Cox DA, et al: Comparison of angioplasty with stenting, with or without abciximab, in acute myocardial infarction. N Engl J Med 2002;346:957–966.
6. Efficacy and safety of tenecteplase in combination with enoxaparin, abciximab, or unfractionated heparin: The ASSENT-3 randomised trial in acute myocardial infarction. Lancet 2001;358:605–613.
7. Topol EJ, GUSTO V Investigators: Reperfusion therapy for acute myocardial infarction with fibrinolytic therapy or combination reduced fibrinolytic therapy and platelet glycoprotein IIb/IIIa inhibition: The GUSTO V randomised trial. Lancet 2001;357:1905–1914.
8. Schomig A, Mehilli J, Antoniucci D, et al: Mechanical reperfusion in patients with acute myocardial infarction presenting more than 12 hours from symptom onset: A randomized controlled trial. JAMA 2005;293:2865–2872.
9. Hochman JS, Sleeper LA, Webb JG, et al: Early revascularization in acute myocardial infarction complicated by cardiogenic shock: SHOCK Investigators. Should we emergently revascularize occluded coronaries for cardiogenic shock? N Engl J Med 1999;341:625–634.
10. Keeley EC, Boura JA, Grines CL: Comparison of primary and facilitated percutaneous interventions for ST-elevation myocardial infarction: Quantitative review of randomized trials. Lancet 2006;367:579–588.
11. Sabatine MS, Cannon CP, Gibson M, et al: Addition of clopidogrel to aspirin and fibrinolytic therapy for myocardial infarction with ST-segment elevation. N Engl J Med 2005;352:1179–1189.
12. COMMIT (ClOpidogrel and Metoprolol in Myocardial Infarction Trial) collaborative group: Early intravenous then oral metoprolol in 45 of 852 patients with acute myocardial infarction: Randomised placebo-controlled trial. Lancet 2005;366:1622–1632.
13. Montalescot G, Borentain M, Payot L, et al: Early vs late administration of glycoprotein IIb/IIIa inhibitors in primary percutaneous coronary intervention of acute ST-segment elevation myocardial infarction: A meta-analysis. JAMA 2004;292:362–366.
14. Antman EM, Morrow DA, McCabe CH, et al: Enoxaparin versus unfractionated heparin with fibrinolysis for ST-elevation myocardial infarction. N Engl J Med 2006;354:1477–1488.
15. Yusuf S, Mehta SR, Chrolavicius S, et al: Effects of fondaparinux on mortality and reinfarction in patients with acute ST-segment elevation myocardial infarction: The OASIS-6 randomized trial. JAMA 2006;295:1519–1530.
16. ISIS-4 (Fourth International Study of Infarct Survival) Collaborative Group: A randomised factorial trial assessing early oral captopril, oral mononitrate, and intravenous magnesium sulphate in 58,050 patients with suspected acute myocardial infarction. Lancet 1995;345:669–685.
17. Yusuf S, Sleight P, Pogue J, et al: Effects of an angiotensin-converting enzyme inhibitor, ramipril, on cardiovascular events in high-risk patients: The Heart Outcomes Prevention Evaluation Study Investigators. N Engl J Med 2000;342:145–153.
18. Pitt B, Remme W, Zannad E, et al: Eplerenone, a selective aldosterone blocker, in patients with left ventricular dysfunction after myocardial infarction. N Engl J Med 2003;348:1309–1321.

19. Cannon CP, Steinberg BA, Murphy SA, et al: Meta-analysis of cardiovascular outcomes trials comparing intensive versus moderate statin therapy. J Am Coll Cardiol 2006;48:438–445.
20. Mehta SR, Yusuf S, Diaz R, et al: Effect of glucose-insulin-potassium infusion on mortality in patients with acute ST-segment elevation myocardial infarction: The CREATE-ECLA randomized controlled trial. JAMA 2005;293:437–446.
21. Moss AJ, Zareba W, Hall J, et al: Prophylactic implantation of a defibrillator in patients with myocardial infarction and reduced ejection fraction. N Engl J Med 2002;346:877–883.

SUGGESTED READINGS

Antman EM, Anbe DT, Armstrong PW, et al: 2004 Update: ACC/AHA Guidelines for the Management of Patients with ST-Elevation Myocardial Infarction—executive summary. A Report of the American College of Cardiology/American Heart Association Task Force on Practice Guidelines. Circulation 2004;110:588–636. Available at www.acc.org/clinicalguidelines. *Consensus treatment guidelines and comprehensive background, rationale, and references for management of ST segment elevation acute MI.*

Bradley E, Herrin J, Wang Y, et al: Strategies for reducing the door-to-balloon time in acute myocardial infarction. N Engl J Med 2006;355:2308–2320. *A comparative study.*

Eagle KA, Montoye CK, Riba AL, et al: Guideline-based standardized care is associated with substantially lower mortality in Medicare patients with acute myocardial infarction: The American College of Cardiology's Guidelines Applied in Practice (GAP) projects in Michigan. J Am Coll Cardiol 2005; 46:1242–1248. *Embedding acute MI guidelines into practice was associated with improved 30-day and 1-year mortality.*

Inglessis I, Shin JT, Lepore JJ, et al: Hemodynamic effects of inhaled nitric oxide in right ventricular myocardial infarction and cardiogenic shock. J Am Coll Cardiol 2004;44:793–798. *Nitric oxide inhalation resulted in acute hemodynamic improvement.*

Keeley EC, Hillis LD: Primary PCI for myocardial infarction with ST-segment elevation. N Engl J Med 2007;356:47–54. *A comprehensive review.*

Wijeysundere HC, Vijayaraghavan R, Nallamothu BK, et al: Rescue angioplasty or repeat fibrinolysis after failed therapy for ST-segment myocardial infarction: A meta-analysis of randomized trials. J Am Coll Cardiol 2007;49:422–430. *Rescue PCI is associated with improved clinical outcomes for STEMI patients after failed fibrinolytic therapy.*

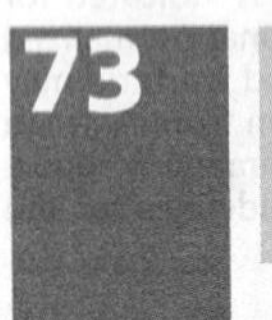

73 PERCUTANEOUS CORONARY INTERVENTIONS

Paul S. Teirstein

PERCUTANEOUS TRANSLUMINAL CORONARY ANGIOPLASTY

Percutaneous coronary intervention (PCI) is applicable to most forms of coronary artery disease, including multivessel disease, total occlusions, saphenous vein graft disease, unstable angina (Chapter 71), and acute myocardial infarction (MI) (Chapter 72). An estimated 2 million PCIs are performed worldwide each year, making it one of the most widely used medical procedures. Its popularity is based largely on its simplicity, the need for only local anesthesia, a short (approximately 1 day) hospitalization, and negligible postprocedure recovery time. Continued technologic advances are likely to create an even greater demand for PCI in the future.

Mechanisms and Technical Considerations

Under local anesthesia, a hollow-bore needle is inserted percutaneously into a peripheral artery (usually the femoral or radial artery). A guidewire (approximately 0.038 inch) is placed through this needle and advanced into the aorta. The needle is removed, leaving the guidewire, over which a small-caliber (approximately 3 mm), specially shaped catheter (called a guiding catheter) is advanced under fluoroscope guidance into the ostium of the obstructed coronary artery. By use of radiographic contrast injections that provide fluoroscopic visualization of the coronary artery lumen, a thin (approximately 0.014 inch), highly steerable guidewire is directed down the coronary artery and across the stenotic lesion. This guidewire becomes a "rail" over which therapeutic tools such as inflatable balloons, stents, and atherectomy catheters are passed to the diseased segment (Fig. 73–1).

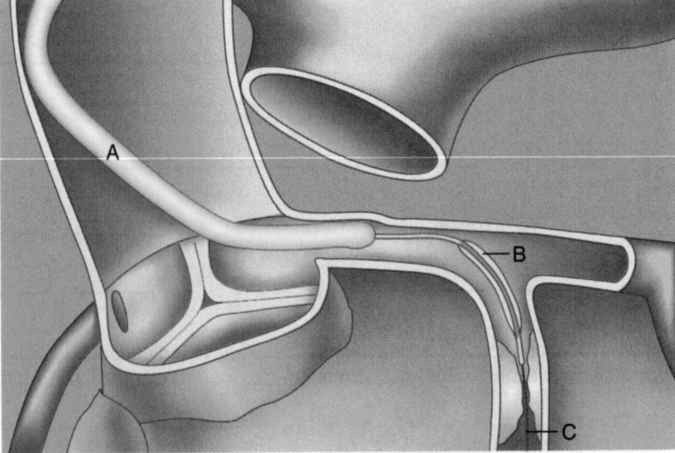

FIGURE 73–1 • Schematic view of coronary angioplasty technique. A guide catheter (A) is inserted into the orifice of the coronary artery (in this figure, the left main); a balloon catheter (B) is advanced over a thin guidewire (C) into the lesion. Balloon inflation dilates the stenotic region. (Modified from Baim DS: Percutaneous balloon angioplasty and general coronary intervention. *In* Baim DS [ed]: Grossman's Cardiac Catheterization, Angiography, and Intervention, 7th ed. Philadelphia, Lippincott Williams & Wilkins, 2005.)

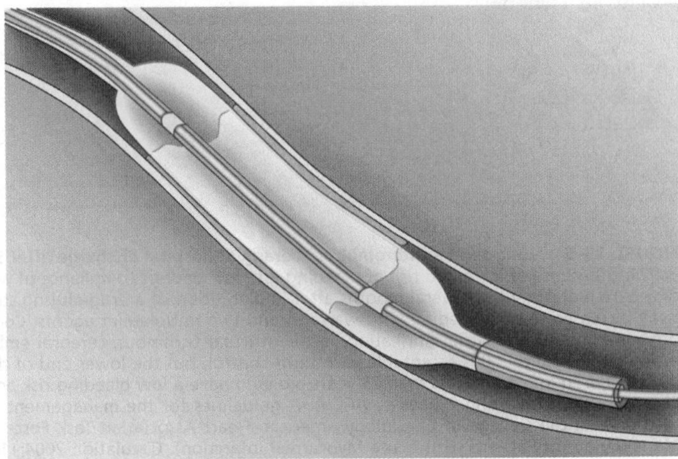

FIGURE 73–2 • Balloon angioplasty catheter. The catheter consists of two lumens, an inflation lumen and a guidewire lumen. Two radiopaque markers, indicating the lateral balloon margins, aid in positioning of the balloon before inflation.

Balloon catheters (Fig. 73–2) typically have two lumens, one to allow passage over the guidewire and another to carry a mixture of saline and radiographic contrast material to inflate a balloon at the distal catheter tip. Under fluoroscopy, the balloon is centered across the lesion and inflated to 3 to 20 atmospheres of pressure. Balloon inflation widens the narrowed lumen by stretching the vessel and, in most cases, causing a tear (a therapeutic dissection) at the edges of the plaque, where the atheroma meets the nondiseased media. Atherectomy catheters, which also are passed over a guidewire to the diseased segment, remove plaque by a shaving, grinding, slicing, or suction mechanism. Coronary stents are metallic (usually 316L stainless steel or nitinol) scaffolding devices that are crimped onto a deflated balloon catheter before insertion into the diseased vessel. During balloon inflation, the collapsed stent expands to support the vessel lumen (Fig. 73–3). Whereas balloons and atherectomy devices create an adequate, albeit rough channel through diseased arteries, the supporting structure of the stent can widen the lumen to near its predisease dimensions. With a stent, tissue flaps are "pinned" against the wall, and recoil is limited. Most stents are designed so that the metallic struts compose only about 20% of the surface area to allow a rapid endothelialization (during about 2 weeks) and a reduced risk of thrombosis. Because coronary stents are able to obtain a larger and more secure lumen, resist restenosis, and elute beneficial medications, they are now used in more than 95% of PCIs.

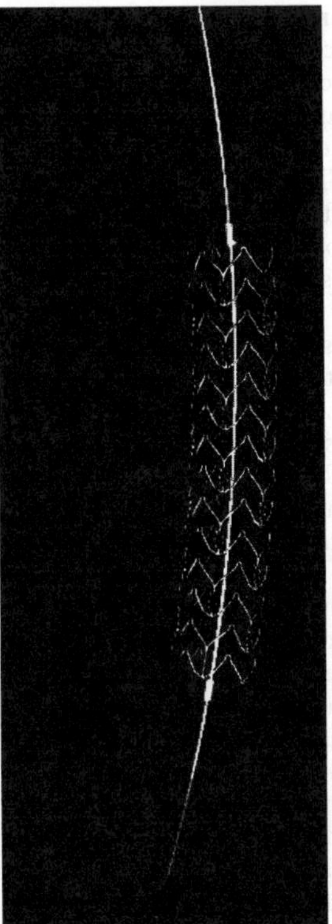

FIGURE 73–3 • Balloon-expandable coronary stent. The stainless steel stent is crimped onto a balloon catheter to allow low-profile passage through the coronary artery. When it is positioned across the lesion, the balloon is inflated, expanding the stent. After balloon deflation and removal, the stent remains, providing a scaffold that supports the vessel lumen.

During the PCI procedure, the interventional cardiologist is able to assess the target vessel fluoroscopically by injections of contrast material through the guiding catheter (Fig. 73–4). When the coronary artery has been opened successfully, all catheters are withdrawn, and the arterial access site is sealed by mechanical pressure, an absorbable plug, or a remote suturing device. Patients without comorbidity ambulate in 3 to 6 hours. Discharge from the hospital usually occurs on the morning after the procedure, after stability of the arterial access site, cardiac biomarkers, and electrocardiogram is confirmed. Selected patients in some medical centers are treated as outpatients and released 6 to 12 hours after the procedure without an overnight stay.

Selection of Patients

Any decision to perform PCI must include a review of the coronary angiogram (Chapter 56) by an experienced interventional cardiologist to assess the lesion's technical suitability for the procedure. The disease must narrow the coronary artery lumen by at least 60%, and the quantity of myocardium subtended by the vessel should not be trivial. High-risk lesion characteristics (Table 73–1), such as longer lesion length, vessel tortuosity, lesion calcification, or the presence of thrombus, must be taken into consideration. Subtle angiographic findings, such as the presence of collateral vessels that supply a different myocardial territory and that originate distal to the target, should be appreciated. For each patient, the benefits of PCI must be weighed against the procedural risk. Characteristics of the patient conveying increased risk include advanced age (i.e., older than 75 years), diabetes, smaller vessels that are often found in women, prior MI, significant impairment of left ventricular function, and renal insufficiency.

Procedural Success and Complications

With use of modern techniques in appropriately selected patients, most PCI procedures have a greater than 95% success rate. The single

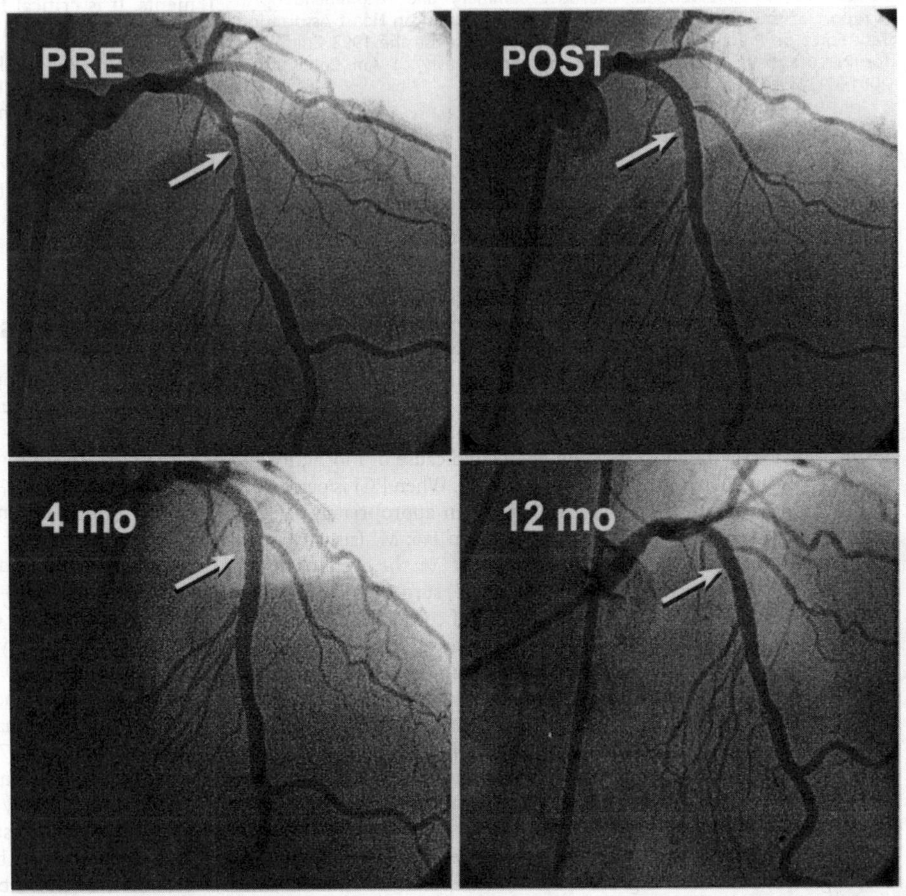

FIGURE 73–4 • Angiographic images before, after, and at late follow-up after placement of a sirolimus-eluting stent. The left anterior descending artery contains a tight stenosis (arrow, upper left panel). After stent implantation (upper right panel), the stenosis is abolished (arrow). Follow-up at 4 and 12 months (bottom panels) reveals a completely open lumen, with no evidence of restenosis (arrows).

TABLE 73-1 LESION CHARACTERISTICS ASSOCIATED WITH AN INCREASED RISK OF PERCUTANEOUS CORONARY INTERVENTIONS

LOW RISK
Discrete (length <10 mm)
Concentric
Readily accessible
Nonangulated segment (<45°)
Smooth contour
Little or no calcification
Less than totally occlusive
Not ostial in location
No major side branch involvement
Absence of thrombus
MODERATE RISK
Tubular (length 10–20 mm)
Eccentric
Moderate tortuosity of proximal segment
Moderately angulated segment (>45°, <90°)
Irregular contour
Moderate or heavy calcification
Total occlusions <3 months old
Ostial in location
Bifurcation lesions requiring double guidewires
Some thrombus present
HIGH RISK
Diffuse (length >20 mm)
Excessive tortuosity of proximal segment
Excessive angulated segments (>90°)
Total occlusion >3 months old and/or bridging collaterals
Inability to protect major side branches
Degenerated vein grafts with friable lesions

From Smith SC Jr, Dove JT, Jacobs AK, et al: ACC/AHA guidelines for percutaneous coronary intervention: Executive summary and recommendations: A report of the American College of Cardiology/American Heart Association Task Force on Practice Guidelines (Committee to Revise the 1993 Guidelines for Percutaneous Transluminal Coronary Angioplasty). J Am Coll Cardiol 2001;37:2215–2238.

exception is the totally occluded vessel (100% obstruction of the lumen), in which the interventional cardiologist's ability to negotiate a guidewire through the blockage is only about 50 to 73%. Procedural complications during and after PCI have decreased dramatically with the increased use of coronary stents and adjunctive antiplatelet agents (thienopyridines and platelet glycoprotein IIb/IIIa inhibitors). Abrupt coronary artery closure, previously the most frequent and feared cause of morbidity and mortality during PCI, is now rarely encountered. When PCI is performed by an experienced interventional cardiologist in appropriately selected patients, the risk of in-hospital death is less than 1%; MI (usually small, non–ST segment elevation MI) is approximately 5%; the need for urgent or emergent coronary artery bypass graft (CABG) surgery is less than 1%; the risk of stroke is less than 0.1%; the chance of coronary perforation is less than 1%; and morbidity at the arterial access site (i.e., hematoma, pseudoaneurysm, or arteriovenous fistula) occurs in less than 5%. Balloons and filters deployed within a coronary vessel beyond the target lesion to limit distal embolization of plaque, platelet aggregates, and other "debris" can reduce ischemic complications further in selected, high-risk patients.

Restenosis and Thrombosis

Restenosis is a renarrowing of an artery after a PCI procedure, usually resulting from one of two general mechanisms. The first mechanism, unfavorable remodeling and elastic recoil, is a mechanical renarrowing caused by adventitial constriction and shrinkage of the vessel lumen. The second mechanism, neointimal hyperplasia, is due to the proliferation of smooth muscle cells and matrix in response to the injury caused by balloons, stents, or atherectomy devices. Restenosis occurs in 10 to 50% of PCI patients after balloon angioplasty without stenting, usually within the first 6 months after the procedure. Characteristics associated with higher risk of restenosis include longer lesions, small-diameter vessels, diabetes, and multivessel disease. Treatment with either balloon angioplasty or atherectomy devices results in similar rates of restenosis. Coronary stents provide a semirigid scaffolding within the lumen and reduce restenosis by eliminating the mechanical renarrowing caused by unfavorable remodeling and elastic recoil. In randomized trials, bare metal stents reduce restenosis by about one third, from approximately 30 to 40% in patients randomized to balloon angioplasty to 20 to 30% in patients receiving stents. [1]

Although bare metal stents reduce restenosis, they do not eliminate restenosis because the stent struts that embed into the vessel wall increase the intimal proliferative response to injury. With bare metal stents, the mechanical component of restenosis is eliminated, but the proliferative component is enhanced. Smooth muscle cell division and matrix formation migrate through the stent struts to renarrow the vessel lumen. Antiproliferative drugs that are embedded into a polymer stent coating are extremely effective for the control of restenosis. However, drug-eluting stents carry a higher risk of thrombosis later (>1 year), especially if patients cannot or do not continue with aspirin plus clopidogrel. As a result, randomized trials of stents that release the cell cycle inhibitors sirolimus and paclitaxel have reduced the need for early repeated procedures, [2] but have not improved long-term outcome compared with bare metal stents. [3,4]

Choices Related to Stenting

Drug-eluting stents now are almost always the treatment of choice when PCI is performed. Because bare metal stents are relatively inexpensive (approximately one-fourth the cost of drug-eluting stents), a strategy of initial bare metal stenting followed by provisional drug-eluting stenting for restenosis is used in some cost-sensitive environments. It is critical for the clinician to be aware of the need for 3 to 6 months of dual antiplatelet therapy when drug-eluting stents are implanted. In some patients who have a relative or absolute contraindication to antiplatelet therapy (i.e., a planned surgical procedure in the near future), a bare metal stenting is favored. Atherectomy is rarely used, with the exception of the Rotablator (Boston Scientific, Maple Grove, MN), which pulverizes plaque into microparticles that pass through the coronary microcirculation and is particularly helpful for the treatment of heavily calcified lesions. After plaque debulking with the Rotablator, a drug-eluting stent is usually implanted.

Discharge Issues

Discharge planning after PCI represents an important opportunity to emphasize evidence-based medical treatment of atherothrombotic disease and coronary risk factor modification. All patients should receive aspirin (81 to 325 mg/day) indefinitely. For patients receiving bare metal stents, a minimum 2-week course of clopidogrel (75 mg/day) is mandatory. If a drug-eluting stent is deployed, this dual antiplatelet therapy must be extended for 3 to 6 months, depending on the specific medicated stent used. Prolonged use of aspirin, clopidogrel, angiotensin-converting enzyme inhibitors, β-blockers, and lipid-lowering agents should be considered on the basis of randomized trials showing improved long-term outcome, particularly in patients who present with unstable angina syndromes (Chapters 70, 71, and 72). Smoking cessation (Chapter 30), blood pressure control (Chapter 66), stress management, exercise, weight loss, changes in dietary habits, and strict blood glucose control for diabetic patients (Chapter 247) also are important elements of the discharge plan.

Activity restrictions after PCI are modest. If the femoral artery was instrumented, heavy lifting is discouraged for several days. Intense aerobic exercise is usually discouraged for 2 to 4 weeks (especially after stent implantation) because exercise can activate platelets and lead to formation of thrombus at the angioplasty site. Patients may return to

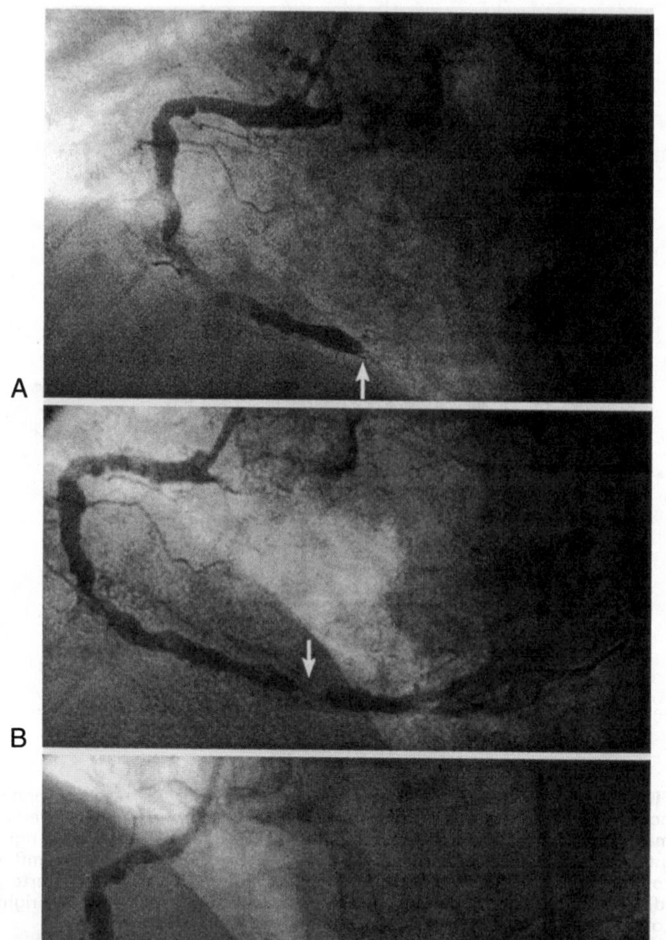

FIGURE 73–5 • Primary coronary angioplasty for acute myocardial infarction. This 50-year-old man presented at midnight with 70 minutes of crushing substernal chest pressure accompanied by inferior ST segment elevation. Emergency angiography performed 45 minutes after arrival found 100% occlusion of the right coronary artery (**A**, arrow). Within 10 minutes, a guidewire was negotiated through the obstruction (presumably caused by fresh thrombus), allowing perfusion into the distal vessel and uncovering a high-grade stenotic lesion (**B**, arrow). After deployment of a coronary stent (**C**, arrow), the stenosis was abolished and significant myocardial damage aborted.

work 1 or 2 days after the procedure if their occupation does not include heavy lifting or excessive physical exercise. There is usually no restriction on driving an automobile.

CORONARY ANGIOPLASTY VERSUS MEDICAL THERAPY

PCI reduces angina, and commonly leads to better treadmill exercise performance and improved quality-of-life measurements. However, PCI has not been shown to reduce the risks of death, MI, or other major cardiovascular events compared with optimal medical therapy in patients with stable angion. [5] When PCI is being considered in truly asymptomatic patients, significant ischemia first should be documented by functional testing, or a large quantity of myocardium should be supplied by the stenotic coronary artery.

Patients experiencing acute MI (Chapters 71 and 72) represent an important subgroup in whom PCI has proved beneficial compared with medical therapy (Fig. 73–5). In ST elevation MI, randomized trials consistently have reported a reduction in mortality, stroke, subsequent MI, and recurrent ischemia with PCI compared with thrombolytic therapy. [6] For non–ST elevation MI and many patients with unstable angina, an early aggressive approach that includes either PCI or CABG in angiographically suitable patients is preferable to a conservative strategy [7] (Chapter 71).

PERCUTANEOUS CORONARY INTERVENTION VERSUS CORONARY ARTERY BYPASS GRAFTING

The decision between PCI and CABG surgery (Chapter 74) largely is determined by anatomic features. Symptomatic patients with one or more total occlusions that cannot be revascularized by PCI techniques will have better relief of angina with CABG surgery. Patients with several lesions in two or three coronary arteries often are referred for CABG surgery because the risk of restenosis is considered unacceptably high. Left main and left main equivalent stenoses often are treated surgically because they are associated with a moderately increased procedural risk, and if restenosis of the left main occurs, it can manifest as sudden death.

Several large, randomized trials of PCI versus CABG surgery in patients with multivessel disease generally show no differences in late (approximately 5 years) death and MI, although the need for repeated revascularization procedures is consistently higher in patients randomized to PCI, [8, 9] and diabetic patients with multivessel coronary disease appear to have better outcomes with CABG surgery. [10] Although the current, nearly universal use of drug-eluting stents may minimize the difference in repeated revascularization rates between PCI and CABG surgery, randomized trials to test this hypothesis have not been completed.

FUTURE DIRECTIONS

Restenosis, the Achilles heel and most significant limitation of PCI, has been vastly reduced by drug-eluting stents. With this lower risk of restenosis, patients with some of the classic contraindications to PCI, such as multivessel disease, diabetes, left main coronary artery stenosis, small-diameter vessels, long lesions, saphenous vein grafts, and bifurcation lesions, may become excellent candidates for this minimally invasive procedure. If randomized trials support this hypothesis, the number of PCI procedures is likely to grow, and the use of CABG surgery may diminish.

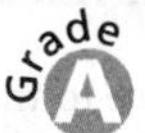

1. Fischman DL, Leon MB, Baim DS, et al: A randomized comparison of coronary-stent placement and balloon angioplasty in the treatment of coronary artery disease. N Engl J Med 1994;331:496–501.
2. Moses JW, Leon MB, Popma JJ, et al: Sirolimus-eluting stents versus standard stents in patients with stenosis in a native coronary artery. N Engl J Med 2003;349:1315–1323.
3. Kastrati A, Mehilli J, Pache J, et al: Analysis of 14 trials comparing sirolimus-eluting stents with bare-metal stents. N Engl J Med 2007;356:1030–1039.
4. Spaulding C, Daemen J, Boersma E, et al: A pooled analysis of data comparing sirolimus-eluting stents with bare-metal stents. N Engl J Med 2007;356:989–997.
5. Boden WE, O'Rourke RA, Teo KK, et al: Optimal medical therapy with or without PCI for stable coronary disease. N Engl J Med 2007;356:1503–1516.
6. Keeley EC, Boura JA, Grines CL: Primary angioplasty versus intravenous thrombolytic therapy for acute myocardial infarction: A quantitative review of 23 randomised trials. Lancet 2003;361:13–20.
7. Mehta SR, Cannon CP, Fox KA, et al: Routine vs selective invasive strategies in patients with acute coronary syndromes: A collaborative meta-analysis of randomized trials. JAMA 2005;23:2908–2917.
8. Serruys PW, Ong ATL, van Herwerden LA, et al: Five-year outcomes after coronary stenting versus bypass surgery for the treatment of multivessel disease: The final analysis of the Arterial Revascularization Therapies Study (ARTS) randomized trial. J Am Coll Cardiol 2005;46:575–581.
9. Hannan EL, Racz MJ, Walford G, et al: Long-term outcomes of coronary-artery bypass grafting versus stent implantation. N Engl J Med 2005;352:2174–2183.
10. The BARI Investigators: The final 10-year follow-up results from the BARI randomized trial. J Am Coll Cardiol 2007;49:1600–1606.

SUGGESTED READINGS

Smith SC Jr, Feldman TE, Hirshfeld JW Jr, et al: ACC/AHA/SCAI 2005 Guideline Update for Percutaneous Coronary Intervention. A Report of the American College of Cardiology/American Heart Association Task Force on Practice Guidelines (ACC/AHA/SCAI Writing Committee to Update the 2001 Guidelines for Percutaneous Coronary Intervention). Available at: http://www.acc.org/clinical/guidelines/percutaneous/update/index.pdf. Accessed February 9, 2006. *Cousensus guidelines.*

Stroupe KT, Morrison DA, Hlatky MA, et al: Cost-effectiveness of coronary artery bypass grafts versus percutaneous coronary intervention for revascularization of high-risk patients. Circulation 2006;114:1251–1257. *PCI was more cost-effective over the long-term, even including the likely need for subsequent revascularization.*

74 SURGICAL TREATMENT OF CORONARY ARTERY DISEASE

Bruce W. Lytle

Coronary artery bypass grafting (CABG) is based on the premise that the morbidity and mortality associated with coronary atherosclerosis are largely related to atherosclerotic coronary stenoses that can be demonstrated by coronary angiography (Chapter 56) and that if grafts are constructed to route blood flow around these stenoses, myocardial blood supply can be improved or preserved, cardiac symptoms relieved, cardiac events diminished, and survival prolonged. Over time, the fundamentals of that concept have been shown to be correct.

CORONARY BYPASS OPERATION

The most common types of grafts for coronary artery bypass have been reversed segments of saphenous vein and the internal thoracic arteries. Saphenous vein grafts are anastomosed to the aorta (proximal anastomosis) and to the coronary artery distal to the major obstruction (Fig. 74–1). Saphenous vein grafts have the advantages of availability, larger size than most coronary arteries, and favorable handling characteristics. However, with time, saphenous vein grafts may develop intrinsic pathologic changes, intimal fibroplasia, and vein graft atherosclerosis, each of which may lead to narrowing or occlusions. By 10 years postoperatively, approximately 30% of saphenous vein grafts become occluded, and 30 to 35% of those remaining exhibit angiographic evidence of vein graft atherosclerosis. Treatment with platelet inhibitors and hydroxymethylglutaryl coenzyme A inhibitors (statins; Chapter 217) decreases the risk of vein graft failure but does not eliminate it.

Internal thoracic artery grafts, on the other hand, are resistant to the development of late atherosclerosis. When it is used as an in situ (subclavian origin intact) graft to the left anterior descending (LAD) coronary artery, the left internal thoracic artery graft has a more than 90% patency rate up to 20 years after operation. Because the LAD coronary artery has a strong prognostic influence, the left internal thoracic artery to LAD graft is a clinically important part of myocardial revascularization. Patients who receive a left internal thoracic artery to LAD graft with or without saphenous vein grafts have a better long-term survival rate, fewer reoperations, and fewer cardiac events compared with patients receiving only saphenous vein grafts. The right internal thoracic artery may also be used for revascularization as an in situ graft, as an aorta to coronary graft, or as a composite arterial graft from the left internal thoracic artery to a coronary artery. Use of both internal thoracic arteries as grafts provides incremental benefit over a single internal thoracic artery graft strategy and produces an improved survival with a lower risk of reoperation. By comparison, 1-year patency rates are somewhat better with radial artery grafts than with saphenous vein grafts.

Most CABG operations have been performed with a full median sternotomy incision, historically with the aid of cardiopulmonary bypass, aortic cross-clamping, and cardioplegic solution—techniques that allow exposure and arrest of the heart such that detailed microsurgical anastomoses can be constructed while myocardial function is effectively protected. By comparison, strategies for performing operations through smaller incisions (minimally invasive surgery) have had limited application for coronary revascularizations. However, beating heart ("off-pump") surgery without cardiopulmonary bypass has become a standard surgical option, with equivalent outcomes. 1 Off-pump surgery offers some clear advantages for patients with comorbidities but is technically more difficult for patients with severe and diffuse coronary artery disease.

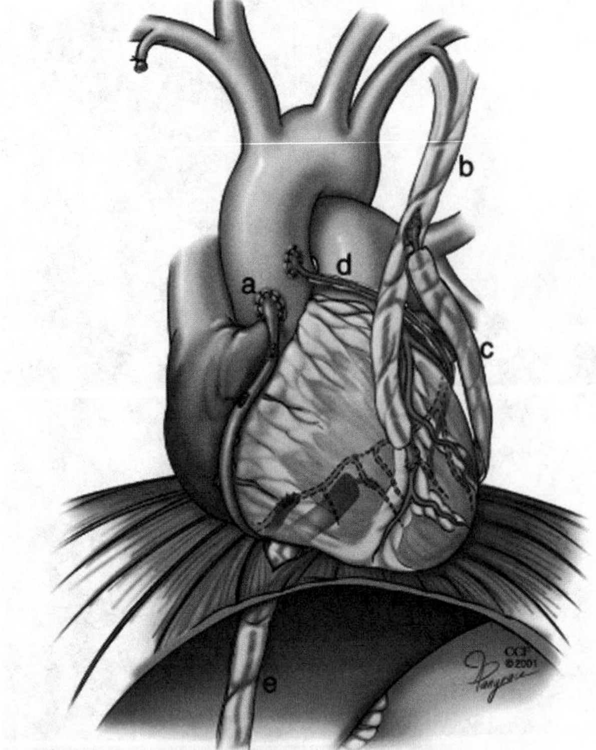

FIGURE 74–1 • Types of bypass grafts. Bypass grafts include reversed saphenous vein graft from aorta to right coronary artery (a), in situ left internal mammary artery graft to anterior descending coronary artery (b), Y graft of right internal mammary artery from left internal mammary artery to circumflex coronary artery (c), radial artery graft from aorta to circumflex coronary artery (d), and in situ gastroepiploic graft to posterior descending branch of the right coronary artery (e).

Perioperative Risks

The risk of mortality associated with CABG correlates with ischemia at the time of operation, left ventricular function, extent of coronary stenoses, noncardiac atherosclerosis, and comorbid conditions and with the experience, skill, and judgment of the surgeon. Effective myocardial protection has diminished much of the incremental risk based on the severity of cardiac disease. For patients younger than 70 years without serious comorbid conditions, the mortality risk of primary CABG surgery is less than 1% in experienced hands regardless of the number of coronary arteries that are stenotic, and left ventricular dysfunction only slightly increases risk. Nevertheless, CABG surgery in the presence of ongoing myocardial ischemia due to acute myocardial infarction, unstable angina, or vessel closure associated with percutaneous coronary intervention (PCI; Chapter 73) is still associated with increased risk. National data on primary CABG operations show a 1.7% mortality rate for elective operations, a 2.6% rate for "urgent" operations, a 6% rate for "emergency" procedures, and a 23% rate for "salvage" operations. Noncardiac comorbid conditions (aortic atherosclerosis, renal function, chronic obstructive pulmonary disease, and coagulation system disorders) increase perioperative risk when these conditions are severe.

The most serious postoperative morbidity after CABG is stroke, often related to aortic or cerebrovascular atherosclerosis and atherosclerotic embolization. Heightened awareness of the importance of aortic and carotid atherosclerosis and improved management strategies, including off-pump surgery and ascending aortic replacement, appear to have decreased the risk of focal stroke for patients previously at high risk. Serious wound complications of median sternotomy are uncommon (1 to 2%). Obesity, diabetes, and bilateral internal thoracic artery grafting (particularly in combination with diabetes) are associated with higher rates of wound complications.

TABLE 74–1 INDICATIONS FOR CORONARY ARTERY BYPASS SURGERY

Randomized Trials Available: Initial CABG versus Initial Medical Treatment	Level of Evidence
Chronic stable angina (mild to moderate angina)	
To prolong survival	
Left main coronary stenosis (≥50% diameter)	A
Three-vessel disease (EF ≥50%)	A
Two-vessel disease with proximal LAD stenosis and either EF ≥ 50% or ischemia	A
Single proximal LAD stenosis with ischemia	A
To relieve symptoms	
Significant angina (with significant coronary stenoses and objective evidence of ischemia) despite alternative therapy	A
Unstable angina	
To prolong life and relieve symptoms	
Multivessel disease (EF ≥50%)	A
Randomized Trials Not Available: CABG versus Medical Treatment	**Level of Evidence**
To prolong survival	
Severe angina, multivessel disease, normal LV function	B
Previous CABG with late stenoses in multiple SVGs or SVG-LAD	B
ST elevation acute myocardial infarction not responsive to other therapy	C
Life-threatening ventricular arrhythmias	C
Failed PTCA with ongoing ischemia	C
CABG in conjunction with surgery for other cardiac conditions	C
To relieve symptoms	
Previous CABG with disabling angina despite medical management	B

A = data derived from multiple randomized trials; B = data derived from a single randomized trial or from nonrandomized studies; C = consensus opinion of experts, case studies, or standard-of-care; CABG = coronary artery bypass graft; EF = ejection fraction; LAD = left anterior descending coronary artery; LV = left ventricular; PTCA = percutaneous transluminal coronary angioplasty; SVG = saphenous vein graft.

Late Outcomes

The late outcomes after CABG are related to age, severity of cardiac disease before operation, noncardiac comorbid conditions, progression of atherosclerosis, and the operation itself. Many of these factors can be influenced by treatment choices. CABG tends to diminish but not to eliminate long-term survival differences based on the number of diseased coronary vessels, left main stenosis, and different levels of left ventricular function. The achievement of complete revascularization (bypass grafts to all stenotic coronary vessels) and the use of internal thoracic artery grafts improve long-term survival rates and symptomatic status.

Patients often have prolonged survival after CABG; more than 80% of patients are alive more than 10 years after operation. Over the long term, control of the progression of atherosclerosis by lifestyle modifications, pharmacologic treatment of hypertension (Chapter 66) and lipids (Chapter 217), and platelet inhibitors (Chapter 35) appears to extend the benefits of CABG.

INDICATIONS FOR BYPASS SURGERY

The goals of CABG are to relieve symptoms and to prolong life expectancy (Table 74–1). On the basis of randomized trials and the emergence of alternative medical treatments and PCI, the surgical population has evolved toward patients with complex conditions, often involving left main or triple-vessel disease, diffuse coronary stenoses, totally obstructed vessels, abnormal left ventricular function, and diabetes. Surgically treated patients with single-vessel disease usually have LAD stenoses or have failed alternative treatments.

Symptom Relief

If patients who experience angina have severe stenoses in graftable coronary arteries that supply areas of myocardium ischemic at rest or with stress, CABG will reliably relieve angina. Randomized trials have shown that the relief of angina after CABG is more consistent than that achieved with alternative treatments. When intermittent heart failure symptoms represent an “anginal equivalent” that is also caused by ischemia, such symptoms also respond well to relief of that ischemia by CABG. Patients with symptoms of heart failure at rest are more complex, but dobutamine echocardiography (Chapter 53) and positron emission tomography (Chapter 54) can identify segments of viable but hibernating myocardium (ischemic at rest) that may improve with bypass grafting, thus reducing symptoms of heart failure.

Survival

Randomized Trials

Chronic Stable Angina

In randomized trials of patients with mild to moderate chronic stable angina, an improved survival rate has been documented for patients treated with initial CABG compared with initial medical treatment in the presence of a left main stenosis of more than 50% of the diameter, triple-vessel disease, double-vessel disease with a proximal LAD lesion, abnormal left ventricular function, or a strongly positive exercise test result (Chapter 70). Meta-analysis of these randomized trials also suggests a survival benefit of CABG for any patient with a proximal LAD lesion and myocardial ischemia. [2] These are subgroups of patients for whom bypass surgery should be strongly considered even in the absence of severe symptoms. During these trials, patients with severe angina were not randomized but were included in observational studies that noted improved survival rates with CABG for patients with double- and triple-vessel disease and normal or abnormal left ventricular function. Medical, interventional, and surgical treatments have all advanced since these trials were completed.

Unstable Angina or Non–ST Elevation Myocardial Infarction

Current data suggest an aggressive strategy, including CABG when indicated, in patients with unstable angina or non–ST elevation acute myocardial infarction (Chapters 71 and 73). [3]

Ischemic Syndromes without Randomized Trials

ST Elevation Acute Myocardial Infarction

For patients with ST segment elevation acute myocardial infarction, CABG may be indicated in the acute setting when thrombolytic therapy or PCI has not been effective, ischemia is ongoing, and large areas of myocardium remain jeopardized. CABG after a completed myocardial infarction may be indicated in patients in whom persistent ischemia in noninfarcted areas of myocardium produces post-infarction angina or hemodynamic instability. Mechanical complications of myocardial necrosis, including papillary muscle rupture, ventricular septal rupture, and myocardial free wall rupture, are acute life-threatening situations that usually require urgent operation for repair of the defect, often combined with CABG (Chapter 72).

Failed PCI

The availability of intracoronary stents has decreased the need for emergency CABG to treat acute failure of PCIs (Chapter 73). Current indications for emergency CABG include closure or threatened closure of a vessel supplying a significant amount of myocardium.

Coronary Bypass Reoperations

Patients in whom new stenoses develop in native arteries or in bypass grafts may have recurrent ischemic syndromes. Observational study of patients with severe vein graft atherosclerosis indicate that this is an unstable lesion often leading to serious cardiac events, particularly if the LAD or multiple vessels are jeopardized; reoperation appears to improve the survival rate of these patients. Reoperations are more difficult and dangerous than primary procedures, but the risk now approaches that for primary procedures in institutions performing a large number of reoperations. PCI is sometimes an alternative for the treatment of vein graft disease (Chapter 73).

Coexisting Cardiac Disease

During cardiac operations performed for valvar (Chapter 75) or aortic (Chapter 78) disease, the standard treatment is to perform bypass grafts to major coronary arteries with angiographic stenoses of more than 50% of the luminal diameter. No randomized trials have addressed this issue, and these indications, although logical given the natural history of atherosclerosis, remain practice patterns based on consensus but not on definitive data.

CORONARY ARTERY BYPASS GRAFTING VERSUS PERCUTANEOUS CORONARY INTERVENTIONS

CABG and PCIs are alternative anatomic treatments for coronary artery disease, each with different advantages and disadvantages. After 7 years of follow-up in the Bypass Angioplasty Revascularization Investigation (BARI), the patients treated with balloon angioplasty without stenting experienced more angina and underwent significantly more repeated revascularization procedures (PCI 60% versus CABG 13%), and 34% of PCI patients had "crossed over" to CABG. The survival rates for these selected patients in the BARI trial were equivalent for balloon angioplasty and CABG except for patients with treated diabetes, who had a significantly worse survival rate with PCI than with CABG. [4]

Randomized trials of bare metal stenting versus CABG have shown either no survival differences or an advantage for CABG. [5,6] Furthermore, large observational studies comparing survival rates after bypass surgery and PCI have shown a better prognosis for patients treated with surgery. Recent technologic improvements in PCI (e.g., drug-eluting stents) have decreased the rate of restenosis from about 50% at 1 year after PCI to approximately 10%, but it is not yet known whether the survival rate after PCI will now match CABG across the full spectrum of patients, especially because late events after PCI are often related to progression of disease in nonstented areas. By comparison, CABG bypasses longer areas of coronary atherosclerosis.

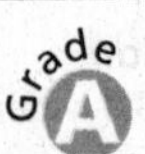

1. Khan NE, De Souza A, Mister R, et al: A randomized comparison of off-pump and on-pump multivessel coronary-artery bypass surgery. N Engl J Med 2004;350:21–28.
2. Yusuf S, Zucker D, Peduzzi P, et al: Effect of coronary artery bypass graft surgery on survival: Overview of 10-year results from randomized trials by the Coronary Artery Bypass Graft Surgery Trialists Collaboration. Lancet 1994;344:563–570.
3. Mehta SR, Cannon CP, Fox KA, et al: Routine vs selective invasive strategies in patients with acute coronary syndromes: A collaborative meta-analysis of randomized trials. JAMA 2005;23: 2908–2917.
4. BARI Investigators: The final 10-year follow-up results from the BARI randomized trial. J Am Coll Cardiol 2007;49:1600–1606.
5. Legrand VMG, Serruys PW, Unger F, et al: Three-year outcome after coronary stenting versus bypass surgery for the treatment of multivessel disease. Circulation 2004;109:1114–1120.
6. Hannan EL, Racz MJ, Walford G, et al: Long-term outcomes of coronary-artery bypass grafting versus stent implantation. N Engl J Med 2005;352:2174–2183.

SUGGESTED READINGS

ACC/AHA 2004 Guideline Update for Coronary Artery Bypass Graft Surgery. A report of the American College of Cardiology/American Heart Association Task Force on Practice Guidelines (Committee to Update the 1999 Guidelines for Coronary Artery Bypass Graft Surgery). Circulation 2004;110:1168–1176. *Guidelines for the indications for coronary bypass surgery in a variety of clinical situations.*

Goldman S, Zadina K, Moritz T, et al: Long-term patency of saphenous vein and left internal mammary artery grafts after coronary artery bypass surgery: Results from a Department of Veterans Affairs Cooperative Study. J Am Coll Cardiol 2004;44:2149–2156. *Patency at 10 years was 61% for saphenous vein grafts compared with 85% for internal mammary artery grafts.*

Martens TP, Argenziano M, Oz MC: New technology for coronary revascularization. Circulation 2006;114:606–614. *Review of the various techniques and procedures.*

Sabik JF III, Blackstone EH, Houghtaling PL, et al: Is reoperation still a risk factor in coronary artery bypass surgery? Ann Thorac Surg 2005;80:1719–1727. *Yes, but not as big a risk as in the past.*

van Dijk D, Spoor M, Hijman R, et al: Cognitive and cardiac outcomes 5 years after off-pump vs on-pump coronary artery bypass graft surgery. JAMA 2007;297:701–708. *In low-risk patients undergoing CABG surgery, avoiding the use of cardiopulmonary bypass had no effect on 5-year cognitive or cardiac outcomes.*

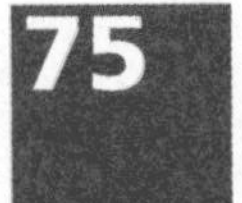

VALVULAR HEART DISEASE

Blase A. Carabello

The cardiac valves permit unobstructed forward blood flow through the heart when they are open while preventing backward flow when they are closed. Most valvular heart diseases cause either valvular stenosis with obstruction to forward flow or valvular regurgitation with backward flow. Valvular stenosis imparts a pressure overload on the left or right ventricle because these chambers must generate higher than normal pressure to overcome the obstruction to pump blood forward. Valvular regurgitation imparts a volume overload on the heart, which now must pump additional volume to compensate for what is regurgitated. When valve disease is severe, these hemodynamic burdens can lead to ventricular dysfunction, heart failure, and sudden death (Table 75–1). In almost every instance, definitive therapy for severe valvular heart disease is mechanical restoration of valve function.

AORTIC STENOSIS

Epidemiology

Bicuspid and Other Congenitally Abnormal Aortic Valves

Approximately 1% of the population is born with a bicuspid aortic valve, with a male preponderance (Chapter 68). Although this abnormality does not usually cause a hemodynamic disturbance at birth, bicuspid aortic valves tend to deteriorate with age. Approximately a third of these valves become stenotic, another third become regurgitant, and the remainder cause only minor hemodynamic abnormalities. When stenosis develops, it usually occurs when patients are in their 40s, 50s, and 60s.

Sometimes, congenital aortic stenosis from a unicuspid, bicuspid, or even abnormal tricuspid valve causes symptoms during childhood and requires correction by adolescence. Occasionally, these congenitally stenotic aortic valves escape detection until adulthood.

Tricuspid Aortic Valve Stenosis

In some patients born with apparently normal tricuspid aortic valves, thickening and calcification develop similar to what occurs in bicuspid

TABLE 75–1 SUMMARY OF SEVERE VALVAR HEART DISEASE

	Aortic Stenosis	Mitral Stenosis	Mitral Regurgitation	Aortic Regurgitation
Etiology	Idiopathic calcification of a bicuspid or tricuspid valve Congenital Rheumatic	Rheumatic fever Annular calcification	Mitral valve prolapse Ruptured chordae Endocarditis Ischemic papillary muscle dysfunction or rupture Collagen vascular diseases and syndromes Secondary to LV myocardial diseases	Annuloaortic ectasia Hypertension Endocarditis Marfan syndrome Ankylosing spondylitis Aortic dissection Syphilis Collagen vascular disease
Pathophysiology	Pressure overload on the LV with compensation by LV hypertrophy As disease advances, reduced coronary flow reserve causes angina Hypertrophy and afterload excess lead to systolic and diastolic LV dysfunction	Obstruction to LV inflow increases left atrial pressure and limits cardiac output, thus mimicking LV failure. Mitral valve obstruction increases the pressure work of the right ventricle Right ventricular pressure overload is augmented further when pulmonary hypertension develops	Places volume overload on the LV. Ventricle responds with eccentric hypertrophy and dilation, which allow increased ventricular stroke volume Eventually, however, LV dysfunction develops if volume overload is uncorrected	*Chronic* Total stroke volume causes hyperdynamic circulation, induces systolic hypertension, and causes pressure and volume overload. Compensation is by concentric and eccentric hypertrophy *Acute* Because cardiac dilation has not developed, hyperdynamic findings are absent. High diastolic LV pressure causes mitral valve preclosure and potentiates LV ischemia and failure
Symptoms	Angina Syncope Heart failure	Dyspnea Orthopnea PND Hemoptysis Hoarseness Edema Ascites	Dyspnea Orthopnea PND	Dyspnea Orthopnea PND Angina Syncope
Signs	Systolic ejection murmur radiating to the neck Delayed carotid upstroke S_4, soft or paradoxical S_2	Diastolic rumble after an opening snap Loud S_1 Right ventricular lift Loud P_2	Holosystolic apical murmur radiating to the axilla, S_3 Displaced PMI	*Chronic* Diastolic blowing murmur Hyperdynamic circulation Displaced PMI Quincke pulse DeMusset's sign *Acute* Short diastolic blowing murmur Soft S_1

Continued

TABLE 75–1 SUMMARY OF SEVERE VALVAR HEART DISEASE—cont'd

	Aortic Stenosis	Mitral Stenosis	Mitral Regurgitation	Aortic Regurgitation
Electrocardiogram	LAA LVH	LAA RVH	LAA LVH	LAA LVH
Chest radiograph	Boot-shaped heart Aortic valve calcification on lateral view	Straightening of left heart border Double density at right heart border Kerley B lines Enlarged pulmonary arteries	Cardiac enlargement	*Chronic* Cardiac enlargement Uncoiling of the aorta *Acute* Pulmonary congestion with normal heart size
Echocardiographic findings	Concentric LVH Reduced aortic valve cusp separation Doppler shows mean gradient ≥50 mm Hg in most severe cases	Restricted mitral leaflet motion Valve area ≤1 cm^2 in most severe cases Tricuspid Doppler may reveal pulmonary hypertension	LV and LAA in chronic severe disease Doppler: large regurgitant jet	*Chronic* LV enlargement Large Doppler jet PHT <400 msec *Acute* Small LV Mitral valve preclosure
Catheterization findings	Increased LVEDP Transaortic gradient 50 mm Hg AVA ≤0.7 in most severe cases	Elevated pulmonary capillary wedge pressure Transmitral gradient usually >10 mm Hg in severe cases MVA <1 cm^2	Elevated pulmonary capillary wedge pressure Ventriculography shows regurgitation of dye into LV	Wide pulse pressure Aortography shows regurgitation of dye into LV Usually unnecessary
Medical therapy	Avoid vasodilators Digitalis, diuretics, and nitroglycerin in inoperable cases	Diuretics for mild symptoms Anticoagulation in atrial fibrillation Digitalis, β-blockers, verapamil, or diltiazem for rate control	Vasodilators in acute disease No proven therapy in chronic disease (but vasodilators commonly used)	*Chronic* Vasodilators in chronic asymptomatic disease with normal left ventricular function *Acute* Vasodilators
Indications for surgery	Appearance of symptoms in patients with severe disease (see text)	Appearance of more than mild symptoms Development of pulmonary hypertension Appearance of persistent atrial fibrillation	Appearance of symptoms EF <0.60 ESD ≥45 mm	*Chronic* Appearance of symptoms EF <0.55 ESD ≥55 mm *Acute* Even mild heart failure Mitral valve preclosure

AVA = aortic valve area; EF = ejection fraction; ESD = end-systolic diameter; LAA = left atrial enlargement; LV = left ventricle; LVEDP = left ventricular end-diastolic pressure; LVH = left ventricular hypertrophy; MVA = mitral valve area; PHT = pressure half-time; PMI = point of maximal impulse; PND = paroxysmal nocturnal dyspnea; RVH = right ventricular hypertrophy.

valves. When aortic stenosis develops in previously normal tricuspid aortic valves, it usually does so in the 60s to 80s. Although stenosis and calcifications of bicuspid and tricuspid aortic valves were formerly considered to be degenerative processes, it is clear that this type of aortic stenosis arises from an active inflammatory process similar to that of coronary heart disease. This concept is supported by many pieces of evidence. First, the initial lesion of aortic stenosis is similar to the plaque of coronary disease. Second, both diseases have hypertension and hyperlipidemia as risk factors. Third, there is excellent correlation between calcification of the aortic valve and calcification of the coronary arteries. Fourth, patients with the most severe aortic stenosis have the highest levels of C-reactive protein.

Rheumatic Valvular Heart Disease

Rheumatic valve disease is now a rare cause of aortic stenosis in developed countries. In virtually every case, the mitral valve is also detectably abnormal.

Pathobiology

Relationship to Symptoms

The presence or absence of the classic symptoms of aortic stenosis—angina, syncope, and the symptoms of heart failure—is the key to the natural history of the disease. Before the onset of symptoms, survival is similar to that for the normal population, and sudden death is rare, occurring in less than 1% of asymptomatic patients. When the classic symptoms develop, however, survival declines precipitously. Approximately 35% of patients with aortic stenosis are initially evaluated for angina. Of these, 50% are dead in 5 years unless aortic valve replacement is performed. Approximately 15% have syncope; of these, 50% are dead in only 3 years unless the aortic valve is replaced. Of the 50% with symptoms of heart failure, 50% are dead in 2 years without aortic valve replacement. In all, only 25% of patients with symptomatic aortic stenosis survive 3 years in the absence of valve replacement, and the annual risk for sudden death ranges from 10% in patients with angina to 15% with syncope to 25% with heart failure. Prompt recognition of symptoms and evaluation for possible severe aortic stenosis are crucial in managing the disease.

The normal aortic valve area is 3 to 4 cm^2, and little hemodynamic disturbance occurs until the orifice is reduced to about a third of normal, at which point a systolic gradient develops between the left ventricle and aorta. Left ventricular (LV) and aortic pressure is normally nearly equal during systole. In aortic stenosis, intracavitary LV pressure must increase above aortic pressure, however, to produce forward flow across the stenotic valve and to achieve acceptable downstream pressure (see Fig. 56–1). There is a geometric progression in the magnitude of the gradient as the valve area narrows. Given a normal cardiac output, the gradient rises rapidly from 10 to 15 mm Hg at valve areas of 1.5 to 1.3 cm^2 to about 25 mm Hg at 1.0 cm^2, 50 mm Hg at 0.8 cm^2, 70 mm Hg at 0.6 cm^2, and 100 mm Hg at 0.5 cm^2. The rate of progression of aortic stenosis varies widely from patient to patient; it may remain stable for many years or increase by more than 15 mm Hg per year.

A major compensatory response to the increased LV pressure associated with aortic stenosis is the development of concentric LV hypertrophy. The Laplace equation—stress (s) = pressure (p) × radius (r)/2 × thickness (th)—indicates that the force on any unit of LV myocardium (afterload) varies directly with ventricular pressure and radius and inversely with wall thickness. As pressure increases, it can be offset by increased LV wall thickness (concentric hypertrophy). The determinants of LV ejection fraction are contractility, preload, and afterload. By normalizing afterload, the development of concentric hypertrophy helps preserve ejection fraction and cardiac output despite the pressure overload. Although hypertrophy clearly serves a compensatory function, it also has a pathologic role and is in part responsible for the classic symptoms of aortic stenosis.

Angina

In general, angina (Chapter 70) results from myocardial ischemia when LV oxygen (and other nutrient) demand exceeds supply, which is predicated on coronary blood flow. In normal subjects, coronary blood flow can increase five- to eightfold under maximum metabolic demand, but in patients with aortic stenosis this reserve is limited. Reduced coronary blood flow reserve may be caused by a relative diminution in capillary ingrowth to serve the needs of the hypertrophied left ventricle or by a reduced transcoronary gradient for coronary blood flow because of the elevated LV end-diastolic pressure. Restricted coronary blood flow reserve appears to be responsible for angina in many patients who have aortic stenosis despite normal epicardial coronary arteries. In other patients, angina is due to increased oxygen demand when inadequate hypertrophy allows wall stress, a key determinant of myocardial oxygen consumption, to increase.

Syncope

Syncope (Chapters 61 and 427) generally occurs because of inadequate cerebral perfusion. In aortic stenosis, syncope is usually related to exertion. It may result when exertion causes a fall in total peripheral resistance that cannot be compensated by increased cardiac output because output is limited by the obstruction to LV outflow; this combination reduces systemic blood pressure and cerebral perfusion. In addition, high LV pressure during exercise may trigger a systemic vasodepressor response that lowers blood pressure and produces syncope. Cardiac arrhythmias, possibly caused by exertional ischemia, also cause hypotension and syncope.

Heart Failure

In aortic stenosis, contractile dysfunction (systolic failure) and failure of normal relaxation (diastolic failure) occur and cause symptoms (Chapter 57). The extent of ventricular contraction is governed by contractility and afterload. In aortic stenosis, contractility (the ability to generate force) is often reduced. The mechanisms of contractile dysfunction may include abnormal calcium handling, microtubular hyperpolymerization causing an internal viscous load on the myocyte, and myocardial ischemia. In some cases, contractile function is normal, but the hypertrophy is inadequate to normalize wall stress and excessive afterload results. Excessive afterload inhibits ejection, reduces forward output, and leads to heart failure.

The increased wall thickness that helps normalize stress increases diastolic stiffness. Even if muscle properties remain normal, higher filling pressure is required to distend a thicker ventricle. As aortic stenosis advances, collagen deposition also stiffens the myocardium and adds to the diastolic dysfunction.

Diagnosis

Physical Examination

The diagnosis of aortic stenosis is usually first suspected when the classic systolic ejection murmur is heard during physical examination (Chapter 48). The murmur is loudest in the aortic area and radiates to the neck. In some cases, the murmur may disappear over the sternum and reappear over the LV apex, thereby giving the false impression that a murmur of mitral regurgitation is also present (Gallivardan's phenomenon). The intensity of the murmur increases with cycle length because longer cycles are associated with greater aortic flow. In mild disease, the murmur peaks in intensity in early or mid-systole. As the severity of stenosis worsens, the murmur peaks progressively later in systole. Perhaps the most helpful clue to the severity of aortic stenosis by physical examination is the characteristic delay in the carotid pulse with a diminution in its volume (see Fig. 48–2); in elderly patients, however, increasing carotid stiffness may pseudonormalize the carotid upstrokes. The LV apical impulse in aortic stenosis is not displaced but is enlarged and forceful. The simultaneous palpation of a forceful LV apex beat and a delayed and weakened carotid pulse is a persuasive clue that severe aortic stenosis is present. The S_1 in aortic stenosis is generally normal. In congenital aortic stenosis when the valve is not calcified, S_1 may be followed by a systolic ejection click. In calcific disease, S_2 may be single and soft when the aortic component is lost because the valve neither opens nor closes well. In some cases, delayed LV emptying secondary to LV dysfunction may create paradoxical splitting of S_2. An S_4 gallop is common. In advanced disease, pulmonary hypertension and signs of right-sided failure are common.

Because of the dire consequences of missing the diagnosis of aortic stenosis, the physician must have a low threshold for obtaining an echocardiogram whenever aortic stenosis cannot be excluded by physical examination. In asymptomatic patients with suspicious murmurs, early diagnosis allows the patient and physician to be more vigilant regarding possible early signs and symptoms and to guide the use of prophylactic regimens to prevent bacterial endocarditis (Chapter 76).

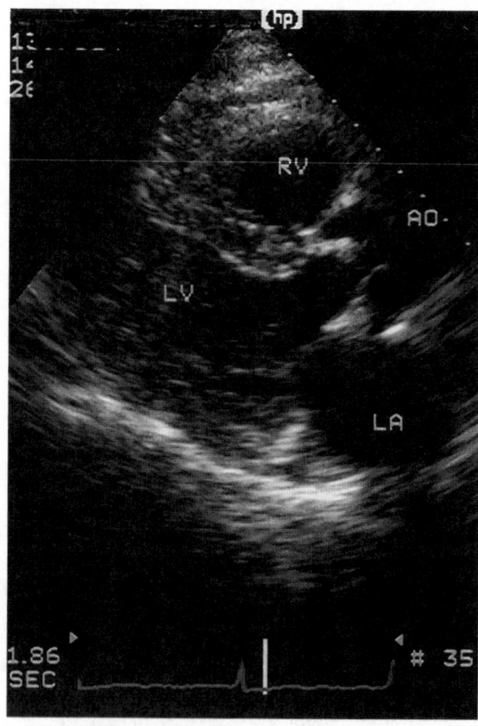

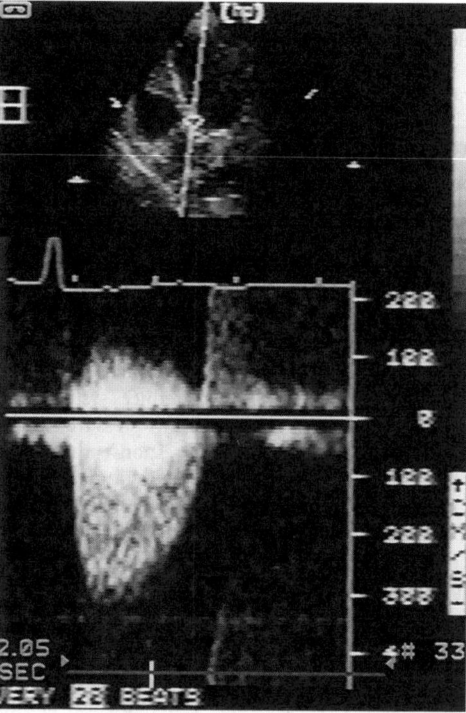

FIGURE 75–1 • Doppler echocardiogram from a patient with aortic stenosis. The left panel shows thickened aortic valve leaflets that dome into the aorta with restricted opening in systole. The right panel shows a miniaturized apical four-chamber view at the top with a Doppler cursor through the aorta, whereas the bottom panel shows a continuous-wave spectral Doppler signal with a peak velocity of 3 m/sec. The peak valve gradient can be calculated as 4×3^2, or 36 mm Hg. AO = aorta; LA = left atrium; LV = left ventricle; RV = right ventricle. (Courtesy of Dr. Anthony DeMaria.)

Diagnostic Testing

The electrocardiogram (ECG) in patients with aortic stenosis usually shows LV hypertrophy (Chapter 52). In some cases of even severe aortic stenosis, however, LV hypertrophy is absent on the ECG, possibly because of the lack of LV dilation. Left atrial abnormality is common because the stiff left ventricle increases left atrial afterload and causes the left atrium to dilate.

The chest radiograph in aortic stenosis is generally nondiagnostic. The cardiac silhouette is not usually enlarged but may assume a boot-shaped configuration. In advanced cases, there may be signs of cardiomegaly and pulmonary congestion; aortic valve calcification may be seen in the lateral view.

Echocardiography (Chapter 53) is indispensable to assess the extent of LV hypertrophy, systolic ejection performance, and aortic valve anatomy (Fig. 75–1). Doppler interrogation of the aortic valve makes use of the modified Bernoulli equation (gradient = $4 \times \text{velocity}^2$) to assess the severity of the stenosis (Chapter 53). As blood flows from the body of the left ventricle across the stenotic valve, the flow rate must accelerate for the volume to remain constant. Doppler interrogation of the valve can be performed to detect this increase in velocity for estimation of the valve gradient. The peak aortic flow velocity in patients with preserved LV systolic function is a useful clinical guide to prognosis. In patients with a flow velocity of 3.0 mL/sec or less, symptoms are unlikely to develop in the next 5 years; by comparison, in patients with a flow velocity of 4.0 mL/sec or greater, symptoms usually develop within 2 years.

Although exercise testing is contraindicated in symptomatic patients with aortic stenosis because of the high risk for complications, cautious exercise testing is gaining favor in asymptomatic patients. Such testing often reveals latent symptoms or hemodynamic instability that have gone unrecognized during the patient's normal daily activities. Exercise-induced hypotension or symptoms are indications for aortic valve replacement in patients with severe aortic stenosis; in patients with mild to moderate aortic stenosis, another source of exercise limitation should be sought.

Brain natriuretic peptide levels may be higher in patients who will become symptomatic in a short time span. However, use of this biomarker to indicate the need for valve replacement is premature.

Cardiac catheterization for performance of coronary arteriography is usually undertaken before surgery because most patients with aortic stenosis are of the age at which coronary disease is common. When echocardiography shows severe aortic stenosis and the patient has one or more of the classic symptoms of the disease, formal invasive documentation of the severity of the stenosis is not necessary, and coronary angiography need not be performed in young adults. When the hemodynamic diagnosis is unclear, however, right-sided and left-sided heart catheterization should be performed to determine the transaortic valvular pressure gradient and cardiac output, which are used to calculate the aortic valve area by the Gorlin formula:

$$A = \frac{CO/SEP \times HR}{44.3\sqrt{h}}$$

where CO is cardiac output (mL/min), SEP is the systolic ejection period (sec), HR is the heart rate, and h is the mean gradient.

Treatment

Invasive Therapy

Valve Replacement Surgery

The only proven effective therapy for aortic stenosis is aortic valve replacement. Once the symptoms of aortic stenosis develop, the 3-year mortality is 75% without aortic valve replacement. When the valve is replaced, however, survival returns nearly to normal. Even octogenarians benefit from valve replacement unless other comorbid factors preclude surgery, so aortic valve replacement should not be denied simply on the basis of age. Valve replacement should also not be denied because the ejection fraction is reduced; the excess afterload imposed by the stenotic valve is relieved with valve replacement, and a depressed ejection fraction usually improves dramatically after surgery. The exception to this rule is a severely reduced ejection fraction in the face of only a small aortic valve gradient; in this case the severity of the aortic stenosis may be overestimated because the failing left ventricle has difficulty opening a mildly to moderately stenotic valve. In such patients, LV muscle dysfunction either has another cause or is often so severe that it does not recover after valve replacement. Evidence indicates, however, that even some well-selected patients in this category, such as patients who demonstrate increased cardiac output during dobutamine infusion, may benefit from aortic valve replacement.

Balloon Aortic Valvotomy

In acquired calcific aortic stenosis, leaflet restriction results from heavy calcium deposition in the leaflets themselves and is not due to commissural fusion. Balloon aortic valvotomy is relatively inef-

Rx

fective in improving aortic stenosis; it generally results in a residual gradient of 30 to 50 mm Hg and a valve area of 1.0 cm^2. Mortality after this procedure is similar to that in untreated patients. The only occasional indication for balloon aortic valvotomy is palliative in cases in which aortic valve replacement is impossible because of comorbidity or is impractical when immediate temporary relief is required because of the demands of other noncardiac conditions.

Percutaneous Aortic Valve Replacement

Early trials indicate the feasibility of replacing the aortic valve percutaneously in patients too ill to undergo surgery. In this procedure, the native valve is dilated as described earlier. After dilation, a stented valve is inserted over a balloon into the aortic annulus. The balloon is expanded to secure the valve and its stent, which is intended to help prevent restenosis.

Medical Therapy

The only medical therapy indicated in patients with aortic stenosis is antibiotic prophylaxis to prevent bacterial endocarditis (Chapter 76). Otherwise, the patient is either asymptomatic and requires no therapy or is symptomatic and requires surgery. In patients with heart failure awaiting surgery, diuretics can be used cautiously to relieve pulmonary congestion. Nitrates may also be used cautiously to treat angina pectoris. Although vasodilators, especially angiotensin-converting enzyme inhibitors, have become a cornerstone of therapy for heart failure, they are not recommended for aortic stenosis. With fixed valvular obstruction to outflow, vasodilation reduces pressure distal to the obstruction without increasing cardiac output and may cause syncope. Statins do not slow the progression of calcific aortic stenosis. When surgery and valvoplasty are unsuccessful or impossible, digitalis and diuretics can be used to improve symptoms with the understanding that they will not improve life expectancy.

MITRAL STENOSIS

Epidemiology

In almost all cases of acquired mitral stenosis, the cause is rheumatic heart disease. Occasionally, severe calcification of the mitral annulus can lead to mitral stenosis in the absence of rheumatic involvement. Mitral stenosis is three times more common in women and usually develops in the 40s and 50s. Although the disease has become rare in developed countries because of the waning incidence of rheumatic fever, mitral stenosis is still prevalent in developing nations, where rheumatic fever is common.

Pathobiology

At the beginning of diastole, a transient gradient between the left atrium and left ventricle normally initiates LV filling. After early filling, left atrial and LV pressures equilibrate. In mitral stenosis, obstruction to LV filling increases left atrial pressure and produces a persistent gradient between the left atrium and the left ventricle (see Fig. 56–1). The combination of elevated left atrial pressure (and pulmonary venous pressure) and restriction of inflow into the left ventricle limits cardiac output. Although myocardial involvement from the rheumatic process occasionally affects LV muscle function, the muscle itself is normal in most patients with mitral stenosis. However, in approximately a third of patients with mitral stenosis, LV ejection performance is reduced despite normal muscle function because of reduced preload (from inflow obstruction) and increased afterload as a result of reflex vasoconstriction caused by reduced cardiac output.

Because the right ventricle generates most of the force that propels blood across the mitral valve, the right ventricle incurs the pressure overload of the transmitral gradient. In addition, secondary but reversible pulmonary vasoconstriction develops, thus further increasing pulmonary artery pressure and the burden on the right ventricle. As mitral stenosis worsens, right ventricular (RV) failure develops.

Diagnosis

History

Patients with mitral stenosis usually remain asymptomatic until the valve area is reduced to about a third its normal size of 4 to 5 cm^2. Then the symptoms typical of left-sided failure—dyspnea on exertion, orthopnea, and paroxysmal nocturnal dyspnea—develop. As the disease progresses and RV failure occurs, ascites and edema are common. Hemoptysis, which is common in mitral stenosis but uncommon in other causes of left atrial hypertension, develops when high left atrial pressure ruptures the anastomoses of small bronchial veins. In some cases, a large left atrium may impinge on the left recurrent laryngeal nerve and cause hoarseness (Ortner's syndrome) or may impinge on the esophagus and cause dysphagia.

Physical Examination

Although mitral stenosis produces typical and diagnostic findings on physical examination, the diagnosis is missed frequently because the auscultatory findings may be subtle. Palpation of the precordium finds a quiet apical impulse. If pulmonary hypertension and RV hypertrophy have developed, the examiner notes a parasternal lift. S_1 is typically loud and may be the most prominent physical finding of the disease. A loud S_1 is present because the transmitral gradient holds the mitral valve open throughout diastole until ventricular systole closes the fully opened valve with a loud closing sound. In far-advanced disease, the mitral valve may be so damaged, however, that it neither opens nor closes well, so S_1 may become soft. S_2 is normally split; the pulmonic component is increased in intensity if pulmonary hypertension has developed. Left-sided S_3 and S_4 gallop sounds, which represent the ventricular and atrial components of rapid LV filling, are exceedingly rare in mitral stenosis because obstruction at the mitral valve prevents rapid filling. S_2 is usually followed by an opening snap. The distance between S_2 and the opening snap provides a reasonable estimation of left atrial pressure and the severity of the mitral stenosis. The higher the left atrial pressure, the sooner the left atrial pressure and the falling LV pressure of early ventricular relaxation equilibrate. At this equilibration point, the mitral valve opens, and the opening snap occurs. When left atrial pressure is high, the opening snap closely (0.06 second) follows S_2. Conversely, when left atrial pressure is relatively normal, the snap occurs later (0.12 second) and may mimic the cadence of an S_3 gallop. The opening snap is followed by the classic low-pitched early diastolic mitral stenosis rumble, which increases in length as the mitral stenosis worsens. This murmur may be inaudible if the patient has a relatively low resting cardiac output. Modest exercise, such as isometric handgrip, may accentuate the murmur's intensity. If the patient is in sinus rhythm, atrial systole may produce a presystolic accentuation of the murmur. If pulmonary hypertension has developed, the pulmonic component of S_2 increases in intensity to become as loud or louder than the aortic component. With pulmonary hypertension, a diastolic blowing murmur of pulmonary insufficiency (Graham Steell's murmur) is often heard, although in many cases a coexistent murmur of mild aortic insufficiency is mistaken for this murmur. Neck vein elevation, ascites, and edema are present if RV failure has developed.

Noninvasive Evaluation

If the patient is in sinus rhythm, left atrial abnormality is generally present on the ECG. Atrial fibrillation is common, however. If pulmonary hypertension has developed, there is often evidence of RV hypertrophy.

On the chest radiograph, left atrial enlargement produces straightening of the left heart border and a double density at the right heart border as a result of the combined silhouettes of the right atrium and left atrium. Pulmonary venous hypertension produces increased vascularity. Kerley B lines, which represent thickening of the pulmonary septa secondary to chronic venous engorgement, may also be seen.

The echocardiogram produces excellent images of the mitral valve and is the most important diagnostic tool in confirming the diagnosis (Fig. 75–2). Transthoracic echocardiography or, if necessary, transesophageal echocardiography makes the diagnosis in nearly 100% of cases and accurately assesses severity. Mitral stenosis, similar to aortic stenosis, can be quantified by assessing the transvalvular gradient with the modified Bernoulli principle. The stenosis is considered mild when the calculated or planimetered valve area is more than 1.75 cm^2, moderate at 1.25 to 1.75 cm^2, moderately severe at 1.0 to 1.25 cm^2, and severe at less than 1.0 cm^2.

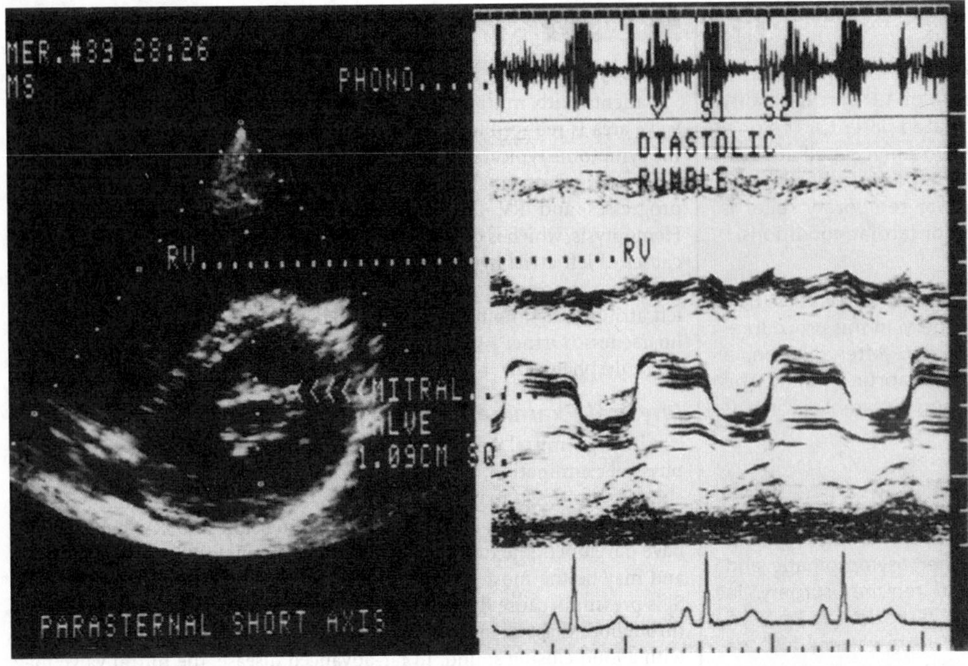

FIGURE 75–2 • Mitral stenosis. An en fosse view of a stenotic mitral valve in the short-axis view of the left ventricle is shown on the left. Planimetry for the mitral valve orifice yielded an area of 1.09 cm^2. The M-mode echocardiogram on the right has been aligned with the appropriate structures on the left. It shows the restricted opening of the mitral valve in diastole associated with the classic diastolic rumbling murmur. RV = right ventricle. (From Assey ME, Usher BW, Carabello BA: The patient with valvular heart disease. *In* Pepine CJ, Hill JA, Lambert CR [eds]: Diagnostic and Therapeutic Cardiac Catheterization, 3rd ed. Baltimore, Williams & Wilkins, 1998, p 709.)

During echocardiography, the suitability of the valve for balloon valvotomy can also be assessed (see later). If even mild tricuspid regurgitation is present, the systolic gradient across the tricuspid valve can be used to gauge pulmonary artery pressure, which is an important prognostic factor in mitral stenosis because the prognosis worsens as pulmonary pressure increases.

Invasive Evaluation

Cardiac Catheterization

Cardiac catheterization is usually unnecessary to assess the severity of mitral stenosis. Because many patients with mitral stenosis are of an age when coronary disease might be present, however, coronary arteriography is generally performed if cardiac surgery is anticipated or if the patient has coexistent angina. In these cases, it is common to perform left-sided and right-sided heart catheterization to confirm the transmitral gradient and to calculate the valve area from the Gorlin formula (see earlier).

Prevention and Treatment

Mitral stenosis can be prevented by appropriate antibiotic treatment of β-hemolytic streptococcal infections (Chapters 312 and 313).

Medical Therapy

Asymptomatic patients with mitral stenosis and sinus rhythm require no therapy. Symptoms of mild dyspnea and orthopnea can be treated with diuretics alone. When symptoms worsen to more than mild or if pulmonary hypertension develops, mechanical correction of the stenosis is preferable to medical therapy because it improves longevity in severely symptomatic patients.

Patients with mitral stenosis in whom atrial fibrillation develops usually decompensate because the rapid heart rate reduces diastolic filling time, increases left atrial pressure, and decreases cardiac output. The heart rate must be controlled promptly, preferably with an infusion of diltiazem or esmolol for acute atrial fibrillation or with a β-blocker, a calcium-channel blocker, or oral digoxin in chronic atrial fibrillation (Chapter 63).

Conversion to sinus rhythm is routinely recommended either pharmacologically or with direct-current countershock (Chapter 63) after anticoagulation is therapeutic. It should be noted that patients with rheumatic atrial fibrillation have been excluded from trials of echocardiogram-guided cardioversion without anticoagulation and trials of rate control versus rhythm control for the chronic management of atrial fibrillation. If sinus rhythm cannot be maintained, mechanical therapy for the mitral stenosis is generally recommended in the hope that sinus rhythm can be restored after the obstruction to atrial outflow is corrected. However, the cause of atrial fibrillation in patients with mitral stenosis probably includes atrial rheumatic inflammation, so restoration of sinus rhythm is unpredictable even after mechanical intervention.

Because patients with concomitant mitral stenosis and atrial fibrillation have an extraordinarily high risk for systemic embolism, they should undergo chronic anticoagulation with warfarin at an international normalized ratio (INR) target of 2.5 to 3.5. Anticoagulation is warranted in all patients unless there is a serious contraindication to its use.

Mechanical Therapy

When symptoms progress past early functional class II, that is, symptoms with more than ordinary activity, or if pulmonary hypertension develops, the prognosis is worse unless the mitral stenosis is relieved. In most instances, an excellent result can be achieved with percutaneous balloon valvotomy. In contrast to aortic stenosis, in mitral stenosis there is fusion of the valve leaflets at the commissures. Balloon dilation produces a commissurotomy and a substantial increase in valve area that appears to persist for at least a decade and provides improvement comparable to that of closed or open commissurotomy in suitable patients. 1 Suitability for balloon valvotomy is determined partially during echocardiography. Patients with pliable valves, little valvular calcification, little involvement of the subvalvular apparatus, and less than moderate mitral regurgitation are ideal candidates. Even when valve anatomy is not ideal, however, valvotomy may be attempted in patients with advanced age or in situations in which comorbid risk factors increase surgical risk. In otherwise healthy patients with unfavorable valve anatomy, surgery to perform an open commissurotomy or valve replacement is undertaken.

MITRAL REGURGITATION

Epidemiology

The mitral valve is composed of the mitral annulus, the leaflets, the chordae tendineae, and the papillary muscles. Abnormalities in any of these structures may lead to mitral regurgitation. The most common cause of mitral regurgitation in the United States is mitral valve prolapse, which is responsible for approximately two thirds of all cases and comprises many diseases, including myxomatous degeneration of the valve. Myocardial ischemia leading to papillary muscle dysfunction or infarction is the next most common cause and accounts for approximately a fourth of all cases. Annular calcification, endocarditis, collagen vascular disease, and rheumatic heart disease are less common causes. Use of the weight loss agents dexfenfluramine and fenfluramine has been implicated in causing valve damage in a few patients who received these drugs.

Mitral regurgitation can be subdivided on the basis of chronicity. Common causes of severe acute mitral regurgitation include ruptured chordae tendineae, ischemic papillary muscle dysfunction or rupture, and infective endocarditis. Chronic severe mitral regurgitation is more likely to be due to myxomatous degeneration of the valve, rheumatic heart disease, or annular calcification.

Pathobiology

The pathophysiology of mitral regurgitation can be divided into three phases (Fig. 75–3). In acute mitral regurgitation of any cause, the sudden option for ejection of blood into the left atrium "wastes" a portion of the LV stroke volume as backward rather than forward flow. The combined regurgitant and forward flow causes volume overload of the left ventricle and stretches the existing sarcomeres toward their maximum length. Use of the Frank-Starling mechanism is maximized, and end-diastolic volume increases concomitantly. The regurgitant pathway unloads the left ventricle in systole because it allows ejection into the relatively low-impedance left atrium and thereby reduces end-systolic volume. Although increased end-diastolic volume and decreased end-systolic volume act in concert to increase total stroke volume, forward stroke volume is subnormal because a large portion of the total stroke volume is regurgitated into the left atrium. This regurgitant volume increases left atrial pressure, so the patient experiences heart failure with low cardiac output and pulmonary congestion despite normal LV contractile function.

In many cases, severe acute mitral regurgitation necessitates emergency surgical correction. Patients who can be managed through the acute phase may enter the phase of compensation. In this phase, eccentric LV hypertrophy and increased end-diastolic volume, combined with normal contractile function, allow ejection of a sufficiently large total stroke volume to permit forward stroke volume to return toward normal. Left atrial enlargement allows accommodation of the regurgitant volume at a lower filling pressure. In this phase, the patient may be relatively asymptomatic even during strenuous exercise.

Although severe mitral regurgitation may be tolerated for many years, the lesion eventually causes LV dysfunction. The now damaged ventricle has impaired ejection performance, and end-systolic volume increases. Greater LV residual volume at end-systole increases end-diastolic volume and end-diastolic pressure, and the symptoms of pulmonary congestion may reappear. Additional LV dilation may worsen the amount of regurgitation by causing further enlargement of the mitral annulus and malalignment of the papillary muscles. Although there is substantial contractile dysfunction, the increased preload and the presence of the regurgitant pathway, which tends to normalize afterload despite ventricular enlargement, augment the ejection fraction and may maintain it in a relatively normal range.

The causes of LV contractile dysfunction in patients with mitral regurgitation may relate to loss of contractile proteins and abnormalities in calcium handling. In at least some cases, contractile dysfunction is reversible by timely mitral valve replacement.

Diagnosis

The standard symptoms of left-sided heart failure should be sought (Chapter 57). An attempt to discover potential causes should be made by questioning for a prior history of a heart murmur or abnormal findings on cardiac examination (Chapter 48), rheumatic heart disease, endocarditis (Chapter 76), myocardial infarction (Chapter 72), or the use of anorexigenic drugs.

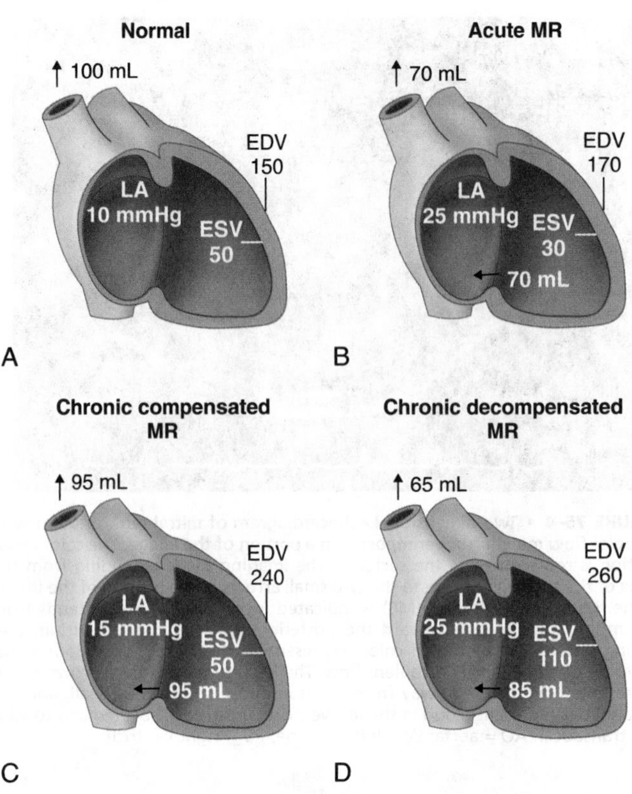

	Preload SL (μ)	Afterload ESS (Kdyne/cm²)	CF	EF	RF	FSV (mL)
N	2.07	90	N	.67	.0	100
AMR	2.25	60	N	.82	.50	70
CCMR	2.19	90	N	.79	.5	95
CDMR	2.19	120	↓	.58	.57	65

FIGURE 75–3 • Mitral regurgitation. A and B, Normal physiology (N) **(A)** is compared with the physiology of acute mitral regurgitation (AMR) **(B)**. Acutely, the volume overload increases preload (sarcomere length [SL]), and end-diastolic volume (EDV) increases from 150 to 170 mL. Unloading of the left ventricle by the presence of the regurgitant pathway decreases afterload (end-systolic stress [ESS]), and end-systolic volume (ESV) falls from 50 to 30 mL. These changes result in an increase in the ejection fraction (EF). Because 50% of the total left ventricular (LV) stroke volume (regurgitant fraction [RF]) is ejected into the left atrium (LA), however, forward stroke volume (FSV) falls from 100 to 70 mL. At this stage, contractile function (CF) is normal. **C,** Chronic compensated mitral regurgitation (CCMR). In CCMR, eccentric cardiac hypertrophy has developed, and EDV has increased substantially. Increased EDV combined with normal contractile function permits ejection of a larger total stroke volume and a larger forward stroke volume than in the acute phase. Left atrial enlargement permits lower left atrial pressure. Because the radius term in the Laplace equation has increased with increasing LV volume, afterload and ESV return to normal. **D,** Chronic decompensated mitral regurgitation (CDMR). In this stage, contractile dysfunction causes a large increase in ESV with a fall in total and forward stroke volume. Additional LV enlargement leads to worsening mitral regurgitation. The relatively favorable loading conditions in this phase still permit a normal EF, however, despite contractile dysfunction. (From Carabello BA: Mitral regurgitation: Basic pathophysiologic principles. Mod Concepts Cardiovasc Dis 1988;57: 53–57.)

Physical Examination

Volume overload of the left ventricle displaces the apical impulse downward and to the left. S_1 may be reduced in intensity, whereas S_2 is usually physiologically split. In severe mitral regurgitation, S_2 is followed by S_3, which does not indicate heart failure but reflects rapid filling of the left ventricle by the large volume of blood stored in the left atrium during systole. The typical murmur of mitral regurgitation is a holosystolic apical murmur that often radiates toward the axilla (Chapter 48). There is a rough correlation between the intensity of the murmur and the severity of the disease, but this correlation is too weak to use in clinical deci-

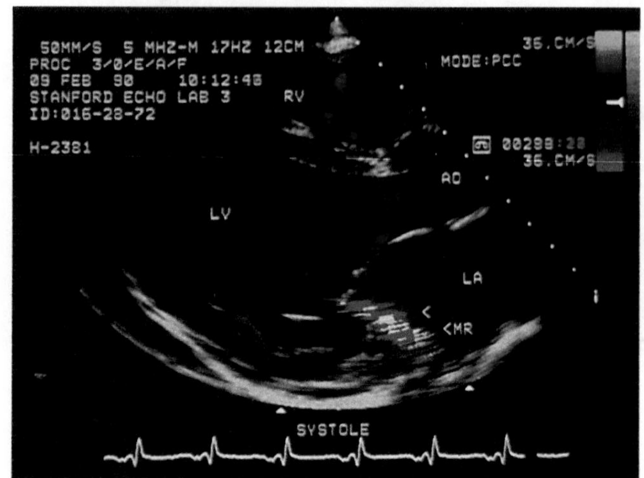

FIGURE 75–4 • Two-dimensional echocardiogram of mitral regurgitation with Doppler flow mapping superimposed on a portion of the image. The color information is represented in the sector of the imaging plane extending from the apex of the triangular plane to the two small arrows at the bottom of the image plane. Mitral regurgitation (MR) is indicated (open arrows) and extends from the mitral valve leaflets toward the posterior aspect of the left atrium (LA) during systole. The mosaic of colors representing the mitral regurgitant signal is typical of high-velocity turbulent flow. The low-intensity orange-brown signal represents flow directed away from the transducer on the chest wall, and the blue shades represent blood in the left ventricular outflow tract moving toward the transducer. AO = aorta; LV = left ventricle; RV = right ventricle.

sion making because the murmur may be soft when cardiac output is low. In contrast to aortic stenosis, murmur intensity does not usually vary with the RR interval. In acute mitral regurgitation, the presence of a large v wave may produce rapid equilibration of left atrial and LV pressure, thereby reducing the driving gradient and shortening the murmur. Pulmonary hypertension may develop and produce right-sided signs, including an RV lift, an increased P_2, and if RV dysfunction has developed, signs of right-sided heart failure.

Noninvasive Evaluation

The ECG usually shows LV hypertrophy and left atrial abnormality. The chest radiograph typically shows cardiomegaly; the absence of cardiomegaly indicates either that the mitral regurgitation is mild or that it has not been chronic enough to allow cardiac dilation to occur.

Echocardiography shows the extent of left atrial and LV enlargement (Chapter 53). Ultrasonic imaging of the mitral valve is excellent and offers clues to the mitral valve abnormalities responsible for the regurgitation. Color flow Doppler interrogation of the valve (Fig. 75–4) helps assess the severity of regurgitation, but because this technique images flow velocity rather than actual flow, it is subject to errors in interpretation. The Doppler technique is excellent for excluding the presence of mitral regurgitation and for distinguishing between mild and severe degrees. Although newer techniques may quantify regurgitation more precisely, they are not yet in widespread use, and standard color flow Doppler examination may not be sufficient for exact quantification of mitral regurgitation or to determine whether the severity of the lesion is sufficient to cause eventual LV dysfunction. When the severity of mitral regurgitation is in doubt or if mitral valve surgery is being contemplated, cardiac catheterization (Chapter 56) is helpful in resolving the severity of the lesion; coronary arteriography should be included in patients older than 40 years or with symptoms suggesting coronary disease (Chapter 70).

Treatment

Medical Therapy

Severe Acute Mitral Regurgitation

In severe acute mitral regurgitation, the patient is usually symptomatic with heart failure or even shock. The goal of medical therapy is to increase forward cardiac output while concomitantly reducing regurgitant volume (Chapter 58). Arterial vasodilators reduce systemic resistance to flow and preferentially increase aortic outflow and simultaneously decrease the amount of mitral regurgitation and left atrial hypertension. If hypotension already exists, vasodilators such as nitroprusside lower blood pressure further and cannot be used. In these cases, intra-aortic balloon counterpulsation (Chapter 108) is preferred if the aortic valve is competent. Counterpulsation increases forward cardiac output by lowering ventricular afterload while augmenting systemic diastolic pressure.

Chronic Symptomatic Mitral Regurgitation

In patients with *symptomatic* mitral regurgitation, angiotensin-converting enzyme inhibitors reduce LV volume and improve symptoms. Mitral valve surgery rather than medical therapy is generally preferred, however, in most symptomatic patients with mitral regurgitation. When atrial fibrillation is present, long-term anticoagulation should achieve the same INR goal as for mitral stenosis.

Chronic Asymptomatic Mitral Regurgitation

Vasodilators have had little effect in reducing LV volume or improving normal exercise tolerance in patients with mitral regurgitation, perhaps because afterload is not usually increased in those with chronic asymptomatic mitral regurgitation. Thus, there is no definitive indication to begin afterload reduction before symptoms appear.

Surgical Therapy

The timing of mitral valve surgery must weigh the risks of the operation and placement of a prosthesis, if one is inserted, versus the risk for irreversible LV dysfunction if surgery is delayed unwisely. For most other types of valve disease, surgical correction usually requires placement of a prosthetic valve, but in patients with mitral regurgitation the native valve can often be repaired. Because conservation of the native valve obviates the risks associated with a prosthesis, the option of mitral valve repair should influence the patient and physician toward earlier surgery.

Types of Mitral Valve Surgery

Mitral Valve Repair

When feasible, mitral valve repair is the preferred operation. Repair restores valve competence, maintains the functional aspects of the apparatus, and avoids the insertion of a prosthesis. Repair is most applicable in cases of posterior chordal rupture; anterior involvement and rheumatic involvement make repair more difficult. Currently, the percentage of mitral valve surgeries that are valve repair varies from 0 to 95% at different hospital centers. In all cases, the feasibility of repair depends on the pathoanatomy that is causing the mitral regurgitation and the skill and experience of the operating surgeon.

Mitral Valve Replacement with Preservation of the Mitral Apparatus

In this procedure, a prosthetic valve is inserted, but continuity between the native leaflets and the papillary muscles is maintained. This procedure has the advantage of ensuring mitral valve competence while preserving the LV functional aspects of the mitral apparatus. Even if only the posterior leaflets and chordae are preserved, the patient benefits from improved postoperative ventricular function and better survival. In many cases it is possible to preserve the anterior and posterior chordal attachments, although anterior continuity can be associated with LV outflow tract obstruction. Although the patient benefits from restored mitral valve competence and maintenance of LV function, insertion of a prosthesis still carries all prosthesis-associated risks.

Mitral Valve Replacement without Preservation of the Mitral Apparatus

When the native valve cannot be repaired or the chordae preserved, such as in severe rheumatic deformity, the mitral valve leaflets and its apparatus are removed and a prosthetic valve is inserted. Although this operation almost guarantees mitral valve competence, the mitral valve apparatus is responsible for coordinating LV contraction and for helping maintain the efficient prolate ellipsoid shape of the left ventricle. Destruction of the apparatus leads to a sudden fall in LV function and a decline in postoperative ejection fraction that is often permanent.

Rx

Timing of Surgery

Symptomatic Patients

Most patients with symptoms of dyspnea, orthopnea, or fatigue should undergo surgery regardless of which operation is performed because they already have lifestyle limitations from their disease. The mere presence of symptoms may worsen the prognosis despite relatively well preserved LV function. The onset or worsening of symptoms is a summary of the patient's pathophysiology and may give a broader view of cardiovascular integrity than possible with any single measurement of pressure or function.

Asymptomatic Patients with Normal Left Ventricular Function

Surgery has increasingly been considered in asymptomatic patients who have normal LV function but echocardiographic findings indicating that valve *repair* is likely to be successful. Although these patients are at low risk without surgery, the risk associated with valve repair is less than 1%, and this approach avoids the risks of later valve *replacement*, which may be required if the valvular disease progresses. Valve repair obviates the need for protracted, expensive follow-up and provides a durable correction of the lesion. This approach is sensible, however, only if it is certain that valve repair can be performed because insertion of a prosthesis carries unacceptable risk in this low-risk group.

Asymptomatic Patients with Left Ventricular Dysfunction

The onset of LV dysfunction in patients with mitral regurgitation may occur without causing symptoms. Early surgery is warranted to prevent the muscle dysfunction from becoming severe or irreversible. Regardless of whether valve repair or replacement is eventually performed, survival is prolonged to or toward normal if surgery is performed before the ejection fraction declines to less than 0.60 or before the left ventricle is unable to contract to an end-systolic dimension of 45 mm. Patients with severe mitral regurgitation should be monitored yearly with a history, physical examination, and echocardiographic evaluation of LV function. When the patient reports symptoms or echocardiography shows the onset of LV dysfunction, surgery should be undertaken.

Asymptomatic Elderly Patients

Patients older than 75 years may have poor surgical results, especially if coronary disease is present or if mitral valve replacement rather than repair must be performed. Although elderly patients with symptoms refractory to medical therapy may benefit from surgery, there is little compelling reason to commit elderly *asymptomatic* patients to a mitral valve operation.

MITRAL VALVE PROLAPSE

Definition

Mitral valve prolapse occurs when one or both of the mitral valve leaflets prolapse into the left atrium superior to the mitral valve annular plane during systole. The importance of mitral valve prolapse varies from patient to patient. In some cases, prolapse is simply a consequence of normal LV physiology without significant medical impact, such as in situations that produce a small left ventricle (e.g., the Valsalva maneuver or an atrial septal defect), in which reduction of ventricular volume causes relative lengthening of the chordae tendineae and subsequent mitral valve prolapse. At the other end of the spectrum, severe redundancy and deformity of the valve, which occurs in myxomatous valve degeneration, increases the risk for stroke, arrhythmia, endocarditis, and progression to severe mitral regurgitation.

Diagnosis

History

Most patients with mitral valve prolapse are asymptomatic. In some cases, however, mitral valve prolapse is associated with symptoms, including palpitations, syncope, and chest pain. In some cases, chest pain is associated with a positive thallium scintigram indicating the presence of true ischemia despite normal epicardial coronary arteries, perhaps because excessive tension on the papillary muscles increases oxygen consumption and causes ischemia. Palpitations, syncope, and presyncope, when present, are linked to autonomic dysfunction (Chapters 61, 427, and 445), which seems to be more prevalent in patients with mitral valve prolapse.

Physical Examination

On physical examination, the mitral valve prolapse syndrome produces the characteristic findings of a midsystolic click and a late systolic murmur. The click occurs when the chordae tendineae are stretched taut by the prolapsing mitral valve in midsystole. As this occurs, the mitral leaflets move past their coaptation point, permit mitral regurgitation, and cause the late systolic murmur (see Table 48–6). Maneuvers that make the left ventricle smaller, such as the Valsalva maneuver, cause the click to appear earlier and the murmur to be more holosystolic and often louder (see Table 48–6). In some cases of echocardiographically proven mitral valve prolapse, neither the click nor the murmur is present; in other cases, only one of these findings is present.

Noninvasive Evaluation

Echocardiography is useful to prove that prolapse is present, to image the amount of regurgitation and its physiologic effects, and to discern the pathoanatomy of the mitral valve. Although an echocardiogram is not necessary to diagnose prolapse in patients with the classic physical findings, the echocardiogram adds significant prognostic information because it can detect patients who have specifically abnormal valve morphology and in whom most of the complications of the disease occur.

In the 1990s it became clear that the mitral annulus did not exist in a single plane but had a saddleback shape. Prolapse shown in the four-chamber echocardiographic view should be confirmed in the parasternal long-axis view. Echocardiographic diagnoses made before the understanding that the mitral valve plane was multidimensional (circa 1987) may have been made in error.

Treatment

Rx

Because most patients with mitral valve prolapse are asymptomatic, therapy is unnecessary. Patients with mitral valve prolapse and its characteristic murmur should observe standard endocarditis prophylaxis (Chapter 76). Those with otherwise normal valve leaflets who are shown to prolapse during echocardiography and who do not have a heart murmur do not require endocarditis precautions. Patients with clearly abnormal valves but no murmur fall into a middle category of endocarditis risk in which a firm recommendation about prophylaxis cannot be made. In patients with palpitations and autonomic dysfunction, β-blockers are often effective in relieving symptoms. Low-dose aspirin therapy has been recommended for patients with redundant leaflets because these patients have a slightly increased risk for stroke. No data from large studies are available to support this contention, however. If severe mitral regurgitation develops, the therapy is the same as for other causes of mitral regurgitation.

Prognosis

Most patients with mitral valve prolapse have a benign clinical course; even for complication-prone patients with redundant and misshapen mitral leaflets, complications are relatively rare. Approximately 10% of patients with thickened leaflets experience infective endocarditis, stroke, progression to severe mitral regurgitation, or sudden death. The progression to severe mitral regurgitation varies with gender and age, and men are approximately twice as likely to progress as women. By 50 years of age, only approximately 1 in 200 men requires surgery to correct mitral regurgitation. By the age of 70, the risk increases to approximately 3%.

AORTIC REGURGITATION

Definition

Aortic regurgitation is caused either by abnormalities of the aortic leaflets or by abnormalities of the proximal aortic root. Leaflet abnormalities causing aortic regurgitation include a bicuspid aortic valve, infective endocarditis, and rheumatic heart disease; anorexigenic drugs have also been implicated. Common aortic root abnormalities that cause aortic regurgitation include Marfan syndrome (Chapter 281), hypertension-induced annuloaortic ectasia, aortic dissection (Chapter 78), syphilis (Chapter 341), ankylosing spondylitis (Chapter 286), and psoriatic arthritis (Chapter 286). Acute aortic regurgitation is usually caused by infective endocarditis (Chapter 76) or aortic dissection.

Pathobiology

As with mitral regurgitation, aortic regurgitation imparts a volume overload on the left ventricle because the left ventricle must pump the forward flow entering from the left atrium and the regurgitant volume returning through the incompetent aortic valve. Also as with mitral regurgitation, the volume overload is compensated for by the development of eccentric cardiac hypertrophy, which increases chamber size and allows the ventricle to pump a greater total stroke volume and a greater forward stroke volume. Ventricular enlargement also allows the left ventricle to accommodate the volume overload at a lower filling pressure. In contrast to mitral regurgitation, the entire stroke volume is ejected into the aorta in aortic regurgitation. Because pulse pressure is proportional to stroke volume and elastance of the aorta, the increased stroke volume increases systolic pressure. Systolic hypertension leads to afterload excess, which does not generally occur in mitral regurgitation. Ventricular geometry also differs between mitral and aortic regurgitation because the afterload excess in aortic regurgitation causes a modest element of concentric hypertrophy, as well as severe eccentric hypertrophy.

In acute aortic insufficiency, such as might occur in infective endocarditis, severe volume overload of the previously unprepared left ventricle results in a sudden fall in forward output while precipitously increasing LV filling pressure. It is probably this combination of pathophysiologic factors that leads to rapid decompensation, presumably because the severely diminished gradient for coronary blood flow causes ischemia and progressive deterioration in LV function. In acute aortic insufficiency, reflex vasoconstriction increases peripheral vascular resistance. In compensated chronic aortic insufficiency, vasoconstriction is absent, and vascular resistance may be reduced and contribute to the hyperdynamic circulation observed in these patients.

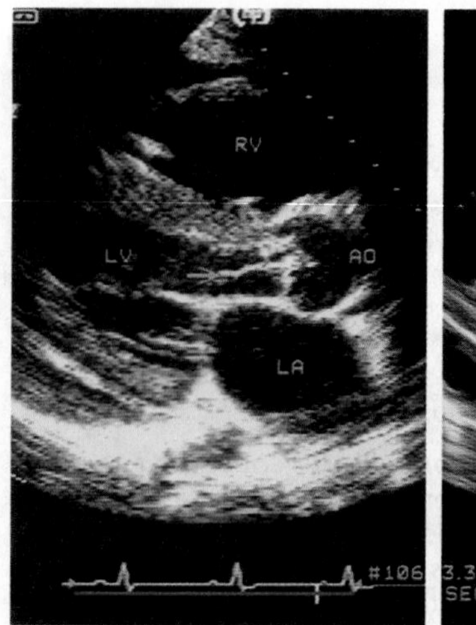

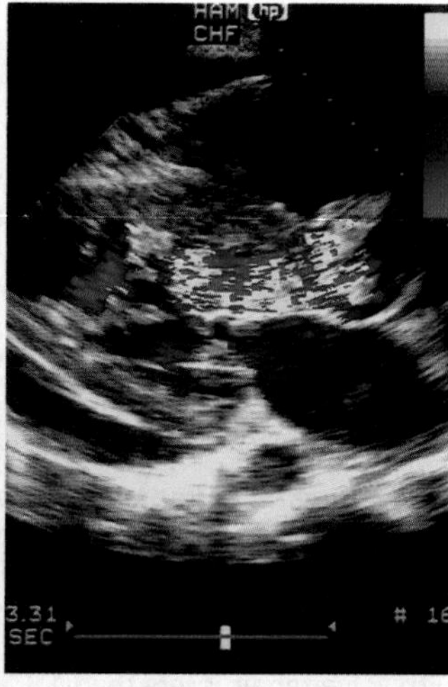

FIGURE 75–5 • Echocardiogram of a patient with aortic regurgitation caused by infective endocarditis. The left panel shows a linear vegetation (arrow) prolapsing into the left ventricular outflow tract from the aortic valve leaflet in diastole. AO = aorta; LA = left atrium; LV = left ventricle; RV = right ventricle. The right panel is a color flow Doppler exhibiting turbulent blood flow filling the left ventricular tract during diastole. (Courtesy of Dr. Anthony DeMaria.)

Clinical Manifestations

The most common symptoms from chronic aortic regurgitation are those of left-sided heart failure, that is, dyspnea on exertion, orthopnea, and fatigue. In acute aortic regurgitation, cardiac output and shock may develop rapidly. The onset of symptoms in patients with chronic aortic regurgitation usually heralds the onset of LV systolic dysfunction. Some patients with symptoms have apparently normal systolic function, however, and the symptoms may be attributed to diastolic dysfunction. Other patients may have ventricular dysfunction yet remain asymptomatic.

Angina may also occur in patients with aortic insufficiency but less commonly than in those with aortic stenosis. The cause of angina in aortic regurgitation is probably multifactorial. Coronary blood flow reserve is reduced in some patients because diastolic runoff into the left ventricle lowers aortic diastolic pressure while increasing LV diastolic pressure—these two influences lower the driving pressure gradient for flow across the coronary bed. When angina occurs in aortic regurgitation, it may be accompanied by flushing. Other symptoms include carotid artery pain and an unpleasant awareness of the heartbeat.

Diagnosis

Physical Examination

Aortic regurgitation produces a myriad of signs because a hyperdynamic, enlarged left ventricle ejects a large stroke volume at high pressure into the systemic circulation. Palpation of the precordium finds a hyperactive apical impulse displaced downward and to the left. S_1 and S_2 are usually normal. S_2 is followed by a diastolic blowing murmur heard best along the left sternal border with the patient sitting upright. In mild disease, the murmur may be short and heard only in the beginning of diastole when the gradient between the aorta and the left ventricle is highest. As the disease worsens, the murmur may persist throughout diastole. A second murmur, a mitral valve rumble, is heard at the LV apex in patients with severe aortic insufficiency. Although the cause is still debated, this Austin Flint murmur is probably produced as the regurgitant jet impinges on the mitral valve and causes it to vibrate.

In chronic aortic regurgitation, the high stroke volume and reduced systemic arterial resistance result in a wide pulse pressure, which may generate a number of signs, including Corrigan's pulse (sharp upstroke and rapid decline of the carotid pulse), de Musset's sign (head bobbing), Duroziez's sign (combined systolic and diastolic bruits created by compression of the femoral artery with the stethoscope), and Quincke's pulse (systolic plethora and diastolic blanching in the nail bed when gentle traction is placed on the nail). Perhaps the most reliable of physical signs indicating severe aortic regurgitation is Hill's sign, an increase in femoral systolic pressure of 40 mm Hg or more when compared with systolic pressure in the brachial artery.

In contrast to chronic aortic insufficiency with its myriad of clinical signs, acute aortic insufficiency may have a subtle manifestation. The eccentric hypertrophy, which compensates for chronic aortic insufficiency, has not yet had time to develop, and the large total stroke volume responsible for most of the signs of chronic aortic insufficiency is absent. The only clues to the presence of acute aortic insufficiency may be a short diastolic blowing murmur and reduced intensity of S_1. This latter sign occurs because high diastolic LV pressure closes the mitral valve early in diastole (mitral valve preclosure) so that when ventricular systole occurs, only the tricuspid component of S_1 is heard.

Noninvasive Evaluation

The ECG in patients with aortic insufficiency is nonspecific but almost always demonstrates LV hypertrophy. The chest radiograph shows an enlarged heart, often with uncoiling and enlargement of the aortic root.

Echocardiography (Chapter 53) is the most important noninvasive tool for assessing the severity of aortic insufficiency and its impact on LV geometry and function (Fig. 75–5). During echocardiography, the LV end-diastolic dimension, end-systolic dimension, and fractional shortening are determined. Aortic valve anatomy and aortic root anatomy can be assessed and the cause of the aortic regurgitation can often be determined. Color flow Doppler examination of the aortic valve helps quantify the severity of aortic regurgitation by assessing the depth and width to which the diastolic jet penetrates the left ventricle. Another way to assess the severity of aortic regurgitation is the pressure half-time method: continuous-wave Doppler interrogation of the aortic valve displays the decay of the velocity of retrograde flow across the valve. In mild aortic insufficiency, the gradient across the valve is high throughout diastole, and its rate of decay is slow, with production of a long Doppler half-time (the time that it takes the velocity to decay from its peak to that value divided by the square root of 2). In severe aortic regurgitation, there is rapid equilibration between pressure in the aorta and pressure in the left ventricle, and the Doppler half-time is short. If mitral valve preclosure is detected in acute aortic insufficiency, urgent surgery is necessary. In cases in which the severity of aortic insufficiency is in doubt, catheterization to perform aortography is useful in resolving the issue.

Treatment

Rx

Medical Therapy

Asymptomatic Patients with Normal Left Ventricular Function

Because aortic regurgitation increases LV afterload, which decreases cardiac efficiency, afterload reduction with nifedipine and other vasodilators, including angiotensin-converting enzyme inhibitors and hydralazine, improves hemodynamics in the short term. Although initial data suggested that such therapy could delay or reduce the need for aortic valve surgery without any adverse effects when surgery is finally performed, more recent data suggest no benefit from such therapy. These discrepant results from relatively small trials preclude firm recommendations.

Symptomatic Patients or Patients with Left Ventricular Dysfunction

Patients who are symptomatic or manifest LV dysfunction should not be treated medically, except for short-term stabilization, but should undergo aortic valve surgery as soon as feasible.

Surgical Therapy

Acute Aortic Regurgitation

When any of the symptoms or signs of heart failure develop, even if mild, medical mortality is high and approaches 75%. Therapy with vasodilators, such as nitroprusside, may temporarily improve the patient's condition before surgery but is never a substitute for surgery. In patients with acute aortic regurgitation caused by bacterial endocarditis (Chapter 76), surgery may be delayed to permit a full or partial course of antibiotics, but persistent, severe aortic regurgitation requires emergency valve replacement. Even when blood cultures have been positive recently and antibiotic therapy has been of brief duration, the valve reinfection rate is low, 0 to 10%, with valve replacement or valve repair. Emergency surgery should not be withheld simply because the duration of antibiotic therapy has been brief.

Chronic Aortic Regurgitation

Asymptomatic patients who manifest evidence of LV dysfunction benefit from surgery. Because loading conditions differ between aortic and mitral regurgitation, the objective markers for the presence of LV dysfunction also differ. In aortic regurgitation, when the ejection fraction is less than 0.55 or the end-systolic dimension is greater than 55 mm, postoperative outcome is impaired, presumably because these markers indicate that LV dysfunction has developed. Surgery should be performed before these benchmarks are reached.

Patients with advanced symptoms are at increased risk for a suboptimal surgical outcome regardless of whether they have evidence of LV dysfunction. Patients should undergo aortic valve replacement before symptoms impair lifestyle.

Although some patients may be able to undergo successful aortic valve repair to restore aortic valve competence, most patients require insertion of an aortic valve prosthesis.

TRICUSPID REGURGITATION

Definition

Tricuspid regurgitation is usually secondary to a hemodynamic load on the right ventricle rather than a structural valve deformity. Diseases that cause pulmonary hypertension, such as chronic obstructive airway disease or intracardiac shunts, lead to RV dilation and subsequent tricuspid regurgitation. Because most of the force that is needed to fill the left ventricle is provided by the right ventricle, LV dysfunction leading to elevated LV filling pressure also places the right ventricle under a hemodynamic load and can eventually lead to RV failure and tricuspid regurgitation. In some instances, tricuspid regurgitation may be caused by pathology of the valve itself. The most common cause of primary tricuspid regurgitation is infective endocarditis, usually stemming from drug abuse and unsterile injections. Other causes include carcinoid syndrome, rheumatic involvement of the tricuspid valve, myxomatous degeneration, RV infarction, and mishaps during endomyocardial biopsy.

Diagnosis

The symptoms of tricuspid regurgitation are those of right-sided heart failure and include ascites, edema, and occasionally right upper quadrant pain. On physical examination, tricuspid regurgitation produces jugular venous distention accentuated by a large v wave as blood is regurgitated into the right atrium during systole. Regurgitation into the hepatic veins causes hepatic enlargement and liver pulsation. RV enlargement is detected as a parasternal lift. Ascites and edema are common.

The definitive diagnosis of tricuspid regurgitation is made during echocardiography. Doppler interrogation of the tricuspid valve shows systolic disturbance of the right atrial blood pool. Echocardiography (Chapter 53) can also be used to determine the severity of pulmonary hypertension, measure RV dilation, and assess whether the valve itself is intrinsically normal or abnormal.

Treatment

Therapy for secondary tricuspid regurgitation is generally aimed at the cause of the lesion. If LV failure has been responsible for RV failure and tricuspid regurgitation, the standard therapy for improving LV failure (Chapter 58) lowers LV filling pressure, reduces secondary pulmonary hypertension, relieves some of the hemodynamic burden of the right ventricle, and partially restores tricuspid valve competence. If pulmonary disease is the primary cause, therapy is directed toward improving lung function. Vasodilators, so useful in the treatment of left-sided heart failure, are often ineffective in treating pulmonary hypertension itself. Medical therapy directed at tricuspid regurgitation is usually limited to diuretic use.

Surgical intervention for the tricuspid valve is rarely entertained in isolation. However, if other cardiac surgery is planned in a patient with severe tricuspid regurgitation, ring annuloplasty or tricuspid valve repair is frequently attempted to ensure postoperative tricuspid competence. Tricuspid valve replacement is often not well tolerated and is rarely performed except when severe deformity, as is often seen in endocarditis or carcinoid disease, precludes valve repair.

PULMONIC STENOSIS

Definition

Pulmonic stenosis is a congenital disease resulting from fusion of the pulmonic valve cusps (Chapter 68). It is usually detected and corrected during childhood, but occasionally cases are diagnosed for the first time in adulthood. Symptoms of pulmonic stenosis include angina and syncope. Occasionally, symptoms of right-sided heart failure develop. During physical examination, the uncalcified valve in pulmonic stenosis produces an early systolic ejection click on opening. During inspiration, the click diminishes or disappears because increased flow into the right side of the heart during inspiration partially opens the pulmonic valve in diastole so that systole causes less of an opening sound. The click is followed by a systolic ejection murmur that radiates to the base of the heart. If the transvalvular gradient is severe, RV hypertrophy develops and produces a parasternal lift.

The diagnosis of pulmonic stenosis is confirmed by echocardiography, which quantifies the transvalvular gradient and the degree of RV hypertrophy and dysfunction.

Treatment

In asymptomatic patients with a gradient less than 25 mm Hg, no therapy is required. If symptoms develop or the gradient exceeds 50 mm Hg, balloon commissurotomy is effective in reducing the gradient and relieving symptoms.

Postoperative Care of Patients with Substitute Heart Valves

Different types of prosthetic valves (Fig. 75–6) have different advantages and disadvantages (Table 75–2). After a prosthetic valve

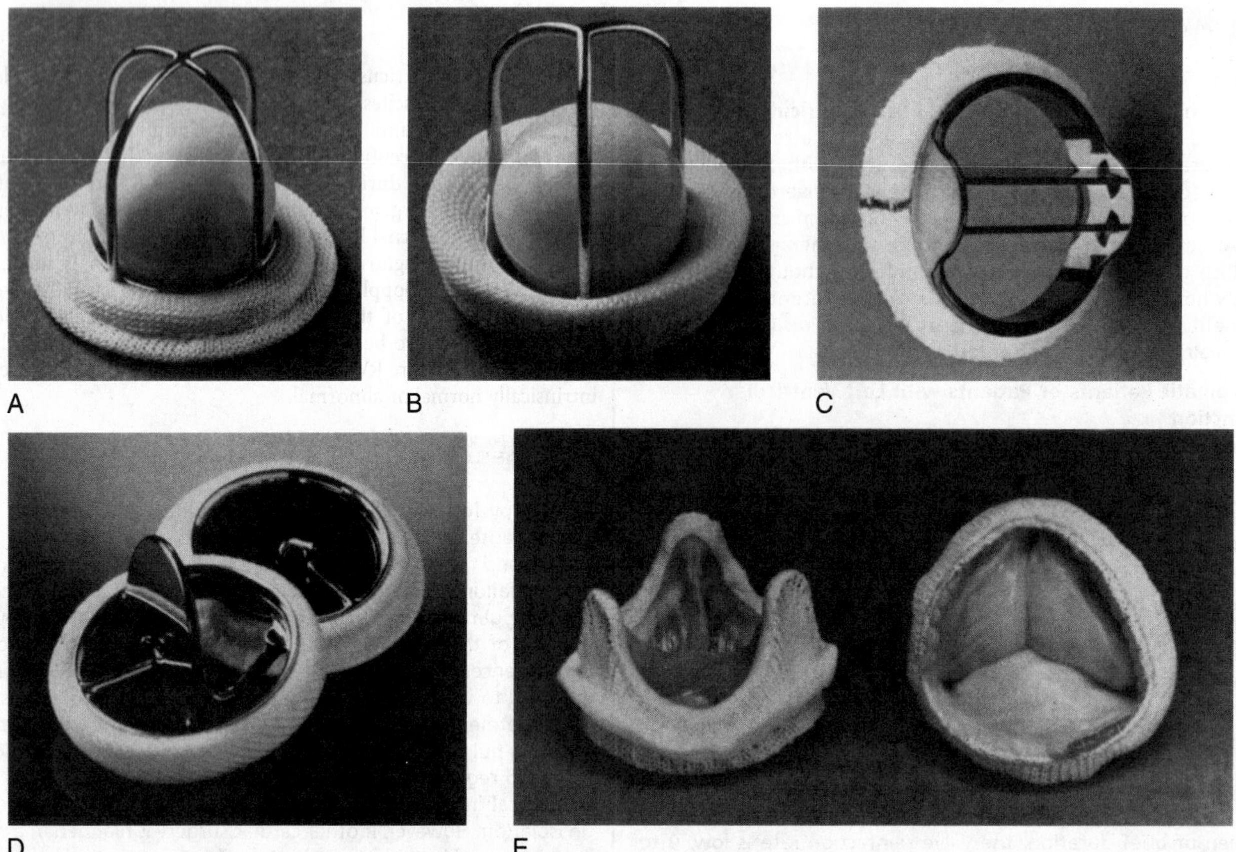

FIGURE 75–6 • Different types of commonly used prosthetic valves. A, Starr-Edwards caged ball mitral prosthesis. **B,** Starr-Edwards aortic prosthesis. **C,** St. Jude Medical bileaflet prosthesis. **D,** Medtronic-Hall tilting disc valve. **E,** Carpentier-Edwards bioprosthesis. (From Wernly JA, Crawford MH: Choosing a prosthetic heart valve. Cardiol Clin 1991;9:329–338.)

TABLE 75–2 ADVANTAGES AND DISADVANTAGES OF SUBSTITUTE CARDIAC VALVES

Type of Valve	Advantages	Disadvantages
Bioprosthesis (Carpentier-Edwards, Hancock)	Avoids anticoagulation in patients with sinus rhythm	Durability limited to 10–15 yr Relatively stenotic
Mechanical valves (St. Jude, Medtronic-Hall, Starr-Edwards)	Good flow characteristics in small sizes Durable	Require anticoagulation
Homografts and autografts	Anticoagulation not required Durability increased over that of bioprostheses	Surgical implantation technically demanding

Rx

has been inserted, a baseline echocardiogram should be obtained to provide a reference point in the event that valve dysfunction is suspected at a later date. Echocardiography does not need to be repeated unless there is a change in clinical status or physical findings. The major causes of valve dysfunction are infective endocarditis, clot, and valve degeneration. Dysfunction is manifested most commonly by valvular regurgitation, but valvular stenosis can also occur with a clot, vegetations, or degeneration, especially degeneration of a bioprosthesis.

Whenever a patient with a prosthetic heart valve has a temperature higher than 100° F, endocarditis must be excluded by blood culture; for fever with signs of sepsis, broad-spectrum antibiotics must be begun while awaiting culture results. For patients with bioprosthetic valves, mechanical prostheses, and homografts, endocarditis prophylaxis should be instituted at the time of procedures that are associated with a high risk for bacteremia (Chapter 76). Whether prophylaxis is necessary for pulmonary autografts is currently unclear, but physicians usually prescribe prophylaxis for these patients.

By 15 years after surgery, a randomized trial showed no differences in mortality in patients with mechanical valves versus tissue valves in the mitral position. In the aortic position, all-cause mortality was worse for bioprostheses (79%) than for mechanical prostheses (66%), with much of the increased mortality related to a higher rate of bioprosthetic valve failure. 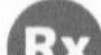

All patients with a mechanical heart valve require anticoagulation. Recommended INR values range from 2.0 for a young normotensive patient in sinus rhythm with an aortic valve prosthesis to 3.5 for a patient with atrial fibrillation and a mitral valve prosthesis. Aspirin, 325 mg, is recommended in addition to warfarin to reduce the risk for valve thrombosis in patients who have mechanical prosthetic valves that are at higher risk for thromboembolic complications.

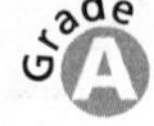
1. Ben Farhat M, Ayari M, Maatouk F, et al: Percutaneous balloon versus surgical closed and open mitral commissurotomy: Seven-year follow-up results of a randomized trial. Circulation 1998;97:245–250.
2. Hammermeister K, Sethi GK, Henderson WG, et al: Outcomes 15 years after valve replacement with a mechanical versus a bioprosthetic valve: Final report of the Veterans Affairs randomized trial. J Am Coll Cardiol 2000;36:1152–1158.

SUGGESTED READINGS

ACC/AHA 2006 guidelines for the management of patients with valvular heart disease: Executive summary. Circulation 2006;114:450–527. *A consensus overview.*

Bekeredjian R, Grayburn PA: Valvular heart disease: Aortic regurgitation. Circulation 2005;112:125–134. *A comprehensive review.*

Elkayam U, Bitar F: Valvular heart disease and pregnancy: Part I: Native valves. J Am Coll Cardiol 2005;46:223–230; Elkayam U, Bitar F: Valvular heart disease and pregnancy: Part II: Prosthetic valves. J Am Coll Cardiol 2005;46:403–410. *Two comprehensive reviews.*

Enriquez-Sarano M, Avierinos J-F, Messika-Zeitoun D, et al: Quantitative determinants of the outcome of asymptomatic mitral regurgitation. N Engl J Med 2005;352:875–883. *A calculated regurgitant orifice above 40 mm² portends a poorer prognosis and may warrant surgery.*

Hayek E, Gring CN, Griffin BP: Mitral valve prolapse. Lancet 2005;365:507–518. *A comprehensive overview.*

Otto CM: Valvular aortic stenosis: Disease severity and timing of intervention. J Am Coll Cardiol 2006;47:2141–2151. *A thorough review.*

Pellikka PA, Sarano ME, Nishimura RA, et al: Outcome of 622 adults with asymptomatic, hemodynamically significant aortic stenosis during prolonged follow-up. Circulation 2005;111:3290–3295. *Symptoms typically developed within 5 years.*

Soltesz EG, Cohn LH: Minimally invasive valve surgery. Cardiol Rev 2007;15:109–115. *An updated review.*

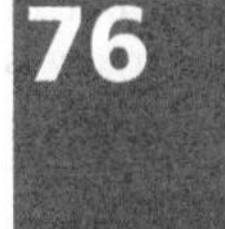

76 INFECTIVE ENDOCARDITIS

Vance G. Fowler, Jr., and Arnold S. Bayer

Definition

Infective endocarditis is defined as an infection, usually bacterial, of the endocardial surface of the heart. Infective endocarditis primarily affects the cardiac valves, although the septa between the chambers or the mural endocardium may be involved in some cases. Traditionally, infective endocarditis has been categorized as acute or subacute, depending on the length of symptoms before presentation; however, this distinction is somewhat arbitrary. A classification that considers the causative organism and the valve involved is more clinically relevant.

Epidemiology

The incidence of infective endocarditis is difficult to determine because of the criteria for diagnosis and the methods of reporting. An analysis based on strict case definitions often reveals that only a relatively small proportion (~20%) of clinically diagnosed cases are categorized as definite. Nevertheless, in 10 large surveys, infective endocarditis accounted for approximately 1 case per 1000 U.S. hospital admissions, with a range of 0.16 to 5.4 cases per 1000 admissions. This incidence has not changed appreciably during the past 30 years. Estimates from the American Heart Association place the annual incidence of infective endocarditis in the United States at 10,000 to 20,000 new cases.

Men are affected more commonly than women are (mean male-to-female ratio of 1.7:1 in 18 large series). However, in patients younger than 35 years, more cases occur in women. More than 50% of patients with infective endocarditis in the United States are now older than 50 years; this is due to the low incidence of acute rheumatic fever (Chapter 277) and low subsequent prevalence of rheumatic heart disease compared with prior eras and with developing countries, as well as a simultaneous rise in the prevalence of degenerative heart disease as the population lives longer.

TABLE 76–1 PREDISPOSING CONDITIONS ASSOCIATED WITH INCREASED RISK OF ENDOCARDITIS

More Common	Less Common
Mitral valve prolapse with murmur	Rheumatic heart disease
Degenerative valvular disease	Hypertrophic obstructive cardiomyopathy
Intravenous drug use*	
Prosthetic valve*	Pulmonary-systemic shunts*
Congenital abnormalities (valvular or septal defect)	Coarctation of the aorta
	Previous endocarditis*
	Complex cyanotic congenital heart disease*

*Indicates lesions with highest risk for endocarditis.

Although some patients have no clearly definable risk factor for endocarditis, cardiac conditions that cause turbulent flow at the endocardial surface or across a valve (Chapter 75) have been found to predispose patients to infective endocarditis (Table 76–1). Historically, rheumatic heart disease with valvular dysfunction has been the most common underlying condition, although its contribution is diminishing in the antibiotic era, especially in developed countries. Degenerative valvular disease is also associated with infective endocarditis, particularly in elderly patients; the increasing relevance of senile calcification as a risk factor is reflected in the increasing proportion of aortic valve involvement in infective endocarditis. Most significant congenital heart defects (Chapter 68) confer an increased risk of infective endocarditis, particularly complex cyanotic disease such as single-ventricle states, transposition of the great vessels, and tetralogy of Fallot. Similarly, surgically constructed pulmonary-systemic shunts and ventricular septal defects place patients at high risk for infective endocarditis.

Mitral valve prolapse is currently the most common underlying cardiac condition in infective endocarditis, a statistic that reflects its prevalence in the general population (4%). Notably, mitral valve prolapse is a risk only in patients with thickened mitral leaflets or regurgitation, in which case the risk of endocarditis increases by about 10-fold above that of the general population. In addition, patients with hypertrophic cardiomyopathy are at increased risk of infective endocarditis, particularly in the presence of outflow obstruction. Finally, previous endocarditis is among the highest risk factors for infective endocarditis.

Prosthetic cardiac valves represent an important risk factor for infective endocarditis. More than 150,000 heart valves are implanted annually worldwide, and prosthetic valve infective endocarditis develops in 1 to 4% of prosthetic valve recipients in the first year after valve replacement and in approximately 0.8% of recipients annually thereafter. Mechanical prosthetic valves may initially be more susceptible to infective endocarditis, but bioprosthetic valves are more likely to develop infective endocarditis after 1 year; overall, the rate is similar with either type of valve.

The incidence of infective endocarditis in injection drug users (Chapter 32) may be 30 times higher than in the general population and 4 times higher than the risk in adults with rheumatic heart disease. In some areas of the United States, injection drug use is the most common predisposing cause of infective endocarditis in patients younger than 40 years. *Staphylococcus aureus* is the predominant organism, and tricuspid valve involvement is noted in 78% of cases, mitral involvement in 24%, and aortic involvement in 8%. More than one valve is infected in approximately 20% of cases, and some of these infections are polymicrobial.

Health care–associated infective endocarditis arises primarily as a consequence of invasive therapies, including intravenous catheters, hyperalimentation lines, pacemakers, and dialysis shunts. For example, in a prospective multinational cohort study of 1779 prospectively enrolled patients with definite infective endocarditis from 39 referral and nonreferral centers in 16 countries, 24% had health care–associated infective endocarditis. Patients with health care–associated infective endocarditis are typically older and have other comorbid conditions. Health care–associated infective endocarditis in industrialized nations is commonly caused by *S. aureus* (Chapter 310), which frequently causes bacteremia and increasingly is antibiotic resistant.

Systemic medical conditions predispose patients to the development of infective endocarditis. For example, human immunodeficiency virus infection is an independent risk factor for the development of infective endocarditis in injection drug users, with the risk increasing as the CD4^{+} count decreases. Catheter-related bacteremia is an important risk factor for nosocomial infective endocarditis. Patients with end-stage renal disease, particularly those receiving long-term hemodialysis, and patients with diabetes mellitus are also at increased risk, presumably because of the recurrent vascular access associated with hemodialysis and the low-level immunosuppression associated with both conditions.

The mitral valve has classically been the most commonly affected valve, followed by the aortic valve. Although mitral valve relapse remains the most common underlying condition, the decreasing frequency of rheumatic mitral disease and increasing senescence of the population may account for the increase in aortic valve endocarditis reported in many studies. The next most commonly affected valves in descending order of prevalence are the mitral and aortic valves together, the tricuspid valve, mixed right- and left-sided infection, and the pulmonic valve.

Microbiology

About 90% of community-acquired, native valve infective endocarditis is due to staphylococci, streptococci, or enterococci, each of which is a normal inhabitant of the skin, oropharynx, and urogenital tract with frequent access to the blood stream. These organisms express specific receptors for attachment and adherence to damaged valve surfaces. Streptococcal species (Chapter 311) are the most common cause in community-dwelling patients with no history of injection drug use or health care contact. In patients with either of these epidemiologic risk factors, *S. aureus* (Chapter 310) is the predominant cause of infective endocarditis. Because of the emergence of health care contact as the predominant risk factor for blood stream infections, *S. aureus* is now the most common cause of infective endocarditis in many regions of the world.

Viridans streptococci (Chapter 311) are the most common streptococci implicated in native valve infective endocarditis. This group of organisms, which normally inhabit the oropharynx, includes species such as *Streptococcus sanguis, Streptococcus mutans,* and *Streptococcus mitis.* Group B streptococci, β-hemolytic organisms that are also normal oropharyngeal and urogenital flora, most frequently cause infective endocarditis in patients with cirrhosis or diabetes mellitus and in injection drug users. By contrast, group A streptococci, although also β-hemolytic, rarely cause infective endocarditis. *Streptococcus bovis,* a group D streptococcus, is now a leading cause of infective endocarditis in some parts of the world; for example, its incidence in France has increased significantly in recent years. Its presence should prompt endoscopic evaluation for adenocarcinoma of the colon or other malignant lesions of the gastrointestinal tract. Pneumococcal endocarditis is decreasing in incidence but is fulminant when present; it may occur as part of Austrian's (or Osler's) triad of endocarditis, meningitis, and pneumonia and is associated with high morbidity and mortality.

As noted, *S. aureus* (Chapter 310) is now the most common cause of infective endocarditis in many parts of the world, and it is the pathogen of primary concern among injection drug users or patients with health care contact. The clinical course of *S. aureus* endocarditis is typically acute, with a rapid progression during the course of several days. Because approximately 12% of nonselected patients with *S. aureus* bacteremia will have infective endocarditis, the possibility of cardiac involvement should always be considered in any patient with *S. aureus* bacteremia. Patients with *S. aureus* bacteremia who manifest clinical risk factors, including persistent bacteremia or fever, community acquisition, and cutaneous findings, are at particular risk for infective endocarditis and other complications. Coagulase-negative staphylococci are an unusual cause of native valve disease but important pathogens in prosthetic valve endocarditis; presentation is usually subacute.

Enterococcal bacteremia is far more common, particularly in hospitalized patients, than enterococcal endocarditis; however, enterococci are still responsible for a significant number of cases of both community-acquired and nosocomial endocarditis. In most cases, the source of the bacteria is thought to be the genitourinary tract, and the presentation is usually subacute. Enterococcal endocarditis, as opposed to enterococcal bacteremia, is suggested by community acquisition of infection, absence of a clear source of infection, preexistent valvular heart disease, and absence of polymicrobial bacteremia. As in most enterococcal infections, the overwhelming majority of cases (>90%) are due to *Enterococcus faecalis.*

TABLE 76–2 ETIOLOGY OF PROSTHETIC VALVE ENDOCARDITIS*

Early (<2 Months)	Intermediate (2–12 Months)	Late (>12 Months)
Coagulase-negative staphylococci	Coagulase-negative staphylococci	Streptococci
		S. aureus
S. aureus	Enterococci	Coagulase-negative staphylococci
Gram-negative bacilli	*S. aureus*	
Enterococci	Fungi	Enterococci
Fungi	Streptococci	
Diphtheroids		

*Listed in order of relative frequency on the basis of time at onset after surgery.

The HACEK group of gram-negative organisms (*Haemophilus* species, *Actinobacillus actinomycetemcomitans, Cardiobacterium hominis, Eikenella corrodens,* and *Kingella* species) accounts for about 5% of cases of endocarditis. Because these fastidious organisms will usually grow in blood cultures within 7 days by current methods, prolonged incubation is generally no longer required to isolate HACEK strains. Many other gram-negative bacilli have been reported to cause infective endocarditis but are even more unusual.

Fungal endocarditis is difficult to diagnose and to treat; it is most commonly found in patients with a history of injection drug use, recent cardiac surgery, or prolonged use of indwelling vascular catheters, especially those used for total parenteral nutrition. The most common fungi found in infective endocarditis are *Aspergillus* and *Candida* species. *Aspergillus* (Chapter 360) rarely grows in blood cultures and must usually be cultured from a pathologic specimen (either an embolic site or vegetation); by contrast, *Candida* (Chapter 359) frequently grows out of blood cultures. Mortality is very high, and valve replacement surgery is usually necessary.

Special Situations: Health Care–Associated Infective Endocarditis and Prosthetic Valves

Health care–associated infective endocarditis is defined as endocarditis occurring in the presence of extensive health care contact. Traditionally, this definition was synonymous with nosocomial in-hospital acquisition; however, the increased complexity of outpatient therapy and the increase in the number of patients in long-term care facilities have resulted in a growing number of nonhospitalized patients with health care–associated bacteremia and infective endocarditis. Such patients retain many of the same risk factors as in patients with nosocomial infection (e.g., long-term intravascular catheters, extensive instrumentation) and are infected with the same array of pathogens (e.g., high rates of methicillin-resistant *S. aureus*). Health care–associated infective endocarditis now constitutes about 25% of all cases and is most frequently associated with indwelling vascular catheters; as a result, the most common organisms implicated in nosocomial infective endocarditis are *S. aureus* and coagulase-negative staphylococci.

Prosthetic valve endocarditis can be classified into one of three groups on the basis of time at onset after valve surgery (Table 76–2): early (less than 2 months after surgery), intermediate (2 to 12 months), and late (more than 12 months). Staphylococci, particularly *S. aureus,* predominate during the early period, when most episodes of infective endocarditis are thought to be related to perioperative infection. The intermediate period has a fairly similar microbiologic spectrum, with unusual gram-negatives and diphtheroids decreasing and streptococci increasing. In the late period, 1 year and more after surgery, the spectrum of organisms becomes more akin to that of community-acquired native valve disease, in which *S. aureus* and streptococci predominate. Of note, approximately 50% of prosthetic valve recipients with *S. aureus* bacteremia will develop infective endocarditis.

Pathobiology

Experimental models of infective endocarditis have demonstrated that development of the disease follows a predictable sequence: endocardial damage, aggregation of platelets and fibrin to form a sterile vegetation, transient bacteremia resulting in seeding of the vegetation, microbial proliferation on and invasion of the endocardial surface, and metastatic infection to visceral organs and brain.

Most cases of infective endocarditis begin with a damaged endocardial surface. Damage to the endocardium may be caused by a number of factors, ranging from rheumatic disease to senile degeneration and calcification; indeed, any excessive turbulence or high-pressure gradient may cause injury to the nearby endocardium. Next, fibrin-platelet aggregates develop at the site of damage to form sterile vegetations, also termed nonbacterial thrombotic endocarditis. Nonbacterial thrombotic endocarditis may occur spontaneously in patients with systemic illnesses (for instance, the marantic endocarditis of malignant disease or other wasting diseases and Libman-Sacks endocarditis in systemic lupus erythematosus). When transient bacteremia occurs, for example, as a result of distant infection or gingival disease, the previously sterile vegetation may be seeded. Some bacterial species, such as staphylococci and streptococci, are more avidly adherent than others to vegetations and therefore more frequently cause endocarditis. The bacteria then proliferate within the vegetation and ultimately may achieve an organism load of 10^9 to 10^{11} colony-forming units per gram of tissue. The surfaces of cardiac valves and vegetations are avascular, thereby making antibiotic therapy and healing difficult.

Clinical Manifestations

History

The initial presentation of infective endocarditis varies enormously from patient to patient, so sometimes it is difficult to make the diagnosis. Some cases develop acutely, with symptoms progressing rapidly during several days. Other cases develop insidiously and present with nonspecific symptoms that have been progressing for weeks or months. In patients thought to have infective endocarditis, the initial history should include a complete review of systems, a travel history, and a thorough discussion of health-related behaviors such as illicit drug use and sexual activity. Most patients complain of fever and nonspecific constitutional symptoms, such as fatigue, malaise, and weight loss. Nearly 50% of patients complain of musculoskeletal symptoms ranging from frank arthritis to diffuse myalgias; 5 to 10% of patients have low back pain as their chief complaint, even in the absence of osteomyelitis or epidural abscess. Many intravenous drug users with endocarditis complain of pleuritic chest pain because tricuspid valve endocarditis mimics pneumonia. Health care–associated infective endocarditis is more likely to be clinically occult and requires a high index of suspicion.

Physical Examination

A thorough physical examination should be performed, including a search for the peripheral stigmata of infective endocarditis (Table 76–3). Fever is present in nearly 50% of patients in most studies; however, elderly patients and patients with renal failure or heart failure may be less likely to mount a febrile response. A widened pulse pressure should alert the clinician to the possibility of acute aortic insufficiency (Chapter 78). The skin and nails should be carefully examined for embolic phenomena, such as petechiae, Osler's nodes, Janeway lesions, and splinter hemorrhages; these findings are uncommon in infective endocarditis in the current era but are extremely helpful diagnostic clues when they are present. Petechiae are most often found on the conjunctiva, palate, and extremities; like the other peripheral stigmata of infective endocarditis, they are a nonspecific but suggestive finding (Fig. 76–1). Osler's nodes are small, painful nodules found most often on the palmar surfaces of the fingers and toes; they frequently wax and wane (Fig. 76–2). Classically considered to be an immunologic phenomenon, Osler's nodes may have an immune complex–mediated component but are most likely initiated by microemboli. Janeway lesions are hemorrhagic, nonpainful macules also found primarily on the palms and soles; they are embolic in origin and are less frequently noted than the other cutaneous stigmata. Splinter hemorrhages are nonblanching, linear, brownish red lesions in the nail beds perpendicular to the direction of growth of the nail; they are nonspecific and may also be found in a significant percentage of hospitalized patients without infective endocarditis.

Funduscopic examination should be performed to look for Roth's spots, chorioretinitis, and endophthalmitis, the last two of which are present in a substantial proportion of cases of fungal endocarditis. A careful cardiac examination should be performed to detect any systolic or diastolic murmurs or evidence of heart failure, which is an ominous sign. Of note, injection drug users and patients with health care–associated infective endocarditis are less likely than other patients to have a pathologic murmur on initial presentation. The abdomen should be examined for evidence of splenomegaly (Chapter 174), a finding that is more common in patients with a subacute form of infective endocarditis. Finally, a thorough neurologic examination should be performed, both to assess the patient for any focal neurologic deficit and to serve as a baseline during the hospital stay. The neurologic examination may demonstrate evidence of major vessel embolism, cranial nerve palsies, visual field defects, or a generalized toxic-metabolic encephalopathy with altered mental status.

TABLE 76–3 PHYSICAL EXAMINATION AND LABORATORY FINDINGS IN INFECTIVE ENDOCARDITIS

Finding	% of Cases
Fever	80–95
Audible murmur	85
New or changed murmur	15–47
Neurologic abnormalities	20–40
Splenomegaly	0–60
Petechiae	20–40
Splinter hemorrhages	15
Osler's nodes	10–25
Janeway lesions	<10
Roth's spots	<5
Anemia of chronic disease	50–90
Leukocytosis	20–66
Elevated erythrocyte sedimentation rate	90–100
Microscopic hematuria	50–70
Presence of rheumatoid factor	40–50
Abnormal chest x-ray (effusion, infiltrate, septic emboli)	67–85 (right-sided infective endocarditis)

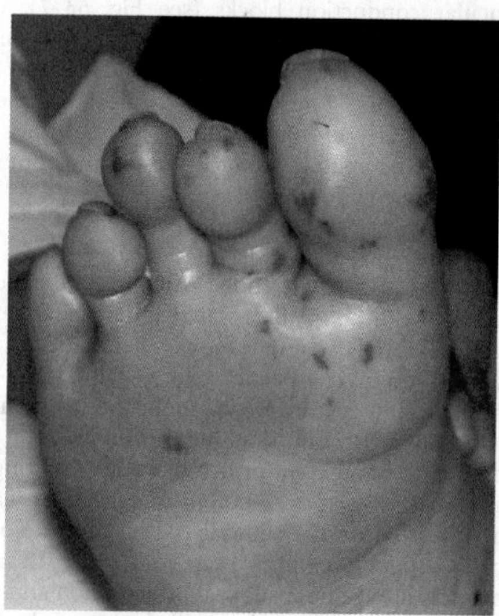

FIGURE 76–1 • Petechiae in infective endocarditis.

Laboratory Findings

Initial laboratory tests should include a complete blood count with differential, electrolyte determinations, measurement of renal function, urinalysis, chest radiography, and electrocardiography. All patients should receive at least three sets of blood cultures as well, and many require echocardiography during their admission (see later).

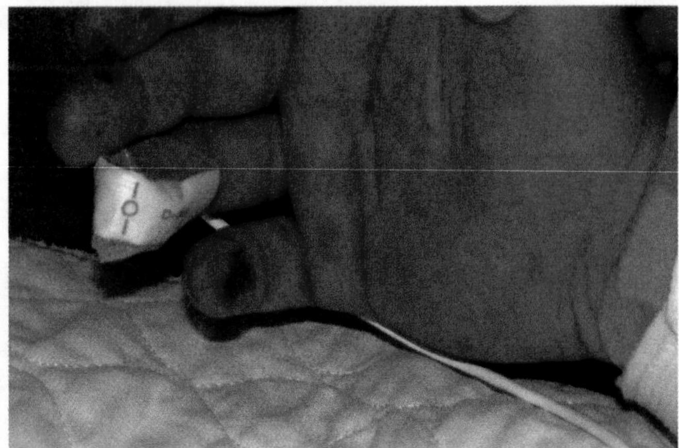

FIGURE 76–2 • Osler's node in infective endocarditis.

Most patients with subacute infective endocarditis have anemia of chronic disease. The white blood cell count may or may not be elevated; it is more frequently elevated in cases of acute infective endocarditis, particularly if *S. aureus* or a fungus is the causative organism. Microscopic hematuria is noted in many cases, as is proteinuria. The chest radiograph is abnormal, demonstrating consolidation, atelectasis, pleural effusion, or clear septic emboli in the overwhelming majority of patients with right-sided endocarditis; in others, it may provide evidence of congestive heart failure. The electrocardiogram should be carefully examined for evidence of atrioventricular conduction blocks (see Fig. 63–7), which might suggest an aortic ring abscess or other myocardial involvement, or frank myocardial infarction (see Figs. 72–1 and 72–2).

Other ancillary tests might include an erythrocyte sedimentation rate, which is elevated in nearly all cases of infective endocarditis with a mean value of 57 mm/hr. Rheumatoid factor is present in about half of cases, particularly in subacute endocarditis.

Complications

The complications of infective endocarditis may be divided into four groups for ease of classification: direct valvular damage and consequences of local invasion, embolic complications, metastatic infections from bacteremia, and immunologic phenomena. Local damage to the endocardium or myocardium is a dreaded complication that can be difficult to diagnose and to treat. Infection may directly erode through the involved cardiac valve or adjacent myocardial wall, resulting in hemodynamically significant valvular perforations or cardiac fistulas. Such local complications typically present clinically with the acute onset of heart failure and carry a poor prognosis, even with prompt cardiac surgery. Valve ring abscesses also require surgical intervention and are more frequent in patients with prosthetic valves. Although a conduction defect on electrocardiography may suggest the diagnosis, transesophageal echocardiography is the diagnostic technique of choice for paravalvular abscesses, valve perforation, or intracardiac fistulas. Frank myocardial abscess has been found in up to 20% of cases at autopsy; *Aspergillus* endocarditis invades the myocardium in more than 50% of cases. Pericarditis is rare and is associated with myocardial abscess in most cases. Myocardial infarction, thought to be due to embolism of vegetative material in the coronary arteries, has been found in 40 to 60% of cases at autopsy, although most cases are clinically silent and without characteristic electrocardiographic changes. However, up to 16% of elderly patients may present with clinical evidence of acute myocardial infarction, with potentially disastrous complications if the myocardial infarction is thought to be the primary event and the patient is given thrombolytic therapy. Heart failure is the leading cause of death in infective endocarditis, usually related to direct valvular damage.

Embolic events are less common now than in the preantibiotic era; nevertheless, about 35% of patients have at least one clinically evident embolic event. In fungal endocarditis, the *majority* of patients have at least one embolic event, frequently with a large embolus. The presence of large (>10 mm), mobile vegetations on the echocardiogram, particularly involving the anterior mitral valve leaflet, predicts a high risk of embolic complications. Most of the classic "peripheral stigmata" of infective endocarditis are probably embolic in nature; patients may also have frank infarction of cutaneous tissue from emboli. In addition to the skin, emboli most commonly lodge in the lungs (in right-sided endocarditis), kidneys, spleen, large blood vessels, or central nervous system (CNS). Vegetations of right-sided endocarditis usually embolize to the lungs, resulting in an abnormality on the chest radiograph.

Renal abscesses are rare in infective endocarditis, but renal infarction is seen in more than 50% of cases at autopsy. Similarly, splenic infarction occurs in up to 44% of autopsy-confirmed cases; although frequently silent, such emboli may cause left upper quadrant pain radiating to the left shoulder, sometimes as the presenting symptom of infective endocarditis. Splenic infarction progressing to abscess may be a cause of persistent fevers in patients with infective endocarditis; patients with infective endocarditis and unexplained persistent fever should undergo abdominal computed tomographic imaging to exclude this complication. Vascular aneurysms, which frequently occur at bifurcation points, may be clinically silent until they rupture (which may be months to years after apparently successful antibiotic treatment of infective endocarditis) and have been found in 10 to 15% of cases at autopsy. The presence of large emboli occluding major vessels can suggest fungal infective endocarditis. Peripheral mycotic aneurysms require surgical resection; intracerebral aneurysms should be resected if they bleed or if they are causing a mass effect.

Finally, many patients have evidence of cerebrovascular emboli, which have a predilection for the middle cerebral artery distribution and may be devastating. Most emboli to the CNS occur early in the course of the disease and are evident at the time of presentation or shortly thereafter. Cerebrovascular accidents related to these emboli are prone to catastrophic hemorrhagic transformation. The possibility of right-sided infective endocarditis leading to a paradoxical CNS embolism through a patent foramen ovale (Chapter 68) should not be neglected. Of note, the majority of patients with fungal endocarditis have a CNS embolic event.

Some complications of infective endocarditis are a result of bacteremic seeding causing metastatic infection at a distant site. Patients may present with osteomyelitis, septic arthritis, or epidural abscess. Purulent meningitis (Chapter 437) is a rare complication except in pneumococcal endocarditis, although many patients with *S. aureus* infective endocarditis who undergo lumbar puncture will have a pleocytosis. Importantly, the finding of one metastatic complication of infective endocarditis does not exclude the possibility of additional sites of hematogenous infection, particularly in *S. aureus* endocarditis. Thus, the need for additional diagnostic evaluations should be guided by the patient's clinical course. Intracranial abscesses are uncommon in bacterial endocarditis but frequent in *Aspergillus* endocarditis; such a finding in the setting of culture-negative endocarditis should prompt consideration of *Aspergillus* as an etiologic agent.

Multiple immunologic phenomena may occur, many of which are directly related to the circulating immune complexes characteristic of the disease. Renal biopsies performed in the setting of active infective endocarditis show some abnormality in nearly all cases. Infective endocarditis classically causes a hypocomplementemic glomerulonephritis. On histopathologic examination, the glomerular changes may be focal, diffuse, or membranoproliferative or may be akin to the immune complex disease found in systemic lupus erythematosus. In addition, many of the musculoskeletal conditions associated with infective endocarditis, including monarticular and oligoarticular arthritides, are probably immune mediated.

Diagnosis

The "gold standard" for the diagnosis of infective endocarditis is culture of a pathologic organism from a valve or other endocardial surface. However, unless the patient undergoes valve replacement or postmortem examination, the diagnosis is made clinically. As a result, various clinical criteria have been proposed; the most widely accepted are the modified Duke criteria (Table 76–4), which have an estimated 76 to 100% sensitivity and 88 to 100% specificity, with a negative predictive value of at least 92%.

The Duke criteria rely heavily on the appropriate use of blood cultures and echocardiographic data. At least three sets of blood cultures should be obtained from separate sites; each set consists of one aerobic and one anaerobic bottle, with careful attention paid to aseptic technique. Ideally, these sets are collected at least 1 hour apart to document continuous

TABLE 76–4 MODIFIED DUKE CRITERIA FOR THE DIAGNOSIS OF INFECTIVE ENDOCARDITIS

MAJOR CRITERIA

Blood culture positive
- Typical organism (α-hemolytic streptococcus, *Streptococcus bovis,* HACEK organisms, or community-acquired *Staphylococcus aureus* or enterococcus without a primary focus) from two separate blood cultures
- *or*
- Persistent bacteremia with any organism (two positive cultures >12 hr apart or three positive cultures or a majority of four or more cultures >1 hr apart)
- *or*
- Bacteremia with *S. aureus,* regardless of whether the bacteremia was nosocomially acquired or whether a removable focus of infection is found

Evidence of endocardial involvement
- Echocardiographic findings: mobile mass attached to valve or valve apparatus, or abscess, or new partial dehiscence of prosthetic valve
- New valvar regurgitation

Serology
- Single positive blood culture for *Coxiella burnetii* or antiphase 1 immunoglobulin G antibody titer >1 : 800

MINOR CRITERIA

Predisposing condition: intravenous drug use or predisposing cardiac condition
Temperature ≥38° C
Vascular phenomena: arterial embolism, septic pulmonary emboli, mycotic aneurysm, intracranial hemorrhage, conjunctival hemorrhages, Janeway lesions
Immunologic phenomena: glomerulonephritis, Osler's nodes, Roth's spots, rheumatoid factor
Echocardiogram findings consistent with endocarditis but not meeting major criteria
Microbiologic evidence: positive blood cultures not meeting major criteria or serologic evidence of active infection consistent with endocarditis

DEFINITE INFECTIVE ENDOCARDITIS

Pathologically proven infective endocarditis
or
Clinical criteria meeting either
- Two major criteria *or*
- One major and one minor criteria *or*
- Three minor criteria

POSSIBLE INFECTIVE ENDOCARDITIS

Findings that fall short of definite infective endocarditis but not rejected

REJECTED INFECTIVE ENDOCARDITIS

Firm alternative diagnosis
or
Resolution of infective endocarditis syndrome with antibiotic therapy of ≤4 days
or
No pathologic evidence of infective endocarditis at surgery or autopsy with antibiotic therapy of ≤4 days

Modified from Durack DT, Lukes AS, Bright DK, et al: New criteria for diagnosis of infective endocarditis. Am J Med 1994;96:200–209; and Li JS, Sexton DJ, Mick N, et al: Proposed modifications to the Duke criteria for the diagnosis of infective endocarditis. Clin Infect Dis 2000;30:633–638.

bacteremia; however, in cases in which patients are critically ill, this may not be feasible.

In most cases of endocarditis, in the absence of prior antibiotic therapy, every blood culture is positive because the bacteremia of endocarditis is continuous. Blood cultures are truly negative in less than 5% of cases of endocarditis; however, prior antibiotic administration may decrease the yield of blood cultures by up to 35%. Accordingly, most "culture-negative" cases of endocarditis occur in patients who have recently received antimicrobial agents. These cases are probably caused by the same organisms responsible for most native valve endocarditis; viridans streptococci and the HACEK organisms are the most likely suspects as they are much more fastidious than staphylococci and enterococci and therefore more likely to be affected by previous antibiotic administration. Ultimately, however, when blood cultures are negative and endocarditis is suspected, especially when a history of recent antimicrobials is lacking, consideration should be given to fastidious organisms, fungi, and noncultivatable organisms (Table 76–5). This possibility should receive particular attention when the patient's history reveals a suggestive exposure: farm animals or unpasteurized milk *(Coxiella burnetii, Brucella),* cats *(Bartonella henselae),* body lice *(Bartonella quintana),* or contact with birds or frequent lawn mowing *(Chlamydia psittaci).* Notification of the microbiology laboratory that endocarditis is suspected is an important step in diagnosis; special culture techniques can increase the yield for the HACEK species, nutritionally variant streptococci (*Abiotrophia* species), *Brucella, Legionella,* and some fungi. The traditional practice of "holding" blood cultures for 2 to 4 weeks to investigate culture-negative endocarditis does not appear to be required routinely. Specific serologic tests can be used to diagnose endocarditis related to *C. burnetii* (the agent of Q fever), *Brucella* species, *Bartonella,* and *C. psittaci. Tropheryma whipplei,* the etiologic agent in Whipple's disease, and multiple other organisms may be diagnosed by polymerase chain reaction. If the search for a causative organism remains fruitless, consider noninfectious etiologies such as marantic or Libman-Sacks endocarditis and atrial myxoma.

Both transthoracic echocardiography (TTE) and transesophageal echocardiography (TEE) (Chapter 53) are highly specific tests (~98%) as part of the diagnostic evaluation of suspected endocarditis. By contrast, TEE has a sensitivity of 90 to 95% in this setting, significantly better than the sensitivity of 48 to 63% usually found with TTE. Significant controversy still exists about whether the diagnostic approach to suspected infective endocarditis should begin with TTE or TEE. In most cases in which endocarditis is a serious diagnostic consideration, evaluation should begin with TEE because normal TTE is not sensitive enough to exclude endocarditis (Fig. 76–3). In some cases, however, TEE is unavailable, technically impossible, or considered too invasive by the patient, in which case it is reasonable to begin with TTE.

Some special situations may also dictate whether to begin with TTE or TEE. TEE is the only relatively noninvasive means of detecting perivalvular extension of infection as the esophageal probe's proximity to the aortic root and basal septal wall of the myocardium allows better visualization of these structures most frequently involved in local spread of infection. For this reason, any patient with a new conduction system abnormality or persistent fever—clinical predictors of perivalvular extension—should be initially evaluated with TEE. Likewise, the heightened sensitivity of TEE is especially important in the evaluation of suspected prosthetic valve endocarditis, in which TEE provides superior definition of prosthetic valve vegetations and valve ring abscesses. Finally, it has been suggested that the high sensitivity of TEE in detecting vegetations on native valves can be used in combination with clinical parameters (e.g., prompt resolution of bacteremia and defervescence) to support the clinical decision to abbreviate therapy in patients with vascular catheter–associated *S. aureus* bacteremia.

The combination of normal TTE and normal TEE has a negative predictive value of 95%. Nevertheless, when clinical suspicion of endocarditis is high and the initial TEE is normal, repeating the TEE in 7 to 10 days may reveal the diagnosis.

Treatment

Definitive antibiotic treatment of infective endocarditis (Table 76–6) is guided by antimicrobial susceptibility testing of the responsible pathogen isolated from clinical culture specimens. Frequently, however, it is advisable to begin empirical treatment before

TABLE 76–5 ORGANISMS CAUSING "CULTURE-NEGATIVE" ENDOCARDITIS*

Organism	Epidemiology	Diagnostic Tests
HACEK spp.	Mostly oral flora, so often preceded by dental work or history of periodontal disease	Prolonged incubation of standard blood cultures; may need to be subcultured onto blood or chocolate agar
Nutritionally variant streptococci	Slow and indolent course	Supplemented culture media or growth as satellite colonies around *S. aureus* streak
Coxiella burnetii (Q fever)	Worldwide; exposure to raw milk, farm environment, or rural areas	Serologic tests (high titers of antibody to both phase 1 and phase 2 antigens); also PCR on blood or valve tissue
Brucella spp.	Ingestion of contaminated milk or milk products; close contact with infected livestock	Bulky vegetations usually seen on echocardiography; blood cultures positive in 80% of cases with incubation time of 4–6 weeks; lysis-centrifugation technique may expedite growth; serologic tests are available
Bartonella spp.	*B. henselae*—transmitted by cat scratch or bite or by cat fleas *B. quintana*—transmitted by human body louse; predisposing factors include homelessness and alcohol abuse	Bulky vegetations usually seen on echocardiography; serologic testing (may cross-react with *Chlamydia* spp.) PCR of valve or emboli is best test; lysis-centrifugation technique may be useful
Chlamydia psittaci	Exposure to birds; lawn mowing	Serologic tests available, but must exclude *Bartonella* because of cross-reactivity; monoclonal antibody direct stains on tissue may be useful; PCR now available
Whipple's disease (*Tropheryma whipplei)*	Systemic symptoms include arthralgias, diarrhea, abdominal pain, lymphadenopathy, weight loss, CNS involvement; however, endocarditis may be present without systemic symptoms	Histologic examination of valve with PAS stain; valve cultures may be done with fibroblast cell lines; also PCR on vegetation material
Legionella spp.	Contaminated water distribution systems; often nosocomial outbreaks; usually prosthetic valves	Lysis-centrifugation technique; also periodic subcultures onto buffered charcoal yeast extract medium; serologic tests are available, as is PCR
Aspergillus and other noncandidal fungi	Prosthetic valve	Lysis-centrifugation technique; also culture and direct examination of any emboli

*Listed in approximate order of relative frequency.
CNS = central nervous system; HACEK = *Haemophilus* species, *Actinobacillus actinomycetemcomitans*, *Cardiobacterium hominis*, *Eikenella corrodens*, and *Kingella* species; PAS = periodic acid–Schiff; PCR = polymerase chain reaction.

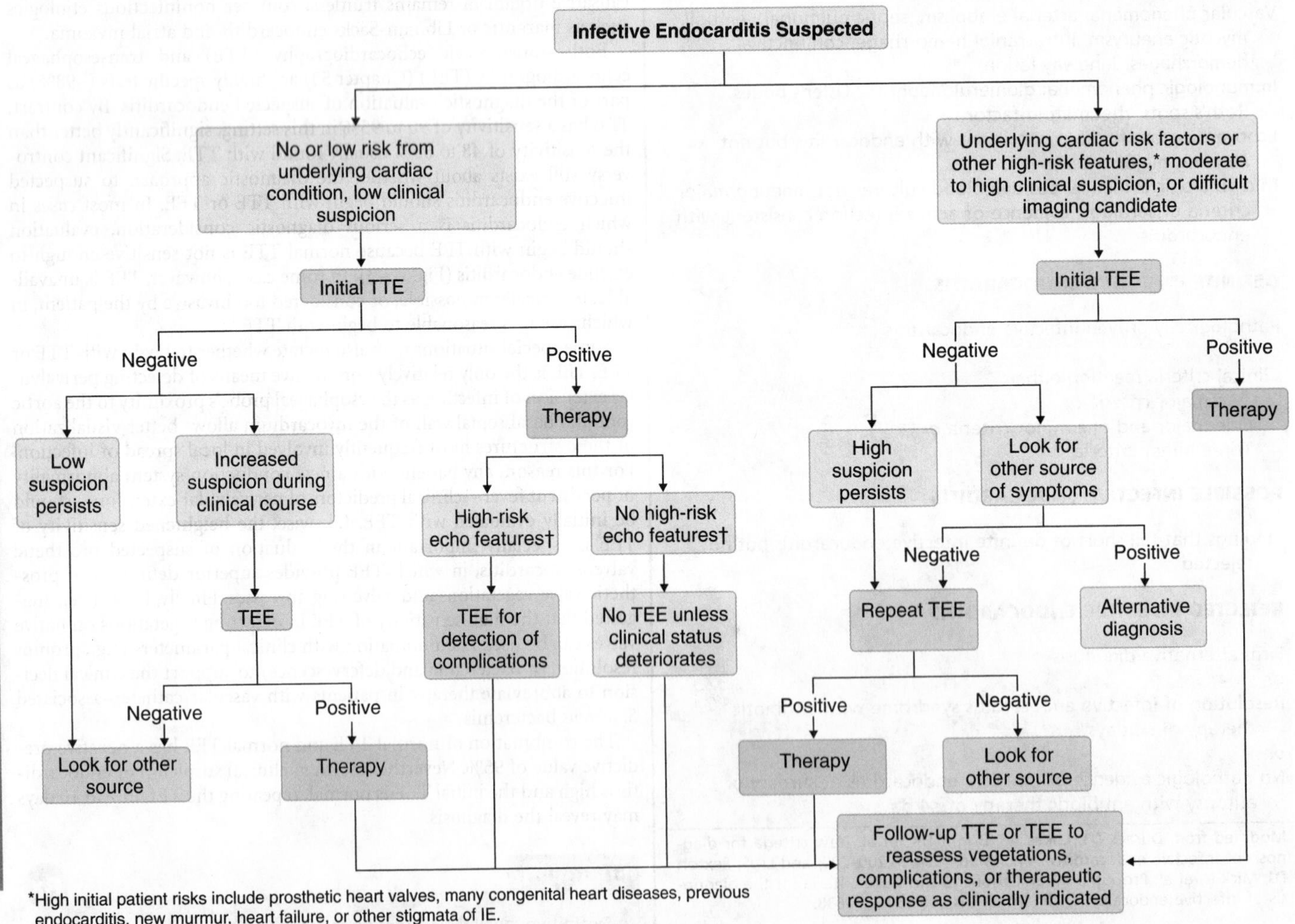

*High initial patient risks include prosthetic heart valves, many congenital heart diseases, previous endocarditis, new murmur, heart failure, or other stigmata of IE.

†High-risk echocardiographic features include large and/or mobile vegetations, valvular insufficiency, suggestions of perivalvular extension, or secondary, ventricular dysfunction.

FIGURE 76–3 • Algorithm for diagnostic use of echocardiography in suspected cases of infective endocarditis. IE = infective endocarditis; TEE = transesophageal echocardiography; TTE = transthoracic echocardiography. (Modified from Bayer AS, Bolger AF, Taubert KA, et al: Diagnosis and management of infective endocarditis and its complications. Circulation 1998;98:2936–2948.)

TABLE 76–6 DEFINITIVE THERAPY FOR BACTERIAL ENDOCARDITIS*

Organism and Regimen	Comments
PCN-susceptible viridans streptococci (MIC ≤0.1 μg/mL) and *S. bovis*	
PCN 2–4 million units IV q4h × 4 wk	Also effective for other PCN-susceptible non-viridans streptococci
Ceftriaxone 2 g IV qd × 4 wk	Uncomplicated infection with viridans streptococci, candidate for outpatient therapy; also PCN allergy
PCN 2–3 million units IV q4h × 2 wk *plus* Gentamicin 1 mg/kg IV q8h × 2 wk	Uncomplicated infection with none of the following features: renal insufficiency, eighth cranial nerve deficit, prosthetic valve infection, CNS complications, severe heart failure, or age older than 65 years; also not acceptable for nutritionally variant streptococci
PCN 2–4 million units IV q4h × 4 wk *plus* Gentamicin 1 mg/kg IV q8h × 2 wk	Nutritionally variant strain; for prosthetic valve, 6 weeks of PCN
Vancomycin 1 g IV q12h × 4 wk	For PCN allergy
Relatively PCN-resistant viridans group streptococci (MIC 0.12 to ≤0.5 μg/mL)	
PCN 4 million units IV q4h × 4 wk *plus* Gentamicin 1 mg/kg IV q8h × 2 wk	
Vancomycin 1 g IV q12h × 4 wk	For PCN allergy, or to avoid gentamicin
Enterococci[†] and PCN-resistant viridans group streptococci (MIC >1 μg/mL)	
PCN[‡] 18–30 million units IV per day in divided doses ×4–6 wk *plus* Gentamicin 1 mg/kg IV q8h × 4–6 wk	Increase duration of both drugs to 6 weeks for prosthetic valve infection or symptoms longer than 3 months in enterococcal infection
Vancomycin 1 g IV q12h × 6 wk *plus* Gentamicin 1 mg/kg q8h × 6 wk[§]	For PCN allergy; PCN desensitization is also an option; high risk of nephrotoxicity with this regimen
Staphylococcus aureus	
Nafcillin 2 g IV q4h × 4–6 wk with *optional* addition of gentamicin 1 mg/kg IV q8h × 3–5 days	Methicillin-susceptible strain; omit gentamicin if significant renal insufficiency
Vancomycin 1 g IV q12h × 6 wk	PCN allergy (immediate hypersensitivity or anaphylaxis) or MRSA
Nafcillin 2 g IV q4h × 2 weeks *plus* Gentamicin 1 mg/kg IV q8h × 2 wk; *or* Daptomycin 6 mg/kg 1V qd	Methicillin-susceptible strain; 2-week regimen for use only in IV drug abuser with tricuspid valve–only infection with no renal insufficiency and no extrapulmonary infection susceptible strain
Nafcillin 2 g IV q4h × ≥6 wk *plus* Gentamicin 1 mg/kg IV q8h × 2 wk *plus* Rifampin 300 mg PO/IV q8h × ≥6 wk	Prosthetic valve infection with MRSA—use vancomycin instead of nafcillin
Cefazolin 2 g IV q8h for 4–6 wk with *optional* addition of gentamicin 1 mg/kg IV q8h × 3–5 days	PCN allergy other than immediate hypersensitivity
Coagulase-negative staphylococci, prosthetic valve infection	
Vancomycin 1 g IV q12h × ≥6 wk *plus* Gentamicin 1 mg/kg IV q8h × 2 wk *plus* Rifampin 300 mg PO/IV q8h × ≥6 wk	Nafcillin (2 g IV q4h × >6 wk) can be substituted for vancomycin if the isolate is methicillin sensitive.
HACEK strains	
Ceftriaxone 2 g IV qd × 4 wk; 6 wk for prosthetic valves	
Ampicillin-sulbactam 3 g IV q6h × 4 wk; 6 wk for prosthetic valves	HACEK strains increasingly may produce β-lactamase.
Non-HACEK gram-negative bacilli	
Enterobacteriaceae	
Extended-spectrum penicillin or cephalosporin *plus* aminoglycosides for susceptible strains	Treat for a minimum of 6–8 weeks. Some species of Enterobacteriaceae exhibit inducible resistance to third-generation cephalosporins. Valve surgery is required for most patients with left-sided endocarditis caused by gram-negative bacilli. Consultation with a specialist in infectious diseases is recommended.
Pseudomonas aeruginosa	
High-dose tobramycin (8 mg/kg/day IV or IM in once-daily doses) with maintenance of peak and trough concentrations of 15–20 μg/mL and ≤2 μg/mL, respectively, in combination with (1) an extended-spectrum penicillin (e.g., ticarcillin, piperacillin, azlocillin), (2) ceftazidime, cefepime, or imipenem in full doses, or (3) imipenem	Treat for a minimum of 6–8 weeks. Early valve surgery is usually required for left-sided *Pseudomonas* endocarditis. Consultation with a specialist in infectious diseases is recommended.
Fungi	
Treatment with a parenteral antifungal agent (usually an amphotericin B–containing product) and valve replacement	Long-term or lifelong suppressive therapy with oral antifungal agents is often required. Consultation with a specialist in infectious diseases is recommended.

*Dosages are for patients with normal renal function; adjustments must be made for renal insufficiency for all drugs except nafcillin, rifampin, and ceftriaxone. Gentamicin doses should be adjusted to achieve a peak serum concentration of approximately 3 μg/mL 30 minutes after dosing and a trough level of less than 1 μg/mL.

[†]Enterococci must be tested for antimicrobial susceptibility. These recommendations are for enterococci sensitive to penicillin, gentamicin, and vancomycin.

[‡]Ampicillin, 12 g/day, may be used instead of PCN.

[§]Need for addition of aminoglycoside has not been demonstrated for PCN-resistant streptococci.

CNS = central nervous system; HACEK = *Haemophilus* species, *Actinobacillus actinomycetemcomitans, Cardiobacterium hominis, Eikenella corrodens,* and *Kingella* species; IV = intravenous; MIC = minimum inhibitory concentration; MRSA = methicillin-resistant *Staphylococcus aureus;* PCN = penicillin.

Modified from Baddour LM, Wilson WR, Bayer AS, et al: Infective endocarditis: Diagnosis, antimicrobial therapy, and management of complications. Circulation 2005;111:e394–e433.

TABLE 76–7 EMPIRICAL TREATMENT OF ENDOCARDITIS*

Characteristics of Patients	Treatment Regimen
Native valve, community acquisition of infection, MRSA unlikely	Nafcillin 2 g IV q4h *plus* Penicillin 4 million units IV q4h *plus* Gentamicin 1 mg/kg IV q8h
Any of the following: health care–associated infection or other reason to suspect MRSA; severe penicillin allergy	Vancomycin 1 g IV q12h *plus* Gentamicin 1 mg/kg IV q8h
Prosthetic valve	Vancomycin 1 g IV q12h *plus* Gentamicin 1 mg/kg IV q8h *plus* Rifampin 300 mg PO or IV q8h

*Dosages are for patients with normal renal function; adjustments must be made for renal insufficiency for all drugs except nafcillin.
MRSA = methicillin-resistant *Staphylococcus aureus.*

Rx

definitive culture results are available. Not all patients admitted to rule out endocarditis need to be empirically treated; patients who are clinically stable, with a subacute presentation of disease and without evidence of congestive heart failure or other end-organ complications, may be closely observed without antibiotics so that serial blood cultures may be performed. Likewise, stable patients who were empirically prescribed antibiotics before hospitalization without blood being drawn for cultures may have their antibiotics discontinued so that blood culture specimens may be obtained, preferably as long as is feasible after the antibiotics are stopped. By contrast, acutely ill patients, patients with evidence of sequelae of endocarditis, and patients who are at high risk for endocarditis should be empirically treated with antibiotics pending culture results. In most cases of infective endocarditis, it is advisable to seek consultation with an infectious diseases specialist to assist in design of an appropriate antibiotic regimen.

Either of two regimens provides appropriate empirical coverage for patients with suspected native valve endocarditis: nafcillin-penicillin-gentamicin or vancomycin-gentamicin (Table 76–7). Nafcillin-penicillin-gentamicin is suitable in most cases of suspected native valve endocarditis, providing optimal coverage for streptococci, staphylococci, enterococci, and HACEK organisms. If methicillin-resistant *S. aureus* is an important consideration, as it is for injection drug users, patients with health care contact, and patients with a prior history of such infections, empirical therapy should be with vancomycin and gentamicin. This regimen is also acceptable for patients with a severe penicillin allergy. Patients with prosthetic valves should be empirically treated with vancomycin, gentamicin, and rifampin for adequate coverage of *S. aureus* (including methicillin-resistant *S. aureus*), coagulase-negative staphylococci, and gram-negative organisms.

Treatment of Specific Organisms

When the organism is definitively identified, antibiotic treatment must be narrowed accordingly. Standardized regimens have been developed and validated for the most common organisms, and these protocols should be assiduously followed (see Table 76–6). More controversy exists about the treatment of unusual organisms, and consultation with infectious disease specialists is advisable in such circumstances. Of note, the gentamicin recommended in these regimens is so-called low dose, which reduces the risk of toxicity while providing adequate levels for synergism. In cases in which the risk of aminoglycoside toxicity is significantly increased (for instance, elderly people, patients with preexisting renal disease or hearing impairment, and diabetic patients), exposure to gentamicin should be minimized or avoided entirely. In fact, for the organisms listed in Table 76–6, gentamicin has been established as truly critical for cure only in cases of enterococcal endocarditis. As a result, current guidelines classify even low-dose, short-course gentamicin therapy as optional for the treatment of native valve *S. aureus* endocarditis.

In uncomplicated viridans streptococcal endocarditis, outpatient therapy with once-daily dosing of ceftriaxone has been shown to be as effective as more complex regimens, provided the patient has been observed in the hospital for a time for the development of complications. [1] The decision to administer antimicrobial therapy in the outpatient setting must, of course, take into account the patient's social situation, likelihood of compliance, and other risks involved with either an indwelling intravenous line or recurrent peripheral intravenous placement.

Standard therapy for infective endocarditis caused by fully susceptible enterococci includes penicillin or ampicillin plus either streptomycin or gentamicin. Although gentamicin is preferred to streptomycin, the choice of a specific aminoglycoside should be based on in vitro susceptibility testing, and the duration of aminoglycoside therapy can be as short as 2 to 3 weeks. Although the optimal therapy for infective endocarditis due to ampicillin-sensitive aminoglycoside-resistant enterococci is undefined, in vitro and experimental data have suggested the potential efficacy of double β-lactam combinations of third-generation cephalosporins and ampicillin for such infections.

Optimal therapy for enterococci that are resistant (to aminoglycosides or vancomycin) is not well defined. Some authorities suggest that high-dose ampicillin (20 to 30 g/day, administered by continuous infusion) plus surgical treatment may be effective in cases of enterococci with high-level aminoglycoside resistance. Endocarditis caused by vancomycin-resistant strains of enterococci may be treatable with daptomycin, quinupristin-dalfopristin, or linezolid; however, clinical experience with these agents is limited. In this situation, relapse or failure rates are likely to be high, and many cases require surgical intervention (discussed later).

Data suggest that patients with methicillin-sensitive *S. aureus* endocarditis treated with vancomycin have higher rates of bacteriologic failure than do those treated with nafcillin. Therefore, every attempt should be made to treat methicillin-sensitive *S. aureus* endocarditis with an antistaphylococcal β-lactam. If vancomycin must be used because of methicillin resistance or severe penicillin allergy and the patient has failed to respond clinically and remains bacteremic a week or more into therapy, the addition of a second antistaphylococcal agent (e.g., rifampin, quinupristin-dalfopristin, or an aminoglycoside) should be considered as this approach has been anecdotally effective. In a randomized trial, daptomycin (6 mg/kg once daily for 10 to 42 days, depending on the severity of the infection) was as effective as either semisynthetic antistaphylococcal penicillin or vancomycin for the treatment of *S. aureus* bacteremia and right-sided infective endocarditis. [2]

In cases of presumed culture-negative endocarditis in which unusual organisms (see Table 76–5) and other infections have been reasonably excluded, and when clinical suspicion of endocarditis remains high, an empirical course of treatment for culture-negative endocarditis may be undertaken. In this situation, most authorities recommend a 4- to 6-week regimen of ceftriaxone alone, vancomycin-ceftriaxone, or vancomycin-gentamicin (if the clinical setting suggests enterococcus).

Continuing Care of the Patient with Endocarditis

In addition to antibiotics, appropriate care of the inpatient with endocarditis requires careful surveillance for the development of any complications. Repeated echocardiography and serial electrocardiograms should be obtained to look for the development of conduction system disease that might herald perivalvular extension, especially in patients with prosthetic valves and persistent fever. Widening pulse pressure should alert the clinician to the possible development of acute aortic insufficiency (Chapter 78). Similarly, a careful cardiac examination should be performed on a daily basis to assess for new regurgitant murmurs. Any new neurologic findings should prompt a search for CNS complications. Renal function

TABLE 76–8 INDICATIONS FOR SURGERY IN ENDOCARDITIS

Indication	Class*
NATIVE VALVE ENDOCARDITIS	
Acute aortic insufficiency or mitral regurgitation with heart failure	I
Acute aortic insufficiency with tachycardia and early closure of the mitral valve on echocardiogram	I
Fungal endocarditis	I
Evidence of annular or aortic abscess; sinus or aortic true or false aneurysm; valve dehiscence, rupture, perforation, or fistula	I
Evidence of valve dysfunction and persistent infection after a prolonged period (7–10 days) of appropriate therapy, provided there are no noncardiac causes for infection	I
Recurrent emboli after appropriate antibiotic therapy	I
Infection with gram-negative organisms or organisms with a poor response to antibiotics in patients with evidence of valve dysfunction	I
Anterior mitral leaflet vegetation (especially >10 mm) or persistent vegetation after systemic embolization	IIa
Increase in vegetation size despite appropriate antimicrobial therapy	IIb
Early infections of the mitral valve that can probably be repaired	III
Persistent fever and leukocytosis with negative blood cultures	III
PROSTHETIC VALVE ENDOCARDITIS	
Early prosthetic valve endocarditis (<2 months after surgery)	I
Heart failure with prosthetic valve dysfunction	I
Nonstreptococcal endocarditis	I
Evidence of perivalvar leak, annular or aortic abscess, sinus or aortic true or false aneurysm, fistula formation, or new-onset conduction disturbances	I
Persistent bacteremia after 7–10 days of appropriate antibiotic therapy without noncardiac causes for bacteremia	IIa
Recurrent peripheral embolus despite therapy	IIa
Vegetation of any size seen on or near the prosthesis	IIb

*Definitions:
Class I: Conditions for which there is evidence and/or general agreement that a given procedure or treatment is useful and effective.
Class II: Conditions for which there is conflicting evidence and/or a divergence of opinion about the usefulness/efficacy of a procedure or treatment. IIa: Weight of evidence/opinion is in favor of usefulness/efficacy. IIb: Usefulness/efficacy is less well established by evidence/opinion.
Class III: Conditions for which there is evidence and/or general agreement that the procedure/treatment is not useful and in some cases may be harmful.
Modified with permission from Bonow RO, Carabello B, de Leon AC, et al: Guidelines for the management of patients with valvular heart disease. Circulation 1998;98:1949–1984.

should be closely monitored so that antibiotic doses may be adjusted if necessary. If gentamicin is to be used for more than a few days, the patient should be alerted to the signs and symptoms of vestibular or otic toxicity. Audiometric testing at baseline and periodically thereafter should be considered in patients at high risk for aminoglycoside-induced ototoxicity, including the elderly, patients with preexisting renal dysfunction or hearing damage, and patients receiving prolonged courses of gentamicin. Serum gentamicin trough concentrations should also be assayed at regular intervals (e.g., twice weekly and more often if renal function is changing) and should be less than 1 μg/mL. Higher concentrations suggest underlying renal insufficiency and accumulation of the drug, indicating that a lower dose should be used. Follow-up blood cultures may be indicated toward the end of the first week of therapy in patients with infective endocarditis related to organisms for which first-line treatment commonly fails, such as *S. aureus* and enterococci. Positive cultures in this setting might suggest the need for a change in therapy or surgical intervention, and negative cultures would be reassuring.

Patients with infective endocarditis may continue to be febrile for some time after the institution of appropriate antibiotic treatment. About half of patients defervesce within 3 days of starting antibiotics, and 75% have defervesced at 1 week. By 2 weeks, 90% of patients have defervesced. Patients with endocarditis caused by *S. aureus,* gram-negative organisms, or fungi tend to defervesce more slowly than do patients with infective endocarditis related to other organisms. Prolonged fever (more than 1 week after institution of appropriate antibiotics) should prompt consideration of several possibilities other than treatment failure: myocardial abscess, extracardiac infection (e.g., mycotic aneurysm, psoas or splenic abscess, vertebral osteomyelitis or septic arthritis), immune complex–mediated tissue damage, or a complication of hospitalization and therapy (e.g., drug fever, nosocomial superinfection, or pulmonary embolism). Appropriate studies might include TEE, computed tomographic scan of the abdomen, bone scan, and urinalysis with microscopy (to elicit evidence of interstitial nephritis). Intravenous line sites should be carefully examined for evidence of infection, and indwelling central lines should be changed. In addition, blood cultures are useful at this point to document the absence of persistent bacteremia and prompt a search for other sources.

Anticoagulation in individuals with infective endocarditis is controversial. Although anticoagulation in the setting of native valve endocarditis does not appear to provide benefit, some authorities recommend continuing anticoagulation in patients with mechanical prosthetic valve endocarditis. However, it is generally advised to discontinue all anticoagulation in patients with *S. aureus* prosthetic valve endocarditis who have experienced a recent CNS embolic event for at least the first 2 weeks of antibiotic therapy to allow the thrombus to organize and potentially prevent the acute hemorrhagic transformation of embolic lesions. Reintroduction of anticoagulation in these patients must be cautious, and the international normalized ratio must be monitored carefully. The best option for patients with other indications for anticoagulation, such as deep venous thrombosis, major vessel embolization, or atrial fibrillation, is less clear and should be decided in a multidisciplinary fashion that balances the risks and benefits for each individual patient.

Surgery

Some patients require surgical treatment, either to establish cure or to prevent death from the complications of infective endocarditis. The American College of Cardiology and the American Heart Association published an evidence-based set of recommendations for selection of patients for surgical intervention (Table 76–8). Patients with evidence of direct extension of infection to myocar-

TABLE 76–9 CARDIAC LESIONS ASSOCIATED WITH ENDOCARDITIS

ENDOCARDITIS PROPHYLAXIS RECOMMENDED	
High risk	Prosthetic valves Previous endocarditis Complex cyanotic congenital heart disease, e.g., single-ventricle states, transposition of the great vessels, tetralogy of Fallot Surgically constructed systemic-pulmonary shunts
Moderate risk	Other congenital heart defects except as below Acquired valve dysfunction as follows: valvar stenosis, at least mild aortic insufficiency, at least moderate mitral regurgitation or tricuspid regurgitation, and thickened mitral valve with at least mild mitral regurgitation Hypertrophic cardiomyopathy Mitral valve prolapse with regurgitation and/or thickened leaflets
PROPHYLAXIS NOT RECOMMENDED	
Negligible risk	Isolated secundum atrial septal defect Surgical repair of atrial septal defect, ventricular septal defect, or patent ductus arteriosus without residua beyond 6 months Previous coronary artery bypass grafting Mitral valve prolapse without mitral regurgitation or thickened leaflets Physiologic, functional, or innocent heart murmurs Previous rheumatic fever without valvar dysfunction Pacemakers and implanted defibrillators

Modified from Dajani AS, Taubert KA, Wilson W, et al: Prevention of bacterial endocarditis: Recommendations of the American Heart Association. JAMA 1997;277:1794–1801.

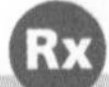

dial structures, prosthetic valve dysfunction, or heart failure from endocarditis-induced valve damage should in most cases undergo surgery. In addition, many cases of endocarditis caused by fungi or by gram-negative or resistant organisms (e.g., vancomycin- or gentamicin-resistant enterococci) require surgical management. Progression of disease or persistence of fever and bacteremia for more than 7 to 10 days in the presence of appropriate antibiotic therapy may indicate the need for surgery; however, a thorough search must first be conducted to exclude other foci of infection. Surgical management should also be considered for patients with recurrent (two or more) embolic events or large vegetations (>10 mm) on echocardiography with one embolic event, although the data in these situations are less convincing. The triad of *S. aureus* endocarditis involving the anterior mitral valve leaflet and large vegetations (>10 mm) may be a special circumstance for early surgical interventions to reduce the high risk of CNS emboli.

Delaying surgery in patients with deteriorating cardiac function in an attempt to "sterilize" the affected valve is ill-advised; the risk of progressive congestive heart failure or further complications usually outweighs the relatively small risk of recurrent infective endocarditis after prosthetic valve implantation. Relative contraindications to valve replacement include recent CNS emboli or bleed (because of the risk of bleeding in the perioperative period when anticoagulation is required), multiple prior valve replacements (because of the difficulty of sewing a new valve into tissue already weakened from previous surgeries), and ongoing injection drug use.

After definitive surgical treatment, most patients should receive some amount of further antibiotic therapy unless a full course of antibiotics has been administered before surgery and there is no evidence of ongoing infection. If the patient has received less than 1 week of antibiotics before surgery and the Gram stain or culture from the operative site is positive, an additional 4- to 8-week course of antibiotics after surgery is reasonable. If the patient has received 2 weeks or more of therapy and the Gram stain and culture of the operative site are negative, at least 2 more weeks of antibiotic therapy are probably sufficient (depending on the organism).

Prevention

Although the current standard of care is to administer prophylactic antibiotics to patients with known risk factors for infective endocarditis before procedures known to cause bacteremia, no large-scale, prospective, randomized controlled trials have addressed the efficacy of this practice. Several small case-control studies have suggested that the practice of prescribing prophylactic antibiotics may prevent only 1 to 10% of cases of infective endocarditis. Animal studies suggest that antibiotic prophylaxis is effective, but retrospective epidemiologic studies have produced conflicting results. Moreover, most experts now think that the cumulative risk of daily oral bacteremias far outweighs the risk of a single dental procedure for inducing infective endocarditis. Nevertheless, in the absence of clear data showing that antibiotic prophylaxis is ineffective and with the high morbidity and mortality associated with endocarditis, antibiotic prophylaxis for selected patients continues to be recommended.

Predisposing cardiac lesions can be stratified on the basis of the relative risk of endocarditis into high risk, moderate risk, and negligible risk, with the first two groups requiring prophylaxis (Table 76–9). Prophylaxis is recommended for patients with mitral valve prolapse only if they have turbulent flow, that is, patients with an audible murmur, echocardiographic demonstration of significant regurgitation, or thickened mitral leaflets on echocardiography.

Preprocedure prophylaxis is recommended for procedures that tend to cause bleeding that introduces organisms capable of attachment to the endocardial surface, that is, staphylococci, streptococci, and enterococci (Table 76–10). Thus, many oral and genitourinary procedures require prophylaxis, as do most procedures involving infected tissues. As an additional precaution, fastidious oral hygiene should be maintained by patients at high risk for endocarditis, both to decrease the rate of spontaneous bacteremia from gingival disease and to obviate more invasive periodontal work.

The antibiotics chosen for preprocedure prophylaxis should be active against the organisms most likely to be released into the blood stream by the procedure (Table 76–11). For dental, oral, respiratory tract, and esophageal procedures, antibiotics that cover primarily oral flora are recommended. Prophylactic regimens for genitourinary and nonesophageal gastrointestinal procedures need to cover enterococci as well and are therefore more complicated.

Prognosis

Untreated, infective endocarditis is uniformly fatal. Aggressive medical and surgical management, however, has dramatically improved the outcome. Mortality overall from both native and prosthetic valve endocarditis remains fairly high, ranging from 17 to 36%. Certain subgroups carry a lower risk of death (endocarditis related to viridans streptococci);

TABLE 76–10 PROCEDURES AND THE NEED FOR ENDOCARDITIS PROPHYLAXIS

ENDOCARDITIS PROPHYLAXIS RECOMMENDED*

Dental
- Dental and oral procedures likely to cause significant bleeding, periodontal surgery, scaling, and professional teeth cleaning
- Intraligamentary oral local anesthetic injections

Respiratory tract
- Surgical operations that involve respiratory mucosa
- Bronchoscopy with a rigid bronchoscope
- Tonsillectomy or adenoidectomy

Gastrointestinal tract†
- Sclerotherapy for esophageal varices
- Esophageal stricture dilation
- Endoscopic retrograde cholangiography with biliary obstruction
- Biliary tract surgery
- Surgical operations that involve intestinal mucosa

Genitourinary tract
- Prostatic surgery
- Cystoscopy

Other
- Incision and drainage of infected tissue

ENDOCARDITIS PROPHYLAXIS NOT RECOMMENDED*

Dental
- Restorative dentistry (including filling cavities and replacement of missing teeth)
- Oral local anesthetic injections
- Placement of removable prosthodontic or orthodontic appliances
- Taking of oral impressions or radiographs
- Orthodontic appliance adjustment

Respiratory tract
- Endotracheal intubation
- Bronchoscopy with flexible bronchoscope, with or without biopsy‡
- Tympanostomy tube insertion

Gastrointestinal tract
- Transesophageal echocardiography‡
- Endoscopy with or without biopsy‡

Genitourinary tract
- Vaginal hysterectomy‡
- Vaginal delivery‡
- Cesarean section
- Uninfected urethral catheterization, uterine dilation and curettage, therapeutic abortion, sterilization procedures, placement or removal of intrauterine devices

Other
- Cardiac catheterization, including angioplasty
- Implanted cardiac pacemakers, implanted defibrillators, and coronary stents
- Incision or biopsy of surgically scrubbed skin
- Circumcision

*Recommendations apply to high- and moderate-risk patients only (see Table 76–9), except where noted.
†Prophylaxis is recommended for high-risk patients, optional for moderate-risk patients.
‡Prophylaxis is optional for high-risk patients.
Modified from Dajani AS, Taubert KA, Wilson W, et al: Prevention of bacterial endocarditis: Recommendations of the American Heart Association. JAMA 1997;277:1794–1801.

endocarditis due to *S. aureus*, fungal endocarditis, and zoonotic endocarditis have higher mortalities. Heart failure and CNS events are the most frequent causes of death.

Endocarditis recurs in 12 to 16% of patients and is more common in injection drug users, elderly people, and patients with prosthetic valves. The rate of relapse also varies according to the causative organism. Easily treated infections, such as those with α-hemolytic streptococci, have a low rate of relapse (~5%), whereas infections with organisms that are more difficult to eradicate may have significantly higher rates.

TABLE 76–11 SUGGESTED ANTIBIOTICS FOR ENDOCARDITIS PROPHYLAXIS

DENTAL, ORAL, RESPIRATORY TRACT, AND ESOPHAGEAL PROCEDURES

Patient able to take oral medications; medication should be administered 1 hour before procedure
- First-line therapy:
  - Amoxicillin 2 g PO
- For penicillin allergy:
  - Cephalexin 2 g PO (not immediate-type hypersensitivity) *or*
  - Clindamycin 600 mg PO *or*
  - Azithromycin 500 mg PO *or*
  - Clarithromycin 500 mg PO

Patient unable to take oral medications; medication should be administered within 30 minutes before procedure
- First-line therapy:
  - Ampicillin 2 g IV or IM
- For penicillin allergy:
  - Cefazolin 1 g IV (not for immediate-type hypersensitivity) *or*
  - Clindamycin 600 mg IV

GENITOURINARY AND NONESOPHAGEAL GASTROINTESTINAL PROCEDURES

High-risk patients
- First-line therapy:
  - Within 30 minutes of starting procedure:
    - Ampicillin 2 g IM or IV *plus*
    - Gentamicin 1.5 mg/kg IV or IM, not to exceed 120 mg
  - *plus*
  - Six hours after procedure:
    - Ampicillin 1 g IM or IV *or*
    - Amoxicillin 1 g PO
- For penicillin allergy:
  - Completed within 30 minutes of starting procedure:
  - Vancomycin 1 g IV during 1–2 hours *plus*
  - Gentamicin 1.5 mg/kg IV or IM, not to exceed 120 mg
- No postprocedure dose necessary

Moderate-risk patients
- First-line therapy:
  - Amoxicillin 2 g PO 1 hour before procedure
- For penicillin allergy:
  - Vancomycin 1 g IV during 1–2 hours within 30 minutes of starting procedure

Modified from Dajani AS, Taubert KA, Wilson W, et al: Prevention of bacterial endocarditis: Recommendations of the American Heart Association. JAMA 1997;277:1794–1801.

Future Directions

As cardiac imaging technology continues to improve, the duration of treatment of endocarditis may be dictated in part by the characteristics of visualized vegetations. In addition, now that large vegetations have been demonstrated to cause more embolic events, interventions to remove vegetations "prophylactically" (e.g., valve repair and vegectomy) or to introduce agents that prevent the formation or promote the dissolution of vegetations may be feasible. Finally, novel therapeutic approaches (for instance, antibacterial antibodies and cell wall–specific enzymes) that act as adjuncts to antibiotics in facilitating bacteriologic clearance are in development.

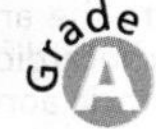

1. Sexton DJ, Tenenbaum MJ, Wilson WR, et al: Ceftriaxone once daily for four weeks compared with ceftriaxone plus gentamicin once daily for two weeks for treatment of endocarditis due to

Section VIII Cardiovascular

penicillin-susceptible streptococci. Endocarditis Treatment Consortium Group. Clin Infect Dis 1998;27:1470–1474.
2. Fowler, VG Jr, Boucher HW, Corey GR, et al: Daptomycin versus standard therapy for *Staphylococcus aureus* bacteremia and endocarditis. N Engl J Med 2006;355:653–665.

SUGGESTED READINGS

Baddour LM, Wilson WR, Bayer AS, et al: Infective endocarditis: Diagnosis, antimicrobial therapy, and management of complications. Circulation 2005;111:e394–e433. *An American Heart Association Scientific Statement providing a thorough summary of the treatment and management of infective endocarditis.*

Baddour LM, Wilson WR, Bayer AS, et al: Infective endocarditis: Diagnosis, antimicrobial therapy, and management of complications. Circulation 2005;111:3167–3184. *Detailed recommendations on treatment.*

Breitkopf C, Hammel D, Scheld HH, et al: Impact of a molecular approach to improve the microbiological diagnosis of infective heart valve endocarditis. Circulation 2005;111:1415–1421. *Molecular methods improved the diagnostic sensitivity.*

Fowler VG Jr, Miro JM, Hoen B, et al: *Staphylococcus aureus* endocarditis: A consequence of medical progress. JAMA 2005;293:3012–3021. *Demonstrates the emergence of* S. aureus *as the most common cause of infective endocarditis throughout much of the developed world.*

Petti CA, Bhally HS, Weinstein MP, et al: Utility of extended blood culture incubation for isolation of *Haemophilus, Actinobacillus, Cardiobacterium, Eikenella,* and *Kingella* organisms: A retrospective multicenter evaluation. J Clin Microbiol 2006;44:257–259. *Extended incubation of blood cultures to recover HACEK bacteria is unnecessary.*

Petti CA, Fowler VG Jr: *Staphylococcus aureus* bacteremia and endocarditis. Cardiol Clin 2003;21:219–233. *Suggestions for distinguishing the two entities clinically.*

Wang A, Athan E, Pappas PA, et al: Contemporary clinical profile and outcome of prosthetic valve endocarditis. JAMA 2007;297:1354–1361. *A comprehensive review of prosthetic valve endocarditis.*

Wilson W, Taubert KA, Gewitz M, et al: Prevention of infective endocarditis. Guidelines from the American Heart Association. J Am Dent Assoc 2007;138:739–760. *The updated guidelines on the prevention of infective endocarditis.*

77 PERICARDIAL DISEASE

Warren J. Manning

The pericardium is composed of two distinct layers. The fibrous parietal pericardium provides a protective sac around the heart to prevent sudden cardiac dilation and to minimize bulk cardiac motion. The inner, visceral pericardium is intimately related to the surface of the heart. These two layers are normally separated by 10 to 50 mL of clear fluid, an ultrafiltrate of plasma that is produced by the visceral pericardium and functions as a lubricant to minimize frictional forces between the heart and the pericardium. In health, the intrapericardial pressure is slightly negative.

Although congenital total absence of the pericardium is not associated with clinical disease, partial or localized absence of pericardium, specifically around the left atrium, may be associated with focal herniation and subsequent strangulation. This condition, usually diagnosed by thoracic computed tomography (CT) or magnetic resonance imaging (MRI), has been associated with atypical chest pain or sudden death; surgical repair often is recommended when a partial pericardial defect is confirmed. Benign pericardial cysts are rare and often seen as rounded or lobulated structures adjacent to the usual cardiac silhouette on the chest radiograph or adjacent to the right atrium on transthoracic echocardiography (Chapter 53). Thoracic CT and MRI (Fig. 77–1) are useful for the diagnosis of these cysts.

Acquired pericardial disease may have numerous causes, most of which produce responses that are pathophysiologically and clinically similar. These responses most frequently result in acute pericarditis, pericardial effusion, or constrictive pericarditis.

ACUTE PERICARDITIS

Definition

The most common clinical pathologic process involving the pericardium is acute pericarditis. Although multiple causes are possible (Table 77–1), the most common are viral infection and unknown (idiopathic). Classically, this disorder is characterized by chest pain, pericardial friction rub, diffuse electrocardiographic changes, and pericardial effusion, although sometimes neither electrocardiographic changes nor a pericardial effusion is present. The clinical syndrome is often relatively brief (days to weeks) in duration and uncomplicated, although vigilance for progression to tamponade is always prudent.

Clinical Manifestations

Chest pain of acute infectious (viral) pericarditis typically develops in young adults (18 to 30 years) 1 to 2 weeks after a "viral illness." The symptoms are sudden and severe in onset, characteristically with retrosternal or left precordial pain and referral to the back and trapezius ridge. Pain may be *preceded* by low-grade fever (in contrast to myocardial infarction, in which the pain precedes the fever). Although radiation to the arms in a manner similar to myocardial ischemia also may occur, it is less common. The pain is often pleuritic (e.g., accentuated by inspiration or coughing) and may be aggravated (supine or left lateral decubitus posture) or relieved (upright posture) by changes in posture.

The physical examination in patients with acute pericarditis is most notable for a pericardial friction rub. Although classically described as

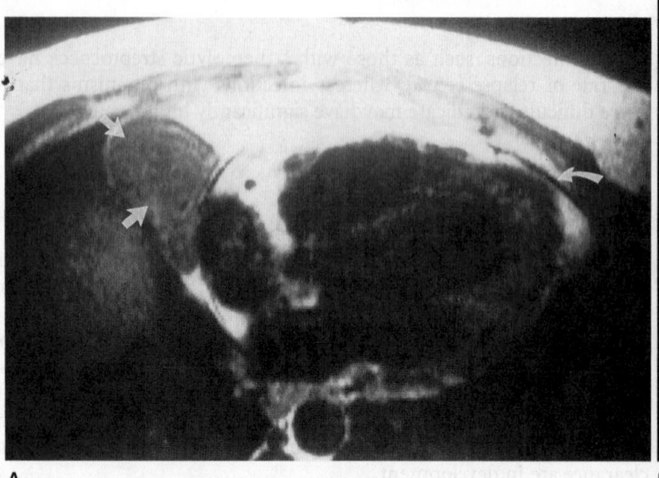
A

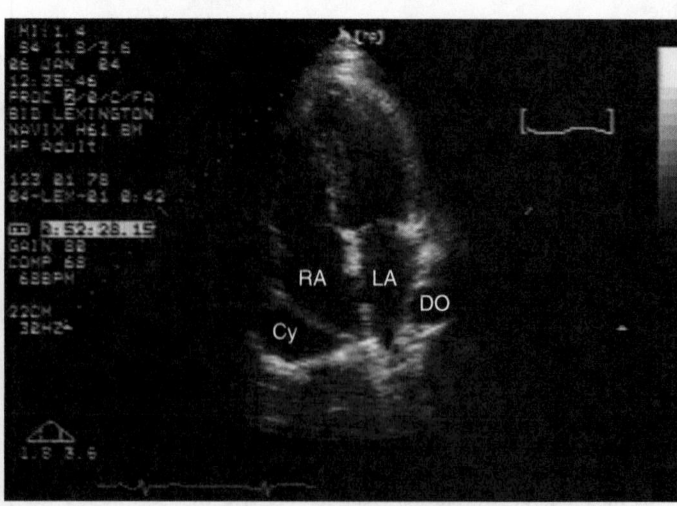

B

FIGURE 77–1 • A, Transverse (axial) magnetic resonance image. Note the anterior pericardial cyst (straight white arrows) and the normal pericardium (curved white arrow). (Courtesy of Robert R. Edelman, MD). **B,** Transthoracic echocardiogram from the apical four-chamber view demonstrating a pericardial cyst (Cy) anterior to the right atrium (RA). The left atrium (LA) and descending thoracic aorta (DO) are also seen in this view.

TABLE 77–1 ETIOLOGY OF PERICARDITIS

INFECTIOUS PERICARDITIS
Viral (coxsackieviruses A and B, echovirus, mumps, adenovirus, Epstein-Barr, human immunodeficiency virus, influenza)
Mycobacterium tuberculosis
Bacterial (*Pneumococcus, Streptococcus, Staphylococcus, Legionella*)
Fungal (histoplasmosis, coccidioidomycosis, candidiasis, blastomycosis)
Other (syphilis, parasites, Q fever)
NONINFECTIOUS PERICARDITIS
Idiopathic
Neoplasm
Metastatic (lung cancer, breast cancer, melanoma, lymphoma)
Primary (mesothelioma)
Renal failure
Trauma
Irradiation (especially for breast cancer, Hodgkin's disease)
Myocardial infarction
Hypothyroidism
Aortic dissection with hemopericardium
Chylopericardium (thoracic duct injury)
Trauma
Post pericardiotomy
Chest wall injury or trauma
Pneumonia
HYPERSENSITIVITY PERICARDITIS
Collagen vascular disease (systemic lupus erythematosus, rheumatoid arthritis, scleroderma, acute rheumatic fever, Sjögren's syndrome, Reiter's syndrome, ankylosing spondylitis)
Drug induced (procainamide, hydralazine, isoniazid; smallpox vaccine)
Post myocardial infarction (Dressler's syndrome)
Familial Mediterranean fever

triphasic, with systolic and early (passive ventricular filling) and late (atrial systole) diastolic components, more commonly a biphasic (systole and diastole) or a monophasic rub may be heard. The rub may be transient and positional, often best appreciated in the supine or left lateral decubitus posture. Low-grade fever, resting tachycardia, and atrial ectopy are common, but atrial fibrillation is unusual.

Diagnosis

Diagnosis must proceed expeditiously to exclude emergent problems (Fig. 77–2). Electrocardiographic changes (Fig. 77–3) are common, particularly with an infectious etiology because of associated inflammation of the superficial epicardium. During the initial few days, diffuse (limb leads and precordial leads) ST segment elevations occur in the absence of reciprocal ST segment depression. PR segment depression also is common and reflects atrial involvement. After several days, the ST segments normalize and then the T waves become inverted (in contrast to the electrocardiographic changes seen with myocardial infarction, in which the temporal relationship of the T wave inversions is earlier and precedes normalization of the ST segment changes). In a large pericardial effusion, tachycardia, loss of R wave voltage (absolute R wave magnitude of 5 mm or less in all limb leads and 10 mm or less in all precordial leads), and electrical alternans (Fig. 77–4) also may be seen (see Pericardial Effusion). Blood tests reflect an inflammatory state, with an elevated sedimentation rate, C-reactive protein level, and usually, leukocyte count. A mildly increased creatine kinase MB fraction and elevated troponin level occur in up to half of patients and are thought to represent epicardial inflammation rather than myocardial necrosis. If the biomarker elevation persists for several weeks or is associated with ventricular dysfunction, myocarditis with or without concomitant pericarditis should be considered.

If the pericardial effusion is minimal, the chest radiograph is often unrevealing, although a small left pleural effusion may be seen. With larger effusions (see Pericardial Effusion), there may be a loss of distinct cardiac contours and "water bottle" appearance to the cardiac silhouette (Fig. 77–5).

Treatment

In the absence of significant pericardial effusion (see later), treatment that is directed primarily at relieving the patient's symptoms can be successful in 85% or so of cases on an outpatient basis. Among nonsteroidal anti-inflammatory drugs, indomethacin (25 to 50 mg three times daily) is commonly prescribed, but ibuprofen (300 to 800 mg three or four times a day) or aspirin (325 to 650 mg three times daily) also may be used. Glucocorticoids (prednisone, 20 to 60 mg/day) may be useful for resistant situations. Anti-inflammatory drugs should be continued at a constant high dose until the patient is afebrile and asymptomatic for 5 to 7 days, followed by a gradual taper during the next several weeks. The use of warfarin or heparin should be avoided to minimize the risk of hemopericardium, but anticoagulation may be required in atrial fibrillation or in the presence of a coexistent prosthetic valve. Avoidance of vigorous physical activity is recommended during the acute and early convalescent periods. For patients with a first episode of viral or idiopathic pericarditis, colchicine (0.6 to 1.2 mg/day for 3 to 12 months) reduces the recurrence rate from about 32% to about 11%. [1] Colchicine is also effective in patients with familial Mediterranean fever (Chapters 175 and 297).

Viral and idiopathic pericarditis usually is self-limited, but a quarter of patients may have recurrent pericarditis. For this group, prolonged treatment with nonsteroidal anti-inflammatory drugs (e.g., ibuprofen, 300 to 600 mg three times a day) plus colchicine (0.6 mg twice daily, declining to once daily after a year) should be considered. [2] For the 10 to 14% of patients who are intolerant of colchicine and have recurrent episodes despite high-dose nonsteroidal anti-inflammatory drugs (e.g., indomethacin, 50 mg three times a day, or ibuprofen, 800 mg four times a day), oral steroids (e.g., prednisone, 60 mg with a 2- to 4-week taper) and pericardiectomy should be considered. Patients with recurrent pericarditis are at increased risk for progression to constrictive pericarditis (see later).

PERICARDIAL EFFUSION

Excess fluid may develop in the pericardial space in all forms of pericardial disease (Table 77–2). Most commonly, the fluid is exudative and reflects pericardial injury or inflammation. Serosanguineous effusions are typical of tuberculous and neoplastic disease but also may be seen in uremic and viral or idiopathic disease or in response to mediastinal irradiation. Hemopericardium is seen most commonly with trauma, myocardial rupture after myocardial infarction, catheter-induced myocardial or epicardial coronary artery rupture, aortic dissection with rupture into the pericardial space, or primary hemorrhage in patients receiving anticoagulant therapy (often after cardiac valve surgery). Chylopericardium is rare and results from leakage or injury to the thoracic duct.

Although the presence of pericardial effusion indicates underlying pericardial disease, the clinical relevance of the pericardial effusion is associated most closely with the *rate* of fluid collection, intrapericardial pressure, and subsequent development of tamponade physiology. A rapidly accumulating effusion, as in hemopericardium caused by trauma or aortic dissection, may result in tamponade physiology with collection of only 100 to 200 mL. By comparison, a more slowly developing effusion (hypothyroidism or chronic renal failure) may allow gradual stretching of the pericardium, with effusions exceeding 1500 mL in the absence of hemodynamic embarrassment.

Diagnosis

Pericardial effusion often is suspected clinically when the patient has symptoms and signs of tamponade physiology (see later), but it also may be suggested first by unsuspected cardiomegaly on the chest radiograph, especially if loss of the customary cardiac borders and a water bottle con-

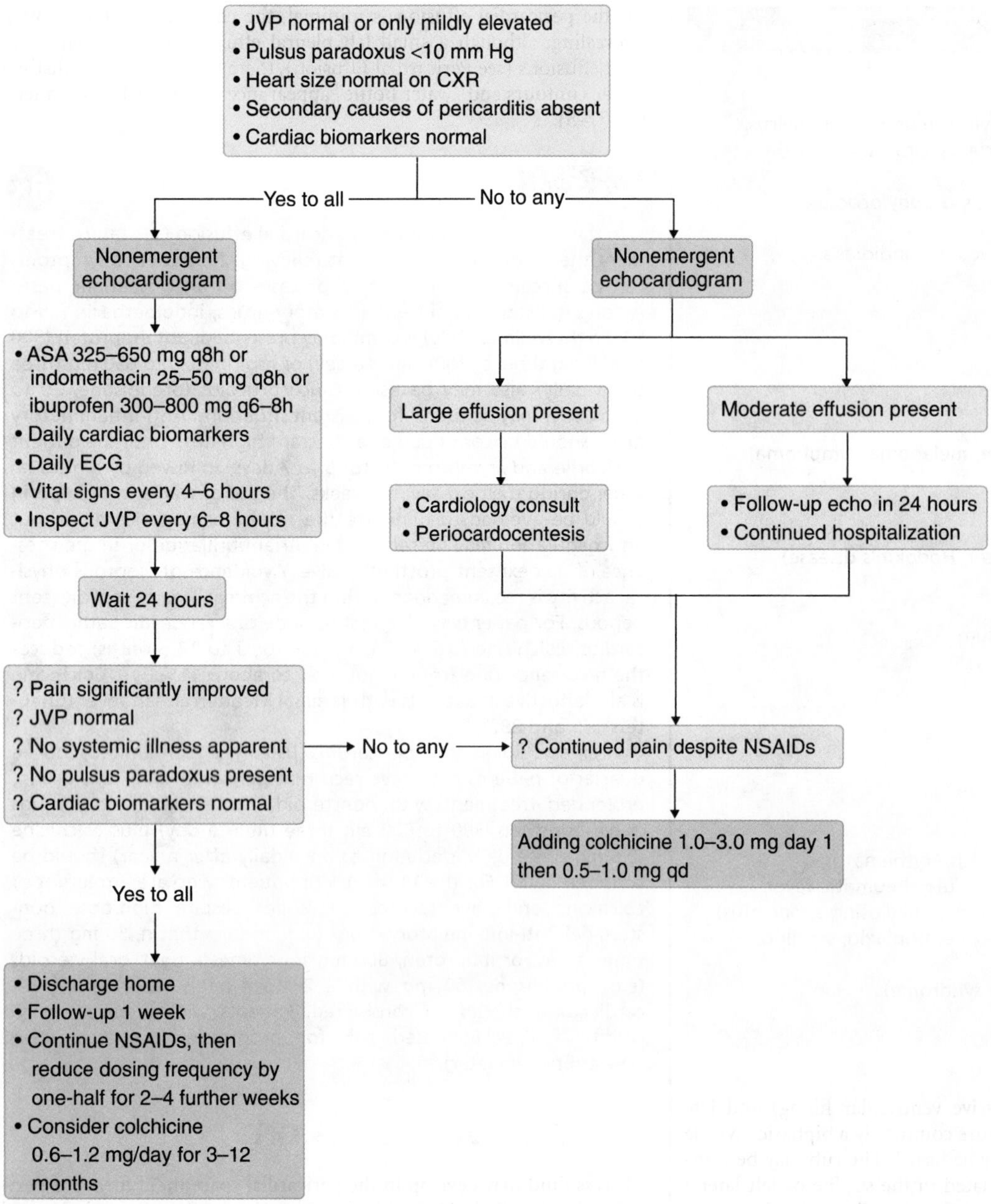

- JVP normal or only mildly elevated
- Pulsus paradoxus <10 mm Hg
- Heart size normal on CXR
- Secondary causes of pericarditis absent
- Cardiac biomarkers normal

Yes to all →

Nonemergent echocardiogram

- ASA 325–650 mg q8h or indomethacin 25–50 mg q8h or ibuprofen 300–800 mg q6–8h
- Daily cardiac biomarkers
- Daily ECG
- Vital signs every 4–6 hours
- Inspect JVP every 6–8 hours

→ Wait 24 hours

- ? Pain significantly improved
- ? JVP normal
- ? No systemic illness apparent
- ? No pulsus paradoxus present
- ? Cardiac biomarkers normal

Yes to all →

- Discharge home
- Follow-up 1 week
- Continue NSAIDs, then reduce dosing frequency by one-half for 2–4 further weeks
- Consider colchicine 0.6–1.2 mg/day for 3–12 months

No to any → ? Continued pain despite NSAIDs

No to any →

Nonemergent echocardiogram

Large effusion present →
- Cardiology consult
- Periocardocentesis

Moderate effusion present →
- Follow-up echo in 24 hours
- Continued hospitalization

→ ? Continued pain despite NSAIDs

→ Adding colchicine 1.0–3.0 mg day 1 then 0.5–1.0 mg qd

FIGURE 77–2 • Initial management of patients with pericarditis. ASA, aspirin; CXR, chest radiograph; ECG, electrocardiogram; JVP, jugular venous pressure; NSAIDs, nonsteroidal anti-inflammatory drugs. (Modified from Malik F, Foster E: Pericardial disease. *In* Wachter RM, Goldman L, Hollander H [eds]: Hospital Medicine, 2nd ed. Philadelphia, Lippincott Williams & Wilkins, 2005, p 448.)

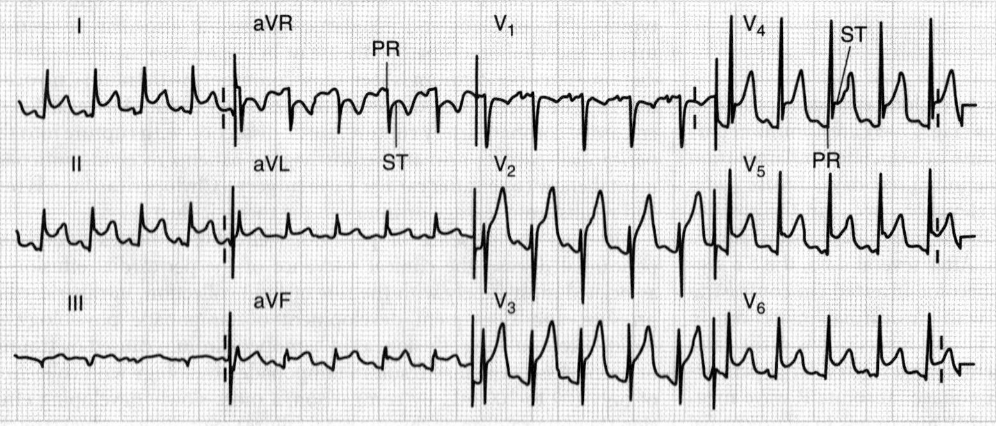

FIGURE 77–3 • A 12-lead electrocardiogram from a patient with acute pericarditis. Note the diffuse ST-T wave changes and PR elevation in lead aVR and PR segment depression in leads II and aVF and in the precordial leads. (Courtesy of Ary L. Goldberger, MD.)

figuration are noted (Fig. 77–5). Fluoroscopy, which may display minimal or absent motion of cardiac borders, is performed commonly when myocardial or epicardial coronary artery perforation is suspected during a diagnostic or interventional percutaneous procedure.

In most situations, two-dimensional transthoracic (surface) echocardiography is the diagnostic imaging procedure of choice for the evaluation and qualitative assessment of suspected pericardial effusion (Fig. 77–6). In emergency situations, it can be performed at the bedside. The subcostal four-chamber view is the most informative imaging plane; it is particularly relevant because it allows the size and location of the effusion to be assessed from an orientation that determines whether the effusion can be drained percutaneously. Transudative effusions typically appear relatively echolucent (see Fig. 77–6), whereas organized-exudative and hemorrhagic effusions have an echo-filled or a ground-glass appearance (Fig. 77–7). Stranding, which may be appreciated in organized or chronic effusions, suggests loculation and an inability to drain the effu-

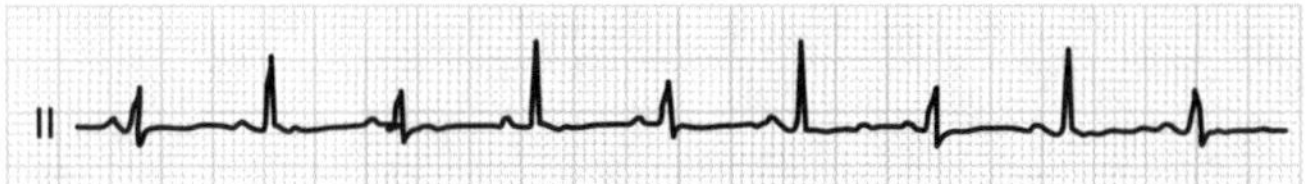

FIGURE 77–4 • Lead II rhythm strip taken from a patient with acute pericarditis complicated by a large pericardial effusion and tamponade physiology. Note the resting sinus tachycardia with relatively low voltage and electrical alternans. (Courtesy of Ary L. Goldberger, MD.)

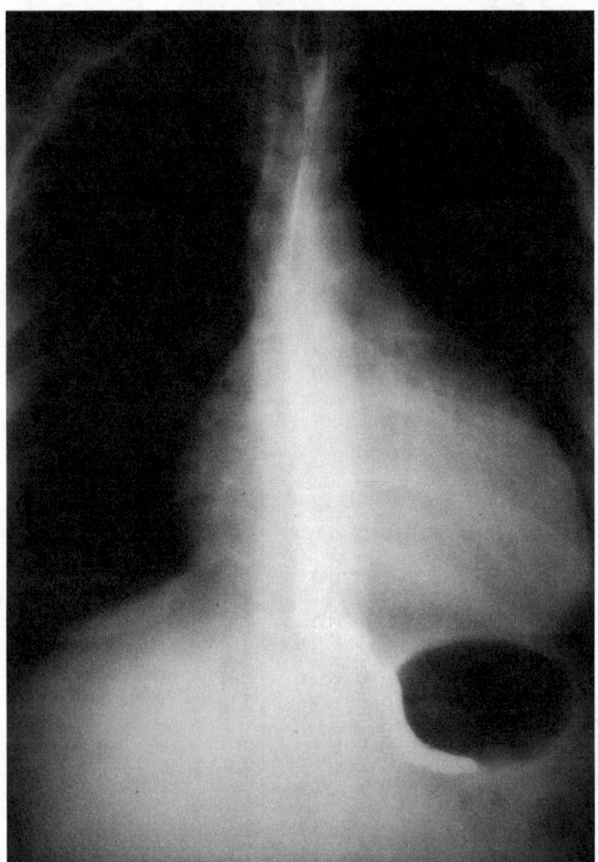

FIGURE 77–5 • Posteroanterior chest radiograph in a patient with a large pericardial effusion. Note the loss of customary heart borders and a "water bottle" configuration. (Courtesy of Sven Paulin, MD.)

sion fully by percutaneous approaches. In patients with large effusions, which are associated with electrical alternans (see Fig. 77–4), the heart may appear to swing freely within the pericardial sac.

Cardiac Tamponade

Accumulation of fluid in the pericardium with a resultant increase in pericardial pressure and impairment of ventricular filling results in cardiac tamponade. Although progression to tamponade, which may be fatal if it is not recognized quickly and treated aggressively, occurs in 10 to 15% of patients with idiopathic pericarditis, it develops in more than 50% of patients with oncologic, tuberculous, or purulent pericarditis. The hallmarks of cardiac tamponade are increased intracardiac pressure and the resulting impaired ventricular filling and depressed cardiac output. In tamponade, ventricular filling is impaired throughout diastole; by comparison, early diastolic filling is relatively normal with pericardial constriction. Invasive hemodynamic assessment reveals equalization of right and left atrial and right and left ventricular diastolic pressures. Tamponade may not be an "all-or-none" phenomenon; mild or "low-pressure" tamponade can be seen when intrapericardial pressures are only modestly elevated, with resultant equalization of atrial pressures but not diastolic ventricular pressures.

Clinical Manifestations

The clinical features of cardiac tamponade may mimic those of heart failure, with dyspnea on exertion, orthopnea, and hepatic engorgement. Many clinical features help distinguish cardiac tamponade from constrictive pericarditis and restrictive cardiomyopathy (Table 77–3). The typical physical examination with tamponade includes jugular venous distention with a prominent *x* descent (Fig. 77–8), sinus tachycardia with hypotension, narrow pulse pressure, elevated (>10 mm Hg) pulsus paradoxus, and distant heart sounds. The pulsus paradoxus may be apparent with palpation, but more commonly it is measured with a sphygmomanometer during slow respiration; direct arterial monitoring is not generally necessary for quantification. A small (<10 mm Hg) pulsus is normal and is related to the ventricles being confined within the pericardium and sharing a common septum. With inspiration, right ventricular filling is enhanced, displacing the interventricular septum toward the left ventricle and exaggerating the reduction in left ventricular filling and resultant stroke volume. The exaggerated pulsus is not specific for tamponade; it also may be present with hypovolemic shock, chronic obstructive pulmonary disease, and bronchospasm.

Diagnosis

For patients in whom the history or physical examination suggests tamponade, emergency transthoracic echocardiography is imperative and generally diagnostic. Echocardiographic evidence of tamponade physiology includes a compressed or small right ventricular chamber with late diastolic invagination of the right atrial and right ventricular free wall on two-dimensional imaging (Chapter 53). Because of the frequent coexistence of tachycardia, diastolic invagination sometimes is appreciated best with higher temporal resolution M-mode echocardiography. In addition to diastolic invagination, M-mode echocardiography also may show exaggerated inspiratory septal motion and variation in the duration of aortic valve opening. Localized right atrial, left atrial, and left ventricular diastolic collapse also may be seen and is particularly relevant for loculated effusions, such as effusions after trauma and cardiac surgery. Pseudoprolapse of the mitral valve may be seen because of the compressed left ventricular cavity. When surface echocardiography is inadequate, as in a post-thoracotomy patient or a patient with chest wall trauma, transesophageal echocardiography may be helpful. Thoracic CT and MRI may be particularly valuable for delineation of loculated pericardial effusions. Finally, Doppler echocardiography may be used to assess transtricuspid and transmitral flow profiles, with an exaggerated peak E wave respiratory variation seen in tamponade. Many of these typical echocardiographic findings may be absent in patients who have significant pulmonary artery hypertension or are on a ventilator.

Treatment

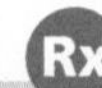

When tamponade is suggested clinically and confirmed on echocardiography, acute management includes maintenance of systolic blood pressure with volume resuscitation. In dire circumstances, immediate pericardiocentesis may be life-saving (Fig. 77–9). When time allows, right-sided heart catheterization should be performed to confirm elevated intrapericardial pressure and "equalization" of right atrial, left atrial, pulmonary capillary wedge, right ventricular diastolic, and left ventricular diastolic pressures. If echocardiography shows at least 1 cm of fluid anterior to the mid right ventricular free wall throughout diastole, percutaneous pericardiocentesis generally can be performed safely. During this procedure, a small catheter is advanced over a needle inserted into the pericardial cavity. Echocardiographic guidance is particularly useful for smaller effusions or if percutaneous pericardiocentesis is performed by less experienced operators. As much fluid as possible should be removed, with monitoring of filling pressures. Unless the cause already has been identified, pericardial fluid should be sent for evaluation (including pH, glucose, lactate dehydrogenase, protein, cell count, and cytology as well as staining and culture for bacteria, fungi, and tuberculosis). A flexible drainage catheter may be left in the pericardial space for several days to avoid early reaccumulation. Before the catheter is removed, serial echocardiography should be performed to confirm that the fluid has not reaccumulated.

Hemodynamically significant effusions of less than 1 cm, organized or multiloculated effusions, and focal effusions confined to the posterior or lateral cardiac borders or around the atria should

TABLE 77–2 PRESENTATION AND TREATMENT OF THE MOST COMMON SPECIFIC CAUSES OF PERICARDITIS

Type of Cause	Pathogenesis or Etiology	Diagnosis	Treatment	Complications	Comments
Viral	Coxsackievirus B Echovirus type 8 Epstein-Barr virus	Leukocytosis Elevated erythrocyte sedimentation rate Mild cardiac biomarker elevation	Symptomatic relief, NSAIDs	Tamponade Relapsing pericarditis	Peaks in spring and fall
Tuberculosis	*Mycobacterium tuberculosis*	Isolation of organism from biopsy fluid Granulomas not specific	Triple-drug antituberculosis regimen Pericardial drainage followed by early (4–6 wk) pericardiectomy if signs of tamponade or constriction develop	Tamponade Constrictive pericarditis	1–8% of patients with tuberculosis pneumonia; rule out HIV infection
Bacterial	Group A streptococcus *Staphylococcus aureus* *Streptococcus pneumoniae*	Leukocytosis with marked left shift Pericardial fluid purulent	Pericardial drainage by catheter or surgery Systemic antibiotics Pericardiectomy if constrictive physiology develops	Tamponade in one third of patients	Very high mortality rate if not recognized early
Post myocardial infarction	12 hours–10 days after infarction	Fever Pericardial friction rub Echo: effusion	Aspirin Prednisone	Tamponade rare	More frequent in large Q wave infarctions Anterior > inferior
Uremic	Untreated renal failure: 50% Chronic dialysis: 20%	Pericardial rub: 90%	Intensive dialysis Indomethacin: probably ineffective Catheter drainage Surgical drainage	Tamponade Hemodynamic instability on dialysis	Avoid NSAIDs About 50% respond to intensive dialysis
Neoplastic	In order of frequency: lung cancer, breast cancer, leukemia and lymphoma, others	Chest pain, dyspnea Echo: effusion CT, MRI: tumor metastases to pericardium Cytologic examination of fluid positive in 85%	Catheter drainage Subxiphoid pericardiectomy Chemotherapy directed at underlying malignant neoplasm	Tamponade Constriction	

CT = computed tomography; HIV = human immunodeficiency virus; MRI = magnetic resonance imaging; NSAIDs = nonsteroidal anti-inflammatory drugs.
Modified from Malik F, Foster E: Pericardial disease. *In* Wachter RM, Goldman L, Hollander H (eds): Hospital Medicine, 2nd ed. Philadelphia, Lippincott Williams & Wilkins, 2005, p 449.

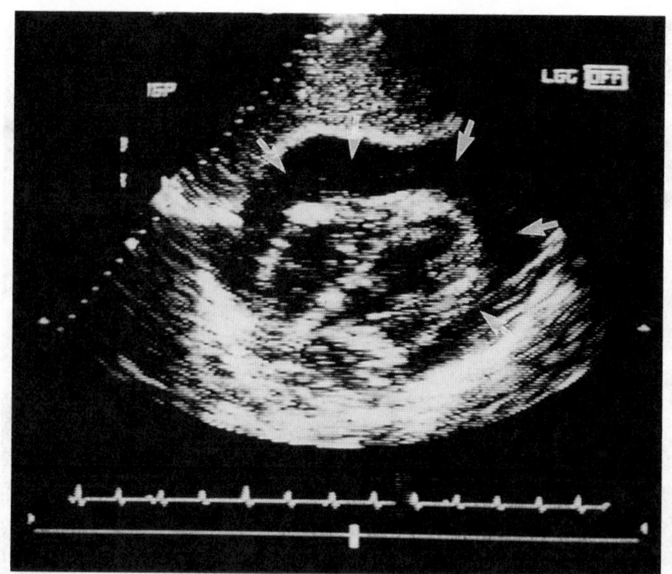

FIGURE 77–6 • Transthoracic echocardiogram from the subcostal approach. Note the large echolucent area/pericardial effusion (arrows) surrounding the heart. The right ventricle is compressed.

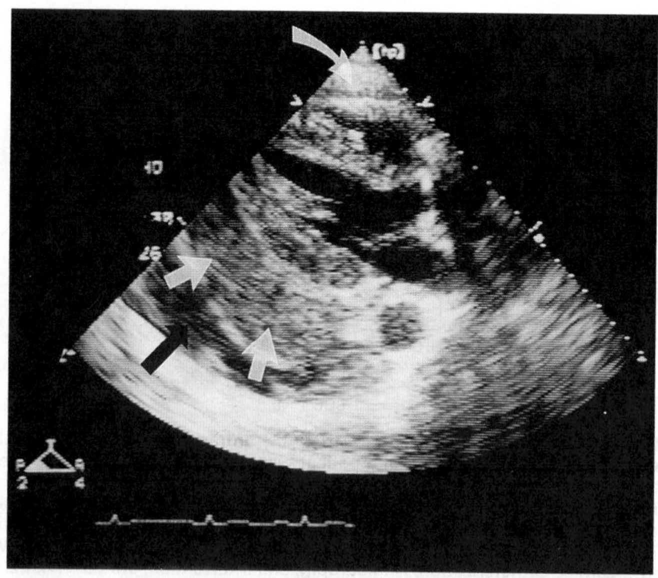

FIGURE 77–7 • Transthoracic echocardiogram from the parasternal long-axis window in a different patient than the one in Figure 77-6. Note the large echo-filled pericardial effusion posterior (straight white arrows) to the left ventricle and anterior (curved white arrow) to the right ventricle. This patient had a hemorrhagic pericardial effusion that developed several weeks after aortic valve replacement and long-term warfarin treatment. A pleural effusion (black arrow) also is seen.

TABLE 77–3 COMPARISON OF PHYSICAL EXAMINATION FINDINGS AND DIAGNOSTIC TEST RESULTS FOR CARDIAC TAMPONADE, CONSTRICTIVE PERICARDITIS, AND RESTRICTIVE CARDIOMYOPATHY

Characteristic	Cardiac Tamponade	Constrictive Pericarditis	Restrictive Cardiomyopathy
CLINICAL			
Pulsus paradoxus	+	+/–	–
Prominent y descent	–	+	–
Prominent x descent	+	+	–
Kussmaul's sign	–	+	–
S_3 or pericardial "knock"	–	+	+
S_4	–	–	+
ELECTROCARDIOGRAPHY			
Low voltage	+	+	+
Abnormal P waves	–	+	+/–
Electrical alternans	+	–	+
CHEST RADIOGRAPHY			
Cardiomegaly	+	–	–
Pericardial calcification	–	+	–
ECHOCARDIOGRAPHY			
Pericardial effusion	+	–	–
Pericardial thickening	–	+	–
Small right ventricle	+	–	–
Thickened myocardium	–	–	+
Enhanced respiratory variation in E wave	+	+	–
COMPUTED TOMOGRAPHY, MAGNETIC RESONANCE IMAGING			
Pericardial thickening	–	+	–
Pericardial calcification	–	+	–
CARDIAC CATHETERIZATION			
Equalization of pressures	+	+	–
Abnormal myocardial biopsy	–	–	+

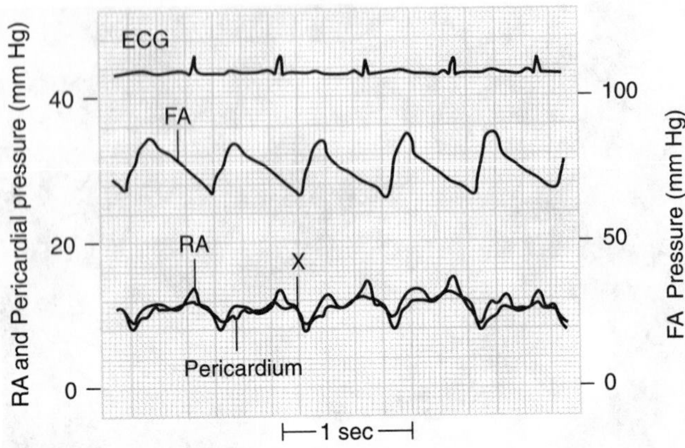

FIGURE 77–8 • Simultaneous right atrial (RA), intrapericardial, and femoral artery (FA) pressure recordings in a patient with cardiac tamponade. Note the elevated and equilibrated intrapericardial and right atrial pressures with a prominent *x* descent and blunted *y* descent suggestive of impaired right atrial emptying in early diastole. The arterial pulse pressure is narrowed. (From Lorell BH: Profiles in constriction, restriction and tamponade. *In* Baim DS, Grossman W [eds]: Cardiac Catheterization, Angiography, and Intervention, 6th ed. Philadelphia, Williams & Wilkins, 2000, p 840.)

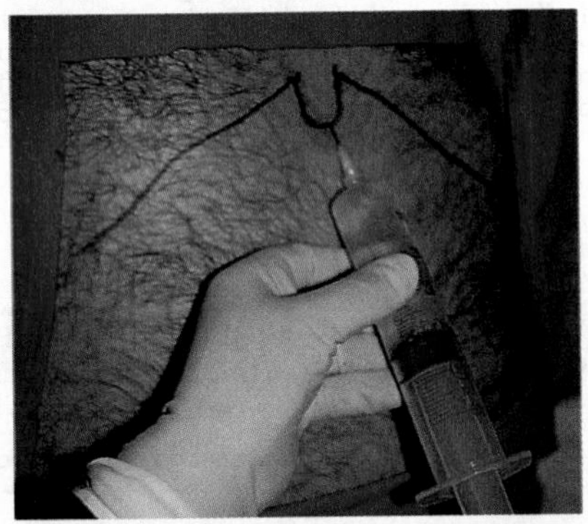

FIGURE 77–9 • Aspiration of pericardial fluid is indicated in cardiac tamponade or to obtain fluid for diagnostic purposes. A wide-bore needle is inserted in the epigastrium below the xiphoid process and advanced in the direction of the medial third of the right clavicle. The procedure is preferably performed in a catheterization laboratory under echocardiographic guidance, but it may need to be performed emergently for life-saving purposes in other settings. If the needle is connected to the V lead of an electrocardiographic monitor, ST elevation usually is seen if the needle touches the epicardium. This can be useful in distinguishing a bloody pericardial effusion from accidental puncture of the heart. Other complications of the procedure may include arrhythmias, vasovagal attack, and pneumothorax. (From Forbes CD, Jackson WF: Color Atlas and Text of Clinical Medicine, 3rd ed. London, Mosby, 2003, with permission.)

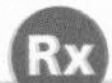

be approached surgically through a limited thoracotomy-mediastinoscopy and pericardial window. For all effusions related to a malignant neoplasm and for which aggressive chemotherapy is *not* being administered, reaccumulation in the ensuing weeks or months is the norm, and elective surgery (pericardial window) should be considered before hospital discharge. Hemorrhagic effusions related to cardiac trauma or aortic dissection also are managed best by emergency surgery (if it is available) or in combination with temporizing pericardiocentesis. If the patient is in extremis, emergency pericardiocentesis should be performed at the bedside.

Approach to Effusion without Tamponade

For patients with suspected pericardial effusion, transthoracic echocardiography is the initial test of choice and in most patients is definitive in confirming the presence or absence of a significant pericardial effusion (loculated effusions may be identified better by CT or MRI). If a small (0.5 to 1 cm) echolucent or "organized" pericardial effusion is seen, the patient generally can be observed with a follow-up echocardiogram in 1 to 2 weeks (sooner if clinical deterioration is evident). If the follow-up study shows a smaller effusion, subsequent echocardiograms are not

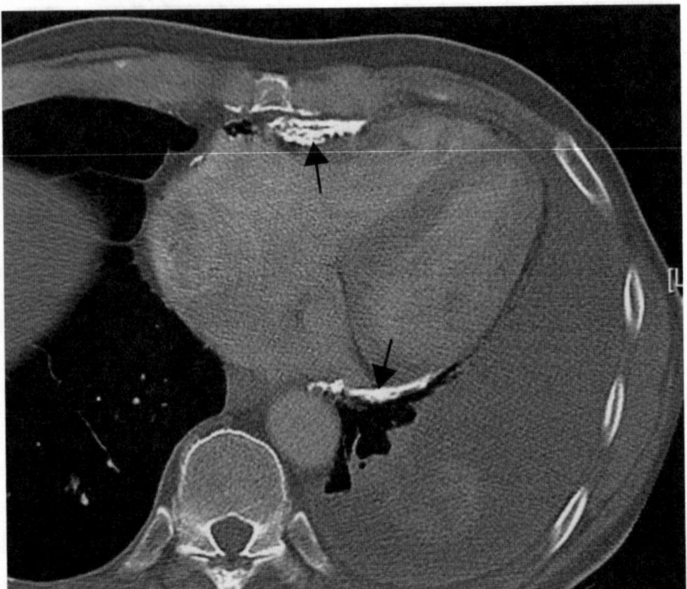

FIGURE 77–10 • Transverse computed tomography of a 32-year-old patient with anterior and posterior pericardial calcification (arrows). (Courtesy of Noriko Oyama, MD.)

necessary (unless the patient's clinical condition changes). Assuming a clinical history of "viral" pericarditis, assessment of renal function and thyroid-stimulating hormone is reasonable, but the results probably will be normal. A tuberculin skin test should be performed routinely. One also should exclude a drug-induced etiology (e.g., cromolyn, hydralazine, isoniazid, phenytoin, procainamide, reserpine).

In a moderate (1 to 2 cm) or large (>2 cm) pericardial effusion, treatment and follow-up depend on the clinical scenario and echocardiographic findings. If the patient is clinically unstable and tamponade is suggested (see earlier), urgent cardiology consultation and diagnostic or therapeutic pericardiocentesis should be planned. If the patient is hemodynamically stable and tamponade is not suggested, the patient can be observed with a follow-up echocardiographic study performed in 1 to 7 days. The initial evaluation is the same as listed earlier for a small effusion. Follow-up echocardiographic studies should be continued until the size of the effusion is minimal, but echocardiograms need not be repeated until complete resolution. If bacterial or malignant pericarditis is suspected, diagnostic pericardiocentesis should be performed even in the absence of clinical instability or suggestion of tamponade; tuberculous pericarditis is diagnosed best by pericardial biopsy. A tuberculin skin test, complete blood count with differential, platelet count, and coagulation parameters also should be assessed. Anticoagulation with heparin or warfarin should be discontinued unless the patient has a mechanical heart valve or atrial fibrillation. Blood cultures are indicated if an infectious cause is suspected. Complement, antinuclear antibodies, and the sedimentation rate may be helpful if systemic lupus erythematosus is being considered, although isolated pericardial effusion is unlikely to be the first manifestation of this disorder. Pericarditis after myocardial infarction (Dressler's syndrome) is now unusual; given experimental laboratory evidence that some of the nonsteroidal drugs promote left ventricular aneurysm formation in this setting, aspirin is the preferred agent to relieve pain in Dressler's syndrome. The presence of an echo-filled effusion should raise concern for hemorrhagic or organized pericarditis, which may progress to constriction.

Chronic or Recurrent Pericardial Effusions

With chronic or recurrent pericarditis from any cause, pericardial calcification develops and can be appreciated by thoracic CT (Fig. 77–10). Symptoms are those of a chronic systemic illness and include weight loss, fatigue, and dyspnea on exertion (Chapter 345).

The evaluation of chronic pericarditis should exclude the possibility of tuberculosis; a tuberculin skin test, chest radiograph, and (when highly suspicious) analysis of gastric aspirates should be performed (Chapter 345). Pericardial biopsy is more commonly diagnostic of tuberculous pericarditis than is pericardial fluid staining or culture. Aggressive drug treatment is indicated (Chapter 345).

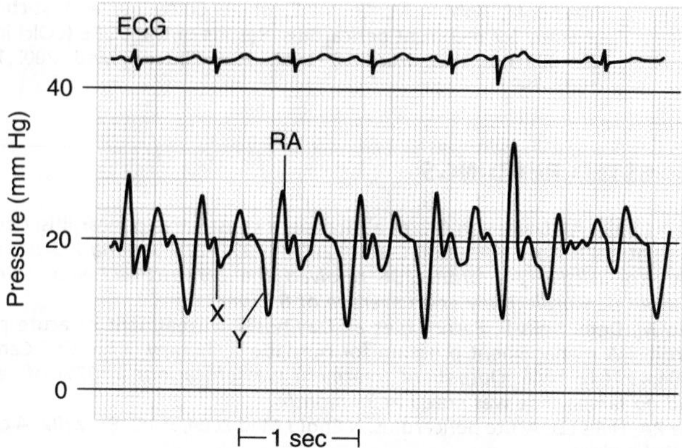

FIGURE 77–11 • Right atrial (RA) pressure recording from a patient with constrictive pericarditis. Note the elevation in pressure and prominent *y* descent corresponding to rapid early diastolic right atrial emptying. (From Lorell BH: Profiles in constriction, restriction and tamponade. *In* Baim DS, Grossman W [eds]: Cardiac Catheterization, Angiography, and Intervention, 6th ed. Philadelphia, Williams & Wilkins, 2000, p 832.)

Hypothyroidism-myxedema is another common cause of large pericardial effusions, especially in the elderly (Chapter 244). The effusion commonly is identified first on a chest radiograph and often is seen in the absence of resting tachycardia. Measurement of thyroid-stimulating hormone is diagnostic. The effusion and coexistent cardiomyopathy respond to hormone replacement, but sometimes slowly during several months. In the absence of hemodynamic compromise, pericardiocentesis often is not needed in this situation as the effusion has developed slowly and does not present hemodynamic compromise. Uremic pericardial effusions also are common and often respond to initiation of or more intensive dialysis (Chapter 131).

Treatment of chronic or recurrent idiopathic effusions is similar to the treatment of recurrent pericarditis. If medical therapy is unsuccessful, creation of a pericardial window is indicated.

CONSTRICTIVE PERICARDITIS

Constrictive pericarditis is an uncommon condition with impairment of mid and late ventricular filling from a thickened or noncompliant pericardium. In the classic form, fibrous scarring and adhesions of both pericardial layers lead to obliteration of the pericardial cavity. Early ventricular filling is unimpeded, but diastolic filling subsequently is reduced abruptly as a result of the inability of the ventricles to fill because of physical constraints imposed by a rigid, thickened, and sometimes calcified pericardium. In less developed countries, tuberculosis is the most common cause of chronic constrictive pericarditis, whereas in the United States, tuberculosis is infrequently the culprit. Constriction may be associated with malignant disease (lung cancer, breast cancer, lymphoma), histoplasmosis, mediastinal irradiation, purulent or recurrent viral pericarditis, rheumatoid arthritis, uremia, chest trauma or hemopericardium, and cardiac surgery. Constriction may follow cardiac surgery by several weeks to months and may occur decades after chest wall irradiation. The "cause" may not be identified in many patients.

Pathobiology

The normal pericardium is 3 mm or less thick. With chronic constriction, especially from tuberculosis, the pericardium may thicken to 6 mm or more, calcify, and intimately involve the epicardium. In subacute constriction, calcification is less prominent, and the pericardium may be only minimally thickened. As with cardiac tamponade, the pathophysiologic process of constriction includes impaired diastolic ventricular filling, which leads to elevated venous pressure. Tamponade and constriction have many important differences (see Table 77–3), however. With constriction, the impairment in ventricular filling is minimal in early diastole, and a prominent *y* descent is present (Fig. 77–11). Subsequently, diastolic pressure rises abruptly when cardiac volume reaches the anatomic limit set by the noncompliant pericardium; by comparison, in tamponade, ventricular filling is impaired throughout diastole. Diastolic pressure remains elevated until the onset of systole. This prominent *y* descent with an elevated plateau of ventricular pressure has been termed the "dip and plateau" or "square root" sign (Fig. 77–12); by comparison, in tamponade, the *y* descent is absent. Stroke volume and cardiac output are reduced because of impaired filling, whereas intrinsic systolic function of the ventricles may be normal or only minimally impaired.

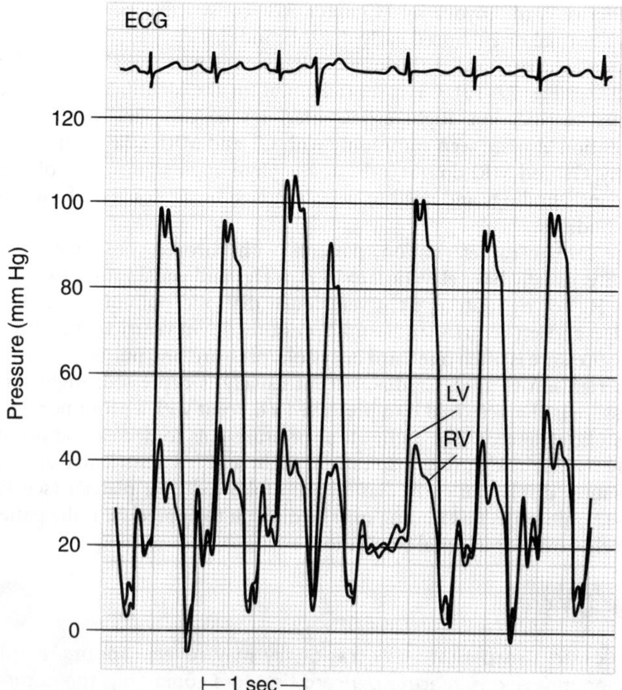

FIGURE 77–12 • Simultaneous left ventricular (LV) and right ventricular (RV) pressure recordings in a patient with constrictive pericarditis. Note the equilibration of LV and RV diastolic pressures and the "dip and plateau" most apparent with the prolonged diastole. (From Lorell BH: Profiles in constriction, restriction and tamponade. *In* Baim DS, Grossman W [eds]: Grossman's Cardiac Catheterization, Angiography, and Intervention, 6th ed. Philadelphia, Lippincott Williams & Wilkins, 2000, p 832.)

Clinical Manifestations

In constriction, the most prominent physical finding is an abnormal jugular venous pulse (Chapter 48). Central venous pressure is elevated and displays prominent *x* and *y* descents. For patients in sinus rhythm, the *x* descent is coincident with the carotid pulse. The *y* descent, which is absent or diminished in tamponade, is most prominent and abbreviated because of a rapid rise in pressure in mid-diastole. A diagnosis of constriction always should be suspected in patients with a prominent *y* descent with dyspnea, weakness, anorexia, peripheral edema, hepatomegaly, splenomegaly, and ascites. The pulse pressure is often narrowed, but pulsus paradoxus is usually absent. Pleural effusions are common. The clinical picture may mimic hepatic cirrhosis, but with distended neck veins. Venous pressure often fails to fall with inspiration (Kussmaul's sign), and arterial pulse pressure is normal or reduced. The apical pulse is often poorly defined, and heart sounds may be distant. A loud S_3, the pericardial knock, may be audible early after aortic valve closure because of the sudden deceleration in ventricular filling.

Diagnosis

The electrocardiogram of patients with constriction is often abnormal and displays low QRS voltage (especially in the limb leads), P mitrale, and nonspecific ST-T wave changes. Atrial fibrillation may be present in one third of patients. The chest radiograph may show pericardial calcification in tuberculous constriction. Though suggestive, the finding of pericardial calcification is not diagnostic of constriction. Cardiac size may be small, normal, or enlarged. Transthoracic echocardiography is less helpful than with cardiac tamponade, but it may display pericardial thickening or calcification, abrupt posterior deflection of the interventricular septum at end diastole, and M-mode posterior wall "flat tiring." Enhanced transmitral and transtricuspid Doppler E wave variation with respiration may be particularly helpful in establishing the diagnosis. The inferior vena cava and hepatic veins often are markedly dilated with blunted respiratory variability in caval diameter. Newer tissue Doppler imaging is also helpful to distinguish constrictive pericarditis from restrictive cardiomyopathy (Chapter 59); constrictive pericarditis displays normal or enhanced early diastolic indexes.

Increased pericardial thickness is diagnosed most reliably by CT or MRI (see Fig. 77–10). CT is more helpful for the identification of pericardial calcification. Right atrial, inferior vena cava, and hepatic vein distention also are seen commonly with CT and MRI. Like chest radiography, CT and MRI do not indicate the physiologic significance of these anatomic findings and need to be interpreted in the context of the clinical findings.

At cardiac catheterization, patients with chronic constrictive pericarditis usually have elevation (>15 mm Hg) and equalization (within 5 mm Hg) of right atrial, right ventricular diastolic, pulmonary capillary wedge, and left ventricular diastolic pressures. Right ventricular end-diastolic pressure is often one third of systolic pressure, and pulmonary artery hypertension is mild. Cardiac output usually is depressed. Right atrial pressure is characterized by a preserved *x* descent with a prominent early diastolic *y* descent. The right atrial pressure fails to decrease appropriately or may rise during inspiration. Right and left ventricular diastolic pressures display an early diastolic dip followed by a plateau (see Fig. 77–12), although this finding may be difficult to appreciate if the patient is tachycardic or in atrial fibrillation.

Treatment

Rx

Constrictive pericarditis occasionally may reverse spontaneously when it develops in acute pericarditis. More commonly, the natural history of this disease is one of progression with declining cardiac output and progressive renal and hepatic failure. Surgical stripping or removal of both layers of the adherent pericardium is the definitive therapy. The benefits of pericardial stripping may be modest initially but continue to be manifested in the ensuing months. Operative mortality is generally low but may exceed 5 to 15% in the most advanced cases. The surgical risk is related to the extent of myocardial involvement and the severity of secondary hepatic or renal dysfunction. For patients with suspected tuberculous constriction, antituberculosis therapy should be administered before and after pericardial surgery. In addition to advanced age and systolic dysfunction, postirradiation constriction is a predictor of worse prognosis.

Effusive-Constrictive Pericarditis

Effusive-constrictive pericarditis is a rare disorder occurring in about 1% of patients who have pericarditis and approximately 7% of patients with tamponade. It is characterized by the combination of a tense pericardial effusion in the presence of visceral pericardial constriction and may represent an intermediate stage in the development of constrictive pericarditis. Causes of effusive-constrictive pericarditis are the same as those associated with constriction, and the clinical features resemble those of tamponade and constriction. Physical examination shows pulsus paradoxus and a prominent *x* descent in the absence of a *y* descent. The cardiac silhouette is generally enlarged because of the associated pericardial effusion, whereas the electrocardiogram displays low QRS voltage and nonspecific ST-T wave changes. Surface echocardiography may show an echo-filled pericardial effusion with thickened pericardium and fibrinous pericardial bands. Although this echocardiographic appearance should heighten suspicion, the diagnosis generally is made after successful pericardiocentesis. Rather than normalizing after pericardiocentesis, intracardiac pressures remain elevated with a square root sign in the ventricular tracings and development of a prominent *y* descent in the atrial and jugular venous pressure pulses. Kussmaul's sign also may be evident. Treatment by excision of visceral and parietal pericardium is usually effective. A transient, self-limited form of effusive-constrictive pericarditis has also been reported.

Future Directions

Access to the pericardial space may provide a new means to deliver novel gene or pharmacologic therapies for myocardial (angiogenesis, antiarrhythmics) or pericardial disease.

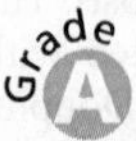

1. Imazio M, Bobbio M, Cecchi E, et al: Colchicine in addition to conventional therapy for acute pericarditis: Results of the COlchicine for acute PEricarditis (COPE) trial. Circulation 2005;112:2012–2016.
2. Imazio M, Bobbio M, Cecchi E, et al: Colchicine as first-choice therapy for recurrent pericarditis. Results of the CORE (COlchicine for REcurrent pericarditis) trial. Arch Intern Med 2005;165:1987–1991.

SUGGESTED READINGS

Haley JH, Tajik AJ, Danielson GK, et al: Transient constrictive pericarditis: Causes and natural history. J Am Coll Cardiol 2004;43:271–275. *Among 212 patients with constrictive pericarditis, 36 resolved the constrictive hemodynamics without pericardiectomy at an average of 8.3 weeks.*

Imazio M, Demichelis B, Parrini I, et al: Day-hospital treatment of acute pericarditis: A management program for outpatient therapy. J Am Coll Cardiol 2004;43:1042–1046. *Outpatient treatment was efficacious in 87% of cases, and no tamponade was noted at 38 months.*

Lange RA, Hillis LD: Acute pericarditis. N Engl J Med 2004;351:2195–2202. *A case-based review.*

Little WC, Freeman GL: Pericardial disease. Circulation 2006;113:1622–1632. *A comprehensive review.*

Mayosi BM, Burgess LJ, Doubell AF: Tuberculous pericarditis. Circulation 2005;112:3608–3616. *A comprehensive review.*

Roy CL, Minor MA, Brookhart MA, et al: Does this patient with a pericardial effusion have cardiac tamponade? JAMA 2007;297:1810–1818. *A review of the accuracy of the history, physical examination, and basic diagnostic tests for the diagnosis of cardiac tamponade.*

Sagristà-Sauleda J, Angel J, Sanchez A, et al: Effusive-constrictive pericarditis. N Engl J Med 2004;350:469–475. *The largest reported series of patients with effusive-constrictive pericarditis.*

Troughton RW, Asher CR, Klein AL: Pericarditis. Lancet 2004;363:717–727. *Comprehensive review with good figures.*

78 DISEASES OF THE AORTA

Eric M. Isselbacher

The aorta is composed of three tissue layers. The intima is a thin inner layer lined with endothelial cells. The middle layer, or media, is the thickest layer of the aortic wall and is composed of sheets of elastic tissue that give the aorta tremendous tensile strength. The outermost layer, or adventitia, is composed mostly of collagen and carries the vasa vasorum, which nourish the aortic wall.

The ascending aorta is about 3 cm wide and 5 cm long and is located in the anterior mediastinum. Its most proximal portion (just above the aortic valve) is called the *aortic root* and is composed of the three sinuses of Valsalva. In the superior mediastinum, the ascending aorta meets the aortic arch and gives rise to the brachiocephalic arteries. The descending thoracic aorta courses posteriorly and is about 2.5 cm in diameter and 20 cm in length. After crossing the diaphragm, it becomes the abdominal aorta, which is normally 2 cm in width and about 15 cm in length before it bifurcates into the two common iliac arteries.

AORTIC ANEURYSMS

Definition

An aortic aneurysm is pathologic dilation of the aorta. Aneurysms are described in terms of their location, size, shape, and etiology. The shape of an aneurysm is *fusiform* when there is symmetrical dilation of the aorta and *saccular* when the dilation involves mainly one wall. In addition, there may be a *false aneurysm* or *pseudoaneurysm* when the aorta is enlarged as a consequence of dilation of only the outer layers of the vessel wall, such as occurs with a contained rupture of the aortic wall.

Epidemiology

Aneurysms may involve any part of the aorta, but abdominal aortic aneurysms are much more common than thoracic aneurysms. Abdominal aortic aneurysms are 5 to 10 times more frequent in men than in women and have a prevalence of at least 3% in persons older than 50 years. Among thoracic aortic aneurysms, aneurysms of the ascending aorta are most common, followed by aneurysms involving the descending aorta; aneurysms of the aortic arch are uncommon. If a descending thoracic aortic aneurysm extends distally and involves the abdominal aorta, a thoracoabdominal aortic aneurysm is created.

Smoking is the strongest risk factor associated with the development of an abdominal aortic aneurysm, followed by age, hypertension, and hyperlipidemia. In addition, there appears to be a genetic predisposition to the development of abdominal aortic aneurysms because up to 28% of first-degree relatives of patients with abdominal aortic aneurysms may be similarly affected.

Pathobiology

Atherosclerosis has long been considered the common underlying cause of abdominal aortic aneurysms. Indeed, the infrarenal aorta tends to be most severely affected by the atherosclerotic process and is accordingly the common site for aortic aneurysm formation. However, although aortic atherosclerosis clearly contributes to the process, the pathogenesis of abdominal aortic aneurysms is multifactorial, with genetic, environmental, hemodynamic, and immunologic factors all contributing to the development and progressive growth of aneurysms.

The strength of the aortic wall lies in its extracellular matrix, the most important components of which are elastin and collagen. Consequently, degradation of these structural proteins weakens the aortic wall and in turn allows aneurysms to develop. There is histologic evidence of inflammatory infiltrates—in particular, macrophages and T lymphocytes—within the media and adventitia of aneurysms, and this inflammation may lead to degradation of the extracellular matrix. Furthermore, matrix metalloproteinases—enzymes produced by smooth muscle and inflammatory cells that can degrade elastin and collagen—are significantly elevated in the walls of abdominal aortic aneurysms and thus probably contribute to the formation of aneurysms. As the wall begins to dilate, tension on the wall increases according to Laplace's law (tension is proportional to the product of pressure and the radius), thereby promoting further expansion of the aneurysm.

Atherosclerosis is also a common cause of aneurysms of the descending thoracic aorta. However, the most important cause of aneurysms of the ascending thoracic aorta is a process known as cystic medial degeneration, which histologically appears as smooth muscle cell necrosis and degeneration of elastic layers within the media. Cystic medial necrosis is found in almost all patients with Marfan syndrome (Chapter 281), who are at very high risk for thoracic aortic aneurysms. Among patients without overt evidence of connective tissue disease, a bicuspid aortic valve (Chapter 68) and familial thoracic aortic aneurysm syndrome are important congenital causes. A long-standing history of hypertension is a common risk factor in older patients. Syphilis (Chapter 340), once a common cause of thoracic aortic aneurysms, is now rarely a factor. Other uncommon causes of thoracic aortic aneurysms include infectious aortitis (Chapter 76), great vessel arteritis, aortic trauma (Chapter 113), and aortic dissection (see later). Many thoracic aortic aneurysms are idiopathic.

Clinical Manifestations

The large majority of abdominal and thoracic aortic aneurysms are asymptomatic and discovered incidentally on a routine physical examination or imaging study. When patients with abdominal aortic aneurysms experience symptoms, pain in the hypogastrium or lower part of the back is the most frequent complaint. The pain tends to have a steady gnawing quality that may last hours or days. Expansion or impending rupture of an aneurysm may be heralded by new or worsening pain, often of sudden onset. With rupture, the pain is frequently associated with hypotension and a pulsatile abdominal mass.

Patients with thoracic aortic aneurysms may have chest pain or, less often, back pain. Vascular complications include aortic insufficiency (sometimes with secondary heart failure), hemoptysis, and arterial thromboembolism. An enlarging aneurysm may produce local mass effects as a result of compression of adjacent mediastinal structures, with symptoms including coughing, wheezing, dyspnea, hoarseness, recurrent pneumonia, or dysphagia.

Diagnosis

Abdominal aortic aneurysms may be palpable on physical examination, although obesity may obscure even large aneurysms. Typically, abdominal aortic aneurysms are hard to size accurately by physical examination alone because adjacent structures frequently make an aneurysm feel larger than it really is. Thoracic aortic aneurysms cannot usually be palpated at all.

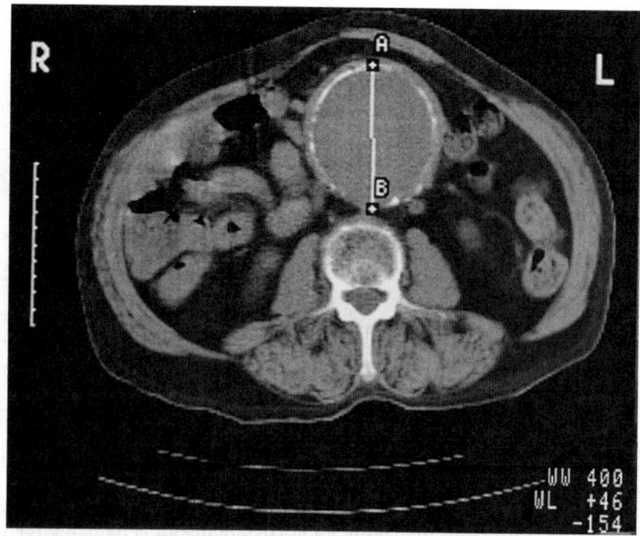

FIGURE 78–1 • Abdominal aortic aneurysm on computed tomography. This sensitive imaging method allows precise measurement of size (point A to point B) and demonstrates the thickened wall of the aneurysm. (From Forbes CD, Jackson WF: Color Atlas and Text of Clinical Medicine, 3rd ed. London, Mosby, 2003.)

Definitive diagnosis of an aortic aneurysm is made by radiographic examination. Abdominal aortic aneurysms can be detected and sized by either abdominal ultrasonography or computed tomography (CT). Ultrasound is extremely sensitive and is the most practical method to use in screening for aortic aneurysms. Screening programs using ultrasound reduce mortality in men ages 65 to 79. [1] CT is even more accurate (Fig. 78–1) and can size an aneurysm to within a diameter of 2 mm. Although CT is less practical than ultrasound as a screening tool, when the diagnosis has been made, it is the preferred modality for monitoring serial changes in size over time.

Thoracic aortic aneurysms are frequently recognized on chest radiographs; they often produce widening of the mediastinal silhouette, enlargement of the aortic knob, or displacement of the trachea from midline. CT is an excellent modality for detecting and sizing thoracic aneurysms and is particularly useful for monitoring size over time. Transthoracic echocardiography, which generally visualizes the aortic root and ascending aorta well, is useful for screening patients with Marfan syndrome because this group is at particular risk for aneurysms involving this portion of the aorta.

Treatment

Rx

The goal of therapy for patients with aortic aneurysms is to attempt to reduce the risk for expansion and rupture of the aneurysm. Although blood pressure control is generally recommended, β-blockers do not reduce the rate of growth of abdominal aortic aneurysms. Aneurysms should be monitored closely with serial imaging studies (e.g., CT) to detect any progressive enlargement over time, which may indicate the need for surgical repair.

Aortic aneurysms that produce symptoms secondary to expansion, vascular complications, or compression of adjacent structures should be repaired. Size is the major indicator for repair of asymptomatic aortic aneurysms. Abdominal aortic aneurysms larger than 5.5 cm should be repaired, [2,3] as should aneurysms larger than 5 cm in good operative candidates. Abdominal aneurysms larger than 4 cm should be monitored every 6 months. Descending thoracic aortic aneurysms larger than 6 cm should undergo surgical repair. Aneurysms of the ascending thoracic aorta should be repaired at 5.5 cm or larger, except that patients with Marfan syndrome or a bicuspid aortic valve should undergo repair when the aneurysm is 5 cm or larger because of the high risk for rupture in these patients.

Open surgical repair consists of insertion of a synthetic prosthetic tube graft. When aneurysms involve branch vessels, such as the renal

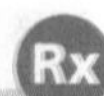

or mesenteric arteries, the vessels must be reimplanted into the graft. Similarly, when a dilated aortic root must be replaced in the repair of an ascending thoracic aortic aneurysm, the coronary arteries must be reimplanted. An alternative approach for repair of abdominal aortic aneurysms (and some descending thoracic aneurysms) is the percutaneous placement of an expandable endovascular stent graft inside the aneurysm. This endovascular technique is associated with a better short-term outcome but a similar outcome at 2 years when compared with open repair. [4,5] In patients who are not candidates for open repair because of comorbid diseases or high surgical risk (Chapter 457), endovascular repair is no better than conservative medical management in terms of survival. [6]

Prognosis

The chief concern in managing an aortic aneurysm is its tendency to rupture. Most aneurysms expand over time, and the risk for rupture increases with size.

Abdominal aortic aneurysms less than 4.0 cm have only a 0.3% annual risk for rupture, whereas aneurysms 4.0 to 4.9 cm have a 1.5% annual risk for rupture, and aneurysms 5.0 to 5.9 cm have a 6.5% annual risk for rupture. The overall mortality in patients in whom an abdominal aortic aneurysm ruptures is 80%, including a mortality of 50% even for patients who reach the hospital.

Thoracic aneurysms smaller than 5 cm typically expand slowly and rarely rupture, but the rate of growth and risk of rupture increase significantly when thoracic aneurysms are 6 cm or larger. Similar to what is seen with abdominal aneurysms, rupture of thoracic aneurysms has a high early mortality of 76% at 24 hours.

INTRAMURAL AORTIC HEMATOMA AND AORTIC DISSECTION

Definition

An intramural aortic hematoma occurs when bleeding from the vasa vasorum causes a hematoma within the aortic media. Aortic dissection occurs when the media of the blood vessel is cleaved longitudinally to form a false lumen that communicates with the true lumen.

The location of an intramural aortic hematoma or dissection may be described according to one of several classification systems (Fig. 78–2). Two thirds of aortic dissections are type A (proximal) and the other third are type B (distal). The classification schemes all serve the same purpose, which is to distinguish dissections that involve the ascending aorta from dissections that do not. Involvement of the ascending aorta carries a high risk for early rupture and death from cardiac tamponade, so the prognosis and management differ according to the extent of aortic involvement. Hematomas and dissections are also classified according to their duration: less than 2 weeks is considered acute, whereas 2 weeks or more is considered chronic.

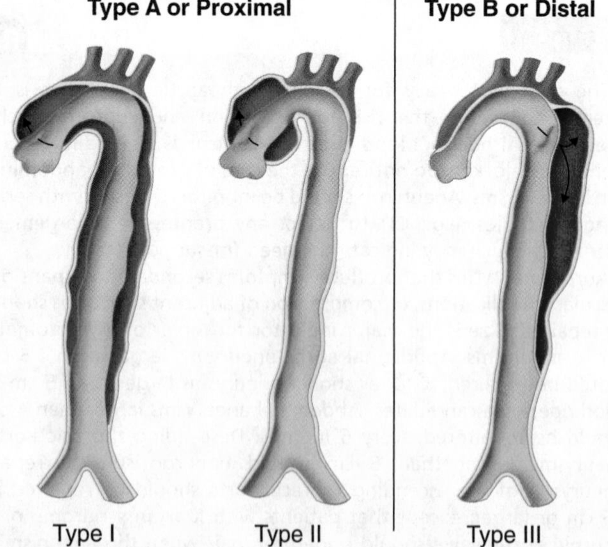

FIGURE 78–2 • Classification systems for aortic dissection. (From Isselbacher EM: Diseases of the aorta. *In* Braunwald E, Zipes DP, Libby P, Bonow RO [eds]: Braunwald's Heart Disease: A Textbook of Cardiovascular Medicine, 7th ed. Philadelphia, Saunders, 2004, p 1416.)

The peak incidence of aortic dissection in patients without Marfan syndrome is in their 60s and 70s, and men are affected twice as often as women. A history of hypertension is present in most cases, whereas a bicuspid aortic valve or known preexisting thoracic aortic aneurysm is less common. Rarely, aortic dissection may occur in a young woman during the peripartum period. Iatrogenic trauma from intra-aortic catheterization procedures or cardiac surgery may also cause aortic dissection.

Pathobiology

Disease of the aortic media, with degeneration of the medial collagen and elastin, is the most common predisposing factor for aortic dissection. Patients with Marfan syndrome have classic cystic medial degeneration and are at particularly high risk for aortic dissection at a relatively young age. Aortic dissection classically begins either with a tear in the aortic intima, thereby exposing the diseased medial layer to the systemic pressure of intraluminal blood, or with an intramural hematoma caused by bleeding in the vasa vasorum of the arterial wall. This hematoma may propagate longitudinally along a variable length of the aorta. If the intimal layer remains intact, the hematoma does not communicate with the aortic lumen, but if it does, it will become no different than a dissection that began with an intimal tear. The result will be cleavage of the media into two layers longitudinally, thereby producing a blood-filled false lumen within the aortic wall. This false lumen propagates distally (or sometimes retrogradely) a variable distance along the aorta from the site of the intimal tear.

Clinical Manifestations

Pain, which occurs in 96% of cases of both aortic intramural hematoma and dissection and is typically severe, is the most common initial symptom. The pain may be retrosternal, in the neck or throat, interscapular, in the lower part of the back, abdominal, or in the lower extremities, depending on the location of the aortic hematoma or dissection. The pain may migrate as dissection propagates distally. Thoracic pain is often of sudden onset and most severe at the start. It sometimes is described as "tearing," "sharp," or "stabbing." Although an isolated hematoma rarely causes symptoms other than pain, a dissection, regardless of how it started, may also result in acute aortic insufficiency (Chapter 75), right coronary artery occlusion, hemopericardium (Chapter 77), syncope (Chapter 427), a cerebrovascular accident (Chapter 430), mesenteric ischemia (Chapter 146), or ischemic peripheral neuropathy (Chapter 446).

Hypertension is a common finding on physical examination and is present in 70% of patients with distal aortic dissection. Hypotension may also occur, particularly in patients with proximal dissections, and is usually due to rupture into the pericardium or severe aortic insufficiency. *Pseudohypotension* occurs when a falsely low measure of upper extremity blood pressure is obtained because of involvement of the subclavian artery by the dissection. Similarly, pulse deficits are a common finding on physical examination, particularly in patients with proximal aortic dissections, when there is involvement of the subclavian, carotid, or femoral arteries. Aortic insufficiency occurs in more than a third of patients with a proximal dissection; paradoxically, however, when acute aortic insufficiency is severe, the murmur may not be appreciable, so finding a widened pulse pressure and heart failure should raise suspicion of its presence.

Vascular complications from aortic dissection include compromise of a coronary artery with subsequent myocardial ischemia or infarction. Involvement of the brachiocephalic arteries may produce a stroke or coma, whereas compromise of the spinal arteries may produce paraplegia. When a dissection extends into the abdominal aorta, flow to one or

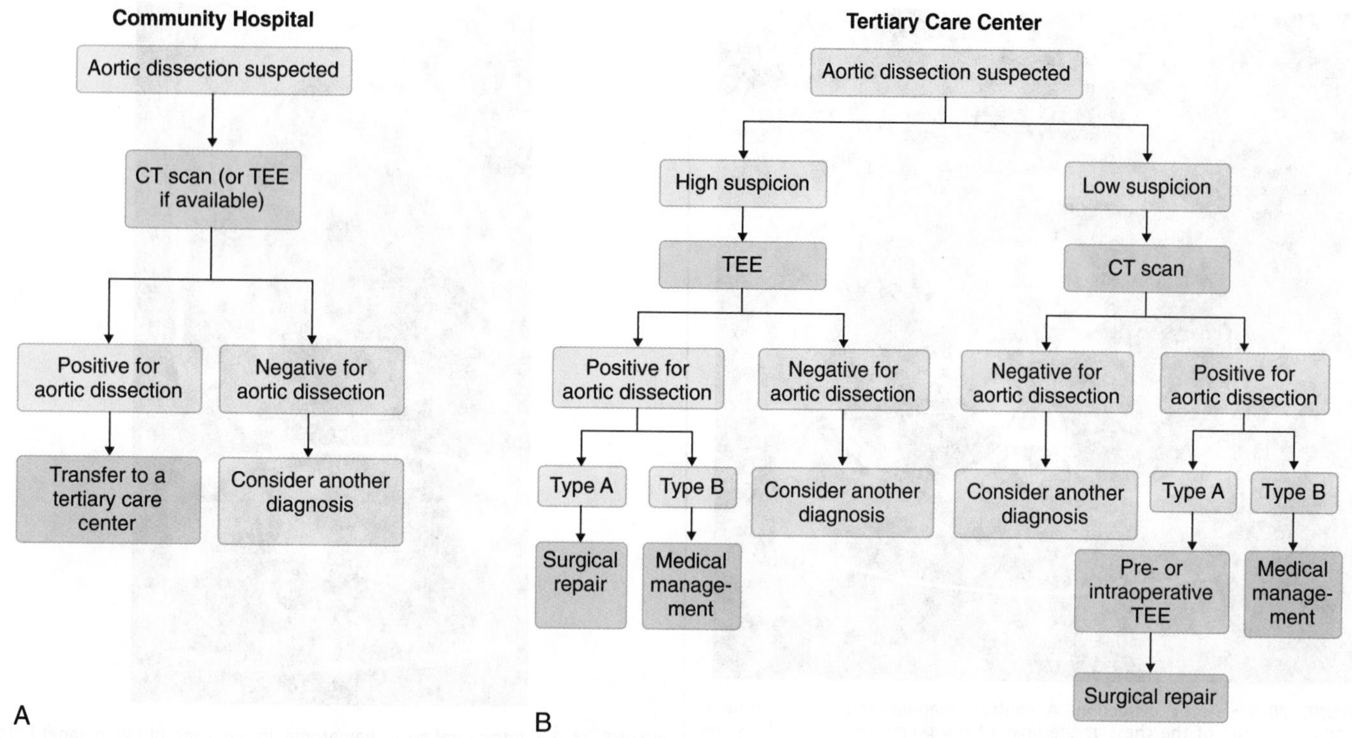

FIGURE 78–3 • Suggested algorithms for the evaluation of suspected acute aortic dissection. A, Approach used in many community hospitals where cardiac surgery is not performed. **B,** Approach used in many tertiary care centers where transesophageal echocardiography (TEE) and cardiac surgery are available. CT = computed tomography.

both renal arteries may be compromised and produce acute renal failure, which may exacerbate the hypertension. Mesenteric ischemia or frank infarction may be manifested as abdominal pain. Finally, the dissection may extend distally to the aortic bifurcation and compromise or occlude one of the common iliac arteries and thereby produce a femoral pulse deficit and ischemia of the lower extremities.

An abnormality on a chest radiograph often first raises the suspicion of aortic dissection. The findings on chest radiography are nonspecific, however, and rarely diagnostic. An enlarged mediastinal silhouette is the most common finding, but it may be present in as few as 65% of patients in whom dissection is ultimately diagnosed. A left pleural effusion is commonly seen in patients with involvement of the descending thoracic aorta and, when small, typically represents an exudate from the inflamed aortic wall. A normal chest radiograph does not exclude the diagnosis of aortic dissection. Electrocardiographic findings in aortic dissection are nonspecific.

Diagnosis

When there is clinical suspicion of aortic dissection, it is essential to confirm or exclude the diagnosis promptly with an imaging study (Fig. 78–3). Several imaging modalities can be used to diagnose the presence of aortic dissection accurately, including aortography, CT (Chapter 54), magnetic resonance imaging (Chapter 55), and transesophageal echocardiography (TEE) (Chapter 53). Each institution must determine which of these modalities is most appropriate as an initial diagnostic approach based on the availability of each and the skill and experience of the clinicians who perform and interpret the diagnostic studies.

Nevertheless, when suspicion of aortic dissection is high, TEE (Fig. 78–4) is the most rapid means of providing sufficient detail to enable the surgeon to take the patient directly to the operating room. When clinical suspicion is low (i.e., when one wants to rule out aortic dissection), contrast medium–enhanced CT (Fig. 78–5) is preferred because it is entirely noninvasive. If TEE is not readily available, contrast medium–enhanced CT is the imaging modality of choice in high-probability and low-probability patients.

On cross-sectional imaging, an isolated intramural hematoma appears as a crescentic thickening around the aortic wall rather than a true and false lumen separated by an intimal flap (Fig. 78–6). The presence of an intramural hematoma may be missed on aortography.

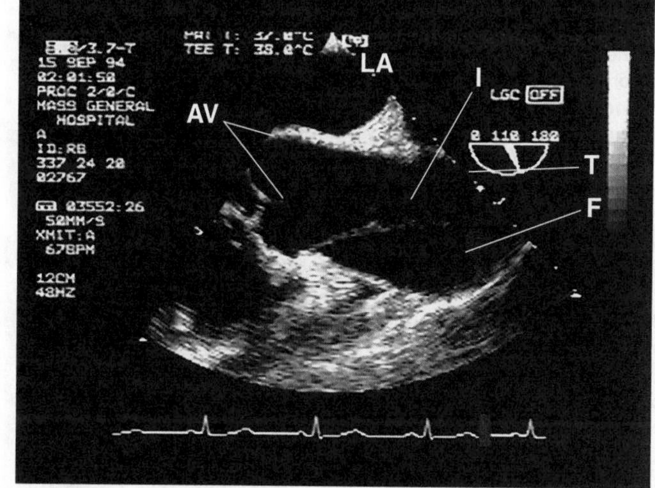

FIGURE 78–4 • Transesophageal echocardiogram of the ascending aorta in the long axis in a patient with type A aortic dissection. The aortic valve (AV) is on the left, and the ascending aorta extends to the right. Within the aorta is an intimal flap (I) that originates at the level of the sinotubular junction. The true (T) and the false (F) lumens are separated by the intimal flap. LA = left atrium. (From Isselbacher EM: Diseases of the aorta. *In* Braunwald E, Zipes DP, Libby P, Bonow RO [eds]: Braunwald's Heart Disease: A Textbook of Cardiovascular Medicine, 7th ed. Philadelphia, Saunders, 2004, p 1423.)

Treatment

The goal of initial medical therapy for an acute aortic intramural hematoma or dissection is to halt any further progression and reduce the risk for rupture. Acute management of an isolated hematoma should be the same as for dissection because of the risk that the hematoma will propagate.

Whenever there is suspicion of an aortic intramural hematoma or dissection, therapy should be instituted immediately while imaging studies are ordered rather than waiting until the diagnosis is confirmed. The initial goal is to reduce the force of ventricular con-

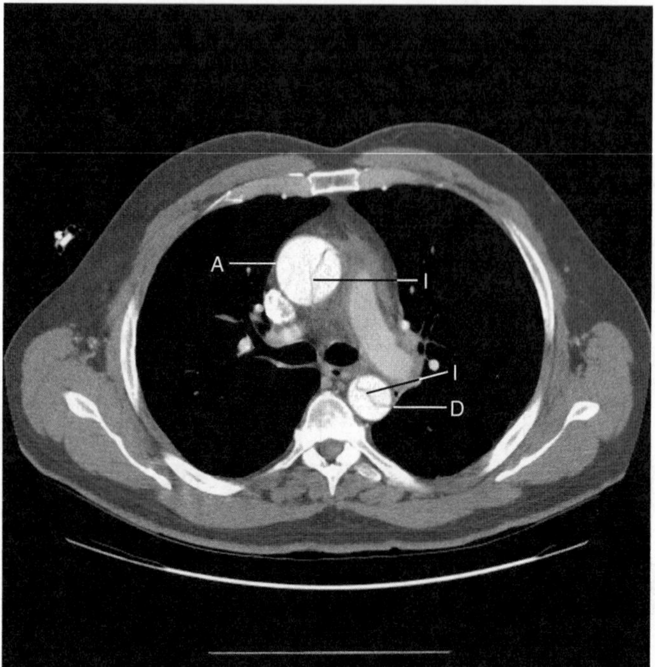

FIGURE 78–5 • **Aortic dissection.** A contrast medium–enhanced computed tomography scan of the chest at the level of the pulmonary artery shows an intimal flap (I) separating the two lumens of the ascending (A) and descending (D) thoracic aorta in a type A aortic dissection.

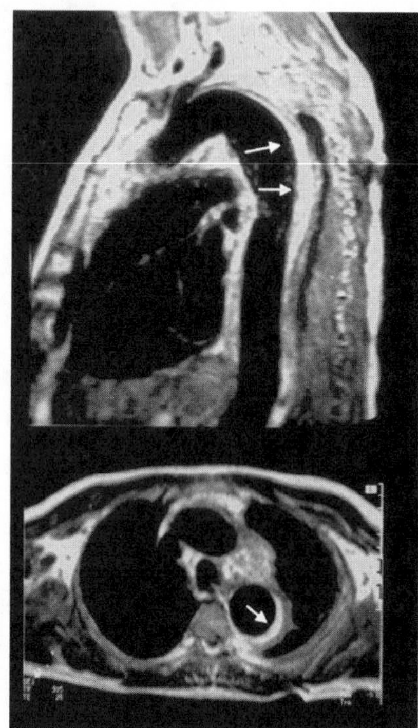

FIGURE 78–6 • **Intramural aortic hematoma.** In the acute phase, magnetic resonance imaging shows high signal intensity suggestive of intramural hematoma. **Top,** A sagittal view demonstrates the hematoma in the upper and middle thirds of the descending thoracic aorta. **Bottom,** The intramural hematoma is seen as a crescent in the axial view. This particular hematoma, which was observed without surgical treatment, later progressed (over 4 years of follow-up) to localized dissection and the formation of a pseudoaneurysm. (Reproduced with permission from Evangelista A, Dominguez R, Sebastia C, et al: Long-term follow-up of aortic intramural hematoma: Predictors of outcome. Circulation 2003; 108:583–589.)

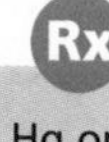

traction and reduce systolic blood pressure to 100 to 120 mm Hg or to the lowest level that maintains cerebral, cardiac, and renal perfusion. Intravenous labetalol (20 mg administered over a 2 minute period, followed by additional doses of 20 to 80 mg every 10 to 15 minutes up to a maximum total dose of 300 mg, and then a continuous infusion at 2 to 20 mg/min), which acts as an α-blocker and a β-blocker, may be particularly useful in aortic dissection for controlling hypertension and contractile force. After labetalol or a pure β-blocker (e.g., intravenous propranolol at 1-mg boluses every 3 to 5 minutes to start, followed by a continuous infusion at rates up to 20 mg/hr) has been administered, intravenous nitroprusside (0.5 to 8 μg/kg/min) should be added to titrate blood pressure minute by minute as needed. If β-blockers are contraindicated, calcium-channel blockers (e.g., intravenous diltiazem with an initial bolus of 20 mg over a 2-minute period, followed by a continuous infusion of 5 to 15 mg/hr) may be useful.

When patients have significant hypotension, pseudohypotension should be carefully excluded first. True hypotension may be due to hemopericardium and cardiac tamponade as a result of rupture of the dissection into the pericardium. These patients should be treated with volume expansion and taken to surgery as quickly as possible because their early mortality is extremely high. Pericardiocentesis should be performed only as a last resort because it may precipitate hemodynamic collapse and death.

After initial medical therapy has been instituted and the diagnosis of aortic dissection confirmed, definitive therapy must be determined. Whenever an acute dissection involves the ascending aorta, surgical repair is indicated to minimize the risk for life-threatening complications such as rupture, cardiac tamponade, severe aortic insufficiency, or stroke. Patients with acute dissections confined to the descending aorta are at much lower risk for these complications and tend to fare as well with medical therapy as with surgical repair. When a type B dissection is associated with a serious complication, however, such as end-organ ischemia, surgery is indicated. Patients with chronic type A dissections can be managed medically because they already have survived the early period of high mortality associated with acute proximal dissections.

For an isolated intramural hematoma, the likelihood of progressive dissection or other complications is lower than in patients who are initially seen with a frank dissection, especially those who have smaller hematomas and normal aortic dimensions. Although the 25 to 50% risk of progression may warrant early surgery, serial imaging with surgery reserved for progressive disease is reasonable in patients who are at increased risk with surgery. For *distal* intramural hematomas, management is generally the same as for distal dissection.

Prognosis

Acutely, the mortality rate from untreated aortic dissection is about 1% per hour. Patients with acute aortic dissection who survive the initial hospitalization generally do well thereafter, whether treated medically or surgically. Late complications such as aortic insufficiency, recurrent dissection, aneurysm formation, and aneurysm rupture can occur, however. Medications to control hypertension and reduce ventricular contractility can dramatically reduce the incidence of late complications and should be continued indefinitely. β-Blockers (e.g., metoprolol, 25 to 200 mg twice daily, or atenolol, 25 to 200 mg daily) are the drugs of choice in this setting, but typically a second (e.g., lisinopril, 5 to 40 mg daily) or third (amlodipine, 2.5 to 10 mg daily, or hydrochlorothiazide, 12.5 to 50 mg daily) agent needs to be added to achieve the goal of a systolic blood pressure less than 120 mm Hg (Chapter 66).

Patients are at highest risk for complications during the first 2 years after an intramural hematoma or aortic dissection. Progressive expansion typically occurs without symptoms, so patients must be observed closely with serial aortic imaging at 6-month intervals for the first 2 years and annually thereafter, provided that the anatomy is stable.

TAKAYASU'S ARTERITIS

Definition

Takayasu's arteritis is a chronic inflammatory disease of unknown etiology that involves the aorta and its branches. The mean age at onset is 29, with women affected eight times as often as men. It occurs more often in Asia and Africa than in Europe or North America. An early stage characterized by active inflammation involving the aorta and its branches progresses at a variable rate to a later sclerotic stage with intimal hyperplasia, medial degeneration, and obliterative changes. Most of the resulting arterial lesions are stenotic, but aneurysms may also occur. The aortic arch and brachiocephalic vessels are affected most often, and the disease tends to be most pronounced at branch points in the aorta. The abdominal aorta is also commonly involved, and the pulmonary artery is sometimes involved. The disease may be diffuse or patchy, with affected areas separated by lengths of normal aorta.

Clinical Manifestations

Most patients are initially seen with symptoms of a systemic inflammatory process, such as fever, night sweats, arthralgia, and weight loss. There is often a delay of months to years, however, between the onset of symptoms and the time when the diagnosis is made. At the time of diagnosis, 90% of patients have entered the sclerotic phase and have symptoms of vascular insufficiency, typically with pain in the upper (or less often lower) extremities. There are often absent pulses and diminished blood pressure in the upper extremities, and the condition has earned the name *pulseless disease.* There may be bruits over affected arteries. Significant hypertension (secondary to renal artery involvement) occurs in more than half the patients, but its presence may be difficult to recognize because of the diminished pulses. Aortic insufficiency may result from proximal aortic involvement. Heart failure may result from either hypertension or aortic insufficiency. Involvement of the ostia of the coronary arteries may cause angina or myocardial infarction. Carotid artery involvement may cause cerebral ischemia or stroke. Abdominal angina may result from mesenteric artery compromise.

The overall 15-year survival rate in patients in whom Takayasu's arteritis is diagnosed is 83%, with most deaths being caused by stroke, myocardial infarction, or heart failure. The survival rate in patients with major complications of the disease is 66%; the survival rate in patients without a major complication is 96%.

Diagnosis

Laboratory abnormalities during the acute phase include an elevated erythrocyte sedimentation rate, mild leukocytosis, anemia, and elevated immunoglobulin levels. The diagnosis is best made by aortography, which reveals stenosis of the aorta and stenosis or occlusion of its branch vessels, often with post-stenotic dilation or associated aneurysms.

Treatment

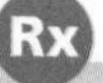

Corticosteroids (e.g., prednisone, 60 to 100 mg daily, often for months and tapered after symptoms or evidence of inflammation subside) are the primary therapy for the acute inflammatory stage and may be effective in improving constitutional symptoms, lowering the erythrocyte sedimentation rate, and slowing disease progression. Cyclophosphamide (2 mg/kg/day) or methotrexate (15 to 25 mg/wk) may be used when corticosteroid therapy alone is ineffective. It is unknown whether medical therapy reduces the risk for major complications or prolongs life.

Balloon angioplasty can dilate stenotic lesions of the aorta and renal arteries. Surgery may be necessary to bypass or reconstruct key segments, such as the coronary, carotid, or renal arteries, or to treat aortic insufficiency. Ideally, when possible, surgery should not be performed during the inflammatory phase.

GIANT CELL ARTERITIS

Giant cell arteritis (Chapter 292) is more common than Takayasu's arteritis. Its cause is also unclear, but it tends to occur in an older population with a mean age of 67 years. It typically affects medium-sized arteries, but in 15% of cases it involves the aorta and branches of the aortic arch. Narrowing of the aorta is rare, but weakening of the ascending aortic wall may lead to localized thoracic aortic aneurysms and secondary aortic insufficiency. Narrowing of the branches of the aortic arch produces symptoms similar to those seen in Takayasu's arteritis. Because the temporal artery is commonly involved, the diagnosis is usually made by temporal artery biopsy. Management involves the use of high-dose corticosteroid therapy (e.g., prednisone, 60 to 100 mg daily, often for months and tapered after symptoms or evidence of inflammation subside), to which the disease is usually responsive.

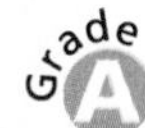

1. Cosford P, Leng G: Screening for abdominal aortic aneurysm. Cochrane Database Syst Rev 2007;CD002945.
2. United Kingdom Small Aneurysm Trial Participants: Long-term outcomes of immediate repair compared with surveillance of small abdominal aortic aneurysms. N Engl J Med 2002;346:1445–1452.
3. Ashton HA, Buxton MJ, Day NE, et al: The Multicentre Aneurysm Screening Study (MASS) into the effect of abdominal aortic aneurysm screening on mortality in men: A randomised controlled trial. Lancet 2002;360:1531–1539.
4. Blankensteijn JD, de John SECA, Prinssen M, et al: Two-year outcomes after conventional or endovascular repair of abdominal aortic aneurysms. N Engl J Med 2005;352:2398–2405.
5. EVAR Trial Participants: Endovascular aneurysm repair versus open repair in patients with abdominal aortic aneurysm (EVAR trial 1): Randomised controlled trial. Lancet 2005;365:2179–2186.
6. EVAR Trial Participants: Endovascular aneurysm repair and outcome in patients unfit for open repair of abdominal aortic aneurysm (EVAR trial 2): Randomised controlled trial. Lancet 2005;365:2187–2192.

SUGGESTED READINGS

Brady AR, Thompson SG, Fowkes GR, et al: Abdominal aortic aneurysm expansion: Risk factors and time intervals for surveillance. Circulation 2004;110:16–21. *Annual or less frequent screening is recommended for aneurysms 4.5 cm or less; smoking is a key risk factor for progression.*

Hackam DG, Thiruchelvam D, Redelmeier DA: Angiotensin-converting enzyme inhibitors and aortic rupture: A population-based case-control study. Lancet 2006;368:659–665. *Patients who received ACE inhibitors before admission were significantly less likely to present with ruptured aneurysm.*

Isselbacher EM: Thoracic and abdominal aortic aneurysms. Circulation 2005;111:816–828. *A comprehensive review.*

Liang P, Hoffman GS: Advances in the medical and surgical treatment of Takayasu arteritis. Curr Opin Rheumatol 2005;17:16–24. *A comprehensive review.*

Sakalihasan N, Limet R, Defawe OD: Abdominal aortic aneurysm. Lancet 2005;365:1577–1589. *A detailed update.*

Tsai TT, Nienaber CA, Eagle KA: Acute aortic syndromes. Circulation 2005;112:3802–3813. *A comprehensive review.*

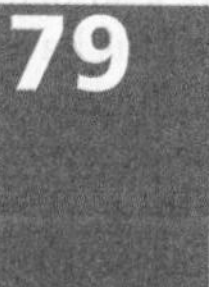

ATHEROSCLEROTIC PERIPHERAL ARTERIAL DISEASE

William R. Hiatt

Definition

Peripheral arterial disease (PAD), due to atherosclerotic occlusions of the arterial circulation to the lower extremities, is part of a systemic disorder of atherosclerosis affecting other major circulations. The disease may initially be asymptomatic and then become manifested by intermittent claudication or severe critical leg ischemia. These clinical manifestations are related to the severity of the hemodynamic obstruction and reduced perfusion to skeletal muscle and skin of the lower extremity.

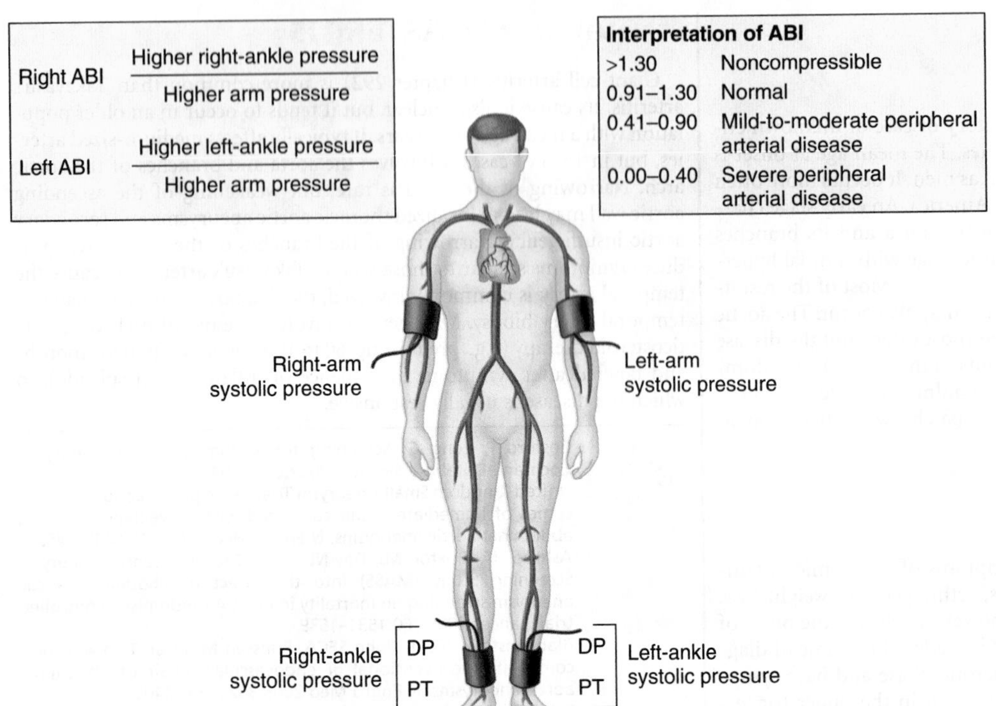

FIGURE 79–1 • Measurement and interpretation of the ankle-brachial index (ABI). DP = dorsalis pedis; PT = posterior tibial. (From Hiatt WR: Medical treatment of peripheral arterial disease and claudication. N Engl J Med 2001;344:1608–1621, with permission.)

Epidemiology

The incidence of intermittent claudication in men ranges from 6 per 10,000 at 30 to 44 years of age to 61 per 10,000 at 65 to 74 years of age. In women, the incidence ranges from 3 per 10,000 at 30 to 44 years of age to 54 per 10,000 at 65 to 74 years of age. The prevalence of PAD based on ankle-brachial blood pressure ratios is approximately 3% in persons younger than 60 years and increases to 20% in those older than 70 years. In these same studies, the prevalence of symptomatic claudication was less than half the prevalence of PAD. Severe critical leg ischemia affects fewer than 1 million adults in the United States. A screening program conducted in primary care offices identified a 29% prevalence of PAD in patients who were 50 to 69 years of age with diabetes or smoking or who were older than 70 years.

When patients with PAD are assessed by history alone, the physician recognizes the presence of significant coronary disease only 20 to 40% of the time. However, when these patients are evaluated with noninvasive testing, such as dipyridamole–stress thallium, the prevalence of coexistent significant coronary disease is 60%; when these patients are evaluated by angiography, the prevalence is as high as 90%. The prevalence of critical cerebrovascular disease is also markedly increased in patients with PAD. These strong associations with atherosclerosis in the coronary and carotid circulation place the patient with PAD at high risk for fatal and nonfatal cardiovascular events.

In contrast to coronary heart disease, women and men have a similar risk for development of PAD. Patients with type 2 diabetes mellitus have a four-fold increased risk of PAD compared with a two-fold increased risk of myocardial infarction or stroke. In patients with diabetes, every 1% increase in the hemoglobin A_{1c} level is associated with a 28% increased risk for development of PAD. The risk of PAD increases 10% with an increase of 10 mg/dL in total cholesterol value. Whereas an elevated low-density lipoprotein cholesterol level is highly associated with the development of coronary disease, reduced high-density lipoprotein cholesterol and increased triglyceride levels are more often associated with PAD. Cigarette smoking is associated with a three- to four-fold increased risk for PAD and is synergistic with other risk factors; the prevalence of cigarette smoking in the PAD population is approximately twice that in the general population. As with coronary heart disease, risk of PAD is doubled in hypertensive patients. Elevated homocysteine levels promote PAD as well as coronary heart disease. Systemic markers of inflammation, such as C-reactive protein, are also strongly predictive of PAD. Patients with hypercoagulable states more commonly have venous thrombosis and thromboembolism, but they may also have peripheral arterial thrombosis, particularly younger patients.

Pathobiology

PAD is caused by atherosclerosis and is similar to atherosclerosis in other circulations in etiology and pathogenesis (Chapter 69). Atherosclerosis in the peripheral circulation has a pathophysiology similar to that of coronary atherosclerosis. However, coronary artery disease is often associated with acute cardiovascular events, whereas peripheral atherosclerosis is associated with relatively stable, chronic symptoms of claudication, which rarely progress to critical leg ischemia.

Hemodynamics

The hemodynamic significance of arterial stenosis is a function not only of the percentage of stenosis but also of flow velocity across the lesion. For example, resting blood flow velocity in the femoral artery may be as low as 20 cm/sec; at this velocity, a stenosis does not become hemodynamically significant until it is 90% occlusive, after which flow and pressure rapidly decrease across the stenosis with increasing obstruction. With exercise in a normal extremity, flow velocity may increase to as high as 150 cm/sec. At these higher flow velocities, about a 50% stenosis becomes hemodynamically significant in a patient with PAD. Thus, patients with claudication have normal flow to skeletal muscle at rest but markedly impaired flow to meet metabolic demand with exercise.

The hemodynamic significance of arterial occlusive disease can be assessed easily by measuring the systolic blood pressure in the ankle and forming a ratio of that pressure to the systolic blood pressure in the arm (the ankle-brachial index, or ABI; Fig. 79–1). Because blood pressures are normally higher in the leg than in the arm, a resting ABI below 0.90 is considered diagnostic of PAD. In a normal extremity, exercise increases the ankle blood pressure in proportion to the increase in arm blood pressure. With PAD, however, ankle blood pressure becomes markedly reduced after exercise. Thus, if a patient with claudication has a normal resting ABI, a decrease in the ABI after exercise would be an alternative way to diagnose PAD.

When blood flow in the extremity is reduced at *rest,* symptoms of severe critical leg ischemia develop. In contrast to claudication (in which the supply-demand mismatch involves skeletal muscle with exercise), severe leg ischemia affects the most distal portion of the extremity with ischemia to the skin and subcutaneous tissues of the forefoot. These patients have ischemic rest pain, distal ulceration, and gangrene.

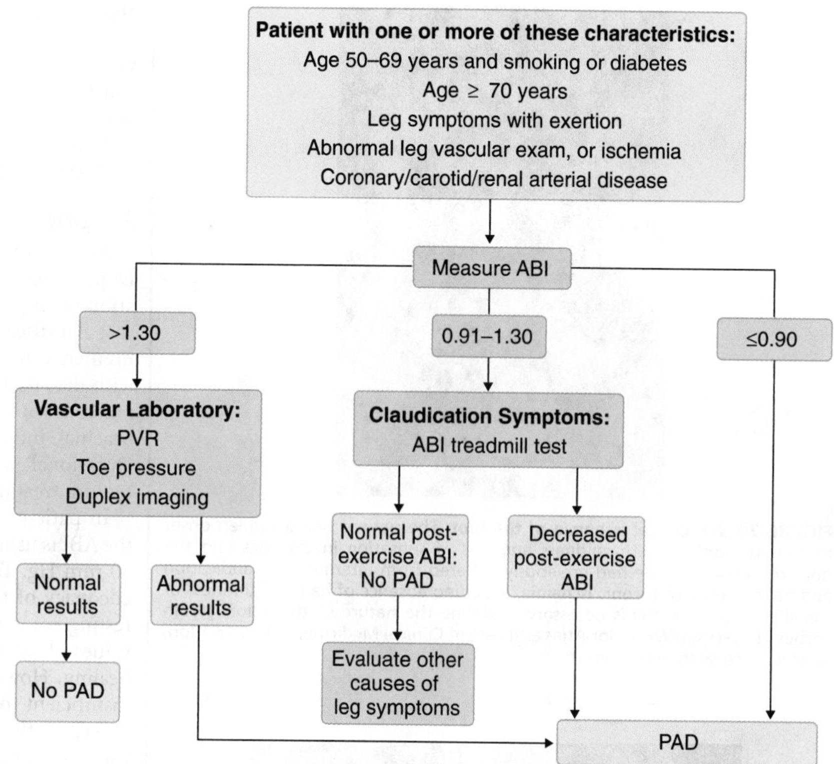

FIGURE 79–2 • Diagnosis of peripheral arterial disease. ABI = ankle-brachial index; PAD = peripheral arterial disease; PVR = pulmonary vascular resistance. (Modified from Hiatt WR: Medical treatment of peripheral arterial disease and claudication. N Engl J Med 2001;344:1608–1621, with permission.)

Metabolic and Neurologic Abnormalities

The marked impairment in exercise performance, walking ability, and physical functioning in patients with claudication cannot be fully explained by the reduction in blood pressure and blood flow to the extremities. Although the pathogenesis of claudication is initiated by atherosclerotic occlusion of the major conduit vessels, denervation of skeletal muscle leads to atrophy and weakness in the affected limbs. More important, oxidative metabolism and the capacity to generate high-energy phosphates are severely impaired in patients with PAD beyond what can be explained simply by the reduction in blood flow. Treatment should focus not only on improving the hemodynamic state of the patient but also on modifying these alterations in skeletal muscle metabolism and function.

Clinical Manifestations

Chronic arterial insufficiency of the lower extremity causes two characteristic types of pain, intermittent claudication and ischemic rest pain, often with ulceration or gangrene. Claudication is derived from the Latin word meaning to limp, which accurately describes the gait pattern of the patient at the onset of symptoms during exercise. Depending on the level and extent of the PAD, the patient may have claudication affecting the buttock and thigh (iliac occlusive disease), calf (most commonly), or foot (rarely).

Claudication is caused by reversible muscle ischemia and is characterized by cramping, aching, or fatigue in the affected muscle. The discomfort develops only during exercise and steadily increases with walking until the patient has to stop because of intolerable discomfort. The discomfort is quickly relieved by rest without change of position. Claudication may occur in one leg only (40% of the time) or affect both legs (60% of the time). The physician should ascertain severity by the distance that the patient can walk before experiencing discomfort (initial claudication distance) and before being forced to stop (absolute or maximal claudication distance). Any recent change in walking distance should be determined.

Foot claudication is rare and is usually seen in thromboangiitis obliterans (Chapter 80) rather than in atherosclerotic PAD. The complaint is usually of a painful ache or cramp in the forefoot associated only with walking. Patients also have the otherwise nonspecific complaint of a persistently cold foot at night.

Ischemic (or nocturnal) rest pain is a severe form of pain that diffusely involves the foot distal to the tarsal bones, although it may be localized to the vicinity of an ischemic ulcer or gangrenous toe. The progression from claudication to rest pain reflects severe arterial occlusive disease with inadequate blood flow to the distal extremity at rest. The pain typically occurs at night when the patient assumes the horizontal position without gravity to help arterial flow. The pain may become so severe that it is not relieved even by substantial doses of narcotics.

Diagnosis

An approach to the diagnostic evaluation of the patient with PAD is suggested in Figure 79–2. All patients should have a smoking history to define current smoking status and previous pack years (Chapter 30).

Physical Examination

A complete physical examination should be performed to evaluate the patient for systemic hypertension, cardiac murmurs or arrhythmias, carotid bruits, or an abdominal aortic aneurysm. The skin of the legs, especially the foot, should be inspected for color changes, ulceration, infection, or trauma from poorly fitting shoes.

All arterial pulses should be palpated, including the brachial, femoral, and pedal arteries. Absence of a femoral pulse indicates inflow disease of the iliac arteries. Patients with a palpable femoral pulse but absent pedal pulses have disease confined to the femoropopliteal or tibial arteries. Bruits of the aorta or femoral vessels reflect turbulent flow and are markers of systemic atherosclerosis. A femoral bruit or absent pedal pulses should suggest PAD, and ankle blood pressure should be measured.

With severe claudication or ischemic rest pain, calf muscles atrophy, hair is lost over the dorsum of the toes and foot, and toenails thicken. More advanced ischemic atrophy results in a shiny, "skeletonized" appearance. Severely affected limbs also display pallor on elevation because of inadequate arterial pressure and flow; rubor on dependency occurs with restricted arterial inflow and chronic dilation of the peripheral vascular bed.

Severe critical leg ischemia (Fig. 79–3) can cause ulceration initially affecting the most distal aspect of the toes. These ulcers are painful, do not bleed when they are manipulated, and often have a dark necrotic base (Fig. 79–4). The foot may be edematous from being continually kept in the dependent position in an attempt to relieve the ischemic pain. Gangrene usually begins with the toes and forefoot and may occur separately from ulceration.

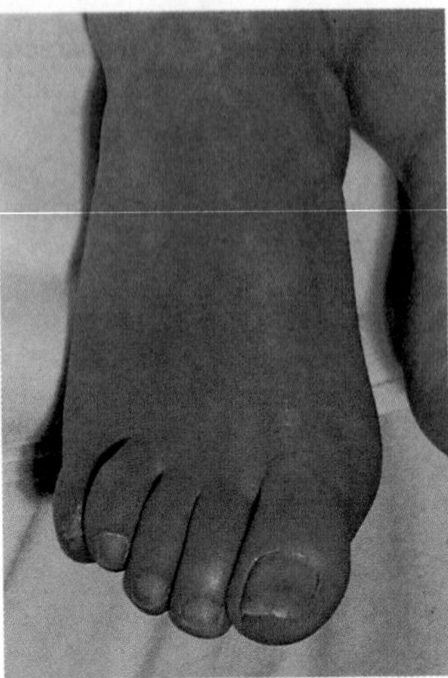

FIGURE 79–3 • Critical ischemia of the foot. The patient had a sudden onset of foot discomfort, with coldness and loss of sensation in the toes and the dorsum of the foot. He had previously suffered from intermittent claudication and has evidence of chronic ischemia, including absence of hair and thinness of the skin. Arteriography is necessary to define the nature of the lesion. (From Forbes CD, Jackson WF: Color Atlas and Text of Clinical Medicine, 3rd ed. London, Mosby, 2003, with permission.)

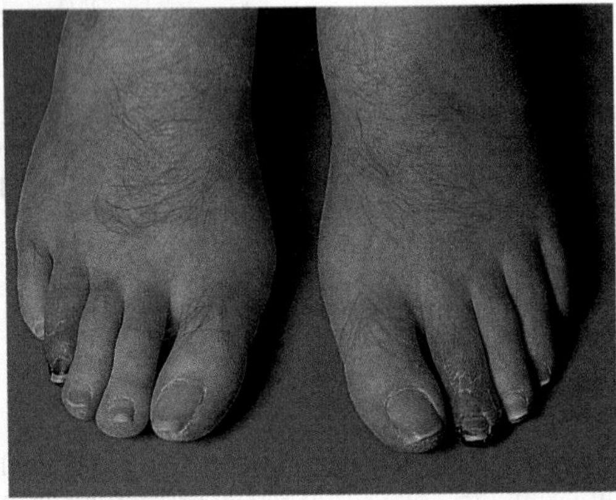

FIGURE 79–4 • Typical dry gangrene of two toes in a patient with diffuse atheroma. The patient had a history of intermittent claudication. Note the chronic nail changes that are also seen (resembling onycholysis). The residual hair on the dorsum of the feet is unusual in chronic ischemia; usually the hair is lost. (From Forbes CD, Jackson WF: Color Atlas and Text of Clinical Medicine, 3rd ed. London, Mosby, 2003, with permission.)

General Evaluation

An electrocardiogram should be obtained to evaluate for evidence of coronary artery disease. Elevations in the hematocrit or platelet count can result in hyperviscosity with an associated decrease in peripheral perfusion. Significant anemia reduces the oxygen content and decreases oxygen delivery. In patients with significant lung disease, arterial saturation should be measured to determine whether a low saturation could exacerbate peripheral oxygen delivery. Renal function should be evaluated because chronic renal failure is a significant risk factor for PAD, and patients with PAD are at risk for renovascular hypertension and renal insufficiency.

An occasional patient with PAD may develop an acute thrombotic occlusion of a peripheral vessel from in situ thrombosis or an embolus from a more proximal site. These patients may need a coagulation screen consisting of (but not limited to) factor V Leiden, protein S, protein C, antithrombin III, and other tests of coagulation.

Risk Factor Evaluation

Diabetes should be evaluated by determination of a fasting and postprandial glucose concentration or hemoglobin A_{1C} level (Chapter 247). A complete lipid profile should be obtained, including measurements of low-density lipoprotein cholesterol, high-density lipoprotein cholesterol, and triglycerides (Chapter 217). Blood pressure should be routinely measured and any history of hypertension ascertained. Screening for elevated homocysteine levels is generally not recommended but should be considered in patients with an early age at onset or a history of thrombotic events (Chapters 49 and 70). Measurement of high-sensitivity C-reactive protein may be useful in assessing the patient's risk not only for PAD but also for ischemic cardiac events (Chapters 49 and 70).

Peripheral Vascular Studies

Measurement of systolic blood pressure in the ankle and arm by Doppler ultrasonography has become the standard for the initial evaluation of all patients thought to have vascular disease (see Fig. 79–1). The vascular disease can be further localized by taking several pressure measurements in the thigh and calf (segmental limb pressures). In patients with iliac occlusive disease, the thigh-brachial index is reduced, whereas patients with disease more distal in the leg may have a normal thigh-brachial index but reduced calf-brachial and ankle-brachial indices. Occasional patients with claudication but normal ABIs (≥0.90) at rest require treadmill testing to document a fall in the ABI to below 0.90.

In patients with severe critical limb ischemia and nonhealing ulcers, the ABI is usually less than 0.40 and the ankle systolic pressure is less than 50 mm Hg. Transcutaneous oximetry also provides information on the adequacy of the peripheral circulation for wound healing. The normal resting transcutaneous oxygen tension is greater than 60 mm Hg, but values of 40 mm Hg or greater are usually associated with good wound healing. However, when values are less than 20 mm Hg, blood flow is insufficient to heal a wound, and additional measures must be taken to reperfuse the extremity. Measurement of toe pressures is particularly useful in patients with noncompressible ankle vessels (ABI above 1.40 as may be seen in patients with diabetes). In this situation, a toe-brachial index of less than 0.70 is diagnostic of PAD.

Vascular Imaging

Color-assisted duplex ultrasonography can detect stenoses and measure flow velocity at a particular arterial segment or bypass graft. Invasive arteriography, which is the most accurate means of defining arterial anatomy, is indicated only when the patient is being considered for angioplasty or vascular surgery. Magnetic resonance angiography and computed tomographic angiography are newer noninvasive tests that provide excellent anatomic definition of arterial lesions and are indicated in planning a revascularization.

Assessment of Functional Status

Compared with healthy individuals of the same age, patients with claudication have a 50 to 60% reduction in peak treadmill performance, a severity similar to that of patients with severe heart failure. Treadmill testing can quantify the functional limitations in patients with claudication and can also serve as an objective measure of response to therapy. Patients with claudication are typically tested at a slow speed not to exceed 2 miles per hour, with the treadmill grade beginning at 0% and increasing 2% every 2 minutes until maximal symptoms prevent further exercise. The time or distance at which claudication pain is first noted is termed the initial claudication distance, and the maximal walking performance is termed the absolute claudication distance; therapy to improve claudication results in an increase in both. A 25 to 50% increase in treadmill performance after treatment is considered clinically significant. Several questionnaire measures of functional status, such as the Walking Impairment Questionnaire, have been developed and validated in patients with PAD and are useful adjuncts to treadmill testing.

Differential Diagnosis

Pain from arthritis of the hip or knee is often present at rest and exacerbated by exercise. With cessation of exercise, the pain may not improve unless the patient rests and unloads the joint. Claudication-like symptoms may also arise from spinal stenosis, which is due to osteophytic narrowing of the lumbar neurospinal canal (Chapter 423). These symptoms usually consist of lower extremity numbness and weakness produced by standing or increasing lumbar lordosis rather than just by ambulation. The symptoms are relieved not simply by rest but also by sitting down or leaning forward to straighten out the lumbar spine.

Venous insufficiency (the sequela of thrombophlebitis) causes swelling and discomfort in the calf with standing and often worse swelling with prolonged walking (Chapter 81). Patients with severe venous insuffi-

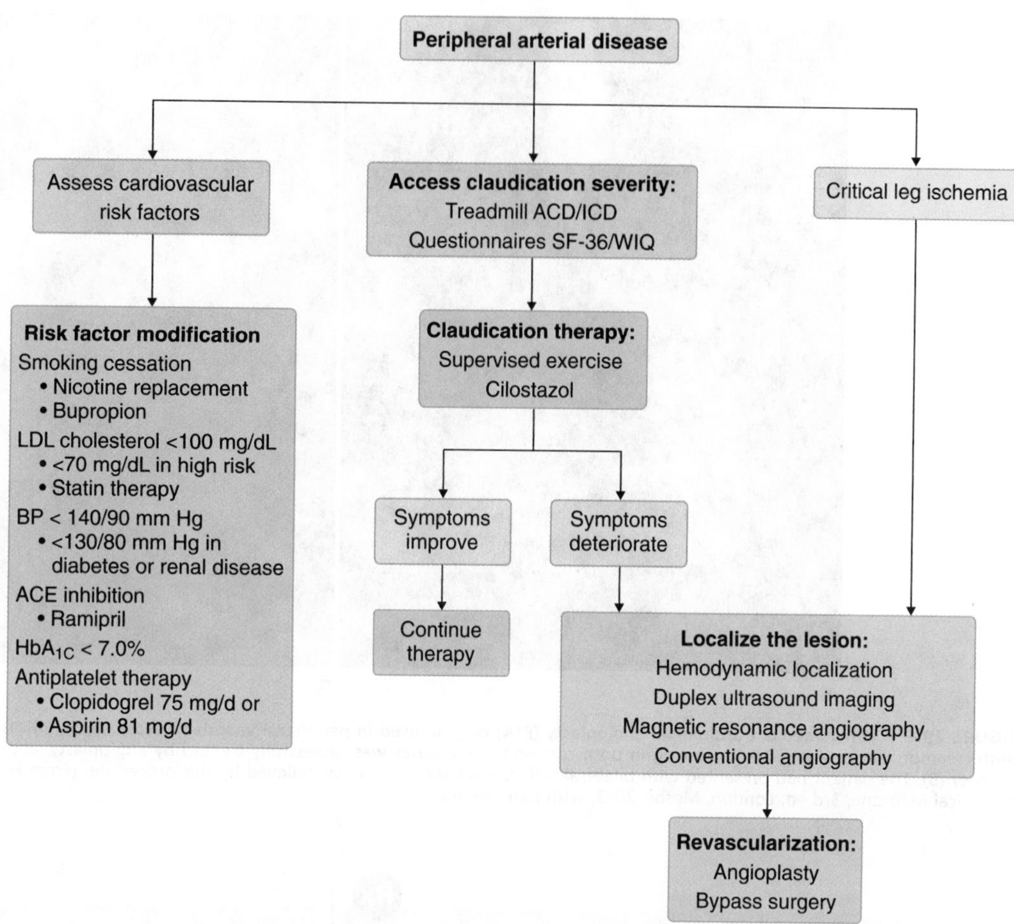

FIGURE 79–5 • Therapy for peripheral arterial disease. ACD/ICD = absolute claudication distance/initial claudication distance; ACE = angiotensin-converting enzyme; BP = blood pressure; LDL = low-density lipoprotein; WIQ = Walking Impairment Questionnaire. (Modified from Hiatt WR: Medical treatment of peripheral arterial disease and claudication. N Engl J Med 2001;344:1608–1621, with permission.)

ciency may complain of venous claudication from calf swelling (not ischemic cramping) with exercise. Peripheral neuropathies are common in the elderly but are associated with a continuous burning sensation in the foot that is unaffected by exercise; a history of diabetes or alcoholism is common. Older individuals also complain of nocturnal cramps in the calf that are not vascular in origin. Tightness and discomfort in the calf precipitated by exercise may sometimes result from a chronic compartment compression syndrome; such patients are often athletes with large calf muscles. Calf claudication may also develop in athletes from popliteal entrapment caused by external muscle compression of the popliteal artery.

Treatment

Rx

Medical Therapy

Medical therapy in patients with PAD has two important objectives. First, patients should undergo aggressive risk factor modification and be prescribed antiplatelet therapy to reduce the risk of cardiovascular morbidity and mortality by treatment of systemic atherosclerosis. Second, medical therapy is indicated to treat claudication, to improve functional status, and to prevent limb loss (Fig. 79–5). Smoking cessation is critical to delay the progression of PAD and to reduce cardiovascular morbidity and mortality (Chapter 30).

Several large clinical trials have shown the benefit of lowering low-density lipoprotein cholesterol levels in patients with coronary atherosclerosis. The Heart Protection Study demonstrated that 40 mg of simvastatin significantly reduced the risk of myocardial infarction, ischemic stroke, revascularization, and death in patients with PAD but no other clinical evidence of cardiovascular disease. [1] Current guidelines recommend lowering low-density lipoprotein cholesterol to below 100 mg/dL in all patients with PAD and to below 70 mg/dL (Chapters 70 to 72 and 217) in patients with PAD who have evidence of coronary disease.

Rx

Aggressive control of blood glucose concentration has not been shown to modify the natural history of PAD, but current guidelines recommend controlling the hemoglobin A_{1c} level to less than 7.0% to mitigate the complications of this disease in other circulations.

To lower blood pressure (Chapter 66), use of the angiotensin-converting enzyme inhibitor ramipril leads to a significant reduction in myocardial infarction, stroke, and vascular death. [2] In patients with both diabetes and PAD, reduction in blood pressure to 125/75 mm Hg with either an angiotensin-converting enzyme inhibitor or a calcium-channel blocker reduces cardiovascular events compared with a blood pressure of 135/85 mm Hg. [3] Well-designed studies have not found any adverse effects on claudication with β-blocker use. Aggressive blood pressure reduction with any medication reduces perfusion pressure into the limb and may result in a slight worsening of claudication, but this side effect should not alter the blood pressure goal.

Antiplatelet therapy in patients with PAD reduces the risk of myocardial infarction, stroke, and vascular death by 23%. [4] Clopidogrel, an antagonist of adenosine diphosphate–induced platelet aggregation, provides a 24% relative risk reduction in the incidence of vascular death, myocardial infarction, and stroke compared with aspirin in patients with PAD. [5] Thus, clopidogrel may be more effective than aspirin for secondary prevention in PAD.

In terms of symptomatic relief, an established agent is cilostazol, which has antiplatelet and vasodilating properties. A meta-analysis of cilostazol demonstrated an approximate 50% improvement in exercise performance over placebo as well as improvements in quality of life and functional status. [6] Ramipril can also significantly improve pain-free walking time. [7] Safety concerns prohibit the use of this drug in patients with heart failure. Meta-analyses of pentoxifylline indicate minimal clinical benefit, so it is not recommended for the treatment of claudication.

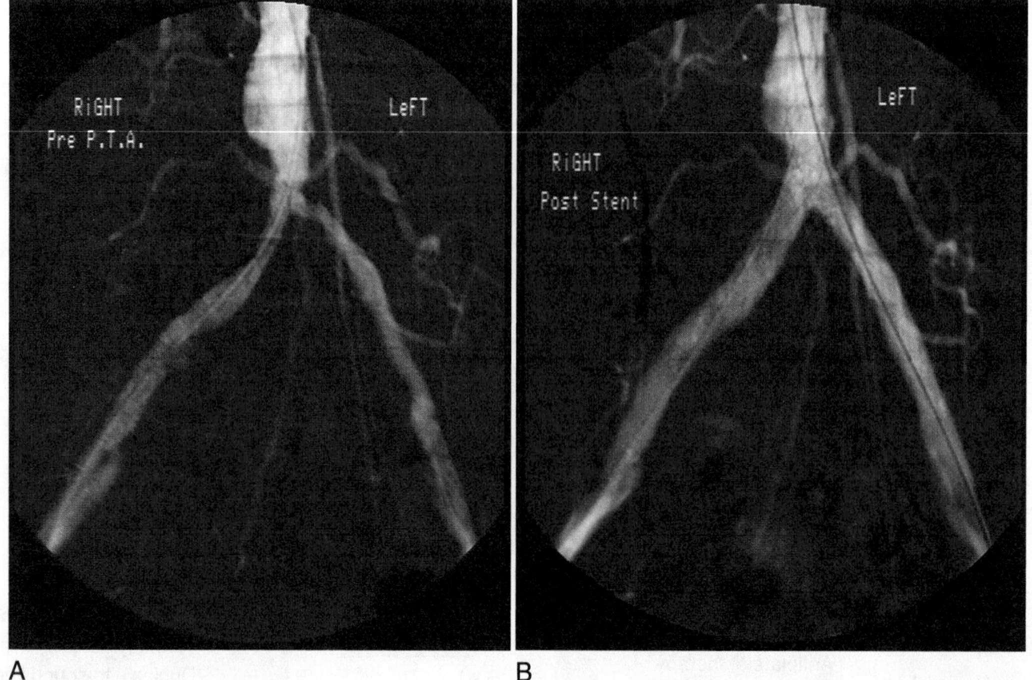

FIGURE 79–6 • Percutaneous transluminal angioplasty (PTA) may be used in peripheral vascular disease. A, Significant narrowing of the aortic bifurcation and both common iliac arteries. The narrowing in both common iliac arteries was successfully treated by angioplasty, and bilateral stents were inserted to maintain patency **(B).** The patient had presented with bilateral calf claudication, which was relieved by this procedure. (From Forbes CD, Jackson WF: Color Atlas and Text of Clinical Medicine, 3rd ed. London, Mosby, 2003, with permission.)

Rx

For severe critical leg ischemia, medical treatments are limited. Prostaglandin drugs may help heal ischemic ulcers and reduce the risk of amputation, but these benefits are not fully established. Analgesics, in particular narcotics, may also be needed, and spinal cord stimulation may reduce ischemic pain. Topical antibiotics, growth factors, and débriding agents have not been effective in treating ulcerated lesions of the lower extremity. Patients in whom cellulitis develops around an ischemic ulceration should be treated with systemic antibiotics. Chelation therapy has no benefit.

Exercise Therapy

Supervised exercise training is a well-documented treatment to relieve claudication and to improve exercise performance. Typically, exercise training is performed on a treadmill or a track, three times a week. The initial workload on the treadmill is set at the speed and grade that precipitated claudication during the evaluation treadmill test. For training purposes, patients should be able to walk between 3 and 5 minutes at this workload until they achieve a moderately severe level of claudication pain. The patient steps off the treadmill and rests until the pain subsides and then repeats this activity for approximately 40 to 60 minutes per training session. The speed and grade of the treadmill are increased on a regular basis to induce a training effect. Results of this program are typically a 100 to 200% increase in peak exercise performance, an improvement comparable to that achieved with surgery or angioplasty without the side effects of pharmacologic therapy and without the morbidity and mortality of interventional procedures. However, the training benefit is maintained only if patients continue with their exercise program. Home-based exercise and simple recommendations to exercise are much less effective than supervised programs. There are few supervised training programs across the country, and third-party payers often do not reimburse for exercise training.

Invasive Therapies

Indications for Surgery or Angioplasty

Invasive therapies should be limited to claudicating patients whose initial medical treatment fails, patients who have severe disability, and patients who have an appropriate anatomic lesion for

Rx

bypass or angioplasty (Fig. 79–6; see also Fig. 79–5). In contrast, patients with critical leg ischemia should be considered for immediate vascular surgery and angioplasty, which is necessary to heal ischemic lesions, to relieve ischemic rest pain, and to prevent amputation.

Angioplasty

Angioplasty guidelines emphasize that more proximal lesions (e.g., the aortoiliac segment, and short occlusions of the femoral and superficial femoral artery) have better patency rates and durability than do more distal popliteal and tibial lesions (Table 79–1). Below the inguinal ligament, the initial success and long-term patency rates have been less well studied but are not as good as for more proximal lesions. Stenting is superior to balloon angioplasty: restenosis rates are reduced from 63% to 37% at 6 months, and exercise tolerance is also better. [8]

Surgery

Surgery is principally used to treat severe critical leg ischemia rather than claudication because of the associated morbidity and mortality of surgery, the relatively benign natural history of claudication, and the efficacy of medical (particularly exercise) therapies. In aortoiliac disease, prosthetic materials are usually implanted. Aortoiliac surgery is associated with an average mortality of 3% and morbidity of 8%. In patients with femoropopliteal disease, the best conduit is saphenous vein. Femoropopliteal surgery with vein bypass is associated with a mortality of 2%, a morbidity of 5 to 10%, and a 5-year patency rate of 70 to 80%. The use of prosthetic material (required if a vein is not available) reduces 5-year patency rates to 50% or less. Distal femorotibial operations for limb salvage have morbidity and mortality similar to femoropopliteal surgery but slightly lower 5-year patency rates of 50 to 60%.

In patients with stable coronary artery disease, additional cardiac evaluation is generally not indicated before peripheral vascular surgery. When vascular surgery is considered in the patient at high risk of cardiac complications, however, further evaluation is appropriate (Chapter 457). Unless it is contraindicated, all vascular surgery patients should be prescribed a β-adrenergic blocker perioperatively.

TABLE 79–1 RESULTS OF ANGIOPLASTY AND SURGERY FOR PERIPHERAL ARTERIAL DISEASE

			Patency Rates (%)		
Treatment	**Mortality (%)**	**Morbidity (%)**	**3 Years**	**5 Years**	**10 Years**
Aortoiliac					
Angioplasty with stent	<1	5–14	70–78	58	—
	<1	3–13	81	—	—
Surgery	3	8	—	88–91	82–87
Femoropopliteal					
Angioplasty with stent	<1	7	56	51	—
	<1	2	67	—	—
Surgery (vein)	2	5–10	—	70–80	—
Surgery (prosthetic)	2	5–10	—	50	—
Femorotibial	3–5	10–20	—	50–60	—

Prognosis

In patients with PAD, all-cause mortality is increased in both men and women, and cardiovascular mortality is six-fold higher than in age-matched control patients. This mortality risk is almost exclusively due to death from myocardial infarction and stroke. In one study of persons with an average age of 66 years, healthy individuals had an approximate 80% 10-year survival rate, patients with asymptomatic PAD (defined as an ABI below 0.95 but without symptoms of claudication) had an approximate 55% 10-year survival rate, patients with intermittent claudication resulting from peripheral atherosclerosis had a 40% 10-year survival rate, and those with severe symptoms had only a 25% 10-year survival rate. In addition, the severity of PAD in the legs is closely associated with the risk of myocardial infarction, ischemic stroke, and vascular death. The lower the ABI, the greater the risk of cardiovascular events.

In contrast to the marked increased risk of mortality, patients with claudication have little risk of limb loss. The risk of amputation during 5 years is estimated at 4%. In addition, most patients with claudication have stable symptoms during 5 years and do not require a revascularization procedure. In contrast, patients with critical leg ischemia have a 20% annual mortality risk and a 35% annual risk of amputation.

ACUTE ARTERIAL ISCHEMIA

Definition

Acute arterial ischemia can be caused by occlusion of an existing bypass graft, embolism, or native vessel thrombosis. Patients may have sudden onset of claudication, rest pain, or a cool or cold extremity. The physician must assess the current circulation status and the limb's viability as well as the nature of previous operations.

Diagnosis and Treatment

The extremity is often pale and cool to palpation; pulses are absent. It is particularly important to palpate the femoral as well as pedal pulses. The ability to palpate pedal pulses is often limited, even in the hands of experienced vascular surgeons. Therefore, unless pulses are grossly obvious, Doppler study should be used to determine signals at the three major tibial arteries in the ankle. Any audible Doppler signal should prompt measurement of ankle pressure at that site to calculate an ABI.

The most important initial assessment is viability. Most acutely ischemic limbs are salvageable; skeletal muscle can generally tolerate 6 hours of warm ischemia before irreversible loss. Paralyzed, insensate extremities with fixed skin mottling and hard calf musculature are not salvageable and require primary amputation as soon as the patient is medically prepared for the procedure. The decision to proceed with limb salvage in marginal cases usually relies on the judgment of the vascular surgeon.

Graft Occlusion

The most common cause of acute arterial ischemia is occlusion of an existing bypass graft. Patients have either rest pain or increasing claudication, depending on the degree of acute change in ischemia.

Initial management requires rapid therapeutic heparin anticoagulation to prevent propagation of thrombus. A vascular surgeon should be consulted immediately to assess the timing of arteriography and surgery. Management of comorbid diseases such as heart failure, respiratory insufficiency, and infection should be initiated, and central venous access should be obtained while arm veins are preserved as potential conduits for vascular reconstruction.

Embolism (Cardiac or Arterial)

Cardiac embolism is most commonly encountered in patients who have preexisting valvar heart disease, mural thrombus of the ventricle or atrium, or underlying rhythm disturbances (e.g., atrial fibrillation). The most frequent sites of lower extremity embolization are the aortic and femoral bifurcations. Patients may suffer severe ischemia because of a lack of existing collateral circulation at the time of occlusion. The decision to proceed directly to surgery for embolectomy versus angiography with catheter-directed thrombolysis depends on the severity of the ischemia. Thrombolysis takes more time to relieve the occlusion but offers the advantage of complete thrombus removal (often incomplete with blind catheter extraction) and avoids endothelial balloon trauma, which often leads to later fibrointimal hyperplasia and branch stenosis or occlusion of the involved arteries.

Arterial-arterial embolization (atheroembolism) may be spontaneous or iatrogenic. Patients with spontaneous atheroembolism have painful, cyanotic digits of acute onset. If embolization is ipsilateral, iliac or femoral artery sources are more likely; bilateral findings indicate an aortic source. Aneurysms of the aorta and femoral and popliteal arteries are also causes. The patient has a normal or only slightly diminished ABI because the circulation from the digital arteries to the embolic source must be relatively uninterrupted. Cases of iatrogenic atheroembolism occur after aortic catheterization procedures. The clinical picture of limb atheroembolism in this setting can vary from mild livedo reticularis to severe limb pain or cyanosis and eventual tissue loss with concurrent elevated plasma muscle enzymes and myoglobinuria (Chapter 126). The diagnosis of cholesterol emboli can be confirmed by skin biopsy of peripheral lesions demonstrating cholesterol crystals in the capillaries. Elevated creatinine, oliguria, and urine eosinophils are present in patients with renal atheroemboli. Arteries that are occluded by atheroembolic material usually cannot be reopened surgically because of the small particle or vessel size. Similarly, most patients with catheter-induced atheroembolism have diffuse aortic disease not amenable to surgical treatment. An exception occurs when catheter-induced atheroembolism calls attention to an arterial aneurysm as the suspected source of the embolic material.

Native Artery Thrombosis

Native artery thrombosis occurs in two common scenarios: (1) a native artery becomes acutely occluded in a patient with a known or unknown hypercoagulable state (frequently with previous subclinical thromboses of small arteries) and (2) acute thrombosis in the iliac artery secondary to catheter trauma from coronary angiography develops in a patient with severe aortoiliac occlusive disease (as a result of either dissection of the iliac artery from the catheter or overzealous compression and occlusion of the groin after catheterization). The primary goals in this setting are to make the diagnosis (baseline ABI before cardiac catheterization is critical), to determine the level of ischemia, to determine the viability of the distal end of the limb, to achieve rapid therapeutic heparin anticoagulation, and to make appropriate plans for diagnostic angiography (usual) or urgent surgical exploration (unusual).

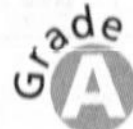

1. Heart Protection Study Collaborative Group: MRC/BHF Heart Protection Study of cholesterol lowering with simvastatin in 20,536 high-risk individuals: A randomised placebo-controlled trial. Lancet 2002;360:7–22.
2. Yusuf S, Sleight P, Pogue J, et al: Effects of an angiotensin-converting-enzyme inhibitor, ramipril, on cardiovascular events in high-risk patients. The Heart Outcomes Prevention Evaluation Study Investigators. N Engl J Med 2000;342:145–153.
3. Mehler PS, Coll JR, Estacio R, et al: Intensive blood pressure control reduces the risk of cardiovascular events in patients with peripheral arterial disease and type 2 diabetes. Circulation 2003; 107:753–756.
4. Antithrombotic Trialists' Collaboration: Collaborative meta-analysis of randomised trials of antiplatelet therapy for prevention of death, myocardial infarction, and stroke in high-risk patients. BMJ 2002;324:71–86.
5. CAPRIE Steering Committee: A randomised, blinded trial of clopidogrel versus aspirin in patients at risk of ischaemic events (CAPRIE). Lancet 1996;348:1329–1339.
6. Regensteiner JG, Ware JE Jr, McCarthy WJ, et al: Effect of cilostazol on treadmill walking, community-based walking ability, and health-related quality of life in patients with intermittent claudication due to peripheral arterial disease: Meta-analysis of six randomized controlled trials. J Am Geriatr Soc 2002;50:1939–1946.
7. Ahimastos AA, Lawler A, Rein CM, et al: Ramipril markedly improves walking ability in patients with peripheral arterial disease: A randomized trial. Ann Intern Med 2006;144:660–664.
8. Schillinger M, Sabeti S, Loewe C, et al: Balloon angioplasty versus implantation of nitinol stents in the superficial femoral artery. N Engl J Med 2006;354:1879–1888.

SUGGESTED READINGS

Aboyans V, Criqui MH, Denenberg JO, et al: Risk factors for progression of peripheral arterial disease in large and small vessels. Circulation 2006;113:2623–2629. *Emphasizes importance of typical cardiovascular risk factors.*

Hankey GJ, Norman PE, Eikelboom JW: Medical treatment of peripheral arterial disease. JAMA 2006;295:547–553. *A practical overview.*

Hirsch AT, Haskal ZJ, Hertzer NR, et al: ACC/AHA 2005 Practice guidelines for the management of patients with peripheral arterial disease (lower extremity, renal, mesenteric, and abdominal aortic): Executive summary. Circulation 2006;113:e463–654. *Also available at http://www.circulationaha.org.*

Khan NA, Rahim SA, Anand SS, et al: Does the clinical examination predict lower extremity peripheral arterial disease? JAMA 2006;295:536–546. *The physical examination is of limited utility, emphasizing the importance of symptoms and the ankle-brachial index.*

Marso SP, Hiatt WR: Peripheral arterial disease in patients with diabetes. J Am Coll Cardiol 2006;47:921–929. *A comprehensive review.*

White C: Intermittent claudication. N Engl J Med 2007;356:1241–1250. *A scholarly review.*

80 OTHER PERIPHERAL ARTERIAL DISEASES

Jeffrey W. Olin

LIVEDO RETICULARIS

Livedo reticularis is characterized by a reticular, fishnet, or lacy pattern on the skin of the lower extremities and other parts of the body. This pattern is red or blue and is caused by deoxygenated blood in the surrounding horizontally arranged venous plexus.

Primary or benign livedo reticularis occurs most commonly in young women between the ages of 20 and 40 years. Ulceration generally does not occur with this form of the disease, which may result from vasomotor instability or increased sensitivity of the dermal blood vessels. It is intensified by cold exposure and is relieved by rewarming, and it may occur in association with Raynaud's phenomenon. The benign variety of livedo reticularis often needs no treatment other than measures to keep the body part as warm as possible.

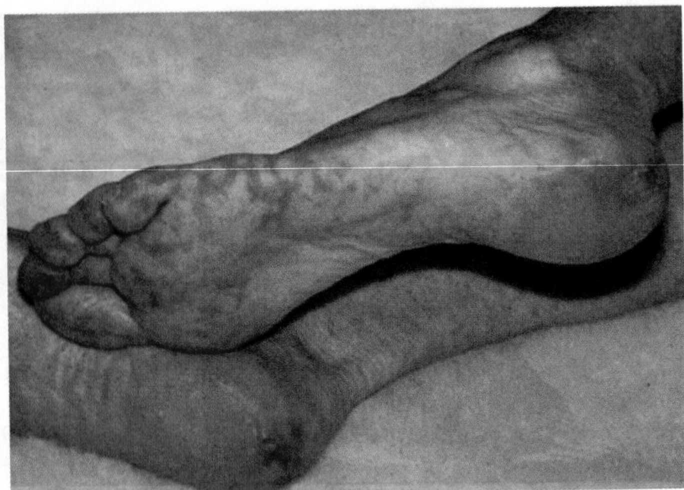

FIGURE 80–1 • Typical livedo reticularis on the lateral portion of the left foot and both heels. The second and fourth toes are cyanotic. These findings are typical of atheromatous embolization, and the fact that both feet are involved indicates a source above the aortic bifurcation. (From Bartholomew JR, Olin JW: Atheromatous embolization. *In* Young JR, Olin JW, Bartholomew JR [eds]: Peripheral Vascular Diseases, 2nd ed. St. Louis, Mosby, 1996.)

Secondary livedo reticularis occurs in association with atheromatous embolization (Fig. 80–1), polyarteritis nodosa (Chapter 291), systemic lupus erythematosus (Chapter 287), leukocytoclastic vasculitis (Chapter 291), other connective tissue diseases, therapy with amantadine, and various neurologic or endocrine diseases and in patients receiving large doses of vasopressors such as epinephrine, norepinephrine, and dopamine. Livedo reticularis is also one of the many skin manifestations of the anti–phospholipid antibody syndrome. In patients with secondary livedo reticularis, therapy should be directed at the underlying cause.

Livedoid Vasculopathy

In livedoid vasculopathy or livedoid vasculitis, extensive livedo reticularis surrounds a painful, ischemic-appearing ulceration located on the anterior or posterior portion of the lower leg (Fig. 80–2). Pathologically, thrombosis of the microvasculature occurs, with little or no active inflammatory component. Small doses of tissue plasminogen activator (10 mg intravenously daily for 14 days) may be effective in treating the ulcerations. Atrophie blanche is a variant of livedoid vasculopathy. These ulcerations generally occur around the ankle or foot. They have a white or yellowish base with poor granulation tissue and are exquisitely painful and difficult to heal.

ATHEROMATOUS EMBOLIZATION

Definition

Atheromatous embolization (cholesterol embolization) refers to the embolization of cholesterol crystals or platelet fibrin aggregates to the extremities or one or more organs. Atheromatous emboli usually originate from ulcerated or stenotic atherosclerotic plaques or from aneurysms that are primarily in the thoracic or abdominal aorta, iliac artery, or carotid artery.

Epidemiology and Pathobiology

Atheromatous embolization of the kidneys is a common histologic finding and may occur in 15 to 30% of patients with severe aortic atherosclerosis or aneurysm of the abdominal aorta. Increasing aortic plaque thickness, protruding aortic atheroma, and mobile aortic atheroma are associated with a high likelihood of atheromatous embolization. Atheromatous embolization may be spontaneous, but it occurs most often after percutaneous coronary, peripheral, or cerebrovascular intervention. Pathologically, biconvex cholesterol crystals lodge in the arterioles and lead to a foreign body reaction in which polymorphonuclear leukocytes, macrophages, and multinucleated giant cells appear several days to several weeks after the inciting event.

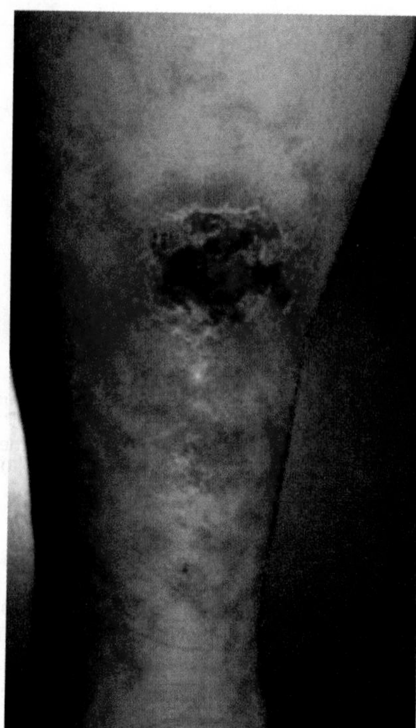

FIGURE 80–2 • Livedoid vasculitis. Ischemic ulceration is evident on the posterior portion of the calf surrounded by a livedoid pattern to the skin.

Clinical Manifestations

The most common clinical manifestations are skin changes. These changes occur in more than one third of patients and are generally found in the lower extremities, but they may also be seen in the trunk, over the buttocks, and rarely in the upper extremities. These manifestations include livedo reticularis (embolization to the dermal blood vessels), purple or blue toes (see Fig. 80–1), splinter hemorrhages, gangrenous digits or ulcerations, and nodules in the presence of palpable foot pulses. The pain associated with ischemic lesions is disproportionate to the amount of tissue involvement.

Atheroembolic renal disease is a small vessel occlusive disease leading to uncontrolled hypertension and advanced or end-stage renal disease (Chapter 115). Atheromatous embolization may also involve the gastrointestinal tract and may produce ischemic bowel with generalized abdominal pain, nausea, vomiting, melena, or hematochezia. Cholesterol emboli to the gallbladder may produce acute gangrenous cholecystitis, whereas emboli to the pancreas can cause acute pancreatitis.

Cardiac manifestations of atheroemboli include angina pectoris (Chapter 70) and myocardial infarction (Chapter 72). Patients may develop amaurosis fugax or blindness caused by retinal artery occlusion. A Hollenhorst plaque (yellow, highly refractile atheromatous material) may be present at the bifurcation of retinal blood vessels. Stroke, headache, confusion, organic brain syndrome, dizziness, and spinal cord infarction can occur. Constitutional signs and symptoms such as fever, weight loss, anorexia, fatigue, myalgias, headache, nausea, vomiting, or diarrhea may suggest necrotizing vasculitis, infection, or malignant disease.

Diagnosis

Atheromatous embolization is frequently overlooked or misdiagnosed. No single laboratory test is diagnostic. Nonspecific findings such as elevation in the erythrocyte sedimentation rate, leukocytosis, or anemia may be present. Increased levels of serum amylase, hepatic transaminases, blood urea nitrogen, or serum creatinine may be noted if the pancreas, liver, or kidney is involved. The urine sediment may be abnormal but is nonspecific. Eosinophilia and eosinophiluria may be present early in the course, and hypocomplementemia has been reported in a small number of series. Biopsy remains the most specific way to make the diagnosis, but it is often not required because the clinical findings may be highly suggestive of atheromatous embolization.

On arteriography, a markedly irregular and shaggy aorta may be demonstrated. Transesophageal echocardiography may detect mobile, protruding atheroma, which are associated with a very high risk for future embolization.

Atheromatous embolization may mimic vasculitis, such as polyarteritis nodosa or leukocytoclastic vasculitis, or it may suggest an underlying malignant disease, nonbacterial thrombotic endocarditis, subacute bacterial endocarditis, multiple myeloma, the anti–phospholipid antibody syndrome, or atrial myxoma. A cardiac source of emboli should always be excluded.

Treatment

Rx

The treatment of atheromatous embolization should be directed toward three goals: (1) removal of the source of atheromatous material (by surgical exclusion and bypass, percutaneous transluminal angioplasty, stent implantation, or stent grafting), (2) symptomatic care of the end organs in which the emboli are located, and (3) risk factor modification to prevent the progression of atherosclerosis.

Pain control and local care of ischemic ulcers are critical to the management of patients with atheromatous embolization. Intravenous prostaglandin analogues (iloprost, 0.5 ng/kg/minute to 2.0 ng/kg/minute continuously for 10 to 14 days followed by 8-hour infusions three times a week for an additional 2 to 3 weeks) may be useful in the healing of ischemic ulcerations and in controlling pain secondary to atheromatous embolization. Patients should be given antiplatelet therapy with aspirin (81 mg/day) and clopidogrel (75 mg/day). Use of anticoagulants such as heparin or warfarin should be avoided unless a compelling reason exists to use this class of drugs. If a vasospastic component is present, a dihydropyridine calcium-channel blocker (amlodipine, 2.5 to 10 mg/day, or nifedipine extended release, 30 to 120 mg/day) may be effective in relieving some of the symptoms. Chemical or surgical sympathectomy or spinal cord stimulators have been helpful for ulcer healing and pain relief in some patients.

Covered stents or stent grafts, which can be inserted in the thoracic or abdominal aorta for aneurysms or occlusive disease, are now the treatment of choice to prevent future embolic events when such approaches are technically feasible. In other cases, surgical bypass therapy is the next alternative, although patients who are poor surgical risks may require ligation of the common femoral arteries followed by an extra-anatomic bypass such as an axillobifemoral bypass.

Patients with atheromatous embolization generally have advanced atherosclerosis and a poor prognosis. Patients should receive appropriate risk factor modification (Chapter 70) to slow the progression of atherosclerosis and to improve overall cardiac and cerebrovascular morbidity and mortality. Statins may reduce the risk of embolic events.

THROMBOANGIITIS OBLITERANS (BUERGER'S DISEASE)

Definition

Thromboangiitis obliterans (Buerger's disease) is a nonatherosclerotic, segmental, inflammatory disease that most commonly affects the small and medium-sized arteries and veins in the upper and lower extremities. The origin of Buerger's disease is unknown, but an extremely strong association exists with heavy tobacco use, and progression of the disease is closely linked to continued tobacco use.

Epidemiology

Buerger's disease has a worldwide distribution, but it is more prevalent in the Middle East, Near East, and Far East than in North America and Western Europe. The prevalence of Buerger's disease is decreasing as the consumption of tobacco products declines.

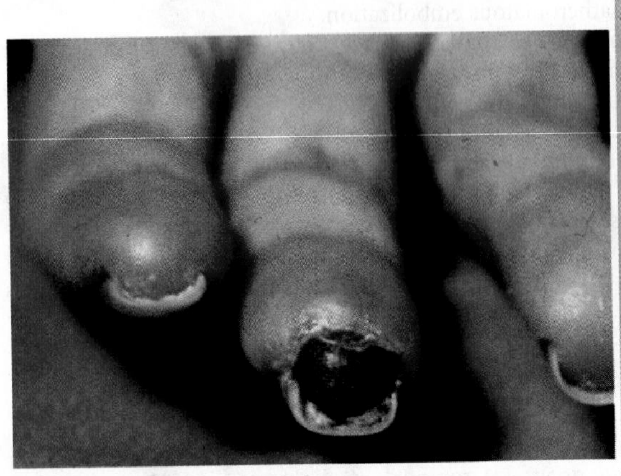

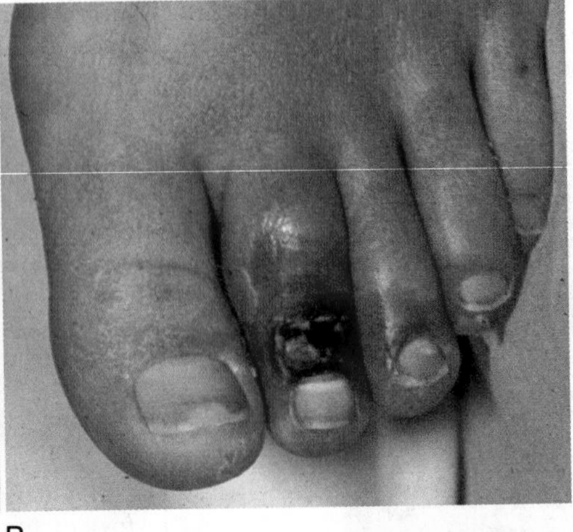

FIGURE 80–3 • Buerger's disease. Ischemic finger of a young male patient **(A)** and ischemic toe of a 28-year-old woman **(B)** with Buerger's disease.

Pathobiology

Patients with Buerger's disease may be hypercoagulable, and some patients have anti–endothelial cell antibodies, anticollagen antibodies, circulating immune complexes, and/or impaired endothelial-dependent vasorelaxation. Patients with thromboangiitis obliterans also have an increase in cellular sensitivity to type I and III collagen (normal constituents of human arteries).

In the acute phase of thromboangiitis obliterans, a highly inflammatory thrombus may affect both the arteries and veins. The lesion is characterized by acute inflammation involving all layers of the vessel wall in association with occlusive inflammatory cellular thrombosis. Around the periphery of the thrombus, one may see polymorphonuclear leukocytes with karyorrhexis, the so-called microabscess in which one or more multinucleated giant cells may be present. The acute phase lesion is followed by an intermediate phase characterized by progressive organization of the acute occlusive thrombus in the arteries and veins; a prominent, inflammatory cellular infiltrate may persist within the thrombus. The chronic phase or end-stage lesion is characterized by complete organization of the occlusive thrombus with extensive recanalization, prominent vascularization of the media and adventitia, and perivascular fibrosis.

Clinical Manifestations

Classically, Buerger's disease occurs in young male smokers, with the onset of symptoms before the age of 40 to 45 years, but 20 to 30% of patients with Buerger's disease may be women. Buerger's disease usually begins with ischemia of the toes, feet, fingers, and hands (Fig. 80–3). As the disease progresses, it may involve more proximal arteries, but involvement of large arteries is unusual.

Patients may present with claudication of the foot, the legs, and occasionally the arms and hands. Foot or arch claudication may be the presenting manifestation and is often mistaken for an orthopedic problem. Seventy-five to 80% of patients present with ischemic rest pain and/or ulcerations. Two or more limbs are always involved, and angiographic abnormalities are consistently found in limbs that are not yet clinically involved. Superficial thrombophlebitis and Raynaud's phenomenon each occur in approximately 40% of patients.

A positive Allen test indicates the distal nature of thromboangiitis obliterans and its involvement of the lower and upper extremities, to help differentiate it from atherosclerosis. In this test, the physician simultaneously occludes both the radial and the ulnar arteries. When pressure is released from either artery, one should note prompt filling from that artery, with the return of color to the hand. A positive test result is indicated when color does not return to the blanched hand.

Diagnosis

No specific laboratory tests aid in the diagnosis of Buerger's disease, but tests should exclude vasculitis, hypercoagulable states, anti–phospholipid antibodies, and a proximal source of emboli. On arteriography, the proximal arteries are normal, and the disease is most often infrapopliteal in the lower extremities and distal to the brachial artery in the upper extremities. Multiple vascular occlusions with collateralization around the obstruction (corkscrew collaterals) may occur, similar to what may be seen in other small vessel occlusive diseases such as the CREST (calcinosis cutis, Raynaud's phenomenon, esophageal motility disorder, sclerodactyly, and telangiectasias) syndrome or scleroderma (Chapter 288). However, the arteriographic appearance of Buerger's disease may also be identical to that seen in patients with systemic lupus erythematosus (Chapter 287), rheumatoid vasculitis (Chapter 291), mixed connective tissue diseases (Chapter 281), and anti–phospholipid antibody syndrome (Chapter 182), although the diagnosis of these other diseases can usually be established or excluded by other tests. Patients with Takayasu's arteritis (Chapter 75) or giant cell arteritis (Chapter 292) present with proximal vascular involvement and can readily be distinguished from patients with Buerger's disease.

Treatment

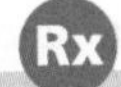

The cornerstone of therapy for thromboangiitis obliterans is the complete discontinuation of cigarette smoking or tobacco use in any form. Patients who stop using tobacco almost always avoid amputations, whereas 40% or more of patients who continue tobacco use progress to one or more amputations.

In a randomized trial, intravenous iloprost was superior to aspirin at 28 days in relieving rest pain and in healing all ischemic ulcerations. At 6 months, 88% of patients receiving iloprost (0.5 to 2.0 ng/kg/minute, maintaining hemodynamic stability for 6 hours daily for up to 28 days) responded to therapy, compared with 21% in the aspirin-treated group; only 6% underwent amputation in the iloprost-treated group, compared with 18% in the aspirin-treated group. [1] Other treatments such as calcium-channel blockers (amlodipine, 2.5 to 10 mg/day, or nifedipine extended release, 30 to 120 mg/day), antibiotics, and anticoagulants, as well as sympathectomy, are palliative.

Surgical bypass is not a viable option in most patients because they may not have a distal target vessel with which to bypass. Sympathectomy and implantable spinal cord stimulators may help some patients. Vascular endothelial growth factor has helped in healing ischemic ulcers and in preventing amputation in patients with Buerger's disease. Other therapies that have been used with some success include placing a Kirschner wire in the medullary canal of the tibia to stimulate angiogenesis, the use of intermittent pneumatic compression to enhance blood flow to the foot, and the use of endothelin antagonists such as bosentan.

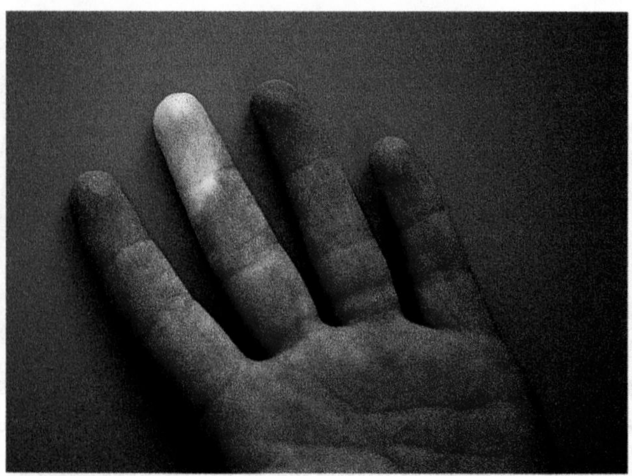

FIGURE 80–4 • Raynaud's phenomenon in the acute phase, with severe blanching of the tip of one finger. (From Forbes CD, Jackson WF: Color Atlas and Text of Clinical Medicine, 3rd ed. London, Mosby, 2003.)

TABLE 80–1 DIFFERENTIATING PRIMARY FROM SECONDARY RAYNAUD'S PHENOMENON

Characteristics	Primary	Secondary
Associated diseases	No	Yes
Age at onset	Younger (<30 yr)	Older (>30 yr)
Nailfold capillaries	Normal	Large, tortuous with "dropout"
Autoantibodies	Negative or low titers	Frequent
Endothelial cell activation	Yes	Yes
Endothelial damage	No	Frequent
Structural occlusion	No	Yes
Digital gangrene	Rare; only superficial	Common
α_2-Adrenergic activity	High	High
Calcitonin gene–related peptide	Low	Low

From Block JA, Sequeira W: Raynaud's phenomenon. Lancet 2001;357:2042–2048.

VASCULAR DISEASES ASSOCIATED WITH CHANGES IN TEMPERATURE

Raynaud's Phenomenon

Definition

Raynaud's phenomenon is the abrupt onset of a triphasic color response: well-demarcated pallor of the digits progressing to cyanosis with pain and often numbness followed by reactive hyperemia on rewarming. This vasospastic phenomenon is often precipitated by cold exposure or stress. *Primary Raynaud's phenomenon* denotes patients who have no underlying cause, whereas *secondary Raynaud's phenomenon* is associated with or caused by some other systemic illness or disease process (Fig. 80–4).

Epidemiology

Raynaud's phenomenon is common in patients with connective tissue diseases. Approximately 90% of patients with scleroderma (Chapter 288) experience Raynaud's phenomenon, and it may be a presenting manifestation in many patients with scleroderma. Raynaud's phenomenon is also a component of the CREST syndrome. These patients have small vessel occlusive disease that may lead to digital pitting or ulceration and eventual amputation.

The β-adrenergic receptor antagonists are the most common drugs associated with Raynaud's phenomenon because they block the vasodilatory β-receptors and thus leave the vasoconstrictive α-receptors unopposed. Ergotamine preparations, polyvinyl chloride, and several cancer chemotherapeutic agents can also cause Raynaud's phenomenon.

Raynaud's phenomenon is common in individuals who use vibratory tools such as pneumatic hammers, chain saws, sanders, and grinders. This syndrome has been termed the *hand-arm vibration syndrome,* and the prevalence of Raynaud's phenomenon may exceed 90% at 10 years in individuals with heavy exposure. Continued use of vibratory tools can lead to chronic occlusive small vessel vascular disease. The syndrome has also been described in typists, pianists, meat cutters, and sewing machine operators.

Trauma to the distal ulnar artery (several centimeters distal to the wrist) may occur with activities such as pounding with the palm of the hand, karate, or other activities that traumatize the hypothenar eminence and lead to an aneurysm or pseudoaneurysm of the distal ulnar artery (hypothenar hammer syndrome). Thrombus within the aneurysm may then embolize to the fingers, or the distal ulnar artery may thrombose.

Pathobiology

The initial manifestation of Raynaud's phenomenon occurs when the digits turn white as a result of the intense vasoconstriction or spasm of the digital arteries. At this point, blood flow ceases totally, and the digits are often numb. As the arterial vasoconstriction becomes less severe, postcapillary venule constriction causes the blood in the capillaries and veins to become deoxygenated, thus producing the cyanotic appearance. When rewarming occurs, blood flow is markedly increased, producing reactive hyperemia to the digits (red color).

The pathophysiologic factors operative in Raynaud's phenomenon include vascular, neural, and intravascular abnormalities. Vascular factors include small vessel occlusive disease, such as seen in scleroderma, and functional abnormalities, such as impaired endothelium-dependent and endothelium-independent vasodilatation, reduced production of vasodilators, and increased vasoconstriction. Neural abnormalities include impairment in sympathetic nervous system activity that disturbs the balance between vasoconstriction and vasodilatation. Intravascular factors such as platelet activation, impaired fibrinolysis, white blood cell activation, reduced red blood cell deformability, and oxidative stress may play important roles in some patients.

Clinical Manifestations

The symptoms of Raynaud's phenomenon may include pallor (see Fig. 80–4), cyanosis, and reactive hyperemia. The triphasic color response occurs in 4 to 65% of patients. Exposure to the cold is the typical precipitating factor, but emotional lability may also cause or exacerbate attacks in some patients. Vasospastic attacks usually occur only in the fingers, but vasospasm can occur in the toes, nose, ears, lips, and other body parts.

In primary Raynaud's disease, the physical examination is normal between attacks. However, in patients with secondary Raynaud's phenomenon, pits or ulcerations on the fingertips may be present in patients with scleroderma, CREST syndrome, or thromboangiitis obliterans. An abnormal result of the Allen test on physical examination indicates fixed arterial obstruction.

Diagnosis

The diagnosis of Raynaud's phenomenon is not difficult when it is based on the patient's description of the attacks. Patients with persistent cyanosis or persistent hyperemia generally have some condition other than Raynaud's phenomenon. In primary Raynaud's phenomenon, vasospastic attacks are precipitated by exposure to the cold or emotional stimuli, there is bilateral involvement of the extremities without gangrene, and, after a careful search, no evidence indicates underlying systemic diseases that could be responsible for the vasospastic attacks (Table 80–1).

To evaluate systemic illnesses, a serologic evaluation should include a complete blood cell count, multiphasic serologic analysis, urinalysis,

Westergren sedimentation rate, C-reactive protein, antinuclear antibody, extractable nuclear antigen (anti-Smith and ribonuclear protein), anti-DNA, cryoglobulins, complement, anticentromere antibodies, and SCL70 scleroderma antibodies. In addition, nailfold capillaroscopy can be performed to help confirm a diagnosis of CREST syndrome or scleroderma in patients in whom the symptoms are not clear. An abnormal nailfold capillaroscopy result indicates that the patient does not have primary Raynaud's phenomenon.

The noninvasive vascular laboratory (pulse volume recordings) is useful in identifying the degree of digital arterial occlusive disease (fixed ischemia) and in predicting whether ischemic ulcerations on the digits will heal. Arteriography is not routinely performed.

Treatment

Rx

In patients with mild vasospastic attacks, reassurance about the benign nature of the disease and instructions on how to prevent attacks are often all that is needed. Patients should limit the amount of exposure to the cold and should dress warmly and protect not only their extremities but also their entire body. Smoking should be avoided because nicotine causes intense vasoconstriction. β-Blocking agents may exaggerate the symptoms of Raynaud's phenomenon. Mittens are better than gloves for keeping the hands warm. Patients need to be especially careful when they handle cold objects. Hand- and foot-warming devices (battery operated or chemical) may be helpful. Conditioning techniques and biofeedback are sometimes helpful in controlling vasospastic episodes.

The dihydropyridine calcium-channel blocking drugs are the most effective pharmacotherapeutic agents for Raynaud's phenomenon. Patients who have infrequent attacks may benefit from a short-acting calcium-channel blocker such as nifedipine, 10 to 20 mg, given 30 minutes to 1 hour before cold exposure. When vasospasm occurs more frequently, the extended-release preparations of nifedipine (0 to 90 mg/day) or amlodipine (2.5 to 10 mg/day) should be used. α_1-Adrenergic receptor antagonists such as prazosin (1 to 10 mg twice daily) or terazosin (2 to 20 mg/day) are also highly effective in decreasing the severity, frequency, and duration of vasospastic attacks in patients.

Nitroglycerin can be used topically (0.1 to 0.8 mg/hour), whereas prostacyclin can be given intravenously. The angiotensin-converting enzyme inhibitors and the angiotensin receptor antagonists have shown some benefit in uncontrolled trials, but other vasodilators such as niacin and papaverine are not beneficial. Several reports have suggested a beneficial effect from selective serotonin reuptake inhibitors such as fluoxetine. Small case series suggest that cilostazol (100 mg twice daily one half hour before breakfast and one half hour before dinner) may improve ulcer healing in patients with secondary Raynaud's phenomenon. In a small randomized trial, sildenafil (50 mg/day) decreased the frequency and severity of Raynaud's episodes. 2

Although sympathectomy may be beneficial in the short term, with about a 50% improvement rate, the vasospastic attacks may recur in 6 months to 2 years. Some patients with severe disease have had success with digital sympathectomy.

Prognosis

The prognosis in patients with primary Raynaud's phenomenon is excellent. No mortality is associated with this condition. In a long-term study involving 307 patients with primary Raynaud's disease, 38% had stable disease, 36% were improved, 16% were worsened, and the syndrome disappeared in 10%. The prognosis associated with secondary Raynaud's phenomenon depends on the underlying condition that caused it.

Pernio (Chilblains)

Definition and Epidemiology

Pernio (a Latin word that literally means "frostbite," although its synonym *chilblains* is an Anglo-Saxon term that means "cold sore") is a localized inflammatory lesion of the skin as a result of abnormal response to the cold. Up to 50% of women developed pernio in wartime conditions in northern Europe. Pernio is now less common but is still seen in the temperate, humid climates of northwestern Europe and in the northern United States.

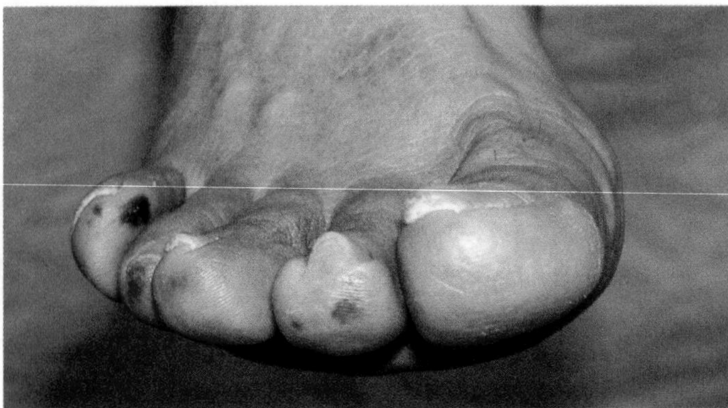

FIGURE 80–5 • Pernio on the toes of the right foot. The lesions on the second, third, and fourth toes are the typical red, brown, and yellow scaling lesions. The lesion on the fifth toe can be confused with atheromatous embolization.

Pathobiology

Pernio develops in susceptible individuals who are exposed to nonfreezing cold. The pathologic changes include edema of the papillodermis, vasculitis characterized by perivascular infiltration (with lymphocytes) of the arterioles and venules of the dermis, thickening and edema of the blood vessel walls, fat necrosis, and chronic inflammatory reaction with giant cell formation.

Clinical Manifestations and Diagnosis

Pernio most commonly occurs in young women between the ages of 15 and 30 years, but it may occur in older individuals or in children. Acute pernio may develop 12 to 24 hours after exposure to the cold. Single or multiple erythematous, purplish, edematous lesions appear, accompanied by intense itching or burning. These lesions may have a yellowish or brownish discoloration and may be associated with some flaking. They tend to affect the toes and dorsum of the proximal phalanges. The lesions of acute pernio are usually self-limited, although they may lead to recurrent disease. The arterial circulation is normal on physical examination and in the noninvasive vascular laboratory. Chronic pernio occurs when repeated exposure to the cold results in the persistence of lesions with subsequent scarring and atrophy. Characteristically, the lesions begin in the fall or winter and disappear in the spring or early summer. In advanced cases, the seasonal variation may disappear, and chronic occlusive vascular disease may develop.

In the typical form, the patient develops violet or yellow-brown blisters and shallow toe ulcers that burn and itch (Fig. 80–5). The lesions first appear in the fall or winter and disappear each spring. The differential diagnosis of pernio includes recurrent, erythematous, nodular, and ulcerative lesions such as erythema induratum, nodular vasculitis, erythema nodosum, and cold panniculitis. The skin lesions of pernio may resemble those of atheromatous embolization (see earlier), and an arteriogram may sometimes be required.

Prevention and Treatment

Prevention is the best form of therapy. Cold exposure should be minimized as much as possible. In a randomized trial, nifedipine reduced the pain and facilitated the healing process. 3 The severe itching may be treated with local application of an antipruritic agent.

Acrocyanosis

Acrocyanosis, which is a persistent blue or cyanotic discoloration of the digits, occurs most commonly in the hands and may worsen with exposure to cold and improve with rewarming. The primary form is a benign cosmetic condition, but it may also be seen in patients with connective tissue diseases, thromboangiitis obliterans, and diseases associated with central cyanosis. The exact pathophysiologic abnormality is not clear but may be vasospasm in the cutaneous arteries and arterioles with compensatory dilatation in the postcapillary venules.

Ulceration or tissue loss is unusual, and the overall prognosis is excellent. Patients should be advised to keep their extremities warm. Drugs such as α-adrenergic blocking agents (prazosin, 1 to 10 mg twice daily, or terazosin, 2 to 20 mg/day) or calcium-channel blockers (amlodipine, 2.5 to 10 mg/day, or nifedipine extended release, 30 to 120 mg/day) may be helpful.

Frostbite

Epidemiology and Pathobiology

Frostbite is freezing of tissues resulting from exposure to cold. It may occur in above-freezing temperatures under circumstances such as wetness, strong wind, or high altitude.

A person's response to cold is aimed at conserving the core (internal body) temperature as well as the viability of the extremity. Heat loss is reduced by peripheral vasoconstriction caused by sympathetic stimulation and catecholamine release. Maintenance or augmentation of body heat is accomplished by muscular activity such as shivering. However, the heat production from shivering cannot be sustained for more than a few hours because of the depletion of glycogen, which is the source of heat during shivering. The extremities are also protected by the "hunting reaction," which consists of irregular, 5- to 10-minute cycles of alternating periods of vasoconstriction and vasodilatation that protect the extremities against excessive sustained vasoconstriction at minimal loss of internal body temperature. However, when the body is exposed to cold of a magnitude or duration that threatens the internal body temperature, this mechanism fails. Because the disruption of core temperature is more deleterious to the body than peripheral vasoconstriction, conservation of core temperature takes precedence over rewarming of the extremities, and the hunting response is replaced by continuous and more intense vasoconstriction that promotes frostbite by means of ice crystal formation, cellular dehydration, and thrombosis of the microvasculature.

Clinical Manifestations and Diagnosis

Soon after exposure to the cold, pain develops and gradually progresses to numbness; the frozen part turns white because of intense vasoconstriction (Fig. 80–6). With rewarming or thawing, the circulation is restored, and the affected parts become hyperemic. Edema may first occur within hours of thawing and remains for days or weeks. Blisters appear within the first 24 hours and are reabsorbed within 1 to 2 weeks, after which a black eschar may persist. Overactivity of the sympathetic nervous system is manifested by hyperhidrosis or a burning sensation.

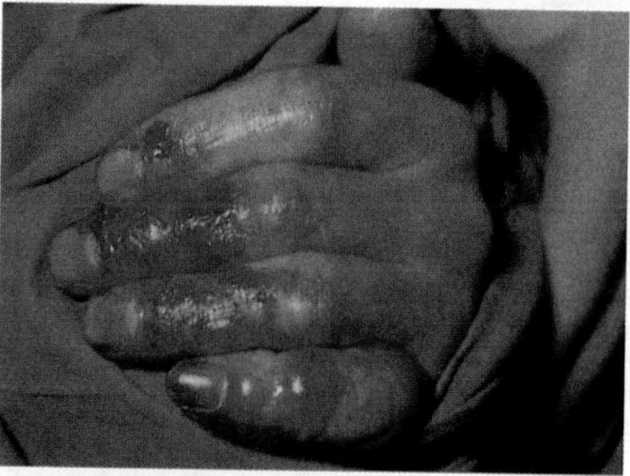

FIGURE 80–6 • Frostbite of the hand in a mountaineer. On rewarming, the hand became painful, red, and edematous, with signs of probable gangrene in the fifth finger. (From Forbes CD, Jackson WF: Color Atlas and Text of Clinical Medicine, 3rd ed. London, Mosby, 2003.)

Seventy percent of victims develop chronic sequelae including cold sensitivity, pain, and sensory disturbances, often resembling reflex sympathetic dystrophy. Frostbite arthritis may occur in particularly severe cases.

It is important to establish the depth of the frostbite and to determine whether the tissue is viable. This may not be obvious on initial clinical examination but is usually determined weeks or months after the cold injury, when the demarcation zone appears and the dead tissue is sloughed.

Treatment

Rx

In mild cases of frostbite, the only necessary treatment may be daily whirlpool baths with bedrest. However, treatment of deep frostbite should be considered a medical emergency because the early institution of medical therapy may reduce the amount of subsequent tissue loss. Thawing, the mainstay of therapy, should not be implemented if the patient may be exposed to cold again because refreezing of thawed tissue promotes further tissue damage. Walking on a frozen limb produces substantially less damage than walking on a thawed limb.

After transfer to a medical facility, frozen tissue should be rapidly rewarmed in a water bath of 40 to 42° C (104 to 108° F) for 15 to 30 minutes until complete thawing has occurred. After thawing, reappearance of normal color signifies the reestablishment of blood flow. Thawing is often a painful process and may require the administration of narcotics.

After thawing, the extremity should be cleansed twice daily in a whirlpool bath with an aseptic solution at 35 to 37° C (95 to 99° F). Care should be taken to prevent and treat secondary infections. Tetanus prophylaxis should be administered. A frostbite protocol consisting of débridement of clear blisters with a topical application of aloe vera, oral ibuprofen, and daily hydrotherapy is highly effective. An important principle is to avoid early débridement or amputation, which is indicated only when infected gangrene or generalized sepsis occurs.

ERYTHROMELALGIA

Definition and Epidemiology

Erythromelalgia literally means red, painful extremities. It may be classified as primary (or idiopathic), which may be nonfamilial or familial. A secondary category is associated with other diseases, the most common being myeloproliferative disorders such as polycythemia vera and essential thrombocythemia. Other diseases associated with secondary erythromelalgia include hypertension, diabetes, rheumatoid arthritis, gout, spinal cord disease, multiple sclerosis, systemic lupus erythematosus, cutaneous vasculitis, and viral infection; it also may result from therapy with various drugs (e.g., nifedipine, nicardipine, verapamil, bromocriptine, and pergolide).

Pathobiology

Families with autosomal dominant erythromelalgia have demonstrated mutations in the sodium channel $Na_v1.7$, which is selectively expressed within the nociceptive dorsal root ganglion and sympathetic ganglion neurons. The histologic features vary from normal findings to arterial occlusion with thrombus formation.

Clinical Manifestations and Diagnosis

Erythromelalgia is characterized by the clinical triad of erythema, burning pain, and increased temperature usually of the extremities. The feet, especially the soles, are more commonly involved than the hands. The peripheral pulses are generally normal in the primary type and variable in secondary erythromelalgia. The symptoms may occur in "attacks" that last for minutes to hours and occasionally days and are precipitated by a warm environment. Exercise and dependency tend to exacerbate symptoms. Patients seek relief by exposing the affected extremity to a cooler environment, such as placing the extremity in cold water, walking on a cold floor barefoot, or running an air conditioner even in the winter. This response often leads to a cold-induced vascular injury superimposed on the erythromelalgia. Erythromelalgia may precede the clinical appearance of a myeloproliferative disorder by several years, so patients older than age 30 years should be monitored periodically with blood cell counts.

Treatment

The treatment of erythromelalgia is often difficult and frustrating. Symptoms can be so debilitating that they lead to suicide. In secondary erythromelalgia, treatment of the underlying disease (phlebotomy in patients with polycythemia vera and normalization of the platelet count in patients with thrombocythemia) may relieve the symptoms. Aspirin (81 to 325 mg/day) is the most effective treatment available, particularly for patients with erythromelalgia secondary to myeloproliferative disorders. Other therapies with variable success in case reports include methysergide, ephedrine, nonsteroidal anti-inflammatory drugs, phenoxybenzamine, nitroglycerin, sodium nitroprusside, corticosteroids, and surgical sympathectomy. Lidocaine transdermal (Lidoderm) patches on the feet and thalamic stimulation have also been used anecdotally.

POPLITEAL ARTERY ENTRAPMENT SYNDROME

In the *popliteal artery entrapment syndrome*, the popliteal artery is compressed as a result of a congenital anatomic abnormality or an abnormal muscle or fibrous band. In the most frequent abnormality, the medial head of the gastrocnemius muscle compresses the popliteal artery and causes medial deviation of the artery.

The clinical presentation is in a healthy, "athletic-type" male patient complaining of typical claudication symptoms in the absence of premature atherosclerosis. Disappearance of the pulse with passive dorsiflexion of the foot or active plantar flexion against resistance may suggest the diagnosis. Duplex ultrasound may help, and computed tomography or magnetic resonance imaging can confirm the diagnosis. On arteriography, the characteristic finding is medial deviation of the popliteal artery with post-stenotic dilation. Other diseases that can cause mid-popliteal occlusion include cystic adventitial disease, thrombosed popliteal artery aneurysm, and atherosclerosis of the superficial femoral and popliteal arteries. The primary treatment of popliteal artery entrapment syndrome is surgical.

CYSTIC ADVENTITIAL DISEASE

In *cystic adventitial disease*, gelatinous fluid accumulates in an arterial wall cyst, and then the cyst encroaches on the vessel lumen, with resulting stenosis or occlusion. The cyst arises in the outer portion of the media or subadventitial layer, most commonly in the popliteal artery. Cystic adventitial disease is an isolated lesion not associated with a systemic process, and the precise pathophysiologic mechanism is unknown.

The disease predominates in men, with an approximate ratio of 5 : 1, and the mean age at diagnosis is about 45 years. Claudication is the most frequent symptom. The pulses may disappear on flexion of the knee (Ishikawa's sign). However, if the artery is occluded, no pulses are palpable.

Pulse volume recordings may show the characteristic decrease in blood pressure and the change in waveform configuration in the affected limb. A perivascular cystic structure may be visualized on duplex ultrasound. Computed tomography or magnetic resonance imaging can show the anatomy in the popliteal region. Computed tomography–guided needle aspiration can partially but usually not completely remove the highly viscous and gelatinous fluid. If arterial occlusion has occurred, catheter-directed thrombolytic therapy and surgical resection are indicated.

FIBROMUSCULAR DYSPLASIA OF THE EXTREMITIES

Although *fibromuscular dysplasia* (in particular, medial fibroplasia) is most common in the renal and carotid arteries (Chapter 126), it may also occur in peripheral arteries of the extremity (iliac, superficial femoral, popliteal, tibial, subclavian, axillary, radial, and ulnar). These lesions may be asymptomatic, or they may produce a difference in blood pressure between the two limbs, with paresthesias, claudication, or critical limb ischemia.

The typical arteriographic appearance of a "string of beads" is virtually pathognomonic of medial fibroplasia. Long, smooth areas of narrowing are characteristic of intimal fibroplasia, but they may also be seen in Takayasu's arteritis (Chapter 78) and giant cell arteritis (Chapters 78 and 292).

Therapy should be reserved for symptomatic disease. Under most circumstances, percutaneous balloon dilatation is the treatment of choice.

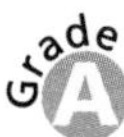

1. Fiessinger JN, Schafer M: Trial of iloprost versus aspirin treatment for critical limb ischaemia of thromboangiitis obliterans: The TAO Study. Lancet 1990;335:555–557.
2. Fries R, Shariat K, von Wilmowsky H, et al: Sildenafil in the treatment of Raynaud's phenomenon resistant to vasodilatory therapy. Circulation 2005;112:2894–2895.
3. Rustin MH, Newton JA, Smith NP, et al: The treatment of chilblains with nifedipine: The results of a pilot study, a double-blind placebo-controlled randomized study and a long-term open trial. Br J Dermatol 1989;120:267–275.

SUGGESTED READINGS

Boin F, Wigley FM: Understanding, assessing and treating Raynaud's phenomenon. Curr Opin Rheumatol 2005;17:752–760. *Current pathophysiology and treatment in patients with Raynaud's phenomenon.*

Davis JD, O'Fallon WM, Rogers RS 3rd, et al: Natural history of erythromelalgia: Presentation and outcome in 168 patients. Arch Dermatol 2000;136:406–409. *A large series of patients with erythromelalgia describing the clinical presentation as well as the natural history of the disease.*

Olin JW, Shih A: Thromboangiitis obliterans (Buerger's disease). Curr Opin Rheumatol 2006;18:18–24. *A contemporary review of the clinical manifestations, pathogenesis, and treatment of thromboangiitis obliterans.*

Slovut DP, Olin JW: Fibromuscular dysplasia. N Engl J Med 2004;350:1862–1871. *Classification, clinical manifestations, and treatment options in patients with fibromuscular dysplasia of the renal, carotid, and peripheral arteries.*

81 PERIPHERAL VENOUS DISEASE

Jeffrey Ginsberg

DEEP VENOUS THROMBOSIS

Definition

Deep venous thrombosis (DVT), which is the most important disease affecting the peripheral veins, has an estimated annual incidence of 0.1% in white populations. Most pulmonary emboli (Chapter 99) arise from DVT of the legs. In fact, DVT and pulmonary embolism are usually considered to be different clinical manifestations of one disease, venous thromboembolism (VTE), because up to 50% of patients who present with proximal (popliteal vein or more proximal) DVT will have abnormal lung scans suggestive of clinically silent pulmonary emboli, whereas up to 90% of patients with proven pulmonary emboli will have DVT, even though only 15% of them have leg symptoms. For the most part, the cornerstones of management of DVT and pulmonary embolism are the same, immediate and long-term anticoagulation.

Superficial thrombophlebitis consists of thrombosis and inflammation of one or more superficial veins. Provided the associated thrombus has not extended into the deep veins, affected patients have a negligible risk for development of pulmonary emboli and can often be effectively managed conservatively with ice, elevation, and anti-inflammatory medication.

Epidemiology

DVT usually originates in one of the distal or calf veins, where it has little or no potential to cause clinically important pulmonary emboli. The true incidence of calf vein thrombosis is not known because many affected patients remain asymptomatic while the thrombus forms and spontaneously resolves. On the basis of results of studies of *symptomatic* patients with suspected DVT, about 10 to 25% actually have a diagnosable DVT, of whom about 15% have isolated calf DVT. Approximately one quarter of these thrombi that are initially isolated to a calf vein will subsequently extend into the proximal veins, usually within a week of presentation, where they *then* have the potential to cause pulmonary emboli.

From a clinical perspective, risk factors can be subdivided by duration, that is, transient and finite duration (e.g., fractured fibula treated with plaster immobilization) compared with permanent or long term (e.g., congenital antithrombin deficiency, metastatic cancer), and according to the magnitude of the risk, that is, major (hip or knee replacement surgery) or minor (long-distance air travel, use of oral contraceptives). Classification of patients according to the presence or absence and type of risk factor is predictive of the risk of recurrence after a prolonged (≥3 months) course of anticoagulant therapy and provides key information that helps determine the optimal duration of anticoagulant therapy. Patients in whom DVT develops in association with a major risk factor that has resolved have a much lower risk of recurrence after a 3-month course of anticoagulants than do patients whose DVT was associated with a transient minor risk factor that has resolved or patients whose DVT was apparently idiopathic or associated with an ongoing risk factor.

Pathobiology

Virchow's triad of hypercoagulability, venous stasis, and injury to the vessel wall provides a useful model for understanding many of the risk factors that lead to the formation of thrombosis. For example, in patients who have total hip or knee replacement surgery, there is venous endothelial injury caused by surgery, venous stasis due to perioperative immobilization, and hypercoagulability as a result of postoperative fibrinolytic shutdown. In other patients, an identifiable "thrombophilia" or "tendency to clot," such as congenital antithrombin (formerly antithrombin III) deficiency or the presence of factor V Leiden (Chapter 182), combined with use of oral contraceptives results in DVT in women of childbearing age. However, a relatively high proportion of patients have unexplained DVT without "clinical" risk factors that cause endothelial damage or venous stasis or identifiable thrombophilias that cause hypercoagulability. Undoubtedly some of these patients have yet to be determined thrombophilias, but the DVT currently is labeled idiopathic.

Clinical Manifestations

The clinical features of lower extremity DVT include leg pain, tenderness, swelling (Fig. 81–1), palpable cord, discoloration, venous distention, prominence of the superficial veins, and cyanosis. In most patients in whom DVT is clinically suspected, the symptoms and signs are nonspecific; in more than 50% of these patients, the clinical suspicion of DVT is not confirmed by objective testing. Conversely, patients with relatively minor symptoms and signs may have extensive DVT.

In some patients, DVT may be asymptomatic, but the patient will present with pulmonary embolism. Conversely, pulmonary embolism occurs in 50% of patients with objectively documented proximal leg vein thrombosis, but many of the emboli are asymptomatic. Usually, only part of the thrombus embolizes, so 50 to 70% of patients with angiographically documented pulmonary emboli have detectable DVT of the legs at the time of initial evaluation.

Diagnosis

By itself, clinical diagnosis of DVT is inaccurate because no individual symptom or sign is sufficiently sensitive or specific for the diagnosis to be made or excluded. Clinical assessment can categorize patients according to their pretest probability of DVT with reasonable accuracy. By combining a validated prediction rule (Table 81–1) to assess this pretest probability with the results of noninvasive tests, diagnostic accuracy can be improved, thereby often limiting or eliminating the need for further investigation (Fig. 81–2).

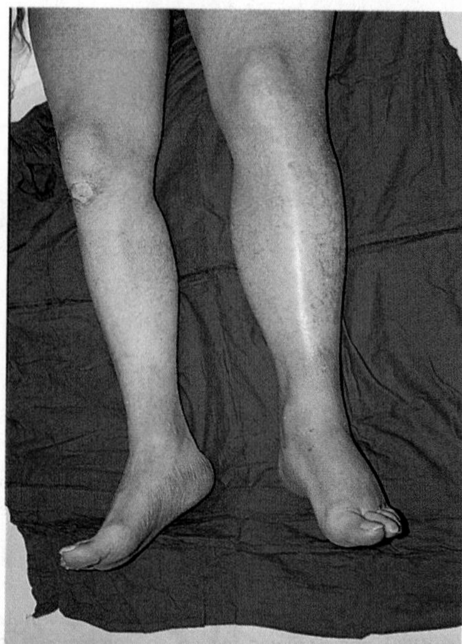

FIGURE 81–1 • Deep venous thrombosis (DVT) presenting as an acutely swollen left leg. Note the dilation of the superficial veins. The leg was hot to the touch, and palpation along the line of the left popliteal and femoral veins caused pain. Less than 50% of DVTs present in this way, and other conditions may mimic DVT, so further investigation is always indicated. Note the coincidental psoriatic lesion below the patient's right knee. (From Forbes CD, Jackson WF: Color Atlas and Text of Clinical Medicine, 3rd ed. London, Mosby, 2003, with permission.)

TABLE 81–1 PREDICTION RULE FOR DEEP VENOUS THROMBOSIS

Clinical Characteristic	Score
Active cancer (treatment ongoing within previous 6 months or palliative)	1
Paralysis, paresis, or recent plaster immobilization of the lower extremities	1
Recent bedrest >3 days or major surgery within 3 months requiring anesthesia	1
Localized tenderness of the deep veins of the leg	1
Entire leg swollen	1
Calf swelling >3 cm larger than asymptomatic side measured 10 cm below tibial tuberosity	1
Pitting edema confined to the symptomatic leg	1
Collateral superficial veins (not varicosed)	1
Previously documented DVT	1
Alternative diagnosis as likely as or more likely than DVT	−2

A score of 0 or less indicates low probability, 1 or 2 indicates moderate probability, and 3 or more indicates high probability.
Modified from Wells PS, Anderson DR, Bormanis J, et al: Value of assessment of pretest probability of deep-vein thrombosis in clinical management. Lancet 1997;350:1795–1798.

Imaging

Contrast Venography

Ascending contrast venography remains the "gold standard" for diagnosis, but because of its expense, discomfort to the patient, and potential for adverse experiences, venography is currently indicated in symptomatic patients only when diagnostic uncertainty persists after noninvasive testing or if noninvasive testing is unavailable. A constant

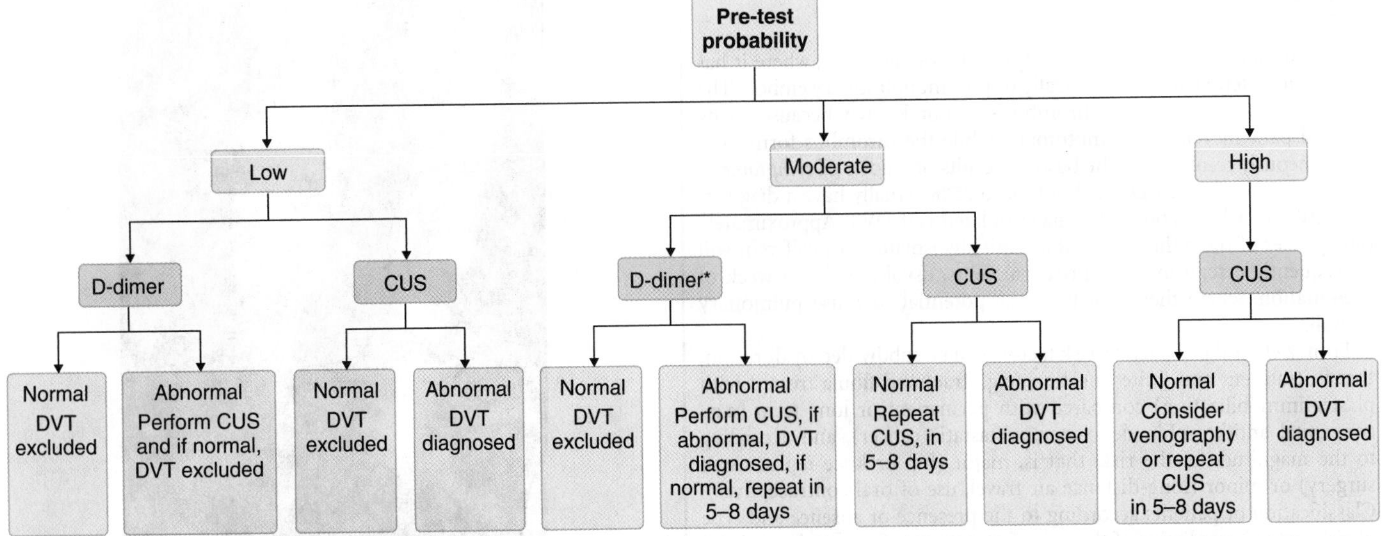

FIGURE 81–2 • Diagnostic algorithm for suspected deep venous thrombosis. This algorithm uses evaluation of pretest probability based on a clinical prediction rule (see Table 81–1) and D-dimer testing to complement compression ultrasonography (CUS). The asterisk indicates use of a highly sensitive (>95%) D-dimer.

intraluminal filling defect is diagnostic of acute thrombosis (Fig. 81–3), and DVT can essentially be excluded in patients who have a normal, adequately performed venogram. Minor side effects of local pain, nausea, and vomiting are not uncommon, whereas more serious adverse reactions, such as bronchospasm, are rare; however, venography itself can also induce DVT.

Compression Ultrasonography

Compression venous ultrasonography is currently the most widely used noninvasive test for suspected DVT because of its accuracy in detection of thrombus involving the popliteal or more proximal veins; absence of compressibility (Fig. 81–4) of the proximal leg veins on ultrasonography has a sensitivity of 97% and a specificity of 96% for symptomatic patients with suspected DVT. Thus, the finding of a noncompressible venous segment, particularly in the popliteal or common femoral vein, has a high positive predictive value for DVT in symptomatic patients and is an indication for treatment. Of patients with symptoms suggestive of DVT but with normal findings on initial ultrasound examination of the proximal veins, about 15% will have undetected isolated calf DVT; progression into the proximal veins occurs in a minority of patients, usually within a week of presentation. Isolated calf DVT that does not extend into the proximal veins is rarely if ever associated with clinically important pulmonary embolus. The sensitivity of ultrasonography for calf DVT is well below 90%, with a wide range of accuracies reported for different populations of patients.

Imaging of the calf veins is time-consuming, potentially inaccurate, and generally not recommended. Rather, two-point (common femoral and popliteal) or three-point (two-point plus the calf "trifurcation") ultrasonography should be performed and, if the results are normal, repeated in 1 week after the initial examination. This approach will identify the 20 to 25% of patients who have had proximal extension of distal clot in the calf veins. If the repeated ultrasound examination is normal, further investigation and therapy can be safely withheld. In centers with highly skilled operators, however, normal ultrasonography of the proximal and calf veins at presentation may be sufficiently accurate to exclude clinically important DVT; in these settings, further testing is unwarranted. The need for repeated testing can also be limited by either D-dimer testing or clinical assessment in conjunction with the ultrasound examination (see later).

Magnetic Resonance Venography

Magnetic resonance venography, which uses the difference in magnetic resonance signals between flowing blood and stationary clot, has a high sensitivity and specificity for proximal DVT but has not yet been used broadly in management trials. Recent interest has focused on magnetic resonance for direct imaging of the thrombus because a thrombus produces a positive image without the use of contrast material owing to its methemoglobin content.

Laboratory Findings

D-Dimer

D-dimer is a plasma protein specifically produced after lysis of cross-linked fibrin by plasmin. Levels are almost invariably elevated in the presence of acute VTE, so measurement of D-dimer levels is a sensitive test for recent DVT and pulmonary emboli. Unfortunately, numerous nonthrombotic conditions, including sepsis, pregnancy, surgery, and cardiac or renal failure, can also cause elevated levels. As a result of this nonspecificity, the role of D-dimer assays is limited to helping exclude VTE when levels are not raised.

Laboratory tests for D-dimer use enzyme-linked immunosorbent assay (ELISA) or agglutination techniques, both involving specific monoclonal antibodies. Sensitivity and cut points vary among assays, so results cannot be generalized. Highly sensitive tests, consisting of new rapid ELISA or immunoturbidimetric assays, have sensitivities of 95 to 100% for acute VTE but in general have low specificities (20 to 50%). Moderately sensitive tests, of which the SimpliRED red cell agglutination assay is the main example, have a reported sensitivity of approximately 90% but a higher specificity (~75%) for acute VTE. Highly sensitive D-dimer assays can be employed as "stand-alone tests" for exclusion of DVT, but clinicians must be aware of the accuracy of the assay in their institution before using the D-dimer assay to make management decisions.

Algorithms for Diagnosis of Deep Venous Thrombosis

A number of diagnostic algorithms have been tested in prospective management trials (see Fig. 81–2).

Clinical Assessment and Venous Ultrasonography

It is safe to perform only a single ultrasound examination in patients with a low pretest probability by a validated clinical prediction rule (Table 81–2). Other patients require serial ultrasonographic testing if only clinical assessment and ultrasonography are used. Venography should be considered in patients with a high pretest probability and normal compression ultrasonography because the probability of DVT is still approximately 20% in such patients.

Clinical Assessment, D-Dimer Testing, and Venous Ultrasonography

A normal D-dimer test result should not yet be used in isolation to exclude DVT. However, diagnostic imaging and treatment can be safely withheld in patients who have (1) a low pretest probability based on a validated clinical prediction rule and a negative value on a moderately sensitive D-dimer assay or (2) a low or intermediate pretest probability and a negative value on a highly sensitive D-dimer assay. Patients with a high pretest probability require ultrasonography regardless of the D-dimer result. A normal D-dimer result with use of either a moderately or highly sensitive assay can safely obviate the need for repeated imaging in patients with normal findings on initial ultrasound examination.

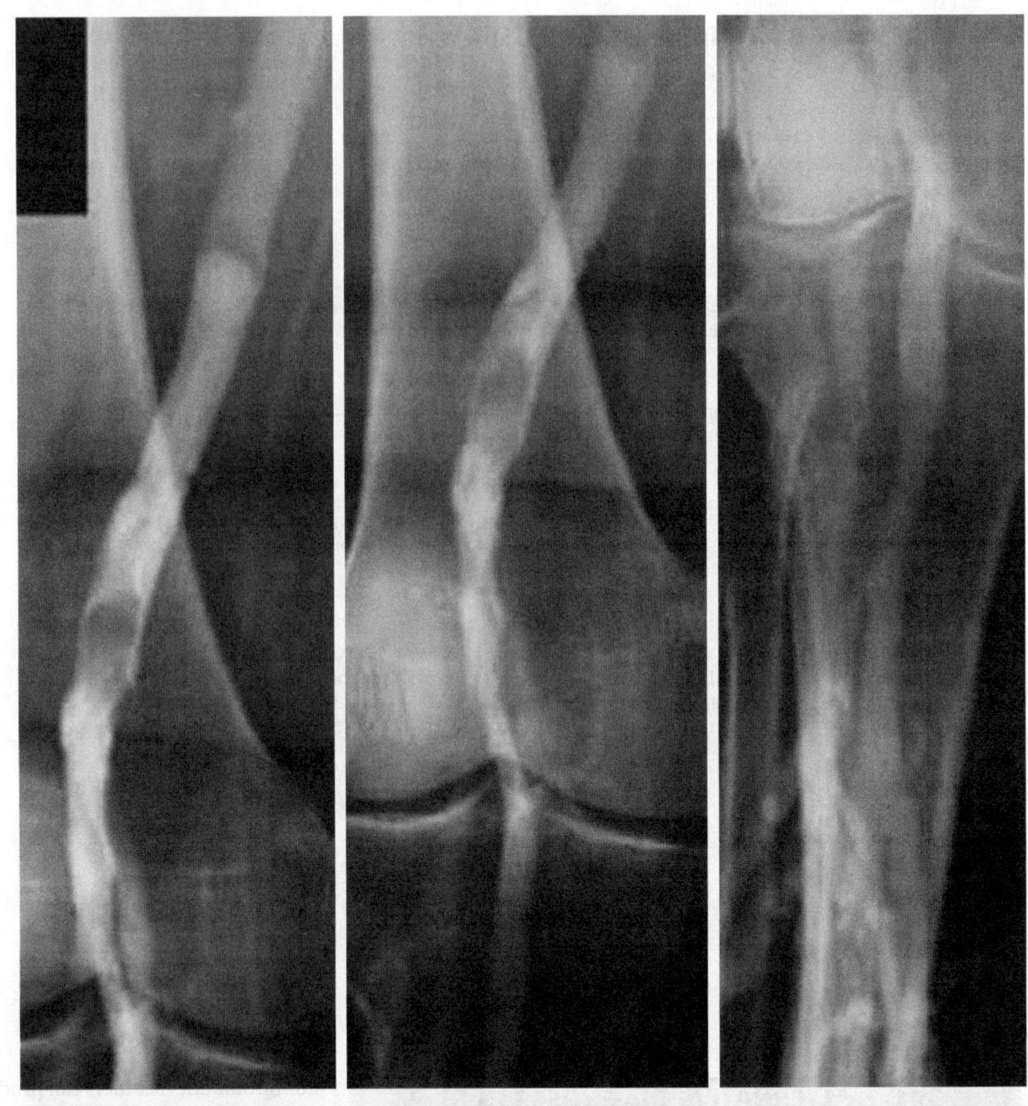

FIGURE 81–3 • Abnormal venogram demonstrates a persistent (two or more different views) intraluminal filling defect in the popliteal vein.

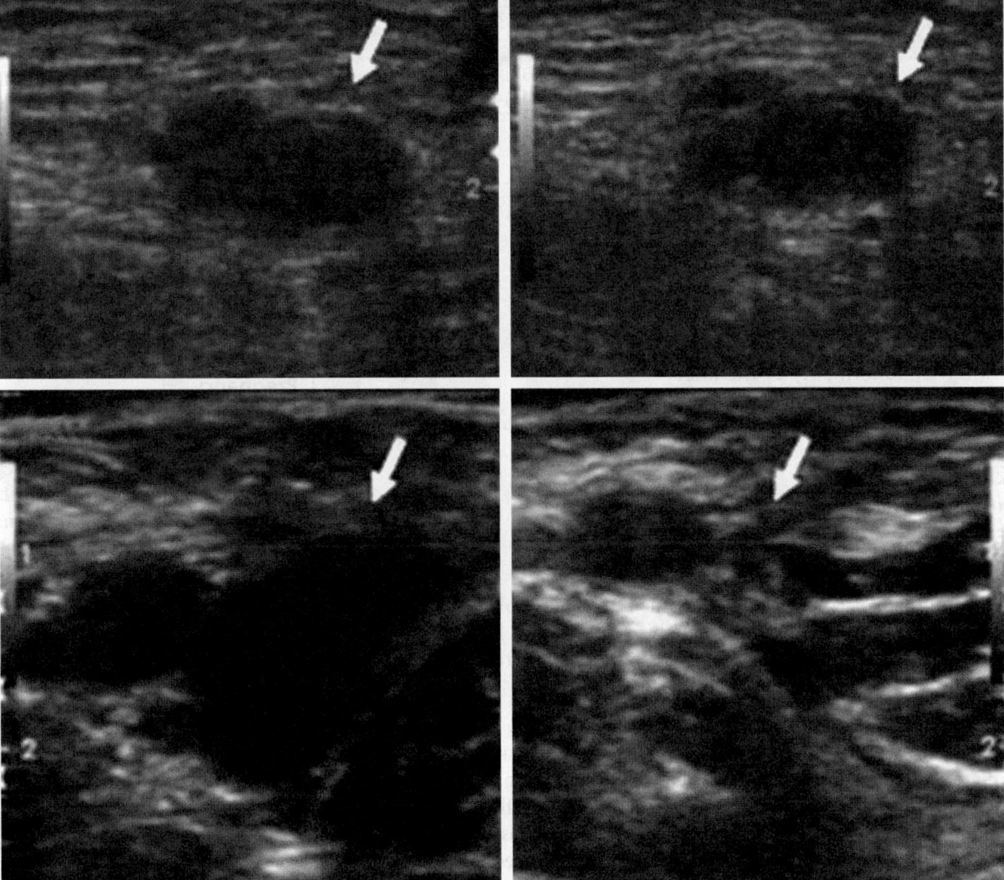

FIGURE 81–4 • Compression venous ultrasonography demonstrates thrombosis of the popliteal vein. The sonograms in the top row demonstrate examination without (left side) and with (right side) gentle probe compression of the skin overlying the popliteal vein. The lack of compressibility is diagnostic of deep venous thrombosis. The bottom row shows analogous views of the femoral vein, which shows partial compressibility.

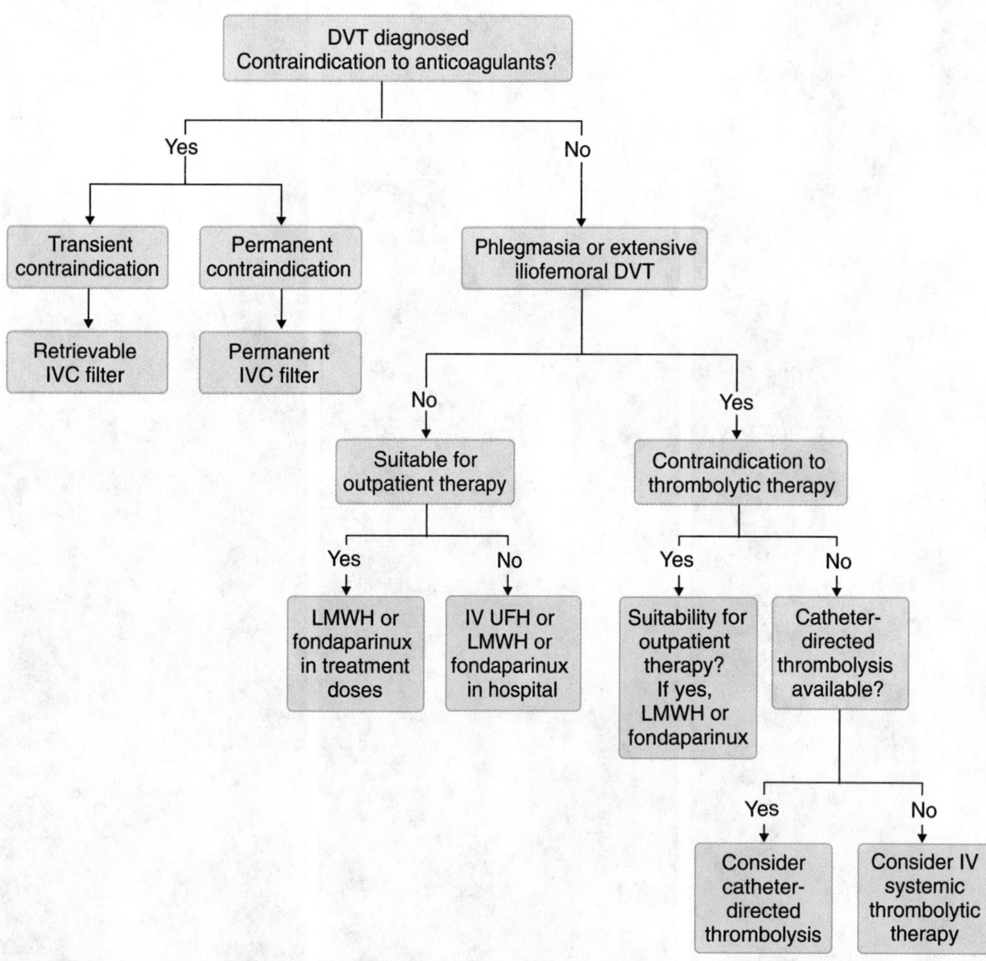

FIGURE 81–5 • Guidelines for treatment of deep venous thrombosis. IVC = inferior vena cava; LMWH = low-molecular-weight heparin; UFH = unfractionated heparin.

TABLE 81–2 ALTERNATIVE DIAGNOSES IN 87 CONSECUTIVE PATIENTS WITH CLINICALLY SUSPECTED VENOUS THROMBOSIS AND NORMAL VENOGRAMS*

Diagnosis	Patients (%)
Muscle strain	24
Direct twisting injury to the leg	10
Leg swelling in paralyzed limb	9
Lymphangitis, lymphatic obstruction	7
Venous reflux	7
Muscle tear	6
Baker's cyst	5
Cellulitis	3
Internal abnormality of the knee	2
Unknown	26

*The diagnosis was made once venous thrombosis was excluded by venography.

Differential Diagnosis

A number of conditions can mimic DVT (see Table 81–2), but DVT often can be excluded only by objective testing. In some patients, however, the cause of pain, tenderness, and swelling remains uncertain.

Suspected Recurrent Deep Venous Thrombosis

Approximately 10% of patients with unprovoked VTE will experience recurrent thromboembolism in the first year after ceasing anticoagulant therapy. In addition, many patients will have positional leg swelling and pain early during treatment as a result of venous outflow obstruction or later (≥6 months after diagnosis) because of the post-thrombotic syndrome when venous valvar incompetence is manifested. These and other nonthrombotic disorders can produce symptoms that are similar to acute recurrent DVT, so accurate diagnostic testing to confirm recurrence is mandatory. However, residual venous abnormalities are common after an initial event; persistent abnormalities are seen on compression ultrasonography in approximately 80% of patients at 3 months and 50% of patients at 1 year after a documented proximal DVT. Therefore, comparison with previous ultrasound images is required in patients with suspected recurrence. Although an increase in diameter of 4 mm or more in the compressed vein strongly suggests recurrent DVT, a new noncompressible proximal venous segment is the most reliable criterion for the diagnosis of recurrence. When compression ultrasonography is inconclusive, venography should be considered; a new intraluminal filling defect is diagnostic of acute DVT, and the absence of a filling defect excludes the diagnosis. Nonfilling of venous segments may mask recurrent DVT and is considered a nondiagnostic finding. A normal D-dimer test result is useful in excluding recurrent DVT.

Pregnancy

Symptoms of leg pain or swelling, shortness of breath, and atypical chest pain are common during pregnancy, so objective testing is needed to diagnose VTE. As in nonpregnant patients, compression ultrasonography is the initial test of choice. Because isolated iliac DVT is thought to be more common in pregnancy, venography should be considered when clinical suspicion is high even if the findings of the initial ultrasound examination are normal. Magnetic resonance venography, which is sensitive for pelvic DVT, may be useful in this circumstance.

Treatment

Anticoagulant therapy, which is the treatment of choice in most patients with VTE, reduces the extension and recurrence of symptomatic proximal and calf DVT and reduces mortality in patients with pulmonary emboli (Fig. 81–5). Coumarin derivatives (e.g., warfarin) are usually the drugs of choice for long-term anticoagulant

TABLE 81–3 GUIDELINES FOR ANTICOAGULATION WITH LOW-MOLECULAR-WEIGHT HEPARIN AND FONDAPARINUX

Indications	Guidelines
VTE suspected	Obtain baseline aPTT, PT, CBC Check for contraindication to heparin therapy Order imaging study; consider giving IV unfractionated heparin (5000 IU) or LMWH
VTE confirmed	Give LMWH (dalteparin,* enoxaparin,† nadroparin,‡ tinzaparin,§ fondaparinux**) Start warfarin therapy on day 1 at 5 mg and adjust the subsequent daily dose according to INR Check platelet count between days 3 and 5 Stop LMWH therapy after at least 4 or 5 days of combined therapy when the INR is >2 Anticoagulate with warfarin for at least 3 months at an INR of 2.5, range of 2–3

*Dalteparin sodium, 200 anti-Xa IU/kg/day subcutaneously. A single dose should not exceed 18,000 IU. (Approved in Canada.)
†Enoxaparin sodium, 1 mg/kg q12h subcutaneously, or enoxaparin sodium, 1.5 mg/kg/day subcutaneously. A single daily dose should not exceed 180 mg. (Approved in both the United States and Canada.)
‡Nadroparin calcium, 86 anti-Xa IU/kg two times a day subcutaneously for 10 days (approved in Canada), or nadroparin calcium, 171 anti-Xa IU/kg subcutaneously daily. A single dose should not exceed 17,100 anti-Xa IU.
§Tinzaparin sodium, 175 anti-Xa IU kg/day subcutaneously daily. (Approved in Canada and the United States.)
**Fondaparinux subcutaneously according to weight: <50 kg, 5 mg once daily; 50–100 kg, 7.5 mg; and >100 kg, 10 mg.
aPTT = activated partial thromboplastin time; CBC = complete blood count; INR = international normalized ratio; LMWH = low-molecular-weight heparin; PT = prothrombin time; VTE = venous thromboembolism.
Modified from Hyers TM, Agnelli G, Hull RD, et al: Antithrombotic therapy for venous thromboembolic disease. Chest 2001;119:176S–193S.

therapy, but such drugs have a delayed onset of anticoagulant effect (Chapter 35). Therefore, initial short-term therapy with a rapid-acting heparin or heparin derivative for approximately 1 week is necessary to provide an immediate antithrombotic effect and to reduce the risk of thrombus growth or embolization in patients with acute DVT. Initial outpatient therapy with a low-molecular-weight heparin (LMWH) or fondaparinux is preferred to inpatient treatment with intravenous unfractionated heparin whenever feasible in patients with DVT. Rarely, medical therapy is unsuccessful or cannot be tolerated; such patients may require procedural therapy.

Initial Treatment

LMWH preparations, which are produced by either enzymatic or chemical depolymerization of unfractionated heparin, have lower mean molecular weights ranging from 4000 to 6000. The reduced molecular size provides a sufficient pentasaccharide moiety to antithrombin to inhibit factor Xa but reduces the ability of LMWH to inhibit thrombin in comparison to unfractionated heparin. Therefore, LMWH has an increased ratio of anti–factor Xa to anti–factor IIa (thrombin) inhibitory activity. The reduced size of LMWH also decreases charge-related nonspecific protein binding, thereby resulting in improved subcutaneous bioavailability, more predictable anticoagulant response, and predominantly dose-independent renal clearance. These qualities have made outpatient management of DVT with unmonitored, weight-based subcutaneous LMWH feasible and preferable.

LMWH products differ in their method of production, molecular weight, and anticoagulant effect. Few trials have directly compared different LMWH preparations for treatment of acute VTE, and definitive conclusions with regard to comparative efficacy and safety cannot be made. Dosage regimens differ for the various LMWH formulations (Table 81–3), but once-daily administration of LMWH is thought to be as safe and effective as twice-daily administration.

Rx

Because the antithrombotic response to weight-based dosing of LMWH is predictable, laboratory monitoring during LMWH treatment is usually unnecessary. There are, however, three populations of patients in whom anti–factor Xa monitoring should be considered: (1) patients with renal insufficiency (calculated creatinine clearance of less than 30 mL/min); (2) obese patients, in whom the volume of distribution of LMWH might be different, so weight-adjusted dosing might not be appropriate; and (3) pregnant women, in whom it is unclear whether the dose should be adjusted according to the woman's weight change. Levels are usually determined on blood samples drawn 4 hours after subcutaneous injection; therapeutic ranges of 0.6 to 1.0 U/mL for twice-daily administration and 1.0 to 2.0 U/mL for once-daily treatment have been proposed.

Meta-analyses have documented that unmonitored, fixed-dose subcutaneous injection of LMWH is as effective and safe as adjusted-dose intravenous administration of unfractionated heparin for the treatment of acute DVT, [1] with a trend toward a significant difference in mortality benefit favoring LMWH, probably because of improved survival in patients with malignant disease. However, patients with extensive iliofemoral DVT have often been excluded from trials of LMWH, and extended-duration (i.e., more than 5 days) intravenous unfractionated heparin therapy is often administered to such patients. Outpatient therapy with LMWH is as good as inpatient treatment, thereby making LMWH more cost-effective than intravenous unfractionated heparin in most health care settings.

Fondaparinux

Fondaparinux is a synthetic analogue of the critical pentasaccharide sequence required for binding of heparin molecules to antithrombin (Chapter 35). Chemically engineered, it has minor modifications from the natural pentasaccharide moiety, thereby improving stability and resulting in enhanced binding to antithrombin. Given subcutaneously, fondaparinux demonstrates 100% bioavailability, with peak plasma concentrations occurring 1.7 hours after dosing. Once-daily subcutaneous administration of fondaparinux (5.0 mg daily if weight is less than 50 kg; 7.5 mg daily if weight is 50 to 100 kg; 10 mg daily if weight is more than 100 kg) is an effective and safe alternative to LMWH for the initial 5 to 10 days of treatment of DVT. [2] Clearance is predominantly renal, with approximately 70% of the initial dose recovered in the urine in an unchanged form. Patients with reduced creatinine clearance, such as the elderly, have higher peak drug levels and longer drug half-life, so their dose may need to be adjusted downward.

Unfractionated Heparin

Unfractionated heparin is a sulfated glycosaminoglycan that exerts its anticoagulant effect predominantly by binding to antithrombin and inducing a conformational change that accelerates the rate at which antithrombin inhibits coagulation enzymes (Chapter 35). It consists of a heterogeneous group of molecules ranging in molecular weight from 3000 to 30,000, and only one third of unfractionated heparin molecules contain the unique pentasaccharide sequence required for binding to antithrombin. This molecular heterogeneity, along with variable charge-related nonspecific binding of unfractionated heparin to other plasma proteins such as von Willebrand factor and platelet factor 4, contributes to the large variability in the anticoagulant response in individual patients.

Unfractionated heparin is usually administered by continuous intravenous infusion, a route that has been shown to be effective in reducing recurrence and extension of thrombus. Much larger doses of subcutaneous unfractionated heparin are required for therapeutic anticoagulation, but adequate-dose subcutaneous unfractionated heparin is likely to be as effective and safe as intravenous unfractionated heparin for treatment of acute DVT.

It is standard practice to monitor unfractionated heparin therapy by measurement of the activated partial thromboplastin time (aPTT), aiming for an aPTT of 1.5 to 2.5 times the control value to reduce the risk of recurrent VTE. However, plasma heparin levels, not aPTT, are the more accurate measure of the "biologic effect" of therapy with unfractionated heparin, so individual institutions

TABLE 81–4 WEIGHT-BASED NOMOGRAM FOR INITIAL INTRAVENOUS HEPARIN THERAPY

aPTT	Dose (IU/kg)
Initial dose	80 bolus, then 18/hr
<35 sec (<1.2×)*	80 bolus, then 4/hr
35–45 sec (1.2–1.5×)	40 bolus, then 2/hr
46–70 sec (1.5–2.3×)	No change
71–90 sec (2.3–3×)	Decrease infusion rate by 2/hr
>90 sec (>3×)	Hold infusion 1 hr, then decrease infusion rate by 3/hr

*Figures in parentheses show comparison with control.
aPTT = activated partial thromboplastin time. In general, with contemporary aPTT reagents, the target therapeutic range is more than 1.2 to 2.3 times control.
Modified from Raschke RA, Reilly BM, Guidry JR, et al: The weight-based heparin dosing nomogram compared with a "standard care" nomogram. A randomized controlled trial. Ann Intern Med 1993;119:874–881.

should establish their own therapeutic aPTT range that correlates with a therapeutic heparin level of 0.3 to 0.7 IU/mL anti–factor Xa activity, which often results in therapeutic aPTT ranges that are 2 to 3.5 times the control value.

An initial bolus dose of unfractionated heparin followed by a constant intravenous infusion is standard treatment for acute VTE. The use of validated nomograms (Table 81–4), with either fixed initial dosing or dosing according to a patient's weight, results in more rapid achievement of therapeutic aPTT levels and improves outcome, although adjustment according to the sensitivity of local aPTT methods is required. The initial aPTT level should be measured 6 hours after therapy is commenced. Up to 25% of patients with acute VTE have resistance to heparin, defined as a requirement for greater than expected doses of unfractionated heparin to achieve a "therapeutic" aPTT. If it is available, anti–factor Xa monitoring is recommended in patients with heparin resistance.

Transition to Oral Treatment

Coumarin Derivatives (Warfarin)

Warfarin is a vitamin K antagonist that inhibits the production of clotting factors II (prothrombin), VII, IX, and X as well as the naturally occurring anticoagulants protein C and protein S. In patients with DVT, the drug should be started within 24 to 48 hours of initiation of heparin with a goal of achieving international normalized ratio (INR) results between 2.0 and 3.0 (Chapter 35). A higher target INR of 3.0 to 4.0 is associated with more bleeding but no better efficacy, even in patients with the antiphospholipid antibody syndrome (Chapter 182), [3] and lower intensity warfarin therapy (target INR, 1.5 to 1.9) is significantly less effective at preventing recurrent VTE despite similar rates of major bleeding. [4]

The dose is empirical, but a starting dose of 5 to 10 mg is suitable for most patients. Warfarin doses are adjusted according to the prothrombin time, expressed as the INR, performed daily or every other day until the results are in the therapeutic range for at least 24 hours. After initial dosing, warfarin can be monitored two or three times per week for 1 to 2 weeks and then less frequently, depending on the stability of INR results, up to intervals as long as 4 to 6 weeks. If dose adjustment is needed, such as when medications that can interact with warfarin are introduced, the cycle of more frequent monitoring is repeated until a stable dose response is again achieved.

Side Effects of Anticoagulants

Bleeding is the most common side effect of anticoagulant therapy. Major bleeding (e.g., intracranial [Chapter 432], gastrointestinal [Chapter 137], or retroperitoneal) leading to hospitalization or transfusion or death occurs in approximately 2% of patients treated with intravenous unfractionated heparin for acute VTE. Factors such as recent surgery, trauma, and concurrent aspirin or thrombolytic therapy increase the risk of bleeding.

Rx

The risk of major bleeding with warfarin in doses adjusted to achieve a target INR of 2.0 to 3.0 ranges from 1 to 3% per year and appears to be highest soon after treatment is started or if anticoagulation is difficult to control. The risk of major bleeding increases according to individual characteristics, such as older age, the presence of comorbid conditions (e.g., diabetes, hypertension, renal insufficiency, previous gastrointestinal bleeding, or cancer), and the use of concomitant drugs, in particular antiplatelet therapy.

Heparin-induced thrombocytopenia, which is a nonhemorrhagic complication of therapy with unfractionated heparin and LMWH, is manifested typically with thrombocytopenia and new thrombosis (Chapter 35). Monitoring of the platelet count is recommended every other day until day 14 in patients receiving therapeutic unfractionated heparin but is not routinely recommended with LMWH or fondaparinux because of the extremely low risk with these newer medications.

Long-Term Treatment

The preferred long-term treatment of DVT for most patients is warfarin or another coumarin derivative (e.g., acenocoumarol), continued until the benefits of treatment for reducing recurrent VTE no longer outweigh its risks of major bleeding. The decision to prolong or to stop anticoagulation should be individualized, and a patient's preferences should be considered.

Patients with symptomatic proximal DVT or pulmonary emboli should be treated for at least 3 months, even if the VTE was associated with a transient risk factor, [5] but the optimal duration of treatment for patients whose VTE is not associated with a transient risk factor is controversial. Three months of treatment is associated with a 10 to 27% risk of a recurrence during the 12 months after anticoagulant therapy is stopped, whereas 6 months of anticoagulant therapy reduces the risk of recurrence in the first year after stopping to about 10%. In patients whose VTE developed in association with minor risk factors (e.g., air travel, pregnancy, within 6 weeks of estrogen therapy, after leg injury or immobilization), the risk of recurrence is probably lower than 10%. Continuation of treatment beyond 6 months reduces the risk of recurrent VTE during the course of therapy, but the benefit is lost after warfarin is discontinued.

The most convincing association of thrombophilia with the risk of recurrent VTE is the antiphospholipid antibody (lupus anticoagulant or anticardiolipin antibody; Chapter 182), which is associated with a two-fold increase in the risk of recurrence. Homozygous factor V Leiden, elevated levels of homocysteine, and deficiencies of antithrombin, protein C, and protein S also have been associated with an increased risk of recurrence in some reports, but other data suggest that testing for heritable thrombophilia does not predict recurrent VTE in the first 2 years after anticoagulant therapy is stopped. In the absence of randomized trials to assess different durations of anticoagulation in patients with VTE and thrombophilia, routine testing for thrombophilias need not be performed but should be considered in young (<50 years) patients, patients with venous thrombosis in unusual sites, and patients with a strong family history of VTE (i.e., one or more first-degree relatives with a history of VTE).

The decision to extend anticoagulant therapy beyond 3 months must balance the risk of recurrent VTE with the risk of bleeding. The annual risk of major bleeding when warfarin is adjusted to achieve a target INR of 2.0 to 3.0 is 1 to 3%, with a case-fatality rate of 10% when major bleeding occurs in patients who received treatment for more than 3 months. By comparison, the case-fatality rate for recurrent VTE is about 5%. In patients whose VTE was associated with a transient risk factor or who are at high risk of bleeding, treatment for 3 months is generally adequate because the risk of fatal recurrent VTE is lower than the risk of fatal bleeding if warfarin treatment is prolonged. Among patients without a reversible or transient cause, however, prolonged warfarin therapy for more than 6 months can be considered because the risk of fatal hemorrhage is counterbalanced by the risk of fatal recurrence. The argument to prolong therapy is stronger in patients with high-risk thrombophilia

Rx

(e.g., homozygous factor V Leiden; antiphospholipid antibody; deficiency of antithrombin, protein C, or protein S; or combined heterozygous state for factor V Leiden and the prothrombin gene mutation). Indefinite therapy (preferably with LMWH) should be considered in patients with cancer-related VTE (Chapter 189) if the risk of bleeding is not high because the risk of recurrent VTE is more than 10% in the first year after anticoagulation is stopped. In motivated and capable patients, self-management of warfarin therapy is better than management by a physician or nurse. 6

Alternatives to Coumarin Derivatives

For patients in whom warfarin is impractical or contraindicated and for those who have recurrent VTE while being treated with appropriate doses of oral anticoagulants, therapeutic doses of LMWH are as effective as warfarin. For patients with cancer-related VTE (DVT, pulmonary embolus, or both), weight-based LMWH decreased to 75% of the initial dose after 1 month of treatment reduces the risk of recurrent VTE compared with warfarin, with similar bleeding rates. 7

Therapeutic strategies to manage patients in whom symptomatic VTE recurs while they are receiving conventional-intensity warfarin include unfractionated heparin, LMWH, higher intensity warfarin (e.g., INR range of 3.0 to 4.0), and insertion of a vena caval filter. However, the optimal management of such patients is unknown because no randomized studies have been performed.

Thrombolytic Therapy

Although thrombolytic therapy results in increased rates of early patency of leg veins after DVT, it has not been conclusively shown to decrease the subsequent rate of post-thrombotic syndrome or pulmonary emboli. Except for patients who have life-threatening limb ischemia due to massive thrombosis, thrombolysis is not recommended in patients with DVT.

Vena Caval Filters

In a randomized trial of 400 patients with DVT, the incidence of pulmonary emboli at day 12 was lower in patients who received an inferior vena caval filter plus therapeutic anticoagulation than in those who received anticoagulation alone. However, filters did not reduce early or late mortality and are not recommended in patients who can receive therapeutic anticoagulation because this benefit did not persist at 2 years and was offset by an almost doubling of the risk of recurrent DVT. Inferior vena caval filters should be used in patients who have contraindications to anticoagulant therapy or develop major bleeding while receiving it as well as in patients who develop recurrent VTE while receiving appropriate anticoagulation. Retrievable or removable inferior vena caval filters can be retrieved and removed within 14 days to several weeks after insertion or can be left in permanently. These filters are ideal for a patient who has a reversible cause of or the potential for major bleeding (e.g., DVT after craniotomy, DVT late in pregnancy).

Oral Direct Thrombin Inhibitors

Ximelagatran is an oral direct thrombin inhibitor that does not require anticoagulant monitoring. When it is used for the acute and long-term treatment of patients with acute VTE, ximelagatran is as effective and safe as unfractionated heparin or LMWH followed by warfarin in preventing recurrent VTE. 8 However, elevation in liver enzyme activities (especially alanine aminotransferases) has been reported in 5 to 10% of patients with long-term use. Although the clinical implications of these elevated levels, which may decrease to normal with continued treatment, are unclear, the drug has been removed from the market by the manufacturers.

Compression Stockings

The use of below-knee graduated compression stockings for 2 years after acute DVT reduces the risk of the post-thrombotic syndrome by 50%. 9 Some experts recommend routine stocking therapy in all patients with DVT. Others recommend waiting until the acute inflammatory process and acute outflow obstruction have subsided (usually up to 6 months) and then prescribing stockings if the patient's symptoms persist at that time.

Prevention

Despite the plethora of large randomized trials demonstrating the efficacy and safety of mechanical and pharmacologic measures in reducing the risk of VTE in a wide range of hospitalized populations of patients, prophylaxis remains grossly underused. Factors that increase the risk of DVT include surgery (particularly major hip and knee surgery as well as neurosurgery; Chapters 457 and 459), major trauma (Chapter 113), prolonged bedrest or immobilization, previous episodes of VTE, presence of malignant disease, paralysis, morbid obesity, and increasing age. In general, mechanical prophylaxis (antiembolic stockings and intermittent pneumatic compression) should be used as an adjunct to pharmacologic prophylaxis (see Table 35–2) or in patients with a high risk of bleeding. For general medical patients admitted to the hospital with a major illness and in whom mobility is likely to be reduced for 72 hours or longer, low-dose unfractionated heparin or LMWH (see Table 35–2) should be considered. In patients who undergo major hip or knee surgery, warfarin (to an INR of 2.0 to 3.0), subcutaneous LMWH (see Table 81–4), or fondaparinux (2.5 mg once daily) should be used for at least 7 to 14 days postoperatively. In patients with continued immobility, prophylaxis should be considered until they regain their preoperative mobility. Comprehensive consensus guidelines have been developed for the prevention of VTE in different populations of patients.

Management of Deep Venous Thrombosis in Pregnancy

The management of pregnant women with DVT (Chapter 259) is problematic because all coumarin derivatives cross the placenta and have the potential to cause warfarin embryopathy, consisting of nasal hypoplasia and epiphyseal stippling, if the newborn is exposed to warfarin between 6 and 12 weeks of gestation. Consequently, parenteral unfractionated heparin and LMWH, which do not cross the placenta and are safe for the fetus, are the agents of choice. The easiest approach is to initiate therapy with weight-adjusted "treatment" doses of LMWH (see Table 81–3), continued for the duration of the pregnancy. Although it is not proved, it is likely that the dose of LMWH can be safely decreased to approximately 80% of the therapeutic dose after 3 months of therapy. As pregnancy progresses, women normally gain weight and generally require higher doses of LMWH to achieve an anti–factor Xa level similar to that achieved at the time of diagnosis. The adequacy of the dose can be assessed by measuring a 4-hour post-injection anti–factor Xa level and targeting the dose to achieve a level of 0.5 to 1.0 U/mL for twice-daily LMWH and 0.8 to 1.5 U/mL for once-daily LMWH. Alternatively, the dose of LMWH can simply be adjusted periodically on the basis of the woman's weight.

Unfractionated heparin is less attractive than LMWH because it is associated with a greater reduction of bone density and a higher risk of heparin-induced thrombocytopenia. Unfractionated heparin can be initiated either by continuous intravenous infusion in doses adjusted to maintain an aPTT in the therapeutic range, followed by 12-hourly subcutaneous injections, or simply with 12-hourly subcutaneous injections throughout the course of pregnancy. The dose should be adjusted to target a midinterval (6-hour postinjection) aPTT in the therapeutic range.

Pregnant women with a DVT should probably be treated for the duration of pregnancy and for at least 6 weeks post partum. If the DVT occurred early in pregnancy, elective induction of delivery at about 37 weeks with discontinuation of the heparin 24 hours prior is recommended. If the DVT occurs in the latter part of the third trimester, intravenous heparin should be administered by continuous infusion until approximately 6 hours before the expected time of delivery. Intravenous unfractionated heparin or subcutaneous LMWH should be started post partum as soon as hemostasis has been achieved. Maternal warfarin therapy is safe for the breast-fed infant because warfarin and its metabolites are not secreted into breast milk in doses sufficient to cause an anticoagulant effect. Consequently, warfarin (with bridging LMWH or unfractionated heparin until the INR is 2.0 or higher) can be used after delivery.

Venous Thrombosis of the Upper Extremities

DVT of the upper extremities (including the arm and the axillary, subclavian, and internal jugular veins as well as the superior vena cava) is

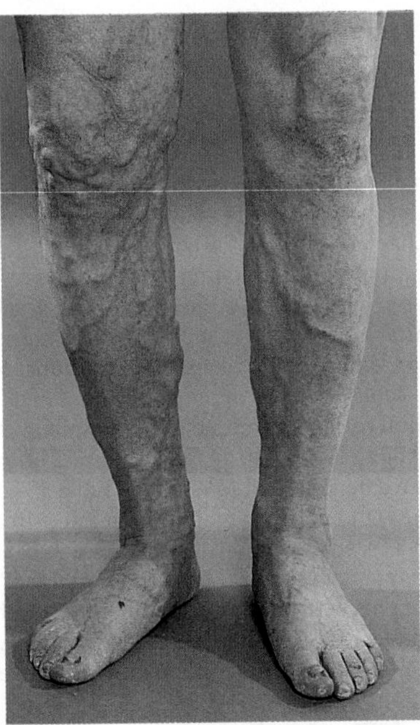

FIGURE 81–6 • Varicose veins are a risk factor for deep venous thrombosis and may result from it. (From Forbes CD, Jackson WF: Color Atlas and Text of Clinical Medicine, 3rd ed. London, Mosby, 2003, with permission.)

much less common than DVT of the legs, but it is not rare. Factors associated with upper extremity DVT include central venous catheters, acquired or hereditary thrombophilias, and anatomic (cervical rib) and physiologic (muscular individuals) impingement of the vein. The incidence of clinically important post-thrombotic syndrome is not high if patients are treated with anticoagulants alone.

Contrast venography is the gold standard for the diagnosis of upper extremity DVT, but venous ultrasonography is accurate and less invasive. Because it is not feasible to test for compression of the subclavian vein, a diagnosis of subclavian DVT by ultrasonography is based on flow abnormalities or direct visualization of thrombus by B-mode ultrasonography. Upper extremity DVT can cause pulmonary emboli, although the exact frequency is not known.

Considerable controversy exists about the management of patients in whom DVT develops in association with a central venous catheter. If the line is not necessary or is nonfunctional, some recommend simply removing the line without subsequent anticoagulant therapy, whereas others treat with full-dose anticoagulants (a heparin-related compound, followed by 1 to 3 months of warfarin). If the line is functional and must stay in place (e.g., no alternative venous access), full-dose anticoagulants should be given. Otherwise, anticoagulant therapy should be given in all patients with upper extremity DVT, with medications, doses, regimens, and durations identical to those for treatment of DVT of the leg.

SUPERFICIAL THROMBOPHLEBITIS

Superficial thrombophlebitis usually presents with pain, swelling, redness, and tenderness of superficial veins. Varicose veins (Fig. 81–6) can be red, warm, and clustered in a circumscribed area. When superficial thrombophlebitis occurs in the short or long saphenous veins, there is usually redness, tenderness, and often linear induration that follows the course of the involved vein (medial calf or thigh). Superficial thrombophlebitis can also occur at the insertion site of an intravenous catheter. Invariably, superficial thrombophlebitis is associated with thrombosis of the corresponding vein, and particularly when the long saphenous vein is involved, venous ultrasonography should be performed to exclude extension into the deep veins, which occurs in up to 19% of patients.

Randomized trials comparing nonsteroidal anti-inflammatory drugs with moderate or full doses of LMWH show that either dose of LMWH relieves symptoms more quickly and prevents growth of thrombus more effectively than do nonsteroidal anti-inflammatory drugs. Thus, it is reasonable to use moderate doses of LMWH for the initial treatment of acute, symptomatic superficial thrombophlebitis. Alternatively, and particularly for intravenous catheter–induced superficial thrombophlebitis, a nonsteroidal anti-inflammatory drug can be tried.

POST-THROMBOTIC SYNDROME

The initial pain and swelling in many patients with DVT are due to the venous obstruction or the inflammatory process mediated by the acute thrombus. Once anticoagulant therapy is initiated, the acute obstruction usually resolves during a period of several months as recanalization occurs and collateral venous channels develop, thereby leading to initial improvement in pain and swelling. However, in the long term, probably because of venous valvar incompetence produced when the thrombosed venous segments recanalize and sometimes because of residual chronic obstruction, venous hypertension and sometimes pain and swelling can recur.

This post-thrombotic syndrome develops in up to 50% of patients with proximal DVT, usually within the first 1 to 2 years after DVT. The syndrome is often a chronic, progressive disease with pain, swelling, and occasionally ulceration of the leg in patients with previous DVT.

Prevention and Treatment

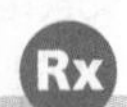

Graduated compression stockings reduce the risk of the post-thrombotic syndrome by about 50%. [9] These benefits have led to the widespread practice in Europe (and to some extent in North America) of using graduated compression stockings routinely in *all* patients with DVT. However, stockings are hot in the summer, relatively expensive, difficult for many patients to put on in the morning, and cosmetically unappealing to many patients. In addition, simple lifestyle alteration (such as frequent leg elevation, avoidance of prolonged standing or sitting, and occasional use of analgesics) suffices in relieving symptoms in many patients. If symptoms are severe, it is usually because of extensive thrombus causing massive edema. In such patients, a lightweight stocking (such as support hose) can be helpful until the edema improves. If symptoms persist or worsen despite these measures, or if ulceration seems imminent (as evidenced by severe skin changes), a full-strength stocking (30 to 40 mm Hg of pressure at the ankle) can be prescribed. However, if symptoms subside and the patient remains asymptomatic or has only trivial persistent signs or symptoms with little or no effect on quality of life, stockings can be avoided and the patient can be observed for clinically important signs and symptoms of the post-thrombotic syndrome.

VENOUS ULCERS

Venous ulcers, which are the most severe complication of post-thrombotic syndrome, typically occur in the perimalleolar area of the leg. The best management is prevention by application of graduated compression stockings either at the time of diagnosis of DVT or, at the latest, when skin changes develop in association with leg swelling. When an ulcer occurs, treatment with an emollient and regular wrapping should be commenced. Once the ulcer heals, the patient should be prescribed graduated compression stockings and watched for recurrent ulceration. Surgical closure or removal of the incompetent saphenous veins plus dressing management in patients with chronic venous ulceration does not reduce healing time of the acute ulcer compared with dressing management alone but significantly reduces the rate of recurrent ulceration at 1 year. [10]

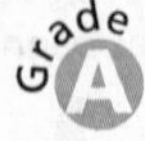

1. Gould MK, Dembitzer AD, Doyle RL, et al: Low-molecular-weight heparins compared with unfractionated heparin for treatment of acute deep venous thrombosis. A meta-analysis of randomized, controlled trials. Ann Intern Med 1999;130:800–809.
2. Buller HR, Davidson BL, Decousus H, et al: Fondaparinux or enoxaparin for the initial treatment of symptomatic deep venous thrombosis: A randomized trial. Ann Intern Med 2004;140:867–873.
3. Crowther MA, Ginsberg JS, Julian J, et al: A comparison of two intensities of warfarin for the prevention of recurrent thrombosis in patients with the antiphospholipid antibody syndrome. N Engl J Med 2003;349:1133–1138.
4. Kearon C, Ginsberg JS, Kovacs MJ, et al: Comparison of low-intensity warfarin therapy with conventional-intensity warfarin

therapy for long-term prevention of recurrent venous thromboembolism. N Engl J Med 2003;349:631–639.

5. Kearon C, Ginsberg JS, Anderson DR, et al: Comparison of 1 month of anticoagulation with 3 months of anticoagulation for a first episode of venous thromboembolism provoked by a transient risk factor. J Thromb Haemost 2003;2:743–749.
6. Menéndez-Jándula B, Souto JC, Oliver A, et al: Comparing self-management of oral anticoagulant therapy with clinical management: A randomized trial. Ann Intern Med 2005;142:1–10.
7. Lee AY, Levine MN, Baker RI, et al: Randomized comparison of low-molecular-weight heparin versus oral anticoagulant therapy for the prevention of recurrent venous thromboembolism in patients with cancer. N Engl J Med 2003;349:109–111.
8. Fiessinger JN, Huisman MD, Davidson BL, et al: Ximelagatran vs low-molecular-weight heparin and warfarin for the treatment of deep-vein thrombosis: A randomized trial. JAMA 2005;293: 681–689.
9. Prandoni P, Lensing AW, Prins MH, et al: Below-knee elastic compression stockings to prevent the post-thrombotic syndrome: A randomized, controlled trial. Ann Intern Med 2004;141:249–256.
10. Barwell JR, Davies CE, Deacon J, et al: Comparison of surgery and compression with compression alone in chronic venous ulceration (ESCHAR study): Randomised controlled trial. Lancet 2004;363: 1854–1859.

SUGGESTED READINGS

Bergan JJ, Schmid-Schonbein GW, Coleridge Smith PD, et al: Chronic venous disease. N Engl J Med 2006;355:488–498. *Chronic venous disease is extremely common, although the prevalence estimates vary.*

Geerts WH, Pineo GF, Heit JA, et al: Prevention of venous thromboembolism. The Seventh ACCP Conference on Antithrombotic and Thrombolytic Therapy. Chest 2004;126:338s–400s. *A comprehensive review.*

Joffe HV, Kucher N, Tapson VF, et al: Upper-extremity deep vein thrombosis: A prospective registry of 592 patients. Circulation 2004;110:1605–1611. *An indwelling catheter explained more than 50% of cases.*

Kyrle PA, Eichinger S: Deep vein thrombosis. Lancet 2005;365:1163–1174. *A scholarly review.*

Segal JB, Streiff MB, Hofmann LV, et al: Management of venous thromboembolism: A systematic review for a practice guideline. Ann Intern Med 2007;146:211–222. *A meta-analysis examining the type and duration of anticoagulation, as well as the role of vena cava filters.*

Wells PS, Owen C, Doucette S, et al: Does this patient have deep vein thrombosis? JAMA 2006;295:199–207. *A case-based review. In low-probability patients with a negative D-dimer, DVT can be excluded without ultrasound.*

82 CARDIAC TRANSPLANTATION

Mariell Jessup

Cardiac transplantation is the treatment of choice for suitable patients with refractory heart failure (Chapters 58, 59, and 108). The number of heart transplant procedures worldwide reached a peak of about 4500 in 1994 but has subsequently declined because the rate of identification of potential donors has not kept pace with the increased number of patients on waiting lists, where the annual mortality is 10 to 20% (Fig. 82–1). Because newer therapeutic options have usually failed and they now lack other alternatives, patients referred for heart transplantation are becoming progressively older and more ill, with increasing medical comorbidities, which have significantly increased the risk of cardiac transplantation. At the same time, the selection criteria for donors have been broadened to increase the number of organs available. As a result, sicker recipients are now receiving less ideal organs than in the past.

POPULATION OF PATIENTS

Evaluation of the Potential Recipient

The purpose of heart transplantation is to prolong life and to improve quality of life, so the referring physician must understand the potential benefits of transplantation as well as comorbidities that may portend an unsatisfactory outcome. Suitable patients for consideration have cardiogenic shock requiring mechanical support or high-dose inotropic or pressor drugs (Chapter 108); stage D heart failure symptoms despite maximal therapy (Chapter 58); recurrent life-threatening arrhythmias despite maximal interventions, including implanted defibrillators (Chapters 62 and 64); or, rarely, refractory angina without the potential for revascularization (Chapter 70) (Table 82–1). The most potent predictor of outcome in ambulatory patients with heart failure is a symptom-limited metabolic stress test to calculate peak oxygen consumption; a peak of less than 10 mL/kg/min indicates a lower survival with medical therapy than after transplantation.

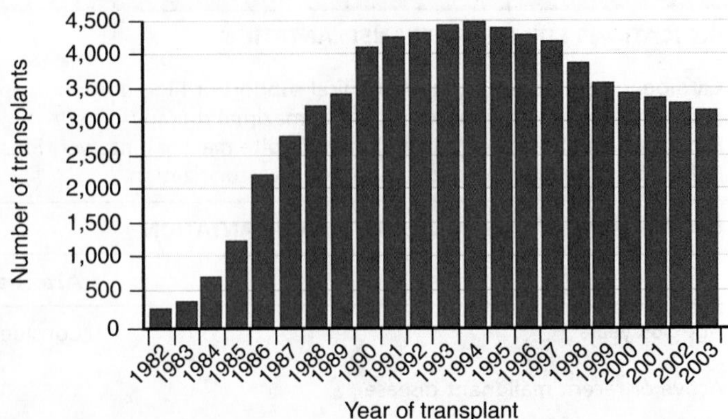

FIGURE 82–1 • The number of heart transplant procedures by year. (Data from the Registry of the International Society for Heart and Lung Transplantation. Reproduced with permission.)

An extensive medical and psychosocial evaluation must be performed to exclude contraindications to transplantation. In the setting of fixed pulmonary hypertension, such patients are occasionally considered for combined heart-lung transplantation.

An immunologic evaluation includes determination of ABO blood type, antibody screen, panel-reactive antibody level, and human leukocyte antigen (HLA) typing. Patients with a panel-reactive antibody value above 10% should have a full crossmatch at the time of transplantation because elevated levels increase the risk of rejection.

Management of the Patient Waiting for Cardiac Transplantation

A patient's priority status according to the United Network for Organ Sharing is based on the recipient's status level, blood type, body size, and duration of time at a particular status level. Patients who can be managed successfully outside the hospital are the lowest priority. Intermediate priority is given to patients who require hospitalization and some continuous inotropic support. The highest priority, status 1A, is given to patients requiring high-dose inotropic support or mechanical support, such as intra-aortic balloon counterpulsation or ventricular assist device. Hearts are offered geographically, by the location of the donor, and limited by an ischemic time of approximately 4 hours. Patients who are waiting for transplantation are regularly re-evaluated for a change in status or the development or worsening of a comorbidity that would preclude transplantation.

THE CARDIAC TRANSPLANT PROCEDURE

The Cardiac Donor

Relevant history for the assessment of cardiac donors includes the presence or absence of thoracic trauma, hemodynamic stability, pressor and inotropic requirements, duration of cardiac arrest, need for cardiopulmonary resuscitation, and assessment of hypotensive episodes. In many potential donors, brain death causes hemodynamic deterioration that requires inotropic support and substantial fluid administration. Donors up to the age of 50 to 55 years are considered safe by most centers. The final decision to accept a heart for transplantation is made at the time of harvest, after direct examination for myocardial infarction, trauma, and coronary calcification.

Currently, the acceptable cold ischemia time between explant and implant is approximately 4 hours. One of the main reasons for early graft failure after transplantation is inadequate myocardial protection during prolonged ischemic periods.

TABLE 82–1 EVALUATION OF THE POTENTIAL HEART TRANSPLANT RECIPIENT

INDICATIONS FOR HEART TRANSPLANTATION		
Cardiogenic shock requiring mechanical support or high-dose inotropic drugs		
Stage D heart failure symptoms despite maximal therapy		
Recurrent life-threatening arrhythmias despite maximal interventions and implanted defibrillator		
Refractory angina without potential for revascularization		
CONTRAINDICATIONS TO HEART TRANSPLANTATION		
	Alternative Treatment	**Options**
Age >65 years	Consider permanent mechanical support	End-of-life considerations or investigational therapy
Active or recent malignant disease		End-of-life considerations or investigational therapy
Diabetes with severe end-organ damage	Consider permanent mechanical support	End-of-life considerations or investigational therapy
FEV/FVC <40%	Consider heart-lung transplantation	End-of-life considerations or investigational therapy
BMI <20 or BMI >35	Nutritional modification; BMI >35, consider permanent mechanical support or weight loss	
Irreversible pulmonary hypertension (≥4 Wood units)	Consider heart-lung transplantation	End-of-life considerations or investigational therapy
Other comorbidities: cirrhosis, vascular disease, addictions, hepatitis C, human immunodeficiency virus infection, social or psychiatric disorders	Individual transplant team decisions	

BMI = body mass index; FEV = forced expiratory volume; FVC = forced vital capacity.

Surgical Considerations

The biatrial anastomosis technique consists of four suture lines: left atrium, pulmonary artery, aorta, and right atrium. The bicaval anastomosis technique, introduced to minimize distortion of the heart and to preserve atrial conduction, has five anastomoses: left atrium, pulmonary artery, aorta, inferior vena cava, and superior vena cava. To date, there has been no prospective trial to establish the superiority of either technique. Failure to wean a heart transplant patient from cardiopulmonary bypass is most commonly the result of right-sided heart failure, which is evidenced by low cardiac output in the face of a rising central venous pressure. Native heart pacemakers and cardiac defibrillators are usually surgically removed at the end of the operation after the chest has been closed.

POSTOPERATIVE MANAGEMENT

Early Postoperative Management

Cardiovascular Issues

Management of the heart transplant patient early after surgery does not differ substantially from management after other cardiac procedures (Chapter 74). Cardiac transplant patients typically need chronotropic and inotropic support for a few days in the intensive care unit.

Because the donor heart is denervated, bradycardia is a frequent problem. It is usually treated with titrated isoproterenol to maintain a heart rate above 90 beats per minute for the first several days after transplantation. Temporary pacing leads are necessary for all patients, and as many as 10 to 15% of patients require a permanent pacemaker after transplant surgery.

Inhaled nitric oxide, in a usual dose of 20 to 60 parts per million, is a potent vasodilator that has a selective effect on the pulmonary vasculature, reduces pulmonary vascular resistance, and improves right ventricular function in patients with pulmonary hypertension. Intravenous epoprostenol, an alternative, is typically used at 5 to 50 ng/kg/min.

Immunosuppression

Most immunosuppressive regimens begin with the simultaneous use of three classes of drugs: glucocorticoids, calcineurin inhibitors, and antiproliferative agents. In addition, patients may receive a variety of drugs during induction therapy (Chapter 46).

Perioperative Induction Therapy

The goal of perioperative induction therapy is to inhibit only those T cells that respond to donor antigen, thus achieving immunologic unresponsiveness to the transplant in the face of a fully functioning immune system, called donor-specific tolerance. Agents include the anti-CD3 antibody OKT3 and the interleukin-2 receptor antagonists daclizumab and basiliximab.

Acute and Maintenance Immunosuppression

Patients initially receive high doses of intravenous corticosteroids (e.g., 500 mg of IV methylprednisolone at the end of cardiopulmonary bypass, followed by 150 mg IV every 8 hours for three additional doses), then oral steroids that are gradually tapered during the next 6 months in an attempt to minimize side effects (Chapter 33). Corticosteroids also are usually the drug of first choice to treat acute rejection.

The calcineurin inhibitors cyclosporine and tacrolimus act specifically on the immune system and do not affect other rapidly proliferating cells. Important and often limiting side effects include nephrotoxicity, which occurs in up to 40 to 70% of patients, and hypertension. Target therapeutic levels 2 hours after a dose improve outcome.

Mycophenolate mofetil has replaced azathioprine as the first-line antiproliferative drug, with several randomized trials demonstrating superiority to azathioprine. [1] Mycophenolate mofetil may cause leukopenia, debilitating diarrhea, and nausea.

Sirolimus (often called rapamycin) and everolimus are complementary to calcineurin inhibitors, and both drugs have been used as alternatives to standard maintenance immunosuppression and as rescue drugs for rejection. In one randomized trial using cyclosporine and steroids, addition of sirolimus halved the number of patients with acute rejection and reduced the development of vasculopathy in the donor heart compared with addition of azathioprine. [2]

Other Potential Management Issues

The transplant recipient is often debilitated or malnourished. Depression (Chapter 420) is common, and many patients exhibit a marked emotional lability that is aggravated by high-dose steroids. Successful heart transplant teams must include dedicated physical therapists, nutritionists, and social workers or psychologists, in addition to the nurses and physicians, so that all these needs may be addressed.

Long-Term Care of the Cardiac Transplant Patient

Rejection

Rejection is categorized histologically and immunologically into three major types: hyperacute, acute (cellular or humoral), and chronic. Hyperacute rejection, which results when an abrupt loss of allograft function occurs within minutes to hours after circulation is established in the allograft, is rare in modern-day transplantation. The phenomenon is mediated by preexisting antibodies to allogeneic antigens on the vascular endothelial cells of the donor organ. These antibodies fix complement, which promotes intravascular thrombosis, leading to rapid occlusion of graft vasculature and swift rejection.

Acute cellular rejection, which is a predominantly lymphocytic mononuclear inflammatory response directed against the cardiac allograft, commonly occurs from the first week to several years after transplantation. The key event in both the initiation and the coordination of the rejection is T-cell activation. The risk of acute cellular rejection in the first 6 months is 40 to 70%. Acute cellular rejection after 6 months occurs most often in patients who have had substantial rejection early after transplantation, recent reduction in immunosuppression, intercurrent infection, or noncompliance with medication.

Acute humoral rejection occurs days to weeks after transplantation and is initiated by alloantibodies directed against donor HLA or endothelial cell antigens rather than by T cells. Patients at greatest risk for humoral rejection are women and patients with a high panel-reactive antibody screen or a positive crossmatch. It is estimated that significant humoral rejection occurs in about 7% of patients, but the rate may be as high as 20%.

Chronic rejection, or late graft failure, is an irreversible gradual deterioration of graft function occurring in many allografts months to years after transplantation. It is characterized by intimal thickening and fibrosis, which lead to luminal occlusion of the graft vasculature; it is often called cardiac allograft vasculopathy.

Diagnosis

Allograft rejection is most frequent within the first month after cardiac transplantation and declines progressively thereafter. Clinical symptoms of rejection are often vague and relatively late in terms of immune injury to myocytes. Unlike for renal and liver transplants, there are no reliable serologic markers for rejection of cardiac transplants. Although gene expression assays have the potential to identify patterns of gene activation that may correlate with allograft rejection, it is not yet clear how the information obtained can be best used in post-transplantation patients. Therefore, endomyocardial biopsy remains the "gold standard" for the diagnosis of rejection. Biopsies are performed by a transjugular approach weekly for 3 or 4 weeks, then every other week for several months; monthly biopsies continue for 6 to 12 months in many transplant programs.

Biopsy grading of cellular rejection is based on the severity of lymphocyte infiltration and myocyte necrosis (Table 82–2). Humoral rejection is usually suspected clinically when there is evidence of suboptimal graft function but the endomyocardial biopsy specimen shows either no evidence of cellular rejection or only mild rejection. The pathologic markers of humoral rejection identifiable in endomyocardial biopsy tissue include deposits of immunoglobulin M, immunoglobulin G, or complement in the microvasculature or myocytes. Evidence for antibodies in the circulation with specificity for non-HLA antigens on the graft also supports the diagnosis of humoral rejection.

Prognosis

Acute rejection causes only 12% of deaths in the first year after transplantation, but cardiac allograft vasculopathy represents a substantial portion of annual mortality beyond 3 years. Moreover, efforts to avert rejection with potent immunosuppressive therapy are responsible for other common complications after cardiac transplantation.

TABLE 82–2 STANDARDIZED CARDIAC BIOPSY GRADING: ACUTE CELLULAR REJECTION*

	2004
Grade 0 R	No rejection
Grade 1 R, mild	Interstitital and/or perivascular infiltrate with up to 1 focus of myocyte damage
Grade 2 R, moderate	Two or more foci of infiltrate with associated myocyte damage
Grade 3 R, severe	Diffuse infiltrate with multifocal myocyte damage, ± edema, ± hemorrhage, ± vasculitis

*International Society for Heart and Lung Transplantation.

Infection

Infections cause approximately 20% of deaths within the first year after transplant surgery and continue to be a common cause of morbidity and mortality throughout the recipient's life. Infections of any type during the first month after transplantation also increase the risk of a subsequent fatal cytomegalovirus (CMV) infection (Chapter 399).

Prophylaxis against CMV infection, *Pneumocystis carinii* pneumonia, herpes simplex virus infection, and oral candidiasis is now routine during the first 6 to 12 months after transplantation. As a result, the most common infections seen in the first month after surgery are nosocomial bacterial and fungal infections related to mechanical ventilation, catheters, and the surgical site.

The prophylactic use of trimethoprim-sulfamethoxazole, typically for the first year after transplantation, has virtually eliminated *P. carinii* pneumonia (Chapter 362) and also prevents nocardial infections and toxoplasmosis. The combination drug is generally reinstituted during subsequent episodes of increased risk, such as enhanced immunosuppression. Aspergillosis and candidiasis (Chapters 359 and 360) are the most common fungal infections after heart transplantation; oral nystatin solution or clotrimazole troches are routinely used in the first 6 to 12 months. Viral infections, especially CMV infection (Chapter 399), can increase immunosuppression, resulting in additional opportunistic infections. Prophylactic intravenous ganciclovir or oral valganciclovir is generally given for variable amounts of time in the CMV-seronegative recipient of a CMV-positive donor.

Health Maintenance

After 5 years, 95% of recipients have hypertension, 81% have hyperlipidemia, and 32% have diabetes. In addition, 25% to 50% have cardiac allograft vasculopathy, and up to 33% have renal insufficiency. Lifelong immunosuppression makes all recipients more susceptible to a number of malignant neoplasms, so careful follow-up is mandatory (Chapters 6 and 191).

In many centers, recipients are given daily aspirin to reduce vascular disease, but no randomized trial has evaluated the benefits of antiplatelet therapy in heart transplant patients. Likewise, most recipients are given vitamins, stool softeners, iron supplements, and proton pump inhibitors early after surgery on an empirical basis.

Surveillance

New Health Problems

Because osteoporosis (Chapter 264) is a major problem, in part related to use of corticosteroids, prophylaxis with calcium and vitamin D is usually initiated. Depression occurs in up to 25% of recipients. A number of antidepressants may be used, but the potential for adverse drug interactions must be considered. The management of gout is difficult because colchicine may increase the risk of myoneuropathy, nonsteroidal anti-inflammatory drugs often worsen renal insufficiency and hyperkalemia, and allopurinol used with azathioprine can cause life-threatening neutropenia. Minimizing diuretic use and judicious use of colchicine with allopurinol will usually alleviate most patients' symptoms.

Risk factors for malignant disease (Chapter 185) include impaired immunoregulation, a synergistic effect with other carcinogens such as nicotine or ultraviolet light exposure, and oncogenic causes such as the Epstein-Barr virus and papillomavirus. The cumulative amount of immunosuppression is positively correlated with risk of malignant change. Lymphoproliferative diseases, skin and lip cancers, and Kaposi's sarcoma are particularly common. Malignant neoplasms account for 24% of deaths after 5 years.

TRANSPLANT VASCULOPATHY

Epidemiology and Pathobiology

Transplant vasculopathy remains the most daunting long-term complication of heart transplantation, with an annual incidence rate of 5 to 10%. After the first postoperative year, cardiac allograft vasculopathy becomes increasingly important as a cause of death. Despite advances in immunosuppression, the average half-life of the cardiac allograft increased only 6 months (8.8 years to 9.4 years) from 1986–1990 to 1991–1997.

The risk of transplant vasculopathy increases as the number of HLA mismatches and the number and duration of rejection episodes increase. CMV infection and ischemia-reperfusion injury also increase the risk, as do classic risk factors for atherosclerotic disease (Chapter 49), such as smoking, obesity, diabetes, dyslipidemia, and hypertension. Transplant vasculopathy can develop as early as 3 months after transplantation and is detected angiographically in 20% of grafts at 1 year and in 40 to 50% at 5 years.

Clinical Manifestations

In contrast to eccentric lesions seen in atheromatous disease, cardiac allograft vasculopathy produces concentric narrowing from neointimal proliferation of vascular smooth muscle cells and affects the entire length of the coronary tree, from the epicardial to the intramyocardial segments, leading to rapid tapering, pruning, and obliteration of third-order branch vessels. The majority of patients will not experience anginal symptoms because of denervation of coronary arteries, so the first clinical manifestation may be myocardial infarction, heart failure, ventricular arrhythmia, or sudden death. As a result, most transplant centers screen patients annually for possible transplant vasculopathy.

Diagnosis

Intravascular ultrasonography, which is currently the most sensitive imaging technique to study early transplant vasculopathy, provides quantitative data on intimal thickness, luminal cross-sectional area, and external elastic membrane cross-sectional area. An increase in intimal thickness of at least 0.5 mm in the first year after transplantation is a reliable indicator of both cardiac allograft vasculopathy and 5-year mortality. However, increased invasiveness and cost of intravascular ultrasonography preclude its widespread application. Dobutamine stress echocardiography (Chapter 53) has a high sensitivity (83 to 95%) and specificity (between 53 and 91%) compared with angiography. Most transplant centers do one of the screening tests on an annual basis to assess the risk of new cardiac allograft vasculopathy.

Treatment

Rx

The only definitive treatment of transplant vasculopathy is repeated transplantation. The statins pravastatin and simvastatin repress the induction of class II major histocompatibility complex antigen expression by interferon-γ and thereby inhibit T-cell proliferation and have a direct influence on the expression of genes for growth factors that are essential for the proliferation of smooth muscle cells. Randomized controlled trials have shown that either drug significantly reduces rates of severe rejections and transplant vasculopathy while also significantly reducing cholesterol levels and improving survival (see later). 3, 4 It is not clear whether all statin drugs have the same benefit in this population. Sirolimus and everolimus are also being evaluated to prevent the development or progression of cardiac allograft vasculopathy, but their role has not yet been determined.

Diabetes

Diabetes (Chapter 248) occurs in 32% of transplant recipients, and patients who develop new-onset diabetes mellitus after transplantation are at increased risk for morbidity and mortality. Although impaired B-cell function appears to be the primary mechanism of calcineurin inhibitor–induced new-onset diabetes, impaired peripheral glucose use also appears to contribute to insulin resistance and abnormal glucose metabolism. Risk factors include obesity, increased age, family history of diabetes, abnormal glucose tolerance, and African American or Hispanic descent. Management is generally similar to that of the non-transplant patient.

Hypertension and Renal Insufficiency

The 5-year incidence of hypertension (Chapter 66) in the population of cardiac transplant recipients is 95%. Excess risk of hypertension is attributable primarily to the use of calcineurin inhibitors because of both direct effects and the associated renal insufficiency. Treatment often requires a combination of agents and is generally as in the non-transplant patient.

The risk of chronic renal failure is about 16% at 10 years, largely related to direct calcineurin inhibitor–mediated renal arteriolar vasoconstriction, increased levels of endothelin-1, decreased nitric oxide production, and alterations in the kidney's ability to adjust to changes in serum tonicity. Once early renal insufficiency occurs, no single treatment has yet been shown to be effective.

Hyperlipidemia

Hyperlipidemia (Chapter 217) occurs in more than 80% of cardiac transplant recipients and is associated with the development of cardiac allograft vasculopathy, cerebrovascular disease, and peripheral vascular disease. Characteristically, total cholesterol, low-density lipoprotein cholesterol, apolipoprotein B, and triglyceride levels increase by 3 months after transplantation and then generally fall somewhat after the first year. Corticosteroids, cyclosporine, sirolimus, and mycophenolate mofetil all have unfavorable effects on lipid levels, whereas tacrolimus probably causes less hyperlipidemia.

In heart transplant recipients, pravastatin and simvastatin have been associated with better outcomes, but there are no long-term data in this population demonstrating that lowering of low-density lipoprotein cholesterol levels to less than 100 mg/dL (compared with 100 to 130 mg/dL) with more potent or higher dose statin therapy improves outcomes. Different statins are metabolized differently, so caution must be exercised in the prescription of statins beyond the doses used in the randomized trials: simvastatin, 20 to 40 mg daily, and pravastatin, 10 to 20 mg daily.

OUTCOME OF TRANSPLANTATION

During the first year after transplantation, early causes of death are graft failure, infection, and rejection, with an overall survival of 87% at 1 year and 78% at 3 years (Fig. 82–2). The percentage of patients dying of early graft failure, malignant disease, and infection has remained rel-

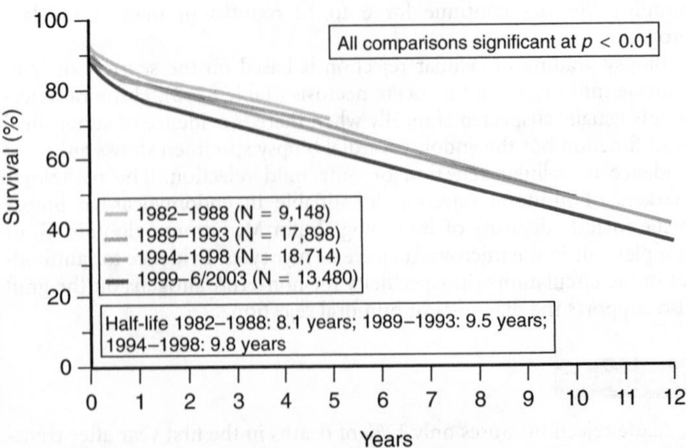

FIGURE 82–2 • The Kaplan-Meier survival by era for heart transplants performed between January 1982 and June 2003. The graph shows a significant improvement in survival over time. (Data from the Registry of the International Society for Heart and Lung Transplantation. Reproduced with permission.)

atively stable during the past decade. After 5 years, cardiac allograft vasculopathy and late graft failure (31% together), malignant disease (24%), and non-CMV infection (10%) are the most prominent causes of death.

Hemodynamic and Functional Outcomes

The transplanted heart markedly improves cardiac hemodynamics, but there may be a slightly diminished maximal cardiac output during exercise secondary to denervation, limited atrial function, decreased myocardial compliance from rejection or ischemic injury, and donor-recipient size mismatch. Immediately after surgery, a restrictive hemodynamic pattern is frequently observed, but it gradually improves during a few days to weeks. Some 10 to 15% of recipients develop a chronic restrictive cardiomyopathy (Chapter 59) that may produce fatigue and breathlessness during exercise. Because parasympathetic innervation, which normally lowers the heart rate, is absent, the typical resting heart rate of a recipient is 90 to 115 beats per minute.

At 1 year, 90% of surviving patients report no functional limitations, and approximately 35% return to work. Adapting to life after transplantation depends on many factors, including the patient's condition and duration of illness before transplantation and the patient's personality, intelligence, social support, and financial well-being.

Other Key Long-Term Issues for the Nontransplant Physician

Drug Interactions

The physician outside the transplanting hospital may be reluctant to interact at all with the heart transplant recipient, a fear that complicates the comprehensive care of these patients. Often a phone call placed to the transplant center to clarify any proposed medications or new symptoms will obviate the need for the recipient to travel to the transplant hospital. The most common errors made by non-transplant physicians are the addition of new drugs that result in adverse drug interactions; examples include acyclovir, allopurinol, amlodipine, antacids, antidepressants, cimetidine, clarithromycin, clotrimazole, colchicine, diltiazem, erythromycin, felodipine, ganciclovir, grapefruit juice, iron, ketoconazole, phenobarbital, phenytoin, primidone, rifampin, statin drugs, St. John's wort, trimethoprim-sulfamethoxazole, valganciclovir, and verapamil. In addition, the index of suspicion must be higher in evaluating the possibility of infection in a transplant recipient (Chapter 303).

FUTURE DIRECTIONS IN CARDIAC TRANSPLANTATION

It is not surprising that uniform agreement has not been achieved among transplant centers regarding the precise indications for and timing of listing for cardiac transplantation. The basic tenet of organ allocation embraces two axioms that are at times contradictory: equity, or equal access of all patients to donor organs, with priority given to patients closest to death; and utility, an allocation policy for organs that maximizes survival of the patient and graft. As newer therapies, such as cell transplantation and better permanent mechanical devices, become available, the role of heart transplantation will need to be redefined.

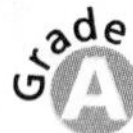

1. Eisen HJ, Kobashigawa J, Keogh A, et al: Three-year results of a randomized, double-blind, controlled trial of mycophenolate mofetil versus azathioprine in cardiac transplant recipients. J Heart Lung Transplant 2005;24:517–525.
2. Keogh A, Richardson M, Ruygrok P, et al: Sirolimus in de novo heart transplant recipients reduces acute rejection and prevents coronary artery disease at 2 years: A randomized clinical trial. Circulation 2004;110:2694–2700.
3. Wenke K, Meiser B, Thiery J, et al: Simvastatin reduces graft vessel disease and mortality after heart transplantation: A four-year randomized trial. Circulation 1997;96:1398–1402.
4. Kobashigawa JA, Katznelson S, Laks H, et al: Effect of pravastatin on outcomes after cardiac transplantation. N Engl J Med 1995;333:621–627.

SUGGESTED READINGS

Boyle A, Colvin-Adams M: Recipient selection and management. Semin Thorac Cardiovasc Surg 2004;16:358–363. *Summarizes the issues involved in evaluating a potential transplant candidate.*

Goldstein DJ, Smego D, Michler RE: Surgical aspects of congestive heart failure. Heart Fail Rev 2006;11:171–192. *A practical review.*

Grady KL, Naftel DC, Kobashigawa J, et al: Patterns and predictors of quality of life at 5 to 10 years after heart transplantation. J Heart Lung Transplant 2007;26:535–543. *QOL remained positive and stable. Biopsychosocial variables predicted satisfaction and QOL.*

Hosenpud JD: Immunosuppression in cardiac transplantation. N Engl J Med 2005;352:2749–2750. *An honest appraisal of the difficulties in gathering evidence-based recommendations in heart transplantation.*

Lindenfeld J, Miller GG, Shakar SF, et al: Drug therapy in the heart transplant recipient: Parts I to IV. Circulation 2004;110:3734–3740, 2004;110:3858–3865, 2005;111:113–117, and 2005;111:230–239. *An excellent summary of drug therapy in cardiac transplantation.*

Taylor DO, Edwards LB, Boucek MM, et al: Registry of the International Society for Heart and Lung Transplantation: Twenty-second Official Adult Heart Transplant Report—2005. J Heart Lung Transplant 2005;24:945–955. *Summary of international data.*

Section IX

Respiratory Diseases

APPROACH TO THE PATIENT WITH RESPIRATORY DISEASE

Monica Kraft

Respiratory symptoms, which are among the most common reasons that patients seek medical care, represent about 20% of office visits to a primary care physician. Key common respiratory complaints include cough, wheezing, dyspnea, and hemoptysis.

APPROACH TO THE PATIENT WITH COUGH

Cough is the single most common respiratory complaint for which patients seek care. Referrals of patients with persistently troublesome chronic cough of unknown etiology account for 10 to 38% of outpatient visits to respiratory specialists.

For acute cough, defined as coughing that has been present for less than 8 weeks, a careful medical history and physical examination will usually reveal the diagnosis (Table 83–1). Although most acute coughs are of minor consequence, cough can occasionally be a sign of a potentially life-threatening illness, such as pulmonary embolism (Chapter 99), pneumonia (Chapter 97), or heart failure (Chapter 57). Nonspecific treatment of acute cough is discussed in Grade A reference 1.

Up to 98% of all cases of chronic cough, defined as a cough that persists for more than 8 weeks, in immunocompetent adults are caused by eight common conditions: postnasal drip syndrome from a variety of rhinosinus conditions (Chapter 272), asthma (Chapter 87), gastroesophageal reflux disease (Chapter 140), chronic bronchitis (Chapter 88), eosinophilic bronchitis, bronchiectasis (Chapter 90), use of angiotensin-converting enzyme inhibitors, and postinfectious cough. Postinfectious cough is usually nonproductive and lasts for 3 to 8 weeks after an upper respiratory infection; patients have a normal chest radiograph. Uncommon causes of chronic cough include bronchogenic carcinoma (Chapter 201), chronic interstitial pneumonia (Chapter 92), sarcoidosis (Chapter 95), left ventricular failure (Chapter 57), and aspiration (Chapter 94).

Diagnosis

In chronic cough (Fig. 83–1), the character and timing are not of diagnostic help. A chest radiograph should be obtained in all patients, but other tests should not be ordered in current smokers or patients taking angiotensin-converting enzyme inhibitors until the response to smoking cessation or discontinuation of the drug for at least 4 weeks can be assessed. Sinus radiographs, barium esophagography, methacholine challenge, esophageal pH, and bronchoscopy can be ordered as part of the initial evaluation, depending on the history and physical examination findings (see Fig. 83–1 and Table 83–2). If a test result points toward a possible diagnosis, a trial of treatment for that condition is needed to confirm the diagnosis.

The specific cause of cough can be diagnosed and treated successfully 84 to 98% of the time, so nonspecific therapy aimed to suppress the cough is rarely indicated. There is no strong evidence that nonspecific therapies such as antitussives, mucolytics, decongestants, or antihistamine-decongestant combinations are efficacious for acute cough in the setting of an upper respiratory tract infection. [1] An empirical trial of a proton pump inhibitor may sometimes be warranted for chronic cough because it may be caused by otherwise asymptomatic gastroesophageal reflux [2] (Chapter 140).

APPROACH TO THE PATIENT WITH WHEEZING

Wheeze is a continuous musical sound that lasts longer than 80 to 100 msec, probably generated by flow though critically narrowed collapsible bronchi. Although expiratory wheezing is a common physical finding in asthma (Chapter 87), the many causes of wheezing (Table 83–3), such as chronic obstructive pulmonary disease (Chapter 88), pulmonary edema (Chapter 91), bronchiolitis (Chapter 87), bronchiectasis (Chapter 90), and less common entities like carcinoid (Chapter 251) and parasitic infections, often can be distinguished on the basis of the history, physical examination, and pulmonary function testing (Chapter 85). The shape of inspiratory and expiratory flow-volume loops provides key information about whether the obstruction is extrathoracic or intrathoracic (Fig. 83–2). Vocal cord lesions are an important cause of extrathoracic obstruction (Chapters 200 and 455). Variable intrathoracic obstruction can be caused by tracheomalacia, whereas fixed upper airway obstruction can be caused by a proximal tracheal tumor.

APPROACH TO THE PATIENT WITH DYSPNEA

Dyspnea is the sensation of difficult, labored, or unpleasant breathing. The word *unpleasant* is important to this definition; the labored or difficult breathing encountered by healthy individuals during exercise does not qualify as dyspnea because it is at the level expected for the degree of exertion. The sensation of dyspnea is often poorly or vaguely described by the patient. The physiology of dyspnea remains unclear, but multiple neural pathways can be involved in processes that lead to dyspnea.

Diagnosis

Dyspnea should be approached in a systematic manner (see Fig. 48–1). In acute dyspnea, or shortness of breath of sudden onset, the history, physical examination, and laboratory testing must first focus on potential life-threatening conditions, including pulmonary embolism (Chapter 99), pulmonary edema (Chapters 57 and 58), acute airway obstruction from anaphylaxis or foreign bodies, pneumothorax (Chapter 100), and pneumonia (Chapter 97). Treatment of each is determined by the nature and severity of the underlying cause.

For chronic dyspnea, specific conditions to consider include chronic obstructive pulmonary disease (Chapter 88), asthma (Chapter 87), interstitial lung disease (Chapter 92), heart failure (Chapter 57), cardiomyopathy (Chapter 59), gastroesophageal reflux disease (Chapter 140), other respiratory diseases, and the hyperventilation syndrome. A chest radiograph, an electrocardiogram, pulmonary function tests, and an exercise test with electrocardiographic monitoring and pulse oximetry at rest and during exercise are key to assessment of patients with unexplained dyspnea (Table 83–4). The utility of more detailed pulmonary testing with maximal inspiratory and expiratory pressures, flow-volume loops, or methacholine challenge and of computed tomographic screening of the chest and echocardiography depends on the history and physical examination and the results of these tests. When gastroesophageal reflux disease is a suspected cause of dyspnea, a modified barium esophagogram or 24-hour esophageal pH monitoring should be considered (Chapter 140). Other more invasive tests, such as cardiac catheterization and lung biopsy, may be indicated when the results of less invasive tests have not been conclusive. Whenever possible, the final determination of the cause of dyspnea is made by observing which specific therapy eliminates it. Because dyspnea may be simultaneously due to more than one condition, it may be necessary to treat more than one condition.

APPROACH TO THE PATIENT WITH HEMOPTYSIS

Hemoptysis is the expectoration of blood from the lung parenchyma or airways. Hemoptysis may be scant, with just the appearance of streaks of bright red blood in the sputum, or massive, with the expectoration of a large volume of blood. Massive hemoptysis, which is defined as the expectoration of more than 600 mL of blood in 24 to 48 hours, may occur in 3 to 10% of patients with hemoptysis. Dark red clots may also be expectorated when the blood has been present in the lungs for days.

Pseudohemoptysis, which is the expectoration of blood from a source other than the lower respiratory tract, may cause diagnostic confusion when patients cannot clearly describe the source of their bleeding. Pseudohemoptysis can occur when blood from the oral cavity, nares, pharynx, or tongue clings to the back of the throat and initiates the cough reflex or when patients who have hematemesis aspirate into the lower respiratory tract. When the oropharynx is colonized with *Serratia marcescens*, a red pigment–producing aerobic gram-negative rod, the sputum can also be red and be confused with hemoptysis.

Hemoptysis can be caused by a wide variety of disorders. Virtually all causes of hemoptysis (Table 83–5) may result in massive hemoptysis, but massive hemoptysis is most frequently caused by infection, for example, tuberculosis (Chapter 345), bronchiectasis (Chapter 90), lung abscess

TABLE 83–1 SPECTRUM OF CAUSES AND FREQUENCIES OF COUGH IN IMMUNOCOMPETENT ADULTS

Common	Less Common
ACUTE COUGH	
Common cold	Asthma
Acute bacterial sinusitis	Pneumonia
Pertussis	Heart failure
Exacerbations of chronic obstructive pulmonary disease	Aspiration syndromes
Allergic rhinitis	Pulmonary embolism
Environmental irritant rhinitis	Exacerbation of bronchiectasis
CHRONIC COUGH	
Rhinosinus conditions	Bronchogenic carcinoma
Asthma	Chronic interstitial pneumonia
Gastroesophageal reflux	Sarcoidosis
Chronic bronchitis	Left-sided heart failure
Eosinophilic bronchitis	
Bronchiectasis	
Angiotensin-converting enzyme inhibitors	
Postinfectious	

(Chapter 98), and cancer (Chapter 201). Infections with aspergilloma (Chapter 360) and in patients with cystic fibrosis (Chapter 89) also are associated with massive hemoptysis. Iatrogenic causes of massive hemoptysis include rupture of a pulmonary artery after less than 0.2% of cases of balloon-guided flotation catheterization and tracheal artery fistula as a complication of tracheostomy.

In nonmassive hemoptysis, the etiology is bronchitis in more than one third of cases (Chapter 88), bronchogenic carcinoma (Chapter 201) in one fifth of cases, tuberculosis (Chapter 345) in 7%, pneumonia (Chapter 97) in 5%, and bronchiectasis in 1% (Chapter 90). By a systematic diagnostic approach (see later), the cause of hemoptysis can be found in 68 to 98% of cases. The remaining 2 to 32% have idiopathic or central hemoptysis, which occurs most commonly in men between the ages of 30 and 50 years. Prolonged follow-up of idiopathic hemoptysis almost always fails to reveal the source of bleeding even though 10% continue to have occasional episodes of hemoptysis.

Diagnosis

The diagnostic evaluation for hemoptysis begins with a detailed medical history and a complete physical examination. Information on the amount of bleeding as well as details about the frequency, timing, and duration of hemoptysis should be obtained. For example, repeated episodes of hemoptysis occurring during a period of months to years suggest a bronchial adenoma or bronchiectasis as the cause, whereas small amounts of hemoptysis occurring every day for weeks are more likely to be caused by bronchogenic carcinoma. A travel history can suggest coccidioidomycosis (Chapter 354) and histoplasmosis (Chapter

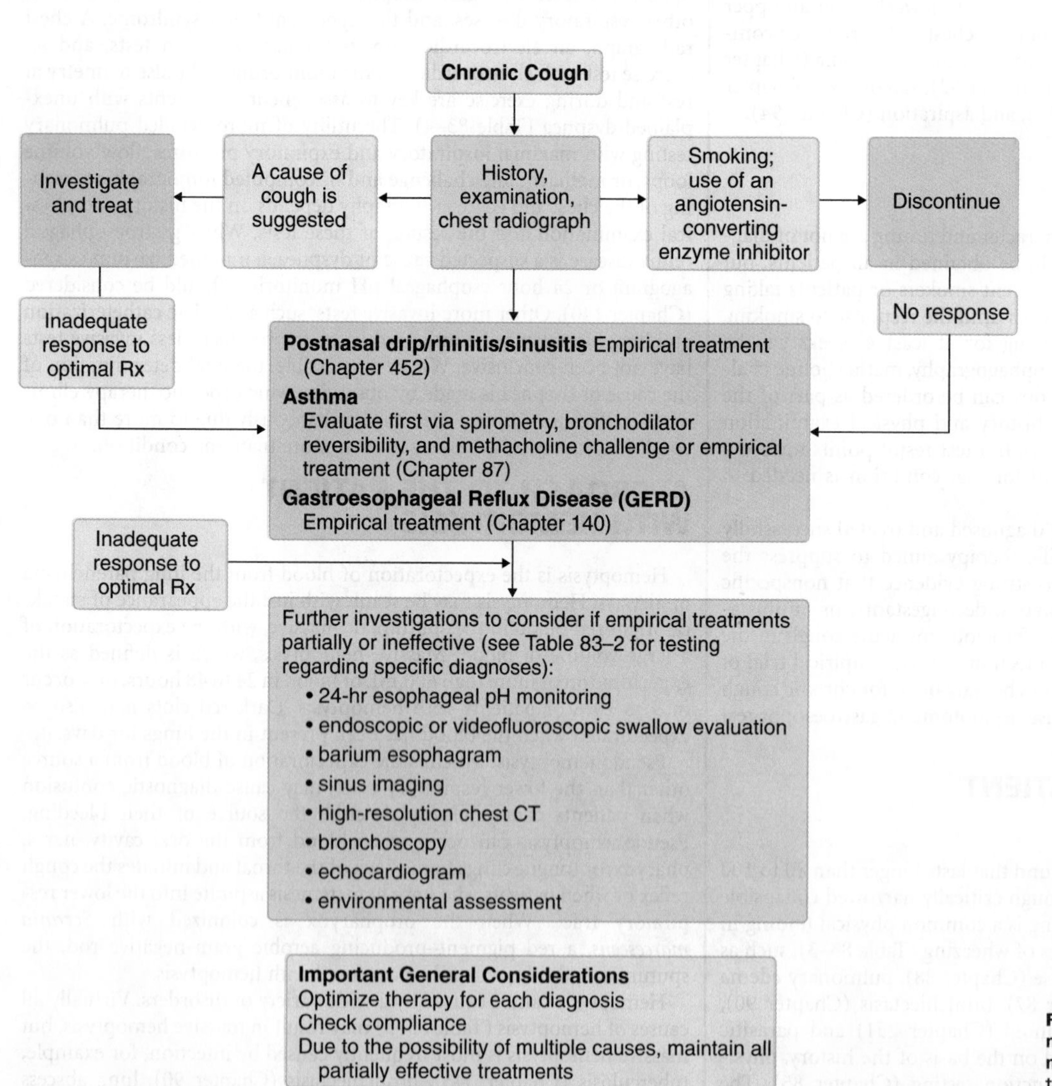

FIGURE 83–1 • Algorithm for the management of chronic cough lasting more than 8 weeks. CT = computed tomography.

TABLE 83–2 TESTING CHARACTERISTICS OF DIAGNOSTIC PROTOCOL FOR EVALUATION OF CHRONIC COUGH

Tests	Diagnosis	Positive Predictive Value (%)	Negative Predictive Value (%)
Sinus radiography	Sinusitis	57–81	95–100
Methacholine inhalation challenge	Asthma	60–82	100
Modified barium esophagography	GERD, esophageal stricture	38–63	63–93
Esophageal pH	GERD	89–100	<100
Bronchoscopy	Endobronchial mass or lesion	50–89	100

Esophageal pH = 24-hour esophageal pH monitoring; GERD = gastroesophageal reflux disease.

TABLE 83–3 DIAGNOSIS OF SELECTED WHEEZING ILLNESSES OTHER THAN ASTHMA

	Distinguishing Features
UPPER AIRWAY DISEASES	
Postnasal drip syndrome	History of postnasal drip, throat clearing, nasal discharge; physical examination shows oropharyngeal secretions or cobblestone appearance to mucosa
Epiglottitis	History of sore throat out of proportion to pharyngitis; evidence of supraglottitis on endoscopy or lateral neck radiographs
Vocal cord dysfunction syndrome	Lack of symptomatic response to bronchodilators, presence of stridor plus wheeze in absence of increased $P(A - a)O_2$; extrathoracic variable obstruction on flow-volume loops; paradoxical inspiratory or early expiratory adduction of vocal cords on laryngoscopy during wheezing; this syndrome can masquerade as asthma, be provoked by exercise, and often coexists with asthma
Retropharyngeal abscess	History of stiff neck, sore throat, fever, trauma to posterior pharynx; swelling noted by lateral neck or CT radiographs
Laryngotracheal injury due to tracheal cannulation	History of cannulation of trachea by endotracheal or tracheostomy tube; evidence of intrathoracic or extrathoracic variable obstruction on flow-volume loops, neck and chest radiographs, laryngoscopy, or bronchoscopy
Neoplasms	Bronchogenic carcinoma, adenoma, or carcinoid tumor is suspected when there is hemoptysis, unilateral wheeze, or evidence of lobar collapse on chest radiograph or combinations of these; diagnosis is confirmed by bronchoscopy
Anaphylaxis	Abrupt onset of wheezing with urticaria, angioedema, nausea, diarrhea, and hypotension, especially after insect bite, in association with other signs of anaphylaxis such as hypotension or hives, with the administration of drug or intravenous contrast agent, or with family history
SMALL AIRWAY DISEASES	
COPD	History of dyspnea on exertion and productive cough in cigarette smoker; because productive cough is nonspecific, it should be ascribed to COPD only when other cough-phlegm syndromes have been excluded, forced expiratory time to empty more than 80% of vital capacity is >4 sec, and there is decreased breath sound intensity, unforced wheezing during auscultation, and irreversible, expiratory airflow obstruction on spirometry
Pulmonary edema	History and physical examination consistent with passive congestion of the lungs, ARDS, impaired lung lymphatics; abnormal chest radiograph, echocardiogram, radionuclide ventriculography, cardiac catheterization, or combinations of these
Aspiration	History of risk for pharyngeal dysfunction or gastroesophageal reflux disease; abnormal modified barium swallow study or 24-hour esophageal pH monitoring
Pulmonary embolism	History of risk for thromboembolic disease, positive confirmatory test results
Bronchiolitis	History of respiratory infection, connective tissue disease, transplantation, ulcerative colitis, development of chronic airway obstruction during months to few years rather than during many years in a nonsmoker; mixed obstructive and restrictive pattern on PFTs and hyperinflation; may be accompanied by fine nodular infiltrates on chest radiograph
Cystic fibrosis	Combination of productive cough, digital clubbing, bronchiectasis, progressive COPD with *Pseudomonas* colonization or infection, obstructive azoospermia, family history, pancreatic insufficiency, and two sweat chloride determinations >60 mEq/L; some patients are not diagnosed until adulthood, in one instance as late as the age of 69 years; when sweat test is occasionally normal, definitive diagnosis may require nasal transepithelial voltage measurements and genotyping
Carcinoid syndrome	History of episodes of flushing and watery diarrhea; elevated 5-hydroxyindoleactic acid level in 24-hour urine specimen
Bronchiectasis	History of episodes of productive cough, fever, or recurrent pneumonias; suggestive chest radiographs or typical chest CT findings; ABPA should be considered when bronchiectasis is central
Lymphangitic carcinomatosis	History of dyspnea or prior malignant neoplasm; reticulonodular infiltrates with or without pleural effusions; suggestive high-resolution chest CT scan; confirmed by bronchoscopy with biopsies
Parasitic infections	Consider in a nonasthmatic who has traveled to an endemic area and complains of fatigue, weight loss, fever; peripheral blood eosinophilia; infiltrates on chest radiograph; stools for ova and parasites for nonfilarial causes; blood serologic studies for filarial causes

ABPA = allergic bronchopulmonary aspergillosis; ARDS = acute respiratory distress syndrome; COPD = chronic obstructive pulmonary disease; CT = computed tomography; $P(A - a)O_2$ = alveolar-arterial oxygen tension gradient; PFTs = pulmonary function tests.

353) in the United States, paragonimiasis and ascariasis (Chapter 378) in the Far East, and schistosomiasis (Chapter 376) in South America. Orthopnea and paroxysmal nocturnal dyspnea suggest heart failure (Chapter 57), especially from mitral stenosis (Chapter 75). In patients who have occupational exposure to trimellitic anhydride, which occurs when heated metal surfaces are sprayed with a corrosion-resistant epoxy resin, hemoptysis can be part of the postexposure syndrome. In a patient with the triad of upper airway disease, lower airway disease, and renal disease, Wegener's granulomatosis (Chapter 92) should be suspected. Pulmonary hemorrhage may also be a presenting manifestation of systemic lupus erythematosus (Chapter 287). Goodpasture's syndrome, which typically occurs in young men, is also associated with renal disease (Chapter 115). Diffuse alveolar hemorrhage occurs in 20% of cases during autologous bone marrow transplantation (Chapter 184) and should be suspected in patients who have undergone recent bone marrow transplantation (Chapter 184) when they present with cough, dyspnea, hypoxemia, and diffuse pulmonary infiltrates.

On physical examination, inspection of the skin and mucous membranes may show telangiectasias suggesting hereditary hemorrhagic telangiectasia (Chapter 466) or ecchymoses and petechiae suggesting a hematologic abnormality (Chapter 179). Pulsations transmitted to a tracheostomy cannula should heighten suspicion of a tracheal artery fistula. Inspection of the thorax should show evidence of recent or old chest trauma, and unilateral wheeze or rales may herald localized disease such as a bronchial adenoma or carcinoma. Although pulmonary embolism (Chapter 99) cannot be definitively diagnosed on physical examination, tachypnea, phlebitis, and pleural friction rub suggest this disorder. If rales are heard on the chest examination, heart failure as well as other diseases causing diffuse pulmonary hemorrhage (see earlier) or idiopathic pulmonary hemosiderosis (Chapter 92) should be considered. Careful cardiovascular examination may help diagnose mitral stenosis (Chapter 75), pulmonary artery fistulas, or pulmonary hypertension (Chapter 67).

Routine laboratory studies should include a complete blood count, urinalysis, and coagulation studies. The complete blood count may suggest an infection, hematologic disorder, or chronic blood loss. Urinalysis may reveal hematuria and suggest the presence of a systemic disease (e.g., Wegener's granulomatosis, Goodpasture's syndrome, systemic lupus erythematosus) associated with renal disease. Coagulation studies may uncover a hematologic disorder that is primarily responsible for hemoptysis or that contributes to excessive bleeding from another disease. The electrocardiogram may help suggest the presence of a cardiovascular disorder. Although as many as 30% of patients with hemoptysis have a normal chest radiograph, routine chest radiographs may be diagnostically valuable.

Bronchoscopy can localize the bleeding site in up to 93% of patients by fiberoptic bronchoscopy and in up to 86% with rigid bronchoscopy.

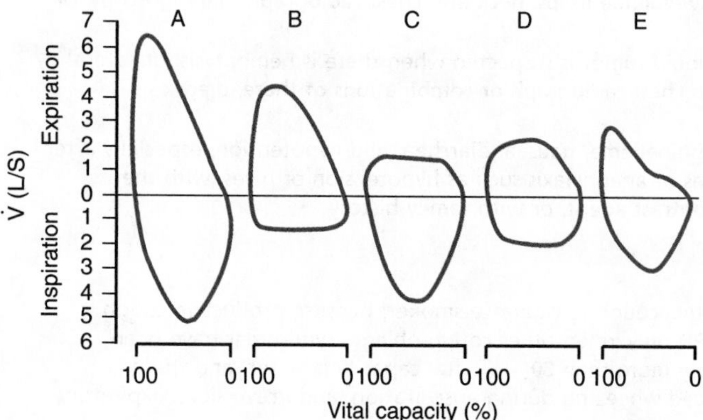

FIGURE 83–2 • Schematic flow-volume loop configurations in a spectrum of airway lesions. A is normal; B is variable extrathoracic upper airway obstruction; C is variable intrathoracic upper airway lesion; D is fixed upper airway obstruction; and E is small airway obstruction. (Reproduced with permission from the American College of Chest Physicians, Pulmonary Board Review Syllabus, 2003.)

TABLE 83–5 COMMON CAUSES OF MASSIVE HEMOPTYSIS

Cardiovascular
- Arterial bronchial fistula
- Heart failure, especially from mitral stenosis
- Pulmonary arteriovenous fistula

Diffuse intrapulmonary hemorrhage

Diffuse parenchymal disease

Iatrogenic
- Malposition of chest tube
- Pulmonary artery rupture after pulmonary arterial catheterization
- Tracheal artery fistula

Infections
- Aspergilloma
- Bronchiectasis
- Bronchitis
- Cystic fibrosis
- Lung abscess
- Sporotrichosis
- Tuberculosis

Malignant neoplasms
- Bronchogenic carcinoma
- Leukemia
- Metastatic cancer

Trauma

TABLE 83–4 REPORTED PREDICTIVE VALUES OF DIAGNOSTIC TESTS IN THE EVALUATION OF CHRONIC DYSPNEA

Test	Diagnosis	Positive Predictive Value (%)	Negative Predictive Value (%)
Spirometry	COPD	32	100
Spirometry	Asthma	18	72
Spirometry	All diagnoses	80	56
Methacholine challenge	Asthma	95	100
Diffusing capacity	ILD	79	95
Echocardiogram	Cardiac	44	0
Barium esophagram	GERD	33	83
Comprehensive ETT	All diagnoses	93	0
Chest radiograph	All diagnoses	75	91

COPD = chronic obstructive pulmonary disease; ETT = exercise tolerance test; GERD = gastrointestinal reflux disease; ILD = interstitial lung disease.
Modified from Pratter MR, Curley FJ, Dubois J, Irwin RS: Cause and evaluation of chronic dyspnea in a pulmonary disease clinic. Arch Intern Med 1989;149:2277–2282.

TABLE 83–6 EXAMPLES OF SPECIAL EVALUATIONS FOR HEMOPTYSIS ACCORDING TO CATEGORY OF DISEASE*

Tracheobronchial disorders
Expectorated sputum for TB, parasites, fungi, and cytology
Bronchoscopy (if not done)
Bronchography
High-resolution chest CT scan
Localized parenchymal diseases
Expectorated sputum for TB, parasites, fungi, and cytology
Chest CT scan
Lung biopsy with special stains
Diffuse parenchymal diseases
Expectorated sputum for cytology
Assess renal function; urinalysis; evaluation for systemic disease (e.g., ANA, RF, complement, cryoglobulins, ANCA, anti-GBM antibody)
Lung or kidney biopsy with special stains
Cardiovascular disorders
Echocardiogram
Arterial blood gas on room air and 100% oxygen
Ventilation-perfusion scans
Pulmonary arteriogram
Aortogram, contrast-enhanced CT scan
Hematologic disorders
Coagulation studies
Bone marrow

*This table is not meant to be all-inclusive.
ANA = antinuclear antibody; ANCA = antineutrophil cytoplasmic antibodies; CT = computed tomographic; GBM = glomerular basement membrane; RF = rheumatoid factor; TB = tuberculosis.

It may establish sites of bleeding different from those suggested by the chest radiograph. The best results are obtained when bronchoscopy is performed during or within 24 hours of active bleeding, and rates of diagnosis fall to about 50% by 48 hours after bleeding. When there is no active bleeding, bronchoscopy with bronchoalveolar lavage can be helpful in patients thought to have diffuse intrapulmonary hemorrhage. Typical findings are bright red or blood-tinged lavage fluid from multiple lobes in both lungs and a substantial number of hemosiderin-laden macrophages (i.e., at least 20% of the total number of alveolar macrophages).

Depending on the results of the initial evaluation and the likely categories of hemoptysis, additional diagnostic tests can be helpful (Table 83–6). Bronchoscopy may not be needed in patients who have stable chronic bronchitis (Chapter 88) with one episode of blood streaking or who have acute tracheobronchitis (Chapter 88). Bronchoscopy may also not be needed with obvious cardiovascular causes of hemoptysis, such as heart failure and pulmonary embolism.

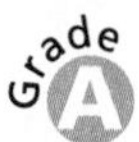

1. Schroeder K, Fahey T: Over-the-counter medications for acute cough in children and adults in ambulatory settings. Cochrane Database Syst Rev 2004;4:CD001831.
2. Chang AB, Lasserson TJ, Kiljander TO, et al: Systematic review and meta-analysis of randomised controlled trials of gastro-oesophageal reflux interventions for chronic cough associated with gastro-oesophageal reflux. BMJ 2006;332:11–17.

SUGGESTED READINGS

Bidwell JL, Pachner RW: Hemoptysis: Diagnosis and management. Am Fam Physician 2005;72:1253–1260. *A review emphasizing risk factors, etiology, diagnostic strategies, and management.*

Irwin RS: Assessing cough severity and efficacy of therapy in clinical research: ACCP evidence-based clinical practice guidelines. Chest 2006;129 (1 Suppl): 232S–237S. *Review on evaluation and treatment of cough, with algorithms.*

Irwin RS, Madison JM: Diagnosis and treatment of cough. N Engl J Med 2000;343:1715–1721. *A concise review.*

Scano G, Ambrosino N: Pathophysiology of dyspnea. Lung 2002;80:131–148. *A comprehensive review.*

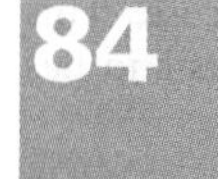

IMAGING IN PULMONARY DISEASE

Paul Stark

IMAGING OF THE LUNGS, MEDIASTINUM, AND CHEST WALL

Epidemiology

Worldwide, chest radiography is the most commonly performed imaging procedure; more than 75 million chest radiographs are performed every year in the United States alone. Chest radiographs provide useful information about the patient's anatomy and disease at a minimal monetary cost and with radiation exposure that most experts agree is negligible. Although many novel imaging techniques are available, the plain chest radiograph remains invaluable in the initial assessment of disorders of the lung, pleura, mediastinum, and chest wall.

Imaging Techniques

Chest radiographs, although classically obtained with cassettes and x-ray film, are now commonly acquired by digital imaging with electronic display at workstations and distribution of data through networks. Regardless of the image processing approach used, the standard chest radiograph is performed at 2 m from the x-ray tube focal spot to the image detector, in frontal and lateral projections. If possible, the films should be obtained with the patient inhaling to total lung capacity. These images provide views of the lungs, mediastinum, and chest wall simultaneously.

Portable Radiography

Although bedside or portable radiography accounts for a large number of chest radiographs, the images obtained are generally of lower technical quality, cost more, and are more difficult to interpret. Lung volumes are low, thereby leading to crowding of vascular structures, and the low kilovoltage technique required for the portable equipment yields films with overexposed lungs and an underpenetrated mediastinum. The anteroposterior projection and the slightly lordotic angulation of the x-ray beam combine to distort the basilar lung structures and magnify the cardiac silhouette. Recumbent studies also make recognition of pleural effusions or pneumothoraces more difficult.

Computed Tomography

Computed tomography (CT) has multiple advantages over conventional radiography. It displays cross-sectional anatomy free of superimposition, with a 10-fold higher contrast resolution. Multislice CT scanners acquire a continuous, volumetric, isotropic data set with possibilities for high-quality two-dimensional or three-dimensional reformatting (volume rendering) in any plane. High-resolution CT of the lung parenchyma is an important application; narrow collimation of the beam combined with an edge-enhancing high spatial frequency algorithm results in exquisite detail of normal and abnormal lungs, and correlation with pathologic anatomy is high.

Magnetic Resonance Imaging

Magnetic resonance imaging (MRI) depends on the magnetic properties of hydrogen atoms. Magnetic coils and radio frequency coils lead to induction, excitation, and eventual readout of magnetized protons. The molecular environment of hydrogen atoms will affect the rate at which they release energy; this energy yields a spatial distribution of signals that is converted into an image by computer algorithms, similar to CT. Because of its soft tissue specificity, MRI has applications in the assessment of chest wall invasion, mediastinal infiltration, and diaphragmatic involvement by lung cancer or malignant mesothelioma.

Positron Emission Tomography

Fluorodeoxyglucose positron emission tomography (FDG-PET) uses labeled fluorodeoxyglucose to image the glycolytic pathway of tumor cells or other metabolically active tissues with affinity for glucose. This technique has proved helpful in studying intrathoracic tumors and has facilitated the work-up of solitary pulmonary nodules.

Ultrasonography

Outside the heart, ultrasonography plays only a limited role in thoracic imaging. Its primary use is to localize pleural effusions and to guide their drainage.

Evaluation of Chest Images

Images of the chest are best evaluated by examining regions of the lung for specific findings and relating these findings to known diagnostic groups. A number of critical radiographic features should be considered, with an appreciation for the known causes of these changes.

Diffuse Lung Disease

Diffuse lung disease is an overall term for a number of related abnormal parenchymal radiographic patterns. Although radiologists have attempted to separate alveolar from interstitial lung disease radiographically, this distinction is no longer recommended because the correlation between the radiographic localization to a compartment and the actual histopathologic findings is relatively poor. For example, nodular patterns can be produced by either interstitial or alveolar disease. Conversely, so-called alveolar disease processes can induce an interstitial reaction. Ground-glass opacities can be induced by either alveolar or interstitial disease. Air bronchograms, the presumed paradigm of air space disease, can be identified in a small percentage of patients with predominantly interstitial lung disease, such as sarcoidosis, pulmonary lymphoma, and pulmonary calcinosis.

Because of such limitations, a graphically descriptive approach that combines analysis of predominant opacities, assessment of lung expansion, and distribution and profusion of disease yields a differential diagnosis. The term *infiltrate* should be avoided; instead, pulmonary opacities are classified as large (i.e., exceeding 1 cm in largest dimension) or small (i.e., less than 1 cm in diameter).

Large Opacities

Large opacities (Table 84–1) are characterized according to their distribution. Diffuse homogeneous opacities are typical for diffuse alveolar damage (Fig. 84–1A), increased permeability (noncardiogenic) pulmonary edema, diffuse viral pneumonia, or *Pneumocystis jiroveci* pneumonia. Multifocal patchy opacities (see Fig. 84–1B) are found in multifocal bronchopneumonia, recurrent aspiration, or vasculitis. Lobar opacities without atelectasis are typically seen in lobar pneumonia. Lobar opacities with atelectasis often result from obstruction of a lobar bronchus by foreign bodies, tumors, or mucus plugs. Perihilar opacities are seen in hydrostatic pulmonary edema due to left-sided heart failure (Fig. 84–2), renal failure, volume overload, or pulmonary hemorrhage.

TABLE 84–1 CLASSIFICATION OF LARGE PULMONARY OPACITIES

Diffuse homogeneous
Multifocal patchy
Lobar without atelectasis
Lobar with atelectasis
Perihilar
Peripheral

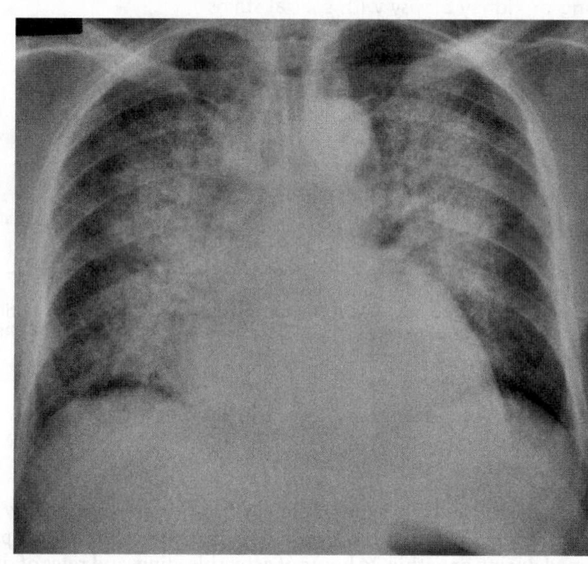

FIGURE 84–2 • Patient with hydrostatic pulmonary edema due to left-sided heart failure. Chest frontal radiograph demonstrates classic "batwing" distribution of pulmonary edema.

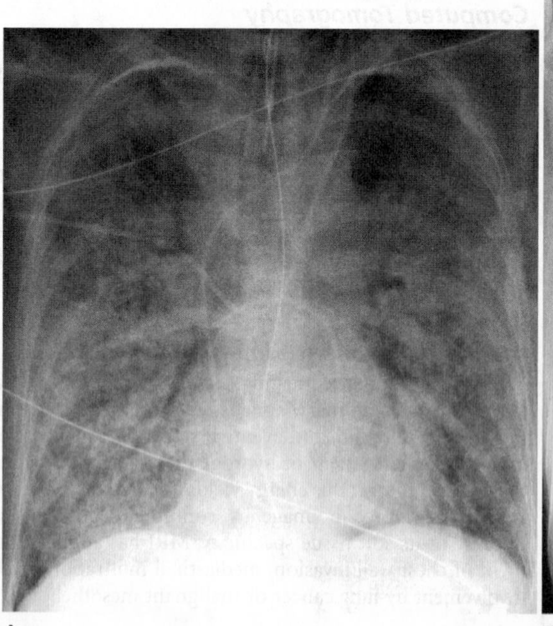

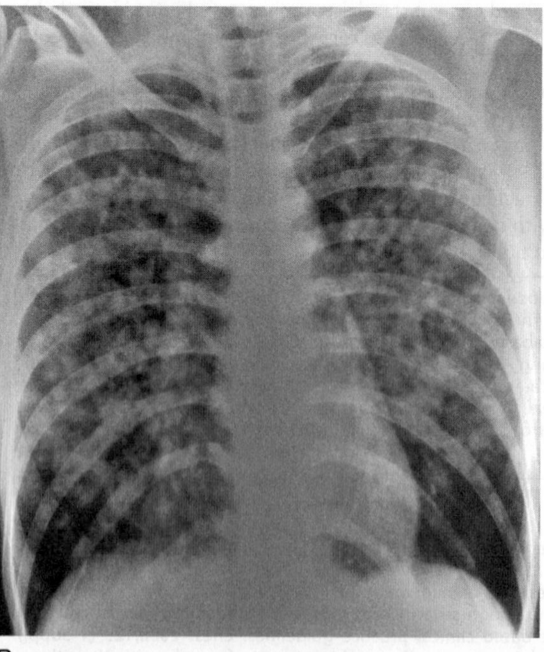

FIGURE 84–1 • A, Patient with diffuse alveolar damage. Chest radiograph shows diffuse homogeneous opacification of both lungs with clearly visible air bronchograms. **B, Patient with acute varicella pneumonia.** Chest radiograph demonstrates multiple "acinar" nodules with tendency for confluence, yielding multifocal patchy parenchymal opacification.

TABLE 84–2 PATTERNS OF SMALL PULMONARY OPACITIES

Micronodular
Acinar
Linear
Reticular
Bronchial
Arterial
Destructive

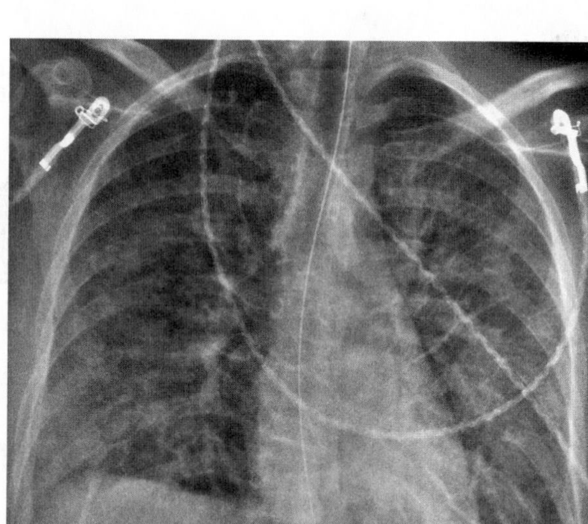

FIGURE 84–3 • Patient with known transfusion reaction. Chest radiograph displays ground-glass opacification of both lungs and bilateral Kerley's A lines, presenting as long linear structures extending from the hilar regions into the pulmonary periphery.

Small Opacities

In contrast to the large pulmonary opacities, a number of radiographic patterns characterize small pulmonary opacities in diffuse lung disease. It is helpful to differentiate small nodular, linear, reticular, or combined patterns (Table 84–2). Micronodular opacities, which include nodules 1 mm and smaller in diameter, can result from talc granulomatosis in intravenous drug abusers (Chapter 32), alveolar microlithiasis, rare cases of silicosis, talcosis, coal workers' pneumoconiosis (Chapter 93), and beryllium-induced lung diseases (Chapter 93) as well as from occasional cases of sarcoidosis (Chapter 95) or hemosiderosis. The nodular pattern includes nodules up to 1 cm in diameter. Frequent causes include infections or inflammatory granulomas such as miliary tuberculosis (Chapter 345), sarcoidosis (Chapter 95), fungal diseases, extrinsic allergic alveolitis, and Langerhans cell histiocytosis (Chapter 92).

Linear Patterns

Linear patterns, also called Kerley's lines, are mostly a reflection of thickened interlobular septa. Kerley's A lines, which radiate 2 cm to 4 cm from the hilum toward the pulmonary periphery and particularly toward the upper lobes (Fig. 84–3), reflect thickening of the axial interstitial compartment and can be a feature of left ventricular failure or allergic reactions. Kerley's B lines, which reflect thickening of the subpleural interstitial compartment, typically are about 1 cm in length and 1 mm in thickness and usually found in the periphery of the lower lobes, abutting the pleura. The B lines are characteristic of subacute and chronic left ventricular failure (Chapter 57), mitral valve disease (Chapter 75), lymphangitic carcinomatosis, viral pneumonia, and pulmonary fibrosis (Chapter 92). Kerley's C lines, which are rarely diagnosed by radiologists, result from thickening of the lung parenchymal interstitium and form a reticular pattern on chest radiographs.

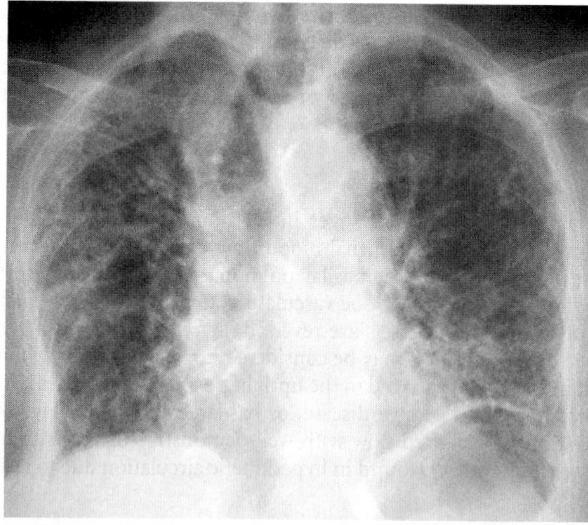

FIGURE 84–4 • Diffuse reticular lung disease. Chest radiograph in a 94-year-old patient with diffuse reticular opacities due to idiopathic pulmonary fibrosis with honeycombing and traction bronchiectases. The lung volumes are typically reduced by a decreased pulmonary compliance.

Reticular Patterns

Reticular patterns are small polygonal, irregular, or curvilinear opacities on chest radiographs (Fig. 84–4). The differential diagnosis varies according to the timeline of the pathologic change. Acute onset of a reticular pattern can occur in interstitial edema (e.g., due to left-sided heart failure), atypical pneumonitides (e.g., viral or mycoplasmal pneumonia), early exudative changes in a connective tissue disorder (e.g., systemic lupus erythematosus; Chapter 287), and acute allergic reactions (e.g., transfusion reactions [Chapter 183] or reactions to Hymenoptera stings). The common chronic processes resulting in a reticular pattern are idiopathic interstitial pneumonias (Chapter 92), connective tissue diseases (particularly scleroderma and rheumatoid lung), asbestosis (Chapter 93), radiation pneumonitis, end-stage hypersensitivity pneumonitis, drug reactions, lymphangitic spread of cancer, end-stage granulomatous infection, lymphoma in its bronchovascular form, Kaposi's sarcoma in its bronchovascular manifestation, and sarcoidosis.

Honeycombing

Honeycombing, which is an indication of end-stage interstitial lung disease (Chapter 92), reflects a restructuring of pulmonary anatomy accompanied by bronchiolectasis. Honeycombs form a multilayer of small subpleural spaces between 3 and 10 mm in diameter. They can be distinguished from paraseptal emphysema by their thicker wall and multiple layers.

Alveolar Pattern

An alveolar (Chapter 91) or air space pattern is characterized by acinar nodules, 0.6 to 1 cm in diameter. These nodules encompass an acinus, in the strict anatomic sense, and surrounding peribronchiolar lung tissue. Other patterns include ground-glass opacities (a reflection of incomplete alveolar filling), coalescent large opacities, consolidation involving whole lobes or segments, opacification in a bronchocentric distribution, air bronchograms, and air alveolograms. These radiographic features are helpful in placing a disease into a particular radiologic category, but the radiographic pattern called alveolar does not simply correspond to exclusive histologic alveolar filling because the interstitial compartment is involved as well in most cases. A more accurate description is parenchymal rather than alveolar opacification or consolidation.

Bronchial Patterns

Bronchial patterns, as best depicted by diffuse bronchiectasis (Chapter 90), are seen on conventional radiographs as linear, tubular, or cystic lucencies and opacities that follow the expected path of bronchi, so-called tramlines because they resemble tram tracks. Mucoid impaction, as seen in patients with asthma, allergic bronchopulmonary aspergillosis, or plastic bronchitis, leads to opacities described as toothpaste, cluster of grapes, or finger-in-glove. The "dirty lung" pattern seen in smokers with chronic bronchitis (Chapter 88) results from bronchial wall thickening, peribronchial fibrosis, respiratory bronchiolitis, and pulmonary arterial hypertension.

Vascular Patterns

Arterial patterns reflect changes in pulmonary perfusion. The term *caudalization* reflects the normal blood flow distribution pattern in an upright person in which the basilar pulmonary vessels are two to three times wider than the upper lobe vasculature. *Cephalization,* in which the ratios of diameters of vessels are reversed, is frequently seen in recumbent persons, in whom it may be considered normal; however, when it is present in individuals imaged in the upright position, it indicates left ventricular failure, mitral valve disease, or basilar emphysema (Fig. 84–5). Equalization, or balanced flow with well-demonstrated vessels to upper and lower lung zones, is found in hyperkinetic circulation due to anemia, obesity, pregnancy, Graves' disease, or left-to-right shunts. Equalization or balanced flow with oligemia can be seen in hypovolemia, diffuse emphysema, or right-to-left shunts. Centralization reflects dilation of central pulmonary vessels, with accompanying normal or diminished peripheral circulation. Typically, it is seen in pulmonary arterial hypertension (Fig. 84–6). Lateralization of flow, favoring one lung over the other, also called asymmetrical perfusion, is visible with unilateral emphysema, unilateral bronchiolitis obliterans (Swyer-James-McLeod syndrome), or unilateral obstruction of the pulmonary artery. Locally enlarged vessels occur in patchy emphysema, multiple pulmonary emboli, arteriovenous malformations, and nonuniform bronchiolitis obliterans. This pattern produces a mosaic perfusion on high-resolution CT scanning.

Lung Volume

Conventional radiographs and CT scans are taken during a breath hold at full inspiration. Lung volume is inferred from the relative size of the

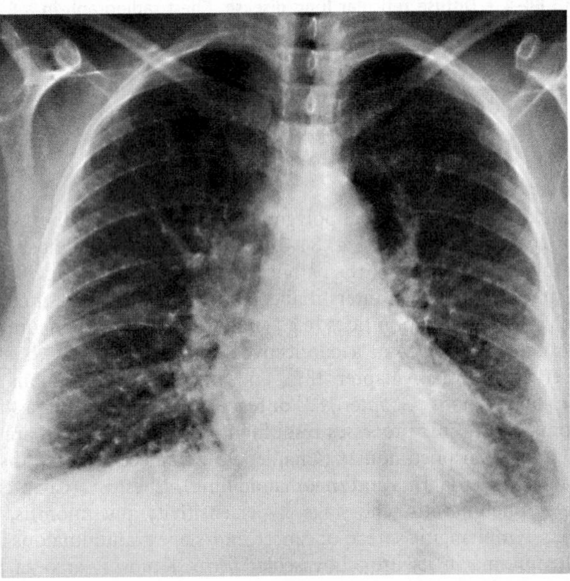

FIGURE 84–5 • Patient with left ventricular failure. Chest frontal radiograph shows cephalization of pulmonary blood flow.

TABLE 84–3 CONDITIONS ASSOCIATED WITH VARIOUS LUNG VOLUMES IN PATIENTS WITH AN UNDERLYING DIFFUSE LUNG DISEASE PATTERN

Large lung volumes
Emphysema
Chronic asthma
Diffuse bronchiolitis obliterans
Highly trained athletes
Lymphangioleiomyomatosis
Small lung volumes
End-stage lung fibrosis
Bilateral diaphragmatic paralysis
Massive ascites
Normal lung volumes
Sarcoidosis
Langerhans cell histiocytosis
Neurofibromatosis
Emphysema with pulmonary fibrosis

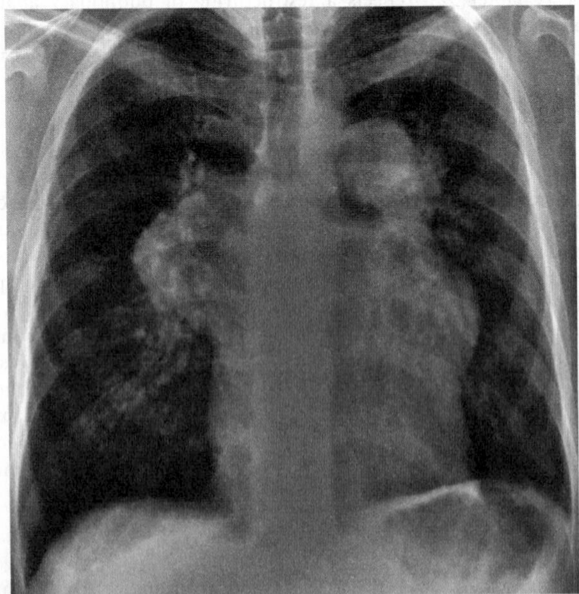

FIGURE 84–6 • Patient with primary pulmonary arterial hypertension. Chest frontal radiograph shows centralization of flow with pulmonary artery aneurysms and peripheral pulmonary oligemia.

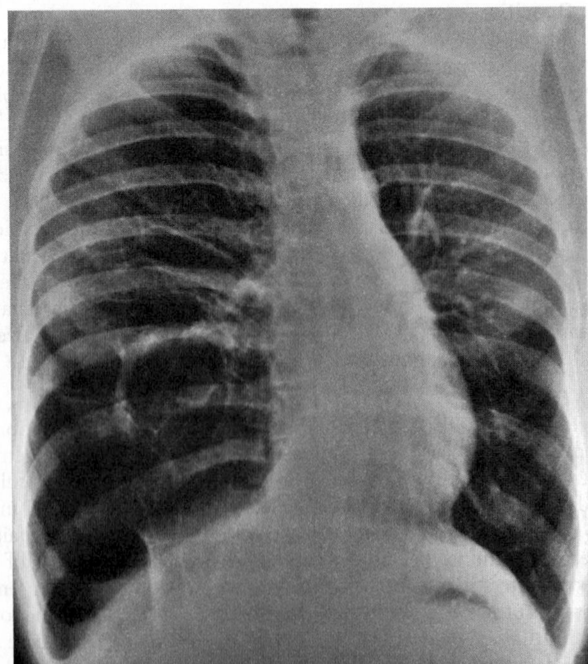

FIGURE 84–7 • Patient with severe emphysema. Chest radiograph shows hyperexpansion of both lungs with bullous changes at the right lung base and leftward mediastinal shift.

low-attenuation gas-containing regions compared with what one would expect for an equivalently sized chest wall (Table 84–3). Lung volumes larger than expected are commonly found in patients with diffuse emphysema (Fig. 84–7) (Chapter 88), chronic asthma (Chapter 87), or diffuse bronchiolitis and in highly trained athletes. With a few rare exceptions, chronic diffuse infiltrative lung diseases (Chapter 92) lead to loss of volume.

Anatomic Distribution

The anatomic distribution of disease can significantly facilitate the approach to diagnosis (Table 84–4 and Fig. 84–8). Upper zone lung disease predominates in tuberculosis, fungal disease, sarcoidosis, pneumoconiosis (except asbestosis), Langerhans cell histiocytosis, ankylosing spondylitis, cystic fibrosis, cystic *P. jiroveci* pneumonia, radiation pneumonitis, and end-stage hypersensitivity pneumonitis. Basilar lung disease is preferentially found in bronchiectases, aspiration, desquamative interstitial pneumonia, nonspecific interstitial pneumonitis, usual interstitial pneumonitis, drug reactions, asbestosis, scleroderma, and rheumatoid arthritis. However, any diffuse lung process will eventually progress to involve both lungs irrespective of zonal boundaries.

TABLE 84–4 CONDITIONS ASSOCIATED WITH DISEASE DISTRIBUTION PATTERNS

Upper zone lung disease
Tuberculosis
Fungal disease
Sarcoidosis
Pneumoconioses
Langerhans cell histiocytosis
Cystic fibrosis
End-stage hypersensitivity pneumonitis
Ankylosing spondylitis
Radiation pneumonitis
Basilar lung disease
Bronchiectases
Aspiration
Drug reactions
Interstitial pulmonary fibrosis, nonspecific interstitial pneumonitis, desquamative interstitial pneumonitis, cryptogenic organizing pneumonia, bronchiolitis obliterans with organizing pneumonia
Asbestosis
Scleroderma

Lymph Nodes

Enlarged lymph nodes that are visible on chest CT scans and, when larger, on chest radiographs can provide diagnostic information (Table 84–5). The following entities can be associated with diffuse lung disease and concurrent enlarged lymph nodes: sarcoidosis (Chapter 95); lymphoma; fungal disease; tuberculosis (Chapter 345); pneumoconioses (Chapter 93), particularly silicosis and beryllium-associated lung disease; lung cancer; and metastatic malignant disease other than lung cancer.

Pulmonary Nodules

Solitary pulmonary nodules are covered in Chapter 201. The majority of patients with multiple pulmonary nodules have metastatic disease from primary cancers either within or outside the lung (Fig. 84–9). These lesions have a predilection for subpleural lung regions, including the

TABLE 84–5 CONDITIONS ASSOCIATED WITH HILAR AND MEDIASTINAL LYMPH NODE ENLARGEMENT

Sarcoidosis
Lymphoma
Fungal disease
Tuberculosis
Metastatic cancer
Silicosis, coal worker's pneumoconiosis, beryllium lung

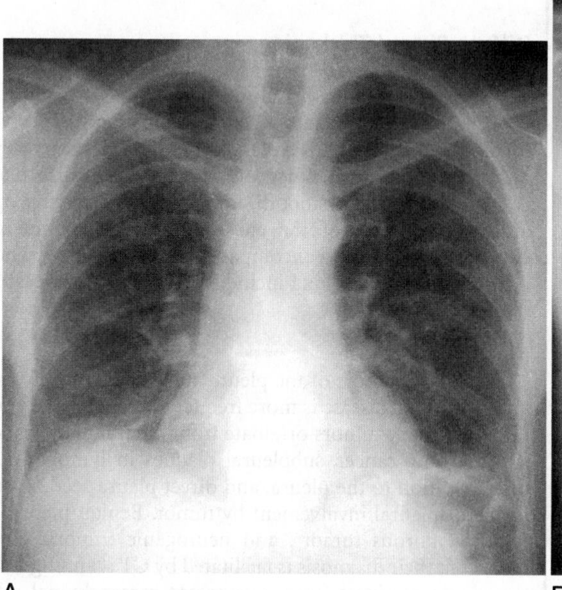

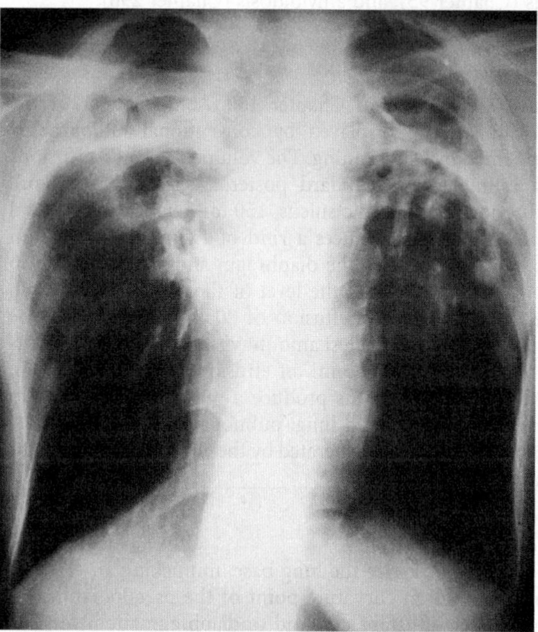

FIGURE 84–8 • A, Basilar pulmonary disease. Chest radiograph in a 48-year-old patient with known scleroderma. Bibasilar fine reticular opacities and parenchymal bands are visible in both lower lobes. **B, Apical lung disease.** Chest radiograph in a 42-year-old patient with ankylosing spondylitis. Severe architectural distortion with cicatrizing atelectasis of both upper lobes, retraction of both pulmonary arteries cephalad, and bilateral bulla formation containing fungus balls are evident.

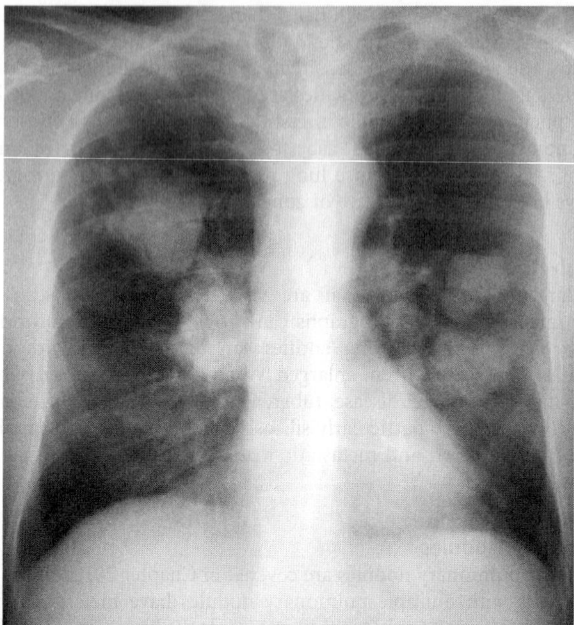

FIGURE 84–9 • Multifocal pulmonary opacities. Chest radiograph in a 70-year-old patient with known carcinoma of the thyroid gland widening the superior mediastinum and displacing the cervical trachea to the right. Bilateral large and small pulmonary nodules and masses due to metastatic tumor are present.

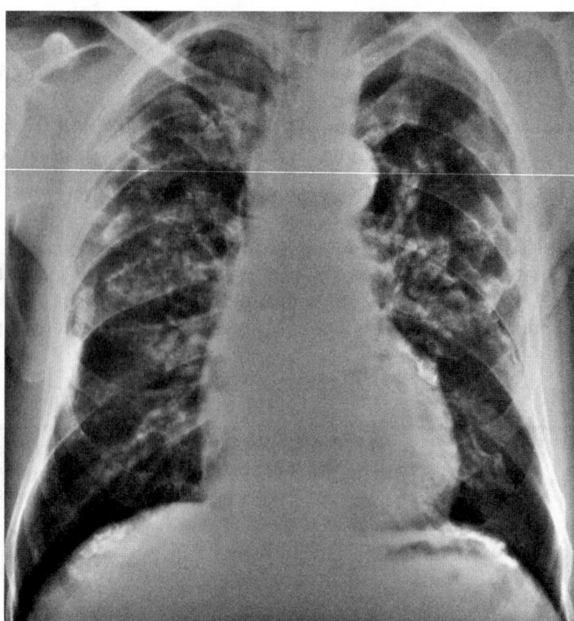

FIGURE 84–10 • Patient with known prior occupational asbestos exposure. Chest radiograph shows extensive bilateral calcified plaques seen en face, in profile, and along the diaphragmatic contour.

interlobar fissures. In patients with human immunodeficiency virus infection, Kaposi's sarcoma and lymphoma can induce the formation of such nodules. Infectious processes that present with multiple nodules include multiple abscesses from recurrent aspiration (Chapter 94) or septic emboli (Chapter 76); tuberculous and nontuberculous mycobacterial granulomas (Chapters 345 and 346); fungal processes, including histoplasmosis (Chapter 353), coccidioidomycosis (Chapter 354), and cryptococcosis (Chapter 357); and infection with flukes, such as *Paragonimus westermani* (Chapter 377). Noninfectious inflammatory conditions that can present with multiple pulmonary nodules include Wegener's granulomatosis (Chapter 291), rheumatoid nodules (Chapter 285), sarcoidosis (Chapter 95), and amyloidosis (Chapter 296).

Pleural Disease

Pleural diseases are covered in Chapter 100. Abnormalities of the pleural space easily can be displayed by conventional radiographic methods supplemented by CT scanning. The volume of pleural effusions can be reliably estimated on standard posteroanterior films: 75 mL obscures the posterior costophrenic sulcus, 150 mL obscures the lateral costophrenic sulcus, 200 mL produces a rind of 1 cm in thickness on decubitus films, 500 mL obscures the diaphragm and is also visible on supine films, and 1000 mL reaches the level of the fourth anterior rib on upright chest radiographs. An effusion of 200 mL or more can be sampled by thoracentesis. The smallest amount visible on decubitus films is 10 mL. With care, as little as 175 mL of effusion can be detected on supine films. Free layering effusions produce a veil of opacity or filter effect superimposed on the aerated lung; pulmonary vessels are clearly visible through the added opacity generated by the effusion, and air bronchograms are absent.

Subpulmonic Effusions

Subpulmonic effusions elevate the lung base, mimicking an elevated hemidiaphragm. The highest curvature point of the pseudodiaphragm is shifted laterally. Large effusions can lead to diaphragmatic inversion. Separation of the lung base from the gas-containing stomach is indicative of a subpulmonic effusion, particularly when the stomach gas bubble is displaced inferomedially. Loculated pleural effusions suggest the presence of pleural adhesions. Such encapsulated collections have obtuse angles of interface with the chest wall and have a sharply defined border with the adjacent lung.

Pleural Plaques

Pleural plaques result from parietal pleural accumulation of hyalinized collagen fibers (Fig. 84–10); their presence suggests asbestos exposure (Chapter 93). Plaques preferentially involve the parietal pleura adjacent to ribs six through nine and the diaphragm. They are less pronounced in the intercostal spaces and spare the costophrenic sulci as well as the apices. Calcifications are visible on chest radiographs in 20% and on CT scans in 50% of individuals with plaques. Imaged in profile, pleural plaques produce focal areas of apparent pleural thickening. Over the diaphragm, they appear as curvilinear calcifications or scalloping. Pleural plaques viewed en face can simulate lung disease. Their appearance has been likened to holly leaves, sunburst patterns, "geographic" patterns, or stippled or irregular structures. Rare visceral pleural plaques that occur in interlobar fissures can mimic pulmonary nodules.

Diffuse Pleural Thickening

Diffuse pleural thickening is a response observed after exposure to any of a number of stimuli including infection, inflammation, trauma, tumor, thromboembolism, radiation, and asbestos. Severe involvement results in formation of a generalized pleural peel with smooth margins and usually less than 2 cm in thickness. Radiologically diffuse pleural thickening is characterized by a smooth, noninterrupted pleural opacity involving at least a quarter of the chest wall circumference, obliterating the costophrenic sulci and encompassing also the apices. The CT criteria for diffuse pleural thickening include a thickness of at least 3 mm.

Malignant Disease

Malignant tumors of the pleura are more common than benign ones, and metastatic disease is more frequent than a primary pleural mesothelioma. Primary tumors originate from pleural membranes. Pleural invasion by lung cancer, subpleural plaques in lymphoma, hematogenous dissemination to the pleura, and direct pleura seeding are other mechanisms of pleural involvement by tumor. Benign pleural tumors include lipomas, fibrous tumors, and neurogenic tumors. Lipomas are most common; their diagnosis is facilitated by CT scanning. Fibrous tumors of the pleura originate from pluripotent mesenchymal cells found in the visceral pleura or, less commonly, in the parietal pleura. They can induce paraneoplastic syndromes such as hypertrophic osteoarthropathy (Chapter 189) or hypoglycemia and only rarely invade or metastasize. In nearly half of these patients, the tumor can be on a pedicle and be mobile as a patient changes position.

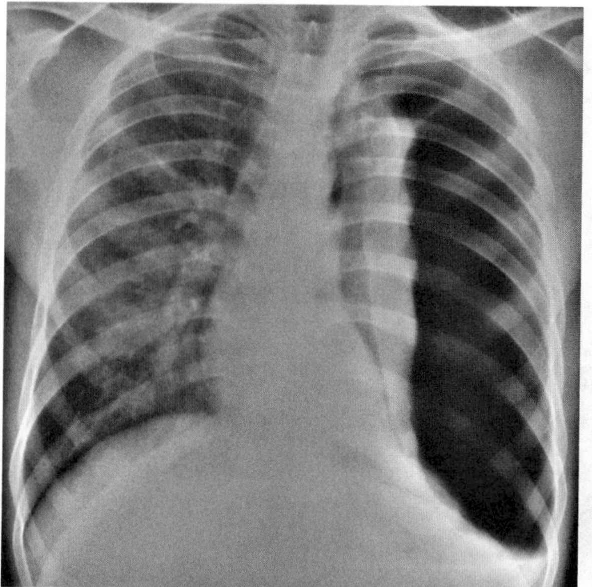

FIGURE 84–11 • Patient with spontaneous tension hydropneumothorax. Chest radiograph shows complete atelectasis of the left lung with a large pneumothorax and a left basilar gas-liquid level. The patient had primary tuberculosis.

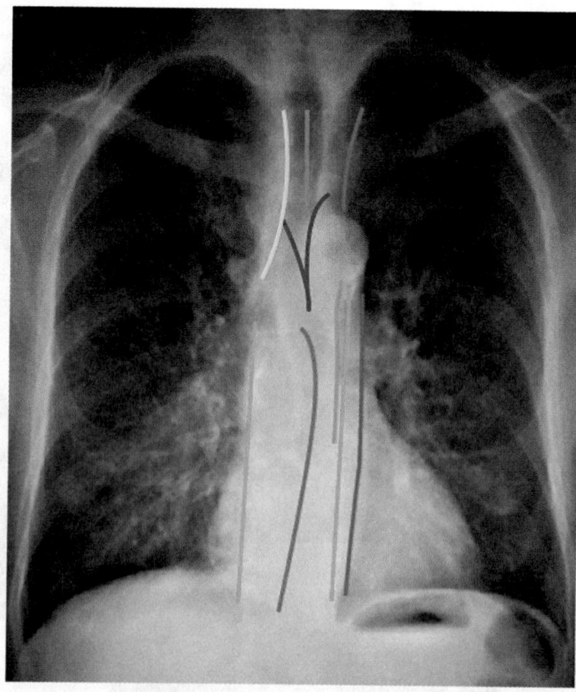

FIGURE 84–12 • Chest radiograph with superimposed mediastinal stripes. Yellow: right paratracheal stripe. Light blue: right and left paraspinal stripes. Red: azygoesophageal stripe. Brown: pleuroesophageal stripe. Purple: anterior junction line complex. Pink: left subclavian artery border. Light green: posterior-superior junction line. Dark green: para-aortic line.

TABLE 84–6 CLASSIFICATION OF MEDIASTINAL COMPARTMENTS

Anterior mediastinum
Retrosternal
Middle mediastinum—visceral compartment
Subcarinal space
Paratracheal region
Retrotracheal space
Aortic-pulmonic window
Retrocardiac space
Posterior mediastinum
Paraspinal region

Pneumothorax

Pneumothorax means gas in the pleural space (Chapter 100). The most important radiologic feature of a pneumothorax is a visceral pleural line or edge that is convex or straight toward the chest wall and produces a lucent separation of the visceral and parietal pleura (Fig. 84–11). In a majority of cases, no pulmonary vascular structures are visible beyond the visceral pleura. On upright chest radiographs, gas is primarily found in the apicolateral pleural space. Expiratory chest radiographs are not necessary for the detection of small pneumothoraces because all pneumothoraces are visible on inspiratory films. On supine chest radiographs, pleural gas accumulates in a subpulmonic location; it outlines the costophrenic sulcus, forming the deep sulcus sign. A tension pneumothorax leads to marked shift of the mediastinum to the contralateral side and to flattening or inversion of the ipsilateral hemidiaphragm.

Imaging of the Mediastinum

The mediastinum encompasses midline thoracic structures that are delineated by mediastinal pleura, the diaphragm, the sternum, the spine, and the thoracic inlet. The mediastinum is commonly divided into an anterior compartment, a visceral middle compartment, and a paraspinal, posterior mediastinal compartment (Table 84–6). Each compartment contains specific pathologic entities.

Imaging Techniques

On well-penetrated chest radiographs, the anterior junction line, the posterior-superior junction line, the azygoesophageal stripe, the pleuroesophageal stripe, the paratracheal stripe, and the para-aortic and the paraspinal stripes or lines should be assessed (Fig. 84–12). Mediastinal masses need to be detected and localized first. Their obtuse angles of interface with the mediastinal pleura as well as extension into both hemithoraces indicate the mediastinal origin of such lesions.

CT facilitates localization of a mass to a specific mediastinal compartment. Once it is known whether the mass is predominantly fat, cystic, soft tissue, or calcified, the differential diagnosis can be limited. MRI of the mediastinum has a role in diagnosis of vertebral disease or neurogenic tumors with extension into the spinal canal. It is as good as CT in diagnosis of aortic aneurysms and dissections (Chapter 78).

Mediastinal Compartments

The anterior mediastinum is actually a potential space that may contain the fatty replaced thymus and small normal lymph nodes. Space-occupying lesions in this compartment typically include thymomas, lymphomas, teratomas and other germ cell tumors, substernal thyroid goiters, lipomas, and other connective tissue tumors as well as hemangiomas or lymphangiomas (Fig. 84–13A).

The middle mediastinum is subdivided into the subcarinal space, paratracheal region, retrotracheal region, aortic-pulmonic window region, and retrocardiac space. Characteristic lesions are enlarged lymph nodes and bronchopulmonary foregut malformations (see Fig. 84–13B).

In the retrotracheal region, aberrant right subclavian arteries, posterior descending goiters, esophageal tumors, diverticula, or thoracic duct cysts can be found. In the aortic-pulmonic window, ductus diverticula, bronchopulmonary foregut malformations, or aortic or pulmonic artery aneurysms can form compartment-specific space-occupying lesions.

The paraspinal region is considered radiologically to belong to the posterior mediastinum. Important masses in that space include neurogenic tumors that originate from the sympathetic chain or from segmental nerve roots (see Fig. 84–13C). Extramedullary hematopoiesis in patients with severe anemia can result in paravertebral masses formed

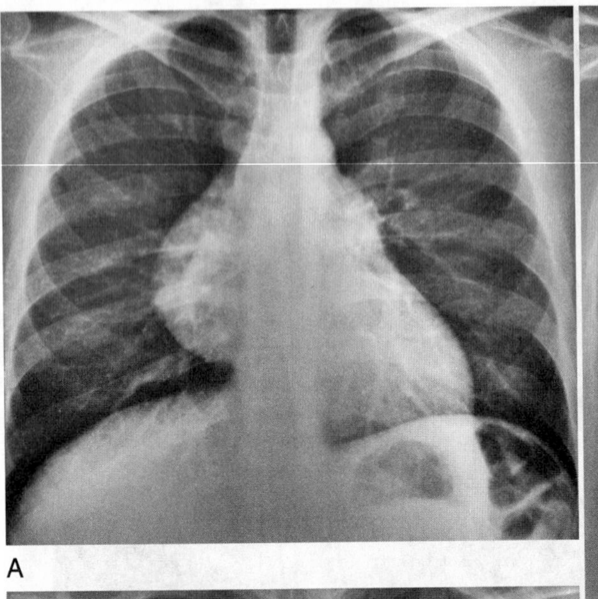

A

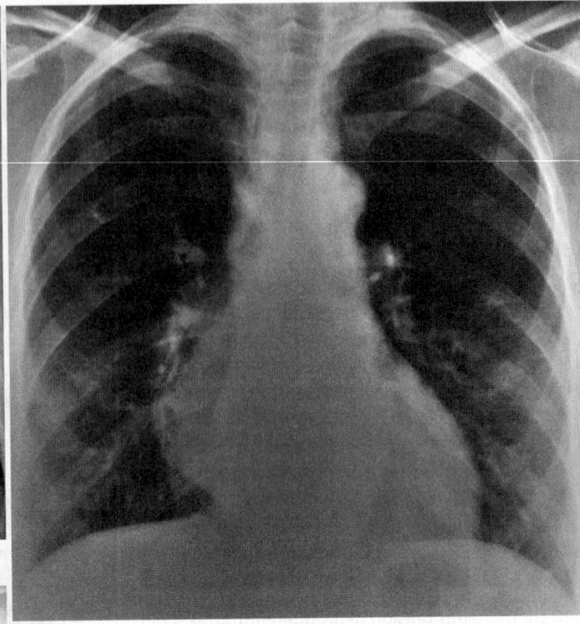

B

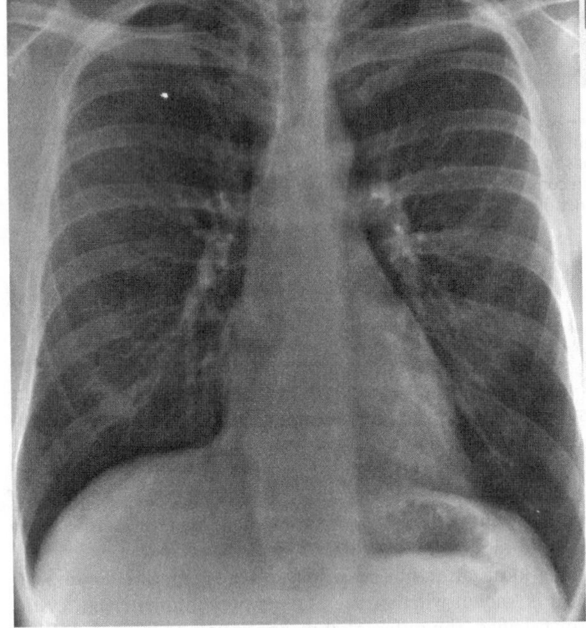

C

FIGURE 84–13 • A, Patient with anterior mediastinal teratoma. Chest radiograph shows a mediastinal contour abnormality due to projection of the mass into the right hemithorax. Note the obtuse angle of interface formed by the pleura covering the mass with the mediastinum. **B,** Patient with Castleman's giant lymph node hyperplasia. Chest frontal radiograph shows large subcarinal middle mediastinal mass that projects lateral to the right atrium. **C,** Patient with paraspinal ganglioneuroma. Chest radiograph shows right lower paraspinal contour abnormality widening the right paraspinal region and encompassing the height of three thoracic vertebrae.

by hypertrophied bone marrow that extrudes from ribs or vertebral bodies. Enlarged lymph nodes due to lymphoma or metastatic disease are occasionally seen in a paraspinal location. Vertebral disease, including bacterial or tuberculous spondylitis, tumors, and post-traumatic hematomas, can widen the paraspinal region and produce contour abnormalities.

SUGGESTED READINGS

Friedman PJ, Stark P: Pulmonary diagnostic techniques, radiographic evaluation of lung disease. *In* Bordow RA, Ries AL, Morris TA (eds): Manual of Clinical Problems in Pulmonary Medicine, 6th ed. Philadelphia, Lippincott Williams & Wilkins, 2005.

Friedman PJ, Stark P: Advanced imaging and image-guided intervention in chest radiology. *In* Bordow RA, Ries AL, Morris TA (eds): Manual of Clinical Problems in Pulmonary Medicine, 6th ed. Philadelphia, Lippincott Williams & Wilkins, 2005.

Katsuragawa S, Doi K: Computer-aided diagnosis in chest radiograpy. Comput Med Imaging Graph 2007;31:212–223. *Radiologists' readings improve when aided by computer interpretations.*

Sharma S, Maycher B, Eschun G: Radiological imaging in pneumonia: Recent advances. Curr Opin Pulm Med 2007;13:159–169. *A practical approach using pattern recognition.*

85 RESPIRATORY STRUCTURE AND FUNCTION: MECHANISMS AND TESTING

Herbert Y. Reynolds

The lungs are designed for gaseous exchange (oxygen uptake and carbon dioxide elimination) through the process of ventilation and molecular diffusion. To maintain health, purified air must be presented to the alveolar epithelial surface to aerate pulmonary capillary blood. Ambient air, which contains environmental debris, microbes, and possibly solubilized toxins and is admixed at times with aspirated oropharyngeal secretions, must be cleansed. Inspired ambient air encounters a system of host defenses that usually removes these contaminants mechanically (by sneezing, rhinorrhea, coughing, and mucociliary clearance), through innate (natural) immunity mechanisms, or immunologically through adaptive (acquired) immunity. This nonventilatory function can be missing (primary host defects) or compromised by systemic illness or the side effects of other medical therapy. Because ventilation and nonventilatory function are so intertwined, both are described together; methods for assessment of clinical function then follow.

RESPIRATORY STRUCTURE

Respiratory Tract Structure

Although the respiratory tract is a continuum of branching tubes leading to the air exchange–alveolar surface, it functionally has four distinct anatomic segments: naso-oropharynx or upper airways, conducting airways (larynx, trachea, and bronchi that branch to terminal bronchioles), respiratory bronchioles, and alveolar ducts and alveoli. Vascular and neural structures are integral to each segment; lymphatic channels begin at the level of respiratory bronchioles and flow upward or cephalad into the hilar nodes.

The airways and their accompanying blood supply develop from an evagination of the foregut and primitive esophagus. The conducting airways form a continuum of approximately 14 generations of branches, which are extended by another 10 or so branches within the acinar airways, finally ending as alveolar sacs. This anatomic structure has been described as a tree with irregular, dichotomously branching tubes. Later developments in the fetus initiate progressive thinning of the mucosal epithelial layer in distal bronchi and then the respiratory bronchioles to a single cell surface, which defines the beginning of the gas exchange unit within the acinar-alveolar structures. Because this mucosal surface that lines the airways down to the respiratory bronchioles is in breath-to-breath contact with the external environment, mechanisms to cleanse inspired air are dispersed along the entire tract.

The *naso-oropharynx* includes the upper airways and associated sinuses (Chapter 452). It begins at the nares and lips and extends back through a richly vascular, undulant mucosal covering of the nasal passage, through the glottis, into the extrathoracic trachea. Nasal hairs and turbinates filter out large particles (>10 μm diameter) as turbulent air passes over the nasal surface; also, air is humidified and warmed as necessary. These climatologic adjustments occur as air passes through the nose and over the soft palate and are completed before air reaches the posterior pharynx. Sinus and posterior nasal secretions can collect in the posterior pharynx, where salivary and parotid fluids stimulated by mastication also accumulate. Deglutition and respiration are coordinated exquisitely by the epiglottis and laryngeal musculature to direct fluids and food into the esophagus and air into the subglottic trachea. Control is not perfect, however, and aspiration can occur in normal persons during sleep; also, esophageal reflux causing cough and asthma symptoms is common (Chapters 87 and 140). The surface of the nasal mucosa is similar to that in the lower conducting airways with respect to ciliary function and immunologic components. Mucociliary clearance declines with age, explaining in part the more frequent occurrence of respiratory infections in the elderly.

The *conducting airways* begin with the trachea, a flexible tube held open by cartilaginous, horseshoe-shaped rings with a posterior muscular face that abuts the esophagus. The trachea is oval, is about 10 cm in length, and contains about 15 rings. At the carina, it divides into two major bronchi, and thereafter multiple smaller bronchial branches diverge through many generations of smaller divisions. In aggregate, however, the branching creates a much greater overall cross-sectional area that not only reduces resistance to airflow but also decelerates the velocity of air molecules as they prepare to enter the acinar ducts and alveolar sacs. Although airflow is laminar, the slower movement further cleanses the air by allowing the settling out of any 0.5- to 3-μm particulates that still are present and would be impacted at branching points. This action seems especially important in the respiratory bronchioles, which serve as the transition segment between the conducting airways and alveoli, where several adaptations facilitate further removal of particulates or antigens. Throughout the conducting airways (Fig. 85–1), the mucosal surface provides a barrier function because of the tight apical junctions between epithelial cells. About half of the epithelial cells are ciliated; a fluid film and mucus cover the beating cilia, creating the mucociliary apparatus. The thickness of the mucosal surface attenuates as the pseudostratified cell layer flattens to become a single cell layer in the terminal bronchioles. Here the less protected surface may become more vulnerable to injury from inhaled toxins and microbes and more susceptible to ravages of chronic inflammation (bronchiolitis).

The *respiratory bronchioles*, which are positioned between the distal conducting airways and the alveolized air exchange surface, functionally separate the upper and lower respiratory tracts. This segment is a bottleneck for airflow and a last surface to capture small particulates and microbial or antigenic debris before the alveolar space; immune responses can be initiated here. The respiratory bronchioles can be the site of airway obstruction, however, due to inflammation typical of bronchiolitis obliterans (Chapter 92) and associated with several lung diseases, such as chronic graft rejection after lung transplantation (Chapter 102) and lung involvement by collagen vascular diseases (Chapter 92). In this transition segment, several changes occur: the single-layer cuboidal epithelial surface further differentiates into alveolar type I cells that cover the alveolar lining surface; mucus-secreting cells disappear, although goblet cells can develop in cigarette smokers; and another secretory cell type emerges, the Clara cells. Pulmonary brush cells with a tuft of squat microvilli are dense in this area and may be involved with chemosensing or trapping of inhaled particles and pollutants as well as with regulation of fluid and solute absorption. Also, many dendritic macrophage-like cells, which may constitute 1% of the cells, are present to capture antigens. Surface host defenses change from a focus on mucociliary clearance to an emphasis on featuring macrophage phagocytes, inflammatory cells (neutrophils or eosinophils), and opsonins. Lymphatic channels form to collect the lymphatic fluid squeezed up from the interalveolar interstitial spaces into lymphatic capillaries that course along pulmonary capillaries and venules in the alveolar walls. Finally, the changeover is made from the bronchial arterial blood supply for the conducting airways to the pulmonary artery–pulmonary capillary blood that courses around the alveoli for aeration.

The *air exchange* compartment, or the alveolar space, is composed of about 480 million alveoli supported by a fibrous scaffolding and intertwined with a meshwork of pulmonary artery capillaries that permit air-blood contact. Oxygen uptake and carbon dioxide elimination occur across a thin tissue layer of type I epithelial cells and capillary endothelium that in aggregate creates a large surface area of approximately 130 square feet. To increase the likelihood that respiratory function will support a healthy human lifespan despite pollutants, infections, or systemic diseases that affect the lungs, an intricate system of host defenses has evolved. The system specialized for the alveoli is different from the system described in the proximal airways. Although an alveolus is reasonably protected from airborne debris by aerodynamic filtration that occurs in the upper respiratory tract, small particles (<0.5 μm) can remain suspended in air or toxic gases can gain access to the alveoli directly.

Respiratory host defenses balance two mechanisms that eliminate or detoxify microbes and other antigens that enter the airways. First is an innate or quick response reaction that produces inflammation as an end point (bronchitis or pneumonitis) with subsequent apoptosis of neutrophils and suppression of inflammation to limit the reaction. Second is a more deliberate approach that stimulates lymphocytic pathways, creating a versatile and adaptive response involving specific T-cell activity or production of immunoglobulins (antibodies).

Microbes can be contained in aspirated fluid or carried intravascularly to the parenchyma (septicemia). A microbe entering an alveolus may encounter an antigen-presenting cell or several opsonins in the epithelial lining fluid, including immunoglobulin (Ig) G antibodies (IgG1 and IgG3 subtypes) and nonimmune substances (type II cell–secreted surfactant protein A and D, fibrinogen, and complement fragments [C3b]) that can promote receptor-mediated uptake or phagocytosis by macrophages. Alveolar T lymphocytes can stimulate the macrophage with cytokines, such as interleukin (IL)-1 and interferon-γ, that enhance its bactericidal activity or, if microbes are too numerous or too virulent, can create an inflammatory response quickly. Chemokines, derived from macrophages or epithelial cells, including IL-8, leukotriene B_4, and tumor necrosis factor, can attract neutrophils and other inflammatory products from adjacent capillaries into the alveolus. If inflammation, or pneumonitis, is successful in eradicating infection, neutrophils undergo apoptosis, the inflammation resolves, and normal lung tissue function is restored. If the inflammatory process is prolonged, a smoldering, chronic inflammatory response can persist and lead to tissue injury that causes fibrosis and scarring or, depending on the antigen-particle or microbe involved, a granulomatous reaction. If this wound-type healing occurs after substantial injury, respiratory function can be lost permanently.

Cellular Structure

The airway layer of pseudostratified epithelial cells creates a physical barrier by forming tight apical junctions that control permeability and

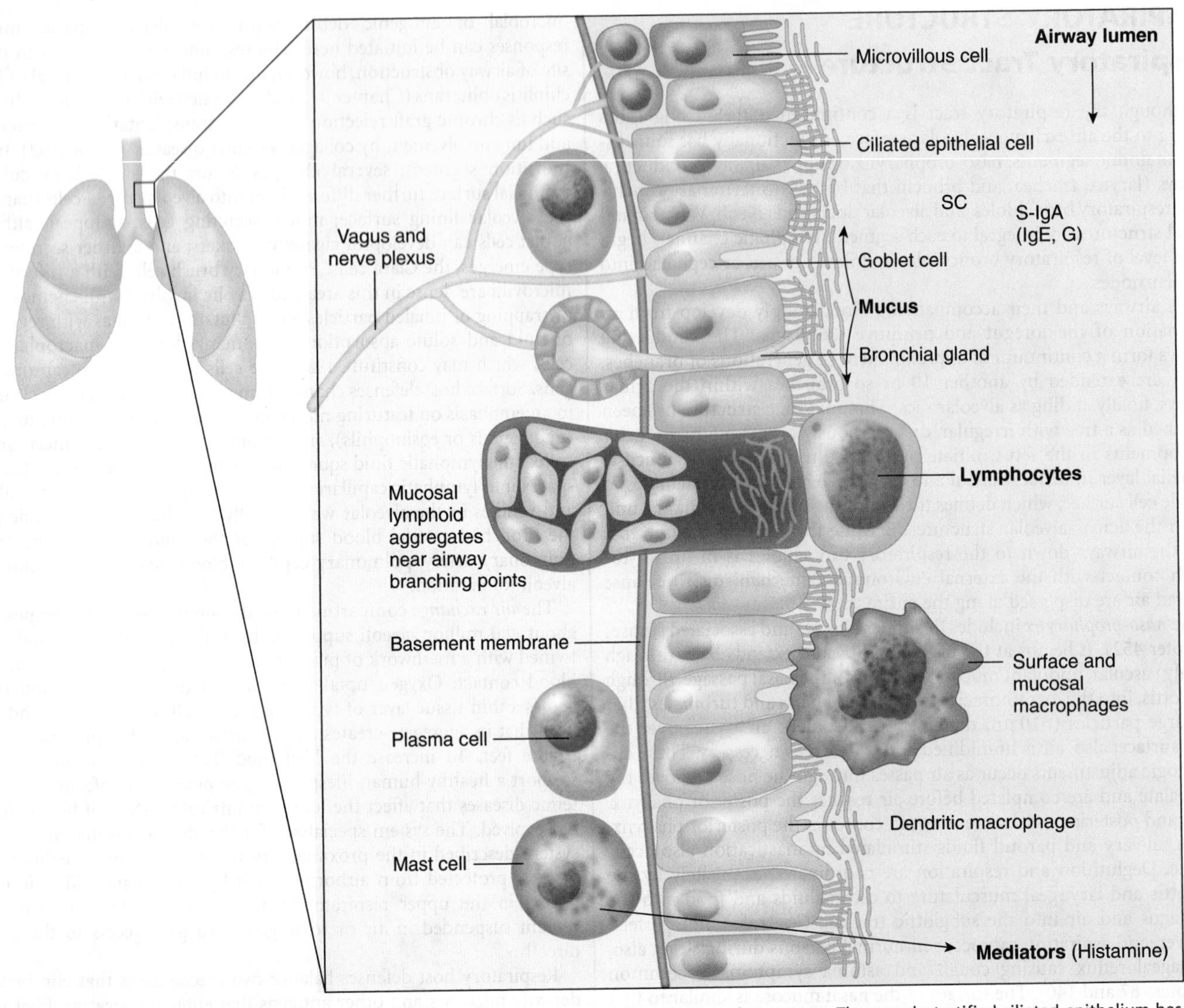

FIGURE 85–1 • A portion of the bronchial airway surface depicts the mucosa and its submucosal structures. The pseudostratified ciliated epithelium has a covering layer of mucus (produced by goblet cells and bronchial glands) and a film of fluid that contains various proteins, including immunoglobulins and free secretory component (SC). A few surface cells may be present, such as lymphocytes (from bronchial-associated lymphoid aggregates) and macrophages. Among the epithelial cells are absorptive microvillous cells and dendritic cells, whose cellular processes interdigitate with the mucosal surface. The epithelial cells can produce inflammatory cytokines that affect mucosal swelling and permeability. In the submucosa below the basement membrane, mast cells and plasma cells reside that secrete mediators (e.g., histamine) and local immunoglobulins (e.g., IgA). Interacting with all of these glandular and cellular networks are nerves, exerting their control through neuropeptides and by adrenergic and cholinergic nerve fibers. A rich bronchial arterial vascular supply exists also. (Modified from Reynolds HY: Pulmonary host defenses. Chest 1989;95:223S–230S.)

promote pericellular ion and fluid flux in addition to the usual transepithelial uptake and secretion. About half of the epithelial cells have cilia to propel a covering layer of fluid and admixed mucus that can collect airway debris and eliminate it by mucociliary clearance. These epithelial cells have dynamic turnover of several days, with continuous self-renewal from progenitor stem cells, but the normal replication rate may vary at different locations along the airways. If airway injury has destroyed epithelial cells and denuded the surface, regeneration begins quickly from reservoirs of self-renewing stem cells found in niches in the ducts of submucosal glands in the trachea or bronchi and within the surface epithelium of more distal airways.

Epithelial cells have about the same repertoire of proinflammatory chemokines as alveolar macrophages do, including IL-8, leukotriene B_4, transforming growth factor-β, monocyte chemotactic protein 1, and RANTES. They also can inhibit or downregulate inflammation. This dual capability to help initiate inflammation and then suppress it makes the epithelium crucial for the pathogenesis of diseases such as asthma (Chapter 87), bronchitis, and emphysema (Chapter 88). Chronic inflammatory changes can cause bronchiectasis (Chapter 90) or cell atypia that leads to endobronchial cancer (Chapter 201).

Dendritic cells or surface macrophages process antigens, using Toll-like receptors such as TLR2 and TLR4, and present them to major histocompatibility complex–compatible but naive $CD4^+$ lymphocytes, a process facilitated with the stimulatory cytokine IL-12. IL-2 produced by $CD4^+$ T cells subsequently can direct T_H1 lymphocytes to develop and proliferate. T_H1 cells can produce IL-1 and interferon-γ, which can stimulate macrophages for heightened activity (phagocytic uptake) in the inflammatory pathway. Also, IL-2 can induce clonal expansion of $CD4^+$ lymphocytes that contributes to creating granulomas for containment of certain microbes, such as mycobacteria, or particles (silica or beryllium).

Another subset of dendritic cells (or macrophages) can produce IL-10, an inhibitory cytokine that promotes the T_H1 response preferentially in normal subjects and suppresses the T_H2 cellular pathway. T_H2 lymphocytes stimulate mast cells and eosinophils and the production of reaginic antibodies (IgE, IgG4). The host usually needs to suppress this response so that not every inhaled, environmental antigen entering the airways elicits an allergic response.

Dendritic cells or macrophages also interact with other lymphocytes to create a delayed or more protracted cellular immune response (adaptive). Stimulation of $CD8^+$ suppressor lymphocytes creates cytotoxic functioning cells or natural killer cells that can destroy aberrant cells, destroy cells containing intracellular microbes, or program another cell's death. Finally, antigens can be presented to B lymphocytes that become plasma cells.

ASSESSMENT OF DYNAMIC PULMONARY FUNCTION

Documentation of the working capacity and condition of the overall respiratory tract, or some of its individual components, requires lung function tests, arterial blood gas analyses, imaging studies, or measurements of secretions from specific sites. The goal is to correlate physiologic respiratory measurements, which are obtained from spirometry tests, with functional activity, which can be assessed by an exercise or timed walking test that measures exercise capacity or the distance that can be walked in a prespecified amount of time (typically 6 minutes). Another goal of functional tests is to reproduce clinical symptoms, such as breathlessness or dyspnea, and to correlate these symptoms with the degree of physical limitation. These tests are useful to measure baseline status, to monitor treatment, and to estimate prognosis.

Pulmonary Function Tests

Lung function tests (Table 85–1) are essential to measure a person's objective ability to move the ventilatory apparatus in comparison with normal subjects, adjusted for sex, height, ethnicity, and age. Basic tests for preliminary assessment and for monitoring disease progression include spirometry, which is a record of exhaled volume versus time during a forced exhalation (with or without determination of the response to an inhaled bronchodilator for possible reversible airflow); diffusion capacity, which measures the transfer of carbon monoxide to indicate how well inspired gases cross the alveolar-interstitial-capillary endothelial interface into blood; and noninvasive pulse oximetry, for oxygen saturation measured at rest or during ambulation. Pulmonary function testing performed after graduated exercise on a treadmill or a timed walking test on a level surface provides a more dynamic assessment of pulmonary function and correlates well with prognosis in patients with chronic pulmonary conditions such as lung fibrosis and chronic obstructive disease. More specialized tests include body plethysmography to determine total lung volumes and airway resistance, as well as maximal cardiopulmonary exercise testing to assess cardiac function and oxygen uptake and consumption. The clinical utility of these tests can be appreciated by understanding how they can be applied to representative types of patients (Table 85–2).

Spirometry

Spirometry is used to document baseline lung function, to make a preliminary diagnostic assessment, or to monitor patients as lung or cardiac disease evolves and responds to treatment. Although measurements are made with the patient at rest, considerable physical effort and attentiveness are required for spirometry to be performed well. Patients, especially during hospitalization, after procedures, or if they are still deconditioned, often cannot give maximum effort or cooperate or coordinate well, and test results are not optimal. Too often, patients who are responding to therapy for an exacerbation of chronic obstructive pulmonary disease (COPD) or asthma but who are not yet back to preillness status are sent prematurely for lung function tests in an attempt to reestablish a baseline for future reference. Recent nebulizer or metered-dose inhaler treatment with a bronchodilator also may confuse results. Reproducibility of several test attempts (at least three) is important and is a criterion for valid interpretation of test results. Other medical problems that can confuse spirometric testing include pulmonary congestion, coughing, thyroid dysfunction, neurologic illness, poor nutrition, and corticosteroid-associated muscle weakness.

Spirometry is recorded by having a seated subject breathe calmly several times at tidal volume, then draw a maximum inhalation followed by a forced exhalation that is continued for at least 6 seconds or more with sustained vigorous effort (forced vital capacity [FVC]) and completed by a vigorous full inspiration (inspiratory vital capacity). These maneuvers are represented as a volume-time loop or as a flow-volume loop (plotting flow against FVC and inspiratory vital capacity). Flow-volume loops are scrutinized for special patterns that can indicate various clinical or anatomic conditions (Fig. 85–2).

Among the most helpful spirometric values are FVC (liters), forced expiratory volume in the first second of exhalation (FEV_1, liters), ratio of FEV_1 to FVC (percentage), and forced expiratory flow in the middle of expiration ($FEF_{25-75\%}$, liters/sec). Residual volume (liters) cannot be determined by spirometry and often is measured by helium dilution or plethysmographic methods. Residual volume is necessary to compute total lung capacity (liters), which is a measure of the air capacity of the maximally inflated lung. FEV_1, although recorded as a volume, is equated with a measure of airflow and is effort dependent. Because FEV_1 represents the most effective portion of the breathing volume, it usually correlates well with the amount of physical activity a patient can sustain. For

TABLE 85–1 PULMONARY FUNCTION TESTS

LUNG VOLUME	
TLC	Total lung capacity (volume of gas in lungs at the end of maximal inspiration)
FRC	Functional residual capacity (volume of gas in the lungs when elastic inward pull is balanced by outward pull of the chest wall and diaphragm)
ERV	Expiratory reserve volume (volume of gas expired from FRC to maximal expiration)
RV	Residual volume (FRC – ERV)
EXPIRATORY FLOW	
FEV_1	Forced expiratory volume (in 1 second)
FVC	Forced vital capacity
$FEV_1\%$	FEV_1/FVC ratio (expressed as percentage)
DIFFUSING CAPACITY	
DLCO	Diffusing capacity for carbon monoxide
ARTERIAL BLOOD GASES	
PaO_2	Arterial oxygen pressure
$PaCO_2$	Arterial carbon dioxide pressure
pH	

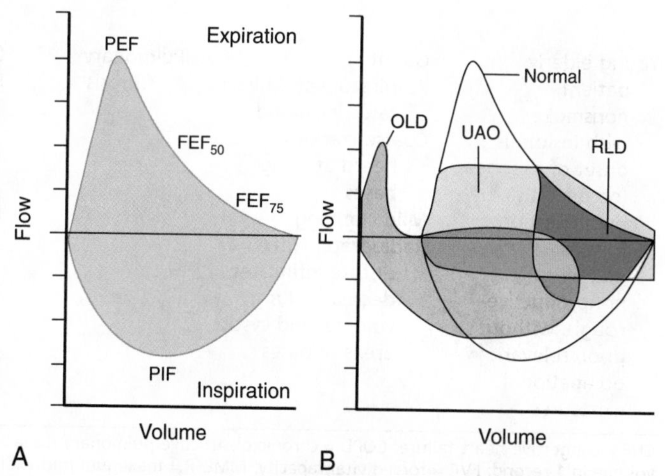

FIGURE 85–2 • Flow-volume curve. A, The maximum expired flow-volume curve in a normal subject. The peak expiratory flow (PEF) and forced expiratory flows at 50% and 75% of the exhaled vital capacity (FEF_{50} and FEF_{75}) are indicated. **B,** In obstructive lung disease (OLD), hyperinflation pushes the position of the curve to the left, and there is characteristic scalloping on expiration. In restrictive lung disease (RLD), lung volumes are reduced, but flow for any point in volume is normal. The flow-volume curve displays different patterns with various forms of upper airway obstruction (UAO), with reduction in respiratory flow if the obstruction is outside the thoracic cavity and reduction in expiratory flow if the obstruction is caused by a fixed deformity. PIF = peak inspiratory flow. (From Diagnostic techniques and their indications. *In* Andreoli T, et al [eds]: Cecil Essentials of Medicine, 5th ed. Philadelphia, WB Saunders, 2001, p 183.)

TABLE 85–2 CLINICAL UTILITY OF TESTING IN REPRESENTATIVE TYPES OF PATIENTS WITH COMMON PULMONARY COMPLAINTS

Clinical Presentation	Physical Findings and Chest Radiograph	Diagnosis	Pulmonary Function Tests	Characteristic Abnormalities	Monitoring or Predictive Use of Tests
Young adult with episodic attacks of cough, wheezing, and anxiety	Rapid respiratory rate Wheezing and prolonged expiration Thorax hyperresonant Radiograph normal or hyperinflated	Asthma	Spirometry (but cough and dyspnea may preclude complete results) Oximetry Arterial blood gas analysis (only if the episode is prolonged or severe)	Decreased PEFR, FEV_1, MMEFR to grade as mild, moderate, or severe attack Hypoxemia, hypocapnia, and pH changes on blood gas analysis during an attack	Spirometry after bronchodilator treatment or challenge testing Daily peak flow measurements (keep diary of results) FEV_1 may return to normal range after episode or therapy
Middle-aged adult, moderate smoker (20 cigarettes per day), mild dyspnea, occasional cough and sputum	Examination findings and radiograph are likely to be normal	Normal smoker with occasional episodes of acute bronchitis	Baseline spirometry and oximetry Optional baseline cardiorespiratory exercise test	Slight decrease in FEV_1 and perhaps FVC	Spirometry with health maintenance visit/yearly Daily peak flow monitoring Reduce or stop smoking
Older middle-aged adult, moderate smoker for 30–40 years, dyspnea (with moderate exertion), morning cough and phlegm, mild weight loss	Respiratory rate is likely to be increased at rest Thorax hyperinflated Breath sounds decreased Scattered wheezes and crackles Nail bed cyanosis Radiograph normal or hyperinflated; no mass lesions evident	COPD is suspected	Spirometry and oximetry or arterial blood gas analysis Timed walk test Cardiopulmonary exercise testing (especially if heart failure is evident)	Decreased FEV_1 (usually <40% predicted), FVC, and FEV_1/FVC (<0.70); increased residual volume and total lung capacity DLCO decreased Hypoxemia CO_2 retention perhaps	Spirometry yearly and after exacerbations on return to baseline Daily peak flow monitoring Blood gas analysis yearly (if FEV_1 < 40% predicted) Echocardiogram with signs of CHF Chest radiograph yearly Reduce or stop smoking Observe nutritional status and weight
Young elderly patient, nonsmoker, with insidious onset of dyspnea (occurs only with exertion for past 2 years) and mild nonproductive cough, without prior, relevant occupational exposures	Gaunt Respiratory and heart rates increased Coarse crackles heard at lung bases Mild clubbing Radiograph with diffuse infiltrates, decreased lung volume, and cystic areas at bases	Pulmonary fibrosis	Spirometry DLCO Timed walking, with oximetry and arterial blood gas analysis Cardiopulmonary exercise test advised	Reduced lung volumes (vital capacity, total lung capacity) FEV_1/FVC ratio increased DLCO reduced Hypoxemia, but normal CO_2 Exercise tolerance limited	Spirometry at each visit every 6–12 months Oximetry Timed velocity walk (with oxygen if O_2 < 88% at rest) Echocardiogram with signs of CHF

CHF = congestive heart failure; COPD = chronic obstructive pulmonary disease; DLCO = diffusing capacity of lung for carbon monoxide; FEV_1 = forced expiratory volume in 1 second; FVC = forced vital capacity; MMEFR = maximum mid-expiratory flow rate; PEFR = peak expiratory flow rate.

patients with significant airway obstruction, a slow expiratory vital capacity is obtained. Peak flow measured with portable devices is used often for outpatient monitoring of lung function in subjects with asthma, COPD, or interstitial lung diseases. Encouraging a patient to keep a daily log can improve compliance with the testing protocol and yield helpful information about variations in effort and related symptoms. Although a healthy young person can produce a peak flow of 500 to 600 L/min, many people with COPD are unable to achieve a peak flow greater than 200 to 350 L/min and experience significant exertional dyspnea when peak flow decreases to less than 200 L/min. Patients whose peak flow is around 150 L/min are usually sedentary.

From analysis of measured values for FEV_1 and FVC (and their ratio) and total lung capacity, the main categories of ventilatory lung disease—obstructive and restrictive—can be defined (Fig. 85–3). A reduced FEV_1 and low FEV_1/FVC ratio combined with a large total lung capacity indicate obstructive disease of large airways and bronchi, a pattern typically observed in patients with COPD and asthma. FVC is preserved, but the time of exhalation is prolonged. After the administration of bronchodilators, the FEV_1 and FVC may increase by 10 to 15%, especially in asthma, indicating reversibility of airway obstruction. A lesser degree of improvement often is found, however, in patients who are already using inhaled bronchodilators regularly. A decrease in the $FEF_{25-75\%}$ typically is found in patients with obstruction of small airways. If a person's post-bronchodilator FEV_1 is less than 80% of the predicted value and FEV_1/FVC is less than 70%, airflow limitation is not fully reversible—the defining characteristic of COPD (Chapter 88). In patients with restrictive lung disease, the FEV_1 and FVC are reduced, as is total lung capacity, but the FEV_1/FVC ratio is usually normal or increased. Causes of restrictive interstitial lung disease include fibrosis of the lung parenchyma due to many toxic and inhalation exposures and toxic drug reactions (Chapter 94) and idiopathic interstitial lung diseases (Chapter 92). Restrictive physiology with a normal or low FEV_1 may reflect the chest wall habitus, chest wall muscle weakness or deformity, and pleural thickening (Chapter 100).

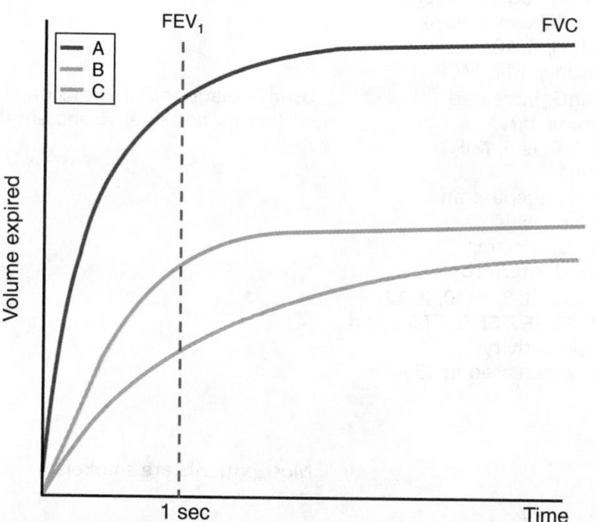

FIGURE 85–3 • Typical results of spirometry in a normal patient (A), a patient with a restrictive defect (B), and a patient with an obstructive defect (C). In a patient with a restrictive defect, the FEV_1/FVC ratio is preserved at the normal level, but both absolute values are reduced. In a patient with an obstructive defect, both absolute values are again reduced, but the FEV_1/FVC ratio is considerably reduced as the forced expiratory time required to reach the FVC is greatly prolonged. (Redrawn from Forbes CD, Jackson WF: Color Atlas and Text of Clinical Medicine, 3rd ed. London, Mosby, 2003, with permission.)

Diffusion Capacity

Measurement of diffusion capacity assesses how well gas in inspired air can cross the two tissue layers and one tissue space that make up the alveolar-capillary exchange surface (i.e., the alveolar type I epithelial cells, the interstitial space [not continuously present], and the vascular endothelial cells). The test measures the absorption of a low concentration of carbon monoxide in inhaled air by hemoglobin in red blood cells that circulate through pulmonary capillaries. Results must be corrected for reduced lung volumes, anemia, increased carbon monoxide levels in cigarette smokers, and high altitude. The diffusion capacity provides a general assessment of the air-blood interface; reduced values are obtained when interstitial fibrosis is extensive or when the capillary surface is compromised by vascular obstruction or nonperfusion (e.g., pulmonary embolism; Chapter 99) or destroyed as in emphysema (Chapter 88).

Site-Specific Sampling, Including Bronchoalveolar Lavage

Pulmonary function tests measure the effectiveness of breathing and air exchange but not the health of the respiratory tract's structure or cells or the metabolic and immunologic activity of inflammatory cells that accumulate in airways. Noninvasive methods can assess in situ airway inflammation by measuring breath pH and endogenously produced biomarkers of oxidative stress (i.e., reactive oxygen and nitrogen species or aldehydes of lipid peroxides damaged in cell membranes) in exhaled air and breath condensate and by assaying mediators in induced sputum (e.g., IL-8, leukotriene B_4, myeloperoxidase, IL-6, and elastase products). For example, as COPD worsens, induced sputum specimens or exhaled breath condensates provide evidence of neutrophilic inflammation with higher concentrations of exhaled nitric oxide, tumor necrosis factor-α, IL-6, transforming growth factor-β, IL-8, and growth-related oncogene-α as well as more leukotriene B_4.

Site-specific sampling to detach cells by washing or abrading the mucosal surface coupled with endobronchial or transbronchial biopsy can provide contiguous samples containing viable cells, noncellular secretions, and adjacent tissue. Multiple sites can be sampled; mucosal cell function can be compared between the nose and lower airways to assess allergic diseases. Bronchoalveolar lavage retrieves cells and secretions from the distal airways and the alveolar space surface. In combination with a thorough clinical evaluation and lung imaging studies, distinctive cellular patterns sometimes can obviate the need for lung biopsy (Table 85–3). Lung biopsy tissue can be microdissected with laser capture of specific cell types, and cells recovered in bronchoalveolar lavage fluid can be prepared for microarray analysis; gene chips created specifically for

TABLE 85–3 BRONCHOALVEOLAR LAVAGE CELL AND FLUID FINDINGS

Status or Illness	Cell Profile	Noncellular Components	Other Illnesses in the Differential Diagnosis with Overlapping Findings
Normal nonsmokers	Differential cell count (mean %): AM, 85%; lymphocytes, 7–12%; PMN, 1–2%; eosinophils-basophils, <1%; ciliated cells, 1–5% Lymphocyte subsets: CD4 helper, 50%; CD8 suppressor or cytotoxic, 30%; CD4/CD8 ratio, 1.5; B lymphocytes (plasma cells), 5%	95% as IgA (40% as IgA2), almost no IgM, IgG (IgG1–3/albumin ratios similar to serum), increased IgG4 Low concentrations of cytokines (IL-6, IL-8) Adhesion molecules detectable Histamine Surfactant	

Continued

TABLE 85–3 BRONCHOALVEOLAR LAVAGE CELL AND FLUID FINDINGS—cont'd

Status or Illness	Cell Profile	Noncellular Components	Other Illnesses in the Differential Diagnosis with Overlapping Findings
Healthy moderate smokers	3-fold increase of total cells, 95% AM, 3- to 5-fold increased AM PMN approximately 3% Lymphocytes 3% in differential cell count	Increased IgG as IgG/albumin ratio with serum, increased IgG3 and IgG4, decreased FSC, less surfactant recovered (lipid component profile same as that of nonsmoker) Decreased A_1AT elastase inhibitory activity Increased ACE (in AM) may be found	
DIFFUSE INTERSTITIAL LUNG DISEASES			
Sarcoidosis	Lymphocytes >20% total cells, increased CD4 cells, increased CD4/CD8 ratio AM-lymphocytes (T cells) form spontaneous rosettes	Increased IL-2, IL-6, IL-8, IL-10, IL-12, MCP-1 ACE level can be increased Increased adhesion molecule ICAM-1 Increased fibronectin	Extrathoracic granulomatous diseases (e.g., Crohn's disease), primary biliary cirrhosis, extrinsic allergic alveolitis, idiopathic pulmonary fibrosis, collagen vascular disease
Extrinsic allergic alveolitis (hypersensitivity pneumonitis)	Increased lymphocytes to >40–60% of total cells, often increased CD8 Foamy cytoplasm of AM Increased plasma cells, sometimes increased mast cells or basophils	Increased IgM and IgG; IgG fraction may have specific precipitating antibody activity against etiologic antigens (thermophilic microbes) Increased IL-4, IL-10, interferon-γ, MIF, MCP	Drug-induced hypersensitivity
Idiopathic pulmonary fibrosis	Increased PMN, approximately 5–15% of cells Increased eosinophils, approximately 3–6% Increased lymphocytes, 15% in some cases	Increased IgG, increased monomeric IgA Increased IL-6, IL-8, MIF, galactin-1 Increased collagenase and histamine levels Increased fibronectin, decreased interferon-γ	Usually diagnosis of exclusion (occupational, environmental)
Systemic sclerosis	Increased PMNs to approximately 3–10% of cells Increased eosinophils to approximately 2% of cells Lymphocytes about 10%, but CD8 cells may be increased Myofibroblasts can be recovered	Increased IL-4, IL-8, IL-10, IL-12, MCP-1, PDGF, TGF-β, CTGT, and thrombin activity Interferon-γ increased in 15%	
Langerhans cell histiocytosis	Cell profile similar to that of smokers: Increased $CD1^+$ cells (>4% AM) Cytoplasmic X body or Birbeck granule on EM		Most patients are smokers
Alveolar lipoproteinosis	Foamy cytoplasm of AM	Milky, turbid fluid with altered phospholipid proportions; increased surfactant protein A	Extrinsic allergic alveolitis, lipoid pneumonia, drug-induced hypersensitivity (e.g., amiodarone), silicosis
Eosinophilic pneumonia	Increased percentage of eosinophils to 40% of cells		Churg-Strauss, allergic bronchopulmonary aspergillosis, drug-induced hypersensitivity
Alveolar hemorrhage (Goodpasture's, Wegener's)	Hemosiderin-laden AM		
Inhalation exposure (asbestosis, fiber, silica)	Asbestos bodies or fiber in AM		Subclinical exposure must be considered in asymptomatic subjects

A_1AT = α_1-antitrypsin protease; ACE = angiotensin-converting enzyme; AM = alveolar macrophages; CD4 = T-helper lymphocyte subset; CD8 = T-suppressor lymphocyte; CTGT = connective tissue growth factor; EM = electron microscopy; FSC = free secretory component; ICAM-1 = intercellular adhesion molecule 1; Ig = immunoglobulin; IL = interleukin; PDGF = platelet-derived growth factor; PMN = polymorphonuclear neutrophils; MCP = monocyte chemotactic protein; MIF = macrophage migration inhibition factor; TGF-β = transforming growth factor-β.

gene expression patterns may prove helpful for determining genetic susceptibility, aiding diagnosis, and monitoring clinical activity.

SUGGESTED READINGS

Hallstrand TS, Boitano LJ, Johnson WC, et al: The timed walk test as a measure of severity and survival in idiopathic pulmonary fibrosis. Eur Respir J 2005;25:96–103. *The 6-minute walk test modified to be a timed test that incorporates the velocity of walking to reflect the impact of hypoxemia may be the best way to assess exercise function.*

Mannino DM, Reichert MM, Davis KJ: Lung function decline and outcomes in an adult population. Am J Respir Crit Care Med 2006;173:985–990. *Declines in lung function independently predict COPD hospitalizations and death.*

Reynolds HY: Lung inflammation and fibrosis. Am J Respir Crit Care Med 2005;171:98–102. *Details of the cells and cytokines/chemokines that participate in these processes.*

Silkoff PE, Erzurum SC, Workshop members: ATS/ERS Recommendations for standardized procedures for online and offline measurement of exhaled lower respiratory nitric oxide and nasal oxide, 2005. Am J Respir Crit Care Med 2005;171:912–930. *This emerging technology can measure products reflecting inflammation noninvasively in lung biologic specimens.*

86 DISORDERS OF VENTILATORY CONTROL

Steven A. Shea and David P. White

NORMAL VENTILATORY CONTROL SYSTEM

The human ventilatory control system (Fig. 86–1) determines the neural output to the respiratory muscles, thereby dictating the quantity and pattern of ventilation in an attempt to maintain arterial blood gas values within fairly tight constraints despite substantial alterations in metabolic rate (exercise), the work of breathing (underlying cardiopulmonary or chest wall disease), or disease of the respiratory muscles. Although the respiratory rhythm emerges primarily from neurons in the medulla and pons, these neurons receive afferent input from a number of sources that provide constant information about blood gases (e.g., arterial oxygen partial pressure [Pa_{O_2}], arterial carbon dioxide partial pressure [Pa_{CO_2}]), lung and chest wall inflation, and respiratory muscle function. The principal sources of this afferent input include the carotid bodies (responsive to changes in Pa_{O_2}, Pa_{CO_2}, and pH), the medullary chemoreceptor (Pa_{CO_2} and pH), muscle spindles and Golgi tendon organs (responsive to respiratory muscle activity and chest wall inflation), and receptors in the airways and lungs (responsive to temperature, stretch, and pressure). During wakefulness, ventilation is also substantially influenced by behavioral activities such as speech, swallowing, and anxiety. The principal focus of this chapter is disorders of the chemoreceptor mechanisms (Pa_{O_2}, Pa_{CO_2}) because these are more common and clinically important.

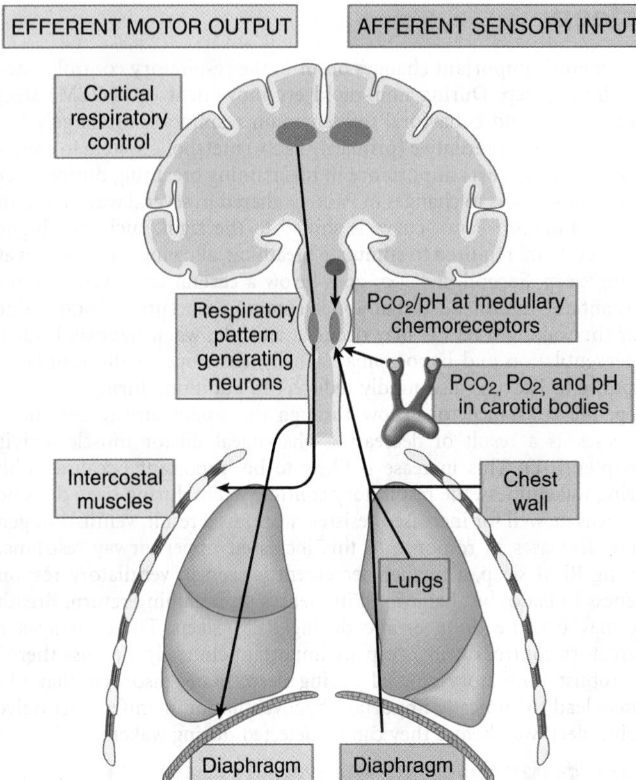

FIGURE 86–1 • A simplified diagram of the principal efferent (left) and afferent (right) respiratory control pathways. A section through the brain, brain stem, and spinal cord is shown (with pertinent respiratory areas indicated by shading), as are the central nervous system links with the respiratory apparatus.

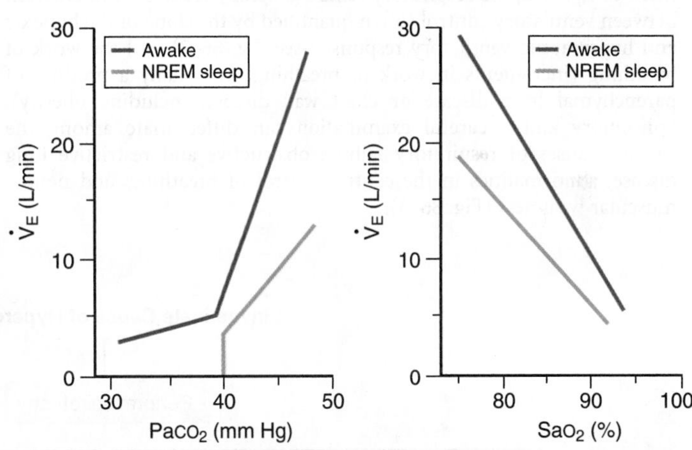

FIGURE 86–2 • Typical ventilatory responses to hypercapnia (left) and hypoxia (right). Compared with wakefulness, the ventilatory responses decline during non–rapid eye movement (NREM) sleep and decline even further during REM sleep (not shown). $\dot{V}_E$ = expired minute ventilation.

Awake

In awake resting individuals, Pa_{CO_2} is generally stable, varying by less than 2 to 4 mm Hg (slightly more in premenopausal adult women because progesterone stimulates breathing during the luteal phase of the menstrual cycle). Ventilation increases briskly if Pa_{CO_2} is acutely elevated above this resting level but does not decline significantly if Pa_{CO_2} decreases. This "dog-leg" appearance of the awake hypercapnic ventilatory response (Fig. 86–2) has led to the concept of a "wakefulness drive to breathe" that persists in the absence of chemoreceptive (Pa_{CO_2}, Pa_{O_2}) stimulation of breathing. Similarly, decreases in Pa_{O_2} from 500 mm Hg to approximately 65 mm Hg have a negligible effect on breathing; at less than 65 mm Hg, a hyperbolic relationship occurs between decreasing Pa_{O_2} and increasing ventilation (yielding a roughly linear relationship between decreasing arterial oxyhemoglobin saturation and increasing ventilation). Within the normal range, the fairly weak chemical control system permits relatively unfettered behavioral control of breathing. However, if the Pa_{CO_2} increases to more than about 42 mm Hg or the Pa_{O_2} decreases to less than about 65 mm Hg, ventilation increases rapidly. Because of the shapes of the ventilatory response curves relative to those of normal blood gases, hypercapnia rather than hypoxia elicits the greater response to hypoventilation and thereby normalizes blood gases. Nonetheless, in clinical situations in which Pa_{CO_2} and Pa_{O_2} change simultaneously, hypoxia does accentuate the ventilatory response to hypercapnia in a synergistic fashion.

During mild exercise, ventilation normally increases in direct proportion to carbon dioxide production, such that Pa_{CO_2} changes minimally. Surprisingly, the chemoreceptive feedback system seems unlikely to be responsible for such tight Pa_{CO_2} control, in that no detectable change in Pa_{CO_2} or Pa_{O_2} is generally noted during mild exercise. Other proposed mechanisms that may contribute to hyperpnea during exercise include stimulation of breathing by afferents in the moving limbs, afferents from receptors detecting carbon dioxide flow to the lungs, mixed venous chemoreceptors, and conditioned responses. However, ventilatory control during exercise remains poorly understood, partly because redundant control mechanisms are involved.

Asleep

Numerous important changes occur in the respiratory control system on falling asleep. During non–rapid eye movement (non-REM) sleep, both wakeful and behavioral influences on respiration are largely lost, leaving the chemoreceptive (primarily $Paco_2$) metabolic system to control breathing. Despite its importance in maintaining breathing during sleep, the responsiveness to changes in $Paco_2$ is altered in several ways. First, the entire ventilation-$Paco_2$ curve is shifted to the right, such that higher $Paco_2$ levels are required to stimulate breathing, allowing $Paco_2$ to elevate during sleep. Second, if $Paco_2$ goes below a certain level, ventilation is substantially inhibited, so that apnea commonly occurs at $Paco_2$ values near the waking level (as may occur at altitude, when hypoxia leads to hyperventilation and hypocapnia). Finally, the slope of the ventilatory response to $Paco_2$ is also mildly reduced. In addition, during non-REM sleep, the resistance to airflow through the upper airway commonly increases as a result of decreasing pharyngeal dilator muscle activity (Chapter 101). This increase is likely to be important because unlike during wakefulness, the respiratory control system during sleep does not compensate well for increased resistive work. As a result, ventilation generally decreases in response to this increased upper airway resistance. During REM sleep, a further decrement is seen in ventilatory responsiveness to $Paco_2$ but behavioral influences on breathing return. Breathing may become quite erratic during REM sleep. These changes in ventilatory control during sleep are important clinically. Because there is less robust ventilatory control during sleep, many disorders that ultimately lead to clinically important hypoventilation manifest themselves during sleep well before they can be detected during wakefulness.

DISORDERS OF VENTILATORY CONTROL

Relationship to Respiratory Failure

Ventilatory control disorders that cause respiratory failure are more commonly hypercapnic than hypoxic (Chapter 105). First, the development of hypercapnic respiratory failure generally reflects an interaction between ventilatory control (often quantified by the slope of the hypoxic and hypercapnic ventilatory responses; see Fig. 86–2) and the work of breathing (increments in work of breathing are usually a product of parenchymal lung disease or chest wall disease, including obesity). Spirometry and a careful examination can differentiate among the various causes of respiratory failure: obstructive and restrictive lung disease, abnormalities in the central control of breathing, and neuromuscular weakness (Fig. 86–3).

When chemoresponsiveness is markedly diminished or absent, hypercapnia may develop in an individual with a normal respiratory apparatus and normal work of breathing. Conversely, when the work of breathing is extraordinarily high (as might occur with severe chronic obstructive pulmonary disease; Chapter 88), respiratory failure may develop despite normal or robust ventilatory control. Therefore, although low or diminished chemoresponsiveness may predispose an individual to hypercapnia, the work required to maintain ventilation often determines when hypercapnia actually occurs. Second, individual variability in chemoresponsiveness is substantial, with slopes varying seven-fold from one individual to another because of genetic differences, previous neurologic disease (e.g., encephalitis, meningitis), prolonged exposure to hypoxia and hypercapnia, and other poorly understood influences. Studies are beginning to identify the numerous genes underlying this chemosensitivity and may eventually explain the differences in ventilatory chemosensitivity and disease vulnerability among individuals. Regardless of the cause, low chemoresponsiveness in combination with increased work of breathing contributes to the development of hypercapnic respiratory failure. Finally, the speed of development of respiratory failure (Chapter 105) is variable. Acute changes in blood gas values, such as occur with a respiratory infection, can generally be detected quickly by a patient (e.g., by sensing shortness of breath) and lead to effective early treatment. Conversely, with diminished ventilatory control, hypercapnia and hypoxia may develop slowly, with little sensation of dyspnea, making the early detection of respiratory failure difficult, potentially leading to more severe and more chronic disease.

Hypoventilation Associated with "Pure" Control of Breathing Abnormalities (without Increased Work of Breathing or Cardiopulmonary Disease)

Hypoventilation can develop in an individual with normal lungs and respiratory muscle function but with a markedly diminished ability to respond to hypoxia or hypercapnia. In children, the most common cause is the congenital "central" hypoventilation syndrome; recent data suggest specific gene mutations as the cause (e.g., *PHOX2B;* see Suggested Readings). The most common such disorder in adults is acquired central alveolar hypoventilation, which is defined by markedly diminished ventilatory chemoresponsiveness, normal respiratory apparatus (normal pulmonary function), and absence of obesity or chest wall disease.

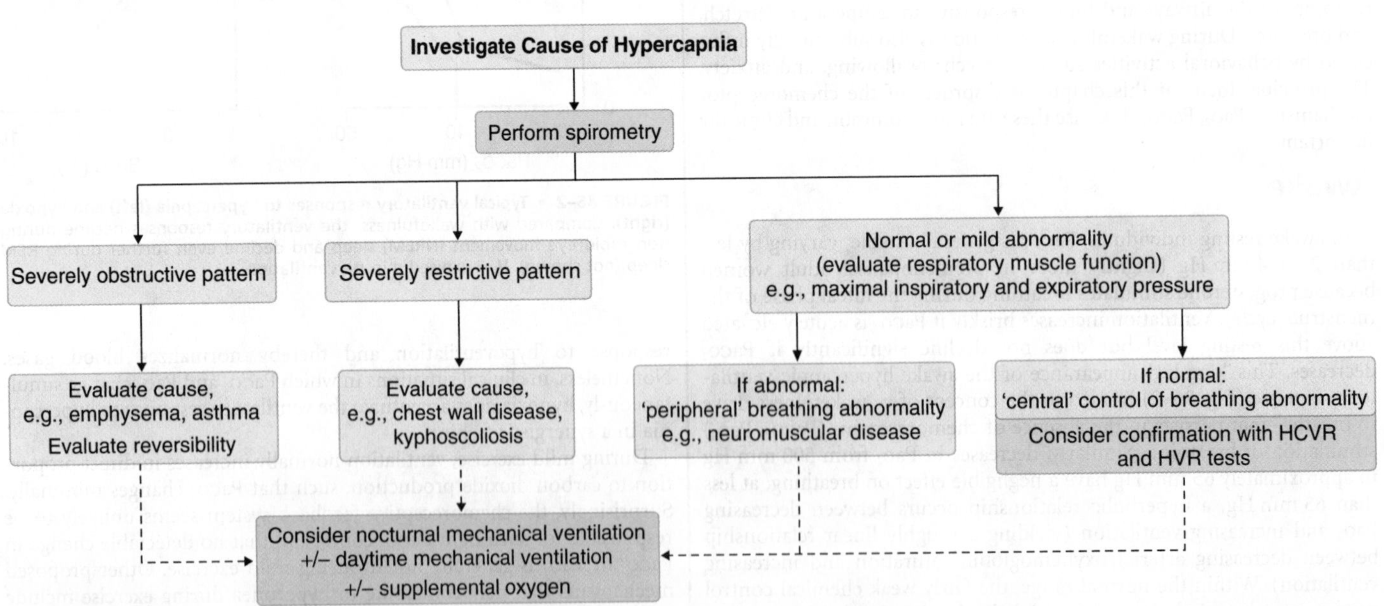

FIGURE 86–3 • A flow diagram. The flow diagram demonstrates the various causes of respiratory failure with hypercapnia and delineates how obstructive and restrictive lung disease, abnormalities in the central control of breathing, and neuromuscular weakness can be distinguished. Mechanical ventilation is usually initiated only during sleep (nocturnal ventilation), but severe cases may also require daytime mechanical ventilation or oxygen supplementation. HCVR = hypercapnic ventilatory response; HVR = hypoxic ventilatory response.

TABLE 86–1 APPROACHES TO THERAPY FOR THE MOST COMMON DISORDERS OF VENTILATORY CONTROL

Diagnosis	Approach	Specific Therapy	Time until Response
COPD "blue bloaters"	Reduce work of breathing	Bronchodilators	Hours to days
		Nocturnal ventilation	Days to weeks
	Improve oxygenation	Oxygen supplementation	Immediate
	Ventilatory stimulants*	Rarely used	
Central alveolar hypoventilation	Improve oxygenation	Oxygen supplementation	Immediate
	Nocturnal ventilation	Nasal ventilator	Days to weeks
		Diaphragmatic pacers	Days to weeks
	Ventilatory stimulants*	Progesterone (20 mg tid)	~1 wk
		Acetazolamide (250 mg qid; 500 mg bid)	~1 wk
Obesity hypoventilation	Reduce work of breathing	Weight loss	Months
		Nasal CPAP	Days to weeks
		Nocturnal ventilation	Days to weeks
	Improve oxygenation	Oxygen supplementation	Immediate
	Ventilatory stimulants*	Progesterone (20 mg tid)	~1 wk
		Acetazolamide (250 mg qid; 500 mg bid)	~1 wk

*Ventilatory stimulants, although used occasionally in the disorders listed, are generally of limited efficacy, particularly compared with nocturnal ventilation. COPD = chronic obstructive pulmonary disease; CPAP = continuous positive airway pressure.

Because of their decreased chemoresponsiveness, patients with the central hypoventilation syndrome (without increased work of breathing or cardiopulmonary disease) have arterial blood gas values that are labile when they are awake and that worsen substantially with sleep—particularly during non- REM sleep when breathing is almost totally dependent on negative feedback control of arterial blood gases through chemoreceptive reflexes. Ventilation also may deteriorate during respiratory infections, even if the work of breathing increases only minimally. Therefore, most of these individuals are chronically hypoxic and hypercapnic, often with cor pulmonale. Despite these severe blood gas abnormalities, patients rarely complain of dyspnea or respiratory discomfort and can often correct the hypercapnia with voluntary hyperventilation. Some patients with acquired central hypoventilation have previously documented neurologic disease as the explanation for their diminished chemoresponsiveness.

Hypoventilation with Increased Work of Breathing

Hypercapnia may also develop in patients with increased work of breathing in whom chemoresponsiveness may be diminished but is not necessarily absent; the most common example is chronic obstructive pulmonary disease (Chapter 88). As airflow obstruction worsens (increasing work of breathing), the incidence of respiratory failure increases, although the relationship between pulmonary function and increasing $Paco_2$ is certainly not linear. Such patients are sometimes classified as either "pink puffers" (high chemoresponsiveness and a general maintenance of blood gas homeostasis) or "blue bloaters" (low chemoresponsiveness and frequent respiratory failure), implying an important role for individual variability in chemosensitivity. However, overlap between groups is considerable, and hypercapnia in chronic obstructive pulmonary disease has a multifactorial etiology.

The obesity hypoventilation (pickwickian) syndrome is characterized by morbid obesity, diminished to absent ventilatory chemoresponsiveness during wakefulness, hypoxia and hypercapnia during wakefulness, absence (generally) of parenchymal lung disease, and severe obstructive sleep apnea (Chapter 101). Although the diminished responsiveness to hypoxia and hypercapnia almost certainly contributes to the blood gas abnormalities when the patient is awake and asleep, the cause of this abnormal ventilatory control is controversial. Some argue that genetically diminished chemoresponsiveness leads to the entire syndrome, whereas others contend that the obstructive apnea desensitizes the chemoreceptors and ultimately culminates in waking hypercapnia.

Hypoventilation with Neuromuscular Disease

Hypoventilation is also commonly observed in patients with neuromuscular weakness (e.g., motor neuron disease, muscular dystrophy, myasthenia gravis, poliomyelitis, Guillain-Barré syndrome, and quadriplegia). In these patients, the neural output from the brain stem respiratory center cannot always fully compensate for the defects in neuromuscular function, particularly during REM sleep, when chemoreceptor responsiveness is substantially reduced and a general loss of accessory respiratory muscle activity occurs (skeletal hypotonia characterizes this stage of sleep). Therefore, REM sleep becomes a potentially vulnerable time for patients with diaphragmatic dysfunction. Other rare neurologic disorders that influence ventilatory control include Ondine's curse (patients lack the ability to breathe automatically but are able to breathe voluntarily) and the locked-in syndrome (patients lack the ability to breathe voluntarily but are able to breathe automatically).

Treatment

Treatment of ventilatory control disorders includes (1) therapy to reduce the work of breathing (e.g., with bronchodilators or weight loss), (2) ventilatory stimulants, such as acetazolamide and progesterone, (3) supplemental oxygen, and (4) assisted ventilation (Table 86–1). There is no "grade A" evidence from randomized controlled trials addressing any of these therapeutic approaches. Nonetheless, it is always advisable to reduce the work of breathing (although it is not always possible). Ventilatory stimulants are often of only limited effectiveness, particularly in patients with central neural defects. Supplemental oxygen may improve oxygenation but rarely corrects hypercapnia; in some situations, oxygen may actually worsen hypercapnia. Assisted ventilation is most often the treatment of choice, particularly for patients with central neural defects and neuromuscular disease. Positive-pressure assisted ventilation is usually applied noninvasively by a nose mask, but it may be administered through tracheotomy, depending on the clinical situation. Currently, positive-pressure ventilation is predominantly administered during sleep so the patient can have a more normal waking existence; however, improved nocturnal ventilation also often leads to diminished daytime hypercapnia, which suggests a role for nocturnal hypoventilation in the development of waking hypercapnia. In severe cases, daytime ventilatory assistance may also be required.

SUGGESTED READINGS

Bales MJ, Timpe EM: Respiratory stimulant use in chronic obstructive pulmonary disease. Ann Pharmacother 2004;38:1722–1725. Epub 2004 Aug 17. *Review of the effect of ventilatory stimulants on arterial blood gases in chronic obstructive pulmonary disease.*

Homer RL, Bradley TD: Update in sleep and control of ventilation. Am J Respir Crit Care Med 2007;175:426–431. *Review of latest advances.*

Perrin C, D'Ambrosio C, White A, et al: Sleep in restrictive and neuromuscular respiratory disorders. Semin Respir Crit Care Med 2005;26:117–130. *Review of the role of noninvasive positive-pressure ventilation in the management of patients with restrictive thoracic disorders.*

87 ASTHMA

Jeffrey M. Drazen

Definition

Asthma is a clinical syndrome of unknown etiology characterized by three distinct components: (1) recurrent episodes of airway obstruction that resolve spontaneously or as a result of treatment; (2) exaggerated bronchoconstrictor response to stimuli that have little or no effect in nonasthmatic subjects, a phenomenon known as airway hyperresponsiveness; and (3) inflammation of the airways as defined by a variety of criteria. Although airway obstruction is largely reversible, it is currently thought that changes in the asthmatic airway may be irreversible in some settings.

Epidemiology

Asthma is an extremely common disorder affecting boys more commonly than girls and, after puberty, women slightly more commonly than men; approximately 7% of the adult population of the United States has signs and symptoms consistent with a diagnosis of asthma. Although most cases begin before the age of 25 years, asthma may develop at any time throughout life.

The worldwide prevalence of asthma has increased more than 45% since the late 1970s. The greatest increases in asthma prevalence have occurred in countries that have recently adopted an "industrialized" lifestyle. Although a variety of theories have been proposed, the reasons for the overall increase in prevalence of asthma are not known.

Asthma is among the most common reasons to seek medical treatment. In the United States, it is responsible for about 15 million annual outpatient visits to physicians and for nearly 2 million annual inpatient hospital days of treatment. The yearly direct and indirect costs of asthma care are more than $8 billion; more than 80% of these costs are attributable to direct expenditures on medical care encounters or asthma medications.

Pathobiology

Genetics

In twin studies, asthma has about 60% heritability, indicating that both genetic and environmental factors are important in its etiology. Despite this evidence for a substantial genetic contribution to the biology of asthma and identification of a number of candidate genes, no discovered genetic variant has enhanced risk for the asthma phenotype across all populations. These data suggest that multiple genetic variants account for the heritability of asthma in a given individual and that variations in different genes contribute to expression of the phenotype across a population. Genetic variants that influence the response to treatment also have been identified.

Pathology

The pathology of mild asthma, as delineated by bronchoscopic and biopsy studies, is characterized by edema and hyperemia of the mucosa and by infiltration of the mucosa with mast cells, eosinophils, lymphocytes bearing the T_H2 phenotype, and a newly identified subset of T cells, CD1d-restricted natural killer T cells. These last cells express a conserved (invariant) T-cell receptor and have potent immunoregulatory function. These cells create an environment that promotes the synthesis of immunoglobulin E (IgE), an important allergic effector molecule. Chemokines such as eotaxin, RANTES, macrophage inflammatory protein 1α, and interleukin-8, produced by epithelial and inflammatory cells, and the loss of the T-cell signaling molecule T-bet serve to amplify and to perpetuate the inflammatory events within the airway. As a result of these inflammatory stimuli coupled with the mechanical deformation of the epithelium from airway smooth muscle constriction, the airway wall is thickened by the deposition of type III and type V collagen below the true basement membrane. In addition, in severe chronic asthma, there is hypertrophy and hyperplasia of airway glands and secretory cells as well as hyperplasia of airway smooth muscle. Morphometric studies of airways from asthmatic subjects have demonstrated airway wall thickening of sufficient magnitude to increase airflow resistance and enhance airway responsiveness. During a severe asthmatic event, the airway wall is thickened markedly; in addition, patchy airway occlusion occurs by a mixture of hyperviscous mucus and clusters of shed airway epithelial cells.

The episodic airway narrowing that constitutes an asthma attack results from obstruction of the airway lumen to airflow. Although it is now well established that asthma is associated with infiltration of the airway by inflammatory cells, the links between these cells and the pathobiologic processes that account for asthmatic airway obstruction have not been clearly delineated. Three possible but not mutually exclusive links have been postulated: (1) the constriction of airway smooth muscle, (2) the thickening of airway epithelium, and (3) the presence of liquids within the confines of the airway lumen. Among these mechanisms, the constriction of airway smooth muscle due to the local release of bioactive mediators or neurotransmitters is the most widely accepted explanation for the acute reversible airway obstruction in asthma attacks. Several bronchoactive mediators are thought to be the agents that initiate the airway obstruction characteristic of asthma.

Mediators of the Acute Asthmatic Response

Acetylcholine

Acetylcholine released from intrapulmonary motor nerves causes constriction of airway smooth muscle through direct stimulation of muscarinic receptors of the M_3 subtype. The potential role for acetylcholine in the bronchoconstriction of asthma primarily derives from the observation that atropine and its congeners have some bronchodilator action, albeit less than β-agonists, when they are administered by inhalation for the treatment of asthma.

Histamine

Histamine, or β-imidazolylethylamine, was identified as a potent endogenous bronchoactive agent nearly 100 years ago. Mast cells, which are prominent in airway tissues obtained from patients with asthma, constitute the major pulmonary source of histamine. Clinical trials with novel potent antihistamines indicate a minor role for histamine as a mediator of airway obstruction in asthma.

Leukotrienes and Lipoxins

The cysteinyl leukotrienes, namely, LTC_4, LTD_4, and LTE_4, as well as the dihydroxy leukotriene LTB_4 are derived by the lipoxygenation of arachidonic acid released from target cell membrane phospholipids during cellular activation. 5-Lipoxygenase, the 5-lipoxygenase–activating protein, and LTC_4 synthase make up the cellular protein and enzyme content needed to produce the cysteinyl leukotrienes. The production of LTB_4 requires 5-lipoxygenase, the 5-lipoxygenase–activating protein, and LTA_4 epoxide hydrolase. Mast cells, eosinophils, and alveolar macrophages have the enzymatic capability to produce cysteinyl leukotrienes from their membrane phospholipids, whereas polymorphonuclear leukocytes produce exclusively LTB_4, which is predominantly a chemoattractant molecule; LTC_4 and LTD_4 are among the most potent contractile agonists ever identified for human airway smooth muscle. Clinical trials with leukotriene receptor antagonists or synthesis inhibitors have shown significant clinical efficacy in the treatment of chronic persistent asthma, leading to the conclusion that the leukotrienes are important but not exclusive mediators of the asthmatic response. Lipoxins are double lipoxygenase products of arachidonic acid metabolism and are thought to be endogenous downregulators of the inflammatory response. Their role in human asthma remains inferential.

Nitric Oxide

Nitric oxide (NO•) is produced enzymatically by airway epithelial cells and by inflammatory cells found in the asthmatic lung. Free NO• has a half-life on the order of seconds in the airway and is stabilized by conjugation to thiols to form RS-NO. Both NO• and RS-NO have bronchodilator actions and may play a homeostatic role in the airway. Paradoxically, high levels of NO•, when it is coavailable with superoxide anion, may form toxic oxidation products, such as peroxynitrite ($OONO^-$), which could damage the airway. Patients with asthma have higher than normal levels of NO• in their expired air, and these levels decrease after treatment with corticosteroids. Placebo-controlled trials have demonstrated that the fraction of nitric oxide in the exhaled air can serve as a marker for changes in the airway that necessitate escalation of asthma treatment.

Physiologic Changes in Asthma

An increased resistance to airflow is the consequence of the airway obstruction induced by smooth muscle constriction, thickening of the airway epithelium, or free liquid within the airway lumen. Resistance to airflow is manifested by increased airway resistance and decreased flow rates throughout the vital capacity. At the onset of an asthma attack, obstruction occurs at all airway levels; as the attack resolves, these changes are reversed—first in the large airways (i.e., mainstem, lobar, segmental, and subsegmental bronchi) and then in the more peripheral airways. This anatomic sequence of onset and reversal is reflected in the physiologic changes observed during resolution of an asthmatic episode (Fig. 87–1). Specifically, as an asthma attack resolves, flow rates first normalize at a high point in the vital capacity and only later at a low point in the vital capacity. Because asthma is an airway disease, not an air space disease, no primary changes occur in the static pressure-volume curve of the lungs. However, during an acute attack of asthma, airway narrowing may be so severe as to result in airway closure, with individual lung units closing at a volume that is near their maximal volume. This closure results in a change of the pressure-volume curve such that for a given contained gas volume within the thorax, elastic recoil is decreased, which in turn further depresses expiratory flow rates.

Additional factors influence the mechanical behavior of the lungs during an acute attack of asthma. During inspiration in an asthma attack, the pleural pressure becomes more negative than the 4 to 6 cm H_2O subatmospheric pressure usually required for tidal airflow. The expiratory phase of respiration also becomes active as the patient tries to force air from the lungs. As a consequence, peak pleural pressures during expiration, which normally are, at most, only a few centimeters of water above atmospheric pressure, may be as high as 20 to 30 cm H_2O above atmospheric pressure. The low pleural pressures during inspiration tend to dilate airways, whereas the high pleural pressures during expiration tend to narrow airways. During an asthma attack, the wide pressure swings coupled with alterations in the mechanical properties of the airway wall lead to a much higher resistance to expiratory airflow than to inspiratory airflow.

The respiratory rate is usually rapid during an acute asthmatic attack. This tachypnea is driven not by abnormalities in arterial blood gas composition but rather by stimulation of intrapulmonary receptors with subsequent effects on central respiratory centers. One consequence of the combination of airway narrowing and rapid airflow rates is a heightened mechanical load on the ventilatory pump. During a severe attack, the load can increase the work of breathing by a factor of 10 or more and can predispose to fatigue of the ventilatory muscles. The patchy nature of asthmatic airway narrowing results in a maldistribution of ventilation (V) relative to pulmonary perfusion (Q). A shift occurs from the normal preponderance of V/Q units, with a ratio of near unity, to a distribution with a large number of alveolar-capillary units, with a V/Q ratio of less than unity. The net effect is to induce arterial hypoxemia. In addition, the hyperpnea of asthma is reflected as hyperventilation with a low arterial P_{CO_2}.

Clinical Manifestations

History

During an acute asthma attack, patients seek medical attention for shortness of breath accompanied by cough, wheezing, and anxiety. The degree of breathlessness experienced by the patient is not closely related to the degree of airflow obstruction but is often influenced by the acuteness of the attack. Dyspnea may occur only with exercise (exercise-induced asthma), after aspirin ingestion (aspirin-induced asthma), after exposure to a specific known allergen (extrinsic asthma), or for no identifiable reason (intrinsic asthma). Variants of asthma exist in which cough, hoarseness, or inability to sleep through the night is the only symptom. Identification of a provoking stimulus through careful questioning helps establish the diagnosis of asthma and may be therapeutically useful if the stimulus can be avoided. Most patients with asthma complain of shortness of breath when they are exposed to rapid changes in the temperature and humidity of inspired air. For example, during the winter months in less temperate climates, patients commonly become short of breath on leaving a heated house; in warm humid climates, patients may complain of shortness of breath on entering a cold dry room, such as an air-conditioned theater.

An important factor to consider in taking a history from a patient with asthma is the potential for occupational exposures leading to the asthmatic diathesis (Table 87–1). In such cases, preexisting asthma may be exacerbated or asthma may occur de novo after workplace exposure; it is this clue that eventually leads to the diagnosis of occupational asthma. However, one cannot depend on a reversal of asthmatic symptoms when the patient is removed from the offending environment.

Physical Examination

Vital Signs

Common features noted during an acute attack of asthma include a rapid respiratory rate (often 25 to 40 breaths per minute), tachycardia, and pulsus paradoxus (an exaggerated inspiratory decrease in the systolic pressure). The magnitude of the pulsus is related to the severity of the attack. Pulse oximetry, with the patient respiring ambient air, commonly reveals an oxygen saturation near 90%.

Thoracic Examination

Inspection may reveal that patients experiencing acute attacks of asthma are using their accessory muscles of ventilation; if so, the skin over the thorax may be retracted into the intercostal spaces during inspiration. The chest is usually hyperinflated, and the expiratory phase is prolonged relative to the inspiratory phase. Percussion of the thorax demonstrates hyperresonance, with loss of the normal variation in dullness due to diaphragmatic movement; tactile fremitus is diminished.

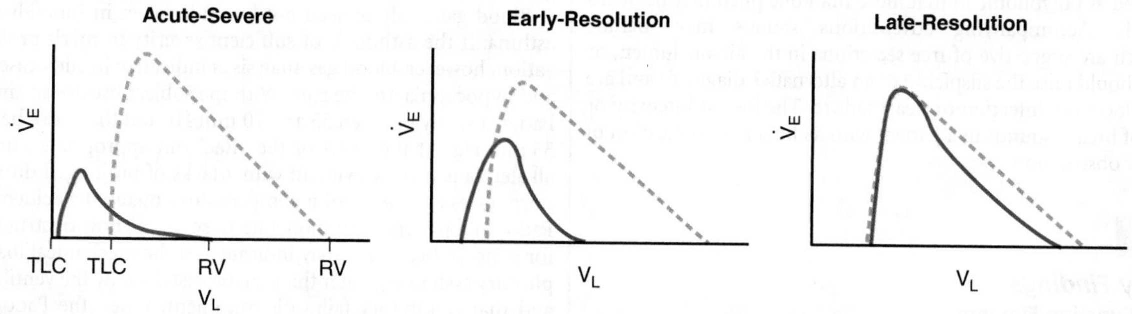

FIGURE 87–1 • Schematic flow-volume curves in various stages of asthma; in each figure, the dashed line depicts the normal flow-volume curve. Predicted and observed total lung capacity (TLC) and residual volume (RV) are shown at the extremes of each curve. $\dot{V}_E$ = expiratory flow rate; V_L = lung volume.

TABLE 87–1 COMMON OCCUPATIONAL CAUSES OF ASTHMA

Agent	Occupation	Prevalence*
HIGH-MOLECULAR-WEIGHT COMPOUNDS†		
Animals		
Laboratory animals (rats, mice, rabbits, guinea pigs)	Laboratory workers, veterinarians	Moderate
Chicken	Poultry workers	
Crab	Crab processing	Moderate
Prawns	Prawn processing	High
Hoya	Oyster farmers	High
River fly	Contact with riverside power plants	Low
Screwworm fly	Flight crews	High
Bee moth	Fish bait breeders	Moderate
Plants and vegetables		
Grain dust	Grain handlers	
Wheat or rye flour	Bakers, millers	
Gum acacia	Printers	High
Biologic enzymes		
Bacillus subtilis	Detergent industry	High
Trypsin	Plastics, pharmaceutical	High
Papain	Packing	High
LOW-MOLECULAR-WEIGHT COMPOUNDS‡		
Metals		
Platinum	Platinum refining	High
Vanadium	Hard metal industry	High
Other		
Trimetallic anhydride	Epoxy resin, plastics	High
Toluene diisocyanate	Polyurethane industries, varnishing, plastics	Moderate
Western red cedar	Carpenters, cabinet makers, sawmill workers	Low-moderate
Azidocarbonamide	Plastic and rubber workers	Moderate
Formalin	Hospital workers	
Urea formaldehyde	Insulation workers, affected homeowners	

*Prevalence is indicated by low (<3% of exposed individuals), moderate (3 to 20% of exposed individuals), or high (>20% of exposed individuals).
†High-molecular-weight compounds are usually considered to induce occupational asthma by an allergic mechanism.
‡Asthma induced by low-molecular-weight compounds that act as haptens; other mechanisms also exist but are not clearly elucidated.
Modified from Chan-Yeung M: Occupational asthma. Chest 1990;98:148S–161S.

Auscultation reveals wheezing, which is the cardinal physical finding in asthma but does not establish the diagnosis (Chapter 83). Wheezing, commonly louder during expiration but heard during inspiration as well, is characterized as polyphonic in that more than one pitch may be heard simultaneously. Accompanying adventitious sounds may include rhonchi, which are suggestive of free secretions in the airway lumen, or rales, which should raise the suspicion of an alternative diagnosis and are indicative of localized infection or heart failure. The loss of intensity or the absence of breath sounds in a patient with asthma is an indication of severe airflow obstruction.

Diagnosis

Laboratory Findings

Pulmonary Function Findings

A decrease in airflow rates throughout the vital capacity is the cardinal pulmonary function abnormality during an asthmatic episode. The peak expiratory flow rate (PEFR), the forced expiratory volume in the first second (FEV_1), and the maximal mid-expiratory flow rate (MMEFR) are all decreased in asthma (Chapter 85). In severe asthma, dyspnea may be so severe as to prevent the patient from performing a complete spirogram. In this case, if 2 seconds of forced expiration can be recorded, useful values for PEFR and FEV_1 can be obtained. Gradation of attack severity (Table 87–2) *must* be assessed by objective measures of airflow; no other methods yield accurate and reproducible results. As the attack resolves, the PEFR and the FEV_1 increase toward normal in concert while the MMEFR remains substantially depressed; as the attack resolves further, the FEV_1 and the PEFR may normalize while the MMEFR remains depressed (see Fig. 87-1). Even when the attack has resolved clinically, residual depression of the MMEFR is not uncommon; this depression may resolve during a prolonged course of treatment. If the patient is able to cooperate such that more complete measurements of lung function can be made, lung volume measurements demonstrate an increase in both total lung capacity and residual volume; the changes in total lung capacity and residual volume resolve with treatment.

TABLE 87–2 RELATIVE SEVERITY OF AN ASTHMATIC ATTACK AS INDICATED BY PEFR, FEV_1, AND MMEFR

Test	Predicted Value	Severity of Asthma
PEFR	>80%	
FEV_1	>80%	No spirometric abnormalities
MMEFR	>80%	
PEFR	>80%	
FEV_1	>70%	Mild asthma
MMEFR	55–75%	
PEFR	>60%	
FEV_1	45–70%	Moderate asthma
MMEFR	30–50%	
PEFR	<50%	
FEV_1	<50%	Severe asthma
MMEFR	10–30%	

FEV_1 = forced expiratory volume in the first second; MMEFR = maximal mid-expiratory flow rate; PEFR = peak expiratory flow rate.

Exhaled NO•

The fraction of NO• in the exhaled air (FENO) is elevated in patients with asthma. Although the exact concentration considered "elevated" will vary with the details of the technique, a concentration of 15 parts per billion is a convenient and reliable level that can be used to distinguish normal subjects from patients with untreated asthma. Because inhaled steroids suppress FENO levels, these values can guide titration of the dose of inhaled corticosteroids and are better than use of symptoms for this purpose. 1 In this approach, patients who have greater than a certain level of NO• in their exhaled air (the exact proportion will vary with the sampling technique) are considered to lack asthma control, and the dose of inhaled corticosteroids is increased. If the level of NO• in the exhaled air is low and the patient is clinically stable, attempts at dose reduction can be made.

Arterial Blood Gases

Blood gas analysis need not be undertaken in individuals with mild asthma. If the asthma is of sufficient severity to merit prolonged observation, however, blood gas analysis is indicated; in such cases, hypoxemia and hypocapnia are the rule. With the subject breathing ambient air, the PaO_2 is usually between 55 and 70 mm Hg and the $PaCO_2$ between 25 and 35 mm Hg. At the onset of the attack, an appropriate pure respiratory alkalemia is usually evident; with attacks of prolonged duration, the pH normalizes as a result of a compensatory metabolic acidemia. A normal $PaCO_2$ in a patient with moderate to severe airflow obstruction is reason for concern because it may indicate that the mechanical load on the respiratory system is greater than can be sustained by the ventilatory muscles and that respiratory failure is imminent. When the $PaCO_2$ increases in such settings, the pH decreases quickly because the bicarbonate stores have become depleted as a result of renal compensation for the prolonged preceding respiratory alkalemia. Because this chain of events can take place rapidly, close observation is indicated for asthmatic patients with "normal" Pa_{CO_2} levels and moderate to severe airflow obstruction.

Other Blood Findings

Asthmatic subjects are frequently atopic; thus, blood eosinophilia is common. In addition, elevated serum levels of IgE are often documented; epidemiologic studies indicate that asthma is unusual in subjects with low IgE levels. If indicated by the patient's history, specific radioallergosorbent tests, which measure IgE directed against specific offending antigens, can be conducted. In rare instances during severe asthma attacks, serum concentrations of aminotransferases, lactate dehydrogenase, muscle creatine kinase, ornithine transcarbamylase, and antidiuretic hormone may be elevated.

Radiographic Findings

The chest radiograph of a subject with asthma is often normal. Severe asthma is associated with hyperinflation, as indicated by depression of the diaphragm and abnormally lucent lung fields. Complications of severe asthma, including pneumomediastinum or pneumothorax, may be detected radiographically. In mild to moderate asthma without adventitious sounds other than wheezing, a chest radiograph need not be obtained; if the asthma is of sufficient severity to merit hospital admission, a chest radiograph is advised.

Electrocardiographic Findings

The electrocardiogram, except for sinus tachycardia, is usually normal in acute asthma. However, right axis deviation, right bundle branch block, "P pulmonale," or even ST-T wave abnormalities may arise during severe asthma and resolve as the attack resolves.

Sputum Findings

The sputum of the asthmatic patient may be either clear or opaque with a green or yellow tinge. The presence of color does not invariably indicate infection, and examination of a Gram-stained and Wright-stained sputum smear is indicated. The sputum often contains eosinophils, Charcot-Leyden crystals (crystallized eosinophil lysophospholipase), Curschmann's spirals (bronchiolar casts composed of mucus and cells), or Creola bodies (clusters of airway epithelial cells with identifiable cilia), which can affect color without the presence of infection.

Diagnosis

Differential Diagnosis

Asthma is easy to recognize in a young patient without comorbid medical conditions who has exacerbating and remitting airway obstruction accompanied by blood eosinophilia. A rapid response to bronchodilator treatment is usually all that is needed to establish the diagnosis. However, in the patient with cryptic episodic shortness of breath, an elevated FENO can help establish a diagnosis of asthma. However, in the absence of an elevated FENO, other causes of wheezing (see Table 83–3) should be investigated.

Prevention and Treatment

Rx

There is currently no way to prevent a patient from developing an asthmatic diathesis. If a patient has such a diathesis with an allergic component, avoidance of allergens can reduce the frequency of asthma attacks.

The treatment of asthma is directed at the airway obstruction and the propensity for the airways to narrow too much and too easily in response to inhaled bronchoconstrictors. Resolution of airway obstruction should be documented by objective measures, such as FEV_1 or PEFR. Inexpensive and easy-to-use peak flowmeters make the measurement feasible in virtually all cases. Treatment of asthma has two components. The first is the use of acute reliever (rescue) agents (i.e., bronchodilators) for acute asthmatic airway obstruction. The second is the use of controller treatments, which modify the asthmatic airway environment so that acute airway narrowing, requiring rescue treatments, occurs much less frequently.

In a given individual, the intensity of asthma treatment is adjusted, for the most part, to achieve four goals:

Rx

1. to allow the patient to pursue the activities of his or her daily life without excessive interference from asthma;
2. to allow the patient to sleep without awakening because of asthmatic symptoms;
3. to minimize the use of rescue bronchodilator treatments; and
4. to prevent the need for unscheduled medical care.

Recommendations for chronic control of asthma are based on the Global Initiative for Asthma, 2006 revision (Fig. 87–2). Based on a directed history and physical examination, the patient's current degree of control can be determined, and then recommendations for future treatment can be made.

Rescue Treatments

All patients with asthma should be prescribed a rescue inhaler to use if they develop acute asthmatic airway obstruction.

β-Adrenergic Agents

β-Adrenergic agents given by inhalation are the mainstay of bronchodilator treatment of asthma. Constricted airway smooth muscle relaxes in response to stimulation of β_2-adrenergic receptors. β-Adrenergic agonists with varying degrees of β_2-selectivity are available for use in inhaled (by nebulizer or metered-dose inhaler; Fig. 87–3), oral, or parenteral preparations. Most patients with mild intermittent asthma should be treated with a moderate-duration β_2-selective inhaler on an as-needed basis. Regardless of the specific type of medication used, rescue treatment should consist of two "puffs" from the inhaler, with the first and second puffs separated by a 3- to 5-minute interval, which is thought to allow enough time for the first puff to dilate narrowed airways, thus giving the agent better access to affected areas of the lung. Patients should be instructed to exhale to a comfortable volume, to breathe in very slowly (such as they would when sipping hot soup), and to actuate the inhaler as they inspire. Inspiration to near total lung capacity is followed by holding the breath for 5 seconds to allow the deposition of smaller aerosol particles in more peripheral airways. This treatment can be repeated every 4 to 6 hours; patients should be instructed to "advance" their asthma treatment as noted in Figure 87–2 if they need to use more than 18 puffs of a β-agonist in a 72-hour period.

Patients should receive specific instructions for correct inhaler use. Aerosol "spacers" are available from many manufacturers for patients who have difficulty coordinating their inspiratory effort and inhaler actuation. There is definitive evidence from prospective, randomized, placebo-controlled trials that the regularly scheduled use of prophylactic inhaled β-agonists has no deleterious effects in most patients with asthma.

In 2008, inhalers containing chlorofluorocarbon propellants will be withdrawn from the market and replaced by inhalers powered by hydrofluoroalkanes. These new inhalers have a lower velocity aerosol plume, so patients will notice a subjective difference in how the aerosol feels as it is dissipated into the mouth; nevertheless, clinical trials document that most hydrofluoroalkane inhalers will have nearly identical therapeutic effects.

Depending on the population, about one of six people is homozygous for the arginine 16 allele of the β_2-adrenergic receptor. A genotype-stratified, randomized trial demonstrated that the regularly scheduled use of albuterol in patients homozygous for this β_2-adrenergic receptor variant is associated with tachyphylaxis (a loss of physiologic and symptomatic asthma control) compared with persistent benefit in patients homozygous for the glycine 16 allele. 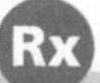 On the basis of these data, it is appropriate to prescribe a nonadrenergic rescue inhaler for patients who are homozygous for the arginine 16 genotype at this locus. Implementation of this recommendation will require widespread availability of genetic testing at this locus; this test is currently available only on a limited basis.

Anticholinergics

Atropinic agents inhibit the effects of acetylcholine released from the intrapulmonary motor nerves that run in the vagus and innervate airway smooth muscle. Ipratropium bromide, the atropinic

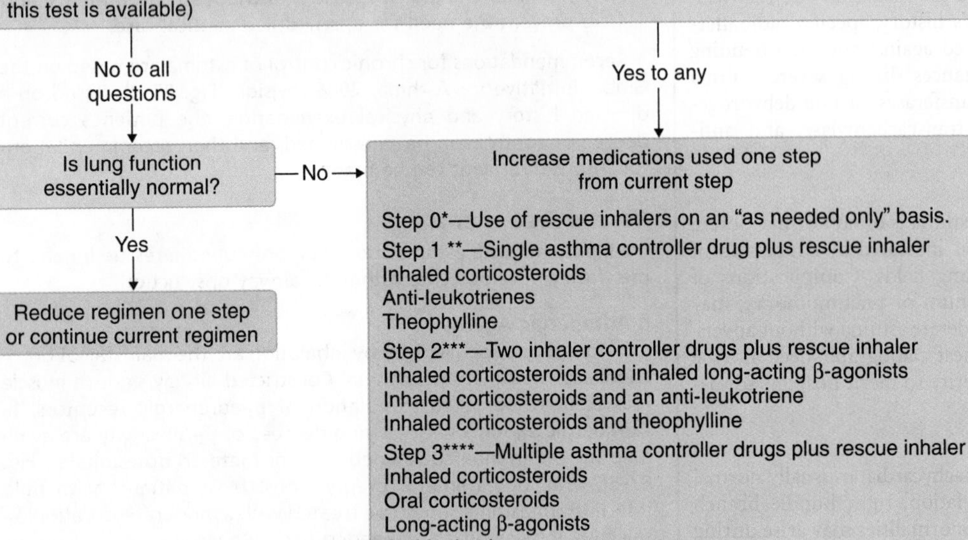

FIGURE 87–2 • Approach to chronic control of asthma and rescue from increased symptoms.
*Inhaled albuterol or, in patients predisposed to adverse effects from this treatment, inhaled ipratropium bromide.
**The choice between these two agents as "first-line" therapy is up to the patient and provider. Inhaled corticosteroids are more potent for improving lung function but have adverse effects when they are used at high doses for extended periods. Efforts should be made to use the lowest doses possible. Although antileukotrienes are less effective, some patients prefer oral to inhaled treatment and wish to avoid the potential side effects of inhaled steroids. If a response to one treatment is not achieved, it makes sense to try the other.
***The best documented combination is a long-acting β-agonist plus an inhaled steroid, but the dose of inhaled steroids should be at least the median dose (see Table 87–3) before long-acting β-agonists are added.
****The use of multiple medications indicates asthma of substantial severity. Unless success is easily achieved, consultation with an asthma specialist may be appropriate.

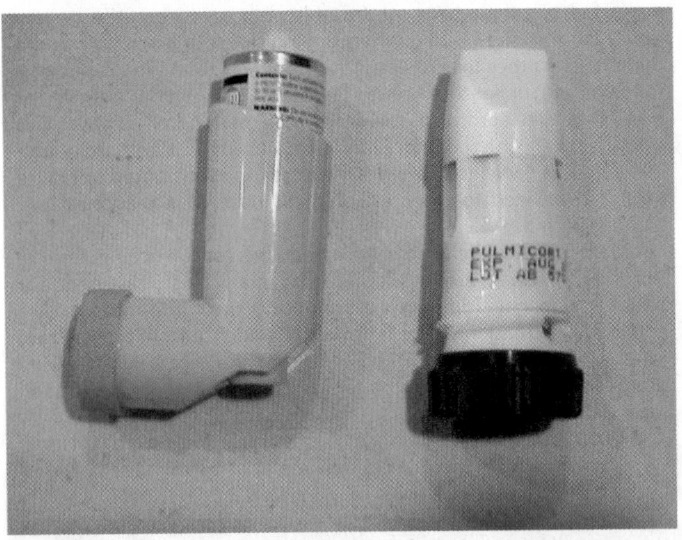

FIGURE 87–3 • Commonly used inhalers. Left, a pressurized metered-dose inhaler for a branded form of albuterol. Such inhalers propel the medication by means of a pressurized gas. Because of environmental concerns, the use of chlorofluorocarbons as propellants is being phased out; these agents are being replaced by propellants without an adverse effect on the ozone layer. Right, one of many types of dry powder inhalers; the one shown is a Turbuhaler and dispenses budesonide. In these inhalers, the patient creates the energy for airflow by means of an inspiratory effort that is directed through the device and that entrains medication into the inhaled airway to "rain out."

Rx

agent used therapeutically in asthma, is available in a metered-dose inhaler; the recommended dose is two puffs from a metered-dose inhaler every 4 to 6 hours. Although ipratropium bromide is not approved for this indication by the Food and Drug Administration, it is an appropriate first-line reliever treatment for patients homozygous for the arginine 16 allele of the β_2-adrenergic receptor; these are the patients, as noted before, whose lung function deteriorates when β-agonists are used on a regular basis.

Controller Treatments

Inhaled Corticosteroids

Inhaled corticosteroids (see Fig. 87–3), which have less systemic impact for a given level of therapeutic effect than systemic steroids, are effective controller treatments for improving lung function and preventing asthmatic exacerbations in patients with persistent asthma. [3, 4] However, inhaled corticosteroids do not change the natural history of asthma. A wide variety of inhaled corticosteroid products are on the market (Table 87–3). All available products are effective treatments of persistent asthma but differ in terms of the magnitude of adrenal suppression and the potential for systemic effects, including growth retardation in children, loss of bone mineralization, cataracts, and glaucoma. Overall, no convincing data are available to suggest that there is reason to prefer one corticosteroid over the others. An adverse effect common to all inhaled corticosteroids, at recommended doses, is oral thrush and hoarseness of voice (from myopathy of the laryngeal muscles); the risk and severity of this complication can be reduced by use of aerosol spacers and good oropharyngeal hygiene (i.e., rinsing out the mouth by gargling after dosing).

Antileukotrienes

Agents with the capacity to inhibit the synthesis of the leukotrienes (zileuton [Zyflo], 600 mg four times daily; liver function should be monitored for the first 3 to 6 months of treatment; if levels rise to more than three times the upper limit of normal, the drug should be stopped) or the action of leukotrienes at the $CysLT_1$ receptor (montelukast [Singulair], 10 mg once a day; pranlukast [Onon, Ultair], 225 mg twice a day, available in Japan only; zafirlukast [Accolate], 20 mg twice a day) are effective oral controller medications for patients with mild or moderate persistent asthma. These treatments can be used on their own for mild persistent asthma or in combination with inhaled steroids for more severe asthma.

TABLE 87–3 ESTIMATED EQUIPOTENT DAILY DOSE FOR INHALED GLUCOCORTICOSTEROIDS FOR ADULTS

Drug	Low Daily Dose (μg)	Median Daily Dose (μg)	High Daily Dose (μg)
Beclomethasone dipropionate	200–500	500–1000	>1000
Budesonide*	200–400	400–800	>800
Ciclesonide*	80–160	160–320	>320
Flunisolide	500–1000	1000–2000	>2000
Fluticasone	100–250	250–500	>500
Mometasone furoate*	200–400	400–800	>800
Triamcinolone acetonide	400–1000	1000–2000	>2000

Note: Some doses may be outside package labeling. Metered-dose inhaler doses are expressed as the amount of drug leaving the valve, not all of which is available to the patient. Dry powder inhaler doses are expressed as the amount of drug in the inhaler after activation.
*Once-a-day dosing is acceptable.
Modified from 2006 Global Initiative for Asthma guidelines.

Long-Acting β-Agonists

In contrast to medium-acting β-agonists, long-acting β-agonists currently available in the United States (salmeterol [Serevent, 42 μg per puff; the same dose is labeled 50 μg per puff outside of the United States; one or two puffs should be delivered every 12 hours] and formoterol [Foradil, 12 μg through a proprietary dry powder inhaler every 12 hours]) have a duration of action of nearly 12 hours; they are considered a controller rather than a bronchodilator agent. Randomized controlled trials demonstrate that long-acting β-agonists should not be used as a sole controller agent. Other trials have shown that there are excess asthma deaths (about one for every 650 patient years of treatment) when long-acting β-agonists are used. Therefore, long-acting β-agonists should be used only when they are given in concert with inhaled corticosteroids. 5 Combination products with both inhaled steroids and long-acting β-agonists in the same aerosol device are available. These agents provide benefit because the patient needs to use only a single device, but they may not be cost-effective and do not allow variation in the proportions of medications delivered.

Theophylline

Theophylline and its more water soluble congener aminophylline are bronchodilators of moderate potency that are useful in both inpatient and outpatient management of asthma. Theophylline is sold in a large number of formulations that allow therapy to proceed with daily or twice-daily dosing. The mechanism by which theophylline exerts its effects has not been established with certainty but is probably related to the inhibition of certain forms of phosphodiesterase. The utility of theophylline is limited by its toxicity and by wide variations in the rate of its metabolism, both in a single individual over time and among individuals in a population. There are multiple preparations of theophylline available on the market that vary in their duration of action. As a result of this variability, the starting dose should be about 300 mg/day; the frequency will depend on the preparation used.

Plasma theophylline levels should be monitored to ensure that patients are treated appropriately. Acceptable plasma levels for therapeutic effects are between 10 and 20 μg/mL; higher levels are associated with gastrointestinal, cardiac, and central nervous system toxicity, including anxiety, headache, nausea, vomiting, diarrhea, cardiac arrhythmias, and seizures. These last catastrophic complications may occur without antecedent mild side effects when plasma levels exceed 20 μg/mL. Because of these potentially life-threatening complications of treatment, plasma levels need to be measured with great frequency in hospitalized patients receiving intravenous aminophylline and less frequently in stable outpatients receiving one of the long-acting theophylline preparations. Most asthma care providers use dosing amounts and intervals to achieve steady-state theophylline levels of 10 to 14 μg/mL, thereby avoiding the toxicity associated with decrements in metabolism. Treatment with theophylline is recommended only for patients with moderate or severe persistent asthma who are receiving controller medications, such as inhaled steroids or antileukotrienes, but whose asthma is not adequately controlled.

Systemic Corticosteroids

Systemic corticosteroids are effective for the treatment of moderate to severe persistent asthma as well as for occasional severe exacerbations of asthma that occur in a patient with otherwise mild asthma, but the mechanism of their therapeutic effect has not been established. No consensus has been reached on the specific type, dose, or duration of corticosteroid to be used in the treatment of asthma. In nonhospitalized patients with asthma refractory to standard therapy, a steroid "pulse" with initial doses of prednisone on the order of 40 to 60 mg/day, tapered to zero during 7 to 14 days, is recommended. For patients who cannot stop taking steroids without having recurrent uncontrolled bronchospasm despite the addition of multiple other controller treatments, alternate-day administration of oral steroids is preferable to daily treatment. For patients whose asthma requires in-hospital treatment but is not considered life-threatening, an initial intravenous bolus of 2 mg/kg of hydrocortisone, followed by continuous infusion of 0.5 mg/kg/hr, has been shown to be beneficial within 12 hours. In attacks of asthma that are considered life-threatening, the use of intravenous methylprednisolone (125 mg every 6 hours) has been advocated. In each case, as the patient improves, oral steroids are substituted for intravenous steroids, and the oral dose is tapered during 1 to 3 weeks; addition of inhaled steroids to the regimen is strongly recommended when oral steroids are started.

Anti-IgE Treatment

Subcutaneous administration of omalizumab, a humanized murine monoclonal antibody that binds circulating IgE, is associated with decreased serum free (not total) IgE levels. In patients who have moderate to severe allergic asthma with elevated levels of serum IgE and who are receiving inhaled corticosteroids, omalizumab treatment improves asthma control even as doses of inhaled steroids are decreased. Dosing is guided by weight and by pretreatment IgE levels: a monthly subcutaneous dose of 0.016 mg × body weight (kg) × IgE level (IU/mL). For example, in a patient weighing 70 kg with a pretreatment total IgE level of 300 IU/mL, 336 mg of omalizumab would be administered monthly by subcutaneous injection. Anti-IgE antibodies can reduce exacerbations and improve quality of life in severe allergic asthma, but their place in treatment schema has not been established.

Other Controller Drugs

Cromolyn sodium (one or two puffs from a metered-dose inhaler three or four times a day) and nedocromil sodium (two puffs from a metered-dose inhaler three or four times a day) are nonsteroid inhaled treatments that have proved beneficial in the management of mild to moderate persistent asthma. They appear to be most useful in pediatric populations or when an identifiable stimulus (such as exercise or allergen exposure) elicits an asthmatic response.

The use of systemic gold (as in rheumatoid arthritis), methotrexate, or cyclosporine has been suggested as adjunctive treatment of patients with severe chronic asthma who cannot otherwise discontinue high-dose corticosteroid treatment. However, these agents are experimental, and their routine use is not advocated.

Control-Driven Asthma Therapy

The approach to the management of asthma is to titrate treatment to achieve an adequate level of control. If a patient's asthma is well controlled, treatment can be continued or "stepped down" (see Fig. 87–2). If a patient's asthma is poorly controlled, treatment intensity should be stepped up. At the mild end of the spectrum, a patient who has rare limitations in activities of daily life, has nearly normal lung function, and sleeps without interruption from asthma can be prescribed nothing more than inhaled rescue treatment on an as-needed basis. In general, if a patient can control his or her asthma with the use of a single metered-dose inhaler of rescue treatment dispensed every 7 to 8 weeks or less frequently, there is no need for background controller treatment. If a patient has a requirement for more rescue treatment, has symptoms that interfere with sleeping through the night, or has moderately deranged lung function, controller therapy should be added.

Single-agent controller therapy should consist of an inhaled corticosteroid or an antileukotriene. If control is not achieved with one of these agents, the patient can be switched to the other or have a second agent added. [6] The best studied two-agent combination is inhaled corticosteroids and a long-acting inhaled β_2-adrenergic agonist, [5] a combination that provides excellent disease control and should allow a reduction in the dose of inhaled corticosteroids. Data indicate that another combination, an antileukotriene and inhaled steroid, is more effective than either treatment alone, but this regimen does not have as substantial an evidence base as the combination of inhaled corticosteroids and a long-acting β-agonist.

Specific Treatment Scenarios

Concurrent Pulmonary Infection

In some patients, acute exacerbations of asthma may be due to concurrent infection, which requires targeted therapy (Chapters 88, 90, and 97).

Aspirin-Induced Asthma

Approximately 5% of patients with moderate to severe persistent asthma develop asthma when they ingest agents that inhibit cyclooxygenase, such as aspirin and other nonsteroidal anti-inflammatory drugs (Chapter 34). Inhibitors of cyclooxygenase 2 are less likely to cause these reactions, but aspirin-type reactions have been reported in sensitive patients treated with selective cyclooxygenase 2 inhibitors. Although the physiological manifestations of laboratory-based aspirin challenge can be blocked by leukotriene pathway inhibitors, these agents do not prevent clinical aspirin-induced asthma. Thus, patients with this form of asthma must avoid aspirin and other nonsteroidal anti-inflammatory drugs.

Asthma in the Emergency Department

When a patient with asthma presents for acute emergency care, objective measures of the severity of the attack, including quantification of pulsus paradoxus and measurement of airflow rates (PEFR or FEV_1), should be evaluated in addition to the usual vital signs. If the attack has been prolonged and failed to respond to treatment with bronchodilators and high-dose inhaled steroids before arrival at the emergency department, intravenous steroids (40 to 60 mg of methylprednisolone or its equivalent) should be administered. If the patient has not been receiving treatment with a leukotriene receptor antagonist, such agents should be administered (10 mg of montelukast or 20 mg of zafirlukast) as soon as possible. [7] Treatment with inhaled β-agonists should be repeated at 20- to 30-minute intervals until the PEFR or FEV_1 increases to greater than 40% of the predicted values. If this point is not reached within 2 hours, admission to the hospital for further treatment is strongly advocated.

When patients have PEFR and FEV_1 values that are greater than 60% of their predicted value on arrival in the emergency department, treatment with inhaled β_2-agonists alone, albuterol (0.5 mL of an albuterol 0.083% solution) or equivalent, is likely to result in an objective improvement in airflow rates. If significant improvement takes place in the emergency department, such patients can usually be treated as outpatients with inhaled β_2-agonists and a controller agent (see Fig. 87–2). A good strategy is to add inhaled corticosteroids if the patient has not been receiving this treatment or has been using a single controller therapy.

For patients whose PEFR and FEV_1 values are between 40% and 60% of the values predicted at the time of initial evaluation in the emergency care setting, a plan of treatment varying in intensity between these two plans is indicated. Failure to respond to treatment by objective criteria (PEFR or FEV_1) within 2 hours of arrival at the emergency department is an indication for the use of systemic corticosteroids.

Status Asthmaticus

The asthmatic subject whose PEFR or FEV_1 does not increase to greater than 40% of the predicted value with treatment, whose $Paco_2$ increases without improvement of indices of airflow obstruction, or who develops major complications such as pneumothorax or pneumomediastinum should be admitted to the hospital for close monitoring. Frequent treatments with inhaled β-agonists (0.5 mL of an albuterol 0.083% solution every 2 hours), intravenous aminophylline (at doses to yield maximal acceptable plasma levels, that is, 15 to 20 μg/mL; 500 to 1000 mg loading dose given during an hour followed by an infusion of 30 to 60 mg/hr), and high-dose intravenous steroids (methylprednisolone, 40 to 60 mg every 4 to 6 hours) are indicated. Oxygen should be administered by face mask or nasal cannula in amounts sufficient to achieve Sao_2 values between 92% and 94%; a higher Fio_2 promotes absorption atelectasis and provides no therapeutic benefit. If objective evidence of an infection is present, appropriate treatment should be given for that infection. If no improvement is seen with treatment and if respiratory failure appears imminent, bronchodilator treatment should be intensified to the maximum tolerated by the patient as indicated by the maximum tolerated heart rate, usually 130 to 140 beats per minute. If indicated, intubation of the trachea and mechanical ventilation can be instituted; in this case, the goal should be to provide a level of ventilation just adequate to sustain life but *not sufficient to normalize arterial blood gases*. For example, a $Paco_2$ of 60 to 70 mm Hg, or even higher, is acceptable for a patient in status asthmaticus.

Asthma in Pregnancy

Asthma may be exacerbated, remain unchanged, or remit during pregnancy (Chapter 259). There need not be substantial departures from the ordinary management of asthma during pregnancy. However, no unnecessary medications should be administered; systemic steroids should be used sparingly to avert fetal complications, and certain drugs should be avoided, including tetracycline (as a treatment of intercurrent infection), ipratropium bromide (which may cause fetal tachycardia), terbutaline (which is contraindicated during active labor because of its tocolytic effects), and iodine-containing mucolytics (such as saturated solution of potassium iodide). Moreover, use of prostaglandin $F_{2\alpha}$ as an abortifacient should be avoided in asthmatic patients.

Prognosis

Asthma is a chronic relapsing disorder. Most patients have recurrent attacks without a major loss in lung function for many years. A minority of patients experience a significant irreversible loss in lung function over and above the normal pulmonary senescence.

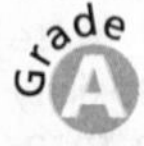

1. Smith AD, Cowan JO, Brassett KP, et al: Use of exhaled nitric oxide measurements to guide treatment in chronic asthma. N Engl J Med 2005;352:2163–2173.
2. Israel E, Chinchilli VM, Ford JG, et al: Use of regularly scheduled albuterol treatment in asthma: Genotype-stratified, randomised, placebo-controlled cross-over trial. Lancet 2004;364:1505–1512.

3. Boushey HA, Sorkness CA, King TS, et al: Daily versus as-needed corticosteroids for mild persistent asthma. N Engl J Med 2005;352:1519–1528.
4. Bateman ED, Boushey HA, Bousquet J, et al: Can guideline-defined asthma control be achieved? The Gaining Optimal Asthma Control study. Am J Respir Crit Care Med 2004;170:836–844.
5. Obyrne PM, Bisgaard H, Godard PP, et al: Budesonide/formoterol combination therapy as both maintenance and reliever medication in asthma. Am J Respir Crit Care Med 2005;171:129–136.
6. Szefler SJ, Phillips BR, Martinez FD, et al: Characterization of within-subject responses to fluticasone and montelukast in childhood asthma. J Allergy Clin Immunol 2005;115:233–242.
7. Silverman RA, Nowak RM, Korenblat PE, et al: Zafirlukast treatment for acute asthma—evaluation in a randomized, double-blind, multicenter trial. Chest 2004;126:1480–1489.

SUGGESTED READINGS

American Lung Association Asthma Clinical Research Centers: Randomized comparison of strategies for reducing treatment in mild persistent asthma. N Engl J Med 2007;356:2027–2039. *Patients with well-controlled asthma using twice-daily inhaled fluticasone can be switched to once-daily fluticasone plus salmeterol, but switching to montelukast increases treatment failure.*

Eder W, Ege M, von Mutius E: The asthma epidemic. N Engl J Med 2006; 355:2226–2235. *An overview of the rising prevalence of asthma worldwide.*

Holgate ST, Polosa R: The mechanisms, diagnosis, and management of severe asthma in adults. Lancet 2006;368:780–793. *A comprehensive overview.*

Papi A, Canonica GW, Maestrelli P, et al: Rescue use of beclomethasone and albuterol in a single inhaler for mild asthma. N Engl J Med 2007;356: 2040–2052. *Symptom-driven inhaled beclomethasone (250 μg) and albuterol (100 μg) in a single inhaler is as effective as regular use of inhaled beclomethasone (250 μg twice daily), with a lower cumulative steroid dose.*

88 CHRONIC OBSTRUCTIVE PULMONARY DISEASE

Nicholas Anthonisen

Definition

Chronic obstructive pulmonary disease (COPD) is the term used to describe slowly progressive airways obstruction, usually associated with smoking, that is not reversible and is not due to another specific cause. Patients with COPD have varying degrees of three pathologic processes, each associated with smoking: chronic bronchitis, small airways obstruction, and emphysema. Whereas chronic bronchitis can be defined clinically, small airways obstruction and emphysema cannot be reliably diagnosed during life. COPD results in airways obstruction, which is easily measured, and current therapy is largely aimed at reducing obstruction. Physicians, therefore, can commonly focus on the COPD syndrome and not its specific pathologic causes.

Although patients with COPD may improve with treatment, especially when an acute infection or exposure precipitates decompensation, COPD by definition implies some degree of fixed, irreversible disease. By comparison, patients with pure asthma (Chapter 87) have intermittent airway obstruction that may revert to normal after treatment and in between exacerbations.

Epidemiology

COPD is common, affecting about 16 million Americans. It is the fourth most common cause of death in the United States, and mortality from COPD is increasing. The economic burden of COPD is enormous, although it is extremely difficult to assess accurately and inclusively.

The prevalence of COPD reflects societal smoking habits, increasing steadily in men in the United States until the early 1990s and then leveling off. In women, COPD was previously uncommon, but the prevalence has increased and is still rising owing to increased smoking rates in women. It is unusual for a person to have clinically apparent COPD without a history of smoking for at least 20 pack years, and most patients have at least 40 pack years of exposure. A pack year is the equivalent of smoking 20 cigarettes per day for a year (Chapter 30).

Figure 88–1 shows a well-validated model of the development of COPD in terms of the most commonly used index of airways obstruction, which is the forced expiratory volume in 1 second, or FEV_1 (Chapter 85). In normal nonsmoking men, FEV_1 declines by about 30 mL per year after the age of 30 years, and disability due to dyspnea does not occur. In the "average" smoker, FEV_1 declines at a rate that is approximately twice as fast but still slow enough so that disability due to dyspnea is unlikely until late in life. About 15 to 20% of smokers, however, have more rapid declines of up to 100 mL per year, and it is these patients in whom symptomatic COPD develops in middle age. These individuals are in some way "sensitive" to tobacco products and constitute a high-risk group. A variety of additional risk factors have been identified, but all have relatively weak effects, and no currently known combination of factors satisfactorily explains why some smokers fare so much worse than others (Chapter 30).

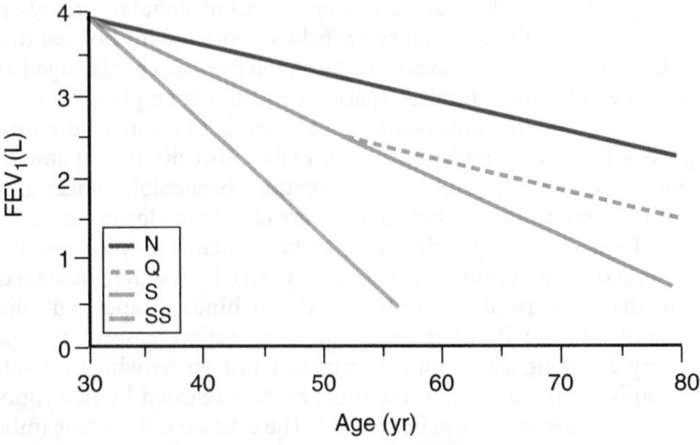

FIGURE 88–1 • Course of lung function decline through adulthood. The vertical axis is forced expiratory volume in 1 second (FEV_1); the horizontal axis is age. The course of decline is shown in a normal nonsmoker (N), in an average smoker (S), in a smoker who is sensitive to tobacco smoke (SS), and in an individual who quits smoking (Q, dashed line). Dyspnea first occurs when the FEV_1 is less than 2 L (50% of the normal value) and becomes severe when the FEV_1 is about 1 L.

Quitting smoking often alters the subsequent loss of lung function to the same rate as in nonsmokers during a few years' time. Thus, smoking cessation early enough in life can prevent the onset of clinical disease in middle age. However, severe COPD may progress even in patients who stop smoking.

Pathobiology

Chronic Bronchitis

Chronic bronchitis is a clinical diagnosis, defined as the presence of chronic cough and sputum production for at least 3 months of the year for at least 2 consecutive years in the absence of any other disease. At least one third of smokers aged 35 to 59 years have chronic bronchitis, and its prevalence increases with age.

The anatomic basis of chronic bronchitis is hypertrophy and hyperplasia of the mucus-secreting glands normally found in the epithelium of larger airways. These cells increase in size and number; as a consequence, they are found in smaller diameter airways than in nonsmokers. This expansion of mucus-secreting cells is accompanied by low-grade neutrophilic inflammation and increased airway smooth muscle. Chronic bronchitis is not necessarily associated with airways obstruction, and smokers can develop severe COPD in the absence of bronchitis. However, chronic bronchitis is associated with an increased tendency to develop repetitive episodes of acute bronchitis, which result in morbidity and may contribute to the progression of airways obstruction.

Peripheral Airway Disease

In COPD, the most striking increase in the resistance to airflow occurs in peripheral airways or bronchioles. Smokers have increased bronchiolar smooth muscle, inflammation, and fibrosis that narrow the airway lumens and thicken their walls. The degree of abnormality in these airways is correlated with lung function. The mechanisms involved in these changes are unknown.

Emphysema

Emphysema is defined as the enlargement of air spaces distal to the conducting airways, that is, respiratory bronchioles and alveoli, due to destruction of the walls of these air spaces. There are two important types of emphysema, centrilobular and panacinar. Centrilobular emphysema primarily involves the respiratory bronchioles, often with normal distal alveoli; however, in severe disease, distal alveoli may also be damaged and incorporated into the central air space. Centrilobular emphysema is seen almost exclusively in smokers, in whom it tends to occur in the upper lung lobes. Panacinar emphysema involves the entire distal lung unit, distorting and destroying alveoli and respiratory bronchioles alike; it can occur throughout the lung but may involve chiefly the lower lobes.

Some families develop early-onset, severe panacinar emphysema associated with α_1-antitrypsin (AAT) deficiency. AAT is an acute phase serum protein that is secreted by the liver and that binds to and neutralizes neutrophil elastase; it is the most abundant antiprotease in the lung periphery. Smoking causes an inflammatory process by which activated neutrophils are recruited into the lung; elastase released by neutrophils digests lung tissue in the absence of AAT. The elastase-antielastase imbalance present in patients with AAT deficiency might also occur in people without the deficiency under the proper conditions, such as oxidation of AAT, but it is not clear that this is the case.

There are a number of abnormal alleles of the gene *AAT*, the most common and important of which is termed Z. Patients homozygous for the Z allele (ZZ), a rare condition, have very low serum AAT levels and develop severe panacinar emphysema early in life if they smoke. Patients who do not smoke may not develop significant lung disease. Heterozygotes (AZ) are more common, representing about 2 to 3% of North European populations, and have serum levels of AAT that are intermediate between those of normals and homozygotes. Although it is not certain, it is likely that these individuals are predisposed to airways obstruction if they smoke.

Reduction in Maximum Expiratory Flow

Reduced expiratory flow is the hallmark of COPD (Chapter 85). Figure 88–2 shows a maximum expiratory flow-volume curve and a diagrammatic representation of the lungs and airways inside the thorax. In the maximum expiratory flow-volume curve, flow from the lungs is plotted against lung volume during expiration at maximum effort, beginning with the lung expanded to total lung capacity. In the model, expiratory effort is generated by compression of the thorax, causing an increase in pleural and alveolar pressure. During expiration, the pressure that drives flow down the airways is the alveolar pressure. As air flows down the airways, pressure is lost because of frictional resistance and the acceleration of gas particles as the airway narrows.

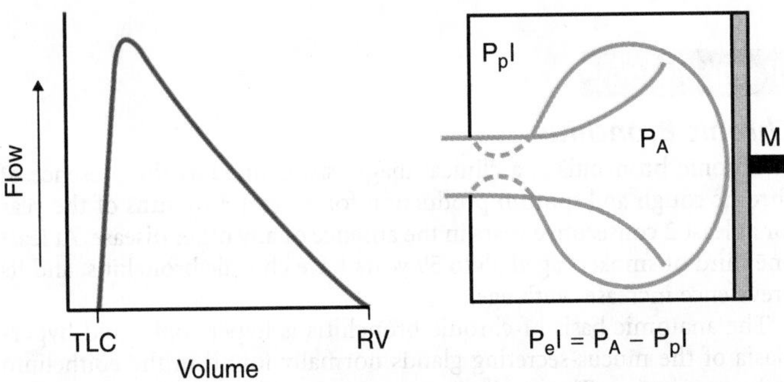

FIGURE 88–2 • Maximum expiratory flow-volume curve (left) with an explanatory model (right). The left panel shows flow as a function of expired volume during forced expiration at maximum effort, from the total lung capacity (TLC) before expiration to the residual volume (RV) after expiration in a normal individual. Flow rises to a maximum and then declines as lung volume decreases. Flow over much of the declining limb is independent of expiratory effort, provided a threshold effort is achieved. In the model, the thorax is represented by a box and the expiratory muscles by a piston (M). The lung is a balloon inside the box, and the airways are represented as a tube that branches as it goes from outside the lung to the inside. The expiratory muscles compress the thoracic contents and raise pleural pressure (P_pl). Alveolar pressure (P_A) in the lung increases by the same amount because it is related to P_pl by the elastic recoil of the lung (P_el). Because of the increase in P_pl and P_A, gas flows out of the lung, reaching a peak (peak flow) and declining thereafter. The pressure driving flow is P_A, and the flow achieved is related to the resistance of the airways. As lung volume decreases, P_el decreases, so P_A decreases in relation to P_pl. Also, as lung volume decreases, resistance increases. Because of the reduced P_A and increased resistance, as lung volume decreases, the pressure in a major airway becomes less than P_pl, and the airway is compressed (dashed lines), thereby limiting flow. Further increases in effort (P_pl) simply further compress the airway and do not increase flow. Flow limitation occurs after about 30% of the vital capacity is expired. When this limitation occurs, maximum expiratory flow is dependent on lung elastic recoil (P_el), which determines P_A, the resistance of the airways upstream from the flow-limiting segment, and the mechanical properties of the flow-limiting segment.

At the onset of the expiration, flow rises sharply to a maximum (peak flow) related to the properties of the lung and the intensity of effort. Thereafter, flow declines as lung volume decreases. After about 30% of the vital capacity is expired, expiratory flow becomes effort independent, that is, unchanged over a variety of expiratory efforts and pleural pressures, because of flow-related pressure losses down the airway. As a result, pressure in a central airway is less than the pleural pressure, the airway is compressed, and flow attains a maximum value after which further increases in pleural pressure compress the airway further. These so-called flow-limiting segments are initially found only in large central airways, but such segments exist in intrapulmonary airways at low lung volumes. Under the condition of flow limitation, the maximum flow attained depends on the upstream or alveolar pressure, the resistance of the airways, and the properties of the compressed, flow-limiting segment. If the lung's elastic recoil is reduced (e.g., as in emphysema), alveolar pressures are reduced relative to pleural pressure, and so is maximum expiratory flow. Increases in airways resistance (e.g., as in chronic bronchitis) increase pressure losses down the airway and decrease maximum expiratory flow. Finally, abnormally "floppy" segments of airway, a rare phenomenon, undergo premature collapse and cause abnormal limitation of flow.

In normal lungs, flow decreases as lung volume decreases because the lung's elastic recoil decreases and resistance increases. In COPD, the lung's elastic recoil is reduced by emphysema, and airways resistance is increased. Maximum expiratory flow is reduced, and even less effort than normal causes limitation of flow. Tests of maximum expiratory flow, such as the flow-volume curve and the FEV_1, are of clinical value because they reflect major pathologic processes in COPD and are relatively insensitive to a patient's effort and cooperation beyond a threshold minimum effort.

Clinical Manifestations

Lung Function

The decrease in maximum expiratory flow that characterizes COPD is most easily identified in terms of a reduction in FEV_1 that is larger than the reduction in vital capacity, measured in the same forced expiratory maneuver and termed the forced vital capacity (FVC) (Chapter 85). Both FEV_1 and FVC decline with normal aging (see Fig. 87–1), but their ratio, FEV_1/FVC, normally exceeds 0.7; lower ratios indicate airways obstruction. Both the FEV_1 and the FVC may increase after treatment with an inhaled bronchodilator, but the FEV_1 does not attain normal values in COPD, whereas it can return to normal in patients with asthma (Chapter 87).

Hyperinflation of the lungs, which is often manifested as an increase in total lung capacity, is characteristic of COPD and reflects loss of lung recoil and limitation of expiratory flow. Residual volume, the lung volume after a maximum expiration, often is increased even in mild cases of COPD. Functional residual capacity, the lung volume at the end of a normal expiration, is routinely increased in moderate and severe COPD. The diffusing capacity for carbon monoxide, which measures the alveolar uptake of trace amounts of carbon monoxide, is reduced in emphysema because of loss of alveolar surface area. It is the most reliable physiologic method for assessing the presence of emphysema.

Arterial hypoxemia with or without carbon dioxide retention is common in severe COPD. Hypoxemia generally precedes carbon dioxide retention, rarely occurs in patients with an FEV_1 in excess of 40% of the predicted normal value, and is common when the FEV_1 is less than 30% of the predicted value. Gas exchange abnormalities in COPD are due to abnormally large differences in ventilation-perfusion ratios among units in the lung.

Dyspnea

Dyspnea is the major cause of disability in COPD. It arises from a sense of increased muscle effort to breathe in relation to the level of ventilation achieved (Chapter 83). Normal subjects, even at the most strenuous levels of exercise, use only 60 to 70% of their maximum voluntary ventilation and never experience dyspnea comparable to that of diseased patients.

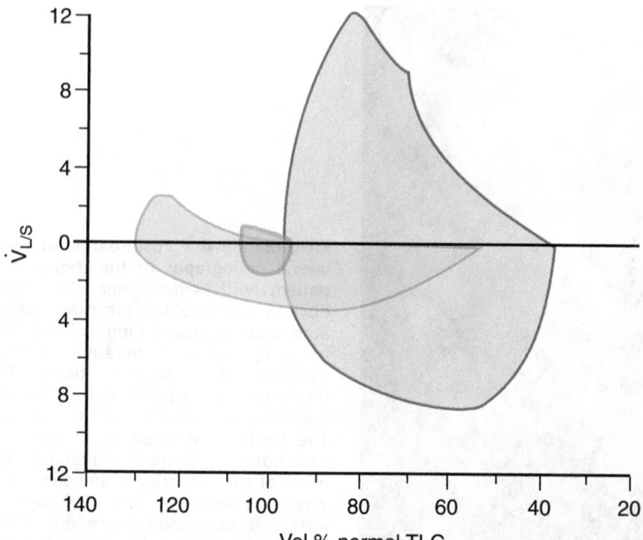

FIGURE 88–3 • Flow-volume relationships during quiet resting breathing (small inner loop) and maximum forced expiration in a patient with severe COPD. The vertical axis is flow in liters per second ($\dot{V}_{L/S}$); the horizontal axis is lung volume, expressed as a percentage of the normal total lung capacity (TLC). The shaded area shows normal maximal inspiration and expiration. The patient has substantial increases in the maximum lung volume (TLC) and the minimum lung volume attained (residual volume). Expiratory flow during maximal expiration is grossly reduced and is similar to the flow used during resting breathing. With exercise, the only way for this patient to increase expiratory flow and thereby increase ventilation is to breathe at higher lung volumes than at rest.

Patients with obstructive airways disease usually characterize dyspnea as difficulty in inspiring because airways obstruction changes the shape of the chest wall and puts the inspiratory muscles at a mechanical disadvantage. Expiratory flow limitation does not permit adequate expiration at normal lung volumes, so patients breathe at increased lung volumes. This hyperinflation renders inspiratory muscles relatively ineffective, so that greater inspiratory effort is required to achieve the needed ventilation, as illustrated in Figure 88–3, which shows flow-volume plots in a patient with COPD during resting breathing and forced expiration after full inspiration. At the same lung volume, expiratory flows during resting breathing are similar to flows during a maximum effort. The only way this patient can increase expiratory flow, and therefore ventilation, is to breathe at higher lung volumes than at rest.

The degree of dyspnea in patients with COPD generally correlates inversely with the FEV_1, but patients with similar degrees of airways obstruction may complain of different degrees of dyspnea. Careful assessment of dyspnea is a useful way to follow the progress of patients with COPD.

Diagnosis

History

COPD is insidious. Although the diagnosis can be made in any smoker with airways obstruction, most people are first seen only when they experience dyspnea. Dyspnea typically does not occur until the FEV_1 is about 50% of normal, when the disease has usually been present for decades.

Patients with COPD often have a history of chronic bronchitis that has antedated the onset of dyspnea. Dyspnea usually is first experienced during episodes of acute bronchitis. Eventually, dyspnea becomes consistent, and during approximately 10 to 15 years, dyspnea progresses from occurring only with extreme exertion to being present with any effort and finally to being present at rest. Wheezing is also common in COPD, usually with exertion, but may occur at rest in severe disease.

Patients with COPD have periodic exacerbations, marked by increased dyspnea, wheezing, cough, and sputum production. The sputum often changes in color from the usual white (mucoid) to yellow or green, sometimes with blood streaking. Exacerbations usually occur in the winter, often with upper respiratory infections, and are more common in patients with symptomatic chronic bronchitis and in those with severe obstruction. The causes vary from patient to patient and from time to time, but many are associated with bacterial infection of the airways. Exacerbations of COPD are the most common cause of hospitalization and result in substantial morbidity.

Some patients with COPD lose weight and muscle mass especially in the presence of severe emphysema. Weight loss is an ominous prognostic sign in COPD.

Physical Examination

In mild to moderate COPD, the physical examination is usually normal. In severe disease, signs are often apparent but are not specific. The breathing rate is increased, often to more than 20 breaths per minute at rest in patients with hypoxemia or carbon dioxide retention. Physical signs related to hyperinflation include the appearance of a barrel chest with increased anteroposterior diameter, relatively low-lying diaphragms, and faint heart sounds. Patients with severe disease use the strap muscles of the neck during inspiration. Breath sounds are often diminished, and both crackles and wheezes may be heard. Hypoxemic patients may be cyanotic.

In advanced disease, secondary pulmonary hypertension (Chapter 67) leads to right-sided heart failure, which commonly is termed cor pulmonale. Signs of cor pulmonale include an increased pulmonic second sound, jugular venous distention, hepatic congestion, and ankle edema.

Spirometry

Spirometry, the measurement of the FEV_1 and FVC, is the "gold standard" for diagnosis of COPD and is easy to perform in the office setting (Chapter 85). Airways obstruction ($FEV_1/FVC < 0.70$) in a person with at least 20 pack years of tobacco exposure is a presumptive diagnosis of COPD.

Radiologic Studies

Routine chest radiographs are insensitive for detecting COPD (Chapter 84). In advanced cases, patients develop hyperinflation with flattened diaphragms, increased retrosternal air space, and an apparently small, vertical heart (Fig. 88–4). Increased or decreased lung markings and thin-walled bullae may be seen. Signs of pulmonary hypertension, including fullness of the main pulmonary arteries, are occasionally observed. The chief value of the chest radiograph is to assess other causes of airways obstruction and to look for evidence of lung cancer (Chapter 201).

Computed tomographic (CT) scans are of considerable value in assessing the presence, distribution, and extent of emphysema. There are no standard grading systems. Emphysematous spaces are seen as "holes" in the lung (Fig. 88–5).

Serial Evaluation

Patients thought to have COPD should undergo full pulmonary function testing at least once (Chapter 85). Testing should also include repeated spirometry at yearly intervals and when the patient is acutely ill. If the FEV_1 is less than 40% of the predicted normal value, arterial blood gas analysis is advisable (Chapter 104). Annual chest radiographs should be performed only if the patient is a candidate for cancer surgery. Finally, the degree of dyspnea should be documented carefully, as should dietary intake, weight loss, and occurrence of exacerbations.

Differential Diagnosis

The most difficult disease to differentiate from COPD is asthma (Chapter 87), although the distinction can be made on the basis of history alone in most cases. Asthma typically begins early in life with episodes of dyspnea and wheezing of rapid onset and that reverse rapidly and completely. However, patients with asthma can develop chronic airways obstruction that reverses little with therapy, and some smokers with chronic airways obstruction demonstrate substantial reversibility with therapy. In these instances, the difference between asthma and COPD can become a matter of semantics. Fortunately, the therapies for asthma and COPD are similar enough so that diagnostic uncertainties between these two entities should have little impact on management of the patient.

Several other diseases cause chronic airways obstruction but differ from COPD in important ways. Cystic fibrosis (Chapter 89) and bronchiectasis (Chapter 90) occur at an earlier age and are normally

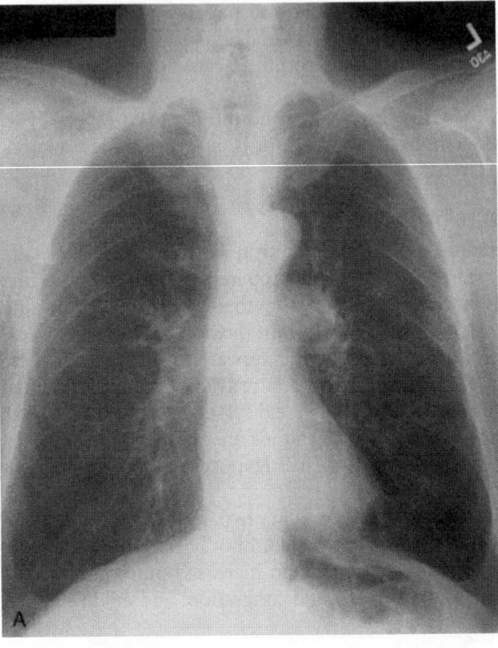

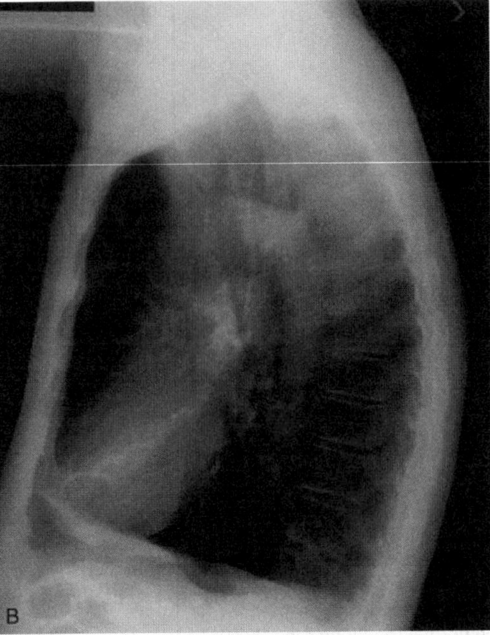

FIGURE 88–4 • Posteroanterior and lateral radiographs of the thorax in a patient with emphysema. The most obvious abnormalities are those associated with increased lung volume. The lungs appear dark because of their increased air relative to tissue. The diaphragms are caudal to their normal position and appear flatter than normal. The heart is oriented more vertically than normal because of caudal displacement of the diaphragm, and the transverse diameter of the rib cage is increased; as a result, the width of the heart relative to the rib cage on the posteroanterior view is decreased. The space between the sternum and heart and great vessels is increased on the lateral view.

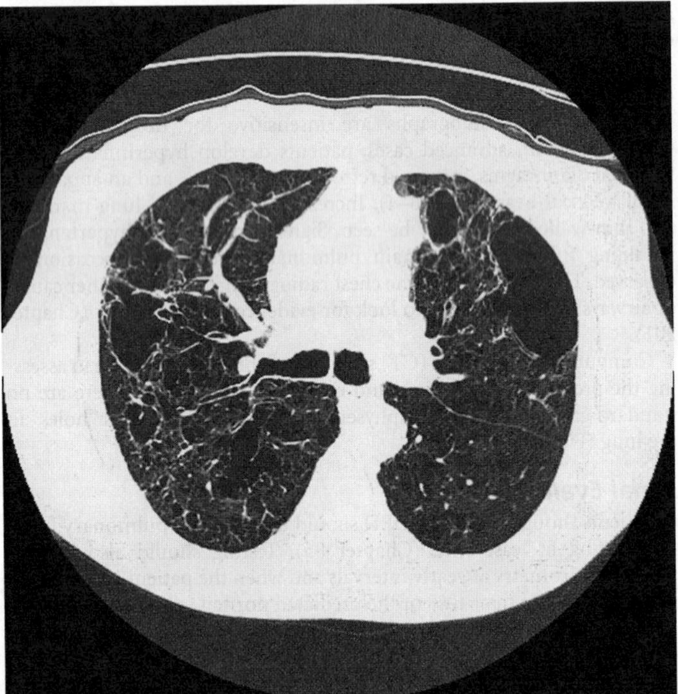

FIGURE 88–5 • High-resolution axial CT scan of a 1-mm section of the thorax of a patient with emphysema at the level of the tracheal carina. The right lung is on the left. Multiple large bullae—black holes—are evident. Many smaller areas of similar tissue destruction are also present in both lungs. The right upper lobe bronchus is seen entering the lung; its walls are thickened, suggesting chronic inflammation. (Courtesy of Dr. Bruce Maycher.)

accompanied by specific radiologic abnormalities. Eosinophilic granuloma (Chapter 241), which is associated with cigarette smoking, and lymphangioleiomyomatosis (Chapter 92) cause airways obstruction, but both present with abnormal chest radiographs and have characteristic abnormalities on CT scan. Bronchiolitis obliterans (Chapter 92) also causes airways obstruction; however, bronchiolitis obliterans usually occurs in a setting different from that of COPD, and it may be accompanied by more radiographic changes than in COPD.

It is important to differentiate upper or central airways obstruction from COPD. Extrathoracic airways obstruction (Chapters 101 and 452) is accompanied by stridor and compromised inspiratory flow. Intrathoracic tracheal obstruction produces characteristic changes in the maximum expiratory flow-volume curve.

Prevention and Treatment

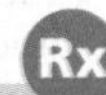

Stable COPD

Smoking cessation is the only treatment that has been shown to alter the course of COPD. [1] Smoking cessation when the FEV_1 exceeds 50% of the predicted normal value either averts or greatly delays the onset of symptomatic disease. It is probably never too late for patients with COPD to stop smoking.

Inhaled bronchodilators afford symptomatic relief in COPD and should be prescribed for all patients who find them helpful (Fig. 88–6). There are a number of effective agents with few side effects. Short-acting β_2-agonists have rapid onset of action and are useful as rescue agents on a discretionary basis. Albuterol is the prototypical short-acting β_2-agonist; the normal dose is 200 µg (two puffs from a metered-dose inhaler). Ipratropium bromide is an inhaled anticholinergic drug that is as effective as β_2-agonists in COPD. Because it has a slower onset of action, it is usually given on a schedule of three or four times a day at a dose of 36 µg (two puffs from a metered-dose inhaler). Higher doses of these drugs are of benefit in some patients, and many use both; a combination inhaler is available. Longer acting β_2 agents, such as salmeterol (50 µg) and formoterol (12 µg), have durations of action up to 12 hours. A very long acting (once a day) inhaled anticholinergic drug, tiotropium (18 µg), is available. Long-acting bronchodilators are unquestionably effective and tend to control symptoms better than short-acting agents do. They also may prevent exacerbations. [2] Metered-dose and powdered formulations of these drugs are less expensive than those used in wet nebulizers and are equally effective.

Theophylline is less effective, although some patients receive symptomatic benefit when theophylline is added to inhaled agents, and a trial of theophylline is reasonable in patients with severe dyspnea. Theophylline has a relatively narrow dosage range in which it is effective and nontoxic, and many drugs and conditions influence theophylline metabolism. Serum levels should be measured, and a target of about 10 µg/mL is usually achieved with a dose of approximately 300 mg twice a day.

Inhaled steroids do not change the long-term rate of decline in lung function in COPD, but inhaled steroid therapy may produce a small (about 200 mL) one-time increase in FEV_1. Of greater

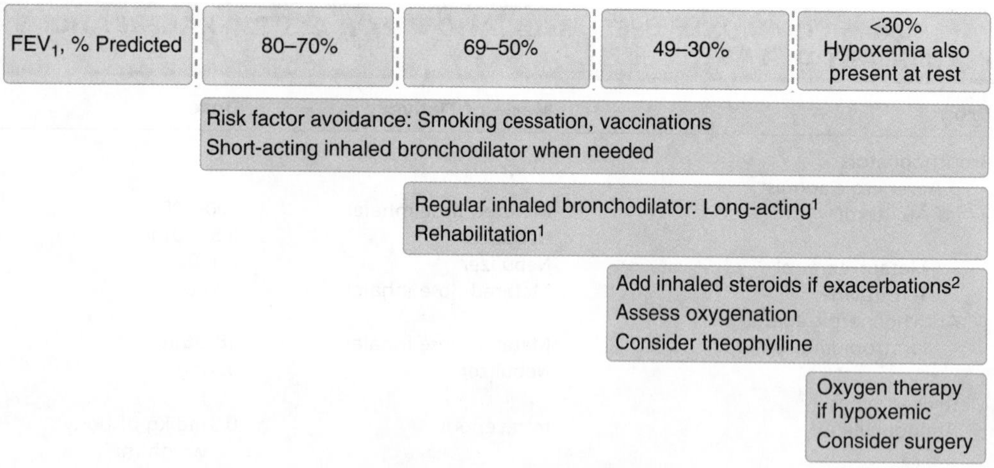

FEV$_1$, % Predicted	80–70%	69–50%	49–30%	<30% Hypoxemia also present at rest

Risk factor avoidance: Smoking cessation, vaccinations
Short-acting inhaled bronchodilator when needed

Regular inhaled bronchodilator: Long-acting[1]
Rehabilitation[1]

Add inhaled steroids if exacerbations[2]
Assess oxygenation
Consider theophylline

Oxygen therapy if hypoxemic
Consider surgery

FIGURE 88–6 • Flow diagram for the management of stable COPD. FEV$_1$ levels are approximate; the level of symptoms is equally important in determining treatment. As patients become more severely ill, therapies are added; for example, virtually all patients should receive a short-acting "rescue" inhaled bronchodilator. [1]If the patient's normal daily activities are accompanied by dyspnea. [2]The patient averages 1.5 exacerbations per year.

Rx

importance is evidence that inhaled steroids reduce the frequency and severity of exacerbations and reduce mortality in COPD. [3] Patients with severe disease and multiple exacerbations should be given inhaled steroids in relatively high doses, such as 500 to 1000 μg of fluticasone per day. The combined use of a long-acting β-agonist with an inhaled steroid produces better control of symptoms without increased side effects compared with either used alone. [4]

Many older COPD guidelines recommend trials of high-dose oral steroids in patients who are not doing well. The evidence cited earlier has largely superseded these recommendations, and at present there is not convincing evidence for the use of oral steroids in stable COPD, although many current guidelines recommend trials of oral steroids.

COPD patients benefit from pulmonary rehabilitation. The major component of rehabilitation programs is exercise training. Regular exercise improves exercise tolerance and quality of life in patients with COPD. In addition, rehabilitation programs teach coping skills and self-reliance, and they tend to reduce anxiety and depression.

In hypoxemic COPD, home oxygen therapy prolongs life, and home oxygen should be prescribed for stable patients with arterial Po_2 below 60 mm Hg. Acceptable blood gas levels (Po_2 of 65 to 80 mm Hg) can usually be achieved with oxygen flows of 2 L/min delivered by nasal cannula. There is no good evidence that oxygen therapy benefits COPD patients who do not have continuous hypoxemia. However, some patients who are not hypoxemic during the day exhibit hypoxemia while asleep, and many patients with severe COPD develop significant hypoxemia with exercise. As a result, oxygen therapy may be considered in such patients during sleep or exercise. Oxygen delivery systems vary greatly in terms of mobility and cost, and the choice among systems should be individualized.

Surgical approaches to COPD include lung transplantation and lung volume reduction surgery (Chapter 102). Lung transplantation is falling out of favor because it is not clear that it prolongs useful life. Lung volume reduction surgery involves removal of substantial amounts of emphysematous lung as identified by CT scan. In patients with emphysema predominantly in the upper lung zones, surgery improves exercise tolerance and also reduces mortality in those with poor initial exercise tolerance. On the other hand, surgery is dangerous in very ill patients, defined as those with FEV$_1$ less than 20% of the predicted normal and either a diffusing capacity below 20% of the predicted normal or homogeneous emphysema distribution. [5]

Influenza vaccine should be administered annually to all patients with COPD to prevent exacerbations. Pneumococcal vaccination is also recommended because pneumococcal pneumonia is devastating in these patients (Chapters 16 and 311).

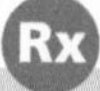

Exacerbations of COPD

Exacerbations of COPD are associated with transient decreases in lung function, which account for the increased dyspnea. Increased bronchodilator therapy with short-acting agents is rational and recommended. When exacerbations are accompanied by increases in sputum volume or purulence, antibiotic therapy is associated with measurable benefit (Tables 88–1 and 88–2). Sputum smear and culture are not usually helpful, and empirical treatment is the rule. In low-risk patients, inexpensive antibiotics such as amoxicillin and trimethoprim-sulfamethoxazole may be used for 10 days, but bacterial resistance to these agents is common. In high-risk patients, the newer macrolides (e.g., azithromycin, 500 mg on day 1, 250 mg on days 2 to 5) or fluoroquinolones (e.g., levofloxacin, 500 mg/day for 7 to 10 days) may be advisable. In severe exacerbations, systemic steroid therapy has been shown to result in a relatively rapid recovery, [6] and the equivalent of 40 mg of prednisone per day for 10 to 14 days is justifiable. It is reasonable to give compliant patients with COPD a supply of antibiotics and steroids so they self-treat exacerbations.

In severe exacerbations seen in the hospital or emergency department, other diagnoses must be considered. Exacerbations of COPD must be distinguished from pneumonia (Chapter 97), pneumothorax (Chapter 100), and pulmonary embolism (Chapter 99). Pneumonia and pneumothorax usually can be diagnosed by the chest radiograph. In patients with signs and symptoms typical of pneumonia, especially substantial fevers or elevated white blood cell counts, empirical treatment of pneumonia is appropriate until it can be excluded. Pulmonary embolism can be difficult to diagnose in patients with COPD, and spiral CT angiography should be used if embolic disease is suspected (Chapter 99).

Exacerbations of COPD may be difficult to distinguish from acute heart failure (Chapters 57 and 58), and many elderly smokers may have both conditions concurrently. The distinction can be especially difficult in patients with right-sided heart failure, in whom the cause may be cor pulmonale from advanced COPD or worsening right-sided heart failure caused by worsening left-sided heart failure. The chest radiograph and the electrocardiogram are the best tools for differentiation here. A careful physical examination may reveal left-sided murmurs or a left-sided S_3 gallop typical of left-sided heart failure. An electrocardiogram is occasionally helpful, whereas a chest radiograph may provide diagnostic information. An echocardiogram can detect left ventricular systolic dysfunction, valvar heart disease, and sometimes diastolic dysfunction causing heart failure (Chapter 53). Brain natriuretic peptide levels have been shown to be a reliable way to distinguish an exacerbation of heart failure (elevated levels) from a worsening of COPD or other conditions (Chapter 57). [7]

Exacerbations of COPD are often accompanied by hypoxemia, which can precipitate heart failure (Chapters 57 and 58), angina

TABLE 88–1 COMMONLY USED MEDICATIONS FOR ACUTE EXACERBATIONS OF CHRONIC OBSTRUCTIVE PULMONARY DISEASE

Drug	Mode of Delivery	Dose	Frequency
Bronchodilators			
β-Adrenergic agonist			
Albuterol	Metered-dose inhaler	100–200 μg	4 times daily
	Nebulizer	0.5–2.0 mg	4 times daily
Metaproterenol	Nebulizer	0.1–0.2 mg	4 times daily
Terbutaline	Metered-dose inhaler	400 μg	4 times daily
Anticholinergic agent			
Ipratropium bromide	Metered-dose inhaler	18–36 μg	4 times daily
	Nebulizer	0.5 mg	4 times daily
Methylxanthines			
Aminophylline*	Intravenous	0.9 mg/kg of body weight/hr	Infusion
Theophylline	Pill (sustained-release preparations)	150–450 mg†	Twice daily
Corticosteroids			
Methylprednisolone succinate	Infusion, then pill	125 mg	Every 6 hours for 3 days, then
		60 mg	Daily for 4 days
		40 mg	Daily for 4 days
		20 mg	Daily for 4 days
Prednisone (for outpatients)	Pill	30–60 mg	Daily for 5 to 10 days
Limited-spectrum antibiotics			
Trimethoprim-sulfamethoxazole	Pill	160 mg and 800 mg	Twice daily for 5 to 10 days
Amoxicillin	Pill	250 mg	4 times daily for 5 to 10 days
Doxycycline	Pill	100 mg	2 tablets first day, then 1 tablet/day for 5 to 10 days

*Aminophylline is sometimes administered after a loading dose; the dose should be determined on the basis of serum levels of theophylline.
†The dose varies among and within patients.
From Stoller JK: Acute exacerbations of chronic obstructive pulmonary disease. N Engl J Med 2002;346:988–994.

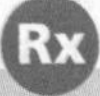

(Chapter 70), an acute coronary syndrome (Chapter 71), or hypoxic death in susceptible individuals. Hypoxemia may also cause an acute worsening of pulmonary hypertension (Chapter 67) or systemic hypertension (Chapter 66). It is essential to measure the arterial P_{O_2} and to treat hypoxemia with oxygen.

Severe exacerbations of COPD require hospitalization and should be treated with bronchodilator therapy, intravenous antibiotics, and steroids. Arterial blood gases should be measured and oxygen therapy instituted. In COPD, uncontrolled high-flow oxygen carries the risk of precipitating carbon dioxide narcosis, and the initial goals should be to maintain arterial P_{O_2} at levels of about 60 mm Hg (Chapters 103 to 106). In patients who can be discharged from the emergency department, a 10-day course of 40 mg of prednisone per day improves symptoms and reduces the relapse rate. [8]

Prognosis

Even though the average patient with COPD suffers relentless progression of the disease, the course may be variable in different individuals. The two most important predictors of the course of COPD are age and severity of airways obstruction as evidenced by FEV_1. Other key prognostic factors include weight loss, degree of dyspnea, and exercise capacity.

The need for hospital admission for an exacerbation, especially if intensive care is required, is an ominous prognostic sign in COPD; at least half such patients do not survive a year after admission. In patients with severe COPD, the issue of intensive care and artificial ventilation should be raised to ascertain the patient's attitudes with regard to these interventions and end-of-life care, and the results of these discussions must be documented (Chapters 3 and 103).

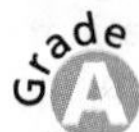

1. Anthonisen NR, Connett JC, Kiley JP, et al: Effects of smoking intervention and the use of an inhaled anticholinergic bronchodilator on the rate of decline of FEV_1: The Lung Health Study. JAMA 1994;272:1497–1505.
2. Niewoehner DE, Rice K, Cote C, et al: Prevention of exacerbations of chronic obstructive lung disease with tiotropium, a once-daily inhaled anticholinergic bronchodilator. Ann Intern Med 2005;143:317–326.
3. Sin DD, Anderson JA, Anthonisen NR, et al: Inhaled corticosteroids and mortality in chronic obstructive lung disease. Thorax 2005;60:992–997.
4. Aaron SD, Vandemheen KL, Fergusson D, et al: Tiotropium in combination with placebo, salmeterol, or fluticasone-salmeterol for treatment of chronic obstructive pulmonary disease: A randomized trial. Ann Intern Med 2007;146:545–555.
5. National Emphysema Treatment Trial Research Group: A randomized trial comparing lung-volume-reduction surgery with medical therapy for severe emphysema. N Engl J Med 2003;348:2059–2073.
6. Niewoehner DE, Erbland ML, Deupree RH, et al: Effect of systemic glucocorticoids on exacerbations of chronic obstructive pulmonary disease. Department of Veterans Affairs Cooperative Study Group. N Engl J Med 1999;340:1941–1947.
7. Mueller C, Scholer A, Laule-Kilian K, et al: Use of B-type natriuretic peptide in the evaluation and management of acute dyspnea. N Engl J Med 2004;350:647–654.
8. Aaron SD, Vandemheen KL, Hebert P, et al: Outpatient oral prednisone after emergency treatment of chronic obstructive pulmonary disease. N Engl J Med 2003;348:2618–2625.

SUGGESTED READINGS

Bradley JM, Laserson T, Elborn S, et al: A systematic review of randomized controlled trials examining the short-term benefit of ambulatory oxygen in COPD. Chest 2007;131:278–295. *A modest benefit is seen, but long-term benefits are less clear.*

Calverley P, Anderson J, Cell B, et al: Salmeterol and fluticasone propionate and survival in chronic obstructive pulmonary disease. N Engl J Med 2007;356:775–789. *Symptoms improved significantly with combination therapy, but all-cause mortality did not.*

TABLE 88–2 RECOMMENDATIONS BY PROFESSIONAL SOCIETIES REGARDING THE MANAGEMENT OF ACUTE EXACERBATIONS OF CHRONIC OBSTRUCTIVE PULMONARY DISEASE

Variable	British Thoracic Society	American College of Chest Physicians and American College of Physicians–American Society of Internal Medicine	European Respiratory Society	American Thoracic Society	Global Initiative for Chronic Obstructive Lung Disease
Date of statement	2004	2001	2004	2004	2005
Type of statement	Consensus	Evidence-based systematic review	Consensus	Consensus	Evidence-based review
Diagnostic testing	Recommended for patients being admitted: chest radiography, arterial blood gases, complete blood count, electrolytes, blood urea nitrogen, electrocardiography, and FEV_1 or peak flow or both; sputum culture and sensitivity	Recommended for patients admitted from emergency department: chest radiography Not recommended: spirometry	Recommended for hospitalized patients: FEV_1, arterial blood gases, chest radiography, complete blood count, sputum Gram stain and culture, electrolytes, electrocardiography	Recommended: determine the cause of exacerbation; sputum culture in severe exacerbations, if condition has worsened despite use of antibiotics, or for residents of a nursing home	Recommended: chest radiography, electrocardiography, arterial blood gases, sputum culture and sensitivity testing (if no response to initial antibiotics), electrolytes, hematocrit
Bronchodilator therapy	Recommended: For outpatients: β-adrenergic agonists, anticholinergic agents, or both For inpatients: β-adrenergic agonists and anticholinergic agents; add IV aminophylline if no response	Recommended: anticholinergic agent in maximal dose as first-line agent; then add β-adrenergic agonist Not recommended: methylxanthines	Recommended: β-adrenergic agonists, anticholinergic agents, or both in increased dose or frequency; consider IV aminophylline in severe exacerbations	Recommended: β-adrenergic agonist as first-line agent, possibly in combination with anticholinergic agent; IV aminophylline if aerosol therapy cannot be given or proves inadequate	Recommended: β-adrenergic agonist as first-line agent; add anticholinergic agent if prompt response not evident; consider oral or IV methylxanthine in severe exacerbation
Bronchodilator delivery	For outpatients: metered-dose inhaler (with instruction) For inpatients: nebulizer	Insufficient evidence for a preferred delivery device	Metered-dose inhaler can generally achieve good response; some patients prefer nebulizer during exacerbations	No preference	Not discussed

Continued

TABLE 88–2 RECOMMENDATIONS BY PROFESSIONAL SOCIETIES REGARDING THE MANAGEMENT OF ACUTE EXACERBATIONS OF CHRONIC OBSTRUCTIVE PULMONARY DISEASE—cont'd

Variable	British Thoracic Society	American College of Chest Physicians and American College of Physicians–American Society of Internal Medicine	European Respiratory Society	American Thoracic Society	Global Initiative for Chronic Obstructive Lung Disease
Antibiotics	Recommended for moderate or severe exacerbations: oral route; "common" antibiotic (e.g., tetracycline, amoxicillin) as first-line agent; broader spectrum cephalosporin or macrolide if no response	Optimal duration of therapy unclear	Recommended: 7- to 14-day course of inexpensive antibiotic (e.g., amoxicillin or tetracycline)	Recommended for abnormal mucus: "simple" antibiotic (e.g., doxycycline or amoxicillin) unless severe exacerbation, in which case consider extended-spectrum penicillin or cephalosporin	Recommended with increased sputum volume and purulence: choice should reflect local sensitivity for *Streptococcus pneumoniae, Haemophilus influenzae,* and *Moraxella catarrhalis*
Corticosteroids	Not recommended for outpatients unless already receiving, known response, or failure to achieve response to increased bronchodilator dose Recommended for inpatients: e.g., 30 mg of prednisone daily for 7–14 days	Recommended for patients not receiving long-term oral corticosteroids: systemic corticosteroids for up to 2 wk	Recommended: 0.4–0.6 mg/kg/day of oral corticosteroids for outpatients; IV for severe exacerbation in hospitalized patients	Recommended: reassess use after 1–2 wk	Recommended: 30–40 mg of oral or IV prednisolone per day for 10–14 days
Supplemental oxygen	Recommended: to achieve $Pa{O_2}$ ≥50 mm Hg without pH <7.26; initial treatment with face mask with $F{IO_2}$ ≤0.28	Recommended	Recommended: to raise $Pa{O_2}$ ≥60 mm Hg without raising $Pa{CO_2}$ by ≥10 mm Hg	Recommended: to raise $Pa{O_2}$ just above 60 mm Hg	Recommended: target $Pa{O_2}$ >60 mm Hg or $Sa{O_2}$ <90%; measure arterial blood gases 30 minutes after the initiation of oxygen
Chest physiotherapy and clearance of secretions	Not recommended	Not recommended	Recommended: coughing to clear sputum; physiotherapy at home	Recommended for hospitalized patients with ≥25 mL of sputum/day	Manual or mechanical chest percussion and postural drainage possibly beneficial for patients with lobar atelectasis or >25 mL of sputum/day; facilitate sputum clearance by stimulating coughing

FEV_1 = forced expiratory volume in 1 second; $F{IO_2}$ = inspired concentration of oxygen.
Modified from Stoller JK: Acute exacerbations of chronic obstructive pulmonary disease. N Engl J Med 2002;346:988–994.

Rennard SI: Treatment of stable chronic obstructive pulmonary disease. Lancet 2004;364:791–802. *Detailed, well-referenced review, including smoking cessation.*

Stoller JK, Aboussouan LS: α_1-Antitrypsin deficiency. Lancet 2005;365:2225–2236. *A comprehensive review.*

Sutherland ER, Cherniack RM: Management of chronic obstructive pulmonary disease. N Engl J Med 2004;350:2689–2697. *A compact, comprehensive summary focusing on stable disease.*

Wouters EFM: Management of severe COPD. Lancet 2004;364:883–895. *Detailed, well referenced review including exacerbation management, end-of-life issues, and extrapulmonary manifestations.*

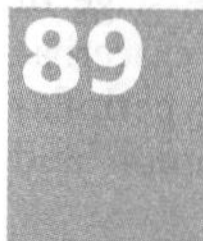

89 CYSTIC FIBROSIS

Michael J. Welsh

Definition

Cystic fibrosis is an autosomal recessive genetic disease caused by mutations in the gene encoding the cystic fibrosis transmembrane conductance regulator (CFTR). It is relatively common, with an incidence of 1 in 2000 to 3000 whites; approximately 30,000 persons in the United States are affected. About 1 in 20 to 25 whites carry mutations in the *CFTR* gene; carriers are completely asymptomatic. The disease affects several different organs, but most current morbidity and 90 to 95% of mortality result from chronic pulmonary infections. Pancreatic insufficiency is also a common cause of morbidity.

Pathobiology

The *CFTR* gene encodes a 1480–amino acid protein that belongs to a family of proteins called *a*denosine triphosphate (ATP)-*b*inding *c*assette (ABC) transporters. Several members of this family are clinically important, including the multidrug resistance protein (MDR), the sulfonylurea receptor (SUR), lipid transport proteins that are defective in sitosterolemia (ABCG8 and ABCG5) and Tangier disease (ABC1), and the Stargardt macular dystrophy protein (ABCR). Although most ABC transporters form membrane pumps, CFTR forms an anion-permeable channel that is regulated by phosphorylation. It contains five domains. Two membrane-spanning domains, each composed of six membrane-spanning sequences, form the Cl^- conducting pore. Two nucleotide-binding domains gate the channel by binding ATP and then manifesting adenylate kinase or ATPase enzymatic activity. A regulatory (R) domain stimulates the channel to open when it is phosphorylated by cyclic adenosine monophosphate–dependent protein kinase. The intracellular N- and C-termini interact with several other proteins to influence function and cellular localization. CFTR is located in the apical (lumen-facing) membrane of epithelium in the pulmonary airways, pancreatic duct, intestine, biliary ducts, and the apical and basolateral membranes of the sweat gland duct.

The most common cystic fibrosis mutation is a three–base pair deletion that causes loss of phenylalanine at position 508 (ΔF508). The ΔF508 mutation occurs on about 70% of cystic fibrosis chromosomes; the percentage is somewhat higher in persons of northern European descent. More than 1000 other mutations and variations have been discovered in the gene, with only a handful accounting for more than 1% of mutations. CFTR protein with the ΔF508 mutation is made in the endoplasmic reticulum but is misfolded. As a result, it is recognized by the cellular quality control system, which prevents its traffic to the Golgi complex and then the apical membrane and instead targets it for degradation by the proteosome. Although it is not normally delivered to the cell membrane, the ΔF508 protein retains significant Cl^- channel activity. Thus, correction of the defective processing could provide a novel approach to treatment. It is now appreciated that there are four general classes of mutation (Fig. 89–1). Class I mutations in the *CFTR* gene cause loss or reduction of CFTR Cl^- channel activity by generating an incomplete messenger RNA (mRNA) with premature stop signals, frame shifts, and abnormal splice sites or reduced amounts of CFTR mRNA. Class II mutations, such as ΔF508, cause misfolding. Class III and IV mutations generate correctly localized proteins that either do not open appropriately or form pores

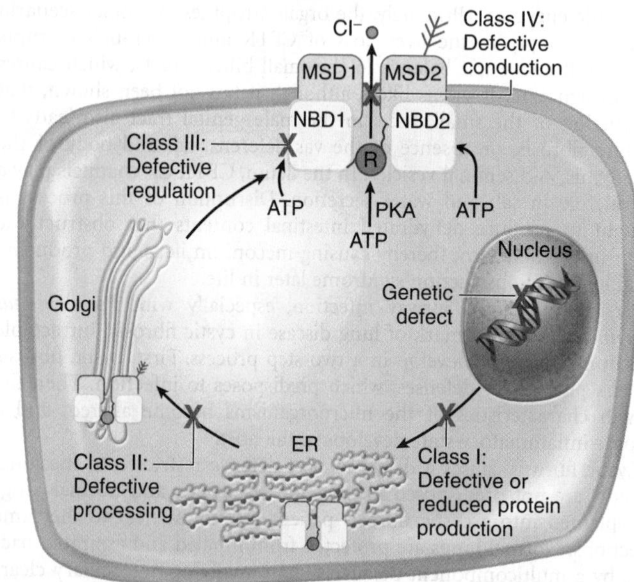

FIGURE 89–1 • Biosynthesis and function of CFTR in an epithelial cell. Glycosylation is indicated by the orange branched structure. Domains of CFTR are labeled as MSD, membrane-spanning domains; NBD, nucleotide-binding domains; and R, regulatory domain. Loss of CFTR function can result from four different classes of mutation. The ΔF505 mutation is a class II defect. ATP = adenosine triphosphate; ER = endoplasmic reticulum; PKA = protein kinase A. (From Welsh MJ, Smith AE: Molecular mechanisms of CFTR chloride channel dysfunction in cystic fibrosis. Cell 1993;73:1251–1254.)

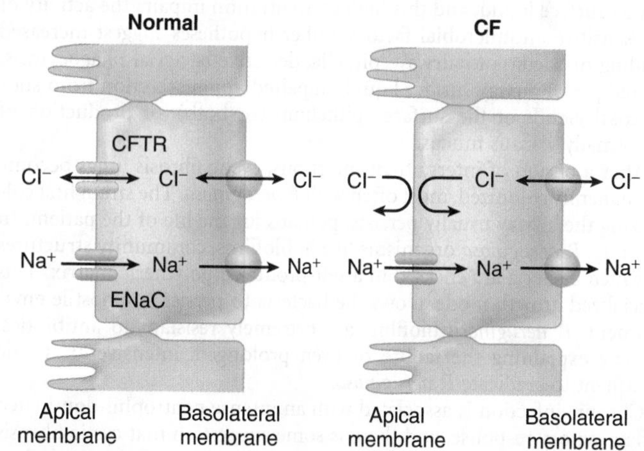

FIGURE 89–2 • Model of electrolyte transport by normal and cystic fibrosis airway epithelia. The apical membrane of normal epithelia contains CFTR Cl^- channels (which can also conduct HCO_3^-) and epithelial Na^+ channels (ENaC). The complex transport processes at the basolateral membrane are not shown in detail. The paracellular pathway between the cells through the tight junctions also shows some permeability to ions.

that do not allow normal passage of Cl^-, respectively. Much of the variability in clinical disease can be explained by variations in the severity of specific *CFTR* gene mutations. Nevertheless, other genes and environmental factors also modify the clinical course. A search is under way to identify modifier genes because they might suggest novel therapeutic strategies.

Knowledge that CFTR is an epithelial Cl^- channel combined with an appreciation of the epithelial physiology of organs affected by the disease has provided some insight into the pathogenesis and manifestations of the disease (Fig. 89–2). The water-impermeable sweat gland duct absorbs NaCl through ENaC Na^+ channels and CFTR Cl^- channels as sweat flows from the secretory coil to the surface of the skin. In cystic fibrosis, loss of CFTR prevents absorption of Cl^- and, because of the requirements for electroneutrality, absorption of Na^+. As a result, sweat emerges onto the skin with high Cl^- and Na^+ concentrations. In the pancreatic ducts, CFTR anion channels are important for alkalinization and hydration of pancreatic secretions as they flow from the pancreatic acinar cells to the intestine. In cystic fibrosis, loss of CFTR prevents this process and causes obstruction of the small pancreatic ducts, thereby blocking the output of pancreatic enzymes. Ultimately, the organ atrophies. A similar scenario appears to apply in the liver: loss of CFTR anion channels disrupts normal salt and water balance in the small biliary ducts, which causes their obstruction. It seems likely, although it has not been shown, that obstruction of the small ducts in the male genital tract also leads to atrophy, fibrosis, or absence of the vas deferens, tail and body of the epididymis, and seminal vesicles. In the ileum, CFTR Cl^- channels play a central role in salt and water secretion. Disruption of this process is thought to produce dehydrated intestinal contents that obstruct the ileum in the newborn, thereby causing meconium ileus and producing distal intestinal obstruction syndrome later in life.

Persistent bacterial airway infection, especially with *Pseudomonas aeruginosa,* is the hallmark of lung disease in cystic fibrosis. Intractable infections appear to develop in a two-step process. First, cystic fibrosis impairs pulmonary defenses, which predisposes to infection. Then the growth characteristics of the microorganisms become altered, and a chronic inflammatory state develops in the host.

Cystic fibrosis causes a defect in host defense restricted to the lung; patients are not predisposed to infection elsewhere, and normal lungs transplanted into a cystic fibrosis patient are not subject to the same infections. Normal lungs are protected from inhaled and aspirated bacteria by a multicomponent defense system involving mucociliary clearance, phagocytic cells (macrophages and neutrophils), and the innate immune system. The latter includes lysozyme, lactoferrin, β-defensin, and other antimicrobial proteins contained in the thin layer of liquid covering the airways. Several hypotheses might explain the defect in pulmonary host defense. One hypothesis suggests that loss of CFTR increases Na^+ and liquid absorption, thereby reducing airway surface liquid volume and impairing mucociliary clearance. Another hypothesis suggests that loss of CFTR Cl^- channels leads to increased NaCl concentrations in airway surface liquid, and this high concentration impairs the activity of salt-sensitive antimicrobial factors. Other hypotheses suggest increased binding of bacteria to airway epithelia, defective bacterial phagocytosis, altered pH of airway surface liquid, impaired anion secretion from submucosal glands or the surface epithelium (or both), or production of abnormally viscous mucus.

After a period of intermittent infections, cystic fibrosis lungs become permanently colonized, most often with *P. aeruginosa.* The strain first colonizing the airway usually persists, perhaps for the life of the patient. In the lung, *P. aeruginosa* organisms live in biofilms, community structures in which bacteria are encased in a self-produced polymeric matrix. This specialized growth mode allows the bacteria to persist in a hostile environment. *P. aeruginosa* biofilms are extremely resistant to antibiotics, thereby explaining the failure of even prolonged, intensive antibiotic treatment to eradicate *P. aeruginosa.*

Chronic infection is associated with an intense neutrophil-dominated inflammatory response, and there is some suggestion that cystic fibrosis lungs may have an abnormally profuse inflammatory response when compared with normal lungs. The inflammatory stimulus remodels the airways, causes submucosal gland hypertrophy, and increases mucus output. The combination of increased mucus, abundant neutrophils, and inflammatory debris, including DNA, actin, and other macromolecules, produces thick, purulent sputum that obstructs airways. The resulting damage leads to bronchitis, progressive bronchiectasis, and respiratory failure.

Clinical Manifestations

Patients with cystic fibrosis may initially be seen at several ages with a variety of clinical manifestations. For example, as newborns they may have meconium ileus; as infants or children, failure to thrive; and from childhood to adulthood, recurrent respiratory tract infections. These and other symptoms can mimic those found in a variety of other diseases. As the care of cystic fibrosis patients has improved, cystic fibrosis has increasingly become a disease of adults, with approximately 40% of patients in the United States 18 years or older.

LUNG DISEASE

Clinical Mainifestations

Cough is usually the earliest manifestation. At first it is intermittent and occurs with what appears to be an acute respiratory illness. It is worse at night and on awakening. The coughing is sometimes accompanied by wheezing, particularly in infants and young children. Episodes of coughing tend to persist longer than expected for an acute respiratory illness and, with time, occur more and more frequently. As the disease progresses, the cough becomes productive of thick, purulent, often green sputum. Patients may have symptoms of bronchitis for several years or even a decade or two. Eventually, however, exacerbations of cough and sputum production are accompanied by dyspnea, reduced appetite, and weight loss. Exercise tolerance decreases as the disease progresses. Acute exacerbations improve with intensive therapy but tend to increase in frequency and severity until symptoms of bronchiectasis (Chapter 90) develop. Physical findings depend on the stage of the disease. At first crackles are intermittent and occur with exacerbations. Lung sounds may be decreased because of pulmonary hyperinflation. As the disease progresses, rales and rhonchi are common and continuous.

Sputum Culture

Early in the disease, cystic fibrosis airways become colonized with bacteria, which are difficult to eliminate. *Staphylococcus aureus* and *Haemophilus influenzae* are often found initially. With time, however, *P. aeruginosa* becomes common, often as a mucoid species. Although mucoid *P. aeruginosa* is occasionally cultured from patients with other lung diseases, its presence in sputum should immediately alert the physician to the possibility of cystic fibrosis. As the disease progresses, antibiotic-resistant bacteria and concomitant infection with more than one organism, including *Burkholderia cepacia, Stenotrophomonas maltophilia, Achromobacter xylosoxidans,* and nontuberculous mycobacteria, are increasingly observed.

Radiologic Evaluation

With standard chest radiographs, hyperinflation may be the first finding, followed by peribronchial cuffing, which creates linear opacities. Impaction of mucus and changes consistent with bronchiectasis are observed as the disease progresses. For unknown reasons, the right upper lobe is often the first and most severely involved. High-resolution chest computed tomography reveals early changes of bronchiectasis that may be widespread before conventional radiographs show any change. Hilar adenopathy is uncommon. Changes of pulmonary hypertension become obvious late in the disease. Chest imaging should be considered to document the progression of disease and to evaluate hemoptysis (Chapter 83) or symptoms suggestive of pulmonary exacerbations, pneumothorax, or atelectasis.

Pulmonary Function

The first changes consist of airways obstruction, particularly of the small airways. Spirometry shows reduced airflow rates, including a decreased forced expiratory volume in 1 second (FEV_1), FEV_1/forced vital capacity (FVC) ratio, and maximal midexpiratory flow. The ratio of residual volume to total lung capacity is often increased. Changes consistent with airway obstruction may even be present in infants. Evidence of airway hyperreactivity is common. Arterial Po_2 tends to decrease with time as a result of ventilation-perfusion mismatching. Only in late-stage disease is Pco_2 increased and chronic respiratory acidosis apparent. The course of the disease and the response to therapy are often monitored by serial measurement of spirometry, lung volumes, and oxygenation.

Complications

Pneumothorax (Chapter 100) is a well-recognized complication, and the incidence increases with age. Although it is occasionally an incidental finding on a chest radiograph, it is often associated with chest pain, dyspnea, and hemoptysis. Indications for chest tube placement are the same as for pneumothorax from other causes. The rate of recurrence is high; pleural sclerosis may be required to prevent recurrences.

Hemoptysis (Chapter 83) becomes common as bronchiectasis develops (Chapters 90 and 96). Blood-streaked sputum is the most frequent finding. Massive hemoptysis occurs in approximately 1% of patients and is generally associated with an exacerbation of the chronic respiratory infection. Treatment is usually directed at the underlying pulmonary disease, but when hemoptysis is life-threatening, bronchial artery embolization or surgery may be required.

Digital clubbing, which occurs in nearly all patients with cystic fibrosis, is often discovered when the lung disease becomes symptomatic. Hypertrophic pulmonary osteoarthropathy may occur in up to 15% of patients, especially adolescents and adults; its symptoms may correlate with exacerbations of the pulmonary disease.

Loss of CFTR function also affects the upper airway epithelium, and chronic rhinitis is common. The sinuses are almost universally involved, as evidenced by opacification on plain radiography or magnetic resonance imaging, but acute or chronic sinusitis is not common. Nasal polyps occur in 15 to 20% of patients and occasionally require resection to prevent nasal obstruction. Of note, epithelial cells isolated from resected nasal polyps are critical in producing the model systems used in research on pathogenesis and novel therapies. When surgery is scheduled to resect nasal polyps, a cystic fibrosis research center should be contacted because the polyps are a valuable research resource.

Although more than 50% of patients have antibodies to *Aspergillus fumigatus,* in only a small number does allergic bronchopulmonary aspergillosis develop (Chapters 90 and 361). Expectoration of rusty brown sputum plugs is suggestive of this condition. Late in the disease, untreated hypoxemia and progressive loss of functional lung may produce pulmonary artery hypertension and right ventricular failure (Chapter 57). Respiratory failure (Chapter 105) becomes increasingly difficult to manage as the disease worsens. Because patients with cystic fibrosis rely on cough to clear their airways, they often respond poorly to mechanical ventilation, which is generally instituted only if there is an acute or reversible precipitating event.

PANCREATIC DISEASE

Failure of the exocrine pancreas (Chapter 147) occurs in approximately 85% of patients. It is almost universal in patients homozygous for the ΔF508 mutation. Some mutations appear to produce CFTR with sufficient residual function to prevent complete pancreatic failure, although the pancreas is not usually normal. Obstruction of ducts, loss of acinar cells, and pancreatic enzyme deficiency lead to malabsorption of protein, fat, and fat-soluble vitamins. Bulky, foul-smelling stools are often difficult to flush. If left untreated, patients with pancreatic insufficiency may show failure to thrive, weight loss, and growth inhibition. Weight loss can also be associated with severe respiratory disease and increased work of breathing.

Symptoms of pancreatitis (Chapter 147) occur in a small percentage of adolescents and adults, particularly patients who have retained some pancreatic function. Interestingly, the frequency of pancreatic disease in cystic fibrosis led to the discovery that patients with idiopathic and chronic pancreatitis have a higher than expected frequency of abnormal copies of the *CFTR* gene; in patients with two mutations, additional investigation typically reveals laboratory or clinical findings consistent with mild cystic fibrosis.

Although the islets of Langerhans are relatively spared, destruction of the pancreas can cause endocrine pancreatic dysfunction. The incidence of cystic fibrosis–related diabetes mellitus is age related, and approximately 7% of all patients are affected. The manifestation of symptomatic hyperglycemia is similar for patients with cystic fibrosis and type 1 diabetes (Chapter 247). Random serum glucose measurements should be performed annually in all adults with cystic fibrosis. In addition, weight loss or unexplained pulmonary deterioration should prompt assessment of glucose tolerance.

GASTROINTESTINAL DISEASE

Symptoms of gastrointestinal disease are common in patients with cystic fibrosis, although they are rarely life-threatening if properly managed. Meconium ileus, which occurs in approximately 18% of newborns with cystic fibrosis, is virtually diagnostic. Small bowel obstruction, or "distal intestinal obstruction syndrome," occurs in approximately 3% of patients, and intermittent abdominal pain, perhaps from partial obstruction, is much more common. Another cause of abdominal pain is intussusception, which generally requires surgical intervention. Rectal prolapse occurs occasionally in children but infrequently in adults.

GENITOURINARY DISEASE

More than 95% of males are sterile because of atrophy of wolffian duct structures. Spermatogenesis is intact, and retrieval of sperm has been used for in vitro fertilization. Interestingly, male patients with infertility as a result of congenital bilateral absence of the vas deferens, but no other symptoms of cystic fibrosis, also have an increased prevalence of mild mutations in the *CFTR* gene or sequence variations that decrease the number of functional transcripts. It may be that the vas deferens is the tissue most sensitive to a decrease in functional CFTR, followed by the lung and then the pancreas. Female patients with cystic fibrosis also have reduced fertility because of poor nutrition, chronic lung infections, or the presence of a thick plug of mucus at the cervical os. Women with severely compromised pulmonary and nutritional status may show accelerated deterioration during pregnancy.

HEPATOBILIARY DISEASE

Focal biliary fibrosis and cirrhosis (Chapter 157) are increasing in frequency as patients live longer. Data about prevalence vary, but perhaps as many as 24% of patients may have obstructive biliary tract disease, hepatomegaly, or persistently abnormal liver enzymes. The severity varies widely, with the abnormality limited to an elevated alkaline phosphatase level in many patients. In severe cases, hepatosplenomegaly, jaundice, ascites, and edema develop. Hematemesis from esophageal varices is a severe complication that may require endoscopy and sclerosis of affected vessels. Hepatic congestion from cor pulmonale can also cause liver disease. Hepatic insufficiency may require liver transplantation.

OTHER ABNORMALITIES

The increased salt loss in cystic fibrosis sweat can lead to salt depletion, especially with heat stress. Volume depletion and metabolic alkalosis are uncommon, but serious complications. Enlarged submandibular, sublingual, and submucosal glands are commonly observed on physical examination. The parotid glands are not enlarged. Numerous contributing factors may reduce bone mineral density in some adult patients and thus predispose to fracture. Psychosocial issues in dealing with a lethal disease need to be recognized and treated appropriately.

Diagnosis

Meconium ileus, pancreatic insufficiency, typical pulmonary manifestations, or a history of cystic fibrosis in the immediate family should prompt consideration of cystic fibrosis. The diagnosis can be made when a person has one or more of these phenotypic manifestations of cystic fibrosis combined with evidence of CFTR dysfunction. Functional evidence of CFTR dysfunction is usually obtained with a positive sweat Cl^- test or less frequently by measuring the voltage across the nasal epithelium. Alternatively, confirmation can be obtained if DNA testing identifies disease-causing mutations on both alleles.

Laboratory Findings

Sweat Cl^- Test

An increased concentration of Na^+ and Cl^- in sweat is one of the most consistent findings in cystic fibrosis. Sweat Cl^- should be measured by an experienced laboratory using pilocarpine iontophoresis, and it should always be repeated. A sweat Cl^- concentration greater than 60 mEq/L, when accompanied by the major clinical manifestations, is sufficient to make the diagnosis. Only 2% of cystic fibrosis patients have a normal sweat Cl^- level.

Genetic Testing

If the diagnosis is strongly suspected, DNA testing may provide definitive evidence of cystic fibrosis. DNA testing, which is readily available from commercial and university laboratories, is also of value for the detection of carriers, genetic counseling, and prenatal screening. Standard tests that can be performed from buccal swab specimens report on more than 80 of the most common mutations, which yields a detection rate of approximately 90% for northern European whites.

In the absence of a positive sweat test or detection of cystic fibrosis mutations on both chromosomes, evidence for the diagnosis has been established in some research laboratories by measurement of voltage across the nasal epithelium. This test evaluates the function of CFTR Cl^- channels in airway epithelia.

Treatment

Current therapy for cystic fibrosis is targeted at prevention and treatment of the various organ dysfunctions and symptoms. This multifactorial approach has been promoted by a network of Cystic Fibrosis Foundation–accredited care centers that provide multidisciplinary care for these complicated patients.

Antibiotics

Both in early phases of the disease and after infections become intractable, antibiotics remain the mainstay of treatment. Before pulmonary infection becomes chronic, there may be a window of opportunity in which aggressive antibiotic treatment may eliminate bacteria and thereby delay the onset of progressive lung disease. Once infection becomes persistent, however, exacerbations of lung disease usually require an intensive course of parenteral antibiotics for 2 to 3 weeks. The choice of antibiotics is based on sputum cultures to identify and test the susceptibility of organisms. *P. aeruginosa* is a particularly common pathogen, and therefore the combination of an aminoglycoside and a β-lactam antibiotic is commonly used. In general, the highest recommended doses are given to achieve penetration into respiratory secretions. Because clearance of aminoglycosides by the kidney is increased in cystic fibrosis, the required doses are often two to three times higher than in non–cystic fibrosis patients and should be adjusted by serum measurements. Extensive treatment with aminoglycosides makes adult patients susceptible to renal injury and ototoxicity. Therefore, renal function should be tested regularly, and hearing tests should be performed if symptoms develop. Emergence of antibiotic-resistant organisms is a serious problem, especially with *P. aeruginosa* and *B. cepacia*.

Although *P. aeruginosa* is rarely eradicated once it becomes chronic, an important benefit is gained by decreasing the net bacterial load with intensive intravenous antibiotics. As the number of organisms decreases, airway inflammation is reduced, thereby decreasing airway destruction and the accompanying systemic symptoms. Response to therapy is assessed by improvement in symptoms, pulmonary function, and in some cases, quantitative bacterial counts in sputum. During therapy, serum concentrations of aminoglycosides must be measured frequently because cystic fibrosis patients usually require higher than normal antibiotic doses because of increased clearance rates and increased volumes of distribution.

Chronic suppressive antibiotic therapy is increasingly becoming a standard part of care. Administration of antibiotics by inhalation is attractive because high concentrations can be attained at the airway surface and in mucus. Moreover, systemic toxicity can be minimized. Using optimal nebulizers, aerosolized high-dose tobramycin (300 mg twice daily, with 4 weeks of therapy alternating with 4 weeks without it) can reduce the density of *P. aeruginosa,* improve FEV_1, and reduce the number of days that patients are hospitalized. [1] Chronic, continuous low-dose azithromycin (3 days/wk of 250 mg if less than 40 kg and 500 mg if more than 40 kg) also improves lung function and reduces the frequency of exacerbations. [2]

Treatment of Pulmonary Disease

Several approaches can facilitate clearance of purulent secretions from the lungs. Chest percussion and postural drainage are mainstays of treatment, but other approaches to physiotherapy, high-frequency chest compression with an inflatable vest, positive expiratory pressure, and airway oscillation with a flutter valve are of benefit for some patients. Physical activity is encouraged to promote cough, as well as for its effects on the cardiovascular system and physical conditioning.

The DNA released from neutrophils forms long fibrils that contribute to the viscosity of cystic fibrosis sputum. By cleaving the DNA, inhaled recombinant human deoxyribonuclease I can increase the cough clearance of sputum and decrease the frequency of respiratory exacerbations that require intravenous antibiotics. [3] It should be considered for patients with purulent sputum and airway obstruction.

Bronchial hyperreactivity occurs frequently in cystic fibrosis patients, and therefore β-adrenergic agonists and anticholinergic agents (Chapter 87) have become a standard part of therapy. Beneficial effects have been demonstrated in short-term studies, although long-term benefit remains controversial. Bronchodilator therapy should be considered during exacerbations to facilitate airway clearance and in hospitalized patients.

Inhalation of hypertonic (7%) saline administered after a β-adrenergic agonist increases pulmonary function and reduces the frequency of pulmonary exacerbations. [4] It may facilitate clearance of secretions in advanced disease.

Glucocorticoids improve lung function, but their beneficial effects come with significant adverse effects, [5] which have tempered enthusiasm for their use. Long-term oral corticosteroids should be avoided if possible. Very high doses of ibuprofen have been reported to slow the rate of decline in FEV_1, but frequent monitoring of serum concentrations is required, and long-term safety data are not available.

Nutrition

Good nutritional status is associated with long-term survival and a slower decline in pulmonary function. Thus, prevention of malnutrition is an important goal. The fat-soluble vitamins A, D, and E are administered routinely, and vitamin K may be given sporadically for bleeding or to correct a prolonged prothrombin time. Patients are encouraged to eat a balanced diet, and an increase in total calories is encouraged. For some children and for patients with anorexia, supplemental feedings through a percutaneous gastrostomy or duodenostomy is recommended.

The frequency of pancreatic dysfunction means that pancreatic enzymes are critical for nutrition. Enzymes are administered at mealtimes as enteric-coated capsules. The number of capsules is adjusted according to weight gain or loss, abdominal cramping, and the character of stools. High doses of delayed-release pancreatic enzymes have been associated with colonic strictures.

Other Considerations

Attention should be paid to sufficient salt intake during hot weather. Adequate immunizations (Chapter 16), including influenza, are mandatory. Supplemental oxygen should be given to patients with hypoxemia. Cigarette smoke, including passive smoke, should be avoided. Other air pollutants can have adverse effects, although their role in pulmonary deterioration is not certain. Lung transplantation (Chapter 102) should be considered in patients with an FEV_1 less than 30% of predicted.

Insulin therapy (Chapter 247) should be initiated in patients with cystic fibrosis–related diabetes and fasting hyperglycemia. Oral agents are ineffective.

Patients with cholestatic liver disease may benefit from therapy with ursodeoxycholic acid (Chapter 157). Recognition of distal intestinal obstruction (Chapter 138) syndrome is important because surgical intervention can be avoided. Treatment includes correction of dehydration and attempts to relieve obstruction with enemas or polyethylene glycol electrolyte solutions if they can be safely administered by mouth.

Novel Treatments

Conceptually, the simplest approach to treating this disease would be to transfer a normal *CFTR* gene or cDNA into affected cells. Correction of approximately 5 to 10% of airway epithelial cells could correct the electrolyte transport defect, and the airway epithelium is accessible to local inhalant delivery. Studies using recombinant viral and nonviral vectors in animals and humans indicate that gene transfer is possible, but at present it is not efficient enough. Additional problems include limited persistence of expression and development of an immune response to some vectors. Progress in this area of research has been substantial, and it is hoped that successful gene therapy will become a reality. Other experimental

Rx

approaches include attempts to modulate ion transport of the airway epithelium by compensating for the loss of CFTR Cl^- channels. Although amiloride has been evaluated for inhibition of Na^+ transport, in multicenter trials the rate of decline in pulmonary function was no different in control and amiloride groups. Attempts to retarget CFTR containing the ΔF508 mutation to the cell surface (class II mutations), to suppress stop mutations (class I), and to increase the opening of channels present at the cell surface (class III) are under investigation.

Prognosis

The course is punctuated by exacerbations of lung disease followed by improvement with intensive therapy. Exacerbations are characterized by an increased frequency and severity of cough, increased sputum production, a change in the color or appearance of sputum, increased dyspnea (especially with exertion), reduced appetite, and a feeling of chest congestion. These findings are accompanied by an increased respiratory rate, use of accessory muscles of respiration, and increased rales, rhonchi, and wheezes. Laboratory evaluation may show worsening pulmonary function, new infiltrates on chest radiograph, and leukocytosis.

The lung disease is progressive. Patients with an FEV_1 less than 30% of predicted, an arterial Po_2 less than 55 mm Hg, or an arterial Pco_2 greater than 50 mm Hg have 2-year mortality rates greater than 50%. Among patients with the same FEV_1, there is a greater relative risk for female and younger patients.

Marked improvements in diagnosis and management have increased the median predicted survival from 16 years in 1970 to approximately 32 years now. Nearly half the patients with cystic fibrosis are now adults. The dramatic improvement in length and quality of life have been the result of aggressive treatment, attention to the details of treating a complex disease that affects numerous organs, and vigilant monitoring and treatment of early lung disease.

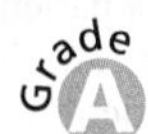

1. Ramsey BW, Pepe MS, Quan JM, et al: Intermittent administration of inhaled tobramycin in patients with cystic fibrosis. N Engl J Med 1999;340:23–30.
2. Saiman L, Marshall BC, Mayer-Hamblett N, et al: Azithromycin in patients with cystic fibrosis chronically infected with *Pseudomonas aeruginosa:* A randomized controlled trial. JAMA 2003;290: 1749–1756.
3. Fuchs HJ, Borowitz DS, Christiansen DH, et al: Effect of aerosolized recombinant human DNase on exacerbations of respiratory symptoms and on pulmonary function in patients with cystic fibrosis. N Engl J Med 1994;331:637–642.
4. Elkins MR, Robinson M, Rose BR, et al: A controlled trial of long-term inhaled hypertonic saline in patients with cystic fibrosis. N Engl J Med 2006;354:229–240.
5. Eigen H, Rosenstein BJ, FitzSimmons S, et al: A multicenter study of alternate-day prednisone therapy in patients with cystic fibrosis. J Pediatr 1995;126:515–523.

SUGGESTED READINGS

Drumm ML, Konstan MW, Schluchter MD: Genetic modifiers of lung disease in cystic fibrosis. N Engl J Med 2005;353:1443–1453. *Describes the effect of modifier genes on the clinical phenotype.*

Gershman AJ, Mehta AC, Infeld M, et al: Cystic fibrosis in adults: An overview for the internist. Cleve Clin J Med 2006;73:1065–1074. *A practical review.*

Ratjen F, Doring G: Cystic fibrosis. Lancet 2003;361:681–689. *Summary of the disease, with an emphasis on pulmonary manifestations.*

Rowe SM, Miller S, Sorscher EJ: Cystic fibrosis. N Engl J Med 2005;352:1992–2001. *Discussion of mechanisms of the disease.*

Yankaskas JR, Marshall BC, Sufian B, et al: Cystic fibrosis adult care: Consensus conference report. Chest 2004;125:1S–39S. *Summary of many aspects of care for adults with cystic fibrosis.*

90 BRONCHIECTASIS, ATELECTASIS, CYSTS, AND LOCALIZED LUNG DISORDERS

Alan F. Barker

BRONCHIECTASIS

Definition

Bronchiectasis is an acquired disorder of the major bronchi and bronchioles; it is characterized by permanent abnormal dilation and destruction of bronchial walls. The affected airways show a variety of changes including transmural inflammation, mucosal edema, cratering and ulceration, bronchial arteriole neovascularization, and distortion due to scarring or obstruction from repeated infection. The obstruction often leads to postobstructive pneumonitis that may temporarily or permanently damage the lung parenchyma. The induction of bronchiectasis requires several factors: (1) an infectious insult, (2) airway obstruction, (3) reduced clearance of mucus and other material from the airways, and/or (4) a defect in host defense.

Pathobiology

Airway Obstruction

Examples of airway obstruction causing bronchiectasis include previous foreign body aspiration or encroaching lymph nodes (middle lobe syndrome). Bronchiectasis as a sequela of foreign body aspiration usually occurs in the right lung and in the lower lobes or the posterior segments of the upper lobes. It is important to identify the presence of airway obstruction (as with foreign body aspiration), because surgical resection often produces a cure. Although witnessed or recognized aspiration (Chapter 97) is uncommon, an episode of choking and coughing or unexplained wheezing or hemoptysis should raise the suspicion of a foreign body.

Particulate aspiration is typically associated with an altered state of consciousness due to stroke, seizures, inebriation, or emergent general anesthesia. The foreign body is often unchewed food or part of a tooth or crown. Delayed or ineffective therapy and poor nutrition may contribute to prolonged pneumonitis with resultant focal bronchiectasis.

Humoral Immunodeficiency

Patients with hypogammaglobulinemia (Chapter 271) usually present in childhood with repeated sinopulmonary infections. In adults, the history may include frequent episodes of "sinusitis" and "bronchitis." Establishing the diagnosis of humoral immunodeficiency is important, because gamma globulin replacement can diminish or even prevent further respiratory tract infections and lung damage. Intravenous immunoglobulin (Ig) augmentation should be administered when levels of IgG, IgA, and IgM are less than 5 to 10% of normal values. In patients with isolated IgG subclass deficiency, tests of humoral competency, such as a serum antibody response to *Haemophilus influenzae* or pneumococcal antigen/vaccine, help decide whether low levels are functional.

Cystic Fibrosis

Major respiratory diseases in cystic fibrosis (CF) are sinusitis and bronchiectasis; the latter may be the sole feature of CF in adults (Chapter 89). Clues suggesting the presence of this disorder are upper lobe radiographic involvement and sputum cultures showing mucoid *Pseudomonas aeruginosa* or *Staphylococcus aureus.* An elevated sweat chloride value is diagnostic; genetic testing is warranted if the clinical findings are suggestive and sweat chloride values are borderline elevated.

Young's Syndrome

Patients with Young's syndrome exhibit clinical features similar to those observed in CF, including bronchiectasis, sinusitis, and obstructive azoospermia. They are often middle-aged men identified during evaluation for infertility. They do not have increased sweat chloride values, pancreatic insufficiency, or genetic abnormalities. No cause has been identified.

Rheumatic Diseases

Rheumatoid arthritis and Sjögren's syndrome can be complicated by bronchiectasis (Chapters 285 and 289). Although most patients have obvious rheumatic features when the bronchiectasis is discovered, some patients have only mild arthropathy. The presence of bronchiectasis increases the mortality rate associated with respiratory infections.

Dyskinetic Cilia

Although immotile cilia were originally described in the respiratory tract and sperm of patients with Kartagener's syndrome (dextrocardia, sinusitis, bronchiectasis), other patients have dyskinetic cilia leading to poor mucociliary clearance, repeated respiratory infections, and subsequent bronchiectasis. Several candidate genes responsible for the abnormal protein involved in the modified motility of cilia have been identified.

Pulmonary Infections

Pulmonary infections have been associated with the development of bronchiectasis. Some individuals with presumed viral or *Mycoplasma* infection develop repeated respiratory infections and bronchiectasis. In addition to direct tissue injury, a sequela of virulent infections (tuberculosis) may result in enlarged and caseous lymph nodes around bronchi or damaged airways that predispose to bacterial colonization (Chapter 345). The recognition of bronchiectasis in acquired immunodeficiency syndrome (AIDS; Chapter 414) illustrates the accelerated destructive interaction between repeated infections and impaired host defense; highly active antiretroviral therapy may alter this cycle of repeated infection and airway damage. Childhood whooping cough (pertussis; Chapter 334) is now of mostly historical interest in the pathogenesis of bronchiectasis, and adult pertussis has not been associated with bronchiectasis. It is unclear whether many of these children had secondary bacterial pneumonia. *Mycobacterium avium-intracellulare* (MAI) has traditionally been considered a secondary pathogen in an abnormal host (AIDS) or in already damaged lung (bullous emphysema). However, presumed normal hosts have developed bronchiectasis with primary MAI infections (Chapter 346). The syndrome has been recognized in white women older than age 55 years with chronic cough and involvement of the middle lobe or lingula.

Allergic Bronchopulmonary Aspergillosis

Aspergillus may also be associated with bronchiectasis (Chapter 360). This disorder should be suspected in patients with a long history of asthma that is resistant to bronchodilator therapy and is associated with a cough productive of sputum plugs or mucopurulence. Allergic bronchopulmonary aspergillosis probably represents a hyperimmune reaction to the presence of the *Aspergillus* organism, airway damage due to mycotoxins and inflammatory mediators, and even direct infection.

Cigarette Smoking

A causal role for cigarette smoking in bronchiectasis has not been shown. However, smoking and repeated infections may worsen pulmonary function and accelerate the progression of disease that is already present.

Clinical Manifestations

Patients often report frequent bouts of "bronchitis" requiring therapy with repeated courses of antibiotics (Chapter 96). Symptoms in most patients include daily cough productive of mucopurulent phlegm, intermittent hemoptysis, pleurisy, and shortness of breath. In bronchiectasis, bleeding can be brisk; it is often associated with acute infective episodes and is produced by injury to superficial mucosal neovascular bronchial arterioles. Physical findings on chest examination include crackles, rhonchi, wheezing, or combinations of these. Digital clubbing is rare.

Diagnosis

The diagnostic evaluation is designed to confirm the diagnosis of bronchiectasis, to identify potentially *treatable* underlying causes, and to provide functional assessment (Table 90–1). However, a defined etiology is found in fewer than 50% of patients with bronchiectasis. Imaging of the chest is always necessary to confirm the diagnosis.

Chest Radiography

The chest radiograph, which is abnormal in most patients with bronchiectasis, in combination with the clinical findings may be sufficient to establish the diagnosis. Suspicious but not diagnostic radiographic findings include platelike atelectasis, dilated and thickened airways (tram or parallel lines; ring shadows on cross section), and irregular peripheral opacities that may represent mucopurulent plugs. The distribution of changes also may be helpful. A central (perihilar) distribution of the abnormal shadowing is suggestive of allergic bronchopulmonary aspergillosis, whereas predominant upper lobe distribution is suggestive of CF.

High-Resolution Computed Tomography

High-resolution computed tomography (HRCT) of the chest is the defining modality for diagnosis of bronchiectasis. The major potentially progressive features of bronchiectasis on HRCT include airway dilatation, lack of airway tapering toward the periphery, bronchial wall thickening, varicose constrictions, and ballooned cysts off the end of a bronchus (Fig. 90–1). HRCT is indicated in the following settings: a patient with suspicious clinical findings but a relatively normal chest radiograph; a patient whose chest radiograph is abnormal (e.g., pneumonic infiltrate) and in whom underlying bronchiectasis is strongly suspected; a patient for whom management decisions, such as surgical resection of the abnormal areas of lung, depend on the extent of bronchiectasis; and a patient in whom the presence or absence of another confounding disease, such as chronic obstructive lung disease or interstitial lung disease, needs to be defined. The HRCT may also demonstrate other findings, such as consolidation of a segment or lobe (from pneumonia), which can be present in bronchiectasis but is not diagnostic as an isolated finding; peripheral irregular branching lines (tree-in-bud) of impacted mucus in small airways; enlarged lymph nodes, which may be indicative of reaction to infection; or areas of low attenuation and vascular disruption, probably

TABLE 90–1 BRONCHIECTASIS: DIAGNOSTIC FEATURES OF ASSOCIATED CONDITIONS

Condition	Diagnostic Test	Abnormal Result
Immunodeficiency	Quantitative IgG, IgA, IgM	All low; rarely, isolated subclass G is low
Ciliary dyskinesia	Respiratory mucosa biopsy (examine by electron microscopy)	Ciliary struts or spokes broken or missing
	Exhaled nitric oxide	Low
Bronchopulmonary aspergillosis	IgE	High, often >1000 IU/mL
	Type I and type III skin tests; precipitins	Positive
	Fungal sputum cultures	Positive about 50% of time
Mycobacterium avium-intracellulare infection	Mycobacterial sputum culture/DNA probe	Positive in about two thirds of patients
Cystic fibrosis	Sweat chloride	>55–60 mEq/L
	Sputum culture	*Pseudomonas aeruginosa*
	Genetic testing	ΔF508 most frequent
Foreign body aspiration	Bronchoscopy	Lobar or segmental obstruction

Ig = immunoglobulin; IU = international units.

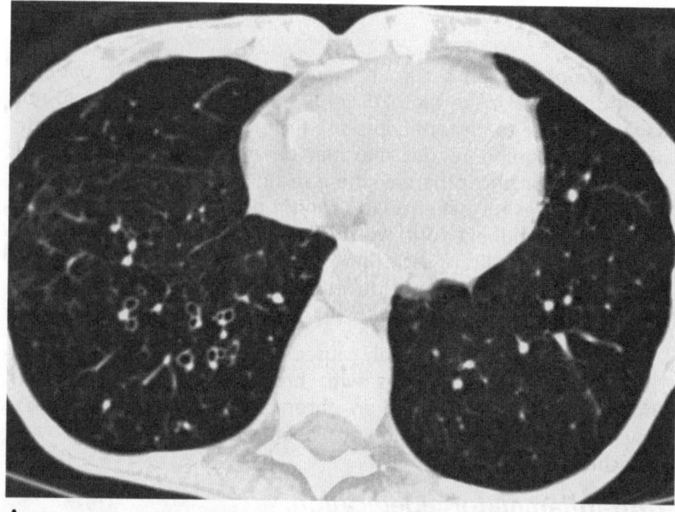

A

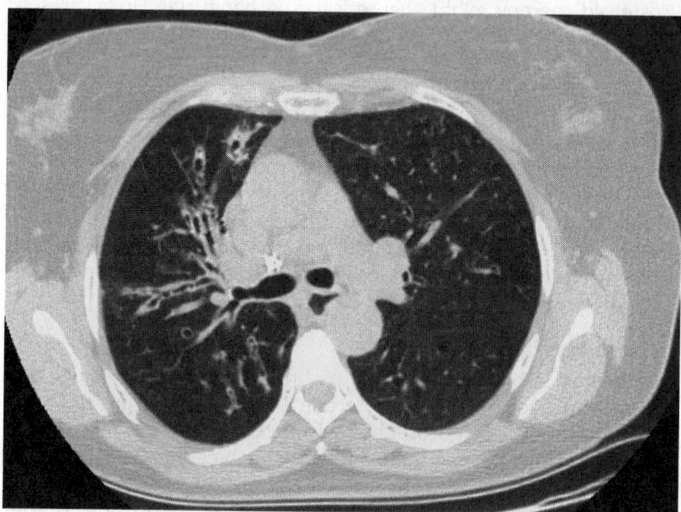

B

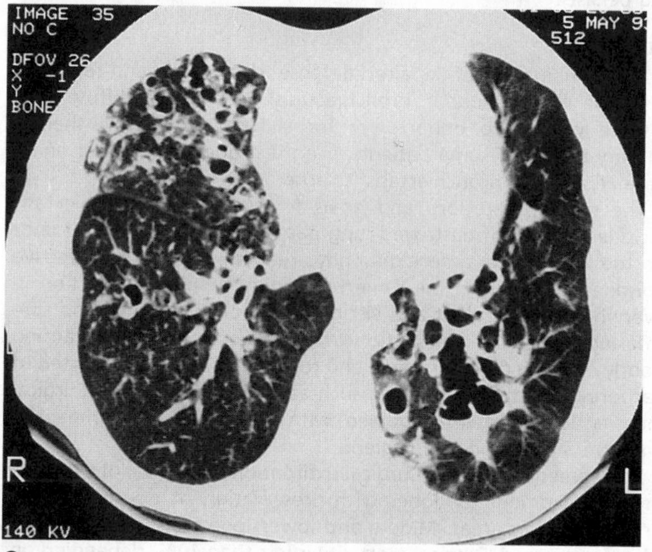

C

FIGURE 90–1 • High-resolution chest computed tomography of patients with bronchiectasis. A, Dilated airways are present in the right lung. **B,** In the right lung are dilated and thickened airways almost to the periphery of the lung, with a beaded appearance of varicose bronchiectasis. **C,** Both lungs show hugely dilated airways that cluster as cystic or saccular bronchiectasis, which is the most severe and damaging form of bronchiectasis.

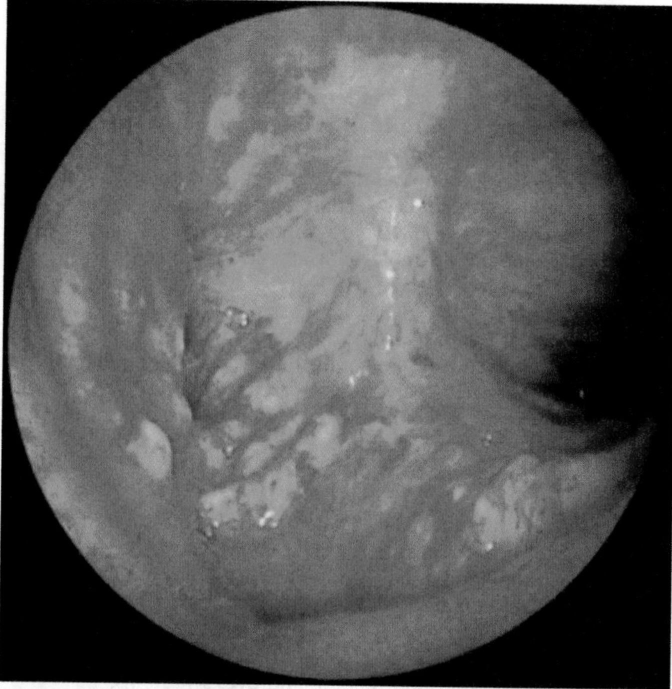

FIGURE 90–2 • Bronchoscopic photograph of endobronchial papillary tumor with complete obstruction leading to distal collapse and subsequent bronchiectasis.

caused by the distorting effect of inflammatory small airways and suggestive of emphysema.

Bronchoscopy

Bronchoscopy is an important diagnostic tool in focal (segmental or lobar) bronchiectasis to examine for obstruction by a foreign body, tumor, structural deformity, or extrinsic compression from lymph nodes (Fig. 90–2). Bronchoscopic lavage may help identify or confirm pathogens such as MAI, and a biopsy specimen can be examined by electron microscopy for the ultrastructural features of ciliary dyskinesia. Bronchoscopy plays a key role in patients with hemoptysis to help localize the bleeding to a lobe so that appropriate intervention can be performed.

Pulmonary Function Tests

Pulmonary function testing allows a functional assessment of the impairment induced by bronchiectasis. Spirometry before and after the administration of a bronchodilator is adequate in most patients. Obstructive impairment (reduced or normal forced vital capacity [FVC], low forced expiratory volume in 1 second [FEV_1], or low FEV_1/FVC ratio) is the most frequent finding, but a very low FVC is also seen in advanced disease in which much of the lung has been destroyed.

Prevention and Treatment

Antibiotics are used to treat an acute exacerbation and to prevent recurrent infection by suppression or eradication of pathogens.

Acute Exacerbation

The diagnosis of an acute exacerbation depends on symptomatic changes rather than any specific laboratory feature. Acute bacterial infections are usually accompanied by increased production of darker and more viscid sputum, shortness of breath, and pleuritic chest pain and are often accompanied by lassitude. Systemic complaints such as fever and chills are usually absent, and the chest radiograph rarely shows new infiltrates. Frequent bacterial pathogens include *H. influenzae* (Chapter 323) and *P. aeruginosa* (Chapter 328), often different from the pathogenic agents in patients with chronic bronchitis. Initial treatment should include a fluoroquinolone such as levofloxacin, 500 mg daily for 14 days or ciprofloxacin, 750 mg every 12 hours for 14 days. For patients who

Rx

are too ill for oral therapy, parenteral therapy with two different classes of antipseudomonal agents (e.g., ceftazidime, 2 g every 8 hours plus tobramycin, 5 to 7 mg/kg/day for 14 days) is needed. The duration of therapy is not well defined, but a minimum of 7 to 14 days has become frequent practice. Sputum culture and sensitivity to help define antibiotic selection and resistance patterns are indicated in patients who have no response to the initial antibiotic or who have repeated symptomatic attacks in a short interval.

Prevention

Less clear is the role of suppressive antibiotic regimens. Chronic macrolide administration (e.g., azithromycin, 500 mg/day three times each week) has been shown to reduce sputum volume and coughing only for *Pseudomonas*. However, three organisms that contribute to symptomatic episodes and are particularly problematic and difficult to eradicate are *P. aeruginosa*, MAI, and *Aspergillus* species.

P. aeruginosa (Chapter 328) is almost impossible to eradicate in patients with bronchiectasis. The quinolones, such as ciprofloxacin or a newer quinolone in doses noted earlier, are the only effective oral agents against *P. aeruginosa*, but resistance often develops after one to two treatment cycles. When *Pseudomonas* causes repeated symptomatic episodes, aerosolized tobramycin reduces the burden of *Pseudomonas* in the sputum and improves symptoms. 1

MAI (Chapter 346) and *Aspergillus* (Chapter 360) species are often harbored in damaged lung tissue and bronchiectatic airways. Guidelines to help decide whether a patient is infected with MAI or *Aspergillus* include (1) symptomatic episodes not responding to antibacterial agents, (2) two or more independent positive sputum cultures, (3) new infiltrates on chest radiograph with sputum culture growing either organism, and (4) HRCT showing nodular opacities with MAI infection. For the treatment of MAI infection, a three- to four-drug regimen is recommended by the American Thoracic Society, including the following: clarithromycin, 500 mg twice daily, or azithromycin, 250 mg/day; rifampin, 600 mg/day; ethambutol, 15 mg/kg/day; and streptomycin, 15 mg/kg two to three times a week for the first 8 weeks as tolerated. Therapy is continued until cultures are negative for 12 months. For patients with allergic bronchopulmonary aspergillosis, a prolonged course of prednisone (beginning at 0.5 mg/kg/day) stabilizes exacerbations. Itraconazole (400 mg/day) allows reduced steroid dosing and improves clinical outcome in some patients. 2

Bronchial Hygiene

Bronchiectasis is the prototypical disease for which secretion loosening or thinning, combined with enhanced removal techniques, should be salutary. This approach is particularly important for patients in whom tenacious secretions are not reduced with appropriate antibiotic administration. Potential therapies include hydration, nebulization with saline solutions and mucolytic agents, mechanical techniques, bronchodilators, and corticosteroids.

Hydration and Nebulization

General hydration with oral liquids and nebulization with saline solutions or mucolytic agents are important considerations in the management of bronchiectasis. The mucolytic agent acetylcysteine is beneficial in some patients when delivered by nebulization. Although recombinant human deoxyribonuclease (rhDNase) is effective in CF, in bronchiectasis it neither reduces pulmonary exacerbations nor improves pulmonary function.

Physiotherapy

Mechanical techniques to loosen viscid secretions, followed by gravitational positioning, should be effective if practiced assiduously. Chest percussion techniques include hand clapping of the chest by an assistant or application of a mechanical vibrator to the chest wall. Because bronchiectasis most often follows a middle or lower lobe distribution, the patient needs to recline prone on a bed with the head over the edge for postural drainage, but this position may be difficult or uncomfortable for many patients. If physiotherapy is performed regularly, three to four times daily, enhanced sputum mobilization occurs in many patients. However, patients often do not take the time (15 to 30 minutes per session), do not have assistance to perform vibratory techniques, or cannot tolerate proper positioning to get maximal benefit. Despite decades of enthusiasm for physiotherapy, these techniques have limited value. 3 Alternatives for patients who cannot perform chest physiotherapy include handheld positive expiratory pressure devices or flutter valves, which facilitate secretion drainage by maintaining airway patency, or a vibratory vest applied to the chest.

Bronchodilators

Airway reactivity, presumably caused by transmural inflammation, is often present in patients with bronchiectasis. Aerosol bronchodilator therapy, as used in chronic bronchitis (Chapter 88), may be appropriate but has not been studied in patients with bronchiectasis.

Anti-inflammatory Medication

Because inflammation plays a major role in bronchiectasis, corticosteroid therapy might theoretically be beneficial. However, systemic steroids can further depress host immunity and promote increased bacterial and fungal colonization and even perpetuation of infection. One practical approach involves oral systemic prednisone therapy (20 to 30 mg/day for 2 days, tapering completely over 10 to 14 days) along with antibacterial therapy at the time of acute exacerbations. Regular inhaled steroids could be considered at other times. In pilot studies of aerosolized beclomethasone (2 puffs of 80 μg each, twice daily), and fluticasone (2 puffs of 220 μg each, twice daily), treated patients had fewer inflammatory mediators in their sputum, less sputum production, reduced coughing, and improved pulmonary function. 4

Hemoptysis

Bleeding in bronchiectasis can be brisk and life-threatening. It is often associated with acute infective episodes and is produced by injury to superficial mucosal neovascular bronchial arterioles. HRCT and bronchoscopy may help localize the bleeding to a lobe or segment. Selective bronchial arterial embolization, when available, is the treatment of choice, because it preserves lung tissue. Thoracotomy and resection (Chapter 102) may still be necessary if bleeding persists.

Surgery

The combination of impaired defense mechanisms and recurrent infection often results in bronchiectasis' becoming a diffuse lung disease with little opportunity for surgical cure. Nevertheless, surgery may help some patients, even if it does not cure or eliminate all areas of bronchiectasis (Chapter 102).

The major indications and goals for surgery in bronchiectasis include removal of destroyed lung partially obstructed by a tumor or the residue of a foreign body; reduction in acute infective episodes occurring in the same pulmonary segment; reduction in overwhelming purulent and viscid sputum production from a specific lung segment; elimination of bronchiectatic airways causing poorly controlled hemorrhage; and removal of an area suspected of harboring resistant organisms, such as MAI or *Aspergillus*. Surgical intervention is often combined with an aggressive regimen of antibiotics and bronchial hygiene.

The immediate goal of surgical extirpation is removal of the most involved segments or lobes with preservation of nonsuppurative or nonbleeding areas. Middle and lower lobe resections are most often performed. Surgical mortality is less than 10%, depending on patient selection. Complications include empyema, hemorrhage, prolonged air leak, and poorly expanding remaining lung due to persistent atelectasis or suppuration.

Lung Transplantation

Patients with suppurative lung disease were initially considered poor candidates for lung transplantation because of the potential persistence of infection that might worsen during prolonged immunosuppression (Chapter 102). Patients with non-CF bronchiec-

Rx

tasis have undergone bilateral lung transplantation. Timing and selection for lung transplantation in patients with bronchiectasis are similar to the guidelines for individuals with CF (Chapter 89). The outcome of lung transplantation in non-CF bronchiectasis includes a 1-year survival rate of 68% and an overall 5-year survival rate of 62%. Double-lung transplantation is required in most patients.

ATELECTASIS

Atelectasis, or collapse, is associated with hypoventilation of the lung (Fig. 90–3). Atelectasis may include the whole lung as the result of an intrinsic mainstem mass or extrinsic compression from lymph node enlargement. Lobar, segmental, or subsegmental regions may be involved. The decreased ventilation and sustained blood flow lead to ventilation-perfusion mismatch and hypoxemia.

Platelike or *discoid* atelectasis refers to the appearance on chest radiography of horizontal or curvilinear lines. This type of atelectasis is seen after surgery or lengthy recumbency with conditions such as stroke or head or spinal injuries. Sustained chest pain of any cause may also lead to splinting and platelike atelectasis.

Patchy atelectasis occurs in any air space–filling disease such as pulmonary hemorrhage, pulmonary edema, or respiratory distress syndrome. Fluid-filled alveoli and loss of surfactant contribute to patchy areas of infiltrate.

Passive, relaxation, or *compression* atelectasis occurs when the lung recoils to a smaller volume due to a process in the adjacent pleural space such as pneumothorax or pleural effusion. Obstructive atelectasis can be caused by an obstructed bronchus due to an intrinsic process, such as a tumor or mucus plug, or an extrinsic process, such as enlargement of peribronchial lymph nodes (middle lobe syndrome).

Rounded atelectasis is a round, masslike density abutting the pleura. It is caused by pleural scar that invaginates and contracts lung tissue. Rounded atelectasis is almost always seen in the setting of asbestos pleural disease.

Diagnosis and Treatment

Rx

Chest imaging is a key diagnostic tool. Volume loss is almost always present on a chest radiograph and involves displacement of a lobar fissure, the mediastinum, or diaphragm to the affected area or side. Diagnosis and management of segmental or lobar obstructive atelectasis includes bronchoscopy. An intrinsic mass can be visualized and biopsied for cytologic analysis. Mucus plugs can be removed by lavage and suctioning.

Rounded atelectasis must be distinguished from a tumor mass; CT may confirm the pleural thickening and the invaginating lung tissue. For patients at bed rest or with other risks for development of platelike atelectasis, attention to deep breathing, mobilization, analgesic medication for chest pain, and bronchial hygiene improves gas exchange and prevents pneumonia. For patchy atelectasis, treatment is directed at the underlying disease and to the types of measures that also enhance lung volume in platelike atelectasis. Passive atelectasis requires attention to the pleural space process, such as evacuation of a pneumothorax or drainage of a pleural effusion.

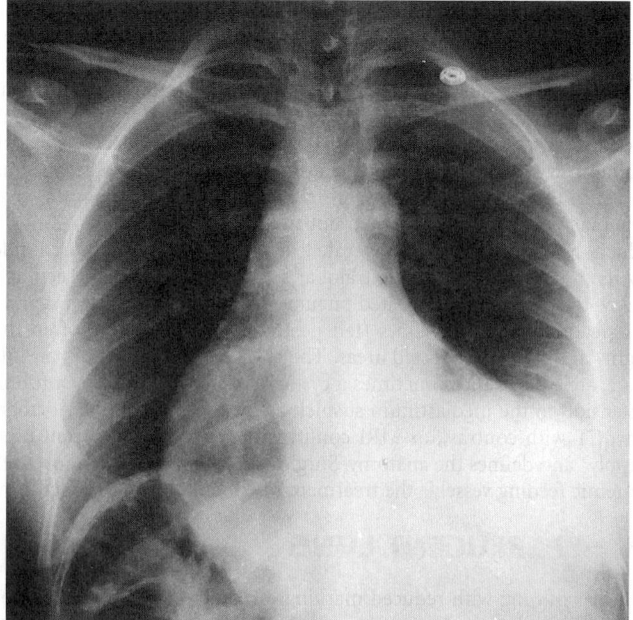

A

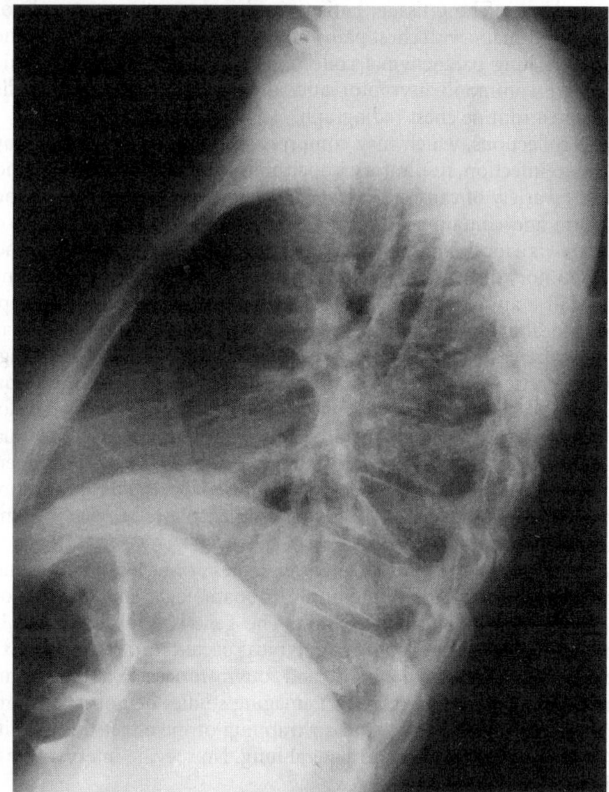

B

FIGURE 90–3 • Chest films of a patient with left lower lobe atelectasis. A, The posteroanterior film shows on the left opacity over the heart, loss of the diaphragmatic contour, and diagonal line of the major fissure. **B,** The lateral projection shows an elevated left diaphragm.

CONGENITAL CYSTIC DISEASES OF THE LUNG

Lung cysts involve abnormal foregut branching or development. The cyst lining contains airway or alveolar epithelium. Cysts communicate poorly with normal airway or lung tissue. Cysts are usually clinically apparent in childhood but occasionally remain unrecognized until later in life. Manifestations include an abnormal chest radiograph with a localized cyst, irregular focal infiltrate, pneumonia that resolves slowly or recurs in the same location, compression of normal lung or mediastinal structure, or hemoptysis. Although the chest radiograph may show a focal abnormality or even a well-developed cyst, CT of the chest with contrast or magnetic resonance imaging (MRI) is needed to define the location (lung, mediastinum, or abdomen), vascular supply, and degree of compression of other structures.

Of these rare disorders, the two that may present in adulthood are bronchogenic cysts and pulmonary sequestration. Bronchogenic cysts rarely produce symptoms. Commonly, an asymptomatic mass is noted on a chest radiograph inferior to the tracheal carina in the middle or posterior mediastinum. CT or MRI of the chest usually distinguishes a bronchogenic cyst from a pericardial or esophageal cyst, diaphragmatic hernia, or tumor. If the cyst becomes infected or compresses other structures, surgical resection via thoracotomy or video-assisted thoracoscopy is warranted.

Pulmonary sequestration is characterized by nonfunctioning pulmonary parenchyma that has no connection to the tracheobronchial airways. The blood supply is from a systemic artery, usually the aorta. Pulmonary sequestrations may be intralobar (75% of all sequestrations), in which the abnormal lung is within a normal lobe and does not have a separate visceral pleura, or extralobar (25% of all sequestrations), in which the abnormal lung is separate from a normal lobe and surrounded by its own visceral pleura. Extralobar sequestrations may be seen at or below the diaphragm. Repeated pneumonia in the same lobe or segment is a feature. The lower lobes (left posterior segments more often than right) are the most affected areas. The chest radiograph shows an infiltrate, atelectasis, and sometimes a cystic mass accompanied by a tubular extension to the mediastinum suspicious for a feeding vessel. Aortography, CT with contrast, or MRI confirms the diagnosis (aberrant blood supply) and defines the anatomy. Surgical resection with attention to the systemic feeding vessel is the treatment of choice and is usually curative.

HYPERLUCENT LUNG

Areas of lung with reduced markings on a chest radiograph are considered hyperlucent. At one extreme is a pneumothorax (Chapter 100), with complete absence of markings due to air in the pleural space that causes collapse of lung tissue; patients with pneumothorax are almost always symptomatic with chest pain and shortness of breath. At the other extreme are lung parenchymal collections of air and sometimes fluid; patients are commonly asymptomatic, and the disorder usually is discovered on a routine chest radiograph.

These collections, which may compress surrounding lung or airways and lead to infection, respiratory impairment, rupture, and pneumothorax have a variety of causes. *Developmental cysts* are lined by respiratory epithelium and contain air and fluid; *congenital lobar hyperinflation* or *emphysema* is a localized anomaly that almost always manifests in infancy with respiratory distress due to compression of an airway or normal lung. Occasionally, an older individual presents with a chest radiograph showing focal hyperlucency. Lobar emphysema usually has areas of vasculature, whereas a pneumothorax has complete absence of markings. Surgical resection of the lobe is indicated in individuals with respiratory impairment from compressed lung or mediastinal shift. *Blebs* develop after traumatic chest injury or barotrauma during mechanical ventilation; *pneumatoceles* are noted after staphylococcal or *Pneumocystis* pneumonia and are similar to blebs; *bullae* are caused by alveolar destruction in severe emphysema and are sometimes amenable to surgical decompression (Chapter 102).

Hyperlucency of an entire lung (Swyer-James or Macleod's syndrome) is unilateral bronchiolitis obliterans. Histopathologic specimens show fibrosis in and around small airways. The genesis is presumed to be remote virulent respiratory viral or atypical bacterial infection or toxic fume inhalation. Exertional dyspnea and cough are occasional symptoms. Inspiratory and expiratory chest CT imaging studies demonstrate complete unilateral hyperlucency and air trapping of the affected lung with normal appearance of the contralateral lung. No specific intervention is required.

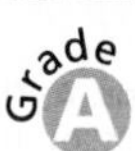

1. Barker AF, Couch L, Fiel SB, et al: Tobramycin solution for inhalation reduces sputum *Pseudomonas aeruginosa* density in bronchiectasis. Am J Respir Crit Care Med 2000;162:481–485.
2. Stevens DA, Schwartz HJ, Lee JY, et al: A randomized trial of itraconazole in allergic bronchopulmonary aspergillosis. N Engl J Med 2000;342:756–762.
3. Jones A, Rowe BH: Bronchopulmonary hygiene physical therapy in bronchiectasis and chronic obstructive pulmonary disease: A systemic review. Heart Lung 2000;29:125–135. *Summary indluding appropriate diagnostic testing.*
4. Tsang KW, Tan KC, Lam WK, et al: Inhaled fluticasone in bronchiectasis: A 12 month study. Thorax 2005;60:239–243.

SUGGESTED READINGS

Barker AF: Bronchiectasis. N Engl J Med 2002;346:1383–1393. *A practical review.*

Beirne PA, Banner NR, Khaghani A, et al: Lung transplantation for non-cystic fibrosis bronchiectasis: Analysis of a 13-year experience. J Heart Lung Transplant 2005;24:1530. *The 5-year survival rate is 63%.*

Bratu I, Flageole H, Chen M-F, et al: The multiple facets of pulmonary sequestration. J Pediatr Surg 2001;36:784–790. *Review mainly of children, but illustrates need to look for other congenital manifestations.*

Duggan M, Kavanagh BP: Atelectasis in the perioperative patient. Curr Opin Anesthesiol 2007;20:37–42. *A clinical and pathophysiologic overview.*

Takeda S, Miyoshi S, Minami M, et al: Clinical spectrum of mediastinal cysts. Chest 2003;124:125–132. *Good clinical update that takes a very aggressive approach; accompanying editorial gives more balance.*

91 ALVEOLAR FILLING DISORDERS

Stephanie M. Levine

Definition

Alveolar filling disorders (Table 91–1) are characterized by chest radiographic findings of alveolar involvement ranging from a ground-glass appearance to consolidation; the pathologic process shows primary involvement of the alveolar air spaces distal to the terminal bronchioles. For example, in pulmonary alveolar proteinosis, the alveoli are filled by proteinaceous fluid; in bronchioloalveolar cell cancer, the alveolar walls are lined by adenocarcinoma cells. In acute interstitial pneumonia, exudative organizing fibroproliferative infiltrates fill the alveolar space; in the alveolar hemorrhage disorders, blood fills the alveolar space. Alveolar spaces filled with acute inflammatory cells, as in bacterial pneumonia (Chapter 97), or water, as in cardiogenic or hydrostatic pulmonary edema (Chapter 58), or high-protein fluid, as in noncardiogenic or increased permeability pulmonary edema (Chapter 105), are also part of the radiographic differential diagnosis of alveolar filling disorders and must be excluded.

A general approach to these suspected alveolar filling diseases (Fig. 91–1) can be stratified by time since the onset of symptoms. The typical patient may present with the onset of cough (usually dry) and dyspnea of variable duration, depending on the disease process. Hemoptysis is a frequent presenting symptom in the alveolar hemorrhagic disorders. With the exception of acute interstitial pneumonia, acute infectious symptoms such as fever, leukocytosis, and productive cough are usually absent. If the initial chest radiograph or chest computed tomographic (CT) scan is consistent with a possible alveolar filling process (Chapter 84), and acute pneumonia and pulmonary edema are excluded, bronchoscopy with bronchoalveolar lavage (Chapter 85) and transbronchial biopsy should be performed, particularly if pulmonary alveolar proteinosis, bronchioloalveolar cell cancer (Chapter 201), or alveolar hemorrhage is suspected. When these tests are nondiagnostic and in most cases of suspected acute interstitial pneumonia, a surgical lung biopsy obtained by thoracoscopy or an open surgical procedure is indicated.

PULMONARY ALVEOLAR PROTEINOSIS

Epidemiology

Pulmonary alveolar proteinosis is a rare alveolar filling disease caused by the accumulation of phospholipoproteinaceous material in the alveoli. The incidence is estimated to be 3.7 cases per million people. Pulmonary alveolar proteinosis in adults is an acquired primary disorder in more than 90% of cases, but similar histopathologic features may be found with identifiable causes, such as acute silicosis (silicoproteinosis; Chapter 93), aluminum dust exposure (Chapter 93), immunodeficiency disorders (e.g., immunoglobulin G monoclonal gammopathy and severe combined immunodeficiency syndrome), hematologic malignant neoplasms (particularly myeloid leukemias; Chapters 194 and 195), and certain infections (e.g., *Pneumocystis* pneumonia). Pulmonary alveolar proteinosis has also been described after bone marrow transplantation (Chapter 184).

Pathobiology

The pathogenesis of pulmonary alveolar proteinosis is related to impaired processing of surfactant by alveolar macrophages due to defects in granulocyte-macrophage colony-stimulating factor (GM-CSF) signal-

TABLE 91–1 ALVEOLAR FILLING DISORDERS

Diseases	Pathophysiology	Radiographic Findings
Pulmonary alveolar proteinosis	Impaired processing of surfactant by alveolar macrophages due to defects in GM-CSF signaling	Bilateral alveolar infiltrates with "crazy paving" and diffuse areas of ground-glass attenuation on CT scan
Acute interstitial pneumonia	Diffuse alveolar damage with temporal uniformity	Diffuse alveolar filling process similar to the acute respiratory distress syndrome
Diffuse alveolar hemorrhage	Bleeding from the pulmonary microcirculation, usually from the capillaries	Acute development of bilateral alveolar infiltrates
Bronchioloalveolar cell carcinoma	Cancer cells growing along the alveolar septa	Pneumonic infiltrate or nodules (either solitary or multiple)

CT = computed tomographic; GM-CSF = granulocyte-macrophage colony-stimulating factor.

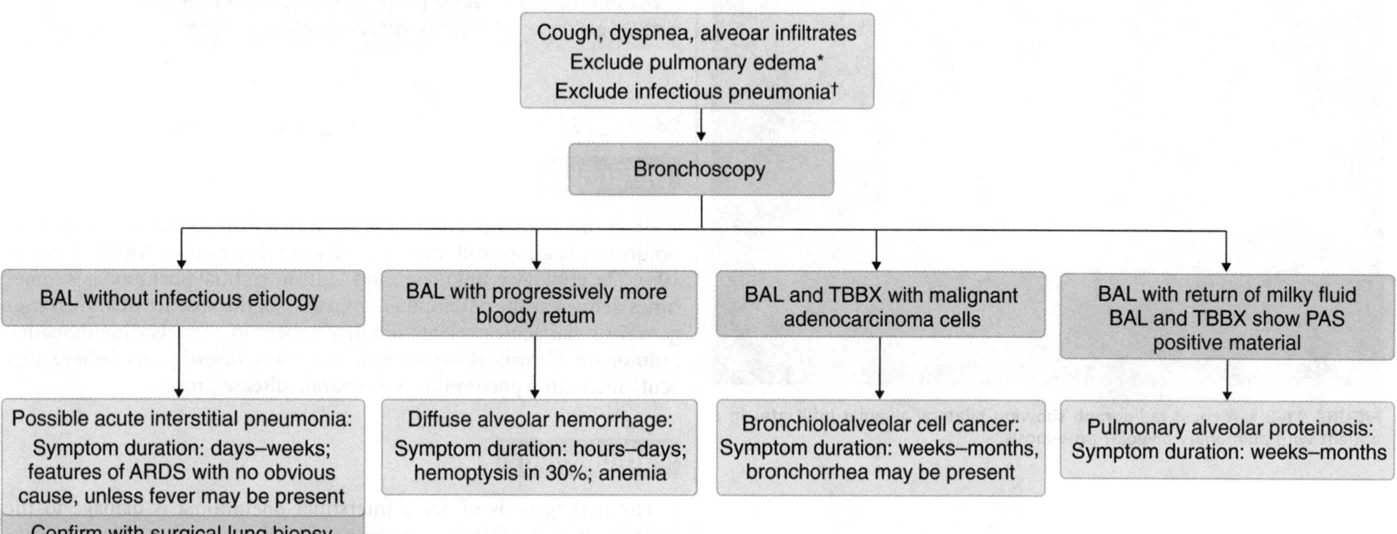

FIGURE 91–1 • A general approach to the alveolar filling disorders. *See Chapter 58; †See Chapter 97. ARDS = acute respiratory distress syndrome; BAL = bronchoalveolar lavage; PAS = periodic acid–schiff; TBBX = transbronchial biopsy.

ing. This impairment may be due to autoantibodies against GM-CSF or GM-CSF receptor gene mutations, but it is not thought to be due to a problem with GM-CSF production. An autosomal recessive congenital form of pulmonary alveolar proteinosis, caused by a mutation in the genes encoding surfactant protein B or C, results in abnormal surfactant function and severe respiratory distress in homozygous infants. The result of this impairment is accumulation of surfactant-rich material and progressive dysfunction in phagocytosis due to excessive production or diminished clearance of surfactant by alveolar macrophages.

Histologic examination in pulmonary alveolar proteinosis reveals alveoli filled with lipoproteinaceous material that stains pink (positive reaction) with periodic acid–Schiff stain. Classically, there is no destruction of alveolar architecture. Electron microscopy reveals lamellar (phospholipid-containing) myelin bodies.

Clinical Manifestations

Pulmonary alveolar proteinosis presents in patients in the third to fourth decade with a 2 : 1 male predominance. The majority of patients (72%) are smokers. Patients present with the insidious onset of dyspnea and cough, which may be dry or occasionally productive of grayish material. The duration of symptoms before diagnosis is typically 6 weeks to 6 to 8 months. Low-grade fevers, malaise, and weight loss may also be present. Hemoptysis is unusual. On physical examination, rales are present in 50% of cases. Clubbing is an unusual finding until later stages of disease.

Diagnosis

Mildly elevated leukocyte counts and mildly to moderately elevated lactate dehydrogenase levels may be found in more than 80% of patients; lactate dehydrogenase levels may correlate with the severity of disease. The chest radiograph (Fig. 91–2) and chest CT scans demonstrate a diffuse symmetrical alveolar filling process with predominance in the lower two thirds of the lung fields; the radiographic appearance may mimic pulmonary edema. The characteristic CT pattern is often described as "crazy paving," which is due to scattered or diffuse areas of ground-glass attenuation with thickening of intralobular structures and interlobular septa in polygonal shapes (Fig. 91–3). This radiographic pattern is not specific for this disorder and can be seen with acute respiratory distress syndrome (ARDS; Chapter 105), *Pneumocystis jiroveci* pneumonia (Chapter 362), bronchioloalveolar cell carcinoma (Chapter 201), lipoid pneumonia (Chapter 94), sarcoidosis (Chapter 95), organizing pneumonia (Chapter 92), drug reactions, and pulmonary hemorrhage as well as with cardiogenic pulmonary edema (Chapter 58) and acute interstitial pneumonias. Pulmonary function tests often but not always show a restrictive pattern, with a reduced diffusing capacity. Arterial blood gas analyses reveal hypoxemia.

Bronchoscopy should be the initial procedure when pulmonary alveolar proteinosis is suspected. The diagnosis of pulmonary alveolar proteinosis can be established in the majority of cases by the recovery of milky white to sandy-colored or light brown fluid on bronchoalveolar lavage. When it is subjected to microscopic analysis, the bronchoalveolar lavage fluid has a positive reaction on periodic acid–Schiff staining.

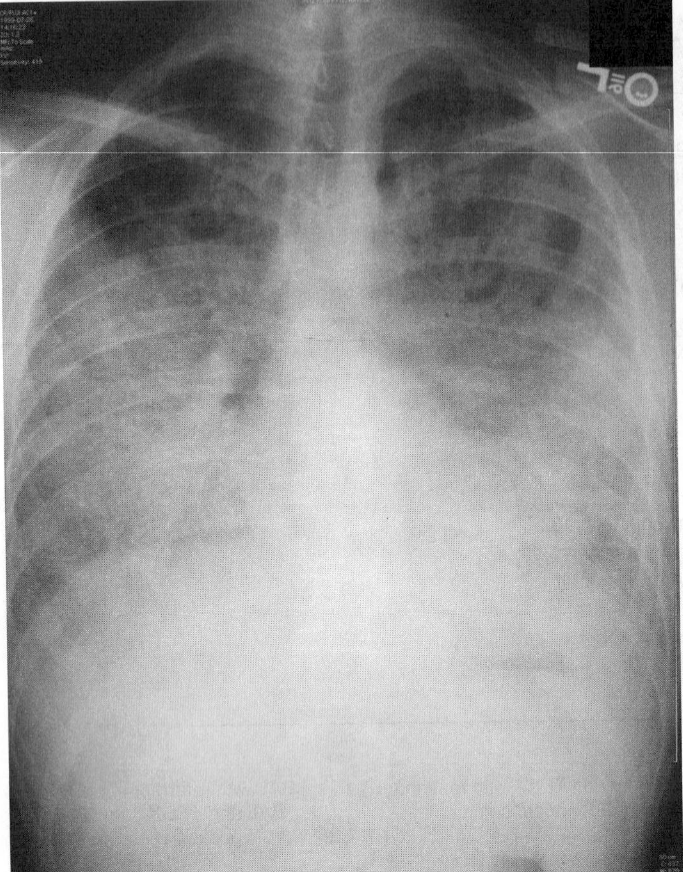

FIGURE 91–2 • A chest radiograph showing bilateral alveolar infiltrates in a patient with pulmonary alveolar proteinosis.

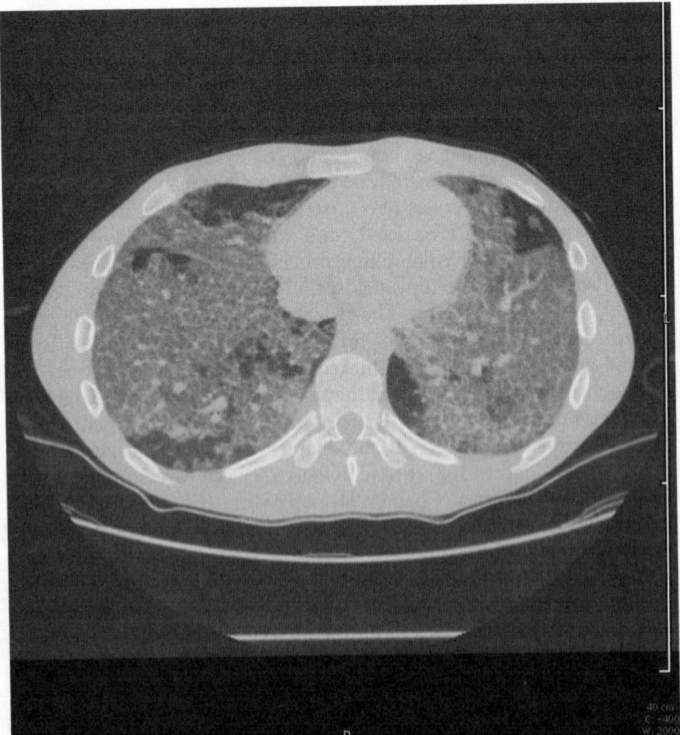

FIGURE 91–3 • A chest computed tomographic scan showing the "crazy paving" pattern characteristic of pulmonary alveolar proteinosis.

Transbronchial biopsy or thoracoscopic biopsy can confirm the diagnosis by providing tissue that has similar staining characteristics.

Treatment

About 8 to 30% of cases of pulmonary alveolar proteinosis resolve spontaneously, and smoking cessation may contribute to spontaneous resolution. A second group of patients will progress to respiratory failure. The remainder will have stable disease. Superinfection with *Nocardia,* atypical mycobacteria, and other opportunistic organisms can occur in more than 15% of patients as a result of macrocyte phagocytic dysfunction.

Therapy begins with multistage or sequential whole lung lavage performed under general anesthesia with a double-lumen endotracheal tube. This procedure may have to be repeated at variable intervals. Recent data suggest that GM-CSF therapy may be helpful in some cases. Lung transplantation can be performed, but recurrent pulmonary alveolar proteinosis has been reported.

Survival rates at 5 years approach 75%.

ACUTE INTERSTITIAL PNEUMONIA

Definition

Acute interstitial pneumonia, also referred to as the Hamman-Rich syndrome, is a rare and often fatal disease that mimics ARDS (Chapter 105). The etiology is unknown, and acute interstitial pneumonia is sometimes defined as the development of ARDS in the absence of known triggers. A similar acute presentation may be seen in patients with idiopathic pulmonary fibrosis (Chapter 92), but most investigators believe that acute interstitial pneumonia is a separate disease process.

Pathobiology

The pathogenesis of acute interstitial pneumonia is damage to the epithelium of the alveolar membranes by a neutrophil-mediated mechanism; the result is pouring of exudate into the air space in the initial exudative phase of disease. Histologic examination reveals diffuse alveolar damage with intra-alveolar hyaline membrane formation, interstitial and intra-alveolar edema, acute inflammation, and epithelial cell necrosis with a nonspecific distribution and temporal uniformity. This process progresses to the organizing phase, characterized by alveolar septal thickening, type II pneumocyte hyperplasia, and fibroblast proliferation along the interstitium and alveolar spaces. In situ thrombi of small pulmonary arteries may be present. Finally comes a fibrotic phase with alveolar septal thickening from organizing fibrosis. One of the key pathologic findings in acute interstitial pneumonia is the temporal uniformity of the diffuse alveolar damage and of organizing and proliferating connective tissue. This uniformity supports a single acute injury at a particular point in time. Long-standing fibrosis is not a typical pathologic finding in acute interstitial pneumonia.

Clinical Manifestations

Acute interstitial pneumonia manifests with equal frequency in men and women, typically in previously healthy individuals in the 50- to 55-year age range. It develops acutely to subacutely during a few days to a few weeks. The mean duration of symptoms is 15 days. Dry cough, shortness of breath, malaise, and fever (in 50% of patients) are typical clinical findings. A virus-like prodrome period has been described. Pulmonary rales are heard on physical examination, and hypoxemia is characteristic. Acute interstitial pneumonia often progresses to hypoxemic ventilatory failure, and intensive care unit admission with mechanical ventilation is usually required. Early mortality is high. Radiographic features of acute interstitial pneumonia are diffuse alveolar infiltrates and air space consolidation similar to the appearance of ARDS; CT scans reveal bilateral air space consolidation with areas of ground-glass opacities with little honeycombing. Septal thickening and a subpleural distribution of the opacities may also be present.

Diagnosis

The diagnosis of acute interstitial pneumonia is made in the appropriate clinical setting in a patient who has a clinical presentation compatible with ARDS but without a clear etiology. The differential diagnosis histologically and clinically includes other causes of ARDS (Chapter 105), such as severe infection, trauma, and sepsis, and other causes of acute lung injury (Chapter 94), such as drug toxicity, inhalation injury, and collagen vascular diseases. The presentation is clinically and radiographically similar to that of diffuse alveolar hemorrhage, acute hypersensitivity pneumonitis, acute exacerbation of pulmonary fibrosis, acute eosinophilic pneumonia, and cryptogenic organizing pneumonia. Bronchoscopy with bronchoalveolar lavage is often performed to exclude alveolar hemorrhage, eosinophilic pneumonias, and infectious causes of lung injury. In a small number of cases, transbronchial biopsy may yield the diagnosis, but definitive diagnosis in the majority of cases of acute interstitial pneumonia requires a surgical lung biopsy.

Treatment

Rx

Treatment includes supportive intensive care unit management. In small case series, corticosteroids at doses of 1 g of methylprednisolone intravenously per day for three consecutive days followed by prednisone or equivalent at 1 mg/kg/day with a taper during several weeks to months, with or without cyclophosphamide, may be of benefit, but mortality remains higher than 60% during the subsequent 6 months. Patients also can have recurrences in months to years. Some cases of acute interstitial pneumonia may resolve without sequelae, but in some series, more than 50% of survivors may be left with residual fibrosis.

DIFFUSE ALVEOLAR HEMORRHAGE

Definition

The alveolar hemorrhage syndromes cause alveolar filling disease, usually with an acute onset and often with life-threatening severity. They can be associated with vasculitides, such as microscopic polyangiitis (Chapter 291) and Wegener's vasculitis (Chapter 291); immunologic diseases, such as Goodpasture's syndrome (anti–glomerular basement membrane antibody disease; Chapter 122); collagen vascular diseases, such as systemic lupus erythematosus (Chapter 287); cocaine inhalation (Chapter 32); drugs (including penicillamine, mitomycin C, trimellitic anhydride, all-*trans* retinoic acid, propylthiouracil, and isocyanates); bone marrow transplantation (Chapter 184); coagulopathy (Chapter 180); and mitral stenosis (Chapter 75). A small percentage of idiopathic and recurrent cases are termed idiopathic pulmonary hemosiderosis. In Goodpasture's syndrome, there is a strong association with tobacco use and a male predominance, with young men most frequently affected. A viral syndrome and exposure to hydrocarbons may simulate Goodpasture's disease. Idiopathic pulmonary hemosiderosis most often occurs in children and young adults.

Pathobiology

Alveolar hemorrhage is caused by bleeding from the pulmonary microcirculation, including the capillaries, arterioles, and venules. It may be associated with injury or neutrophilic inflammation of the capillaries or a capillaritis, usually when it is associated with collagen vascular or vasculitic processes. In Goodpasture's syndrome, for example, the circulating anti–glomerular basement membrane antibodies are directed against the α_3 chain of type IV collagen in the glomerular basement membrane, where they cause glomerulonephritis; these core antibodies can cross-react with the alveolar capillary basement membranes, resulting in alveolar hemorrhage. Alternatively, alveolar hemorrhage may be associated with relatively bland pathologic changes with red blood cells in the alveolar spaces. Idiopathic pulmonary hemosiderosis is an example of bland hemorrhage.

Clinical Manifestations

Patients present acutely (usually in hours to a week) with dyspnea, shortness of breath, hemoptysis (which may not be present in all patients), and cough. Some patients also have low-grade fever. Lung examination reveals rales.

Laboratory examination may reveal anemia. In Goodpasture's syndrome and Wegener's granulomatosis, hematuria and renal insufficiency due to glomerulonephritis are typically present.

Radiographic features include the acute development of bilateral alveolar filling disease similar to pulmonary edema but without cardiomegaly or pleural effusions. Rapid remission and recurrences are seen with repeated episodes of bleeding, which also may result in chronic interstitial changes on the chest radiograph. Pulmonary function testing may reveal an increase in the diffusion capacity for carbon monoxide because of the presence of hemoglobin in the alveolar spaces.

Diagnosis

The diagnosis of alveolar hemorrhage is usually made in the appropriate clinical setting by the triad of diffuse alveolar infiltrates, hemoptysis (in two thirds of patients), and anemia. Bronchoalveolar lavage typically demonstrates the return of progressively more bloody aliquots of fluid, and cytologic analysis reveals that more than 20% of the macrophages are hemosiderin laden. Goodpasture's syndrome is diagnosed by circulating anti–glomerular basement membrane antibodies, which are present in more than 90% of patients, or by the demonstration of linear deposition of immunoglobulin G antibodies along the alveolar or renal capillary basement membrane tissue when it is viewed by direct immunofluorescence. Wegener's granulomatosis causes a focal, segmental, necrotizing glomerulonephritis and is associated with the presence of proteinase 3 antineutrophilic cytoplasmic antibodies in 90% of active cases (Chapter 291). Necrotizing granulomatous inflammation is often found in the upper airway in addition to the lungs and kidneys. A perinuclear myeloperoxidase antineutrophilic antibody is often present in association with microscopic polyarteritis (Chapter 291). Patients with systemic lupus erythematosus usually have antinuclear antibodies (Chapter 287). Idiopathic pulmonary hemosiderosis is a diagnosis of exclusion after other causes of diffuse alveolar hemorrhage have been eliminated.

Treatment

Treatment of alveolar hemorrhage varies according to its underlying cause. Massive hemoptysis from any cause of alveolar hemorrhage should be managed as needed. In the case of drug- or toxin-related alveolar hemorrhage, the offending agent should be withdrawn, and supportive care is indicated. In Goodpasture's syndrome, Wegener's granulomatosis, and other vasculitides (Chapter 291), treatment typically includes immunosuppressant agents such as corticosteroids (methylprednisolone, 500 to 2000 mg/day in divided doses for 3 to 5 days followed by a prednisone taper beginning at 1 mg/kg/day during the next 6 to 9 months) and cyclophosphamide (2 mg/kg/day orally or 0.75 g/m^2 intravenously for one dose). In Goodpasture's syndrome, plasmapheresis is also a mainstay of therapy to remove the offending circulating antibody.

Prognosis

Recurrent alveolar hemorrhage from any cause, such as idiopathic pulmonary hemosiderosis, can be associated with the development of pulmonary fibrosis. Alveolar hemorrhage related to collagen vascular disease, vasculitides, and idiopathic pulmonary hemosiderosis can have mortality rates ranging from 25 to 50%. With Goodpasture's syndrome, renal failure is common, and degree of renal impairment may correlate with outcome.

BRONCHIOLOALVEOLAR CELL CARCINOMA

Definition

Bronchioloalveolar cell carcinoma, which is a bronchogenic adenocarcinoma, is characterized by well-differentiated, malignant cells lining the alveolar cell wall (Chapter 201). Of bronchogenic carcinomas, bronchioloalveolar cell carcinoma is the least strongly associated with tobacco use, with a higher relative risk in nonsmoking individuals. There is a female-to-male predominance of 1.4 : 1, and younger patients may be affected.

Pathobiology

Bronchioloalveolar cell carcinoma usually arises in the periphery of the lung and is characterized by lepidic growth, which means contiguous growth along the intact alveolar septa, without stromal, pleural, or lymphatic invasion and without a known primary adenocarcinoma elsewhere. Bronchioloalveolar cell carcinoma can be categorized into mucinous and nonmucinous forms histologically; the mucinous type is thought to derive from respiratory goblet cells, and the nonmucinous type from type II pneumocytes or Clara cells.

Clinical Manifestations

Patients present with the gradual onset of shortness of breath and cough. The duration of symptoms is usually several months. Constitutional symptoms such as malaise and weight loss may be present. An unusual but unique clinical finding is bronchorrhea, with patients reporting the production of copious amounts of clear sputum daily. This finding is more common in the pneumonic form of disease.

Diagnosis

Radiographic patterns vary and can include localized disease with peripheral solitary or multiple nodules or masses in 60% of cases or a persistent pneumonic pattern in 40% of cases (Fig. 91–4). The radiographic findings are often thought to be consistent with pneumonia, and a typical clinical presentation is that of a nonresolving peripheral density on chest radiograph. Positron emission tomography may be normal because of the low glucose uptake of this lesion. The diagnosis of bronchioloalveolar cell carcinoma is most often made by bronchoscopy with transbronchial biopsy.

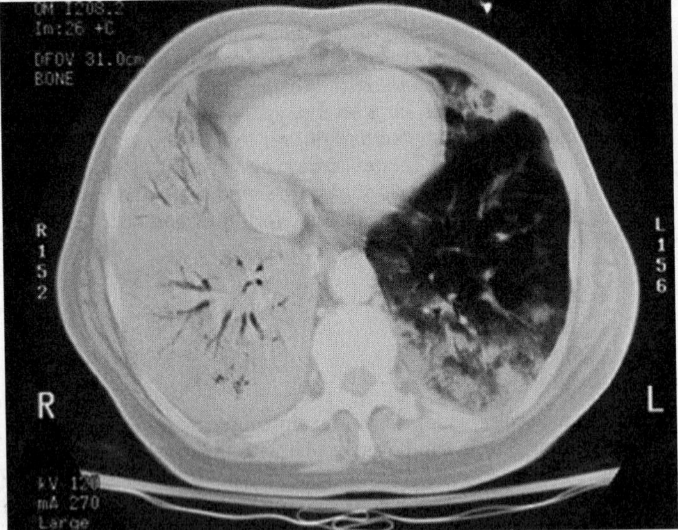

FIGURE 91–4 • A chest computed tomographic scan in a patient with bronchioloalveolar cell cancer revealing the pneumonic form of the disease.

Treatment

For staging and treatment, bronchioloalveolar cell carcinoma is approached like other types of non–small cell lung cancer (Chapter 201). Bilateral lung transplantation has been performed, but recurrence in the transplanted lungs has been reported.

Prognosis

Prognosis correlates with disease stage and probably with the histologic and radiographic patterns. Patients with a single focus of disease (i.e., a solitary nodule) who undergo surgical resection have a prognosis better than that of patients with non-bronchioloalveolar adenocarcinomas of like stage. Multinodular, pneumonic, and diffuse forms of disease have a worse prognosis, as does the mucinous histologic subtype.

SUGGESTED READINGS

Collard HR, Schwarz MI: Diffuse alveolar hemorrhage. Clin Chest Med 2004;25:583–592. *An excellent review of this topic.*

Swigris JJ, Brown KK: Acute interstitial pneumonia and acute exacerbations of idiopathic pulmonary fibrosis. Semin Respir Crit Care Med 2006;27:659–667. *Each has a case-fatality rate approaching 70%.*

Trapnell BC, Whitsett JA, Nakata K: Pulmonary alveolar proteinosis. N Engl J Med 2003;349:2527–2539. *A comprehensive review of this topic.*

92 INTERSTITIAL LUNG DISEASE

Ganesh Raghu

Definition

In an apparent immunocompetent host, interstitial lung disease (ILD) is a clinical term for a heterogenous group of lower respiratory tract disorders with many potential causes. Common initial features include exertional dyspnea, a restrictive pattern of physiologic abnormality on pulmonary function testing (Chapter 85), decreased diffusing capacity (DLCO), increased alveolar-arterial oxygen difference ($PAO_2 - PaO_2$) at rest or during exertion, and absence of pulmonary infection or neoplasm. ILDs comprise several acute and chronic lung disorders with variable degrees of pulmonary fibrosis (Table 92–1). The term *interstitial* in the commonly used acronym ILD is a misnomer because the pathophysiologic processes are not restricted to the interstitium, which is the microscopic space bounded by the basement membranes of epithelial and endothelial cells. Rather, all of the several cellular and soluble constituents that make up the gas exchange units (alveolar wall, capillaries, alveolar space, and acini), bronchiolar lumen, terminal bronchioles, and pulmonary parenchyma beyond the gas exchange units (as well as the pleura, lymphatics, and sometimes the lymph nodes) are involved in the pathogenesis and manifestations of ILD.

Epidemiology

A population-based registry in New Mexico of patients 18 years or older derived a prevalence of all ILDs in the United States of 80.9 per 100,000 men and 67.2 per 100,000 women. The overall incidence was also higher in men (31.5 per 100,000 per year) than in women (26.1 per 100,000 per year). Moreover, the prevalence of undiagnosed or early ILD is estimated to be 10 times that of clinically recognized disease; as physicians' awareness of these entities increases, it is expected that the frequency of the diagnosis of ILD will rise. Among the ILDs, the most common is idiopathic pulmonary fibrosis, which represents at least 30% of incident cases. In the United States, the annual incidence is estimated to be 6.8 to 16.3 per 100,000, with a prevalence of 14.0 to 42.7 per 100,000.

TABLE 92–1 CLINICAL CLASSIFICATION OF INTERSTITIAL LUNG DISEASE

IDIOPATHIC INTERSTITIAL PNEUMONIAS
Idiopathic pulmonary fibrosis
Nonspecific pulmonary fibrosis
Respiratory bronchiolitis–associated interstitial lung disease
Desquamative interstitial pneumonia
Acute interstitial pneumonia
Cryptogenic organizing pneumonia
Lymphoid interstitial pneumonia
INTERSTITIAL LUNG DISEASE ASSOCIATED WITH COLLAGEN VASCULAR DISEASE
Progressive systemic sclerosis
Rheumatoid arthritis
Systemic lupus erythematosus
Dermatomyositis/polymyositis
Sjögren's syndrome
Mixed connective tissue disease
Ankylosing spondylitis
HYPERSENSITIVITY PNEUMONITIS
Occupational and environmental interstitial lung disease
Drug-induced/iatrogenic interstitial lung disease
ALVEOLAR FILLING DISORDERS (Chapter 91)
Goodpasture's syndrome
Pulmonary alveolar proteinosis
Pulmonary hemosiderosis
Pulmonary hemorrhage
Chronic eosinophilic pneumonia
INTERSTITIAL LUNG DISEASE ASSOCIATED WITH PULMONARY VASCULITIS
Wegener's granulomatosis
Churg-Strauss syndrome
OTHER FORMS OF INTERSTITIAL LUNG DISEASE
Sarcoidosis
Langerhans cell histiocytosis (histiocytosis X)
Lymphangioleiomyomatosis
INHERITED FORMS OF INTERSTITIAL LUNG DISEASE
Familial idiopathic pulmonary fibrosis or interstitial pneumonia
Tuberous sclerosis
Neurofibromatosis
Gaucher's disease
Niemann-Pick disease
Hermansky-Pudlak syndrome

Pathobiology

ILDs result from tissue injury and attempted repair in the lung in a genetically predisposed person, but how genetic factors determine the host/lung response in concert with risk factors is unknown. As a result, *the inciting cause is obscure in several ILDs.*

In *idiopathic pulmonary fibrosis,* the varying degrees of acute, subacute, and chronic fibroproliferation that are present in the lungs at the time of diagnosis are thought to be due to abnormal parenchymal wound healing resulting in intraluminal and interstitial fibrosis, with progressive loss of the alveolar surface area. Ultimately, progressive fibrosis will result in honeycombing, an end-stage finding that is often associated with increased pulmonary vascular resistance and secondary pulmonary hypertension. As a reflection of these dynamic processes, histopathologic examination of lung tissue often reveals highly heterogeneous findings; for example, a single biopsy specimen may show normal alveoli adjacent to abnormal areas of inflammation and fibrosis, with or without granulomas, vasculitis, or secondary vascular changes within the pulmonary parenchyma.

Clinical Manifestations

ILDs are typically characterized by progressive dyspnea. Nonproductive cough and fatigue are also common complaints. Pleuritic chest pain may occur with certain collagen vascular or drug-induced ILDs, whereas acute pleuritic chest pain with dyspnea may represent a spontaneous pneumothorax (Chapter 100) in association with lymphangioleiomyomatosis, tuberous sclerosis (Chapter 444), neurofibromatosis, or Langerhans' cell histiocytosis. Hemoptysis suggests a diffuse alveolar hemorrhagic syndrome, systemic lupus erythematosus (Chapter 287), lymphangioleiomyomatosis, Wegener's granulomatosis (Chapter 291), or Goodpasture's syndrome (Chapter 122); it is rare in other ILDs. In patients with existing ILD, new hemoptysis should prompt consideration of a superimposed malignancy, pulmonary embolus, or infection such as aspergillosis.

In some patients, the first clue may be the finding of coarse rales (crackles) on auscultation of the lungs. These coarse crackles must be distinguished from the finer rales typical of heart failure (Chapter 57) or noncardiogenic pulmonary edema (Chapter 105). Unlike patients with obstructive lung disease, wheezes are not common. A history of wheezing suggests the coexistence of occult hyperactive airways/airflow obstruction and raises the possibility of allergic bronchopulmonary aspergillosis (Chapter 360), Churg-Strauss syndrome (Chapter 291), chronic eosinophilic pneumonia (see later), or parasitic infection (Chapter 365). In some patients, the initial presentation may be with peripheral cyanosis, clubbing, or the signs and symptoms of an underlying systemic disease (see below).

Diagnosis

The first key in patients with an ILD is to establish the syndromic diagnosis and then pursue the differential diagnosis of its specific cause (Fig. 92–1). However, a conclusive cause may not often be identified despite exhaustive medical history taking and invasive diagnostic interventions, including sufficiently large and multiple lung biopsy specimens. Thus, the cause/etiology of several of the ILDs, even when diagnosed as specific entities, remains unknown.

History

The patient's age, sex, and cigarette smoking history may provide useful clues to the diagnosis. Idiopathic pulmonary fibrosis is an adult disorder that usually occurs in patients older than 50 years of age. Pulmonary sarcoidosis (Chapter 95), in contrast, is more common in young adults and middle-aged persons. Pulmonary Langerhans cell histiocytosis (previously known as pulmonary histiocytosis X or eosinophilic granuloma) characteristically occurs in young cigarette-smoking males, whereas lymphangioleiomyomatosis occurs exclusively in women of childbearing age. Respiratory bronchiolitis–associated interstitial lung disease is seen almost exclusively in cigarette smokers but occurs in both men and women of all ages.

The medical history also should focus on environmental factors, especially changes in environmental exposure (domestic, recreational, hot tub, Jacuzzi, indoor swimming pool, ventilation system at home, automobiles, and workplace), occupational exposure, medication, and drug use (Chapters 93 and 94). A family medical history should address possible familial ILD. Environmental risk factors that may suggest the diagnosis of hypersensitivity pneumonitis include farming or exposure to birds (bird fancier's lung or pigeon breeder's lung) or humidifiers in the domestic environment (hypersensitivity to thermophilic actinomycetes). Other at-risk occupations include mining (pneumoconioses), machine tool grinding, sandblasting and working with granite (silicosis), welding and working in a shipyard (asbestosis), and working in the aerospace or electronic industries (berylliosis) (Chapters 93 and 94). Because of the long interval between the exposure and the onset of symptoms in many occupations associated with ILD, it is important to take a lifelong occupational history (Chapter 17), as well as establish the interval between exposure and the onset of symptoms. Because the list of medications

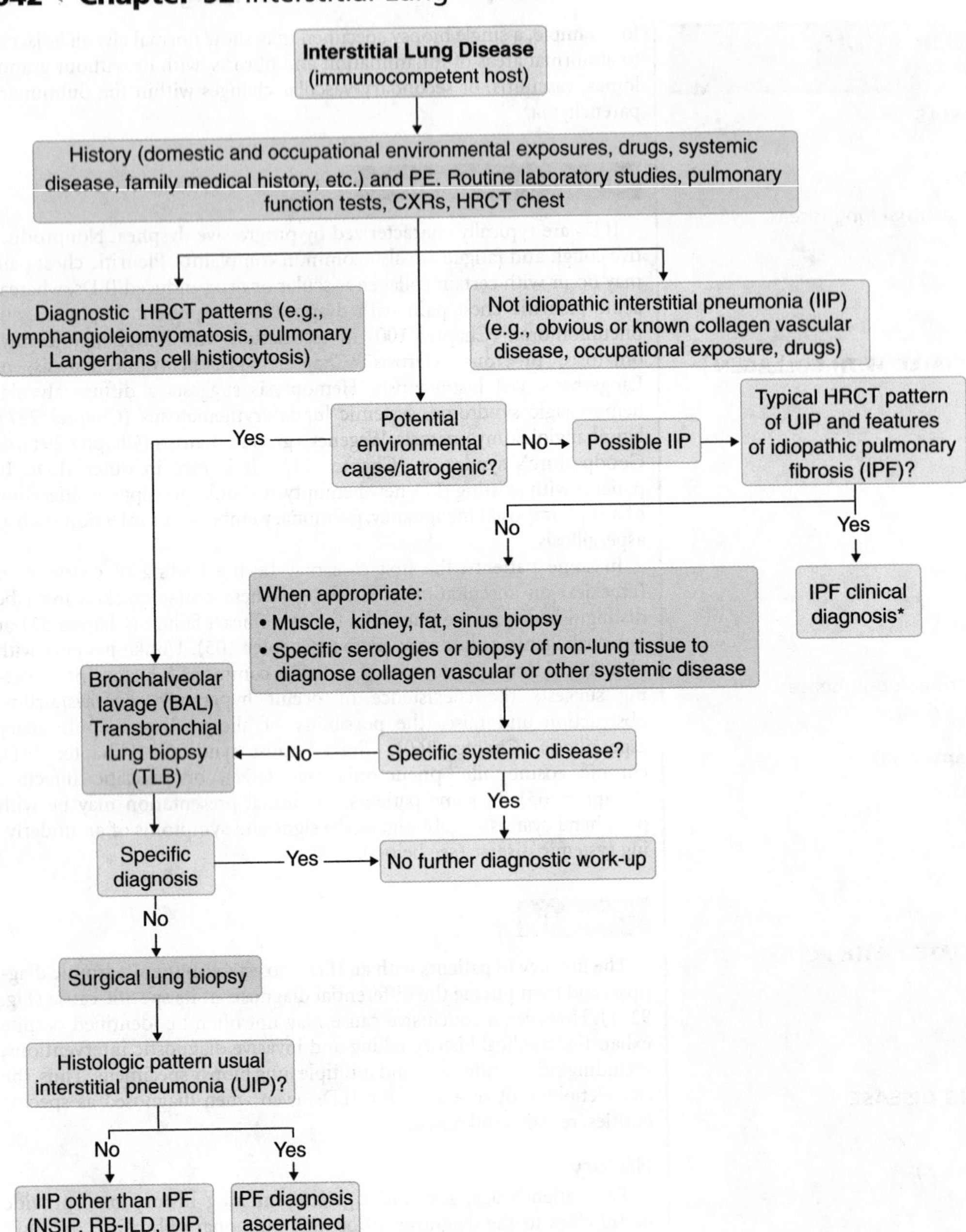

FIGURE 92–1 • An approach to interstitial lung disease. *American Thoracic Society/European Respiratory Society Criteria: Idiopathic pulmonary fibrosis: Diagnosis and treatment. International consensus statement. Am J Respir Crit Care Med 2000;161:646–664. **American Thoracic Society/European Respiratory Society: International multidisciplinary consensus classification of idiopathic interstitial pneumonias. Am J Respir Crit Care Med 2002;165:277–304. HRCT = high-resolution computed tomography; PE = physical examination.

known to cause ILD is long and continues to grow (Table 92–2), a careful history regarding recent use of prescription and over-the-counter products is essential. Risk factors for immunosuppression, including infection with human immunodeficiency virus, raise the possibility of opportunistic lung infections (Chapter 414), neoplasm (Chapter 201), and transplant-related pulmonary complications.

Particular attention should be paid to the onset and duration of symptoms, the rate of disease progression, and association with hemoptysis, fever, or extrathoracic symptoms. Symptoms lasting 4 weeks or less and the presence of fever suggest cryptogenic organizing pneumonia, drug-induced pulmonary injury, or hypersensitivity pneumonitis, whereas idiopathic pulmonary fibrosis, ILD associated with connective tissue diseases, and Langerhans cell histiocytosis tend to have a more subacute onset. Extrathoracic symptoms such as dysphagia, dry eyes or mouth, or arthritis may suggest a collagen vascular disorder (Chapters 287 and 291) or sarcoidosis (Chapter 95). Proximal muscle weakness suggests the possibility of polymyositis/dermatomyositis (Chapter 290), and recurrent sinusitis suggests Wegener's granulomatosis (Chapter 291). Extrathoracic manifestations present in tuberous sclerosis (Chapter 444) include hematuria, epilepsy, and mental retardation.

Physical Examination

Physical examination of the respiratory system is rarely helpful in the diagnostic evaluation of ILD because findings such rhonchi and rales on auscultation or digital clubbing are nonspecific. Findings on cardiac examination, such as an accentuated P_2, a right ventricular heave, or tricuspid insufficiency, are suggestive of pulmonary hypertension (Chapter 67) and cor pulmonale in patients with advanced lung disease. However, extrathoracic findings such as skin abnormalities, peripheral lymphadenopathy, and hepatosplenomegaly may be more specifically associated with underlying sarcoidosis (Chapter 95); muscle tenderness and proximal muscle weakness may point to coexisting polymyositis (Chapter 290); and signs of arthritis may indicate collagen vascular disease (Chapters 285, 287, and 291) or sarcoidosis (Chapter 95). Characteristic rashes occur in several collagen vascular diseases, disseminated Langerhans cell histiocytosis, tuberous sclerosis, and neurofibromatosis. Ophthalmologic

TABLE 92–2 COMMON DRUG-INDUCED/IATROGENIC INTERSTITIAL LUNG DISEASE

ANTIMICROBIAL AGENTS
Cephalosporins
Isoniazid
Nitrofurantoin
Penicillins
Sulfonamides
ANTI-INFLAMMATORY AGENTS
Aspirin
Gold
Methotrexate
Nonsteroidal anti-inflammatory agents
Penicillamine
Phenylbutazone
Zafirlukast
CARDIOVASCULAR DRUGS
Amiodarone
Angiotensin-converting enzyme inhibitors
β-Blockers
Hydralazine
Hydrochlorothiazide
Procainamide
Protamine sulfate
Tocainide
ANTINEOPLASTIC AGENTS
Bleomycin
Busulfan
Chlorambucil
Cyclophosphamide
Melphalan
Mercaptopurine
Mitomycin
Mitomycin C
Nitrosoureas
Procarbazine
CENTRAL NERVOUS SYSTEM DRUGS
Carbamazepine
Chlorpromazine
Imipramine
Phenytoin
ORAL HYPOGLYCEMIC AGENTS
Chlorpropamide
Tolazamide
Tolbutamide
ILLICIT DRUGS
Cocaine
Heroin
Methadone
Propoxyphene
OTHER AGENTS
High FIO_2 (fraction of inspired oxygen) with mechanical ventilation
Interferon alfa
Irradiation

findings (Chapter 449) such as iridocyclitis, uveitis, or conjunctivitis may be a clue to the diagnosis of sarcoidosis or a collagen vascular disease, whereas central nervous system abnormalities may be present in sarcoidosis, systemic lupus erythematosus, Langerhans cell histiocytosis, or tuberous sclerosis.

Laboratory Testing

Routine laboratory testing should include a complete blood count, leukocyte differential, erythrocyte sedimentation rate, chemistry panel (calcium, liver enzymes, electrolytes, creatinine), and urinalysis. Although these data rarely yield a specific diagnosis, they may provide helpful clues. When appropriate, patients should be screened for systemic lupus erythematosus (e.g., antinuclear antibodies), rheumatoid arthritis (rheumatoid factor), polymyositis (creatine kinase, aldolase, and anti–Jo-1 antibody), Wegener's granulomatosis (antineutrophil cytoplasmic antibodies), and Goodpasture's syndrome (anti–basement membrane antibodies).

Mild hypoxemia is typically present on arterial blood gas analysis because of abnormal ventilation-perfusion ratios, especially in moderate to severe cases of ILD. However, carbon dioxide retention is rare and suggests possible coexisting emphysema (Chapter 88) or a hypoventilatory disorder (Chapter 86).

Noninvasive Evaluation

Chest Radiograph

The distribution and appearance of radiographic abnormalities (Chapter 84) may prove useful in differentiating the clinicopathologic syndromes in patients with ILD (Table 92–3). Comparison of previous chest radiographs with the current one is important in establishing the rate of progression of the patient's disease. A diffuse ground-glass pattern is often observed early in the course of ILD, followed by progression to reticular (linear) infiltrates with nodules (reticulonodular infiltrates) or, in the case of alveolar filling disorders, ill-defined nodules (acinar rosettes) with air bronchograms. The majority of ILDs cause infiltrates in the lower lung zones, but upper lobe predominance is typically present in sarcoidosis, berylliosis, Langerhans cell histiocytosis, silicosis, chronic hypersensitivity pneumonitis, cystic fibrosis, and ankylosing spondylitis, whereas the middle and lower lung zones show the most prominent abnormalities in lymphangitic carcinomatosis, idiopathic pulmonary fibrosis, subacute eosinophilic pneumonia, asbestosis, and pulmonary fibrosis caused by rheumatoid arthritis or progressive systemic sclerosis. Hilar adenopathy and mediastinal adenopathy are not common in ILDs; their presence should suggest sarcoidosis, berylliosis, silicosis, lymphocytic interstitial pneumonia, amyloidosis, or Gaucher's disease. A pattern of peripherally located pulmonary infiltrates in the upper and middle lung zones with relatively clear perihilar and central zones is a clue to chronic eosinophilic pneumonia. Recurrent infiltrates raise the possibility of cryptogenic organizing pneumonia, chronic eosinophilic pneumonia, or drug- or radiation-induced pneumonitis, whereas fleeting or migratory infiltrates may occur in Churg-Strauss syndrome (allergic angiitis), allergic bronchopulmonary aspergillosis, tropical eosinophilic pneumonia, or Löffler's syndrome. Localized pleural plaques may indicate asbestosis, whereas diffuse pleural thickening can result from asbestosis, rheumatoid arthritis, progressive systemic sclerosis, radiation pneumonitis, nitrofurantoin, or malignancy. In the absence of left ventricular failure, the presence of a pleural effusion (Chapter 100) raises the possibility of rheumatoid arthritis, systemic lupus erythematosus, acute hypersensitivity pneumonitis, sarcoidosis, asbestosis, amyloidosis, lymphangioleiomyomatosis, or lymphangitic carcinomatosis. Reduction of lung volumes is typical in the majority of ILDs; the presence of preserved lung volumes or hyperinflation should raise suspicion for chronic hypersensitivity pneumonitis, Langerhans cell histiocytosis, lymphangioleiomyomatosis, neurofibromatosis, sarcoidosis, or tuberous sclerosis. Finally, in about 10% of patients with biopsy-proven ILD, plain chest radiographs are normal despite "microscopic ILD."

High-Resolution Computed Tomography

Because of its increased sensitivity and ability to distinguish active, reversible areas of lung disease from irreversible fibrotic and honeycomb changes, high-resolution computed tomography (HRCT) is essential in both the diagnosis and staging of ILD. Although microscopic ILD cannot be excluded by a normal HRCT, HRCT allows earlier diagnosis, helps narrow the differential diagnosis patterns (Table 92–4), aids in selecting the site or sites for bronchoalveolar lavage and lung biopsy, and assists in choosing among therapeutic options and in estimating the response to treatment. The presence of patchy subpleural reticular and basilar septal fibrosis, traction bronchiectasis, and honeycombing increases the level of diagnostic confidence for idiopathic pulmonary fibrosis. The finding of bilateral cysts, including their size, configuration, distribution, and

TABLE 92–3 CHARACTERISTIC CHEST RADIOGRAPHIC PATTERNS IN PATIENTS WITH INTERSTITIAL LUNG DISEASE

Pattern	Suggested Diagnoses*
Decreased lung volumes	Idiopathic pulmonary fibrosis, nonspecific interstitial pneumonia, desquamative interstitial pneumonia, collagen vascular disease, chronic eosinophilic pneumonia, asbestosis, chronic hypersensitivity pneumonitis or drug-induced ILD
Increased or preserved lung volumes	Idiopathic pulmonary fibrosis with emphysema, respiratory bronchiolitis–associated ILD, cryptogenic organizing pneumonia, hypersensitivity pneumonitis, lymphangioleiomyomatosis, Langerhans cell histiocytosis, sarcoidosis, neurofibromatosis, tuberous sclerosis
Micronodules	Infection, hypersensitivity pneumonitis, sarcoidosis, respiratory bronchiolitis–associated ILD
Septal thickening	Malignancy, infection, chronic congestive heart failure, pulmonary veno-occlusive disease
Honeycombing	Idiopathic pulmonary fibrosis, fibrotic nonspecific interstitial pneumonia, collagen vascular disease, asbestosis, chronic hypersensitivity pneumonitis, sarcoidosis
Recurrent infiltrates	Cryptogenic organizing pneumonia, chronic eosinophilic pneumonia, drug- or radiation-induced ILD
Migratory or fleeting infiltrates	Cryptogenic organizing pneumonia, hypersensitivity pneumonitis, Churg-Strauss syndrome, Löffler's syndrome, allergic bronchopulmonary aspergillosis
Pleural disease	Collagen vascular disease, asbestosis, malignancy, radiation-induced ILD, amyloidosis, sarcoidosis, lymphangioleiomyomatosis, nitrofurantoin-induced ILD
Pneumothorax	Langerhans cell histiocytosis, lymphangioleiomyomatosis, tuberous sclerosis, neurofibromatosis
Mediastinal and/or hilar adenopathy	Lymphocytic interstitial pneumonia, collagen vascular disease, silicosis, chronic berylliosis, malignancy, infection, sarcoidosis, amyloidosis, Gaucher's disease
Normal (rare)	Cellular nonspecific interstitial pneumonia, respiratory bronchiolitis–associated interstitial lung disease, collagen vascular disease, hypersensitivity pneumonitis, sarcoidosis
Location of Radiographic Abnormality	**Suggested Diagnoses***
Mid to upper lung zone	Hypersensitivity pneumonitis, chronic berylliosis, ankylosing spondylitis, silicosis, Langerhans cell histiocytosis, sarcoidosis, cystic fibrosis
Lower lung zone	Idiopathic pulmonary fibrosis, collagen vascular disease, asbestosis, chronic hypersensitivity pneumonitis
Peripheral	Idiopathic pulmonary fibrosis, cryptogenic organizing pneumonia, chronic eosinophilic pneumonia

*This list is not intended to be comprehensive.
ILD = interstitial lung disease.
Adapted from Raghu G, Brown K: Clinical issues: Patient evaluation. *In* Baughman RP, du Bois RM (eds): Diffuse Lung Disease. A Practical Approach. New York, Oxford University Press, 2004.

TABLE 92–4 RADIOGRAPHIC FEATURES OF THE IDIOPATHIC INTERSTITIAL PNEUMONIAS

Clinical Diagnosis	Usual Radiographic Features	Typical Findings on HRCT
Idiopathic pulmonary fibrosis	Basal-predominant reticulation abnormality with volume loss	Peripheral, basal, subpleural reticulation with honeycombing, traction bronchiectasis, and focal ground-glass attenuation
Nonspecific interstitial pneumonia	Ground-glass and reticular opacification	Peripheral, basal, subpleural, symmetrical ground-glass attenuation with irregular lines and consolidation
Cryptogenic organizing pneumonia	Patchy bilateral consolidation	Subpleural or peribronchial patchy consolidation and/or nodules
Acute interstitial pneumonia	Diffuse ground-glass density/consolidation	Diffuse consolidation and ground-glass opacification, often with lobular sparing and late traction bronchiectasis
Desquamative interstitial pneumonia	Ground-glass opacity	Peripheral, lower lung zone ground-glass attenuation with reticulation and/or small cysts
Respiratory bronchiolitis–associated interstitial lung disease	Bronchial wall thickening, ground-glass opacification	Diffuse bronchial wall thickening with poorly defined centrilobular nodules and patchy ground-glass opacification
Lymphocytic interstitial pneumonia	Reticular opacities and nodules	Diffuse centrilobular nodules, ground-glass attenuation, septal and bronchovascular wall thickening, and thin-walled cysts

HRCT = high-resolution computed tomography.
Adapted from American Thoracic Society/European Respiratory Society: International multidisciplinary consensus classification of the idiopathic interstitial pneumonias. Am J Respir Crit Care Med 2002;165:277–304.

appearance, helps differentiate among lymphangioleiomyomatosis, tuberous sclerosis, and pulmonary Langerhans cell histiocytosis. HRCT can detect ILD despite normal chest radiographs in patients with asbestosis, silicosis, sarcoidosis, and scleroderma. Patients with respiratory bronchiolitis–associated interstitial lung disease typically have patchy ground-glass attenuation on HRCT in concert with bilateral interstitial prominence/fine nodular radiographic infiltrates and normal lung volumes.

Pulmonary Function Tests

The most characteristic physiologic abnormalities in patients with ILD, regardless of etiology, are a restrictive lung defect and decreased DLCO

(Chapter 85). Forced expiratory volume in 1 second (FEV_1) and forced vital capacity (FVC) are decreased proportionally such that the ratio of the two remains normal or may even be increased. Both total lung capacity and lung volumes measured by body plethysmography are reduced. Pulmonary function tests (PFTs) may be useful in monitoring the progression of disease and prognosis; significant changes in FVC, DLCO (corrected to hemoglobin), and physiologic measurements (FVC, DLCO) at 1 year portend a worse survival in patients with idiopathic pulmonary fibrosis.

Certain PFT findings may also aid in the differential diagnosis. A mixed obstructive-restrictive pattern occurs in patients with Churg-Strauss syndrome, allergic bronchopulmonary aspergillosis, endobronchial sarcoidosis, cryptogenic organizing pneumonia, tropical pulmonary interstitial eosinophilia, coexisting chronic obstructive pulmonary disease or asthma, or secondary bronchiectasis. Diseases associated with respiratory muscle weakness, such as polymyositis, progressive systemic sclerosis, and systemic lupus erythematosus, may exhibit a decrease in maximal voluntary ventilation and increased residual volume out of proportion to the decrease in FEV_1.

Exercise Testing

The magnitude of the increase in $PAO_2 - PaO_2$ on exercise correlates well with the severity of disease and the degree of pulmonary fibrosis in patients with idiopathic pulmonary fibrosis. Other exercise-induced physiologic abnormalities in ILD include a decrease in work rate and maximal oxygen consumption, abnormally high minute ventilation at submaximal work rates, decreased peak minute ventilation, and failure of tidal volumes to increase at submaximal levels of work while the respiratory rate increases disproportionately. The 6-minute walk test, performed on a flat surface, may be sensitive in detecting clinically relevant variables such as walk distance covered, walk velocity, and oxygen desaturation with exercise.

Invasive Evaluation

Bronchoscopy

Findings on bronchoalveolar lavage (BAL) can be diagnostic in patients with ILD. Examples include the identification of an infectious or neoplastic process, a predominance of eosinophils in the setting of clinical and radiographic findings consistent with eosinophilic pneumonia, Langerhans cells in a patient with pulmonary Langerhans cell histiocytosis, an asbestos body count greater than 1 fiber per milliliter of BAL fluid in a patient with asbestosis, or specially staining surfactant material in a patient with pulmonary alveolar proteinosis (see Table 85–3). A transbronchial lung biopsy may reveal distinctive pathologic abnormalities in sarcoidosis (noncaseating granulomas), hard metal pneumoconiosis (giant cell granulomas), or lymphangioleiomyomatosis (smooth muscle proliferation identified with special stains). However, failure to establish a diagnosis on BAL and transbronchial lung biopsy does not exclude these entities.

Surgical Lung Biopsy

Video-assisted thoracoscopic biopsy (Chapter 102) or open lung biopsy may be required to obtain an adequate sample for histologic evaluation of a patient with unexplained signs and symptoms when other studies have failed to establish a diagnosis. The mortality rate for the procedure is less than 1%, and the morbidity is less than 3%. Patients with typical clinical, radiographic, and HRCT features of idiopathic pulmonary fibrosis generally do not benefit from biopsy given the high likelihood of an accurate diagnosis based on a thorough assessment of the findings of all recommended clinical tests. A collegial interaction among the pulmonary clinician, radiologist, thoracic surgeon, and pathologist can help decide on the best approach for complicated patients (see Fig. 92–1).

Treatment

When the cause of the ILD is clearly known (e.g., acute/subacute hypersensitivity pneumonitis, occupational ILD, iatrogenic), further avoidance of the inciting agent or agents is essential. Although systemic corticosteroids are generally indicated and are associated with good response in some ILDs, the dosage and duration are unclear and essentially based on anecdotal experience (Table 92–5).

Supportive oxygen supplementation is dictated by clinical needs. For selected patients with end-stage ILDs, such as those associated with significant pulmonary fibrosis and pulmonary hypertension, lung transplantation (Chapter 102) may be a feasible and viable option.

TABLE 92–5 INTERSTITIAL LUNG DISEASE: CLINICAL RESPONSE TO SYSTEMIC CORTICOSTEROIDS*

Generally Responsive	Unresponsive
Sarcoidosis	Idiopathic interstitial pneumonia
Acute hypersensitivity pneumonitis	Idiopathic pulmonary fibrosis (usual interstitial pneumonia)
Drug induced	Desquamative interstitial pneumonia (subset)
Environmental causes (some)	Chronic secondary and advanced pulmonary fibrosis
Idiopathic interstitial pneumonia	Cryptogenic organizing pneumonia (subset)
Cryptogenic organizing pneumonia	Chronic pulmonary hemorrhage syndromes
Nonspecific interstitial pneumonia (cellular)	Pulmonary veno-occlusive disease
Respiratory bronchiolitis–associated ILD	Environmental (e.g., asbestosis, pneumoconiosis)
Lymphocytic interstitial pneumonia	End-stage ILDs/pulmonary fibrosis coexisting/associated with pulmonary hypertension
Desquamative interstitial pneumonia (subset)	Pulmonary Langerhans cell histiocytosis
Acute interstitial pneumonia(?)	Lymphangioleiomyomatosis
Acute pulmonary capillaritis	ILD in inherited disorders(?)
Eosinophilic pneumonia (acute and chronic)	
Acute radiation pneumonitis†	
Organizing pneumonia associated with collagen vascular diseases	

*The dosage plus duration of corticosteroids used is variable and based on anecdotal experience, individual expert opinion, clinical judgment, and response as judged by objective measurements (clinical, radiologic, and/or physiologic). Most patients who respond during the first few weeks of 20 to 60 mg of prednisone per day require maintenance low-dose oral prednisone at 5 to 10 mg/day beyond 6 months. There is no evidence to recommend a specific regimen. Patients should be monitored carefully and regularly for known side effects of corticosteroid use (e.g., osteoporosis, glucose intolerance), and preventive/therapeutic measures must be undertaken appropriately.

†Although most patients respond to modest doses of oral prednisone (initially, 40 to 60 mg/day), it is important to taper the prednisone slowly to reach a maintenance dose of 5 to 10 mg/day beyond 6 months; rapid taper of oral prednisone has been associated with "rebound"—an exaggerated lung injury beyond the irradiated segment of the lung and in the contralateral lung.

ILD = interstitial lung disease.

SPECIFIC TYPES OF INTERSTITIAL LUNG DISEASE

Idiopathic Interstitial Pneumonias

Idiopathic interstitial pneumonias, which are a subset of acute or chronic ILDs of unknown etiology, are characterized by the presence of varying degrees of interstitial and alveolar inflammation and fibrosis. A recent consensus statement by the American Thoracic Society and the European Respiratory Society recognized several distinct clinicopathologic forms of idiopathic interstitial pneumonia, including idiopathic pulmonary fibrosis, nonspecific interstitial pneumonia (NSIP), respiratory bronchiolitis–associated ILD, desquamative interstitial pneumonia, acute interstitial pneumonia, cryptogenic organizing pneumonia, and lymphocytic interstitial pneumonia.

Although clinical severity may vary, the idiopathic interstitial pneumonias tend to be manifested as an insidious onset of exertional dyspnea and a nonproductive cough. Chest pain and systemic symptoms such as weight loss and fatigue may be present. Bibasilar end-inspiratory crackles are often heard on auscultation. Clubbing, though not specific, is found in 25 to 50% of patients with idiopathic pulmonary fibrosis. Findings on the chest radiograph are most often nonspecific, and the presence of normal lung markings on the chest radiograph does not exclude ILD. On HRCT, many pathologic entities have characteristic image patterns that have greatly aided diagnosis (see Table 92–4).

Idiopathic Pulmonary Fibrosis

Epidemiology and Clinical Manifestations

Idiopathic pulmonary fibrosis, also known as cryptogenic fibrosing alveolitis, accounts for 50 to 60% of all idiopathic interstitial pneumonias. Idiopathic pulmonary fibrosis occurs in adult men and women with a mean age at onset of 57 years. It is defined as a distinct entity limited to the lungs in adults, usually older than 50 years. Typical manifestations include a gradual onset and progression of exertional dyspnea, restrictive physiologic abnormalities on PFTs, and a distinct pattern of bilateral pulmonary fibrosis on HRCT in patients who have otherwise been in good health with no known collagen vascular disease or exposure to drugs or environmental factors known to cause pulmonary fibrosis.

Diagnosis

Chest radiographs show basal-predominant reticular abnormalities with low lung volumes. The diagnostic features on HRCT are peripheral, predominantly basilar patchy intralobular reticulation, often with subpleural honeycomb cysts, traction bronchiectasis, and traction bronchiolectasis as the disease becomes more advanced (Fig. 92–2A). Reticulation may progress to honeycombing, although neither alveolar consolidation nor parenchymal nodules are present. When compared with the other idiopathic interstitial pneumonias, the HRCT appearance of idiopathic pulmonary fibrosis is distinguished by a greater extent of fibrotic abnormality, by its hallmark honeycombing, and by a notable absence of extensive ground-glass opacification, micronodules, cysts, consolidation, and extensive mediastinal adenopathy.

The cellular pattern in BAL fluid, which is nonspecific, is marked by an excess of neutrophils in proportion to the extent of reticular change on HRCT; the percentage of eosinophils may be mildly increased. The histopathologic pattern termed *usual interstitial pneumonia* consists of patchy interstitial changes alternating with zones of honeycombing, fibrosis, inflammation, collagen deposition, and normal lung (see Fig. 92–2B). Subepithelial fibroblastic foci, small aggregates of myofibroblasts, and fibroblasts within myxoid matrix are invariably present and represent areas of active fibrosis. The presence of temporal heterogeneity, or areas at different stages of fibrosis transitioning with normal areas and honeycomb cysts, along with fibrotic foci within the lung, is an essential feature of usual interstitial pneumonia that distinguishes it from other processes such as NSIP. Interstitial cellular inflammation is minimal in usual interstitial pneumonia. Although usual interstitial pneumonia characterizes the histologic abnormality in idiopathic pulmonary fibrosis, the same histologic and radiologic pattern can also be seen in patients with rheumatologic lung diseases and asbestosis (Chapter 93).

In the appropriate clinical setting (and after exclusion of other known clinical conditions associated with ILD) (see later), a definitive diagnosis of idiopathic pulmonary fibrosis is based on the presence of a pattern of

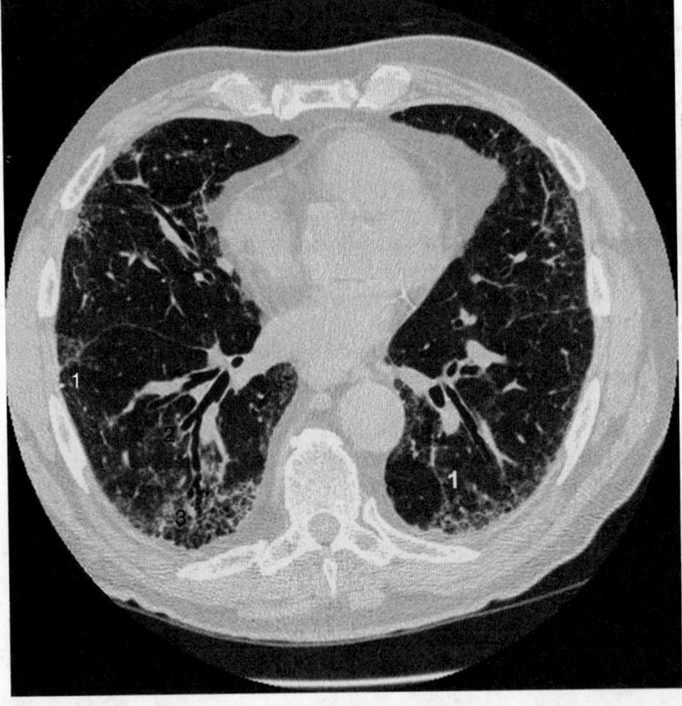

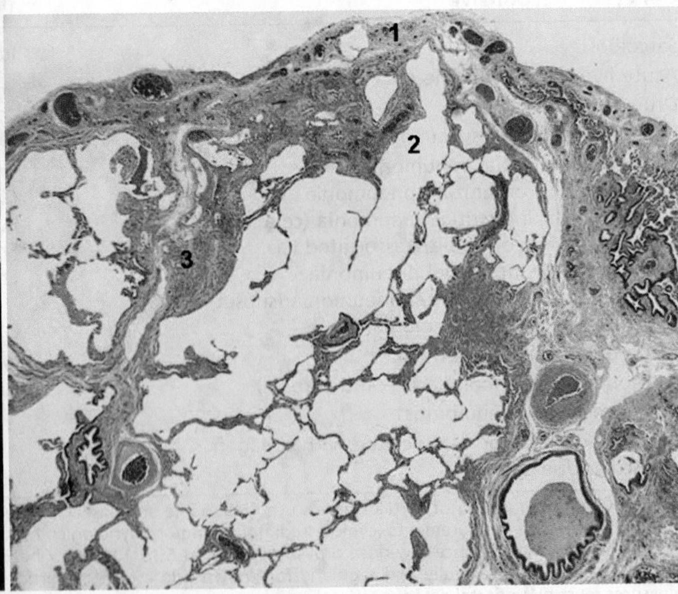

FIGURE 92–2 • Diagnosis of idiopathic pulmonary fibrosis. A, The usual interstitial pneumonia pattern of idiopathic pulmonary fibrosis in the lower lobes on high-resolution computed tomography consists of (1) subpleural fibrotic changes with (2) traction bronchiectasis and (3) honeycomb cysts in the lower lobes. **B,** Usual interstitial pneumonia pattern of idiopathic pulmonary fibrosis. Note the presence of (1) subpleural fibrosis with (2) traction emphysema, (3) fibroblastic foci, and temporal heterogeneity of microscopic abnormalities at low magnification. (Courtesy of Kevin Leslie, MD.)

TABLE 92–6 DIAGNOSIS OF IDIOPATHIC PULMONARY FIBROSIS IN THE ABSENCE OF SURGICAL LUNG BIOPSY

MAJOR CRITERIA (ALL FOUR MUST BE PRESENT)
Exclusion of other known causes of ILD, such as certain drug toxicities, environmental exposures, and connective tissue diseases
Abnormal pulmonary function studies that include evidence of restriction (reduced FVC often with an increased FEV_1/FVC ratio) and impaired gas exchange (increased $PAO_2–PaO_2$ at rest or during exercise or decreased DLCO)
Bibasilar reticular abnormalities with minimal or absent ground-glass opacity on HRCT scans
Transbronchial lung biopsy or BAL fluid showing no features to support an alternative diagnosis
MINOR CRITERIA (THREE OF FOUR MUST BE PRESENT)
Age >50 years
Insidious onset of otherwise unexplained dyspnea on exertion
Duration of illness ≥3 months
Bibasilar, inspiratory crackles (dry or "Velcro" type in quality)

BAL = bronchoalveolar lavage; DLCO = diffusion capacity of lung for carbon monoxide (corrected to hemoglobin); FEV_1 = forced expiratory volume in 1 second; FVC = forced vital capacity; HRCT = high-resolution computed tomography; ILD = interstitial lung disease; VC = vital capacity.
From American Thoracic Society/European Respiratory Society: Idiopathic pulmonary fibrosis: Diagnosis and treatment. International consensus statement. Am J Respir Crit Care Med 2000;161:646–664.

usual interstitial pneumonia on lung biopsy or HRCT. Fulfillment of all of the four major and three of the four minor clinical criteria (Table 92–6) may obviate the need for surgical lung biopsy.

Treatment

The current clinical course in patients with idiopathic pulmonary fibrosis is typically one of progressive impairment of lung function and gas exchange with an ultimately fatal outcome despite the use of currently available therapies. Additionally, acute exacerbations of respiratory impairment in the absence of infection or other complications usually necessitate hospitalization and supportive care in an intensive care unit and are associated with high mortality despite aggressive supportive care and empirical intravenous corticosteroids.

Because no treatment regimen to date has demonstrated improvement in survival and clinically relevant outcomes, all treatments should be considered experimental for idiopathic pulmonary fibrosis. The most commonly prescribed agent is an oral corticosteroid, and it is often given with an adjunctive immunosuppressive, azathioprine. A recent clinical trial demonstrated better preservation of PFT results after 1 year of treatment with combined oral prednisone (initiated at 0.5 mg/kg ideal body weight per day during the first month and tapered to a maintenance dose of 0.1 to 0.2 mg/kg of ideal body weight per day, or ≈10 mg/day, over the subsequent 3 to 4 months), azathioprine (maintenance dose of 2 mg/kg of ideal body weight per day, or 100 to 150 mg/day), and *N*-acetylcysteine (600 mg three times daily) than with prednisone and azathioprine. [1] To date, however, no randomized trials have compared the results of an experimental treatment regimen with no treatment at all. Other immunosuppressive/immune-modulating agents, such as cyclophosphamide, and antifibrotic agents, such as colchicine and D-penicillamine, are not beneficial. Interferon gamma-1b may be useful and is undergoing further study. Several new agents, including etanercept, pirfenidone, bosentan, *N*-acetylcysteine, and agents to block/modulate specific cellular, cytokine, molecular, and oxidant processes implicated in the pathogenesis of pulmonary fibrosis and vascular modeling, are currently under investigation.

Ancillary treatment measures, including supplemental oxygen based on clinical and physiologic needs, prompt detection and treatment of respiratory tract infections and pulmonary emboli, pulmonary rehabilitation, and immunization for influenza and pneumococcus, are appropriate interventions. Lung transplantation (Chapter 102) is indicated in selected patients, but about two thirds of patients with idiopathic pulmonary fibrosis are older than 60 to 65 years, which is a relative contraindication to lung transplantation.

Prognosis

The median survival of patients with idiopathic pulmonary fibrosis is 3 to 5 years after the time of diagnosis, with or without currently available/used treatment regimens. Patients who survive longer generally have less fibrosis on HRCT, less functional impairment, and no significant oxygen desaturation during a modified version of the 6-minute walk test.

Nonspecific Interstitial Pneumonia

NSIP is a recently described entity that is often associated with collagen vascular diseases or hypersensitivity pneumonitis, but it may also occur as an idiopathic entity. Two subgroups have been described: the cellular (NSIP, cellular) and the fibrotic (NSIP, fibrotic) variety. Because several clinical features of idiopathic fibrotic NSIP are very similar to early cases of idiopathic fibrotic pulmonary fibrosis and some patients with idiopathic pulmonary fibrosis may have coexisting histologic evidence of NSIP and usual interstitial pneumonia patterns in the same lung, it is unclear whether idiopathic fibrotic NSIP is a separate clinical entity or whether it represents an early form of idiopathic interstitial pneumonia that precedes the clinical manifestation of idiopathic pulmonary fibrosis. The average age at onset is about 10 years earlier in NSIP than in idiopathic pulmonary fibrosis.

Diagnosis

Chest radiographs show bilateral patchy pulmonary infiltrates with a lower lung zone predominance. HRCT reveals a predominance of ground-glass attenuation, usually bilateral and subpleural and often associated with loss of volume in the lower lobe. Cellular NSIP is characterized by mild to moderate lymphoplasmacytic interstitial chronic inflammation with ground-glass opacification or consolidation, or both, on HRCT. The major differential diagnosis to consider as an alternative to cellular NSIP is acute/subacute hypersensitivity pneumonitis, so a thorough history regarding environmental exposures is crucial. In contrast, fibrotic NSIP has uniformly dense interstitial fibrosis histopathologically and a bilateral lower lobe distribution with architectural derangement on HRCT; it may sometimes be difficult to distinguish from idiopathic pulmonary fibrosis/usual interstitial pneumonia in the early clinical stages. In these circumstances, the diagnosis of NSIP can be ascertained only by the histologic features in a surgical lung biopsy specimen.

Treatment and Prognosis

Patients with cellular NSIP usually respond to treatment with corticosteroids (Table 92–5), and their prognosis is generally better than that of patients with idiopathic pulmonary fibrosis. In some cases,

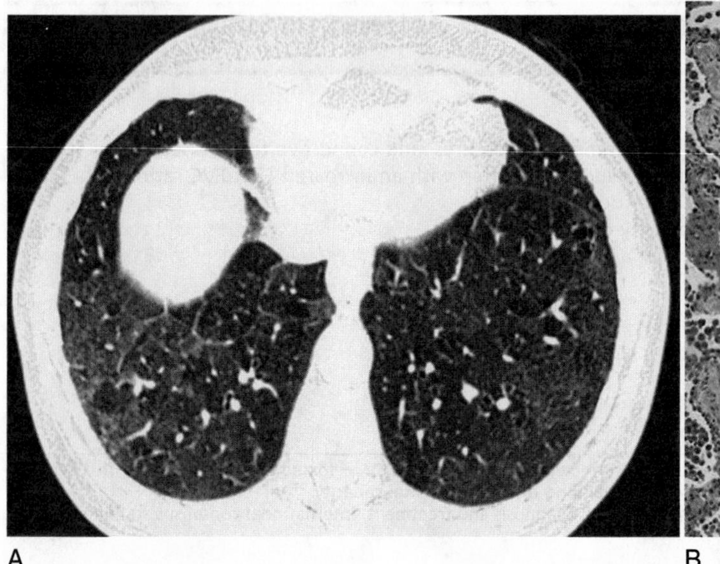

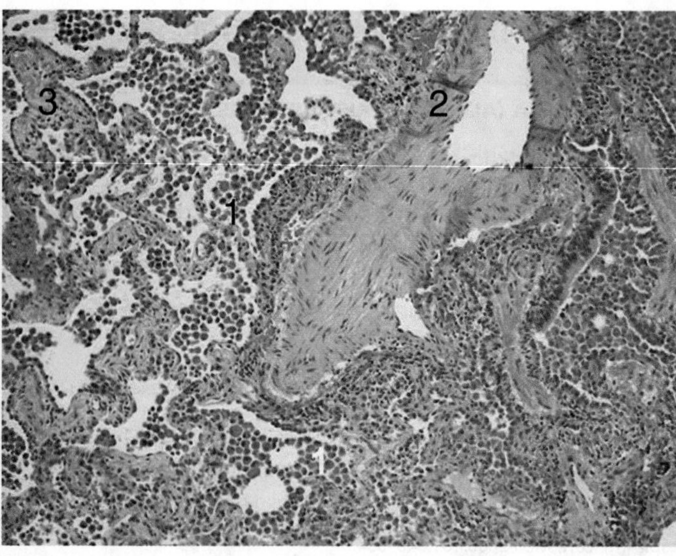

FIGURE 92–3 • Respiratory bronchiolitis–associated interstitial lung disease. A, Ground-glass attenuation with a mosaic pattern on high-resolution computed tomography. **B,** Note the dense aggregates of (1) pigmented macrophages present in the air spaces around the terminal airways with (2) variable bronchiolar metaplasia and (3) interstitial fibrosis.

Rx

the prognosis of fibrotic NSIP may be similar to that of idiopathic pulmonary fibrosis, but no studies/clinical trials have investigated a treatment regimen for idiopathic fibrotic NSIP. Given the similarities of the clinical manifestation of fibrotic NSIP and idiopathic pulmonary fibrosis, treatment approaches to fibrotic NSIP have been extrapolated from studies in idiopathic pulmonary fibrosis.

Respiratory Bronchiolitis–Associated Interstitial Lung Disease

This ILD is almost invariably associated with chronic and current cigarette smoking, and it usually manifests clinically during the fourth or fifth decade of life. However, it may also be detected incidentally on radiographs in relatively younger and asymptomatic persons with a previous history of cigarette smoking or in people passively exposed to chronic cigarette smoke.

Diagnosis

PFTs show varying degrees of airway obstruction, mildly decreased or preserved total lung capacity, and decreased DLCO. Coexistent centrilobular emphysema is frequent. The chest radiograph typically reveals bronchial wall thickening and areas of ground-glass attenuation. HRCT reveals centrilobular nodules with an upper lobe predominance, patchy ground-glass attenuation, and peribronchial alveolar septal thickening (Fig. 92–3A). Areas of hypoattenuation (mosaic attenuation) represent air trapping as a result of small airways disease. The characteristic finding on BAL is numerous brown-pigmented alveolar macrophages, often with a modest increase in neutrophils. The hallmark histopathologic feature on biopsy is the accumulation of pigmented alveolar macrophages with glassy eosinophilic cytoplasm and granular pigmentation within respiratory bronchioles, typically with a chronic inflammatory cell infiltrate in the bronchioles and surrounding alveolar walls (see Fig. 92–3B). Fibroblastic foci and honeycomb change are not present.

Treatment and Prognosis

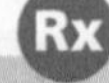

Progression to honeycomb lung and end-stage fibrosis seldom occurs, and the prognosis is good with cessation of smoking. Discontinuation of cigarette smoking is essential, and patients may benefit from low-dose corticosteroids (e.g., prednisone, 10 to 20 mg/day) for a few months.

Desquamative Interstitial Pneumonia

Desquamative interstitial pneumonia is a rare entity (<3% of all ILDs) that may represent a more extensive form of respiratory bronchiolitis–associated ILD. Although the vast majority of affected individuals are cigarette smokers, the histologic pattern of desquamative interstitial pneumonia may also occur in pneumoconiosis, rheumatologic disease, and drug-associated ILD. Patients are often initially seen with advanced disease and striking hypoxemia.

Diagnosis

PFTs reveal a restrictive lung defect and decreased DLCO with or without coexisting airway obstruction. The chest radiograph shows patchy basal consolidation with a lower lobe and peripheral predominance. HRCT shows bilateral symmetrical ground-glass opacities with a predominantly basal and peripheral distribution, as well as diffuse alveolar septal thickening (Fig. 92–4A). Irregular linear opacities, typically associated with traction bronchiectasis, may be noted. The finding of small discrete cysts, believed to represent trapped air in dilated bronchioles, within areas of ground-glass changes and intervening normal lung parenchyma is highly suggestive of desquamative interstitial pneumonia. Fluid recovered from BAL quite often shows increased numbers of pigmented alveolar macrophages, frequently with increased inflammatory cells. Histopathologic findings on biopsy include diffuse alveolar septal thickening, hyperplasia of type II pneumocytes, and intense accumulation of intra-alveolar granular pigmented macrophages in a uniform manner (see Fig. 92–4B); fibrosis is minimal.

Treatment and Prognosis

Therapeutic outcomes are generally good, particularly with cessation of smoking and administration of oral corticosteroid therapy (see Table 92–5); the estimated overall survival rate is 70% at 10 years.

Acute Interstitial Pneumonia

Acute interstitial pneumonia is seen in otherwise healthy persons immediately after an apparent viral upper respiratory infection (Fig. 92–5). The syndrome, historically known as Hamman-Rich syndrome (Chapter 91), mimics the acute respiratory distress syndrome.

Cryptogenic Organizing Pneumonia

Cryptogenic organizing pneumonia, previously referred to as bronchiolitis obliterans organizing pneumonia of unknown cause (BOOP), is an idiopathic pneumonia that is most commonly manifested as a flulike illness with a nonproductive cough, followed by exertional dyspnea.

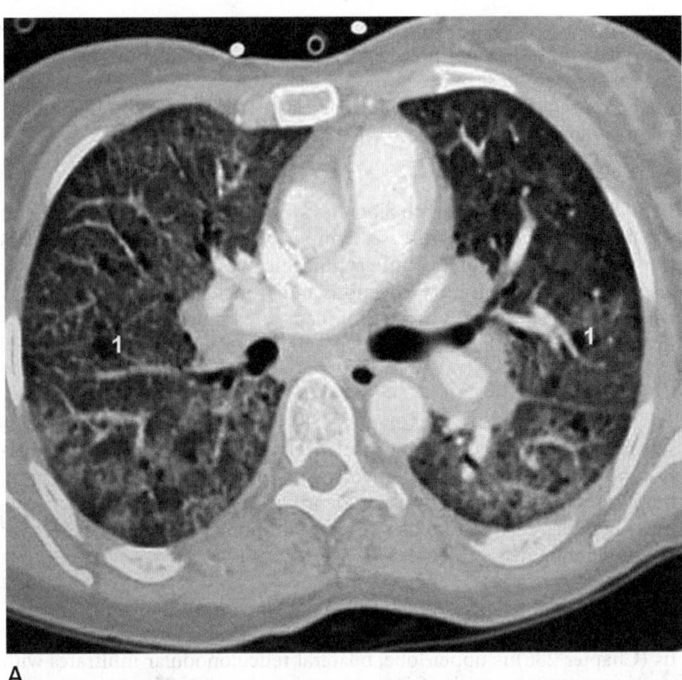

A

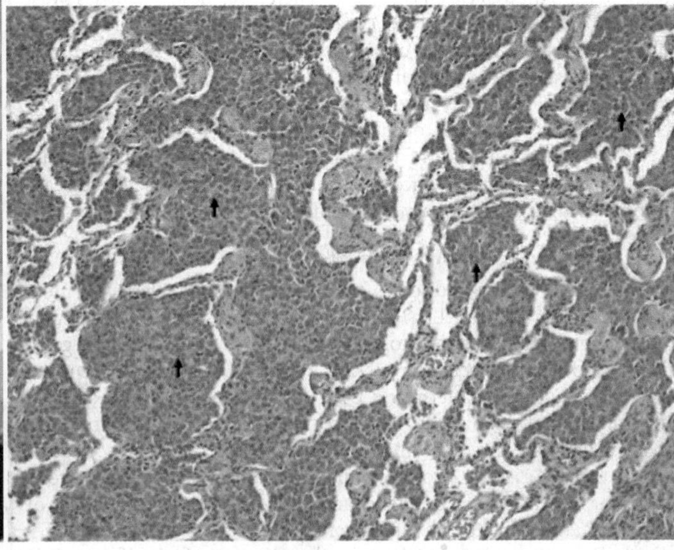

B

FIGURE 92–4 • Desquamative interstitial pneumonia. A, Ground-glass attenuation with (1) cystic spaces on high-resolution computed tomography. **B,** Note that the alveolar spaces are densely filled with macrophages (arrowheads).

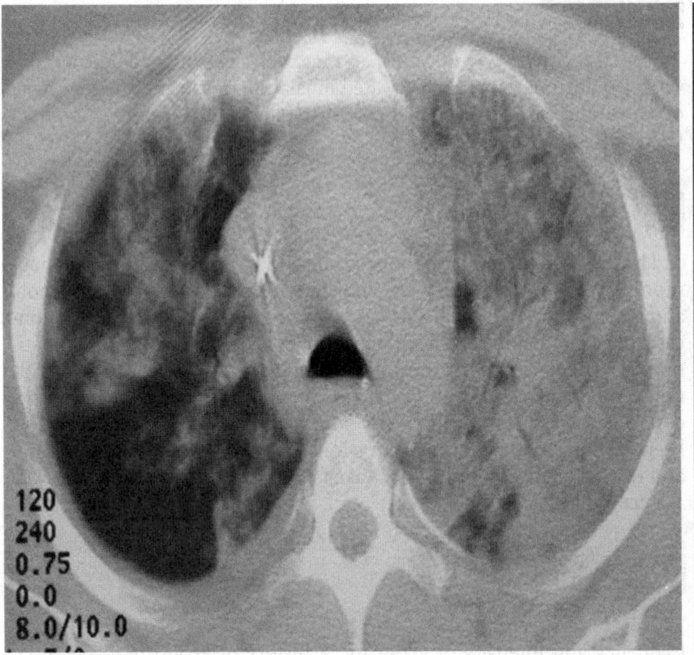

FIGURE 92–5 • Acute interstitial pneumonia with diffuse alveolar damage histologically. Note the dense air space consolidation.

Diagnosis

PFTs show a restrictive defect, but 20% of patients, most of whom are current or past smokers, also have an obstructive defect. Chest radiography reveals patchy unilateral or bilateral alveolar opacities that may be peripheral or migratory; small nodular opacities are seen in 10 to 50% of cases. In about 90% of patients, HRCT shows areas of air space consolidation with lower lung zone predominance. Other frequent features are a subpleural or peribronchial distribution, small nodules along bronchovascular bundles, and ground-glass attenuation. BAL is nonspecific; increased lymphocytes, neutrophils, and eosinophils may be seen. On biopsy, key histologic features are excessive proliferation of granulation tissue within the small airways and alveolar ducts, as well as chronic inflammation in the surrounding alveoli.

Treatment and Prognosis

The majority of patients recover rapidly and completely with oral corticosteroids (see Table 92–5) for 6 months but may relapse after discontinuation and require oral corticosteroids indefinitely, often with adjunct immunosuppressive agents such as azathioprine. A small subset of patients in whom pulmonary fibrosis develops despite corticosteroids and azathioprine behave similarly to patients with idiopathic pulmonary fibrosis. Spontaneous remissions are known to occur.

Lymphoid/Lymphocytic Interstitial Pneumonia

This condition is more common in women, especially in the fifth decade of life, but it may occur at any age. Concurrent collagen vascular disease or an autoimmune disorder (especially Sjögren's syndrome) should be sought because idiopathic lymphocytic interstitial pneumonia is very rare. Symptoms are nonspecific and include a gradual onset of cough and exertional dyspnea.

Diagnosis

Chest radiographs show a reticular or reticulonodular pattern predominantly involving the lower lung zones. HRCT reveals bilateral ground-glass attenuation, small or large nodules, and scattered cysts; perivascular honeycombing and reticular abnormalities may also be seen. Increased numbers of lymphocytes are found on BAL, and biopsy reveals a dense interstitial lymphocytic infiltrate.

Treatment and Prognosis

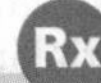

Some patients respond to or stabilize with oral corticosteroids (see Table 92–5). The prognosis is variable, with more than a third of patients progressing to diffuse pulmonary fibrosis.

Interstitial Lung Disease Associated with Collagen Vascular Disease

Many of the collagen vascular diseases, including progressive systemic sclerosis (Chapter 288), rheumatoid arthritis (Chapter 285), systemic lupus erythematosus (Chapter 287), dermatomyositis/polymyositis

(Chapter 290), Sjögren's syndrome (Chapter 289), and mixed connective tissue disorder (Chapter 288), may have ILD as one of their manifestations. In fact, up to 20% of patients with collagen vascular disease may initially be thought to have an ILD alone. Therefore, these diagnoses must be considered in patients with ILD, even in the absence of extrathoracic findings. Conversely, because pulmonary involvement is a major cause of death in patients with collagen vascular disease, the presence of ILD should be carefully sought in affected patients. All forms of idiopathic interstitial pneumonia can occur in patients with collagen vascular disease. The natural history of ILD complicating collagen vascular diseases is variable, especially since coexisting pulmonary vascular disease or nonparenchymal pulmonary involvement may be present.

Progressive Systemic Sclerosis

Of the collagen vascular diseases, progressive systemic sclerosis is most frequently associated with ILD. Pulmonary symptoms may antedate cutaneous or digital manifestations of the disease by several years. The great majority of patients affected have NSIP, with a minority having a usual interstitial pneumonia pattern, and DLCO levels correlate with mortality. Pulmonary hypertension, which can occur in the absence of pulmonary fibrosis, may result in cor pulmonale. The chronic pulmonary fibrosis also increases the risk for bronchogenic carcinoma, usually either bronchoalveolar cell carcinoma or adenocarcinoma. Treatment with 1 year of cyclophosphamide (50 to 100 mg/day orally) appears to stabilize the PFT findings. Pulmonary hypertension in the absence of significant ILD responds to treatment with prostacyclin analogues and other agents (Chapter 67), but it is unknown whether these agents can also stabilize the ILD.

Rheumatoid Arthritis

Although rheumatoid arthritis is more common in women, (2 : 1 to 4 : 1 ratio), ILD associated with rheumatoid arthritis is more common in men (3 : 1 ratio). Most cases occur at 50 to 60 years of age, and pulmonary symptoms most often follow the onset of arthritis (≈75%). Lung involvement in rheumatoid arthritis may take many forms, but bronchiectasis, bronchiolitis, idiopathic interstitial pneumonias, and pleural effusions or pleural thickening are some of the most common. Early in the course, the histologic changes are similar to those of idiopathic interstitial pneumonias, including pulmonary fibrosis, but are distinguished by a prominent lymphocytic infiltrate that may contain germinal follicles adjacent to vessels and airways. As the disease progresses, the infiltration becomes less pronounced and is replaced by fibrous tissue or honeycomb changes, or both. Other pulmonary manifestations include pulmonary nodules, vasculitis, pulmonary hypertension, and Caplan's syndrome (progressive upper lobe nodular pulmonary fibrosis in a miner with rheumatoid arthritis) but are relatively rare. Treatment is directed at the underlying rheumatoid arthritis (Chapter 285).

Systemic Lupus Erythematosus

Pulmonary abnormalities complicating systemic lupus erythematosus may vary greatly. Pleural disease or pleural effusions (or both) are commonly present in lung disease that complicates systemic lupus erythematosus. Acute lupus pneumonitis may mimic acute interstitial pneumonia, with widespread ground-glass attenuation admixed with consolidation, or it may be manifested as diffuse alveolar hemorrhage. Chronic ILD may also occur. Infection must always be considered in acutely ill patients who have received steroids or other immunosuppressive therapy. Rarely, the restrictive lung defect may be predominantly a result of diaphragmatic weakness, and the small-appearing lungs on chest radiographs may appear progressively smaller over time, the so-called shrinking lung that is generally resistant to corticosteroids or other immunosuppressive agents used for systemic lupus erythematosus. Otherwise, treatment of the ILD is similar to treatment of the underlying systemic lupus erythematosus.

Dermatomyositis/Polymyositis

In contrast to progressive systemic sclerosis, the pattern of lung involvement in dermatomyositis/polymyositis is more heterogeneous. Usual interstitial pneumonia, NSIP, and organizing pneumonia have all been reported. Most patients have anti–Jo-1 antibody, and the disease is typically progressive over time. An acute interstitial pneumonia–like syndrome occurs in a subset of patients and is associated with high mortality despite aggressive immunosuppressive agents and high-dose corticosteroids. ILD may precede the muscular manifestations by months to years or be superimposed on established muscle disease. The severity of the muscular disease does not correlate with that of the ILD. Treatment is directed at the underlying disease (Chapter 290).

Sjögren's Syndrome

ILD is seen in patients with Sjögren's syndrome, particularly those with the primary form of the disease. Lymphocytic interstitial pneumonia is the most frequent subtype, but cryptogenic organizing pneumonia may also be present. Respiratory infections and bronchiectasis are common in advanced stages, perhaps because of inspissated mucus. Response to corticosteroid or immunosuppressive therapy is usually good (Chapter 288).

Mixed Connective Tissue Disease

This overlap syndrome (Chapter 288) combines features of progressive systemic sclerosis, systemic lupus erythematosus, rheumatoid arthritis, and polymyositis/dermatomyositis. Pulmonary disease is common, but it is most often subclinical and identified only radiographically. Treatment includes corticosteroids and other immune-modulating agents for the underlying disease.

Ankylosing Spondylitis

The most common pulmonary manifestation of ankylosing spondylitis (Chapter 286) is upper lobe, bilateral reticulonodular infiltrates with cyst formation as a result of parenchymal destruction. There is no known effective therapy for this apical fibrobullous disease.

Hypersensitivity Pneumonitis

Definition

Hypersensitivity pneumonitis, also known as extrinsic allergic alveolitis, is a syndrome caused by repeated inhalation of specific antigens from occupational or environmental exposure (Chapters 93 and 94) in sensitized individuals.

Pathobiology

The acute response after inhalation is a nonspecific diffuse pneumonitis with inflammatory cell infiltration of the bronchioles, alveoli, and interstitium. In the subacute and chronic stages, loosely formed, noncaseating, epithelioid cell granulomas may be dispersed in the interstitium. Hypersensitivity pneumonitis can occur with exposure to a wide range of inhaled antigens (Chapters 93 and 94). Some of the more common exposures are farmer's lung, bird fancier's lung, parakeet keeper's lung, and pigeon breeder's lung. Hobbies (wood worker's lung) and recreational activities (sauna taker's lung) may be implicated, as well as occupations.

Clinical Manifestations

The clinical features and severity of symptoms vary according to the frequency and intensity of exposure. A history of exposure to potential agents or changes in the domestic and other environments (or both) is essential to diagnosis and treatment (Chapter 17). The interval between exposure to the antigen and the clinical manifestations of lung disease is unknown, although symptoms can occur as soon as 4 to 12 hours after exposure. In such cases, fever and chills are common symptoms, are often temporally related to the workplace or to hobbies, and may actually disappear on vacations or during absence from the site of exposure, only to recur when exposure is resumed. In more chronic and low-level exposures, however, the onset is insidious.

Diagnosis

Findings on chest radiography are diverse, with focal patchy consolidation or a diffuse ground-glass appearance in acute hypersensitivity pneumonitis, micronodular and reticular shadowing in subacute forms, and diffuse, predominantly upper lung zone reticulation with honeycombing in the chronic form. Chest radiographs may be normal in up to 30% of patients with significant physiologic abnormalities. On HRCT, small centrilobular ill-defined nodules of ground-glass densities are seen, along with evidence of mosaic attenuation (trapped air) as a result of concomitant bronchiolitis. Chronically, findings of lung fibrosis may be indistinguishable from the patterns seen in usual interstitial pneumonia/idiopathic pulmonary fibrosis.

BAL may be quite helpful by showing the most marked increase in lymphocytes of any of the ILDs, as well as increased numbers of plasma cells. The characteristic histologic triad in hypersensitivity pneumonitis is cellular NSIP, cellular bronchiolitis, and granulomatous inflammation; however, this triad is seen in no more than 75% of affected patients. Differentiation from cellular NSIP may be challenging.

Treatment and Prognosis

Rx

Further avoidance of exposure to the antigen or antigens and treatment with corticosteroids (see Table 92–5) are important if improvement is to be obtained. Continued exposure to the unidentifiable antigens or prolonged exposure to antigens, or both, have led to chronic hypersensitivity pneumonitis and irreversible fibrosis that may not respond to any treatment regimen.

Occupational Interstitial Lung Diseases

ILDs associated with specific occupations generally involve the inhalation and deposition of dust in the lungs, followed by a tissue reaction that ultimately results in fibrosis. Examples include silicosis (inhalation of silica in crystalline form or silicon dioxide as quartz, cristobalite, or tridymite; at-risk occupations include sandblasting and working with granite), coal workers' pneumoconiosis (inhalation of coal dust), asbestosis (deposition of fibers during mining, milling, or other handling of asbestos; welding and working in a shipyard are two at-risk occupations), berylliosis (seen in aerospace workers and in electronic industries), and hard metal disease (Chapter 93). Radiographic features are specific to the inhalant. Cessation of the exposure is important, but the fibrosis is generally irreversible.

Drug-Induced Interstitial Lung Disease

More than 300 drugs, biomolecules, or homeopathic remedies (see Table 92–2) can cause acute, subacute, or chronic ILD. The clinical and radiographic manifestations are quite varied. Examples of known syndromes include chronic nitrofurantoin-induced ILD that mimics idiopathic pulmonary fibrosis (and is fatal in approximately 8% of cases), granulomatous pneumonitis secondary to methotrexate (<5%), sarcoid-like granulomatous ILD induced by interferon alfa, nonspecific bilateral alveolar and interstitial inflammatory and fibrotic abnormalities caused by bleomycin and other chemotherapeutic agents, and alveolar and interstitial abnormalities and nodular densities in acute and chronic amiodarone pulmonary toxicity. Most drug-induced ILD is reversible if recognized early and if use of the responsible drug is discontinued. In addition to discontinuing the implicated drug, treatment with corticosteroids (see Table 92–5) is indicated in patients with moderate to severe functional impairment.

Alveolar Filling Disorders

In alveolar filling disorders (Chapter 91), air spaces distal to the terminal bronchioles are filled with blood, lipid, protein, water, or inflammatory cells. The radiographic appearance is that of an alveolar infiltrate with small nodular densities and ill-defined margins; hence, the radiographic picture is similar to an ILD, and virtually all the alveolar filling disorders may result in ILD, including Goodpasture's syndrome, pulmonary alveolar proteinosis (primary and secondary), alveolar hemorrhage syndromes (Chapter 91), acute interstitial pneumonia, and bronchoalveolar cell carcinoma (Chapter 201).

Idiopathic Pulmonary Hemosiderosis

This rare disorder of children and young adults is characterized by intermittent, diffuse alveolar hemorrhage without evidence of vasculitis, inflammation, granulomas, or necrosis. The etiology is poorly understood. Anemia and hepatosplenomegaly may be present. Hemosiderin-laden macrophages in BAL fluid and lung tissue are part of the diagnostic picture. The chest radiograph reveals diffuse, bilateral alveolar infiltrates. A chronic interstitial infiltrate may develop after repeated episodes, infrequently with hilar and mediastinal adenopathy. Systemic corticosteroids (see Table 92–5) may be beneficial in treating acute disease.

Chronic Eosinophilic Pneumonia

The clinical manifestation of chronic eosinophilic pneumonia varies over a wide spectrum, from asymptomatic to respiratory failure. The disease often occurs in women in the second to fourth decades of life; such women often manifest constitutional symptoms of fevers, sweats, weight loss, fatigue, dyspnea, and cough. Peripheral blood eosinophilia (Chapter 176), usually at levels of 10 to 40%, is common but may be absent in up to a third of affected patients at initial evaluation. On chest radiography and HRCT, the cardinal feature is peripheral multifocal consolidation, predominantly in the upper and mid-lung zones. These dense peripheral infiltrates, which have sometimes been termed the "photographic negative of pulmonary edema," often resolve dramatically after treatment with corticosteroids. Ground-glass attenuation commonly accompanies the consolidation. BAL fluid may show greater than 40% eosinophils during exacerbations. Treatment with corticosteroids (see Table 92–5) results in rapid response, frequently within hours; in fact, such a dramatic resolution of symptoms with radiographic clearance of infiltrates shortly after initiation of corticosteroid therapy is considered "diagnostic." However, the rate of relapse is high, so most patients require prolonged treatment with low-dose corticosteroids (prednisone, 5 to 10 mg/day) to stay in remission.

Interstitial Lung Disease Associated with Pulmonary Vasculitides

Wegener's Granulomatosis

Wegener's granulomatosis (Chapter 291) is the most common form of vasculitis that involves the lung. The systemic necrotizing granulomatous inflammation and small-vessel vasculitis are often manifested first in the upper respiratory tract as chronic rhinitis or sinusitis (or both), epistaxis, oropharyngeal ulcerations, gingival hyperplasia with clefting, or serous otitis media. Destruction of the nasal cartilage may lead to septal perforation or a saddle nose deformity. Ulcerative lesions of the tracheobronchial tree, cavitating nodules within the lung parenchyma, and diffuse alveolar hemorrhage caused by pulmonary capillaritis are lower respiratory tract manifestations. Focal segmental necrotizing glomerulonephritis is the most common extrathoracic manifestation, although pulmonary involvement may occur without renal disease. Chest radiography usually reveals multiple nodular or cavitating infiltrates, but single nodules may be found as well. The diagnosis is most commonly made serologically, with demonstration of antineutrophil cytoplasmic antibodies, although a negative test does not exclude the disease. Treatment is usually with cyclophosphamide (50 to 100 mg/day or 2 mg/kg of ideal body weight per day, but not more than 150 mg/day) in conjunction with oral corticosteroids (prednisone, 10 to 40 mg/day). Initial remission occurs in more than 90% of patients, but most patients require treatment for several years. Relapses may occur in up to 30% of patients, especially when treatment is tapered; such patients may need treatment indefinitely. Prophylaxis for *Pneumocystis carinii* infection is indicated in patients receiving chronic treatment.

Churg-Strauss Syndrome (Allergic Angiitis)

This systemic necrotizing vasculitis (Chapter 291) affects both the upper and lower respiratory tracts and is almost invariably preceded by allergic disorders such as asthma, allergic rhinitis, sinusitis, or a drug reaction. Peripheral and lung eosinophilia, bronchospasm, increased immunoglobulin (Ig) E levels, and rashes are common manifestations. The pulmonary radiographic findings are bilateral patchy, fleeting infiltrates, diffuse nodular infiltrates, or diffuse reticulonodular disease. Histopathologic examination of lung tissue is generally diagnostic with features of granulomatous angiitis/vasculitis. Although treatment with corticosteroids is indicated, the dosage and duration are unclear (see Table 92–5).

Idiopathic Pulmonary Capillaritis

Idiopathic pulmonary capillaritis may involve the pulmonary vasculature within the alveolar walls and be manifested as ILD. Patients may also have subclinical alveolar hemorrhage, often associated with the presence of perinuclear antineutrophilic cytoplasmic antibodies. Corticosteroids are the mainstay of treatment, but the doses and duration of treatment are unclear. Frequently, patients need adjunctive treatment with cyclophosphamide, similar to patients with vasculitis and Wegener's granulomatosis (Chapter 291).

Other Forms of Interstitial Lung Disease

Sarcoidosis

See Chapter 95.

Pulmonary Langerhans Cell Histiocytosis

This condition, previously known as pulmonary histiocytosis X or eosinophilic granuloma of the lung, is an idiopathic, granulomatous ILD that typically occurs in the second or third decade of life; there is a male preponderance. The currently accepted term is Langerhans cell histiocytosis. Pulmonary Langerhans cell histiocytosis is rare, with an estimated incidence of two to five cases per million population. The large majority (>90%) of those affected are smokers, and current evidence suggests that the disorder results from an abnormal immune response to cigarette smoke.

Clinical Manifestations

The clinical findings are variable and range from an abnormal chest radiograph in an asymptomatic patient to progressive dyspnea with a nonproductive cough. Systemic symptoms of malaise, fever, and weight loss may be present. Hemoptysis is rare. Spontaneous pneumothorax, which occurs in approximately 25% of patients and is due to rupture of subpleural cysts, may be an initial finding. Langerhans cell histiocytosis may be confined to the lung or may be a component of a multisystem disease that includes painful cystic bone lesions and diabetes insipidus (Chapter 243).

Diagnosis

The chest radiograph shows diffuse symmetrical reticulonodular opacities superimposed on multiple small cysts in the upper and mid lung zones. HRCT reveals subpleural nodules, scattered ground glass densities, and irregular cysts of varying number, size, and configuration in both lungs, with sparing of the lung bases; in the appropriate clinical setting this pattern may be pathognomonic. As the disease progresses, the increase in fibrosis and cysts may lead to honeycombing of the lung. PFTs are characterized by a mixed restrictive and obstructive pattern, including a reduction in diffusing capacity. Vital capacity is disproportionately reduced in comparison to total lung capacity because of air trapping within the cysts; the result is an increased residual volume. BAL reveals Langerhans cells (atypical histiocytes) that have the characteristic "x-body" (i.e., Birbeck granule) on electron microscopy; immunostaining shows CD1 antigen on the cell surface and S-100 protein in the cytoplasm. However, the absence of these findings does not exclude the diagnosis. The diagnosis is usually made by transbronchial biopsy or open lung biopsy, which reveals interstitial and peribronchiolar collections of histiocytes, eosinophils, and lymphocytes; peribronchiolar nodules; and cysts with areas of central stellate fibrosis.

Treatment and Prognosis

Rx

Although definitive regression after discontinuation of smoking has not been proved, small series report improvement, so patients should be encouraged to discontinue smoking. The prognosis in pulmonary Langerhans cell histiocytosis is usually favorable, with approximately 75% of patients improving or stabilizing, especially with cessation of smoking; some patients, however, may progress to end-stage lung disease. In patients with progressive disease, corticosteroids (see Table 92–5) with or without vincristine, cyclosporine, cyclophosphamide, and azathioprine have been used with some anecdotal reports of success. Lung transplantation has been performed, but recurrent disease has been reported in the allograft.

Lymphangioleiomyomatosis

This rare interstitial lung disease is limited to women, primarily of childbearing age. Proliferation of abnormal smooth muscle around bronchioles leads to bilateral small cysts, which give an appearance of ILD on chest radiographs, and progressive impairment of lung function. Hemoptysis, pneumothorax (from rupture of subpleural cysts), and chylothorax (from lymphatic obstruction) may be initial symptoms that distinguish this disorder from other diffuse lung diseases. Although lymphangioleiomyomatosis is usually limited to the lungs, an association with angiomyolipomas of the mediastinal and retroperitoneal lymph nodes and kidney has been described, so the disease may mimic the manifestations of tuberous sclerosis (Chapter 444). Coarse reticulonodular infiltrates, often with cysts or bullae, are typically seen on chest radiographs. In contrast to the majority of other ILDs, increased lung volumes may be present and should prompt consideration of this diagnosis in a nonsmoking woman of reproductive age. HRCT shows characteristic diffuse thin-walled cysts, generally less than 2 cm in diameter. BAL may show occult alveolar hemorrhage. Lung biopsy reveals abnormal smooth muscle cells lining the airways, lymphatics, and blood vessels, with concurrent airflow obstruction and replacement of the lung parenchyma with cysts.

Treatment and Prognosis

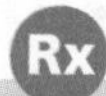

Treatment with progesterone or tamoxifen has been tried in some patients, but there are no randomized trials to support the use of interventions to alter the estrogen-progesterone balance. There is no cure. Although lung transplantation is indicated as the patient reaches severe functional impairment, the disease may recur in the transplanted lung. Most patients die of respiratory failure about 10 years after the onset of symptoms.

Inherited Disorders

Several rare genetic disorders are associated with ILD and pulmonary fibrosis. Inheritance is autosomal dominant with variable penetrance for most cases of familial idiopathic pulmonary fibrosis/idiopathic interstitial pneumonia and for tuberous sclerosis (Chapter 444), neurofibromatosis (Chapter 444), and familial hypocalciuric hypercalcemia (Chapter 266). Inheritance is autosomal recessive for Gaucher's disease (Chapter 223), Niemann-Pick disease (Chapter 223), and Hermansky-Pudlak syndrome (Chapter 223). The congenital form of the alveolar filling disorder pulmonary alveolar proteinosis also is inherited in an autosomal recessive manner.

Tuberous sclerosis (Chapter 444), which is an autosomal dominant disease of variable penetrance, is characterized pathologically by the presence of hamartomas in multiple organs. The most well known clinical manifestations include epilepsy, mental retardation, adenoma sebaceum, and renal angiomyolipomas. ILD occurs in only 1% of patients with tuberous sclerosis, usually in women older than 30 years with little or no mental retardation. The pulmonary involvement, which is indistinguishable from lymphangioleiomyomatosis both radiographically and histopathologically, may be manifested as exertional dyspnea, recurrent pneumothorax, and hemoptysis. HRCT reveals thin-walled cysts and a diffuse reticulonodular infiltrate. Recurrent parenchymal hemorrhage may lead to hemosiderin deposition and interstitial pulmonary fibrosis. There is no cure, and treatment is supportive.

Neurofibromatosis (Chapter 444) may affect all age groups and both sexes. Type 1 (von Recklinghausen's disease) is characterized by cafe au lait spots, neurofibromas, optic glioma, and bony lesions; the more rare type 2 is associated with bilateral acoustic neuromas. Diffuse ILD is manifested as bilateral lower lobe fibrosis, as well as bullae or cystic changes. Interstitial fibrosis and alveolitis with thickening of the alveolar septa, accompanied by a cellular infiltrate, are seen on lung biopsy. Management is as for idiopathic pulmonary fibrosis.

Gaucher's disease (Chapter 223), a lysosomal glycolipid storage disorder, has a predilection for the Ashkenazi Jewish population. Pulmonary manifestations, which occur most frequently in type 2 disease, may be a result of interstitial infiltration by Gaucher cells with fibrosis, alveolar consolidation, and filling of alveolar spaces; capillary plugging by

Gaucher cells may cause secondary pulmonary hypertension. Treatment is as for the systemic disease, and the general approaches for idiopathic interstitial pneumonias and pulmonary arterial hypertension may be followed for these patients.

Niemann-Pick disease (Chapter 223) is a rare lipid storage disease that may cause infiltration of the characteristic "foam cell" throughout the pulmonary lymphatics, the pulmonary arteries, and the pulmonary alveoli. Patients with type B may survive into adulthood. Treatment is as for the systemic disease.

Hermansky-Pudlak syndrome (Chapter 223) is characterized by oculocutaneous albinism, a bleeding diathesis, and ceroid inclusions in macrophages. Most patients are of Puerto Rican ancestry, and women are affected more frequently than men. Pulmonary fibrosis, with onset in the third or fourth decade, is slowly progressive. Treatment principles and interventions are largely supportive and extrapolated from other related conditions, especially idiopathic pulmonary fibrosis.

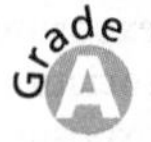

1. Demedts M, Behr J, Buhl R, et al: High dose acetyl cysteine in idiopathic pulmonary fibrosis. N Engl J Med 2005;353:2229–2242.

SUGGESTED READINGS

American Thoracic Society/European Respiratory Society: International multidisciplinary consensus classification of the idiopathic interstitial pneumonias. Am J Respir Crit Care Med 2002;165:277–304. *An approach to differentiating among these various conditions.*

Raghu G, Weycker D, Edelsberg J, et al: Incidence and prevalence of idiopathic pulmonary fibrosis. Am J Respir Crit Care Med 2006;174:810–816. *Incidence is 6.8 to 16.3 per 100,000; prevalence is 14.0 to 42.7 per 100,000.*

Flaherty KR, King TE, Raghu G, et al: Idiopathic interstitial pneumonia—what is the effect of a multidisciplinary approach to diagnosis? Am J Respir Crit Care Med 2004;170:904–910. *Supports the multidisciplinary approach.*

Martinez FJ, Safrin S, Weycker D, et al: The clinical course of patients with idiopathic pulmonary fibrosis. Ann Intern Med 2005;142:125–133. *The common acute deterioration of otherwise stable mild to moderate idiopathic pulmonary fibrosis has important implications for monitoring and supports timely referral for lung transplantation.*

Park JH, Kim DS, Park IN, et al: Prognosis of fibrotic interstitial pneumonia: Idiopathic versus collagen vascular disease–related subtypes. Am J Respir Crit Care Med 2007;175:705–711. *Patients with idiopathic disease generally had a worse prognosis.*

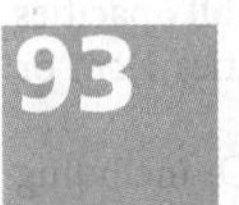

93 OCCUPATIONAL PULMONARY DISORDERS

Jonathan M. Samet

Definition

Interstitial lung disease (ILD) damages the pulmonary interstitium by disrupting alveolar structures and the small airways (Chapter 92). Occupational diseases affecting the pulmonary interstitium include primarily the pneumoconioses, or dust diseases of the lung (Table 93–1), and hypersensitivity pneumonitis. The principal pneumoconioses—asbestosis, coal workers' pneumoconiosis, and silicosis—typically occur after sustained exposures to dust concentrations that are no longer legally permissible in many developed countries, including the United States.

TABLE 93–1 PRINCIPAL PNEUMOCONIOSES CAUSED BY MINERAL DUSTS

Agent	Disease	Radiographic Appearance
Asbestos	Asbestosis	Reticular, basilar predominance
Coal dust	Coal workers' pneumoconiosis	Nodular, upper lobe predominance
Cobalt	Hard metal disease	Reticular, basilar predominance
Silica	Silicosis	Nodular, upper lobe predominance
Talc	Talcosis	Rounded, irregular, or both

Epidemiology

Although these diseases are declining, cases still occur in locales where industries have been historically associated with high dust exposures; "sentinel" cases signal unsuspected and uncontrolled occupational exposures (Chapter 17). During the period 1968–2000, mortality from most pneumoconioses dropped substantially but increased nearly four-fold for asbestosis. In many developed countries, these diseases remain common. Beryllium, originally linked to lung disease in workers making fluorescent lamps, now has widespread use in high-technology applications and the nuclear weapons industry (Chapter 20). New agents introduced into the workplace may also cause unanticipated diseases, as in a 1999 example of workers in a nylon flocking plant and a 2000 report of bronchiolitis obliterans in workers in a microwave popcorn plant. People with occupational ILD may present to health care providers through diverse paths. Physicians may evaluate previously undiagnosed patients with occupational ILD who present with dyspnea or unexplained radiographic infiltrates or previously diagnosed patients who present for assessment of the extent of associated physiologic impairment, often in the context of a legal proceeding or a claim for disability. Current or former workers exposed to agents causing lung disease may ask to be screened for possible adverse effects.

Pathobiology

Although this chapter focuses on occupational ILD, occupational exposures have also been linked to narrowing in the airways, including asthma (Chapter 87), bronchitis (Chapter 96), and bronchiolitis (Chapter 90). Some occupational agents, including coal dust, and fume- and dust-contaminated workplaces, generally increase the natural rate of decline of lung function with age (Chapter 92).

The occupational ILDs result when dusts are inhaled and retained, inducing inflammation and fibrosis. Dust particles in the respirable size range, about 10 μm mass median aerodynamic diameter or less as detailed later, are generated in workplaces by diverse processes; power-driven equipment, such as drills and grinders, place their operators at risk for diseases caused by dust; nearby workers, even if they are not working directly with the materials, may be secondarily exposed. The lung is defended against dust particles by a system including the physical barrier posed by the upper airway that filters out larger particles, the mucociliary escalator that removes inhaled particles, and the alveolar macrophages that scavenge inhaled and deposited particles in the small airways and alveoli (Chapter 85). Particle size determines the likelihood and site of deposition in the respiratory tract. During quiet breathing, most particles larger than 10 μm in aerodynamic diameter are deposited in the upper respiratory tract, although some particles in this size range may enter the lung during exertion. Particles between approximately 3 and 10 μm tend to be deposited in the larger airways of the lung, whereas smaller particles down to about 0.1 μm are preferentially deposited in the small airways and alveoli.

Pathogenesis

Inflammation and subsequent fibrosis are central in the pathogenesis of the occupational ILDs, although the mechanisms underlying the distinctive pathologic responses found in the different pneumoconioses are still not fully characterized. Present concepts of pathogenetic mechanisms for the pneumoconioses emphasize the roles of alveolar macrophages in the initial response to dust inhalation, of cytokine release, and of interactions among macrophages, lymphocytes, neutrophils, and fibroblasts. Hypersensitivity pneumonitis reflects cell-mediated immune responses to inhaled antigens. As for idiopathic pulmonary fibrosis, genetic susceptibility has been postulated as a determinant of the response to inhaled occupational agents. To date, however, a genetic linkage has been found for only one agent and disease—beryllium and chronic beryllium disease.

Diagnosis

Diagnostic Evaluation

Diagnosis of an occupational ILD is based on an appropriate clinical picture and documentation of exposure, related in a temporally appropriate fashion to the occurrence of the disease. In addition to the exposure history, chest radiography, lung function testing, and high-resolution computed tomography (HRCT) are the key components of the diagnostic evaluation (Fig. 93–1). Further evaluation may also be needed to exclude other disorders associated with a comparable clinical picture. For example, in an elderly man with a history of underground mining and of cigarette smoking, a lung nodule might represent complicated silicosis or a primary cancer of the lung. The clinical history should cover the cardinal respiratory symptoms—cough, phlegm production, dyspnea, and wheezing; emphasis should be placed on quantifying the degree of dyspnea. Graded questions used for this purpose inquire, for example, about having dyspnea while hurrying on level ground or walking up a slight hill, about walking more slowly than same-age peers on level ground, about stopping for breath after walking about 100 yards, and about having dyspnea during such routine activities as dressing and bathing. On physical examination, the physician should look for clubbing of the fingers (Chapter 48) or cyanosis, indicative of advanced disease.

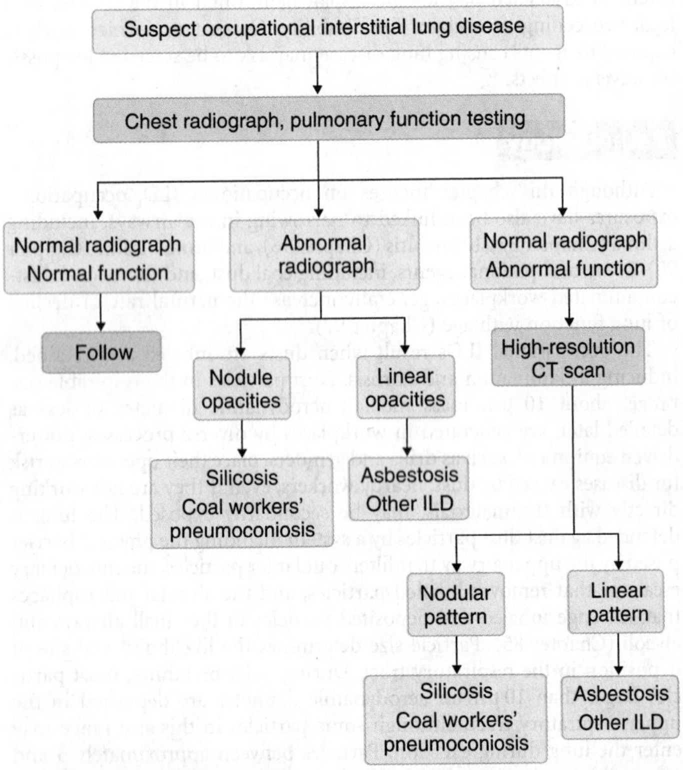

Suspect occupational interstitial lung disease

Chest radiograph, pulmonary function testing

Normal radiograph Normal function → Follow

Abnormal radiograph → Nodule opacities → Silicosis, Coal workers' pneumoconiosis; Linear opacities → Asbestosis, Other ILD

Normal radiograph Abnormal function → High-resolution CT scan → Nodular pattern → Silicosis, Coal workers' pneumoconiosis; Linear pattern → Asbestosis, Other ILD

FIGURE 93–1 • Diagnostic approach to occupational interstitial lung disease (ILD). CT = computed tomography.

On examining the chest, the physician should note the quality of the breath sounds and the timing (early or late) and the type (fine or coarse) of any crackles (Chapter 83).

History

A comprehensive occupational history should be taken from all patients with suspected occupational disease (Chapter 17; see Fig. 17–1). The history needs to cover each job systematically, describing the industry in which the patient worked, the specific occupation and job duties, the materials handled, the required and actual use of respiratory protective equipment, and the occurrence of disease in fellow workers. Seasonal, part-time, and temporary jobs should not be omitted as such jobs may have a greater likelihood of hazardous exposure. The dates of specific jobs may also be relevant because exposures for many agents were higher during past decades. Although the frequency of the more common pneumoconioses is now declining, some exposures (e.g., beryllium) are still widespread, and newer exposures may cause ILD. The history should inquire about specific materials (e.g., asbestos) and about exposure through hobbies and the jobs of family members. A temporal association between entering the workplace and symptoms may indicate an exposure that triggers hypersensitivity pneumonitis.

The history should also cover cigarette smoking and other tobacco use (Chapter 30). Chronic bronchitis and chronic airflow obstruction associated with smoking may explain cough and dyspnea or complicate the diagnosis of a distinct occupational lung disease.

Noninvasive Evaluation

In addition to a comprehensive occupational history, the diagnostic evaluation of patients with suspected occupational ILD also includes imaging of the lungs to establish the presence of disease and the characteristics of any abnormalities (Chapter 84). All patients thought to have an occupational ILD need to have standard posteroanterior and lateral radiographs. Most patients with pneumoconiosis have an abnormal chest radiograph, but 10 to 20% do not. The type of infiltrates, nodular or reticular, and the distribution provide an indication of the underlying disease (see Table 93–1). By use of the standardized system for classifying the abnormalities found on the posteroanterior radiograph in pneumoconioses, small parenchymal opacities are classified by shape (irregular or rounded), size, distribution, and profusion or concentration. The profusion, scored on a 12-point scale, is indicative of the degree of histopathologic derangement. The pneumoconiosis is termed simple if all opacities are smaller than 1 cm in diameter and complicated if opacities 1 cm or larger are present.

HRCT is increasingly used to evaluate patients with ILD, including occupational diseases. The narrow slice thickness of 1 to 2 mm provides visualization of fine parenchymal detail and detects interstitial changes and emphysema. For example, in berylliosis, the chest radiograph shows hilar adenopathy and extensive infiltrates, whereas the HRCT scan documents extensive air space destruction and infiltration (Fig. 93–2). In silicosis, the typical nodular opacities are evident in the chest radiograph,

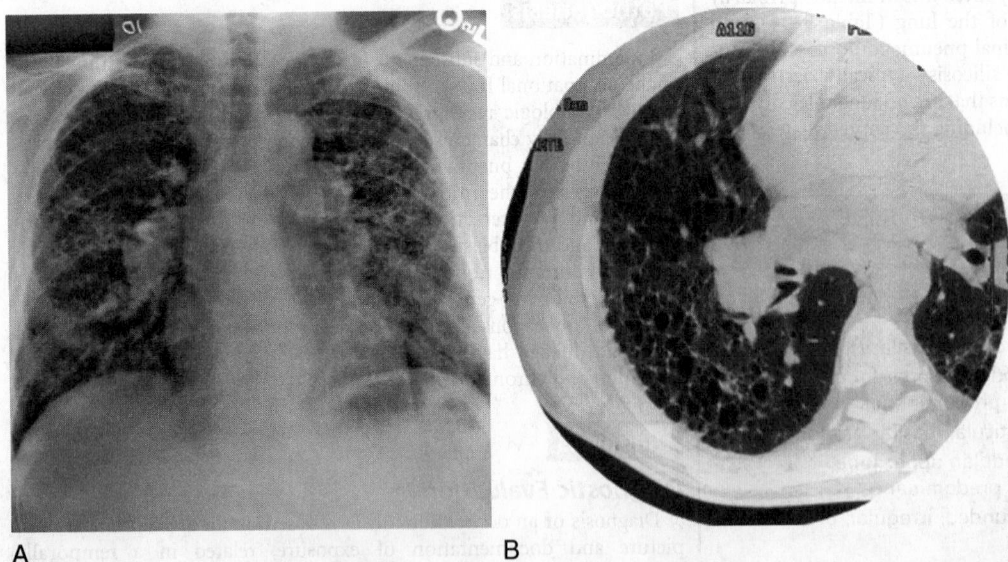

FIGURE 93–2 • Posteroanterior chest radiograph (A) and HRCT scan (B) from a patient with berylliosis. The chest radiograph demonstrates hilar adenopathy and extensive infiltrates, and the HRCT scan shows extensive air space destruction and infiltrates.

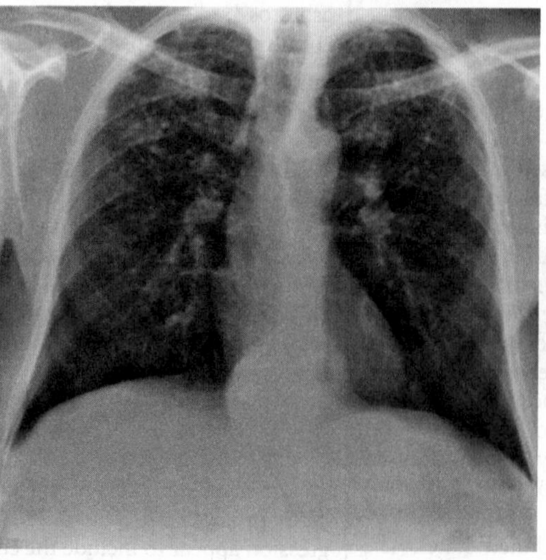

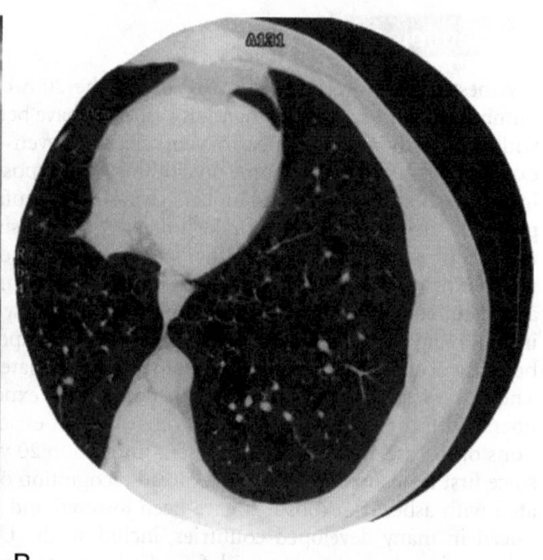

FIGURE 93–3 • Posteroanterior chest radiograph (A) and HRCT scan (B) from a patient with silicosis. The chest radiograph demonstrates the typical nodular opacities, and the HRCT scan shows the nodules as well as air space enlargement.

whereas the HRCT scan shows the nodules as well as air space enlargement (Fig. 93–3). Although the role of HRCT is still evolving, it should be considered for patients who have a normal chest radiograph but are thought to have an occupational ILD. HRCT may also prove valuable for quantifying the degree of abnormality and the extent of coexisting emphysema, but it cannot be recommended for these purposes at present.

Pulmonary Function Testing

Spirometry should be performed for all patients at risk for an occupational ILD and the results compared with predicted values based on gender, race, age, and height (Chapter 85). If the results are within the limits of normal, further testing is not indicated except for patients complaining of dyspnea or having radiographic abnormalities indicative of pneumoconiosis. Those patients as well as patients with abnormal spirometry should have measurements of the single-breath diffusing capacity for carbon monoxide and lung volumes (total lung capacity and residual volume). Exercise testing with measurement of blood gases and gas exchange parameters may be needed to evaluate dyspnea and to quantitate exercise impairment.

Invasive Evaluation

Invasive procedures are rarely indicated to establish the diagnosis of an occupational ILD, although biopsy may be warranted on clinical grounds to exclude alternative diagnoses. Bronchoalveolar lavage, the least invasive approach, provides fluid that can be analyzed for dusts and fibers and for cell populations; it is primarily a research tool. Transbronchial lung biopsy specimens obtained through the fiberoptic bronchoscope may yield a specific diagnosis, and the specimens can be analyzed for dusts and fibers, as can those obtained by open lung biopsy. Polarized light microscopy, which is routinely available, can detect crystals, and ferruginous bodies (ferritin-coated fibers) can be identified with routine optical microscopy. More sophisticated techniques can be used to quantify and to identify particles in lung tissue for medicolegal purposes.

Prevention and Treatment

Rx

Prevention of these diseases rests largely on controlling exposures in the workplace through regulations that limit exposures to levels considered to be safe and that specify respiratory protection. Medical screening for early evidence of disease represents a complementary but secondary control approach. In the United States, the standard-setting agencies are the Occupational Safety and Health Administration and the Mine Safety and Health Administration. Physicians who make a diagnosis indicating a failure of control measures should follow through by contacting relevant agencies and, with permission and possibly preservation of confidentiality, the employer or the union, as appropriate. The burden of respiratory morbidity and mortality in workers at risk for occupational lung disease can also be reduced by preventing and stopping smoking (Chapter 30). For the nonmalignant occupational lung diseases, the adverse effects of cigarette smoking on lung function appear additive to those of the occupational agents, whereas for lung cancer, synergism with smoking has been found for most occupational carcinogens. New genetic approaches may eventually provide strategies to identify workers with the greatest susceptibility; however, prevention continues to be based on workplace controls for the foreseeable future.

For patients with clinically significant impairment, supportive treatment, as for other chronic lung diseases, is warranted. Patients should receive pneumococcal and influenza vaccines and oxygen therapy, as needed. Physical activity should be encouraged, and a comprehensive pulmonary rehabilitation program may benefit some patients. As for other patients with advanced chronic lung diseases, lung transplantation may be a consideration (Chapter 102). Adequate controlled clinical trials to test agents that might retard or reverse the loss of function that occurs in these diseases have not been performed.

PNEUMOCONIOSES

Asbestosis

Definition

Asbestosis refers to fibrosis of the lung parenchyma and not to the pleural fibrosis and plaques that are frequently found in asbestos-exposed workers (Chapters 20 and 100). Asbestos exposure is also associated with mesothelioma of the pleura and peritoneum, lung cancer (Chapter 201), laryngeal cancer, and possibly gastrointestinal cancers.

Asbestos refers to several fibrous silicate minerals having unique physical-chemical properties that make them effective for insulation, reinforcing materials, and friction products. All types of asbestos fibers are associated with asbestosis, pleural disease, and lung cancer. Chrysotile, the type primarily used in the United States, is a serpentine mineral that undergoes gradual physical and chemical dissolution in tissues. Crocidolite, anthophyllite, and amosite, the other principal asbestos types used, are in the amphibole mineral group and are more needle-like than the curly chrysotile fibers and not as prone to dissolution. Chrysotile asbestos appears to be a weaker cause of mesothelioma than the amphiboles.

Epidemiology

Asbestos fibers were widely used during the 20th century, and large numbers of workers directly handling asbestos have been exposed, along with indirectly exposed nearby workers and even family members exposed to fibers brought home on clothing. The exposed worker groups include asbestos miners and millers, workers manufacturing asbestos products such as textiles and brake linings, workers using asbestos products such as insulators, and other construction trades. With a large number of buildings now having asbestos-containing materials, custodial and maintenance workers may also be exposed, as may workers involved in removing asbestos and demolishing buildings. Exposures for general building occupants are low and in a range not associated with asbestosis. The risk of asbestosis increases with cumulative exposure to asbestos fibers; with the exception of extraordinarily high exposures, manifestations of disease are not usually present until 15 to 20 years have elapsed since first exposure. With the widespread recognition of the risks associated with asbestos, exposures have been lowered and substitutes introduced in many developed countries, including the United States. The cohort of workers at greatest risk for asbestosis was exposed through the early 1970s, after which asbestos use was sharply reduced; the incidence of asbestosis should diminish as these workers age.

Pathobiology

In experimental models of asbestosis, the earliest lesions are found in the alveolar ducts and peribronchiolar regions, where deposited asbestos fibers attract alveolar macrophages. The lungs of asbestos-exposed workers show an inflammatory and fibrotic lesion of the small airways, termed mineral dust–induced small airways disease. As the disease progresses, the fibrotic process becomes more extensive and may ultimately involve the entire lung. In advanced cases, extensive fibrosis may destroy the normal architecture of the lung to cause honeycombing, cystic spaces bounded by fibrosis. In advanced disease, the lungs are small and stiff with macroscopically visible fibrosis and honeycombing. Asbestos, or ferruginous, bodies are typically visible with conventional microscopy.

Clinical Manifestations

Patients with asbestosis present with the same clinical picture found in other ILDs: cough and exertional dyspnea. Some cases of asbestosis may also be detected by screening exposed worker populations. Bibasilar fine crackles are heard on auscultation of the chest in most patients, and clubbing may be present in advanced cases. The chest radiograph shows irregular opacities that are typically most prominent in the lung bases; pleural disease, particularly in the form of localized and often calcified plaques, is often present as well. The degree of physiologic impairment on lung function testing varies with the severity of the asbestosis. The small airways lesions produce airflow obstruction, manifested by changes in the shape of the expiratory flow-volume curve, with corresponding reduction of flow rates at lower lung volumes. Airflow obstruction cannot be readily attributed to asbestos exposure in individual patients who have smoked cigarettes. In patients with clinically significant dyspnea, spirometry typically shows a reduced forced vital capacity (FVC), with preservation of the ratio of the forced expiratory volume in 1 second (FEV_1) to FVC, and reduced total lung capacity and diffusing capacity; however, this typical physiologic profile is not invariably observed, and obstruction secondary to smoking may complicate interpretation of pulmonary function findings. Progressive exercise testing shows pulmonary limitation of exercise capacity and desaturation in many patients with asbestosis.

Diagnosis

Asbestosis can be diagnosed with confidence if there is a history of significant exposure to asbestos; radiographic, clinical, and physiologic evidence of ILD compatible with asbestosis; and no indication of another disease process associated with a comparable clinical picture of ILD, such as scleroderma (Chapter 288). At typical levels, the exposure should have started at least 15 years before the disease developed. Pleural plaques provide a strong indication of past asbestos exposure. In patients with biopsy-proven ILD without a firm history of exposure, the presence of asbestos bodies should increase suspicion for asbestosis. More formal counting of asbestos bodies or of fibers may be warranted.

Prevention and Treatment

At present, no effective treatment for asbestosis is available, other than appropriate supportive care, including vaccination against influenza and pneumococci, as well as oxygen therapy as needed. Lung transplantation may be considered for selected patients. Because of the increased risk of asbestos-exposed individuals for lung cancer, perhaps particularly those with asbestosis, smoking cessation (Chapter 30) should be emphasized.

Prognosis

The course of radiographically identified asbestosis is variable; some cases progress, whereas others remain static. Factors influencing progression appear to include the cumulative exposure to asbestos, the duration of exposure, and the type of asbestos exposure. Early identification and cessation of exposure may improve prognosis. The extent of radiographic fibrosis is a strong predictor of mortality.

Coal Workers' Pneumoconiosis

Definition

Coal workers' pneumoconiosis is the parenchymal lung disease caused by inhalation of coal mine dust. The disease is termed simple if all radiographic opacities are smaller than 1 cm in diameter. Progressive massive fibrosis complicates simple coal workers' pneumoconiosis if any nodular opacities 1 cm or larger are present on the chest radiograph. Exposure to coal mine dust is also associated with industrial bronchitis and loss of lung function at a rate beyond that associated with aging; these consequences of such exposure are not considered coal workers' pneumoconiosis, although they do contribute to the respiratory morbidity experienced by coal miners. The group of lung diseases caused by coal mine dust are commonly referred to as black lung.

Coal refers to a group of carbonaceous materials characterized by the hardness or "rank," ranging from peat, the softest, to anthracite, the hardest. Inhalation of coal dust causes coal workers' pneumoconiosis, but inhalation of more pure carbon materials (lampblack and carbon black) has also been associated with a comparable lung disease. Silica in the coal dust may also contribute to the development of coal workers' pneumoconiosis.

Epidemiology

Extensive epidemiologic information shows that the risk of coal workers' pneumoconiosis increases with dust level in the mine and cumulative exposure to coal mine dust. Risk also increases with the rank of the coal, being greatest for the harder coals. In studies of the mortality of underground coal miners, progressive massive fibrosis increases risk of death, whereas simple coal workers' pneumoconiosis has a lesser adverse effect. Reduced exposure for U.S. miners since the passage of the Coal Mine Health and Safety Act of 1969 has reduced risks.

Pathobiology

The characteristic lesion of coal workers' pneumoconiosis is the coal macule, an inflammatory lesion consisting of focal collections of coal mine dust–laden macrophages surrounding respiratory bronchioles. The coal macule may extend to the alveoli and be accompanied by fibrosis of the small airways and alveoli and by focal emphysema. Larger "coal nodules," which are grossly firm and contain dust-filled macrophages in collagen and reticulin, may develop. Progressive massive fibrosis is diagnosed pathologically if nodules reach at least 2 cm in diameter, although the radiographic definition is based on opacities of at least 1 cm. These lesions also contain collagen and tend to disrupt the lung's architecture. In Caplan's syndrome, or rheumatoid pneumoconiosis (Chapter 285), multiple lung nodules ranging from 1 to 5 cm are present, typically in the periphery.

Clinical Manifestations

Coal mine dust–exposed miners may present with cough and sputum production reflecting industrial bronchitis and dyspnea associated with pulmonary function impairment, whether it is secondary to progressive massive fibrosis involving the parenchyma or accelerated loss of ventilatory function related to dust-induced airways disease. Other than characteristic radiographic findings, there are no specific clinical manifestations of simple coal workers' pneumoconiosis. Despite widespread radiographic abnormalities, many miners are asymptomatic or have only mild adverse changes in lung function, whereas some may have significant impairment with little or no radiographic abnormality. In simple disease, the chest radiograph typically shows small nodules that tend to predominate in the upper lung zones. Reticular opacities may also be present, more often in cigarette smokers.

Progressive massive fibrosis is associated with worsening dyspnea, pulmonary hypertension, and even respiratory failure. The chest radiograph shows the characteristic nodules of progressive massive fibrosis, often with contraction of the affected lung (typically upper lobes) and compensatory hyperinflation (typically lower lobes). The nodules may cavitate and produce melanoptysis. In progressive massive fibrosis, lung function is typically impaired, particularly if larger nodules are present. Both airflow obstruction (reduced FEV_1 and FEV_1/FVC ratio) and lung restriction (reduced total lung capacity) can occur. The single-breath diffusing capacity for carbon monoxide is also reduced, and resting hypoxemia or desaturation with exercise may be present. Caplan's syndrome should be considered in miners with multiple peripheral nodules; this uncommon syndrome may develop in miners with rheumatoid arthritis or with circulating rheumatoid factor without arthritis (Chapter 285).

Diagnosis

Coal workers' pneumoconiosis is diagnosed on the basis of an appropriate history of exposure and characteristic radiographic abnormalities. In patients with probable progressive massive fibrosis, consideration should be given to alternative causes of lung masses, including lung cancer.

Prevention and Treatment

No effective treatment is currently available for coal workers' pneumoconiosis. Appropriate supportive care and rehabilitation should be provided for those with impaired lung function, as for asbestosis.

Prognosis

Total coal mine dust exposure, type of coal exposure, and increasing severity of simple pneumoconiosis predict the development of progressive massive fibrosis, which is associated with more severe morbidity and increased overall mortality. Simple pneumoconiosis alone does not increase mortality.

Silicosis

Definition

Silicosis refers to the parenchymal lung diseases associated with crystalline silica exposure, including acute, accelerated, and chronic or classic silicosis. These entities are distinguished by their clinical pictures and time course in relation to silica exposure. In acute silicosis, an alveolar filling process (Chapter 91) follows heavy exposure within a few years. Accelerated silicosis occurs within 5 to 10 years of exposure and has a clinical picture comparable to that of chronic silicosis, which develops after a longer latent period.

Epidemiology

Crystalline silicon dioxide, the causal agent, is abundant and ubiquitous in the earth's crust and is used in a variety of industrial applications. Quartz is the most common form. Consequently, large numbers of workers, probably millions in the United States, are still exposed (Table 93–2).

TABLE 93–2 PRINCIPAL OCCUPATIONS ASSOCIATED WITH SILICON EXPOSURE

Abrasives workers	Silica flour workers
Foundry workers	Silica millers
Glassmakers	Stone workers
Pottery workers	Surface mine drillers
Quarriers	Underground miners
Sandblasters	

As for the other pneumoconioses, the risk for development of disease increases with the level and duration of exposure. Although the hazard posed by silica exposure has long been recognized and exposure standards have been promulgated, new cases continue to occur, even of acute silicosis, which has been recently reported in sandblasters, ground silica workers, and rock drillers.

Pathobiology

Like coal workers' pneumoconiosis, chronic silicosis occurs in a simple form and as progressive massive fibrosis. The earliest lesions are collections of dust-laden macrophages in the peribronchiolar and paraseptal or subpleural areas. The silicotic nodule has an acellular core composed of collagen surrounded by a cellular capsule with macrophages, lymphocytes, and fibroblasts. Silicotic nodules may also involve the hilar lymph nodes. Silicotic nodules coalesce to form the lesions of progressive massive fibrosis, masses of dense hyalinized connective tissue with little inflammation. Accelerated silicosis progresses rapidly to progressive massive fibrosis, whereas acute silicosis has a distinct pattern with few or no nodules and alveolar filling with proteinaceous material. Polarized light microscopy may show birefringent particles indicative of silica in the lungs of silica-exposed persons, including those with silicosis.

Clinical Manifestations

Chronic silicosis without progressive massive fibrosis is associated with little physiologic impairment. Cough and sputum production may reflect underlying bronchitis related to dust exposure or cigarette smoking. As in coal workers' pneumoconiosis, progressive massive fibrosis can be associated with significant impairment on lung function testing and clinically significant dyspnea. Both airflow obstruction and lung restriction may be present. Acute silicosis presents with rapidly progressive dyspnea. Persons with silicosis are at increased risk for mycobacterial infection (Chapters 345 and 346), and they may present with manifestations of infection such as fever and weight loss.

In chronic silicosis, the chest radiograph shows small nodules that tend to predominate in the upper lobes (see Fig. 93–3). Calcification of the nodules is rare, as is so-called eggshell calcification of enlarged hilar nodes. In progressive massive fibrosis, the mass lesions are typically in the upper lobes and are often associated with compensatory hyperinflation of the lower lobes. Widespread consolidation is present on the chest radiograph in acute silicosis. Caplan's syndrome (silicosis and rheumatoid arthritis) may also occur in silica-exposed workers, but it is rare.

Diagnosis

The diagnosis of chronic silicosis is made on the basis of characteristic radiographic findings and history of employment in a job associated with exposure to silica-containing dust. Before a diagnosis of progressive massive fibrosis is accepted in a silica-exposed worker, other causes of lung masses should be considered, including, specifically, lung cancer (Chapter 201) and mycobacterial infection (Chapters 345 and 346). Acute silicosis should be considered in heavily exposed individuals with a diffuse consolidating process. Unless the epidemiologic features of the case make the diagnosis of acute silicosis certain, lung biopsy may be indicated to establish the diagnosis and to exclude other diseases.

Prevention and Treatment

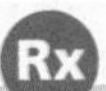

As in any chronic lung disease, supportive therapy, oxygen, and rehabilitation may be indicated. One report suggested possible short-term benefits of corticosteroid therapy, but steroid therapy cannot be recommended at present. Because of the increased risk of mycobacterial diseases, particularly *Mycobacterium tuberculosis* infection, all persons with silicosis should receive yearly tuberculin skin tests and evaluation for active tuberculosis if the test result is positive. Isoniazid prophylaxis (300 mg/day) is recommended if the test result is positive and active disease is not present. Some studies indicate that prolonged antituberculous therapy may be indicated in patients with silicosis and active tuberculosis (Chapter 346).

Prognosis

The prognosis of accelerated silicosis and acute silicosis is poor; both are associated with progressive loss of function, and acute silicosis may be rapidly fatal. Progressive massive fibrosis has a more variable course, which may also lead to progressive impairment and respiratory failure. Factors determining progression from chronic silicosis to progressive massive fibrosis are uncertain.

Other Pneumoconioses

Inhalation of other minerals and metals may also cause pneumoconioses (see Table 93–1). Silicates other than asbestos have been linked to ILD, including talc, kaolinite, mica, and vermiculite. Benign pneumoconioses are associated with inhalation of forms of barium (baritosis) and tin (stannosis). Hard metal disease occurs in workers exposed to cobalt in applications involving its use in alloys and abrasives. This diffuse interstitial disease, which can be associated with clinically significant impairment, should be considered in workers in foundries and in industries involving grinding of metals, gems, and other materials. Some workers exposed to man-made fibers develop small opacities, but a distinct pneumoconiosis has not yet been identified from exposure to these newer fibers. Mixed-dust pneumoconiosis is a nonspecific label often used for the presence of both rounded and irregular opacities on the chest radiograph of a worker with exposure to several types of dust. Typically, there is exposure to crystalline silica and to an additional mineral.

BERYLLIUM DISEASE

Beryllium disease is a granulomatous lung disease that results from inhalation of beryllium, a rare metal now widely used in high-technology applications (Table 93–3). The typical cases currently observed present with gradual onset and are referred to as chronic beryllium disease (Chapter 20); a more acute form was reported with past higher levels of exposure. When it was first recognized, the disease was found in workers who extracted and produced beryllium and in workers making fluorescent lamps containing a beryllium phosphor. Cases have been reported in bystanders not working directly with the metal and in persons residing in the vicinity of beryllium processing plants. More contemporary industries place a large number of workers at risk. In a study of nuclear weapons workers, about 5% of exposed workers were shown to be sensitized to beryllium. Cases of chronic beryllium disease continue to be identified, even though an exposure standard promulgated by the Occupational Safety and Health Administration is in place.

TABLE 93–3 CURRENT INDUSTRIES USING BERYLLIUM

Aerospace	Nuclear reactors
Beryllium extraction, fabrication, smelting	Nuclear weapons
Ceramics	Plating
Dental alloys and prostheses	Telecommunications
Electronics	Tool and die
Foundries	

Advances in understanding of the pathogenesis of beryllium disease are providing insights into the immunologic basis of the disease and the genetic basis of susceptibility. Beryllium, a metal, acts as an antigen or hapten, sensitizing T cells when it is presented in the context of a major histocompatibility complex class II molecule (Chapter 43). A specific genetic marker, human leukocyte antigen (HLA)-DPB1 Glu69, has been linked to increased susceptibility for chronic beryllium disease; this marker may affect binding to receptors in the T cells of the lung. Homozygotes may have particularly high risks, and this marker may eventually prove useful to identify workers at greatest risk. Sensitization to beryllium can be shown by the beryllium lymphocyte transformation test. In this in vitro assay, blood lymphocytes or lung lymphocytes obtained by bronchoalveolar lavage are exposed to beryllium salts; cells from sensitized individuals show proliferation. This test can identify workers who are sensitized but without evidence of chronic beryllium disease as well as those having disease.

The lymphocyte transformation test can confirm beryllium exposure, but the metal can also be measured in tissue specimens and urine. Patients with beryllium disease may have both respiratory and systemic symptoms and chest radiograph findings ranging from normal to diffuse interstitial infiltrates and hilar adenopathy. Corticosteroid therapy may be beneficial, but lifelong treatment is needed.

HYPERSENSITIVITY PNEUMONITIS

Hypersensitivity pneumonitis, typically a granulomatous ILD, results from inhalation of diverse environmental antigens and chemicals. Although interstitial fibrosis is classically considered to be a granulomatous disorder, some patients may have interstitial fibrosis without granulomas. If granulomas are present in lung or other tissue specimens, the differential diagnosis includes sarcoidosis and hypersensitivity pneumonitis. Hypersensitivity pneumonitis may present as an acute illness, but it may also present in a chronic form with pulmonary fibrosis. The workplace is often a site of exposure to antigens generated by microbial contaminants of heating, ventilating, and air-conditioning systems or other moist devices or materials. Chemical agents associated with hypersensitivity pneumonitis include isocyanates and trimellitic anhydride. The diagnosis is made on the basis of the clinical picture, exposure history, and demonstration of precipitating antibodies to antigens. Researchers are exploring polymorphisms in immune response genes for hypersensitivity pneumonitis.

SUGGESTED READINGS

American Thoracic Society: Diagnosis and initial management of nonmalignant diseases related to asbestos. Am J Respir Crit Care Med 2004;170:691–715. *Provides an extensive discussion of criteria for making a diagnosis of asbestosis.*

Balmes J, Becklake M, Blanc P, et al; Environmental and Occupational Health Assembly, American Thoracic Society: American Thoracic Society Statement: Occupational contribution to the burden of airway disease. Am J Respir Crit Care Med 2003;167:787–797. *A comprehensive review.*

Dominici F, Peng RD, Bell ML, et al: Fine particulate air pollution and hospital admission for cardiovascular and respiratory diseases. JAMA 2006;295: 1127–1134. *Short-term exposure increases the risk of hospital admission for cardiovascular and respiratory diseases.*

McCanlies EC, Kreiss K, Andrew M, et al: HLA-DPB1 and chronic beryllium disease: A HuGE review. Am J Epidemiol 2003;157:388–398. *A comprehensive review of HLA-DPB1 and chronic beryllium disease.*

94 PHYSICAL AND CHEMICAL INJURIES OF THE LUNG

David C. Christiani

SUBMERSION INCIDENTS: DROWNING

Definition

Drowning is defined as "the process of experiencing respiratory impairment from submersion/immersion in liquid." The term *near-drowning* was previously used to describe individuals who survived a submersion incident, at least temporarily, but it has been abandoned on the basis of recommendations of the First World Congress of Drowning in Amsterdam in 2002.

Epidemiology

The estimated annual number of deaths worldwide due to drowning is 500,000. About 4200 persons are treated per year for nonfatal drowning in U.S. emergency departments, and about another 3400 suffer fatal drowning. Alcohol use, age younger than 4 years, and male gender are associated with increased rates of nonfatal and fatal drowning.

Pathobiology

The initial response to submersion/immersion is apnea, followed almost invariably by aspiration. Laryngospasm may result in aspiration of a variable quantity of liquid medium into the lungs. Hypoxemia, hypercapnia, and acidemia develop acutely. Aspiration of either fresh or salt water results in occlusion of the airway, reduced surfactant activity, direct alveolar injury, and bronchospasm. Acute lung injury or the acute respiratory distress syndrome (ARDS), associated with noncardiogenic pulmonary edema and severe hypoxemia, may develop hours or days after the incident. Mortality is primarily due to cardiovascular effects as a result of severe early or late hypoxia. The most serious secondary consequence of hypoxia is anoxic brain injury. Acute renal failure may also occur. Alcohol consumption also increases the risk of hypothermia. Changes to serum electrolytes with drowning in either fresh water or salt water are not clinically significant.

Clinical Manifestations

The initial presentation of a drowning victim varies widely. Hypothermia, which is common in drowning victims, may be associated with bradycardia or cardiac arrest due to asystole or ventricular fibrillation. Tachypnea, tachycardia, and low-grade fever are typical in nonhypothermic patients. Cyanosis may be present, and a coughing patient may produce pink frothy sputum. Neurologic evaluation may reveal agitation with or without intoxication or coma. The patient should be examined carefully for signs of associated trauma.

Expected laboratory findings include mild electrolyte abnormalities independent of whether submersion occurs in salt water or fresh water, moderate leukocytosis, slight decrease in hematocrit in the first 24 hours or slight increase in free hemoglobin with a stable hematocrit in fresh water submersion due to hemolysis, severe hypoxemia, and metabolic acidosis. Evidence of disseminated intravascular coagulation may occur. Initial electrocardiographic changes include sinus tachycardia and nonspecific ST segment and T wave changes, which revert to normal within hours. Life-threatening ventricular arrhythmias, complete heart block, or evidence of myocardial infarction can occur early or late in the course. Chest radiographs may initially be normal, despite severe respiratory impairment. Bilateral patchy alveolar infiltrates indicating progression to acute lung injury or ARDS may develop.

Diagnosis

The diagnosis of drowning is made on clinical history of submersion in liquid medium with resulting respiratory impairment. Patients with unusual presenting circumstances should be carefully examined for evidence of trauma or assault.

Prevention

Drowning incidents are largely preventable, particularly in children. Pool fencing is a proven, effective strategy to prevent drowning. The primary cause of drowning of infants and toddlers is lack of adult supervision, and supervision of all young children near any form of water is recommended. The role of alcohol in teenage and adult drowning incidents is substantial, and all individuals participating in water-based activities should restrict alcohol intake. The use of personal flotation devices is recommended for children and adults.

Treatment

Rx

Once the victim has been recovered from submersion, treatment should focus on basic life support algorithms, including notification of emergency response personnel and establishment of an adequate airway and cardiopulmonary resuscitation, if necessary (Chapter 62). If the victim is apneic, rescue breathing should occur immediately, even before removal from the water. Cervical spine stabilization is needed if there is a history of diving, use of a water slide, signs of injury, or signs of alcohol intoxication. Spinal cord injury (Chapter 422) is otherwise unlikely, and cervical spine stabilization techniques and equipment may impede timely and effective treatment. Attempts to remove water from the airway are unnecessary. Cardiac arrhythmias should be treated with Advanced Cardiac Life Support (ACLS) protocols, including the use of automated external defibrillators when appropriate (Chapter 62). A majority of drowning victims who receive cardiopulmonary resuscitation or rescue breathing will vomit; if vomiting occurs, the head should be turned to the side and the vomitus removed with a finger. When vomiting occurs in patients who may have spinal cord injury, log rolling techniques are recommended for turning the patient to the side.

All victims of a submersion incident should be transported to a hospital for further evaluation, treatment (Chapter 105), and monitoring for up to 24 hours. Bronchoscopy may be required to evaluate localized wheezing or persistent atelectasis. Prophylactic antibiotics are not useful, but evidence of pneumonia (Chapter 97) should be treated with appropriate antibiotics. Because unusual microorganisms may be isolated from the lower airways, efforts should be made to identify specific microbial flora pertinent to the locus of the drowning incident.

Treatment of neurologic injury is focused on supportive care while the extent of cerebral edema is minimized. Empirical therapies to decrease cerebral edema include oxygen and positive end-expiratory pressure at the lowest possible levels, mannitol (1 g/kg bolus of 20% solution initially, with repeated doses of 0.25 to 0.5 g/kg every 6 to 8 hours), hyperventilation to a $Pa{CO_2}$ of 30 to 35 mm Hg, corticosteroids (typically with a loading dose of 8 mg/kg of dexamethasone, followed by 4 mg/kg every 6 hours), and monitoring of intracranial pressure, but there is no established evidence for any of these therapies. Intracranial pressure may increase in response to shivering or purposeless movements, which should be reduced. Induced therapeutic hypothermia improves neurologic outcome after cardiac arrest, and current recommendations for drowning victims who remain comatose after rescue are to avoid rewarming to core or tympanic temperatures above 34° C and to maintain temperature of 32° to 34° C for 24 to 48 hours. Hyperthermia should be avoided at all times.

Prognosis

The mortality rate for drowning victims who present alive to an emergency department is about 25%. Long-term neurologic deficits persist in approximately 6% of nonfatal drowning victims. Although prolonged duration of submersion is associated with a worse prognosis, young children who are hypothermic when they are rescued after submersion times of up to 60 minutes have recovered without neurologic damage. Other factors associated with poor prognosis include hypotension, persistent apnea, coma, more than a 10-minute delay in receiving basic life support, and duration of resuscitation of more than 25 minutes.

DISEASES OF HIGH ALTITUDE

Definition

Neurologic and pulmonary disturbances, primarily due to direct tissue effects of hypoxia, occur in individuals who either ascend to or reside at altitudes of 7000 feet (2133 meters) or more (Table 94–1).

Epidemiology

Acute mountain sickness is the most common high-altitude syndrome. It occurs in approximately 20% of individuals who ascend to altitudes of

TABLE 94–1 HIGH-ALTITUDE SYNDROMES

Syndrome	Clinical Description
Acute mountain sickness	Recent ascent to altitudes above 7,000 feet; headache, anorexia, and malaise; common
Chronic mountain sickness	Dwelling above 10,000 feet; headache, fatigue, dyspnea, and digestive disturbances; incidence: 5–18%
High-altitude cerebral edema	Above 15,000 feet; confusion, ataxia, hallucinations, coma, or death; rare
High-altitude pulmonary edema	Above 9,500 feet; dyspnea, cough, and tachycardia; incidence: 2–6%
High-altitude retinal hemorrhage	Above 15,000 feet; asymptomatic or reversible vision changes; common

7000 to 9000 feet, 40% at 10,000 to 14,000 feet, and more than 50% above 14,000 feet. The incidence of chronic mountain sickness, also known as Monge's disease, is thought to be between 5 and 18%. More severe neurologic disturbances due to high-altitude cerebral edema are rare, occurring in approximately 1 to 2% of individuals who ascend to altitudes above 15,000 feet. High-altitude pulmonary edema occurs in approximately 2 to 6% of otherwise healthy individuals who ascend to altitudes of 8000 to 15,000 feet. However, the incidence in individuals with a prior history of high-altitude pulmonary edema may be as high as 60%, or higher during rapid ascents. The occurrence of high-altitude retinal hemorrhage is approximately 33% among individuals who ascend to very high altitudes (up to 19,000 feet) and is thought to be common at lower altitudes as well. High-altitude retinal hemorrhage is not associated with high-altitude cerebral edema or long-term visual consequences.

Pathobiology

Clinically significant hypoxemia is the underlying factor in all high-altitude diseases. The decrease in barometric pressure during an ascent to altitude causes a decrease in the alveolar pressure of oxygen (P_{AO_2}). For example, P_{AO_2} drops from 105 mm Hg at sea level to 60 mm Hg at 10,000 feet and to 40 mm Hg at 18,000 feet. Below 60 mm Hg, oxygen dissociates from hemoglobin more readily (see Fig. 168-2), thereby decreasing oxygen saturation and oxygen delivery to tissues. The effect is even more noticeable in individuals with impaired diffusion capacity, for example, emphysema or heart failure. Furthermore, increased ventilatory drive induces an acute respiratory alkalosis. In the brain, hypoxia causes cerebral vasodilation, whereas hypobaria causes cerebral vasoconstriction. In severe hypoxia, vasodilation is the likely cause of cerebral edema in susceptible individuals. The response to hypoxia in the lungs is primarily increased pulmonary arterial pressures due to hypoxic pulmonary vasoconstriction, which results in reversible injury to pulmonary capillaries, increased capillary permeability, and eventually pulmonary edema. Reduced oxygen consumption also occurs, perhaps from impaired mitochondrial function in the presence of hypoxia. Periodic breathing of sleep is also noted but has minimal if any clinical significance.

Clinical Manifestations

Symptoms of acute mountain sickness begin 2 to 3 hours after ascent and include breathlessness, lightheadedness, fatigue, nausea, anorexia, headache, and insomnia. Most symptoms resolve within 2 to 3 days, although insomnia may persist. Chronic symptoms of headache, fatigue, sleep disturbances, dyspnea, and digestive complaints are seen with chronic mountain sickness in individuals residing at higher elevations. Chronic mountain sickness may be associated with polycythemia (hemoglobin concentrations above 21 g/dL). Severe neurologic symptoms with high-altitude cerebral edema include ataxia and confusion that may proceed to coma or death. Symptoms of high-altitude pulmonary edema that usually begin 2 to 4 days after ascent to higher altitudes include dyspnea, cough, and tachycardia. Funduscopic changes of flame-shaped hemorrhages are seen with high-altitude retinal hemorrhage.

Diagnosis

Diagnosis of most high-altitude disease is made on the basis of clinical manifestations at high altitude. Diagnosis of chronic mountain sickness, and a milder form often termed subacute mountain sickness, is more challenging as it may mimic other cardiopulmonary, neurologic, or psychiatric disease. Individuals with chronic mountain sickness typically have higher hemoglobin concentrations, higher serum erythropoietin levels, higher nocturnal heart rates, lower nocturnal oxygen saturation, and higher systolic and diastolic arterial pressure than do normal individuals living at similar altitude.

Prevention

Prevention of high-altitude disease can be achieved by avoidance in high-risk individuals, such as young children and persons with a history of high-altitude disease. Gradual ascent and acclimatization are crucial to prevention of high-altitude illness, particularly at extreme altitudes. At altitudes up to 10,000 feet, 2 to 3 days or more may be needed for adjustment to the effects of hypoxia. For mountaineers, current recommendations are to ascend no more than approximately 984 feet (300 meters) per day at altitudes higher than 9843 feet (3000 meters).

When rapid ascent is unavoidable, such as flights to high-altitude locales, the carbonic anhydrase inhibitor acetazolamide (250 mg orally once or twice daily) provides effective prophylaxis of acute mountain sickness, and 125 mg at night may improve sleep. Dexamethasone (given in doses of 4 mg twice daily) and prednisolone (20 mg daily) have been shown to decrease the severity of acute mountain sickness. The calcium-channel blocker nifedipine (20 mg of slow-release formulation) is useful for preventing recurrent high-altitude pulmonary edema in individuals with previous episodes. The long-acting β-adrenergic agonist salmeterol (125 μg inhaled twice daily) also reduces the risk of high-altitude pulmonary edema. [1]

Treatment Rx

Several pharmacologic therapies have been investigated for treatment of high-altitude disease. Acetazolamide (250 mg or 500 mg once daily) is also useful in treating symptoms of chronic mountain sickness. [2] Sildenafil (50 mg) can increase exercise capacity at altitude by 10 to 35%. [3] Increasing inspired oxygen concentrations in high-altitude working facilities also improves productivity and quality of sleep. Milder forms of acute mountain sickness, such as headache, can be treated with typical doses of nonsteroidal anti-inflammatory medications, including aspirin and acetaminophen. Immediate treatment of hypoxemia is essential for acute, life-threatening diseases such as high-altitude pulmonary edema and high-altitude cerebral edema: immediate descent, if possible, with supplemental oxygen therapy and, if needed, use of a portable hyperbaric chamber.

Prognosis

Symptoms of high-altitude disease respond rapidly to immediate descent. However, high-altitude cerebral edema and high-altitude pulmonary edema can be fatal, particularly at extreme altitudes and weather when descent may be impossible.

DECOMPRESSION ILLNESS: DECOMPRESSION SICKNESS, BAROTRAUMA, AND ARTERIAL GAS EMBOLISM

Definition

Exposures to changes in ambient pressure cause a spectrum of illness, either (1) by increasing or decreasing the volume of gas in air-filled body cavities or (2) by causing the release of inert gas bubbles from solution in tissues or blood vessels. Symptoms associated with decreasing ambient pressure, which occur most commonly with ascent from depth during recreational or occupational diving, are known as decompression illness. The most common form of decompression illness is decompression sickness, which is classified as either type I (mild symptoms, such as general fatigue or joint pain) or type II (more severe neurologic or cardiopulmonary disturbances). Life-threatening forms of decompression illness include pulmonary barotrauma and arterial gas embolism syndromes. During the descent of a dive, increasing ambient pressure may cause mild symptoms of facial or sinus pain, often called "the squeezes."

Epidemiology

In addition to the approximately 9 million recreational divers in the United States, aviators, astronauts, and compressed air workers are also exposed to changes in ambient pressure that may cause decompression illness. Among recreational divers, the annual incidence rate for either type I or type II decompression sickness is estimated at 1 case per 5000 to 10,000 dives. Approximately 1000 episodes of decompression illness severe enough to warrant recompression therapy occur each year, up to 10% of which are fatal. Well-recognized risk factors for decompression illness include long duration of dives, deep dives, repetitive dives, heavy exertion at depth, cold water, and rapid ascent. Additional risk occurs in individuals who experience further decreases in ambient pressure after the dive, such as on commercial or private aircraft or driving over mountainous areas.

Pathobiology

The principles of Boyle's law and Henry's law describe the properties of gases during changes in ambient pressure. Boyle's law states that the volume of a gas varies inversely to changes in pressure, $P_1V_1 = P_2V_2$. During the descent of a dive, pain due to the "squeezes" is caused by increasing ambient pressures that are not equalized by an increase in gas volume. The resulting negative pressure causes a vacuum effect in the mask associated with engorgement of the blood vessels in adjacent tissues, such as periorbital and ocular vessels, and may result in swelling, pain, and subconjunctival hemorrhages. Facial sinuses, the middle ear, and the external auditory canal may also be affected.

Barotrauma in sinus, otic, or pulmonary tissues may be due to changes in ambient pressures and the resulting increase or decrease in the volume of gas. During descent, the decreasing volume of gas causes vascular engorgement in the sinuses and otic compartments and may result in rupture of the tympanic or inner ear membranes. During ascent, breath-holding, particularly with compressed air devices (SCUBA diving), and the presence of obstructive lung disease with delayed exhalation times and air trapping impair equilibration and increase the risk of pulmonary barotrauma. If the expanding volume of gas causes a pressure gradient between the alveoli and pulmonary interstitium that exceeds the compliance of the lung, alveolar disruption will lead to pulmonary interstitial emphysema. Further extension of gas along pulmonary tissues may cause additional barotrauma, leading to pneumothorax, mediastinal emphysema, pneumopericardium, and soft tissue emphysema.

Arterial gas embolism, which is a serious consequence of pulmonary barotrauma, results in the development of free gas in the pulmonary arterial circulation. The resulting bubbles may then enter the systemic circulation by overwhelming the filtering mechanism of the pulmonary capillaries or through a right-to-left intracardiac shunt (Chapter 68). Bubbles may then migrate to the brain, spinal cord, heart, lung, or kidney and lead to tissue ischemia or infarct.

Henry's law states that the solubility of a gas in liquid is proportional to the partial pressure of that gas above the liquid. An increase in partial pressure of gases during descent will therefore cause the amount of gas dissolved in the pulmonary capillaries to increase. Dissolved oxygen is used during normal body metabolism; however, inert nitrogen, which is abundant in inspired air, becomes dissolved in the blood and tissues, particularly in fat, where it is five-fold more soluble than in water. During ascent, decreasing ambient pressure causes tissues to become supersaturated with nitrogen, and nitrogen is subsequently released into blood vessels and tissues as gas bubbles. Decompression-induced gas bubbles cause decompression illness by either mechanical compression of tissues or embolization through blood vessels to end organs. Bubbles that obstruct capillaries or venules damage the endothelium and cause tissue ischemia, which leads to activation of inflammatory mediators or tissue reperfusion injury. Although not well understood, toxic effects due to increased partial pressure of gases also are likely to contribute to symptoms of decompression illness, possibly by denaturing of proteins and release of fatty acids from cell membranes.

Clinical Manifestations and Diagnosis

Symptoms of decompression illness can occur within minutes and up to 24 hours or more after exposure to changes in ambient pressure associated with dives of 20 feet in depth or more. The severity of symptoms depends on the rate and the magnitude of the change of ambient pressure and can vary among individuals. Diagnosis is based on clinical manifestations, which can be classified according to whether they are caused by formation of inert nitrogen gas bubbles or the localized toxic effects of gas (associated with decompression sickness), barotrauma associated with descent (sinus or otic barotrauma), barotrauma associated with ascent (pulmonary barotrauma), or more severe arterial gas embolism syndromes.

Symptoms vary according to location of bubble formation. For example, type I decompression sickness, also known as the bends or caisson disease, is typically associated with pain in the joints, from mild to severe, and numbness of the extremities. Rashes and lymphedema may also occur. Symptoms of type II decompression sickness may be systemic (fatigue, hypovolemic shock), cardiopulmonary (cough, substernal chest pain, tachypnea, asphyxia), otic (vertigo, hearing loss), or neurologic (ataxia, aphasia, speech disturbances, incontinence, confusion, personality changes, depression, paralysis, and loss of consciousness).

Otic barotrauma, which typically occurs during descent, can affect the external, middle, or inner ear (Chapter 452). External ear symptoms, such as a sensation of ear fullness or otalgia, are caused by a blockage of the canal, for example, with the use of ear plugs or presence of cerumen. Middle ear symptoms of otalgia, vertigo, tinnitus, transient conductive hearing loss, and facial nerve palsy occur when inadequate equalization of pressures results from blocked eustachian tubes, typically in association with allergic rhinitis or upper respiratory infections. Inner ear barotrauma, which is a more serious form of otic barotrauma, is associated with elevated intracranial pressure and rupture of the inner ear membrane. Inner ear barotrauma causes symptoms of sensorineural deafness, tinnitus, vertigo, nausea, and vomiting. Sinus barotrauma typically occurs during descent, is associated with facial pain and epistaxis, and occurs more frequently in individuals with mucosal inflammation from allergies or infection.

Pulmonary barotrauma, which is the second leading cause of death among divers, should be suspected in post-dive individuals, particularly at-risk individuals, with symptoms of sudden pleuritic pain, dyspnea, or coughing. Physical examination findings include tachypnea, subcutaneous emphysema, and dullness to percussion or decreased breath sounds over a pneumothorax. Development of tension pneumothorax (Chapter 100) or severe pneumomediastinum may lead to decreased venous return of systemic blood and reduced cardiac preload, a situation that is characterized by hypotension and may lead to refractory shock or cardiac arrest. Chest and neck radiographs are recommended for diagnosis, particularly because pneumothoraces must be treated with chest tube thoracostomy before recompression therapy.

Because arterial gas embolism syndromes are caused by pulmonary barotrauma, careful neurologic assessment is critical. The neurologic findings are similar to those of an acute cerebrovascular accident (Chapter 430), with manifestations of focal or unilateral motor deficits, visual disturbances, sensory deficits, speech difficulties, and cognitive disturbances, including loss of consciousness. Symptoms typically occur within 10 minutes after ascent. Delayed neurologic symptoms are more likely to be due to type II decompression sickness.

Prevention

Education is the most effective method of preventing decompression illness. Before participation in diving-related activities, all individuals should undergo a thorough and intensive training program. Instruction of proper pressure equalization techniques is critical in the prevention of decompression illness. Persons with asthma who wish to dive should be assessed by a physician (preferably knowledgeable in the field of diving medicine), have no wheezing on physical examination, and have normal spirometry before and after exercise. The presence of structural lung disease (e.g., lung cysts or bullae) is associated with a significant increase in the risk of pneumothorax and is a contraindication to diving. Presence of a known right-to-left intracardiac shunt, such as a patent foramen ovale, is not an absolute contraindication to diving, although conservative diving is recommended, and patients should be cautioned that they are at increased risk of decompression illness.

Treatment

Rx

Symptoms of decompression illness at altitude should be treated with supplemental oxygen and return to the lowest attainable altitude. Serious decompression illness associated with diving requires immediate medical evaluation by emergency personnel, including basic and advanced life support (Chapter 62) when hemodynamic instability is present. Pneumothorax (Chapter 100) should be treated immediately with needle decompression or chest tube thoracostomy.

Symptoms that persist for more than 2 hours or increase in intensity require recompression therapy, preferably with 100% oxygen or transfer to a facility with a hyperbaric chamber, where standard protocols should be followed.

Prognosis

Survival of patients with decompression illness depends on prompt medical evaluation and treatment. Immediate hyperbaric oxygen therapy per standard protocols is associated with resolution of symptoms in 95% of cases. However, symptoms of decompression illness, even neurologic deficits, may respond to recompression therapy after delays of 24 hours or more.

SMOKE INHALATION

Smoke Inhalation and Thermal Injury

Definition

Pulmonary complications, largely caused by smoke inhalation, occur in a large proportion of burn victims (Chapter 113) and account for a substantial number of deaths in these patients. Even patients who do not sustain surface burns in a fire can inhale sufficient smoke to result in injury to the lungs or airways.

Epidemiology

Modern building codes and the widespread presence of firefighting personnel in communities have decreased the importance of fire as a cause of death in the United States. However, fire continues to cause several thousand deaths annually. Also, larger scale fires with mass casualties and wildfires that affect large geographic areas still occur occasionally.

Pathogenesis

Smoke loses heat rapidly as it traverses the upper airway, so direct thermal injury is often limited to the mucosa of the supraglottic airway. A notable exception is steam inhalation, which can produce thermal injury throughout the airways. Smoke inhalation injury affects the entire respiratory tract. The pathogenesis of smoke inhalation is complicated by the wide variety of pulmonary irritants in smoke, many of which are directly toxic to respiratory epithelial or alveolar cells: aldehydes such as acrolein, acetaldehyde, and formaldehyde; acids such as hydrochloric, hydrofluoric, and hydrocyanic acid; and ammonia, nitrogen oxides, and phosgene.

Irritants can rapidly induce intense neutrophilic inflammation, which evolves during 12 to 24 hours after injury and is characterized by mucosal edema and ulceration, abnormally increased permeability of pulmonary capillaries with resultant capillary leak, and epithelial, alveolar, and immune cellular dysfunction. Bronchospasm or bronchorrhea may occur, and the processes may result in ARDS. In addition, because oxygen is consumed in fires, breathing of hypoxic air for prolonged periods may potentiate other injuries or cause clinically significant hypoxia in its own right.

Clinical Manifestations

Thermal injury to upper airway mucosa can cause airway compromise, particularly due to laryngeal edema, sometimes rapidly and sometimes during 12 to 24 hours. Burns to the face, mouth, and neck can externally damage and distort structures of the upper airway and cause airway compromise, both subacutely and late in the course. Inhalation injury manifests primarily with bronchospasm and bronchorrhea, which cause cough, dyspnea, or wheezing and may progress rapidly to respiratory failure. Accumulation of secretions, failure of mucociliary clearance and immune mechanisms, and epithelial necrosis predispose to pulmonary infection, particularly 3 to 5 days after injury. Late pulmonary complications can also be caused indirectly by eschar formation and restriction of thoracic motion.

Diagnosis

Patients with apparent or suspected burn injuries should be assessed emergently for airway patency. Head or neck burns, respiratory distress, stridor, or visibly erythematous or edematous oral mucosa should prompt immediate laryngoscopic evaluation of the oropharynx and supraglottic airway. Hypoxemia may develop and may be severe enough to meet criteria for ARDS. Chest radiography should be performed serially to detect the evolution of lung injury or superinfection.

Treatment

If airway patency is threatened, endotracheal intubation should be performed immediately. Delay can result in increased edema and greater technical difficulty of intubation. Patients who cannot be intubated should have emergent tracheostomy performed surgically. Because of the risk of ARDS, mechanical ventilation with a goal tidal volume of 3 to 6 mL per kilogram of ideal body weight should be considered. All patients should receive supplemental oxygen with the goal of providing a high fractional concentration of inspired oxygen (FIO_2) to reverse the effects of hypoxia and carbon monoxide inhalation (see later).

Pulmonary toilet is essential to maintain secretion clearance in the face of bronchorrhea and epithelial sloughing. Because of the risk of superinfection, surveillance for infection should be vigilant, including diagnostic bronchoscopy if ventilator-associated pneumonia is suspected.

Prognosis

Patients who survive burns and recover generally do not have long-term pulmonary sequelae. Tracheostomies placed at the time of injury can usually be removed later, unless airway structures are damaged or distorted. Impaired pulmonary function is uncommon but may be manifested as airway hyperresponsiveness that has been termed reactive airway dysfunction syndrome.

Carbon Monoxide Poisoning

Definition and Epidemiology

Carbon monoxide is a colorless, odorless gas produced by the combustion of carbon-based fuels. Because of the ubiquity of these substances, carbon monoxide inhalation is often coincident with smoke inhalation in fires or may occur accidentally in association with malfunctioning equipment or improper venting of emissions from heaters, stoves, combustion motors, or other similar devices. In addition, intentional inhalation of carbon monoxide is a method commonly used in suicide attempts (Chapter 420). Carbon monoxide inhalation is the leading cause of death from poisoning (Chapter 111) worldwide.

Pathobiology

Carbon monoxide readily diffuses across the alveolar-capillary interface and binds to hemoglobin with extremely high affinity. When the resulting carboxyhemoglobin molecule undergoes an allosteric change at oxygen-binding sites, the ability of bound oxygen to dissociate and to be delivered to peripheral tissues is greatly reduced. This tissue hypoxia can cause severe functional impairment and ischemic injury of oxygen-sensitive tissues, particularly in the brain and heart.

Clinical Manifestations

Mild carbon monoxide intoxication may go unrecognized as the symptoms are nonspecific and may include headache, nausea, malaise, fatigue, and dizziness. With more severe intoxications, neuropsychiatric symptoms may range from minor disturbances in attention and cognition to agitation, confusion, hallucination, or, in the worst intoxications, seizures or frank coma. Physical findings, which are generally nonspecific, can include tachycardia or hyperthermia. The classic "cherry-red" skin thought to be associated with carbon monoxide intoxication is rarely seen. Other manifestations of severe intoxications may include lactic acidosis, cardiac dysfunction with arrhythmia or ischemia, pulmonary edema, and rhabdomyolysis.

Diagnosis

A high index of suspicion is required for diagnosis because clinical findings are nonspecific. All patients known to have been involved in fires, suicide attempts, or other scenarios compatible with exposures should have arterial carboxyhemoglobin levels checked by co-oximetry. Although levels do not correlate well with clinical findings or risk of complications, symptoms generally occur at carboxyhemoglobin concentrations of 10% or higher.

Treatment

Rx

All patients should be treated with 100% supplemental oxygen, which competes with carbon monoxide for hemoglobin-binding sites and gradually eliminates it from the blood. If patients require mechanical ventilation because of depressed neurologic status or respiratory problems, 100% oxygen should be administered by endotracheal tube. Treatment with hyperbaric oxygen at a pressure of 2.5 to 3.0 atm can increase the dissolved oxygen content of blood by more than 10-fold, and at least one treatment of approximately 2 hours should be considered in severe cases to reverse the effects of acute intoxication; three hyperbaric oxygen treatments within 24 hours of diagnosis reduce neurocognitive sequelae. 4

Prognosis

The mortality rate is highly variable according to the severity of intoxication but can approach 30% in severe cases. Approximately two thirds of patients who survive acute intoxication will recover without sequelae. Many of the remainder will suffer from long-term neuropsychiatric symptoms including cognitive dysfunction, abnormal mood or affect, memory disturbances, and other motor or sensory abnormalities, which can often occur within the first month but may be delayed for up to 6 to 9 months.

Cyanide and Other Gases

Pathobiology

In addition to carbon monoxide and pulmonary irritants, cyanide gas may be formed when a number of commonly found substances, particularly plastics and textiles, are combusted. This gas is highly toxic and can rapidly cause morbidity and death by binding to cytochrome enzymes and inhibiting cellular respiration.

Other inhaled gases that can injure the lungs in occupational settings include ammonia, chlorine, nitrogen dioxide, organic dust, paraquat, phosgene (which has also been used as a chemical weapon), sulfur dioxide, and toxic metal fumes such as cadmium and mercury.

Clinical Manifestations and Diagnosis

Cyanide intoxication typically includes shock, lactic acidosis, and coma; it can rapidly lead to death before results of laboratory studies are available. In the setting of possible exposure, an elevated venous oxygen saturation indicates that cyanide is preventing cells from extracting oxygen from arterial blood.

Other inhaled gases that can produce potent irritant responses include ammonia, chlorine, and nitrogen dioxide ("silo-filler's lung"). Phosgene is notable for its propensity to cause delayed symptoms, up to 24 hours after exposure. Other inhalants may produce an acute chemical pneumonitis with respiratory distress (Chapter 93). A diverse group of inhaled toxins can cause syndromes of inhalational fever, including heavy metal fumes, polymer fumes, and organic dust fumes that contain thermophilic bacteria or fungal elements. These inhalations are characterized by fever and malaise with mild respiratory symptoms and are also notable for tachyphylaxis with repeated exposure (and thus referred to as Monday morning fever in some professions). The herbicide paraquat is typically ingested, not inhaled, but is unique in its ability to cause a rapidly progressive syndrome of pulmonary fibrosis.

Treatment

Cyanide intoxication is treated by use of a Lilly kit, which contains amyl nitrate gas ampules (one 0.3-mL ampule each minute until sodium nitrate infusion begins) for inhalation. This treatment is followed by intravenous administration of sodium nitrite (300 mg), which acts by converting hemoglobin to methemoglobin. Finally, patients are treated with intravenous sodium thiosulfate (12.5 g), which converts cyanide to less harmful thiocyanate ions. If carboxyhemoglobinemia is present, sodium thiosulfate should be used alone because of the additive toxicity of this condition with methemoglobinemia (Chapter 168).

The mainstay for treatment of other irritating inhalations is to remove the patient immediately from the toxic environment and to provide supportive care for respiratory injury. Depending on the intensity and duration of exposure, most patients will recover completely without sequelae.

OXYGEN TOXICITY

Definition

Hypoxic respiratory failure often requires treatment with supplemental oxygen to maintain tissue oxygenation. In some settings, such as ARDS, patients may require high F_{IO_2} for prolonged periods to combat severe hypoxia. However, it has long been recognized that oxygen may be toxic to the lungs when it is present in concentrations higher than those found in ambient air.

Pathobiology

When the concentration of oxygen in the airways is high, formation of reactive oxygen species and free radicals is increased. Under normal circumstances, innate antioxidant mechanisms in airway epithelia and alveoli are sufficient to abrogate the effect of these molecules. However, under conditions of critical illness, prolonged exposure to increased concentrations of these toxins may overwhelm these defenses. Superoxide, hydrogen peroxide, and hydroxyl radicals may directly oxidize cellular components. Cellular damage potentiates inflammation and may be synergistic with inflammatory processes already under way in the diseased lung; the result can be alveolar edema, formation of hyaline membranes, hypoxemia, and progression to fibrosis and obliteration of alveolar and capillary structures. In addition, washout of nitrogen from air spaces can result in absorptive atelectasis if oxygen is removed by the circulation faster than it can be replenished by ventilation (especially in the setting of ventilation-perfusion mismatch). Hyperoxia can also worsen hypercapnia through multiple mechanisms, as occurs in patients with chronic obstructive pulmonary disease who suffer from carbon dioxide retention.

Clinical Manifestations and Diagnosis

Although the exact levels of hyperoxia that cause lung injury are unclear, it appears to occur with exposure to FIO_2 of 50 to 60% after exposures as short as 6 hours in duration. Because of the high flow of supplemental oxygen required to deliver this FIO_2, oxygen toxicity is observed primarily in mechanically ventilated patients being treated for hypoxic respiratory failure. This level of exposure can cause a clinically detectable tracheobronchitis, demonstrable by symptoms of cough and dyspnea, as well as airway erythema that is visible macroscopically on bronchoscopy. This syndrome may impair mucociliary clearance and result in impaction of secretions, especially in conjunction with absorptive atelectasis.

Patients who may be susceptible to oxygen toxicity generally already have a significant degree of parenchymal injury from other processes. Thus, although some patients may appear to display a syndrome of worsening air space disease, atelectasis, consolidation, hypoxia, and diffuse alveolar damage, it is not clear when these changes are related to oxygen therapy or merely occur as part of the acute lung injury from other causes.

Treatment

Rx

Because the threshold level for oxygen toxicity is unknown, a general guideline for treatment of hypoxemic respiratory failure (Chapter 105) is that patients be ventilated with the lowest possible FIO_2 that is required to restore an acceptable oxygen saturation. An SaO_2 of 90%, corresponding to PaO_2 of 55 to 60 mm Hg, is generally considered the minimum acceptable level. Unfortunately, under conditions of severe hypoxia, as in ARDS, patients often require FIO_2 approaching 100% to achieve this oxygen level. Maneuvers to improve oxygenation without increasing FIO_2 include red blood cell transfusion to improve delivery of oxygen; alternative ventilatory strategies, such as high-frequency oscillatory ventilation, airway pressure–release ventilation, inverse-ratio ventilation, and prone positioning; and alveolar recruitment maneuvers using positive end-expiratory pressure or transiently increased inflation pressures.

Prognosis

Patients who sustain oxygen toxicity in the setting of prior bleomycin exposure may be left with residual pulmonary fibrosis. In other patients, the incremental impact of oxygen toxicity on prognosis is unknown.

LUNG INJURY

Radiation Lung Injury

Definition

Accidental or occupational radiation exposures (Chapter 18) are generally characterized by systemic toxicity that outweighs any injury to the lungs. As such, radiation lung injury refers to a pneumonitis that can progress to pulmonary fibrosis and that results from therapeutic use of ionizing radiation, usually in the treatment of malignant neoplasms.

Epidemiology

As many as 50% of patients receiving thoracic radiation will display radiographic abnormalities after treatment; duration and dose of therapy affect the odds for development of lung injury. However, most of these patients will never have clinically significant radiation lung injury. For unclear reasons, the incidence of lung injury appears to vary by the type of underlying malignant disease and modality of treatment. The highest frequency appears to be found in lung cancer (10 to 15%).

Pathobiology and Clinical Manifestations

The pathogenesis of radiation lung injury is often divided into three or four phases on the basis of time course. Typically, the early phase occurs immediately after exposure and is characterized by injury to alveolar cells, resulting in mild alveolitis, recruitment of inflammatory cells, capillary leak, and pulmonary edema. These changes are usually asymptomatic; patients do not usually come to clinical attention, although the chest radiograph will be abnormal if it is performed. In most patients, these changes resolve without progression within 1 to 3 months.

A minority of patients will progress to the next phase, in which alveolar cells desquamate and the air spaces fill with protein-rich fluid. In this phase, referred to as radiation pneumonitis, patients will complain of cough, dyspnea, and occasionally fever or pleuritic chest pain. Severe cases may present with hypoxemic respiratory failure. This phase generally resolves within 3 to 6 months after exposure and is followed by an organizing phase, in which alveolar edema resolves and the damaged alveoli heal. Clinically, patients generally show improvement in symptoms during this period. However, this phase is also characterized by fibroblast proliferation and deposition of collagen in the lung. In a minority of patients, this process will proceed unchecked and result in clinically significant fibrosis, with progressive loss of alveolar-capillary surface and development of restrictive lung disease.

Diagnosis

Clinical history and radiographic evaluation are often sufficient for diagnosis of radiation lung injury as patients typically present with respiratory symptoms and opacities on chest radiography after undergoing radiation therapy. Radiography may show air space disease with alveolar filling or consolidation during the pneumonitis phase, which may progress to an interstitial pattern and eventual honeycombing with parenchymal distortion in the chronic phase. Because radiation characteristically causes injury only within directly affected lung tissue, radiography may show opacities that are well delineated and form straight lines that cross anatomically distinct regions of lung. This finding is rarely if ever seen in other conditions.

The differential diagnosis may include pneumonia, recurrence, and metastatic malignant disease. On occasion, invasive evaluation with bronchoalveolar lavage or even biopsy is required to exclude these possibilities if the clinical history and imaging do not provide a diagnosis.

Treatment and Prevention

Corticosteroids such as prednisone, 1 mg/kg body weight/day, followed by a slow taper during several weeks or months, are the mainstay of therapy. Patients often show a dramatic response to treatment, and symptoms may recur after treatment is discontinued. Other immunosuppressive agents have been used successfully in case reports of patients who failed to respond to corticosteroids.

One small trial suggested that the tumor necrosis factor inhibitor pentoxifylline (400 mg orally, three times daily for the duration of radiation therapy) was effective in reducing the incidence and severity of radiation lung injury in patients who received radiotherapy for breast or lung cancer.

Prognosis

Within 2 years after initial exposure, progression will usually slow, and symptoms and lung function will stabilize and improve. After this time, further improvement or worsening is uncommon. In severe cases that become chronic, patients may develop features of advanced interstitial lung disease, including pulmonary hypertension and hypoxic respiratory failure.

Aspiration Injury

Definition

Aspiration, which is defined as the inhalation of any nongaseous foreign substance into the lungs, generally refers specifically to the inhalation of gastric contents or secretions from the oropharynx. Aspiration is a common occurrence, and in most cases it resolves spontaneously without clinical manifestations. Clinically significant aspiration can range from acute pneumonitis and respiratory failure caused by a single massive aspiration to chronic symptoms of respiratory disease caused by recurrent small-scale aspiration. These syndromes may overlap with pneumonia that occurs when the lungs are exposed to bacteria from the gastrointestinal tract (Chapter 97).

Pathobiology

The common element of clinically significant aspiration is impairment of normal airway protective mechanisms. Under normal circumstances, the airway is protected by the normal swallowing mechanism, the cough reflex, and the anatomy of the supraglottic airway. However, even healthy individuals experience microaspiration despite having functional protective mechanisms. These secretions are handled by normal pulmonary clearance mechanisms.

Any disturbance of these protective mechanisms can result in aspiration injury to the lungs. An altered level of consciousness can impair normal swallowing and suppress the cough reflex. Even in patients who are alert, neurologic injury can result in dysphagia and concomitant aspiration, as in patients who have bulbar neurologic deficits in association with ischemic stroke. Patients with altered airway or oropharyngeal anatomy, such as patients who have received surgical or radiation therapy for head and neck malignant neoplasms, may also be highly susceptible to aspiration of oral secretions.

The nature of the aspirated material is also important in determining whether an injury occurs. Materials with a pH lower than 2.5, such as acidic gastric contents, are much more likely to cause a significant chemical pneumonitis. Particulate matter also increases the likelihood for development of clinically significant inflammation. A large-volume aspiration with distribution throughout the lungs is more likely to produce an acute, severe pneumonitis.

Once material has been aspirated into the lungs, the injury that occurs is similar to a chemical burn. Acid rapidly injures airway epithelial and alveolar cells; within hours, cells become dysfunctional and capillary leak occurs, resulting in profound noncardiogenic pulmonary edema. In severe cases, diffuse alveolar damage may result.

Clinical Manifestations

The classic eponym applied to aspiration pneumonia is Mendelsohn's syndrome, which refers to a single, large-volume aspiration of gastric contents followed by rapidly progressive hypoxemic respiratory failure that develops within hours. Patients may suffer from cough, dyspnea, fever, and respiratory distress. Physical examination may reveal diffuse crackles, wheezing, cyanosis, and hypotension. Chest radiography may show a pattern of alveolar filling with diffuse bilateral involvement or involvement of dependent regions, particularly the right lower lobe. In many patients, this period of acute deterioration is followed by stabilization and resolution within 2 or 3 days. In other patients, deterioration may continue, and patients may meet clinical criteria for ARDS. If the volume of aspirated material is large enough, the initial aspiration may be sufficient to cause tracheal obstruction and asphyxiation.

In patients who initially improve, a small percentage will show further deterioration after 2 or 3 days. This deterioration should prompt an investigation for bacterial superinfection.

Diagnosis

The clinical history and presentation are generally sufficient for diagnosis of aspiration pneumonitis. Bacterial pneumonia and other causes of ARDS also should be considered, as should cardiogenic pulmonary edema. Airway erythema and edema on bronchoscopy can be suggestive of aspiration. Bronchoalveolar lavage may help evaluate for the presence of bacterial infection.

Prevention

Prevention should focus on identification of patients who are at risk for aspiration and then use of strategies to minimize the risk. Patients with swallowing dysfunction or airway abnormalities can work with speech pathologists to learn effective strategies for swallowing. Patients who are unsuccessful or not suitable for this approach may benefit from tracheostomy or enteral tube feedings, which do not prevent microaspiration but can prevent large-volume aspiration. In hospitalized patients, particularly patients with an altered mental status due to illness or sedation, simple strategies such as avoidance of oral feeding and semirecumbent positioning can effectively reduce the risk of aspiration. Use of H_2 blockers or proton pump inhibitors (Chapter 142) can alter gastric pH to reduce the risk of injury from acidic secretions.

Treatment

Rx

Because of the acuity and severity of this aspiration pneumonitis, immediate attention should be paid to maintaining a patent airway. The oropharynx and trachea should be suctioned to clear any potentially obstructing material, and endotracheal intubation should be performed if necessary (Chapter 106). Bronchoscopy is often performed to clear residual particulate or solid matter, but it cannot remove acidic secretions, which damage airways and parenchyma quickly and then are rendered neutral. Oxygen supplementation should be provided as needed for hypoxia. Corticosteroids have not been shown to be beneficial. Antibiotics should be reserved for patients who appear to have developed bacterial superinfection (Chapter 97).

Prognosis

For patients with severe respiratory failure or ARDS, mortality can be high. In others, improvement should be expected within days. If the underlying factor that led to aspiration is irreversible, patients have an increased likelihood of recurrent episodes.

Lipoid Pneumonia

Definition

Lipoid pneumonia is a chronic inflammatory reaction of the lungs to the presence of lipid substances. Exogenous lipoid pneumonia results from the aspiration of vegetable, animal, or (most commonly) mineral oils.

Pathobiology

The most frequently implicated agent is mineral oil used as a laxative and to reduce dysphagia, either in clear liquid form or as petroleum jelly. Mineral oil is bland and, when introduced into the pharynx, can enter the bronchial tree without eliciting the cough reflex. It also mechanically impedes the ciliary action of the airway epithelium. The risk of mineral oil aspiration is increased in debilitated or senile patients, in those with neurologic disease that interferes with deglutition, and in patients with esophageal disease. Mineral oil taken as nose drops to relieve nasal dryness can also cause lipoid pneumonia. Inhalation of mineral oil mist by airplane and automobile mechanics has also been implicated as a cause.

Mineral oils, which cannot be hydrolyzed in the body, provoke a chronic inflammatory reaction that may not become clinically overt until years later. In the alveolar spaces, macrophages accumulate and phagocytose the emulsified oil. Some macrophages disintegrate, releasing their lysosomal enzymes and oil. The alveolar septa become thickened and edematous, containing lymphocytes and lipid-laden macrophages. Oil droplets are seen in the pulmonary lymphatics and hilar nodes. Later, fibrosis develops, and the normal lung architecture is effaced. A single pathologic specimen may include both the early inflammatory and the later fibrotic picture, in keeping with repetitive aspirations during many months or years. Nodular lesions may grossly resemble tumor and be called paraffinomas.

Clinical Manifestations

Most patients are asymptomatic and come to the physician's attention because of an abnormal chest radiograph. When patients are symptomatic, cough and exertional dyspnea are the most frequent complaints. Chest pain (sometimes pleuritic), hemoptysis, fever (usually low grade), chills, night sweats, and weight loss may occur. Findings on physical examination may be completely normal, but fever, tachypnea, dullness on percussion of the chest, bronchial or bronchovesicular breath sounds, rales, and rhonchi may be found. Clubbing and cor pulmonale are rare.

Diagnosis

In mild lipoid pneumonia, arterial blood gas values may be normal with the patient at rest but may show hypoxemia after exercise. In more severe disease, resting hypoxemia, hypocapnia, and mild respiratory alkalosis develop. Pulmonary function testing reveals a restrictive ventilatory defect; lung compliance is decreased. The only specific laboratory finding is the presence in sputum of macrophages with clusters of vacuoles that are 5 to 50 μm in diameter and that stain deep orange with Sudan IV; extracellular droplets may stain similarly.

On radiographic examination, the earliest abnormalities are air space infiltrates, most often in the dependent portions of the lung. The infiltrates may be unilateral or bilateral, localized or diffuse. Air bronchograms may be seen. Hilar adenopathy and pleural reaction are rare. As fibrosis develops, volume loss occurs, and linear and nodular infiltrates appear. A solid lesion that closely resembles bronchogenic carcinoma may develop. High-resolution computed tomography usually shows consolidated areas of low attenuation and "crazy paving" (Fig. 94–1).

The differential diagnosis is extensive, particularly in the late phase, when multiple other causes of pulmonary fibrosis must be considered. The key to the correct diagnosis before biopsy is the history of chronic oral or intranasal use of an oil- or a lipid-based product or an occupational exposure to oil mists. The presence of lipid-laden macrophages in sputum or bronchoalveolar lavage fluid also can be used to confirm the diagnosis, particularly in conjunction with typical findings on high-resolution computed tomography.

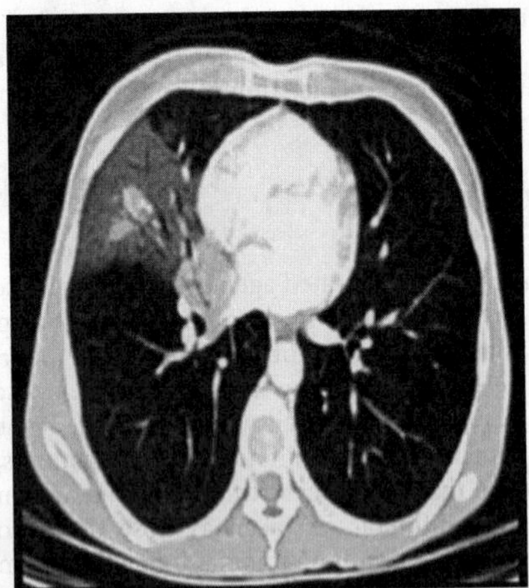

FIGURE 94–1 • Lipoid pneumonia on a computed tomographic scan.

Treatment and Prevention

Rx

Once the diagnosis has been made and the aspiration stopped, the subsequent course is variable. Because the only way the lung can dispose of mineral oil is by expectoration, the patient should be instructed in coughing exercises to be performed many times each day for months. Expectorants have not been shown to help. Systemic corticosteroids have been recommended on the basis of improvement seen in a few uncontrolled reports. Because of the well-recognized side effects of systemic corticosteroids, their use for lipoid pneumonia should be limited to patients who have significant symptoms, and then for as brief a period as possible.

Transfusion-Related Acute Lung Injury

Definition

The syndrome of transfusion-related acute lung injury (TRALI; Chapter 183) involves the rapid onset of respiratory distress within minutes to hours after the transfusion of blood products (fresh-frozen plasma, platelets, and red blood cells). The initial clinical picture is indistinguishable from acute lung injury or ARDS due to other causes, such as sepsis, multiple trauma, and lung injury. TRALI may similarly be confused with pulmonary edema due to volume overload (Chapter 57).

Epidemiology

The true incidence of TRALI is unknown; incidence rates are underestimated because of the difficulty in distinguishing TRALI from other causes of acute respiratory failure and the labor-intensive and costly diagnostic evaluation required. Reported incidences range from 1 : 1000 to 1 : 100,000 units of blood products transfused. The risk of TRALI varies according to the type of blood product transfused, with pooled products associated with a higher incidence. Only 8 to 21 TRALI-related deaths are reported to the Food and Drug Administration annually, and even liberal estimates accounting for underreporting suggest the number may be only as high as 300 per year of an estimated 25 million transfusions in the United States.

Pathobiology

The physiologic manifestations of TRALI are caused by alveolar filling with fluid and protein. This alveolar process is the result of increased microvascular permeability due to pulmonary endothelial damage mediated by either leukocyte antibodies or the priming and activation of neutrophils in the pulmonary circulation by bioactive substances.

TRALI most commonly occurs when human leukocyte antigen (HLA) type I or II or neutrophil-specific antigen antibodies from the donor attach to the recipient's leukocytes, leading to the release of injurious oxidative and nonoxidative products. Development of HLA antibodies occurs commonly in women during pregnancy, and increasing parity in female blood donors is associated with an increased risk of TRALI.

Episodes of TRALI occurring in patients without HLA or neutrophil-specific antigen antibodies in either the donor or recipient are thought to be caused by a two-hit process of neutrophil priming and activation. Neutrophils are primed and sequestered in the lung by conditions that often occur in patients requiring blood products, such as multiple trauma, surgery, or sepsis. Primed neutrophils are then activated by bioactive lipids and cytokines stored in the blood products, thereby leading to lung injury and alveolar damage. Levels of these bioactive lipids or cytokines may increase after prolonged storage of blood products.

Clinical Manifestations

Although most cases of TRALI present within 1 to 2 hours after the transfusion of blood products, tachypnea, hypoxemia, cyanosis, dyspnea, and fever can develop during the transfusion or up to 6 hours later. Hypertension or hypotension commonly occurs, depending on the severity of the reaction. Copious amounts of pink, frothy edema fluid may be present. Lung auscultation generally reveals bilateral crackles and decreased breath sounds in dependent lung zones.

Diagnosis

Bilateral patchy infiltrates consistent with alveolar edema are found on plain chest radiographs, typically without effusions. Arterial blood gas analysis demonstrates reduced Po_2, and further laboratory testing may reveal thrombocytopenia or a transient leukopenia. Diagnosis of TRALI requires the presence of the following:

1. acute onset of hypoxemia with $Pao_2/Fio_2 \leq 300$ or room air oxygen saturation <90%;
2. bilateral infiltrates on frontal chest radiographs;
3. no evidence of left atrial hypertension;
4. no preexisting acute lung injury before transfusion;
5. appearance during or within 6 hours of transfusion; and
6. no temporal relationship to an alternative risk factor for acute lung injury.

The diagnosis of "possible TRALI" is made in patients who have a concurrent diagnosis of another risk factor for acute lung injury, including (1) direct lung injury due to aspiration, pneumonia, toxic inhalation, lung contusion, or nonfatal drowning and (2) indirect lung injury due to severe sepsis, shock, multiple trauma, burn injury, acute pancreatitis, cardiopulmonary bypass, or drug overdose. Absolute confirmation of the diagnosis requires testing for HLA and neutrophil-specific antigen antibodies, usually performed first in female donors, then in male donors, and finally in the recipient.

Treatment

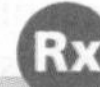

Most cases are self-limited and resolve within hours to days with supplemental oxygen and supportive care. Volume resuscitation, with or without vasopressors, is required for hypotension. Mechanical ventilation should be managed as for any other case of acute lung injury, with the implementation of a low tidal volume ventilation strategy to prevent further ventilator-induced lung injury. Diuresis should be attempted cautiously and may even be detrimental because intravascular filling pressures are often low.

Prognosis

The mortality rate of TRALI is approximately 5%. If an implicated donor can be identified, the recipient should not receive any further transfusions from that donor, but patients are not at increased risk for further episodes of TRALI from nonimplicated donor transfusions.

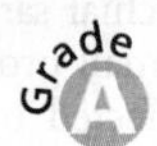

1. Sartori C, Allemann Y, Duplain H, et al: Salmeterol for the prevention of high-altitude pulmonary edema. N Engl J Med 2002;346:1631–1636.
2. Richalet JP, Rivera M, Bouchet P, et al: Acetazolamide: A treatment for chronic mountain sickness. Am J Respir Crit Care Med 2005; 72:1427–1433.
3. Ghofrani HA, Reichenberger F, Kohstall MG, et al: Sildenafil increased exercise capacity during hypoxia at low altitudes and at Mount Everest base camp: A randomized, double-blind, placebo-controlled crossover trial. Ann Intern Med 2004;141:169–177.
4. Weaver LK, Hopkins RO, Chan KJ, et al: Hyperbaric oxygen for acute carbon monoxide poisoning. N Engl J Med 2002;347: 1057–1067.

SUGGESTED READINGS

2005 American Heart Association guidelines for cardiopulmonary resuscitation and emergency cardiovascular care. Part 10.3: Drowning. Circulation 2006; 112:IV-133–IV-135. *Recommendations include early initiation of rescue breathing while the victim is in the water, initiation of cardiopulmonary resuscitation once the victim is removed from the water, and stabilization of the cervical spine only if traumatic injury is likely.*

British Thoracic Society guidelines on respiratory aspects of fitness for diving. Thorax 2003;58:3–13. *Includes level of evidence and grading of recommendations for the assessment of fitness to dive for patients with respiratory conditions.*

Camus P, Costabel U: Drug-induced respiratory disease in patients with hematological diseases. Semin Respir Crit Care Med 2005;26:458–481. *Review of radiation lung injury as well as other pulmonary complications of cancer therapy.*

Divers Alert Network. Available at http://www.diversalertnetwork.org/index.asp. *This website includes a link to a 24-hour hotline for diving emergencies.*

Gajic O, Moore B: Transfusion-related acute lung injury. Mayo Clin Proc 2005;80:766–770. *A clinical review.*

Henry CR, Satran D, Lindgren B, et al: Myocardial injury and long-term mortality following moderate to severe carbon monoxide poisoning. JAMA 2006;295:398–402. *Myocardial injury occurs frequently and is a significant predictor of mortality.*

Kales SN, Christiani DC: Acute chemical emergencies. N Engl J Med 2004;350:800–808. *Review of various inhalation injuries, including carbon monoxide poisoning.*

Maggiorini M, Brunner-La Rocca H, Path S, et al: Both tadalafil and dexamethasone may reduce the incidence of high-altitude pulmonary edema. Ann Intern Med 2006;145:497–506. *Both decrease systolic pulmonary artery pressure and may reduce HAPE.*

95 SARCOIDOSIS

Steven E. Weinberger

Definition

Sarcoidosis is a disease of unknown cause that is characterized by the presence of noncaseating granulomas in multiple organ systems. Although the lungs and the lymph nodes in the mediastinum and hilar regions are the most common sites of involvement, the disorder is considered a systemic disease, and a variety of other organ systems or tissues may be the source of either primary or concomitant clinical manifestations and morbidity. The clinical course is variable and ranges from asymptomatic disease with spontaneous resolution to progressive disease with organ system failure and even death.

Epidemiology

Although sarcoidosis has a worldwide distribution, its reported incidence and prevalence vary considerably in different geographic areas and among disparate population subgroups. However, the accuracy and comparability of the data available are suspect because of a high frequency of asymptomatic cases and widely differing methods of case identification.

Sarcoidosis appears to be relatively common in northern Europe (especially Scandinavia, Ireland, and Great Britain), North America, and Japan, whereas regions with a reportedly low incidence include China, Africa, India, and Russia. Even in these presumed low-incidence regions it is likely that more cases of sarcoidosis have been present but have been misdiagnosed, especially as tuberculosis or leprosy. In a number of countries, such as Italy and Japan, the incidence of the disease is significantly greater in the northern than the southern part of the country, thus raising the possibility that climate affects the likelihood of the disease.

The peak age at onset of sarcoidosis is in the 20s and 30s, and women are affected slightly more often than men. Approximately 50% of patients are younger than 30 years at initial evaluation, and approximately 75% are younger than 40. In some countries, such as Sweden and Japan, a second peak in incidence has been noted in middle age, especially in women.

In the United States, sarcoidosis is more frequent in blacks than in whites, with the age-adjusted annual incidence reported as 35.5 and 10.9 per 100,000, respectively. Worldwide, however, nearly 80% of affected patients are white.

There are also geographic, ethnic, and racial differences in the mode of manifestation and the clinical features of sarcoidosis. Erythema nodosum is common in Scandinavian and British patients with sarcoidosis but is rare in African Americans and Japanese. Cardiac and ocular involvement is particularly prevalent in Japan, where cardiac involvement is the most common cause of death from sarcoidosis.

Pathobiology

The cause of sarcoidosis is unknown. A substantial body of information has suggested that immune mechanisms are important in pathogenesis of the disease, and it has been presumed that one or more causal antigens trigger a cascade of immunologic events in a genetically susceptible individual. However, neither a single antigen nor a particular genetic factor is known to be common to all patients with this disease.

Several observations have suggested that one or more exogenous agents may be responsible for sarcoidosis:

1. Identification of case clusters of sarcoidosis (e.g., in nurses and firefighters and in specific geographic regions) supports the possibility of either person-to-person transmission of an infectious agent or shared exposure to an environmental agent.
2. The disease berylliosis, which is due to exposure to beryllium, produces a histologic pattern and clinical features that are quite similar to those seen with sarcoidosis.
3. The disease can recur in the transplanted lung of patients who receive a transplant for end-stage sarcoidosis. In addition, sarcoidosis has been reported to develop in the recipient of tissue from a donor with sarcoidosis.

A variety of exogenous agents, both infectious and noninfectious, have been hypothesized as being possible causes of sarcoidosis. Proposed infectious causes include mycobacteria (both *Mycobacterium tuberculosis* and nontuberculous mycobacteria), cell wall–deficient mycobacteria (called *L-forms*), *Propionibacterium acnes, Borrelia burgdorferi*, viruses, fungi, spirochetes, and the agent associated with Whipple's disease. Although the diagnosis of sarcoidosis depends on the absence of organisms that are known to be associated with granuloma formation (e.g., mycobacteria and fungi on stain or culture), the possibility remains that sarcoidosis may represent a variant host response to an infectious agent and that the organism may not be readily identifiable or recoverable at the time of manifestation of the disease. For example, a number of studies have used polymerase chain reaction to identify mycobacterial DNA from biologic specimens obtained from patients with sarcoidosis, but the results are inconclusive.

Environmental or occupational exposure to noninfectious agents has been an important alternative theory of the etiology of sarcoidosis. Based on the model provided by berylliosis, it has been suggested that an exogenous agent induces immunologic sensitization, perhaps by acting as a "hapten" that binds to peptides or alters major histocompatibility complex (MHC) molecules. Noninfectious agents proposed to be causally related to sarcoidosis have included beryllium and other metals, organic antigens (e.g., pine pollen, peanut dust), and inorganic dust (e.g., clay). A large case-control study exploring occupational and environmental exposure found that agricultural employment and exposure to insecticides or microbial aerosols were associated with an increased risk. Nevertheless, the current weight of evidence does not adequately support exposure to any particular agent as a primary cause of sarcoidosis.

It is believed, though not proved, that genetic factors may influence the development of sarcoidosis by affecting the nature of the cellular and immune response to the exogenous agents. Familial sarcoidosis, in which an individual with sarcoidosis is found to have a first- or second-degree relative with the disease, has been noted in up to 15% of patients. In the aforementioned large case-control study, the relative risk of sarcoidosis for the sibling of an individual with sarcoidosis was 5.8; the overall familial risk in first- or second-degree relatives of patients with sarcoidosis was 18 in white and 2.8 in African American individuals. However, the comparative roles of genetics versus shared environmental exposure in explaining the familial occurrence of sarcoidosis remain undefined. MHC genes located on the short arm of chromosome 6, especially HLA genes, as well as non-MHC genes, have been implicated as risk factors for sarcoidosis, but the results of studies involving a variety of candidate genes have not been consistent.

Despite the lack of definitive evidence about intrinsic and extrinsic factors that initiate sarcoidosis, a substantial body of information has been accumulated about the intermediate pathogenesis of the disease (i.e., the role played by cellular responses, immune mechanisms, and elaboration of cytokines). Antigen processing by macrophages is believed to trigger an oligoclonal expansion of CD4 (helper-inducer) lymphocytes of the T_H1 phenotype, with production of interleukin-2 (IL-2) and interferon-γ. IL-2 causes the proliferation of more CD4 cells, which elaborate cytokines that recruit macrophages into the granuloma. A variety of cytokines, adhesion molecules, and growth factors that amplify the inflammatory response and have the potential to induce fibrosis are released from both lymphocytes and macrophages. Tumor necrosis factor-α (TNF-α), released from alveolar macrophages involved in the inflammatory process, is believed to be a particularly important cytokine mediator involved in the formation of granulomas.

Although B lymphocytes do not appear to play a primary role in the disease, their function is altered secondarily by mediators released from activated T lymphocytes. Polyclonal hyperglobulinemia results, with the formation of antibodies reactive against a variety of microbial agents and self-antigens.

Clinical Manifestations

Sarcoidosis is notable for its protean manifestations and variable course. Not only can almost any organ system be affected, but the clinical features and natural history of disease affecting a particular organ system are also quite variable. The respiratory system is most commonly affected, with approximately 90% of patients demonstrating intrathoracic involvement on a chest radiograph. Extrathoracic disease can develop with or without concomitant intrathoracic involvement and can be the predominant component of the clinical picture or can be either subclinical or less problematic than the intrathoracic disease.

As many as 30 to 60% of patients have no symptoms at the time of diagnosis, with the disease being identified because of abnormalities on a chest radiograph. Alternatively, patients are commonly seen with respiratory symptoms, such as dyspnea and cough; nonspecific retrosternal chest discomfort is sometimes present. Approximately a third of patients may have constitutional symptoms, including fever, weight loss, malaise, and fatigue. As many as 10 to 20% of patients have a syndrome of bilateral hilar adenopathy and erythema nodosum, a constellation of findings that is called *Löfgren's syndrome;* fever or arthralgias (or both) may also accompany this type of manifestation. Findings related primarily to extrathoracic involvement are less common; the specific signs and symptoms depend on the particular organ systems involved.

Respiratory System Disease

Intrathoracic nodal involvement and parenchymal lung disease are the two most common ways in which sarcoidosis affects the respiratory system. Both hilar and mediastinal lymph nodes may be affected; involvement of the hilar nodes is usually bilateral and relatively symmetrical. The pulmonary parenchyma demonstrates well-defined, noncaseating granulomas within the pulmonary interstitium, typically in a pattern that preferentially follows the bronchovascular bundles. The upper lobes of the lung tend to be more involved than the lower lobes. The granulomatous inflammation is often accompanied by nonspecific mononuclear cell infiltration; in severe disease, parenchymal involvement may progress to irreversible fibrosis and honeycombing. Cystic lesions may be complicated by colonization with *Aspergillus* and the development of intracavitary aspergillomas.

Granulomatous involvement of the airways (i.e., endobronchial sarcoidosis) is common and may lead to bronchostenosis in a small proportion of patients. The upper respiratory tract may be affected by sarcoidosis, with involvement taking the form of nasal mucosal, nasal bone, or laryngeal disease. Pleural disease is relatively infrequent, with effusions occurring in less than 5% of patients.

Dyspnea and cough, typically nonproductive, are the primary symptoms that accompany either pulmonary parenchymal or endobronchial sarcoidosis. Examination of the chest can reveal crackles resulting from parenchymal lung involvement, although such examination is often notable for the paucity or even absence of findings despite the extent of radiographic changes. Wheezing may be present in a small proportion of cases and results from either endobronchial involvement or airway distortion as a consequence of end-stage fibrotic disease.

Pulmonary function tests (Chapter 85) in patients with parenchymal lung disease often demonstrate a pattern of restrictive disease with a relatively symmetrical decrease in lung volumes, although they can remain normal despite parenchymal changes on the chest radiograph. Obstructive changes may also be seen in some patients as a result of airway involvement. The diffusing capacity of the lung for carbon monoxide may be either normal or abnormal and does not necessarily follow the presence or absence of abnormal lung volumes.

Skin Disease

Cutaneous manifestations of sarcoidosis resulting from granulomatous involvement of the skin affect 15 to 25% of patients. A variety of

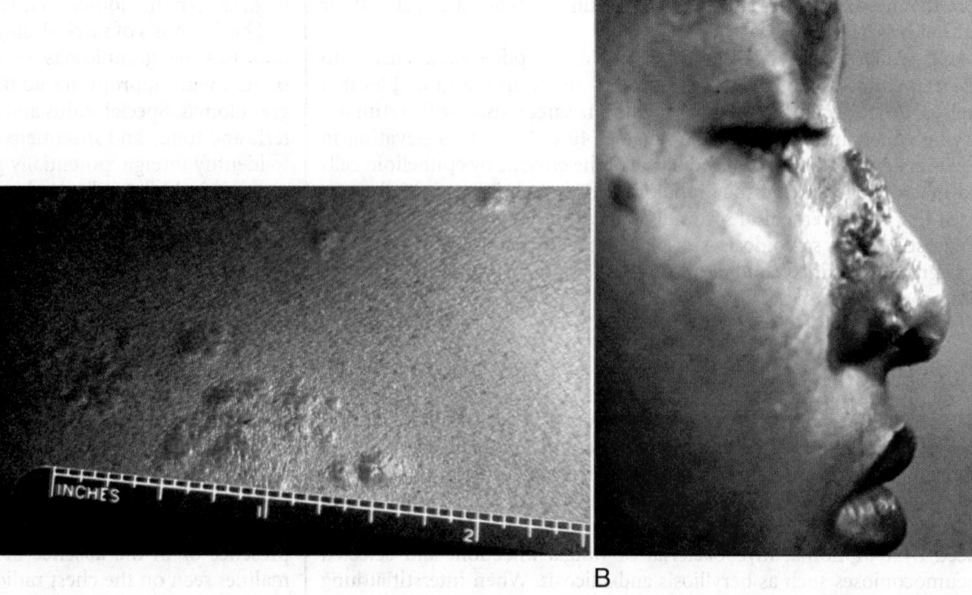

FIGURE 95–1 • Skin lesions of sarcoidosis. A, Sarcoid lesions may occur at any site, and they may take a nodular, papular, or plaque form. This patient's papules have a waxy appearance and are located on the upper part of the back. B, Lupus pernio is the term used to describe infiltrative skin lesions affecting the nose, cheeks, or ears in chronic sarcoidosis.

lesions can be seen, including papules, plaques, nodules, infiltration of old scars, and lupus pernio (Fig. 95–1). Old scars or tattoos often become infiltrated with granulomas, so previously atrophic scars can assume an appearance of keloid formation. *Lupus pernio* is a chronic, violaceous, often disfiguring lesion primarily affecting the nose, cheeks, and ears. It tends to affect women older than 40 years, especially African Americans and individuals from the West Indies.

Erythema nodosum commonly occurs in combination with bilateral hilar adenopathy as part of Löfgren's syndrome. These raised, red, tender nodular lesions, generally but not exclusively on the anterior surface of the lower part of the leg, do not represent granulomatous involvement of the skin. Rather, the histopathology is primarily that of a panniculitis, with cellular inflammation and edema of the deep dermis and subcutaneous tissue, especially involving the connective tissue septa of adipose tissue.

Eye Disease

Ocular sarcoidosis can take a number of forms, including anterior or posterior uveitis, conjunctival involvement, and papilledema. Overall, 15 to 25% of patients have some form of ocular involvement. Anterior uveitis, the most common form of ocular sarcoidosis, is often associated with the relatively acute onset of a red eye, photophobia, and ocular discomfort. *Heerfordt's syndrome,* or uveoparotid fever, is a form of sarcoidosis in which anterior uveitis is accompanied by parotid gland enlargement and frequently fever and facial palsy. Posterior uveitis, which may be obscured on examination by anterior chamber involvement, can be manifested as vitreous infiltrates, choroidal nodules, periphlebitis, retinal hemorrhage, and papilledema. Conjunctival involvement can produce small, pale yellow nodules that demonstrate granulomatous inflammation on biopsy (Fig. 95–2).

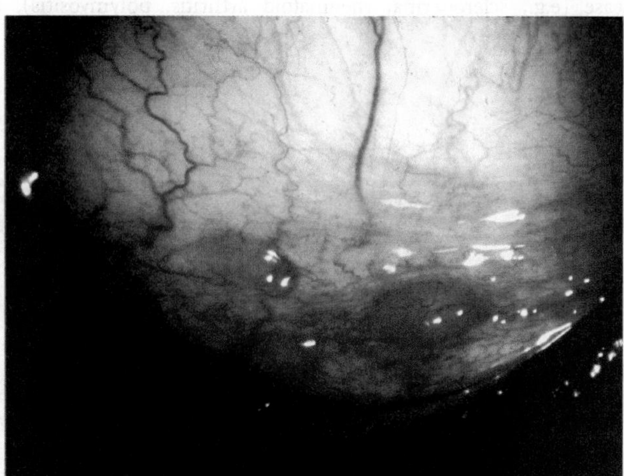

FIGURE 95–2 • Raised or nodular areas on the conjunctiva may indicate granulomatous involvement of the conjunctiva.

Cardiac Disease

Approximately 5 to 10% of patients with sarcoidosis have symptomatic cardiac involvement, whereas 20 to 30% have histologic involvement at postmortem examination. Potential clinical consequences include conduction defects (e.g., first-, second-, or third-degree heart block or a bundle branch block), ventricular or supraventricular arrhythmias, and heart failure (Chapter 59).

Neurologic Disease

Neurologic complications of sarcoidosis develop in 5 to 10% of patients. Although involvement of the base of the brain is particularly common, virtually any part of the nervous system can be involved, including the cranial nerves, peripheral nerves, meninges, cerebrum, spinal cord, and the hypothalamic-pituitary axis. The most common form of clinically apparent neurologic involvement is unilateral facial nerve palsy, but other clinical consequences include seizures, meningitis, peripheral neuropathy, and psychiatric symptoms. Involvement of the hypothalamic-pituitary axis can cause hyperprolactinemia and diabetes insipidus.

Other Extrathoracic Disease

Although granulomas are commonly found on histologic examination of the liver in patients with sarcoidosis, symptoms related to hepatic involvement are uncommon, and clinical evidence is usually limited to abnormalities in one or more hepatic enzymes (Chapter 155). In addition to intrathoracic lymph node involvement, peripheral lymph nodes may be enlarged because of granulomatous infiltration, but they rarely produce important clinical consequences. Parotid gland enlargement, lacrimal gland infiltration, bone lesions, splenomegaly, and myopathy as a result of granulomas within muscle tissue may also be seen.

Biochemical Changes

Biochemical changes noted in many patients with sarcoidosis include alterations in calcium metabolism and elevated levels of angiotensin-converting enzyme (ACE). Hypercalcemia, a potentially important complication of sarcoidosis, occurs in less than 10% of patients and is due to elevated levels of 1,25-dihydroxyvitamin D (calcitriol) produced by macrophages within the granulomas. As a result, calcium absorption from the intestine is increased, thereby leading to hypercalciuria with or without hypercalcemia.

ACE, which catalyzes breakdown of the decapeptide angiotensin I to the octapeptide angiotensin II, is normally found in the lung. Elevated levels of ACE occur relatively frequently in sarcoidosis, with estimates varying widely but usually in the range of 40 to 90%. This elevation in ACE is believed to be due to production of the enzyme by epithelioid cells and macrophages within the granulomas. Although it was initially proposed that measurement of serum ACE might be a useful diagnostic and prognostic test in sarcoidosis, subsequent experience has shown its lack of diagnostic specificity and poor prognostic value in identifying patients with progressive disease.

Diagnosis

The initial consideration of sarcoidosis is usually based on the clinical or chest radiographic findings, or both. When intrathoracic disease is the primary mode of manifestation, the differential diagnosis generally depends on the radiographic findings. Hilar or mediastinal adenopathy, with or without associated parenchymal lung disease, can also be produced by lymphoma, mycobacterial or fungal infection, and selected pneumoconioses such as berylliosis and silicosis. When interstitial lung disease is present in the absence of intrathoracic lymphadenopathy, a much broader differential diagnosis is raised, including idiopathic pulmonary fibrosis, pulmonary fibrosis associated with systemic rheumatic disease (e.g., scleroderma, rheumatoid arthritis, polymyositis), and disease secondary to a broad range of inorganic dust (i.e., pneumoconiosis), organic antigens (i.e., hypersensitivity pneumonitis), and drugs (e.g., cancer chemotherapeutic agents).

The diagnosis of sarcoidosis is confirmed by the finding of well-formed noncaseating granulomas in one or more affected organ systems or tissues, with appropriate additional studies to exclude other causes of granulomas. Special stains and cultures must be performed for mycobacteria and fungi, and specimens should be examined under polarized light to identify foreign, potentially granulomagenic material. In patients with symmetrical bilateral hilar lymphadenopathy, either in association with erythema nodosum (Löfgren's syndrome) or in the absence of any symptoms, physical findings, or screening laboratory data that might indicate another cause, many clinicians believe that a clinical diagnosis of sarcoidosis can be made without needing histologic confirmation. Estimates of the likelihood of finding a diagnosis other than sarcoidosis in a patient with asymptomatic bilateral hilar lymphadenopathy suggest that the risk and cost of an invasive procedure outweigh its benefit.

Chest Radiography and Other Imaging Procedures

The plain chest radiograph is an important component of the diagnostic evaluation of patients with sarcoidosis; the diagnosis is frequently suspected initially from the radiographic abnormalities, either in the presence or in the absence of symptomatic disease. The major abnormalities seen on the chest radiograph include lymphadenopathy, usually involving both hila in a relatively symmetrical fashion, as well as the right paratracheal region, and involvement of the pulmonary parenchyma (Fig. 95–3). Although the pattern of parenchymal involvement is typically described as interstitial, alveolar and nodular patterns may also be

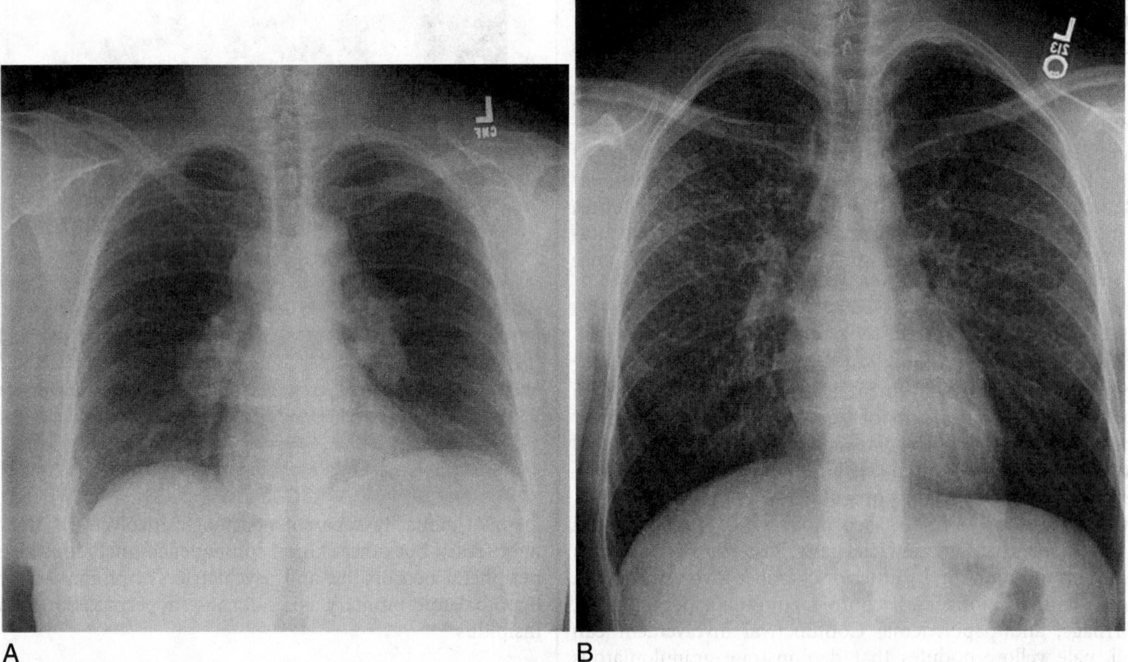

FIGURE 95–3 • Typical chest radiographs in sarcoidosis. A, Stage I sarcoidosis is characterized by bilateral hilar and often mediastinal adenopathy without visible parenchymal lung disease. **B,** In stage III sarcoidosis, the radiograph shows parenchymal lung involvement without hilar adenopathy.

TABLE 95–1 RADIOGRAPHIC STAGING OF INTRATHORACIC SARCOIDOSIS

Stage	Hilar Adenopathy	Parenchymal Disease	Percentage at Onset	Percentage with Resolution
0		No	No	<10 NA
1	Yes	No	50	65 (<10% progress to parenchymal disease)
2	Yes	Yes	30	20–50
3 or 4	No	Yes (with fibrosis in stage 4)	10–15	<20

NA = not applicable.

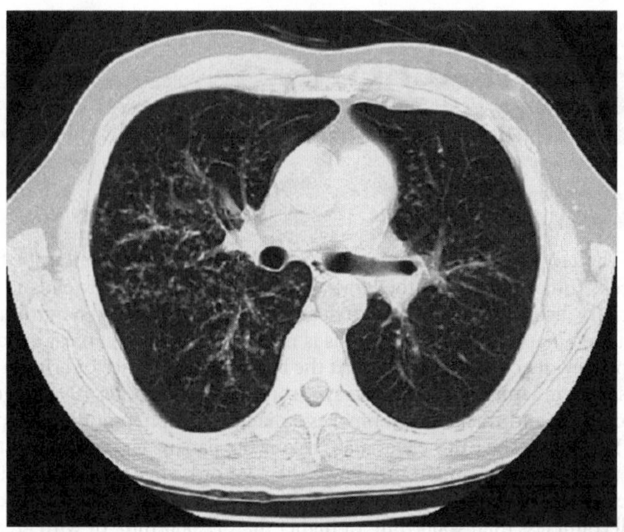

FIGURE 95–4 • High-resolution chest computed tomography scan in a patient with pulmonary parenchymal involvement by sarcoidosis. There are numerous small nodules in a predominantly bronchovascular distribution.

seen. A commonly used radiographic staging system considers the pattern of involvement seen on the chest radiograph (Table 95–1).

Computed tomography (CT) of the chest is often not necessary for the evaluation of suspected sarcoidosis, especially when typical findings are seen on plain chest radiography. However, when the findings are atypical or better definition of mediastinal lymph node involvement or the pattern of parenchymal lung disease is needed, CT may be beneficial. In addition to bilateral hilar lymphadenopathy, the chest CT scan frequently shows much more mediastinal involvement than was suspected on the chest radiograph, especially involving the right paratracheal, subcarinal, and aortopulmonary lymph nodes. High-resolution CT commonly demonstrates that pulmonary parenchymal involvement is localized around bronchovascular structures, with an appearance resembling budding branches on a tree (Fig. 95–4).

Scanning with gallium citrate Ga 67 may demonstrate uptake of this isotope in regions involved with granulomatous inflammation. However, because tracer uptake is nonspecific and because the correlation with other indices of disease activity or involvement is not particularly good, gallium scanning is not generally recommended as part of the routine evaluation of patients with suspected sarcoidosis.

Imaging studies are, however, important when attempting to confirm extrapulmonary involvement of the heart or nervous system because neither system is readily amenable to biopsy. Several types of imaging studies have been used to suggest or document myocardial sarcoidosis, including thallium scans, gallium scans, contrast-enhanced cardiac magnetic resonance imaging (MRI), positron emission tomography (PET), and single-photon emission computed tomography (SPECT). The preferred imaging study for neurosarcoidosis is MRI, which typically shows gadolinium enhancement of affected areas.

Tissue Biopsy

Noncaseating granulomas found on biopsy of an affected organ or tissue are generally well formed and consist of a localized collection of epithelioid histiocytes surrounded by a rim of variable numbers of lymphocytes. Multinucleated giant cells are typically present within the granulomas. Additional findings of mononuclear cell alveolitis and variable amounts of fibrosis are diagnostically nonspecific. Although noncaseating granulomas may also be seen in hypersensitivity pneumonitis, the granulomas are generally less discrete and well formed than in sarcoidosis.

The pulmonary parenchyma, intrathoracic lymph nodes, and skin are the most common sites for diagnostic biopsy in sarcoidosis. Flexible bronchoscopy provides a number of options to obtain diagnostic material from the pulmonary parenchyma, airways, or mediastinal lymph nodes. Transbronchial biopsy of the lung parenchyma is particularly useful, with a yield of 60 to 95%, depending on the radiographic stage of the disease and the number of biopsy specimens. Even when pulmonary parenchymal involvement is not grossly visible on plain chest radiography (e.g., in radiographic stage 1 disease), transbronchial lung biopsy is positive in more than 60% of patients. Biopsy of the bronchial mucosa (endobronchial biopsy) may sometimes demonstrate noncaseating granulomas, particularly when mucosal nodularity is seen on visualization of the airways through the bronchoscope. Transbronchial needle aspiration performed through the bronchoscope can also aspirate diagnostic cellular material from enlarged mediastinal lymph nodes. Finally, bronchoalveolar lavage, which samples the inflammatory cell population within the lung, is not diagnostic for sarcoidosis but characteristically shows an increased proportion of lymphocytes, with the ratio of $CD4^+$ to $CD8^+$ cells typically being elevated to greater than 3.5 : 1.

More invasive intrathoracic procedures are typically used when less invasive procedures have not been diagnostic or if more tissue is needed. Mediastinoscopy is sometimes performed in the presence of isolated mediastinal adenopathy without parenchymal lung disease, particularly when another diagnosis such as lymphoma is strongly being considered. Thoracoscopic lung biopsy is sometimes used when a broader differential diagnosis of parenchymal lung disease has been raised and more tissue is believed to be necessary than can be obtained by transbronchial lung biopsy.

Biopsy of tissue other than the lung or mediastinal lymph nodes is performed primarily because of clinical evidence of involvement. Skin biopsy, a relatively noninvasive procedure, is useful when findings suggestive of cutaneous sarcoidosis are present and when the overall clinical picture is compatible with sarcoidosis. Similarly, biopsy of peripheral lymph nodes, conjunctiva, parotid glands, skeletal muscle, and myocardium can be performed in selected cases. Liver biopsy is generally thought to be less useful because of the nonspecificity of granulomatous liver disease.

Prevention and Treatment

Because sarcoidosis follows a variable natural history, with many patients experiencing spontaneous resolution, it is often difficult to decide whether and when to institute therapy. Consequently, serial evaluation of symptoms, signs, laboratory findings, and radiographic abnormalities is often useful before beginning treatment, provided that severe disease does not obligate immediate therapy.

Whenever there is significant ocular, myocardial, or neurologic involvement, treatment is generally instituted promptly. For pulmonary disease, intrathoracic nodal involvement is not an indication for treatment, but parenchymal lung disease is a potential indication, depending on its effects on pulmonary function and symptoms rather than on the severity of radiographic involvement alone. The manifestation of Löfgren's syndrome does not warrant therapy, except as needed for symptoms (e.g., nonsteroidal anti-inflammatory drugs for associated joint symptoms).

Corticosteroids acutely suppress the manifestations of sarcoidosis and, overall in a meta-analysis, improve the chest radiograph, symptoms, and spirometry for 3 to 24 months. 1 However, it has never been clearly demonstrated that they alter its long-term natural history. Typically, prednisone is started at a dose of 0.5 mg/kg/day, although occasionally up to 1.0 mg/kg/day and continued at that dose for several weeks in an attempt to suppress the disease acutely. The dose can then be tapered, with the goal of using the lowest possible dose that keeps the disease under adequate control. Many clinicians taper to 10 to 30 mg every other day. Patients requiring systemic corticosteroid therapy for hypercalcemia can often be treated with relatively low doses of prednisone even initially, such as 10 to 20 mg/day.

The optimal overall duration of therapy is unknown and needs to be customized for each patient according to the response to therapy and the effect of drug tapering. Treatment durations of 6 to 12 months are typical, and premature discontinuation of therapy may lead to recurrence of symptomatic and functional disease. Patients must be advised about and monitored for the myriad potential side effects observed with systemic corticosteroids (Chapter 33).

Rx

Alternative agents when systemic corticosteroids are ineffective or not tolerated include methotrexate, generally at a dose of 10 to 15 mg/wk, or other immunosuppressive or cytotoxic agents, especially azathioprine. However, data are inconclusive regarding their benefit. 2 Although methotrexate has been used mostly as a corticosteroid-sparing agent, it can be administered as the sole agent, particularly for musculoskeletal or cutaneous sarcoidosis. Hydroxychloroquine has been used for serious and disfiguring cutaneous sarcoidosis. Topical corticosteroid preparations are used for anterior uveitis, but refractory disease may require treatment with systemic corticosteroids. Given the presumed role of TNF-α in granuloma formation, there has recently been interest in the potential benefit of TNF-α blockade with agents such as infliximab, accompanied by anecdotal reports of therapeutic success in steroid-refractory cases. However, such therapy is not currently approved for the treatment of sarcoidosis. In patients with severe, end-stage pulmonary disease refractory to therapy, lung transplantation is an important option (Chapter 102), but the disease may recur in the allograft.

Prognosis

The natural history of sarcoidosis is variable and ranges from spontaneous resolution to either smoldering or progressive disease. The prognosis is good for the majority of patients, with approximately two thirds experiencing resolution of their disease, whereas 10 to 30% have a chronic or progressive course. Resolution typically occurs within 2 years of disease onset, so persistence of disease beyond that time often predicts a more chronic course.

Patients with Löfgren's syndrome tend to have a good prognosis characterized by spontaneous resolution of disease. The chest radiographic stage of disease is also a useful prognostic indicator inasmuch as patients with radiographic stage 1 disease are much more likely to experience spontaneous resolution than are patients with higher radiographic stages (see Table 95–1).

Assessment of functional involvement of an organ and its course over time provides the general framework for monitoring the natural history of the disease. For pulmonary disease, monitoring includes symptoms, pulmonary function tests, and chest radiographs; conversely, gallium scanning, bronchoalveolar lavage (using lavage lymphocytosis as a marker of alveolitis), and measurement of serum ACE level are not recommended.

Progressive disease can lead to significant organ system involvement and to disability, particularly respiratory failure from severe interstitial lung disease. Less than 5% of patients die of sarcoidosis, with pulmonary, neurologic, and cardiac involvement being the major reasons for disease-related mortality.

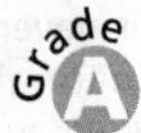

1. Paramothayan S, Lasserson TJ, Jones PW: Corticosteroids for pulmonary sarcoidosis. Cochrane Database Syst Rev 2005;2:CD001114.
2. Paramothayan S, Lasserson TJ, Walters EH: Immunosuppressive and cytotoxic therapy for pulmonary sarcoidosis. Cochrane Database Syst Rev 2005;2:00075320.

SUGGESTED READINGS

American Thoracic Society: Statement on sarcoidosis. Am J Respir Crit Care Med 1999;160:736–755. *A comprehensive review of sarcoidosis, including recommendations regarding diagnosis and treatment that represent a consensus statement of the American Thoracic Society, the European Respiratory Society, and the World Association of Sarcoidosis and Other Granulomatous Disorders.*

Doty JD, Mazur JE, Judson MA: Treatment of sarcoidosis with infliximab. Chest 2005;127:1064–1071. *A report of 10 patients who failed traditional therapy for sarcoidosis but responded to infliximab.*

Judson MA: Extrapulmonary sarcoidosis. Semin Respir Crit Care Med 2007;28:83–101. *A practical overview.*

Nunes H, Soler P, Valeyre D: Pulmonary sarcoidosis. Allergy 2005;60:565–582. *An excellent review article covering all aspects of pulmonary sarcoidosis.*

96 ACUTE BRONCHITIS AND TRACHEITIS

Richard P. Wenzel

Definition

The term *acute bronchitis and tracheitis* defines a self-limited (1 to 3 weeks) inflammation of the large airways of the lung that extends to the tertiary bronchi (Fig. 96–1). In patients with a primary symptom of cough (Chapter 83), the diagnosis is made if there is no clinical or radiologic evidence of pneumonia. At the bedside, the absence of criteria for systemic inflammatory response syndrome (SIRS) (Chapter 109) suggests bronchitis and tracheitis and makes a diagnosis of pneumonia (Chapter 97) unlikely. The SIRS criteria are met if the patient has more than two of the following: temperature lower than 36° or higher than 38° C, pulse greater than 90/min, respiratory rate higher than 20/min, or white blood cell count less than 4000/mm^3 or higher than 12,000/mm^3 or with greater than 10% bands.

The definition of acute bronchitis and tracheitis also seeks to differentiate the illness from acute inflammation of the small airways (bronchiolitis), even though the accompanying symptoms with the former may include sputum production, wheezing, and shortness of breath. Among patients with primarily small airways disease, some might be expected to have prominently decreased breath sounds in the areas involved. Acute bronchitis and tracheitis is also different from bronchiectasis (Chapter 90), which is associated with permanent dilatation of bronchi and a chronic cough. Furthermore, a diagnosis of chronic bronchitis (Chapter 88) is reserved for patients who have prolonged cough and sputum production: at least 3 months of the year for 2 consecutive years.

Epidemiology

Occurring at a rate of 44 per 1000 adults per year, acute bronchitis and tracheitis affects approximately 5% of adults annually. A higher incidence is observed in the winter and fall than in the summer and spring. In the

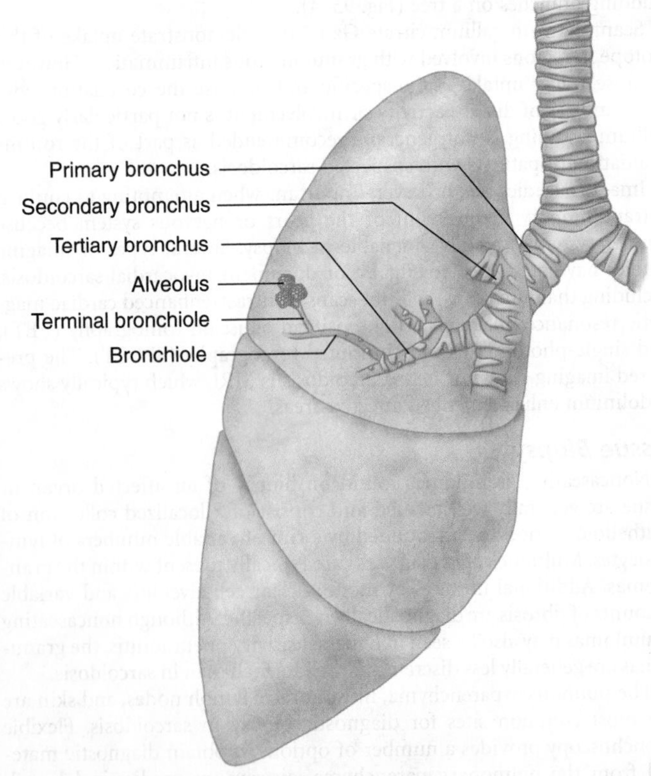

FIGURE 96–1 • Many infecting agents that cause bronchitis and tracheitis can infect both large and small airways of the lung and occasionally the alveoli. Not surprisingly, a wide spectrum of signs and symptoms are associated with bronchitis, including cough, wheezing, and shortness of breath.

United States, acute bronchitis and tracheitis is the ninth most common illness in outpatients as reported by physicians.

The disorder is thought to be viral in origin almost all the time. However, viruses have been isolated in only 8 to 37% of patients. Thus, the true causes of the illness are unknown in most cases. Nevertheless, at least 70% of patients with acute bronchitis and tracheitis in the United States receive antibacterial antibiotics after visiting a physician. Importantly, although the same bacteria that are commonly implicated in community-acquired pneumonia are also isolated from the sputum in half the patients, their role in the pathobiology of acute bronchitis and tracheitis or its attendant symptoms is unclear, and bronchial biopsies have not shown bacterial invasion.

Pathobiology

Infections of the epithelium of the bronchi and trachea are thought to incite an inflammatory response. Pathologically, there is an accompanying microscopic thickening of bronchial and tracheal mucosa corresponding to the inflamed areas. Such pathologic findings are also consistent with the occasional case report of upper airway inflammation confined to the bronchi and trachea detected by ^{18}F-labeled fluorodeoxyglucose positron emission tomography (FDG-PET).

In human experimental rhinovirus infections (Chapter 384), virus was detected in all subjects in induced sputum samples and also in approximately a third of bronchial biopsy specimens, almost a quarter of bronchoalveolar lavage samples, and over a third of biopsy and brushing samples. Such data indicating viral infection of the lower airways may help explain the relationship observed between rhinovirus infection and exacerbations of asthma (Chapter 87). Furthermore, pathologic islands of inflammation have been found in the trachea with rhinovirus infection, thus supporting the idea of a patchy distribution. The viruses implicated in acute bronchitis and tracheitis include influenza A and B (Chapter 387), parainfluenza (Chapter 386), respiratory syncytial virus (Chapter 385), coronavirus (Chapter 389), adenovirus (Chapter 388), and rhinoviruses (Chapter 384), usually in this order from the most to the least common. However, a recent French study of influenza-vaccinated adults found a viral cause in 37% of 164 cases of acute bronchitis, 21% of which were rhinovirus. Thus, at least three variables can influence the yield of specific pathogens: the presence of epidemics, the season of the year, and the population's influenza vaccination status. More recently, human metapneumovirus (Chapter 384) has been identified as an etiologic agent.

Up to 10% of cases of acute bronchitis and tracheitis may be due to "atypical" bacterial: *Bordetella pertussis* (Chapter 173), *Chlamydophila (Chlamydia) pneumoniae* (Chapter 97), and *Mycoplasma pneumoniae* (Chapter 97). Severe bronchiolitis has also been reported with *M. pneumoniae,* even though this pathogen is usually associated with either pneumonia or acute bronchitis and tracheitis in adults. In children, bronchiolitis has been associated with respiratory syncytial virus, influenza virus, parainfluenza virus, and metapneumovirus. Thus, there are probably wide variations in the anatomic distribution of all pathogens causing acute bronchitis and tracheitis, extending from the nasal mucosa to the bronchiolar epithelium.

Clinical Manifestations

The cardinal clinical symptom is cough (Chapter 83) of recent onset. Because most upper respiratory infections resolve within a week, a more extended period of cough is useful for considering the diagnosis of acute bronchitis. Patients usually seek care from their physician after 4 to 7 days of coughing that is not resolving. With acute bronchitis, there is often a continued cough and sometimes a worsened cough that lasts an initial 1 to 3 weeks. Associated symptoms vary and include sputum production, fever, malaise, wheezing, and dyspnea. Adults with pertussis may exhibit paroxysms of coughing, whooping, or vomiting, though less commonly than seen in children with this infection.

Diagnosis

Acutely ill patients may not be able to distinguish their early symptoms from those accompanying very mild upper respiratory infections. However, with acute bronchitis and tracheitis, a protracted phase of coughing persists beyond 1 to 5 days, during which time pulmonary function tests may become abnormal. A substantial proportion of patients will have significant declines in forced expiratory volume (FEV_1).

Rapid diagnostic tests exist for most viruses linked to acute bronchitis and tracheitis. However, their value lies in identifying a virus for which there is therapy or avoiding antibacterial antibiotics if any virus is identified. Not all rapid tests are widely available, and they are expensive and rarely cost-effective in an outpatient setting.

When "atypical" bacteria are identified by culture or serology, patients tend to be seen later in the course of their illness than patients with viral causes and more often have wheezing. In some studies, 12 to 32% of patients with coughing that persists for longer than 1 week had pertussis. In other studies, however, pertussis has been confirmed in only 1% of such patients.

Polymerase chain reaction (PCR) testing of nasopharyngeal swabs or aspirates is the easiest and most sensitive way to diagnose infections by *B. pertussis, M. pneumoniae,* and *C. pneumoniae;* most experts recommend calcium alginate swabs for pertussis because cotton inhibits growth. Dacron swabs with aluminum handles are preferred for specimens used to diagnose *Chlamydophila* because cotton, calcium alginate, and the wooden shaft can all inhibit growth of the organism. Cultures for *M. pneumoniae* are slow and insensitive. In general, testing for atypical organisms should not be done because of the cost of PCR and both the insensitivity and slowness of cultures. However, if the clinician suspects an outbreak in the community or the likelihood of pertussis, rapid testing with PCR may be quite beneficial.

Treatment

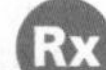

In a meta-analysis of nine randomized trials of antibacterial antibiotics for acute bronchitis, patients receiving antibiotics were significantly less likely to have a cough, but their 0.58 fewer days with cough, 0.52 fewer days of productive cough, and 0.58 fewer days of feeling ill were not statistically significant. [1] These results are not surprising because at most about 50% of cases are probably caused by bacterial pathogens. Nevertheless, antibiotics are used in 50 to 85% of cases worldwide.

Antibiotics may be used in patients with known atypical pathogens, but even then their effect on outcomes is not clear except to limit the spread of pertussis, especially during a defined outbreak. In adults suspected of having pertussis, erythromycin, 500 mg four times a day for 14 days, is thought to be most effective. However, many patients cannot tolerate erythromycin, and either doxycycline, 100 mg every 12 hours, or a newer macrolide such as azithromycin, 500 mg on day 1 and 250 mg/day thereafter, is effective. The latter two drugs are also active against *C. pneumoniae* and *M. pneumoniae,* although the optimal duration of therapy for acute bronchitis is unknown. A useful range is 5 to 14 days.

During influenza season, anti-influenza agents may be useful in decreasing symptoms by approximately 1 day and may lead to a 0.5-day earlier return to normal activity in patients with influenza. The first-generation drugs amantadine and rimantadine are ineffective against H3N2 influenza A viruses and are not recommended. Second-generation drugs such as zanamivir (two inhalations of 5 mg each—twice a day) or oseltamivir (75 mg twice a day) can be given for 5 days. Up to 20% of patients given oseltamivir will have nausea or vomiting.

Antihistamines or over-the-counter antitussives or expectorants have no apparent value. Subsets of patients with bronchial hyperresponsiveness may benefit from β-agonists, but no data support the use of inhaled steroids.

In experimental rhinovirus colds, nonsteroidal drugs, alone or in combination with antihistamines, reduce the severity of symptoms, including cough. However, the widespread use of either type of drug alone or as a combination in naturally occurring, community-acquired bronchitis and tracheitis has not been evaluated. In patients with acute bronchitis, a single randomized trial of an extract of *Pelargonium sidoides* roots, used in Europe and Mexico, showed a significantly improved severity of illness on day 7 and a reduced duration of the inability to work. [2]

Prognosis

Coughing usually lasts 10 to 14 days, during which time the illness causes significant transient decrements in vitality and social functioning. Limited data on short- and long-term outcomes show that up to 20% of patients have persistent or recurrent symptoms for a month. Antibiotics may reduce symptoms by a fraction of a day, but side effects, the emergence of antibiotic resistance, and cost must be weighed against their modest benefits. The mean duration of an office visit for adults in the United States with upper respiratory tract infections is 14.2 minutes when patients are prescribed antibiotics versus 15.2 minutes without prescription of antibiotics, but antibiotic use is not an independent predictor of visit length. Future widespread use of rapid diagnostic tests for specific bacterial and viral pathogens will be useful in targeting effective therapies.

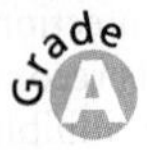

1. Smucny J, Fahey T, Becker L, et al: Antibiotics for acute bronchitis. *In* The Cochrane Collaboration. New York, J Wiley & Sons, 2005, pp 1–26. Available at www.cochrane.org/reviews/en/ab000245.html.
2. Matthys H, Eisebitt R, Seith B, et al: Efficacy and safety of an extract of *Pelargonium sidoides* (EPs 7630) in adults with bronchitis. A randomized double-blind, placebo-controlled trial. Phytomedicine 2003;10:7–17.

SUGGESTED READINGS

Aagaard E, Gonzales R: Management of acute bronchitis in healthy adults. Infect Dis Clin North Am 2004;18:919–937. *A practical review emphasizing that antibiotics are often overused.*

Linder JA, Singer DE: Health-related quality of life of adults with upper respiratory tract infections. J Gen Intern Med 2003;18:802–807. *Document decrements from baseline quality-of-life measures, presumed to be transient, associated with acute bronchitis.*

Wenzel RP, Fowler AA: Acute bronchitis. N Engl J Med 2006;355:2125–2130. *A clinical overview.*

97 OVERVIEW OF PNEUMONIA

Andrew H. Limper

It is a useful distinction to separate pneumonias, which are infections of the lung parenchyma and thus distinct from infections limited to the trachea or large bronchi (Chapter 96), into those acquired in the community (community-acquired pneumonia) as opposed to those arising in institutional settings, with the second group being composed of hospital-acquired pneumonia, ventilator-associated pneumonia, and health care–associated pneumonia. These two major pneumonia categories will be considered separately. Additional consideration should also be given to pneumonia caused by recurrent gross aspiration of oropharyngeal contents.

The term *pneumonia* itself, however, includes other causes of inflammation of the lower respiratory air spaces, particularly the alveoli, such as acute or chronic eosinophilic pneumonia, bronchiolitis obliterans with organizing pneumonia, and usual interstitial pneumonia, all of which are presented in more detail elsewhere (Chapter 92).

COMMUNITY-ACQUIRED PNEUMONIA

Definition

Community-acquired pneumonia includes cases of infectious pneumonia in patients living independently in the community. Patients who have been hospitalized for other reasons for less than 48 hours before the development of respiratory symptoms are also considered to have community-acquired pneumonia because it is likely that the inoculation had occurred before admission. However, patients who have previously been hospitalized for at least 2 days within the 90 days before infection, patients from nursing homes who received intravenous antibiotic therapy, chemotherapy, or wound care within the past 30 days, and patients from hemodialysis centers are considered to have health care–associated pneumonia and are therefore excluded from the case definition of community-acquired pneumonia. Patients contracting pneumonia greater than 48 hours after the institution of endotracheal intubation and mechanical ventilation are also excluded inasmuch as they are considered to have ventilator-associated pneumonia. These distinctions are important because they help define the most likely infectious agents and hence strongly influence appropriate choices for the initial antibiotic therapy.

Epidemiology

Between 5 and 10 million cases of infectious pneumonia occur annually in the United States and result in more than 1 million hospitalizations. Pneumonia is a leading cause of death worldwide, the sixth leading cause of death in the United States, and the most common lethal infectious disease. The mortality of community-acquired pneumonia ranges from less than 5% in mildly ill outpatients to somewhat greater than 12% overall in patients who are admitted to a hospital. Mortality is even greater in patients who have severe invasive disease, which is often associated with bacteremia, and in elderly nursing home patients. Mortality from pneumonia can exceed 40% in patients who require management in the intensive care unit (ICU). It costs approximately $7000 to manage an uncomplicated case of pneumonia in the hospital, or about 20-fold more than treating it in the outpatient setting.

Pathobiology

Aspiration of Oropharyngeal Contents

The most common mechanism by which the lung is inoculated with pathogenic organisms is through microaspiration of oropharyngeal contents, a process that occurs in otherwise healthy individuals during sleep (Chapter 94). Colonization of the oral pharynx with pathogenic organisms, such as *Streptococcus pneumoniae* (Chapter 312), can thereby lead to delivery of sufficient quantities of organisms to infect the lung. In contrast, gross aspiration normally occurs only in individuals with altered sensorium, depressed consciousness, abnormalities in protective cough or gag reflexes, or substantial gastroesophageal reflux. Gross aspiration, which can also deliver large numbers of anaerobic bacteria to the lower respiratory tract, is a major contributing factor to anaerobic lung infection and abscess formation (Chapter 98).

Inhalation of Aerosolized Droplets

The second most frequent mechanism of lung infection is the inhalation of small, suspended aerosolized droplets ranging in size from 0.5 to 1 μm that may contain microorganisms. In view of the limited number of organisms delivered in such a manner, only relatively aggressive pathogenic organisms such as *Mycobacterium tuberculosis* (Chapter 345), *Legionella pneumophila* (Chapter 335), *Yersinia pestis* (plague; Chapter 333), *Bacillus anthracis* (anthrax; Chapter 317), and some viral infections can be transmitted in this manner.

Blood Stream Infection

Less commonly, the lung may become infected as a consequence of a blood stream infection. Blood-borne pneumonia is seen especially in staphylococcal sepsis (Chapter 310) or right-sided endocarditis (Chapter 76), which are more common in intravenous drug users (Chapter 32), and in gram-negative bacteremias, particularly in an immunocompromised host. The lung may also rarely be inoculated directly by penetrating chest trauma or by local spread from a nearby infected organ (paragonimiasis or amebic liver abscess; Chapters 373 and 377) or a contiguous soft tissue infection.

Fortunately, the lung is well equipped to defend against inoculation with most microbes. When large droplets of infected material reach the airways, they are removed by the mucociliary escalator, which sweeps entrapped contents up to the oropharynx, where they are swallowed or expectorated. Smaller particles, in the range of 0.5 to 2.0 μm, are deposited in the alveoli, where alveolar macrophages phagocytize and destroy most pathogens. These macrophages are further activated to release potent cytokines and chemokines, including tumor necrosis factor-α, interleukin-8, and leukotriene B_4, which help recruit neutrophils from the blood stream into the alveolar spaces, where they par-

TABLE 97–1 HOST FACTORS ASSOCIATED WITH SPECIFIC PATHOGENIC CAUSES OF PNEUMONIA

Underlying Condition	Associated Microorganism
Active smoking/chronic obstructive lung disease	*Streptococcus pneumoniae, Haemophilus influenzae, Legionella pneumophila*
Nursing home residents	*S. pneumoniae*, gram-negative bacilli, *H. influenzae, Staphylococcus aureus, Chlamydia pneumoniae*, anaerobes, tuberculosis
Alcoholism	*S. pneumoniae* (including drug-resistant strains), gram-negative bacilli, anaerobes, tuberculosis
Gross aspiration/poor dentition	Anaerobes
Travel to southwestern United States	*Coccidioides immitis*
Exposure to bats	*Histoplasma capsulatum*
Exposure to birds	*Cryptococcus neoformans, Chlamydia psittaci, H. capsulatum*
Exposure to rabbits	*Francisella tularensis*
Exposure to farm animals	*Coxiella burnetii* (Q fever)
Viral influenza	Influenza, *S. aureus, S. pneumoniae, H. influenzae*
Bronchiectasis, cystic fibrosis	*Pseudomonas aeruginosa, Pseudomonas cepacia, S. aureus, Aspergillus* species, *Mycobacterium avium* complex
Intravenous drug use	*S. aureus*, anaerobes, tuberculosis, *Pneumocystis jiroveci*
Endobronchial obstruction	Anaerobes
Recent antibiotic therapy	Drug-resistant *S. pneumoniae, P. aeruginosa*

Adapted from American Thoracic Society: Guidelines for management of adults with community-acquired pneumonia: Diagnosis, assessment of severity, initial antimicrobial therapy, and prevention. Am J Respir Crit Care Med 2001:163:1730–1754.

ticipate in the uptake and degradation of microorganisms. For many microorganisms such as *S. pneumoniae* (Chapter 311), clearance of infection is greatly facilitated by the development of specific immunoglobulin G that binds the surface of the organisms or their polysaccharide capsule. These specific antibodies, which act as immune opsonins, greatly augment the ability of neutrophils and macrophages to phagocytize and destroy the bacteria. In addition, pattern recognition receptors and other nonimmune opsonins, including surfactant proteins A and D, fibronectin, and vitronectin, also bind to specific epitopes on the surface of organisms that reach the lower respiratory tract and assist in their recognition and elimination. Only when organisms overwhelm or evade these multiple host defense systems does inoculation of the lung result in clinically significant pneumonia.

Clinical Manifestations

The possibility of pneumonia should be considered in any patient who has new respiratory symptoms, including cough, sputum, or dyspnea, particularly when these symptoms are accompanied by fever or abnormalities on physical examination of the chest, such as rhonchi and rales. The initial manifestation is frequently more subtle in patients who are elderly or have an altered immunologic status; in such patients, nonspecific symptoms, including loss of appetite, confusion, dehydration, worsening of symptoms or signs of other chronic illnesses, or failure to thrive, may be the initial manifestation of pneumonia. Pneumonia is also increasingly prevalent in patients with specific comorbid conditions, including smoking, chronic obstructive pulmonary disease (COPD, Chapter 88), diabetes mellitus, malignancy, heart failure, neurologic diseases, narcotic and alcohol use, and chronic liver disease.

The initial symptoms and signs are often variable from patient to patient and cannot be reliably used to establish a specific (microbiologic) diagnosis. The classic physical findings in lobar pneumonia include evidence of consolidation with altered transmission of breath sounds, egophony, crackles, and changes in tactile fremitus. However, in many patients, the physical findings are more subtle and may be limited to scattered rhonchi. A thorough physical examination, posteroanterior and lateral chest radiographs, and a blood leukocyte count with a differential cell count should be performed when pneumonia is suspected. An assessment of gas exchange (oximetry or arterial blood gas determination) should be obtained for all patients who are admitted to the hospital. The clinician needs to be mindful of competing diagnoses that can mimic the findings of pneumonia, such as pulmonary embolism (Chapter 99), bronchogenic and bronchoalveolar carcinoma (Chapter 201), drug-induced lung diseases (Chapter 94), and idiopathic interstitial lung diseases (Chapter 92).

Diagnosis

Even with intensive laboratory investigation, the specific microbiologic cause can be established with certainty only in approximately 50% of patients with pneumonia. The probable predominant organism varies with the host's epidemiologic factors, the severity of illness, and which laboratory approach is used to establish the diagnosis.

Bacterial Pneumonia

S. pneumoniae (Chapter 312) is the organism most frequently detected by culture of sputum or blood. In contrast, *Mycoplasma pneumoniae* (Chapter 338) is frequently detected with serologic tests. Additional bacterial agents include *Haemophilus influenzae* (Chapter 323), *Staphylococcus aureus* (Chapter 310), enteric gram-negative bacilli (Chapters 304 and 328), and *L. pneumophila* (Chapter 335). *Chlamydia* and respiratory viruses have also been implicated in up to 10% of cases (Chapters 353, and 384 through 389). The so-called atypical pathogens, including *M. pneumoniae, Chlamydia pneumoniae*, and *Legionella* species, are increasingly being recognized as important and prevalent causes of pneumonia. Mixed infections, particularly those related to coinfection with these "atypical" pathogens in addition to the usual bacterial pathogens, have been reported in up to a third of patients with lower respiratory tract infection.

Specific host factors also influence the relative risk for infection with specific microorganisms (Table 97–1). For instance, smokers and those with COPD are at increased risk for invasive *S. pneumoniae*, as well as *H. influenzae, Moraxella catarrhalis* (Chapter 323), and *Legionella*. Alcoholism is associated with increased risk for drug-resistant *S. pneumoniae*, anaerobic lung infection, and tuberculosis.

The clinician also should solicit information about household and workplace exposure, such as to other ill persons. The clinician should ask about recent travel to specific geographic regions, such as the central United States, where histoplasmosis is endemic (Chapter 353), the Southwest, where coccidioidomycosis is found (Chapter 354), and selected northern and central regions of the United States, where blastomycosis is found (Chapter 355). Recent travel to Asia or other regions with epidemic viral respiratory infections, including influenza and severe acute respiratory syndrome (SARS), or travel to Asia, Africa, and central and eastern Europe, which are highly endemic for tuberculosis, should be considered (Chapter 345). In addition, environmental exposure, such as to birds (psittacosis), bird droppings (histoplasmosis), bats (histoplasmosis), rabbits (tularemia, Chapter 338), and farm animals (Q fever, Chapter 349), is additional data that should be obtained during the history.

Virals Pneumonia

Although most attention traditionally focuses on bacterial causes of severe community-acquired pneumonia, viruses can also cause serious lower respiratory tract infections. The predominant respiratory viruses that can cause severe pneumonia include influenza and respiratory syncytial virus (RSV) (Chapters 386 and 388). Both influenza virus and RSV can be detected in respiratory secretions, which should be obtained in suspected cases. It is estimated that influenza infections are responsible for in excess of 36,000 respiratory- and circulatory-related deaths annually in the United States, predominantly in elderly patients and those with underlying cardiopulmonary or metabolic disease. Influenza-associated pneumonia should be considered in the differential diagnosis of respiratory infections in high-risk patients with underlying disease and in residents of nursing homes or other chronic care facilities during the season of October through May, especially in patients who have not received appropriate vaccination.

It is also increasingly being appreciated that RSV and parainfluenza viruses, though formerly considered mainly infections of pediatric populations, can lead to serious lower respiratory tract infections in adults during the winter season. Host immunity to RSV infection in childhood is incomplete, and recurrent infections can occur in both immune-competent and immune-impaired adults, particularly in the elderly. It is estimated that RSV is associated with more than 11,000 deaths each year in the United States, with most deaths occurring in the elderly and in patients with chronic cardiopulmonary disease.

Severe Acute Respiratory Syndrome

SARS has emerged as a newly appreciated form of life-threatening atypical pneumonia that was first detected in the Guangdong Province of China in late 2002, with major outbreaks in Hong Kong, Guangdong, Singapore, and Toronto and Vancouver, Canada. The disease is caused by a novel coronavirus (Chapter 390) with an incubation period of 2 to 10 days. The initial source of the infection remains uncertain, although palm civet cats and Chinese ferret badgers harbor a coronavirus with greater than 99% similarity to human SARS isolates. Worldwide, however, the illness is largely a nosocomial disease, with health care workers representing a significant fraction of the infected individuals. SARS is characterized by an insidious onset of fever, chills, headache, cough, malaise, and dyspnea, with radiologic evidence of pneumonia. Although upper respiratory symptoms are uncommon, voluminous watery diarrhea without mucus or blood develops in up to 70% of patients. SARS is believed to be principally transmitted by respiratory droplets. Current treatment is supportive, with no antiviral agent yet having been proved to be efficacious. SARS pneumonia tends to resolve slowly and spontaneously, usually by the third week of illness. However, the estimated case-fatality rate remains at approximately 10%.

SARS should be considered in any patient who within the past 10 days has traveled (including transit in an airport) to an area with documented or suspected SARS or had close contact with a person known or suspected to have SARS. Signs and symptoms of SARS include temperature higher than 100.4° F (>38° C) and one or more clinical findings of respiratory illness (e.g., cough, shortness of breath, difficulty breathing, or hypoxia), particularly if there is radiographic evidence of pneumonia or clinical evidence of respiratory distress syndrome without another identifiable cause. The Centers for Disease Control and Prevention (CDC) maintains updated lists of regions with community transmission of SARS and recommended management of SARS through their website *(www.cdc.gov)*.

SARS is highly contagious, and lethal transmission to health care workers has been documented. Isolation procedures and equipment appropriate for SARS include standard, contact, and airborne isolation precautions such as scrupulous hand hygiene, gowning, disposable gloves, the use of N95 respirators, and eye protection. Suspected cases of SARS require notification of local public health departments and the CDC.

Agents of Bioterrorism

Physicians should also be vigilant for clues of pneumonia related to agents of bioterrorism (Chapter 19). These clues can include outbreaks of severe illness and pneumonia in multiple, otherwise healthy individuals or the isolation of unusual organisms in patients with pneumonic illness. The microorganisms most likely to be associated with severe pneumonia during bioterrorism-related inhalation exposure include *B. anthracis* (Chapter 318), *Francisella tularensis* (Chapter 333), and *Y. pestis* (Chapter 334). Inhalational anthrax always indicates a bioterrorism threat, whereas pneumonic plague or tularemia may or may not be associated with bioterrorism.

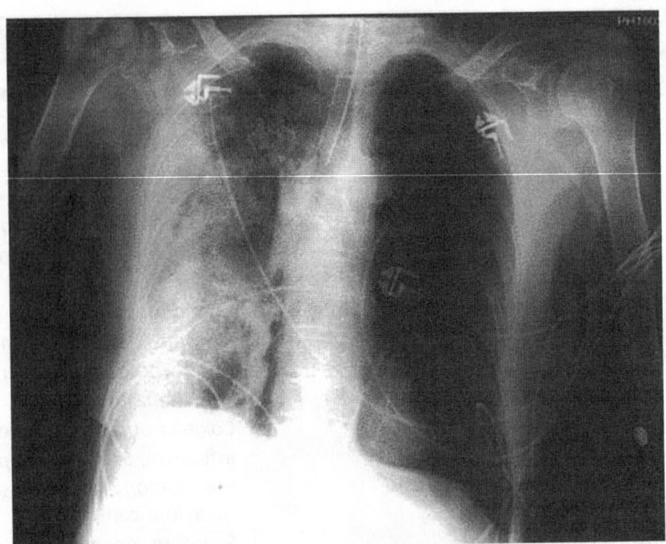

FIGURE 97–1 • Radiologic diagnosis of pneumonia. A standard posteroanterior radiograph in a 70-year-old woman demonstrates chronic obstructive pulmonary disease complicated by right multilobar *Streptococcus pneumoniae* pneumonia and empyema.

Radiography

Clinical suspicion of pneumonia should prompt standard posteroanterior and lateral chest radiography. Although the pattern of infiltration can rarely establish a specific microbiologic etiology, chest films are most useful for providing essential information on the distribution and extent of involvement, as well as potential pneumonic complications. Many bacterial pneumonias result in localized alveolar infiltrates and consolidation. Even though pneumococcal pneumonia is classically described as having a lobar distribution, the pattern can be multilobar (Fig. 97–1) or bilateral. The "bulging" fissure sign, which represents lobar filling and consolidation, has traditionally been attributed to *Klebsiella pneumoniae*, but this finding is not specific and can be observed with *S. pneumoniae* and other bacteria and even with bronchoalveolar carcinoma. Diffuse interstitial and alveolar infiltrates should suggest viral infections (cytomegalovirus, influenza virus, or RSV), *L. pneumophila*, or enteric gram-negative pneumonia, particularly in neutropenic patients. These diffuse pulmonary infiltrations can be indistinguishable from other causes of adult respiratory distress syndrome. Diffuse alveolar and interstitial infiltration can also be observed in patients with *Pneumocystis jiroveci* pneumonia (Chapter 363) related to immune suppression, such as in those with acquired immunodeficiency syndrome. Cavitary lesions often indicate a necrotizing infection related to *S. aureus, M. tuberculosis* (Fig. 97–2), and certain endemic fungi such as *Coccidioides immitis*, *Aspergillus* infection in an immunocompromised patient (Chapter 361), or anaerobic lung infection with abscess formation. Mediastinal adenopathy and widening have been observed in inhalational anthrax infections.

The chest radiograph provides further important information about potential infectious complications of pneumonia. Pleural effusions (Chapter 100), which occur in a variety of respiratory infections, are best documented with lateral decubitus views or with computed tomography (CT) imaging of the thorax. The discovery of any pleural effusion greater than 10-mm in thickness on a lateral decubitus film or any loculated effusion should prompt thoracentesis to aid in the identification of a complicated parapneumonic effusion or empyema, which may require definitive drainage (Chapter 100). Enlargement of mediastinal and hilar lymph nodes, which is rare in acute bacterial infection, suggests fungal

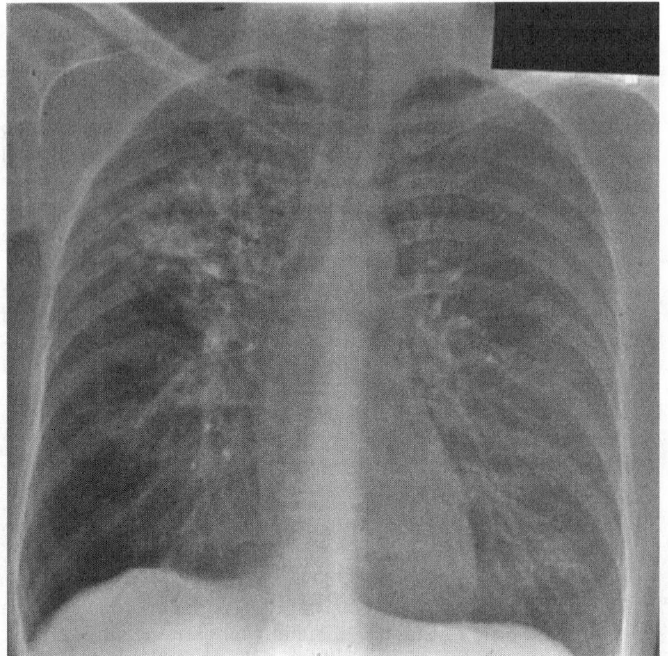

FIGURE 97-2 • Cavitary lesions. A posteroanterior radiograph in a 54-year-old man with cough and fever shows a right upper lobe cavitary process caused by *Mycobacterium tuberculosis* infection.

or mycobacterial infection or an underlying lung cancer. Loss of volume of a lung segment or lobe should raise suspicion of postobstructive pneumonia distal to an endobronchial lesion caused by a neoplasm, occult foreign body, or broncholithiasis.

Laboratory Findings

Sputum Gram Stain and Culture

Considerable controversy exists over the appropriate microbiologic evaluation of patients with suspected pneumonia. Despite intensive microbiologic evaluation, a specific organism may not be discovered in half the patients with pneumonia. Furthermore, the majority of patients with pneumonia satisfactorily respond to simple, relatively nontoxic antibiotic regimens based on the most likely organisms causing infection. Thus, the necessity to document the precise cause of the process remains uncertain.

Debate continues over the need to perform a sputum examination with Gram staining in every patient with community-acquired pneumonia. An American Thoracic Society consensus panel has recommended that a sputum Gram stain and culture be obtained primarily if an organism that is resistant to the usual empirical treatment regimens is suspected. To be useful, sputum should contain fewer than 10 squamous cells and more than 25 leukocytes per low-power field; a well-performed Gram stain may reveal a single, predominant organism such as encapsulated gram-positive cocci (pneumococci) or small pleomorphic gram-negative coccobacilli *(Haemophilus)*. However, current data have not clearly correlated Gram stain findings with the results of culture of alveolar materials in large numbers of patients with community-acquired pneumonia. Nevertheless, sputum examination can strongly support the diagnosis of certain specific infections, including *M. tuberculosis* (acid-fast stain), endemic fungi (KOH preparations), *P. jiroveci* (methenamine silver or fluorescent antibody stain), or *Legionella* species (direct fluorescent antibody staining). In most cases of community-acquired pneumonia, the general intent of sputum Gram stain examination, if it is performed, should be to detect additional or unusual pathogens and hence to expand rather than narrow the initial antibiotic therapy. All too often, an adequate sputum specimen cannot be obtained, and the Gram stain interpretation may be equivocal. Therefore, the initial therapeutic plan must be based on the most likely pathogens responsible for the pneumonia.

If unusual or drug-resistant pathogens are suspected, sputum specimens should be sent for culture before antibiotic therapy is initiated. When the culture results are available, they should be compared with the predominant organisms observed on Gram stain. Unfortunately, the sensitivity and specificity of sputum culture are not optimal, each being roughly 50%. Antibiotic susceptibility information on an isolated pathogenic organism can, however, be useful both for epidemiologic surveillance and for management of patients who do not respond to initial empirical therapy.

Other Bacterial Cultures

Cultures of normally sterile body fluids such as blood, pleural fluid, or occasionally cerebrospinal fluid (CSF) are highly specific when positive. Approximately a fourth of patients with bacterial pneumonia have demonstrable bacteremia. Blood should be drawn for culture before administration of antibiotics in patients with serious illness attributable to pneumonia, and diagnostic thoracentesis should be performed if an effusion is large enough to be aspirated safely. CSF examination is generally reserved for patients with additional signs and symptoms of meningeal irritation (Chapter 312) or abnormalities on neurologic examination.

Testing for Suspected Bioterrorism

Recommended testing for suspected anthrax includes blood culture and chest CT scanning. For the diagnosis of pneumonic plague, blood culture as well as sputum Gram stain and culture are advised. For tularemic pneumonia, cultures should be obtained from blood, sputum, and the pharynx. Culture of these extremely virulent organisms should be undertaken in a level 3 (BL3) biocontainment laboratory.

Immunologic Studies

Immunologic techniques such as immunofluorescence, enzyme-linked immunosorbent assay, antigen detection, polymerase chain reaction, and DNA hybridization may be considered when specific organisms are strongly suspected on clinical grounds, but these tests are not routinely indicated in most cases of community-acquired pneumonia. For example, *Legionella* urinary antigen screening and acute and convalescent serologic evaluation may be helpful when *L. pneumophila* pneumonia is suspected (Chapter 336). *Legionella* urinary antigen testing may underdiagnose infections caused by organisms other than *Legionella* serogroup 1. Furthermore, the judicious use of fungal serology can detect endemic mycoses, particularly histoplasmosis and coccidioidomycosis (Chapters 354, 355, and 356). Histoplasmosis can also be confirmed by urinary antigen testing with high sensitivity. Bronchoscopy with lavage for immunostaining may, in selected circumstances, provide enhanced sensitivity, such as in the diagnosis of *P. jiroveci* pneumonia (Chapter 363).

Viral Studies

Rapid antigen detection tests are now available, with tests that distinguish between influenza A and B being preferred. These tests are currently recommended for epidemiologic purposes in the community and also help direct individual therapy. RSV antigen detection tests are likewise available, but they are insensitive when applied to sputum in adult patients.

Diagnosis of SARS includes culture of the SARS coronavirus; detection of antibody during the acute phase of the illness or at any time after the onset of symptoms; and detection of SARS coronavirus RNA, which must be confirmed with a second polymerase chain reaction assay on a second aliquot of the specimen or with a different set of primers.

Bronchoscopy

Invasive sampling of respiratory secretions is not usually necessary in patients with community-acquired pneumonia. Flexible fiberoptic bronchoscopy with a protected catheter brush and bronchoalveolar lavage (BAL) sampling has largely supplanted transtracheal and transthoracic needle aspiration. Bronchoscopy is indicated in selected clinical situations in which a delay in accurate diagnosis may have serious consequences, such as in immunocompromised hosts or patients whose condition has worsened despite initial antimicrobial therapy. Other indications for bronchoscopy in the setting of apparent community-acquired pneumonia include either lung abscess detected on a chest radiograph (Chapter 84) or evidence of volume loss and distal consolidation suggesting endobronchial obstruction.

Prevention

In light of the significant morbidity and potential mortality of pneumonia, appropriate measures should be instituted to reduce the possibility of lung infection. Important but often neglected interventions include smoking cessation (Chapter 30) and avoidance of illicit drugs (Chapter 32) or excess alcohol (Chapter 31), which may impair consciousness. Optimizing the patient's nutritional status is also important in that markedly underweight or obese patients are at increased risk. Finally, the appropriate and consistent use of vaccines can strongly reduce the risk for pneumonia in appropriate patient populations (Chapter 16). The current pneumococcal vaccine contains 23 purified capsular polysaccharides from the serotypes of *S. pneumoniae* that are responsible for more than 85% of invasive pneumococcal infections. Overall, this vaccine is approximately 50 to 80% effective in preventing death from invasive infection. Accordingly, current recommendations are that it should be administered to all patients older than 65 years and to patients younger than 65 who have chronic pulmonary disease, heart disease, diabetes mellitus, alcoholism, chronic liver disease, CSF leaks, or asplenia and to patients who live in certain settings, including Alaskan natives, high-risk Native American populations, and patients in long-term care facilities. Current pneumococcal vaccines have little toxicity, limited mainly to local site irritation. Individuals generally receive one dose of vaccine, but a single revaccination 5 years later should be considered in those who received their vaccination before 65 years of age or who are at increased risk for severe pneumonia. Pneumococcal vaccine can safely be administered at the time of hospitalization for community-acquired pneumonia.

Vaccination (Chapter 16) should also be considered for viral influenza (Chapter 388). Though usually manifested as an upper respiratory tract infection, influenza can itself cause pneumonia in both immunocompetent and immunosuppressed individuals. More commonly, influenza may precipitate a subsequent bacterial infection, often with *S. aureus.* Influenza vaccines are developed annually against the current influenza strains, so annual revaccination is necessary (Chapter 16). Influenza vaccines are estimated to be roughly 80% effective in preventing mortality related to influenza. [1] The vaccine should be considered in all patients older than 50 years; residents of nursing homes and chronic care facilities; persons with chronic pulmonary, cardiac, or other diseases requiring ongoing medical care; pregnant women in the second or third trimester during influenza season; and all health care workers with direct patient contact.

Contraindications to influenza vaccine include allergy to raw eggs or thimerosal. Side effects are generally self-limited and include injection site soreness, myalgia, mild fever, and malaise. The vaccine does not contain live virus and therefore cannot cause influenza. The vaccine should be administered in the fall of the year, but it can also be administered during local epidemics.

Treatment

Rx

Initial Empirical Therapy

Because the microbiologic etiology of community-acquired pneumonia is determined in only approximately 50% of cases and the diagnosis may take a day or two, the clinician must institute appropriate empirical therapy based on the most likely agents contributing to the lung infection (Table 97–2). When possible, empirical therapy should be initiated within the first 4 hours of diagnosis, an interval that appears to reduce the 30-day mortality. Empirical antimicrobial therapy is based on the severity of illness (inpatient or outpatient setting) and should broadly cover the most likely organisms (Fig. 97–3). [2] The most common bacterial pathogens are *S. pneumoniae* (Chapter 312) and *H. influenzae* (Chapter 324); however, the so-called atypical pathogens, including *M. pneumoniae, C. pneumoniae,* and *Legionella* species (Chapters 336, 339, and 340), can be the primary or coinfecting agents in up to 40% of community-acquired pneumonia and must be covered in empirical antibiotic regimens. Therapy can be narrowed later after any relevant culture information is obtained.

Guidelines for Hospital and Intensive Care Unit Admission

Under current guidelines, patients are stratified with respect to where treatment is initiated (outpatient, inpatient, or ICU setting), the presence of underlying cardiopulmonary disease, and other modifying factors, such as whether the patient is likely to be infected with drug-resistant *S. pneumoniae,* gram-negative enteric bacilli, or *Pseudomonas aeruginosa.* Following these guidelines reduces the number of hospital admissions without adversely affecting outcomes (Table 97–3). [3]

The decision to admit a patient to the hospital must be made on clinical grounds. Patients can be effectively and safely managed as outpatients if they are mildly ill, are younger than 50 years, and do not have coexisting cardiopulmonary disease, malignancy, immune compromise, or renal, liver, or other significant systemic diseases. Features such as a respiratory rate greater than 30 breaths per minute, a diastolic blood pressure less than 60 mm Hg, evidence of poor perfusion or end-organ dysfunction (e.g., confusion or an elevated blood urea nitrogen or creatinine level), multilobar disease on the chest radiograph, or hypoxemia predict a more severe course and generally require inpatient management.

In general, outpatients who are mildly ill and do not have any underlying cardiopulmonary disease or other modifying factors are usually infected with *S. pneumoniae, M. pneumoniae, C. pneumoniae, H. influenzae,* respiratory viruses, or *Legionella* species. These uncomplicated outpatient cases can be managed with an oral advanced-generation macrolide, such as azithromycin or clarithromycin, which are better tolerated and provide better coverage of *Haemophilus* than erythromycin does. Alternatively, doxycycline can be used in patients who are intolerant of macrolides, although this option is less optimal because increasing levels of tetracycline resistance are being observed in *S. pneumoniae* isolates.

TABLE 97–2 COMMON MICROBIOLOGIC CAUSES OF COMMUNITY-ACQUIRED PNEUMONIA IN APPROXIMATE ORDER OF FREQUENCY

Outpatients	Hospitalized Patients	Severe Pneumonia/ICU
Streptococcus pneumoniae	*S. pneumoniae*	*S. pneumoniae*
Mycoplasma pneumoniae	*H. influenzae*	*Legionella* sp
Chlamydia pneumoniae	*M. pneumoniae*	*H. influenzae*
Haemophilus influenzae	*C. pneumoniae*	*M. pneumoniae*
Respiratory viruses	Mixed infections	Enteric gram-negative organisms
Miscellaneous, including *Legionella* sp and endemic fungi	Enteric gram-negative organisms	*Pseudomonas aeruginosa*
	Aspiration (anaerobes)	Respiratory viruses
	Respiratory viruses	Miscellaneous, including *C. pneumoniae, M. tuberculosis,* and endemic fungi
	Legionella sp	
	Miscellaneous, including *Mycobacterium tuberculosis, Pseudomonas jiroveci,* and endemic fungi	

Adapted from American Thoracic Society: Guidelines for management of adults with community-acquired pneumonia: Diagnosis, assessment of severity, initial antimicrobial therapy, and prevention. Am J Respir Crit Care Med 2001;163:1730–1754.

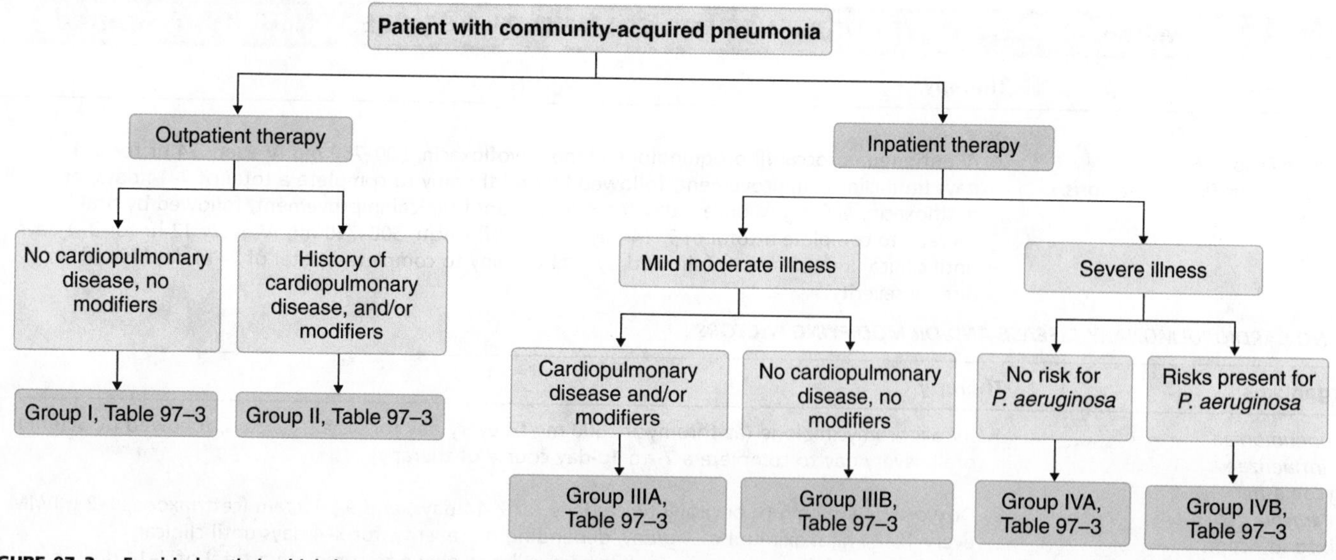

FIGURE 97–3 • Empirical antimicrobial therapy. Initial empirical therapy for community-acquired pneumonia is based on the severity of illness, underlying cardiopulmonary disease, and location of treatment. (Modified from American Thoracic Society: Guidelines for management of adults with community-acquired pneumonia: Diagnosis, assessment of severity, and antimicrobial therapy and prevention. Am J Respir Crit Care Med 2001;163:1730–1754.)

TABLE 97–3 EMPIRICAL TREATMENT GUIDELINES FOR COMMUNITY-ACQUIRED PNEUMONIA

GROUP I: OUTPATIENTS WITHOUT CARDIOPULMONARY DISEASE OR MODIFYING FACTORS

Organisms	Therapy
Streptococcus pneumoniae *Mycoplasma* *Chlamydia pneumoniae* *Haemophilus influenzae* Respiratory viruses *Legionella* sp *Mycobacterium tuberculosis* Endemic fungi	1. Advanced-generation oral macrolide (azithromycin, 500 mg orally on day 1, followed by 250 mg on days 2 through 5, or clarithromycin, 250 mg orally twice daily for 7–14 days) *or* 2. Doxycycline (100 mg orally twice daily for 7–14 days)

GROUP II: OUTPATIENTS WITH CARDIOPULMONARY DISEASE OR OTHER MODIFYING FACTORS

Organisms	Therapy
S. pneumoniae (consider drug resistance—DRSP) *Mycoplasma* *Chlamydia* Mixed infection (±atypical) *H. influenzae* Gram-negative organisms Respiratory viruses Miscellaneous (*Moraxella*, *Legionella* sp, aspiration, *anaerobes, M. tuberculosis*, fungi)	1. Oral or parenteral β-lactam (cefpodoxime, 200 mg orally every 12 hr for 14 days; cefuroxime, 500 mg orally twice a day for 10 days; high-dose amoxicillin, amoxicillin-clavulanate, 2000 mg [2 tablets of the extended-release tablets] orally every 12 hr for 7–10 days; or parenteral ceftriaxone, 1–2 g IV/IM every 12–24 hr, maximum of 4 g/day, for 3 or 4 days until clinical improvement, then followed by oral cefpodoxime at the doses listed above to complete a total of 14 days of treatment) plus a macrolide (azithromycin, 500 mg orally on day 1, followed by 250 mg on days 2 through 5; or clarithromycin, 250 mg orally twice daily for 7–14 days) or doxycycline (100 mg orally twice daily for 7–14 days) *or* 2. Antipneumococcal fluoroquinolone (levofloxacin, 500 mg orally every 24 hr for 7–14 days; gatifloxacin, 400 mg orally once a day for 7–14 days; or ciprofloxacin, 500–750 mg orally every 12 hr for 7–14 days based on disease severity)

GROUP III: HOSPITALIZED INPATIENTS NOT REQUIRING ICU CARE
A. PRESENCE OF CARDIOPULMONARY DISEASE AND/OR OTHER MODIFYING FACTORS (INCLUDING NURSING HOME)

Organisms	Therapy
S. pneumoniae (including DRSP) *H. influenzae* *Mycoplasma* *Chlamydia* Mixed infection Enteric gram-negative organisms Aspiration (anaerobes)	1. IV β-lactam (ceftriaxone, 1–2 g IV/IM every 12–24 hr, maximum of 4 g/day, depending on severity, for 3–4 days until clinical improvement, followed by an oral β-lactam as listed above to complete a total of 7–14 days; or cefotaxime, 1–2 g IV/IM every 8 hr, depending on severity, for 3–4 days until clinical improvement, followed by an oral β-lactam as listed above to complete a total of 7–14 days) plus either a macrolide (azithromycin, 500 mg IV every day for at least 2 days, followed by 500 mg orally every day to complete a 7- to 10-day course of therapy) or doxycycline (100 mg IV or orally twice daily for 7–14 days)

Continued

TABLE 97–3 EMPIRICAL TREATMENT GUIDELINES FOR COMMUNITY-ACQUIRED PNEUMONIA—cont'd

Organisms	Therapy
Viruses *Legionella* sp Miscellaneous (*M. tuberculosis,* fungi, PcP)	*or* 2. IV antipneumococcal fluoroquinolone alone (levofloxacin, 500–750 mg IV every 24 hr for 3–4 days until clinical improvement, followed by oral therapy to complete a total of 7–14 days; or gatifloxacin, 400 mg IV once a day for 3–4 days until clinical improvement, followed by oral therapy to complete a total of 7–14 days; or ciprofloxacin, 500–750 mg IV every 12 hr for 3–4 days until clinical improvement, followed by oral therapy to complete a total of 7–14 days based on disease severity)

B. NO CARDIOPULMONARY DISEASE AND/OR MODIFYING FACTORS

Organisms	Therapy
S. pneumoniae *H. influenzae* *Mycoplasma* *Chlamydia* Mixed infection Viruses *Legionella* sp Miscellaneous (*M. tuberculosis,* fungi, PcP)	1. IV azithromycin alone (azithromycin, 500 mg IV every day for at least 2 days, followed by 500 mg orally every day to complete a 7- to 10-day course of therapy) *or* 2. Doxycycline (100 mg IV or orally twice daily for 7–14 days) and a β-lactam (ceftriaxone, 1–2 g IV/IM every 12–24 hr, maximum of 4 g/day, depending on severity, for 3–4 days until clinical improvement, followed by an oral β-lactam as listed above to complete a total of 7–14 days; or cefotaxime, 1–2 g IV/IM every 8 hr, depending on severity, for 3–4 days until clinical improvement, followed by an oral β-lactam as listed above to complete a total of 7–14 days) *or* 3. IV antipneumococcal fluoroquinolone alone (as listed above)

GROUP IV: ICU-ADMITTED PATIENTS

A. NO RISK FOR PSEUDOMONAS AERUGINOSA

Organisms	Therapy
S. pneumoniae (±DRSP) *Legionella* sp Enteric gram-negative rods *Staphylococcus aureus* *Mycoplasma* Respiratory viruses Miscellaneous (*Chlamydia, M. tuberculosis,* fungi, PcP)	IV β-lactam (cefotaxime, 2 g IV every 8 hr for 3–4 days until clinical improvement, followed by an oral β-lactam as listed above to complete a total of 7–14 days; or ceftriaxone, 2 g IV every 12 hr for 3–4 days until clinical improvement, followed by an oral β-lactam as listed above to complete a total of 7–14 days) *plus* either a. IV macrolide (azithromycin, 500 mg IV every day for at least 2 days, followed by 500 mg orally every day to complete a 7- to 10-day course of therapy) *or* b. IV fluoroquinolone (levofloxacin, 500–750 mg IV every 24 hr for 3–4 days until clinical improvement, followed by oral therapy to complete a total of 7–14 days; or gatifloxacin, 400 mg IV once a day for 3–4 days until clinical improvement, followed by oral therapy to complete a total of 7–14 days; or ciprofloxacin, 500–750 mg IV every 12 hr for 3–4 days until clinical improvement, followed by oral therapy to complete a total of 7–14 days based on disease severity)

B. RISKS FOR PSEUDOMONAS AERUGINOSA

Organisms	Therapy
Same as above *P. aeruginosa*	1. IV antipseudomonal β-lactam (cefepime, 1–2 g IV every 12 hr for 10 days; imipenem, 1 g IV every 6–8 hr, depending on severity of infection, maximum of 50 mg/kg/day or 4 g/day, whichever is lower, for 10 days; meropenem, 1 g IV every 8 hours for 10 days; or piperacillin/tazobactam, 4.5 g IV every 6 hr for 10 days) plus IV antipseudomonal fluoroquinolone (ciprofloxacin, 500–750 mg IV every 12 hr for 3–4 days until clinical improvement, followed by oral therapy to complete a total of 7–14 days based on disease severity) *or* 2. IV antipseudomonal β-lactam (as listed above) plus IV aminoglycoside (amikacin, 20 mg/kg/day in divided doses, with monitoring to maintain trough levels lower than 4–5 μg/mL; gentamicin, 7 mg/kg/day in three divided doses, with monitoring to maintain trough levels lower than 1 μg/mL; or tobramycin, 7 mg/kg/day in three divided doses, with monitoring to maintain trough levels lower than 1 μg/mL) *plus* a. IV macrolide (azithromycin, 500 mg IV every day for at least 2 days, followed by 500 mg orally every day to complete 10 days) *or* b. IV fluoroquinolone (as listed above)

Adapted from American Thoracic Society: Guidelines for management of adults with community-acquired pneumonia: Diagnosis, assessment of severity, initial antimicrobial therapy, and prevention. Am J Respir Crit Care Med 2001;163:1730–1754.
DRSP = drug-resistant *S. pneumoniae*; ICU = intensive care unit; PcP = *Pneumocystis jiroveci* pneumonia.

Rx

Outpatients who have underlying cardiopulmonary conditions or other modifying factors but whose pneumonia is sufficiently severe to warrant admission can be managed either with an extended-spectrum oral β-lactam (such as cefpodoxime, cefuroxime, high-dose amoxicillin, or amoxicillin-clavulanate) or with parenteral ceftriaxone followed by oral cefpodoxime, plus either an advanced-generation macrolide or doxycycline. Alternatively, such patients can also be managed with an oral antipneumococcal fluoroquinolone, such as levofloxacin, gatifloxacin, or ciprofloxacin. Such outpatients merit careful monitoring to be certain that they respond over the first 72 hours of therapy. The clinician must maintain vigilance about the need to hospitalize patients who deteriorate or fail to respond to the initial empirical therapy.

Patients who require hospitalization but not intensive care and who do not have history of underlying cardiopulmonary disease or modifying factors may be treated initially with intravenous azithromycin alone or may be started on doxycycline plus a β-lactam if they cannot tolerate macrolides. Alternatively, single-agent treatment can be instituted with an intravenous antipneumococcal fluoroquinolone [4] such as levofloxacin, gatifloxacin, or ciprofloxacin. Although fluoroquinolones remain effective against the most likely bacterial causes of community-acquired pneumonia, the widespread increase in fluoroquinolone use has been accompanied by occasional resistance to fluoroquinolones in some geographic regions. The empirical approach in each hospital can be tailored within the published guidelines to suppress the emergence of drug resistance.

Inpatients who do not require intensive care but who also have underlying cardiopulmonary disease or are elderly are at risk for infection with enteric gram-negative bacteria and are more likely to be infected with drug-resistant *S. pneumoniae* or *M. catarrhalis* (Chapter 324). Such patients should be managed initially not only with a macrolide or doxycycline to cover atypical organisms but also with an intravenous β-lactam (such as ceftriaxone or cefotaxime). Alternatively, single-agent treatment can be instituted with an antipneumococcal fluoroquinolone such as levofloxacin, gatifloxacin, or ciprofloxacin.

Patients who have respiratory insufficiency, septicemia, or significant multiorgan dysfunction require management in an ICU and evaluation to exclude infection with *P. aeruginosa* (Chapter 329). Patients at high risk for *P. aeruginosa* infection include those with structural lung disease (particularly bronchiectasis), greater than 10 mg/day of previous corticosteroid therapy, neutropenia, malnutrition, or previous broad-spectrum antibiotics for more than 7 days in the last month. ICU patients who are not considered at risk for *P. aeruginosa* infection can be treated initially with an intravenous β-lactam (such as cefotaxime or ceftriaxone) combined with either an intravenous macrolide (azithromycin) or an intravenous fluoroquinolone. Fluoroquinolone monotherapy is not considered appropriate in the setting of severe community-acquired pneumonia. In the ICU population considered to be at risk for *P. aeruginosa* infection, combination antipseudomonal therapy should be used, including intravenous antipseudomonal β-lactams (e.g., cefepime, imipenem, meropenem, or piperacillin/tazobactam) plus an intravenous antipseudomonal fluoroquinolone (e.g., ciprofloxacin). Alternatively, an intravenous antipseudomonal β-lactam can be administered along with an aminoglycoside plus either an intravenous macrolide (azithromycin) or an intravenous nonpseudomonal fluoroquinolone.

Oversight agencies are increasingly focused on objective measures of optimal care for community-acquired pneumonia, particularly in the hospital setting. Although recommendations are evolving and sometimes vary, current recommendations are that hospitalized patients with community-acquired pneumonia should undergo assessment of oxygenation, initiation of antibiotic therapy within 4 hours of admission and drawing of blood for culture, a smoking cessation intervention, and review and update of immunization status. Most experts also advise chest radiography at the time of admission.

Suspected or Proven Viral Infection

Therapies for suspected and proven viral infection are markedly limited when compared with those for bacterial infections. Early treatment of influenza A or B within the first 48 hours of symptoms with oseltamivir (75 mg orally taken twice daily for 5 days), or zanamivir (two inhalations of 5 mg per inhalation every 12 hours for 5 days) is effective in reducing symptoms and the duration of illness (Chapter 388). These agents are preferred over amantadine and rimantadine, which were effective only against influenza A, but this virus is now often resistant to them. Empirical antibiotic treatment of possible bacterial superinfection in addition to influenza should include agents effective against *S. pneumoniae, S. aureus,* and *H. influenzae.* In these considerations, amoxicillin-clavulanate, cefpodoxime, cefprozil, cefuroxime, or a respiratory fluoroquinolone would be appropriate. Pneumonias caused by varicella-zoster and herpes simplex virus should be treated with parenteral acyclovir (10 mg/kg intravenously every 8 hours for 7 days) (Chapters 398 and 399). No antiviral agents have established efficacy against RSV in adults, parainfluenza virus, adenovirus, metapneumovirus, the SARS coronavirus, or *Hantavirus.* Treatment is largely supportive, with oxygen and ventilator therapy as necessary.

Duration of Therapy

Most patients respond to empirical antibiotic regimens over the first 3 days of therapy. In general, it is not advisable to alter the antibiotic program in the first 72 hours unless the patient is deteriorating or culture results indicate alternative therapy. Patients initially begun on parenteral therapy may be switched to an oral regimen when they are afebrile (temperature less than 100° F on two occasions 8 hours apart) and demonstrate improvement in cough, dyspnea, and leukocytosis.

The optimal duration of antibiotic therapy for community-acquired pneumonia has received little formal study, with most recommendations ranging between 5 and 14 days of therapy. Accordingly, the total duration of antimicrobials should be individualized to the patient's clinical response. Initial multiagent regimens of a β-lactam with the addition of macrolides for the coverage of *Legionella* and *Mycoplasma* can frequently be de-escalated after several days to the β-lactams alone if *Legionella* urinary antigen and *Mycoplasma* serology prove negative. The clinical caveat remains, however, that macrolides may still be required in clinical situations in which a strong clinical suspicion for *Legionella* persists because urinary antigen testing does not detect organisms other than *Legionella* serogroup 1. Furthermore, in situations in which a causative organism is isolated from a normally sterile site, such as blood or pleural fluid, antibiotic therapy should be simplified and directed by susceptibility testing. Finally, when alternative clinical diagnoses other than pneumonia are proved to be the cause of the respiratory symptoms and all cultures remain negative over the first 72 hours, antibiotic therapy may be safely discontinued.

Treatment Failure

Treatment failures occur in approximately 10% of patients with community-acquired pneumonia, and complications occur in roughly 25% of patients. Adherence to treatment guidelines, such as those described earlier, increases the likelihood of a good outcome.

For patients who do not respond to initial empirical coverage, an aggressive search should be undertaken to detect unusual pathogens, alternative diagnoses such as pulmonary embolism (Chapter 99), or complications of pneumonia such as a complicated pleural effusion (Chapter 100), empyema, or lung abscess (Chapter 98). Additional diagnostic testing may include a chest CT scan, sampling of pleural fluid, and bronchoscopy with collection of respiratory secretions, brushings, and BAL fluid for microbiologic analysis.

Follow-up after Treatment

Even when the patient appears to respond to the initial antibiotic regimen, the chest radiograph signs resolve more slowly (over a period of 6 to 8 weeks) than other clinical signs and symptoms. The physician must document that abnormalities on the chest radiograph have resolved completely or, in some cases, have led to the formation of a fibrotic scar. Usual practice includes performing repeat radiography 6 to 8 weeks after completion of the antibiotic

Rx

regimen. Persistence of abnormalities on the chest radiograph or the development of recurrent pneumonia in a similar distribution should prompt a careful search for an underlying endobronchial obstruction such as an occult neoplasm (Chapter 201), foreign body, bronchostenosis, or broncholithiasis. Follow-up CT scanning is usually the prelude to formal pulmonary consultation for consideration of bronchoscopy and other further diagnostic tests.

ASPIRATION PNEUMONIA

Epidemiology and Pathobiology

Although microaspiration is the mechanism underlying most cases of pneumonia, the clinician is occasionally confronted with recurrent bacterial pneumonia in a patient experiencing repeated gross aspiration of oropharyngeal contents. Most of these patients have difficulty swallowing related to either underlying neuromuscular disorders or altered sensorium as a result of medications, drugs or alcohol, or underlying neurologic diseases. Common clinical scenarios associated with recurrent aspiration pneumonia include tracheobronchial fistulas secondary to esophageal or tracheal malignancies, esophageal obstruction related to esophageal cancer and its treatment (Chapter 202), and a wide variety of neurologic disorders, including amyotrophic lateral sclerosis (Chapter 435), multiple sclerosis (Chapter 436), stroke (Chapter 431), and other myopathic processes. Other patients with severe esophageal reflux (Chapter 140) may also experience significant aspiration during sleep despite apparently normal deglutition mechanisms and protective reflexes during wakefulness. Patients with neuromuscular disorders tend to have greater difficulty swallowing thin or liquid materials, whereas patients with obstruction from either malignancy or benign strictures tend to have the greatest difficulty swallowing solid food.

Clinical Manifestations

Aspiration pneumonias tend to have a less acute manifestation than the usual bacterial pneumonias do, with the onset of fever, dyspnea, purulent sputum, malaise, and other systemic symptoms, including loss of appetite, evolving over a number of days. Physical examination of the chest generally reveals only coarse rhonchi in the lower lobes or dependent lung regions.

Diagnosis

The diagnosis of aspiration pneumonia relies foremost on maintaining a high clinical index of suspicion. Recovery of tracheal secretions containing food particles or lipid-laden macrophages strongly supports the diagnosis. In patients receiving tube feedings, the respiratory secretions should be tested for glucose because these secretions normally contain low levels of glucose. Alternatively, methylene blue or similar tracer dyes can be added to tube feeding materials to confirm the presence of aspiration. Additional diagnostic modalities include the use of cineradiographic swallowing studies with thin liquid water-soluble contrast agents to confirm the aspiration event. Radionuclide imaging studies may also document aspiration in adults whose neurologic status precludes them from cooperating fully with the cineradiographic studies. Overnight esophageal pH monitoring may be undertaken in individuals who are suspected of having recurrent esophageal reflux and aspiration events at night. However, except in the most severe cases, it remains difficult to predict which patients with gastroesophageal reflux will actually experience aspiration pneumonia.

Chest radiographs should be reviewed in light of the patient's probable position during aspiration. The lower lobes, particularly the superior segments of the right lower lobe, and the posterior segments of the upper lobes are frequently involved. However, unilateral aspiration or aspiration into virtually any pulmonary segment has been reported, depending on the patient's position during the aspiration event. The radiographic appearance usually reflects a parenchymal bronchopneumonia process. Pleural involvement is uncommon initially, unless aggressive anaerobic infection is present. Nonresolving or inadequately treated aspiration pneumonia can result in lung abscess and empyema formation.

Bronchoscopy, though not routinely necessary, can confirm the presence of aspiration by recovering food particles or lipid-laden macrophages derived from fats present in the aspirated food. Bronchoscopy with BAL can be useful in providing quantitative counts of aerobic bacteria, and protected specimen brush sampling can document anaerobic organisms, although negative cultures do not exclude the presence of anaerobes.

Microbiology

Oropharyngeal secretions contain massive numbers of microorganisms, with counts of aerobic bacteria ranging between 10^6 and 10^8 and anaerobic organisms being as high as 10^9 per milliliter of saliva. Accordingly, aspiration pneumonia should be viewed as a polymicrobial infection, with the clinical manifestations being driven by the predominant and most aggressive organisms in the mixture. Oropharyngeal colonization is strongly influenced by the clinical setting in which the patient was dwelling at the time of aspiration (outpatient versus hospital or institutional). In otherwise healthy outpatients, aggressive organisms such as *S. pneumoniae*, *S. aureus*, and *H. influenzae* may be present. In contrast, the oropharyngeal secretions of hospitalized patients and resident of long-term care facilities include aerobic gram-negative bacteria and *P. aeruginosa*. Anaerobic organisms, which are a major consideration in both settings, include anaerobic and microaerophilic streptococci, *Bacteroides* species, *Fusobacterium nucleatum*, and *Prevotella* species. Cultures of sputum and tracheal secretions probably document such mixed flora.

Treatment

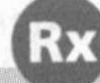

Empirical antibiotic therapy should be initiated rapidly once the diagnosis of aspiration pneumonia is made; the regimen can be modified later after culture information from sputum, tracheal secretions, or bronchoscopic sampling is available. Otherwise healthy individuals with isolated aspiration pneumonia related to trauma, seizures, or oversedation may be treated initially with either oral amoxicillin-clavulanate or intravenous ampicillin-sulbactam, depending on the severity of illness. Alternatively, intravenous clindamycin alone can be used. For patients with underlying chronic diseases, intravenous ampicillin-sulbactam or intravenous fluoroquinolones that cover anaerobes, such as moxifloxacin or gatifloxacin, can be considered. In seriously ill individuals, particularly patients requiring intubation and mechanical ventilation, as well as patients experiencing aspiration in the hospital or long-term care setting, coverage must be extended to aerobic gram-negative bacteria and *Pseudomonas* species, including extended-spectrum β-lactam/β-lactamase inhibitor combinations such as piperacillin-tazobactam or ticarcillin-clavulanate or carbapenems such as imipenem. Intravenous clindamycin can also be added in these settings, or alternatively, intravenous clindamycin can be given in combination with ciprofloxacin or aztreonam. In patients with concern about organisms with high levels of antibiotic resistance, such as *P. aeruginosa*, an antipseudomonal β-lactam such as ceftazidime or cefepime can be combined with an antipseudomonal fluoroquinolone such as ciprofloxacin or an aminoglycoside. Again, addition of extended anaerobic coverage with clindamycin should be considered. Finally, if the patient is known or suspected to harbor methicillin-resistant *S. aureus* (MRSA), intravenous vancomycin or linezolid should be added to the regimen.

Surgical Therapy

Adequate nutrition is a concern in patients with multiple episodes of aspiration pneumonia and underlying neurologic disease or malignancy. Endoscopic or surgical placement of a gastrostomy or jejunostomy feeding tube can be considered to aid in providing nutrition, fluids, and medications in the palliation of such patients. Of greater challenge are patients who continue to have pneumonia related to aspiration of saliva, sometimes around cuffed endotracheal and tracheostomy tubes. If aggressive therapy is considered appropriate, ligation of the submaxillary and parotid salivary ducts can decrease the production of saliva.

TABLE 97–4 HOST RISK FACTORS ASSOCIATED WITH DEVELOPMENT OF MULTIDRUG-RESISTANT INFECTION DURING HAP, VAP, AND HCAP

Antibiotic therapy in the past 90 days
High incidence of antibiotic resistance in the community or in the specific hospital unit
Current hospitalization for 5 or more days
Immunosuppressive disease or therapy
Presence of risk factors for HCAP
Hospitalization for 2 or more days in the past 90 days
Resident in a nursing home or extended care facility
Home infusion therapy (including antibiotics)
Chronic dialysis within the past 30 days
Home wound care
Family member with an MDR pathogen

HAP = hospital-associated pneumonia; HCAP = health care–associated pneumonia; MDR = multidrug resistant; VAP = ventilator-associated pneumonia.
Adapted from American Thoracic Society and Infectious Diseases Society of America: Guidelines for management of adults with hospital-acquired, ventilator-associated, and health care–associated pneumonia. Am J Respir Crit Care Med 2005:171:388–416.

HOSPITAL-ACQUIRED PNEUMONIA, VENTILATOR-ASSOCIATED PNEUMONIA, AND HEALTH CARE–ASSOCIATED PNEUMONIA

Epidemiology

Hospital-acquired pneumonia, ventilator-associated pneumonia, and health care–associated pneumonia represent the second most common nosocomial infection in the United States. Hospital-acquired pneumonia on average increases the length of hospital stay from 7 to 9 days, at an additional cost of more than $40,000 per patient; it is responsible for a quarter of all ICU infections and half of all antibiotic use. Early-onset hospital-acquired pneumonia and ventilator-associated pneumonia, defined as infections occurring within the first 4 hospital days, tend to be caused by antibiotic-susceptible bacteria, whereas late-onset infections are more frequently caused by multidrug-resistant (MDR) organisms (Table 97–4), which are associated with greater morbidity and mortality. The overall mortality attributed to hospital-acquired pneumonia may be as high as 30 to 50%.

Pathobiology

Gram-negative bacterial pneumonias are fairly uncommon in previously healthy outpatients, except in patients with impaired immunity or underlying structural lung disease such as COPD. However, aerobic gram-negative bacilli, including *P. aeruginosa*, *Escherichia coli*, *K. pneumoniae*, and *Acinetobacter* species, play major roles in patients with hospital-acquired pneumonia, ventilator-associated pneumonia, and health care–associated pneumonia. Many cases are polymicrobial, and gram-positive agents such as *S. aureus*, particularly MRSA strains, are also common. The frequency of MDR bacteria varies by the patient population, hospital, ICU, and local use of antimicrobial agents, so routine surveillance and monitoring of local pathogens and drug susceptibilities are key to appropriately adjusting antibiotic use.

P. aeruginosa, *Acinetobacter* species, *Stenotrophomonas maltophilia*, and *Burkholderia cepacia* are of particular concern because these organisms rapidly become resistant to multiple classes of antibiotics. MDR organisms are most commonly found in patients with severe underlying chronic disease, in patients with health care–associated pneumonia, and in those with late-onset hospital-acquired pneumonia and ventilator-associated pneumonia. Although considerable emphasis is placed on gram-negative bacteria in the hospital setting, more traditional bacterial pathogens such as *S. pneumoniae* and *H. influenzae* must also be considered as potential causes. *L. pneumophila* also occasionally occurs as a nosocomial infection, particularly where there is contaminated water or during construction.

Clinical Manifestations

Hospital-acquired pneumonia, ventilator-associated pneumonia, and health care–associated pneumonia are often first suspected with the demonstration of new or worsening radiographic infiltrates along with other clinical signs of infection, including fever, leukocytosis, and purulent sputum. Oxygenation may have also worsened. In general, two of the three major clinical features (fever, leukocytosis, purulent sputum) should be present. In patients with acute respiratory distress syndrome, however, a single clinical factor alone should prompt additional investigation and microbiologic culture.

Diagnosis

All patients with suspected hospital-acquired pneumonia, ventilator-associated pneumonia, and health care–associated pneumonia should receive a comprehensive history and physical examination to define the severity of disease and potential sources of infection. Chest radiography is essential to determine the extent of pneumonia, particularly whether it is focal or multilobar. Some patients without new or evolving radiographic infiltrates but with other signs of infection may have purulent tracheobronchitis (Chapter 96), which may require antibiotic therapy if clinical signs of infection are present. Arterial blood gases, complete blood count, electrolytes, and liver and renal function should also be evaluated. Blood should be obtained for culture, although it is positive in only a minority of patients, before instituting new antibiotics whenever possible.

Lower respiratory tract secretions should be obtained for culture from all patients by endotracheal aspiration, BAL, or protected specimen brush whenever possible before changes in antibiotic therapy; a reliable Gram stain can help direct initial empirical therapy. A sterile culture of lower respiratory tract secretions in the absence of a new antibiotic in the past 72 hours essentially excludes most bacterial pneumonias with a 94% negative predictive value, although *Legionella* and viral infection are still possible in this situation. The quantitative diagnostic threshold for significant bacterial infection, in the absence of recent (<72 hours) changes in antibiotic regimens, is as follows: greater than 10^6 colony-forming units (cfu)/mL for tracheal aspirates, greater than 10^4 or 10^5 cfu/mL for quantitative BAL fluid, and greater than 10^3 cfu/mL for protected specimen brushings. The use of bronchoscopically obtained specimens and quantitative bacterial culture in directing therapy reduces the 14-day mortality in suspected ventilator-associated pneumonia. 

Treatment

Rx

Initial Empirical Therapy

If the patient is unstable or has evidence of sepsis or if there is a high suspicion for hospital-acquired pneumonia, ventilator-associated pneumonia, or health care–associated pneumonia, prompt antibiotic therapy is required regardless of whether bacteria are found on the initial microscopic examination of lower respiratory tract samples because delays in antimicrobial therapy increase mortality. The choice of initial empirical therapy is based on several factors, including whether the pneumonia is early onset, whether there are risk factors for MDR bacterial infections (Table 97–5), and local surveillance data on bacterial prevalence and susceptibilities.

Suspected or Early-Onset Disease

For patients with suspected hospital-acquired or ventilator-associated pneumonia, with early-onset disease, and with no identifiable risk factors for MDR organisms, initial empirical therapy can include either ceftriaxone, an intravenous fluoroquinolone (levofloxacin, moxifloxacin, or ciprofloxacin), ampicillin/sulbactam, or ertapenem. These options will cover *S. pneumoniae*, *H. influenzae*, methicillin-sensitive *S. aureus*, and most antibiotic-sensitive gram-negative bacilli, including *E. coli*, *K. pneumoniae*, *Proteus* species, *Enterobacter* species, and *Serratia marcescens*.

Late-Onset Disease

In contrast, with late-onset hospital-acquired pneumonia, ventilator-associated pneumonia, or health care–associated pneumonia

TABLE 97–5 EMPIRICAL ANTIBIOTIC TREATMENT OF HOSPITAL-ACQUIRED PNEUMONIA (HAP), VENTILATOR-ASSOCIATED PNEUMONIA (VAP), AND HEALTH CARE–ASSOCIATED PNEUMONIA (HCAP)

GROUP A: PATIENTS WITH EITHER HAP OR VAP, WITHOUT RISK FACTORS FOR MDR PATHOGENS, AND WITH EARLY-ONSET PNEUMONIA

Potential Pathogens	Recommended Therapy
Streptococcus pneumoniae *Haemophilus influenzae* Methicillin-sensitive *Staphylococcus aureus* Antibiotic-sensitive enteric gram-negative bacilli *Escherichia coli* *Klebsiella pneumoniae* *Enterobacter* sp *Proteus* sp *Serratia marcescens*	Ceftriaxone (1–2 g IV/IM every 12–24 hr, maximum of 4 g/day, with duration dependent on clinical response and individualized, as discussed in text) *or* Levofloxacin (500–750 mg IV every day, with duration dependent on clinical response and individualized), ciprofloxacin (400 mg IV every 8 hr, with duration dependent on clinical response and individualized), or moxifloxacin (400 mg IV or orally every 24 hr, with duration dependent on clinical response and individualized) *or* Ampicillin/sulbactam (1.5–3 g [1–2 g ampicillin and 0.5–1 g sulbactam] IV/IM every 6 hr, maximum of 4 g sulbactam/day, depending on type and severity of infection, with duration dependent on clinical response and individualized) *or* Ertapenem (1 g IV/IM once a day, with duration dependent on clinical response and individualized)

GROUP B: PATIENTS WITH HAP, VAP, OR HCAP AND WITH LATE-ONSET PNEUMONIA OR WITH RISK FACTORS FOR MDR PATHOGENS

Organisms	Therapy
Streptococcus pneumoniae *Haemophilus influenzae* Methicillin-sensitive *S. aureus* Antibiotic-sensitive enteric gram-negative bacilli *E. coli* *K. pneumoniae* *Enterobacter* sp *Proteus* sp *S. marcescens* *PLUS* MDR pathogens *Pseudomonas aeruginosa* *K. pneumoniae* (extended spectrum β-lactamase producing) *Acinetobacter* sp Methicillin-resistant *S. aureus* *Legionella pneumophila*	Antipseudomonal cephalosporin (ceftazidime, 2 g IV every 8 hr, or cefepime, 1–2 g every 8–12 hr, with duration dependent on clinical response and individualized) *or* Antipseudomonal carbapenems (meropenem, 1 g every 8 hr, or imipenem, 500 mg every 6 hr or 1 g every 8 hr, with duration dependent on clinical response and individualized) *or* β-Lactam/β-lactamase inhibitor (piperacillin/tazobactam, 4.5 g IV every 6 hr, with duration dependent on clinical response and individualized) *PLUS* Antipseudomonal fluoroquinolone (levofloxacin, 750 mg IV every day, or ciprofloxacin (400 mg IV every 8 hr, with duration dependent on clinical response and individualized) or Aminoglycoside (amikacin, 20 mg/kg/day, with monitoring to maintain trough levels lower than 4–5 μg/mL; gentamicin, 7 mg/kg/day in three divided doses, with monitoring to maintain trough levels lower than 1 μg/mL; or tobramycin, 7 mg/kg/day in three divided doses, with monitoring to maintain trough levels lower than 1 μg/mL and duration dependent on clinical response and individualized) *PLUS* Vancomycin (15 mg/kg every 12 hr, with monitoring to maintain trough levels at 15–20 μg/mL and duration dependent on clinical response and individualized) or linezolid (600 mg every 12 hr, with duration dependent on clinical response and individualized)

MDR = multidrug-resistant.
Adapted from American Thoracic Society: Guidelines for management of adults with hospital-acquired ventilator associated, and healthcare-associated pneumonia. Am J Respir Crit Care Med 2005:171:388–416.

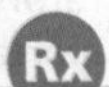

or when risk factors for MDR infection have been identified, multiagent regimens should be used initially. Options include an antipseudomonal cephalosporin such as ceftazidime or cefepime, an antipseudomonal carbapenem (meropenem or imipenem), or a β-lactam/β-lactamase inhibitor agent such as piperacillin-tazobactam; in addition, either an antipseudomonal fluoroquinolone (ciprofloxacin or levofloxacin) or an aminoglycoside such as amikacin, gentamicin, or tobramycin should be used. In combination, these agents should empirically address most MDR pathogens, including *P. aeruginosa*, *Acinetobacter* species, and *K. pneumoniae* strains with extended-spectrum β-lactamase production. Most *L. pneumophila* isolates will also be covered, but if *Legionella* is strongly suspected, a macrolide such as azithromycin should be included. Finally, either vancomycin or linezolid should be added for coverage of MRSA if risk factors are present or the risk for MRSA is high locally.

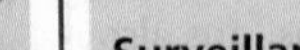

Surveillance

The initiation of empirical antibiotic therapy mandates careful daily reassessment. If the patient improves over the first 48 to 72 hours, strong consideration should be given to de-escalating antibiotic therapy based on culture results. If lower respiratory cultures remain negative but the patient has not improved, an extrapulmonary site of infection should be considered. Additional radiographic imaging and cultures from the lung, pleura, and other sites may be helpful.

Duration of Treatment

The total duration of therapy should also be individualized. In general, aminoglycoside use should be limited to 5 to 7 days. Overall antibiotic therapy can be as short as 7 days if the patient has improved, but patients with sluggish improvement may require 14 to 21 days of therapy.

Prevention

Sources of pathogens for hospital-acquired pneumonia include the environment, health care devices, and transfer of microbes by patients, staff, and visitors. Thus, scrupulous hand hygiene is essential for reducing these infections. Colonization plus aspiration of oropharyngeal pathogens or leakage of secretions around endotracheal tubes is the usual route of inoculation. The stomach and sinuses may be additional sites harboring pathogens. Infected biofilms on endotracheal tubes may also serve as an important reservoir for these infections.

In this light, aggressive measures should be enforced to reduce the risk for hospital-acquired pneumonia and ventilator-associated pneumonia. Prevention centers first on staff education and compliance with alcohol-based hand disinfection, which must be used before and after each patient interaction. In addition, patients with documented MDR organisms should be isolated to reduce the risk for patient cross-contamination. Microbiologic surveillance within the hospital environment is also necessary to identify MDR organisms and determine antibiotic use and susceptibility patterns. Within the ICU, intubation and reintubation rates should be monitored and reduced as feasible, the duration of mechanical ventilation should be minimized to reduce the risk for ventilator-associated pneumonia, and methods known to reduce infection rates should be followed (Chapter 106).

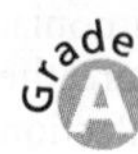

1. Harper SA, Fukuda K, Uyeki TM, et al: Prevention and control of influenza. Recommendations of the Advisory Committee on Immunization Practices. MMWR Recomm Rep 2005;54(RR-8):1–40.
2. van der Eerden MM, Vlaspolder F, de Groot CS, et al: Comparison of pathogen directed antibiotic treatment and empirical broad-spectrum antibiotic treatment in patients with community-acquired pneumonia: A prospective randomized study. Thorax 2005;60:672–678.
3. Yealy DM, Auble TE, Stone RA, et al: Effect of increasing the intensity of implementing pneumonia guidelines: A randomized, controlled trial. Ann Intern Med 2005;143:881–894.
4. Marrie TJ, Lau CY, Wheeler SL, et al: A controlled trial of a critical pathway for treatment of community-acquired pneumonia. CAPITAL Study Investigators. Community-Acquired Pneumonia Intervention Trial Assessing Levofloxacin. JAMA 2000;283:749–755.
5. Fagon JY, Chastre J, Wolff M, et al: Invasive and non-invasive strategies for the management of suspected ventilator-associated pneumonia: A randomized trial. Ann Intern Med 2000; 132:621–630.

SUGGESTED READINGS

American Thoracic Society and Infectious Diseases Society of America: Guidelines for the management of adults with hospital-acquired, ventilator-associated, and health care associated pneumonia. Am J Respir Crit Care Med 2005; 171:388–416. *A comprehensive guide to the diagnosis and management of hospital-acquired pneumonia, ventilator-associated pneumonia, and health care–associated pneumonia.*

Falguera M, Martín M, Ruiz-González A, et al: Community-acquired pneumonia as the initial manifestation of serious underlying diseases. Am J Med 2005;118:378–383. *Among 660 patients, 45% had prior underlying diseases, whereas 6% had one or more new comorbid conditions.*

Kyaw MH, Lynfield R, Schaffner W, et al: Effect of introduction of the pneumococcal conjugate vaccine on drug-resistant *Streptococcus pneumoniae*. N Engl J Med 2006;354:1455–1463. *Rates of resistant disease caused by vaccine serotypes fell 87%, whereas serotype 19A, which was not included in the vaccine, increased.*

Mandell LA, Wunderink RG, Anzueto A, et al: Infectious Diseases Society of America/American Thoracic Society consensus guidelines on the management of community-acquired pneumonia in adults. Clin Infect Dis 2007;44(Suppl 2):S27–S72. *Consensus guidelines.*

Menendez R, Torres A, Rodriguez de Castro P, et al: Reaching stability in community acquired pneumonia: The effects of the severity of disease, treatment and characteristics of the patients. Clin Infect Dis 2004;239:1783–1790. *Empirical treatment that follows guidelines is associated with earlier clinical stability.*

Skowronski DM, Astell C, Brunham RC, et al: Severe acute respiratory syndrome (SARS): A year in review. Annu Rev Med 2005;56:357–381. *Overview of clinical, virologic, and epidemiologic factors related to infection with the SARS-associated coronavirus.*

The Canadian Critical Care Trials Group: A randomized trial of diagnostic techniques for ventilator-associated pneumonia. N Engl J Med 2006;355: 2619–2630. *Two diagnostic strategies showed similar clinical outcomes and similar overall antibiotic use.*

98 LUNG ABSCESS

Sydney M. Finegold

Definition

A lung abscess is a cavity containing pus and necrotic debris. Although mycobacterial, fungal, and parasitic infections can cause cavitary lesions, the term *lung abscess* is usually reserved for other bacterial infections and is distinguished from empyema (Chapter 100), which is a collection of pus within the pleural space rather than the lung parenchyma. Many different microorganisms can produce a lung abscess, and a number of conditions can simulate it radiographically (Table 98–1). Lung abscess

TABLE 98–1 ORGANISMS AND CONDITIONS WITH THE RADIOGRAPHIC APPEARANCE OF LUNG ABSCESS

INFECTIOUS
BACTERIAL ASPIRATION/PNEUMONIA
Anaerobes: pigmented and nonpigmented *Prevotella, Porphyromonas, Fusobacterium, Peptostreptococcus* (now divided into four additional genera—*Anaerococcus, Finegoldia, Gallicola,* and *Peptoniphilus*), *Bacteroides fragilis, Clostridium perfringens, Actinomyces, Eubacterium lentum, Propionibacterium, Veillonella*
Aerobes: streptococci, *Enterococcus, Staphylococcus aureus,* Enterobacteriaceae, including *Klebsiella pneumoniae* and *Klebsiella oxytoca, Proteus mirabilis, Pseudomonas aeruginosa, Legionella* sp, *Nocardia asteroides, Haemophilus influenzae, Haemophilus parainfluenzae, Eikenella corrodens, Pasteurella multocida, Moraxella, Acinetobacter, Stenotrophomonas maltophilia, Salmonella* sp, *Burkholderia pseudomallei, Burkholderia mallei, Rhodococcus, Treponema pallidum, Mycoplasma pneumoniae*
BACTERIAL EMBOLIC
Staphylococcus aureus, P. aeruginosa, Fusobacterium necrophorum
MYCOBACTERIA (OFTEN MULTIFOCAL)
Mycobacterium tuberculosis, Mycobacterium avium complex, *Mycobacterium kansasii,* other mycobacteria
FUNGI
Aspergillus sp, Mucoraceae, *Histoplasma capsulatum, Pneumocystis carinii, Coccidioides immitis, Blastomyces dermatitidis, Cryptococcus neoformans, Candida albicans, Candida glabrata*
PARASITES
Entamoeba histolytica, Paragonimus westermani, Strongyloides stercoralis (postobstructive)
Empyema (with air-fluid level)
Septic embolism (endocarditis)
PREDISPOSING CONDITIONS
Fluid-filled cysts or bullae
Infarction without infection
Pulmonary embolism
Vasculitis
Goodpasture's syndrome
Wegener's granulomatosis
Polyarteritis nodosa
Bronchiectasis
Postobstructive pneumonia (neoplasm, foreign body)
Necrotizing carcinoma
Pulmonary sequestration
Pulmonary contusion
Neoplasm

formation usually reflects infection with an unusual microbial burden (e.g., acute aspiration), an especially virulent organism (e.g., *Staphylococcus aureus*), or failure of microbial clearance mechanisms (e.g., bronchial obstruction).

Epidemiology

Most lung abscesses involve the indigenous flora of the oropharynx. Abscesses involving *S. aureus* or gram-negative bacilli are most often nosocomial (Chapter 304). *Nocardia* and *Rhodococcus* are found almost exclusively in immunocompromised hosts (Chapter 303). Septic pulmonary emboli are generally due to *S. aureus*, primarily in intravenous drug abusers with tricuspid valve endocarditis (Chapter 76). Lung abscesses caused by infection with *Paragonimus westermani* and melioidosis are usually acquired in the Far East or Indonesia. The incidence of lung abscess has decreased since the advent of antimicrobial therapy, but larger U.S. hospitals see 10 to 25 cases per year.

Pathobiology

Conditions that predispose to lung abscess include any cause of aspiration or decreased ciliary action, such as reduced levels of consciousness, alcoholism, seizure disorders, general anesthesia, cerebrovascular accidents, drug addiction, dysphagia, esophageal reflux, and mechanical interference with the cardiac sphincter, such as caused by nasogastric tubes and endotracheal intubation (Chapters 97 and 311). Periodontal disease, gingivitis, sinus infection, and bronchiectasis provide a source for anaerobic infection and are other important background factors. Another cause of lung abscess is septic pulmonary embolism, most commonly with *S. aureus* and most frequently in intravenous drug users. Unlike lung abscesses related to aspiration, which are usually solitary, the lung abscesses seen with septic pulmonary emboli are commonly multiple or are associated with other septic embolic lesions in various stages of development. Any necrotizing pneumonia can also be associated with areas of abscess, which are commonly small and multiple and are less likely to be defined clearly as abscesses by chest radiograph than by pathologic specimen. When bronchial obstruction develops distal to a pulmonary neoplasm (Chapter 201), drainage is difficult and abscess formation is common. For all causes of abscess, however, diabetes, malignancy, and other immunocompromising conditions are common predisposing factors.

Although most cases involve anaerobic bacteria, half include aerobes as well. The principal anaerobes are pigmented and nonpigmented *Prevotella, Fusobacterium,* and *Peptostreptococcus. Bacteroides fragilis* group strains are found in 7% of cases. Among the aerobes, streptococci, staphylococci, and gram-negative bacilli are prominent. One study reported that *Klebsiella pneumoniae* was the single most common isolate in lung abscesses in Taiwan.

Small numbers of oropharyngeal bacteria are commonly aspirated during sleep but are readily cleared by host defense mechanisms (Chapters 85, 97, and 311). Defense mechanisms are not as efficient in handling larger numbers of aspirated bacteria.

Counts of anaerobes in oral flora are lower than usual in edentulous subjects and higher in patients with periodontal disease. Alcoholics and patients who are acutely or chronically ill (especially if hospitalized) often demonstrate oropharyngeal colonization with aerobic or facultative gram-negative bacilli and *S. aureus.* Among the anaerobes, organisms more likely to cause infection as sole agents are *Fusobacterium nucleatum, Fusobacterium necrophorum, B. fragilis,* and *Clostridium perfringens.* Both the size of the bacterial inoculum and the role of associated organisms and host defenses are important. Organisms such as *S. aureus* and *K. pneumoniae,* which produce extracellular toxins or enzymes, often produce abscesses.

The various types of aspiration-related pleuropulmonary infections—pneumonitis (the initial stage), necrotizing pneumonia (multiple excavations <2 cm in diameter), lung abscess (one or more cavities >2 cm in diameter communicating with a bronchus), and empyema—should be considered one process with a continuum of changes. A predilection for infection in dependent segments is seen, particularly the posterior segments of the upper lobes and the superior segments of the lower lobes, but the location of the abscess depends on gravity and the position of the subject (Fig. 98–1). Normally, the aspirated material is handled effectively by ciliary action, cough, and alveolar macrophages (Chapters 85 and 97). Endotracheal tubes impair coughing, impede pulmonary clearance mechanisms, and allow leakage of oropharyngeal secretions into the tracheobronchial tree. Thick or particulate matter and foreign bodies, which are not easily removed by standard techniques used in intensive care units, can produce bronchial obstruction and atelectasis. In pneumonia, after aspiration of gastric contents, gastric acid and enzymes are the primary offending agents (Chapter 311). Subdiaphragmatic infection may extend to the lung by way of lymphatic vessels, directly through the diaphragm, or by way of the blood stream.

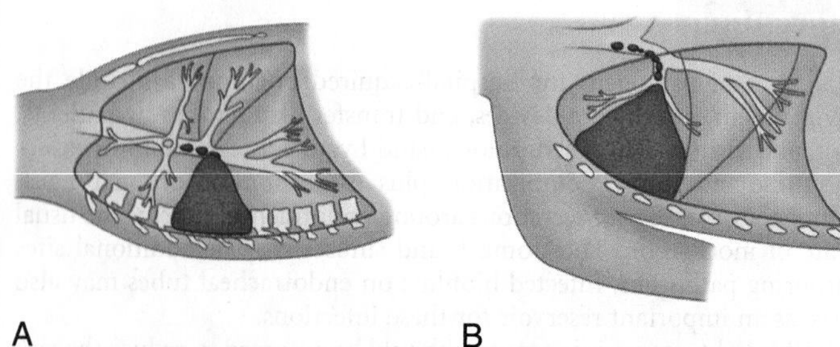

FIGURE 98–1 • Relationship between posture and location of lung abscess. With patient lying face up **(A)**, aspiration occurs into the superior segment of the lower lobe. With patient lying on the side **(B)**, aspiration occurs into the posterior segment of the upper lobe. (From Brock RC: Lung Abscess. Oxford, Blackwell, 1952.)

Clinical Manifestations

A relatively insidious onset of infection is seen in many patients; additional clues are involvement of dependent segments of lung, predisposition to aspiration, and frequently, periodontal disease. After 1 to 2 weeks, tissue necrosis with abscess formation or empyema occurs. After cavitation, putrid sputum is noted in 50% or more of patients, and hemoptysis may be seen. Weeks to months of malaise and low-grade fever may be associated with cough, weight loss, and anemia. Neoplasia is a serious diagnostic consideration in such patients. On occasion, the picture is acute, with fever, malaise, cough, and pleurisy. Patients with lung abscess as a result of infection with *S. aureus* or gram-negative bacilli and those with secondary lung abscess as a result of septic pulmonary emboli may have a more fulminant course. In edentulous persons with intact oropharyngeal function, lung abscesses are uncommon and suggest the presence of an obstructing lesion of the bronchus (carcinoma or other) or a pulmonary embolus.

Diagnosis

The classic radiographic appearance of lung abscess is a cavity with an air-fluid level, with or without surrounding infiltrate (Fig. 98–2); in some patients, however, repeat chest radiographs or computed tomography (CT) may be needed to detect the cavity. A similar radiographic appearance can be seen with a variety of conditions other than bacterial lung abscess (see Table 98–1), so definitive bacterial confirmation is required. Because radiography occasionally reveals mediastinal lymphadenopathy, the differential diagnosis includes tuberculosis, fungal infection, and lung cancer. Infected cysts or bullae and pulmonary sequestration are often evident with radiography. CT can readily distinguish between lung abscess and an air-fluid level in an empyema cavity.

The spectrum of organisms causing lung abscess has widened as patients are seen with more complex medical and surgical conditions. Antibiotic resistance has emerged and the number of immunocompromised persons has increased. Thus, microbiologic studies are increasingly desirable to guide therapy. Expectorated sputum cannot be used for anaerobic culture because large numbers of anaerobes are present in the indigenous flora. Even for infection with *S. aureus* and gram-negative bacilli, use of expectorated sputum is a problem because of frequent oropharyngeal colonization with such organisms in institutionalized patients. Bacteremia is uncommon in aspiration pneumonia, and all

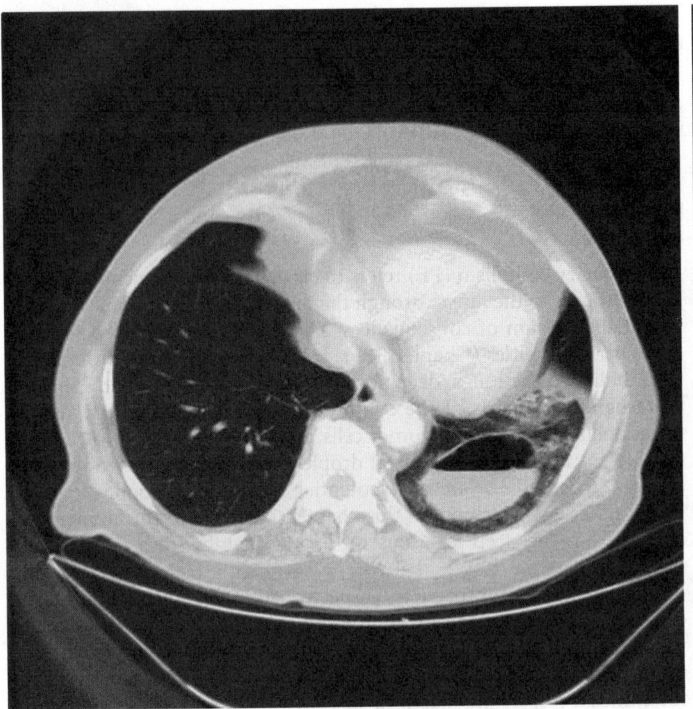

FIGURE 98–2 • Left upper lobe lung abscess distal to bronchographic carcinoma in the left hilum. Note the loss of volume in the left upper lung and the air-fluid level.

organisms involved in the lung abscess may not be recovered in blood cultures. Empyema fluid is an excellent source for anaerobic (and aerobic) culture. Transtracheal aspiration bypasses the normal flora of the upper respiratory tract, but contamination with indigenous flora can be a problem, and the procedure is now seldom performed. Two approaches for obtaining samples that are relatively free of upper airway contamination include use of a protected specimen brush and bronchoalveolar lavage. The protected specimen brush procedure involves sampling with a bronchial brush protected within a telescoping plugged double catheter via a fiberoptic bronchoscope. It is essential that the technique be performed exactly as described and that cultures be done quantitatively. For the protected specimen brush procedure, 10^3 to 10^4 or more colony-forming units per milliliter is significant. The small volume of material obtained and the difficulty associated with anaerobic transport are concerns. Quantitative culture of fluid obtained by bronchoalveolar lavage, during or without bronchoscopy, also provides reliable results. Counts of 10^4 or more organisms per milliliter are considered significant. Demonstration of bacteria intracellularly in at least 3 to 5% of cells in bronchoalveolar lavage fluid is good evidence of active pulmonary infection, and the morphology of these bacteria is extremely useful in directing therapy. Specimens must be maintained in anaerobic conditions immediately after being obtained. In patients who are intubated or who have a tracheotomy, there is typically contamination of the upper airways with oropharyngeal flora. In these settings and in general, when bronchoscopy can be performed, directed aspiration of the involved pulmonary segment can provide excellent access to material for reliable culture. Bronchoscopy is also often important to exclude cavitating or obstructing malignancy or the presence of a foreign body.

Prevention and Treatment

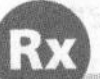

Precautions should be taken to minimize aspiration, particularly in feeding feeble or confused patients and those with swallowing difficulties (Chapter 97). In the case of gross aspiration, immediate clearing of the airway by postural drainage and suctioning, preferably by bronchoscopy, is important. Proper treatment of periodontal disease and gingivitis and early treatment of pneumonia minimize the risk for bacterial lung abscess.

Rx

Antimicrobial therapy and drainage are the keystones of treatment, but identification plus treatment of underlying or primary processes is also important. Prolonged therapy is essential to prevent relapse; the actual duration of treatment must be individualized, but periods of 1 to 3 months or more may be required. The approach to a specific patient is based on the clinical status of the patient, as well as the microbiologic features of the infection. The initial choice of antimicrobial agents is empirical but should be guided by Gram stain and the probable bacteriologic source of the infection, and then it should be adjusted as culture and susceptibility data become available. A small to moderate-sized abscess in an otherwise healthy person may respond to conservative management: antimicrobial therapy and aggressive pulmonary toilet through positioning and other drainage maneuvers. A rapidly expanding pulmonary abscess in an immunocompromised host (e.g., caused by one of the Mucoraceae) requires urgent lung resection in addition to antimicrobial therapy. Surgery may also be required for massive hemoptysis (Chapter 102). Secondary lung abscesses may require more intensive antimicrobial therapy.

Therapy for infections caused by aerobic bacteria (Chapters 97 and 309), mycobacteria (Chapters 345 and 346), fungi (Chapter 352), and parasites (Chapter 365) is based on their susceptibilities to specific agents. Anaerobic agents, which include *Prevotella* and *Bacteroides* species, fusobacteria, anaerobic cocci, clostridia, and *B. fragilis* and which predominate in bacterial lung abscesses, produce β-lactamases and demonstrate resistance to penicillin G in up to 40% of cases. Clindamycin, given initially at a dose of 600 mg every 6 hours intravenously, then when the patient is afebrile and improved, 300 mg orally every 6 hours, is more effective than penicillin. When penicillin is used, it should be administered in high doses (12 million U/day intravenously in average-sized adults with normal renal function) and in combination with clindamycin or metronidazole (2 g/day intravenously in four divided doses). Metronidazole alone may be ineffective because of resistance of aerobic bacteria, *Actinomyces*, and microaerophilic streptococci. After improvement, one option is to give ampicillin or amoxicillin plus metronidazole orally, each in a dose of 500 mg every 6 to 8 hours. Imipenem or meropenem and β-lactam/β-lactamase inhibitor combinations such as ticarcillin and clavulanic acid are active against essentially all anaerobes and many of the aerobes important in nosocomial aspiration pneumonia. If a specific anaerobe or set of anaerobes is identified in the lung abscess, antibiotic therapy can be targeted on the basis of general susceptibility characteristics (Table 98–2) while awaiting the results of local susceptibility testing.

Postural drainage is important in the treatment of lung abscess. Bronchoscopy may help in effecting good drainage, removal of foreign bodies, and the diagnosis of tumor. Experience dictates caution with the bronchoscopic drainage of closed cavities; spillage of cavity contents into other lung segments may occur and be catastrophic.

Persistence of bacteremia or high-grade fever after 72 hours or the absence of change in sputum production or character or in radiographic images during a period of 7 to 10 days suggests undiagnosed obstruction, empyema, or resistant organisms. Progression of pulmonary infiltrates may occur after the initiation of appropriate therapy as a result of poorly ventilated and underperfused infected lung tissue. Surgical resection of necrotic lung may occasionally be needed if the response to antibiotics is poor or if airway obstruction limits drainage. In patients who are poor surgical risks, percutaneous or CT-guided drainage via catheters may be helpful. Bronchoscopic balloon dilatation and stent placement may be useful for malignant disease with post-stenotic abscess.

End-of-Life Care

In patients at the end of life, the goal is not to cure a lung abscess. Nevertheless, antimicrobial therapy is sometimes useful to eliminate the foul odor of secretions, to minimize cough and sputum production, and to avoid high fevers.

TABLE 98–2 DRUGS OF CHOICE FOR ANAEROBES INVOLVED IN LUNG ABSCESS*

PRINCIPAL PATHOGENS

Prevotella: Metronidazole, clindamycin, β-lactam/β-lactamase inhibitor combinations, carbapenems
Fusobacterium: As for *Prevotella*
Peptostreptococcus (see Table 98–1): β-lactam/β-lactamase inhibitor combinations, carbapenems, penicillin (high dosage)
Streptococcus (anaerobic, microaerophilic strains): penicillin (high dosage), β-lactam/β-lactamase inhibitor combinations, carbapenems

LESS COMMON PATHOGENS

Bacteroides: Metronidazole, β-lactam/β-lactamase inhibitor combinations, carbapenems
Clostridium: Metronidazole, β-lactam/β-lactamase inhibitor combinations, carbapenems, penicillin
Actinomyces: Penicillin (high dosage), clindamycin
Eikenella corrodens (microaerophilic): Penicillin, β-lactam/β-lactamase inhibitor combinations, carbapenems

UNKNOWN BACTERIOLOGY

Metronidazole plus penicillin, β-lactam/β-lactamase inhibitor combinations, carbapenems

*Drugs listed for each group of organisms are roughly comparable in activity and are the drugs that are most active. Other drugs (e.g., cefoxitin or clindamycin, alone or with penicillin) may be useful in patients with abscess of unknown bacteriologic origin who are only mildly to moderately ill.

Prognosis

Mortality occurs in 5 to 10%. Patients with large abscesses (>6 cm), progressive pulmonary necrosis, obstructing lesions, aerobic bacterial infection, immune compromise, old age, and systemic debility and those in whom major delays have occurred in seeking medical attention have higher mortality and a higher incidence of complications. The most common complication is empyema, with or without bronchopleural fistula. Spillover of pus from a large lung abscess sometimes leads to spread of infection and even to asphyxiation. Other complications, which are rare, include brain or other distal abscesses, generalized infection, severe hemorrhage, and pulmonary gangrene. Superinfection by other bacteria or by fungi can occur in relation to antimicrobial therapy. In patients with chronic lung abscess, chronic bronchitis, localized emphysema, or bronchiectasis may be present, with subsequent recurrence of acute pneumonitis in the involved area.

SUGGESTED READINGS

Bartlett JG: The role of anaerobic bacteria in lung abscess. Clin Infect Dis 2005;40:923–925. *A nice summary.*

Fernandez-Sabé N, Carratalà J, Dorca J, et al: Efficacy and safety of sequential amoxicillin-clavulanate in the treatment of anaerobic lung infections. Eur J Clin Microbiol Infect Dis 2003;22:185–187. *A good study of 40 consecutive anaerobic pulmonary infections, 25 with lung abscess, with an excellent response to amoxicillin-clavulanate.*

Moreira J da S, Camargo J da J, Felicetti JC, et al: Lung abscess: Analysis of 252 consecutive cases diagnosed between 1968 and 2004. J Bras Pneumol 2006;32:136–143. *An instructive case series.*

Wang J-L, Chen K-Y, Fang CT, et al: Changing bacteriology of adult community-acquired lung abscess in Taiwan: *Klebsiella pneumoniae* versus anaerobes. Clin Infect Dis 2005;40:915–922. *This large study's finding of so many* Klebsiella *infections may be a unique geographic problem because a large number of* Klebsiella *liver abscesses have also been reported from Taiwan.*

99 PULMONARY EMBOLISM

Victor F. Tapson

THROMBOTIC PULMONARY EMBOLISM

Definitions

Pulmonary embolism (PE) refers to exogenous or endogenous material that travels to the lungs through the pulmonary circulation, causing a potential spectrum of consequences. Thrombus from the deep veins of the lower extremities (Chapter 81) is by far the most common material to embolize to the lungs; deep venous thrombosis (DVT) and PE must be recognized as parts of the continuum of one disease entity, venous thromboembolism (VTE). Tumor cells, air bubbles (Chapter 94), carbon dioxide, intravenous catheters, fat droplets, and talc in intravenous drug abusers (Chapter 32) are also potential sources of emboli. However, unless otherwise specified, in this chapter, PE refers to thromboemboli arising from the deep leg veins or, less frequently, from the axillary-subclavian system.

The diagnostic approach to suspected acute DVT or PE generally depends on which of the two is the initial cause of symptoms. VTE is usually but not always associated with specific risk factors that help guide prophylaxis and together with compatible symptoms and signs also help the clinician *suspect* the diagnosis of DVT or PE. Both DVT and PE are frequently unsuspected clinically, thereby resulting in significant diagnostic and therapeutic delays that account for substantial morbidity and mortality. Even though VTE is diagnosed and treated in as many as 260,000 patients in the United States each year, more than half of the cases that actually occur are never diagnosed, and as many as 600,000 cases may therefore occur. Many patients who die of acute PE have coexisting terminal illnesses, but this disease entity appears to be responsible each year in the United States for the deaths of at least 100,000 to 200,000 patients who have an otherwise good prognosis and whose deaths are otherwise preventable. Autopsy studies have repeatedly documented the high frequency with which PE has gone unsuspected and undetected; furthermore, prophylaxis continues to be underused. The incidence of VTE is especially high in hospitalized patients, whether on a medical service or in the postoperative setting.

Pathobiology

Venous thrombi develop most commonly in the leg veins (Chapter 81). One or more components of Virchow's triad (stasis, hypercoagulability, and intimal injury) are present in the majority of patients. The risk increases with age. Calf vein thrombi often propagate into the proximal veins, including and above the popliteal veins, from which they are more likely to embolize. More than 95% of these emboli arise from the deep veins of the legs. Emboli from axillary-subclavian vein thromboses often develop in patients with central vein catheters, particularly those with malignant neoplasms, but may also result from effort-induced upper extremity thrombosis (Paget von Schroetter syndrome).

In acute PE, minute ventilation acutely increases with resulting tachypnea, and hypoxemia develops in most patients. The obstruction of blood flow creates alveolar dead space with regions of high ventilation-perfusion ratios as well as shunting due to perfusion of atelectatic areas. This imbalance appears to be the principal explanation for hypoxemia in acute PE.

When emboli obstruct a substantial portion of the pulmonary arterial bed, profound hemodynamic alterations occur. The impact of the embolic event depends on the extent of reduction of the cross-sectional area of the pulmonary vasculature as well as on the presence or absence of underlying cardiopulmonary disease. Hypoxemia stimulates an increase in sympathetic tone, with resulting systemic vasoconstriction, increased venous return, and increase in stroke volume. With more massive emboli, the increase in pulmonary vascular resistance impedes right ventricular outflow and reduces left ventricular preload. In the absence of underlying cardiopulmonary disease, occlusion of 25 to 30% of the vascular bed by emboli is associated with a significant increase in pulmonary artery pressure. With increasing vascular obstruction, hypoxemia worsens, stimulating vasoconstriction and a further increase in pulmonary artery pressure. More than 50% obstruction of the pulmonary arterial bed is usually present before there is substantial elevation of the mean pulmonary artery pressure. When the extent of obstruction of the pulmonary circulation approaches 75%, the right ventricle must generate a systolic pressure in excess of 50 mm Hg to preserve pulmonary perfusion. A normal right ventricle is rarely able to achieve this pressure acutely and thus may fail. Patients with underlying cardiopulmonary disease often experience a more substantial deterioration in cardiac output than do normal individuals in the setting of massive embolism. Although supportive measures may sustain a patient with massive PE, any additional increment in embolic burden may be fatal.

The pathologic findings of PE vary according to the age and extent of the emboli. In general, both lungs are involved, and the lower lobes are involved more often than the upper lobes. An embolus generally has blunt, nontapering ends and may be folded over on itself. When unfolded, emboli often appear as casts of the originating venous segment and may have imprints of venous valve cusps. In cases of massive embolism with rapid deterioration and death, the autopsy may reveal large emboli obstructing the right ventricular outflow tract, the main pulmonary artery, or the pulmonary artery bifurcation. Smaller, more peripheral emboli of various ages and in various stages of organization usually indicate emboli predating the terminal event. Pulmonary infarction is characterized histologically by intra-alveolar hemorrhage and necrosis of alveolar walls and is usually evident in peripheral lung supplied by smaller vessels. Because of the dual pulmonary circulation arising from the pulmonary and bronchial arteries, infarction is not present in most cases.

Clinical Manifestations

The history and physical examination are notoriously insensitive and nonspecific for both DVT and PE. Patients with lower extremity venous thrombosis often do not exhibit erythema, warmth, pain, swelling, or tenderness (Chapter 81). When these signs are present, they are nonspecific but still may merit further evaluation. Homans' sign (pain with dorsiflexion of the foot) may be present in the setting of DVT, but this finding is neither sufficiently sensitive nor specific enough to be relied on. The most common symptom of acute PE is dyspnea (Table 99–1), which is often sudden in onset. Pleuritic chest pain and hemoptysis occur more commonly with pulmonary *infarction*. Palpitations, cough, anxiety, and lightheadedness may all be associated with acute PE but may also result from a number of other entities, thereby contributing to difficulty in making the diagnosis. Syncope or sudden death may occur with massive PE. PE should be considered whenever unexplained symptoms including dyspnea, syncope, hypotension, and hypoxemia are present. Tachypnea and tachycardia are the most common signs of PE but are also nonspecific. Other physical findings may include fever, wheezing, crackles, pleural rub, loud pulmonic component of the second heart sound, right-sided third or fourth heart sound, and right ventricular lift. Both the cardiac and pulmonary physical examinations are nonspecific in patients with PE. Findings such as dyspnea, cough, tachypnea, crackles, and hypoxemia in patients with concomitant cardiopulmonary disease (such as heart failure, pneumonia, or chronic obstructive pulmonary disease) may be caused by the underlying disease or by superimposed acute PE. Symptoms and signs consistent with PE should be particularly heeded in the setting of significant risk factors for VTE, such as concomitant malignant disease, immobility, and the postoperative state.

TABLE 99–1 SYMPTOMS AND SIGNS IN PATIENTS WITH ACUTE PULMONARY EMBOLISM WITHOUT PREEXISTING CARDIAC OR PULMONARY DISEASE

Symptoms*	% of Patients	Signs*	% of Patients
Dyspnea	73	Tachypnea (≥20/min)	70
Pleuritic pain	66	Rales (crackles)	51
Cough	37	Tachycardia (>100/min)	30
Leg swelling	28	Fourth heart sound	24
Leg pain	26	Increased pulmonary component of second sound	23
Hemoptysis	13	Deep venous thrombosis	11
Palpitations	10	Diaphoresis	11
Wheezing	9	Temperature >38.5° C	7
Angina-like pain	4	Wheezes	5
		Homans' sign	4
		Right ventricular lift	4
		Pleural friction rub	3
		Third heart sound	3
		Cyanosis	1

*Whereas these symptoms and signs have been documented in the setting of acute pulmonary embolism, their presence does not necessarily imply that the symptom is due to acute pulmonary embolism. Dyspnea and chest pain, for example, may be due to underlying pneumonia, which places the patient at risk for acute pulmonary embolism.

Modified from Stein PD, Terrin ML, Hales CA, et al: Clinical, laboratory, roentgenographic and electrocardiographic findings in patients with acute pulmonary embolism and no pre-existing cardiac or pulmonary disease. Chest 1991;100:598–603.

Diagnosis

The differential diagnosis of acute PE (Table 99–2) depends on the clinical presentation and concomitant disease. When patients present with dyspnea (Chapter 83) or chest pain (Chapter 48), the differential diagnosis may include pneumonia (Chapter 97), a flare of asthma or chronic obstructive lung disease (Chapters 87 and 88), anxiety with hyperventilation, pneumothorax (Chapter 100), heart failure (Chapters 57 and 58), angina or myocardial infarction (Chapters 70 to 73), musculoskeletal pain, pericarditis (Chapter 77), pleuritis from infection or connective tissue disease, herpes zoster, rib fracture, intrathoracic cancer, and, occasionally, intra-abdominal processes such as acute cholecystitis (Chapter 134). Acute PE can be superimposed on another underlying cardiopulmonary disease, on which new or worsening symptoms are sometimes blamed.

Blood Tests

Hypoxemia on respiration of ambient air is common in acute PE. Some individuals, particularly young patients without underlying lung disease, may have a normal arterial oxygen tension (Pao_2) and, rarely, a normal alveolar-arterial difference. A sudden decrease in the Pao_2 or in the oxygen saturation in a patient unable to communicate an accurate history (e.g., a mechanically ventilated patient) may be evidence of acute PE.

A circulating D-dimer (a specific derivative of cross-linked fibrin) positive test result (i.e., above a designated threshold value) by enzyme-

TABLE 99–2 DIFFERENTIAL DIAGNOSIS OF ACUTE PULMONARY EMBOLISM*

Myocardial infarction
Pericarditis
Heart failure
Pneumonia
Asthma
Chronic obstructive pulmonary disease
Pneumothorax
Pleurodynia
Pleuritis from connective tissue disease
Thoracic herpes zoster ("shingles")
Rib fracture
Musculoskeletal pain
Primary or metastatic intrathoracic cancer
Infradiaphragmatic processes (e.g., acute cholecystitis, splenic infarction)
Hyperventilation syndrome

*Diagnoses that commonly present with chest pain or dyspnea and, in a few cases, hemoptysis and that might be considered along with acute pulmonary embolism, depending on the clinical setting.

TABLE 99–3 DICHOTOMIZED CLINICAL DECISION RULE FOR SUSPECTED ACUTE PULMONARY EMBOLISM*

Variable	Points
Symptoms and signs of deep venous thrombosis†	3.0
Alternative diagnosis less likely than pulmonary embolism‡	3.0
Heart rate >100 beats/min	1.5
Immobilization (>3 days) or surgery in previous 4 weeks	1.5
Previous deep venous thrombosis or pulmonary embolism	1.5
Hemoptysis	1.0
Malignancy (current therapy, or in previous 6 months, or palliative)	1.0

*See Figure 99–2. Clinical probability of pulmonary embolism is unlikely with a score of 4 points or less; clinical probability is likely with a score of more than 4 points. This clinical decision scoring system was previously used with three separate likelihood categories (low, intermediate, and high). In that trial, a low-probability score (<2) together with a negative result of the SimpliRED D-dimer assay excluded the need for further evaluation (Wells PS, Anderson DR, Rodger M, et al: Ann Intern Med 2001;135:98–107).
†Minimum of leg swelling and pain with palpation of the deep veins.
‡Pulmonary embolism as likely as or more likely than an alternative diagnosis. Physicians were told to use clinical information along with chest radiography, electrocardiography, and laboratory tests.
From van Belle A, Buller HR, Huisman MV, et al: Christopher Study Investigators: Effectiveness of managing suspected pulmonary embolism using an algorithm combining clinical probability, D-dimer testing, and computed tomography. JAMA 2006;295:172–179.

linked immunosorbent assay (ELISA) is 96 to 98% sensitive for acute PE, but its positive predictive value is much lower. In one prospective study, for example, only 1 of 437 patients presenting to the emergency department with suspected PE and with a negative result of the D-dimer test (SimpliRED assay, a non-ELISA, qualitative test) and low clinical probability (score < 2) by the Wells clinical decision rule (Table 99–3) developed PE during follow-up; thus, the negative predictive value for this strategy was 99.5%. A number of D-dimer assays are available, and the sensitivity and specificity of these assays vary. A positive D-dimer test result means that DVT or PE is possible, but it is by no means proof of VTE. Similarly, although a negative D-dimer test result may strongly suggest that VTE is absent, D-dimer testing should not be ordered in the setting of a high clinical suspicion for acute VTE; one should instead proceed straight to imaging. Troponin levels may be elevated in acute PE, especially in more massive embolism, when myocyte injury due to right ventricular strain might be expected. Troponin levels cannot, however, be used like D-dimer testing; that is, they are not sensitive enough to exclude PE, even when the clinical suspicion is relatively low, without additional diagnostic testing.

Imaging

Electrocardiography

Electrocardiographic findings, which are present in the majority of patients with acute PE, include ST segment abnormalities, T wave changes, and left or right axis deviation. Only one third of patients with massive or submassive emboli have manifestations of acute cor pulmonale, such as an S_1-Q_3-T_3 pattern, right bundle branch block, P wave pulmonale, or right axis deviation. All of these findings are also nonspecific. Thus, the utility of electrocardiography in suspected acute PE arises more from its ability to establish or to exclude alternative diagnoses, such as acute myocardial infarction (Chapter 72) or pericarditis (Chapter 77), rather than from diagnosis or exclusion of PE.

Chest Radiography

The chest radiograph is often abnormal in patients with acute PE, but it is nearly always nonspecific. Common findings include pleural effusion, atelectasis, pulmonary infiltrates, and mild elevation of a hemidiaphragm. Classic findings of pulmonary infarction, such as Hampton's hump and decreased vascularity (Westermark's sign), are suggestive of the diagnosis but are infrequent. PE should be considered in patients who

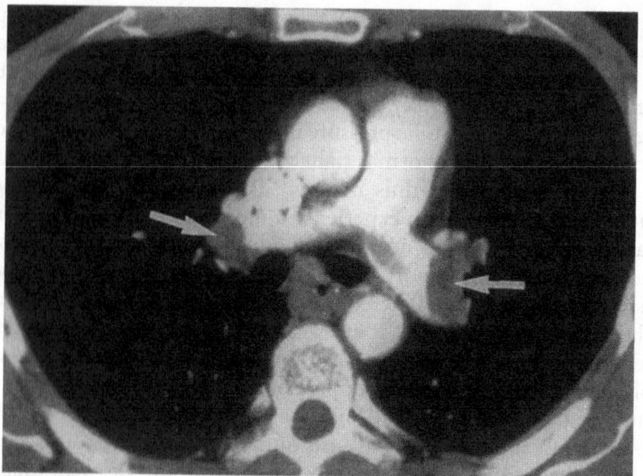

FIGURE 99–1 • Spiral computed tomographic image of acute pulmonary emboli in both main pulmonary arteries in a postoperative patient with the sudden onset of dyspnea, hypoxemia, and hypotension.

have dyspnea and hypoxemia with a normal chest radiograph in the absence of bronchospasm or anatomic cardiac shunt. Under most circumstances, however, the chest radiograph cannot be used for conclusive diagnosis or exclusion. Although the radiograph may exclude other processes, such as pneumonia, pneumothorax, or rib fracture, which may cause similar symptoms, acute PE may frequently coexist with other underlying heart or lung diseases.

Spiral Computed Tomography

Spiral (helical) computed tomography (CT) can be used for diagnosis of both acute and chronic PE and has replaced ventilation-perfusion (VQ) scanning at many centers (Fig. 99–1). This technique involves continuous movement of the patient through the CT scanner and allows concurrent scanning by a constantly rotating gantry and detector system. Rapid scanning is performed with continuous acquisitions obtained during a single breath. Retrospective reconstructions can be performed. An intravenous injection of contrast material is required for imaging of the pulmonary vasculature.

Increased experience and advances in multislice scanning provide rapid images with a sensitivity in the 80 to 90% range and specificity to consistently above 90%. By also including images of the legs without additional contrast material, the sensitivity for VTE was increased from about 83% to about 90% in one large study, in which the specificity was 95%. The imperfect results should not be surprising because even the "gold standard" test, pulmonary arteriography, is not perfect for smaller, peripheral emboli. Spiral CT is most sensitive for detecting emboli in the main, lobar, or segmental pulmonary arteries; its specificity for clot in these vessels is also excellent. For subsegmental emboli, spiral CT appears to be less accurate, but the importance of emboli of this size has been questioned. An advantage of spiral CT over VQ scanning and arteriography is the ability of CT to define nonvascular conditions such as lymphadenopathy, lung tumors, emphysema, and other parenchymal abnormalities as well as pleural and pericardial disease. A second advantage of spiral CT over other diagnostic methods is the rapidity with which the scan can be performed. Conversely, disadvantages of CT include its poor sensitivity for detecting clots in small vessels, the fact that it is not portable at present, and the fact that patients with significant renal insufficiency cannot be scanned without risk of renal failure.

Stable patients with suspected acute PE, nondiagnostic CT scans, and adequate cardiopulmonary reserve (absence of hypotension or severe hypoxemia) may undergo noninvasive lower extremity testing in an attempt to diagnose DVT (Chapter 81). An abnormal compression ultrasound finding (in the absence of prior DVT) presents the opportunity to treat without further testing.

Data suggest that the outcome after a normal spiral CT scan is excellent, with the risk of recurrence (development of acute VTE) being exceedingly low. For example, a strategy using a dichotomized version of the Wells score (see Table 99–3), D-dimer testing, and CT imaging can reduce the need for expensive testing and provide good outcomes at 3 months (Fig. 99–2).

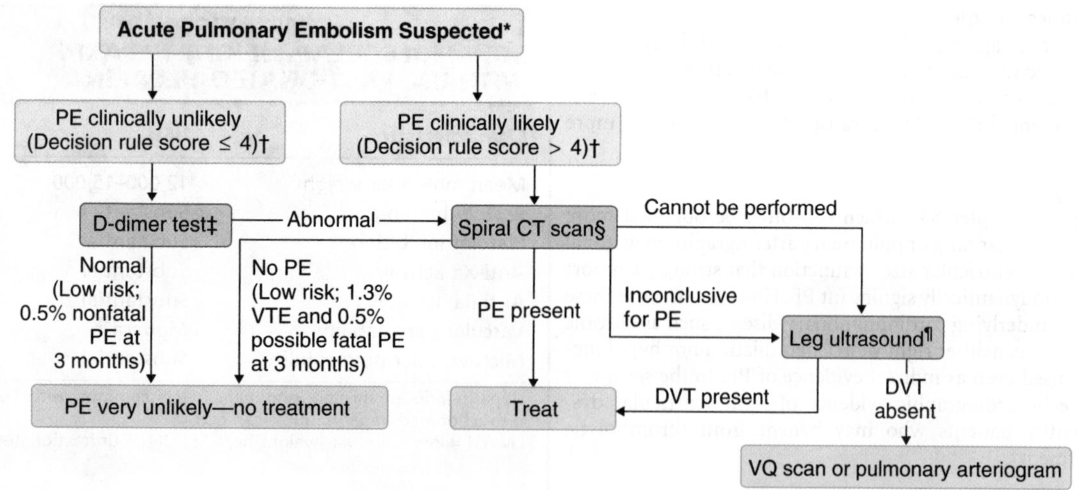

FIGURE 99–2 • A CT scan–based algorithm for the diagnostic approach to suspected acute pulmonary embolism. CT = computed tomography; DVT = deep venous thrombosis; PE = pulmonary embolism; VQ = ventilation-perfusion.
*The evidence base for the use of this decision rule score with D-dimer testing and CT scanning is derived from a large multicenter clinical trial (Christopher Study; JAMA 2006;295:172–179). In the study, not all patients with inconclusive CT scans underwent further testing or received treatment, but only 20 such patients were studied. Thus, additional testing in these individuals is recommended in the algorithm, pending confirmatory data.
†See Table 99–3.
‡Rapid enzyme-linked immunosorbent assays provide excellent sensitivity and are favored.
§Contrast-enhanced spiral CT of the chest with timed contrast including leg imaging could be considered, but more limited data are available. A VQ scan–based algorithm could be considered instead of CT, but the VQ scan is much more frequently nondiagnostic. The VQ scan may be particularly useful when the chest radiograph is clear and when no underlying cardiopulmonary disease is present. When PE is deemed clinically likely but findings on CT are normal, compression ultrasonography could also be considered.
¶Pulmonary arteriography could be considered instead. Although it is invasive, arteriography remains the gold standard test for suspected acute PE. Because CT offers the advantage of potentially identifying alternative disease processes, it should be performed before arteriography is considered.

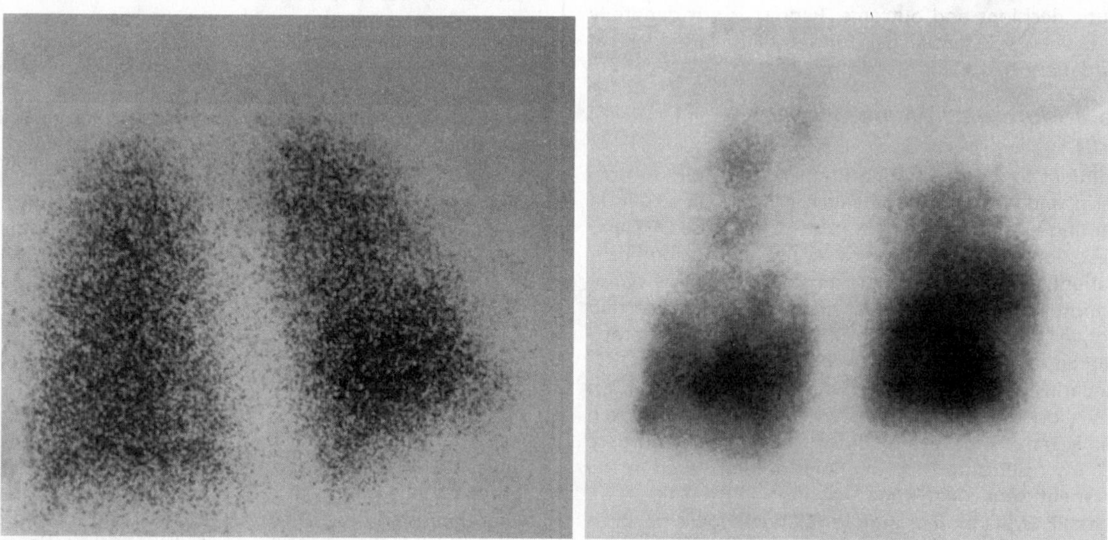

FIGURE 99–3 • High-probability ventilation-perfusion scan.

Ventilation-Perfusion Scanning

A normal perfusion scan (Fig. 99–3) excludes PE with a high enough degree of certainty that further diagnostic evaluation is almost never necessary. Although large, central, nonocclusive emboli might transiently permit tracer to perfuse the lungs normally, this phenomenon is exceedingly unusual, and PE should be pursued only when the clinical suspicion is exceptionally high. Matching areas of decreased ventilation and perfusion in the presence of a normal chest radiograph generally represent a process other than PE. However, low- or intermediate-probability (nondiagnostic) VQ scans are commonly found with PE, and further evaluation with pulmonary arteriography or leg studies is often appropriate in such situations.

The specificity of high-probability scans is 97%, but the sensitivity is only 41%. When the clinical suspicion of PE is considered very high, PE is present in 96% of patients with high-probability VQ scans, 66% of patients with intermediate scans, and 40% of patients with low-probability scans. Thus, the diagnosis of PE should be rigorously pursued even when the lung scan is of low or intermediate probability if the clinical setting strongly suggests the diagnosis. Although the VQ scan either may be diagnostic of PE in higher risk patients or may exclude the possibility with sufficient certainty in low-risk patients, it is often nondiagnostic. Even in the latter circumstance, however, it may serve as a guide for the interventional radiologist by directing selective dye injection to minimize the contrast load and to limit the duration of pulmonary arteriography.

Pulmonary Arteriography

Pulmonary arteriography, which remains the gold standard for the diagnosis of acute PE, is an extremely sensitive and specific test. Major nonfatal complications occur with 1% of angiograms, and death occurs in 0.5%. Its clinical role has been for patients in whom PE must be diagnosed or excluded, but preliminary testing has been nondiagnostic. However, with the advent of CT, pulmonary angiography is now used infrequently.

Magnetic Resonance Imaging

Magnetic resonance imaging can be used in suspected PE, but the main advantage of magnetic resonance imaging at present is its excellent sensitivity and specificity for the diagnosis of DVT (Chapter 81). Disadvantages include the potential difficulty in transporting and studying more critically ill patients.

Echocardiography

Echocardiography (Chapter 53), which can often be obtained more rapidly than either lung scanning or pulmonary arteriography, may reveal abnormalities of right ventricular size or function that strongly support the diagnosis of hemodynamically significant PE. However, because these patients often have underlying cardiopulmonary disease such as chronic obstructive lung disease, neither right ventricular dilation nor hypokinesis can be reliably used even as indirect evidence of PE. In the setting of documented PE, echocardiographic evidence of right ventricular dysfunction can identify patients who may benefit from thrombolytic therapy (see Treatment).

TABLE 99–4 A COMPARISON OF LOW-MOLECULAR-WEIGHT HEPARIN WITH UNFRACTIONATED HEPARIN

Characteristic	UFH	LMWH
Mean molecular weight	12,000–15,000	4000–6000
Protein binding	Substantial	Minimal
Platelet inhibition	Substantial	Minimal
Anti-Xa activity	Substantial	Substantial
Anti-IIa activity	Substantial	Minimal
Vascular permeability	Moderate	None
Microvascular permeability	Substantial	Minimal

Heparin-induced thrombocytopenia is less common with LMWH than with unfractionated heparin, but it can occur.
LMWH = low-molecular-weight heparin; UFH = unfractionated heparin.

Treatment

Rx

Therapy for acute PE overlaps substantially with treatment of DVT (Chapter 81). Parenteral anticoagulation with low-molecular-weight heparin (LMWH) or with standard, unfractionated heparin is initiated unless it is contraindicated. Depending on the clinical setting, thrombolytic therapy, inferior vena cava filter placement, or surgical embolectomy may be considered. Each approach has specific indications as well as advantages and disadvantages. The unstable patient requires a rapid evaluation and integration of data to optimize therapeutic decisions and outcome. Bedrest is not generally helpful, except when substantial pain and swelling are present. Otherwise, outpatient therapy is often appropriate.

Heparin, Low-Molecular-Weight Heparin, and Warfarin

Recommendations for treatment of acute PE with LMWH, unfractionated heparin, and warfarin are based largely on clinical trials in patients presenting with acute DVT (Chapter 81) because DVT and PE are manifestations of a single clinical entity, and a significant minority of patients presenting with proximal DVT also have symptomatic or asymptomatic PE. However, therapy may differ in certain specific settings, including massive PE, in which thrombolytic therapy may be considered.

Although heparins (Chapter 35) do not directly dissolve thrombus or emboli, they allow the fibrinolytic system to proceed unopposed and more readily reduce the size of the thromboembolic burden. Nevertheless, early recurrence can sometimes develop, even in the setting of therapeutic anticoagulation.

When DVT or PE is diagnosed, anticoagulation should be instituted immediately unless contraindications are present. [1] It is also appropriate to initiate therapy in patients in whom there is a high index of suspicion for acute PE even while diagnostic testing is under way, as long as the risk of anticoagulation is not excessive. If possible, warfarin therapy should be initiated within the first 24 hours, but premature initiation of warfarin without LMWH or heparin may intensify hypercoagulability and increase the clot burden because of the short half-life of anticoagulation factors that are inhibited by warfarin. At least 5 days of subcutaneous LMWH or intravenous unfractionated heparin is generally recommended because definitive anticoagulation requires the depletion of factor II (thrombin), a process that takes approximately 5 days. Ideally, the parenteral anticoagulant should be maintained until the international normalized ratio (INR) is stable at 2.0 to 3.0. [1]

LMWH preparations have greater bioavailability, more predictable dosing, fewer side effects, and the advantage of being administered subcutaneously once or twice per day; they do not require monitoring of the activated partial thromboplastin time (aPTT) and are less likely to cause heparin-induced thrombocytopenia (Chapters 35 and 179). As a result, they are preferred to unfractionated heparin

TABLE 99–5 POTENTIAL ADVANTAGES OF LOW-MOLECULAR-WEIGHT HEPARIN OVER UNFRACTIONATED HEPARIN

- Similar or superior efficacy
- Similar or superior safety
- Superior bioavailability
- Once- or twice-daily dosing
- No laboratory monitoring; thus, less phlebotomy*
- Potential for earlier ambulation
- Subcutaneous administration†
- Lower incidence of heparin-induced thrombocytopenia
- Home therapy in certain subsets of patients

*No monitoring needed for either prophylaxis or treatment. With body weight below 40 kg or above 150 kg or with unstable renal insufficiency, anti-factor Xa levels can be measured to aid in dosing. With stable, abnormal renal function (creatinine clearance of less than 30 mL/min), a lower dose of enoxaparin (1 mg/kg once daily for treatment, or 30 mg subcutaneously once daily) can be used. In the therapeutic setting, when the creatinine is changing significantly over time, unfractionated heparin should be considered.
†For both prophylaxis and treatment.

(Tables 99–4 and 99–5). [2,3] Anti–factor Xa levels performed approximately 4 hours after the subcutaneous administration of a weight-adjusted dose of LMWH may be used to monitor LMWH in certain settings, such as in morbidly obese patients, very small patients (<40 kg), pregnant patients, and patients with renal insufficiency. For twice-daily administration, a conservative therapeutic range for the assay is 0.6 to 1.0 IU/mL. The target range is less clear in patients treated with LMWH once daily, but a level between 1.0 and 2.0 IU/mL appears reasonable. Because LMWHs are renally metabolized, they should be used with caution when the creatinine clearance is significantly reduced; enoxaparin can be administered at a lower therapeutic dose (1 mg/kg once daily, instead of the usual 1 mg/kg every 12 hours) when the creatinine clearance is less than 30 mL/min.

Although outpatient therapy for acute DVT (Chapter 81) is proved to be safe, outpatient therapy for acute, symptomatic PE is not routinely recommended. However, patients with mild PE who are minimally symptomatic can be treated successfully in the outpatient setting or after a brief hospitalization. No data strongly support a search for asymptomatic PE in patients who present with acute symptomatic DVT.

In the United States, three LMWH preparations are currently approved by the Food and Drug Administration (FDA) for treatment

Rx

of patients with proven DVT with or without acute PE. Enoxaparin is approved for both inpatients and outpatients at a dose of 1 mg/kg subcutaneously every 12 hours or as a once-daily dose of 1.5 mg/kg for inpatient use (see Table 35–3). Both doses have proved as effective and safe as unfractionated heparin. The second preparation, tinzaparin, is administered as 175 units once daily, with the FDA approval being based on therapy for inpatients with DVT. The third drug, a pentasaccharide or "ultra-LMWH" called fondaparinux, is approved for treatment of DVT and PE.

The only advantage of standard heparin over LMWH is when the short half-life of intravenous unfractionated heparin is beneficial and when its complete reversibility with protamine is potentially advantageous. When continuous intravenous unfractionated heparin is initiated, the aPTT should be observed at 6-hour intervals until it is consistently in the therapeutic range of 1.5 to 2.5 times control values. This range corresponds to a heparin level of 0.2 to 0.4 U/mL as measured by protamine sulfate titration. Achieving a therapeutic aPTT within 24 hours after PE has been documented to reduce recurrences. Heparin dosing should be weight based; one approach is an intravenous bolus of 80 IU/kg followed by a maintenance dose of 18 IU/kg/hr by continuous infusion (see Table 81–4). 1 Further adjustment of the heparin dose should also be based on weight.

Patients with acute PE require long-term anticoagulant treatment to prevent a high frequency (as high as 50%) of symptomatic extension of thrombosis or recurrent VTE. The recommendations about long-term anticoagulation for PE are the same as for DVT; documented PE in the setting of transient risk factors should be treated for 3 to 6 months, but more extended treatment is appropriate when significant risk factors persist, when thromboembolism is idiopathic, or when previous episodes of VTE have been documented. For idiopathic VTE, standard-dose warfarin (INR goal of 2.0–3.0) is recommended. 1 Bleeding related to warfarin increases with the intensity and duration of therapy. Warfarin-induced skin necrosis is a rare but serious complication mandating immediate cessation of the drug. Warfarin crosses the placenta and may cause fetal malformations if it is used during pregnancy.

Unlike heparin and LMWH, which work indirectly and require antithrombin III as a cofactor, newer antithrombotic agents are effective against clot-bound thrombin (Chapter 35). Like heparin, these direct thrombin inhibitors have narrow therapeutic indices. Ximelagatran, an oral direct thrombin inhibitor, is efficacious for the treatment of acute VTE; however, because of potential hepatic toxicity and rebound thrombosis, it was not approved by the FDA.

Bleeding is the major complication of anticoagulation (Chapters 35 and 179). Heparin-induced thrombocytopenia typically develops 5 days or more after the initiation of heparin therapy (Chapters 35 and 179). The primary problem is not bleeding but rather venous or arterial thrombosis as a result of platelet and thrombin activation by heparin-dependent immunoglobulin G antibodies that activate the platelets through their Fc receptors. If a patient is prescribed heparin for acute PE and the platelet count progressively decreases to 100,000/mm^3 or less, or to 50% of the initial value, all heparin therapy (including LMWH) should be discontinued, and heparin-induced thrombocytopenia should be considered. Both argatroban and lepirudin have been FDA approved for use in the setting of VTE with heparin-induced thrombocytopenia (Chapter 35). These drugs are not reversible but have relatively short half-lives. Warfarin should not be initiated until the heparin-induced thrombocytopenia is clearly controlled because of the potential for further thrombotic complications, including venous limb gangrene and warfarin-induced skin necrosis.

Argatroban should be initiated at a dose of 2 μg/kg/min. The aPTT should be rechecked 2 hours after initiation and adjusted until a target aPTT value of 1.5 to 3.0 times baseline is attained (not to exceed 100 seconds). Doses above 10 μg/kg/min should not be administered. No adjustment is necessary in renal failure. Lepirudin is administered as an intravenous bolus of 0.4 mg/kg up to a maximum of 44 mg during 15 to 20 seconds; no bolus is necessary if the aPTT is 1.5 to 2 times baseline. A continuous intravenous infusion at 0.15 mg/kg/hr up to a maximum of 16.5 mg for 2 to 10 days is used with an aPTT goal of 1.5 to 2.5 above baseline. Lepirudin is excreted by the kidneys, so the dose must be reduced in renal insufficiency (creatinine clearance of less than 60 mL/min or a serum creatinine concentration above 1.5 mg/dL). The circulating half-life is only 1.3 hours in patients with normal renal function but may be as long as 2 days in patients with advanced renal failure, so patients on dialysis should receive lepirudin with caution and at a reduced dose.

Vena Cava Interruption

When a patient cannot be anticoagulated in the setting of proven DVT or PE, inferior vena cava filter placement is indicated to prevent lower extremity thrombi from embolizing. The primary indications for filter placement include contraindications to anticoagulation, significant bleeding complications during anticoagulation, and recurrent embolism with adequate therapy. Inferior vena cava filters are sometimes placed in the setting of massive PE when it is believed that any further emboli might be lethal, particularly if thrombolytic therapy is contraindicated; however, this indication is not based on firm clinical trial data. Although filters are effective in reducing PE, they increase DVT and have not been shown to increase overall survival. 3 Filters inserted through the jugular or femoral vein are effective, and complications including insertion-related problems and migration of the filter are unusual. Retrievable filters can be used when the risk of bleeding appears to be short term; such devices can be removed up to 2 weeks later, and some can be removed as late as 90 days after placement.

Thrombolytic Therapy

Because anticoagulants do not actively lyse emboli, thrombolytic therapy is indicated when PE causes hemodynamic instability with hypotension. 1 Other settings in which thrombolytic therapy might be considered include echocardiographic right ventricular dysfunction without hypotension, 4 severely compromised oxygenation, massive radiographic embolic burden even without clear hemodynamic instability, and extensive DVT accompanying nonmassive embolism. In the United States, currently approved drugs for thrombolysis in acute PE include streptokinase (administered as a 250,000-unit bolus during 30 minutes followed by 100,000 units per hour for 12 to 24 hours) and recombinant tissue-type plasminogen activator (100 mg administered intravenously during a 2-hour period) (Table 99–6). When thrombolytics appear reasonable but are contraindicated (Table 99–7), low-dose direct intraembolic infusion of tissue-type plasminogen activator or mechanical fragmentation appears reasonable. Heparin is generally withheld until the thrombolytic infusion is completed, but several large clinical trials have continued heparin during the thrombolytic infusion without adverse consequences.

The most devastating complication associated with thrombolytics is intracranial hemorrhage, which occurs in approximately 1 to 3%

TABLE 99–6 THROMBOLYTIC THERAPY FOR ACUTE PULMONARY EMBOLISM: REGIMENS APPROVED FOR USE IN THE UNITED STATES

Streptokinase: 250,000 units IV (loading dose during 30 minutes), then 100,000 units/hr for 24 hours*

Tissue-type plasminogen activator: 100 mg IV during 2 hours†

*Streptokinase administered during 24 to 72 hours (at this loading dose and rate) has also been approved for use in patients with extensive deep venous thrombosis.

†The American College of Chest Physicians has recommended that agents with shorter infusion times (i.e., tissue-type plasminogen activator) be used. This is not, however, based on conclusive evidence (see Buller HR, Agnelli G, Hull RD, et al: Chest 2004;126;401S–428S).

TABLE 99–7 CONTRAINDICATIONS TO THROMBOLYTIC THERAPY IN PULMONARY EMBOLISM*

Absolute
- Intracranial surgery or disease
- Active or recent internal bleeding

Relative
- Bleeding diathesis or thrombocytopenia
- Uncontrolled severe hypertension
- Cardiopulmonary resuscitation
- Surgery within the previous 7–14 days†
- Pregnancy

*The use of thrombolytic therapy depends on the severity of pulmonary embolism; resultant hypotension is the clearest indication. There should be a lower threshold to administer thrombolytic therapy in the setting of a contraindication when a patient is extremely unstable from life-threatening pulmonary embolism.
†The waiting time after surgery needed to permit safe administration of thrombolytic therapy depends on the type of surgery performed and its associated bleeding risk.

Rx

of patients. In the setting of imminent death due to massive PE, a clinician may elect to use thrombolytic therapy even in the setting of a relative contraindication such as recent surgery or bleeding. Pulmonary embolectomy is appropriate in patients who have massive embolism with hypotension and cannot receive thrombolytic therapy.

Hemodynamic Management of Massive Pulmonary Embolism

Massive PE should always be considered in the setting of the sudden onset of hypotension, extreme hypoxemia, electromechanical dissociation, or cardiac arrest. Once massive PE associated with hypotension or severe hypoxemia is suspected, supportive treatment is immediately initiated (Fig. 99–4). Intravenous saline should be infused rapidly but cautiously because right ventricular function is often markedly compromised. Dopamine (initial dose of 1 μg/kg/min, titrated to 10 to 20 μg/kg/min) or norepinephrine (initial dose of 0.05 μg/kg/min and increased as tolerated) appears appropriate in massive PE and should be administered if the blood pressure is not rapidly restored. In general, upper dose limits for these pressor agents are not set in the presence of severe hypotension due to acute PE, but cautious monitoring is required. Because death due to PE results from right ventricular failure, dobutamine (5 to 20 μg/kg/min) can be considered to augment right ventricular output; however, this drug may also worsen hypotension. Oxygen therapy is administered, and thrombolytic therapy is considered as described before. Intubation and mechanical ventilation are instituted when necessary to support respiratory failure.

Prognosis

Most patients with PE who receive adequate anticoagulation survive. However, patients who are treated for PE are almost four times more likely (1.5% vs. 0.4%) to die of recurrent VTE in the next year than are those treated only for DVT. The 3-month mortality rate is about 15 to 18%. In some series, PE itself has been the principal cause of death, whereas other series report that only 10% of deaths during the first year are attributable to PE. The presence of shock defines a three-fold to seven-fold increase in mortality; a majority of deaths appear to occur within the first hour of presentation. A potential long-term sequela from acute DVT is chronic leg pain and swelling (postphlebitic syndrome), which may result in significant morbidity (Chapter 81).

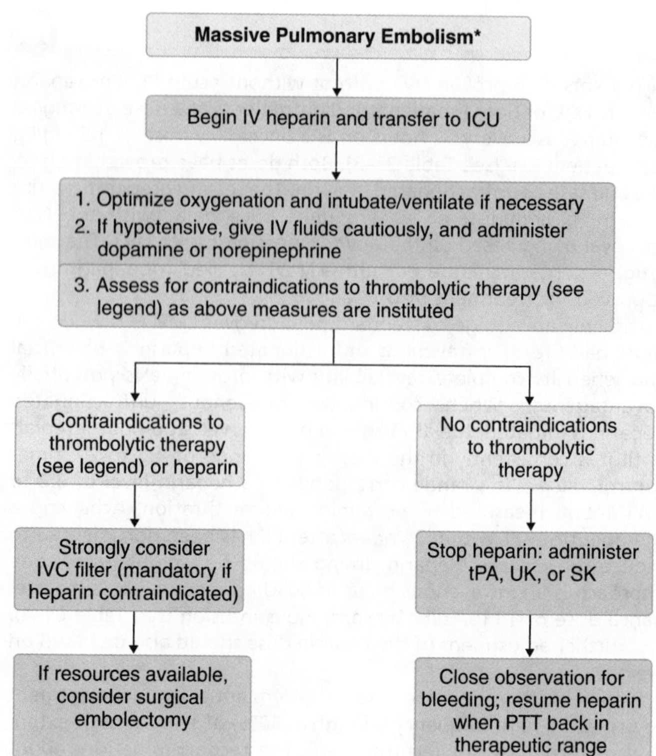

FIGURE 99–4 • An algorithm for the approach to the patient with massive acute pulmonary embolism. Contraindications to thrombolytic therapy include intracranial abnormality, gastrointestinal or other bleeding, bleeding diathesis, surgery within the previous 10 days, and pregnancy (see text). ICU = intensive care unit; IV = intravenous; IVC = inferior vena cava; PTT = partial thromboplastin time; SK = streptokinase; tPA = tissue-type plasminogen activator; UK = urokinase.

Chronic Thromboembolic Pulmonary Hypertension

Although most cases of acute PE resolve with therapy, a substantial residual thromboembolic burden occasionally persists or develops over time. The risk of pulmonary hypertension from chronic PE may be as high as 3 to 4% during 2 to 3 years after an acute PE. However, at least 50% of patients who develop chronic thromboembolic pulmonary hypertension have no documented history of previous thromboembolic disease.

Clinical Manifestations and Diagnosis

If the obstruction becomes extensive, pulmonary hypertension develops (Chapter 67). Fatigue and dyspnea with exertion are the most common complaints. The nonspecific nature of these findings may substantially delay the correct diagnosis. The physical examination generally reveals a right ventricular heave, a loud P_2, and tricuspid regurgitation consistent with pulmonary hypertension. In 20% of patients, murmurs due to partially occluded and remodeled vessels may be auscultated over the lung fields. The chest radiograph usually shows right ventricular enlargement and enlarged main pulmonary arteries. The electrocardiogram often reveals changes consistent with pulmonary hypertension (Chapter 67). Arterial blood gas analysis generally reveals hypoxemia with a widened alveolar-arterial difference, although some patients may demonstrate hypoxemia only with exercise. Echocardiography documents pulmonary hypertension and enlargement of the right ventricle. Spiral CT scanning may reveal evidence of chronic thromboembolism but occasionally may be normal. At present, it is not believed that chronic thromboembolic pulmonary hypertension can be definitively excluded by CT; a VQ scan should always be considered. The VQ scan is usually high probability for PE but occasionally is less impressive. Pulmonary arteriography should be performed to establish the diagnosis with certainty, to aid in characterizing severity, and to determine operability. Pulmonary angioscopy frequently has proved complementary to arteriography in assessing these patients.

Treatment

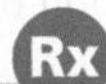

When chronic thromboembolic pulmonary hypertension is diagnosed, anticoagulation should be instituted and an inferior vena cava filter placed. Pulmonary thromboendarterectomy through median sternotomy on cardiopulmonary bypass should be considered in selected cases; the overall mortality rate is less than 5% at centers with considerable experience. Treatment of nonoperable chronic thromboembolic pulmonary hypertension with medications such as the oral endothelin antagonist bosentan (initial dose of 62.5 mg twice daily, increased to 125 mg twice daily after 1 month) may effectively address small vessel vasculopathy associated with this disease. In more severely ill patients, epoprostenol (initial dose inglkglmin increasing to 30–40 ng/kg/min by continuous intravenous) infusion should be considered. Lung transplantation can be considered in selected patients with severe pulmonary hypertension in whom thrombi are too distal to be extracted, if appropriate criteria are met (Chapter 67).

Prevention

The risk of DVT and subsequent PE is substantial in hospitalized patients, but the risk can be reduced significantly when patients receive appropriate prophylaxis. Such preventive measures appear to be grossly underused. Anticoagulant prophylaxis appears more effective than mechanical prophylaxis, but the risk of both thrombosis and bleeding must be considered.

After total hip or knee replacement, the risk of DVT is 50% or greater without prophylaxis. The superiority of LMWH over standard, unfractionated heparin has been clearly demonstrated in these settings as well as in trauma (Chapter 113) and spinal cord injury (Chapter 422). In other settings, low-dose standard heparin appears adequate. In general medical patients, the risk of DVT without prophylaxis may be as high as 15%, and LMWH (enoxaparin, at 40 mg subcutaneously once daily, or dalteparin or fondaparinux) is superior to placebo in preventing acute DVT. These drugs appear to be at least as effective and as safe as standard heparin prophylaxis with 5000 units every 8 hours in the general medical patient. 5

Three LMWH preparations (enoxaparin, dalteparin, and fondaparinux) are available for specific prophylactic indications. At present, enoxaparin has the most FDA-approved prophylactic indications, including patients undergoing total hip replacement, total knee replacement, and general abdominal surgery as well as general medical patients. Fondaparinux, a pentasaccharide (an ultra-LMWH), is approved for abdominal surgery and several orthopedic prophylactic settings, including total hip and knee replacement and hip fracture surgery. It is a pure anti–factor Xa inhibitor with a longer half-life than that of other larger LMWH preparations, but at present, there is not a way to reverse this drug. Other LMWHs, although not as easily reversed as standard heparin, are approximately 70% reversible with protamine sulfate. The appropriate dosage for all surgical and medical prophylactic indications for enoxaparin is 40 mg subcutaneously once daily except in the setting of total knee replacement (30 mg every 12 hours). When the creatinine clearance is less than 30 mL/min, the dose is reduced to 30 mg once daily. In the setting of surgical prophylaxis, the drug is initiated 12 to 24 hours after surgery. The prophylactic dose of dalteparin is 2500 units once daily for moderate-risk surgical patients and medical patients. For high-risk patients (e.g., orthopedic surgery or patients with a malignant neoplasm undergoing abdominal or gynecologic surgery), 5000 units is recommended. Finally, the recommended dose for prophylaxis with fondaparinux is 2.5 mg once daily, initiated no sooner than 6 hours after surgery.

Intermittent pneumatic compression devices should be used when prophylactic doses of LMWH or heparin are contraindicated. Both methods combined are reasonable in patients deemed at exceptionally high risk, but combination regimens have not been studied in large populations of such individuals.

Every hospitalized patient should be assessed for the need for prophylactic measures. All hospitals should formulate their own written guidelines for each particular clinical setting based on the available medical literature. 5

NONTHROMBOTIC PULMONARY EMBOLISM

Because of venous blood return to the lungs, the pulmonary vascular bed is exposed to a wide variety of potentially obstructing and detrimental substances. These substances, which may be exogenous or endogenous in origin, may result in a number of consequences, including dyspnea, chest pain, hypoxemia, and sometimes death.

Fat Embolism

Epidemiology

Fat embolism generally occurs in the setting of traumatic fracture of long bones (Chapter 113) and is usually a more impressive clinical syndrome when larger bones and multiple fractures are involved. However, orthopedic procedures and trauma to other fat-rich tissues such as the liver or subcutaneous tissue can occasionally result in similar consequences.

Pathobiology

The physiologic consequences of fat embolism derive from both the obstruction of multiple vessels by neutral fat particles and the deleterious effects of free fatty acids released from neutral fat by lipases. These free fatty acids appear to cause diffuse vasculitis with capillary leak from cerebral, pulmonary, and other vascular beds.

Clinical Manifestations

After the traumatic event, there is generally a delay of 24 to 48 hours before symptoms develop. As neutral fat enters the vascular system, a characteristic syndrome of dyspnea, petechiae, and mental confusion often develops. It is not clear why the syndrome develops in some patients and not in others, even when the extent of injury is comparable, but it is possible that the presence of a patent foramen ovale could render patients more susceptible to the sequelae.

Diagnosis

The diagnosis is made from the clinical and radiographic findings in the setting of risk factors such as surgery and trauma. Although fat droplets (by oil red O stain) in bronchoalveolar lavage fluid may be suggestive of fat embolism, this finding does not appear to be sensitive or specific. The diagnosis of fat embolism syndrome remains a diagnosis of exclusion and is based on clinical criteria. Whereas clinically apparent fat embolism syndrome is uncommon, it also may be masked by the effects of concomitant injuries in more severely injured patients (Chapter 113).

Treatment

Treatment is supportive, including oxygen and mechanical ventilation, and the prognosis is generally good. Corticosteroid therapy remains controversial and is generally not recommended.

Amniotic Fluid Embolism

Epidemiology and Pathobiology

Amniotic fluid embolism is an uncommon syndrome but still represents one of the leading causes of maternal death in the United States. It occurs during or after delivery when amniotic fluid gains access to uterine venous channels and then to the pulmonary and general circulations. The delivery may be either spontaneous or by cesarean section and usually has been without complication. There are no identifiable risk factors in either the mother or the baby. The primary mechanism of injury appears to involve the thromboplastic activity of amniotic fluid, which leads to extensive fibrin deposition in the pulmonary vasculature and sometimes in other organs.

Clinical Manifestations

The syndrome is heralded by the sudden onset of severe respiratory distress; hypotension and death frequently result. A severe consumptive coagulopathy develops, with marked hypofibrinogenemia. After the acute event, an enhanced fibrinolytic state often is present. Left ventricular dysfunction may occur, possibly due to the myocardial depressant effect of amniotic fluid. The resulting pulmonary edema may be both hydrostatic and noncardiogenic.

Diagnosis

The diagnosis may be suspected on the basis of the clinical picture. The differential diagnosis includes PE, septic and hemorrhagic shock, venous air embolism, aspiration pneumonia, heart failure (from acute myocardial infarction or other causes), abruptio placentae, and ruptured uterus. Examination of the pulmonary arterial blood may or may not reveal the amorphous fragments of vernix caseosa, squamous cells, or mucin. Although administration of heparin, antifibrinolytic agents such as ε-aminocaproic acid, and cryoprecipitate has been suggested, the primary treatment is supportive, with oxygen, mechanical ventilation, and any necessary hemodynamic support.

Air Embolism

Epidemiology and Pathobiology

The incidence of this entity reflects the variety of invasive surgical and medical procedures now available, the frequent use of indwelling venous and arterial catheters, and the frequency of thoracic and other forms of trauma. With venous embolism in the setting of a patent foramen ovale, embolization to the coronary or cerebral circulation is of most concern. In the absence of a patent foramen ovale, the lungs can filter modest amounts of air, but large single or continuous episodes of air embolism can still gain access to the systemic arterial circulation.

Clinical Manifestations and Diagnosis

Symptoms and signs are dependent on the severity of the episode, and the consequences of venous air embolism range from none to death. Air in the systemic circulation may be difficult to recognize because only small quantities may cause significant symptoms, yet intravascular air clears quickly. Dyspnea, wheezing, chest pain, cough, agitation, confusion, tachycardia, and hypotension may be evident. A "mill wheel murmur" from air in the right ventricle may sometimes be auscultated. Hypoxemia and hypercapnia are present in severe cases, and the chest radiograph may reveal pulmonary edema or air-fluid levels.

Treatment

Rx

The treatment of venous air embolism includes immediate placement of the patient in the Trendelenburg–left lateral decubitus position and administration of 100% oxygen. If a central venous catheter is in place near the right atrium, air aspiration should be attempted. Hyperbaric oxygen should be considered. Anticonvulsants are administered in the presence of seizures.

Schistosomiasis

Schistosomiasis (Chapter 376) causes severe pulmonary vascular obstruction and pulmonary hypertension from both anatomic obstruction by the organism itself and an inflammatory vasculitic response. In endemic areas such as Egypt, schistosomal disease is a common cause of cor pulmonale. The liver is always involved, usually extensively, before pulmonary involvement occurs. The disease is refractory to treatment unless it is detected before extensive hepatic and pulmonary inflammation occurs.

Septic Embolism

Septic embolism was first noted as a complication of septic pelvic thrombophlebitis due to septic abortion or postpartum uterine infection. In recent years, however, intravenous drug abuse (Chapter 32), infections caused by indwelling intravenous catheters (Chapter 304), and right-sided infective endocarditis (Chapter 76) are the most common causes.

Other Emboli

A variety of other substances can also embolize to the lungs. Cancer cells may enter and adhere to pulmonary vessels, occasionally mimicking PE. Brain tissue has been discovered in the lungs after head trauma, and liver cells have been found after abdominal trauma. Bone marrow has been reported in lung tissue after cardiopulmonary resuscitation.

Noninfectious vasculitic-thrombotic complications also occur in intravenous drug users. Materials such as talc, used to "cut" heroin or cocaine, and occasionally the drugs themselves may provoke vascular inflammation and secondary thrombosis (Chapter 32). Perfusion scans occasionally demonstrate segmental or smaller defects. Distinguishing these from VTE can be difficult.

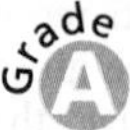

1. Buller HR, Agnelli G, Hull RD, et al: Antithrombotic therapy for venous thromboembolic disease. The Seventh American College of Chest Physicians on antithrombotic and thrombolytic therapy. Chest 2004;126;401S–428S.
2. Quinlan DJ, McQuillan A, Eikelboom JW: Low-molecular-weight heparin compared with intravenous unfractionated heparin for treatment of pulmonary embolism: A meta-analysis of randomized, controlled trials. Ann Intern Med 2004;140:175–183.
3. The PREPIC Study Group: Eight-year follow-up of patients with permanent vena cava filters in the prevention of pulmonary embolism. Circulation 2005;112:416–422.
4. Konstantinides S, Geibel A, Heusel G, et al: Heparin plus alteplase compared with heparin alone in patients with submassive pulmonary embolism. N Engl J Med 2002;347:1143–1150.
5. Geerts WH, Pineo GF, Heit JA, et al: Prevention of venous thromboembolism. The Seventh American College of Chest Physicians on Antithrombotic and Thrombolytic Therapy. Chest 2004;126: 338S–400S.

SUGGESTED READINGS

Francis CW: Prophylaxis for thromboembolism in hospitalized medical patients. N Engl J Med 2007;356:1438–1444. *A practical review.*

Goldhaber SZ: Pulmonary embolism. Lancet 2004;363:1295–1305. *A comprehensive review.*

Moores LK, Jackson WL, Shorr AF, et al: Meta-analysis: Outcomes in patients with suspected PE managed with computed tomographic pulmonary angiography. Ann Intern Med 2004;141:866–874. *In the setting of suspected acute PE, when the contrast-enhanced chest CT is normal, the outcome appears to be good, with a very low risk of recurrence.*

Pengo V, Lensing AWA, Prins MH, et al: Incidence of chronic thromboembolic pulmonary hypertension after pulmonary embolism. N Engl J Med 2004; 350:2257–2264. *Cumulative incidence was 3.8% at 2 years, but no cases developed later.*

Stein PD, Fowler SE, Goodman LR, et al: Multidetector computed tomography for acute pulmonary embolism. N Engl J Med 2006;354:2317–2327. *In patients with suspected PE, multidetector CT angiography of the chest together with CT venous-phase imaging of the legs has a higher diagnostic sensitivity than does CT angiography alone.*

Tillie-Leblond I, Marquette CH, Perez T, et al: Pulmonary embolism in patients with unexplained exacerbation of chronic obstructive pulmonary disease: Prevalence and risk factors. Ann Intern Med 2006;144:390–396. *PE may be the cause of up to 25% of otherwise unexplained exacerbations.*

van Belle A, Buller HR, Huisman MV, et al: Christopher Study Investigators: Effectiveness of managing suspected pulmonary embolism using an algorithm combining clinical probability, D-dimer testing, and computed tomography. JAMA 2006;295:172–179. *A diagnostic management strategy using a dichotomized version of the Wells clinical decision rule, D-dimer testing, and computed tomography was effective in evaluating and managing patients with suspected acute PE.*

100 DISEASES OF THE DIAPHRAGM, CHEST WALL, PLEURA, AND MEDIASTINUM

Bartolome R. Celli

THE DIAPHRAGM

The diaphragm, the most important muscle of respiration, is shaped like a thin dome and separates the thoracic and abdominal cavities. It has two components—the central noncontractile tendon and the muscle fibers that arise from it and radiate down and outward to insert distally in the circumferential caudal limits of the rib cage. There is a hiatus for the structures that pass from the thorax to the abdomen. The diaphragm is neurologically controlled by the phrenic nerve, the motor neurons of which arise in the cervical spinal cord at levels C3 to C5. The anatomic arrangement of the diaphragm and its coupling to the rib cage and abdomen explain its mechanical action. Diaphragmatic contraction displaces the abdominal contents downward and raises the ribs outward, thereby resulting in the negative intrapleural inspiratory pressure. Like the heart, the diaphragm and, to a lesser degree, the other respiratory muscles must intermittently contract throughout a person's life. Unlike the heart, it has no intrinsic contractile mechanism, and the respiratory cycle is regulated by a complex set of centrally organized neurons and several peripheral feedback mechanisms that synchronize the diaphragm with many other muscles. The diaphragm serves other nonrespiratory functions such as speech, defecation, and parturition. The blood supply to the diaphragm is rich and is arranged to minimize interruption during contraction. Nevertheless, the muscle itself is highly oxygen dependent.

Dysfunction and Fatigue

Diaphragmatic dysfunction is most frequently caused by lung hyperinflation—acute as in asthma or chronic as in chronic obstructive pulmonary disease (COPD). Hyperinflation shortens the diaphragm and changes its shape to a flatter one in which the horizontal fibers do not generate the normal expanding action on the thorax but rather an inward retraction of the lower part of the rib cage (i.e., Hoover's sign in COPD). These changes, coupled with increased airway resistance and decreased lung and chest wall compliance, result in increased work of breathing. If the increased energy demand outstrips the energy supply, the muscle fatigues and ventilation may fail.

Diaphragmatic fatigue can be determined by pressure measurements across the diaphragm (transdiaphragmatic pressure) or by the more elaborate power spectrum analysis of electromyographic signals. Both correlate well with the simpler clinical sign of rapid and shallow breathing. As fatigue progresses, ventilation is maintained by intermittent expansion of the rib cage and abdomen (respiratory alternans) and then paradoxical inward abdominal motion during inspiration (abdominal paradox). A number of strategies can improve diaphragmatic function in patients with impending fatigue (Table 100–1); if fatigue results in hypercapnia and acidosis, the respiratory muscles must be rested with noninvasive or invasive mechanical ventilation. 1

TABLE 100–1 THERAPEUTIC MODALITIES TO IMPROVE DIAPHRAGMATIC FUNCTION

REDUCE MECHANICAL LOAD
Decrease airway resistance (administer bronchodilators, treat infection, decrease inflammation)
Reduce hyperinflation
Decrease ventilatory requirement (administer oxygen, control fever, avoid caloric loads)
IMPROVE RESPIRATORY MUSCLE CONTRACTILITY AND ENDURANCE
Administer oxygen therapy
Improve nutrition
Improve cardiovascular performance
Correct electrolytes (sodium, potassium, calcium, phosphorus)
Administer drugs that improve contractility (β_2-agonist, caffeine)
Check for hypothyroidism or drugs that impair contractility (aminoglycosides)
Provide ventilatory muscle training
IMPROVE RESPIRATORY MUSCLE COORDINATION AND ENERGY CONSERVATION
REHABILITATION
RESPIRATORY MUSCLE RESTING

Disorders of Diaphragmatic Motion

Unilateral diaphragmatic paralysis is usually secondary to phrenic nerve involvement by a tumor, with bronchogenic carcinoma being the most frequent. Paralysis may result from neurologic diseases such as myelitis, encephalitis, poliomyelitis, or herpes zoster; from trauma to the thorax or cervical spine; or from compression by benign processes such as a substernal thyroid, aortic aneurysm, or infectious collections. With the advent of cardiac surgery, paralysis secondary to phrenic nerve cooling has increased. Occasionally, the paralysis may be idiopathic. The diagnosis is suspected when the diaphragmatic leaflet is elevated on the chest radiograph and is confirmed fluoroscopically by observing paradoxical diaphragmatic motion with sniffing and coughing. In patients with normal lungs, unilateral paralysis is usually asymptomatic and rarely requires treatment. Irreversible symptomatic unilateral paralysis may be treated by surgical plication of the affected hemidiaphragm. Bilateral paralysis generally results from high cervical trauma (C3 to C5), neuropathies, or myopathies. The myopathy may be generalized (muscular dystrophy, polymyositis, hypothyroidism) or limited and primarily affecting the diaphragm (acid maltase deficiency, collagen vascular disorders). In many cases, the cause remains unknown. Patients become symptomatic early. The dyspnea is characteristically worsened by the supine position because the abdominal contents displace the diaphragm into the thorax, which results in a significant (>500 mL) decrease in vital capacity and oxygen saturation. Fluoroscopy is not reliable because the flaccid diaphragm may lag behind the rib cage expansion when accessory muscles contract, thus giving the impression of diaphragmatic contraction. The diagnosis is suspected by the presence of inspiratory abdominal paradoxical retraction. It is confirmed by measuring transdiaphragmatic pressure with and without electromyographic recording. Phrenic nerve conduction establishes the diagnosis of neuropathy. Treatment of ventilatory failure secondary to bilateral paralysis consists of intermittent mechanical ventilation. In some cases, such as cardiac surgery, the paralysis recovers, and ventilation may be discontinued. In permanent paralysis with intact muscle function (e.g., high quadriplegics), diaphragmatic pacing has been life-saving.

Hiccup (singultus) is a disorder produced by spasm of the diaphragm followed by closure of the glottis during an inspiratory effort. Hiccups are usually self-limited but may persist for days or weeks. In most patients a cause is never found, but hiccups may occasionally be a sign of serious disease such as a central nervous system disorder (encephalitis, stroke, tumor), uremia, herpes zoster, or pleural or abdominal processes that irritate the diaphragm. Prolonged hiccups are sometimes psychogenic. In general, hiccups subside spontaneously or when the initiating disease improves. When hiccups are chronic or debilitating, local anesthesia or phrenic nerve crushing may be required (permanent paralysis may occur with the latter). Diaphragmatic flutter is a rare disorder in which rhythmic contractions of the diaphragm occur at a rate of 1 to 8 per second; the cause and treatment are similar to those of hiccups.

Diaphragmatic hernias occur through congenitally weak or incompletely fused areas of the diaphragm, through the esophageal hiatus (>70% of all hernias), or because of traumatic rupture of the muscle. Anterior hernias occur through the foramina of Morgagni, are rare, and tend to occur in obese patients; they are usually visualized as a rounded density in the right cardiophrenic angle. Posterior hernias through the foramina of Bochdalek are more common, especially in infants; they occur more frequently on the left. Traumatic diaphragmatic hernias may result from penetrating injuries or abdominal compression. Diaphragmatic hernias generally contain omentum but may also contain stomach, bowel, or liver anteriorly or kidney and spleen posteriorly. Symptom severity depends on the extension of abdominal contents into the thorax and the presence of strangulation. Hernias may be asymptomatic for several years before respiratory and abdominal symptoms occur.

Eventration may resemble a hernia but consists of a localized elevation of the diaphragm resulting from impaired muscle development or weakness. Eventration is more frequent in the right anteromedial portion and tends to occur in middle-aged obese persons; once differentiated from neoplasm, it rarely requires surgical treatment.

A diaphragmatic hernia is suspected on chest radiography and in some cases when there is borborygmus over the chest. Computed tomography (CT) scans, gastrointestinal contrast films, radioisotope scan of the liver, and induction of pneumoperitoneum with a follow-up film help establish the diagnosis. In infants, large hernias may compromise ventilation and thus require immediate surgical correction. In an asymptomatic adult with previous evidence of a hernia, observation is indicated. Surgery may be needed for diagnosis or to relieve strangulation of the sac contents.

THE CHEST WALL

The chest wall, an integral part of the ventilatory pump, consists of the bony thoracic cage (ribs, sternum, and vertebrae) and the various muscles of respiration. Besides the diaphragm, the intercostal and scalene muscles are active even during quiet breathing in normal persons. Other muscles such as the sternocleidomastoid, pectoralis minor and major, serratus anterior, latissimus dorsi, and trapezius partake in respiration during increased ventilatory demand. Even the abdominal muscles can participate in ventilation by contracting during exhalation. The thoracic cage is a major determinant of ventilation and static and dynamic lung volumes. Diseases that disrupt the system alter the ventilation and ventilation-perfusion relationship, thus causing hypoxemia or hypercapnia. Primary disorders of the chest wall may occur from impairment of the neuromuscular apparatus or the bony thoracic cage. Alterations in the neuromuscular apparatus are discussed elsewhere in this textbook; primary alterations of the bony thoracic cage are discussed in this section.

Diseases of the bony thoracic cage (Table 100–2) are all linked by a similar pathophysiologic process: (1) changes in chest wall compliance, (2) variable lung compression, (3) ventilation-perfusion imbalance, (4) alveolar hypoventilation, and (5) pulmonary hypertension and cor pulmonale. Clinical symptoms include dyspnea without significant cough, sputum, or pain. Physical examination usually establishes the diagnosis and helps determine the presence of cor pulmonale.

Kyphoscoliosis

Deformities of the dorsolumbar spine are the most common cause of symptomatic derangements of the chest wall. Scoliosis consists of lateral angulation and rotation of the spine and is categorized as right (most frequent) or left according to the direction of the convexity of the curvature. Kyphosis is less important and consists of anteroposterior angulation of the spine.

The severity of scoliosis is quantified by measuring the angle (Cobb's angle) between the upper and lower portions of the spinal curve on a radiograph. Only when this angle exceeds 70 degrees is any abnormality of respiratory function detectable. When the angle is more than 120 degrees, dyspnea and respiratory failure are expected. The ribs over the convex side are separated and rotated posteriorly, thus giving rise to the kyphoscoliotic hump. On the concave side, the ribs are crowded, displaced anteriorly, and combined with decreased thoracic height. These abnormalities produce forward bulging of the anterior wall.

Kyphoscoliosis is usually idiopathic and begins in childhood. Ventilatory failure may result in death in the fourth to sixth decade. If the scoliosis is not severe and progressive, life expectancy may be normal. Static lung volumes and chest wall and, to a lesser degree, lung compliance are also decreased. Ventilation-perfusion imbalances result in hypoxemia. When the mechanical load caused by progressive scoliosis or superimposed infection is such that the muscles fail, the hypoxemia may be associated with hypercapnia. Blood gases may worsen during sleep and cause frequent deterioration in some patients with otherwise stable kyphoscoliosis.

Several therapeutic approaches are available. Surgical correction includes traction, plaster, and rods; the effects are mostly cosmetic, and improvement in pulmonary function is usually minimal. In hypoxemic patients, oxygen is beneficial. Intermittent positive pressure ventilation increases tidal volume, thereby temporarily improving compliance and lung volumes. In chronic ventilatory failure, nighttime ventilatory assistance is beneficial. Effort must be made to induce the patient to stop smoking. Bronchospasm and respiratory infections must be treated aggressively. If obese, the patient should lose weight.

TABLE 100–2 MOST IMPORTANT RIB CAGE DERANGEMENTS

SPINE
Scoliosis (idiopathic, congenital, paralytic)
Kyphosis
Ankylosing spondylitis
STERNUM, RIBS, OR PLEURA
Pectus excavatum
Thoracoplasty
Fibrothorax

Ankylosing Spondylitis

This inflammatory disease results in fusion of the costotransverse and vertebral joints but may also involve the sternomanubrial and clavicular joints (Chapter 286). With relative fixation of the rib cage in an inspiratory position, most of the ventilatory movement is performed by the diaphragm-abdomen, which is already placed at a mechanical disadvantage because of normal or increased functional residual capacity. In contrast to kyphoscoliosis, cor pulmonale and ventilatory failure are rare in ankylosing spondylitis. In some patients, upper lobe fibrosis may develop with minimal alterations in gas exchange.

Pectus Excavatum

This congenital deformity of the lower portion of the sternum produces symmetrical bowing of the anterior ribs. In infants it tends to occur with multiple abnormalities and is associated with high mortality. It may also be associated with mitral valve prolapse. With severe deformity, the heart and mediastinal structures are laterally displaced. Although some patients may fail to increase cardiac output normally during exercise, the functional impairment is generally mild. Surgical correction is mainly cosmetic.

Thoracoplasty

Surgical procedures used from 1940 to 1950 to treat tuberculosis included resection of several ribs with collapse of the underlying lung. This procedure results in paradoxical retraction of that portion of the chest wall. Thoracoplasty was originally thought to have minimal physiologic consequences, but the incidence of cardiorespiratory failure is increased in these patients.

Fibrothorax

Resulting from pleural diseases such as hemothorax or asbestosis, fibrothorax is also considered a primary disease of the chest wall because the lung itself may not be affected. It may result in ventilatory and cardiac failure. Treatment is similar to that for kyphoscoliosis. Pleurectomy may help patients with fibrothorax secondary to pleural fibrosis.

Flail Chest

A flail chest is produced by double fractures of three or more adjacent ribs or by combined sternal and rib fractures. The flail segment paradoxically moves inward during inspiration. The inefficient ventilation increases the work of breathing, which may worsen ventilation because of the frequent association with neuromuscular impairment. Flail chest occurs most frequently with accidental chest trauma or after cardiopulmonary resuscitation. The ventilation-perfusion mismatch and lung contusion cause hypoxemia. In most cases, supportive care with attention to oxygenation, clear airways, and prevention of infection is the preferred therapy. Artificial ventilation should be reserved for patients with ventilatory failure. When the flail segment is large, chest fixation may be considered.

THE PLEURA

Definition

The parietal pleura covers the surface of the chest wall, diaphragm, and mediastinum; it is supplied with blood from the systemic circulation and contains sensory nerves. The visceral pleura covers the surface of the lungs, including the interlobar fissures; its blood supply arises from the low-pressure pulmonary circulation, and it has no sensory nerves.

The pleura consists of a layer of mesothelial cells with a smooth semitransparent appearance. It is supported by a network of connective and fibroelastic tissue, lymphatics, and vessels. The mesothelial cells are rich in microvilli, and their most important function is to deliver glycoproteins rich in hyaluronic acid to decrease friction between the lung and chest wall.

Physiology

The two layers of the pleura are separated by a virtual cavity, which is lubricated by 5 to 10 mL of fluid, facilitates lung expansion, and helps maintain lung inflation by coupling the lungs with the chest wall.

Pleural fluid has a low protein concentration (<2 g/dL) with a pH and glucose value similar to that of blood. Pleural fluid is formed primarily from the parietal pleura, and part of its turnover depends on the same Starling forces that govern vascular and interstitial fluid exchange. The parietal pleura has a hydrostatic pressure similar to that of the systemic circulation (30 cm H_2O), whereas that of the visceral pleura depends on the pulmonary circulation (10 cm H_2O). Oncotic pressure is similar in both (25 cm H_2O), but the pressure within the pleural cavity is affected by the gravity gradient. Thus, the pleural space is heterogeneous with a nondependent portion in which Starling forces favor outpouring of fluid into the cavity and the parenchymal capillaries. The stomas, or "lacunae," that are present over the parietal surface of the low mediastinum, low chest wall, and diaphragm seem to empty into the lymphatics. These subpleural lymphatics represent the major pathway for liquid and solute drainage. Alterations in this formation-resorption mechanism frequently result in the accumulation of pleural fluid. Increases in hydrostatic force or decreases in oncotic pressure result in low-protein "transudates." Increased outpouring by capillaries or cells or blocking of lymphatics (or both) results in high-protein "exudates" (Table 100–3).

Clinical Manifestations

Though suggestive, a patient's history of pain, dyspnea, or cough is neither sensitive nor specific. These symptoms may be absent in some large effusions and in critically ill patients. When present, the pain is generally unilateral and sharp and worsens with inspiration or cough. It may radiate to the shoulder, neck, or abdomen. Dyspnea may result from compression of lung tissue and from mechanical alterations in the respiratory muscles as the fluid changes their length-tension relationship. The degree of dyspnea relates to fluid volume and intrathoracic pressure and their effect on mechanics and gas exchange. Pleural effusions in patients with minimal lung compromise are well tolerated, whereas similar effusions in patients with lung disease may cause ventilatory failure.

Physical examination reveals decreased breath sounds and excursions in the affected hemithorax (splinting). Percussion reveals dullness with absent tactile fremitus over the area. Frequently, there are E to A changes (egobronchophony) at the upper fluid border where underlying lung parenchyma is compressed.

TABLE 100–3 MECHANISMS THAT LEAD TO ACCUMULATION OF PLEURAL FLUID

Increased hydrostatic pressure in the microvascular circulation (heart failure)
Decreased oncotic pressure in the microvascular circulation (severe hypoalbuminemia)
Decreased pressure in the pleural space (lung collapse)
Increased permeability of the microvascular circulation (pneumonia)
Impaired lymphatic drainage from the pleural space (malignant effusion)
Movement of fluid from the peritoneal space (ascites)

Diagnosis

Radiologic Examination

An effusion is suspected when there is blunting and medial displacement of the sharp costophrenic angle. Fluid accumulation between the lung and the diaphragm (subpulmonic effusion) is suspected when there is apparent elevation of the hemidiaphragm or widening of the shadow between the gas-containing stomach and the lower left lung margin. Up to 300 mL of fluid may fail to be seen on a posteroanterior chest radiograph, whereas as little as 150 mL may be seen on a lateral decubitus view. A supine film (frequent in patients in intensive care units) may obscure the diagnosis because the fluid layers posteriorly. A pseudotumor occurs when fluid loculates in an interlobar fissure, most commonly in the minor fissure, and gives the radiologic appearance of a tumor; a clue to the diagnosis is the presence of pleural fluid elsewhere and a biconvex lenticular configuration of the mass.

A collection of pleural air and fluid (hydropneumothorax) usually produces horizontal and not concave margins. A pneumothorax is identified by the contrast between the water density of the visceral pleura centrally and the gas radiolucency without vascular markings laterally. Small pneumothoraces may be harder to diagnose, but an expiratory film may help outline them.

Pleural plaques may be seen when calcified or may be detected when viewed tangentially but not en face. Ultrasonography (Fig. 100–1) and CT (Fig. 100–2) provide better definition of pleural and parenchymal abnormalities.

Diagnostic Procedures

A variety of diagnostic procedures can be used to determine the cause of a pleural effusion and sometimes be therapeutic as well.

Thoracentesis and Pleural Fluid Analysis

Thoracentesis may be performed for diagnosis or therapy. Thoracentesis is diagnostic in approximately 75% of patients; even when not diagnostic, it helps exclude other important diagnoses such as empyema. Diagnostic thoracentesis (Fig. 100–3) requires a relatively small amount of material (30 to 50 mL). As a rule, newly discovered effusions should

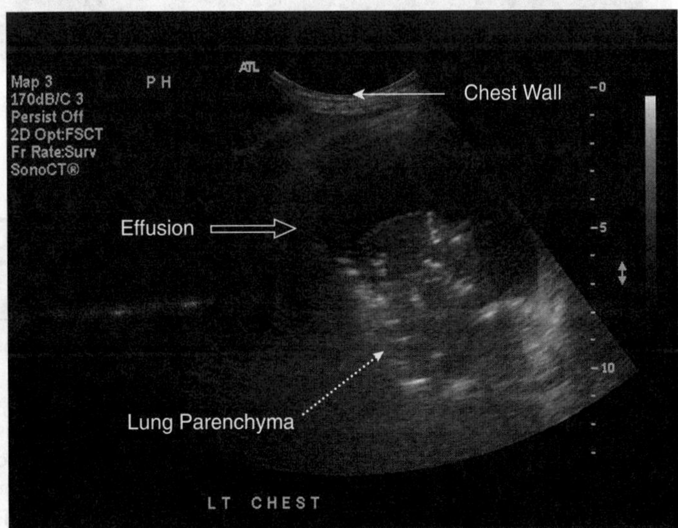

FIGURE 100–1 • Ultrasound image of the left hemithorax. Bilateral pleural effusions from pneumonia are apparent in the patient whose computed tomography scan is shown in Figure 100–2. The chest wall is indicated by the thin arrow, the effusion by the thick arrow. The underlying consolidated lung is evident by the echolucent area outlined by the dotted arrow. (Courtesy of David Lee, MD, Department of Radiology, Caritas-St. Elizabeth's Medical Center, Boston.)

be tapped. Although there are no absolute contraindications to diagnostic thoracentesis, relative contraindications include a bleeding diathesis, anticoagulation, a small volume, mechanical ventilation, and a low benefit-to-risk ratio. Therapeutic thoracentesis involves removing larger amounts of fluid (no more than 1000 to 1500 mL at one time because edema may occur in the re-expanded underlying lung, especially in cases of tension effusion).

Although the classification of "transudate" or "exudate" is not absolute, the distinction is helpful in suggesting further evaluation and possible diagnoses. To differentiate transudates and exudates, it is cost-effective to determine total protein, lactate dehydrogenase (LDH), the white blood cell count with differential, and either glucose or pH (Table 100–4). *Transudates* are due to imbalances in hydrostatic and oncotic pressure such as is seen in heart failure or hypoalbuminemia; they may result from movement of fluid from the peritoneum to the pleural space. *Exudates* (Table 100–5) are defined by the presence of at least one of the following criteria: (1) pleural fluid–serum protein ratio greater than 0.5, (2) pleural fluid–serum LDH ratio greater than 0.6, and (3) pleural fluid LDH concentration greater than 200 IU/L. A fluid cholesterol level greater than 45 mg/dL may also be helpful.

Diagnoses that can be established by thoracentesis include malignancy, empyema (pus), tuberculosis (positive acid-fast bacilli in smears or culture; Chapter 345), fungal infection (positive potassium hydroxide stains or culture), the pleuritis of suptemic lupus erythematosus (LE cells; Chapter 287), chylothorax (high triglycerides or the presence of chylomicrons), urinothorax (pleural fluid–serum creatinine ratio >1), and esophageal rupture (increased pleural fluid amylase and pH around 6.0).

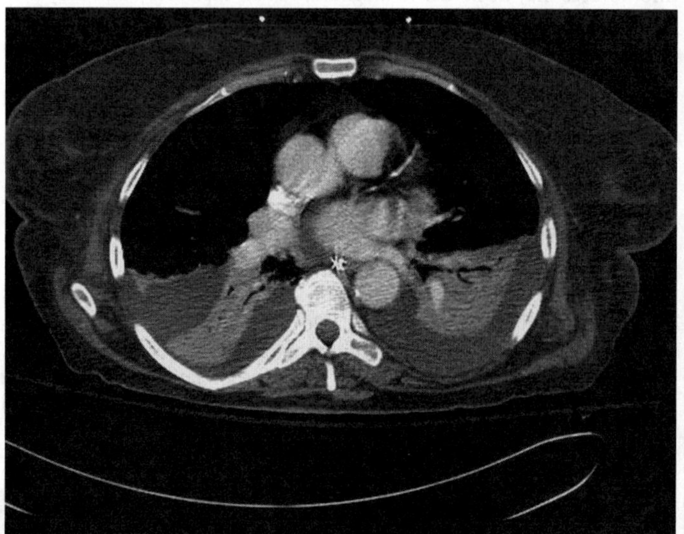

FIGURE 100–2 • Computed tomography of the patient shown in Figure 100–1. Bilateral pleural effusions are present as a result of pneumonia. (Courtesy of David Lee, MD, Department of Radiology, Caritas-St. Elizabeth's Medical Center, Boston.)

Because many diagnoses produce overlapping values, acid-fast and Gram stains, aerobic and anaerobic cultures, cell count and differential, and cytologic analysis should be included in the study of these effusions. A predominance of polymorphonuclear leukocytes (PMNs) is most compatible with bacterial infection, whereas lymphocytes (particularly with a paucity of mesothelial cells) suggest tuberculosis. Lymphocytes are also seen in lymphoma and leukemic effusions. Eosinophils are nonspecific and suggest long-standing fluid or air, sometimes even in small amounts, as from a previous thoracentesis. A bloody effusion that is not due to trauma is most likely due to malignancy or pulmonary infarction (Chapters 99 and 201). A white effusion suggests chyle, cholesterol, or lymphoma; black fluid suggests aspergillosis (Chapter 360); and a yellow-green color may be seen in rheumatoid pleurisy (Chapter 285). A putrid odor is diagnostic of anaerobic empyema, whereas an ammonia odor suggests urinothorax. The value of other diagnostic markers is uncertain, except for adenosine deaminase, which is useful for tuberculosis (see later

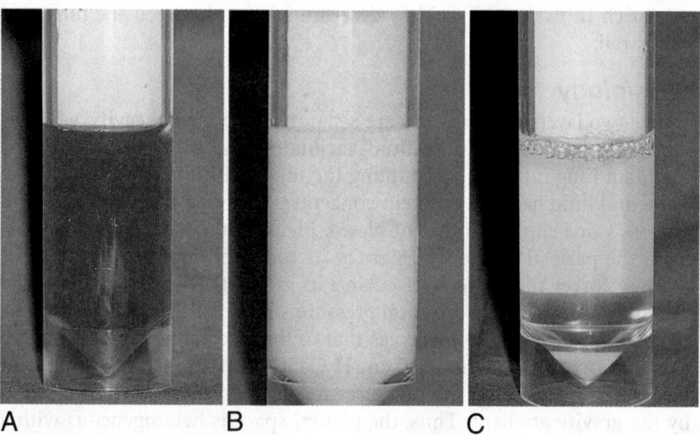

FIGURE 100–3 • Pleural effusion. A, Blood-stained pleural aspirate. This patient had pleural metastases from carcinoma of the breast. **B,** Chylous pleural effusion. This patient had bronchial carcinoma that had invaded and obstructed the thoracic duct. **C,** Pleural transudate. This pale effusion is typically found in patients with heart failure or other causes of generalized edema. (From Forbes CD, Jackson WF: Color Atlas and Text of Clinical Medicine, 3rd ed. London, Mosby, 2003.)

TABLE 100–4 CHARACTERISTICS OF PLEURAL FLUID TRANSUDATES

	Absolute Value	Pleural Fluid/Serum Value
Protein	<3 g/dL	<0.5
Lactate dehydrogenase	<200 IU/L	<0.6
Glucose	>60 mg/dL	1.0
White blood cell count	<1000/mm^3	—
Cholesterol	<45 mg/dL	

TABLE 100–5 CORRELATION OF PLEURAL FLUID EXUDATE FINDINGS AND CAUSATIVE DISEASE

Tests	Diseases
pH <7.2	Empyema, malignancy, esophageal rupture; rheumatoid, lupus, and tuberculous pleuritis
Glucose (<60 mg/dL)	Infection, rheumatoid pleurisy, tuberculous and lupus effusions, esophageal rupture
Amylase (>200 μg/dL)	Pancreatic disease, esophageal rupture, malignancy, ruptured ectopic pregnancy
Rheumatoid factor, antinuclear antibody, LE cells	Collagen vascular disease
Complement (decreased)	Lupus erythematosus, rheumatoid arthritis
Red blood cells (>5000/μL)	Trauma, malignancy, pulmonary embolus
Chylous effusion (triglycerides >110 mg/dL)	Tuberculosis, violation of the thoracic duct (trauma, malignancy)
Biopsy (+)	Malignancy
Adenosine deaminase (>40 μg/L)	Tuberculosis

LE = lupus erythematosus.

text). β_2-Microglobulin, pleural/serum cholinesterase, and lysozyme remain to be determined. Complications of thoracentesis include pain, bleeding (local, pleural, or abdominal), pneumothorax, infection, and spleen or liver puncture. With therapeutic thoracentesis, up to 50% of patients experience a temporary decrease in Pa_{O_2} of as much as 20 mm Hg.

Percutaneous Pleural Biopsy

Biopsy is indicated to evaluate patients with an undiagnosed exudative effusion (particularly those with lymphocytic predominance) because the most frequently diagnosed disease is malignancy or tuberculosis. The procedure is performed under local anesthesia with a hook-type needle (Cope or Abrams). Contraindications are a small or loculated pleural effusion, an uncooperative patient, and anticoagulation or a bleeding diathesis, including azotemia with an abnormal bleeding time. Because pleural seeding may not be uniform, multiple samples are needed. The overall diagnostic yield is about 60% for malignancy and 75% for tuberculosis.

Exploration of the Pleura

In most of the 5 to 10% of patients with undiagnosed effusion, the effusion itself disappears spontaneously or the cause becomes evident. When it is considered necessary to make a diagnosis, a biopsy specimen can be obtained through thoracoscopy (usually video-assisted thoracoscopy [VATS]; Chapter 102). Thoracoscopy can be performed under local anesthesia and has a high yield (>85%). In some cases, it is necessary to perform an open pleural biopsy under general anesthesia. The main advantage is the possibility of obtaining larger specimens and concomitant lung tissue.

Differential Diagnosis

Transudative Effusion

Biventricular failure with venous hypertension is the most common cause of a transudative effusion (Chapters 57 and 58). Effusions are often bilateral, usually larger on the right, and on the chest radiograph are associated with vascular congestion and cardiomegaly (Chapter 51). In chronic heart failure (months) or as the effusion is in the process of resolving as the heart failure is treated, total protein may be higher than 3 g/dL. Thoracentesis is indicated if the patient is febrile, the effusion is large and unilateral, or there is pain or unexplained hypoxemia. Transudates occur in 5 to 10% of patients with liver cirrhosis (Chapter 157) secondary to movement of ascitic fluid through diaphragmatic defects or lymphatic channels; the effusion is more frequent on the right (70%). If in doubt, radioactive tracer injected in the ascitic fluid appears in the chest. The effusion often improves with improvement of the ascites (Chapter 145). Occasionally, chemical pleurodesis has effectively relieved symptomatic, recurrent effusions. A transudate is seen in up to 20% of patients with nephrotic syndrome (Chapter 122) because of decreased oncotic pressure (hypoalbuminemia) and increased hydrostatic forces; frequently bilateral, it is improved by correcting the protein-losing nephropathy. Peritoneal dialysis (Chapter 133) and atelectasis may also cause transudative effusions. Urinothorax is a rare ipsilateral pleural transudate that occurs with obstruction of the urinary system; the effusion has the characteristic odor of urine, and relief of the obstruction promptly resolves the effusion.

Exudative Effusions

Infections

Parapneumonic effusion (pleural fluid associated with pneumonia or lung abscess; Chapters 97 and 98) is the most common cause of exudates. They may be uncomplicated and resolve spontaneously with antibiotics or may be complicated and require drainage. Complicated effusions are rich in white blood cells (empyema) or have positive Gram stains or cultures. Uncomplicated effusions are generally small and contain moderate amounts of PMNs, a glucose value similar to that of blood, a pH greater than 7.30, and an LDH level less than 500 U/L. In contrast, complicated effusions have large numbers of PMNs, often more than 100,000/mm^3, a pH less than 7.20, a glucose value less than 40 g/dL, and LDH greater than 1000 U/L. If the effusion is also purulent and has bacteria, immediate drainage is necessary and is best achieved with a chest tube. If a fever persists for more than 48 to 72 hours in patients with complicated effusions, either the drainage is inadequate (such as when fluid becomes loculated), the antibiotic is inappropriate, or the diagnosis is wrong. If drainage is not effective, existing data favor the early use of VATS, with intrapleural streptokinase reserved for patients who are poor surgical risks for settings in which VATS is not available. [2] Poorly treated empyemas may result in communication with the bronchial tree (bronchopleural fistula) or skin (bronchopleurocutaneous fistula) and require open drainage with rib resection, decortication, and extensive reconstruction. In some patients with uncontrolled pleural sepsis, thoracotomy with drainage and decortication may be life-saving. Pleural involvement by nonbacterial, nontuberculous infection is uncommon and, when present, is usually limited. Fungal diseases rarely affect the pleura except for coccidioidomycosis, which may cause a hypersensitivity pleuritis.

Other Infective-Inflammatory Disorders

Exudative effusions may result from subdiaphragmatic processes such as an upper abdominal abscess, of which a subphrenic site is the most common location. Frequently postoperative in origin, subphrenic abscesses may result from hepatic diseases and gastrointestinal perforations. Patients are generally febrile and dyspneic and have an elevated hemidiaphragm with ipsilateral splinting. Abscesses may also arise in the liver or spleen. Antibiotics alone may not be sufficient; drainage may be necessary.

Pancreatitis and pancreatic pseudocysts (Chapter 147) can cause pleural effusions, more often on the left or bilaterally. The amylase level is higher than that in serum, and the exudate may be blood tinged; the exudate tends to resolve as the pancreatic problem improves.

Esophageal rupture (Chapter 140) is an urgent cause of pleural effusion. Close to half of cases are secondary to endoscopy (Chapter 136) or esophageal dilation, whereas others are secondary to a foreign body or trauma or occur spontaneously (Boerhaave's syndrome). Patients complain of chest pain, dyspnea, and dysphagia. Fever is universal, and half of patients have subcutaneous emphysema. The radiograph may confirm the emphysema and may show pneumothorax, more frequent on the left. Pleural effusion occurs in 75% of patients, with the findings dependent on the time of thoracentesis. Early in the course, the exudate has abundant PMNs, followed by high concentrations of salivary amylase. Later, anaerobic mouth organisms seed the space, and the pH approaches 6.0. The diagnosis is established by using barium sulfate or water-soluble compounds (Chapter 140). Early diagnosis and prompt surgical correction result in a greater than 90% survival rate. If surgical closure is delayed, antibiotics for anaerobes, parenteral nutrition, and mediastinal and pleural drainage are necessary.

Tuberculosis

Pleural effusion occurs in most cases of pulmonary tuberculosis (Chapter 345) but is frequently inapparent. The effusion may accompany the primary infection, in which case it is an exudate, is commonly unilateral, and results from a hypersensitivity phenomenon. These patients, who are generally febrile, may recover without treatment, but in close to two thirds active tuberculosis develops within 5 years. A second form occurs when a subpleural focus of *Mycobacterium tuberculosis* ruptures into the pleural space. The clinical findings simulate an acute pneumonia (60% of cases) with a subacute or chronic fever, nonproductive cough (80%), or chest pain (75%). Chest radiography shows a small to moderate effusion (4% are large), and parenchymal disease is seen in a third of cases. Intermediate-strength purified protein derivative testing is positive in 70% of patients, and if repeated after 6 to 8 weeks, it may become positive in those with a previous negative test. The fluid is usually rich in protein (>4 g/dL), with a leukocyte count of about 5000 cells/mm^3 (90 to 95% lymphocytes). A PMN predominance may occur after the first few days. The glucose level may be low, but rarely lower than 20 mg/dL. The pH ranges between 7.00 and 7.30, with a pH higher than 7.40 virtually excluding tuberculosis. The fluid is characteristically free of mesothelial cells. Recently, the presence of an adenosine deaminase level greater than 40 μg/L and lysozyme has been found to correlate with tuberculosis. An enzyme-linked immunosorbent assay or polymerase chain reaction to demonstrate mycobacterial antigen may be helpful diagnostically and may provide a more rapid diagnosis in the more than 90% of cases in which acid-fast bacilli are not seen on smear. Multiple samples from closed pleural biopsy are positive in 50 to 80% of cases, whereas cultures are positive in 30 to 70%. With all methods combined, the yield is close to 95%. The fever typically resolves within 2 weeks of instituting treatment but may persist for 6 or 8 weeks. The effusion usually resolves by 6 weeks but may persist for 3 to 4 months. Very ill patients may be helped by short-term corticosteroid treatment. Rarely, surgical drainage or decortication may be necessary.

Other Infectious Effusions

Actinomycosis (Chapter 350) caused by the anaerobic organism *Actinomyces israelii* may cause purulent effusions that may bulge the thoracic wall and drain through the chest. Sulfur granules (whitish yellow or brown interwoven filaments) can be identified in the fluid. Pleural effusions are also common in *Nocardia* infection (Chapter 351); the effusion is generally purulent with abundant PMNs, and sulfonamides are the treatment of choice. Aspergillosis (Chapter 360) of the pleura is uncommon, but a thickened pleura is frequently seen in progressive invasive aspergillosis. Pleural effusions secondary to parasitic diseases are uncommon but increasing in immigrants from developing countries. Paragonimiasis (Chapter 377) causes pleural thickening or effusion in up to 48% of patients; the effusion has a triad of low glucose (<10 g/dL), high LDH (>1000 U/L), and low pH (<7.10); complement fixation antibodies greater than 1:64 are diagnostic. Amebiasis and echinococcosis are rare causes of pleural effusion.

Immunologic Causes of Pleural Effusion

Clinical pleurisy occurs in close to 5% of patients with *rheumatoid arthritis* (Chapter 285), even though autopsy studies suggest up to 50% involvement. It has a male preponderance and appears within 5 years after onset of the disease; nevertheless, effusions have occurred up to 20 years before the onset of joint disease. The fluid is an exudate with low glucose (<30 mg/dL), low pH, and high LDH. The complement level is generally low, with high titers of rheumatoid factor. The patient may complain of pleuritic pain or dyspnea. Fever is not common, in contrast to lupus pleuritis. The effusion usually resolves over a period of months but occasionally persists for years. The major complication is fibrosis with lung trapping. Anti-inflammatory agents and corticosteroids are the recommended therapy. Pleuritic pain or effusion can be the initial manifestation in 5% of patients with *systemic lupus erythematosus* (Chapter 287) and occurs at some point in the course in up to 50% of patients. Pain (86%), cough (64%), dyspnea (50%), pleural friction rub (71%), and fever (57%) are common. The effusions are exudates that in the majority of cases have normal pH and glucose. Hemolytic complement, especially C3 and C4 components, is low, and classic LE cells may be present. Lupus pleuritis is likely if the antinuclear antibody ratio in the fluid is greater than 1:160. Spontaneous resolution of lupus pleuritis is uncommon, but it generally disappears within 2 weeks after beginning therapy with corticosteroids. Sarcoidosis (Chapter 95), Wegener's granulomatosis (Chapter 291), Sjögren's syndrome (Chapter 289), and immunoblastic lymphadenopathy are rare causes of pleural effusion.

Other Conditions

Asbestosis (Chapter 92) is frequently associated with pleural disease; the effusion is often unilateral, small, and serosanguineous. The cell count is less than 6000 cells/mm^3, with either PMN or mononuclear predominance. Eosinophilia (up to 50%) has been described. The diagnosis is suspected with known exposure. Exclusion of malignant mesothelioma in the presence of pleural plaques may be difficult and requires follow-up. The effusion tends to resolve in 1 month to 1 year, with a blunted costophrenic angle left in more than 90% of patients and diffuse pleural thickening in about 50%. Calcification of the plaques occurs late (20 to 40 years after exposure). About 5% of patients may have underlying pulmonary parenchymal asbestosis.

Meigs' syndrome is the triad of benign fibroma or other ovarian tumors with ascites and large pleural effusions (usually on the right side). Most frequent after menopause, its symptoms are malaise, chest pain, and increased abdominal girth. Fluid moves from the abdomen through small diaphragmatic defects or lymphatics. The fluid is usually an exudate with a paucity of mononuclear cells. When suspected, a pelvic examination or abdominal-pelvic CT scan documents the ovarian tumor. Removal of the tumor resolves the effusion within 2 to 3 weeks.

Uremia (Chapter 131) causes a polyserositis and generally a bloody pleural exudate that resolves with treatment of the uremia. The diagnosis must be distinguished from a urinothorax or hydrothorax caused by the nephrotic syndrome. Repeated thoracentesis may be needed if the patient is symptomatic (dyspnea, cough, chest pain).

Other causes of inflammatory effusions include radiation therapy, esophageal sclerotherapy, enteral feeding misplacement, and drug-induced pleural disease from medications such as nitrofurantoin, dantrolene, methysergide, methotrexate, procarbazine, amiodarone, mitomycin, bleomycin, and minoxidil. Pleuritis with a lupus-like syndrome has been associated with procainamide, hydralazine, isoniazid, and quinidine; the signs and symptoms usually resolve after discontinuing use of the medication, but corticosteroids may occasionally be required.

Malignancy

Malignant effusions are probably the most common cause of exudate in patients older than 60 years. Invasion by lung cancer is the most frequent (Chapter 201), whereas spread from liver metastasis or invasion of chest wall lymphatics is the most frequent mechanism in breast cancer (Chapter 208). Ovarian cancer (Chapter 209) and gastric cancer (Chapter 202) represent close to 5% of cases, whereas 7% may have an unknown primary lesion at the time of diagnosis. Patients may be asymptomatic or exhibit cough, pain, and dyspnea. The effusion is an exudate with abundant red cells (30,000 to 50,000/mL) and mononuclear cells (lymphocytes >50%). Occasionally, they are transudative (5 to 10%), and about a third may have pH less than 7.3 or a glucose value less than 60 mg/dL. Cytology is positive in close to 60% of cases, but biopsy increases the yield only to 70%. Thoracentesis should be repeated if the diagnosis is still suspected. Malignant pleural effusion carries a very poor prognosis, with the exception of breast cancer and small cell carcinoma of the lung, both of which may respond temporarily to therapy. The best method, short of pleurectomy or pleural abrasion, to control recurrent malignant effusion is to instill tetracycline, talc, or medroxyprogesterone intrapleurally after chest tube drainage.

Lymphomas, especially non-Hodgkin's lymphoma (Chapter 196), may cause exudative effusions because of tumor spread to the pleura. Mediastinal invasion with lymphatic blockage and effusion is more common in Hodgkin's lymphoma (Chapter 197). Although the prognosis is uncertain when lymphoma causes pleural effusion, patients frequently respond to chemotherapy.

Hemothorax

Frank blood in the pleural space (hematocrit >20%) is usually the result of trauma, hematologic disorders, pulmonary infarction, or pleural malignancies. Left-sided hemothorax, particularly with a widened mediastinum, may indicate rupture of the aorta. Pleural blood often does not clot and can readily be removed by lymphatics if the volume is small. Larger effusions require tube drainage. Persistent bleeding necessitates surgical correction.

Chylothorax

Leakage of lymph (chyle) from the thoracic duct most commonly results from mediastinal malignancy (50%), especially lymphoma. Chylothorax may also result from thoracic surgery (20%) or trauma (5%). The triad of slow-growing yellow nails, lymphedema, and pleural effusion (yellow nail syndrome) is due to hypoplastic or dilated lymphatics. Because chyle collects within the posterior mediastinum, the chylothorax may not appear for days until the mediastinal pleura ruptures. The usual milky appearance of the effusion may be confused with a cholesterol effusion or an effusion with many leukocytes. The best diagnostic criterion for chylothorax is the presence of a triglyceride concentration greater than 110 mg/dL, with rare instances of values between 50 and 110 mg/dL. The major complications are malnutrition and immunologic compromise because fat, protein, and lymphocytes are depleted with repeated thoracentesis or chest tube drainage. Treatment should include pleural drainage and attempts to decrease chyle formation by intravenous hyperalimentation, decreased oral fat intake, and intake of medium-chain triglycerides, which are absorbed directly into the portal circulation. For traumatic effusions, ligation of the thoracic duct should be considered; when secondary to tumor, treatment should focus on the primary cause.

Malignant Mesothelioma

Asbestos exposure precedes 80 to 90% of malignant mesotheliomas (Chapters 93 and 201). Patients may complain of dyspnea, cough, weight loss, and pain. Smoking is not a risk factor. The tumors often encase the underlying lung. The effusion may be massive and is often bloody; in 70% of cases, the pH is less than 7.30. Cytologic evaluation is controversial because even when positive it may be difficult to differentiate mesothelioma from metastatic carcinoma. Elevated levels of hyaluronic acid and special stains and electron microscopy of biopsy tissue may help in the diagnosis. Median survival is 8 to 12 months after diagnosis. Malignant mesothelioma may be confused with benign mesothelioma, which has the histology of a fibroma. Benign mesotheliomas may reach a large size and be pedunculated (migrating with position changes); they are often associated with hypertrophic pulmonary osteoarthropathy and clubbing.

Treatment of mesothelioma involves surgical removal and, in malignant cases, chemotherapy.

Pneumothorax

Pneumothorax is defined as an accumulation of gas in the pleural space. It may be caused by (1) perforation of the visceral pleura and entry of gas from the lung; (2) penetration of the chest wall, diaphragm, mediastinum, or esophagus; or (3) gas generated by microorganisms in an empyema. When gas originates in the lung, rupture may occur in the absence of known disease (simple pneumothorax) or as a result of parenchymal disease (secondary pneumothorax).

Simple spontaneous pneumothorax occurs most commonly in previously healthy men between 20 and 40 years of age and is due to spontaneous rupture of subpleural blebs at the apex of the lungs. The right lung is more frequently involved, and recurrence is frequent (30% ipsilateral, 10% contralateral). Patients usually have acute pain, dyspnea (related to the size of the pneumothorax), and cough. Physical examination shows decreased breath sounds and tactile fremitus with ipsilateral hyperresonance. The chest radiograph classically shows the visceral pleural line, but small pneumothoraces may become evident only on an expiratory or lateral decubitus film. Small amounts of fluid (sometimes blood) are present in 25% of patients. *Tension pneumothorax* (caused by increased positive pressure through a "ball valve" air leak) can result in mediastinal shift and compromise circulation. For a small pneumothorax (<20% of the hemithorax) in an asymptomatic patient, observation may suffice because the air may be reabsorbed in 7 to 14 days. Larger pneumothoraces can be treated by air aspiration. A chest tube, which can be connected to suction or placed under water seal, is required for a pneumothorax that occupies more than 50% of the hemithorax, for symptomatic patients, or for a tension pneumothorax. The tube should be left in place until the leak seals. Because of frequent recurrences, chemical pleurodesis or surgical correction, usually by VATS, may be necessary.

Secondary or complicated pneumothorax results from trauma or pulmonary diseases. Widespread emphysema (Chapter 88) is the most common cause, but rupture of an abscess with spillage of pus into the pleural space can cause a pyopneumothorax. Less frequent underlying conditions are asthma (Chapter 87), certain interstitial lung diseases (idiopathic fibrosis, eosinophilic granulomatosis, sarcoidosis, tuberous sclerosis; Chapters 92 and 95), neoplasms (sarcoma, bronchogenic carcinoma; Chapter 201), some rare diseases such as Marfan and Ehlers-Danlos syndromes (Chapter 281), and endometriosis (catamenial pneumothorax). Iatrogenic injuries (e.g., insertion of central lines) and barotrauma (Chapter 106) are seen in the intensive care unit. The patient should be hospitalized and a chest tube inserted because spontaneous expansion is rare and the decreased reserve resulting from the pneumothorax may cause ventilatory compromise. Surgery must not be taken lightly because the rate of complications is high, but it may be life-saving in some patients. In patients maintained on ventilatory support, a pneumothorax is always under tension and requires immediate insertion of a chest tube. If a bronchopleural fistula persists, a portion of the minute ventilation exits through it; hence, it is necessary to increase ventilation to compensate for this loss. For a severe leak, high-frequency low-pressure ventilation may be helpful. Frequent complications of chest tube insertion include re-expansion pulmonary edema, lung trauma or infarction, subcutaneous emphysema, bleeding, and infection.

THE MEDIASTINUM

Definition

The mediastinum is the anatomic space that lies in the midthorax and separates the two pleural cavities. It is limited by the diaphragm below and the suprasternal thoracic outlet above. The mediastinum contains several vital structures in a small space, so mediastinal abnormalities can produce important symptoms. For clinical purposes, it is convenient to divide the mediastinum into anterior, middle, and posterior compartments (Fig. 100–4). The anterior compartment contains the thymus, substernal extensions of the thyroid and parathyroid glands, blood vessels, pericardium, and lymph nodes. The middle compartment contains the heart, great vessels, trachea, main bronchi, lymph nodes, and phrenic and vagus nerves. The posterior compartment contains the vertebrae, descending aorta, esophagus, thoracic duct, azygous and hemizygous veins, lower portion of the vagus, sympathetic chains, and posterior mediastinal nodes.

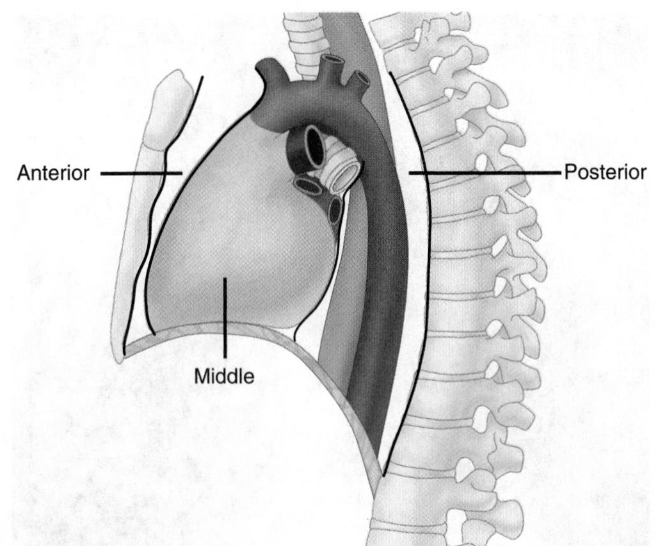

FIGURE 100–4 • Anatomic compartments of the mediastinum. The anterior compartment is bounded posteriorly by the pericardium, ascending aorta, and brachiocephalic vessels and anteriorly by the sternum. The middle compartment extends from the posterior limits of the anterior compartment to the posterior pericardial line. The posterior compartment extends from the pericardial line to the dorsal chest wall.

Clinical Manifestations

Most patients with mediastinal masses are asymptomatic, and the mass is found incidentally on a chest radiograph obtained for another reason. The most common symptoms are chest pain, cough, hoarseness, and dyspnea, whereas stridor, dysphagia, and Horner's syndrome are less frequent. Occasionally, some syndromes are associated with a primary mediastinal lesion. Myasthenia gravis (Chapter 448) is present in nearly 50% of patients with thymoma. Hypoglycemia has been seen in patients with mesothelioma, fibrosarcoma, and teratoma. Parathyroid tumors (Chapter 266) may induce hypercalcemia, whereas neurogenic tumors may cause neurologic symptoms. The physical examination is usually nonspecific. The mass may produce superior vena cava obstruction with facial edema, dilated veins, and arm edema. The masses may erode the trachea, esophagus, and great vessels with life-threatening consequences.

Diagnosis

Most mediastinal masses are detected on a plain chest radiograph (Figs. 100–5 and 100–6). Chest CT is the initial procedure of choice (Fig. 100–7) because it provides good definition of mediastinal structures. If the patient is asymptomatic and the noninvasive information obtained by CT, with and without enhancement by contrast medium, suggests a benign process, careful follow-up is justified. The radiologic evaluation may include angiography and esophagography. The role of magnetic resonance imaging is being investigated, specifically for evaluating vessels and blood flow without the need for contrast medium enhancement. In some patients it may be necessary to obtain tissue for histologic diagnosis. Classically, anterior and middle compartment lesions are reached through mediastinoscopy or mediastinotomy. Thoracotomy may be needed for middle and posterior compartment lesions or when surgery is the treatment of choice for the suspected lesion (i.e., lung cancer). Direct sampling by CT-guided needle aspiration has become the procedure of choice in many centers.

Tumors

The most common cause of a mediastinal mass in older patients is a metastatic carcinoma (most commonly bronchogenic carcinoma). In young adults, primary mediastinal pathology is more frequent (Table 100–6).

In the posterior mediastinum, neurogenic tumors are most common (20%). Nonspecific chest pain and nonproductive cough with occasional compression of the intercostal nerves, trachea, and bronchi are the most frequent symptoms. Most tumors are benign and originate in the nerve

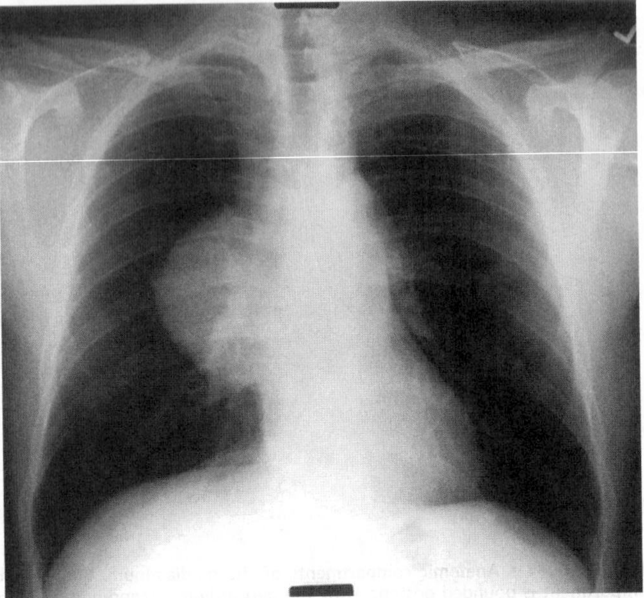

FIGURE 100–5 • Posteroanterior radiograph of a patient with a mass in the anterior mediastinum.

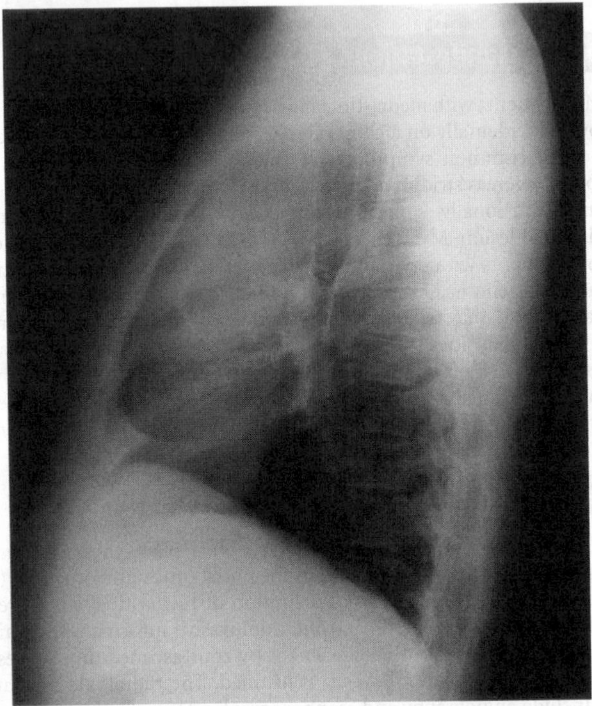

FIGURE 100–6 • Lateral chest radiograph of the patient in Figure 100–5.

sheath (neurilemoma, neurofibroma) or sympathetic ganglion cells (ganglioneuroma). Neuroblastoma (malignant tumor of sympathetic ganglion cells) has a better prognosis than the same tumor occurring in the adrenals. Neurofibromas may occur in association with von Recklinghausen's disease (Chapter 444). Ganglioneuromas and neuroblastomas may secrete hormones that cause flushing, diarrhea, and hypertension. Pheochromocytomas (Chapter 246) may occasionally arise in the mediastinum. Neurogenic tumors should be resected; neuroblastomas require postoperative radiation therapy.

Thymomas (Chapter 448) account for 20% of mediastinal tumors and are located in the superior portion of the anterior mediastinum. Two thirds of them are malignant. Myasthenia gravis is seen in 40% of cases, and other paraneoplastic syndromes such as Cushing's syndrome, refractory anemia, and hypogammaglobulinemia have been reported. All thymomas should be regarded as malignant, and surgical resection should be followed by radiation therapy.

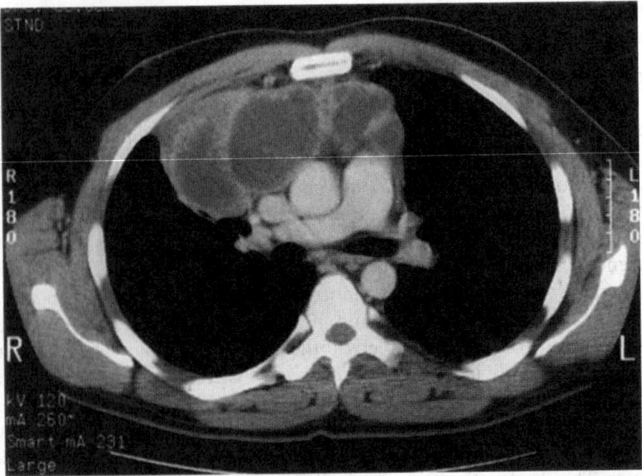

FIGURE 100–7 • Computed tomography scan of the patient in Figures 100–5 and 100–6. The mass proved to be a dermoid cyst. (Courtesy of Paul Palefsky, MD, and Barbara Balkin, MD, Department of Radiology, Caritas-St. Elizabeth's Medical Center, Boston.)

TABLE 100–6 MOST FREQUENT CAUSES OF MEDIASTINAL MASSES

Anterior	Middle	Posterior
Thymoma	Lymphoma	Neurogenic tumors
Lymphoma	Cancer	Enteric cysts
Teratogenic tumors	Cysts	Esophageal lesions
Thyroid aneurysms	Aneurysms	Diaphragmatic hernias (Bochdalek)
Parathyroid aneurysms	Hernia (Morgagni)	

Lymphatic tumors (17%) also arise in the anterior mediastinum. Hodgkin's lymphoma (Chapter 197) is the most frequent and carries the best prognosis. Non-Hodgkin's lymphoma (Chapter 196), plasmacytomas (Chapter 198), and angiomatous lymphoid hamartomas with similar clinical features carry a worse prognosis.

Teratomatous tumors, also located in the anterior compartment, account for 10% of mediastinal tumors, and a third of them are malignant. They are embryologically and histologically linked to the thymus. Cystic teratomas are more frequent and may contain squamous cells, hair follicles, sweat glands, cartilage, and linear calcifications.

An intrathoracic goiter (10%) is usually a benign nodular or follicular enlargement of the thyroid gland (Chapter 244). Three fourths of patients complain of stridor, cough, and dyspnea. Most frequently located in the anterior mediastinum, intrathoracic goiters occasionally cause superior vena cava syndrome.

Benign cysts are generally asymptomatic and occur as an incidental radiographic finding. Bronchogenic cysts develop around the paratracheal area or carina and are seen in the middle and posterior compartments; they are filled with liquid and are lined with respiratory epithelium and cartilage but do not communicate with the tracheobronchial tree. Pericardial cysts (Chapter 77) occur in the anterior compartment and cardiophrenic angle; they contain clear liquid and a flattened endothelial or mesothelial lining with a bland fibrous wall. Enteric cysts are located in the posterior mediastinum and are lined by gastric or intestinal epithelium. All cysts may become infected, bleed, or rupture into the mediastinum or pleural cavity.

Vascular tumors may originate in the mediastinum. Vascular hamartomas, lymphangiomas, and hemangiomas are benign tumors, whereas hemangiopericytomas are malignant. Mesenchymal benign (lipoma) or malignant (liposarcoma, mesothelioma, rhabdomyosarcoma, and mesenchymoma) tumors rarely cause mediastinal masses.

Hernias through the diaphragm may also be manifested as mediastinal masses. They may be retrosternal through the foramen of Morgagni, posterolateral through the foramen of Bochdalek, or most commonly

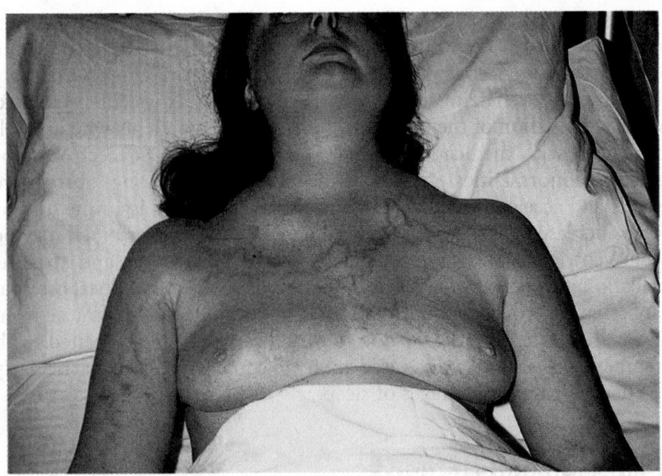

FIGURE 100–8 • Superior vena cava obstruction in bronchial carcinoma. Note the swelling of the face and neck and the development of collateral circulation in the veins of the chest wall. (From Forbes CD, Jackson WF: Color Atlas and Text of Clinical Medicine, 3rd ed. London, Mosby, 2003.)

through the esophageal hiatus. When gas is contained in the herniated organ, the presumptive diagnosis is easily made.

Pneumomediastinum

Air may enter the mediastinum through a tear in the esophagus or tracheobronchial tree or as dissecting air from ruptured alveoli. Tears in the esophagus and tracheobronchial tree commonly have a traumatic origin, whereas alveolar rupture may occur spontaneously or as a complication of artificial ventilation. Air may track to the neck and body and produce subcutaneous emphysema or pneumothorax, or both. The patient complains of retrosternal pain and dyspnea. Subcutaneous emphysema may cause classic crepitus. Auscultation may reveal a crunching sound synchronous with the heartbeat (Hamman's sign). Rarely, cardiac function is compromised. A lateral chest radiograph is usually diagnostic. Simple spontaneous pneumomediastinum generally resolves without treatment. When severe or resulting from organ rupture, surgical drainage and repair are required.

Superior Vena Cava Syndrome

Obstruction of blood flow through the superior vena cava causes dilation of the collateral veins of the upper thorax and neck and edema and congestion of the face (Fig. 100–8); patients may have headache, dyspnea, dysphagia, and wheezes. Malignancy is the most frequent cause of this syndrome, with bronchogenic carcinoma being responsible for more than 70% of cases and lymphoma a distant second. Fibrosing mediastinitis after granulomatous diseases such as histoplasmosis (Chapter 353) or tuberculosis (Chapter 345) or associated with methysergide ingestion can also be seen. Aortic aneurysm (Chapter 78) and a retrosternal thyroid (Chapter 244) are relatively benign causes of superior vena cava syndrome. Because of vessel dilation, invasive procedures are contraindicated. When the obstruction is thought to be caused by tumor, effort must be made to obtain tissue elsewhere. Irradiation, chemotherapy, or stent placement should be initiated before attempts are made to obtain mediastinal tissue.

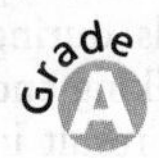

1. Evans TW: International Consensus Conferences in Intensive Care Medicine: Non-invasive positive pressure ventilation in acute respiratory failure. Organised jointly by the American Thoracic Society, the European Respiratory Society, the European Society of Intensive Care Medicine, and the Societe de Reanimation de Langue Française. Intensive Care Med 2001;27:166–178.
2. Maskell N, Davies C, Nunn A, et al: U.K. controlled trial of intrapleural streptokinase for pleural infection. N Engl J Med 2005;351:865–874.

SUGGESTED READINGS

ATS/ERS Statement of Respiratory Muscle Testing. Am J Respir Crit Care Med 2002;166:518–624. *Review of the available tests of respiratory muscle function.*

Giacomini M, Iapichino G, Armani S, et al: How to avoid and manage a pneumothorax. J Vasc Access 2006;7:7–14. *Clear lessons on safe techniques.*

Laghi F, Tobin M: Disorders of the respiratory muscles. Am J Respir Crit Care Med 2003;168:10–48. *The pathophysiology of respiratory muscle dysfunction.*

Maskell NA, Butland RJ: Pleural Diseases Group, Standards of Care Committee, British Thoracic Society. BTS guidelines for the investigation of a unilateral pleural effusion in adults. Thorax 2003;58:ii8–ii17. *Consensus guidelines.*

Schiza S, Siafakas NM: Clinical presentation and management of empyema, lung abscess and pleural effusion. Curr Opin Pulm Med 2006;12:205–211. *A practical overview.*

Tan C, Sedrakyan A, Browne J, et al: The evidence on the effectiveness of management for malignant pleural effusion: A systematic review. Eur J Cardiothorac Surg 2006;29:829–838. *A systematic review.*

101 OBSTRUCTIVE SLEEP APNEA-HYPOPNEA SYNDROME

Robert C. Basner

Definition

Obstructive sleep apnea-hypopnea syndrome (OSAHS) is a chronic condition of cyclic obstruction of the upper airway during sleep combined with associated symptoms or signs of disturbed sleep (Chapter 429), the most common being excessive daytime sleepiness. A frequency of at least five obstructive events per hour of sleep is a minimal criterion for diagnosing OSAHS in adults, and its presence carries an increased risk for cardiovascular and neurocognitive sequelae regardless of the presence of symptoms.

Epidemiology

OSAHS is under-recognized by clinicians and under-reported by patients, and it is estimated that in the vast majority of adults, moderate to severe OSAHS remains undiagnosed. In adults, OSAHS is characteristically found in overweight persons, although anatomic (upper airway, craniofacial, and chest wall) and ventilatory abnormalities may also predispose to development of the syndrome. The presence of at least five obstructive events per hour of sleep has been found in 9 to 28% of persons without specific risk factors for or symptoms of OSAHS. Its prevalence appears to be much greater in men than women; for example, at least five obstructive events per hour have been found to be present in 27% and 9% of middle-aged community dwelling men and women, respectively. Postmenopausal and obese women tend to have a similar prevalence as their male counterparts. Populations that carry a particularly high prevalence of OSAHS include individuals older than 60 years; patients with systemic hypertension, particularly those with poorly controlled hypertension (Chapter 66); patients who have had strokes (Chapter 431); patients with heart failure (Chapter 57); and patients with medically refractory epilepsy (Chapter 426). African Americans, particularly those younger than 25 and older than 65 years, adult Hispanics, and Asians have been found to have a higher incidence or greater severity of OSAHS than whites. There is a strong familial disposition to OSAHS such that the presence of OSAHS in a given patient more than doubles the chance of family members having the disorder when compared with controls. Mean annual medical costs for untreated OSAHS patients are almost double that of controls. It is estimated that untreated OSAHS costs the United States $3.4 billion annually in excess health costs.

Pathobiology

Genetics

Most of the identified candidate genes linked to OSAHS are shared with linkages to body mass index (BMI). Similarly, most polymorphism expression related to OSAHS appears to be linked to characteristics that are likely to predispose to the disorder, including obesity, serotonin transport, and craniofacial structure, or to correlates of the disorder, such as elevated blood pressure. Therefore, no specific genetic transmission for OSAHS has been identified to date.

Pathogenesis

OSAHS characteristically involves complete or partial closure of the collapsible segments of the pharynx, including the velopharynx, oropharynx, and hypopharynx. Obstructive apnea is defined by absent airflow for at least 10 seconds associated with continued ventilatory effort. Partial obstruction is referred to as "hypopnea" and is recognized functionally by a discrete decrease rather than cessation of airflow through the upper airway for at least 10 seconds associated with either a pathologic decrease in the oxygen saturation of hemoglobin (Sao_2) or an abrupt arousal from sleep. Hypopnea is considered obstructive when a progressive pattern of upper airway flow limitation or crescendo snoring (or both) is apparent.

Both excess weight and increasing weight are closely linked to the development of OSAHS and worsening of existing OSAHS in adults. For example, gain of as little as 1% of body weight has been associated with an increased apnea plus hypopnea per hour index (AHI) of 3%; conversely, weight loss of as little as 1% is associated with a similarly decreased AHI (see Treatment). Anatomic and physiologic explanations exist for the contribution of increased weight to OSAHS, including restriction of chest wall movement with resultant mechanical and reflex upper airway narrowing, increased compliance and narrowing of the upper airway, ventilatory instability, and impaired ability to compensate for increased upper airway resistance at sleep onset.

The final common pathway in each obstructive event is attainment of a critical pharyngeal closing pressure; that is, because of inherent anatomic and respiratory control in a given patient, the threshold for upper airway dilator activity sufficient to allow patency of the upper airway appears to be exceeded as the patient transitions into sleep. Once collapsed, the pharynx is more difficult to expand during the next inspiratory effort, thereby resulting in the characteristic progressive generation of increasingly forceful inspiratory effort against the obstructed upper airway with resultant increasingly negative intrathoracic pressure. An abrupt and transient change in the state of sleep (so-called arousal) characteristically follows, probably because of a complex set of interactions at the brain stem level, associated with subsequent reopening of the airway. Transition into sleep typically follows after several hyperpneic breaths, and this cycling of blood gases and behavioral state interferes with the respiratory controllers' need to find a set point during sleep, which results in exaggerated and asynchronous cycling of neural input to the diaphragm and upper airway muscles. Thus, OSAHS is not strictly an "anatomic" or "peripheral" disorder, but rather a form of periodic breathing.

The inherent importance of respiratory periodicity in the pathogenesis of OSAHS is apparent in the distinct responses of patients to different stages of sleep (Chapter 429). The transition into "light" stages of sleep, termed stages 1 and 2 non–rapid eye movement (NREM) sleep, is characterized by a tendency to arousal and cyclic sleep/wake cycles, and these stages are most likely to demonstrate the periodic obstructive events characteristic of OSAHS. In contrast, "deep" NREM sleep, termed stages 3 and 4 or slow-wave sleep, is characteristically a time of relatively regular central nervous system output with a decreased tendency to arousal, regularization of breathing, and a relative paucity of obstructive events, even though it is associated with generally increased upper airway resistance when compared with light NREM sleep. During rapid eye movement (REM) sleep, descending inhibition of inspiratory motor neurons to accessory respiratory muscles may lead to severe alveolar hypoventilation. Severe hypoxemia, probably caused by an exaggerated ventilation-perfusion mismatch and lengthening of obstructive events, is a characteristic finding during REM sleep in patients with OSAHS.

Pathophysiology

With each obstructive event, the combination of progressive asphyxia, generation of increasingly negative intrathoracic pressure, and sudden autonomic and behavioral arousal results in characteristic acute cardiac and cerebrovascular perturbations: increased afterload of both the left and right ventricles, decreased left ventricular compliance, increased pulmonary artery pressure, decreased coronary artery blood flow, and increased myocardial oxygen demand (Chapter 50). The abrupt arousal at the termination of the majority of obstructive events results in sympathetic discharge with peripheral vasoconstriction and an abrupt increase in the heart rate and in systolic and diastolic blood pressure even as cardiac output continues to fall when ventilation resumes after the airway reopens. Accordingly, systemic blood pressure characteristically fluctuates between being low during the apnea and being acutely elevated at the termination of the obstructive event, even in patients who are well controlled with medications while awake (Chapter 66). Electrocardiographic abnormalities include sinus bradycardia during obstructive events and acceleration at arousal; in REM sleep, which is a time of tonically increased vagal tone, sinoatrial and atrioventricular block may be seen. Ventricular and supraventricular ectopy is common, and atrial fibrillation may develop. At the termination of obstructive apnea, cerebral blood flow and oxygenation are decreased. Abrupt transient arousal from sleep at the termination of an obstructive event is associated with fragmented sleep and a decreased ability to consolidate sleep, particularly the deeper, restorative stages of sleep.

Clinical Manifestations

Symptoms and Signs

The cardinal manifestations of OSAHS include loud, chronic snoring, excessive daytime somnolence, and witnessed apneas. Snoring in OSAHS reflects the partially occluded pharynx with vibratory noise from these soft tissues, usually with the mouth opened, and it typically occurs in a crescendo pattern, with a burst of louder noise at resolution of the event. Primary snoring without OSAHS may progress to OSAHS, particularly if the patient gains weight.

OSAHS is first diagnosed in some patients because of apnea or refractory decreases in Sao_2 during surgical or endoscopic procedures that require sedation or anesthesia. In others, the diagnosis is made when hospital staff note nocturnal heart block or arrhythmias.

Excessive Daytime Somnolence

Patients with excessive daytime somnolence fall asleep unexpectedly but often suffer from microsleeps rather than reaching consolidated sleep on such occasions. Excessive daytime somnolence may be quantified by laboratory tests that monitor the propensity to fall asleep during the day or by questionnaires or subjective scales that assess decrements in quality of life and hypersomnolence. Resolution of OSAHS does not necessarily resolve the excessive daytime somnolence completely, thus suggesting the possibility of sustained neurologic perturbation from chronic intermittent hypoxemia. Many patients with significant OSAHS do not complain of excessive daytime somnolence, nor are patients typically aware of their degree of nighttime sleep fragmentation. Mood disorders, including depression and irritability, as well as perturbations in visual memory and working memory, are related to the severity of sleep fragmentation and hypoxemia.

Obstructed Breathing

The bed partner will often describe the patient as suffering from breathing cessation rather than obstructed breathing; close questioning will usually elicit the obstructive nature of the breathing. Patients may be aware of their own snoring or complain of choking or dyspnea, particularly an inability to sleep supine. Morning headache is common, probably because of mechanical effects, as well as intermittent hypercapnia and hypoxemia.

Insomnia and Parasomnia

Insomnia, which is the subjective complaint of difficulty falling asleep or staying asleep (Chapter 429), is associated with the consistent sleep interruption characteristic of the disorder. Transient arousals during sleep may result in confusional parasomnias, such as sleep walking and sleep talking. Arousals and increased work of breathing may result in restless sleep and night sweats. Nocturia often resolves with treatment of OSAHS.

Upper Airway Abnormalities

Nasal congestion, rhinitis, chronic sinusitis, and nasopharyngeal anatomic abnormalities are often associated with OSAHS, as are craniofacial abnormalities such as micrognathia and retrognathia. Large tonsils, redundant soft palate tissue, and a large tongue may all be associated with a "crowded oropharynx," but the precise role of any of these upper airway abnormalities in the pathogenesis of OSAHS is unclear.

Diagnosis

The spectrum of sleep-disordered breathing includes hypoventilation and gas exchange disorders that may worsen with sleep, including nocturnal asthma (Chapter 87), chronic obstructive pulmonary disease (Chapter 88), neuromuscular and chest wall disorders (Chapter 100), and obesity-hypoventilation syndrome (Chapter 239), as well as other disorders in which central apnea (Chapter 429) is prominent (idiopathic central apnea, Cheyne-Stokes respiration with central sleep apnea, and congenital and acquired central alveolar hypoventilation [Chapter 86]). The majority of patients with OSAHS do not hypoventilate while awake, unlike patients with other disorders of hypoventilation.

Algorithms for diagnosing OSAHS include such features as male sex, chronic snoring, higher BMI, advancing age, increased neck circumference, presence of systemic hypertension, and witnessed apnea or struggling to breathe. Other causes of hypersomnia, such as narcolepsy, insufficient sleep, poor sleep hygiene, periodic limb movement disorder, and circadian rhythm disorders such as shift work sleep disorder, must be considered (Chapter 429).

Polysomnography

The definitive diagnostic study is polysomnography (Fig. 101–1), which involves all-night monitoring in a sleep laboratory via electroencephalography, electro-oculography (to determine eye movements during REM sleep), respiratory effort, airflow, Sao_2, estimates of alveolar or arterial carbon dioxide (usually end-tidal or transcutaneous CO_2), electrocardiography, and leg and chin electromyography. Audiovisual recordings help differentiate obstructive from nonobstructive hypopnea and can detect abnormal motor activity that may disrupt sleep and mimic respiratory events.

The severity of OSAHS is generally described by the AHI, which is the number of obstructive events per hour of sleep. A "respiratory disturbance index" may also include obstructive events that did not meet the threshold for hypopnea but nevertheless resulted in a discrete arousal that appeared to be associated with abnormally increased respiratory effort. Indices of oxygen desaturation, such as the frequency of events that result in a decrease in Sao_2 of 4% or more, are also commonly used. However, the clinician cannot rely on a specific set of polysomnographic criteria to define a patient's risk for either cardiovascular or neurocognitive dysfunction. Treatment is indicated for all patients who have an elevated frequency of obstructive events during sleep and who have associated symptoms or signs.

If diagnosis in a sleep laboratory cannot be conducted expeditiously, as an alternative a sleep consultant can arrange for the outpatient use of an autotitrating positive airway pressure (PAP) machine, which continuously self-adjusts the level of positive pressure delivered to the airway on a breath to breath basis in response to upper airway impedance changes. Such monitoring allows immediate diagnosis and treatment of a patient suspected of having severe OSAHS, with a high level of efficacy.

Treatment

Rx

The goal of treatment is to decrease sleep fragmentation and the repetitive asphyxia, cardiovascular stress, and increased work of breathing associated with OSAHS.

Rx

Mechanical Therapy

Positive Airway Pressure

PAP is the mainstay of therapy and the only treatment other than tracheostomy that has consistently been shown to decrease morbidity and mortality. The major equipment is an interface with appropriate headgear or anchoring straps, hosing, and a compact airflow generator that delivers a fixed level of positive pressure to the upper airway and acts as a physiologic splint throughout the respiratory cycle, thereby allowing the patient to achieve normal ventilation, as well as more continuous and deeper sleep. Continuous positive airway pressure (CPAP) does not supply ventilation over and above this splinting; the end-expiratory pressure may, however, result in improved oxygenation.

Prescribing Pap

A prescription for PAP is typically made after therapeutic titration in the sleep laboratory, beginning with minimal CPAP of 2 to 4 cm H_2O and increasing by 1- to 2-cm H_2O increments to the minimum level that eliminates obstructive events and other evidence of increased upper airway resistance and work of breathing (e.g., snoring, use of accessory inspiratory muscles, and thoracoabdominal paradoxical respiration), as well as improves sleep. Typically, CPAP is prescribed in the 8- to 12-cm H_2O range, although it is not uncommon for patients with severe OSAHS to need pressures up to 20 cm H_2O. However, as pressures increase above the 12- to 14-cm H_2O range, the likelihood of air leak and discomfort rise. When titration is not available, CPAP at a level of 10 cm H_2O is about as good a treatment as can be determined from more rigorous in-laboratory titration. Outcomes at 12 weeks, including adherence, are similar whether the use of CPAP is guided by titration at a sleep center, by autotitration using a machine, or by following an algorithm that takes into account the patient's AHI, BMI, and neck circumference. [1]

The first night of CPAP is generally associated with "rebound" of deeper sleep stages (slow-wave NREM sleep and REM sleep), along with amelioration of acute fluctuations in heart rate and blood pressure. Daytime sleepiness and vigilance consistently improve with chronic use of CPAP; diurnal and nocturnal blood pressure and catecholamine levels decrease, whereas left ventricular ejection fraction and diastolic function also improve. [2] PAP does not ameliorate the sleep-disordered breathing itself and must therefore be used nightly rather than intermittently.

Bilevel Pap

In some cases, a more ventilatory mode (generally bilevel PAP, wherein inspiratory pressure is higher than expiratory pressure) may be optimal after the degree of expiratory positive pressure necessary to prevent closure of the airway during expiration is established. Bilevel PAP is particularly useful in hypoventilation syndromes that overlap OSAHS or in very obese patients who continue to have significant hypoventilation or ventilation-perfusion mismatch–related hypoxemia despite CPAP. Bilevel PAP may be delivered with a backup rate, similar to assist/control mode ventilation. However, bilevel PAP is neither better tolerated by patients nor more effective in the vast majority of cases than CPAP is.

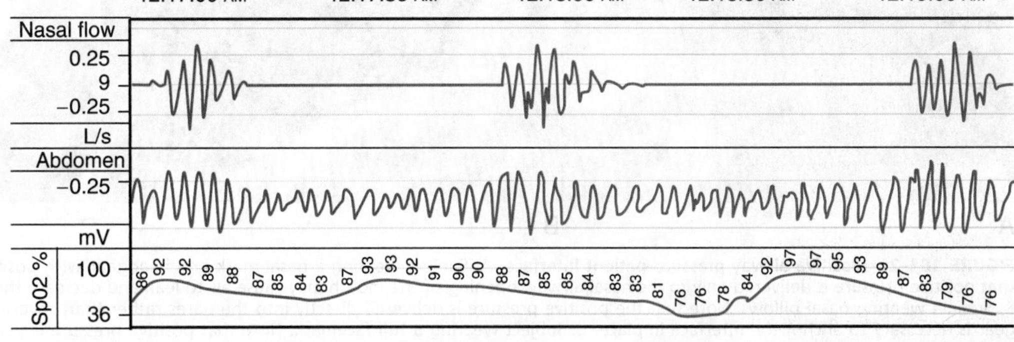

FIGURE 101–1 • Representative polysomnographic tracing of a patient with obstructive sleep apnea during 2 minutes of NREM sleep. Displayed are airflow in the upper airway ("nasal flow") recorded with a nasal pressure transducer, respiratory effort ("abdomen") recorded by inductance plethysmography, and oxygen saturation of hemoglobin (Spo_2) recorded with pulse oximetry.

Rx

Supplemental oxygen may be needed if Sa_{O_2} remains less than 90% despite CPAP. Oxygen is usually added directly to the mask, and higher flow rates are necessary as PAP levels increase, particularly if bilevel PAP is being used.

Pap-Patient Interface

The choice of interface is important for achieving optimal efficacy and adherence of nasally delivered PAP. Aside from many different shapes, sizes, and consistencies of nasal masks (Fig. 101–2A), there are flexible nasal "pillows" (see Fig. 101–2B) that fit directly into the nares, thereby avoiding the discomfort of a mask over the nose, particularly in claustrophobic patients, and avoiding pain and pressure at the bridge of the nose and over the upper teeth. Although nasal CPAP is most commonly used, nasal delivery is often ineffective because of nasal congestion, nasopharyngeal anatomic abnormalities, or inability of the patient to keep the mouth closed, thereby allowing air to leak from the mouth so that ineffective pressure is delivered to the collapsible airway. Full facemasks (see Fig. 101–2C) improve the efficacy in such situations, but gastrointestinal bloating is a common side effect, and the risk of vomiting and aspiration is a theoretical concern. Humidification may be added directly to the circuit and often greatly improves comfort and adherence. The patient must be vigilant to keep the interface on properly throughout sleep, particularly after changes in position.

Adherence and Outcome

Adherence with PAP is generally similar to that of treatments for other chronic medical disorders, although most studies suggest that CPAP is not consistently used optimally for maximizing restorative sleep. Adherence may be improved by education and strategies to address the specific issues of individual patients. Treatment with PAP can be objectively monitored by tracking the amount of time that physiologically successful PAP levels are delivered, as well as the residual number of obstructive events.

Rx

Oxygen

Oxygen alone may be successful in ameliorating hypoxemia in OSAHS and in some cases may improve sleep quality. However, such treatment alone may lengthen apneas and cause paradoxical worsening of Sa_{O_2} with obstruction; furthermore, such treatment does not reliably improve sleep fragmentation. Therefore, prescription of oxygen for suspected OSAHS and documented nocturnal hypoxemia without nocturnal monitoring is not recommended.

Other Mechanical Ways to Relieve or Bypass Obstruction

Mandibular advancement devices, or devices worn in the mouth that protrude the jaw forward, are generally more useful in milder forms of OSAHS and in patients with predominantly supine OSAHS. Such devices are less effective than CPAP for decreasing AHI and symptoms. Moreover, long-term adherence with these devices appears to be low.

General Measures

Sleep Positioning

Sleep positioning may be of definitive benefit in many patients who tend to have more severe obstruction when supine or prone than in lateral decubitus positions. Treatment of chronic nasal congestion and inflammation with nasal steroids, saline washes, and systemic antihistamine/decongestant regimens may ameliorate OSAHS in many cases.

Weight Loss

Weight loss is a primary treatment in an overweight patient in whom OSAHS has been diagnosed because it not only may definitively affect the severity of the breathing disorder during sleep but may also contribute to regression of the deleterious metabolic and cardiovascular perturbations associated with OSAHS. In obese patients with a BMI greater than 35 kg/m^2, loss of weight in the range of 24 to 80% of excess weight, whether achieved medically

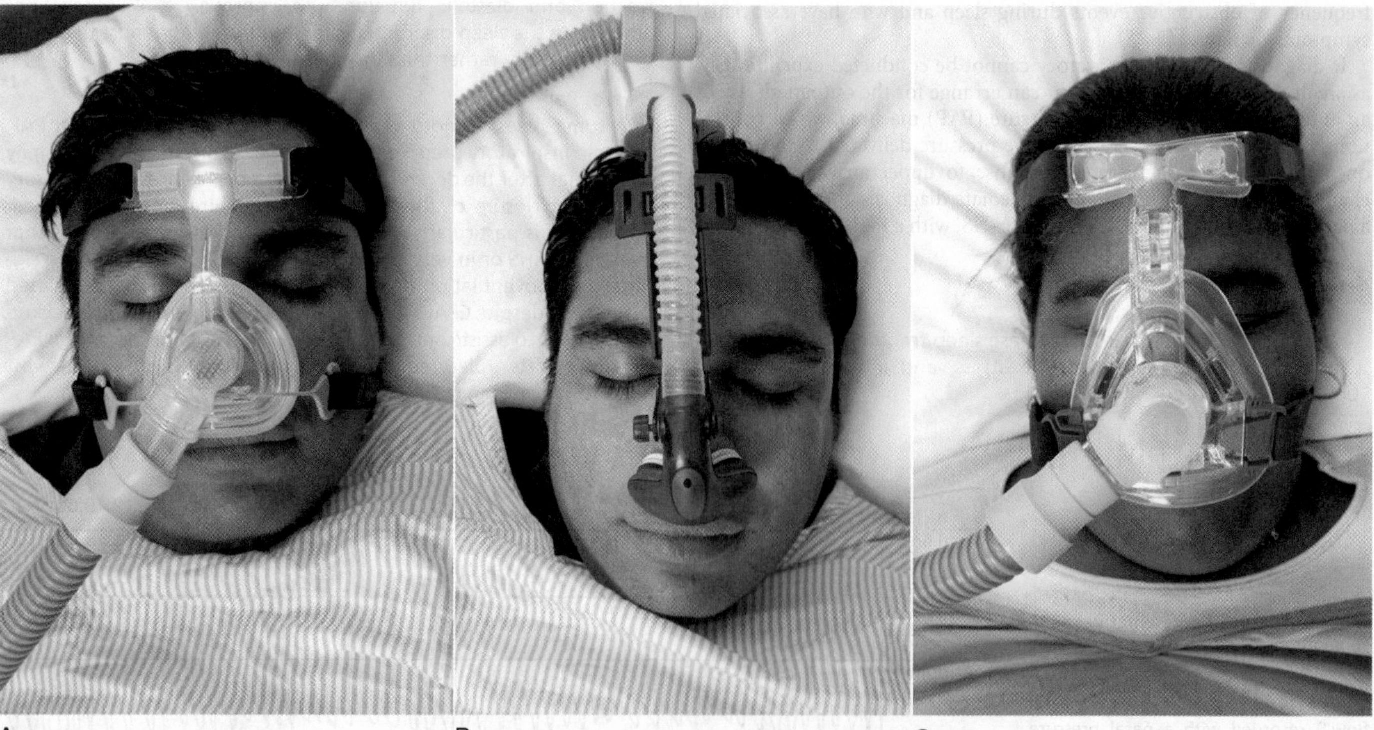

FIGURE 101–2 • Positive airway pressure–patient interface. A, Subject wearing a nasal mask and headgear with positive airway pressure being delivered. Note that positive pressure is delivered only to the nasal airway; opening of the mouth may cause air to leak and decrease the efficacy of the positive pressure regimen. **B,** Subject wearing nasal pillows. Note that the positive pressure is delivered directly into the nares rather than covering the nose or mouth; only minimal headgear is necessary to anchor the interface in place. **C,** Subject wearing a full facemask. Note that positive pressure is delivered to both the nose and mouth based on the subject's own breath to breath partitioning of nasal and oral airflow.

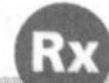

or surgically, ameliorates OSAHS so that CPAP may be decreased or discontinued. Even a decrease in BMI from a mean of 38 to 35 kg/m^2, representing a weight loss of about 8%, results in a significant decrease in the number of apneic-hypopneic events per hour and the degree of O_2 desaturation during sleep. Weight loss has also been associated with regression of many of the metabolic and cardiovascular disturbances associated with OSAHS.

The safety and efficacy of bariatric surgery for weight loss in patients with OSAHS are unclear, although weight loss by any means decreases the severity of OSAHS. Nevertheless, bariatric surgery is not considered first-line therapy at the present time.

Surgery

Tracheostomy

Tracheostomy, which bypasses the site of upper airway obstruction, decreases morbidity and mortality and improves blood gas abnormalities in OSAHS. However, tracheostomy is currently reserved for the most severe cases and for patients whose concomitant obesity-hypoventilation syndrome does not respond to less invasive forms of PAP.

Uvulopalatopharyngoplasty

Palatal procedures, including surgical uvulopalatopharyngoplasty, are not generally curative, particularly in obese patients, and often are no better than mandibular devices. Radio frequency volumetric tissue reduction of the palate or tongue (or both), palatal stiffening, and laser-assisted uvuloplasty are not generally first-line treatments but may be physiologically rational in individual patients with craniofacial or florid velopharyngeal or oropharyngeal abnormalities, particularly those who are not obese. Otolaryngologic consultation is particularly useful in identifying nasopharyngeal lesions, including the rare nasopharyngeal neoplasm.

Medical Therapy

Medications

Selective serotonin reuptake inhibitors, including fluoxetine and paroxetine at 20 mg/day for 4 to 6 weeks, have been associated with a decreased apnea index during NREM but not REM sleep in a small number of patients. Respiratory stimulants, including medroxyprogesterone and acetazolamide, in contrast, have not proved to be effective in patients with normal $Paco_2$ levels. Tricyclic antidepressants have had some utility in predominantly REM sleep–associated OSAHS by decreasing the REM volume, although side effects have hindered the use of such agents. Hormone replacement therapy may ameliorate the breathing disorder in postmenopausal women. Promising pharmacologic therapies include adenosine receptor analogues, which may stimulate respiration while decreasing sleep fragmentation, and agents that increase slow-wave sleep, such as gabapentin and its analogues; however, the efficacy of these agents remains to be investigated.

Prognosis

An AHI as low as five per hour has been associated with an increased risk for arterial hypertension, heart failure, stroke, coronary artery disease, and probably pulmonary hypertension independent of any concomitant obesity. Data suggest that untreated OSAHS is associated with increased mortality, particularly in patients with an apnea index of at least 20 events per hour of sleep. Patients with OSAHS are at increased risk for sudden death during sleep and suffer a threefold increased risk for morbidity and mortality from motor vehicle accidents. The clinician must advise a patient suspected of having OSAHS of the driving risk, particularly if there is a history of drowsy driving or accidents or if the patient is a frequent or professional driver.

Successful treatment leads to regression of daytime sleepiness. CPAP decreases diurnal and nocturnal blood pressure and biochemical markers of increased cardiovascular risk, and it leads to improvement in left ventricular function and baroreflex sensitivity, [3] as well as a reduction in ventricular ectopy during sleep in patients with heart failure. [4] Seizure control has improved in treated epileptic patients with OSAHS, and subsequent hospitalization may also be reduced. It is not clear, however, whether any treatment fully reverses the increased medical risks of patients with OSAHS.

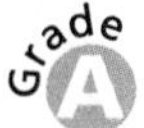

1. Masa JF, Jimenez A, Duran J, et al: Alternative methods of titrating continuous positive airway pressure. A large multicenter study. Am J Respir Crit Care Med 2004;170:1218–1224.
2. Arias MA, Garcia-Rio F, Alonso-Fernandez A, et al: Obstructive sleep apnea syndrome affects left ventricular diastolic function. Circulation 2005;112:375–383.
3. Kaneko Y, Floras J, Usui K, et al: Cardiovascular effects of continuous positive airway pressure in patients with heart failure and obstructive sleep apnea. N Engl J Med 2003;348:1233–1241.
4. Ryan CM, Usui K, Floras JS, et al: Effect of continuous positive airway pressure on ventricular ectopy in heart failure patients with obstructive sleep apnoea. Thorax 2005;60:781–785.

SUGGESTED READINGS

Caples SM, Gami AS, Somers VK: Obstructive sleep apnea. Ann Intern Med 2005;142:187–197. *A comprehensive overview.*

Hailey D, Jacobs P, Mayers I, et al: The current status of autotitrating continuous positive airway pressure systems in the management of obstructive sleep apnea. Can Respir J 2005;12:271–276. *A comprehensive review of the use of autotitrating CPAP.*

Hunsaker DH, Riffenburgh RH: Snoring significance in patients undergoing home sleep studies. Otolaryngol Head Neck Surg 2006;134:756–760. *Percent time snoring during sleep and loudness of snoring correlated with measures of severity of OSAHS.*

Mulgrew AT, Fox N, Ayas NT, et al: Diagnosis and initial management of obstructive sleep apnea without polysomnography: A randomized validation study. Ann Intern Med 2007;146:157–166. *In high-risk patients, treatment with CPAP and ambulatory oximetry was as good as screening polysomnography in terms of 3-month outcomes.*

102 SURGICAL APPROACH TO LUNG DISEASE

John J. Reilly, Jr., and Steven J. Mentzer

The role of surgery in the diagnosis and treatment of lung disease has expanded greatly as lung transplantation has gained acceptance as a therapeutic option for selected patients with advanced lung disease. In addition, the concept of surgery to reduce lung volume in patients with emphysema has been reintroduced and is an area of active clinical investigation. Minimally invasive thoracic surgery has also created new options for lung biopsy and pulmonary resection.

LUNG TRANSPLANTATION

Human lung transplantation was first attempted in the 1960s, but little success was achieved until the availability of more effective immunosuppressive drugs (cyclosporine) and improved surgical techniques in the early 1980s. The annual number of lung transplant procedures increased steadily from 1982 through 1995 but has increased modestly over the last 9 years to the current level of about 1700 transplants per year.

Types of Transplants

Currently, four types of lung transplantation procedures are performed.

Single-Lung Transplantation

Single-lung transplantation is typically performed through a posterolateral thoracotomy incision and requires three anastomoses: the mainstem bronchus, pulmonary artery, and pulmonary veins/left atrium. The contralateral lung is not removed, so single-lung transplantation is not performed in patients with bilaterally infected lungs (e.g., patients with cystic fibrosis).

Bilateral Lung Transplantation

Bilateral lung transplantation was initially performed as an en bloc procedure but is currently performed in a sequential fashion that is functionally equivalent to two single-lung transplantations completed during a single operation, most commonly through a transverse sternotomy ("clamshell") incision. It requires six anastomoses: both mainstem bronchi, both pulmonary arteries, and both sets of pulmonary veins. It is the procedure of choice for patients with bilaterally infected lungs and is also performed in certain patients with emphysema, primary pulmonary hypertension, and other diseases.

Heart-Lung Transplantation

Heart-lung transplantation was initially the most common type of lung transplant procedure but is now performed infrequently (approximately 75 cases in 2003). It is an en bloc procedure with right atrial, aortic, and distal tracheal anastomoses. It is performed in patients with advanced lung disease and coexistent cardiac disease, such as those with Eisenmenger's syndrome (Chapter 68) who have uncorrectable intracardiac defects, end-stage lung disease, and irreversible cor pulmonale, or in patients who have advanced lung disease and left ventricular dysfunction as a result of coronary artery disease.

Living Donor Lobar Transplantation

The most recently introduced lung transplant procedure is *living donor lobar transplantation.* This procedure involves the removal of a lower lobe from each of two living donors, with the implantation of one in each hemithorax of the recipient in a manner similar to bilateral lung transplantation.

Indications

The most common indications for transplantation are diseases or conditions that share the following common features: they produce extreme disability in affected patients, they are unresponsive to medical therapy, and they are responsible for limited life expectancy in affected patients (Table 102–1). With the exception of a small number of cases of sarcoidosis and lymphangioleiomyomatosis, the original lung disease does not recur after lung transplantation.

Evaluation of Potential Transplant Recipients

The ideal candidate for lung transplantation has lung disease unresponsive to medical therapy but is in otherwise good health. In contrast to cardiac transplantation (Chapter 82), patients who are critically ill are not usually appropriate candidates for lung transplantation. Patients who experience critical illness as a result of lung disease often have poor nutritional status, coexistent major organ dysfunction, refractory infection, or other contraindications to transplantation (Table 102–2). Older patients have higher mortality after transplantation, which has led to the current recommendations that single-lung transplant recipients be younger than 65 years and bilateral transplant recipients be younger than 60 years; nevertheless, policies concerning age limits vary between programs. The specific recommendations for referral for transplant evaluation vary with the underlying disease (Table 102–3). The lung allograft allocation system was changed in May 2005 in the United States to a utility-based system, but the impact of this change on waiting times and the proportion of transplants performed for specific indications remain to be determined.

Post-transplant Issues

Most of the medical issues that patients and physicians face after lung transplantation are the consequence of the transplant and post-transplant medication rather than the underlying disease for which the transplantation was performed. Examples include immunosuppression, infections and their prophylaxis, acute allograft rejection, chronic allograft rejection, and nonpulmonary complications of transplantation.

Immunosuppression

The standard chemotherapeutic regimen for immunosuppression after lung transplantation consists of cyclosporine or tacrolimus, azathioprine or mycophenolate mofetil, and corticosteroids. Conclusive data demonstrating the superiority of the newer agents over cyclosporine or azathioprine are not available, but most centers use a regimen of prednisone (typically beginning at 60 mg/day and tapering over a period of several months to 5 to 10 mg/day), tacrolimus (dosing based on trough measurements of drug level), and mycophenolate mofetil (typically 1 g twice daily indefinitely) as their standard regimen. Some centers add an antilymphocyte antibody preparation in the first days after transplantation, although this addition has not been demonstrated to improve outcome. Experience with rapamycin is limited, but reports of airway complications associated with its use have limited its prescription.

Infections and Prophylaxis after Lung Transplantation

Lung transplant recipients are at high risk for bacterial, viral, fungal, and protozoal infections; infections are the leading causes of death during the early post-transplant period. Predisposing factors include the susceptibility of the allograft after ventilator-induced damage, severing of lymphatic drainage at the time of the procedure, and ischemia or reperfusion injury (or both). Additionally, patients are pharmacologically immunosuppressed, are in a catabolic state, have impaired defenses as a result of endotracheal intubation, and have arterial and central venous catheters, chest tubes, and a large surgical incision.

TABLE 102–2 CONTRAINDICATIONS TO LUNG TRANSPLANTATION

ABSOLUTE CONTRAINDICATIONS

Major organ dysfunction (other than lung)
Recent active malignancy
Infection with human immunodeficiency virus
Hepatitis B antigen positivity
Hepatitis C with histologic evidence of active liver disease
Active substance abuse (including cigarettes)
Severe musculoskeletal disease affecting the thorax

RELATIVE CONTRAINDICATIONS

Poor nutritional status (<70% or >130% of ideal body weight)
Symptomatic osteoporosis
Colonization with fungi, atypical mycobacteria, or pan-resistant bacteria
Requirement for invasive ventilation
Psychosocial problems likely to affect the outcome adversely
High-dose (>20 mg of prednisone daily) corticosteroid use

Adapted From Joint Statement of American Society of Transplant Physicians/American Thoracic Society/International Society of Heart and Lung Transplantation: International guidelines for the selection of lung transplant candidates. Am J Respir Crit Care Med 1998;158:335–339.

TABLE 102–1 INDICATIONS FOR LUNG TRANSPLANTATION

Single-Lung Transplant	Patients (%)	Double-Lung Transplant	Patients (%)
COPD	53	Cystic fibrosis	32
Idiopathic pulmonary fibrosis	24	Emphysema	23
α_1-Antitrypsin deficiency	8	α_1-Antitrypsin deficiency	9
Primary pulmonary hypertension	1	Primary pulmonary hypertension	7
Other	11	Other	29

COPD = chronic obstructive pulmonary disease.
From Trulock EP, Edwards LB, Taylor DO, et al: Registry of the International Society for Heart and Lung Transplantation: Twenty-second Official Adult Lung and Heart-Lung Transplant Report—2005. J Heart Lung Transplant 2005;24:956–967.

TABLE 102–3 GUIDELINES FOR LUNG TRANSPLANT REFERRAL

Disease	Pulmonary Function	Arterial Blood Gas Values	NYHA Class	Other Considerations
Chronic obstructive lung disease	FEV_1 <25% of predicted	PCO_2 >55 mm Hg		Pulmonary hypertension, progressive deterioration
Cystic fibrosis	FEV_1 <30% of predicted or rapid decline	PCO_2 >50 mm Hg or PO_2 <55 mm Hg		Increasing admissions or rapid deterioration
Idiopathic pulmonary fibrosis	VC <60% of predicted or DLCO <50% of predicted	Exertional desaturation		Lack of response to therapy
Pulmonary hypertension			Functional class III or IV despite vasodilator therapy	CI, <2 L/min/m²; RAP, >15 mm Hg; mean PAP, >55 mm Hg
Eisenmenger's syndrome			Functional class III or IV	

CI = cardiac index; FEV_1 = forced expiratory volume in 1 second; NYHA = New York Heart Association; PAP = pulmonary artery pressure; RAP = right atrial pressure; VC = vital capacity.
Adapted from Joint Statement of American Society of Transplant Physicians/American Thoracic Society/International Society of Heart and Lung Transplantation: International guidelines for the selection of lung transplant candidates. Am J Respir Crit Care Med 1998;158:335–339.

In the first 3 months after transplantation, bacterial infections are responsible for most deaths. In approximately a third of patients, pneumonia is diagnosed in the first weeks after transplantation, with gram-negative organisms being the etiology in 75% of cases. Colonization and recurrent infections, usually with *Pseudomonas* species, often develop in patients with chronic rejection.

Among potential viral pathogens, *cytomegalovirus* (CMV) is the most important in lung transplant recipients. Seronegative patients who receive an allograft from a seropositive donor are at particularly high risk for the development of a clinically significant CMV infection. Seronegative patients who have a seronegative donor are at low risk for infection, as long as they are treated with seronegative blood products. The CMV syndrome includes fever, bone marrow suppression, hepatitis, enteritis, and pneumonitis. Most programs use prophylactic ganciclovir or valganciclovir in patients at risk, although the optimal dosing regimen and duration of treatment are as yet undetermined.

Epstein-Barr virus (EBV) has been associated with the development of post-transplant lymphoproliferative disorder. *Herpes simplex* infections are relatively unusual, in part because of the standard use of prophylactic antiviral medication (valganciclovir or acyclovir). There are reports of *paramyxovirus* and *respiratory syncytial virus* infection after lung transplantation.

Aspergillus species are the most common cause of invasive fungal infection. Predisposing factors for such infection include preoperative colonization with *Aspergillus*, stenotic airways, or the presence of an airway stent.

Because of the nature of the immunosuppressive chemotherapeutic regimen used, patients are at high risk for infection by the protozoan *Pneumocystis carinii*. The use of trimethoprim-sulfamethoxazole prophylaxis (typically 1 double-strength tablet three times weekly indefinitely) has virtually eliminated *Pneumocystis* pneumonia.

Acute Rejection

Histologically, the initial manifestation of acute rejection is a lymphocyte-predominant inflammatory response, usually centered around blood vessels, airways, or both. The vascular inflammation is accompanied by endothelial inflammation, and the lymphocyte infiltration can progress to involve the alveolar walls. By convention, acute rejection is graded from 0 (normal) to 4 (severe), with subclasses defined by the presence or absence of airway inflammation.

The risk for acute allograft rejection is highest in the early months after transplantation and declines with time. Multiple episodes of acute rejection are the major risk factor for the subsequent development of chronic rejection. Because up to 25% of surveillance bronchoscopies reveal asymptomatic rejection, some programs perform surveillance biopsies at regular intervals with the goal of reducing the incidence of chronic rejection; however, the efficacy of this approach has not been established.

Clinically, patients may have fever, cough, and exertional dyspnea. Evaluation may demonstrate rales or rhonchi on chest examination, a decline in pulmonary function by spirometry, leukocytosis, opacities on chest radiography, and exertional desaturation. The clinical manifestation is often indistinguishable from infectious pneumonia, and the clinical impression is accurate in only 50% of cases. Bronchoscopy with bronchoalveolar lavage or transbronchial biopsy (or both) is commonly needed to clarify the diagnosis.

Treatment of acute rejection most often consists of high-dose corticosteroids (typically, 1 g/day of methylprednisolone [Solu-Medrol] administered intravenously for 3 days). In patients with persistent or recurrent acute rejection, therapeutic strategies include antilymphocyte antibodies, changing maintenance immunosuppressive drugs, and other attempts to augment immunosuppression.

Chronic Rejection

Pathobiology

The bronchiolitis obliterans syndrome is thought to be a manifestation of chronic rejection. Risk factors for development of the syndrome include the number of acute rejection episodes and, in some series, previous symptomatic CMV infection. Evidence supporting the conclusion that it is a manifestation of chronic rejection includes the association with the number of acute rejection episodes, the association with donor or recipient HLA locus mismatch, the similarity to the syndrome seen after bone marrow transplantation (graft-versus-host disease), and laboratory evidence of donor-specific alloreactivity in certain allograft recipients.

Pathologically, "early" lesions demonstrate inflammation and disruption of the epithelium of small airways, followed by growth of granulation tissue into the airway lumen and subsequent complete or partial obstruction. The granulation tissue then organizes in a stereotypical pattern with resultant fibrosis that obliterates the lumen of the airway.

Clinical Manifestations

Clinically, bronchiolitis obliterans is accompanied by nonspecific symptoms. Progressive exertional breathlessness typically develops, and pulmonary function testing usually demonstrates evidence of progressive airflow obstruction. Bronchiolitis obliterans is classified according to the forced expiratory volume in 1 second (FEV_1): 0 (no significant abnormality) if FEV_1 is greater than 80% of baseline; 1 (mild) if FEV_1 is 65 to 80% of baseline; 2 (moderate) if FEV_1 is 50 to 65% of baseline; and 3 (severe) if FEV_1 is 50% or less of baseline. In early stages, chest radiography is notable only for hyperinflation, but it may show bronchiectasis as the syndrome progresses. Later stages of bronchiolitis obliterans may include a syndrome of bronchiectasis with chronic productive cough and airway colonization with *Pseudomonas* species.

Diagnosis

The diagnosis of bronchiolitis obliterans is made on both clinical and pathologic grounds. Transbronchial biopsy has a low yield for demonstrating histologic evidence of bronchiolitis obliterans, but when such evidence is seen, it is diagnostic. In patients with a compatible clinical syndrome, exclusion of anastomotic stenosis and occult pulmonary infection is sufficient to establish the diagnosis.

Treatment

Rx

A variety of types of therapy have been tried, including pulse corticosteroids, antilymphocyte antibodies, total lymphoid irradiation, photopheresis, and nebulized cyclosporine, but none has been clearly established as effective. Uncontrolled reports suggest that azithromycin may slow progression, as may surgical fundoplication in patients with documented gastroesophageal reflux. Most patients with bronchiolitis obliterans experience a progressive decline in pulmonary function despite augmentation of immunosuppression.

Prognosis

Bronchiolitis obliterans is the leading cause of late mortality after lung transplantation.

Nonpulmonary Medical Complications of Lung Transplantation

Most of the nonpulmonary medical complications that arise in patients after lung transplantation are the result of immunosuppressive therapy. One or more of these complications develop in virtually all lung transplant recipients.

Osteoporosis is common because of the long-term use of corticosteroids and cyclosporine. Bone density should be monitored periodically, and pharmacologic therapy should be instituted if excessive bone loss is identified (Chapter 265).

Chronic renal insufficiency is common and is the result of therapy with cyclosporine or tacrolimus, both of which affect afferent vascular tone in the kidneys and result in an average 50% drop in the glomerular filtration rate in the 12 months after lung transplantation. Hypertension is also common and is caused by corticosteroids and cyclosporine. Calcium-channel blockers, which are often used to treat hypertension, raise serum cyclosporine levels; appropriate monitoring and dose adjustment are needed when starting such therapy. Both corticosteroids and tacrolimus contribute to the development of diabetes mellitus and hyperlipidemia.

Organ transplantation is associated with an increased incidence of malignancy, thought to be due to pharmacologic immunosuppression and alteration in immune surveillance. Patients are at increased risk for lymphoproliferative malignancies and other types of cancer. *Posttransplant lymphoproliferative disorders* occur in about 4% of patients after organ transplantation; most are associated with EBV. These syndromes can be polyclonal or monoclonal. Reduction in immunosuppression is sometimes therapeutic in those with polyclonal disease. The prognosis in patients with monoclonal disease is poor, with little response to modification of immunosuppression or antineoplastic chemotherapy. Patients are also at increased risk for skin, cervical, anogenital, and hepatobiliary malignancy after solid organ transplantation.

Outcomes after Lung Transplantation

One-year survival rates after lung transplantation have improved significantly over time. The current approximately 8 to 10% annual mortality rate largely reflects the effects of bronchiolitis obliterans on patient survival. Median survival after lung transplantation is approximately 4 years (Fig. 102–1).

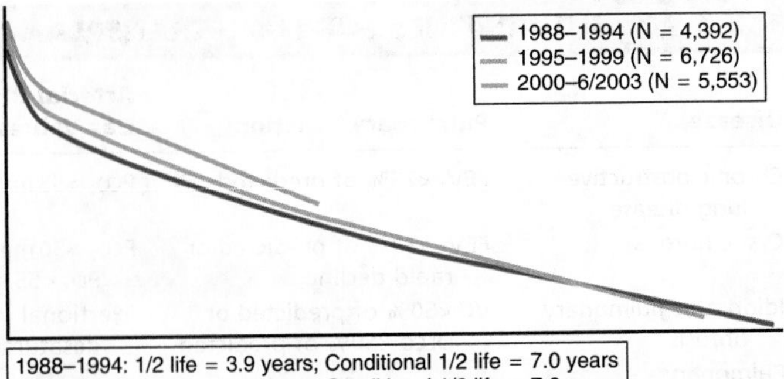

FIGURE 102–1 • Survival after lung transplantation. Kaplan-Meier survival by era for adult lung transplantations performed between January 1988 and June 2003. Conditional half-life is the time to 50% survival for the subset of recipients who were alive at 1 year after transplantation. (From Trulock EP, Edwards LB, Taylor DO, et al: Registry of the International Society for Heart and Lung Transplantation: Twenty-second Official Adult Lung and Heart-Lung Transplant Report—2005. J Heart Lung Transplant 2005;24:956–967.)

LUNG VOLUME REDUCTION SURGERY

Types of Lung Volume Reduction Surgery

A variety of approaches may be taken in the common goal of reducing lung volume by about 30%. The current concept is that physiologic benefit results from increasing lung elastic recoil and resizing of the lung in relation to the chest wall. In the absence of a specific contraindication, bilateral lung volume reduction surgery is currently the procedure of choice. Currently favored techniques include stapled resection of peripheral lung tissue, with or without the use of exogenous material to buttress the suture lines, via either a median sternotomy or thoracoscopic approach. Early clinical trials of endobronchial approaches, both mechanical and biologic, to lung volume reduction are currently under way.

Evaluation of Potential Candidates for Lung Volume Reduction Surgery

In general terms, the principles of evaluation are similar to those before lung transplantation. In addition, pulmonary hypertension and marked deconditioning are contraindications to lung volume reduction surgery. The ideal candidate has severe airflow obstruction as a result of emphysema but is otherwise in good health. Patients undergo computed tomography (CT), pulmonary function testing (with lung volumes by plethysmography), echocardiography to assess pulmonary artery pressure, and some form of noninvasive screening for significant coronary artery disease. If a candidate appears suitable for lung volume reduction surgery, most programs require completion of a 6- to 10-week course of pulmonary rehabilitation before surgery. After completion of rehabilitation, patients should undergo a cardiopulmonary exercise test to allow assessment of risk and benefit.

The ideal candidate for this procedure has anatomic evidence of emphysema, severe obstruction not reversed by bronchodilators on spirometry, pulmonary artery systolic pressure less than 45 mm Hg, and no significant cardiac, hepatic, or renal disease; in addition, ideal candidates do not smoke cigarettes, have completed pulmonary rehabilitation, have no significant pleural disease, and have not previously undergone thoracic surgery. Contraindications include severe deconditioning (6-minute walk <150 m), use of parenteral corticosteroids (e.g., prednisone >20 mg/day), clinically significant bronchiectasis, pulmonary artery systolic pressure greater than 45 mm Hg, or need for invasive mechanical ventilation. Hypercapnia, age older than 75 years, marked anatomic deformity of the thorax, and marked pleural scarring are relative contraindications.

Outcomes of Lung Volume Reduction Surgery

The National Emphysema Treatment Trial, a randomized trial of lung volume reduction surgery compared with medical therapy, categorized patients into five groups based on preoperative assessment of functional capacity, physiologic tests, and imaging procedures. Among the 608 patients assigned to surgery, 90-day mortality was 7.9%. The 69 patients who had an FEV_1 less than 20% of predicted and either a homogeneous distribution of emphysema on CT or diffusing capacity less than 20% of predicted had a 29% 90-day mortality, whereas the 90-day operative mor-

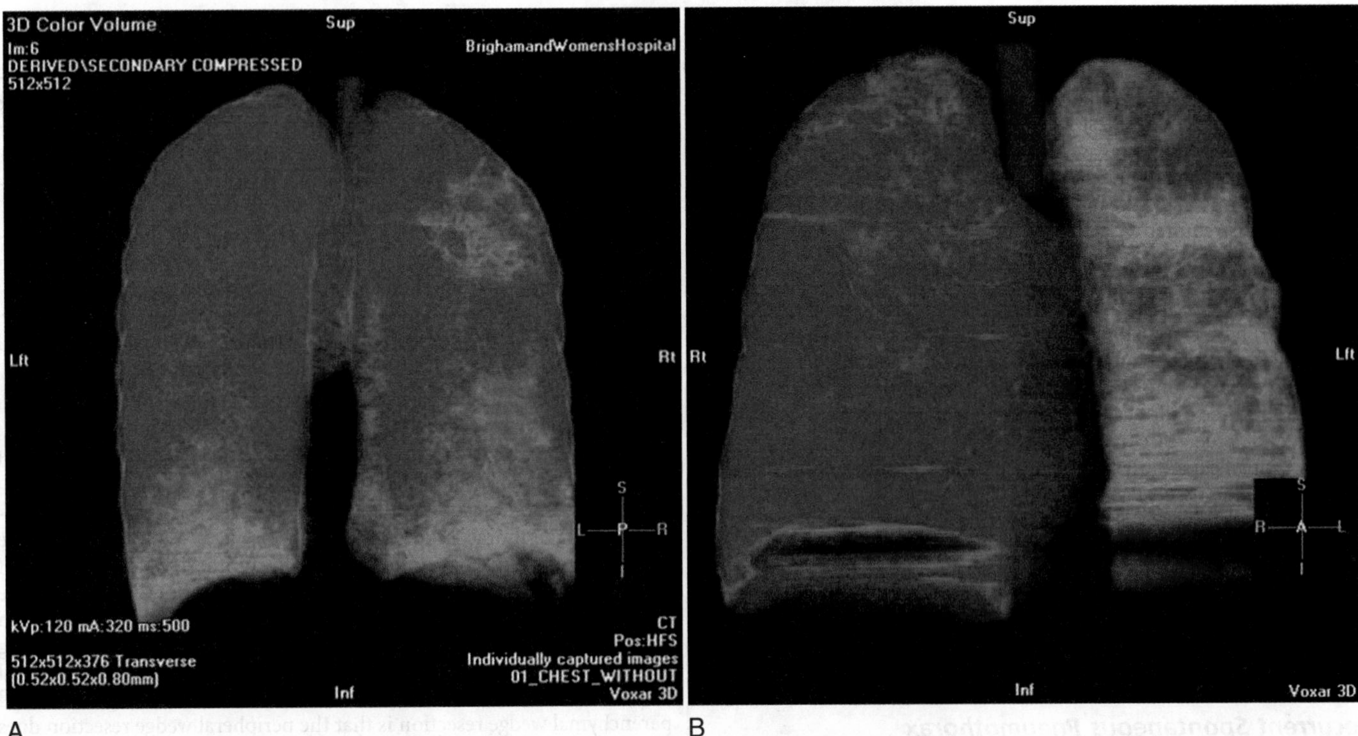

FIGURE 102–2 • Anatomic distribution of emphysema assessed by volume-rendered computed tomography. A, Patient with upper lobe–predominant emphysema (in blue) with preserved basilar lung tissue (in pink). **B,** Patient with a previous right lung transplant. The left lung shows hyperinflation and diffuse emphysema (in blue) with relatively little normal (in pink) lung tissue. (Images and reconstruction courtesy of Andetta Hunsaker and Jean Allen of the Brigham and Women's Hospital 3D and Image Processing Laboratory.)

tality was 5.2% in the remaining patients. The trial identified two characteristics that classify patients into four groups with differing benefits from lung volume reduction surgery: upper lobe distribution of emphysema and exercise capacity. Patients with upper lobe–predominant emphysema (Fig. 102–2) were more likely to experience significant improvements in health-related quality of life and exercise capacity than were patients with a non–upper lobe–predominant pattern. Among patients with "low" preoperative exercise capacity (<25 watts for women, <40 watts for men), there was also a significant reduction in mortality (relative risk [RR] = 0.47) with surgery, whereas mortality was not improved in patients with "high" preoperative exercise capacity. Among patients with non–upper lobe–predominant disease, patients with low exercise capacity had no change in mortality or exercise capacity but were more likely to report improved health-related quality of life. Patients with non–upper lobe distribution and high exercise capacity had no improvement in quality of life or exercise capacity and had increased early mortality (RR = 2.06). Based on these findings and others reported in the literature, lung volume reduction surgery has a reasonable chance of offering physiologic and symptomatic benefit in patients with upper lobe–predominant disease; among those with poor exercise capacity, it may offer a substantial reduction in mortality. Conversely, in patients without upper lobe–predominant emphysema, the most disabled may note some symptomatic benefit, and the more functional are unlikely to benefit and have a higher risk for death with surgery.

THORACOSCOPY AND VIDEO-ASSISTED THORACIC SURGERY

Thoracoscopy was originally limited to pleural biopsies and the drainage of empyemas or pleural effusions (Chapter 100). The recent improvement in light sources and video-optic instrumentation has led to integration of the thoracoscope into most thoracic surgical procedures. The coincident development of advanced endoscopic surgical instrumentation has facilitated the performance of these operations through "minimally invasive" thoracic incisions. Widespread application of the thoracoscope in thoracic surgery has led to the more inclusive term *video-assisted thoracic surgery.*

Video-Assisted Thoracic Surgery Procedures

Video-assisted thoracic surgery generally involves at least three small incisions or "access ports" placed in any intercostal space: one port for the video thoracoscope and two ports for endoscopic instrumentation. Although the access ports are small, the rigid instruments result in trauma to the intercostal nerves and rib periosteum that can result in regional postoperative discomfort.

The size of video-assisted surgical incisions depends on the goals of the procedure and the anatomic findings at the time of exploration. Unexpected pleural symphysis or incomplete lobar fissures may require extension of the incision to facilitate visualization. In patients undergoing anatomic resection, such as segmentectomy or lobectomy, at least one of the incisions is extended to permit extraction of the resected lung from the hemithorax. For most video-assisted thoracic procedures, the operation requires single-lung ventilation. The requirement for selective ventilation excludes many patients with severe pulmonary hypertension or acute respiratory failure. In contrast, many patients with chronic respiratory insufficiency and preserved ventilation-perfusion matching tolerate periods of selective lung ventilation. The ability of many patients with severe emphysema to tolerate selective ventilation has led to the application of thoracoscopy for lung volume reduction surgery. Obliteration of the pleural space, either from infection or as a result of previous surgery, is a relative contraindication to thoracoscopic surgery.

Indications

Benign Lung Disease

A variety of benign lung diseases are manifested as focal parenchymal lesions that require a tissue biopsy for diagnosis. The traditional approach to lung biopsy has been a limited thoracotomy and wedge resection. As an alternative to limited thoracotomy, thoracoscopy has proved to be an effective approach to the diagnosis of localized disorders of the lung. Thoracoscopy can provide a more complete view of the ipsilateral hemithorax, including the visceral, parietal, and mediastinal pleura. In addition, subpleural nodules that are too small to be visualized by preoperative radiography can be identified so that representative biopsy samples can be obtained.

Diffuse lung diseases can often be diagnosed clinically on the basis of the history, characteristic chest radiographs, physical findings, and pulmonary function testing. In cases that require histopathologic confirmation, lung tissue can be obtained by transbronchial biopsy. Thoracoscopy plays a limited role in diffuse lung disease but may be helpful when a large tissue sample is required.

Bullous Lung Disease

Most patients with chronic obstructive pulmonary disease (COPD) (Chapter 88) have diffuse parenchymal disease, but in a small number of patients with COPD, heterogeneous disease with dominant bullae and relatively preserved lung parenchyma can develop. In some cases, rapid expansion of these bullae can be associated with a substantial increase in dyspnea and a decrease in expiratory airflow. Chest radiographs of patients with an expanding bulla frequently demonstrate compression of surrounding lung tissue. Patients with bullous lung disease may also have an infected bulla that requires drainage before definitive surgery.

The indications for thoracoscopic bullectomy are similar to those for lung volume reduction surgery for emphysema. Patients who benefit most from surgery are those who have rapidly progressive symptoms associated with the expansion of a single bullous lesion combined with radiographic demonstration of compression of the surrounding lung parenchyma. Either excision or plication can remove the bullous lesion.

Recurrent Spontaneous Pneumothorax

Primary spontaneous pneumothorax (Chapter 100) is caused by rupture of subpleural blebs of the lung. In more than 95% of cases, the blebs are located at the apex of the lung. In approximately 5% of cases, associated subpleural blebs are found at the margin of the lower lobe, usually in the superior segment. In an otherwise healthy patient with less than a 20% pneumothorax, observation without intervention is appropriate. In patients with larger pneumothoraces, a tube may be necessary to evacuate the pleural air and re-expand the lung. In most cases of primary spontaneous pneumothorax the inflammation associated with a pleural rupture heals, and patients do not have an ongoing air leak after re-expansion of the lung.

Although most spontaneous pneumothoraces are uncomplicated, 3 to 20% of patients with pneumothoraces experience complications such as tension pneumothorax, persistent air leaks, or recurrent pneumothoraces. Patients in whom a second pneumothorax develops have a 70 to 80% chance of a third recurrence within 2 years. The current surgical approach to the treatment of recurrent pneumothoraces is removal of the subpleural blebs. Although some surgeons combine bleb resection with pleurodesis, pleurodesis alone has an unacceptably high rate of recurrence. Subpleural blebs can be effectively removed via a thoracoscopic approach or through a more traditional axillary incision.

Solitary Pulmonary Nodules

Solitary pulmonary nodules, or "coin lesions," defined as spherical lesions less than 3 cm in diameter, occur in the outer third of the lung (Chapter 83). Although most solitary pulmonary nodules do not represent cancer (Chapter 201), the diagnosis must be considered in all patients, especially those with a smoking history.

Transthoracic needle biopsy is associated with low morbidity: post-procedure pneumothorax develops in less than 10% of normal patients and in a slightly higher percentage of patients with emphysema. However, a small but tangible false-negative rate occurs with transthoracic needle biopsies. Furthermore, in the absence of a malignant diagnosis, transthoracic needle biopsies rarely establish a benign diagnosis definitively.

Thoracoscopic resection of a solitary pulmonary nodule is an alternative to transthoracic needle biopsy. Because thoracoscopic resection excises the entire nodule, there are no false-negative diagnoses. Furthermore, thoracoscopy can positively establish a diagnosis of benign disease. The disadvantage of thoracoscopic resection is that it requires general anesthesia; however, the hospital stay is generally less than 24 hours.

Anatomic Lung Resections

In most cases of primary lung cancer (Chapter 201), a standard anatomic resection is indicated to decrease the incidence of local recurrence. Patients who can tolerate general anesthesia and single-lung ventilation for the thoracoscopic resection are generally able to tolerate the segmentectomy or lobectomy. Although thoracoscopic resection of primary lung cancer has not been studied in a randomized setting, the available evidence indicates that a parenchymal margin within 2 cm results in a 20% incidence of local recurrence. In addition, a recent Lung Cancer Study Group report demonstrated a 2.5-fold increase in local recurrence rates with limited resection. Another disadvantage of limited parenchymal wedge resection is that the peripheral wedge resection does not provide segmental or lobar lymph node staging. In patients with isolated regional metastases, this staging information could provide important data to guide possible adjuvant therapy.

Anatomic resections can be performed with a variety of techniques, including video-assisted surgical techniques. The difference between standard lobectomy and thoracoscopic lobectomy has become less distinct in recent years. Thoracoscopic instruments have become commonplace in the resection of a lobe of the lung, even when performed through a standard thoracotomy. The improved visualization and smaller instruments have resulted in smaller incisions and less morbidity.

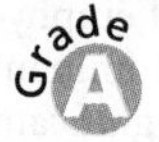

1. NETT Research Group: Patients at high risk of death after lung-volume-reduction surgery. N Engl J Med 2001;345:1075–1083.
2. Fishman A, Martinez F, Naunheim K, et al: A randomized trial comparing lung-volume-reduction surgery with medical therapy for severe emphysema. N Engl J Med 2003;348:2059–2073.

SUGGESTED READINGS

Corris PA, Christie JD: Update in transplantation 2006. Am J Respir Crit Care Med 2007;175:432–435. *A review of current clinical practice and clinical research in lung transplantation.*

Miller JD, Malthaner RA, Goldsmith CH, et al: A randomized clinical trial of lung volume reduction surgery versus best medical care for patients with advanced emphysema: A two-year study from Canada. Ann Thorac Surg 2006;81:314–321. *A small trial, not powered to assess mortality, showed significant improvements from lung volume reduction surgery that persisted for 24 months.*

Section X

Critical Care Medicine

103 APPROACH TO THE PATIENT IN A CRITICAL CARE SETTING

Deborah J. Cook

ASPECTS OF THE INTENSIVE CARE UNIT SETTING

Patients with critical illness in the intensive care unit (ICU) usually require advanced life support with mechanical ventilation, inotropic medications, or dialysis. Morbidity associated with critical illness includes complications of both acute and chronic diseases, nosocomial and iatrogenic consequences, and impaired quality of life among survivors. Critically ill patients are at a higher risk of death than any other hospital population. Accordingly, the goals of critical care are to reduce the morbidity and mortality, to maintain organ function, and to restore health. Unlike many other specialties, critical care medicine is not limited to a particular population, disease, diagnosis, or organ system.

The Intensivist-Led Multidisciplinary Team

Staffing of ICUs with critical care physicians, often referred to as intensivists, who provide mandatory consultation or are responsible for all care is associated with a significantly lower ICU and hospital mortality and a shorter ICU and hospital length of stay. These findings may be due to the on-site availability of trained physicians dedicated to appropriate triage, prevention, diagnosis, monitoring, treatment, and palliation of critically ill patients.

In addition, daily rounds by an ICU physician who leads a multidisciplinary team appears to improve outcomes, probably because leadership, communication, and organizational culture can streamline the process of critical care. These favorable findings may be due to the intensivist-coordinated teamwork of nurses, respiratory therapists, dietitians, and pastoral care workers.

Applying Evidence to Prevent Complications of Critical Illness

Considerable randomized trial evidence about effective preventive and therapeutic interventions has emerged in the ICU during the last decade. However, barriers to the application of this evidence reflect the ICU setting itself, which is characterized by fast-paced decision making by many clinicians, sometimes leading to a lack of responsibility and decision-making authority as well as errors of omission. Effective strategies to encourage implementation of evidence-based recommendations include interactive education, audit and feedback, written or computerized reminders, involvement of local opinion leaders, and multifaceted approaches.

In the ICU setting, preprinted physician orders may help guide but should never dictate management. Sample physician orders for a previously healthy, mechanically ventilated patient with community-acquired pneumonia and the acute respiratory distress syndrome (Table 103–1) emphasize evidence-based management, including low tidal volume ventilation, daily interruption of sedation infusion, early enteral small bowel nutrition, elevation of the head of the bed to decrease aspiration pneumonia, stress ulcer prophylaxis, thromboprophylaxis, and intensive insulin therapy if stress hyperglycemia develops. [1,2]

Fluid Resuscitation

Intravenous fluids to maintain or to restore intravascular volume are an important component of ICU therapy. Crystalloids are readily available and inexpensive, whereas colloids generally require less volume to achieve a specific physiologic goal. Albumin is a naturally occurring protein colloid that increases intravascular oncotic pressure, but its use also carries a small risk of infection. In a randomized trial of 7000 patients allocated to fluid replacement with either normal saline or 4% albumin, mortality was 21% in each group, and there were no differences in organ failure, duration of mechanical ventilation, need for renal replacement therapy, or length of ICU or hospital stay. [3] On the basis of these data, either crystalloid- or albumin-based fluid resuscitation can be recommended for most critically ill patients, although crystalloids may be preferred for patients with head injuries.

Intravenous Sedation and Analgesia

Endotracheal intubation, central venous catheterization, postoperative pain management, and other ICU procedures require that most patients receive sedation, analgesia, or both. In a randomized trial, transient daily interruption of sedatives was associated with a shorter duration of mechanical ventilation and ICU length of stay compared with continuous infusion. [4] A standardized, nurse-implemented approach to sedation and analgesia by use of a validated sedation scale can target specific physiologic goals, shorten the duration of mechanical ventilation, and potentially reduce resource consumption compared with a continuous infusion.

Stress Ulcer Prophylaxis

A complex interplay of systemic and local factors, such as impaired microcirculation, decreased mucosal integrity, and *Helicobacter pylori* infection, may predispose to bleeding for upper gastrointestinal stress ulceration in critically ill patients. In patients who are mechanically ventilated for at least 48 hours or who have a coagulopathy, the incidence of clinically important bleeding is at most 4%; in this group, H_2-receptor antagonists are the only agents that have been shown to reduce the risk of clinically important bleeding in randomized trials. [5] Because this treatment is associated with a trend toward an increased risk of ventilator-associated pneumonia, patients should also receive effective strategies to prevent pneumonia, such as minimal ventilator circuit changes, use of heat and moisture exchangers and filters, and elevation of the head of the bed.

Thromboprophylaxis

Due to immobility, inflammation, and procedures, venous thromboembolism is a common complication of critical illness. Anticoagulant thromboprophylaxis is clearly beneficial in patients who do not have contraindications. Either low-dose unfractionated heparin or low-molecular-weight heparin [6] is suitable, but low-molecular-weight heparin is more effective in orthopedic trauma patients. [7] Mechanical devices (such as antiembolic stockings or pneumatic compression devices) are recommended for patients with contraindications to anticoagulants.

Long-Term Outcomes for Survivors

For survivors of critical illness, triggers for ICU discharge are restoration of hemodynamic stability, ability to protect the airway, and spontaneous breathing. However, biomarkers of inflammation, residual organ dysfunction, and functional disabilities persist in most ICU survivors. Treatments administered in the ICU also have serious sequelae. For example, neuromuscular blockers and corticosteroids may contribute to polyneuropathy. These problems have particularly serious adverse consequences for elderly critically ill patients who are deconditioned before hospitalization.

In addition, anxiety, post-traumatic stress, and major mood disorders are common among patients and their caregivers. Therefore, although ICU discharge and hospital discharge are milestones in a patient's trajectory, critical illness has rarely completely resolved when patients leave the ICU or the hospital. Accordingly, multidimensional rehabilitation may be necessary to optimize the long-term outcomes among survivors of critical illness.

Predictions, Preferences, and End-of-Life Care

Prognostic information, which can help clinicians make better triage and treatment decisions, is generally welcomed by families. Options include the Acute Physiology and Chronic Health Evaluation score, the Simplified Acute Physiology Score, and the Mortality Prediction Model. More recently, specific measures of organ dysfunction at the time of ICU admission (the Logistic Organ Dysfunction score) and serially during the course of critical illness (the Multiple Organ Dysfunction score and the Sequential Organ Failure Assessment score) have helped describe baseline and evolving organ dysfunction. Despite the ubiquity of these scoring

TABLE 103–1 INTENSIVE CARE UNIT BEST PRACTICE ADMISSION ORDERS: A PATIENT WITH COMMUNITY-ACQUIRED PNEUMONIA AND ARDS

Community-Acquired Pneumonia and ARDS Management	Orders	Re-evaluate
Mechanical ventilation	Target tidal volume, 5–7 mL/kg of ideal body weight; pressure control, 14 cm; rate, 12; FIO_2, 0.5; PEEP, 14 cm	As needed
Maintenance fluid	Lactated Ringer's solution, 75 mL/hr IV	As needed
Sedation	Midazolam, 2–8 mg/hr IV, bolus 2–4 mg as needed; daily interruption 0700 until 0900; restart at half prior infusion at 0900 unless instructed otherwise	Daily
Analgesia	Morphine, 1–4 mg IV as needed	As needed
Antibiotics	Moxifloxacin, 400 mg IV once daily; cefotaxime, 1 g IV tid	Daily
Head of bed	45-Degree elevation from horizontal	As needed
Small bowel enteral nutrition	10 mL/hr of a commercial balanced feeding containing about 1 kcal/mL; increase by 10 mL q6h to maximum of 70 mL/hr	Daily
Stress ulcer prophylaxis	Ranitidine, 50 mg IV q8h	Daily
Thromboprophylaxis	Unfractionated heparin, 5000 U SC q12h	Daily
Intensive insulin therapy: if glucose level >200 mg/dL	50 U insulin in 50 mL NS; start 0.5 U/hr, repeat measurement of glucose q1h for 4 hours; treat according to intensive insulin therapy algorithm	As per algorithm
Calibrate capillary glucometer with laboratory glucose values	Every morning	—
Laboratory and radiology tests	Glucose level q4h when stable; arterial blood gas analysis with each ventilator change; other tests as per ICU team	As needed
Monitoring	Electrocardiography, oximetry, arterial catheter, central venous catheter, Foley catheter, as per monitoring protocols	As needed

ARDS = acute respiratory distress syndrome; FIO_2 = fraction of inspired oxygen; ICU = intensive care unit; IV = intravenously; NS = normal saline; PEEP = positive end-expiratory pressure; SC = subcutaneously.

systems, their utility as prognostic tools for individual patients is limited. Furthermore, an intensivist's prediction of survival for a mechanically ventilated patient is generally a better estimate of ICU mortality than are baseline measures of the severity of illness, the use of inotropic agents, or evolving and resolving organ dysfunction scores.

As the population ages and new technologies are developed, use of basic and advanced life support will increase. Because demand for ICU beds is outstripping supply, selection of patients to receive critical care is challenging. Three common but not mutually exclusive approaches to rationing of ICU beds are admission of the sickest patients; admission on a first-come, first-served basis; and triage on the grounds of likely relative benefit. Patients who are refused ICU admission because of a perceived minimum potential to benefit have a three-fold higher hospital mortality than patients who are admitted to the ICU. However, when ICU beds are reduced because of bed closures, admitted patients are generally sicker, are less frequently admitted for monitoring, and have shorter stays without adverse effects. These data suggest that physicians can ration ICU beds to maximize benefit by adapting admission and discharge thresholds.

The prognosis of many critically ill patients improves once they are in the ICU. For others, responses are delayed or not realized, organ dysfunction evolves but does not resolve, and complications arise. Despite the best efforts of the multidisciplinary ICU team, critical illness proves fatal in 5 to 40% of adults. When a therapeutic trial of critical care is started, and particularly when it is failing, it is crucial to discuss prognosis openly with families. Families bring key information to meetings about patients' prior function and preferences. In the shared decision-making model that dominates today, these exchanges often result in plans to withhold or to withdraw basic or advanced life support (Chapter 3).

Mechanical ventilation (Chapter 106) is the most frequent life support administered to and withdrawn from critically ill patients. Withdrawal of mechanical ventilation often precedes death in the ICU, and patients from whom ventilation is withdrawn now have a shorter ICU length of stay than do patients successfully weaned from the ventilator. The traditional biomedical model of withdrawal of life support on the basis of age, severity of illness, and other physiologic characteristics has been replaced by a contemporary life support model that considers the patient's values as well as the physician's predictions about future quality of life. This approach underscores the need for ICU teams to be expert communicators, sensitive to eliciting patients' preferences, timely in relieving suffering, and compassionate in providing dignity to decedents while ministering culturally competent family-centered end-of-life care (Chapter 3).

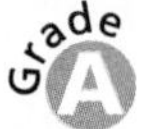

1. Dodek P, Keenan S, Cook DJ, et al: Evidence-based clinical practice guideline for the prevention of ventilator-associated pneumonia. Ann Intern Med 2004;141:305–313.
2. Van den Berghe G, Wilmer A, Hermans G, et al: Intensive insulin therapy in the medical ICU. N Engl J Med 2006;354:449–461.
3. The SAFE Study Investigators: A comparison of albumin and saline for fluid resuscitation in the intensive care unit. N Engl J Med 2004;350:2247–2256.
4. Kress JP, Pohlman AS, O'Connor MF, et al: Daily interruption of sedative infusions in critically ill patients undergoing mechanical ventilation. N Engl J Med 2000;342:1471–1477.
5. Cook DJ, Reeve BK, Guyatt GH, et al: Stress ulcer prophylaxis in critically ill patients: Resolving discordant meta-analyses. JAMA 1996;275:308–314.
6. Fraisse F, Holzapfel L, Couland JM, et al: Nadroparin in the prevention of deep vein thrombosis in acute decompensated COPD. Am Rev Respir Crit Care Med 2000;161:1109–1114.
7. Geerts WH, Jay RM, Code KI, et al: A comparison of low-dose heparin with low-molecular-weight heparin as prophylaxis against venous thromboembolism after major trauma. N Engl J Med 1996;335:701–707.

SUGGESTED READINGS

Berge KH, Maiers DR, Schreiner DP, et al: Resource utilization and outcome in gravely ill intensive care unit patients with predicted in-hospital mortality rates of 95% or higher by APACHE III scores: The relationship with physician and family expectations. Mayo Clin Proc 2005;80:166–173. *Unrealistic family expectations were associated with higher costs but not better outcome.*

Davidson JE, Powers K, Hedayat KM, et al: Clinical practice guidelines for support of the family in the patient centered intensive care unit: American College of Critical Care Medicine Task Force 2004–2005. Crit Care Med 2006;35:605–622. *Recommendations based on evidence in the literature.*

McMillan TR, Hyzy RC: Bringing quality improvement to the critical care unit. Crit Care Med 2007;35(2 Suppl):S59–S65. *Emphasizes how to reduce errors and complications.*

Sinuff T, Khanamoui K, Cook DJ, et al: Acute care bed triaging and rationing: A systematic review. Crit Care Med 2004;32:1588–1597. *A systematic review outlining the process of critical care delivery and associated outcomes in the face of scarce ICU bed resources.*

RESPIRATORY MONITORING IN CRITICAL CARE

John M. Luce

The word *respiration* describes the exchange of oxygen (O_2) and carbon dioxide (CO_2) between humans (or other animals) and the environment. Human respiration may be divided into the following four processes: (1) *ventilation,* in which O_2 is inhaled and CO_2 is excreted into the atmosphere; (2) *arterial oxygenation,* in which O_2 is transferred from the alveoli into mixed venous blood in the pulmonary capillaries in exchange for CO_2; (3) *oxygen transport* or *delivery,* in which O_2 is carried in systemic arterial blood to the tissues; and (4) *oxygen extraction* and *utilization,* in which the tissues take up O_2 from blood and give up CO_2, which is transported in venous blood to the lungs.

ASSESSMENT OF VENTILATION

Physical Examination

Ventilation requires the rhythmic use of the respiratory muscles to pump gases in and out of the lungs. Measurement of the respiratory rate is particularly important in assessing the adequacy of ventilation. The respiratory rate at rest usually ranges from 12 to 22 breaths/min; a respiratory rate substantially less than 12 breaths/min suggests that ventilation is inadequate to meet metabolic needs, whereas a respiratory rate substantially greater than 22 breaths/min may reflect incipient ventilatory failure. In fact, patients may require mechanical ventilation if their respiratory rate exceeds 35 breaths/min over a prolonged period.

Whereas the respiratory rate can easily be measured by direct observation, tidal volume (V_T), which is the amount of gas that enters and leaves the lungs with each breath (Chapter 85), can only be approximated. Such approximation may be useful, for example, when the respiratory rate and V_T are so low or high that ventilation must be impaired and medical intervention is necessary. Nevertheless, clinicians should avoid using words such as hypoventilation and hyperventilation for patients whose respiratory rates and V_T appear low or high because these words refer to specific abnormalities in systemic arterial CO_2 tension ($Pa{CO_2}$) that can be diagnosed only by blood gas analysis.

In the presence of increased airway resistance or decreased lung or chest wall compliance, patients must expend more respiratory muscle work to achieve adequate ventilation (Chapter 86). The work of breathing in such patients is the product of V_T and the pressure required to generate that V_T. This pressure, the transpulmonary pressure, is the difference between airway and pleural pressure. Transpulmonary pressure cannot be measured on physical examination. Recession of the suprasternal and intercostal spaces during inspiration suggests a greater than normal negative swing in pleural pressure and hence an increase in the work of breathing. Another manifestation of increased breathing effort is forceful contraction of the sternocleidomastoid muscles.

Finally, a marked increase in the work of breathing, along with probable ventilatory inadequacy, may be suggested by certain abnormal breathing patterns. The first, an asynchrony between the peak excursions of the chest wall and abdomen, is called respiratory muscle asynchrony (Fig. 104–1). The second, respiratory muscle paradox, is seen when the abdomen moves inward rather than outward during inspiration, thus indicating that the chest wall muscles are being recruited more than the diaphragm.

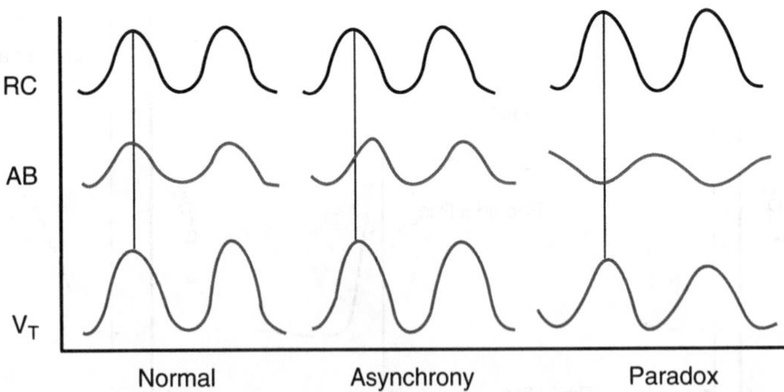

FIGURE 104–1 • Tracings of the movements of the rib cage (RC), the abdomen (AB), and their sum (VT) recorded by inductance plethysmography. The dashed lines are drawn at the time of maximum inspiratory volume. (From Dantzker DR, Tobin MJ: Monitoring respiratory muscle function. Respir Care 1985;30:422–428.)

Systemic Arterial Blood Gas Analysis

Samples of systemic arterial blood may be obtained by repeated percutaneous arterial puncture or from indwelling arterial catheters for measurement of $Pa{CO_2}$, pH, arterial O_2 tension ($Pa{O_2}$), and bicarbonate (HCO_3^-) concentration. Miniature intra-arterial sensors may also be placed through the catheters for continuous analysis of blood gases, although this technology is not sufficiently accurate for clinical use.

$Pa{CO_2}$ is used to assess the adequacy of ventilation and to diagnose hypercapnic respiratory failure, also called failure of ventilation. At sea level, $Pa{CO_2}$ normally ranges from 35 to 45 mm Hg. Hyperventilation and respiratory alkalosis are said to be present if $Pa{CO_2}$ is less than 35 mm Hg. Hypoventilation, hypercapnia, and respiratory acidosis are present if $Pa{CO_2}$ is greater than 45 mm Hg, and ventilatory failure exists when $Pa{CO_2}$ exceeds 50 mm Hg.

pH and HCO_3^- concentration measurements can be used to determine whether hypercapnia and hypocapnia and respiratory acidosis and respiratory alkalosis are acute or chronic. Such determination is based on the Henderson-Hasselbalch equation for the HCO_3^- buffer system:

$$pH = 6.1 + \log_{10} [HCO_3^-]/0.003\ Pa{CO_2} \quad (1)$$

In keeping with this equation, acute increases or decreases in $Pa{CO_2}$ cause the pH to fall or rise until the kidneys gradually retain or release HCO_3^- to buffer the fall or rise in pH (Chapter 119).

pH normally ranges from 7.35 to 7.45. An acute increase in $Pa{CO_2}$ causes pH to fall below 7.35, a condition called acute respiratory acidosis. If $Pa{CO_2}$ is increased, pH is below normal, and the HCO_3^- concentration is increased, the patient has either a chronic respiratory acidosis with a compensatory metabolic alkalosis or a respiratory acidosis of unknown duration with a concurrent but not compensatory metabolic alkalosis.

Conversely, an acute decrease in $Pa{CO_2}$ causes pH to rise above 7.45, thereby creating an acute respiratory alkalosis. If $Pa{CO_2}$ is decreased, pH is above normal, and the HCO_3^- concentration is decreased, the patient has either a chronic respiratory alkalosis with a compensatory metabolic acidosis or a respiratory alkalosis of unknown duration with a concurrent metabolic acidosis.

Measurement of Transcutaneous Carbon Dioxide Tension

$Pa{CO_2}$ can be estimated by measuring transcutaneous CO_2 tension through an electrode placed on the skin. Because the electrode is heated, this value is generally higher than $Pa{CO_2}$, although transcutaneous CO_2 tension can be adjusted to obtain a close approximation of $Pa{CO_2}$. In contrast to transcutaneous O_2 values, transcutaneous CO_2 tension is relatively insensitive to alterations in skin perfusion and does not change significantly with age. Transcutaneous monitoring of CO_2 tension is performed most commonly in neonates, in whom repeated percutaneous arterial puncture and arterial catheters are impractical.

Measurement of End-Tidal Carbon Dioxide Tension

In intubated patients of all ages, $Pa{CO_2}$ may be approximated by measuring the end-tidal CO_2 tension in expired gas. End-tidal CO_2 tension can be measured either by a capnometer, which displays its value breath by breath, or by a capnograph, which also displays its waveform.

The capnogram (Fig. 104–2A) reflects the sequential measurement of CO_2 tension from several dead-space compartments that do not participate in CO_2 exchange—apparatus, anatomic, and alveolar—in addition to the CO_2 tension in alveolar gas that is in equilibrium with end-capillary blood. When a plateau is reached, indicative of the presence of CO_2 in alveolar gas and minimal amounts of gas from areas of dead space, end-tidal CO_2 tension should be similar to $Pa{CO_2}$, albeit usually 1 to 5 mm Hg less. If CO_2 tensions in samples of systemic arterial blood and end-tidal gas obtained simultaneously are measured, the correlation of CO_2 tensions can be known.

When alveolar ventilation decreases in comparison to perfusion, as might occur in a patient with chronic obstructive pulmonary disease (COPD; Chapter 88), there may not be a plateau on the capnogram and

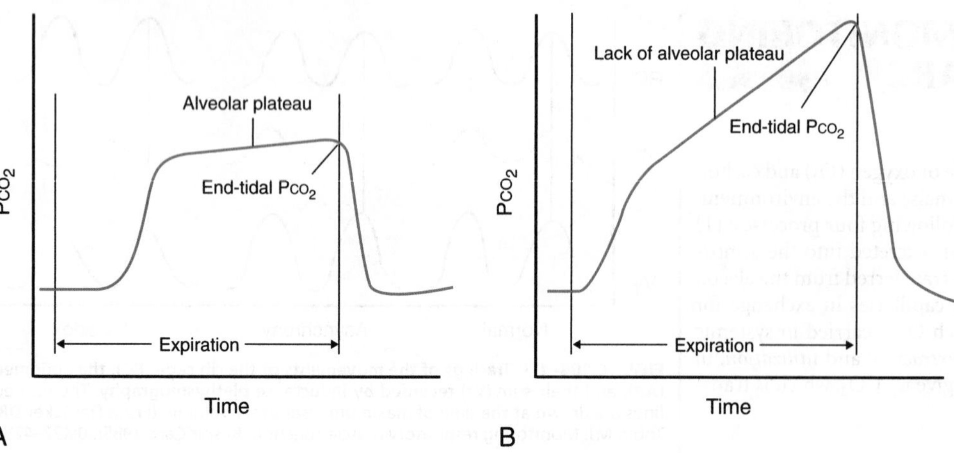

FIGURE 104–2 • Capnogram. A, Illustration of a normal capnogram in which the carbon dioxide tension (PCO_2) rises as dead-space gas from the apparatus, the airways, and the alveoli is supplanted by alveolar gas with a high concentration of CO_2. The high point of this "alveolar plateau" represents the end-tidal PCO_2. **B,** Capnogram of patient with chronic obstructive pulmonary disease in whom end-tidal PCO_2 does not reach a plateau because of delayed CO_2 excretion. See text for further discussion.

the gradient between end-tidal CO_2 tension and $PaCO_2$ may decrease (Fig. 104–2B). Conversely, when perfusion decreases in comparison to ventilation, as might occur in a patient with pulmonary embolism or another dead space–producing disease, end-tidal CO_2 may be considerably less than $PaCO_2$.

Measurement of Dead Space

Dead space is usually expressed as a fraction of VT. The ratio of dead space to VT (VD/VT) per breath can be calculated in patients whose $PaCO_2$ and mean expired PCO_2 ($PECO_2$) are known by using the modified Bohr equation:

$$V_D/V_T = (PaCO_2 - PECO_2)/PaCO_2 \quad (2)$$

VD/VT is usually 0.30 to 0.40 in healthy persons breathing spontaneously. In patients with normal lungs being ventilated mechanically, it approaches 0.50 because gas is stored transiently in compressible portions of the ventilator circuit. VD/VT may rise to values of 0.7 or more in patients with significant respiratory disease.

Measurement of Ventilatory Variables

Ventilatory variables such as the respiratory rate and VT may be measured by respiratory inductance plethysmography, which uses wire coils embedded in bands that fit around the chest and abdomen to detect movement in these areas. These variables may also be measured with a pneumotachograph or other types of spirometers in patients who are breathing through endotracheal tubes. In healthy persons in a hospital setting and in the absence of metabolic abnormalities, VT is approximately 400 mL. A patient with a VT less than 300 mL or 5 mL/kg during spontaneous breathing is unlikely to be weaned from mechanical ventilation.

The product of the respiratory rate and VT is the minute ventilation ($\dot{V}E$). $\dot{V}E$ is approximately 6 L/min in normal adults (at rest) and is usually increased in critically ill patients because of increases in CO_2 production, increases in VD/VT, or both. In hospitalized patients, values in excess of 10 L/min are difficult to maintain without mechanical ventilatory support (Chapter 106).

The ratio of the respiratory rate to VT increases as patients breathe rapidly and shallowly. This breathing pattern is inefficient in excreting CO_2 when VD/VT is normal and is associated with CO_2 retention when this ratio is increased. Studies have demonstrated that weaning from mechanical ventilation is unlikely in patients whose ratio of respiratory rate to VT exceeds 105 breaths/min/L (Chapter 106).

Measurement of Carbon Dioxide Production

The body's CO_2 production can be measured in patients breathing spontaneously or receiving mechanical ventilation by closed systems that compare the difference in CO_2 in inspired (with virtually no CO_2) and expired gases. Newer systems such as indirect calorimeters allow rapid calculation of CO_2 production at the bedside. The CO_2 production of a healthy adult is approximately 200 mL/min, and it varies with body temperature and metabolism.

Use of the Alveolar Ventilation Equation

Although measurement or approximation of $PaCO_2$ helps determine the adequacy of ventilation, the explanation of why ventilation is inadequate in a given patient can be derived only by using the alveolar ventilation equation:

$$PaCO_2 = (K)\ \dot{V}CO_2/\dot{V}A \quad (3)$$

where K is a constant, $\dot{V}CO_2$ is the body's CO_2 production, and $\dot{V}A$, or alveolar ventilation, is equal to minute ventilation minus dead space. From Equation 3 it follows that hypercapnia and ventilatory failure can occur if the body's CO_2 production increases and alveolar ventilation does not, if alveolar ventilation decreases and CO_2 production does not, or if dead space increases out of proportion to minute ventilation.

An example of the first situation might be a patient who becomes septic and thereby increases CO_2 production but cannot increase minute ventilation (and alveolar ventilation) because of respiratory muscle weakness. Patients with severe asthma (Chapter 87) and COPD (Chapter 88) may have ventilatory failure because alveolar ventilation is reduced by airway obstruction, especially when CO_2 production is increased. A primary reduction in alveolar ventilation is seen in cases of narcotic or sedative drug overdose. Diseases such as acute respiratory distress syndrome (ARDS; Chapters 107 and 109) and pulmonary embolism (Chapter 99), in which dead space may increase because of vascular obstruction in the lungs, can cause ventilatory failure if patients cannot increase alveolar ventilation, for example, because of oversedation.

Measurement of Respiratory Mechanics

Vital capacity (VC) is the greatest amount of gas that can be exhaled after a maximum inspiration. Normal VC is approximately 70 mL/kg, but there is wide variation depending on sex, age, and race. VC is reduced in most obstructive and restrictive respiratory diseases (Chapter 85), and VC less than 10 mL/kg is generally associated with inadequate ventilation. VC can be measured by a variety of spirometers in intubated or nonintubated patients.

The volume change per unit of pressure change across the lungs and chest cavity is termed the compliance of the respiratory system. When determined in a patient who is being mechanically ventilated, effective respiratory system compliance (CEFF) is VT divided by the maximum or peak airway pressure (PMAX) required to deliver a given VT minus the amount of positive end-expiratory pressure (PEEP) that the patient is receiving. Thus,

$$C_{EFF} = V_T/(P_{MAX} - PEEP) \quad (4)$$

Because it is a dynamic measurement made when gas is flowing, CEFF includes the resistance to gas flow in the airways and ventilator tubing, as well as the volume and pressure characteristics of the lungs and chest wall. Normal CEFF is 50 to 80 mL/cm H_2O; it is decreased by airway obstruction, secretions, and a small-diameter endotracheal tube.

Static respiratory system compliance (CSTAT) is a measure of the airway pressure required to distend the lungs and chest wall and maintain the increase in volume after a VT has been delivered and gas is not flowing in or out of the lungs. This pressure is called the plateau pressure or static recoil pressure (PSTAT) and is measured while temporarily occluding the expiratory port of a mechanical ventilator for approxi-

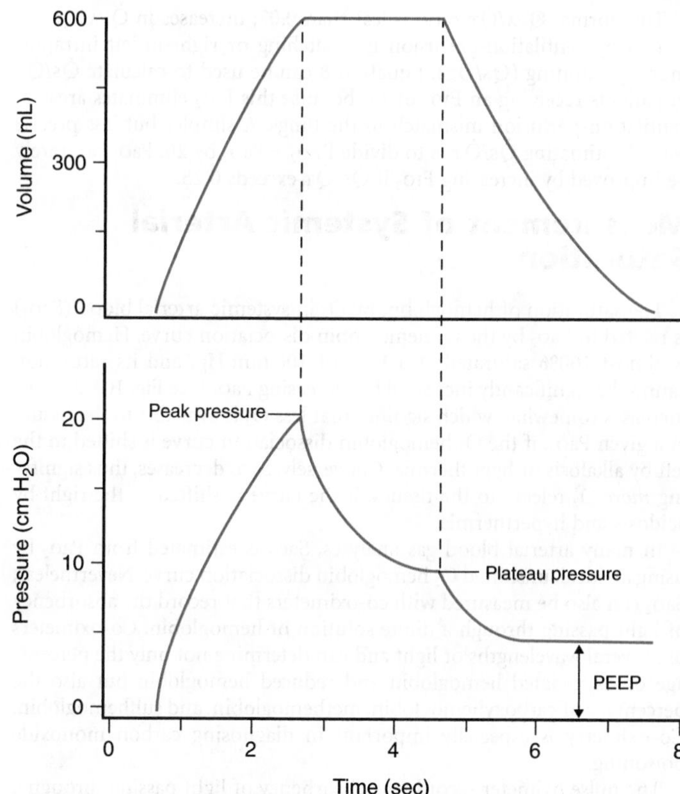

FIGURE 104–3 • Relationship between tidal volume and airway pressure in a mechanically ventilated patient. Peak pressure is used to calculate effective respiratory system compliance, whereas plateau pressure is used to calculate static compliance. PEEP = positive end-expiratory pressure. (From Tobin MJ: Respiratory monitoring in the intensive care unit. Am Rev Respir Dis 1988;138: 1625–1642.)

mately 2 seconds (Fig. 104–3). The amount of PEEP should be subtracted from PSTAT. Thus,

$$C_{STAT} = V_T/(P_{STAT} - PEEP) \quad (5)$$

Because it is a static measurement, CSTAT reflects the compliance of the lungs and chest wall and is not affected by resistance to gas flow. It is decreased (normal level is 60 to 100 mL/cm H_2O) by conditions that decrease lung volume, such as ARDS (Chapter 107). Weaning from mechanical ventilation is difficult if CSTAT is less than 25 mL/cm H_2O (Chapter 106).

Intrinsic or auto-PEEP occurs in patients with airway obstruction and other disorders who fail to complete expiration during either spontaneous breathing or mechanical ventilation. The result is air trapping that produces positive pressure at end expiration. The positive pressure in turn can decrease cardiac filling and increase vascular pressure in the chest, as intentional PEEP can. Auto-PEEP can be measured in mechanically ventilated patients by stopping airflow at end expiration just before the next breath, allowing pressure in the airways and the ventilator tubing to equilibrate, and reading the pressure from the ventilator manometer or airway pressure tracing (Fig. 104–4). Auto-PEEP should be taken into account when calculating effective respiratory system compliance and CSTAT.

Measurement of Ventilatory Drive

The drive to breathe is responsible in large part for the sensation of dyspnea and determines how avidly patients attempt to achieve adequate ventilation. Ventilatory drive can be estimated in intubated patients by measuring the inspiratory pressure developed at the end of the first 100 msec of surreptitious airway occlusion. This measurement provides only an estimate because the inspiratory pressure developed in the first 100 msec of surreptitious airway occlusion, which is normally less than 2 cm H_2O, is influenced somewhat by respiratory muscle strength and, hence, by lung volume. Values greater than 4 cm H_2O are thought to reflect the need for ventilatory support, and values less than 4 cm H_2O are associated with successful discontinuation of ventilatory support.

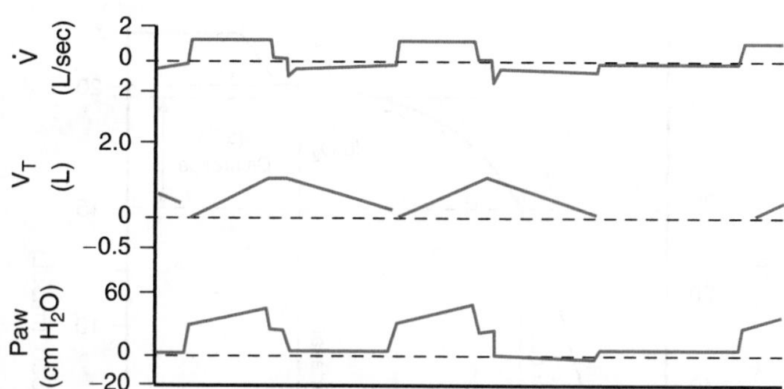

FIGURE 104–4 • As airflow ($\dot{V}$) is stopped at end expiration after a tidal volume (VT) is given and pressures in the airways and ventilator tubing equilibrate, auto-PEEP can be measured as an increase in airway pressure (Paw). PEEP = positive end-expiratory pressure. See text for further discussion.

Measurement of Respiratory Muscle Strength

Respiratory muscle strength can be assessed by measuring with a manometer the maximum airway pressures developed during inspiration from a low lung volume and during expiration from a high lung volume. At functional residual capacity, healthy adults have a maximum inspiratory pressure more negative than −100 cm H_2O and a maximum expiratory pressure more positive than 150 cm H_2O. A maximum inspiratory pressure that is less negative than −30 cm H_2O suggests the need for ventilatory support, whereas a value that is more negative than −30 cm H_2O, especially if it can be sustained for 3 to 5 seconds, correlates with successful weaning from mechanical ventilation.

Measurement of the Work of Breathing

As noted earlier, the work of breathing is the product of transpulmonary pressure (the difference between airway and pleural pressure) and VT. Although pleural pressure is impractical to measure and varies regionally, it can be approximated by measuring pressure in the esophagus with a balloon. Changes in this pressure can be used to compute the work of breathing in spontaneously breathing and mechanically ventilated patients.

ASSESSMENT OF ARTERIAL OXYGENATION

Physical Examination

Cyanosis of the tongue and oral mucosa, which is called central cyanosis, provides a crude estimate of the adequacy of arterial oxygenation. Central cyanosis reflects the presence of 3 g/dL or more of reduced (i.e., deoxygenated) hemoglobin. However, the blue discoloration of tissues caused by deoxygenated hemoglobin may also be caused by dyshemoglobins such as sulfhemoglobin. Furthermore, clinicians vary in their ability to detect cyanosis when it actually occurs.

Arterial Blood Gas Analysis

The systemic arterial O_2 tension (Pa_{O_2}) obtained by arterial blood gas analysis is the standard for assessing the adequacy of arterial oxygenation. Normal Pa_{O_2} at sea level is approximately 100 mm Hg (Fig. 104–5). However, Pa_{O_2} is inversely correlated with age, as expressed in the following equation:

$$\text{Normal } Pa_{O_2} = 100 \text{ mm Hg} - (0.3) \text{ age in years} \quad (6)$$

Equation 6 does not correct for the effects of barometric pressure.

Measurement of Transcutaneous Oxygen Tension

As with CO_2, the transcutaneous tension of O_2 can be measured with a heated electrode on the skin. However, the correlation between Pa_{O_2} and transcutaneous tension of O_2 is affected by both age and perfusion status, which is not the case with the correlation between Pa_{CO_2} and transcutaneous CO_2 tension.

Use of the Alveolar Gas Equation

Although alveolar O_2 tension (PA_{O_2}) cannot be measured directly, it can be estimated from the alveolar gas equation:

$$PA_{O_2} = FI_{O_2}(P_B - 47) - Pa_{CO_2}/R \quad (7)$$

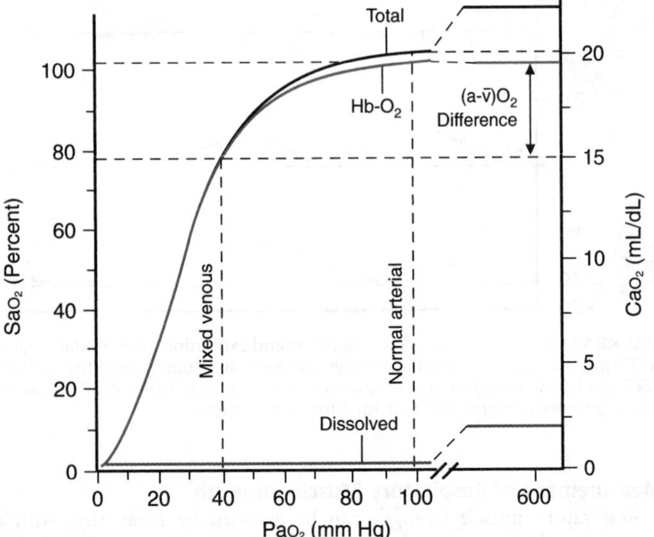

FIGURE 104–5 • Normal oxyhemoglobin dissociation curve showing the relationship between systemic arterial O_2 saturation (SaO_2), tension (PaO_2), and content (CaO_2). See text for further discussion.

where FIO_2 is the fraction of inspired O_2 (0.21 when breathing ambient air), PB is barometric pressure, 47 is the vapor pressure of water at 37° C, and R is the respiratory exchange ratio, which represents the ratio of CO_2 production to O_2 consumption (usually assumed to be 0.8). Normally, a difference or gradient of 10 mm Hg or less exists between PAO_2 and PaO_2. This difference, $PAO_2 - PaO_2$, increases to 30 mm Hg with age and increases further with respiratory disease.

The word *hypoxemia* is used to describe a PaO_2 of less than normal; hypoxemic respiratory failure, also called failure of arterial oxygenation, exists when PaO_2 is below 50 to 60 mm Hg. As indicated by the alveolar gas equation and the relationship between PaO_2 and PAO_2, hypoxemia can be caused by a decrease in FIO_2, as might result from breathing air in a fire in which O_2 has been consumed; a decrease in barometric pressure, as occurs at altitude; an increase in $PaCO_2$, as might happen during a drug overdose; or an increase in the alveolar-arterial gradient of oxygen, as caused, for example, by a mismatch of ventilation and perfusion in the lungs.

Even if the PaO_2 of a patient with hypoxemic respiratory failure is normalized by the administration of supplemental O_2, O_2 exchange in the lungs may remain abnormal. In this situation, the inadequacy of O_2 exchange is reflected by an increased alveolar-arterial gradient of oxygen, which remains a helpful indicator of respiratory function at all but the highest levels of FIO_2, where it may change unpredictably.

Other Indicators of Arterial Oxygenation

The arterial-to-alveolar PO_2 ratio (PaO_2/PAO_2) can be calculated by using the alveolar gas equation. PaO_2/PAO_2 is relatively stable with changing levels of FIO_2 and can be used to predict the expected PaO_2 when FIO_2 is altered. The normal PaO_2/PAO_2 is 0.9. The PaO_2/FIO_2 ratio is easier to calculate because it does not require use of the alveolar gas equation. The normal PaO_2/FIO_2 is 460. Although PaO_2/FIO_2 does not account for changes in $PaCO_2$, this limitation is not important at high levels of FIO_2.

Measurement of Venous Admixture and Shunt Fraction

Venous admixture ($\dot{Q}VA/\dot{Q}T$) is the fraction of mixed venous blood that does not become oxygenated as it courses through the lungs. It can be calculated with the equation

$$\dot{Q}VA/\dot{Q}T = (Cc'O_2 - CaO_2)/(Cc'O_2 - C\bar{v}O_2) \quad (8)$$

where $\dot{Q}T$ is cardiac output and $Cc'O_2$, CaO_2, and $C\bar{v}O_2$ are the O_2 contents of end-capillary, arterial, and mixed venous blood, respectively. Although end-capillary blood cannot be sampled routinely, the end-capillary O_2 content can be calculated by assuming that the tension of end-capillary blood is the same as PAO_2.

The normal $\dot{Q}VA/\dot{Q}T$ ratio is less than 0.07; increases in $\dot{Q}VA/\dot{Q}T$ are caused by ventilation-perfusion mismatching or right-to-left intrapulmonary shunting ($\dot{Q}S/\dot{Q}T$). Equation 8 can be used to calculate $\dot{Q}S/\dot{Q}T$ in patients receiving an FIO_2 of 1.0 because this FIO_2 eliminates areas of ventilation-perfusion mismatch in the lungs. A simpler but less precise way of estimating $\dot{Q}S/\dot{Q}T$ is to divide $PAO_2 - PaO_2$ by 20. PaO_2 can rarely be improved by increasing FIO_2 if $\dot{Q}S/\dot{Q}T$ exceeds 0.25.

Measurement of Systemic Arterial Saturation

The saturation of hemoglobin by O_2 in systemic arterial blood (SaO_2) is related to PaO_2 by the O_2 hemoglobin dissociation curve. Hemoglobin is almost 100% saturated at a PaO_2 of 100 mm Hg, and its saturation cannot be significantly increased by increasing PaO_2 (see Fig. 104-5). SaO_2 increases somewhat, which signifies that less O_2 is available to the tissues at a given PaO_2, if the O_2 hemoglobin dissociation curve is shifted to the left by alkalosis or hypothermia. Conversely, SaO_2 decreases, thus signifying *more* O_2 release to the tissues, if the curve is shifted to the right by acidosis and hyperthermia.

In many arterial blood gas analyses, SaO_2 is estimated from PaO_2 by using an ideal, unshifted O_2 hemoglobin dissociation curve. Nevertheless, SaO_2 can also be measured with co-oximeters that record the absorbency of light passing through a dilute solution of hemoglobin. Co-oximeters use several wavelengths of light and can determine not only the percentage of oxygenated hemoglobin and reduced hemoglobin but also the percentage of carboxyhemoglobin, methemoglobin, and sulfhemoglobin. Co-oximetry is especially important in diagnosing carbon monoxide poisoning.

The pulse oximeter records the absorbency of light passing through a pulsatile tissue bed such as a fingertip. The absorption characteristics of oxygenated hemoglobin and reduced hemoglobin are different at the two wavelengths of light used. Pulse oximetry accurately measures SaO_2 values above 80% in persons with adequate peripheral arterial flow. This technique is particularly helpful in patients who are hemodynamically stable and in whom a nonshifted O_2 hemoglobin dissociation curve allows good correlation between SaO_2 and PaO_2. SaO_2 measured by pulse oximetry does not account for hemoglobin that is saturated by substances other than O_2, such as carbon monoxide; consequently, SaO_2 is falsely elevated in patients with carbon monoxide poisoning. In addition, SaO_2 provides no information about $PaCO_2$ or pH. Nevertheless, the accuracy, ease, and low expense of pulse oximetry make it a useful substitute for analysis of PaO_2 in many situations.

ASSESSMENT OF OXYGEN DELIVERY AND UTILIZATION

Physical Examination

The adequacy of O_2 delivery and utilization may be appreciated by examination of the skin. For example, the presence of normal skin color and warmth suggests adequate peripheral flow of oxygenated blood in some circumstances. Such adequacy is also suggested by normal capillary refill, in which skin color returns to baseline 2 to 3 seconds after the skin is blanched. Nevertheless, although these findings may help exclude significant hypovolemia or impairment of cardiac output, which are associated with increased systemic vascular resistance, they do not exclude sepsis and other processes in which systemic vascular resistance is decreased.

When skin findings are unreliable, O_2 delivery and utilization may be assessed in other organs where blood supply is maintained despite hypoperfusion elsewhere. In this regard, the onset of confusion or obtundation in a previously healthy patient may signify a significant decrease in cerebral oxygenation. Similarly, a decrease in urine output below 0.5 mL/kg/hr may result from a reduction in renal blood flow from sepsis and other causes.

Measurement of Oxygen Delivery

The amount of O_2 delivered to the tissues ($\dot{D}O_2$) is the product of cardiac output ($\dot{Q}T$) and the content of O_2 in systemic arterial blood (CaO_2). Thus,

$$\dot{D}O_2 = (\dot{Q}T)(CaO_2) \quad (9)$$

Cao_2 (mL O_2/dL blood) can be calculated from the following equation:

$$CaO_2 = (1.39)(Hb)\left(\frac{Sao_2}{100}\right) + (0.003)(Pao_2) \quad (10)$$

where 1.39 is the oxygen-carrying capacity of hemoglobin in milliliters of O_2 per gram, Hb is the hemoglobin concentration in grams/dL, and 0.003 is the solubility coefficient of O_2 in plasma. Most of the O_2 in blood is bound to hemoglobin (see Fig. 104-5), although additional O_2 can be dissolved in blood if Pao_2 is raised to supranormal levels. At a normal Sao_2 of approximately 100%, a Pao_2 of 100 mm Hg, and a hemoglobin concentration of 14 g/dL, Cao_2 is 20 mL O_2/dL of blood.

Cardiac output can be measured via the thermodilution technique with a pulmonary artery catheter. In this technique, a bolus of cold liquid, usually dextrose in water, is rapidly injected into the right atrium through the proximal catheter port, which causes the negative heat to be diluted by mixing with blood as it passes into the pulmonary artery. A thermistor senses the temperature of blood on passing the distal catheter port, and the temperature change is used to compute cardiac output, which averages 5 L/min in healthy persons. If arterial O_2 content is normal, the amount of O_2 delivered to the tissues normally averages 1000 mL O_2/min.

Measurement of Mixed Venous Oxygen Saturation

Placement of a pulmonary artery catheter allows the collection of samples for determination of O_2 tension, saturation, and the content of mixed venous blood. Saturation can also be measured continuously with an oximetric pulmonary artery catheter containing fiberoptic bundles that transmit and receive light from the catheter tip.

Normal persons have a mixed venous O_2 saturation of approximately 75%, which corresponds to a mixed venous O_2 tension of 40 mm Hg on an unshifted O_2 hemoglobin dissociation curve. Reductions in mixed venous O_2 saturation to below 60%, corresponding to mixed venous O_2 tension values less than 28 mm Hg, are associated with a severely impaired amount of O_2 delivered to the tissues. Indeed, anaerobic metabolism commonly develops when mixed venous O_2 saturation falls below 50%.

Although a low mixed venous O_2 saturation may be clinically alarming, inadequate O_2 transport and utilization may exist in the presence of normal or supranormal values. For example, a mixed venous O_2 saturation greater than 80% may be seen in sepsis, when the tissues either cannot extract O_2 from the blood or perform aerobic metabolism or when blood is redistributed to metabolically inactive organs such as the skin.

Measurement of Oxygen Consumption

Total body O_2 consumption, which reflects the amount of O_2 used during aerobic metabolism, can be measured in closed systems by comparing the difference in O_2 in inspired and expired gases, which is difficult to accomplish in patients with a high minute ventilation and FIO_2. Alternatively, total body O_2 consumption can be measured by indirect calorimetry and calculated with the Fick equation.

Use of the Fick Equation

The Fick equation holds that total body O_2 consumption ($\dot{V}O_2$) is equal to the product of cardiac output ($\dot{Q}T$) and the amount of O_2 extracted by the tissues, which is the difference in O_2 content in systemic arterial (Cao_2) and mixed venous ($C\bar{v}o_2$) blood. Thus,

$$\dot{V}O_2 = (\dot{Q}T)(Cao_2 - C\bar{v}o_2) \quad (11)$$

The mixed venous O_2 content is normally 15 mL O_2/dL of blood. Because the mixed arterial content is usually 20 mL/dL, the normal difference is 5 mL O_2/mL blood. With this value and a cardiac output of 5 L/min, total body O_2 consumption averages 250 mL O_2/min in healthy persons.

In addition to allowing calculation of total body O_2 consumption, the Fick equation provides insight into physiologic function during stress and exercise. It reveals, for example, that normally only 25% of the O_2 in systemic arterial blood is extracted by the tissues, thus leaving a large O_2 reserve. Patients characteristically call on this reserve when the amount of O_2 delivered to the tissues decreases because of a fall in cardiac output, a fall in the content of O_2 in systemic arterial blood (and its major components Sao_2 and hemoglobin), or both. Nevertheless, a shift to anaerobic metabolism generally occurs when more than 50% of the O_2 is extracted, and lactic acidosis may result.

Measurement of Other Indicators of Oxygen Transport and Utilization

Clinicians commonly monitor serum lactate levels as a sign of the development and progression of anaerobic metabolism. This approach is supported by studies demonstrating that lactate levels above 2 mEq/L correspond to a mixed venous O_2 tension less than 28 mm Hg, with an increased mortality rate among critically ill patients. Nonetheless, elevated lactate levels may result from decreased lactate degradation rather than increased production, and they should be interpreted with caution.

Assessment of oxygenation of the gastrointestinal tract may provide an early indication of inadequate tissue perfusion in the critically ill. Such assessment can be derived from measurement of gastric intramucosal pH by passing a saline-filled balloon into the lumen of the stomach. After approximately 30 minutes, gastric CO_2 tension equilibrates with the CO_2 tension in the balloon; the equilibrated CO_2 tension can then be combined with the HCO_3^- concentration in blood to calculate intramucosal gastric pH by using the Henderson-Hasselbalch equation.

Studies have suggested that a gastric intramucosal pH lower than the normal level of 7.35 correlates with a high mortality rate in patients admitted to a critical care unit and that such mortality can be reduced by therapy designed to restore intraluminal pH to normal. Nevertheless, this approach has not been verified in large groups of patients. In fact, it is not clear whether any method of assessing O_2 delivery and utilization is superior to monitoring urine output and changes in the physical examination.

SUGGESTED READINGS

Huang Y-HT: Monitoring oxygen delivery in the critically ill. Chest 2005;128:554S–560S. *Discusses approaches to monitoring oxygen delivery.*

Levy MM: Pathophysiology of oxygen delivery in respiratory failure. Chest 2005;128:547S–553S. *A review of the variables of oxygen delivery.*

Nuckton TJ, Alonso JA, Kallet RH, et al: Pulmonary dead-space fraction as a risk factor for death in the acute respiratory distress syndrome. N Engl J Med 2002;346:1281–1286. *Dead space was the most powerful predictor of death.*

105 ACUTE RESPIRATORY FAILURE

Leonard D. Hudson and Arthur S. Slutsky

ACUTE RESPIRATORY FAILURE

Definition

Acute respiratory failure occurs when dysfunction of the respiratory system results in abnormal gas exchange that is potentially life-threatening. Each element of this definition is important to understand. The term *acute* implies a relatively sudden onset (from hours to days) and a substantial change from the patient's baseline condition. Dysfunction of the respiratory system indicates that the abnormal gas exchange may be caused by abnormalities in any element of the respiratory system (e.g., a central nervous system abnormality affecting regulation of breathing or a musculoskeletal thoracic abnormality affecting ventilation; Chapter 83) in addition to abnormalities of the lung itself. The term *respiration* in its broad sense refers to the delivery of oxygen (O_2) (Table 105–1) to metabolically active tissues for energy usage and the removal of carbon dioxide (CO_2) from these tissues. Respiratory failure is a failure of the process of delivering O_2 to the tissues and/or removing CO_2 from the tissues. Abnormalities in the periphery (e.g., cyanide poisoning, pathologic distribution of organ blood flow in sepsis) also can lead to tissue hypoxia; although these conditions represent forms of respiratory failure in the broadest terms, this chapter focuses on respiratory failure resulting from dysfunction of the lungs, chest wall, and control of respiration.

TABLE 105–1 ABBREVIATIONS COMMONLY USED IN ACUTE RESPIRATORY FUNCTION

ABG	Arterial blood gas or arterial blood gas analysis
ALI	Acute lung injury
ARDS	Acute respiratory distress syndrome
ARF	Acute respiratory failure
cm H_2O	Centimeters of water
Cao_2	Content of oxygen in the arterial blood
Cco_2	Content of oxygen in end-capillary blood
CO_2	Carbon dioxide
COPD	Chronic obstructive pulmonary disease
CPAP	Continuous positive airway pressure (used when positive pressure during exhalation is applied with spontaneous ventilation)
Cvo_2	Content of oxygen in mixed venous blood
Fio_2	Fraction of inspired oxygen
g/dL	Grams per deciliter
HbO_2	Saturation of hemoglobin by oxygen
L/min	Liters per minute
mL/kg	Milliliters per kilogram
mL/min	Milliliters per minute
mm Hg	Millimeters of mercury
NIPPV	Noninvasive positive-pressure ventilation
O_2	Oxygen
$P(A-a)o_2$	Difference of partial pressure of oxygen between alveolar gas and arterial blood (alveolar-to-arterial oxygen difference)
$PAco_2$	Partial pressure of carbon dioxide in alveolar gas
$Paco_2$	Partial pressure of carbon dioxide in arterial blood
PAo_2	Partial pressure of oxygen in alveolar gas
Pao_2	Partial pressure of oxygen in arterial blood
Pao_2/Fio_2	Ratio of partial pressure of oxygen in arterial blood to fraction of inspired oxygen
PBW	Predicted body weight
$Pcco_2$	Partial pressure of carbon dioxide in end-capillary blood
Pco_2	Partial pressure of oxygen in end-capillary blood
PEEP	Positive end-expiratory pressure (used when positive pressure during exhalation is applied with mechanical ventilation)
P/F	Pao_2/Fio_2 ratio
Pio_2	Partial pressure of oxygen in inspired gas
Po_2	Partial pressure of oxygen
$Pvco_2$	Partial pressure of carbon dioxide in mixed venous blood
Pvo_2	Partial pressure of oxygen in mixed venous blood
Q	Blood flow or perfusion
RR	Respiratory rate
Sao_2	Percentage of saturation of hemoglobin by oxygen in arterial blood
$\dot{V}$	Ventilation
$\dot{V}/\dot{Q}$	Ventilation-to-perfusion ratio
V_T	Tidal volume

Pathobiology

Abnormal gas exchange is the physiologic hallmark of acute respiratory failure, which can be classified in several ways (Table 105–2). Although gas exchange can be abnormal either for oxygenation or for CO_2 removal, significant hypoxemia is nearly always present in patients with acute respiratory failure. If CO_2 retention is present at a level that is potentially life-threatening, it usually is accompanied by significant hypoxemia (see later). The *life-threatening* aspect of the definition places the degree of abnormal gas exchange in a clinical context and calls for urgent treatment.

The diagnosis of acute respiratory failure requires a significant change from baseline. Many patients with chronic respiratory problems can function with blood gas tensions that would be alarming in a physiologically normal individual. Over time, these patients with so-called chronic respiratory failure or chronic respiratory insufficiency have developed mechanisms to compensate for inadequate gas exchange. Conversely, the chronic condition makes these patients vulnerable to insults that could be tolerated easily by a previously healthy individual.

In acute respiratory failure, the O_2 content in the blood (available for tissue use) is reduced to a level at which the possibility of end-organ dysfunction increases markedly. The value of the partial pressure of O_2 in the arterial blood (Pao_2) that demarcates this vulnerable zone is the point of the oxyhemoglobin dissociation relationship at which any further decrease in the Pao_2 results in sharp decreases in the amount of hemoglobin that is saturated with O_2 (Sao_2) and in the arterial blood O_2 content (Cao_2). Although arbitrary, acute respiratory failure often is defined in practice as occurring when the Pao_2 is less than 55 mm Hg (Fig. 105–1). In general, the locus on the curve that indicates the partial pressure at which O_2 is being unloaded to the tissues is the most important determinant of how much O_2 is available for the cells and their mitochondria. Usually, the ability to unload O_2 at the tissue level more than compensates for small decreases in the amount of O_2 that is picked up in the lungs when the oxyhemoglobin dissociation curve is shifted rightward. With a leftward shift in the curve, O_2 is bound more tightly to hemoglobin, so less O_2 is available for tissue delivery.

These clinical considerations imply that any definition of acute respiratory failure based on an absolute level of Pao_2 is arbitrary. A healthy, young, conditioned individual climbing at high altitude may have a Pao_2 of less than 50 mm Hg because of the reduction in inspired O_2 pressure. This individual is not in acute respiratory failure even though the Pao_2 may be in the low 40s. A patient who has chronic obstructive pulmonary disease (COPD) and whose usual range of Pao_2 is 50 to 55 mm Hg would not be considered to be in acute respiratory failure if the Pao_2 was 50 mm Hg. However, if a patient's usual Pao_2 was 60 to 70 mm Hg, a Pao_2 of 50 mm Hg would be associated with a substantial risk for a further life-threatening reduction in oxygenation; this patient should be considered to have acute respiratory failure.

The level of arterial CO_2 partial pressure ($Paco_2$) that defines acute respiratory failure traditionally has been 50 mm Hg or greater if accompanied by arterial acidosis with a pH of 7.30 or less. The $Paco_2$ is linked to pH in the definition because it generally is thought that the acidosis leads to tissue dysfunction and symptoms. Patients with severe COPD may have chronic CO_2 retention, but their compensated respiratory acidosis protects them against abnormalities related to the elevation in CO_2. A further acute rise in $Paco_2$ can precipitate symptoms and other organ dysfunction, however. By comparison, respiratory acidosis (even as severe as a pH of 7.1) seems to be well tolerated in most previously healthy individuals if arterial and tissue oxygenation is adequate.

Pathophysiology

Five mechanisms can lead to a reduction in Pao_2: (1) decreased inspired partial pressure of O_2 (Pio_2) (e.g., at high altitude or when breathing a reduced percent O_2 mixture); (2) hypoventilation; (3) ventilation-perfusion ($\dot{V}/\dot{Q}$) mismatch; (4) a shunting of blood from the pulmonary to systemic circulation, bypassing the alveoli anatomically or functionally; and (5) abnormal diffusion of O_2 from the alveoli into the capillary blood. In essence, a shunt is an extreme $\dot{V}/\dot{Q}$ mismatch in which blood perfuses alveoli with *no* ventilation; it is differentiated clinically from other $\dot{V}/\dot{Q}$ mismatching by the response to breathing supplemental O_2 (see later).

For clinical purposes, diffusion abnormalities are not an important cause of hypoxemia at sea level because there is sufficient time for adequate diffusion during the transit of a red blood cell through the pulmonary capillary bed, even in the presence of severe lung disease. Even when diffusion abnormalities are present and contribute to hypoxemia, $\dot{V}/\dot{Q}$ mismatch and shunting nearly always coexist and are quantitatively more important causes of hypoxemia. Except at high altitude or when a subject is breathing a gas mixture low in O_2, hypoventilation, $\dot{V}/\dot{Q}$ mismatch, and shunting are the dominant causes of acute respiratory failure.

If only hypoventilation is present, the resulting hypoxemia is associated with a normal difference between the calculated alveolar and the measured arterial oxygenation levels ($P(A-a)o_2$). In this setting, an

TABLE 105–2 SYSTEMS TO CLASSIFY ACUTE RESPIRATORY FAILURE

HYPOXIC VERSUS HYPERCAPNIC-HYPOXIC ARF	**ARF: WITH AND WITHOUT CHRONIC LUNG DISEASE**
Causes of Hypoxic ARF	**With Chronic Lung Disease**
Acute lung injury/ARDS	COPD
Pneumonia	Asthma
Pulmonary thromboembolism	Parenchymal lung diseases
Acute lobar atelectasis	Restrictive lung/chest wall diseases
Cardiogenic pulmonary edema	**Without Lung Disease (These also can be Superimposed on Chronic Disease)**
Lung contusion	Acute lung injury/ARDS
Acute collagen vascular disease (Goodpasture's syndrome, systemic lupus erythematosus)	Pneumonia
Causes of Hypercapnic-Hypoxic ARF	Pulmonary thromboembolism
Pulmonary disease	**ARF BY ORGAN SYSTEM INVOLVED**
COPD	**Respiratory (Lungs and Thorax)**
Asthma: advanced acute severe asthma	Airways/airflow obstruction
Drugs causing respiratory depression	COPD
Neuromuscular	Asthma
Guillain-Barré syndrome	Pulmonary parenchyma
Acute myasthenia gravis	Pneumonia
Spinal cord tumors	Acute lung injury/ARDS
Metabolic derangements causing weakness (including hypophosphatemia, hypomagnesemia)	Acute flare of chronic collagen vascular disease (e.g., Goodpasture's syndrome or systemic lupus erythematosus)
Musculoskeletal	**Central Nervous System**
Kyphoscoliosis	Respiratory depression
Ankylosing spondylitis	Increased sedatives, tranquilizers with respiratory effect, opiates, alcohol
Obesity hypoventilation syndrome (often with acute superimposed additional abnormality as cause of ARF)	Brainstem and spinal cord involvement
ETIOLOGIC MECHANISMS OF HYPOXEMIA	Tumors, trauma, vascular accidents
Normal $P(A - a)O_2$*	Neuromuscular
$\downarrow PIO_2$	Guillain-Barré syndrome
High altitude; inadvertent administration of low FIO_2 gas mixture hypoventilation	Myasthenia gravis
See causes of hypercapnic-hypoxic ARF above	**Cardiovascular**
Increased $P(A - a)O_2$*	Cardiogenic pulmonary edema
Ventilation-perfusion ($\dot{V}/\dot{Q}$) mismatch	Pulmonary thromboembolism
Airway disease	**Renal/Endocrine**
Vascular disease including pulmonary thromboembolism	Volume overload
Shunt	Metabolic abnormalities
Acute lung injury/ARDS	
Pneumonia	
Parenchymal lung disease	
Cardiogenic pulmonary edema	
Pulmonary infarction	
Diffusion limitation†	

*Calculated using the alveolar-air equation; see text for description.
†See text for discussion.
ARDS = acute respiratory distress syndrome; ARF = acute respiratory failure; COPD = chronic obstructive pulmonary disease; FIO_2 = fraction of inspired oxygen; $P(A - a)O_2$ = alveolar-to-arterial oxygen difference; PIO_2 = partial pressure of inspired oxygen; $\dot{V}/\dot{Q}$= ventilation-to-perfusion ratio.

elevated $PaCO_2$ suggests disease processes that affect nonpulmonary respiratory function (e.g., central respiratory depression resulting from drug overdose, neuromuscular diseases such as Guillain-Barré syndrome, or chest wall disease such as flail chest; Chapter 86). In contrast, $\dot{V}/\dot{Q}$ mismatch and shunting are associated with an elevated $P(A - a)O_2$, which may or may not coexist with hypoventilation.

When $\dot{V}/\dot{Q}$ mismatch or shunting is the cause of hypoxemia, some alveolar regions have increased $PACO_2$ and reduced PAO_2; the blood in the vessels perfusing these alveoli reflects these abnormal gas tensions. The increased $PACO_2$ usually can be reversed by increasing overall ventilation, but hyperventilation does not correct the decreased PaO_2.

$\dot{V}/\dot{Q}$ mismatch is distinguished from shunting by assessing the PaO_2 response to enhanced O_2 administration. Hypoxemia caused by $\dot{V}/\dot{Q}$ mismatch can be corrected to a nearly complete O_2 saturation of the hemoglobin in most patients by a relatively small increase in the fraction of inspired O_2 (FIO_2), such as an increase in FIO_2 from 0.21 to 0.24 to 0.28 or 1 to 2 L/minute O_2 (by nasal prongs) in patients with acute exacerbations of COPD. If the airways to poorly ventilated alveoli remain open and the enriched O_2 mixture is administered for an adequate length of time (ranging from a few minutes to 20 minutes, depending on the degree of $\dot{V}/\dot{Q}$ inequality), the increased PIO_2 is reflected by an increased PAO_2 and an increased PaO_2. When a shunt is present (no ventilation but continued perfusion), a relatively small increase in the FIO_2 has little or no effect on the PaO_2, and even large increases in FIO_2 up to 1.0 result in only modest increases in PaO_2 (Fig. 105–2).

Clinical Manifestations

The hallmark of acute respiratory failure from any cause is the inability to maintain adequate oxygenation or the inability to maintain an appropriate $PaCO_2$. Patients are typically dyspneic and tachypneic, unless progressive respiratory failure causes fatigue—sometimes leading to respiratory arrest—or a drug overdose or neuromuscular condition prevents an appropriate respiratory response to hypoxia and/or the hypercapnic acidosis. Neurologic function may deteriorate, and myocardial ischemia or even infarction may be precipitated by the hypoxemia. In addition, each cause has its own specific manifestations (see later).

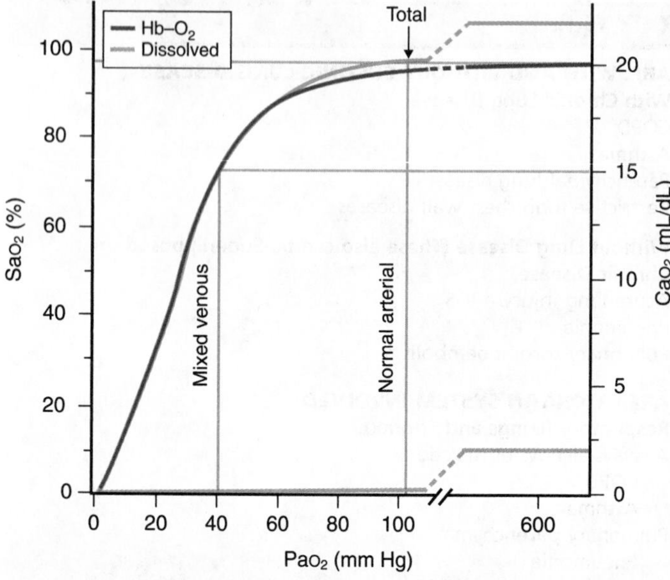

FIGURE 105–1 • The oxyhemoglobin association-dissociation curve. The axis for oxygen saturation (Sao_2) is on the left, and the axis for arterial content of oxygen (Cao_2) is on the right. Cao_2 is the sum of the oxygen dissolved in plasma (denoted as "Dissolved" in the figure) plus the oxygen bound to hemoglobin (Hb-O_2). At a normal hemoglobin, most of the oxygen is carried in combination with hemoglobin (Hb-O_2), with only a relatively small amount of oxygen dissolved in plasma. When the value of the arterial partial pressure of oxygen (Pao_2) is on the "flat" portion of the curve ($Pao_2 \geq 60$ to 65 mm Hg, normal partial pressure of carbon dioxide [Pco_2], and normal pH), raising the Pao_2 further has relatively little effect on total oxygen content. Increases in temperature, Pco_2, hydrogen ion concentration, or 2,3-diphosphoglycerate cause a rightward shift in the oxyhemoglobin association-dissociation curve. Sao_2 = percentage of saturation of hemoglobin by oxygen in the arterial blood.

Diagnosis

As part of the diagnosis of acute respiratory failure, the physician should address three objectives: (1) confirm the clinical suspicion that acute respiratory failure is present; (2) classify the type of acute respiratory failure (e.g., hypoxemia caused by hypoventilation versus hypoxemia caused by $\dot{V}/\dot{Q}$ mismatch or shunting); and (3) determine the specific cause (e.g., acute lung injury secondary to sepsis or decompensated COPD because of acute bronchitis). Defining the type of acute respiratory failure and determining the specific cause are prerequisites to optimal management.

The initial approach to diagnosis consists of consideration of information from four sources: (1) the clinical history and physical examination; (2) the physiologic abnormalities, particularly the arterial blood gas derangements, which help to establish the pathophysiologic mechanisms of hypoxemia; (3) the chest radiographic findings; and (4) other tests aimed at elucidating specific causes. In many cases, the clinical picture from the history is so clear that the presumptive type of acute respiratory failure (and sometimes the cause) is obvious, so treatment can be started while confirmatory laboratory studies are ordered. In other cases, the clinician may be asked to see the patient because of an abnormal chest radiograph or abnormal arterial blood gases that were ordered by someone else and may elicit the pertinent history based on these clues. When the degree of hypoxemia is life-threatening, therapeutic decisions must be made quickly, even if data are limited. The clinician must obtain updated information continually and view most therapeutic decisions as therapeutic trials, with careful monitoring to assess desired benefits and possible detrimental effects.

Clinical Evaluation

The presentation often reflects one of three clinical scenarios: (1) the effects of hypoxemia and/or respiratory acidosis, (2) the effects of primary (e.g., pneumonia) or secondary (e.g., heart failure) diseases involving the lungs, and (3) the nonpulmonary effects of the underlying disease process. The clinical effects of hypoxemia and/or respiratory acidosis are manifest mainly in the central nervous system (e.g., irritability, agitation, changes in personality, a depressed level of consciousness, or coma) and the cardiovascular system (e.g., arrhythmias, hypotension, or hypertension) (Table 105–3). In patients with underlying COPD (Chapter 88) with gradual onset of acute respiratory failure, central nervous system abnormalities may be the major presenting findings. Cyanosis, which requires at least 5 g/dL of unsaturated hemoglobin to be detectable, may not be seen before serious tissue hypoxia develops, especially in patients with underlying anemia.

Pulmonary symptoms and signs often reflect the respiratory disease that is causing the acute respiratory failure. Examples include cough and sputum with pneumonia (Chapter 97) or chest pain from pulmonary thromboembolism with infarction (Chapter 99). Conversely, dyspnea and respiratory distress are nonspecific reflections of increased demands on the respiratory system from pulmonary and nonpulmonary diseases.

Physical findings may be associated with a particular pathologic lung process, such as pneumonia, causing bronchial breathing and crackles on auscultation, or the crackles (rales) of cardiogenic pulmonary edema (Chapter 57). Abnormal findings may be minimal or absent in patients with acute lung injury or pulmonary thromboembolism.

In some patients, the clinical picture is dominated by the underlying disease process, particularly with diseases that cause acute lung injury, such as sepsis (Chapter 109), severe pneumonia (Chapter 97), aspiration of gastric contents (Chapter 94), and trauma. In these conditions, the physical examination is often nonspecific, without obvious clues except, for example, fever with sepsis or pneumonia or hypotension with septic shock.

Assessment of Physiologic Abnormalities

The clinical suspicion of acute respiratory failure must be addressed by arterial blood gas analysis to answer several questions.

1. *Is hypoxemia present?* The answer is largely based on the value of the Pao_2 or Sao_2, and the degree of the hypoxemia not only confirms the diagnosis of acute respiratory failure but also helps to define its severity.
2. *Is hypoventilation present?* If the $Paco_2$ is elevated, alveolar hypoventilation is present.
3. *Does the degree of hypoventilation explain the hypoxemia?* If the $P(A-a)o_2$ is normal, hypoventilation explains the presence and degree of hypoxemia. In this circumstance, the most likely causes of acute respiratory failure are central nervous system abnormalities and a chest wall abnormality. If the $P(A-a)o_2$ is increased, hypoventilation does not explain all of the hypoxemia, and another condition must be present: Common diagnoses include COPD, severe asthma, and early-stage acute respiratory distress syndrome (ARDS).
4. If hypoxemia exists without hypoventilation, an elevated $P(A-a)o_2$ should be confirmed, and the response to breathing an enhanced O_2 mixture would answer this question: *Is the increase in $P(A-a)o_2$ the result of a $\dot{V}/\dot{Q}$ abnormality or of shunting?* If hypoxemia is primarily the result of a $\dot{V}/\dot{Q}$ abnormality, the likely cause is an airway disease, either COPD or acute severe asthma, or a vascular disease, such as pulmonary thromboembolism. If shunting is the major explanation for the hypoxemia, then processes that fill the air spaces (e.g., cardiogenic pulmonary edema, noncardiogenic pulmonary edema in early acute lung injury or ARDS, or purulent pulmonary secretions in acute pneumonia) or, less commonly, an intracardiac or anatomic intrapulmonary shunt are the likely causes. Conditions that fill air spaces should be confirmed by an abnormal chest radiograph; if the radiograph is normal, an intracardiac shunt should be considered by echocardiography.

Chest Radiography

The chest radiograph in acute respiratory failure is likely to show one of three patterns (Fig. 105–3): (1) normal (or relatively normal), (2) localized alveolar filling opacities, and (3) diffuse alveolar filling opacities. Diffuse interstitial opacities are also possible, but diseases that cause this pattern are usually of more gradual onset and are associated with chronic respiratory failure. If the chest radiograph is normal (i.e., it is clear or relatively clear), airway diseases, such as COPD and asthma, or pulmonary vascular diseases, such as thromboembolism, are more likely. If a localized alveolar filling abnormality is present, pneumonia is the major consideration, but pulmonary embolism and infarction also should be considered. When diffuse (bilateral) alveolar filling abnormalities are present, cardiogenic pulmonary edema, acute lung injury (e.g., as seen in sepsis, trauma, or aspiration of gastric contents), and diffuse pneumonia are the major considerations. The combination of the chest

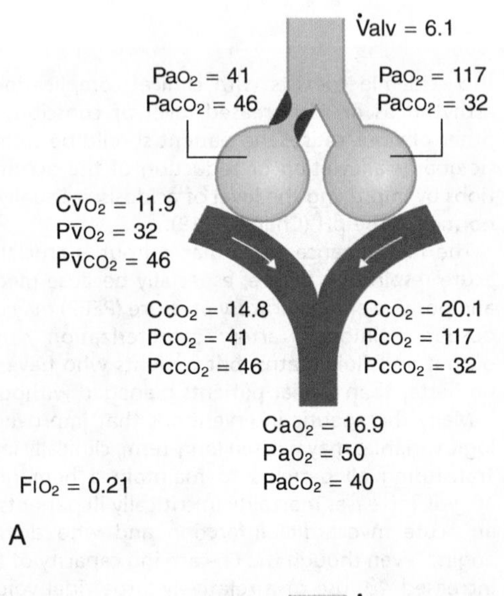

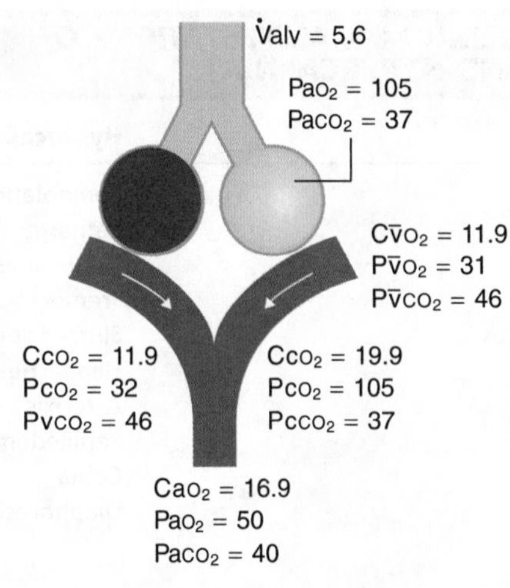

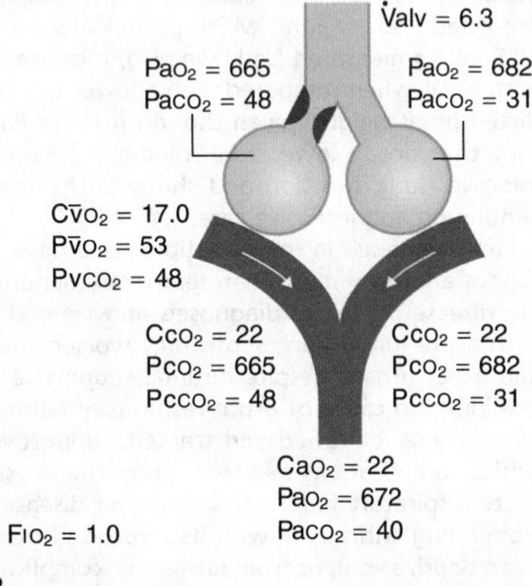

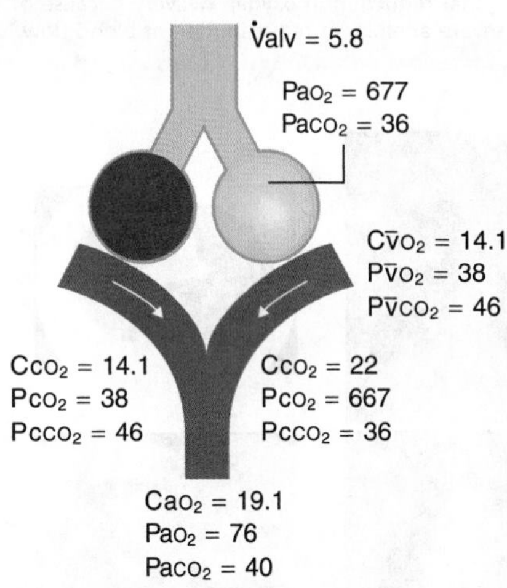

FIGURE 105–2 • The difference in the effect on arterial oxygenation of increasing fraction of inspired oxygen (FIO_2) from breathing room air (FIO_2 = 0.21) (A) compared with breathing 100% oxygen (FIO_2 = 1.0) (B) between low ventilation-to-perfusion ratio ($\dot{V}/\dot{Q}$) (left) and shunt (right), using a two-compartment lung model. Shunt and decreased $\dot{V}/\dot{Q}$ can lead to identical arterial blood gases (partial pressure of oxygen in the arterial blood [PaO_2] = 50 mm Hg; partial pressure of carbon dioxide in the arterial blood [$PaCO_2$] = 40 mm Hg); the response to supplemental oxygen administration is markedly different. Hypoxemia is only partially corrected by breathing 100% oxygen when a shunt is present because arterial oxygenation represents an average of the end-capillary oxygen contents (CcO_2) from various parts of the lung, not an average of the partial pressures of oxygen (partial pressure of carbon dioxide in the end-capillary blood [$PaCO_2$]). When the CcO_2 values are mixed, the PaO_2 is determined from the resultant content of oxygen in the arterial blood (CaO_2) by the oxyhemoglobin association-dissociation relationship (see Fig. 105-1). With low $\dot{V}/\dot{Q}$ (as is often the case in patients with chronic obstructive pulmonary disease), an increase in FIO_2 increases the alveolar PO_2 of the low $\dot{V}/\dot{Q}$ unit and leads to a marked increase in arterial PO_2. The values in this figure were generated from modeling to result in the same $PaCO_2$ ($PaCO_2$ = 40 mm Hg) for all four situations shown, and this is the reason for slight changes in alveolar ventilation ($\dot{V}alv$) for some of the conditions. Several assumptions are made: (1) No diffusion limitation is present; (2) oxygen consumption = 300 mL/minute and CO_2 production = 240 mL/minute; (3) cardiac output = 6.0 L/minute; (4) the low $\dot{V}/\dot{Q}$ region in the left panels represents 60% of the cardiac output perfusing alveoli with $\dot{V}/\dot{Q}$ of 25% of normal; and (5) the shunt in the right panels represents a 37% shunt (i.e., 37% of the cardiac output is perfusing alveoli with no ventilation). $PcCO_2$ = partial pressure of carbon dioxide in the end-capillary blood; PO_2 = partial pressure of oxygen.

radiograph with the arterial blood gas interpretation can be helpful. The finding of a significant shunt may suggest acute lung injury in a patient in whom this diagnosis was not otherwise clinically obvious; the chest radiograph should help to confirm that possibility.

Other Evaluations

All patients with acute respiratory failure should have a complete blood count, including a platelet count, routine blood chemistry tests, a prothrombin time, and a urinalysis to screen for possible underlying causes and comorbid conditions. Other blood tests should be guided by the clinical picture. Examples include a serum amylase level if pancreatitis is a possible cause of ARDS and thyroid indices if severe hypothyroidism is a possible cause of hypoventilation. Blood cultures are recommended whenever sepsis is suspected.

Any abnormal fluid collections, especially pleural effusion (Chapter 100), should be aspirated for diagnostic purposes. Sputum Gram stain and culture are indicated when pneumonia is suspected.

Other specific tests should be directed by the history, physical examinations, arterial blood gas levels, and chest radiograph. An abdominal computed tomography (CT) scan may be indicated to search for the source of infection in a patient with sepsis and acute lung injury. A chest CT scan may help to define pulmonary disease if the chest radiograph is not definitive. A spiral CT arteriogram of the pulmonary circulation may diagnose pulmonary thromboembolism (Chapter 99). A head CT scan may be indicated if a stroke involving the respiratory center is suspected. Routine blood chemistry studies can detect diabetic ketoacidosis or renal failure as contributing causes.

Treatment Rx

General Measures

The management of acute respiratory failure depends on its cause, its clinical manifestations, and the patient's underlying status. Certain goals apply to all patients: (1) improvement of the hypoxemia to eliminate or reduce markedly the acute threat to life, (2) improvement of the acidosis if it is considered life-threatening, (3)

TABLE 105–3 CLINICAL MANIFESTATIONS OF HYPOXEMIA AND HYPERCAPNIA

Hypoxemia	Hypercapnia
Tachycardia	Somnolence
Tachypnea	Lethargy
Anxiety	Restlessness
Diaphoresis	Tremor
Altered mental status	Slurred speech
Confusion	Headache
Cyanosis	Asterixis
Hypertension	Papilledema
Hypotension	Coma
Bradycardia	Diaphoresis
Seizures	
Coma	
Lactic acidosis*	

*Usually requires additional reduction in oxygen delivery because of inadequate cardiac output, severe anemia, or redistribution of blood flow.

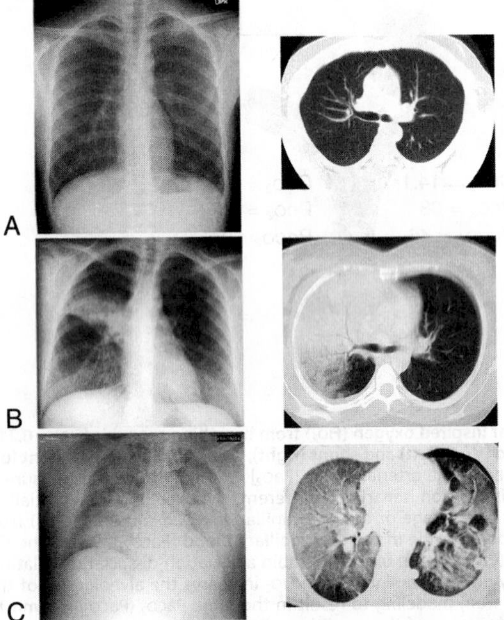

FIGURE 105–3 • Chest radiographs (left) and computed tomography (CT) (right) scans of the three most common findings in diseases causing acute respiratory failure. A, A relatively clear chest, consistent with airway disease with an acute exacerbation (i.e., asthma and chronic obstructive pulmonary disease) or a central nervous system or neuromuscular disease cause of acute respiratory failure. **B,** A localized alveolar filling opacity, most commonly seen with acute pneumonia. **C,** Diffuse bilateral alveolar filling opacities consistent with acute lung injury and acute respiratory distress syndrome. The CT scan in **C** shows a small left pneumothorax and cavities or cysts that are not apparent on the anteroposterior chest radiograph.

maintenance of cardiac output or improvement if cardiac output is compromised, (4) treatment of the underlying disease process, and (5) avoidance of predictable complications.

The precise methods for improving hypoxemia depend on the cause of the acute respiratory failure. An increase in the inspired O_2 concentration is a cornerstone of treatment for nearly all patients, however.

The level of acidosis that requires treatment other than for the underlying disease process is not clear. Although normalization of the arterial pH has been suggested in the past, respiratory acidosis is apparently well tolerated in many patients with severe ARDS, so a patient with a pH of 7.15 may not require bicarbonate therapy. If the acidemia coexists with clinical complications, such as cardiac arrhythmias or a decreased level of consciousness, that have no other obvious cause, the patient should be treated. The therapeutic goal is alleviation or reduction of the accompanying complications by improving the level of acidosis; it usually is not necessary to normalize the pH (Chapter 119).

The maintenance of cardiac output is crucial for O_2 delivery in acute respiratory failure, especially because mechanical ventilation and positive end-expiratory pressure (PEEP) may compromise cardiac output. Pulmonary artery catheterization can measure cardiac output and fluid status, but patients who have these catheters do no better than similar patients managed without them. [1]

Many therapeutic interventions that improve short-term physiologic variables may worsen long-term, clinically important outcomes. Transfusing all patients to maintain a hemoglobin greater than 10 g/dL increases mortality in critically ill patients who have not had an acute myocardial infarction and who do not have unstable angina, even though the O_2-carrying capacity of the blood is acutely increased [2]; use of a relatively large tidal volume (i.e., 12 mL/kg predicted body weight, which is equivalent to approximately 10 to 10.5 mL/kg measured body weight), increases mortality in patients with ARDS when compared with a lower tidal volume (6 mg/kg predicted body weight), even though it raises $Pa{O_2}$ more in the short term than does a lower tidal volume. [3] Conservative use of fluids improves lung function and shortens the duration of mechanical ventilation and intensive care. [4]

Improvements in oxygenation, acid-base status, and cardiac output are of no more than temporary benefit, unless the underlying disease process is diagnosed and treated properly. In patients with acute lung injury, sepsis may worsen the injuries to the lung and other organs despite optimal supportive care. Similarly, if the precipitating cause of acute respiratory failure in the patient with COPD is not identified and treated, supportive care is likely to be futile. Complications may arise from the physiologic effects of the acute respiratory failure and whatever disease process is causing it, from being critically ill with its associated treatment settings (e.g., sleep deprivation), or from iatrogenic complications associated with therapy.

Mechanical Therapy to Improve Oxygenation

A $Pa{O_2}$ of greater than 60 mm Hg is usually adequate to produce an $Sa{O_2}$ in the low to middle 90s. The $Pa{O_2}$ can be increased by administration of supplemental O_2, by pharmacologic manipulations, by continuous positive airway pressure (CPAP), by mechanical ventilation with or without maneuvers such as PEEP, and by use of the prone position. PEEP, pharmacologic manipulations, and positioning are used primarily in patients with acute lung injury (see later).

The initial choice of the concentration and amount of supplemental O_2 likely to be needed is based on the severity of the hypoxemia, the clinical diagnosis, the likely mechanism causing the hypoxemia, and the O_2 delivery systems available. For the tracheal $F{IO_2}$ to be the same as the delivered $F{IO_2}$, the O_2 delivery system must deliver a flow that is able to match the patient's peak inspiratory flow rate with gas of a known $F{IO_2}$. High-flow O_2 blenders can achieve this goal by delivering gas at equal to or greater than 80 L/minute or with any $F{IO_2}$ to a nonintubated patient. These systems require a large flow of O_2 (from a wall unit or tank), however, and are not universally available. Other systems for nonintubated patients (including nasal prongs, simple face masks, and nonrebreather and partial-rebreather masks) use a simple regulator that mixes room air with O_2 at 12 L/minute from a wall unit or tank, with resulting flows that frequently are not able to match the patient's peak inspiratory flow rate. The patient entrains more air from the environment, and the resulting tracheal $F{IO_2}$ or partial pressure of oxygen in inspired gas ($P{IO_2}$) is unknown. The amount of air entrained depends on the patient's inspiratory pattern and minute ventilation. Although the resulting $F{IO_2}$ is unknown, these systems are satisfactory if the delivery is constant and if they result in adequate arterial O_2 saturation, as monitored by arterial blood

Rx

gases or oximetry. Nasal prongs are able to deliver a tracheal FIO_2 of approximately 0.50, and nonrebreather masks can deliver 50 to 100% O_2, in both cases depending on the inspiratory pattern and flow rate. If only hypoventilation or $\dot{V}/\dot{Q}$ mismatch is present, only a small increment in FIO_2 (e.g., an FIO_2 of 0.24 or 0.28 delivered by a Venturi principle face mask or by mechanical ventilation or 1 to 2 L/minute O_2 delivered by nasal prongs) is likely to be required. By comparison, if marked shunting is the cause of hypoxemia, a considerably higher FIO_2 (e.g., >0.7) is required; a common practice when a significant shunt is suspected is to give an FIO_2 of 1.0, then to adjust the FIO_2 downward as guided by the resulting PaO_2 or SaO_2.

The concentration of O_2 that is toxic to the lungs in critically ill patients is not known, but prior injury may provide tolerance to O_2 toxicity, whereas other conditioning agents, such as bleomycin, may enhance oxidative injury. An FIO_2 of 0.8 or higher generally is considered injurious to the human lung, at least the normal human lung. Because it is unknown what lower concentration is safe, however, patients should be given the lowest FIO_2 that provides an adequate SaO_2 (≥90%). If an FIO_2 equal to or greater than 0.5 to 0.7 is required for adequate oxygenation, other measures described subsequently, especially PEEP or CPAP, should be considered. Even a lower FIO_2 of about 0.5 may be associated with impaired ciliary action in the airways and impaired bacterial killing by alveolar macrophages, but the clinical importance of these effects is not known.

A low concentration of supplemental O_2 can be administered by nasal prongs or nasal cannula, which are generally well tolerated and allow the patient to cough, speak, eat, and drink while receiving O_2. When the nasal passages are open, the PIO_2 does not depend greatly on whether the patient breathes through the nose or mouth because O_2 is entrained from the posterior nasal pharynx during a breath taken through the mouth. The level of O_2 can be adjusted by the flow rate to the nasal prongs. In patients with COPD, flows as low as 0.5 to 2 L/minute are usually adequate, unless an intrapulmonary shunt is contributing to the hypoxemia, as usually occurs in acute pneumonia. At flows greater than approximately 6 L/minute, only a small further augmentation in the PIO_2 can be achieved. Because gas flow through the nose has a drying and irritating effect, a face mask should be considered at high flow rates. O_2 face masks using the Venturi principle allow regulation of the FIO_2 and can be particularly useful when COPD is suspected and it is important to avoid the CO_2 retention that can be associated with the unregulated administration of O_2. A higher FIO_2 of 0.5 to nearly 1.0 can be administered through a non-rebreathing face mask with an O_2 reservoir. If an FIO_2 equal to or greater than 0.70 is required for more than several hours, particularly in an unstable patient, endotracheal intubation should be considered so O_2 can be administered by a closed system with reliable maintenance of the patient's SaO_2. Indications for placing an artificial airway in the patient with acute respiratory failure include airway protection against massive aspiration of gastric contents, delivery of an increased FIO_2, facilitation of prolonged mechanical ventilation, and aid in the control of respiratory secretions (Chapter 106).

Ventilatory maneuvers that may increase arterial oxygenation include mechanical ventilation itself and the administration of PEEP or CPAP, all of which allow ventilation of areas of lung that previously were poorly ventilated or unventilated. Although large tidal volumes with mechanical ventilation may open areas of atelectasis and may improve oxygenation initially, these higher tidal volumes can cause lung injury, particularly if the lung is already injured. The mechanism of injury is related to overdistention, which is related to the distending pressure (i.e., alveolar pressure minus pleural pressure). Pleural pressure is not routinely estimated clinically, and the alveolar pressure is usually estimated by the plateau pressure (the pressure measured at the end of inspiration during a period of no flow with any given tidal volume), which can serve as a surrogate for the possibility of injury. What level of plateau pressure can be considered safe is unknown. In the past, a plateau pressure less than 30 cm H_2O was considered relatively noninjurious, but current data suggest that this may not be the case. Conditions other than an overdistending tidal volume, such as abdominal distention, pleural effusion, or pneumothorax, also may contribute to increases in plateau pressure, but under such conditions, the distending pressure may not be elevated because pleural pressure is also elevated.

CPAP refers to the maintenance of positive pressure during the expiratory cycle with spontaneous breathing. *PEEP* refers to the maintenance of positive pressure throughout the expiratory cycle when it is applied together with mechanical ventilation (Chapter 106). CPAP and PEEP can result in recruitment of microatelectatic regions of the lung that are perfused but were not previously ventilated. CPAP and PEEP have the theoretical advantage of keeping some of these regions open during exhalation, thus preventing cyclic closure and reopening of lung units, which can result in alveolar wall stress and injury. The optimal tradeoff between the use and level of CPAP/PEEP compared with the risk of O_2 toxicity from the administration of a higher FIO_2 is not known. PEEP results in an increased intrathoracic pressure, which can diminish venous return to the heart and decrease cardiac output. PEEP should be titrated to a level that allows adequate O_2 saturation at a nontoxic FIO_2 without impairing cardiac output.

Supportive Measures

Every patient with acute respiratory failure is at risk for deep venous thrombosis, pulmonary thromboembolism, and gastric stress ulceration. Prophylactic anticoagulation generally is recommended in patients who are not at high risk of bleeding complications; sequential leg compression therapy may be preferred for patients who are at high risk (Chapter 81).

The best means of preventing stress ulceration is not known; current evidence indicates that the use of an H_2-blocker is superior to gastric administration of sucralfate, based on a large randomized controlled trial that found a higher incidence of significant bleeding in patients receiving sucralfate than in patients receiving ranitidine. Evidence also indicates that proton pump inhibitors may be useful in the acute care setting. There is little firm evidence to guide nutritional management in patients with acute respiratory failure (Chapters 233 and 236).

Current evidence supports maintaining the head of the bed in the critically ill patient at a 45-degree angle to reduce aspiration. Attempts should be made to ensure a normal day/night sleep pattern, including minimizing activity and reducing direct lighting at night. The patient should change position frequently, including sitting in a chair and walking short distances if possible, even while still receiving mechanical ventilatory support. Mobilization can enhance the removal of secretions, help to maintain musculoskeletal function, reduce the risk of deep venous thrombosis, and provide psychological benefits.

Specific Acute Respiratory Failure Syndromes

Chronic Obstructive Pulmonary Disease

Epidemiology and Pathobiology

The epidemiology and pathobiology of COPD are discussed in Chapter 88.

Clinical Manifestations

When COPD causes acute respiratory failure, patients commonly have a history of increasing dyspnea and sputum production. Acute respiratory failure may manifest in more cryptic ways, however, such as changes in mental status, arrhythmias, or other cardiovascular abnormalities. Acute respiratory failure must be considered whenever patients with COPD have significant nonspecific clinical changes.

Diagnosis

The diagnosis can be confirmed or excluded by arterial blood gas analysis. The pH is helpful in assessing whether the hypoventilation is partly or exclusively acute: The pH drops by approximately 0.08 for each 10 mm Hg rise in the $Paco_2$ in acute respiratory acidosis without renal compensation. By comparison, in chronic respiratory acidosis with normal renal compensation, the pH drop is only about approximately 0.03 for each 10 mm Hg rise in the $Paco_2$.

Treatment

Rx

General Care

As soon as acute respiratory failure is confirmed in a patient with COPD, attention must focus on detecting any precipitating events (Table 105–4). Examples include the following: decreased ventilatory drive, commonly because of oversedation; decreased muscle strength or function, often related to electrolyte abnormalities including hypophosphatemia and hypomagnesemia; decreased chest wall elasticity, possibly related to rib fracture, pleural effusion, ileus, or ascites; decreased lung capacity for gas exchange, related to atelectasis, pneumonia, or pulmonary edema; increased airway resistance, caused by bronchospasm or increased secretion; or increased metabolic O_2 requirements, such as with systemic infection. Many of these abnormalities can impair the cough mechanism, diminish the clearance of airway secretions, and precipitate acute respiratory failure.

Infection

The most common specific precipitating event is airway infection, especially acute bronchitis. The role played by viral agents, *Mycoplasma pneumoniae*, chronic contaminants of the lower airway such as *Haemophilus influenzae* and *Streptococcus pneumoniae*, and other acute pathogens is difficult to determine on a clinical or even microbiologic basis. Acute exacerbations of COPD commonly result from new infections rather than recurrent emergence of an infection from preexisting colonization. Antibiotics modestly shorten the duration of the exacerbation without a significant increase in toxicity compared with placebo; the impact of antibiotics on the subsequent emergence of resistant organisms is not known. It is standard practice, however, to use antibiotics to treat the patient with COPD who has an exacerbation severe enough to cause acute respiratory failure and who has evidence consistent with acute tracheobronchitis (Chapters 88 and 96). Pneumonia may account for 20% of cases of acute respiratory failure in patients with COPD. Compared with the physiologically normal population, patients with COPD who have community-acquired pneumonia are more likely to have gram-negative enteric bacteria or *Legionella* infections and are more likely to have antibiotic-resistant organisms.

Other Precipitating Causes

Other common precipitating causes of acute respiratory failure include heart failure and worsening of the underlying COPD, often related to noncompliance with medications. Less common and often difficult to diagnose in this setting is pulmonary thromboembolism. The severe acute respiratory syndrome (SARS) requires supportive care; no specific antiviral therapies are currently available (Chapters 97 and 389).

Site of Care

Many patients with COPD and acute respiratory failure can be managed on a general medical hospital floor rather than in an intensive care unit if the precipitating cause of acute respiratory failure has been diagnosed and is potentially responsive to appropriate therapy, if any blood gas abnormalities respond to O_2 therapy and are not life-threatening, if the patient can cooperate with the treatment, and if appropriate nursing and respiratory care can be provided (Chapter 88). An unstable patient who requires closer observation and monitoring should be admitted to an intensive care unit.

TABLE 105–4 KEY PRINCIPLES IN THE MANAGEMENT OF CHRONIC OBSTRUCTIVE PULMONARY DISEASE PATIENTS WITH ACUTE RESPIRATORY FAILURE

1. Monitor and treat life-threatening hypoxemia (these measures should be performed virtually simultaneously).
   a. Assess the patient clinically, and measure oxygenation by arterial blood gases and/or oximetry
      (1) If the patient is hypoxemic, initiate supplemental oxygen therapy with nasal prongs (low flows [0.5–2. L/min] are usually sufficient) or by Venturi face mask.
      (2) If the patient needs ventilatory support, consider noninvasive ventilation.
      (3) Determine whether the patient needs to be intubated; this is almost always a clinical decision; immediate action is required if the patient is comatose or severely obtunded.
   b. A reasonable goal in most patients is Pao_2 of 55–60 mm Hg or an Sao_2 of 88–90%.
   c. After changes in Fio_2, check blood gases and check regularly for signs of carbon dioxide retention.
2. Start to correct life-threatening acidosis.
   a. The most effective approach is to correct the underlying cause of ARF (e.g., bronchospasm, infection, heart failure).
   b. Consider ventilatory support, based largely on clinical considerations.
   c. With severe acidosis, the use of bicarbonate can be considered, but it is often ineffective, and little evidence exists for clinical benefit.
3. If ventilatory support is required, consider noninvasive mechanical ventilation.
   a. The patient must have intact upper airway reflexes and be alert, cooperative, and hemodynamically stable.
   b. Careful monitoring is required; if patient does not tolerate the mask, becomes hemodynamically unstable, or has deteriorating mental status, consider intubation.
4. Treat airway obstruction and underlying disease process that triggered the episode of ARF.
   a. Treat airway obstruction with pharmacologic agents: systemic corticosteroids and bronchodilators (ipratropium and/or β-adrenergic agents).
   b. Improve secretion clearance: encourage the patient to cough, administer chest physical therapy if cough is impaired and a trial appears effective.
   c. Treat the underlying disease process (e.g., antibiotics, diuretics).
5. Prevent complications of the disease process and minimize iatrogenic complications.
   a. Pulmonary thromboembolism prophylaxis: use subcutaneous heparin if no contraindications exist.
   b. Gastrointestinal complications: Administer prophylaxis of gastrointestinal bleeding.
   c. Hemodynamics: If the patient is ventilated, monitor and minimize auto-PEEP.
      (1) Treat the underlying obstruction.
      (2) Minimize minute ventilation; use controlled hypoventilation.
      (3) Use small tidal volumes; increase the inspiratory flow rate to decrease the inspiratory time and to lengthen the expiratory time.
   d. Cardiac arrhythmias: Maintain oxygenation, and normalize electrolytes.

ARF = acute respiratory failure; Fio_2 = fraction of inspired oxygen; Pao_2 = partial pressure of oxygen in arterial blood; PEEP = positive end-expiratory pressure; Sao_2 = oxygen saturation.

Rx

Mechanical Therapy

The decision to use mechanical ventilation in patients with COPD and acute respiratory failure must be made on clinical grounds and is not dictated by any particular arterial blood gas values. In general, if the patient is alert and is able to cooperate with treatment, mechanical ventilation is unlikely to be necessary. If ventilatory support is required (Chapter 106), the decision is whether to use noninvasive positive pressure ventilation therapy (without endotracheal intubation) or endotracheal intubation with positive pressure ventilation. Many studies have demonstrated that noninvasive positive pressure ventilation is preferred for patients with COPD and can decrease mortality if applied in appropriate patients without factors that are likely to lead to complications. [5] Patients must be able to tolerate the nasal or facial mask, must be cooperative and hemodynamically stable, and must have intact upper airway reflexes to prevent aspiration. Noninvasive ventilation is usually more comfortable for the patient, and it reduces the need for sedation. The correction of blood gases is slower with noninvasive ventilation, and gastric distention can occur. Patients must be monitored carefully, and endotracheal intubation is required if the patient's condition deteriorates or the patient cannot tolerate the face mask.

Complications

Auto-PEEP or intrinsic PEEP with air trapping is a common and dangerous complication of ventilation in the patient with COPD. For any given increase in alveolar pressure, patients with significant emphysema and increased lung compliance have a greater increase in lung volume and a greater increase in pleural pressure. The result is a greater risk of decreasing venous return and of impairing cardiac output. This complication must be considered and looked for when mechanical ventilation is used in the patient with COPD.

Prognosis

Acute respiratory failure in patients with severe COPD is associated with an in-hospital mortality of 6 to 20%. The severity of the underlying disease and the severity of the acute precipitating illness are important determinants of hospital survival. Hospital mortality is higher if the respiratory failure is associated with a pH less than 7.25. The pH, the $Pa{CO_2}$, and other clinical characteristics cannot be used, however, to predict a particular patient's chances of survival reliably. It is unclear whether an episode of acute respiratory failure changes the long-term prognosis if the patient survives the acute episode.

Acute Lung Injury/Acute Respiratory Distress Syndrome

Definition

ARDS was first described in 1967 as the abrupt onset of diffuse lung injury characterized by severe hypoxemia (shunting) and generalized pulmonary infiltrates on the chest radiograph in the absence of overt cardiac failure. In the early 1990s, the term *acute lung injury* officially was introduced to include traditional ARDS and less severe forms of lung injury. The definitions of acute lung injury and ARDS require bilateral pulmonary infiltrates compatible with pulmonary edema in the absence of clinical heart failure (usually as determined by no evidence of elevated left atrial pressures), but the two are differentiated by the degree of abnormal oxygenation: Patients are defined as having acute lung injury if the $Pa{O_2}$ divided by the $F{IO_2}$ ($Pa{O_2}/F{IO_2}$, also called the P/F ratio), is less than or equal to 300. When the $Pa{O_2}/F{IO_2}$ is less than or equal to 200, the patient meets criteria for ARDS.

Epidemiology

Current data suggest an annual incidence of acute lung injury of 40 to 75 cases per 100,000 population annually. These incidence figures, taken together with the associated case-fatality rates, which currently are 30 to 50% but are highly dependent on the severity of disease, make acute lung injury and ARDS major public health problems and major causes of death.

Etiology

Acute lung injury should be considered a clinical syndrome secondary to some other cause (Table 105–5). This underlying clinical disorder may affect and injure the lungs directly, such as in diffuse pneumonia or aspiration of gastric contents, or may affect the lungs indirectly, such as in severe sepsis (Chapter 109) or severe nonthoracic trauma (Chapter 113). Severe sepsis is the most common precipitating cause of acute lung injury worldwide. The organisms vary widely, ranging from gram-negative and gram-positive bacteria and viruses, to leptospiral infections, or to malaria. It may be difficult to determine whether pneumonia is diffuse, with endobronchial spread involving most of the lungs, or whether localized pneumonia has precipitated a sepsis syndrome with secondary injury to other parts of the lung.

Pathobiology

Pathology

Despite the variety of underlying disease processes leading to acute lung injury, the response to these insults in the lung is monotonously characteristic, manifest by similar clinical findings, physiologic changes, and morphologic abnormalities. The pathologic abnormalities in acute lung injury and ARDS are nonspecific and are described as *diffuse alveolar damage* by pathologists. Abnormalities of epithelial cells, particularly type 1 alveolar cells and pulmonary vascular endothelial cells, are seen. The initial process is inflammatory, with neutrophils usually predominating in the alveolar fluid. Hyaline membranes develop, similar to those seen in premature infants with infant respiratory distress syndrome, presumably related to the presence of large-molecular-weight proteins that

TABLE 105–5 DISORDERS ASSOCIATED WITH ACUTE LUNG INJURY AND ACUTE RESPIRATORY DISTRESS SYNDROME

COMMON

Sepsis (gram-positive or gram-negative bacterial, viral, fungal, or parasitic)
Diffuse pneumonia (bacterial, viral, or fungal)
Aspiration of gastric contents
Trauma (usually severe)

LESS COMMON

Near-drowning (fresh or salt water)
Drug overdoses
- Acetylsalicylic acid
- Heroin and other narcotic drugs

Massive blood transfusion (likely a marker of severe trauma but also seen with severe gastrointestinal bleeding, especially in patients with severe liver disease)
Leukoagglutination reactions
Inhalation of smoke or corrosive gases (usually requires high concentrations)
Pancreatitis
Fat embolism

UNCOMMON

Miliary tuberculosis
Aspiration of paraquat
Central nervous system injury or anoxia (neurogenic pulmonary edema)
Cardiopulmonary bypass
Severe acute respiratory syndrome (SARS)

have leaked into the alveolar space. Alveolar flooding leads to impairment of surfactant, which is abnormal in quantity and quality. The result is microatelectasis, which may be associated with an impairment of immune function. Cytokines and other inflammatory mediators usually are markedly elevated, although with different patterns over time in the bronchoalveolar lavage and the systemic blood. Lung repair also is disturbed; early evidence of profibrotic processes is manifest by the appearance of breakdown products of procollagen in the bronchoalveolar lavage fluid, followed by subsequent scarring. The pulmonary fibrosis observed on lung biopsy or at autopsy is identical to that seen in patients with idiopathic pulmonary fibrosis (Chapter 92). Because lung function improves over time in survivors of ARDS, however, it has been assumed that this scarring is potentially reversible.

Pathophysiology

The physiologic abnormalities are dominated by severe hypoxemia with shunting, decreased lung compliance, decreased functional residual capacity, and increased work of breathing. Initially, the $PaCO_2$ is low or normal, usually associated with increased alveolar ventilation. The initial abnormalities in oxygenation are thought to be related to alveolar flooding and collapse. As the disease progresses, especially in patients who require continued ventilatory support, fibroproliferation develops; the lungs (including alveoli, blood vessels, and small airways) remodel and scar, with a loss of microvasculature. These changes may lead to pulmonary hypertension and increased dead space; marked elevations in minute ventilation are required to achieve a normal $PaCO_2$ even as oxygenation abnormalities are improving.

Clinical Manifestations

Most cases of acute lung injury have an onset that either coincides with the recognition of the underlying disease process or occurs within 72 hours of its onset; the mean time from onset of the underlying cause to onset of acute lung injury is 12 to 24 hours. The presenting picture is dominated by respiratory distress and the accompanying laboratory findings of severe hypoxemia and generalized infiltrates or opacities on the chest radiograph, or it is dominated by the manifestations of the underlying disease process, such as severe sepsis with hypotension and other manifestations of systemic infection.

Diagnosis

The key to diagnosis is to distinguish ARDS from cardiogenic pulmonary edema (Table 105–6). No specific biochemical test exists to define ARDS. Certain blood or bronchoalveolar lavage (Chapter 85) abnormalities are frequent but are not sufficiently specific to be useful clinically.

Treatment

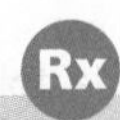

Treatment for acute lung injury and ARDS consists predominantly of respiratory support and treatment of the underlying disease (Fig. 105–4).

Mechanical Therapy

Current recommendations for mechanical ventilation via endotracheal intubation (Table 105–7) emphasize lower tidal volumes based on a patient's predicted body weight (Chapter 106). 3 PEEP remains a mainstay in the ventilatory strategy for acute lung injury, although the method for determining the optimal level of PEEP has not been established. PEEP may allow a lower FIO_2 to provide adequate oxygenation, thus avoiding O_2 toxicity. It also may prevent the cyclic collapse and reopening of lung units, a process that is thought to be a major cause of ventilator-induced lung injury, even when adequate oxygenation can be obtained at relatively low levels of FIO_2.

Inhaled nitric oxide is a potent vasodilator and bronchodilator that can enhance arterial oxygenation. It has not been shown to improve outcome in clinical trials, however, so its routine use cannot

TABLE 105–6 FEATURES ASSOCIATED WITH NONCARDIOGENIC AND CARDIOGENIC PULMONARY EDEMA*

Noncardiogenic Edema (ARDS)	Cardiogenic Edema/Volume Overload
PRIOR HISTORY	
Younger	Older
No history of heart disease	Prior history of heart disease
Appropriate fluid balance (difficult to assess after resuscitation from shock or trauma)	Hypertension, chest pain, new-onset palpitations; positive fluid balance
PHYSICAL EXAMINATION	
Flat neck veins	Elevated neck veins
Hyperdynamic pulses	Left ventricular enlargement, lift, heave, dyskinesis
Physiologic gallop	S_3 and S_4; murmurs
Absence of edema	Edema: flank, presacral, legs
ELECTROCARDIOGRAM	
Sinus tachycardia, nonspecific ST-T wave changes	Evidence of prior or ongoing ischemia, supraventricular tachycardia, left ventricular hypertrophy
CHEST RADIOGRAPH	
Normal heart size	Cardiomegaly
Peripheral distribution of infiltrates	Central or basilar infiltrates; peribronchial and vascular congestion
Air bronchogram common (80%)	Septal lines (Kerley's lines), air bronchograms (25%), pleural effusion
HEMODYNAMIC MEASUREMENTS	
Pulmonary artery wedge pressure <15 mm Hg, cardiac index >3.5 L/min/m^2	Pulmonary capillary wedge pressure >18 mm Hg, cardiac index <3.5 L/min/m^2 with ischemia, may be >3.5 L/min/m^2 with volume overload

*These features generally are neither highly sensitive nor specific. Although the findings more commonly are associated with the types of pulmonary edema as listed, they have not been shown to have high positive or negative predictive values.

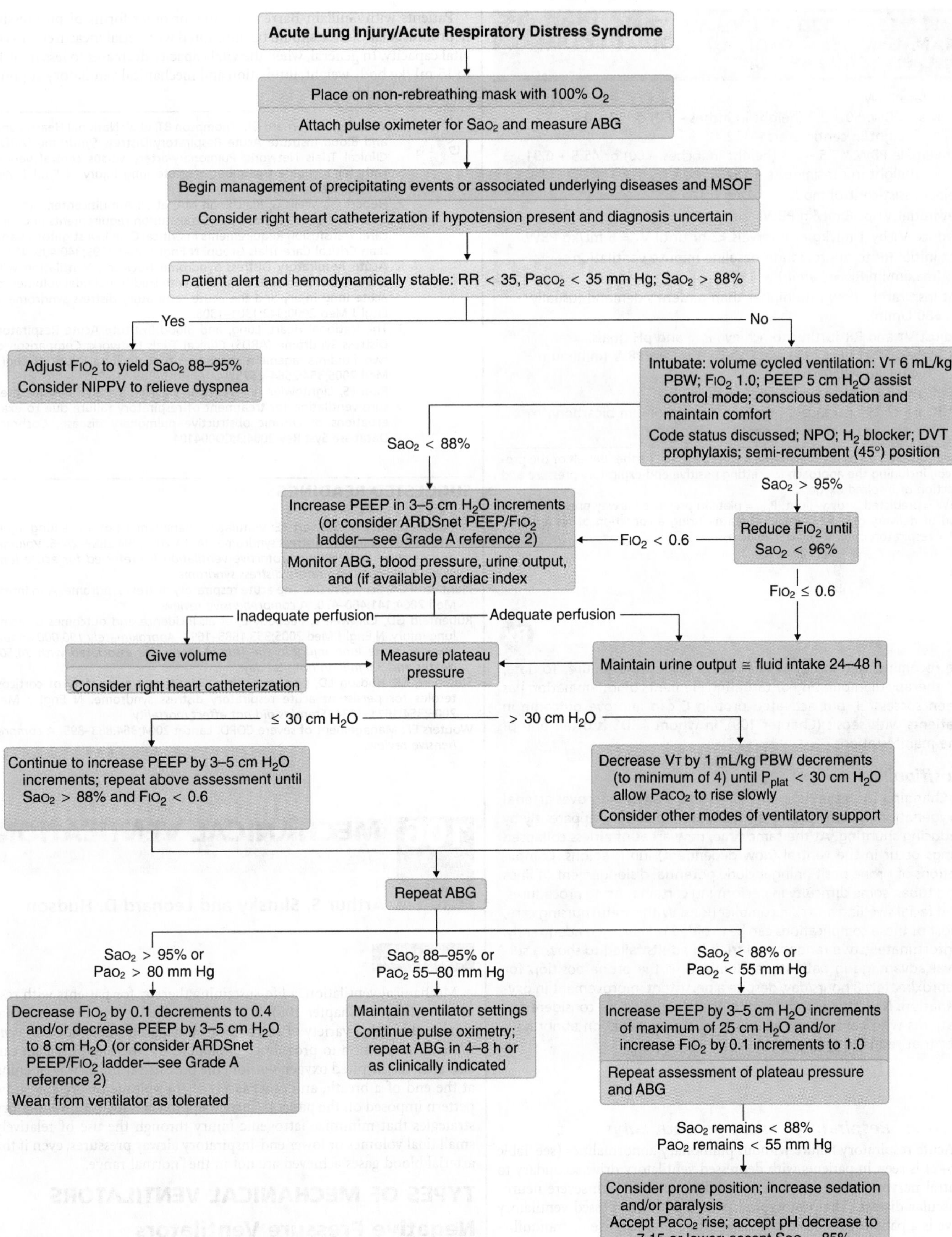

FIGURE 105–4 • An algorithm for the initial management of acute respiratory distress syndrome. ABG = arterial blood gas analysis; CO_2 = carbon dioxide; DVT = deep venous thrombosis; Fio_2 = inspired oxygen concentration; MSOF = multisystem organ failure; NIPPV = noninvasive intermittent positive-pressure ventilation; O_2 = oxygen; $Paco_2$ = arterial partial pressure of carbon dioxide; Pao_2 = arterial partial pressure of oxygen; PBW = predicted body weight; PEEP = positive end-expiratory pressure; P_{plat} = plateau pressure; RR = respiratory rate; Sao_2 = arterial oxygen saturation; V_T = tidal volume.

TABLE 105–7 ARDSNet VENTILATORY MANAGEMENT PROTOCOL FOR TIDAL VOLUME AND PLATEAU PRESSURE*

Calculate PBW.
- Male PBW: 50 + 2.3 (height in inches – 60) or 50 + 0.91 (height in centimeters – 152.4).
- Female PBW: 45.5 + 2.3 (height in inches – 60) or 45.5 + 0.91 (height in centimeters – 152.4).

Select assist-control mode.

Set initial VT at 8 mL/kg PBW.

Reduce VT by 1 mL/kg at intervals <2 hr until VT = 6 mL/kg PBW.

Set initial RR to approximate baseline minute ventilation (maximum RR = 35/min).

Set inspiratory flow rate higher than patient's demand (usually >80 L/min).

Adjust VT and RR further to achieve P_{plat} and pH goals.
- If P_{plat} >30 cm H_2O: decrease VT by 1 mL/kg PBW (minimum = 4 mL/kg PBW).
- If pH ≤7.30, increase RR (maximum = 35).
- If pH <7.15, increase RR to 35; consider sodium bicarbonate administration or increase VT.

*See ARDSNet website (http://www.ardsnet.org) for further details of the protocol, including the approach for setting positive end-expiratory pressure and fraction of inspired oxygen.
PBW = predicted body weight; P_{plat} = plateau pressure (airway pressure at the end of delivery of a tidal volume breath during a condition of no airflow); RR = respiratory rate; VT = tidal volume.

be recommended in adults with acute respiratory failure. To date, no therapy manipulating or targeting elements of inflammation has been successful, but activated protein C can improve outcome in patients with sepsis (Chapter 109), in whom ARDS is often one of the manifestations.

Positioning

Changing from the supine to the prone position improves arterial oxygenation in many patients with acute lung injury, apparently by reducing shunting. At the same time, new areas of airless collapsed lungs occur in the ventral (now dependent) lung regions. Complications of prone positioning include potential dislodgement of lines and tubes, some difficulty in performing certain nursing procedures, and facial swelling and skin complications. With careful nursing care, most of these complications can be avoided or managed adequately. Unfortunately, two randomized trials in adults failed to show a survival advantage in patients randomized to the prone position for approximately 8 hours/day, despite a persistent improvement in oxygenation. Nevertheless, the prone position should be considered in patients who have life-threatening severe oxygenation abnormalities that require high FIO_2 and PEEP.

Acute Respiratory Failure without Lung Disease

Acute respiratory failure without pulmonary abnormalities (see Table 105–2) is seen in patients with depressed ventilatory drive secondary to central nervous system dysfunction and in patients with severe neuromuscular disease. The prototypical patient with suppressed ventilatory drive is a patient who has taken an overdose of a sedative or tranquilizing medication (Chapter 111). The prototypical patient with neuromuscular disease is the patient with Guillain-Barré syndrome (Chapter 446). The treatment for both these types of patients is supportive. In the patient with a sedative overdose, the threshold for intubation with mechanical ventilatory support should be low because this temporary condition should be quickly reversible when the responsible drug is eliminated. The patient with a sedative overdose may require intubation for airway protection against aspiration of gastric contents.

Patients with Guillain-Barré syndrome or other forms of progressive neuromuscular disease should be monitored with serial measurements of vital capacity. In general, when the vital capacity decreases to less than 10 to 15 mL/kg body weight, intubation and mechanical ventilatory support should be considered.

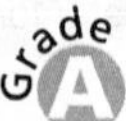

1. Wheeler AP, Bernard GR, Thompson BT, et al: National Heart, Lung, and Blood Institute Acute Respiratory Distress Syndrome (ARDS) Clinical Trials Network: Pulmonary-artery versus central venous catheter to guide treatment of acute lung injury. N Engl J Med 2006;354:2213–2224.
2. Hebert PC, Wells G, Blajchman MA, et al: A multicenter, randomized, controlled clinical trial of transfusion requirements in critical care: Transfusion Requirements in Critical Care Investigators, Canadian Critical Care Trials Group. N Engl J Med 1999;340:409–417.
3. Acute Respiratory Distress Syndrome Network: Ventilation with lower tidal volumes as compared with traditional tidal volumes for acute lung injury and the acute respiratory distress syndrome. N Engl J Med 2000;342:1301–1308.
4. The National Heart, Lung, and Blood Institute Acute Respiratory Distress Syndrome (ARDS) Clinical Trials Network: Comparison of two fluid-management strategies in acute lung injury. N Engl J Med 2006;354:2564–2575.
5. Ram FS, Lightowler JV, Wedzicha JA: Non-invasive positive pressure ventilation for treatment of respiratory failure due to exacerbations of chronic obstructive pulmonary disease. Cochrane Database Syst Rev 2004;3:CD004104.

SUGGESTED READINGS

Fan E, Needham DM, Stewart TE: Ventilatory management of acute lung injury and acute respiratory distress syndrome. JAMA 2005;294:2889–2896. *Volume- and pressure-limited lung-protective ventilation is preferred for acute lung injury and acute respiratory distress syndrome.*

Piantadosi CA, Schwartz DA: The acute respiratory distress syndrome. Ann Intern Med 2004;141:460–470. *A comprehensive review.*

Rubenfeld GD, Caldwell E, Peabody E, et al: Incidence and outcomes of acute lung injury. N Engl J Med 2005;353:1685–1693. *Approximately 190,000 annual cases of acute lung injury in the United States are associated with 74,500 deaths and 3.6 million hospital days.*

Steinberg KP, Hudson LD, Goodman RB, et al: Efficacy and safety of corticosteroids for persistent acute respiratory distress syndrome. N Engl J Med 2006;354:1671–1684. *Steroids did not affect mortality.*

Wouters EF: Management of severe COPD. Lancet 2004;364:883–895. *A comprehensive review.*

106 MECHANICAL VENTILATION

Arthur S. Slutsky and Leonard D. Hudson

Definition

Mechanical ventilation, a life-sustaining therapy for patients with respiratory failure (Chapter 105), is provided partially or fully by external sources through a variety of mechanical strategies termed *modes of ventilation.* In addition to providing ventilation, the treating physician can also alter the inspired oxygen tension, the pressure at the airway opening at the end of a breath, and other facets of the volume or pressure time pattern imposed on the patient. Current approaches focus on ventilatory strategies that minimize iatrogenic injury through the use of relatively small tidal volumes or lower end-inspiratory airway pressures, even if the arterial blood gases achieved are not in the "normal range."

TYPES OF MECHANICAL VENTILATORS

Negative Pressure Ventilators

Delivery of gas to the lungs requires a pressure gradient across the airways and alveoli. During spontaneous breathing, this pressure gradient is generated by development of a negative pleural pressure as a result of contraction of the respiratory muscles. Some ventilators operate by generating negative pressure around the chest wall (e.g., cuirass) or the entire body below the neck (e.g., iron lung). Such ventilators have two major advantages: there is no need to intubate the patient to apply mechanical ventilation, and the detrimental hemodynamic consequences are minimized if the ventilators generate negative pressure solely around the chest wall. However, several difficulties have been reported with these ventilators. First, the seal must be adequate to couple the output of the ventilator to the chest wall. Second, the nursing care of patients in such ventilators can be difficult, especially with iron lungs, which enclose the entire patient from the neck down in the ventilator. Although this type of ventilator was widely used during the polio epidemic of the mid-1950s, its only current use is for patients who have relatively normal lungs but who require long-term ventilation for neuromuscular problems.

Positive Pressure Ventilators

The most widely used mechanical ventilation approach is to deliver gas to the lung using positive pressure ventilation (PPV) applied through an endotracheal tube, a tracheostomy, or a tight-fitting mask. The approach using a mask is considered noninvasive ventilation (NIV) and is considered separately.

The most basic mode of PPV is *controlled ventilation,* in which a preset tidal volume and rate are delivered to the patient regardless of the patient's requirements or efforts. This form of ventilation is usually used in patients who cannot initiate spontaneous breaths (e.g., heavily sedated or paralyzed patients) or in those who need full ventilatory support because of extremely severe pulmonary or cardiovascular disease (e.g., severe shock). This mode is not routinely used in patients who are able to make spontaneous ventilatory efforts because it can lead to asynchrony between the patient's efforts and the breaths generated by the ventilator. *Assisted ventilation* is the term used when spontaneous ventilatory efforts are present; the onset of a breath is triggered by the patient's respiratory efforts, rather than being based strictly on the time between breaths.

Mechanical ventilation can be applied using either volume-controlled or pressure-controlled modes. In volume-controlled ventilation, the desired tidal volume and respiratory rate are programmed into the ventilator, and the airway pressure is the dependent variable that changes with the mechanical properties of the patient's respiratory system and with the flow settings on the ventilator. In pressure-controlled ventilation, the pressure imposed at the airway opening and the respiratory rate are programmed into the ventilator, and the tidal volume becomes the dependent variable.

Positive End-Expiratory Pressure

A key characteristic that can be used with any of the modes of ventilation is the level of the end-expiratory pressure. Positive pressure in the airway is used in patients with diffuse pulmonary diseases (e.g., pulmonary edema, acute respiratory distress syndrome [ARDS]) to recruit collapsed alveolar regions and to maintain them in a recruited state, to reopen collapsed airways, to redistribute fluid in the lung, to increase functional residual capacity, and to redistribute ventilation to dependent regions. All these changes can improve the ratio of ventilation to perfusion as well as oxygenation, thereby allowing the fractional inspiratory concentration of oxygen (FIO_2) to be reduced. Positive end-expiratory pressure (PEEP) does not usually improve alveolar ventilation and, in fact, may increase dead space by overdistending alveoli, with a concomitant decrease in alveolar capillary blood flow. PEEP can also be administered to spontaneously breathing subjects by using a technique termed *continuous positive airway pressure.* Continuous positive airway pressure and PEEP can be used in patients with exacerbations of chronic obstructive pulmonary disease (COPD) to overcome auto-PEEP (see later) and to minimize the work of breathing, provided the magnitude of the PEEP is low enough that it does not cause additional hyperinflation.

Volume-Controlled Ventilation

The term *volume-controlled ventilation* (or *volume-limited ventilation*) refers to mechanical ventilation in which the tidal volume is preset. The major advantage is that the delivered tidal volume is maintained even if lung mechanics change, thereby ensuring a more constant partial pressure of arterial carbon dioxide ($PaCO_2$). The potential disadvantage is that if lung mechanics deteriorate, higher pressures may be required to achieve the tidal volume goal, and regions of overinflation with lung injury may result. Although controlled ventilation as described earlier can be either volume limited (preset tidal volume) or pressure limited, clinicians usually use the term *controlled mechanical ventilation* to refer to volume-limited ventilation with a set rate. An upper limit to applied airway pressure is commonly included for safety reasons.

The most common form of volume-controlled ventilation is one in which the patient assists the ventilator, thus triggering at least some of the breaths. The term *assisted mechanical ventilation* can refer either to volume-limited ventilation or to pressure-limited ventilation when the patient triggers some or all of the breaths, but the ventilator will always deliver a minimum number of breaths if apnea occurs. This mode is also referred to as *assist/control* (A/C).

Intermittent Mandatory Ventilation

The term *intermittent mandatory ventilation* (IMV) refers to a mode in which the patient is allowed to breathe spontaneously through an endotracheal tube or tracheostomy but also receives some preset (and thus mandatory) volume-limited breaths from the ventilator. In current ventilators, the mandatory breaths are triggered by the patient and thus are synchronized (synchronized IMV); however, if the patient ceases spontaneous ventilatory efforts, breaths at the rate set on the ventilator will still be delivered. Synchronized IMV is a form of partial ventilatory support, because some breaths are spontaneous, rather than full ventilatory support, in which all breaths are delivered by the ventilator. This mode allows the patient to do a variable amount of the respiratory work but with the security of a set minimal backup rate should spontaneous ventilatory efforts stop.

Pressure Control Ventilation

Pressure control ventilation is a mode of ventilation in which gas is delivered by the ventilator at a set pressure relative to atmospheric pressure; delivered volume becomes a dependent variable. The initiation of each breath may be triggered by the patient (assisted breaths) or may be initiated by the ventilator (controlled breaths). The delivered tidal volume depends on the preset pressure, the ventilatory rate, the inspiratory-to-expiratory ratio, and the patient's respiratory mechanics (resistance, compliance, and auto-PEEP). At a fixed preset pressure and inspiratory-to-expiratory ratio, tidal volume decreases as respiratory frequency increases. In patients with COPD, the tidal volume at low frequencies is relatively high but decreases substantially as the respiratory rate is increased, whereas in patients with stiff respiratory systems (e.g., ARDS), the tidal volume does not change much with respiratory frequency because the lung fills with gas quickly.

Pressure Support Ventilation

Pressure support ventilation is a pressure-limited, patient-triggered ventilatory mode. Once the patient triggers the ventilator, by creating either a small negative pressure or a low inspiratory flow at the airway, the ventilator cycles on and provides the airflow needed to maintain a preset level of pressure. In contrast to pressure control ventilation, inspiration terminates when the inspiratory airflow decreases to a threshold level (the specific algorithm varies from ventilator to ventilator). This mode provides flexibility for the patient with respect to tidal volume, inspiratory flow, and ratio of time allowed for inspiration as compared with expiration. Tidal volume depends on patient-related factors (effort), respiratory system mechanics, and the set pressure level. Pressure support ventilation is a form of partial ventilatory support in which the size of each breath is determined partially by the patient's muscular effort and partially by the ventilator. This mode can compensate for the added work of breathing imposed by the resistance of the endotracheal tube compared with the natural airway. Pressure support ventilation has largely been used to wean patients from ventilatory support because it provides a simple way to reduce the magnitude of mechanical support while the patient assumes a larger fraction of the ventilatory work than with most other modes of assisted ventilation.

High-Frequency Ventilation

The term *high-frequency ventilation* refers to certain ventilatory modes that have the common feature of providing ventilation using frequencies that are substantially greater than those used during normal breathing. Several different approaches are used for the delivery of high-frequency ventilation: high-frequency PPV, high-frequency jet ventilation, and high-frequency oscillatory ventilation. During high-frequency ventilation, tidal volumes may be less than the dead space, so adequate gas transport takes place by various convective and diffusive mechanisms. Interest in using these modes of ventilation has waxed and waned over the past 2 decades. In recent years, interest in high-frequency ventilation has had a resurgence, based on the concept that it may be the ideal way to minimize ventilator-induced lung injury because the small tidal volumes make it easier to avoid both overdistention of lung units and injury at low lung volumes. Animal data in support of this approach are very strong in models of acute lung injury. Recent data in infants with respiratory distress syndrome and in adults with ARDS that suggest that high-frequency ventilation may be as effective as conventional mechanical ventilatory assistance.

Noninvasive Positive Pressure Ventilation

Since the mid-1990s, interest in providing PPV through a mask rather than through an endotracheal tube has increased. The NIV method has been termed *noninvasive* because the patient is not intubated, and hence the approach is relatively noninvasive. This approach, although conceptually simple, requires appropriate implementation and monitoring for its successful application. Of particular importance are the selection of patients and the appropriate training of hospital personnel. Patients must be alert, cooperative, and hemodynamically stable. Patients must also have intact upper airway reflexes, so they do not aspirate upper airway materials into the lung, and they must not have any facial trauma that would preclude the use of a mask. Once patients are started on NIV, they should be carefully monitored, and NIV should be discontinued if the patient does not tolerate the mask, if it becomes clear from clinical examination that the patient may aspirate, if cardiovascular instability exists, or if the patient's mental status is deteriorating.

NIV has certain potential advantages compared with invasive ventilation. It is relatively easy to apply and can be used for short intervals because it can be started and stopped very easily. The major advantages are that it avoids the complications associated with intubation, it is usually more comfortable for the patient, and it reduces the need for sedation. Patients receiving NIV are able to communicate verbally with medical staff and family members, are likely able to sleep better, and are able to eat if they are sufficiently stable to remove the mask for short periods of time.

However, NIV has several disadvantages. Implementation of NIV takes more time from caregivers at the bedside initially, and the time course of correction of blood gases is slower than usually occurs in patients who are intubated and ventilated. Gastric distention is an unusual occurrence; medical staff should be aware of this complication and should watch for signs of abdominal distention. Data strongly support the use of NIV for patients with COPD (see later), but whether it provides better outcomes in other forms of respiratory failure is uncertain.

COMPLICATIONS

Intubation

Endotracheal intubation can be used to secure a patient's airway, to act as a conduit to deliver gas from the ventilator to the patient, to prevent aspiration, and/or to help with pulmonary toilet when secretions are increased. However, intubation can be associated with a certain complications, including upper airway trauma, disruption of normal host defense mechanisms, and the risk of aspiration during intubation. Pressure from the cuff of the endotracheal tube, which achieves a pneumatic seal between the tube and trachea, can lead to regions of tracheal ischemia that, as a result of injury-repair processes, may eventually cause tracheal stenosis. Because the endotracheal tube is smaller than the airway into which it is inserted, an increase in airway resistance occurs, the magnitude of which depends on the length, radius, and shape of the tube. Furthermore, the upper airway is normally a very effective means of heating and humidifying inspiratory gases. This natural system is bypassed by an endotracheal tube; inadequately humidified inspiratory gases can reduce mucociliary clearance and can even lead to inspissation of tracheal secretions.

Cough is impaired in patients in whom an endotracheal tube has been placed. Normally, cough involves an increase in airway pressure as respiratory muscles are contracted against a closed glottis. When the glottis opens, expiratory flow sharply increases, resulting in dynamic compression of major airways. The presence of an endotracheal tube limits the buildup of airway pressure and alters the dynamics of expiratory flow, thereby greatly impairing the efficacy of the patient's cough.

A cuffed endotracheal tube helps to prevent gross aspiration, but pharyngeal secretions that pool at the top of the cuff often seep into the lungs and increase the probability of developing nosocomial pneumonia (Chapter 97). Endotracheal tubes also make swallowing and communication difficult.

Hemodynamic Compromise

The major mechanical determinants of cardiovascular hemodynamics during mechanical ventilation are intrathoracic pressure, changes in lung volume, and the patient's circulatory volume status. An increase in lung volume can cause a beneficial decrease in pulmonary vascular resistance, if lung units that had been closed are opened as a result of mechanical ventilation, or it can lead to a detrimental increase in pulmonary resistance related to overdistention of the lung with concomitant compression and lengthening of alveolar vessels.

PPV can have a major impact on cardiovascular hemodynamics through its effect on pleural pressure, an effect that is directly related to changes in lung volume and not necessarily directly reflected in measurements of airway pressure, because the relation between alveolar pressure and lung volume depends on respiratory system mechanics. For example, in a patient with stiff lungs (e.g., ARDS), a given increase in plateau pressure (Pplat) will lead to much less of an increase in lung volume than in a patient with COPD, so the increase in pleural pressure will be much less in the patient with ARDS. As a result, patients with ARDS tolerate relatively high PEEP levels, whereas similarly high levels in patients with normal lungs (e.g., in a drug overdose) or in COPD would markedly reduce cardiac output. At very high lung volumes, a direct effect of the pressure of the lung on the heart can increase pericardial pressure and can thereby decrease cardiac filling.

Auto-PEEP and Dynamic Hyperinflation

A key factor that affects cardiovascular hemodynamics and other physiologic variables during mechanical ventilation is the development of *auto-PEEP,* defined as the difference between alveolar pressure and airway pressure at the end of expiration. Auto-PEEP leads to dynamic hyperinflation, which is an increase in the end-expiratory lung volume higher than the value that would be obtained if there were complete exhalation to the static functional residual capacity. This phenomenon occurs whenever time is insufficient for a complete exhalation to occur; the respiratory system is thus prevented from reaching its static end-expiratory volume. The major determinants of auto-PEEP and hence dynamic hyperinflation are increased expiratory airway resistance, high minute ventilation, increased respiratory system compliance, and decreased expiratory time.

Auto-PEEP is more likely to occur in patients with airway obstruction. It is good practice to use approaches such as controlled hypoventilation to prevent its occurrence when mechanical ventilation is provided to such patients.

Auto-PEEP may not be detected by routine measurements of pressure at the airway opening, because the major pressure drop occurs across the airways. Moreover, measurements of auto-PEEP are difficult to make in spontaneously breathing patients. When patients are not making spontaneous breathing efforts, auto-PEEP can be assessed as the difference in pressure between the set PEEP and the pressure obtained when the airway opening is occluded at the end of expiration (Fig. 106–1). It can also be assessed using the change in Pplat after a prolonged pause during volume cycle ventilation. If it is considered safe for the patient, a rapid estimate of the effect of auto-PEEP on cardiovascular hemodynamics can be obtained by transiently disconnecting the ventilator and allowing the auto-PEEP to approach zero during a long expiration. If the auto-PEEP is less than 5 cm H_2O, it is unlikely to cause clinically important changes in the measured intravascular pressures.

If auto-PEEP is not considered in the interpretation of respiratory mechanics, measurements of respiratory system compliance will be falsely low. Dynamic hyperinflation can be measured as the volume of gas that is released when the expiratory time of a given breath is lengthened by 20 to 30 seconds. These techniques are based on the assumptions that no respiratory efforts are made and that the alveoli communicate with the airway opening, thereby allowing equilibration of pressures or exhalation of trapped gas. However, this assumption is not necessarily correct in patients with very severe airways obstruction (e.g., status asthmaticus).

Auto-PEEP should be suspected whenever flow at the end of expiration is detectable or when a patient fails to trigger the ventilator consistently with inspiratory efforts. This failure to trigger the ventilator occurs because the patient must generate sufficient pressure to overcome the level of auto-PEEP before a negative deflection of pressure is sensed at the airway opening.

Auto-PEEP and dynamic hyperinflation have numerous detrimental consequences. In a patient who is not breathing spontaneously, the dynamic hyperinflation increases pleural pressure and right atrial pressure, thereby leading to a decrease in the driving pressure for venous return, with a concomitant decrease in cardiac output. This effect can be magnified in the patient with airway obstruction immediately after intubation and initiation of mechanical ventilation, because compensatory mechanisms are impaired by pharmacologic agents that are often used to prepare the patient for endotracheal tube insertion and that also reduce venous and arterial tone. In such patients, auto-PEEP can also lead to gross misinterpretation of vascular pressures. For example, the absolute value of capillary wedge pressure will be directly affected by the increase in intrathoracic pressure during auto-PEEP. The clinician may interpret this high (absolute) capillary wedge pressure as indicating adequate ventricular filling, when, in fact, transmural capillary wedge pressure is low because intrathoracic pressure is also high. This misinterpretation coupled with the decreased cardiac output related to the high intrathoracic pressure may suggest the diagnosis of cardiogenic shock, rather than the correct diagnosis of auto-PEEP.

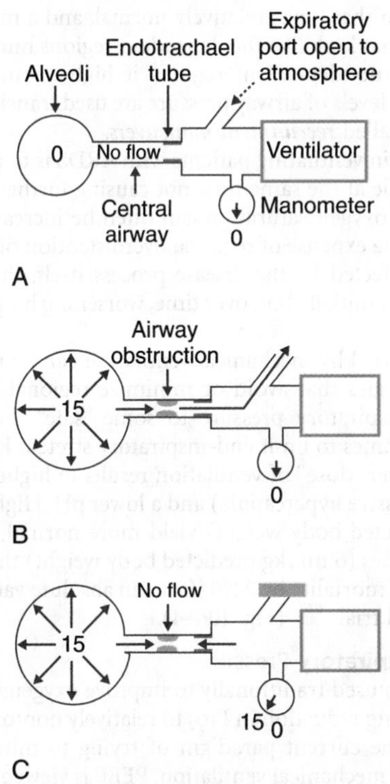

FIGURE 106–1 • The relationships among alveolar, central airway, and ventilator circuit pressure at the end of exhalation under the following conditions: (A) normal conditions (no auto–positive end-expiratory pressure [auto-PEEP]); **(B)** severe dynamic airway obstruction with the expiratory port open; and **(C)** severe dynamic airway obstruction with the expiratory port occluded at the end of exhalation. The auto-PEEP level is identified by creating an end-expiratory hold, thereby allowing the alveolar, central airway, and ventilator circuit pressures to equilibrate, because there is no flow in the circuit. During equilibration, the level of auto-PEEP can be read on the manometer in the ventilator circuit. (Adapted from Pepe PE, Marini JJ: Occult positive end-expiratory pressure in mechanically ventilated patients with airflow obstruction: The auto-PEEP effect. Am Rev Respir Dis 1982;126:166–170.)

Treatment of the detrimental hemodynamic consequences of auto-PEEP include decreasing the level of auto-PEEP by increasing the expiratory time, decreasing airway resistance (e.g., bronchodilators, when appropriate), or decreasing minute ventilation. The last approach is usually the most effective ventilatory maneuver. Cardiovascular hemodynamics can also usually be restored by infusion of fluids.

In a spontaneously breathing patient, dynamic hyperinflation can markedly increase the oxygen cost of breathing for two reasons. First, because the respiratory system is stiffer at higher lung volumes, more energy is required to complete each ventilatory cycle. Second, to initiate flow into the lung, the patient must generate a pressure in the alveolar zone that is lower than atmospheric pressure. However, if dynamic hyperinflation is present, the patient first has to generate an inspiratory effort sufficient to overcome the (positive) end-expiratory alveolar pressure before he or she begins to lower alveolar pressure to less than atmospheric pressure to initiate airflow. The increase in lung volume associated with dynamic hyperinflation also has an impact on the effectiveness of the ventilatory muscles: at high lung volumes, the diaphragm is relatively flat, so it is at a mechanical disadvantage in producing changes in pleural pressure.

Ventilator-Induced Lung Injury

Mechanical ventilation itself can lead to numerous types of lung injury (Fig. 106–2). The term *barotrauma* refers to large pulmonary air leaks, such as pneumothorax and pneumomediastinum. However, a much more subtle injury, *diffuse alveolar damage* presenting as pulmonary edema, also can be caused by overdistention of the lung. For both types of injury, the critical factor is the degree of overdistension of the lung, best assessed by the transpulmonary pressure (Ptp = alveolar minus pleural pressure). The esophageal pressure, measured using an esophageal balloon, estimates pleural pressure (Ppl), although this measurement is not routinely performed in clinical practice.

The usual pressures measured during mechanical ventilation are airway pressures referenced to atmospheric pressure. The peak inspiratory pressure (PIP) is easy to measure, but its interpretation is not always simple. PIP includes the pressure needed to overcome the resistance to flow, and thus a high PIP does not necessarily indicate an increased propensity to the development of ventilator-induced lung injury. For example, if inspiratory flow is constant and a smaller endotracheal tube is used, PIP will increase even though the danger of pulmonary overdistention is no greater than would be present with ventilation using a larger-bore tube. The Pplat, which is the airway pressure at the end of an end-inspiratory pause (>0.5 second), is the pressure that can be most easily measured at the bedside and that bears some relationship, depending on Ppl, to the development of overdistension; however, the "danger-

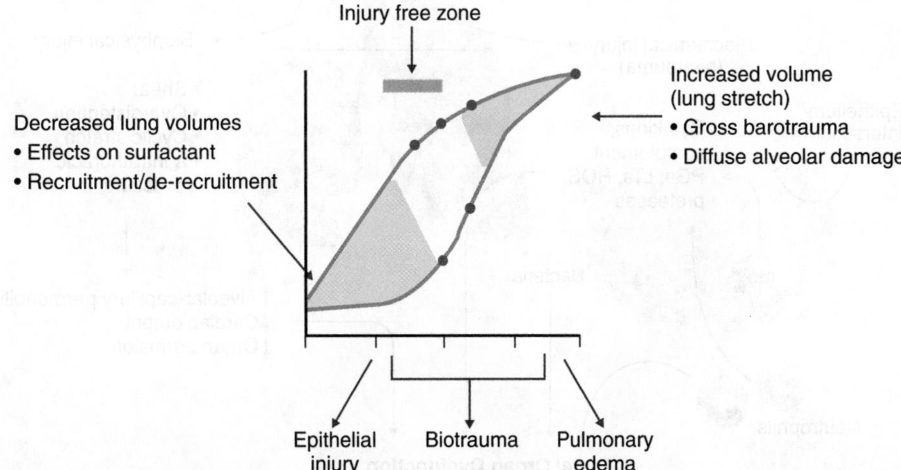

FIGURE 106–2 • Schematic representation of the pressure-volume curve of a lung with diffuse alveolar edema. Mechanical ventilation can induce or worsen lung injury by numerous mechanisms when ventilation occurs at high lung volumes and/or when ventilation occurs at low lung volumes. Lung-protective strategies during ventilation of patients with acute respiratory distress syndrome should try to keep the ventilatory pattern in the *injury-free zone.* Data in patients confirm the benefit of ensuring that overdistention does not occur.

ous" level of Pplat is not known, but based on the ARDSNet study, this level is almost certainly less than 30 cm H_2O. [1] In addition, certain caveats should be noted in interpreting Pplat and PIP, related to associated changes in Ppl. If the patient is breathing spontaneously, Ppl will be negative, and overdistention may occur even with a Pplat lower than 30 cm H_2O. Conversely, in a patient who is either paralyzed or not making ventilatory efforts and who has a very stiff chest wall (e.g., due to ascites, obesity, pregnancy), as airway pressure increases, most of the pressure drop will be dissipated across the chest wall, thus leading to values of Ppl that are positive. In this setting, a high Pplat may not be indicative of a high Ptp and hence may not indicate increased lung distention. Thus, the physician caring for a patient receiving mechanical ventilatory support must analyze the measured airway pressures within their clinical context. Measurement of Ppl, as noted earlier, can resolve these difficulties.

During mechanical ventilation, some areas of the lung may undergo cyclic recruitment and derecruitment. This process, which is of particular importance in patients who have acute lung injury or ARDS, has been termed *atelectrauma* and can cause significant lung injury. The precise mechanisms of injury are not entirely clear but are thought to result from shear stress owing to opening and closing of lung units, regional hypoxia in atelectatic lung units, and effects on surfactant. Prevention of this type of injury provides part of the rationale for the use of PEEP to maintain recruitment of lung units during tidal ventilation.

Finally, evidence suggests that mechanical ventilation strategies that promote overdistention and/or atelectrauma can lead to an inflammatory response in the lung, a mechanism of injury termed *biotrauma*, through the release of certain pro-inflammatory cytokines and chemokines. To the extent that these mediators can translocate from the lung into the systemic circulation, they could potentially lead to dysfunction of other organs (Fig. 106–3). This concept suggests that optimal ventilatory strategies are important not only for maintenance of lung function, but also for preventing the development of multiple organ dysfunction (Chapter 107) that commonly occurs in this setting. This hypothesis may explain the decreased mortality recently observed with a strategy designed to avoid overdistention in a large randomized trial of mechanical ventilation in patients with ARDS. [1]

SPECIFIC COMMON TREATMENT SCENARIOS

Initiation of Mechanical Ventilation

The initiation of mechanical ventilation involves several steps in clinical decision making (Table 106–1). Despite the utility of such guidelines, each patient must be evaluated for specific factors that could modify the recommendation or mandate an alternative.

Acute Respiratory Distress Syndrome

Patients with ARDS (Chapter 105) have noncardiogenic pulmonary edema, with a reduced functional residual capacity and a mortality rate of 30 to 60%. Although therapy may be available for the underlying disease process that led to the development of ARDS (e.g., antibiotics for a predisposing pneumonia), no effective therapy is directly aimed at the diffuse alveolar damage. These patients require mechanical ventilation as supportive therapy to improve oxygenation and to decrease the oxygen cost of breathing until their lungs recover from the primary insult that led to the alveolar damage.

The lungs in a patient with ARDS are stiff and are characterized on computed tomographic scans by patchy, heterogeneous infiltrates that consist of airless atelectatic or consolidated regions. Many patients have a dependent region that is consolidated, atelectatic, or fluid filled, a nondependent region that looks relatively normal, and a middle region that has some areas that look like the dependent regions but can be recruited to resemble the nondependent regions if high enough tidal volumes and/or increased levels of airway pressure are used transiently; these latter approaches are called *recruitment maneuvers*.

The challenge in ventilating patients with ARDS is to provide adequate gas exchange while at the same time not causing further lung injury (see earlier). Arterial oxygen saturation can often be increased by high tidal volumes but at the expense of regional overdistention of those lung units that were not affected by the disease process itself, thereby improving oxygen saturation initially but, over time, worsening lung injury and clinical outcome.

The injury caused by mechanical ventilation can be reduced by using ventilatory strategies that avoid or minimize regional lung overdistention: limiting inspiratory pressure to some "safe" level and/or using smaller tidal volumes to limit end-inspiratory stretch. However, in some patients, this lower "dose" of ventilation results in higher levels of $Paco_2$ (so-called permissive hypercapnia) and a lower pH. Higher tidal volumes (12 mL/kg predicted body weight) yield more normal blood gases, but lower tidal volumes (6 mL/kg predicted body weight) that permit hypercapnia decreased mortality by 22% (from an absolute value of 40 to 31%) in a large clinical trial [1] (Fig. 106–4).

Positive End-Expiratory Pressure

PEEP has been used traditionally to improve oxygenation while at the same time allowing reduction in Fio_2 to relatively nontoxic levels. Within the context of the current paradigm of trying to minimize iatrogenic complications of mechanical ventilation, PEEP is viewed as a therapy that potentially can abrogate or minimize the injury caused by ventilation at low lung volumes, by recruiting lung units and keeping them open. No definitive answer exists regarding how PEEP levels should be set in

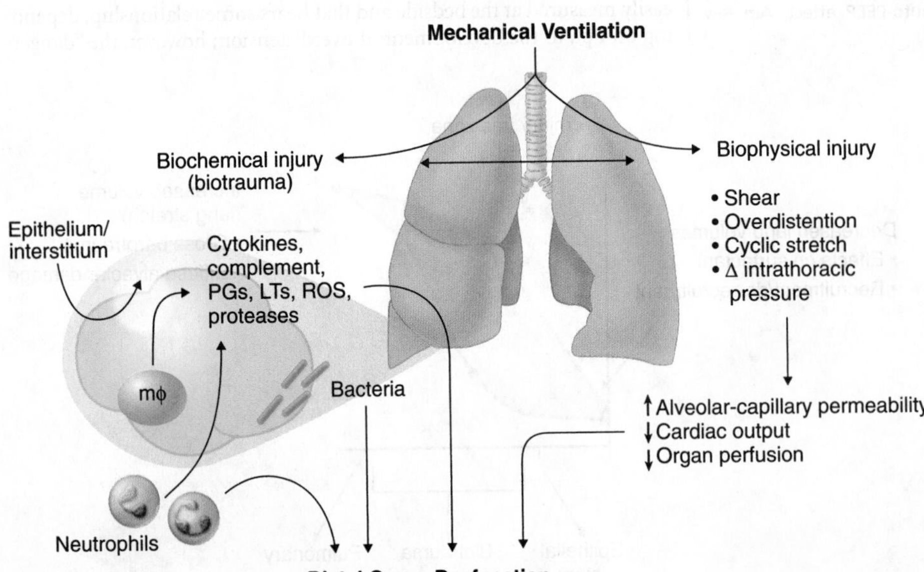

FIGURE 106–3 • Mechanisms by which mechanical ventilation may lead to distal organ dysfunction. LTs = leukotrienes; mϕ = macrophages; ROS = reactive oxygen species. (Adapted from Slutsky AS, Tremblay LN: Multiple system organ failure: Is mechanical ventilation a contributing factor? Am J Respir Crit Care Med 1998;157:1721–1725.)

TABLE 106–1 STEPS AND GUIDELINES FOR INITIATING MECHANICAL VENTILATION*

1. Ventilatory mode
   Unintubated patients:
   - NIPPV for patients with COPD and acute hypercapnic respiratory failure if alert, cooperative, and hemodynamically stable
   - NIPPV not routinely recommended for acute hypoxemic respiratory failure

   Intubated patients:
   - Assist/control with volume-limited ventilation as initial mode
   - Consider specific indications for PCV or HFOV (see text) in acute lung injury
   - SIMV: consider if some respiratory effort, dyssynchrony
   - PSV: consider if patient's effort good, ventilatory needs moderate to low, and patient more comfortable during PSV trial
2. Oxygenation
   - If infiltrates on chest radiograph, then
     FIO_2: begin with 0.8–1.0, reduce according to SpO_2
     PEEP: begin with 5 cm H_2O, increase according to PaO_2 or SpO_2, FIO_2 requirements, and hemodynamic effects; consider PEEP/FIO_2 "ladder" (see Fig. 106-4); goal of SpO_2 >90%, FIO_2 ≤0.6
   - No infiltrates on chest radiograph (COPD, asthma, PTE),
     FIO_2: start at 0.4 and adjust according to SpO_2 (consider starting higher if pulmonary embolism is strongly suspected)
3. Ventilation
   - Tidal volume: begin with 8 mL/kg PBW (see Fig. 106-4 for formulas); decrease to 6 mL/kg PBW over a few hours if acute lung injury present (see Fig. 106-4)
   - Rate: begin with 10–20 breaths/min (10–15 if not acidotic; 15–20 if acidotic); adjust for pH; goal pH >7.3 with maximal rate of 35; may accept lower goal if minute ventilation high
4. Secondary modifications
   - Triggering: in spontaneous modes, adjustment of sensitivity levels to minimize effort
   - Inspiratory flow rate of 40–80 L/min; higher if tachypneic with respiratory distress or if auto-PEEP present, lower if high pressure in ventilator circuit leads to a high-pressure alarm
   - Assessment of auto-PEEP, especially in patients with increased airways obstruction (e.g., asthma, COPD)
   - I : E ratio: 1 : 2, either set or as function of flow rate; higher (1 : 3 or more) if auto-PEEP present
   - Flow pattern: decelerating ramp reduces peak pressure
5. Monitoring
   - Clinical: blood pressure, ECG, observation of ventilatory pattern including assessment of dyssynchrony, effort or work by the patient; assessment of airflow throughout expiratory cycle
   - Ventilator: tidal volume, minute ventilation, airway pressures (including auto-PEEP), total compliance
   - Arterial blood gases, pulse oximetry

*Decisions within this algorithm will be influenced by the specific conditions of the individual patient.
COPD = chronic obstructive pulmonary disease; ECG = electrocardiogram; FIO_2 = fraction of inspired oxygen; HFOV = high-frequency oscillatory ventilation; I:E ratio = inspiratory-to-expiratory ratio; NIPPV = noninvasive positive pressure ventilation; PaO_2 = partial pressure of oxygen in arterial blood; PBW = predicted body weight; PCV = pressure control ventilation; PEEP = positive end-expiratory pressure; PSV = pressure support ventilation; PTE = pulmonary thromboembolism; SIMV = synchronized intermittent mandatory ventilation; SpO_2 = arterial oxygen saturation by pulse oximetry.

patients with ARDS; outcomes appear to be similar with the routine use of higher (~13 cm H_2O) and lower (~8 cm H_2O) levels of PEEP. 2 The critical issues are how to assess the level of PEEP in an individual patient and how to determine whether the procedures to recruit the lung units and keep them open are less harmful than allowing the lung units to remain de-recruited. One experimental option is chest computed tomography to assess whether areas of the lung are recruited, but this technique is not practical for routine assessment. A second approach is to measure the mechanical properties of the respiratory system by generating a pressure-volume curve (see Fig. 106-2). Investigators have suggested that the optimal strategy is to set PEEP just higher than the lower inflection point, which is thought to represent the opening pressure of the lung, and to adjust tidal volume so Pplat is just lower than the upper inflection point, where compliance decreases. Although lung continues to be recruited well above the lower inflection point, and the upper inflection point may not indicate overdistention, two clinical studies that based their lung protection strategies on the pressure-volume curve demonstrated reductions in mortality; however, both studies also included other features to reduce lung injury, so use of the pressure-volume curve to set PEEP levels and tidal volume (or pressure limits) cannot be recommended at this time. In the trial that demonstrated the benefit of lower tidal volumes, PEEP levels were individualized based on a PEEP/FIO_2 table (see Fig. 106–4); a subsequent trial using PEEP about 5 cm H_2O higher found no additional benefit. 2

Obstructive Airways Diseases

The major pathophysiologic abnormality in patients with obstructive airways diseases is an increase in airway resistance leading to expiratory airflow limitation; patients may also have a concomitant increase in minute ventilation. These factors may lead to dynamic hyperinflation, which is associated with numerous complications, including respiratory muscle compromise, an increased oxygen cost of breathing, and hemodynamic compromise. Thus, the main goals in the ventilatory support of patients with obstructive airway diseases (COPD, asthma) are to rest the respiratory muscles, to maintain adequate gas exchange, and to decrease the oxygen cost of breathing while simultaneously minimizing the iatrogenic complications of mechanical ventilation and allowing time for the successful diagnosis and treatment of the primary cause of the exacerbation and the resulting increase in airway obstruction (Chapters 87 and 88).

Noninvasive Ventilation

For patients with acute respiratory failure resulting from an exacerbation of COPD, the preferred approach is NIV using a mask if the patient is hemodynamically stable, alert, and cooperative and does not need to be intubated to protect the airway. 3 It is important to choose a comfortable mask and to reassure the patient because some people find the mask difficult to tolerate. This strategy may be applied using several ventilation modes, including pressure support or bilevel positive airway pressure. The ventilation settings are adjusted to improve gas exchange and to ensure the patient's comfort. Despite this approach, some patients with COPD require intubation and ventilation because of cardiac or respiratory arrest, agitation, increased sputum, or other concomitant severe disorders.

Intubation and Ventilation

The key goal after intubation is to minimize the detrimental effects of dynamic hyperinflation. The most effective way to minimize dynamic hyperinflation is to decrease the minute ventilation, even if this means an increase in $PaCO_2$, a strategy known as *permissive hypercapnia* or *controlled hypoventilation.* Judicious use of sedation may decrease carbon dioxide production and improve patient-ventilator dyssynchrony. Care must be taken in the use of paralytic agents, especially when patients with asthma are also receiving corticosteroids, because such patients may have an increased risk of myopathy. The duration of use of paralytic agents should be minimized to reduce the risk of myopathy.

Increasing expiratory time by using a higher peak inspiratory flow may be somewhat helpful, but it is not nearly as effective as decreasing minute ventilation. What level of $PaCO_2$ (and pH) should be tolerated is not known with certainty, but maintaining pH higher than approximately 7.15 is a reasonable target, although much lower values have been reported in clinical studies.

In patients with COPD who are spontaneously breathing, the addition of external (set) PEEP at a level that is just less than what is necessary to overcome the auto-PEEP fully will decrease the inspiratory effort that the patient needs to generate to initiate inspiratory airflow and will not increase Pplat. This strategy does not appear to be as effective in patients with status asthmaticus, in whom it may cause an increase in Pplat. Measurements of auto-PEEP by airway occlusion may be inaccurate in some

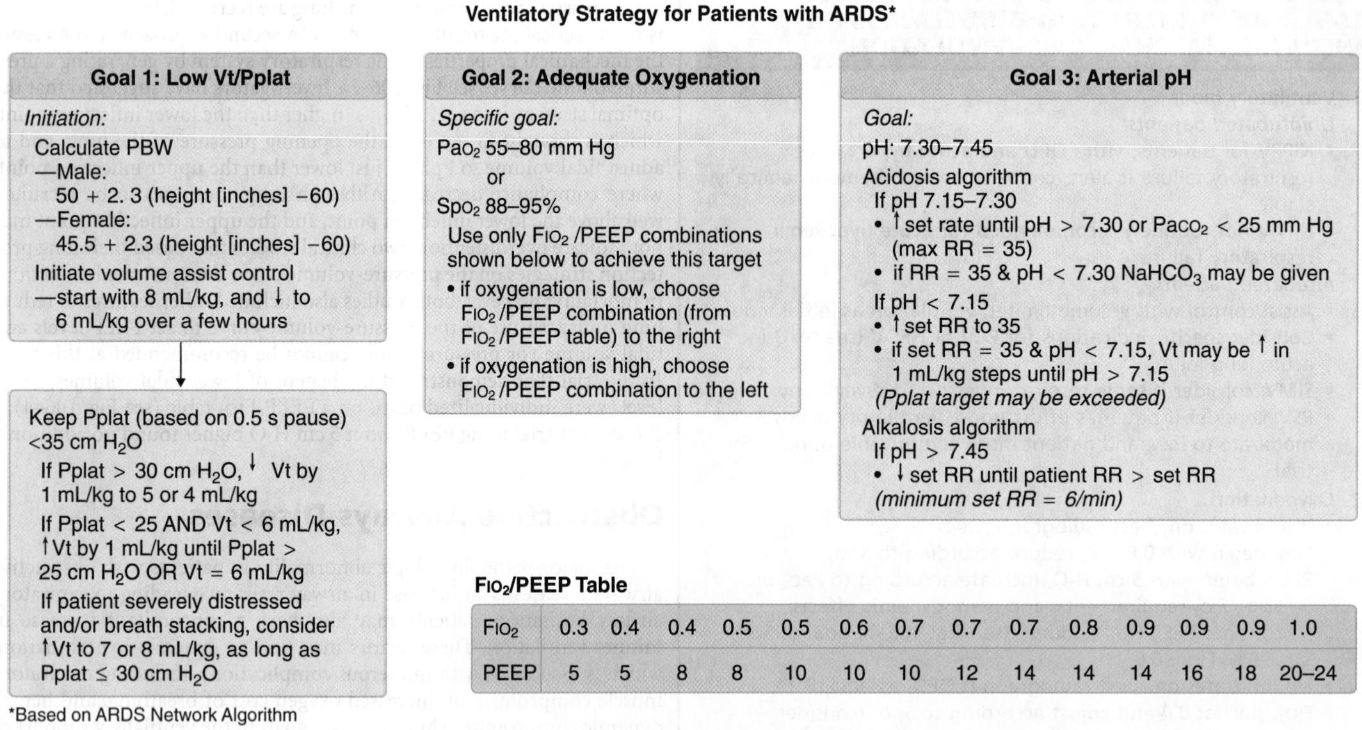

Ventilatory Strategy for Patients with ARDS*

Goal 1: Low Vt/Pplat

Initiation:

Calculate PBW
—Male:
50 + 2. 3 (height [inches] −60)
—Female:
45.5 + 2.3 (height [inches] −60)

Initiate volume assist control
—start with 8 mL/kg, and ↓ to 6 mL/kg over a few hours

↓

Keep Pplat (based on 0.5 s pause) <35 cm H_2O

If Pplat > 30 cm H_2O, ↓ Vt by 1 mL/kg to 5 or 4 mL/kg

If Pplat < 25 AND Vt < 6 mL/kg, ↑Vt by 1 mL/kg until Pplat > 25 cm H_2O OR Vt = 6 mL/kg

If patient severely distressed and/or breath stacking, consider ↑Vt to 7 or 8 mL/kg, as long as Pplat ≤ 30 cm H_2O

Goal 2: Adequate Oxygenation

Specific goal:

Pa_{O_2} 55–80 mm Hg
or
Sp_{O_2} 88–95%

Use only F_{IO_2} /PEEP combinations shown below to achieve this target

- if oxygenation is low, choose F_{IO_2} /PEEP combination (from F_{IO_2} /PEEP table) to the right
- if oxygenation is high, choose F_{IO_2} /PEEP combination to the left

Goal 3: Arterial pH

Goal:

pH: 7.30–7.45

Acidosis algorithm

If pH 7.15–7.30
- ↑ set rate until pH > 7.30 or Pa_{CO_2} < 25 mm Hg (max RR = 35)
- if RR = 35 & pH < 7.30 $NaHCO_3$ may be given

If pH < 7.15
- ↑ set RR to 35
- if set RR = 35 & pH < 7.15, Vt may be ↑ in 1 mL/kg steps until pH > 7.15

(Pplat target may be exceeded)

Alkalosis algorithm

If pH > 7.45
- ↓ set RR until patient RR > set RR

(minimum set RR = 6/min)

F_{IO_2}/PEEP Table

F_{IO_2}	0.3	0.4	0.4	0.5	0.5	0.6	0.7	0.7	0.7	0.8	0.9	0.9	0.9	1.0
PEEP	5	5	8	8	10	10	10	12	14	14	14	16	18	20–24

*Based on ARDS Network Algorithm

FIGURE 106–4 • Ventilatory strategy for patients with the acute respiratory distress syndrome (ARDS). Several caveats should be considered when using the low tidal volume strategy: (1) tidal volume (VT) is based on predicted body weight (PBW),[1] not actual body weight; PBW tends to be about 20% lower than actual body weight; (2) the protocol mandates decreases in the VT lower than 6 mL/kg of PBW if the plateau pressure (Pplat) is greater than 30 cm H_2O and allows for small increases in VT if the patient is severely distressed and/or if there is breath stacking, as long as Pplat remains at 30 cm H_2O or lower; (3) because arterial carbon dioxide (CO_2) levels will rise, pH will fall; acidosis is treated with increasingly aggressive strategies dependent on the arterial pH; (4) the protocol has no specific provisions for the patient with a stiff chest wall, which in this context refers to the rib cage and abdomen; in such patients, it seems reasonable to allow Pplat to increase to more than 30 cm H_2O, even though it is not mandated by the protocol; in such cases, the limit on Pplat may be modified based on analysis of abdominal pressure, which can be estimated by measuring bladder pressure. RR = respiratory rate; Sp_{O_2} = oxygen saturation based on pulse oximeter.

patients with status asthmaticus, likely because of gas trapping at the end of expiration with closed off lung regions that do not communicate with the central airways.

ADJUNCTS

Tracheal gas insufflation involves washing out the carbon dioxide–rich gas in the anatomic dead space with fresh gas via a special catheter or endotracheal tube, thereby allowing a reduction in tidal volume while maintaining the same Pa_{CO_2}. A clinically significant outcome benefit has not yet been demonstrated with tracheal gas insufflation.

The prone position compared with the supine position in patients with acute lung injury results in improved oxygenation in approximately 70% of patients and has a rationale (through more even distribution of pleural pressure) for preventing ventilator-induced lung injury. Trials in adults have not demonstrated an outcome benefit but have been limited to prone positioning for approximately 8 hours per day; studies of more prolonged periods of the prone position in ARDS patients are ongoing. Until results of these studies are available, the prone position should be considered for patients with severe gas exchange abnormalities who require high PEEP and high F_{IO_2}.

DISCONTINUATION

To minimize the iatrogenic consequences of intubation and mechanical ventilation, discontinuation of ventilatory support and extubation should occur as expeditiously as possible. However, if discontinuation is attempted too early, patients may deteriorate and require urgent reintubation.

From the moment that mechanical ventilation is instituted, it is important for the clinician to start planning for eventual discontinuation of ventilatory support. A key aspect of this approach is serial evaluation, with aggressive treatment of the factors contributing to the patient's ventilatory dependence, including respiratory systems factors (e.g., respiratory muscles), cardiovascular factors (e.g., myocardial ischemia), neurologic factors (e.g., respiratory muscle weakness), and metabolic factors (e.g., increased oxygen consumption).

Two major types of weaning strategy have been used historically: (1) a ventilatory mode thought to hasten the weaning process and (2) daily monitoring of the patient for criteria to suggest the likelihood of successful weaning and a trial of spontaneous breathing for those deemed likely to succeed. Studies of ventilatory modes of weaning have included trials in which patients are allowed to breathe spontaneously from a fresh gas supply delivered to the endotracheal tube (a so-called T-tube), trials of IMV, and studies of pressure support ventilation. With all approaches, the level of support is gradually decreased until extubation is tolerated by the patient. These methods have been compared in randomized controlled trials, with mixed results, although weaning with IMV appeared less favorable in most trials. Likewise, using ventilatory criteria to predict weaning success has been disappointing, mainly because some patients who fail to meet the criteria will be successfully weaned if they are given the opportunity to breathe spontaneously. The criterion with the greatest predictive accuracy is the so-called rapid shallow breathing index, in which the respiratory rate is divided by tidal volume (in liters), with a value less than 105 suggesting the ability to wean; however false-negative and false-positive test results occur.

More recently, the approach to weaning has been based on the concept that a patient is ready to be removed from ventilatory support when the underlying disease process that led to the intubation has resolved or improved substantially. Rather than applying rigorous ventilatory criteria, the only requirements are that the patient be clinically stable (i.e., has shown improvement in the underlying process), be hemodynamically stable, and have oxygen requirements that can be met by face mask once the patient is extubated. If the patient meets these general criteria, then a spontaneous breathing trial is recommended (Fig. 106–5). A corollary is that a gradual weaning is not necessary; instead, patients should be assessed on a daily basis regarding their suitability to be removed from ventilatory support, and, if they are not ready, a comfortable, nonfatiguing form of mechanical ventilation should be used in between the assessments. Assisted modes of ventilation are preferred in between the spontaneous breathing trials.

Another major issue to assess is whether the patient has a patent airway and can adequately clear secretions following extubation. Assessment of

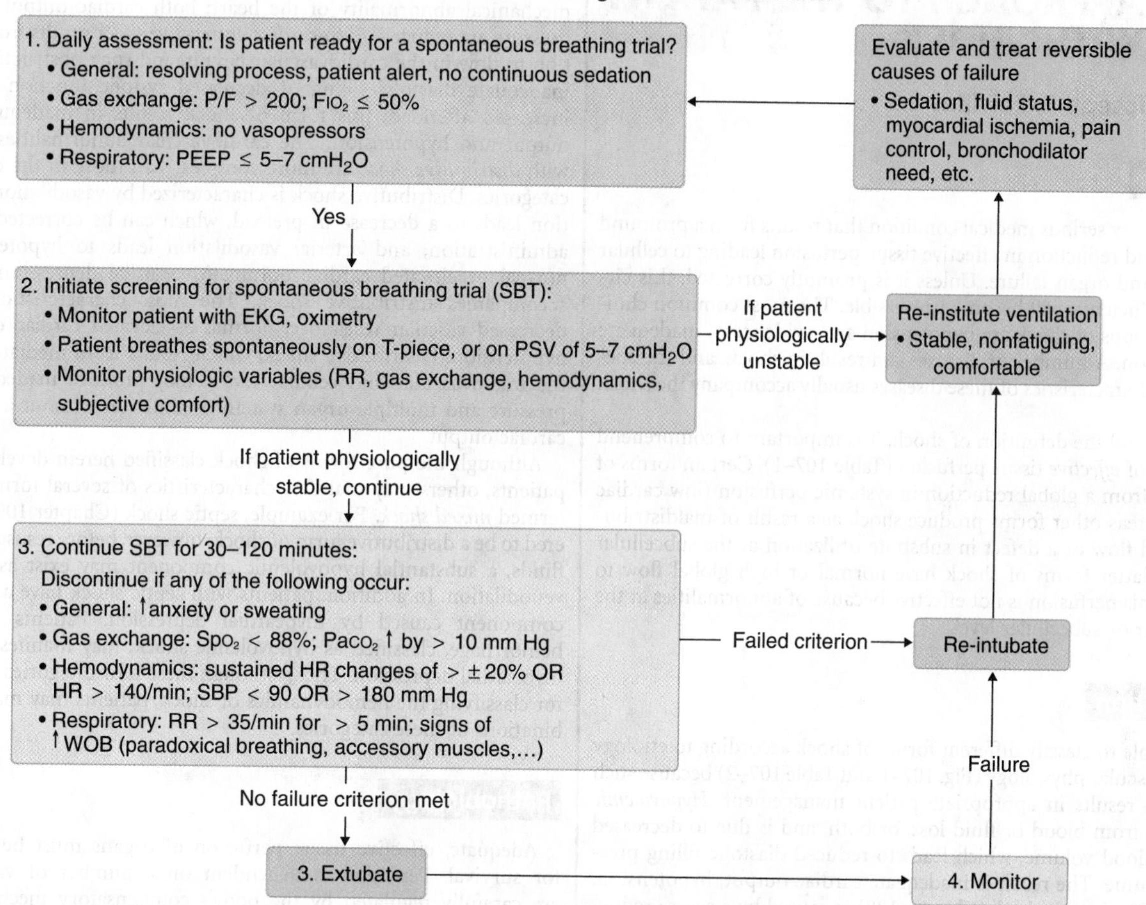

FIGURE 106–5 • Algorithm for assessing whether a patient is ready to be liberated from mechanical ventilation and extubated. HR = heart rate; P/F = PaO_2/FIO_2 ratio; PSV = pressure support ventilation; RR = respiratory rate; SBP = systolic blood pressure; SpO_2 = oxygen saturation based on pulse oximeter; WOB = work of breathing.

the likely patency of the upper airway can be achieved using the *cuff-leak volume,* which is the difference between the inspiratory and expiratory tidal volume when the cuff of the endotracheal tube is deflated. If this volume is greater than 110 mL, it is usually an indication that major upper airway obstruction will not occur following extubation. Although this test is not required before extubation, a low *cuff-leak volume* warrants added precautions, such as the availability of equipment and personnel for managing a difficult intubation, when extubating the patient.

Despite the use of all these techniques, approximately 5 to 25% of patients will have to be reintubated and have mechanical ventilation reinstituted. Once a patient is reintubated, it is again necessary to reevaluate the respiratory and nonrespiratory reasons for the failure.

An important recommendation in relation to weaning or discontinuing mechanical ventilation relates to evidence that intensive care units should develop weaning or discontinuation protocols that are designed to be implemented by health care professionals other than physicians. Three large randomized trials have demonstrated that protocols implemented by health care professionals other than physicians improved care and were associated with substantial savings in costs compared with standard management approaches, even though the specifics of the protocols were different. 4 The choice of the specific protocol should be left to the individual institution and should be individualized to the specific group of patients considered. In instituting such protocols, several key issues should be recognized. First, protocols are guides that should not replace clinical judgment. If a clinician does not follow some aspect of the protocol, there should be a mechanism in place for keeping track of what recommendations were not accepted, with an explanation of the rationale; these data should be collated and used to reassess the protocol. Second, protocols should be viewed as dynamic structures that are open to change and should be reevaluated on a regular basis. Third, implementation of a protocol requires adequate resources, and an institution must make a commitment not only to develop protocols, but also to implement and assess them.

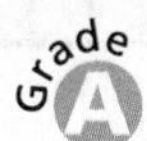

1. Acute Respiratory Distress Syndrome Network: Ventilation with lower tidal volumes as compared with traditional tidal volumes for acute lung injury and the acute respiratory distress syndrome. N Engl J Med 2000;342:1301–1308. Available at www.ardsnet.org.
2. National Heart, Lung, and Blood Institute: ARDS Clinical Trials Network: Higher versus lower positive end-expiratory pressures in patients with the acute respiratory distress syndrome. N Engl J Med 2004;351:327–336.
3. Plant PK, Owen JL, Elliott MW: Non-invasive ventilation in acute exacerbations of chronic obstructive pulmonary disease: Long term survival and predictors of in-hospital outcome. Thorax 2001; 56:708–712.
4. Ely EW, Meade MO, Haponik EF, et al: Mechanical ventilator weaning protocols driven by nonphysician health-care professionals: Evidence-based clinical practice guidelines. Chest 2001;120: 454S–463S.

SUGGESTED READINGS

Fan E, Needham DM, Stewart TE: Ventilatory management of acute lung injury and acute respiratory distress syndrome. JAMA 2005;294:2889–2896. *Volume- and pressure-limited lung-protective ventilation is preferred for acute lung injury and ARDS.*

Girard TD, Bernard GR: Mechanical ventilation in ARDS: A state-of-the-art review. Chest 2007;131:921–929. *Practical recommendations.*

MacIntyre NR, Cook DJ, Ely EW Jr, et al: Evidence-based guidelines for weaning and discontinuing ventilatory support: A collective task force facilitated by the American College of Chest Physicians; the American Association for Respiratory Care; and the American College of Critical Care Medicine. Chest 2001;120:375S–395S. *A comprehensive review of the weaning literature, with 12 recommendations and a discussion of the rationale and grade of evidence for each.*

Peter JV, Moran JL, Phillips-Hughes J, et al: Effect of non-invasive positive pressure ventilation (NIPPV) on mortality in patients with acute cardiogenic pulmonary oedema: A meta-analysis. Lancet 2006;367:1155–1163. *CPAP reduces mortality and both reduce the need for subsequent mechanical ventilation compared with standard therapy.*

Tremblay LN, Slutsky AS: Ventilator induced lung injury: From the bench to the bedside. Intensive Care Med 2006;32:24–33. *A scientific and practical review.*

APPROACH TO THE PATIENT WITH SHOCK

Joseph E. Parrillo

Definition

Shock is a very serious medical condition that results from a profound and widespread reduction in effective tissue perfusion leading to cellular dysfunction and organ failure. Unless it is promptly corrected, this circulatory insufficiency will become irreversible. The most common clinical manifestations of shock are hypotension and evidence of inadequate tissue perfusion. A number of diseases can result in shock, and the specific clinical characteristics of these diseases usually accompany the shock syndrome.

To understand the definition of shock, it is important to comprehend the meaning of *effective* tissue perfusion (Table 107–1). Certain forms of shock result from a global reduction in systemic perfusion (low cardiac output), whereas other forms produce shock as a result of maldistribution of blood flow or a defect in substrate utilization at the subcellular level. These latter forms of shock have normal or high global flow to tissues, but this perfusion is not effective because of abnormalities at the microvascular or subcellular level.

Classification

It is valuable to classify different forms of shock according to etiology and cardiovascular physiology (Fig. 107–1 and Table 107–2) because such classification results in appropriate patient management. *Hypovolemic shock* results from blood or fluid loss, or both, and is due to decreased circulating blood volume, which leads to reduced diastolic filling pressure and volume. The result is inadequate cardiac output, hypotension, and shock. *Cardiogenic shock* (Chapter 108) is caused by a severe reduction in cardiac function resulting from direct myocardial damage or a mechanical abnormality of the heart; both cardiac output and blood pressure are reduced. *Extracardiac obstructive shock* results from obstruction to flow in the cardiovascular circuit, and such obstruction leads to inadequate diastolic filling or decreased systolic function because of increased afterload; this form of shock results in inadequate cardiac output and hypotension. The cardiovascular abnormalities associated with *distributive shock* are more complex than those in the other shock categories. Distributive shock is characterized by vasodilation: venodilation leads to a decrease in preload, which can be corrected with fluid administration, and arterial vasodilation leads to hypotension with normal or elevated cardiac output. Myocardial depression frequently accompanies distributive shock. The most characteristic pattern is decreased vascular resistance, normal or elevated cardiac output, and hypotension. Distributive shock, which results from mediator effects at the microvascular and cellular levels, may produce inadequate blood pressure and multiple organ system dysfunction without a decrease in cardiac output.

Although the pure forms of shock classified herein develop in many patients, others may manifest characteristics of several forms of shock, termed *mixed shock.* For example, septic shock (Chapter 109) is considered to be a distributive form of shock; however, before resuscitation with fluids, a substantial hypovolemic component may exist as a result of venodilation. In addition, patients with septic shock have a cardiogenic component caused by myocardial depression. Patients with severe hemorrhage, classified as hypovolemic shock, may manifest significant myocardial depression. Thus, although these four categories are valuable for classifying the hemodynamics of shock, patients may manifest combinations of these categories.

TABLE 107–1 DETERMINANTS OF EFFECTIVE TISSUE PERFUSION

ARTERIAL PRESSURE/CARDIAC PERFORMANCE
- Cardiac function
  - Preload
  - Afterload
  - Contractility
  - Heart rate
- Venous return

VASCULAR PERFORMANCE
- Distribution of cardiac output
  - Extrinsic regulatory systems
    - Sympathetic nervous system
    - Adrenal hormone release
  - Intrinsic regulatory systems
  - Anatomic vascular disease
  - Exogenous vasoactive agents
- Microvascular function
  - Pre- and postcapillary sphincter function
  - Capillary endothelial integrity
- Microvascular obstruction

CELLULAR FUNCTION
- Oxygen unloading and diffusion
  - Red blood cell 2,3-diphosphoglycerate
  - Blood pH
  - Temperature
- Cellular energy generation/substrate utilization
  - Citric acid (Krebs) cycle
  - Oxidative phosphorylation
  - Other energy metabolism pathways

Pathobiology

Adequate, effective tissue perfusion of organs must be maintained for survival. Perfusion is dependent on a number of variables that are carefully regulated by the body's compensatory mechanisms (see Table 107–1).

Control of Arterial Pressure

One excellent physiologic and clinical measure of perfusion is arterial pressure, which is determined by cardiac output and vascular resistance and can be defined by the following equation:

$$MAP - CVP = CO \times SVR$$

where MAP is mean arterial pressure, CVP is central venous pressure, CO is cardiac output, and SVR is systemic vascular resistance.

MAP and cardiac output can be measured directly, and these two variables are frequently used to describe tissue perfusion. SVR can be calculated as a ratio of MAP minus central venous pressure divided by cardiac output.

Arterial pressure is regulated by changes in cardiac output or SVR, or both. These regulatory mechanisms consist of neural and hormonal reflexes and local factors. Blood flow to the heart and brain is carefully regulated and maintained over a wide range of blood pressure (from an MAP of 50 to 150 mm Hg); this autoregulation results from reflexes in the local vasculature and ensures the perfusion of these especially vital organs. Failure to maintain the minimal arterial pressure required for autoregulation during shock indicates a severe abnormality that may produce inadequate coronary perfusion and a further reduction in cardiac function as a result of myocardial ischemia.

Cardiac Performance

Cardiac output is a product of heart rate and stroke volume. Stroke volume is determined by preload, afterload, contractility, and ventricular size, whereas preload is dependent on adequate venous return (Chapter 50).

Vascular Performance

Effective perfusion requires appropriate resistance to blood flow to maintain arterial pressure. Resistance to flow of blood in a vessel is proportional to the length of the vessel and the viscosity of blood and inversely proportional to the radius of the vessel raised to the fourth power. Therefore, the cross-sectional area of a vessel is by far the most important determinant of resistance to flow. In the systemic vasculature,

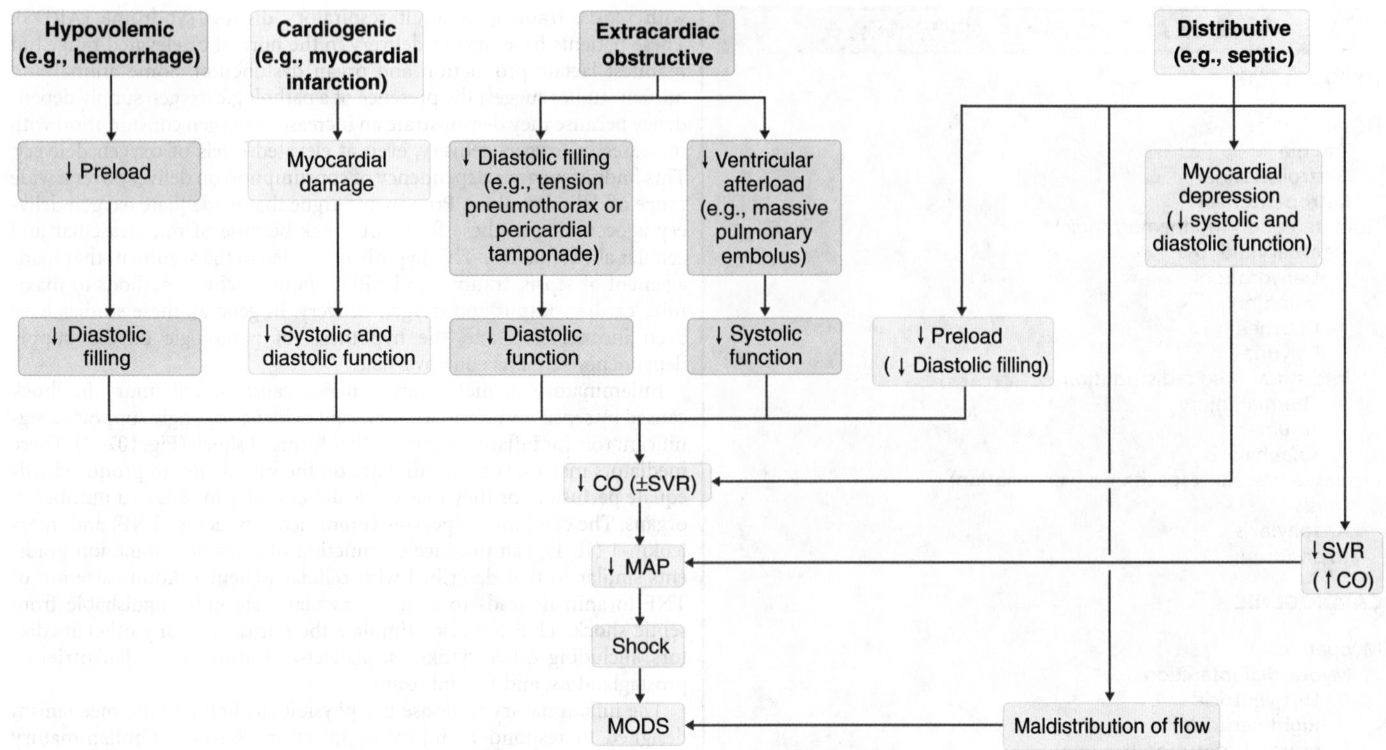

FIGURE 107–1 • Classification of shock showing interrelationships among the different forms of shock. CO = cardiac output; MAP = mean arterial pressure; MODS = multiple organ dysfunction syndrome; SVR = systemic vascular resistance.

the major (>80%) site of resistance is at the arteriolar sphincter, and regulation of this arteriolar tone constitutes the major determinant of vascular resistance.

Arteriolar smooth muscle tone is regulated by extrinsic and intrinsic factors. The extrinsic factors consist of sympathetic nervous system innervation of arterioles, which are largely regulated by arterial and cardiopulmonary baroreceptors. Circulating epinephrine and norepinephrine are released into the circulation by stimulation of the adrenal medulla. The intrinsic mechanisms include a vascular smooth muscle (myogenic) response in which blood vessels relax or constrict in response to changes in transmural vessel pressure to maintain vessel blood flow at a constant level despite changes in perfusion pressure. Other intrinsic mechanisms are a metabolic response that results from release of vasodilators in response to increased metabolic activity and an oxygen tension response that results in vasodilation with low oxygen tensions. Vasodilators released locally and systemically include nitric oxide, prostacyclin, eicosanoids, kinins, and adenosine. Vasoconstrictor molecules include norepinephrine, epinephrine, endothelin-1, renin, angiotensin II, thromboxane, vasopressin, and oxygen free radicals.

In addition to vascular tone, the microvasculature also affects perfusion by obstruction to microvascular flow. In shock, this obstruction can be caused by adhesion of leukocytes or platelets to the endothelium, with subsequent sludging and occlusion of microvessels. Leukocyte adhesion and rolling are mediated by integrins and selectins on the surface of activated neutrophils and endothelial cells. Activation of the coagulation system with fibrin deposition and microthrombi can contribute to this process. Shunting around these occluded vessels may occur. Decreased red or white blood cell deformability can also aggravate this microvascular dysfunction. Therapeutic success using activated protein C, an anticoagulant, in severe septic shock emphasizes the importance of the coagulation cascade in the pathogenesis of septic shock (Chapter 109). [1]

Microvascular permeability to fluids or other substances may also be altered by vasoactive mediators, activated leukocytes, and damaged endothelial cells. Because intravascular and extravascular fluid is determined by a balance between hydrostatic pressure and colloid osmotic pressure, damage to the endothelium may cause increased extravasation of fluid into the interstitial space and result in tissue edema. This fluid accumulation may further worsen organ dysfunction.

Cellular Function

At the cellular level, a number of factors regulate the unloading of oxygen and other substrates to cells. Shock produces cellular dysfunction through three major mechanisms: cellular ischemia, inflammatory mediators, and free radical injury. Cellular ischemia is probably the major cause of cell damage in shock with low cardiac output. In hypovolemic shock, inadequate perfusion and the resultant lack of oxygen lead to increasing dependence on anaerobic glycolysis, which produces only two adenosine triphosphate (ATP) molecules during the breakdown of one glucose molecule as opposed to 36 ATP molecules produced by aerobic metabolism through the citric acid (Krebs) cycle; the result is depletion of ATP and intracellular energy reserves. Intracellular acidosis occurs, and anaerobic glycolysis leads to the accumulation of lactate. Lack of adequate energy results in failure of energy-dependent ion transport pumps and an inability to maintain normal transmembrane gradients of potassium, chloride, and calcium; the result is mitochondrial dysfunction, abnormal carbohydrate metabolism, and failure of many energy-dependent enzyme reactions. Ultrastructural changes in mitochondria ensue, and the cell dies (cellular necrosis). In addition, shock can damage cells and organs by accelerating cellular apoptosis (programmed cell death).

One important, but controversial hypothesis regarding cellular ischemia in shock is the degree of dependence on oxygen supply. In normal humans, oxygen delivery to tissues (CO × O_2 content of arterial blood) is maintained at a high level so that tissue oxygen consumption [CO × (O_2 content of arterial blood − O_2 content of mixed venous blood)] is not altered or dependent on changes in oxygen delivery. However, if systemic flow drops below a critical value of oxygen delivery, tissues must switch from aerobic metabolism to the less efficient anaerobic metabolism. This deficiency of energy production may lead to multiple organ system dysfunction and death. Below this critical value (estimated to be 8 to 10 mL of oxygen/min/kg in anesthetized humans), oxygen consumption is dependent on oxygen delivery (or supply), a relationship termed *physiologic oxygen supply dependency.* This process is believed to be an important mechanism of cellular damage in forms of shock that are characterized by low oxygen as a result of inadequate cardiac output, low oxygen saturation, or decreased hemoglobin concentration. The controversy regarding this mechanism stems from the hypothesis that a *pathologic oxygen supply dependency* exists in patients

TABLE 107–2 CLASSIFICATION OF SHOCK

HYPOVOLEMIC

- Hemorrhagic
  - Trauma
  - Gastrointestinal
  - Retroperitoneal
- Fluid depletion (nonhemorrhagic)
  - External fluid loss
    - Dehydration
    - Vomiting
    - Diarrhea
    - Polyuria
  - Interstitial fluid redistribution
    - Thermal injury
    - Trauma
    - Anaphylaxis
- Increased vascular capacitance (venodilation)
  - Sepsis
  - Anaphylaxis
  - Toxins/drug

CARDIOGENIC

- Myopathic
  - Myocardial infarction
    - Left ventricle
    - Right ventricle
  - Myocardial contusion (trauma)
  - Myocarditis
  - Cardiomyopathy
  - Postischemic myocardial stunning
  - Septic myocardial depression
  - Pharmacologic
    - Anthracycline cardiotoxicity
    - Calcium-channel blockers
- Mechanical
  - Valvular failure (stenotic or regurgitant)
  - Hypertrophic cardiomyopathy
  - Ventricular septal defect
- Arrhythmic
  - Bradycardia
  - Tachycardia

EXTRACARDIAC OBSTRUCTIVE

- Impaired diastolic filling (decreased ventricular preload)
  - Direct venous obstruction (vena cava)
    - Intrathoracic obstructive tumors
  - Increased intrathoracic pressure
    - Tension pneumothorax
    - Mechanical ventilation (with excessive pressure or volume depletion)
    - Asthma
  - Decreased cardiac compliance
    - Constrictive pericarditis
    - Cardiac tamponade
- Impaired systolic contraction (increased ventricular afterload)
  - Right ventricle
    - Pulmonary embolus (massive)
    - Acute pulmonary hypertension
  - Left ventricle
    - Aortic dissection

DISTRIBUTIVE

- Septic (bacterial, fungal, viral, rickettsial)
- Toxic shock syndrome
- Anaphylactic, anaphylactoid
- Neurogenic (spinal shock)
- Endocrinologic
  - Adrenal crisis
  - Thyroid storm
- Toxic (e.g., nitroprusside, bretylium)

with sepsis, trauma, or adult respiratory distress syndrome (ARDS). These patients have oxygen delivery in the normal or elevated range but manifest lactate production and organ dysfunction. Some animal and human studies suggest the presence of a pathologic oxygen supply dependency because they demonstrate an increase in oxygen consumption with increases in oxygen delivery, even at elevated levels of oxygen delivery. This finding suggests dependency of consumption on delivery over a wide range of delivery values. Proponents argue that inadequate oxygen delivery is occurring in these forms of shock because of microvascular and cellular abnormalities. This hypothesis has led to the argument that management of sepsis, trauma, and ARDS should include methods to maximize cardiac output and oxygen delivery. In general, these studies have been inconclusive, and the hypothesis of pathologic oxygen supply dependency remains controversial.

Inflammatory mediators are a major cause of cell injury in shock caused by sepsis and trauma, and recent evidence strongly supports a significant role for inflammation in other forms of shock (Fig. 107–2). These mediators may exert their influence on the vasculature to produce inadequate perfusion, or they may cause direct injury to cells in a number of organs. The cytokines, especially tumor necrosis factor (TNF) and interleukin-1 (IL-1), can produce dysfunction of transmembrane ion gradients similar to that described with cellular ischemia. Administration of TNF to animals leads to a cardiovascular state indistinguishable from septic shock. TNF can also stimulate the release of many other mediators, including other cytokines, platelet-activating factor, leukotrienes, prostaglandins, and thromboxane.

The inflammatory response is a physiologic, homeostatic mechanism designed to respond to injury or infection. Release of inflammatory mediators usually provides beneficial effects such as activating host defense systems and enhancing blood flow to damaged tissues. With a self-limited insult, the inflammatory reaction is carefully controlled by counter-regulatory, anti-inflammatory mechanisms. In shock, the inflammatory response becomes excessive and unregulated, and it contributes to cell injury and tissue damage (see Fig. 107–2).

Free radicals are highly reactive oxygen intermediates that can occur after ischemia with subsequent reperfusion. Cellular ischemia and intracellular accumulation of calcium can result in the formation of xanthine oxidase, which can oxidize purines with formation of the highly toxic superoxide radical. These oxygen products can inactivate proteins, damage DNA, induce lipid peroxidation of cell membranes, and lead to cell lysis and tissue injury.

Altered gene expression may also play a role in the cellular dysfunction during shock. For example, generation of cytokines, adhesion proteins, and inducible nitric oxide synthase enzymes represents upregulation of gene expression. The heat shock proteins may be an especially important genetic response in shock. These proteins are involved in the genetic program of cell death known as *apoptosis*, a physiologic mechanism that normally functions to remove senescent cells. During shock, the induction of heat shock proteins may interfere with cell synthetic pathways and initiate a heightened activation of programmed cell death. Inappropriate initiation of this mechanism may be an important contributor to cell demise in shock. Recent genetic studies in septic shock have documented an association between the presence of the *TNF2* allele, a polymorphism promoter of TNF-α, and a very high relative risk for septic shock and high mortality from this disease. This finding demonstrates the potential predictive ability of genetic studies in shock.

Compensatory Mechanisms

With the onset of hemodynamic dysfunction in shock, homeostatic compensatory mechanisms attempt to maintain effective tissue perfusion, and many of the manifestations of shock represent the body's attempt to correct abnormalities. Most compensatory mechanisms are dependent on various sensing mechanisms designed to recognize hemodynamic or metabolic dyshomeostasis. The sensing mechanisms consist of pressure receptors located in the cardiovascular system (right atrium, pulmonary artery, aortic arch, carotid, and splanchnic baroreceptors) and the kidney (juxtaglomerular apparatus), as well as chemoreceptors sensitive to concentrations of carbon dioxide or oxygen and located in the central nervous system (mostly in the medulla).

The compensatory responses in shock maintain mean circulatory pressure, maximize cardiac performance, redistribute perfusion to the most vital organs, and optimize the unloading of oxygen to tissues. These effects are produced by stimulation of the sympathetic nervous system,

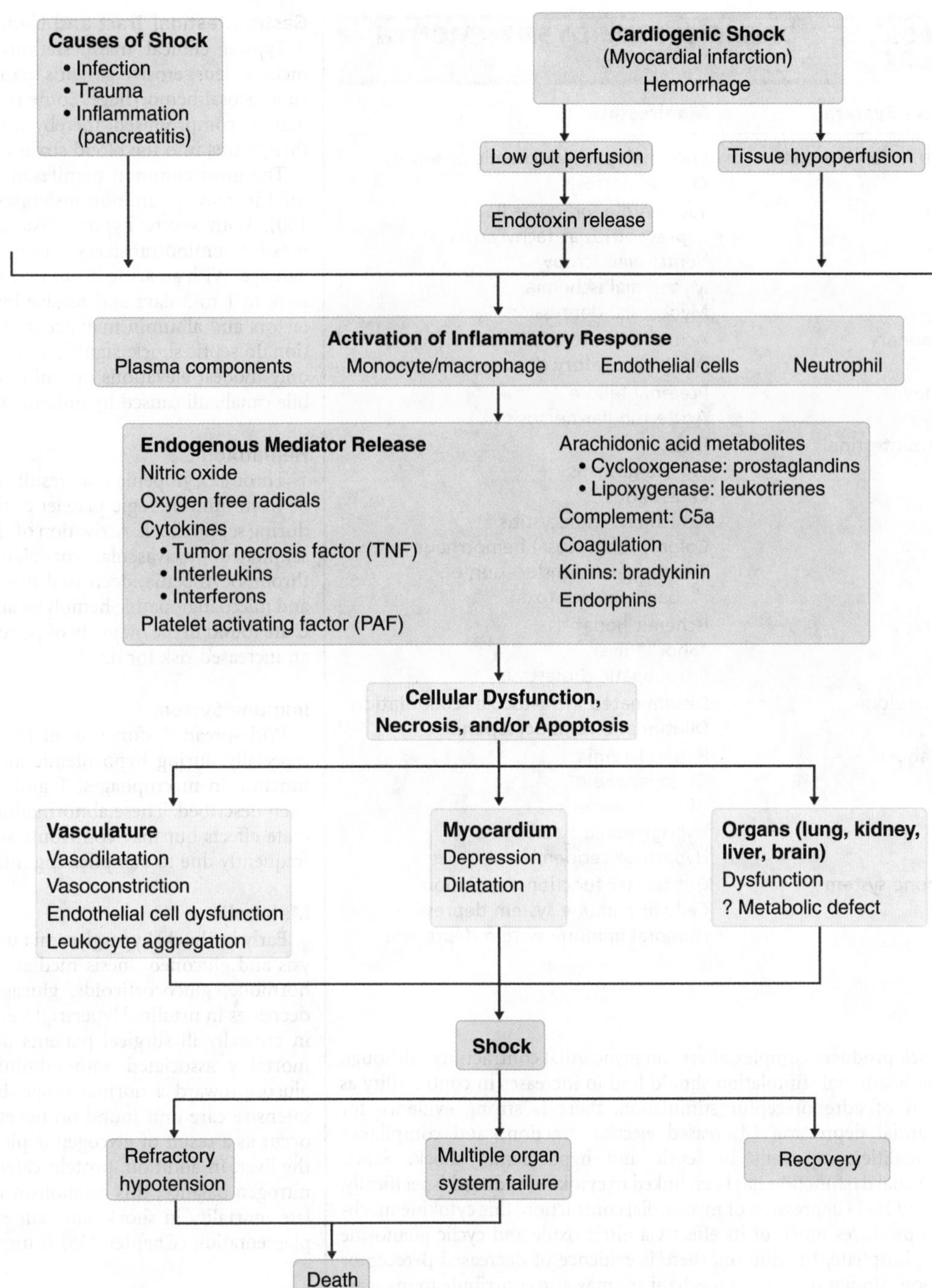

FIGURE 107–2 • Pathogenesis of different causes of shock.

release of hormones (angiotensin II, vasopressin, epinephrine, and norepinephrine), and creation of a local tissue environment that enhances the unloading of oxygen to tissues due to acidosis, pyrexia, and increased red blood cell 2,3-diphosphoglycerate. The magnitude of these compensatory mechanisms is dependent on the severity of the hemodynamic or metabolic derangements. Compensation is effective at restoring tissue perfusion for a period during shock; however, if the initiating process is not reversed during this period, shock becomes irreversible as a result of widespread cellular damage.

Clinical Manifestations

Multiple Organ Dysfunction Syndrome

The clinical manifestation of shock is variable and depends on the initiating cause and the response of multiple organs (Table 107–3). Different organs may be affected minimally, mildly, moderately, or severely. This diffuse damage leads to multiple organ dysfunction syndrome (see Fig. 107–1), which is one of the major causes of death in shock.

Central Nervous System

The most frequent findings in shock are alterations in the level of consciousness ranging from confusion to coma. Autoregulation protects the ischemia-sensitive neurons by maintaining adequate blood flow down to an MAP of approximately 50 to 60 mm Hg. Below this level, however, tissue ischemia ensues. Acid-base and electrolyte abnormalities also contribute to neuronal damage. Sepsis-related central nervous system dysfunction may occur at a higher MAP as a result of the effects of inflammatory mediators.

Heart

Many of the clinically apparent manifestations of cardiac involvement in shock result from sympathoadrenal stimulation, with tachycardia being the most sensitive indicator that shock is present. As in the brain, autoregulation ensures good coronary perfusion down to an MAP of approximately 50 mm Hg. In low cardiac output forms of shock, myocardial ischemia is prominent and leads to a vicious cycle in which ischemia produces a further reduction in cardiac output, which further aggravates the ischemia. This cycle is believed to be important in producing the high mortality (70 to 90%) rate of cardiogenic shock (Chapter 108).

TABLE 107–3 ORGAN SYSTEM DYSFUNCTION IN SHOCK

Organ System	Manifestations
Central nervous system	Encephalopathy (ischemic or septic) Cortical necrosis
Heart	Tachycardia, bradycardia Supraventricular tachycardia Ventricular ectopy Myocardial ischemia Myocardial depression
Pulmonary	Acute respiratory failure Adult respiratory distress syndrome
Kidney	Prerenal failure Acute tubular necrosis
Gastrointestinal	Ileus Erosive gastritis Pancreatitis Acalculous cholecystitis Colonic submucosal hemorrhage Transluminal translocation of bacteria/endotoxin
Liver	Ischemic hepatitis "Shock" liver Intrahepatic cholestasis
Hematologic	Disseminated intravascular coagulation Dilutional thrombocytopenia
Metabolic	Hyperglycemia Glycogenolysis Gluconeogenesis Hypoglycemia (late) Hypertriglyceridemia
Immune system	Gut barrier function depression Cellular immune system depression Humoral immune system depression

Shock produces complex effects on myocardial contractility. Although sympathoadrenal stimulation should lead to increases in contractility as a result of adrenoreceptor stimulation, there is strong evidence for myocardial depression (decreased ejection fraction) and compliance abnormalities, especially in septic and hypovolemic shock. Septic myocardial dysfunction has been linked to cytokine-induced (specifically, TNF and IL-1) depression of myocardial contraction; this cytokine mechanism produces much of its effect via nitric oxide and cyclic guanosine monophosphate. In addition, there is evidence of decreased β-receptor function. Similar depressant mechanisms may also contribute to myocardial dysfunction in hypovolemic and cardiogenic shock.

Lungs

Acute lung injury causes impaired gas exchange, decreased compliance, and shunting of blood through underventilated areas. The pathologic findings are fibrin-neutrophil aggregates within the pulmonary microvasculature, inflammatory damage to the interstitium and alveoli, and exudation of proteinaceous fluid into the alveolar space; the result is severe hypoxemia with bilateral pulmonary infiltrates, a condition termed *adult respiratory distress syndrome* (Chapter 105). The work of breathing is increased, and respiratory muscle fatigue and ventilatory failure ensue, often requiring mechanical ventilation.

Kidney

Acute renal failure (Chapter 121) is a major complication of shock and is associated with a high mortality rate. Hypoperfusion of the renal vasculature occurs frequently in shock, in part as a result of preferential direction of blood flow to the brain and heart. Initially, vasoconstriction may maintain glomerular perfusion, but when this compensatory mechanism fails, acute tubular necrosis and renal insufficiency occur. An important clinical challenge is to differentiate between acute tubular necrosis and hypovolemia because both are associated with oliguria.

Gastrointestinal Tract and Liver

Typical clinical manifestations of gut involvement during shock include ileus, erosive gastritis, pancreatitis, acalculous cholecystitis, and submucosal hemorrhage. Some studies suggest that gut barrier integrity may be compromised, thereby leading to translocation of bacteria and their toxins into the blood stream.

The most common manifestation of liver involvement in shock is a mild increase in aminotransferases and lactate dehydrogenase (Chapter 150). With severe hypoperfusion, shock liver may be manifested by massive aminotransferase elevations and extensive hepatocellular damage. With an acute insult that resolves, these transaminase elevations peak in 1 to 3 days and resolve by 10 days. Decreased levels of clotting factors and albumin may occur as a result of decreased synthetic function. In septic shock, significant elevations of bilirubin may be seen with only modest elevations of aminotransferases because of dysfunction of bile canaliculi caused by inflammatory mediators or bacterial toxins.

Hematologic

Thrombocytopenia may result from dilution during volume repletion or from immunologic platelet destruction, which is especially common during septic shock. Activation of the coagulation cascade can lead to disseminated intravascular coagulation (Chapter 181), which results in thrombocytopenia, decreased fibrinogen, elevated fibrin split products, and microangiopathic hemolytic anemia. Reduced blood levels of protein C are found in the majority of patients with sepsis and are associated with an increased risk for death.

Immune System

Widespread dysfunction of the immune system has been described, especially during hypovolemic and traumatic shock. Abnormalities of function in macrophages, T and B lymphocytes, and neutrophils have been described. These abnormalities are not thought to produce immediate effects but may contribute significantly to late mortality, which is frequently due to complicating infection.

Metabolic

Early in shock, hyperglycemia usually occurs as a result of glycogenolysis and gluconeogenesis mediated by increases in adrenocorticotropic hormone, glucocorticoids, glucagon, and catecholamines, as well as decreases in insulin. Hypertriglyceridemia may also occur. A clinical trial in critically ill surgical patients demonstrated reduced morbidity and mortality associated with administration of insulin to lower blood glucose toward a normal range, but a subsequent study in a medical intensive care unit found no benefit. Later in shock, hypoglycemia may occur as a result of glycogen depletion or failure of glucose synthesis in the liver. In addition, protein catabolism ensues and results in negative nitrogen balance; this catabolism may be an important determinant of late mortality in shock, and some studies suggest that nutritional supplementation (Chapter 236) is important in shock therapy.

Specific Forms of Shock

Inadequate tissue perfusion results from low cardiac output in hypovolemic, cardiogenic, and extracardiac obstructive forms of shock (Chapter 109). In distributive shock, although low cardiac output may occur infrequently as a result of inadequate preload or myocardial depression, most commonly, low SVR and maldistribution of blood flow lead to low blood pressure and shock despite normal or increased cardiac output.

Hypovolemic Shock

Hypovolemic shock is characterized by a decrease in ventricular preload that results in decreased ventricular diastolic pressure and volume, decreased stroke volume and cardiac output, and reduced blood pressure. Patients have pale, cool, clammy skin; tachycardia; a decreased jugular venous pulse; decreased urine output; and altered mental status. The severity of hypovolemic shock is clearly associated with both the magnitude and the rate of fluid loss. Acute loss of 10% of circulating blood volume results in tachycardia and increased SVR with maintenance of blood pressure. Compensatory mechanisms begin to fail with a 20 to 25% volume loss: mild to moderate hypotension and decreased cardiac output occur, SVR is markedly increased, and lactate production may begin. With loss of 40% of circulating blood volume, severe hypotension develops with signs of shock, and cardiac output and tissue perfusion are severely decreased. Hypoperfusion activates the inflammatory cascade (see Fig. 107–2), thereby leading to widespread cellular damage. If this shock state persists for more than 2 hours, sufficient tissue damage occurs that adequate fluid repletion is no longer effective in reversing the shock; that is, the shock is irreversible.

If volume is lost at a slower rate, the compensatory mechanisms are more effective, and similar amounts of volume depletion are better tolerated. Furthermore, a patient's underlying disease, especially a limited cardiac reserve, also influences the response to a hypovolemic insult.

Cardiogenic Shock

Cardiogenic shock is caused by failure of the heart as a pump as a result of myocardial, valvular, or structural abnormalities. Hemodynamically, ventricular filling pressure and volume are increased; cardiac output, stroke volume, and MAP are reduced. Patients manifest signs of peripheral hypoperfusion coupled with evidence of ventricular failure (Chapters 57 and 108). Recent evidence supports a role for activation of the inflammatory cascade during cardiogenic shock (see Fig. 107–2).

Extracardiac Obstructive Shock

This form of shock results from obstruction to flow in the cardiovascular circuit. Pericardial tamponade and constrictive pericarditis (Chapter 74) impair diastolic filling of the right ventricle. Massive pulmonary emboli (Chapter 99) may lead to shock as a result of a severe increase in right ventricular afterload. The hemodynamic pattern is similar to that of other low-output shock states with decreased cardiac output, stroke volume, and MAP. Other hemodynamic variables depend on the site of the obstruction. With pericardial tamponade, increased and equalized right and left ventricular diastolic pressure usually develops. Constrictive pericarditis may produce a similar pattern. Acute pulmonary embolism results in right heart failure with elevated pulmonary artery and right heart pressure and low or normal left heart filling pressure.

The tempo of the disease process influences the clinical manifestations. With pericardial tamponade secondary to myocardial rupture after myocardial infarction (Chapter 72), for example, immediate tamponade and shock can occur within minutes with as little as 150 mL of blood in the pericardium. Survival requires immediate drainage and surgery. In patients with malignant or inflammatory causes of pericardial tamponade, fluid accumulates more slowly, and 1 or 2 L of fluid may be necessary to produce shock.

Distributive Shock

The major feature of distributive shock is decreased peripheral resistance. Although anaphylaxis (Chapter 274), drug overdose, neurogenic insults, and addisonian crisis can produce this form of shock, the most important and prevalent cause is septic shock (Chapter 109). In this form of shock, tissue hypoperfusion results from either microvascular abnormalities (maldistribution or shunting of blood flow) or a mediator-induced metabolic block that prevents cells from adequately using oxygen and other nutrients delivered through the vasculature.

Early in distributive shock, venodilation and leakage of fluid from the microvasculature lead to inadequate intravascular volume and reduced preload. Volume resuscitation corrects this preload abnormality and produces the usual hemodynamic pattern of distributive shock: normal or elevated cardiac output, normal stroke volume, tachycardia, decreased SVR, and decreased MAP. Left and right heart filling pressures are variable and depend on the amount of fluid resuscitation.

In addition, most patients with distributive shock also manifest myocardial depression, which is characterized by a decreased stroke work response to volume loading, biventricular reduction in the ejection fraction, and ventricular dilation. The dilation allows patients to compensate for a depressed ejection fraction and maintain stroke volume, which combined with a high heart rate leads to elevated cardiac output. In approximately 10 to 15% of septic shock patients, the myocardial dysfunction is dominant and severe and results in a hypodynamic low-cardiac output form of shock (see Fig. 107–1).

Clinical Approach to Shock

Shock is a life-threatening emergency. Diagnosis, evaluation, and management most often occur simultaneously, and speed in evaluation is important to achieve a good outcome. The clinical approach must balance two important goals: (1) the need to initiate therapy before shock causes irreversible damage to organs and (2) the need to perform a diagnostic evaluation to determine the cause of the shock (Fig. 107–3). A reasonable approach is to make a rapid clinical evaluation initially based on a directed history and physical examination and to perform diagnostic tests aimed at determining the cause. In severe shock, initiation of therapy should be based on the initial clinical impression. Certain symptoms and signs are common to all forms of shock. Most patients have hypotension, tachycardia, cool extremities, oliguria, and a clouded sensorium. In general, an MAP less than 60 mm Hg in an adult is considered hypotension. However, blood pressure must be evaluated in terms of previous chronic blood pressure readings. A patient with chronic hypertension may experience shock pathophysiology at higher blood pressure values. A decrease of 50 mm Hg or more from chronic elevated levels is frequently sufficient to produce tissue hypoperfusion. Conversely, in some patients with chronically low blood pressure, shock may not develop until the MAP drops to less than 50 mm Hg.

Other clinical manifestations may be useful in differentiating the cause of the shock. Patients with hypovolemic shock frequently manifest evidence of gastrointestinal hemorrhage, bleeding from another site, or vomiting or diarrhea. Patients with cardiogenic shock may have manifestations of heart disease with prior angina or myocardial infarction and often have elevated filling pressure, cardiac gallops, or pulmonary edema (Chapter 57). Cardiac murmurs may suggest mechanical causes of cardiogenic shock (Chapters 72 and 108). Elevated jugular venous pressure and a quiet precordium suggest pericardial tamponade (Chapter 77). A site of infection with prominent fever should raise the possibility of septic shock (Chapter 109).

Even though the brief history and physical examination are directed at potential causes and signs of shock, blood should be drawn to evaluate hemoglobin, platelets, coagulation, oxygenation and ventilation, electrolytes, kidney function, and blood lactate levels. An electrocardiogram and chest radiograph should be taken.

Simultaneously, venous access with one or two large-bore catheters should be established, and central venous and arterial catheters should be inserted (see Fig. 107–3). Electrocardiographic monitoring and continuous pulse oximetry are usually valuable. If MAP is less than 60 mm Hg or evidence of tissue hypoperfusion is present, an intravenous fluid challenge with 500 to 1000 mL of crystalloid or colloid should be given rapidly (if hemorrhage is likely, blood should be the volume replacement). If the patient remains hypotensive, vasopressors such as dopamine or norepinephrine (or both) should be administered to restore adequate blood pressure while the diagnostic evaluation continues. The shock patient should be admitted to an intensive care unit.

If the diagnosis remains undefined or the hemodynamic status requires repeated fluid challenges or vasopressors, a flow-directed pulmonary artery catheter should be placed to determine cardiac output and ventricular filling pressure (Table 107–4), and echocardiography should be performed. Echocardiography is valuable in identifying the presence of pericardial fluid, tamponade physiology, ventricular function, valvular heart disease, and intracardiac shunts (Chapter 53). Based on these data, patients can usually be classified and managed according to the specific form of shock.

Treatment

Rx

In all forms of shock, restoration of blood pressure and tissue perfusion is a critical goal and commonly requires fluids, vasopressors, inotropic agents (Table 107–5), mechanical ventilation, and repeated monitoring.

Hypovolemic Shock

The major goal is to infuse adequate volume to restore perfusion before the onset of irreversible tissue damage without raising cardiac filling pressure to a level that produces hydrostatic pulmonary edema, which usually begins at a pulmonary artery occlusion (capillary wedge) pressure greater than 18 mm Hg. In hemorrhagic shock, restoration of oxygen delivery is achieved by transfusion of packed red blood cells with the goal of maintaining the hemoglobin concentration at greater than 10 g/dL. Restoration

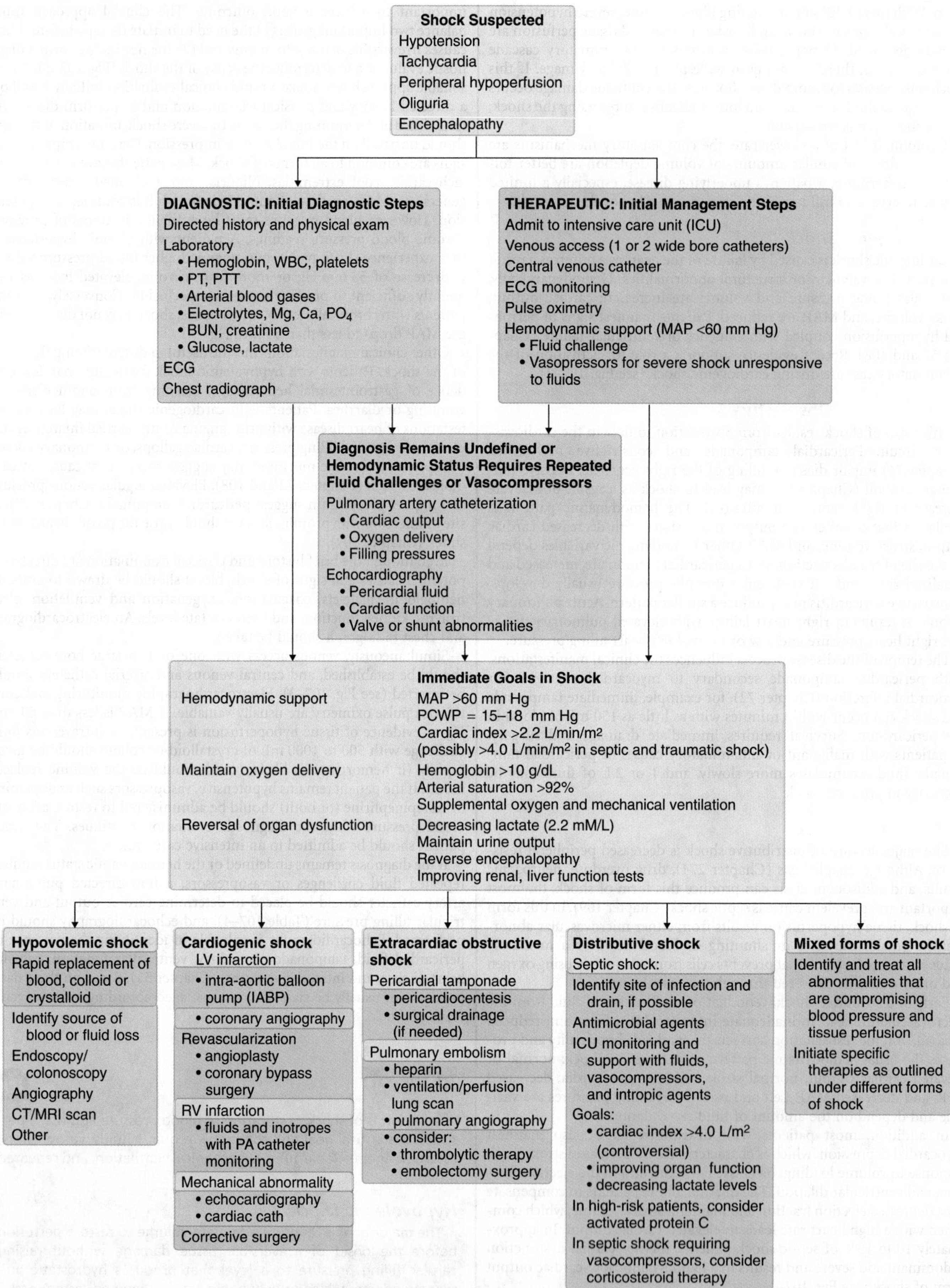

FIGURE 107–3 • An approach to the diagnosis and treatment of shock. BUN = blood urea nitrogen; CT = computed tomography; ECG = electrocardiogram; LV = left ventricular; MAP = mean arterial pressure; MRI = magnetic resonance imaging; PA = pulmonary artery; PCWP = pulmonary capillary wedge pressure; PT = prothrombin time; PTT = partial thromboplastin time; RV = right ventricular; WBC = white cell blood.

TABLE 107–4 DIAGNOSIS OF SHOCK ETIOLOGY VIA PULMONARY ARTERY CATHETERIZATION

Diagnosis	Pulmonary Capillary Wedge Pressure	Cardiac Output	Miscellaneous Comments
CARDIOGENIC SHOCK			
Cardiogenic shock caused by myocardial dysfunction	↑↑	↓↓	Usually occurs with evidence of extensive myocardial infarction (40% of the LV infarcted), severe cardiomyopathy, or myocarditis
Cardiogenic shock caused by a mechanical defect			
Acute ventricular septal defect	↑	LVCO ↓↓ and RVCO > LVCO	Predominant shunt is left to right, pulmonary blood flow is greater than systemic blood flow: oxygen "step-up" occurs at the RV level
Acute mitral regurgitation	↑↑	Forward CO ↓↓	V waves in pulmonary capillary wedge pressure tracing
Right ventricular infarction	Normal or ↓	↓↓	Elevated RA and RV filling pressure with low or normal pulmonary capillary wedge pressure
EXTRACARDIAC OBSTRUCTIVE FORMS OF SHOCK			
Pericardial tamponade	↑	↓ or ↓↓	Mean RA, end-diastolic RV, and mean pulmonary capillary wedge pressures are elevated and within 5 mm Hg of one another
Massive pulmonary embolism	Normal or ↓	↓↓	Usual finding is elevated right-sided pressure
HYPOVOLEMIC SHOCK			
DISTRIBUTIVE FORMS OF SHOCK			
Septic shock	↓ or normal	↑ or normal, rarely ↓	
Anaphylactic shock	↓ or normal	↑ or normal	

CO = cardiac output; LV = left ventricular; RV = right ventricular; RA = right atrial.
Adapted from Parrillo JE, Ayres SM (eds): Major Issues in Critical Care Medicine. Baltimore, Williams & Wilkins, 1984.

TABLE 107–5 RELATIVE POTENCY OF VASOPRESSORS AND INOTROPIC AGENTS IN SHOCK

Agent	Dose	Cardiac: Heart Rate	Cardiac: Contractility	Peripheral Vascular*: Vasoconstriction	Peripheral Vascular*: Vasodilatation	Peripheral Vascular*: Dopaminergic
Dopamine	1–4 µg/kg/min	1+	1+	0	1+	4+
	4–20 µg/kg/min	2+	2–3+	2–3+	0	2+
Norepinephrine	2–20 µg/min	1+	2+	4+	0	0
Dobutamine	2.5–15 µg/kg/min	1–2+	3–4+	0	2+	0
Isoproterenol	1–5 µg/min	4+	4+	0	4+	0
Epinephrine	1–20 µg/min	4+	4+	4+	3+	0
Phenylephrine	20–200 µg/min	0	0	3+	0	0
Milrinone	37.5–75 µg/kg via bolus; then 0.375–0.75 µg/kg/min	1+	3+	0	2+	0
Vasopressin	0.1–0.4 U/min	0	0	4+	0	0

*The 1 to 4+ scoring system is an arbitrary system to allow a judgment of comparative potency among these vasopressor agents.
Adapted from Parrillo JE, Ayres SM (eds): Major Issues in Critical Care Medicine. Baltimore, Williams & Wilkins, 1984.

Rx

of intravascular volume must be accompanied by aggressive evaluation to identify a bleeding source and treatment to prevent further bleeding.

In other forms of hypovolemic shock, crystalloid solutions such as normal saline or Ringer's lactate are equivalent to albumin for restoring volume depletion.  Because colloids such as albumin and hetastarch are more expensive, crystalloids should be favored unless the serum albumin concentration is low and specific albumin repletion is required. Hypertonic saline, which can provide volume repletion with small volumes of fluid, may be therapeutically useful in burns (Chapter 113) and head trauma (Chapter 422), in which case limitation of free water is often important.

Cardiogenic Shock

In hypotensive patients with cardiogenic shock, pulmonary capillary wedge pressure should be maintained at 14 to 18 mm Hg, and medications should be given in an attempt to restore MAP to greater than 60 mm Hg and the cardiac index (cardiac output divided

Rx

by body surface area in meters squared) to more than 2.2 L/min/m^2 (Chapters 58 and 108). Appropriate patients benefit from an intra-aortic balloon pump or from surgical correction of valvular abnormalities or septal defects. In patients with acute myocardial infarction and cardiogenic shock as a result of myocardial damage, emergency coronary revascularization has been shown to be superior to medical therapy. 3

Extracardiac Obstructive Shock

In pericardial tamponade, blood pressure can be maintained with fluids and vasopressors in a fashion similar to the method used for cardiogenic shock. However, these measures are only temporizing, and one should move quickly to drain pericardial fluid by needle pericardiocentesis or surgery (Chapter 77).

In patients with severe pulmonary embolism (Chapter 99) producing right ventricular failure and shock, thrombolytic therapy should be considered in addition to conventional anticoagulation with heparin and warfarin. If thrombolysis is contraindicated, emergency surgical pulmonary embolectomy can sometimes produce a successful outcome.

Distributive Shock

For septic shock (Chapter 109), principles of management include eliminating the nidus of infection with surgical drainage and antimicrobial therapy, early restoration of blood pressure with fluids and vasopressor agents, and maintenance of adequate tissue perfusion with fluids, inotropic agents, and other supportive measures. Aggressive therapy with fluids, blood transfusions, and inotropic agents in the emergency department significantly lowers the mortality of patients with severe sepsis and septic shock. 4 In patients with a high risk of death, activated protein C therapy also improves survival. 1 Arginine vasopressin appears to be useful in catecholamine-resistant vasodilatory shock. 5

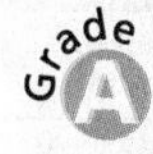

1. Bernard GR, Vincent JL, Laterre PF, et al: Efficacy and safety of recombinant human activated protein C for severe sepsis. N Engl J Med 2001;344:699–709.
2. SAFE Study Investigators: A comparison of albumin and saline for fluid resuscitation in the intensive care unit. N Engl J Med 2004;350:2247–2256.
3. Hochman JS, Sleeper LA, Webb JG, et al: Early revascularization in acute myocardial infarction complicated by cardiogenic shock. SHOCK Investigators. Should we emergently revascularize occluded coronaries for cardiogenic shock. N Engl J Med 1999;341:625–634.
4. Rivers E, Nguyen B, Havstad S, et al: Early goal-directed therapy in the treatment of severe sepsis and septic shock. N Engl J Med 2001;345:1368–1377.
5. Dünser MW, Mayr AJ, Ulmer H, et al: Arginine vasopressin in advanced vasodilatory shock: A prospective, randomized controlled study. Circulation 2003;107:2313–2319.

SUGGESTED READINGS

Beale RJ, Hollenberg SM, Vincent J-L, Parrillo JE: Vasopressor and inotropic support in septic shock: An evidence-based review. Crit Care Med 2004;32 (Suppl.):S455–S465. *An evidence-based review of the hemodynamic support of septic shock.*

Dutton RP: Current concepts in hemorrhagic shock. Anesthesiol Clin 2007;25:23–34. *A practical overview of pathophysiology and management.*

Shah MR, Hasselblad V, Stevenson LW, et al: Impact of the pulmonary artery catheter in critically ill patients: Meta-analysis of randomized clinical trials. JAMA 2005;294:1664–1670. *Use of the PAC neither increased overall mortality or days in the hospital nor conferred benefit.*

108 CARDIOGENIC SHOCK

David R. Holmes, Jr.

Definition

Cardiogenic shock describes tissue hypoperfusion as a result of an acute myocardial infarction (MI) or end-stage heart failure from any cause. Cardiogenic shock can be defined by clinical parameters alone (Chapter 107), including the manifestations of a low–cardiac output state with peripheral hypoperfusion and cool, clammy extremities, cyanosis, oliguria, and altered central nervous system function. An obligate requirement is the presence of hypotension. The degree of hypotension required to fulfill the criteria for shock has varied but is usually a systolic blood pressure less than 90 mm Hg; an alternative definition is a systolic blood pressure more than 30 mm Hg *below* the patient's basal level. A confounding variable is the requirement for and use of vasopressors to maintain blood pressure. A previously normotensive patient who now requires vasopressors to maintain a systolic blood pressure of 90 mm Hg is also typically characterized as having cardiogenic shock. Although the clinical manifestations of hypoperfusion and systolic blood pressure less than 90 mm Hg are the hallmarks of shock, other important hemodynamic manifestations include an elevated left ventricular (LV) filling pressure greater than 15 mm Hg and a reduction in cardiac index to less than approximately 2.2 L/min/m^2. In addition, many patients with end-stage heart failure, especially if treated with afterload-reducing agents (Chapter 58), may have blood pressure readings chronically less than 90 mm Hg but not be in shock.

Epidemiology

Acute Cardiogenic Shock

The incidence of cardiogenic shock after an acute MI has varied from 5 to 19%. The incidence may be underestimated because some reports may exclude patients with shock on admission or may not represent the full spectrum of those with both ST segment elevation and non–ST segment elevation MI. When compared with patients with ST segment elevation, those with ST segment depression have approximately half the incidence of cardiogenic shock. The incidence of cardiogenic shock has also varied over time; earlier recognition of the symptoms of MI, earlier initiation of medical care, and the administration of thrombolytic therapy may have reduced the incidence. Typically, only a minority of patients with shock (approximately 10 to 15%) have it on admission. Shock develops in most patients within the next 48 hours. In a multicenter, country-wide survey from Denmark, shock developed in about 60% of patients within 48 hours, but in 30%, shock developed more than 4 days after the MI. In another study, only about 30% of patients had cardiogenic shock on admission, whereas it developed in the remainder later. When cardiogenic shock develops in patients without ST segment elevation, it usually develops relatively later, commonly as a result of reinfarction. As might be expected, previous MI, older age, diabetes mellitus, female gender, and a history of angina pectoris, stroke, or peripheral vascular disease have been associated with an increased incidence of cardiogenic shock, but the predictive power of these factors in an individual patient is limited. In a registry of more than 24,000 patients with acute coronary syndrome from 14 countries between 1999 and 2002, the incidence of cardiogenic shock increased from 1.6% in patients younger than 45 years to 10% in those 85 years or older. Patients with preexisting LV dysfunction are also at higher risk. Occasionally, cardiogenic shock develops in patients with severe myocarditis, especially postpartum cardiomyopathy.

Refractory Chronic Heart Failure

Many of the chronic causes of refractory heart failure result in sudden death as often as or more often than they result in hospitalization or home treatment for refractory low-output heart failure. Essentially every cause of heart failure (Chapter 57), however, can result in a refractory low-output state with congestion and systemic hypoperfusion.

Section X Critical Care

TABLE 108–1 CARDIOGENIC SHOCK

Acute myocardial infarction
Pump failure
Mechanical complication
Ventricular septal defect
Mitral regurgitation
Ventricular rupture
Tachyarrhythmia
Valvular heart disease
Acute mitral regurgitation
Acute aortic regurgitation
Aortic or mitral stenosis and acute comorbid condition, e.g., infection, anemia, tachyarrhythmia
Prosthetic valve dysfunction
Traumatic cardiac injury—penetrating or blunt
Myocarditis
Orthotopic transplant rejection
Peripartum cardiomyopathy
Pericardial disease with effusion
End-stage low-output heart failure

TABLE 108–2 RISK FACTORS FOR CARDIOGENIC SHOCK COMPLICATING ACUTE MYOCARDIAL INFARCTION

Factors Associated with the Development of Shock	Factors Associated with Increased Mortality from Shock
Older age	Older age
Diabetes mellitus	Previous infarction
History of previous MI, stroke, or peripheral vascular disease	Altered sensorium
	Peripheral vasoconstriction
	Baseline systolic blood pressure
Female gender	Lower cardiac output
Reinfarction	Higher heart rate
Initial EF <35%	
Lack of compensatory hyperkinesis in remote segments	

EF = ejection fraction; MI = myocardial infarction.

Pathobiology

Acute Cardiogenic Shock

Acute cardiogenic shock is typically the result of an extensive MI associated with damage to 40% or more of the LV myocardium, but other causes include a wide range of cardiac conditions (Table 108–1). It does not seem to matter whether this loss of LV myocardium is the result of a single ischemic insult, with occlusion of a single artery that supplies a large region of myocardium, or a series of multiple previous MIs. The sequence of ischemic insults (i.e., a single catastrophic event or a series of multiple previous infarctions) may affect the time course of the shock, however. A single catastrophic event may result either in early shock or in sudden death, in contrast to patients with multiple smaller previous infarctions, in whom shock may develop after hospital admission. Multiple clinical factors have been associated with the development or outcome of shock (Table 108–2). Autopsy and angiographic studies have documented that multivessel coronary artery disease is almost universally present, particularly involving the left main and left anterior descending coronary artery.

Infarct extension or reinfarction is common in patients with shock and is often the mechanism responsible for shock. Among the multiple factors that may be involved in infarct extension or expansion are impaired collateral flow, increased myocardial oxygen consumption, thrombus propagation or embolization, and passive collapse or vasoconstriction at a second site within the coronary circulation as a result of low coronary perfusion pressure during diastole. In patients with hypertensive cardiovascular disease and LV hypertrophy or aortic stenosis, the hypotension and elevated LV end-diastolic pressure may cause or aggravate diffuse subendocardial ischemia. Other important factors that can aggravate shock include anemia, poor oxygenation, and in some patients, inappropriately decreased peripheral arterial resistance.

TABLE 108–3 REASONS WHY CHRONIC HEART FAILURE MAY DECOMPENSATE WITH CARDIOGENIC SHOCK

Development of new comorbid condition
Infection/sepsis
Renal insufficiency
Uncontrolled diabetes
Anemia
Pulmonary embolism
Hypothyroidism/hyperthyroidism
Cardiac rhythm disorders—atrial fibrillation, bradycardia
Progression of underlying disease
Myocardial ischemia
Chronic renal insufficiency
Uncontrolled hypertension
Patient compliance
Poor compliance with the drug therapy regimen
Dietary indiscretion
Alcohol
Drug therapy
Inadequate doses of beneficial drugs
Failure to prescribe beneficial drugs
Over- or under-diuresis
Sudden alteration in drug therapy
Drug interactions
Cardiotoxic medications

The mechanical complications of mitral regurgitation, ventricular septal defect (VSD), or rupture of the LV myocardium account for 15 to 25% of cases of acute cardiogenic shock. The underlying MI may be only small or moderate in size but can involve crucial structures, such as the interventricular septum or papillary muscle. Free wall rupture accounts for 10% of all deaths from MI and is typically associated with an ST segment elevation anterior MI. In this setting, shock may develop abruptly and be followed by circulatory collapse with electromechanical dissociation. Rupture of the interventricular septum may result in a single direct perforation or many complex serpentine tracts; this defect is also seen with ST segment elevation anterior MI. Partial or complete rupture of one of the papillary muscles may result in severe mitral regurgitation; the posteromedial papillary muscle is involved more frequently than the anterolateral papillary muscle because the former usually receives its blood supply from just one source, the posterior descending coronary artery. Cardiogenic shock is a distinct and well-recognized complication of a right ventricular MI, which is always associated with posterobasal infarction of the left ventricle. With occlusion of the proximal right coronary artery, right ventricular pump function decreases and the right ventricle dilates, thereby leading to a decrease in LV preload and subsequent hypotension.

Refractory Chronic Heart Failure

End-stage refractory heart failure can be the final stage of any of the diseases that cause chronic heart failure (Chapter 57). In these patients, key issues include evaluation of the underlying disease process, the development of new comorbid conditions, compliance with medication, and the adequacy of long-term therapy (Table 108–3).

Clinical Manifestations

Cardiogenic shock is manifested as tissue hypoperfusion. Hypotension is usually defined as systolic blood pressure less than 90 mm Hg or more than a 30-mm Hg decrease in systolic blood pressure from baseline, although the latter criterion includes a larger group of patients who may not have shock or who have a milder form of shock. The term *preshock* has been used to define some of these patients. The prognosis of patients with preshock may be substantially better than that of patients with full-blown shock. Hypoperfusion is recognized by altered sensorium, cyanosis, oliguria, and cool, clammy extremities. Attendant dyspnea and ongoing ischemic chest pain may be present.

This constellation of findings may be noted at the initial evaluation for acute MI, but they more frequently develop later, 48 hours after the onset of MI. Either bradycardia, usually a manifestation of the Bezold-Jarisch reflex, or tachycardia may be present. Acute myocarditis with shock is also characterized by hypoperfusion; marked fluid retention may be prominent if the myocarditis has been present for several days to weeks. When accompanied by low blood pressure and systemic hypoperfusion, the clinical manifestations of refractory heart failure may be indistinguishable from those of acute cardiogenic shock.

Physical Examination

The physical examination should be focused on identification of hypoperfusion, volume status, and secondary causes of shock. Typically, venous pressure is elevated. The presence of low venous pressure identifies a group of patients who usually have hypovolemia rather than cardiogenic shock as a predominant cause; correction by fluid administration may lead to an improved outcome (Chapter 107). Concomitant pulmonary edema (Chapter 58) may be present, which in a hypotensive patient establishes the diagnosis of cardiogenic shock. In patients with a mechanical complication resulting in shock, the physical findings may not be typical of the underlying cause. Patients with acute mitral regurgitation may not have a systolic murmur because of equalization of pressure between the left ventricle and left atrium (Chapter 75); in these patients, a high index of suspicion is required so that appropriate tests (e.g., LV angiography or echocardiography) can be performed to make the definitive diagnosis. In patients with a VSD, the systolic murmur may be at the lower left sternal border without a thrill. Patients with a free wall rupture commonly demonstrate electromechanical dissociation, which is almost uniformly fatal. In patients with myocarditis, a pericardial or pleuropericardial rub may be present.

Diagnosis

Noninvasive Evaluation

Electrocardiogram

In patients with circulatory collapse, an initial electrocardiogram (ECG) is essential. In acute cardiogenic shock caused by acute MI, ST segment elevation is the most common finding, although cardiogenic shock can occur without it. ST segment depression or nonspecific ST segment changes may occur in approximately 25% of patients. The ECG also provides information on previous MI and rhythm disorders. Isolated elevation of the ST segment in lead aVR in a patient with acute MI and shock suggests the possibility of left main coronary artery involvement. In patients in whom right ventricular MI is suspected, modified right precordial leads are helpful (Chapter 52). In acute myocarditis, ECG abnormalities are usually diffuse. Tachyarrhythmias are common, especially sinus tachycardia or atrial fibrillation; in some patients, new intraventricular conduction defects may be seen. When cardiogenic shock complicates end-stage heart failure, the ECG may reflect extensive previous MI, interventricular conduction defects, or bundle branch blocks.

Echocardiography

Echocardiography (Chapter 53) is extremely useful in the evaluation of a patient with shock (Fig. 108–1). It can make the diagnosis of a mechanical complication, such as a ruptured papillary muscle or a VSD. In addition, echocardiography can assess overall LV function, including compensatory hyperkinesis of noninfarcted segments. Patients with cardiogenic shock from a large MI can be expected to have severe regional wall motion abnormalities. Severe diffuse hypokinesis may suggest cardiomyopathy as the cause of shock, whereas a flail mitral leaflet would suggest acute mitral regurgitation (Chapter 75). Both short- and long-term mortality are associated with worse initial LV function and more mitral regurgitation as assessed by echocardiography. In patients in whom free wall rupture is suspected, echocardiography can document a pericardial effusion (Chapter 77).

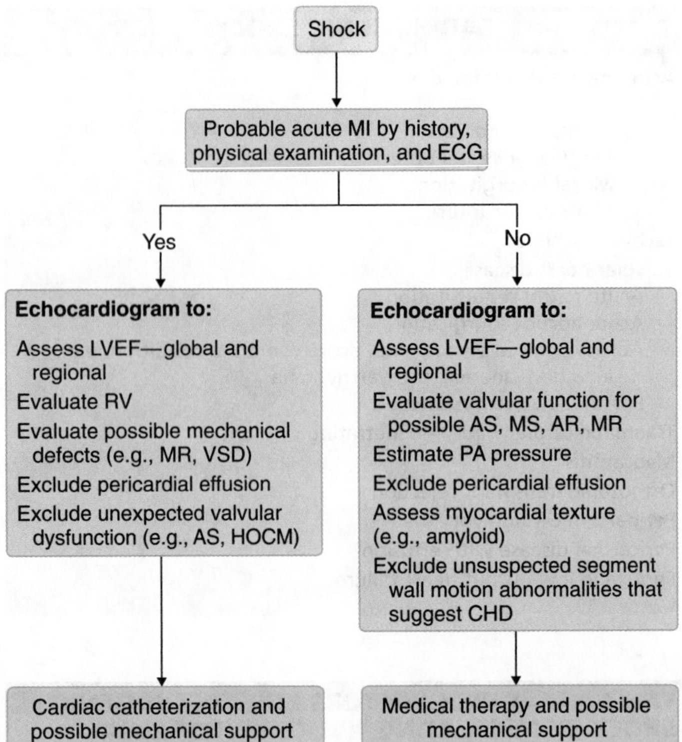

FIGURE 108–1 • Role of echocardiography in assessing the cause of cardiogenic shock. AR = aortic regurgitation; AS = aortic stenosis; CHD = coronary heart disease; ECG = electrocardiogram; HOCM = hypertrophic obstructive cardiomyopathy; LVEF = left ventricular ejection fraction; MI = myocardial infarction; MR = mitral regurgitation; MS = mitral stenosis; PA = pulmonary artery; RV = right ventricle; VSD = ventricular septal defect.

Although echocardiography is a vital tool, it must be performed expeditiously, particularly in the setting of an acute ischemic event. Other procedures, most importantly urgent cardiac catheterization in patients with acute MI (Chapter 56), should not be delayed excessively while echocardiography is being considered or performed. LV angiography can yield extremely important data on ventricular and valvular function.

Invasive Evaluation

Pulmonary Artery Catheterization

Right heart catheterization with flow-directed catheters can sometimes be useful by documenting low LV filling pressure in patients with hypovolemic shock or right ventricular infarction, giant v waves in patients with unsuspected severe mitral regurgitation, or an oxygen saturation gradient in a patient with a VSD.

Differential Diagnosis

Acute Cardiogenic Shock

In the acute setting, cardiogenic causes of shock must be distinguished from septic and other causes of shock (see Fig. 107–2). Even in cardiac patients, shock can be due to noncardiogenic causes, including hypotension caused by medications such as nitrates, angiotensin-converting enzyme inhibitors, other vasodilators, or streptokinase; hemorrhage from anticoagulant or thrombolytic drugs; pulmonary embolism (Chapter 99); or hypovolemia. The diverse causes of cardiogenic shock must be kept in mind (see Table 108–1). Although the classic cause is pump failure secondary to extensive LV damage, right ventricular infarction can also lead to cardiogenic shock if associated posterior LV infarction is present (Chapter 72). In addition, the differential diagnosis of *acute* cardiogenic shock includes the mechanical causes of mitral regurgitation from papillary muscle rupture or dysfunction, rupture of the LV free wall, and VSD. In a large registry, acute shock was due to predominantly LV failure in 74.5% of patients but was related to acute severe mitral regurgitation in 8.3%, ventricular septal rupture in 4.6%, and isolated right ventricular shock in 3.4%. Cardiogenic shock may also result from other cardiac conditions, such as aortic stenosis (Chapter 75) or pericardial tamponade (Chapter 77), the latter of which may be the result of an ascending aortic dissection (Chapter 78) that propagates in retrograde fashion, with shearing of the right coronary artery and then creation of a rupture into the pericardium. Cardiac arrhythmias, such as atrial fibrillation with a rapid ventricular response (Chapter 63) or ventricular tachycardia (Chapter 64), may contribute to hypotension. Myocarditis (Chapter 59) can also result in shock.

The clinical circumstances and time course of shock often provide important clues to specific causes. Given the diverse number of disease states that may cause shock (Chapter 107), identifying the specific cause is important because it may mandate a different treatment strategy and may affect the prognosis.

Refractory Chronic Heart Failure

Patients with end-stage refractory heart failure (Chapters 57 and 58) may also have severe hypoperfusion, but in general, shock develops more slowly than in patients with acute MI. In patients with chronic heart failure, blood pressure may be less than 90 mm Hg in the absence of shock, especially if aggressive afterload reduction therapy is being administered; in these individuals, fluid overload may precipitate cardiogenic shock.

Treatment

Medical Therapy

The prognosis of patients with cardiogenic shock is poor. Supportive measures, such as maintenance of adequate oxygenation and treatment of arrhythmias, are essential, and documentation of volume status is important. Attempts to improve blood pressure are crucial to break the vicious cycle of progressive hypotension leading to further myocardial ischemia. If LV filling pressure is elevated as assessed by either hemodynamic monitoring or the presence of pulmonary edema, further volume expansion is not beneficial and may be harmful. If volume status is uncertain, a trial of volume expansion is warranted with careful monitoring. Monitoring of left-sided heart pressure with periodic wedge recordings can help optimize filling pressure during the initial attempts at stabilization. Hemodynamic monitoring is also extremely useful for initiating aggressive afterload reduction. Nevertheless, routine use of pulmonary artery catheters to guide therapy does not improve the outcome. [1] Furthermore, in some patients the relationship between central venous pressure and pulmonary capillary wedge pressure may be sufficiently consistent to allow the physician to monitor only central venous pressure. Urine output should also be monitored.

Vasopressor therapy (see Table 107–5) is usually essential to improve cardiac performance and stabilize the patient; its risks include aggravation of arrhythmias and, even more importantly, an increase in myocardial oxygen demand. Dopamine, which is generally the initial drug given, can increase systemic pressure and cardiac output. Dobutamine may be used in combination with dopamine to augment cardiac output, but it does not usually increase arterial pressure further. Levosimendan, a calcium sensitizer, may be better than dobutamine in low-output heart failure. [2] In patients who have severe or resistant hypotension, norepinephrine is commonly given and may be effective. In general, myocardial oxygen demand can be minimized by titrating vasopressive agents to the lowest dose required to optimize blood pressure and maintain adequate cardiac output. Vasodilators, such as intravenous nitroglycerin or nitroprusside, are not generally used initially because they can aggravate hypotension; however, they may be given later in combination with vasopressors and inotropic agents. The effectiveness of all inotropic agents may diminish over time, so these drugs are not usually definitive therapies. Milrinone, a second-generation phosphodiesterase inhibitor, should not be used because of its substantial vasodilatory properties.

In patients with acute MI, aspirin and heparin are important and serve as baseline treatments. Thrombolytic drugs have been used widely for acute MI, but most trials have not included patients with preexisting cardiogenic shock. The benefit of thrombolysis has been equivocal, with some trials showing no benefit and others showing a small benefit. This equivocal benefit may be related to multiple factors, including (1) poor delivery or penetrance of lytic agents to the thrombus because of the hypotension and (2) impaired transformation of plasminogen to plasmin because of acidosis. To negate the effect of these factors as much as possible, thrombolytic therapy in patients with shock or preshock should be accompanied by vigorous attempts to augment blood pressure and treat acidosis. Thrombolysis may reduce the subsequent development of shock, perhaps because of a decrease in reinfarction or limitation of the size of the initial infarct.

Inhaled nitric oxide, 80 ppm, can result in a significant decrease in right atrial and mean pulmonary arterial pressure and an increase in the cardiac index. However, a large randomized trial showed that use of a nitrous oxide synthetase inhibitor was of no clinical benefit.

Mechanical Therapy

Insertion of an intra-aortic balloon pump (IABP) for counterpulsation increases diastolic coronary artery perfusion pressure, decreases LV afterload, improves cardiac output, and decreases myocardial oxygen demand. An IABP can stabilize hemodynamics and improve survival at 30 days and 1 year in acute cardiogenic shock complicating acute MI. [3] However, the currently available data suggest that IABP is underused.

A variety of percutaneous partial cardiopulmonary bypass techniques can be performed in the acute or chronic setting, but these devices are used only in specialized centers because of the need for special equipment. Partial LV assist devices decrease myocardial oxygen demand while maintaining or augmenting perfusion and may provide an important adjunct to myocardial salvage. In one randomized trial of patients with end-stage heart failure, an implantable LV assist device improved survival and quality of life. [4] Clinical trials are also under way to test whether devices that lower body temperature to approximately 33° C can improve outcome.

Surgical Therapy

Revascularization

Urgent percutaneous intervention (PCI) (Chapter 73) has been advocated for cardiogenic shock in the setting of acute MI based on nonrandomized data and subset analysis of large randomized trials. In the one randomized trial that focused exclusively on cardiogenic shock in acute MI, early coronary revascularization within 6 hours was compared with medical stabilization and IABP followed by delayed coronary revascularization. The primary end point, 30-day mortality, was not significantly different in the two groups (46.7% in the early revascularization group vs. 56.0% in the initial medical stabilization group). At 6 months, however, mortality in the revascularization group was significantly lower (50.3 vs. 63.1%, $P = .027$), and the benefit was greatest in patients younger than 75 years. [5] Other nonrandomized data also suggest improved survival in patients older than 75 years.

In clinical trials and in clinical practice, PCI is generally combined with other adjunctive therapies, such as IABP, which is typically placed before treatment. Historically, only the infarct-related artery was treated at the initial PCI, unless the patient had multivessel disease with other critical lesions and was not helped by PCI of the infarct-related artery. With the advent of coronary stents (Chapter 73), it may be possible to treat all significant stenoses and provide more complete revascularization. Adjunctive therapy with glycoprotein IIb/IIIa inhibitors may be helpful, although these drugs may complicate the situation by increasing the potential for bleeding in patients in whom surgery is subsequently required.

Coronary stents provide improved angiographic success for PCI, and this higher angiographic success rate has been associated with improved 30-day survival. The additional benefit, if any, of newer adjunctive pharmacologic agents and new devices that prevent distal embolization is unknown, but they are currently being tested.

Coronary artery bypass graft (CABG) surgery (Chapter 74) has potential advantages, including the ability to achieve complete revascularization and the opportunity to vent the ventricle and cool the heart with cardioplegia to limit ongoing ischemia and reduce myocardial oxygen consumption. There are currently no randomized studies, however, comparing CABG surgery with PCI or medical

Rx

therapy. Despite the likelihood that aggressive revascularization with either PCI or surgery will improve survival in cardiogenic shock, these approaches appear to be underused, particularly in older patients.

Other Surgical Procedures

In patients with mechanical complications, surgery often provides the only therapeutic approach. If possible, these patients should be stabilized before surgery, often with an IABP. In patients with a VSD or severe mitral regurgitation, surgery can improve the outcome dramatically despite high operative mortality rates. Free wall rupture is commonly accompanied by electromechanical dissociation and is almost always fatal. Subacute rupture with false aneurysm formation is rare, but it can be treated surgically with suture or patch closure when it is diagnosed in time. In patients with shock from mechanical causes not related to acute MI, such as ruptured chordae or severe acute aortic regurgitation, surgical approaches are required. In some patients (e.g., those with ruptured chordae), placement of an IABP may improve cardiac performance substantially and reduce the risk associated with surgery.

Recommended Current Approach

Acute Myocardial Infarction

At present, an aggressive approach seems to have the most potential to improve outcome (Fig. 108–2). Management requires rapid evaluation of the multiple potential causes of shock in parallel with supportive therapy designed to improve perfusion and optimize right ventricular and LV pressure. An IABP and right heart catheterization are helpful for stabilization, management, and diagnosis. Catheterization can detect an increase in oxygen saturation in the right ventricle as found in a post-MI VSD (Chapters 68 and 72). Revascularization with either emergency percutaneous transluminal coronary angioplasty or CABG surgery seems to confer early and longer-term survival benefits in eligible patients, although the problem of selection bias and its effect on outcome must be kept in mind.

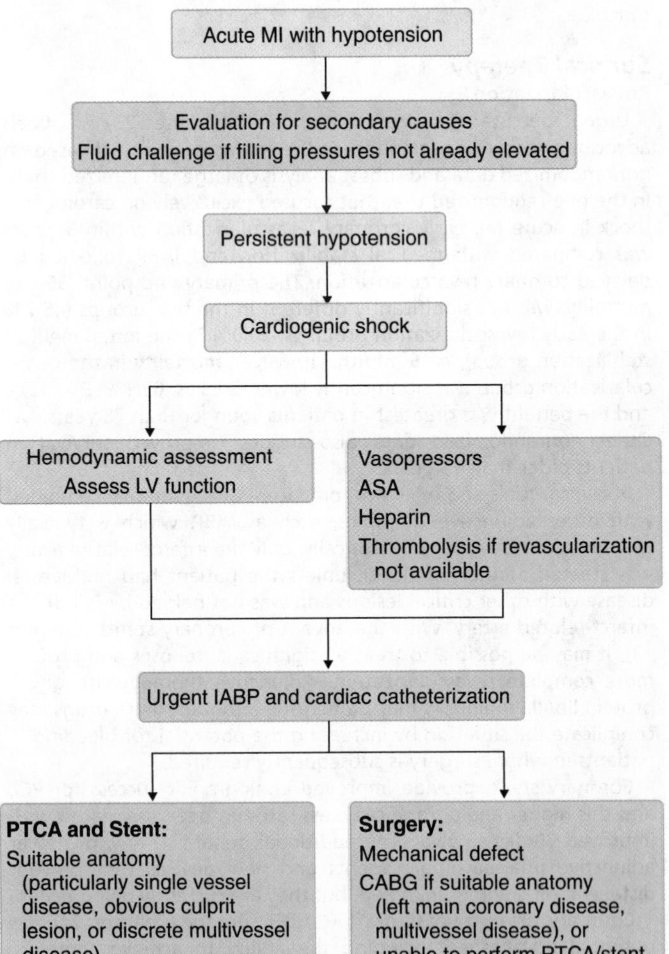

FIGURE 108–2 • Acute myocardial infarction with hypotension: an aggressive approach. ASA = acetylsalicylic acid (aspirin); CABG = coronary artery bypass graft; IABP = intra-aortic balloon pump; LV = left ventricular; MI = myocardial infarction; PTCA = percutaneous transluminal coronary angioplasty.

Rx

Acute Myocardial Disease

General supportive measures (Chapter 58) are the cornerstone of therapy for severe heart failure. If the patient is in shock despite supportive measures, circulatory support with either an IABP or LV or biventricular assist devices should be considered. Some patients may have spontaneous recovery of ventricular function; alternatively, circulatory support may be used as a bridge to heart transplantation (Chapter 82). Specific therapies, such as steroids and cyclosporine or azathioprine, may be helpful in specific patient groups (e.g., those with idiopathic giant cell myocarditis or sarcoidosis), but not in patients with nonspecific myocarditis (Chapter 59).

Refractory Chronic Heart Failure

In patients with refractory chronic heart failure, medical therapy is generally similar to therapy for acute cardiogenic shock. Mechanical and surgical interventions, including cardiac transplantation (Chapter 82), can benefit selected patients (Chapter 58).

Prognosis

Acute Cardiogenic Shock

Cardiogenic shock now accounts for most deaths related to acute MI. Before the era of reperfusion, mortality from cardiogenic shock approximated 80%. In the larger thrombolytic trials, mortality rates remain at 51 to 70%. Although findings such as altered sensorium and peripheral vasoconstriction are important predictors of prognosis, cardiac output and wedge pressure measurements add essential independent information regarding prognosis and increase the ability to identify patients at greatest risk of dying of cardiogenic shock. Cardiac power, which is a function of the product of cardiac output times mean arterial pressure, measures the rate of energy input that the systemic vasculature receives from the heart and is also a strong predictor of outcome in cardiogenic shock.

In selected series of shock patients, an aggressive strategy consisting of placement of an IABP followed by revascularization, either by PCI or by CABG surgery, may reduce 30-day mortality to 30 to 40%. The outlook in patients who survive for 1 month is good; among 1-month survivors, 85 to 90% are alive at 1 year. This survival rate is better in patients who have undergone coronary revascularization.

The prognosis in patients with myocarditis and shock is variable and depends on the underlying cause (Chapter 59). Some patients can be supported by a mechanical circulatory device until spontaneous recovery occurs or a heart transplant is available (Chapter 82).

Refractory Chronic Heart Failure

Except in patients who may benefit from specific mechanical or surgical interventions, the prognosis of patients with refractory chronic heart failure is bleak (Chapter 58).

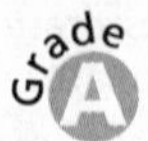

1. The ESCAPE Investigators and ESCAPE Study Coordinators: Evaluation study of congestive heart failure and pulmonary artery catheterization effectiveness: The ESCAPE trial. JAMA 2005;294:1625–1633.
2. Follath F, Cleland JGF, Just H, et al: Efficacy and safety of intravenous levosimendan compared with dobutamine in severe low-output heart failure (the LIDO study): A randomised double-blind trial. Lancet 2002;360:196–202.
3. Stone GW, Marsalese D, Brodie BR, et al: A prospective, randomized evaluation of prophylactic intra-aortic balloon counterpulsation in high-risk patients with acute myocardial infarction treated with primary angioplasty: Second Primary Angioplasty in Myocardial Infarction (PAMI-II) Trial Investigators. J Am Coll Cardiol 1997;29:1459–1467.

4. Rose EA, Gelijns AC, Moskowitz AJ, et al: Long-term use of a left ventricular assist device for end-stage heart failure. N Engl J Med 2001;345:1435–1443.
5. Hochman JS, Sleeper LA, White HD, et al: One-year survival following early revascularization for cardiogenic shock. JAMA 2001;285:190–192.

SUGGESTED READINGS

Avezum A, Makdisse M, Spencer F, et al: Impact of age on management and outcome of acute coronary syndrome: Observations from the Global Registry of Acute Coronary Events (GRACE). Am Heart J 2005;149:67–73. *A large registry from 14 countries and 102 hospitals describing suboptimal use of evidence-based therapy for cardiogenic shock.*

Iakobishvili Z, Behar S, Boyko V, et al: Does current treatment of cardiogenic shock complicating the acute coronary syndromes comply with guidelines? Am Heart J 2005;149:98–103. *Many patients do not receive recommended therapies.*

Mann HJ, Nolan PE Jr: Update on the management of cardiogenic shock. Curr Opin Crit Care 2006;12:431–436. *A pactical overview.*

TRIUMPH Investigators, Alexander JH, Reynolds HR, et al: Effect of tilarginine acetate in patients with acute myocardial infarction and cardiogenic shock. JAMA 2007;297:1657–1666. *No benefit from a maneuver to raise nitric oxide levels.*

109 SHOCK SYNDROMES RELATED TO SEPSIS

James A. Russell

Definition

Sepsis is defined by presence of at least two of four signs of the systemic inflammatory response syndrome (SIRS): (1) fever (>38° C) or hypothermia (<36° C); (2) tachycardia (>90 beats per minute); (3) tachypnea (>20 breaths per minute), hypocapnia (partial pressure of carbon dioxide <32 mm Hg), or the need for mechanical ventilatory assistance; and (4) leukocytosis (>12,000 cells/mm^3), leukopenia (<4000 cells/mm^3), or a left shift (>0% immature band cells) in the white cell differential and suspected or proven infection. *Bacteremia* is defined as growth of bacteria in blood cultures, but infection does not have to be proven to diagnose sepsis at onset. *Severe sepsis* is sepsis in addition to dysfunction of one or more organ systems (e.g., hypoxemia, oliguria, lactic acidosis, thrombocytopenia, decreased Glasgow Coma Score). *Septic shock* is defined as severe sepsis in addition to hypotension (systolic blood pressure <90 mm Hg or a decrease of >40 mm Hg from baseline) despite adequate fluid resuscitation.

Epidemiology

Approximately 750,000 cases of severe sepsis or septic shock occur every year in the United States. Sepsis causes as many deaths as acute myocardial infarction, and septic shock and its complications are the most common causes of death in noncoronary intensive care units. The medical care costs associated with sepsis are approximately $16.7 billion/year in the United States alone. The frequency of septic shock is increasing as physicians perform more aggressive surgery, as more resistant organisms are present in the environment, and as the prevalence immune compromise resulting from disease and immunosuppressive drugs increases.

Septic shock may be caused by gram-positive or gram-negative bacteria, fungi, and, very rarely, protozoa or rickettsiae. Increasingly common causes of septic shock are gram-positive bacteria, especially methicillin-resistant *Staphylococcus aureus,* vancomycin-resistant enterococci, penicillin-resistant *Streptococcus pneumoniae,* and resistant gram-negative bacilli.

The common sites of infection causing septic shock are pneumonia, peritonitis, pyelonephritis, abscess (especially intra-abdominal), primary bacteremia, cholangitis, cellulitis, necrotizing fasciitis, and meningitis. Nosocomial pneumonia is the most common cause of death from nosocomial infection.

Pathobiology

Initially, septic shock activates inflammation, thereby leading to enhanced coagulation, activated platelets, increased neutrophils and mononuclear cells, and diminished fibrinolysis (Table 109–1). After several days, a compensatory anti-inflammatory response with immunosuppression may contribute to death. Several pathways amplify one another: inflammation triggers coagulation, and coagulation triggers inflammation, thereby resulting in a positive feedback loop that is pro-inflammatory and pro-coagulant. Tissue hypoxia in septic shock also amplifies inflammation and coagulation. Many mediators that are critical for the homeostatic control of infection may be injurious to the host (e.g., tumor necrosis factor-α [TNF-α]), so therapies that fully neutralize such mediators are largely ineffective.

Widespread endothelial injury is an important feature of septic shock; an injured endothelium is more permeable, so fluid flux of protein-rich edema fluid into tissues such as the lung increases. Injured endothelial cells release nitric oxide, a potent vasodilator that is a key mediator of septic shock. Septic shock also injures epithelial cells of the lung and intestine. Intestinal epithelial injury increases intestinal permeability, and this leads to translocation of intestinal bacteria and endotoxin, which further augment the inflammatory phenotype of septic shock.

Early Infection, the Innate Immune Response, Inflammation, and the Endothelium

Host defense is organized into innate and adaptive immune responses. The innate immune system responds by using pattern recognition receptors (e.g., toll-like receptors) to pathogen-associated molecular patterns, which are extremely well-conserved molecules of microorganisms. Surface molecules of gram-positive and gram-negative bacteria (peptidoglycan and lipopolysaccharide, respectively) bind to toll-like receptor-2 (TLR-2) and TLR-4, respectively (Fig. 109–1). TLR-2 and TLR-4 binding initiates an intracellular signaling cascade that culminates in nuclear transport of transcription factor nuclear factor kappa B (NFκB), which triggers transcription of cytokines such as TNF-α and interleukin-6 (IL-6). Cytokines upregulate adhesion molecules of neutrophils and endothelial cells, and neutrophil activation leads to bacterial killing. However, cytokines also directly injure host endothelial cells. Activated neutrophils, monocytes, and platelets also injure endothelial cells. Inhibition of early cytokine mediators of sepsis, such as TNF-α and IL-1β, has not proven successful likely, in part, because TNF-α and IL-1β peak and then decline quickly before these antagonist therapies were applied clinically.

The early cytokine inflammatory response is followed by release from immune cells, including macrophages and neutrophils, of later mediators such as high-mobility group box-1 (HMGB-1). HMGB-1 activates neutrophils, monocytes, and endothelium. Unlike TNF-α antagonists, inhibitors of HMGB-1 decrease mortality even when they are given 24 hours after induction of experimental peritonitis.

Adaptive Immunity Adds Specificity and Amplification of the Immune Response

Microorganisms stimulate specific humoral and cell-mediated adaptive immune responses that amplify innate immunity. B cells release immunoglobulins that bind to microorganisms and thereby facilitate delivery of microorganisms to natural killer cells and neutrophils. In sepsis, type 1 helper T (T_H1) cells generally secrete pro-inflammatory cytokines (TNF-α, IL-1β), and type 2 helper T (T_H2) cells secrete anti-inflammatory (IL-4, IL-10) cytokines.

Coagulation Response to Infection

Septic shock activates the coagulation system (Fig. 109–2) and ultimately converts fibrinogen to fibrin, which is bound to platelets to form microvascular thrombi. Microvascular thrombi further amplify endothelial injury by release of mediators and by tissue hypoxia because of obstruction to blood flow.

Normally, natural anticoagulants (protein C, protein S, antithrombin, and tissue factor pathway inhibitor) dampen coagulation, enhance fibrinolysis, and remove microthrombi. Thrombin-α binds to throm-

TABLE 109–1 PATHWAYS, MEDIATORS, AND POSITIVE, NEGATIVE, AND POTENTIALLY ATTRACTIVE TRIALS IN SEPTIC SHOCK

Pathways	Mediators	Positive RCTs*	Negative RCTs	Examples of Potential Therapies
Organism features	Superantigens: TSST-1			Anti-TSST1
	Streptococcal exotoxins (pyrogenic exotoxin A)			Anti-exotoxins
	Lipopolysaccharide (endotoxin)		Anti-lipopolysaccharide	
Innate immunity	TLR-2, TLR-4			TLR agonists; TLR antagonists
	Monocytes, macrophages			GM-CSF, interferon-γ
	Neutrophils			G-CSF†
Adaptive immunity	B cells, plasma cells, immunoglobulin			Immunoglobulin G
	T cells: CD4 T_H1, T_H2			
Pro-inflammatory pathway	TNF-α		Anti–TNF-α	
	IL-1β		IL-1 receptor antagonist	
	IL-6			IL-6 antagonist
	Prostaglandins, leukotrienes		Ibuprofen, high-dose corticosteroids	
	Bradykinin		Bradykinin antagonist	
	Platelet-activating factor		Platelet-activating factor Acetyl hydrolase	
	Proteases (e.g., elastase)		Elastase inhibitor‡	
	Oxidants			Antioxidants (e.g., *N*-acetylcysteine)
	Nitric oxide		Nitric oxide synthase inhibitor	
Pro-coagulant pathway	↓ Protein C	Activated protein C[1]		
	↓ Protein S			Protein S [3,4]
	↓ Antithrombin		Antithrombin	
	↓ Tissue factor pathway inhibitor		Tissue factor pathway inhibitor	
	↑ Tissue factor			Tissue factor antagonist
	↑ Plasminogen activator inhibitor (PAI-1)			Tissue plasminogen activator
Anti-inflammatory pathway	IL-10		IL-10§	
	TNF-α receptors		TNF-α receptors	
Tissue hypoxia	HIF-1α, VEGF	Early goal-directed therapy [1]	Supernormal oxygen delivery	Erythropoietin
Immunosuppression/apoptosis	Lymphocyte apoptosis			Anti-caspases
	Intestinal epithelial cell apoptosis			Anti-caspases
Endocrine dysfunction	Adrenal insufficiency			Corticosteroids‖
	Vasopressin deficiency			Vasopressin
	Hyperglycemia			Intensive insulin¶

*Positive RCTs means pivotal randomized controlled trials powered for mortality as the primary end point.
†G-CSF is effective in septic patients who have profound neutropenia.
‡Elastase inhibitor was ineffective in a phase II trial in acute lung injury.
§IL-10 was ineffective in a phase II trial in acute lung injury.
‖Corticosteroids had no effect on overall 28-day mortality but deceased mortality in a subgroup of nonresponders to corticotropin. [5]
¶Intensive insulin decreased mortality in critically ill surgical patients but has not yet been evaluated in sepsis or septic shock.
↑ = increased; ↓ = decreased; HIF-1α: hypoxia-inducing factor-1α; GM-CSF = granulocyte-macrophage colony-stimulating factor; G-CSF = granulocyte colony-stimulating factor; IL = interleukin; RCT = randomized controlled trial; T_H1 and T_H2 = T-helper cell 1 and 2, respectively; TNF-α: tumor necrosis factor-α; TLR = toll-like receptor; TSST-1 = toxic shock syndrome toxin-1; VEGF = vascular endothelial growth factor.

bomodulin, which activates protein C when protein C is bound to the endothelial protein C receptor (EPCR). Activated protein C dampens the pro-coagulant phenotype because it inactivates factors Va and VIIIa and inhibits synthesis of plasminogen activator inhibitor-1 (PAI-1). Activated protein C also decreases apoptosis, leukocyte activation and adhesion, and the production of cytokines.

Septic shock decreases the levels of the natural anticoagulants protein C, protein S, antithrombin, and tissue factor pathway inhibitor. Furthermore, lipopolysaccharide and TNF-α decrease thrombomodulin and EPCR, thereby limiting activation of protein C. Lipopolysaccharide and TNF-α also increase levels of PAI-1, thus inhibiting fibrinolysis.

Tissue Hypoxia in Septic Shock

Tissue hypoxia independently activates inflammation (by activation of NFκB and cytokines, by synthesis of nitric oxide, and by activation of HMGB-1), induces coagulation (through tissue factor and PAI-1), and activates neutrophils, monocytes, and platelets. Hypoxia induces hypoxia-inducing factor-1α (HIF-1α), which upregulates erythropoietin,

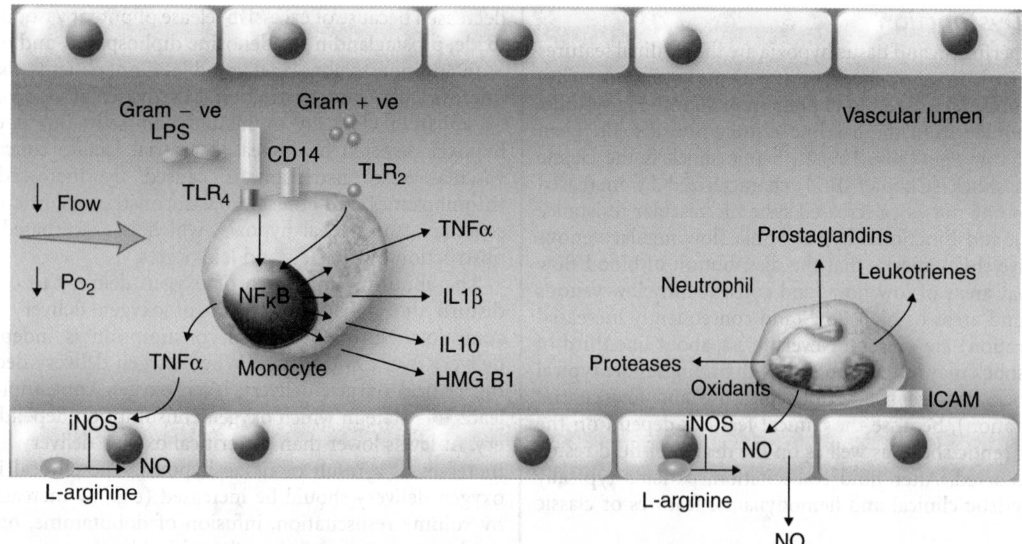

FIGURE 109–1 • Inflammatory responses to sepsis. Gram-positive and gram-negative bacteria, viruses, and fungi have unique cell wall molecules called pathogen-associated molecular patterns that bind to pattern recognition receptors (called toll-like receptors [TLRs]) on the surface of immune cells. Lipopolysaccharide (LPS) of gram-negative bacilli binds to LPS-binding protein, CD14 complex. Peptidoglycan of gram-positive bacteria and lipopolysaccharide of gram-negative bacteria bind to TLR-2 and TLR-4, respectively. TLR-2 and TLR-4 binding activates intracellular signal transduction pathways that lead to activation of the cytosolic transcription factor nuclear factor kappa B (NFκB). Activated NFκB moves from the cytoplasm to nucleus, binds to transcription start sites, and increases transcription of cytokines such as tumor necrosis factor-α (TNF-α), interleukin-1β (IL-1β) and interleukin-10 (IL-10). TNF-α and IL-1β are pro-inflammatory cytokines that activate the adaptive immune response but also cause both direct and indirect host injury. IL-10 is an anti-inflammatory cytokine that inactivates macrophages and has other anti-inflammatory effects. Sepsis increases activity of inducible nitric oxide synthase (iNOS), which increases synthesis of nitric oxide (NO), a potent vasodilator. Cytokines activate endothelial cells by upregulating adhesion receptors such as intercellular adhesion molecule (ICAM), and injure endothelial cells by activation and binding of neutrophils, monocytes, macrophages and platelets to endothelial cells. These effector cells release mediators such as proteases, oxidants, prostaglandins, and intercellular adhesion molecule (ICAM) leukotrienes. Cytokines also activate the coagulation cascade.

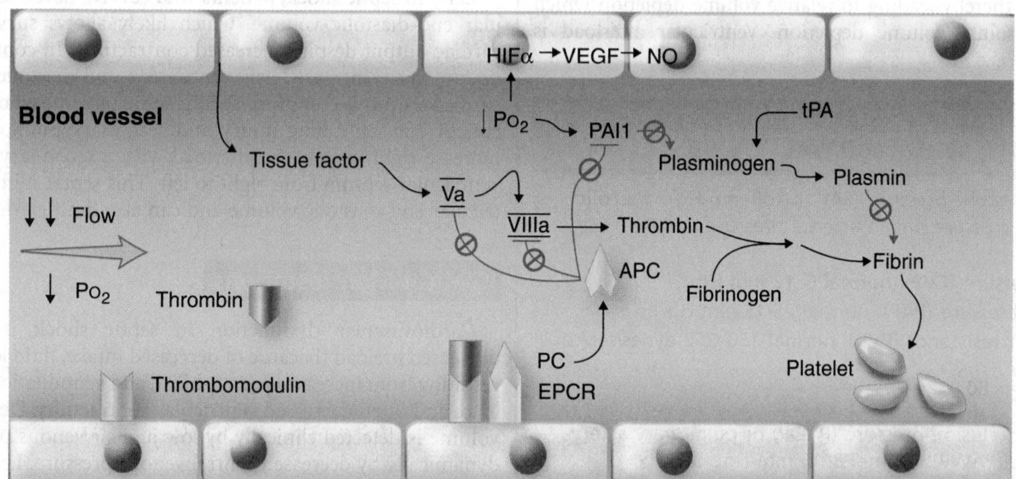

FIGURE 109–2 • Procoagulant response in sepsis. Sepsis activates coagulation by activating endothelium to increase tissue factor. Activation of factors Va and VIIIa leads to formation of thrombin-α, which converts fibrinogen to fibrin. Fibrin binds to platelets that adhere to endothelial cells forming microvascular thrombi. Microvascular thrombi amplify injury by release of mediators and by microvascular obstruction, which causes distal ischemia and tissue hypoxia. Normally, natural anticoagulants (protein C [PC], protein S [PS], antithrombin, and tissue factor pathway inhibitor [TFPI]) dampen coagulation, enhance fibrinolysis, and remove microthrombi. Thrombin-α binds to thrombomodulin on endothelial cells and thus activates binding of PC to endothelial PC receptor (EPCR). PC forms a complex with its cofactor PS. PC binding to EPCR increases activation of PC to activated PC (APC). APC proteolytically inactivates factors Va and VIIIa and decreases synthesis of plasminogen activator inhibitor-1 (PAI-1). Sepsis decreases levels of PC, PS, antithrombin, and TFPI. Lipopolysaccharide and tumor necrosis factor-α (TNF-α) decrease thrombomodulin and EPCR, thus decreasing activation of PC. Lipopolysaccharide and TNF-α also inhibit PAI-1, so fibrinolysis is inhibited.

and vascular endothelial growth factor (VEGF). Erythropoietin is protective to brain and other tissues. VEGF inhibits fibrinolysis and increases inducible nitric oxide synthase, which augments nitric oxide–induced vasodilation. Nitric oxide has a further injurious effect: excessive nitric oxide inhibits the beneficial actions of HIF-1α (e.g., upregulating synthesis of erythropoietin) during hypoxia.

Late Septic Shock, Immunosuppression, and Apoptosis of Immune and Epithelial Cells

Death after about 1 week of septic shock can be the result of immunosuppression, which is suggested by anergy, lymphopenia, hypothermia, and nosocomial infection. Multiple organ dysfunction could be an anti-inflammatory phenotype because of apoptosis of immune, epithelial, and endothelial cells. Activated CD4⁺ T cells evolve into either a T_H1 pro-inflammatory (TNF-α, IL-1β) or T_H2 anti-inflammatory (IL-4, IL-10) phenotype. Sepsis leads to migration from a T_H1 to T_H2 phenotype; for example, persistent elevation of IL-10 is associated with increased risk of death. Immunosuppression also develops because of apoptosis of lymphocytes. Pro-inflammatory cytokines, activated B and T cells, and glucocorticoids induce lymphocyte apoptosis, whereas TNF-α and endotoxin induce apoptosis of lung and intestinal epithelial cells.

Death from infectious disease appears to be highly heritable. Sepsis is a prime example of a polygenic disease related to the interaction of multiple genes with an environmental insult (infection). Studies of individual single nucleotide polymorphisms of cytokines (TNF-α, IL-6, and IL-10) and innate immunity genes (CD-14, TLR-2) have been variably associated with an increased risk of death from sepsis.

Cardiovascular Dysfunction

Inadequate tissue perfusion and tissue hypoxia are the cardinal features of all types of shock. Early in septic shock, most patients have sinus tachycardia and, by definition, decreased blood pressure (<90 mm Hg systolic, a decrease of ≥40 mm Hg from the baseline systolic pressure, or mean arterial pressure <65 mm Hg; Table 109–2). Septic shock is the classic form of distributive shock (Chapter 107), characterized by increased pulse pressure (bounding pulses), decreased systemic vascular resistance (warm flushed skin), and functional hypovolemia (low jugular venous pressure). Distributive shock means that the distribution of blood flow is abnormal such that areas of low flow (and consequently low venous oxygen saturation) and areas of high flow (and consequently increased venous oxygen saturation) are present. Nevertheless, about one third of patients with septic shock may initially present with findings more typical of hypovolemic shock (low central venous pressure and low central venous oxygen saturation), because the clinical features depend on the stage and severity of septic shock as well as on the degree of fluid resuscitation that has occurred. After fluid resuscitation, patients typically develop the characteristic clinical and hemodynamic features of classic distributive shock.

Ventricular preload is commonly decreased in early septic shock for several reasons. First, patients may be volume depleted because of decreased fluid intake and because of increased fluid losses as a result of fever, vomiting, and diarrhea if gastrointestinal disease is present. Second, fluid loss from the intravascular to the interstitial space (capillary leak) is caused by mediators that induce widespread endothelial injury, which increases capillary permeability. Increased capillary permeability leads to loss of protein-rich edema fluid into the interstitial space. In the lung, increased permeability is a key component of acute lung injury. A third reason that ventricular preload is decreased in septic shock is venodilation induced by mediators such as nitric oxide. Venodilation increases venous capacitance, thereby leading to relative volume depletion which compounds the absolute volume depletion. Ventricular afterload is decreased because of excessive release of potent vasodilators such as nitric oxide, prostaglandin I_2, adenosine diphosphate, and other vasodilators.

In addition to abnormal vasodilatation, patients also have concurrent microvascular vasoconstriction. Microvascular vasoconstriction may not be apparent clinically or hemodynamically, but it can lead to tissue hypoxia detected by increased arterial lactate concentrations. Microvascular vasoconstriction is caused by increased norepinephrine, thromboxanes, and other local vasoconstrictors. Microvascular vasoconstriction causes focal hypoxia, which is exacerbated by microvascular obstruction by platelets and leukocytes.

The abnormal mismatch of oxygen delivery to oxygen demand can disturb the global relationship of oxygen delivery with oxygen consumption. Normally, oxygen consumption is independent of oxygen delivery over a wide range. When oxygen delivery decreases to less than the critical oxygen delivery level, oxygen consumption decreases and leads to a state in which oxygen consumption depends on oxygen delivery. At levels lower than the critical oxygen delivery level, arterial lactate increases as a result of tissue hypoxia. The clinical implication is that oxygen delivery should be increased (e.g., by increasing cardiac output by volume resuscitation, infusion of dobutamine, or by transfusion of erythrocytes) to more than the critical level.

Cardiovascular function is further compromised in septic shock because of decreased ventricular contractility. Decreased ventricular contractility may be difficult to detect clinically and may be diagnosed only by hemodynamic or echocardiographic assessment. Numerous circulating mediators of sepsis including cytokines (e.g., IL-6, TNF-α) and nitric oxide (locally released into the coronary circulation) decrease contractility. Coronary ischemia resulting from microvascular obstruction by leukocytes and oxygen free radicals, which are released by neutrophils adherent to the coronary capillary endothelium, is another mechanism of decreased contractility.

Early in septic shock, patients who survive have increased left ventricular end-diastolic volume, which likely allows survivors to maintain cardiac output despite decreased contractility. In contrast, nonsurvivors do not have increased left ventricular end-diastolic volume, so their cardiac output is compromised. In some patients who have septic shock, concurrent acute lung injury and secondary pulmonary hypertension increase right ventricular afterload with a secondary shift of the interventricular septum from right to left. This septal shift decreases left ventricular end-diastolic volume and can also limit cardiac output.

TABLE 109–2 HEMODYNAMIC VARIABLES, ABBREVIATIONS, AND NORMAL VALUES

Arterial pressure: systolic pressure (SAP) (>100 mm Hg), diastolic pressure, pulse pressure, mean arterial pressure (MAP) (>65 mm Hg)
Central venous pressure (CVP): normal 6–12 mm Hg
Pulmonary artery pressure (PAP): normal 25/15 mm Hg
Pulmonary vascular resistance (PVR): normal 150–250 dynes/sec/cm $\left(\equiv \frac{PAP - PAOP}{CO} \times 80\right)$
Pulmonary artery occlusion pressure (PAOP) or pulmonary artery wedge pressure (PAWP): normal 8–15 mm Hg
Systemic vascular resistance (SVR): normal 900–1400 dynes/sec/cm $\left(\equiv \frac{MAP - CVP}{CO} \times 80\right)$
Cardiac output (CO): normal 5 L/min
Left ventricular stroke work (LVSW): normal xx = SV × (MAP – PAWP)
Oxygen delivery (Do_2): normal 1 L/min (= CO × [Hg × 1.38 × Sao_2] + [0.003 × Po_2])
Oxygen consumption (Vo_2): normal 250 mL/min (= CO × Hg × 1.38 × [Sao_2 – Svo_2] + [0.003 × (Pao_2 – Pvo_2)])
Oxygen extraction ratio: normal 0.23–0.32 (= Vo_2/Do_2)
Hemodynamic variables are often normalized to account for different body mass by dividing by body surface area (BSA):
Pulmonary vascular resistance index (PVRI): normal (= PVR/BSA)
Systemic vascular resistance index (SVRI): normal (= SVR/BSA)
Cardiac index (CI): normal 2.5–4.2 L/min/m^2 (= CO/BSA)
Left ventricular stroke work index (LVSWI): normal (= LVSW/BSA)
Oxygen delivery index (Do_2I): normal 460–650 mL/min/m^2 (= Do_2/BSA)
Oxygen consumption index (Vo_2I): normal 95–170 mL/min/m^2 (= Vo_2/BSA)

Clinical Manifestations

Cardiovascular dysfunction in septic shock is characterized by decreased preload (because of decreased intake, fluid losses, third spacing resulting from increased permeability, and venodilation), decreased afterload, and often decreased ventricular contractility. Decreased ventricular volume is detected clinically by low jugular venous pressure and hemodynamically by decreased central venous pressure. Left ventricular resistance, or afterload, is also commonly decreased and is detected clinically by warm, flushed skin and hemodynamically by decreased systemic vascular resistance.

Diagnosis

Even as the diagnostic evaluation is beginning, the initial assessment of a critically ill patient must focus immediately on the airway (need for intubation), breathing (respiratory rate, respiratory distress, pulse oximetry), circulation (heart rate, blood pressure, jugular venous pressure, skin perfusion), and rapid initiation of resuscitation (Fig. 109–3). Vital signs and the leukocyte count will establish quickly whether the patient has SIRS (two of four criteria required to establish the presence of SIRS). Arterial blood gases and lactate levels are useful immediate complementary tests. A secondary survey is designed to determine the likely source of infection and the status of organ function. Pneumonia (Chapter 97) is suggested by cough, sputum, and respiratory distress; empyema (Chapter 100) is suggested by pleuritic chest pain. Signs of peritonitis, an abdominal mass, and right upper quadrant tenderness suggest abdominal sepsis. Pyelonephritis (Chapter 307) is likely in patients with dysuria and costovertebral angle tenderness. Integumentary assessment for erythema (cellulitis), line site erythema (line sepsis), tenderness (necrotizing fasciitis), crepitus (anaerobic myonecrosis), and petechiae

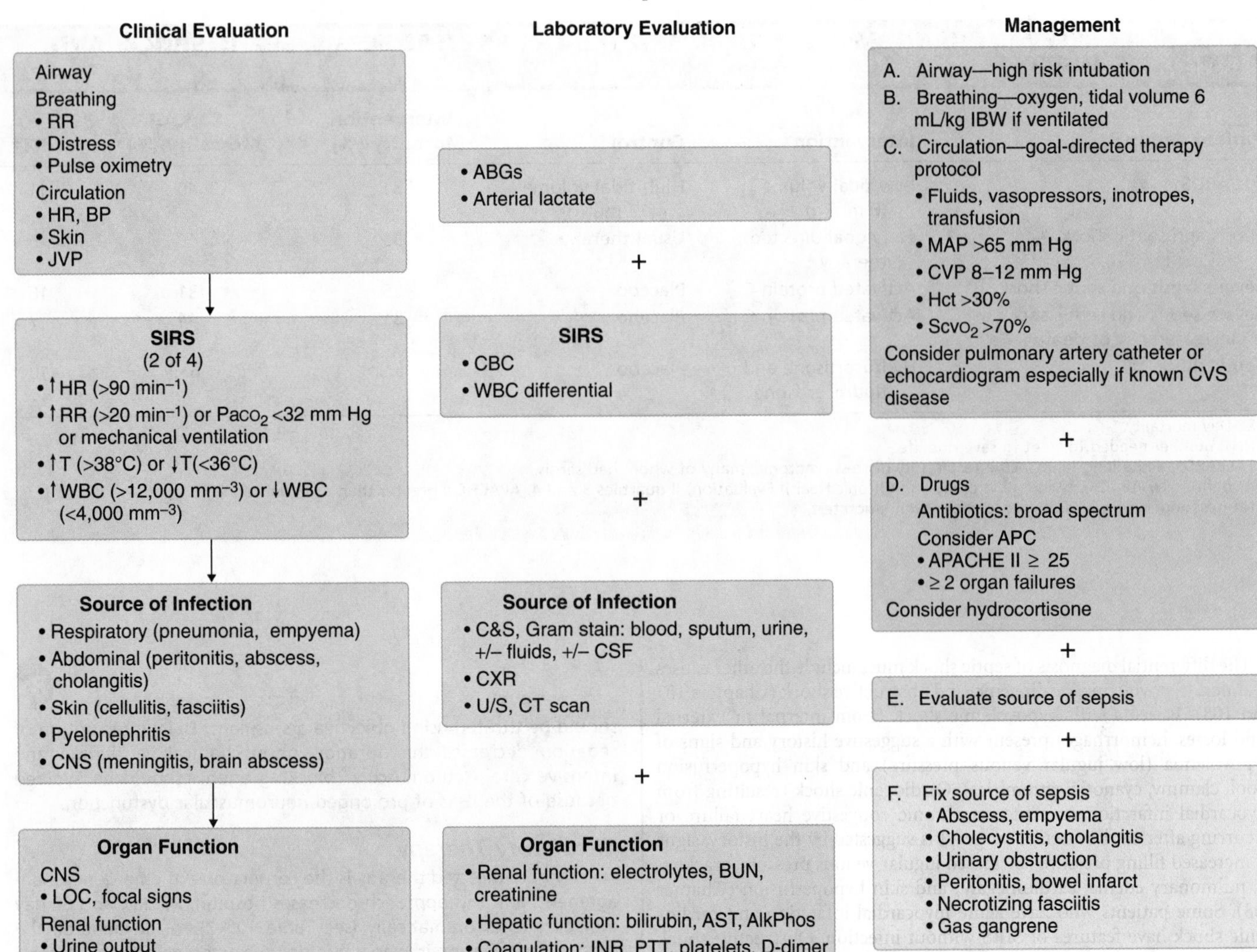

FIGURE 109–3 • Algorithm for clinical and laboratory evaluation and management approach to septic shock. ABG = arterial blood gases; Alk Phos = alkaline phosphatase; APC = activated protein C; AST = aspartate aminotransferase; BP = blood pressure; BUN = blood urea nitrogen; C&S = culture and sensitivity; CBC = complete blood count; CNS = central nervous system; CT = computed tomography; CVP = central venous pressure; CXR = chest radiograph; HCT = hematocrit; IBW = ideal body weight; INR = international normalized ratio; LOC = level of consciousness; MAP = mean arterial pressure; $Paco_2$ = partial pressure of carbon dioxide; PTT = partial thromboplastin time; RR = respiratory rate; $Scvo_2$ = central venous oxygen saturation; SIRS = systemic inflammatory response syndrome; U/S = ultrasound; WBC = white blood cell count.

(meningococcemia) can be illuminating. Headache, neck stiffness, and signs of meningismus raise suspicion of meningitis (Chapter 437). Focal neurologic signs suggest brain abscess (Chapter 438).

Laboratory investigations that are helpful to identify the source of infection include appropriate cultures and Gram stains (blood, sputum, urine, fluids, and cerebrospinal fluid). Blood cultures are positive in 40 to 60% of patients who have septic shock. The chest radiograph will aid in the diagnosis of pneumonia, empyema, and acute lung injury. Abdominal ultrasound and CT scanning are indicated if abdominal sepsis is suspected.

Hemodynamic assessment of the patient includes insertion of a central venous or pulmonary artery catheter. In early septic shock, central venous pressure is usually low and usually increases in response to volume resuscitation. Central venous oxygen saturation, cardiac output, and ventricular filling pressures may be determined continuously. Pulmonary artery pressure is usually normal but may be increased because septic shock can cause pulmonary hypertension. Pulmonary artery occlusion (or wedge) pressure is usually low before resuscitation, but it may be normal or increased if the patient has underlying preexisting heart disease (e.g., heart failure or coronary artery disease with prior myocardial infarction) or if left ventricular contractility is decreased by sepsis. Cardiac output may be low or normal before fluid resuscitation and typically increases to higher than normal after fluid resuscitation. If fluid resuscitation increases central venous pressure and pulmonary artery occlusion pressure but cardiac output does not increase, left ventricular dysfunction presumably is present.

Echocardiographic features of decreased ventricular contractility include decreased right and left ventricular ejection fraction and increased end-diastolic and end-systolic volumes. Early in septic shock, the left ventricular ejection fraction is decreased, and it remains low in nonsurvivors. In survivors, left ventricular ejection fraction returns to normal over 5 to 10 days.

Renal, hepatic, and coagulation function tests are helpful to evaluate organ function. After determining the source of sepsis, it is crucial to address that source by drainage of abscesses and empyemas, by radiologic or surgical correction of urinary tract obstruction, and by surgical management of peritonitis, bowel infarction, cholecystitis, cholangitis, necrotizing fasciitis, and gas gangrene.

Differential Diagnosis

The major differential diagnoses of classic septic shock are other nonseptic causes of SIRS, such as acute pancreatitis (Chapter 147), acute respiratory distress syndrome (Chapter 105), aspiration pneumonitis (Chapter 94), multiple trauma (Chapter 113), and recent major surgery without infection (Chapter 459). Other causes of distributive shock are anaphylactic shock (suggested by angioedema and hives; Chapter 466), spinal shock (recent trauma and paraplegia; Chapter 422), acute adrenal insufficiency ("tanned skin," hyperkalemia, metabolic alkalosis; Chapter 245), and acute or acute on chronic hepatic failure (jaundice, ascites, encephalopathy; Chapters 158 and 159).

TABLE 109–3 RELEVANT RANDOMIZED CONTROLLED TRIALS IN SEVERE SEPSIS, SEPTIC SHOCK, AND ACUTE LUNG INJURY

Patient Group	Intervention	Control	Intervention Mortality (%)*	Control Mortality (%)*	NNT†
ALI/ARDS†† [2]	Low tidal volume (6 mL/kg)	High tidal volume (12 mL/kg)	31	40	11
Sepsis and septic shock [1]	Early goal-directed therapy	Usual therapy	33	49	6
Severe sepsis and septic shock [3]	Activated protein C	Placebo	25	31	16
Severe sepsis and septic shock at increased risk of death§ [3]	Activated protein C	Placebo	31	44	7.7
Septic shock [8]	Hydrocortisone and fludrocortisone	Placebo	53¶	63¶	10

*28-Day mortality.
†NNT: number needed to treat to save one life.
††ALI/ARDS: acute lung injury/acute respiratory distress syndrome, many of whom had sepsis.
§As defined by APACHE (Acute Physiology and Chronic Health Evaluation) II quartiles 3 and 4, APACHE II greater than or equal to 25.
¶Nonresponders to a 250-µg corticotropin stimulation test.

The differential diagnosis of septic shock must include the other causes of shock: hypovolemic, cardiogenic, and obstructive shock (Chapters 107 and 108). Patients with hypovolemic shock (from internal or external fluid losses, hemorrhage) present with a suggestive history and signs of hypovolemia (low jugular venous pressure) and skin hypoperfusion (cool, clammy, cyanotic extremities). Cardiogenic shock (resulting from myocardial infarction or acute on chronic congestive heart failure or occurring after cardiovascular surgery) is suggested by the history, signs of increased filling pressure (increased jugular venous pressure, crackles, S_3, pulmonary edema, cardiomegaly) and skin hypoperfusion (Chapter 108). Some patients who have acute myocardial infarction and cardiogenic shock have features of SIRS without infection. Obstructive shock (from pulmonary thromboembolism, cardiac tamponade, pneumothorax) manifests similarly to cardiogenic shock.

Prevention

Measures to prevent sepsis include hand washing, elevation of the head of the bed, scrupulous sterile techniques for insertion of catheters, and possibly, use of antibiotic-impregnated catheters. New catheter insertion sites for catheter changes, isolation of patients who have resistant organisms, and isolation of patients who are significantly immunocompromised may also prevent infection.

Prevention of progression from sepsis to septic shock requires early diagnosis and aggressive resuscitation of severe sepsis before progression to overt hypotension. Early goal-directed therapy, [1] lung protective ventilation, [2] antibiotics, and consideration of activated protein C [3, 4] are critical therapies in early septic shock (Table 109–3).

Treatment

Rx

Respiratory Therapy

All patients in septic shock require oxygen initially, and many will require mechanical ventilation. Mechanical ventilation is required in most patients who have septic shock because acute lung injury is the most common complication. Lung protective ventilation (mechanical ventilation that minimizes lung injury by using relatively low tidal volume, i.e., ~6 mL/kg of predicted body weight) decreases mortality of acute lung injury and acute respiratory distress syndrome (Chapter 106). [2]

Patients who require ventilation need adequate but not excessive sedation, which can worsen hemodynamic instability, prolong ventilation, and increase the risks of nosocomial pneumonia. Sedation should be titrated using objective assessment. Daily interruption of sedation decreases the duration of mechanical ventilation and intensive care. Neuromuscular blocking agents should be avoided because of the risks of prolonged neuromuscular dysfunction.

Circulatory Therapy

Early goal-directed therapy is the cornerstone of emergency management, and this approach decreases hospital, 28-day, and 60-day mortality rates dramatically (see Table 109–3). [1] In general, the goal of resuscitation is to increase tissue oxygen delivery by increasing profoundly low blood pressure, by increasing inadequate blood flow, by increasing low arterial oxygen saturation, and by increasing mixed venous oxygen saturation. Although oxygen delivery is higher in survivors than in nonsurvivors, it is not clear that a specific oxygen delivery target is more beneficial than clinical end points. Several trials have shown that supernormal global oxygen delivery does not decrease mortality of sepsis and septic shock. Goal-directed therapy requires continuous monitoring of central venous oxygen saturation, with resuscitation directed to increase and then maintain central venous oxygen saturation greater than 70%.

In patients who have acute lung injury, no difference in outcomes is seen when comparing management using a pulmonary artery catheter versus a central venous catheter; this finding suggest that no advantage exists to using a pulmonary catheter to guide hemodynamic management of acute lung injury. [5] Patients whose acute lung injury is managed after 24 to 48 hours with a conservative fluid strategy (as compared with a liberal fluid strategy) have significantly improved lung function and shorter duration of ventilation and intensive care unit stay. [6]

Fluids should be used to maintain a central venous pressure 8 to 12 mm Hg; at present, no convincing data indicate that albumin is better than normal saline solution. Vasopressors (e.g., norepinephrine, 1 to 50 µg/minute; epinephrine, 1 to 30 µg/minute) should be added if the mean arterial pressure is less than 65 mm Hg. If central venous oxygen saturation is less than 70%, packed red cell transfusions should be used to maintain a hematocrit greater than 30%. Dobutamine (2.5 to 20 µg/kg/minute) is required if central venous pressure, mean arterial pressure, and hematocrit are optimized yet the central venous oxygen saturation remains less than 70%.

In general, patients require fluid resuscitation to achieve a central venous pressure of 8 to 12 mm Hg. If hypotension persists despite adequate fluid resuscitation, then vasopressors such as norepinephrine (1 to 50 µg/minute) are added. If the cardiac index is low or if the mixed venous oxygen saturation is low (<70 %) despite an adequate central venous pressure, then an inotropic agent such as dobutamine should be added, initially at approximately 2 to 5 μg/kg/minute and increasing until the mixed venous oxygen saturation is adequate. In some patients in septic shock, the cardiac index is inadequate, as reflected by a low mixed venous oxygen saturation despite a high central venous pressure (>12 mm Hg) and/or pulmonary artery wedge pressure (>18 mm Hg) because of underlying cardiovascular dysfunction or because of acute left ventricular dysfunction resulting from sepsis. In such patients, earlier use of an inotropic agent such as dobutamine should be considered to increase left ventricular contractility. The overall goal is to achieve an adequate mean arterial pressure (>65 mm Hg), central venous pressure, and mixed venous oxygen saturation while other indices of adequate perfusion are monitored such as hourly urine output (>0.5 mL/kg/hour), arterial lactate levels (<2 mmol/L), mental status, and skin perfusion.

Transfusion of Erythrocytes and Erythropoietin

Anemia is common in septic shock, but the optimal hemoglobin level for resuscitation in septic shock is controversial. Goal-directed therapy aims for a hematocrit of 30%, whereas a randomized trial of transfusion in critically ill patients found that a hemoglobin range of 7 to 9 g/dL was equivalent to or better than a higher hemoglobin (10 to 12 g/dL), except possibly in patients with acute myocardial infarction or unstable angina. [7] A reasonable approach is to use a hematocrit level of 30% as a threshold to erythrocyte transfusion for the first 6 hours and then to lower the threshold to a hemoglobin of 7 to 9 g/dL for the rest of the hospital course, except in patients with underlying cardiac disease. Recombinant erythropoietin decreases the need for transfusion in critically ill patients, but it does not decrease mortality.

Drugs

Antibiotics

The infected site and infecting organisms of septic shock are often not known initially. After appropriate cultures are obtained, intravenous broad-spectrum antibiotics should be administered on an emergency basis while considering host factors such as immune and allergic status (Chapters 302 and 303; see Fig. 109-3). Outcomes in patients with septic shock are worse if the organisms that caused sepsis are not sensitive to the initial antibiotic regimen.

Emergency, empirical antibiotic therapy (Table 109–4) should be guided by the greater frequency of gram-positive bacteria, the possibility of resistant organisms, and local bacteriologic features. If a causative organism is identified (~20% of septic patients have negative cultures), then the antibiotic regimen should be narrowed to decrease the emergence of resistant organisms. The duration of antibiotics should be guided by the cause of septic shock, but patients generally require 10 to 14 days of therapy.

Corticosteroids

High-dose corticosteroids do not improve outcomes in the full spectrum of patients with sepsis or acute respiratory distress syndrome, but these drugs may increase survival in septic patients who have an increase in their serum cortisol levels to 9 μg/dL or less after a 250-μg corticotropin stimulation test. [8] In addition, hydrocortisone may decrease the duration of required vasopressor support in septic shock. The recommended treatment is hydrocortisone (50 mg intravenously every 6 hours) plus fludrocortisone (50 μg tablet per nasogastric tube or orally daily) for 7 days. Corticosteroids administered before antibiotics also decrease neurologic sequelae of bacterial, especially pneumococcal, meningitis (Chapter 437). Enthusiasm for corticosteroid therapy must be tempered by knowledge of complications such as neuromyopathy, hyperglycemia, immune suppression, and impaired wound healing.

Recombinant Human Activated Protein C

Activated protein C infusion (24 μg/kg/hour for 96 hours) decreases mortality, improves organ dysfunction, and decreases biomarkers of inflammation and coagulation in severe sepsis and septic shock. [3] Activated protein C is approved for patients who have severe sepsis and a high risk of death, as defined by an APACHE (Acute Physiology and Chronic Health Evaluation) II score of 25 or higher and/or two or more dysfunctional organs (see Fig. 109–3). By comparison, activated protein C is not beneficial in low-risk patients. [4] Activated protein C also has not been tested in patients with major trauma, recent surgery (within 12 hours), active hemorrhage, coagulopathy, thrombocytopenia, or recent stroke because of the increased risk of hemorrhage. Even in patients without these risk factors, treatment increases serious hemorrhage nearly twofold, and about 0.5% of treated patients develop intracranial hemorrhage. Activated protein C should not be used in surgical patients who have severe sepsis with single organ dysfunction.

Controversial Therapies in Septic Shock

Vasopressin Deficiency and Use of Vasopressin

Vasopressin deficiency and downregulation of vasopressin receptors are common in septic shock. Vasopressin selectively dilates renal afferent but not efferent glomerular arterioles, as well as pulmonary, cerebral, and coronary arterioles. Low-dose vasopressin infusion (0.03 to 0.04 U/minute) increases blood pressure, urine output, and creatinine clearance while dramatically decreasing the doses of norepinephrine required to maintain blood pressure in patients with septic shock. Complications of vasopressin include gastrointestinal ischemia, decreased cardiac output, skin or digital necrosis, and cardiac arrest (especially at doses >0.04 units/minute). Virtually all studies of vasopressin in septic shock have been small, used acute (hours) infusions, and did not evaluate efficacy or safety of prolonged (days) infusion of vasopressin. Inducing nitric oxide synthase inhibition with N^{w}-methyl-L-arginine hydrochloride also can decrease the use of vasopressors, but this approach also significantly increases mortality in septic shock.

Hyperglycemia and Intensive Insulin Therapy

Hyperglycemia and insulin resistance are common in septic shock. Hyperglycemia is pro-coagulant and pro-apoptotic, it impairs neutrophil function, it increases the risk of infection, it impairs wound healing, and it is associated with increased mortality. However, the risks of unrecognized hypoglycemia and cerebral injury may be increased in septic shock because of the instability of endocrine function and the use of sedation. In addition, brain ischemia and hypoxia increase sensitivity to even transient hypoglycemia. At present, the appropriate glucose range and insulin doses are unknown, and intensive insulin therapy to control hyperglycemia is not of benefit in patients in medical intensive care units. [9]

Renal Dysfunction and Dialysis

Acute renal failure is an important complication of septic shock because of its associated morbidity, mortality, and resource utilization (Fig. 109–4). Continuous renal replacement therapy induces less hemodynamic instability compared with intermittent hemodialysis, but no conclusive evidence indicates that continuous renal replacement therapy or more intensive dialysis changes the mortality of acute renal failure.

Low-dose dopamine (2 to 4 μg/kg/minute) does not decrease the need for renal support, does not improve outcomes, and is not recommended. Lactic acidosis is a common complication of septic shock, but administration of sodium bicarbonate in the setting of lactic acidosis does not improve hemodynamics or the response to vasopressors.

Other Therapies

Deep venous thrombosis prophylaxis using low-dose heparin, which may be administered in combination with activated protein C, is recommended for patients who do not have active bleeding, coagulopathy, or a contraindication to heparin (see Fig. 109-4). Stress ulcer prophylaxis using H_2-receptor antagonists decreases the risk of gastrointestinal hemorrhage. Proton pump inhibitors may also be effective, but they have not been as fully evaluated in septic shock.

TABLE 109–4 ANTIBIOTICS FOR PATIENTS WHO HAVE SEPTIC SHOCK*

Source of Sepsis	Initial Antibiotic Regimen	Alternative Antibiotic Regimen
Community-acquired pneumonia	Third-generation cephalosporin: cefotaxime 2 g IV q6h; ceftriaxone 2 g IV q12h; ceftizoxime 2 g IV q8h) PLUS Fluoroquinolone (e.g., ciprofloxacin 400 mg IV q12h; levofloxacin 750 mg IV q24h; moxifloxacin 400 mg IV q24h) OR Macrolide (e.g., azithromycin 500 mg IV q24h)	Piperacillin-tazobactam (3.375 g IV q6h) PLUS Fluoroquinolone OR Macrolide
Hospital-acquired pneumonia	Imipenem (0.5 g IV q6h) OR Meropenem (1 g IV q8h)	Fluoroquinolone (ciprofloxacin 400 mg IV q12h) PLUS Vancomycin (1.5 g IV q12h) OR Piperacillin/tazobactam (3.375 g IV q6h) PLUS Tobramycin (1.5 mg/kg q8h) PLUS Vancomycin
Abdominal (mixed aerobic/anaerobic)	Piperacillin/tazobactam (3.375 g IV q6h) OR Imipenem (0.5 g IV q6h) (or meropenem 1 g IV q8h)	Ampicillin (2 g IV q4h) PLUS Metronidazole (500 mg IV q8h) PLUS Fluoroquinolone (ciprofloxacin 400 mg IV q12h)
Urinary tract	Fluoroquinolone (ciprofloxacin 400 mg IV q12h)	Ampicillin (2 g IV q4h) PLUS Gentamicin (1.5 mg/kg IV q8h) OR Third-generation cephalosporin (cefotaxime 2 g IV q6h; OR ceftriaxone 2 g IV q12h; OR ceftizoxime 2 g IV q8h)
Necrotizing fasciitis	Imipenem (0.5 g IV q6h)	Penicillin G (if confirmed group A streptococci)
Primary bacteremia (normal host)	Piperacillin/tazobactam (3.375 g IV q6h) PLUS Vancomycin (1.5 g IV q12h)	Imipenem (0.5 g IV q6h) PLUS Vancomycin (1.5 g IV q12h)
Primary bacteremia (intravenous drug user)	Vancomycin (1.5 g IV q12h) PLUS Fluoroquinolone (e.g., ciprofloxacin 400 mg IV q12h)	Piperacillin/tazobactam (3.375 g IV q6h) PLUS Vancomycin (1.5 g IV q12h)
Febrile neutropenia	Cefepime (2 g IV q8h) PLUS Vancomycin (1.5 g IV q12h)	Piperacillin/tazobactam (3.375 g IV q6h) PLUS Gentamicin (1.5 mg/kg q8h) OR Imipenem (0.5 g IV q6h) PLUS Gentamicin (1.5 mg/kg q8h)
Bacterial meningitis	Ceftriaxone (2 g IV q12h) PLUS Ampicillin (3 g IV q6h) PLUS Vancomycin (1.5 g IV q12h) PLUS Dexamethasone (0.15 mg/kg IV q6h for 2–4 days)	Gram-positive cocci: Vancomycin PLUS Ceftriaxone (2 g IV q12h) Gram-negative diplococci: Cefotaxime (2 g IV q4–6h) Gram-positive bacilli: Ampicillin (3 g IV q6h) PLUS Gentamicin Gram-negative bacilli: Ceftazidime (2 g IV q8h) PLUS Gentamicin (1.5 mg/kg IV q8h) All above PLUS Dexamethasone
Cellulitis	Ciprofloxacin (400 mg IV q12h) PLUS Clindamycin (900 mg IV q8h)	Imipenem (0.5 g IV q6h)

*Most antibiotic doses must be adjusted if there is hepatic or renal dysfunction. Some antibiotics require adjustment based on levels (e.g., gentamicin). In drug selection, consider carefully the patient's history of antibiotic (especially penicillin) allergy.
IV = intravenously.

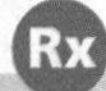

Enteral nutrition is generally safer and more effective than total parenteral nutrition, but total parenteral nutrition is sometimes required in patients who have had abdominal sepsis, surgery, or trauma. The use of sedation, neuromuscular blocking agents, and corticosteroids should be minimized because they can exacerbate septic encephalopathy and the polyneuropathy/myopathy of sepsis. Neutropenic patients may benefit from granulocyte colony-stimulating factor (Chapter 173). The risk of nosocomial infection is decreased by narrow spectrum antibiotics, early weaning from ventilation, and periodic removal and replacement of catheters (Chapter 304).

Prognosis

The 28-day mortality rate of septic shock is 40 to 70%. Early deaths (in the first 72 hours) are usually the result of refractory, progressive shock despite escalating life support. Later deaths from septic shock (after day 3) are usually secondary to multiple organ dysfunction. The number of dysfunctional organs and the progression or lack of improvement of organ dysfunction are indicators of increased risk of death. Other factors that portend a poor prognosis are increased age, underlying medical condition, high APACHE II score, increased arterial lactate concentrations, and lack of response to vasopressors. Furthermore, recent evidence indicates that delay in achieving the goals of early goal-directed therapy is associated with increased mortality. Survivors of sepsis who also had acute lung injury (Chapter 105) can have weakness, fatigue, and dyspnea on exertion after hospital discharge owing to pulmonary dysfunction, neuromuscular dysfunction, or other persistent organ dysfunction.

B. Breathing—Oxygen, with a tidal volume 6 mL/kg IBW if ventilated. Wean according to ARDSnet protocol (Chapters 105 and 106)

C. Circulation
- Fluids, vasopressors, inotropes, transfusion; goals include:
  - MAP > 65 mm Hg
  - CVP 8–12 mm Hg
  - Hg 70–90 G/L
  - $Scvo_2$ > 70%

Consider pulmonary artery catheter or echocardiogram especially if known cardiovascular disease; goals include:
- Wedge pressure 8–15 mm Hg
  - Cardiac index: normal or increased

D. Drugs:
- Antibiotics: Narrow spectrum to cause of infection
- APC (if indicated): 24 μg/kg/hour infusion for 96 hours
- Hydrocortisone (if evidence of relative adrenal insufficiency (see text)): hydrocortisone 50 mg intravenous every 6 hours and fluorocortisone 50 μg tab orally or per NG tube daily for 7 days

Other Organ Support
- Renal function: Continuous renal replacement
- DVT Prophylaxis: Low dose heparin 5000 IU subcutaneous every 12 hours
- Stress Ulcer Prophylaxis: H2 receptor antagonist (e.g., ranitidine 50 mg intravenous every 8 hours)
- Nutrition: Enteral preferred
- Sedation: Intermittent with daily awakening

FIGURE 109–4 • Ongoing critical care support and management in septic shock.

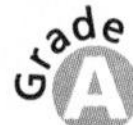

1. Rivers E, Nguyen B, Havstad S, et al: Early goal-directed therapy in the treatment of severe sepsis and septic shock. N Engl J Med 2001;345:1368–1377.
2. Acute Respiratory Distress Syndrome Network: Ventilation with lower tidal volumes as compared with traditional tidal volumes for acute lung injury and the acute respiratory distress syndrome. N Engl J Med 2000;342:1301–1308.
3. Bernard GR, Vincent JL, Laterre PF, et al: Efficacy and safety of recombinant human activated protein C for severe sepsis. N Engl J Med 2001;344:699–709.
4. Abraham E, Laterre PF, Garg R, et al: Drotrecogin alfa (activated) for adults with severe sepsis and a low risk of death. N Engl J Med 2005;353:1332–1341.
5. Wheeler AP, Bernard GR, Thompson BT, et al: National Heart, Lung, and Blood Institute Acute Respiratory Distress Syndrome (ARDS) Clinical Trials Network: Pulmonary-artery versus central venous catheter to guide treatment of acute lung injury. N Engl J Med 2006;354:2213–2224.
6. Wiedemann HP, Wheeler AP, Bernard GR, et al: Comparison of two fluid management strategies in acute lung injury. N Engl J Med 2006;354:2564–2575.
7. Hebert PC, Wells G, Blajchman MA, et al: A multicenter, randomized, controlled clinical trial of transfusion requirements in critical care. N Engl J Med 1999;340:409–417.
8. Annane D, Sebille V, Charpentier C, et al: Effect of treatment with low doses of hydrocortisone and fludrocortisone on mortality in patients with septic shock. JAMA 2002;288:862–871.
9. van den Berghe G, Wilmer A, Hermans G, et al: Intensive insulin in the medical ICU. N Engl J Med 2006:354:449–461.

SUGGESTED READINGS

Hamrahian AH, Oseni TS, Arafah BM: Measurements of serum free cortisol in critically ill patients. N Engl J Med 2004;350:1629–1638. *Demonstrates the complexity in interpreting total cortisol (measured clinically) because of marked changes in serum free cortisol in the critically ill.*

Hotchkiss RS, Karl IE: The pathophysiology and treatment of sepsis. N Engl J Med 2003;348:138–150. *A thorough review.*

Lauzier F, Levy B, Lamarre P, Lesur O: Vasopressin or norepinephrine in early hyperdynamic septic shock: A randomized clinical trial. Intensive Care Med 2006;32:1782–1789. *Vasopressin use improved hemodynamics and decreased norepinephrine requirements, but, as in other trials, mortality was not reduced.*

Martin GS, Mannino DM, Eaton S, et al: The epidemiology of sepsis in the United States from 1979 through 2000. N Engl J Med 2003;348:1546–1554. *Shows rising incidence of sepsis in the U.S.*

Russell JA: Management of sepsis. N Engl J Med 2006;355:1699–1713. *Sepsis requires early, goal-directed therapy; lung-protective ventilation; antibiotics; and possibly activated protein C.*

Schrier RW, Wang W: Acute renal failure and sepsis. N Engl J Med 2004; 351:159–169. *A comprehensive review.*

110 DISORDERS DUE TO HEAT AND COLD

William Winkenwerder and Michael N. Sawka

TEMPERATURE REGULATION

Body temperature is regulated through two parallel processes that modify body heat balance: behavioral (clothing, shelter, physical activity) and physiologic (skin blood flow, sweating, shivering). Both peripheral (skin) and central (core) thermal receptors provide afferent input to a central nervous system integrator (hypothalamic thermoregulatory center), and any deviation between the controlled variable (body temperature) and a reference variable ("set point" temperature) results in a heat loss or conservation response (Fig. 110–1).

Humans normally regulate body (core) temperature at about 37° C (98.6° F), and fluctuations within the narrow range of 35° C (95° F) to 41° C (105.8° F) can be tolerated by healthy acclimatized persons; core temperatures outside this range can induce morbidity and mortality. There is no single core temperature because temperature varies at different deep body sites, and these relationships vary during rest and physical exercise. Arterial blood temperature provides the "best" invasive measurement of core temperature. The most accurate noninvasive index of core temperature is esophageal temperature, followed in preference by rectal, gastrointestinal tract (telemetry pill), and oral temperature. Ear (tympanic and auditory meatus) temperature should not be relied on for clinical judgment.

HEAT ILLNESS

Definitions

Heat-related illnesses are named relative to severity. Minor heat-related illnesses include miliaria rubra, heat syncope, and heat cramps. Serious heat illness represents a continuum from heat exhaustion to heat injury and stroke.

Epidemiology

Body temperature can increase from exposure to environmental heat (impeded heat dissipation), physical exercise (increased heat production), and fever (elevated set point). Febrile persons have accentuated elevations in core temperature when exposed to high ambient temperature or physical exercise, or both. Serious heat illness is associated with a variety of individual factors, health conditions, medications, and environmental factors (Table 110–1). *Anticholinergic and sympathomimetic poisoning* (Chapter 111) can induce hyperthermia. *Malignant hyperthermia* (Chapter 447) is caused by rapid and massive skeletal muscle contraction from exposure to anesthesia. *Neuroleptic malignant syndrome* is hyperthermia caused by skeletal muscle rigidity from treatment with neuroleptic medications (e.g., antipsychotics, antidepressants, antiemetics).

However, heat illness can also occur even in low-risk individuals who have taken appropriate precautions for situations to which they have been exposed before. Historically, such unexpected cases were attributed to dehydration (which impairs thermoregulation and increases hyperthermia and cardiovascular strain), but it is now suspected that a previous heat exposure or event (e.g., sickness or injury) might make victims more susceptible to serious heat illness. One theory is that previous heat injury or illness might prime the acute phase response and augment the hyperthermia of exercise, thus inducing unexpected serious heat

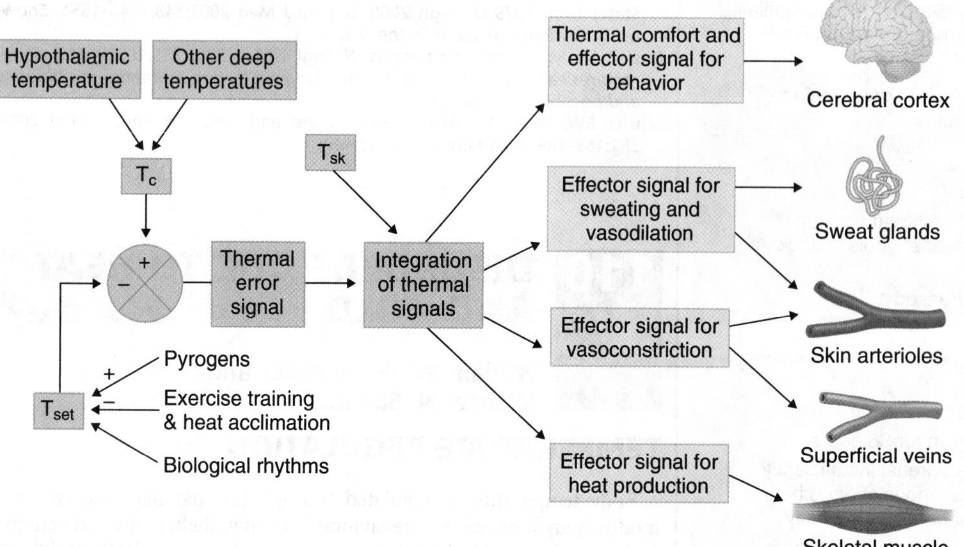

FIGURE 110–1 • Control of human thermoregulation. (From Sawka MN, Young AJ: Physiological systems and their responses to conditions of heat and cold. *In* Tipton CM, Sawka MN, Tate CA, Terjung RL [eds]: ACSM's Advanced Exercise Physiology. Baltimore, Lippincott Williams & Wilkins, 2005, pp 535–563.)

illness. Another theory is that previous infection might produce pro-inflammatory cytokines that deactivate the ability of cells to protect against heat shock.

Pathobiology

Environmental and exercise heat stress challenge the cardiovascular system to provide high blood flow to the skin, where blood pools in warm compliant vessels, such as found in the extremities. When blood flow is diverted to the skin, reduced perfusion of the intestines and other viscera can result in ischemia, endotoxemia, and oxidative stress. In addition, excessively high tissue temperatures (heat shock >41° C, 105.8° F) can produce direct tissue injury; the magnitude and duration of the heat shock influence whether cells respond by adaptation (acquired thermal tolerance), injury, or death (apoptotic or necrotic). Heat shock, ischemia, and systemic inflammatory responses can result in cellular dysfunction, disseminated intravascular coagulation, and multiorgan dysfunction syndrome. In addition, reduced cerebral blood flow, combined with abnormal local metabolism and coagulopathy, can lead to dysfunction of the central nervous system.

Clinical Manifestations and Diagnosis

Mild heat illness is common and can be recognized by its clinical features. *Miliaria rubra* (heat rash) results from occlusion of eccrine sweat gland ducts and can be complicated by secondary staphylococcal infection. *Heat syncope* (fainting) is caused by temporary circulatory insufficiency as a result of pooling of blood in the peripheral veins—especially those of the lower extremity. *Heat cramps* (skeletal muscles cramps) occur during and after intense exercise and are believed to result from excessive loss of sodium in sweat.

Serious heat illness is often not apparent at initial evaluation. Patients who exhibit symptoms (e.g., dizziness, unsteady gait, ataxia, headache, confusion, weakness, fatigue, nausea, vomiting, diarrhea) should undergo immediate assessment of their mental status, core (rectal) temperature, and other vital signs. Heat stroke should be the working diagnosis in anyone who is a heat casualty and has altered mental status.

Heat exhaustion is a mild to moderate illness characterized by an inability to sustain cardiac output with moderate (>38.5° C, 101° F) to high (>40° C, 104° F) body temperatures. It is frequently accompanied by hot skin and dehydration. *Heat injury* is a moderate to severe illness characterized by organ (e.g., liver, renal) and tissue (e.g., gut, muscle) injury with high body temperatures, usually but not always greater than 40° C (104° F).

Heat stroke is a severe illness characterized by central nervous system dysfunction with high body temperatures, usually but not always greater than 40° C (104° F). However, patients with a core temperature higher than 40° C do not universally have a heat injury or heat stroke, and the entire clinical picture, including mental status and laboratory results, must be considered together. Heat stroke is often categorized as "classic" or "exertional," with the former observed primarily in otherwise sick and compromised individuals and the latter observed primarily in apparently healthy and physically fit individuals (Table 110–2). Heat stroke victims have profound neuropsychiatric impairments that develop early and universally. In addition, heat stroke can be complicated by liver damage, rhabdomyolysis, disseminated intravascular coagulation, water and electrolyte imbalance, and renal failure.

Prevention, Treatment, and Prognosis

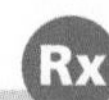

Heat illness can be prevented by inducing heat acclimatization and acquired thermal tolerance, maintaining adequate hydration, and avoiding overwhelming heat exposure.

Management of serious heat illness includes cooling, rehydration, and monitoring (Table 110–3). Body cooling should be initiated immediately and continued until the core temperature falls below 38.8° C. Body cooling lowers tissue temperatures and reduces cardiovascular stress by causing vasoconstriction in the skin. Immersion or soaking skin in cool or iced water with skin massage is the most effective method, but ice sheets and ice packs are also effective in dissipating the body heat load. Cooling can induce shivering, which is not usually sufficient to increase body temperature, so shivering need not be treated.

Fluid and electrolyte deficits should be corrected; restoration of plasma volume with isotonic fluids sufficient to sustain adequate perfusion, as judged by urine output, is a priority. Rapid overcorrection of serum electrolytes (e.g., sodium) should be avoided. If rhabdomyolysis and myoglobinuria (Chapters 114 and 447) are present, maintaining urine flow will help minimize renal injury. Patients should be monitored for cardiac arrhythmia and acute respiratory failure. Medications to be avoided include antipyretics and some sedatives with hepatic toxicities. Lorazepam (2 to 4 mg administered intravenously over a 2- to 5-minute period) is a safe sedative because of its low hepatotoxicity and rapid metabolism.

A single episode of heat exhaustion does not imply any predisposition to heat illness, and most patients recover within several hours after cooling and rehydration. In contrast, heat injury and stoke patients should not be re-exposed to heat until recovery is complete, and about 10% of heat stroke patients remain intolerant of heat.

TABLE 110–1 FACTORS PREDISPOSING TO SERIOUS HEAT ILLNESS

INDIVIDUAL FACTORS
Lack of acclimatization
Low physical fitness
Excessive body weight
Dehydration
Advanced age
Young children
HEALTH CONDITIONS
Inflammation and fever
Cardiovascular disease
Diabetes mellitus
Gastroenteritis
Rash, sunburn, and previous burns to large areas of skin
Seizures
Thyroid storm
Neuroleptic malignant syndrome
Malignant hyperthermia
Sickle cell trait
Cystic fibrosis
Spinal cord injury
MEDICATIONS
Anticholinergic properties (atropine)
Antiepileptic (topiramate)
Antihistamines
Glutethimide (Doriden)
Phenothiazines (a class of antipsychotic drugs, including chlorpromazine [Thorazine], trifluoperazine [Stelazine], and perphenazine [Trilafon])
Tricyclic antidepressants (e.g., imipramine, amitriptyline)
Amphetamines, cocaine, "Ecstasy"
Ergogenic stimulants (e.g., ephedrine, ephedra)
Lithium
Diuretics
β-Blockers (e.g., propranolol and atenolol)
Ethanol
ENVIRONMENTAL FACTORS
High temperature
High humidity
Little air motion
Lack of shade
Heat wave
Physical exercise
Heavy clothing
Air pollution (nitrogen dioxide)

COLD INJURY

Definitions

Cold injuries are classified as hypothermia and peripheral cold injuries. Hypothermia is whole body cooling, whereas peripheral cold injuries are localized to the extremities and exposed skin. Peripheral cold injuries can be divided into nonfreezing (chilblain, trench foot) and freezing (frostbite). Both hypothermia and peripheral cold injuries often occur simultaneously.

Epidemiology

A variety of individual factors, health conditions, medications, and environmental factors are associated with a predisposition to cold injury (Table 110–4). In trauma patients (Chapter 103), hypothermia is associated with increased morbidity and mortality.

Pathobiology

Cold exposure elicits peripheral vasoconstriction to reduce heat transfer between the body's core and shell (skin, subcutaneous fat). If sufficiently cold, the underlying tissues (e.g., muscle) constrict to thicken the isolative shell while reducing the body core area. This vasoconstrictor response defends core temperature, but at the expense of declining peripheral tissue temperatures, which contribute to peripheral cold injuries. Hypothermia depresses enzymatic activity, interferes with physiologic functions (e.g., clotting, respiration, cardiac conduction and rhythm), impairs expression of cytokines, and can induce cellular injury and death.

Clinical Manifestations and Diagnosis

Hypothermia is a core temperature below 95° F (35° C), and clinical manifestations are related to the core temperature achieved (Table 110–5). *Chilblain* (Chapter 80) appears as localized inflammatory lesions of the skin that most often involve the dorsal surface of fingers, but the ears, face, and exposed shins are common areas. "*Trench foot*" is caused by prolonged cold-wet (e.g., wet socks or gloves) exposure, which can cause skin breakdown and nerve damage. Trench foot is often accompanied by infection and increased sensitivity to pain. *Frostbite* is the freezing of tissues and can be categorized as first degree (superficial, "*frostnip*"), second degree (full skin), third degree (subcutaneous tissue), and fourth degree (extensive tissue and bone). The severity of frostbite may take many days to weeks to determine. Frostbite requires early surgical consultation once the diagnosis is made. The classic J wave on the electrocardiogram appears at a core temperature below about 93° F (Fig. 110–2).

Provention, Treatment, and Prognosis

Rx

Humans demonstrate minimal cold acclimatization, so prevention primarily depends on avoiding cold exposure and having adequate protection and caloric intake to support metabolism. Management of hypothermia depends on the core temperature (Table 110–6). Patients should have wet clothing removed and be provided dry insulation. Shivering is an effective physiologic rewarming mechanism and should not be pharmacologically suppressed. Moderately and profoundly hypothermic patients will require active rewarming. Rewarming at a rate of 0.5° C to 1.0° C (0.9° F to 1.8° F) per hour is acceptable, except that aggressive rewarming is warranted in patients with significant trauma (because coagulation is hindered by hypothermia) or cardiac arrest.

Patients should be warmed gently because ventricular fibrillation is easily precipitated. When ventricular fibrillation is present, repeated electrical shocks should not be attempted until victims are rewarmed to a core temperature higher than 30° C (86° F); instead, cardiopulmonary resuscitation should be maintained during this period. Arrhythmias can be treated with lidocaine, propranolol, or bretylium. Body cooling induces cold diuresis, so plasma volume needs to be re-established to support adequate perfusion: patients should receive an intravenous infusion of 250 to 1000 mL of heated (104° F to 108° F; 40° C to 42° C) 5% dextrose in normal saline. Lactated Ringer's solution should be avoided because the liver cannot metabolize lactate efficiently during hypothermia. Patients should be monitored for disturbances in potassium and glucose. If hypoglycemia, alcohol, or opiate intoxication is contributing to hypothermia, intravenous glucose (10 to 25 g), thiamine (100 mg), or naloxone (1 to 2 mg) may be indicated.

Frostbitten tissues should be protected from friction or trauma and be gently rewarmed in a water bath (100° F to 108° F or 38° C to 43° C). Patients should receive ibuprofen, antibiotics, and possibly an analgesic.

TABLE 110–2 COMPARISON OF CLASSIC AND EXERTIONAL HEAT STROKE

Patient Characteristics	Classic	Exertional
Age	Young children or elderly	15–55 yr
Health	Chronic illness	Usually healthy
Fever	Unusual	Common
Prevailing weather	Frequent in heat waves	Variable
Activity	Sedentary	Strenuous exercise
Drug use	Diuretics, antidepressants, anticholinergics, phenothiazines	Ergogenic stimulants or cocaine
Sweating	Often absent	Common
Acid-base disturbances	Respiratory alkalosis	Lactic acidosis
Acute renal failure	Uncommon	Common (≈15%)
Rhabdomyolysis	Uncommon	Common (≈25%)
CK	Mildly elevated	Markedly elevated (500–1000 U/L)
ALT, AST	Mildly elevated	Markedly elevated
Hyperkalemia	Uncommon	Common
Hypocalcemia	Uncommon	Common
DIC	Mild	Marked
Hypoglycemia	Uncommon	Common

ALT = alanine aminotransferase; AST = aspartate aminotransferase; CK = creatine kinase; DIC = disseminated intravascular coagulation.

TABLE 110–3 MANAGEMENT OF HEAT ILLNESS

HEAT EXHAUSTION

Rest and shade
Loosen and remove clothing
Supine and elevate legs
Actively cool skin
Fluids by mouth
Monitor core temperature
Monitor mental status

HYPERTHERMIA

Protect the airway
Insert at least two large-bore intravenous lines
Monitor core temperature; options include pulmonary artery, rectal probe, esophageal probe
Actively cool the skin until core temperature reaches 39° C
- Exposure to cool environment
- Wetting with water (avoid alcohol rubs)
- Continuous fanning
- Ice baths or immersion (22° C)
- Axillary/perineal ice packs
- Infusion of room-temperature saline
- Gastric/colonic iced saline lavage
- Peritoneal lavage with cool saline

If shivering occurs, administer chlorpromazine, 10–25 mg IM
Monitor for seizures
Monitor electrocardiogram for arrhythmia
Obtain serial diagnostic studies*

*Electrocardiogram, chest radiograph, complete blood count with differential, platelet count, urinalysis, aminotransferases, alkaline phosphatase, bilirubin, creatine kinase, blood urea nitrogen, creatinine, phosphate, calcium, glucose, electrolytes, uric acid, prothrombin time and partial thromboplastin time, fibrin split products, fibrinogen, arterial blood gases, toxicology screen.

TABLE 110–4 FACTORS PREDISPOSING TO COLD INJURY

INDIVIDUAL FACTORS

Inadequate clothing and shelter
Lean and low body fat
Low physical fitness
Advanced age
Young children
Black men and women

HEALTH CONDITIONS

Burns
Diabetes
Hypoglycemia
Neurologic lesions
Dementia
Hypoadrenalism, hypopituitarism, and hypothyroidism
Raynaud's phenomenon
Sickle cell trait
Trauma
Spinal cord injury

MEDICATIONS

Alcohol
Anesthetics
Antidepressants
Antithyroid agents
Sedatives and narcotics

ENVIRONMENTAL FACTORS

Cold temperatures
High air motion
Rain and immersion
Skin contact with metal and fuels
Repeated cold exposure
Physical fatigue
Immobility
High-altitude and low–oxygen tension environments

TABLE 110–5 HYPOTHERMIA: STAGES AND ASSOCIATED CLINICAL MANIFESTATIONS

Stage	Core Temperature ° F	° C	Clinical Manifestations
Normothermia	98.6	37.0	
Mild hypothermia	95.0	35.0	Cold diuresis, maximal shivering
	93.0	33.8	Ataxia, poor judgment, J wave
	91.0	32.7	Amnesia, blood pressure difficult to measure
Moderate hypothermia	89.0	31.6	Stupor, pupils dilated
	87.0	30.5	Shivering ceases
	85.0	30.0	Cardiac arrhythmias, insulin inactive
	82.0	27.8	Unconsciousness, ventricular fibrillation likely
	80.0	26.6	No muscle reflexes
Profound hypothermia	78.0	25.5	Acid-based disturbances, no response to pain
	75.0	23.8	Pulmonary edema, mortality from exertional hypothermia
	73.0	22.7	No corneal reflexes
	66.0	18.8	Heart standstill
	62.0	16.6	Isoelectric electrocardiogram
	57.6	14.2	Lowest infant survival from accidental hypothermia
	48.2	9.0	Lowest adult survival from accidental hypothermia

TABLE 110–6 TREATMENT OF HYPOTHERMIA

Stage	Management	Body Rewarming
Mild hypothermia	Monitor vital signs Warm intravenous saline Oxygen Monitor electrocardiogram for arrhythmia	Insulate Shivering Warm bath
Moderate hypothermia	Diagnostic studies* Intensive care Anticipate infection and multiorgan dysfunction	Prevent extra heat loss by supplementing with airway rewarming Colonic irrigation Peritoneal dialysis
Profound hypothermia	Diagnostic studies	Central rewarming

*See Table 110–3. Also lactate dehydrogenase, serum lactate, cortisol, thyroid-stimulating hormone, T3, and T4.

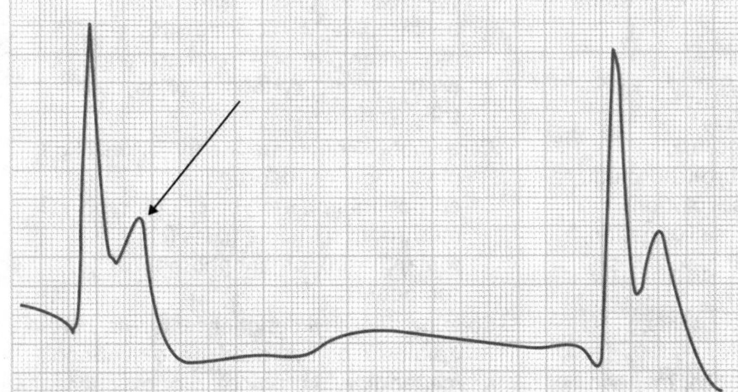

FIGURE 110–2 • J (Osborne) wave.

Hypothermic Syndromes

Exercise-induced bronchospasm (Chapter 87) can be triggered by exercise in cold air, particularly in patients with asthma. *Livedo reticularis* (Chapter 80) is patchy mottling of the limbs with cold exposure. *Cryoglobulinemia* (Chapter 198) occurs when immunoglobulins (IgM, IgG) reversibly precipitate after being cooled and contribute to impaired capillary blood flow in hypothermic tissues. *Cold urticaria* (Chapters 273 and 466) is the development of localized and general erythema and wheals in skin exposed to cold. *Paroxysmal hypothermia* is periodic lowering of the thermoregulatory set point and is often associated with hypothalamic abnormalities. *Raynaud's phenomenon* (Chapter 288) is intense vasoconstriction with sensitivity to pain in limbs exposed to cold.

SUGGESTED READINGS

Aslam AF, Aslam AK, Vasavada BC, et al: Hypothermia: Evaluation, electrocardiographic manifestations, and management. Am J Med 2006;119:297–301. *A comprehensive review.*

Carter R, Cheuvront SM, Williams JO, et al: Epidemiology of hospitalizations and deaths from heat illness in soldiers. Med Sci Sports Exerc 2005;37:1338–1344. *Provides epidemiologic data on all U.S. Army heat illness hospitalizations from 1980 through 2002.*

Inter-Association Task Force on Exertional Heat Illnesses Consensus Statement. Available at http://www.the-aps.org/news/heat.htm. *A consensus document regarding treatment of exertional heat illness.*

Smith JE: Cooling methods used in the treatment of exertional heat illness. Br J Sports Med 2005;39:503–507. *Ice water immesion appears to be the best treatment.*

Sonna LA, Wenger CB, Flinn S, et al: Exertional heat injury and gene expression changes: A DNA microarray analysis study. J Appl Physiol 2004;96:1943–1953. *Provides molecular evidence that heat injury can result from the cumulative effects of multiple adverse stimuli.*

Wang HE, Callaway CW, Peitzman AB, et al: Admission hypothermia and outcome after major trauma. Crit Care Med 2005;33:1296–1301. *In 681 trauma patients, hypothermia was independently associated with increased mortality.*

ACUTE POISONING

Marsha D. Ford

Epidemiology

Each year, an estimated 4 million poisoning cases, suspected or verified, and 300,000 related hospital admissions occur in the United States. Poisoning-related deaths total more than 30,000 per year and are increasing. Nevertheless, almost all patients who reach the hospital alive survive with appropriate care; inpatient mortality rates of 0.2 to 0.5% have been reported. The incidence of recurrent, purposeful self-poisoning is 12 to 18%, with most occurring within 3 months of the original attempt. These facts emphasize the need for aggressive treatment of poisoned patients, including early psychiatric intervention for suicidal behavior, to reduce fatalities and repeat attempts (Chapter 420).

Diagnosis

Diagnosis and management of poisoned patients require knowledge and skill in five areas to identify and treat the factors that contribute to the risk for death or long-term disability: (1) history taking; (2) physical examination, with recognition of specific toxic syndromes, or *toxidromes*; (3) appropriate use of diagnostic tests; (4) treatment, including initial stabilization and critical care, decontamination, and administration of antidotes for specific poisonings; and (5) use of methods to enhance the elimination of specific toxicants.

History

Details elicited about toxic exposures should include the involved drugs and other toxicants, including their estimated or known amounts, the time and routes of exposure, the patient's symptoms and signs, and any treatment already administered. Intoxication may result from acute, chronic, or acute-on-chronic exposure. A *toxicant* is defined as a chemical capable of harming a biologic organism; this definition encompasses toxins, which are derived from living organisms, as well as drugs and industrial and other chemicals. Determination of chronicity is important because signs and symptoms of chronic intoxication (Chapter 20) can differ from those of acute and acute-on-chronic intoxication. For example, a history of acute collapse narrows the toxicant possibilities to a few gases, chemicals, and drugs. A listing of available medications (e.g., medications of the patient, spouse, relative, or friend); use of nonprescription medications, herbal/dietary supplements, or ethnic remedies; and occupational and avocational activities should be obtained. Occupational and avocational histories should include present and all past jobs and hobbies with a focus on chemicals, metals, and gases. Known medical conditions may suggest classes of medications available to the patient. The patient's history, which may be incomplete if the patient is confused or suicidal, should be correlated with the clinical manifestations and course. Further history from relatives and friends and findings from the scene as reported by the transporting emergency medical services personnel may be relevant.

Physical Examination

The physical examination should focus on vital signs; the eye, ear, nose, and throat examination; and the neurologic, cardiopulmonary, gastrointestinal, and dermatologic systems. Findings can suggest certain toxicants by recognition of toxidromes, which are clusters of signs and symptoms typical of poisoning with adrenergic, anticholinergic, cholinomimetic, opioid, and sedative-hypnotic agents (Table 111–1). Patients may have

TABLE 111–1 TOXIDROMES AND ASSOCIATED DRUGS AND TOXICANTS

	Syndrome Features		
Toxidrome	**Vital Signs**	**End Organ**	**Drugs/Toxicants**
Adrenergic	Hypertension, hyperthermia, tachycardia, tachypnea	Agitation, arrhythmias, diaphoresis, mydriasis, seizures	Amphetamines, caffeine, cocaine, ephedrine/pseudoephedrine/*Ephedra* sp, phenylpropanolamine,* theophylline
Anticholinergic	Hyperthermia, tachycardia	Agitation/delirium, decreased/absent bowel sounds, dry flushed skin/mucous membranes, mydriasis/blurred vision, seizures, urinary retention	First-generation H_1-receptor antagonists (e.g., classic antihistamines), belladonna alkaloids (e.g., scopolamine, hyoscyamine) from plants (e.g., *Datura* sp—deadly nightshade, henbane), benztropine, cyclic antidepressants, dicyclomine, muscle relaxants (e.g., orphenadrine, cyclobenzaprine), trihexyphenidyl
Cholinomimetic	Tachycardia/bradycardia†	Agitation/delirium/coma, bronchorrhea, bronchospasm, diaphoresis, fasciculations, lacrimation, miosis, urination, diarrhea/vomiting, seizures	Carbamates, cholinesterase inhibitors (e.g., physostigmine, neostigmine, edrophonium), *Inocybe* or *Clitocybe* mushroom sp, nerve gases (e.g., soman, sarin), organophosphorus compounds
Opiate/opioid	Bradycardia, bradypnea/apnea, hypotension (rare), hypothermia	CNS depression, hypotonia, miosis, mydriasis (dextromethorphan, meperidine, pentazocine)	Codeine, fentanyl/designer fentanyls, heroin, opioids (e.g., hydrocodone, oxycodone, meperidine, morphine), propoxyphene, central α_2-agonists (e.g., clonidine, imidazolines)
Sedative-hypnotic	Bradypnea/apnea, hypotension, hypothermia	Ataxia, CNS depression, hyporeflexia, slurred speech, stupor/coma	Barbiturates, benzodiazepines, bromides, chloral hydrate, ethanol, ethchlorvynol, etomidate, glutethimide, meprobamate, methaqualone, methyprylon, propofol, zolpidem

*Reflex bradycardia can occur as a result of a pure α-adrenergic agonist effect.
†Tachycardia can occur early as a result of a preganglionic nicotinic effect; as toxicity progresses, postganglionic muscarinic effects predominate, and bradycardia develops.
CNS = central nervous system.

some or all of these signs and symptoms; an incomplete clinical picture does not exclude a particular toxidrome but can still assist the clinician in identifying the correct category of toxicant involved.

Vital Signs

Tachycardia can occur with numerous toxicants and with anxiety and other nontoxicologic conditions and is not a helpful finding. The limited differential diagnosis for toxicant-induced *bradycardia* includes baclofen, β-adrenergic receptor antagonists, L-type calcium-channel antagonists (diltiazem or verapamil), cardiac glycosides, α-adrenergic receptor agonists (e.g., phenylpropanolamine, whose effects are mediated by baroreceptor reflexes), γ-hydroxybutyric acid, opioids, some sedative-hypnotics, central α_2-agonists, organophosphorus compounds, carbamates, cyanide, muscarine-containing mushrooms (*Clitocybe, Inocybe* sp), therapeutic cholinesterase inhibitors (e.g., physostigmine), cyclic antidepressants (bradycardia is a preterminal sign), and some antiarrhythmic drugs (e.g., procainamide, flecainide, and other class IA and IC drugs).

Many toxicants cause *hypotension* (Chapter 7). The primary pathophysiologic mechanisms are decreased peripheral vascular resistance, decreased myocardial contractility, hypovolemia secondary to vomiting or loss of intravascular volume, and occasionally, arrhythmias. Common causes of *hypertension* (Chapter 66) include amphetamines, cocaine, ephedrine and similar agents, ergots, phencyclidine, nicotine, phenylpropanolamine, thyroid hormones, and chronic lead toxicity. Blood pressure can rise early in poisoning with cyclic antidepressants, central α_2-adrenergic agonists, and monoamine oxidase inhibitors.

Hyperthermia (Chapter 110) occurs with toxicants that cause agitation or excessive motor activity (e.g., cocaine, phencyclidine, monoamine oxidase inhibitors, strychnine), uncouple oxidative phosphorylation (e.g., salicylates, dinitrophenol), increase the metabolic rate (thyroid hormones), impair sweating (e.g., antihistamines, anticholinergics, cocaine, phenothiazines, zonisamide), cause vasoconstriction (e.g., amphetamines, ephedrine), or impair vasodilation and alter perception of heat (cocaine). Other toxicant-induced states associated with hyperthermia include malignant hyperthermia, neuroleptic malignant syndrome, serotonin syndrome, metal fume fever, and hydrocarbon aspiration. Toxicant-induced *hypothermia* is typically due to sedative-hypnotics, opioids, barbiturates, ethanol, phenothiazines, or hypoglycemic agents such as insulin, sulfonylureas, meglitinides, or unripe akee fruit. Oxygen saturation, as measured by *pulse oximetry*, decreases with true hypoxemia or methemoglobinemia (Chapter 168) but remains normal or may be increased in carbon monoxide poisoning (Chapter 94).

Eyes, Ears, Nose, and Throat

Toxicant-induced bilateral miosis (Fig. 111–1) has a limited differential diagnosis that includes central α_2-agonists, such as clonidine and the imidazolines; olanzapine; opioids; organophosphorus compounds/carbamates; therapeutic cholinesterase inhibitors (e.g., physostigmine); topical miotic ophthalmic drugs (e.g., pilocarpine); and variably, phencyclidine, phenothiazines, ethanol, and some sedative-hypnotics (Chapter 450). Pontine hemorrhage is the major nontoxicologic diagnosis to consider in a comatose patient with miotic pupils (Chapter 432). Mydriasis is a nonspecific finding. A unilateral dilated pupil may be due to topical ocular application of sympathomimetics (e.g., phenylephrine), antihistamines, or anticholinergic agents (e.g., dust or sap from *Datura* species) and can be caused by a postauricular scopolamine patch. Failure of topical 4% pilocarpine ophthalmic drops to constrict the pupil supports the diagnosis of pupillary dilation from a topical mydriatic agent. Visual disturbances, including partial or total blindness as a result of systemic toxicity, have been reported with anticholinergic agents, carbon monoxide, digitalis, ethambutol, methanol, methyl bromide, quinine, and agents that are associated with pseudotumor cerebri, including antimicrobials (e.g., ampicillin, metronidazole, nalidixic acid, nitrofurantoin, sulfa drugs, and tetracycline), glucocorticosteroids, lead, lithium, oral contraceptives, phenothiazines, phenytoin, and vitamin A. Nonarteritic anterior ischemic optic neuropathy has developed after the use of sildenafil and other related drugs (Chapter 253); the causal relationship is unknown.

Acute hearing loss (Chapter 454) can occur as a toxic effect of aminoglycosides, bromates, chloroquine, cisplatin, carboplatin, high-dose loop diuretics, nitrogen mustard, quinine, salicylates, vinblastine, and vincristine. Nasal septal erosions and perforations may be due to chronic exposure to intranasal cocaine (Chapter 32) or inhalation of fumes from chromium and nickel (Chapters 93 and 94).

Neurologic Signs

Many toxicants affect the central nervous system (CNS) and can produce agitated delirium, depression, or seizures (Table 111–2). Distinguishing features of various toxicants may assist in making the correct diagnosis. Patients withdrawing from opioids are alert and oriented, whereas patients withdrawing from alcohol, barbiturates, benzodiazepines, and other sedative-hypnotics can be disoriented. Initial CNS depression can also develop with large ingestions of acetaminophen or ibuprofen. Isoniazid and theophylline are noted for producing seizures refractory to the usual doses of benzodiazepines and barbiturates. Pyridoxine treats isoniazid-induced seizures by increasing CNS γ-aminobutyric acid; phenytoin is relatively ineffective for theophylline-induced seizures. Plant or mushroom ingestion can also produce CNS depression (e.g., species of *Rhododendron, Solanum* [bittersweet], *Taxus* [yew], and *Sophora* [mescal bean]), CNS stimulation (e.g., *Catha edulis* [khat], *Strychnos nux vomica* [contains strychnine], species of *Cicuta* [water

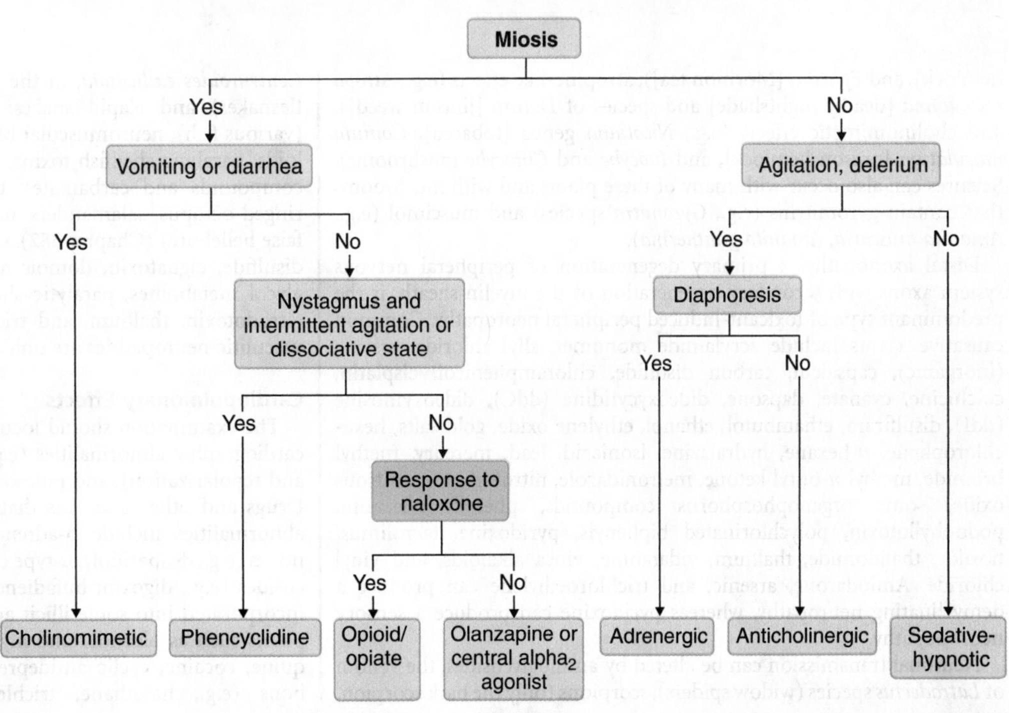

FIGURE 111–1 • Diagnostic algorithm using the size of the pupils.

TABLE 111–2 CENTRAL NERVOUS SYSTEM EFFECTS OF TOXICANTS

Toxicant Categories/Agents	CNS Effects		
	Agitated Delirium	**Decreased Level of Consciousness**	**Seizures**
CATEGORIES			
Adrenergic agonists	•		•
Anticholinergic agents	•	•	•
Anticonvulsants		•	• (Paradoxical with some agents)
Antipsychotic drugs	•	•	•
β-Adrenergic receptor antagonists		•	•
Hallucinogenic agents	•		
Monoamine oxidase inhibitors	•	•	•
Opioids	• (Propoxyphene, normeperidine, tramadol)	•	• (Propoxyphene, normeperidine, tramadol)
Sedative-hypnotics		•	• (Rare)
Serotonin agonists	•	•	•
AGENTS			
Amphetamines, cocaine	•	•	•
Antihistamines (first generation, e.g., diphenhydramine)	•	•	•
Barbiturates		•	
Benzodiazepines		•	
Cyclic antidepressants	•	•	•
Cytochrome oxidase inhibitors (e.g., carbon monoxide, cyanide, hydrogen sulfide, and azides)		•	•
Ephedra alkaloids and similar agents			•
γ-Hydroxybutyrate and precursors	•	•	• (Rare)
Lithium	•	•	•
Organophosphorus compounds/carbamates (e.g., diazinon, malathion, fenthion/carbaryl)		•	•
Salicylates	•	•	•
SSRIs/SRIs	•	•	• (Uncommon)
Withdrawal from alcohol, barbiturates, benzodiazepines, and other sedative-hypnotics	•	•	•
Withdrawal from opioids			• (Reported only in neonates)

SRIs = serotonin re-uptake inhibitors; SSRIs = selective serotonin re-uptake inhibitors.

hemlock], and *Ephedra* [Mormon tea]), atropine-like effects (e.g., *Atropa belladonna* [deadly nightshade] and species of *Datura* [jimson weed]), and cholinomimetic effects (e.g., *Nicotiana* genus [tobacco], *Conium maculatum* [poison hemlock], and *Inocybe* and *Clitocybe* mushrooms). Seizures can also occur with many of these plants and with mushrooms that contain gyromitrins (e.g., *Gyromitra* species) and muscimol (e.g., *Amanita muscaria, Amanita pantherina*).

Distal axonopathy, a primary degeneration of peripheral nervous system axons with secondary degeneration of the myelin sheath, is the predominant type of toxicant-induced peripheral neuropathy. Common causative agents include acrylamide monomer, allyl chloride, arsenic (inorganic), capsaicin, carbon disulfide, chloramphenicol, cisplatin, colchicine, cyanate, dapsone, dideoxycytidine (ddC), dideoxyinosine (ddI), disulfiram, ethambutol, ethanol, ethylene oxide, gold salts, hexachlorophene, *n*-hexane, hydralazine, isoniazid, lead, mercury, methyl bromide, methyl *n*-butyl ketone, metronidazole, nitrofurantoin, nitrous oxide, some organophosphorus compounds, phenol, platinum, podophyllotoxin, polychlorinated biphenyls, pyridoxine, tacrolimus, taxoids, thalidomide, thallium, vidarabine, vinca alkaloids, and vinyl chloride. Amiodarone, arsenic, and trichloroethylene can produce a demyelinating neuropathy, whereas pyridoxine can produce a sensory neuronopathy.

Neuronal transmission can be altered by aminoglycosides; the venom of *Latrodectus* species (widow spiders), scorpions (only the bark scorpion, *Centruroides exilicauda*, in the United States), and crotaline (e.g., rattlesnakes) and elapid snakes; brevetoxin (shellfish) and ciguatoxin (various fish); neuromuscular blocking drugs; nicotine and related alkaloids; paralytic shellfish toxins, saxitoxin (shellfish); organophosphorus compounds and carbamates; tetrodotoxin (puffer fish [fugu], blue-ringed octopus, salamanders, newts, and others); and veratridine (e.g., false hellebore) (Chapter 382). Cranial nerves can be affected by carbon disulfide, ciguatoxin, domoic acid (shellfish), elapid venom, ethylene glycol metabolites, paralytic shellfish toxins, bark scorpion, saxitoxin, tetrodotoxin, thallium, and trichloroethylene. Mononeuropathies and vasculitic neuropathies are unlikely to be induced by toxicants.

Cardiopulmonary Effects

The examination should focus on blood pressure, heart rate, electrocardiographic abnormalities (e.g., rhythm, conduction, depolarization, and repolarization), and pulmonary findings, including pulse oximetry. Drugs and other toxicants that can cause arrhythmias or conduction abnormalities include β-adrenergic receptor antagonists, butyrophenones (e.g., droperidol), L-type calcium-channel antagonists, cardiac glycosides (e.g., digoxin; bufadienolides, found in toxic toad venom and incorporated into some illicit aphrodisiacs; and cardenolides, found in plants such as oleander and lily of the valley), chloral hydrate, chloroquine, cocaine, cyclic antidepressants, ethanol, halogenated hydrocarbons (e.g., halothane, trichloroethylene), magnesium, potassium, propoxyphene, thioridazine/mesoridazine, and antiarrhythmics and other agents that affect the myocardial voltage-gated sodium channels (e.g., bupivacaine, chloroquine, cocaine, cyclic antidepressants, flecainide, mexiletine, quinidine, procainamide, propafenone) and potassium channels (e.g., astemizole, cisapride, citalopram, and erythromycin [especially when taken concomitantly with cytochrome P-4503 A inhibitors; see Chapter 27]), quinidine, sotalol, and terfenadine). Bedside echocardiography may reveal depressed myocardial contractility as a result of agents that block the myocardial voltage-gated sodium channel, β-adrenergic receptor antagonists, calcium-channel antagonists, cyclic antidepressants, magnesium, arsenic, ciguatoxin, cyanide, ethanol, iron, scorpion venom, and tetrodotoxin.

Toxicants can produce myriad pulmonary effects, including parenchymal, pleural, and vascular diseases and airway irritation and barotrauma. Immediate life-threatening toxic effects include acute lung injury and pulmonary edema, acute respiratory distress syndrome (ARDS), and rapidly developing pulmonary fibrosis or bronchiolitis obliterans. Typical syndromes and etiologic agents include pulmonary edema (β-adrenergic receptor antagonists, calcium-channel antagonists, antiarrhythmics, daunorubicin, and doxorubicin), acute lung injury/ARDS (amphetamines, cadmium, chlorine, cocaine, ethchlorvynol, methotrexate, opioids/heroin, paraquat, salicylates, and inhalation of smoke, zinc chloride, methyl bromide, and methyl chloride), and rapidly developing pulmonary fibrosis/bronchiolitis obliterans (nitrogen dioxide and paraquat).

Gastrointestinal Effects

Symptoms of nausea, vomiting, diarrhea, and abdominal pain are nonspecific and must be interpreted in the context of other findings. Agents that produce severe or life-threatening toxicity with early gastrointestinal findings include acid or large alkali ingestions; cardiac glycosides, colchicines, and other microtubular toxicants; iron; metals such as arsenic, acute high-level lead, mercury salts, or thallium; mushrooms containing amanitine (*Amanita phalloides*, *Amanita virosa*, *Amanita verna*, *Lepiota chlorophyllum*), gyromitrins (*Gyromitra esculenta*), orellanines (*Cortinarius orellanus*), or allenic norleucine (*Amanita smithiana*); nicotine; organophosphorus compounds; and theophylline. Severe abdominal pain and rigidity can occur with envenomation by *Latrodectus* species (widow spiders). Right upper quadrant tenderness develops with toxic hepatitis. Hepatotoxicity can occur as an adverse effect of the therapeutic use of many drugs; in the United States, acetaminophen and ethanol are the most common causes of toxicant-induced hepatotoxicity (Chapters 153 and 157). Other notable hepatotoxicants include aflatoxins (in food contaminated with *Aspergillus flavus*), arsenicals, carbon tetrachloride, copper sulfate, cyclopeptide mushrooms (e.g., *Amanita phalloides*), *Ephedra* species (e.g., ma huang), iron, methamphetamine, pennyroyal oil, pyrrolizidine alkaloids (various plant species used in herbal teas), and vitamin A in chronic excessive doses.

Dermatologic Signs

The skin, hair, nails, and mucous membranes should be examined for evidence of intravenous drug use; the presence or absence of skin and mucous membrane moisture; abnormal skin coloration, including erythema and cyanosis; alopecia; and nail abnormalities. Bullous skin lesions have been reported with chronic barbiturate use, glutethimide, carbon monoxide, meprobamate, methadone, and valproic acid. Cyanosis may reflect hypoxia or methemoglobinemia. Commonly used agents that can cause methemoglobinemia include aniline dyes, benzocaine and other amide anesthetics, dapsone, naphthalene, nitrates, nitrites, phenazopyridine, rifampin, and sulfonamides (Chapter 168). Skin erythema or flushing occurs with anticholinergic agents, boric acid ingestion, monosodium glutamate, niacin, scombroid toxicity (Chapter 382) as a result of the ingestion of inadequately refrigerated fish with a high histidine content (e.g., tuna, mahi-mahi, amberjack), vancomycin, and interactions between ethanol and numerous agents that produce disulfiram or disulfiram-like reactions (e.g., carbon disulfide, some cephalosporins, *Coprinus atramentarius* mushroom, disulfiram, griseofulvin, metronidazole, thiuram herbicides, and trichloroethylene).

Specific Toxicants

Some common toxicants can be suspected from their characteristic manifestations (Table 111–3). These suspicions should guide specific diagnostic and therapeutic strategies that complement general decontamination and supportive treatments.

Diagnostic Tests

Drug testing should be guided by the history and physical examination, with emphasis on tests that can influence management. Rapid qualitative urine drug screening tests are readily available in most hospitals, but their clinical value is limited by the number of drugs that can be tested and the reliability of the tests themselves. A positive test result may be unrelated to the patient's condition because drug analytes may be detectable within hours to more than 30 days after drug use, depending on the drug, dose, and frequency of use. False-positive and false-negative results occur (Table 111–4), and the screening result must be verified with a second method, such as gas chromatography–mass spectrometry. Varying drug use in a population should be considered when determining the drugs to be screened in order to decrease the incidence of false-positive results. A test with 99% specificity for a drug with a prevalence of 0.1% in a population would produce 10 false-positive results for every true-positive result. Clinically irrelevant true-positive findings also occur, such as when poppy seeds produce a positive opiate test. Failure to consider these limitations of drug screens can result in misdiagnosis.

For a limited number of drugs and toxicants, levels in blood or urine are useful for diagnosis, therapy, or monitoring (Table 111–5). Threshold levels of certain toxicants indicate the need for specific therapies: acetaminophen (*N*-acetylcysteine), ethylene glycol (fomepizole and hemodialysis), iron (deferoxamine), methanol (fomepizole and hemodialysis), methemoglobin (methylene blue), salicylates (urine alkalinization and hemodialysis), and theophylline (hemoperfusion/hemodialysis). In chronic poisoning with some drugs, such as salicylates or theophylline, these therapies may be indicated at lower drug levels. In general, any end-organ toxicity that is evident or anticipated (based on the toxicant, amount ingested, and time required to produce toxic effects) is more important than a specific level in determining the need for treatment.

Occult acetaminophen ingestion with toxic serum levels occurs in 0.3 to 1.9% of intentional ingestions. Given that these patients may be asymptomatic until hepatotoxicity develops and that administration of an antidote can prevent this hepatotoxicity, the current recommendation is to test for acetaminophen in all patients with intentional ingestions.

Other Blood Tests

Anion gap metabolic acidosis resulting from primary lactic acidosis can be caused by cyanide, hydrogen sulfide, iron, isoniazid, metformin, phenformin, sodium azide, and rarely, acetaminophen with high serum levels. Anion gap metabolic acidosis not related to lactic acidosis occurs with diethylene glycol, ethylene glycol, nonsteroidal anti-inflammatory drugs (NSAIDs), methanol, salicylates, theophylline, and toluene. In poisonings resulting from ethylene glycol, ibuprofen, methanol, propylene glycol, and salicylates, lactic acid can also be produced, but the level is insufficient to account for the anion gap. Anion gap metabolic acidosis can also develop in patients with ongoing agitation, hyperthermia, and muscle rigidity, such as in neuroleptic malignant syndrome (Chapters 110 and 445), or in some cases of rhabdomyolysis (Chapter 114) secondary to toxicants such as doxylamine, phencyclidine, strychnine, cocaine, and amphetamines. Elevated serum creatinine and blood urea nitrogen levels indicative of declining renal function may be seen with numerous toxicants. Direct toxicity occurs with acetaminophen, aminoglycosides, cadmium, Chinese weight loss botanicals (containing *Stephania tetrandra* or *Magnolia officinalis*), chromium, *Crotalus durissus* venom, diethylene glycol, diquat, ethylene glycol, fluorinated anesthetics, gold, heroin, lithium (diabetes insipidus), mercury salts, mushrooms (*Amanita smithiana* and *Cortinarius* sp), paraquat, radiocontrast agents, solvents (e.g., carbon tetrachloride, trichloroethylene and tetrachloroethylene, toluene), and sulfonamides. Agents that decrease glomerular perfusion by reducing renal blood flow include amphotericin, angiotensin-converting enzyme inhibitors, angiotensin receptor blockers, cocaine, cyclosporine, mannitol (excessive chronic doses), methotrexate, and NSAIDs.

Imaging

A computed tomographic scan of the head can detect life-threatening cerebral edema secondary to toxicant-induced hepatic failure, ethylene glycol, and methanol. It also detects intracranial bleeding caused by anticoagulant drugs and rodenticides, scorpion venom, and sympathomimetics (e.g., amphetamines, cocaine, phenylpropanolamine). An abdominal radiograph can reveal radiopaque ferrous sulfate tablets or metals such as arsenic, lead, mercury, and thallium.

Text continued on p. 778.

TABLE 111–3 PATHOPHYSIOLOGY, CLINICAL EFFECTS, AND MANAGEMENT OF SPECIFIC DRUGS AND TOXICANTS**

Drug or Toxicant	Pathophysiology	Clinical Effects	Laboratory	Specific Therapy
Acetaminophen	*NAPQI* (*toxic metabolite*) binds hepatic and renal tubular cells; acetaminophen itself induces transient decrease in functional factor VII	*Initial:* nausea/vomiting, coma, lactic acidosis in severe cases *Days 1–3:* elevated INR, aminotransferase, and bilirubin levels; RUQ tenderness; increased creatinine level in severe cases *Days 4–14:* gradual recovery or continued increase in INR and creatinine, lactic acidosis, coma, cerebral edema, death	Potentially toxic level ≥150 μg/mL 4 hr after ingestion* INR may be transiently elevated in first 24 hr because of decrease in functional factor VII; further increases indicate hepatic necrosis; elevated aminotransferase and bilirubin levels not predictive of hepatic failure Creatinine elevated in severe cases	N-*acetylcysteine* (NAC): See dosing guidelines in Table 111–6. NAC can increase the INR but not the aPTT.
Amphetamines	Increase release of presynaptic norepinephrine and dopamine Increase serotonin release (especially MDMA, PMA, DOB, other synthetic amphetamines)	*Mild:* euphoria, decreased appetite, repetitive behavior *Moderate:* vomiting, agitation, hypertension, tachycardia, mydriasis, bruxism, diaphoresis *Severe:* hypertension/ hypotension, arrhythmias, hyperthermia, seizures, coma, hepatotoxicity, rhabdomyolysis, DIC, hyponatremia (SIADH), renal failure, cerebral infarction/hemorrhage	Not helpful, many false-positives and false-negatives on screening tests (see Table 111–4)	IV crystalloids External cooling Benzodiazepines or barbiturates to control agitation/ seizures Benzodiazepines or nitroprusside for hypertension See SSRIs/SRIs for features and treatment of serotonin syndrome
β-Adrenergic receptor antagonists	Block catecholamines from β-adrenergic receptors α and β Adrenergic receptor antagonism: carvedilol, labetalol Delayed rectifier potassium-channel blockade: sotalol	Bradyarrhythmias; decreased myocardial contractility; hypotension; respiratory depression; decreased consciousness with seizures, coma (liphophilic agents, e.g., propranolol); prolonged QT interval (sotalol)	ECG No specific tests	Glucagon, 3.5–5 mg IV over 1-min period. If no increase in BP or HR, can repeat up to 10 mg; if effective, immediately, start continuous infusion at 1–10 mg/hr If still unstable, options include (1) regular insulin, 1 U/kg by IV bolus, followed by 1 U/kg/hr, plus dextrose to maintain euglycemia; (2) norepinephrine or dobutamine infusion titrated to desirable BP and HR; (3) milrinone, 50 μg/kg IV over 10-min period, then 0.375–0.75 μg/kg/min based on hemodynamic status Electrical pacing and IABP in refractory cases

L-type calcium-channel antagonists	Block L-type voltage-sensitive calcium channels, thereby decreasing calcium entry into myocardial and vascular smooth muscle cells Decrease pancreatic insulin release and increase insulin resistance	Bradyarrhythmias (verapamil and diltiazem) Hypotension Hyperglycemia	ECG No specific tests	10% calcium chloride, 10–20 mg/kg (0.1–0.2 mL/kg) IV; can repeat once. If BP improves, continuous infusion at 0.2–0.5 mL/kg/hr (20–50 mg/kg/hr) Ionized Ca^{2+} levels should not exceed 2× normal (severe cases will be refractory to calcium therapy) Glucagon, high-dose insulin and dextrose, catecholamines, and milrinone (as for β-adrenergic antagonists)
Cardiac glycosides, including digoxin, bufadienolides (toxic toad venom), or cardenolides (e.g., oleander, lily of the valley, dogbane)	Inhibits Na^+,K^+-ATPase Decreased CNS sympathetic output Decreased baroreceptor sensitivity Increased vagal acetylcholine discharge	Bradyarrhythmias including second- and third-degree AV block and asystole Ventricular ectopy, tachycardia, fibrillation Junctional tachycardia, paroxysmal atrial tachycardia with block Weakness, visual disturbances, nausea, vomiting	Serum digoxin level Serum potassium (hyperkalemia occurs in acute poisoning; hypokalemia may be present in chronic poisoning), magnesium, and creatinine levels	Correct hypokalemia and hypomagnesemia; do not give calcium Digoxin-specific antibody fragments (Fab) indicated if patient has hemodynamically significant arrhythmias, serum potassium ≥5 mg/L, Mobitz II or third-degree AV block, ingestion of bufadienolide- or cardenolide-containing agents, or renal insufficiency *(1) Empirical dose* Chronic: 2–5 vials Acute: 10–20 vials *(2) Calculated dose* Chronic: number of vials = 2 × serum digoxin level (ng/mL) × 5.6 × weight (kg)/1000 Acute: number of vials = 2 × oral digoxin dose (mg) × 0.8
Cyclic antidepressants	Myocardial sodium- and potassium-channel blockade Blockade of α-adrenergic and cholinergic muscarinic receptors Inhibition of norepinephrine re-uptake	Decreased level of consciousness (can develop rapidly), myoclonus, seizures, coma Anticholinergic toxidrome (see Table 111–1) Sinus tachycardia, ventricular conduction delays, ventricular arrhythmias, asystole Hypotension	Serum levels not helpful in management	Intermittent IV boluses of $NaHCO_3$ (1 mEq/kg) to maintain arterial pH at 7.5 because acidemia can worsen cardiovascular complications Intubation and neuroparalytic drugs may be useful to ameliorate acidemia from muscular hyperactivity while seizures are being treated Contraindicated drugs: types IA and IC antiarrhythmic agents, physostigmine, flumazenil

Continued

TABLE 111–3 PATHOPHYSIOLOGY, CLINICAL EFFECTS, AND MANAGEMENT OF SPECIFIC DRUGS AND TOXICANTS—cont'd

Drug or Toxicant	Pathophysiology	Clinical Effects	Laboratory	Specific Therapy
Ethylene glycol/methanol (e.g., antifreeze, window cleaners, camping stove fuels)	*Ethylene glycol*—toxic metabolites produce cytotoxicity in CNS, kidneys, lungs, heart, liver, muscles; metabolic acidosis is due to glycolate accumulation; oxalate complexes with calcium, so hypocalcemia can develop *Methanol*—metabolized to formic acid, which is responsible for the metabolic acidosis and inhibition of cytochrome *aa_3*; target organs include retina, optic nerve, CNS	*Ethylene glycol* CNS depression, cerebral edema, seizures Anion gap metabolic acidosis Renal failure with acute tubular necrosis Pulmonary edema Myositis *Methanol* Nausea, vomiting Cerebral edema, hemorrhage, infarcts Anion gap metabolic acidosis Visual disturbances, papilledema, hyperemic optic disc, nonreactive pupils	Serum ethylene glycol and methanol levels Levels may be low or undetectable if significant metabolism has occurred *Ethylene glycol*—serum calcium, creatinine, and BUN levels; examine urine for calcium oxalate crystals	*Both* Fomepizole (which inhibits alcohol dehydrogenase and blocks the formation of toxic metabolites): 15-mg/kg IV loading dose, then 10 mg/kg IV for 5 doses during the next 48 hours, then 15 mg/kg for subsequent doses; interval dosing is q12h (q4h during hemodialysis with dosing interval adjustments at start and finish); continue until ethylene glycol or methanol is no longer detectable Use of ethanol is no longer recommended Hemodialysis: initiate if level ≥50 mg/dL or metabolic acidosis with end-organ toxicity; continue until acidosis resolves and serum level of ethylene glycol or methanol is undetectable Monitor for cerebral edema with possible herniation *Ethylene glycol* IV calcium for symptomatic hypocalcemia *Methanol* Folinic acid, 50 mg IV q4h until methanol not detectable and acidosis cleared
γ-Hydroxybutyrate (GHB) and its precursors (γ-butyrolactone and 1,4-butanediol [1,4-BD])	Agonist effect on CNS GHB receptors; indirect action with opioid receptors (may increase proenkephalins); metabolized to GABA, interacts with $GABA_B$ receptors Decreases dopamine release	CNS: rapid loss of consciousness, with recovery typical within 2–4 hr; myoclonus (possible seizures) Respiratory depression Bradycardia Nausea, vomiting	No specific tests	Supportive care, including respiratory support as needed Withdrawal resembles sedative-hypnotic withdrawal and can be treated with benzodiazepines or pentobarbital
Lithium	Decreases brain inositol Alters CNS serotonin, dopamine, and norepinephrine Inhibits adenylate cyclases, including those that mediate vasopressin-induced renal concentration and thyroid function	*Chronic toxicity* usually more severe than acute toxicity: Tremor, hyperreflexia, drowsiness, incoordination, clonus, confusion, ataxia, and in severe cases, seizures, coma, death; recovery may take weeks, and CNS deficits may persist	Peak serum levels: *Normal dose* 2–3 hr; up to 5 hr for sustained-release lithium *Acute overdose* Peak may be delayed ≥4–12 hr	Replete intravascular volume, maintain urinary output at 1–2 mL/kg/hr Consider GI decontamination with oral polyethylene glycol electrolyte solution within 1–2 hr after acute overdose of sustained-release drug Hemodialysis‡ in patients with altered mental status, ataxia, seizures, or coma or in patients with mild symptoms in the setting of acute overdose or renal insufficiency

		Sinus node dysfunction, QT prolongation, T wave abnormalities, U waves Nephrogenic diabetes insipidus, hypothyroidism and hyperthyroidism, hypercalcemia, pseudotumor cerebri *Acute toxicity:* nausea, vomiting, diarrhea, and milder neurologic findings		Ineffective or contraindicated therapies include oral activated charcoal, diuretics, and aminophylline
Opioids (e.g., heroin, morphine, oxycodone, fentanyl)	Agonist effect at CNS μ, κ, and δ opioid receptors; result is cell hyperpolarization and decreased neurotransmitter release	CNS depression Respiratory depression Miosis (see Table 111–1) Dextromethorphan increases CNS serotonin and inhibits NMDA receptors, which causes hallucinations Propoxyphene and its metabolite norpropoxyphene block sodium channels and can cause seizures and wide-complex arrhythmias similar to cyclic antidepressants; $NaHCO_3$ treats arrhythmias Seizure risk with tramadol, meperidine, propoxyphene Rapid powerful heroin-like effect when sustained-release oxycodone is crushed before ingestion, snorting, or smoking	Rapid urine drug screens detect morphine and codeine but may not detect semisynthetic and synthetic opioids; some interferents/irrelevants (see Table 111–4)	*Naloxone* 0.4–2 mg IV; can repeat up to 10 mg if no response Continuous infusion for recurrent symptoms or sustained-release opioid ingestion; give 50% of the dose that produces desired effect 15 min after initial effect is obtained, then infuse two thirds of this dose every hour; infusion rate can be increased or decreased to maintain normal respiration and avoid withdrawal symptoms *Contraindicated therapies* Nalmefene and naltrexone should not be used for acute opioid reversal
Organophosphorus compounds and carbamates (e.g., diazinon, mevinphos, fenthion, aldicarb)	Inhibit acetylcholinesterase, thereby resulting in excessive acetylcholine stimulation of nicotinic and muscarinic receptors in the autonomic and somatic motor nervous systems and CNS	*Nicotinic-mediated effects:* tachycardia, mydriasis, hypertension, delirium, coma, seizures, muscle weakness, fasciculations *Muscarinic-mediated effects:* salivation, lacrimation, urination, vomiting, defecation, miosis, bronchorrhea, bronchospasm, bradycardia	Serum (butyrylcholinesterase) or RBC (acetylcholinesterase) activity <50% of normal (see Table 111–6) Clinical recovery occurs before serum cholinesterase levels normalize	*Atropine* 1–2 mg by initial IV bolus, double the dose every 5 min (2 mg, 4 mg, 8 mg, 16 mg, etc.) until achieve drying of bronchial secretions and adequate oxygenation; continuous infusion at 0.2–0.8 mg/kg/hr if needed *Pralidoxime* 1–2 g by IV bolus over 30–60 min, then 500-mg/hr continuous infusion; administer as soon as possible after poisoning; wean after 24–48 hr if patient improved

Continued

TABLE 111–3 PATHOPHYSIOLOGY, CLINICAL EFFECTS, AND MANAGEMENT OF SPECIFIC DRUGS AND TOXICANTS—cont'd

Drug or Toxicant	Pathophysiology	Clinical Effects	Laboratory	Specific Therapy
Salicylates	Inhibit cyclooxygenase; decrease formation of prostaglandins and thromboxane A_2 Stimulate CNS medullary respiratory receptor and chemoreceptor trigger zone Impair platelet function Disrupt carbohydrate metabolism Uncouple oxidative phosphorylation Increase vascular permeability	*Acute toxicity* *Mild:* nausea, vomiting, diaphoresis, tinnitus, decreased hearing, hyperpnea, tachypnea *Moderate/severe:* confusion, delirium, coma, seizures, hyperthermia, ALI; death can occur within hours of an overdose *Chronic toxicity* Same as acute but may not have diaphoresis or vomiting Consider diagnosis in patients with new-onset confusion, anion gap metabolic acidosis, or ALI	Serum salicylate level: toxic ≥30 mg/dL; level ≥100 mg/dL indicates life-threatening toxicity with possible sudden, rapid clinical deterioration; in chronic toxicity, levels may be minimally elevated (>30 mg/dL), and clinical evaluation is more reliable for gauging the degree of toxicity Arterial blood gases: respiratory alkalosis with metabolic acidosis Anion gap metabolic acidosis Prolonged PT and PTT, ketonuria, ketonemia	Multidose activated charcoal q2–3h in acute overdose with progressive symptoms or rising salicylate level Urinary alkalinization to increase renal elimination if level >40 mg/dL (except if ALI, cerebral edema, or renal failure) $NaHCO_3$, 1–2 mEq/kg by IV bolus, followed by infusion of 132–150 mEq in 850 mL of D_5W at 1.5–2.0 × maintenance rate (see Table 111–6); adjust rate to maintain urine pH >7.5 while avoiding blood pH >7.55 Replace potassium Avoid respiratory depression; hypercapnia can worsen acidemia Frequent monitoring of clinical status and salicylate levels is essential to gauge progression of toxicity and need for hemodialysis Hemodialysis if level ≥100 mg/dL regardless of clinical condition or if severe end-organ toxicity (e.g., CNS dysfunction, seizures, ALI, renal failure, severe and ongoing acid-base disorder, regardless of level)
SSRIs/SRIs	Inhibit re-uptake of serotonin SRIs have additional effects (e.g., duloxetine inhibits norepinephrine re-uptake, nefazodone inhibits serotonergic 5-HT2 receptors, trazodone inhibits peripheral α-adrenergic receptors, venlafaxine inhibits norepinephrine and dopamine re-uptake)	Vomiting, blurred vision, CNS depression, tachycardia Seizures and coma rare Torsades de pointes reported with citalopram *Serotonin syndrome:* clonus, agitation, tremor, diaphoresis, hyperreflexia; hyperthermia, and hypertonicity in severe cases	No specific tests If serotonin syndrome suspected: electrolytes, BUN, glucose, liver enzymes, coagulation panel, blood gases, chest radiograph	Respiratory support as needed Benzodiazepines for agitation or seizures *Serotonin syndrome:* Consider cyproheptadine, 4–8 mg PO q1–4h to a maximum of 32 mg/day Critical care therapies for hyperthermia, rhabdomyolysis, DIC, ARDS, renal and hepatic dysfunction, torsades de pointes

*Rumack BH, Matthew H: Acetaminophen poisoning and toxicity. Pediatrics 1975; 55:871–876. Provides a nomogram to evaluate the potential toxicity of levels drawn more than 4 hours after ingestion. The nomogram is valid only for levels drawn after a single acute ingestion.

†*N*-acetylcysteine can be discontinued in patients with uncomplicated disease after a loading dose plus six maintenance doses if hepatic aminotransferase levels and the INR are normal; otherwise, the full regimen should be administered.

‡Continue hemodialysis until the serum lithium level is less than 1 mEq/L. Recheck the level 8 hours after dialysis, and restart hemodialysis if the level is higher than 1 mEq/L. Repeat this cycle until the serum lithium level remains lower than 1 mEq/L.

ALI = acute lung injury; aPTT = activated partial thromboplastin time; ARDS = acute respiratory distress syndrome; AV = atrioventricular; BP = blood pressure; BUN = blood urea nitrogen; CNS = central nervous system; DIC = disseminated intravascular coagulation; DOB = 4-bromo-2,5-dimethoxyamphetamine; D_5W = 5% dextrose in water; ECG = electrocardiogram; GABA = γ-aminobutyric acid; GI = gastrointestinal; HR = heart rate; IABP = intra-aortic balloon counterpulsation; INR = international normalized ratio; IV = intraveous; MDMA = 3,4-methylenedioxymethamphetamine; Na^+,K^+-ATPase = sodium, potassium adenosine triphosphatase; NAPQI = *N*-acetyl-*p*-benzoquinone imine; NMDA = *N*-methyl-d-aspartate; PMA = paramethoxyamphetamine; PT = prothrombin time; PTT = partial thromboplastin time; RBC = red blood cell; RUQ = right upper quadrant (abdomen); SIADH = syndrome of inappropriate antidiuretic secretion; SRI = serotonin reuptake inhibitor; SSRI = selective serotonin reuptake inhibitor.

TABLE 111–4 QUALITATIVE URINE DRUG SCREENS: CAUSES OF ERRONEOUS RESULTS

Drug/Toxicant	Interferents/Irrelevants*	Comments
Amphetamines	Chlorpromazine, ephedrine/pseudoephedrine, desoxyephedrine, *Ephedra* sp, mexiletine, phenylephrine, phenylpropanolamine, selegiline	Vicks nasal inhaler (desoxyephedrine) and selegiline also cause positive GC-MS findings; chiral confirmation is required. Interferents in older assays include labetalol and ranitidine
Benzodiazepines	Oxaprozin—false-negative result	Poor detection of parent drugs with absent or low concentration of oxazepam metabolite, e.g., alprazolam, lorazepam, triazolam
Cocaine	Coca leaf teas	Urine is must reliable for detecting true positives
Opiates/opioids	Poppy seeds, ofloxacin, rifampin	Does not detect semisynthetic or designer opioids (e.g., fentanyls, meperidine, methadone, propoxyphene)
Phencyclidine	Dextromethorphan, diphenhydramine, ketamine, thioridazine, venlafaxine	
Tetrahydrocannabinol	Dronabinol, hemp consumables	Positive result is seldom clinically relevant
Tricyclic antidepressants	Cyclobenzaprine, diphenhydramine, phenothiazines, quetiapine	

*Irrelevants are agents causing true-positive but clinically irrelevant results on laboratory screening tests and vary depending on the screening method. Positive screening results should be verified by GC-MS.
GC-MS = gas chromatography–mass spectrometry.

TABLE 111–5 CLINICALLY IMPORTANT QUANTITATIVE DRUG LEVELS

Drug or Toxicant	Levels: Therapeutic	Levels: Toxic
SOURCE: BLOOD/SERUM		
Acetaminophen*	10–30 μg/mL	≥150 μg/mL 4 hr after ingestion†
Carbamazepine	4–12 μg/mL	>15 μg/mL
Carboxyhemoglobin	Nonsmoker: 0.5–1.5% Smoker: 4–9%	>20%‡
Cholinesterase§		
Serum (butyrylcholinesterase)	3100–6500 U/L	<50% of normal value
Red blood cell (acetylcholinesterase)	26.7–49.2 U/g of hemoglobin	<50% of normal value
Digoxin (≥12 hr after dose for long-term therapy)	0.8–2.0 ng/mL	>2.0 ng/mL‖
Ethanol	None measured	>80–100 mg/dL
Ethylene glycol	None measured	>25 mg/dL
Iron	50–175 μg/dL	>350 μg/dL
Lead	<10 μg/dL	>25 μg/dL
Lithium	0.6–1.2 mEq/L	>1.2 mEq/L¶
Methanol	None measured	>20 mg/dL
Methemoglobin	1–2%	>15%
Phenobarbital	15–40 μg/mL	>40 μg/mL
Phenytoin	10–20 μg/mL	>20 μg/mL
Salicylates	≤30 mg/dL	>30 mg/dL
Theophylline	8–20 μg/mL	>20 μg/mL
Valproic acid	50–100 μg/mL	>100 μg/mL
SOURCE: URINE		
Arsenic	None measured	>100 μg/24 hr urine¶
Mercury	None measured	>20 μg/L¶
Thallium	None measured	>200 μg/L¶

*False-positive levels ranging 16 to 28μg/mL have been reported in patients with bilirubin levels greater than 17mg/dL.
†Levels drawn more than 4 hours after ingestion should be plotted on the nomogram provided by Rumack and Matthew (Rumack BH, Matthew H: Acetaminophen poisoning and toxicity. Pediatrics 1975;55:871–876) to assess the potential for toxicity.
‡Lower levels may be toxic in pregnant patients and in those exposed to carbon monoxide for a prolonged time.
§Consult a reference laboratory for normal values; results are assay dependent.
‖Some patients may require levels above the therapeutic range to control symptoms.
¶Lower values may indicate toxicity if appropriate clinical findings are present.

Diagnostic Syndromes

Given the myriad combinations of signs, symptoms, and laboratory findings, making the correct diagnosis in a noncommunicative patient can be daunting. A thorough history from bystanders, friends, and prehospital medical personnel may yield crucial information. Additionally, the diagnostic possibilities can be narrowed by noting a finding to limit that list. For example, consider a patient with sudden loss of consciousness, anion gap metabolic acidosis, and bradycardia without hypoxia. Among the possible causes of anion gap metabolic acidosis (see earlier), agents that can cause sudden loss of consciousness include hydrogen sulfide, cyanide, and severe poisoning with sodium azide; however, the sinus bradycardia, in the absence of acute ischemic injury, is typical only of cyanide poisoning.

Treatment

Rx

Initial Stabilization

Intubation and Respiratory Support

Appropriate airway management should be instituted to correct hypoxemia and respiratory acidosis and to protect against pulmonary aspiration (Fig. 111–2); intubation should be considered if the patient has depressed consciousness and a decreased gag reflex. Rapid-sequence intubation facilitates airway management. Anatomic difficulties should be anticipated in patients with caustic ingestions (hypopharyngeal burns that may perforate), angioedema caused by angiotensin-converting enzyme inhibitor therapy or

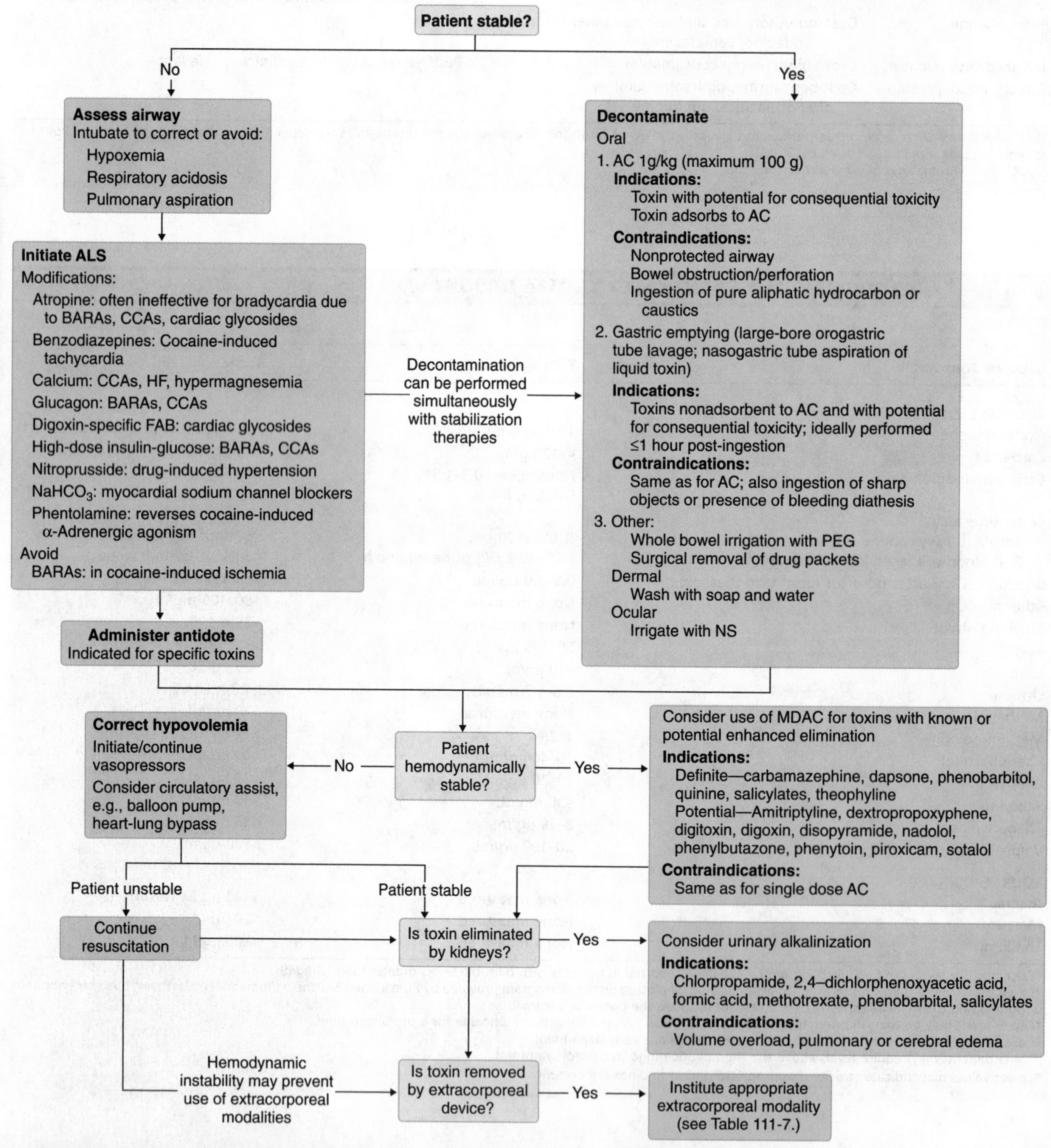

FIGURE 111–2 • Algorithm for the management of acute poisoning. AC = activated charcoal; BARAs = β-adrenergic receptor antagonists; CCAs = L-type calcium-channel antagonists; HF = hydrofluoric acid; MDAC = multidose activated charcoal; NS = 0.9% saline solution; PEG = nonabsorbable polyethylene glycol solution.

Rx

envenomation by some rattlesnakes such as the canebrake (*Crotalus horridus atricaudatus*) and eastern diamondback (*Crotalus adamanteus*), and swelling secondary to direct tissue injury (e.g., huffing Freon, snake bite on the tongue) or secondary to anaphylactoid and anaphylactic reactions. Endotracheal intubation via flexible fiberoptic nasopharyngoscopy may be indicated in these cases. Hypoxemia can occur with toxicants that produce CNS depression, such as antidepressants, barbiturates, sedative-hypnotics, and central α_2-adrenergic receptor agonists (clonidine), or agents causing peripheral neuromuscular impairment, such as nicotine, organophosphorus compounds, strychnine, tetrodotoxin (puffer fish, blue-ringed octopus), botulinum, or envenomation from elapids (coral snake), Mojave rattlesnakes, or certain coelenterates (box jellyfish, Portuguese man-of-war).

Respiratory acidosis can rapidly worsen the toxicities of cyclic antidepressants and salicylates; sedation of these patients should be immediately accompanied by airway support. Intoxicated patients may have an increased risk for pulmonary aspiration because of concomitant CNS depression, attenuated airway reflexes, full stomachs, and delayed gastric emptying.

Succinylcholine can cause prolonged paralysis in patients with organophosphorus poisoning and can exacerbate hyperkalemia from cardiac glycosides, hydrofluoric acid, or rhabdomyolysis. Rhabdomyolysis has been reported with adrenergic agents, doxylamine, phencyclidine, heroin, *Tricholoma equestre* mushrooms, and envenomation by crotaline snakes, scorpions, or widow spiders (*Lactrodectus* species); short-acting nondepolarizing agents, such as vecuronium and rocuronium, are preferable in these cases.

Advanced Life Support

Standard emergency cardiovascular care algorithms (Chapter 62) must be modified for effects caused by specific poisons. Atropine often does not reverse bradycardia secondary to β-adrenergic receptor antagonists, L-type calcium-channel antagonists, or cardiac glycosides. In these cases, more specific therapy with intravenous calcium (calcium-channel antagonists), high doses of glucagon (β-adrenergic receptor antagonists, calcium-channel antagonists), or digoxin-specific Fab antibody (cardiac glycosides) is indicated. High-dose insulin-glucose therapy can successfully reverse myocardial depression and conduction abnormalities in humans poisoned with β-adrenergic receptor antagonists and calcium-channel antagonists. Intravenous sodium bicarbonate may reverse cardiac conduction delays caused by antiarrhythmic drugs with sodium-channel blockade recovery rates of greater than 1 second (Vaughn-Williams classification IA and IC), cocaine, cyclic antidepressants, diphenhydramine, propoxyphene, and quinine. β-Adrenergic receptor antagonists are contraindicated in patients with cocaine-induced myocardial syndromes, but phentolamine can reverse the agonistic effects of cocaine on α-adrenergic receptors. Benzodiazepines can reverse significant sinus tachycardia from sympathomimetic agents. Calcium may also be life-saving in systemic hydrofluoric acid poisoning and severe hypermagnesemia, and it is indicated for symptomatic hypocalcemia caused by ethylene glycol toxicity. Drug-induced hypertension may be transitory; nitroprusside should be used if treatment is clinically indicated. In patients with toxicant-induced circulatory collapse refractory to maximal therapy, including vasopressors, circulatory assist devices may support the patient until sufficient toxicant is eliminated (Chapter 108).

Decontamination

Activated Charcoal

Single-dose activated charcoal without prior gastric emptying is the preferred method for ingestion of substances that have the potential to cause moderate to life-threatening toxicity and that are known to adsorb to activated charcoal. The absence of clinical signs and symptoms does not preclude administering activated charcoal because drug absorption and toxicity can be delayed. Activated charcoal can also be administered when the ingested toxicant cannot be identified but significant toxicity is a concern. Activated charcoal consists of pyrolysis products that have been specially cleaned to produce an internal pore structure to which substances can reversibly adsorb, thus preventing their absorption by the gastrointestinal tract. Activated charcoal can be administered with antiemetic drugs or given through a nasogastric tube, when necessary. The oral dose is approximately 1 g/kg body weight, with a maximum single dose of 100 g. Efficacy in preventing toxicant absorption declines with time, so activated charcoal should be given as soon as possible after ingestion. Activated charcoal should not be used in patients with CNS depression until the airway is secure to minimize aspiration; the patient's head should also be elevated unless contraindicated. Activated charcoal is contraindicated in patients with a perforated bowel, functional/mechanical bowel obstruction, ingestion of a pure aliphatic hydrocarbon such as gasoline or kerosene (no benefit and increased risk for aspiration), and ingestion of caustic acid and alkali (no benefit and obscures endoscopy). Certain agents, such as lithium, iron, metals, and ethanol, do not adsorb significantly to activated charcoal but also do not preclude its use if the patient has concomitantly ingested toxicants that do adsorb to activated charcoal. Pulmonary aspiration and bowel obstruction from inspissated activated charcoal are the most common complications; both occur more frequently when multidose activated charcoal is administered but can be avoided by withholding treatment in patients who have suboptimal bowel function or decreased fecal elimination.

Gastric Emptying

Two methods of gastric emptying, syrup of ipecac and orogastric lavage via a large-bore tube, are no longer routinely used. Both are relatively ineffective therapies that potentially increase the risk for aspiration. One prospective study of gastric emptying showed clinical benefit in a few overdose patients who were obtunded and underwent lavage within 1 hour of ingestion, but other studies have shown no benefit of gastric emptying, either by lavage or by syrup of ipecac, when compared with the use of activated charcoal alone. Gastric emptying via lavage or rarely by syrup of ipecac may be of benefit and should be performed in patients who have ingested toxicants that do not adsorb to activated charcoal, that are known to produce significant morbidity, or for which aggressive decontamination may offer the best chance for survival (e.g., colchicine, sodium azide, sodium fluoroacetate). Removal of a liquid toxicant, such as ethylene glycol, may be accomplished by aspiration of gastric contents via a nasogastric tube. Contraindications to gastric emptying include those for activated charcoal, a bleeding diathesis, and the ingestion of sharp objects. Placement of an endotracheal tube before gastric lavage may be necessary to protect the airway in patients who have a decreased level of consciousness and impaired gag reflex; major complications of gastric emptying include pulmonary aspiration, esophageal tears and perforations, and laryngospasm (with lavage).

Whole Bowel Irrigation

Whole bowel irrigation with a nonabsorbable polyethylene glycol solution has been recommended for iron and sustained-release medications, for agents not adsorbed to activated charcoal, and for body packers (smugglers who swallow packets of illicit drugs). The most common complication is vomiting, and whole bowel irrigation is contraindicated in patients with bowel perforation, obstruction, hemorrhage, or hemodynamic or respiratory instability. An initial dose of 500 mL/hr given orally or via nasogastric tube, with titration to 2000 mL/hr as tolerated, is recommended; treatment continues until the rectal effluent clears. Rarely, surgery may be necessary to remove packets in smugglers who have symptoms of drug toxicity; endoscopic removal of these packets should never be attempted because of the risk of packet rupture.

Antidotes

Few toxicants have specific therapies (Table 111–6). Although antidotes may be essential in treating certain toxicants, their use does not preclude the need for ongoing supportive care and, in some cases, extracorporeal elimination.

Text continued on p. 787.

TABLE 111–6 ANTIDOTES AND INDICATIONS FOR USE

Antidote	Indication for Use	Dose*	Treatment End Point	Comments†
Antivenom (equine), crotalid (Crotalidae polyvalent antivenin)‡	Crotalines: rattlesnakes (*Crotalus* sp and *Sistrurus* sp), cottonmouth (*Agkistrodon* sp), copperhead (*Agkistrodon* sp)	Based on severity of envenomation: *Mild:* none *Moderate:* 10–20 vials *Severe:* 20–40+ vials	Halt in progression of circumferential and proximal swelling Resolving systemic effects	Dosing based on severity of envenomation. Adverse effects include urticaria, bronchospasm, hypotension, serum sickness (delayed)
Antivenom, elapid‡	Eastern *(Micrurus fulvius fulvius)* and Texas *(Micrurus fulvius tenere)* coral snakes	3–5 vials, administer prophylactically for suspected bite; repeat for persistent or worsening clinical condition	Unknown Neurologic effects may not resolve with antivenom polyvalent antivenin	Decision to administer in asymptomatic patient is based on bite history. Coral snakes must chew to envenom and usually require forcible removal. Be prepared to manage airway despite antivenom therapy Same adverse effects as Crotalidae
Antivenom (Fab)‡	Crotalines	4–6 vials, repeat for persistent or worsening clinical condition. Repeat doses of 2 vials at 6, 12, and 18 hr after initial antivenom dose(s) are recommended*	Halt in progression of circumferential and proximal swelling Resolving systemic effects	Better safety profile than equine-derived antivenom Repetitive dosing indicated for recurrent soft tissue swelling
Antivenom, *Latrodectus* (equine)‡	Black widow spider (*Latrodectus* sp)	1 vial diluted in 100 mL of NS, infuse over period of 1 hr; can repeat	Resolution of symptoms, vital signs normal	Dilution and slow infusion rate are **critical** to avoid anaphylactoid reaction. Indications include severe pain unresponsive to opioids and severe hypertension. Serum sickness can occur. IV calcium ineffective
Antivenom, scorpion (goat)‡	Scorpions (*Centruroides* sp)	1 vial diluted in 100 mL of NS, infuse over period of 1 hr; can repeat	Resolution of pain and systemic symptoms, vital signs normal	Available only in Arizona
Atropine	Carbamates Nerve agents Organophosphorus compounds	2 mg IV; double the dose every 5 min to achieve atropinization	Cessation of excessive oral and pulmonary secretions is best indication of atropinization	Doubling of the dose every 5 min (e.g., 2 mg, 4 mg, 8 mg, 16 mg) estimated to achieve atropinization within 30 min
Calcium§	Calcium-channel antagonists	Calcium chloride 10%, 20–50 mg (0.2–0.5 mL)/kg/hr	Reversal of hypotension; may not reverse bradycardia	*All indications:* Monitor ionized calcium levels. IV extravasation causes tissue necrosis especially with calcium chloride. Can administer faster than stated rates for immediate life-threatening conditions Taper infusions and monitor for relapse of toxicity when discontinuing therapy Calcium chloride contains three times more elemental calcium than calcium gluconate does *Calcium-channel antagonists:* may be ineffective in severe toxicity

	Hydrofluoric acid	*Systemic toxicity:* Calcium gluconate 10%, 1–3 g (10–30 mL) per dose IV over 10-min period. Repeat as needed every 5–10 min	Reverse life-threatening manifestations of hypocalcemia and hyperkalemia	Can dilute and give intra-arterially or IV with a Bier block for extremity exposures and burns
	Hyperkalemia (except cardiac glycosides)	Calcium gluconate 10%, 1 g (10 mL) per dose IV over 10-min period Repeat as needed every 5–10 min	Reversal of myocardial depression and conduction delays	*Cardiac glycosides:* may precipitate ventricular arrhythmias
	Hypermagnesemia	Calcium gluconate 10%, 1–2 g (10–20 mL) per dose IV over 10-min period. Repeat as needed every 5–10 min	Reversal of respiratory depression, hypotension, and cardiac conduction blocks	Simultaneous therapies to increase magnesium elimination should be instituted
	Hypocalcemia, e.g., ethylene glycol	Calcium gluconate 10%, 0.5–1.0 g (5–10 mL) per dose over 10-min period. Repeat as needed every 10 min	Reversal of tetany	Correct symptomatic hypocalcemia; avoid excessive administration that may increase production of calcium oxalate crystals in ethylene glycol poisoning
Cyanide antidote kit Amyl nitrite Sodium nitrite Sodium thiosulfate	Cyanide	Amyl nitrite: 0.3-mL pearls, crush and inhale over 30-sec period Sodium nitrite 3%: 10 mL IV over 10-min period Sodium thiosulfate 25%: 50 mL IV over 10-min period	Resolution of lactic acidosis and moderate to severe clinical signs and symptoms: seizures, coma, dyspnea, apnea, hypotension, bradycardia	Coordinate amyl nitrite with continued oxygenation and give only until sodium nitrite infusion is begun; nitrites may produce hypotension and excess methemoglobinemia; sodium nitrite dose must be adjusted if patient has hemoglobin <12 g/dL. Sodium thiosulfate dosing can be repeated
Deferoxamine	Iron	15 mL/kg/hr IV *Mild to moderate:* Administer for 6–12 hr *Severe toxicity:* Administer 24 hr on, 12 hr off, 12 hr on. Continue 12 hr off, 12 hr on for ongoing toxicity	Resolution of clinical signs and symptoms. Do not use urine color, which is an unreliable marker for iron clearance	Indications: symptomatic patients with lethargy, severe abdominal pain, hypovolemia, acidosis, shock; any symptomatic patient with peak serum iron level >350 µg/dL; prolonged therapy can cause pulmonary toxicity. Initial therapy of 15 mg/kg/hr IV should not exceed 24 hr. If further deferoxamine required, 12-hr drug-free intervals should be alternated with 12-hr infusions of deferoxamine
Digoxin-specific antibody fragments (Fab)	Digoxin Digitalis Other cardiac glycosides, e.g., bufodienalides (*Bufo* toads), oleander	*Unknown digoxin dose or serum level or for plant/toad source:* Acute toxicity—20 vials; chronic toxicity—6 vials *Digoxin dose known:* number of vials = mg ingested × 0.8 ÷ 0.5 *Digoxin serum level known*: number of vials = serum level (ng/mL) × weight (kg) ÷ 100	Resolution of hyperkalemia, symptomatic bradydysrhythmias, ventricular arrhythmias, Mobitz II or third-degree heart block	Each vial contains 38 mg of Fab that binds 0.5 mg of digoxin or digitoxin Monitor ECG and potassium levels. Digoxin serum levels unreliable after antidote administered unless test is specific for *free* serum digoxin

Continued

TABLE 111–6 ANTIDOTES AND INDICATIONS FOR USE—cont'd

Antidote	Indication for Use	Dose*	Treatment End Point	Comments†
Dimercaprol (BAL)	Arsenic Lead Mercury, elemental and inorganic	*Arsenic:* 3–5 mg/kg IM every 4 hr *Lead:* 75 mg/m^2 (4 mg/kg) IM every 4 hr for 5 days *Inorganic mercury:* 3–5 mg/kg IM every 4 hr for 2 days, then 2.5–3 mg/kg IM every 6 hr for 2 days followed by every 12 hr for 1 to 3 days	*Arsenic:* 24-hr urinary arsenic <50 μg/L *Lead:* encephalopathy resolved, blood lead level <100 μg/dL, and succimer therapy can be started *Mercury, elemental and inorganic:* 24-hr urinary mercury <20 μg/L	Maximum adult dose is 3 g/day BAL started 4 hr before initiation of concomitant $CaNa_2EDTA$ for lead encephalopathy Dosing not well established for arsenic and elemental or inorganic mercury toxicity. Not used for organic mercury poisoning Adverse effects: painful injections, fever, diaphoresis, agitation, headache, salivation, nausea/vomiting, hemolysis in G6PD-deficient patients, chelation of essential metals. Check essential metal levels if chelation prolonged Succimer is replacing BAL for many indications except lead encephalopathy Treatment end points for arsenic and mercury include improving clinical condition
Edetate calcium disodium ($CaNa_2EDTA$)	Lead	1500 mg/m^2/24 hr by continuous infusion	Treat for 5 days, followed by 2-day hiatus; repeat until encephalopathy resolved, lead level <100 μg/dL, and succimer therapy can be started	Use in patients with lead encephalopathy or lead level >100 μg/dL. Administer BAL 4 hr before initiating $CaNa_2EDTA$ Hydrate patient and establish good urinary output before starting therapy Avoid thrombophlebitis by diluting in NS or D_5W to a concentration ≤0.5% Substitution of Na_2EDTA can cause fatal hypocalcemia
Flumazenil	Benzodiazepines Venlafaxine	0.1 mg/min IV to a total dose of 1 mg	Reversal of respiratory depression	Limit use to reversal of inadequate respiration in benzodiazepine-toxic patients; increases intracranial pressure and risk for seizures in presence of underlying seizure disorder or ingestion of seizure-producing toxicants Monitor for resedation up to 2 hr after last dose
Folinate (tetrahydrofolic acid [leucovorin])	Methanol Methotrexate	*Methanol:* 50 mg IV every 4 hr *Methotrexate:* 100 mg/m^2 IV every 6 hr	*Methanol:* methanol undetectable, metabolic acidosis cleared *Methotrexate:* serum level $<1 \times 10^{-8}$ mol/L	Essential therapy for both toxicants *Methotrexate*: large ingestions may require increased dose

Fomepizole	Ethylene glycol Methanol	**Dose amount** *Dose 1:* 15 mg/kg IV *Doses over next 48 hours:* 10 mg/kg IV *All subsequent doses:* 15 mg/kg IV **Dose timing** Every 12 hr, except when HD performed*:* *(1) HD initiation*—½ next dose if more than 6 hr since last dose; *(2) HD ongoing*—every 4 hr *(3) End of HD* (based on time of last dose)—<1 hr, no dose; 1–3 hr, ½ next dose; >3 hr, next dose	*For both:* serum level <20 mg/dL and metabolic acidosis resolved	Start immediately if toxic alcohol suspected without waiting for confirmatory levels The dose amount is not affected by the interval timing of the doses
Glucagon	β-Adrenergic receptor antagonists Calcium-channel antagonists	Bolus of 3.5–5 mg IV; can repeat to achieve clinical effect, then infusion of 1–10 mg/hr	Reversal of hypotension and bradycardia; taper infusion	Can precipitate vomiting; be prepared to protect airway. Mild hyperglycemia occurs Maximum dosing amounts unknown; bolus doses up to 30 mg reported Duration of effect is 15 min; thus infusion must be started immediately
Insulin-glucose	Calcium-channel antagonists β-Adrenergic receptor antagonists	Regular insulin, 1 U/kg bolus, followed by 0.5–1 U/kg/hr. Titrate 50% dextrose IV to avoid hypoglycemia	Reversal of myocardial depression	Beneficial in case series and reports. Initiate if glucagon and vasopressor/inotropic drugs fail to reverse myocardial depression. More effective if used before onset of cardiogenic shock Monitor glucose and potassium; hypoglycemia can occur during and after therapy Hyperglycemia results from toxicant-induced insulin resistance, and initial dextrose requirements may be less than anticipated. Recovery may be heralded by normalization of glucose levels with increased dextrose required to avoid hypoglycemia
Hyberbaric oxygen (HBO)	Carbon monoxide Experimental: carbon tetrachloride, cyanide, hydrogen sulfide	3.0 atm pressure for 70 min (30 min O_2, 5 min air, 30 min O_2, 5 min air), then 2.0 atm for 65 min (30 min O_2, 5 min air, 30 min O_2), then "surface" to 1.0 atm	One treatment	*Carbon monoxide:* treatment protocols may vary slightly HBO indicated for coma, neurologic symptoms/signs, chest pain, arrhythmias, hypotension, pregnancy, or acidosis, regardless of carboxyhemoglobin level Second treatment rarely administered (controversial) *Experimental indications:* treatment protocols not established
Methylene blue	Methemoglobin-producing agents	1–2 mg/kg body weight (0.1–0.2 mL/kg) of 1% methylene blue is administered over period of 5 min; repeat dose for persistent or recurrent symptoms or signs	Resolution of dyspnea and altered mental status	Use if patient is symptomatic (i.e., dyspneic, altered mental status) Maximum dose should not exceed 7 mg/kg (0.7 mL/kg) Contraindicated in G6PD-deficient patients; may cause hemolysis Some toxicants, e.g., dapsone, may require prolonged therapy

Continued

TABLE 111–6 ANTIDOTES AND INDICATIONS FOR USE—cont'd

Antidote	Indication for Use	Dose*	Treatment End Point	Comments†
N-acetylcysteine (NAC)	Acetaminophen Experimental: carbon tetrachloride, chloroform, pennyroyal oil	*Oral:* *Load*—140 mg/kg *Maintenance* (starting 4 hr after load)—70 mg/kg every 4 hr *IV:* *Load*—150 mg/kg over 1-hr period *Maintenance infusion*—12.5 mg/kg over 4-hr period, then 6.25 mg/kg as continuous infusion	Administer 24 hr of NAC and repeat AST and APAP levels: AST normal, APAP not detected—stop NAC AST normal, APAP detected—continue NAC for 12 hr, reassess AST and APAP levels AST elevated, continue NAC for total of 72 hr of therapy If INR <2.0—stop NAC If INR ≥2.0 or severe hepatotoxicity present—continue NAC until INR <2.0	Most effective if initiated within 8 hr after ingestion; may be started at any time after ingestion and is beneficial in severe hepatotoxic states. Use IV in patients unable to tolerate PO or with severe hepatotoxicity. The dose and timing differ from the oral regimen Dosage and administration of FDA-approved IV formulation must be altered in patients with hepatotoxicity Treatment end points simplified for ease of use INR result not valid indicator if FFP recently administered
Naloxone	Opioids	*Bolus:* 0.4–2 mg via IV, sublingual injection, or endotracheal instillation; 0.4–0.8 mg SC *Continuous infusion:* Establish bolus dose required to reverse respiratory depression Begin infusing two thirds of reversal dose every hour and titrate to maintain adequate respirations Rebolus with half of reversal dose 15 min after reversing respiratory depression	*Initial:* reversal of respiratory depression with resolution of hypoxia and hypercapnia *Final:* resolution of CNS and respiratory depression	Preventilate patients with respiratory depression by bag-valve mask or intubation before administration. Use smaller doses in opioid-dependent patients. Some opioids (e.g., propoxyphene, pentazocine, fentanyls) may require larger doses of naloxone; use continuous infusion for recurrent symptoms and prolonged action of some formulations, e.g., sustained-release morphine, methadone Resedation can occur Do not use nalmefene or naltrexone to reverse acute toxicity
Octreotide	Sulfonylureas	50 mg SC every 12 hr	Resolution of hypoglycemia and dextrose not required	Maintain dextrose infusion as needed
Physostigmine	Anticholinergic agents, e.g., diphenhydramine, jimsonweed (*Datura* sp), scopolamine	1–2 mg IV over 5-min period, can repeat once if no effect	Reversal of anticholinergic effects	Duration of effect is 60–90 min. Benzodiazepine used for subsequent treatment of agitation and seizures; additional physostigmine used rarely (e.g., refractory seizures or agitation) Adverse effects include seizures, excessive oral secretions, and bradyarrhythmias; contraindicated in cyclic antidepressant toxicity

Pralidoxime	Organophosphorus compounds Nerve agents—sarin, VX	1–2 g IV in NS over period of 30–60 min, followed by continuous infusion of 500 mg/kg/hr	Resolution of signs and symptoms and atropine no longer required	Can give initial dose over 2-min period for life-threatening clinical effects Administer early when diagnosis known or strongly suspected Efficacy variable, depending on the organophosphate Fat-soluble organophosphates may require prolonged treatment
Pyridoxine	Ethylene glycol (theoretical efficacy)	50 mg IV	One dose	Efficacy theoretical
	Isoniazid Monomethylhydrazine mushrooms	5 g IV, repeat for refractory seizures	Resolution of seizures	Pyridoxine may stop seizures, but patient can remain comatose (isoniazid, mushrooms); use benzodiazepines and phenobarbital concomitantly to manage seizures Other dosing regimens include 1 g IV for each gram of isoniazid ingested Excessive dosing can cause neuropathy
Sodium bicarbonate ($NaHCO_3$)	Reversal of myocardial sodium-channel blockers, e.g., cyclic antidepressants, cocaine, propoxyphene, sodium-channel–blocking antiarrhythmics with $\tau_{recovery}$ >1 sec, piperidine phenothiazines (thioridazine, mesoridazine)	1–2 mEq $NaHCO_3$/kg via intermittent bolus; repeat as needed	Narrowing of prolonged QRS, resolution of ventricular arrhythmias, reversal of hypotension	Monitor blood pH (optimal pH approximately 7.50); avoid pH >7.55
	Altered tissue distribution/enhanced elimination: salicylates; may be used in chlorophenoxy herbicides, chlorpropamide, formic acid, methotrexate, phenobarbital	1–2 mEq $NaHCO_3$/kg, followed by 3 ampules (150 mL) $NaHCO_3$ (44 mEq per 50 mL) in 850 mL of D_5W, infused at 2–3 times normal maintenance fluid rate		Monitor urinary pH hourly, adjust infusion to maintain urine pH of 7.5–8.0 (avoid blood pH >7.55); monitor ABGs Maintain normokalemia

Continued

TABLE 111–6 ANTIDOTES AND INDICATIONS FOR USE—cont'd

Antidote	Indication for Use	Dose*	Treatment End Point	Comments†
Succimer (DMSA)	Arsenic Lead Mercury, all forms	10 mg/kg per dose every 8 hr for 5 days, followed by every 12 hr for 14 days. Drug holiday for 2 wk, repeat if treatment end point not reached	*Arsenic:* 24-hr urinary arsenic less than 50 μg/L *Lead:* resolution of encephalopathy, gastrointestinal symptoms, neuropathy, nephropathy, arthralgias, and myalgias and blood lead level <70 μg/dL *Mercury, elemental and inorganic:* 24-hr urinary mercury <20 μg/L *Mercury, organic:* end point not well established	Oral chelator; adverse effects include rash, transient AST and alkaline phosphatase elevations, and gastrointestinal distress; minimal chelation of essential metals occurs Dosing for arsenic and mercury not well established Therapeutic end point for organic mercury not established; neurotoxicity not responsive to chelation therapy. Suggest chelation until blood mercury level within normal value range for reference laboratory
Vitamin K	Anticoagulants, e.g., warfarin, long-acting anticoagulant rodenticides (LAARs)	*Subcutaneous*—AquaMEPHYTON (K_1), 10–25 mg, repeat every 6–12 hr until oral vitamin K_1 started *Oral*—25–50 mg every 6 hr; larger doses may be required	INR is normal 48–72 hr after stopping vitamin K_1 therapy. Can also monitor factor VII activity	Anaphylactoid reaction can occur with IV administration Severe bleeding may also require FFP or factor concentrates Base decision to treat on finding of elevated INR; do not administer prophylactic vitamin K_1 Oral therapy has been required for months with LAAR poisoning because of lipophilicity of toxicant with slow body clearance

*Dose concentrations and infusion times not given. Drug dosages may require adjustment in patients with renal or hepatic failure.
†Standard critical care therapies also required to treat many intoxications.
‡Administer antivenom in a monitored setting; antivenom must be reconstituted and then diluted; initially infuse at a rate of 2 to 5 mL/hr, and double the infusion rate every 5 minutes as tolerated to administer antivenom over a 1-hour period.
§Ten percent calcium chloride solution = 100 mg/mL (27.2 mg/mL elemental calcium); 10% calcium gluconate solution = 100 mg/mL (9 mg/mL elemental calcium).
ABG = arterial blood gas; APAP = acetyl-*para*-aminophenol (acetaminophen); AST = aspartate aminotransferase; BAL = British antilewisite; CNS = central nervous system; DMSA = 2,3-dimercaptosuccinic acid; D_5W = 5% dextrose in water; ECG = electrocardiogram; FDA = Food and Drug Administration; FFP = fresh-frozen plasma; G6PD = glucose-6-phosphate dehydrogenase; HD = hemodialysis; IV = intravenous; IM = intramuscular; INR = international normalized ratio; NS = normal saline; $\tau_{recovery}$ = drug blockade recovery rate; SC = subcutaneous.

TABLE 111–7 COMMON TOXICANTS REMOVED BY HEMODIALYSIS

Toxicant	Indications	Comments
Ethylene glycol	Serum level ≥50 mL/dL or lower levels with concomitant metabolic acidosis and evidence of end-organ toxicity	May not be required in a patient with normal creatinine clearance and acid-base status who is receiving fomepizole
Lithium*	Clinical indications	Clinical indication is CNS toxicity (e.g., decreased mental status, ataxia, coma, seizures)
Methanol	Serum level ≥50 mL/dL or lower levels with concomitant metabolic acidosis and evidence of end-organ toxicity	Usually required because of slow elimination half-life in presence of fomepizole (mean, 52 hr; range, 22–87 hr), even in patients with no metabolic acidosis or evidence of end-organ toxicity
Phenobarbital	Clinical indications	Rarely necessary except when the patient is hemodynamically unstable despite aggressive support
Salicylates	*Acute toxicity:* serum level ≥100 mL/dL or <100 mg/dL in the presence of a clinical indication *Chronic toxicity:* any clinical indication	Serum protein binding decreases with increasing toxic levels, increasing the amount of free salicylate available for HD removal; clinical indications are one or more of the following: altered mental status, seizures, pulmonary edema, intractable acidosis, renal failure
Theophylline	*Acute toxicity:* serum level ≥90 μg/mL or <90 μg/mL plus any clinical indication *Chronic toxicity:* serum level ≥40 μg/dL and not declining despite MDAC; any clinical indication	Clinical indications for HD: seizures, hypotension, ventricular arrhythmias

*Hemodiafiltration removes lithium; clinical benefit with this technique is unknown.
CNS = central nervous system; MDAC = multidose activated charcoal.

Rx

Enhanced Elimination

Three methods are used to accelerate elimination of toxicants or drugs from the body: (1) multiple doses of oral activated charcoal, (2) urinary alkalinization, and (3) extracorporeal removal. A fourth method using the oral ion exchange resins sodium polystyrene sulfonate and cholestyramine has experimentally enhanced the elimination of lithium, digoxin, digitoxin, and organochlorines but has limited clinical usefulness.

Multiple Doses of Oral Activated Charcoal

The rationale for administering multiple doses of oral activated charcoal includes the adsorption of any toxic agent remaining in the gastrointestinal tract (e.g., sustained-release drugs, drugs that retard their absorption); interfering with the enterohepatic and enteroenteric recirculation of toxicants; and enhancing the elimination of drugs with a long half-life, a volume of distribution less than 1.0 L/kg body weight, and low protein binding. The existing evidence shows enhanced elimination of carbamazepine, dapsone, phenobarbital, quinine, salicylates, and theophylline, but multiple doses of activated charcoal may also be effective for amitriptyline, dextropropoxyphene, digitoxin, digoxin, disopyramide, nadolol, phenylbutazone, phenytoin, piroxicam, and sotalol. Whether enhanced elimination translates into decreased morbidity and mortality has not been examined in controlled clinical trials. The usual recommendations are an average dose of 12.5 g of activated charcoal (after the initial dose) administered every 1, 2, or 4 to 6 hours after the previous dose. The contraindications to single-dose activated charcoal also apply to multidose activated charcoal. Reported complications include pulmonary aspiration, bowel obstruction, and fluid and electrolyte imbalance from multiple doses of a simultaneously administered cathartic.

Urinary Alkalinization

Alkalinization of the urine, which increases the renal elimination of weak acids, is used primarily to enhance elimination of salicylates, but elimination of chlorpropamide, 2,4-dichlorophenoxyacetic acid, formic acid, methotrexate, and phenobarbital may be increased with this method. Urinary alkalinization is accomplished by an intravenous bolus of 1 to 2 mEq of sodium bicarbonate per kilogram body weight, followed by three ampules (150 mL) of sodium bicarbonate (44 mEq/50 mL) in 850 mL of 5% dextrose in water infused at two to three times the normal maintenance fluid rate. Urinary pH should be checked hourly, and the infusion should be adjusted to maintain a urine pH of 7.5 to 8.0. Potassium should be administered simultaneously to avoid hypokalemia, which would result in urinary acidification because the distal tubule excretes hydrogen ion in exchange for potassium (Chapter 113). Serum pH should be monitored to avoid excessive alkalemia. Contraindications to this therapy include volume overload and cerebral or pulmonary edema. Urinary acidification is no longer recommended to enhance the elimination of weak bases, such as amphetamines, because of the danger of precipitating tubular myoglobin in patients with rhabdomyolysis.

Extracorporeal Removal

Extracorporeal techniques enhance the elimination of a few drugs and toxicants that exhibit single-compartment kinetics, a volume of distribution less than 1 L/kg, and endogenous clearance of less than 4 mL/min/kg (Table 111–7). For hemodialysis, the toxicant must be water soluble, have a molecular weight less than 500 D, and exhibit low protein binding. For hemoperfusion, the toxicant must adsorb to activated charcoal. For continuous renal replacement therapy, the toxicant must have a molecular weight less than the permeability limit of the filter membrane. Rarely, extracorporeal removal has been used for aminoglycosides, atenolol, bromide, carbamazepine, diethylene glycol, isopropanol, magnesium, metformin, methotrexate, *N*-acetylprocainamide, phenobarbital, procainamide, sotalol, trichloroethanol (chloral hydrate), and valproic acid.

SUGGESTED READINGS

Eddleston M, Buckley NA, Checketts H, et al: Speed of initial atropinisation in significant organophosphorus pesticide poisoning—a systematic comparison of recommended regimens. Clin Toxicol 2004;42:865–875. *Suggests that rapid IV bolus doses of atropine are preferred.*

Isbister GK, Bowe SJ, Dawson A, et al: Relative toxicity of selective serotonin reuptake inhibitors (SSRIs) in overdose. Clin Toxicol 2004;42:277–285. *Among 469 poisoned patients, 14% had the serotonin syndrome, 2% had seizures, and 2.4% were in coma.*

Schmidt LE, Larsen FS: MELD Score as a predictor of liver failure and death in patients with acetominophen-induced liver injury. Hepatology 2007;45: 789–796. *The INR was as good for prognosis.*

112 ELECTRIC INJURY

Basil A. Pruitt, Jr.

ELECTRIC CURRENT INJURY

Definition

The tissue damage caused by electric current ranges from a transient increase in cell membrane permeability to immediate coagulation necrosis of large volumes of tissue. The clinical consequences include disturbances in the physiologic electrical conduction systems, a process that may cause cardiopulmonary arrest; tetanic muscle contractions, with resulting compression fractures of vertebrae; and delayed tissue damage, such as cataract formation.

Epidemiology

As the use of electricity has increased worldwide, the number of electric injuries has increased. The precise incidence of electric injury is unknown, but the National Centers for Health/Centers for Disease Control and Prevention have estimated that 52,000 trauma admissions take place in the United States each year for electric injuries. Four percent of patients admitted to the U.S. Army Burn Center during a recent 20-year period had high-voltage electric injury; at other burn centers, the percentage of admissions related to electric injury has ranged from 0.04 to 6.7%.

Pathobiology

Environmental conditions, duration of contact, pathway of the current, type of current (and if alternating current, the frequency of the current), and voltage all influence the effects of electricity on tissue. Voltage greater than 40 is potentially dangerous, and the likelihood of sudden death and remote tissue injury increases as voltage increases to 1000. Voltages greater than 1000 are considered to be high tension and are associated with immediate severe tissue damage. Alternating current is more dangerous than direct current because of its likelihood of producing cardiac arrest or cessation of respiration and its tetanic effect, which may prevent the patient from breaking contact with the source of electricity. As the frequency of alternating current increases to greater than 60 cps, tissue injury decreases. The path of the current through the body between the points of contact is important in determining tissue damage; a course through the heart or the respiratory center of the brain is especially dangerous. Ventricular fibrillation can be produced by current flow of only 100 mA from a hand to the feet. Rapid separation of a patient from the source of electricity is crucial because tissue damage increases in proportion to the duration of contact. Resistance to current flow at the point of contact is influenced by environmental conditions; dry and thickened palmar or plantar skin is more resistant to the passage of current than is skin moistened by perspiration or other liquid.

Heat is the principal mediator of tissue damage in electric injury, the severity of which is related to voltage and duration of contact. Tissue-specific differences in resistance to the flow of current (neural tissue least; blood vessels, muscle, and skin intermediate; and bone greatest) may explain differences in tissue injury caused by low-voltage current. Because all body tissues and fluids are conductive, the soft tissues between bone and skin can be viewed as a volume conductor. Heat is produced in tissues as a function of voltage drop and current flow per unit of cross-sectional area (i.e., density of the current). The inverse relationship between the density of the current and the tissue's cross-sectional area accounts for the frequency of severe injury to the digits and extremities and the rarity of major injury to the trunk in patients with high-tension electric injury (Fig. 112–1). Contact with less than 1000 V causes injuries that are self-limited because at contact points, where the density of the current is greatest, the skin is severely injured and chars, which results in a rapid increase in resistance and reduction of the passage of current. When the source is greater than 1000 V, arcing is so intense that tissue destruction is increased markedly as relatively constant levels of current are maintained. Arcing, which may occur across the flexor surfaces of joints, can char the skin in these areas and ignite the patient's clothing. After cessation of the flow of current, the heated tissue acts like a volume radiator and cools unevenly, with the superficial portions cooling more rapidly than the deeper portions; deeper tissues are therefore more prone to severe injury.

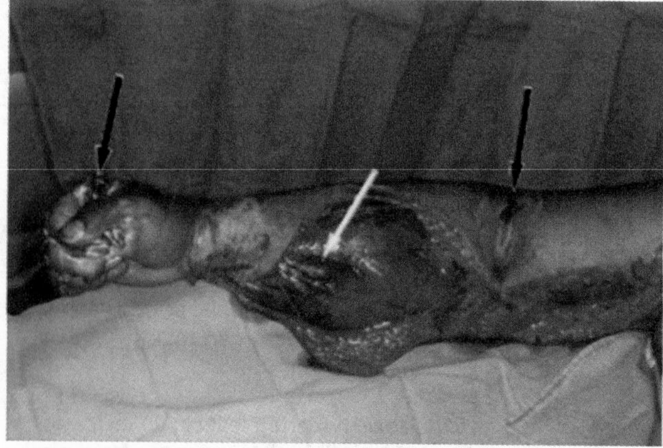

FIGURE 112–1 • Charring at the contact site in the first web space and at the site of arcing in the antecubital space (black arrows) of a victim of electric injury. The fixed flexion deformity of the thumb and other digits is characteristic of severe high-voltage injury to the hand and forearm. The severity of injury is indexed by the marked edema of the forearm muscles bulging above the cut edges of the fasciotomy incision and by the patchy dark discoloration of the muscles of the arm and the forearm, particularly the deeper muscle exposed in the central portion of the forearm incision (white arrow).

Tissue damage can also be caused by low-voltage direct current (i.e., contact with automobile battery terminals or with defective or inappropriately used medical equipment, such as electrosurgical devices, external pacing devices, or defibrillators). Direct current injuries have been reported to be particularly common during laparoscopy with high-voltage coagulation.

Clinical Manifestations

Cardiopulmonary arrest can be caused by low-voltage electric injury but is more common with high-voltage electric injury. Extensive tissue necrosis may also liberate enough potassium to cause cardiac dysfunction. Because cardiac arrhythmias may recur after resuscitation or develop 24 to 48 hours after injury, all patients who have sustained high-voltage electric injury should undergo continuous electrocardiogram (ECG) monitoring for at least 48 hours after the last ECG-documented arrhythmia. Renal failure may occur in patients with high-voltage electric injury if inapparent deep tissue injury with accompanying occult edema results in an underestimation of fluid requirements, inadequate resuscitation, and oliguria. Additionally, the destruction of muscle and red blood cells liberates hemochromes that may precipitate in the renal tubules unless adequate urinary output is maintained (Chapter 121).

Muscle Damage

High-voltage electric injury commonly causes edema beneath the investing fascia of the involved muscle compartments, thereby compromising nutrient blood flow to muscles within the compartments and to distal unburned tissue. Clinical indications for surgical release of intracompartmental pressure by fasciotomy and surgical exploration of a limb include impaired capillary refilling of distal unburned skin or nails, cyanosis of distal unburned skin, stony hardness of a muscle compartment on palpation, and diminished or absent pulsatile flow in the distal arteries as assessed by Doppler ultrasound. Tissue pressures 30 mm Hg or higher above atmospheric pressure, as measured by a catheter placed in the compartment, indicate the need for immediate decompression. If clinical signs are consistent with deep tissue injury but large vessel pulses are intact, arteriography can determine the need for operative intervention, including amputation of the affected limb. "Pruning" of the arterial tree, with a decrease in the density of nutrient branches in the muscles of an involved limb, identifies the level of amputation needed to remove muscle that has been irreversibly damaged. Muscle blood flow of 1 mL/min/100 g of tissue, as determined by xenon 133 "washout," has been proposed as the minimum level required for ultimate tissue viability. In patients with high-voltage electric injury, myoglobinemia and elevation of serum creatine phosphokinase reflect significant muscle damage, and myoglobinuria is a strong predictor of the need for fasciotomy in the first 24 hours after injury.

Neurologic Examination

On admission and at scheduled intervals thereafter, a detailed neurologic examination must be performed on all patients with high-voltage electric injury; all nerve deficits should be documented fully. Central nervous system or peripheral nerve dysfunction may be apparent immediately after electric injury or may appear later. Recovery of function after direct electrical nerve damage is rare. Conversely, spontaneous resolution of immediate and early functional deficits of nerves not injured directly (motor nerves are more sensitive to nondestructive injury than sensory nerves are) is common. A polyneuritic syndrome of relatively late onset can induce deficits in the function of peripheral nerves far removed from the points of electric contact. Direct nerve damage of the spinal cord causes immediate deficits, which are more often transient than deficits of later onset. Delayed-onset spinal cord deficits can be manifested as quadriplegia, hemiplegia, localized nerve deficits with signs of ascending paralysis, transverse myelitis, and even an amyotrophic lateral sclerosis–like syndrome. The cause of delayed paresthesias and nerve dysfunction after electric injury is unknown, but an increase in permeability of the cell membrane and associated loss of cell contents induced by exposure to a millivoltage electric field (electroporation) have been implicated. The greater improvement in neurologic function in children than in adults has been attributed to their greater neurologic plasticity.

Remote Organ Injury

Direct liver injury, focal pancreatic and gallbladder necrosis, and intestinal perforation have been reported after electric injury, but all are uncommon. Delayed hemorrhage from moderate to large blood vessels has been ascribed to an arteritis caused by the electric injury, but this hemorrhage seems to be most closely related to inadequate débridement of injured tissue or to vascular wall necrosis as a consequence of exposure after débridement.

Compression fractures of vertebral bodies may be produced by tetanic contractions of the paraspinous muscles. Fractures of the skull and the long bones of both the upper and lower extremities may be caused by falls after the electric shock.

Delayed Organ Damage

High-voltage electric injury has been associated with the subsequent formation of cataracts, most frequently in patients in whom the contact site was on the head or neck. Cataracts may form rapidly, but they more commonly develop 3 or more years after the injury. Rarely, exfoliative debris may be evident in the anterior chamber of the eye immediately after injury. Cholelithiasis and gastrointestinal dysfunction have been reported after high-voltage injury, but most centers have not noted an increased rate of either of these problems.

Treatment

Rx

Cardiopulmonary arrest must be treated by immediate institution of cardiopulmonary resuscitation (Chapter 62). In patients with high urinary hemochrome concentrations, a urinary output of 75 to 100 mL/hr should be maintained (Chapter 114). If the hemochromes do not clear promptly or the patient remains oliguric despite the administration of resuscitation fluids at more than twice the required rate as estimated on the basis of the extent of the burn and the patient's weight (Chapter 113), 25 g of mannitol should be given as an intravenous bolus and 12.5 g of mannitol should be added to each liter of intravenous fluid until the pigment has cleared from the urine. Hyperkalemia is treated as in any other patient (Chapter 118).

If the electric injury is limited to the skin and subcutaneous tissue, an antibacterial cream such as Sulfamylon burn cream should be applied twice daily to the burned tissue until débridement is performed. The antimicrobial (mafenide acetate) in Sulfamylon readily diffuses into the nonviable tissue to limit microbial proliferation. As soon as resuscitation has restored hemodynamic stability, severely damaged limbs or other areas of tissue necrosis should be surgically explored. The viability of vital structures and the extent of deep tissue damage are assessed to determine the need for amputation. If amputation is not required, all necrotic tissue should be débrided to eliminate the source of hyperkalemia and reduce the risk for infection. It is imperative to examine the periosseous muscles, which may be necrotic because of delayed heat dissipation yet be overlain by more superficial viable muscles. After débridement or amputation, the operative wound should be dressed but not surgically closed, and the patient should be scheduled for re-exploration of the wound 24 to 72 hours later. At that time, residual necrotic tissue is débrided, and the wound is closed by skin grafts, tissue transfer, or the use of biologic dressings, depending on the condition, extent, and site of the wound. Overall, current treatment is associated with a 96% survival rate.

LIGHTNING INJURY

An estimated 300 to 350 persons are struck by lightning each year, and about 30% of these patients die. The duration of a lightning bolt is $^1/_{100}$ to $^1/_{1000}$ of a second, but it may have a voltage of approximately 1 billion V and induce currents ranging from 12,000 to 200,000 A. The temperature in a lightning bolt, which may be 30,000 K, dissipates in a few microseconds.

Clinical Manifestations

Cardiopulmonary arrest, which can be secondary to either asystole or ventricular fibrillation, is common in patients struck by lightning. Cardiopulmonary resuscitation must be instituted immediately; recovery has been reported in some patients who were apparently without life signs for 15 minutes or longer. Although signs of acute myocardial damage may become evident later, persistent or recurrent ECG abnormalities are uncommon. Coma is common immediately after injury and typically resolves in a few hours. Abdominal signs of peritonitis with free air in the peritoneal cavity of a patient struck by lightning should alert one to the possibility of intestinal perforation, which if present must be treated by prompt primary closure. Keraunoparalysis (lightning paralysis), which is characterized by paresthesias and paralysis, usually involves the lower limbs, often develops over a period of several days after lightning injury, is typically associated with vasomotor disorders, and is usually transient. Myoglobinuria is uncommon; when present, it is treated as described earlier for other electric injuries. Tympanic membrane rupture and hearing loss may also be caused by lightning injury. Cutaneous burns of the trunk and proximal areas of the limbs caused by lightning injury typically have a "splashed on" arborescent and spidery appearance and are generally superficial (Fig. 112–2). Small, circular, full-thickness burns of the tips of the toes are also common and have been termed the *tiptoe sign.* Mottling of the skin and other signs of vasoconstriction previously considered to be specific to lightning injury generally resolve with adequate resuscitation.

Treatment

Current treatment, which emphasizes immediate cardiopulmonary resuscitation, has decreased mortality significantly to the point at which two thirds of lightning-injured patients now survive. Persistent nerve deficits and long-term problems are relatively uncommon in survivors.

Prognosis

Cardiopulmonary and fluid resuscitation combined with monitoring of limb tissue pressure and wound care has maximized tissue salvage, reduced renal failure, and increased survival of patients with lightning and high-voltage electric injuries. In a 10-year period, only 28 (22%) of 127 patients admitted to the U.S. Army Burn Center with high-voltage electric injury had permanent neurologic deficits at discharge.

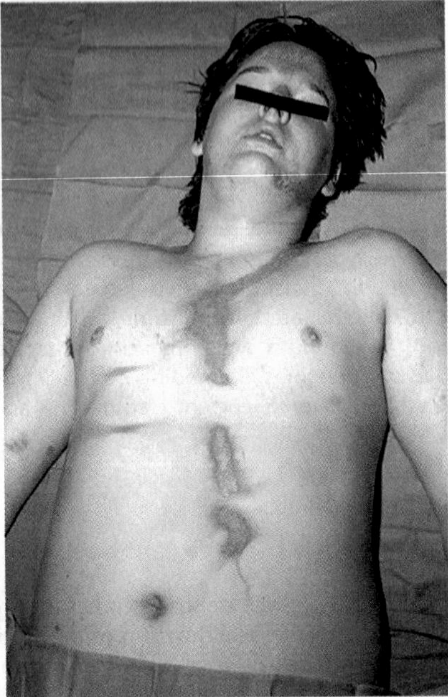

FIGURE 112-2 • The arborescent current markings shown on the face, neck, and anterior aspect of the trunk of this young patient, which are characteristic of lightning injury, healed without need for grafting. Note the focal lesions on the right arm indicating spread of the current that produced the markings on the right anterolateral aspect of the chest wall.

SUGGESTED READINGS

Cancio LC, Jimenez-Reyna JF, Barillo DJ, et al: One hundred ninety-five cases of high-voltage electric injury. J Burn Care Rehabil 2005;26:331–340. *Comprehensive review of current management.*

Maghsoudi H, Adyani Y, Ahmadian N: Electrical and lightning injuries. J Burn Care Res 2007;28:255–261. *A review of more than 200 cases.*

Spies C, Trohman R: Electrocution and life-threatening electrical injuries. Ann Intern Med 2006;145:531–537. *Overview of electrical injuries.*

113 MEDICAL ASPECTS OF TRAUMA AND BURN CARE

Robert H. Demling and Jonathan D. Gates

MEDICAL ASPECTS OF TRAUMA

Epidemiology

Trauma is the third leading cause of death in people of all ages in the United States (Chapter 15), surpassed only by cancer and atherosclerosis. Trauma is the leading cause of death in children, adolescents, and young adults aged 1 to 44 years.

More than 140,000 deaths and twice as many permanent disabilities occur annually in the United States from injuries. Fatal injuries have a trimodal distribution. Half of all fatalities occur within minutes of the injury as a result of massive hemorrhage from the heart, lacerations of large blood vessels, or catastrophic neurologic injury. In such cases there is insufficient time for medical intervention to alter the outcome; the only method to reduce this category of trauma-related morbidity and mortality is prevention and education programs (Chapter 15). Of fatalities, 30% occur within a few hours after injury from airway obstruction, shock, or neurologic dysfunction. This interval represents an opportunity during which appropriate and timely medical or surgical intervention is most likely to influence outcome. Fatalities within this second peak occur as a result of epidural and subdural hematomas, chest injuries, liver lacerations, splenic rupture, pelvic fractures, or the accumulation of multiple injuries resulting in significant blood loss. The third peak of trauma fatalities is due to multisystem organ dysfunction or overwhelming infection weeks later. This delayed systemic response is related to the degree of the initial insult, the individual response to the injury, and the cumulative effect of any additional complications that arise after injury.

Motor vehicle crashes, firearms, and falls are major contributors to injury in the United States. Four million injuries from motor vehicle crashes occur annually and result in 500,000 admissions to the hospital and approximately 42,000 fatalities. About 50% of all traffic deaths in 15- to 34-year-olds are alcohol related (Chapter 31). About 35,000 gun-related deaths, unintentional and intentional, occur annually (Chapter 15). Of all injury deaths, 8% are related to falls, and fall from a height is responsible for a third of all injury-related hospitalizations.

Pathobiology

Mechanism of Injury

Trauma produces a structural or physiologic alteration as a result of an external force, whether it be mechanical, chemical, electrical, or thermal energy. The force that initiated the motion of an object must be absorbed or dissipated in an effort to decelerate that object. When an automobile traveling at a given speed strikes an immobile object, a tremendous amount of energy in the moving vehicle is transmitted to the immobile object and the structure of the vehicle, deforming both until the automobile stops. These same forces are imparted to the occupants of the vehicle with potentially dire consequences. In a head-on impact, the driver continues to move forward until impeded by objects inside the automobile or until the energy is dissipated by the restraint of a seat belt or air bag. Deceleration forces are imparted to individual organs. These same physical principles apply to injury after a fall from a height. Compression, shear, and overpressure from these and other forces injure internal organs.

Penetrating injuries, which are described as either low velocity or high velocity, result from the kinetic energy of the missile. In the case of a bullet discharged from a gun, the tissue immediately contacted by the bullet is crushed to create a permanent cavity. Transfer of energy farther away from the bullet path creates a temporary cavity beyond the boundary of the permanent tract, the so-called blast effect. A simple stab wound from a knife or sharp object is considered a low-velocity injury in which the wound is confined to the tract itself. Virtually no temporary cavity is created, but the consequences may be just as devastating as a high-velocity injury if a vital structure is affected.

Pathophysiology of Injury

Shock (Chapter 107) is an abnormality of the circulatory system that results in inadequate organ perfusion and subsequent failure to deliver sufficient oxygen to maintain aerobic metabolism. Poor peripheral perfusion results in cellular hypoxia and slowing of oxidative phosphorylation, with the accumulation of H^+ ion in the extracellular fluid resulting in metabolic acidosis. The initial step in managing shock associated with trauma is to recognize inadequate organ perfusion. The second step is to identify and treat the probable cause. The four general categories of shock in trauma are hemorrhagic, compressive, neurogenic, and cardiogenic; however, most shock is hypovolemic in nature. Adrenal insufficiency (Chapter 245), anaphylaxis (Chapter 274), and septic shock (Chapter 109) are less common but may occur during the recovery period. The goal of treatment is restoration of cellular and organ perfusion with adequately oxygenated blood volume.

Hemorrhagic Shock

Hemorrhagic shock results from a decline in cardiac filling pressure as blood is lost (Chapter 107). Cardiac output is preserved through compensatory mechanisms when the loss of blood is about 10% of blood volume. Endogenous neurogenic and endocrine responses result in peripheral vasoconstriction and shunting of blood from the nonessential areas of skin, muscle, and abdominal viscera to maintain perfusion to the heart and brain. Cardiac output decreases with a blood volume loss of 20 to 40%, with a resultant decrease in systolic blood pressure. Additional compensatory mechanisms to maintain perfusion pressure in the face of a sudden decrease in intravascular volume result in a shift of proteins and fluids from the extracellular space to the intravascular compartment. The relative decrease in volume and increase in osmolarity of the extracellular space stimulate movement of fluid out of the cells to replace it.

It is imperative to identify a patient in shock or compensated shock. A normal systemic arterial blood pressure or absence of tachycardia may lead an inexperienced physician to believe that the patient is hemodynamically stable when in fact the patient may be in the precarious situation of partially compensated shock. A high index of suspicion and early aggressive diagnostic evaluation and treatment minimize the possibility that occult blood loss may be missed and lead to appropriate volume resuscitation and possible surgical correction.

Compressive Shock

Compressive shock arises when external compression of the lungs or heart from air, fluid, or blood either compromises diastolic filling of the right ventricle or prevents adequate ventilation and oxygenation. The two most notable forms of compressive shock are tension pneumothorax (Chapter 100) and pericardial tamponade (Chapter 77).

In tension pneumothorax, air within the pleural space impedes expansion of the ipsilateral lung and shifts the mediastinum. Compression of the inferior and superior vena cavae leads to inadequate filling of the right atrium and ventricle, which decreases cardiac output. Identification of the injury is paramount; typical findings include absence of breath sounds in the ipsilateral chest, jugular venous distention, and tracheal deviation to the ipsilateral side. Appropriate intervention involves release of air under tension in the hemothorax by means of needle or tube thoracentesis.

Cardiac tamponade occurs because of extrinsic compression of the chambers of the heart from blood in the pericardial space, which is normally a potential space filled with less than 50 mL of pericardial fluid (Chapter 77). An external chest wound that penetrates the pericardium and the heart may create a rent in the pericardium too small to vent the accumulated blood; as a result, blood collects in the noncompliant pericardial sac, and pressure is directed inward into the hollow chambers of the heart. The external compression inhibits diastolic filling of the chambers and reduces stroke volume. Pericardial tamponade should be suspected in patients who have wounds in the vicinity of the precordium and epigastrium, hypotension, tachycardia, jugular venous distention, and muffled heart sounds. Treatment is immediate evacuation of the pericardial space by needle pericardiocentesis, followed by sternotomy or left thoracotomy.

Neurogenic Shock

Complete injury to the cervical or upper thoracic spinal cord may result in sympathetic denervation manifested as loss of vasomotor tone in the periphery. Neurogenic shock should be considered in any trauma patient who is hypotensive but not actively bleeding. Only about 20% of patients with a complete high spinal cord injury have neurogenic shock, however, and patients with incomplete motor or sensory deficits (or both) rarely have hypotension directly caused by neurologic injury.

Cardiogenic Shock

Cardiogenic shock (Chapter 108) implies inadequate peripheral perfusion as a result of pump failure. It may be caused by arrhythmias, valvar dysfunction, or failing myocardial contraction. The latter may be seen with cardiac contusion or ischemic dysfunction of a previously damaged myocardium with marginal reserve.

Diagnosis and Treatment

Rx

An organized approach to a trauma patient is mandatory to avoid confusion or missing life-threatening injury. The standardized response is divided into the primary survey for rapid diagnosis and treatment of life-threatening injuries and the secondary survey for a more complete, in-depth evaluation of the whole patient for definitive therapy.

The initial management of a trauma patient requires immediate intravenous access for volume resuscitation. The type and rapidity of solution delivered are determined by the patient's hemodynamic stability as reflected by the degree of intravascular depletion or blood loss. Four classes of hemorrhage are widely accepted (Table 113–1). Intravenous access also allows the administration of analgesics, sedatives, and antibiotics. The rapidity of volume resuscitation with isotonic crystalloid and blood products is determined by the initial degree or class of shock. The guidelines are based on the "three-to-one" rule, which derives from the empirical observation that most patients in hemorrhagic shock require 300 mL of electrolyte solution for each 100 mL of blood loss because crystalloid equilibrates in the entire extracellular space.

Primary Survey

The primary survey (airway, breathing, circulation) is the same whether the mechanism of injury was blunt, penetrating, or thermal. Evaluation of the airway is paramount. Supplemental oxygen is given to all trauma patients to maximize delivery of oxygen to the periphery. If the patient is hemodynamically unstable or is unable to maintain a patent airway because of mental status changes or airway debris, endotracheal intubation should be performed. There is little role for the use of oral airways or nasal trumpets in a trauma patient. Care must be taken to avoid movement of the cervical spine during intubation so that exacerbation of an undiagnosed cervical spine fracture or ligamentous disruption is avoided. Inability to perform endotracheal intubation in a trauma patient should lead to rapid surgical control of the airway by cricothyroidotomy. Tracheostomy is a poor second choice because it is more time-consuming and potentially bloody, especially if the landmarks are obscured by trauma.

The primary survey should observe the symmetry of chest wall movement, determine whether breath sounds are equal bilaterally and adequate, and assess the chest wall for crepitus, instability, or tenderness. If a tension pneumothorax or massive hemothorax is suspected (and the findings are not caused by intubation of the right mainstem bronchus), a large-bore chest tube is placed in the ipsilateral anterolateral fifth intercostal space. Chest tube insertion is diagnostic and therapeutic. Return of greater than 1500 mL of blood suggests a significant injury within the ipsilateral hemothorax; this magnitude of initial output or ongoing hourly blood loss of 200 to 250 mL through the chest tube may warrant urgent thoracic surgical exploration.

Adequacy of the circulation is determined clinically by noting the presence of carotid, radial, and femoral pulses. Brisk capillary refill,

TABLE 113–1 CATEGORIZATION AND INITIAL TREATMENT OF HEMORRHAGIC SHOCK*

	Class I	Class II	Class III	Class IV
Blood loss (mL)	≤750	750–1500	1500–2000	≥2000
Blood loss (% of blood volume)	≤15	15–30	30–40	≥40
Pulse rate	<100	>100	>120	≥140
Blood pressure	Normal	Normal	Decreased	Decreased
Capillary refill test	Normal	Positive	Positive	Positive
Respiratory rate	14–20	20–30	30–40	>35
Urine output (mL/hr)	≥30	20–30	5–15	Negligible
Mental status	Slightly anxious	Mildly anxious	Anxious and confused	Confused and lethargic
Fluid replacement (3:1 rule)	Crystalloid	Crystalloid	Crystalloid + blood	Crystalloid + blood

*Based on a 70-kg adult.

Rx

as elicited by transient compression of the nail bed, and a warm, well-perfused patient suggest good peripheral perfusion. A patient in extremis may have a barely palpable carotid pulse, mental status changes, and mottled, cold clammy skin. During this evaluation, simultaneous insertion of short, large-caliber intravenous catheters into the antecubital veins is recommended for the initial administration of normal saline or lactated Ringer's solution.

The primary survey should include an evaluation of neurologic function. The Glasgow Coma Scale (Chapter 422) grades the patient's eye movement, best motor response, and best verbal response on a scale from 1 to 5; the score is the sum of the individual results.

The patient should be assessed for all evidence of traumatic injury. This assessment should include an examination of the back with the patient log-rolled under cervical spine precautions.

Secondary Survey

The secondary survey is the head-to-toe physical examination of the patient to evaluate the airway, reassess the adequacy of breathing and circulation, and look for any injuries or underlying conditions that were not immediately apparent during the primary survey. At this stage, pertinent radiographs, blood tests, and other tests (e.g., an electrocardiogram) are obtained, and a Foley catheter is inserted.

Head and Neck

Evaluation of neurologic function should determine whether there is evidence of closed head injury (Chapter 422). Physical examination should assess for skull and facial fractures and eye and ear injuries. The physician should have a low threshold for performing computed tomography (CT) of the head, which is preferred over magnetic resonance imaging in this situation.

Management of penetrating wounds to the anterior aspect of the neck is controversial. The neck is anatomically divided into three zones corresponding to ease of surgical access. Zone I is from the clavicles downward to the thoracic outlet. In a stable patient, injuries in this area require an arteriogram to define the injury and plan the surgical approach; hemodynamically unstable patients should undergo immediate surgical exploration. Zone III extends from the angle of the mandible to the base of the skull. Most patients with injuries in this region are hemodynamically stable. Arteriography, bronchoscopy, esophagoscopy, and sometimes direct laryngoscopy should be performed to evaluate the type and extent of injury. Zone II is located between the other zones, from the cricoid cartilage to the angle of the mandible. Any stab wound in the neck must be evaluated locally to determine whether the platysma muscle has been penetrated; if so, operative exploration is performed. It is controversial whether patients with penetrating wounds deep to the platysma should undergo mandatory neck exploration or nonoperative evaluation with arteriography and diagnostic upper endoscopy and bronchoscopy, with operative intervention reserved for situations when the evaluation reveals pathology. Spiral CT with intravenous contrast material can help define arterial injuries, but angiography remains the "gold standard." Hemodynamically unstable patients should be resuscitated and explored surgically without further testing.

Chest

Life-threatening injuries of the chest include tension pneumothorax, massive hemothorax, cardiac tamponade (see earlier), flail chest, open pneumothorax, and disruption of the thoracic aorta. Flail chest implies an unstable segment of the chest wall as a result of multiple rib fractures. The negative pleural pressure required for inspiration pulls the unstable segment of the chest wall inward while the remainder of the chest moves in the opposite direction. An open pneumothorax implies air entering the pleural space through an external chest wound. The wound should be covered with a partially occlusive dressing, and a chest tube should be inserted to prevent the accumulation of air and the development of tension pneumothorax. Large open chest wounds require endotracheal intubation, operative débridement, chest tube drainage, chest wall stabilization, and closure. Though not usually considered life-threatening, there are a myriad of chest injuries, including simple pneumothorax, pulmonary contusions (Fig. 113–1), rib fractures, and minor to moderate hemothorax, that may play a major role in the duration of lung dysfunction or the need for ventilatory support, or both.

All trauma patients should have a supine chest radiograph taken to examine the lung fields, the mediastinal contour, and the chest wall. Thoracic aortic injury, which is a feared complication of severe acceleration-deceleration injury, results in the immediate death of 90% of persons with this injury. Survivors who reach medical care often have a contained mediastinal hematoma that appears as a widened superior mediastinum or loss of the aortic contour on the chest radiograph, or both (Fig. 113–2). These patients have historically been evaluated by arteriography (Fig. 113–3), but now chest CT is used to screen for this injury. A contained mediastinal hematoma is an unstable condition that demands timely evaluation and possible operative intervention.

Myocardial Injury

Myocardial contusion results from transmission of force to the myocardium in the form of compression, blast, or sudden deceleration. The true incidence is difficult to define given the absence of consensus on a reliable test to identify myocardial contusion. A high degree of suspicion is needed because there are no specific clinical signs of myocardial injury. Sternal fracture, anterior rib fractures,

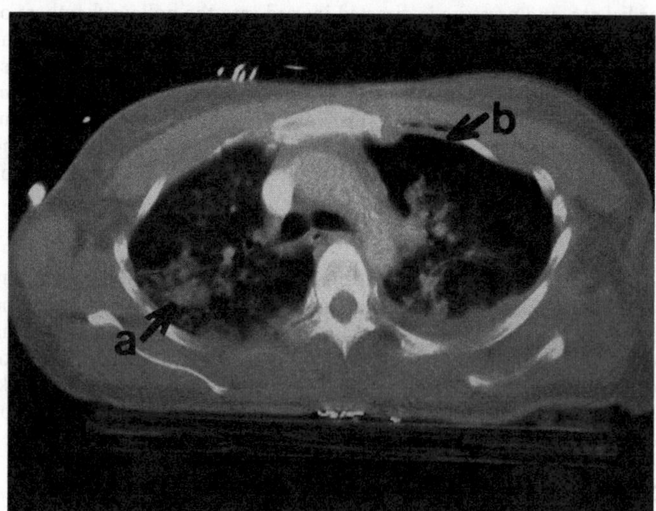

FIGURE 113–1 • Chest evaluation. A chest computed tomographic scan shows bilateral pulmonary contusions (arrow a) and effusions with a small pneumothorax on the left (arrow b).

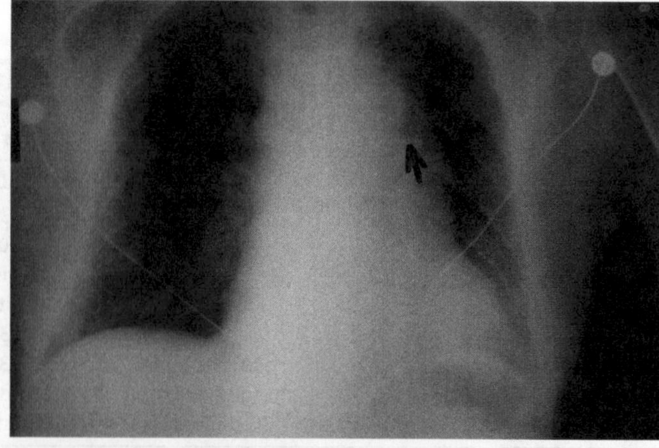

FIGURE 113–2 • Widened superior mediastinum on an upright chest radiograph. Note the loss of normal contour of the aortic knob (arrow).

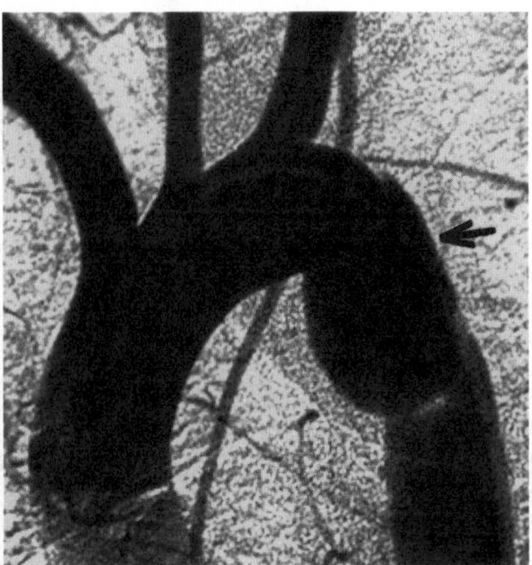

FIGURE 113–3 • Arteriography of the chest. An arteriogram shows thoracic aortic disruption (arrow) beyond the left subclavian artery in the patient depicted in Figure 113–2.

Rx

and aortic injuries are all examples of trauma that may suggest underlying cardiac contusion. Life-threatening myocardial contusion (5%) is manifested within the first 6 to 12 hours after injury as malignant arrhythmias or, if enough of the left ventricle is damaged, cardiogenic shock. Myocardial rupture is uncommon and typically involves the right ventricle because of the thin muscular wall and close proximity to the sternum. More commonly, arrhythmias or conduction disturbances may occur with elevation of cardiac biomarkers. Electrocardiographic findings include ST-T wave anomalies, supraventricular and ventricular arrhythmias, and atrioventricular nodal dysfunction. The echocardiogram may show left ventricular wall motion abnormalities, valvar dysfunction, or pericardial effusion. There is no evidence to support prophylactic treatment of arrhythmias, and emergency surgery for other injuries does not seem to carry a risk for increased morbidity or mortality in the presence of minor abnormalities.

Commotio cordis is sudden cardiac arrest after acute blunt trauma to the chest. The so-called concussion to the heart is one of the more common causes of sudden death in youth sports. By definition, there is no preexisting cardiac disease or identifiable morphologic change in the heart. The precordial impact, most commonly from softballs, baseballs, and hockey pucks, presumably occurs during an electrically vulnerable period between 30 and 15 msec before the T wave peak and produces ventricular fibrillation. The mortality rate is 90%, and nearly all survivors require resuscitation (Chapter 62) initiated within 1 minute of the insult. Education, improved chest protective equipment, and personnel competent in the use of automatic external defibrillators at youth sporting events may reduce the incidence of this infrequent, but feared injury.

Injuries to the coronary arteries are uncommon. Potential vascular injuries include laceration, intimal disruption with dissection, and vasospasm. The sequelae and treatment are similar to that for myocardial ischemia from atherosclerotic occlusion (Chapter 72).

Back

Palpation of the thoracic and lumbar spine combined with a thorough history is sufficient to exclude a thoracolumbar spine fracture in an alert patient. Ongoing back discomfort or a mechanism suggestive of the possibility of injury should lead to radiographic examination of the spine.

Abdomen

The abdominal contents may be injured by blunt or penetrating mechanisms. The ability to identify intra-abdominal injury is limited on physical examination. If the patient is hemodynamically stable, has a normal abdominal examination, and has sustained no other injuries that warrant operative repair, serial abdominal examination, a complete blood count, and amylase/lipase levels suffice. If there is any question about the normality of the abdominal examination or the ability to monitor the patient reliably, further evaluation is warranted.

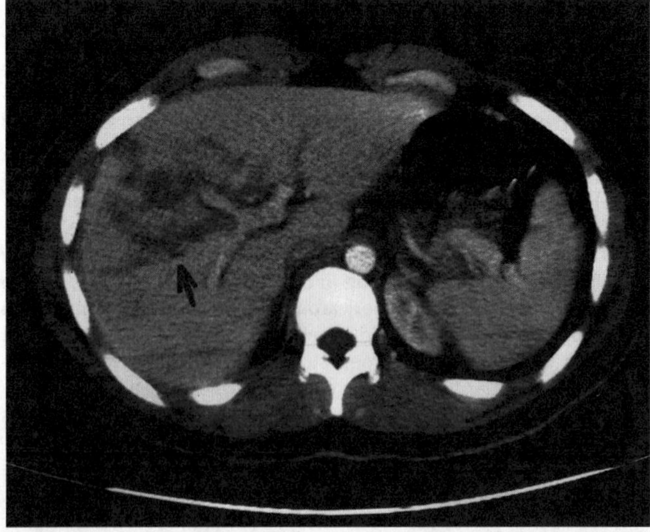

FIGURE 113–4 • Abdominal injury. An abdominal computed tomographic scan shows an injury to the right lobe of the liver (arrow).

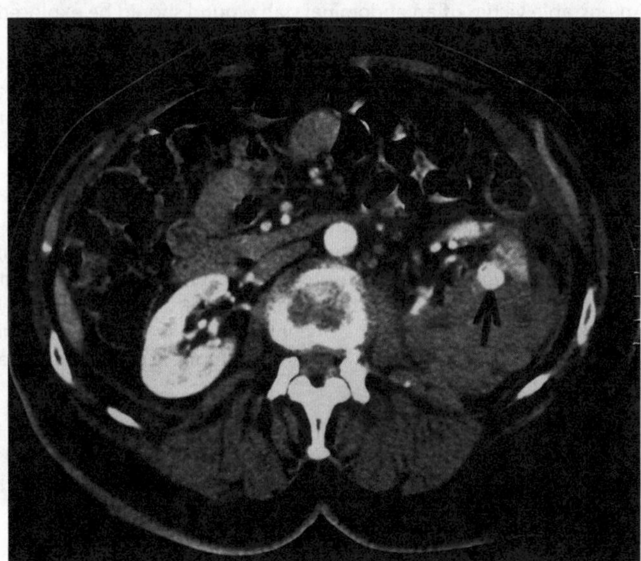

FIGURE 113–5 • Intraperitoneal and retroperitoneal injury. An abdominal computed tomographic scan shows blood in the retroperitoneum surrounding a shattered left kidney, with pooling of contrast (arrow) in the kidney parenchyma. These findings are consistent with a pseudoaneurysm of a branch of the left renal artery.

Rx

Abdominal CT has proved to be a reliable determinant of intra-abdominal injury in a stable patient (Fig. 113–4). It identifies both intraperitoneal and retroperitoneal injury (Fig. 113–5). CT evaluation can identify sources of blood loss and help decide whether the problem requires operative exploration.

The most frequently injured intra-abdominal organ is the spleen. Left-sided rib fractures, left upper quadrant pain or tenderness, and pain referred to the left shoulder secondary to diaphragmatic irritation are suggestive of splenic injury. CT allows definition of the grade of splenic injury and detection of free intraperitoneal blood. Hemodynamic instability, ongoing blood loss, and CT findings of a high-grade injury to the spleen are all indications for splenectomy or, preferably, splenorrhaphy for salvage of the damaged spleen with preservation of splenic function.

Rx

Blunt injury to the liver is often associated with right-sided rib fractures and right upper quadrant tenderness with or without peritonitis. An abdominal CT scan with intravenous contrast material allows classification of the liver injury according to the location, depth, and extent of the hematoma or laceration. Currently, most (85%) blunt liver injuries are managed successfully nonoperatively if other intra-abdominal injuries do not require surgery.

Focused abdominal sonography in trauma (FAST) has a sensitivity of 95% for detecting free blood in the abdomen (Fig. 113–6). It also enables evaluation of the pericardium for blood and tamponade physiology. FAST is limited in its ability to identify the source of bleeding and the retroperitoneal structures. It is effective in a pregnant trauma patient and allows evaluation of the fetus.

An alternative to FAST is diagnostic peritoneal lavage. In this approach, a small midline infraumbilical incision is made in the peritoneum to allow sampling of fluid in the peritoneal cavity. If blood is found, laparotomy is necessary to identify and correct the source.

Wounds that penetrate the anterior abdominal region are further divided into low-velocity stab wounds and gunshot wounds, each of which has a different management algorithm. Because mandatory laparotomy for stab wounds results in a high number of negative explorations, many institutions have adopted a selective approach. An unstable victim of an abdominal stab wound should be explored immediately in the operating room. In contrast, a stable patient can undergo local exploration of the wound to determine the depth of penetration. If the wound is superficial, it is irrigated and the patient is observed; if the wound extends beneath the fascia, the patient should undergo exploratory laparotomy to exclude intra-abdominal injury. All gunshot wounds to the anterior abdominal region are explored routinely except for injuries with tangential trajectories.

In an unstable patient or a patient with clinical signs of peritonitis, penetrating wounds to the flanks and posterior abdominal region require exploratory laparotomy. In a stable patient without peritoneal signs, a CT scan with oral, intravenous, and occasionally rectal contrast material may help identify injury to retroperitoneal structures, the ascending and descending colon, the duodenum, the pancreas, and the kidneys.

Pelvis, Perineum, and Buttocks

Clinical evaluation of the pelvis is accomplished through compression of the lateral and anterior aspect of the pelvis to elicit tenderness or bony instability. Rectal examination is essential to exclude bony fragments or blood. Bladder catheterization can identify hematuria and monitor urinary output as a reflection of intravascular volume. Scrotal hematoma, meatal blood, or a high-riding boggy prostate indicates potential urethral injury and requires a urethrogram before insertion of a Foley catheter. All patients with major trauma require an anteroposterior plain film of the pelvis to exclude pelvic or hip fractures. A wound in the perineum in the presence of a pelvic fracture represents an open fracture until proved otherwise.

Penetrating wounds of the buttocks should not be overlooked or underestimated. The likelihood of concomitant peritoneal penetration is 25%, with a mortality rate of 5%. Structures at risk include the retroperitoneal rectum, bladder, ureters, and major arterial and venous structures within the pelvis.

Extremities

Palpation of the long bones is performed to determine whether there is any tenderness or deformity. Range of motion should be assessed in all joints of the upper and lower extremities. Areas of concern on examination should be evaluated radiographically. If there is any suspicion of vascular injury, angiographic examination should be performed.

The compartments of the lower part of the leg are most prone to intracompartmental swelling from direct trauma, long bone fracture, or arterial injury with ischemia or bleeding. Palpation of rigid compartments suggests elevated compartment pressures, which may be measured directly; if pressures are elevated, four-compartment fasciotomies should be performed.

Penetrating wounds to an extremity require operative exploration if they are associated with an enlarging hematoma, active arterial bleeding, or absent arterial pulses. Penetrating wounds resulting in diminished or fluctuating pulses require arteriography to document arterial injury. Otherwise, extremity wounds in proximity to major arterial structures do not require an arteriogram, but the vascular territory should be observed for 24 hours.

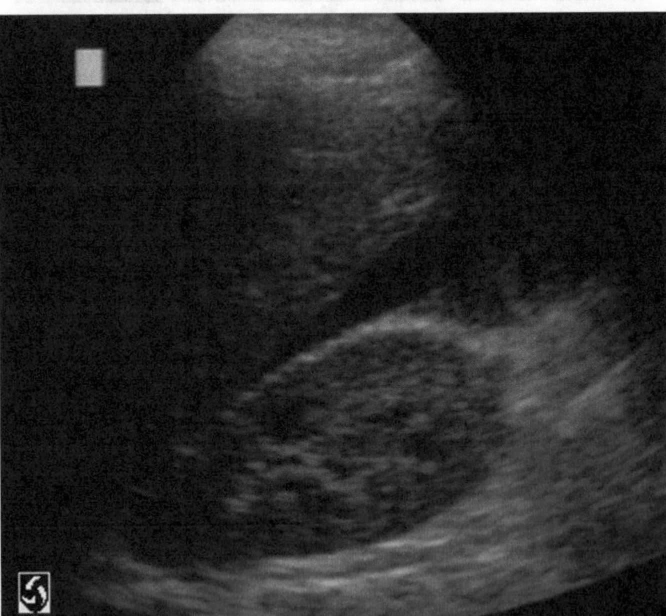

FIGURE 113–6 • Positive focal abdominal sonography in trauma (FAST) study. There is a collection of fluid that shows up as a black strip between the liver and kidney. The white appearance is fat around the kidney. These findings are consistent with a fluid collection in Morrison's pouch.

MEDICAL ASPECTS OF BURNS

Epidemiology

Each year, about 1% of the U.S. population sustains a burn injury. More than 2 million burns occur annually, a quarter of which require medical care and produce significant disability.

Approximately 100,000 burn patients require hospital admission, and more than 10,000 persons die of burn-related causes annually in the United States. The most common age groups involved are toddlers (2 to 4 years), for whom scalding is the most common cause, and young adults (17 to 25 years), usually male, for whom the most common cause is a flammable liquid. Structural fires account for less than 5% of hospital admissions but are responsible for more than 45% of burn-related deaths. The National Fire Prevention and Control Administration estimates that 2.6 million fires are reported annually.

Burns can be categorized as scalds, contact burns, and flame burns. Scald burns are the predominant injury in children, whereas contact and flame burns are most common in adults. The major cause of the injury to the skin is exposure to high temperature, which destroys surface tissue. Flames result in temperatures of several thousand degrees Fahrenheit, especially in a closed space. Because water can conduct heat 1000 times better than air can, a much lower temperature (120 to 130° F) is required to produce a deep burn from hot liquid.

Chemical and electrical burns (Chapter 112), though often severe, account for less than 5% of burn admissions. The mechanism of a chemical burn is protein coagulation of skin caused by the acid or alkali. The injury progresses until the chemical is removed by aggressive water lavage. An electrical burn produces tissue coagulation along the course of passage of the current. This deeper injury is hidden from view and must be anticipated to make an early diagnosis and initiate effective treatment.

TABLE 113–2 SMOKE INHALATION COMPLEX

Carbon monoxide (cyanide) toxicity
Onset of peak symptoms is immediate
Symptoms are systemic
Supraglottic injury
Onset of peak symptoms is delayed (hours)
Problem is upper airway edema
Infraglottic injury
Onset of peak symptoms is delayed (days)
Problem is lower airway mucosal injury

Pathobiology

The skin is the largest organ of the body and ranges from 0.25 m^2 in a newborn to more than 2 m^2 in an adult (Chapter 461). The outermost layer of the epidermis is composed of dead, cornified cells that act as a tough protective barrier against the environment. The second, thicker layer, the corneum (0.06 to 0.12 mm), is composed chiefly of fibrous connective tissue. The dermis contains the blood vessels and nerves to the skin and the epithelial appendages of specialized function. The nerve endings that mediate pain are found in the dermis. Partial-thickness injuries are extremely painful because the nerve endings are exposed. Full-thickness burns are usually anesthetic because of destruction of the nerves.

The skin is also the barrier that prevents loss of body heat and fluids by evaporation. Sweat glands help maintain body temperature by controlling the amount of heat lost by evaporation. Increased loss of water and heat through burned skin is a major problem early after a burn. In addition, the skin is the primary protective barrier against invasive infection. The skin also detects the sensations of touch, pressure, pain, cold, and heat; loss of this function leads to long-term impairment.

Treatment

Rx

A burned patient undergoes many dramatic physiologic and metabolic changes over the course of the injury. These changes are so marked that the physician may have the feeling of treating a different patient every several days as the process evolves. The burn injury is divided into four phases, each of which has many different physiologic and metabolic characteristics: (1) resuscitation phase (0 to 36 hours), (2) postresuscitation phase (2 to 6 days), (3) inflammation and infection phase (7 days to wound closure), and (4) rehabilitation and wound-remodeling phase (admission to 1 year afterward).

Resuscitation Phase (0 to 36 hours)

Life-threatening airway and breathing problems are of major immediate concern, with the effects of smoke inhalation injury being the most concerning problem (Chapter 94). The initial phase is also characterized by hypovolemia as plasma volume is lost into the burned tissue. The burn itself is of less immediate concern except for initial assessment regarding its severity and depth and the selected need for escharotomy. Wound management becomes a higher priority in later phases. The adequacy of initial treatment of pulmonary and circulatory abnormalities sets the stage for subsequent management.

Smoke Inhalation Injury

The first priority in managing a burn victim is recognition and treatment of smoke exposure. Inhalation injury can be divided into three components based on the onset of symptoms and pathophysiology (Table 113–2).

Carbon Monoxide Toxicity

Carbon monoxide and sometimes cyanide toxicity is evident immediately, with peak symptoms occurring at the scene of the inhalation (Chapter 94). Carbon monoxide rapidly displaces oxygen

Rx

from hemoglobin and produces carboxyhemoglobin, which impairs oxygen delivery to tissues. The peak level of carboxyhemoglobin also occurs at the scene of the burn; its half-life is about 20 minutes. Treatment is 100% oxygen. Symptoms, which range from confusion to coma, resolve with oxygen therapy unless the patient also suffered severe anoxic injury. The use of hyperbaric oxygen remains controversial in this situation.

Cyanide, which is present in smoke, is absorbed rapidly through the lung and causes systemic toxicity. Cyanide levels are difficult to obtain, but an unexplained base deficit can be assumed to be due to cyanide mitochondrial toxicity; treatment consists of oxygen along with sodium thiosulfate and hydroxycobalamin.

Supraglottic Injury

Smoke injures the mucosa above the glottis because of the combination of superheated air and the toxins in smoke. Mucosal edema, which usually develops over a period of several hours, impedes and potentially obstructs the upper airway. Early endotracheal intubation is indicated if significant edema is evident on direct laryngoscopy, especially if the edema is increasing on subsequent examinations. Upper airway edema generally resolves in 3 to 4 days.

Infraglottic Injury

Toxins in the inhaled air or coating the inhaled soot particles damage the tracheobronchial mucosa, but heat does not usually reach this level. The extent of damage depends on the toxicity of the chemicals and the duration of exposure. Symptoms vary from transient bronchospasm to sloughing of the airway mucosa, which results in plugging and infection. Bronchoscopic evidence of erythema and edema indicates that an injury has occurred but does not predict the degree of injury or time course to recovery.

Endotracheal intubation and positive pressure ventilation are indicated if symptoms increase, especially if there is an early and progressive impairment in gas exchange. Aggressive pulmonary toilet is necessary to avoid respiratory failure. The time course to resolution may be days or weeks.

Burn Shock and Resuscitation

Adequate volume resuscitation is crucial to survival of the victim of a major body burn. Hypovolemia can also rapidly lead to conversion of viable burned tissue to a nonviable, full-thickness burn, thus further increasing mortality. With modern treatment in burn centers, the failure rate of initial volume restoration is less than 5%, even for large burns involving greater than 85% of the total body skin surface.

Two processes lead to postburn hypovolemia: an increase in microvascular permeability in the burn wound and an increase in the osmolarity of surface burn tissue. A large intravascular to extravascular plasma shift occurs. The phase of rapid loss of intravascular fluid persists for about 24 to 36 hours.

Isotonic crystalloid, preferably lactated Ringer's solution, is used in the first 24 hours. Normal saline in large amounts predictably leads to hyperchloremic metabolic acidosis. A volume of 4 mL/kg is given for each percent of body surface burned, with 50% given in the first 8 hours and 50% in the subsequent 16 hours. Isotonic crystalloid is used for the first 24 hours in view of the change in skin capillary permeability for protein. Albumin can be added to the resuscitation fluid to maintain a serum albumin level greater than 2.5 g/dL. After the acute injury, the major fluid loss is water from the injured skin surface, which is no longer able to act as a barrier to the evaporation of water.

Burn Wound

The initial management of a burn wound is based on knowledge of the anatomy of the skin and the functional losses with injury. The major objectives are to decrease the potential for further local damage and the systemic abnormalities that can be produced by loss of the barrier function. Early treatment focuses on neutralizing the source of burn injury, avoiding excess heat loss, determining the extent of the injury, cleaning and débriding the wound, controlling infection with topical antibiotics, and maintaining tissue perfusion.

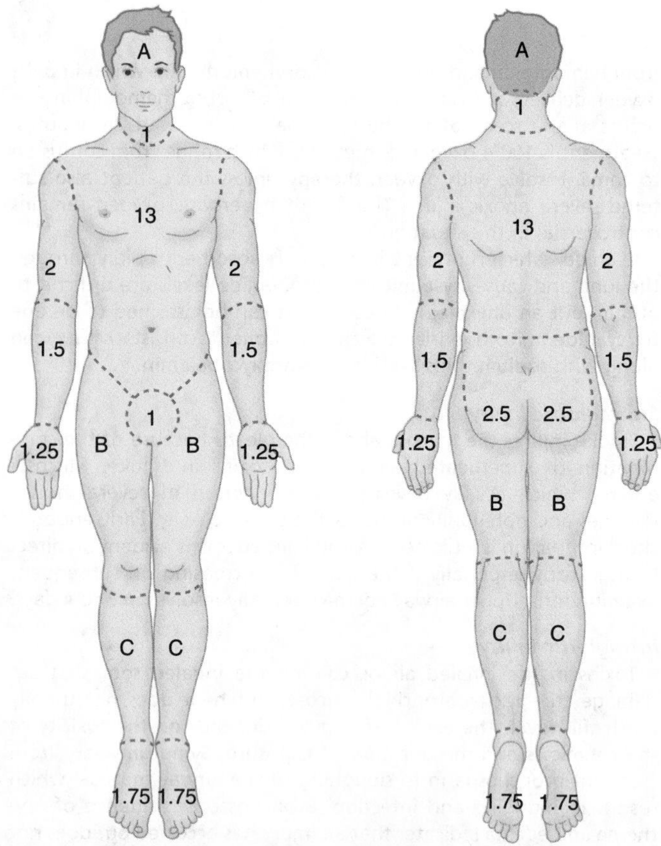

Relative percentages of areas affected by growth			
	Age		
Area	10	15	Adult
A = half of head	5.5	4.5	3.5
B = half of one thigh	4.25	4.5	4.75
C = half of one leg	3	3.25	3.5

FIGURE 113–7 • Assessment tool for assessing burn size as a percentage of total body surface area.

Rx

Assessment of Burn Depth and Size

Burns are categorized into partial thickness and full thickness. A partial-thickness burn is defined by destruction of the epidermis and a portion of the dermis; a superficial partial-thickness burn is confined to the upper third of the dermis, a mid partial-thickness burn involves the middle third, and a deep partial-thickness burn leaves only a portion of the dermis viable. For management purposes, a deep partial-thickness burn is managed similar to a full-thickness burn: wound excision and skin grafting are required. The approach to superficial partial-thickness burns is to provide for optimal healing, which is initiated by the remaining viable epidermal cells in the hair follicles. Burn size in older children and adults is determined by the percentage of total skin surface area that is involved by the burn (Fig. 113–7).

Postresuscitation Phase (2 to 6 days)

The early postresuscitation phase is a period of transition from the shock phase to the hypermetabolic phase. In general, cardiopulmonary stability is optimal during this period because wound inflammation and infection have not yet developed. Early wound excision and grafting are initiated during this period. Operative risks, especially blood loss and septicemia, are substantially less than later, when inflammation and infection are common.

Rx

Pulmonary Support

Continued upper airway maintenance with an endotracheal tube may be required. Placement of the patient with the head elevated 30 to 45 degrees allows faster resolution of edema. The decision when to extubate is difficult, and the degree of lower airway injury dictates the timing. Laryngoscopy to determine the presence of cord edema is helpful. Extubation should not be performed unless reintubation is feasible. Lower airway injury is managed by aggressive pulmonary toilet for increased sputum production and microbial overgrowth. Progressive tracheobronchitis and bronchopneumonia are common. The predicted extravascular to intravascular fluid shift results in an increased risk for pulmonary edema. Increased levels of antidiuretic stress hormones can prevent appropriate diuresis.

Hemodynamic Stability

The postresuscitation period is characterized by major fluid shifts mainly from the extravascular to the intravascular fluid space. Edema in burned tissue is maximal between 24 and 30 hours after injury in patients with well-controlled fluid resuscitation. The red blood cell mass continues to decrease. Electrolyte and acid-base changes are prominent.

Evaporation from the surface of the burn is a major source of water loss that persists until the wound is closed. The loss is measured in terms of water vapor pressure at the surface. In normal skin, vapor pressure is 2 to 3 mm Hg, whereas the pressure is about 32 mm Hg in a full-thickness burn in which the eschar is soft and hydrated. The rate of loss is increased with increasing surface blood flow. A reasonable estimate of the average loss per hour can be obtained from the following formula: evaporative water loss (mL/hr) = (25 + % total body surface burn) × body surface area (m^2).

Burn Wound

The wound undergoes dramatic changes during the next several days as inflammation develops. Of particular importance is the potential for change in the zone of injured, but still viable tissue. Changes in local wound microcirculatory blood flow as a result of vasoactive inflammatory agents or local infection can convert this zone of ischemia to a zone of necrosis.

Hypermetabolic-Sepsis Phase (7 days to Recovery)

The generalized inflammation of the final phase alters organ function and magnifies any preexisting organ dysfunction. The burn wound is now colonized with bacteria, so wound sepsis is of prominent concern. Infection, whether lung or wound, becomes increasingly difficult to diagnose because of the continued presence of a non–infection-induced hyperdynamic state. Multisystem organ failure, if it is to occur, is seen during this period.

Burn Wound Infection

Burn wounds are never sterile, even with the administration of topical agents or systemic antibiotics. The presence of bacteria just on the wound surface is termed colonization. Colonization may be with a single type of organism or with multiple types. Infection of the wound (Table 113–3) indicates invasion of the underlying viable tissue; this process is diagnosed by eschar biopsy and quantitative culture showing greater than 10^5 organisms per gram of tissue. With progression, viable tissue and its blood vessels are invaded, and septicemia develops. Wound infections require systemic antibiotics. Because all patients have a hyperdynamic state with an elevated temperature and leukocytosis, it is difficult to make a diagnosis of infection based on systemic symptoms. Optimally, most of the eschar should be removed in the first week to avoid burn wound sepsis. *Staphylococcus aureus* is the most common organism isolated from the burn, especially during the first week.

Hypermetabolic State

Beginning at day 5 or 6, there is a gradual increase in the metabolic rate from a normal of 35 to 40 cal/m^2/hr (25 cal/kg/day) to levels twice this value at about 10 days. The increase in metabolic rate after burns is far in excess of that seen after any other severe injury, including sepsis. The magnitude of the increase is related to the size

TABLE 113–3 MOST COMMON ORGANISMS IN BURN INFECTIONS

	Staphylococcus aureus	*Pseudomonas aeruginosa*	*Candida albicans*
Wound appearance	Loss of wound granulation	Surface necrosis, patchy black	Minimal exudates
Course	Slow onset, 2–5 days	Rapid onset, 12–36 hr	Slow onset, days
Central nervous system	Disorientation	Modest changes	Often no change
Temperature	Marked increase	High or low	Modest changes
White blood cells	Marked increase	High or low	Modest changes
Hypotension	Modest	Often severe	Minimal change
Mortality	5%	20–30%	30–50%

Rx

of the burn. The hypermetabolic state is characterized by increased oxygen consumption, increased heat production, increased body temperature, and increased protein catabolism. Body temperature increases from normal to 100 to 101° F (38 to 38.5° C) because of resetting of the hypothalamic temperature center as a result of the altered hormonal environment (Chapter 302).

Marked and sustained increases in circulatory catecholamines lead to hypermetabolism, and treatment with β-blockers may be protective. Sustained increases in glucagon and glucocorticoids result in excessive gluconeogenesis and an insulin-resistant state. Increased glucocorticoids also lead to a severe catabolic state, especially because anabolic hormones (growth hormone and testosterone) are decreased after a burn injury.

Nutritional Support

Optimal nutritional support is essential and can decrease net catabolism by about 50%. Currently, there is no recognized ideal nutritional program because of evolving changes with new research findings on postburn nutrient processing. Decreasing stress by wound closure and control of pain, heat loss, and hypovolemia further controls the hypermetabolism. Caloric requirements can be measured with indirect calorimetric techniques. Because more than 95% of the energy generated requires oxygen, there is a direct relationship between oxygen consumption and the metabolic rate. Caloric needs can be estimated by the formula whereby energy requirements = basal metabolic rate × 1.25 × stress factor; the stress factor is 1.2 for a 10% burn, 1.5 for a 20% burn, 1.7 for a 30% burn, 1.8 for a 40% burn, and 2.0 for a 50% or greater burn. If the activity level is increased markedly or additional stress (e.g., severe pain) is present, the metabolic rate can be increased further.

Nutrients Required

Carbohydrate is the preferred fuel for most tissues, but there is a limit to the amount that is used, especially in a hypermetabolic or septic patient (Chapters 233, 235, and 236). Current recommendations are that carbohydrate infusions not exceed 5 to 7 mg/kg/min, or approximately 1800 to 2200 carbohydrate calories per day. Excess carbohydrate results in the formation of fat, which requires energy rather than produces energy. Approximately 50% of the estimated calorie requirements is usually given as glucose to spare nitrogen. Fat is used as a calorie source, but fat should account for no more than 30% of the total calories. Protein represents 20 to 25% of infused calories. A standard estimate of 1.5 to 2 g of protein per kilogram of body weight can be used for all major burns. Necessary vitamins and trace elements should be provided in the form of high-potency multivitamin-mineral pills or liquid.

Route of Administration of Nutrition

Nutritional support is best managed during this period by the enteral route, generally through a combination of balanced tube feeding and voluntary intake (Chapter 235). Parenteral hyperalimentation (Chapter 236) through a central vein is occasionally required if for some reason the gastrointestinal tract is not functioning adequately, as sometimes occurs in a patient on a ventilator or a patient with sepsis.

Rx

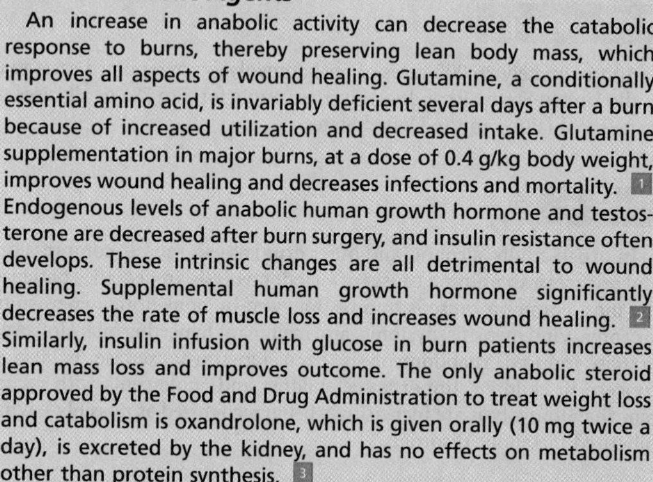

Use of Anabolic Agents

An increase in anabolic activity can decrease the catabolic response to burns, thereby preserving lean body mass, which improves all aspects of wound healing. Glutamine, a conditionally essential amino acid, is invariably deficient several days after a burn because of increased utilization and decreased intake. Glutamine supplementation in major burns, at a dose of 0.4 g/kg body weight, improves wound healing and decreases infections and mortality. 1 Endogenous levels of anabolic human growth hormone and testosterone are decreased after burn surgery, and insulin resistance often develops. These intrinsic changes are all detrimental to wound healing. Supplemental human growth hormone significantly decreases the rate of muscle loss and increases wound healing. 2 Similarly, insulin infusion with glucose in burn patients increases lean mass loss and improves outcome. The only anabolic steroid approved by the Food and Drug Administration to treat weight loss and catabolism is oxandrolone, which is given orally (10 mg twice a day), is excreted by the kidney, and has no effects on metabolism other than protein synthesis. 3

Oxandrolone acts on androgenic receptors in lean mass, especially on skin fibroblasts. A number of studies have demonstrated its ability to preserve lean mass after burn injury and thereby improve local healing. In addition, several recent studies have demonstrated direct wound-healing properties.

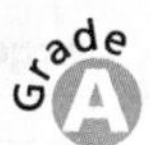

1. Garrel D, Patenaude J, Nedelec B, et al: Decreased mortality and infectious morbidity in adult burn patients given enteral glutamine; a prospective controlled randomized clinical trial. Crit Care Med 2003;10:2444–2449.
2. Ramirez R, Wolf S, Herndon D: Growth hormone treatment in pediatric patients; a safe therapeutic approach. Ann Surg 1998;4:439–448.
3. Demling R, Orgil D: The anticatabolic and wound-healing effects of the testosterone analog oxandrolone after severe burn injury. J Crit Care 2000;15:12–17.

SUGGESTED READINGS

Branas CC, MacKenzie EJ, Williams JC, et al: Access to trauma centers in the United States. JAMA 2005;293:2626–2633. *There is generally an oversupply in urban areas and undersupply in rural areas.*

Herndon D, Tompkins R: Support of the metabolic response to burn injury. Lancet 2004:363:1895–1902. *A practical overview.*

Kirkpatrick AW, Simons RK, Brown R, et al: The hand-held FAST: Experience with hand-held trauma sonography in a level-I urban trauma center. Injury 2002;33:303–308. *Handheld portable ultrasound examinations facilitate rapid evaluation of victims of abdominal trauma.*

Lehmann RK, Arthurs ZM, Cuadrado DF, et al: Trauma team activation: Simplified criteria safely reduce overtriage. Am J Surg 2007;193:630–634. *Glasgow coma score <14, hypertension, altered respiratory effort, and penetrating truncal injury were high-risk features.*

Pham TN, Eibran NS: Thermal and electrical injuries. Surg Clin North Am 2007;87:185–206. *A comprehensive review.*

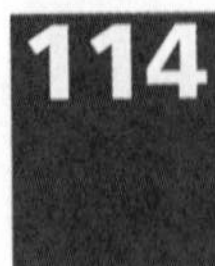

RHABDOMYOLYSIS

Francis G. O'Connor and Patricia A. Deuster

Definition

Rhabdomyolysis, the dissolution and disintegration of striated muscle, is an acute, potentially fatal clinical syndrome. Myoglobinemia and myoglobinuria are common. Skeletal muscle destruction can cause systemic effects mediated by substances released from affected muscle cells (e.g., myoglobin, calcium, potassium). Prerenal azotemia, complicated by the toxicity of free myoglobin on the renal tubules, may lead to acute renal failure, which exacerbates other metabolic abnormalities. At the extreme, arrhythmias, caused by the release of intracellular potassium and organic acids, coupled with hypocalcemia may be fatal.

Epidemiology

Approximately 26,000 cases of rhabdomyolysis are reported each year in the United States. Rhabdomyolysis accounts for 5 to 7% of all cases of acute renal failure in the United States.

Etiology

In urban adults, alcohol (and other drug) abuse, muscle compression, and seizures are common causes of rhabdomyolysis. In pediatric patients, the most common cause is trauma, followed by nonketotic hyperosmolar coma, viral myositis, dystonia, and malignant hyperthermia. However, exercise-induced rhabdomyolysis from repetitive exercise is also a concern in children. Importantly, children and adolescents with recurrent rhabdomyolysis are increasingly being recognized as possibly having inherited metabolic disorders.

Drugs and Intoxications

Intoxications are a common cause of rhabdomyolysis (Table 114–1). The most frequent illegal drug–associated causes are cocaine and heroin (Chapter 32), with nearly 20% of cocaine overdoses complicated by rhabdomyolysis. Other substances that can induce rhabdomyolysis include ethanol (Chapter 31), amphetamines, phenylalkylamine derivatives, statins (Chapter 217), caffeine, and many others. The incidence of hospitalization for rhabdomyolysis in patients treated with lipid-lowering agents in a cohort of more than 250,000 patients was 0.44 when statins were used as monotherapy. The incidence increased to 5.98% when statin therapy was combined with a fibrate.

Exertional Rhabdomyolysis

Rhabdomyolysis is also seen as a consequence of excessive exertion, prolonged heat exposure (Chapter 110), coexisting sickle cell trait (Chapter 167), and the use of dietary supplements (e.g., ephedra). In one series, 35 of 225,000 emergency department visits to an urban tertiary care center were for exertional rhabdomyolysis. The average creatine kinase (CK) level was 40,000 U/L, but in no patient did acute renal failure develop. In another series, 57% of participants in an ultramarathon had evidence of myoglobinemia, but none progressed to acute renal failure. Rhabdomyolysis has also been diagnosed in other sports settings (e.g., baseball, football, track, wrestling), but none with a higher frequency than seen with endurance events.

In the military, acute exertional rhabdomyolysis occurs in 2 to 40% of individuals undergoing basic training, usually within the first 6 days. Resolution of myoglobinuria typically occurs within 2 to 3 days, with clinical improvement within 1 week. Consistent risk factors are low levels of physical fitness and early introduction of repetitive exercises (e.g., squats, push-ups, and sit-ups). Although most cases are self-limited with no long-term evidence of renal or muscle injury, patients who demonstrate systemic signs, generalized clinical findings, or acute renal failure often have an underlying metabolic myopathy. Importantly, 25% of all cases of heat stroke ($N = 944$) in the military between 1980 and 2000 were associated with rhabdomyolysis; of those, acute renal failure developed in 33%. A retrospective review of deaths in a military basic trainee population found an increased risk for nontraumatic exertional sudden death in African Americans with sickle cell trait.

The extreme exertion characteristics of military service also carry over to the population of correctional inmates and civil servants. Reports indicate that unsupervised repetitive exercise in prison populations has led to exertional rhabdomyolysis. Among New York City firefighters, 32 (0.2%) of 16,506 candidates were hospitalized for rhabdomyolysis after a physical fitness test, with 4 requiring hemodialysis. In a group of 50 prospective policemen from Massachusetts, 13 trainees were hospitalized with rhabdomyolysis and CK levels greater than 32,000 U/L; 6 required dialysis, and 1 died 44 days later as a result of complications of heat stroke, rhabdomyolysis, and renal and hepatic failure.

TABLE 114–1 INHERITED AND ACQUIRED CAUSES OF RHABDOMYOLYSIS

Inherited	Acquired
Glycolytic/glycogenolytic, e.g., McArdle's disease (myophosphorylase deficiency)	**Exertion,** e.g., exercise, status epilepticus, delirium, electrical shock, status asthmaticus, cardiopulmonary resuscitation (see also Table 114–2)
Fatty acid oxidation, e.g., carnitine palmitoyl transferase II deficiency	**Crush,** e.g., external weight, prolonged immobility, bariatric surgery
Krebs cycle, e.g., aconitase deficiency	**Ischemia,** e.g., arterial occlusion, compartment syndrome, sickle cell disease, disseminated intravascular coagulation
Pentose phosphate pathway, e.g., glucose-6-phosphate dehydrogenase deficiency	**Extremes of body temperature,** e.g., fever, exertional heat stroke, burns, malignant hyperthermia, hypothermia, lightning
Purine nucleotide cycle, e.g., myoadenylate deaminase deficiency	**Metabolic,** e.g., hypokalemia, hypernatremia/hyponatremia, hypophosphatemia, pancreatitis, diabetic ketoacidosis, renal tubular acidosis, hyperthyroidism/hypothyroidism, nonketotic hyperosmolar states
Mitochondrial respiratory chain, e.g., succinate dehydrogenase deficiency	**Drugs/toxins,** e.g., anticholinergics, amphetamines, antihistamines, arsenic, ethanol, opiates, statins, cocaine, succinylcholine, halothane, corticosteroids, cyclosporine, itraconazole, phenothiazines
Malignant hyperthermia susceptibility, e.g., familial malignant hyperthermia *(RYR1)* mutations, myotonic dystrophy, Duchenne's and Becker's dystrophies	**Infections,** e.g., Epstein-Barr virus, human immunodeficiency virus, herpes simplex, influenza A and B, *Borrelia burgdorferi*, tetanus
Other, e.g., familial recurrent myoglobinuria	**Inflammatory and autoimmune disorders,** e.g., polymyositis, dermatomyositis

Adapted and reproduced with permission from Warren JD, Blumbergs PC, Thompson PD: Rhabdomyolysis: A review. Muscle Nerve 2002;25:332–347.

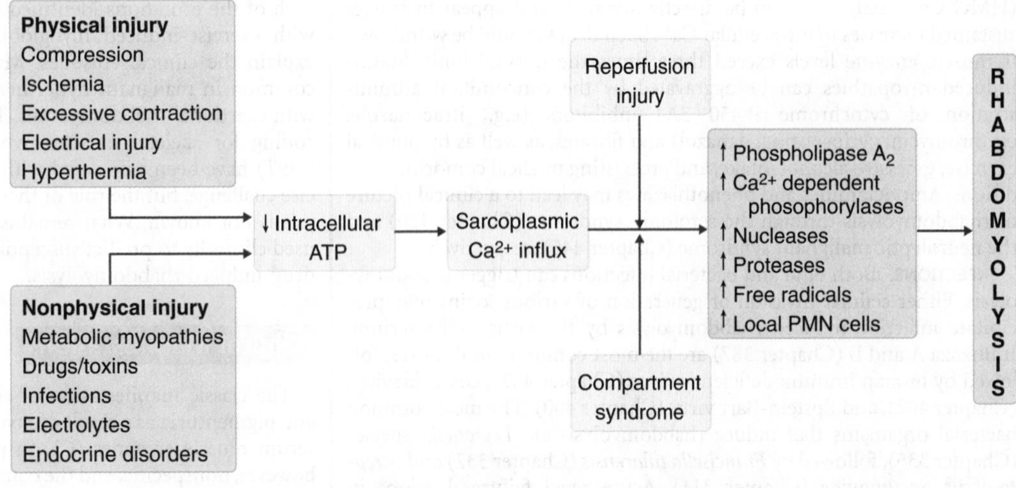

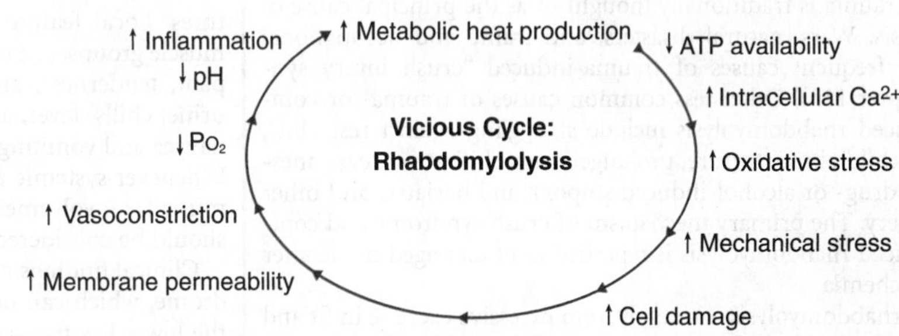

FIGURE 114–1 • **A,** Pathogenesis of rhabdomyolysis. ATP = adenosine triphosphate; PMN = polymorphonuclear. **B,** Vicious cycle of rhabdomyolysis.

Pathobiology

Pathophysiology

The final common pathway for all cases of rhabdomyolysis is destruction of muscle cells as a result of direct or indirect injury with displacement of their intracellular contents into extracellular fluid or the circulation, or both (Fig. 114–1). Cell function is critically dependent on the relationship between intracellular calcium (Ca^{2+}) and sodium (Na^+) concentrations. Sarcolemmal Na^+,K^+-ATPase regulates extracellular Ca^{2+} concentrations by exchanging Na^+ for Ca^{2+} across the sarcolemma. A low intracellular Na^+ concentration creates a gradient that actively results in efflux of Ca^{2+} as it is exchanged for Na^+ ions. This process maintains intracellular Ca^{2+} levels at several orders of magnitude lower than extracellular Ca^{2+}.

When the cell is subjected to mechanical stress, stretch-activated channels in the sarcolemma can open and cause an influx of Na^+ and Ca^{2+}. With excessive intracellular Ca^{2+}, several pathologic processes begin. Excessive intracellular Ca^{2+} results in persistent contraction of myofibers, depletion of adenosine triphosphate (ATP), production of free radicals, activation of vasoactive molecules, release of proteases, and ultimately, cell death. Cell death is followed by an invasion of neutrophils, which amplify the damage by further release of proteases and increased production of free radicals. Rather than simple necrosis, a self-sustaining, inflammatory myolytic reaction develops.

Rhabdomyolysis can be further complicated by reperfusion injury and compartment syndrome. In reperfusion injury, ischemia for a prolonged period is followed by restoration of vascular flow. The increase in blood flow results in the delivery of activated neutrophils in combination with an abundance of oxygen, which contributes to the development of highly reactive free radicals. Because most muscle groups are contained within rigid fascial compartments, rhabdomyolysis can quickly precipitate a secondary acute compartment syndrome. The swelling associated with traumatized tissue can also lead to increased intracompartmental pressure, which can provoke additional damage by compromising both venous and arterial blood flow. Thus, compartment syndrome can also lead to rhabdomyolysis.

Inherited and Acquired Rhabdomyolysis

Rhabdomyolysis can be classified into two major categories: inherited and acquired (see Table 114–1). Metabolic myopathies, though not the most common etiology, should be carefully considered in patients who have recurrent episodes that are triggered by low levels of stress or exertion. A number of pathways that lead to the formation of ATP can be disrupted by genetic defects (e.g., inherited disorders of glycogenolysis, glycolysis, and lipid and purine metabolism). In one series of 77 patients who underwent biopsy for idiopathic myoglobinuria, 47% were found to have enzymatic defects. The most common disorders were deficiencies of carnitine palmitoyltransferase II and myophosphorylase.

Inherited Rhabdomyolysis

Malignant hyperthermia is a potentially fatal, heterogeneous, pharmacogenetic disorder triggered by volatile anesthetics in predisposed individuals (Chapter 458). The disorder is most commonly inherited in an autosomal dominant pattern. Evidence from molecular studies indicates that 25% of patients who are susceptible to malignant hyperthermia have mutations in the ryanodine receptor (*RyR1*) gene, a gene that is responsible for coding proteins for one of the primary Ca^{2+} release channels involved in triggering muscle contraction. When a susceptible patient is exposed to a triggering agent, excessive release of Ca^{2+} into the myoplasm leads to a hypermetabolic state manifested by hypercapnia, tachycardia, and metabolic acidosis. Whether the genetic predisposition to malignant hyperthermia may be related to exertional rhabdomyolysis and exercise-induced heat injury is not yet proved.

Acquired Rhabdomyolysis

DRUGS AND TOXINS. Drugs and toxins, also common causes of rhabdomyolysis, operate through a number of mechanisms, including direct membrane toxicity (e.g., herbicides), indirect metabolic derangements (e.g., anticholinergics), ischemia (e.g., cocaine), and agitation (e.g., hemlock). The most commonly cited drugs precipitating rhabdomyolysis are alcohol, statins, cocaine, amphetamines, and phenothiazines. Alcohol can induce rhabdomyolysis through a combination of mechanisms, including immobilization, direct myotoxicity, and electrolyte abnormalities. Statins, which inhibit 3-hydroxy-3-methylglutaryl–coenzyme A

(HMG-CoA) reductase, can be directly myotoxic and appear to trigger sustained increases in intracellular Ca^{2+}. Such drugs should be withdrawn if muscle enzyme levels exceed three times the normal limit. Statin-induced myopathies can be aggravated by the concomitant administration of cytochrome P-450 3A4 inhibitors (e.g., itraconazole, erythromycin, cyclosporine, danazol) and fibrates, as well as by physical exercise, excessive alcohol intake, and preexisting medical comorbid conditions. Amphetamines and phenothiazines may lead to a clinical picture of rhabdomyolysis through the serotonin syndrome (Chapter 420) and the neuroleptic malignant syndrome (Chapter 445), respectively.

INFECTIONS. Both viral and bacterial infections can trigger rhabdomyolysis. Either cellular invasion or generation of various toxins may precipitate infection-induced rhabdomyolysis by the virus or bacterium. Influenza A and B (Chapter 387) are the most common viral causes, followed by human immunodeficiency virus (Chapter 407), coxsackievirus (Chapter 402), and Epstein-Barr virus (Chapter 400). The most common bacterial organisms that induce rhabdomyolysis are *Legionella* species (Chapter 335), followed by *Francisella tularensis* (Chapter 332) and *Streptococcus pneumoniae* (Chapter 311). Acute renal failure develops in approximately 57% (33 to 100%) of bacterial-induced and 34% (0 to 100%) of viral-induced cases of rhabdomyolysis.

TRAUMA. Trauma is traditionally thought of as the principal cause of rhabdomyolysis. Wars, natural disasters, and traffic and occupational accidents are frequent causes of trauma-induced "crush injury syndrome" (Chapter 113). Other less common causes of trauma- or compression-induced rhabdomyolysis include struggling against restraints, direct blows, child abuse, torture, prolonged immobilization (e.g., anesthesia, coma, drug- or alcohol-induced stupor), and bariatric and other forms of surgery. The primary mechanism of crush syndrome and compression-induced rhabdomyolysis is reperfusion of damaged tissue after a period of ischemia.

Exertional rhabdomyolysis can result from excessive exercise in fit and unfit individuals, particularly eccentrically based activities (lengthening contractions, such as lowering a weight), but it can also be triggered by exertion in combination with thermal stress, sickle cell trait, altitude, or the use of medications (e.g., anticholinergics) or ergogenic substances (e.g., caffeine, ephedra). Exertional rhabdomyolysis may also reveal or provide evidence of an underlying inherited disorder in certain individuals. The spectrum of exertional rhabdomyolysis is broad and can range from a subclinical event to catastrophic collapse and death. The underlying mechanisms may be either mechanical or metabolic in nature, but exertional rhabdomyolysis is associated with elevated myoplasmic Ca^{2+} concentrations.

A number of genetic mutations (Table 114–2) have been identified in association with metabolic myopathies, and exercise usually precipitated the rhabdomyolysis. Multiple mutations in the carnitine palmitoyltransferase II and myophosphorylase genes have been found, and although each of the mutations identified in these two genes has been associated with exercise-induced myoglobinuria, the mutations alone may not explain the clinical episodes. Mutations in the *RyR1* gene, which are common in malignant hyperthermia, have also been noted in persons with exertional rhabdomyolysis. Two single point mutations in the gene coding for skeletal muscle myosin light-chain kinase (*C37885A* and *C49T*) have been associated with exaggerated CK responses to an exercise challenge, but the role of these mutations in exertional rhabdomyolysis is not known. What remains to be identified are genes that can be used clinically to predict susceptibility to infection-, toxin-, exertion-, or drug-induced rhabdomyolysis.

TABLE 114–2 GENETIC MUTATIONS ASSOCIATED WITH EXERTIONAL RHABDOMYOLYSIS

Gene	
Ryanodine receptor 1	*RyR1*
Myoadenylate deaminase	*AMPDA1*
Carnitine palmitoyltransferase II	*CPT2*
Myophosphorylase	*PYGM*
Phosphofructokinase	*PFKM*
Phosphorylase *b* kinase	*PHKA1*
Very-long-chain acyl coenzyme A dehydrogenase	*ACAD9*
Phosphoglycerate mutase	*PGAMM*
Phosphoglycerate kinase	*PGK1*
Lactate dehydrogenase	*LDHA*
Cytochrome *c* oxidase	*COX I, II,* and *III*
Cytochrome *b* (complex III)	*CYTB*
Mitochondrial tRNA	*Mt-tRNA*
β-Sarcoglycan	*SGCB*

Clinical Manifestations

The classic manifestation of rhabdomyolysis includes acute myalgia and pigmenturia as a result of myoglobinuria in association with elevated serum muscle enzymes (CK in particular). Many clinical features are, however, nonspecific, and the course and initial signs, symptoms, and laboratory abnormalities are clearly dependent on the underlying cause and severity of the event.

Rhabdomyolysis can be accompanied by both local and systemic features. Local features, generally noted in the area of the traumatized muscle groups, can occur within hours of the trauma and include muscle pain, tenderness, and swelling. Systemic features include tea-colored urine, chills, fever, and malaise. In extreme cases, patients complain of nausea and vomiting and demonstrate confusion, agitation, or delirium. Whenever systemic features such as chills, fever, malaise, or generalized muscular involvement are observed, an underlying metabolic myopathy should be considered.

Clinical findings may also include the possibility of compartment syndrome, which can occur in muscle groups encased by fascia, especially the lower leg, forearm, and thigh muscle groups. Sensory abnormalities caused by nerve compression are an early manifestation of compartment syndrome; the loss of a pulse as a result of vascular compromise is a later finding. If compartment syndrome is not addressed within 6 to 8 hours, irreversible ischemic muscle and nerve damage may occur.

Laboratory findings are related to the degree of muscle involvement. Early findings include elevated blood levels of CK, myoglobin, potassium, urea, and phosphorus. CK levels typically peak 2 to 5 days after the initial insult; levels higher than 16,000 U/L are more likely to be associated with renal failure than lower levels are. Hypocalcemia, caused by the influx and deposition of Ca^{2+} in damaged muscle tissue, may accompany rhabdomyolysis. Moreover, an anion gap metabolic acidosis may develop because of release of organic acids from damaged muscle. With resolution of rhabdomyolysis, sequestered Ca^{2+} may be released back into the circulation and cause hypercalcemia.

Diagnosis

Creatine Kinase Levels

A diagnosis of rhabdomyolysis is made when there is clinical evidence of myonecrosis with release into the systemic circulation of muscle cell contents, including myoglobin, creatinine, CK, organic acids, potassium, aldolase, lactate dehydrogenase, and hydroxybutyrate dehydrogenase. The skeletal muscle subtype CK-MM of the CK enzyme is abundantly present in skeletal muscle and released as a result of muscle destruction. Serum levels exceeding 100,000 U/L are not uncommon with rhabdomyolysis. Because CK remains in the circulation longer than myoglobin does and is both easy and efficient to detect clinically, it is the most frequently used marker to diagnose rhabdomyolysis. Levels in excess of five times normal are accepted as evidence of significant muscle breakdown and are generally considered to be consistent with a diagnosis of rhabdomyolysis.

Myoglobin Testing

Myoglobin should be the best marker and the diagnostic cornerstone because myoglobinuria does not occur in the absence of rhabdomyolysis. However, testing for serum or urine myoglobin is problematic and not always consistent. Myoglobin is normally bound to plasma globulins, and therefore only a small fraction reaches the glomeruli. In the face of severe muscle damage, blood levels of myoglobin overwhelm the binding capacity of the circulating proteins, so free myoglobin reaches the glomeruli and eventually the renal tubules. Elevations in serum myoglobin occur before a rise in serum CK, but the elimination kinetics of serum myoglobin is more rapid than that of CK, which makes the often evanescent rises in serum myoglobin a less reliable marker of muscle injury. Furthermore, the liver can quickly metabolize myoglobin. Diagnostic tests for urine myoglobin are often not readily available, and it may take more than 24 hours to obtain results. However, urine screening for rhabdomyolysis may be performed by dipstick if the urine sediment is also examined. The orthotoluidine portion of the dipstick turns blue in the presence of hemoglobin or myoglobin, so if the urine sediment does not contain erythrocytes, one can assume, in the appropriate clinical setting, that the positive dipstick reading reflects the presence of myoglobin. Other associated laboratory findings in acute rhabdomyolysis can include hypocalcemia or hypercalcemia, hyperphosphatemia, metabolic (lactic) acidosis, thrombocytopenia, and disseminated intravascular coagulation.

Differential Diagnosis

The clinical findings of acutely swollen muscles or muscle weakness (or both) with reddish brown urine are not always the result of rhabdomyolysis, and the examining clinician must be careful to scrutinize all information. The differential diagnosis includes disorders that may indirectly affect myocytes, such as Guillain-Barré syndrome and periodic paralysis. Guillain-Barré syndrome (Chapter 446) is distinguished from rhabdomyolysis in that it is characterized as a fulminant polyneuropathy, usually after an antecedent viral infection. Periodic paralysis (Chapter 446) is frequently associated with transient electrolyte disturbances and is unique from rhabdomyolysis in that most cases follow periods of rest or sleep.

Myoglobinuria causes the urine to be reddish brown, but tea (or cola) colored urine does not necessarily indicate the presence of myoglobin. Other conditions associated with discoloration of urine include hemoglobinuria from hemolysis, intrinsic renal disease, porphyria, acute glomerulonephritis, "athletic pseudonephritis," or external factors such as ingestion of beets and various drugs (e.g., phenytoin, rifampin, vitamin B_{12}).

Diagnosing rhabdomyolysis is complete when the clinician determines the cause. This step, though frequently established during the history and physical examination, may require further diagnostic assessment after initiating clinical treatment during the acute phase. Clinical issues that are not only controversial but also poorly defined include who warrants further testing and what tests to perform. Individuals with recurrent rhabdomyolysis, a positive family history of rhabdomyolysis or malignant hyperthermia, low exercise tolerance, no apparent etiology, or a fulminant/explosive form of rhabdomyolysis appear to warrant further testing.

Testing may include a nonischemic forearm test, which involves isometric exercise at 70% of maximal voluntary contraction for 30 seconds under nonischemic conditions; electromyography; a muscle disease enzyme panel (e.g., mitochondrial myopathies [Chapter 447], fatty acid transport defects [Chapter 119], glycogen storage diseases [Chapter 219], diseases associated with myoglobinuria); muscle biopsy to investigate specific metabolic myopathies and other enzyme or genetic defects; or any combination of such testing. The forearm exercise test may help identify metabolic and genetic causes of rhabdomyolysis. Patients who have had an episode of malignant hyperthermia or exertional heat illness may be candidates for a caffeine halothane contracture test, which evaluates the force produced in small muscle biopsy samples after exposure to caffeine and separately to halothane in the laboratory. Isolated, perfused muscle fibers must show an increase in tension of at least 0.2 g when exposed to 2 mM of caffeine or at least 0.7 g of tension after exposure to 3% halothane. Additionally, genetic investigation for mutations of the *RYR1* receptor gene may be warranted.

Prevention

Approaches for preventing rhabdomyolysis induced by infections, medications, toxins, heat stress, or exercise may emerge in the future, but no definitive guidelines can be presented. To prevent further muscle injury, blood flow to ischemic areas must be promptly restored to minimize ischemia-reperfusion damage. Administration of free radical scavengers to prevent rhabdomyolysis may prove useful in the future.

Treatment

Treatment of rhabdomyolysis begins with a careful history and physical examination to identify and manage any underlying illness and then focuses on preserving renal function. All patients require aggressive, early management because it is difficult to stratify risk initially. Careful observation plus treatment of potential early and late complications is critical. Accordingly, vital signs, urine output, serial electrolyte levels, and CK levels should be obtained as soon as possible. Intensive care monitoring may be required, depending on the clinical situation.

Hydration

Hydration is the cornerstone of preserving renal function in patients with rhabdomyolysis. Providing fluids addresses the early threats to survival: hypovolemic shock and hyperkalemia. Currently, no clinical prediction rule exists for risk-stratifying patients with rhabdomyolysis or for determining in whom acute renal failure will develop, but CK levels greater than 15,000 U/L are thought to portend an increased risk. Patients with mild symptoms and serum CK levels less than 3000 U/L are considered to be at low risk and may be treated as outpatients with hydration, limited physical activity, and careful follow-up. Victims of collapse, trauma, or exertional heat injury or patients who demonstrate moderate early symptoms with more than mild elevations in CK or an abnormal metabolic panel should be treated with intravenous hydration in an inpatient setting. Hydration is accomplished by aggressive intravenous fluid therapy with isotonic fluids at a rate that will result in a urine output of 200 mL/hr until CK levels begin to decrease. When fluid resuscitation fails to correct intractable hyperkalemia and acidosis, dialysis should be considered.

Specific Therapeutic Measures

Several retrospective clinical studies and case reports, as well as animal models, promote the addition of bicarbonate and mannitol, but no prospective clinical trials have been conducted to support or refute their benefits in managing rhabdomyolysis. Alkalinization of urine is advocated for the purpose of decreasing cast formation, minimizing the toxic effects of myoglobin on the renal tubules, inhibiting lipid peroxidation, and decreasing the risk for hyperkalemia. However, this approach can cause Ca^{2+} to precipitate and be deposited in the soft tissues, as well as contribute to a hyperosmolar state. Mannitol serves as an osmotic diuretic, volume expander, and free radical scavenger; it should be used very carefully in patients with marginal cardiac function and only after adequate renal function is established.

For rhabdomyolysis caused by crush syndrome, both mannitol and a forced alkaline diuresis are recommended when CK levels are greater than 20,000 U/L. The treatment goals of this algorithm are to (1) achieve a urine output of 200 mL/hr, (2) maintain urine pH between 6 and 7, (3) keep serum pH below 7.50, and (4) achieve hemodynamic stability and prevent volume overload. The fluid resuscitation recommendation begins with a bolus of 1 L of 5% dextrose plus 0.22% NaCl and 100 mEq $NaHCO_3$ over a 30-minute period, followed by an infusion at 2 to 5 mL/kg/hr. A 20% mannitol infusion at a dose of 0.5 g/kg is given over a 15-minute period and subsequently followed by an infusion at 0.1 g/kg/hr. Adjustments are made to maintain urine output at greater than 200 mL/hr. Urinary and serum pH levels are monitored, with acetazolamide added if the serum pH exceeds 7.45 or urinary pH remains below 6.0. However, the use of mannitol and forced alkaline diuresis in patients with crush syndrome, as well as other clinical manifestations of rhabdomyolysis, has not been tested in randomized trials.

Managing Metabolic Abnormalities

Deposition of Ca^{2+}, which occurs early in rhabdomyolysis, is directly related to the degree of muscle destruction and administration of Ca^{2+}. Reversal of hypocalcemia may in fact worsen ectopic calcification and exacerbate hypercalcemia during the resolution phase. Accordingly, hypocalcemia should be treated only when clinical symptoms, signs of tetany, or severe hyperkalemia develops.

Rx

Management of Compartment Syndrome

Compartment syndrome (Chapter 113) is a well-described late complication as well as a potential cause of rhabdomyolysis. Compartment syndrome can occur as a direct consequence of muscle injury with increased vascular permeability, aggressive fluid resuscitation, or restoration of reperfusion. In patients in whom a compartment syndrome is suspected, such as when the muscles are tense and swollen or there is evidence of neurovascular compromise, compartment pressures should be promptly measured; in the proper clinical setting, pressures in excess of 30 mm Hg should prompt consideration of fasciotomy. However, late fasciotomy (>12 hours after the onset of symptoms) may be counterproductive by converting a closed injury to an open wound with an increased risk for uncontrollable infection. Accordingly, late fasciotomy is relatively contraindicated.

Management of Crush Injury

Management of crush injury victims (Chapter 113) is unique in that many individuals have the opportunity for treatment before extrication and reperfusion. Current recommendations for on-site management of trauma victims before extrication include aggressive hydration with intravenous normal saline. In the event of massive damage, amputation of the extremity may be required to protect the patient's overall health. A Mangled Extremity Severity Score (MESS) may be used to identify nonsalvageable extremities prospectively. The MESS is a grading system based on four groups of clinical criteria, including the degree of skeletal/soft tissue injury, rating of blood pressure (shock) and pulse (ischemia), and age. Scores from each group are added to obtain a total score that ranges from 0 to 14; higher scores indicate more severe involvement, and a score of 7 or greater has a positive predictive value of nearly 100% for amputation. Ongoing clinical trials in this population will, it is hoped, elucidate the role of antioxidant therapy (glutathione and vitamin E) in scavenging free radicals, dantrolene sodium in inhibiting Ca^{2+} release, and deferoxamine in reducing the direct toxic effects of myoglobin on the kidneys.

Malignant Hyperthermia

One cause of rhabdomyolysis that requires rapid and aggressive management is malignant hyperthermia (Chapter 458). Episodes of malignant hyperthermia occur most commonly in the operating room and are recognized by the anesthesiologist. The typical clinical features represent an uncontrolled, exaggerated, hypermetabolic state; an increase in end-tidal CO_2 during ventilation is the most sensitive sign. On clinical recognition of impending malignant hyperthermia, anesthetics should be discontinued, and the patient should be treated with dantrolene sodium; the usual initial dose is 2.5 to 4.0 mg/kg, followed by about 1 mg/kg every 4 hours for up to 48 hours to avoid recrudescence.

Prognosis

The most serious consequence of rhabdomyolysis is acute renal failure, which occurs in up to 67% of all cases of rhabdomyolysis, regardless of etiology. Although acute renal failure may be relatively benign, the mortality rate from myoglobinuric renal failure is reported to range from 3 to 80%. Various clinical factors are used to predict the risk for acute renal failure, including serum CK, creatinine, potassium, and Ca^{2+}, as well as the urine myoglobin level, but no single parameter has been established. However, mortality appears to be significantly higher in patients with CK values in excess of 75,000 U/L and in those with hyperkalemia or hypocalcemia. For compartment syndrome, a poor prognosis is associated with an ischemic period lasting longer than 6 hours.

The prognosis of patients with rhabdomyolysis improves markedly when treatment is started soon after the diagnosis has been made. With mild episodes, the prognosis is customarily excellent, and the patient can typically resume usual activities within several weeks after CK levels have normalized. However, some patients do not return to normal and continue to experience extreme fatigue and muscle pain on exertion. These patients will require additional testing (a nonischemic forearm test, electromyography, a muscle disease enzyme panel, muscle biopsy) to determine whether an underlying metabolic myopathy exists. The results of these tests will help determine future recommendations, but the patient's tolerance and response to light and more strenuous exercise will also be very important in providing recommendations.

Future Directions

Although a number of genetic mutations have already been defined, the prevalence of such mutations is unknown. Moreover, a genetic linkage for individuals susceptible to exertional or drug-induced rhabdomyolysis (or both) has not been investigated. It is also likely that the greatest progress will come from prospective trials that evaluate treatment modalities for myoglobinuric renal failure.

SUGGESTED READINGS

Antons KA, Williams CD, Baker SK, et al: Clinical perspectives of statin-induced rhabdomyolysis. Am J Med 2006;119:400–409. *A practical overview.*

Fine DM, Gelber AC, Melamed ML, et al: Risk factors for renal failure among 72 consecutive patients with rhabdomyolysis related to illicit drug use. Am J Med 2004;117:607–610. *Renal failure was more likely in patients with higher initial creatinine levels, leukocytosis, and hypotension.*

Giannoglu GD, Chatzizisis YS, Misirli G: The syndrome of rhabdomyolysis: Pathophysiology and diagnosis. Eur J Intern Med 2007;18:90–100. *A clinical review.*

Malinoski DJ, Slater MS, Mullins RJ: Crush injury and rhabdomyolysis. Crit Care Clin 2004;20:171–192. *A comprehensive review.*

Warren JD, Blumbergs PC, Thompson PD: Rhabdomyolysis: A review. Muscle Nerve 2002;25:332–347. *A comprehensive review.*

Cecil Medicine 23

Section XI

Renal and Genitourinary Diseases

APPROACH TO THE PATIENT WITH RENAL DISEASE

Hasan Bazari

Diagnosis

The patient with renal dysfunction exhibits signs and symptoms of renal disease regardless of etiology and features of any accompanying systemic illness. Clinical presentation highlights the central role that the kidney plays in a variety of physiologic functions. These functions include the clearance of nitrogenous waste products, regulation of electrolytes and pH, maintenance of blood pressure, regulation of volume, synthesis of active forms of vitamin D, and synthesis of erythropoietin.

Most of the diagnoses of renal disease can be made with a careful history and physical examination supplemented by review of basic laboratory tests, especially the urinary sediment. The specificity of the diagnosis can be improved by the use of serologic analysis, imaging, and, occasionally, invasive procedures such as angiography and renal biopsy.

History

The history reviews potential factors that contribute to the development of renal disease and identifies the systemic features of diseases that may affect the kidney. These factors include

- Medication use
- Family history of renal disease
- The time of onset of symptoms of renal dysfunction
- Changes in bladder function, including nocturia, polyuria, and hesitancy
- Fatigue and weakness
- Dyspnea on exertion, a manifestation of fluid overload or acidosis

A systemic vasculitis may present in a variety of ways, with skin manifestations including petechial rash, purpura, digital gangrene, and splinter hemorrhages. Otitis, sinusitis, epistaxis, hemoptysis, and nasal septal ulcers are common manifestations of Wegener's granulomatosis. Pulmonary hemorrhage can be a catastrophic manifestation of Goodpasture's syndrome or anti–glomerular basement membrane (anti-GBM) disease. Abdominal distention may be seen in nephrotic syndrome with ascites, as well as in autosomal polycystic kidney disease. Abdominal pain and tenderness may be observed in Henoch-Schönlein purpura and classic polyarteritis nodosa. Lower extremity edema is common in cirrhosis, congestive heart failure, and nephrotic syndrome. Neurologic symptoms may be a manifestation of vasculitis, such as microscopic polyangiitis and cryoglobulinemia.

Physical Examination

The vital signs are crucial. A patient with a "normal blood pressure" may be relatively hypotensive in the setting of renovascular disease. Pulsus paradoxus may reflect cardiac tamponade.

The eyes may exhibit conjunctivitis, episcleritis, or uveitis. In the abdomen, ascites may be seen in cirrhosis, nephrosis, and congestive heart failure. Hepatomegaly is seen in passive congestion and amyloidosis. Splenomegaly may be seen in amyloidosis, endocarditis, and lymphoma. Kidney and liver enlargement may be seen in autosomal dominant polycystic kidney disease. Lower extremity edema can be seen in cirrhosis, nephrotic syndrome, and congestive heart failure. Splinter hemorrhages as well as Osler's nodes and Janeway lesions may represent bacterial endocarditis. Rashes can be seen in many of the vasculitides.

Cardiovascular Signs

Assessment of the jugular venous pressure plays a crucial role in the bedside evaluation of volume status and, perhaps more than any other part of the examination, should be assessed daily. The presence of a pericardial friction rub can be observed in the serositis associated with systemic lupus erythematosus (SLE) or the pericarditis associated with uremia. Infiltrative diseases, such as amyloidosis and sarcoidosis, can lead to restrictive cardiomyopathy with associated congestive heart failure. The presence of a fourth heart sound (S_4) may be a sign of cardiac hypertrophy, and S_3 may be a sign of congestive heart failure. Vascular bruits reflect generalized atherosclerosis, and the presence of an abdominal bruit may be an important clue to the presence of renovascular disease.

Neurologic Signs

Peripheral neuropathy may be seen in vasculitis with involvement of the nerves as mononeuritis multiplex. Frank cerebrovascular accidents may be seen in SLE and in the antiphospholipid antibody syndrome.

The signs and symptoms of chronic renal failure are shown in Figure 115–1.

Laboratory Findings

Urinalysis is central to the renal evaluation of the patient. The following aspects of the assessment of the urine are important in the approach to the patient with renal disease.

Twenty-four Hour Urine Collection for Protein Excretion

Proteinuria (as albuminuria) of greater than 3.5 g in 24 hours indicates glomerular disease. Lesser quantities do not preclude glomerular disease, and electrophoresis gives valuable insight into the composition of the proteinuria. Occasionally, overflow proteinuria of a small-molecular-weight protein, such as light chains in Bence Jones proteinuria, can be greater than 3.5 g/day without any of the manifestations or implications of the nephrotic syndrome. A urine protein electrophoresis study is important in making the distinction. Collection must be done by discarding the first morning void and collecting the voids for the next 24 hours, including the first morning void the next day.

Protein-to-Creatinine Ratio

The 24-hour urine collection for protein excretion is cumbersome and subject to inaccuracies. A spot urine sample for protein and creatinine can be used to estimate the amount of protein excreted. A protein-to-creatinine ratio of 3 estimates that the 24-hour protein excretion is about 3 g. The ratio may be inaccurate in patients with orthostatic proteinuria.

Urine for Microalbumin

The excretion of abnormal quantities of albumin below the level detectable by the urine dipstick is called *microalbuminuria*. Normal albumin excretion is less than 30 mg/day. This is detected by radioimmunoassay or enzyme immunoassay. Microalbuminuria is the earliest clinically detectable stage of diabetic nephropathy.

Fractional Excretion of Sodium

The excretion of sodium in the setting of oliguria and acute renal failure often gives insight into the appropriateness of tubular function. The fractional excretion of sodium (Fe_{Na}) is calculated as follows:

$$Fe_{Na} = (\text{urine Na/plasma Na})/(\text{urine Cr/plasma Cr}) \times 100$$

where *Na* is the urine sodium concentration (in millimoles per liter [mmol/L]), and *Cr* is the creatinine concentration (in mmol/L). In the setting of oliguria, an Fe_{Na} of less than 1% often denotes prerenal azotemia, whereas an Fe_{Na} of greater than 1% denotes intrinsic renal failure. Although this measurement is generally useful, there are instances when an Fe_{Na} of less than 1% may be seen in cases without a prerenal component, including contrast nephropathy, hepatorenal syndrome, obstructive uropathy, interstitial nephritis, glomerulonephritis, and rhabdomyolysis. Conversely, a high Fe_{Na} can be seen in cases in which there is a prerenal component, including diuretic use, adrenal insufficiency, cerebral salt wasting, and salt-wasting nephropathy. The Fe_{Na} must be evaluated in the context of the clinical situation, because it can be low or high in a normal patient or in a patient with chronic kidney disease. Ultimately, volume assessment is done best at the bedside, assessing the patient, and cannot be deduced from a measurement of electrolytes.

Fractional Excretion of Urea

If diuretics are being used, the Fe_{Na} is unreliable, and the fractional excretion of urea can be used as a surrogate for the assessment of volume status. Urea reabsorption varies with the volume status, increasing in the setting of volume depletion. A fractional excretion of less than 30% indicates a state of decreased effective circulating volume. The formula for calculation of the fractional excretion of urea is the same as that for Fe_{Na}.

Twenty-four Hour Urine Collection for Calcium, Uric Acid, Oxalate, Citrate, Sodium, and Creatinine

These studies are performed in the evaluation of the patient with recurrent kidney stones. Depending on the laboratory, the calcium measurement may made on a different collection from the others. These measurements should be conducted with the patient on a normal diet and with normal activity and should not be done during a hospitalization.

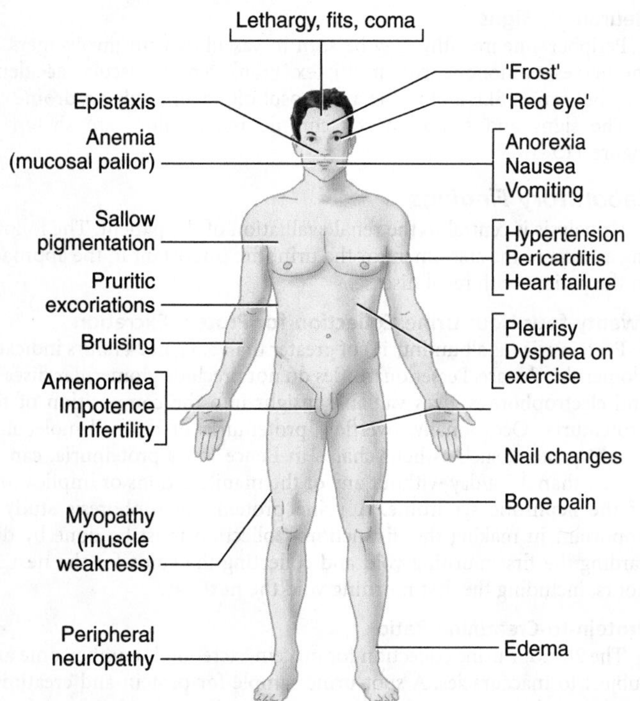

FIGURE 115–1 • Common symptoms and signs of chronic renal failure. (Redrawn from Forbes CD, Jackson WF: Color Atlas and Text of Clinical Medicine, 3rd ed. London, Mosby, 2003, with permission.)

Often these tests need to repeated before therapeutic decisions are made. The 24-hour urine sodium and creatinine excretion should be determined with each measurement to ensure adequacy of collection.

Urine Potassium Excretion and the Transtubular Potassium Gradient

Potassium is handled differently from sodium. It is completely reabsorbed and excreted in a flow-dependent manner. Potassium excretion depends on adequate distal sodium delivery and reabsorption to provide a sufficient electrochemical gradient for tubular potassium excretion. Failure to excrete potassium is seen in volume depletion. The excretion of less than 15 mmol/day of potassium in the face of hyperkalemia suggests an inadequate renal response. The transtubular potassium gradient (TTKG) is an approximation of the gradient of potassium before the effect of antidiuretic hormone on the concentration of potassium in the urine. The formula for the measurement of the TTKG is as follows:

$$\text{TTKG} = (\text{urine K}/\text{plasma K})/(\text{urine Osm}/\text{plasma Osm})$$

where *K* is the potassium concentration, and *Osm* is osmolality. A TTKG ratio of less than 4 in the setting of hyperkalemia implies either inadequate distal sodium delivery or inadequacy of the distal potassium excretion system. A TTKG ratio of greater than 10 in the setting of hypokalemia supports the presence of renal potassium wasting, and further elucidation of the exact stimulus for potassium loss is warranted.

Urine Net Charge

Urine net charge measures the ability of the kidney to synthesize ammonia (NH_4^+) and to excrete acid in non–anion gap metabolic acidosis. The difference between the concentration of urine cations (Na^+ and K^+) and that of urine anions (mainly Cl^-) represents the urine net charge:

$$\text{Urine net charge} = (\text{urine Na}^+ + \text{urine K}^+) - (\text{urine Cl}^-)$$

A negative urine net charge indicates NH_4^+ in the urine. This formula does not apply when there is an anion gap metabolic acidosis. The unmeasured anion complicates this measurement of ammonium ion in the urine.

Urinalysis

The analysis of the urine sample involves simple observation and separate measurements using specific tools or commercially available dipsticks.

TABLE 115–1 MACROSCOPIC APPEARANCE OF URINE

Appearance	Cause
Milky	Acid urine: urate crystals Alkaline urine: insoluble phosphates Infection: pus Spermatozoa Chyluria
Smoky pink	Hematuria (>0.54 mL blood/L urine)
Foamy	Proteinuria
Blue or green	*Pseudomonas* urinary tract infection Bilirubin Methylene blue
Pink or red	Aniline dyes in sweets Porphyrins (on standing) Blood, hemoglobin, myoglobin Drugs: phenindione, phenolphthalein Anthocyaninuria (beetroot-"beeturia")
Orange	Drugs: anthraquinones (laxatives), rifampicin Urobilinogenuria
Yellow	Mepacrine Conjugated bilirubin Phenacetin Riboflavin
Brown or black	Melanin (on standing) Myoglobin (on standing) Alkaptonuria
Green or black	Phenol Lysol
Brown	Drugs: phenazopyridine, furazolidone, L-dopa, niridazole Hemoglobin and myoglobin (on standing) Bilirubin

From Forbes CD, Jackson WF: Color Atlas and Text of Clinical Medicine, 3rd ed. London, Mosby, 2003.

Appearance and Color

The normal color of the urine is derived from urochromes, which are pigments excreted in the urine. Abnormal color or appearance of the urine may be explained by many conditions, as listed in Table 115–1.

Specific Gravity

The specific gravity of the urine can be raised by the presence of an increased number of solutes or by molecules with a high molecular weight, such as glucose or contrast dye. There is a linear relationship between specific gravity and osmolality, unless there is glycosuria or excretion of contrast media, in which case the specific gravity is higher. A fixed specific gravity of 1.010 is characteristic of chronic kidney disease.

pH

Urine pH is often 5 as a result of daily net acid excretion. An alkaline pH often is noted after meals, when an "alkaline tide" associated with gastric acid excretion causes a high urine pH. A high urine pH also is seen in patients who are on a vegetarian diet or who have an infection with a urea-splitting organism, such as *Proteus*. An inappropriately high urine pH in the setting of systemic non–anion gap metabolic acidosis may be seen in certain forms of renal tubular acidosis (RTA). In a proximal RTA, the urine pH is high until the tubular threshold for bicarbonate, which is reset, is reached. At this point, the urine pH decreases to 5. In distal RTA, there is usually an inability to create a sufficient gradient for hydrogen ion (H^+) excretion, and the urine pH is always higher than 5.5. The urine net charge gives complementary and confirmatory information. In type 4 RTA, the urine pH is often 5, and the urine net charge is often positive, confirming the absence of significant amounts of ammonium in the urine, a defect that is exacerbated by the accompanying hyperkalemia.

Glucose

Glucose in the urine is detected by an assay using dipsticks impregnated with the enzyme glucose oxidase. Glycosuria is seen in diabetes

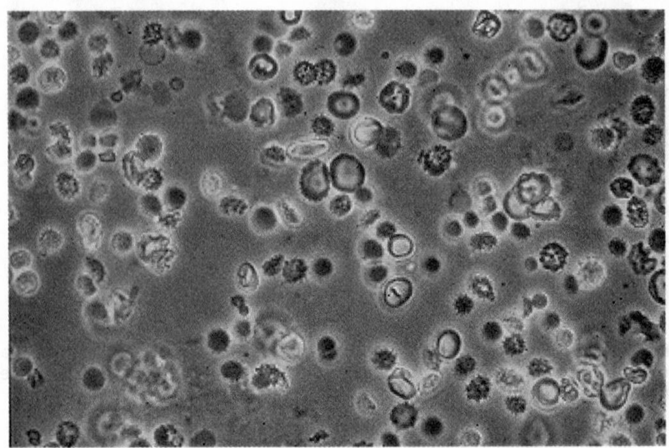

FIGURE 115–2 • Dysmorphic erythrocytes. These dysmorphic erythrocytes vary in size, shape, and hemoglobin content and reflect glomerular bleeding. (From Johnson RJ, Feehally J: Comprehensive Clinical Nephrology. London, Mosby, 2000, with permission.)

mellitus, when pregnancy causes the tubular threshold for glucose reabsorption to change, and in tubular diseases that affect the proximal convoluted tubule and cause tubular glycosuria. Evidence for panproximal tubular dysfunction (e.g., glycosuria, aminoaciduria, phosphaturia) indicates that Fanconi's syndrome is present.

Protein

The dipstick for protein is a sensitive assay based on color change induced by the presence of proteins at a given pH. It is most sensitive to the presence of albumin and is much less sensitive to other proteins, such as the light chains of Bence Jones protein. The presence of 1+ protein correlates with about 30 mg/dL of albuminuria, and 3+ protein correlates with greater than 500 mg/dL of proteinuria. Because the dipstick is not a quantitative measurement, small amounts of proteinuria in an oliguric patient may give the false appearance of high-grade proteinuria.

Heme

The dipstick uses the peroxidase-like activity of the hemoglobin and myoglobin molecules to detect the presence of heme pigment. The reaction occurs on exposure to hemoglobin, myoglobin, or intact red blood cells (RBCs). The presence of myoglobin or hemoglobin is suspected if the heme reaction is intensely positive and there is a paucity of cellular elements in the sediment.

Leukocytes

The detection of leukocytes depends on the presence of leukocyte esterase in leukocytes. They usually are present in infections and in inflammatory conditions.

Urine Sediment

Cells

The urine sediment is the most crucial step in the evaluation of renal disease. The sediment gives an insight through the cellular elements resulting from activity within the kidney. The cells that may be seen include RBCs, white blood cells (WBCs), tubular cells, transitional cells, and squamous epithelial cells. Casts are formed in tubules and may contain cells or be acellular.

RBCs may originate from intrarenal vessels, glomeruli, tubules, or anywhere in the urogenital tract. Dysmorphic RBCs are cells that have been deformed by transit through glomeruli, as opposed to RBCs from the remainder of the genitourinary tract (Figs. 115–2 and 115–3). The cells are often lysed and less refractile than nonglomerular RBCs. They often fragment with poikilocytosis and with blebs, forming so-called Mickey Mouse RBCs. Phase contrast microscopy aids in the identification of dysmorphic RBCs. The presence of a majority of dysmorphic RBCs in a urine sediment points to a glomerular origin for the hematuria. The presence of RBC casts is often conclusive evidence for the presence of glomerulonephritis. WBCs are seen most commonly in urinary tract infections. They also can be seen in acute interstitial nephritis, with *Legionella* and *Leptospira* infections, chronic infections such as tuberculosis, allergic interstitial nephritis, atheroembolic diseases, and granulomatous diseases such as sarcoidosis and tubulointerstitial nephritis

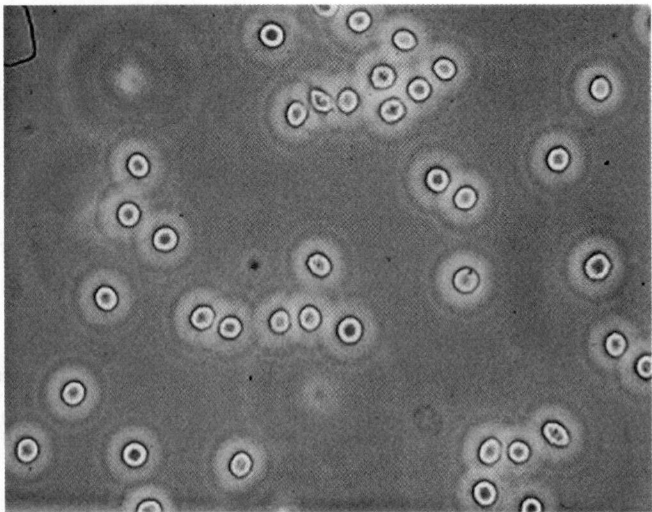

FIGURE 115–3 • Isomorphic erythrocytes. These erythrocytes are similar in size, shape, and hemoglobin content. Isomorphic cells reflect nonglomerular bleeding from lesions such as calculi or papillomas or hemorrhage from cysts in polycystic renal disease. (From Johnson RJ, Feehally J: Comprehensive Clinical Nephrology. London, Mosby, 2000, with permission.)

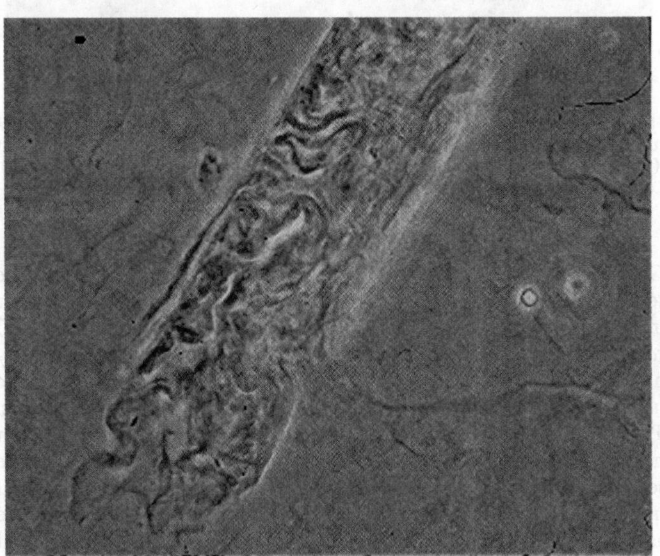

FIGURE 115–4 • Hyaline cast of the type seen in small numbers in normal urine. (From Johnson RJ, Feehally J: Comprehensive Clinical Nephrology. London, Mosby, 2000, with permission.)

syndrome. Mononuclear cells often appear with transplant rejection. Tubular cells are seen in many conditions involving tubulointerstitial diseases. They also are seen in ischemic and nephrotoxic injury, such as with myeloma kidney or cast nephropathy. Eosinophils require special stains, with the Giemsa stain being much less sensitive than the Hansel stain. Urine eosinophils are seen in a variety of conditions. Classically associated with allergic interstitial nephritis, they also have been documented in atheroembolic disease, prostatitis, and vasculitis.

Other Elements

Other elements that may be seen in the urine sediment are bacteria. A spun urine sediment may show rods or cocci in chains, but these are identified best by Gram staining of the urine sediment. In the sediment, one may see budding yeast forms, which are highly refractile, and spermatozoa.

Casts

Casts are formed in tubules and are characterized by the arrangement of the cells in a clearly formed matrix composed of Tamm-Horsfall protein. Because casts are formed in the renal parenchyma, they may give a clue to the origin of accompanying cellular elements.

Hyaline casts are casts of Tamm-Horsfall proteins that are formed normally and are seen in increased numbers after exercise (Fig. 115–4).

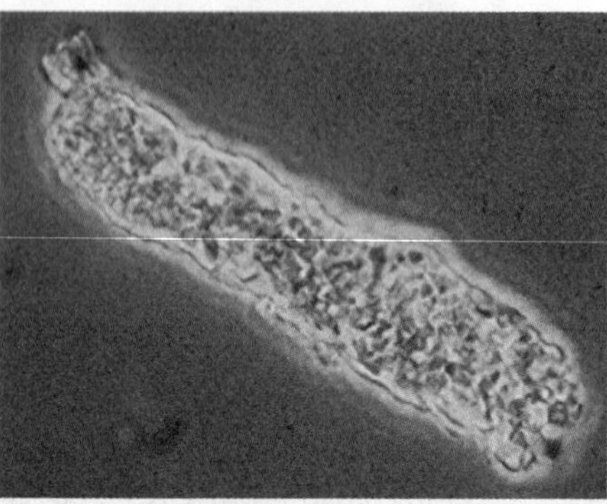

FIGURE 115–5 • Number and type of granules and their density in the cast vary in different casts. The presence of erythrocytes in this cast may mean that the granules are derived partly from disrupted erythrocytes. (From Johnson RJ, Feehally J: Comprehensive Clinical Nephrology. London, Mosby, 2000, with permission.)

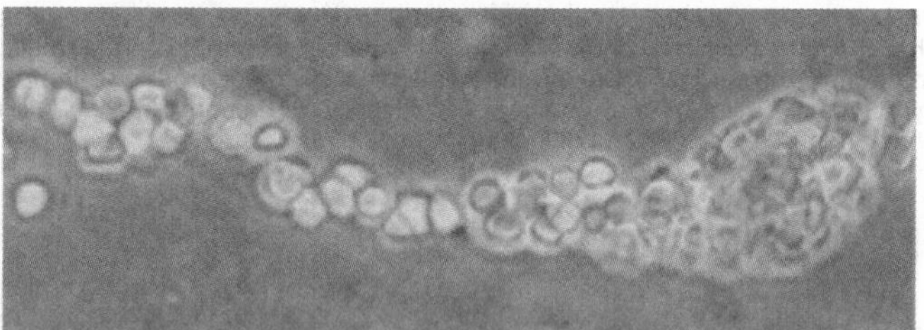

FIGURE 115–6 • A cast composed entirely of erythrocytes reflects heavy hematuria and active glomerular disease. Crescentic nephritis is likely to be present if erythrocyte cast density is greater than 100/mL. (From Johnson RJ, Feehally J: Comprehensive Clinical Nephrology. London, Mosby, 2000, with permission.)

Granular casts are degenerated tubular cell casts that are seen in the setting of tubular injury (Fig. 115–5). *Pigmented granular casts* are seen in rhabdomyolysis with myoglobinuria or, rarely, hemoglobinuria. *RBC casts* are diagnostic of glomerulonephritis (Fig. 115–6). Although they have been reported in allergic interstitial nephritis and diabetic nephropathy, they almost always are seen in acute glomerulonephritis. The presence of RBC casts in a patient with microscopic hematuria can narrow the focus of the work-up to a glomerular lesion. *WBC casts* are seen commonly in pyelonephritis and in acute and chronic nonbacterial infections. They also are seen in other conditions in which WBCs are associated with parenchymal renal processes, such as allergic interstitial nephritis, atheroembolic diseases, and granulomatous diseases such as sarcoidosis. Rarely, they can be a dominant feature of many diseases that traditionally are thought of as glomerular diseases, such as SLE and Wegener's granulomatosis. *Tubular cell casts* are seen with any acute tubular injury and are the dominant cellular casts in ischemic acute tubular necrosis. They also can be seen with nephrotoxic injury, such as with aminoglycosides and cisplatin. Casts may have leukocytes and tubular cells or be difficult to distinguish.

Crystals

Crystals often can be a normal finding in the urine or serve as clues to pathophysiologic processes. Certain crystals, such as the hexagonal crystals seen with cystinuria, are always abnormal (Fig. 115–7). Others, such as calcium oxalate crystals (Fig. 115–8), may be a normal finding or may be evidence for ethylene glycol intoxication in a patient with anion gap metabolic acidosis, acute renal failure, or hypocalcemia and mental status change. Triple phosphate crystals are composed of ammonium magnesium phosphate and are coffin shaped (Fig. 115–9). These are seen in urinary tract infections with urea splitting organisms. Uric acid crystals, sodium urate crystals (Fig. 115–10), and calcium phosphate amorphous crystals all are common and do not denote any pathologic significance.

Measurement of Renal Function

In clinical practice, renal function is measured by serum creatinine. It is normally a relatively fixed value in a given patient. Creatine is released as a waste product from myocytes and converted to creatinine in the liver. The normal range of serum creatinine is 0.6 to 1.5 mg/dL. About 10% of the daily creatinine is excreted through tubular secretion. Mild elevations of the plasma creatinine concentration can occur during treatment with cimetidine or trimethoprim, both of which interfere with the tubular secretion of creatinine. They are unlikely to cause significant elevations of the plasma creatinine. Ketoacids cause an artifactual increase in the plasma creatinine by interfering with the creatinine assay. The relationship between the glomerular filtration rate (GFR) and serum creatinine is such that there can be substantial loss of renal function while the serum creatinine concentration remains in the normal range. The concentration of blood urea nitrogen (BUN), which is a product of protein catabolism, is about 10-fold higher than creatinine concentration, and the BUN-to-creatinine ratio commonly is used as a marker of volume status. There

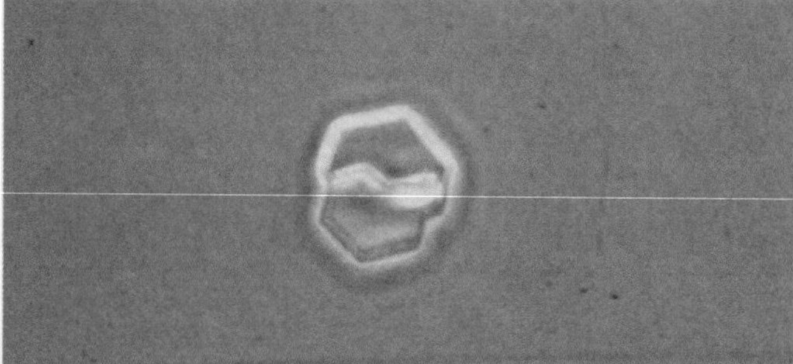

FIGURE 115–7 • Typical hexagonal cystine crystal. A single crystal provides a definitive diagnosis of cystinuria. (From Johnson RJ, Feehally J: Comprehensive Clinical Nephrology. London, Mosby, 2000, with permission.)

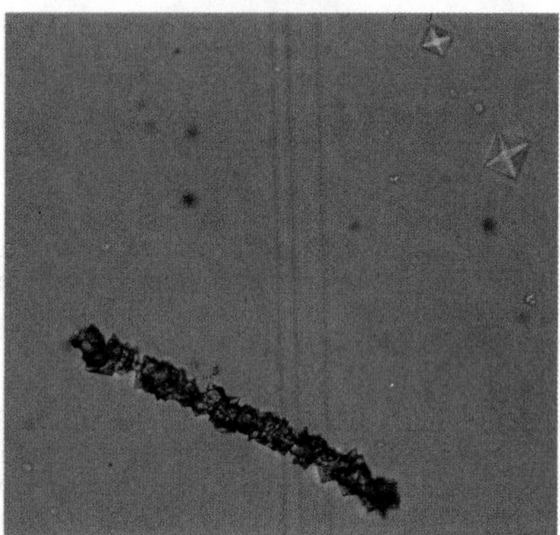

FIGURE 115–8 • Oxalate crystals. A pseudocast of calcium oxalate crystals accompanied by crystals of calcium oxalate dehydrate. (From Johnson RJ, Feehally J: Comprehensive Clinical Nephrology. London, Mosby, 2000, with permission.)

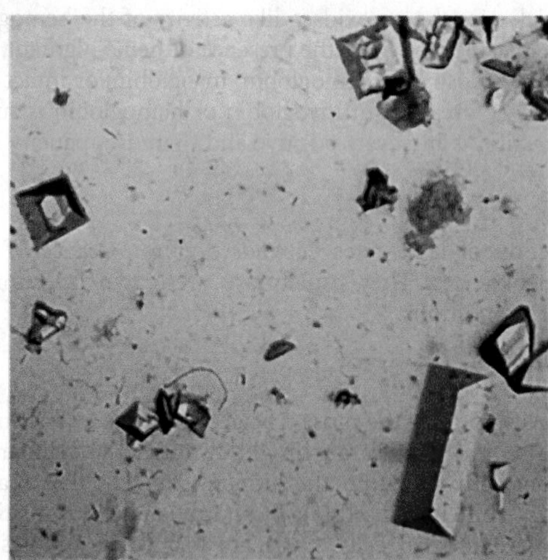

FIGURE 115–9 • Coffin-lid crystals of magnesium ammonium phosphate (struvite). (From Johnson RJ, Feehally J: Comprehensive Clinical Nephrology. London, Mosby, 2000, with permission.)

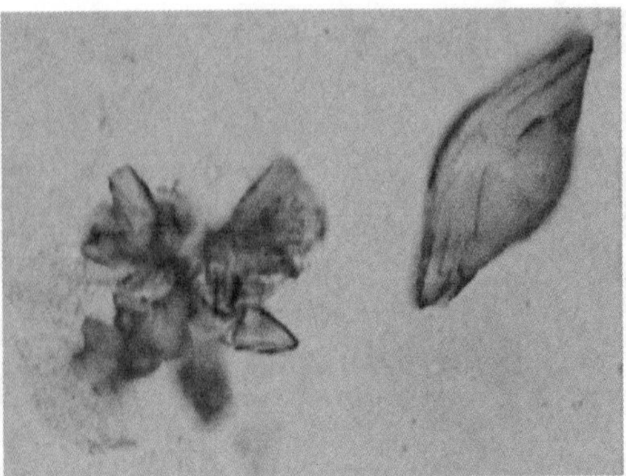

FIGURE 115–10 • Urate crystals. Complex crystals suggestive of acute urate nephropathy or urate nephrolithiasis. (From Johnson RJ, Feehally J: Comprehensive Clinical Nephrology. London, Mosby, 2000, with permission.)

are circumstances, however, in which the BUN may be inappropriately high, such as with gastrointestinal bleeding or the use of steroids or tetracyclines. The BUN may be low if there is poor dietary intake of protein and in liver disease.

The creatinine clearance can be estimated from the serum creatinine concentration by the Cockcroft-Gault formula:

$$GFR = \frac{(140 - age) \times wt\,[in\ kg]}{72 \times serum\ creatinine} (\times .85\ if\ female)$$

Creatinine clearance is calculated often using a 24-hour urine collection for measurement of the creatinine concentration. The patient needs to be instructed to discard the first morning urine before initiating the collection and to conclude the collection by including the next morning void. The formula for calculating creatinine clearance is as follows:

$$CCr = urine\ Cr \times V/plasma\ Cr$$

where *CCr* is creatinine clearance, *urine Cr* is urine creatinine concentration, *V* is urine flow rate, and *plasma Cr* is plasma creatinine. The creatinine clearance overestimates GFR by about 10% owing to tubular secretion of creatinine. This secretion can be modified by the use of cimetidine, which is a competitive inhibitor of tubular creatinine secretion.

Inulin, a 5200-D uncharged polymer of fructose, is an ideal marker for the measurement of GFR because it is not reabsorbed, secreted, synthesized, or metabolized. It is not available for routine clinical assessment, however. Iothalamate clearance is an accurate measurement of GFR and is available as a diagnostic tool in clinical studies. Other agents that are used for the measurement of GFR include technetium-99m diethylenetriaminepentaacetic acid (^{99m}Tc-DPTA) and sodium chromate chromium 51-labeled ethylenediaminetetraacetic acid.

Serology and Urine Tests for the Evaluation of Renal Disease

The evaluation of renal dysfunction has to follow a stepwise progression from noninvasive serologic evaluation to a definitive or confirmatory diagnostic evaluation, such as a renal biopsy. Sometimes an expeditious diagnosis is needed, and a biopsy may be done relatively early in the evaluation. The advent of improved serologic diagnostic markers for certain diseases such as Wegener's granulomatosis has made the role of biopsy less mandatory than in the past. The following serologic tests are used commonly in the evaluation of renal insufficiency.

Antinuclear Antibody

The antinuclear antibody (ANA) is one of the most commonly used tests in the evaluation of acute renal failure and chronic kidney disease, when there is the presumption of a glomerular disease, and in the evaluation of the cause of idiopathic nephrotic syndrome. Although a high titer, especially if it is accompanied by a more specific finding such as anti-double-stranded DNA (anti-dsDNA) antibody or anti-Smith antibody, can be highly specific for the diagnosis of SLE, the usual titers are lower and have less specificity. The diagnosis of SLE still hinges on classic clinical criteria and often requires a renal biopsy, although there have been arguments in the literature regarding the utility of renal biopsy in the therapeutic decision making.

Rheumatoid Factor

The role of rheumatoid factor (RF) is even less clear than that of ANA. Vasculitis in rheumatoid arthritis is a relatively late and rare event. RF can be detected in cases of cryoglobulinemia; immunoglobulin M (IgM) has RF activity in type II and type III cryoglobulinemia. RF can be seen as a nonspecific finding in diseases such as endocarditis and systemic vasculitis.

Complement

The levels of complement components C3 and C4 and the 50% hemolyzing dose of complement (CH_{50}) usually are measured in the evaluation of suspected rapidly progressive glomerulonephritis (RPGN). Complement levels are usually low in active SLE, poststreptococcal glomerulonephritis, endocarditis, membranoproliferative glomerulonephritis, cryoglobulinemia, shunt nephritis, and glomerulonephritis associated with visceral abscesses. A particularly depressed C4 compared with C3 should raise the suspicion of cryoglobulinemia.

Serum Immunoelectrophoresis

Elevated polyclonal IgA levels are seen in about half of the cases of IgA nephropathy and Henoch-Schönlein purpura. Polyclonal elevation of IgG may occur in a variety of systemic diseases and is a nonspecific finding. The presence of a monoclonal protein in the serum should raise the suspicion for a monoclonal gammopathy–associated disease. The differential diagnosis includes monoclonal gammopathy of uncertain significance, myeloma kidney, lymphomas, amyloidosis, light chain deposition disease, heavy chain deposition disease, immunotactoid glomerulonephritis, and cryoglobulinemia. The concentration of the monoclonal protein is higher when the diagnosis of multiple myeloma is made, but even small quantities of Bence Jones proteins in the serum can have clinical significance. Because a substantial fraction of multiple myelomas can have no heavy chain excretion, and small quantities of light chains may be hard to detect by serum immunoelectrophoresis, a sample for urine immunoelectrophoresis always must be sent with a serum immunoelectrophoresis sample to ensure a complete evaluation.

Urine for Bence Jones Protein

This test complements the serum immunoelectrophoresis and may reveal Bence Jones protein even in the absence of an M-component in the serum immunoelectrophoresis. Bence Jones proteinuria may be present in myeloma kidney, amyloidosis, light chain deposition disease, lymphoma, or, occasionally, monoclonal gammopathy of uncertain significance. One must be cautious not to use these tests to exclude completely a diagnosis of amyloidosis, because many patients with systemic amyloidosis have a normal serum immunoelectrophoresis result and no Bence Jones proteinuria.

Antineutrophil Cytoplasmic Antibody

The antineutrophil cytoplasmic antibody (ANCA) assay has allowed for earlier and more definitive recognition of one of the most common causes of RPGN. The ANCA test, when confirmed by enzyme-linked immunosorbent assay (ELISA), is highly sensitive and specific for a group of vasculitides. The antibodies are present in the serum of the affected patient and cause two different patterns of staining: perinuclear staining (p-ANCA) and cytoplasmic staining (c-ANCA). Both antigens have cytoplasmic distribution, and the former pattern is an artifact of the fixation method. The antigen for p-ANCA is myeloperoxidase, and the antigen for c-ANCA is proteinase-3. The former often is associated with positive staining in the clinical setting of microscopic polyangiitis, idiopathic crescentic glomerulonephritis, or Churg-Strauss syndrome. The c-ANCA serology result often correlates with the classic disease of Wegener's granulomatosis, but the relationship is not definitive. No cases have been reported with antibodies to both antigens. Immunofluorescence, although highly sensitive, is not specific, but it gains specificity when used with ELISA and Western blotting and precludes the need for renal biopsy in the appropriate clinical setting. Anti-GBM antibody staining also may occur in the presence of a positive ANCA, the significance of which is unclear. It is speculated that exposure of the Goodpasture antigen, as a result of the glomerular injury, leads to anti-GBM antibody formation as a secondary process.

Anti-Glomerular Basement Membrane Antibody

The identification of the presence of autoantibodies to the Goodpasture antigen, which resides in a domain of the α chain of type 4 collagen, was an important step in elucidating the mechanism of renal injury in Goodpasture's syndrome. The availability of this test provides early and accurate diagnosis of a disease that, if left untreated, can lead to irreversible renal failure. Recovery is rare when renal failure is advanced to the point of requiring dialysis at the time of presentation. The initial diagnosis can be made by immunofluorescence and confirmed by Western blot analysis.

Cryoglobulins

Cryoglobulins are thermolabile immunoglobulins of single monoclonal type (type I cryoglobulinemia); in type II and type III cryoglobulinemia, there is a mixture of immunoglobulins in which one of the components has RF activity against IgG. The identification of cryoglobulins does not prove their role in a disease process unless the clinical and pathologic features are characteristic. Type I and type II cryoglobulins are more likely to be associated with clinical disease, especially at higher titers. In type II cryoglobulinemia, the monoclonal component has the RF activity and is often an IgM κM component. Type III cryoglobulinemia is often of less clinical significance. Type I cryoglobulinemia is seen with Waldenström's macroglobulinemia and multiple myeloma; type II, with hepatitis C infection, Sjögren's syndrome, lymphomas, and SLE; and type III, with hepatitis C, chronic infections, and inflammatory conditions. In cryoglobulinemia that is associated with hepatitis C, the hepatitis C viral (HCV) RNA is concentrated in the cryoprecipitate. This may warrant an assay for HCV RNA in the cryoprecipitate to rule out hepatitis C as the offending agent. The sample must be transported warm (37° C) to the laboratory to avoid precipitation of the cryoglobulins at room temperature. The samples are handled warm in the laboratory before cryoprecipitate is allowed to form at 4° C. The precipitate is identified by immunofixation and double-diffusion in agar.

Hepatitis B Serology

Membranous nephropathy is associated with hepatitis B infection and always denotes chronic infection with hepatitis B surface antigenemia. Classic polyarteritis nodosa occasionally has been seen in the setting of hepatitis B infection, often with surface antigenemia and hepatitis B e-antigenemia.

Hepatitis C Serology

This is associated with a variety of renal entities, including cryoglobulinemia, membranoproliferative glomerulonephritis, and membranous nephropathy. The evaluation may include the antibody test and an assay for HCV RNA. Occasionally, the HCV RNA analysis may have to be conducted on the cryoprecipitate, as discussed previously, to verify that hepatitis C is the cause of the cryoglobulinemia.

Human Immunodeficiency Virus Serology

Human immunodeficiency virus (HIV)-associated nephropathy is associated with nephrotic syndrome and acute renal failure. In the appropriate clinical setting, HIV serology and viral titers are appropriate tests for both clinical syndromes.

Anti-Dnase B or Antistreptolysin O

Streptococcal infection is determined in the evaluation of poststreptococcal glomerulonephritis. Acute and convalescent serology assays are used to confirm recent infection.

Erythrocyte Sedimentation Rate

The erythrocyte sedimentation rate (ESR) is a relatively nonspecific test in the evaluation of renal disease. However, a high ESR often points to systemic vasculitis, multiple myeloma, or malignancy as the underlying cause. One must use caution in pursuing an elevated ESR as the only finding in the setting of renal failure. The ESR often is elevated in nephrotic syndrome, including in diabetic nephropathy.

Imaging

A variety of renal imaging techniques have been developed to assist in the evaluation of diseases of the kidney.

Plain radiography of kidney, ureter, and bladder (KUB) was used in the past for estimation of renal size and in the evaluation of calcium stones. It has been largely replaced by other studies. Intravenous pyelography has been largely replaced by computed tomography (CT) scanning for the evaluation of renal size and the detection of stones and masses.

Renal Ultrasonography

Renal ultrasonography has become the most commonly used imaging study (Fig. 115–11). It is expedient, is noninvasive, and gives reliable information regarding obstruction, renal size, and the presence of masses and renal echotexture. The study has only 90% sensitivity for the detection of hydronephrosis, however, and should not be relied on to rule out hydronephrosis with certainty. Additionally, it cannot detect stones in the ureters and bladder and has limited utility in the evaluation for kidney stones. Doppler imaging permits evaluation of the renal vessels and resistive index.

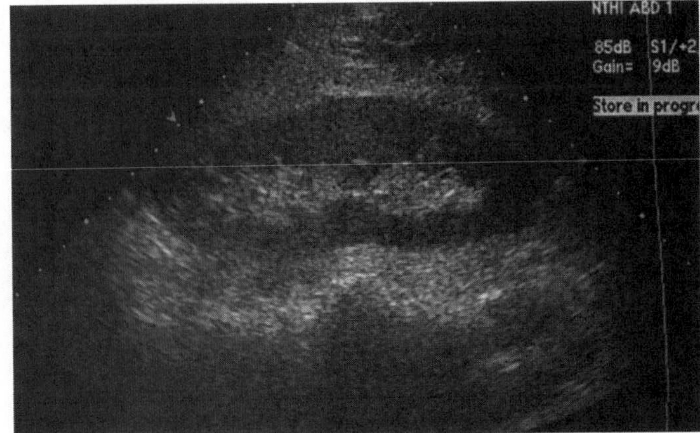

FIGURE 115–11 • Normal sagittal renal ultrasound. The cortex is hypoechoic compared with the echogenic fat containing the renal sinus. (From Johnson RJ, Feehally J: Comprehensive Clinical Nephrology. London, Mosby, 2000, with permission.)

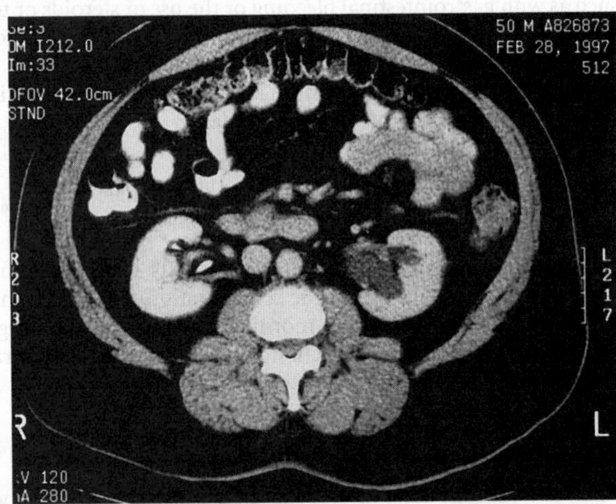

FIGURE 115–12 • Delayed excretion in the left kidney secondary to a distal calculus. Contrast-enhanced computed tomography scan shows dilated left renal pelvis (arrow). (From Johnson RJ, Feehally J: Comprehensive Clinical Nephrology. London, Mosby, 2000, with permission.)

Computed Tomography

A stone protocol CT scan of the kidneys, ureter, and bladder has become the study of choice for the detection of kidney stones because of its ability to detect stones of all kinds, including uric acid stones and the nonobstructing stones in the ureters (Fig. 115–12). Masses in the kidney can be evaluated using either contrast CT or a renal ultrasound study.

CT angiography is used for the study of renal artery stenosis and is emerging rapidly as a useful study. Although it is comparable to magnetic resonance (MR) angiography as a noninvasive tool, it requires the use of iodinated contrast material, which may cause renal dysfunction in patients with chronic kidney disease.

Magnetic Resonance Imaging with Magnetic Resonance Angiography

The use of magnetic resonance imaging (MRI) with MR angiography has revolutionized the evaluation of renovascular disease (Fig. 115–13). The test is highly sensitive but tends to overestimate the degree of stenosis. Its accuracy in detecting fibromuscular dysplasia causing renal artery stenosis has not been well validated. MRI also can be used to evaluate renal masses. Its main advantages are that it is a noninvasive test and does not require the use of iodinated contrast material. Claustrophobic patients may not tolerate this study.

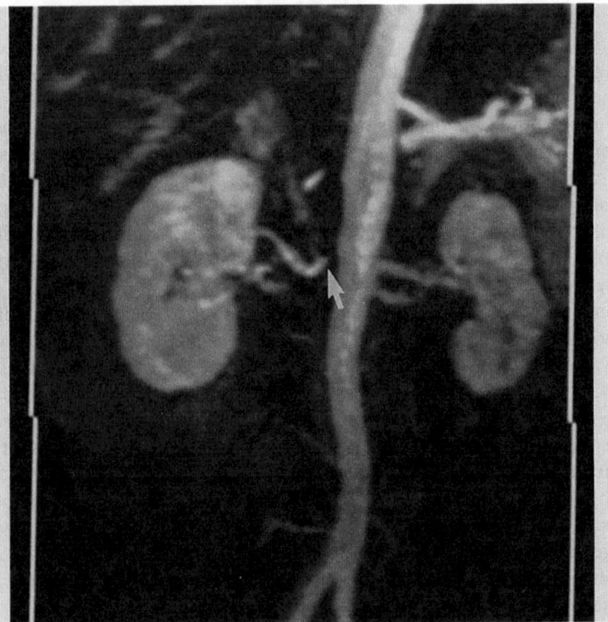

FIGURE 115–13 • Magnetic resonance angiography. Coronal three-dimensional image shows right renal artery stenosis (arrow). (From Johnson RJ, Feehally J: Comprehensive Clinical Nephrology. London, Mosby, 2000, with permission.)

Renography

The uptake by the kidneys of ^{99m}Tc-DPTA and mercaptoacetyl triglycine, the former as a marker of GFR and the latter as a marker of renal blood flow, has been used to evaluate for renovascular disease. The first component reflects perfusion, whereas the second component evaluates renal function by the assessment of radiotracer uptake and excretion by the kidneys. The rate of uptake of the radioisotope often is decreased and delayed when there is renal artery stenosis, and the excretion is markedly delayed if captopril is administered before the study. There is also a decrease in the GFR of the affected kidney after the administration of captopril. Although the renogram is useful for the evaluation of unilateral renal artery stenosis, it is of limited use in the evaluation of bilateral renal artery stenosis or in the setting of significant renal dysfunction.

If dilation of the collecting system is present, furosemide renography is used to investigate whether there is an obstructive component to the dilation. A renogram is done, after which furosemide is administered intravenously. Rapid washout of the isotope suggests that there is no anatomic obstruction.

Renal Angiography

Renal arteriography is the gold standard in the evaluation of renal artery stenosis. It also is used for the evaluation of arteriovenous malformations, polyarteritis nodosa, and other vascular lesions of the kidneys. The study is invasive, uses iodinated contrast material, and incurs a small risk of atheroembolic disease. Therapeutic angioplasty and stenting can be done at the time of the angiogram.

Renal vein renins are predominantly of historical interest. The measurement of renins from each of the renal veins is used to determine whether the presence of renal artery stenosis causes a physiologic response of higher renin secretion on the ipsilateral side. A ratio of 1.5 on the affected side compared with the contralateral side gives support to a physiologically important stenosis.

Invasive Evaluation

Renal Biopsy

Renal biopsy is an invaluable tool in the evaluation of renal disease. This technique has identified new entities, such as the collapsing variant of focal and segmental sclerosis and immunotactoid glomerulonephritis. Most biopsies are done percutaneously with realtime ultrasound guidance or with CT-guided localization. More recently, the transjugular approach is being used in patients in whom the risks of bleeding are high. The current indications for renal biopsy include the following:

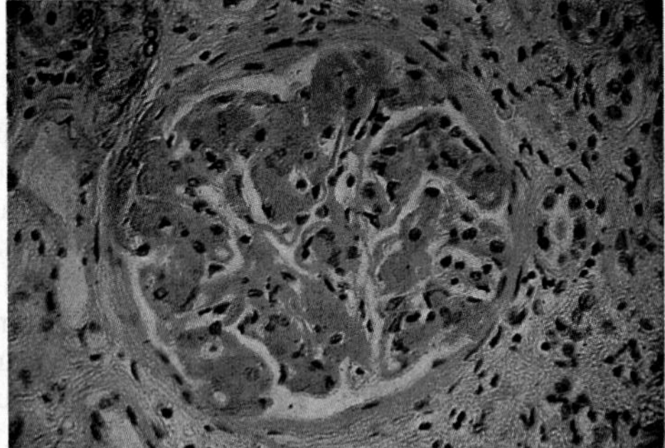

FIGURE 115–14 • Renal amyloidosis. The glomerulus shows amyloid deposition, stained by Congo red, in the glomerular capillaries (magnification, 330×). (From Johnson RJ, Feehally J: Comprehensive Clinical Nephrology. London, Mosby, 2000, with permission.)

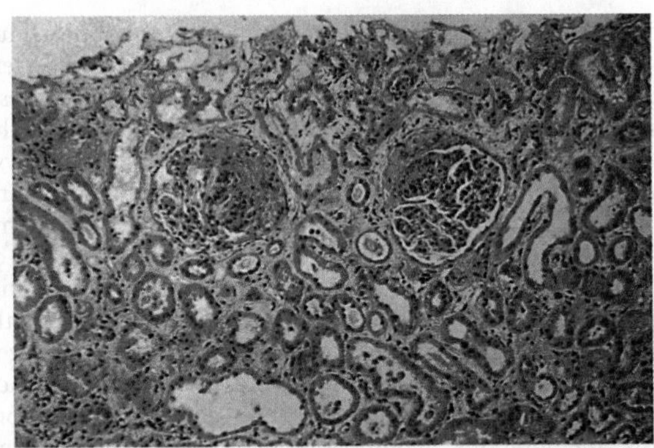

FIGURE 115–15 • Systemic lupus erythematosus. This renal biopsy specimen shows proliferative change and crescent formation in both glomeruli (hematoxylin and eosin stain; magnification, 115×). (From Johnson RJ, Feehally J: Comprehensive Clinical Nephrology. London, Mosby, 2000, with permission.)

1. RPGN without a serologic diagnosis. Although some use serology alone for ANCA-related vasculitis, others still seek pathologic confirmation. For many other entities, such as cryoglobulinemia and SLE, the biopsy is valuable for stratifying patients before therapy and for follow-up on therapy.
2. Nephrotic syndrome without an obvious cause. In childhood nephrotic syndrome, empirical steroid therapy is used routinely because of the high prevalence of steroid-responsive minimal change disease. In adults, the approach is often to proceed with a biopsy followed by initiation of appropriate therapy based on the pathology (Fig. 115–14).
3. SLE with renal involvement, in which more proliferative glomerulonephritis, such as ISN class IV SLE nephritis (Fig. 115–15), may be treated more aggressively with immunosuppression.
4. Unexplained renal failure of any cause. Although it is uncommon to perform a biopsy in patients with hospital-acquired renal failure, the biopsy can be useful, especially if steroid therapy is contemplated, such as in allergic interstitial nephritis.
5. Renal transplantation with acute and chronic renal failure, in which the biopsy information can be crucial in guiding diagnosis and treatment.
6. Proteinuria, below the nephrotic range. This is less established as an indication for renal biopsy. Other factors, such as the presence of hypertension, renal insufficiency, and the age and preference of the patient, are included in the decision to pursue a renal biopsy.

A renal biopsy is generally a safe procedure in the hands of an experienced operator using real-time ultrasound guidance. The bleeding risk is 1 to 2% in patients without coagulopathy.

MAJOR RENAL SYNDROMES

Renal disease can be divided logically into major overlapping categories, which are used to characterize the most common renal syndromes.

Nephritic Syndrome

Acute nephritic syndrome is an uncommon but dramatic presentation of an acute glomerulonephritis. Some of the diseases that manifest with acute nephritic syndrome cause necrotizing crescentic glomerulonephritis with rapid and irreversible renal dysfunction, creating a narrow therapeutic window; others are more forgiving. This group contains all of the causes of RPGN. The hallmark of acute nephritic syndrome is the presence of RBC casts, but their absence does not rule out the syndrome. Dysmorphic RBCs can be identified accurately by the trained eye under phase contrast microscopy and can be characterized to be of glomerular origin. The diseases that make up this group are detailed later in the description of the RPGN group. This group warrants urgent and usually inpatient evaluation. The nephritic syndrome often is accompanied by avid sodium and water retention, occasionally leading to a diagnosis of congestive heart failure.

Nephrotic Syndrome

Nephrotic syndrome is characterized by the presence of proteinuria of greater than 3.5 g/day/1.73 m^2, with accompanying edema, hypertension, and hyperlipidemia. It leads to a multitude of other consequences, such as predisposition to infection and hypercoagulability. In general, the diseases associated with nephrotic syndrome cause chronic kidney dysfunction, but they only rarely cause acute renal failure. Acute renal failure may be seen with minimal change disease, HIV-associated nephropathy, and bilateral renal vein thrombosis. The causes of nephrotic syndrome can be divided into primary and secondary causes. The latter include diabetic nephropathy, amyloidosis, and SLE with membranous nephropathy. Of these, diabetic nephropathy is the most prevalent cause of end-stage renal disease in the United States. The causes of idiopathic nephrotic syndrome in decreasing order of prevalence are focal and segmental glomerulosclerosis, membranous nephropathy, minimal change disease, and membranoproliferative glomerulonephritis. In the 1990s, focal and segmental glomerulosclerosis emerged as the leading cause of idiopathic nephrotic syndrome in the United States, replacing membranous nephropathy.

Tubulointerstitial Diseases

Tubulointerstitial diseases vary in presentation from acute renal failure to chronic kidney dysfunction that manifests as asymptotic mild renal insufficiency. It is more challenging to diagnose the cause of a mild chronic kidney disease than it is to determine the cause of RPGN. Because specific therapeutic options are much more limited for chronic kidney disease, it is less likely to be evaluated. The urine sediment often contains small-to-moderate amounts of proteinuria, usually less than 1g/day. The sediment often contains tubular cells, WBCs, RBCs, and casts. Casts are composed of tubular cells, WBCs, granular casts, and waxy casts, the last-mentioned being seen in chronic kidney disease. RBC casts are rare in acute interstitial nephritis and are more characteristic of glomerular disease. The major causes of tubulointerstitial disease are listed in Table 115–2.

TABLE 115–2 MAJOR CAUSES OF TUBULOINTERSTITIAL DISEASE

Ischemic and toxic acute tubular necrosis.
Allergic interstitial nephritis
Interstitial nephritis secondary to immune complex–related collagen vascular disease, such as Sjögren's disease or systemic lupus erythematosus
Granulomatous diseases: sarcoidosis, tubulointerstitial nephritis with uveitis
Pigment-related tubular injury: myoglobulinuria, hemoglobinuria
Hypercalcemia with nephrocalcinosis
Tubular obstruction: drugs such as indinavir, uric acid in tumor lysis syndrome
Myeloma kidney or cast nephropathy
Infection-related interstitial nephritis: *Legionella, Leptospira*
Infiltrative diseases, such as lymphoma

Vascular Diseases of the Kidney

Vascular diseases of the kidney can be divided into large vessel obstruction and medium-to-small vessel diseases. Renovascular disease is a common cause of hypertension, congestive heart failure, and renal insufficiency. The most common cause of renal artery stenosis is atherosclerotic renal artery stenosis. Fibromuscular dysplasia is much less prevalent, causing only about 10% of renal artery stenosis. The latter cause is more common in women 20 to 50 years of age. Variants of fibromuscular dysplasia affect men and women and are associated with renal artery dissections and infarcts.

Small vessel diseases, although they have similar effects on the kidney, vary greatly in terms of pathophysiology and etiology. One is classic polyarteritis nodosa, which is seen in patients with hepatitis B, HIV infection, or, rarely, hepatitis C. The symptoms include abdominal pain, hypertension, and mild renal insufficiency, often with a benign sediment. The diagnostic findings include demonstration of microaneurysms at the bifurcation of medium-sized arteries in the visceral organs by arteriography. Other diseases involving small vessels include atheroembolic disease, which is seen either spontaneously or after arteriography or surgery. This syndrome affects the kidneys, gastrointestinal tract, and lower extremities. Central nervous system involvement is seen when angiography or surgery affects the aortic arch.

The thrombotic microangiopathies include hemolytic-uremic syndrome (HUS) and thrombotic thrombocytopenic purpura (TTP). TTP is associated with an acquired inhibitor to, or the congenital inherited absence of, a protease that cleaves large-molecular-weight von Willebrand multimers. HUS is caused by endothelial injury induced by Shiga's toxin from *Escherichia coli* 057:H7 infection. The antiphospholipid antibody syndrome can affect the kidney in many ways. There can be large vessel thrombosis and stenosis as well as a thrombotic microangiopathy with proteinuria, hypertension, and renal insufficiency. Scleroderma renal crisis is a manifestation of systemic sclerosis, often with an inexorable progression to end-stage renal insufficiency if untreated.

Acute Renal Failure

Acute renal failure is a syndrome in which there is a decline in glomerular filtration over a period of days. Most cases of acute renal failure in the hospital have hemodynamic or toxic etiologies. Other causes include obstruction, tubulointerstitial diseases such as myeloma kidney, vascular diseases such as HUS and TTP, scleroderma kidney, atheroembolic diseases, antiphospholipid antibody syndrome, and the glomerular diseases that cause RPGN. The patient with acute renal failure is approached best by evaluation for prerenal, renal, and postrenal causes. The careful and systematic evaluation of the patient should start with a thorough history and physical examination. This should be followed by selected laboratory and radiographic tests. The urinalysis is often a key element in determining the cause.

Rapidly Progressive Glomerulonephritis

RPGN usually manifests with dramatic acute renal failure, often associated with the systemic features of vasculitis, a nephritic sediment, and a rapid decrement of GFR. There are four major groups of diseases in this category.

Anti-Glomerular Basement Membrane Disease

Anti-GBM disease may manifest with or without pulmonary hemorrhage. Anti-GBM disease is the most dramatic of the causes of RPGN. An acquired autoantibody to an epitope in type IV collagen leads to a necrotizing crescentic glomerulonephritis and rapid deterioration in renal function. Because recovery is unlikely if the creatinine is greater than 6.8 mg/dL or if the patient is anuric, diagnosis and treatment cannot be delayed. Serologic diagnosis is sensitive and specific, and occasionally a positive serology result obviates the need for tissue diagnosis.

Antineutrophil Cytoplasmic Antibody–Associated Vasculitis

The ANCA-associated vasculitides include Wegener's granulomatosis, microscopic polyangiitis, Churg-Strauss syndrome, and idiopathic pauci-immune crescentic glomerulonephritis. Wegener's granulomatosis is a necrotizing granulomatous vasculitis that affects the upper airways, sinuses, lungs, and kidneys. The lung lesions classically are cavitating nodules. The renal pathology is common to all ANCA-associated glomerulonephritis and shows pauci-immune necrotizing and crescentic glomerulonephritis. Microscopic polyangiitis is associated with skin lesions, mononeuritis multiplex, and pulmonary hemorrhage, which can be life-threatening. Churg-Strauss syndrome has the unique feature of eosinophilia and asthma. Idiopathic pauci-immune crescentic glomerulonephritis has the renal features of the disease, is ANCA positive, but does not have the extrarenal manifestations of the systemic vasculitides.

Hypocomplementemic Immune Complex Glomerulonephritis

These are a group of diseases associated with low complement concentrations and an immune complex glomerulonephritis. They include SLE, poststreptococcal glomerulonephritis, infective endocarditis, shunt nephritis, membranoproliferative glomerulonephritis, cryoglobulinemia, and glomerulonephritis associated with visceral abscesses.

Immune Complex Glomerulonephritis Associated with Normal Complement

This category includes IgA nephropathy and Henoch-Schönlein purpura. IgA nephropathy is the most common glomerulonephritis and is associated with mesangial deposits, predominantly of IgA. The disease is variable in severity and encompasses a range from incidental asymptomatic hematuria to cases of RPGN caused by crescentic IgA nephropathy. Henoch-Schönlein purpura is often self-limited and is associated with gastrointestinal involvement and palpable purpura of the extensor surfaces of the lower extremities.

Chronic Kidney Disease

The National Kidney Foundation has defined the stages of chronic kidney disease (Table 115–3). Chronic kidney disease is defined as either kidney damage or a GFR of less than 60 mL/min/1.73 m^2 for longer than 3 months. Kidney damage is defined as pathologic abnormalities or markers of kidney damage, including abnormalities in the composition of blood or urine or abnormalities in the imaging tests. The excretion of 30 to 300 mg of albumin in a 24-hour period defines microalbuminuria. It is estimated that 11.7% of the adult U.S. population have abnormal albumin excretion in the urine, and the frequency increases with age. Kidney failure is defined as either a GFR of less than 15 mL/min/1.73 m^2 that is accompanied by signs and symptoms of uremia or a need for initiation of kidney replacement therapy for treatment of complications of decreased GFR. End-stage renal disease includes all cases requiring treatment by dialysis or transplantation regardless of the level of GFR.

Patients with chronic kidney disease warrant referral to a nephrologist. Care of these patients should focus on efforts to slow disease progression, optimize medical management, and make a seamless transition to renal replacement therapy. The care should include optimal blood pressure control, use of angiotensin-converting enzyme inhibitors and angiotensin receptor blockers if indicated, dietary counseling, careful management of calcium and phosphorus levels, monitoring of the parathyroid hormone level, and management of anemia with the use of erythropoietin and iron supplements. Early-access placement and initiation of transplant evaluation are important components of the care of patients with chronic kidney disease. The quality of life can be well maintained, and the transition to renal replacement therapy can be made smooth with well-timed nephrology care.

TABLE 115–3 STAGES OF CHRONIC KIDNEY DISEASE*

Stage	Description	GFR (mL/min/1.73 m^2)
1	Kidney damage with normal or ↑GFR	≥90
2	Kidney damage with mild or ↓GFR	60–89
3	Moderate ↓GFR	30–59
4	Severe ↓GFR	15–29
5	Kidney failure	<15 (or dialysis)

*Chronic kidney disease is defined as either kidney damage or GFR <60 mL/min/1.73 m^2 for ≥3 months. Kidney damage is defined as pathologic abnormalities or markers of damage, including abnormalities in blood or urine tests or image studies.
GFR = glomerular filtration rate.
From www.kidney.org/professionals/doqi/kdoqi/Gif_File/kck_t10.gif (accessed July 12, 2006).

SUGGESTED READINGS

Kidney Foundation Disease Outcomes Quality Initiative (DOQI) Guidelines. Available at: www.kidney.org/professionals/KDOQI/index.cfm. *A periodically updated source of consensus guidelines for the management of chronic kidney disease.*

Whitfield HN: ABC of urology: Urological evaluation. BMJ 2006;333:432–435. *Practical recommendations for nonurologists.*

116 STRUCTURE AND FUNCTION OF THE KIDNEYS

C. Craig Tisher

The complex multicellular composition of the kidney reflects the complicated nature of its functional properties. This organ is responsible for maintaining the volume and ionic composition of body fluids; excreting fixed or nonvolatile metabolic waste products such as creatinine, urea, and uric acid; and eliminating exogenous drugs and toxins. In addition, the kidney serves as a major endocrine organ that produces renin, erythropoietin, 1,25-dihydroxycholecalciferol, prostaglandins, and kinins; it also serves as a target organ for many hormones. Finally, the kidney catabolizes low-molecular-weight proteins and is responsible for a host of metabolic functions (e.g., ammoniagenesis and gluconeogenesis).

DEVELOPMENT

The kidney originates from two sources: (1) the ureteral bud, which gives rise to the ureter, pelvis, calyces, and collecting ducts, and (2) the metanephric blastema, which develops into the glomerulus and tubules. During embryogenesis, three successive sets of excretory organs evolve: the pronephros, mesonephros, and metanephros. The permanent kidney is derived from the metanephros. Cellular and molecular mechanisms that underlie renal morphogenesis include cell proliferation, expression of nuclear proto-oncogenes and homeobox genes, the actions of peptide growth factors, and alterations in cell adhesion and the composition of the extracellular matrix.

GROSS ANATOMY

The kidneys are located in the retroperitoneal space and extend from the 12th thoracic vertebra to the 3rd lumbar vertebra. The right kidney is usually more caudad, and the left tends to be slightly larger. Each adult human kidney weighs 115 to 170 g, measures approximately 11 × 6 × 2.5 cm, and is surrounded by a tough, fibroelastic capsule.

The cut surface of a bisected kidney reveals a darker inner region, the medulla, and a pale outer region approximately 1 cm in thickness, the cortex. The human kidney has a multipapillary configuration in which the medulla is divided into 8 to 18 striated, conical masses called *pyramids* (Fig. 116–1). The base of each pyramid is positioned at the corticomedullary junction, and the apex extends toward the renal pelvis and forms a papilla. On the tip of each papilla are numerous small openings that represent the distal ends of the collecting ducts (of Bellini). Extending downward between the pyramids are portions of cortex, the septa of Bertin. Close examination of the cut surface reveals fine longitudinal striations, the medullary rays (of Ferrein), which extend into the cortex. Despite their name, the medullary rays are part of the cortex and are formed by the straight segments of the proximal tubule, the thick ascending limbs, and the collecting ducts.

The renal pelvis is the saclike dilation of the upper ureter. Two or three major calyces extend from the pelvis and divide into the minor calyces that surround individual papillae.

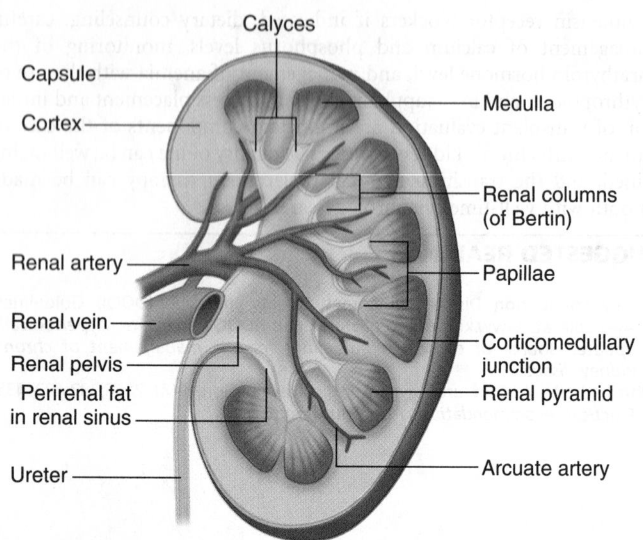

FIGURE 116–1 • Sagittal section of the human kidney illustrating its gross anatomic features.

NEPHRON

Each human kidney contains about 0.8 to 1.2 × 10^6 nephrons—the functional units of the kidney. A nephron consists of the glomerulus or renal corpuscle, the proximal tubule, the thin limbs of Henle, and the distal tubule, all of which originate from the metanephric blastema (Fig. 116–2). The connecting tubule, a transitional segment also believed to be derived from the metanephric blastema, joins the nephron to the collecting duct system.

ARCHITECTURE

In the renal cortex two architectural regions can be distinguished, the *cortical labyrinth* and the *medullary rays* (see Fig. 116-1). The cortical labyrinth is a continuous zone of parenchyma that surrounds the medullary rays. Glomeruli, proximal and distal convoluted tubules, connecting tubules, initial collecting tubules, interlobular veins, and a rich capillary network are located in the cortical labyrinth. Ascending connecting tubules of juxtamedullary nephrons fuse to form arcades within the cortical labyrinth. The medullary rays contain the proximal and distal straight tubules and collecting ducts, all of which enter the medulla.

In the medulla, specific nephron segments are found at precise levels and divide the medulla into an inner and an outer zone, with the latter subdivided into an inner and an outer stripe (see Fig. 116–2). In the outer stripe of the outer medulla are the terminal portions of the proximal straight tubules, the thick ascending limbs, and the collecting ducts. The thicker inner stripe of the outer medulla contains thin descending limbs, thick ascending limbs, and collecting ducts. The thin descending and thin ascending limbs of long loops and the collecting ducts are located in the inner medulla. This intricate arrangement of the parenchyma in the cortex and medulla provides an anatomic basis for integration of many of the complex functions of the kidney.

VASCULATURE

Structure

The kidney has an extensive vasculature that accommodates 20 to 25% of the cardiac output. The main renal artery branches to form anterior and posterior divisions, which divide into five segmental arteries. The *segmental arteries* traverse the renal sinus and divide into the *interlobar arteries.* The latter pierce the parenchyma and course toward the cortex along the septa of Bertin between adjacent renal pyramids (see Fig. 116–1). At the corticomedullary junction, the interlobar arteries branch into the *arcuate arteries*, which follow a gently curved course along the base of the pyramids. The arcuate arteries give rise to the *interlobular arteries*, which ascend in the cortex toward the renal surface.

The *afferent arterioles* are branches of the interlobular arteries, and each supplies a single glomerulus (renal corpuscle) (Fig. 116–3). The *efferent arterioles* exit the glomeruli and divide to form an intricate peritubular microcirculation. The capillary networks formed by the efferent arterioles of the superficial and midcortical glomeruli supply the cortical labyrinth and medullary rays, whereas the efferent arterioles of the juxtamedullary glomeruli are responsible for the entire medullary blood supply. In the outer stripe of the outer medulla these vessels divide to form the *descending vasa recta*, which are located in vascular bundles. At various levels in the medulla, the descending vasa recta exit the bundles to form capillary networks. The *ascending vasa recta* drain the medulla.

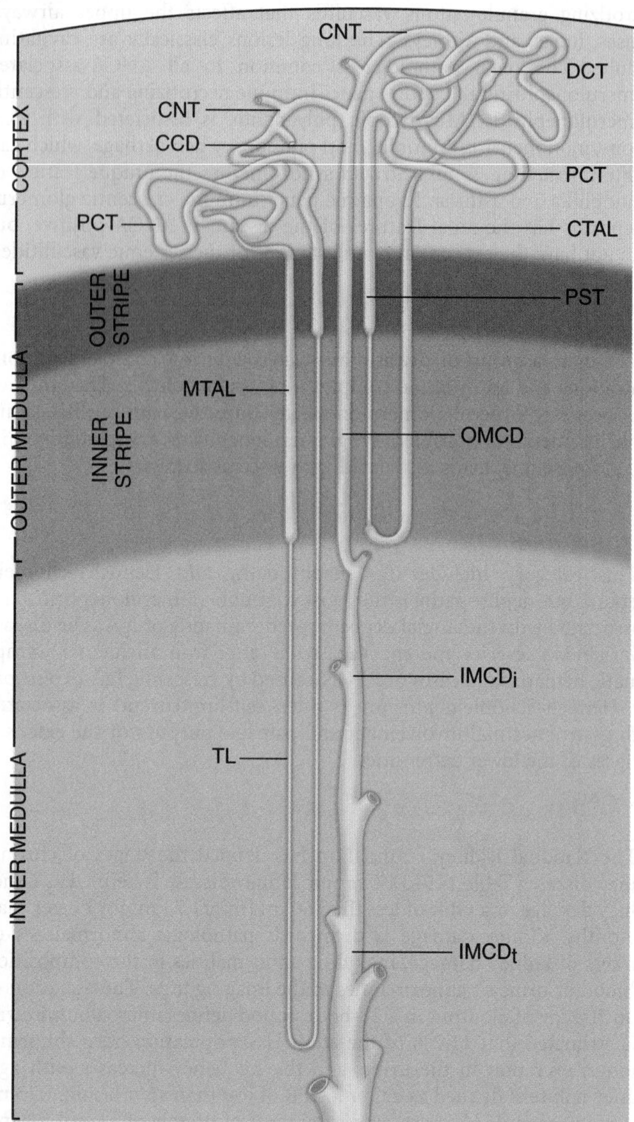

FIGURE 116–2 • Diagram illustrating the superficial and juxtamedullary nephrons. CCD = cortical collecting duct; CNT = connecting segment; CTAL = cortical thick ascending limb; DCT = distal convoluted tubule; $IMCD_i$ = initial inner medullary collecting duct; $IMCD_t$ = terminal inner medullary collecting duct; MTAL = medullary thick ascending limb; OMCD = outer medullary collecting duct; PCT = proximal convoluted tubule; PST = proximal straight tubule; TL = thin limb of Henle's loop. (Modified from Madsen KM, Tisher CC: Structural-functional relationships along the distal nephron. Am J Physiol 1986;250:F1–F15.)

Function

In a 70-kg person, renal blood flow (RBF) amounts to a fourth to a fifth of the resting cardiac output, or approximately 1.2 L/min. The renal cortex receives 85 to 90% of this flow as compared with 10% to the outer medulla and 1 to 2% to the inner medulla, including the papilla. With one kidney removed, blood flow to the remaining kidney nearly doubles within a few weeks.

RBF and the glomerular filtration rate (GFR) remain relatively constant over a wide range of perfusion pressures, a process that is termed *autoregulation.* An intrinsic property of smooth muscle cells in the renal vasculature—the myogenic reflex—permits instantaneous alterations in the tone of the vessel wall to maintain RBF and GFR constant over a pressure range of 80 to 180 mm Hg.

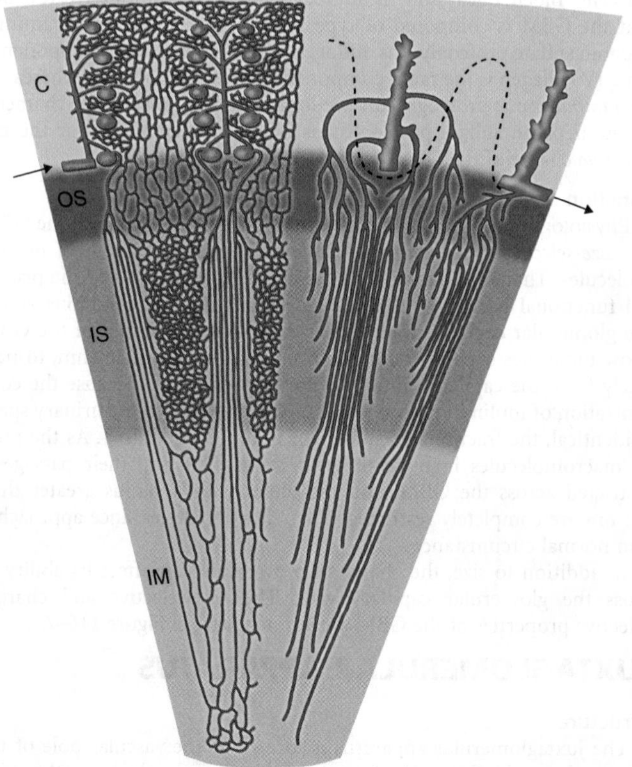

FIGURE 116–3 • Diagram illustrating the vascular arrangement in the renal cortex and medulla. (Reproduced with permission from Kriz W, Kaissling B: Structural organization of the mammalian kidney. *In* Seldin DW, Giebisch G [eds]: The Kidney: Physiology and Pathophysiology, 2nd ed. New York, Raven Press, 1992, p 709.)

A host of hormonal and neural factors can alter RBF. Renal vasoconstrictors that reduce RBF include endothelin, angiotensin II, thromboxane, stimulation of the α-adrenergic system, vasopressin, and catecholamines. Vasodilating agents include prostaglandins I_2 and E_2, atrial peptides, bradykinin, and endothelial-derived relaxing factor, or nitric oxide.

GLOMERULUS

Structure

The anatomically correct name for the glomerulus is the *renal corpuscle.* Because of common usage, however, this structure is generally called the *glomerulus.* The glomerulus includes the glomerular tuft and Bowman's capsule (Fig. 116–4). The glomerular tuft contains three specialized cells, a basement membrane, and a supporting framework, the mesangium. The specialized cells include the *endothelial cells* lining the lumens of the capillaries, the *mesangial cells* located in the centrilobular region of the glomerular tuft, and the *visceral epithelial cells* situated on the outer surfaces of the capillaries (Fig. 116–5). A fourth cell type, the *parietal epithelial cell,* lines Bowman's capsule. At the vascular pole where the afferent and efferent arterioles enter and exit the glomerulus, the visceral epithelium is continuous with the parietal epithelium. The glomerulus resembles an epithelial-lined sac invaginated by a tuft of capillaries. Bowman's space, also called the *urinary space,* is the area between the visceral epithelial cells and the parietal epithelial layer lining Bowman's capsule. It receives the glomerular filtrate, which exits Bowman's space at the urinary pole to enter the proximal tubule (see Fig. 116–4). A filtration barrier is formed between the blood and the urinary space by the fenestrated endothelium lining the capillary loops, the peripheral glomerular basement membrane (GBM), and the overlying visceral epithelial cell (Fig. 116–6). In humans, the mean area of the filtration surface per glomerulus is approximately 0.136 mm^2.

Function

In a 70-kg person, the kidney forms approximately 180 L of glomerular filtrate each day through a process termed *ultrafiltration.* This is the initial step in urine formation. The driving force to move fluid from the glomerular capillaries across the glomerular capillary wall to the urinary

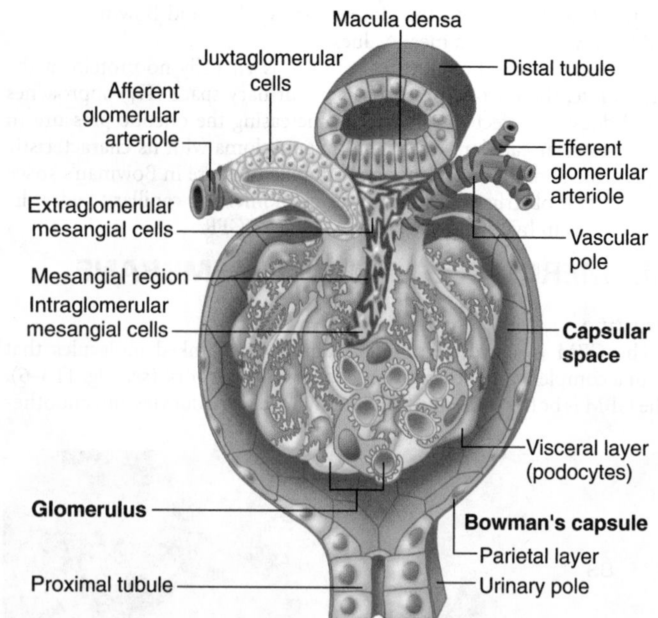

FIGURE 116–4 • Schematic three-dimensional depiction of the glomerulus. (From Bargmann W: Histologie und Mikronscopische Anatomie des Menschen. Stuttgart, Germany, Georg Thieme, 1977, p 86.)

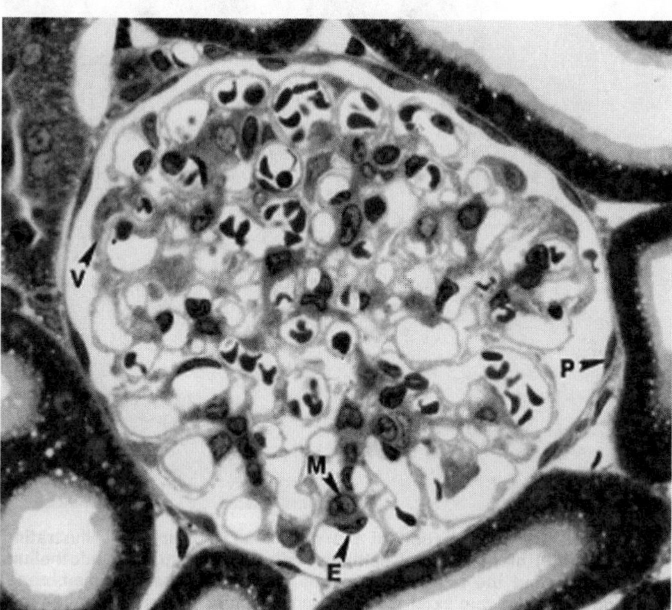

FIGURE 116–5 • Cross-sectional view of the glomerulus depicting endothelial cells (E), mesangial cells (M), visceral epithelial cells (V), and parietal epithelial cells (P) (×480).

space (Bowman's space) is derived from hydraulic pressure generated by the pumping action of the heart. Each glomerulus has a filtration rate (single-nephron glomerular filtration rate [SNGFR]) of 60 nL/min, which is much higher per unit surface area than in other capillary beds in the body. The rate of filtration is proportional to the net ultrafiltration pressure (P_{UF}) that is present across the glomerular capillary wall and is determined by the balance of hydraulic (P) and oncotic (Π) pressures (Starling's forces) that are operative between the glomerular capillary lumen and Bowman's space. The intrinsic water permeability of the capillary wall (k) and the surface area (A), which together define the ultrafiltration coefficient (K_f), are also important determinants of ultrafiltration. Thus,

$$\begin{aligned} SNGFR &= K_f \cdot \bar{P}_{UF} \\ &= K_f \cdot [(\bar{P}_{GC} - P_T) - (\Pi_{GC} - \Pi_T)] \\ &= k \cdot A(\Delta\bar{P} - \Delta\bar{\Pi}) \end{aligned}$$

where *GC* and *T* refer to the glomerular capillary and Bowman's space and the *overbar* denotes mean values.

Because in normal circumstances there is virtually no protein in the ultrafiltrate, the oncotic pressure in the urinary space (Π_T) approaches 0 and does not affect ultrafiltration. Increasing the oncotic pressure in the glomerular capillary (as in multiple myeloma with its characteristic hyperproteinemia), increasing the hydraulic pressure in Bowman's space (via ureteral obstruction), and lowering glomerular capillary hydraulic pressure (as in hypotension) all reduce the SNGFR.

GLOMERULAR BASEMENT MEMBRANE

Structure

The GBM is a hydrated gel containing cross-linked molecules that form a complex, three-dimensional lattice-like network (see Fig. 116–6). The GBM is both synthesized and maintained by podocytes and endothelial cells. Biochemical and immunocytochemical studies have revealed that the GBM is composed of type IV and type V collagens, laminin, heparan sulfate proteoglycans, nidogen, entactin, and other components. Type IV collagen is the main component in the *lamina densa*, whereas in the *laminae rarae* proteoglycans predominate. The polyanionic character of the heparan sulfate proteoglycans is largely responsible for the net negative charge of the GBM.

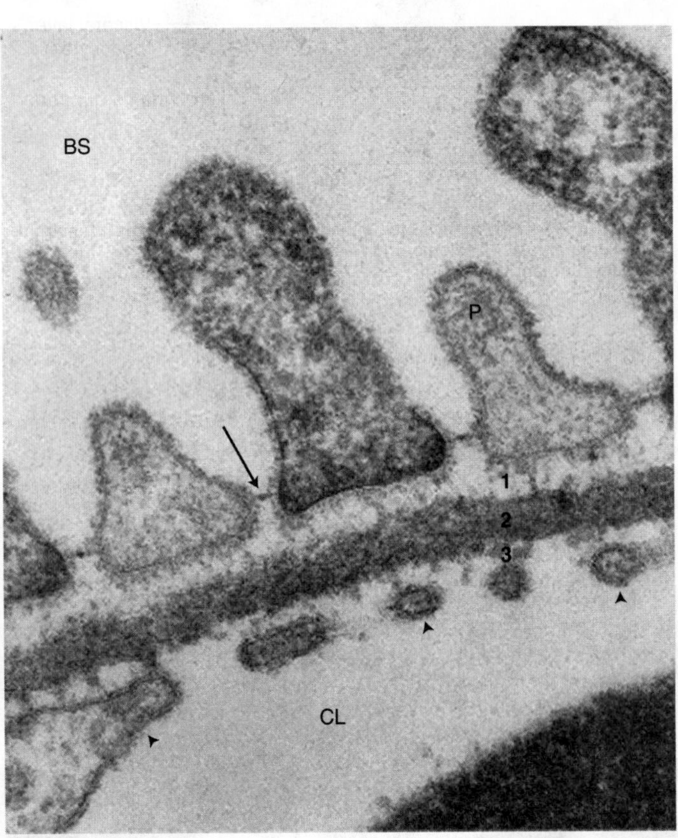

FIGURE 116–6 • Cross section of the glomerular capillary wall illustrating the pedicels (P) of the visceral epithelial cells, the fenestrated endothelium (arrowheads), and the three layers of the glomerular basement membrane, including the lamina rara externa (1), the lamina densa (2), and the lamina rara interna (3). BS = Bowman's space; CL = capillary lumen; arrow = filtration slit diaphragm (×120,000). (From Tisher CC, Madsen KM: Anatomy of the kidney. *In* Brenner BM, Rector FC Jr [eds]: The Kidney, 4th ed. Philadelphia, Saunders, 1991, p 14.)

Function

Physiologic and ultrastructural studies have established that the GBM is a *size-selective* and a *charge-selective* barrier to the passage of macromolecules. The GBM, along with the endothelium, serves as the principal functional barrier to the passage of circulating polyanions across the glomerular capillary wall. The size-selective properties of the GBM allow molecules such as inulin, with a radius of about 1.4 nm, to pass freely from the capillary lumen to the urinary space. Because the concentration of inulin in plasma water and in the fluid in the urinary space is identical, the fractional clearance of inulin is equal to 1. As the radii of macromolecules increase to greater than 2.0 nm, their passage is restricted across the GBM, and molecules with a radius greater than 4.2 nm are completely restricted. Their fractional clearance approaches 0 in normal circumstances.

In addition to size, the charge of a molecule can affect its ability to cross the glomerular capillary wall. The size-selective and charge-selective properties of the GBM are summarized in Figure 116–7.

JUXTAGLOMERULAR APPARATUS

Structure

The juxtaglomerular apparatus is located at the vascular pole of the glomerulus and is formed by four structures: the macula densa, the afferent and efferent arterioles, and the extraglomerular mesangium (see Fig. 116–4). In the wall of the afferent arteriole are modified smooth muscle cells, the so-called granular cells, which secrete renin.

The macula densa is a plaquelike configuration of specialized cells within the cortical thick ascending limb (TAL) of Henle that is in contact with the extraglomerular mesangium (see Fig. 116–4).

Function

The juxtaglomerular apparatus is believed to be responsible for *tubuloglomerular feedback*, in which the composition of tubular fluid delivered to the macula densa changes the filtration rate of the associated glomerulus, presumably by altering renin secretion, which ultimately regulates glomerular hemodynamics.

PROXIMAL TUBULE

Structure

The proximal tubule includes an initial convoluted portion, the *pars convoluta*, located in the cortical labyrinth, and a straight portion, the *pars recta*, located in the medullary ray. Proximal tubule cells are tall and possess a prominent brush border that markedly increases the surface area of the luminal membrane. The cells contain a well-developed endocytic-lysosomal apparatus that has an important role in the absorption and degradation of macromolecules, such as albumin from the glomerular filtrate.

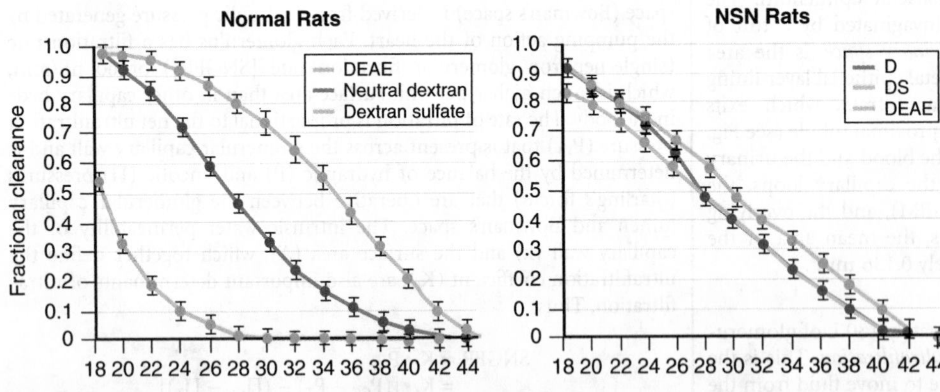

FIGURE 116–7 • Fractional clearances of diethylaminoethyl (DEAE) dextran (positively charged molecule), neutral dextran (D) (neutral charge), and dextran sulfate (DS) (negatively charged molecule), plotted as a function of effective molecular radius in normal rats (left) and in rats with nephrotoxic serum nephritis (NSN, right). Values are expressed as means ± 1 SEM. (From Bohrer MP, Baylis C, Humes HD, et al: Permselectivity of the glomerular capillary wall: Facilitated filtration of circulating polycations. J Clin Invest 1978;61:72–78, by copyright permission of the American Society for Clinical Investigation.)

TABLE 116–1 TRANSPORT OF IONS IN THE PROXIMAL TUBULE

Ion	Principal Site of Transport	Process
Potassium	Early proximal tubule	Freely filtered by the glomerulus; 70% reabsorbed by a passive process that parallels sodium and water and is regulated in part by the transepithelial potential difference
Bicarbonate	Early proximal tubule	Filtered by the glomerulus; 90% of the 4500 mEq filtered each day is reabsorbed secondary to proton secretion
Hydrogen	Proximal convoluted tubule	Approximately 65% secreted via the Na^+/H^+ antiporter; 35% secreted by an electrogenic sodium-independent H^+-ATPase
Chloride	S_2 segment of the proximal tubule	Coupled to active transport of sodium; passive transport driven by a favorable lumen-to-peritubular concentration gradient for Cl^-
Calcium	Entire proximal tubule	Can exit the tubule lumen through a paracellular pathway via passive voltage-dependent diffusion; active transport via Na^+-Ca^{2+} exchange and Ca^{2+}-ATPase

The basolateral plasma membranes are markedly amplified because of extensive interdigitations of basal and lateral cytoplasmic processes between adjacent cells. Localization of Na^+,K^+-ATPase (the sodium pump) in the basolateral membranes explains the active transport of sodium characteristic of this tubule segment. Numerous elongated mitochondria are located close to the interdigitating basolateral membrane processes and provide a source of the cellular energy required for active transport. There is an excellent correlation along the length of the proximal tubule between the elaborate basolateral membrane expressed as surface area, the high Na^+,K^+-ATPase activity localized to this membrane, and the capacity to transport sodium and other ions. The intrinsic rates at which solutes and fluid are transported decrease along the length of the proximal tubule.

Function

The proximal tubule is the first component of the nephron that modifies the volume and ionic composition of the glomerular ultrafiltrate. Through iso-osmotic fluid reabsorption, fluid volume is reduced by 60% or more under normal conditions. The principal driving force for the reabsorption of solutes is the Na^+,K^+-ATPase located along the basolateral plasma membrane. By maintaining a low intracellular sodium concentration, there is passive entry of sodium into the cell across the luminal plasma membrane and down its electrochemical gradient. In the early proximal tubule, this leads to a small electrical potential difference that is lumen negative. Sodium is pumped out of the cell actively at the basolateral surface via Na^+,K^+-ATPase. This process also creates a slight osmotic gradient that facilitates the reabsorption of fluid. The balance between osmotic and hydraulic pressure (Starling's forces) in the peritubular capillaries and the surrounding interstitium determines the extent of the back-leak of sodium and water into the tubule lumen via the intercellular space through the nonoccluding tight junction and the net reabsorption of sodium, water, and other solutes. Water permeability of the proximal tubule is due largely to the presence of a transmembrane protein, aquaporin-1 (AQP-1), that functions as a molecular water channel and is located in the luminal and basolateral membranes.

Each day, approximately 25,000 mEq of sodium (140 mEq/L × 180 L) is filtered, whereas less than 1% is excreted in urine by a euvolemic individual. Normally, about 65% of the filtered sodium is reabsorbed by the proximal tubule, 20% by the TAL, 7 to 10% by the distal convoluted tubule (DCT), and the remainder by the collecting duct. With a salt load, there is a progressive increase in urine sodium excretion until a new steady state is achieved in which output matches intake. Until a steady state is attained, however, the individual goes into positive sodium balance, retains water, and gains weight. Restricting sodium intake produces the opposite effect until the kidney fully compensates over a 3- to 5-day period.

Several factors influence normal sodium balance. The kidney is extremely sensitive to changes in effective arterial blood volume. Dehydration or acute volume depletion secondary to blood loss leads to a fall in RBF and GFR secondary to a decrease in cardiac output, activation of the renin-angiotensin-aldosterone system, and an increase in renal sympathetic nerve activity. As the filtered load of sodium decreases, the proximal tubule increases sodium reabsorption. Because the vasoconstrictive effect of angiotensin II affects the efferent glomerular arteriole to a greater degree than the afferent arteriole, the filtration fraction is increased, which increases oncotic pressure in the peritubular capillaries. This enhances proximal tubule sodium and fluid reabsorption. An increase in the plasma level of aldosterone from activation of the renin-angiotensin-aldosterone system stimulates sodium reabsorption in the collecting duct. Expansion of the effective arterial blood volume, as occurs with excessive sodium intake or the administration of intravenous saline, has the opposite effect.

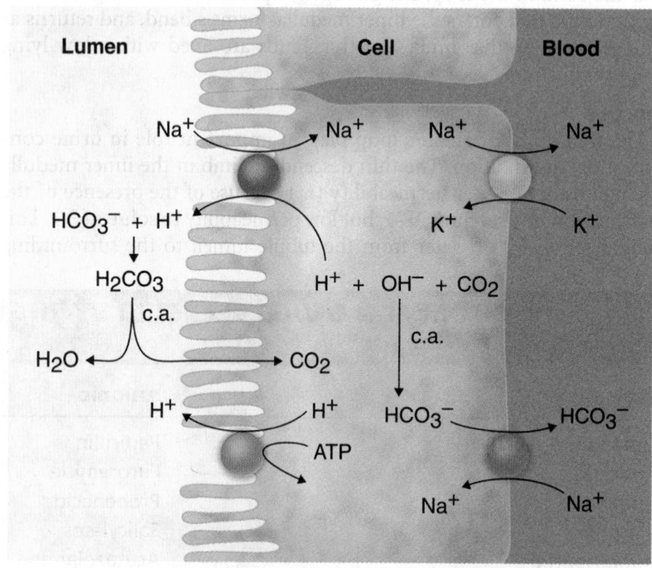

FIGURE 116–8 • Diagram depicting the major mechanism for bicarbonate reclamation in the proximal convoluted tubule. c.a. = carbonic anhydrase.

Other factors also control renal sodium excretion. Several hormones lead to retention of sodium by acting at the tubular level (e.g., growth hormone, cortisol, insulin, and estrogen). Parathyroid hormone (PTH), progesterone, and glycogen inhibit the tubular reabsorption of sodium. Atrial natriuretic peptide—a 28–amino acid peptide produced in the atria of the heart and released in the circulation in response to atrial stretch from, for example, expansion of the central blood volume—also enhances sodium excretion, in part by inhibiting sodium reabsorption by the collecting duct.

Reabsorption of glucose, amino acids, citrate, lactate, acetate, and phosphate also occurs early in the proximal tubule by sodium-coupled active transport processes. Other transported ions are listed in Table 116–1. The crucial elements of bicarbonate reabsorption are depicted in Figure 116–8.

The proximal tubule is also an important site for *ammoniagenesis*, in which glutamine serves as the substrate. Ammonia combines with protons to form the ammonium ion (NH_4^+), which is secreted into the tubule lumen. This process is enhanced in patients with metabolic acidosis and hypokalemia.

The proximal tubule also modifies the composition of the tubular fluid through many well-defined secretory processes. The liver produces many cationic and anionic organic waste products that must be eliminated by the kidney, such as urate, hippurate, oxalate, and bile salts. Certain exogenous compounds and drugs are also removed from plasma in a single pass through the kidney. The S_2 segment of the proximal tubule, which includes the distal half of the pars convoluta and the early pars recta, represents the prime, though not exclusive site for organic ion secretion. The initial step in the secretory process involves active transport against a concentration gradient at the basolateral surface of the cell, followed by passive diffusion across the luminal plasma membrane into the tubule fluid. Table 116–2 lists several common drugs that are secreted by the proximal tubule.

THIN LIMBS OF HENLE'S LOOP

Structure

There is an abrupt transition from the terminal proximal tubule to the descending thin limb of Henle's loop at the junction between the outer and inner stripes of the outer medulla (see Fig. 116–2). Short-looped nephrons have a short descending thin limb that continues into the TAL near the bend in the loop. Long-looped nephrons have a long descending thin limb that enters the inner medulla, forms a bend, and returns as a long ascending thin limb. The thin limbs are lined with a low-lying simple epithelium.

Function

The thin limbs of Henle's loop play an important role in urine concentration and dilution. The thin descending limb in the inner medulla has high osmotic water permeability (L_p) because of the presence of the transmembrane protein AQP-1, but low permeability to solutes (P_S). This facilitates transfer of water from the tubule lumen to the surrounding hypertonic medullary interstitium and raises the concentration of NaCl and urea in the tubule fluid (Fig. 116–9). In humans, the tonicity of the tubule fluid can reach 1200 mOsm/kg H_2O with severe water restriction.

The thin ascending limb of Henle has low osmotic water permeability, moderate permeability for urea, and high permeability for NaCl. The surrounding interstitium has an NaCl concentration that is lower and a urea concentration that is higher than in the tubule fluid at the hairpin turn. These characteristics favor the formation of a dilute tubule fluid because the passive movement of NaCl out of the tubule exceeds the passive entry of urea into the tubule. At any given level in the inner medulla, the tonicity of the surrounding interstitial fluid is greater than that of the tubule fluid in the thin ascending limb of Henle (see Fig. 116–9). Overall, the thin limbs of the loop of Henle reabsorb about 15% of the glomerular ultrafiltrate and 25% of the sodium and chloride.

TABLE 116–2 COMMON DRUGS SECRETED BY THE PROXIMAL TUBULE

Cationic	Anionic
Cimetidine	Penicillin
Paraquat	Furosemide
Quinine	Probenecid
Morphine	Salicylates
Trimethoprim	Acetazolamide
Atropine	Chlorothiazides
Epinephrine	Cephalothin
	Ethacrynic acid

DISTAL TUBULE

Structure

The distal tubule includes two morphologically distinct segments: the *thick ascending limb* of Henle's loop and the *distal convoluted tubule* (see Fig. 116–2). The TAL traverses the outer medulla upward into the cortex near its glomerulus of origin and ends just beyond the macula densa. The TAL can be divided into a medullary and a cortical segment.

The TAL is composed of cuboidal cells with extensive basolateral plasma membrane invaginations and interdigitations between adjacent cells that enclose elongated mitochondria. These ultrastructural features are typical of epithelial cells involved in active solute transport. The *macula densa* is a specialized region of the cortical TAL that is in contact with the extraglomerular mesangium (see Fig. 116–4).

The DCT is the terminal part of the distal tubule and begins at a variable distance beyond the macula densa. The cells of the DCT resemble those of the TAL.

Function

The TAL actively reabsorbs NaCl, which is mediated by a Na^+-K^+-$2Cl^-$ cotransport mechanism in the apical plasma membrane (see Fig. 116–9). The energy for this process is provided by the Na^+,K^+-ATPase localized on the basolateral plasma membrane. A major function of the medullary TAL is to generate and maintain a hypertonic medullary interstitium that permits maximally concentrated urine to form, whereas the cortical segment continues to dilute the tubule fluid, thereby permitting the formation of maximally dilute urine. The tubule fluid that exits the cortical TAL has an osmolality of less than 150 mOsm/kg H_2O. At this point the total volume of the original glomerular ultrafiltrate in the nephron has been reduced by 85%.

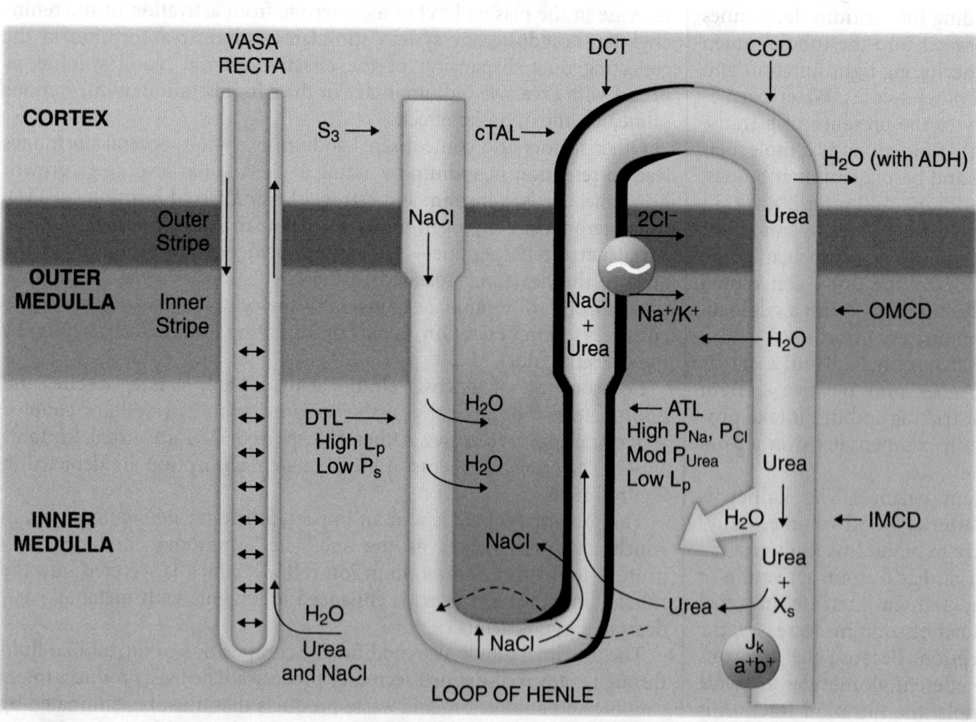

FIGURE 116–9 • Diagram illustrating the essential components of the countercurrent multiplication and exchange systems in the kidney (see text for explanation). The heavy black line indicates water-impermeable segments of the nephron, and shading denotes a progressive increase in tonicity of the medullary interstitium. ADH = antidiuretic hormone; ATL = ascending thin limb; CCD = cortical collecting duct; cTAL = cortical thick ascending limb; DCT = distal convoluted tubule; DTL = descending thin limb; IMCD = inner medullary collecting duct; ; $J_Ka^+b^+$ = Kidd antigen and urea transporter; L_p = osmotic water permeability; OMCD = outer medullary collecting duct; P_S, P_{Na}, P_{Cl}, P_{Urea} = permeability to solutes, Na^+, Cl^-, and urea; S_3 = third segment of the proximal tubule; X_S = nonreabsorbable solutes. (Modified from Brenner BM, Coe FL, Rector FC Jr [eds]: Renal Physiology in Health and Disease. Philadelphia, Saunders, 1987, pp 53 and 160.)

The TAL also reabsorbs about 15% of the filtered load of *calcium* (Ca^{2+}) from the tubular fluid. Throughout the TAL, a significant component of calcium transport is passive, presumably paracellular and driven by the transepithelial potential difference (PD_1). In addition, active transport that is independent of Ca^{2+}-ATPase activity, sodium transport, and anaerobic metabolism has been identified in the cortical TAL. Calcium transport is enhanced in the cortical TAL by PTH and cyclic adenosine monophosphate (AMP) and in the medullary TAL by calcitonin and cyclic AMP.

Bicarbonate transport is present along the entire TAL through a sodium-coupled HCO_3^- transport mechanism located on the basolateral plasma membrane. Active and passive transport of NH_4^+ out of the lumen and into the interstitium for subsequent transport in the form of NH_3 into the lumen of the collecting duct also occurs in the TAL. Thus, this region of the nephron also plays a role in acidification of the tubule fluid.

The cortical TAL is a major site for reabsorbing *magnesium*. The passive component of magnesium transport is facilitated by the Na^+-K^+-$2Cl^-$ cotransport mechanism, which establishes a favorable lumen-positive electrochemical gradient, whereas the active magnesium transport mechanism is incompletely understood.

In the DCT, *sodium chloride* continues to be reabsorbed through an ouabain-sensitive Na^+,K^+-ATPase–driven active transport process. Because the DCT is also impermeable to water, there is further dilution of the tubule fluid to an osmolality of approximately 50 to 100 mOsm/kg H_2O. This segment is also a site for active *calcium* reabsorption stimulated by calcitonin and PTH.

The distal tubule is the principal target for the action of several commonly prescribed diuretic drugs. The so-called loop diuretics, such as furosemide, bumetanide, and ethacrynic acid, block sodium chloride reabsorption in the TAL. Thiazide diuretics, including hydrochlorothiazide, chlorthalidone, and metolazone, act on the DCT.

CONNECTING TUBULE

Structure

The connecting tubule or connecting segment joins the DCT with the collecting duct system (see Fig. 116–2). Representing a transitional segment in the human kidney, the connecting tubule is composed of four specific cell types resulting from an intermixing of cells from the adjacent DCT and the initial collecting tubule. The most characteristic cell type is the connecting tubule cell, which is intermediate in appearance between the DCT cell and the principal cell of the collecting duct. Intercalated cells involved in proton and bicarbonate transport vary considerably in structure in the connecting tubule.

Function

PTH affects *calcium* transport in this segment, whereas vasopressin (antidiuretic hormone) has no effect on adenylate cyclase activity or water permeability. This segment is responsible for reabsorbing *sodium* and secreting *potassium*. The latter is believed to be controlled at least partially by mineralocorticoids. The connecting segment is also involved in *proton* and *bicarbonate* transport and is a major site for kallikrein production and secretion in the kidney.

COLLECTING DUCT

Structure

The collecting duct begins in the cortex and descends through the medulla to the tip of the papilla. It can be divided into cortical, outer medullary, and inner medullary segments (see Fig. 116–2). There is remarkable cellular heterogeneity along the collecting duct.

The *cortical collecting duct* (CCD) can be subdivided into the initial collecting tubule and the medullary ray portion. The CCD is composed of principal cells and intercalated cells. The principal cells, which represent approximately two thirds of the total cell population, have a light-staining cytoplasm and relatively few organelles but prominent infoldings of the basal plasma membrane. The intercalated or "dark" cells constitute approximately a third of the cells in the CCD.

There is evidence for the presence of two distinct configurations of intercalated cells in the CCD, type A and type B. Type A or α cells have prominent microprojections on the apical plasma membrane and extensive tubulovesicular structures in the apical cytoplasm. Type B or β cells have a denser cytoplasm, more mitochondria, more spherical vesicular structures in the cytoplasm, and a larger basolateral membrane surface area. The type B cell is localized to the CCD.

The *outer medullary collecting duct* (OMCD) is composed of both principal cells and intercalated cells. The latter represent a third of the cells in the OMCD and resemble the type A cells in the CCD.

The *inner medullary collecting duct* (IMCD) is subdivided into two regions: the initial IMCD, located in the outer third of the inner medulla, and the terminal IMCD, situated in the distal two thirds of the inner medulla (see Fig. 116-2). The initial IMCD is formed mainly of principal cells and a few intercalated cells, whereas the terminal IMCD is composed of one cell type, the IMCD cell.

Function

The collecting duct is the final site in the renal tubule that modifies the volume and solute composition of the tubule fluid.

Water Transport

AQP-2, AQP-3, and AQP-4 function as molecular water channels in the collecting duct (see Fig. 116–9). AQP-2 is located predominantly in the apical plasma membrane of all principal cells and IMCD cells, whereas AQP-3 is found in the basolateral membrane throughout the collecting duct system from the cortex to the papillary tip. AQP-4 is limited to the basolateral plasma membrane of principal cells in the inner stripe of the outer medulla and the basolateral plasma membrane of IMCD cells in the outer third of the inner medulla. In all segments of the collecting duct, osmotic water permeability is controlled largely by vasopressin. In the absence of vasopressin, only the papillary collecting duct manifests some residual permeability. In the presence of vasopressin, the principal cells and all cells in the IMCD are highly permeable to water (see Fig. 116–9). It should be emphasized that in vasopressin-induced antidiuresis, the bulk of the tubule fluid is actually reabsorbed in the CCD.

Proton and Bicarbonate Transport

The entire collecting duct is involved in proton transport and the "fine-tuning" of acid secretion by the kidney. The presence of high levels of carbonic anhydrase II in the intercalated cells suggested initially that they were involved in urine acidification. Immunocytochemical studies have localized a vacuolar-type H^+-ATPase in the apical membrane and a Cl^-/HCO_3^- exchanger in the basolateral membrane of type A intercalated cells (Fig. 116–10A). These findings implicate the type A cell in proton or hydrogen ion secretion in the CCD. The immunolocalization of H^+-ATPase to the basolateral membrane of type B cells and the functional evidence for an apical Cl^-/HCO_3^- exchanger in these cells provide evidence that type B intercalated cells are involved in bicarbonate secretion (see Fig. 116–10B). Recent immunolocalization of a Cl^-/HCO_3^- exchanger in the apical membrane of type B cells confirms the functional evidence for Cl^-/HCO_3^- exchange.

The intercalated cells in the OMCD are responsible for hydrogen ion secretion, which is an active mineralocorticoid-stimulated, sodium-independent process driven in part by H^+-ATPase. The IMCD is also involved in urine acidification. Acid-secreting intercalated cells are present in the initial IMCD, and microcatheterization studies have documented a decrease in luminal pH along the IMCD.

Urea Transport

The cortical and outer medullary segments of the collecting duct are largely impermeable to urea in the presence and absence of vasopressin. In the terminal IMCD, urea reabsorption occurs by means of a vasopressin-sensitive, phloretin-inhibitable, facilitated transport pathway that helps maintain a high urea concentration in the deep inner medulla to facilitate urea recycling, which is important for maximum urine concentration (see Fig. 116–9).

Sodium and Potassium Transport

Virtually all sodium transport and much of the potassium transport in the collecting duct are controlled by aldosterone. Although it is this region of the renal tubule that "fine-tunes" sodium excretion, it is estimated that less than 10% of the filtered load of sodium is controlled by aldosterone. The target for aldosterone is the principal cell. This hormone increases sodium reabsorption by increasing the number of sodium channels in the apical plasma membrane of the principal cell. The sodium channels permit electrogenic sodium entry down a concentration gradient, which creates a lumen-negative potential difference. The increase in intracellular sodium concentration stimulates basolateral Na^+,K^+-ATPase activity to maintain a concentration gradient for sodium entry while

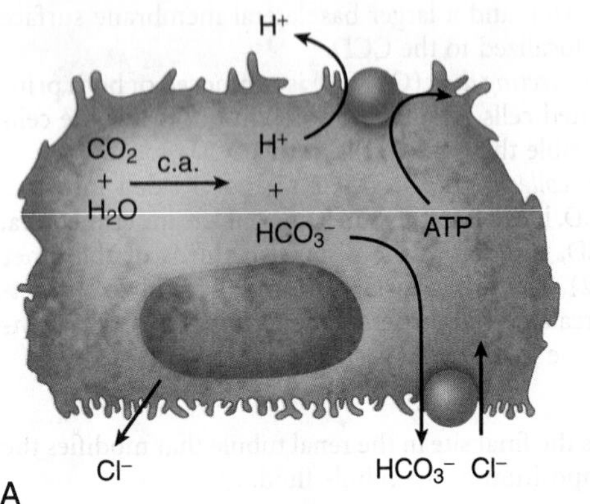

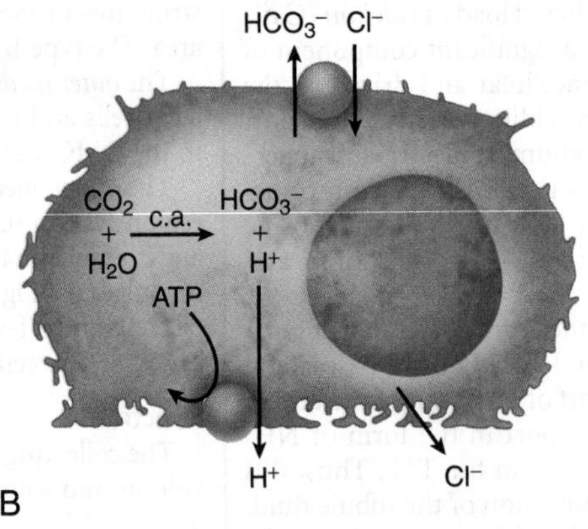

FIGURE 116–10 • Diagrams illustrating the transport characteristics of type A (left) and type B (right) intercalated cells of the cortical collecting duct. c.a. = carbonic anhydrase. (Used with permission from Madsen KM, Verlander JW, Kim J, Tisher CC: Morphological adaptation of the collecting duct to acid-base disturbances. Kidney Int 1991;33:S57–S63.)

increasing the intracellular potassium concentration. Potassium secretion across the luminal membrane through aldosterone-sensitive potassium channels is also enhanced by the lumen-negative potential difference. Conditions that increase plasma aldosterone levels enhance sodium absorption and potassium secretion.

The kidney is chiefly responsible for maintaining potassium homeostasis. The total body potassium content of a 70-kg individual is estimated to be approximately 3500 mEq, 98 to 99% of which resides in the intracellular compartment at a concentration of 125 mEq/L. The concentration of potassium in the extracellular fluid ranges from 3.5 to 4.5 mEq/L. Each day approximately 720 mEq of potassium (4.0 mEq/L × 180 L) is filtered, whereas only 10 to 15% is excreted in urine by an individual with normal body potassium stores. In general, potassium excretion equals potassium ingestion. With a normal potassium intake of approximately 100 mEq/day, the kidney excretes all but about 10 mEq. Approximately 70% of the filtered load of potassium is reabsorbed in the proximal tubule, and another 15 to 20% is reabsorbed in the loop of Henle. The kidney can respond quickly to increase potassium excretion 10-fold when potassium intake is increased. With potassium deprivation, however, it takes up to 14 days to reach a new steady state, a period of time sufficient for a considerable potassium deficit to develop.

The collecting duct is also responsible for fine-tuning potassium excretion. As noted earlier, the principal cells secrete potassium under the control of mineralocorticoids, whereas intercalated cells reabsorb potassium. Several factors influence renal potassium secretion, including the rate of distal tubule fluid flow, acid-base balance, aldosterone, and the electronegativity of the distal tubule. The flow dependence of potassium secretion in the collecting duct is well documented. With an increase in flow (such as that induced by diuretics), there is a parallel increase in sodium delivery to the collecting duct, which facilitates sodium reabsorption and potassium secretion. With metabolic acidosis and to a lesser extent with respiratory acidosis, potassium secretion is suppressed. An opposite effect is observed in metabolic alkalosis. With an increase in the circulating aldosterone level (such as induced by hyperkalemia), there is a parallel increase in the exchange of sodium for potassium by the principal cells that leads to enhanced potassium secretion. Finally, an increase in the lumen-negative potential, a decrease in the luminal potassium concentration, an increase in the intracellular potassium concentration, and an increase in luminal membrane permeability to potassium all favor potassium secretion by the principal cell.

The kidney also can protect against hypokalemia. The presence of H^+,K^+-ATPase has been documented in the intercalated cell of the collecting duct, and data suggest that with potassium deprivation there is enhanced reabsorption of potassium in exchange for protons in these cells.

Intercalated cells also help maintain potassium balance by the collecting duct. During states of potassium deprivation, an H^+,K^+-ATPase located in the apical cell membrane facilitates potassium reabsorption in exchange for hydrogen ions throughout the CCD and OMCD.

SUGGESTED READINGS

Lee DB, Huang E, Ward HJ: Tight junction biology and kidney dysfunction. Am J Physiol Renal Physiol 2006;290:F20–F34. *Overview of contributions to renal failure, polycystic disease, ischemic injury, and magnesium and calcium wasting.*

Nielson S, Kwon TH, Frokiaer J, et al: Regulation and dysregulation of aquaporins in water balance disorders. J Intern Med 2007;261:33–64. *A scientific review.*

Pallone TL, Zhang Z, Rhinehart K: Physiology of the renal medullary microcirculation. Am J Physiol Renal Physiol 2003;284:253–266. *Emphasizes the role of the renal medulla in salt and water balance.*

Sekine T, Miyazai H, Endou H: Molecular physiology of renal organic ion transporters. Am J Physiol Renal Physiol 2006;290:F251–F261. *A scholarly review.*

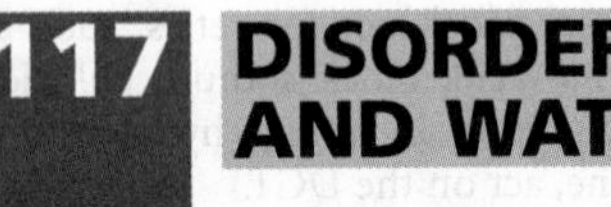

117 DISORDERS OF SODIUM AND WATER HOMEOSTASIS

Karl Skorecki and Dennis Ausiello

SODIUM AND WATER HOMEOSTASIS

Physiology

Disturbances in sodium and water balance or distribution, with attendant perturbations in the volume or solute composition of body fluid compartments, are among the most frequently encountered abnormalities and occur in a wide variety of clinical settings and disease states. The principal clinical manifestations of these disturbances are *hypovolemia, hypervolemia, dysnatremia (hyponatremia* or *hypernatremia),* and *polyuria.* Disturbances in body tonicity, reflected by hyponatremia or hypernatremia, are estimated to affect up to 15 to 20% of hospitalized patients. Only in about 5% of these patients are the abnormalities severe (>10% deviation from normal values). Prevalence rates for these abnormalities in ambulatory populations are lower, with elderly individuals and patients treated with multiple medications being the most susceptible.

Approximately 60% of body mass is composed of solute-containing fluid solutions that are divided into extracellular fluid (ECF) and intracellular fluid (ICF) compartments. Water flows freely across cell membranes according to the dictates of osmotic forces, thus maintaining near equality of the solute-water ratio (osmolality) in the ICF and ECF. However, the composition of the major solutes differs between the ECF and ICF, as shown in Figure 117–1. Sodium and potassium are the major cations in the ECF and ICF, respectively. Chloride and bicarbonate are the major accompanying anions in the ECF, and negative charges on organic molecules maintain electroneutrality with potassium in the ICF. The difference in cationic solute composition between these two compartments is maintained by a pump-leak mechanism involving the activity of Na^+,K^+-adenosine triphosphate (ATPase) operating in concert with cell membrane sodium and potassium conductance pathways. The free movement of water ensures that the sodium concentration in ECF is nearly equivalent to the potassium concentration in ICF. *Osmolality* refers to the concentration of all solutes, whereas *tonicity* refers to the concentration of solutes that are "effective" in eliciting a water shift between body fluid compartments. Addition or removal of solutes causes a sustained shift of water to restore the near equality of concentrations, and they are thus considered *"effective solutes"* (sometimes referred to as "tonomoles") that contribute to body fluid tonicity. Solutes that are permeant across most cell membranes, such as urea, do not elicit such a

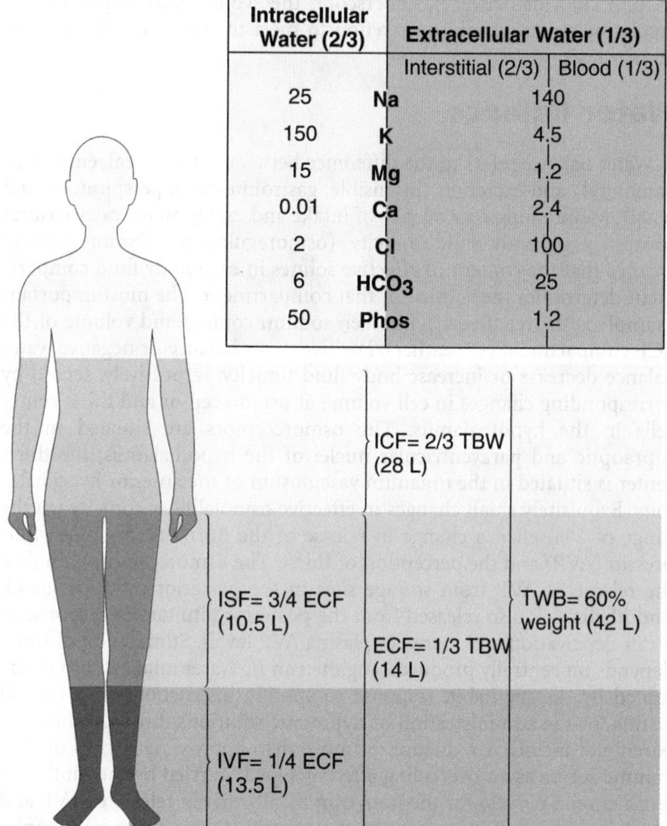

FIGURE 117–1 • Composition of body fluid compartments. **A,** Schematic representation of body fluid compartments in humans. The shaded areas depict the approximate size of each compartment as a function of body weight. The figures indicate the relative sizes of the various fluid compartments and the approximate absolute volumes of the compartments (in liters) in a 70-kg adult. **B,** Relative volumes of various body fluid compartments. In a normally built individual, the total body water content is roughly 60% of body weight. Because adipose tissue has a low concentration of water, the relative water–to–total body weight ratio is lower in obese individuals. Intracellular electrolyte concentrations are in millimoles per liter and are typical values obtained from muscle. ECF = extracellular fluid; ICF = intracellular fluid; ISF = interstitial fluid; IVF = intravascular fluid; TBW = total body water. **(A,** From Verbalis JG: Body water osmolality. *In* Wilkinson B, Jamison R [eds]: Textbook of Nephrology. London, Chapman & Hall, 1997, pp 89–94. Reproduced with permission of Hodder Arnold.)

sustained shift in water and are therefore not considered effective solutes, although they do contribute to the laboratory measurement of fluid osmolality. The addition or removal of water without solutes results in a proportionate reduction or increase, respectively, in both osmolality and tonicity of all body fluid compartments.

The restriction of sodium to the ECF compartment by virtue of the pump-leak mechanism, together with maintenance of osmotic equilibrium between the ECF and ICF, ensures that ECF volume is determined principally by the total body fluid sodium content and governs the partitioning of fluid between the ECF and ICF compartments. This is an important nuance that will be discussed in greater detail later in the chapter.

The mechanisms that govern body fluid homeostasis preserve near constancy of the volumes of the ECF and ICF compartments despite variations in dietary intake and extrarenal losses of sodium and water and adjust this balance in response to variations in the capacity of these compartments. Thus, the overriding principle of body fluid and solute homeostasis is mass balance of total body intake and output of water, as well as balance of osmotically active particles. Such balance is achieved through the integrated action of a number of sensing and effector mechanisms whose aim is to safeguard hemodynamic stability, cellular volume, and solute composition. Even the slightest perturbations in these parameters activate neural and hormonal mediators for restoration of balance. This balance is achieved through adjustments in the urinary excretion of sodium and water in response to perceived changes in ECF or ICF volume. Constancy of ECF volume, together with control of vascular capacitance, ensures a high degree of circulatory stability.

TABLE 117–1 MECHANISMS FOR SENSING REGIONAL CHANGES IN BODY FLUID VOLUME

Cardiopulmonary volume sensors
Atria (neural/humoral pathways)
Ventricular and pulmonary sensing sites
Arterial volume sensors
Carotid and aortic arch baroreceptors
Renal volume sensors
Central nervous system sensors
Hepatic volume sensors

Constancy of ICF volume is necessary to prevent brain cell swelling or shrinkage and its attendant adverse neurologic effects.

Sodium Balance

Sodium balance refers to the difference between intake (dietary or intravenous) and excretion (gastrointestinal, perspiratory, or renal). In the nonclinical setting, sodium intake is controlled by dietary habits. In the clinical setting, prescribed adjustments in sodium intake or the administration of sodium-containing medications or solutions cause variation to overall sodium intake. Although nonrenal sources of sodium loss are under some regulatory influence (e.g., aldosterone-mediated regulation of sodium concentration in stool and sweat), the fine adjustment of sodium balance in response to changes in intake is mediated by regulation of urinary sodium excretion. Thus, in the steady state, urinary excretion of sodium is closely matched to dietary salt intake. This balance depends on a series of afferent mechanisms that sense the volume of the ECF compartment relative to its capacitance and trigger effector mechanisms that modify the rate of renal sodium excretion to maintain ECF volume homeostasis. Normal functioning of these mechanisms in turn is impacted by the partitioning of the ECF into two subcompartments: intravascular and extravascular (interstitial) (see Fig. 117–1). The composition and concentration of small, noncolloid electrolyte solutes in these two subcompartments are nearly equivalent (with the exception of slight differences as a result of the Gibbs-Donnan effect). However, there is a higher concentration of colloid osmotic particles in the intravascular compartment (mostly molecules of albumin and globulin proteins). Opposing transcapillary hydraulic and colloid osmotic (oncotic) pressure gradients (Starling forces) favor the net transudation of fluid from the intravascular to the interstitial compartment. At the same time, lymphatic fluid movement from interstitial sites back to the circulation via the thoracic duct ensures that the intravascular subcompartment is replenished and maintains a nearly constant proportion of approximately 25% of the overall ECF, which corresponds to 3.5 L of plasma. The remaining approximately 75% of ECF volume (equivalent to 10.5 L in a normal 70-kg male) is contained in the interstitial spaces. Because intravascular volume is one of the key determinants of circulatory integrity, preservation of the constancy of ECF volume and appropriate partitioning of the ECF volume between the intravascular and interstitial subcompartments is critical for hemodynamic stability. ECF volume—in particular, the volume of the plasma compartment relative to overall vascular capacitance—determines such fundamental indices of cardiovascular performance as mean arterial blood pressure and left ventricular filling volume.

Effective Arterial Blood Volume

The circulatory network can be regarded as being composed of central and peripheral venous compartments, as well as renal and extrarenal arterial compartments. Each compartment reflects a unique characteristic of overall circulatory function (e.g., cardiac filling, tissue perfusion, renal perfusion, and transudation of fluid into the interstitial space. Table 117–1). The combination of characteristics provides an integrated picture of the state of "fullness" of the intravascular volume relative to capacitance.

The concept of effective arterial blood volume (EABV) is crucial to understanding the afferent mechanisms governing regulation of sodium homeostasis. Unlike ICF, ECF, and intravascular volume, EABV is not measurable as an anatomically defined space but rather is best understood in functional terms as an integration of hemodynamic parameters emanating from specific sites in the arterial circuit that monitor tissue perfusion and trigger appropriate changes in urinary sodium excretion. These sites include the carotid baroreceptor and intrarenal mechanisms located at the glomerular afferent arterioles, the juxtaglomerular apparatus, and peritubular capillaries. EABV often, but not always, varies directly with actual ECF volume. Deviations from this correlation are responsible for abnormalities in sodium balance, as described later. Taken together, the integrated ECF volume–sensing signals elicit an appropriate response for modulating urinary sodium excretion in an effort to maintain constancy of ECF volume. Low-pressure sensors (e.g., cardiac atrial transmural stretch and tension receptors) respond to the state of cardiac filling and tend to protect against overfilling of the ECF compartment, but they also have a role in renal sodium retention in states of perceived underfilling. The filtered load of sodium vastly exceeds net intake such that under most circumstances, it is tubular reabsorption that serves as the principal arbiter of adjustments in urinary sodium excretion that are necessary to preserve sodium balance and constancy of ECF volume (Chapter 116). Adjustments in urinary sodium excretion depend on the relationship between the filtered load of sodium and the fraction of that filtered load that is reabsorbed along the length of the tubule.

Specific luminal membrane sodium transporters or channels at each tubule segment mediate movement of sodium from the luminal fluid into the cell in a carefully regulated manner, followed by extrusion of sodium across the basolateral surface via Na^+, K^+-ATPase and other sodium transporters. Among others, these regulated luminal transporters include the Na/H exchanger (proximal tubule), the Na-K-2Cl (NKCC2) cotransport pathway (loop of Henle), the NaCl cotransporter (NCCT) along the distal convoluted tubule, and the apical sodium channel (ENaC) along the connecting and cortical collecting tubule. At some nephron sites, sodium reabsorption is isotonic (e.g., proximal tubule), whereas at other sites, sodium reabsorption exceeds that of water in relation to body tonicity, and tubule fluid is generated with a sodium concentration less than that of plasma (e.g., thick ascending limb of the loop of Henle). These and additional sodium reabsorptive transport pathways are subject to a series of different neural and hormonal regulatory influences, and the levels of transport or channel activity respond to the afferent limb signals for sensing the fullness of the circulation. Hormonal regulatory factors include the circulating and intrarenal renin-angiotensin-aldosterone pathways acting at multiple nephron sites and circulating peptides such as atrial and brain natriuretic peptides, among others. Numerous additional systemic and local paracrine mediators have been identified, including, for example, the nitric oxide and eicosanoid/prostaglandin systems. The redundancy of multiple hormonal mediators, acting together with modulation of renal neural stimulation and intrarenal physical factors (e.g., peritubular capillary Starling forces, tubule lumen sodium chloride delivery), underscores the evolutionary importance of regulating urinary sodium excretion to meet the needs of ECF volume homeostasis.

Water Balance

Water balance refers to the difference between intake (oral, enteral, or parenteral) and excretion (insensible, gastrointestinal, perspiratory, and renal). Maintaining equivalency of intake and excretion of water ensures constancy of body fluid tonicity (osmoregulation). Osmoregulation ensures that the content of effective solutes in each body fluid compartment determines the volume of that compartment. The most important example is the relationship between sodium content and volume of the ECF compartment (see earlier). Positive water balance or negative water balance decrease or increase body fluid tonicity, respectively, sensed by corresponding changes in cell volume at osmoreceptor and thirst center cells in the hypothalamus. The osmoreceptors are situated in the supraoptic and paraventricular nuclei of the hypothalamus; the thirst center is situated in the organum vasculosum of the anterior hypothalamus. Exquisitely small changes in effective osmolality or tonicity (in the range of 2%) elicit a change in release of the hormone arginine vasopressin (AVP) and the perception of thirst. The osmoreceptors stimulate the release of AVP from storage sites in the posterior pituitary gland. Endothelin-1 is also released from the posterior pituitary in response to water deprivation and increases plasma AVP levels. Stimulation of thirst depends on centrally produced angiotensin II. Water intake is also determined by dietary habit, response to specific instructions in a clinical setting, or the administration of hypotonic solutions through enteral or parenteral means. A reduction of more than approximately 8% of ECF volume serves as an overriding afferent signal (carried by the ninth and tenth cranial nerves) for the non–osmotically driven release of AVP and also stimulates thirst by means of angiotensin II, even when body tonicity is not elevated. The relationship between tonicity and volume stimuli to AVP release is shown in Figure 117–2A).

AVP is the final arbiter of urinary excretion of hypotonic fluid, which depends on three sequential renal processes: delivery of isotonic sodium-containing filtrate to the thick ascending limb of the loop of Henle, reabsorption of sodium and accompanying electrolytes without water in the thick ascending limb of the loop of Henle to generate a hypotonic luminal fluid, and reabsorption of solute-free water along the length of the collecting tubule. The latter is regulated in response to AVP, which acts by binding to its V_2 receptors on the basolateral membrane of principal cells and triggering a signaling cascade that eventuates in the synthesis and insertion of aquaporin-2 water channels into the luminal membrane of these cells. In the *presence* of AVP, the hydro-osmotic movement of water from the collecting tubule lumen to the hyperosmotic milieu of the

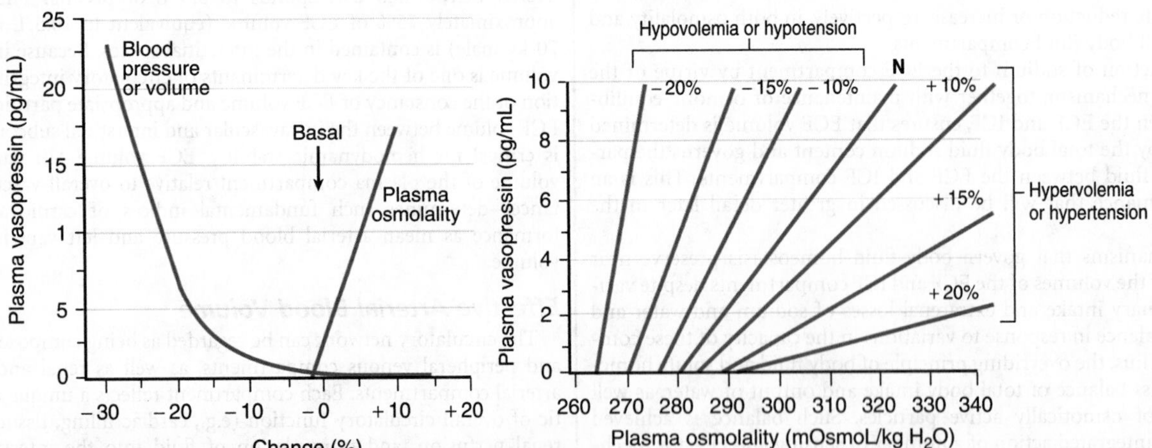

FIGURE 117–2 • Relationship between arginine vasopressin (AVP) and osmolality. A, Comparative sensitivity of AVP secretion in response to increases in plasma osmolality versus decreases in blood volume or blood pressure in human subjects. The arrow indicates the low plasma AVP concentrations found at basal plasma osmolality. Note that AVP secretion is much more sensitive to small changes in blood osmolality than to changes in volume or pressure. **B,** The relationship between the osmolality of plasma and the concentration of AVP in plasma is modulated by blood volume and pressure. The line labeled N shows plasma AVP concentrations across a range of plasma osmolality in an adult with normal intravascular volume (euvolemic) and normal blood pressure (normotensive). The lines to the left of N show the relationship between plasma AVP concentration and plasma osmolality in adults whose low intravascular volume (hypovolemia) or blood pressure (hypotension) is 10%, 15%, and 20% below normal. Lines to the right of N are for volumes and blood pressure 10%, 15%, and 20% above normal. Note that hemodynamic influences do not disrupt the osmoregulation of AVP but rather raise or lower the set point and possibly also the sensitivity of AVP secretion in proportion to the magnitude of the change in blood volume or pressure.

renal medulla minimizes urinary excretion of the hypotonic fluid generated in the thick ascending limb of the loop of Henle, and thereby promotes positive water balance. In the *absence* of AVP, this hypotonic fluid is excreted, which promotes negative water balance. Under normal physiologic conditions, these adjustments in urinary water excretion represent the appropriate response to changes in net water intake. However, when adjustments are inappropriate, they may lead to states of positive or negative water balance with corresponding hypotonicity or hypertonicity. The typical levels of urine osmolality that can be achieved in the human kidney by fluctuations in AVP action range between 50 and 1200 mOsm/kg, but this range narrows at the extremes of age or in the presence of intrinsic renal disease. Laboratory measurement of urine osmolality reflects overall renal concentrating ability, including the hydro-osmotic action of AVP. However, not all solutes that contribute to the laboratory measurement of urine osmolality correspond to effective solutes in terms of body fluid tonicity. Thus, excretion of urine with high concentrations of urea and low concentrations of sodium, potassium, and chloride indicates a strong renal concentrating capacity but contributes less to positive water balance than does excretion of urine with the same measured osmolality and higher concentrations of these electrolytes.

Pathobiology

Disturbances in sodium balance primarily affect ECF volume and disturbances in water balance primarily affect body fluid tonicity. A cumulative negative balance of sodium (sodium deficit) in the absence of a change in tonicity results in ECF volume contraction (hypovolemia), whereas a cumulative positive balance of sodium (sodium surfeit) results in ECF volume expansion (hypervolemia). In contrast, a cumulative positive body water balance (water surfeit) results in volume expansion of all the body fluid compartments, whereas negative water balance (water deficit) results in volume contraction of all the body fluid compartments. However, because ICF volume is double that of ECF at baseline, the more prominent expansion or contraction in absolute volume terms involves the ICF compartment. Furthermore, maintenance of a surfeit or deficit of water relative to solutes results in a respective uniform decrease or increase in body fluid tonicity in all fluid compartments and therefore a disturbance in osmoregulation. Because the solute composition of the plasma component of the ECF compartment is sampled, a disturbance in tonicity is most commonly detected as an abnormality in plasma sodium concentration (hyponatremia for water surfeit and hypernatremia for water deficit). Frequently, disturbances in water and sodium balance occur together, and all combinations of surfeit or deficit can occur (Table 117–2). The clinical approach to a patient with a sodium or water balance disturbance (or both) can be facilitated by careful consideration of which states apply.

SODIUM BALANCE DISORDERS

Hypovolemia

Definition

Hypovolemia refers to a reduction in the volume of the ECF compartment in relation to its capacitance. In states of absolute hypovolemia, a deficit in sodium reflects past or ongoing negative sodium balance. In states of relative hypovolemia, there is no deficit of sodium; rather, the capacitance of the ECF compartment is increased. Both processes may occur simultaneously. The volume of the ECF intravascular and extravascular (interstitial) subcompartments may vary in the same or opposite directions. ICF volume is reflected by the measurement of plasma osmolality and sodium concentration and may be concomitantly disturbed, thus allowing designation of the appropriate clinical category as indicated in Table 117–2.

In *relative hypovolemia,* ECF volume is not reduced in absolute terms, but the capacitance of the ECF or intravascular compartment is expanded, which leads to clinical manifestations that mimic those of absolute hypovolemia. Relative hypovolemic states can be classified into two categories: states of vasodilation and states of generalized edema. Vasodilation occurs in response to drugs that induce arteriolar vasodilation (e.g., hydralazine, minoxidil) and is also characteristic of certain phases of sepsis with peripheral vasodilation and low systemic vascular resistance. The ensuing perception of reduced intravascular volume can be accompanied by clinical manifestations suggestive of absolute hypovolemia, such as tachycardia and hypotension. Renal responses, including renal sodium and water conservation, are triggered as well. Peripheral vasodilation also occurs in normal pregnancy and accounts for the characteristic sodium retention.

The other category of relative hypovolemia consists of patients with generalized edema states in the context of reduced EABV. As noted previously, EABV is that component of intravascular volume that effectively perfuses tissues, is detected by arterial and renal pressure and flow sensors, and elicits changes in hemodynamic settings and renal transport functions. EABV often, but not always, correlates directly with actual ECF volume. Deviations from a direct correlation are responsible for many of the so-called edema states in patients with cardiac failure, those with decompensated cirrhosis with ascites, and some patients with nephrotic syndrome.

Pathobiology

Causes of absolute and relative hypovolemia are listed in Table 117–3 and can be categorized into extrarenal and renal causes.

Extrarenal Causes of Absolute Hypovolemia

Bleeding is the most frequent and direct cause of a reduction in the volume of the intravascular subcompartment of the ECF. The immediate effect of bleeding is a proportionate net loss in plasma and erythrocytes and hence an isotonic reduction in ECF volume. Compensatory hemodynamic responses include tachycardia and vasoconstriction, followed by a shift of fluid from the interstitial to the intravascular compartment secondary to altered transcapillary Starling hydraulic forces. Additional neural and hormonal responses result in renal sodium and water retention, with the aim of restoring intravascular volume and stabilizing the circulation. Other extrarenal causes of absolute hypovolemia include fluid loss from the gastrointestinal, integumentary, or respiratory systems. Besides dietary intake, approximately 7 L of isotonic fluid enters the gastrointestinal tract on a daily basis, the bulk of which is reabsorbed to minimize fecal fluid loss. Because these fluids contain varying concentrations of sodium and accompanying anions, enhanced secretion or

Section XI Renal

TABLE 117–2 PATHOGENIC PROCESSES LEADING TO DISORDERS OF BODY SODIUM AND FLUID HOMEOSTASIS

Clinical State	Extracellular Fluid Volume	Body Fluid Tonicity	Pathogenic Process
Normal	↔	↔	
Hypervolemic normonatremia	↑	↔	Isotonic net gain of sodium and water
Hypervolemic hyponatremia	↑	↓	Hypotonic net gain sodium and water
Hypervolemic hypernatremia	↑	↑	Hypertonic net gain of sodium and water
Normovolemic hyponatremia	↔	↓	Net water gain ± sodium loss
Normovolemic hypernatremia	↔	↑	Net water loss ± sodium gain
Hypovolemic hypernatremia	↓	↑	Net loss of water in excess of sodium
Hypovolemic normonatremia	↓	↔	Isotonic net loss of sodium and water
Hypovolemic hyponatremia	↓	↓	Net loss of sodium in excess of water

↔ = unchanged.

TABLE 117–3 CAUSES OF ABSOLUTE AND RELATIVE HYPOVOLEMIA

EXTRARENAL

Absolute
- Bleeding
- Gastrointestinal fluid loss (diarrhea, vomiting, ileostomy or colostomy secretions)
- Fluid loss from skin (burns, sweat)
- Respiratory fluid loss

Relative
- "Third-space" loss
- Sepsis
- Edema states (congestive heart failure, cirrhosis)

RENAL

Absolute
- Diuretics
- Inherited sodium-wasting tubulopathies
- Tubulointerstitial diseases
- Partial obstruction or postobstruction etiology
- Endocrine disorders (e.g., hypoaldosteronism, adrenal insufficiencies)

Relative
- Nephrotic syndrome

impaired reabsorption causes absolute ECF volume depletion. The composition of the fluid loss (and accompanying anions and other cations such as potassium) differs according to the cause and source of gastrointestinal fluid loss (vomiting, different causes of diarrhea, ileostomy or colostomy secretions). These in turn affect both the consequent renal response and body fluid composition (pH, potassium and sodium concentrations, osmolality). Infectious diarrhea remains a leading cause of death from hypovolemia in many areas of the world.

Given its large surface area, it is not surprising that fluid losses from the integumentary system can be an important cause of hypovolemia. Burns allow the loss of large volumes of plasma and interstitial fluid and can rapidly lead to degrees of profound hypovolemia similar to those seen with bleeding. In the absence of medical intervention, hemoconcentration and hypoalbuminemia are expected. Given the isotonic composition of the lost fluid, no changes in plasma osmolality or sodium concentration are expected. Exertion in hot environments increases thermoregulatory fluid losses from the skin in the form of sweat. Fluid loss through perspiration can reach 1 L/hr or more, depending on exertion and environment. The sodium concentration in sweat varies among individuals (range of approximately 20 to 50 mmol/L). Thus, although the fluid loss is hypotonic, a significant sodium deficit and ECF volume contraction can ensue. The extent of hypovolemia and the resulting body fluid composition (plasma osmolality and sodium concentration) will depend on fluid replacement, which is determined primarily by thirst and availability.

Enhanced evaporative water loss from the respiratory tract can occur in febrile states and in patients undergoing mechanical ventilation with inadequate humidification. Though frequently listed as a cause of hypovolemia, the volumes of fluid (and in particular the sodium concentration) are such that this does not serve as a major source of sodium deficit and is more relevant in consideration of water deficit. In the special case of dialysis patients, excessive ultrafiltration is a frequent cause of hypovolemia.

In addition, pathologic conditions exist in which ECF can be sequestered into compartments within the body without an evident history of loss. In such cases, the clinical manifestations mimic those of absolute hypovolemia because the sequestered compartment is not in hemodynamic equilibrium with the ECF. Such pathologic conditions are often referred to as *"third-space"* loss and include gastrointestinal obstruction, sequestration of fluids in subcutaneous tissue after trauma or burns, and sequestration in the retroperitoneal or peritoneal space in patients with pancreatitis or peritonitis, respectively. The accumulation of malignant ascites or peritoneal fluid may also compromise intravascular volume. These extrarenal causes of absolute hypovolemia are expected to invoke a renal response whose hallmark is sodium and fluid conservation. Obviously, this expected response is absent when the kidney itself is responsible for sodium loss, whether due to the effect of pharmacologic or hormonal influences or due to intrinsic renal disease.

Renal Causes of Hypovolemia

When the glomerular filtration rate (GFR) and plasma sodium concentration are normal, approximately 24,000 mmol of sodium are filtered per day. Even when the GFR is markedly impaired, the quantities of sodium filtered far exceed normal dietary intake. Thus, the small quantities of sodium excreted in urine relative to the filtered load depend on the integrity of tubular sodium reabsorptive mechanisms to match urinary sodium excretion to dietary intake through volume sensing and effector mechanisms. Impairment in the integrity of one or more of these sodium reabsorptive mechanisms can result in a profound sodium deficit and absolute volume depletion. This occurs in response to a number of pharmacologic agents and in numerous renal and endocrine disorders (see Table 117–3). Most of the widely used diuretic medications inhibit specific pathways for sodium reabsorption at various sites along the nephron. These agents are often used to treat hypervolemic states, but their overuse or inappropriate use can result in hypovolemia. Loop diuretics (furosemide, bumetanide, torsemide, and ethacrynic acid) are the most potent pharmacologic agents in this regard, and their potential to induce renal sodium loss (natriuresis) is augmented when they are combined with other classes of diuretic agents (thiazides, carbonic anhydrase inhibitors, aldosterone antagonists, distal epithelial sodium-channel blockers).

Tubular sodium reabsorption may also be disrupted in certain inherited or acquired renal tubulopathies, such as various forms of proximal tubulopathy and different forms of Bartter's and Gitelman's syndromes (Chapter 129). In most cases, the disorder is brought to medical attention because of an accompanying electrolyte or acid-base disturbance (e.g., hypokalemic metabolic alkalosis in the case of Bartter's and Gitelman's syndromes) or by the family history. Impairment of renal tubule sodium reabsorption at various sites along the nephron may also be one of the components of overall tubule dysfunction in a variety of acquired renal injury states. The most common of such acquired renal injury states in hospitalized patients are nonoliguric acute kidney injury and the recovery phase after oliguric acute kidney injury or after release of urinary obstruction (Chapter 121 and 124). In addition, the causes of interstitial renal disease may result in fluid and electrolyte abnormalities, which can include renal sodium wasting. In any form of kidney disease, whenever tubular reabsorption of the filtered sodium load does not match the sum of this filtered load plus dietary intake, a renal sodium-wasting state may ensue. The frequent use of diuretic agents in patients with chronic kidney disease can unmask or accelerate such a process. Filtration of nonelectrolyte solutes of exogenous or endogenous origin also can impair tubular sodium reabsorptive capacity. This explains in part the polyuric state frequently observed after recovery from acute renal injury or obstruction, wherein urea is the endogenous solute. Other frequently encountered nonelectrolyte urinary solutes are glucose (in severe hyperglycemia) and mannitol or glycerol, which are administered to patients with increased intracranial pressure to induce translocation of fluid from the ICF to the ECF compartment, with the aim of decreasing brain swelling. These conditions are accompanied by evident polyuria. The plasma solute composition in these hypovolemic states depends on the complex interplay of intercompartmental fluid shifts and fluid intake.

In addition to intrinsic defects in tubule function, hormonal and other systemic disturbances may disrupt the function of sodium reabsorption transporters. Mineralocorticoid deficiency and resistance states are most important in this regard, and adrenal insufficiency should always be considered in a patient with evidence of urinary sodium loss in the face of hypovolemia. In cerebral salt wasting (an as yet unidentified systemic factor) is thought to impair tubular sodium reabsorption in the setting of acute head injury or intracranial hemorrhage. Hyponatremia is a frequent concomitant manifestation of this syndrome and is generally what leads to its diagnosis.

Another underappreciated but frequent clinical setting for renal sodium loss occurs after the iatrogenic administration of high volumes of volume-expanding, salt-containing solutions to hospitalized patients. Such patients are usually in the postoperative or post-trauma setting and are frequently administered many liters of saline or other sodium-containing maintenance intravenous fluids for several consecutive days, during which tubule reabsorption of sodium is downregulated. There may be a lag in the restoration of full tubule reabsorptive capacity, when intravenous fluids are discontinued, and high volumes of urine rich in sodium continue to be excreted. During this lag phase, the patient may become mildly, but transiently, hypovolemic. This scenario can be avoided by a graduated reduction in administered sodium-containing fluids, at a pace that allows sodium reabsorptive tubular pathways to be upregulated and restored to their normal reabsorptive levels.

Diabetes insipidus represents a spectrum of conditions resulting from deficiency or tubular resistance to the action of AVP. However, since it is the tubule reabsorption of water and not solutes that is impaired, and consequently the impact on ECF volume is generally a minor consideration in comparison to the impact on ICF and body fluid tonicity. Therefore, this spectrum of disorders will be considered later.

Clinical Manifestations

The clinical manifestations of hypovolemia depend on the magnitude and rate of volume loss, the solute composition of the net fluid loss (taking into account ingested or administered fluids), and vascular and renal responses. Clinical manifestations should be considered in terms of (1) underlying pathophysiologic process, (2) the hemodynamic consequences of volume depletion of various degrees, and (3) the related perturbations in acid-base and electrolyte concentrations that attend the renal response to hypovolemia.

A detailed history is often helpful in determining the cause of hypovolemia (bleeding, vomiting, diarrhea, polyuria, medications, diaphoresis). It is important to note that the absence of symptoms does not exclude mild to moderate hypovolemia, especially if the volume loss has occurred gradually. Intravascular volume contraction of less than 5% does not usually elicit symptoms and readily escapes detection by physical examination. With greater degrees of absolute hypovolemia (corresponding to intravascular volume contraction in the 5 to 15% range), symptoms and signs begin to appear. Patients may exhibit nonspecific symptoms related to end-organ hypoperfusion, including weakness, muscle cramps, and postural lightheadedness. Thirst may be an early manifestation but more likely reflects a concomitant hypertonic state.

A number of clinical scenarios can be illustrative of the relationship of clinical manifestations to causes of hypovolemia.

A patient with an acute *gastrointestinal hemorrhage* of 0.5 L of whole blood can experience tachycardia, postural hypotension, peripheral vasoconstriction with cool extremities, lightheadedness, and oliguria, with high urine osmolarity and low urine sodium concentration. Hemoglobin and albumin will probably remain constant initially, and then a drop in hemoglobin will ensue after movement of ECF from the interstitial to the intravascular compartment. The plasma solute composition (sodium and potassium concentration, acid-base parameters) is not likely to change initially. The plasma concentration of urea may rise somewhat as a result of both reduced renal plasma flow and the effects of destruction of erythrocytes in the gastrointestinal tract. Jugular venous pressure is expected to fall, and central venous pressure (CVP) will generally be less than 5 cm H_2O in the absence of confounding factors. Urine output is expected be low, with a high specific gravity and osmolality and a low urine sodium concentration.

In another scenario, a patient inappropriately receiving potent *loop diuretics* over a period of many days for localized peripheral edema may suffer a cumulative net ECF loss of 3 L (≈20%). Approximately a third of this volume originates in the intravascular compartment the remainder from the interstitial compartment. The degree of intravascular loss is expected to induce weakness, tachycardia, low jugular venous pressure, and hypotension. However, because the deficit may have accumulated over time, a degree of adaptation would attenuate the severity of these clinical manifestations and lead the clinician to underestimate the extent of hypovolemia. The plasma sodium concentration may remain unaltered because disruption of the urine-concentrating mechanism by loop diuretics attenuates the tendency to water retention, and an intact thirst mechanism prevents hypertonicity. Because loop diuretics enhance urinary potassium and ammonium excretion, hypokalemic metabolic alkalosis is expected. The ongoing effect of the loop diuretic would mitigate oliguria and lead to inappropriately high concentrations of solutes including sodium and potassium in urine. After cessation of the loop diuretic, the appropriate renal response of oliguria, high urine osmolality, and sodium concentration would be expected.

A third scenario is a patient with relative hypovolemia secondary to *bacteremic sepsis.* No source of fluid loss would be identified in the history. Nevertheless, the patient would manifest symptoms of weakness extending to prostration, accompanied by compromised vital signs with tachycardia and hypotension. The severity of clinical manifestations reflects the effect of systemic inflammatory mediators on the peripheral circulatory endothelium. Inflammatory mediators of sepsis and other factors also reduce cardiac output. The extremities may be warm, although reduced tissue perfusion would be reflected in a reduced level of consciousness, oliguria, elevated plasma urea and creatinine, and lactic acidosis.

Diagnosis

The most readily appreciated physical findings are those related to contraction of the intravascular compartment and include tachycardia, orthostatic hypotension, and reduced jugular venous pressure. It should be noted that jugular venous pressure provides a crude estimate of CVP, which can also be measured directly. However, a number of confounding factors obfuscate the reliability of CVP as a measure of hypovolemia. Although low CVP often reliably reflects intravascular volume contraction, elevated CVP does not necessarily exclude hypovolemia because of the possible confounding influence of conditions such as cardiac or lung disease. Severe degrees of hypovolemia (corresponding to intravascular volume contraction exceeding 10 to 20%) cause hypotension (even in the supine position), peripheral cyanosis, cold extremities, and reduced levels of consciousness (extending even to coma) as a result of end-organ and cerebral hypoperfusion. Hemodynamic collapse (hypovolemic shock) (Chapter 107) can also occur in this range of intravascular volume contraction, depending on the rate of volume loss and comorbid conditions, and is certainly expected with greater degrees of hypovolemia. When the source of volume loss is purely extrarenal, oliguria is expected. Traditional physical findings such as reduced skin or eyeball turgor and dry mucous membranes are no longer considered reliable indicators of hypovolemia.

Laboratory Findings

Laboratory measurements may serve as an adjunct to clinical assessment.

Decreases in *hemoglobin* indicate past or ongoing bleeding. However, stable hemoglobin does not rule out bleeding as a source of hypovolemia. A reduction in hemoglobin depends on translocation of fluid from the interstitial to the intravascular compartment, which in turn, mitigates the degree of hemodynamic compromise and accompanying physical findings. Hemoconcentration is often observed when hypovolemia is not the consequence of bleeding; however, concomitant disease processes that produce anemia may mitigate this rise.

The *albumin* concentration may vary depending on the underlying disease process and therefore often provides a clue to the underlying causes and pathophysiologic processes rather than pointing to a diagnosis of hypovolemia per se. For example, gastrointestinal, urinary, or skin losses of albumin-free fluids may result in a rise in albumin concentration. Fluid losses accompanied by albumin loss (proteinuria, catabolic state, hepatic disease, protein-losing enteropathy) may mitigate this rise or even result in hypoalbuminemia. Similarly, burns and third-space sequestration are often accompanied by hypoalbuminemia as a result of loss of protein-rich fluid rather than a plasma ultrafiltrate.

Sodium and *other electrolytes* can also vary widely, depending on the underlying and concomitant disease processes and intake of fluids. Thus, the sodium concentration reflects the body fluid tonicity state and the composition of the fluid loss, as well as the solute composition of self- or physician-administered fluids. Even subtle and subclinical degrees of hypovolemia trigger urinary water retention and result in a hypotonic hyponatremic plasma composition if there is exposure to solutions that are more hypotonic than that of the fluid lost. In contrast, loss of hypotonic fluids with inadequate water ingestion or replacement results in a hypertonic plasma composition and hypernatremia.

Acid-base and *potassium* changes indicate a number of possible scenarios. Hypokalemia with metabolic alkalosis frequently accompanies vomiting and some forms of diarrheal fluid loss. More often, diarrheal fluid loss is associated with a non–anion gap type of metabolic acidosis. Loop and thiazide diuretic–induced hypovolemia is often associated with hypokalemic metabolic alkalosis, as are the inherited tubulopathies (Bartter's and Gitelman's syndromes) (Chapter 129), which disrupt sodium reabsorptive mechanisms at the loop of Henle and distal convoluted tubule, respectively. Degrees of hypovolemia that induce circulatory compromise and tissue hypoperfusion are accompanied by lactic acidosis.

Increases in *plasma urea* and *creatinine* concentrations are frequently observed in hypovolemic states and reflect reduced renal plasma flow. If acute tubule injury does not supervene, the rise in plasma urea concentration is often disproportionate to the rise in plasma creatinine concentration (see Prerenal Azotemia in Chapter 121). The rise in plasma urea and creatinine concentrations is particularly indicative when hypovolemia is a consequence of urinary fluid losses. In such conditions, the patient is not oliguric, even though renal plasma flow and GFR are compromised. Other forms of urinary sodium loss, such as occur with adrenal insufficiency or aldosterone unresponsiveness, are accompanied by a tendency to hyperkalemia and mild metabolic acidosis.

Urinary biochemical parameters may also help in the clinical assessment of hypovolemic states. When fluid loss is extrarenal, the expected renal response of water and sodium conservation results in oliguria with an elevated urine specific gravity (>1.020) and osmolality (>400 mOsm/kg) and a sodium concentration less than 20 mmol/L because of enhanced renal tubule reabsorptive activity. More complex indices of the appropriate renal response to hypovolemia include fractional excretion of sodium less than 1% and fractional excretion of urea less than 30 to 35%. Intrinsic renal injury confounds the diagnostic value of these urinary indices.

Differential Diagnosis

Relative hypovolemia secondary to arterial vasodilation mimics some, but not all of the clinical manifestations of absolute hypovolemia. Thus, tachycardia and hypotension are frequently observed. However, the extremities may be warm and seem to be well perfused, as is frequently observed in states of sepsis. This finding is misleading because tissues are actually underperfused, as reflected by reduced renal and cerebral function and lactic acidosis. As noted earlier, generalized edema states are really states of ECF volume expansion; however, reduced EABV sometimes leads to a confusing overlap of clinical manifestations.

Treatment

Rx

Absolute Hypovolemia

The major goal in treatment of hypovolemia is to restore hemodynamic integrity and tissue perfusion. The clinical parameters described in the preceding section serve as appropriate end points. The treatment approach can be divided into the following components: (1) treatment of the underlying disease state when possible, (2) fluid replacement of the volume deficit, and (3) fluid administration to maintain ECF volume in the event of continuing losses. Beyond the specific treatments, the mainstay of therapy involves fluid administration. The important issues are the volume, rate of administration, and composition of the replacement and maintenance fluids. These decisions may vary during different stages of treatment and should be adjusted according to the patient's response as determined by closely monitored clinical parameters.

The choice of oral or intravenous replacement fluids (or both) for hypovolemic states is dictated principally by the disturbances in other electrolyte and acid-base parameters. The rate of replacement is a function of the urgency of the threat to circulatory integrity and consideration of complications related to overzealous or too rapid correction.

Fluid therapy for hypovolemic states sometimes begins with a "diagnostic fluid challenge." In situations in which clinical parameters do not permit a firm diagnosis of hypovolemia, the response to a fluid challenge can be informative and serve as the initial treatment step. For example, a patient with known long-standing compensated cardiac failure who is being maintained on a therapeutic

Rx

regimen that includes diuretics may have tachycardia, a reduction in blood pressure from baseline values, poor cognition, and renal dysfunction. Such a clinical scenario could have a number of different explanations, including volume depletion with inadequate left ventricular filling volume. CVP, whether measured directly or assessed via jugular venous pressure, may be misleading in the face of right ventricular dysfunction. More invasive monitoring by direct measurement of pulmonary capillary wedge pressure has not been shown to confer a significant clinical outcome advantage. In such a case, a carefully monitored and diagnostic fluid challenge can minimize the risk for fluid overload. Obviously, such monitoring should include clinical assessment of parameters indicating pulmonary venous hypertension (pulmonary congestion or edema by physical examination or chest radiograph). Reversal of the disturbed clinical parameters would support the diagnosis of volume depletion.

Another example is a patient with hyponatremia in the setting of suspected volume depletion. Often the degree of volume depletion is too subtle to be detected by clinical examination, and a therapeutic challenge with fluid of the appropriate composition can be informative, as outlined later in the section on hyponatremia.

The initial volume and rate of therapeutic replacement fluid should be determined by ongoing monitoring of clinical parameters rather than a priori estimates of volume deficit. In some settings, the clinical state will dictate rapid fluid replacement, as in a patient with unambiguous hypovolemic shock and life-threatening circulatory collapse. In such cases, fluids can be administered at the most rapid rate possible, limited only by intravenous access, until blood pressure and tissue perfusion are restored. However, in most cases, much slower rates are indicated, especially in elderly patients, patients whose medical background is unclear, or those with known comorbid conditions. It is important to note that replacement fluids of different compositions have quite disparate volumes of distribution in the body fluid compartments and therefore differ in their efficiency of restoring ECF volume. *Crystalloid solutions* with sodium as the principal cation are the mainstay in fluid replacement therapy for hypovolemic states and are indicated primarily for hypovolemic states secondary to renal, gastrointestinal, or sweat-based sodium losses. These solutions also are useful initial agents and adjuncts to therapy for the hypovolemia of hemorrhage and burns. *Isotonic saline* is confined to the ECF compartment (except in cases of severe dysnatremia). Thus, retention of 1 L of infused isotonic saline increases plasma volume by about 300 mL, with the remaining portion distributed in the interstitial subcompartment of the ECF. In contrast, a solution of *5% dextrose in water (D_5W)* is equivalent to administering solute-free water and distributes uniformly throughout all body fluid compartments (a third of the retained volume of infusate remains in the ECF compartment and only approximately 10 to 15% in the intravascular compartment). Infusing a given volume of *half isotonic saline (0.45% sodium chloride plus 5% glucose)* can be considered equivalent to infusing half that volume as solute-free water (distributed throughout body fluid compartments) and the other half as isotonic saline (confined to the ECF compartment). The retained solute-free volume reduces body tonicity and the plasma sodium concentration, potential benefit in the follow-up treatment of patients whose hypovolemia is accompanied by hypertonicity and hypernatremia, but a detriment for patients with normotonic or hypotonic hypovolemia.

When hypovolemia is accompanied by hypobicarbonatemia (metabolic acidosis), it may be appropriate to design a solution in which a portion of the sodium is accompanied by bicarbonate. For example, it is possible to add a given quantity of hypertonic sodium bicarbonate to a solution of half isotonic saline or D_5W (in which chloride is the anion accompanying sodium) to obtain an isotonic replacement fluid appropriate for the given acid-base status of the patient. Similarly, in patients with concomitant potassium depletion, especially when accompanied by metabolic alkalosis, addition of potassium chloride to the replacement solution may be indicated. Details regarding quantities and cautions in the administration of sodium bicarbonate or potassium chloride in intravenous solutions are provided in Chapters 118 and 119. A number of crystalloid

Rx

solutions with predetermined concentrations of potassium, lactate (converted to bicarbonate by the liver), and other electrolytes are commercially available, but it is more appropriate to begin with a sodium chloride–containing solution at a concentration appropriate to body tonicity, then add other solutes as indicated or at a separate intravenous administration site. This approach provides maximum flexibility in tailoring individualized fluid replacement therapy to patient needs.

Colloid-containing solutions include albumin or large-molecular-weight carbohydrate molecules (e.g., hydroxyethyl starch or dextran) at concentrations that exert a colloid osmotic pressure equal to or greater than that of plasma. Banked human plasma itself is also considered a colloid solution. Because large molecules such as albumin and high-molecular-weight carbohydrates do not readily cross the transcapillary barrier, they are thought to expand the intravascular compartment more rapidly and efficiently than crystalloid solutions. However, this is the case only if the transcapillary barrier partitioning the intravascular and extravascular (interstitial) compartments is not disrupted by a capillary leak state, as often occurs in patients with multiorgan system failure and systemic inflammatory response syndrome (Chapter 109). Nevertheless, albumin-containing solutions may be useful in hypovolemia associated with burns, where cutaneous protein losses are appreciable. Furthermore, because of the capacity for rapid intravascular volume expansion with just a small volume of replacement fluid, colloid-containing solutions are frequently used when rapid intravascular expansion is desired. These solutions are often used at trauma sites outside the hospital setting because they are more conveniently transported and stored. However, except for the traume site consideration, studies have not shown an outcome advantage for colloid-containing solutions in the treatment of hypovolemic states. In the case of albumin-containing solutions, this lack of advantage may be attributed to the more rapid catabolism of infused albumin or increased leakage across the transcapillary barrier in patients. Some large-molecular-weight carbohydrates are nephrotoxic and should be used with caution in patients with renal impairment. In fact, in patients with capillary leakage, redistribution of albumin into the interstitial compartment might aggravate interstitial edema without providing an intravascular volume repletion benefit. It is for these reasons that crystalloid-containing solutions remain the mainstay of volume replacement therapy.

Blood products are also often listed among the solutions available for volume replacement in hypovolemic states. Indeed, a unit of packed red blood cells remains entirely in the vascular compartment. However, erythrocytes are actually considered part of the intracellular compartment and do not contribute to organ plasma flow. The role of packed red cells in the treatment of hemorrhage is to restore the principal function of the erythrocyte in oxygen carriage and delivery, not as a means of ECF volume replacement.

In addition to replacement fluids, maintenance fluids must be provided to counteract ongoing losses. Such ongoing losses may be a continuation of the underlying disease state (e.g., continued vomiting, diarrhea, polyuric states, or severe burns). The volume, rate of administration, and composition of these replacement fluids are best determined by actual measurements of the corresponding ongoing fluid losses, with appropriate adjustments for the patient's clinical assessment parameters.

Relative Hypovolemia

The treatment approach to relative hypovolemia is more complex than for absolute hypovolemia. When relative hypovolemia is the result of peripheral vasodilation, therapy should be directed toward reversal of the underlying cause and restoration of normal vascular reactivity. Bridging to maintain circulatory integrity until the underlying cause is successfully reversed can be achieved by infusion of an *isotonic crystalloid solution* such as normal saline. In such situations, selection of volumes and rates must be extremely cautious because there is no absolute deficit and the administered volume will have to be excreted or removed once systemic vascular resistance and vascular capacitance are restored to normal. Furthermore, it is more difficult to estimate an increase in vascular capacitance than it is to estimate an absolute volume deficit. Occasionally, it is appropriate to consider the use of vasoconstrictor agents. When relative hypovolemia occurs in the setting of an edema state, therapy must take into account the fact that the patient actually has a total body sodium surfeit with excess ECF volume, but a maldistribution of that volume away from the EABV. When crystalloid solutions are provided to such patients, a variable, but usually substantial, proportion of administered fluid is distributed into the interstitial compartment and consequently does not contribute to restoration of EABV. This vicious cycle emphasizes the importance of treatment directed at the underlying disease state.

Hypervolemia

Definition

Hypervolemia refers to expansion of ECF volume. It should be recalled that ECF volume varies, even in normal individuals, with dietary sodium intake. Thus, an individual in steady state with low daily dietary sodium intake (e.g., 20 mmol/L, corresponding to ≈1.2 g of table salt per day) will have correspondingly low urinary sodium excretion, equivalent to dietary intake minus extrarenal losses. A shift to much higher sodium intake (e.g., 200 mmol/day, corresponding to ≈12 g of table salt per day) will bring the individual to a new steady state characterized by a correspondingly higher urinary sodium excretion rate. This shift is accompanied by an increase in ECF volume, which triggers the sensor and effector mechanisms for increased urinary sodium excretion (described earlier). In most individuals this increase in ECF volume is not clinically detectable and does not have pathologic consequences. However, in a subset of individuals, this upward shift in ECF volume moves the individual into pathologic ranges of systemic arterial blood pressure. It is debated whether this degree of increased ECF volume, which accompanies a habitually high daily sodium intake typical of diets in many global populations, presents a public health concern. When the sodium surfeit expands the ECF volume beyond the range necessary for the adjustment needed to restore sodium balance, a state of pathologic hypervolemia is considered to be present. Such hypervolemic states result from past or ongoing sodium retention, inappropriate to the prevailing ECF volume.

Pathobiology

Conceptually, two categories of pathophysiologic mechanisms can lead to pathologic states of sodium retention with ECF volume expansion. The first involves renal sodium retention that is primary and unrelated to the activation of afferent sensor mechanisms. This category includes primary renal diseases and endocrine disorders characterized by excess mineralocorticoid action, such as progressive stages of congestive heart failure and cirrhosis with ascites. In the second category, EABV is reduced and afferent sensory mechanisms activate effector responses driving renal sodium retention. In these conditions, ECF volume is expanded, intravascular volume may be expanded, normal, or contracted, but the volume homeostatic mechanisms of the body mimic those of hypovolemia because of the perception of reduced EABV. The degree of solute-free water retention that accompanies the sodium surfeit has a relatively small influence on the extent of hypervolemia but certainly influences the accompanying tonicity state and determines whether the hypervolemia is hypotonic or isotonic.

When the ECF volume is expanded, the relative distribution between the intravascular and extravascular (interstitial) compartments depends on a number of factors. When cardiac and hepatic functions are normal and peripheral transcapillary Starling forces are intact, the excess ECF volume is evenly distributed between the intravascular and interstitial fluid compartments. In such cases, edema does not occur until there is a substantial surfeit of sodium, and hypertension is expected. In contrast, concomitant disruption of transcapillary Starling forces in a given microcirculatory bed would favor the accumulation of retained fluid at one or more such interstitial locations (e.g., dependent edema progressing to anasarca, ascites, pleural effusion, pulmonary congestion).

TABLE 117–4 PRIMARY AND SECONDARY RENAL SODIUM-RETAINING STATES
Oliguric renal failure
Chronic kidney disease
Glomerular disease, including nephrotic syndrome
Severe bilateral renovascular obstruction
Mineralocorticoid excess
Inherited sodium-retaining tubulopathies
Cardiac failure
Cirrhosis
Idiopathic edema

Primary Renal Sodium Retention

Causes of primary and secondary renal sodium retention states are listed in Table 117–4. Patients with oliguric renal failure of any cause have a limited ability to excrete both sodium and water. Such patients retain ingested or administered sodium and water loads and suffer expansion of ECF volume. In patients with chronic kidney disease, the filtered load of sodium remains well above dietary intake until very late stages of severely reduced GFR. As previously noted, even when the GFR is decreased by as much as 90%, the daily filtered load of approximately 2400 Osm still greatly exceeds dietary intake. However, the relationship between tubular absorption and filtered load may be disrupted, and this varies greatly with the type of kidney disease. Urinary sodium retention can be one of the cardinal manifestations of certain primary glomerular diseases, even when the GFR is well preserved; this is particularly striking in certain forms of nephrotic syndrome (Chapter 122). Two major pathophysiologic mechanisms may be involved. In some patients there is clear evidence of intravascular volume depletion with activation of the renin-angiotensin-aldosterone axis. In these patients, the intravascular volume depletion results from disruption of capillary Starling forces and transudation of fluid from the intravascular to the interstitial compartment. Decreased plasma colloid osmotic pressure as a result of *hypoalbuminemia* may be one of the main causes of a disruption in Starling forces. In other patients, both the interstitial and intravascular compartments are expanded, and the renin-angiotensin-aldosterone axis is relatively suppressed for the degree of ECF volume expansion. In such patients, glomerular disease is thought to be associated with primary renal sodium retention. The nephron site of enhanced sodium reabsorption relative to glomerular filtration (glomerulotubular imbalance) is the distal nephron, although details of the mechanism remain to be elucidated. In other forms of chronic kidney disease, sodium retention may not present a severe problem until the most advanced stages. Renovascular disease is not generally associated with hypervolemia unless there is severe bilateral renovascular obstruction, usually sufficient to compromise GFR as well.

States of *mineralocorticoid excess* or enhanced activity are associated with a phase of sodium retention. However, because of the phenomenon of "mineralocorticoid escape," the clinical manifestation is generally that of hypertension rather than hypervolemia. A number of monogenic disorders cause or mimic enhanced mineralocorticoid activity or are associated with enhanced activity of the distal nephron sodium reabsorptive pathways. Included in these disorders are several inherited tubulopathies, among which Liddle's syndrome and pseudohypoaldosteronism type II have been well characterized at the molecular level (Chapters 118 and 129). As in the case of mineralocorticoid excess, often the only clue to mild hypervolemia is the presence of hypertension, which can be severe. The plasma potassium concentration may be increased or reduced, depending on the molecular mechanism involved. Mineralocorticoid excess, glucocorticoid remediable hypertension, apparent mineralocorticoid excess, and Liddle's syndrome are associated with hypokalemia. Pseudohypoaldosteronism type II or Gordon's syndrome are often accompanied by hyperkalemia. Because of their prominent associated disturbances in blood pressure and potassium homeostasis, these disorders are discussed in detail in Chapters 66, 118, and 129.

Secondary Renal Sodium Retention

Both cardiac failure and cirrhosis are associated with renal sodium retention. In the case of cardiac failure, both low-output and high-output forms and both systolic and diastolic dysfunction with congestive heart failure are associated with sodium retention. The pathophysiologic components of the syndrome of congestive heart failure consist of low cardiac output (or in the case of high-output heart failure, relatively low cardiac output in comparison to tissue needs) and systemic or pulmonary venous hypertension (or both). Among these pathophysiologic components, low cardiac output (or diversion of cardiac output from arterial intravascular volume–sensing sites) appears to be a necessary and sufficient condition for initiating renal sodium retention. In the case of cirrhosis with ascites, hepatic intrasinusoidal hypertension is a sufficient and necessary condition for initiating renal sodium retention. These pathophysiologic disturbances in cardiac or hepatic function disrupt afferent signals for governing normal sodium homeostasis and trigger effector mechanisms leading to enhanced tubular reabsorption of sodium at multiple nephron sites. Experimental evidence indicates that at the very earliest stages of disease, sodium retention occurs independently of any measurable or detectable reduction in the volume of the intravascular compartments or any of its measurable subcompartments. At more advanced stages of disease, reduced intravascular volume serves as the overriding stimulus for renal sodium retention and thereby leads to a decompensated state of intractable ECF volume accumulation. The more advanced stages are often accompanied by a disproportionate degree of positive water balance and consequent hyponatremia, and herald imminent compromise of the GFR. Among the many neuronal and humoral abnormalities that characterize the sodium retention associated with cardiac failure and cirrhosis are enhanced sympathetic nerve activity, activation of the renin-angiotensin-aldosterone axis, and resistance to the natriuretic action of elevated levels of atrial natriuretic peptide at the latter's site of action in the cortical collecting tubule. In the case of cirrhosis with ascites, portosystemic shunting together with translocation of intravascular volume to the splanchnic and venous circulation further compromise EABV. In addition, synthetic dysfunction resulting in hypoalbuminemia favors transudation of fluid into the interstitial compartment. At the level of intrahepatic hemodynamics, intrasinusoidal hypertension results in enhanced hepatic lymph formation. When the rate of enhanced hepatic lymph formation exceeds the capacity for return to the intravascular compartment via the thoracic duct, hepatic lymph accumulates in the form of ascites, and the intravascular compartment is further compromised.

Clinical Manifestations

In addition to the clinical manifestations of the underlying disease, the clinical manifestations of *hypervolemia* depend on the amount and relative distribution of accumulated fluid in the various ECF subcompartments, including the venous and arterial components of the intravascular compartment (jugular venous distention and hypertension), the interstitial spaces of the extremities, subcutaneous tissues of the lower back and the periorbital region (peripheral pitting edema, whose predominant location depends on the patient's position), the peritoneal and pleural spaces (ascites and pleural effusion, respectively), and the alveolar space (pulmonary edema). When cardiac and hepatic function is normal and the transcapillary Starling forces are not disrupted, the excess volume is distributed proportionately throughout the ECF compartment. *Hypertension* is the earliest manifestation, and only very severe degrees of sodium surfeit will induce additional clinical findings, such as jugular venous distention or peripheral edema formation. The presence of clinically detectable peripheral edema usually signifies the accumulation of at least 3 L of excess interstitial volume. Because intravascular plasma volume is itself only 3 L, any state of generalized peripheral edema must signify ECF volume expansion and therefore past or ongoing renal sodium retention, or both.

When cardiac function is impaired because of myocardial disease, valvular disease, or pericardial disease, pulmonary and systemic venous hypertension predominates and systemic arterial pressure may be low as a result of disproportionate accumulation of intravascular volume in the venous as opposed to the arterial circulation. The presence of transudative ascites signifies the substantial accumulation of excess ECF volume in the peritoneal cavity, most commonly secondary to disruption of intrahepatic hemodynamics in the setting of liver disease. Pleural effusions can also be a manifestation of hypervolemia, particularly in the setting of heart failure or advanced cirrhosis with ascites.

Diagnosis

Hypervolemia is usually easily detected by findings of generalized edema, ascites, elevated jugular venous pressure, inspiratory pulmonary crepitations, or evidence of the presence of pleural effusion. The prevailing systemic arterial blood pressure often provides a clue about whether the hypervolemic state is secondary to reduced EABV or instead due to primary renal sodium retention. The history and physical examination are often sufficient to yield the diagnosis of an underlying secondary cause of sodium retention, such as congestive heart failure or cirrhosis. Adjunctive laboratory tests providing evidence of cardiac dysfunction or liver disease may be helpful. The presence of glomerular-range proteinuria with hypoalbuminemia indicates a glomerular cause of the sodium retention and hypervolemia. Elevated creatinine points to renal failure, which can be intrinsic or may occur in association with advanced stages of some of the aforementioned conditions, such as congestive heart failure (cardiorenal failure) or hepatic cirrhosis (hepatorenal failure). Hypoalbuminemia is characteristic of both cirrhosis and nephrotic syndrome.

A low urine sodium concentration and low fractional excretion of sodium confirm renal sodium retention secondary to a perceived decrease in EABV in the edema states, even in the face of overall hypervolemia. More recently, elevated concentrations of brain natriuretic peptide have been used to support the diagnosis of hypervolemia, particularly in the setting of cardiac failure and renal disease.

Treatment

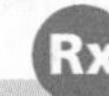

Recognition plus treatment of the underlying disease is the most important step in ameliorating renal sodium retention. Thus, optimization of hemodynamic parameters in cardiac failure, improvement of liver function, or remission of nephrotic syndrome improves or reverses sodium retention. Therapeutic intervention to reduce ECF volume without addressing the underlying disease is often met by complications, especially when ECF volume expansion is associated with decreased intravascular volume or EABV. Nevertheless, three treatment modalities are available to reduce ECF volume directly by inducing negative sodium balance: dietary sodium restriction, diuretics, and extracorporeal fluid removal by ultrafiltration. The modality and the desired rate of sodium removal vary with the clinical setting and depend on the relative distribution of the sodium surfeit and excess volume in the body fluid compartments. Therefore, before initiating any treatment, the clinician should identify the specific disturbances that are harmful to the patient in clinical parameters and monitor the improvement in these parameters during the course of treatment. Manifestations of hypervolemia that may be harmful include hypertension, pulmonary congestion and edema or pleural effusions with compromised respiratory function, hepatic congestion and ascites, and degrees of peripheral edema that compromise skin integrity and predispose the patient to cellulitis. Once ECF volume reduction has removed these threats to the patient's well-being, rates of sodium removal should be slowed significantly. Thus, a patient with mild peripheral edema, small pleural effusions, minimal ascites, jugular venous distention, and normal blood pressure might be managed with sodium restriction and limited use of diuretic medications to induce a gradual negative sodium balance over a period of many days to weeks. In contrast, a patient with limb- or life-threatening anasarca, pulmonary congestion, or hypervolemia-induced hypertension might require the continuous intravenous infusion of diuretics or possibly extracorporeal ultrafiltration therapy in the event of renal resistance to diuretic action.

Sodium Restriction

It has been shown that other modalities are futile if not accompanied by restriction of sodium intake because renal sodium avidity results in the reaccumulation of ECF fluid as soon as the influence of diuretics has ceased. Dietary sodium restriction in the range of 20 to 40 mmol/day is often recommended and requires abstention from added salt, as well as from foods rich in sodium. Sodium substitutes can be useful, although caution needs to be exercised in patients with a tendency to hyperkalemia because some salt substitutes contain potassium. Caloric intake and nutritional parameters should be monitored to ensure that an overly draconian diet does not induce protein-energy malnutrition. In hospitalized patients, it is particularly important to ensure that the sodium content of administered intravenous fluids and sodium-containing medications is monitored and reduced to the minimum possible. The practice of infusing sodium-containing solutions on the one hand and simultaneously treating with diuretics has no sound physiologic or therapeutic basis. Furthermore, water restriction is not appropriate in hypervolemic edema states unless severe (plasma sodium concentration <135 mmol/L) or symptomatic hyponatremia supervenes.

Diuretics

Diuretic medications are classified according to their sites of action in the nephron (Fig. 117–3).

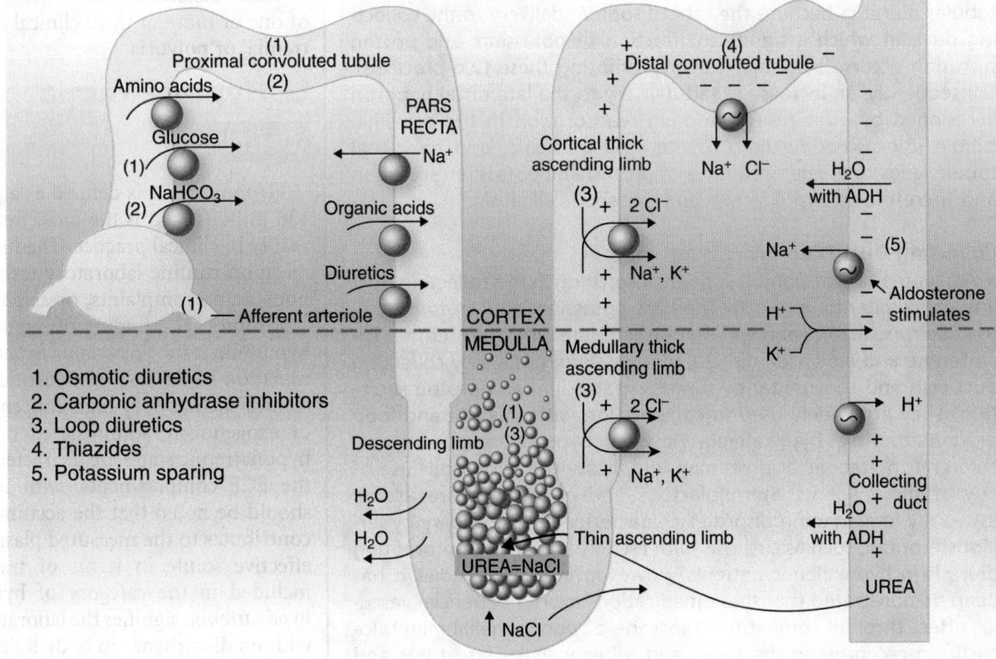

FIGURE 117–3 • Major transport processes along the nephron segment and primary sites of action of diuretics. The numbers next to the diuretics in the insert refer to the site of action along the nephron. ADH = antidiuretic hormone. (From Kokko JP: Diuretics. *In* Alexander RW, Schlant RC, Fuster V [eds]: The Heart, 9th ed. New York, McGraw-Hill, 1998, with permission of The McGraw-Hill Companies.)

Rx

Proximal Tubule Diuretics

The cardinal example of a proximal tubule diuretic is acetazolamide, a carbonic anhydrase inhibitor that blocks proximal reabsorption of sodium bicarbonate. Consequently, prolonged use of acetazolamide may lead to hyperchloremic acidosis, in contrast to all other diuretics, which act at loci before the late distal nephron. Metolazone, a congener of the thiazide class of diuretics, blocks sodium chloride absorption at two nephron sites. Specifically, in addition to action on the early distal tubule, metolazone also inhibits proximal tubular sodium chloride absorption. Because the major locus for phosphate absorption is in the proximal nephron, the phosphaturia accompanying metolazone administration considerably exceeds that observed with other thiazide-class diuretics. Proximal tubule diuretics are rarely used as primary diuretic therapy in modern practice. More commonly, these diuretics, particularly metolazone, are used as supplements to loop diuretics in instances in which loop diuretics alone are ineffective in producing diuresis. Mannitol also inhibits proximal tubule reabsorption, but it is induced mainly in the treatment of increased intracranial pressure.

Loop Diuretics

Loop diuretics, such as furosemide, bumetanide, torsemide, and ethacrynic acid, induce diuresis by inhibiting the coupled entry of Na^+, Cl^-, and K^+ across apical plasma membranes in the thick ascending limb of the loop of Henle, which is responsible for the reabsorption of approximately 25% of filtered sodium. For practical purposes, loop diuretics are the most potent diuretics and are commonly referred to as *high-ceiling diuretics.*

Distal Tubule Diuretics

Distal tubule diuretics, such as hydrochlorothiazide, chlorthalidone, and metolazone, interfere primarily with sodium chloride absorption in the earliest segments of the distal convoluted tubule by blocking the sodium chloride cotransport mechanism across apical plasma membranes. In general, distal tubule diuretics are used for the same circumstances as loop diuretics. The major exception occurs in chronic renal failure and in disorders of calcium metabolism. Loop diuretics are calciuric and are valuable for managing acute hypercalcemia. In contrast, thiazide diuretics promote hypocalciuria and calcium retention and are useful in managing hypercalciuric states, but not hypercalcemia. Loop diuretics are much more effective in chronic renal failure than are thiazide diuretics.

With the exception of acetazolamide (which impairs bicarbonate absorption), hypokalemia and metabolic alkalosis may complicate the administration of proximal diuretics, loop diuretics, and distal tubular diuretics because the rate of sodium delivery to the collecting duct, in which a significant fraction of potassium and proton secretion occurs, is a major factor promoting these two processes. Consequently, an increase in salt delivery to the late distal nephron occasioned by inhibition of sodium reabsorption in the proximal tubule, the ascending limb of the loop of Henle, and the distal tubule leads to accelerated rates of proton and potassium secretion and therefore to hypokalemia and metabolic alkalosis.

Collecting Duct Diuretics

A group of agents inhibit sodium absorption in the collecting duct and concomitantly indirectly suppress potassium and proton secretion. Spironolactone and eplerenone compete with aldosterone. Triamterene and amiloride directly block sodium uptake by collecting duct cells and concomitantly suppress potassium and proton secretion. They are widely used in combination with thiazide and loop diuretics to offset hypokalemia. However, hyperkalemia and hyperchloremic metabolic acidosis may complicate the injudicious use of any of these agents. Spironolactone and eplerenone are useful, especially in managing disorders characterized by secondary hyperaldosteronism, such as cirrhosis with ascites, as well as in promoting diuresis in hypokalemic patients. However, in recent studies it has been demonstrated that these medications exert a beneficial vascular effect through competitive blockade of nonepithelial mineralocorticoid receptors in the heart and other vascular structures and improve the survival of patients with left ventricular dysfunction (Chapter 58).

Rx

Nesiritide is a naturally occurring brain natriuretic peptide that has been introduced primarily for the treatment of hypervolemia in the setting of cardiac failure. Recent reports indicate that treatment with nesiritide may compromise renal function, and therefore caution must be exercised in its use, with frequent monitoring of plasma urea and creatinine concentrations.

Patients with severe degrees of renal sodium avidity might be resistant to conventionally recommended doses of individual classes of diuretic agents. In such patients, combining diuretic agents acting at different sites along the nephron may overcome this resistance and induce a natriuretic response. The continuous intravenous infusion of furosemide, sometimes in conjunction with intermittent bolus infusions of albumin, has also been shown to overcome diuretic resistance in certain subsets of hospitalized patients. Certainly, improving the underlying disease process causing sodium retention is the most helpful means of reversing diuretic resistance. When using any class of diuretic agents, the expected or actually measured urine composition should be taken into account in considering associated effects on body tonicity and the balance of other electrolytes. Monitoring of plasma sodium, potassium, magnesium, calcium, and phosphate concentrations is mandatory in patients treated with high or frequent doses or continuous infusions of diuretic agents. Besides body tonicity and electrolyte disturbances, other adverse consequences of diuretic use include intravascular hypovolemia (overdiuresis) with a concomitant decreased GFR. Drug-specific idiosyncratic adverse responses such as allergic cutaneous reactions, interstitial nephritis, pancreatitis, and blood dyscrasias are much less common.

Extracorporeal Ultrafiltration

In a small subset of patients, either superimposed renal impairment or extreme resistance to diuretic action requires the direct removal of excess ECF volume by hemofiltration or peritoneal dialysis. The use of these modalities is discussed in greater detail in Chapter 133. Chronic ambulatory peritoneal dialysis has been used for the symptomatic relief of pulmonary congestion and anasarca in some patients with chronic congestive heart failure who are unresponsive to other therapeutic modalities and are not candidates for cardiac transplantation.

WATER BALANCE DISORDERS

Water balance disorders generally come to medical attention because of one or more of three clinical manifestations: hyponatremia, hypernatremia, or polyuria.

Hyponatremia

Definition

Hyponatremia is defined as a plasma sodium concentration less than 136 mmol/L and is the most frequently encountered electrolyte abnormality in clinical practice. The finding of hyponatremia is often incidental upon routine laboratory testing, laboratory testing of patients with nonspecific complaints, or as part of the investigation of other clinical syndromes. The finding of hyponatremia does not necessarily signify a hypotonic state. *Hypertonic hyponatremia* occurs when there is an accumulation in the ECF compartment of non–sodium-containing effective solutes such as very high concentrations of glucose in diabetic patients or exogenously administered mannitol or glycerol. These hypertonic hyponatremic states are characterized by a shift of water from the ICF to the ECF compartments, with ICF shrinkage rather than swelling. It should be noted that the accumulation of a solute such as urea, which contributes to the measured plasma osmolality but is not an osmotically effective solute in terms of transcellular water shift, should not be included in the category of hypertonic hyponatremic states. *Isotonic hyponatremia* signifies the laboratory finding of hyponatremia in patients with no disturbance in body fluid tonicity and almost always reflects the interference of marked hyperlipidemia or marked hyperglobulinemia with certain laboratory techniques in the measurement of plasma sodium concentration. These latter situations are termed *pseudohyponatremia* and should not prompt diagnostic or therapeutic measures targeted to alter water balance or body tonicity.

Hyponatremia, *hypotonic hyponatremia* is of concern to the clinician for two major reasons: it always reflects an important underlying disorder leading to abnormal body water balance, and the hypotonic state indicates either past or ongoing expansion of ICF volume with the possibility of life-threatening brain cell swelling and attendant neurologic manifestations. Even in chronic hypotonic hyponatremic states where cell volume has been restored to normal through osmotic adaptive mechanisms, this occurs at the price of loss of intracellular solutes—a state that compromises optimal cell function.

Clinical Manifestations

The symptoms of hypotonic hyponatremia depend on its duration. In the first hours to days, the major clinical manifestations are neurologic and are due to acute brain swelling or cerebral edema. Symptoms include headache, lethargy, seizures, and a progressively decreased level of consciousness eventuating in coma and death. The severity of these neurologic manifestations depends more on the rate of the hypotonic decline in plasma sodium concentration than on the absolute concentration. In addition, it has been found that young women in the age group between menarche and menopause are particularly susceptible to the life-threatening neurologic manifestations of acute hyponatremia, even of relatively mild degree. Adaptive mechanisms designed to protect cell volume are engaged over a period of hours to days. Such mechanisms include the extrusion of intracellular solutes, including potassium, sodium, and organic osmolytes from brain cells. Thus, if a patient has survived the acute hyponatremia, osmotic adaptation tends to mitigate the symptoms of cerebral edema. However, patient well-being continues to be compromised, probably because of the loss of intracellular solutes combined with the clinical manifestations of the underlying disease state.

Diagnosis

After immediate assessment of the clinical urgency of the situation, the first step in the diagnostic approach to a patient with the laboratory finding of hyponatremia is to confirm the presence of true hypotonic hyponatremia. This requires a repeat set of plasma determinations, including electrolytes, osmolality, urea, and glucose, to allow comparison of the measured with the calculated plasma osmolality according to the following equation:

$$\text{Plasma osmolality (mOsm/kg)} = 2\text{Na}^+ \text{ (mmol/L)} + (\text{Blood urea nitrogen [mg/dL]}/2.8) + (\text{Glucose [mg/dL]}/18)$$

Marked elevation in the plasma glucose concentration increases both measured and calculated plasma osmolality and indicates a state of hypertonic hyponatremia that should be approached as a state of body fluid hypertonicity with cell shrinkage (see later) rather than hypotonicity. The plasma sodium concentration declines by approximately 1.6 mmol/L for each 100 mg/dL (5.5-mmol/L) increase in plasma glucose concentration. However, recent studies have shown that the value of approximately 1.6 is quite variable and is greater in states of progressively severe hyperglycemia. In contrast to hyperglycemia, when the urea concentration is elevated, it should not be considered as contributing to plasma or ECF tonicity, even though urea does contribute to the laboratory measurement of plasma osmolality. Thus, a hyponatremic patient with a normal or elevated laboratory measurement of plasma osmolality, which can be fully attributed to an increased urea concentration, should be considered as having hypotonic hyponatremia. A discrepancy in which measured plasma osmolality exceeds calculated plasma osmolality and cannot be attributed to either glucose or urea indicates the presence of an unidentified small solute (osmolar gap). In such cases, a history of the administration of mannitol should be sought, and if present, the patient should then be considered in the category of hypertonic hyponatremia. In the absence of such a history, additional occult small solutes should be sought by a history of exposure or laboratory measurements. These solutes include alcohols such as ethanol, methanol, ethylene glycol, and isopropyl alcohol and the organic anions of weak acids, which raise the plasma anion gap. Because these small solutes are not effective solutes in terms of water movement, the water balance and tonicity status of the patient is determined by the plasma sodium concentration. Just as for urea, a patient with hyponatremia and normal or elevated measured plasma osmolality as a result of one of these small solutes should be approached as a patient with true hypotonic hyponatremia, notwithstanding the normal or elevated plasma osmolality measurement. However, the finding of such an osmolar gap should prompt a thorough investigation for poisoning, intoxication, or an organic acidosis (Chapters 20 and 119).

Once a state of true hypotonic hyponatremia has been established, determination of the cause and further diagnostic approach follows a classification into one of three categories based on assessment of the volume status of the patient (Fig. 117–4). A sequential analysis of hyponatremic inpatients revealed that approximately 85% had true hypotonic hyponatremia. Among these, approximately a quarter were hypovolemic, a quarter had an edema state, a third were normovolemic, and most of the remainder suffered from renal failure.

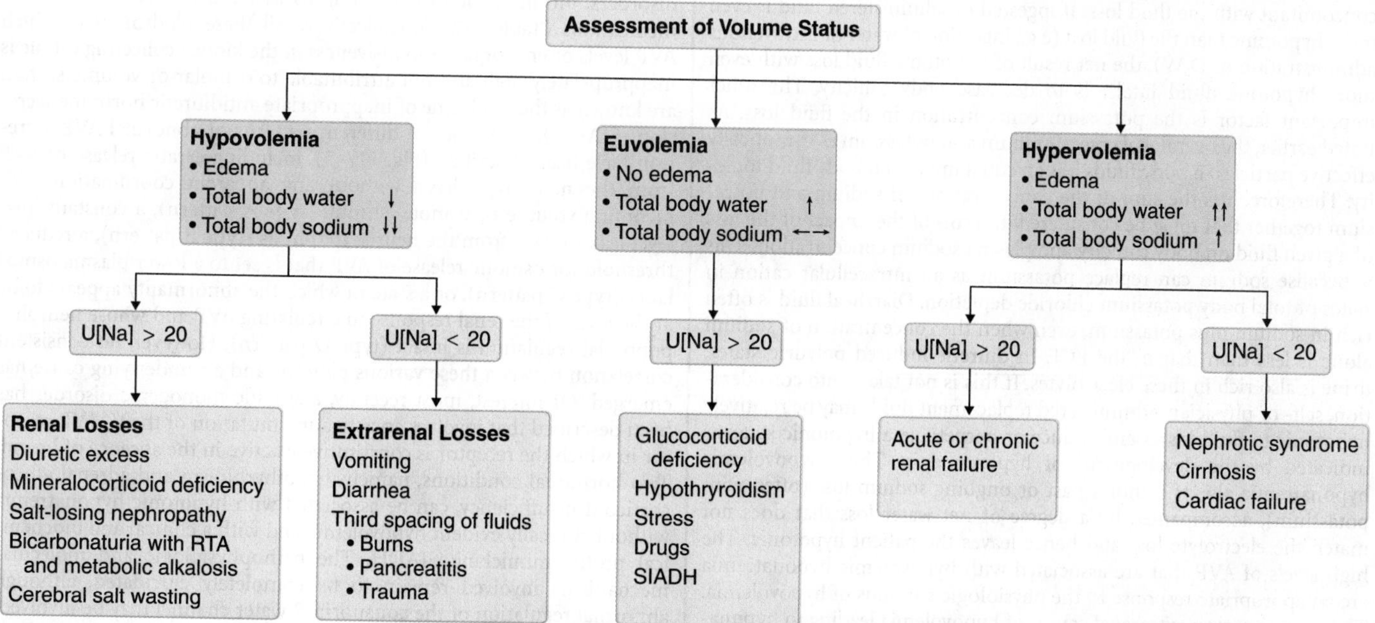

FIGURE 117–4 • Diagnostic approach to hyponatremia. RTA = renal tubular acidosis; SIADH = syndrome of inappropriate antidiuretic hormone secretion. (Modified from Halterman R, Berl T: Therapy of dysnatremic disorders. *In* Brady H, Wilcox C [eds]: Therapy in Nephrology and Hypertension. Philadelphia, Saunders, 1999, p 256.)

Hypervolemic Hyponatremia

A patient with hypervolemic hyponatremia suffers from a surfeit of both sodium and water, but the surfeit of water is disproportionate to that of sodium in tonicity terms. The clinical approach described earlier for hypervolemia is used to establish that the patient is hypervolemic and to determine the cause of the sodium surfeit. The most frequently diagnosed causes are congestive heart failure, decompensated cirrhosis with ascites, and renal failure. The occurrence of hyponatremia in any of these conditions is often an ominous prognostic finding signifying either a more advanced stage of disease or overzealous medical intervention (diuretics and sodium restriction). In the case of congestive heart failure and cirrhosis with ascites, reduced EABV stimulates the release of AVP and may also limit the delivery of glomerular ultrafiltrate to the diluting segments of the nephron. As described in the section on hypervolemia, these patients experience avid renal sodium retention with urine sodium concentrations less than 20 mmol/L and fractional sodium excretion less than 1% in the face of clear-cut clinical evidence of ECF volume expansion, usually with generalized edema. However, these urine parameters can be masked by the ongoing influence of diuretic agents. The edema state of nephrotic syndrome is less commonly associated with hyponatremia, unless the patient has been exposed to severe salt restriction and diuretic therapy. Water retention with hyponatremia is a feature of renal failure only in its more advanced stages (stages IV and V chronic kidney disease, Chapter 131).

Normovolemic and Hypovolemic Hyponatremia

These categories are considered together because of the frequently encountered difficulty in distinguishing between them clinically. This difficulty occurs because a mild degree of hypovolemia, which can easily escape clinical detection, is nevertheless sufficient to limit excretion of maximally dilute urine by nonosmotic stimulation of AVP release and by limiting the delivery of glomerular ultrafiltrate to the diluting segment of the nephron. The initial approach is to use the history and physical examination to try to establish or exclude a diagnosis and cause of the hypovolemia. When the hypovolemia is of extrarenal origin, in the absence of intrinsic renal disease or the ongoing influence of diuretics a low urine sodium concentration and low fractional excretion of sodium provide an important clue. Unlike extrarenal urinary volume losses, when the hypovolemia is due to urinary loss, the urine sodium concentration is usually elevated rather than decreased. It should be noted that in most sources of fluid loss from the body, the sodium concentration in the fluid is hypotonic to that of plasma. This is true of sweat, most gastrointestinal losses, and even many cases of urinary fluid loss. Therefore, two important factors must be taken into acount when considering the extent, if any, to which a given renal or extrarenal source of fluid loss is likely to induce hyponatremia and the extent of that hyponatremia. The first and most obvious factor is the nature of the fluid ingested or administered concomitant with the fluid loss. If ingested or administered fluid is even more hypotonic than the fluid lost (e.g., ingestion of water or intravenous administration of D_5W), the net result of hypotonic fluid loss with even more hypotonic fluid intake is to decrease body tonicity. The other important factor is the potassium concentration in the fluid loss. As noted earlier, the overall balance of sodium and potassium as osmotically effective particles in body fluids has an equal impact on body fluid tonicity. Therefore, it is the sum of the concentrations of sodium and potassium together that must be considered in terms of the impact of the loss of a given fluid on body tonicity and plasma sodium concentration. This is because sodium can replace potassium as an intracellular cation in states of total body potassium chloride depletion. Diarrheal fluid is often rich in sodium plus potassium, even when the concentration of sodium alone is less than that in the ECF. In diuretic-induced polyuric states, urine is also rich in these electrolytes. If this is not taken into consideration, self- or physician-administered replacement fluids may be relatively hypotonic to fluid losses and induce or perpetuate a hypotonic state, as indicated by the development of hyponatremia. Thus, hypovolemic hyponatremia always signifies past or ongoing sodium loss (often with potassium), accompanied by a degree of net water loss that does not match the electrolyte loss and hence leaves the patient hypotonic. The high levels of AVP that are associated with hypovolemic hyponatremia are an appropriate response to the physiologic stimulus of hypovolemia. The most common extrarenal causes of hypovolemia leading to hyponatremia are gastrointestinal fluid losses and excessive sweating. In the case of gastrointestinal fluid losses, vomiting may be particularly prominent, and nausea and vomiting serve as independent triggers for the central release of AVP. Besides the history, clues to vomiting include the characteristic plasma and urine biochemical parameters of metabolic alkalosis, with higher than expected concentrations of sodium in urine accompanied by bicarbonate and a low urine chloride concentration (see Metabolic Alkalosis in Chapter 119). The plasma and urine biochemical parameters accompanying hyponatremia in patients with fecal losses depend on the composition of the diarrhea fluid. Hyponatremia as a complication of diarrhea is more common when the diarrheal fluid is secretory and rich in electrolytes. Sweating-induced hyponatremia is particularly evident in high-endurance athletic sports or among military personnel undergoing training in the heat. Such individuals are often instructed to ingest high volumes of hypotonic fluid, often pure water, while losing sodium in sweat.

The renal causes of hypovolemia that can be associated with hyponatremia are listed in Figure 117–4; many overlap those already discussed in the section on hypovolemia.

Special mention should be made of two particular clinical settings in the category of hypovolemic hyponatremia. The first is diuretic-induced hyponatremia, which is far more common with thiazide diuretics than after loop and other classes of diuretic agents. Though less potent than loop diuretics, thiazide diuretics do not disrupt the medullary countercurrent concentrating mechanism. Thus, patients with impaired urinary diluting capacity who are treated with thiazide diuretics can excrete concentrated urine containing high concentrations of sodium plus potassium. This renders them particularly susceptible to hyponatremia when ingesting or receiving hypotonic solutions that exceed their maximum capacity for excretion of electrolyte-free water in urine. An additional special setting is that of cerebral salt wasting, also mentioned in the section on hypovolemia. As noted, head injury and intracranial hemorrhage can induce a state of negative sodium balance through urinary losses, with clinical parameters consistent with hypovolemia. The hypovolemia-induced release of AVP coupled with the ingestion or administration of hypotonic fluids tends to produce hyponatremia that is often quite severe. In these patients, urine sodium concentrations can be impressively high, thereby increasing the tendency to hyponatremia. Because of the setting of intracranial pathology and because the degree of hypovolemia may escape clinical detection, this condition is frequently difficult to distinguish from hyponatremia caused by the syndrome of inappropriate secretion of AVP (see later).

In normovolemic hypotonic hyponatremia there is neither an osmolar nor a volume stimulus to the release of AVP. Thus, concentrated urine, usually containing high concentrations of sodium (often >40 mmol/L as a result of dietary intake plus the effects of mild ECF volume expansion), indicates either inappropriate secretion or an augmented renal response to AVP. The conditions that can result in such inappropriate AVP secretion or responsiveness include tumors, central nervous system lesions or disorders, intrathoracic or chest wall disease, and numerous drugs and medications (Table 117–5). Collectively, all these syndromes in which AVP levels or end-organ responsiveness in the kidney collecting tubule is inappropriately high and not attributable to osmolar or volume stimuli are known as the syndrome of inappropriate antidiuretic hormone secretion (SIADH). A number of different patterns of abnormal AVP secretion have been described (Fig. 117–5), including erratic release of AVP from the neurohypophysis without any apparent coordination with incoming volume or osmotic stimuli (type A pattern), a constant low-level leak of AVP from the neurohypophysis (type B pattern), a reduced threshold for osmotic release of AVP that is set to a lower plasma osmolality (type C pattern), or a state in which the abnormality appears to be at the level of the renal response to circulating AVP and whose neurohypophysial regulation is intact (type D pattern). However, no consistent correlation between these various patterns and an underlying cause has emerged. Of interest, most recently, a specific monogenic disorder has been described that involves an activating mutation of the V_2 AVP receptor in which the receptor is constitutively active in the absence of ligand. Two hormonal conditions, namely, hypothyroidism and adrenal glucocorticoid insufficiency, can be associated with hypotonic hyponatremia without clinically evident hypovolemia and with a clinical and biochemical profile mimicking SIADH. The pathophysiologic and molecular mechanisms involved remain to be completely elucidated, although abnormal regulation of the aquaporin-2 water channel may be involved, along with the contribution of hypovolemia or reduced GFR in adrenal insufficiency and hypothyroidism, respectively. Pregnancy is also associ-

TABLE 117–5 CAUSES OF THE SYNDROME OF INAPPROPRIATE ANTIDIURETIC HORMONE SECRETION

MALIGNANT NEOPLASIA
Carcinoma: bronchogenic, pancreatic, duodenal, ureteral, prostatic, bladder
Lymphoma and leukemia
Thymoma and mesothelioma
CENTRAL NERVOUS SYSTEM DISORDERS
Trauma
Infection
Tumors
Porphyria
PULMONARY DISORDERS
Tuberculosis
Pneumonia
Fungal infections
Lung abscesses
Mechanical positive pressure ventilation
DRUG INDUCED
Carbamazepine
Desmopressin
Oxytocin
Vincristine
Chlorpropamide
Nicotine
Cyclophosphamide
Morphine
Amitriptyline
Selective serotonin re-uptake inhibitors

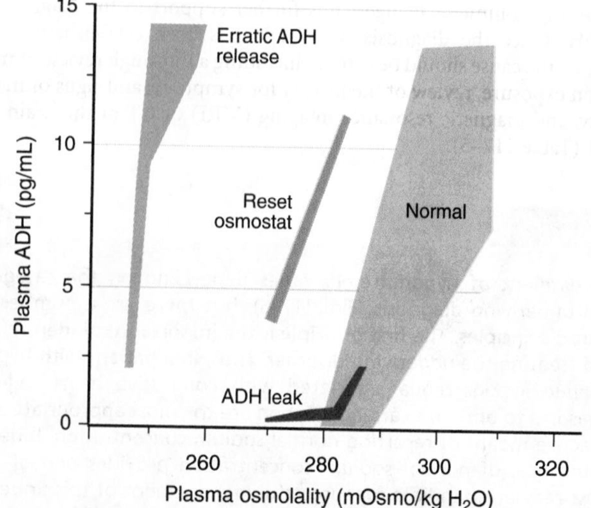

FIGURE 117–5 • Patterns of serum antidiuretic hormone (ADH) abnormalities in the syndrome of inappropriate ADH secretion (SIADH). The shaded areas indicate the normal relationship between increases in effective extracellular osmolality and ADH levels; the normal osmotic threshold is lower than the normal serum osmolality. The three shaded areas indicate ADH patterns in SIADH. (Adapted from Zerbe R, Strope L, Robertson G: Vasopressin function in the syndrome of inappropriate diuresis. Annu Rev Med 1980;31:315–327.)

ated with a reduction in both the osmotic threshold for AVP release and thirst and results in a mild degree of hyponatremia (Chapter 259). Another unusual setting for normovolemic hyponatremia is the "beer potomania" syndrome. Because the minimum urine osmolarity, even in the absence of AVP, is 30 to 50 mOsm/L, the upper limit of solute-free water excretion depends on total obligate solute excretion. Thus, a paucity of available urinary solutes sets an upper limit on the total water intake that can be tolerated without inducing hyponatremia. Patients with very low levels of sodium intake and little urea excretion fall into this category. Among others, this group includes patients who consume large volumes of beer (rich in carbohydrates and water, but poor in sodium and electrolytes). The ingestion of carbohydrates in the absence of protein intake limits urea production and excretion, thus limiting nonelectrolyte urinary solutes and hence urinary water excretion. Together with the large volumes of beer ingested, this results in the unusual combination of a normovolemic hypotonic hyponatremic state with low urine osmolality.

Clinical Evaluation

When faced with a patient with hyponatremia, a careful history, including a search of the medical record for previous measured concentrations of plasma sodium, is critical. The history together with the physical examination usually provides important clues to underlying disorders, disease states, or medication exposures that can inform the diagnosis. A history of the patient's weight gain or loss can also be helpful in the assessment of recent fluid mass balance. The patient's gender and age and the presence and extent of neurologic involvement helps dictate the urgency of therapy. Physical examination should also focus on attempts to establish the state of ECF volume. The presence of generalized edema with jugular venous distention and ascites, especially in the setting of heart or liver disease, points quite clearly to a hypervolemic hyponatremic state. The presence of clear-cut orthostatic hypotension and tachycardia, particularly in the setting of a history of diuretic use or gastrointestinal fluid losses, tends to support hypovolemia as a contributing cause. However, the absence of these findings does not rule out hypovolemia.

Laboratory tests should include a repeat set of plasma electrolyte concentrations, including potassium, chloride, and bicarbonate. It is often useful to measure acid-base parameters, including pH and P_{CO_2}, which point to processes not in the history, such as vomiting, diarrhea, or diuretic use. Other laboratory tests should include liver function tests and measurement of plasma urea, creatinine, uric acid, thyroid-stimulating hormone, and cortisol concentrations and, if indicated, an adrenocorticotropic hormone stimulation test. High levels of both urea and creatinine point to intrinsic renal disease, whereas a disproportionate elevation of urea over creatinine might support hypovolemia with a tendency to prerenal azotemia (Chapter 121). In contrast, very low levels of urea and uric acid are typical of SIADH. Interestingly, these parameters may also be low in the cerebral salt-wasting syndrome, although there is no convincing explanation for this observation.

Abnormal liver function test results can provide adjunctive support for hepatic disease and a hypervolemic hyponatremic state. The diagnosis of congestive heart failure should be made clinically, but it can be assisted by echocardiographic assessment of cardiac function. A chest radiograph or chest computed tomography (CT) scan is usually indicated to look for intrathoracic lesions that may be associated with SIADH, for the assessment of congestive heart failure, and if volume repletion is being considered as a diagnostic/therapeutic intervention in patients with suspected hypovolemic hyponatremia. Measurement of the urine sodium concentration can be helpful in many cases. In the absence of a clinically obvious edema state, a low urine sodium concentration (<20 mmol/L) or a low fractional excretion of sodium (<1%) supports the diagnosis of hypovolemic hyponatremia secondary to extrarenal losses or past renal losses that have since abated. If hypovolemia is due to ongoing renal losses, the urine sodium concentration may remain high in the face of hypovolemia. High concentrations of potassium in urine point to ongoing diuretic use or vomiting. In SIADH, the urine sodium concentration often reflects sodium intake, as well as mild volume expansion, and is therefore most often greater than 40 mmol/L and frequently higher than 100 mmol/L. The combination of hypotonic hyponatremia in a patient without evidence of either hypovolemia or hypervolemia, together with low plasma urea and uric acid concentrations without hypothyroidism or adrenal insufficiency, strongly suggests SIADH. If there is any doubt about the presence of hypovolemia, a carefully monitored volume challenge can be of diagnostic as well as therapeutic benefit (see later). Lack of sustained improvement after an adequate salt-containing volume challenge lends further support to the diagnosis of SIADH. Once the diagnosis of SIADH has been established in this manner, the cause should be sought, including a thorough review of medication exposure, review of the history for symptoms and signs of malignancy, and magnetic resonance imaging (MRI) or CT of the brain and chest (Table 117–5).

Treatment

Rx

Treatment of hyponatremia varies depending on the category and underlying diagnosis (Fig. 117–6), but there are a number of shared principles. The first principle is the importance of identifying and treating the underlying disorder. Thus, in a patient with hypervolemic hyponatremia associated with congestive heart failure, measures to optimize cardiac function are the most appropriate and effective means of resorting normal sodium concentration. Indeed, restoration of normal sodium concentration provides one of the most reassuring indices for successful management of this underlying disorder. Another principle common to all causes of hypotonic hyponatremia, irrespective of the underlying cause is that the sodium concentration and the rate of correction should be guided by the clinical neurologic status of the patient, age and gender considerations, and any information about recent past plasma sodium concentrations or osmolality values. Delayed or too slow a rate of correction of hyponatremia can perpetuate cerebral edema and result in irreversible neurologic damage and death. As noted earlier, this risk is greater in young women of reproductive age and in all patients in whom hyponatremia has developed rapidly at a pace that outstrips the rate of osmotic adaptation by brain cells. In contrast, too rapid correction or correction to a sodium concentration that is above the level needed to safeguard the patient from the neurologic sequelae of cerebral edema can result in a different adverse outcome known as *osmotic demyelination syndrome*. This devastating and often irreversible syndrome is characterized clinically by findings expected with brain stem demyelinating injury, including fluctuating levels of consciousness, pseudobulbar palsy, ataxia, dysarthria, difficulty swallowing, and characteristic MRI abnormalities in the region of the brain stem. Osmotic demyelination syndrome can be fatal, and in nonfatal cases recovery is either slow or incomplete, often with irreversible residual neurologic sequelae.

The overall treatment approach can be divided into the immediate approach to newly appreciated hypotonic hyponatremia and long-term management of chronic persistent hyponatremia.

Hypotonic Hyponatremia

Current guidelines suggest that if the hyponatremia is known to be acute (<24 to 48 hours) by documentation of previous sodium concentration or osmolality and if the hyponatremia is accompanied by severe neurologic symptoms such as seizures or decreased level of consciousness, correction should be rapid and should reach a target sodium concentration based on amelioration of neurologic symptoms. However, even under these circumstances, the desired rise in sodium concentration should not exceed 2 mmol/L/hr, and the total increase in sodium concentration during the first 12 to 24 hours of treatment should not exceed 12 mmol/L. The only exceptions to these guidelines would be an unusual patient who has suffered documented severe acute water intoxication, such as occurs during the inadvertent instillation of a glycine-containing irrigation solution during prostate surgery or the administration of hypotonic solutions to a patient who is anuric.

Chronic Hyponatremia

In cases in which the rate of decline in plasma sodium concentration has been slow, it can be assumed that brain cells have had the opportunity to undergo osmotic adaptation and have extruded or eliminated intracellular solutes. It is this subgroup of patients who are most susceptible to osmotic demyelination after too rapid or overzealous correction of hyponatremia. Patients in whom there is no previous record of sodium concentration or osmolality should be considered in the same category and treated accordingly. In such cases the targeted rate of increase in sodium concentration should not exceed 0.5 mmol/L/hr, and the total rise in sodium concentra-

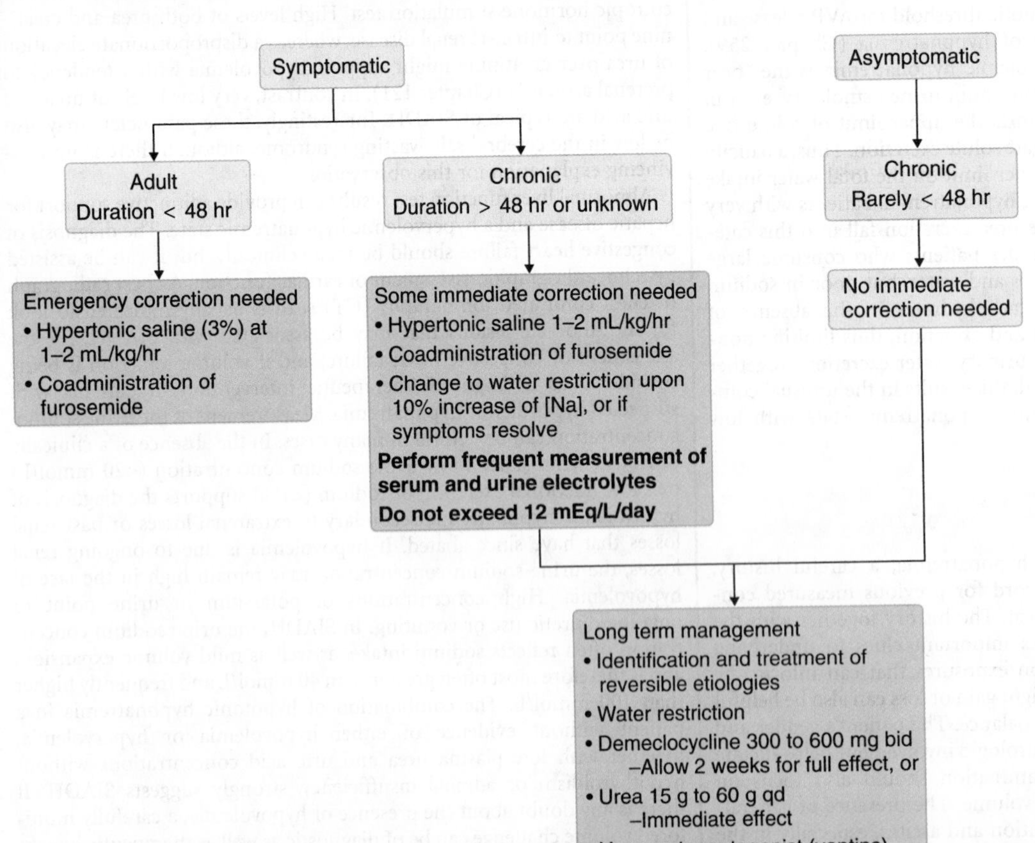

FIGURE 117–6 • Treatment of severe normovolemic hyponatremia. (From Thurman J, Halterman R, Berl T: Therapy of dysnatremic disorders. *In* Brady H, Wilcox C [eds]: Therapy in Nephrology and Hypertension, 2nd ed. Philadelphia, Saunders, 2003.)

Rx

tion should not exceed 8 mmol/L in the first 24 hours. This is true even and especially if the initial sodium concentration is extremely low (<110 mmol/L), as long as the hyponatremia is not accompanied by severe neurologic symptoms. Patients with severe degrees of chronic hyponatremia in the setting of malnutrition, alcoholism, or chronic illness are particularly susceptible to osmotic demyelination.

Having established a target goal and rate of correction, the specific approach varies with the underlying diagnosis. It should be recalled that although signifying a serious underlying perturbation in body fluid homeostasis, mild degrees of hyponatremia can be tolerated over long periods, and only symptomatic hyponatremia or sodium concentrations below 125 to 130 mmol/L require specific additional treatment. In hypervolemic hyponatremia, there is a surfeit of both sodium and water, but in tonicity terms the excess water is disproportionate to the excess sodium. Thus, the goal of treatment is to remove both sodium and water, but to replace proportionately less water than sodium. In this regard, water restriction always contributes to the management of hyponatremia. However, water restriction alone is often inadequate or impractical for several reasons. Patients frequently have thirst driven by a combination of perceived EABV contraction, the action of angiotensin II and other mediators, and hypokalemia. Furthermore, adequate nutrition requires caloric intake that is accompanied by obligate water ingestion and metabolic water production. Accordingly, interventions beyond water restriction are generally required to alleviate hyponatremia. Overall correction can be facilitated by the use of loop diuretics to increase overall urine flow, together with judicious replacement of sodium and potassium by dietary means or parenterally, with caution to avoid untoward changes in ECF volume or potassium concentration. Potassium replacement also contributes to the correction of hyponatremia. Recently, AVP V_2-receptor antagonists called vaptans have been introduced and show great promise in inducing an aquaretic (water diuretic) response that ameliorates hyponatremia. Vaptans are low-molecular-weight, nonpeptide compounds that are structurally related to benzazepines, benzodiazepines, or oxindoles (Fig. 117–7). Tolvaptan and lixivaptan are V_2 receptor selective, whereas conivaptan is nonselective for V_{1a} and V_2 receptors. In clinical trials, these agents have been shown to increase urine volume, decrease urine osmolality, increase free water clearance, and increase serum sodium in a variety of hyponatremic states (see later).

Hypovolemic Hypotonic Hyponatremia

As noted previously, a frequent diagnostic dilemma is the distinction between hypovolemic and normovolemic hypotonic hyponatremia. When hypovolemia is clearly evident (appropriate clinical history, orthostatic hypotension, low urine sodium concentration in the setting of extrarenal fluid losses, elevated plasma urea and uric acid concentrations), administration of volume repletion in the form of isotonic saline is the treatment of choice. The salutary effect of saline derives from the effect of volume repletion to remove the hypovolemic stimulus to release of AVP, thereby inducing a water diuresis rather than the osmolar effect of the infused solute. However, great caution should be exercised in the administration of isotonic saline to these patients, a subgroup in whom the administration of small volumes of isotonic saline can induce a brisk and rapid decrease in urine osmolality and accompanying water diuresis with overly rapid correction of hyponatremia. Accordingly, whenever isotonic saline or other forms of volume repletion therapy are administered to patients with known or suspected hypovolemic hyponatremia, careful hour-by-hour monitoring of urine output, urine osmolality, the plasma concentration of sodium, and plasma osmolality are required. A rapid drop in urine osmolality accompanied by water diuresis should prompt cessation of volume repletion and, in some cases, administration of hypotonic solutions or even AVP itself to halt or reverse the rapid rise in sodium concentration. If an overly rapid rise in sodium concentration has occurred, the patient's sodium concentration should be brought back down to a safer level within the recommended guidelines, through the same measures of administration of hypotonic solutions with AVP, to prevent the complication of osmotic demyelination. When hypovolemia is not clearly evident but cannot be ruled out, a brisk drop in urine osmolality in response to a saline challenge confirms the suspicion of hypovolemia and simultaneously initiates therapy. In contrast, failure to induce such a response lends support instead to a diagnosis of normovolemic hyponatremia.

Normovolemic Hyponatremia

In patients with normovolemic hyponatremia, the appropriate therapeutic approach is to address the underlying disease. Hypothyroidism and adrenal insufficiency should be corrected with appropriate hormonal replacement therapy. Medication-induced SIADH mandates identification and cessation of the offending medication when possible. In cases in which the underlying disease cannot be identified or reversed, treatment is aimed at removing the water surfeit. The therapeutic outcome depends on the minimum urine osmolality that can be achieved, which in turn depends on the severity of SIADH. In many cases, when urine osmolality cannot be suppressed below certain high levels, water restriction alone, though contributory, is not an adequate management strategy for reasons noted previously.

The severity of water restriction required would not be consistent with the need for caloric intake nor compatible with reasonable expectations for patient adherence. In such cases, maneuvers to generate a gradual net negative water balance are required. In rare cases in which there is an urgent need to correct the hyponatremia acutely because of a neurologic emergency or available clear-cut documentation that the sodium concentration has decreased acutely (over a 24- to 72-hour period), three possible approaches are available. The first is the use of a loop diuretic together with isotonic or hypertonic saline. The loop diuretic induces the excretion of large volumes of urine containing sodium, potassium, and other electrolytes. Concomitant infusion of hypertonic saline returns the sodium to a concentration exceeding that in urine, thereby raising the plasma sodium concentration and increasing overall body fluid tonicity. The other electrolytes lost in urine (especially potassium and

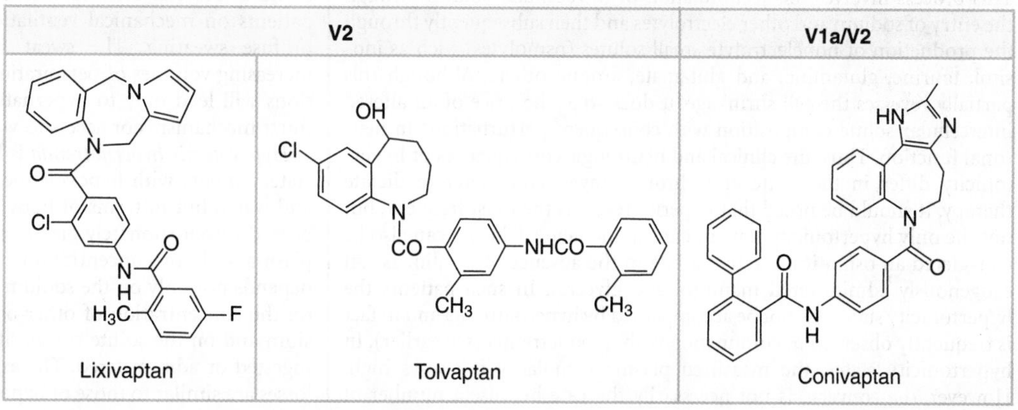

Section XI Renal

FIGURE 117–7 • Structure of nonpeptide, orally available vasopressin V_2 or V_1/V_2 mixed-receptor (YM 097) antagonists in clinical development. (From Quittnat F, Gross P: Vaptans and the treatment of water-retaining disorders. Semin Nephrol 2006;26:234–243.)

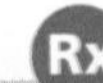

magnesium) must also be replaced. The second approach is to use an AVP V_2-receptor antagonist. As noted earlier, conivaptan is the first vaptan approved by the Food and Drug Administration for the treatment of normovolemic hyponatremia. 1 This approach carries the risk of too rapid correction and mandates careful monitoring of the response. Furthermore, when in doubt about volume status assignment for a given patient, these agents are better avoided until the possibility of hypovolemic hyponatremia has been ruled out. Finally, in the case of an extreme hyponatremic emergency with severe life-threatening neurologic complications, hemodialysis therapy can rapidly raise the plasma sodium concentration. For ambulatory patients with chronic persistent hyponatremia in whom the underlying disease process cannot be reversed, water excretion can be enhanced by one of several approaches, which can be coupled to an appropriate degree of water restriction. Both lithium and demeclocycline impair collecting tubule responsiveness to AVP and thus increase solute-free water excretion, thereby allowing greater volumes of water intake in patients with chronic SIADH. The AVP V_2-receptor antagonists may now be added to this armamentarium of therapeutic agents, although experience in their use for chronic SIADH remains limited at this time. Because all these agents induce a state of diabetes insipidus (Chapter 243), titration of dosing and reliance on an intact thirst mechanism are crucial for avoidance of polyuria or hypernatremia. An alternative approach is to provide the patient with an osmotic agent to ingest, such as urea or glycerol. By increasing total available urinary nonelectrolyte solutes at a given fixed urine osmolality, a greater water load can be tolerated by the patient without inducing hyponatremia. However, all these approaches, especially use of the novel aquaretic agents, must be accompanied by frequent monitoring of urine output, body weight, and plasma sodium and osmolality to avoid adverse water balance and electrolyte outcomes.

Hypernatremia

Definition

Hypernatremia, defined as a plasma sodium concentration greater than 144 mmol/L, always reflects a state of hypertonicity because sodium is an osmotically effective ECF solute. Hypertonicity refers to an increase in the ratio of the concentration of osmotically active solutes to water throughout all body fluid compartments. Osmotically effective solutes are those that cause a shift of water between the ICF and ECF body fluid compartments. Therefore, although sodium is distributed primarily in the ECF compartment, an elevated ECF sodium concentration reflects an increased solute-water ratio in all body fluid compartments. Hypernatremic patients have undergone a process whereby water has moved from the ICF to the ECF compartment, accompanied by a reduction in ICF volume and cell shrinkage. Cell shrinkage in the brain is associated with neurologic sequelae reflecting intracerebral hemorrhage, often punctate, but sometimes with major disruption of blood vessels, particularly at the brain surface and arachnoid interface. With time, brain cells undergo a process of osmotic adaptation in an effort to restore their cell volume. This process involves the accumulation of intracellular solutes through the entry of sodium and other electrolytes and then subsequently through the production of nonelectrolyte small solutes (osmolytes) such as inositol, taurine, glutamine, and glutamate, among others. Although this partially reverses the cell shrinkage, it does so at the price of an altered intercellular solute composition with consequent perturbations in neuronal function. Thus, the clinical and neurologic consequences of hypertonicity differ in the acute and chronic stages, and therefore dictate therapy. It should be noted that hypernatremia is the most frequent, but not the only hypertonicity state in clinical medicine. Glucose can also be considered an osmotically active solute in the absence of insulin, as can exogenously administered mannitol and glycerol. In such patients the hypertonicity state may not be accompanied by hypernatremia and in fact is frequently observed in conjunction with hyponatremia (see earlier). In hypertonicity states, the measured plasma osmolality is always high. However, the converse is not necessarily the case because a number of solutes that contribute to the measured plasma osmolality are not osmotically effective in terms of movement of water from the ICF to the ECF compartment. Thus, patients with high concentrations of urea or small alcohols (e.g., methanol, ethylene glycol, ethanol) often have elevated plasma osmolality but should not be considered to have a hypertonicity state.

TABLE 117–6 CAUSES OF HYPERNATREMIA CLASSIFIED BY TOTAL BODY SODIUM CONTENT

Hypervolemia	Hypertonic saline excess Hypertonic sodium bicarbonate solutions
Hypertonicity with near normovolemia	Diabetes insipidus Febrile fluid loss
Hypovolemia	Gastrointestinal loss (diarrhea, vomiting) Skin fluid loss (burn, sweat) Loop diuretics Osmotic diuresis Impaired thirst perception

Although hypernatremia can be diagnosed as an incidental laboratory abnormality, it most commonly occurs in the setting of a severe underlying disease with other accompanying disturbances in body fluid homeostasis. Three categories of patients with hypernatremia can be identified based on total body sodium content as estimated by ECF volume (Table 117–6).

In *hypervolemic hypernatremia*, there is a disproportionate excess of sodium as opposed to water in the ECF compartment. Despite the expansion of ECF volume, ICF volume is decreased with shrinkage of cells. This usually occurs in the hospital setting after exposure to sodium-rich parenteral or enteral dietary supplements. The inadvertent or overzealous administration of hypertonic saline, the administration of hypertonic sodium bicarbonate solutions during cardiopulmonary resuscitation, or dialysis against a hypertonic dialysate can lead to hypervolemic hypernatremia in the clinical setting.

In normovolemic hypernatremia a pure water deficit with no disturbance in body sodium content does not generally result in a clinically perceptible decrease in ECF volume because the predominant (approximately two thirds) origin of the water deficit is in the ICF rather than the ECF compartment. Thus, for example, a 3-L pure net water deficit will reduce ECF volume by only 1 L, approximately 300 mL of which emanates from plasma water. Yet a 3-L or greater deficit certainly increases body fluid tonicity and the measured plasma sodium concentration. Therefore, such pure net water deficits with no change in body sodium content are often considered to be approximately normovolemic. Clinical conditions that fit this category require a source of fluid loss that has a relatively low content of osmotically effective solutes (principally sodium and potassium and their accompanying anions), such as the various forms of diabetes insipidus. In these conditions, profuse volumes of urine with low osmolality are excreted. However, hypernatremia is actually uncommon as long as thirst perception and availability of water remain intact. The principal clinical manifestation is polyuria and polydipsia (see later). Insensible evaporative losses from the skin and respiratory tract are also a source of hypotonic fluid loss. Increased volumes of fluid loss can arise in febrile patients (skin and respiratory tract), patients on mechanical ventilation (respiratory tract), and those with profuse sweating. The sweat sodium concentration decreases with increasing volumes of perspiration in the heat. Once again, these conditions will lead only to hypernatremia with body fluid hypertonicity if thirst mechanisms or access to water is impaired.

Hypovolemic hypernatremia is by far the most common hypertonicity state. Patients with hypovolemic hypernatremia have lost both sodium and water, but in terms of body fluid tonicity, the net loss of water has been disproportionately greater than the net loss of sodium. The actual plasma sodium concentration resulting from loss of hypotonic fluid depends not only on the sodium concentration of the fluid lost but also on the concentration of other osmotically active solutes such as potassium and on the solute composition in volumes of fluid concomitantly ingested or administered. The extrarenal and renal causes of such fluid losses are similar to those of hypovolemia. Among gastrointestinal causes of hypovolemic hypernatremia, diarrhea is more common than vomiting. More specifically, osmotic diarrheas result in disproportionately greater loss of water than electrolytes and therefore a greater propensity to hypernatremia than is the case with secretory diarrheas. Among the renal sources of sodium and water loss, the two most common causes are loop diuretics and osmotic diuresis. Loop diuretics interfere with the countercurrent mechanism and generate large volumes of urine with an iso-osmolar composition. Because some of the solutes are nonelectrolyte (urea), the impact on body tonicity may be to increase tonicity, unless there is concomitant intake or administration of hypotonic fluids. In contrast to loop diuretics, thiazides do not interfere with the countercurrent mechanism and therefore rarely promote hypernatremia. The presence of nonelectrolyte solutes in urine causes an osmotic diuresis. Such solutes can be of either endogenous origin (e.g., urea or glucose) or exogenous origin (e.g., mannitol or glycerol). The presence of these solutes in tubular fluid impairs both sodium and water reabsorption, but the excretion of urine whose composition is relatively rich in nonelectrolyte solutes tends to promote body fluid hypertonicity, unless sufficient hypotonic fluids are ingested or administered concomitantly.

Failure to replace hypotonic fluid losses generally reflects either impairment in thirst, disability or infirmity that prevents the patient from responding to thirst, or failure of the medical practitioner to recognize the need for hypotonic fluid replacement. Rarely, impaired thirst in patients who are awake and alert can be caused by damage to the hypothalamic osmoreceptors that control thirst perception and response, a condition known as primary hypodipsia. Usually this tends to be associated with an abnormality in the osmotic regulation of AVP secretion. However, cases have been described in which the osmotic regulation of AVP secretion has been dissociated from the osmotic regulation of thirst. Such patients suffer hypernatremia only when extrarenal fluid losses exceed their habitual water intake, as might occur in settings of thermal stress or exercise. Rare patients have a very specific defect in the nonosmotic regulation of AVP secretion (essential hypernatremia). In such patients, volume loading suppresses AVP and results in the excretion of dilute urine, which can lead to hypernatremia if not appreciated and replaced with appropriate oral intake.

Clinical Manifestations

The clinical features of patients with hypernatremia can be divided into those associated with the underlying disease state, those associated with a concomitant disturbance in ECF volume, and those associated with an increase in body fluid tonicity. The main clinically relevant consequence of increased body fluid tonicity is decreased brain cell volume, with the attendant risk for intracerebral hemorrhage. Thus, the major symptoms are neurologic and include confusion, seizures, focal neurologic deficits, and progressively decreasing level of consciousness eventuating in coma. In the absence of an underlying neurologic problem or disturbance in the thirst mechanism and if neurologic injury secondary to hypernatremia has not yet disturbed consciousness, the patient would be expected to complain of thirst.

In patients with hypernatremia of longer duration that is sufficient to enable brain cells to undergo osmotic adaptation, the risk for intracerebral hemorrhage from cell shrinkage is decreased, but a hypertonic intracellular environment with the accumulation of new intracellular solutes is expected to perturb normal cellular function. Furthermore, as outlined later, such accumulation of intracellular osmolytes strongly influences the recommended management approach.

Diagnosis

The diagnosis of hypernatremia is made by laboratory testing of the sodium concentration. Testing should always be repeated to confirm accuracy and corroborated by measurement of plasma osmolality, which is expected to be elevated in all cases. The underlying cause of the hypernatremia is usually evident from the history and physical examination. The history should include a review of recent and current medication use and questions regarding exercise, heat exposure, sweating, vomiting, diarrhea, urine output, recent fluid intake, and the presence of thirst. Physical examination should include an assessment of ECF volume and a complete neurologic evaluation. Urine volume should be monitored, urine osmolality should be measured in several spot urine samples, and 24-hour urine osmolar excretion should also be measured if polyuria is present. In the less common situation of hypervolemic hypernatremia, there is often an antecedent history of medical intervention that includes the administration of sodium-containing solutions, and the findings on physical examination are consistent with ECF volume expansion. In the absence of underlying intrinsic renal disease or diuretic action, urine osmolality should be high because of the hypertonic stimulus to AVP release, which overrides the attenuating effect of hypervolemia. In such patients the urine sodium concentration should be elevated in response to hypervolemia.

In the more common condition of hypovolemic hypernatremia, when the source of fluid loss is extrarenal, urine output should be reduced to less than 500 mL/day and urine osmolality should be the maximum expected for age (urine osmolality >1000 mOsm/kg in young adulthood and decreasing to >600 mOsm/kg by the seventh decade of life and beyond). Preexisting or underlying intrinsic renal disease or exposure to diuretic agents will mask this expected response. Polyuria with a submaximal urine osmolality in the presence of hypernatremia suggests impaired urine-concentrating ability. In such settings, a timed collection for measurement of total urine solute excretion is helpful (see the later section on polyuria). Thus, spot urine osmolality measurements less than 100 to 200 mOsm/kg or polyuria (>3 L/day), together with 24-hour urine solute excretion less than 600 mOsm/day in the face of hypernatremia, suggests a state of diabetes insipidus. In contrast, daily solute excretion exceeding 800 to 1000 mOsm/day suggests osmotic diuresis as the cause of hypovolemic hypernatremia with polyuria. The cause of osmotic diuresis can be confirmed by measuring glucose and urea in urine. Once again it should be recalled that in all these conditions, the presence of hypernatremia indicates an associated abnormality in thirst or access to water.

Treatment

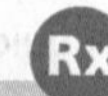

The main components of treatment are to (1) treat the underlying disorder, (2) correct the abnormality in ECF volume, (3) replace the water deficit, and (4) provide maintenance fluids to match continuing ongoing fluid losses if they persist.

The therapeutic approach to serious symptomatic hypovolemic hypernatremia is challenging and often controversial. It is best to divide the therapeutic approach into two separate phases: rapid correction of severe ECF volume depletion when present, followed by gradual replacement of the water deficit, including provision for ongoing fluid losses. When ECF volume contraction is severe (evidence of tissue hypoperfusion and shock), it makes sense to choose a fluid with a sodium concentration as close as possible to that of the patient and whose volume of distribution is confined to the ECF or even the intravascular compartment. This ensures the most efficient treatment of hypovolemia while avoiding overly rapid correction of hypertonicity. Isotonic saline is generally the fluid of choice, and the volume and rate of administration should be guided by clinical parameters related to reversal of hypovolemia. Once the patient has emerged from the danger of hypovolemic tissue hypoperfusion, further fluid replacement should be aimed at correcting the estimated water deficit. This estimate begins with a simple calculation of the percent deficit based on the measured sodium concentration:

$$\text{Total body water deficit} = 0.6 \times \text{Premorbid weight} \times (1 - [140/\text{Na}^+])$$

Total body water is used because the sodium concentration reflects tonicity in all body fluid compartments, including the ICF. Unlike the isotonic fluid replacement for ECF volume, the water replacement should be administered gradually over a period of hours to days, unless there is clear documentation that the hypernatremia has itself evolved over minutes to hours. The necessity for gradual replacement is dictated by the process of osmotic adaptation described previously, and ideally, the rate of water replacement should match the rate at which brain intracellular solutes can be adaptively extruded or removed. More rapid rates of administration could result in brain cell swelling with attendant dangerous neurologic consequences. It is recommended that the estimated volume

of the water deficit be replaced at a rate that will lead to an approximately 0.5- to 1.0-mmol/L reduction in measured plasma sodium concentration per hour. In addition to the estimated water deficit, the estimated ongoing water loss during the hours of replacement should be added. This includes at least 1 L per 24 hours of insensible fluid losses (greater volumes in patients who are febrile or mechanically ventilated), supplemented with any ongoing water losses (renal or gastrointestinal) resulting from continuation of the underlying disease process. Because of the need to distribute replacement of the initial water deficit (which can amount to several liters), over a number of days, during which ongoing water losses continue, it is not unusual to have to deliver large volumes of water, sometimes reaching 5 to 10 L, over the duration of the correction period. This water deficit together with ongoing losses can be replaced through the dietary ingestion of tap water if the patient's condition is suitable or through an enteral feeding tube when feasible. If a gastrointestinal or other disease process precludes these preferred routes, a hypotonic intravenous solution such as D_5W or half-normal saline can be used. When D_5W is used, the glucose is either stored as glycogen or fat or metabolized into carbon dioxide and water, thus effectively providing the patient with solute-free water replacement. In the case of half-normal saline, for any given liter administered, only half can be considered as replacement of the water deficit, and the sodium content will either replace any remaining sodium deficit that has not been fully corrected in the first phase of treatment or will be excreted if there is no impairment in urinary sodium excretion. In elderly patients with known or possible underlying cardiac, hepatic, or renal disease, caution should be exercised in the provision of excessive volumes of salt-containing solutions. In any case, the sodium concentration should be monitored at regular intervals of no less than every 4 hours to avoid too slow or too rapid correction, and ECF volume parameters should be monitored to avoid hypervolemic complications. The route of administration should change in accordance with the patient's response. Although an initial parenteral or nasogastric enteral route might be appropriate when the patient's neurologic status is compromised, subsequent therapy can consist of simple dietary intake of water. Once a patient is awake and alert and if thirst mechanisms are intact, the patient will generally correct the hypertonic state by spontaneous oral fluid intake. Special considerations apply for hypertonic states in the setting of uncontrolled diabetes with hyperglycemia (Chapter 248). The unusual cases of patients with hypervolemic hypernatremia in the hospital setting also need special attention and sometimes require continuous infusions of loop diuretics together with the administration of hypotonic solutions or, in some cases, extracorporeal means to remove both the sodium and water excess in a controlled and safe manner under careful monitoring, often in the intensive care unit.

Polyuria

Polyuria is defined as a urine output greater than 3 L/day and should be distinguished from frequency of urination, which can occur with frequent voiding of small volumes totaling less than this amount per day. The reason for this choice of 3 L is based on physiologic principles related to average daily solute excretion and renal concentrating ability. Because average daily urine solute excretion is approximately 600 mOsm/day, the corresponding average daily urine osmolality with a urine output of 3 L is hypotonic (≈200 mOsm/L). Thus, a daily urine volume exceeding this value of 3 L suggests the possibility that urine-concentrating mechanisms are not being used at any time during the day (water diuresis) or that urine solute excretion is excessive (solute diuresis). These two possibilities also provide a convenient classification of the causes of polyuric states (Table 117–7).

Solute Diuresis

Solute diuresis is defined as the excretion of greater than 800 to 1000 mOsm of urinary solute per day. The composition of these excess solutes can be electrolyte or nonelectrolyte. Electrolyte solute diuresis usually occurs in response to the iatrogenic administration of high volumes of electrolyte-containing solutions, which are disposed of by the kidney through normal physiologic mechanisms. Nonelectrolyte solute diuresis is equivalent to osmotic diuresis in which the presence of a nonreabsorbable nonelectrolyte solute in the tubule fluid prevents reabsorption of sodium and other electrolytes, as well as water. This results in the excretion of large volumes of urine with a urine osmolality close to that of plasma osmolality.

TABLE 117–7 CAUSES OF POLYURIA CLASSIFIED BY WATER AND SOLUTE DIURESIS

SOLUTE DIURESIS (ABNORMALLY INCREASED EXCRETION OF SOLUTE)*			
Electrolyte			
	Sodium driven		
		Sodium chloride load: oral, enteral, parenteral	
		Renal sodium wasting	
	Anion driven†		
		Chloride	
			Loop diuretic
			Bartter's syndrome
		Bicarbonate	
			Exogenous bicarbonate loading
			Inhibition of carbonic anhydrase
		Ketoanion	
			Diabetic ketoacidosis‡
Nonelectrolyte			
	Glucose		
		Exogenous loading	
		Diabetic ketoacidosis	
		Hyperglycemic hyperosmolar syndrome	
		Renal glycosuria	
	Urea		
		Exogenous urea loading	
		Protein or amino acid loading	
		Hypercatabolic states	
		Postrhabdomyolysis	
		Massive hematoma reabsorption or gastrointestinal tract bleeding	
		Diuretic phase of acute tubular necrosis	
		Postobstructive diuresis	
	Sugar alcohols (exogenous loading)§		
		Mannitol	
		Glycerol	
WATER DIURESIS (ABNORMALLY INCREASED EXCRETION OF WATER)			
Excessive water intake			
	Iatrogenic		
	Psychogenic		
	Defect in thirst center		
	Hyperangiotensinemia		
Diabetes insipidus			
	Central		
	Nephrogenic		
	Excessive vasopressinase		

*Other solutes, such as radiocontrast agents (which can produce a very high urine specific gravity), may induce transient increases in urine output.
†Usually sodium will be the associated cation; rarely, the cation will be ammonium, arginine, or cationic medication.
‡Probably contributes to the diuresis caused predominantly by glucose.
§Urinary excretion of ethanol, an "ineffective" solute, does not result in solute diuresis.
From Oster JR, Singer I: The polyuria of solute diuresis. Arch Intern Med 1997;157:721–729.

Water Diuresis

When polyuria is associated with 24-hour urine solute excretion greater than 600 mOsm/day, a defect in urine concentrating ability is generally suggested. In some cases, this defect occurs in association with a more general state of intrinsic renal injury and can be part of the spectrum of interstitial injury in chronic renal disease. More specific defects in urine-concentrating ability fall into the category of the diabetes insipidus disorders, which are discussed in detail in Chapter 243.

Treatment

Once a patient with polyuria has been classified as having abnormally increased excretion of solute (solute diuresis) or water (water diuresis) (Table 117–7), the clinical manifestations and treatment will be those of the underlying disease, and the consequences of changes in ECF volume and tonicity are the same as discussed earlier. Depending on the nature of fluid intake and medications (e.g., diuretics) at the onset of polyuria, a significant percentage of polyuric patients will have alterations in serum sodium and ECF volume and will need attention to the underlying disease, as well as correction of fluid and electrolyte abnormalities. Thus for example, although antihyperglycemic treatment effectively corrects the solute diuresis and polyuric state of uncontrolled diabetes mellitus, initial correction of the concomitant electrolyte and ECF volume disorders takes precedence (Chapter 248).

Future Directions

Given the importance of total body fluids and electrolytes to organ and organism well-being and survival, it is no surprise that a large number of complex and redundant regulatory mechanisms for salt and water balance exist, largely focused on the kidney as the response organ. With the rapidly developing molecular understanding of these regulatory pathways, new drug-accessible targets are now known to modify salt and water balance. Such increased knowledge will improve on the efficacy and specificity of diuretics, the mainstay of therapy in this area for several decades. The vaptans (aquaretics) are just the first class of novel drugs to be available for such use, and novel applications for their use have already been discovered based on detailed molecular understanding of their modes of action.

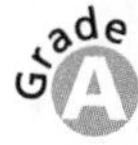

1. Udelson JE, Smith WB, Hendrix GH, et al: Acute hemodynamic effects of conivaptan, a dual V1a and V2 vasopressin receptor antagonist, in patients with advanced heart failure. Circulation 2001;104:2417–2423.

SUGGESTED READINGS

Robertson GL: Regulation of arginine vasopressin in the syndrome of inappropriate antidiuresis. Am J Med 2006;119(7 Suppl. 1):S36–S42. *Comprehensive overview.*

Schrier RW: Body water homeostasis: Clinical disorders of urinary dilution and concentration J Am Soc Nephrol 2006;17:1820–1832. *A clinical review.*

118 POTASSIUM DISORDERS

Julian L. Seifter

Definition

Potassium is ubiquitous in both plant and animal sources of nutrition. It is difficult to avoid eating potassium in a normal diet. Plant cells have cytosolic potassium concentrations of approximately 80 mmol/L, whereas animal cells may have as much as 140 mmol/L. Within the body, potassium is not equally distributed in the total body water. Approximately two thirds of body water is intracellular, and within that compartment potassium is the major cation. Most cells express sodium-potassium adenosine triphosphatase (Na^+, K^+-ATPase) on the cell plasma membranes and through this enzyme utilize metabolic energy in the form of ATP to establish gradients of potassium and sodium. As a result, the potassium concentration of the cell may reach 140 mmol/L, compared with the extracellular potassium concentration of approximately 4 mmol/L. These established ion gradients, and the associated electrical gradients that follow, provide the essential mechanisms for electrical activity in excitable cells such as muscle and neural tissue, cellular nutrient uptake, and transcellular solute transport in polarized epithelial cells in the kidney and intestine. Therefore, maintenance of a normal and narrow range of serum potassium, usually in the order of 3.5 to 5.0 mmol/L, is vital for health. The actual concentration may vary during the day according to a circadian rhythm of decreased excretion in the morning, and dietary intake.

If there is a ratio of 35 : 1 intracellular-to-extracellular potassium and a 2 : 1 ratio of intracellular-to-extracellular water, then it is apparent that more than 98% of potassium resides within cells. The total amount of potassium is usually on the order of 50 mmol/kg of body weight, so that a 70 kg individual has a store of about 3500 mmol of potassium. In the entire extracellular fluid, which is approximately 20% of body weight, or 14 L in a 70-kg person, the total potassium content is 50 to 60 mmol.

From these calculations, several important issues of potassium homeostasis emerge. First, total body potassium balance may be poorly reflected by the extracellular or serum potassium concentration. This fact dissociates hypokalemia from potassium depletion, or hyperkalemia from potassium excess. Changes in the distribution between the cells and extracellular fluid can occur rapidly, within minutes, in contrast to the matching of dietary intake of potassium to potassium elimination from the body, which occurs within hours. It is also apparent that potassium ingestion at the time of a meal may be equal to a large fraction of the total extracellular potassium. An average daily consumption may be on the order of 50 to 100 mmol. Because this potassium cannot be eliminated instantaneously, there exists a potential danger of rapid rises in extracellular potassium concentration after meals. Protection against this eventuality is the ability of potassium to distribute from the extracellular to intracellular spaces. The intracellular space, given its large volume and potassium content, can accommodate, or buffer, an extra load of potassium without significant changes in concentration. Distribution of potassium from extracellular to intracellular spaces is known as *internal balance*, and the matching of intake to losses from the body is known as *external balance*.

The Importance of Potassium

Potassium is essential for a number of critical body functions. Examples include enzymatic reactions that regulate protein synthesis, glycogen synthesis, cell growth, and cell division. The ability of cells to take up potassium or extrude potassium contributes to the important function of cell volume regulation during periods of osmotic stress. In excitable cells, such as cardiac myocytes, the relationship of intracellular to extracellular potassium concentrations is critical in establishing the resting membrane potential, which normally may approach the Nernst equilibrium potential for potassium. Because larger percentage changes can occur in the extracellular potassium concentration compared with the intracellular concentration (due to the relative concentrations), it follows that changes in extracellular potassium have the greatest impact on the electrical potential difference across cell membranes.

The serum potassium itself has effects on conductance of potassium through specific K^+ channels, effects that also are critical to cardiac conduction velocity and therefore, if abnormal, could contribute to arrhythmogenesis. Among the major effects of changes in potassium are serious cardiac arrhythmias, which can cause sudden death. A very dramatic consequence of potassium abnormalities is complete skeletal muscle paralysis, which can occur with either a severe increase or a severe decrease in serum levels of potassium. Growth states are associated with greater need for potassium; for example, in normal pregnancy, the maternal potassium concentration may fall as the developing fetus grows. Potassium is also an important local mediator of vascular tone in muscle beds. During exercise, local extracellular potassium concentrations may rise to as high as 10 mmol/L, causing local vasodilation to allow more blood supply to the exercising muscle. Very little of that potassium remains within the total extracellular fluid, so severe hyperkalemia does not usually occur with exercise. The trained athlete develops an adaptive increase in Na^+, K^+-ATPase, allowing for efficient re-uptake of potassium into muscle cells. The importance of adequate potassium stores to muscle function is well known to experienced marathoners, and overexertion of muscles in a state of potassium depletion can lead to rhabdomyolysis.

Pathobiology

Consequences of Potassium Depletion and Excess

Some consequences of potassium depletion include hypertension, decreased growth, and muscle symptoms such as weakness, cramps, fasciculations, and even paralysis. In severe cases, the diaphragm may be paralyzed, leading to respiratory failure. Cardiac arrhythmias are a critical component of low potassium states and are usually seen when the serum potassium falls below 3 mmol/L or when ischemia, hypercalcemia, and/or drugs such as digoxin are simultaneously present. Low serum potassium not only hyperpolarizes most cells, leading to an increase in the resting potential, but also has effects on certain potassium channels required for repolarization. Thus, hypokalemia decreases or slows potassium conductance, the prolonged repolarization phase accounting for the characteristic electrocardiographic findings of broad, flattened T waves. U waves are also indicative of this delay in repolarization (Fig. 118–1). The patient is prone to tachyarrhythmias, including ventricular tachycardia.

In the intestine, hypokalemia may result in a paralytic ileus, which may interfere with oral replacement. Hypokalemia may result in acute skeletal muscle paralysis. In one such syndrome, there is an inability to raise the arms from the side.

Hypokalemia has been implicated as a cause of hyponatremia due to thiazide diuretics. Potassium is as important a body fluid osmole as sodium, and losses of potassium can be thought of as obligating sodium to replace it in the intracellular space, resulting in hyponatremia. Isotonic losses of potassium and sodium salts in watery diarrhea may result not only in extracellular volume depletion but also in hyponatremia. Similarly, if potassium chloride is added to isotonic saline, a hypertonic solution results, and potassium may enter cells as sodium exits, contributing to hypernatremia.

In addition to these systemic effects of potassium imbalance, the kidney is particularly sensitive to depletion of potassium. Structural changes in the glomeruli and tubules are noted, and functional disruption includes a decreased glomerular filtration rate (GFR), increased proximal tubule ammoniagenesis, increased sodium bicarbonate reabsorption, and net acid excretion. A condition of nephrogenic diabetes insipidus results from an effect of potassium depletion that decreases expression of vasopressin-dependent water channels (aquaporin-2) in the collecting duct luminal plasma membranes.

Hypokalemia is also a stimulus to renin production by the kidney and has a negative effect on aldosterone synthesis in the zona glomerulosa cells of the adrenal cortex. Hyperkalemia has the opposite effect: it is an important stimulus to aldosterone synthesis and release, particularly when volume expansion and low angiotensin-II coexist, as in patients with renal failure. The feedback mechanism coupling aldosterone with serum potassium is important in regulating the degree of potassium losses in the urine.

Excess potassium is often asymptomatic, but it can result in skeletal muscle weakness or paralysis, and it has serious potential cardiac implications. In hyperkalemia, there is a depolarizing effect on the resting membrane potential and potassium channel conductance is increased, leading to the classic electrocardiographic changes of hyperacute peaked T waves associated with rapid repolarization (Fig. 118–2). Because of the increased potassium conductance, hyperkalemia antagonizes the normal slow depolarization of pacemaker tissue that is usually associated with a decrease in potassium conductance. Hyperkalemia, like acetylcholine, commonly results in sinus bradycardia. Heart block, loss of P waves on the electrocardiogram, and prolonged QRS intervals are all seen in cases

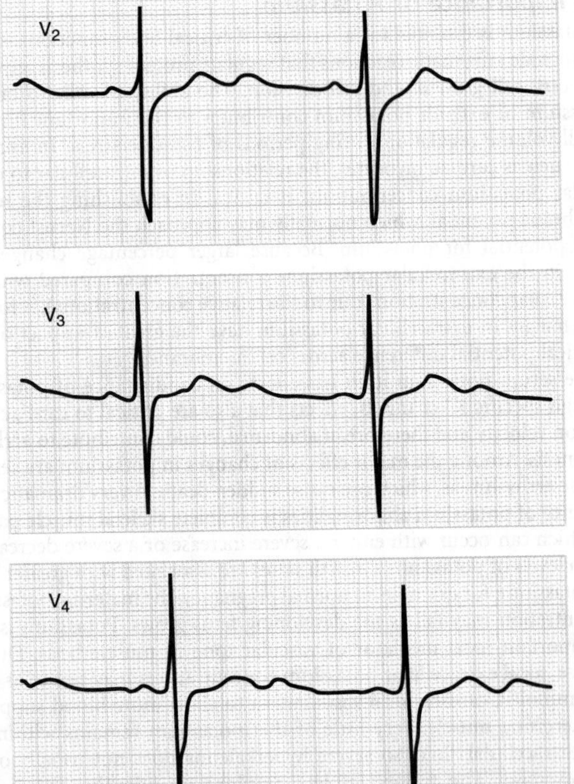

FIGURE 118–1 • The electrocardiographic manifestations of hypokalemia. The serum potassium concentration was 2.2 mEq/L. The ST segment is prolonged, primarily because of a U wave following the T wave, and the T wave is flattened.

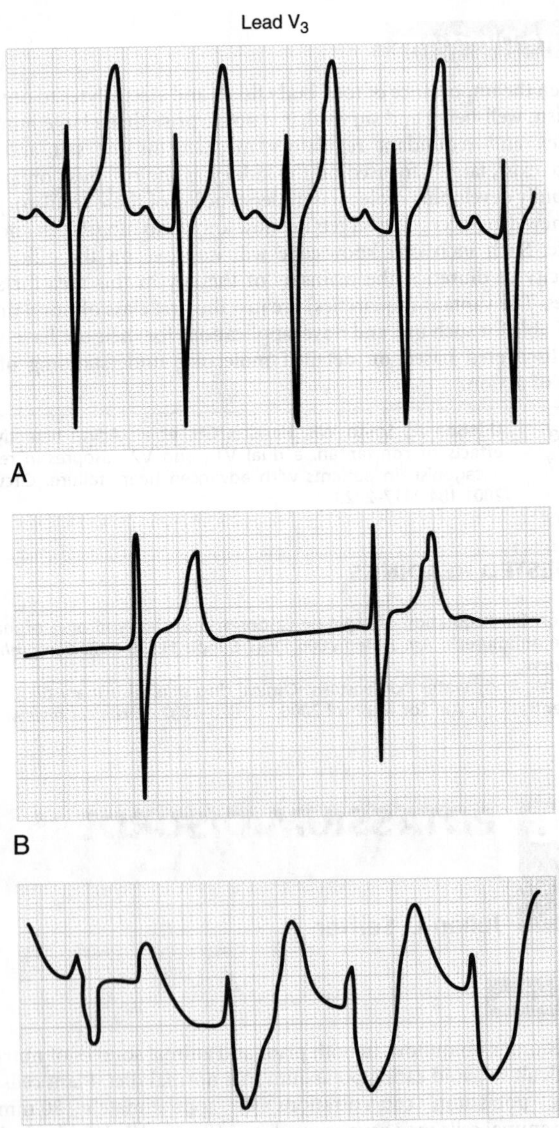

FIGURE 118–2 • The effects of progressive hyperkalemia on the electrocardiogram. All of the illustrations are from lead V_3. **A,** Serum potassium concentration ($[K^+]$) = 6.8 mEq/L; note the peaked T waves together with normal sinus rhythm. **B,** Serum $[K^+]$ = 8.9 mEq/L; note the peaked T waves and absent P waves. **C,** Serum $[K^+]$ = >8.9 mEq/L; note the classic sine wave with absent P waves, marked prolongation of the QRS complex, and peaked T waves.

of severe hyperkalemia, usually in excess of 6 mmol/L. The electrocardiogram, however, is not a sensitive indicator of severe hyperkalemia. Cardiac arrest may occur suddenly and without warning. Certain muscle depolarizing anesthetic agents, such as succinylcholine, may potentiate effects of hyperkalemia. The aminoglycoside gentamicin may also do this, particularly in the patient with renal failure. Like hypokalemia, severe hyperkalemia can also cause skeletal muscle paralysis; unlike hypokalemic paralysis, it is often ascending in nature.

Internal Potassium Balance and Associated Disorders

Because of the delay in hours before renal excretion matches dietary intake, and because potassium first enters the extracellular fluid from the gastrointestinal tract, it is critical that the process of cellular buffering be effective. Essentially, increases in postprandial blood potassium are minimized, before potassium is eliminated from the body. A major factor in this regulation after meals is the feedback loop involving insulin and potassium. An increase in serum potassium stimulates insulin release from the beta cells of the pancreatic islets. Insulin increases potassium uptake into cells, primarily muscle, independently of its effect on glucose uptake. Potassium uptake is chiefly the result of increased Na^+, K^+-ATPase trafficking to the plasma membranes in these cells. It is apparent that insulin-deficient diabetics have a greater tendency to develop hyperkalemia, especially if other factors, such as a high-potassium diet, renal disease, or treatment with medications that interfere with renal excretion, are also at work. Hypokalemia diminishes insulin secretion and may be associated with glucose intolerance.

Another important mechanism of regulating the distribution of potassium between extracellular and cellular spaces involves the sympathoadrenal system. β-Adrenergic activation, particularly through the β_2-receptor, increases potassium uptake into muscle and fat cells. Importantly, epinephrine, which also has α-adrenergic effects, is associated with a transient increase in potassium release from the liver before a more prolonged period of decreased serum potassium mediated by the β_2-receptor. Phenylephrine, an α-adrenergic agonist, increases serum potassium. As with insulin, potassium uptake is the consequence of increased Na^+, K^+-ATPase activity associated with an increased intracellular concentration of cyclic AMP. Other potassium uptake mechanisms, including K^+-Cl^- and Na^+-K^+-Cl^- cotransporters, may also be involved. The adrenergic effect is important in regulating the serum potassium concentration during exercise and is independent of the additional effect that catecholamines may have on blood sugar with the expected increases in insulin. In the trained athlete, there is chronic increase in Na^+, K^+-ATPase on cell membranes such that, after exertion, there may be a transient lowering of the serum potassium concentration. Such athletes may have chronically mild decreases in serum potassium. β-Blockers may be associated with increased potassium during exercise, particularly in patients with renal failure. On the other hand, a severe stress may contribute to hypokalemia, through both direct β_2 effects and insulin action secondary to the blood sugar rise. A patient who has a chronically low potassium level (e.g., due to diuretic use) may be particularly vulnerable to cardiac arrhythmias during periods of stress, such as head trauma, or during the acute coronary syndrome, to which cardiac ischemia also contributes.

Other mechanisms that govern the distribution of potassium between cells and the extracellular space are particularly important in pathologic states. For example, the acid-base balance has an influence on distribution. The mechanisms for changes in potassium in acid-base disturbances are not completely understood, but the general rules are that metabolic acidosis has a greater impact to raise the potassium level than does respiratory acidosis, and that metabolic alkalosis a greater impact to lower the potassium level than does respiratory alkalosis, although the latter can also do it. Anion gap acidosis does not raise potassium, probably because of the movement of the organic anion (e.g., lactate) from cells into the extracellular space with an accompanying proton, whereas the ingestion of chloride salts has the most profound effect, because chloride is restricted to the extracellular space and protons enter cells with an electroneutral exchange for the potassium cation. Not only hydrochloric acid addition, but also the ingestion of excessive chloride salts of arginine and lysine have been associated with hyperkalemic acidosis. ε-Aminocaproic acid has also been associated with hyperkalemia and is hypothesized to exchange for cellular potassium, much like the other cationic amino acids.

Often in an acid-base disorder, where there is disruption of other electrolytes through losses or inputs into the body, the serum potassium does not depend solely on one factor. For that reason, whether the serum potassium level is low, normal, or high, it is important to consider the various processes that may influence that level. Just as multiple acid-base disturbances may be present simultaneously, leading to a single blood pH, many processes that affect potassium can be simultaneously present. Metabolic acidosis may be associated with diarrheal or urinary losses of potassium, such that the potassium concentration is low, not high. However metabolic acidosis in the diabetic could also be associated with insulin deficiency and renal failure, in which case the serum potassium level might be elevated despite increased osmotically driven urinary losses.

Other hormonal effects on potassium include thyroid and growth hormone, but patients with disorders of these hormones do not usually manifest significant changes in blood potassium levels. Some patients with hyperthyroidism may have mild hypokalemia, but this could be related to the increased sympathetic activity in that condition. Thyroid hormone increases the activity of Na^+, K^+-ATPase.

Hypomagnesemia frequently accompanies hypokalemia. Both magnesium and potassium are found predominantly in cells, but the Na^+, K^+-ATPase requires magnesium for function. If magnesium is deficient, potassium distributes more to the extracellular fluid, masking the degree of potassium deficiency. Moreover, magnesium deficiency leads to renal potassium wasting, and until magnesium is repleted, potassium depletion is hard to correct. Factors involved in the internal balance of potassium are shown in Table 118–1.

Patients with pernicious anemia, who receive vitamin B_{12} to stimulate erythropoiesis, may deplete extracellular potassium and suffer from hypokalemia as a cost to producing new red blood cells. Certain leukemias with rapid rates of growth also may cause a drop in serum potassium. Some forms of myelogenous leukemias are associated with a high level of lysozyme, which leads to urinary potassium loss as well. Familial hypokalemic periodic paralysis is caused by genetic defects in a cellular calcium channel, with resulting reduced activity of an ATP-regulated K^+ channel that extrudes potassium from skeletal muscle cells. Without the ability to effectively recycle potassium to the extracellular space, the hypokalemic effect of the Na^+, K^+-ATPase is unopposed. A form is seen in Asian patients with hyperthyroidism; it manifests as episodic paralysis brought out by high-carbohydrate meals (insulin secretion). Another aggravating factor is rest after exercise, a time when blood potassium falls due to reuptake of potassium by the ATP pumps. The condition is treated by dietary means, as well as with β_2-blockers and acetazolamide, which, by creating hyperchloremic acidosis, offsets the urinary potassium wasting it causes.

Barium salt toxicity is associated with profound hypokalemia through inhibition of cellular K^+ channels that normally function to transport potassium from cells to the extracellular space.

The abnormal distribution of potassium between cells and extracellular space may also result in hyperkalemia. Acidosis has already been mentioned, as have insulin-deficient states and β-adrenergic blockade with drugs such as labetalol. Acute increases in serum osmolality with a rapid rise in glucose in the diabetic patient, infusions of mannitol, or, rarely, administration of intravenous contrast material causes osmotic shifts of water from cells. The cellular potassium concentration rises, favoring the movement of potassium into the extracellular space. Although it is not always possible, it is best to know the levels of serum glucose and potassium in an unconscious diabetic before infusing concentrated glucose solutions, because of the risk of aggravating an already elevated potassium concentration.

TABLE 118–1 FACTORS REGULATING INTERNAL POTASSIUM BALANCE

Insulin
β-Adrenergic activity
Acid-base balance
Magnesium
Osmolality
Thyroid hormone
Potassium

Familial hyperkalemic periodic paralysis a myopathy caused by a genetic defect in voltage-gated Na^+ channels in skeletal muscle, is treated with β_2-agonists and diuretics. Exercise or dietary increases in plasma potassium result in mild depolarization of skeletal muscle that then unmasks the sodium channel defect, rendering the cells inexcitable.

Potassium competes with digoxin-binding sites on the Na^+, K^+-ATPase, so that, if hypokalemia coexists, digoxin will have an intensified effect and may lead to drug toxicity. Only in extreme cases of digitalis overdose will severe hyperkalemia develop due to generalized blockade of Na^+, K^+-ATPase.

External Potassium Balance and Associated Disorders

Normally, no more than 10 to 20% of total potassium excretion is accomplished by the gastrointestinal tract, but in renal failure colonic excretion is increased, primarily through potassium-induced increases in epithelial Na^+, K^+-ATPase activity and aldosterone. In renal failure, the normal mechanisms to distribute potassium acquire increased importance.

The usual requirement of the kidneys in potassium balance is to excrete a net amount of potassium to maintain balance with dietary intake. As mentioned, there is a variable amount of gastrointestinal potassium loss that adapts to levels of kidney function and to potassium excesses, but losses can be increased in the presence of liquid stools. Because of the ubiquity of potassium in the diet, it is less common in humans for the kidneys to be called upon to conserve potassium due strictly to a low potassium intake. However, under conditions of anorexia or extrarenal potassium loss, the kidneys will be enlisted to retain potassium. More often, there are identifiable sources of potassium loss. Some conditions that cause the greatest losses of gastrointestinal potassium include secretory diarrheas of the colon, the result of infection or laxative abuse. Disorders of the small intestine may lead to large quantities of liquid stool with low potassium concentration, engendering favorable gradients for marked potassium secretion by the colon. A syndrome of watery diarrhea and hypokalemia is associated with neuroendocrine tumors secreting vasoactive intestinal peptide. Rectosigmoid secretion of potassium may result in particularly high potassium losses, and is the likely explanation for the potassium deficiency seen with ureterosigmoidostomies and for the effectiveness of potassium exchange resins used to treat hyperkalemia. Potassium can be lost from a variety of other sources, including excess sweat or salivation, vomiting, and diarrhea.

Hypokalemia usually results from an imbalance between intake and excretion. If intake is low compared with excretion, hypokalemia will develop. Potassium can be lost from vomiting or diarrhea. In gastric alkalosis, the predominant potassium losses are urinary, and the same holds in diarrhea if excessive chloride is lost in the stool, resulting in metabolic alkalosis. Urinary losses may exceed intake if diuretics are used, in renal tubular disorders, or when excessive quantities of osmotic or anionic products are excreted in the urine.

It is unusual for hyperkalemia to be caused by excessive potassium intake unless the patient has renal dysfunction. In such a case, it is mandatory to restrict dietary potassium. However, patients who have brisk hemolysis, internal hemorrhage, or rhabdomyolysis, particularly if the hemoglobinuria or myoglobinuria also results in acute renal failure, can quickly develop life-threatening hyperkalemia due to rapid release of cellular potassium stores.

In the kidney, potassium excretion begins with filtration, which is dependent on the GFR and the plasma potassium concentration. Because the extracellular potassium concentration is approximately 4 mmol/L, and that of sodium is 140 mmol/L, far less potassium is filtered than sodium (about 3%).

The renal proximal tubule reabsorbs potassium passively in the process of reabsorbing sodium and water by both transcellular and paracellular mechanisms. In the loop of Henle, particularly in the thick ascending limb, potassium is reabsorbed both by the apical sodium-potassium-chloride cotransporter (NKCC) and, like calcium and magnesium, by paracellular reabsorption of the cation. The latter mechanism is a consequence of the luminal electropositivity created by recycling of potassium through K^+ channels from the cell to the lumen. Importantly, luminal ammonium ($NH4^+$) can substitute for potassium on the NKCC cotransporter, accounting for the observation that in hyperkalemic states less $NH4^+$ appears in the urine; it is the reabsorption of $NH4^+$ by the thick limb, and establishment of a multiplication effect to raise medullary interstitial fluid $NH4^+$ concentrations, that eventually leads to increasing medullary collecting duct fluid $NH4^+$ and net acid excretion. High luminal potassium competes with $NH4^+$ for reabsorption in the thick limb and thereby decreases net acid excretion. $NH4^+$ not reabsorbed by the NKCC stays in the lumen and diffuses as ammonia (NH_3) into the highly perfused renal cortex rather than remaining within the urinary space for excretion. As a consequence, a renal mechanism exists for metabolic acidosis to develop in hyperkalemic states, and this in part accounts for the success in treating certain types of hyperkalemic acidosis by lowering the serum potassium level. Another mechanism for a competition between acid excretion and potassium exists in the principal cells of the cortical collecting duct. Cellular acidification, as in metabolic acidosis, inhibits potassium secretion via an effect on potassium secretory channels, resulting in hyperkalemia during metabolic acidosis.

In hypokalemia, whether through proximal tubule intracellular acidosis attending cellular hyperpolarization or other mechanisms, glutaminase enzymes are increased and greater quantities of ammonia are produced. This ammonia leads to greater medullary interstitial fluid ammonia/ammonium concentrations and therefore to enhanced net acid elimination. Ammonium production in this condition could be considered an adaptation to allow for both sodium and potassium to be reabsorbed as the expendable cation, $NH4^+$, accompanies excreted anions into the urine. The increase in ammonia production can have a deleterious effect, in that ammonia is thought to contribute to the chronic tubulointerstitial nephritis of chronic hypokalemia.

By the time the tubular fluid reaches the distal tubule and collecting duct, more than 90% of potassium has been reabsorbed. In the unusual condition in which potassium needs to be more completely retained (e.g., in potassium depletion), reabsorptive mechanisms in the distal nephron and collecting duct are increased, most importantly the apical membrane hydrogen-potassium (H^+, K^+)-ATPase, allowing for near-complete restriction of potassium from the urine. However, potassium reabsorption is seldom as complete as that of sodium. Because the potassium concentration in the medullary interstitium is raised due to the process of countercurrent multiplication accompanying potassium reabsorption in the thick ascending limb, it is difficult for the collecting duct fluid to move potassium outward against such a steep gradient. In fact, some potassium may leak from the medullary cells into the lumen. It is unusual to see potassium concentrations in the urine lower than 5 to 10 mmol/L.

In the more common circumstance, when dietary potassium is abundant, the reabsorption of 90% of filtered potassium by the proximal and distal nephron is followed by net potassium secretion. The urinary potassium most closely reflects potassium secreted by the distal nephron. Although there is some potassium secretion coupled to chloride secretion in the distal tubule, the major regulatory site for potassium secretion resides in the principal cells of the cortical collecting duct. Three major mechanisms control overall potassium secretion (Fig. 118–3), which may vary depending on the need by as much as 400%. Those three mechanisms are (1) development of a lumen-negative transepithelial potential difference that provides the driving force for potassium secretion into the lumen, (2) adequacy of a variety of apical membrane secretory potassium channels, and (3) flow-dependent movement of fluid through the lumen.

Mechanism of Potassium Secretion

Development of Transepithelial Potential Difference in the Cortical Collecting Duct

First, sodium must be delivered in ample amounts (depending on the flow rate and sodium concentration of the tubular fluid) to result in sodium reabsorption through the apical epithelial sodium channel (ENaC) in the principal cell. In severely prerenal states of avid proximal and loop sodium reabsorption, sodium delivery may become rate limiting for potassium secretion. A sign of this condition is urinary sodium concentrations as low as 1 mmol/L. This might be the case in hepatorenal syndrome or severe heart failure. Assuming that sodium delivery is not limiting, reabsorption of the sodium cation creates a lumen-negative transepithelial potential difference. The reabsorption of sodium in turn is a secondary active transport process that depends on low intracellular sodium concentrations resulting from the energy-requiring Na^+, K^+-

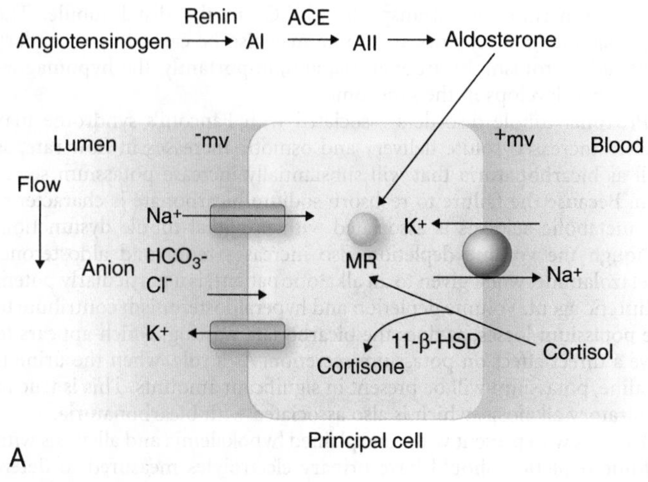

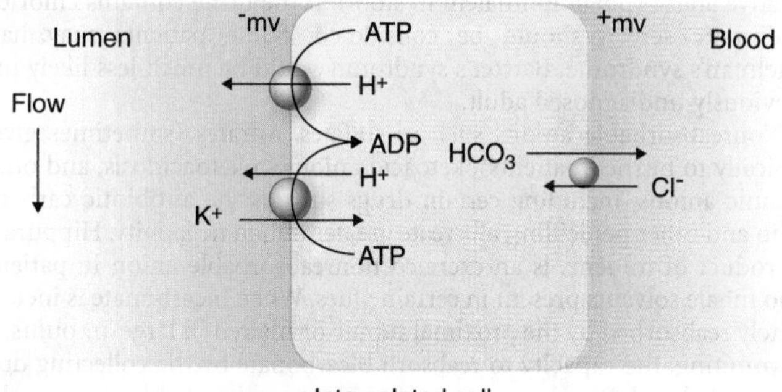

FIGURE 118–3 • Two cell types in the cortical collecting duct. A, The principal cells mediate sodium (Na^+) reabsorption energized by the basolateral Na^+, K^+ pump. Entry from the lumen is through the epithelial Na^+ channel (ENaC), which renders the lumen negatively charged (–mv). This transepithelial voltage stimulates secretion of potassium (K^+) through K^+ channels. Reabsorbable anions such as chloride (Cl^-) lessen the luminal negativity and decrease K^+ secretion. Bicarbonate (HCO_3^-) has an effect to increase K^+ secretion. High flow rates increase net K^+ secretion by preventing development of high lumen K^+ concentrations. The effects of the renin-angiotensin-aldosterone axis are shown: increased mineralocorticoid receptor (MR) activation increases ENaC, the Na^+, K^+ pump, and K^+ channels, thereby increasing Na^+ reabsorption and K^+ secretion. Cortisol would also increase MR activity, but it is inactivated by the enzyme, 11β-hydroxysteroid dehydrogenase (11β-HSD). AI = angiotensin I; AII = angiotensin II; ACE = angiotensin-converting enzyme; mv, millivolts. **B,** Intercalated cells are carbonic anhydrase–rich cells that secrete acid and reabsorb HCO_3^-. The H^+ ATPase secretes H^+ in a way favored by the negatively charged lumen in conjunction with the aldosterone-stimulated effect on Na^+ reabsorption in neighboring principal cells. The K^+, H^+-ATPase is an electroneutral pump. The K^+/H^+ exchanger, reabsorbing K^+, is important in states of K^+ depletion when urinary K^+ is decreased. ADP = adenosine diphosphate; ATP = adenosine triphosphate.

ATPase on the basolateral membrane. Most of the potassium that enters the principal cell from the extracellular fluid via this Na^+, K^+-ATPase is recycled back to the extracellular fluid by basolateral potassium transport mechanisms rather than being secreted into the urine. This explains the magnitude of difference by which sodium reabsorption exceeds potassium secretion by these cells.

Extracellular potassium is also a regulator of potassium secretion in the kidney. As plasma potassium increases, Na^+, K^+-ATPase increases, bringing more potassium into the cells for transepithelial secretion. In peripheral cells as well, the higher the potassium, the more potassium will be taken up into cells through this mechanism.

Other factors that determine the transepithelial potential difference include the effects of anions in the lumen. For example, nonreabsorbable anions present in the lumen maximize the lumen negativity that accompanies sodium reabsorption through the ENaC. To the extent that anions such as chloride are reabsorbed in the collecting duct cells, the effect on luminal negativity will be reduced as sodium is reabsorbed. As a consequence, there will be less driving force for potassium (and hydrogen) secretion.

Aldosterone affects the transepithelial potential difference in a few ways. It has an intracellular mineralocorticoid receptor that results in increased density of ENaC, as well as increased basolateral expression of Na^+, K^+-ATPase enzymes. Cortisol, which is normally present in higher concentrations than aldosterone, has equal affinity for the aldosterone receptor and therefore could lead to enhanced potassium secretion. However, an enzyme known as 11β-hydroxysteroid dehydrogenase type 2 is present in the collecting duct cells and converts cortisol to inactive cortisone. This is similar to the enzymatic step that converts cortisone to cortisol in the adrenal gland.

Role of Potassium Secretory Channels

The second mechanism for collecting duct potassium secretion is adequate function of the several types of potassium secretory channels on the luminal membrane of the principal cell. Although many factors regulate the function of these channels, antidiuretic hormone (ADH) and intracellular pH are among the clinically significant regulators. The increase in K^+ channel activity in response to ADH, combined with an ADH effect to increase ENaC, may be important in elaborating the highest potassium concentration in the urine under circumstances of low flow that accompanies increased water reabsorption.

Intracellular acidity in metabolic acidosis and hypokalemic states may play a role in turning down potassium secretion through inhibitory effects on the potassium channels. This mechanism would allow more of the cation secretion required to balance sodium reabsorption to be in the form of hydrogen, via the secretory and electrogenic proton ATPases that are abundant in the neighboring α-intercalated cell of the collecting duct.

In addition to the predominant effects on the sodium transporters, ENaC, and the ATP pump, aldosterone also increases potassium channel and proton ATPase activity.

Flow Rate Dependence of Potassium Secretion

The final mechanism for potassium secretion in the collecting duct is the flow rate of urine. Increasing flow allows for greater sodium delivery and, hence, greater sodium reabsorption via ENaC; it also diminishes the buildup of K^+ concentration in the collecting duct fluid. This allows the maintenance of optimal K^+ gradients for further secretion into the lumen. On the other hand, in conditions of water diuresis, the decreased ADH diminishes the net amount of potassium secreted. Yet, because the urine cannot fully be free of potassium, polyuria over a prolonged period, from whatever cause, is likely to lead to significant potassium losses. Because potassium excretion is highly dependent on flow rate, conditions in which high urine flow rates are accompanied by high aldosterone levels may result in substantial potassium losses. Such is the case with diuretic use (e.g., acetazolamide, thiazide and loop diuretics). Increased urinary flow rates contribute to the hypokalemia in osmotic diuresis. On the other hand, low urinary flow rates make potassium excretion difficult and may contribute to hyperkalemic states.

Excretion Mechanisms and Normal Function

Taken together, three feedback loops are relevant to normal function. First, drinking excessive water does not usually lead to large losses of potassium, because there is a simultaneous decrease in ADH. Second, expansion of the extracellular fluid with isotonic sodium chloride does not necessarily result in potassium depletion, because the renin-angiotensin-aldosterone axis is suppressed. Third, in metabolic acidosis, intracellular acidification limits potassium secretion, favoring more acid secretion to compensate for the acidosis.

Diuretics such as furosemide and thiazides are well known and common causes of hypokalemia. The potassium-losing effects of thiazides are greater than those of loop diuretics, an observation that seems counterintuitive given the increased potency and direct inhibition of potassium reabsorption that accompany inhibition of the NKCC transporter. It is likely that the decreased reabsorption of calcium by loop diuretics counterbalances the electronegativity in the collecting duct associated with sodium reabsorption, and less potassium is secreted. Calcium presented to the principal cells of the collecting duct after furosemide inhibition may also activate luminal calcium sensors, decreasing expression of ENaC on the apical membranes. Thiazide inhibition increases calcium reabsorption in the distal tubule, thereby delivering less calcium to the collecting duct and allowing for more potassium secretion.

HYPOKALEMIC DISORDERS

Hypokalemic, Hypertensive Syndromes

Several disorders are associated with failure to achieve the required transepithelial electrical gradient to maintain potassium balance. Those conditions that result in increased luminal negativity may produce hypokalemia in association with metabolic alkalosis, because not only potassium but also hydrogen secretion via the H^+-ATPase depends on this developed voltage. If the abnormality is related to a primary increase in sodium reabsorption, then hypertension or extracellular volume expansion will also develop. In this category, there are both common and rare disorders. Urinary potassium wasting, inappropriate to the blood potassium level, is observed. Evaluation of the plasma renin and aldosterone values may be helpful in distinguishing the individual diagnoses.

Primary hyperaldosteronism is associated with high aldosterone and low renin levels due to the volume expansion. If corrected for serum potassium, an aldosterone-to-renin ratio of 30 : 1 suggests a primary adrenal cortical tumor (aldosteronoma) or hyperplasia. The tubular delivery of large amounts of sodium chloride in a setting of volume expansion and nonsuppressible aldosterone results in hypokalemia. This explains the improvement in serum potassium concentration with sodium restriction in hyperaldosteronism, and it provides the basis of a provocative test for adrenal adenomas, in which intravenous saline expansion produces hypokalemia. Certain forms of congenital adrenal hyperplasia, such as 11β-hydroxylase deficiency, may lead to hypokalemic alkalosis associated with characteristics of excessive androgen production. Aldosterone may be increased by high renin and angiotensin and may cause increased sodium reabsorption, hypertension (with angiotensin II contributing), and hypokalemic metabolic alkalosis in renin-secreting tumors and unilateral renal artery stenosis.

In some cases in which adrenocorticotropic hormone (ACTH) is overproduced, as in ectopic production from certain malignancies, the amount of cortisol present may overwhelm the aldosterone receptor and result in hypertensive hypokalemic alkalosis. The patient will probably show signs of Cushing's syndrome. Though ACTH is a minor stimulus to aldosterone secretion, there is a condition known as glucocorticoid remediable aldosteronism (GRA) in which episodes of hypokalemia develop with hypertension. In this condition, a chimeric gene duplication couples the ACTH-responsive 11β-hydroxylase promoter to the coding region of aldosterone synthase. GRA is remediable by dexamethasone because of the suppression of ACTH at the level of the pituitary.

A curious syndrome of licorice or anisette use depends on an active sweet substance known as glycyrrhizic acid that inhibits the enzyme 11β-hydroxysteroid dehydrogenase and thereby causes hypokalemia, metabolic alkalosis, and hypertension. A rare genetic disorder known as apparent mineralocorticoid excess syndrome (AME) produces the same effect as a result of deficiency of 11β-hydroxysteroid dehydrogenase. The cause of the syndrome is activation of the mineralocorticoid receptor by endogenous cortisol that is not inactivated to cortisone. The AME syndrome produces a high ratio cortisol to cortisone. As a feedback response, renin and aldosterone are suppressed by the volume expansion.

Activating mutations of ENaC likewise appear as mineralocorticoid excess (Liddle's syndrome). The syndrome of primary increases in ENaC can be distinguished from primary or secondary hyperaldosteronism by a decrease in renin and aldosterone levels.

Hypokalemic, Hypotensive Syndromes

In contrast to the hypokalemic, hypertensive syndromes, in which sodium reabsorption is increased as a primary event, very common disorders of hypokalemic alkalosis are associated with extracellular volume depletion and secondary high renin and hyperaldosteronism seen in extracellular volume depletion of nonrenal causes. Diuretic use, Bartter's syndrome, and Gitelman's syndrome are renal tubular causes of extracellular volume depletion, hypotension, and hypokalemic alkalosis, but sodium and chloride losses are found in the urine and secondary rises in renin and aldosterone are also observed. Increased urinary flow rates are important contributors to the increased potassium losses in each of these examples. Bartter's syndrome affects the function of the thick ascending limb through mutations in NKCC or in K^+ or Cl^- channels, as does Gitelman's syndrome through inactivating mutations or dysregulation of the sodium-chloride cotransporter (NCC) in the distal tubule. The hypokalemia in Gitelman's syndrome may also be caused by secondary hyperaldosteronism, bicarbonaturia, and, importantly, the hypomagnesemia that develops in the syndrome.

Proximal tubule disorders associated with Fanconi's syndrome may lead to increased solute delivery and osmotic increases in flow rate, as well as bicarbonaturia that will substantially increase potassium secretion. Because the failure to reabsorb sodium bicarbonate is characteristic, metabolic acidosis is associated with proximal tubule dysfunction, although the volume depletion also increases renin and aldosterone. Acetazolamide, when given to an alkalotic patient, is a particularly potent kaliuretic agent. Volume depletion and hyperaldosteronism contribute to the potassium losses, as does the bicarbonate wasting, which appears to have a direct effect on potassium secretion. As a rule, when the urine is alkaline, potassium will be present in significant amounts. This is true in respiratory alkalosis, which is also associated with bicarbonaturia.

Patients who present with unexplained hypokalemia and alkalosis with volume depletion should have urinary electrolytes measured to determine whether the urine chloride is low, as in surreptitious vomiting or laxative abuse (phenolphthalein in stool). If the urine contains chloride, a diuretic screen should be considered. Some patients may have Gitelman's syndrome. Bartter's syndrome would be much less likely in a previously undiagnosed adult.

Nonreabsorbable anions such as sulfates, nitrates (sometimes given topically to burned patients), ketoacid anions in ketoacidosis, and other organic anions, including certain drugs such as the antibiotic carbenicillin and other penicillins, all create greater lumen negativity. Hippurate, a product of toluene, is an excreted nonreabsorbable anion in patients who inhale solvents present in certain glues. When bicarbonate is incompletely reabsorbed by the proximal tubule or filtered in large amounts, as in vomiting, the capacity to reabsorb bicarbonate by the collecting duct is overwhelmed. Bicarbonate may act as a nonreabsorbable anion in this segment, but it most likely has additional effects to stimulate potassium secretion. The marked potassium wasting associated with vomiting is caused by renal losses, not losses in the gastrointestinal tract.

Other forms of renal tubular acidosis may result from disorders of the H^+, K^+-ATPase or chloride-bicarbonate exchange, in which case potassium can be lost in the urine and the urine pH may be alkaline. Classic distal renal tubular acidosis, type 1, is often associated with hypokalemia, which may improve with correction of the acidemia. In contrast, proximal renal tubular acidosis, when corrected with bicarbonate, often results in worsening of the hypokalemia due to greater bicarbonate wasting associated with increases in the filtered bicarbonate load.

Certain tubular toxins may be associated with severe potassium losses, including aminoglycosides, cisplatinum, and ifosfamide. Amphotericin B results in significant potassium wasting accompanied by renal tubular acidosis. In many of these conditions, simultaneous use of amiloride may diminish potassium losses by as much as 50%. Causes of hypokalemia and potassium depletion are summarized in Table 118–2.

HYPERKALEMIC DISORDERS

Hyperkalemic, Hypotensive or Normotensive Syndromes

Disorders that affect the transepithelial potential difference and can result in hyperkalemia, acidosis, and extracellular volume depletion include inactivating mutations of ENaC (pseudohypoaldosteronism type 1), which may be accompanied by high renin and aldosterone levels. Primary selective hypoaldosteronism or complete adrenal cortical deficiency is associated with elevated renin and low aldosterone. Secondary hypoaldosteronism may be seen in hyporenin states caused by use of β-blockers or nonsteroidal anti-inflammatory drugs (NSAIDs), or by autonomic neuropathies in diabetes, analgesic nephropathy, sickle cell anemia, systemic lupus erythematosus (SLE), and amyloidosis. Hypopituitarism does not characteristically result in a disorder of potassium. Commonly used angiotensin-converting enzyme inhibitors and angiotensin II type I–receptor blockers can decrease aldosterone and increase renin, particularly when given to patients who have renal dysfunction or low urine volumes. These drugs can cause hyperkalemia.

The ENaC may also be inhibited by potassium-sparing diuretics, amiloride, triamterene, and certain medications secreted by the proximal tubule cation transporter, such as trimethoprim and pentamidine, as well

TABLE 118–2 CAUSES OF HYPOKALEMIA AND POTASSIUM DEPLETION

NONRENAL CAUSES
Dietary deficiency
Gastrointestinal losses
RENAL CAUSES
Osmotic diuresis
Diuretics: acetazolamide, furosemide, and thiazides
Renal tubular disorders: Fanconi's syndrome, Bartter's syndrome, Gitelman's syndrome
Toxic medications: aminoglycosides, carboplatinum, amphotericin
Nonreabsorbable anions
Hypertensive syndromes with alkalosis:
Liddle's syndrome—low renin, low aldosterone
Licorice ingestion and apparent mineralocorticoid excess—low renin, low aldosterone
Renal artery stenosis and renin-secreting tumors—high renin, high aldosterone
Adrenal hyperfunction or tumor—low renin, high aldosterone
Ectopic ACTH—low renin, high cortisol

as by lithium. Inhibition of the aldosterone receptor may be the result of antagonists such as spironolactone and eplerenone. Because these drugs have been used for cardiac protection, a marked increase in serious hyperkalemic events has been noted among patients with heart failure. Spironolactone is a progesterone derivative. In pregnancy progesterone, by blocking the aldosterone receptor, may protect against excessive renal losses of potassium, despite the marked hyperaldosteronemic state. Most progesterone analogs do not, however, result in hyperkalemia.

Heparin, including low-molecular-weight and fractionated forms, can lead to hyperkalemia even in small subcutaneous doses, presumably as a result of decreased production of adrenal aldosterone. A number of important diseases disrupt cortical nephron function, including SLE, urinary tract obstruction, amyloidosis, kidney and bone marrow transplant nephropathy, and sickle cell nephropathy. Males who present with hyperkalemia and renal insufficiency of unknown cause should have prostatic obstruction excluded. Each of these conditions may also be associated with failure to concentrate the urine (nephrogenic diabetes insipidus) or with a hyperchloremic metabolic acidosis caused by abnormalities in acid secretion. Collectively, they are known as type 4 renal tubular acidoses and may be associated with inability to acidify the urine. By comparison, hypoaldosteronism is associated with normally acidic urine but less ammonium excretion, which accounts for the decreased renal acid excretion.

Hyperkalemic, Hypertensive Syndromes

A genetic disorder known as Gordon's syndrome (pseudohypoaldosteronism type 2) is associated with hyperkalemia, volume expansion, and metabolic acidosis and is highly responsive to thiazide diuretics. It is associated with increased sodium chloride reabsorption in the distal nephron. The increased reabsorption of electroneutral sodium chloride diminishes the transepithelial lumen-negative voltage and therefore the driving force for potassium secretion, as well as hydrogen secretion.

Treatment with cyclosporine or tacrolimus may also produce a form of hyperkalemic acidosis. The mechanism may involve inhibition of cyclooxygenase 2 (COX2) and therefore hyporenin-hypoaldosteronism. There may also be a decrease in the apical potassium secretory channel in the collecting duct. NSAIDs can cause hyperkalemia, particularly in renal patients by several mechanisms. There is decreased sodium delivery, increased water reabsorption leading to low flow, and a decrease in renin and aldosterone. Hypertension with the NSAIDs is most likely caused by interference with peripheral circulatory vasodilating prostaglandins as well as renal salt and water retention.

Causes of hyperkalemia and potassium excess are shown in Table 118–3.

TABLE 118–3 CAUSES OF HYPERKALEMIA AND POTASSIUM EXCESS

Cell breakdown—hemolysis and rhabdomyolysis
Excessive intake
Decreased excretion
Renal failure
Hypotension and metabolic acidosis:
Pseudohypoaldosteronism type I—high renin, high aldosterone
Potassium-sparing diuretics—amiloride and triamterene
Drug effects of sodium channel inhibition—trimethaprim
Hypoaldosteronism—high renin, low aldosterone
Hyporenin-hypoaldosteronism—low renin, low aldosterone
Hypertension and metabolic acidosis
Gordon's syndrome (pseudohypoaldosteronism, type 2)
Cyclosporine

Diagnosis

It may be difficult to determine exactly the state of total body potassium stores from the serum potassium level. As much as 100 to 300 mmol of potassium may be lost from the body with a fall in serum potassium of only 1 mmol/L. However, it is useful to take a detailed medical history, attending to medications, family history, and sources of potassium excess or loss. It is also important to perform a complete physical examination, with particular attention to blood pressure, extracellular volume status, heart rate and rhythm, and muscle strength and reflexes. Finally, assessment of a 12-lead electrocardiogram and evaluations of renal function, acid-base balance, osmolar status, and the concentrations of other important electrolytes, such as magnesium, should be performed. Certain syndromes are associated with hypokalemia and alkalosis or acidosis; some with hypotension or hypertension; and some with hyperosmolality or hypo-osmolality.

Usually, the first clue to a disorder in potassium balance is an abnormal serum potassium concentration. Hypokalemia may be the most common electrolyte disorder discovered in practice. When the potassium is elevated above normal, it is imperative to exclude some common artifacts, known as pseudohyperkalemia. Hemolysis in the test tube that releases potassium is a common artifact, usually recognized in the laboratory. A particular challenge in some patients with autoimmune hemolytic anemia is to distinguish between hyperkalemia that may exist in vivo and laboratory artifact due to hemolysis in the test tube. In some cases of cold-induced hemolysis, it is important to collect the blood and allow it to clot in a warm environment. Some patients have pseudohyperkalemia resulting from high platelet counts, usually in excess of 1 million/μL, or severe cases of myelogenous leukemias; serum potassium can increase due to release of potassium as the blood clots. In such cases, it is reasonable to obtain a plasma potassium level, which should be within the normal range. Normally, the increase in serum versus plasma potassium levels is less than 0.5 mmol/L. Many elderly patients have high potassium due to poor venipuncture sites or ischemia related to application of the tourniquet and clenching of the fist. In such cases, blood may need to be drawn without a tourniquet.

The urine chemistry is important in that it can give insight into the appropriateness of renal potassium handling, given an abnormality in the serum potassium. In general, in a state of potassium deficiency, a low urinary potassium excretion value would be expected, unless the urine was the source of the potassium depletion. In a hypokalemic patient, a urinary potassium concentration greater than 30 mEq/L suggests renal potassium wasting, whereas extrarenal losses are usually reflected by concentrations lower than 20 mEq/L. In a state of potassium excess, the kidney retains a high capacity to eliminate potassium, so that urinary potassium excretion can be expected to be maximal, unless urinary underexcretion was the cause of the hyperkalemia. A common finding in the urine when high aldosterone is present is a high potassium-to-sodium relationship, whereas in a patient with hypoaldosteronism it may be the opposite. Another frequently used tool to determine the appropriateness of urinary potassium content is known as the transtubular potassium gradient (TTKG). What is indirectly being estimated in this case is the gradient between the plasma potassium (P_k) and the fluid in the distal cortical collecting duct segments. Measurements are made when the urine is hyperosmotic to plasma, because under those conditions it is assumed that the osmolality in the cortical collecting duct lumen will have equilibrated with plasma osmolality, owing to the effects of ADH-dependent water reabsorption in the cortex. An analysis of the urine osmolality (Uosm) and urinary potassium concentration (UK) is used to approximate the concentration of potassium in the inaccessible cortical collecting duct lumen. For example, if the Uosm is twice the plasma osmolality (Posm), then it is assumed that the urinary potassium concentration is twice the collecting duct luminal potassium concentration. Of course, this depends on an assumption of minimal potassium transport within the medulla. Although imperfect in assumptions, these calculations can be used based on empirical information gained from patients with known disturbances in aldosterone.

The equation, (UK/PK)/(Uosm/Posm) = TTKG, has been useful in the following situations. In a hyperkalemic patient, a TTKG greater than 8 to 10, would be expected. Lower values would lead to suspicion of renal underexcretion as the cause of the hyperkalemia. In such a case, a dose of mineralocorticoid could be given and the TTKG repeated, to determine whether there is potential benefit in treatment with mineralocorticoid. In a hypokalemic patient, the normal kidney should be conserving potassium, so the TTKG should be less than 3. If it is greater than 3, urinary potassium wasting would be suspected as the cause of the hypokalemia.

Treatment

Rx

Most hospitals regulate the rate at which potassium can be given to patients intravenously. The reason is the recognition that potassium must traverse the extracellular space before repleting intracellular stores, and it is easy to dangerously elevate the serum potassium. Such guidelines usually suggest that oral potassium be given if possible, and that intravenous potassium be given slowly at a rate that usually does not exceed 10 to 20 mmol/hour. However, in cases of severe hypokalemia, greater amounts may be required, particularly if there are cardiac arrhythmias, and a central venous catheter may be required. In these unusual circumstances, it is best to consult with a specialist and the pharmacy.

Oral potassium replacement should be in the form of chloride salts, particularly if hypokalemia is associated with chloride-depletion metabolic alkalosis. If severe phosphate deficiency is present, solutions of potassium phosphate may be used. Giving potassium with a nonreabsorbable anion such as gluconate may inadequately replace a potassium deficit. In patients who have prerenal azotemia associated with hyperglycemia or severe metabolic alkalosis, it should be realized that volume expansion with sodium chloride solutions alone could result in life-threatening potassium losses, despite improvement in the extracellular volume. This is the result of improved GFR, which increases urinary glucose excretion (osmotic diuresis) in the hyperglycemic patient and bicarbonaturia in the alkalotic patient. Potassium must be given in anticipation of such events. Attention to the urine output and ongoing losses is crucial. In a hypokalemic patient, care must be exercised when glucose-containing solutions are given, because the resulting increase in insulin may further decrease the blood potassium level.

If the potassium level is less than 3 mmol/L, it may be best to treat the patient in a monitored setting to observe for cardiac complications. If ongoing losses of potassium are severe, it may be necessary to provide a potassium-sparing diuretic or to treat the cause of the ongoing losses (e.g., diarrhea). Magnesium should be measured and replaced, if necessary, in any hypokalemic patient.

Treatment of hyperkalemia follows an understanding of the regulators of internal and external potassium balance. If hyperkalemia is severe, the most immediate requirement is to achieve a rapid reduction in potassium concentration. However, if hyperkalemia is associated with cardiac arrhythmias, calcium gluconate, 10 mL of a 10% solution over 10 to 20 minutes, is often administered to stabilize electrical effects on cardiac excitation. If calcium chloride is used, it should be administered through a central access line, because extravasation of the chloride salt may result in tissue necrosis. Calcium will not lower the potassium concentration. To do so, one can take advantage of the known effects of insulin to distribute potassium into cells, usually with a time course of 10 to 15 minutes. In the nonhyperglycemic patient, 10 units of regular insulin should be given with glucose, whereas in the hyperglycemic patient, diabetic glucose may be avoided. Glucose administration should be spread out over 1 hour and is best given as a 10% solution for a total of 30 to 50 g. The blood glucose level should be monitored. Fifty-percent glucose may worsen hyperkalemia if given so rapidly as to create a hyperosmolar state. The β_2-agonist effect to distribute potassium may be utilized by treating with albuterol nebulizers. Higher doses are required than are usually used in the treatment of asthma. In some cases, intravenous β-adrenergic agonists have been used. Epinephrine, with its early α-adrenergic effects, should not be used. Although sodium bicarbonate has been a method of treatment, it should be reserved for acidemic patients who otherwise require alkalinization, and attention should be paid to other simultaneous electrolyte disorders, particularly hypocalcemia. Complications of sodium bicarbonate infusions include hypernatremia, volume expansion, and decreased ionized calcium, resulting in tetany.

Over the longer term, potassium loss from the body should be achieved. Cation exchange resins such as sodium polystyrene sulfonate can be given by mouth or as an enema with an osmotic agent such as sorbitol. A dose of 30 to 50 g may achieve a decline in potassium levels over several hours. It should be noted that this resin will provide a sodium load to the patient. Caution about prolonged use of these resins includes the possibility of colonic ulcerations; in addition, if given by mouth, they may bind other medications such as lithium and thyroxine, limiting their absorption. The resins should not be given in combination with aluminum-based antacids such as aluminum hydroxide, because the resulting concretions could obstruct the gastrointestinal tract. If the patient is volume expanded, potassium-losing diuretics such as furosemide and Diuril (chlorothiazide), or acetazolamide if alkalotic, may enhance renal potassium clearance. If the patient is volume depleted, isotonic saline expansion may improve urine output and, with it, potassium excretion. Diabetic patients who may be potassium depleted but present oliguric with hyperkalemia may become hypokalemic as urine output increases and require potassium replacement. Patients who are treated with angiotensin blockers, particularly if diabetic and with renal insufficiency, may be particularly prone to hyperkalemia. They should have a repeat potassium measurement within several days after starting one of these medications or with a change in dose and should be counseled about the potential dangers of hyperkalemia should they become volume depleted.

The patient who has renal failure with hyperkalemia is unlikely to have access to dialysis within the time frame of need to lower the potassium concentration; therefore, the previously mentioned procedures should be followed until dialysis can be mobilized. In the patient with renal failure, it is extremely important to be cautious with blood transfusions, which provide a large potassium load to a patient who will not be able to excrete it.

SUGGESTED READINGS

Alfonzo AV, Isles C, Geddes C, et al: Potassium disorders—clinical spectrum and emergency management. Resuscitation 2006;70:10–25. *Review with practical algorithms.*

Cohn JN, Cowey PR, Whelton PK, Prisant LM: New guidelines for potassium replacement in clinical practice: A contemporary review by the National Council on Potassium and Clinical Practice. Arch Intern Med 2000;160:2429–2436. *Consensus guidelines.*

Perezella MA: Drug-induced hyperkalemia: Old culprits and new offenders. Am J Med 2000;109:307–314. *Review of drug-induced causes.*

Section XI Renal

ACID-BASE DISORDERS

Julian L. Seifter

Definition

Normal Acid-Base Physiology

Many of the body's metabolic and physiologic functions are pH dependent or pH sensitive. The range of normal arterial pH is 7.38 to 7.42. Intracellular pH is lower than extracellular pH because cells are electronegative with respect to extracellular fluid and metabolically produced acids are constantly being transported to extracellular fluid for eventual elimination from the body. In severe disease states, arterial pH may fall as low as 6.8 and rise as high as 7.8. Strenuous exercise with the metabolic production of lactate may transiently, but severely lower pH, even in normal healthy individuals.

pH is equal to minus the log of the hydrogen ion concentration. At a pH of 7.40, the hydrogen ion concentration is 40 nanoequivalents (nEq) per liter, a very small concentration in comparison to serum sodium at 140 mEq/L. The hydrogen ion concentration of body fluids is in equilibrium with each of multiple buffers, such as proteins, phosphate, and hemoglobin (the isohydric principle), but acid-base equilibria in the body are often analyzed by using the CO_2/HCO_3^- system and the relationship of the proton concentration (thus pH) to the ratio of HCO_3^- to CO_2. The Henderson-Hasselbalch equation is a logarithmic expression of the relationship.

$$CO_2 + H_2O \rightarrow H_2CO_3 \rightarrow H^+ + HCO_3^-$$
$$pH = pK + \log [HCO_3]/0.03(Pco_2)$$

In this equation, pK, or the dissociation constant, is 6.1; 0.03 (mM/mm Hg) is the solubility factor for CO_2 in solution. The product of $0.03 \times Pco_2$ represents the carbonic acid concentration; the total CO_2 in plasma is the sum of HCO_3^-, normally about 25 mM, and $0.03 \times Pco_2$, normally about 1.2 mM. It is important to note that pH is a function of the *ratio* of HCO_3^- to Pco_2. The HCO_3^- concentration in the numerator is regulated by the kidney, and Pco_2 is regulated by the lung, the major organ systems involved in acid-base balance.

Production of Acids and the Elimination of CO_2 by the Lung

Volatile acid is the term used for the carbon dioxide produced by metabolic processes in all tissues, an amount that approximates 20,000 mmol/day. This CO_2 is carried to the lung, where it is eliminated by alveolar ventilation. Steady-state Pco_2 is normally 38 to 42 mm Hg.

Nonvolatile acid is a term used to describe acids other than carbonic acid that are formed primarily from protein metabolism. The usual amount of formation is approximately 1 to 2 mEq of H^+ per kilogram of body weight per day. Most diets that contain animal protein have a net positive quantity of nonvolatile acids, primarily from the sulfur-containing amino acids cysteine and methionine; phosphate from phosphoproteins, phospholipids, phosphonucleotides, and inorganic sources; and chloride salts of lysine, arginine, and histidine. The addition of protons to body fluids by these acid end products can be seen as consuming bicarbonate, which then needs to be replenished by the kidney as it eliminates the proton. Oxidation of carbohydrates and fats results in the production of water and CO_2, but not nonvolatile acids. High-protein diets increase the metabolic acid load. Under pathologic conditions, other acids are produced in the body, such as ketoacids in diabetes and lactic acid in states of increased anaerobic metabolism.

In most humans, particularly those who eat animal protein or an acid-ash diet, the requirement for net acid excretion dominates. However, vegetarians could have an overall alkaline-ash diet, which means that to maintain a steady-state normal serum HCO_3^- concentration, net alkali would need to be excreted to match intake. It is the role of the kidney to excrete this acid or alkali load to maintain a steady-state serum HCO_3^- concentration, normally in the range of 22 to 28 mM.

As for sodium, water, and potassium balance, the concept of steady state is important to acid-base regulation. The amount of acid or base produced per day must be equivalent to that excreted. If CO_2 production exceeds CO_2 excretion by the lungs, a state of respiratory acidosis characterized by a high Pco_2 will develop. If the rate of CO_2 excretion exceeds production, a state of respiratory alkalosis exists. The following equation shows the inverse relationship of alveolar ventilation, $\dot{V}a$, to Pco_2:

$$\dot{V}a = CO_2 \text{ elimination} \div Pco_2$$

Note the similarity of this relationship to a clearance expression in which the clearance of CO_2 is a pulmonary function (alveolar ventilation) directly related to the rate of CO_2 eliminated and inversely related to Pco_2. The steady-state principle here is that CO_2 production by tissues must equal CO_2 elimination by the lungs for a constant Pco_2 to be maintained. The changes in Pco_2 are almost always caused by changes in $\dot{V}a$ rather than production of CO_2. Thus, respiratory acidosis is nearly always a consequence of decreased pulmonary ventilation from lung or central nervous system (CNS) disease rather than only increased production of CO_2. Respiratory alkalosis develops from hyperventilation rather than decreased CO_2 production. In either case, when the elimination rate of CO_2 (the product of $\dot{V}a \times Pco_2$) again equals CO_2 production, a new steady state will prevail with no net carbonic acid retention or loss.

In metabolic disorders, if metabolic production of acid exceeds elimination, a state of metabolic acidosis exists, whereas if elimination exceeds production, metabolic alkalosis will develop. In the case of metabolic acidosis, production could exceed excretion via a marked excess in the production rate, as might be seen with diabetic ketoacidosis (DKA) or lactic acidosis, or it could develop even with a normal rate of metabolic acid production if the kidney were unable to eliminate acid normally, as in kidney failure.

Bicarbonate and the Kidney in Acid-Base Balance

The first role of the kidney in acid-base balance is to reabsorb all the filtered HCO_3^- (Fig. 119–1). At a normal glomerular filtration rate (i.e., 180 L/day in an adult) and serum HCO_3^- concentration of 25 mEq/L, it follows that 4500 mEq of HCO_3^- is filtered in 1 day. Loss of even a small fraction of that HCO_3^- would result in metabolic acidosis, so the necessity for reabsorption is clear.

The Proximal Tubule

The bulk of HCO_3^- reabsorption is accomplished in the proximal tubule, where 80 to 90% is reabsorbed. The mechanism for reabsorption is a proton secretory process that works as follows. The brush border membranes of the proximal tubule cell contain transporters known as Na/H exchangers (NHE3 is the abundant isoform). Through the normal function of basolateral membrane Na^+, K^+-adenosine triphosphatase (ATPase), cell Na^+ is kept at low concentration so that filtered Na^+ in the lumen will be favored to enter the cell in exchange for H^+ secreted into the lumen. This H^+ will combine with filtered HCO_3^- to rapidly form H_2CO_3, which will then dehydrate in the lumen to form CO_2 and H_2O. This process is greatly facilitated by luminal carbonic anhydrase (CA_{IV}). The CO_2 next enters the proximal cell, where it reforms HCO_3^-, also helped by intracellular carbonic anhydrase (CA_{II}). The HCO_3^- is then transported back to the blood by a cotransporter coupling Na and $3HCO_3^-$ (NBC), thereby accomplishing net HCO_3^- reabsorption. Note that the entire process requires a source of adenosine triphosphate (ATP) (mitochondrial) for the Na/K pump, intact NHE3 and NBC, and two isoforms of carbonic anhydrase. A disturbance at any of these sites may disrupt proximal HCO_3^- reabsorption enough to cause loss of HCO_3^- in urine.

There is continued HCO_3^- reabsorption in the thick limb of Henle via a similar mechanism of Na/H exchange on the luminal membrane.

The Cortical Collecting Duct

The cortical collecting duct (CCD) continues to reabsorb HCO_3^-—about 5 to 10% of the filtered load—by the following mechanism. In principal cells, Na^+ is reabsorbed by the epithelial Na^+ channel (ENaC) driven by secondary active transport (as a result of lowering the cell Na^+ level by the ATP-dependent active transport of Na^+ by Na^+, K^+-ATPases at the blood side). The lumen becomes electronegative, thus favoring the secretion of both K^+, through K^+ channels, and H^+, through H^+-ATPases on the luminal surface of the intercalated cells, which are the acid-secreting cells (α-intercalated cells). The secreted H^+ will combine with the remaining HCO_3^- in the lumen to generate CO_2, with subsequent reabsorption of CO_2, re-formation of cellular HCO_3^- with the help of cellular carbonic anhydrase (CA_{II}), and then exchange of HCO_3^- from cell to blood and entry of Cl^- via Cl/HCO_3 exchangers. These exchangers

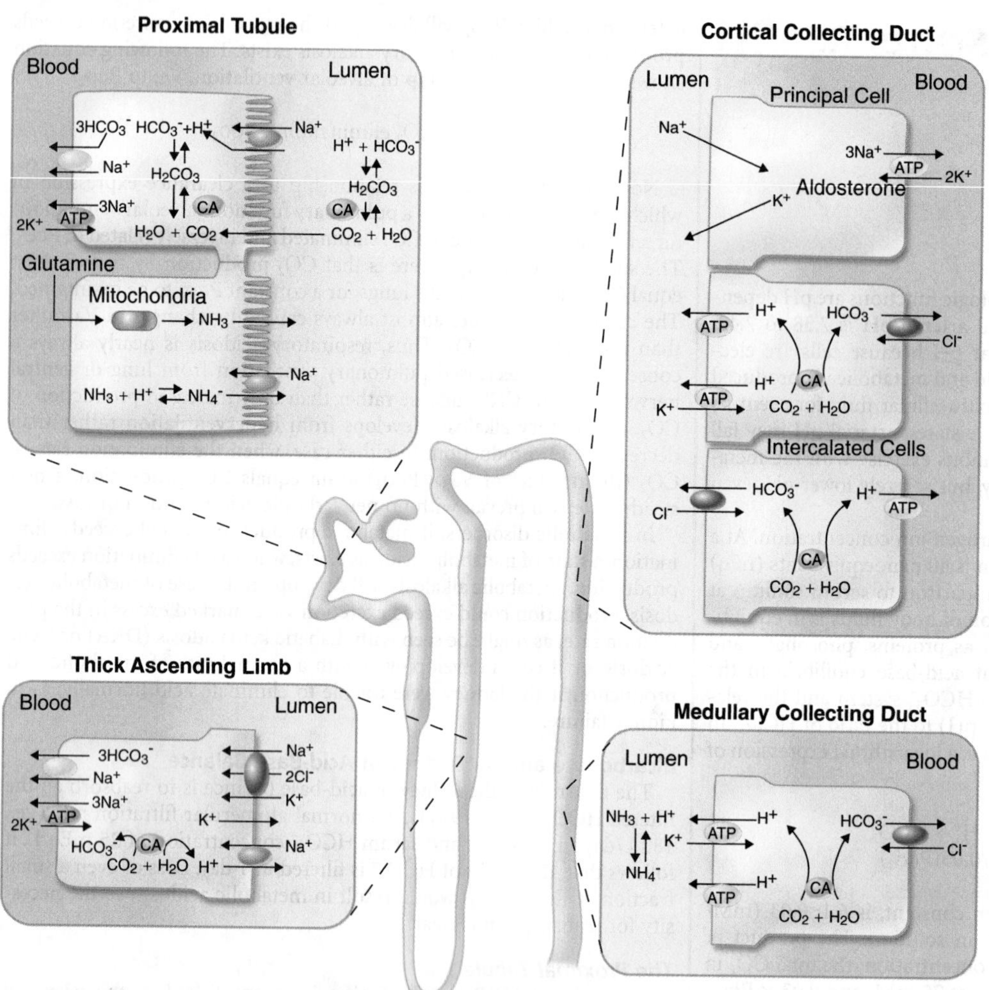

FIGURE 119–1 • Renal acidification mechanisms. ATP = adenosine triphosphate; CA = carbonic anhydrase.

belong to a family of HCO_3^--transporting proteins (SLC4) that includes the red blood cell, band 3, Cl/HCO_3 exchanger, and epithelial anion exchangers mediating Cl/HCO_3 transport (AE1–3). It is at this distal site that tubular fluid pH starts to fall to levels below pH 6.0.

There are some collecting duct cells that have reverse polarity such that they secrete HCO_3^- into the lumen in exchange for Cl^- entry into the cell, and the H^+-ATPase faces the blood side of the cell (β-intercalated cells). These cells may be important when a net amount of HCO_3^- needs to be excreted, as with an alkaline-ash diet. An elevated extracellular HCO_3^- concentration will increase HCO_3^- secretion by these cells, in contrast to an inhibitory effect on HCO_3^- reabsorption in both proximal and α-CCD cells.

The Medullary Collecting Duct

The medullary collecting duct continues to secrete protons into the luminal fluid, where the pH reaches its lowest values of close to 5.0. The mechanism is due to continued function of H^+-ATPases with an additional role of an ATP-dependent K/H exchanger, a member of the family of K^+, H^+-ATPases found in the stomach and colon.

Once the filtered HCO_3^- is fully reabsorbed, the kidney is still required to eliminate an additional net amount of acid equivalent to that produced in metabolism. The majority of this net acid excretion is in the form of ammonium, NH_4^+, derived from the renal synthesis of ammonia from glutamine in the proximal tubule and the titration of filtered phosphate to acid phosphate (titratable acidity).

$$NH_3 + H^+ \rightarrow NH_4^+ \text{ pK } 9.1, \text{ and}$$
$$HPO_4^{2-} + H^+ \rightarrow H_2PO_4^- \text{ pK } 6.8$$

Urinary Buffers

As the collecting duct cells continue to secrete H^+ with a diminishing luminal HCO_3^- concentration and lowering of pH, H^+ is captured by the urinary buffers. The resulting alkalinization of the cells after H^+ leaves results in the formation of HCO_3^- ready for transport into blood. This is considered "new" HCO_3^- generation because it is not a result of filtered HCO_3^- reabsorption. The amount of new HCO_3^- matches the amount of net acid eliminated and results in a return to normal acid-base equilibrium.

The ability of the kidney to lower urinary pH to values as low as 5.0 enables the buffers to capture a proton. Net acid excretion in urine is accomplished not simply by a decrease in urine pH but also by titration of these important urinary buffers. For example, a liter of urine at pH 5.0 contains only 10^{-5} molar hydrogen ion, or 0.01 mmol/L. Note how this compares with the need to excrete 70 mmol of hydrogen ion daily in an average person. In fact, it is the failure to produce enough ammonium in chronic renal failure that leads to a poorly buffered, though acid urine and an inability to excrete enough net acid to stay in normal balance.

Regulation of Urinary Acid Secretion

Renal mechanisms of urinary acidification are adaptable. Transport processes such as H^+-ATPases, Na/H exchange, and Cl/HCO_3 exchange can increase or decrease their capacity to handle acid-base equivalents, depending on the challenge presented, and the renal ammoniagenic mechanisms are also critically regulated to serve the acid-base needs of the individual. Metabolic acidosis and respiratory acidosis increase the capacity to reabsorb HCO_3^-, including increased expression of the transporters involved in acidifying the urine. At the same time, increased ammonia production enables increased acid excretion and new HCO_3^- generation. Metabolic alkalosis and respiratory alkalosis have the opposite effects.

In the end, net acid production must equal net acid excretion. When the diet calls for excretion of acids, urine pH will fall and urine will become nominally free of bicarbonate. When there is an alkaline load, the kidney will reject the excess filtered HCO_3^- and urine pH may approach a maximum value of 8.0 to 8.5.

Carbonic anhydrase is important in acid-secreting epithelia, as well as in other cells such as red blood cells, in which conversion of large quantities of CO_2 to HCO_3^- is required. In the proximal tubule, carbonic anhydrase exists not only within cells but also on the luminal brush border membrane, where it functions to accelerate the dehydration of carbonic acid to CO_2, thereby allowing the large amount of reabsorption necessary in that segment. The distal nephron, which has a smaller requirement for bicarbonate reabsorption, lacks luminal carbonic anhydrase. However, intracellular carbonic anhydrase is present in all acid-handling cells.

Note that in acid-secreting cells, as protons exit across the apical membrane, bicarbonate exits across the basolateral membrane, back to blood. These processes could be reversed in bicarbonate-secreting cells. In addition, the mechanism of proton secretion and bicarbonate reabsorption may vary in different cell types. Compare Na/H exchange in the proximal tubule with the proton ATPase of the distal tubule. Also recall that the luminal sodium concentration is high and equivalent to the extracellular Na^+ level in the proximal luminal fluid and that pH has not usually fallen below 6.8 because of incomplete bicarbonate reabsorption. Therefore, the gradients can generate enough energy to support exchange of Na^+ for H^+. In the distal nephron, the Na^+ concentration may decrease because of Na^+ reabsorption without water in the diluting segments, and the pH of the luminal fluid falls as bicarbonate is cleared from its contents. In these conditions, it is likely that further proton secretion will require the additional energy of an ATPase.

As previously mentioned, ammoniagenesis is a key element in urinary acid excretion by providing the major buffer for protons. Ammonia is produced predominantly in the proximal tubule cell by mitochondrial glutaminase enzymes. Production is increased by increasing the acid load in the body and by other mechanisms of acidifying the intracellular milieu (hypokalemia and respiratory acidosis). In particular, hypokalemia, like metabolic acidosis, stimulates excretion of ammonium. This is useful to body economy because NH_4^+ can preserve scarce potassium in the hypokalemic state as a counter-ion for anion excretion. Similarly, in response to metabolic acidosis, the kidney would ideally excrete chloride with ammonium and preserve Na^+ and K^+.

Ammonia can be secreted by nonionic diffusion into the proximal fluid, where it will pick up a proton and form ammonium (NH_4^+), or it could form ammonium within the proximal tubule cell and be secreted via Na/NH_4 exchange, a mode of operation of the Na/H exchanger. Ammonium may be reabsorbed by the thick ascending limb of Henle on the Na/K/2Cl transporter, where it can substitute for K^+. By countercurrent multiplication, the medullary interstitial fluid will contain large concentrations of NH_4^+. Less ammonium will therefore reach the highly perfused renal cortex, where it could otherwise dissipate into renal venous blood; the countercurrent mechanism also allows for ammonia to diffuse into the lumen of the collecting duct, where it will be trapped as ammonium in the acid tubular fluid. Collecting duct cells also secrete NH_3 by way of glycoproteins that are in the family of the Rh factor, red blood cell ammonia transporters.

Regulation is accomplished at a number of levels. Hormones such as angiotensin II and catecholamines stimulate Na^+ reabsorption in the proximal tubule by increasing Na/H exchange. Aldosterone increases proton ATPase in the distal collecting duct cell and stimulates Na^+ reabsorption, with the result being increasing proton secretion. Low extracellular fluid volume increases proximal HCO_3^- reabsorption, as does hypokalemia and high Pco_2. These factors also stimulate distal proton secretion.

Hyperkalemia may limit urinary acidification by several mechanisms, including decreased ammonia synthesis, decreased NH_3 entering the countercurrent multiplier in the loop of Henle, and decreased H^+ secretion by ATPases in the collecting duct as the need to secrete K^+ predominates.

Diagnosis

Assessment of clinical acid-base disturbances usually begins with measurement of arterial blood gases. In some situations, venous blood can be used as an alternative to the more invasive arterial puncture if one recalls that normal venous pH is approximately 0.05 pH units more acid than arterial pH and Pco_2 is 5 to 6 mm Hg higher than that of arterial blood. Except in conditions of low cardiac output, these assumptions are reasonable. Venous bicarbonate concentrations are normally greater than arterial concentrations. Tissue CO_2 is transported to the lungs as venous bicarbonate, so a rise in this quantity will depend on tissue CO_2 production and the capacity to convert CO_2 to HCO_3^- by erythrocytes.

If arterial pH is below normal, acidemia is said to exist. If pH is greater than normal, alkalemia exists. This does not exclude the possibility of many processes simultaneously present that would drive the pH in an upward or downward direction. The individual processes are known as *acidoses* or *alkaloses.* Because multiple processes may coexist (for example, it would not be unusual for a patient to be vomiting and have diarrhea), an abnormal pH is not required for there to be acid-base disturbances. Because pH is related to the ratio of HCO_3^- to Pco_2, the finding of an abnormal bicarbonate level alone cannot define acidemia or alkalemia.

It is customary to define acid-base balance in terms of the hydrogen ion concentration and the buffer pair bicarbonate and Pco_2. The following equation is an expression of the overall equilibrium of CO_2 and water with protons and bicarbonate:

$$CO_2 + H_2O \rightarrow H_2CO_3 \rightarrow H^+ + HCO_3^-$$

The addition of CO_2, as in respiratory acidosis, can be seen to increase hydrogen and bicarbonate concentrations. Removal of CO_2 in respiratory alkalosis will decrease CO_2, protons, and bicarbonate. The addition of protons with an anion other than HCO_3^- in metabolic acidosis will lead to an increased proton and decreased bicarbonate concentration. The CO_2 can be rapidly removed by the lungs. Removal of HCO_3^- with a cation such as Na^+, also a cause of metabolic acidosis, will increase the proton concentration and lower the HCO_3^- concentration. Metabolic alkalosis might be caused by the addition of $NaHCO_3$ with a resulting decrease in the proton concentration or by removal of H^+ with chloride, thereby leading to a decreased proton concentration and increased HCO_3^-.

Compensatory Changes

When an acid-base disturbance develops, the initial response to modulate its severity depends on the titration of various body buffer pairs. For example, phosphate, hemoglobin, and other proteins (including albumin) change in protonated and unprotonated concentrations. The body will then further attempt to correct the extracellular pH toward normal (but not to normal). For metabolic disturbances caused by increased or decreased nonvolatile acid, the response is respiratory; for primary respiratory acidosis and alkalosis, the compensation is renal. The degree of this compensation cannot be calculated without the input of empirically obtained data indicating normal human responses (Table 119–1). Note that the direction of change in HCO_3^- and Pco_2 is the same when the primary disturbance is compensated; the ratio of HCO_3^- to Pco_2 and thus pH becomes more normal. In Table 119–1, also note that these compensations tend to take time to develop to their fullest, and therefore acid-base disturbances, particularly the respiratory conditions, are classified as acute or chronic (lasting longer than 24 to 48 hours).

In cases of metabolic acidosis resulting in acidemia, the CNS, through chemoreceptors, will stimulate ventilation with a subsequent fall in Pco_2.

TABLE 119–1 EXPECTED DEGREES OF COMPENSATION IN ACID-BASE DISORDERS

Disorder	Expected Compensation
Metabolic acidosis	Steady state in 12–36 hours Expected Pco_2 = 1.5 (measured HCO_3) + 8 ± 2
Metabolic alkalosis	Less predictable Expected Pco_2 increases 0.5 mm Hg per 1-mEq/L increase in HCO_3
Respiratory acidosis	
Acute	Expected 1-mEq/L increase in HCO_3 per 10-mm Hg rise in Pco_2
Chronic, 24–36 hours	Expected 3- to 5-mEq/L increase in HCO_3 per 10-mm Hg rise in Pco_2
Respiratory alkalosis	
Acute	Expected 1- to 2-mEq/L fall in HCO_3 per 10-mm Hg fall in Pco_2
Chronic, after 24–36 hours	Expected 5-mEq/L fall in HCO_3 per 10-mm Hg fall in Pco_2

When the bicarbonate concentration increases as a result of metabolic alkalosis, there will be a hypoventilatory response that raises P_{CO_2}. Clinically, one should not equate the respiratory rate with the ventilation rate because the typical Kussmaul respirations in metabolic acidosis, a sign of respiratory compensation, are due to increased minute ventilation rather than increased respiration frequency. Rapid breathing may not be associated with increased minute ventilation or decreased P_{CO_2}.

The acute stimulus of hypercapnia to increase renal acid excretion disappears in chronic respiratory acidosis when, at the elevated P_{CO_2}, carbonic acid production and elimination are again equal. However, the hypochloremia and elevated serum HCO_3^- maintained by the high P_{CO_2} remains. In respiratory alkalosis, the primary event is a fall in P_{CO_2} because of increased $\dot{V}a$. In the transition from acute to chronic respiratory alkalosis, the compensatory mechanisms that initially helped maintain a more normal systemic pH are no longer required when CO_2 production and elimination become equal. Thus, the initial decreased renal acid excretion in compensation for respiratory alkalosis ceases, but low serum HCO_3^- and high serum Cl^- concentrations are still maintained.

In identifying whether an acid-base disturbance is simple (a single disturbance with its compensation) or complex, it is useful to compare the expected compensation with the observed parameters of the blood gases (Table 119–2). For example, if P_{CO_2} is lower in a patient with metabolic acidosis than would be predicted for the simple disorder, an additional process has to be present that must be a respiratory alkalosis because it drives P_{CO_2} down. If P_{CO_2} were higher than what would be predicted for a low bicarbonate level in a patient with metabolic acidosis, there would be coexistence of a respiratory acidosis.

Because there is no reason that multiple acid-base disturbances could not coexist, one should be able to expect a specific process by eliciting a proper history. For example, hypochloremic alkalosis would be suggested by a history of vomiting or the use of thiazide or loop diuretics. The process of metabolic acidosis might be anticipated in hypotensive shock, sepsis, diarrhea, and renal failure. A history of chronic lung disease could be associated with respiratory acidosis, whereas fever, infection, stroke, or acute pulmonary disease may be a cause of acute respiratory alkalosis. It is important to follow up on the history and physical examination with laboratory clues to detect the presence of these independent disturbances. Furthermore, an abnormal acid-base balance should always alert the clinician to the possible presence of an underlying condition rather than be considered an isolated problem.

TABLE 119–2 LABORATORY STEPS IN IDENTIFYING ACID-BASE DISORDERS

Evaluate pH	Acidemic	Alkalemic
Elevated P_{CO_2}	Respiratory acidosis	Metabolic alkalosis
Elevated HCO_3	Respiratory acidosis	Metabolic alkalosis
Decreased P_{CO_2}	Metabolic acidosis	Respiratory alkalosis
Decreased HCO_3	Metabolic acidosis	Respiratory alkalosis

EVALUATE FOR EXPECTED COMPENSATION

Meets expectation: Simple disorder with compensation or could be offsetting metabolic alkalosis and acidosis

Does not meet expectation: Complex disorder but pH indicates whether acidosis or alkalosis is dominant

If a metabolic disorder is dominant, a P_{CO_2} greater than predicted indicates an additional respiratory acidosis. A P_{CO_2} less than predicted indicates an additional respiratory alkalosis.

If a respiratory disorder is dominant, an HCO_3 concentration greater than predicted indicates additional metabolic alkalosis. An HCO_3 concentration less than predicted indicates an additional metabolic acidosis.

ASSESS ANION GAP

Elevated: Metabolic acidosis is present whether acidemic or alkalemic. If alkalemic, an additional metabolic or respiratory alkalosis is present.

If the gap is greater than the fall in HCO_3, consider an additional metabolic alkalosis or respiratory acidosis.

If the gap is less than the fall in HCO_3, consider an additional non-gap acidosis or respiratory alkalosis.

Adaptations

In addition to the aforementioned compensations, which usually involve the lung for metabolic disturbances and renal excretion for respiratory disturbances, it should be pointed out that the lung adjusts to respiratory disturbances and the kidney will compensate for metabolic disturbances, that is, help modify the pH toward normal. In respiratory acidosis, the peripheral arterial chemosensors and the CNS chemosensors both signal the lung to hyperventilate. Although this signal is unlikely to remove the initial stimulus to CO_2 retention, it will modify the degree of hypercapnia that has developed. Respiratory alkalosis will have the opposite effect on the chemosensors, again modifying the resultant degree of hypocapnia. In the kidney, structural and functional changes may occur in an adaptive way to a disturbed environment. In cases of metabolic acidosis of extrarenal origin, the renal response will be to increase net acid excretion by increasing ammoniagenesis. Bicarbonate reabsorptive processes under the influence of hormones such as glucocorticoids, angiotensin II, and aldosterone will increase, thereby maximizing net acid excretion. In fact, at the membrane transport level, metabolic acidosis itself may result in an increased number of transporters, such as Na/H exchange or proton ATPases, to maximize HCO_3^- reabsorption. Limitation of the effectiveness of bicarbonate reabsorption in metabolic acidosis is due to already low serum levels and therefore a low filtered HCO_3^- concentration and the nearly complete clearance of HCO_3^- from urine. In metabolic alkalosis, the kidney may modulate the degree of alkalemia by enhancing urinary bicarbonate loss. These responses may be limited by mitigating factors such as extracellular volume depletion and hypokalemia (see later).

The Acid-Base Status of the Brain

Peripheral blood does not usually undergo complete compensation for most acid-base disturbances, with the occasional exception of chronic respiratory alkalosis. Yet the CNS closely regulates its pH with nearly full correction occurring within 1 to 2 days. Acute disturbances in acid-base status, before compensation occurs, and rapid treatment of acidemia or alkalemia may have profound effects on brain function. Acute alkalemia may be associated with cerebral vasoconstriction and ischemia, whereas acidemia may result in vasodilation and cerebral edema. Rapid changes in P_{CO_2} affect the CNS chemosensors more quickly than changes in HCO_3^- do because of the more rapid movement of nonionic P_{CO_2} across the blood-brain barrier. It is important to consider the effects of brain pH when approaching an acid-base problem.

METABOLIC ACIDOSIS

Pathobiology

In metabolic acidosis, the primary change is a fall in serum bicarbonate. The compensatory response is increased ventilation with a fall in P_{CO_2}. Worsening acidosis elicits increasing alveolar ventilation.

Primary metabolic acidosis results from an imbalance between net acid production and net acid excretion (NAE) in the form of urinary ammonium and acid phosphate. Consider the following relationship, where U_x represents the urinary concentration and $\dot{V}$ the urinary flow rate:

$$NAE = (U_{NH4^+}\dot{V}) + (U_{phos}\dot{V}) - (U_{bicarb}\dot{V})$$

In a normal steady-state condition, the rate of excretion of net acid must be equal to the rate of production. The normal production rate depends on diet. Metabolic acidosis can develop if there is an inequality in the relationship between net acid production and net acid excretion. Thus, if net acid production were normal, metabolic acidosis could occur because of either failure of bicarbonate reabsorption leading to high bicarbonate excretion rates or failure to elaborate enough urinary buffers, as is the case in renal failure and renal tubular acidosis. In contrast, an inequality could develop if net acid production were excessive or if large extrarenal bicarbonate losses were unable to be matched by maximal adaptive increases in net acid excretion. Endogenous sources of acid include ketoacidosis and lactic acidosis, whereas some exogenous sources are metabolic products of ingested ethylene glycol or methanol. On occasion, strong inorganic acids may be ingested. When net acid is retained in body fluids, the serum bicarbonate concentration falls. However, maintenance of a constant serum HCO_3^- concentration does not guarantee that there is a new steady state in which net acid production is equal to net acid excretion because body buffers such as carbonate salts of bone may become depleted by relentless acid retention. Such is the case in renal failure and distal renal tubular acidosis.

The causes of metabolic acidosis are usually categorized according to the presence of either a normal or an elevated serum anion gap. The serum anion gap is the net charge difference when the sum of chloride and bicarbonate is subtracted from the serum sodium concentration.

$$\text{Anion gap} = Na^+ - (Cl^- + HCO_3^-)$$

The normal anion gap is due to the unmeasured anionic charge associated predominantly with albumin. When acidemia is present, albumin is in a more protonated form, which lowers the normal gap. In alkalemia, the effect of pH is to increase the gap attributed to albumin. Each 1 g/dL of albumin contributes approximately 2.8 mEq/L to the normal anion gap. The anion gap may be low with hypoalbuminemia or with an increase in an unmeasured cation such as IgG myeloma proteins, calcium, lithium, or magnesium. When the anion gap is increased above the normal value of approximately 10 to 12 mEq/L, an anion gap metabolic acidosis is said to exist. The anion gap reflects the presence of a nonchloride acid anion. The accompanying proton is responsible for lowering the serum bicarbonate concentration. The degree of increase in the anion gap, sometimes referred to as the *gap delta,* may be estimated by the difference between the observed gap and a normal value of 12 mEq/L. A similar calculation for a change in serum HCO_3^- can be made by subtracting the observed HCO_3^- from the normal value of 25 mEq/L. Comparison of the two values may help identify more complicated acid-base disorders. Much larger increases in the anion gap than decreases in serum HCO_3^- may indicate coexisting metabolic alkalosis, and larger decreases in serum HCO_3^- than increases in the anion gap may signify the existence of an additional hyperchloremic acidosis or respiratory alkalosis.

It is important to consider the individual causes of anion gap acidosis; some common examples will be discussed (Table 119–3). Other substances may be detectable by screening for additional organic anions; rare metabolic disturbances, such as methylmalonicaciduria or oxoprolinuria, may be detected in such a way. 5-Oxoprolinuria may be an acquired form of anion gap acidosis in patients ingesting acetaminophen with resulting depletion of intracellular glutathione.

Clinical Manifestations

The effects of metabolic acidosis depend on its rapidity of onset and severity. Patients are often tired and disposed to dyspnea, particularly on exertion. Nausea and vomiting are common. On examination, deep respirations, often labored with the use of accessory muscles, may be detected in acute states, but signs of hyperventilation may be noted only by careful inspection of the respiratory pattern in patients with longstanding metabolic acidemia. Altered hemodynamics may accompany metabolic acidemia, such as vasodilation associated with tachycardia and hypotension. Acidemia may exert a negative inotropic effect on the heart. The stress of either an underlying illness or an increase in adrenergic and corticosteroid activity associated with acidemia may elevate the peripheral white blood cell count and cause hyperglycemia. Other laboratory findings include variable degrees of hyperkalemia, hyperphosphatemia, and hyperuricemia (in lactic acidosis), as well as hypocalcemia as a result of decreased renal 1,25-dihydroxyvitamin D synthesis.

TABLE 119–3 CAUSES OF INCREASED ANION AND OSMOLAL GAPS

Anion Gap Metabolic Acidosis	Osmolal Gap
Uremia	No
Lactic acidosis	Variable/no
D-Lactic acidosis	No
Diabetic ketoacidosis	No
Starvation ketoacidosis	No
Alcoholic ketoacidosis	If ethanol is present
Ethylene glycol	Yes
Methanol	Yes
Salicylates	No

Anion Gap Metabolic Acidoses

Uremic Acidosis

The metabolic acidosis of kidney failure may be due to tubular leakage of HCO_3^-, but it is often present when inadequate ammonia production is unable to facilitate excretion of the normal metabolic acid load. Many patients with renal failure can acidify their urine, but because of the lack of buffering capacity, net acid excretion is diminished. Many organic and inorganic anions, such as phosphate and sulfates, are retained at glomerular filtration rates of less than 25 mL/min and constitute an increased anion gap in association with the metabolic acidosis. The magnitude of the gap is usually less than 20 mEq/L.

The systemic acid-base disturbance in renal failure is attributable to the kidney's inability to excrete hydrogen and to generate and reabsorb HCO_3^-. It is particularly pronounced in oliguric acute renal failure and is exacerbated by hypercatabolic states such as infection. Treatment of the metabolic acidosis of chronic renal failure is directed at maintaining the plasma HCO_3^- concentration and potassium balance and includes oral bicarbonate administration and furosemide if fluid overload and hyperkalemia are present.

Overproduction of Endogenous Acids

Lactic Acidosis

Pathobiology

Lactic acidosis is caused by an imbalance in the rates of lactate production and clearance from the circulation. When production exceeds utilization of lactate, primarily in the liver, the anion gap increases and a state of lactic acidosis exists. Lactic acidosis is most often due to circulatory failure, hypoxia, and mitochondrial dysfunction resulting in decreased tissue ATP (type A lactic acidosis). The result is increased anaerobic glycolysis and rate of reaction of pyruvate to lactate. Other causes are thiamine deficiency, hypophosphatemia, isoniazid toxicity, and hypoglycemic states. Metformin may cause lactic acidosis, particularly in elderly patients with cardiac, hepatic, or renal dysfunction. Nucleoside antivirals, including zidovudine, may cause lactic acidosis and abnormal liver function as a result of toxic mitochondrial effects. Abnormal mitochondrial function is also a feature of toxicity with hypoglycin from ingestion of the unripe akee fruit (Jamaican vomiting sickness), as well as aspirin. Lactic acidosis may accompany hepatic failure because of reduced hepatic lactate clearance.

Type B lactic acidosis is associated with overproduction, which might be caused by severe exertion and malignancies, particularly those with a large tumor burden such as lymphoma and widely metastatic cancer. The Warburg phenotype refers to the capacity of malignant cells to upregulate glycolytic activity, which may increase glucose uptake and utilization by tumor cells and decrease tumor dependence on mitochondrially derived energy. Mechanisms proposed may involve hypoxia-inducible transcription factor-1 and other regulators of phosphofructokinase activity.

Lactate, the final product in the anaerobic pathway of glucose metabolism, is produced from pyruvate by the following reaction catalyzed by lactate dehydrogenase:

$$\text{NADH} + \text{pyruvate} + H^+ \rightarrow \text{lactate} + \text{NAD}$$

A high reduced nicotinamide adenine dinucleotide (NADH)/NAD ratio will favor lactate formation. Conversion of ethanol to acetaldehyde and the ketoacid β-hydroxybutyrate to acetoacetate each uses NAD and produces NADH. Alcohol metabolism may be associated with excessive β-hydroxybutyrate and lactic acidosis.

Sepsis is associated with elevated lactate related to poor clearance and impaired gluconeogenesis. The level of lactate is predictive of mortality in patients with acquired lactic acidosis. Symptoms are those of metabolic acidosis in addition to those of the underlying cause.

Treatment

Rx

Lactic acidosis can result from seizure activity when lactate is released from muscle cells that have undergone a period of anaerobic metabolism. The lactate is quickly metabolized to HCO_3^- by the liver and kidneys, and the acidosis often resolves within 60 minutes. Therefore, administration of HCO_3^- is usually unnecessary and may in fact precipitate an overshoot metabolic alkalosis, a development of particular concern in a patient with seizures because it lowers the seizure threshold. Seizures have also been associated with cerebral lactic acidosis.

Controversy exists regarding the treatment of lactic acidosis with $NaHCO_3$. Arguments against its use concern the potential for hypertonicity, volume expansion, worsened hemodynamics, lactic acidosis, and intracellular acidosis from increased CO_2 production. It has been argued, however, that severe systemic acidosis carries greater risk for cardiac function and hemodynamics and that intracellular acidosis is less likely when adequate ventilation is provided. A trial of $NaHCO_3$ versus NaCl for lactic acidosis in an intensive care unit found that the acidemia could be decreased with $NaHCO_3$, although no difference in hemodynamics was demonstrated. Treatment of lactic acidosis is aimed at correcting the underlying cause. Tissue perfusion and ventilation should be restored if possible. Bicarbonate therapy should be considered when arterial pH is below 7.1 or 7.2.

In patients with intestinal bacterial overgrowth, a syndrome of disorientation, ataxia, and anion gap metabolic acidosis may develop after a carbohydrate meal because of bacterial production of D-lactate. This isomer of the mammalian L-lactate can be measured only by a specific D-lactate assay. The condition is treated with oral antibiotics and appropriate diet.

Diabetic Ketoacidosis

Definition

DKA is defined as hyperglycemia with metabolic acidosis resulting from generation of the ketones β-hydroxybutyrate and acetoacetate in response to insulin deficiency and elevated counter-regulatory hormones such as glucagon. Glucagon has an additional effect of increasing hepatic ketogenesis. It is most commonly seen in cases of type 1 diabetes mellitus.

Clinical Manifestations

Symptoms include nausea and vomiting, anorexia, polydipsia and polyuria, and occasionally, abdominal pain. Patients often exhibit Kussmaul respirations and volume depletion. Neurologic symptoms include fatigue and lethargy with depression of the sensorium.

In this state, lack of insulin leads to increased lipolysis in adipose tissue with the transport of free fatty acids to the liver, where hepatic mitochondria produce ketone bodies from acetyl coenzyme A with the formation of acetoacetate. In the presence of high NADH/NAD, the more reduced form of β-hydroxybutyrate is produced. The brain may use ketoacids as a fuel in this condition. Acetoacetate may also form the nonketoacid acetone. Direct measurements of β-hydroxybutyrate and acetoacetate are available, but tests that depend on a nitroprusside test, such as the urinary dipstick, may underestimate the degree of ketosis if the predominant form is β-hydroxybutyrate, which goes undetected by this test. In fact, the ketone test may become more positive with treatment as the β-hydroxybutyrate is metabolized to acetoacetate. Unusually, in some cases of type 2 diabetes mellitus with severe infection or stress, the counter-regulatory hormones epinephrine and glucagon may be increased such that lipolysis is enhanced, even without complete insulin deficiency, thereby leading to ketoacidosis. In addition to ketoacids increasing the anion gap, diabetic patients are more prone to lactic acidosis because of an increase in NADH favoring the formation of lactate from pyruvate, inhibition of pyruvate dehydrogenase in the absence of insulin, and increased pyruvate generation from alanine. Of note, some of the ketoacids will spill into urine with cations, including sodium and potassium, and thereby contribute to volume depletion and potassium depletion. The loss of ketoacids in urine with sodium will lead to relative chloride retention and give the appearance of a mixed anion gap and hyperchloremic acidosis. The "delta HCO_3^-" will exceed the "delta anion gap." This is more likely to be true when the glomerular filtration rate and therefore the filtered load of ketoacids are high. The serum anion gap in general will be greatest when renal failure is present because the additional anions cannot be cleared from extracellular fluid.

Ketoacidosis is also observed in cases of starvation, in which it is generally mild and not associated with hyperglycemia.

Treatment

Treatment of DKA may precipitate acid-base disturbances in the CNS with potentially devastating results. Administration of HCO_3^- to these patients occasionally results in cerebral edema significant enough to lead to loss of consciousness and even death. This intracellular acidosis may be related to decreased oxygen delivery to brain tissue resulting from withdrawal of the compensatory effect of acidemia on hemoglobin's affinity for oxygen. Hemoglobin's affinity for oxygen is generally in the normal range in metabolic acidosis despite systemic phosphate depletion and the resultant decrease in 2,3-diphosphoglycerate activity because acidemia counteracts this effect. With the removal of acidemia, oxygen delivery to tissues decreases.

Treatment of DKA consists of volume repletion, insulin administration with dextrose if necessary to avoid hypoglycemia, and potassium replacement. Bicarbonate administration should be considered only if DKA is accompanied by shock or coma or if arterial pH is less than 7.1 or 7.2, and bolus infusion should be avoided.

Cerebrospinal fluid (CSF) exhibits a change in acid-base status with treatment of DKA. Even without bicarbonate administration, CSF pH falls as a result of the ventilatory response to correction of acidosis and sudden rise in P_{CO_2}. However, no correlation between decreased CSF pH and depression of sensorium has been established in DKA.

Salicylate Intoxication

Salicylate intoxication is most often seen as a result of accidental overdose, therapeutic overdose, or suicide attempt and produces a complex acid-base picture. The most common manifestation is a combined metabolic acidosis and respiratory alkalosis, although the condition can be manifested as either one or the other or as a combined respiratory and metabolic acidosis.

Manifestations of intoxication include hemorrhage, fever, nausea and vomiting, hyperventilation, diaphoresis, tinnitus, and occasionally polyuria followed by oliguria. Noncardiogenic pulmonary edema is sometimes seen in adults. An anion gap metabolic acidosis may develop and in severe cases has led to seizures, respiratory depression, and coma. Respiratory alkalosis is the result of a direct stimulatory effect of salicylate on the medullary respiratory control center. Another characteristic of salicylate intoxication is an increase in the metabolic rate. Salicylate functions as an uncoupler of oxidative phosphorylation and consequently results in increased oxygen consumption and CO_2 production. However, the increase in alveolar ventilation resulting from stimulation of central chemoreceptors overcomes this increase in CO_2. Children are often seen with metabolic acidosis, whereas adults often have respiratory alkalosis.

Treatment of salicylate intoxication is aimed at correcting the metabolic acidosis and removing salicylate. Bicarbonate should be administered if metabolic acidosis predominates. Salicylates are removed by alkaline diuresis. In cases of severe intoxication, other methods include gastric lavage, osmotic diuresis, and dialysis. Urinary alkalinization with acetazolamide is controversial because it may impair CO_2 transport from tissue to blood and potentially worsen acidosis in the respiratory center.

Alcoholic Ketoacidosis

Ethanol

Pathobiology

The pathophysiology of this disorder is thought to be overproduction of β-hydroxybutyrate and, to a lesser extent, acetoacetate secondary to increased free fatty acids produced in the altered hormonal milieu. The increase in the ratio of β-hydroxybutyrate to acetoacetate is believed to result from oxidation of ethanol, which increases the ratio of NADH to NAD^+ and favors β-hydroxybutyrate production. Damage to mitochondria by alcohol could further elevate this ratio by preventing reoxidation of NADH.

Clinical Manifestations

Alcoholic ketoacidosis usually follows binge drinking and may be associated with withdrawal symptoms and the associated hyperadrenergic state. Alcoholic ketoacidosis is associated with abdominal pain, vomiting, starvation, and volume depletion. In contrast to DKA, coma is rare. Alcohol inhibits the conversion of lactate to glucose in the liver. Blood glucose levels are generally low or normal, and insulin is frequently low, with elevated glucagon and cortisol levels. Some patients have hyperglycemia because of the increased catecholamine response. Blood alcohol levels may be absent or elevated on initial evaluation.

Diagnosis

Patients typically have a high osmolal gap initially (defined as the difference between the measured and the calculated serum osmolality).

$$\text{Calculated osmolality} = 2(Na^+) + (\text{Glucose [mg/dL]} \div 18) + (\text{Blood urea nitrogen [mg/dL]} \div 2.8)$$

This gap should be equal to the ethanol concentration in milligrams per deciliter divided by 4.6; if it is not, ingestion of another alcohol such as methanol, isopropanol, or ethylene glycol should be suspected (see Table 119–3). Patients with toxic alcohol levels are at increased risk for ingestion of these alcohol substitutes. A clue to the diagnosis of toxic alcohol ingestion is the simultaneous presence of an anion gap metabolic acidosis and an osmolal gap. Serum osmolality should be measured by a freezing point depression technique and compared with the calculated osmolality. Direct measurement of ethanol, ethylene glycol, and methanol should be performed when possible. Metabolic acidosis is associated with the ingestion of these other alcohols.

Treatment

Treatment of alcoholic metabolic acidosis consists of volume repletion and thiamine and glucose administration, with correction of hypophosphatemia, hypokalemia, and hypomagnesemia if present. The acid-base disturbance usually resolves after several hours. Hypophosphatemia may be manifested 12 to 24 hours after the initiation of treatment in an undernourished patient and is exacerbated by glucose administration.

Ethylene Glycol

Ethylene glycol is commonly found in antifreeze and is used as an industrial solvent. It has a sweet taste and patients are occasionally seen clinically after ingestion as a substitute for ethanol. Intoxication is characterized by profound CNS symptoms, including seizures and coma, severe metabolic acidosis, and cardiac, pulmonary, and renal failure.

Although ethylene glycol itself does not appear to be particularly damaging, its metabolites are highly toxic and include glyoxylate and glycolate, as well as oxalic acid and ketoaldehydes. The increased anion gap seen in ethylene glycol intoxication is attributable to ethylene glycol metabolites. A high osmolal gap will also be present because of the uncharged alcohol. Glycolic acid appears to be primarily responsible for the metabolic acidosis observed in this condition. Calcium oxalate crystals may be seen in urine and may be responsible for intratubular obstruction and acute renal failure. Patients are often dehydrated because of osmotic diuresis from the renal excretion of alcohol. Treatment is aimed at rehydration and competitive inhibition of alcohol dehydrogenase by the use of ethanol and fomepizole (recently shown to be safe and effective). Hemodialysis is required in severe cases.

Methanol

Methanol, a component of wood alcohol and windshield wiper fluid, is highly toxic to the CNS after metabolism to formaldehyde and formic acid. Optic papillitis may cause blindness. Treatment consists of competitive inhibitors for alcohol dehydrogenase, including ethanol or fomepizole, which will reduce the formation of acid anions and the anion gap while maintaining a higher level of methanol in the blood. Hemodialysis may be necessary to increase elimination.

Isopropyl Alcohol

Toxic ingestion of isopropyl alcohol, as in rubbing alcohol, does not cause an increased anion gap or ketoacidosis because the metabolite is acetone, but tests for ketones are positive and a high osmolal gap will be present.

Propylene Glycol

Occasionally, patients in the intensive care unit setting are given high doses of intravenous benzodiazepines, such as lorazepam. A high osmolal gap may develop because of the diluent propylene glycol and lead to the clinical picture of sedation, failure to wean from the respirator, and increased lactate, a metabolite of propylene glycol.

Normal Anion Gap or Hyperchloremic Acidosis

Hyperchloremic Metabolic Acidosis of Nonrenal Origin Associated with Normal or Increased Potassium

These acidoses can develop as a result of the addition of chloride salts such as NaCl, KCl, $CaCl_2$, NH_4Cl, arginine and lysine hydrochlorides, or HCl itself (Table 119–4). If the quantity of Cl^- introduced exceeds the ability of the kidney to eliminate Cl^- salts in urine, hyperchloremia will develop. Electroneutrality is maintained by a decrease in the serum HCO_3^- concentration, and a hyperchloremic acidosis ensues. Renal production of NH_3 will increase in an attempt to improve HCl excretion. Hyperkalemia can occur in this situation because the acidemia favors the exit of K^+ from cells. Hyperchloremic acidosis has a greater effect in causing cellular K^+ efflux than the organic acidoses and respiratory acidosis do. Another mechanism for hyperkalemia may be an inhibitory effect of intracellular acidity on K^+ secretion in the collecting duct cell.

Hyperchloremic Metabolic Acidosis of Nonrenal Origin Associated with Hypokalemia

Hypokalemic, hyperchloremic acidosis may result from loss of a body fluid that is low in Cl^- relative to Na^+ and K^+ when compared with the ratio of Na^+ to Cl^- in extracellular fluid. For example, stool losses of Na^+ and K^+ with HCO_3^- in small bowel diarrhea or organic acid anions of bacterial origin in colonic diarrhea lead to hyperchloremic acidosis. Pancreatic secretions or heavy losses from ileostomy sites may lead to loss of bicarbonate-containing fluids. Secretagogues such as vasoactive intestinal peptide (VIP), when associated with neoplasms of the pancreas or sympathetic chain (VIPomas), cause large HCO_3^- losses in stool and hypokalemic, hyperchloremic metabolic acidosis. Concomitant gastric achlorhydria is part of the syndrome known as "watery diarrhea, hypokalemic, hypochlorhydric, acidosis." Urinary diversions such as ureterosigmoidostomies and ileal loops may result in increased chloride absorption in exchange for bicarbonate in the intestinal segment and lead to hyperchloremic acidosis. As will be discussed next, renal tubular

TABLE 119–4 CAUSES OF HYPERCHLOREMIC ACIDOSIS

Type	Cause
Renal with hypokalemia	Proximal RTA, type 2 Distal RTA, type 1 Some anion gap acidoses with high anion clearance
Renal with hyperkalemia	Type 4 RTA; hyporeninism-hypoaldosteronism
Nonrenal with hypokalemia	Diarrhea Urinary diversions
Nonrenal with hyperkalemia	NaCl, KCl, NH_4Cl, $CaCl_2$, Arg-HCl, Lys-HCl

RTA = renal tubular acidosis.

acidosis causes the cations Na^+ and K^+ to be lost in the urine with HCO_3^- rather than Cl^-, thereby leading to hyperchloremia.

Hyperchloremic Metabolic Acidosis of Renal Origin Associated with Hypokalemia

Proximal renal tubular acidosis (type II) is characterized by a decreased threshold for bicarbonate reabsorption, in which case initial HCO_3^- wasting occurs until a new low level of serum bicarbonate develops. At that point, the filtered HCO_3^- is reduced, and the renal tubule can completely reabsorb the filtered load so that the new steady state allows for a normally acid urine pH. In proximal renal tubular acidosis, urine pH is usually less than 5.3, the acidosis is not severe, and there is not relentless acid retention because acid excretion may balance acid production at this new steady state. In children, however, the acidosis may have effects on growth and may need to be treated with bicarbonate supplements. It is characteristic of proximal renal tubular acidosis that large quantities of HCO_3^- need be administered to correct the acidosis because attempts to give alkali are associated with prompt renal excretion and an alkaline urine. Another characteristic related to the alkaline urine is the hypokalemia brought out by HCO_3^- replacement.

Isolated proximal renal tubular acidosis may result from mutations of specific transporters of the proximal tubule such as the Na-HCO_3 cotransporter, or it could be due to hereditary deficiency of carbonic anhydrase. The latter would resemble the effects of carbonic anhydrase inhibitors such as acetazolamide.

More commonly, proximal renal tubular acidosis is associated with generalized proximal tubule dysfunction: the Fanconi syndrome. Glycosuria, phosphaturia, aminoaciduria, and uricosuria may be present. Causes include genetic diseases such as the glycogen storage disease glucose-6-phosphatase deficiency, cystinosis, hereditary fructose intolerance, and Wilson's disease. Multiple myeloma and Sjögren's syndrome should be considered in an adult patient. Primary hyperparathyroidism results in proximal renal tubular acidosis and hypophosphatemia secondary to inhibition of Na/H exchange and Na-phosphate cotransport in the proximal tubule. Drug toxicity with aminoglycosides, cisplatin, and ifosfamide may cause proximal tubule dysfunction. The syndrome may be seen after kidney transplantation.

In contrast to proximal renal tubular acidosis, distal renal tubular acidosis (type 1) is generally a more severe metabolic disorder and may be accompanied by hypercalciuria, nephrocalcinosis, kidney stones, and bone disease. The degree of acidemia is often more severe and urine pH usually exceeds 5.3. This observation is the basis of the NH_4Cl loading test in which plasma bicarbonate is lowered by an acid challenge. If urine pH remains above 5.3, a distal abnormality is suspected. This test is rarely indicated to distinguish between proximal and distal acidosis.

In distal renal tubular acidosis there is failure to produce ammonia and therefore an inability to adequately excrete net acid, which leads to continuous retention of acid in the body. This disorder must be treated but can usually be managed with small amounts of bicarbonate or citrate salts equal to the daily production of acid, generally 1 to 2 mEq/kg/day. Hypokalemia often accompanies distal renal tubular acidosis and may improve with treatment.

Kindreds have been described with mutations in genes for the distal H^+-ATPase causing an autosomal recessive distal renal tubular acidosis with deafness, and mutations resulting in defective Cl/HCO_3 exchange protein (AE1) have been linked to an autosomal dominant form of distal renal tubular acidosis.

Distal renal tubular acidosis is also associated with autoimmune disorders, including systemic lupus erythematosus and Sjögren's syndrome, and genetic diseases, including sickle cell anemia, Wilson's disease, Fabry's disease, cystic kidney diseases, and hereditary elliptocytosis. Hypercalciuria and hyperoxaluria may cause distal renal tubular acidosis; nephrocalcinosis may be present. Amyloidosis may be manifested as severe acidemia and other tubular dysfunction, including nephrogenic diabetes insipidus. Tubulointerstitial disease of the kidney, including reflux nephropathy and urinary obstruction, may result in renal tubular acidosis with hypokalemia or hyperkalemia. Drugs such as amphotericin B can cause hypokalemic distal renal tubular acidosis.

Hyperchloremic Metabolic Acidosis of Renal Origin Associated with Hyperkalemia

Hyperkalemic, hyperchloremic acidosis (type 4) suggests dysfunction of the CCD, where acidification of urine and disorders in potassium secretion may occur. Some patients with high blood potassium and hyperchloremic acidosis can lower urinary pH below 5.5, whereas others appear to have defects in both potassium balance and urinary acidification. Causes include hyporeninism-hypoaldosteronism, as seen in diabetic renal disease; other tubulointerstitial diseases, usually with some renal impairment; sickle cell anemia; or the use of drugs such as β-blockers and nonsteroidal anti-inflammatory drugs. Low renin and aldosterone levels can also be found in cases of volume expansion with hypertension. Cyclosporine may increase distal Cl^- reabsorption as Na^+ is reabsorbed, thereby leading to decreased electrical driving forces for K^+ and H^+ secretion. Increases in Na^+ and Cl^- reabsorption lead to hypertension, hyperkalemic acidosis, volume expansion, and consequently, low renin and aldosterone in the autosomal dominant condition known as Gordon's syndrome. Increased activity of the distal thiazide-sensitive NaCl transporter is suspected. Hyperkalemic acidosis with elevated renin and low aldosterone is found in cases of adrenal insufficiency, isolated hypoaldosteronism, and the use of angiotensin-converting enzyme inhibitors or angiotensin II receptor blockers. High renin and aldosterone levels are anticipated when the renal collecting duct cell is insensitive to aldosterone, as in urinary tract obstruction, sickle cell anemia, amyloidosis, and systemic lupus erythematosus. Inhibition of aldosterone action with spironolactone will cause hyperkalemic acidosis, as would ENaC inhibition by amiloride and triamterene. Pseudohypoaldosteronism is due to inactivating mutations of the Na^+ channel.

Hyperkalemia itself may worsen metabolic acidosis by decreasing NH_3 accumulation by countercurrent multiplication in the medullary interstitium. Often, treatment of hyperkalemia improves urinary acidification without the use of bicarbonate salts.

The Urinary Anion Gap in Hyperchloremic Acidosis

An important means of distinguishing between renal tubular acidosis and extrarenal bicarbonate loss (e.g., from diarrhea) is to look at the urinary anion gap. Because the normal renal response to metabolic acidosis is an increase in ammoniagenesis, the urine in the case of diarrhea should normally contain large amounts of NH_4Cl while the kidney retains sodium and potassium. The urinary anion gap, which is $(Na^+ + K^+) - Cl^-$, should then be strongly negative because of the unmeasured NH_4^+. This test is superior to measurement of urine pH because decreased Na^+ delivery to the distal nephron in the Na^+ avid state of diarrhea and hypokalemia may impair urinary acidification and pH will not be maximally acid. In renal diseases in which there is either failure of ammoniagenesis or excretion of sodium plus potassium with bicarbonate, the urinary anion gap will be zero or positive. This is characteristic of distal renal tubular acidosis.

When other unmeasured anions such as ketoacids and lactate are present in urine, a positive urinary anion gap does not indicate renal tubular acidosis. These situations are usually associated with an elevated serum anion gap, but on occasion, prompt renal excretion of organic anions with sodium and potassium may minimize an increase in the serum gap. This is particularly possible in cases of DKA and D-lactic acidosis because D-lactate is not absorbed by the renal tubule. In the metabolic acidosis of glue sniffers, hippurate, a product of toluene, is excreted, thus giving the appearance of a non-gap metabolic acidosis with a positive urinary anion gap.

Treatment

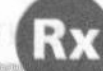

If possible, treatment of metabolic acidosis should focus on correcting the underlying cause and permitting the body's homeostatic mechanisms to correct the acid-base disturbance. It is often recommended that one consider treating patients whose pH is less than 7.2 with alkali infusion. Sodium bicarbonate is most frequently used. However, rapid correction of arterial pH can lead to complications, including a paradoxical CSF acidosis and continued hyperventilation, hypokalemia, and hypocalcemia. Formulas have been developed that allow the physician to estimate the base deficit in milliequivalents roughly based on the serum HCO_3^- concentration in milliequivalents per liter:

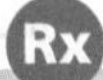

$$\text{Amount of } HCO_3^- = (25 - [HCO_3^-]) \times \text{wt (kg)}/2$$

In general, only partial correction of the deficit should be attempted before recalculations with this formula. Moreover, this equation represents an estimate of deficit only, so ongoing losses need to be considered.

METABOLIC ALKALOSIS

Pathobiology

In metabolic alkalosis, the primary event is elevation of the plasma bicarbonate concentration. In response to increased systemic pH, alveolar ventilation is decreased in order to increase P_{CO_2} and thereby decrease pH. However, compensation is generally believed to be less effective in cases of metabolic alkalosis than in cases of metabolic acidosis. Contributing factors may include the fact that hypoventilation also decreases P_{O_2}, a potent stimulus for the peripheral chemoreceptors to increase alveolar ventilation. A second mechanism that may blunt respiratory compensation is intracellular acidosis in the brain in the setting of hypokalemia. In acute metabolic alkalosis, there is an initial paradoxical acidotic shift in CSF pH secondary to a sudden increase in P_{CO_2}, similar to the alkaline shift in CSF pH in acute metabolic acidosis. This may contribute to the unpredictable respiratory response to metabolic alkalosis by activating central chemoreceptors and increasing ventilatory drive in the face of peripheral stimulation to decrease alveolar ventilation. In chronic metabolic alkalosis, CSF pH may return to normal values such that the respiratory drive derives entirely from the peripheral chemoreceptors. Whatever the causes, the result is that the ventilatory response to metabolic alkalosis is highly varied. Many patients with metabolic alkalosis maintain nearly normal P_{CO_2} levels, and the level rarely rises above 60 mm Hg.

Metabolic alkalosis requires a generation phase, in which new HCO_3^- is added to the extracellular fluid, and a maintenance phase, by which the new elevated serum HCO_3^- concentration is sustained. Without the latter phase, a kidney with normal filtration and tubular function has a high capacity to excrete HCO_3^-, thereby preventing alkalosis. Maintenance of a high HCO_3^- concentration usually occurs because of volume depletion, a reduced glomerular filtration rate, hypokalemia, or low chloride levels.

Metabolic alkalosis is generally divided into two categories based on its responsiveness to chloride (Table 119–5). Chloride-responsive metabolic alkalosis is associated with extracellular fluid and chloride depletion and is seen in cases of gastric fluid loss and diuretic use. A diagnostic clue comes from the serum electrolytes. HCO_3^- is increased with a corresponding fall in serum chloride (hypochloremic alkalosis). Chloride-unresponsive metabolic alkalosis is seen in patients with extracellular fluid expansion in conditions such as primary aldosteronism and hypokalemia. Entry of hydrogen ions into cells can also lead to metabolic alkalosis, as seen in hypokalemia.

TABLE 119–5 CAUSES OF METABOLIC ALKALOSIS

Type	Causes
Renal, hypochloremic alkalosis: Cl responsive with urine Cl >20	Loop and distal tubule diuretics Bartter's syndrome Gittelman's syndrome Posthypercapnic status Vomiting/nasogastric suction
Nonrenal, hypochloremic alkalosis: Cl responsive with urine Cl <20	Chloridorrhea
Renal, alkalosis with extracellular expansion: Cl unresponsive with urine Cl >20	Hyperaldosteronism, primary and secondary Liddle's syndrome
Nonrenal alkalosis, Cl unresponsive	$NaHCO_3$, acetate, citrate, lactate
Other causes of metabolic alkalosis	Excessive non-reabsorbable anion excretion Hypoproteinemia

Metabolic Alkalosis of Renal Origin Associated with Volume Depletion

Metabolic alkalosis of renal origin may be the result of excessive urinary chloride excretion. The most common causes are diuretics that inhibit reabsorption of Cl^- proportionately more than Na^+. Most often it is due to potent diuretics that inhibit the Na-K-2Cl cotransporter in the thick ascending limb, such as furosemide and bumetanide, or due to thiazides, which inhibit the Na-Cl cotransporter in the distal tubule, and metolazone. In each case the urine is found to be rich in Cl^- relative to Na^+ when one compares the concentrations with the starting point in the extracellular fluid of roughly 140 Na^+ to 100 Cl^-. The Cl^- loss results in hypochloremia and increases in plasma HCO_3^- to maintain electroneutrality. Extracellular volume depletion results in stimulation of the renin-angiotensin-aldosterone pathway, and high aldosterone superimposed on increased distal urinary flow rates results in increased K^+ excretion and hypokalemia. The volume depletion and hypokalemia enhance proximal HCO_3^- reabsorption, thereby maintaining the alkalosis, and the prerenal fall in the glomerular flow rate limits HCO_3^- filtration. Correction of this type of metabolic alkalosis requires replacement with NaCl and KCl solutions. Replacement with saline alone is potentially dangerous because the consequently increased glomerular filtration and decreased proximal reabsorption will allow large quantities of alkaline urine to interact with the aldosterone-sensitive distal sites and thus worsen the hypokalemia.

Several important, but rare genetic syndromes characterized by urinary chloride wasting have been described. Bartter's syndrome is an autosomal recessive salt-losing state associated with extracellular volume depletion and excessive urinary chloride loss that results in hypokalemia and hypochloremic metabolic alkalosis. There are secondary increased levels of plasma renin and aldosterone and renal juxtaglomerular cell hyperplasia. The syndrome is reminiscent of effects of the diuretic furosemide on the thick ascending limb of Henle. Gene mutations associated with Bartter's syndrome have been described for the Na-K-2Cl cotransporter, K^+ channel, and Cl^- channels that take part in loop of Henle Cl^- transport. Because calcium reabsorption occurs in this segment, Bartter's syndrome, like furosemide, causes hypercalciuria. Polyuria is present because of the important role of the thick ascending limb of Henle in urinary concentration. Indomethacin has been used to treat Bartter's syndrome by interfering with prostaglandin E_2 and thus allowing greater Na-Cl reabsorption in the thick ascending limb.

Like Bartter's syndrome, the more common Gitelman's syndrome is an autosomal recessive cause of extracellular volume depletion, urinary chloride wasting, and hypokalemic metabolic alkalosis. It is due to inactivating mutations in the *SLC12A3* gene encoding the thiazide-sensitive NaCl cotransporter of the renal distal tubule. In contrast to Bartter's syndrome but similar to the thiazide diuretics, urinary concentration is spared and patients are hypocalciuric because decreased NaCl reabsorption in this segment is associated with a decrease in calcium excretion. Hypomagnesemia may also be severe.

Metabolic Alkalosis of Nonrenal Origin with Extracellular Volume Depletion

Metabolic alkalosis may develop as a result of Cl^- loss in gastrointestinal secretions. In such cases, extracellular volume is usually contracted, hypochloremia develops, and because the loss of Cl^- is nonrenal, the urinary chloride level is low, usually less than 20 mEq/L.

The most common disorder in this category is gastric alkalosis secondary to vomiting or nasogastric suctioning. Gastric juice is higher in Cl^- than Na^+, the reverse state of the extracellular fluids.

It is not uncommon for secretory diarrheas to lead to disproportionate Cl^- loss as opposed to Na^+. In Zollinger-Ellison syndrome, excessive gastrin-induced gastric acid secretion may result in an acidic stool with high chloride, a distinguishing feature from VIPomas. Infectious gastroenteritis, congenital chloridorrhea, and villous adenomas are other causes of stool chloride loss. Congenital chloridorrhea is an autosomal recessive disorder of defective colonic, apical Cl/HCO_3 exchange associated with the downregulated adenoma *(DRA)* gene. Villous adenomas or adenocarcinomas, particularly of the rectosigmoid colon, also cause a secretory diarrhea (McKittrick-Wheelock syndrome) with high chloride content that is mediated by excessive prostaglandin E_2. Diarrhea should not be equated with the development of metabolic acidosis. Alkalosis is most likely to develop when the stool electrolytes $[(Na^+ + K^+) - Cl^-]$ are less than plasma HCO_3^-.

In gastric alkalosis, the initiating event is loss of HCl. In acid-secreting epithelia, when protons are secreted into the lumen, HCO_3^- is transported back to blood. Thus, in gastric alkalosis, secretion of HCl into the stomach lumen by the parietal cell is coupled to the absorption of HCO_3^- in exchange for chloride at the basolateral membrane. Normally, when gastric acid is secreted, a mild increase in serum HCO_3^- occurs, and this spills into urine and causes an "alkaline tide." With vomiting, a net loss of HCl is removed from the body, thereby generating the alkalosis.

Initially, the increased HCO_3^- is filtered by the glomeruli, and because the proximal tubule is not yet poised to increase reabsorption, the HCO_3^- flows distally and is excreted in urine. The accompanying cations are Na^+ and K^+, and urine pH is alkaline. At this stage the kidney appears to be protecting the body from alkalosis, but at the expense of Na^+ and K^+ loss. The presence of Na^+ in the HCO_3^--containing urine belies the volume depletion that begins to develop. Clinically, low urinary Cl^- is more indicative of the volume depletion than urinary Na^+ is. As vomiting continues, extracellular volume depletion worsens and renal responses begin to change. Glomerular filtration falls, thus limiting HCO_3^- filtration. Volume depletion increases the renin–angiotension II–aldosterone system, and as a consequence, proximal volume and HCO_3^- reabsorption increase. Distal Na^+ reabsorption increases under the influence of aldosterone, and greater H^+ secretion enhances HCO_3^- reabsorption. These effects begin to prevent renal Na^+ loss, but at the expense of maintaining metabolic alkalosis; it becomes harder to excrete the HCO_3^-. Significant K^+ losses occur as a result of the bicarbonaturia and hyperaldosteronism and lead to hypokalemia. The K^+ depletion associated with vomiting is actually due to renal, not gastrointestinal losses. The loss of K^+ is a consequence of mechanisms to maintain extracellular volume. The hypokalemia further increases proximal $NaHCO_3$ reabsorption and distal H^+ secretion, effects that also maintain the alkalosis. Hypokalemia leads to increased K^+ reabsorption, probably through increased K^+, H^+-ATPase activity in the collecting duct. Note that the mechanisms for conserving K^+ at this stage do so at the expense of further reabsorption of HCO_3^-. At the new steady state after vomiting or nasogastric suctioning ceases, the urine has low levels of Na^+, K^+, and Cl^- and is acid as a result of complete HCO_3^- reabsorption. At this stage the paradoxical aciduria of metabolic alkalosis is noted. In the end, the patient may be hypovolemic, hypokalemic, and alkalemic, but because Na^+, K^+, and acid-base balance are intrinsically linked, life-threatening volume depletion, K^+ depletion, and alkalemia are usually avoided. The overlap of Na^+, K^+, and acid-base balance is obvious at both the clinical level and the cellular level, where transporters such as Na/H exchange, K^+, H^+-ATPase, and Cl/HCO_3 exchange are at work. Additionally, there is overlap in hormonal regulation, with angiotensin II influencing Na/H exchange and aldosterone exerting effects on Na^+, K^+, and H^+ transport.

From the standpoint of the renal tubule, similarities exist in the initial bicarbonaturia leading to K^+ wasting in gastric alkalosis and in the development of proximal tubular acidosis; the difference is in the source of HCO_3^-. The source is a high filtered load in an alkalemic patient and a decreased reabsorptive component in a patient with proximal renal tubular acidosis.

Metabolic Alkalosis of Renal Origin with Volume Expansion and Hypertension

The renal conditions that cause metabolic alkalosis and volume expansion are due to the primary increase in Na^+ reabsorption above that required to maintain a steady state of Na^+ balance rather than primary loss of the Cl^- anion. Reabsorption of Na^+ is proportionately greater than that of Cl^-. As Na^+ is reabsorbed, electroneutrality is maintained by an increase in plasma HCO_3^-. The plasma Na^+ concentration may be increased and Cl^- balance is normal; Cl^- appears in urine and hypochloremia is not present. In the kidney, the loss of net acid as NH_4Cl in excess of the acid produced would generate metabolic alkalosis, where again the new bicarbonate generated is due to proton secretion by the distal nephron through H^+-ATPases. The H^+ then combines with NH_3 to form NH_4^+ in urine.

The site in the nephron where Na^+ is reabsorbed independently of Cl^- is the CCD through the aldosterone-sensitive cells containing the ENaC. When Na^+ is reabsorbed by the principal cells of the CCD, the tubule lumen becomes electronegative. This will stimulate both K^+ and H^+ secretion by the electrogenic H^+-ATPases. To the extent that HCO_3^- remains in the lumen, the secreted protons will complete HCO_3^- reabsorption. Additional secreted protons will combine with NH_3 and phosphates and lead to net acid excretion. If there is an increase in the distal H^+ secretory mechanism caused by disease, more urinary net acid will be produced, more "new" HCO_3^- will be generated and returned to the now expanded extracellular fluid, and metabolic alkalosis will develop. The increased plasma HCO_3^- will be filtered, but in the absence of a stimulus to increase proximal HCO_3^- reabsorption, the HCO_3^- will flow distally to be reabsorbed by the increased H^+ secretion of the collecting duct. At first the alkalosis in such a case is mild. However, increased CCD Na^+ reabsorption will also lead to increased K^+ secretion, and hypokalemia will develop. Hypokalemia will increase the capacity for proximal HCO_3^- reabsorption, thus opposing the effect of volume expansion, so that distal delivery of HCO_3^- decreases. This allows the higher than normal distal H^+ secretion to titrate urinary buffers rather than complete HCO_3^- reabsorption, so further "new" HCO_3^- is formed and the alkalosis worsens. This is the process by which hypermineralocorticoid syndromes cause and sustain alkalosis; there is an important role for hypokalemia in the process. Hypokalemia will develop in patients with suspected hyperaldosteronism when given a salt load because of increased Na^+ delivery to distal sites and more K^+ loss. Metabolic alkalosis can be lessened in hyperaldosteronism by potassium replacement or by blocking Na^+ reabsorption with aldosterone antagonists or amiloride.

Specific causes of this type of renal alkalosis can be classified according to levels of renin and aldosterone. Primary increases in renin resulting in high aldosterone can be seen in patients with unilateral renal artery stenosis, renin-secreting tumors of the kidney, and malignant hypertension. A low renin and elevated aldosterone level is characteristic of primary hyperaldosteronism from adrenal adenoma or hyperplasia. Hypertension and hypokalemic alkalosis could result from increased function of the aldosterone receptor in the CCD driving greater Na^+ reabsorption even without increased aldosterone levels. Because cortisol can also stimulate the receptor, patients with hypercortisolism or adrenocorticotropic hormone–secreting tumors are subject to development of the syndrome, with suppression of renin and aldosterone by the volume expansion. Inhibition of the intracellular enzyme 11β-hydroxysteroid dehydrogenase, which normally inactivates cortisol to form cortisone in the CCD, will also result in low renin levels, low aldosterone levels, and hypokalemic alkalosis. Such is the effect of a substance found in licorice or anisette when taken in excess. Another cause of hypertension with hypokalemic alkalosis but with low renin and aldosterone levels is Liddle's syndrome, in which an activating mutation in the CCD Na^+ channel (ENaC) leads to increased Na^+ reabsorption.

Metabolic alkalosis may also develop without volume expansion when a non-reabsorbable anion is presented to the CCD lumen. Nitrates, sulfates, and certain antibiotics such as carbenicillin may obligate K^+ and H^+ secretion as Na^+ is reabsorbed. Topical administration of silver nitrate to burn victims may result in alkalosis.

Metabolic Alkalosis of Nonrenal Origin Associated with Normal or Expanded Volume

Sometimes inspection of serum electrolytes fails to reveal hypochloremia. To maintain electroneutrality, there must be either an alternative anion that is depleted or an excessive concentration of a cation. An example of metabolic alkalosis associated with depletion of a nonchloride anion is hypoproteinemic alkalosis, recognized by hypoalbuminemia and a small anion gap. Chloride balance is normal and chloride appears in urine.

Alkalosis may be a result of the addition of alkali salts of non-Cl^- organic anions. The normal response to the ingestion of $NaHCO_3$ is rapid urinary alkalinization because there is an unaltered threshold for HCO_3^- reabsorption. However, marked excesses of HCO_3^- may be administered such that volume expansion and alkalemia will result. It is more likely to occur in a patient with volume depletion or low glomerular filtration because the low filtered load prevents HCO_3^- excretion. In practice, this is important whenever an effort is made to alkalinize a patient's urine, as for example in tumor lysis syndrome or myoglobinuria. When the glomerular filtration rate is low, such alkalinization may not occur until severely elevated plasma bicarbonate concentrations develop. Milk-alkali syndrome is a form of alkalosis usually seen in renal failure patients that is associated with the ingestion of milk or calcium antacids. The result is hypercalcemia and alkalemia with normal Cl^-.

Other situations in which intake of alkali salts results in metabolic alkalosis include infusion of large quantities of sodium salts of metabolizable organic compounds such as acetate, citrate, lactate, or bicarbonate; hyperalimentation with acetate salts; chronic peritoneal dialysis with acetate or lactate dialysate; or excessive transfusions or plasmapheresis, in which large quantities of citrate, used as an anticoagulant, are delivered.

Clinical Manifestations

Metabolic alkalosis has a profound effect on the CNS and is frequently associated with metabolic encephalopathy. This is the result of the alkalosis itself and the compensatory hypoventilation that leads to changes in blood flow and oxygenation. Significant cerebral tissue hypoxia is a consequence of cerebral vasoconstriction and increased hemoglobin affinity for oxygen. Symptoms include confusion, obtundation, delirium, and coma. The seizure threshold is lowered, and tetany, paresthesias, muscular cramping, and other symptoms reflecting low free calcium levels are observed. Neurologic manifestations are generally seen when the pH exceeds 7.55, although patients with hypocalcemia may exhibit signs at lower pH values. Other findings include cardiac arrhythmias and hypotension. Lactate production increases as a result of the increased anaerobic glycolysis.

Treatment

In treating metabolic alkalosis, it is important to distinguish whether the condition is chloride responsive or chloride unresponsive, as discussed earlier.

In chloride-responsive patients, treatment is directed at increasing urinary excretion of bicarbonate. In patients with mild to moderate alkalosis, administration of NaCl and KCl is effective in suppressing renal acid excretion and increasing renal HCO_3^- excretion. Unless KCl is also replenished, the improvement in filtration and proximal reabsorption will result in severe K^+ wasting as bicarbonaturia develops and aldosterone's effects remain. In addition, complete resolution of alkalosis will not occur until K^+ is normalized. In a patient with renal failure and vomiting, the elevation in HCO_3^- may be more severe because of poor HCO_3^- filtration. In cases of volume expansion and alkalosis, acetazolamide may be attempted with care, given the potential for losing K^+. If this agent fails to work, dilute solutions of HCl may be cautiously administered.

In patients with more severe alkalemia and volume expansion, mineral acids (e.g., HCl or arginine monohydrochloride) may be necessary. In the absence of renal failure, acetazolamide may be effective but may greatly increase K^+ losses.

Chloride-unresponsive patients include those with mineralocorticoid excess. The hypokalemia and hyperaldosteronism lead to increased hydrogen secretion and bicarbonate reabsorption in the kidney. These patients respond to potassium replacement, which reverses the intracellular shift of hydrogen ions and increases bicarbonate excretion, and to agents that reduce aldosterone activity, such as spironolactone and amiloride.

RESPIRATORY ACIDOSIS

Pathobiology

Respiratory acidosis is characterized by a primary elevation in Pco_2 as reflected by reduced arterial pH with variable elevation in the HCO_3^- concentration. It is most frequently caused by a decrease in alveolar ventilation.

Respiratory acidosis is seen clinically in cases of pulmonary insufficiency and can be the result of pulmonary disease, respiratory muscle fatigue, or abnormalities in ventilatory control. Disorders include central effects of drugs, stroke, and infection; airway obstruction; primary parenchymal processes such as chronic obstructive pulmonary disease and acute respiratory distress syndrome; and neuromuscular diseases such as myasthenia gravis and muscular dystrophies. The slow time course of many of these diseases allows the kidney to compensate adequately as the disease progresses by increasing its excretion of hydrogen ion as ammonium and generating and reabsorbing bicarbonate to restore systemic pH toward normal values. This process is not maximal until 3 to 5 days after the onset of respiratory acidosis.

Permissive hypercapnia has been used clinically in patients with acute respiratory distress syndrome to limit pulmonary damage secondary to mechanical ventilation. Clinically significant respiratory acidosis can result from elevations in Pco_2 when using this approach, however. Effects are most commonly seen when Pco_2 is allowed to rise precipitously and include increased intracranial pressure, increased cardiac output, and increased organ perfusion in some studies. The dangers of this technique rest in the fact that many patients have significant comorbid conditions that make the complications of respiratory acidosis particularly dangerous. By controlling peripheral pH with bicarbonate infusions, many of these potentially lethal effects can be lessened.

Clinical Manifestations

Clinical findings in respiratory acidosis are related to the degree and duration of the respiratory acidosis and whether hypoxemia is present. Neurologic symptoms figure prominently in this disorder. A precipitous rise in Pco_2 can lead to confusion, anxiety, psychosis, asterixis, seizures, and myoclonic jerks, with progressive depression of the sensorium to coma at an arterial Pco_2 greater than 60 mm Hg (CO_2 narcosis). Hypercapnia has been shown to increase cerebral blood flow and volume. As a result, hypercapnia can lead to symptoms and signs reflecting elevated intracranial pressure, including headaches and papilledema. Other findings in acute respiratory acidosis include signs of catecholamine release, such as skin flushing, diaphoresis, and increased cardiac contractility and output.

Symptoms of chronic hypercapnia include fatigue, lethargy, and confusion, in addition to the findings seen in acute hypercapnia.

It can be difficult to distinguish the signs of hypercapnia from those of hypoxemia clinically because the two often appear together. In many patients, however, correction of the hypoxemia does not improve the clinical picture; as a result, it can be surmised that hypercapnia is responsible for many of the findings seen.

Treatment

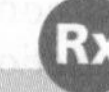

Treatment of both chronic and acute respiratory acidosis is aimed primarily at correcting the underlying cause and ensuring adequate ventilation. Acute respiratory acidosis can be very dangerous, and measures to relieve severe hypoxemia and acidemia should be instituted immediately, including intubation and assisted mechanical ventilation if necessary.

Two complications can be seen in patients with chronic respiratory acidosis as a result of treatment. In patients breathing spontaneously, oxygen should be carefully titrated; ventilation may be driven by hypoxemia, and correction of the hypoxemia can result in worsening of the hypercapnia.

In patients with compensated chronic respiratory acidosis, rapid and complete correction of hypercapnia can also result in posthypercapnic metabolic alkalosis. Patients recovering from an acute-on-chronic respiratory acidosis should be monitored carefully to correct for hypokalemia, hypochloremia, and hypovolemia so that adequate renal excretion of bicarbonate can occur.

Bicarbonate therapy should not be considered for respiratory acidosis unless the pH falls below 7.1 and the patient is about to be intubated; in such cases it can be used transiently until the patient is ventilated. There is also a role for bicarbonate therapy in patients with renal failure, in whom adequate compensatory acid excretion cannot take place.

RESPIRATORY ALKALOSIS

Pathobiology

Respiratory alkalosis is characterized by a primary decrease in P_{CO_2} reflected by an increased arterial pH and variably decreased plasma bicarbonate concentration. It is most commonly the result of alveolar hyperventilation rather than underproduction of CO_2.

Alveolar hyperventilation leading to respiratory alkalosis may have multiple causes, including those secondary to hypoxemia, such as pulmonary disease, congestive heart failure, and high-altitude living, or anemia. Mechanical ventilation is also a common cause of respiratory alkalosis.

Primary stimulation of the central chemoreceptor is a common cause of respiratory alkalosis, as seen in endotoxemia, hepatic cirrhosis, salicylate intoxication, correction of metabolic acidosis, hyperthermia, and pregnancy, as well as cortical hyperventilation from anxiety and pain. In these cases, the signals from central and peripheral chemoreceptors will be in opposition to each other, with central signals overriding peripheral input until the primary stimulus is removed. However, in cases in which the primary stimulus is the result of systemic conditions such as hypoxia secondary to pulmonary disease or anemia, the peripheral and central chemoreceptors initially receive similar signals to reduce ventilation from an increase in both peripheral and CSF pH.

Primary neurologic diseases have also been shown to stimulate alveolar hyperventilation. The causes include acute stroke, infection, trauma, and tumors. Two patterns of respiration are seen: central hyperventilation and Cheyne-Stokes respiration. Central hyperventilation associated with lesions at the pontine-midbrain level is regular, but with an increased rate and tidal volume, whereas Cheyne-Stokes breathing is characterized by periods of hyperventilation alternating with apnea in patients with bilateral cortical and upper pontine lesions and may be related to increased sensitivity of the respiratory center to P_{CO_2}. This mechanism may contribute to the central sleep apnea associated with congestive heart failure and may respond to the application of positive airway pressure.

Renal compensation for sustained hypocapnia is complete in 36 to 72 hours. The mechanism rests primarily in the kidney's net reduction of hydrogen ion excretion, which it accomplishes largely by decreasing ammonium and titratable acid excretion. The threshold for bicarbonate excretion is also lowered, and bicarbonaturia develops. As a result, systemic bicarbonate levels decrease and arterial pH returns toward normal values.

Clinical Manifestations

The clinical manifestations of respiratory alkalosis depend on the degree and duration of the condition but are primarily those of the underlying disorder. Symptoms of acute hypocapnia are largely attributable to the alkalemia and include dizziness, perioral or extremity paresthesias, confusion, asterixis, hypotension, seizures, and coma. Most symptoms are manifested only when the P_{CO_2} has fallen below 25 or 30 mm Hg and can be related to decreased cerebral blood flow or reduced free calcium (because alkalosis increases calcium's protein-bound fraction). Some symptoms frequently seen in the hyperventilation syndrome secondary to pain or anxiety do not appear to be related to hypocapnia and include shortness of breath and chest wall pain. Chronic hypocapnia does not appear to be associated with significant clinical symptoms.

Cerebral blood flow is significantly decreased by hypocapnia, which is a potent vasoconstrictor. This phenomenon is used clinically to decrease intracranial pressure by hyperventilating patients with cerebral edema. As in respiratory acidosis, the CNS is immediately affected by decreases in systemic P_{CO_2} because of the blood-brain barrier's permeability to CO_2. In addition, as in respiratory acidosis, CSF and intracellular pH show an initial short-lived response that parallels the systemic increase in pH.

Acute hypocapnia results in an initial increase in the pH of both CSF and the brain's intracellular environment. However, this increase is quickly offset by a decrease in bicarbonate levels. In acute respiratory alkalosis, one of the primary mechanisms of this fall in bicarbonate appears to be the generation of lactate as a result of vasoconstriction, hypoxia, and increased hemoglobin affinity for oxygen. The combination of increased oxygen demand and decreased oxygen delivery may contribute to adverse clinical outcomes in hypocapnic alkalosis.

Adaptation to High Altitude

Acute exposure to high altitude results in hypoxia-induced hyperventilation. Compensation requires at least several days to take effect and is characterized by a gradual increase in hyperventilation. The result of this continuing increased hyperventilation is a steadily decreasing P_{CO_2} and increasing P_{O_2}. This phenomenon may be the result of conflicting signals from peripheral and central chemoreceptors. The effect of the hypoxic stimulus to ventilate is initially modulated by the effects of alkalosis, both peripherally and centrally. However, as HCO_3^- in CSF falls, inhibition of the central stimulus to ventilate decreases. Therefore, the changing balance between hypoxemia, alkalosis, and CSF pH in adaptation to high altitude may be responsible for this gradual increase in hyperventilation over time. Once a steady state is achieved, the drive to ventilate is determined by the effects of hypoxemia and alkalemia on the peripheral chemoreceptors.

Treatment

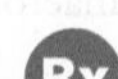

Treatment of respiratory alkalosis must address the underlying cause of the disturbance. Hyperventilation syndrome is a diagnosis of exclusion, but patients who exhibit symptoms, such as tetany and syncope, and do not have more serious causes of hyperventilation can be treated with a rebreathing mask. Hypophosphatemia can be seen in these patients, but it usually improves with treatment of the alkalosis. Patients with respiratory alkalosis associated with mountain sickness can be pretreated with acetazolamide to induce a metabolic acidosis, thereby preventing extreme elevations in pH.

SUGGESTED READINGS

Androgue HJ: Metabolic acidosis: Pathophysiology, diagnosis and treatment. J Nephrol 2006;19(Suppl 9):S62–S69. *A comprehensive review.*

Calabrese AT, Coley KC, DaPos SV, et al: Evaluation of prescribing practices: Risk of lactic acidosis with metformin therapy. Arch Intern Med 2002;162:434–437. *Renal insufficiency and the concomitant administration of cationic agents were risk factors for lactic acidosis.*

De Backer D: Lactic acidosis. Intensive Care Med 2003;29:699–702. *A practical review.*

Gauthier PM, Szerlip HM: Metabolic acidosis in the intensive care unit. Crit Care Clin 2002;18:289–308. *An approach to diagnosis and therapy.*

Laffey JG, Kavanagh BP: Medical progress: Hypocapnia. N Engl J Med 2002; 347:43–53. *A practical review of pathogenesis, diagnosis, and therapy.*

Laing CM, Unwin RJ: Renal tubular acidosis. J Nephrol 2006;19(Suppl 9):S46–S52. *Review of the clinical presentation and therapy.*

Laski ME, Sabatini S: Metabolic alkalosis, bedside and bench. Semin Nephrol 2006;26:441–446. *Review of basic science, diagnosis, and treatment.*

Moviat M, van Haren F, van der Hoeven H: Conventional or physicochemical approach in intensive care unit patients with metabolic acidosis. Crit Care 2003;7:R41–R45. *There was an excellent relationship between the strong ion gap and the albumin-corrected and lactate-corrected anion gap, so calculation of the more time-consuming strong ion gap according to Stewart was unnecessary.*

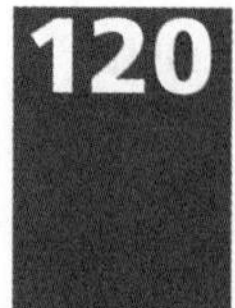

120 DISORDERS OF MAGNESIUM AND PHOSPHORUS

Alan S. L. Yu

MAGNESIUM METABOLISM

Magnesium is an important mineral component of the bony skeleton, a cofactor for many metabolic enzymes, and a regulator of ion channels and transporters in excitable tissues.

Normal Magnesium Metabolism

The majority of total body magnesium is intracellular, or in bone, with only 1% in extracellular fluid. The normal serum magnesium concentration is 1.8 to 2.3 mg/dL (1.5 to 1.9 mEq/L). The average daily intake of magnesium is 300 mg, the main sources of which are green vegetables, nuts, whole grain cereals, milk, and seafood. Magnesium is absorbed mainly in the jejunum and ileum. In the kidney, 70 to 80% of serum magnesium is filtered at the glomerulus, with the majority being reabsorbed along the length of the tubule, particularly in the thick ascending limb of Henle. In states of magnesium deficiency or excess, renal tubule reabsorption is tightly regulated so that magnesium excretion is adjusted accordingly.

Magnesium Deficiency

Pathobiology

Magnesium deficiency is usually detected when hypomagnesemia becomes evident. However, because magnesium is primarily stored intracellularly, substantial depletion of total body magnesium can occur before serum magnesium levels drop appreciably.

Magnesium deficiency may be due to nutritional deficiency, intestinal malabsorption, redistribution into bone, or losses via cutaneous, lower gastrointestinal, or renal routes (Table 120–1). Approximately 25% of alcoholics are chronically hypomagnesemic because of a combination of poor nutritional intake and increased renal loss. Magnesium deficiency can rarely occur in protein-calorie malnutrition and be associated with acute hypomagnesemia during refeeding because of rapid cellular magnesium uptake. Fat malabsorption in conditions such as celiac disease, Crohn's disease, and small intestinal resection causes magnesium deficiency as a result of accumulation of free fatty acids in the intestinal lumen that combine with magnesium to form insoluble soaps. Lower gastrointestinal secretions are rich in magnesium, so diarrhea of colonic origin is a common cause of hypomagnesemia. Sweat contains significant amounts of magnesium, and transient hypomagnesemia can occur after prolonged, intense exercise such as marathon runs. Magnesium is also lost from burned skin surfaces, and 40% of patients with severe burns are hypomagnesemic. In patients with severe hyperparathyroidism and high bone turnover, continued sequestration of minerals within bone may continue for several days after parathyroidectomy and cause transient hypocalcemia, hypomagnesemia, and hypophosphatemia. Renal magnesium losses can occur in any polyuric state, including the recovery phase of acute tubular necrosis or urinary tract obstruction, or in uncontrolled diabetes mellitus. Failure of sodium reabsorption in the thick ascending limb of Henle as a result of Bartter's syndrome or loop diuretic use and failure in the distal convoluted tubule as a result of Gitelman's syndrome or thiazide diuretic use inhibits tubular magnesium reabsorption and leads to urinary magnesium wasting. Drugs that are tubular toxins are also common causes of renal magnesium wasting. Cisplatin causes frequent, dose-dependent hypomagnesemia and hypokalemia. Amphotericin B can cause renal potassium and magnesium wasting, often in association with distal renal tubular acidosis. Significant potassium and magnesium wasting also occurs with aminoglycosides, but only at high cumulative doses. These tubular wasting disorders do not generally correlate with the occurrence of drug-induced acute renal failure.

TABLE 120–1 CAUSES OF MAGNESIUM DEFICIENCY

Nutritional deficiency
Alcoholism*
Malnutrition
Refeeding syndrome
Intestinal malabsorption*
Lower gastrointestinal losses
Colonic diarrhea*
Intestinal fistula
Laxative abuse
Cutaneous losses
Burns*
Exercise-induced sweating
Redistribution into bone
Hungry bone syndrome
Renal losses
Polyuria*
Volume expansion
Hyperaldosteronism
Bartter's/Gitelman's syndrome
Hypercalcemia
Loop and thiazide diuretics*
Nephrotoxins (cisplatin, amphotericin, aminoglycosides, pentamidine, cyclosporine)*

*Common causes.

Clinical Manifestations

Mild to moderate hypomagnesemia or magnesium deficiency is frequently asymptomatic. Manifestations of increased neuronal excitability are the most common symptoms, including paresthesias, tetany, and seizures, which may be associated with the Chvostek or Trousseau signs. Cardiac disturbances may also occur and range in severity from mild electrocardiographic abnormalities (nonspecific T wave changes, U waves, prolonged QT interval, and repolarization alternans) to ventricular tachycardia, torsades de pointes, and ventricular fibrillation. Coexistent hypokalemia is very common, both because many of the causes of hypomagnesemia are also causes of potassium loss and because hypomagnesemia itself causes renal potassium wasting. Severe hypomagnesemia also impairs parathyroid hormone secretion and induces tissue resistance to its actions, thereby leading to hypocalcemia.

Diagnosis

The cause of the magnesium deficiency is often obvious from the history. In difficult diagnostic cases, 24-hour urinary magnesium excretion should be measured. With extrarenal magnesium loss (usually malabsorption or laxative abuse), urinary magnesium excretion is appropriately suppressed (<25 mg/day). Higher urinary magnesium levels indicate renal magnesium wasting, often secondary to surreptitious diuretic use or one of the familial magnesium-wasting disorders.

Treatment

It is unclear whether mild, asymptomatic hypomagnesemia needs to be treated. Magnesium repletion is recommended in hypomagnesemic patients if they are symptomatic, have underlying cardiac or seizure disorders, exhibit concurrent severe hypocalcemia or hypokalemia, or have severe hypomagnesemia (<1.4 mg/dL). In mild cases or in the outpatient setting, oral magnesium salts such as magnesium oxide may be used for repletion, but these substances frequently cause diarrhea, particularly at high doses. In the inpatient setting, intravenous magnesium sulfate may be used for repletion. Because redistribution of magnesium from extracellular to intracellular compartments is relatively slow, the serum magnesium concentration may normalize before total body magnesium stores are replete. It is therefore prudent to continue intravenous magnesium repletion for an additional 1 to 2 days after restoration of normo-

magnesemia. In patients with normal renal function, any excess magnesium is simply excreted renally. Adverse effects from intravenous magnesium administration are primarily due to transient hypermagnesemia and include flushing, hypotension, and flaccid paralysis. Amiloride abrogates renal magnesium wasting in some patients with this problem, but the mechanism of this effect is unknown.

Hypermagnesemia

Transient hypermagnesemia can occur in patients given large doses of intravenous magnesium, for example, in the setting of preeclampsia. It has also been reported in individuals taking large doses of magnesium-containing antacids or cathartics, particularly in settings in which intestinal absorption is enhanced, such as inflammatory bowel disease and intestinal obstruction. However, the kidney has a very large capacity to excrete excess magnesium. Thus, persistent hypermagnesemia is seen almost exclusively in patients with chronic renal insufficiency who are also taking excessive amounts of magnesium in the form of antacids, cathartics, or enemas.

Clinical Manifestations

Magnesium toxicity is a serious and potentially fatal condition. Mild hypermagnesemia (serum magnesium level >4 to 6 mg/dL) causes hypotension, nausea, vomiting, facial flushing, urinary retention, and ileus. Above serum magnesium levels of 8 to 12 mg/dL, flaccid skeletal muscular paralysis and hyporeflexia may ensue, together with bradyarrhythmias, respiratory depression, coma, and cardiac arrest. A low, or even negative serum anion gap may sometimes be seen.

Treatment

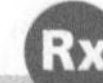

Mild hypermagnesemia in a patient with good renal function usually requires no treatment because renal clearance is rapid and the normal serum half-life of magnesium is about 1 day. In the event of serious toxicity, the effects of magnesium can be temporarily antagonized by the administration of intravenous calcium salts. Renal magnesium excretion can be enhanced by saline diuresis with concomitant administration of furosemide. In patients with advanced renal insufficiency, the most effective method of magnesium removal is hemodialysis.

PHOSPHORUS METABOLISM

Phosphorus has many critical roles. It is a major component of bone mineral, of phospholipids in cell membranes, and of nucleic acids. It forms high-energy phosphate bonds in compounds such as adenosine triphosphate (ATP), is post-translationally bound to proteins as an intracellular signal, and acts as a major pH buffer in serum and urine.

Normal Phosphorus Metabolism

Of the total body phosphorus content, 85% is in bone, 14% is in intracellular compartments, and only 1% is in extracellular fluid. The normal concentration of phosphorus in plasma is 3 to 4.5 mg/dL (1 to 1.5 mM). Daily intake of phosphorus is 800 to 1500 mg. Phosphorus is present in many foods, including dairy products, meat, and grains, and is absorbed in the small intestine. The kidneys excrete excess phosphorus, which is the principal mechanism by which the body regulates extracellular phosphate balance. Ninety percent of serum phosphate is filtered at the glomerulus, of which 80 to 97% is reabsorbed along the nephron, primarily in the proximal tubule. Parathyroid hormone increases renal phosphate excretion by inhibiting the sodium-phosphate cotransporter in the proximal tubule, whereas vitamin D enhances intestinal phosphate absorption.

TABLE 120–2 CAUSES OF HYPOPHOSPHATEMIA

Nutritional deficiency
Alcoholism*
Impaired intestinal absorption
Antacids
Vitamin D deficiency*
Redistribution into cells
Respiratory alkalosis*
Insulin*
Refeeding syndrome
Burns*
Redistribution into bone
Hungry bone syndrome
Renal losses
Hyperparathyroidism*
Renal tubulopathy
Fanconi's syndrome
Drugs (pentamidine, foscarnet, acetazolamide)
Phosphatonin excess syndrome
Oncogenic osteomalacia
Familial hypophosphatemic rickets

*Common causes.

Hypophosphatemia

Pathobiology

Hypophosphatemia may be caused by decreased intake, impaired intestinal absorption, redistribution into cells or bone, and renal losses (Table 120–2). Alcoholics are frequently phosphate depleted because of intake of a carbohydrate-rich, phosphate-poor diet, as well as renal phosphate wasting. Divalent cation–containing antacids bind phosphate in the intestinal lumen to form insoluble salts, thus preventing their absorption. Vitamin D deficiency also leads to decreased intestinal phosphate absorption and hence to hypophosphatemia. Respiratory (but not metabolic) alkalosis may cause transient hypophosphatemia. In this disorder, intracellular pH is increased, thereby stimulating glycolysis, which depletes the intracellular inorganic phosphate pool and leads to a shift of phosphate into cells. Insulin is also a strong stimulus for shifting phosphate into cells. Patients with diabetic ketoacidosis are often hyperphosphatemic because of a shift of phosphate out of cells under insulinopenic conditions, but they are actually total body phosphate depleted as a result of urinary losses. Subsequent treatment with insulin may uncover severe hypophosphatemia. Similarly, in malnourished patients whose total body phosphate stores may be depleted, overzealous intravenous refeeding with carbohydrate-rich fluids may stimulate insulin release and cause acute hypophosphatemia.

Renal phosphate wasting is usually due to impaired proximal tubule phosphate reabsorption. In primary hyperparathyroidism, hypercalcemia is typically associated with hypophosphatemia. Fanconi's syndrome is a generalized proximal tubule disorder characterized by hypophosphatemia in association with glycosuria, aminoaciduria, hypokalemia, and type II renal tubular acidosis; it can be caused by a variety of inherited metabolic disorders, multiple myeloma, heavy metal intoxication, and drugs such as ifosfamide, cidofovir, and tenofovir. Phosphaturia can also occur with diuretics, particularly carbonic anhydrase inhibitors, and with antimicrobial agents such as pentamidine and foscarnet. Oncogenic osteomalacia is a paraneoplastic syndrome associated primarily with mesenchymal tumors that secrete a variety of phosphaturic factors collectively known as phosphatonins. A similar phenotype is found in X-linked and autosomal dominant hypophosphatemic rickets, inherited disorders characterized by an increase in a circulating phosphatonin, fibroblast growth factor-23. Phosphatonins inhibit both renal tubular phosphate reabsorption and 1α-hydroxylation of 25-hydroxycholecalciferol, thus leading to hypophosphatemia, rickets or osteomalacia, and inappropriately low serum levels of 1,25-dihydroxycholecalciferol.

Clinical Manifestations

Clinical complications are usually observed only with severe hypophosphatemia (<1 mg/dL) and are thought to be due to disruption of cell membrane composition, depletion of ATP (which particularly affects high energy-consuming tissues such as skeletal and cardiac muscle), and in erythrocytes, depletion of 2,3-diphosphoglycerate, thus impairing tissue oxygen delivery. Manifestations of severe hypophosphatemia include encephalopathy, dilated cardiomyopathy, generalized muscle weakness that can lead to respiratory failure, rhabdomyolysis, and hemolysis. Hypophosphatemia also impairs renal ammoniagenesis and reduces the availability of urinary buffer, thereby impairing renal acid excretion and causing metabolic acidosis. Chronic hypophosphatemia leads to resorption of bone and osteomalacia.

Diagnosis

The cause of hypophosphatemia is often evident from the history and examination. If not, measurement of either 24-hour urinary phosphate excretion or fractional excretion of phosphate (F_EPO_4) in a spot urine sample is often helpful.

$$F_EPO_4 = \frac{\text{Uring phosphate} \times \text{Serum creatinine}}{\text{Serum phosphate} \times \text{Urine creatinine}}$$

In the setting of hypophosphatemia, the normal response of the kidney is to reduce urinary phosphate excretion to less than 100 mg/day or reduce F_EPO_4 to less than 5%. Values above these suggest one of the causes of renal phosphate wasting.

Treatment

Rx

Patients with asymptomatic, mild to moderate hypophosphatemia, normal total body phosphorus stores, and minimal ongoing phosphorus losses (e.g., a patient with hypophosphatemia as a result of acute respiratory alkalosis) do not require treatment. Phosphate should be repleted in patients who are symptomatic, suspected to have severe depletion of intracellular phosphorus stores (malnourished or alcoholic patients), have ongoing gastrointestinal or renal losses, or have severe hypophosphatemia (<1 mg/dL). Oral repletion can be performed with sodium or potassium phosphate salts or with skimmed milk. Intravenous phosphorus repletion at rates of up to 15 mmol/hr (465 mg/hr) for 1 to 3 hours is recommended for severe hypophosphatemia but contraindicated in patients with renal insufficiency. Complications of phosphate therapy include hypocalcemia, metastatic calcification, hypotension, acute renal failure, and arrhythmias, as well as concomitant hypernatremia or hyperkalemia, depending on which salt is administered.

Hyperphosphatemia

Pathobiology

Pseudohyperphosphatemia may occur in blood specimens that are hemolyzed or hyperglobulinemic, such as in multiple myeloma. True hyperphosphatemia is caused by excessive phosphate intake, increased intestinal absorption, redistribution from intracellular stores, or impaired renal excretion (Table 120–3). Overzealous phosphate repletion can obviously cause hyperphosphatemia. The phosphorus in some laxatives and enemas may be absorbed and cause hyperphosphatemia. Intoxication with vitamin D or its analogues increases intestinal absorption of both calcium and phosphorus. Conditions associated with massive cell lysis, such as rhabdomyolysis and tumor lysis syndrome, cause release of intracellular phosphate into the extracellular fluid. Patients with diabetic ketoacidosis are often hyperphosphatemic at initial evaluation because of redistribution out of cells in the insulin-deficient state. Decreased phosphate excretion is most commonly due to acute or chronic renal failure. With a normal diet, serum phosphate levels can be maintained within the normal range until the glomerular filtration rate falls below 25 mL/min. However, even mild degrees of renal insufficiency may predispose to hyperphosphatemia if there is concurrent excessive intake of phosphate-containing compounds such as laxatives. Finally, because parathyroid hormone stimulates proximal tubule phosphate excretion, primary hypoparathyroidism is often associated with mild hyperphosphatemia together with hypocalcemia.

TABLE 120–3 CAUSES OF HYPERPHOSPHATEMIA

Phosphate intake
Phosphate repletion
Phosphate-containing laxatives and enemas*
Increased intestinal absorption
Vitamin D toxicity
Redistribution from intracellular stores
Rhabdomyolysis
Tumor lysis syndrome
Diabetic ketoacidosis
Decreased renal excretion
Renal failure*
Hypoparathyroidism

*Common causes.

Clinical Manifestations

Acute hyperphosphatemia increases the risk of precipitation of calcium phosphate and subsequent metastatic calcification in soft tissues, including the kidney, which may cause acute renal failure. The resultant hypocalcemia can cause tetany, hypotension, seizures, and cardiac arrhythmias. In the chronic hyperphosphatemia of chronic renal insufficiency, patients with a serum phosphate concentration greater than 6.5 mg/dL or a calcium-phosphate product greater than 72 mg^2/dL^2 have higher mortality. Hyperphosphatemia in this setting is a risk factor for coronary calcification, thus suggesting that this may be the underlying mechanism for the increased mortality.

Treatment

Rx

Acute hyperphosphatemia in an asymptomatic patient with normal renal function often resolves spontaneously as excess phosphate is excreted. In symptomatic patients and those with impaired renal function, phosphate should be removed by extracorporeal therapy. Because of the slow rate of mobilization of phosphate from intracellular stores, continuous venovenous hemodiafiltration is considerably more effective than intermittent hemodialysis. Chronic hyperphosphatemia can be managed by minimizing dietary phosphorus intake and administering oral phosphate binders such as calcium salts, lanthanum carbonate, or sevelamer during meals. Aluminum hydroxide is also a very effective phosphate binder, but prolonged use leads to aluminum accumulation and results in encephalopathy and osteomalacia. Cinacalcet, a calcimimetic used in patients with chronic renal insufficiency for the treatment of secondary hyperparathyroidism, also reduces the serum phosphate concentration and calcium-phosphate product.

SUGGESTED READINGS

Block GA, Port FK: Re-evaluation of risks associated with hyperphosphatemia and hyperparathyroidism in dialysis patients: Recommendations for a change in management. Am J Kidney Dis 2000;35:1226–1237. *Discussion of topical issues in the management of hyperphosphatemia in patients with chronic renal insufficiency.*

Charron T, Bernard F, Skrobik Y, et al: Intravenous phosphate in the intensive care unit: More aggressive repletion regimens for moderate and severe hypophosphatemia. Intensive Care Med 2003;29:1273–1278. *Evidence supporting the safety and efficacy of relatively aggressive intravenous phosphate regimens.*

Konrad M, Weber S: Recent advances in molecular genetics of hereditary magnesium-losing disorders. J Am Soc Nephrol 2003;14:249–260. *Nice discussion* of inherited hypomagnesemia and recent insights into the mechanisms for renal tubular magnesium transport.*

Schiavi SC, Kumar R: The phosphatonin pathway: New insights in phosphate homeostasis. Kidney Int 2004;65:1–14. *Highlights this novel pathway for phosphate regulation.*

Tenenhouse HS: Phosphate transport: Molecular basis, regulation and pathophysiology. J Steroid Biochem Mol Biol 2007;103:572–577. *A comprehensive, scholarly review.*

121 ACUTE KIDNEY INJURY

Bruce A. Molitoris

Definition

Acute kidney injury (AKI) was recently suggested as the new nomenclature for acute renal failure (ARF) by an international group of nephrologists and critical care specialists. The impetus for this change in nomenclature arose not only to ameliorate the historical lack of consensus on a concise definition of ARF but also to encompass the diverse causes of ARF better. This new nomenclature defines AKI as a functional or structural abnormality of the kidney manifested within 48 hours as determined by blood, urine, or tissue tests or imaging studies. Diagnostically, the reduction in kidney function in AKI is associated with either an absolute increase in serum creatinine of 0.3 mg/dL or a percent increase in serum creatinine of 50%. In addition, a reduction in urine output consisting of oliguria of less than 0.5 mL/kg/hr for longer than 6 hours fulfills the diagnostic criteria for AKI.

Epidemiology

Most episodes of AKI occur in the hospital with an incidence ranging from 5 to 7%. By contrast, the incidence of community-acquired AKI was 1% in a recent study. Regardless of the setting, however, the impact of AKI on patient mortality is profound, with mortality rates ranging from 36% to as high as 86%. The magnitude of mortality depends on the setting in which AKI is acquired, the age of the patient, and the acuity of the illness. Higher mortality rates occur in older patients with hospital-acquired AKI admitted to an intensive care unit. Furthermore, mortality in patients with AKI is incremental, and seemingly modest increases in serum creatinine can result in marked increases in the mortality rate. In three studies, an increase in serum creatinine of only 0.3 mg/dL resulted in a markedly increased risk for mortality.

Pathobiology

The etiology of AKI is diverse and it can arise from a number of physiologic insults. Decreased renal perfusion with or without cellular injury; toxic, ischemic, or obstructive injury to the renal tubule; inflammation and edema of the tubulointerstitium; and a primary glomerular disease process can all confer kidney injury and result in a reduced glomerular filtration rate (GFR). Both conceptually and diagnostically, the various causes of AKI are divided broadly into three anatomic categories: prerenal, intrarenal or intrinsic, and postrenal (Fig. 121–1). Each of these categories represents a unique pathophysiologic process with distinctive diagnostic parameters and prognosis.

Prerenal Acute Kidney Injury

Prerenal azotemia is the most common cause of AKI and accounts for approximately 60 to 70% of community-acquired and 40% of hospital-acquired cases. The precipitating event for prerenal AKI is renal hypoperfusion (Fig. 121–2). It can occur secondary to a reduction in the volume of extracellular fluid or in disease states that have normal extracellular fluid volume but decrements in effective arterial volume such as in sepsis, congestive heart failure (CHF), and advanced cirrhosis. Additionally, medications that reduce glomerular capillary perfusion, such as angiotensin-converting enzyme inhibitors (ACEIs), angiotensin-receptor blockers (ARBs), and nonsteroidal anti-inflammatory drugs (NSAIDs), can also cause prerenal AKI. Early in the course of prerenal AKI the renal parenchyma remains intact and functional. During this initial phase, renal autoregulatory mechanisms attempt to maintain GFR and renal blood flow by altering the vascular tone of the afferent and efferent arterioles of the glomerulus. Specifically, renal hypoperfusion initiates a neurohormonal cascade that results in afferent arteriolar dilation and efferent arteriolar constriction. As a result, the GFR remains largely intact. Because prerenal azotemia is often easily reversible and mortality rates are low, early diagnosis and correction of the underlying pathophysiology are of critical importance. However, without early medical corrective intervention, progression to worsening ischemia results in tubular cell injury and further decreases in GFR. Thus, prerenal azotemia progresses to tubular cell injury and intrinsic AKI. Progression from prerenal azotemia to ischemic renal injury is a continuum that depends on the severity and duration of the physiologic insult.

Intrinsic Acute Kidney Injury

The causes of intrinsic AKI are diverse and can involve any portion of the renal nephron and interstitium (see Fig. 121–2). Intrinsic AKI is classified according to the primary histologic site of injury: tubules, interstitium, vasculature, or glomerulus. Renal tubular cell injury, commonly termed *acute tubular necrosis* (ATN), occurs more commonly in the setting of ischemia, although the renal tubules can also incur damage from specific renal toxins. Ischemia can arise from a number of different clinical scenarios, but the common underlying pathogenesis is reduced renal blood flow (Table 121–1). This progression from prerenal azotemia

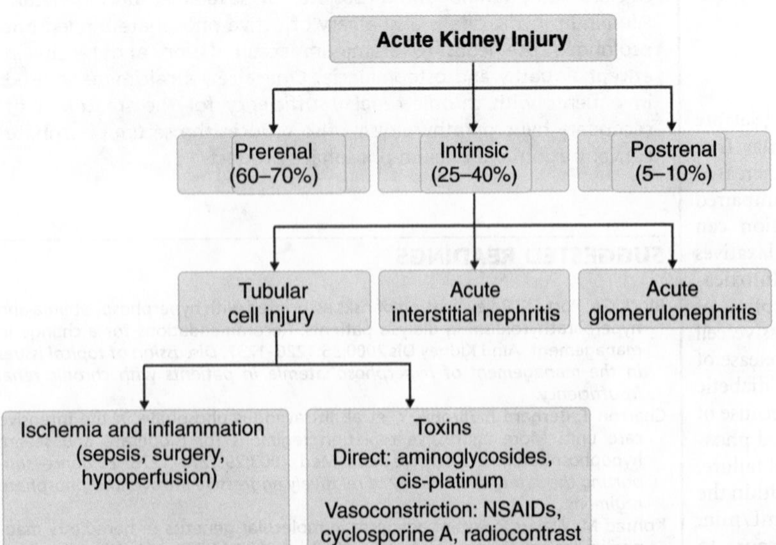

FIGURE 121–1 • Main categories of acute kidney injury. NSAIDs = nonsteroidal anti-inflammatory drugs.

to ischemic AKI occurs in four distinct clinical and cellular phases: initiation, extension, maintenance, and recovery. Each of these phases encompasses distinct cellular events and temporal rates of glomerular filtration that occur as the kidneys respond to the insult and attempt to maintain and re-establish function (Fig. 121–3). The initiation phase, which marks the transition from prerenal to tubular cell injury and dysfunction, is characterized by severe cellular depletion of adenosine triphosphate. Renal tubular epithelial cell injury is a prominent feature during this phase; however, endothelial and vascular smooth muscle cell injury has also been documented. During the extension phase, two major events occur: microvascular congestion with continued hypoxia and inflammation. These events are most pronounced in the corticomedullary junction of the kidney. In this region, limitations to reperfusion occur secondary to endothelial dysfunction with white blood cell adhesion. The GFR is at its ebb during the maintenance phase, but cells continue to undergo repair, migration, and proliferation, and attempts at cellular and tubule integrity are re-established. Finally, during the recovery phase, the GFR begins to improve as cellular differentiation continues and normal cellular and organ function returns.

The S3 segment of the proximal tubule is located in the outer stripe of the medullary region of the nephron. This region is particularly susceptible to continued reduced perfusion following injury, and ongoing or worsening hypoxia results in continued cellular injury. Proximal tubular cell injury during the initiation phase of renal ischemia is first manifested as bleb formation in the apical membranes with loss of the brush border. Proximal tubule cells also lose their surface membrane polarity and integrity of their tight junction. As the injury progresses, both live and necrotic proximal cells detach and enter the tubular lumen and then ultimately form casts in the distal tubule. Casts contribute to a reduction in GFR by obstructing tubular urine flow. In addition, loss of the epithelial cell barrier and cell tight junctions allows back-leakage of the glomerular filtrate into the interstitium, thus further compromising GFR (Fig. 121–2).

Renal toxins can cause tubular damage both directly and indirectly. Common agents that can cause direct tubular cell toxicity (Table 121–2) include the aminoglycoside antibiotics, intravenous radiocontrast agents, and cisplatin. Other agents such as radiocontrast dyes, NSAIDs, and cyclosporine induce vasoconstriction and reduce renal perfusion. Cocaine and the 3-hydroxy-3-methylglutaryl coenzyme A (HMG-CoA) reductase inhibitors can induce skeletal muscle damage and a heme pigment tubular toxicity termed *rhabdomyolysis.* Finally, some compounds, through precipitation of the parent compound or its metabolites, can cause intratubular obstruction. Agents in this category include acyclovir, sulfonamides, ethylene glycol (calcium oxalate metabolite), methotrexate, and multiple myeloma light chains. Fortunately, AKI does not develop in every patient exposed to these agents, but certain patients are more susceptible. Generally, elderly patients, patients with diabetes mellitus, hypotensive patients, and patients with a reduced effective arterial volume (CHF, cirrhosis, hypoalbuminemia) are the most susceptible to toxic renal injury. In fact, the incidence of aminoglycoside antibiotic nephrotoxicity increases from 3 to 5% to 30 to 50% in these high-risk patients.

AKI secondary to injury to the renal interstitium is termed *acute interstitial nephritis* (AIN) (Table 121–3). Commonly implicated medications include penicillins, cephalosporins, sulfonamides, and NSAIDs (Chapter 123). Bacterial and viral infections have also been shown to be causative agents for AIN. Finally, AIN has been associated with a kidney-confined

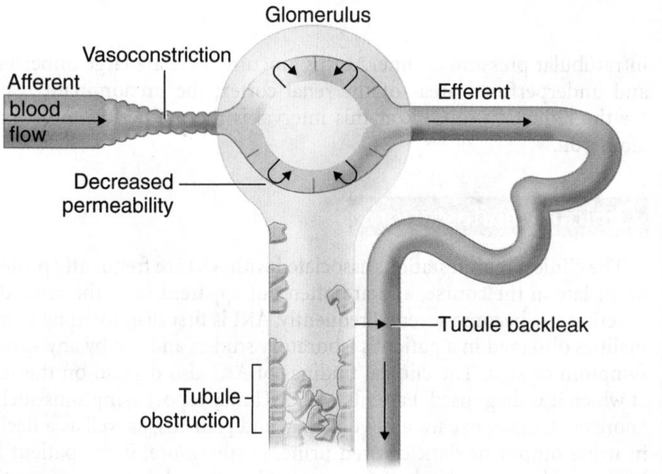

FIGURE 121–2 • Mechanisms of prerenal and intrinsic acute renal injury. See text for descriptions.

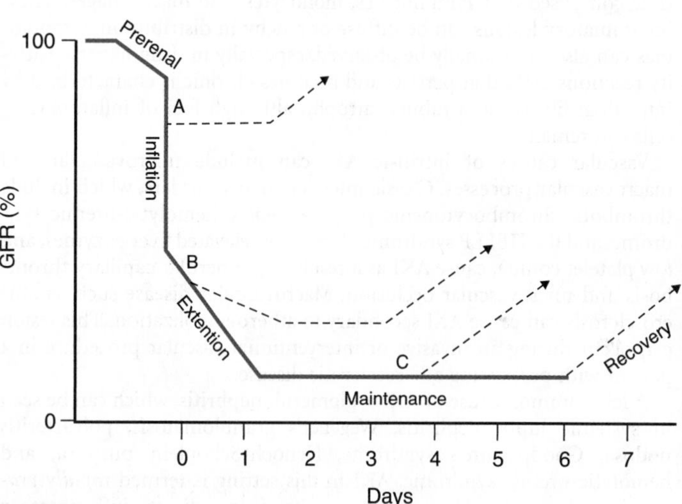

FIGURE 121–3 • Phases of acute kidney injury. GFR = glomerular filtration rate. (Reprinted with permission from Sutton TA, Fisher CJ, Molitoris BA: Microvascular endothelial injury and dysfunction during ischemic acute renal failure. Kidney Int 2002;62:1539–1549.)

TABLE 121–1 CONDITIONS THAT LEAD TO ISCHEMIC ACUTE RENAL FAILURE

Mechanism	Condition
Intravascular volume depletion and hypotension	Hemorrhage; gastrointestinal, renal, and dermal losses
Decreased effective intravascular volume	Congestive heart failure, cirrhosis, hepatorenal syndrome, peritonitis
Systemic vasodilation/renal vasoconstriction	Sepsis, hepatorenal syndrome
Large-vessel renal vascular disease	Renal artery thrombosis or embolism, intraoperative arterial cross-clamping, renal artery stenosis, cholesterol emboli
Small-vessel renal vascular disease	Sepsis, vasculitis, atheroembolism, hemolytic-uremic syndrome, malignant hypertension, scleroderma, preeclampsia, sickle cell anemia, hypercalcemia, transplant rejection
Impaired renal blood flow	Cyclosporine, tacrolimus, ACEIs, ARBs, NSAIDs, radiocontrast agents

ACEIs = angiotensin-converting enzyme inhibitors; ARBs = angiotensin-receptor blockers; NSAIDs = nonsteroidal anti-inflammatory drugs.

TABLE 121–2 COMMON RENAL TUBULAR TOXINS

Aminoglycosides
Radiocontrast agents
Acyclovir
Cisplatin
Sulfonamides
Methotrexate
Cyclosporine
Tacrolimus
Amphotericin B
Methotrexate
Foscarnet
Pentamidine
Ethylene glycol
Toluene
Cocaine
HMG-CoA reductase inhibitors

HMG-CoA = 3-hydroxy-3-methylglutaryl coenzyme A.

or systemic autoimmune process. Disease states implicated in this setting include systemic lupus erythematosus, Sjögren's syndrome, cryoglobulinemia, and primary biliary cirrhosis (Table 121–3). The interstitial injury arising from AIN occurs secondary to a mixed inflammatory infiltrate composed of T lymphocytes, monocytes, and macrophages. These inflammatory lesions can be diffuse or patchy in distribution. Granulomas can also occasionally be observed, especially in drug hypersensitivity reactions. AIN that persists and becomes chronic is characterized by interstitial fibrosis and tubular atrophy, although foci of inflammatory cells can remain.

Vascular causes of intrinsic AKI can include microvascular and macrovascular processes. Classic microvascular disorders, which include thrombotic thrombocytopenic purpura, sepsis, hemolytic-uremic syndrome, and the HELLP syndrome (*h*emolysis, *e*levated *l*iver enzymes, and *l*ow *p*latelet count), cause AKI as a result of glomerular capillary thrombosis and microvascular occlusion. Macrovascular disease such as atherosclerosis can cause AKI secondary to atheroembolization. This lesion can occur during an invasive or interventional vascular procedure in a patient with preexisting atherosclerotic disease.

A less common cause of AKI is glomerulonephritis, which can be seen in systemic lupus nephritis, Wegener's granulomatosis, polyarteritis nodosa, Goodpasture's syndrome, Henoch-Schönlein purpura, and hemolytic-uremic syndrome. AKI in this setting is termed *rapidly progressive glomerulonephritis* and results from direct inflammatory glomerular injury.

Postrenal Acute Kidney Injury

Postrenal AKI can occur in the setting of bilateral urinary outflow obstruction or in a patient with a solitary kidney when a single urinary outflow tract is obstructed (Chapter 124). Most commonly, this type of outflow obstruction is observed in patients with prostatic hypertrophy, prostatic or cervical cancer, or retroperitoneal disorders. A functional obstruction can be observed in those with a neurogenic bladder. In addition, intraluminal obstruction can be seen in patients with bilateral renal calculi, papillary necrosis, blood clots, and bladder carcinoma, whereas extraluminal obstruction can develop in connection with retroperitoneal fibrosis, colon cancer, and lymphomas. Finally, intratubular crystallization of compounds such as uric acid, calcium oxalate, acyclovir, sulfonamide, and methotrexate, as well as myeloma light chains, can result in tubular obstruction.

The pathology seen in postrenal AKI is caused by obstruction to luminal flow of the glomerular filtrate. This obstruction results in a relatively complex pathophysiology that begins with transmission of backpressure to Bowman's space of the glomerulus. Intuitively, this backpressure would be expected to reduce the GFR. However, by dilation of the glomerular afferent arteriole, the GFR remains largely preserved. Unfortunately, such compensation is only transient and the GFR will begin to attenuate if the obstruction is not rapidly relieved. With continued obstruction eclipsing 12 to 24 hours, renal blood flow, GFR, and

TABLE 121–3 MEDICATIONS ASSOCIATED WITH ACUTE INTERSTITIAL NEPHRITIS

β-LACTAM ANTIBIOTICS
Penicillin
Cephalosporins
Ampicillin
Methicillin
Nafcillin
DIURETICS
Furosemide
Hydrochlorothiazide
Triamterene
OTHER ANTIBIOTICS
Sulfonamides
Vancomycin
Rifampin
Acyclovir
Indinavir
NSAIDS
Ibuprofen
Naproxen
Indomethacin

NSAIDs = nonsteroidal anti-inflammatory drugs.

intratubular pressure decline. At this juncture there are large unperfused and underperfused areas of the renal cortex; the predominant reason for the reduction in GFR at this interval is the nonperfusion of many glomeruli.

Clinical Manifestations

The clinical manifestations associated with AKI are frequently protean, occur late in the course, and are often not apparent until the renal dysfunction has become severe. Frequently, AKI is first diagnosed by abnormalities observed in a patient's laboratory studies and not by any specific symptom or sign. The clinical findings of AKI also depend on the stage at which it is diagnosed. Patients with AKI may report symptoms such as anorexia, fatigue, nausea and vomiting, and pruritus, as well as a decline in urine output or dark-colored urine. Furthermore, if the patient has become volume overloaded, shortness of breath and dyspnea on exertion may be noted. On physical examination, findings such as asterixis, myoclonus, or a pericardial rub may be evident. If volume overload is present, peripheral edema, pulmonary crackles, and jugular venous distention may be found. It is also not unusual for a patient to be entirely asymptomatic, with advanced AKI discovered only by laboratory testing.

Diagnosis

The history and physical examination often help reveal the etiology of AKI in a patient. The history must include any potential exposure to nephrotoxins and NSAID use. A thorough physical examination with special emphasis on determination of volume status and effective arterial volume is essential. A systematic approach that considers each of the three major categories in the pathogenesis of AKI will ensure that an accurate diagnosis and an appropriate therapeutic plan will be achieved. Hence, an appropriate diagnostic strategy would be to exclude prerenal and postrenal causes first and then, if needed, begin an evaluation for possible intrinsic causes.

Laboratory analysis of blood and urine samples of patients with AKI reveals the level of dysfunction and will frequently suggest an etiology. It may also direct the rapidity with which a specific therapy needs to be instituted because AKI is usually clinically silent. All patients with clini-

TABLE 121–4 FE_{Na} VALUES FOR THE VARIOUS CAUSES OF ACUTE KIDNEY INJURY

Etiology of Acute Kidney Injury	FE_{Na}	BUN-to-Serum Creatinine Ratio
Prerenal	<1%	>20
Intrarenal		<10–15
Tubular necrosis	≥1%	
Interstitial nephritis	≥1%	
Glomerulonephritis (early)	<1%	
Vascular disorders (early)	<1%	
Postrenal	≥1%	>20

TABLE 121–5 COMMON URINALYSIS FINDINGS IN ACUTE KIDNEY INJURY

Cause of Acute Kidney Injury	Urinalysis
Prerenal	Normal or hyaline casts
Intrarenal	
Tubular cell injury	Muddy-brown, granular, epithelial casts
Interstitial nephritis	Pyuria, hematuria, mild proteinuria, granular and epithelial casts, eosinophils
Glomerulonephritis	Hematuria, marked proteinuria, red blood cell casts, granular casts
Vascular disorders	Normal or hematuria, mild proteinuria
Postrenal	Normal or hematuria, granular casts, pyuria

cal findings of AKI should have a renal panel and complete blood count with differential performed. In addition, urine studies, including sodium, potassium, chloride, and creatinine (Cr) determinations for calculation of the fractional excretion of sodium (FE_{Na}), are important. The formula for calculating FE_{Na} is

$$FE_{Na} = \frac{\text{Urine Na} \times \text{Plasma Cr}}{\text{Plasma Na} \times \text{Urine Cr}} \times 100$$

The numerical value of FE_{Na} can be helpful in determining the potential cause of the AKI (Table 121–4). In some cases it is better to use FE_{Cl} because urinary sodium can be elevated during systemic alkalosis with high urinary bicarbonate obligating loss of sodium. Urine dipstick and microscopy should also be performed. Urine microscopy must be performed on a fresh urine sample because important cellular elements that could indicate potential causes degrade rapidly with time. Table 121–5 lists typical urinalysis findings seen in the various causes of AKI. Finally, renal ultrasound to determine the presence of outlet obstruction should also be included in the initial evaluation.

Prerenal Azotemia

Prerenal azotemia is the most common cause of renal dysfunction and can often be determined by the patient's history. Common historical features in patients with prerenal azotemia include vomiting, diarrhea, and poor oral intake. CHF can suggest a possible prerenal cause secondary to reduced renal perfusion from a concomitant exacerbation in CHF or from diuresis with loop diuretics. Other medications that can attenuate renal perfusion, such as NSAIDs, ACEIs, and ARBs, have also been implicated in the prerenal state. Common physical examination findings include tachycardia, systemic or orthostatic hypotension (or both), and dry mucous membranes.

Laboratory studies in patients with prerenal azotemia demonstrate elevated serum creatinine and blood urea nitrogen (BUN) levels. FE_{Na} is typically less than 1%. However, in a patient taking diuretics such as furosemide, FE_{Na} may be greater than 1% even though the patient has prerenal azotemia. This is secondary to diuretic-induced natriuresis. For these clinical situations, fractional excretion of urea can be used and is calculated in similar fashion:

$$FE_{urea} = \frac{\text{Urine urea} \times \text{Plasma Cr}}{\text{Plasma urea} \times \text{Urine Cr}} \times 100$$

FE_{urea} less than 35% suggests prerenal AKI. Other causes of an FE_{Na} greater than 1% include the presence of a non-reabsorbable solute such as bicarbonate, glucose, or mannitol. Chronic kidney disease, ATN, and late obstructive nephropathy are also associated with an FE_{Na} greater than 1%. However, in these disease states, FE_{Na} cannot be relied on to provide any useful diagnostic information. Moreover, FE_{urea} has not been validated for these clinical entities.

Another laboratory parameter that can assist in diagnosing prerenal AKI is the ratio of BUN to serum creatinine. Commonly, a patient with prerenal azotemia will have a BUN-to–serum creatinine ratio of greater than 20:1.

Intrarenal Acute Kidney Injury

A history of nephrotoxin exposure is a common finding in patients with intrarenal AKI. The nephrotoxin can be a specific tubular toxin causing ATN or can be the result of an allergic reaction as in AIN (see Tables 121–2 and 121–3). Physical examination may reveal signs and symptoms of fluid overload such as pulmonary edema and decreased urine output. Rash may accompany AIN. Cholesterol embolism in patients with severe atherosclerotic disease may be manifested classically as cyanotic digits and AKI. This finding is frequently seen after invasive vascular surgery or an interventional study. Laboratory studies will demonstrate elevated serum creatinine and BUN levels in intrarenal AKI. ATN and AIN are frequently associated with an FE_{Na} greater than 1, whereas in glomerulonephritis and vascular disorders, FE_{Na} is typically less than 1. Peripheral eosinophilia and urinary eosinophils may be present in AIN, although the latter are neither sensitive nor specific for this type of AKI. Urinary eosinophils are also associated with microembolic disease. Intrarenal AKI has specific urinalysis findings that can be helpful in making diagnostic and therapeutic decisions (see Table 121–5).

Postrenal Acute Kidney Injury

A history of prostatic hypertrophy, prostate cancer, lymphoma, cervical cancer, or retroperitoneal disease can often be found in patients with postrenal AKI. Postrenal AKI should always be in the differential diagnosis of patients with severe oliguria (urine output <450 mL/day) or anuria (urine output <100 mL/day). However, many patients with postrenal AKI are not oliguric or anuric. Beyond an elevation in a patient's serum creatinine and BUN, laboratory studies generally yield benign results. Bladder catheterization can be both diagnostic and therapeutic in postrenal AKI; however, renal ultrasound is the diagnostic test of choice. An important caveat is that early in postrenal AKI, renal ultrasound may be falsely negative.

Treatment

The cornerstones of therapy for AKI are rapid recognition and correction of reversible causes, avoidance of any further renal injury, and maintenance of a normal electrolyte and fluid volume milieu. Studies have demonstrated that preventive therapy or medical interventions performed during the initiation and extension phases of AKI provide the greatest chance for minimizing the extent of injury (Fig. 121–3, lines A and B) and hastening renal recovery (Fig. 121–3, line B); interventions provided during the maintenance phase of AKI have not proved beneficial (Fig. 121–3, line C). Hence, correction of the prerenal state, early preventive therapy, and early diagnosis of AKI are imperative for patients with AKI regardless of the cause. Prerenal azotemia in its early stages can be rapidly corrected by aggressive normalization of effective arterial volume. Normalization of the patient's effective arterial volume may involve administering volume (normal saline), improving cardiac output by afterload reduction, or normalizing systemic vascular resistance. More care must be taken during volume resuscitation in patients with a history of CHF. If prerenal AKI is not addressed early in a

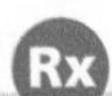

patient's course or if the patient is seen by the physician late in the course, acute tubular cell injury may occur and result in a marked increase in morbidity and mortality. Postrenal AKI secondary to prostatic hypertrophy can frequently be corrected by placement of a bladder catheter. However, outlet obstruction from a neoplastic process will usually require urologic consultation for consideration of ureteral stenting or placement of a percutaneous nephrostomy tube. Intrarenal AKI can often be the most complex and difficult to treat. AKI secondary to glomerulonephritis or vasculitis will frequently require immunosuppressive therapy. For suspected AIN, the offending medication must be determined and discontinued. Often a tapering course of glucocorticoids is given, but definitive data supporting the value of this are lacking. Other general supportive measures that should be instituted include avoiding any further nephrotoxins and paying careful attention to the patient's fluid balance by monitoring weight and input and output daily. In addition, serum electrolytes, creatinine, and BUN should be monitored at least daily, more frequently if the patient's renal function appears to be tenuous. Patients with AKI should also receive a low-sodium and low-potassium diet, which can be liberalized as the patient's renal function improves.

Some patients will initially be seen with severe complications from AKI, and hemodialysis must be considered. Acute indications for hemodialysis include severe metabolic acidosis unresponsive to sodium bicarbonate infusions and electrolyte abnormalities such as hyperkalemia that is unresponsive to medical management. Other indications for emergency hemodialysis include pulmonary edema not responding to diuretic therapy and symptoms of uremia (encephalopathy, seizures, pericarditis). As mentioned, early and prompt nephrology consultation will ensure that the patient receives maximal care.

Prevention

Given the marked increase in morbidity and mortality associated with AKI, especially for critically ill patients, potential measures to prevent AKI are essential. The first step in prevention, however, is being aware of patients who are at highest risk for AKI. This group of patients includes not only those with known kidney disease but also those with known medical comorbid conditions that increase their risk for AKI. This latter group of patients consists of those with diabetes, hypertension, nephrotic syndrome, coronary heart disease, and peripheral vascular disease. These patients may have normal renal function at baseline based on their laboratory studies. Early consultation with a nephrologist before a potentially nephrotoxic exposure is warranted for this high-risk group. The first consideration is to evaluate these patients carefully regarding the necessity for a specific medication or intervention that will expose them to a potential nephrotoxin. Alternative medications or procedures that do not carry the same renal risk must be considered, such as magnetic resonance imaging instead of computed tomography with intravenous radiocontrast agents. If a specific diagnostic or therapeutic procedure does not have any appropriate substitute, these patients must receive renal protective measures. First, all potential nephrotoxins that they are taking before the procedure, such as NSAIDs, should be discontinued and avoided after the procedure when possible. Second, the patient's volume and hemodynamic status must be maximized. Then, in high-risk patients, a renal protective intervention must be instituted before exposure to the agent. Fortunately, two medically supported renal protective interventions have recently gained favor for prevention of AKI associated with intravenous radiocontrast agents. The first of these is the use of *N*-acetylcysteine with an intravenous infusion of 0.45 normal saline. The 0.45 normal saline infusion is given concurrently with the *N*-acetylcysteine. More recently, an intravenous infusion of sodium bicarbonate has also proved efficacious in preventing AKI. [1] These renal protective measures require more effort and coordination with all of the health care staff providing care for the patient, but preventing AKI is critical to avoid the excess morbidity and mortality. Furthermore, patients at risk for AKI require increased surveillance during both routine clinic visits and hospitalizations to reduce the risk for exposure to nephrotoxins. Recent studies have identified several clinical variables that enhance the risk for acquiring AKI. Of all the risk factors identified, having preexisting chronic kidney disease is the most predictive. Appropriate surveillance measures include carefully selecting medications and diagnostic procedures that will minimize nephrotoxin exposure and aggressive monitoring of renal function with frequent determination of serum electrolytes, creatinine, and BUN after any procedures known to induce AKI. These measures are appropriate in both the clinic and hospital settings and regardless of whether exposure to a potential nephrotoxin is anticipated. Additionally, educating the patient regarding common nonprescription nephrotoxins such as NSAIDs can ameliorate the risk for AKI.

Prognosis

Typically, AKI secondary to prerenal causes, if diagnosed and treated early, has the best prognosis for renal recovery. Patients with prerenal AKI commonly return to their baseline level of renal function and have a mortality rate of less than 10%. Similarly, patients with postrenal AKI also have a good prognosis for renal recovery if the outlet obstruction is promptly diagnosed and definitively treated. In contrast, patients with intrarenal AKI have a less predictable renal outcome, and mortality in this group varies between 30 and 80%, depending on the severity of injury. The clinical course after recovery from ATN is subsequent tubular regeneration with recovery of renal function. However, this outcome is less ensured in patients with preexisting kidney disease. In addition, given the frequent systemic nature of their illness, patients with glomerulonephritic and vasculitic causes of AKI may not fully recover to their baseline renal function. Finally, patients who have a severe episode of AKI requiring hemodialysis may not recover their renal function and need hemodialysis indefinitely, especially if they have a preexisting history of chronic kidney disease.

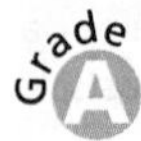

1. Merten GJ, Burgess WP, Gray LV, et al: Prevention of contrast-induced nephropathy with sodium bicarbonate. JAMA 2004;291:2328–2334.

SUGGESTED READINGS

Bagshaw SM, McAlister FA, Manns BJ, et al: Acetylcysteine in the prevention of contrast-induced nephropathy: A case study of the pitfalls in the evolution of evidence. Arch Intern Med 2006;166:1668–1669. *Demonstrates that benefit or lack thereof remains uncertain.*

Bellomo R: The epidemiology of acute renal failure: 1975 versus 2005. Curr Opin Crit Care 2006;12:557–560. *Claims that the outcome of acute renal failure has not changed over time are misleading because patients now are older and have more comorbidities.*

Chertow GM, Soroko SH, Paganini EP, et al: Mortality after acute renal failure: Models for prognostic stratification and risk adjustment. Kidney Int 2006;70:1120–1126. *At the time of consultation, advanced age, oliguria, hepatic failure, respiratory failure, sepsis, and thrombocytopenia are associated with mortality.*

Friedrich JO, Adhikary N, Herridge MS, et al: Meta-analysis: Low-dose dopamine increases urine output but does not prevent renal dysfunction or death. Ann Int Med 2005;142:510–524. *Low-dose dopamine offers transient improvements in renal physiology, but no good evidence shows that it offers important clinical benefits to those with or at risk of renal failure.*

Ho KM, Sheridan DJ: Meta-analysis of frusemide to prevent or treat acute renal failure. BMJ 2006;333:420. *Frusemide is not associated with any significant clinical benefits in the prevention and treatment of acute renal failure in adults.*

Uchino S: The epidemiology of acute renal failure in the world. Curr Opin Crit Care 2006;12:538–543. *A worldwide overview.*

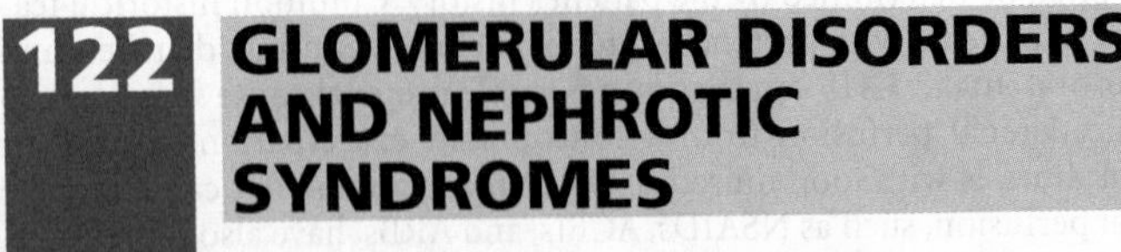

122 GLOMERULAR DISORDERS AND NEPHROTIC SYNDROMES

Gerald B. Appel

GLOMERULAR DISORDERS

Definition

Each *glomerulus*, the basic filtering unit of the kidney, consists of a tuft of anastomosing capillaries formed by branchings of the afferent arteriole. Approximately 1 million glomeruli account for about 5% of the kidney's weight and provide almost 2 m^2 of glomerular capillary filtering surface. The glomerular basement membrane (GBM) provides both a size- and charge-selective barrier to the passage of circulating macromolecules. Renal processes that involve all glomeruli are called *diffuse* or *generalized;* if only some glomeruli are involved, the process is called *focal.* When dealing with the individual glomerulus, a process is *global* if the whole glomerular tuft is involved and *segmental* if only part of the glomerulus is involved. The modifying terms *proliferative, sclerosing,* and *necrotizing* are often used (e.g., focal and segmental glomerulosclerosis [FSGS]; diffuse global proliferative lupus nephritis). Extracapillary proliferation, or crescent formation, is caused by the accumulation of macrophages, fibroblasts, proliferating epithelial cells, and fibrin within Bowman's space. In general, crescent formation in any form of glomerular damage conveys a serious prognosis. Scarring of tissue between the tubules and glomeruli, or interstitial fibrosis, is also a poor prognostic sign in every glomerular disease.

Epidemiology

At present, 20 million people in the United States have proteinuria or renal dysfunction, and many, if not most cases are caused by glomerular diseases. By 2002, the U.S. Renal Data System documented that more than 430,000 persons were in end-stage renal disease (ESRD) programs with an annual cost to the government of billions of dollars, largely as a result of renal involvement by glomerular diseases. Diabetic renal damage alone affects many millions of persons and is the major cause of ESRD in the United States (Chapter 125). Worldwide, glomerular diseases associated with infections such as malaria and schistosomiasis are major health problems. The emergence of glomerular diseases linked to human immunodeficiency virus (HIV) and hepatitis B and C viruses has focused new attention on the patterns and mechanisms of glomerular injury. The manifestations of glomerular injury range from asymptomatic microhematuria and albuminuria to rapidly progressive oliguric renal failure. In some patients, massive fluid retention and edema develop at the onset of their glomerular disease, whereas others have only the slow insidious signs and symptoms of chronic renal failure.

Pathobiology

Certain common mechanisms may underlie key findings in glomerular diseases such as hematuria and proteinuria (e.g., breaks in the glomerular capillary wall and loss of glomerular size and the charge-selective barrier). Nevertheless, the nature of the processes initiating this damage differs. In some glomerular disorders, such as diabetes and amyloidosis, there are structural and biochemical alterations of the glomerular capillary wall. In others, there is immune-mediated renal injury, whether through deposition of circulating immune complexes, localization of anti-GBM antibodies, or other mechanisms.

Clinical Manifestations

Findings that indicate the presence of a glomerular origin of renal disease include erythrocyte casts or dysmorphic erythrocytes in the urinary sediment (or both) and the presence of large amounts of albuminuria. Urinary excretion of more than 500 to 1000 erythrocytes per milliliter is abnormal, and dysmorphic erythrocytes deformed during passage through the glomerular capillary wall and tubules indicate glomerular damage. Red blood cell casts, formed when erythrocytes pass the glomerular capillary barrier and become enmeshed in a proteinaceous matrix in the lumen of the tubules, are also indicative of glomerular disease.

In a normal person, urinary excretion of albumin is less than 50 mg/day. Although increases in urinary protein excretion may come from the filtration of abnormal circulating proteins (e.g., light chains in multiple myeloma) or from deficient proximal tubular reabsorption of normal filtered small-molecular-weight proteins (e.g., β_2-microglobulin), the most common cause of proteinuria—and specifically albuminuria—is glomerular injury. Proteinuria associated with glomerular disease may range from several hundred milligrams to more than 30 g daily. In some diseases, such as minimal change nephrotic syndrome, albumin is the predominant protein found in urine. In others, such as focal sclerosing glomerulonephritis and diabetes, the proteinuria, though still largely composed of albumin, contains many larger-molecular-weight proteins as well.

NEPHROTIC SYNDROME

Definition

The nephrotic syndrome is defined by albuminuria in amounts of more than 3 to 3.5 g/day accompanied by hypoalbuminemia, edema, and hyperlipidemia. In practice, many clinicians refer to "nephrotic-range" proteinuria regardless of whether their patients have the other manifestations of the full syndrome because the latter are consequences of the proteinuria.

Pathobiology

Hypoalbuminemia is in part a consequence of urinary protein loss. It is also due to the catabolism of filtered albumin by the proximal tubule, as well as redistribution of albumin within the body. This in part accounts for the inexact relationship between urinary protein loss, the serum albumin level, and other secondary consequences of heavy albuminuria.

The salt and volume retention in nephrotic syndrome may occur through at least two different major mechanisms. In the classic theory, proteinuria leads to hypoalbuminemia, low plasma oncotic pressure, and intravascular volume depletion. Subsequent underperfusion of the kidney stimulates the priming of sodium-retentive hormonal systems such as the renin-angiotensin-aldosterone axis, which causes increased renal sodium and volume retention. In the peripheral capillaries with normal hydrostatic pressure and decreased oncotic pressure, the Starling forces lead to transcapillary fluid leakage and edema. In some patients, however, intravascular volume has been measured and found to be increased along with suppression of the renin-angiotensin-aldosterone axis. An animal model of unilateral proteinuria shows evidence of primary renal sodium retention at a distal nephron site, perhaps caused by altered responsiveness to hormones such as atrial natriuretic factor. In this situation only the proteinuric kidney retains sodium and volume and at a time when the animal is not yet hypoalbuminemic. Thus, local factors within the kidney may account for the volume retention of nephrotic patients as well.

Diagnosis

Epidemiologic studies clearly define an increased risk for atherosclerotic complications in patients with nephrotic syndrome. Most nephrotic patients have elevated levels of total and low-density lipoprotein cholesterol along with low or normal high-density lipoprotein cholesterol. Lipoprotein(a) levels are elevated as well and return to normal with remission of the nephrotic syndrome. Nephrotic patients often have a hypercoagulable state and are predisposed to deep vein thrombophlebitis, pulmonary emboli, and renal vein thrombosis.

Initial evaluation of a nephrotic patient includes laboratory tests to define whether the patient has primary, idiopathic nephrotic syndrome or a secondary cause related to a systemic disease, toxin, or medication. Common screening tests include the fasting blood sugar and glycosylated hemoglobin tests for diabetes, an antinuclear antibody test for collagen vascular disease, and serum complement, which screens for many immune complex–mediated diseases (Table 122–1). In selected patients, cryoglobulins, hepatitis B and C serology, antineutrophil cytoplasmic antibodies (ANCAs), anti-GBM antibodies, and other tests may be useful.

Treatment

Once secondary causes have been excluded, treatment of an adult nephrotic patient often requires a renal biopsy. In many studies, patients with heavy proteinuria and nephrotic syndrome have been a group highly likely to benefit from renal biopsy in terms of a change in specific diagnosis, prognosis, and therapy. Selected adult nephrotic patients such as the elderly have a slightly different spectrum of disease, but again, renal biopsy is the best guide to treatment and prognosis (Tables 122–2 and 122–3).

TABLE 122–1 SERUM COMPLEMENT LEVELS IN GLOMERULAR DISEASES

DISEASES WITH A REDUCED COMPLEMENT LEVEL
Poststreptococcal glomerulonephritis
Subacute bacterial endocarditis/visceral abscess/shunt nephritis
Systemic lupus erythematosus
Cryoglobulinemia
Idiopathic membranoproliferative glomerulonephritis
DISEASES ASSOCIATED WITH NORMAL SERUM COMPLEMENT
Minimal change nephrotic syndrome
Focal segmental glomerulosclerosis
Membranous nephropathy
IgA nephropathy
Henoch-Schönlein purpura
Anti–glomerular basement membrane disease
Pauci-immune rapidly progressive glomerulonephritis
Polyarteritis nodosa
Wegener's granulomatosis

TABLE 122–2 CAUSES OF IDIOPATHIC NEPHROTIC SYNDROME IN ADULTS

	Incidence (%)
Minimal change disease	5–10
Focal segmental glomerulosclerosis	20–25
Membranous nephropathy	25–30
Membranoproliferative glomerulonephritis	5
Other proliferative and sclerosing glomerulonephritides	15–30

Idiopathic Nephrotic Syndrome

Minimal Change Disease

Minimal change disease is the most common pattern of nephrotic syndrome in children and accounts for 5 to 10% of cases of idiopathic nephrotic syndrome in adults. A similar histologic pattern may be seen as an adverse reaction to certain medications (nonsteroidal anti-inflammatory drugs [NSAIDs], lithium) and in association with certain tumors (Hodgkin's disease and leukemias). Patients typically experience weight gain and periorbital and peripheral edema related to the proteinuria, which is usually well into the nephrotic range. Additional findings in adults are hypertension and microscopic hematuria, each in about 30% of patients. However, active urinary sediment with erythrocyte casts is not found. Many adult patients have mild to moderate azotemia, which may be related to hypoalbuminemia and intravascular volume depletion. Complement levels and serologic test results are normal.

In true minimal change disease, histopathologic examination typically reveals no glomerular abnormalities on light microscopy (LM) (Fig. 122–1). The tubules may show lipid droplet accumulation from absorbed lipoproteins (hence the older term *lipoid nephrosis*). Immunofluorescence (IF) staining and electron microscopy (EM) (Fig. 122–2) show no immune-type deposits. By EM the GBM is normal, and effacement, or "fusion," of the visceral epithelial foot processes is noted along virtually the entire distribution of every capillary loop.

The course of minimal change nephrotic syndrome is often one of remissions, relapses, and responses to additional treatment. When treated with corticosteroids for 8 weeks, 85 to 95% of children experience a remission of proteinuria. In adults, the response rate is somewhat lower, with 75 to 85% of patients responding to regimens of daily (60 mg) or alternate-day (120 mg) prednisone therapy, tapered after 2 months of treatment. The time to clinical response is slower in adults, and they are not considered steroid resistant until they have failed to respond to 16 weeks of treatment. Tapering of the steroid dose after remission should occur gradually over a period of 1 to 2 months. Both children and adults are likely to have at least one relapse of their minimal change disease once corticosteroid therapy has been discontinued. Approximately 30% of adults experience relapse by 1 year, and in 50% it occurs by 5 years. Most clinicians treat the first relapse similarly to the initial episode. Patients who relapse a third time or who become corticosteroid dependent (unable to decrease the prednisone dose without proteinuria recurring) may be treated with a 2-month course of the alkylating agent cyclophosphamide at a dose of up to 2 mg/kg/day. Up to 50% of these patients have

TABLE 122–3 NEPHROTIC SYNDROME ASSOCIATED WITH SPECIFIC CAUSES ("SECONDARY" NEPHROTIC SYNDROME)

SYSTEMIC DISEASES
Diabetes mellitus
Systemic lupus erythematosus and other collagen diseases
Amyloidosis (amyloid AL or AA associated)
Vasculitic-immunologic disease (mixed cryoglobulinemia, Wegener's granulomatosis, rapidly progressive glomerulonephritis, polyarteritis, Henoch-Schönlein purpura, sarcoidosis, Goodpasture's syndrome)
INFECTIONS
Bacterial (poststreptococcal, congenital and secondary syphilis, subacute bacterial endocarditis, shunt nephritis)
Viral (hepatitis B, hepatitis C, HIV infection, infectious mononucleosis, cytomegalovirus infection)
Parasitic (malaria, toxoplasmosis, schistosomiasis, filariasis)
MEDICATION RELATED
Gold, mercury, and the heavy metals
Penicillamine
Nonsteroidal anti-inflammatory drugs, including cyclooxygenase-2 inhibitors
Lithium
Paramethadione, trimethadione
Captopril
"Street" heroin
Others—probenecid, chlorpropamide, rifampin, tolbutamide, phenindione, pamidronate
ALLERGENS, VENOMS, IMMUNIZATIONS, AND ASSOCIATED NEOPLASMS
Hodgkin's lymphoma and leukemia-lymphomas (with minimal change lesion)
Solid tumors (with membranous nephropathy)
HEREDITARY AND METABOLIC DISEASE
Alport's syndrome
Fabry's disease
Sickle cell disease
Congenital (Finnish type) nephrotic syndrome
Familial nephrotic syndrome
Nail-patella syndrome
Partial lipodystrophy
OTHER
Pregnancy related (includes preeclampsia)
Transplant rejection
Serum sickness
Accelerated hypertensive nephrosclerosis
Unilateral renal artery stenosis
Massive obesity–sleep apnea syndrome
Reflux nephropathy

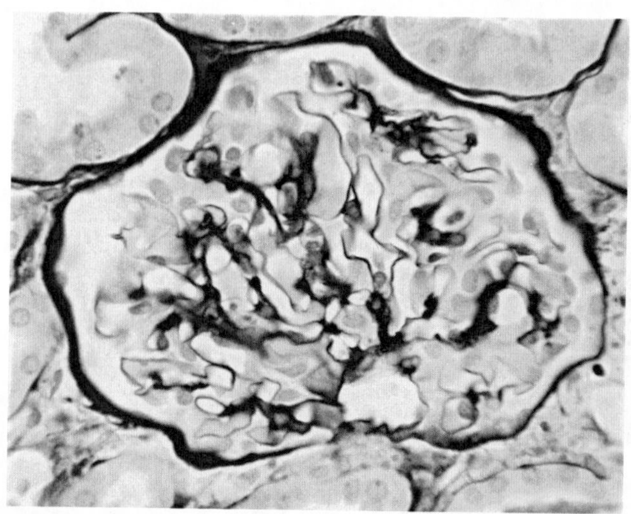

FIGURE 122–1 • Unremarkable light microscopic appearance of minimal change glomerulopathy. Glomerular basement membranes are thin, and there is no glomerular hypercellularity or mesangial matrix expansion (Jones methenamine silver stain, ×300). (From Falk RJ, Jennette JC, Nachman PH: Primary glomerular disease. *In* Brenner BM [ed]: Brenner and Rector's The Kidney, 7th ed. Philadelphia, Elsevier, 2004.)

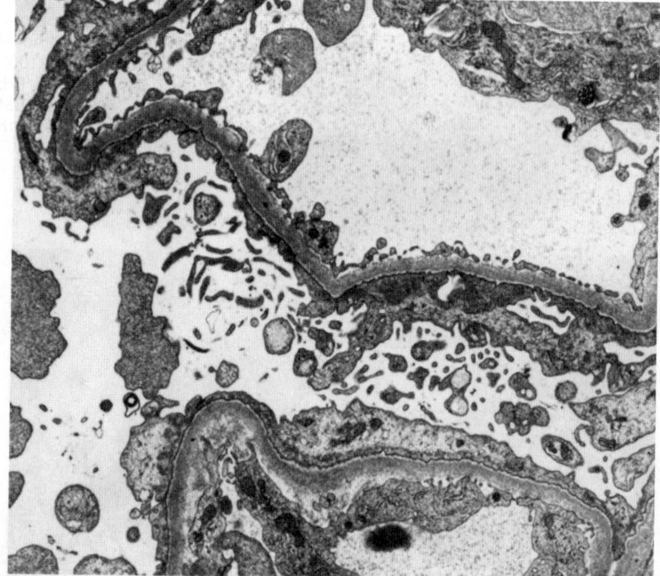

FIGURE 122–2 • Minimal change disease. An electron micrograph shows widespread effacement of the foot processes with microvillous transformation of the visceral epithelium. No electron-dense deposits are present (uranyl acetate, lead citrate stain; original magnification ×6000).

a prolonged remission of nephrotic syndrome (at least 5 years). The response rate is lower in corticosteroid-dependent patients. A commonly used alternative for the treatment of frequently relapsing and steroid-resistant patients is low-dose cyclosporine (4 to 6 mg/kg/day for 4 months), but this therapy carries some risk for nephrotoxicity and a higher relapse rate.

Focal Segmental Glomerulosclerosis

Twenty to 25% of adults with idiopathic nephrotic syndrome are found on biopsy to have FSGS. The incidence of FSGS is increasing in all races; it is the most common form of idiopathic nephrotic syndrome in blacks. FSGS may be either idiopathic or secondary to a number of different causes (e.g., heroin abuse, HIV infection, sickle cell disease, obesity, reflux of urine from the bladder to the kidneys, and lesions associated with a single or remnant kidneys). Recent reports have documented FSGS in multiple family members as a result of genetic defects in structural components of the visceral epithelial cell. Such abnormalities include an autosomal recessive pattern of nephrotic syndrome secondary to mutations in the structural protein podocin and autosomal dominant mutations in the structural protein α-actinin 4, as well as in the TRCP6 glomerular slit diaphragm–associated channel. In general, such patients with genetic forms of the disease are steroid resistant, have a progressive course, and do not experience recurrences of FSGS when they receive a renal transplant.

Patients with idiopathic FSGS typically present with asymptomatic proteinuria or edema. Although nephrotic syndrome is present in two thirds of patients at initial evaluation, proteinuria may vary from less than 1 to more than 30 g/day. Hypertension is found in 30 to 50%, and microscopic hematuria occurs in about half of these patients. The glomerular filtration rate (GFR) is decreased at diagnosis in 20 to 30% of patients. Complement levels and other serologic test results are normal.

By LM, initially only some glomeruli have areas of segmental scarring (Fig. 122–3). As renal function declines, repeat biopsy specimens show more glomeruli with segmental sclerosing lesions and increased numbers of globally sclerotic glomeruli. By IF staining, IgM and C3 are commonly trapped in the areas of glomerular sclerosis. EM shows no deposits and only effacement of visceral epithelial cell foot processes. Recently, several morphologic variants of FSGS have been shown to have either a more benign course and prognosis (e.g., the "tip lesion" variant) or a more progressive course (e.g., the "collapsing" variant).

The course of untreated FSGS is usually one of progressive proteinuria and declining GFR. Only a minority of patients experience spontaneous remission of proteinuria, and ESRD eventually develops in most untreated patients 5 to 20 years after diagnosis.

Although there have been few randomized, controlled trials in adults with FSGS, in general, patients with a sustained remission of their nephrotic syndrome are unlikely to progress to ESRD, whereas those with unremitting nephrotic syndrome are likely to progress. Studies using more intensive and more prolonged immunosuppressive regimens (6 to 12 months) consisting of corticosteroids and cytotoxic agents have achieved up to a 40 to 60% remission rate of nephrotic syndrome with preservation of long-term renal function. Cyclosporine, 4 mg/kg/day for 4 to 6 months, has been associated with greater remissions of nephrotic syndrome and less long-term renal failure in a blinded, randomized controlled trial involving patients who were resistant to steroids and frequently cytotoxic agents. Recent studies are evaluating the role of mycophenolate mofetil in the treatment of FSGS. Focal sclerosis recurs in the transplanted kidney in up to 30% of cases, often in association with elevated levels of a circulating permeability factor. Younger patients, those with a rapid course to renal failure, and patients with a previous recurrence are more likely to have FSGS recur in the allograft.

Membranous Nephropathy

Membranous nephropathy is the most common pattern of idiopathic nephrotic syndrome in white Americans. It may also be associated with infections (syphilis, hepatitis B and C), systemic lupus erythematosus (SLE), certain medications (gold salts, NSAIDs), and certain tumors (solid tumors and lymphomas). It is typically manifested as proteinuria and edema. Hypertension and microhematuria are not infrequent findings, but renal function and GFR are usually normal at diagnosis. Despite the finding of complement in the glomerular immune deposits, serum complement levels are normal. Membranous nephropathy is the most common pattern of the nephrotic syndrome to be associated with a hypercoagulable state and renal vein thrombosis. The presence of sudden flank pain, deterioration of renal function, or symptoms of pulmonary disease in a patient with membranous nephropathy should prompt an investigation for renal vein thrombosis and pulmonary emboli.

On LM, the glomerular capillary loops often appear rigid or thickened (Fig. 122–4), but there is no cellular proliferation. IF and EM show subepithelial immune-type dense deposits all along the glomerular capillary loops (Fig. 122–5).

In most large series the renal survival rate is higher than 75% at 10 years, with a spontaneous remission rate of 20 to 30%. Both the slow progression and the spontaneous remission rate have confounded clinical treatment trials. A number of studies using corticosteroids to treat membranous nephropathy have given conflicting results; proof of their benefit is lacking. In general, older patients, males, and those with heavy persistent proteinuria are most likely to progress to renal failure and hence to benefit from therapy. Controlled trials of alternating months of corticosteroid therapy and oral cytotoxic therapy (either cyclophosphamide

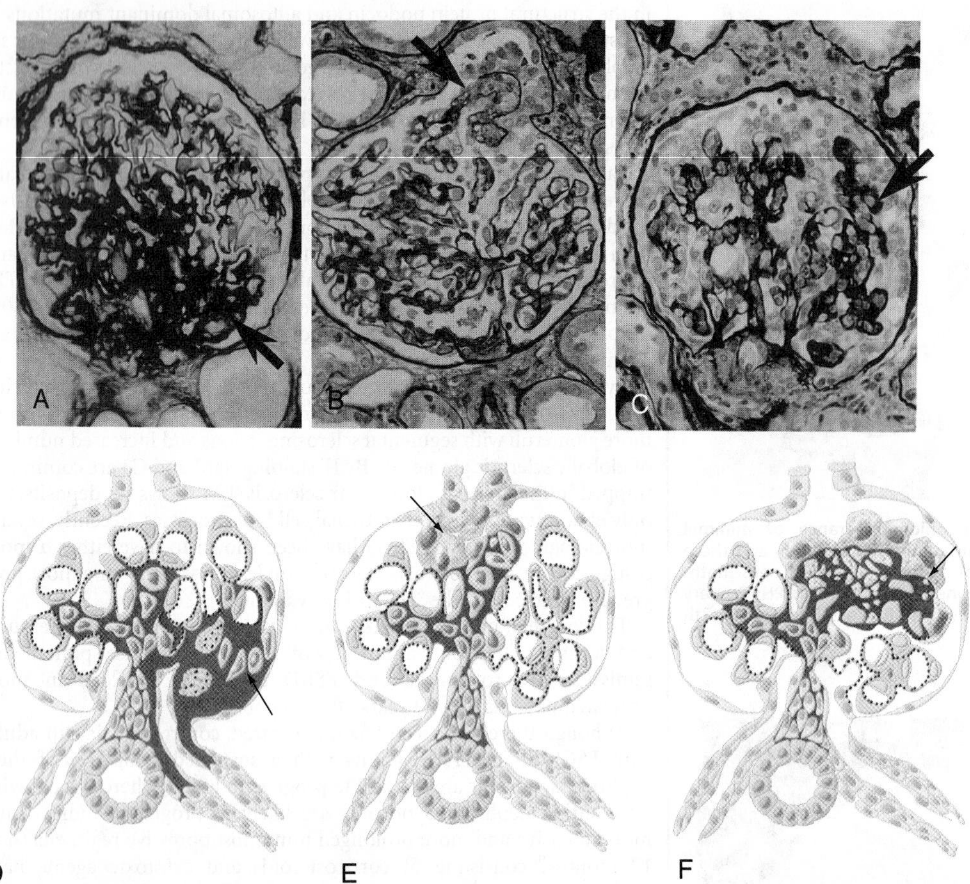

FIGURE 122–3 • Light micrographs and diagrams depicting patterns of focal segmental glomerulosclerosis. One pattern (**A** and **D**) has a predilection for sclerosis in the perihilar regions of the glomeruli. The glomerular tip lesion variant has segmental consolidation confined to the segment adjacent to the origin of the proximal tubule (**B** and **E**). The collapsing glomerulopathy variant has segmental collapse of capillaries with hypertrophy and hyperplasia of overlying epithelial cells (**C** and **F**) (Jones methenamine silver stain, ×100). (From Falk RJ, Jennette JC, Nachman PH: Primary glomerular disease. *In* Brenner BM [ed]: Brenner and Rector's The Kidney, 7th ed. Philadelphia, Elsevier, 2004.)

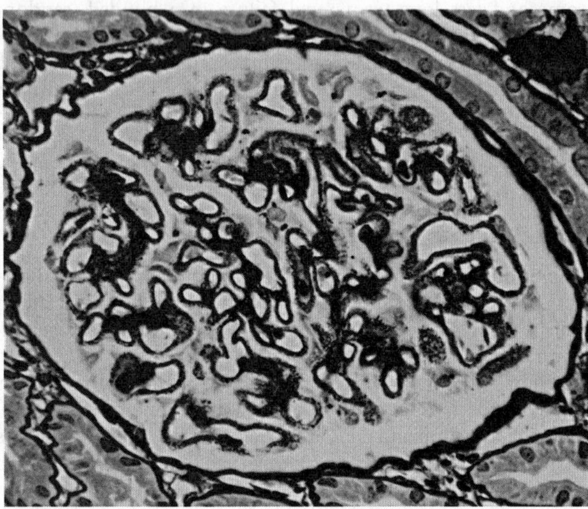

FIGURE 122–4 • Light micrograph of a glomerulus with stage II membranous glomerulopathy demonstrating spikes along the outer aspects of the glomerular basement membrane (see Fig. 122–1). These spikes correspond to projections of basement membrane material between the immune deposits (Jones methenamine silver stain, ×300). (From Falk RJ, Jennette JC, Nachman PH: Primary glomerular disease. *In* Brenner BM [ed]: Brenner and Rector's The Kidney, 7th ed. Philadelphia, Elsevier, 2004.)

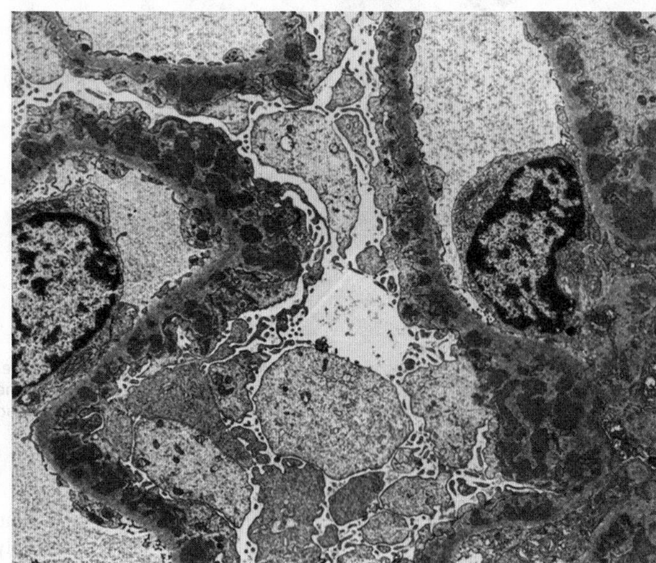

FIGURE 122–5 • Membranous glomerulopathy. On ultrastructural examination there are numerous, closely apposed epimembranous electron-dense deposits separated by basement membrane spikes (uranyl acetate, lead citrate stain; original magnification ×2500).

or chlorambucil) over a 6-month period have achieved greater numbers of total remissions and better preservation of renal function. Meta-analyses have confirmed beneficial results from the use of cytotoxic agents for idiopathic membranous nephropathy. In randomized controlled trials, cyclosporine has led to increased remissions of nephrotic syndrome. Other agents used successfully in uncontrolled trials of membranous nephropathy include mycophenolate mofetil, pentoxifylline, and the monoclonal anti-CD20 antibody rituximab.

Membranoproliferative Glomerulonephritis

Idiopathic type I membranoproliferative or mesangiocapillary glomerulonephritis (MPGN) is an uncommon primary glomerular disease that is found in only a small percentage of renal biopsy specimens. However, by LM, similar patterns of glomerular damage have commonly been seen in association with certain infectious agents (hepatitis C), autoimmune disease (SLE), and diseases of intraglomerular coagulation. All of these stimuli have been proposed to incite the glomerular mesangial cells to grow out along the capillary wall and split the GBM. Type II MPGN, or dense deposit disease, an even less common disease than MPGN type I, is associated with uncontrolled systemic activation of the alternative complement pathway. In most patients it is due to C3 nephritic factor, an autoantibody directed against C3 convertase of the alternative complement pathway. By preventing degradation of the enzyme, there is increased activation and consumption of complement noted in dense deposit disease. It may be associated with partial lipodystrophy.

Most patients with idiopathic MPGN are children or young adults who are initially evaluated for proteinuria or nephrotic syndrome. A low serum complement level is found intermittently in type I MPGN, whereas the C3 level is always reduced in type II MPGN (dense deposit disease). Most studies have found a similar course and prognosis for the various patterns of MPGN, with half the patients progressing to ESRD within 10 years of diagnosis. Attempts to treat MPGN have included the use of corticosteroids and other immunosuppressive medications, as well as anticoagulants and antiplatelet agents. No therapy has proved to be effective in a controlled randomized trial in adults with MPGN, although corticosteroids have had some success in children with the disease.

ACUTE GLOMERULONEPHRITIS AND THE NEPHRITIC SYNDROME

Pathobiology

Known inciting causes of acute glomerulonephritis include infectious agents such as streptococci and bacteria causing endocarditis, deposition of immune complexes in autoimmune diseases such as SLE, and the damaging effect of circulating antibodies directed against the GBM (as in Goodpasture's syndrome). Regardless of the inciting cause, acute glomerulonephritis is characterized on LM by hypercellularity of the glomerulus. It may be secondary to infiltrating inflammatory cells, proliferation of resident glomerular cells, or both. Both invading inflammatory neutrophils and monocytes, as well as resident cells, can damage the glomerulus through a number of mediators, including a host of oxidants, chemoattractant agents, proteases, cytokines, and growth factors. Some factors, such as transforming growth factor-β, have been related to eventual glomerulosclerosis and chronic glomerular damage.

Patients with acute glomerulonephritis often have a nephritic picture characterized by a decreased GFR and azotemia, oliguria, hypertension, and an active urinary sediment. The hypertension is caused by intravascular volume expansion, although renin levels may not be appropriately suppressed for the degree of volume expansion. Patients may note dark, smoky, or cola-colored urine in association with the active urinary sediment. This sediment is composed of erythrocytes, leukocytes, and a variety of casts, including erythrocyte casts. Although many patients with acute glomerulonephritis have proteinuria, sometimes even in the nephrotic range, most patients have lesser degrees of albumin leakage into urine, especially when the GFR is markedly reduced.

IgA Nephropathy

IgA nephropathy was originally thought to be an uncommon and benign form of glomerulopathy (Berger's disease). It is now recognized as the most frequent form of idiopathic glomerulonephritis worldwide (15 to 40% of cases of primary glomerulonephritides in parts of Europe and Asia) and that up to 30% of patients will progress to ESRD in 10 years. In geographic areas where renal biopsy is commonly performed for milder urinary findings, a higher incidence of IgA has been noted. In the United States, some centers report this diagnosis in up to 20% of all cases of primary glomerulopathy. Males outnumber females, and the peak occurrence is in the second to third decades of life.

The diagnosis of IgA nephropathy is established by finding glomerular IgA deposits as either the dominant or codominant immunoglobulin on IF microscopy. Deposits of C3 and IgG are also found frequently. The LM picture varies from the most common situation of mild mesangial proliferation to severe crescentic glomerulonephritis. By EM, immune-type dense deposits are typically found in the mesangial and paramesangial areas. In IgA nephropathy, the predominant antibody is composed of polymeric IgA1, but the antigen—whether infectious, dietary, or other—to which it is directed is unknown in the vast majority of cases. The pathogenesis may involve abnormal *O*-linked galactosylation of the IgA molecule at the hinge region, which allows abnormal binding of IgA complexes to the glomerular mesangial cells.

IgA nephropathy is frequently manifested either as asymptomatic microscopic hematuria or proteinuria or both (most common in adults) or as episodic gross hematuria after upper respiratory tract infection or exercise (most common in children and young adults). The course is variable, with some patients showing no decline in the GFR over decades and, in others, nephrotic syndrome, hypertension, and renal failure. Hypertension is present in 20 to 50% of all patients. Increased serum IgA levels, noted in a third to half of cases, do not correlate with the course of the disease. Serum complement levels are normal.

Factors predictive of a poor outcome in patients with IgA nephropathy have included (1) older age at onset, (2) absence of gross hematuria, (3) hypertension, (4) persistent proteinuria greater than 1 g/day, (5) male sex, (6) an elevated serum creatinine level, and (7) the histologic features of severe proliferation and sclerosis or tubulointerstitial damage and crescent formation, or both. Renal survival rates are estimated at 80 to 90% at 10 years and 70 to 80% at 20 years. A significant percentage of patients who have undergone renal transplantation have a morphologic recurrence in the allograft, but graft loss as a result of the disease is uncommon.

Because the pathogenesis of IgA nephropathy is thought to involve abnormal antigenic stimulation of mucosal IgA production and subsequent immune complex deposition in the glomeruli, treatment has been directed at these sites. Efforts to treat the disease by preventing antigenic stimulation, including broad-spectrum antibiotics (e.g., doxycycline), tonsillectomy, and dietary manipulations (e.g., gluten elimination), have generally been unsuccessful. Most physicians choose to treat only patients at high risk for progression to renal failure. Trials using fish oils to decrease proteinuria and slow progressive disease have provided conflicting results. Controlled studies suggest that glucocorticoids may decrease proteinuria and progressive renal failure in some patients. The benefit of immunosuppressive agents (e.g., cyclophosphamide, azathioprine, mycophenolate mofetil) is far from clear. For the few patients with crescentic IgA nephropathy, cytotoxic agents have been used. Certain antihypertensives, such as angiotensin-converting enzyme (ACE) inhibitors and angiotensin receptor blockers, have been shown to reduce proteinuria and the progression of renal disease in almost every trial studied.

Henoch-Schönlein Purpura

Henoch-Schönlein purpura (HSP) is characterized by small vessel vasculitis with arthralgias, skin purpura, and abdominal symptoms, along with a proliferative acute glomerulonephritis that has histopathologic features similar to those of IgA nephropathy. HSP is predominantly a disease of childhood, although it does occur in adults. Despite the finding of circulating IgA-containing immune complexes, no infectious agent or allergen has been defined as causative, and serum complement levels are normal.

The renal histopathology of HSP is similar to that of IgA nephropathy. In the skin there is small vessel vasculitis, a leukocytoclastic angiitis with immune deposition of IgA. The clinical manifestations of HSP (Chapter 291) include dermatologic, gastrointestinal, rheumatologic, and renal findings. Skin involvement typically starts with a macular rash coalescing into purpuric lesions on the ankles, legs, and occasionally, the arms and buttocks. Gastrointestinal symptoms include cramps, diarrhea, and less frequently, nausea and vomiting. Melena and bloody diarrhea are present in the most severely involved cases. Although arthralgias of the knees, wrists, and ankles are common, true arthritis is uncommon. Symptoms of involvement of different organ systems may occur concurrently or separately, and recurrent episodes are not uncommon during the first year.

Like IgA nephropathy, HSP has no proven therapy. Episodes of rash, arthralgias, and abdominal symptoms usually resolve spontaneously. Some patients with severe abdominal findings have been treated with short courses of high doses of corticosteroids. Patients with severe glomerular involvement may benefit from modalities used to treat patients with severe IgA nephropathy. Although most patients with HSP recover fully, patients with a more severe nephritic or nephrotic manifestation and more severe glomerular damage on renal biopsy have an unfavorable long-term prognosis.

Poststreptococcal Glomerulonephritis

Acute poststreptococcal glomerulonephritis (PSGN) may be manifested as an acute nephritic syndrome or as isolated hematuria and proteinuria. It may occur in either an epidemic or sporadic form. PSGN is largely a disease of childhood, but severe disease in adults has been well documented. The disease is most common after episodes of pharyngitis, but it can follow streptococcal infections at any site, and subclinical cases greatly outnumber clinical cases.

PSGN is an acute immune complex disease characterized by the formation of antibodies against streptococci and localization of immune complexes with complement in the kidney. PSGN occurs only after infection with certain nephritogenic strains of group A β-hemolytic streptococci.

On LM, glomeruli are markedly enlarged and often fill Bowman's space. They exhibit hypercellularity because of an infiltration of monocytes and polymorphonuclear cells and a proliferation of glomerular cellular elements. The capillary lumens are often compressed by the glomerular hypercellularity. Some cases demonstrate extracapillary proliferation with crescent formation. By IF microscopy there is coarse granular deposition of IgG, IgM, and complement, especially C3, along the capillary wall. EM shows large dome-shaped, electron-dense subepithelial deposits resembling the humps of a camel at isolated intervals along the GBM.

Most cases are diagnosed by detecting hematuria, proteinuria, and hypertension, with only some of the findings of nephritic syndrome detected after a latency period of 10 days to several weeks following a streptococcal infection. Throat and skin cultures of suspected sites of streptococcal involvement may often not be positive for group A β-hemolytic streptococci. A variety of antibodies (e.g., antistreptolysin O [ASLO]), antihyaluronidase [AHT]) and a Streptozyme panel of antibodies against streptococcal antigens (including ASLO, AHT, antistreptokinase, and anti-DNase) often show high titer, but a change in titer over time is more indicative of a recent streptococcal infection. More than 95% of patients with PSGN secondary to pharyngitis and 85% of patients with streptococcal skin infections have positive antibody titers. Serum total hemolytic complement levels and C3 levels are decreased in more than 90% of patients during the episode of acute glomerulonephritis.

With a classic acute nephritic episode following a documented streptococcal infection and associated with a change in streptococcal antibody titer and a depressed serum complement level, renal biopsy adds little to the diagnosis. In other cases, biopsy may prove necessary to confirm or refute the diagnosis. In most patients, PSGN is a self-limited disease, with recovery of renal function and disappearance of hypertension in several weeks. Proteinuria and hematuria may resolve more slowly over a period of months. Therapy is symptomatic and directed at controlling the hypertension and fluid retention with antihypertensive agents and diuretics.

Glomerulonephritis with Endocarditis and Visceral Abscesses

Various glomerular lesions have been found in patients with acute and chronic bacterial endocarditis (Chapter 76). Although embolic phenomena can lead to glomerular ischemia and infarction, a common finding is immune complex glomerulonephritis. In the pre-antibiotic era, with most cases of endocarditis being due to *Streptococcus viridans,* both focal and diffuse forms of proliferative glomerulonephritides were common. Recently, with an increased incidence of *Staphylococcus aureus* endocarditis, 40 to 80% of these patients have clinical evidence of an immune complex proliferative glomerulonephritis. Glomerulonephritis is now more common with acute than with subacute bacterial endocarditis, and the duration of illness is not an important determinant of the renal disease.

Patients often have hematuria and erythrocyte casts in their urinary sediment, proteinuria ranging from less than 1 g/day to nephrotic levels, and progressive renal failure. Serum total complement and C3 levels are usually reduced. Renal insufficiency may be mild and reversible with appropriate antibiotic therapy, or it may be progressive and lead to dialysis and irreversible renal failure.

A proliferative immune complex glomerulonephritis has also been noted in patients with deep visceral bacterial abscesses and infections such as empyema of the lung and osteomyelitis. With appropriate antibiotic therapy, most patients' glomerular lesions heal and renal function is restored. Immune complex forms of acute glomerulonephritis have also been noted in patients with pneumonia associated with many bacterial organisms, as well as *Mycoplasma.* Patients with chronically infected cerebral ventriculoatrial shunts for hydrocephalus may have similar glomerular pathology. Many have nephrotic-range proteinuria and only mild renal dysfunction.

Rapidly Progressive Glomerulonephritis

Rapidly progressive glomerulonephritis (RPGN) comprises a group of glomerular diseases that progress to renal failure in a matter of weeks to months along with the presence of extensive extracapillary proliferation (i.e., crescent formation). RPGN thus includes renal diseases with different causes, pathogeneses, and clinical manifestations (Table 122–4). Patients with primary RPGN have been divided into three patterns defined by immunologic pathogenesis: type I, with anti-GBM disease (e.g., Goodpasture's syndrome); type II, with immune complex deposition (e.g., SLE, HSP, poststreptococcal); and type III, without immune deposits or anti-GBM antibodies, so-called pauci-immune. Most of the last group fall into the category of ANCA-positive RPGN. In the past, with the exception of postinfectious RPGN, the prognosis was generally poor for most patients regardless of the pathogenesis. This prognosis has dramatically changed for some patterns of RPGN.

Anti–Glomerular Basement Membrane Disease

Anti-GBM disease (Table 122–5) is caused by circulating antibodies directed against the noncollagenous domain of the α_3-chain of type 4 collagen that damage the GBM. Such injury leads to an inflammatory response, breaks in the GBM, and the formation of a proliferative and often crescentic glomerulonephritis. If the anti-GBM antibodies cross-react with and damage the basement membrane of pulmonary capillaries, pulmonary hemorrhage and hemoptysis develop, an association called *Goodpasture's syndrome.* The disease has two peaks of occurrence: in men in the third decade of life and in women older than 60 years. These patients initially have a nephritic picture. Renal function may deteriorate from normal to dialysis-requiring levels in a matter of days to weeks. Patients with pulmonary involvement may have life-threatening hemoptysis with dyspnea and diffuse alveolar infiltrates on chest radiographs. The course of the disease, once it has progressed to dialysis levels, is usually one of permanent renal dysfunction. If treatment is started before severe renal failure develops, most patients regain considerable kidney function.

The pathology of anti-GBM disease shows a proliferative glomerulonephritis, often with severe crescentic proliferation in Bowman's space. There is linear deposition of immunoglobulin (usually IgG) along the

TABLE 122–4 CLASSIFICATION OF RAPIDLY PROGRESSIVE ("CRESCENTIC") GLOMERULONEPHRITIS

PRIMARY

Type I: Anti–glomerular basement membrane antibody disease (with pulmonary disease—Goodpasture's syndrome)
Type II: Immune complex mediated
Type III: Pauci-immune (usually antineutrophil cytoplasmic antibody positive)

SECONDARY

Membranoproliferative glomerulonephritis
IgA nephropathy—Henoch-Schönlein purpura
Poststreptococcal glomerulonephritis
Systemic lupus erythematosus
Polyarteritis nodosa, hypersensitivity angiitis

TABLE 122-5 COMMON RENAL DISEASES WITH ASSOCIATED PULMONARY DISEASES

Disease	Marker
Goodpasture's syndrome	+Anti–glomerular basement membrane antibodies
Wegener's granulomatosis, polyarteritis	+Antineutrophil cytoplasmic antibodies
Systemic lupus erythematosus	+Anti-DNA antibodies, low complement
Nephrotic syndrome, renal vein thrombosis, pulmonary embolus	+Lung scan
Pneumonia with immune complex glomerulonephritis	−Low complement, circulating immune complexes
Uremic lung	−Elevated creatinine level

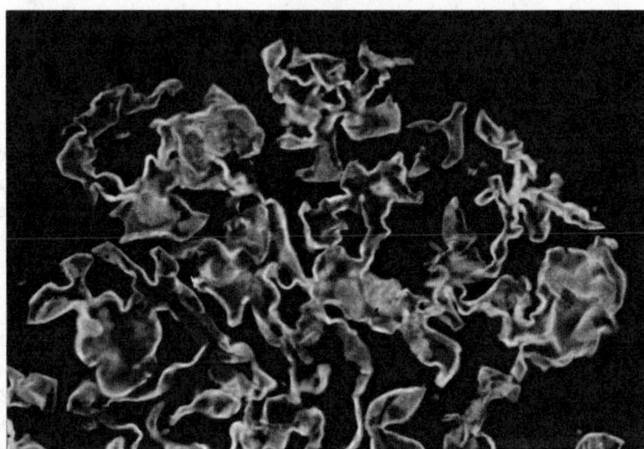

FIGURE 122-6 • Anti–glomerular basement membrane (GBM) glomerulonephritis. An immunofluorescence micrograph of a portion of a glomerulus with anti-GBM glomerulonephritis shows linear staining of GBMs for IgG (fluorescein isothiocyanate anti-IgG stain, ×600). (From Falk RJ, Jennette JC, Nachman PH: Primary glomerular disease. *In* Brenner BM [ed]: Brenner and Rector's The Kidney, 7th ed. Philadelphia, Saunders/Elsevier, 2004.)

GBM by IF (Fig. 122–6), but EM does not show any electron-dense deposits.

Although treatment of this rare disease has not been studied in large controlled trials, intensive immunosuppressive therapy with cyclophosphamide and corticosteroids to reduce the production of anti-GBM antibodies, combined with daily plasmapheresis to remove circulating anti-GBM antibodies, has been successful in many patients. Rapid treatment is necessary to prevent irreversible renal damage and pulmonary hemorrhage. Patients already requiring dialysis support at the time of treatment generally do not regain renal function despite aggressive therapy.

Immune Complex Rapidly Progressive Glomerulonephritis

Type II RPGN is associated with immune complex–mediated damage to the glomeruli and may occur with idiopathic glomerulopathies such as IgA nephropathy and MPGN or diseases of known origin such as postinfectious glomerulonephritis and SLE. Therapy for IgA nephropathy and MPGN was discussed previously. Many cases of crescentic postinfectious glomerulonephritis resolve with successful treatment of the underlying infection. Treatment of severe SLE is considered later.

Pauci-immune and Vasculitis-Associated Rapidly Progressive Glomerulonephritis

Pauci-immune type III RPGN includes patients with and without evidence of systemic vasculitis. Retrospective analyses have found no difference in prognosis between patients with or without documented true arterial vasculitis along with the crescentic and focal segmental necrotizing glomerulonephritis. Patients are often initially found to have progressive renal failure and a nephritic picture. Many patients have circulating antibodies directed against components of neutrophil primary granules (ANCA). Patients who are perinuclear ANCA positive (antibodies usually directed against granulocyte myeloperoxidase) more often have a clinical picture akin to that of microscopic polyarteritis with arthritis, skin involvement with leukocytoclastic angiitis, and constitutional and systemic signs. Patients who are cytoplasmic ANCA positive (antibodies usually directed against a granulocyte serine proteinase—anti-PR3) more often have granulomatous disease associated with their glomerulonephritis, as in Wegener's granulomatosis. There is considerable overlap between these groups. Moreover, some patients have the combination of both ANCA and anti-GBM antibodies. Although there is no direct correlation between ANCA titers and disease activity, patients with high titers (especially high anti-PR3 titers) and those with a fourfold increase in titer are more likely to have flares of their disease.

As in all forms of RPGN, renal function may deteriorate rapidly. Administration of oral cyclophosphamide in addition to corticosteroids has led to markedly improved patient and renal survival in those with Wegener's granulomatosis and polyarteritis nodosa. For example, in a series of 158 patients with Wegener's granulomatosis, more than 90% experienced marked improvement and 75% had a complete remission. These excellent results include patients with true crescentic glomerulonephritis. The use of steroids plus cytotoxic agents has produced successful results in both oliguric and dialysis-dependent patients. Several recent large randomized controlled trials and retrospective reviews have better defined high-risk populations and therapy for pauci-immune RPGN. Older patients, those with severe pulmonary involvement, and patients with severe renal failure may be at higher risk. Intravenous treatment of ANCA-positive RPGN with cyclophosphamide leads to fewer complications but perhaps a higher relapse rate than does treatment with oral cyclophosphamide. Controlled trials have shown that methotrexate is as effective as cyclophosphamide in achieving remission in early or limited disease but that the relapse rate was higher with methotrexate. In severe renal vasculitis, renal survival (but not patient survival) is improved with the addition of plasmapheresis, as opposed to methylprednisolone pulses, to a standard regimen of cyclophosphamide and corticosteroids. Finally, regimens using a long course of cyclophosphamide versus a shorter course followed by the less toxic azathioprine had equal efficacy with a trend toward fewer side effects in the azathioprine group. Ongoing trials are comparing mycophenolate mofetil with azathioprine for maintenance therapy in ANCA-positive vasculitis patients, as well as the appropriate duration of maintenance therapy.

ASYMPTOMATIC URINARY ABNORMALITIES AND GLOMERULAR DISEASES ASSOCIATED WITH GENETIC DEFECTS

Some patients have the asymptomatic urinary abnormalities of microhematuria or proteinuria (or both) discovered through routine evaluations. Microscopic hematuria associated with deformed erythrocytes or erythrocyte casts is likely to be glomerular in origin. Levels of proteinuria less than the nephrotic range may be due to orthostatic proteinuria, hypertension, and tubular disease, as well as glomerular damage.

In patients with asymptomatic urinary abnormalities of glomerular origin, the underlying glomerular lesion may be the early phase of one of the progressive glomerular diseases or be due to a benign, nonprogressive glomerular lesion. Most such patients have a lesion with mild proliferation limited to the mesangial areas of the glomeruli. Some patients have mesangial IgA immune deposits and hence IgA nephropathy, whereas others have deposition of IgM or complement only. In general, for patients with less than 1 g of proteinuria daily or glomerular microhematuria, or both, if the GFR is normal, many clinicians would not proceed to a renal biopsy to establish a diagnosis. Because the vast majority of these patients need no immunosuppressive therapy, they prefer to monitor the patient closely and perform biopsy only on those with progressive proteinuria or evidence of decreasing GFR.

Some patients, often with a history of similar findings in siblings and other relatives, have a hereditary nephritis. A hereditary form of glomerulonephritis that is often accompanied by asymptomatic urinary findings is Alport's syndrome. In approximately 85% of cases it is an X-linked condition with hematuria and proteinuria, frequently in association with high-pitched hearing loss and abnormalities of the lens of the eye (lenticonus). In males, this disease often leads to progressive glomerulosclerosis and ESRD. The defect in most of these cases is localized to a mutation in the α_5-chain of type IV collagen *(COL4A5)*. Other families have different patterns of inheritance, more often with mutations in the α_3- and α_4-chains of type IV collagen *(COL4A3, COL4A4)*. Although LM findings vary from mild mesangial proliferative to advanced sclerosing lesions, depending on the stage of biopsy, EM typically shows areas of thinning of the GBM and areas of splitting of the basement membrane with lamellations. Some other patients with mutations in the collagen IV gene have microhematuria and proteinuria with areas of extreme thinning of the basement membrane on EM of their biopsy specimens. This entity, thin basement membrane disease, was formerly thought to be uniformly benign, but some patients do progress to glomerulosclerosis with time.

Fabry's disease is caused by an X-linked recessive genetic defect in α-galactosidase that leads to the deposition of ceramide trihexose in the kidneys and other organs. It may result in progressive proteinuria and renal insufficiency in males and some female carriers and is associated with telangiectases of the skin, typically in the bathing suit area, acroparesthesias, cardiac abnormalities, and eye changes. Nail-patella syndrome, associated with skeletal and nail deformities, is a rare cause of nephrotic syndrome in children. It is due to an autosomal dominant mutation in the LMX1B transcription factor, which regulates collagen genes and genes for nephrin and podocin.

Systemic Lupus Erythematosus

Renal involvement may greatly influence the course and treatment of SLE (Chapter 287). Although the incidence of clinical renal disease in SLE varies from 15 to 75%, histologic evidence of renal involvement is found in the vast majority of biopsy specimens.

The new International Society of Nephrology (ISN) classification of lupus nephritis is now used widely for both clinical and research activities (Table 122–6). It involves the use of LM, IF, and EM to classify each biopsy specimen by separating the milder mesangial lesions and the bland membranous lupus nephritis from true proliferative lupus nephritis. It is being used and studied as a guide for prognosis and treatment.

In general, patients with ISN class I and II have mild lesions that require no therapy directed at the kidney. All patients with class IV lesions on biopsy deserve some form of vigorous therapy for their lupus nephritis. Many class III patients (especially those with active necrotizing lesions and large amounts of subendothelial deposits; Fig. 122–7) also benefit from such therapy. The optimal therapy for class V patients is less clear; some clinicians treat all membranous lupus nephritis patients vigorously, whereas others reserve such therapy for those with serologic activity or more severe nephrotic syndrome. Vigorous lupus nephritis therapy has included corticosteroids, as well as immunosuppressive therapy, usually with oral or intravenous cyclophosphamide in the past. A series of well-performed randomized studies at the National Institutes of Health (NIH) found that patients treated with cytotoxic agents had less renal failure at 10 years than did those treated with corticosteroids. Intravenous cyclophosphamide appeared to be an effective therapy with fewer side effects than with oral cyclophosphamide. Other NIH studies have documented the superiority of regimens with monthly high-dose intravenous cyclophosphamide therapy (0.5 to 1 g/m^2) for 6 months over monthly pulse methylprednisolone in preventing renal progression and flares of disease. Another controlled trial found that combination therapy with monthly cyclophosphamide along with methylprednisolone was more effective in preventing renal failure than either drug regimen was alone, with no increased long-term side effects.

Recent studies have tried to match the efficacy of cyclophosphamide with newer immunosuppressive agents that have a better safety profile. In recent trials, daily oral mycophenolate mofetil appeared to be equally effective in inducing remissions of severe lupus nephritis but had a better safety profile in several populations, including those at high risk for progressive renal disease (e.g., African Americans). Likewise, in another trial, maintenance therapy with mycophenolate proved to be more effective as cyclophosphamide and was associated with fewer infections and hospitalizations. [2] The precise role of mycophenolate as induction and maintenance therapy in patients with severe lupus nephritis versus cyclophosphamide and the less expensive and relatively nontoxic azathioprine will be decided by future studies. Newer agents such as rituximab, an anti-CD20 monoclonal antibody, and blockers of costimulatory molecules are also currently being studied.

Many patients with lupus nephritis (40 to 50%) produce autoantibodies against certain phospholipids, including anticardiolipin antibodies. Some of these patients have coagulation in the glomeruli and arterioles and require treatment with anticoagulation or antiplatelet agents, or both, as well as immunosuppressive medications.

Diabetes Mellitus

Diabetic nephropathy is the most common form of glomerular damage seen in developed countries. In 2002, it was the most frequent diagnosis in new patients with ESRD in the United States (Chapter 125). Nephropathy develops in 20 to 30% of all patients with type 1 or type 2 diabetes, with a much higher percentage of those with type 1 disease progressing to ESRD. However, because of the much greater prevalence of type 2 disease, the majority of diabetics starting dialysis have this form of the disease.

The histopathologic changes in the kidneys of diabetics involve all components of the kidney, including the glomeruli, vessels, tubules, and interstitium. Changes in the glomeruli consist of thickening of the GBM, mesangial sclerosis, nodular intercapillary glomerulosclerosis (so-called Kimmelstiel-Wilson nodules), lesions caused by insudation of plasma proteins along the glomerular capillary walls, and microaneurysms of the glomerular capillaries.

A current goal of treatment in diabetics is to prevent diabetic renal failure by controlling hyperglycemia and blood pressure, reducing intracapillary glomerular pressure, and preventing the deleterious effects of growth factors and angiotensin II on the kidney. The superiority of ACE

TABLE 122–6 ISN/RPS CLASSIFICATION OF LUPUS NEPHRITIS

Class	Clinical Features
I. Minimal mesangial LN	No renal findings
II. Mesangial proliferative LN	Mild clinical renal disease; minimally active urinary sediment; mild to moderate proteinuria (never nephrotic) but may have active serology
III. Focal proliferative LN (<50% of glomeruli involved) Active A/C: active and chronic Chronic	More active sediment changes; often active serology; increased proteinuria (about 25% nephrotic); hypertension may be present; some evolve into a class IV pattern. Active lesion require treatment, chronic do not
IV. Diffuse proliferative LN (>50% of glomeruli involved); all may be with segmental or global involvement (S or G) Active A/C Chronic	Most severe renal involvement with active sediment, hypertension, heavy proteinuria (frequent nephrotic syndrome), often reduced glomerular filtration rate; serology very active. Active lesions require treatment
V. Membranous LN glomerulonephritis	Significant proteinuria (often nephrotic) with less active lupus serology
VI. Advance sclerosing LN (>90% glomerulosclerosis)	No treatment prevents renal failure

ISN = International Society of Nephrology; LN = lupus nephritis; RPS = Renal Pathology Society.

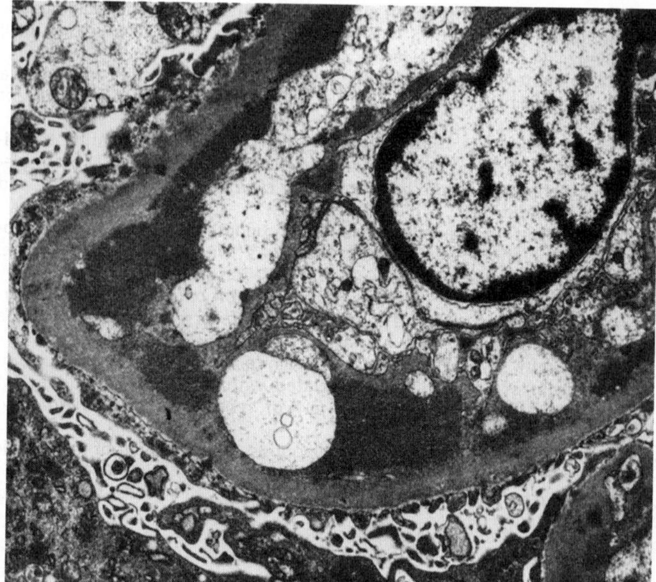

FIGURE 122–7 • Lupus nephritis. At the ultrastructural level, wire loop deposits correspond to large subendothelial electron-dense deposits (uranyl acetate, lead citrate stain; original magnification ×5000).

inhibitors over other antihypertensive agents in preventing the progression of renal disease and renal morbidity and mortality in type 1 diabetics has been documented in controlled trials. In type 2 diabetics with microalbuminuria, ACE inhibitors and angiotensin II receptor blockers also prevent the appearance of clinical proteinuria and progression of renal dysfunction. Studies have documented the efficacy of angiotensin II receptor antagonists in preventing progression of renal disease in type 2 diabetics. In controlled, randomized, double-blind trials, proteinuria is reduced, doubling of creatinine is decreased, and progression to ESRD is diminished by the use of angiotensin II receptor blockers in addition to conventional blood pressure therapy versus conventional therapy alone. Although survival is improving for diabetic patients maintained on dialysis, it is still inferior to that of nondiabetic ESRD patients. Survival in diabetics after living related donor renal transplantation is approaching that of the nondiabetic population.

Amyloidosis

Renal amyloid deposits—whether caused by AL or AA amyloid—are predominantly found within the glomeruli and often appear as amorphous eosinophilic extracellular nodules (Chapter 296). They stain positively with Congo red and, under polarized light, display apple-green birefringence. By EM, amyloid appears as nonbranching rigid fibrils 8 to 10 nm in diameter.

Although almost 80% of patients with AL amyloid have renal disease, amyloidosis is a disease with multisystemic involvement, and hence patients may have symptoms referable to cardiac or neural involvement, as well as renal symptoms. The diagnosis may be made from organ biopsy other than the kidney (e.g., gingival biopsy, rectal biopsy, or fat pad biopsy). Common renal manifestations are albuminuria and renal insufficiency, which are found in almost half of patients. Approximately 25% of patients with AL amyloid are initially found to have nephrotic syndrome, and it eventually develops in up to half the patients. Amyloid is rarely found in association with light chain cast nephropathy. Treatment strategies for renal amyloidosis have focused on combined therapy with melphalan, prednisone, and colchicines. Studies involving stem cell or bone marrow transplantation and ablative therapy to destroy the clone of abnormal plasma cells leading to amyloid production have produced promising results in select patients.

Light Chain Deposition Disease

Light chain deposition disease (LCDD), like AL amyloidosis, is a systemic disease caused by the overproduction and extracellular deposition of a monoclonal immunoglobulin light chain (Chapter 198). However, the deposits do not form β-pleated sheets, do not stain with Congo red, and are granular rather than fibrillar. Most patients with LCDD have a lymphoplasmacytic B-cell disease similar to multiple myeloma. On LM, most glomeruli have eosinophilic mesangial glomerular nodules. Some biopsy specimens from patients with LCDD have associated light chain cast nephropathy with eosinophilic laminated casts obstructing the tubules, as seen in myeloma. By IF, a single class of immunoglobulin light chain (κ in 80% of cases) stains in a diffuse linear pattern along the GBMs, in the nodules, and along the tubular basement membranes, with little or no staining for complement components.

Albuminuria is common, and nephrotic syndrome is found in half the patients at initial evaluation, often accompanied by hypertension and renal insufficiency. Treatment of most patients with LCDD is chemotherapy, similar to that for myeloma, which has led to significant renal and patient survival, although marrow and stem cell transplantation is being tried in select cases.

Fibrillary Glomerulopathy–Immunotactoid Glomerulopathy

Some patients with renal disease have glomerular lesions with deposits of nonamyloid fibrillar proteins ranging in size from 12 to larger than 50 nm. In the past, these lesions were called fibrillary glomerulopathy, immunotactoid glomerulopathy, amyloid-like glomerulopathy, Congo red–negative amyloid-like glomerulonephritis, and nonamyloiditic fibrillary glomerulopathy. Patients with these lesions have been divided into two groups: those with fibrillary glomerulonephritis with fibrils 20 nm in diameter and those with immunotactoid glomerulonephritis, a rare disease often associated with lymphoproliferative disorders in which the fibrils are much larger (30 to 50 nm). Proteinuria is found in almost all patients, and hematuria, nephrotic syndrome, and renal insufficiency are eventually detected in the majority. There is no proven therapy for fibrillary glomerulopathy at this time.

Human Immunodeficiency Virus–Associated Nephropathy

Infection with HIV (Chapter 407) has been associated with a number of patterns of renal disease, including acute renal failure and a unique form of collapsing focal sclerosis now called HIV-associated nephropathy (HIVAN).

Although a number of histologic patterns of glomerulopathy may be seen in HIV-infected patients, by far the most common is HIVAN. HIVAN is characterized by heavy proteinuria and rapid progression to renal failure. The use of ACE inhibitors and highly active antiretroviral therapy (HAART) may slow the progression to renal failure and decrease proteinuria. Studies show that corticosteroid use in selected patients with HIVAN may be beneficial.

The pathology of HIVAN shows features distinct from those of classic FSGS, including, on LM, diffuse global collapse of the glomerular tufts, severe tubulointerstitial changes with interstitial inflammation, edema, microcystic dilation of tubules, and severe tubular degenerative changes and, on EM, tubuloreticular inclusions in the glomerular endothelium.

Mixed Cryoglobulinemia

Cryoglobulinemia is caused by the production of circulating immunoglobulins that precipitate on cooling and resolubilize on warming. Cryoglobulinemia may be found in association with many types of disease, including infections, collagen vascular disease, and lymphoproliferative diseases such as multiple myeloma and Waldenström's macroglobulinemia (Chapter 198). Many patients with what was originally described as glomerulonephritis secondary to essential mixed cryoglobulinemia have been found to have hepatitis C–associated renal disease. An acute nephritic picture with acute renal insufficiency develops in some patients. Most patients have proteinuria, and about 20% of patients are initially found to have nephrotic syndrome. The majority with renal disease have a slow, indolent renal course characterized by proteinuria, hypertension, hematuria, and renal insufficiency. Hypocomplementemia, especially of the early components Clq to C4, is a characteristic and often helpful finding in cryoglobulinemic glomerulonephritis, whether related to hepatitis C or idiopathic.

Thrombotic Microangiopathies

A number of systemic diseases, including HUS, thrombotic thrombocytopenic purpura, and the antiphospholipid syndrome (Chapter 181), as well as microangiopathy associated with drugs such as mitomycin and cyclosporine, are characterized by microthromboses of the glomerular capillaries and small arterioles. The renal findings may be dominant or only part of a more generalized picture of microangiopathy.

The histologic findings in all of the microangiopathies resemble each other. Glomerular capillary thromboses are noted in some glomeruli, whereas others downstream from thrombosed arterioles may have only ischemic damage. Arterioles and small arteries show intimal proliferation with luminal narrowing by thrombus. Renal manifestations of the thrombotic microangiopathies may include gross or microscopic hematuria, proteinuria that is typically less than 2 g/day but may reach nephrotic levels, and renal insufficiency. Patients may have oliguric or nonoliguric acute renal failure. In all thrombotic microangiopathies, treatment includes correcting hypovolemia, controlling hypertension, and providing dialytic support for those with severe renal failure. In thrombotic thrombocytopenic purpura associated with an acquired or hereditary deficiency of the von Willebrand convertase ADAMTS-13 and in some other cases, infusion of fresh plasma with or without plasmapheresis has been beneficial. In the antiphospholipid syndrome, anticoagulation with heparin and then warfarin (Coumadin) has been useful.

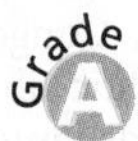

1. Jayne D, Rasmussen N, Andrassy K, et al: European Vasculitis Study Group. A randomized trial of maintenance therapy for vasculitis associated with ANCA. N Engl J Med 2003;349:36–44.
2. Ginzler EM, Dooley MA, Aranow C: Mycophenolate mofetil or intravenous cyclophosphamide for lupus nephritis. N Engl J Med 2006;353:2219–2228.

SUGGESTED READINGS

Amigo MC: Kidney disease in antiphospholipid syndrome. Rheum Dis Clin North Am 2006;32:509–522. *Renal involvement frequently leads to proteinuria, hematuria, nephrotic syndrome, and renal failure; APS patients are at high risk of post-transplant renal thrombosis.*

Appel GB, Cook HT, Hageman G, et al: Membranoproliferative glomerulonephritis Type II—dense deposit disease: An update. J Am Soc Nephrol 2005;16:1392–1403. *A review of the diagnosis, pathology, and pathogenesis of DDD with emphasis on abnormalities in the complement pathways.*

Audard V, Larousserie F, Grimbert P, et al: Minimal change nephrotic syndrome and classical Hodgkin's lymphoma: Report of 21 cases and review of the literature. Kidney Int 2006;69:2251–2260. *The morphology was predominantly nodular sclerosis (71%), and renal disease appeared before the diagnosis of lymphoma in 38%. Effective treatment of Hodgkin's is the best therapy.*

Barratt J, Feehally J: Treatment of IgA nephropathy. Kidney Int 2006;69:1934–1938. *Patients at greatest risk of progressive renal impairment are those with hypertension, proteinuria >1 g/24 h, and reduced glomerular filtration rate at diagnosis. All such patients should be treated to blood pressure of 125/75 mm Hg. There is insufficient evidence for the use of immunosuppressive agents, antiplatelet agents, or anticoagulants.*

Behaescu I, Covic A, Deray G: Treatment of proliferative lupus nephritis—a critical approach. Semin Arthritis Rheum 2007;36:224–237. *Ten-year survival rates now surpass 75% and continue to improve.*

Braun GS, Horster S, Wagner KS, et al: Cryglobulinaemic vasculitis: Classification and clinical and therapeutic aspects. Postgrad Med J 2007;83:87–94. *An overview emphasizing its relationship to hepatitis C.*

Chan TM, Li FK, Tang CSO, et al: Long-term efficacy of mycophenolate mofetil in patients with diffuse proliferative lupus nephritis. J Am Soc Nephrol 2005;16:1076–1084. *Long-term follow-up of a controlled randomized trial of mycophenolate versus oral cyclophosphamide followed by azathioprine showing similar efficacy and low toxicity with mycophenolate.*

Couser WG, Ngaku M: Cellular and molecular biology of membranous nephropathy. J Nephrol 2006;19:699–705. *A scientific overview.*

Crew JR, Radhakrishnan J, Appel GB: The nephrotic syndrome and its complications. Clin Nephrol 2004;62:245–260. *A review of the major manifestations of the nephrotic syndrome with emphasis on their pathogenesis and treatment.*

D'Agati VD, Fogo A, Bruijn JA, Jennette JC: Pathologic classification of focal segmental glomerulosclerosis. Am J Kidney Dis 2004;43:368–382. *Definitions and descriptions of current patterns of FSGS.*

Hass M: IgA nephropathy. Semin Nephrol 2004;24:177–295. *A review of all aspects of this disease.*

Houssiau F: Management of lupus nephritis: An update. J Am Soc Nephrol 2004;15:2694–2704. *A review of recent trials emphasizing less toxic but effective treatment regimens.*

Hudson BG, Tryggvason K, Sundaramoorthy M, et al: Alport's syndrome, Goodpasture's syndrome, and type IV collagen. N Engl J Med 2003;348:2543–2556. *A review of the basic genetic defects of type IV collagen and the clinical renal entities associated with them.*

Jennette JC: Rapidly progressive crescentic glomerulonephritis. Kidney Int 2003;63:1164–1177. *A review of the disease spectrum of RPGN.*

Little MA, Pusey CD: Glomerulonephritis due to ANCA associated vasculitis: An update on approaches to management. Nephrology 2005;10:368–3776. *A review of the diagnosis, pathogenesis, and treatment of ANCA-positive diseases, including Wegener's granulomatosis and microscopic polyarteritis.*

Perna A, Schieppati A, Zamora J, et al: Immunosuppressive therapy for idiopathic membranous nephropathy: A systematic review. Am J Kidney Dis 2004;44:385–401. *A systematic review.*

Pollak M: Inherited podocytopathies: FSGS and nephrotic syndrome from a genetic viewpoint. J Am Soc Nephrol 2002;13:3016–3023. *Review of current genetic defects in FSGS and their clinical features.*

Rosenstack JL, Valeri AM, Appel GB, et al: Fibrillary glomerulonephritis: Definition of the disease spectrum. Kidney Int 2003;63:1450–1462. *A large single-center experience with the manifestations, clinical histologic correlates, and course of the disease.*

Schieppati A, Perna A, Zamora J, et al: Immnosuppressive treatment for idiopathic membranous nephropathy in adults with nephrotic syndrome. Cochrane Database Syst Rev 2004;4:CD004293. *This review failed to show any long-term effect immunosuppressive treatment on patient and/or renal survival. There is weak evidence supporting the efficacy of cyclophosphamide but none for glucocorticoids.*

Szczech LA, Gupta SK, Habash R, et al: The clinical epidemiology and course of the spectrum of renal diseases associated with HIV infection. Kidney Int 2004;66:1145–1152. *An updated review of renal disease in HIV-infected patients.*

Tsai HM: Advances in the pathogenesis, diagnosis, and treatment of thrombotic thrombocytopenic purpura. J Am Soc Nephrol 2003;14:1072–1081. *A review of the new classification and treatment of TTP.*

123 TUBULOINTERSTITIAL DISEASES

Eric G. Neilson

TUBULOINTERSTITIAL NEPHRITIS

Definition

The appearance of tubulointerstitial nephritis in the kidney is especially ominous. Regardless of where the renal inflammation starts, the kidneys do not fail until interstitial nephritis, fibrosis, and tubular atrophy develop. Interstitial nephritis is the pathologic equivalent of clinical progression because it is the final common pathway to structural renal failure.

Tubulointerstitial nephritis can be arbitrarily divided into acute and chronic interstitial nephritis; so-called toxic nephropathy is similar to chronic interstitial nephritis. The acute form of interstitial nephritis often begins abruptly. When the inciting events subside, so does the nephritis, and the glomerular filtration rate returns to nearly normal with little residual damage. Chronic interstitial nephritis is persistent and over time reduces the number of functioning nephrons by encasing and dismantling them with irreversible fibrosis. Sometimes the distinction between acute and chronic injury is difficult to make because global destruction of the tubulointerstitium can occur in a matter of weeks.

Interstitial nephritis can be primary and begin in the tubulointerstitium or appear as a secondary event and spread from blood vessels, including the glomerular capillaries. Although some forms of injury to the tubulointerstitial compartment are the result of autoimmunity, a toxic insult, or exposure to infection or drugs, the inflammatory process always has an immunologic component that leads to the release of tissue cytokines, which eventually converts tubular epithelia into fibroblasts to produce fibrosis.

Pathobiology

Pathophysiology

A decrease in the glomerular filtration rate in nearly all renal diseases correlates best with worsening interstitial injury. There are several potential reasons for this inverse relationship, none of which are mutually exclusive. The simplest explanation is that urinary flow is impeded by tubular obstruction caused by inflammation with the production of aglomerular nephrons. A second explanation is an increase in vascular resistance with progressive tubular injury and fibrosis. For this to be true, a net reduction in the cross-sectional area of peritubular vessels must

TABLE 123–1 WHEN TO CONSIDER A RENAL BIOPSY IN DIAGNOSING NEPHRITIS

The setting, history, or clinical findings do not support a diagnosis of acute tubular necrosis or volume depletion.
The clinical setting warrants a tissue diagnosis to determine the type of lesion, the extent of involvement, or the degree of fibrosis.
The patient is stable enough to undergo biopsy and receive immunosuppressive drugs.
The physician believes that the choice of therapy or the length of treatment is partially determined by the type of tissue injury.

increase postglomerular resistance sufficiently that the compensatory increase in glomerular hydrostatic pressure cannot fully restore filtration to normal levels. Tubuloglomerular feedback, as a third explanation, assumes increasing importance in the transition from acute to chronic glomerulonephritis when autoregulation of renal blood flow is disrupted by tubulointerstitial fibrosis. Loss of autoregulation of tubuloglomerular feedback results from absence or insensitivity of the afferent arteriole. Perhaps more significant is the effect of interstitial pressure on sensitivity of the feedback mechanism. As a fourth explanation, the normal renal osmotic gradient is diminished by decreases in sodium chloride transport along the proximal tubule or thick ascending loop of Henle after tubular atrophy. This leads to poor abstraction of water from the filtrate and results in hyposthenuria and polyuria. Such an increase in solute and water within the tubular fluid decreases glomerular filtration by adaptively downregulating the filtering process in the face of tubular insufficiency.

The antigen targets for the immune system in interstitial nephritis are poorly understood. Drugs either act as haptens, mimic endogenous structures in the interstitium, alter regulation of the immune system, or all of the above. Bacteria, fungi, and viruses can infect the kidney and cause mononuclear cell infiltration or activate toll-like receptors on tubular epithelia, which subsequently educate the adaptive immune response to the interstitium. Autoimmune diseases such as anti–tubular basement membrane disease or spontaneous interstitial nephritis are confined to the kidney, and systemic diseases spread to the kidney and cause a persistent, chronic interstitial nephritis.

Although the adaptive immune response is similar to other tissues, T-cell activation figures highly in interstitial nephritis. Antibodies (anti–tubular basement membrane disease) or immune complexes along the tubular basement membrane (systemic lupus erythematosus) are rarely seen. Antigens presented by class II major histocompatibility complex molecules on macrophages, dendritic cells, and adjacent tubular epithelia in conjunction with associative recognition molecules engage the CD4/CD8 T-cell repertoire. The resultant cytokine and protease activity injures tubular nephrons and basement membranes and causes fibroblasts to form locally by epithelial-mesenchymal transition. Transforming growth factor β (TGF-β), fibroblast growth factor 2, and platelet-derived growth factor are particularly active in this transition. If the nephritis persists, fibrogenesis dismantles nephrons and causes tubular atrophy; in late stages, the inflammatory reaction outgrows its survival factors, and lymphocytes and fibroblasts disappear by apoptosis and leave an acellular fibrotic scar.

Pathology

Although biopsy is performed on only one kidney, both kidneys are typically involved, except in cases of unilateral infection, obstruction, or trauma. The decision to perform a renal biopsy usually depends on meeting one of four conditions (Table 123–1). In primary acute interstitial nephritis, biopsy demonstrates the presence of inflammatory cells that typically spare the glomeruli until last (Fig. 123–1A). Lesions that reduce renal function are usually diffuse, but drug-induced interstitial injury is often patchy, beginning deep in the cortex before spreading. The inflammatory reaction in acute interstitial nephritis consists mainly of T lymphocytes and monocytes, but neutrophils, plasma cells, and eosinophils can be present. The T cells are of a mixed phenotype with a distinct preference for $CD4^+$ lymphocytes. The infiltrative process is associated with interstitial edema, which causes tubules to push away from

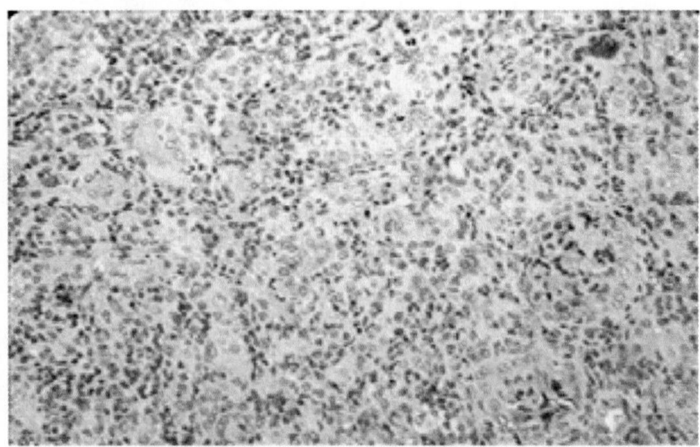

A

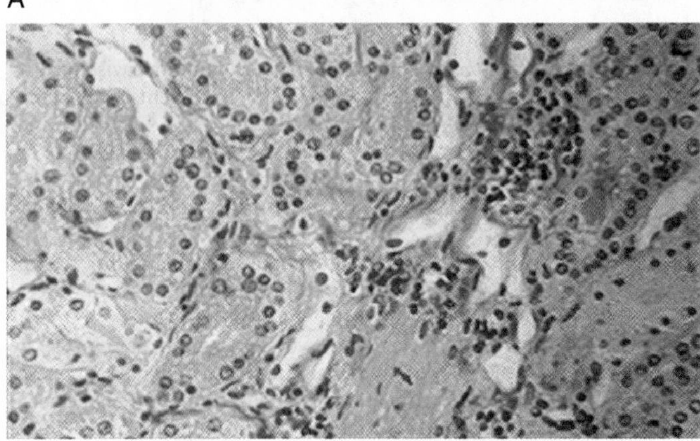

B

FIGURE 123–1 • Tubulointerstitial nephritis on biopsy. A, Acute interstitial nephritis can be most aggressive when the interstitium is crowded with mononuclear cells and giant cells that destroy nearly all tubular nephrons (hematoxylin-eosin). **B,** Chronic interstitial nephritis is slower, with substantial collagen deposition (blue color; trichrome), tubular dropout, and fibroblasts in the interstitial spaces widened by fibrosis.

each other and the kidneys to swell. The tubular basement membrane may be disrupted in more severe cases, but immune deposits are rarely found by immunofluorescence.

In chronic interstitial nephritis, the cellular infiltrate is eventually replaced by tubulointerstitial fibrosis (see Fig. 123–1B), and the kidney assumes an irregular or contracted appearance. The tubular epithelia sit on thickened tubular basement membranes and are often effaced against dilated lumens, and the tubules eventually dismantle and atrophy. Infiltrates of lymphocytes and rare neutrophils are scattered and less abundant than in acute interstitial nephritis. Chronic is a relative term because fibrotic changes can be seen within 7 to 10 days of continuing inflammation. Normal glomeruli in primary interstitial nephritis are eventually surrounded by periglomerular fibrosis and subsequently undergo segmental or global sclerosis. Chronic vascular thickening and glomerular changes are present in advanced stages of disease, so pathologic determination of the primary cause may be difficult in some biopsy samples. Progressive glomerular sclerosis also occurs with aging and must be considered when interpreting the biopsy findings.

A third pathologic category, granuloma formation, can be seen in either acute or chronic interstitial nephritis. In acute granulomatous interstitial nephritis, granulomas are sparse and non-necrotic, and giant cells are rare. The granulomas in chronic interstitial nephritis contain an abundance of giant cells, and if caused by tuberculosis, they may become necrotic. Drugs are a common cause of this lesion in the acute setting, and most of the drugs associated with acute interstitial nephritis have been reported to cause granuloma formation. In the absence of drug exposure, sarcoidosis, Wegener's granulomatosis, histoplasmosis, or tuberculosis, depending on the context, should be considered when numerous granulomas are present. The renal granulomas seen in Wegener's granulomatosis are almost always accompanied by glomerular and vascular pathology.

ACUTE INTERSTITIAL NEPHRITIS

Pathobiology

The development of acute interstitial nephritis is largely due to the use of pharmaceuticals. Other important causes include infection and idiopathic autoimmune diseases (Table 123–2). Penicillin moieties (less so nafcillin and piperacillin), cephalosporins, sulfa-like drugs, and nonsteroidal anti-inflammatory drugs (NSAIDs) top the list. NSAIDs cause both acute interstitial nephritis and chronic analgesic nephropathy. Diphtheria in children, legionellosis, leptospirosis, histoplasmosis, tuberculosis, and DNA viruses such as cytomegalovirus and Epstein-Barr virus are well-recognized agents of acute interstitial nephritis. Anti–tubular basement membrane disease is a rare cause of autoimmune interstitial nephritis, and although sarcoidosis or the tubulointerstitial nephritis and uveitis syndrome can manifest as acute interstitial nephritis on biopsy, they often quickly evolve into chronic disease.

Diagnosis

Acute interstitial nephritis appears unexpectedly in otherwise healthy individuals from a variety of causes. About 1% of patients with hematuria and proteinuria have acute interstitial nephritis, and it is seen in 1 to 15% of autopsy series. These percentages are probably higher today with over-the-counter use of NSAIDs. Because injury is often asymptomatic, patients may have already substantial renal failure when initially seen.

It is important to consider acute interstitial nephritis in any patient with an unexplained precipitous diminution in renal function. Several features may distinguish it from acute tubular necrosis or glomerulonephritis (Table 123–3). Fever and occasional flank pain over the kidneys occur in infection or with drug-induced acute interstitial nephritis. Lumbar pain, sometimes unilateral, is due to distention of the renal capsule. Allergic reactions are associated with maculopapular rash, fever, and eosinophilia. The entire triad is seen in less than 33% of patients, and such signs are uncommon when NSAIDs cause acute interstitial nephritis.

Clinical Course

The course of renal failure in acute interstitial nephritis is several days to weeks and maps with the kinetics of the primary immune response. However, renal failure can be precipitous, especially in patients re-exposed to a previous agent; conversely, it can rarely be protracted, with the glomerular filtration rate declining over a period of months if the diagnosis has gone unnoticed. This protracted course is more common with diuretic-induced interstitial nephritis. The onset of drug-induced nephritis ranges from days to weeks after initiation of therapy, and a previous allergic history is rare. A classic setting for a drug reaction is a febrile patient with an infectious process who defervesces while taking antibiotics, with recurrent fever developing several days later.

Laboratory Findings

Urinalysis is particularly helpful because several features strongly speak for the diagnosis of acute interstitial nephritis. Mild to moderate proteinuria and hematuria are seen in most cases of interstitial nephritis. Gross hematuria is observed occasionally. The sediment will typically show red and white blood cells. White blood cell casts are also seen with some regularity. Red blood cell casts should suggest a glomerular diagnosis. The finding of eosinophils in urine supports the diagnosis of allergic interstitial nephritis. This is best observed by using a Hansel stain on the urine sediment. The absence of eosinophiluria should never discourage the diagnostic pursuit of acute interstitial nephritis.

Serum creatinine is usually the first laboratory test to signal renal failure. The normal range of serum creatinine is 0.6 to 1.3 mg/dL and varies with muscle mass and gender. Without a high index of suspicion, early recognition of acute interstitial nephritis can be missed as the patient's serum creatinine glides through the normal range while the kidneys lose half their renal function. The magnitude of proteinuria in acute interstitial nephritis is nearly always less than 3 g/24 hr and often no more than 1 g/24 hr. Nephrotic-range proteinuria is not seen unless there is a coexisting glomerular lesion or after exposure to NSAIDs. Many patients with acute interstitial nephritis also have a fractional excretion of sodium greater than 1, but occasionally they can be oliguric. In patients with poor histories, it is sometimes difficult to distinguish between non-

TABLE 123–2 CAUSES OF ACUTE INTERSTITIAL NEPHRITIS

DRUGS
Antibiotics
Penicillins
Rifampin/ethambutol
Sulfa
Vancomycin
Ciprofloxacin
Cephalosporins
Erythromycin
Trimethoprim-sulfamethoxazole
Acyclovir
Nonsteroidal anti-inflammatory drugs
Selective and nonselective cyclooxygenase-2 inhibitors
Diuretics
Thiazides
Furosemide
Triamterene
Miscellaneous
Captopril
Ranitidine
Omeprazole
Phenobarbital
Phenytoin
Sodium valproate
Carbamazepine
Allopurinol
Interferon
Interleukin-2
All-*trans* retinoic acid
INFECTION
Bacteria
Legionella
Brucella
Diphtheria
Streptococcus
Staphylococcus
Yersinia
Salmonella
Escherichia coli
Campylobacter
Viruses
Epstein-Barr virus
Cytomegalovirus
Hantaan virus
Human immunodeficiency virus
Herpes simplex virus
Hepatitis B virus
Other
Mycoplasma
Rickettsia
Leptospira
Mycobacterium tuberculosis
Schistosoma mekongi
Toxoplasma
Chlamydia
AUTOIMMUNE DISEASE
Anti–tubular basement membrane disease
Tubulointerstitial nephritis and uveitis (TINU) syndrome
Kawasaki's disease

TABLE 123–3 TYPICAL CLINICAL MANIFESTATION OF ACUTE INTERSTITIAL NEPHRITIS

History of drug hypersensitivity or recent infection and taking antibiotics
Sudden onset of fever lasting several days to weeks
Variable degrees of hypertension
Rise in creatinine with FE_{Na} >1.0; no expected acute tubular necrosis or glomerulonephritis
Kidney size normal or increased
Hematuria with mild proteinuria (<1.0 g)
Presence of WBC casts and WBCs on urinalysis; rarely eosinophils

oliguric acute tubular necrosis and acute interstitial nephritis without a biopsy.

Selective tubular defects and tubular syndromes such as proximal, acquired Fanconi's syndrome (bicarbonaturia with a plasma CO_2 content <20 mEq/L, aminoaciduria, phosphate wasting, uricosuria, and glycosuria) or distal renal tubular acidosis (type 1; urine pH >5.6, plasma CO_2 content <20 mEq/L with low or high potassium) are not typically observed in acute interstitial nephritis if progression to renal failure is rapid. These selective tubular defects are diagnosed more commonly in subacute/chronic interstitial nephritis, if at all.

Imaging

The kidney in acute interstitial nephritis is usually normal or slightly increased in size on echographic or tomographic images. Some reports correlate increased cortical echogenicity with diffuse interstitial infiltrates on renal biopsy. Gallium scanning is not particularly useful because a variety of other renal processes can cause gallium uptake (including minimal-change glomerulonephritis, cortical necrosis, and acute tubular necrosis), and acute interstitial nephritis can be found on biopsy with a normal scan.

Invasive Evaluation

Ultimately, the diagnosis can be established with certainty only by renal biopsy. A biopsy should be performed on patients with acute renal failure who have suggestive signs or symptoms of an interstitial process and in whom prerenal azotemia and obvious acute tubular necrosis can be excluded on clinical grounds.

Treatment

Rx

A renal biopsy helps confirm and assess the extent of interstitial nephritis. Biopsy is important to be sure that the inflammation is acute because chronic disease associated with interstitial fibrosis rarely responds to aggressive treatment. The principal intervention for acute interstitial nephritis is to remove the inciting drug or treat the infection. Switching to different derivatives of a suspected drug is unwise once interstitial nephritis has started with one of them. Concomitantly or after a few days, if the serum creatinine concentration does not fall, steroids (prednisone at 0.75–1.0 mg/kg orally) can be tried for a week or so. If no further improvement is realized, oral cyclophosphamide (1–2 mg/kg) can be added for an additional few weeks. In patients who respond, cyclophosphamide can be steroid sparing, particularly in those with persistent sarcoidosis. It is important not to have patients keep taking high-dose immunosuppression without some evidence of benefit because the combination of immunosuppressive drugs with enduring azotemia can lead to serious infection and even death. It is better to save these drugs for a kidney transplant if the primary disease does not respond quickly.

CHRONIC INTERSTITIAL NEPHRITIS

Pathobiology

All forms of injury to the kidney, regardless of where they start, progress to end stage through a terminal phase of chronic interstitial nephritis. In addition to glomerulonephritides, cystic diseases, and diabetes, a wide variety of renal conditions start slowly in the tubulointerstitium. This process often goes unrecognized until it is too late, and on biopsy it is subsequently diagnosed as primary chronic interstitial nephritis.

Primary chronic interstitial nephritis can be caused by a variety of toxic, metabolic, hematologic, obstructive, and infectious processes. A careful history of drug or toxin exposure, previous renal images, and a family history can often point to a probable diagnosis. A few of the more important causes of chronic interstitial nephritis are mentioned in the following paragraphs; Table 123–4 provides a comprehensive list, and some entities may be discussed in other chapters.

Analgesics

Persistent ingestion of analgesics for headache, back and joint pains, or abdominal discomfort is very common, particularly in women, and because many analgesics can now be bought over the counter, these patients often have advanced renal injury at initial evaluation. Various epidemiologic studies suggest that six or more tablets per day for at least 3 years puts one at some risk for analgesic nephropathy. Acetaminophen, aspirin, and NSAIDs alone or together provide toxic metabolites or induce medullary ischemia and papillary necrosis, sometimes with papillary calcification. The likelihood of analgesic nephropathy from taking acetaminophen alone is much less than with the others. Classic images of analgesic nephropathy on tomography are quite specific (Fig. 123–2) and show a decrease in overall size with atrophic scars and an irregular cortical contour sometimes accompanied by papillary necrosis. Stopping analgesic use can be helpful in reducing progression if it is not found too late. Uroepithelial malignancies occur with increased frequency in this group of patients.

Vascular Disease

Chronic renal ischemia from vascular injury can lead to interstitial nephritis, nephrosclerosis, and fibrosis. This is the classic renal lesion of untreated essential hypertension. Similar injury is seen with aging, diabetes, sickle cell disease, and radiation nephritis. Chronic tubulointerstitial injury from the vascular diseases just mentioned is quite different from the aggressive necrosis seen with acute vasculitis. In patients taking calcineurin inhibitors such as cyclosporine or tacrolimus, renal ischemia can also develop from vasoconstriction. Some evidence suggests a dose effect, and patients with cardiac or lung transplants are kept at higher blood levels than patients with renal transplants and, consequently, have a higher frequency of interstitial fibrosis. Progression to interstitial fibrosis is sometimes hard to distinguish from chronic allograft rejection.

Obstruction

Significant occlusion of both ureters by bladder tumors, cervical carcinoma, ureteral valve disease, or bladder outlet obstruction after prostate enlargement is an important cause of chronic interstitial nephritis. Complete or partial urinary tract obstruction is accompanied by a decline in glomerular filtration and a variety of classic tubular abnormalities, including diminished reabsorption of solutes, impaired excretion of H^+ and K^+, and a vasopressin-resistant concentrating defect in the medulla. The pathophysiology of urinary tract obstruction has been studied thoroughly. Obstruction is associated with a fall in the glomerular filtration rate because of reduced plasma flow and hydraulic pressure associated with the release of angiotensin II, leukotrienes, and nitric oxide, a process leading to mononuclear cell infiltration. Growth factors such as TGF-β, released by infiltrating cells, may in addition contribute to the interstitial and glomerular fibrosis. Obstruction is more common in men than women and is part of the routine assessment of renal failure by renal ultrasound. Almost all obstructed kidneys eventually become infected if the obstruction is not relieved.

Herbal Nephropathy

With the advent of the natural food movement, a growing number of people are taking vitamins and herbal preparations purchased from health food stores. Some of these remedies contain botanicals that produce chronic interstitial nephritis. Aristolochic acid has been implicated in so-called Chinese herbal nephropathy. Women who are dieting often use these remedies and are first seen when they already have late-stage disease. This new risk highlights the importance of taking a good dietary history in patients suspected of having interstitial nephritis. This group of patients is also at higher risk for uroepithelial malignancies.

TABLE 123-4 CAUSES OF CHRONIC INTERSTITIAL NEPHRITIS

HEREDITARY DISEASES
Mitochondrial mutations
METABOLIC DISTURBANCES
Hypercalcemia/nephrocalcinosis
Hyperoxaluria
Hypokalemia
Hyperuricemia
Cystinosis
Methylmalonicacidemia
DRUGS AND TOXINS
Analgesics
Cadmium
Lead
Health food botanicals/herbs
Lithium
Cyclosporine/tacrolimus
Cisplatin/methotrexate
Nitrosoureas
AUTOIMMUNE DISEASE
Renal allograft rejection
Wegener's granulomatosis
Sjögren's syndrome
Systemic lupus erythematosus/vasculitis
Progressive glomerular disease
Sarcoidosis
HEMATOLOGIC DISTURBANCES
Multiple myeloma/light chains
Lymphoma
Sickle cell disease
INFECTION
Complicated pyelonephritis
Human immunodeficiency virus
Epstein-Barr virus
Malacoplakia
Xanthogranulomatous pyelonephritis
OBSTRUCTIVE NEPHROPATHY
Tumors
Stones
Outlet obstruction
Vesicoureteral reflux
MISCELLANEOUS
Aging vascular disease
Hypertension
Ischemia
Balkan (endemic) nephropathy
Radiation nephritis

Hypercalcemia

Hypercalcemia can decrease glomerular filtration through renal vasoconstriction, a decrease in the glomerular ultrafiltration coefficient, and volume depletion as a result of a vasopressin-resistant concentrating defect associated with nephrocalcinosis and calcium deposition around the basement membranes of the distal tubules and collecting ducts. Such deposition secondarily leads to mononuclear cell infiltration and tubular death. Nephrocalcinosis also occurs in normocalcemic disorders of augmented calcium absorption through the gut (sarcoidosis, vitamin D intoxication), skeletal breakdown (neoplasms or multiple myeloma), or classic distal renal tubular acidosis. Therapy is directed toward the primary disease: reduction of the serum calcium concentration when appropriate and correction of acid-base disturbances.

Myeloma

The chronic renal failure of multiple myeloma is caused by multiple overlapping mechanisms, including cast nephropathy ("myeloma kidney"), coexistent volume depletion, hypercalcemia, nephrocalcinosis, and uric acid nephropathy. There are proteinaceous casts in dilated, atrophic distal nephron segments with surrounding multinucleated giant cells in interstitial infiltrates. The casts typically contain both Tamm-Horsfall protein and the pathologic light chain. Interstitial plasma cells and mononuclear infiltrates, calcifications in the interstitium, and amyloid deposits in the vessels and glomeruli are often present. The pathogenesis of cast nephropathy has been an area of investigative interest for many years. Light chains are nephrotoxic by direct injury to tubular cells or through intrarenal obstruction from cast formation. In the setting of excess light-chain production, the proximal tubule reabsorptive capacity is overwhelmed, which leads to the urinary excretion of light chains as "Bence Jones" proteins. Hemodynamic studies suggest that elevated intratubular pressure partly accounts for the decline in glomerular filtration in experimental cast nephropathy. Appropriate therapy for presumed cast nephropathy in multiple myeloma includes chemotherapy to ameliorate excess light-chain production; treatment of hypercalcemia; alkalinization of the urine with the addition of bicarbonate to hypotonic fluids; and avoidance of radiocontrast agents, which may enhance the nephrotoxicity of light chains. Loop diuretics should be used with caution, particularly in the setting of volume depletion.

Lead and Cadmium Toxicity

Exposure to lead in developed countries is restricted by governmental regulations. Exposure still occurs, however, from old water pipes, pottery, crystal, and lead-based paint in older buildings. Several epidemiologic analyses support the association of excess lead burden with chronic renal failure. There are no simple blood tests to easily make this diagnosis; some laboratories can measure delta-aminolevulinic acid dehydratase (ALAD), which is inhibited by lead. Although chelation studies my document the lead burden, this test is difficult to perform in patients with renal failure. X-ray fluorescent measurements of in vivo skeletal lead stores correlate well with ethylenediaminetetraacetic acid (EDTA) chelation tests and have the advantage of being rapid and noninvasive. Blood lead levels reflect only recent, not chronic exposure and can be normal in patients with a significant lead burden. Lead preferentially deposits in the proximal tubule, and nuclear inclusions within proximal tubular cells are characteristic of lead nephropathy. Proximal tubular dysfunction may produce isolated tubule defects or a full Fanconi syndrome. It is unusual to see chronic renal failure from lead in children. In adults, lead nephropathy produces chronic interstitial nephritis, fibrosis, and nephrosclerosis. Patients often have recurrent gout, and hyperuricemia and hypertension may be present. Ingestion of moonshine liquor, with its high lead content, is an important historical clue to the diagnosis. In addition to use as a diagnostic test, EDTA has been advocated as chelation therapy. The goal of chelation is to normalize the EDTA mobilization test. In occasional patients this may arrest or reverse progression of the renal failure.

Cadmium nephropathy is seen in smelters with prolonged low-level exposure. Cadmium is bound to metallothionein, and proximal tubular cells take up these complexes. The liver and kidney are the two major organs in which cadmium accumulates. Its half-life in the body is longer than 10 years. Like blood levels of lead, blood levels of cadmium fall after an acute exposure because of extensive tissue deposition. Once a threshold of renal deposition is exceeded, excess cadmium will be excreted in urine. Cadmium intoxication produces irreversible proximal tubular dysfunction, hypercalciuria, nephrolithiasis, and metabolic bone disease with pain (called "ouch-ouch" disease in Japan). The mechanism by which cadmium and lead elicit chronic inflammation and fibrosis suggests interstitial T-cell injury by reaction to inducible heat shock proteins.

Infection

Viruses have long been suspected of contributing to idiopathic, chronic interstitial nephritis. At least one study found that Epstein-Barr virus could be detected in biopsy samples from a group of nonselected patients

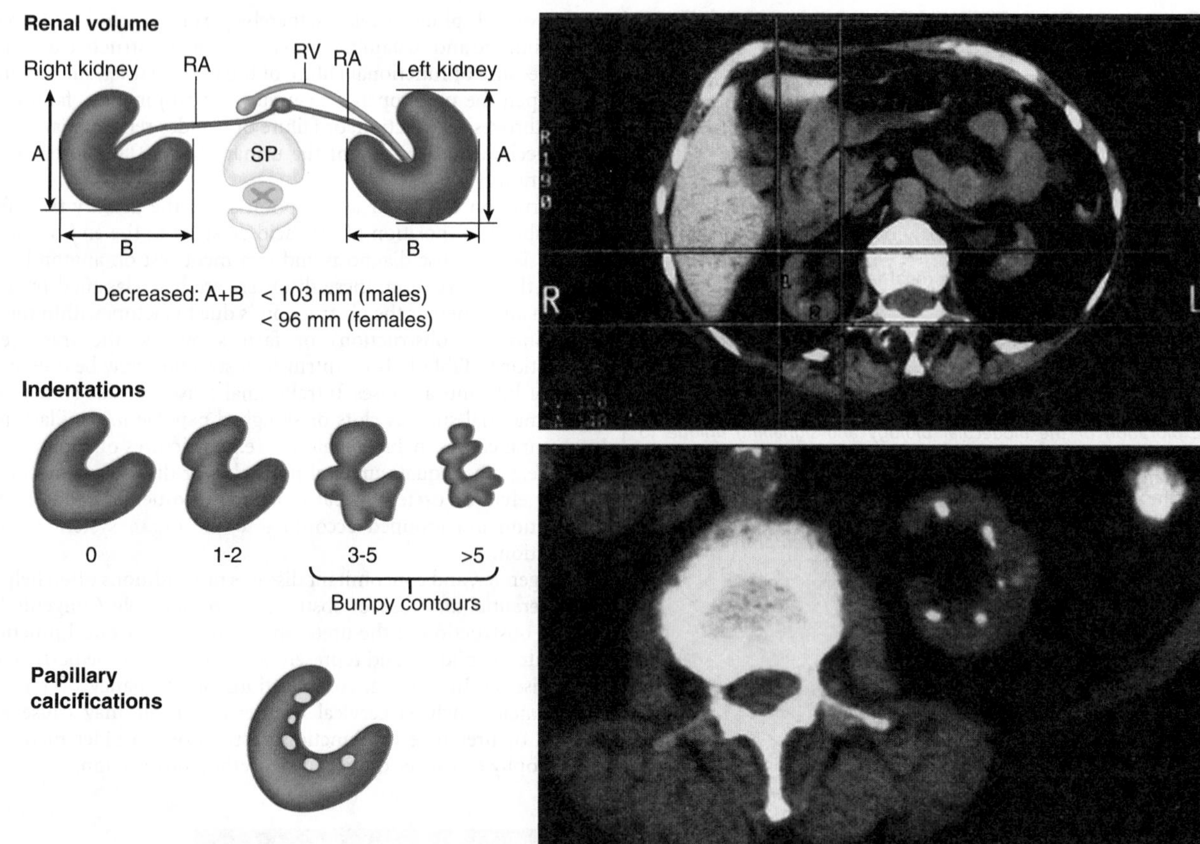

FIGURE 123–2 • Renal changes in analgesic nephropathy seen by tomographic imaging. Structural changes, including reduced volume, nodularity, and calcifications, are seen on computed tomography. RA = right artery; RV = right vein; SP = spinal vertebra. (From Elseviers MM, De Schepper A, Corthouts R, et al: High diagnostic performance of CT scan for analgesic nephropathy in patients with incipient to severe renal failure. Kidney Int 1995;48:1316, with permission.)

with idiopathic interstitial nephritis. Because reactivation typically produces lymphoproliferative disease, it is not clear why the kidney is singled out as a primary target for recrudescent injury in some patients, unless there are host-genetic polymorphisms or infection with new viral cousins as yet unknown. Malacoplakia and xanthogranulomatous pyelonephritis are probably not defects in nephrogenesis, but destructive responses to bacterial inflammation in the interstitium. Focal abnormalities in kidney structure can be a nidus for infection, perhaps confusing the primary etiology. These infections are associated with perinephric, psoas, or peritoneal abscesses and are often identified as primary renal masses in children or in the bladders of immunocompromised adults. Children with vesicoureteral reflux can have chronic or repeating episodes of pyelonephritis, but whether the reflux or the infection is more important to progression of renal failure is unclear. There is also no agreement on whether recurrent pyelonephritis by itself produces chronic interstitial nephritis in adults.

Hyperuricemia

Although it is widely accepted that overproduction of uric acid and hyperuricemia (especially in acutely treated myeloproliferative disease) can cause acute renal failure, it is less clear that chronic hyperuricemia independently results in chronic interstitial nephritis and progressive renal failure. Historically, chronic hyperuricemia associated with chronic interstitial disease was called "gouty nephropathy." Most studies do not demonstrate an association of hyperuricemia with chronic interstitial disease that could not be attributed to hypertension, vascular disease, calculi, or aging. Some of these patients may have undiagnosed lead exposure. Whether chronic hyperuricemia alone leads to interstitial nephritis is an important unanswered question, especially because many patients with chronic renal failure have serum uric acid levels higher than 10 mg/dL, attributable currently to diminished glomerular filtration and the effects of diuretics. If hyperuricemia in chronic renal failure can accelerate progression, lowering the serum uric acid level is most safely accomplished by protein and purine restriction, which is cumbersome to implement.

Clinical Manifestations

Patients with primary chronic interstitial nephritis typically have elevated levels of serum creatinine and signs and symptoms of renal failure, including hematuria, hyposthenuria, nocturia, fatigue, and nausea—all general signs and symptoms of chronic renal failure. Urinalysis shows a fixed specific gravity around 1.010, occasional glycosuria, and non-nephrotic ranges of proteinuria (often under 1 g/L) with red and white blood cells and granular casts. Pyuria and positive urine cultures for bacteria are occasionally seen, and varying degrees of metabolic acidosis and hyperphosphatemia may be present; before the glomerular filtration rate falls below 25 to 30 mL/min, there is non-delta or tubular acidosis. Anemia is often out of proportion to the degree of renal failure, and many patients have hypertension, but not much edema until advanced stages of renal failure. Acquired Fanconi's syndrome can be seen in patients with serum creatinine levels less than 2.5 mg/dL in the setting of drug exposure, myeloma, human immunodeficiency virus infection, lead exposure, and herbal nephropathy.

Treatment

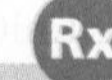

Chronic interstitial nephritis tends to progress slowly. Inciting factors such as obstruction, infection, drugs, or toxins should be removed when possible. Angiotensin-converting enzyme inhibitors or angiotensin-receptor blockers are used early in disease to slow progression, except when hyperkalemia is a problem, and hypertension should be treated aggressively. Early treatment of acidosis with oral citrate, anemia with erythropoietin, and secondary hyperparathyroidism with oral phosphate binders, calcium, and calcitriol can improve performance status and protect against bone loss. There is no clear role for immunosuppressive drugs in the treatment of chronic interstitial nephritis, except perhaps in early sarcoidosis. Generally, it is wiser to save immunosuppression for renal transplantation.

SUGGESTED READINGS

Cosyns JP: Aristolochic acid and 'Chinese herb nephropathy': A review of the evidence to date. Drug Saf 2003;26:33–48. *A good review of an important new problem.*

Harris RC, Neilson EG: Towards a unified theory of renal progression. Annu Rev Med 2006;57:365–380. *Overview of the pathophysiology leading to renal failure.*

Iwano M, Neilson EG: Mechanisms of tubulointerstitial fibrosis. Curr Opin Nephrol Hypertens 2004;13:279–284. *Review of the special mechanisms of interstitial fibrosis.*

Markowitz GS, Perazella MA: Drug-induced renal failure: A focus on tubulointerstitial disease. Clin Chim Acta 2005;351:31–47. *General review of drug-induced nephropathy.*

Nasr SH, Koscica J, Markowitz, GS, D'Agati VD: Granulomatous interstitial nephritis. Am J Kidney Dis 2003;41:714–719. *A good review.*

Rudnicki M, Eder S, Perco P, et al: Gene expression profiles of human proximal tubular epithelial cells in proteinuric nephropathies. Kidney Int 2007;71:325–335. *Exploration of the modecular biology and signalling unique to tubulointerstitial disease.*

Vadivel N, Trikudanathan S, Singh AK: Analgesic nephropathy. Kidney Int 2007 Apr 4. Epub ahead of print. *A comprehensive review.*

Van Vleet TR, Schnellmann RG: Toxic nephropathy: Environmental chemicals. Semin Nephrol 2003;23:500–508. *Overview of environmental injury to the kidney.*

124 OBSTRUCTIVE UROPATHY

Mark L. Zeidel

In the average adult, 1.5 to 2 L of urine flows daily from the renal pelvis to the end of the urethra, a process that requires proper functioning of each renal pelvis, the ureters, bladder, and urethra. *Obstructive uropathy* occurs when a structural or functional defect in the urinary tract interrupts or attenuates urine flow. Obstructive uropathy may impair renal function and lead to *obstructive nephropathy.* Increased hydrostatic pressure from downstream obstruction may cause upstream dilation of elements of the urinary tract, or *hydronephrosis.* Because recovery of renal function is inversely related to the severity and duration of obstruction, prompt recognition and treatment of obstructive uropathy markedly enhance the outcome of this condition.

Incidence and Prevalence

Although few studies of unselected populations have been performed, autopsy series of subjects ranging in age from neonatal to 80 years have revealed a 3.1% (2.9% in females, 3.3% in males) frequency of hydronephrosis. In autopsy series of children younger than 16 years, hydronephrosis was observed in 2.2% of boys and 1.5% of girls; 80% of cases of hydronephrosis were observed in children younger than 12 months. In adults, hydronephrosis is equally common between the sexes below 20 years of age and is more common in women than men between the ages of 20 and 60 years because of pregnancy and uterine cancer. After 60 years of age, obstructive uropathy is more common in men because of prostate disease. In these autopsy series it is unclear how frequently the observed obstruction resulted in clinical sequelae. However, each year in the United States the frequency of hospitalization for obstructive uropathy is 166 per 100,000. In a 3-year period in the 1990s, 6000 patients began treatment of end-stage renal disease with a presumed diagnosis of obstructive nephropathy. Among this group, 3.6% were younger than 20 years, 44% were 20 to 64, and the balance was older than 64 years.

Etiology

Normal movement of urine from the renal tubule requires orderly contraction of the renal pelvis, which feeds the urine into the proximal end of the ureter. The ureter then moves the urine to the bladder by rhythmic peristalsis and opening of the ureterovesical junction. The bladder stores the urine by activating relaxation reflexes that allow the bladder to expand without large increases in intravesicular pressure (Fig. 124–1) (Chapter 24). When voiding is initiated, the bladder contracts and the urethrovesical sphincter relaxes, thereby permitting the build-up of pressure to initiate and sustain the urinary stream. Obstructive uropathy may occur because of functional failure of the urinary tract, such as an inability to open the ureteropelvic or ureterovesical junction, failure to open the urethrovesical junction, or failure of bladder reflexes. Partial or complete mechanical blockade of the urinary tract at any level can lead to obstruction.

Obstruction can occur at any point along the urinary tract from the renal tubules (deposition of uric acid crystals) to the end of the urethra (phimosis). Because diagnosis and treatment rest on anatomic localization of the obstruction, these disorders are best classified by anatomic location and whether the obstruction is due to factors within the urinary tract (intrinsic obstruction) or factors outside the tract (extrinsic obstruction) (Table 124–1). Intrinsic obstruction may be due to intraluminal or intramural causes. Intraluminal causes include stones or sludging of material such as clots or sloughed papillae in papillary necrosis. Intramural causes include anatomic (e.g., strictures or tumors) or functional (e.g., inadequate ureteral peristalsis or disordered motility at the ureteropelvic or ureterovesical junction) disorders. Extrinsic causes of obstruction are grouped according to the organ system causing the obstruction.

Age, gender, and concomitant diseases or conditions often help narrow the differential diagnosis of obstruction considerably. Congenital causes, such as obstruction at the ureteropelvic or ureterovesical junction, predominate in children and represent a major cause of pediatric end-stage renal disease. In women, complications of pregnancy or reproductive malignancies such as cervical or uterine cancer may cause extrinsic ureteral or ureterovesical junction obstruction. In older men, prostatic hypertrophy or cancer often causes urethral obstruction.

Pathology and Pathophysiology

Acute obstructive uropathy reversibly alters renal blood flow, glomerular filtration, and tubular function; more chronic obstruction leads to fibrosis and permanent damage to renal function. Acute unilateral obstruction may cause minimal clinical disease because in the absence of other disease, the contralateral kidney compensates for the loss of function in the affected kidney. Although obstructive uropathy in humans is often partial and of prolonged duration, most studies of renal dysfunction caused by obstruction use models of acute complete obstruction because complete obstruction is reproducible and the short duration avoids confounding chronic changes in renal architecture.

During the initial hours after complete ureteral obstruction, blockade of forward urine flow markedly increases pressure in the lumens of renal tubules. This pressure increase is transmitted to the glomerulus. Initially, glomerular filtration is maintained by dilation of the afferent arteriole. However, afferent vasoconstriction, mediated by increased local production of angiotensin II and thromboxane A_2, soon supervenes and leads to decreases in renal blood flow, glomerular filtration pressure, and the glomerular filtration rate. Angiotensin and thromboxane also contract glomerular mesangial cells, thereby reducing the surface area of the glomerular capillary bed that is available for filtration. At the same time, prostaglandin E_2 and I_2 levels rise and reduce the level of vasoconstriction to some degree.

Obstruction also disrupts the ability of renal tubules, including the proximal tubule, the medullary thick ascending limb of Henle, and the cortical and medullary collecting ducts, to absorb sodium, secrete potassium and acid, and concentrate and dilute the urine. The attenuation of tubular function results from the local release of mediators such as prostaglandin E_2 that inhibit transport, local accumulation of macrophages, and release of inflammatory mediators, as well as mechanisms intrinsic to tubular epithelial cells. When urine flow is halted or markedly slowed, the reduction in delivery of solutes to tubular cells reduces the rate of apical sodium entry, thereby resulting in reduced synthesis and deployment to the plasma membrane of crucial transporter proteins such as Na^+, K^+-adenosine triphosphatase and apical sodium entry pathways such as the sodium channel and Na/K/Cl cotransporter. In addition to attenuation of salt reabsorption, urinary concentration and dilution are markedly inhibited. Because sodium transport is inhibited, the ability of the medullary interstitium to generate a concentration gradient is reduced. In addition, obstruction markedly reduces the synthesis and membrane trafficking of aquaporins, including aquaporin 2.

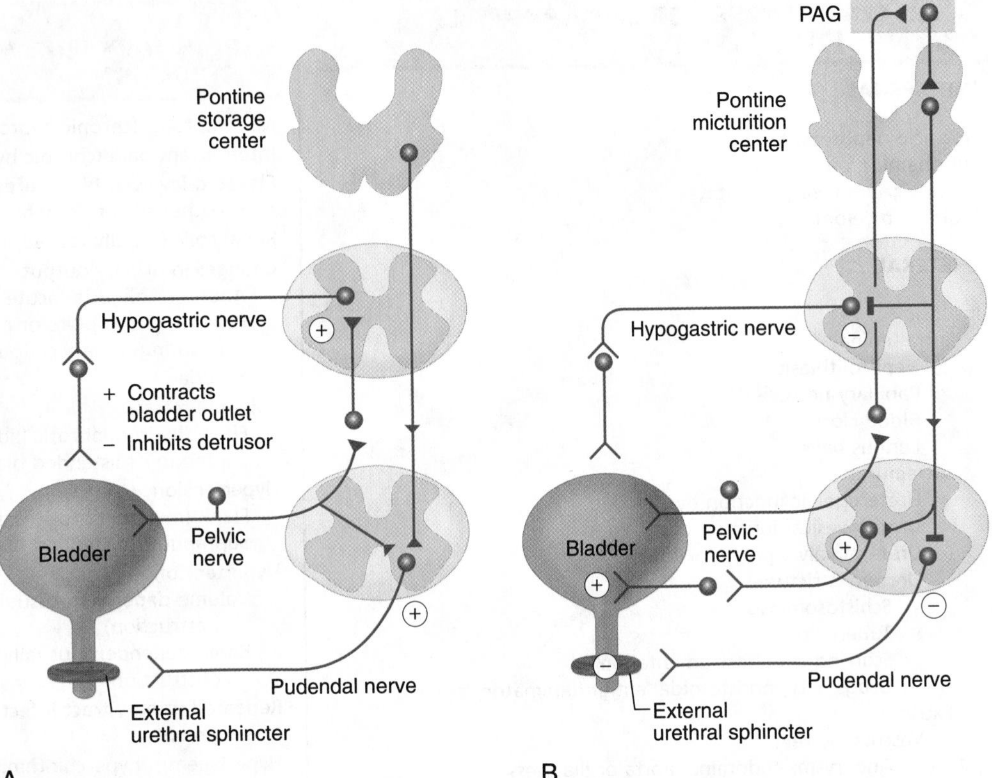

FIGURE 124–1 • Neural circuits controlling continence and micturition. A, Reflexes mediating urine storage and continence. As the bladder fills, distention stimulates low-level firing of vesical afferents (pelvic nerve), which in turn stimulate sympathetic outflow to the bladder outlet (hypogastric nerve to contract the internal sphincter and inhibit detrusor activity) and pudendal outflow to the external urethral sphincter. These responses occur by spinal reflex pathways that promote continence. The pontine storage center in the rostral pons augments pudendal nerve firing to enhance external urethral sphincter activity. **B,** Voiding reflexes. As the bladder becomes fuller, afferents fire more intensely and activate spinobulbospinal reflex pathways passing through the pontine micturition center (PMC). These reflexes stimulate parasympathetic outflow to the bladder and urethral smooth muscle (hypogastric nerve) and inhibit sympathetic and pudendal outflow to the urethral outlet. Ascending afferent input from the spinal cord may pass through the periaqueductal gray (PAG) matter before reaching the cortex, thereby leading to the sensation of urgency. (Modified with permission from DeGroat WC: Integrative control of the lower urinary tract: A preclinical perspective. Br J Phamacol 2006;147[Suppl. 2]:S25–S40.)

The combined impact of absence of medullary solute accumulation and reduced aquaporin activity leads to an inability to concentrate and dilute the urine.

In acute complete obstruction, therefore, glomerular filtration ceases and tubular transport is markedly attenuated. As the obstruction becomes more prolonged, renal fibrosis and permanent damage ensue. The response of the kidney to release of obstruction depends on several factors, including whether the obstruction is unilateral or bilateral, as well as the extent and duration of the obstruction. Release of acute unilateral obstruction leads to gradual release of renal vasoconstriction and rapid recovery of the glomerular filtration rate. Because tubular transport mechanisms may still be attenuated, postobstructive salt wasting, inability to secrete potassium and acid, and inability to concentrate and dilute the urine persist and lead to the production of a high quantity of isosthenuric urine (urine of tonicity similar to that of plasma) from the affected kidney.

During bilateral obstruction, the loss of renal function results in the accumulation of salt, water, and uremic toxins; acidosis; and hyperkalemia. Accumulation of salt and water leads to elevated levels of salt-wasting hormones, such as atrial natriuretic peptide, kinins, and prostaglandins, and reductions in salt-retaining hormones, such as angiotensin II, catecholamines, and aldosterone. This hormonal milieu acts synergistically with the postobstructive state to enhance glomerular filtration and reduce tubular salt reabsorption. As a result, release of acute bilateral obstruction can lead to high volumes of urine output and striking salt wasting.

Chronic partial urethral obstruction such as that caused by prostatic hypertrophy in men can lead to dilation and remodeling of the bladder. Under normal circumstances, as the bladder fills, stretch receptors in the bladder wall detect the filling and stimulate brain stem centers to inhibit contraction of the bladder wall and permit the bladder to fill without a large increase in hydrostatic pressure (see Fig. 124–1). In addition, these bladder-filling reflexes tighten the internal urethral sphincter and permit maintenance of continence without the need for voluntary contraction of the sphincter. However, as the bladder fills to volumes of 200 to 300 mL in women and 300 to 400 mL in men, additional stretch receptors are activated and stimulate micturition centers within the brain stem (see Fig. 124–1). These centers augment reflex contraction of the bladder detrusor musculature, relax the internal sphincter, and send impulses indicating an urge to void to the cortex. As the bladder fills further, the micturition reflex becomes stronger, the urge to void leads to discomfort and urgency, and the bladder begins to contract against the voluntary, external sphincter, thereby rendering it difficult to maintain continence.

In the setting of chronic urethral obstruction, successful micturition requires higher contractile pressure, which leads to hypertrophy of the detrusor muscle. The bladder empties less completely, with significant residual urine volumes. Initially, because of the residual volume left over from incomplete emptying, the capacity of the bladder to hold urine between micturition is diminished, and frequency and nocturia consequently develop. Over time, the transition from bladder accommodation to the micturition reflex may be delayed and occur at ever higher bladder-filling volumes. This leads to bladder dilation and, when the micturition reflex is suddenly activated, urgency, dribbling, and frank incontinence. Some of these features occur as well in women with pelvic floor disturbances that impede normal bladder function.

Clinical Manifestations

The clinical manifestations of obstructive uropathy depend on the location, extent (partial or complete), and duration (acute or chronic) of the obstruction, as well as whether one or both kidneys are affected (Table 124–2). It is important to note that even patients with severe obstruction may be asymptomatic, especially when the obstruction has developed gradually.

Patients with bilateral complete obstruction or complete obstruction of a single functioning kidney may exhibit signs, symptoms, and laboratory evidence of acute renal failure with volume overload, hypertension, and metabolic disturbances. By contrast, in unilateral obstruction with a functioning contralateral kidney, evidence of renal failure is absent, and the functioning kidney may compensate in large part for failure of tubular transport in the obstructed kidney. Patients with chronic partial obstruction may have no symptoms or may have intermittent pain. If the obstruction affects both kidneys, patients may show evidence of impaired renal function, including nocturia and polyuria from failure to concentrate the urine and increased levels of potassium, phosphate, creatinine, and blood urea nitrogen (Chapter 121).

Pain and Renal Colic

The bladder wall and renal and ureteral capsules contain sensitive C pain fibers, so stretching of these structures can result in exquisite pain.

TABLE 124–1 CAUSES OF URINARY TRACT OBSTRUCTION

INTRARENAL
Uric acid nephropathy
Sulfonamide precipitates
Acyclovir, indinavir precipitates
Multiple myeloma
URETERAL
Intrinsic
Intraluminal
Nephrolithiasis
Papillary necrosis
Blood clots
Fungus balls
Intramural
Ureteropelvic junction dysfunction
Ureterovesical junction dysfunction
Ureteral valve, polyp, or tumor
Ureteral stricture
Schistosomiasis
Tuberculosis
Scarring from instrumentation
Drugs (e.g., nonsteroidal anti-inflammatory agents)
Extrinsic
Vascular system
Aneurysm: abdominal aorta or iliac vessels
Aberrant vessels: ureteropelvic junction
Venous: retrocaval ureter
Gastrointestinal tract
Crohn's disease
Diverticulitis
Appendiceal abscess
Colon cancer
Pancreatic tumor, abscess, or cyst
Reproductive system
Uterus: pregnancy, prolapse, tumors, endometriosis
Ovary: abscess, tumors, ovarian remnants
Gartner's duct cyst, tubo-ovarian abscess
Retroperitoneal disease
Retroperitoneal fibrosis (radiation, drugs, idiopathic)
Inflammatory: tuberculosis, sarcoidosis
Hematomas
Primary tumors (e.g., lymphoma, sarcoma)
Metastatic tumors (e.g., cervix, ovarian, bladder, colon)
Lymphocele
Pelvic lipomatosis
BLADDER
Neurogenic bladder
Diabetes mellitus
Spinal cord defect
Trauma
Multiple sclerosis
Stroke
Parkinson's disease
Spinal anesthesia
Anticholinergics
Bladder neck dysfunction
Bladder calculus
Bladder cancer
URETHRA
Urethral stricture
Prostate hypertrophy or cancer
Obstruction from instrumentation

TABLE 124–2 CLINICAL MANIFESTATIONS AND LABORATORY FINDINGS IN URINARY TRACT OBSTRUCTION

No symptoms (chronic hydronephrosis)
Intermittent pain (chronic hydronephrosis)
Elevated levels of blood urea nitrogen and serum creatinine with no other symptoms (chronic hydronephrosis)
Renal colic (usually caused by ureteral stones or papillary necrosis)
Changes in urinary output
Anuria or oliguria (acute renal failure)
Polyuria (incomplete or partial obstruction)
Fluctuating urinary output
Hematuria
Palpable masses
Flank (hydronephrotic kidney, usually in infants)
Suprapubic (distended bladder)
Hypertension
Flank (hydronephrotic kidney, usually in infants)
Suprapubic (distended bladder)
Hypertension
Volume dependent (usually caused by chronic bilateral obstruction)
Renin dependent (usually caused by acute unilateral obstruction)
Repeated urinary tract infections or infection that is refractory to treatment
Hyperkalemic, hyperchloremic acidosis (usually caused by defective tubular secretion of hydrogen and potassium)
Hypernatremia (seen in infants with partial obstruction and polyuria)
Polycythemia (increased renal production of erythropoietin)
Lower urinary tract symptoms: hesitancy, urgency, incontinence, postvoid dribbling, decreased force and caliber of the urinary stream, nocturia

Acute bladder distention caused by sudden loss of the ability to relax the urethral sphincter (e.g., postoperatively) gives rise to sharp pain. By contrast, gradual bladder stretching, as can occur with gradual urethral obstruction from prostatic enlargement, may result in no pain. Abrupt distention of the ureters and renal capsule with acute pain (renal colic) is a common manifestation of acute ureteral obstruction, especially when caused by ureteral calculi. Renal colic is generally experienced as a severe, stabbing pain localized to the flank (when the stone lodges in the upper third of the ureter) or radiating to the groin or pelvic structures (when the stone is located in the lower two thirds of the ureter) and may be associated with vomiting or sweating. The acute episode may last less than 30 minutes (especially if the stone clears rapidly) or as long as a day. Chronic partial ureteral obstruction may cause intermittent flank pain. Abdominal pain radiating to the flank during micturition is said to be indicative of vesicoureteral reflux. Administration of fluid loads or diuretics may elicit pain in some patients with partial obstruction by stretching the ureteral wall. In patients with acute ureteral obstruction, physical examination may be normal or may reveal flank tenderness. In patients with acute obstruction below the bladder, acute bladder distention may be detectable and the bladder may be tender. In the setting of bladder distention, rectal examination in men may reveal prostatic enlargement, whereas pelvic examination in women may reveal pelvic masses. Examination of the sensory and reflex pathways of the sacral nerves may reveal neurologic causes of urinary retention.

Changes in Urine Output

In patients with complete bilateral ureteral obstruction, complete obstruction to urine flow beyond the bladder, or unilateral obstruction of a solitary functioning kidney, anuria and acute renal failure occur. Patients with partial obstruction may manifest normal urine volumes or polyuria. In some cases the major effect of partial obstruction is to prevent urinary concentration, thereby leading to the polyuria and increased thirst of diabetes insipidus; hypernatremia may also be present. Though unusual, a history of oligoanuria alternating with polyuria or the sudden onset of anuria strongly suggests obstructive uropathy.

Lower Urinary Tract Symptoms

Symptoms such as reduced force and caliber of the urine stream, urinary frequency, hesitancy, incontinence, nocturia, postvoid dribbling, and urgency often arise with obstruction of the urethra. Neurogenic bladder disease may alter the process of micturition and result in frequency, urgency, and urinary incontinence. Incontinence may occur because inadequate sensation of bladder fullness or an inability to void properly leads to overfilling of the bladder and reflex emptying (overflow incontinence).

Hematuria

Patients with obstruction may exhibit gross hematuria, especially in the setting of ureteral stones, which may cause bleeding by abrading the ureteral urothelium as they pass. Gross hematuria from any cause may lead to clots, which themselves can cause obstruction.

Hypertension

Any form of renal disease may be associated with hypertension (Chapter 131), which may be due to the renal disease or may be a concomitant condition. Obstructive uropathy may cause hypertension through a variety of mechanisms, including salt and water retention leading to expansion of extracellular volume, as well as increased renin secretion leading to increased circulating levels of angiotensin II. In the setting of unilateral obstruction, it is likely that the associated hypertension is due to increased renin production in the obstructed kidney.

Urinary Tract Infections

Urinary tract infections in nonsusceptible populations such as younger men or repeated urinary tract infections without apparent cause suggest a structural lesion in the urinary tract and are often associated with partial or complete obstruction. Infection occurs more commonly in patients with obstruction involving the bladder or urethra, perhaps because normal defenses against bacterial adherence to the urothelium are disrupted. In addition, the finding of unusual organisms (e.g., *Pseudomonas* or *Proteus* species) in noninstrumented patients again suggests disruption of normal defense mechanisms and possible obstruction.

Polycythemia

Polycythemia occurs rarely in obstructive uropathy. In some obstructed kidneys it appears that vasoconstriction reduces cortical oxygen tension, which leads to increased erythropoietin production. In such cases relief of the obstruction reverses the polycythemia.

Hyperkalemia and Hyperchloremic Metabolic Acidosis

As mentioned, obstructive nephropathy markedly attenuates the ability of distal nephron segments to secrete potassium and acid. Reduced excretion of potassium and acid leads to hyperkalemia and a non–anion gap metabolic acidosis. Failure to acidify the urine may be revealed by a high urine pH (above 5.5) in the setting of acidosis and by a positive urine anion gap (urine sodium and potassium higher than urine chloride), which is indicative of failure by the distal nephron to excrete ammonium in urine despite a low blood pH. In elderly patients, especially those with azotemia, chronic partial obstruction is associated with hyporeninemic hypoaldosteronism. In this condition, hyperkalemia and non–anion gap metabolic acidosis result from a combination of inadequate aldosterone production for the level of potassium and blood pH and inadequate tubular response to aldosterone secondary to tubular dysfunction.

Azotemia

Obstructive uropathy may acutely impair renal function, depending on the extent of obstruction. Chronic and more complete obstruction may lead to permanent renal damage and end-stage renal disease. Any patient with no previous history of renal disease who has significant renal impairment should be evaluated for obstructive uropathy, especially if the urinary sediment is bland. In addition, obstruction should be considered as a potential cause of accelerating deterioration of renal function in patients with known renal disease.

TABLE 124–3 DIAGNOSTIC TESTS USED FOR OBSTRUCTIVE UROPATHY

UPPER URINARY TRACT OBSTRUCTION
Sonography (ultrasound)
Plain films of the abdomen (KUB)
Excretory or intravenous pyelography
Retrograde pyelography
Isotopic renography
Computed tomography
Magnetic resonance imaging
Pressure flow studies (the Whitaker test)
LOWER URINARY TRACT OBSTRUCTION
Some of the tests listed above
Cystoscopy
Voiding cystourethrography
Retrograde urethrography
Urodynamic tests
Debimetry
Cystometrography
Electromyography
Urethral pressure profile

KUB = kidneys, ureter, bladder.
From Klahr S: Obstructive uropathy. *In* Jacobson HR, Striker GE, Klahr S (eds): The Principles and Practice of Nephrology. Toronto, BC Decker, 1991, pp 432–441.

Diagnosis

Because obstructive uropathy may be asymptomatic or may exhibit many different manifestations, the diagnosis may not be apparent. However, early diagnosis (Table 121–3) and prompt treatment are essential because the extent of long-term renal damage depends on the extent and duration of the obstruction.

In the outpatient setting, a history of renal colic, flank pain, or hematuria may suggest stone disease leading to ureteral obstruction. Changes in the volume or frequency of urination, such as anuria, polyuria, or swings from oligoanuria to polyuria, may suggest obstruction. Evidence of bladder dysfunction such as frequency, urgency, and nocturia is suggestive. In addition, a history of conditions that predispose to obstructive uropathy, such as sickle cell disease or chronic ingestion of high levels of pain relievers (papillary necrosis), previous stone disease, or abdominal cancer, should raise suspicion of obstruction. Finally, the presence of a single functioning kidney should raise the possibility that unilateral obstruction may be causing azotemia. In the inpatient setting it is possible to monitor the pattern of urine output to detect oligoanuria or polyuria.

Physical examination may also reveal obstructive uropathy in certain cases. Palpable abdominal masses may represent kidneys enlarged by chronic hydronephrosis; this finding may be accompanied by costovertebral angle tenderness and flank rigidity. Fever and flank tenderness may denote obstruction with complicating pyelonephritis. Abdominal distention and evidence of reduced peristalsis (diminished bowel sounds) may accompany acute renal colic. Finally, a suprapubic mass may represent a bladder that is markedly distended because of bladder outlet obstruction.

Initial laboratory evaluation focuses on careful urinalysis and standard chemistry panels. The urine may reveal hematuria in the case of stones, bacteriuria, numerous granulocytes in the setting of obstruction and infection, or a urine pH greater than 7.5 in the case of chronic infection with urea-splitting organisms. Serum chemistry evaluation may reveal hyperkalemia, non–anion gap acidosis, and in rare cases, hypernatremia, which denotes the failure of tubular secretion of potassium or acid and urinary concentrating mechanisms. Corresponding urine chemistry evaluation may reveal a pH higher than 5.5, lack of a negative anion gap (see earlier), and isosthenuria. The urine sediment may also reveal evidence of crystals (uric acid or calcium oxalate) suggestive of stone disease. In addition, laboratory measurements should include blood urea nitrogen and creatinine to assess the adequacy of glomerular filtration.

When obstructive uropathy is suspected, ultrasonography is the best screening modality because it is highly sensitive, safe, and low in cost and does not expose the patient to the risk of exposure to contrast or ionizing radiation. Because of its safety and low cost, ultrasonography is often used in patients with acute renal failure to "rule out" obstruction. Ultrasound may reveal dilation of the calyces, renal pelvis, and on occasion, the proximal end of the ureter. Earlier studies comparing ultrasound with excretory pyelography demonstrated a sensitivity and specificity of 90%. False-positive findings (dilation in the absence of obstruction) occur in patients with congenital anomalies, during diuresis, and in many patients with ileal conduits. False-negative findings may occur because the pelvis and calyces fail to dilate despite obstruction, as may occur with retroperitoneal fibrosis, volume depletion, or a variety of other conditions. Because of false-negative results, when the clinical setting strongly suggests obstruction and the ultrasound findings are negative, more definitive tests are warranted.

In the setting of renal colic, plain films of the abdomen may visualize ureteral calculi. They may also reveal disparities in renal size and bladder enlargement. Because computed tomography offers resolution far superior to that of plain films, it is often used in renal colic patients in place of plain films. Moreover, computed tomography may define the anatomic location of obstruction in patients found to have hydronephrosis on ultrasound or may identify obstruction in patients with negative ultrasound studies. In the setting of cancer or other structural lesions obstructing the ureters or invading the bladder, computed tomography may define the cause of obstruction.

In the past, intravenous pyelography was used in patients with suspected obstructive nephropathy. However, the risk associated with the administration of contrast to patients with azotemia, combined with poor resolution in many patients and marked improvements in the detection of obstruction by ultrasound and computed tomography, has markedly reduced the use of this modality in obstructive uropathy. Definitive diagnosis of the location of obstruction is often obtained by retrograde pyelography, in which contrast is injected directly into the ureters via catheters inserted into the urethra and bladder, or by antegrade pyelography, in which the contrast is injected into the renal pelvis via a percutaneous catheter.

Finally, when bladder dysfunction or lesions in the bladder have been identified, retrograde cystograms may define the bladder anatomy. In addition, cystometrography with urodynamic testing can define the force of detrusor function, whether the detrusor and the sphincter act in coordinate fashion (lack of coordination is referred to as dyssynergy), and the extent to which pressure within the bladder is elevated and causes obstruction to urine flow.

Differential Diagnosis

Because obstructive uropathy may exhibit subtle manifestations that mimic many other conditions, the differential diagnosis varies in accord with the initial clinical symptoms and signs. Though suggestive of obstructive uropathy, anuria and acute renal failure may result from intrarenal diseases such as glomerulonephritis or acute tubular necrosis (Chapter 121). Patients with polyuria, hypernatremia, and dilute urine may have nephrogenic or central diabetes insipidus. Obstructive uropathy is a rare cause of nephrogenic diabetes insipidus. Patients with hyperkalemic hyperchloremic metabolic acidosis may have hyporeninemic hypoaldosteronism (itself associated with chronic mild obstruction) or other tubular disorders. Renal colic may resemble abdominal pain secondary to diseases of the gastrointestinal or reproductive tracts such as appendicitis or ovarian cyst, especially when the colic is associated with nausea, vomiting, and diaphoresis.

Treatment

Once obstructive nephropathy has been identified, therapy focuses on rapid restoration of normal urine flow, treatment of any accompanying infection, and management of postobstructive complications. The degree to which renal function recovers depends on several factors, including the extent and duration of the obstruction and the extent of previous renal dysfunction.

Rx

Acute Obstruction

Complete obstruction leads to acute renal failure. In this setting, prompt diagnosis and therapy are crucial because the extent and rate of recovery of renal function depend on the speed of relief and prompt recovery obviates the complications of uremia and the need for acute dialysis in patients with bilateral obstruction or obstruction of a single functioning kidney. Because partial obstruction in the setting of antecedent renal disease may lead to further permanent renal damage, prompt relief is again mandatory. In all cases of obstruction, the urine should be examined and cultured to identify and treat infections. In the setting of urinary sepsis and obstruction, the sepsis cannot be treated successfully until the obstruction is relieved. In addition, in urinary sepsis with obstruction it is crucial to look for perinephric abscesses and drain them if present.

The site of the obstruction and its cause determine the therapeutic approach. If the obstruction is in the urethra or is due to bladder dysfunction, placement of a urethral catheter may relieve the obstruction. If catheters cannot be passed through the urethra, suprapubic cystotomy is needed. It then becomes important to develop more permanent approaches to preventing recurrence of obstruction. If the obstruction is in the upper urinary tract, retrograde ureteral catheters or nephrostomy tubes may be needed to relieve the obstruction. Retrograde catheters have the advantage that they can be left in place as internal stents in some cases so that normal voiding is restored, thereby avoiding the need to maintain percutaneous drainage tubes.

Acute Obstruction Caused by Calculi

Calculi are the most common cause of ureteral obstruction; cornerstones of therapy include analgesia, relief of the obstruction, and treatment of concomitant infections. Because stones cause excruciating pain and are often accompanied by nausea and vomiting, parenteral narcotics are generally needed for effective analgesia. Stones smaller than 5 mm often pass without surgical intervention; volume expansion with saline or, if tolerated, oral salt and water may help the patient pass the stone. If the cause of nephrolithiasis in a given patient is not yet known, meticulous straining of urine through gauze often captures the stone and permits chemical analysis.

If the stone is large (7 to 15 mm) and is completely obstructing a ureter, volume expansion is unlikely to dislodge it. If the stone is above the pelvic brim and is less than 15 mm in size, extracorporeal shock wave or ultrasonic lithotripsy may be performed. These modalities use focused electrohydraulic or ultrasonically generated shock waves, respectively, to shatter the stone. These methods are effective in 90% of cases and result in passage of the fragments within 3 months. It is important to increase the volume of urine flow after these approaches to help the patient pass the fragments. For stones located below the pelvic brim or for larger stones, endoureteroscopy with direct removal may be performed via catheters passed through the urethra. In all patients with stone disease, it is crucial to identify the cause and initiate appropriate measures to prevent further stones.

Chronic Partial Obstruction

Although patients with chronic partial obstruction may do well for prolonged periods, the obstructive process should be relieved because it poses a long-term threat to renal function. Prompt relief is mandatory when (1) partial obstruction progresses to frank urinary retention, (2) obstruction is accompanied by urinary sepsis or repeated urinary tract infections, (3) the obstruction is causing renal damage, and (4) the patient has symptoms such as voiding dysfunction, flank pain, or dysuria. Most often, chronic partial obstruction results from lesions in the lower urinary tract, including urethral blockage from prostate enlargement in men and urethral strictures or bladder dysfunction. Chronic obstruction at the bladder neck or urethra can lead to bladder dilation and remodeling, with attendant persistence of dysfunction and symptoms even after relief of the obstruction. On this basis it may be appropriate to relieve the obstruction before infection, major symptoms, or renal dysfunction occur.

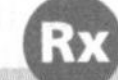

Obstruction caused by benign prostatic hypertrophy may remain stable for long periods or may respond to α_2-agonists. Because hypertrophy is so common and because frequency, urgency, and nocturia can develop insidiously, the physician must inquire carefully for symptoms and be alert for their progression. Therapeutic decisions, including surgery, will depend on the symptoms, the presence of infection, and the risk for permanent bladder or renal dysfunction (Chapter 130). Urethral strictures can be treated by dilation or urethrotomy.

Postobstructive Diuresis

Though usually self-limited, postobstructive diuresis can last several days to a week and may result in clinically important depletion of sodium, potassium, and chloride. Because postobstructive diuresis is prolonged and promoted by excessive fluid replacement, administration of volume is justified only when excessive losses result in clear volume depletion. Proper replacement is guided by measurement of urine chemistry and osmolality. Because the urine is generally isosthenuric with relatively high sodium levels as a result of residual tubular dysfunction, appropriate replacement fluid is often 0.45% saline given at a rate somewhat slower than that of urine output. By careful monitoring of vital signs, volume status, urine output, and serum and urine chemistry and osmolality, coupled with judicious fluid replacement, the diuresis is limited and prevented from causing serious volume or electrolyte abnormalities.

SUGGESTED READINGS

Li C, Klein JD, Wang W, et al: Altered expression of urea transporters in response to ureteral obstruction. Am J Physiol Renal Physiol 2004;286:F1154–F1162. *This paper and the series that precedes it define alterations in tubular epithelial function in the setting of renal obstruction.*

McCrery RJ, Appell RA: Bladder outlet obstruction in women: Iatrogenic, anatomic, and neurogenic. Curr Urol Rep 2006;7:363–369. *A clinical review.*

O'Neil WC: B-mode sonography in acute renal failure. Nephron Clin Pract 2006;103:c19–c23. *Sonography is the key to diagnosing obstruction but cannot diagnose other causes.*

125 DIABETES AND THE KIDNEY

Raymond C. Harris

Epidemiology

In the industrialized world, diabetes mellitus is the single leading cause of end-stage renal disease (ESRD). Both the incidence and prevalence of ESRD secondary to diabetes continue to rise. In the United States, more than 30% of patients undergoing either dialytic therapy or renal transplantation have ESRD as a result of diabetic nephropathy, and 40% of the new (incident) cases of ESRD are attributable to diabetes.

In the United States, Europe, and Japan, more than 90% of patients with diabetes have type 2 (Chapter 248) rather than type 1 (Chapter 247) (insulinopenic). Correspondingly, over 80% of the ESRD secondary to diabetes is also seen in patients with type 2 diabetes. Although it was previously supposed that ESRD secondary to type 2 diabetes was less common than with type 1 diabetes, when cohorts of patients with type 1 and type 2 diabetes are monitored for an extended period, the incidence of renal disease is equivalent. The demographics of ESRD secondary to type 2 diabetes mirror the prevalence of type 2 diabetes in the U.S. population, with a higher incidence in females and in African Americans, Hispanic Americans, Native Americans, and Asian Americans and a peak incidence in the fifth to seventh decade. Given the global epidemic of obesity in developed countries, an increasing incidence of diabetic nephropathy is being widely appreciated.

Pathobiology

Hyperglycemia

Increasing evidence implicates the metabolic sequelae of hyperglycemia as the most important causative factor in the development of diabetic nephropathy. The Stockholm Diabetes Intervention Study and the Diabetes Control and Complications Trial (DCCT) have both clearly demonstrated that aggressive control of blood sugar decreases the development of nephropathy, as well as other microvascular complications, in type 1 diabetes. [1] Furthermore, repeat renal biopsies have documented that the renal lesions of diabetic nephropathy may reverse after long-term (10 years) functioning pancreas transplantation. Hyperglycemia leads to increased generation of reactive oxygen species; depletion of the reduced form of nicotinamide dinucleotide (phosphate) (NAD[P]H); activation of the polyol pathway, which can lead to de novo synthesis of diacylglycerol and increased protein kinase C (PKC) activity; alterations in the hexosamine pathway; and nonenzymatic protein glycation (advanced glycosylation end products [AGEs]), all of which have been implicated in development of diabetic nephropathy, as well as other diabetic microvasculopathies. Aldose reductase inhibitors and AGE inhibitors have shown success in experimental models of diabetes and are currently undergoing clinical trials.

Hemodynamics

Patients with type 1 and, to a lesser extent, type 2 diabetes exhibit an increased glomerular filtration rate (GFR), so-called *hyperfiltration*, that is mediated by proportionately greater relaxation of the afferent arteriole than the efferent arteriole; such hyperfiltration leads to increased glomerular blood flow and elevated glomerular capillary pressure. With poorly controlled diabetes, there is also glomerular hypertrophy with an increased glomerular capillary surface area. These intraglomerular hemodynamic and structural alterations may contribute to the development or progression (or both) of diabetic renal injury. Because angiotensin-converting enzyme (ACE) inhibitors and decreased dietary protein reduce this increased intraglomerular capillary pressure in experimental animals, the hyperfiltration hypothesis provides one rationale for the success of these interventions in resisting the progression of diabetic nephropathy (see later).

Hormones and Cytokines

Studies in experimental animals have implicated a number of cytokines, hormones, and intracellular signaling pathways in either development or progression of diabetic nephropathy, notably transforming growth factor β (TGF-β), connective tissue growth factor, angiotensin II, vascular endothelial growth factor (VEGF), endothelin, prostaglandins, and nitric oxide. Because these factors have also been implicated in a variety of nondiabetic kidney diseases, it is likely that they will not prove to be specific for diabetic nephropathy. However, as discussed later, agents that interrupt angiotensin II production and signaling have proved to be very effective in slowing the progression of diabetic nephropathy. [2] Furthermore, agents that interrupt intracellular pathways activated by these factors or by other consequences of hyperglycemia may provide future therapeutic opportunities. [3] In this regard, the β-isoform of the intracellular signaling protein PKC is increased in the kidney and vascular tissues of diabetics, and specific PKC-β inhibitors have been developed and are currently in clinical trials. [4]

Genetics

At present, it is impossible to predict in which patients diabetic nephropathy will develop. Although poor glycemic and blood pressure control undoubtedly contributes, nephropathy may or may not develop in an individual patient even after many years of hypertension and hyperglycemia. There is evidence for familial clustering of both type 1 and type 2 diabetes. Type 1 diabetics with siblings who have diabetic nephropathy have a greater than 70% lifetime risk of diabetic nephropathy developing in themselves. There also appears to be a hereditary predisposition for the development of diabetic nephropathy in patients with type 2 diabetes. Diabetic nephropathy is likely to be a polygenic disease. Modifier genes have been proposed to be important for the development of diabetic nephropathy, the rate of progression of the injury (from microalbuminuria to ESRD), or both. A number of candidate genes have been tested for association with the development of diabetic nephropathy. A problem with all these studies is that several genes are most likely involved in predisposition to the development of diabetic nephropathy, so the assumptions of simple mendelian genetics do not apply. The complexity is illustrated by examination of various genetic linkage analyses that have provided conflicting results, which may be explained in part by genetic heterogeneity and the relatively small number of cases examined in an individual study. In this regard, an association with ACE insertion (I)/deletion (D) polymorphism has been reported with an increased incidence of the D allele, which predisposes to increased levels of ACE. This polymorphism has been associated with the development or severity of a variety of nondiabetic renal diseases, although negative studies have also been reported. Some, but not all linkage studies have also suggested involvement of angiotensinogen polymorphisms and angiotensin II type 1 (AT1) receptor polymorphisms in the development of diabetic nephropathy.

Endothelial dysfunction is present in diabetes and is associated with impaired vascular nitric oxide synthesis. Linkage studies have suggested an association of polymorphisms in endothelial nitric oxide synthase (eNOS) with nephropathy in Pima Indians with type 2 diabetes, and some but not all linkage studies in other populations of diabetic nephropathy have also identified eNOS polymorphisms. It has likewise been suggested that genetic abnormalities in lipid metabolism may underlie a predisposition to the development of diabetic nephropathy, and in this regard, polymorphisms in apolipoprotein E have also been linked to a predisposition to the development of diabetic nephropathy in some but not all studies. A variety of other genes, including those for the receptor for AGEs (RAGE), the glucose transporter Glut1, plasminogen activator inhibitor 1 (PAI-1), TGF-β, the B2 bradykinin receptor paroxonase, the homocysteine metabolism–related enzyme methylenetetrahydrofolate reductase, atrial natriuretic peptide, RANTES (regulated on activation, T-cell expressed and secreted), superoxide dismutase, lipoprotein lipase, decorin, VEGF, and peroxisome proliferator–activated receptor γ (PPAR-γ), have also been linked in some but not all studies.

Because the "candidate gene" approach has provided such conflicting results, genome-wide scans have recently been used to study the genetic basis of diabetic nephropathy. These scans allow a comprehensive survey of the entire genome for chromosome regions that are linked to diabetic nephropathy. Recent scans in Pima Indians and African Americans have identified susceptibility loci on chromosomes 3q, 7, 18q, and 20p. In addition, there is recent evidence for a susceptibility locus on chromosome 10 in both white and African American persons for the development of ESRD from diabetic nephropathy. The identity of the predisposing genes continues to be the subject of intensive current research, and our understanding of the involved genetic interactions will very probably increase dramatically in the next few years.

Clinical Manifestations

Natural History

Although a minority of patients with diabetic nephropathy have type 1 diabetes, the natural history of the disease is best exemplified in this population because the onset of diabetes is more clearly definable and patients with type 1 diabetes usually do not initially have the comorbid conditions often associated with type 2 diabetes (including essential hypertension, atherosclerotic cardiovascular disease, and obesity) that may independently produce chronic renal injury. Furthermore, the relatively advanced age of onset in patients with type 2 diabetes and the increased cardiovascular mortality in this population may preclude the development of all manifestations of diabetic nephropathy. In this regard, definitive descriptions of diabetic nephropathy in type 2 diabetes have been obtained in studies of Pima Indians, who exhibit a strong genetic predisposition for the development of type 2 diabetes around the fourth decade of life and in whom the diabetic nephropathy progresses in a similar pattern as seen in type 1 diabetic patients.

Stages

In type 1 diabetes, it is possible to characterize the progression of diabetic nephropathy as occurring in four relatively distinct stages (Fig. 125–1).

Stage I

In stage I, which commences soon after the overt manifestations of diabetes, the kidney undergoes hypertrophy in comparison to age- and weight-matched normal control subjects. Both the glomeruli and tubules are hypertrophied. In addition, there is up to a 50% increase in renal blood flow and GFR in the initial phase of diabetic nephropathy. At this stage, no macroalbuminuria is detectable, but transient microalbuminuria (measurable by radioimmunoassay, enzyme-linked immunosorbent assay, or special dipsticks) is occasionally evident, especially when

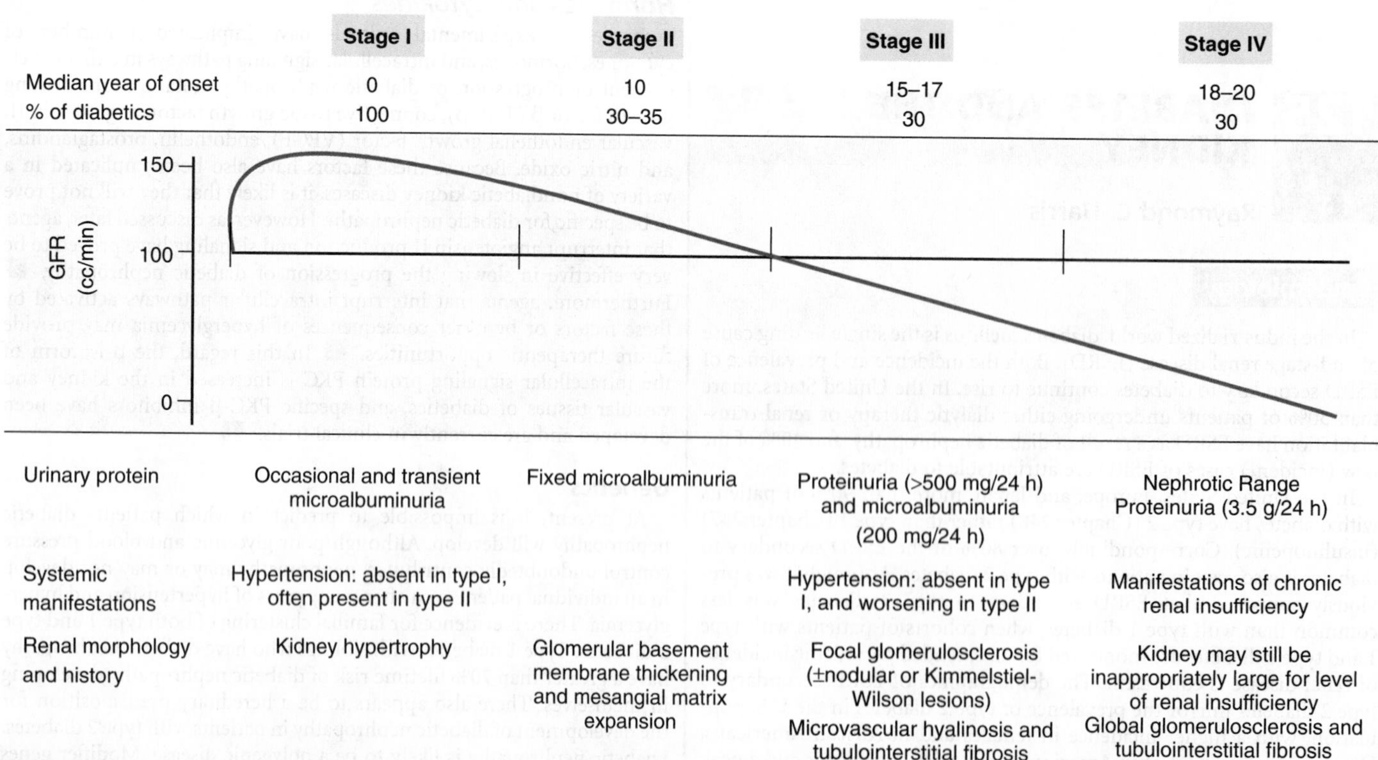

FIGURE 125–1 • Stages of diabetic nephropathy. GFR = glomerular filtration rate.

induced by stress, physical exertion, concurrent illness, or poor glycemic control. In type 1 diabetics, hypertension is usually absent in the early stages of the disease but is often present in type 2 diabetics at initial evaluation.

Stage II

Approximately 30% of type 1 diabetic patients progress to stage 2, which is characterized by fixed microalbuminuria of at least 30 mg/24 hr. The median duration of diabetes for progression to this clinically silent stage is 10 years. Although the GFR either remains elevated or is within the normal range, abnormal renal histology is present and is manifested as glomerular and tubular basement membrane thickening and inception of mesangial matrix expansion. The risk of development of microalbuminuria is greatly increased if other microvascular insults coexist, and in particular, the presence of proliferative retinopathy increases the likelihood that detected microalbuminuria reflects the presence of diabetic nephropathy. In this regard, the predictive value of microalbuminuria for diabetic nephropathy is greater in type 1 than in type 2 diabetics because of the high incidence in the latter population of hypertension, which may itself lead to microalbuminuria.

Stage III

The great majority of patients who are initially seen with fixed microalbuminuria progress to overt nephropathy (stage III) within 5 to 7 years. In this stage, patients manifest overt proteinuria (>500 mg of total protein per 24 hours) and macroalbuminuria (>200 mg/24 hr), which is detectable with a routine urinary protein dipstick. Blood pressure begins to rise in type 1 patients with stage III nephropathy, and in type 2 patients, who frequently have preexistent hypertension, blood pressure control becomes more problematic.

Renal biopsy reveals diffuse or nodular (Kimmelstiel-Wilson) glomerulosclerosis. Although the Kimmelstiel-Wilson lesion is considered pathognomonic of advanced diabetic nephropathy, only approximately 25% of patients manifest this lesion. A nodular pattern of glomerulopathy mimicking Kimmelstiel-Wilson lesions may also be seen in light-chain nephropathy. Older descriptions of "diabetic nephropathy without overt hyperglycemia" that were based solely on light microscopic analysis may have actually represented light-chain disease. Nodular glomerular lesions can also be observed in amyloidosis and membranoproliferative glomerulonephritis type II.

An additional pathognomonic feature of diabetic nephropathy is the finding of both afferent and efferent arteriolar hyalinosis, unlike the arteriolar lesion of essential hypertension, which is restricted to the afferent arteriole. In overt diabetic nephropathy, there is also progressive tubulointerstitial fibrosis, which correlates most closely with the decline in renal function in a number of progressive renal diseases, including diabetic nephropathy. The GFR begins to decline from the normal range, but serum creatinine may remain in the normal range.

Stage IV

Stage IV, or advanced diabetic nephropathy, is characterized by a relentless decline in renal function to end-stage disease. Patients manifest nephrotic-range proteinuria (>3.5 g/24 hr) and systemic hypertension but have no evidence of inflammatory glomerular (red blood cell casts) or tubulointerstitial (white blood cells, white blood cell casts) lesions. The kidneys may be inappropriately large for the observed degree of renal insufficiency.

Although patients with type 2 diabetes also tend to have an elevated GFR during the early course of their disease, the GFR increases are not usually as pronounced as seen with insulin-dependent diabetes mellitus. In addition, there is a greater incidence of hypertension and microalbuminuria at the time of detection of diabetes, with as many as 10 to 25% of patients demonstrating these abnormalities. It is still unclear whether this difference in manifestation represents a fundamental difference in the pathophysiology of the two conditions or, more likely, is due to the fact that type 2 patients may have unrecognized diabetes for many years because they are not ketosis prone and may have other associated conditions predisposing to renal abnormalities.

Other Renal Complications

In addition to the clinical manifestations of diabetic nephropathy described earlier, other kidney and genitourinary abnormalities can ensue in diabetic patients. Type IV (hyporeninemic, hypoaldosteronemic) metabolic acidosis with hyperkalemia is commonly encountered in patients with diabetes and mild to moderate renal insufficiency. These patients should be carefully monitored for the development of severe hyperkalemia in response to volume depletion or after the initiation of drugs that interfere with the renin-angiotensin system, such as ACE inhibitors, AT1 receptor blockers, β-adrenergic blockers, both nonselective and selective cyclooxygenase-2 (COX-2) nonsteroidal anti-inflammatory agents, and heparin, as well as potassium-sparing diuretics.

Patients with diabetes have an increased incidence of bacterial and fungal infections of the genitourinary tract. In addition to lower urinary tract infections, they have an increased risk for pyelonephritis and intrarenal and perinephric abscess formation.

Unilateral or bilateral renal artery stenosis is more frequent in the type 2 diabetic population than in age-matched nondiabetic individuals and should be considered if a diabetic patient has intractable hypertension or a rapidly rising serum creatinine level immediately after initiation of therapy with an ACE inhibitor or AT1 receptor blocker. Other causes of acute deterioration in renal function include papillary necrosis with ureteral obstruction secondary to sloughing of a papilla, obstructive uropathy secondary to bladder dysfunction as a result of autonomic neuropathy, and contrast media–induced acute tubular necrosis. In addition, prerenal azotemia or acute tubular necrosis may develop in diabetic patients as a result of congestive heart failure or volume depletion secondary to vomiting induced by gastroparesis or diarrhea from autonomic neuropathy.

Prevention

As mentioned, studies have convincingly demonstrated that tight glycemic control significantly lessens but does not completely eliminate the incidence of diabetic nephropathy. Furthermore, in the DCCT, the incidence of clinically significant hypoglycemic episodes was increased threefold in patients receiving intensive insulin therapy. Although the role of hypertension in the initiation of diabetic renal lesions remains unresolved (see earlier), it is clear that elevated blood pressure is an important risk factor in the progression of diabetic nephropathy, and blood pressure targets for patients with diabetes are lower (130/80 mm Hg) than those for patients without diabetes. 5 There also is evidence that smoking and elevated cholesterol may be predisposing factors for the development of diabetic nephropathy in type 2 diabetic patients.

Treatment

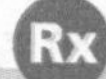

Latent (Stage II) and Overt (Stage III) Diabetic Nephropathy

Although the Stockholm Diabetes Intervention Study and the DCCT demonstrated that strict glycemic control was effective in preventing the development of fixed microalbuminuria, subgroup analysis of DCCT patients who were initially found to have microalbuminuria, as well as a subsequent study by the Microalbuminuria Collaborative Study Group, has determined that tight control in type 1 patients may not prevent progression to macroalbuminuria, although it does prevent other microvascular complications such as retinopathy and peripheral neuropathy (Fig. 125–2). There is increasing evidence that better glycemic control will slow the progression of nephropathy in type 2 as well as type 1 diabetic patients (Chapter 247).

It is clear that optimal blood pressure control will retard progression of diabetic nephropathy. 5 Studies have determined that interfering with the renin-angiotensin system by the administration of either ACE inhibitors or AT1 receptor blockers has additional benefit beyond lowering systemic blood pressure, such as retarding progression in both type 1 and type 2 patients. 6 Conversely, there is evidence that dihydropyridine calcium channel blockers may be less effective or even detrimental in preventing progression of diabetic nephropathy. The underlying pathophysiologic explanation relates to the ability of ACE inhibitors and AT1 receptor blockers to lower intraglomerular capillary pressure by decreasing efferent arteriolar pressure; in contrast, dihydropyridine calcium channel blockers increase intraglomerular capillary pressure by inducing selective afferent arteriolar vasodilation.

Stage I	Tight glucose control; BP control—consider use of ACEI or ARB
Stage II	Tight glucose control; ACEI or ARB; BP control; Smoking cessation; Weight reduction; Exercise; Annual eye examination;
Stage III	ACEI or ARB; BP control; Restriction of dietary protein (to 0.8g/kg of ideal body weight/day); Antihyperlipidemic medications
Stage IV	Treat manifestations of nephrotic syndrome and chronic renal insufficiency; Prepare for renal replacement therapy, including prevention of abnormalities in calcium/phosphorus metabolism and prevention of anemia by early use of erythropoietin

FIGURE 125-2 • Treatment of diabetic nephropathy. ACEI = angiotensin-converting enzyme inhibitor; ARB = angiotensin-receptor blocker; BP = blood pressure.

Rx

When administering ACE inhibitors or AT1 receptor blockers to patients with diabetic nephropathy, serum potassium and creatinine levels should be monitored closely in the first week after initiation because of the associated comorbid conditions of type IV renal tubular acidosis and renal artery stenosis. If blood pressure control is not achieved with these agents, diuretics and other antihypertensive agents, including cardioselective β-blockers, α-blockers, and nondihydropyridine calcium channel blockers, can be added. Smoking cessation and the use of antihyperlipidemic medications by patients with documented lipid abnormalities should be encouraged. Judicial restriction of dietary protein (to 0.8 g/kg of ideal body weight per day) is recommended by the American Diabetes Association. Although some data suggest that further dietary protein restriction may retard the progression of diabetic nephropathy, such an intervention must also take into account the individual nutritional carbohydrate and lipid requirements of the patient.

The efficacy of treatment can be determined by monitoring albuminuria or total proteinuria, or both. For patients with deterioration in renal function, GFR determined by creatinine clearance and plots of the reciprocal of serum creatinine versus time (1/sCr) are effective indicators of whether interventions are affecting the rate of progression of the nephropathy.

Renal Replacement Therapy

More than 80% of patients with end-stage diabetic nephropathy receive dialysis as their modality of renal replacement therapy, with 5.7 times as many of these patients undergoing hemodialysis as peritoneal dialysis. Because of the associated macrovascular complications (cardiovascular, cerebrovascular, peripheral vascular) and the increased risk for infection, the survival of diabetic patients who receive either type of dialysis is lower than that of the nondiabetic dialysis population, with a mortality that is 1.5 to 2.0 times that of nondiabetic patients and a 5-year survival rate of less than 20% in diabetic patients undergoing maintenance dialysis. The survival of diabetic patients is slightly worse with peritoneal dialysis than with hemodialysis. It is not established whether this difference is a consequence of the therapy itself (dialytic adequacy may not be as easily achieved in larger patients, and systemic absorption of the high-glucose solutions used in peritoneal dialysis may lead to poorer glycemic control and accelerate microvascular or macrovascular complications) or a reflection of the patients in whom peritoneal dialysis may be more likely to be initiated (i.e., patients whose associated vascular complications preclude hemodialysis). In general, management of a diabetic patient nearing ESRD is similar to that of a nondiabetic patient. The patient should be under the care of a nephrologist, and planning should be initiated for the modality of dialysis. Although dialysis is generally started when the GFR declines to approximately 10 to 15 mL/min, in diabetic patients, early initiation of dialysis is sometimes necessary when either volume-dependent hypertension or hyperkalemia is not manageable by nondialytic therapy or when uremia, combined with gastroparesis, leads to anorexia and malnutrition or uncontrollable recurrent emesis.

Approximately 25% of the renal transplant recipients in the United States are diabetic patients. The vast majority (>90%) are type 1 diabetic patients because of their younger age and decreased associated macrovascular comorbidity in comparison to type 2 patients. Long-term survival and quality of life after transplantation are generally superior to that in patients who undergo dialytic therapy. However, the other microvascular complications (retinopathy, neuropathy) are not improved by renal transplantation alone. The advent of pancreas and combined kidney-pancreas transplantation has been shown to improve the quality of life of patients with diabetic nephropathy significantly by improving autonomic neuropathy, by either retarding or possibly correcting retinopathy, and by avoiding the potential complications of insulin administration. However, all transplantation options remain limited by organ availability.

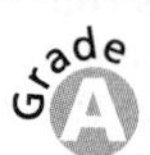

1. The Diabetes Control and Complications Trial Research Group: The effect of intensive treatment of diabetes on the development and progression of long-term complications in insulin-dependent diabetes mellitus. N Engl J Med 1993;329:977–986.
2. Lewis EJ, Hunsicker LG, Bain RP, et al: The effect of angiotensin-converting-enzyme inhibition on diabetic nephropathy. N Engl J Med 1993;329:1456–1462.
3. Lewis EJ, Hunsicker LG, Clarke WR, et al: Collaborative Study Group: Renoprotective effect of the angiotensin-receptor antagonist irbesartan in patients with nephropathy due to type 2 diabetes. N Engl J Med 2001;345:851–868.
4. Brenner BM, Cooper ME, de Zeeuw D, et al: RENAAL Study Investigators: Effects of losartan on renal and cardiovascular outcomes in patients with type 2 diabetes and nephropathy. N Engl J Med 2001;345:861–869.
5. Vijan S, Hayward RA: Treatment of hypertension in type 2 diabetes mellitus: Blood pressure goals, choice of agents, and setting priorities in diabetes care. Ann Intern Med 2003;138:593–602.
6. Chobanian AV, Bakris GL, Black HR, et al: The Seventh Report of the Joint National Committee on Prevention, Detection, Evaluation, and Treatment of High Blood Pressure: The JNC 7 report. JAMA 2003;289:2560–2572.

SUGGESTED READINGS

Alsaad KO, Herzenberg AM: Distinguishing diabetic nephropathy from other causes of glomerulosclerosis: An update. J Clin Pathol 2007;60:18–26. *Immunofluorescence and electron microscopy studies are essential.*

de Zeeuw D: Albuminuria: A target for treatment of type 2 diabetic nephropathy. Semin Nephrol 2007;27:172–181. *The protection from reducing albuminuria is dissociated from blood pressure decreasing effect of drugs.*

Gaston RS, Basadonna G, Cosio FG, et al: Transplantation in the diabetic patient with advanced chronic kidney disease: A task force report. Am J Kidney Dis 2004;44:529–542. *Reviews the outcomes and complications of renal transplantation in the diabetic population.*

Lewis EJ: Treating hypertension in the patient with overt diabetic nephropathy. Semin Nephrol 2007;27:182–194. *In addition to ACE inhibitors and ARBs, some patients may require three or more agents.*

Snow V, Weiss KB, Mottur-Pilson C: Clinical Efficacy Assessment Subcommittee of the American College of Physicians. The evidence base for tight blood pressure control in the management of type 2 diabetes mellitus. Ann Intern Med 2003;138:587–592.

Strippoli GF, Bonifati C, Craig M, et al: Angiotensin converting enzyme inhibitors and angiotensin II receptor antagonists for preventing the progression of diabetic kidney disease. Cochrane Database Syst Rev 2006;4:CD006257. *The 20% or so effects on renal outcomes are similar for both classes of drugs.*

Yuyun MF, Adler AI, Wareham NJ: What is the evidence that microalbuminuria is a predictor of cardiovascular disease events? Curr Opin Nephrol Hypertens 2005;14:271–276.

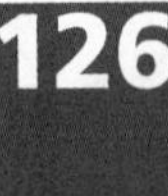

126 VASCULAR DISORDERS OF THE KIDNEY

Thomas D. DuBose, Jr., and
Renato M. Santos

The fact that the kidneys depend on systemic blood pressure to maintain normal renal blood flow, glomerular filtration rate (GFR), and tubular function underscores the vulnerability of the kidneys to diseases involving the renal vasculature. Thrombosis, emboli, atherosclerosis, inflammation, or hypertension may involve the renal vessels. Renal vascular disease can be classified according to anatomic location: arteries, arterioles and microvasculature, and veins.

ARTERIES

Thromboembolic Occlusion of the Renal Arteries

Definition

Thrombosis of the renal arteries and segmental branches may arise as a result of intrinsic pathology of the renal arteries or as a complication of embolization of thrombi arising in distant vessels. In situ thrombosis occurs as a complication of progressive atherosclerosis in elderly patients and may be an important cause of progressive renal insufficiency in this population. In patients younger than 60 years, traumatic thrombosis is the most common etiology. Blunt trauma and deceleration injuries may cause acute thrombosis. Trauma to the renal pedicle may result in an intimal tear with thrombosis in the middle third of the renal artery. Thrombosis may arise in the setting of dissection of the renal artery or as a complication of renal arteriography, angioplasty, stent placement, or endovascular graft placement. Thrombosis may also be associated with thrombophilic states, in particular, the antiphospholipid antibody syndrome. Finally, thrombosis may occur as a consequence of inflammatory disorders that involve the large arteries (Takayasu's arteritis, syphilis, systemic vasculitides, and thromboangiitis obliterans), as well as structural lesions of the renal arteries such as fibromuscular dysplasia (FMD) or renal artery aneurysm. Embolization is a more common cause of renal artery occlusion than in situ thrombosis is and is generally unilateral (bilateral in 15 to 30%). Total infarction of the kidney is much less common than segmental infarction or ischemia. Approximately 90% of thromboemboli to the renal arteries originate in the heart, and a common cause is left atrial thrombi in patients with atrial fibrillation. Valvular heart disease, bacterial endocarditis, nonbacterial (aseptic) endocarditis, and atrial myxomas are other sources of emboli originating in the heart. The diverse causes of occlusion of the renal artery or its segmental branches are summarized in Table 126–1.

Clinical Manifestations

The manifestations of thromboembolic occlusion of the renal arteries depend on the extent and time course of the occlusive event, as well as the preexisting status of the renal circulation. Occlusion of a primary or secondary branch of the renal artery in a patient with preexisting disease and established collateral circulation, such as in long-standing renal artery stenosis (RAS), may produce little or no infarction and minimal symptoms. Acute thrombosis and infarction may result in sudden onset of flank pain (which resembles renal colic), fever, nausea, vomiting, and on occasion, hematuria. Pain may be localized to the abdomen, back, or even the chest, but in more than half the cases, pain is absent. Anuria suggests bilateral involvement or occlusion of a solitary kidney. If infarction occurs, leukocytosis usually develops, and serum enzyme levels may be elevated (aspartate aminotransferase, lactate dehydrogenase, and alkaline phosphatase); urinary lactate dehydrogenase and alkaline phosphatase may also increase. Urinalysis usually reveals microscopic hematuria, but it may be absent and mild proteinuria may be seen. Blood urea nitrogen and creatinine levels typically increase transiently with unilateral infarction, but more severe and protracted renal dysfunction may follow bilateral renal infarction or infarction of a solitary kidney. Hypertension, which usually occurs with infarction, is the result of release of renin from the ischemic renal parenchyma.

TABLE 126–1 CAUSES OF RENAL ARTERY OCCLUSION

THROMBOSIS
Progressive atherosclerosis
Trauma, blunt
Aortic or renal artery aneurysm
Aortic or renal artery dissection
Aortic or renal artery angiography
Superimposed on inflammatory disorders
Vasculitis
Thromboangiitis obliterans
Syphilis
Superimposed on structural lesions
Fibromuscular dysplasia
THROMBOEMBOLISM
Atrial fibrillation
Mitral stenosis
Mural thrombus
Atrial myxoma
Prosthetic valve
Septic or aseptic valvular vegetations
Paradoxical emboli
Tumor emboli
Fat emboli
ATHEROEMBOLI (CHOLESTEROL EMBOLIZATION)
Elderly patients with advanced atherosclerosis
Abdominal aortic surgery
Trauma, blunt
Angiographic catheters
Angioplasty or stent placement
Excessive anticoagulation

Diagnosis

The diagnosis of renal artery occlusion is most reliably established by enhanced and unenhanced computed tomography (CT). CT is accurate, can be performed rapidly, and can identify associated traumatic injury. Magnetic resonance angiography (MRA), renal scintigraphy, duplex ultrasound scanning, and intravenous pyelography can also be used as screening tests for the diagnosis of acute arterial thrombosis. If the diagnosis remains unclear, percutaneous arteriography may be necessary for definitive diagnosis. The advantage of conventional arteriography is that the anatomy, even of subsegmental occlusion, can be most reliably established. In embolic renal artery occlusion, the presence of an intracardiac thrombus must be sought by echocardiography. In nontraumatic thrombotic occlusion, work-up for thrombophilia, vasculitides, or progressive atherosclerosis should be considered.

Treatment

Management of acute arterial thrombosis is initiated with control of hypertension, adequate hydration, anticoagulation, and acute renal replacement therapy when needed. Surgical revascularization is considered, especially with bilateral occlusion or occlusion of a solitary kidney. Medical therapy may be considered for unilateral occlusion with a functioning contralateral kidney. Alternative approaches such as intra-arterial thrombolytic therapy, angioplasty, and rheolytic arterial thrombectomy have been reported with success. Iatrogenic occlusion of the renal artery as a result of angiographic manipulations or angioplasty may be treated with intra-arterial stent placement. Obviously, atheroemboli should not be treated by fibrinolysis. Surgery is also the treatment of choice for

traumatic renal artery thrombosis, which is associated with poor salvage of renal function unless surgery is accomplished immediately. The warm ischemia time beyond which recovery of renal function would not be anticipated is no more than several hours.

Prognosis

Mortality is high in these conditions, particularly because of the severity of underlying and associated conditions. The mortality rate of patients undergoing surgical revascularization for complete acute renal artery occlusion is 11 to 25%. Hypertension may develop as a late sequela of renal artery occlusion and may be treated by angiotensin-converting enzyme inhibitors (ACEIs), angiotensin receptor blocker (ARBs), or nondihydropyridine calcium channel blockers or, if refractory, by balloon angioplasty. Chronic renal replacement therapy may be necessary.

Renal Artery Stenosis and Ischemic Renal Disease

Definition

RAS remains an important cause of secondary hypertension, as well as progressive renal insufficiency. In a general population of hypertensive patients, the prevalence of RAS is only 2 to 4%, but in selected populations, estimates rise to 20 to 40%. In a series of patients being evaluated for cardiac or other vascular diseases, rates of 14 to 45% have been observed. Atherosclerotic disease accounts for 90% of cases and FMD for less than 10%.

Epidemiology

Atherosclerotic disease is more common in the elderly and those with typical cardiovascular risk factors. In several large series of patients undergoing cardiac catheterization, independent risk factors identified by multivariate analysis were increased age, extent of coronary disease, presence of congestive heart failure (CHF), female gender, carotid or peripheral vascular disease, kidney dysfunction, and systolic hypertension. In a population-based study of elderly patients in North Carolina, renal duplex sonography was used to identify asymptomatic patients with RAS. The prevalence of disease in a cohort with a preponderance of female patients (67%) was 6.8%, and no difference in prevalence by ethnicity was noted. Older age, male gender, low high-density lipoprotein cholesterol, and high systolic blood pressure were identified as independent risk factors by multivariate analysis.

Pathobiology

FMD, first described in 1938, is an important cause of treatable hypertension in young patients without cardiovascular risk factors and is angiographically distinct from atherosclerotic disease because of the classic "string of beads" appearance. Furthermore, unlike atherosclerotic disease, which localizes at the ostial and proximal segments of the renal arteries, FMD more commonly involves the mid and distal arterial segments. The four distinct histopathologic types include medial fibroplasia (most common), perimedial fibroplasia, medial hyperplasia, and intimal fibroplasia. Although the cause is yet unknown, there appears to be a genetic predisposition to FMD. Additional risks include hormonal effects, smoking, and hypertension.

Clinical Manifestations

Clinical features suggestive of RAS are listed in Table 126–2. Atherosclerotic disease should be suspected in older patients, especially those with evidence of other cardiovascular disease. RAS should also be considered in patients with unexplained CHF or "flash" pulmonary edema. FMD is more commonly seen in women between the ages of 15 and 50, but diagnosis in patients older than 60 years has been reported. FMD has also been associated with Ehlers-Danlos syndrome.

TABLE 126–2 CLINICAL FEATURES OF RENAL ARTERY STENOSIS

Onset of hypertension <30 or >50 years of age
Absence of a family history of hypertension
Short duration or recent worsening of hypertension
Severe hypertension or retinopathy
Resistance to antihypertensive therapy
Signs of other cardiovascular disease
Deterioration of renal function with angiotensin-converting enzyme inhibitor or angiotensin receptor blocker therapy
Abdominal bruit
Unexplained hypokalemia with or without metabolic alkalosis
Unexplained progression of kidney disease or failure
Neurofibromatosis

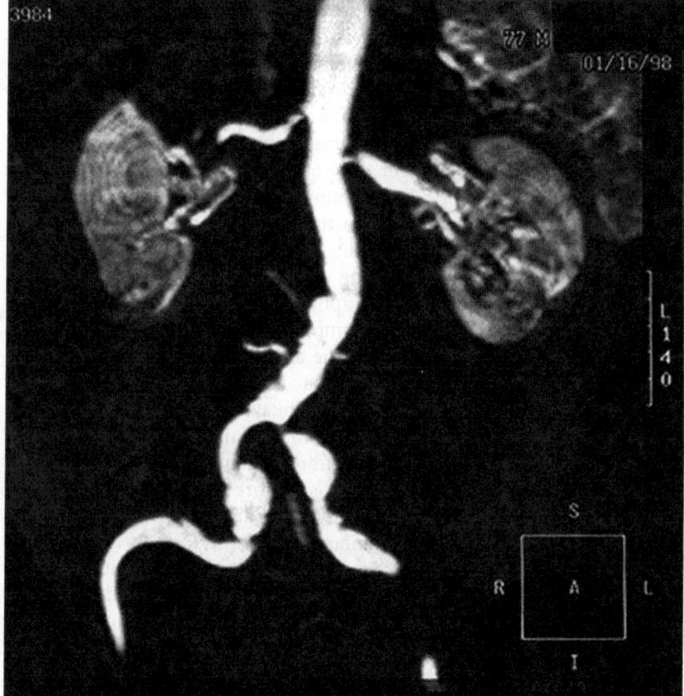

FIGURE 126–1 • Magnetic resonance angiogram of the abdominal aorta showing bilateral renal artery stenosis. Significant iliac stenosis is also demonstrated.

Diagnosis

Although captopril renal scintigraphy has traditionally been the preferred initial noninvasive test for RAS, it has been displaced by other imaging modalities because of reduced sensitivity and specificity in the presence of renal insufficiency, bilateral disease, or disease in a solitary functioning kidney. In a meta-analysis of noninvasive imaging tests, computed tomographic angiography (CTA) and gadolinium-enhanced MRA (Fig. 126–1) were found to have the best diagnostic accuracy, with slightly lower values for unenhanced MRA. These studies were more accurate than ultrasonography or captopril renal scintigraphy. In a separate study that did not include CTA, renal Doppler sonography was found to be more cost-efficient than MRA, albeit less sensitive.

CT is rapid and has good spatial resolution but requires a large contrast load. MRA avoids the need for contrast and can accurately visualize the proximal segment of the renal artery, although motion artifact and spatial resolution limit imaging of the mid and distal segments. Because FMD often affects the mid and distal renal artery, this limitation may reduce diagnostic accuracy. Renal Doppler is the favored noninvasive test for FMD, but it is highly operator dependent. Body habitus and bowel

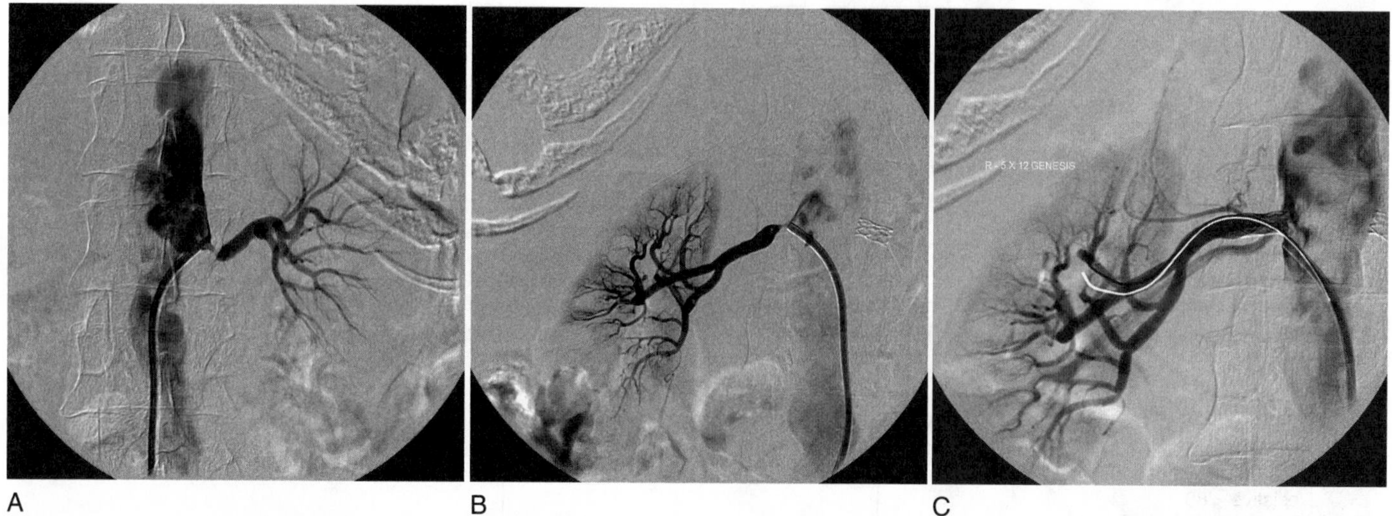

FIGURE 126–2 • Renal angiograms from an elderly patient with heart failure. Cardiac catheterization revealed normal coronary arteries, but after initiation of therapy with an angiotensin-converting enzyme inhibitor and spironolactone, progressive kidney disease with hyperkalemia and poor blood pressure control ensued. Renal Doppler ultrasonography suggested bilateral renal artery stenosis, as confirmed by angiography (**A** and **B**). The patient underwent successful percutaneous revascularization in stages with return to normal left ventricular function and improved blood pressure control (**C**).

gas can also affect image quality, and multiple views such as oblique and flank approaches may be required to visualize the cortical branches. In addition, renal Doppler studies can determine the resistive index. A resistive index less than 80 correlates with a beneficial response to revascularization in patients with atherosclerotic disease. However, others have shown blood pressure improvement and stabilization of renal function even in patients with values higher than 80. When the diagnosis remains unclear or when renal artery revascularization is being considered, digital subtraction renal angiography may be required and is still considered the "gold standard" (Fig. 126–2A and B). Not only is anatomic information acquired, but the translesion gradient can also be measured. Although complication rates are low, the usual risks associated with catheterization should be considered, including access site trauma, contrast reactions, and contrast nephropathy. The risk for contrast nephropathy may be reduced with periprocedural hydration, the administration of acetylcysteine or sodium bicarbonate, and the use of low-osmolar contrast agents. Patients at particularly high risk can be studied by carbon dioxide or gadolinium angiography.

In summary, a reasonable diagnostic approach is to screen with gadolinium-enhanced MRA, especially in patients at risk for contrast nephropathy, or with CTA in patients with implanted metallic devices such as pacemakers or mechanical heart valves. Renal Doppler is favored if FMD is suspected and may be helpful in identifying patients with atherosclerotic disease who would respond to revascularization. Angiography is performed if a definitive diagnosis is required or if renal artery revascularization is planned (Fig. 126–3).

Treatment

Rx

The goals of therapy are to control blood pressure, stabilize renal function, and reduce cardiovascular complications. All patients with atherosclerotic disease should be treated with antiplatelet and cholesterol-lowering agents. Medical therapy for blood pressure control should include ACEIs or ARBs for their proven benefit in renal protection and reduction of cardiovascular mortality. Smoking cessation, weight control, increased exercise, and diabetes control should be universally recommended. The decision for and timing of revascularization, as well as the choice of surgical or percutaneous therapy, remain controversial because of a lack of large-scale randomized trials. A smaller randomized trial of balloon angioplasty versus medical therapy showed no significant difference in blood pressure control at 12 months, although the angioplasty group required fewer medications. This study was criticized for excluding stents in the intervention group and the high crossover (44%) to angioplasty in the medically treated group. There have been several large retrospective studies of both surgical and percutaneous approaches in which improved blood pressure control was observed in 60 to 80%, improved renal function in 25%, and stabilized renal function in 50% of patients. The pervasive limitation has been lack of blood pressure response or deterioration of renal function in up to 25%. Technical success after surgery is high, but mortality rates are 2.3 to 8.6%. Technical success after percutaneous intervention with stent implantation approaches 95 to 100% (see Fig. 126–2C). Complication rates are low and procedural mortality is 0 to 1%. Generally accepted indications for revascularization are (1) hypertension uncontrolled by three or more drugs, sudden acceleration, or association with end-organ damage; (2) unexplained or sudden deterioration in renal function, especially if associated with ACEI or ARB therapy; (3) loss of renal mass or progression of hemodynamically significant RAS while being monitored on adequate medical therapy; and (4) recurrent "flash" pulmonary edema or unstable angina. Relative indications include severe (>75%) bilateral stenosis or stenosis in a solitary kidney, unilateral disease with a low GFR but with split renal function of greater than 10 mL/min, or bilateral disease with a low GFR. The primary treatment of FMD is balloon angioplasty. Stenting is rarely necessary and is reserved for inadequate balloon dilation or flow-limiting dissections. Incidentally discovered FMD without hypertension should be monitored by serial renal duplex ultrasonography and assessment of renal function. In all cases, whether treated medically or after revascularization, close monitoring is required indefinitely.

In summary, medical therapy is recommended for patients with normal renal function and readily controlled hypertension. In selected patients with FMD or atherosclerotic RAS, balloon angioplasty or renal artery stenting has emerged as the treatment of choice. Risk factor modification is essential for reduction of cardiovascular events in patients with atherosclerotic disease.

Prognosis

The progressive nature of atherosclerotic RAS with subsequent decline in renal perfusion has assumed an equal or greater role than the control of hypertension in the justification for renal revascularization. The severity of stenosis is associated with lesion progression. The risk is higher for patients with bilateral disease or disease in a solitary kidney. Stabilization

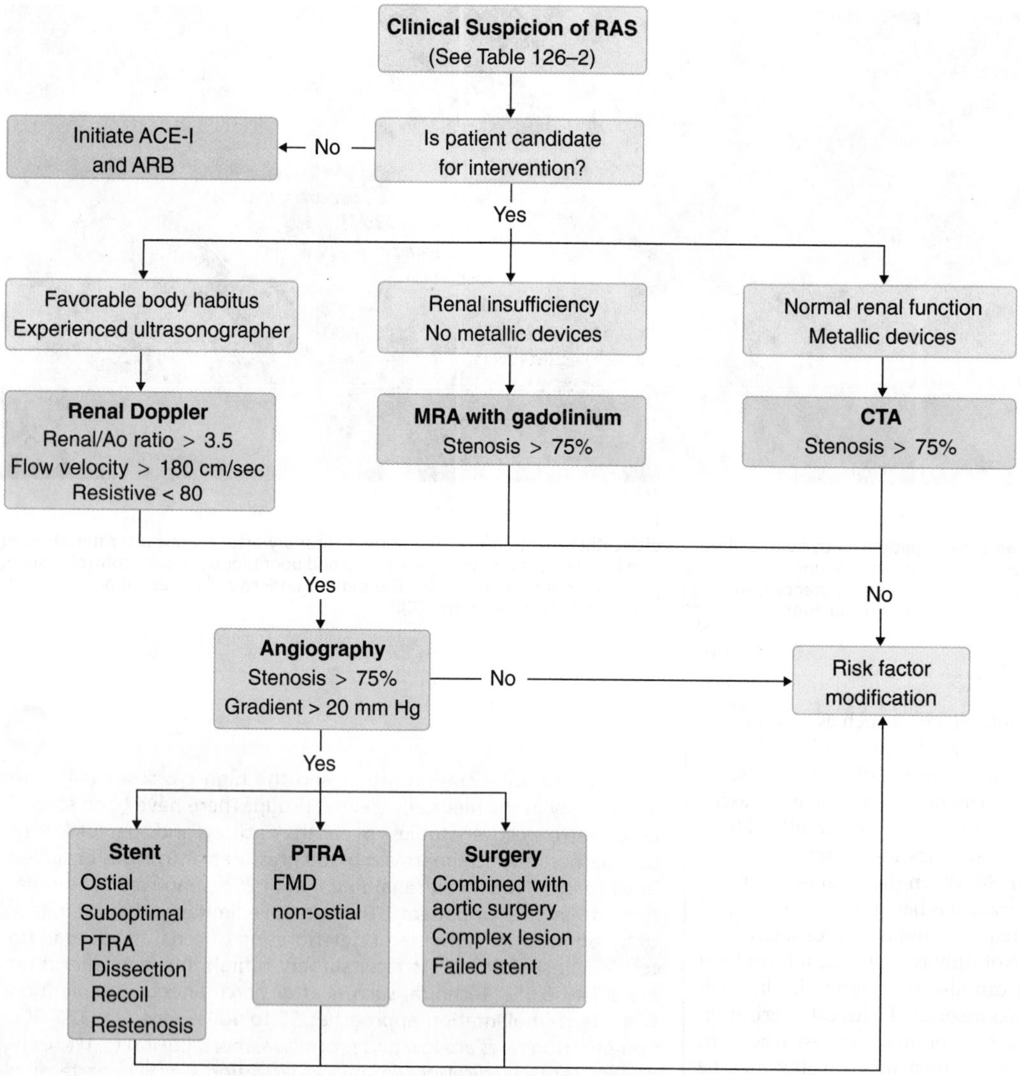

Clinical Suspicion of RAS
(See Table 126–2)

↓

Is patient candidate for intervention? — No → Initiate ACE-I and ARB

Yes ↓

Favorable body habitus
Experienced ultrasonographer
↓
Renal Doppler
Renal/Ao ratio > 3.5
Flow velocity > 180 cm/sec
Resistive < 80

Renal insufficiency
No metallic devices
↓
MRA with gadolinium
Stenosis > 75%

Normal renal function
Metallic devices
↓
CTA
Stenosis > 75%

Yes ↓ / No → Risk factor modification

Angiography
Stenosis > 75%
Gradient > 20 mm Hg
— No → Risk factor modification

Yes ↓

Stent
Ostial
Suboptimal
PTRA
Dissection
Recoil
Restenosis

PTRA
FMD
non-ostial

Surgery
Combined with aortic surgery
Complex lesion
Failed stent

→ Risk factor modification

FIGURE 126–3 • Algorithm for the diagnosis and management of renal artery stenosis. ACE-I = angiotensin-converting enzyme inhibitor; ARB = angiotensin receptor blocker; CTA = computed tomographic angiography; FMD = fibromuscular dysplasia; MRA = magnetic resonance angiography; PTRA = percutaneous transluminal renal angioplasty; RAS = renal artery stenosis.

of renal function and improvement of blood pressure control are similar for patients undergoing surgical or percutaneous revascularization. Reversal of dependence on dialysis has been reported with both surgery and stenting. The long-term durability of angioplasty has improved with stenting, and restenosis rates of 14 to 25% are reported. Favorable response to revascularization has been associated with a resistive index less than 80, recent deterioration in renal function, elevated baseline brain natriuretic peptide (BNP), or a postprocedure drop in BNP levels. Patients with mild to moderate baseline renal insufficiency are more likely to achieve stabilization of renal function. Although those with severe renal dysfunction have a higher risk of progression to end-stage renal disease (ESRD), stabilization has been seen in more than half of these patients. Cardiovascular disease remains the leading cause of death in patients with atherosclerotic RAS. When adjusted for baseline variables, RAS remains an independent predictor of mortality. Factors associated with higher mortality include elevated baseline creatinine, more severe RAS, worsening renal function after revascularization, older age, diabetes, other cardiovascular disease, and CHF. Conversely, improvement of blood pressure control or renal function after revascularization has been associated with improved survival. Patients with FMD respond well to balloon angioplasty, and stenting is rarely needed. Technical success is high, with low restenosis rates. Hypertension is cured in approximately 44% of patients with FMD, and younger age, milder hypertension, and shorter duration of hypertension are associated with successful outcomes. Progression to ESRD or renal artery occlusion is rare.

ARTERIOLES AND MICROVASCULATURE

Atheroembolic Disease of the Renal Arteries

Definition

Embolization of cholesterol crystals as a cause of renal artery occlusion occurs almost exclusively in elderly patients with widespread atherosclerosis. Atheroemboli may also occur as a complication of abdominal aorta or renal artery manipulation or surgery or as a consequence of angiography or transluminal angioplasty, in which atheroemboli may be mistaken for contrast-induced nephropathy. Atheroemboli can also be associated with anticoagulant or thrombolytic therapy and may be accompanied by the finding of a cyanotic toe on physical examination. This entity may be overlooked because patients at risk for this complication often have other chronic illnesses associated with renal failure, hypertension, and atherosclerosis.

Clinical Manifestations

Renal insufficiency, hypertension, or both disorders occur regularly with atheroembolization involving the renal vasculature. Evidence of cholesterol embolization in the retina, muscles, or skin (associated with livedo reticularis) can be helpful and may obviate the need for renal biopsy. Evidence of embolization to other organs resulting in cerebrovascular events, acute pancreatitis, ischemic bowel, and gangrene of the extremities may be noted. Urinalysis may not be helpful because cholesterol crystals are not usually present, but mild proteinuria, eosinophiluria, and increased cellularity are more often observed.

Treatment

Therapy for this disorder is often disappointing inasmuch as cholesterol embolization leads to structural changes in the microvasculature without inflammation. Anticoagulants have not proved to be of value and may delay healing of ulcerating atherosclerotic lesions. Dialysis, treatment of hypertension with attention to avoiding hypotension, and adequate hydration are the mainstays of treatment.

Prognosis

With adequate blood pressure control for several months or years, renal function may recover sufficiently, even in patients requiring chronic renal replacement therapy, to allow nondialytic conservative management.

Hypertensive Arteriolar Nephrosclerosis

Definition

Although autoregulation of renal blood flow and GFR occurs throughout a wide range of systemic blood pressure, the renal vasculature is exquisitely sensitive to damage incurred by systemic hypertension when it is transmitted to the glomerular capillary bed (Chapter 116). Unopposed or sustained increases in glomerular capillary hydrostatic pressure eventually result in sclerosis. In *benign nephrosclerosis,* the kidney is the victim of the adverse effects of chronic hypertension over a prolonged period and does not appear to participate in the pathogenesis of the disorder. The vascular injury in the kidney is nonspecific, but more pronounced than the vascular changes observed systemically. When advanced, such changes can result in ESRD. In *malignant* or *accelerated hypertension,* the vascular changes are unique and severe and lead to renal ischemia, renin production, and exacerbation of the disease, which may terminate in acute renal failure and, if not treated successfully, ESRD. In contrast to benign nephrosclerosis, in which the principal lesion is in the media of the vessels, a unique lesion of the intima characterizes malignant or accelerated hypertension. Renal vascular lesions similar to those seen in malignant hypertension are also observed in scleroderma, thrombotic microangiopathy, and renal transplant rejection.

Epidemiology

The availability of effective antihypertensive medication has sharply reduced the occurrence of this devastating disorder. However, both benign and malignant hypertensive renal disease and the sequelae of these disorders appear to be more prevalent in blacks.

Clinical Manifestations

Patients with benign hypertensive nephrosclerosis have been hypertensive for more than 10 to 15 years. Kidney size is usually reduced, and the urine sediment is unremarkable except for proteinuria, which is generally less than 1.5 g/day. The sudden development of malignant or accelerated hypertension, either in patients with previously established mild to moderate hypertension or in those in whom hypertension had not previously been diagnosed, is manifested by an abrupt increase in blood pressure (diastolic usually greater than 130 mm Hg). Papilledema may develop, and renal function may decline rapidly. The kidneys may be enlarged, or the urinary sediment may be active, with gross or microscopic hematuria, and proteinuria is often in the nephrotic range. Microangiopathic hemolytic anemia may be present. Abnormalities in the central nervous system are usually evident and range from headaches to generalized seizures to coma. Malignant hypertension may coexist with cerebral vascular accidents.

Treatment

Rx

For either benign or malignant hypertension, the primary goal is to control blood pressure to 130/80 or less. In benign hypertensive nephrosclerosis, the renal outcome is dependent on timely initiation of effective therapy, patient compliance, and careful follow-up by a physician. Inadequate treatment may result in irreversible glomerular sclerosis, as well as end-organ damage in the cardiovascular and central nervous systems. Antihypertensives that provide renal protection include ACEIs and ARBs. Nondihydropyridine calcium channel blockers do not afford protection from progression of renal insufficiency and should be used only in patients who cannot tolerate ACEI or ARB therapy. Malignant hypertension, by contrast, is a medical emergency and must be approached aggressively. Controlling the blood pressure can reverse the major manifestations in most patients, including the renal functional impairment. Parenteral antihypertensives, such as nitroprusside infused in the critical care setting, may be necessary initially. Blood pressure should be controlled smoothly and gradually but be in the normal range by 36 to 48 hours. Antihypertensive medications should be continued even if renal function continues to deteriorate and renal replacement therapy is required. Some patients experience partial reversal of vascular lesions and return of renal function to levels compatible with nondialytic, conservative management.

Prognosis

With skillful selection of renal-specific antihypertensive agents (ACEI and ARB therapy) and obsessive control of blood pressure over a period of many years (target of 130/80 or less as tolerated), progression of renal disease can usually be avoided. Hypertension with nephrosclerosis is the second most common cause of ESRD in the United States. The importance of early recognition and aggressive treatment cannot be overemphasized.

Hemolytic-Uremic Syndrome and Thrombotic Thrombocytopenic Purpura

Definition

Renal failure is a common consequence of both hemolytic-uremic syndrome (HUS) and thrombotic thrombocytopenic purpura (TTP). For additional information, see Chapters 122 and 181. These conditions are characterized by platelet and fibrin thrombi within the renal microvasculature, accompanied by thrombocytopenia and microangiopathic hemolytic anemia. Although the vascular lesions are identical, central venous system involvement predominates in TTP, whereas renal involvement is predominant in HUS. Sporadic cases and outbreaks have been reported after exposure to *Escherichia coli* serotype O157 : H7, which produces a Shiga-like cytotoxin. HUS/TTP has also been associated with other bacteria and viruses, and drug-induced cases have been reported.

Clinical Manifestations

TTP is suggested by the co-occurrence of hemolysis, thrombocytopenia, fever, purpura, and alternating mental status changes. HUS may be associated with acute renal failure, thrombocytopenia, and microangiopathic hemolytic anemia, most commonly in children after an acute diarrheal illness. Either disorder may be observed in the setting of cancer and infection and while administering chemotherapeutic agents.

Treatment

Acute implementation of renal replacement therapy has significantly improved survival. For TTP, plasma exchange combined with antiplatelet therapy is recommended and may be required for 1 to 2 weeks. The oliguria and degree of renal failure, as well as the severity of hypertension, are more pronounced in HUS. Early diagnosis, initiation of dialysis, antihypertensives, supportive transfusions, and control of seizures are essential for a good outcome. Up to 85% of children with typical HUS recover with supportive care.

Scleroderma

Clinical Manifestations

The clinical features and progression of scleroderma are highly variable, but mild proteinuria without loss of renal function or evidence of glomerular disease is the most common sign of renal disease in this disorder (see also Chapter 288). Although it is widely appreciated that the mortality associated with scleroderma increases as a function of the number of organ systems involved, significant renal involvement (which has been reported in 50% of patients with systemic sclerosis of 20 or more years' duration) is the most dreaded complication and has the poorest prognosis. A renal crisis may be associated with the use of corticosteroids and can be precipitated in situations that compromise renal blood flow (e.g., dehydration). When the kidneys are involved, the typical manifestation is intimal proliferation, medial thinning, and increased collagen deposition in the adventitial layer of small renal arteries. An increase in vasomotor tone at the level of the renal vasculature is probably a renal manifestation of Raynaud's phenomenon and contributes to the reduction in renal blood flow, hypertension, and progressive impairment in renal function. The increase in renin and angiotensin II elaboration contributes to the development of worsening hypertension and hypertensive nephrosclerosis. Once azotemia develops, hypertension may become more difficult to manage, and dialysis is required within 1 to 2 years. Conversely, patients may initially come to medical attention with a "renal crisis" manifested by the abrupt onset of malignant hypertension and renal failure and commonly associated with heart failure and microangiopathic hemolytic anemia. This manifestation is seen in approximately 2.8% of all patients with scleroderma but in 14 to 18% of those with diffuse cutaneous disease.

Treatment

Rx

Therapy in patients with scleroderma and renal involvement should be directed primarily toward controlling hypertension in an attempt to slow progression of the renal failure. Joint management by a nephrologist and rheumatologist is highly recommended. Adequate control may require several drugs in combination, such as ACEIs or angiotensin II receptor antagonists, nondihydropyridine calcium channel blockers, vasodilators (such as minoxidil), and other agents. Renal crisis is a medical emergency requiring aggressive antihypertensive therapy. Intravenous antihypertensive therapy may be indicated in the critical care setting because of the high mortality without therapy. Successful therapy requires early detection and rapid, aggressive intervention to control hypertension with ACEIs. When accomplished, progression to ESRD may be slowed significantly. Nevertheless, some patients continue to follow a progressive course despite blood pressure control. Additionally, patients who are initially found to have a serum creatinine level of 3.0 mg/dL or greater have a poorer prognosis. In the event that long-term maintenance dialysis is required, there is evidence that with continued aggressive management of hypertension, a small but significant percentage of patients will regain sufficient renal function to allow cessation of renal replacement therapy.

Sickle Cell Nephropathy

Pathobiology

The hypoxemic and hypertonic environment of the renal medulla (vasa recta) encourages the sickling of red blood cells circulating through this region (Chapter 167). When sickle hemoglobin desaturates, polymerization of hemoglobin can impair or interrupt capillary flow. The major manifestations of sickle cell nephropathy can all be explained by the development of papillary infarction.

Clinical Manifestations

A defect in urinary concentration resulting in a tendency toward volume depletion is one of the best-characterized abnormalities in sickle cell nephropathy. Obliteration of the vasa recta compromises operation of the medullary countercurrent system and impairs the ability to generate and maintain medullary solute gradients. The concentrating defect is also observed in sickle trait. A defect in urinary acidification is common and is manifested as distal renal tubular acidosis with hyperkalemia and hyperchloremic metabolic acidosis (type 4 renal tubular acidosis). The acidification defect is not usually observed in patients with sickle trait. Painless gross hematuria has been estimated to occur in up to 50% of patients with sickle cell nephropathy. It also occurs in patients with sickle cell anemia or haemoglobin SC disease. With recurrent papillary infarction, papillary necrosis can occur and progress. Sickle cell "crisis," dehydration, hypoxemia, and the use of nonsteroidal anti-inflammatory drugs predispose to papillary necrosis. Renal papillary necrosis is often "silent," but it may progress to chronic renal insufficiency and predispose the patient to repeated urinary tract infections. Nephrotic syndrome may develop in approximately 4% of patients with sickle glomerulopathy. Microscopic hematuria occurs in most patients with sickle cell anemia, and gross hematuria may be severe in some patients. Findings on renal biopsy usually indicate membranoproliferative glomerulopathy with segmental and global sclerosis. As this disorder progresses, glomerulopathy results in sclerosis and progressive loss of glomerular function. In contrast, papillary infarction can result in persistent hematuria.

Treatment

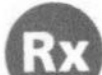

Volume depletion should be corrected by intravenous administration of isotonic or hypotonic saline, as dictated by the serum sodium concentration. Hyperkalemia may require potassium exchange resin (sodium polystyrene [Kayexalate]) per rectum or orally. When acidosis accompanies the hyperkalemia, alkali may help correct the hyperkalemia and the acidosis. Long-term administration of Shohl solution or sodium bicarbonate tablets may be necessary, and loop diuretics may be helpful. Potassium-sparing diuretics, nonsteroidal anti-inflammatory drugs, or potassium supplements should be strictly avoided. Attempts to increase medullary blood flow and reduce medullary tonicity, including the use of distilled water, sodium bicarbonate, and diuretics such as mannitol or loop diuretics, may alleviate the hematuria. Rarely, small doses of ε-aminocaproic acid may be necessary for life-threatening hematuria but can result in thrombosis or ureteral obstruction.

RENAL VEINS

Renal Vein Thrombosis

Definition

Unilateral or bilateral thrombosis of the major renal veins or their segments is a common, but often subtle disorder that may develop in a variety of conditions. The serious risk for thromboembolic complications and vascular occlusion underscores the need for accurate and timely diagnosis and therapy.

Pathobiology

The disparate causes of renal vein thrombosis are outlined in Table 126–3. The reported incidence of renal vein thrombosis in patients with

TABLE 126–3 CAUSES OF RENAL VEIN THROMBOSIS

Nephrotic syndrome
Renal cell carcinoma with renal vein invasion
Pregnancy or estrogen therapy
Volume depletion (especially in infants)
Extrinsic compression (lymph nodes, tumor, retroperitoneal fibrosis, aortic aneurysm)
Corticosteroids

nephrotic syndrome is striking and ranges from 5 to 62%. Although some series emphasize a stronger association with membranous nephropathy, a prospective study of 26 patients with nephrotic syndrome demonstrated an association of renal vein thrombosis with a variety of glomerulopathies, including membranoproliferative, membranous, and proliferative glomerulonephritis and focal glomerular sclerosis. Renal vein thrombosis has also been reported in patients with sickle cell nephropathy, amyloidosis, diabetic nephropathy, renal vasculitis, and lupus nephritis, as well as allograft rejection. Predisposing factors include abnormalities in coagulation or fibrinolysis, and attention has focused on components of clotting parameters in the blood or urine of patients with nephrotic syndrome. Antithrombin III levels are depressed as a result of loss of antithrombin III in the urine of nephrotic patients, and an association between low antithrombin III levels and renal vein thrombosis has been reported in some but not all studies. Circulating levels of proteins S and C may also be altered in nephrotic syndrome and contribute to the tendency toward thromboembolic complications. Renal vein thrombosis in infancy usually occurs in the setting of severe volume depletion and impaired renal blood flow. Extrinsic compression from retroperitoneal sources such as lymph nodes, retroperitoneal fibrosis, abscess, aortic aneurysm, or tumor may lead to renal vein thrombosis as a result of sluggish renal venous flow. Acute pancreatitis, trauma, and retroperitoneal surgery may also predispose to renal vein thrombosis. Renal cell carcinoma characteristically invades the renal vein and compromises venous flow, thereby resulting in renal vein thrombosis. There is also an association of renal vein thrombosis with steroid use, but the mechanism is unknown.

Clinical Manifestations

The manifestations of renal vein thrombosis depend on the extent and rapidity of the development of renal venous occlusion. Patients with acute renal vein thrombosis may have nausea, vomiting, flank pain, leukocytosis, hematuria, compromised renal function, and an increase in renal size. Adult nephrotic patients with chronic renal vein thrombosis may have more subtle findings, such as a dramatic increase in proteinuria or evidence of tubule dysfunction, including glycosuria, aminoaciduria, phosphaturia, and impaired urinary acidification.

Diagnosis

Supportive data may be provided by noninvasive studies such as MRA. Doppler ultrasonography is not adequately sensitive for segmental thrombosis. The diagnosis is established by selective renal venography. Evidence of parenchymal edema, stretching of calyces, and notching of the ureters on intravenous pyelography is much less reliable.

Treatment

Rx

The most widely accepted form of therapy for both acute and chronic renal vein thrombosis is anticoagulation with heparin, which can be converted to oral warfarin (Coumadin) after 7 to 10 days and maintained long-term. Therapy is usually continued for at least 1 year. In patients with recurrence or continued risk factors, anticoagulation might be continued indefinitely. In a pediatric patient with volume depletion and acute renal vein thrombosis, attention to restoration of fluid and electrolyte balance is essential. Fibrinolytic therapy might be considered in patients with acute renal vein thrombosis associated with acute renal failure.

SUGGESTED READINGS

Balk E, Raman G, Chung M, et al: Effectiveness of management strategies for renal artery stenosis: A systematic review. Ann Intern Med 2006;145:901–912. *Evidence suggests no large differences in mortality rates or kidney-related outcomes but better blood pressure outcomes with angioplasty, particularly in patients with bilateral disease.*

Garovic VD, Textor SC: Renovascular hypertension and ischemic nephropathy. Circulation 2005;112:1362–1374. *The most current and comprehensive review on this topic. Provides an inclusive evaluation of the available literature on diagnosis and treatment and a very complete bibliography.*

Silva JA, Chan AW, White CJ, et al: Elevated brain natriuretic peptide predicts blood pressure response after stent revascularization in patients with renal artery stenosis. Circulation 2005;111:328–333. *Interesting observation that an elevated baseline BNP or a greater than 30% drop from baseline after renal artery stenting predicts good blood pressure response.*

Slovut DP, Olin JW: Fibromuscular dysplasia. N Engl J Med 2004;350:1862–1871. *The most current and comprehensive review on FMD. Provides an evaluation of the available literature on diagnosis with a complete bibliography.*

White CJ: Catheter-based therapy for atherosclerotic renal artery stenosis. Circulation 2006;113:1464–1473. *A clinical overview.*

Zalunardo N, Tuttle KR: Atherosclerotic renal artery stenosis: Current status and future directions. Curr Opin Nephrol Hypertens 2004;13:613–621. *Excellent review with cogent recommendations for work-up and management.*

127 NEPHROLITHIASIS

Gary C. Curhan

Definition

A kidney stone is a crystalline mass formed in the kidney that is of sufficient size to be clinically detectable, either by symptoms or imaging. Although stones may also form in other parts of the urinary tract, this chapter focuses on stones that originate in the kidney (but may subsequently move distally to other locations in the urinary tract).

There are many different types of kidney stones, and the composition of the stone determines the clinical evaluation, treatment, and prognosis. The most common component is calcium oxalate; other types are calcium phosphate, uric acid, struvite, and cystine stones (Fig. 127–1). Infrequently, stones may be composed of medications, including acyclovir, indinavir, and triamterene.

Epidemiology

The prevalence of a history of kidney stone disease is increasing in both men and women and in whites and blacks. The lifetime risk of stone formation in the United States is approximately 12% in men and 6% in women. The risk in blacks is one fourth that of whites.

Among men who have never had a stone, the incidence is 3 to 4 cases per 1000 men per year between the ages of 30 and 60 and then slowly declines with age. For women, the incidence is 2 cases per 1000 women per year between the ages of 20 and 30 and then declines to approximately 1 per 1000 women per year for the next 4 decades.

The risk of recurrent stone formation in untreated patients after the first stone remains uncertain. Earlier studies reported stone recurrence rates ranging from 30 to 50% at 5 years. However, control groups in recent randomized controlled trials of incident calcium oxalate stone-formers experienced substantially lower rates of first recurrence (2 to 5 per 100 person years). Unfortunately, no information on sex-specific rates is available from these trials.

Physician office visits for nephrolithiasis increased from 950,000 visits in 1992 to 1,825,000 in 2000—nearly twofold. Despite the increase in visits, the estimated health costs for nephrolithiasis have remained stable at approximately $2 billion per year, in part because of the shift from inpatient to outpatient procedures.

Risk Factors

A variety of influences affect the likelihood of stone formation, including dietary, urinary, and genetic factors, as well as certain medical conditions. It is important to recognize that it is the concentrations, not just the total amounts of relevant urinary factors, that are the key determinants of stone formation. The importance of concentration emphasizes the importance of fluid intake and thereby urinary volume. However, stone formation cannot be perfectly predicted by urinary composition.

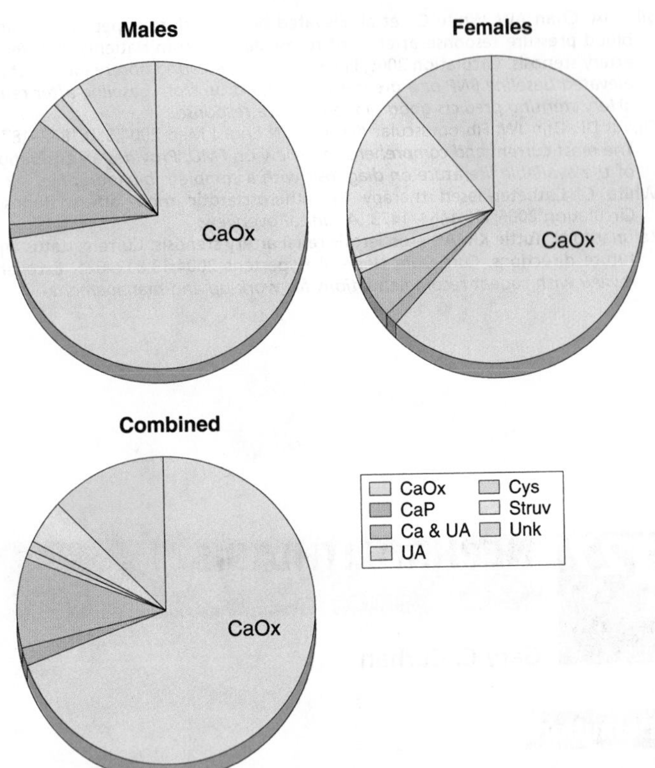

FIGURE 127–1 • Types of stones and frequency in adults. Ca & UA = calcium and uric acid; CaOx = calcium oxalate; CaP = calcium phosphate; Cys = cystine; Struv = struvite; UA = uric acid; Unk = unknown. (From Coe F, Parks J [eds]: Nephrolithiasis: Pathogenesis and Treatment. Chicago, Year Book, 1988. Reprinted in Greenberg A, Cheung AK: Primer on Kidney Diseases. Philadelphia, Elsevier, 2005.)

Therefore, it is important to focus on studies that include actual stone formation rather than changes in the lithogenic composition of the urine.

Dietary Factors

Nutrients

Attention has focused on the role of dietary factors in calcium oxalate stone formation because of rising incidence rates and the recognized impact on urinary composition. Based on physiologic principles and published studies, several dietary factors appear to increase the risk for nephrolithiasis, including animal protein, oxalate, sodium, sucrose, and vitamin C. Higher intake of calcium and increased potassium consumption reduce the risk.

The impact of calcium intake on the risk for stone formation has been clarified over the past decade. A number of prospective studies and a randomized trial [1] found that *lower* calcium intake was associated with an *increased* risk for stone formation. Although the mechanism of this effect is unknown, low calcium intake is known to increase oxalate absorption and urinary excretion. It is also possible that other factors in dairy products, the major source of dietary calcium, may reduce the risk for stone formation.

Several other nutrients may be important in the development of stone formation. Higher animal protein intake may raise urine calcium and uric acid excretion and decrease urinary citrate, thereby increasing the risk for stone formation. Higher sodium or sucrose intake increases urine calcium excretion, and potassium supplementation decreases calcium excretion. In prospective studies, an increased risk for stone formation was observed with higher intake of animal protein only in men and a decreased risk with higher potassium intake in men and women. In women, sucrose was associated with an increased risk. Recently, phytate was also found to reduce the likelihood of stone formation in younger women substantially. These studies suggest that risk factors may vary by age and gender.

There have been few randomized controlled trials of dietary interventions. Notably, in a randomized trial in men with hypercalciuria and recurrent calcium oxalate stones, a low-calcium diet (400 mg/day) was compared with a diet containing 1200 mg of calcium along with low sodium and low animal protein intake. [1] Men assigned to the higher–calcium intake group were less likely to experience stone recurrence.

Although calcium oxalate is the most common stone, insufficient information is available on the role of dietary oxalate, in part because of the lack of complete and reliable information on the oxalate content of many foods. In addition, other contributors to oxalate formation (endogenous generation and metabolism of ingested protein) remain incompletely described.

Fluid Intake

Fluid intake is the primary determinant of urine volume. Daily urine volume is a crucial factor in stone formation, with the risk increasing as urine volume falls, particularly when urine output is less than 1 L/day. The important protective role of fluid intake has been demonstrated in observational studies and a randomized controlled trial. [2] The role of specific beverages is discussed later.

TABLE 127–1 SYSTEMIC DISORDERS ASSOCIATED WITH A HIGHER RISK FOR STONE FORMATION

Crohn's disease
Primary hyperparathyroidism
Gout
Diabetes mellitus
Obesity
Gastric bypass procedure
Renal tubular acidosis

Nondietary Factors

Family History

Individuals with a family history of stone disease have a twofold higher risk of becoming stoneformers. Several rare monogenic causes of nephrolithiasis have been identified, including Dent's disease and cystinuria. Studies of specific genes involved in calcium metabolism, such as the calcium-sensing receptor and the vitamin D receptor, have been unrevealing in humans. It seems clear that the clinically common cases of stone formation are due to polygenic inheritance with substantial environmental influence.

Systemic Conditions

Systemic conditions that increase the risk for formation of calcium-containing stones include primary hyperparathyroidism and renal tubular acidosis (Table 127–1). Primary hyperparathyroidism may be found in 5% of stone formers. In addition, obesity, gout, and diabetes mellitus have been independently associated with a risk for stone formation. The increasing prevalence of obesity may be an important contributor to the rising prevalence of nephrolithiasis.

Pathobiology

Pathogenesis

Supersaturation

Stone formation is the result of a complex physicochemical process leading to crystallization. Although normal individuals can have crystalluria and not actual stones, the presence of crystalluria substantially increases the likelihood of stone formation.

Most stones do not contain one single crystal type but rather are a mixture with one or two types that predominate. Furthermore, kidney stones also contain an organic material upon which the mineral is deposited. The predominant matrix component is protein.

Formation of crystals in urine is largely a function of supersaturation. A solution that contains any material at a concentration above that material's solubility is said to be supersaturated with respect to that material.

Several modifiable factors, other than the specific lithogenic factors (e.g., calcium, oxalate, uric acid), influence supersaturation, including pH, volume, and inhibitors. Uric acid and calcium phosphate crystallization is strongly influenced by urinary pH, but there is little effect on calcium oxalate. Calcium oxalate supersaturation is dependent on urinary volume; increasing daily urine volume to greater than 2 L is of practical benefit in reducing the supersaturation and incidence of stones.

Increasing urine volume is also beneficial in preventing other types of stones.

The urine of most individuals is supersaturated with respect to calcium oxalate, calcium phosphate, and other substances. The remarkable ability of urine to inhibit crystallization prevents the majority of the population from continuously forming stones. The compounds that stabilize and prevent crystallization within the tubules and the urinary tract are incompletely characterized but include citrate and urinary proteins.

Several recent studies suggest that we may need to change our thinking about the initial steps in the process of stone formation. Rather than the traditional belief that the initial events are intratubular crystal formation followed by crystal attachment and stone growth, new evidence suggests that the initial crystal forms in the *medullary interstitium* and is composed of calcium phosphate. The calcium phosphate crystals then erode through the papilla (the classic Randall's plaque) and act as a nidus for calcium oxalate deposition.

Urinary Factors

Twenty-four-hour urine composition provides important prognostic information and directs recommendations for stone prevention. Traditionally, patients have been categorized into "normal" and "abnormal" with respect to the amount of lithogenic substances excreted. However, there is growing appreciation of two important points. First, the measured values for the urinary factors are continuous variables, so dichotomization into "normal" and "abnormal" is somewhat artificial and potentially misleading. Second, stone formation is a disease of *concentration,* not just absolute amounts. Although a patient may have a "normal" amount of calcium in urine, if the volume is low, the concentration of calcium would be abnormally high. Even though terms such as "hypercalciuria" are used in this chapter, these limitations should be remembered.

Hypercalciuria

The common definition of hypercalciuria is urine calcium excretion greater than 300 mg/day in men, 250 mg/day in women, or 4 mg/kg/day on a 1000-mg/day calcium diet. With this definition, approximately 20 to 40% of patients with calcium stone disease will have hypercalciuria. The limitations of this widely used definition deserve discussion. First, it is unclear why the cut point for men is higher than that for women. This is reasonable from a calcium balance perspective, but not for stone formation, because urine volumes in men and women are similar, so the concentrations would be higher in men. Second, a definition based on weight is problematic. For example, if an individual gains 20 kg in weight, the amount of calcium that that person would be "allowed" to excrete would increase by 80 mg. This is difficult to justify from the perspective of stone formation.

Some investigators have proposed subtyping patients with hypercalciuria. The most widely discussed classification divides patients into those with *absorptive* hypercalciuria, *resorptive* hypercalciuria, or *renal* hypercalciuria. Most clinicians do not subtype, however, because a substantial proportion of patients do not fit into one category, an individual's classification may change over time, most of these patients have low bone mineral density (even those classified as absorptive), and subtyping is unlikely to affect therapy.

Hyperoxaluria

Hyperoxaluria is defined as urinary oxalate excretion greater than 45 mg/day. Elevated urinary oxalate excretion may be present in up to 40% of male and 10% of female stoneformers. However, hyperoxaluria is also frequently found in individuals who do not have a history of stone disease.

Hyperuricosuria

The increased frequency of stone disease in persons with gout, as well as a double-blind trial B showing that allopurinol successfully decreased recurrence rates of calcium stones in patients with hyperuricosuria (greater than 800 mg/day in men or 750 mg/day in women), suggests a causative role. However, the mechanism by which uric acid may promote calcium oxalate stone formation remains uncertain.

Hypocitraturia

Citrate inhibits crystal growth and aggregation. Individuals with hypocitraturia (<320 mg/day for men and women) are at increased risk for stone formation. It is unclear whether increasing urinary citrate above the normal range provides additional protection. Although some of the factors that govern citrate in normal individuals are known, they do not completely account for the higher renal tubular reabsorption of citrate that is present in idiopathic calcium stone formers with hypocitraturia.

Formation of Non–Calcium-Containing Stones

Uric Acid Stones

Although uric acid excretion is important, the major determinant of uric acid supersaturation and subsequent uric acid stone formation is urinary pH. The mainstay of treatment is increasing urine pH. Dietary modification should focus on decreasing acid production and increasing alkali-rich foods. If dietary modification is unsuccessful, alkalinization with oral bicarbonate or a bicarbonate precursor (citrate) should be started. The pH goal is 6 to 7 throughout the day and night. Multiple daily doses of alkali, to match the endogenous acid production of approximately 1 mEq/kg/24 hr, are typically needed. However, a urine pH greater than 7 should be avoided to minimize the likelihood of inducing calcium phosphate crystallization. Allopurinol (100 to 300 mg/day) should be prescribed for patients in whom alkalinization fails.

Struvite Stones

Struvite stones, also known as infection or triple-phosphate stones, form only when the upper urinary tract is infected with urease-producing bacteria such as *Proteus mirabilis, Klebsiella pneumoniae,* or *Providencia* species. Hydrolysis of urea by urease results in a supraphysiologic urine pH higher than 8.0 and the formation of struvite ($MgNH_4PO_4$-H_2O). If the infection is inadequately treated, struvite stones may grow quickly, fill the renal collecting system, and result in a staghorn calculus.

Struvite stones require urologic intervention to ensure complete removal. The recommended approach is a combination of percutaneous nephrolithotomy and extracorporeal shock wave lithotripsy (ESWL). Prolonged use of antibiotics alone may slow stone growth but rarely eradicates the infection. Although the medication acetohydroxamic acid inhibits bacterial urease, it is rarely used because of frequent and serious side effects.

Cystine Stones

Cystine stones form in individuals with an uncommon autosomal recessive disorder of defective proximal renal tubular reabsorption of filtered dibasic amino acids. Cystine is clinically significant because of its poor solubility in urine. Normal cystine excretion is less than 18 mg/day, heterozygotes may excrete up to 100 mg/day, and homozygotes may excrete more than 1 g/day. Cystine solubility is about 250 mg/L; thus, heterozygotes do not typically form cystine stones. Cystine stones are visible on plain radiographs and will often be manifested as staghorn calculi or multiple bilateral stones.

The total amount of cystine excreted cannot be easily modified, so treatment is directed at decreasing the urinary cystine concentration below the limit of solubility. Increasing urinary volume is the first approach. However, some patients would need to produce more than 4 L of urine per day, which is impractical. Increasing urine pH above 7.5 will slightly increase cystine solubility, but this pH is often difficult to maintain in the long term. Tiopronin or D-penicillamine will bind cystine and reduce urine supersaturation; however, side effects are common.

Clinical Manifestations

A kidney stone takes weeks to months (and often much longer) to grow to a clinically detectable size. Although stone passage is a dramatic event, stone formation and growth are typically clinically silent. A stone can remain asymptomatic in the kidney for years or even decades. Signs (e.g., hematuria) and symptoms may not become apparent until years after the stone has formed. Thus, it is important to remember that onset of symptoms, typically attributable to a stone moving into the ureter, does not provide insight into when the stone actually formed. The precipitants of stone movement are unknown.

Acute Renal Colic

When a stone moves from the renal pelvis into the ureter, there is typically a sudden onset of unilateral flank pain of sufficient severity that the individual seeks medical attention, often at an emergency department. Although the term "colic" is used, the pain does not completely remit but rather waxes and wanes. The pain, which is often accompanied by nausea and occasionally vomiting, may radiate to different spots, depending on the location of the stone. If the stone lodges in the upper part of the ureter, pain may radiate anteriorly; if the stone is in the lower part of the ureter, pain can radiate to the ipsilateral testicle in men or the ipsilateral labium in women; and if lodged at the ureterovesical junction, the major symptoms may be urinary frequency and urgency. Occasionally, a patient will have gross hematuria without pain.

Diagnosis

Physical examination alone will rarely make the diagnosis, but it may uncover clues to guide the evaluation. The patient will typically be in obvious pain and cannot find a comfortable position. There may be ipsilateral costovertebral tenderness; if there is obstruction with infection, signs of sepsis may be found. In rare cases, the examination may reveal findings of systemic conditions associated with stone formation, but this will rarely be diagnostic for stone disease.

As with the physical examination, laboratory evaluation is rarely diagnostic. Serum chemistry findings are typically normal, but there may be an elevated white blood cell count. Urinalysis should always be performed on fresh urine and will classically reveal red and white blood cells and occasionally crystals. The absence of hematuria does not exclude the diagnosis because if the ureter is completed obstructed, no urine will be flowing from that side into the bladder.

Along with the history, the diagnosis will be made by an appropriate imaging study (Fig. 127–2). The imaging modality of choice is helical computed tomography (CT) because of its high sensitivity, ability to visualize uric acid stones (traditionally considered "radiolucent"), and no need for radiocontrast. Helical CT detects stones as small as 1 mm, thus identifying small stones that may be missed by intravenous urography. Typically, helical CT will reveal a ureteral stone or evidence of recent passage (e.g., perinephric stranding or hydronephrosis), whereas a plain abdominal radiograph (kidney-ureters-bladder) can miss a stone in the ureter or kidney, even if radiopaque, and provides no information on obstruction. Although abdominal ultrasound has the advantage of avoiding radiation, this technique can image only the kidney and possibly the proximal segment of the ureter; thus, most ureteral stones are not seen.

Differential Diagnosis

Stone disease is common; therefore, the presence of a stone in the renal pelvis does not alone determine the diagnosis of a patient with acute abdominal or flank pain. It should also be remembered that signs and symptoms from a ureteral stone may mimic a number of other acute conditions. A stone lodged at the right ureteropelvic junction may mimic acute cholecystitis, one in the distal right ureter may mimic acute appendicitis, one at the ureterovesical junction may mimic acute cystitis, and a stone in the distal left ureter may mimic diverticulitis. An obstructing stone with proximal infection may mimic acute pyelonephritis. Infection in the setting of ureteral obstruction is a medical emergency ("pus under pressure") that requires emergency drainage by placement of either a ureteral stent or a percutaneous nephrostomy tube. Other conditions to consider in the differential diagnosis include muscular or skeletal pain, herpes zoster, duodenal ulcer, abdominal aortic aneurysm, gynecologic causes, ureteral stricture, and ureteral obstruction by materials other than a stone, such as a blood clot or sloughed papilla. Although extraluminal processes can lead to ureteral obstruction, these patients tend not to have colic because of the typical gradual onset of the obstruction.

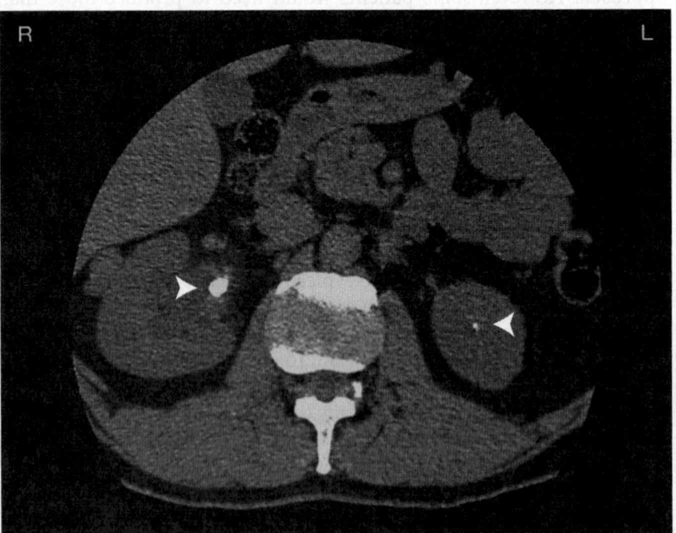

FIGURE 127–2 • High-resolution helical computed tomographic scan of the upper part of the abdomen demonstrating a stone in the right renal pelvis and a smaller stone in the left kidney (arrowheads). There is no hydronephrosis. (From Curhan GC: Clinical crossroads: A 44-year-old woman with kidney stones. JAMA 2005;293:1107–1114.)

Chronic Nephrolithiasis

Among individuals with a documented history of nephrolithiasis, chronic back/flank pain is not infrequently encountered. Clinically, patients with an asymptomatic renal stone often have microscopic hematuria. Because stone disease itself is rarely a cause of chronic pain, the goal should be to determine the source of the pain. The differential diagnosis includes musculoskeletal pain, other intra-abdominal conditions, and drug seeking. A thorough urologic evaluation, including appropriate radiologic studies, may curtail the long-term use of narcotics and avert frequent trips to the emergency room.

Treatment

Rx

Medical Therapy

Renal colic can cause excruciating pain; thus, pain control is a priority after the definitive diagnosis has been made (Fig. 127–3). Nausea and vomiting often prevent the use of oral medication, so parenteral medication is typically required. Narcotics and parenteral nonsteroidal anti-inflammatory drugs (NSAIDs) have been demonstrated to be equally effective, and NSAIDs are preferred because of fewer side effects. [4] However, the risk associated with parenteral NSAIDs needs to be kept in mind because it may be increased in the setting of dehydration, decreased renal function, or the use of radiocontrast. Alkalinization of urine may be effective for acutely treating ureteral uric acid stones, but these are not nearly as common as calcium-based stones. Intravenous fluids are routinely given in the hope that this will increase the likelihood of stone passage, but the status of hydration has little, if any, impact on stone passage. [5]

A urologist should be involved in the following situations: infection, persistent or uncontrollable pain, inability to pass the stone, urinary extravasation detected by imaging, high-grade obstruction with a large stone, a solitary kidney, or pregnancy.

Surgical Therapy

The patient does not require admission if able to tolerate oral analgesics, but instructions should be given to return if fever or uncontrollable pain develops. Most urologists usually wait several days before intervening unless there is evidence of urinary tract infection, a low probability of spontaneous stone passage (e.g., stone >6 mm; anatomic abnormality), or intractable pain. Relief of the obstruction is the initial approach because this will relieve the symptoms. A ureteral stent may be placed cystoscopically but anesthesia is required. Although the stent can be quite uncomfortable and may cause gross hematuria, it may help with stone passage.

The approach to stone removal is dictated by stone size, location, and composition; urinary tract anatomy; availability of technology; and the experience of the urologist. The least invasive approach is ESWL, which can be used in the acute setting, but the success rate depends on the size, location, and composition of the stone. The results of studies of the effectiveness of all stone removal approaches must be compared with caution because of lack of agreement on the definition of success of treatment. Cystoscopic stone removal, both by basket extraction and by fragmentation, is more invasive than ESWL but has a higher stone-free success rate and can remove stones even in the kidney. Percutaneous nephrostolithotomy has the highest likelihood of making a patient stone free but is more invasive than cystoscopic methods. These newer endoscopic approaches have virtually eliminated the need for open surgical procedures such as ureterolithotomy and pyelolithotomy.

The best approach for asymptomatic renal stones is unsettled. Slightly less than 50% of individuals with radiologically documented

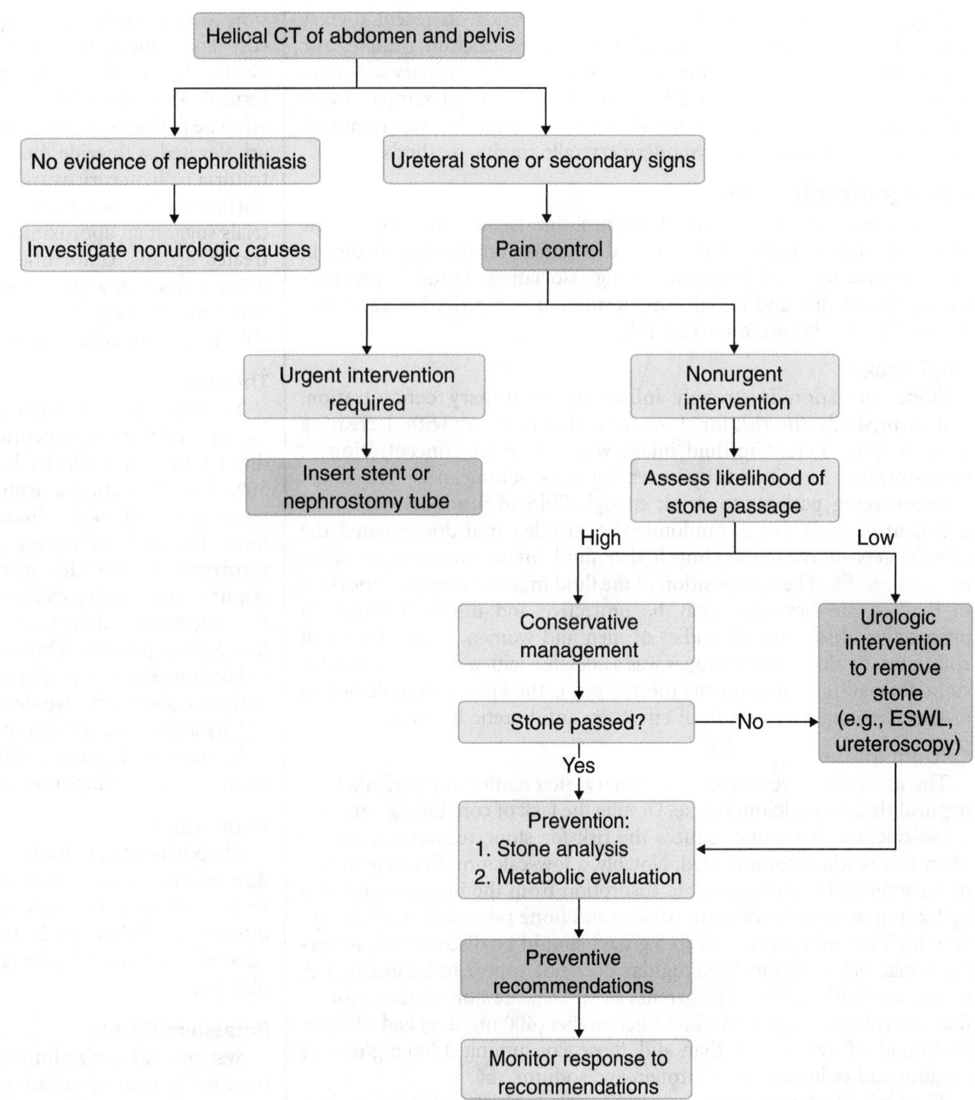

FIGURE 127–3 • Algorithm for evaluation of suspected renal colic. ESWL = extracorporeal shock wave lithotripsy.

Rx

asymptomatic stones will become symptomatic over a 5-year period. With the increasing use of imaging, more incidental stones are being found. Most urologists would not consider removal of a stone that is 6 mm or less. For stones that are 10 mm or larger, many would recommend "prophylactic lithotripsy," but there are no data to support this approach.

Prevention

Evaluation after the First Stone

There is no consensus on the need for an evaluation after the first episode of stone passage. Some authorities believe that cost, low adherence to recommendations, and the relatively low recurrence rate justify no evaluation. However, other experts argue that an evaluation is justified. First, relatively safe and inexpensive interventions are available, such as increasing fluid intake. If an incomplete or no evaluation is performed, the general recommendations may not be appropriate for the individual patient. A common example is recommending a low-oxalate diet, but many patients will already have low urinary oxalate. Second, other potentially clinically important conditions, such as primary hyperparathyroidism, may be identified. Third, there is some evidence that evaluation and subsequent prevention are cost-effective. Other factors influence the decision to proceed with a work-up after the first stone. If there are residual renal stones even though this was the first symptomatic event, the patient could be considered a "recurrent" stone former. Most importantly, if the patient is uninterested in making long-term lifestyle changes or taking medication, an evaluation is not appropriate.

The work-up should include appropriate clinical and laboratory evaluation to identify derangements and predict the likelihood of recurrence. A complete history should include the pace and severity of all stone episodes, previous studies (to distinguish stone passage events from actual new stone formation), previous therapies, surgical interventions, urinary tract infections, bowel disease or surgery, diarrhea or laxative abuse, family history of stone disease, and signs or symptoms suggestive of hyperparathyroidism (Chapter 266). In addition, information should be collected on dietary intake and the use of vitamins (e.g., C and D), minerals, and other supplements, as well as medications (e.g., carbonic anhydrase inhibitors, diuretics). Advice should be deferred until after the evaluation is complete; specifically, patients should be encouraged to resume their usual dietary habits while laboratory studies are completed.

Metabolic Evaluation

The metabolic evaluation for first-time and recurrent stone formers is identical and should include a serum chemistry profile and two 24-hour urine collections (because of substantial day-to-day variability). Even if the content of the stone is known, metabolic evaluation is necessary to identify the abnormalities and guide therapeutic recommendations.

Blood studies should include measurements of creatinine, calcium, phosphorus, albumin, uric acid, potassium, and total CO_2. Routine measurement of plasma parathyroid hormone may be considered optional given the expense; the yield will be higher if serum or urine calcium levels are elevated.

The 24-hour urinary studies should be performed at least six weeks after the stone episode to ensure that patients have resumed their usual diet because the excretion of many factors depends on recent dietary intake. The 24-hour measurements should include calcium, oxalate, uric acid, citrate, sodium, total volume, and creatinine. The urinary sediment should be examined for crystalluria in a freshly voided sample. Every effort should be made to recover a stone that has passed or was removed, and it should be analyzed by modern crystallographic methods.

Dietary Modification

The increasing prevalence of nephrolithiasis and the physiologic impact of dietary factors have focused attention on the role of diet in stone formation. In addition, the strong associations found in prospective studies of diet and initial stone formation (see earlier) suggest that dietary factors play an important role.

Fluid Intake

Stone formation is strongly influenced by urinary concentration. Not surprisingly, the risk for stone formation increases with decreasing urine output. Increasing fluid intake will reduce the concentration of stone-forming constituents by increasing urine volume. A general target is encouraging patients to drink enough fluid to produce more than 2 L of urine each day. A randomized controlled trial documented the effectiveness of recommending higher fluid intake on reducing stone recurrence. [2] The composition of the fluid ingested may be important in that certain beverages may be protective and others harmful. In prospective observational studies of men and women, higher intake of coffee, tea, or alcoholic beverages was associated with a decreased risk for stone formation. The probable mechanism is the known diuretic action of these beverages as a result of effects on antidiuretic hormone.

Calcium Intake

The most controversial topic in dietary intervention for patients with nephrolithiasis is calcium intake. Despite the lack of convincing data that a low-calcium diet alone reduces the risk for stone recurrence, all too often this is still recommended. Notably, a low-calcium diet may in fact be *harmful* by increasing oxalate absorption from the intestine and also by leading to negative calcium balance and bone mineral loss. Although very high calcium intake (>2 to 3 g/day) should be discouraged, lowering intake below 800 to 1200 mg/day does not appear to be justified. A 5-year randomized trial of recurrent calcium oxalate stone formers found that individuals assigned to a low-calcium diet (400 mg/day) had a higher likelihood of recurrence than did those consuming 1200 mg/day of calcium and reduced animal protein and sodium. [1]

The available data support a protective role for higher dietary calcium intake, but this does not hold for calcium from supplements, which either have no effect or slightly increase the risk of stone formation. Because the bioavailability of calcium is the same in dairy and calcium supplements, the differences may be due to timing of ingestion. However, it is also possible that dairy products, the major source of dietary calcium, contain some unidentified protective factor.

Other Dietary Factors

Restriction of nondairy animal protein (e.g., meat, chicken, seafood) is a reasonable option and may result in higher citrate and lower uric acid and calcium excretion. For patients with high oxalate excretion, dietary oxalate restriction may be beneficial. However, reliable and complete data on the oxalate content of many commonly consumed foods are unavailable. Reducing sodium intake to less than 3 g/day may decrease urine calcium and could be particularly important for patients prescribed a thiazide. Sucrose intake may increase urine calcium excretion and thus should be minimized. In contrast, potassium-rich foods should be encouraged. Dietary recommendations should be tailored to the patient's urinary chemistry profile, and the impact of the recommendations can be monitored by repeating the urine collections.

Medical Prevention

Despite nephrolithiasis being a common disease, surprisingly few well-designed prospective double-blind controlled trials have been conducted. Of the published studies, several could be faulted for historical controls, short follow-up, or high dropout rates. Nonetheless, there have been several important studies, both observational and randomized trials, that provide a scientific foundation on which to base preventive recommendations. Additional randomized trials of existing and new medications are needed.

Currently available medications may improve the urinary chemistry profile, but they do not cure the underlying abnormality. Thus, the decision to start medication requires consideration of efficacy, side effects, cost, and adherence of the patient. Certainly, if new stone formation occurs despite dietary recommendations, medication should be prescribed. Most specialists would recommend that a full laboratory evaluation be performed before prescribing medication. If urine calcium levels are elevated, a thiazide diuretic is recommended. For those with hypocitraturia or hyperuricosuria as a sole finding, potassium citrate and allopurinol can be used, respectively. Findings from the available randomized trials suggest an approximately 50% reduction in stone formation in the treated groups. Unfortunately, the optimal duration of required treatment is unclear, a glaring gap in our knowledge about this condition, which affects a substantial number of younger individuals. Understandably, long-term adherence remains suboptimal.

Thiazides

Thiazide diuretics, such as hydrochlorothiazide and chlorthalidone, increase calcium reabsorption in the proximal convoluted tubule and distal tubule and effectively lower urinary calcium excretion by 20 to 50%. In some patients, urine calcium levels may rise after a year despite remaining on therapy. Thiazides can also increase the mineral content of bone. Two trials of 3 years' duration showed a reduction in the risk for recurrence by thiazides over placebo in unclassified patients. The doses required for urinary calcium reduction (25 to 100 mg/day) are higher than those needed for treating hypertension. Side effects are reported in 8 to 35% of patients. Thiazide-induced hypokalemia can be treated with potassium citrate or amiloride. Because of its potential to precipitate, triamterene should be avoided in these patients. Indapamide, though not strictly a thiazide, will also reduce urine calcium.

Monitoring the urine calcium response with subsequent dosage adjustment is clinically important, but there are no studies addressing this issue.

Allopurinol

Allopurinol can reduce urine uric acid excretion by up to 50%. A single double-blind randomized trial found that allopurinol reduced stone recurrence in individuals with hyperuricosuric calcium oxalate stone disease. [3] Other trials of allopurinol in patients not specifically selected for hyperuricosuria showed no benefit when compared with placebo.

Potassium Citrate

Systemic alkalinization with bicarbonate or citrate will lead to an increase in urinary citrate excretion. The most commonly used salt is potassium citrate, which avoids the calciuric effect of a sodium load and restores any potassium deficiency. Only two randomized trials have evaluated the impact of citrate supplementation. One was restricted to individuals with hypocitraturia, but the other was open to all recurrent calcium oxalate stone formers. [6] The latter trial showed a reduction in the stone formation rate when compared with placebo; however, dropout rates were high and adherence to prescribed dosing was suboptimal.

Magnesium

Oral magnesium from supplements may reduce stone risk by forming soluble complexes with oxalate in the bowel or urine. However, in a 3-year double-blind trial, magnesium was no more effective than placebo. Thus, the role of magnesium supplementation remains uncertain.

Future Directions

Research in the next 5 to 10 years will, it is hoped, identify the causes of idiopathic hypercalciuria and hypocitraturia and provide complete information on the oxalate content of foods and the underlying genetic factors that lead to a predisposition to stone formation. Studies exploring nephrolithiasis as a systemic disorder will be important.

New imaging modalities will improve early detection and assist with follow-up. Hopefully, a more complete understanding of conditions predisposing to crystal and stone formation will be possible along with the development of effective and safe interventions, thus avoiding the pain, suffering, and cost associated with recurrent stone disease.

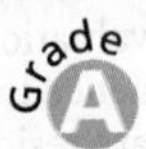

1. Borghi L, Schianchi T, Meschi T, et al: Comparison of two diets for the prevention of recurrent stones in idiopathic hypercalciuria. N Engl J Med 2002;346:77–84.
2. Borghi L, Meschi T, Amato F, et al: Urinary volume, water and recurrences in idiopathic calcium nephrolithiasis: A 5-year randomized prospective study. J Urol 1996;155:839–843.

3. Ettinger B, Tang A, Citron JT, et al: Randomized trial of allopurinol in the prevention of calcium oxalate calculi. N Engl J Med 1986;315:1386–1389.
4. Holdgate A, Pollock T: Systematic review of the relative efficacy of non-steroidal anti-inflammatory drugs and opioids in the treatment of acute renal colic. BMJ 2004;328:1401.
5. Springhart WP, Marguet CG, Sur RL, et al: Forced versus minimal intravenous hydration in the management of acute renal colic: A randomized trial. J Endourol 2006;20:713–716.
6. Ettinger B, Pak CY, Citron JT, et al: Potassium-magnesium citrate is an effective prophylaxis against recurrent calcium oxalate nephrolithiasis. J Urol 1997;158:2069–2073.

SUGGESTED READINGS

Desai RA, Assimos DG: Current opinion in urology: New insights into nephrolithiasis. Curr Opin Urol 2007;17:104–108. *Overview of pathophysiology including Randall's plaques and treatment.*

Hollingsworth JM, Rogers MAM, Kaufman SR, et al: Medical therapy to facilitate urinary stone passage: A meta analysis. Lancet 2006;368:1171–1179. *Findings suggest that medical therapy is a reasonable option.*

Kang DE, Sur RL, Haleblian GE, et al: Long-term lemonade-based dietary manipulation in patients with hypocitraturic nephrolithiasis. J Urol 2007;177:1358–1362. *Lemonade therapy appears to be a reasonable alternative for patients with hypocitraturia.*

Miller NL, Lingeman JE: Management of kidney stones. BMJ 2007;334:468–472. *A practical overview.*

Taylor EN, Curhan GC: Diet and fluid prescription in stone disease. Kidney Int 2006;70:835–839. *A practical overview.*

128 CYSTIC KIDNEY DISEASES

M. Amin Arnaout

Definition

The term *cystic kidney diseases* refers to a heterogeneous group of hereditary and acquired disorders characterized by the presence of unilateral or bilateral renal cysts. Such disorders include polycystic kidney disease (PKD), acquired cystic kidney disease (ACKD), medullary cystic diseases, and rare systemic disorders such as tuberous sclerosis and von Hippel-Lindau (VHL) syndrome. *Renal cysts* are defined as fluid-filled sacs lined by a single layer of epithelial cells. When acquired singly or in small numbers and in the absence of any other pathology, renal cysts are termed *simple cysts.*

Epidemiology

Simple cysts are present in approximately 50% of individuals older than 40 years, are not generally loculated, and tend to bulge out from the renal surface (Fig. 128–1). *Polycystic kidney diseases,* by comparison, constitute a clinically important group of genetically mediated disorders characterized by prominent, expanding, bilateral renal cysts. Classification is based on inheritance pattern as *dominant* or *recessive.* Autosomal dominant PKD (ADPKD), with prevalence rates of 1 in 400 to 1 in 1000, is the most common monogenetic disease in humans. In common with simple cysts, ADPKD develops in an age-dependent manner and affects mainly adults. Autosomal recessive PKD (ARPKD), by contrast, is a relatively rare childhood disorder that appears in 1 in 6000 to 50,000 live births. Collectively, the hereditary PKDs are the fourth leading cause of end-stage renal disease (ESRD) in the United States; they generally affect both genders and all races equally and cost more than $1.5 billion annually to manage in the United States alone. *Acquired cystic kidney disease* refers to the development of multiple bilateral renal cysts in patients who already have kidney disease. ACKD develops in 90% of patients who have been receiving renal replacement therapy for 8 years or longer and is significant mainly for increased rates of development of renal cell carcinoma.

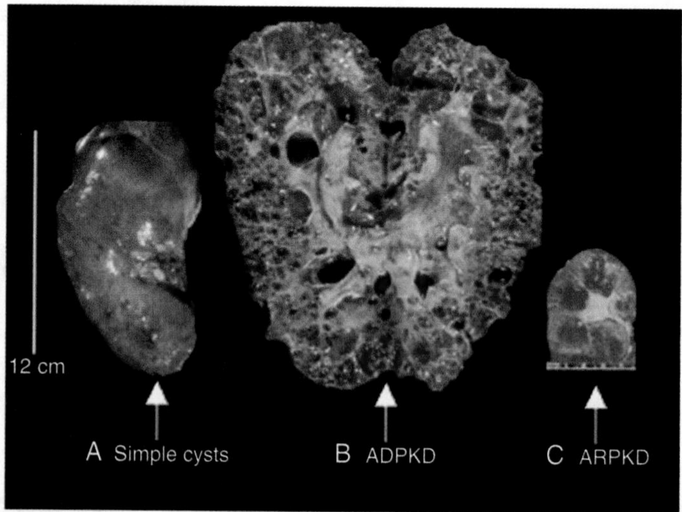

FIGURE 128–1 • Gross pathology of selected cystic kidney diseases. A, Photograph of a kidney with multiple simple cysts. The cysts bulge out from the surface of a normal-sized kidney. **B,** Sagittal cross section of a kidney from an adult with autosomal dominant polycystic kidney disease (ADPKD). Multiple macroscopic cysts have resulted in an enlarged, but still reniform kidney. (Note the evidence of previous hemorrhage within some of the cysts.) **C,** Sagittal cross section of a kidney segment from a neonate with autosomal recessive polycystic kidney disease (ARPKD). The neonatal kidney is enlarged with numerous small cysts. (Courtesy of Dr. Robert Colvin, Massachusetts General Hospital.)

Pathogenesis

Cysts originate as outpouchings of tubules. Any portion of the nephron can undergo this focal dilation, although the preponderance of the tubule site of origin depends on the underlying disease. The impetus for tubular dilation has not been identified but must occur hundreds or even thousands of times because up to 1% of nephrons in kidneys with PKD undergo cystic conversion. The outpouchings expand and eventually separate from the parent tubules and produce cysts (Fig. 128–2). Monoclonal proliferation of the cells lining the cyst, active luminal chloride (and sodium) secretion—which slightly outpaces absorption over time—and remodeling of the extracellular matrix are implicated in cyst initiation and expansion. In most cystic disease models in animals, this propagation is also accompanied by increased apoptotic rates of the epithelial cells lining the cyst, by changes in the amount and distribution of surrounding extracellular matrix and secretory proteins, and by interstitial fibrosis. Altered levels of expression of key regulators of proliferation, apoptosis, extracellular matrix composition, fluid secretion, and fibrosis are documented in animal models of PKD. The contribution of each of these factors to the initiation and propagation of cyst formation varies among the various PKDs. Progressive cyst formation and expansion in the hereditary PKDs lead to enlarged (sometimes massively enlarged) kidneys. When enough normal renal parenchyma has been encroached on by voluminous cysts and by interstitial fibrosis, renal insufficiency and ESRD ensue.

Cyst formation is a complex multistep process that resembles and, in some instances, leads to neoplastic transformation. It represents an abnormality in the developmental and remodeling processes that normally regulate tubular lumen size; hence, any progress made in understanding this process will provide major insight into the normal mechanisms regulating tube size in ductal organs, in addition to its potential for targeted drug development. Major progress has been made in this field in the last 3 years: the vast majority of the human cystogenic genes have been identified, gene-based diagnostics are now available, and coexpression of the gene products in the primary cilium or basal body (or both) has brought to the cell biology front this long-neglected sensory organelle, which is expressed on every kidney cell save the intercalated cell. Future work will focus on elucidating the functions of the proteins encoded by the cloned cystogenic genes at ciliary and extraciliary sites, identifying genetic modifiers responsible for the variable phenotype and course of renal disease, and defining the signal transduction pathways involving the cilium that preserve the delicate balance between cell proliferation and differentiation and thus maintain normal tube structure

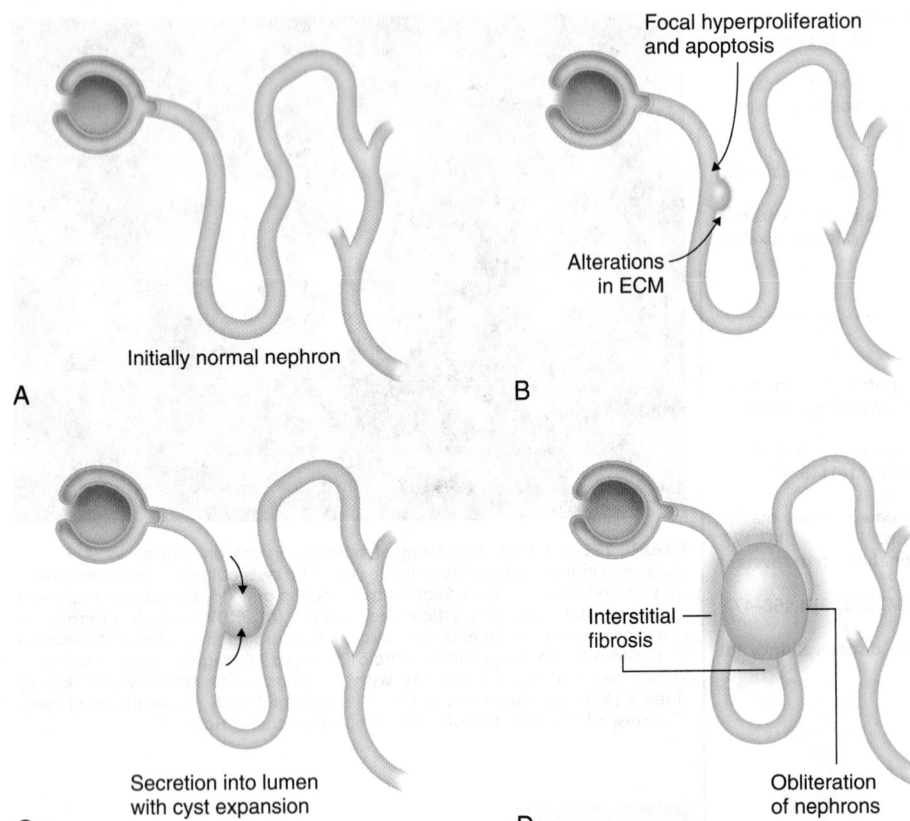

FIGURE 128–2 • A to D, Steps involved in cyst formation: schematic of the sequence of events leading to renal cyst formation. Note that this process occurs hundreds or thousands of times during the natural history of polycystic kidney disease. ECM = extracellular matrix. (Adapted from Arnaout MA: *In* Cooper D [ed]: Nature Encyclopedia of the Human Genome. Nature, 2003.)

and size. New promising therapies addressing secondary pathogenic mechanisms of cyst formation are being tested for efficacy in clinical trials, and novel therapies targeting the primary defect may not be far behind.

AUTOSOMAL DOMINANT POLYCYSTIC KIDNEY DISEASE

Pathobiology

Genetics

ADPKD is a systemic disorder characterized by cyst formation in multiple organs and by the development of abnormalities in the cardiovascular system. Heterogeneous mutations mainly in two genes lead to ADPKD. Mutations in the first identified gene, *PKD1,* account for 85 to 90% of cases. This 54-kilobase (kb) gene is located adjacent to the tuberous sclerosis 2 *(TSC2)* gene on chromosome 16. It has 43 exons and encodes polycystin-1 (PC1), the first described member of an expanding group of proteins termed *polycystins.* More than 200 mutations in this gene have been described to date. They are found throughout the gene but tend to be more common in the 3′ half; mutations in the 5′ half tend to be associated with more severe disease and a higher risk for the development of intracerebral aneurysms. More than 50 heterogeneous mutations in the 68-kb *PKD2,* located on chromosome 4, contribute a further 10 to 15% of ADPKD cases. *PKD2* transcribes 15 exons, which encode polycystin-2 (PC2). Aside from a slower rate of progression, the clinical features of *PKD2*-associated ADPKD are indistinguishable from *PKD1*-associated ADPKD. A small minority of ADPKD cases do not have demonstrable *PKD1* or *PKD2* mutations, thus suggesting that a third gene may be involved.

Polycystin-1 and Polycystin-2

PC1 is composed of 4302 amino acids with 11 predicted membrane-spanning segments connecting a large extracellular amino terminus and a short cytoplasmic carboxyl terminus. Multiple functional motifs are predicted and implicate PC1 in cell-cell or cell-matrix adhesion, or both, as well as in signal transduction (Fig. 128–3). PC2 is a six-transmembrane (6-TM) spanner, nonselective voltage-dependent calcium-permeable ion channel 963 amino acids long with cytoplasmic amino and carboxyl termini. Its 6-TM segment bears topologic and sequence similarity to the 6-TM voltage-activated and transient receptor potential (TRP) channels, which has led to inclusion of PC2 in this protein family. PC1 and PC2 interact through their respective carboxyl-terminal cytoplasmic tails, and such interaction is necessary to stabilize the channel activity of PC2. The last 6-TM segment of PC1 has homology to the 6-TM region of PC2 and, accordingly, has been also included in the TRP channel family (both PC1 and PC2 form a new TRPP subfamily), although it is not known whether PC1, in addition to its putative adhesion function, is also a channel. Other known members of this subfamily are the PC1-like proteins polycystin-REJ, PC1-L1, PC1-L2, PC1-L3, and the PC2-like proteins polycystin-L (also known as polycystin-2L or polycystin-2L1) and polycystin-2L2. None of these proteins appears to be responsible for ADPKD cases in which no identifiable mutation is found in either *PKD1* or *PKD2.* Mouse embryos lacking either PC1 or PC2 die in the perinatal period from a variety of causes that relate to the nature of the mutant alleles. In addition to polycystic kidneys, causes include cardiac abnormalities and vascular fragility, which can lead to generalized edema and widespread hemorrhage.

PC1 and PC2 are widely expressed in tissues, with some overlap consistent with the findings that these two proteins interact directly. PC1 is found in multiple subcellular sites, including the apicolateral and basolateral membranes, intracellular vesicles, and primary apical cilia (organelles that emerge from one of the two basal bodies). PC2 is also found in primary cilia, as well as in the endoplasmic reticulum, the basolateral membrane, and mitotic spindles (Fig. 128–4). PC1 expression is highest in fetal tissue and progressively declines thereafter, whereas PC2 levels are maintained throughout development. This spatiotemporal distribution pattern suggests that the two proteins do not always act as a complex but that each may also function independently. This view is favored by the findings that $Pkd1^{-/-}$ mice display skeletal defects lacking in $Pkd2^{-/-}$ animals and that $Pkd2^{-/-}$ mice exhibit laterality defects not present in $Pkd1^{-/-}$ mice. In addition to PC1 and PC2, the primary apical cilia or basal bodies (or both) also express other proteins that cause polycystic kidneys when mutated, including fibrocystin/polyductin, nephrocystin-1 (NPHP1), nephrocystin-2 (inversin, NPHP2), nephrocystin-3 (NPHP3), nephrocystin-4/nephroretinin (NPHP4), oral-facial-digital syndrome-1 (OFD1) protein, and Bardet-Biedl syndrome (BBS) proteins 1 to 8. In rodents and zebra fish, mutations in the ciliary proteins polaris,

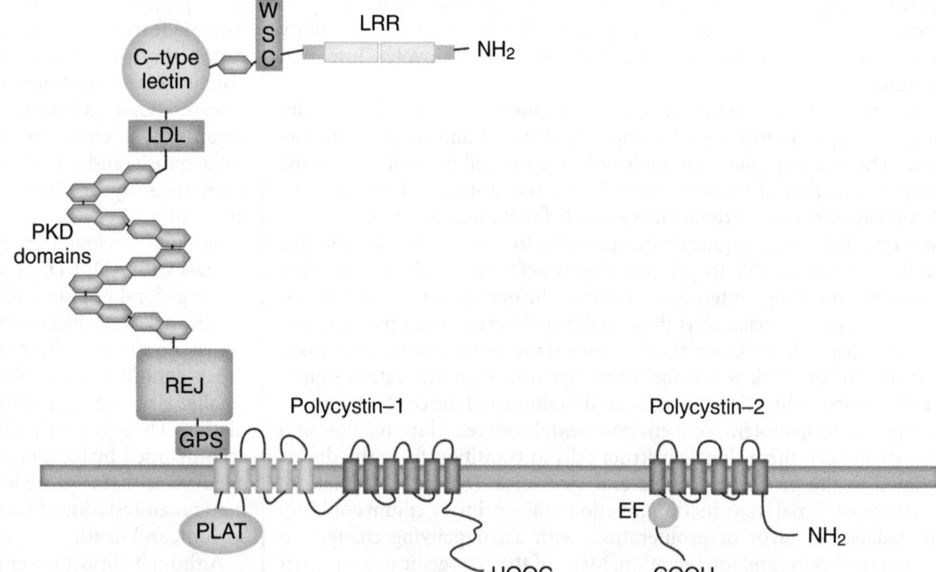

FIGURE 128–3 • Proteins responsible for selected heritable polycystic kidney diseases. *Polycystin-1 domains:* GPS = G protein–coupled receptor proteolytic site; LDL = low-density lipoprotein–like region; LRR = leucine-rich region; PLAT = polycystin-1–lipoxygenase-α toxin; REJ = receptor for egg jelly domain; WSC = cell wall and stress component. *Polycystin-2 domain:* EF = calcium-binding motif consisting of two helixes, E and F. The last six transmembrane regions of polycystin-1 (dark purple) are homologous to those of polycystin-2.

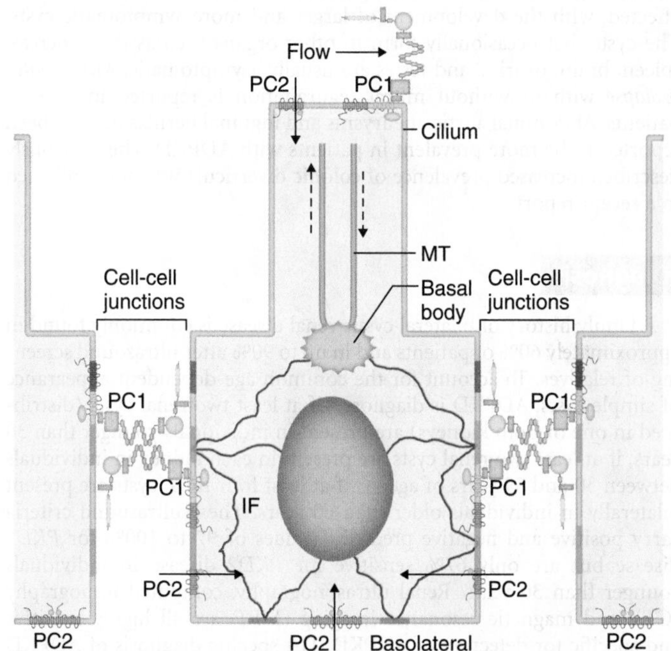

FIGURE 128–4 • Potential sites of action of PC1 and PC2. In primary cilia, the PC1/PC2 complex acts as a flow-sensitive channel that transports calcium intracellularly (solid arrows). At the lateral cell-cell junctions (disproportionately expanded in the figure), PC1 forms homodimers *in trans,* and the PC1/PC2 complex may also act as a mechanosensitive channel. PC1 and PC2 are also expressed in basolateral membranes, where the more abundant PC2 in its multimeric form or in complex with PC1 (not shown) may also transport calcium into cells. PC1 interacts with intermediate filaments (IF, red) and PC2 with microfilaments (not shown), which are anchored respectively to specialized membrane subdomains known as desmosomes (green) and hemidesmosomes (gray) and to adherens junctions (purple). The basal body, a microtubule (MT)-based structure that gives rise to the primary cilium, is also connected to the cytoskeleton. Interrupted arrows indicate the directions of antegrade (toward the cilium) and retrograde (toward the cell body) transport along the ciliary microtubules. Solid arrows indicate movement of calcium across the PC2 channel.

cystin, kinesin-II3a, and several intraflagellar (cilial) transport proteins also cause cystic kidneys; in most of these animal models the apical cilia are structurally deformed.

Pathogenesis

ADPKD-associated cysts develop in organs that are (at least initially) heterozygous for germline mutations in *PKD1* or *PKD2.* Subsequently acquired "somatic" mutations in the remaining normal *PKD1* or *PKD2* allele ("second hits") hasten cyst expansion and progression. Approximately 10% of the germline mutations in patients with ADPKD are believed to have arisen spontaneously. A two-hit mechanism for cyst initiation (consisting of a germline mutation in one allele *and* a somatic mutation in the other) was initially proposed on the basis of epithelial cell clonality within human-derived individual ADPKD cysts and loss of heterozygosity of *PKD1* or *PKD2* in epithelial cells isolated from a proportion of renal or liver cysts. This mechanism could also explain the focal nature of cyst formation and is supported by the finding that renal cysts develop in mice with homozygous knockout of *Pkd1* or *Pkd2* (the murine equivalents of human *PKD1* and *PKD2,* respectively). However, for a second somatic hit affecting the normal allele to be the sole pathogenic mechanism for cyst formation in ADPKD presupposes high somatic mutation rates in *PKD1* and *PKD2,* which have not been demonstrated. Second, mutation analysis of cysts from ADPKD patients has revealed loss of heterozygosity in *PKD1* or *PKD2* in a minority of examined cysts; moreover, such studies have revealed associated chromosomal imbalances, thus suggesting that the identified mutations may also be reflective of the progressive dedifferentiation or increased cell proliferation, or both, that characterize the ADPKD epithelium. Third, ADPKD also develops in mice overexpressing functional PC1 (via a genomic transgene), which is incongruent with the second-hit hypothesis and more suggestive of an imbalance in formation or trafficking of PC1- or PC2-containing multimeric protein complexes (or both). Finally, recent studies show that haplo-insufficiency of *Pkd1 or Pkd2* can itself initiate cysts. Thus, cyst formation appears to require the presence of a germline mutation in *PKD1* or *PKD2,* with expansion and progression of cysts being influenced by a number of additional factors that may include not only a somatic mutation in the normal *PKD1* or *PKD2* allele but also stochastic fluctuations in the level of expression of these alleles (creating a transient homozygous-like state), as well as mutations in "modifier" genes. An example of the latter is the tuberous sclerosis gene *TSC2,* which encodes tuberin; early and aggressive ADPKD develops in individuals with contiguous *PKD1* and *TSC2* mutations, which is probably explained by the role of tuberin in normal trafficking of PC1 to the lateral plasma membrane. PC1 and PC2 are also known to interact directly or indirectly with a number of proteins, including cytoskeletal, adaptor, signaling, adhesion, and ion channel proteins, each of which could serve as a modifier of PC1 or PC2 function (or both).

The key cellular abnormality in ADPKD appears to be increased proliferation, perhaps reflective of an inability to sustain a terminally differentiated state. The observed polarity defects, reflected in abnormal trafficking of proteins such as the epidermal growth factor receptor (EGFR) and the EGFR-related tyrosine kinase receptor Erb-B2 and in increased luminal chloride secretion, may be secondary features. The precise mechanism by which deficiency of either PC1 or PC2 causes defective terminal differentiation of epithelial and endothelial cells is unclear. Because PC2 is a nonselective calcium channel regulated by its interaction with PC1, the cystogenic pathway leading to loss of the ability to sustain terminal cell differentiation appears to involve impaired calcium influx.

The localization of many cystogenic proteins to primary cilia provides an intriguing clue to the pathogenesis of ADPKD and other cystic diseases. The primary cilium (there is only one per cell in most cells of the body) is a marker of the terminally differentiated state and requires one of the two centrioles present in each cell for its formation/sustenance. Because cell division requires both centrioles to form the mitotic spindle, a cell must disassemble its primary cilium before it can divide and then reassemble it through interphase as part of the maturation process. A delicate and dynamic balance is thus established between cell proliferation and terminal differentiation that is centered on the differential use of one centriole for one task versus the other. Dynamic communication signals are channeled bidirectionally between the cilium and the cell body proper in response to spatiotemporal environmental cues (e.g., luminal flow and tube diameter); these signals instruct cells to transition from the differentiated to the proliferative state and vice versa. Defects in formation, structure, or signal transduction function of the primary cilium could tip this balance in favor of proliferation, with accompanying changes in protein trafficking and ion secretion. Many of the cystogenic genes impair the formation or structure of the primary cilium, whereas the ADPKD genes appear to affect its signal transduction component inasmuch as bending of the immobile primary cilia in kidney epithelium in vitro triggers an increase in PC1/PC2-mediated calcium influx, followed by calcium release from inositol-1,4,5-triphosphate stores, subsequent spreading of the calcium signal to neighboring cells, and finally, hyperpolarization of the cell. Defects in several cystogenic genes (e.g., those encoding PC1, fibrocystin, cystin, Bicaudal C, Nek1, and Nek8) are not associated with the laterality defects indicative of abnormal nodal cilia, however, and several ciliary proteins, including PC1, PC2, inversin, and polaris, are also present at extraciliary sites, where they interact with nonciliary proteins (such as the cytoskeletal proteins intermediate filaments and microfilaments in the case of PC1 and PC2, respectively). Cell-cell and cell-matrix sites are known to regulate cell proliferation, polarity, and differentiation; cystogenic proteins could modulate signal transduction at these sites, in part through their known links with the cytoskeleton. Recent evidence suggests that ciliary dysfunction can be dissociated from cyst formation inasmuch as overexpression of polaris in mice corrects the laterality defect but not PKD, thus suggesting that defective function of cystogenic proteins at extraciliary sites may be more relevant to cyst formation. Resolution of this issue will require disruption of cystogenic proteins at selective subcellular compartments and analysis of the resulting phenotype.

Clinical Manifestations

ADPKD has a highly variable manifestation, even within families. Thus, despite an estimated 100% penetrance by 90 years of age, in only half the individuals with heterozygous mutations in *PKD1* or *PKD2* is ADPKD ever diagnosed. Of these, the majority arise in the third or fourth decade of life with symptoms referable to renal cystic disease. However, ADPKD can develop at any age (including infancy) and can have nonrenal manifestations. Renomegaly may predominate in the clinical picture and cause abdominal distention, discomfort, or pain, but it can also be discovered incidentally on physical examination or after radiographic studies of the abdomen. Urinary concentrating defects (manifested as nocturia), recurrent urinary tract infection, and recurrent kidney stone formation (calcium oxalate or uric acid stones) are all more common in patients with ADPKD. Urinary concentrating defects are one of the earliest signs of abnormal renal function in ADPKD. *Hypertension* is present in approximately 70% of cases before renal dysfunction is detected, correlates with activation of the renin-angiotensin system, perhaps as a result of compression of renal vessels, and is associated with poor renal survival. The development of hypertension at a young age in an ADPKD patient is associated with an approximately fourfold increased risk for ESRD. Furthermore, hypertension occurs more frequently and early in the affected offspring of a hypertensive ADPKD parent. Hypertension, which is common in ADPKD, has been postulated to play a causal role in the formation of cerebral aneurysms. However, this link has not been confirmed in cohorts of ADPKD patients screened for cerebral aneurysms, thus suggesting that this vascular defect is primary in nature. Anemia features less prominently than in other renal diseases, an observation that probably stems from the relatively well-preserved erythropoietin secretion. Proteinuria is also less prominent than in other renal diseases. Cyst infection, usually by common urinary tract–infecting organisms, is characterized by flank or abdominal pain, fever, rigors, leukocytosis, and occasionally sepsis. Cyst rupture and hemorrhage occur spontaneously or after trauma and are manifested as sharp pain and hematuria.

Saccular *cerebral aneurysms* develop in an estimated 4 to 15% of individuals with ADPKD, a prevalence rate that is 4 to 10 times greater than in the general population. These aneurysms tend to segregate in families, which makes ADPKD one of a group of diseases characterized by autosomal dominantly inherited familial cerebral aneurysms. As in these other conditions, ADPKD-associated aneurysms tend to rupture at a smaller size and approximately 10 years earlier than in the general population. Though usually clinically silent, intact cerebral aneurysms can be accompanied by focal neurologic symptoms and headaches. By contrast, aneurysms that rupture lead to subarachnoid hemorrhage and have dramatic manifestations that include severe headaches, seizures, altered sensorium, and death.

Although almost never severe enough to cause end-stage liver disease, age-dependent *hepatic cysts* occur in 30 to 80% of patients with ADPKD and can also lead to signs and symptoms of a mass effect, infection, hemorrhage, and rupture. Multiparous women are disproportionately affected, with the development of larger and more symptomatic cysts. The cysts that occasionally form in other organs such as the pancreas, spleen, brain, ovaries, and testes are usually asymptomatic. *Mitral valve prolapse* with or without mitral regurgitation is reported in 25% of patients. Abdominal aortic aneurysms and inguinal hernias have all been reported to be more prevalent in patients with ADPKD. The previously described increased prevalence of colonic diverticula was not confirmed in a recent report.

Diagnosis

A family history of bilateral cystic renal disease is commonly found in approximately 60% of patients and in up to 90% after ultrasound screening of relatives. To account for the common age-dependent appearance of simple cysts, ADPKD is diagnosed if at least two renal cysts (distributed in one or both kidneys) are present in individuals younger than 30 years, if at least two renal cysts are present in each kidney in individuals between 30 and 59 years of age, or if at least four renal cysts are present bilaterally in individuals older than 60 years. These ultrasound criteria carry positive and negative predictive values of 97 to 100% for *PKD1* disease but are only 67% sensitive for *PKD2* disease in individuals younger than 30 years. Renal ultrasonography, computed tomography (CT), and magnetic resonance imaging (MRI) are all highly sensitive and specific for detection of ADPKD. The specific diagnosis of ADPKD requires consideration of the characteristics of associated extrarenal manifestations, age at initial evaluation, and family history (Table 128–1). Because only about 60% of individuals give a family history of PKD, ultrasound screening of asymptomatic parents or grandparents may be required to uncover diagnostically relevant, silent PKD.

DNA-based diagnosis of ADPKD by linkage analysis or direct DNA sequencing is available, though currently expensive, in part because of the length of the transcripts. The marked allelic heterogeneity of the *PKD1* and *PKD2* mutations, as well as the paucity of phenotype-genotype correlations, contributes to the complexity and interpretation of gene-based diagnostics.

Treatment

Management strategies currently aim at monitoring for and treating complications of ADPKD and providing counseling as appropriate.

Blood Pressure Monitoring and Control

Frequent blood pressure monitoring is recommended because hypertension accelerates the decline in renal function. The goals of blood pressure control are the same as for any other patient with

TABLE 128–1 COMPARISON OF THE CLINICAL FEATURES OF CYSTIC KIDNEY DISEASES

Disease	Family History (Inheritance)	Frequency	Gene Product	Age at Onset	Cyst Origin	Renomegaly	Cause of ESRD	Other Manifestations
ADPKD	Yes (AD)	1 in 400–1000	Polycystin-1 Polycystin-2	20s and 30s	Anywhere (including Bowman's capsule)	Yes	Yes	Liver cysts Cerebral aneurysms Hypertension Mitral valve prolapse Kidney stones UTIs
ARPKD	Yes (AR)	1 in 6000–10,000	Fibrocystin/ polyductin	First year of life	Distal nephron, CD	Yes	Yes	Hepatic fibrosis Pulmonary hypoplasia Hypertension
ACKD	No	90% of ESRD patients at 8 yr	—	Years after onset of ESRD	Proximal and distal tubules	Rarely	No	None
Simple cysts	No	50% >age 40 yr	—	Adulthood	Anywhere (usually cortical)	No	No	None
FN	Yes (AR)	1 in 80,000	Nephrocystins (NPHP1–NPHP5)	Childhood, adolescence	Medullary DCT	No	Yes	Retinal, bone, cerebellar anomalies
MCKD	Yes (AD)	Rare	Uromodulin, others	Adulthood	Medullary DCT	No	Yes	Hyperuricemia, gout
MSK	No	1 in 5000 to 20,000	—	30s	Medullary CD	No	No	Kidney stones Hypercalciuria
Tuberous sclerosis	Yes (AD)	1 in 10,000	Hamartin (TSC1), tuberin (TSC2)	Childhood	Loop of Henle, DCT	Rarely	Rarely	Renal cell carcinoma Tubers, seizures Angiomyolipomas Hypertension
VHL syndrome	Yes (AD)	1 in 40,000	VHL protein	20s	Cortical nephrons	Rarely	Rarely	Renal cell carcinoma Pheochromocytoma
OFD syndrome-1	Yes (XD)	1 in 250,000	OFD1 protein	Childhood or adulthood	Renal glomeruli	Rarely	Yes	Malformation of the face, oral cavity, and digits Liver cysts Mental retardation
BBS	Yes (AR)	1 in 65,000 to 160,000	BBS1–BBS8	Adulthood	Renal calyces	Rarely	Yes	Syndactyly and polydactyly, obesity, retinal dystrophy, male hypogenitalism, hypertension, mental retardation

ACKD = acquired cystic kidney disease; AD = autosomal dominant; ADPKD = autosomal polycystic kidney disease; AR = autosomal recessive; ARPKD = autosomal recessive polycystic kidney disease; BBS = Bardet-Biedl syndrome; CD = collecting duct; DCT = distal convoluted tubule; ESRD = end-stage renal disease; FN = familial nephronophthisis; MCKD = medullary cystic kidney disease; MSK = medullary sponge kidney; OFD = oral-facial-digital; UTI = urinary tract infection; VHL = von Hippel-Lindau; XD = X-linked dominant; — = no known genetic susceptibility.

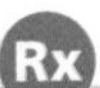

renal disease and include attainment of a symptom-free blood pressure reading of 125/75 mm Hg or less. Although all available antihypertensive agents have been used with roughly equivalent success, theoretical considerations and preliminary data suggest that angiotensin-converting enzyme inhibitors or receptor blockers may be more efficient at delaying the rate of progression to ESRD. However, the effect of these agents on the decline of renal function remains uncertain.

Urinary Tract Infection/Nephrolithiasis

Treatment of urinary tract infection and nephrolithiasis is no different from that in the general population and includes standard antimicrobial therapy and increased fluid intake, respectively. Renal or hepatic cyst infections are optimally treated with lipophilic antibiotics that possess cyst-penetrating capabilities. Such antibiotics include ciprofloxacin, trimethoprim, clindamycin, and vancomycin. The results of blood or urine culture and sensitivities should be used to guide the choice of antibiotic therapy. Cyst hemorrhage and rupture, with resultant pain and hematuria, are usually managed conservatively with rest and non-nonsteroidal anti-inflammatory analgesics. Patients with enlarged kidneys should be advised to avoid playing contact sports, and those with massively enlarged kidneys should refrain even from wearing belts and seat belts. Some patients with unusually painful cysts respond to cyst fluid aspiration, cyst deroofing, or ethanol-induced sclerosis. Nephrectomies are rarely indicated before the onset of ESRD.

Detection and Management of Cerebral Aneurysms

Cerebral aneurysms are increasingly being detected with magnetic resonance angiography (MRA) rather than CT scanning with intravenous contrast. The former is more sensitive for posterior circulation anomalies and does not present a risk for deterioration of renal function. Four-vessel cerebral angiography remains the "gold standard" and is often used for surgical planning. Performance of cerebral MRA in all patients at time of diagnosis of ADPKD was shown to be cost-effective and to lead to reduced morbidity and mortality in a decision analysis model. It was further suggested that individuals with familial cerebral aneurysms (defined as aneurysms in two or more first- to third-degree relatives) undergo screening MRA every 3 years. Individuals shown to have cerebral aneurysms should be referred to a neurosurgeon for consideration of clipping. An annual screening MRA to assess for aneurysmal growth is recommended in all patients with untreated aneurysms. Renal replacement therapies, including renal transplantation for ADPKD, are at least as effective as they are for other causes of ESRD.

Reducing Cyst Formation

Recently, pharmacologic strategies targeting the mislocalized EGFR and Erb-B2 receptors and the cyclic adenosine monophosphate (cAMP) pathway (which is mitogenic in ADPKD) are being developed and tested in animal models of PKD. Inhibiting EGFR kinase activity reduced cyst formation in the *orpk* mouse, defective in the *TgN737Rpw* gene, which encodes polaris; in the *bpk* mouse, defective in the gene encoding the mouse homologue of the *Drosophila* Bicaudal C gene (both are models of ARPKD); and in the *Han-SPRD* rat model of ADPKD. EGFR kinase inhibitors were deleterious, however, in the *pck* murine model of ARPKD, a more relevant model because these mice are defective in the mouse homologue of human *PKHD1*, the gene defective in human ARPKD. A second therapeutic approach is the use of thiazolidinedione peroxisome proliferator–activated receptor γ (PPAR-γ) agonists, which are believed to act in part through the Wnt signaling pathway to increase β-catenin, levels of which are found to be reduced in $Pkd1^{-/-}$ mouse embryos. The thiazolidinedione pioglitazone administered maternally slightly increased the survival of $Pkd1^{-/-}$ mouse embryos and reduced subcutaneous edema, cardiac defects, and renal cystogenesis, as well as endothelial dysfunction. Because the vasopressin V2 receptor (VPV2R) is the major cAMP agonist in the collecting duct, the VPV2R antagonists OPC31260 or OPC41061 (tolvaptan) were tried in the *Pkd2–*, *pcy–*, and *pck* rodent models (orthologous to human ADPKD, adolescent nephronophthisis, and human ARPKD, respectively). In all three models, renal cAMP levels were lowered and cystogenesis reduced in the treated animals. Plans for a multicenter tolvaptan trial to assess the effect of this drug on development/expansion of renal cysts are being developed. Finally, treatment of 13 ADPKD patients for a 6-month period with the somatostatin analogue octreotide, which inhibits active chloride secretion through a reduction in cAMP generation, slowed renal cyst expansion, thus suggesting that longer-term therapy may be renoprotective.

Rx

Counseling

The wide variability in disease manifestations and the tendency to late onset of disease-associated morbidity make consideration of therapeutic abortion less pressing. Still, patients should be advised that their children have a 50% probability of inheriting a disease-causing germline mutation. DNA-based diagnostics are most useful in identifying the germline mutation prenatally or before implantation and in selection of a young transplant donor from an ADPKD family when imaging studies are negative. The decision to screen the children of parents with ADPKD by renal ultrasound is made only after consideration of the potential psychological and economic implications. As DNA-based diagnostics become more widely available and cheaper and as promising treatment options develop, counseling will assume an increasingly important component in prevention and management.

Prognosis

ESRD develops in approximately 50% of patients with ADPKD by 60 years of age. The rate of progression of renal disease is highest in men with poorly controlled hypertension, an early age at diagnosis, and mutations in *PKD1*. Approximately 5% of all ADPKD patients with cerebral aneurysms die of aneurysmal rupture. The longevity of patients with ADPKD is reduced in patients with *PKD1* and *PKD2* mutations, with an average lifespan of approximately 55 and 65 years, respectively.

AUTOSOMAL RECESSIVE POLYCYSTIC KIDNEY DISEASE

Epidemiology

ARPKD is a multisystem childhood disorder that occurs in 1 in 20,000 live births.

Pathogenesis

ARPKD is characterized by severe and early PKD, dominated by dilation of the kidney collecting ducts, biliary dysgenesis, and portal tract fibrosis. It has been linked to heterogeneous mutations in a single gene, *PKHD1*, an orthologue of the rat *pck* gene causing PKD. Located on chromosome 6, *PKHD1* spans approximately 470 kb, includes a minimum of 86 exons, and encodes a complex array of alternatively spliced forms. Its longest approximate 16-kb transcript includes 67 exons and encodes a unique type I membrane protein, fibrocystin/polyductin, composed of 4074 amino acids, with a large extracellular segment and a short cytoplasmic carboxyl terminus. The ectodomain contains at least 10 copies of an immunoglobulin-like domain in addition to plexin- and transcription factor (IPT) domains and multiple parallel β-helix 1 (PβH1) repeats. Alternatively spliced transcripts encode a membrane protein with variable extracellular domains, as well as forms lacking the transmembrane segment, which are therefore probably secreted. *PKHD1* messenger RNA (mRNA) is detected mostly in the kidney (cortical and medullary collecting ducts and thick ascending limbs of Henle), but it is also found in the pancreas, liver, and lung, organs that are affected in ARPKD. In common with other cystogenic proteins, fibrocystin is found subcellularly in the basal bodies and primary apical cilia. Disruption of fibrocystin expression with short interfering RNA (siRNA) reduced ciliary length and structure, thus suggesting that fibrocystin is important in maintaining the structural integrity of this organelle.

Several lines of evidence have suggested that the EGFR and cAMP pathways are important effectors in the pathogenesis of ARPKD. However, as noted earlier, cAMP but not EGFR inhibition is beneficial in the *pcy* and *pck* rodent models of ARPKD.

Clinical Manifestations

In common with ADPKD, ARPKD has a highly variable mode of expression. Although ARPKD can be manifested as radiographically discovered renal cysts antenatally or during adulthood, it is usually associated with bilateral abdominal masses and renal insufficiency in infancy and carries a 30% mortality as a result of severe pulmonary hypoplasia and secondary respiratory failure. Findings related to tubular dysfunction may be present and include polyuria, enuresis, hyponatremia, and hyperchloremic metabolic acidosis. ESRD is expected but can take up to 20 years to develop and may in rare instances never occur. Oligohydramnios, presumably linked to in utero renal disease, is often present and probably accounts for the severe pulmonary hypoplasia that causes most of the deaths in the first year of life. Hepatic fibrosis, a prominent feature of ARPKD, commonly progresses to portal hypertension and its attendant complications of bleeding esophageal varices and hepatosplenomegaly. Pancreatic fibrosis is only rarely a clinical concern. Hypertension is almost universal and probably accelerates the decline in renal function. Cyst complications of infection and rupture also occur, although hematuria is an infrequent finding.

Diagnosis

Abdominal ultrasonography or CT demonstration of both enlarged polycystic kidneys and hepatic fibrosis is sufficient to make the diagnosis of ARPKD. Aside from an occasional affected sibling, a family history is often not elicited. Distinguishing ARPKD from ADPKD may rarely require a liver biopsy to document otherwise undetectable hepatic fibrosis. Gene-based diagnostics are available but currently have approximately 60% sensitivity among all phenotypes.

Treatment

Rx

In the absence of specific therapy for ARPKD, current management goals focus on early detection and treatment of the complications of hypertension, urinary tract or cyst infection, and portal hypertension. Treatment of the latter may require liver transplantation or portosystemic shunting. As in all children with ESRD, attention to issues of nutrition and renal osteodystrophy is paramount.

Prevention

It is hoped that with improving sensitivity of gene-based diagnostics, genetic counseling will play a more active role in prevention. The promising results from the use of VPV2R blockers in animal models of ARPKD will likely be followed by clinical trials in the near future.

Prognosis

ARPKD-affected patients suffer their highest mortality rates during the first year of life. Subsequently, the survival rate to 15 years of age is approximately 50 to 80%.

ACQUIRED CYSTIC KIDNEY DISEASE

Pathobiology

ACKD is largely confined to the ESRD population maintained on dialysis.

Cysts arise from proximal and distal tubule dilations in small, end-stage kidneys, regardless of the etiology, mode of dialysis, or presence of a functioning kidney transplant. Identifiable risk factors include the duration of ESRD, male gender, black race, and chronic hypokalemia.

Clinical Manifestations

ACKD is usually asymptomatic. However, it can occasionally lead to enlarged kidneys with associated abdominal discomfort and pain. Cyst hemorrhage is more common than cyst infection and is manifested as flank pain, anemia, or hematuria. The most significant complication of ACKD is malignant conversion of cysts to renal cell carcinoma. These tumors are frequently associated with hematuria and are 2 to 200 times more common in patients with ACKD than in the general dialysis population.

Diagnosis

Diagnosis of ACKD is relatively straightforward and entails ultrasound or CT demonstration of bilateral renal cysts in a patient with preexistent chronic renal failure or ESRD. In contrast to ADPKD and ARPKD, the kidneys are not usually enlarged and there is no family history of PKD. Renal CT or MRI is preferable for detecting cysts in small kidneys and in assessing in malignant conversion.

Treatment

Alterations in dialysis dose do not modify the course. New or frank hematuria raises concern of renal cell carcinoma and requires both enhanced and nonenhanced CT or MRI to rule it out. Any evidence of septum formation, solid material, or contrast enhancement within a cyst is suspicious for renal cell carcinoma and warrants consideration of nephrectomy.

Prevention

There are no strategies to prevent the appearance or delay the expansion of renal cysts.

Prognosis

Although renal cell carcinoma in patients with ACKD is less often metastatic at time of diagnosis than in other patients with renal cell carcinoma, 5-year mortality rates are greater, probably because of the almost invariable coexistence of ESRD. Asymptomatic ACKD does not affect survival.

MEDULLARY AND MISCELLANEOUS CYSTIC KIDNEY DISORDERS

Medullary cystic diseases of the kidney comprise two rare, but clinically significant hereditary disorders (familial nephronophthisis [FN] and medullary cystic kidney disease [MCKD]) and the common, but usually benign developmental condition medullary sponge kidney (see Table 128–1).

Familial Nephronophthisis

FN develops in early childhood and adolescence with tubular dysfunction that inexorably progresses to ESRD before 20 years of age. Approximately 20% of patients exhibit eye, bone, or cerebellar anomalies. Recessively acquired mutations in at least one of five identified genes *NPHP1* to *NPHP5* (encoding nephrocystin-1 to nephrocystin-5, respectively) result in FN, and cysts develop in kidney distal tubules primarily at the corticomedullay junction, where the encoded respective nephrocystins are expressed. Expression of nephrocystins at extrarenal sites accounts for the associated retinal, skeletal, and neural abnormalities. Mutations in nephrocystin-5 are always associated with retinal involvement, probably explained by the interaction of this protein with the retinitis pigmentosa guanosine triphosphatase (GTPase) regulator in photoreceptor cilia. Nephrocystin-1 (or nephrocystin) interacts with β-tubulin and with nephrocystin-2 to nephrocystin-4 to form protein complexes that may also include the adhesion signaling proteins focal adhesion kinase-2 and p130Cas and the cytoskeletal proteins tensin and filamin. Nephrocystin-3 contains a putative tubulin–tyrosine ligase domain that might tyrosinate α-tubulin, thus regulating the microtubule organization of primary cilia. All five nephrocystins are found in primary cilia. Other isoforms of nephrocystin-2 (inversin) are found at the lateral junctions, in centrosomes, at the poles of the mitotic spindle, and in the nucleus in complex with nonciliary proteins such as β-catenin and the anaphase-promoting complex protein Apc2. The physiologic relevance of all these associations remains to be defined.

Medullary Cystic Kidney Disease

MCKD is similar to FN but is more rare, appears in adulthood, and has an autosomal dominant inheritance pattern. Corticomedullary cysts are present in most of the patients but cannot always be recognized on ultrasonography or CT because they tend to be very small. At least two genes, *MCKD1* and *MCKD2,* cause MCKD. The clinical picture is identical except that gout is more frequent in *MCKD2* disease with more severe hyperuricemia and earlier onset of ESRD. *MCKD1* has not been identified. It is localized on chromosome 1q21, and its position has been further refined to a 2.1-Mb genetic region that houses interesting candidates encoding proteins with known roles in cell-cell adhesion, tubulin assembly, growth and proliferation, and ion transport. *MCKD2* encodes uromodulin (Tamm-Horsfall protein), an 85-kD urinary protein secreted by the thick ascending limb of the loop of Henle and the most abundant protein in human urine.

Medullary Sponge Kidney

Medullary sponge kidney is characterized by congenitally acquired inner medullary and papillary collecting duct dilations and hypercalciuria. Although it can be an incidental finding on intravenous pyelography (with characteristic pooling of contrast within the cystically dilated collecting ducts), it is also manifested as hematuria and recurrent kidney stones. The pathogenesis of medullary sponge kidney is unknown. It may be associated with a variety of congenital anomalies suggestive of a genetic predisposition.

Other Conditions

Renal cyst formation is seen in few other rare inherited conditions. *Tuberous sclerosis* and *VHL syndrome* are both inherited in an autosomal dominant manner. These conditions are systemic disorders whose cardinal features do not usually relate to cystic kidney disease. Cyst formation in tuberous sclerosis is commonly associated with hypertension, can resemble ADPKD (sometimes with severe PKD leading to ESRD), and has an increased incidence of renal cell carcinoma (≈5%). Cyst formation in VHL syndrome can also lead to features of ADPKD but, more importantly, is associated with a 25% incidence of clear cell carcinoma of the kidney. Oral-facial-digital (OFD) syndrome is characterized by malformations in the face, oral cavity, and digits. It is inherited in an X-linked pattern and is caused by defects in the *OFD1* gene, which encodes OFD1 protein expressed in basal bodies but with an otherwise undetermined function. Renal, primarily glomerular, cysts are found in as many as 50% of patients, who are exclusively females (because males carrying the *OFD1* mutation die in utero), thereby distinguishing it from ADPKD. OFD syndrome should also be distinguished from a variety of other glomerulocystic diseases of the kidney, including *tuberous sclerosis, familial juvenile nephronophthisis, short-rib polydactyly syndromes, Zellweger's hepatorenal syndrome, brachymesomelia-renal syndrome, Jeune's asphyxiating thoracic dystrophy syndrome,* and *trisomies* 9, 13, and 18. The Bardet-Biedl syndrome (BBS) is a rare autosomal recessive disease characterized by obesity, hypertension, and dystrophy of the hands, eyes, kidneys, and male genitalia. Calyceal cysts and calyceal clubbing are the predominate renal lesions and are best diagnosed by intravenous urography rather than ultrasound. Renal impairment is frequent and an important cause of death. Eight genes associated with BBS (*BBS1* to *BBS8*) have been identified. The gene products are expressed in basal bodies, thus implicating cilia in the pathogenesis of this pleiotropic syndrome.

SUGGESTED READINGS

Chapman AB, Guay-Woodford LM, Grantham JJ, et al: Renal structure in early autosomal-dominant polycystic kidney disease (ADPKD): The Consortium for Radiologic Imaging Studies of Polycystic Kidney Disease (CRISP) cohort. Kidney Int 2003;64:1035–1045. *Magnetic resonance imaging is an accurate method to detect cysts.*

Grantham JJ, Torres VE, Chapman AB, et al: Volume progression in polycystic kidney disease. N Engl J Med 2006;354:2122–2130. *Kidney volume increased by an average of 5.3% per year.*

Jafar TH, Stark PC, Schmid CH, et al: The effect of angiotensin-converting enzyme inhibitors on progression of advanced polycystic kidney disease. Kidney Int 2005;67:265–271. *Meta-analysis showing improvement in some markers of renal function but not in overall progression of disease.*

Ong AC, Harris PC: Molecular pathogenesis of ADPKD: The polycystin complex gets complex. Kidney Int 2005;67:1234–1247. *A comprehensive review of the types of mutations in ADPKD and the pros and cons of the ciliocentric model in cystogenesis.*

Ruggenenti P, Remuzzi A, Ondei P, et al: Safety and efficacy of long-acting somatostatin treatment in autosomal-dominant polycystic kidney disease. Kidney Int 2005;68:206–216. *A short-term clinical trial showing that a 6-month course of somatostatin therapy in a small number of ADPKD patients is safe and may slow renal volume expansion.*

Torres VE, Harris PC, Pirsm Y, et al: Autosomal dominant polycystic kidney disease. Lancet 2007;369:1287–1301. *A comprehensive overview of pathogenesis, diagnosis, and treatment.*

Torres VE, Wang X, Qian Q, et al: Effective treatment of an orthologous model of autosomal dominant polycystic kidney disease. Nat Med 2004;10:363–364. *Study showing that in a mouse model of PKD2 ADPKD, OPC31260 treatment reduced renal cAMP levels, prevented renal enlargement, inhibited cystogenesis, and was renoprotective.*

129 HEREDITARY NEPHROPATHIES AND ABNORMALITIES OF THE URINARY TRACT

Lisa M. Guay-Woodford

DEVELOPMENT OF THE KIDNEY AND URINARY TRACT

The human kidney and urogenital tract develop from three principal embryonic structures: the metanephric mesenchyme, the mesonephric (wolffian) duct, and the cloaca (Fig. 129–1). At 4 to 5 weeks of gestation, the ureteric bud originates as a diverticulum of the mesonephric duct. Reciprocal interactions between the branching ureteric bud and the metanephric mesenchyme induce kidney development, with the metanephros undergoing an epithelial transformation to form the glomeruli and the proximal and distal tubules. The ureteric bud branches give rise to the collecting ducts, the renal pelvis, the ureter, and the bladder trigone. Nephrogenesis is completed by 34 weeks of gestation.

Concurrent with the initial nephrogenic events, the urorectal fold divides the cloaca into the urogenital sinus and the future rectum. The mesonephric duct opening into the bladder becomes the vesicoureteric orifice of the trigone. Between 5 and 6 weeks of gestation, the second genital duct (müllerian duct) appears and runs in parallel with the wolffian duct. In males, the müllerian duct subsequently regresses, whereas the wolffian duct development proceeds to form the epididymis, the vas deferens, the seminal vesicle, and the ejaculatory duct. In the female, the wolffian duct regresses. The müllerian ducts fuse to form the ureterovaginal primordium, which merges with the urogenital sinus and eventually gives rise to the uterus, the oviducts, and the proximal vagina. The remnants of the allantois form the urachus, a fibrous cord that connects the bladder to the umbilicus.

Developmental abnormalities of the kidney and urinary tract are relatively common, affecting approximately 1 to 1.5% of newborns and accounting for almost one third of all congenital malformations. Some are asymptomatic and inconsequential, but many renal tract malformations are important causes of infant mortality and of morbidity in older children and adults, including the progression to renal failure.

ANOMALIES OF THE URINARY TRACT

Renal Parenchymal Malformations

Congenital defects in renal development may result in the absence of a kidney or abnormalities in kidney size, structure, or position. Irregu-

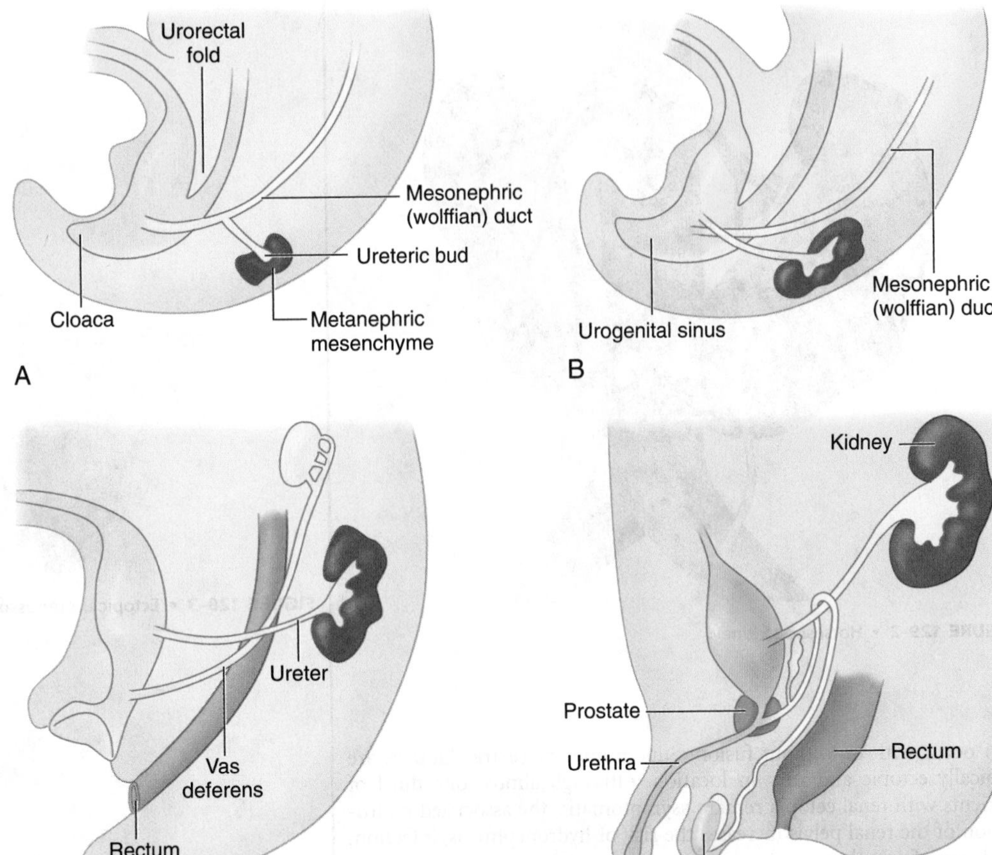

FIGURE 129–1 • Key events in the development of the urinary tract. In the 4-week embryo, the ureteric bud emerges from the wolffian duct **(A)**. Reciprocal interactions between the branching ureteric bud and the metanephric mesenchyme induce kidney development. Concurrently, the cloaca is divided by the urorectal fold into the urogenital sinus and the future rectum **(B)**. In the 8-week male embryo, the wolffian duct begins to give rise to the epididymis, the seminal vesicles, and the caudal part of the vas deferens **(C)**. By 9 weeks, axial growth of the fetal spine prompts the developing kidney to ascend from the pelvis to its final lumbar position. The external genitalia develop between 8 and 16 weeks, and testicular descent begins in month 7 of gestation **(D)**.

larities in the renal contour may arise from the persistence of fetal lobulation or a depression in the midpole of the left kidney by the spleen (a "dromedary hump"). Neither irregularity causes renal functional impairment.

Renal Agenesis

Renal agenesis reflects a complete failure of nephrogenesis. Unilateral agenesis can occur as an isolated abnormality or as a component of syndromic disorders, such as Turner's syndrome. As an isolated entity, the complete absence of one kidney occurs in 1 : 500 to 1 : 1000 individuals. The incidence is higher in males and occurs somewhat more frequently on the left side. Absence of the ipsilateral ureter and hemitrigone occurs in about half the patients. The remaining kidney is usually enlarged due to compensatory hypertrophy, but it may be ectopic or malrotated. Vesicoureteral reflux (VUR) on the contralateral side is observed in about 30% of patients.

Renal agenesis is commonly associated with genital anomalies, suggesting that it represents a developmental field defect. In females, absence of the ipsilateral oviduct and malformation of the uterus and vagina result from maldevelopment of the müllerian duct, whereas in males, wolffian duct–derived structures, such as the vas deferens and the seminal vesicles, are often absent. Other associated anomalies can include cardiovascular malformations, vertebral defects, and imperforate anus.

Bilateral renal agenesis is associated with the "Potter phenotype," which includes pulmonary hypoplasia, a characteristic facies, and deformities of the spine and limbs. At birth, these neonates have a critical degree of pulmonary hypoplasia that is incompatible with survival.

The familial association of unilateral and bilateral renal agenesis, renal dysplasia, and congenital hydronephrosis occurs in hereditary renal adysplasia (HRA) syndrome, an autosomal dominant disorder with variable penetrance.

Renal Hypoplasia

Renal hypoplasia describes small kidneys with apparently normal renal parenchyma. True hypoplasia results from impaired postnatal nephron growth. *Oligomeganephronia* describes a form of bilateral renal hypoplasia with marked reduction in nephron number and associated hypertrophy of individual glomeruli and tubules. This abnormality occurs sporadically as an isolated developmental defect that must be differentiated from acquired renal atrophy and the nephronophthisis–medullary cystic disease complex. Renal function declines slowly, with progression to end-stage renal failure in the second to third decade of life.

Renal Dysplasia

Renal dysplasia can be associated with various abnormalities of kidney size and indicates abnormal metanephric differentiation that causes anomalous and/or incompletely differentiated renal elements. Small dysplastic kidneys are commonly referred to as *aplastic.* Large dysplastic kidneys are often cystic, with the most common type being referred to as *multicystic dysplasia.*

Unilateral dysplasia may be asymptomatic well into adult life. Small aplastic and large multicystic dysplastic kidneys are nonfunctioning and can be distinguished from renal agenesis by imaging studies. The ipsilateral ureter is typically atretic. Contralateral malformations, including obstruction and VUR, are common. Unilateral multicystic kidneys involute over time and often disappear. As noted, unilateral aplasia and multicystic dysplasia may be manifestations of the HRA syndrome.

Renal and Ureteral Structural Anomalies

Renal Malrotation and Ectopia

The metanephric kidney begins developing caudally in the embryo. By 9 weeks of gestation, the kidney has ascended to its normal level (L1–L3), and the renal pelvis has rotated 90 degrees toward the midline. Anomalies of ascent and/or failure of rotation are common. Bilateral renal ectopia is often associated with kidney fusion. The most common renal fusion anomaly is the horseshoe kidney, which occurs in 1 of every 500 births with a 2 : 1 male predominance. Renal ascent is prevented by the root of the inferior mesenteric artery (Fig. 129–2). Crossed renal ectopia

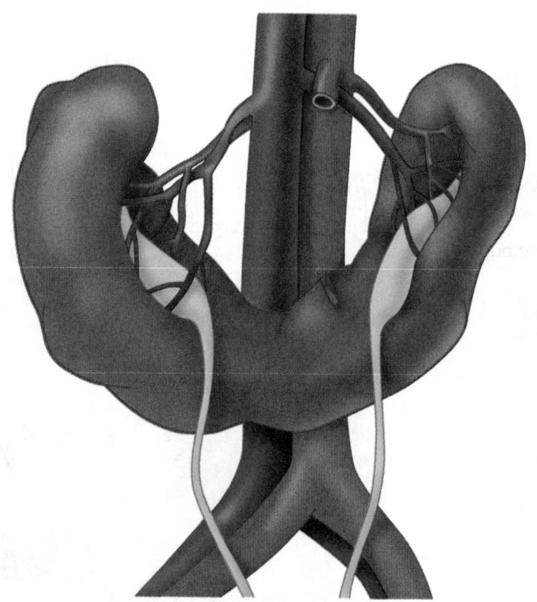

FIGURE 129–2 • Horseshoe kidney.

can occur with or without fusion. Supernumerary (extra) kidneys are typically ectopic and vary in location. Although almost one third of patients with renal ectopia remain asymptomatic, the associated malrotation of the renal pelvis increases the risk of hydronephrosis, infection, and stone formation.

Pelviureteral Abnormalities

Obstruction of the *ureteropelvic junction* (UPJ) impedes the flow of urine from the renal pelvis into the ureter. It is one of the most frequently occurring urinary tract anomalies in children and is the most common cause of collecting system dilatation in the fetal kidney. In congenital UPJ obstruction, urologic anomalies in the contralateral system are common, including renal agenesis, renal dysplasia, multicystic dysplasia, UPJ obstruction, and VUR. UPJ obstruction may also occur in adults secondary to external compression, kinking, or stenosis of the proximal ureter. Surgical intervention is indicated if there is associated renal functional impairment, pyelonephritis, stones, or pain.

Hydrocalyx or *hydrocalycosis* refers to the dilatation of a major calyx that occurs in the context of intrinsic obstruction (as in infundibular stenosis) or extrinsic compression of the pelvis (caused by a vessel or a parapelvic cyst). In comparison, *megacalycosis* represents a nonobstructive, dysplastic lesion, primarily observed in males, in which the calyces are dilated and usually increased in number. Associated renal medullary hypoplasia causes malformation of the renal papillae.

Calyceal diverticula are cystic structures that are connected by a narrow channel to an adjacent minor calyx. In imaging studies, these diverticula typically fill with contrast material, which distinguishes them from renal parenchymal cysts.

Partial duplication of the renal pelvis and ureter is a common anomaly that is more frequent in females, is typically unilateral, and is clinically insignificant.

Ureteric Anomalies

Ectopic ureters usually reflect complete ureteric and renal duplication. Approximately 10% are bilateral. The ectopic ureter typically drains the dysplastic upper pole of a duplex kidney and inserts below the normal vesicoureteral junction into the lower trigone or the proximal urethra. Ectopic ureters occur much more frequently in females, and the insertion sites can include the vagina and the vulva, with resulting incontinence. An ectopic ureter often is associated with a *ureterocele*, a cystic dilatation of the terminal ureter (Fig. 129–3). In children, ureteroceles can be associated with urinary tract infection and obstruction of the bladder neck or even of the contralateral ureter. In adults, the clinical presentation is prompted by associated infection or ureteric stones or both.

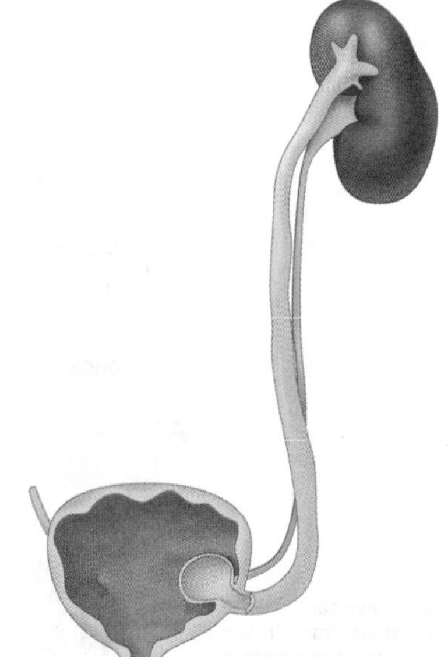

FIGURE 129–3 • Ectopic ureter associated with a ureterocele.

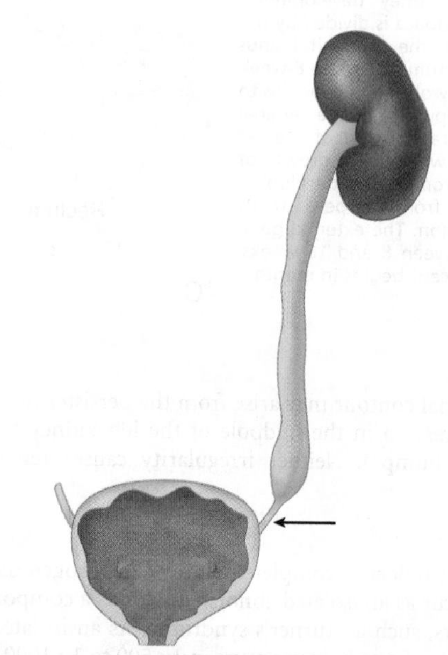

FIGURE 129–4 • Megaureter with the aperistaltic segment (arrow).

A *megaureter*, or grossly dilated ureter, has multiple potential causes, including intrinsic ureteric obstruction by a stone, bladder outflow obstruction, VUR, and external compression of the distal ureter. In contrast, a *primary megaureter* results from a functional obstruction of the distal ureter caused by an aperistaltic segment (Fig. 129–4).

Vesicoureteral Reflux

In the normal urinary tract, urinary reflux from the bladder into the ureters is prevented by a functional valve-like mechanism at the vesicoureteral junction. The competence of this valve is dependent on several critical factors, such as the intramural length of the ureter, the position of the ureteric orifice in the bladder, and the integrity of the bladder wall musculature. Primary VUR results from incompetence of the vesicoureteral junction due to the short length of the ureter's submucosal segment and the lateral, ectopic position of its orifice. As the intramural ureter lengthens with age, primary VUR tends to remit or disappear. Genetic factors appear to contribute to the pathogenesis of primary VUR, as there is a 30- to 50-fold increased risk of VUR in immediate relatives of an index case. VUR also can occur secondary to obstructive maldevelopment of the lower urinary tract, such as in triad syndrome and posterior urethral valves.

In both primary and secondary VUR, intrarenal reflux can lead to the development of *reflux nephropathy,* a tubulointerstitial lesion associated with gross scarring at the renal poles. In addition, the development of a glomerular lesion consistent with focal and segmental glomerulosclerosis can cause proteinuria, hypertension, and a progressive loss of renal function.

Lower Urinary Tract Abnormalities

Triad Syndrome (Prune-Belly Syndrome, Eagle-Barrett Syndrome)

Triad syndrome, also referred to as the *prune-belly syndrome* or *Eagle-Barrett syndrome,* involves a constellation of anomalies including congenital absence/deficiency of the abdominal wall musculature, gross ureteral dilatation, hypotonic bladder, prostatic hypoplasia, and bilateral undescended testes (cryptorchidism). The full syndrome is expressed only in males, and surviving individuals are typically infertile. Patients with an incomplete syndrome can have anomalies of the abdominal wall musculature, bladder, and upper urinary tract; 3% of these patients are females. Although the specific molecular events have yet to be defined, defects in mesenchymal development appear to cause poor prostate and bladder differentiation, ureteral smooth muscle aplasia with consequent ureteral aperistalsis, and varying degrees of renal dysplasia. Three-fourths of patients with triad syndrome have associated malformations in the cardiopulmonary system, the gastrointestinal tract, and the skeleton. In the immediate postnatal period, prognosis depends on the severity of extragenitourinary anomalies. Long-term outcome correlates with the degree of renal dysplasia and the success of urodynamic management.

Bladder Abnormalities

Bladder exstrophy results from a midline closure defect involving the lower anterior abdominal wall, the bladder, and the external genitalia. These abnormalities have been attributed to a primary defect in the differentiation of the cloacal membrane, but the precise molecular events are unclear. In severe cases, bladder exstrophy may be associated with imperforate anus and rectal atresia. However, other congenital anomalies are rarely associated. Clinical studies indicate that there is a correlation between the success of bladder reconstruction and long-term preservation of renal function.

In adults, *neuropathic bladder* has numerous etiologic contributors, such as central nervous system trauma, stroke, disorders such as Parkinson's disease, spinal trauma, multiple sclerosis, and peripheral nerve damage caused by trauma or surgery. In children, myelomeningocele (spina bifida) is the most common cause of neurogenic bladder dysfunction. Other forms of myelodysplasia, such as spinal dysraphism (spina bifida occulta) and sacral agenesis, are less common causes.

Posterior Urethral Valves

In male infants, posterior urethral valves (PUVs) are the most common cause of bladder outflow obstruction with resulting bilateral hydronephrosis and megaureters. However, among all infants with hydronephrosis, only 10% have PUVs. The urethral obstruction results from a defective reabsorption of mucosal folds in the posterior urethra, just distal to the verumontanum. As a result, dilatation of the proximal urethra, bladder wall hypertrophy and trabeculation, associated VUR, and varying degrees of renal dysplasia are present (Fig. 129–5). Patient survival and long-term renal outcome depend on the severity of the associated renal dysplasia.

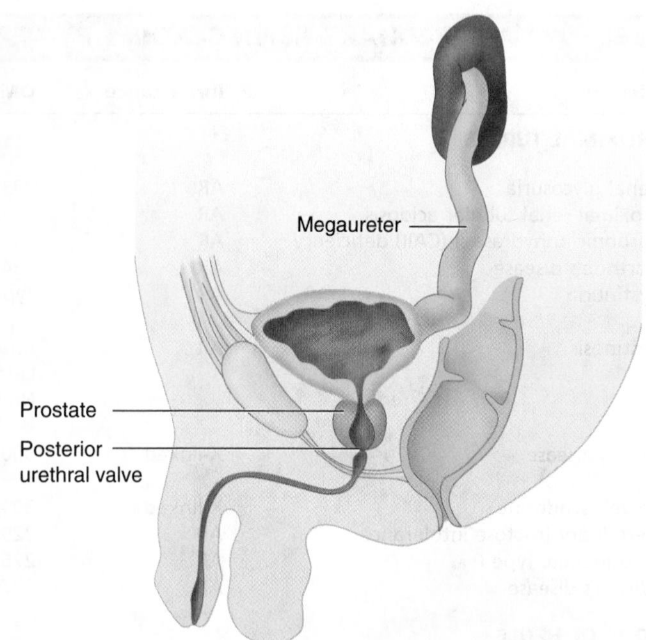

FIGURE 129–5 • Bladder outlet obstruction caused by posterior urethral valves.

HEREDITARY NEPHROPATHIES

Inherited renal tubular disorders are a group of conditions in which the renal tubular reabsorption of ions, organic solutes, and water is disrupted. These defects can be categorized by the nephron segment affected (Table 129–1). As noted in Chapter 123, the proximal tubule is responsible for reclaiming most of the filtered glucose, amino acids, uric acid, phosphate, bicarbonate, and low-molecular-weight proteins. The loop of Henle and the distal nephron reabsorb 25 to 50% of the filtered sodium chloride and divalent cations. The collecting duct, under the regulatory control of aldosterone, fine-tunes sodium reabsorption and secretes hydrogen and potassium ions. In the terminal collecting duct, antidiuretic hormone regulates water reabsorption and urinary concentration.

Disorders of Proximal Tubule Function

Cystinuria

Cystinuria is characterized by defective proximal tubular reabsorption of cystine and dibasic amino acids, resulting in the formation of urinary calculi. Cystinuria is transmitted as an autosomal recessive trait with an estimated prevalence of 1 in 7000 individuals. Clinically, cystinuria is classified based on the level of cystine excretion in heterozygotes: Type I, normal range; Type non-I, high range; and mixed. Stone formation usually becomes evident in the second or third decade of life, and males are typically more severely affected than females. However, the clinical presentation is quite variable and may occur from infancy to the seventh decade. Affected children can be identified by elevated urinary cystine levels, but testing must be performed after tubular transport has fully matured (age 2 years). Cystine stones are radiopaque and often form the nidus for secondary calcium oxalate stone formation. Symptoms include renal colic, which may be associated with urinary tract obstruction and/or infection. Conservative therapy with high urine volume and urinary alkalinization is sufficient for many patients with cystinuria, but recurrent stone formation may cause renal damage and warrants prophylaxis with thiol agents that form mixed disulfides with cystine.

Two cystinuria genes have been identified: *SLC7A9,* which encodes the luminal transport channel itself, and *SLC3A1,* which encodes the transporter regulatory subunit. Several large studies indicate that mutations in *SLC3A1* are more common than mutations in *SLC7A9.* Based on these data, a stepwise algorithm has been developed for genetic screening in patients with cystinuria that provides a low-cost, reliable, and time-saving diagnostic tool.

Cystinosis

Cystinosis is the most common inherited cause of the renal Fanconi's syndrome, as well as a multisystem disorder that affects the eyes, muscles, central nervous system, lungs, and various endocrine organs. Three clinical presentations have been described. The most severe of these is infantile cystinosis, which manifests in the first year of life with renal tubular acidosis (RTA), impaired growth, and evidence of the Fanconi syndrome including aminoaciduria, glycosuria, phosphaturia, and low-molecular-weight proteinuria. Progressive renal failure occurs and reaches end stage in childhood. A less severe, juvenile form involves renal dysfunction that

TABLE 129–1 HEREDITARY NEPHROPATHIES BY NEPHRON SEGMENT

Disorder	Inheritance	OMIM*	Major Renal Features
PROXIMAL TUBULE			
Renal glycosuria	AR	233100	Isolated glycosuria
Proximal renal tubular acidosis	AR	604278	Hyperchloremic, hypokalemic metabolic acidosis
Carbonic anhydrase II (CAII) deficiency	AR	259730	Mixed proximal and distal renal tubular acidosis
Hartnup's disease	AR	234500	Neutral aminoaciduria
Cystinuria	AR	Type A: 220100 Type B: 604144	Urinary calculi
Cystinosis	AR	Infantile: 219800 Late-onset: 219900 Non-nephropathic: 219750	Fanconi's syndrome
Dent's disease	X-linked	300009	Nephrocalcinosis, urinary calculi; low-molecular-weight proteinuria
Lowe's syndrome	X-linked	309000	Fanconi's syndrome
Hereditary fructose intolerance	AR	229600	Fanconi's syndrome
Tyrosinemia, type I	AR	276700	Fanconi's syndrome
Wilson's disease	AR	277900	Fanconi's syndrome
LOOP OF HENLE			
Bartter's syndrome	AR	Type I: 601678 Type II: 241200 Type III: 607364 Type IV: 602522	Hypokalemic, hypochloremic metabolic alkalosis
DISTAL TUBULE			
Gitelman's syndrome	AR	263800	Hypokalemic, hypochloremic metabolic alkalosis
Familial hypomagnesemia with hypercalciuria	AR	248250	Severe renal magnesium and calcium wasting
Isolated hypomagnesemia	AD	154020	Renal magnesium wasting
COLLECTING DUCT			
Glucocorticoid-remediable hyperaldosteronism	AD	103900	Low-renin hypertension
Liddle's syndrome	AD	177200	Low-renin hypertension
Apparent mineralocorticoid excess	AR	218030	Low-renin hypertension
Pseudohypoaldosteronism, type 1	AR, AD	AR: 264350 AD: 177735	Hyponatremic, hypokalemic metabolic acidosis
Pseudohypoaldosteronism, type 2 (Gordon's syndrome)	AD	114300	Low-renin hypertension with hyperkalemia
Distal renal tubular acidosis	AR, AD	AR: 602722 AD: 179800	Hyperchloremic, hypokalemic metabolic acidosis
Carbonic anhydrase II (CAII) deficiency	AR	259730	Mixed proximal and distal renal tubular acidosis
Nephrogenic diabetes insipidus	X-linked, AR, AD	X-linked: 304800 AR and AD: 125800	Urinary concentrating defect

*Entries in Online Mendelian Inheritance in Man, OMIM. Available at: www.ncbi.nlm.nih.gov/omim/ (accessed June 26, 2006).
AD = autosomal dominant; AR = autosomal recessive.

begins later in childhood and involves cystine deposits in the cornea. The mildest form, non-nephropathic cystinosis, features photophobia but no renal problems.

Cystinosis is an autosomal recessive disorder caused by mutations in the gene *CTNS*, which encodes cystinosin, a lysosomal cystine transporter. Defects in this transporter lead to the accumulation of intralysosomal cystine crystals and widespread cellular destruction. The mainstay of cystinosis therapy is oral cysteamine (Cystagon), an aminothiol that can lower intracellular cystine content by 95%. In well-treated adolescent and young adult patients, cysteamine has proven efficacy in delaying renal glomerular deterioration, enhancing growth, preventing hypothyroidism, and lowering muscle cystine content. Therefore, early diagnosis and prompt, proper treatment are critical for preventing, or significantly delaying, the complications of cystinosis.

Disorders of Loop of Henle and Distal Tubule Function

The Bartter-Gitelman Disorders

The Bartter-Gitelman syndromes are a group of disorders characterized by markedly reduced salt transport in the thick ascending limb of Henle (Bartter's syndrome) or in the distal convoluted tubule (Gitelman's syndrome). Individuals with Bartter's syndrome exhibit renal salt wasting and lowered blood pressure, polyuria, hypokalemic metabolic alkalosis, and hypercalciuria with a variable risk of nephrocalcinosis.

Mutations in one of four genes—*SLC12A2*, encoding the sodium-potassium-chloride cotransporter, NKCC2; *KCNJ1*, encoding the ROMK1 potassium ion channel; *CLCNKB*, encoding the ClC-Kb baso-

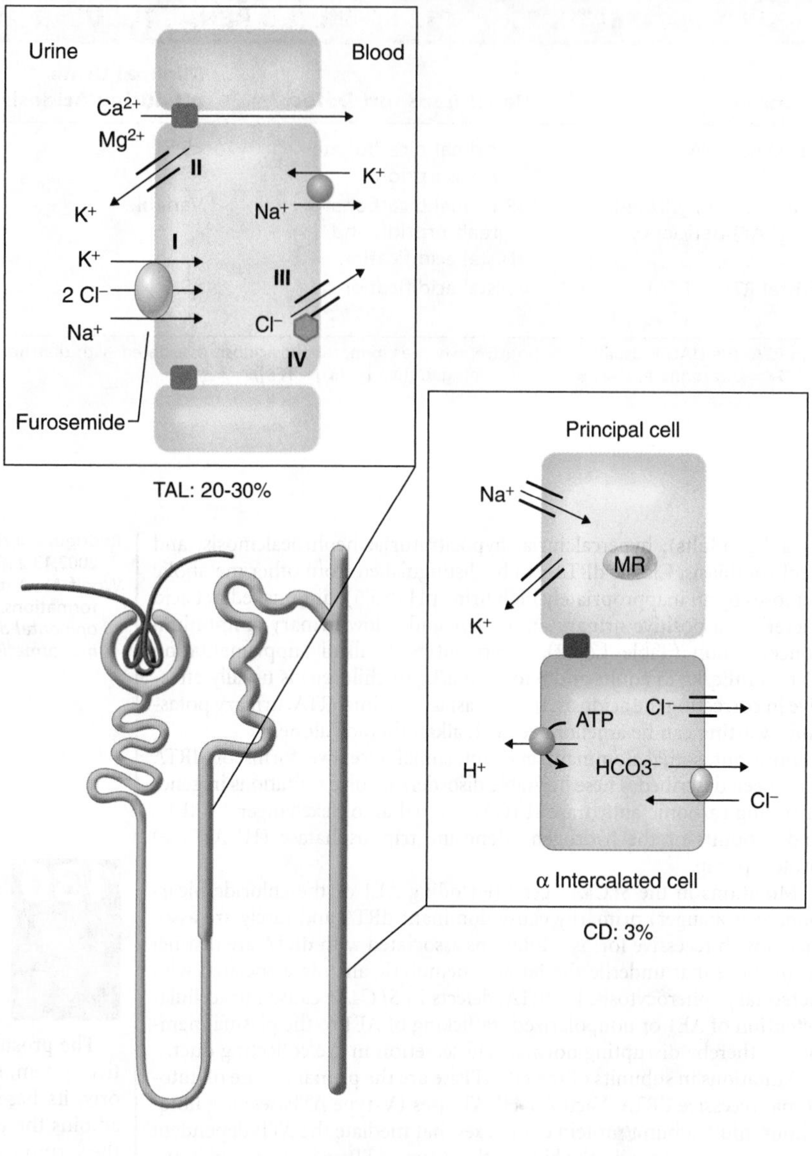

FIGURE 129–6 • Transport in the thick ascending limb (TAL) and the pathophysiology of Bartter's syndrome. Sodium (Na^+), potassium (K^+), and chloride (Cl^-) are reabsorbed across the apical membrane via the sodium-potassium-chloride cotransporter, NKCC2 (defective in Bartter's syndrome type I). NKCC2 can be inhibited by furosemide. The optimal function of this transporter requires the binding of all four ions. Because of the low luminal concentration of potassium, K^+ binding becomes the rate-limiting step. Therefore, to ensure an adequate luminal supply, potassium is recycled through the ROMK1 channel (defective in Bartter's syndrome type II). These apical transport processes result in a relative excess of positive charges in the tubular lumen, providing the driving force for paracellular absorption of calcium (Ca^{2+}) and magnesium (Mg^{2+}). Na^+ exits across the basolateral membrane via the sodium-potassium adenosine triphosphatase (Na^+,K^+-ATPase) pump, whereas Cl^- exits through the chloride channels ClC-Kb (defective in Bartter's syndrome type III) and ClC-Ka. Both channels require barttin (defective in Bartter's syndrome type IV) for proper membrane localization. The TAL reabsorbs approximately 25% of the filtered sodium load, whereas the collecting duct (CD) is responsible for reabsorbing about 3% of the sodium load. The profound defect in TAL sodium reabsorption leads to salt wasting; stimulation of the renin-aldosterone system; and aldosterone-induced increase in potassium and hydrogen ion secretion in the CD, with resultant hypokalemic, metabolic alkalosis. MR = mineralocorticoid receptor.

lateral chloride ion channel; and *BSND*, encoding barttin, a regulatory subunit that is required for basolateral chloride channel targeting to the membrane—cause autosomal recessive Bartter's syndrome types I, II, III, and IV, respectively. Defects in any of these genes disrupt salt transport in the thick ascending limb, causing a furosemide-like effect (Fig. 129–6). In addition, severe gain-of-function mutations in *CASR*, the gene encoding the extracellular calcium ion–sensing receptor (CaSR), can cause a Bartter-like phenotype (referred to as Bartter type V) that is distinguished from Bartter's syndrome types I through IV by autosomal dominant transmission and associated hypocalcemic hypercalciuria.

In comparison, individuals with Gitelman's syndrome exhibit milder renal salt wasting, normal blood pressure, hypokalemic metabolic alkalosis, hypomagnesemia, and hypocalciuria. This clinical disorder resembles the effect of long-term thiazide administration. Most patients have defects in *SLC12A3*, the gene encoding the sodium-chloride cotransporter, NCCT. However, a minority of patients with the Gitelman phenotype have mutations in *CLCNKB*.

Therefore, six genes have been identified as causing Bartter's syndrome (types I through V) and Gitelman's syndrome, with the unifying pathophysiology being defects in salt transport, either in the thick ascending limb or in the distal convoluted tubule. Clinical differences between Bartter's and Gitelman's syndrome relate to the severity of the associated salt wasting; whereas phenotypic differences among Bartter types I through V correlate with the specific physiologic roles that the individual transporters or channels play in the kidney and other organ systems. The mainstay of treatment includes replacing salt and water losses and providing potassium supplementation. In patients with Bartter's syndrome who present in the perinatal period (types I and II), cyclooxygenase inhibitors (ibuprofen, indomethacin, celecoxib) may be beneficial. In patients with Gitelman's syndrome and some of those with Bartter's syndrome type III, oral magnesium supplementation may be required.

Disorders of Collecting Duct Function

Liddle's Syndrome (Pseudoaldosteronism)

Liddle's syndrome is an autosomal dominant form of salt-sensitive hypertension. The severe hypertension typically manifests in childhood, with features of hypokalemic metabolic alkalosis that resemble primary aldosteronism but in which renin and aldosterone secretion are suppressed. The clinical abnormalities can be ameliorated by a low-salt diet plus amiloride or triamterene, which are antagonists of the epithelial sodium channel (ENaC).

The ENaC, composed of α, β, and γ subunits, is expressed at the apical surface of collecting duct cells and plays a critical role in maintaining salt balance and blood pressure. Both the β and the γ subunit regulate the channel activity of the α subunit. Mutations in either of these regulatory subunits result in increased ENaC activity and Liddle's syndrome.

Distal Renal Tubular Acidosis

Distal renal tubular acidosis (dRTA) results from failure of the collecting duct α-intercalated cells to excrete fixed acids (see Fig. 116–10 and Fig. 118–3). Clinical consequences include hypokalemic, hyperchloremic metabolic acidosis; impaired growth and rickets (in children); osteoma-

TABLE 129–2 FEATURES OF THE INHERITED RENAL TUBULAR ACIDOSES (RTAs)

Disorder	Renal Transport Defect	Minimal Urine pH during Acidosis	Alkali Supplementation (HCO_3^-)	UAG during Acidosis*
Proximal RTA	↓Proximal bicarbonate reabsorption	<5.5	Children: 10–15 mEq/kg/d	0 or +
Carbonic anhydrase II (CAII) deficiency	↓Proximal bicarbonate reabsorption and ↓Distal acidification	Variable	Variable	0 or +
Distal RTA (dRTA)	↓Distal acidification	>5.5	Adults: 1–3 mEq/kg/d Children: 3–6 mEq/kg/d	0 or +

*In RTA, the UAG is usually 0 or positive, whereas in metabolic acidosis associated with diarrheal illness, the UAG is negative.
HCO_3^- = bicarbonate; UAG = urinary anion gap ($[Na^+] + [K^+] - [Cl^-]$).

lacia (in adults); hypercalciuria; hypocitraturia; nephrocalcinosis; and nephrolithiasis. Classic dRTA can be distinguished from other metabolic acidoses by an inappropriately high urine pH (>5.5), diminished net acid excretion, a positive urinary anion gap, and a low urinary ammonium concentration (Table 129–2). Treatment with alkali supplementation (1 to 3 mEq/kg in adults and 3 to 6 mEq/kg in children) is usually effective in correcting the acidosis. In contrast to proximal RTA, urinary potassium wasting can be ameliorated with alkali therapy alone.

Both autosomal dominant and autosomal recessive forms of dRTA have been described. These heritable disorders involve mutations in genes encoding carbonic anhydrase II (CAII), renal anion exchanger 1 (AE1), and subunits of the hydrogen–adenosine triphosphatase (H^+-ATPase) proton pump.

Mutations in the *SLC4A1* gene (encoding AE1 or the chloride/bicarbonate exchanger) primarily cause dominant dRTA and rarely are associated with recessive forms. Mutations associated with dRTA are distinct from those that underlie the familial hemolytic anemia associated with hereditary spherocytosis. In dRTA, defects in *SLC4A1* cause intracellular retention of AE1 or nonpolarized trafficking of AE1 to the plasma membrane, thereby disrupting normal acid secretion in the collecting duct.

Mutations in subunits of the H^+-ATPase are the primary cause of autosomal recessive dRTA. Vacuolar H^+-ATPases (V-type ATPases) are ubiquitous, multisubunit protein complexes that mediate the ATP-dependent transport of protons. In the kidney, the V-type ATPase is expressed in the plasma membrane along almost the entire length of the nephron, with apical and/or basolateral localization patterns. V-type ATPases are the major proton-secreting pumps in the distal nephron and are involved in net proton secretion (bicarbonate generation) or proton reabsorption (net bicarbonate secretion). Defects in two genes, *ATP6B1* and *ATP6N1B*, cause dRTA with or without associated sensorineural deafness. The *ATP6B1* gene encodes the B1 subunit of the V-type ATPase, which is expressed in renal tubular epithelia, in the cochlea, and in endolymphatic epithelia. In the ear, the H^+-ATPase regulates the pH of the endolymph, a function that is critical for hair cell survival and normal hearing. The *ATP6N1B* gene encodes the accessory a4 isoform, and mutations in this gene are not associated with deafness.

SUGGESTED READINGS

Atala A, Bauer SB, Soker S, et al: Tissue-engineered autologous bladders for patients needing cystoplasty. Lancet 2006;367:1241–1246. *Engineered bladder tissues can be used in patients who need cystoplasty.*

Dello Strology I, Rizzoni G: Cystinuria. Acta Paediatr Suppl 2006;95:31–33. *A brief review.*

Garofeanu CG, Weir M, Rosas-Arellano MP, et al: Causes of reversible nephrogenic diabetes insipidus: A systematic review. Am J Kidney Dis 2005;45:626–637. *The most common risk factors are lithium, antibiotics, antifungals, antineoplastic agents, antivirals, and metabolic disturbances.*

Laing CM, Unwin RJ: Renal tubular acidosis. J Nephrol 2006;19(Suppl 9):S46–S52. *A clinical overview.*

Murer L, Benetti E, Artifoni L: Embryology and genetics of primary vesico-ureteric reflux and associated renal dysplasia. Pediatr Nephrol 2007;22:788–797. *An overview of the embryology and genetics of primary reflux.*

O'Shaughnessy KM, Karet FE: Salt handling and hypertension. J Clin Invest 2004;113:1075–1081. *An excellent overview of the key gene defects associated with abnormalities of renal salt handling.*

Rodriguez Soriano J: Renal tubular acidosis: The clinical entity. J Am Soc Nephrol 2002;13:2160–2170.

Woolf AS: A molecular and genetic view of human renal and urinary tract malformations. Kidney Int 2000;58:500–512. *An integrated review of the developmental defects and genetic factors that contribute to human urinary tract malformations.*

130 BENIGN PROSTATE DISEASE AND PROSTATITIS

Michael J. Barry and Mary McNaughton-Collins

The prostate gland, the largest accessory gland in the male reproductive system, surrounds the prostatic urethra below the bladder. Superiorly, its base is contiguous with the bladder neck; inferiorly, its apex adjoins the urogenital diaphragm. The prostatic urethra is angulated at the verumontanum, the union with the two ejaculatory ducts. In younger men, the prostate weighs about 20 g. As men age, the prostate enlarges and develops a characteristic zonal anatomy (Fig. 130–1). Its acini communicate with the urethra via prostatic ducts, and it supplies about 20% of the semen volume. Prostatic fluid is rich in citrate, zinc, and polyamines, although their roles in reproduction are poorly defined.

BENIGN PROSTATIC HYPERPLASIA

Definition

Benign prostatic hyperplasia (BPH) is defined histologically by hyperplasia of both epithelial and stromal cells, beginning in the periurethral area. The hyperplasia can be symmetrical or asymmetrical and is generally progressive over time. With aging, multiple small hyperplastic nodules grow, coalesce, and compress normal tissue outward against the true prostatic capsule and create a surgical capsule bounding the expanding adenoma.

Epidemiology

The hyperplastic process often begins in the 30s; by 80 years of age, 85% of men have BPH. The age-specific prevalence of BPH at autopsy is remarkably similar among men of different ethnicities. Aging and functioning testes are the dominant risk factors. The onset of clinical manifestations of BPH before age 65 in a first-degree relative is also a risk factor. The prevalence of clinical manifestations is uncertain because of lack of consensus on a working definition. Nevertheless, about a third of U.S. men aged 40 to 79 years have moderate to severe lower urinary tract symptoms, a majority of which are attributable to BPH.

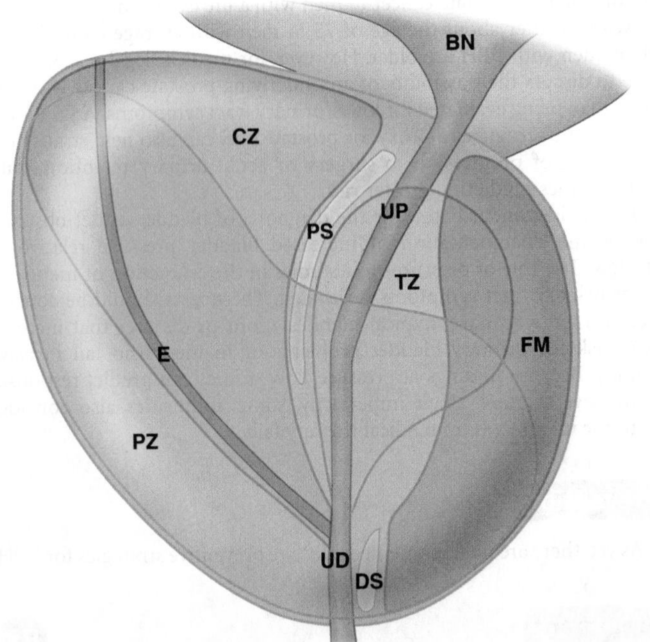

FIGURE 130–1 • Sagittal diagram of the distal prostatic urethral segment (UD), proximal urethral segment (UP), and ejaculatory ducts (E) showing their relationships to a sagittal section of the anteromedial nonglandular tissues (bladder neck [BN], anterior fibromuscular stroma [FM], preprostatic sphincter [PS], and distal striated sphincter [DS]). These structures are shown in relation to a three-dimensional representation of the glandular prostate: central zone (CZ), peripheral zone (PZ), and transitional zone (TZ). (From McNeal J: Normal histology of the prostate. Am J Surg Pathol 1988;12:619–633, with permission.)

Pathobiology

Testosterone is converted by the 5α-reductase enzyme to dihydrotestosterone (DHT), the major intraprostatic androgen. BPH does not develop in men who are castrated before puberty or have 5α-reductase deficiency. Although the type 2 isoenzyme predominates in the prostate, the type 1 isoenzyme predominates elsewhere. An array of peptide growth factors, along with DHT, mediate stromal-epithelial interactions that alter the balance of cell proliferation and apoptosis and thereby lead to BPH. The mechanisms are poorly understood.

The genetics of BPH are also unclear. There may be an autosomal dominant hereditary form accounting for less than 10% of cases.

Clinical Manifestations

The morbidity of BPH is conferred through bothersome lower urinary tract symptoms. Traditionally, voiding symptoms, such as hesitancy, straining, a sense of incomplete emptying, intermittency, a weak stream, and postvoid dribbling, were considered to be a consequence of mechanical bladder outlet obstruction. Filling symptoms, such as frequency, nocturia, urgency, and urge incontinence, were thought to be due to secondary uninhibited detrusor contractions. However, poor correlations among symptom severity, prostate size, degree of obstruction, and detrusor instability suggest that their origin is more complex. The key lower urinary tract symptoms of BPH can be quantified by using the seven symptom questions in the International Prostate Symptom Score (IPSS) (Fig. 130–2).

Bladder outlet obstruction as a result of BPH has both static and dynamic components. The static component is due to the enlarged prostate, whereas the dynamic component is due to increased adrenergic tone in the prostate, where α_2-adrenoreceptors predominate.

	Not at all	Less than 1 time in 5	Less than half the time	About half the time	More than half the time	Almost always
1. Over the past month or so, how often have you had a sensation of not emptying your bladder completely after you finished urinating?	0 ☐	1 ☐	2 ☐	3 ☐	4 ☐	5 ☐
2. Over the past month or so, how often have you had to urinate again less than two hours after you finished urinating?	0 ☐	1 ☐	2 ☐	3 ☐	4 ☐	5 ☐
3. Over the past month or so, how often have you found you stopped and started again several times when you urinated?	0 ☐	1 ☐	2 ☐	3 ☐	4 ☐	5 ☐
4. Over the past month or so, how often have you found it difficult to postpone urination?	0 ☐	1 ☐	2 ☐	3 ☐	4 ☐	5 ☐
5. Over the past month or so, how often have you had a weak urinary stream?	0 ☐	1 ☐	2 ☐	3 ☐	4 ☐	5 ☐
6. Over the past month or so, how often have you had to push or strain to begin urination?	0 ☐	1 ☐	2 ☐	3 ☐	4 ☐	5 ☐

7. Over the past month, how many times did you most typically get up to urinate from the time you went to bed at night until the time you got up in the morning?

0 ☐ none	1 ☐ 1 time	2 ☐ 2 times	3 ☐ 3 times	4 ☐ 4 times	5 ☐ 5 or more times

Total IPSS Score = sum of questions 1–7 = ______

Quality of life due to urinary symptoms

If you were to spend the rest of your life with your urinary condition just the way it is now, how would you feel about that?

Delighted	Pleased	Mostly satisfied	Mixed—about equally satisfied and dissatisfied	Mostly dissatisfied	Unhappy	Terrible
0 ☐	1 ☐	2 ☐	3 ☐	4 ☐	5 ☐	6 ☐

FIGURE 130–2 • International Prostate Symptom Score (IPSS). The seven symptom questions are part of a scale initially developed as the American Urological Association Symptom Index. The eighth question about symptom inconvenience is scored separately. (From Barry MJ, Fowler FJ Jr, O'Leary MP, et al: The American Urological Association symptom index for benign prostatic hyperplasia: The Measurement Committee of the American Urological Association. J Urol 1992;148:1549.)

In the setting of obstruction, increased detrusor pressure can result in detrusor hypertrophy and, eventually, fibrosis. Complications of BPH include acute urinary retention, which may result from prostatic infarction. Postvoid residual urine probably increases the risk for urinary tract infection or stone formation. With long-standing obstruction, hydroureter and hydronephrosis may develop and, eventually, renal failure. Men with BPH may have hematuria because there is often a complex of veins stretched over the enlarged prostate; however, other causes, especially malignancy, need to be considered.

Diagnosis

History

Usually, a working diagnosis of symptomatic BPH is made when an older man is evaluated for lower urinary tract symptoms. These symptoms should be quantified with the IPSS (see Fig. 130–2). Scores of 0 to 7 represent mild symptoms; 8 to 19, moderate symptoms; and 20 to 35, severe symptoms. The pattern of individual responses should be noted. When frequency and nocturia are the dominant symptoms, a voiding diary, in which the patient records the times and amounts of each void over a period of several days, may be helpful. For example, if the diary documents nocturnal polyuria alone, causes other than BPH should be strongly considered. Men with BPH tend to have a balance of voiding and filling symptoms that slowly progress with age. Rapid onset, manifestation before age 50, or filling symptoms without voiding symptoms are "red flags" suggesting alternative causes. A complete list of medications should be obtained because many, especially over-the-counter antihistamines, sympathomimetics, and anticholinergics, can affect the urinary tract.

Differential Diagnosis

Although lower urinary tract symptoms in older men are often due to BPH, the differential includes systemic diseases causing frequency and nocturia, such as diabetes and hypercalcemia, bladder outlet obstruction secondary to urethral strictures, and neurologic diseases affecting the bladder. A general medical history and the pattern of symptoms should provide clues to systemic diseases. Men with strictures have usually undergone genitourinary instrumentation or have had sexually transmitted diseases. Primary bladder problems should be suspected in men with previous stroke, Parkinson's disease, or diabetic neuropathy.

Physical Examination

The physical examination should include a digital rectal examination (DRE) and a focused neurologic examination to look for evidence of peripheral neuropathy or saddle-area anesthesia (the S2–4 segments innervate the bladder), which might suggest an underlying neuropathic bladder. The DRE should assess the size and consistency of the prostate. Classically, BPH causes a symmetrically enlarged, firm prostate, the consistency of the tip of the nose. Asymmetry or frank nodules suggest prostate cancer; however, prostate cancer can be present even when the prostate feels normal. Clinicians tend to underestimate prostate size; if the prostate feels enlarged, it usually is.

Laboratory Findings

Urinalysis should be performed for evidence of pyuria or hematuria. Optional studies include creatinine measurements, uroflow rates, and prostate-specific antigen (PSA) levels. Peak uroflow is often measured in urologists' offices, but it is unreliable with low voided volumes (<150 mL). Peak flows of less than 10 mL/sec are more suggestive of outlet obstruction, whereas flows greater than 15 mL/sec are less suggestive; unfortunately, men can have good flow with obstruction and forceful bladder contractions and poor flow without obstruction with weak bladder contractions.

PSA tests are used for early detection of prostate cancer; however, PSA has relatively poor specificity in this situation. Moreover, early detection of prostate cancer with PSA has not as yet been shown to reduce prostate cancer mortality in randomized trials. If a PSA assay is ordered, generally a level greater than 4 ng/mL should trigger an ultrasonography-guided prostate biopsy. Although about 50% of men with PSA levels greater than 10 ng/mL have prostate cancer at biopsy, about 25% with levels of 4.1 to 10.0 ng/mL have cancer, and 15% with levels of 4.0 ng/mL or less have cancer. Most authorities doubt the value of early detection of nonpalpable prostate cancer in men with a life expectancy of less than 10 years or after about the age of 75 in men with average comorbidity. Many men with BPH are older. However, for medical-legal reasons, it is wise to discuss the possibility of an underlying prostate cancer with any older man being evaluated for lower urinary tract symptoms. A PSA level, probably by serving as a proxy for prostate size, can also help stratify the future risk of progression to surgery or acute urinary retention, with higher values predicting greater risk.

The "gold standard" test for the diagnosis of bladder outlet obstruction is the documentation of increased bladder pressure relative to uroflow. The role of pressure-flow studies in the evaluation of men with lower urinary tract symptoms is debated. These tests should be considered in men who have atypical manifestations or diseases that increase their risk for primary bladder problems or in men who fail invasive therapy. Because findings at pressure-flow studies can predict responses to invasive therapy, albeit imperfectly, some authorities also consider them for men in whom medical therapy fails.

Prevention

As yet, there are no documented effective preventive strategies for BPH.

Treatment

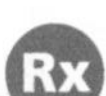

Men with IPSS scores in the mild range are rarely bothered enough to treat. Similarly, an enlarged prostate alone is not an indication for treatment. The key step in decision making for men with moderate or severe symptoms is to assess the degree to which they are bothering the patient. The last IPSS question (see Fig. 130–2) can serve as an entree into this discussion.

For men with little inconvenience, "watchful waiting" is appropriate. The patient's situation should be periodically reassessed. Avoidance of offending medications is also wise.

Medical Therapy

Most men with bothersome symptoms initially choose medical therapy. α_1-Adrenergic blockers and 5α-reductase inhibitors are the available prescription options. α-Blockers (Table 130–1) attack the dynamic component of BPH and have been shown to reduce symptoms in multiple clinical trials of up to 4 years' duration. [A] The response to α-blockers is independent of prostate size. In general, doses should be increased toward the maximum until the therapeutic effect is optimal, unless side effects are limiting. Doxazosin and terazosin are effective for the treatment of both BPH and hypertension; however, α-blocker monotherapy can no longer be consid-

TABLE 130–1 MEDICATIONS USED IN THE TREATMENT OF MEN WITH LOWER URINARY TRACT SYMPTOMS ATTRIBUTED TO BENIGN PROSTATIC HYPERPLASIA

Drug	Tablet/Capsule Sizes (mg)	Recommended Dose Steps
α-BLOCKERS		
Alfuzosin*	2.5	2.5 mg tid
Alfuzosin ER	10	10 mg qd
Doxazosin	1, 2, 4, 8	1, 2, 4, 8 mg qd
Doxazosin XL	4, 8	4, 8 mg qd
Tamsulosin	0.4	0.4, 0.8 mg qd
Terazosin	1, 2, 5, 10	1, 2, 5, 10 mg qd
5α-REDUCTASE INHIBITORS		
Finasteride	5	5 mg qd
Dutasteride	0.5	0.5 mg qd

*This drug has not been approved by the U.S. Food and Drug Administration at the time of publication.

ered optimal for hypertension. The effect of α-blockers on the risk of acute retention or progression to surgery over a period of 4 years is not significant.

In general, side effects of α-blockers include orthostatic hypotension, dizziness, and asthenia. Tamsulosin and alfuzosin appear to be more specific for the α_{1a}-receptor subtype, which dominates in the prostate. Both agents appear to have little or no effect on blood pressure. However, because the dizziness and asthenia seen with α-blockers are not primarily mediated through hypotension, a lack of head-to-head comparisons makes it unclear whether these agents have advantages other than a lower risk for orthostatic hypotension.

Finasteride and dutasteride are the 5α-reductase inhibitors available to date (see Table 130–1). These agents block conversion of testosterone to DHT by the type 2 isoenzyme (finasteride) or both isoenzymes (dutasteride). Prostate size decreases by 15 to 20% over a 1-year period of treatment with either agent. Finasteride and dutasteride reduce lower urinary tract symptoms more than placebo does in trials of 2 to 4 years in duration, although symptom relief is more modest than that seen with α-blockers. [2,3] In addition, these agents reduce the rate of progression to surgery and acute urinary retention in men with larger prostates. PSA levels can be used to stratify the preventive benefit of finasteride. The "number needed to treat" for 4 years to prevent an episode of acute retention or surgery is about 30 for men with PSA levels less than 1.4 ng/mL, about 20 for PSA levels of 1.4 to 3.2 ng/mL, and about 10 for PSA levels greater than 3.2 ng/mL.

The main side effect of finasteride and dutasteride is sexual or ejaculatory dysfunction in about 5% of men. Both agents lower PSA levels by about 50%. Although they do not appear to interfere with the detection of prostate cancer, PSA levels must be interpreted differently. The simplest strategy is to double the measured PSA and interpret it as usual. In a recent randomized trial, finasteride reduced the 7-year cumulative incidence of prostate cancer from 24 to 18% in a group of men who were heavily screened, including routine end-of-study biopsies. [4] However, because finasteride increased the risk for high-grade cancer from 5 to 6%, the ultimate impact of 5α-reductase inhibitors on prostate cancer mortality is uncertain.

Given the different mechanisms of α-blockers and 5α-reductase inhibitors, combination therapy is attractive. In a trial of 1 year's duration, finasteride offered no additional symptomatic benefit over α-blockers in terms of symptom reduction. [5] However, combination therapy was more effective than monotherapy with either doxazosin or finasteride in preventing disease progression, including symptom progression, over a period of 4 years. [2] When men have symptomatic BPH, an α-blocker is a reasonable first choice for medical therapy. Finasteride or dutasteride can be offered as well to men with palpably enlarged prostates or higher PSA levels for added preventive benefit.

Future directions in medical therapy include larger trials of various plant extracts, such as saw palmetto, which men widely use for lower urinary tract symptoms.

Surgical Therapy

Transurethral prostatectomy (TURP) is still considered the "gold standard" for treating BPH because it offers symptom reduction substantially greater than that achieved with medical therapy. TURP generally requires a brief hospital stay and an indwelling catheter at first. In a randomized trial comparing TURP with watchful waiting, both symptoms and BPH complications were substantially reduced with surgery. [6] Moreover, the risks of sexual dysfunction and incontinence were no greater with TURP. Standard TURP uses a wire electrode to resect obstructing tissue. Newer variations use a rolling electrode or laser energy to vaporize or resect prostate tissue. These procedures appear to result in less short-term bleeding and good short-term symptom improvement, but their long-term effectiveness is undefined.

Newer, less invasive surgical therapies, including ethanol injections, high-intensity focused ultrasound, and water-induced thermal therapy, are being developed in an attempt to marry the durable symptom relief of TURP with the ease and minimal side effects of medical therapy.

Ancillary Treatments

Minimally invasive techniques have been developed to relieve symptoms without hospitalization. Transurethral microwave thermotherapy (TUMT) heats and coagulates prostate tissue by using a microwave antenna surrounded by a cooling jacket to protect the urethra. Transurethral needle ablation (TUNA) uses radiofrequency needles placed directly in the prostate to generate heat and cause coagulation. The mechanisms by which these treatments work are poorly understood. However, they appear to produce an initial level of symptom relief intermediate between drug therapy and TURP. Their long-term effectiveness remains unclear.

Prognosis

Lower urinary tract symptoms attributable to BPH generally progress slowly over time, but individuals vary. For example, in one study of men with symptom scores in the moderate range who elected watchful waiting, after 4 years of follow-up, 13% had only mild symptoms, 46% still had moderate symptoms, 17% had severe symptoms, and 24% had opted for surgery. The risk of acute urinary retention in such men is 1 to 2% per year. More serious complications appear to be exceedingly rare.

PROSTATITIS

Definition

The validity of the traditional etiology-based classification of prostatitis has never been confirmed. The current National Institutes of Health (NIH) prostatitis classification system incorporates the terminology "chronic pelvic pain syndrome" to reflect uncertainty over whether chronic nonbacterial prostatitis and prostatodynia are in fact even related to the prostate (Table 130–2).

Epidemiology

Two million outpatient visits for prostatitis are made annually in the United States. The histologic prevalence ranges widely from 6 to 98%. The prevalence of current prostatitis-like symptoms or a previous physician's diagnosis of prostatitis is about 10%.

Pathobiology

Both type I (acute bacterial) and type II (chronic bacterial) prostatitis account for 5 to 10% of cases. Like urinary tract infections, 80% are due to strains of *Escherichia coli;* 10 to 15% are due to *Pseudomonas aeruginosa, Serratia, Klebsiella,* and *Proteus* species; and 5 to 10% are due to enterococci.

The remainder (>90%) of prostatitis cases are type III (chronic abacterial/chronic pelvic pain syndrome) prostatitis, but the pathogenesis of this type remains uncertain. Type III prostatitis is further divided into inflammatory (type IIIA) and noninflammatory (type IIIB) subtypes based on the presence of leukocytes in expressed prostatic secretions and prostatic urine. Given that there appears to be no correlation between the presence of leukocytes and symptoms, the subdivision into types IIIA and IIIB is controversial; many experts believe that both inflammatory and noninflammatory chronic prostatitis/chronic pelvic pain syndrome (CP/CPPS) are the same noninfectious condition, which may or may not be related to the prostate gland.

Theories for the etiology of type III prostatitis include infectious agents, such as *Mycoplasma hominis, Ureaplasma urealyticum, Trichomonas vaginalis, Chlamydia trachomatis,* viruses, anaerobic bacteria, and coagulase-negative staphylococci; pro-inflammatory cytokines; autoimmune mechanisms; neurogenic processes; increased prostate tissue pressure; chemical irritation; and increased tension in the muscles of the bladder neck and prostatic urethra or from tension myalgia of the pelvic floor. Psychological factors have also been implicated.

TABLE 130–2 CLASSIFICATION AND DEFINITION OF PROSTATITIS

Traditional Classification		National Institute of Diabetes and Digestive and Kidney Diseases Classification	
Category	**Definition**	**Category**	**Definition**
Acute bacterial prostatitis	Recovery of bacteria from prostatic fluid, purulence of fluid, and systemic signs of infectious illness (fever, chills, myalgia)	Type I (acute bacterial prostatitis)	Acute infection of the prostate
Chronic bacterial prostatitis	Recovery of bacteria in significant numbers from prostatic fluid in the absence of concomitant urinary infection or significant systemic signs (as in acute bacterial prostatitis)	Type II (chronic bacterial prostatitis)	Recurrent infection of the prostate
		Type III (chronic abacterial prostatitis/chronic pelvic pain syndrome)	No demonstrable infection
Nonbacterial prostatitis	No recovery of significant numbers of bacteria from prostatic fluid, but the fluid consistently reveals microscopic purulence	Type IIIA (inflammatory chronic pelvic pain syndrome)	Leukocytes in semen, expressed prostatic secretions, or post–prostatic massage urine
Prostatodynia	No recovery of significant bacteria or purulence in prostatic fluid, but patients have persistent urinary urgency, dysuria, poor urinary flow, and prostatic discomfort	Type IIIB (noninflammatory chronic pelvic pain syndrome)	No leukocytes in semen, expressed prostatic secretions, or post–prostatic massage urine
		Type IV (asymptomatic inflammatory prostatitis	No subjective symptoms; detected by prostate biopsy or by the presence of leukocytes in expressed prostatic secretions or semen during evaluation for other disorders

Clinical Manifestations

Type I prostatitis is characterized by the acute onset of fever, chills, and malaise; low back or perineal pain; and urinary symptoms, particularly dysuria, frequency, and urgency. The manifestation is generally dramatic, and the patient may appear toxic. DRE often reveals a markedly tender gland.

Type II prostatitis generally occurs in older men in association with recurrent urinary tract infections. The findings are less dramatic but involve similar lower urinary tract symptoms, pelvic pain, and sexual dysfunction. On DRE, the prostate may be normal, swollen, firm, or tender.

Type III prostatitis is characterized by pelvic pain, often associated with lower urinary tract symptoms and pain during or after ejaculation. DRE findings also vary.

Type IV prostatitis is, by definition, asymptomatic.

Because the hallmark of chronic prostatitis is a complex of symptoms that wax and wane, a brief, self-administered index has been developed and validated (NIH Chronic Prostatitis Symptom Index) to quantify them.

Diagnosis

Whereas acute prostatitis is relatively straightforward to diagnose, chronic prostatitis is more challenging. The symptom complexes of chronic prostatitis and BPH overlap such that BPH may be misdiagnosed in older men with chronic prostatitis. Although men can and do get both conditions, pain generally distinguishes chronic prostatitis from BPH. A PSA test is not indicated for the evaluation of chronic prostatitis; however, if a PSA test is performed and found to be elevated, the elevation should not be ascribed to CP/CPPS. In addition to BPH and prostate cancer, the differential diagnosis for chronic prostatitis includes sexually transmitted disease, urethritis, epididymitis, orchitis, urethral stricture, urinary tract infection, kidney stone, bladder cancer, hernia, pudendal artery insufficiency, sphincter dyssynergy, and neurogenic bladder.

Type I prostatitis is diagnosed primarily by clinical findings and a positive urine culture. Prostate massage is not recommended because of concern for bacteremia.

Type II and type III prostatitis are traditionally diagnosed with the four-glass test. This segmented, quantitative culture technique involves culturing initial-stream urine, midstream urine, expressed prostatic secretions after massage, and post–prostate massage urine. The simplified two-glass test involves culture and microscopic examination of urine obtained before and after prostatic massage; it is easier for all concerned, with similar operating characteristics. Although type II prostatitis is characterized by the presence of uropathogenic bacteria, it is the absence of uropathogens in the setting of genitourinary pain that defines type III prostatitis.

Type IV prostatitis is usually diagnosed incidentally by prostate biopsy or by finding leukocytes in prostatic secretions collected for infertility evaluation.

Prevention

There is no proven preventive strategy for any type of prostatitis.

Treatment

Rx

Type I prostatitis is relatively easy to treat. Antibacterial agents that normally diffuse poorly into prostatic fluid work well, probably because intense inflammation enhances penetration. The choice of antimicrobial is driven by culture results. Parenteral antibiotics are necessary for sicker patients, but oral fluoroquinolones or trimethoprim-sulfamethoxazole is adequate for outpatients. Treatment for 4 weeks is generally recommended.

Type II prostatitis is more difficult to treat because prostatic fluid becomes alkaline with chronic inflammation, thereby reducing antibiotic penetration. The fluoroquinolones and trimethoprim-sulfamethoxazole penetrate the prostate, but the penicillins, cephalosporins, aminoglycosides, and nitrofurantoin do not. Recommendations for the duration of therapy range from 6 to 12 weeks. The addition of an α-blocker may improve symptoms and reduce recurrences.

Type III prostatitis often engenders frustration on the part of the physician and confusion and dissatisfaction on the part of the patient. Because the cause is unknown, affected men receive various empirical therapies. The common practice of using antibiotics for chronic abacterial prostatitis is not supported by the existing evidence. [7,8] The effectiveness of α-blocker therapy, another common empirical treatment, remains uncertain. A 6-week trial of tamsulosin did not show symptom improvement [7]; however, pre-

Rx

vious trials had shown a benefit [9, 10]; longer courses of therapy may be more beneficial. Further research is needed to test longer durations of α-blocker therapy, as well as α-blocker therapy in men naïve to previous treatments. In small trials, quercetin, finasteride, [11] pentosan polysulfate sodium, [12] tadalafil, [13] and pelvic floor electromagnetic therapy [14] appear to show possible benefit; further evaluation is merited.

For type IV prostatitis, no treatment is recommended.

Prognosis

The untreated natural history of all types of prostatitis is poorly defined. Most patients with type I prostatitis respond well to antibiotics, but some may progress to chronic prostatitis. Complications of type I prostatitis include prostatic abscess, acute urinary retention, septicemia, and rarely, vertebral osteomyelitis. Type II prostatitis can cause repeated urinary tract infections. Both type II and type III prostatitis have been associated with decreased fertility, although this relationship is not certain.

Future Directions

The Chronic Prostatitis Collaborative Research Network, funded by the NIH/National Institute of Diabetes and Digestive and Kidney Diseases, is a multidisciplinary, multi-institutional effort to provide more information about the etiology, diagnosis, and treatment of prostatitis. Future directions in therapy include trials of medications, such as pregabalin, for treatment of the possible neuropathic pain associated with CP/CPPS. The Urologic Pelvic Pain Collaborative Research Network represents the overarching organization for collaborative research in chronic prostatitis, chronic pelvic pain syndrome, and interstitial cystitis and should serve to provide newer perspectives on chronic pelvic pain of urologic origin.

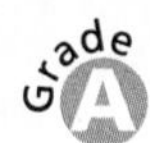

1. Djavan B, Chapple C, Milani S, Marberger M: State of the art on the efficacy and tolerability of alpha-1 adrenoreceptor antagonists in patients with lower urinary tract symptoms suggestive of benign prostatic hyperplasia. Urology 2004;64:1081–1088.
2. McConnell JD, Roehrborn CG, Bautista OM, et al: The long-term effect of doxazosin, finasteride, and combination therapy on the clinical progression of benign prostatic hyperplasia. N Engl J Med 2003;349:2385–2396.
3. Roehrborn CG, Boyle P, Nichol JC, et al: Efficacy and safety of a dual inhibitor of 5-alpha-reductase types 1 and 2 (dutasteride) in men with benign prostatic hyperplasia. Urology 2002;60:434–441.
4. Thompson IM, Goodman PJ, Tangen CM, et al: The influence of finasteride on the development of prostate cancer. N Engl J Med 2003;349:215–224.
5. Lepor H, Williford WO, Barry MJ, et al: The efficacy of terazosin, finasteride, or both in benign prostatic hyperplasia. N Engl J Med 1996;335:533–539.
6. Wasson JH, Reda DJ, Bruskewitz RC, et al: A comparison of transurethral surgery with watchful waiting for moderate symptoms of benign prostatic hyperplasia. N Engl J Med 1995;332:75–79.
7. Alexander RB, Propert KJ, Schaeffer AJ, et al: Ciprofloxacin or tamsulosin in men with chronic prostatitis/chronic pelvic pain syndrome: A randomized, double-blind trial. Ann Intern Med 2004;141:581–589.
8. Nickel JC, Downey J, Clark J, et al: Levofloxacin for chronic prostatitis/chronic pelvic pain syndrome in men: A randomized placebo-controlled multicenter trial. Urology 2003:62:614–617.
9. Cheah PY, Liong ML, Yuen KH, et al: Terazosin therapy for chronic prostatitis/chronic pelvic pain syndrome: A randomized, placebo-controlled trial. J Urol 2003;169:592–596.
10. Mehik A, Alas P, Nickel JC, et al: Alfuzosin treatment for chronic prostatitis/chronic pelvic pain syndrome: A prospective, randomized, double-blind, placebo-controlled, pilot study. Urology 2003;62:425–429.
11. Nickel JC, Downey J, Pontari MA, et al: A randomized placebo-controlled multicenter study to evaluate the safety and efficacy of finasteride for male chronic pelvic pain syndrome (category IIIA chronic nonbacterial prostatitis). BJU Int 2004;93:991–995.
12. Nickel JC, Forrest J, Tomera KM, et al: Effects of pentosan polysulfate sodium in men with chronic pelvic pain syndrome: A multi-center, randomized, placebo-controlled study. J Urol 2005;173:1252–1255.
13. McVary KT, Roehrborn CG, Kaminetsky JC, et al: Tadalafil relieves lower urinary tract symptoms secondary to benign prostatic hyperplasia. J Urol 2007;177:1401–1407.
14. Rowe E, Smith C, Laverick L, et al: A prospective, randomized, placebo-controlled, double-blind study of pelvic electromagnetic therapy for the treatment of chronic pelvic pain syndrome with 1 year of follow-up. J Urol 2005;173:2044–2047.

SUGGESTED READINGS

Connolly SS, Fitzpatrick JM: Medical treatment of benign prostatic hyperplasia. Postgrad Med J 2007;83:73–78. *Review of the natural history and medical treatment.*

Naslund MJ, Miner M: A review of the clinical efficacy and safety of 5alpha-reductase inhibitors for the enlarged prostate. Clin Ther 2007;29:17–25. *An effective therapy, which augments the benefits of therapy with an alpha-blocker.*

Schaeffer AJ: Clinical practice: Chronic prostatitis and the chronic pelvic pain syndrome. N Engl J Med 2006;355:1690–1698. *Review of formal guidelines and clinical recommendations.*

Soliman SA, Wadie BS, Ibrahim el-He, et al: Rotoresection versus transurethral resection of the prostate: Short-term evaluation of a prospective randomized study. J Urol 2007;177:1036–1039. *Rotoresection is a safe and equivalently effective method.*

131 CHRONIC KIDNEY DISEASE

William E. Mitch

Definition

Chronic kidney disease (CKD) refers to the myriad problems that follow loss of kidney function. It results from a large number of diseases that either are systemic and damage the kidney or are intrinsic to the kidney (Table 131–1). CKD has two characteristics. First, there is chronicity because the kidney damage of CKD is rarely repaired and loss of function persists, unlike the course of acute kidney failure. Second, loss of kidney function generates even more kidney damage so that CKD progressively worsens even if the disorder that caused it becomes inactive. CKD is the preferred term because another widely used one, chronic renal failure or insufficiency, is not as easily identifiable by patients as a disorder that affects the kidney. In addition, chronic renal failure suggests that

TABLE 131–1 CAUSES OF CHRONIC RENAL FAILURE

Diabetic glomerulosclerosis*
Hypertensive nephrosclerosis
Glomerular disease
Glomerulonephritis
Amyloidosis, light chain disease*
Systemic lupus erythematosus, Wegener's granulomatosis*
Tubulointerstitial disease
Reflux nephropathy (chronic pyelonephritis)
Analgesic nephropathy
Obstructive nephropathy (stones, benign prostatic hypertrophy)
Myeloma kidney*
Vascular disease
Scleroderma*
Vasculitis*
Renovascular renal failure (ischemic nephropathy)
Atheroembolic renal disease*
Cystic diseases
Autosomal dominant polycystic kidney disease
Medullary cystic kidney disease

*Systemic disease involving the kidney.

Section XI Renal

TABLE 131–2 STAGES OF CHRONIC KIDNEY DISEASE (CKD) WITH PROJECTED NUMBERS OF INDIVIDUALS AND THE FREQUENCY OF COMPLICATIONS

Stage	Description	GFR* (mL/min/1.73 m²)	Projected Number (×1000)	Symptoms or Signs
1	Chronic kidney damage with normal or increased GFR	>90	5900	Anemia 4% Hypertension 40% 5-year mortality 19%
2	Mild GFR loss	60–89	5300	Anemia 4% Hypertension 40% 5-year mortality 19%
3	Moderate GFR loss	30–59	7600	Anemia 7% Hypertension 55% 5-year mortality 24%
4	Severe GFR loss	15–29	400	Hyperphosphatemia 20% Anemia 29% Hypertension 77% 5-year mortality 46%
5	Kidney failure	<15 or dialysis	300	Hyperphosphatemia 50% Anemia 69% Hypertension >75% 3-year mortality 14%

*The formula for estimating the glomerular filtration rate (GFR) of adults with CKD is derived from data obtained during the National Institutes of Health Modification of Diet in Renal Disease trial. GFR = $186 \times [S_{Cr}]^{-1.154} \times [\text{age}]^{-0.203} \times [0.742 \text{ if patient is female}] \times [1.212 \text{ if patient is black}]$.
S_{cr} = serum creatinine.

TABLE 131–3 FUNCTIONS OF THE KIDNEY AND PROBLEMS DUE TO IMPAIRMENT OF KIDNEY FUNCTIONS IN PATIENTS WITH CHRONIC KIDNEY DISEASE

Kidney Functions	Consequences of Dysfunction
Maintain concentrations and body contents of electrolytes and fluid volumes	Hyponatremia, hyperkalemia, low total potassium content, hypocalcemia, hyperphosphatemia, decreased tolerance to electrolyte or mineral loading
Regulate blood pressure	Hypertension, cardiovascular disease
Endocrine mediators	Anemia (low erythropoietin), hypertension (renin system activation), bone disease (secondary hyperparathyroidism), low vitamin D activation, prolonged half-lives of peptide hormones (e.g., insulin)
Waste product excretion	Anorexia, nausea, soft tissue deposition of oxalates and phosphates, neurologic dysfunction, loss of muscle protein

the kidneys have lost all of their function, whereas CKD covers the spectrum of clinical problems beginning with abnormalities detectable only by laboratory testing to a late stage, labeled uremia. Uremia literally means "urine in the blood" and represents the toxic state principally resulting from accumulation of unexcreted waste products derived from metabolism of protein. When the kidney fails to perform most of its function, the clinical state is labeled end-stage renal disease (ESRD), and dialysis or transplantation is required to sustain life. The progressive and chronic nature of CKD is emphasized because treatment can slow or even halt the loss of kidney function, and many symptoms of uremia can be ameliorated or eliminated.

Epidemiology

The increase in the number of patients with ESRD in the United States and other industrialized countries has features of an epidemic. For example, the number of patients with ESRD in the United States increased by an average of 5% between 1980 and 1990, and the incidence of ESRD was 219 per million population in 1991 but grew to 334 per million by 2000. A recent assessment suggests that the rate of increase of patients with ESRD is falling to an annual increase of 1% or less, possibly because of the emphasis on earlier detection of CKD and aggressive treatment of hypertension and especially more widespread treatment with blockers of the renin-angiotensin-aldosterone system (see later).

Population-based studies such as the National Health and Nutrition Survey, a cross-sectional survey of U.S. adults, have uncovered the magnitude of the CKD problem (Table 131–2). Approximately 8 million persons are afflicted with stage 3 or stage 4 CKD and hence are at high risk of progressive kidney failure. Two disorders account for almost 70% of all new ESRD patients; in 2003, 44.8% had diabetes mellitus and 27.1% had hypertension-induced kidney damage. The populations experiencing the highest incidence were the elderly (i.e., >65 years) and African Americans plus Native and Asian Americans. The reasons for the racial susceptibility to CKD are unknown. Besides a racial susceptibility, groups that have been identified as being at high risk for progressing from CKD to ESRD are those with hypertension, diabetes mellitus, or cardiovascular disease and those with family members who have ESRD. Other epidemiologic factors that have been identified as increasing the risk of progressive CKD include smoking, albuminuria, obesity, and hyperlipidemia. The presence of any of these factors should be sought and attempts made to correct them in treating a patient with CKD.

Pathophysiology

Physiologic and metabolic functions of the kidney include the regulation of ion concentrations in the extracellular and intracellular fluids, the regulation of blood pressure, the regulation of several endocrine functions, and the excretion of waste products (Table 131–3). The breadth of these functions yields several predictable and some unpredictable consequences of CKD. For example, it is predictable that limitation of the ability to excrete acid would cause hyperventilation and a decrease in P_{CO_2}, but acidosis also causes less easily predictable losses of muscle mass and bone disease. Although changes in bone metabolism could be predicted from impaired excretion of calcium and phosphates, the discovery that the rate of parathyroid hormone (PTH) secretion varies with activation of calcium-sensitive receptors on parathyroid cells as well as the actions of vitamin D was not predictable. To understand the complex pathophysiologic process of CKD, certain principles must be integrated.

Balance and Steady-State Considerations

The first principle, balance, is the condition in which the intake or production of a substance equals its elimination. For example, a loss of nephrons impairs the ability to excrete sodium, but there is an adjustment by the remaining nephrons to excrete a greater fraction of the sodium that is filtered by each glomerulus. Similar phenomena occur with other ions and substances, allowing the patient with CKD to avoid accumulation of sodium or potassium, for example. The ability to achieve balance has a limit, however, and when this limit is reached, ions and other molecules destined for excretion by the kidney will instead accumulate unless the intake or production of the retained ion or compound is reduced.

A related concept is that of the steady state. A patient is in the steady state when the intake or processes of production and elimination are not changing. Although a patient in balance is also in the steady state, the converse is not necessarily true. A patient can be in the steady state but not be in balance because he or she is gaining or losing an ion or compound at a constant rate. For example, if nitrogen intake is less than the excretion of nitrogen, a patient will be losing protein stores. Such a patient would be in the steady state but in negative nitrogen balance.

The Tradeoff Hypothesis

The second important principle, the tradeoff hypothesis, is that a patient with CKD will achieve balance by activating pathophysiologic responses, but the responses lead to a tradeoff that has the potential of causing adverse consequences. A classic example is the responses activated in CKD to achieve sodium balance. CKD initially reduces salt excretion, leading to sodium retention and expansion of extracellular fluid. The result is high blood pressure. Although a higher blood pressure is beneficial because it increases the filtration and excretion of sodium, the tradeoff for maintaining sodium balance is persistent hypertension. There is experimental evidence that another adjustment that can prevent salt accumulation is an increase in circulating inhibitors of Na^+,K^+-ATPase in patients with CKD. These inhibitors increase the sodium concentration in tubular cells, thereby reducing the ability of the cell to reabsorb filtered sodium. The tradeoff for the ability to increase sodium excretion is that some patients with CKD will not tolerate an abrupt decrease in sodium intake, and persistent sodium excretion will lead to a fall in extracellular volume, impaired perfusion of the kidney, and a decrease in glomerular filtration rate (GFR).

Another CKD tradeoff occurs in response to a decreased ability to excrete potassium. The rise in serum potassium stimulates adrenal aldosterone production, which stimulates potassium excretion by both the damaged kidney and the colon. The tradeoff for this adaptation is an increase in blood pressure caused by aldosterone-mediated sodium retention.

The most intensely studied tradeoff is the adaptation to phosphate retention. When CKD limits the kidney's ability to excrete phosphates, they accumulate in extracellular and intracellular fluids. For example, CKD patients given a challenge dose of phosphates develop supranormal blood phosphorus levels. Accumulated phosphates form calcium-phosphate complexes and decrease the circulating concentration of ionized calcium. This in turn stimulates the production and release of PTH, a beneficial response because it suppresses the reabsorption of phosphates by the proximal tubule. The subsequent increase in phosphate excretion leads to a rise in ionized calcium, but the tradeoff is that the new steady state is maintained only as long as circulating PTH concentration is high (Fig. 131–1). The tradeoff is stimulation of osteoclastic activity in bone that accelerates release of minerals, leading to uremic bone disease (Chapter 132). It follows that restriction of phosphates in the diet plus the use of phosphate binders to increase gastrointestinal excretion of

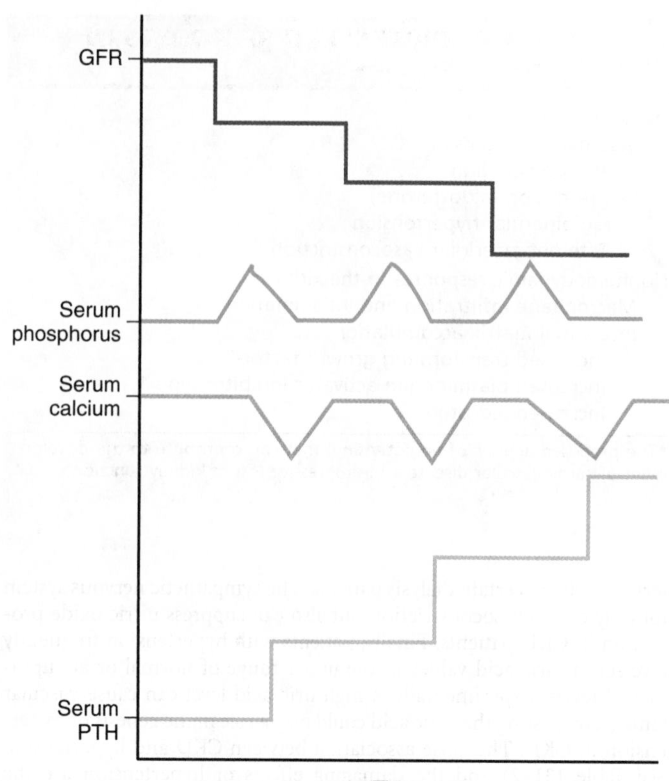

FIGURE 131–1 • A decrease in glomerular filtration rate (GFR) is followed by an increase in serum phosphorus and a decrease in serum calcium. An increase in serum parathyroid hormone (PTH) returns phosphorus and calcium to normal levels.

phosphates will eliminate the increase in circulating PTH concentration. This has been demonstrated experimentally and in CKD patients.

Hypertension

Hypertension, like anemia, is almost universal in CKD patients and often is the first sign of CKD. The coincidence of CKD and high blood pressure is particularly important because hypertension contributes to the development of cardiovascular disease, the leading cause of morbidity and mortality in CKD patients. Hypertension in CKD patients is mainly the result of an expanded extracellular volume from a salt-rich diet and a decreased capacity for excretion of sodium. As discussed earlier, the normal response to an increase in the extracellular volume is a rise in blood pressure that stimulates sodium excretion to achieve a balance between sodium intake and the excretion of salt. In the steady state, however, salt balance can be maintained only as long as blood pressure is high unless dietary salt is restricted and diuretics are used to increase sodium excretion. Two practical implications arise from these relationships. First, they reveal why treatment of hypertensive patients with vasodilating drugs alone is frequently unsuccessful. When vasodilator drugs reduce blood pressure, the fall in sodium excretion leads to sodium retention and expansion of extracellular volume that raises blood pressure. Second, they explain why control of the amount of salt in the diet is required even when diuretics are used to treat hypertension in CKD patients. A salt-rich diet can cancel the benefits of using diuretics, ultimately leading to expansion of extracellular volume and reappearance of hypertension.

Another mechanism for hypertension in CKD patients is activation of the renin-angiotensin-aldosterone (RAA) system and the sympathetic nervous system. Evidence for activation of the RAA system in CKD patients includes circulating levels of renin and aldosterone that are too high for individuals who are hypertensive, suggesting that the vasoconstrictive action of angiotensin II and the salt retention induced by aldosterone contribute to hypertension (Table 131–4). Other evidence includes the beneficial effects of inhibitors of the RAA system in reducing kidney damage and slowing the loss of kidney function. Evidence for activation of the sympathetic nervous system includes higher circulating levels of norepinephrine and the detection of increased sympathetic

TABLE 131–4 ANGIOTENSIN II RESPONSES IN CHRONIC KIDNEY DISEASE*

Hemodynamic responses
- Systemic hypertension
  - Vasoconstriction
- Salt retention (aldosterone)
- Intraglomerular hypertension
  - Efferent arteriolar vasoconstriction

Nonhemodynamic responses in the kidney
- Macrophage infiltration and inflammation
- Interstitial matrix accumulation
  - Increased transforming growth factor-β
  - Increased plasminogen activator inhibitor type 1
  - Increased aldosterone

*The proposed actions of angiotensin II that can contribute to the development of cardiovascular disease and progressive loss of kidney function.

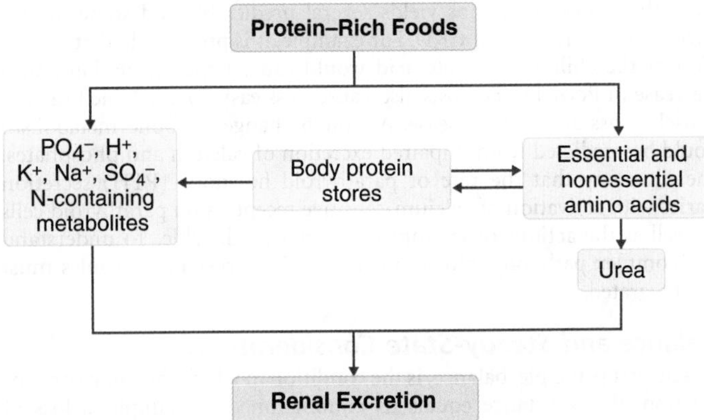

FIGURE 131–2 • Breakdown of dietary protein enlarges the pool of essential and nonessential amino acids that can be used to synthesize body protein. The amino acids are also used to produce urea, which must be excreted. Besides nitrogenous waste products, dietary protein catabolism yields inorganic ions that must be excreted.

nerve activity in certain dialysis patients. The sympathetic nervous system not only causes vasoconstriction but also can suppress nitric oxide production in CKD patients. Finally, patients with hypertension frequently have serum uric acid values in the upper range of normal or at supranormal levels. Experimentally, a high uric acid level can cause vascular damage, suggesting that uric acid could play a role in the genesis of hypertension in CKD. The close association between CKD and hypertension (see Table 131–2) and the damaging effects of hypertension are the reasons that subjects with persistent hypertension (especially those with hypertension and diabetes or other systemic diseases) should be examined yearly for evidence of kidney damage.

Endocrine Disorders

The mechanisms causing bone disease in CKD patients include abnormalities in endocrine responses other than stimulation of PTH secretion. Vitamin D is activated by repeated hydroxylations of the parent molecule, cholecalciferol or vitamin D_3. The initial hydroxylation occurs in the liver, forming 25-hydroxyvitamin D_3. Although 25-hydroxyvitamin D_3 can influence the function of muscle and other organs by poorly defined mechanisms (Chapter 132), it mainly serves as a substrate for a second hydroxylation at the 1α position to form 1,25-dihydroxyvitamin D_3, the most active form of vitamin D. This critical step is catalyzed by 1α-hydroxylase activity in the proximal tubule of the kidney, so loss of kidney function results in decreased function of 1,25-dihydroxyvitamin D_3, including lower absorption of calcium and phosphorus by the gastrointestinal tract and reduced suppression of PTH secretion. The decrease in phosphate absorption plus the persistent stimulation of renal phosphate excretion by the action of PTH accounts for the low values of serum phosphorus that are measured in blood samples obtained after an overnight fast. These considerations indicate why vitamin D should not be given to CKD patients with high serum phosphorus levels. Stimulation of gastrointestinal calcium and phosphate absorption can cause hypercalcemia and, by stimulating the accumulation of phosphates, will initiate the mechanisms that raise circulating PTH concentration (see earlier).

Decades ago, it was shown that CKD causes insulin resistance by reducing the ability of insulin to stimulate glucose uptake by muscle and other organs (Chapter 248). This leads to an increase in circulating insulin concentration, even in CKD patients without type 2 diabetes. In insulin-resistant CKD patients, insulin has been shown to interact normally with its receptor, so the failure to stimulate glucose metabolism is due to a post-receptor defect in cell signaling. The abnormality in insulin-stimulated cell signaling mechanisms is controversial; one possibility is decreased ability to activate phosphatidylinositol 3-kinase and its downstream kinase, Akt. Reduced function of these enzymes in muscle cells impairs the metabolism of both glucose and protein. Clinically, the insulin resistance of nondiabetic CKD patients is rarely associated with blood glucose levels above 200 mg/dL. In fact, blood glucose concentration is usually normal or only slightly high because insulin secretion rises to overcome defects in cell signaling.

One possible initiator of insulin resistance is metabolic acidosis, a frequent complication of CKD. Metabolic acidosis will impair insulin-stimulated glucose uptake in normal adults, and it causes loss of muscle protein, an insulin-sensitive metabolic function. Metabolic acidosis can contribute to other CKD-induced endocrine abnormalities; it impairs the ability of growth hormone to stimulate insulin-like growth factor 1. When this is combined with impaired metabolism of bone minerals, it contributes to the impaired growth of children with CKD. Metabolic acidosis also impairs thyroid function by increasing thyroid-stimulating hormone and depressing circulating levels of thyroxine (T_4) and triiodothyronine (T_3); similar changes are present in the sick euthyroid syndrome (Chapter 244). Metabolic acidosis should be eliminated because its correction largely eliminates these abnormalities in CKD patients.

Another impaired kidney function that affects a patient's endocrine status is the ability to degrade small proteins, including several hormones. For example, diabetic patients treated with their usual dose of insulin can develop hypoglycemia with progressive loss of kidney function because the damaged kidney does not remove enough of the injected insulin. This same function also affects interpretation of circulating PTH concentrations because the damaged kidney leads to accumulation of different fragments of PTH; it is important to know whether the PTH level being measured is the active or one of the inactive fractions of PTH.

In patients with advanced CKD, normochromic, normocytic anemia is almost universal, principally due to another endocrine abnormality, impaired production of erythropoietin by the kidney. Anemia can often be detected in patients with stage 2 CKD who have lost 50% or more of their GFR and have serum creatinine values that are just outside of the normal range. Erythropoietin is produced by interstitial cells in the kidney, and loss of kidney function reduces its production, causing decreased erythropoiesis. Other factors contributing to anemia are a shortened half-life of erythrocytes and vitamin deficiencies. Fortunately, administration of the recombinant hormone erythropoietin eliminates the anemia of CKD. This is therapeutically important because correction of anemia can suppress the development of left ventricular hypertrophy and other factors that contribute to the cardiovascular disease that is so prevalent in CKD patients. The major reasons for an impaired response to erythropoietin are iron deficiency and inflammation, and these should be corrected to achieve optimal responses to erythropoietin therapy (Chapter 160).

Accumulation of Uremic Toxins

The protein in protein-rich foods is metabolized to amino acids that can be used to build body protein stores (Fig. 131–2). The other fate of amino acids is the formation of urea and other potentially toxic products that must be excreted. Besides amino acids, protein-rich foods contain phosphates, sodium, potassium, acid, and other ions that must be eliminated. The principal nitrogen-containing waste product derived from protein metabolism is urea. When a patient is in protein balance, the net production of urea is directly proportional to the amount of protein in the diet; but if a patient is in negative nitrogen balance, urea and other waste products and ions arise from the breakdown of the body stores of protein. It follows that treatment should be directed at maintaining neutral protein balance at the lowest rate of urea production. More than

TABLE 131–5 UREMIA RESULTS FROM THE DYSFUNCTION OF MANY ORGANS SUGGESTING GENERALIZED TOXICITY

Affected System	Cause or Mechanism	Clinical Syndrome
Systemic symptoms	Anemia, inflammation	Fatigue, lassitude
Skin	Hyperparathyroidism, calcium-phosphate deposition	Rash, pruritus, metastatic calcification
Cardiovascular disease	Hypertension, anemia, homocysteinemia, vascular calcification	Atherosclerosis, heart failure, stroke
Serositis	Unknown	Pericardial or pleural pain and fluid, peritoneal fluid
Gastrointestinal	Unknown	Anorexia, nausea, vomiting, diarrhea, gastrointestinal tract bleeding
Immune system	Leukocyte dysfunction, depressed cellular immunity	Infections
Endocrine	Hypothalamic-pituitary axis dysfunction	Amenorrhea, menorrhagia, impotence, oligospermia, hyperprolactinemia
Neurologic	Unknown	Neuromuscular excitability, cognitive dysfunction progressing to coma, peripheral neuropathy (restless leg syndrome or sensory deficits)

135 years ago, it was noted that symptoms of uremia in patients with advanced CKD are ameliorated by reducing the amount of protein in the diet.

The consequences of accumulating ions and uremic toxins include the development of symptoms and problems that involve several organs, including the nervous system, the gastrointestinal system, and the skin (Table 131–5). For example, phosphate accumulation leads to secondary hyperparathyroidism and bone disease (see earlier discussion). Acid accumulation contributes to the bone disease of CKD but also stimulates the breakdown of muscle protein and contributes to hypoalbuminemia. Accumulation of peptides, also known as middle molecules, is associated with disorders that range from anorexia to neurologic abnormalities. Accumulation of indoxyl sulfate, a product of tryptophan metabolism, has been linked to progressive kidney damage; guanidine-containing compounds are associated with neurologic damage. Ideally, the levels of these uremic toxins should be monitored, but measuring the levels of individual products is complicated and impractical. The production of urea, however, is directly proportional to the production of other waste products because urea is the principal end product of protein metabolism (see Fig. 131–2). For this reason, the production of all waste products is approximated by the 24-hour excretion of urea nitrogen as long as the patient is in the steady state (i.e., the serum urea nitrogen [SUN] concentration and body water are stable). The corollary is that the production of urea should be kept to a minimum that is consistent with maintaining body protein stores (see later).

Progression of Chronic Kidney Disease

Persistence of diseases affecting the kidney (e.g., diabetes or inflammatory conditions such as systemic lupus erythematosus) is one factor in the progression of CKD, but other mechanisms progressively damage the kidney in most CKD patients even when the disease that initially damaged the kidney is no longer active. Mechanisms that have been associated with progression of CKD include kidney damage from systemic hypertension, hemodynamic injury to the kidney, proteinuria, and nephrotoxic injury.

Hypertension is suspected to cause progressive loss of kidney function (i.e., progression of CKD) for several reasons. First, hypertension alone can damage the kidney; malignant hypertension damages the endothelial cells of the afferent arteriole and the glomerulus and can even cause thrombosis in these vessels. Second, chronic hypertension is frequently associated with diffuse ischemic injury to the glomerulus and can include collapse of glomerular vessels. The presumed mechanism of progressive kidney damage is direct transmission of the increased blood pressure to the afferent arteriole and the glomerulus, leading to glomerulosclerosis. The degree of hypertension has been directly correlated with the rate of loss of kidney function, and in a multicenter trial, effective treatment of hypertension was associated with slowing of CKD progression. The important question is whether hypertension is a factor contributing to progression or the principal mechanism causing kidney damage. The answer to this question is unsettled. For example, when African American patients with hypertension and kidney disease were studied, progression of CKD continued despite a lowering of blood pressure. Regardless, the close association between the presence of hypertension and the development of cardiovascular diseases mandates control of blood pressure. In multicenter, randomized trials of CKD patients with type 1 or type 2 diabetes or with nondiabetic nephropathy, the major class of drugs with proven effectiveness was the inhibitors of the RAA system, including angiotensin-converting enzyme inhibitors (ACEi) and angiotensin receptor blockers (ARB). The benefits of ACEi or ARB on progression of CKD are additive to their blood pressure–lowering effects.

The association between hypertension and progression extends to another proposed mechanism of progressive glomerular damage (see Table 131–4). The mechanism is based on preferential constriction of the glomerular efferent arteriole to a greater extent than in the afferent arteriole. This imbalance in arteriolar vasoconstriction increases intracapillary pressure to raise filtration (the hyperfiltration mechanism), but the tradeoff for the increase in GFR is damage to glomerular capillaries. Angiotensin II is the mediator of preferential efferent arteriolar constriction, and experimentally, ACEi or ARB administration can prevent both hyperfiltration and damage to the kidney.

The benefits of ACEi or ARB involve more than correction of hyperfiltration. For example, angiotensin II has growth factor properties, and it activates transforming growth factor-β, plasminogen activator inhibitor type 1, and other cytokines, aggravating interstitial damage to the kidney (see Table 131–4). It is also suspected that another product stimulated by angiotensin II, aldosterone, contributes to the development of interstitial damage and collagen deposition. Because ACEi and ARB have been demonstrated to slow the loss of kidney function in patients with diabetes and other types of CKD, they should be considered a major strategy to treat progressive CKD.

It has been repeatedly demonstrated that ACEi or ARB will reduce albuminuria, presumably by decreasing albumin filtration. This is relevant because experimental evidence suggests that albumin or some component of albumin (e.g., lipids or molecules attached to albumin) is toxic to kidney cells. In these experiments with cultured kidney cells, application of albumin increased the expression of cytokines and damage to the cells. In addition, patients with the greatest amounts of albumin in the urine also have the most rapid loss of kidney function, and when the degree of albuminuria is reduced, the loss of kidney function generally slows. These observations raise the possibility that albumin is a major cause of progressive kidney damage. The shortcoming of focusing on albuminuria as the principal cause of progressive kidney damage is that many kidney diseases initiate albuminuria, and as the kidney damage increases, the degree of albuminuria rises. It is possible, therefore, that reducing albuminuria may simply reflect correction or suppression of the mechanism damaging the kidney rather than blocking the ability of albumin to induce kidney damage.

Other proposed mechanisms for progression of CKD can be grouped under a general heading of nephrotoxic damage. It has been known for more than 60 years that animals fed a high-protein diet have more evidence of hypertension and more severe kidney damage, but why this occurs is controversial. Ions or molecules suspected of exerting toxic effects include phosphates and oxalates that lead to deposition of calcium-phosphate or calcium-oxalate salts and toxic responses in the interstitium of the kidney. Other candidates include indoxyl sulfate, generated during the metabolism of the amino acid tryptophan. The mechanisms proposed to explain the toxicity of these ions and compounds include direct damage to kidney cells and stimulation of cytokines (e.g., transforming growth factor-β) and inflammatory pathways that result in damage and fibrosis in the kidney. It has been difficult to assign all of the abnormalities in progressive kidney disease to a single factor.

Clinical Manifestations

CKD may be discovered in patients who develop a urinary abnormality, such as blood in the urine. On occasion, CKD is detected during evaluation of urinary infections, and the ureter or the urinary bladder is found to be obstructed. More frequently, CKD is discovered when the patient is hypertensive or develops edema and is found to have albuminuria and a high SUN or serum creatinine concentration. These depressing facts emphasize the nonspecific nature of signs and symptoms of kidney disease. Even when CKD is advanced, (e.g., stage 4; see Table 131–2), the symptoms are nonspecific. Some patients complain only of exercise intolerance, fatigue, or anorexia. This is unfortunate because problems caused by CKD including cardiovascular disease develop while the patient or physician is unaware of the illness.

There are specific syndromes caused by chronic kidney damage. For example, severe albumin losses (>3 g/day) plus edema and hypercholesterolemia define the nephrotic syndrome. With high degrees of albuminuria, other problems can occur, such as the loss of the relatively small (59 kD) vitamin D–binding protein and its attached 25-hydroxyvitamin D_3. The result is 1,25-dihydroxyvitamin D_3 depletion. Likewise, losses of clotting factors IX, XI, and XII can cause coagulation defects. Contrariwise, losses of antithrombin III can cause thrombosis, especially when accompanied by the hyperfibrinogenemia that occurs with inflammation-induced increases in the levels of other acute phase reactant proteins. The fraction of nephrotic patients who have coagulation disorders varies among studies and averages about 26%, emphasizing that this serious disorder is not rare.

Even with stage 4 or stage 5 CKD (see Staging), individual symptoms are not specific, although when they are grouped together, uremia can be easily recognized. As early as stage 3 CKD, patients can develop several abnormalities in blood chemistry values, such as anemia, metabolic acidosis, hyperkalemia, hyperphosphatemia, hypocalcemia, and hypoalbuminemia. In advanced CKD, so many organs are affected (see Table 131–5) that it is understandable why the uremic syndrome is attributed to toxicity. Symptoms include fatigue, anorexia, gastrointestinal symptoms (e.g., nausea, vomiting, and diarrhea), itching, and muscle wasting; occasionally there is chest pain from pericarditis, and there can be evidence of peripheral neuropathy and diminished mental acuity. Patients with advanced uremia can even develop an ammonia-like smell, and they invariably have anemia, metabolic acidosis, hyperkalemia, hyperphosphatemia, hypocalcemia, or hypoalbuminemia. Dialysis is usually indicated at this stage of CKD.

Diagnosis

Staging

The National Kidney Foundation has proposed five stages of CKD based on an accurate measure of the amount of remaining kidney function, the GFR, and the persistence of an abnormality in kidney function for at least 3 months. Table 131–2 lists the percentage of patients in each stage who will have signs of CKD, demonstrating that these signs become more and more frequent as CKD advances.

The intact nephron hypothesis helps with understanding the importance of GFR as the measure of remaining kidney function. A nephron consists of the glomerulus and the proximal, loop of Henle, and distal tubules plus the collecting duct. Individuals are born with 0.75 to 1.25 million nephrons in each kidney; no additional nephrons are formed in response to loss of nephrons. The intact nephron hypothesis is that each nephron functions as an independent unit, so the sum of the functions of all remaining nephrons determines an individual's kidney function. The most accurate estimate of the remaining kidney function is the GFR. It reflects the number of functioning nephrons and any augmentation of function occurring in individual nephrons that are responding to kidney damage. A GFR persistently below 60 mL/min/1.73 m^2 documents the presence of CKD for three reasons: this value is below the expected decline in kidney function that occurs with aging; most pathophysiologic processes can be detected at this level; and the risk of progression to ESRD rises sharply when a patient has a GFR below 60 mL/min/1.73 m^2.

Other estimates of kidney function are not as accurate in predicting the course of kidney failure. For example, the SUN concentration is determined not only by the remaining kidney function but also by the amount of protein in the diet. Besides reflecting kidney function, the serum creatinine concentration is influenced by creatinine production, which is directly proportional to lean body mass, and a much smaller contribution from dietary meat (see later). A significant problem with interpreting serum creatinine concentration is that it remains in the normal range until both kidneys are damaged and 50% of kidney function is lost; this occurs because of augmentation of the filtering function of individual nephrons and their ability to secrete creatinine. Measurement of GFR is cumbersome, however, so equations to estimate it have been developed on the basis of a patient's serum creatinine concentration, age, body weight, and other characteristics. The widely used equation derived from the National Institutes of Health Modification of Diet in Renal Disease (MDRD) study (see Table 131–2) was developed from characteristics of CKD patients who were participating in a multicenter trial. Notably, when GFR is less than 60 mL/min/1.73 m^2, this equation yields values that are numerically close to the measured GFR, at least when CKD patients in the United States are examined. For unidentified reasons, the equation is less accurate for CKD patients living in China (and probably other regions).

Clinical Evaluation

If CKD is suspected, there should be emphasis placed in the medical history about symptoms related to hypertension, urinary abnormalities, and any family history of kidney disease plus a review of medicines that might affect kidney function or damage the kidney (e.g., nonsteroidal anti-inflammatory drugs). The physical examination should emphasize factors that are associated with CKD, such as hypertension, skin abnormalities caused by itching, evidence of decreased lean body mass, and neurologic abnormalities.

Laboratory Findings

Two measurements of kidney function should be made, the GFR and the degree of albuminuria. The GFR measurement requires infusion or injection of compounds that are eliminated only by glomerular filtration (e.g., iothalamate or radiolabeled compounds). Alternatively, GFR can be estimated by the serum creatinine concentration, the patient's characteristics, and the MDRD equation (see Table 131–2).

The degree of albuminuria can be assessed from a 24-hour urine specimen, but this can introduce errors due to an incomplete collection or incomplete emptying of the bladder (e.g., in diabetic patients with neuropathy). To simplify the measurement, the ratio of albumin to creatinine concentrations in the first morning specimen can be assessed on 3 separate days. The average value yields the same information as does the quantity of albumin in a 24-hour urine collection in terms of the diagnosis of kidney damage and monitoring responses to therapy. Monitoring the degree of albuminuria is important for three reasons: it provides additional information about the rate of loss of GFR (the rate increases as the degree of albuminuria rises); persistence of albuminuria, including microalbuminuria, is associated with an increased risk of cardiovascular disease and ongoing loss of kidney function; and if the goal of achieving a decrease in the degree of albuminuria is achieved, there is evidence that the risk of major cardiovascular events (stroke, myocardial infarction, or congestive heart failure) and progression of CKD are reduced (at least in diabetic patients).

Comparison of Creatinine and Urea Nitrogen Levels

Blood values that should be measured are the serum creatinine and SUN concentrations, electrolyte and mineral concentrations (sodium, potassium, chloride and bicarbonate, calcium, phosphorus), and uric acid level. In addition, tests that might provide information about diseases that could cause or complicate CKD (e.g., blood glucose concentration) are performed. The serum creatinine and SUN concentrations provide an estimate of the degree of kidney function and the accumulation of unexcreted waste products.

Serum Creatinine

Serum creatinine is used to evaluate kidney function because it is cleared predominantly by glomerular filtration, but there also is tubular secretion, and because creatinine production is proportional to lean body mass. Although it can be assumed that lean body mass will vary minimally during prolonged periods in patients with stable body weights, urine collections from outpatients exhibit as much as 25% variability in the amount of creatinine that is excreted by individuals. In hospitalized patients as well, the individual variation in daily rates of creatinine excretion is only slightly better. For these reasons, some have suggested that creatinine clearance should not be used to estimate GFR in patients with CKD. Two causes for the variability in creatinine excretion have been suggested, the influence of dietary meat and the degradation of creatinine (i.e., extrarenal creatinine clearance). Creatinine is formed from creatine, which is highly concentrated in muscle (and other cells), and extensive cooking of meat leads to conversion of creatine to creatinine. Consequently, a meal containing a large amount of well-cooked meat will raise the variability in the amount of creatinine excreted. The enormous reserve of function present in normal kidneys, however, essentially eliminates any detectable rise in serum creatinine concentration. This is not true in patients with advanced CKD as changes in their intake of well-cooked meat will change the serum creatinine concentration. Consequently, if meat is eliminated from the diet of patients with advanced CKD, judgments about changes in the rate of loss of kidney function should be delayed for at least 4 months; but if kidney function continues to decline during and after the 4 months, the serum creatinine concentration will rise in inverse proportion to the loss of GFR. The influence of creatinine degradation is also virtually undetectable in patients with normal kidney function, but when serum creatinine values rise above 5 mg/dL, degradation plays an increasing role in reducing serum creatinine.

Besides disadvantages arising from the variability of creatinine excretion, the use of serum creatinine as an estimate of GFR is relatively insensitive. As noted earlier, a serum creatinine concentration above the normal range of 0.9 to 1.4 mg/dL indicates that there is extensive loss of kidney function, with damage to both kidneys and loss of at least 50% of kidney function. Another problem reflects the production of creatinine in proportion to lean body mass. A serum creatinine concentration of 1.4 mg/dL in an adult with a small muscle mass signifies a much greater loss of kidney function than it does in an individual with a large muscle mass. In spite of these shortcomings, serum creatinine concentration will remain constant as long as GFR is not changing, and it is a relatively inexpensive test that is available on most standard chemistry panels. This availability permits a ready estimation of GFR when it is combined with characteristics of the patient, and changes in the course of CKD (i.e., the loss of GFR) can be detected from plots of changes in GFR or in 1/serum creatinine (Fig. 131–3).

Urea Nitrogen

Urea nitrogen production is directly related to the amount of protein in the diet, and this relationship plus the degree of functional impairment of the kidney determines the SUN concentration (see Fig. 131–2). In general, the ratio of SUN to serum creatinine is 10 to 1 in normal adults or CKD patients. When the SUN concentration is below this ratio, the patient is eating a protein-restricted diet (note that even patients with liver disease will produce urea from dietary protein unless they are so ill that they are unable to eat). If the SUN concentration exceeds 10 times the serum creatinine concentration, three possibilities should be considered. First, the patient may have gastrointestinal bleeding or be suffering from a severely catabolic condition (e.g., trauma or high-dose glucocorticoid administration). Second, the patient may be eating excessive amounts of protein and producing more urea than the impaired kidney can excrete. Finally, there may be extracellular volume depletion that stimulates increased proximal tubular reabsorption of sodium. Enhanced sodium reabsorption produces a concentration gradient of urea leading to the passive reabsorption of urea.

These possibilities can be distinguished by a 24-hour urine collection and measurement of its urea nitrogen and creatinine contents. From these measurements, the urea and creatinine clearances should be calculated and compared because the ratio of the urea to creatinine clearances is 0.6 in normal adults and CKD patients eating a normal diet. If the urea to creatinine clearance ratio is low (i.e., <0.4), it provides evidence that urea reabsorption is increased, leading to a lower urea clearance.

These relationships also explain why neither the GFR nor the creatinine clearance is related to urine flow in contrast to the urea clearance, which is low when urine flow is low. This association occurs because stimulation of sodium (due to extracellular volume depletion or decreased renal perfusion) removes salt and water and reduces urine flow. At the same time, enhanced sodium reabsorption increases urea reabsorption and depresses urea clearance. This diagnostic strategy can be refined by comparing the amount of protein in the diet with the steady-state amount of urea nitrogen excreted (Table 131–6). The comparison is based on the fact that protein is 16% nitrogen and that non-urea nitrogen excretion (i.e., nitrogen in feces, urinary creatinine, uric acid, peptides) averages 0.031 g of nitrogen per kilogram of ideal body weight per day. In a patient who is in nitrogen balance, the amount of dietary protein nitrogen equals the amount of urea nitrogen excreted plus 0.031 g of nitrogen per kilogram per day. If urea nitrogen excretion exceeds the amount of protein nitrogen in the diet, the patient should be examined for gastrointestinal bleeding or the presence of a catabolic illness.

Imaging

The initial evaluation should include an ultrasound examination of the kidney to ensure that there is no obstruction of the ureters or abnormality of the bladder. The ultrasound examination is also helpful diagnostically. Enlarged kidneys suggest diabetes, human immunodeficiency virus–associated nephropathy, or infiltrative diseases (e.g., diseases such as amyloidosis); small kidneys with loss of the kidney cortex suggest the presence of chronic glomerular diseases. If the size of the kidneys differs

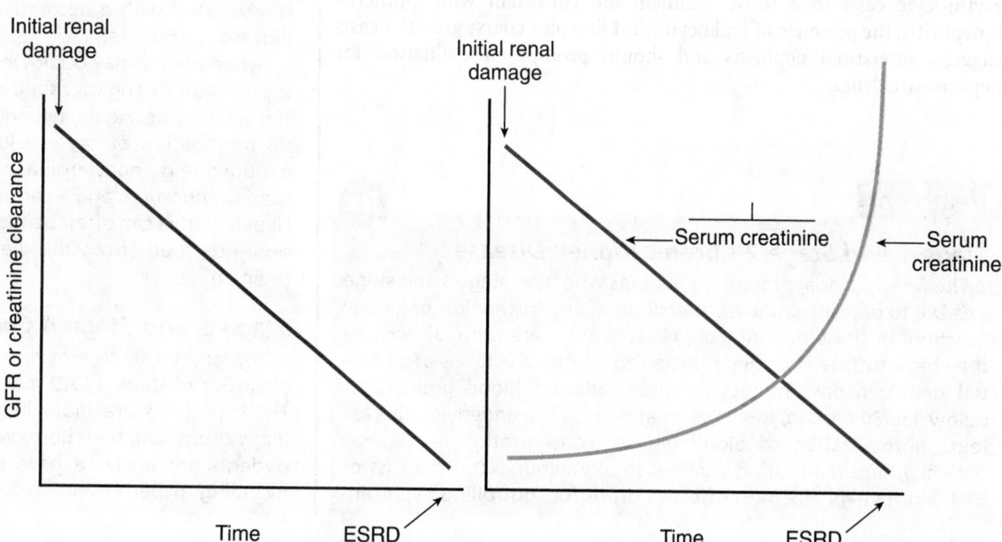

FIGURE 131–3 • The course of renal insufficiency from initial renal damage to ESRD (left panel). The course is estimated most easily as the reciprocal of serum creatinine (right panel). ESRD = end-stage renal disease. (Reprinted, with permission, from the Annual Review of Medicine, Vol. 35, ©1984 by Annual Reviews www.annualreviews.org.)

TABLE 131–6 ESTIMATION OF DIETARY PROTEIN FROM THE 24-HOUR UREA NITROGEN EXCRETION

ASSUMPTIONS

The patient is in the steady state, and neither the serum urea nitrogen concentration nor body weight is changing; there is no edema.

The patient is in nitrogen balance so that nitrogen intake equals nitrogen excretion.

Protein is 16% nitrogen.

The non-urea nitrogen excretion (the nitrogen in urinary creatinine, uric acid, and peptides plus feces) is 0.031 g of nitrogen per kilogram per day.

CASE 1

A 50-year-old patient with a stable weight of 70 kg is prescribed a diet containing 0.8 g of protein per kilogram per day. His 24-hour urea nitrogen excretion is 6.8 g of nitrogen per day. How much protein is he eating?

The diet should contain 70 kg × 0.8 g of protein per kilogram or 56 g of protein. His intake of nitrogen from this diet is approximately 9 g of nitrogen (56 g of protein × 0.16 = 8.96 g of nitrogen). His nitrogen excretion is 6.8 g of urea nitrogen plus 2.17 g of non-urea nitrogen per day (70 × 0.031 g of non-urea nitrogen per kilogram per day). The total nitrogen excretion is 8.97 g of nitrogen, so the patient is compliant with the diet prescription.

CASE 2

A 40-year-old woman weighing 60 kg is confident that she is eating a diet containing 0.6 g of protein per kilogram per day. Her 24-hour urea nitrogen excretion is 10 g of nitrogen per day. Does she require additional investigation?

Her diet should contain 60 kg × 0.6 g of protein per kilogram or 36 g of protein. Therefore, her intake of nitrogen is approximately 5.8 g of nitrogen (36 g of protein × 0.16 = 5.76 g of nitrogen). Her nitrogen excretion is 10 g of urea nitrogen plus 1.86 g of non-urea nitrogen (60 kg × 0.031 g of non-urea nitrogen per kilogram per day). Her total nitrogen excretion is 11.9 g/day, far in excess of the amount of protein she believes she is eating. Consequently, the patient requires investigation for gastrointestinal bleeding.

substantially, renal artery stenosis should be considered, especially in hypertensive patients. Finally, there should be a careful microscopic examination of the urine to document the presence of leukocytes, crystals, or casts. As discussed in Chapters 122 and 123, erythrocytes and erythrocyte casts in a urine sediment are consistent with glomerulonephritis; the presence of leukocytes and fine plus coarse granular casts suggests interstitial nephritis and should prompt an evaluation for nephrotoxic drugs.

Treatment

Stage 1 and Stage 2 Chronic Kidney Disease

The principal goal of treating patients who have stage 1 and stage 2 CKD is to prevent cardiovascular diseases and further loss of kidney function. In these patients, uremic symptoms are unusual because they have sufficient kidney function to control the levels of potential uremic toxins. Therapy involves reducing blood pressure to below 130/80 mm Hg, intensive treatment of the underlying disease (e.g., normalization of blood glucose concentration in diabetic patients), and monitoring changes in albuminuria and the loss of GFR (Fig. 131–4). The most effective drugs for controlling hypertension are ACEi or ARB plus dietary salt restriction and frequently a diuretic. Drugs that block the RAA system are recommended because they have been demonstrated to slow the loss of GFR in patients with CKD from type 1 or type 2 diabetes [1] or nondiabetic causes of CKD. [2,3] In addition, these drugs suppress albuminuria, which is associated with a beneficial effect on the course of CKD. Finally, they are beneficial for patients with cardiovascular disease, a major complication of CKD. The preferred strategy is to begin ACEi or ARB therapy at the lower end of recommended doses and to titrate upward to control blood pressure and albuminuria. Some investigators have advocated use of a combination of ACEi and ARB on the basis of a rationale that the combination would yield a more complete blockade of the RAA system. Certain small-scale studies support this recommendation, but the combination has not been tested in large trials of therapy.

One factor is clear: administration of ACEi or ARB is rarely effective unless steps are taken to avoid salt accumulation. Therefore, a critical factor to monitor in treating hypertension is body weight. If weight increases, it signifies salt retention and the need to reduce dietary salt because excessive sodium intake can overcome the benefits of diuretics. Contrariwise, a rapid loss of weight can be the first clue to the need to reduce diuretic dosage.

Use of ACEi or ARB can be associated, under certain circumstances, with loss of kidney function and hyperkalemia. Rapid loss of kidney function was noted in the early trials of ACEi therapy for patients with bilateral renal artery stenosis. In these patients, GFR fell rapidly because the suppression of angiotensin II production decreased the post-glomerular (efferent) arteriolar vasoconstriction. This resulted in a lower glomerular filtration pressure and a decrease in GFR. The mechanism underlying the decrease in filtration pressure is emphasized for two reasons. First, a decrease in GFR occurring when these classes of drugs are administered is a consequence of changes in glomerular hemodynamics and not due to additional kidney damage. Second, the GFR of patients with congestive heart failure is maintained by these same physiologic responses to angiotensin II. Consequently, the GFR of patients with cardiovascular disorders who begin ACEi or ARB therapy may fall and serum creatinine may increase; but the benefits of blocking the RAA system are substantial for patients with cardiovascular disease, including an improvement in cardiovascular function and slowing of the loss of GFR. In short, an increase in serum creatinine concentration should not trigger an automatic response to stop ACEi or ARB therapy. Instead, if the serum creatinine concentration rises by more than 0.5 mg/dL, other reasons for an increase in the degree of kidney damage should be sought by obtaining a careful history, a review of medications, and a physical examination plus an examination of the urine and consideration of renal artery stenosis. If none of these mechanisms for kidney damage is found, the drug should be continued at a lower dose. This strategy is especially important for patients with albuminuria because ACEi or ARB can suppress albuminuria, which is associated with a decreased risk of progression of CKD and cardiovascular disease.

Hyperkalemia may occur when the RAA system is blocked because suppression of angiotensin II responses includes a decrease in aldosterone release. Again, hyperkalemia is not always an indication for discontinuation of these valuable drugs. Other causes should be excluded (e.g., nonsteroidal anti-inflammatory drugs or potassium-sparing diuretics), and a careful dietary history should be obtained. Hyperkalemia can often be successfully treated by eliminating potassium-rich foods from the diet and adding a loop diuretic to the regimen.

Stage 3 and Stage 4 Chronic Kidney Disease

The greater degree of renal insufficiency found in patients with stage 3 and stage 4 CKD makes their treatment more complicated. These patients are more likely to experience complications from many drugs, and their doses will need adjustment. In addition, these patients are likely to have more familiar complications of CKD, including hypertension, secondary hyperparathyroidism, acidosis,

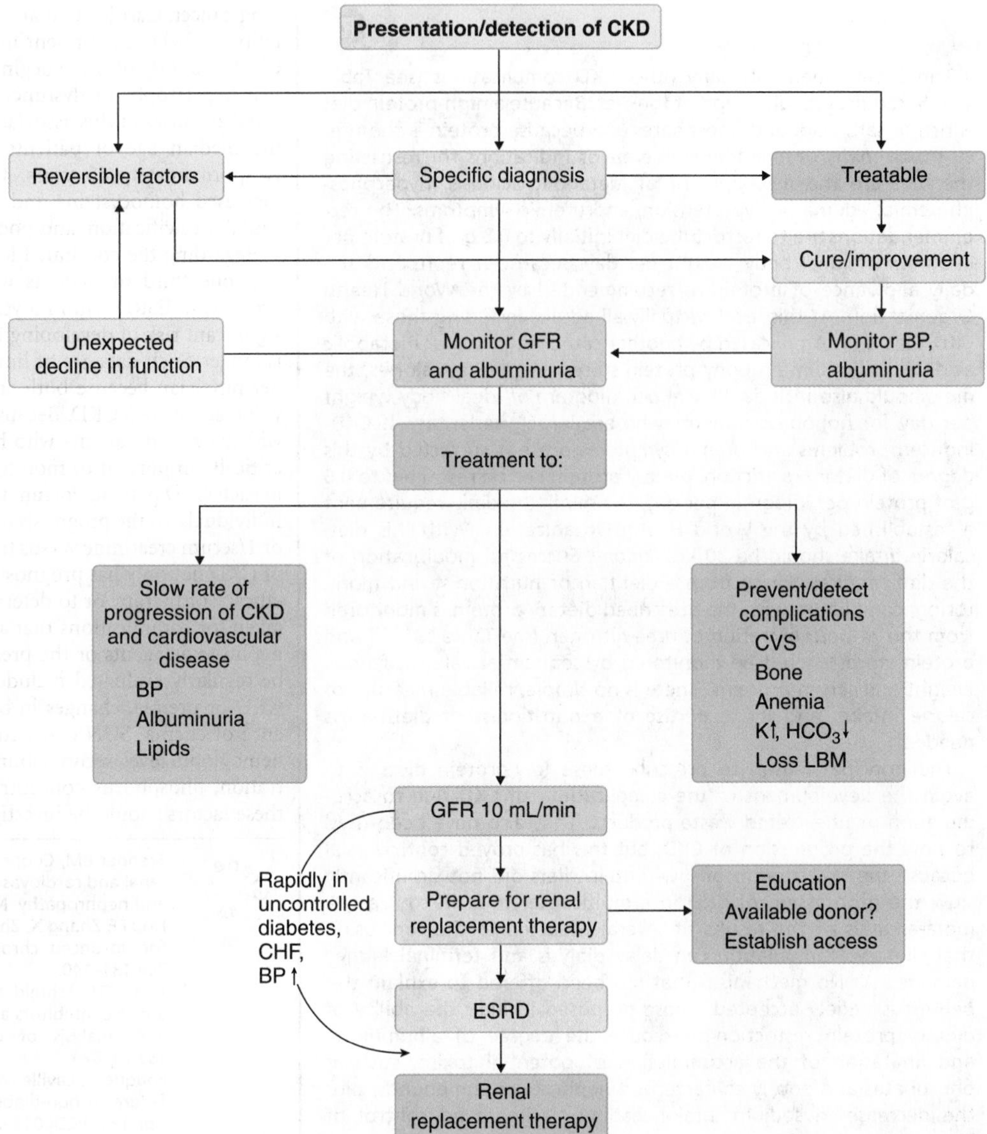

FIGURE 131–4 • Outline of management of patient in the various stages of chronic kidney disease (CKD). BP = blood pressure; CHF = congestive heart failure; CVS = cardiovascular system; ESRD = end-stage renal disease; GFR = glomerular filtration rate.

Rx

and even uremic symptoms. They are at even greater risk of developing cardiovascular disease. It is especially important to monitor the course of CKD in stage 3 and stage 4. If deviations of the linear plot of sequential GFR values versus time occur, there should be an intensive evaluation for changes in blood pressure, the degree of albuminuria, and changes in the urine sediment plus a review of a patient's history and medicines. This is especially important because a radiographic test with contrast dye or drugs such as nonsteroidal anti-inflammatory drugs can accelerate the loss of GFR. Such patients should be referred to a nephrologist to maximize preventive measures and while searching for remediable disorders. When stage 4 CKD is reached, referral to a nephrologist is indicated so the patient can discuss treatment by dialysis or transplantation.

Reducing the risk for development of cardiovascular disease in patients with stage 3 or stage 4 CKD requires maintaining blood pressure at or below 130/80 mm Hg. This level is also recommended for any patient who has a history of CKD or diabetes; the statin drugs may also be useful. Achieving this level will require ACEi or ARB dosing and dietary salt restriction plus a loop diuretic (e.g., furosemide, bumetanide). These diuretics are preferred because unlike thiazide diuretics, which are ineffective at GFR values below 25 mL/min, the loop diuretics are effective even when GFR is below 5 mL/min. In addition, loop diuretics maintain renal blood flow, and unless there is rapid loss of extracellular volume, they exert few adverse effects. Although rapid intravenous administration of large doses has caused ototoxicity, with slower intravenous or oral administration, doses as high as 250 mg of furosemide are tolerated and effective. These drugs have occasionally been associated with interstitial nephritis, but this complication is generally associated with rapid deterioration of kidney function. In short, the loop diuretics are safe and effective, but there are two caveats: excessive dietary salt will cancel their effectiveness, and their dose-response relationship is sigmoidal. High doses are needed for patients with stage 3 or stage 4 CKD; if an effective dose is found, do not divide the dose or the drug will be ineffective.

If blocking the RAA system and diuretics do not correct hypertension, calcium-channel blockers of the non-dihydropyridine type should be added (dihydropyridine drugs are believed to be less effective and cause more side effects). Calcium-channel antagonists can combat hypertension but are not effective in reducing albuminuria, and they can be associated with edema formation. Achieving the blood pressure goal of less than 130/80 mm Hg often requires several classes of antihypertensive drugs in addition to dietary restriction to 2 g of sodium per day.

Rx

The development of many other CKD complications (see Table 131–5) requires modification of the diet. Because a high-protein diet is rich in salt, acid, and phosphates and because protein is the precursor of many uremic toxins, the major indications for restricting the diet are the development of metabolic acidosis, hyperphosphatemia, edema or hypertension, and uremic symptoms. The recommendations are to restrict the diet initially to 0.8 g of protein per kilogram of ideal body weight per day because it represents the daily allowance of protein as recommended by the World Health Organization. At this level, virtually all adults, including those with CKD that is uncomplicated by another catabolic illness or metabolic acidosis, will maintain body protein stores. Regarding calories, the diet should also include 30 kcal per kilogram of ideal body weight per day for nonobese patients who are largely sedentary. If CKD-induced problems and uremic symptoms are not corrected by this degree of dietary restriction, dietary protein can be restricted to 0.6 g of protein per kilogram per day, the minimum daily requirement as established by the World Health Organization. With this diet, calorie intake should be 30 kcal/kg/day. Successful modification of the diet requires advice from a dietitian or nutritionist and monitoring; compliance with the prescribed dietary protein is monitored from the 24-hour excretion of urea nitrogen (see Table 131–6), and protein stores should be monitored by sequential values of body weight and serum proteins. There is no simple, reliable measure of calorie intake, and the expertise of a nutritionist or dietitian is needed.

The principal reason to prescribe these low-protein diets is to avoid the development of the complications of CKD due to accumulation of unexcreted waste products. They also have been used to slow the progression of CKD, but this has proved controversial because the prescription of low-protein diets did not significantly slow the progression of CKD in a multicenter trial. In contrast, a meta-analysis of the results of several trials led to the conclusion that dietary manipulation can delay dialysis and terminal kidney damage. [4] No mechanism that has been offered to explain this benefit is widely accepted. Those proposed include the ability of dietary protein restriction to reduce the degree of albuminuria and limitation of the accumulation of potential toxins, such as phosphates and poorly characterized nephrotoxic compounds, plus the decrease in sodium intake leading to improved control of hypertension.

CKD is associated with high circulating levels of homocysteine and low-density lipoprotein cholesterol, two risk factors for cardiovascular disease in adults without CKD. To reduce the influence of these factors on cardiovascular disease in CKD patients, supplements of folic acid plus vitamin B_6 (pyridoxine) and hydroxymethylglutaryl–coenzyme A reductase inhibitors, the statins, have been tested. With 1 or 5 mg of folic acid and vitamin B_6 supplements, the blood levels of homocysteine in CKD patients are reduced but do not reach normal values. It is not known if such therapy decreases the risk of serious cardiovascular complications. Regardless, with protein-restricted diets, a supplement of water-soluble vitamins should be given; fat-soluble vitamins should be supplied only for specific indications (e.g., vitamin D deficiency). Regarding statin use, recent reports indicate that they provide no statistically significant benefits for patients with stage 5 CKD. However, statin administration did lower the risk for a major cardiovascular event in patients with stage 2 or early stage 3 CKD, even in patients with diabetes and CKD. Thus, in addition to the use of ACEi or ARB, statins should be used in the early stages of CKD.

Prognosis

The prognosis for patients with ESRD is poor; the mortality rate of dialysis patients averages 20% per year and is greater than that of patients with colorectal cancers and only somewhat better than that of those with lung cancer. Cardiovascular disease is the most common cause of mortality in CKD. It is present in many patients even at the early stages of CKD, and 90% of those beginning dialysis therapy will have left ventricular hypertrophy or dysfunction. Several mechanisms have been implicated as causes of this association, including hypertension and older age; the median age of patients beginning dialysis in the United States is approximately 65 years. Other contributors are diabetes, anemia, increased homocysteine and low-density lipoprotein cholesterol levels, vascular calcification, and poorly identified factors.

Regarding the continued loss of GFR, epidemiologic studies indicate that one third of patients with stage 4 CKD (see Table 131–2) will progress to ESRD within 3 years. Patients with stage 3 CKD also have a significant risk of developing ESRD, but the average time to reach ESRD is longer. Such data are of limited value for the CKD patient and his or her physician because both are interested in knowing when the patient will reach stage 5 CKD. Because the rate of loss of kidney function varies widely even in patients who have the same type of kidney disease, it is critically important to monitor the course of declining kidney function in each CKD patient. Fortunately, the rate of progression is linear in most individuals, so the prognosis of CKD can be predicted from a plot of GFR or 1/serum creatinine versus time (see Fig. 131–3). Monitoring the course of CKD not only has prognostic value; it also can be used to evaluate the efficacy of therapy or to determine when investigation should be undertaken for complications that accelerate the loss of kidney function (e.g., nephrotoxic agents or the presence of obstruction). Factors that should be regularly evaluated include the presence of symptoms of advancing CKD or uremia, changes in body weight, blood pressure and the presence of edema, SUN concentration, urine albumin–to-creatinine ratio, hemoglobin level, serum albumin concentration, serum calcium concentration, phosphorus concentration, and electrolyte values. Changes in these factors should be investigated.

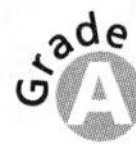

1. Brenner BM, Cooper ME, De Zeeuw D, et al: Effects of losartan on renal and cardiovascular outcomes in patients with type 2 diabetes and nephropathy. N Engl J Med 2001;345:861–869.
2. Hou FF, Zhang X, Zhang GH, et al: Efficacy and safety of benazepril for advanced chronic renal insufficiency. N Engl J Med 2006; 354:131–140.
3. Jafar TH, Schmid CH, Landa M, et al: Angiotensin-converting enzyme inhibitors and progression of nondiabetic renal disease: A meta-analysis of patient-level data. Ann Intern Med 2001; 135:73–87.
4. Fouque D, Laville M, Boissel JP: Low protein diets for chronic renal failure in non-diabetic adults. Cochrane Database Syst Rev 2006 Apr 19;(2):CD001892.

SUGGESTED READINGS

CDC: Racial differences in trends of end-stage renal disease, by primary diagnosis—United States, 1994–2004. MMWR 2007;56:253–256. *ESRD attributed to glomerulonephritis decreased among all races; ESRD attributed to diabetes or hypertension also decreased for American Indians/Alaska Natives and Asians/Pacific Islanders but not for whites or blacks.*

De Jong PE, Brenner BM: From secondary to primary prevention of progressive renal disease: The case for screening for albuminuria. Kidney Int 2004;66: 2109–2118. *Screening for albuminuria detects patients with early kidney disease.*

Go AS, Chertow GM, Fan D, et al: Chronic kidney disease and the risks of death, cardiovascular events, and hospitalization. N Engl J Med 2004;351:1296–1305. *Risks are markedly increased.*

Gooch K, Culleton BF, Manna BJ, et al: NSAID use and progression of chronic kidney disease. Am J Med 2007;120:280.e1–7. *High cumulative NSAID exposure is associated with an increased risk for rapid CKD progression.*

Masud T, Manatunga A, Cotsonis G, Mitch WE: The precision of estimating protein intake of patients with chronic renal failure. Kidney Int 2002; 62:1750–1756. *Compliance with low-protein diet prescriptions can be monitored by 24-hour urine collection of urea nitrogen.*

Meguid El Nahas A, Bello AK: Chronic kidney disease: The global challenge. Lancet 2005;365:331–340. *Examines the epidemiology of CKD worldwide, with emphasis on early detection and prevention.*

Remuzzi G, Benigni A, Remuzzi A: Mechanisms of progression and regression of renal lesions of chronic nephropathies and diabetes. J Clin Invest 2006; 116:288–296. *A scholarly review.*

Stevens LA, Coresh J, Greene T, et al: Assessing kidney function: Measured and estimated glomerular filtration rate. N Engl J Med 2006;354:2473–2483. *A practical approach.*

132 RENAL OSTEODYSTROPHY

Keith A. Hruska

Definition

Renal osteodystrophy (ROD) is a disorder of skeletal remodeling resulting from injury to the kidney, especially as seen in chronic kidney disease (CKD) (Chapter 131). The manifestations of ROD are proportional to the severity of renal injury. In end-stage kidney disease (ESKD) (Chapter 133), stage 5 in the Kidney Disease Outcomes Quality Initiative (K/DOQI) classification, some manifestation of the disorder is expressed in the great majority of patients. ROD encompasses a wide variety of derangements in mineral and bone metabolism, and it directly contributes to the excess cardiovascular mortality associated with CKD.

The earliest histologic abnormalities of bone in ROD are seen after a relatively mild reduction in the glomerular filtration rate (creatinine clearance between 40 and 70 mL/min, stage 2 CKD). By the time that ESKD develops, skeletal histologic pathology is found in virtually all patients. The increasing incidence of CKD and ESKD in the United States and the role of ROD in their high mortality make ROD a major health issue for Americans and all developed societies.

Pathobiology

Pathogenesis

Renal injuries produce a loss of skeletal anabolism manifested as a decrease in bone formation derived from osteoblast activity. The loss of anabolism may represent decreased influence of a hormonal factor or increased activity of an inhibitory principle. The effect is loss of influence of either bone morphogenetic proteins (BMPs) or wingless/ints proteins (Wnts) on osteoblast activity after renal injury. Because osteoblasts are the hematopoietic stem cell niche, an adaptation to the loss of anabolism is required to preserve hematopoiesis. This adaptation is secondary hyperparathyroidism. Three principles—BMPs, Wnts, and parathyroid hormone (PTH)—regulate the hematopoietic stem cell niche. Loss of osteoblastic bone formation secondary to renal injury shrinks the size of the rapidly exchangeable phosphate and calcium pools and causes early secondary hyperparathyroidism as a result of adapting to maintain the niche size; such adaptation is achieved at the expense of high PTH levels and the influence of secondary hyperparathyroidism on skeletal remodeling.

As kidney failure advances, a variety of factors directly stimulate PTH secretion, including hypocalcemia, low levels of circulating calcitriol (the hormonal vitamin D metabolite), hyperphosphatemia, and others. These factors are additive to the initial stimulus produced by renal injury. The initial stimulus to hyperparathyroidism by renal injury is demonstrated in some patients with mild chronic kidney failure who exhibit increased serum PTH levels without alterations in fasting serum levels of calcium, phosphorus, or calcitriol.

Early Kidney Failure

The early sequence of events in ROD remains to be fully defined. However, early stages of kidney failure can be shown to decrease bone formation rates and osteoblast surfaces when normal Ca, Pi, PTH, and vitamin D levels are maintained. This loss of anabolism causes an adaptive hyperparathyroidism in an attempt to maintain normal osteoblastic function. However, higher than normal PTH levels are required in the new abnormal skeletal environment because of loss of osteoblastic anabolism from the BMPs or Wnts. The function of PTH in this setting is to maintain homeostasis of hematopoiesis and the skeleton through regulation of the hematopoietic stem cell niche and skeletal remodeling. The hematopoietic stem cell is the target of another renal hormone, erythropoietin, produced by the kidney in response to its function as the body's oxygen sensor. Thus, it is not surprising that the kidney produces an osteoblast anabolic principle that has yet to be defined because it is necessary to maintain the niche of the erythropoietin target, the hematopoietic stem cell. Disturbances in stem cell function threaten the homeostasis of hematopoiesis and may contribute to the abnormalities in immunity that complicate CKD. The sustained increased PTH levels achieved through adaptation to CKD produce an unwanted disorder of skeletal remodeling, high-turnover ROD, also referred to as osteitis fibrosa.

Advanced Kidney Failure

As renal injuries advance and more significant reductions in the glomerular filtration rate result, classic changes in vitamin D metabolism and divalent ion homeostasis develop and are associated with the pathogenesis of secondary hyperparathyroidism in CKD. These changes are loss of capacity in calcitriol production, decreased calcium absorption leading to hypocalcemia, and a decrease in phosphate excretion leading to hyperphosphatemia.

Pathogenetic Factors in Secondary Hyperparathyroidism

CALCITRIOL DEFICIENCY. As CKD advances, the functioning nephron mass is decreased, which when combined with an increased phosphate load in the remaining nephrons and perhaps increased fibroblast growth factor-23 (FGF-23) levels, results in decreased production of calcitriol by proximal tubular 25-hydroxycholecalciferol 1a-hydroxylase. Calcitriol deficiency in turn decreases intestinal calcium absorption and leads to hypocalcemia. Calcitriol deficiency in cases of advanced kidney failure diminishes tissue levels of vitamin D receptors (VDRs), in particular, VDRs in the parathyroid glands. Because the chief cell VDR suppresses the expression of pre-pro-PTH messenger RNA (mRNA), lower circulating calcitriol levels together with a low number of VDRs in patients with ESKD result in stimulation of both synthesis and secretion of PTH.

HYPOCALCEMIA. As CKD progresses, hypocalcemia develops as a result of decreased intestinal Ca absorption. Low blood levels of ionized calcium stimulate PTH secretion, whereas high calcium concentrations suppress it. The action of calcium on parathyroid gland chief cells is mediated through a calcium sensor—a G protein–coupled plasma membrane receptor expressed in chief cells, in kidney tubular epithelia, and widely throughout the body at lower levels. The short-term stimulation of PTH secretion induced by low calcium is due to exocytosis of the PTH packaged in granules, and longer-term stimulation results from an increase in the number of cells that secrete PTH. More prolonged hypocalcemia induces changes in intracellular PTH degradation and mobilization of a secondary storage pool. Within days or weeks of the onset of hypocalcemia, pre-pro-PTH mRNA expression is stimulated. This effect is exerted through a negative calcium response element located in the upstream flanking region of the gene for PTH. Expression of the calcium receptor is suppressed by calcitriol deficiency and stimulated by calcitriol administration, thus suggesting an additional regulatory mechanism of the active vitamin D metabolite on PTH production. The decreased number of calcium-sensing receptors with low circulating calcitriol levels may, at least in part, explain the relative insensitivity of parathyroid gland cells to calcium in patients undergoing dialysis.

HYPERPHOSPHATEMIA. As renal injury decreases nephron numbers, the stimulus to hyperphosphatemia is reversed through PTH- and perhaps FGF-23–mediated reductions in tubular epithelial phosphate transport. The increase in phosphate excretion per remaining nephron restores phosphate homeostasis at the cost of higher PTH and FGF-23 levels. When renal injury is severe enough that the glomerular filtration rate is less than 30% of normal (stages 4 and 5 CKD), hyperphosphatemia becomes fixed because of insufficient renal excretion despite high PTH and FGF-23 levels. At this reduced renal function, the ability of the remaining nephrons to increase phosphate excretion above roughly 75% of the filtered load fails for unclear reasons. Recent studies have demonstrated that failure of phosphorus deposition in the skeleton or excess resorption of the skeleton also contributes to the hyperphosphatemia seen in patients with CKD and ESKD. Hyperphosphatemia decreases serum calcium through physicochemical binding and suppresses 1α-hydroxylase activity, which results in further lowering of circulating calcitriol levels. Moreover, a direct stimulatory effect of phosphorus on parathyroid gland cells, independent of calcium and calcitriol, produces increased secretion and nodular hyperplasia of parathyroid gland cells. Finally, hyperphosphatemia is a signaling mechanism for induction of heterotopic mineralization of the vasculature in CKD and ESKD.

HYPERPARATHYROIDISM. All of the mechanisms just discussed result in increased production of PTH and increased parathyroid gland mass. The size of the parathyroid glands progressively increases during CKD and in dialyzed patients in parallel with serum PTH levels. This increase in gland size is mainly due to diffuse cellular hyperplasia. Monoclonal chief cell growth also develops and results in the formation of nodules. Nodular hyperplastic glands have fewer VDRs and calcium-sensing receptors than diffusely hyperplastic glands do, thereby promoting parathyroid gland resistance to calcitriol and calcium. Sustained elevations in PTH levels, though adaptive to maintain osteoblast surfaces, produce an abnormal phenotype of osteoblast function with relatively less type 1 collagen and more RANKL ligand production than is the case with anabolic osteoblasts. This leads to high-turnover osteodystrophy, desensitization of PTH receptors, and excess bone resorption.

FIBROBLAST GROWTH FACTOR-23. FGF-23 is the original phosphatonin (phosphate excretion–regulating hormone) discovered in studies of inherited hypophosphatemia and oncogenic osteomalacia. FGF-23 levels progressively rise during the course of CKD, but the role of FGF-23 in regulating phosphate homeostasis in CKD and calcitriol synthesis has not been fully elucidated. Furthermore, FGF-23 is produced mainly by osteoblasts, and it is a mineralization inhibitor. It is unclear whether FGF-23 contributes to the mineralization defects in skeletal remodeling observed in CKD.

INFLAMMATORY MEDIATORS. CKD is well known as an inflammatory state with elevated levels of numerous inflammatory cytokines, chemokines, and their receptors. For instance, interleukin-8 (IL-8) levels are elevated and contribute to PTH secretion. A central inflammatory cytokine, IL-6, is a direct marker of inflammation in CKD and contributes to the pathogenesis of ROD, but the critical roles of inflammatory mediators in ROD remain to be defined.

ALUMINUM. Accumulation of aluminum (Al^{+3}) in bone and other organs such as the parathyroid glands may occur in patients with moderate or severe renal disease or in those undergoing dialysis. Aluminum accumulation in the parathyroid glands results in decreased secretion of PTH and suppression of bone turnover. In addition, Al^{+3} inhibits renal and intestinal 25-hydroxycholecalciferol 1α-hydroxylase activity, and thus Al^{+3} may further contribute to reduced levels of calcitriol. Possible sources of aluminum include high concentrations in the water used for dialysis, prescription of aluminum-containing phosphate binders, and aluminum in drinking water, infant formula, and other liquids or solid food.

ACIDOSIS. As nephron mass declines in CKD, the ability to regenerate bicarbonate consumed in the buffering of metabolic acids is lost. As a result, metabolic acidosis is a uniform finding in stage 4 and 5 CKD. In this setting, bone becomes an important buffer of acid production in patients with ESKD. Metabolic acidosis stimulates bone resorption and suppresses bone formation, thereby resulting in negative bone balance and contributing significantly to the pathogenesis of ROD.

HYPOGONADISM. Patients with ESKD have various states of gonadal dysfunction. Estrogen and testosterone deficiency significantly contributes to the pathogenesis of ROD.

OTHER FACTORS. Some patients with CKD are treated with glucocorticoids, which have an impact on bone metabolism. Patients maintained on chronic dialysis have retention of β_2-microglobulin, which causes a distinct arthropathy. Additionally, alterations in growth factors and other hormones involved in the regulation of bone remodeling may be disordered in CKD/ESRD, thus affecting bone remodeling and contributing to the development of ROD.

Pathology

ROD is not a uniform disease. Depending on the relative contribution of the different pathogenic factors discussed earlier, various pathologic patterns of bone remodeling are expressed in CKD and ESKD.

Predominant Hyperparathyroid Bone Disease, High-Turnover Renal Osteodystrophy, Osteitis Fibrosa

Sustained excess PTH results in increased bone turnover. Osteoclasts, osteoblasts, and osteocytes are found in abundance (Fig. 132–1). Disturbed osteoblastic activity results in a disorderly production of collagen, which leads to the formation of woven bone. Accumulation of fibroblastic osteoprogenitors not in the osteoblastic differentiation program results in collagen deposition (fibrosis) in the peritrabecular and marrow space. The nonmineralized component of bone, osteoid, is increased, and the normal three-dimensional architecture of osteoid is frequently lost. Osteoid seams no longer exhibit their usual birefringence under polarized light; instead, a disorderly arrangement of woven osteoid and woven bone with a typical crisscross pattern under polarized light is seen. The mineral apposition rate and the number of actively mineralizing sites are increased, as documented under fluorescent light after the administration of time-spaced fluorescent (tetracycline) markers.

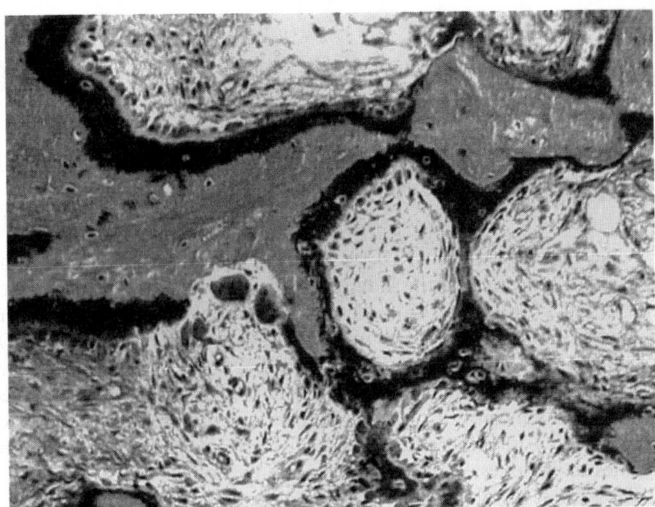

FIGURE 132–1 • Predominant hyperparathyroid bone disease with a high fraction of the trabecular surface covered by osteoid seams, many osteoblasts, and osteoclasts. Peritrabecular marrow fibrosis results from proliferating stromal cells that move efficiently through the osteoblastic differentiation program in an undecalcified 3-μm-thick section of iliac bone (brightfield light microscopy, modified Masson-Goldner stain, original magnification ×125).

Low-Turnover Bone Disease, Adynamic Bone Disorder

Low-turnover uremic osteodystrophy is the other end of the spectrum of ROD. The histologic hallmark of this group is a profound decrease in bone turnover because of a low number of active remodeling sites, suppression of bone formation, and low resorption, which is not as decreased as formation. The result is a low-turnover osteopenic condition. Lining cells with few osteoclasts and osteoblasts cover the majority of trabecular bone. Bone structure is predominantly lamellar, and the extent of mineralizing surfaces is markedly reduced. Usually only a few thin, single tetracycline labels are observed. Two histologic subgroups can be identified in this type of ROD, depending on the cause of events leading to the decline in osteoblast activity: adynamic bone disorder and low-turnover osteomalacia from Al^{+3} intoxication osteomalacia and adynamic bone disease. With Al^{+3}-induced adynamic uremic bone disease, the reduction in mineralization is obscured because of concomitant decreased bone formation. Adynamic uremic bone disease is characterized by few osteoid seams and few bone cells (Fig. 132–2).

Low-turnover osteomalacia is marked by an accumulation of unmineralized matrix in which a diminution in mineralization precedes or is more pronounced than the inhibition of collagen deposition. Unmineralized bone represents a sizable fraction of the trabecular bone volume. The increased lamellar osteoid volume is due to the presence of wide osteoid seams that cover a large portion of the trabecular surface (Fig. 132–3). The occasional presence of woven bone buried within the trabeculae indicates past high bone turnover. When osteoclasts are present, they are usually seen within trabecular bone or at the small fraction of the trabecular surface left without osteoid coating.

Mixed Uremic Osteodystrophy, High-Turnover Renal Osteodystrophy, and a Mineralization Defect

Mixed uremic osteodystrophy is caused primarily by hyperparathyroidism and defective mineralization with or without increased bone formation. These features may coexist in various degrees in different patients. Increased numbers of heterogeneous remodeling sites can be seen (Fig. 132–4). The number of osteoclasts is generally increased. Because active foci with numerous cells, woven osteoid seams, and peritrabecular fibrosis coexist next to lamellar sites with more reduced activity, greater production of lamellar or woven osteoid causes an accumulation of osteoid with a normal or increased thickness of osteoid seams. Whereas active mineralizing surfaces increase in woven bone with a higher mineralization rate and diffuse labeling, mineralization surfaces may be reduced in lamellar bone with a decreased mineral apposition rate.

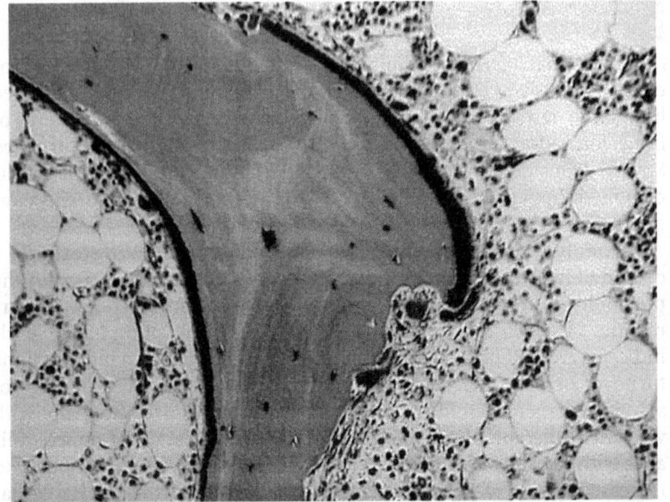

FIGURE 132–2 • Mixed uremic osteodystrophy. Few osteoblasts, several osteoclasts, and mild peritrabecular fibrosis are seen on an undecalcified 3-μm-thick section of human iliac bone (brightfield light microscopy, modified Masson-Goldner stain, original magnification ×125).

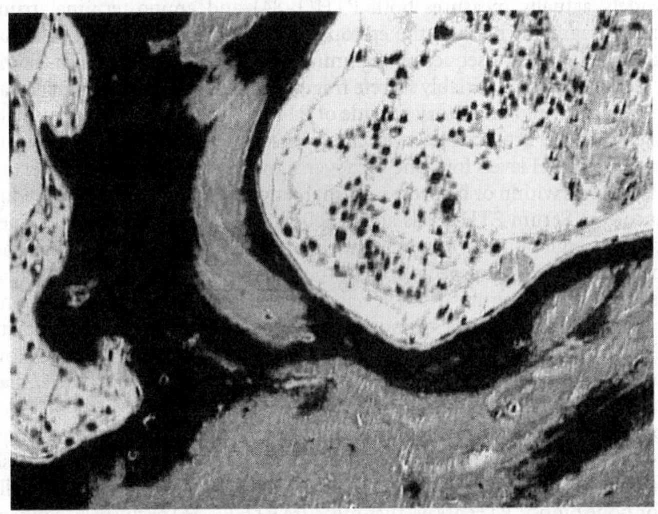

FIGURE 132–3 • Low-turnover osteomalacia. Osteoid has accumulated, and a high ratio of osteoid surface to bone surface, thick osteoid seams, and absence of active osteoblasts or osteoclasts are noted on an undecalcified 3-μm-thick section of iliac bone (brightfield light microscopy, modified Masson-Goldner stain, original magnification ×160).

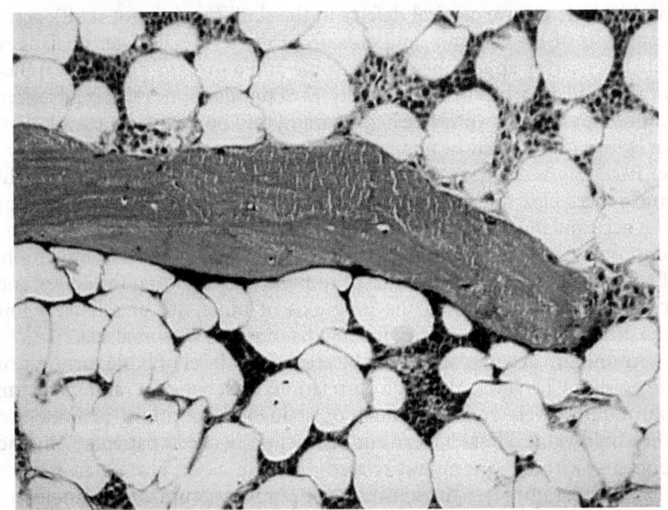

FIGURE 132–4 • Adynamic bone disorder. No accumulation of osteoid and absence of osteoblasts and osteoclasts are seen on an undecalcified 3-μm-thick section of iliac bone (brightfield light microscopy, modified Masson-Goldner stain, original magnification ×125).

Associated Features

Osteoporosis and Osteosclerosis

With progressive loss of renal function, cancellous bone volume may be increased along with loss of cortical bone, but this is in part due to deposition of woven immature collagen fibrils instead of lamellar fibrils. Thus, bone strength suffers despite the increase in mass detected by dual-energy x-ray absorptiometry. Patients undergoing chronic dialysis might have a loss or gain in bone volume depending on bone balance. In the case of negative bone balance, bone loss occurs in cortical and cancellous bone and is more rapid when bone turnover is high. In such cases, bone densitometry will detect osteopenia or osteoporosis. When the bone balance is positive, osteosclerosis may be observed when osteoblasts are active in depositing new bone (especially woven), thus superseding bone resorption. When bone turnover is low, however, positive phosphorus and calcium balance results in hyperphosphatemia and hypercalcemia without an increase in skeletal mineral deposition, but with stimulation of heterotopic mineralization, especially of the vasculature.

Bone Aluminum, Iron, Lanthanum, and Bisphosphonate Accumulation

These substances accumulate in bone at the mineralization front, at cement lines, or diffusely. The extent of stainable aluminum at the mineralization front correlates with histologic abnormalities in mineralization. Aluminum deposition is most severe in cases of low-turnover osteomalacia. However, it can be observed in all histologic forms of ROD. In patients in whom an increased aluminum burden develops, bone mineralization and bone turnover progressively decrease. These abnormalities are reversed with removal of the aluminum. Iron also accumulates at the mineralization front and can cause low-turnover forms of ROD similar to aluminum, although much less is known of iron than aluminum intoxication. Lanthanum has recently been added as a trace metal administered to CKD and ESKD patients. It is poorly absorbed and its levels in bone are much less than those of aluminum. Whether it will prove to have toxic effects remains unknown, but 2-year data suggest not. Lanthanum disappearance from bone deposits is slow, but not as slow as disappearance of bisphosphonate from bone deposits. Bisphosphonates are drugs used for the treatment of osteoporosis and hypercalcemia. There are increasing instances of bisphosphonate use in patients with CKD and ESKD. However, the nature of the bone remodeling abnormalities in CKD, especially with woven bone formation and mineralization defects, creates a high level of risk for skeletal deposition of a substance that once deposited may not be removed. Such a risk for long-term retention of an active drug is now being recognized with the use of bisphosphonates for osteogenesis imperfecta.

Clinical Manifestations

Patients with mild to moderate kidney insufficiency are rarely symptomatic from ROD and its skeletal pathology. However, we must consider vascular calcification a complication of ROD and the appearance of ROD as a cause of vascular stiffness. Vascular stiffness results in an increase in systolic blood pressure, widening of the pulse pressure, and an increase in pulse wave velocity in CKD. Vascular calcification is a clinically important complication of ROD that develops while the patient may be asymptomatic in the musculoskeletal system.

Symptoms of ROD related to the skeleton appear in patients with advanced kidney failure. Clinical manifestations are, however, preceded by an abnormal biochemical profile that should alert the physician and prompt steps to prevent more severe complications. When symptoms related to the skeleton occur, they are usually insidious, subtle, nonspecific, and slowly progressive.

Heterotopic Mineralization, Calciphylaxis, and Tumoral Calcinosis

Vascular calcification is common in patients with ESKD and causes left ventricular hypertrophy, congestive heart failure, and coronary ischemia. The pathogenesis of vascular calcification in CKD is complex, but it involves activation of an osteogenic program in cells of the neointima around atherosclerotic plaques and the tunica media. Diffuse calcification of the tunica media is referred to as Mönckeberg's sclerosis. CKD is the most common cause of Mönckeberg's sclerosis, especially when it complicates diabetes mellitus (Chapter 248). All forms of ROD are associated with vascular calcification, but especially important is the association between low-turnover osteodystrophy and vascular calcification. Here, the decrease in skeletal osteoblast function is associated with osteoblastic differentiation of cells in the vasculature. Furthermore, signals derived from the skeleton are direct causes of the vascular mineralization. One such signal is hyperphosphatemia.

Heterotopic tissue calcification may occur in the eyes and be manifested as band keratopathy in the sclerae or induce an inflammatory response in the conjunctiva known as red eye syndrome. These types of calcification are generally associated with hyperparathyroidism or increased calcium phosphate product. Calcium deposits are also found in the lungs and lead to restrictive lung disease. Deposits in the myocardium might cause arrhythmias, annular calcifications, or myocardial dysfunction. Most soft tissue calcifications are attributed to secondary hyperparathyroidism or to the increased calcium phosphate product associated with it. However, they have also been described in patients with adynamic bone disease. This diversity could be explained by increased calcium or phosphate release (or both) from bone in patients with severe hyperparathyroidism and an inability to maintain normal mineral accretion in patients with adynamic bone disease.

The syndrome of calciphylaxis is characterized by vascular calcification in the tunica media of peripheral arteries. These calcifications induce painful violaceous skin lesions that progress to ischemic necrosis. This syndrome has been linked to serious complications and often death. Calciphylaxis has been associated with high serum calcium phosphate product and severe secondary hyperparathyroidism. However, it can also be seen in patients with normal or mildly elevated serum phosphate or PTH levels. The pathogenesis of calciphylaxis is probably multifactorial because hyperparathyroidism, high calcium phosphate product, steroid therapy, vitamin D therapy, iron overload, aluminum toxicity, and protein C deficiency have all been implicated.

Tumoral calcinosis is a form of soft tissue calcification that usually involves the periarticular tissues. Calcium deposits may grow to enormous size and interfere with the function of adjacent joints and organs. Although this type of calcification is generally associated with high calcium phosphate product, its exact pathogenesis is poorly understood. It may also be associated with certain ill-defined intrinsic factors. Similar to soft tissue calcification, it is observed with severe hyperparathyroidism and low-turnover bone disease.

Bone Pain, Fractures, and Skeletal Deformities

Bone pain is usually vague, ill defined, and deep-seated. It may be diffuse or localized in the lower part of the back, hips, knees, or legs. Weight bearing and changes in position commonly aggravate it. Bone pain may progress slowly to the degree that patients are completely incapacitated. Bone pain in patients with ESKD does not usually cause physical signs; however, local tenderness may be apparent with pressure. Occasionally, pain can occur suddenly at one joint of the lower extremities and mimic acute arthritis or periarthritis not relieved by heat or massage. A sharp chest pain may indicate a rib fracture. Spontaneous fractures or fractures after minimal trauma may also occur in the vertebrae (crush fractures) and tubular bones.

Bone pain and bone fractures can be observed in all patients with ESKD independent of the underlying histologic bone disease, especially when osteoporosis is present. However, low-turnover osteomalacia and aluminum-related bone disease are associated with the most severe bone pain and the highest incidence of fractures and incapacity.

Skeletal deformities can be observed in children and adults. Most children with ESKD have growth retardation, and bone deformities may develop from vitamin D deficiency (rickets) or secondary hyperparathyroidism. In rickets, bowing of the long bones is seen, especially the tibia and femur, along with typical genu valgum that becomes more severe with adolescence. Long-standing secondary hyperparathyroidism in children may be responsible for slipped epiphyses secondary to impaired transformation of growth cartilage into regular metaphyseal spongiosa. This complication most commonly affects the hips, becomes obvious in preadolescence, and causes limping but is usually painless. When the radius and ulna are involved, ulnar deviation of the hands and local swelling may occur. In adults, skeletal deformities can be observed in those with severe osteomalacia or osteoporosis and include lumbar scoliosis, thoracic kyphosis, and recurrent rib fractures.

Diagnosis

ROD is characterized pathologically, and the only unequivocal tool for exact diagnosis is bone biopsy. Histologic examination of mineralized bone after tetracycline double labeling determines the precise level of bone formation, mineralization, bone resorption, and bone turnover. Special stains determine Al, Fe, or La deposition, if present. The results of bone biopsy serve as the basis for appropriate use of tailored therapeutic regimens.

In the absence of bone biopsy, the physician needs to estimate the level of bone turnover, the presence of osteomalacia (Chapter 265), and the possibility of bone toxicity from deposition of an unwanted ion. Abnormalities in serum calcium, phosphorus, and alkaline phosphatase levels indicate severe ROD but are not helpful when used alone to indicate bone turnover or osteomalacia. Hypercalcemia may be observed in cases of severe hyperparathyroidism or adynamic bone disease, especially with vitamin D therapy. Hyperphosphatemia is an indication of noncompliance with phosphate binders or severe hyperparathyroidism secondary to increased release of phosphorus from bone. High serum levels of alkaline phosphatase may be observed in both osteomalacia and predominant hyperparathyroidism.

Serum PTH levels are better indicators of bone turnover. However, the abnormalities in PTH metabolism that accompany CKD have complicated PTH measurements. The "intact" hormone assay currently used widely actually measures both PTH(1–84) and amino-terminal–truncated fragments because the epitope recognized by the amino-terminal antibody detects a sequence beginning with amino acid 13. Because the chief cells in CKD variably secrete fragments such as 7–84, the intact assay may measure an inhibitory peptide of PTH and significantly overestimate biologic PTH activity. However, careful assessment of the predictive value of serum PTH levels for bone turnover shows that all patients with serum PTH levels within or below the normal range (<65 pg/mL) have low bone turnover. Serum PTH levels above 500 pg/mL are 100% and 95.5% specific for high bone turnover in patients maintained on hemodialysis and peritoneal dialysis, respectively. For the majority of dialyzed patients, that is, those with serum PTH levels between 65 and 500 pg/mL, bone turnover unfortunately cannot be predicted accurately by the "intact" PTH assay. In addition to serum PTH values, certain risk factors for low bone turnover have been isolated and include peritoneal dialysis, diabetes, advanced age, high calcium content in the dialysate, high doses of phosphate binders, aggressive vitamin D therapy, or previous parathyroidectomy. However, in individual patients, discrepancies between risk factors, PTH levels, and bone turnover are frequent; this situation calls for bone biopsy. PTH assays that measure PTH(1–84) exclusively confirm that the "intact" PTH assay detects not only PTH(1–84) but also large C-PTH fragments. These large fragments antagonize the effects of PTH(1–84) on serum calcium and bone turnover. However, the value of these PTH assays has not been determined in CKD, and routine implementation of these assays has not been achieved.

Skeletal radiographic abnormalities are seen when ROD is advanced and include erosive cortical defects in the skull (pepper pot skull), acro-osteolysis of the clavicula, and erosion of the terminal finger phalanges. A rugger-jersey appearance of the spine and a ground-glass appearance of the skull, ribs, pelvis, and metaphyses of tubular bones reflect advanced cancellous changes. In severe hyperparathyroid bone disease, pseudocysts or brown tumors may be observed. Radiographs underestimate the extent of ROD. Signs of increased bone resorption may be seen on radiographs and reflect past resorption activity, which may have been succeeded by the accumulation of osteoid. Because osteoid is radiolucent, the superimposed osteomalacia will be missed by radiographic examination. Looser's zones, or straight bands of radiolucency abutting the cortex and running perpendicular to the long axis of bone, are of relatively low sensitivity and low specificity for the diagnosis of osteomalacia.

Aluminum accumulation may be seen at any level of bone turnover or any serum PTH level. Although correlations exist between random serum aluminum levels and the extent of stainable aluminum in bone, no threshold value allows a clear-cut distinction between patients with and patients without aluminum-related bone disease. The deferoxamine infusion test improves the sensitivity of random serum aluminum levels. An increase in serum aluminum levels of greater than 200 μg/L 48 hours after a standardized infusion constitutes a positive result. This test, though improving the sensitivity of predicting aluminum-related bone disease, does not add specificity. Having both a positive deferoxamine test and a PTH level less than 200 pg/mL will make the diagnosis of aluminum-related bone disease with almost absolute certainty. However, the combination test greatly reduces the sensitivity.

Prevention and Treatment

Rx

Medical Therapy

Therapeutic intervention should begin before advanced ROD develops. By the time of institution of dialysis, patients should be receiving therapy for ROD. Avoiding deviations in serum phosphorus and calcium levels from normal can optimize PTH levels.

Control of Serum Phosphorus and Calcium

The available dialytic methods are inefficient in removing phosphorus because of compartmentalization and slow efflux of phosphorus from the exchangeable space. Hemodialysis for 4 hours three times a week removes approximately 3 g of phosphorus per week in the face of roughly 7 g of intake. Nocturnal dialysis for longer periods and daily dialysis are effective in maintaining normal phosphorus levels. Dietary phosphate restriction in ESKD is limited because of nutritional needs. Phosphate is present in most protein-containing food products. The current recommendations for protein intake in dialyzed patients are at least 1.2 g/kg/day (hemodialysis) and 1.3 g/kg/day (peritoneal dialysis), which provide a minimum of 1 g of phosphorus per day. Therefore, the addition of phosphate binders is needed in most patients. Currently used phosphate binders are calcium carbonate, calcium acetate, sevelamer, lanthanum carbonate, and others to a minor degree. Phosphate binders should be taken with meals and in proportion to the size of the meal. Calcium citrate should be avoided because it promotes intestinal aluminum absorption. Aluminum-containing phosphate binders, though more potent than calcium salts, should not be used because of the risk for aluminum-related bone disease. Calcium-containing phosphate binders are effective but increase serum calcium levels and sometimes cause hypercalcemia and an increase in calcium phosphate product. This may suppress bone formation and stimulate vascular calcification. A non–calcium-containing phosphate binder, sevelamer hydrochloride (Renagel), is an alternative to calcium salts. This drug has been shown to be associated with less progression of coronary and aortic calcification than occurs with calcium-containing phosphate binders. Tolerability and cost are limiting factors of sevelamer therapy. Lanthanum carbonate is a newer potent and well-tolerated phosphate binder. It does not appear to accumulate to toxic levels in bone as aluminum does, but only longer-term experience with lanthanum carbonate will determine its role as a therapeutic agent. Ferric citrate is available, but it may share the effects of Al^{+3} on bone remodeling.

Hypocalcemia in CKD may be corrected by control of serum phosphorus and vitamin D treatment. Calcium salt administration between meals as a Ca supplement should be limited to patients with symptomatic hypocalcemia.

Use of Vitamin D and Its Metabolites

Replacement of the deficient hormone calcitriol with active vitamin D analogues may begin in patients with CKD and is routine in those with ESKD. Vitamin D analogues are effective in suppressing secondary hyperparathyroidism. In moderate hyperparathyroidism with or without mineralization defects, oral administration of calcitriol, doxercalciferol, or paricalcitol usually decreases serum PTH levels and improves mineralzation. It is advisable to start with low doses and increase the daily dose in steps to adjust PTH levels to target values after 2 weeks of therapy. Episodes of hypercalcemia may occur and can be circumvented by decreasing oral calcium salts if serum phosphate levels permit or by lowering the dialysate calcium content. Despite these measures, however, hypercalcemia may persist. Intravenous treatment regimens using high doses of one of the vitamin D analogs two or three times per week have become predominant. These measures are effective, but the positive response is clearly reduced if the parathyroid glands undergo monoclonal growth transformation and become refractory to the action of calcitriol. The vitamin D analogues 19-nor-1α, 25-dihydroxyvitamin D_2 (Zemplar) and doxercalciferol (Hectorol) have been introduced for the control of secondary hyperparathyroidism, and their use has largely replaced calcitriol. They have somewhat different profiles of activity at the various tissues affected by calcitriol.

Because expression of the VDR and 25-OH cholecalciferol 1α-hydroxylase is more widespread than initially thought, deficiencies in the precursor vitamin D, 25-hydroxyvitamin D, should be ruled out or corrected if found.

Use of Calcimimetics

Recently, calcimimetic agents have been introduced for the control of PTH levels in CKD and ESKD. This new class of therapeutic agents represents allosteric modulators of the calcium-sensing receptor and allow for suppression of PTH synthesis and secretion while simultaneously lowering serum calcium and phosphorus levels. Therapy with cinacalcet appears to increase the proportion of subjects achieving K/DOQI PTH and Ca × PO_4 targets. However, it remains to be seen whether this will translate into improvement in bone health or cardiovascular outcomes.

Removal of Aluminum

Any therapeutic maneuver that lowers plasma aluminum levels and creates a concentration gradient across the bone–extracellular fluid membrane will be able to move aluminum from bone to blood. Because aluminum is 80% protein bound, only 20% of total aluminum can be removed by ultrafiltration. Elimination of aluminum from bone through normal turnover and by completely withdrawing aluminum sources is very slow and may take years. However, aluminum removal is greatly enhanced with use of the chelator agent deferoxamine. Deferoxamine increases the complex bound fraction of aluminum and facilitates its removal through dialysis. The association between deferoxamine therapy and infection has been a subject of controversy. Numerous case reports of bacteremia and mucormycosis during deferoxamine therapy have been published, but a large survey did not confirm that deferoxamine increases the risk for bacteremia in dialysis patients. The relationship between deferoxamine therapy and mucormycosis represents a very serious complication. Therefore, unequivocal documentation of aluminum overload is required before deferoxamine therapy is begun.

Surgical Therapy

Parathyroidectomy

Despite treatment, overt secondary hyperparathyroidism develops in some patients and may necessitate parathyroidectomy. Indications for parathyroidectomy include (1) persistent hypercalcemia despite no vitamin D treatment and modulation of the dialysate calcium concentration, (2) persistent hyperphosphatemia and a high calcium phosphate product despite aggressive dietary counseling and compliance with prescriptions, (3) progressive and symptomatic soft tissue calcification with high bone turnover (including calciphylaxis), (4) severe progressive and symptomatic hyperparathyroidism when a rapid reduction in PTH is required and vitamin D pulse therapy has failed, and (5) refractory pruritus. Before parathyroidectomy is performed, histologic evidence of severe hyperparathyroidism and absence of aluminum accumulation should be documented.

The most frequently used surgical approaches to parathyroidectomy are subtotal parathyroidectomy and total parathyroidectomy with parathyroid autotransplantation. Subtotal parathyroidectomy risks the possibility of inadequate reduction in parathyroid gland mass or the recurrence of hyperparathyroidism in the remaining tissue. These complications might require re-exploration of the neck, which can be difficult because of the formation of scar tissue. Marking the remaining gland with a metallic clip or a suture may facilitate re-exploration. Total parathyroidectomy with parathyroid autotransplantation in the forearm allows easy access to the residual parathyroid tissue if necessary. However, migration of the transplanted cells into the venous circulation and the muscles of the forearm has been reported. The success of both techniques relies on the expertise and experience of the surgeon.

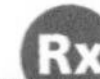

Patients undergoing parathyroidectomy require careful follow-up and meticulous management. Postoperative hypocalcemia should be anticipated and treated with oral and intravenous calcium. The use of calcitriol may minimize the need for large doses of calcium salts; however, its use may interfere with successful function of the transplanted gland. A reasonable approach would be the use of intravenous calcitriol administered at the end of each dialysis treatment for two to three treatments before parathyroidectomy, followed by the lowest dose of oral calcitriol needed.

Treatment of Adynamic Bone Disease

At the present time, adynamic bone disease should be managed by measures to increase PTH levels and increase remodeling. Although no specific treatment is available, effective measures include a reduction in calcium-containing phosphate binders or the dialysate calcium content (or both). Discontinuation of vitamin D analogues and calcimimetics may be necessary. Preventive measures should be carefully considered because of the morbidity of vascular calcification and the threat to the hematopoietic stem cell associated with this form of ROD.

SUGGESTED READINGS

Block GA, Martin KJ, de Francisco AL, et al: Cinacalcet for secondary hyperparathyroidism in patients receiving hemodialysis. N Engl J Med 2004;350:1516–1525. *Reports the efficacy of calcimimetics in the treatment of secondary hyperparathyroidism.*

Bone Metabolism and Disease Workgroup: K/DOQI Clinical Practice Guidelines on bone metabolism and disease in chronic kidney disease. Am J Kidney Dis 2003;42:S52–S57. *This quality improvement initiative establishes clinical practice guidelines for the management of ROD and hyperparathyroidism and represents the basis for treatment recommendations in this chapter, along with the personal opinions of the author.*

Calvi LM, Adams GB, Weibrecht KW, et al: Osteoblastic cells regulate the haematopoietic stem cell niche. Nature 2003;425:841–846. *Identifies the hematopoietic stem cell niche as a target of PTH and offers an explanation for the necessity of PTH adaptation to the loss of skeletal anabolism produced by renal injury.*

Davies MR, Lund RJ, Mathew S, et al: Low turnover osteodystrophy and vascular calcification are amenable to skeletal anabolism in an animal model of chronic kidney disease and the metabolic syndrome. J Am Soc Nephrol 2005;16:917–928. *Presents the critical demonstration that ROD contributes causally to vascular calcification.*

Fukagawa M, Nakanishi S, Kazama JJ: Basic and clinical aspects of parathyroid hyperplasia in chronic kidney disease. Kidney Int Suppl 2006;102:S3–S7.

Go AS, Chertow GM, Fan D, et al: Chronic kidney disease and the risks of death, cardiovascular events, and hospitalization. N Engl J Med 2004;351:1296–1305. *Describes the excess mortality from cardiovascular risk in CKD.*

Gutierrez O, Isakova T, Rhee E, et al: Fibroblast growth factor-23 mitigates hyperphosphatemia but accentuates calcitriol deficiency in chronic kidney disease. J Am Soc Nephrol 2005;16:2205–2215. *Reports early studies of the role of FGF-23 in CKD.*

Lee GH, Benner D, Regidor DC, et al: Impact of kidney bone disease and its management on survival of patients on dialysis. J Rev Nutr 2007;17:38–44. *Bone disease is an independent predictor of adverse outcome.*

Lund RJ, Davies MR, Brown AJ, et al: Successful treatment of an adynamic bone disorder with bone morphogenetic protein-7 in a renal ablation model. J Am Soc Nephrol 2004;15:359–369. *Presents the critical demonstration that renal injury directly impairs bone formation (skeletal anabolism).*

Spasovski GB, Sikole A, Gelev S, et al: Evolution of bone and plasma concentration of lanthanum in dialysis patients before, during 1 year of treatment with lanthanum carbonate and after 2 years of follow-up. Nephrol Dial Transplant 2006;21:2217–2224. *Reports La^{+3} levels and its localization during treatment of ESKD patients with $LaCO_3$.*

Stevens LA, Djurdjev O, Cardew S, et al: Calcium, phosphate, and parathyroid hormone levels in combination and as a function of dialysis duration predict mortality: Evidence for the complexity of the association between mineral metabolism and outcomes. J Am Soc Nephrol 2004;15:770–779. *One of many observational studies suggesting that hyperphosphatemia is a cardiovascular risk factor in ESKD.*

Teng M, Wolf M, Lowrie E, et al: Survival of patients undergoing hemodialysis with paricalcitol or calcitriol therapy. N Engl J Med 2003;349:446–456. *A retrospective analysis of a large dialysis company patient database suggesting that paricalcitol improves survival.*

Zhang J, Niu C, Ye L, et al: Identification of the haematopoietic stem cell niche and control of the niche size. Nature 2003;425:836–841. *Identifies the osteoblast as the hematopoietic stem cell niche and BMPs as anabolic factors regulating the niche. The loss of skeletal anabolic influence through renal injury threatens the niche and explains the necessity of adaptation in bone remodeling to kidney disease.*

133 TREATMENT OF IRREVERSIBLE RENAL FAILURE

Nina Tolkoff-Rubin

Unlike other forms of end-stage organ failure, renal failure is unique in having three modalities of therapy: (1) hemodialysis, (2) peritoneal dialysis, and (3) renal transplantation. Each form of renal replacement therapy (RRT) has its unique risks and benefits.

Kolff first employed hemodialysis in the late 1940s for the treatment of acute renal failure. The development of vascular access by Scribner in the early 1960s enabled the use of hemodialysis as a chronic therapy. However, it was not until 1973, when the U.S. Congress approved Medicare funding for hemodialysis patients, recognizing end-stage renal disease (ESRD) as a "catastrophic illness," that hemodialysis achieved widespread availability. Currently, there are approximately 350,000 patients on dialysis in the United States, and the ESRD population is projected to grow by about 7% per year.

All three modalities of RRT have evolved significantly over the last four decades. The selection of a particular form of RRT is made according to the clinical setting and patient preference. It is important for the physician and the patient to recognize that these modalities should be viewed as alternative and complementary therapies, allowing flexibility of care under different clinical circumstances. The key is to identify patients with progressive renal failure early, so as to enable them to make an educated choice that fits their lifestyle and medical situation. Planning and establishing access early decrease emergency hospitalizations and complications and significantly reduce cost. Early evaluation also enables identification of potential living donors so that preemptive transplantation can be performed.

HEMODIALYSIS

Dialysis substitutes two major renal functions: *solute removal* and *fluid removal.* In hemodialysis, solute removal occurs predominantly by diffusive clearance, which is the movement of solutes from the blood compartment to the dialysate compartment across a semipermeable membrane. The key determinants of clearance of a particular substance are the following:

1. Molecular size: clearance is size dependent and is higher for smaller molecules
2. The concentration gradient of a particular substance between the blood and the dialysis solution: the greater the concentration gradient, the more rapidly diffusion occurs
3. Membrane surface area: the net transfer of solute increases as membrane surface area increases
4. Membrane permeability: this is determined by the specific characteristics of the membrane, such as pore size, charge, and quaternary conformation
5. Blood and dialysate flow rates: higher flow rates allow greater solute removal, especially if the flow of dialysate is countercurrent to blood flow, which permits a maximal gradient across the membrane

Solute removal can also occur by the process of convection, the movement of solutes by bulk flow in association with fluid removal (solvent drag). Although the convective mass transfer of solutes may not play a dominant role in conventional hemodialysis, convection does play a significant role in high flux-dialysis and in continuous venovenous hemofiltration (CVVH).

Fluid removal in hemodialysis occurs by the process of ultrafiltration. The ultrafiltration rate is determined by the hydrostatic pressure gradient across the dialysis membrane, called the *transmembrane pressure.* Ultrafiltration increases if positive pressure is applied to the blood compartment or if negative pressure is applied to the dialysate side of the dialysis membrane. During dialysis, the ultrafiltration rate is adjusted to obtain the desired fluid loss.

The hemodialysis machine has three main components: (1) the dialyzer (i.e., the dialysis membrane); (2) a pump that regulates blood flow; and (3) a dialysate solution delivery system. In addition, the machine has many safety devices to monitor arterial and venous pressures, concentration of ions and temperature in the dialysate, and air and blood leaks (Fig. 133–1).

Under most circumstances, solute removal and fluid removal occur simultaneously. However, if vigorous ultrafiltration is attempted during conventional hemodialysis, patients frequently complain of muscle cramping, nausea, and vomiting. Moreover, during aggressive fluid removal there may be a decrease in systemic vascular resistance, leading to a drop in blood pressure. Separating ultrafiltration from dialysis enables efficient fluid removal with greater hemodynamic stability. Osmotic changes are minimized with isolated ultrafiltration (i.e., fluid removal in the absence of solute removal). As a result, vascular resistance is well maintained, and, consequently, less hypotension occurs in association with large fluid shifts.

Performing Hemodialysis

Hemodialyzers

The hollow-fiber dialyzer is composed of thousands of parallel capillary tubes. Blood flows through the capillary tubes, and dialysate flows in a countercurrent direction, bathing the outside of the capillary tubes (see Fig. 133–1).

The dialysis membrane is an essential component of the dialyzer. The initial membranes were made of cuprophane, a derivative of cellulose, which has excellent clearance of small molecules but very poor clearance of middle-sized molecules. The contact of blood with these membranes leads to activation of inflammatory and clotting cascades. The alternative pathway of complement is also activated by contact with the dialysis membrane, leading to activation of granulocytes. Production of platelet-activating factor is also increased with complement-activating membranes.

The activation of inflammatory and coagulation pathways leads to significant clinical events. Acutely, patients may develop chest pain, back pain, and shortness of breath, especially with cellulose membranes. Chronic activation of inflammatory pathways may also lead to accumulation of β_2-microglobulin and a form of amyloidosis described only in patients undergoing long-term hemodialysis. Dialysis-related amyloidosis is associated with carpal tunnel syndrome, diffuse arthropathy, lytic bone lesions, and pathologic fractures. The newer synthetic membranes made of polycarbonate, polysulfones, polyacrylonitrile, or polymethylmethacrylate are less proinflammatory and also have higher diffusive clearances for larger molecules and higher ultrafiltration rates.

The survival of patients with acute renal failure appears to be affected by the type of membrane employed. Studies comparing cuprophane with synthetic membranes show not only improved patient survival and more rapid recovery of kidney function after acute renal failure but also a decrease in the incidence of death from sepsis in the patients dialyzed with a synthetic membrane.

Access

To perform hemodialysis on a repetitive basis, access to the circulation is essential. The arteriovenous fistula (AVF) is the "gold standard" hemodialysis access and involves anastomosis of the radial artery or brachial artery to the cephalic or basilic veins, with subsequent "arterialization" of the superficial forearm veins to enable blood flow rates up to 400 mL/min. The most frequent problem associated with AVFs is failure to mature, particularly in patients with peripheral vascular disease or diabetes. Therefore, it is important to spare the nondominant arm from venipuncture in all patients with chronic kidney disease (CKD) and to plan the placement of AVFs long in advance of the patient's approach to

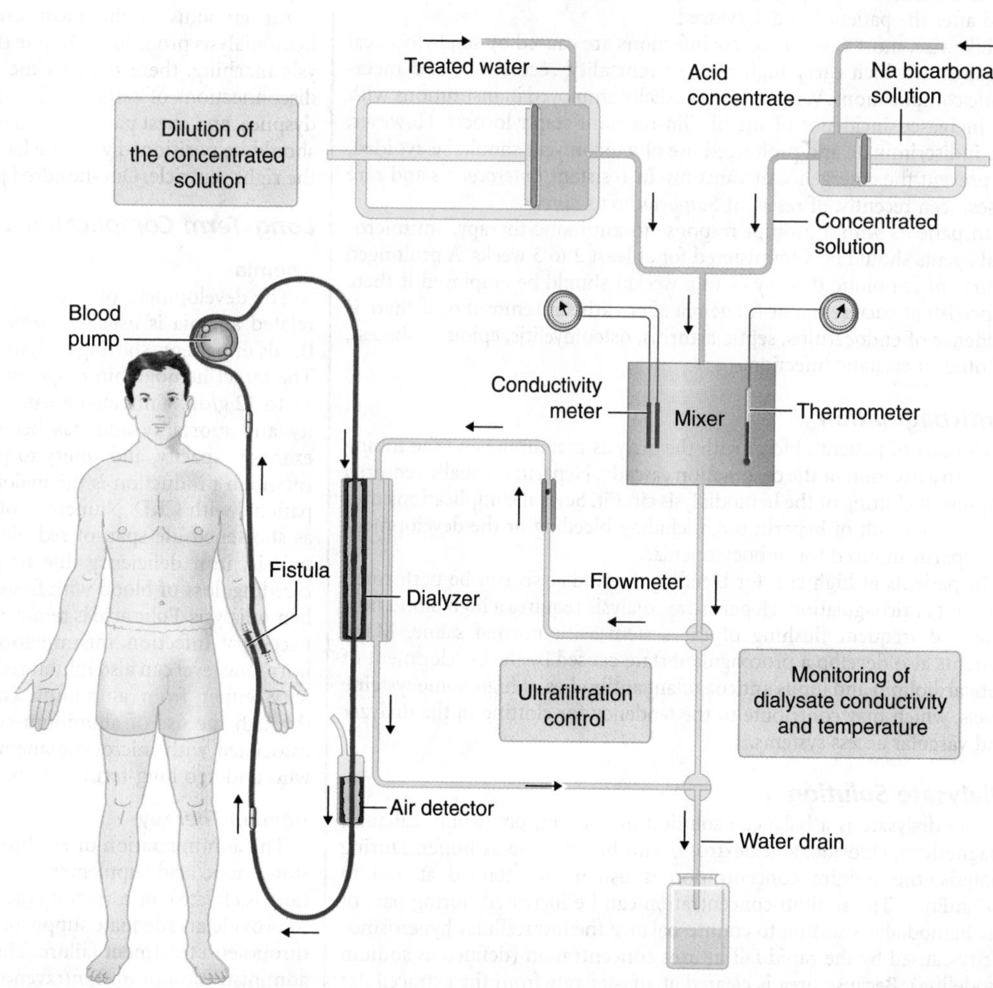

FIGURE 133–1 • Hemodialysis. Treated water is mixed with concentrated dialysate. The dialysate solution flows around the fibers of the hollow-fiber dialyzer counter-current to the blood flow through the dialyzer. A computerized ultra-filtration control device regulates fluid removal.

hemodialysis, because the fistula usually takes 6 to 8 weeks to mature. Less than one half of patients initiating hemodialysis in the United States have a permanent vascular access in place. Elective placement of a permanent access before dialysis initiation reduces morbidity, mortality, and cost. The National Kidney Foundation (NKF) Disease Outcomes Quality Initiative (DOQI) guidelines recommend placement of an AVF if the serum creatinine exceeds 4 mg/dL, creatinine clearance falls to less than 25 mL/min, or hemodialysis initiation is anticipated within one year.

Synthetic arteriovenous grafts (AVGs) can be used when a native AVF cannot be placed. The AVG carries a higher rate of thrombosis and infection than a fistula. The third option is percutaneous dual-lumen catheters, which are placed preferentially in the internal jugular vein with a segment of the line tunneled under the skin. Catheters placed in the subclavian vein are associated with a greater risk of central venous stenosis.

Vascular Access Infections

Although tunneled lines provide immediate and convenient access to the circulation, they have a high rate of infection and clotting. The skin and the catheter hubs are the primary sources of bacteria. Infectious complications of the vascular access are a major source of morbidity and mortality among hemodialysis patients, accounting for up to 73% of all cases of bacteremia in this population.

Over time, the inner surface of indwelling catheters becomes covered by biofilm, a complex of proteoglycans that can act as a nidus for microbial growth. Any approach that aims to limit biofilm formation may help decrease catheter-related infection. Thrombus within the catheter is another significant nidus for pathogens. Therefore, the use of anticoagulants to prevent catheter obstruction may have a beneficial impact on the prevention of catheter-associated infections.

If a patient presents with possible catheter-related bacteremia, blood cultures should be obtained both from the catheter and from a peripheral vein, and empirical antibiotics should be initiated. If the patient has any evidence of systemic sepsis with hemodynamic instability, the line should be pulled promptly; it should be reinserted only after blood cultures are negative under antibiotic administration for at least 48 hours and after the patient has defervesced.

Likewise, most vascular access infections are caused by staphylococcal organisms, which carry high rates of mortality, recurrence, and metastatic complications. Vancomycin is usually employed in institutions with an increased incidence of methicillin-resistant staphylococci. However, the indiscriminate and prolonged use of vancomycin should be avoided, to prevent the emergence of vancomycin-resistant *Enterococcus* and rare cases, seen recently, of resistant *Staphylococcus aureus.*

In patients with a prompt response to antibiotic therapy, antimicrobial agents should be administered for at least 2 to 3 weeks. A prolonged course of antibiotic therapy (4 to 8 weeks) should be employed if there is persistent bacteremia or fungemia after catheter removal or if there is evidence of endocarditis, septic arthritis, osteomyelitis, epidural abscess, or other metastatic infection.

Anticoagulation

Contact of patient's blood with the dialysis membrane and the tubing leads to activation of the coagulation cascade. Heparin is usually required to prevent clotting of the hemodialysis circuit. Several complications may occur as a result of heparin use, including bleeding or the development of heparin-induced thrombocytopenia.

In patients at high risk for bleeding, hemodialysis can be performed without anticoagulation. Heparin-free dialysis requires a high blood flow rate and frequent flushing of the system with normal saline. Many patients also develop a procoagulant state caused by the development of anticardiolipin and lupus anticoagulant antibodies or high homocysteine levels, which may contribute to the tendency for clotting in the dialyzer and vascular access systems.

Dialysate Solution

The dialysate is a balanced solution of sodium, potassium, calcium, magnesium, chloride, and dextrose, with bicarbonate as buffer. During dialysis, the sodium concentration is usually maintained at 135 to 140 mEq/L. The sodium concentration can be increased during part of the hemodialysis session to counterbalance the intracellular hyperosmolarity caused by the rapid fall in urea concentration (defined as sodium modeling). Because urea is cleared at a faster rate from the extracellular space, the intracellular space becomes relatively hyperosmolar during the course of dialysis, causing fluid to shift from the extracellular space into the intracellular space, which may lead to hypotension and central nervous system manifestations (dialysis disequilibrium syndrome). Sodium modeling helps prevent hypotension, muscle cramps, nausea, vomiting, headaches, and seizures during hemodialysis. The sodium concentration is programmed to return to normal range by the end of hemodialysis. Mannitol can also be used to prevent dialysis disequilibrium syndrome.

Water Quality

Because patients are exposed to large volumes of water during each hemodialysis treatment, purity of the water is essential to avoid exposure to aluminum, chloramines, endotoxin, and bacteria. The use of a charcoal filter removes organic toxins such as chloramines, which can cause acute hemolysis.

Aluminum is frequently added to the drinking water supply to precipitate suspended colloidal material. Chronic exposure to aluminum can lead to dialysis dementia. Severe bone disease and erythropoietin-resistant anemia are also associated with aluminum intoxication. Therefore, removal of aluminum from the water used to prepare dialysate is essential. Reverse osmosis or de-ionization of the water effectively removes aluminum, fluoride, and copper.

Complications

Complications during Hemodialysis

In addition to vascular access problems, the most common complications during hemodialysis are hypotension, muscle cramps, nausea, vomiting, headache, and chest pain.

Although excessive fluid removal is the most frequent cause of hypotension, it is critical to rule out other potential causes if the hypotension persists after fluid replacement. These include sepsis, myocardial ischemia, pericardial tamponade, arrhythmias, and active bleeding. Antihypertensive agents may need to be withheld before dialysis to avoid hypotension.

Air embolus is the most dreaded technical complication of the hemodialysis procedure. Despite the presence of air detectors on the dialysis machine, there remains the risk of an air embolus with repeated disconnections of catheters. The patients may develop agitation, cough, dyspnea, and chest pain. As soon as the diagnosis is suspected, the patient should be positioned with the left side down in an attempt to trap air in the right ventricle. One-hundred percent oxygen should be administered.

Long-Term Complications in Hemodialysis

Anemia

The development of anemia parallels the progression of CKD. CKD-related anemia is usually normochromic and normocytic. Almost two thirds of patients starting dialysis have hematocrit levels lower than 30%. The target hemoglobin range established by the NKF/DOQI is between 11 to 12 g/dL. Untreated anemia contributes to cardiovascular morbidity and mortality and has been associated with impaired cognition, exercise capacity, and ability to perform simple tasks. Decreased erythropoietin production is the major factor contributing to anemia among patients with CKD. Numerous other factors contribute to anemia, such as shortened life span of red blood cells, uremic inhibitors of erythropoiesis, iron deficiency due to poor iron absorption, gastrointestinal bleeding, loss of blood with frequent blood sampling, and losses during hemodialysis. Folic acid is removed by dialysis, making folate replacement necessary. Infection, inflammation, malignancy, and a high parathyroid hormone level can also inhibit red blood cell maturation. Aluminum toxicity, either from aluminum contamination of the water supply or through the use of aluminum-containing phosphate binders, has been associated with microcytic anemia in patients with normal iron stores who undergo long-term dialysis.

Anemia Therapy

The administration of erythropoietin, together with repletion of iron stores, folic acid supplementation, and treatment of concomitant infection, is effective in correcting the anemia of chronic renal disease. Failure to provide an adequate supply of iron is the most common cause of erythropoietin treatment failure. The best way to replenish the iron stores is administration of iron intravenously. Some iron preparations have been associated with severe allergic reactions, including anaphylaxis, due to the presence of dextran. The newer iron preparations, which contain sucrose instead of dextran, appear to be associated with fewer side effects. A transferrin saturation level (serum iron ÷ total iron-binding capacity ×100%) lower than 20% and a ferritin level less than 100 ng/mL are considered the point to initiate intravenous iron therapy. Erythropoietin resistance occurs in the presence of ongoing infection, inflammation, hyperparathyroidism, or aluminum toxicity.

A number of adverse effects have been described with erythropoietin therapy, including accelerated hypertension. Erythropoietin therapy has also been associated with seizures and thrombosis of vascular access systems. Hypertension and thrombosis appear to be directly related to the hematocrit and to how rapidly the increase in hematocrit was achieved. The target hemoglobin level, with or without the use of erythropoietin, should be no higher than 12 g/dL because higher levels are associated with higher mortality rates. 1

Malnutrition

Hypoalbuminemia is associated with an increased mortality among patients undergoing dialysis. An albumin level of less than 3.0 g/dL has a 2-year mortality rate of up to 40%, in comparison with the expected mortality rate of 20%. Marked catabolism, anorexia, and severe diet limitations during the predialysis period lead to loss of lean weight. After the initiation of dialysis, patients usually have an improved appetite, and the protein intake recommended should be at least 1.2 g/kg per day for a total caloric intake of 35 cal/kg/day. Water-soluble vitamins, including folic acid, need to be replaced, because they are depleted during dialysis.

Chronic Kidney Disease and Cardiovascular Disease

Cardiovascular disease (CVD) is the most important cause of death among patients with CKD. CVD accounts for approximately 50% of the mortality among patients on dialysis and recipients of renal allografts. Two thirds of patients with CKD have diabetes mellitus or hypertension, but the rates of CVD and mortality are also elevated among patients with primary renal diseases such as glomerulonephritis. The relative hazard is greatest among patients younger than 45 years of age. In this age group, cardiac mortality is 100 times greater than in the general population.

In patients initiating dialysis, the main cardiac abnormality is left ventricular hypertrophy. Ventricular dilation, arterial stiffening (especially aortic), and coronary atherosclerosis with prominent calcification often accompany left ventricular hypertrophy. Although some of the risk factors for CVD in dialysis patients are similar to those in the general population, these patients also have unique risk factors specific to the uremic state, including anemia, hypervolemia, pericardial disease, oxidative stress, hyperhomocystinemia, and increased inflammatory markers such as C-reactive protein.

Disorders of mineral metabolism have also been proposed to play a crucial role in the cardiovascular abnormalities of patients with CKD, as well as contributing to renal osteodystrophy (Chapter 132). A number of studies have shown a direct correlation between an elevated serum phosphorus concentration (>5.5 mg/dL), a calcium-phosphorus product (Ca × P) greater than 56, and mortality in hemodialysis patients. A striking degree of coronary and aortic calcification has been demonstrated in young adults with ESRD using electron-beam tomography. This has been correlated with an elevated calcium-phosphorus product as well as the dose of calcium ingested. These striking findings have raised new questions about the therapy of hyperphosphatemia and have led to a decrease in the use of calcium- versus non–calcium-containing phosphate binders, such as sevelamer and lanthanum carbonate.

Decreased synthesis of the active principle of vitamin D (1,25-$[OH]_2D_3$) contributes to the secondary hyperparathyroidism of dialysis patients, and pulse-dose intravenous activated vitamin D is used to directly suppress synthesis of parathyroid hormone (PTH) and prevent skeletal complications. However, it is now recognized that the biologic consequences of vitamin D extend well beyond absorption of calcium from the intestine and suppression of PTH secretion. For example, vitamin D suppresses renin expression, modulates the immune and inflammatory system, triggers apoptosis, and promotes vascular endothelial integrity. Recent retrospective studies suggest that therapy with pulse-dose activated vitamin D improves the survival of patients undergoing chronic hemodialysis and that paricalcitol in particular may provide a survival advantage over calcitriol. Randomized clinical trials are needed to permit definitive conclusions and further define the mechanism of this effect, particularly in view of recent recommendations to withhold vitamin D injections if serum levels of PTH are low or if serum calcium or phosphorus levels are elevated.

Defining the role of activated injectable pulse-dose vitamin D becomes increasingly important with the recent introduction of the calcimimetic agent cinacalcet. The calcium-sensing receptor regulates the secretion of PTH. Calcimimetic agents increase the sensitivity of the calcium-sensing receptor to extracellular calcium ions, inhibit the release of PTH, and lower PTH levels within hours after administration, but they have not yet been shown to change important clinical outcomes. 2 In addition, the calimimetic cinacalcet lowers the serum calcium and phosphorus levels in patients with secondary hyperparathyroidism. By targeting the molecular mechanism that regulates the secretion of PTH, cinacalcet offers a novel therapeutic approach to the treatment of hyperparathyroidism in chronic renal failure. The question is, however, where does this drug fit into our armamentarium? Long-term studies are needed to define the place of cinacalcet and vitamin D in the treatment of secondary hyperparathyroidism and to explore the role of cinacalcet versus parathyroidectomy for the treatment of tertiary hyperparathyroidism.

Indications for and Frequency of Renal Replacement Therapy

The decision as to when to institute dialysis depends on the patient's signs and symptoms rather than an absolute level of blood urea nitrogen (BUN) or serum creatinine. The current opinion is that patients who begin dialysis at a relatively higher level of residual renal function have less morbidity and mortality. The benefits of early initiation include the avoidance of malnutrition, fluid overload, and the deleterious effects of prolonged exposure to the accumulation of phosphorus, β_2-microglobulin, and other uremic toxins.

There is no question that hyperkalemia (unresponsive to diuretics, ion exchange resins, and dietary restriction) in the face of electrocardiographic changes is an absolute indication for dialysis to avoid life-threatening arrhythmias such as ventricular tachycardia, ventricular fibrillation, or asystole. Likewise, volume overload refractory to intravenous diuretics is an indication to start dialysis. Increasing lethargy, difficulty concentrating, nausea, and anorexia all may reflect advancing renal failure and may be manifestations of the uremic syndrome requiring dialytic therapy. Intervention should occur before the progression of uremic encephalopathy, seizures, and coma or the development of pericarditis or pericardial tamponade. Emergency hemodialysis is more costly, because the patients typically lack vascular access and are sicker, often requiring prolonged hospitalization.

Dialysis Dose

Even though initiation of dialysis acutely prevents death from uremic complications, the mortality rate among patients undergoing chronic dialysis therapy remains high in the United States (~20% per year). Certainly age, comorbid conditions such as diabetes and CVD, nutritional status, and infection all contribute significantly to the high mortality in this population. However, it is also well established that patient outcome on dialysis is related to the dose and adequacy of dialysis.

The National Cooperative Dialysis Study (NCDS) was a landmark prospective, randomized study that demonstrated that the time-averaged concentration of urea and the nutritional status (determined by protein catabolic rate) were important determinants of morbidity and mortality in hemodialysis. It is better for patients to be dialyzed longer and be well nourished than to have a low BUN value and be dialyzed for shorter periods. Therefore, the main lesson is that quantifying and providing an adequate dose of dialysis affects patient outcome. The prescription of hemodialysis is tailored to the patient's size and protein intake. Urea is used as surrogate marker for clearance because it reflects the efficiency of removal of small uremic toxins. Various methods have been proposed to quantify hemodialysis adequacy. The most frequently used methods are the urea reduction ratio (URR) and urea kinetic modeling (Kt/V). The URR (100 × [1 – postdialysis BUN/predialysis BUN]) has the advantage of simplicity but does not account for the facts that urea is removed by ultrafiltration and that urea cannot be used to assess nutritional status. The Kt/V takes into account both of these variables and is the preferred method for determining adequacy for stable chronic dialysis patients.

Kt/V is a dimensionless formula that determines the fractional urea clearance per treatment normalized to the volume of urea distribution.

K is the dialyzer clearance, *t* is the time (duration) of dialysis therapy, and *V* is the volume of distribution of urea, which is approximately equal to the total body water. When supplied with simple clinical information (predialysis and postdialysis weights, ultrafiltration volume, hematocrit, and predialysis and postdialysis BUN as well as the dialyzer clearance), computer software programs perform the calculation. The NKF/DOQI recommends a single pool Kt/V greater than 1.2 and URR greater than 65% to minimize uremic complications and hospitalizations. Increasing the dose of dialysis beyond a Kt/V of 1.4 does not appear to increase survival according to the HEMO study. 3

Continuous Renal Replacement Therapy

Critically ill patients with renal failure are frequently hemodynamically unstable, hypercatabolic (e.g., sepsis, severe burns, brain injury, liver failure, trauma), and require large amounts of fluids (e.g., nutrition, antibiotics). Standard hemodialysis may be attempted to treat patients in the intensive care unit. However, hypotension, due in part to rapid fluid and solute removal, is usually an impediment to conventional dialysis. Moreover, patients with liver failure, traumatic brain injury, or coma do not tolerate the rapid osmolarity changes produced by hemodialysis, which can cause severe brain edema and herniation. In contrast, during continuous RRT, the rate of fluid removal is slow, and solute clearance relies on convection (solvent drag) rather than diffusion, which does not cause osmolarity changes.

CVVH is the most commonly performed method of continuous RRT. This pump-based system requires central venous access (double-lumen catheter) and blood flows between 150 and 200 mL/min. Blood under pressure passes down one side of a highly permeable membrane, allowing both water and solutes up to a molecular weight of about 40 kD to pass across the membrane. During hemofiltration, in contrast to hemodialysis, urea, creatinine, and phosphate are cleared at similar rates (convective clearance). The filtrate is discarded, and the fluid lost is partially replaced with a solution containing the major crystalloid components of the plasma at physiologic levels, which is administered into either the inflow or outflow blood line (predilution versus postdilution mode). However, if further clearance is needed in highly catabolic patients, diffusive dialysis (CVVHD) can be added by passing dialysis solution through the dialysate compartment.

Anticoagulation is usually required to maintain the patency of the CVVH circuit. Although protocols using heparin may be employed, many patients are at high risk for bleeding, which precludes the use of heparin. One effective method of anticoagulation is the use of a calcium-free citrate replacement fluid administered before filtration. Calcium is infused in a separate central line and monitored to avoid hypocalcemia. Citrate chelates calcium in the blood, preventing clotting of the hemofilter. Citrate is metabolized to bicarbonate by the liver. If the patient cannot metabolize citrate, an anion gap metabolic acidosis will develop. The presence of a low ionized calcium and a high total calcium level also should be a clue indicating citrate toxicity. The dissociation between the ionized and total serum calcium occurs because the measurement of total calcium includes calcium bound to citrate. Citrate toxicity often occurs in patients with severe liver failure. Many of these patients with low platelets and coagulopathy can tolerate CVVH without anticoagulation using bicarbonate-containing replacement solution.

Presently, there is no evidence from randomized studies demonstrating that CVVH offers a survival advantage compared with intermittent hemodialysis in patients with acute renal failure, despite the advantages of CVVH in enabling the removal of large amounts of fluid with improved hemodynamic stability and excellent metabolic and acid-base control. However, it appears that the dose of CVVH (ultrafiltration rates >35 mL/kg/hour) correlates with improved survival in critically ill patients with acute renal failure. 4

Nocturnal or daily hemodialysis is associated with marked benefits, including improved solute clearance with excellent control of serum phosphate and medium-sized molecules. It also provides excellent blood pressure control with a reduction in medication requirements. Nocturnal hemodialysis can be performed six or seven nights a week at home for a variable amount of time based on the length of sleep desired (usually 6 to 12 hours in total). A family member can perform the treatment, or the patient can be monitored at a central station through closed-circuit television. It remains to be determined whether increasing the dose of dialysis improves patient outcomes. Studies are underway to determine whether daily hemodialysis improves survival in patients with acute renal failure.

PERITONEAL DIALYSIS

More than 20% of patients with ESRD in the United States and more than 50% of those in the United Kingdom are receiving continuous ambulatory peritoneal dialysis (CAPD). Several studies suggest that CAPD has survival rates comparable to those of hemodialysis, when adjusted for patient age and comorbid conditions. CAPD offers a number of potential advantages. Peritoneal dialysis obviates the need for vascular access, a major challenge in diabetic patients, young children, and patients with severe vascular disease. Moreover, peritoneal dialysis can be performed without anticoagulation, decreasing the possible risk for bleeding. Because peritoneal dialysis is a slow, continuous process, it avoids the marked hemodynamic and osmotic shifts associated with hemodialysis. Moreover, CAPD offers a number of quality-of-life advantages. Patients can be taught to do the procedure at home, giving them a sense of control and independence. Also, peritoneal dialysis enables greater liberalization of diet with respect to salt, potassium, protein, and fluid. Clearly, peritoneal dialysis, when feasible, is the treatment modality of choice in children, because it avoids frequent needlesticks, and, most importantly, allows them to grow.

Performing Peritoneal Dialysis

Peritoneal dialysis uses the patient's own peritoneal membrane for removal of waste products and fluid (Fig. 133–2). During peritoneal dialysis in an adult, 2 to 3 L of dialysate solution containing electrolytes in physiologic concentrations (to correct acid-base and electrolyte disturbances) and varying concentrations of glucose is infused into the peritoneal cavity via a peritoneal catheter. After a specified dwell time varying between 3 and 6 hours per exchange, the fluid is drained and the process is repeated. The removal of solute from the body depends on the development of a concentration gradient between the blood and peritoneal fluid and occurs by diffusion across the peritoneal membrane. Osmotic ultrafiltration is achieved by the addition of increasing concentrations of glucose to the dialysate solution. The osmotic pressure generated by the glucose draws water from the extracellular fluid and the tissues into the peritoneal fluid. However, the net ultrafiltration rate decreases during the exchange, secondary to glucose absorption.

Unlike hemodialysis, where the characteristics of the dialyzer are specified by the manufacturer, in peritoneal dialysis, membrane characteristics vary from one individual to another. To appropriately determine a peritoneal dialysis prescription, it is critical to determine the peritoneal membrane characteristics of an individual patient. The peritoneal equilibration test (PET) is a semiquantitative clinical test commonly used to characterize the transport functions of the peritoneal membrane. The

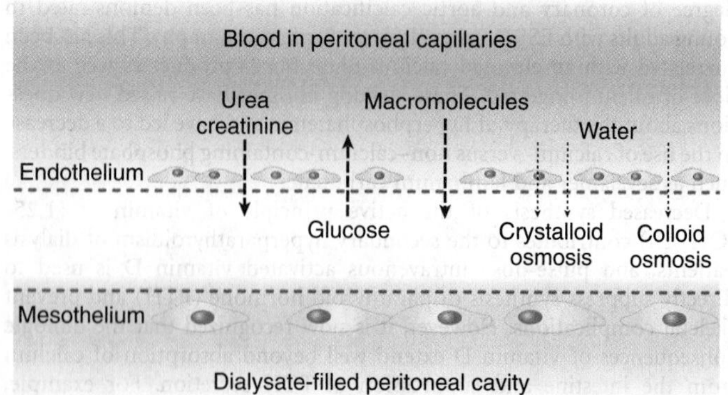

FIGURE 133–2 • Solute and water transport in peritoneal dialysis. Various pore systems in the vascular wall. The small interendothelial pores are involved in the transport of low-molecular-weight solutes and in water transport. Large pores allow the passage of macromolecules. Crystalloid osmosis induces water transport partly across the small pores, but also through ultrasmall transcellular water channels. Colloid osmosis induces fluid transport only across the small pore system. The mesothelium is not an osmotic barrier. (From Andreucci VE, Fine LG: International Yearbook of Nephrology, 1997. Oxford, Oxford University Press, 1998.)

standardized PET procedure consists of a 4-hour dwell using 2 L of 2.5% glucose-containing dialysate solution; equilibration ratios are then determined between plasma and dialysate for creatinine at 0, 2, and 4 hours. The PET also enables measurement of net fluid removal by examining the ratio of dialysate glucose at 4 hours to dialysate glucose at time zero. Patients are classified on the basis of their dialysate-to–plasma creatinine ratio into the following types:

1. ***High transporters:*** These patients have a high dialysate-to–plasma creatinine ratio and achieve rapid equilibration of creatinine and urea across the peritoneal membrane. However, because of their rapid absorption of glucose from the dialysate solution, they also tend to lose their osmotic gradient for fluid removal. Therefore, high or rapid transporters tend to have excellent solute clearance but have difficulty with ultrafiltration. They tend to do well with frequent exchanges and short dwell times that can be achieved with the automated cycler machine. These exchanges can be performed at night while the patient sleeps.
2. ***Low transporters:*** In contrast, these patients have low dialysate-to-plasma ratios for creatinine and urea, reflecting slower solute equilibration across the peritoneal membrane. They tend to do best with long dwells and high volumes of dialysate to maximize diffusion. However, these patients usually have excellent ultrafiltration and excellent fluid removal.
3. **Average transporters:** Patients who are found to be average transporters can do well with either form of peritoneal dialysis—CAPD or automated cycler therapy.

Peritoneal Dialysis Dose

It has been well established by a number of studies that clearance of small solutes is a key predictor of survival in patients undergoing peritoneal dialysis. These results have led to the NKF/DOQI guidelines on peritoneal adequacy, which advocate a target Kt/V for urea of 2 per week and a target creatinine clearance of 60 L/wk/1.73 m^2 body surface area. However, what is emerging is the observation that this relationship between clearance of small solutes and patient outcome in large part is accounted for by residual renal clearance. Nevertheless, a number of investigations have failed to demonstrate an independent effect of peritoneal clearance on outcome, at least within the dose range commonly used in a clinical practice week (Kt/V of 1.8). 5

It also has become clear that residual renal clearance and peritoneal clearances do not have equivalent physiologic significance in prolonging patient survival and that every effort should be made to maintain residual renal function as long as possible by avoiding nephrotoxins such as nonsteroidal anti-inflammatory drugs, iodinated contrast agents, and aminoglycosides.

Complications

Infection

Despite improvements in the technology of peritoneal dialysis, infection remains the most common problem plaguing patients undergoing CAPD, and it represents the most frequent cause for catheter removal and discontinuation of therapy. Infection can occur (1) at the exit site, with purulent or bloody drainage, erythema, tenderness, or induration; (2) around the subcutaneous tunnel of the catheter, with redness, swelling, or tenderness; or (3) in the peritoneal cavity (peritonitis). The diagnosis of peritonitis should be entertained if a patient presents with abdominal pain and cloudy dialysate. These patients frequently have fever, nausea, and vomiting. Abdominal tenderness, often with rebound, is frequently found on physical examination. The major diagnostic criterion is the cell count in the peritoneal fluid. Patients with peritonitis typically show a white blood cell count greater than 100/mm^3 with a predominance of neutrophils. Lymphocytes may predominate with fungal or mycobacterial infections. Prompt recognition and treatment of these infections is critical to avoid relapsing or refractory infections that require catheter removal.

S. aureus is the organism responsible for the majority of exit site and tunnel infections. In contrast, *Staphylococcus epidermidis*, a common cause of peritonitis, is a less frequent cause of exit site and tunnel infection. Initial empirical therapy therefore should cover gram-positive organisms. Oral penicillinase-resistant penicillins, fluoroquinolones, trimethoprim-sulfamethoxazole, or cephalosporins are recommended. Vancomycin should be avoided as first-line therapy except for methicillin-resistant *S. aureus.*

S. aureus nasal carriage is a recognized risk factor for exit site and tunnel infections. Mupirocin nasal ointment used twice daily for 5 days every 4 weeks, or mupirocin ointment applied to the exit site, has significantly reduced the incidence of *S. aureus* exit site infections.

S. epidermidis has been the most common organism causing bacterial peritonitis in CAPD patients, and it usually is the result of contamination, such as in the introduction of skin bacteria due to breaks in sterile technique. The introduction of disconnect systems has led to a reduction in the overall rate of peritonitis, particularly that due to *S. epidermidis. Pseudomonas* accounts for 5 to 8% of the episodes of CAPD peritonitis, which are often difficult to eradicate because of the development of a biofilm on the catheter and are frequently associated with catheter loss. Efforts to prevent the formation of biofilm may be an important future strategy in treating *Pseudomonas.* Likewise, fungal infections are extremely difficult to eradicate despite appropriate antifungal therapy because of the development of biofilm. Consequently, many institutions have made a policy of removing the peritoneal dialysis catheter as soon as the diagnosis of fungal peritonitis is made.

The third major source of peritonitis is intra-abdominal pathology that can occur due to processes such as a perforated diverticulum, ruptured appendix, ischemic bowel, incarcerated hernia, pancreatitis, or gynecologic pathology. The major diagnostic clue is the presence of polymicrobial enteric organisms on culture, particularly the presence of anaerobic organisms in the dialysate. An abdominal computed tomographic (CT) scan may help in identifying the anatomic site of the lesion. Although free air may be seen in asymptomatic patients undergoing peritoneal dialysis, the presence of free air should raise the possibility of a perforated viscus. The key is establishing the diagnosis rapidly and, if appropriate, moving directly to surgery.

A number of antibiotic regimens have been found to be effective in the treatment of CAPD-related peritonitis. The current guidelines recommend vancomycin or a cephalosporin together with a third-generation cephalosporin with antipseudomonal activity (e.g., ceftazidime) or gentamicin intraperitoneally as initial empirical therapy. Once culture and sensitivities results are available, the antibiotic prescription should be tailored to avoid gentamicin, if possible, so as to preserve residual renal function.

Other Complications

Mechanical problems may occur, including catheter malfunction due to omental wraps and blood or fibrin clots in the catheter lumen; catheter migration; and abdominal hernias due to increased intra-abdominal pressure with large volumes of dialysate. A number of metabolic complications may also occur in patients undergoing peritoneal dialysis, including hyperglycemia and hypertriglyceridemia from high glucose loads; weight gain; and protein loss, especially during an episode of peritonitis. Because peritoneal dialysis requires daily multiple exchanges, it is essential to assess for compliance on an ongoing basis and to ensure that the patient has an adequate support system to avoid "burnout."

One of the major advantages of peritoneal dialysis is the biocompatibility of the peritoneal membrane. In contrast, the dialysate solutions are bioincompatible in that they are acidic and hyperosmolar. Moreover, the high glucose concentration has been shown not only to contribute to metabolic abnormalities but also to inhibit the function of leukocytes and affect the long-term function of the peritoneal membrane through the production of advanced glycosylation end products. A dialysate containing 7.5% icodextrin has been approved as a safe and effective substitute for hypertonic glucose as an osmotic agent. This new glucose polymer, which is metabolized to maltose and is not rapidly absorbed, has been particularly effective in patients with ultrafiltration failure (high transporters). The use of glucose alternatives may decrease some metabolic consequences of long-term glucose use as well as preserve peritoneal membrane function. Amino acid–containing solutions are under investigation as a possible source of nutrition as well as an effective osmotic agent.

RENAL TRANSPLANTATION

Successful renal transplantation offers patients the best quality of life. They are liberated from potassium and fluid restrictions, are free to travel and work, and achieve correction of metabolic abnormalities and anemia with restoration of normal renal function. Moreover, in comparison to hemodialysis, renal transplantation also improves long-term survival in both diabetic and nondiabetic patients.

Since 1975, the 1-year cadaver allograft survival rate has dramatically improved, from approximately 50% to 90% in 2000. The 1-year allograft survival for kidneys from living donors has increased from 88 to 93%. Likewise, the half-life for grafts from living donors as well as deceased donors has steadily increased, although the initial projected improvement has not been confirmed with real half-lives based on longer follow-up. Moreover, it remains to be seen what impact the new agents such as tacrolimus, mycophenolate, and sirolimus may have on long-term results.

Many factors have contributed to the extraordinary advances in transplantation over the last 25 years, including widespread improvements in organ preservation and surgical techniques, advances in tissue typing and crossmatching, better immunosuppressive agents, and the recognition that rejection and infection are closely linked and that a concomitant anti-infective prescription is needed to make the immunosuppressive regimen safe (Chapter 303).

Because renal transplantation offers patients the best chance for quality as well as quantity of life, it is essential to evaluate candidates (especially diabetics) early and, if possible, proceed directly to preemptive transplantation if a living donor can be identified. The ideal form of RRT for patients with type 1 diabetes mellitus and nephropathy is renal transplantation from a living related donor, followed by pancreas or islet cell transplantation from a cadaver donor. If a living donor is unavailable, then simultaneous pancreas and kidney transplantation should be pursued from a cadaver donor. Although successful pancreas transplantation does not reverse the established macrovascular and microvascular complications of long-standing diabetes mellitus, it improves blood glucose control and quality of life and may prevent the progression of retinopathy and autonomic neuropathy. Islet cell transplantation after renal transplantation is presently under investigation.

Pretransplantation Evaluation of the Recipient

The potential renal transplant recipient must have irreversible end-stage renal failure and no evidence of active infection or malignancy. In addition to a careful history and physical examination, the evaluation must address the likelihood of compliance and rule out unmanageable patients with psychosis, substance abuse, or alcohol abuse.

Systemic Diseases

Cardiovascular complications have become the main cause of morbidity and mortality in patients undergoing renal transplantation. The high incidence of CVD reflects the combination of pretransplantation factors (e.g., diabetes, hypertension) and post-transplantation factors (e.g., metabolic complications of immunosuppressive agents). A careful cardiovascular workup is critical, including stress testing with imaging and a coronary angiogram if any evidence of ischemia is demonstrated. This is of particular importance in diabetic patients. In view of the increasing recognition of calcific aortic stenosis and hypertension in patients with CKD, an echocardiogram should be obtained to assess valve area as well as systolic and diastolic function.

Likewise, a careful evaluation of carotid and peripheral vessels should be undertaken, because the new kidney is anastomosed to the iliac vessels. The new kidney's ureter may be implanted into the recipient's bladder, or the patient's own ureter may be used. Further urologic testing may be needed if a neurogenic bladder is suspected or if there is a history of obstructive uropathy. Bilateral nephrectomies are required only if there is persistent, smoldering infection unresponsive to chronic suppressive antimicrobial therapy.

It is important to know the underlying cause of the renal failure to help guide the timing of transplantation and to inform the patient as to the risk of recurrence in the new kidney. It is recommended that patients with Goodpasture's syndrome, systemic lupus erythematosus, or antineutrophil cytoplasmic antibody–positive vasculitis become clinically and serologically quiescent before transplantation. A number of primary glomerular diseases have been shown to recur in the renal allograft, including focal segmental glomerulosclerosis, membranous glomerulonephritis, membranoproliferative glomerulonephritis, and immunoglobulin A (IgA) nephropathy. Diabetic nephropathy also may recur after transplantation and can be prevented by combined kidney/pancreas transplantation. Combined kidney/liver transplantation can cure oxalosis.

Infectious Diseases

As part of the evaluation of the recipient, a number of infectious disease issues must be addressed. Serologic determination of human immunodeficiency virus (HIV) and hepatitis B and C virus infection status should be obtained. In this era of highly active antiretroviral therapy, HIV positivity is no longer an absolute contraindication to transplantation. However, transplantation in this setting should be performed only under an experimental protocol, because the long-term impact of immunosuppression on HIV infection is unclear, and dialysis offers a viable alternative. Although patients with hepatitis C do better with renal transplantation than on dialysis, with time liver failure is the major cause of morbidity and mortality. It is therefore critical to stage patients with hepatitis C before transplantation, by means of liver biopsy, viral load determination, measurement of the α-fetoprotein level, and a CT scan looking for hepatocellular carcinoma and portal hypertension. The possibility of a combined kidney and liver transplant needs to be explored. Combined therapy with pegylated interferon and ribavirin may be indicated after transplantation but requires cautious monitoring and usually is not well tolerated. Post-transplantation interferon therapy may trigger allograft rejection, possibly by upregulation of genes for the major histocompatibility complex (MHC) and various cytokines. Severe hemolytic anemia may occur with ribavirin administration.

All patients waiting for renal transplantation should be vaccinated against hepatitis B, although the response rate appears to be less than 50%. If a patient is positive for hepatitis B surface antigen, a DNA viral load determination and liver biopsy should be obtained for staging. Lamivudine therapy may be initiated either before or after transplantation. Once again, if there is significant cirrhosis, consideration should be given to combined kidney/liver transplantation.

Patients with a newly positive purified protein derivative (PPD) skin test should ideally be treated before transplantation. A patient with positive PPD and negative chest radiograph before transplantation may be closely monitored. If the patient has a positive PPD and a history of previous disease or a positive chest radiograph, treatment with isoniazid is indicated starting 1 to 2 months after transplantation.

Likewise, patients should be evaluated for previous exposure to varicella. If the varicella titer is negative before transplantation, an attempt at vaccination may be undertaken. If the patient remains varicella antibody negative or has not been vaccinated, varicella zoster immune globulin should be given on exposure to patients with chickenpox or herpes zoster, because the immunosuppressed host is at risk for fulminant varicella with pulmonary infiltrates, pancreatitis, and liver disease.

Special attention needs to be directed to patients from tropical areas, where *Strongyloides stercoralis* is endemic. A *Strongyloides* titer should be obtained and, if it is positive, the infection should be treated before immunosuppression, because fulminant disease can occur after transplantation. Likewise, if a patient comes from an area where schistosomiasis is endemic, diagnosis and treatment should be initiated before transplantation.

Identifying Donors

Living Donors

There are potentially two ways to obtain a renal transplant: from a living donor or from a deceased donor. The demand for deceased donors far exceeds the supply of organs, and the waiting list for cadaver renal transplants is now 3 to 4 years in all blood groups throughout most of the United States. This is a major impetus for the increase in living donors. Living organ donation accounts for more than 50% of the transplantations now being performed. Living donation is generally safe, although it is not without potential morbidity. Moreover, both short- and long-term outlooks for the recipient are better with a living donor. In addition, data from living but not genetically related donors suggest that the results from a living unrelated donor transplant are equivalent to a one-haplotype parental match, with a 1-year graft survival rate of 92%. This suggests that the quality of the organ is as important or more important than the closeness of the genetic "match." In living unrelated donors, as in all living donors, it is critical that both a complete medical examination and a psychological evaluation be carefully performed by physicians and psychiatrists independent of the recipient, to ascertain the voluntary, altruistic nature of the donor's decision, that is, to ensure no coercion.

The donor must recognize both the short- and long-term risks of donating a kidney. These include the immediate risks of surgery, with a mortality rate of 0.05%, as well as pain, time out of work, and the possibility of phlebitis or pulmonary embolus, urinary tract infection, wound infection, or pneumonia. The long-term risks of having one kidney include the slightly increased risk of proteinuria, chance of trauma, or development of cancer in the one remaining kidney. Although isolated cases of chronic renal failure have been reported after donation, for the most part long-term mortality is not affected by kidney donation.

One impetus for the increase in the living donor pool is the potential for laparoscopic donor nephrectomy in carefully selected patients. This procedure offers the possibility of decreased time in the hospital, potential for faster recovery, and more rapid return to work. However, not all donors are candidates for this procedure because of anatomic variants. All donors must be carefully evaluated and closely monitored long term.

Deceased Donors

The shortage of deceased organs for transplantation has led to the increased use of expanded-criteria donors, such as those older than 55 years of age or with a history of hypertension or cerebrovascular accident. In this situation, a donor biopsy is performed and the degree of fibrosis, sclerosis, and vascular disease is assessed. If deemed appropriate, these kidneys are then offered with informed consent to older potential recipients or patients with multiple access problems. Although there may be a 10% difference in survival between these kidneys and standard deceased donor kidneys at 3 years, the potential benefit to the recipient is the opportunity to terminate dialysis without waiting on the list for 4 years or longer.

Another alternative is the use of organs from donors who die from traditional cardiac death, known as donation after cardiac death (DCD) donors. In the early days of transplantation, such donors were the main source of organs, but this changed with the legal and ethical acceptance of brain death criteria. However, these patients are again emerging as potentially excellent donors in a controlled setting. Usually, the family has decided to withdraw care because of an irreversible and devastating neurologic injury. Once the patient's family and the attending physician have decided that life support will be discontinued, the patient is taken to the operating room, the ventilator is discontinued, and cardiac arrest occurs. The patient is pronounced dead only after all signs of respiration have ceased. At this point, the organs are procured. Studies have shown that patient and graft survival rates of DCD kidneys are not statistically different from rates with traditional brain death donors.

Tissue Typing

A key element in the evaluation for transplantation is tissue typing. The recipient must receive a transplant from a blood group–compatible donor to avoid hyperacute rejection and immediate irreversible graft loss on the operating table. The donor and recipient need not share the same Rh factor.

The genes that code for the MHC are located on the short arm of chromosome 6 and are highly polymorphic (Chapter 43). That is, within a species, there is an extraordinarily large number of alleles (alternative forms of the same gene). These genes encode surface molecules known as human leukocyte antigens (HLA) that contribute to recognition of self as well as antigen binding. Because each individual has at least 12 genes encoding MHC proteins, it is rare for two unrelated individuals to have an identical set of HLA antigens. Inheritance of these genes is codominant (i.e., each parent transmits one set of MHC genes, a haplotype, to his or her child). These antigens appear to be pivotal in the rejection process.

HLA typing is performed on all potential recipients and donors. Although usually this is done by serology, increasingly DNA-based typing techniques are being employed. It is critical to determine the recipient's sensitization (i.e., the level of preformed HLA antibodies in the serum of the recipient). These antibodies typically result from previous transplants, pregnancies, or blood transfusions. The critical test before renal transplantation is the final crossmatch: a complement-dependent cytotoxicity assay performed using the cells of the donor and serum of the recipient. If the crossmatch is positive, the transplantation should not be performed, to avoid hyperacute rejection caused by the presence of preformed antibodies. One of the exciting new options being explored to increase the possibility of transplantation is the donor exchange program, whereby an incompatible ABO (blood group) or sensitized donor-recipient pair in one institution might find a compatible match at another institution through computerized matching.

Rejection

Rejection remains the Achilles heel of transplantation, and acute rejection is the most important predictor of chronic rejection. The introduction of cyclosporine in the early 1980s and mycophenolate mofetil in the 1990s has significantly reduced the incidence of rejection, producing a significant increase in allograft survival.

Allograft rejection is initiated by the recipient's recognition of donor MHC antigens, leading to activation of humoral and cellular immunity (Chapter 46). The clinical manifestations of acute cellular rejection may be minimal with the use of newer immunosuppressive agents but may include fever, allograft swelling and tenderness, or oliguria. The BUN and creatinine concentrations are usually elevated. A Doppler ultrasound study should be performed to rule out obstruction and vascular thrombosis. The diagnosis of acute rejection can be reliably made only with an allograft biopsy. All other potential causes of acute allograft dysfunction should be considered (Table 133–1).

The role of antibodies in the acute rejection process has been increasingly appreciated. Hyperacute humoral rejection is a rare clinical event; however, when it occurs, it usually causes immediate irreversible necrosis of the allograft on the operating table. Hyperacute rejection is caused by preformed alloantibodies in the recipient directed against donor HLA

TABLE 133–1 DIFFERENTIAL DIAGNOSIS OF RENAL ALLOGRAFT DYSFUNCTION

IMMEDIATE/DELAYED GRAFT FUNCTION (1–3 DAYS)
Acute tubular necrosis
Hyperacute humoral rejection
Urinary leak or obstruction
Renal artery or vein thrombosis
Recurrence of disease (e.g., FSGS)
EARLY POST-TRANSPLANTATION PERIOD (FIRST MONTH)
Acute cellular rejection
Acute humoral rejection
Calcineurin inhibitor toxicity
Urinary tract obstruction
Volume depletion
Recurrence of disease
LATE ACUTE DYSFUNCTION
Acute rejection
Cyclosporine or tacrolimus toxicity
Recurrence of primary disease
Tubulointerstitial nephritis, drug-induced
Renal artery stenosis
Infection (bacterial UTI, cytomegalovirus, BK virus)
Hemodynamic (volume; use of ACEI, AIIRB)
CHRONIC DYSFUNCTION
Chronic rejection
Cyclosporine or tacrolimus toxicity
Recurrent renal disease
De novo renal disease
Urinary tract obstruction
Bacterial UTI
Hypertensive nephrosclerosis

ACEI = angiotensin-converting enzyme inhibitor; AIIRB = angiotensin II receptor blocker; FSGS = focal segmental glomerulosclerosis; UTI = urinary tract infection.

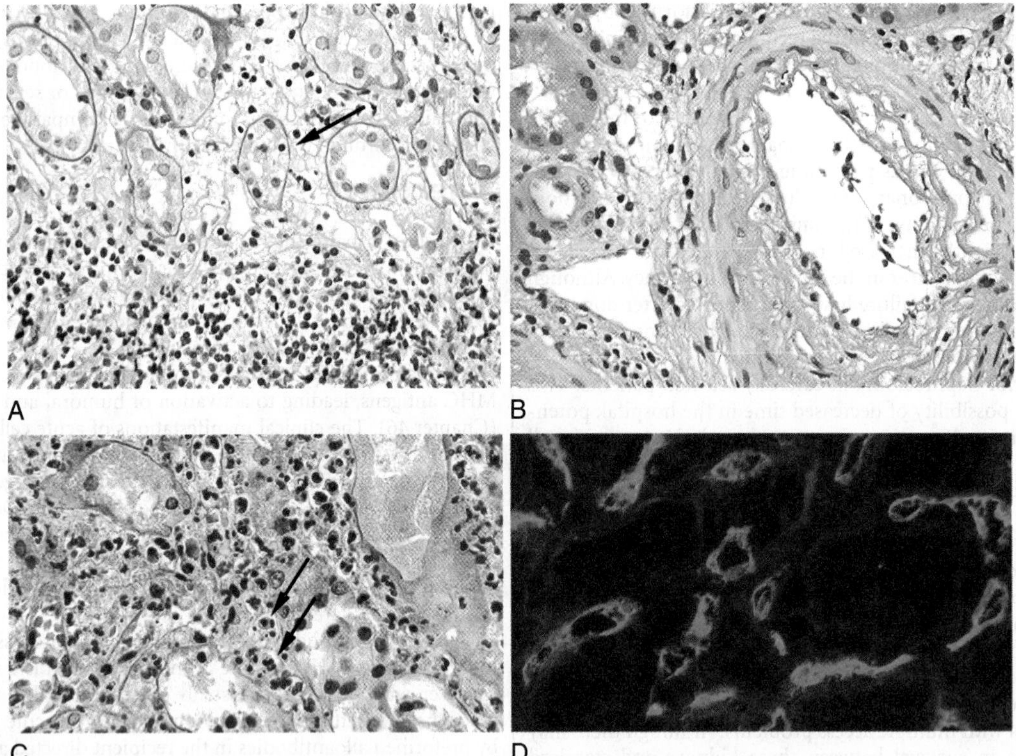

FIGURE 133–3 • Histology of renal allograft with acute cellular rejection (A and B) and acute humoral rejection (C and D). A, Interstitial mononuclear infiltrate. The arrow points to an area with tubulitis. **B,** Arteritis. Note the accumulation of inflammatory cells beneath the intima, which is characteristic of acute cellular rejection type 2 (Banff classification). **C,** Acute humoral rejection. The peritubular space is occupied by an inflammatory infiltrate with the presence of polymorphonuclear neutrophils (arrows). **D,** Positive C4d staining in the peritubular capillaries by immunofluorescence, a hallmark of humoral rejection.

or ABO antigens, and this form of antibody-mediated rejection can usually be prevented by careful crossmatching techniques.

Recently, it was shown that antidonor humoral responses developing after transplantation are associated with severe allograft injury. In other words, the development of de novo donor-reactive cytotoxic antibodies in the serum of the recipient after transplantation that were not present preoperatively (i.e., positive crossmatch after but negative before transplantation) can lead to acute humoral rejection. These alloantibodies may be reactive with HLA class I or II antigens. Acute humoral rejection has been found to have a unique pathologic picture characterized by the presence of neutrophils in peritubular capillaries and glomeruli and the presence of C4d staining, a byproduct of antibody-mediated complement activation deposited strongly in the peritubular capillary region (Fig. 133–3). In the past, patients with this clinicopathologic picture would uniformly lose their allografts. However, early detection and treatment have dramatically changed the prognosis of acute humoral rejection. In those patients with a negative pretransplantation crossmatch but de novo donor-specific antibodies demonstrated after transplantation, treatment with plasmapheresis and pooled human immune globulin in addition to tacrolimus, mycophenolate mofetil, and steroids has led to dramatic reversal of the acute allograft dysfunction in approximately 90% of cases. Protocols using plasma exchange and intravenous immune globulin (IVIG) have also been employed before transplantation in an attempt to lower the levels of preformed HLA antibody in highly sensitized patients. Such protocols convert a previously positive crossmatch to a negative one, thus enabling transplantation from a living donor.

Induction Immunosuppression

The goal of immunosuppression therapy is to prevent allograft rejection but still allow the immune system to fight infection and malignancy. The multiagent strategy allows for a synergistic effect and reduction of specific drug toxicity (Fig. 133–4). Immunosuppression is initiated at high doses (induction) during the initial period after transplantation, when the risk of rejection is highest, and is reduced over time (maintenance immunosuppression). In recipients with a high risk of rejection (children, retransplant recipients, delayed graft function, multiparous women, and multitransfused patients), induction immunosuppression is often employed. Induction therapy consists of a course of (1) polyclonal antilymphocyte-antithymocyte globulin (ATG) or antilymphocyte globulin; (2) monoclonal anti-CD3 antibodies (OKT3); or (3) anti–interleukin-2 receptor monoclonal antibodies (basiliximab or daclizumab). Appropriate antiviral prophylaxis is essential to reduce the risk of severe cytomegalovirus (CMV) infection and Epstein-Barr virus (EBV)–associated post-transplantation lymphoproliferative disease (PTLD). Likewise, prophylaxis with trimethoprim sulfamethoxazole has been effective in preventing urinary tract infections as well as *Pneumocystis carinii* (now *Pneumocystis jiroveci*) infection in these highly immunosuppressed patients.

Polyclonal Antibodies

Polyclonal antibodies are raised in various animals (rabbits, goats, horses) using different antigenic preparations (thymocytes, lymphocytes). Many preparations of polyclonal antibodies are available, and they vary in degree of efficacy, purity, and side effects. Thymoglobulin is prepared by immunizing rabbits with human T thymocytes. The polyclonal antilymphocyte antibodies are used for induction therapy in high-risk recipients (i.e., those with high panel-reactive antibodies (PRA) and those undergoing retransplantation) at the onset of transplantation, for treatment of steroid-resistant acute cellular rejection, and as a calcineurin inhibitor–sparing agent in recipients with delayed graft function. The polyclonal antibodies can cause serum sickness, bone marrow suppression, and hemolysis. The use of these agents may also trigger a potent cytokine response. Most side effects are related either to the degree of purity of the antigenic preparation used to immunize the animals or to the purification of the serum. Serum sickness and anaphylactic reactions are related to previous exposure to the animal species used to raise the antibody.

OKT3

OKT3 is a mouse monoclonal antibody directed against the CD3 antigen. The CD3 complex sits at the cytoplasmic tail of the T-cell receptor (TCR) and transduces signals from the TCR to the cytoplasm. OKT3 interferes with T-cell function through modulation of the TCR and clearance of T cells. OKT3 is used primarily for treatment of steroid-resistant acute cellular rejection and occasionally as an induction agent.

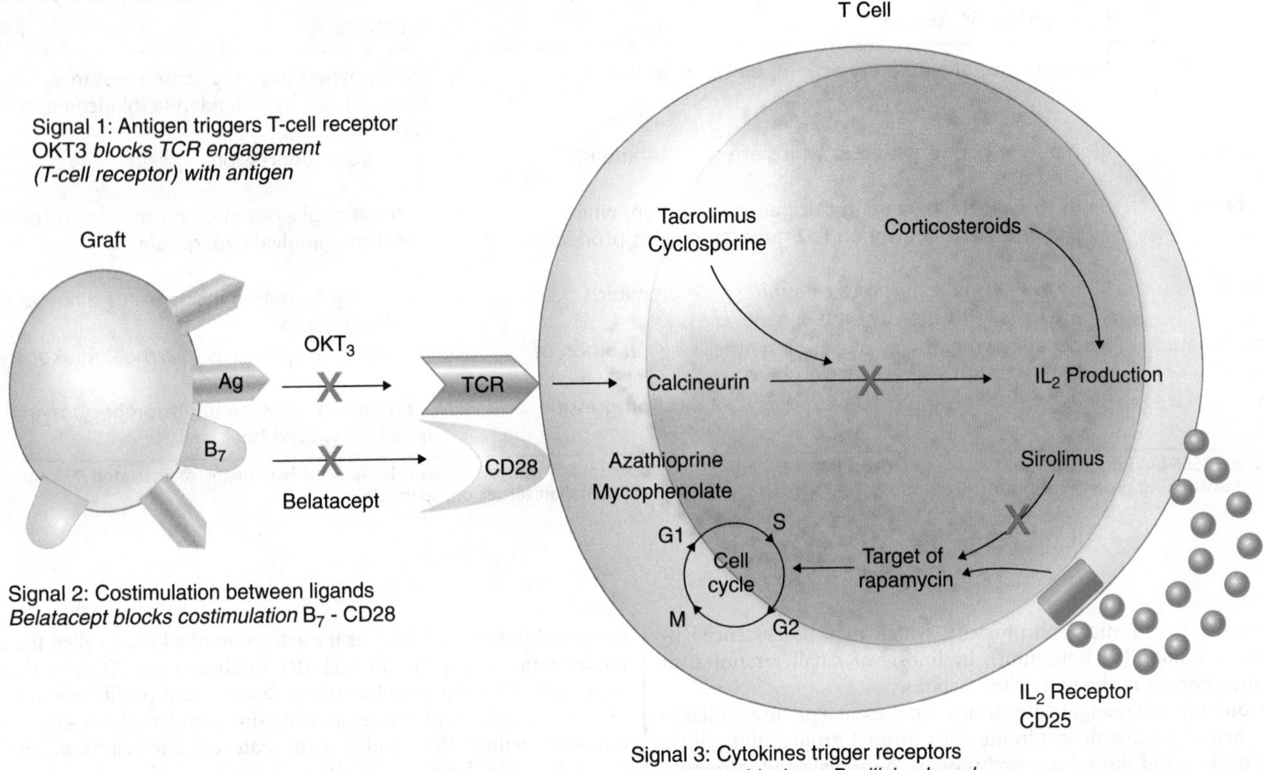

FIGURE 133–4 • **Targets of immunosuppressive agents.** G_1, S, G_2, and M are stages of the cell cycle. Ag = antigen; B_7 = costimulatory molecule; AZA = azathioprine; CsA = cyclosporine; IL = interleukin; MMF = mycophenolate mofetil; SRL = sirolimus; TAC = tacrolimus; TCR = T-cell receptor; TOR = target of rapamycin.

OKT3 can cause myriad side effects, including fever, rigors, nausea, vomiting, diarrhea, severe headache (aseptic meningitis), hypotension, chest pain, dyspnea, wheezing, and, infrequently, pulmonary edema. These symptoms are secondary to massive cytokine release after OKT3 engages the TCR. OKT3 is associated with a higher incidence of severe CMV infections and PTLD. Therefore, appropriate CMV prophylaxis is essential.

Interleukin-2 Receptor Blockers

IL-2 receptor blockers are engineered monoclonal antibodies against the α-chain of the IL-2 receptor. Daclizumab is a humanized molecule consisting of a human IgG1 with antigen-binding regions from a mouse antibody. Basiliximab is a chimeric construct with a murine variable region and human constant regions. The impetus of humanizing these molecules included functional considerations beyond reduction in immunogenicity. Unlike the original mouse antibodies, the humanized antibodies can activate antibody-directed, cell-mediated cytotoxicity without activating complement-mediated cytotoxicity. Daclizumab and basiliximab are used only as induction agents to prevent rather than treat rejection. They both have a safe side effect profile, largely because of their human origin.

New Agents

Alemtuzumab (Campath) is an anti-CD52 monoclonal antibody used as an induction agent at the time of transplantation that leads to prolonged depletion of B and T cells through lysis. Alemtuzumab appears to facilitate minimization of maintenance immunosuppressive protocols (with either sirolimus or low-dose tacrolimus). The dose and frequency of administration remain to be determined. The role of costimulatory blockade with belatacept (LEA29Y), a variant of CTLA4Ig, is also under investigation.

Maintenance Immunosuppression

Many immunosuppressive agents are available for prevention of rejection in the maintenance phase (Table 133–2). Common regimens consist of low-dose steroids, mycophenolate mofetil, or azathioprine plus a calcineurin inhibitor (either cyclosporine or tacrolimus). Corticosteroids have nonspecific immunosuppressive and anti-inflammatory actions. They are used for induction therapy, for maintenance immunosuppression, and in high doses (pulse) for the treatment of acute cellular rejection. Corticosteroids inhibit synthesis of almost all known cytokines and of several surface molecules required for immune function. On crossing the cell membrane, steroids bind to intracellular receptor proteins, which are transferred to the cell nucleus, where they bind to corticosteroid response elements of the target genes. Corticosteroids also inhibit the translocation of nuclear factor-κB (NF-κB) by induction of an inhibitory protein, which traps activated NF-κB in inactive cytoplasmic complexes. This action prevents activation of key cytokine genes, including tumor necrosis factor-α (TNF-α) and IL-1. Corticosteroids cause many metabolic changes, including diabetes, hypercholesterolemia, osteoporosis, increased risk of cardiovascular events, obesity, and hypertension, and they can cause significant mood swings, irritability, and depression.

The calcineurin inhibitors cyclosporine and tacrolimus inhibit the translocation of nuclear factor of activated T lymphocyte (NFAT) from the cytoplasm to the nucleus. Both cyclosporine and tacrolimus bind to a cyclophilin in the cytoplasm; this complex then binds to calcineurin, inhibiting its capacity to dephosphorylate NFAT, and thereby preventing NFAT translocation to the nucleus. NFAT is essential in the activation of IL-2, interferon-γ, IL-4, TNF-α, and granulocyte-macrophage colony-stimulating factor, as well as the gene for CD40 ligand. Cyclosporine and tacrolimus levels must be closely monitored to avoid toxicity as well as rejection. The most important nonimmune toxicity of the calcineurin inhibitors is nephrotoxicity.

The following three distinct patterns of renal dysfunction may be observed with calcineurin inhibitors:

1. An acute hemodynamic effect secondary to afferent arteriolar constriction, which may exacerbate ischemic injury and delayed graft function. This produces a reversible decrease in the glomerular filtration rate, which improves when the dose of the drug is adjusted.

TABLE 133–2 IMMUNOSUPPRESSIVE AGENTS

Agent	Mechanism of Action	Side Effects
Corticosteroids	Multiple anti-inflammatory actions, blockade of IL-1, IL-6, TNF-α	Infection, hypertension, glucose resistance, osteoporosis, hyperlipidemia, glaucoma, adrenal suppression
Azathioprine	Blockade of purine synthesis, which affects DNA and RNA synthesis	Bone marrow suppression
Cyclosporine	Binds to cyclophilin, causing calcineurin inhibition, which prevents NFAT activity on IL-2 gene; stimulates production of TGF-β	Hypertension, glucose intolerance, nephrotoxicity, hirsutism, gingival hyperplasia
Tacrolimus	Binds to FKBP-12, causing calcineurin inhibition, which prevents NFAT activity on IL-2 gene	Neurotoxicity, increased incidence of diabetes mellitus (≈20%)
Mycophenolate mofetil	Blocks de novo pathway of purine synthesis by inhibition of IMPDH, selective for lymphocytes	Gastrointestinal symptoms (diarrhea), leukopenia
Sirolimus	Binds to FKBP-12 and mTOR, blocking cell cycle progression	Hyperlipidemia, leukopenia, thrombocytopenia, impaired wound healing

FKBP-12 = FK506-binding protein 12; IL = interleukin; IMPDH = inosine monophosphate dehydrogenase; NFAT = nuclear factor of activated T lymphocyte; TGF-β = transforming growth factor-β; TNF-α = tumor necrosis factor-α; mTOR = mammalian target of rapamycin.

2. Subacute to chronic nephrotoxicity, which may be evidenced by tubular lesions (vacuolization), hyalinosis of small arterioles, or striped fibrosis in the more chronic phase.
3. Thrombotic microangiopathy, which can present a picture similar to the hemolytic-uremic syndrome with intimal proliferation, fibrin deposition, and thrombotic occlusion of the arcuate and intralobular arteries. The peripheral smear may show evidence of schistocytes. Thrombocytopenia may or may not be present. Switching from cyclosporine to tacrolimus or vice versa may sometimes be beneficial.

Other side effects of the calcineurin inhibitors include neurotoxicity (tremors, mental status changes, irritability, and seizures), hypertension, hyperglycemia, hyperkalemia, hyperuricemia, gout, and an increased incidence of EBV-related B-cell lymphomas (PTLD). Both cyclosporine and tacrolimus are metabolized by the cytochrome P-450 system and excreted by the liver. Therefore, administration of drugs that interact with the P-450 system affects the levels of calcineurin inhibitors. Prescribing physicians need to be aware that inhibitors of the P-450 system, such as macrolide antibiotics, the calcium-channel blocker diltiazem, imidazole, and triazole antifungals among many other drugs, may raise the levels of calcineurin inhibitors. In contrast, agents such as rifampin, phenobarbital, and phenytoin that induce cytochrome P-450 enzymes increase the catabolism of calcineurin inhibitors. Many other significant interactions need to be recognized, including the risk of rhabdomyolysis with statins and interaction with most nephrotoxic agents.

Azathioprine was a cornerstone of transplant immunosuppression until the introduction of mycophenolate mofetil. Azathioprine inhibits DNA synthesis; its main side effect is bone marrow suppression (see Table 133–2). Azathioprine has also been associated with malignancies, especially skin cancers and increased frequency of warts (papillomavirus infection). Azathioprine is metabolized by xanthine oxidase. Concomitant administration of allopurinol, a xanthine oxidase inhibitor, should be avoided, because significant bone marrow toxicity may occur.

Mycophenolate mofetil selectively inhibits lymphocyte proliferation. This is a targeted action on the de novo pathway of purine synthesis, on which lymphocytes, unlike other cell types, are particularly dependent (see Table 133–2). The efficacy of mycophenolate mofetil has been demonstrated in large randomized, multicenter, blinded trials, which showed a 50% reduction in the incidence of acute cellular rejection and a significant reduction in the use of OKT3/ATG. Gastrointestinal symptoms (e.g., nausea, epigastric discomfort, diarrhea) are the main side effects and usually can be improved by dose reduction. The effect of mycophenolate mofetil on the prevention of chronic rejection is currently under study.

Sirolimus binds to the same immunophilin as tacrolimus does (i.e., FK506-binding protein 12 [FKBP-12]), but the sirolimus-FKBP complex does not affect calcineurin activity (see Table 133–2). Rather, this complex binds to and inhibits the activation of a kinase called the mammalian target of rapamycin (mTOR). Inhibition of mTOR by sirolimus suppresses alloantigen and cytokine-driven T-cell proliferation, inhibiting the cell cycle. Regimens employing sirolimus have been shown to significantly reduce the incidence of acute cellular rejection. Sirolimus causes hyperlipidemia and is also associated with thrombocytopenia. Of note, sirolimus interacts with calcineurin inhibitors and may cause an increase in calcineurin inhibitor toxicity.

Outcomes

A number of strategies have been devised to improve long-term outcomes of renal transplantation by preventing chronic rejection and chronic allograft loss, thereby improving long-term survival and life expectancy of renal transplant recipients. These include steroid-sparing protocols using immunosuppressive agents, such as tacrolimus, with mycophenolate mofetil (MMF) or calcineurin inhibitor-sparing protocols using MMF or sirolimus.

Patients may also benefit from aggressive control of coronary risk factors, because coronary disease is a major cause of death in these patients. For example, a statin can reduce nonfatal myocardial infarction and cardiac death in transplant recipients.

The ultimate goal of transplantation is tolerance—unresponsiveness to donor antigens while maintaining the ability to respond to third-party antigens in the absence of ongoing immunosuppression. Although tolerance has been demonstrated in a number of different small animal models, it has been difficult to achieve in large animal models and in humans. In 1990, it was reported that patients who had previously undergone allogeneic bone marrow transplantation for treatment of hematologic disease and subsequently required a kidney transplantation from the same donor demonstrated immunologic nonresponsiveness. In these patients, the kidney was accepted without the need for immunosuppression. Unfortunately, the morbidity associated with the full myeloablative-conditioning regimen required for successful complete bone marrow transplantation, as well as graft-versus-host disease, precludes the routine use of this approach to induce tolerance after transplantation of solid organs. However, the induction of mixed hemopoietic chimerism, using nonmyeloablative conditioning, is a more clinically applicable strategy that has been successfully accomplished in rodents, miniature swine, and nonhuman primates. These observations are now being extended to patients with multiple myeloma and end-stage renal failure and to one-haplotype donor recipient pairs under the National Institutes of Health Immune Tolerance Network Protocol.

Other promising approaches to tolerance induction are presently being investigated, with the hope that chronic rejection can be avoided, as well as long-term immunosuppression and its multiple sequelae: drug toxicity, infection, and the risk of malignancy.

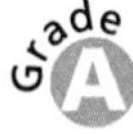

1. Phrommintikul A, Haas SJ, Elsik M, et al: Mortality and target haemoglobin concentrations in anaemic patients with chronic kidney disease treated with erythropoietin: A meta-analysis. Lancet 2007;369:381–388.
2. Strippoli GF, Tong A, Palmer SC, et al: Calcimimetics for secondary hyperparathyroidism in chronic kidney disease patients. Cochrane Database Syst Rev 2006;4:CD006254.
3. Eknoyan G, Beck GJ, Cheung AK, et al: Effect of dialysis dose and membrane flux in maintenance hemodialysis. N Engl J Med 2002;347:2010–2019.
4. Ronco C, Brendolan A, Lupi A, et al: Effects of different doses in continuous veno-venous haemofiltration on outcomes of acute renal failure: A prospective randomised trial. Lancet 2000;356: 26–30.
5. Paniagua R, Amato D, Vonesh E, et al: The Mexican Nephrology Collaborative Study Group. Effects of increased peritoneal clearances on mortality rates in peritoneal dialysis: ADEMEX, a prospective, randomized, controlled trial. Am Soc Nephrol 2002;13: 1307–1320.

SUGGESTED READINGS

Block GA, Raggi P, Bellasi A, et al: Mortality effect of coronary calcification and phosphate binder choice in incident hemodialysis patients. Kidney Int 2007;71:438–441. *In subjects new to hemodialysis, baseline coronary calcification was a significant predictor of all-cause mortality as compared with the use of calcium-containing phosphate binders.*

Delmonico FL: Exchanging kidneys: Advances in living donor transplantation. N Engl J Med 2004;350:1812–1814. *A novel program to increase living related donor transplants in incompatible pairs.*

Halloran PF: Immunosuppressive drugs for kidney transplantation. N Engl J Med 2004;351:2715–2719. *A comprehensive review.*

Ingelfinger JR: Risks and benefits to the living donor. N Engl J Med 2005; 353:447–449. *Thoughtful summary of medical, surgical, and psychological impact of being a living donor.*

Kurella M, Covinsky KE, Collins AJ, et al: Octogenarians and nonagenarians starting dialysis in the United States. Ann Intern Med 2007;146:177–183. *Octogenarians and nonagenarians starting dialysis increased by 9.8%. The rate of dialysis initiation increased by 57% between 1996 and 2003; 1 year mortality for octogenarians and nonagenarians after dialysis initiation was 46%.*

Meier-Kriesche HU, Schold JD, Kaplan B: Long-term renal allograft survival: Have we made significant progress or is it time to rethink our analytic and therapeutic strategies? Am J Transplant 2004;4:1289–1295. *Real half-lives are substantially lower than projected half-lives. Long-term graft survival remains a significant problem.*

Pascual M, Theruvath T, Kawai T, et al: Strategies to improve long-term outcomes after renal transplantation. N Engl J Med 2002;346:580–590. *A comprehensive review.*

Piraino B, Bailie GR, Bernardini J, et al: Peritoneal dialysis-related infections recommendations: 2005 update. Perit Dial Int 2005;25:107–131. *New antibiotic recommendations for peritoneal dialysis infections.*

Rocco MV, Frankenfield DL, Hopson SD, et al: Relationship between clincial performance measures and outcomes among patients receiving long-term hemodialysis. Ann Intern Med 2006;145:512–519. *The risk for death increased for each additional guideline indicator that was not met.*

Rodriguez RA, Sen S, Mehta K, et al: Geography matters: Relationships among urban residential segregation, dialysis facilities, and patient outcomes. Ann Intern Med 2007;146:493–501. *Dialysis facilities in areas with a higher percentage of black residents were more likely to have higher-than-expected mortality rates and were less likely to meet performance targets.*

Tantravahi J, Womer KL, Kaplan B: Why hasn't eliminating acute rejection improved graft survival? Annu Rev Med 2007;58:369–385. *A clinical review.*

Section XII

Gastrointestinal Diseases

APPROACH TO THE PATIENT WITH GASTROINTESTINAL DISEASE

Deborah D. Proctor

Epidemiology

Gastrointestinal (GI) and liver diseases generate 50 million visits to physicians, hospitals, and emergency departments annually in the United States. Non–food-borne gastroenteritis and food-borne illnesses are the most frequent diagnoses. The estimated direct cost for these diseases is approximately $90 billion per year, with a range of above $10 billion for gastroesophageal reflux disease (GERD) (Chapter 140) to about $7 billion for gallbladder disease (Chapter 159) and about $5 to $6 billion for colorectal cancer (Chapter 203). Each disease has a different distribution of costs. For example, pharmaceutical costs account for nearly 60% of the direct costs of GERD, whereas gallbladder disease costs are predominantly related to inpatient stay. GI diseases account for approximately 10% of all deaths annually, with colorectal cancer being the most common cause of mortality.

Function of the Gastrointestinal Tract in Health

The GI tract, pancreas, and liver are responsible for digestion; absorption of fluids, electrolytes, and nutrients; removal of waste products; and metabolism of medications and other exogenous materials.

The epithelial lining of the GI tract is larger than a tennis court. These epithelial cells have a rapid turnover, with a lifespan of 3 to 7 days, and have considerable interaction with endogenous and exogenous materials.

The enteric nervous system (Chapter 138), which is composed of a complex array of neurons and ganglia organized around the myenteric (Auerbach) and submucosal (Meissner) plexus located within the wall of the esophagus, stomach, and intestinal tract, contains between 10 and 100 million neurons—equal to the total number in the spinal cord. Although it is an independent nervous system, complex interactions with the autonomic and central nervous systems are necessary for normal function. Recent evidence suggests abnormal interactions among the enteric, autonomic, and central nervous systems in the development and continuation of symptoms in functional bowel disorders such as irritable bowel syndrome (Chapter 139).

The immunologic system of the GI tract is the largest immune organ in the body (Chapter 42). It consists of luminal and epithelial barrier defenses, cellular components such as T and B cells, and noncellular inflammatory mediators. It has the overwhelmingly complex task of coexisting with luminal antigens (food), host proteins, and commensal bacteria while simultaneously differentiating these "good" antigens from "bad" antigens such as pathogenic bacterial proteins and transformed epithelial cells. The GI immune system plays a role in systemic autoimmune disorders and immune tolerance.

The GI endocrine system is stimulated by the ingestion of food. Secretion of hormones from endocrine cells responds to nutrients and to stimulation from the central nervous system.

The motility of the GI tract depends on a complex interaction between smooth muscle and the enteric nervous system. The interstitial cells of Cajal act as pacemakers of the GI tract and are responsible for the smooth, orderly transport of material from the mouth to the anus (Chapter 138).

With aging, the GI tract undergoes numerous changes. Epithelial cells interact with the environment and, given the appropriate genetic background, may undergo neoplastic transformation. Colon cancer (Chapter 203) is the second most common malignancy in the United States, and the GI tract collectively has more cancers than any other organ in the body.

Diagnosis

History

Even in today's high-tech environment with shortened times for office evaluation, the importance of the history and physical examination (Chapter 6) cannot be overemphasized, particularly when evaluating symptoms that may be related to the GI tract (Table 134–1).

Abdominal Pain

The complaint of abdominal pain (Chapter 145) depends on a complex interaction of sensory neuroreceptors in the abdominal organs, transmission of these impulses through the autonomic nervous system, and then transmission by the spinal cord to the thalamic nuclei, pons, and medulla. The thalamic nuclei sends impulses to the somatosensory cortex, where the discriminative aspects of pain are interpreted within the emotional context of the limbic system and frontal cortex. Inhibitory neurons at the level of the spinal cord and cerebral cortex, in turn, modify afferent pain impulses.

Pain originates from tissue injury, distention, contraction, inflammation, and direct chemical injury. However, the same receptors that respond to these noxious stimuli do not respond to more traditional stimuli such as pinching or burning. Consequently, abdominal pain will be felt by the patient during colonoscopy as a result of colonic distention or stretching of the mesentery, but not during biopsies or removal of a polyp.

The description of the pain will often aid in determining its etiology (Table 134–2). Pain can be either acute (Fig. 134–1) or chronic (Fig. 134–2); intermittent or constant; crampy, sharp, or stabbing; intense; localized or radiating; and burning, gnawing, dull, or achy. Patients should be queried about the duration, character, and intensity of the pain; rapidity of onset; progression of symptoms; location; exacerbating and alleviating factors; coexisting symptoms; past history and previous episodes of any pain; social habits; and family history of diseases and symptoms. The classic five questions are still applicable in current times: where is the pain located, when did it start, does it go anywhere, what does it feel like, and does anything make it better or worse? Appropriate questioning and good listening will give accurate clues to the underlying pathology.

Visceral Pain

Visceral pain is often poorly localized and loosely corresponds to the spinal segment that innervates the involved viscus. Examples include peptic ulcer disease (Chapters 141 and 142), in which pain is localized to the epigastrium, and early appendicitis (Chapter 145), in which pain is localized around the periumbilical region.

Somatoparietal Pain

Somatoparietal pain arises from noxious stimulation of the parietal peritoneum (Chapter 145). This type of pain is more localized and intense and corresponds to the dermatomal distribution that innervates the injured portion of the peritoneum. Somatoparietal pain is aggravated by movement such as coughing or a bumpy car ride. Examples of somatoparietal pain include appendicitis, with localized right lower quadrant pain attributable to localized peritonitis, and an abscess, with localized pain over the perforated viscus and inflammatory collection (Chapter 139).

Referred Pain

Referred pain is perceived by the patient in areas that are remote from the diseased organ and occurs as a result of visceral and afferent neurons from different anatomic regions converging at the same spinal cord segment, such as a diseased gallbladder causing right subscapular pain. Nonabdominal diseases, including myocardial infarction and pneumonia, can cause pain that is centered in or radiates to the abdominal area.

Gastrointestinal Bleeding

Acute Bleeding

GI bleeding can be either acute or chronic, and it can be massive or occult (see Table 137–1). Acute GI bleeding implies a temporally circumscribed event that occurred in the past 24 to 48 hours. The quantity and rapidity of blood loss and the patient's cardiovascular system will determine the degree of hemodynamic instability. Acute GI bleeding is described according to the location: upper GI bleeding is located proximal to the ligament of Treitz; lower GI bleeding is located distal to the

Text continued on p. 957.

TABLE 134–1 APPROACH TO COMMON GASTROINTESTINAL SIGNS AND SYMPTOMS

Symptoms	Abdominal Pain	GI Bleeding	Diarrhea	Steatorrhea	Constipation
History (ask the following questions)	Acute vs. chronic (duration); intermittent vs. constant; crampy, sharp, or stabbing; burning, gnawing, dull, or achy; location; localized or radiating; onset and progression of symptoms; previous episodes; other diseases	Acute vs. chronic (duration); intermittent vs. continuous; quantity; hematemesis, melena, or hematochezia; associated pain and location; symptoms of anemia, e.g., dyspnea, chest pain, lightheadedness; medication use, esp. aspirin/NSAIDs	Acute vs. chronic (duration), fever, weight loss, number of stools/24 hr, large vs. small volume, nocturnal, blood, quality and consistency, change in volume with NPO status, pain, medication use	Weight loss, number of stools/24 hr, duration of symptoms, blood, quality and consistency of stools, pain	Acute vs. chronic (duration), age, weight loss, number of stools per week, incomplete evacuation, bloating or discomfort, blood, chronic illness, mobility of the patient, medication use, previous abdominal surgery
Physical findings (evaluate for the following)	Fever, HR, BP; inspect skin and contour of abdomen; bowel sounds—present or absent; presence of organomegaly or masses (abscess); location of pain; rebound or guarding; peritoneal signs, e.g., shaking, tenderness	HR, BP, orthostatic findings; abdominal pain may or may not be present; look for hepatosplenomegaly, spider angiomas, jaundice, and other signs of portal hypertension, which may indicate varices; examine stool for color, consistency, and blood (Hemoccult)	HR, BP, orthostatic findings; fever; wasting; presence or absence of abdominal pain; extraintestinal symptoms (IBD), e.g., arthritis, erythema nodosum	Wasting, presence or absence of abdominal pain, excessive bruising (vitamin D deficiency), ascites, enlarged lymph nodes (TB, malignancy)	Wasting; assess mobility; abdominal distention; stool in loops of bowel may be palpated; rectal examination—impacted stool; rectal prolapse
Laboratory tests	CBC, BUN, Cr, glucose, amylase, lipase, liver tests (ALT, AST, bilirubin, alkaline phosphatase), albumin, PT, PTT, U/A, stool for pathogens, *Helicobacter pylori* antibodies	CBC (H/H and platelets are most important), BUN, Cr, liver tests, PT, PTT, type and cross; NGT lavage—note color and whether there is clearing with lavage	CBC, BUN, Cr, glucose, electrolytes, liver tests, albumin, stool for culture; ASCA and pANCA antibodies (IBD) may be useful	72-hr stool for fecal fat; carotene; PT; vitamin D; calcium; albumin; celiac disease antibodies, e.g., antigliadin, tTG, antiendomysial antibodies	CBC, Chem-7, calcium, magnesium, phosphate, TFTs
Endoscopy	EGD, colonoscopy, 24-hr pH probe	EGD, colonoscopy, enteroscopy, wireless capsule study	Colonoscopy with biopsies, EGD with duodenal biopsies	EGD with duodenal biopsies	Colonoscopy if recent change in bowel habits
Imaging	CT scan, ultrasound, angiography	Tagged RBC scan, angiography	Small bowel series (strictures in Crohn's disease)	CT of the abdomen (pancreatic calcifications)	Usually not necessary; MRI defecography

ALT = alanine transaminase; ASCA = anti–*Saccharomyces cerevisiae* antibody; AST = aspartate transaminase; BP = blood pressure; BUN = blood urea nitrogen; CBC = complete blood count; Cr = creatinine; CT = computed tomography; DM = diabetes mellitus; EGD = esophagogastroduodenoscopy; GERD = gastroesophageal reflux disease; GI = gastrointestinal; GU = genitourinary; HCG = human chorionic gonadotropin; H/H = hematocrit/hemoglobin; HIV = human immunodeficiency virus; HR = heart rate; IBD = inflammatory bowel disease; MRI = magnetic resonance imaging; NGT = nasogastric tube; NPO = nothing orally; NSAIDs = nonsteroidal anti-inflammatory drugs; pANCA = perinuclear antineutrophil cytoplasmic antibody; PT = prothrombin time; PTT = partial thromboplastin time; RBC = red blood cell; TB = tuberculosis; TFTs = thyroid function tests; tTG = tissue transglutaminase; U/A = urinalysis.

Nausea and Vomiting	Dysphagia	Odynophagia	GERD	Anorexia	Weight Loss
Nausea with or without emesis, acute vs. chronic (duration), intermittent vs. constant, medication use, comorbid illnesses, other symptoms	Oropharyngeal vs. esophageal dysphagia, solids vs. liquids, acute vs. chronic (duration), intermittent vs. progressive, GERD symptoms present or absent, weight loss, skin changes, cold hands (Raynaud's phenomenon)	Duration (acute vs. chronic) of pain with swallowing; underlying immunosuppression, e.g., HIV infection, DM; caustic ingestion; medication use	Duration (acute vs. chronic) of pain, location, burning, dysphagia, extraesophageal manifestations	Acute vs. chronic (duration); association with different foods; psychological factors; underlying disease, e.g., DM, malignancy, HIV infection; medication use	Age; acute vs. chronic (duration); intentional vs. unintentional; quantity; up and down vs. progressively down; anorexia, nausea, vomiting; diarrhea; abdominal pain; blood in stool; cough; GU symptoms; neurologic symptoms; endocrine symptoms; medication use
Presence or absence of abdominal pain; if acute, evaluate for associated causes, e.g., pregnancy, obstruction, GI organ inflammation, medication, head trauma. If chronic, evaluate for associated causes, e.g., pregnancy, medication, diabetes, partial obstruction, intracranial disease, psychogenic disorders	Usually normal, but if malignancy is present, evaluate for lymph nodes and masses, e.g., supraclavicular or in the neck; palpate the thyroid for size and nodules; evaluate the skin for sclerodermatous changes	Usually normal; evaluate for underlying immunosuppression	Usually normal, unless extraesophageal manifestations are present, e.g., chronic cough or asthma (pulmonary wheezing or rhonchi)	Wasting; fever; psychogenic symptoms, e.g., loss of tooth enamel, knuckle ulcerations and calluses; abdominal masses; enlarged lymph nodes	Wasting; malnutrition; poor dentition or poorly fitting dentures; thyromegaly; abdominal masses, enlarged lymph nodes; pelvic masses in women; diabetic neuropathy; psychogenic symptoms, e.g., loss of tooth enamel, knuckle ulcerations and calluses
β-HCG, CBC, serum electrolytes, BUN, Cr, glucose, liver tests, albumin, TFTs, cortisol	CBC	CBC, HIV test, fasting glucose	Usually normal	CBC, Chem-7, liver tests, albumin, HIV test, TFTs	CBC, Chem-7, TFTs, liver tests, calcium, magnesium, phosphate, albumin, HIV test, serum carotene
EGD is usually normal	EGD with biopsies and/or dilation, esophageal motility study, 24-hr pH probe	EGD with biopsies	24-hr pH probe, EGD usually normal	Directed at detecting underlying disease, e.g., if a GI cause is suspected, EGD and/or colonoscopy with biopsies may be helpful	Directed at detecting underlying disease, e.g., if a GI cause is suspected, EGD and/or colonoscopy with biopsies may be helpful
Abdominal ultrasound or CT if acute in onset; if chronic, additionally consider CT of the head	Esophagogram (barium swallow) will show stricture, Schatzki ring, mass, etc.	Usually not necessary	Usually not necessary	Directed at detecting underlying disease, e.g., if a GI cause is suspected, abdominal CT may be helpful	Directed at detecting underlying disease, e.g., a chest or abdominal CT scan may be helpful

TABLE 134–2 TYPICAL MANIFESTATIONS FOR KEY CAUSES OF ACUTE AND CHRONIC ABDOMINAL PAIN

Condition	Location	Quality	Duration	Aggravating or Relieving Factors	Associated Symptoms or Signs	Diagnostic Studies
Peptic ulcer disease (Chapters 141 and 142)	Midepigastric, RUQ, or lower substernal	Burning, gnawing	Days	Relief with food or antacids	Recurrent; associated factors, e.g., *Helicobacter pylori*, aspirin/NSAIDs	Acute or chronic anemia, upper endoscopy, *H. pylori* testing
Acute pancreatitis (Chapter 147)	LUQ, epigastrium, radiates to midback	Intense, localized	Hours	Aggravated by food, better with lying still and narcotics	Nausea, vomiting, lack of bowel sounds; associated factors, e.g., alcohol, gallstones	Elevated amylase and lipase, CT scan
Acute cholecystitis (Chapter 159)	RUQ, radiates to right scapula	Intense, crescendo	Hours	May follow a fatty meal, better with narcotics and surgery	Nausea, vomiting, fever	Elevated WBC count, US or CT
Acute appendicitis Chapter 145)	Periumbilical then moves to RLQ	Intense, localized, deep pain	Hours	Unprovoked, better with narcotics and surgery	Anorexia, nausea, vomiting, fever late	Elevated WBC count, US or CT
Diverticulitis (Chapter 145)	LLQ	Sharp, localized, intense	Hours	Unprovoked, better with narcotics and antibiotics or surgery	Anorexia, nausea, fever late	Elevated WBC count, CT
Ruptured viscus and peritonitis (Chapter 145)	Diffuse	Intense, diffuse	Minutes to hours	Worse with movement; better with lying still, narcotics, and surgery	Anorexia, nausea, vomiting, fever, lack of bowel sounds, rebound, and guarding are present; loath to move	Elevated WBC count, CT
Intestinal ischemia (Chapter 146)	Small intestine—midabdomen; large intestine—right or left side of the abdomen over the colon	Pain out of proportion to physical findings	Minutes	Occurs after eating, or unprovoked; better with narcotics, thrombus dissolution, stenting, or surgical resection	Nausea, bloody diarrhea; associated factors, e.g., cardiac arrhythmias	Elevated WBC count, angiography or colonoscopy (colonic ischemia)
Strangulated hernia (Chapter 146)	Localized	Sharp, localized, intense; may be crampy if obstruction present	Minutes to hours	Previous hernia history; unprovoked; better with narcotics and decompression, including surgery	Anorexia, nausea, vomiting, no stool or flatus passage if obstruction, bowel sounds in hernia sac	Elevated WBC count, CT scan or ultrasound
Small or large bowel obstruction (Chapters 145, 146, and 148)	Small intestine—midabdomen; large intestine—right or left lateral aspect of the abdomen	Colicky, crampy	Hours to days	Aggravated by food; better with narcotics, NGT decompression, and/or surgery	Anorexia, nausea, vomiting, no stool or flatus passage, increased bowel sounds with "rushing"; associated factors, e.g., hernia, previous surgery	Elevated WBC count, CT scan
Abdominal abscess (Chapter 145)	Located over the abscess, usually LLQ or RLQ	Insidious, intense, constant	Days	Aggravated by movement, especially if perforation is not completely walled off	Anorexia, nausea, fever, abdominal mass	Elevated WBC count, CT scan

Acute hepatitis	RUQ	Localized	Days	Worse with deep inspiration	Anorexia, nausea, enlarged liver, jaundice; associated factors, e.g., alcohol, infection	Abnormal liver test results
GERD (Chapter 140)	Retrosternal, substernal, or epigastrium	Burning, gnawing	Days to years	Relief with antacids	Recurrent; may have extraesophageal manifestations, e.g., asthma, chronic cough, or laryngitis	24-hr pH probe, upper endoscopy (usually normal)
Nonulcer dyspepsia (Chapter 139)	Epigastrium	Burning, gnawing	Years	Better with antacids or pain medications	Other IBS symptoms	Normal EGD
Irritable bowel syndrome (Chapter 139)	Lower part of the abdomen	Crampy, bloating, distention	Years	Onset occurs with change in bowel characteristics, e.g., frequency, quality, form; relieved with stool passage	Bloating and abdominal distention	Normal studies, usually not necessary for diagnosis
Chronic pancreatitis (Chapter 147)	Epigastrium, radiates to midback	Intense, localized	Days to years	Aggravated by food, better with narcotics	Anorexia, nausea, vomiting; associated factors, e.g., alcohol	Amylase and lipase may be normal, CT may show calcifications
Inflammatory or infectious enterocolitis (Chapters 143 and 305)	Small intestine—midabdomen; large intestine—right or left side of the abdomen over the colon; rectum—tenesmus	Crampy	Hours to days	Better with stool passage and treatment specific to the underlying cause	Nausea, vomiting, bloody diarrhea; associated factors, e.g., infectious—food transmission, IBD—prolonged duration, family history	Stool studies for culture, colonoscopy with biopsies
Malignancy (Chapter 203)	Variable, depending on cancer location	Intense, localized or diffuse	Days	Better with narcotics and cancer therapy	Primary vs. metastatic disease	CT scan and biopsies, PET scan
Pneumonia/pleurisy (Chapters 97 and 101)	Upper part of the abdomen	Localized, worse with deep breathing	Hours to days	Painful breathing, better with antibiotics	Cough, fever, dyspnea	CXR
Angina and myocardial infarction (Chapters 70–72)	Retrosternal and epigastric	Pressure, squeezing, heaviness	Minutes	Worse with exertion, relief with nitroglycerin	Dyspnea, diaphoresis, murmur	ECG, cardiac enzymes, stress testing
Genitourinary disorders (Chapters 127 and 307)	Bladder—suprapubic; renal colic—LLQ or RLQ radiating to the groin; prostate—suprapubic; kidney—CVA	Constant or colicky; stone passage—restless, cannot find a comfortable position	Minutes to days	Better with antibiotics and pain medications (pyelonephritis or nephrolithiasis)	Hematuria, dysuria, prostate tenderness, fever	Urinalysis, urine culture, CT scan for stone disease

Continued

TABLE 134–2 TYPICAL MANIFESTATIONS FOR KEY CAUSES OF ACUTE AND CHRONIC ABDOMINAL PAIN—cont'd

Condition	Location	Quality	Duration	Aggravating or Relieving Factors	Associated Symptoms or Signs	Diagnostic Studies
Ovarian cysts or torsion (Chapters 209 and 255)	LLQ or RLQ	Constant or colicky	Minutes	Better with NSAIDs or surgery (torsion)	Nausea, vomiting; may be recurrent	Ultrasound
Ruptured ectopic pregnancy (Chapter 259)	LLQ or RLQ	Constant, intense, stabbing	Minutes	Better with surgery	Rebound and guarding present, abnormal menses or amenorrhea	Acute anemia, elevated β-HCG, ultrasound
Musculoskeletal disorders	Specific muscle groups	Aching	Days	Better with heat or NSAIDs, aggravated by movement	History of muscle injury or exertion	Normal laboratory results
Herpes zoster (Chapter 397)	Dermatomal in distribution	Burning, itching, neuropathic, constant	Days	Aggravated by touching the dermatome, better with pain or antiviral medications	Recurrent; rash may or may not be present	Skin culture or biopsy
Metabolic disorders, e.g., diabetes mellitus (Chapter 247)	Epigastric or generalized	Intense, constant	Hours to days	Worse with poor metabolic control, e.g., poor glucose control	Recurrent; nausea, vomiting, diabetic neuropathy	Specific metabolic parameters will be abnormal, e.g., elevated glucose in DM
Abdominal epilepsy (Chapter 426)	Epigastric or umbilical	Constant	Hours to days	Unprovoked, better with antiseizure therapy	Recurrent; may have associated seizure disorder	EEG
Dissecting or leaking abdominal aortic aneurysm (Chapter 78)	Over the aneurysm, radiates to the back or groin	Severe, constant	Minutes to hours to days	History of HTN or CAD	Shock, pulsatile mass; bruit *not* usually present	Acute anemia, CT, angiogram

CAD = coronary artery disease; CT = computed tomography; CVA = costovertebral angle; CXR = chest x-ray; DM = diabetes mellitus; ECG = electrocardiogram; EEG = electroencephalogram; EGD = esophagogastroduodenoscopy; GERD = gastroesophageal reflux disease; HCG = human chorionic gonadotropin; HTN = hypertension; IBD = irritable bowel disease; IBS = irritable bowel syndrome; LLQ = left lower quadrant; LUQ = left upper quadrant; NGT = nasogastric tube; NSAIDs = nonsteroidal anti-inflammatory drugs; PET = positron emission tomography; RLQ = right lower quadrant; RUQ = right upper quadrant; US = ultrasonography; WBC = white blood cell.

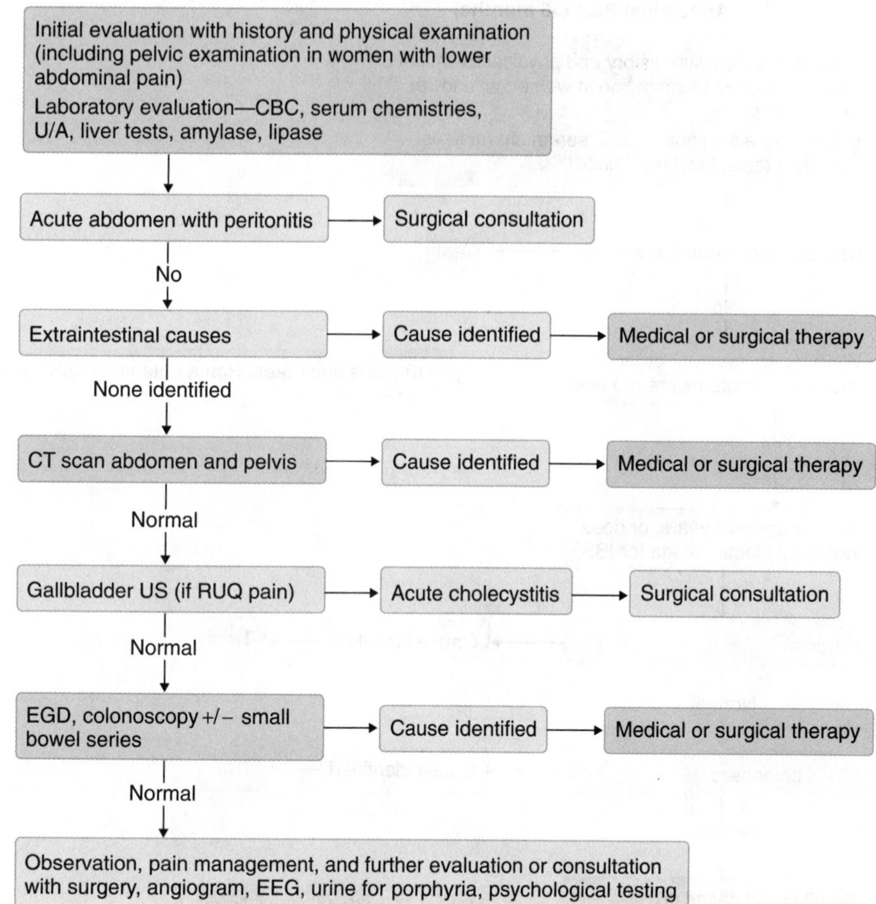

FIGURE 134–1 • Approach to patients with acute abdominal pain. CT = computed tomography; EEG = electroencephalography; EGD = esophagogastroduodenoscopy; RUQ = right upper quadrant; US = ultrasonography.

ileocecal valve; and middle GI bleeding is located in between, for example, the small intestine. Acute upper GI bleeding (see Table 137–1), which may be manifested as hematemesis, melena, or hematochezia, is three times more common than acute lower GI bleeding (see Table 137–4). Upper GI bleeding is further subdivided into variceal and nonvariceal bleeding because treatment of these two conditions differs markedly. The two most common causes of acute lower GI bleeding are diverticulosis and arteriovenous malformations. Whereas upper endoscopy is universally preferred as the first step in the evaluation of acute upper GI bleeding (see Fig. 137–3), the use of colonoscopy as the first diagnostic test for acute lower GI bleeding is more controversial (see Fig. 137–4). Acute GI bleeding from the small intestine, distal to the duodenum, is rare but occurs in 10% of patients with hematochezia.

Chronic Bleeding

Chronic GI bleeding is manifested as Hemoccult-positive stools or iron deficiency anemia, or both (see Fig. 137–6). The most worrisome etiology to exclude is an underlying malignancy of the GI tract, but other diseases can also be accompanied by chronic GI bleeding (see Table 137–5). Endoscopic evaluation is the initial diagnostic test and will yield a diagnosis 95% of the time.

Obscure Bleeding

Obscure GI bleeding occurs when the source of GI bleeding is unidentified (see Table 137–5). The bleeding may be clinically evident or occult in nature, and it may be caused by common conditions such as an arteriovenous malformation or uncommon ones such as Dieulafoy's lesion or Meckel's diverticulum.

Diarrhea and Steatorrhea

Diarrhea

Diarrhea, or an increased number or fluidity of stools, is usually due to an excess of water in stool. Most people have experienced loose stools for a day or two (e.g., viral gastroenteritis), but other causes, such as inflammatory bowel disease (Chapter 144), can be chronic and cause intermittent symptoms for a patient's entire lifetime. Diarrhea results from an increase in secretion, decrease in absorption, or both, and can be classified as secretory or osmotic diarrhea. Although there may be overlap, osmotic diarrhea usually ceases when a patient takes nothing by mouth, whereas secretory diarrhea continues. Large-volume diarrhea generally originates from the small intestine; small-volume diarrhea generally originates from the colon. Blood in the stool always implies an underlying organic abnormality, should always be investigated, and should never be attributed to functional diseases such as irritable bowel syndrome. Bloody diarrhea occurs with mucosal inflammation or erosions or ulcerations secondary to infectious, inflammatory, or ischemic enterocolitis.

Steatorrhea

Steatorrhea, or fatty stools, arises from disruption of fat solubilization, digestion, or absorption in the small intestine (Chapter 143). Maldigestion, or inadequate luminal breakdown of fats, occurs with pancreatic exocrine deficiency (Chapter 147) or lack of bile. Malabsorption (Chapter 143), or inadequate transport of the products of digestion, occurs with mucosal diseases such as celiac sprue or during impaired lymphatic transport.

Constipation

Constipation (Chapter 138) occurs most commonly in the elderly and is often used to describe more than one symptom, including infrequent stools, difficult passage of stool, a sense of incomplete evacuation, and abdominal bloating or discomfort. About 1 to 5% of patients who visit a physician complain of constipation. The causes of constipation are as varied as the complaints and include inadequate stool water or fecal material, decreased colonic motility, reduced mobility, chronic illness, medication use, psychological factors, and functional outlet obstruction. Treatment plans vary, but the simplest and most common starting point is to increase the patient's daily fiber and fluid intake.

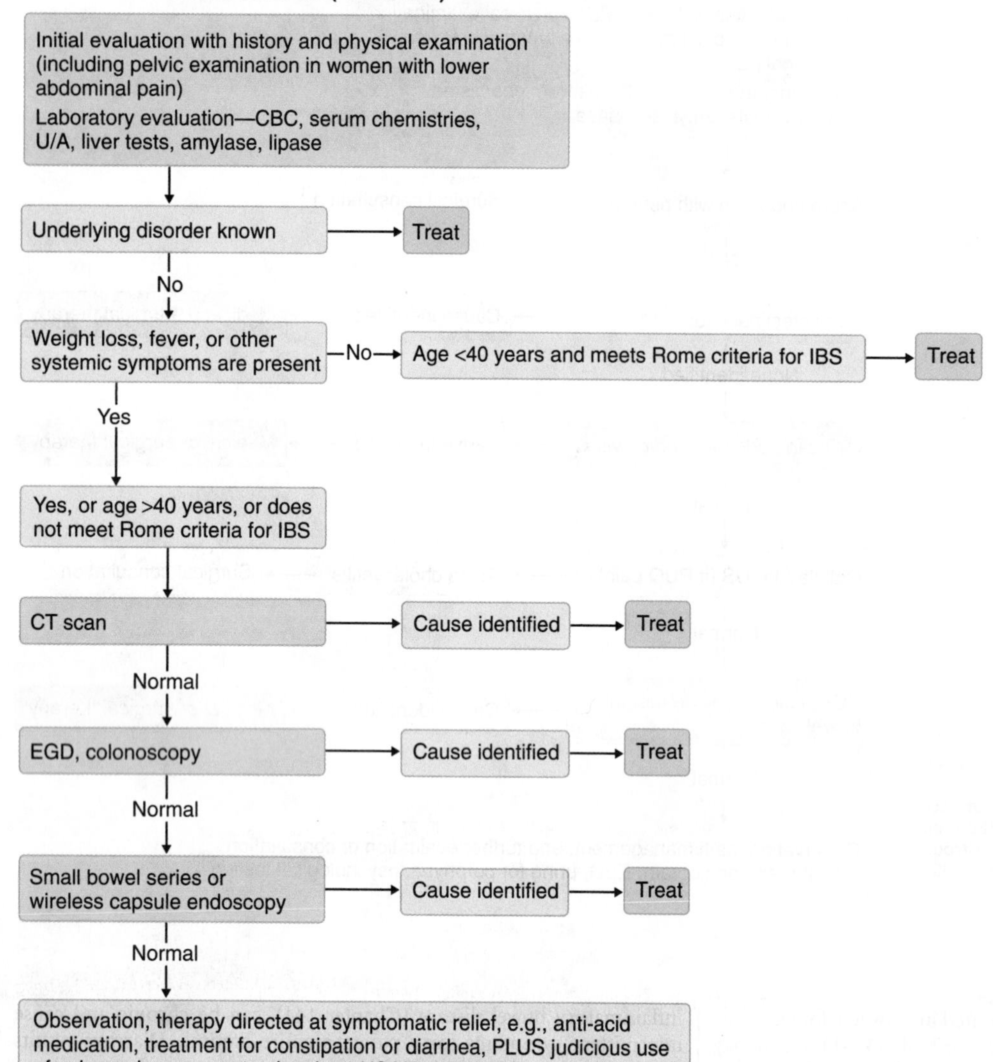

FIGURE 134–2 • Approach to patients with chronic abdominal pain. CBC = complete blood count; CT = computed tomography; EGD = esophagogastroduodenoscopy; ERCP = endoscopic retrograde cholangiopancreatography; IBS = irritable bowel syndrome; NSAIDs = nonsteroidal anti-inflammatory drugs; U/A = urinalysis.

Nausea and Vomiting

Nausea and vomiting may be manifestations of GI diseases or primary non-GI diseases (Table 134–3) and may lead to fluid and electrolyte imbalances, nutritional deficiencies, aspiration pneumonia (Chapter 94), Mallory-Weiss tears (Chapter 140), and esophageal rupture. Nausea is the unpleasant sensation of the desire to vomit. Retching, or "dry heaves," is coordinated voluntary muscle activity of the abdomen and chest without discharge of stomach contents into the mouth.

Vomiting, or the act of emesis, occurs as gastric contents are forcefully ejected out of the mouth. Nausea and vomiting may be acute, such as with acute obstruction, inflammation, or ischemia; other acute infections; medication; pregnancy; or head trauma. Nausea and vomiting that are chronic in nature are usually associated with pregnancy, medications, motility disorders such as diabetic gastroparesis (Chapter 247), partial obstruction, intracranial disease (Chapter 199), psychogenic disorders, or an underlying metabolic or endocrine disturbance. Nausea by itself may be chronic, persistent, or recurrent over a period of months or years. Unless one of the causes mentioned can be identified, evaluation of a patient with chronic nausea, with or without vomiting, is often unrevealing, so treatment must then be aimed at symptomatic relief with antiemetics such as ondansetron, [1] a selective 5-HT_3 receptor antagonist (4 to 8 mg orally every 8 to 12 hours), or prokinetic agents such as tegaserod, a 5-HT_4 receptor partial agonist (2 to 6 mg orally every 12 hours).

Dysphagia, Odynophagia, and Gastroesophageal Reflux

Dysphagia

Dysphagia, or the sensation of solids or liquids not passing from the mouth into the stomach, is a common symptom and can be divided into oropharyngeal dysphagia and esophageal dysphagia. The former may be caused by neuromuscular disease, mechanical obstruction, skeletal muscle disorders, depression, or dementia. Patients are unable to propel their food from the hypopharynx into the upper esophagus and specifically localize their symptoms to the upper cervical region. Coughing or aspiration during meals indicates that food has passed into the tracheobronchial tree. Esophageal dysphagia (Chapter 140) is caused by either a motility disorder, such as achalasia, diffuse esophageal spasm, or scleroderma, or by a mechanical obstruction, such as a benign stricture, ring, or neoplasm. If a motility disorder exists, the patient will complain of difficulty swallowing both liquids and solids; if the major complaint is one of difficulty swallowing solids alone, the underlying cause is mechanical obstruction. A benign stricture will cause intermittent followed by more progressive dysphagia as the esophagus becomes more narrowed. A Schatzki ring will cause intermittent dysphagia, such as "steakhouse

TABLE 134–3 CAUSES OF NAUSEA AND VOMITING

Condition	Quality	Duration	Associated Symptoms or Signs	Diagnostic Studies
NAUSEA AND VOMITING SECONDARY TO GASTROINTESTINAL CAUSES				
Esophageal stricture or motility disorder (Chapters 138 and 140)	Regurgitation, non-acid; liquids and solids	Chronic	Heartburn, dysphagia; weight loss may be present	Esophageal motility study, EGD, esophagogram
Peptic ulcer disease (Chapters 141 and 142)	There may be associated early satiety or emesis of undigested food several hours after eating because of outlet obstruction; acid is present	Chronic	Abdominal pain, hematemesis	Acute or iron deficiency anemia, EGD, UGI series
Alcoholic gastritis (Chapter 142)	Early morning emesis—dry heaves	Acute and recurrent	Intoxicated	Serum alcohol level, abnormal liver test results
Gastric malignancy (Chapter 202)	Non-acid secondary to hypochlorhydria	Chronic	Hematemesis	Iron deficiency anemia, EGD, UGI series
Cholecystitis (Chapter 159)	Nausea > emesis	Acute	RUQ pain radiating to the right scapula	Liver tests, RUQ ultrasound
Pancreatitis (Chapter 147)	Nausea > emesis	Acute or chronic	LUQ or epigastric pain radiating to the back	Elevated amylase and lipase, CT of the abdomen
Small or large bowel obstruction (Chapters 145, 146, and 148)	Emesis of feculent material	Acute	Crampy abdominal pain, no passage of stool or flatus	Acute abdominal series, CT of the abdomen
Diverticulitis (Chapter 145)	Anorexia, nausea, rare emesis	Acute	LLQ pain, fever	Elevated WBC count, CT of the abdomen
Appendicitis (Chapter 145)	Anorexia, nausea, emesis	Acute	Periumbilical, then RLQ pain; fever	CT of the abdomen
Peritonitis (Chapter 145)	Nausea, rare emesis	Acute	Diffuse abdominal pain, fever	Elevated WBC count, CT of the abdomen
Infectious gastroenteritis (Chapter 305)	Nausea; emesis of undigested food 4–6 hr or longer after eating; acid is present	Acute	Diarrhea, fever	CBC; stool cultures if prolonged *or* bloody diarrhea is present
Inflammatory enterocolitis (Chapter 305)	Mild nausea, rare emesis	Acute or chronic	Bloody diarrhea	Colonoscopy with biopsies
Hepatitis (Chapters 151 and 152)	Nausea, rare emesis	Acute or chronic	RUQ pain, jaundice	Abnormal liver test results, RUQ ultrasound
Motility disorders (Chapter 138)	Constant nausea, emesis of undigested food several hours after eating; acid is present	Chronic or acute and recurrent	Crampy abdominal pain, constipation or diarrhea	Gastric emptying study; if prolonged and progressive, full-thickness biopsy of the small/large intestine

Continued

TABLE 134–3 CAUSES OF NAUSEA AND VOMITING—cont'd

Condition	Quality	Duration	Associated Symptoms or Signs	Diagnostic Studies
NAUSEA AND VOMITING SECONDARY TO NONGASTROINTESTINAL CAUSES				
Medication	Nausea > emesis	Chronic	Occurs after taking the medication	None necessary, discontinue medication
Pregnancy	Nausea and emesis	Acute and recurrent	Predominantly in the morning and in the first trimester; amenorrhea	β-HCG, enlarging uterus on examination
Diabetic gastroparesis (Chapter 138)	Undigested food 4–6 hr or longer after eating	Chronic	Elevated fasting glucose	Fasting glucose
Uremia (Chapter 131)	Nausea > emesis	Chronic	Predominantly in the morning; uremic breath	Elevated BUN and creatinine, 24-hr urinary creatinine clearance
Pulmonary disorders	Emesis after coughing, rare nausea	Acute	Cough, dyspnea, fever	Elevated WBC count, chest x-ray
Psychogenic disorders	Self-induced emesis, no associated nausea	Recurrent	Weight loss, loss of tooth enamel, calluses and healing ulcerations of the hand	Psychological testing
Intracranial disease	Nausea > emesis	Chronic	Abnormal neurologic findings	CT of the head
Malignancy	Nausea and emesis	Chronic	Caused by underlying malignancy and/or chemotherapy	Biopsy of the malignancy, CT scan, PET scan
Ovarian torsion (Chapters 209 and 255)	Nausea > emesis	Acute	Lower abdominal pain	Pelvic ultrasound
Non-GI infections	Mild nausea, rare emesis	Acute	Fever, underlying infection	CBC

BUN = blood urea nitrogen; CBC = complete blood count; CT = computed tomography; EGD = esophagogastroduodenoscopy; GI = gastrointestinal; HCG = human chorionic gonadotropin; LLQ = left lower quadrant; LUQ = left upper quadrant; PET = positron emission tomography; RLQ = right lower quadrant; RUQ = left upper quadrant; UGI = upper gastrointestinal; WBC = white blood cell.

syndrome," and an underlying malignancy will cause progressive dysphagia with weight loss. By asking three questions the cause of the dysphagia can usually be identified: (1) Do you have trouble with solids or liquids? (2) Is the dysphagia intermittent or progressive? and (3) Do you have heartburn?

Odynophagia

Odynophagia (Chapter 140) is pain with swallowing and reflects esophageal mucosal inflammation secondary to infectious causes, pill-induced esophagitis, irradiation, or ingestion of caustic substances.

Gastroesophageal Reflux Disease

The terms heartburn, acid regurgitation, sour stomach, and bitter taste are all used to describe GERD (Chapter 140) symptoms. Reflux occurs when the esophageal epithelium is exposed to gastric secretions. Some degree of gastric reflux is considered normal, but symptoms occur when the mucosa's tolerance to acid is exceeded. In addition to the typical symptoms of heartburn or chest pain, extraesophageal manifestations of GERD include laryngitis (Chapter 455), asthma (Chapter 87), and chronic cough (Chapter 83). Patients may or may not have typical esophageal symptoms.

Diagnostic evaluation of a patient with esophageal symptoms includes a careful history. Physical examination is usually unremarkable unless there is an underlying malignancy or systemic disease such as scleroderma. Traditional diagnostic tests that are useful include esophagogastroduodenoscopy (EGD), esophageal motility, 24-hour pH probes, and barium studies (Chapter 140).

Anorexia and Early Satiety

Anorexia, which is loss of the desire to eat, is a major symptom in many GI and non-GI diseases, including central nervous system, systemic, and psychological disorders. Anorexia may be acute, such as that caused by inflammatory GI processes, or chronic, such as that caused by depression. Chronic anorexia may lead to significant weight loss, especially in patients with hypermetabolic states such as malignancy. Anorexia is commonly seen in GI and liver disorders, as well as extraintestinal disorders, and it often precedes identification of the underlying disorder, such as occurs in acute viral hepatitis (Chapter 151) or appendicitis (Chapter 145). Anorexia must be distinguished from the fear of eating because of associated discomfort, such as occurs in intestinal angina or inflammatory bowel disease.

The underlying mechanism of anorexia is complex and includes endocrine and neural regulation in the GI tract and hypothalamus, peptides (e.g., cholecystokinin), and cytokines (e.g., tumor necrosis factor). Anorexia must also be differentiated from early satiety, which refers to the sensation of early gratification of appetite such that an individual consumes less than caloric requirements. Early satiety may be acute or chronic, but it is usually insidious in onset. Patients report that they are simply not hungry at meal time, must often "force" themselves to eat, yet still eat far less than they had in the past. Common causes include delayed gastric emptying such as occurs in long-term diabetes mellitus (Chapters 247 and 248), decreased gastric distention secondary to gastric malignancy (Chapter 202), and gastric outlet obstruction caused by peptic ulcer disease (Chapter 142).

Diagnostic evaluation of anorexia or early satiety includes a careful history and thorough physical examination, including evaluation for abdominal masses and lymph nodes. Diagnostic studies are directed at detecting any underlying diseases. Computed tomography (CT), upper GI endoscopy, or colonoscopy, alone or in combination, may be useful if intra-abdominal pathology is suspected. Therapy is aimed at treating the underlying disorder.

Weight Loss

Many individuals attempt to lose weight by dieting (Chapter 232) or increasing their exercise (Chapter 14), but unintentional weight loss of more than 5% of body weight is an indication of underlying pathology. Diseases of every organ system can cause weight loss, ranging from diseases of the GI tract, such as malignancy, inflammatory bowel disease, or malabsorption, to psychiatric disorders, such as anorexia nervosa or bulimia (Table 134–4). Although most unintentional weight loss occurs over a prolonged period, acute weight loss often occurs in hospitalized patients who are under severe stress and have supranormal caloric requirements, such as after burns or trauma (Chapter 113). The age of the patient can give clues to the underlying cause. Chronic weight loss in the elderly is more commonly caused by malignancy, poor dentition, chronic diseases, depression (Chapter 420), or drugs, whereas weight loss in younger patients is more commonly caused by eating disorders (Chapter 238), endocrine diseases, or human immunodeficiency virus (HIV) infection. The combination of anorexia and weight loss is more common in disorders such as malignancy or depression, whereas an increased appetite with concomitant weight loss is more common in malabsorption (Chapter 143) or hypermetabolic states (Chapter 244). Patients with significant weight loss are fluid and electrolyte depleted, as well as protein-calorie malnourished.

Diagnostic evaluation of a patient with unintentional weight loss includes a thorough history and physical examination to evaluate possible extraintestinal and GI causes (Fig. 134–3). If a good dietary log has been recorded and excessive calories are being ingested, the patient should be evaluated for malabsorption (e.g., steatorrhea) or a hypermetabolic state (e.g., hyperthyroidism). Conversely, if anorexia with decreased caloric intake is the problem, the evaluation should be focused in a different direction. Diagnostic studies and further consultation, including upper GI endoscopy, colonoscopy, CT scanning, angiography, HIV testing, or psychiatric consultation, should each be considered based on pertinent findings in the history and physical examination.

Treatment is based on identification of the underlying disorder but always includes attempts to replete fluids, electrolytes, vitamins, and other nutrients. In the acute setting, total parenteral nutrition (Chapter 236) may be the best option. If adequate treatment of the underlying chronic disorder is not possible, the appetite stimulant megestrol acetate (800 mg orally daily in divided doses) often helps patients with anorexia regain their weight and appropriate nutritional balance.

Physical Examination

The physical examination of a patient with abdominal symptoms is as important as the history. The position of the patient should be noted throughout the examination—a patient loath to move might have peritonitis (somatoparietal pain) because any movement increases irritation of the inflamed peritoneum (Chapter 145), whereas a patient who has colicky pain (visceral pain) cannot get into a comfortable position and often moves about restlessly while attempting to ease the paroxysms of pain. In a patient with acute symptoms, measurement of vital signs is important to determine hemodynamic stability (Chapter 7). A patient's weight should be compared with previous measurements.

Nonabdominal Examination

When examining nonabdominal areas, the focus is on identifying possible clues to underlying or systemic diseases; for example, if jaundice (see Fig. 149–1), spider telangiectases (Fig. 134–4), or other stigmata of chronic liver disease are present, varices should be suspected in a patient with acute upper GI bleeding. Examination of the eyes and skin may give clues to anemia or chronic liver disease. Palpation of lymph nodes (Chapter 174) in the neck, axilla, and groin should be included as part of a routine examination to look for clues to underlying systemic or localized inflammation or malignancy. Examination of the heart and lungs may reveal wheezing, suggestive of esophageal reflux, or an irregular heart rate, S_3 or S_4, suggestive of underlying cardiovascular disease, which is a risk factor for intestinal angina or ischemia (Chapter 146).

Abdominal Examination

The abdominal examination consists of the traditional four parts: inspection, auscultation, percussion, and palpation. Inspection of the abdomen should include evaluation for scars, diffuse or localized distention, or bulging flanks indicating ascites (Chapter 149). In severe necrotizing pancreatitis, Cullen's sign (a faint bluish discoloration around the umbilicus indicative of hemoperitoneum) or Grey Turner's sign (a blue-red or green-brown discoloration of the flanks reflecting tissue catabolism of hemoglobin) may be seen. Auscultation takes place before percussion and palpation so that intestinal activity is not disturbed by the examiner's hands. The pitch, intensity, and frequency of sounds should be elicited. High-pitched, active bowel sounds might indicate an obstruction, whereas a quiet abdomen might indicate peritonitis. If the veracity of the patient's history is in doubt, using the stethoscope for palpation during auscultation may clarify the intensity of the abdominal pain because patients may voluntarily guard their muscles during manual palpation but are less likely to be aware of the depth of abdominal muscle

TABLE 134–4 CAUSES OF INVOLUNTARY WEIGHT LOSS

Condition	Quality	Duration	Aggravating or Relieving Factors	Associated Symptoms or Signs	Diagnostic Studies
WEIGHT LOSS SECONDARY TO GASTROINTESTINAL CAUSES					
GI malignancy (Chapters 202 and 203)	Progressive, fast	Months	Better with cancer therapy, e.g., surgery, XRT, chemotherapy	Metastatic disease; anorexia, nausea, vomiting; abdominal pain; blood in stool	EGD, colonoscopy, abdominal CT scan, PET scan
Malabsorption (Chapter 143) (poor absorption of nutrients)	Progressive, slow	Months to years	Diarrhea/steatorrhea is worse with eating and resolves with NPO status	Hypermetabolic state—always eating	72-hr stool for fecal fat; carotene; PT; vitamin D; calcium; albumin; celiac disease antibodies, e.g., antigliadin, tTG, antiendomysial antibodies
Diarrhea (loss of nutrients) (Chapter 143)	Progressive, slow	Months	Diarrhea continues with fasting	Loose stools, bloody stools, abdominal cramps and pain	Stool culture for pathogens, EGD with duodenal biopsies, colonoscopy with biopsies
GI motility disorders (Chapter 138)	Intermittent, slow	Years	Worse with eating	Diarrhea or constipation may be present	Gastric emptying study, surgical full-thickness intestinal biopsies
Cirrhosis (Chapter 157)	Muscle wasting with edema, so weight can increase	Months to years	Worse with salt/fluid intake	Ascites, peripheral edema	Liver biopsy
Intestinal angina or ischemia (Chapter 146)	Afraid to eat, progressive	Months to years	Worse with eating	Abdominal pain, blood in stool, nausea; associated cardiovascular findings, e.g., arrhythmias	CT angiogram, angiography
WEIGHT LOSS SECONDARY TO NONGASTROINTESTINAL CAUSES					
Non-GI malignancy	Progressive	Months	Better with cancer therapy, e.g., surgery, XRT, chemotherapy	Metastatic disease; anorexia, nausea, vomiting; pain	CT scan for underlying disease, PET scan
Depression (Chapter 420)	Progressive, slow	Months to years		Common in elderly; flat affect	Psychological testing
Medication	Intermittent or progressive	Months	Worse with medication, resolves with discontinuation of offending drug	Anorexia, nausea, vomiting	Review drug profile

Poor dentition or poorly fitting dentures	Intermittent or progressive	Months to years	Worse with solid food	Common in the elderly	Evaluate dentures and dentition
Poor or inadequate caloric intake	Intermittent or progressive, acute (hospitalized) or chronic	Days to months to years	Common in elderly, teenagers, and poor families; occurs with excessive stress, e.g., prolonged hospitalization, burns, trauma	Will eat if enough food is made available to the patient	Review dietary log; if hospitalized, may need TPN
Psychogenic eating disorders—anorexia nervosa and bulimia (Chapter 238)	Intermittent or progressive	Months to years	Worse with stressors	Refuses to eat, loss of tooth enamel, calluses and healing ulcerations of the hand	Psychiatric testing
Endocrine disorders (Chapters 244 and 247)	DM—early satiety; hyperthyroidism—increased appetite	Months to years	Worse with chronicity of the disease	Diabetic neuropathy/retinopathy/nephropathy	Serum glucose, TFT, cortisol
Chronic infections, including HIV and TB (Chapters 345 and 413)	Progressive, fast	Months	Better with directed therapy, Megace	Nausea, anorexia, other infections	HIV test, PPD, cultures, biopsies if necessary
Systemic inflammatory disorders	Progressive, moderate	Months to years	Better with directed therapy, Megace	Arthritis, rash, vasculitis	ANA, RF, ESR, CRP
Chronic renal failure (Chapter 131)	Progressive, slow; edema can increase weight	Months to years	Better with dialysis, Megace	Nausea, anorexia, weight gain	BUN, Cr, 24-hr creatinine clearance
COPD (Chapter 88)	Progressive, slow	Months to years	Better with oxygen, pulmonary therapy	Dyspnea, wheezing, chronic cough, "blue bloater," "pink puffer"	Pulmonary function testing, CXR

ANA = antinuclear antibody; BUN = blood urea nitrogen; COPD = chronic obstructive pulmonary disease; Cr = creatinine; CRP = C-reactive protein; CT = computed tomography; CXR = chest x-ray; DM = diabetes mellitus; EGD = esophagogastroduodenoscopy; ESR = erythrocyte sedimentation rate; GI = gastrointestinal; HIV = human immunodeficiency virus; NPO = nothing orally; PET = positron emission tomography; PPD = purified protein derivative; PT = prothrombin time; RF = rheumatoid factor; TB = tuberculosis; TFT = thyroid function test; TPN = total parenteral nutrition; tTG = tissue transglutamase; XRT = x-ray therapy.

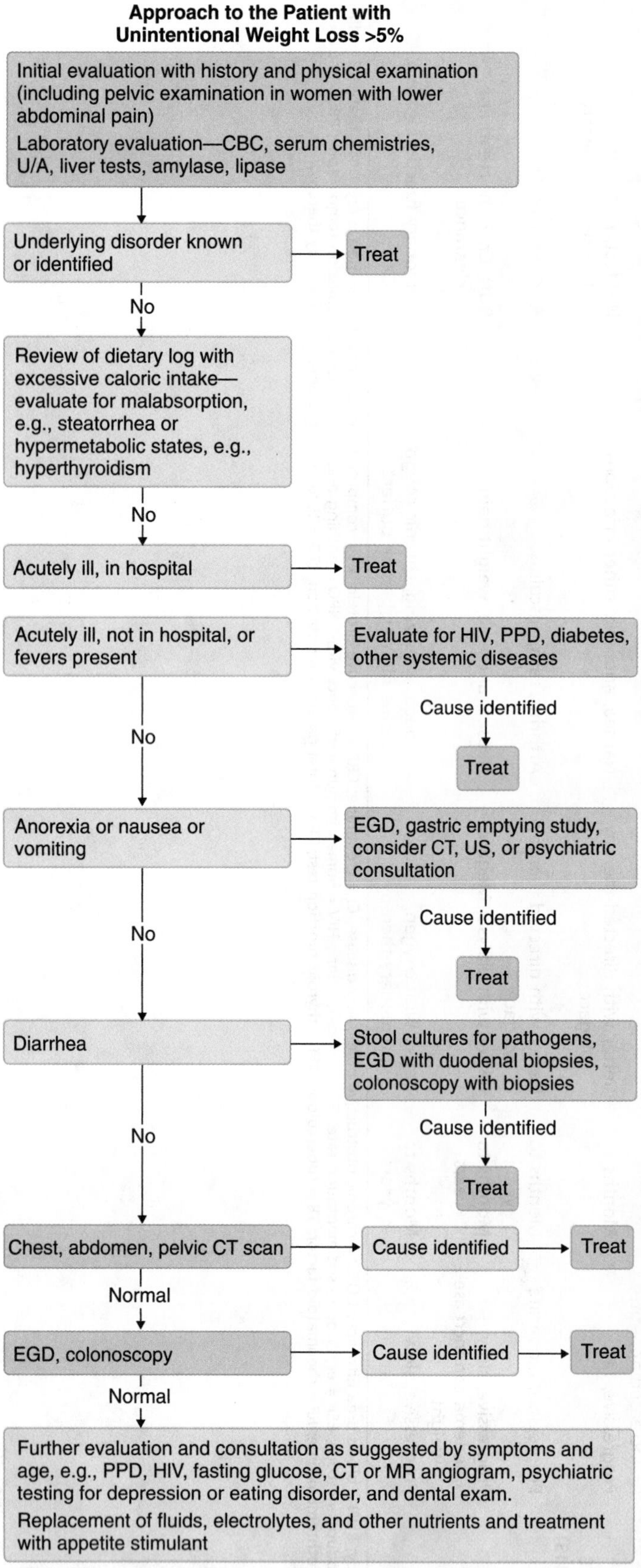

Approach to the Patient with Unintentional Weight Loss >5%

Initial evaluation with history and physical examination (including pelvic examination in women with lower abdominal pain)
Laboratory evaluation—CBC, serum chemistries, U/A, liver tests, amylase, lipase

↓

Underlying disorder known or identified → Treat

No ↓

Review of dietary log with excessive caloric intake—evaluate for malabsorption, e.g., steatorrhea or hypermetabolic states, e.g., hyperthyroidism

No ↓

Acutely ill, in hospital → Treat

Acutely ill, not in hospital, or fevers present → Evaluate for HIV, PPD, diabetes, other systemic diseases → Cause identified → Treat

No ↓

Anorexia or nausea or vomiting → EGD, gastric emptying study, consider CT, US, or psychiatric consultation → Cause identified → Treat

No ↓

Diarrhea → Stool cultures for pathogens, EGD with duodenal biopsies, colonoscopy with biopsies → Cause identified → Treat

No ↓

Chest, abdomen, pelvic CT scan → Cause identified → Treat

Normal ↓

EGD, colonoscopy → Cause identified → Treat

Normal ↓

Further evaluation and consultation as suggested by symptoms and age, e.g., PPD, HIV, fasting glucose, CT or MR angiogram, psychiatric testing for depression or eating disorder, and dental exam.
Replacement of fluids, electrolytes, and other nutrients and treatment with appetite stimulant

FIGURE 134–3 • Approach to patients with unintentional weight loss greater than 5%. CBC = complete blood count; CT = computed tomography; EGD = esophagogastroduodenoscopy; HIV = human immunodeficiency virus; MR = magnetic resonance; PPD = purified protein derivative; TFTs = thyroid function tests; U/A = urinalysis; US = ultrasonography.

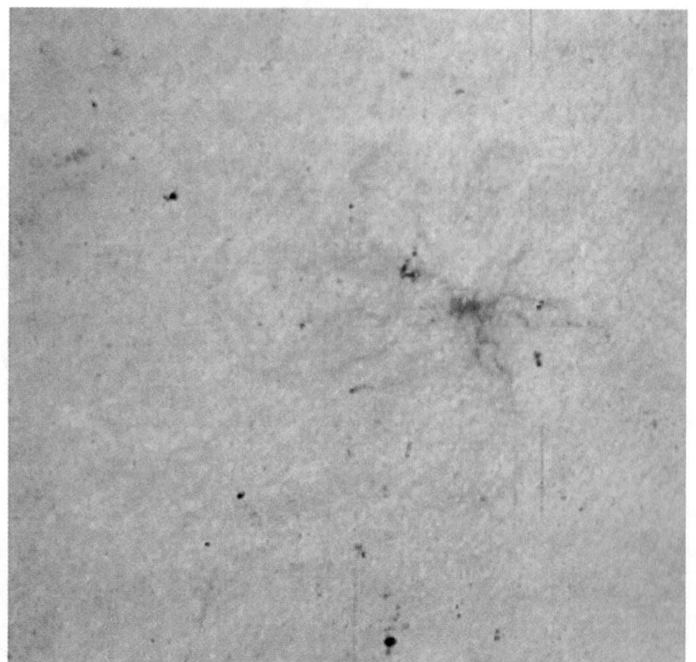

FIGURE 134–4 • Spider telangiectases on the chest of a patient with cirrhosis.

compression during the use of a stethoscope. The physician should listen over the aorta and other arteries for bruits, which indicate stenosis or abnormal blood flow, as occurs with an aortic aneurysm. A rub over the liver capsule indicates inflammation, which may be present with a subcapsular hematoma.

Percussion and palpation are usually performed simultaneously and should involve all four quadrants, the epigastrium, the periumbilical region, and the pelvis. Initial light percussion can indicate where the abdominal pain is most intense. During palpation, one should start with a survey of light palpation in the area farthest away from the point of maximum tenderness, followed by gentle deeper and deeper palpation over the area of greatest tenderness. If the physician immediately palpates the place of maximum tenderness, the patient is unlikely to let the examination continue. Localized or diffuse rebound tenderness and guarding should be gently elicited because even "accidentally" bumping the bed or stretcher will move the patient enough to cause peritoneal irritation and pain in patients who have inflammation of the parietal peritoneum (e.g., peritonitis). The location of any referred pain, such as in the back, should also be examined to exclude extraintestinal diseases (e.g., pyelonephritis [Chapter 306]). Abdominal palpation should include evaluation for any masses, including their size, location, and consistency, as well as for the presence or absence of tenderness. Examination of the right upper quadrant should include a determination of the size, texture, and presence of any liver tenderness or masses, in addition to the presence or absence of a distended gallbladder or evidence of pain on palpation of the gallbladder, such as Murphy's sign, which may be present in acute cholecystitis (Chapter 159). Percussion of the left upper quadrant in inspiration and expiration to evaluate spleen size is useful and will detect splenomegaly at its earliest stages (Chapter 174). The back and costovertebral angles should be inspected and gently percussed to exclude costovertebral angle tenderness, as found in pyelonephritis.

The abdominal examination is not complete without a digital rectal examination. The physician should visually inspect the perianal area and sweep the anorectal area with a finger to feel for any intestinal or pelvic masses or prostate abnormalities (Chapters 148 and 211). Stool color and consistency should be noted, and the stool should be tested for occult blood. Because pelvic abnormalities can mimic abdominal diseases, a female patient with lower abdominal pain should have a pelvic examination performed by a skilled examiner (Chapters 209 and 308).

Finally, to be complete, the extremities should be examined for edema, pulses, and any skin changes that might be present, such as erythema nodosum. A brief neurologic and mental status assessment should be performed because symptoms such as nausea or vomiting may actually be due to underlying neurologic disease, such as an intracranial mass (Chapter 199).

Use of Diagnostic and Therapeutic Tests

The history and physical examination are supplemented by the judicious use of laboratory, radiologic, and endoscopic evaluation (see Table 134–1).

Laboratory Tests

Laboratory tests that may aid in diagnosis include a complete blood count, serum chemistry panel, liver tests, amylase, lipase, urinalysis, and stool examination for pathogens. Increasingly specialized blood tests, such as antibodies for *Helicobacter pylori* (Chapter 141) or celiac disease (Chapter 143), are becoming sensitive and specific enough for diagnosis and monitoring of therapy. Autoimmune markers such as perinuclear antineutrophil cytoplasmic antibody (pANCA) and anti–*Saccharomyces cerevisiae* antibody (ASCA) are helpful, but neither is sufficiently sensitive or specific to be relied on for the diagnosis of inflammatory bowel disease.

Endoscopy

Endoscopic evaluation via EGD or colonoscopy is safe and quick and is increasingly being performed as first line in the diagnosis of many GI complaints (Chapter 136). An added advantage of endoscopic evaluation is the ability to perform therapy during the procedure. Specialized endoscopic evaluation of the pancreaticobiliary tree can be done via endoscopic retrograde cholangiopancreatography. Endoscopic ultrasound can be used to evaluate and stage malignancy. Novel endoscopic evaluation tools include wireless capsule endoscopy, which has made mucosal evaluation of the small intestine routine (Chapter 136); enteroscopy, which can evaluate a third of the small intestine; and double-balloon enteroscopy, which can evaluate the entire small intestine.

Imaging

Radiologic evaluation ranges from traditional barium studies to ultrasound, CT, virtual colonography, magnetic resonance imaging (Chapter 135), and positron emission tomography. Just as therapeutic interventions during endoscopic procedures are commonplace, many interventional radiology procedures can be performed under ultrasound guidance (e.g., fine-needle aspiration of a liver mass), CT guidance (e.g., drainage of an abscess), or fluoroscopic guidance (e.g., angiographic embolization of a bleeding gastroduodenal artery in peptic ulcer disease; Chapter 135).

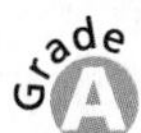

1. Apfel CC, Korttila K, Abdalla M, et al: A factorial trial of six interventions for the prevention of postoperative nausea and vomiting. N Engl J Med 2004;350:2441–2451.

SUGGESTED READINGS

Clouse RE, Mayer EA, Aziz Q, et al: Functional abdominal pain syndrome. Gastroenterology 2006;130:1492–1497. *A helpful review.*

Golash V, Willson PD: Early laparoscopy as a routine procedure in the management of acute abdominal pain: A review of 1,320 patients. Surg Endosc 2005;19:882–885. *A definitive diagnosis was made in 90% of patients after diagnostic laparoscopy, and laparoscopy changed the clinical diagnosis in 30% of cases.*

Lewis LM, Banet GA, Blanda M, et al: Etiology and clinical course of abdominal pain in senior patients: A prospective, multicenter study. J Gerontol A Biol Sci Med Sci 2005;60:1071–1076. *Of 360 patients in the emergency department, 60% were hospitalized, 20% underwent operative or invasive procedures, and 5% died within 2 weeks.*

MacKersie AB, Lane MJ, Gerhardt RT, et al: Nontraumatic acute abdominal pain: Unenhanced helical CT compared with three-view acute abdominal series. Radiology 2005;237:114–122. *Unenhanced helical CT is far superior, with an overall sensitivity, specificity, and accuracy of 96%, 95%, and 96%, respectively.*

Ranji SR, Goldman LE, Simel DL, et al: Do opiates affect the clinical evaluation of patients with acute abdominal pain? JAMA 2006;296:1764–1774. *Opiate administration may alter the physical examination but did not result in a significant increase in management errors.*

Sahyoun NR, Serdula MK, Galuska DA, et al: The epidemiology of recent involuntary weight loss in the United States population. J Nutr Health Aging 2004;8:510–517. *Involuntary weight loss among community-dwelling older adults is independently associated with mortality.*

135 DIAGNOSTIC IMAGING PROCEDURES IN GASTROENTEROLOGY

Perry J. Pickhardt

A wide range of diagnostic imaging modalities are available to evaluate diseases of the gastrointestinal tract and the hepatic-pancreatic-biliary system. Once the workhorse of gastrointestinal radiology, conventional radiography and fluoroscopy are still relevant but have largely given way to more advanced cross-sectional imaging techniques, such as ultrasonography, computed tomography (CT), and magnetic resonance (MR). These imaging techniques may also be applied in a wide variety of interventional procedures. With the emergence of molecular imaging, there has been renewed interest in nuclear medicine, most notably positron emission tomography (PET).

NONINVASIVE EVALUATION

Conventional Radiography

Conventional radiography, often referred to as plain films, remains useful for a limited number of abdominal indications but is generally much less sensitive and specific than the more advanced radiologic techniques, such as CT. Supine and upright frontal abdominal radiographs can rapidly assess for bowel obstruction and pneumoperitoneum in the setting of an acute abdomen (Fig. 135–1). CT, however, not only may demonstrate the underlying cause of obstruction but also may find an alternative diagnosis when plain films are unrevealing. Serial radiographs remain a practical approach for observing patients with an abnormal bowel gas pattern suggestive of either evolving small bowel obstruction or adynamic ileus. Abdominal radiographs can also demonstrate abnormal calcifications and radiopaque foreign bodies, but CT is again more sensitive and specific in this regard. For example, only about 10 to 15% of gallstones are sufficiently calcified to allow radiographic detection, whereas the majority of gallstones can be identified on CT (Chapter 159). Because of its portable nature, conventional radiography remains useful in surgical and critical care settings, where it complements portable ultrasonography for abdominal evaluation.

Fluoroscopic Procedures

Standard double-contrast barium examinations, particularly of the stomach, duodenum, and colon, have been largely supplanted by endoscopy and advanced radiologic techniques. However, a variety of fluoroscopic contrast studies remain useful because of their relatively noninvasive and low-cost nature. Real-time fluoroscopic contrast studies can provide valuable physiologic evaluation, serve as a problem-solving tool when endoscopy is equivocal or contraindicated, and are useful in evaluating for suspected leak, perforation, or fistula. Depending on the specific indication, either barium or water-soluble iodinated contrast material may be used.

The videofluoroscopic swallowing study and barium esophagram are efficient and effective noninvasive means of excluding significant pathologic changes in patients with dysphagia (Chapter 140). Endoscopy (Chapter 136), which is generally indicated when an esophageal stricture or mass is encountered on fluoroscopic examination, can be avoided in many patients who have no concerning findings on fluoroscopy. Fluoroscopic contrast evaluation may also avoid the need for endoscopy in symptomatic patients with suspected esophagitis from *Candida* or herpes infection. In the setting of gastroesophageal reflux disease, the barium esophagram is effective for excluding significant complications, such as peptic stricture and adenocarcinoma, but it cannot be used to detect or to exclude Barrett's esophagus (Chapter 140).

The upper gastrointestinal tract barium series can identify mucosal abnormalities of the stomach and duodenum, such as erosions, ulcers, polyps, and masses (Fig. 135–2), but esophagogastroduodenoscopy is better for these purposes (Chapter 137). Gastroduodenal barium evaluation can still play an important diagnostic role, as in evaluation for sliding or paraesophageal hiatal hernias and pediatric evaluation for malrotation or hypertrophic pyloric stenosis.

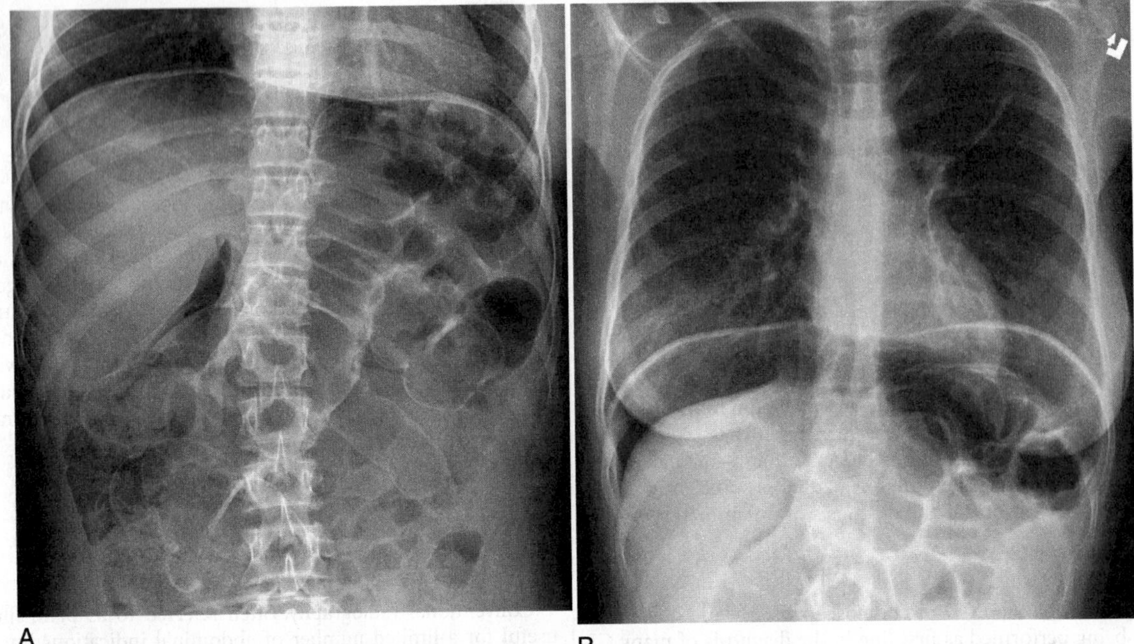

FIGURE 135–1 • Pneumoperitoneum on conventional radiography. A, Supine abdominal radiograph shows abnormal lucency surrounding multiple bowel loops and the liver. Both sides of the bowel wall are outlined by gas in some areas (Rigler's sign), which typically requires a large amount of free peritoneal air to be visible on supine films. **B,** Upright radiograph centered over the diaphragm shows the large amount of free intraperitoneal air to better advantage. This view is more sensitive for detection of pneumoperitoneum.

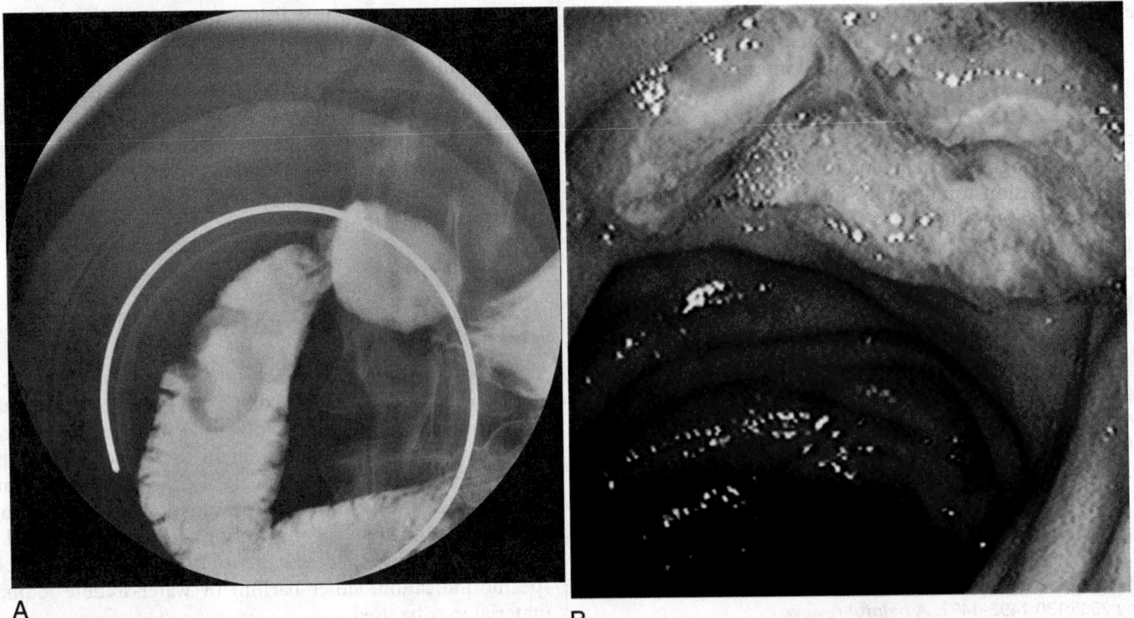

FIGURE 135–2 • Metastatic melanoma on barium study of the upper gastrointestinal tract. A, Fluoroscopic spot film image shows a filling defect within the second portion of the duodenum that has a "bull's-eye" or "target" appearance due to collection of barium in the center of the lesion. This appearance is characteristic of a submucosal mass with central ulceration and is typical of hematogenous metastatic disease from melanoma. **B,** Digital photograph from esophagogastroduodenoscopy confirms the presence of an ulcerated submucosal mass within the duodenum.

Although the small bowel follow-through can provide an effective anatomic roadmap, assess transit time, and detect thickened folds, once-common indications, such as unexplained gastrointestinal tract bleeding and Crohn's disease, are now assessed by CT and capsule endoscopy. Similarly, enteroclysis examination, which involves intubation of the proximal jejunum followed by infusion of barium and methylcellulose, is also being supplanted by these newer (and less invasive) techniques.

The single-contrast enema remains an important diagnostic tool in settings such as suspected sigmoid volvulus, colonic obstruction, postoperative leak or fistula, and ileocolic intussusception in children. The double-contrast barium enema for detection of colorectal polyps, however, has largely been replaced by colonoscopy, either optical or virtual (see later). Fluoroscopic defecography still is used to help delineate functional abnormalities in patients with evacuation disorders (Chapter 138).

Ultrasonography

Ultrasonography is useful for imaging solid organs and fluid-filled structures but is limited by its inability to penetrate gas-filled structures. For example, overlying bowel gas often precludes complete sonographic evaluation of the pancreas. Ultrasound can be applied by many different routes, including transabdominal, endoscopic, transrectal, intravascular, and endovaginal approaches. Ultrasonography also provides an excellent means for many image-guided interventions.

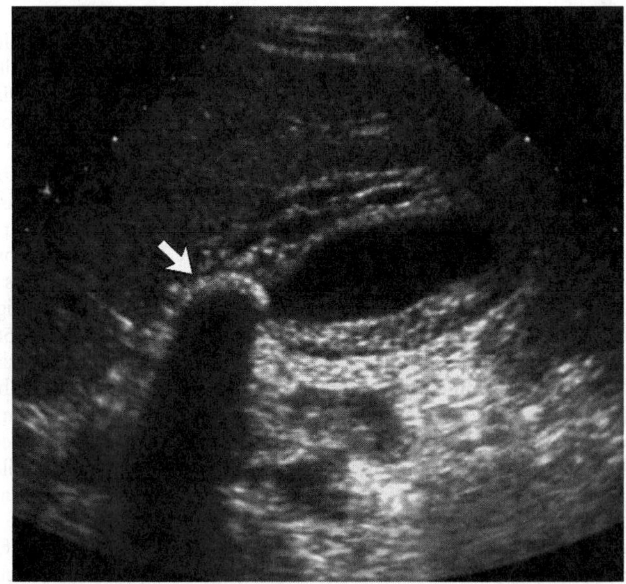

FIGURE 135–3 • Acute cholecystitis on ultrasound examination. Image from right upper quadrant sonography shows diffuse gallbladder wall thickening and a shadowing impacted gallstone (arrow). A sonographic Murphy's sign was present. These findings are diagnostic of acute calculous cholecystitis.

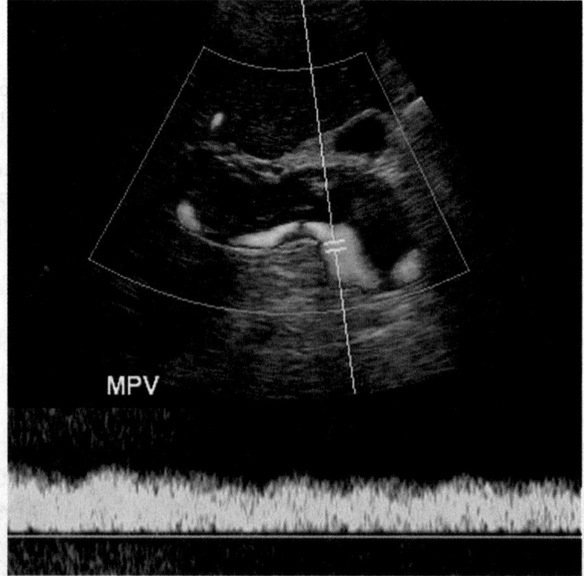

FIGURE 135–4 • Portal vein thrombosis on ultrasound examination. Ultrasound gray-scale image with both power color Doppler and spectral Doppler interrogation shows nonocclusive thrombus filling the majority of the main portal vein (MPV). Flow patency is seen in the peripheral aspect of the vessel.

Ultrasonography is perhaps most frequently used for evaluation of the liver and biliary system. For evaluation of possible acute cholecystitis (Chapter 159), which is a common indication for right upper quadrant sonography, classic findings include cholelithiasis, gallbladder wall thickening, and a "sonographic Murphy's sign" (reproducible pain when the transducer is pressed over the gallbladder) (Fig. 135–3). The sensitivity for detecting gallstones with ultrasonography exceeds 95%. Acalculous cholelithiasis can be a more challenging diagnosis because the findings overlap with nonspecific thickening of the gallbladder wall in critically ill patients. Ultrasonography is typically the first imaging test obtained in patients with new-onset jaundice or cholestatic laboratory findings (Chapter 150); it offers rapid, noninvasive evaluation of the biliary tree to differentiate obstruction from other causes. If biliary ductal dilation is present, the level and cause of obstruction can sometimes be demonstrated on ultrasound examination; common causes include choledocholithiasis and masses in the head of the pancreas. When ultrasonography shows biliary obstruction, additional imaging tests are necessary (e.g., CT, MR cholangiopancreatography [MRCP], endoscopic retrograde cholangiopancreatography [ERCP], or percutaneous transhepatic cholangiography [PTC]), depending on the specific circumstances (Chapter 136).

Ultrasonography can detect or further characterize focal liver lesions, distinguish cystic from solid lesions, and investigate diffuse liver disease. Cavernous hemangiomas are a common incidental liver finding on ultrasound examination; the homogeneous hyperechoic appearance is less specific than on CT or MR but is generally adequate for diagnosis in patients without known malignant neoplasms. Although it is not approved for use in the United States, ultrasound examination combined with intravenous contrast agents may provide information similar to what can be provided with contrast-enhanced CT and MR.

Sonographic findings in cirrhosis (Chapter 157) include heterogeneously coarsened parenchymal echotexture, nodular surface contour, right side–predominant volume loss, and evidence of portal hypertension, including ascites, splenomegaly, and portosystemic collaterals. Focal hepatic lesions in the setting of cirrhosis are concerning for hepatocellular carcinoma (Chapter 206) but may also represent regenerative or dysplastic nodules. Ultrasound screening may sometimes be indicated to observe patients with chronic viral hepatitis (Chapter 152) to detect changes suggestive of cirrhosis or hepatocellular carcinoma. In noncirrhotic patients with elevated liver enzymes, ultrasonography can often suggest the diagnosis of hepatic steatosis (fatty liver; Chapter 149) when the parenchyma demonstrates increased echogenicity and decreased penetration of the sound beam. The findings of steatosis can be focal, multifocal, or diffuse; MR imaging is more specific and can confirm the diagnosis, if it is clinically indicated.

Color Doppler evaluation of the liver in patients with end-stage liver disease can evaluate the portal system and search for portosystemic collaterals. Abnormal portal vein findings include hepatofugal flow and thrombosis (Fig. 135–4). Doppler ultrasound study is also used for evaluation of transjugular intrahepatic portosystemic shunts, both before and after stent placement (Chapter 73). In orthotopic liver transplant recipients (Chapter 158), Doppler evaluation is frequently performed to assess the hepatic vasculature, with particular attention to the hepatic arterial supply.

Computed Tomography

CT, especially helical or spiral CT, provides rapid, reproducible, and comprehensive images. High-resolution scans of the entire chest, abdomen, and pelvis can now be easily acquired during a single held breath. Abdominal CT imaging often uses both oral and intravenous contrast agents for thorough evaluation of the hollow and solid viscera. Dynamic multiphasic imaging of the liver after the administration of contrast material is excellent for characterizing focal hepatic lesions (Fig. 135–5) and obtaining CT angiography, which has largely replaced conventional diagnostic angiography. Commercial software packages for advanced two-dimensional and three-dimensional renderings of the CT data sets are widely available.

The clinical indications for abdominal CT are broad, ranging from unexplained abdominal complaints to blunt trauma to oncologic imaging. For the nontraumatic acute abdomen, common inflammatory conditions such as appendicitis and diverticulitis (Chapter 145) are readily diagnosed by CT. Other common indications include evaluation for intra-abdominal abscess, pancreatitis (Chapter 147), and small bowel obstruction. In cases of relatively high grade bowel obstruction, CT can often localize the transition point, elucidate the underlying cause, and evaluate for vascular compromise. In the setting of blunt trauma (Chapter 113), CT has become invaluable for prompt detection of significant abdominal injury.

Primary abdominal malignant neoplasms, such as pancreatic cancer (Chapter 204) and hepatocellular carcinoma (Chapter 206), are often first detected on CT. Abdominal staging to detect metastatic disease, including hematogenous, lymphatic, peritoneal, and local spread, is commonly performed with CT, as is assessment of the response to various therapies.

CT enterography often combines neutral (i.e., water density) oral contrast media with dynamic, high-resolution imaging to obtain detailed multiplanar evaluation of the small bowel. Concurrent capsule endoscopy (Chapter 134) provides a complementary and comprehensive evaluation of the small bowel. CT colonography, also referred to as virtual colonoscopy, generally combines two-dimensional and three-dimensional evaluation of the distended colon for detection of colorectal polyps and masses (Fig. 135–6). CT colonography holds great promise for colorectal evaluation, particularly if it can improve adherence with screening recommendations. [1] Optical colonoscopy for polypectomy is still required for patients who have large polyps detected at screening CT colonography, but most patients who undergo CT colonographic screening will not need to undergo this more invasive procedure.

Magnetic Resonance

Advantages of MR imaging over CT for abdominal evaluation include superior soft tissue contrast resolution and lack of ionizing radiation.

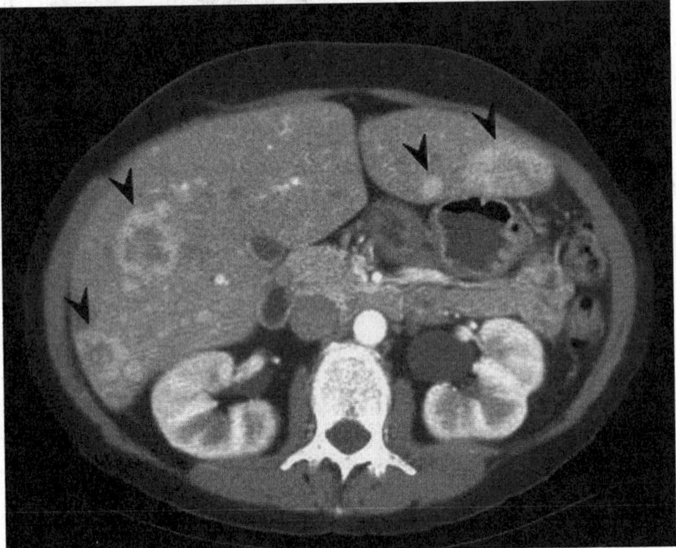

FIGURE 135–5 • Multiple hypervascular liver lesions on CT. Dynamic contrast-enhanced CT image obtained during the arterial phase shows multiple hypervascular liver lesions (arrowheads), which represent hepatic adenomas in this patient with von Gierke's disease.

However, MR remains primarily a problem-solving tool for the abdomen because of its many drawbacks, which include decreased spatial resolution, longer examination times, increased expense, decreased availability, and inability to scan patients with claustrophobia or implanted cardiac pacemakers. Imaging artifacts also can make interpretation of MR more difficult and less uniform across different readers.

Contrast-enhanced MR imaging offers dynamic evaluation comparable with CT for the solid abdominal organs. MR imaging is particularly valuable in patients with impaired renal function, for whom the intravenous administration of contrast material for CT is relatively contraindicated. MR with gadolinium-based intravenous contrast agents is excellent for evaluation of focal hepatic lesions (Fig. 135–7). The high accuracy of MR imaging for diagnosis of hepatic steatosis (Chapter 156) can sometimes prevent unnecessary biopsy, particularly when nodular focal fatty infiltration simulates metastatic disease on ultrasonography. MR is also sensitive for detection of iron overload within the liver and other organs related to primary hemochromatosis (Chapter 231) and secondary hemosiderosis (most often due to multiple transfusions). Similar to CT, MR can provide arterial and venous angiography, so conventional angiography can be reserved for therapeutic interventions.

MRCP, which represents a heavily T2-weighted imaging technique for noninvasive diagnostic evaluation of the biliary and pancreatic ductal systems (Chapter 147), relies not on the administration of contrast material but rather on the presence of static fluid. MRCP can select appropriate candidates for more invasive therapeutic procedures, such as ERCP and PTC. MRCP has proved useful for diagnosis of biliary and pancreatic ductal obstruction (Chapter 147), choledocholithiasis (Chapter 159), primary sclerosing cholangitis (Chapter 159), and cystic lesions (Fig. 135–8). T1-weighted MR cholangiography with intravenous contrast agents that undergo biliary excretion can be useful to evaluate bile leaks.

INTERVENTIONAL EVALUATION

Ultrasonography, CT, fluoroscopy, and even MR techniques have been used for imaging guidance in a wide variety of abdominal interventional procedures.

Biopsy

Percutaneous image-guided biopsy, whether by fine-needle aspiration or core biopsy, is a relatively safe procedure that is commonly performed for tissue diagnosis and has drastically reduced the need for open

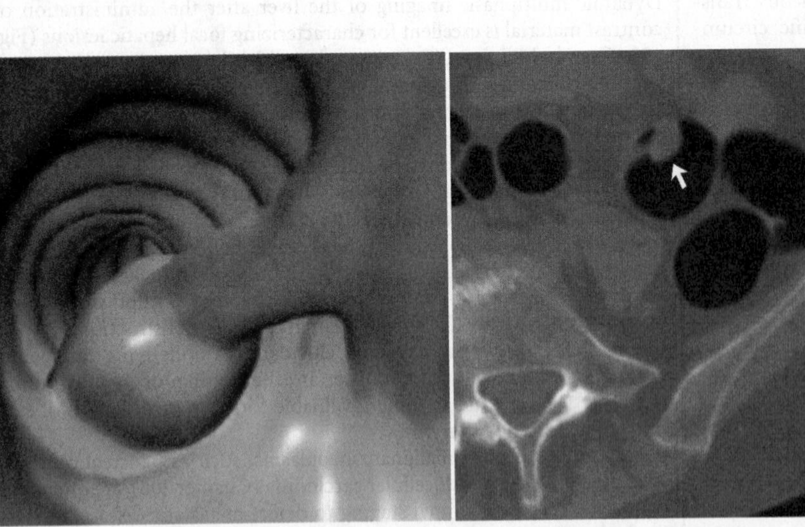

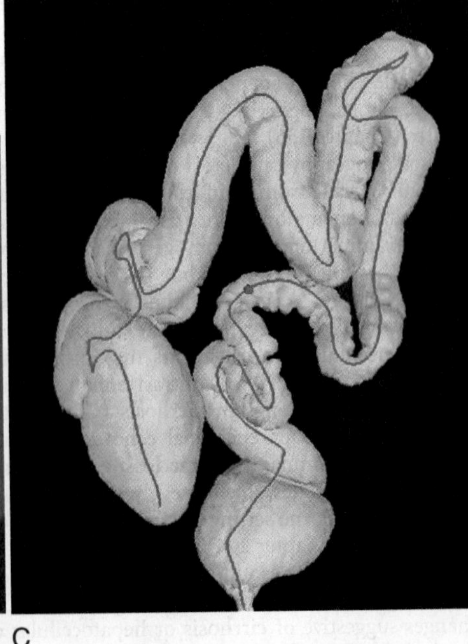

FIGURE 135–6 • Pedunculated polyp (tubulovillous adenoma) on virtual colonoscopy (CT colonography). A, Three-dimensional endoluminal image shows a large polyp on a prominent stalk. This view simulates conventional colonoscopy and allows reliable detection of such lesions. **B,** Transverse two-dimensional image confirms that lesion is composed of soft tissue (arrow). **C,** Colon map generated by the virtual colonoscopy software system allows precise localization of the polyp (red dot in sigmoid colon). The green line represents the centerline for automated navigation.

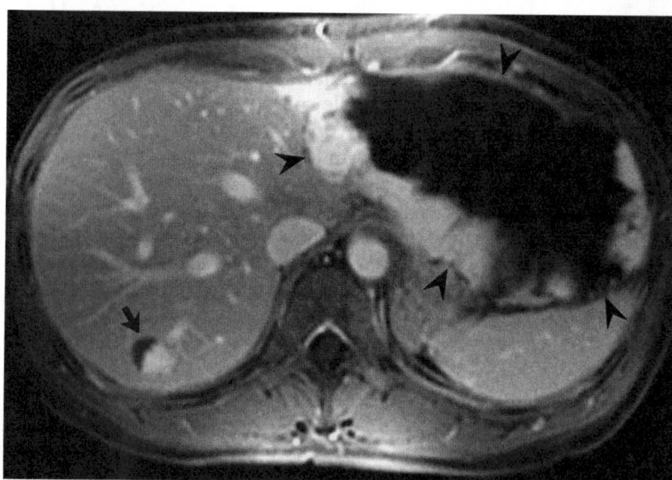

FIGURE 135–7 • Hepatic cavernous hemangiomas on MR. Contrast-enhanced fat-suppressed gradient-echo MR image shows characteristic findings of cavernous hemangiomas, including a giant left hepatic lobe lesion (arrowheads) and smaller right hepatic lobe lesion (arrow). Note the peripheral enhancement of the lesions that matches the signal intensity of the aortic blood pool. The findings are diagnostic, and tissue biopsy is unnecessary.

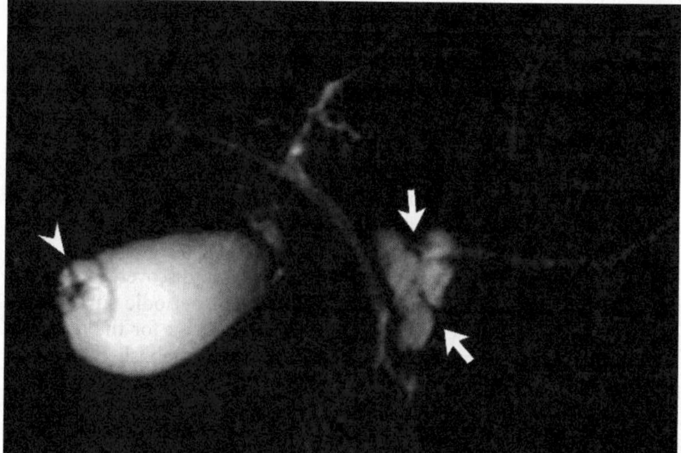

FIGURE 135–8 • Pancreatic intraductal papillary mucinous neoplasm on MRCP. Heavily T2-weighted MR image shows a lobulated cystic lesion in the pancreatic head region (arrows) that represents a side branch intraductal papillary mucinous neoplasm. Note also mild focal irregularity of the gallbladder (arrowhead), consistent with the fundal form of adenomyomatosis. The intrahepatic and extrahepatic biliary ducts are normal.

surgical biopsy. For peridiverticular and periappendiceal abscesses, CT-guided drainage can often simplify the ultimate operative approach and turn high-risk emergent surgery into a safer elective procedure.

Ablation and Other Procedures

Biliary interventions include transhepatic access to an obstructed system for stenting or external drainage as well as placement of a cholecystostomy tube. Percutaneous CT- or ultrasound-guided tumor ablation is a rapidly evolving technique that is particularly useful in poor operative candidates or in conjunction with surgical resection of other lesions. Ablation methods include radio frequency, alcohol, microwave, and cryoablation.

Angiography

Diagnostic conventional angiography has been largely replaced by noninvasive CT and MR techniques, but direct catheter angiography remains an important procedure for directing various therapies. Vascular interventions include angioplasty, stenting, embolization, and thrombolysis. Placement of a transjugular intrahepatic portosystemic shunt stent, which creates a low-pressure communication between the portal and hepatic venous systems, is a commonly performed angiographic procedure in patients whose portal hypertension is complicated by variceal bleeding or intractable ascites (Chapter 149). Chemoembolization can provide palliative care for advanced hepatic malignant disease, whether it is primary or metastatic (Chapter 206).

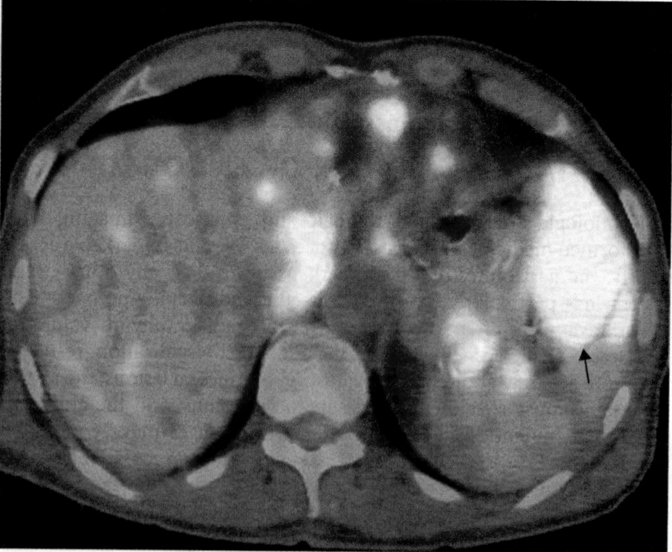

FIGURE 135–9 • Metastatic gastrointestinal stromal tumor on fused PET-CT. Transverse fused PET-CT image shows a dominant hypermetabolic mass (arrow) representing a gastric gastrointestinal stromal tumor. Multiple smaller peritoneal and hepatic hypermetabolic foci are consistent with metastatic deposits. Note the utility in combining the functional information from PET with the anatomic localization provided by CT.

NUCLEAR MEDICINE (RADIONUCLIDE SCINTIGRAPHY)

PET functional imaging is useful for both initial staging and evaluation of response to therapy for a wide range of primary malignant tumors, especially in combination with anatomic CT imaging (Fig. 135–9). Current clinical PET imaging most often uses [^{18}F]fluorodeoxyglucose, but other positron-emitting agents may be employed for specific purposes.

Injection of red blood cells labeled with technetium (Tc) 99m provides a noninvasive, highly sensitive method to detect active gastrointestinal bleeding (Chapter 137), with the ability to scan the patient again hours later without repeated injection; however, anatomic localization is relatively poor, and angiography has the advantage of being potentially therapeutic as well as diagnostic. Hepatobiliary scintigraphy (HIDA scan) remains useful in equivocal cases of cholecystitis (Chapter 159), particularly acalculous disease, and can confirm suspected biliary leaks. Scintigraphic imaging with indium (In) 111 octreotide is valuable for diagnosis, staging, and follow-up of gastrointestinal neuroendocrine tumors (Chapter 251), such as carcinoid and pancreatic islet cell tumors.

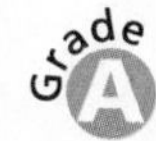

1. Pickhardt PJ, Choi JR, Hwang I, et al: CT virtual colonoscopy to screen for colorectal neoplasia in asymptomatic adults. N Engl J Med 2003;349:2191–2200.

SUGGESTED READINGS

American College of Radiology, Expert Panel on Gastrointestinal Imaging: ACR Appropriateness Criteria. Available at: http://www.acr.org/s_acr/sec.asp?CID=1207&DID=15048. *Recommended imaging approaches for various clinical presentations.*

Rosman AS, Korsten MA: Meta-analysis comparing CT colonography, air contrast barium enema, and colonoscopy. Am J Med 2007;120:203–210. *CT colonography is less accurate than endoscopic colonoscopy for detecting smaller polyps.*

GASTROINTESTINAL ENDOSCOPY

Pankaj Jay Pasricha

IMPORTANCE AND USE OF ENDOSCOPY

Technologic advances in radiologic and endoscopic imaging have transformed medicine in the past few decades. With its remarkable accessibility, the gastrointestinal tract, perhaps more than any other organ system, has particularly benefited from the endoscopic approach. The major advantages of endoscopy over contrast radiography in evaluation of diseases of the alimentary tract include direct visualization, resulting in a more accurate and sensitive evaluation of mucosal lesions; the ability to obtain biopsy specimens from superficial lesions; and the ability to perform therapeutic interventions. These advantages make endoscopy the procedure of choice in most cases in which mucosal lesions or growths are suspected. Conversely, contrast radiography may be indicated when extrinsic or intrinsic distortions of anatomy are suspected, such as volvulus, intussusception, subtle strictures, or complicated postsurgical changes. For most upper gastrointestinal lesions, however, the sensitivity (about 90%) and specificity (nearly 100%) of endoscopy are far higher than those of barium radiography (about 50 and 90%, respectively).

Diagnostic endoscopy (Table 136–1) is usually a remarkably safe and well-tolerated procedure. However, complications do occur and need to be carefully explained to the patient as part of the informed consent process; patients must also be prepared appropriately to reduce complication rates (Table 136–2). In general, diagnostic and uncomplicated therapeutic endoscopy can be done in most patients with a combination of benzodiazepines and narcotics to produce moderate (conscious) sedation (Chapter 458). Propofol, which provides faster and deeper sedation with rapid recovery but is generally administered by an anesthesiologist, is increasingly popular, especially for prolonged procedures such as endoscopic retrograde cholangiopancreatography and endoscopic ultrasonography.

LUMINAL ENDOSCOPY

Specific Indications

Most indications for gastrointestinal endoscopy are based on the presenting symptoms of the patient (e.g., dysphagia, bleeding, diarrhea). In other instances, endoscopy is required to evaluate specific lesions found by other diagnostic imaging, such as a gastric ulcer or colon polyp discovered by barium radiography. Finally, screening endoscopy is often performed in asymptomatic individuals on the basis of their risk for commonly occurring and preventable conditions, such as colon cancer (see later).

Implicit in the decision to perform endoscopy is the assumption that it will have a bearing on future management strategy. In dealing with the evaluation of gastrointestinal symptoms, several questions need to be addressed by the referring physician and the endoscopist. Which patients need endoscopy? When should the endoscopy be done? What is the endoscopist looking for? What endoscopic therapy, if any, should be planned?

Gastroesophageal Reflux and Heartburn (Chapters 139 and 140)

Gastroesophageal reflux disease (GERD) is an extremely common condition in the general population. The fact that its cardinal symptom, heartburn, is relatively specific for this condition justifies an empirical approach to treatment by a combination of lifestyle modifications and over-the-counter or even prescription drugs. Endoscopy is not therefore necessary to make the diagnosis of GERD. Indeed, normal findings on endoscopy do not rule out the diagnosis of GERD because the overall sensitivity of endoscopy in GERD is only about 70%. If necessary, further evaluation with ambulatory pH monitoring may be indicated to establish the diagnosis. However, there are several circumstances in which endoscopy should be considered for patients with reflux, including patients with associated warning symptoms ("red flags") such as dysphagia, odynophagia, regurgitation, weight loss, gastrointestinal bleeding, or frequent vomiting (Fig. 136–1). These symptoms imply either the development of a GERD-related complication (erosive esophagitis, stricture, or adenocarcinoma) or another disorder masquerading as GERD (esophageal cancer or a gastric-duodenal lesion such as cancer or peptic ulcer). Another group of patients who are candidates for endoscopy are those with severe or persistent or frequently recurrent symptoms that suggest significant esophagitis and hence a risk for complications, such as stricture or Barrett's esophagus (intestinal metaplasia of the esophageal lining).

If a significant length of Barrett's esophagus is discovered (see Fig. 136–1), most experts recommend some form of periodic surveillance endoscopy because these patients are at increased risk for the development of adenocarcinoma. Barrett's esophagus, once established, does not generally regress despite adequate control of reflux by either pharmacologic or surgical means. To eliminate the small but definite risk of cancer associated with this lesion, various methods to ablate this epithelium have

TABLE 136–1 ENDOSCOPIC PROCEDURES AND GENERAL APPLICATIONS

Endoscopic Procedure	Therapeutic Applications
LUMINAL ENDOSCOPY	

Common procedures
  Esophagogastroduodenoscopy
  Colonoscopy
  Flexible sigmoidoscopy
Less common procedures
  Enteroscopy
  Capsule endoscopy
	Hemostasis
	Luminal restoration (dilation, ablation, stenting)
	Lesion removal (e.g., polypectomy, mucosal ablation)
	Provision of access (percutaneous endoscopic gastrostomy and jejunostomy)
	Barrier strengthening (antireflux procedures)

PANCREATOBILIARY IMAGING	
Endoscopic retrograde cholangiopancreatography	Lesion (stone) removal Luminal restoration (dilation, stenting) Provision of access (sphincterotomy) Drainage (bile, pancreatic pseudocyst)
TRANSLUMINAL IMAGING	
Endoscopic ultrasonography	Analgesic block Delivery of therapeutic agents (experimental)

TABLE 136–2 COMPLICATIONS OF ENDOSCOPY

Endoscopic Complication	Incidence (%)	Specific Prophylaxis
GENERAL COMPLICATIONS		
Complications related primarily to sedation (cardiovascular and respiratory depression, aspiration)	0.6–0.7	Airway protection with massive upper gastrointestinal bleeding Preprocedure medical evaluation, intraprocedure and postprocedure monitoring Anesthesiology consultation for high-risk patients
Perforation	0.1–0.3 (upper endoscopy) 0.14–0.25 (colonoscopy)	None (except careful technique)
Bleeding	0.3 (upper endoscopy) 0.7–2.5 (polypectomy)	Carefully balance risk and benefits Discontinue or reduce anticoagulant use before high-risk procedures
Bacteremia and infectious complications (endocarditis, bacterial ascites)	<0.1	Antibiotics for patients at risk for endocarditis (patients with artificial valves, pulmonary-systemic shunts, previous history of endocarditis), with synthetic vascular grafts, and with bacterial ascites (cirrhotics)
Death	0.6 (upper endoscopy) 0.2 (colonoscopy)	
COMPLICATIONS ASSOCIATED WITH SPECIALIZED PROCEDURES		
Pancreatitis (ERCP)	3–20	Not well established/experimental
Cholangitis (ERCP)	0.1–2	Preprocedure antibiotics
Wound infections (PEG)	3–4	Preprocedure antibiotics

ERCP = endoscopic retrograde cholangiopancreatography; PEG = percutaneous endoscopic gastrostomy.

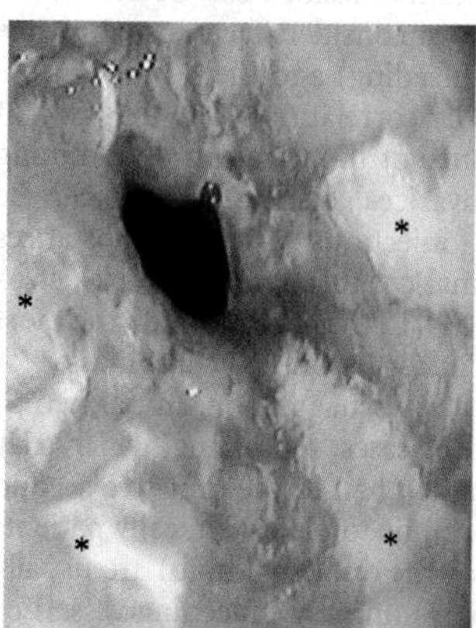

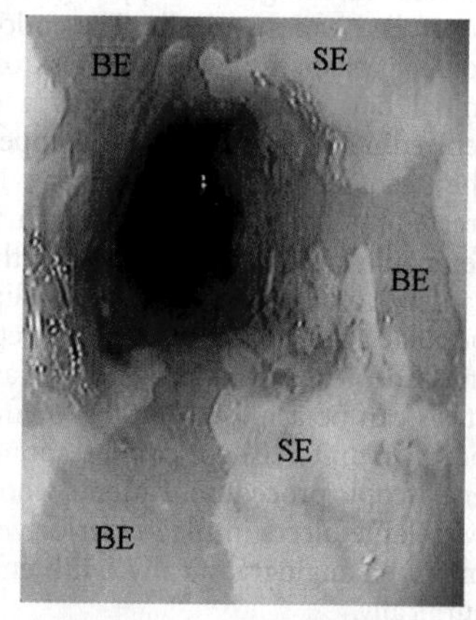

FIGURE 136–1 • Severe reflux esophagitis (left) with mucosal erythema and linear ulcers with yellow exudates (*). It is thought that such changes eventually lead to Barrett's esophagus (right), in which the normal white squamous epithelium (SE) is replaced by red columnar epithelium (BE). These pictures are from different patients.

been attempted, with the rationale that the esophageal lining is reconstituted by squamous epithelium under conditions of acid suppression. For patients who have high-grade dysplasia associated with Barrett's esophagus and who are at high risk for surgery or wish to avoid it, endoscopic ablation or resection may provide a potentially curative alternative to esophagectomy. In patients without dysplasia, the benefit (i.e., reduction in the risk of cancer) remains to be established, and ablation should be considered experimental in this setting. Ablation can be achieved by electrical cautery, argon plasma coagulation, high-energy laser, radio frequency, and photodynamic therapy. However, these approaches do not allow a full pathologic examination and are associated with a small risk of regrowth of Barrett's tissue in ectopic locations, such as the submucosa, where it may subsequently escape detection. An evolving technique is en bloc resection of the mucosa, a procedure that allows complete removal and pathologic analysis.

Endoscopic techniques of therapy for GERD itself include radio frequency to produce a scar and to tighten the lower esophageal sphincter, suturing or plication devices to restructure the area below the sphincter, and injection of different polymers to "bulk up" the gastroesophageal junction. Although initial results were promising, long-term outcomes have been less positive.

Heartburn in immunocompromised patients often indicates an esophageal infection. The most common causes in patients with human immunodeficiency virus (HIV) infection are *Candida*, cytomegalovirus, herpesvirus, and idiopathic esophageal ulcers. Because most patients with the acquired immunodeficiency syndrome and esophagitis have candidiasis, an empirical 1- to 2-week course of antifungal therapy may be justified. Patients who do not respond to this approach, however, should almost always have endoscopy and biopsy so that more specific therapy can be instituted.

The PillCam is a capsule capable of taking bidirectional digital photographs and transmitting 14 wireless images per second to an external data recorder. Patients can swallow this capsule easily and, within seconds, have a nearly complete noninvasive examination of the esophageal lining. This technique has the potential to replace traditional endoscopy for indications such as GERD and cirrhosis, in which screening for complications (Barrett's esophagus or varices, respectively) is of value.

Dysphagia (Chapter 140)

Dysphagia can often be categorized as oropharyngeal on the basis of the clinical features of nasal regurgitation, laryngeal aspiration, or difficulty in moving the bolus out of the mouth. These symptoms are usually associated with a lesion in the central or peripheral nervous system. Although endoscopy is often performed in these patients, videofluoroesophagography (modified barium swallow or cine-esophagogram) is the procedure of choice as it allows a frame-by-frame evaluation of the rapid sequence of events involved in transfer of the bolus from the mouth to the esophagus. Common causes of esophageal dysphagia include malignant as well as benign processes (peptic strictures secondary to reflux, Schatzki's rings) and motility disturbances of the esophageal body or the lower esophageal sphincter. Endoscopic examination is considered mandatory in all patients with esophageal dysphagia. However, contrast esophagography may also be helpful; it can provide guidance for endoscopy that is anticipated to be difficult (e.g., a patient with a complex stricture), suggest a disturbance in motility, and occasionally detect subtle stenoses that are not appreciated on endoscopy (the scope diameter is typically 10 mm or less, whereas some symptomatic strictures can be considerably wider).

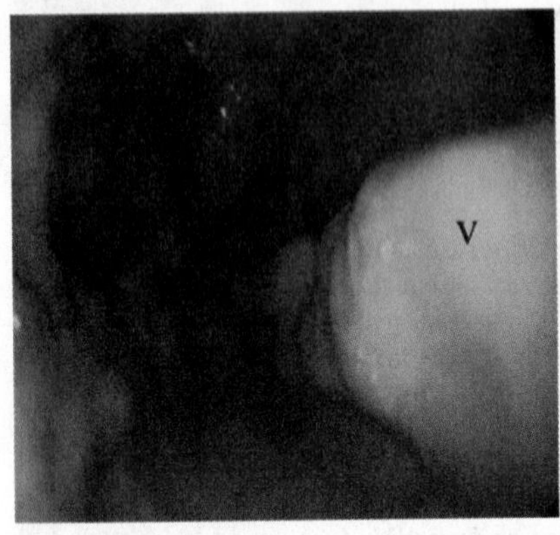

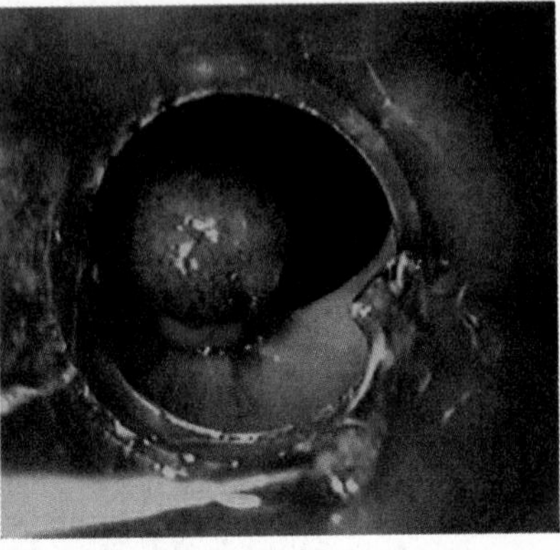

FIGURE 136–2 • Endoscopic view of esophageal varices (left) in the wall of the esophagus (V). Right, image of a varix that has been endoscopically ligated with a band.

Endoscopic treatment options are available for many causes of esophageal dysphagia. Tumors may be dilated mechanically, ablated by thermal means (cautery or laser), or stented with prosthetic devices. Metallic expandable stents have become the palliative procedure of choice for most patients with symptomatic esophageal cancer. Benign lesions of the esophagus, such as strictures or rings, can also be dilated endoscopically, usually with excellent results. Finally, some motility disturbances, such as achalasia, are best approached endoscopically with the use of large balloon dilators for the lower esophageal sphincter or with the local injection of botulinum toxin.

Dyspepsia (Chapter 139)

Dyspepsia, which is chronic or recurring pain or discomfort centered in the upper abdomen, is a common condition that can be caused by a variety of disorders, including peptic ulcer, reflux esophagitis, gallstones, gastric dysmotility, and, rarely, gastric or esophageal cancer. However, up to 60% of patients with chronic (>3 months) dyspepsia belong to the so-called functional category in which there is no definite structural or biochemical explanation for the symptoms. Although *Helicobacter pylori* gastritis is found frequently in these patients, there is no definite evidence to prove a cause-and-effect relationship between these two findings. The optimal diagnostic approach to dyspepsia is somewhat controversial and is still evolving (see Fig. 139–2). If a diagnostic test is to be performed, endoscopy, sometimes with biopsies to detect *H. pylori,* is clearly the procedure of choice, with an accuracy of about 90% (compared with about 65% for double-contrast radiography). There has been a move toward empirical approaches to dyspepsia because only a minority of patients with dyspepsia have peptic ulcers, and gastric cancer is extremely rare in Western countries. However, dyspepsia is a recurrent condition, and patients who do not respond to empirical therapy eventually almost always undergo endoscopy. Many gastroenterologists therefore opt for early endoscopy, if only for the reassurance that a normal examination provides.

Upper Gastrointestinal Bleeding (Chapter 137)

Acid peptic disease (including ulcers, erosions, and gastritis), variceal bleeding, and Mallory-Weiss tears account for most cases of upper gastrointestinal bleeding. Other less common but important lesions are angiomas, gastric vascular ectasia ("watermelon" stomach), and the rarer Dieulafoy's lesion (a superficial artery that erodes through the gut mucosa). Finally, upper gastrointestinal cancers are occasionally associated with significant bleeding. Endoscopy is mandatory in all patients with upper gastrointestinal bleeding, with the rare exception being the terminally ill patient in whom the outcome is unlikely to be affected. Endoscopy is able to detect and to localize the site of the bleeding in 95% of cases and is clearly superior to contrast radiography (with an accuracy of only 75 to 80%). The endoscopic appearance of bleeding lesions can also help predict the risk of rebleeding, thus facilitating the triage and treatment process. Bleeding can be effectively controlled during the initial endoscopic examination itself in the majority of cases. The risk of recurrent bleeding is diminished, resulting in a shorter duration of hospital stay as well as a reduction in the need for surgery.

In general, endoscopy should be performed only after adequate stabilization of hemodynamic and respiratory parameters. The role of gastric lavage before endoscopy is controversial; some endoscopists prefer that it be done, occasionally even with use of a large-bore tube, whereas others avoid such preparation because of the fear of producing artifact. The timing of subsequent endoscopy depends on two factors: the severity of the hemorrhage and the risk status of the patient. Patients with active, persistent, or severe bleeding (>3 units of blood) require urgent endoscopy. Endoscopy in these patients is best performed in the intensive care unit because they are at particular risk for aspiration and may require emergent intubation for respiratory protection and ventilation. Patients with slower or inactive bleeding may be evaluated by endoscopy in a "semielective" manner (usually within 12 to 20 hours), but a case can be made to perform endoscopy early even in these stable patients (perhaps in the emergency department itself) to allow more confident triage and efficient resource management.

Most bleeding from upper gastrointestinal lesions can be effectively controlled endoscopically. The endoscopist considers factors such as age (older patients have a higher risk of rebleeding) and the severity of the initial hemorrhage (which has a direct correlation with the risk of rebleeding) in addition to the appearance of the lesion in determining the need for endoscopic therapy. Nonvariceal bleeding vessels can be treated by a variety of means, including injections of various substances (epinephrine, saline, sclerosants), thermal coagulation (laser or electrocautery), and mechanical means (clipping). In the United States, the most popular approach to a bleeding peptic ulcer lesion is a combination of injection with dilute epinephrine and electrocoagulation. Initial hemostasis can be achieved in 90% or more of cases; rebleeding, which may occur in up to 20% of cases, responds about half of the time to a second endoscopic procedure. Patients who continue to bleed (typically patients with large ulcers in the posterior wall of the duodenal bulb) are usually managed angiographically (with embolization of the bleeding vessel) or surgically.

Variceal bleeding is also effectively managed endoscopically, with a success rate similar to that with bleeding ulcers (Fig. 136–2). Hemostasis is achieved by band ligation (Fig. 136–3), sclerotherapy, or a combination of both. Increasingly, patients who do not respond to endoscopic treatment are considered candidates for a transjugular intrahepatic portosystemic shunt; traditional shunt surgery for bleeding varices is rarely performed. Even if initial endoscopic hemostasis is successful, long-term prevention of rebleeding requires a program of ongoing endoscopic sessions until variceal obliteration is complete. Ligation is the preferred approach in this setting because it is associated with fewer side effects. An ongoing area of investigation is whether endoscopic therapy, in the form of ligation, should be performed in patients whose large esophageal varices have never bled (primary prophylaxis). Currently, β-blockers are considered first-line treatment in this scenario, but there is increasing evidence to suggest that endoscopic band ligation may be useful in selected patients.

Acute Lower Gastrointestinal Bleeding (Chapter 137)

The most common cause of acute lower gastrointestinal bleeding is angiodysplasia, followed by diverticulosis, neoplasms, and colitis. In about 10% of patients presenting with hematochezia, a small bowel lesion may be responsible. In contrast to upper gastrointestinal bleeding, there is no single best test for acute lower gastrointestinal bleeding (Fig. 136–4). In young patients (<40 years) with minor bleeding, features that are highly suggestive of anorectal origin (e.g., blood on the surface of the

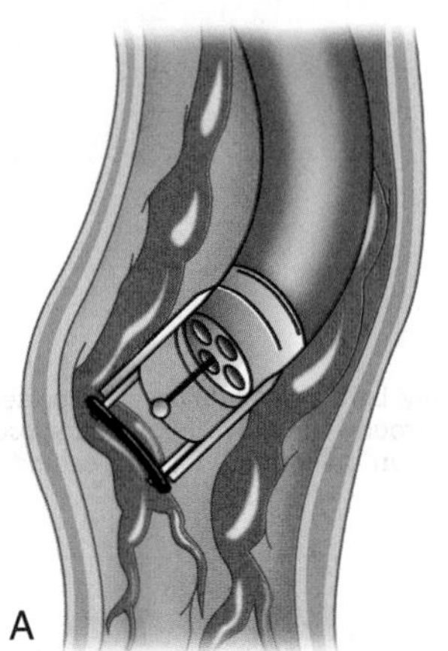

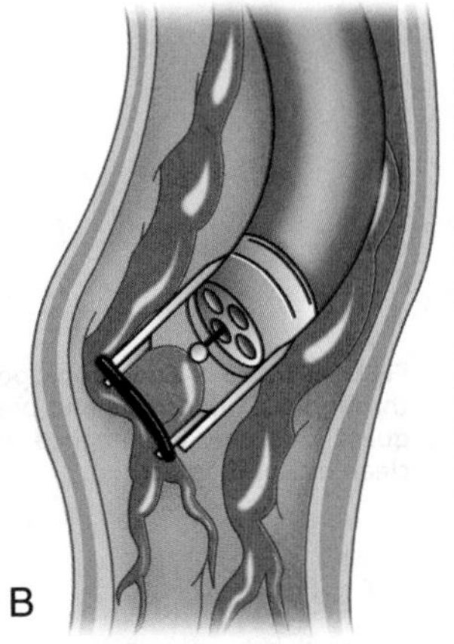

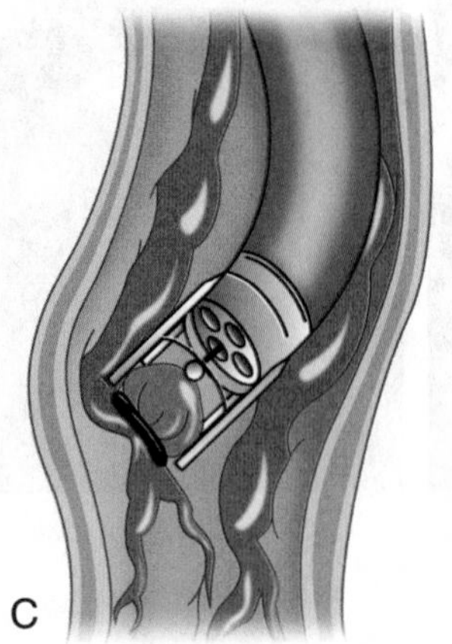

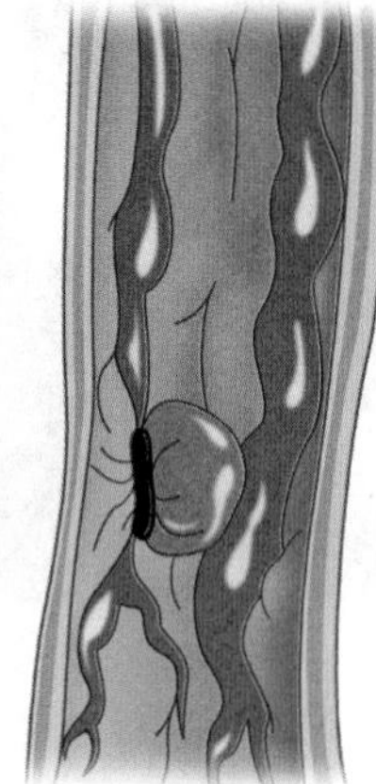

FIGURE 136–3 • Endoscopic variceal ligation technique. A, The endoscope, with attached ligating device, is brought into contact with a varix just above the gastroesophageal junction. **B,** Suction is applied, drawing the varix-containing mucosa into the dead space created at the end of the endoscope by the ligating device. **C,** The tripwire is pulled, releasing the band around the aspirated tissue. **D,** Completed ligation.

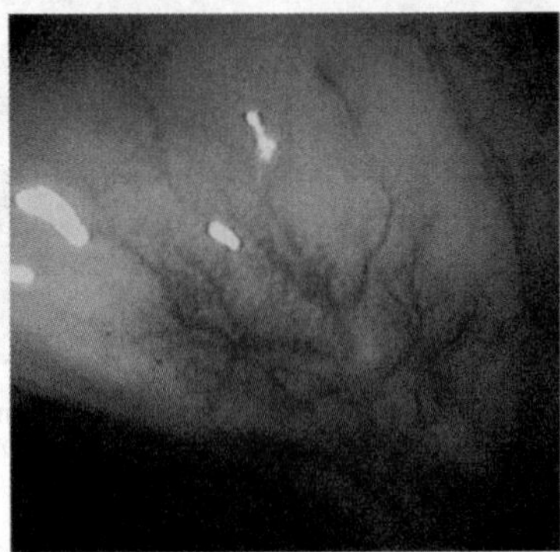

FIGURE 136–4 • Mucosal telangiectasia (arteriovenous malformation) in the colon. The patient presented with hematochezia. The lesion was subsequently cauterized endoscopically.

stool or on the wipe) may warrant only flexible sigmoidoscopy. Conversely, patients presenting with hemodynamic compromise may need upper endoscopy first to exclude a lesion in the upper gastrointestinal tract (typically postpyloric) bleeding so briskly that it arises as hematochezia. Colonoscopy has traditionally been recommended after bleeding has slowed or stopped and the patient has been given an adequate bowel purge. However, a disadvantage of delaying endoscopy is that when a pathologic lesion such as an arteriovenous malformation (see Fig. 136–4) or diverticulum is found, it may be impossible to implicate it confidently as the site of bleeding (complementary information by radiography or scintigraphy becomes particularly important in this situation). Some experts therefore recommend urgent diagnostic endoscopy with little or no preparation for acute lower gastrointestinal hemorrhages and have reported significant diagnostic as well as therapeutic success rates. However, such recommendations have not been universally accepted and remain logistically difficult to implement in most hospital settings.

It is not uncommon for gastrointestinal bleeding to develop or to be discovered in hospitalized patients who have had a recent myocardial infarction. In many cases, the bleeding is of a microscopic nature, and endoscopic evaluation can be deferred until the patient has fully recovered from the cardiac event. In other cases, however, bleeding is more significant, and its risks outweigh the potential adverse effects of endoscopic intervention. In patients with recent myocardial infarctions, upper endoscopy and colonoscopy are associated with a higher risk of cardiovascular complications, but they are usually transient and minor.

Occult Gastrointestinal Bleeding or Iron Deficiency Anemia (Chapter 137)

Normal fecal blood loss is usually less than 2 to 3 mL/day. Most standard fecal occult blood tests detect only blood loss of 10 mL/day or more. Therefore, even if this test result is negative, patients with iron deficiency anemia and no other obvious source of blood loss should always undergo aggressive gastrointestinal evaluation, which uncovers a gastrointestinal lesion in the majority of cases. Although most lesions that cause overt gastrointestinal bleeding can also cause occult blood loss, occult bleeding should almost never be ascribed to diverticulosis or hemorrhoids. Endoscopy is always preferable to radiographic studies for evaluation of occult blood loss or iron deficiency anemia because of its ability to detect flat lesions, particularly vascular malformations, which may be found in 6% or more of patients. If the findings on both upper and lower endoscopy are normal, a small bowel radiographic series (preferably enteroclysis) to look for gross lesions often completes the evaluation. If the patient continues to have symptomatic bleeding, enteroscopy (the use of a long upper endoscope to intubate the small bowel) and capsule endoscopy may be helpful to detect small bowel lesions, such as tumors or angiomas.

An innovation has been the development of capsule endoscopy, which consists of a disposable capsule that can be swallowed and that takes color video images as it travels through the digestive tract. These images are received and recorded by a device that the patient wears as a belt while carrying out his or her routine activities. At the end of the procedure, the information is downloaded to a computer, processed, and scanned for detectable abnormalities. The capsule itself passes out harmlessly in the stool. The capsule is not useful, in its present form, as a method for imaging the upper gastrointestinal tract or the colon; further, it is contraindicated in patients with suspected narrowing or strictures of the small bowel. Nevertheless, capsule endoscopy has become the diagnostic procedure of choice in patients with obscure gastrointestinal bleeding (with normal findings on upper and lower endoscopies) and when mucosal lesions of the small bowel are suspected. Diagnosis is limited by the inability to obtain tissue for histologic analysis, and treatment typically requires open surgery. A double-balloon endoscopy approach potentially allows observation and treatment of the entire small bowel, so in the future, most if not all small bowel lesions may be treated effectively by endoscopy.

Colorectal Neoplasms (Chapter 203)

Colonoscopy is the most accurate test for detecting mass lesions of the large bowel that are suspected on clinical or radiologic grounds. However, the greatest impact of endoscopy on colorectal neoplasia may be in the area of screening and prevention. The adenoma to carcinoma sequence of progression in colorectal cancer provides a unique opportunity for prophylaxis. Thus, if screening programs can identify patients with polyps and if these polyps are removed, cancer can largely be prevented. Various techniques are available for safe and effective polypectomy, depending on the size, presence of a stalk, and location (Fig. 136–5). Colonoscopy is being increasingly accepted as the procedure of choice for screening patients at average risk, that is, anybody older than 50 years. When patients have been found to harbor adenomatous polyps, they

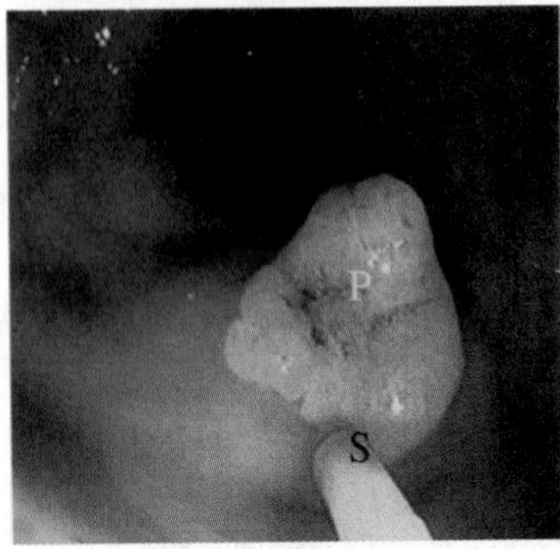

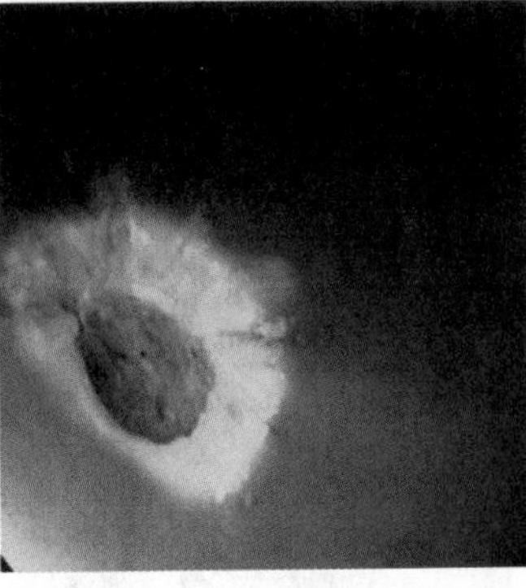

FIGURE 136–5 • Endoscopic polypectomy. Left, a snare (S) has been passed through the endoscope and positioned around the polyp (P). Right, subsequently, cautery was applied and the polyp guillotined, leaving behind a clean mucosal defect.

should be entered into a surveillance program; the frequency of colonoscopic examinations is still not settled but varies in practice from 1 to 3 years.

More aggressive screening strategies are required for patients considered at high risk for colorectal cancer, including patients with well-defined hereditary syndromes as well as those with a history of colorectal cancer in a first-degree relative. In addition, patients with ulcerative colitis with long-standing (more than 8 years) disease affecting the entire colon have an increased risk for development of colon cancer, about 0.5 to 3% after 20 years. Periodic colonoscopic surveillance (every 1 to 2 years with biopsies) is therefore recommended for patients with long-standing disease (8 years with pancolitis, 12 to 15 years with left-sided colitis); the discovery of dysplasia or cancer is an indication for colectomy.

"Virtual colonoscopy" (Chapter 135), which involves the digital construction of an endoluminal view of the colon on the basis of data from abdominal computed tomography, is not yet accurate enough for general screening. However, technical advances in this procedure may change this in the near future.

Chronic Diarrhea (Chapter 143)

Endoscopy may be a valuable aid in the evaluation of patients with persistent diarrhea. The timing of the endoscopy in these patients often depends on the clinical features of the illness. Patients with bloody diarrhea should have lower endoscopy as part of their initial evaluation to look for inflammatory bowel disease (Chapter 144). In most patients with chronic diarrhea, endoscopy is often done when initial routine testing does not yield a specific diagnosis. Both upper and lower endoscopies may be used, depending on the clinical presentation. Thus, the patient suspected of having a malabsorptive process may require upper endoscopy with jejunal or duodenal biopsies to look for celiac sprue or rarer lesions such as lymphoma or Whipple's disease (endoscopic biopsy has largely replaced blind intestinal biopsies for these conditions). Conversely, patients thought to have a secretory cause of diarrhea require a colonoscopy with biopsies to look for overt inflammatory bowel disease or more subtle variants such as microscopic or lymphocytic colitis, in which cases the diagnosis requires careful examination of the biopsy specimens.

The endoscopic approach to diarrhea in immunocompromised patients, such as those with HIV infection, is guided by the degree of immunosuppression and the need to find treatable infections. When results of routine stool tests are negative, patients with CD4 counts less than 100/mm^3 should undergo endoscopic evaluation to detect pathogens such as cytomegalovirus, *Mycobacterium avium* complex, and microsporidiosis. Small-volume stools with tenesmus suggest a proctocolitis, for which sigmoidoscopy (rather than a full colonoscopy) with biopsies is usually adequate. In patients with upper gastrointestinal symptoms (large-volume diarrhea, bloating, and dyspepsia), upper endoscopy with biopsy may be attempted first.

Miscellaneous Indications

The upper endoscope has provided a relatively quick and noninvasive means for removal of accidentally or deliberately ingested foreign bodies. Timing is critical for removal, however, because objects are usually beyond endoscopic retrieval when they reach the small bowel. Any foreign object that is causing symptoms should be removed, as should

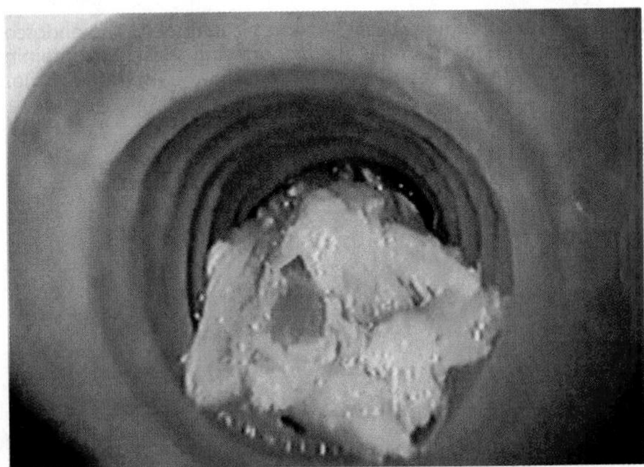

FIGURE 136–6 • Impacted food bolus in a young male patient who was found to have a ringed esophagus on endoscopy. This presentation is characteristic and may be either congenital or acquired secondary to reflux-induced or eosinophilic esophagitis.

potentially dangerous devices such as batteries and sharp objects. In general, objects larger than 2.5 cm in width or 13 cm in length are unlikely to leave the stomach and so should also be removed. On occasion, patients with food impacted in the esophagus require endoscopic removal (Fig. 136–6). This condition almost always indicates an underlying functional or structural problem (Chapter 140) and should prompt a thorough diagnostic evaluation after the acute problem has been addressed.

Because of the relatively poor correlation between oropharyngeal lesions and more distal visceral injury, upper endoscopy is usually recommended urgently in patients with corrosive ingestion (Chapter 111). Endoscopy allows patients to be divided into high- or low-risk groups for complications, with institution of appropriate monitoring and therapy.

Among the myriad causes of nausea and vomiting, a few, such as mucosal lesions and unsuspected reflux disease, are amenable to endoscopic diagnosis. Patients with new-onset constipation (Chapter 138), particularly those who are older than 40 years, should also undergo a colonoscopic evaluation to exclude an obstructing carcinoma. Colonoscopy is also useful in patients with pseudo-obstructive (nonobstructive) colonic dilation or Ogilvie's syndrome (Chapter 138); such patients are at risk for colonic rupture at diameters above 9 to 12 cm, and colonoscopic decompression is often required, sometimes on an emergent basis.

Malignant obstruction of the gastrointestinal lumen including the esophagus (Fig. 136–7), pylorus or duodenum, and colon can now be safely and effectively palliated endoscopically by expandable metal stents, avoiding the need for surgery in these patients. A major advance in enteral feeding has been the introduction of percutaneous endoscopic gastrostomy (PEG), a relatively quick, simple, and safe endoscopic procedure that has virtually eliminated surgical placement of gastric tubes. A variation of PEG is percutaneous endoscopic jejunostomy (PEJ), in which a long tube is passed through the gastric tube, past the pylorus, and into the jejunum. The most common indication for these procedures is the need for sustained nutrition in patients with neurologic impairment of swallowing or with head and neck cancers. Patients with a short life expectancy are not suitable candidates for PEG and can be managed by nasoenteral tubes. Further, despite its intuitive appeal, there is little or no evidence that PEG feeding alters clinical or nutritional outcomes or significantly improves quality of life.

PEJ was originally introduced to prevent aspiration, but it does not prevent this complication; the major indication for PEJ is significant impairment of gastric emptying. Retrograde tube migration with PEJ is common, however, and PEJ may require frequent replacement.

PANCREATOBILIARY ENDOSCOPY (IMAGING)

Endoscopic retrograde cholangiopancreatography (ERCP) involves a special side-viewing endoscope (the duodenoscope) that is used to gain access to the second part of the duodenum. A small catheter is then introduced into the bile or pancreatic duct, and radiographic contrast medium is injected under fluoroscopic monitoring. Successful cannulation and imaging can be achieved in up to 95% of cases. In some centers, a fine-caliber "baby" endoscope can also be introduced into the duct of interest (cholangioscopy or pancreaticoscopy), allowing the direct visualization of intraductal disease. ERCP is perhaps the technically most demanding of gastrointestinal endoscopic procedures, and it is associated with the highest risk of serious complications (notably pancreatitis, in about 5% of cases).

Suspected Biliary Disease (Chapters 149 and 159)

The diagnostic approach to patients with cholestasis begins with an attempt to differentiate obstructive from hepatocellular causes. The most common causes of obstructive jaundice are common bile duct stones and tumors of the pancreatic and bile ducts. Less invasive conventional imaging with ultrasonography, computed tomography, or magnetic resonance imaging demonstrates dilated bile ducts and mass lesions but is not sensitive or specific in detecting or delineating pathologic change in the distal common bile duct and pancreas, two regions where the majority of obstructing lesions are found. Furthermore, some biliary diseases, such as sclerosing cholangitis, do not result in dilated ducts but have a characteristic appearance on cholangiography. Finally, the ability to use devices such as cytology brushes and biopsy forceps during cholangiography provides an additional aid in the diagnosis of biliary lesions. Both percutaneous and endoscopic cholangiographic techniques are associated with a high rate of success in experienced hands, but the endoscopic approach allows visualization of the ampullary region and the performance of sphincterotomy, and it also avoids the small risk of a biliary leak associated with puncture of the liver capsule.

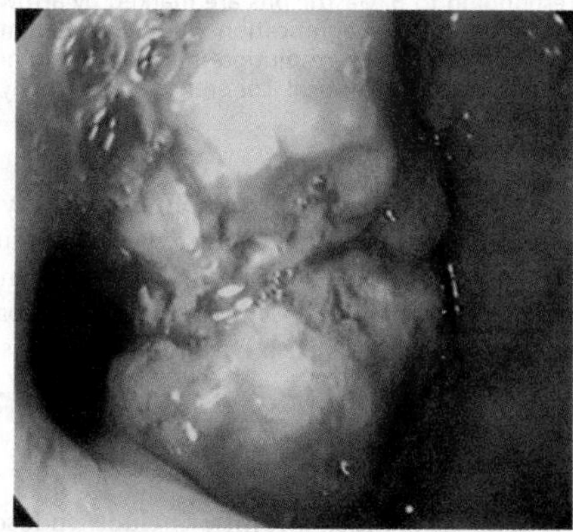

FIGURE 136–7 • Large malignant mass at the gastroesophageal junction as seen endoscopically.

In the last few years, magnetic resonance cholangiopancreatography, a digital reconstruction technique based on an abdominal magnetic resonance imaging scan, has become popular as an imaging modality for the pancreatobiliary system, with excellent sensitivity and specificity. Because of its relative safety, many experts now advocate this procedure for screening patients with a low likelihood of disease. In those with a higher probability, ERCP is still the procedure of choice because of its therapeutic options.

Of the approximately 600,000 patients undergoing cholecystectomy in this country, 5 to 10% may present with bile duct stones before or after the surgery. Endoscopic stone removal is successful in 90% or more of these cases and usually requires a sphincterotomy (Fig. 136–8). The sphincter of Oddi is a band of muscle that encircles the distal common bile duct and pancreatic duct in the region of the ampulla of Vater; cutting of this muscle, or sphincterotomy, is one of the mainstays of endoscopic biliary treatment and is accomplished with a special tool called a papillotome or sphincterotome. This procedure is often sufficient for the treatment of small stones in the bile ducts, but larger stones may require additional procedures, such as mechanical, electrohydraulic, or laser lithotripsy, which can be performed endoscopically. In addition to stone disease, sphincterotomy can be curative for patients with papillary stenosis or muscle spasm (termed sphincter of Oddi dysfunction). Finally, by enlarging the access to the bile duct, sphincterotomy facilitates the passage of stents and other devices into the bile duct. Sphincterotomy carries an additional small risk of bleeding, but its associated morbidity is about one third that of surgical exploration and its cost is only about 20% as high.

Endoscopic therapy has also revolutionized the palliative approach to malignant biliary obstruction. The technique, which requires the placement of indwelling stents, is superior to both radiologic and surgical techniques. Plastic stents have been the mainstay of treatment, but metal stents last longer and are perhaps preferred in patients with longer life expectancies.

Pancreatic Disease (Chapters 147 and 205)

ERCP is also useful in patients with pancreatic diseases that do not always arise with obstructive jaundice, such as pancreatic cancer of the body and tail and, less commonly, chronic pancreatitis. It is also indicated for patients with acute or recurrent pancreatitis without any obvious risk factors on history or routine laboratory evaluation. Imaging of the pancreatic duct may delineate anatomic abnormalities that may be responsible for the pancreatitis, such as congenital variants (pancreas divisum, annular pancreas), intraductal tumors, or possibly sphincter of Oddi dysfunction. In such cases, bile can be collected from the bile duct for microscopic examination for crystals (so-called microlithiasis) that can result in pancreatitis in some patients even in the absence of macroscopic stones. In patients with chronic pancreatitis, which is most often due to excessive alcohol intake, pancreatography can confirm the diagnosis,

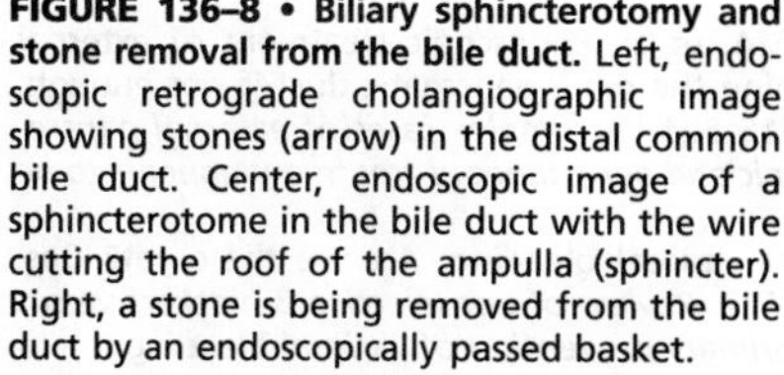

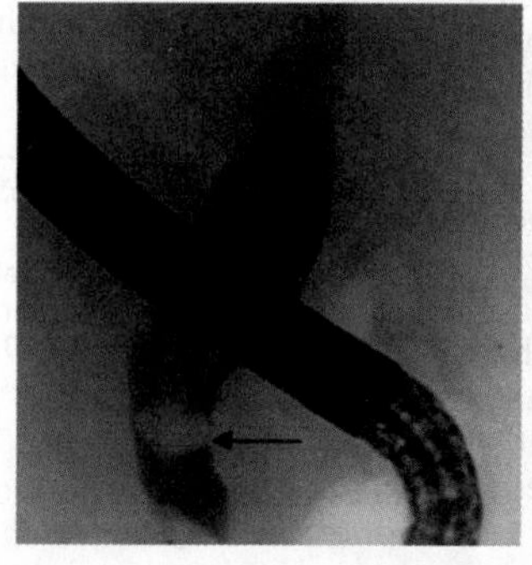

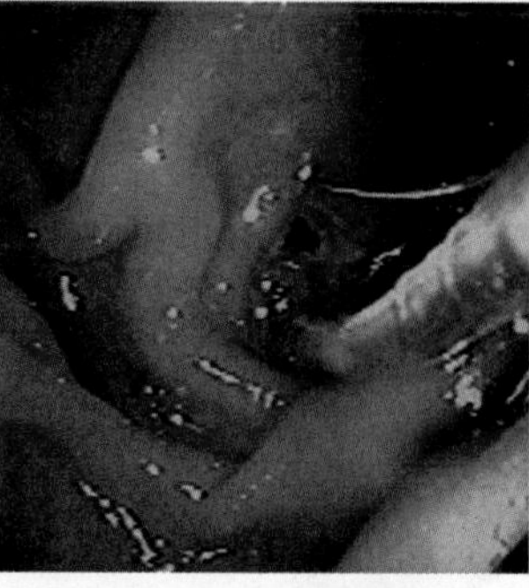

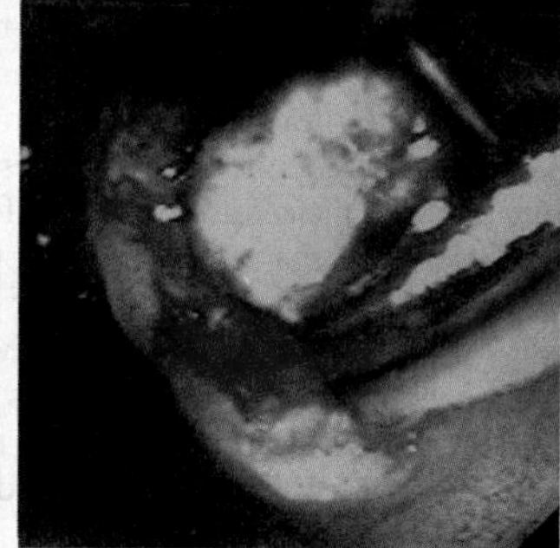

FIGURE 136–8 • Biliary sphincterotomy and stone removal from the bile duct. Left, endoscopic retrograde cholangiographic image showing stones (arrow) in the distal common bile duct. Center, endoscopic image of a sphincterotome in the bile duct with the wire cutting the roof of the ampulla (sphincter). Right, a stone is being removed from the bile duct by an endoscopically passed basket.

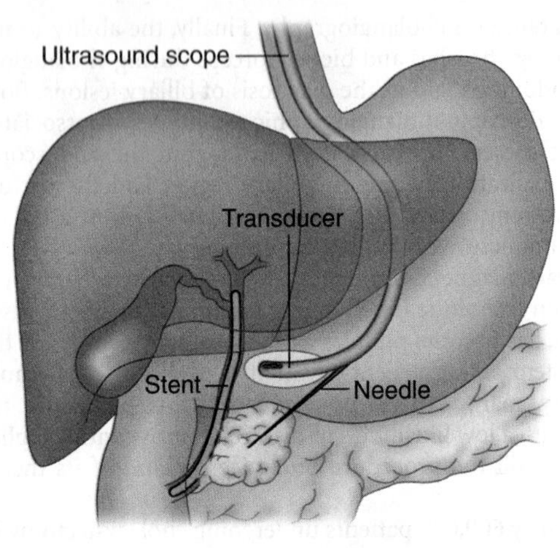

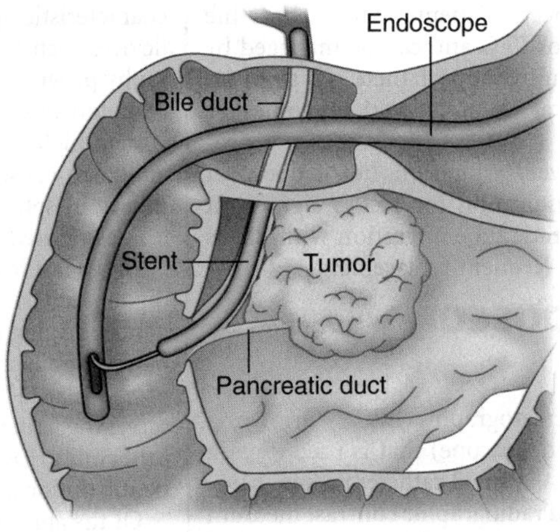

FIGURE 136–9 • Biopsy of a pancreatic mass guided by endoscopic ultrasonography (A) and the placement of a stent into a malignant bile duct stricture with endoscopic retrograde cholangiopancreatography (B). (From Brugge WR, Van Dam J: Pancreatic and biliary endoscopy. N Engl J Med 1999;341:1808–1816.)

provide useful information about the severity of the disease, and identify ductal lesions that may be amenable to therapy by either endoscopic or surgical means. In more subtle cases, collection and analysis of pancreatic juice after stimulation with secretin may be useful in establishing exocrine impairment and hence in confirming chronic pancreatic injury.

ERCP also has a role in some patients with acute pancreatitis (Chapter 147) that is probably caused by obstructing biliary stones. Patients presenting with severe biliary pancreatitis may benefit from urgent ERCP early in their course, with the intention of detecting and removing stones from the common bile duct. Similarly, patients who have smoldering acute pancreatitis that does not appear to be improving satisfactorily with conservative treatment may require ERCP for identification and treatment of any obstructing lesions in the pancreatic or distal biliary duct.

Therapeutic endoscopy for chronic pancreatic disease is still evolving. Relief of ductal obstruction (e.g., by endoscopic removal of pancreatic stones or dilation of strictures) can provide short to intermediate pain relief in some patients with chronic pancreatitis. Endoscopic pseudocyst drainage by a variety of techniques is now technically feasible, with results that appear to be comparable to those of surgical or radiologic techniques. Patients with ductal disruptions (e.g., those with pancreatic ascites) can often be treated successfully with endoscopic stent placement. Pancreatic papillotomy may also be useful for some patients with recurrent pancreatitis, such as when pancreas divisum is thought to play a role. Although the ability to approach these difficult clinical entities by the relatively less invasive endoscopic techniques represents a major accomplishment, the treatment of pancreatic diseases remains a multidisciplinary process with important and in some cases dominant roles played by surgeons and interventional radiologists.

TRANSLUMINAL IMAGING: ENDOSCOPIC ULTRASONOGRAPHY

The incorporation of an ultrasonic transducer in the tip of a flexible endoscope or the use of stand-alone ultrasound probes has now made it possible to obtain images of gastrointestinal lesions that are not apparent on superficial views, including lesions within the wall of the gut as well as those that lie beyond (e.g., pancreatic or lymph node lesions). A further role of endoscopic ultrasonography (EUS) is to guide fine-needle aspiration, which often provides pathologic confirmation of suspicious lesions (Fig. 136–9). In many cases, this approach appears to be even more accurate than conventional radiologic techniques like abdominal ultrasonography and computed tomography. Thus, EUS is probably the single best test for diagnosis of pancreatic tumors (Chapter 205), particularly the small endocrine varieties, with sensitivities approaching 95%. It is also the procedure of choice for imaging of submucosal and other wall lesions of the gastrointestinal tract (overall accuracy of 65 to 70%) as well as for staging of a variety of gastrointestinal tumors (overall accuracy of 90% or more). Preoperative staging is a critical element in the management strategy for tumors such as esophageal and pancreatic cancer, and EUS can complement more conventional radiologic tests to help determine the resectability and curative potential of surgery in these cases.

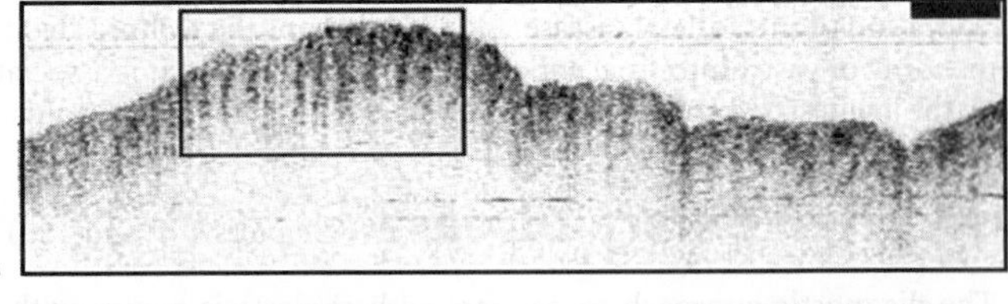

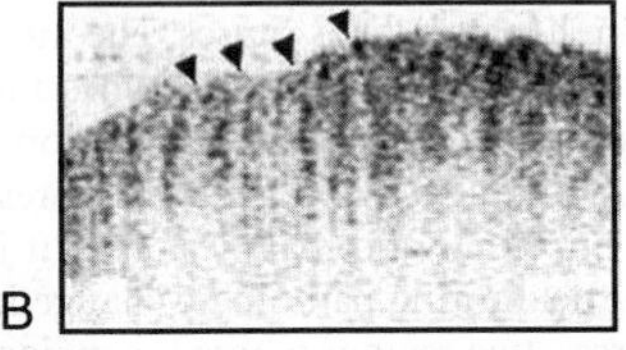

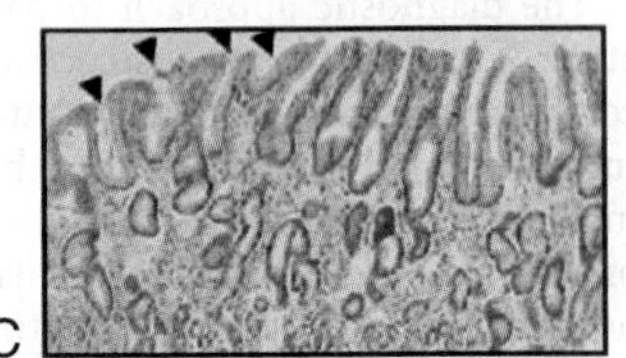

FIGURE 136–10 • A, Optical coherence tomography of the stomach, an endoscopic procedure currently under investigation that provides high-resolution images of the superficial epithelium comparable to those of microscopy. Scale bar = 500 μm. **B,** Magnified view of A. Gastric pits can be clearly identified as areas of relatively low reflectance within the glandular epithelium (arrowheads). **C,** Histology corresponding to **B.** Gastric pits are marked by arrowheads (hematoxylin and eosin stain, original magnification ×40). (From Bouma BE, Tearney GJ, Compton CC, Nishioka NS: High-resolution imaging of the human esophagus and stomach in vivo using optical coherence tomography. Gastrointest Endosc 2000;51:467–474.)

In addition to its valuable diagnostic role, EUS is rapidly emerging as a therapeutic tool. One example is EUS-directed celiac plexus neurolysis, a technique that appears to be effective for the treatment of pain in patients with pancreatic cancer. Unfortunately, this approach does not appear to work as well in patients with chronic pancreatitis.

EVOLVING TECHNIQUES AND FUTURE DIRECTIONS

Recent innovations with much promise include endoscopic optical coherence tomography (Fig. 136–10) and confocal microscopy. These techniques have the ability to provide microscopic images of cells at the surface as well as within deeper layers, thereby providing virtual real-time histology.

Intraluminal or, potentially, transluminal (i.e., entering the peritoneal cavity through a deliberate incision in the wall of the stomach or other organ) endoscopic approaches may provide less invasive treatment of a variety of diseases including obesity, gastrointestinal anastomoses, and even organ resection.

SUGGESTED READINGS

Arvanitakis M, Delhaye M, Bali MA, et al: Endoscopic treatment of external pancreatic fistulas: When draining the main pancreatic duct is not enough. Am J Gastroenterol 2007;102:516–524. *In complex cases of external pancreatic fistuals, combined endoscopic and percutaneous treatment appears to be safe and effective.*

Boyer TD: Primary prophylaxis for variceal bleeding: Are we there yet? Gastroenterology 2005;128:1120–1122. *Review of nonselective ß-blockers versus variceal band ligation for the primary prevention of variceal bleeding.*

Capell MS: Safety and efficacy of colonoscopy after myocardial infarction: An analysis of 100 study patients and 100 control patients at two tertiary cardiac referral hospitals. Gastrointest Endosc 2004;60:901–909. *Risks and complications of performing endoscopy soon after a myocardial infarction.*

Eliakim R, Yassin K, Shlomi I, et al: A novel diagnostic tool for detecting oesophageal pathology: The PillCam oesophageal video capsule. Aliment Pharmacol Ther 2004;20:1083–1089. *Description of a novel noninvasive device for esophageal screening.*

Rex DK: Maximizing detection of adenomas and cancers during colonoscopy. Am J Gastroenterol 2006;101:2866–2877. *An excellent review.*

Saperas E, Dot J, Videla S, et al: Capsule endoscopy versus computed tomographic or standard angiography for the diagnosis of obscure gastrointestinal bleeding. Am J Gastroenterol 2007;102:731–737. *In patients with obscure GI bleeding, capsule endoscopy detects more lesions than CTA or standard mesenteric angiography.*

Sivak MV: Gastrointestinal endoscopy: Past and future. Gut 2006;55:1061–1064. *A review of the past and future of endoscopy.*

Sturniolo GC, Di Leo V, Vettorato MG, et al: Small bowel exploration by wireless capsule endoscopy: Results from 314 procedures. Am J Med 2006;119:341–347. *Visualization of the small bowel (96%) and cecum (80%) identified the source of 58% of obscure gastrointestinal bleeds and 31% of cases of suspected small bowel disease.*

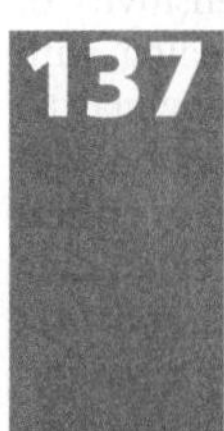

137 GASTROINTESTINAL HEMORRHAGE AND OCCULT GASTROINTESTINAL BLEEDING

David J. Bjorkman

GASTROINTESTINAL HEMORRHAGE

Epidemiology

Gastrointestinal hemorrhage is a common clinical disorder, with an annual incidence of 100 per 100,000 population. Bleeding from the gastrointestinal tract may manifest clinically as acute upper tract bleeding (proximal to the ligament of Treitz), as acute lower tract bleeding (distal to the ligament of Treitz), or as evidence of occult blood loss by iron deficiency anemia or a stool test positive for blood.

Upper Gastrointestinal Bleeding

Epidemiology

Upper gastrointestinal bleeding (proximal to the ligament of Treitz) is responsible for 250,000 to 300,000 hospital admissions and $2.5 billion in costs in the United States each year. The most common causes of upper gastrointestinal bleeding are peptic ulcers (Chapter 141) and esophagogastric varices. Variceal bleeding (Fig. 137–1) most commonly occurs in the setting of portal hypertension (Chapter 157). Less common causes of upper gastrointestinal bleeding are Mallory-Weiss tears (Fig. 137–2), malignant disease, erosive disease, and vascular abnormalities (Table 137–1).

Diagnosis

Most cases of acute upper gastrointestinal bleeding present as hematemesis, although brisk bleeding can present as hematochezia. Gastrointestinal endoscopy (Chapter 136) remains both the diagnostic and the therapeutic procedure of choice for upper gastrointestinal bleeding. Despite progressive advances in diagnosis, the mortality from acute upper gastrointestinal bleeding requiring hospitalization remains near 4% for young patients and has been reported to be as high as 15% in the elderly.

Emergency Evaluation and Treatment

The initial focus for any patient with significant blood loss should be the evaluation and restoration of intravascular volume, which begins with careful evaluation of blood pressure and pulse, including special attention to any orthostatic changes. Blood hemoglobin concentration and hematocrit are unreliable markers of acute blood loss, but they are helpful as baseline values. Intravenous access and vigorous volume replacement decrease the morbidity of acute upper gastrointestinal bleeding and should be initiated immediately in all patients with significant gastrointestinal bleeding. Initial volume restoration can be accomplished with the infusion of isotonic electrolyte solutions until vital signs become stable. Blood products should be based on the patient's clinical condition.

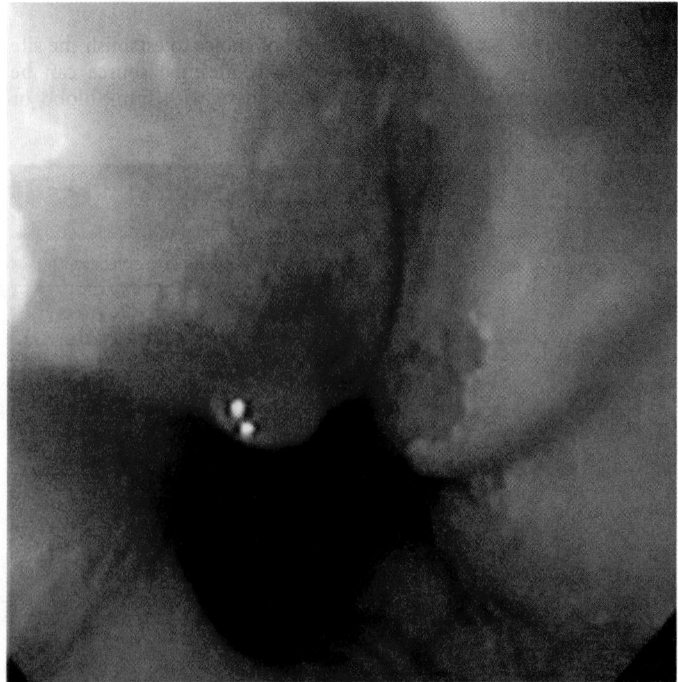

FIGURE 137–1 • Bleeding esophageal varix at the gastroesophageal junction. (Courtesy of Pankaj Jay Pasricha, MD.)

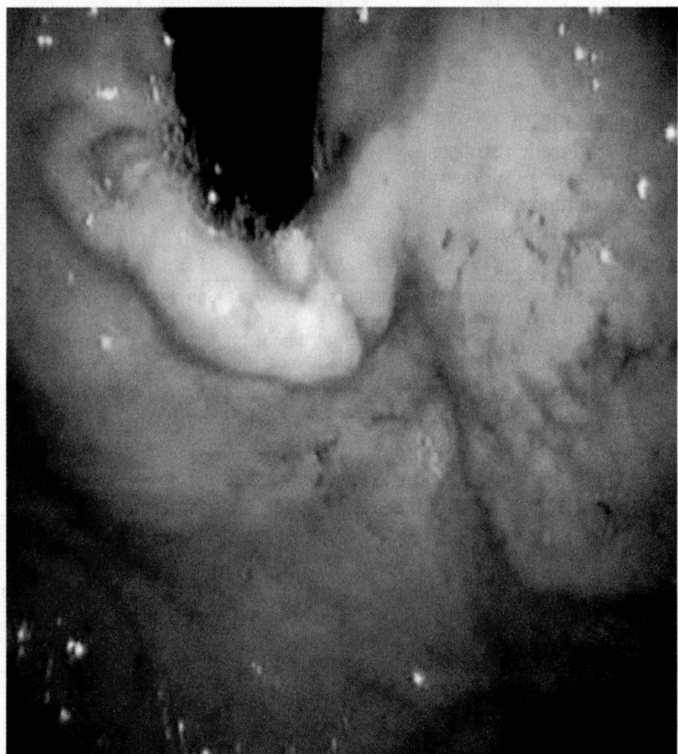

FIGURE 137–2 • Retroflexed endoscopic image of a Mallory-Weiss tear at the gastroesophageal junction.

Assessing the Level of Bleeding

Endoscopy (Chapter 136) is the method of choice to establish the site of gastrointestinal bleeding. An upper gastrointestinal source can be assumed when there is a history of hematemesis with frank blood or coffee grounds–like material. A history of melena alone is suggestive but not pathognomonic of a bleeding source proximal to the ligament of Treitz. In patients with a small bowel or a proximal colonic source of bleeding, delayed colonic transit may result in dark stool that may be difficult to distinguish from melena. Hematochezia is more suggestive of a bleeding site in the lower gastrointestinal tract, but in as many as 10% of cases, it may also result from vigorous upper gastrointestinal bleeding.

When an acute bleeding source is thought to be in the upper gastrointestinal tract, nasogastric aspiration is 80% sensitive for the presence of an actively bleeding lesion, and evidence of blood in a nasogastric aspirate suggests bleeding proximal to the ligament of Treitz. False-negative aspirates may occur in 20% of patients because the tube is improperly positioned or the reflux of blood from the duodenum is prevented by pylorospasm or obstruction. Nasogastric suction is also useful to determine whether bleeding is persistent or recurrent and to estimate the rapidity of bleeding.

TABLE 137–1 ETIOLOGY AND SEVERITY OF UPPER GASTROINTESTINAL TRACT HEMORRHAGE*

	Severity of Hemorrhage	
Source of Hemorrhage	**Mild-Moderate (246 Patients)**	**Severe (140 Patients)**
Esophagus		
Esophagitis	12%	7%
Ulcer	2%	2%
Mallory-Weiss tear	5%	19%
Esophageal varices	5%	31%
Total esophagus	24%	59%
Stomach		
Gastric ulcer	15%	14%
Prepyloric ulcer	2%	4%
Pyloric channel ulcer	4%	2%
Gastric erosions	2%	0
Gastritis	7%	0
Varices	1%	2%
Portal-hypertensive gastropathy	2%	0
Gastric cancer	2%	0
Polyp	0	2%
Dieulafoy's lesion	0	0
Total stomach	35%	24%
Duodenum		
Ulcer	30%	15%
Duodenitis	8%	0
Aortoenteric fistula	0	2%
Pancreatic pseudocyst	2%	0
Post-sphincterotomy	1%	0
Total duodenum	41%	17%
	100%	100%

*All patients underwent diagnostic endoscopy at San Francisco General Hospital during 3 years.
Modified from Cello JP: Gastrointestinal hemorrhage and occult gastrointestinal bleeding. In Goldman L, Bennett JC (eds): Cecil Textbook of Medicine, 21st ed. Philadelphia, WB Saunders, 2000.

Diagnostic Endoscopy

After hemodynamic stabilization, endoscopy is indicated in consenting patients unless the risks of the procedure outweigh its potential benefits, at least temporarily (e.g., patients in shock), or its results would not alter the outcome or care of the patient. Endoscopy has a sensitivity of 92% for identification of the site of upper gastrointestinal bleeding, with a specificity that approaches 100%. The sensitivity of endoscopy may be limited by retained blood and clots in the stomach. In this situation, vigorous gastric lavage with use of a large-bore orogastric tube is critical before the procedure. Endoscopy has the added advantage of guiding biopsies to test for *Helicobacter pylori* infection (Chapters 141 and 142) and to diagnose malignant disease (Chapter 202). By comparison, barium radiography has a sensitivity of only 54%. Barium radiography is contraindicated in acute upper gastrointestinal bleeding because it interferes with subsequent endoscopy, angiography, or surgery.

Careful endoscopic examination not only identifies the source of upper gastrointestinal bleeding but also is the most accurate predictor of prognosis (probability of rebleeding, morbidity, and mortality). Additional clinical risk factors for higher morbidity and mortality include older age, shock, volume of bleeding, need for transfusion, onset of bleeding in the hospital, and presence of comorbid clinical conditions. A scoring system (Table 137–2) that uses clinical factors to predict rebleeding and mortality has been developed and validated. Other scoring systems have also been developed. The most predictive factors for rebleeding appear to be the volume of the initial bleeding episode, comorbid conditions, and endoscopic appearance of the lesion.

Endoscopic classification of ulcers has been shown repeatedly to predict accurately the rates of rebleeding, morbidity, and mortality (Table 137–3). Patients without high-risk stigmata (those with a clean ulcer base

TABLE 137–2 CLINICAL RISK SCORE*

	Score for Finding				
Characteristic	**0**	**1**	**2**	**3**	**Points for This Variable**
Age	<60 years	≥60 and ≤79 years	≥80 years		(maximum = 2)
Shock	Heart rate <100 beats per minute and systolic blood pressure ≥100 mm Hg	Heart rate ≤100 beats per minute and systolic blood pressure ≥100 mm Hg	Systolic blood pressure <100 mm Hg		(maximum = 2)
Comorbidity	None	None	Heart failure Myocardial or ischemia Malignant disease (not disseminated) Other comorbidity	Renal failure Liver disease Disseminated malignant disease	(maximum = 3)
Total score					(maximum = 7)

*Mortality of acute upper gastrointestinal bleeding based on characteristics assessed at the initial presentation. A score of 3 or less indicates a low clinical risk (mortality ≤12%), whereas a score of 4 or more indicates a high clinical risk (mortality >20%).
Modified from Rockall TA, Logan FRA, Devlin HB, et al: Risk assessment after acute upper gastrointestinal haemorrhage. Gut 1996;38:316–321.

or flat, pigmented spots) have an extremely low rate of rebleeding and a negligible mortality.

Endoscopic Triage: Cost-Effective Care for Low-Risk Patients

Although it may seem intuitively obvious that endoscopy would improve outcomes, randomized trials have indicated that *diagnostic* endoscopy alone does not improve mortality, rebleeding rates, need for surgery, or hospital stay. The overwhelming majority (75 to 80%) of patients with bleeding ulcers stop bleeding spontaneously, limiting the impact of early endoscopy for these patients. Nevertheless, prospective studies show that urgent endoscopy in all patients with acute nonvariceal upper gastrointestinal bleeding identifies 20 to 30% of patients who meet both clinical and endoscopic criteria for a low risk of rebleeding and morbidity (see Tables 137–2 and 137–3); these patients can be safely treated as outpatients, thereby dramatically reducing the cost of care. Conversely, patients with a high risk of rebleeding, by the same criteria, can undergo early endoscopic therapy, ideally before admission, and be triaged to more intensive hospital care. Urgent endoscopy as a triage tool is cost-effective care for upper gastrointestinal bleeding (Fig. 137–3). 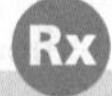

Treatment

Rx

Endoscopic Therapy

In the 20% of patients with nonvariceal upper gastrointestinal bleeding who have persistent or recurrent bleeding as determined by nasogastric lavage or endoscopy, endoscopic therapy reduces both morbidity and mortality. All available endoscopic techniques appear to have similar results but vary in their approach to sealing the bleeding vessel and maintaining hemostasis. The major methods may be divided into thermal coagulation, injection therapy, and mechanical compression. The most common thermal methods use electrical current (multipolar or bipolar electrode) or direct application of a heated device (heater probe) to seal the vessel with thermal energy. With these methods, hemostasis can be achieved in 90% of patients with active bleeding, and rebleeding rates are significantly reduced by more than 50%. [2,3]

The least expensive method of endoscopic therapy for upper gastrointestinal bleeding is to inject the bleeding site with saline or diluted epinephrine. This approach yields initial results that are generally similar to those of thermal therapy but is not as effective for long-term hemostasis. Thermal therapy and injection can be combined to control bleeding and to treat the lesion definitively. Mechanical methods to treat bleeding include hemostatic clips and the use of rubber band ligation. Both of these methods appear to have an efficacy similar to that of thermal therapy. In patients who have recurrent bleeding after initial endoscopic therapy, a second attempt has a significant success rate and can reduce the need for surgery.

TABLE 137–3 RISK OF REBLEEDING AND DEATH BASED ON ENDOSCOPIC FINDINGS

Endoscopic Finding	Risk of Rebleeding (%)	Mortality (%)
Active bleeding	55	11
Visible vessel	43	11
Adherent clot	22	7
Flat spot	10	3
Clean base	5	2

Modified from Laine L, Peterson WL: Bleeding peptic ulcer. N Engl J Med 1994;331:717–727.

Medical Therapy

The most common causes of peptic ulcer disease are *H. pylori* infection and nonsteroidal anti-inflammatory drug (NSAID) use (Chapter 141). NSAIDs should be discontinued and *H. pylori* infection should be treated in all patients with bleeding ulcers. High-dose proton pump inhibition should be started acutely in upper gastrointestinal bleeding because it may reduce the need for emergency endoscopy. [4]

Data are now compelling that profound acid suppression reduces rebleeding in patients with high-risk endoscopic stigmata for rebleeding. Studies with high doses of both intravenous and oral proton pump inhibitors have demonstrated a significant improvement in outcome (rebleeding, hospital stay, transfusion requirement) compared with H_2-receptor antagonists. [5] This effect is likely due to improvement of coagulation and platelet aggregation by increasing intragastric pH. Vigorous acid suppression should be provided to all patients with acute upper gastrointestinal bleeding.

Nonulcer Acute Upper Gastrointestinal Bleeding

Variceal bleeding is the most common cause of nonulcer upper gastrointestinal hemorrhage. The approach to variceal bleeding is a

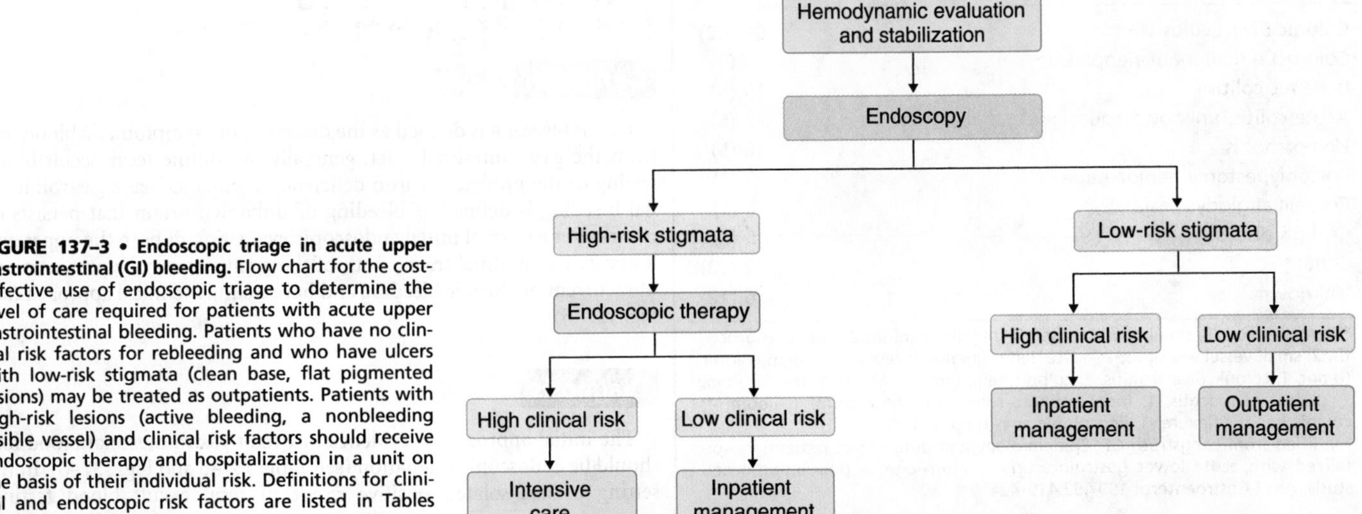

FIGURE 137–3 • Endoscopic triage in acute upper gastrointestinal (GI) bleeding. Flow chart for the cost-effective use of endoscopic triage to determine the level of care required for patients with acute upper gastrointestinal bleeding. Patients who have no clinical risk factors for rebleeding and who have ulcers with low-risk stigmata (clean base, flat pigmented lesions) may be treated as outpatients. Patients with high-risk lesions (active bleeding, a nonbleeding visible vessel) and clinical risk factors should receive endoscopic therapy and hospitalization in a unit on the basis of their individual risk. Definitions for clinical and endoscopic risk factors are listed in Tables 137–2 and 137–3.

Rx

combination of pharmacologic (octreotide, somatostatin), endoscopic (band ligation, sclerotherapy), and mechanical (balloon tamponade) approaches (Chapter 157).

Most non–peptic ulcer, nonvariceal causes of upper gastrointestinal bleeding can be treated by the same endoscopic modalities described earlier with similar success. The most common of these causes is a tear at the gastroesophageal junction, called a Mallory-Weiss tear (Chapter 140), which accounts for 5 to 14% of upper gastrointestinal bleeding. Mallory-Weiss bleeding usually stops spontaneously, but persistent bleeding should be treated in a manner similar to bleeding from peptic ulcers. Dieulafoy's lesion, which is an aberrant submucosal artery that erodes into the lumen of the stomach, is a rare cause of recurrent vigorous upper gastrointestinal bleeding. Tumors also are rare (<1%) causes of acute upper gastrointestinal bleeding. Vascular lesions may rarely present as acute bleeding, but more commonly they cause chronic, low-grade blood loss. Bleeding from diffuse gastric erosions, which can occur in critically ill patients, does not respond to endoscopic therapy but can usually be prevented by prophylactic treatment.

Lower Gastrointestinal Bleeding

Epidemiology

Lower gastrointestinal bleeding occurs at a rate of 20 per 100,000 population, which is about one fifth as frequently as upper gastrointestinal bleeding. Hematochezia, which is the most common presenting symptom for lower gastrointestinal hemorrhage, can be variously described as bloody diarrhea, blood and clots per rectum, maroon-colored stool, or blood mixed with the stool. Hematochezia can occur from bleeding anywhere in the gastrointestinal tract, and as noted previously, about 10% of patients who present with hematochezia have an upper gastrointestinal source of bleeding.

Pathobiology

The most common causes of lower gastrointestinal bleeding (Table 137–4) are colonic diverticula (Chapter 145), vascular ectasias (Chapter 146), and tumors (Chapter 203), all of which increase in prevalence with age. As a result, lower gastrointestinal bleeding is most commonly a disorder of the elderly, with a dramatically increased incidence with advancing age. The initial approach to the patient should be the same as in upper gastrointestinal bleeding, with careful assessment of vital signs and vigorous volume replacement. A history of prior bleeding, inflammatory bowel disease, radiation therapy, and NSAID use may be helpful but does not identify the bleeding lesion.

TABLE 137–4 FINAL DIAGNOSIS IN 219 PATIENTS HOSPITALIZED FOR ACUTE LOWER GASTROINTESTINAL BLEEDING

Diagnosis	n (%)
Colonic diverticulosis	91 (42)
Colorectal malignant neoplasm	20 (9)
Ischemic colitis	19 (9)
Acute colitis, unknown cause	11 (5)
Hemorrhoids	10 (5)
Postpolypectomy hemorrhage	9 (4)
Colonic angiodysplasia	6 (3)
Crohn's disease	5 (2)
Other*	22 (10)
Unknown	26 (12)

*Stercoral ulcer, 3; small bowel tumor, 3; infectious colitis, 2; radiation proctitis, 2; small vessel vasculitis, 2; acute ileitis, unknown cause, 1; benign colonic tumor, 1; colonic diverticulitis, 1; colonic hematoma, 1; Meckel's diverticulum, 1; ulcerative proctitis, 1; indeterminate sources in the rectum, 1; ileum, 1; colonic hepatic flexure, 1; ileocolonic anastomosis, 1.

Modified from Longstreth GF: Epidemiology and outcome of patients hospitalized with acute lower gastrointestinal hemorrhage: A population-based study. Am J Gastroenterol 1997;92:419–424.

Diagnosis

Identification and treatment of the bleeding lesion should be attempted after the patient is hemodynamically stable (Fig. 137–4). It may be difficult to diagnose colonic angiodysplasia, which is as common a cause of lower gastrointestinal bleeding as are colonic diverticula in some studies. Because many elderly patients have colonic diverticula, bleeding due to undiagnosed angiodysplasia may sometimes be mistakenly attributed to diverticula. Urgent colonoscopy after a vigorous cleansing of the colon can help determine whether the bleeding is from diverticula or angiodysplasia. In many cases, the bleeding lesion may be identified by the presence of a fresh clot or active bleeding. Endoscopic therapy for these lesions, similar to the methods described earlier for upper gastrointestinal bleeding, reduces the rate of rebleeding and the need for surgery. Vascular lesions can be treated with injection, contact thermal methods, or endoscopic laser therapy. Early colonoscopy identifies lesions, facilitates treatment, and decreases hospital stay. There is no role for barium enema in the setting of acute lower gastrointestinal bleeding because it is unlikely to provide a definitive diagnosis and prevents or delays more accurate diagnostic modalities with potential therapeutic benefits.

When urgent colonoscopy does not identify a bleeding source or if bleeding is too rapid to permit colonoscopy, angiography may identify the bleeding site. The yield of angiography ranges from 40 to 80%, but to be successful, angiography requires a bleeding rate of at least 1 mL/min. When a bleeding site is identified, the bleeding can be slowed or stopped by local infusion of vasoconstrictors or by selective embolization of the bleeding artery, with success rates exceeding 80%. Both approaches carry a substantial (>10%) risk of causing local ischemia.

In settings in which bleeding is not rapid enough for angiography, nuclear scintigraphy may be helpful in identifying the site but not the cause of the lesion. The bleeding rate required for identification is at least 0.1 mL/min. In optimal conditions, the sensitivity of scintigraphy is 85%, and its specificity is 70%. One advantage of tagged red blood cell scintigraphy is the ability to detect intermittent bleeding by serial scans performed over the lifetime of the radionuclide.

Surgical consultation and comanagement are appropriate in all cases of gastrointestinal bleeding and are most critical in the setting of severe lower gastrointestinal bleeding. Vigorous efforts should be made to diagnose the bleeding lesion or, if that is not possible, at least the involved segment of the colon to guide surgical therapy. Surgery directed at a lesion identified endoscopically or radiographically is often curative. Empirical total colectomy or right hemicolectomy should be reserved for life-threatening bleeding that cannot be localized and has not responded to available therapeutic approaches.

OCCULT AND OBSCURE GASTROINTESTINAL BLEEDING

Definition

Occult bleeding is defined as the detection of asymptomatic blood loss from the gastrointestinal tract, generally by routine fecal occult blood testing or the presence of iron deficiency anemia. *Obscure* gastrointestinal bleeding is defined as bleeding of unknown origin that persists or recurs after a normal initial endoscopic evaluation of both the upper and lower gastrointestinal tracts. Both of these entities may be presentations of recurrent or chronic bleeding and have a similar clinical approach (see Fig. 137–6).

Diagnosis

The initial approach to evidence of occult gastrointestinal blood loss should be endoscopic evaluation (see Table 137–5 and Fig. 137–6). In the setting of an isolated positive result of fecal occult blood testing, colonoscopy is indicated as the first test (Chapter 203). The yield of

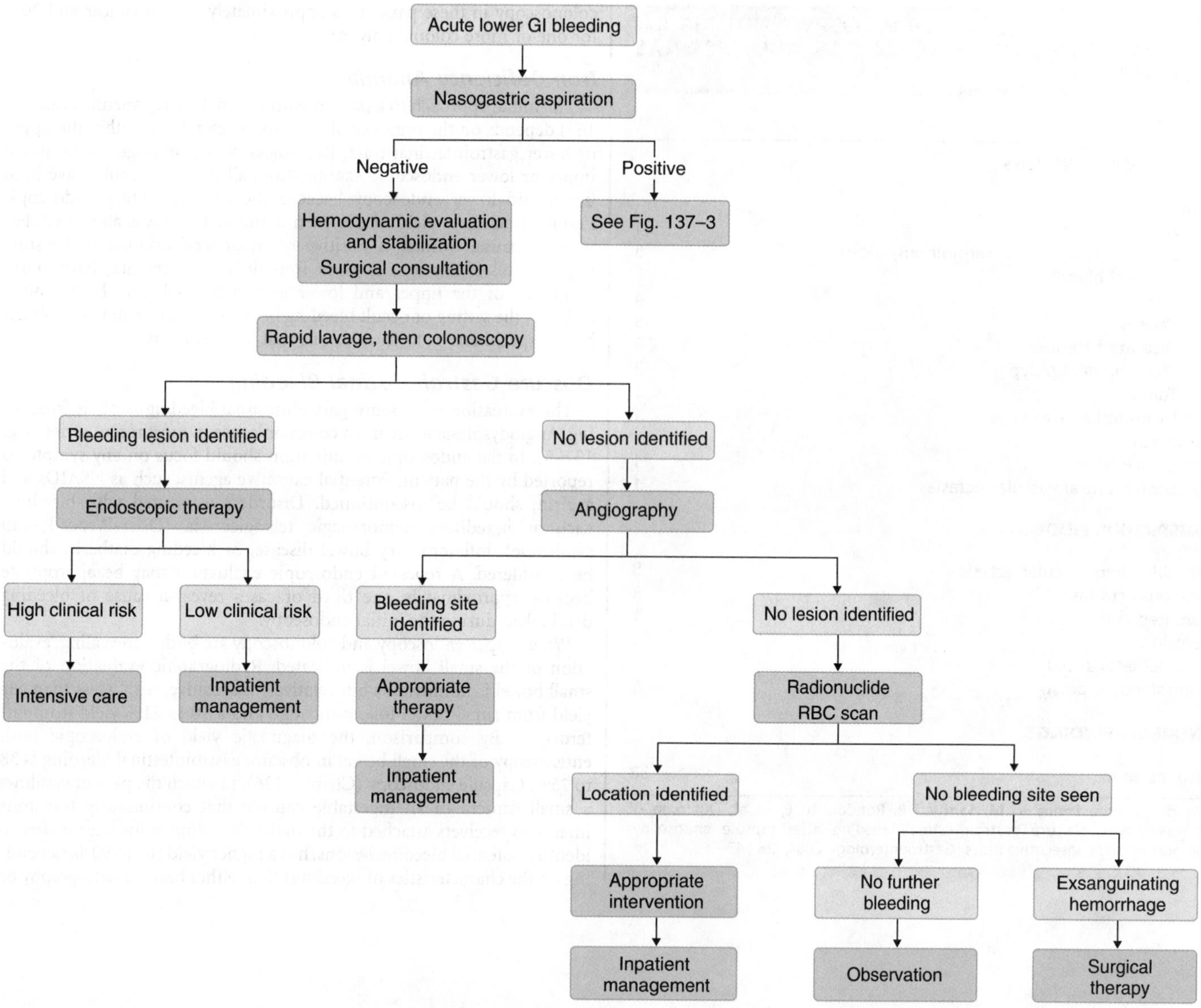

- Acute lower GI bleeding
  - Nasogastric aspiration
    - Positive
      - See Fig. 137–3
    - Negative
      - Hemodynamic evaluation and stabilization
        Surgical consultation
        - Rapid lavage, then colonoscopy
          - Bleeding lesion identified
            - Endoscopic therapy
              - High clinical risk
                - Intensive care
              - Low clinical risk
                - Inpatient management
          - No lesion identified
            - Angiography
              - Bleeding site identified
                - Appropriate therapy
                  - Inpatient management
              - No lesion identified
                - Radionuclide RBC scan
                  - Location identified
                    - Appropriate intervention
                      - Inpatient management
                  - No bleeding site seen
                    - No further bleeding
                      - Observation
                    - Exsanguinating hemorrhage
                      - Surgical therapy

FIGURE 137–4 • Approach to acute lower gastrointestinal (GI) bleeding. Nasogastric aspiration is indicated to exclude an upper gastrointestinal source. The optimal diagnostic approach is rapid colonic lavage followed by colonoscopy, which can also be therapeutic. When colonoscopy does not reveal the bleeding lesion and bleeding persists at a brisk volume, angiography may identify and control the bleeding vessel. In the absence of vigorous bleeding, a radionuclide red blood cell (RBC) scan may identify the site of more slowly bleeding lesions and guide further evaluation and therapy. Close observation is indicated in patients whose bleeding has stopped spontaneously without a definitive diagnosis. Surgical consultation early in the course is indicated. Surgical therapy, however, should be reserved for patients with an identified lesion or those with exsanguinating bleeding that cannot be controlled any other way.

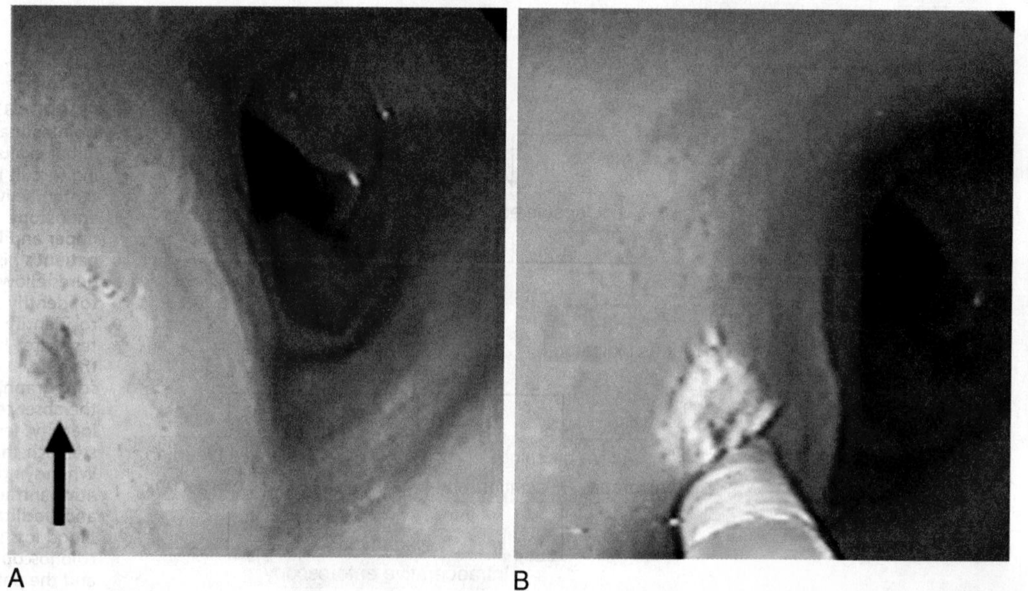

FIGURE 137–5 • Obscure gastrointestinal bleeding. A, Telangiectasia in duodenum (arrow) in a patient presenting with microcytic anemia. **B,** It was subsequently cauterized. (Courtesy of Pankaj Jay Pasricha, MD.)

TABLE 137–5 CAPSULE ENDOSCOPY FINDINGS IN 100 PATIENTS WITH OBSCURE GASTROINTESTINAL BLEEDING

Diagnosis	n
ABNORMAL FINDINGS	
Small bowel	
Angiodysplasia	21
Shallow (aphthoid or serpiginous) ulcers	5
Mucosal bleeding	5
Ulcers	4
Varices	3
Ulcerated stenosis	3
Bleeding ileal polyp	2
Tumor	1
Ulcerated anastomosis	1
Stomach	
Gastric ulcers	1
Gastric antral vascular ectasias	1
SUSPICIOUS FINDINGS	
Nonbleeding vascular ectasias	8
Venous ectasias	3
Isolated clot	1
Erosion	1
Erythematous fold	1
Nonbleeding polyp	1
NORMAL FINDINGS	
No lesion	38

Modified from Pennazio M, Santucci R, Rondonotti E, et al: Outcome of patients with obscure gastrointestinal bleeding after capsule endoscopy: Report of 100 consecutive cases. Gastroenterology 2004;126:643–653.

colonoscopy in these patients is approximately 2% for cancer and 30% for one or more colonic polyps.

Iron Deficiency Anemia

The initial approach to a patient with iron deficiency anemia (Chapter 163) depends on the presence of symptoms referable to either the upper or lower gastrointestinal tract. Regardless of the findings on the initial upper or lower endoscopic examination, all patients should have both upper and lower endoscopy because the complementary endoscopic examination has a yield of 6% even if the first one was abnormal. For premenopausal women, a positive result of fecal occult blood testing requires full evaluation, as does iron deficiency anemia. Barium radiographs of the upper and lower gastrointestinal tract have limited utility in the setting of occult bleeding because of their inability to obtain biopsy specimens or to treat lesions that are identified.

Obscure Gastrointestinal Bleeding

The evaluation of obscure gastrointestinal bleeding is often frustrating. Angiodysplasia is the most common cause in most recent series (Fig. 137–5). Initial endoscopic examination should focus on any symptoms reported by the patient. Potential causative agents, such as NSAIDs and aspirin, should be discontinued. Disorders associated with bleeding, such as hereditary hemorrhagic telangiectasia (Osler-Weber-Rendu syndrome), inflammatory bowel disease, or bleeding diathesis, should be considered. A repeated endoscopic evaluation may be appropriate because approximately one third of cases reveal a cause of bleeding overlooked during the initial endoscopy.

When upper endoscopy and colonoscopy are both unrevealing, evaluation of the small bowel is indicated. Radiographic evaluation of the small bowel is noninvasive but relatively insensitive, with a less than 6% yield from small bowel follow-through and a 10 to 21% yield from enteroclysis. By comparison, the diagnostic yield of endoscopic push enteroscopy of the small bowel in obscure gastrointestinal bleeding is 38 to 75%. Capsule endoscopy (Chapter 136), in which the patient swallows a small camera in an ingestable capsule that continuously transmits images to receivers attached to the patient's abdomen for later review to identify potential bleeding lesions, has a higher yield (60 to 90%, depending on the characteristics of bleeding) than either barium radiography or

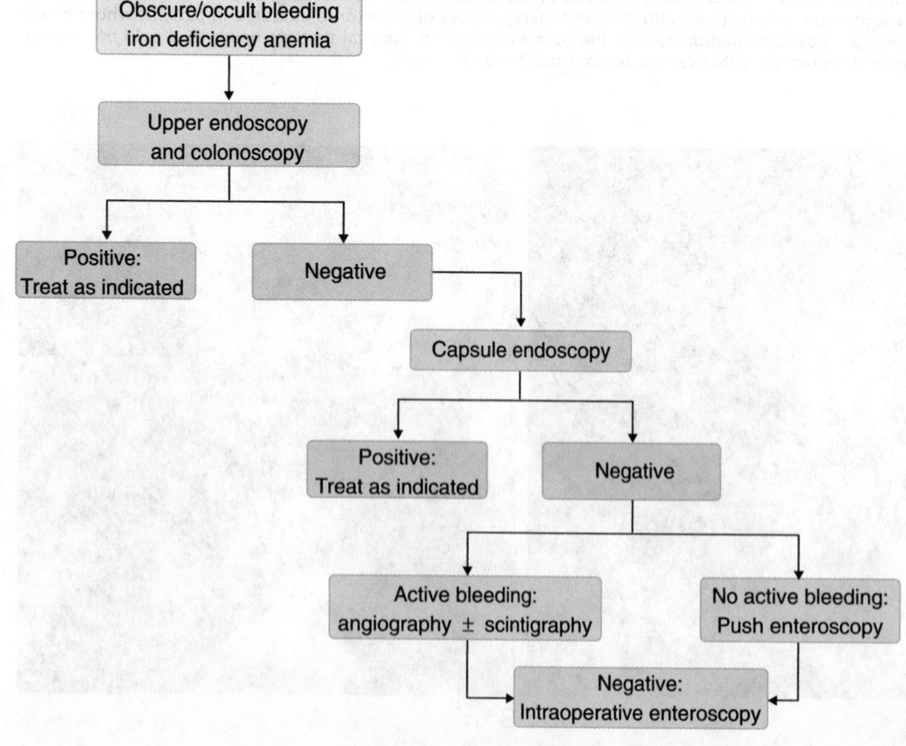

FIGURE 137–6 • Approach to obscure or occult gastrointestinal blood loss and iron deficiency anemia. Initial evaluation of low-grade gastrointestinal bleeding (occult blood, iron deficiency anemia) or intermittently active (obscure) bleeding should be upper endoscopy and colonoscopy. The choice between upper and lower endoscopy should be tailored to the patient's history and clinical condition. If these procedures allow good visualization of the mucosa and fail to identify a source, capsule endoscopy is more likely to identify a potential source than other diagnostic tests are. If capsule endoscopy is not revealing and there is evidence of active bleeding, angiography (or scintigraphy, if appropriate) may identify the lesion. In the absence of active bleeding, push enteroscopy may identify lesions in the proximal small bowel and stomach that may have been missed by prior studies. When symptoms persist after this investigation is negative, intraoperative endoscopy can identify the lesion and facilitate appropriate surgical therapy. If the blood loss stops after a normal upper endoscopy and colonoscopy, further investigations may be delayed and the patient closely observed for further bleeding.

push enteroscopy (Table 137–5). Capsule endoscopy has become the preferred method to evaluate occult and obscure bleeding when upper and lower endoscopic procedures are not revealing (Fig. 137–6).

When endoscopic evaluation does not detect the cause of blood loss, radiographic procedures such as scintigraphy and angiography should be considered. Provocative angiography with use of heparin or thrombolytic agents has been suggested by some authorities, but this approach has the potential risk of precipitating major bleeding.

In the face of continued blood loss and no identified etiology, intraoperative endoscopy may provide simultaneous diagnosis and therapy. During the procedure, the surgeon plicates the bowel over the endoscope. As the scope is withdrawn, endoscopic findings can be identified for surgical resection or treatment. The yield of this procedure exceeds 70%. In some clinical situations, the site of bleeding cannot be identified, and the patient requires long-term transfusion therapy.

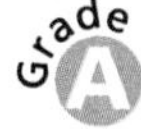

1. Lee JG, Turnipseed S, Romano PS, et al: Endoscopy-based triage significantly reduces hospitalization rates and costs of treating upper GI bleeding: A randomized controlled trial. Gastrointest Endosc 1999;50:755–761.
2. Cook DJ, Guyatt GH, Salena BJ, et al: Endoscopic therapy for acute nonvariceal upper gastrointestinal hemorrhage: A meta-analysis. Gastroenterology 1992;102:139–148.
3. Lau JYW, Sung JJY, Lam Y-H, et al: Endoscopic retreatment compared with surgery in patients with recurrent bleeding after initial endoscopic control of bleeding ulcers. N Engl J Med 1999; 340:751–756.
4. Lau JY, Leung WK, Wu JC, et al: Omeprazole before endoscopy in patients with gastrointestinal bleeding. N Engl J Med 2007;356: 1631–1640.
5. Leontiadis GI, Sharma VK, Howden CW: Proton pump inhibitor therapy for peptic ulcer bleeding: Cochrane collaboration meta-analysis of randomized controlled trials. Mayo Clin Proc 2007; 82:286–296.

SUGGESTED READINGS

Lewis JD, Brown A, Localio AR, et al: Initial evaluation of rectal bleeding in young persons: A cost-effectiveness analysis. Ann Intern Med 2002;136:99–110. *Evaluation of the colon of persons 25 to 45 years of age with otherwise asymptomatic rectal bleeding increases the life expectancy at a cost comparable to that of colon cancer screening.*

Romagnuolo J, Barkun AN, Enns R, et al: Simple clinical predictors may obviate urgent endoscopy in selected patients with nonvariceal upper gastrointestinal tract bleeding. Arch Intern Med 2007;167:265–270. *Selected patients may not require urgent endoscopy.*

Strate LL, Syngal S: Timing of colonoscopy: Impact on length of hospital stay in patients with acute lower intestinal bleeding. Am J Gastroenterol 2003;98:317–322. *A prospective study indicating that early colonoscopy decreases the length of hospital stay in patients with acute lower gastrointestinal bleeding.*

Sturniolo GC, Di Leo V, Vettorato MG, et al: Small bowel exploration by wireless capsule endoscopy: Results from 314 procedures. Am J Med 2006;119:341–347. *Visualization of the small bowel (96%) and cecum (80%) identified the source of 58% of obscure gastrointestinal bleeds and 31% of cases of suspected small bowel disease.*

138 DISORDERS OF GASTROINTESTINAL MOTILITY

Michael Camilleri

Definition

Motility disorders result from impaired control of the neuromuscular apparatus of the gastrointestinal tract. Associated symptoms include recurrent or chronic nausea, vomiting, bloating, abdominal discomfort, and constipation or diarrhea in the absence of intestinal obstruction.

Pathobiology

Normal Physiology

Neuroenteric Control

Motor function of the gastrointestinal tract depends on the contraction of smooth muscle cells and their integration and modulation by enteric and extrinsic nerves. Neurogenic modulators of gastrointestinal motility include the central nervous system, autonomic nerves, and enteric nervous system.

Extrinsic neural control of gastrointestinal motor function consists of the cranial and sacral parasympathetic outflow (excitatory to nonsphincteric muscle) and the thoracolumbar sympathetic supply (excitatory to sphincters, inhibitory to nonsphincteric muscle). The cranial outflow is predominantly through the vagus nerve, which innervates the gastrointestinal tract from the stomach to the right colon. Sympathetic fibers to the stomach and small bowel arise from T5 to T10 of the intermediolateral column of the spinal cord. The prevertebral ganglia play an important role in the integration of afferent impulses between the gut and the central nervous system and in the reflex control of abdominal viscera.

The enteric nervous system is an independent nervous system consisting of approximately 100 million neurons organized into ganglionated plexuses. The larger myenteric or Auerbach's plexus is situated between the longitudinal and circular muscle layers of the muscularis externa; this plexus contains neurons responsible for gastrointestinal motility. The submucosal or Meissner's plexus controls absorption, secretion, and mucosal blood flow. The enteric nervous system also plays an important role in visceral afferent function.

Myogenic factors regulate the electrical activity generated by gastrointestinal smooth muscle cells. Interstitial cells of Cajal form a non-neural pacemaker system at the interface of the circular and longitudinal muscle layers of the intestine and function as intermediaries between the neurogenic enteric nervous system and the myogenic control system. Electrical control activity spreads through the contiguous segments of the gut via neurochemical activation by excitatory (e.g., acetylcholine, substance P) and inhibitory (e.g., nitric oxide, somatostatin) transmitters.

Gastric and Small Bowel Motility

The motor functions of the stomach and small intestine are characterized by distinct manometric patterns of activity in the fasting and postprandial periods (Fig. 138–1). The fasting or interdigestive period is characterized by a cyclic motor phenomenon, the interdigestive migrating motor complex. In healthy individuals, one cycle of this complex is completed every 60 to 90 minutes. The complex has three phases: a period of quiescence (phase I), a period of intermittent pressure activity (phase II), and an activity front (phase III) during which the stomach and small intestine contract at highest frequencies (3 per minute in the stomach, 12 per minute in the duodenum, 8 per minute in the ileum). Another characteristic interdigestive motor pattern in the distal small intestine is the giant migrating complex, or power contraction, which empties residue from the ileum into the colon in bolus transfers.

With eating, the proximal stomach accommodates food by a vagally mediated reduction in its tone, thereby facilitating the ingestion of food without an increase in pressure. Liquids empty from the stomach in an exponential manner. The half-emptying time for non-nutrient liquids in healthy individuals is usually less than 20 minutes. Solids are retained selectively in the stomach, where they undergo acid and peptic digestion as well as "churning" or trituration by high liquid shearing forces in the antrum. Digestible food particles are emptied after their size is less than 2 mm. Gastric emptying of solids is characterized by an initial lag period followed by a linear postlag emptying phase. Secretion of hormones that mediate the motor and digestive process (e.g., gastrin for acid secretion; cholecystokinin for gallbladder contraction and bile and pancreatic secretion; and insulin, glucagon, and incretins for glucose regulation) is integrated with the arrival of food or chyme at different levels of the gut to ensure optimal digestion.

The small intestine transports solids and liquids at approximately the same rate. As a result of the lag phase for the transport of solids from the stomach, liquids typically arrive in the colon before solids. Chyme moves from ileum to colon intermittently in boluses.

In the postprandial period, the interdigestive migrating motor complex is replaced by an irregular pattern of variable amplitude and frequency. This pattern, which enables mixing and absorption, is observed

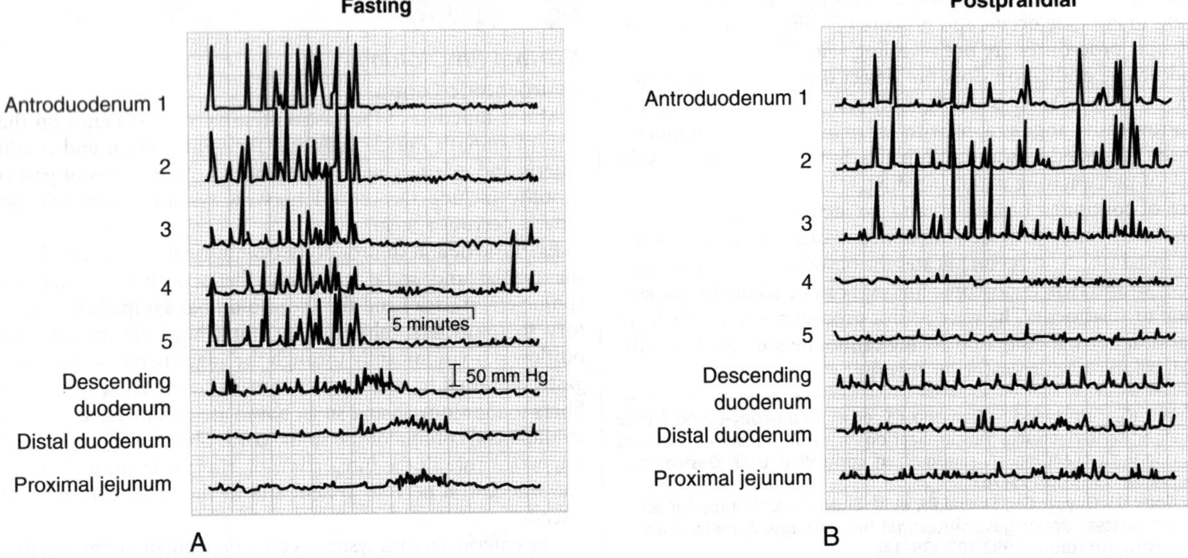

FIGURE 138–1 • Fasting and postprandial gastroduodenal manometric recordings in a healthy volunteer. A 535-kcal meal is ingested during the study. Note the cyclic interdigestive migrating motor complex **(A)** and the sustained, high-amplitude but irregular pressure activity after a meal **(B)**. (From Coulie B, Camilleri M: Intestinal pseudo-obstruction. Annu Rev Med 1999;50:37–55.)

in the regions in contact with food. The maximum frequency of contractions is lower than during phase III of the interdigestive motor complex, and the duration of this period is proportional to the number of calories consumed during the meal (about 1 hour for each 200 kcal ingested). Segments of the small intestine that are not in contact with food continue with interdigestive motor patterns.

Vomiting is characterized by a stereotypic sequence of motor events, including contractions of the stomach, abdominal muscles, and diaphragm. In humans, this sequence is followed immediately by a process similar to the migrating motor complex in the proximal small bowel.

Colonic Motility

The normal colon displays short-duration (phasic) contractions and a background contractility or tone. Nonpropagated phasic contractions have a role in segmenting the colon into haustra, which compartmentalize the colon and facilitate mixing, retention of residue, and formation of solid stool. High-amplitude propagated contractions, which are characterized by an amplitude greater than 75 mm Hg, propagation over a distance of at least 15 cm, and a propagation velocity of 0.15 to 2.2 cm/sec, contribute to the mass movements in the colon. In health, these contractions occur on average five or six times per day, most often postprandially and between 6 AM and 2 PM.

Colonic transit is a discontinuous process, slow most of the time and rapid at other times. Residue may be retained for prolonged periods in the right colon, and a mass movement may deliver the contents to the sigmoid colon in seconds. Movement of colonic content is stimulated by feeding (gastrocolonic response). In health, the average mouth-to-cecum transit time is about 6 hours, and transit times through the right colon, left colon, and sigmoid colon are about 12 hours each. As dietary fiber is increased, mean colonic transit time decreases, stool frequency increases, and stool consistency becomes softer. Decreased calorie intake slows colonic transit. Outlet obstruction in patients with pelvic floor dysfunction or voluntary suppression of defecation often is associated with slow colonic transit and decreased motor response to feeding.

Fluid reabsorption influences gastrointestinal transit. Approximately 9 L of fluid enter the gut from oral intake and endogenous secretions. The small intestine delivers about 1.5 L of fluid to the colon, where most is reabsorbed, leaving a maximum of 200 mL of water excreted in normal stool. Up to 3 L of fluid can be reabsorbed by the colon in a 24-hour period, unless the rate of ileocolonic flow or colonic motility overwhelms the colon's capacity or reabsorptive ability.

Defecation and Continence

Normal defecation requires a series of coordinated actions of the colon, rectum, pelvic floor, and anal sphincter muscles (Fig. 138–2). Filling of the rectum by a volume of 10 mL may be sensed, although the rectum can accommodate 300 mL before a sense of fullness and urge to defecate develop. Distention of the rectum results in the relaxation of the internal anal sphincter (rectoanal inhibitory reflex) and simultaneous contraction of the external anal sphincter to maintain continence. The anal transition zone can sense the difference between solid or liquid stool and gas.

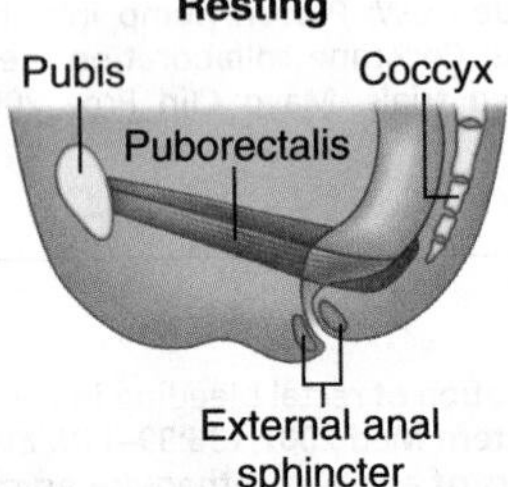

FIGURE 138–2 • Pelvic floor and anorectal functions during continence and defecation. Sagittal view through the pelvis in the resting **(A)** and straining **(B)** postures. Coordinated functions of pelvic floor (puborectalis) and anal sphincter are essential for continence and defecation.

DISEASES OF SLOW TRANSIT THROUGH THE STOMACH AND SMALL BOWEL

Pathobiology

Gastrointestinal motility disturbances (Table 138–1) result from disorders of the extrinsic nervous system, enteric nervous system, interstitial cells of Cajal (or intestinal pacemakers), or smooth muscle. Neuropathic patterns are characterized by normal amplitude but incoordinated contractions, whereas myopathies are characterized by low-amplitude contractions (average of less than 40 mm Hg in the antrum and less than 10 mm Hg in the small bowel). Combined disorders occur in systemic sclerosis (Chapter 288), amyloidosis (Chapter 296), and mitochondrial cytopathy (Chapter 447), which initially can manifest with neuropathic patterns and later display myopathic characteristics with disease progression.

TABLE 138–1 CLASSIFICATION OF GASTROPARESIS AND PSEUDO-OBSTRUCTION

Type	Neuropathic	Myopathic
Infiltrative	Progressive systemic sclerosis Amyloidosis	Progressive systemic sclerosis Amyloidosis Systemic lupus erythematosus Ehlers-Danlos syndrome Dermatomyositis
Familial	Familial visceral neuropathies	Familial visceral myopathies Metabolic myopathies
Idiopathic	Sporadic hollow visceral myopathy	Idiopathic intestinal pseudo-obstruction
Neurologic	Porphyria Heavy metal poisoning Brain stem tumor Parkinson's disease Multiple sclerosis Spinal cord transection	Myotonia Other dystrophies
Infectious	Chagas' disease Cytomegalovirus Norwalk virus Epstein-Barr virus	
Drug induced	Tricyclic antidepressants Narcotic agents Anticholinergic agents Antihypertensives Dopaminergic agents Vincristine Laxatives	
Paraneoplastic	Small cell lung cancer Carcinoid syndrome	
Postsurgical	Postvagotomy with or without pyloroplasty or gastric resection	
Endocrine	Diabetes mellitus Hypothyroidism or hyperthyroidism Hypoparathyroidism	

Genetic defects that result in congenital dysmotilities include abnormalities of *c-ret*, the gene that encodes the tyrosine kinase receptor, and abnormalities in the endothelin B system. The latter serves to retard maturation of migrating neural crest cells, thus facilitating colonization of the entire gut with nerve cells. Other abnormalities resulting in congenital dysmotility involve other transcription factors, such as Sox10, which enhances maturation of neural precursors, and *c-kit*, a marker for the interstitial cells of Cajal. Defects of *c-ret*, endothelin B, and Sox10 are associated with the phenotypic picture recognized as Hirschsprung's disease, whereas *c-kit* defects have been associated with idiopathic hypertrophic pyloric stenosis and congenital megacolon.

Extrinsic Neuropathic Disorders

Extrinsic neuropathic processes include vagotomy, trauma, Parkinson's disease (Chapter 433), diabetes (Chapter 247), amyloidosis (Chapter 296), and a paraneoplastic syndrome usually associated with small cell carcinoma of the lung (Chapter 201). Another common "neuropathic" problem in clinical practice results from the effect of medications, such as α_2-adrenergic agonists and anticholinergics, on neural control.

Damage to the autonomic nerves by trauma, infection, neuropathy, and neurodegeneration may lead to motor, secretory, and sensory disturbances, most frequently resulting in constipation. Patients with spinal cord injury (Chapter 422) above the level of the sacral segments have delayed proximal and distal colonic transit attributable to parasympathetic denervation. In these patients, fasting colonic motility and tone are normal, but the response to feeding generally is reduced or absent. Spinal cord lesions involving the sacral segments and damage to the efferent nerves from these segments disrupt the neural integration of rectosigmoid expulsion and anal sphincter control. In patients with these injuries, there is loss of contractile activity in the left colon and decreased rectal tone and sensitivity, which may lead to dilation and fecal impaction. Parkinson's disease (Chapter 433) and multiple sclerosis (Chapter 436) frequently are associated with constipation.

Enteric and Intrinsic Neuropathic Disorders

Disorders of the enteric nervous system are usually the result of a degenerative, immune, or inflammatory process. Virus-induced gastroparesis (e.g., rotavirus, Norwalk virus [Chapter 403], cytomegalovirus [Chapter 399], or Epstein-Barr virus [Chapter 400]) is associated with infiltration of the myenteric plexus with inflammatory cells. In idiopathic chronic intestinal pseudo-obstruction, there is no disturbance of the extrinsic neural control and no identified cause of the enteric nervous system abnormality.

Smooth Muscle Disorders

Disturbances of smooth muscle may result in significant disorders of gastric emptying and of transit through the small bowel and colon. These disturbances include, in descending order of prevalence, systemic sclerosis (Chapter 288), amyloidosis (Chapter 296), dermatomyositis (Chapter 290), myotonic dystrophy (Chapter 447), and metabolic muscle disorders (Chapter 447). Motility disturbances may be the result of metabolic disorders, such as hypothyroidism (Chapter 244) and hyperparathyroidism (Chapter 244), but these patients more commonly present with constipation. Scleroderma may result in focal or general dilation, diverticula, and delayed transit. The amplitude of contractions is reduced, and bacterial overgrowth may result in steatorrhea or pneumatosis intestinalis. Mitochondrial neurogastrointestinal encephalomyopathy, or familial visceral myopathy type II, is an autosomal recessive condition that may present with hepatic failure in neonates, seizures or diarrhea in infants, and hepatic failure or chronic intestinal pseudo-obstruction in adults.

Gastroparesis and Pseudo-obstruction

Clinical Manifestations

The clinical features of gastroparesis and chronic intestinal pseudo-obstruction are similar and include nausea, vomiting, early satiety, abdominal discomfort, distention, bloating, and anorexia. In severe cases, there may be considerable weight loss, with depletion of mineral and vitamin stores. Diarrhea and constipation indicate that the motility disorder extends beyond the stomach. Vomiting may be complicated by aspiration pneumonia or Mallory-Weiss esophageal tears, and patients with a generalized motility disorder may have abnormal swallowing or delayed colonic transit.

A careful family and medication history is essential. Review of systems may reveal an underlying collagen vascular disease (e.g., scleroderma) or disturbances of extrinsic neural control, including orthostatic dizziness, difficulties with erection or ejaculation, recurrent urinary tract infections, dry mouth, dry eyes, dry vagina, difficulties with visual accommodation in bright lights, and absence of sweating.

On physical examination, a succussion splash indicates stasis, typically in the stomach. The hands and mouth may show signs of Raynaud's phenomenon (Chapter 288) or scleroderma. Testing of pupillary responses (to light and accommodation), external ocular movements, blood pressure in the lying and standing positions, and general features of a peripheral neuropathy can identify patients with an associated neurologic disturbance (e.g., diabetic neuropathy) or with the oculogastrointestinal dystrophy that typically is found with mitochondrial cytopathies (see under Smooth Muscle Disorders).

The differential diagnosis includes mechanical obstruction, functional gastrointestinal disorders, anorexia nervosa, and the rumination syndrome. The rumination syndrome is a relatively common, underdiagnosed condition that presents with early (0 to 30 minutes) postprandial, effortless regurgitation of undigested food after virtually every meal.

Diagnosis

A motility disorder of the stomach or small bowel should be suspected whenever large volumes are aspirated from the stomach, particularly after an overnight fast, or when undigested solid food or large volumes of liquids are observed during esophagogastroduodenoscopy. The clinician should assess the acuity of the symptoms and the patient's state of hydration and nutrition. The goals of the evaluation are to determine what regions of the digestive tract are malfunctioning and whether the symptoms are due to a neuropathy or a myopathy (Fig. 138–3). Key steps include the following:

1. *Suspect and exclude mechanical obstruction.* In symptomatic patients with pseudo-obstruction, plain radiographs of the abdomen typically show dilated loops of small bowel with associated air-fluid levels. Mechanical obstruction should be excluded by upper gastrointestinal endoscopy and barium studies, including a small bowel follow-through. Barium studies may suggest the presence of a motor disorder, particularly if there is gross dilation, dilution of barium, or retained solid food within the stomach. These studies rarely identify the cause, however, except for systemic sclerosis, which is characterized by megaduodenum.
2. *Assess gastric and small bowel motility.* After mechanical obstruction and alternative diagnoses such as Crohn's disease (Chapter 144) have been excluded, a transit profile of the stomach or small bowel should be performed. In a gastric emptying study, ingestion of a radiolabeled meal is followed by scanning at 0, 1, 2, 3, 4, and 6 hours. If the cause of the motility disturbance is obvious, such as gastroparesis in a patient with long-standing diabetes mellitus, it is usually unnecessary to pursue further diagnostic testing. If the cause is unclear, gastroduodenal manometry by use of a multilumen tube with sensors in the distal stomach and proximal small intestine can differentiate a neuropathic process (normal-amplitude contractions but abnormal patterns of contractility) from a myopathic process (low-amplitude contractions in the affected segments).
3. *Identify the pathogenesis* (see Table 138–1). In patients with neuropathic causes of uncertain origin, tests should assess autonomic dysfunction (Chapter 445), measure type 1 antineuronal nuclear autoantibodies associated with paraneoplastic syndromes, and consider the possibility of a brain stem lesion. In patients with a myopathic disorder of unclear cause, the evaluation should consider amyloidosis (immunoglobulin electrophoresis, fat aspirate, or rectal biopsy; Chapter 296), systemic sclerosis (topoisomerase I; Chapter 288), and thyroid disease (Chapter 244). In appropriate settings, porphyria (Chapter 229) and Chagas' disease (Chapter 368) may need to be excluded. In refractory cases, referral to a specialized center may result in genetic testing or full-thickness biopsy of the small intestine (Fig. 138–4) to identify metabolic muscle disorders and mitochondrial myopathies.

   Diabetes mellitus (Chapter 247) is associated with gastroparesis, pylorospasm, intestinal pseudo-obstruction, diarrhea, constipation, and fecal incontinence. All of these manifestations may be caused by autonomic dysfunction, although more recent evidence points to acute changes in glycemia and, more important, changes in the structure and function of the enteric nervous system. The prevalence of constipation is 22% among diabetic patients with neuropathy but only 9.2% in diabetic patients without neuropathy, a rate that is not significantly different from that of healthy controls.
4. *Identify complications of the motility disorder, including bacterial overgrowth, dehydration, and malnutrition.* In patients presenting with diarrhea, it is important to assess nutritional status and to exclude bacterial overgrowth by culture of small bowel aspirates (Chapter 143). Bacterial overgrowth is relatively uncommon in neuropathic disorders but is found more often in myopathic conditions, such as scleroderma, that are associated more often with dilation or low-amplitude contractions. An empirical trial of antibiotics (see later) often is used instead of formal testing.

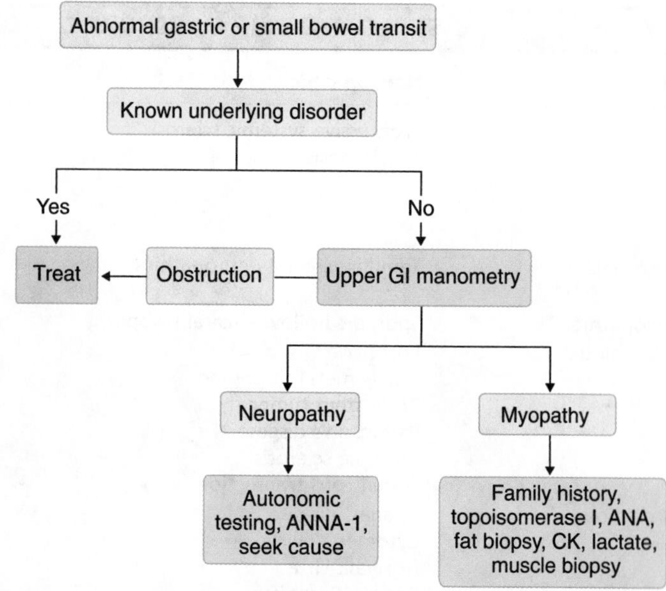

FIGURE 138–3 • Flow diagram outlines steps in diagnosis of idiopathic gastroparesis and intestinal pseudo-obstruction. ANA = antinuclear antibody; ANNA-1 = type 1 antineuronal nuclear antibody; CK = creatine kinase; GI = gastrointestinal.

Treatment

Rx

Rehydration, electrolyte repletion, and nutritional supplementation are particularly important during acute exacerbations of gastroparesis and chronic intestinal pseudo-obstruction. Initial nutritional measures include low-fiber supplements with the addition of iron, folate, calcium, and vitamins D, K, and B_{12} at the usually recommended daily levels. In patients with more severe symptoms, enteral or parenteral supplementation may be required. If it is anticipated that enteral supplementation may be needed for more than 3 months, a jejunostomy tube is recommended. Gastrostomy tubes should be avoided in patients with gastroparesis except for venting purposes.

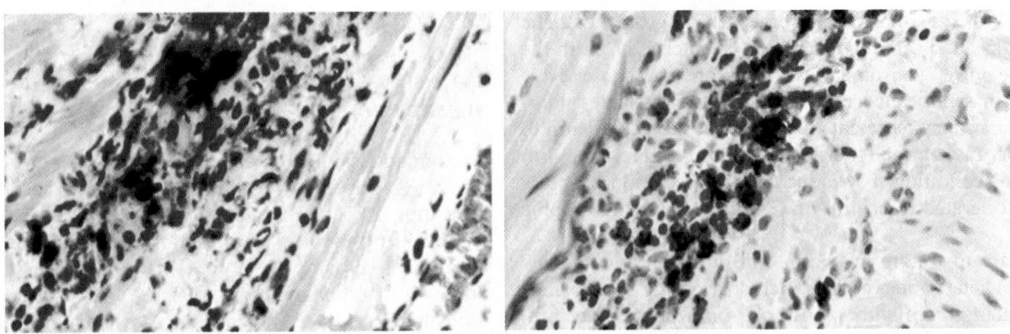

FIGURE 138–4 • Micrographs showing both types of T lymphocytes, CD4 (A) and CD8 (B), detectable within the myenteric plexus of the small intestine (proximal ileum) of a 20-year-old man with chronic intestinal pseudo-obstruction. Note the intense CD4 and CD8 immunoreactivities that represent the predominant component of the immune infiltrate observed in cases of lymphocytic ganglionitis. Alkaline phosphatase anti–alkaline phosphatase immunohistochemical technique. Original magnification ×120 in **A** and **B.** (Reproduced from De Giorgio R, Camilleri M: Human enteric neuropathies: Morphology and molecular pathology. Neurogastroenterol Motil 2004;16:515–531.)

Rx

Medical Therapy

Medications increasingly are being used to treat neuromuscular motility disorders, but there is little evidence of effectiveness in myopathic disturbances except for the rare case of dystrophia myotonica affecting the stomach and for small bowel systemic sclerosis. Metoclopramide is a dopamine antagonist with prokinetic and antiemetic properties. Antiemetic effects are due in part to its anti–5-hydroxytryptamine type 3 (HT_3) antagonist actions. Long-term use of metoclopramide is limited by the side effects of tremor and Parkinson-like symptoms. It is available in tablet or elixir form and typically is taken 30 minutes before meals and at bedtime. Usual doses are 5 to 20 mg four times daily, but patients may experience side effects (changes in affect, anxiety) at relatively low doses (30 to 40 mg/day).

Erythromycin, a macrolide antibiotic that stimulates motilin receptors at higher doses (250 to 500 mg) and cholinergic mechanisms at lower doses (40 to 80 mg), results in the dumping of solids from the stomach, accelerates gastric emptying in gastroparesis, increases the amplitude of antral contractions, and improves antroduodenal coordination. Erythromycin is most effective when it is used intravenously (3 mg/kg every 8 hours) during acute exacerbations of gastroparesis. For oral erythromycin, tolerance and gastrointestinal side effects often prevent use for longer than 1 month, but sometimes liquid erythromycin can be tolerated at 40 to 80 mg three times daily before meals.

Octreotide, a cyclized analogue of somatostatin, induces small intestinal activity that mimics phase III of the interdigestive migrating motor complex. It retards gastric emptying, decreases postprandial gastric motility, and inhibits small bowel transit. Octreotide seems to be useful in the treatment of dumping syndromes associated with accelerated transit. Octreotide may be used at night to induce migrating motor complex activity and to avoid bacterial overgrowth. If it is required during the daytime, octreotide often is combined with oral erythromycin to "normalize" the gastric emptying rate.

Antiemetics, including diphenhydramine, trifluoperazine, and metoclopramide, can treat nausea and vomiting in patients with gastroparesis and intestinal pseudo-obstruction. The more expensive serotonin 5-HT_3 antagonists (e.g., ondansetron) have not proved to be of greater benefit than these less expensive alternatives.

Antibiotic therapy is indicated in patients with documented, symptomatic bacterial overgrowth. Although formal clinical trials have not been conducted, it is common practice to use different antibiotics for 7 to 10 days each month, in an attempt to avoid resistance. Common antibiotics include doxycycline, 100 mg twice daily; metronidazole, 500 mg three times daily; ciprofloxacin, 500 mg twice daily; and double-strength trimethoprim-sulfamethoxazole, two tablets twice daily. Use of antibiotics in patients with diarrhea and fat malabsorption secondary to bacterial overgrowth results in significant symptomatic relief.

Rx

Surgical Therapy

Surgical decompression is rarely necessary in patients with chronic pseudo-obstruction. Venting enterostomy (jejunostomy) is effective, however, in relieving abdominal distention and bloating and in reducing the frequency with which nasogastric intubations and hospitalizations are required for acute exacerbations relative to the period before vent placement. Access to the small intestine by enterostomy also provides nutrients and should be considered in patients with intermittent symptoms. Surgical treatment should be considered whenever the motility disorder is localized to a resectable portion of the gut: duodenojejunostomy or duodenoplasty for patients with megaduodenum, completion gastrectomy for patients with post–gastric surgical stasis syndrome, and colectomy with ileorectostomy for intractable constipation associated with chronic colonic pseudo-obstruction.

Gastric electrical stimulation, an approved treatment, may improve gastric emptying and symptoms in patients with severe gastroparesis, but data on efficacy are inconclusive. Small bowel transplantation currently is limited to patients with intestinal failure who have reversible liver disease induced by total parenteral nutrition or who have life-threatening or recurrent catheter-related sepsis.

DISEASES OF RAPID TRANSIT THROUGH STOMACH AND SMALL BOWEL

Dumping Syndrome and Accelerated Gastric Emptying

Dumping syndrome and accelerated gastric emptying typically follow truncal vagotomy and gastric drainage procedures (Chapter 142). With the widespread use of highly selective vagotomy and the advent of effective antacid secretory therapy, these problems are becoming rare. A high calorie (usually carbohydrate) content of the liquid phase of the meal evokes a rapid insulin response with secondary hypoglycemia. These patients also may have impaired antral contractility and gastric stasis of solids, which paradoxically may result in a clinical picture of gastroparesis (for solids) and dumping (for liquids).

The management of dumping syndrome and accelerated gastric emptying emphasizes dietary maneuvers, such as avoidance of high-nutrient liquid drinks and possibly addition of guar gum or pectin to retard gastric emptying of liquids. Rarely, pharmacologic treatment with octreotide, 25 to 100 μg subcutaneously before meals, is needed to retard intestinal transit and to inhibit the hormonal responses that lead to hypoglycemia.

Rapid Transit Dysmotility of the Small Bowel

Rapid transit of material through the small bowel may occur in the setting of the irritable bowel syndrome (Chapter 139), postvagotomy diarrhea (Chapter 143), short bowel syndrome (Chapter 143), diabetic diarrhea (Chapter 143), and carcinoid diarrhea (Chapter 251). With the exception of irritable bowel syndrome, these conditions may cause severe diarrhea and result in significant losses of fluid and electrolytes. Idiopathic bile acid catharsis may represent an inability of the distal ileum to reabsorb bile acids because of rapid transit and reduced contact time with the ileal mucosa; this condition may induce colonic secretion and secondary diarrhea. Accelerated transit may be confirmed by scintigraphic studies.

Treatment goals are to restore hydration and nutrition and to slow small bowel transit. Dietary interventions include avoiding hyperosmolar drinks and replacing them with iso-osmolar or hypo-osmolar oral rehydration solutions. The fat content in the diet should be reduced to approximately 50 g/day to avoid delivery of unabsorbed fat to the colon. All electrolyte and nutritional deficiencies of calcium, magnesium, potassium, and water-soluble and fat-soluble vitamins should be corrected. In patients with less than 1 m of residual small bowel, it may be impossible to maintain fluid and electrolyte homeostasis without parenteral support. In patients with a longer residual segment, oral nutrition, pharmacotherapy, and supplements are almost always effective.

The opioid agent loperamide (4 mg 30 minutes before meals and at bedtime for a total dose of 16 mg/day) suppresses the motor response to feeding and improves symptoms but may be ineffective or cause side effects (e.g., hypotension). Verapamil (40 mg twice daily) and/or clonidine (0.1 mg twice daily) may be used in addition to loperamide. Octreotide (50 μg subcutaneously three times daily before meals) may be used in patients for whom the oral agents are ineffective or poorly tolerated. 5-HT_3 antagonists (e.g., alosetron) may be efficacious in the treatment of carcinoid diarrhea and diarrhea-predominant irritable bowel syndrome.

COLONIC MOTILITY DISORDERS

Constipation

Epidemiology

Constipation is a common clinical problem, reported by about 20% of the population, and 40% of Americans report needing to strain excessively to pass their bowel movements.

Pathobiology

In functional constipation, transit is normal, and there is no evacuation disorder. These patients may have pain in association with constipation, and there may be overlap with constipation-predominant irritable bowel syndrome (Chapter 139). In patients with acquired slow-transit constipation, unassociated with colonic dilation, the number of interstitial cells of Cajal in the different layers of the sigmoid colon is reduced compared with controls.

Idiopathic megarectum and megacolon can be either congenital or acquired; an enteric nervous system defect is suspected. In megacolon, the dilated segment shows normal phasic contractility but decreased colonic tone, with smooth muscle hypertrophy and fibrosis of the muscularis mucosa, circular muscle, and longitudinal muscle layers.

Acquired defects in the enteric nervous system may result in constipation in Chagas' disease (Chapter 368), which is caused by infection with *Trypanosoma cruzi* and results in the destruction of myenteric neurons. Acquired aganglionosis also has been reported with circulating antineuronal antibodies, with or without associated neoplasm.

Diagnosis

It is essential to distinguish an evacuation disorder, also called functional outlet obstruction (Table 138–2), from constipation resulting from slow transit or other causes. In one study in a tertiary center, 50% of 70 patients with severe, unresponsive constipation had impaired evacuation, and the remainder had constipation associated with either normal transit (also called functional constipation) or delayed colonic transit (also called slow-transit constipation). Characterization of constipated patients (Fig. 138–5) relies on the measurement of transit with radiopaque markers.

TABLE 138–2 CLINICAL CLUES SUGGESTIVE OF AN EVACUATION DISORDER

HISTORY

Prolonged straining to expel stool
Taking up unusual postures on the toilet to facilitate stool expulsion
Support of perineum or digitation of rectum or vagina to facilitate rectal emptying
Inability to expel enema fluid
Constipation after subtotal colectomy for constipation

RECTAL EXAMINATION (with patient in left lateral position)

Inspection
- Anus "pulled" forward during attempts to simulate strain during defecation
- Anal verge descends <1 cm or >4 cm during attempts to simulate strain during defecation
- Perineum balloons down during straining, and rectal mucosa prolapses through anus

Palpation
- High anal sphincter tone at rest precludes easy entry of examining finger (in absence of painful perianal condition, e.g., anal fissure)
- Anal sphincter pressure during voluntary squeeze is minimally higher than tone at rest
- Perineum descends <1 cm or >4 cm during attempts to simulate strain during defecation
- Puborectalis muscle palpable through posterior rectal wall is tender
- Palpable mucosal prolapse during straining
- "Defect" in anterior wall of the rectum, suggestive of rectocele

ANORECTAL MANOMETRY AND BALLOON EXPULSION (with patient in left lateral position)

Average anal sphincter resting tone >80 cm H_2O *or* squeeze pressure >240 cm H_2O
Failure of balloon expulsion despite addition of 200 g weight

Treatment Rx

The average daily fiber intake is around 12 g/day. In patients with normal-transit constipation, 12 to 30 g/day is effective in relief of constipation. In patients with slow-transit constipation, drug-induced constipation, or evacuation disorders, however, supplementation of 30 g of fiber per day does not result in any improvement in constipation. A second step is to add an osmotic laxative, such as a magnesium salt, to enhance the retention of fluid within the lumen by osmotic forces, to increase the fluidity, and to ease aboral transport of colonic content. Polyethylene glycol solutions (such as GoLYTELY, NuLytely, MiraLax, OCL solution) are used frequently as a second-line therapy. [1] If these measures do not suffice, a prokinetic or stimulant agent, such as bisacodyl (5 to 10 mg every 1 to 2 days) may be added.

Newer medications include the 5-HT_4 agonist tegaserod, which accelerates colonic transit and relieves constipation in patients with functional disorders. [2,3] Experimental medications that accelerate colonic transit time and relieve constipation include renzapride, a 5-HT_4 agonist; alvimopan, a mu opiate antagonist with significant potential for opiate-induced constipation; and lubiprostone, a chloride channel activator that induces fluid secretion.

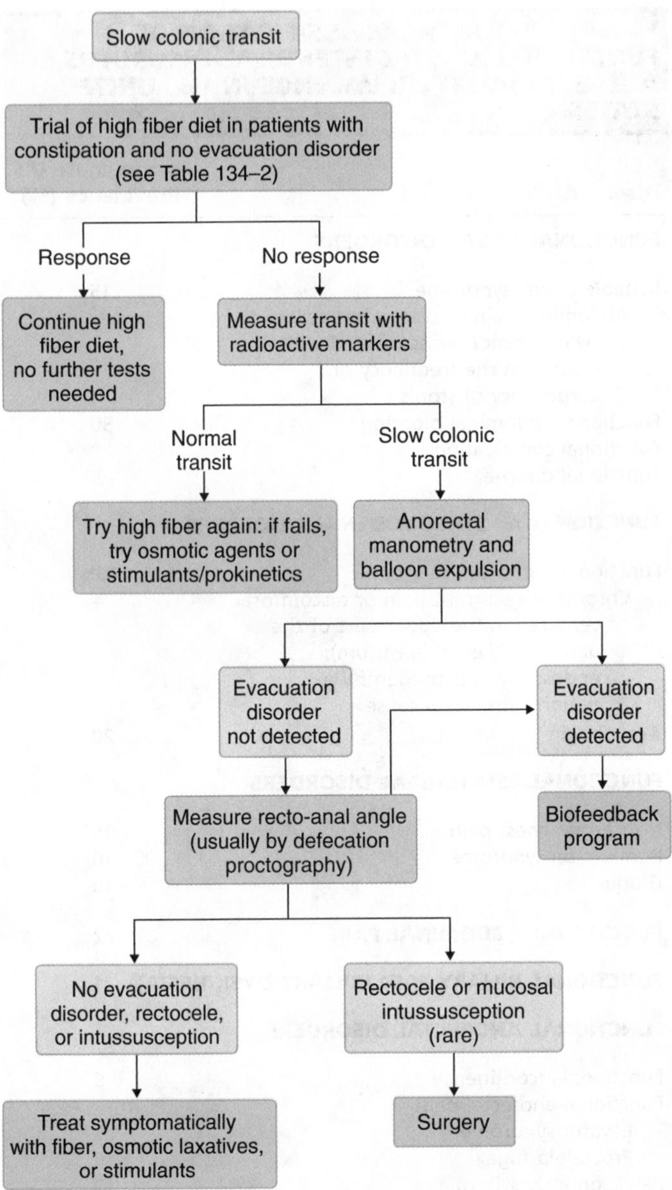

FIGURE 138–5 • Flow diagram outlines steps in the management of constipation.

Rx

When these approaches do not work, the patient should be reassessed to exclude an evacuation disorder. For evacuation disorders, a biofeedback treatment program with muscle relaxation of the anal sphincters and pelvic floor results in a 70% or greater cure rate for the constipation. The response to this treatment program is influenced by comorbidity, such as the coexistence of eating disorders or a psychological or psychiatric diagnosis.

Surgical Therapy

In patients whose constipation is not associated with an evacuation disorder and does not respond to aggressive medical therapies (including combinations described earlier), subtotal colectomy with ileorectostomy is effective in relieving constipation. Laparoscopic colectomy with ileorectostomy may achieve the same success rate with less morbidity compared with open colectomy with ileorectostomy.

Hirschsprung's Disease

Definition

Hirschsprung's disease occurs in 1 in 5000 live births. It is characterized by a localized segment of narrowing of the distal colon as a result of failure of local development of intrinsic nerves in the myenteric plexus.

Pathobiology

A relative deficiency of c-*kit*–positive interstitial cells of Cajal has been reported in Hirschsprung's disease and chronic intestinal pseudo-obstruction. Hirschsprung's disease is well characterized histologically by the absence of ganglion cells in the myenteric and submucosal plexus and the presence of hypertrophied nerve trunks in the space normally occupied by the ganglion cells. The lack of nerve growth factor receptors in the muscle layers of the colon involved with Hirschsprung's disease has been shown. The narrowing and failure of relaxation in the aganglionic segment are thought to be due to the lack of neurons containing nitric oxide synthase.

Clinical Manifestations

Hirschsprung's disease is usually diagnosed at birth because of failure to pass meconium or the presence of megacolon, although it may be identified in childhood as a result of fecal retention, constipation, or abdominal distention. Onset of symptoms or diagnosis after the age of 10 years is rare.

Diagnosis

Diagnosis is based on the typical focal narrowing of the colon, the absence of the rectoanal inhibitory reflex (relaxation of anal sphincter pressure at rest during distention of a balloon in the rectum depends on natural preservation and maturation of intrinsic nerves in the distal bowel), and a deep rectal biopsy specimen showing absence of submucosal neurons with hypertrophied nerve trunks.

Treatment

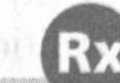

Treatment involves excision of the affected bowel segment or a pull-through procedure by which normal bowel is anastomosed to the cuff of the rectum, just above the anal sphincters.

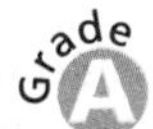

1. Dipalma JA, Cleveland MV, McGowan J, et al: A randomized multicenter, placebo-controlled trial of polyethylene glycol laxative for chronic treatment of chronic constipation. Am J Gastroenterol 2007;102:1436–1441.
2. Fried M, Johanson JF, Gwee KA, et al: Efficacy of tegaserod in chronic constipation in men. Am J Gastroenterol 2007;102: 362–370.
3. Tack J, Muller-Lissner S, Bytzer P, et al: A randomised controlled trial assessing the efficacy and safety of repeated tegaserod therapy in women with irritable bowel syndrome with constipation. Gut 2005;54:1707–1713.

SUGGESTED READINGS

Camilleri M: Diabetic gastroparesis. N Engl J Med 2007;356:820–829. *Clinical recommendations for treating a patient with diabetic gastroparesis.*

Connor FL, Di Lorenzo C: Chronic intestinal pseudo-obstruction: Assessment and management. Gastroenterology 2006;130(2 Suppl 1):S29–36. *A clinical review.*

Lembo A, Camilleri M: Chronic constipation. N Engl J Med 2003;349:1360–1368. *Review of the causes, mechanisms, diagnosis, and treatment of constipation.*

139 FUNCTIONAL GASTROINTESTINAL DISORDERS: IRRITABLE BOWEL SYNDROME, DYSPEPSIA, AND NONCARDIAC CHEST PAIN

Nicholas J. Talley

In clinical practice, most patients with chronic or recurrent gastrointestinal symptoms do not have a structural or biochemical explanation identified by routine diagnostic tests. These patients are labeled as having a functional gastrointestinal disorder. Functional does not imply a psychiatric disturbance or absence of disease but rather a known or suspected underlying disorder of gut function. Based on clinical and epidemiologic studies, functional gastrointestinal disorders have been classified according to the presumed anatomic site of the disorder (Table 139–1). The most widely recognized functional gastrointestinal disorders are irritable bowel syndrome (IBS), functional (or nonulcer) dyspepsia, and functional (or noncardiac) chest pain.

IRRITABLE BOWEL SYNDROME

Definition

Previously, most patients with unexplained abdominal pain or bowel dysfunction were labeled as having IBS, but IBS is now thought to be characterized by chronic or recurrent abdominal pain or discomfort and an erratic disturbance in defecation. Bloating is also common.

Epidemiology

Symptoms consistent with IBS are reported by one in six Americans; similar prevalence rates have been found in Europe, Australia, and Asia. The prevalence is greater in women, may be higher in whites than in blacks, and is lower in people older than 60 years. Approximately 30% of persons with IBS become asymptomatic over time.

Only about a third of persons with IBS consult a physician, but the condition still accounts for about 12% of primary care visits. The first manifestation typically occurs between the ages of 30 and 50 years. Persons who seek care for IBS tend to have more severe abdominal pain; a greater frequency and severity of nongastrointestinal symptoms such as headache, fatigue, or menstrual pain; and greater psychological distress.

TABLE 139–1 ROME CLASSIFICATION OF FUNCTIONAL GASTROINTESTINAL DISORDERS AND ESTIMATED PREVALENCE IN THE UNITED STATES

Disorder	Approximate U.S. Prevalence (%)
FUNCTIONAL BOWEL DISORDERS	
Irritable bowel syndrome	15
Abdominal pain or discomfort relieved by defecation or associated with a change in the frequency or consistency of stools	
Functional abdominal bloating	30
Functional constipation	20
Functional diarrhea	<5
FUNCTIONAL GASTRODUODENAL DISORDERS	
Functional (nonulcer) dyspepsia	15*
Chronic or recurrent pain or discomfort centered in the upper part of the abdomen (i.e., epigastrium); endoscopy fails to identify a definite structural cause	
Aerophagia	20
FUNCTIONAL ESOPHAGEAL DISORDERS	
Noncardiac chest pain	15
Rumination syndrome	10
Globus	10
FUNCTIONAL ABDOMINAL PAIN	<2
FUNCTIONAL BILIARY PAIN (BILIARY DYSKINESIA)	<1
FUNCTIONAL ANORECTAL DISORDERS	
Functional incontinence	5
Functional anorectal pain	
Levator syndrome	5
Proctalgia fugax	10
Pelvic floor dyssynergia	10

*Assumes that one third with dyspepsia have a structural explanation and are excluded.

Pathobiology

Accumulating evidence suggests that IBS represents a true disorder of function, but some patients also have abnormal structure. The symptoms are neither imagined nor the result of a psychiatric disorder.

Abnormal Motor Function

IBS is associated with a generalized disorder of smooth muscle function; the colon, small bowel, upper gastrointestinal tract, gallbladder, and urinary tract may all be affected. Basal colonic motility is normal in IBS, but these patients tend to have an abnormally responsive colon to meals, drugs, gut hormones (e.g., cholecystokinin), and stress. The motility of the distal end of the colon after meals (the gastrocolonic response) is augmented in patients with IBS and may explain why postprandial cramps or discomfort is common. Increased fasting colonic contractions and rapid colonic transit in the proximal part of the colon have been linked to diarrhea, whereas a reduction in high-amplitude propagated contractions in the left colon has been linked to constipation (Chapter 138).

Abdominal pain in IBS has been associated with an exaggerated ileal response with high postprandial pressure waves (prolonged propagated contractions). Fasting clusters of jejunal pressure waves (discrete clustered contractions) occur in some patients with IBS, appear to coincide with abdominal pain, and disappear during sleep.

Disturbed Sensation

The vagal (and spinal) afferent nerves conduct sensory information from the gut through the dorsal horn neurons to the brain. Abnormal perception of gut sensation (visceral hypersensitivity) is a characteristic finding in IBS. In response to rectal or colonic distention by a balloon, a subset of patients with IBS sense the distention at lower volumes or pressures (or both) than healthy persons do. Many patients complain of unsatisfactory defecation or incomplete rectal emptying, which may be a direct result of excess rectal sensitivity. Repetitive rapid sigmoid distention induces rectal hypersensitivity in patients with IBS but not in healthy controls. The mechanisms that lead to increased gut visceral sensitivity are unclear, and patients with IBS do not have generalized lower pain thresholds in other parts of their bodies.

Central Nervous System

The brain modulates gut sensory and motor function and vice versa. In response to rectal distention, patients with IBS have increased activation of the limbic or emotional motor system compared with normal control subjects. These abnormalities may help explain why patients with IBS have visceral hypersensitivity.

A high proportion of patients with a diagnosis of IBS in tertiary referral centers (40 to 60%) have coexisting psychiatric disease, including depression or panic disorder, or a history of sexual or physical abuse.

Patients seen by primary care physicians and persons with IBS who do not seek medical help have a lower prevalence of psychiatric comorbidity. Psychosocial stress, particularly at a young age, may predispose to IBS based on animal models, but convincing human data are not available. Personality, level of social support, and childhood experiences influence how a patient responds to a chronic illness such as IBS.

Infection

From 5 to 30% of patients have persistent colonic symptoms after a history of traveler's diarrhea or gastroenteritis (e.g., *Salmonella* or *Campylobacter*). Prospective studies of patients in whom severe, acute gastroenteritis develops suggest that IBS may develop in up to one in eight. *Candida* does not cause new-onset IBS. Based on breath testing, some centers have reported high rates of bacterial overgrowth in IBS, but this finding remains controversial.

Inflammation

Low-grade colonic inflammation, including a small increase in the number of activated T cells, is seen on biopsy specimens from a subset of patients with IBS, either after acute infection or de novo. Increased mast cells close to colonic nerves may correlate with abdominal pain.

Serotonin

In postinfectious IBS, some patients have increased numbers of serotonin-containing (enterochromaffin) cells, and plasma levels of serotonin may be increased. Moreover, the amount of serotonin transporter in the colonic mucosa may be reduced, thus supporting the concept that excess serotonin contributes to this disorder. Excess serotonin could induce diarrhea until receptor desensitization occurs, followed by constipation.

Diet

True food allergy seems to be rare, but food intolerance may be more important. Lactase deficiency may coexist with IBS and exacerbate symptoms. Excess ingestion of sorbitol or fructose induces diarrhea and bloating. Short-chain fatty acids stimulate prolonged propagated contractions in the ileum. Dietary exclusion has resulted in symptomatic improvement in approximately 50% of patients with functional diarrhea (in whom pain is not a prominent feature), but a response is probably less frequent in those with IBS. No single food group has been implicated, although foods such as wheat, yeast, nuts, eggs, and dairy products may be most important.

Genetics

There is increasing evidence that IBS has a genetic predisposition based on family aggregation and twin studies. Gene associations have been reported, but these findings remain to be confirmed.

Clinical Manifestations

Symptoms and Signs

Chronic or recurrent abdominal pain or discomfort is always a feature of IBS. The pain commonly occurs in the lower part of the abdomen but may be present at any location and tends to be variable in quality, severity, and duration. Classically, the pain is cramplike or aching and occurs in episodes. The pain of IBS is relieved by defecation or is associated with a change in stool frequency or consistency. Pain from IBS rarely awakens the patient from sleep. Pain related to exercise, urination, or menstruation is unlikely to be due to IBS. Chronic unremitting pain for more than 6 months unrelated to defecation is never due to IBS but most often represents a chronic pain syndrome (functional abdominal pain).

An irregular disturbance in defecation (predominant constipation or diarrhea or an alternating bowel pattern) is also a key feature of IBS, and its absence excludes the diagnosis. Constipation may refer to a decreased frequency of stools, passage of hard stools or lumps, excessive straining, or an inability to empty the rectum adequately. To a patient, diarrhea may mean loose or watery stools, increased stool frequency, passage of mucus, urgency, or even fecal incontinence.

Bloating is a common symptom in IBS. There may be visible abdominal distention such that patients can see that their abdomen is distended or feel that they have to loosen their clothes. Sometimes, women complain that they look pregnant.

Symptoms of gastroesophageal reflux (heartburn or acid regurgitation) are reported by a third of patients with IBS. A third of patients also report dyspepsia (epigastric pain or discomfort). Nausea, usually without vomiting, is common. Some patients have difficulty swallowing, but the complaint is most often the sensation of a lump in the throat between meals (globus). Urinary frequency, dysuria, nocturia, and urinary urgency may occur, as may dyspareunia and dysmenorrhea. Fatigue, headache, and back pain are common. None of these extraintestinal symptoms, however, is helpful diagnostically.

Transient bowel symptoms should not be confused with IBS. Patients who have recently had to rest in bed, have undergone a surgical procedure, or have lost weight may become constipated. Similarly, in patients who have been under acute stress, "nervous diarrhea" may develop. Pregnancy, various dietary indiscretions, traveler's diarrhea, food poisoning, and viral or bacterial gastroenteritis may all cause temporary bowel disturbances.

Physical Examination

Physical examination is useful to exclude organic disease. Patients with IBS may have abdominal scars as a result of their higher rates of cholecystectomy, appendectomy, and hysterectomy, in part because of failure to recognize the condition. Abdominal tenderness is a common, nonspecific finding; localized abdominal tenderness that persists after tensing the abdominal wall muscles (e.g., by asking the patient to do a half sit-up) usually indicates abdominal wall pain (e.g., from nerve entrapment, muscle strain, or myositis), which should not be confused with functional gastrointestinal pain, and typically responds to infiltration of a local anesthetic or steroid, or both.

Diagnosis

Clinical Examination

It is important to make a positive clinical diagnosis of IBS by a careful history and physical examination. The Rome criteria for IBS are specific for the syndrome: two or more of (1) pain (or discomfort) relieved by defecation, (2) pain associated with increased or decreased stool frequency, or (3) pain associated with harder or looser stools.

In older patients and those with "red flags" (e.g., unexplained weight loss, persistent vomiting, prominent diarrhea, bleeding, anemia, steatorrhea, fever, strong family history of colon cancer), investigations are mandatory to exclude important diseases that may be confused with IBS (Fig. 139–1). Otherwise, investigations have a low yield and may be omitted based on clinical judgment; exhaustive testing before making IBS the diagnosis of exclusion should be discouraged. Flexible sigmoidoscopy is useful to exclude ulcerative colitis but is not required routinely. Rectal biopsy specimens may be obtained from patients with predominant diarrhea to exclude collagenous or microscopic colitis, but the yield is low and unlikely to be cost-effective. In patients older than 50 years with new-onset symptoms, either colonoscopy or a double-contrast barium enema with flexible sigmoidoscopy is mandatory.

Laboratory Findings

The yield from laboratory tests is low in patients with typical symptoms and no red flags. Of those with typical IBS symptoms, up to 5% may have undiagnosed celiac disease (Chapter 143). Screening for celiac disease (e.g., tissue transglutamase antibodies) should be considered, especially if the patient has predominant diarrhea or bloating. Less commonly, celiac disease can be manifested as constipation-type IBS symptoms. Positive screening tests are an indication for performing small bowel biopsy. Thyroid-stimulating hormone levels should be measured if there is clinical suspicion of hyperthyroidism (diarrhea) or hypothyroidism (constipation). Lactose intolerance causes diarrhea and bloating and is common in certain racial groups (e.g., blacks, Asians, Native Americans, and Jews); however, a substantial amount of lactose generally needs to be ingested to induce symptoms. Resolution of symptoms with a 2-week trial of a lactose-free diet suggests clinically relevant lactase deficiency; the diagnosis can be confirmed with a lactose hydrogen breath test. Testing for bacterial overgrowth is not routine.

If severe pain is predominant, a plain abdominal radiograph is indicated during an acute episode to exclude bowel obstruction or another pathologic process. Gynecologic examination may detect evidence of endometriosis or fibroids. Endometriosis classically causes mid–

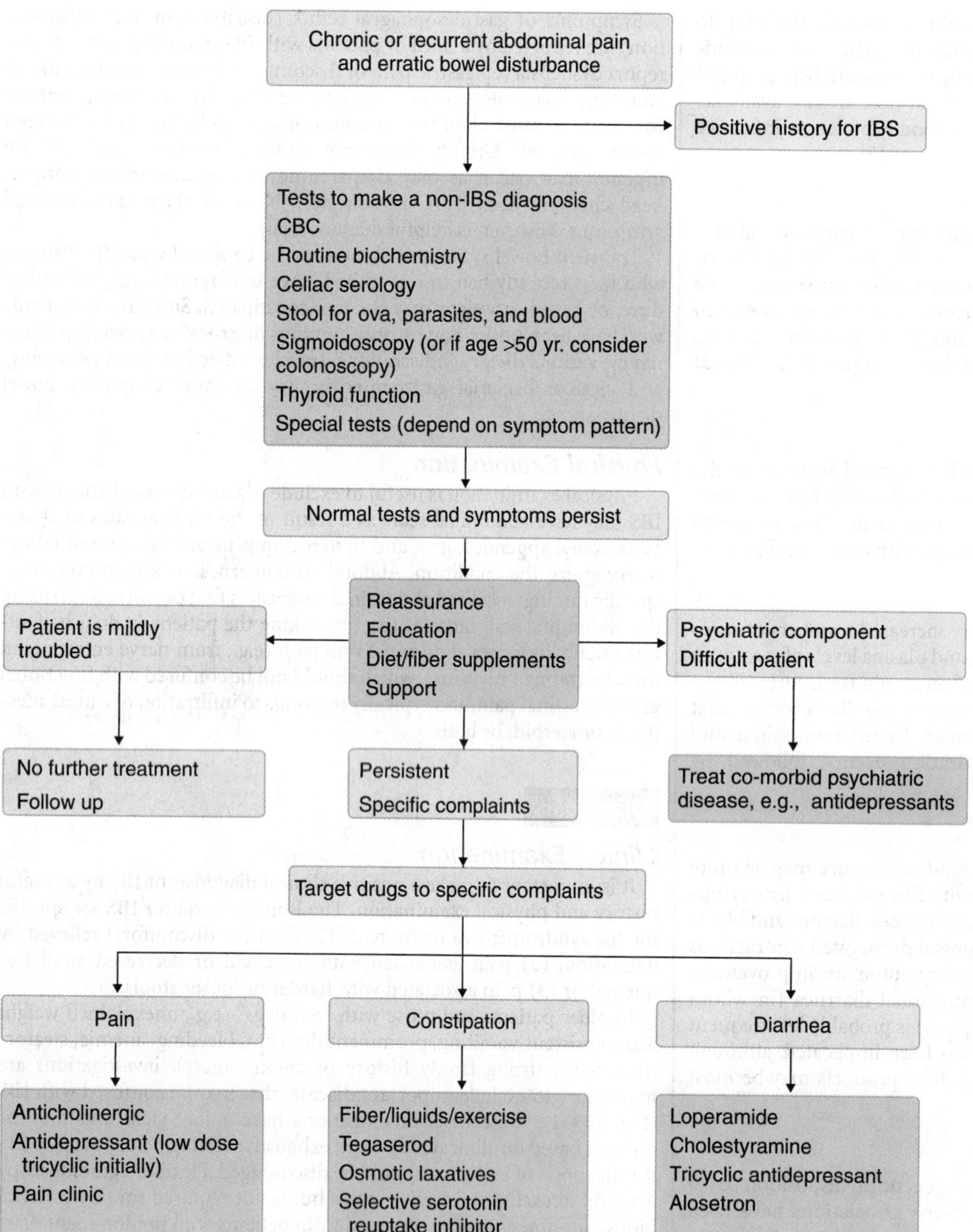

FIGURE 139–1 • Algorithm for the evaluation of suspected irritable bowel syndrome (IBS). CBC = complete blood count.

menstrual cycle pain that can be associated with disturbed defecation; pelvic ultrasonography is a helpful screening test, but laparoscopy is often required. Pelvic inflammatory disease should be considered if a vaginal discharge is present. When a firm diagnosis of IBS has been made, subsequent testing has an extremely low yield and should not be undertaken unless symptoms have changed.

Differential Diagnosis

Constipation

Colonic Inertia

Colonic inertia (Chapter 138) is characterized by the passage of stools once a week or less, usually affects women, and may be diagnosed by a radiopaque marker study, such as having the patient ingest 24 radiopaque markers on 3 separate days and obtaining a single plain abdominal radiograph on the fourth day. By counting the number of markers retained, total colonic transit can be calculated in hours (by multiplying by 1.2). A total colonic transit time greater than 72 hours is grossly abnormal and suggests colonic inertia.

Pseudo-obstruction

Patients with chronic idiopathic intestinal pseudo-obstruction typically have recurrent abdominal pain, visible distention, vomiting, and either constipation (because of colonic or small bowel inertia, or both) or diarrhea (because of bacterial overgrowth). This diagnosis must be considered in patients with colonic inertia. A small bowel barium follow-through to look for dilation of the small intestine is the initial investigation of choice. Small bowel and colonic transit can be measured scintigraphically and is usually delayed in intestinal pseudo-obstruction. Small bowel manometry is confirmatory. Definitive diagnosis requires a full-thickness small intestinal biopsy specimen at laparoscopy or laparotomy.

Dyschezia

Dyschezia refers to difficult defecation, which the patient may describe as straining, feelings of incomplete evacuation or anal blockage, or having to assist defecation by digitally pressing in or around the anus. The symptoms may be part of IBS. Dyschezia may occasionally also be due to mechanical causes, such as rectal prolapse or disease (e.g., aganglionosis of the bowel in Hirschsprung's disease [Chapter 138]) or, more commonly, pelvic floor dysfunction.

Pelvic Floor Dysfunction

Pelvic floor dysfunction refers to paradoxical contraction or failure of relaxation of the pelvic floor during attempts to defecate. Failure to relax the external anal sphincter or puborectalis muscle (or both) obstructs defecation and causes constipation. Pelvic floor function can be evaluated by anorectal manometry and by the inability to expel a balloon. Stool softeners and habit retraining are the first steps in management. Biofeedback to teach relaxation of the pelvic floor during straining is efficacious but expensive.

Diarrhea

Patients with persistent diarrhea (Chapter 143) should have stools screened for ova, cysts, and parasites, although the yield is low. Stool testing for fecal white cells, a Gram stain, bacterial culture, fecal fat, and blood should also be considered. If stool volume is increased (>400 mL/24 hr), additional tests are indicated. Laxative abuse must be excluded, especially in women with recalcitrant symptoms. Osmotic laxatives can be detected by measuring stool electrolytes and osmolality and detecting an osmotic gap. A small bowel barium radiograph or computed tomographic enterography is useful to rule out Crohn's disease (Chapter 144). Bacterial overgrowth, detectable by hydrogen breath testing and confirmed by a small bowel aspirate and quantitative culture, may occur in patients with small bowel diverticula or impaired small bowel motility.

Anal Pain

Sudden severe pain in the anal area persisting for seconds or minutes and then completely resolving is usually due to proctalgia fugax, which should not be confused with IBS. The attacks are typically infrequent and require no treatment. Local application of heat or pressure to the perianal area may be helpful. Inhaled salbutamol (90 µg/puff, two puffs as needed), topical nitroglycerin (0.3% as needed), and injection of botulinum toxin have been used. Proctalgia fugax should be distinguished from levator ani syndrome, which is characterized by chronic or recurrent rectal pain or aching in episodes typically lasting 20 minutes or longer. Treatment is difficult, but sitz baths, digital massage of the levator ani muscle, muscle relaxants, or biofeedback may be helpful. Levator ani syndrome can be distinguished from coccygodynia, in which there is tenderness on pressing over the coccyx.

Treatment

Rx

General Measures

Physician-Patient Relationship

A good physician-patient relationship is therapeutic in IBS. Reassurance and explanation remain essential components of management. It is important to provide the patient with a positive diagnosis and explain the probable pathogenesis. Although there is some debate whether IBS is a real disease, most clinicians accept that it is and patients should be so advised. It is important to tell the patient that the symptoms are real. Patients need to be advised that IBS is not life-threatening and does not cause cancer. Although symptoms may be lifelong, they tend to come and go, sometimes with prolonged remissions. Physicians who order an extensive battery of tests without explanation and then tell their patients that they do not believe there is a serious underlying disease are likely to engender confusion.

Aggravating Medications or Drugs

A change in medications may improve symptoms, and unnecessary drugs should be avoided. Constipation may be aggravated by anticholinergics, opiates, psychotropics, aluminum-containing antacids, bile acid–binding resins, calcium-channel blockers, or nonsteroidal anti-inflammatory drugs (NSAIDs). Diarrhea may be exacerbated by magnesium-containing antacids, sorbitol-containing cough syrups, antibiotics, and laxatives. Heavy alcohol use and caffeine or decaffeinated products may precipitate symptoms. Persons who chew gum may ingest enough sorbitol to induce symptoms.

Stress and Psychiatric Symptoms

Reduction of stress may be helpful. Fear of serious disease or coexistent psychiatric disease frequently precipitates the decision to seek medical attention and must be identified and addressed. Panic disorder is characterized by abrupt discrete episodes of extreme fear or apprehension associated with other symptoms, which may include abdominal pain, nausea, palpitations, chest pain, dyspnea, dizziness, flushing, a choking or smothering sensation, sweating, and fainting. Depression may cause sleep disturbances, mood alterations, and weight loss and may coexist with IBS. If gastrointestinal symptoms are a minor component in patients with a multitude of generalized symptoms, somatization disorder should be considered.

Dietary Recommendations

Increasing dietary fiber with unprocessed bran makes stools bulkier, softer, and easier to pass and can relieve constipation. Urgency may also improve. The effect is maximal if at least 30 g of fiber is taken daily, approximately double the normal American dietary fiber intake. Fiber content must be increased slowly to reduce the bloating and flatulence that are often induced initially. Some patients with IBS and diarrhea or abdominal pain also improve with increased dietary fiber, whereas others may get worse. However, the available clinical trial evidence suggests that wheat bran is no better than placebo in IBS. A bulking agent (e.g., psyllium fiber supplement) is effective [1] and should be started at a low once-daily dose of approximately 3 to 6 g and increased slowly every 1 to 2 weeks until a total of 15 to 20 g is being ingested in divided doses two to three times per day. A gluten-free diet is of uncertain value in IBS in the absence of celiac disease, although the few patients with latent sprue should respond. In one randomized trial, a diet excluding IgG-positive foods (vs. a sham diet) resulted in an improved global symptom score in IBS over a period of 3 months.

Fad diets and high-fat diets should be avoided. Cabbage, beans, legumes, and lentils may be worth avoiding because they are fermented in the colon and may increase flatus.

Avoidance of milk products may be helpful, even in some patients without lactose intolerance. An elimination diet and double-blind reintroduction of foods may be undertaken in patients with suspected food sensitivity and diarrhea, but compliance is often poor. Regular exercise and adequate fluid intake are recommended in patients with predominant constipation, although any benefit is uncertain. Follow-up in 3 to 6 weeks allows the physician to determine the response to initial therapy, reassess psychosocial issues, and continue to support the patient.

Medical Therapy

The placebo response in IBS is 30 to 60%, in part because of the fluctuating nature of IBS symptoms and the tendency for patients to seek care when their symptoms are worse and then improve spontaneously. Drugs must be used sparingly in IBS because at best they provide symptomatic, not disease-modifying therapy.

In patients who complain of postprandial abdominal pain, antispasmodics may be useful when administered 30 to 60 minutes before meals to reduce the gastrocolonic response. Alternatives include hyoscyamine (e.g., one to two sustained-release capsules twice daily), belladonna (0.6 mL four times daily), dicyclomine (20 to 40 mg four times daily), and propantheline bromide (7.5 or 15 mg four times daily). However, there is little evidence that anticholinergics are superior to placebo in IBS. Anticholinergic side effects, including dry mouth, blurred vision, and urinary retention, may require dose reduction. Peppermint oil may also be modestly useful for IBS symptoms in some patients.

Patients who do not respond to dietary fiber for treatment of constipation may benefit from the 5-HT_4 agonist tegaserod (6 mg twice daily), which is a prokinetic agent that is well tolerated and has shown a 5 to 15% improvement in global relief over placebo in women with constipation-predominant IBS. [2] Alternatively, polyethylene glycol (e.g., MiraLax, 17 g of powder once daily) can improve constipation but probably not pain. Lactulose, sorbitol, or milk of magnesium can be titrated to treat constipation, depending on the clinical response. In severe cases, lubiprostone (24 µg twice daily) can help constipation. Stimulant laxatives, such as bisacodyl, senna, and docusate, should generally be avoided because of potential harmful effects such as water and electrolyte loss and aggravation of pain; the theoretical concern that long-term use would predispose to damage to the colonic myenteric plexus has almost

certainly been exaggerated. Colchicine (0.6 mg up to three times daily) sometimes improves constipation but may rarely cause a neuromyopathy. Metoclopramide and domperidone are not efficacious in constipation.

The pharmacologic agent of choice for predominant diarrhea is initially loperamide at a dose of 2 to 4 mg three to four times per day. Loperamide slows intestinal transit and increases intestinal water absorption; it is best taken to prevent diarrhea and not after the event. It causes rebound constipation on cessation in some cases. Abdominal pain is not relieved by loperamide. Diphenoxylate is an alternative but can cause sedation. A bile acid–sequestering agent such as cholestyramine (4 g two to four times daily) may be helpful, particularly in postcholecystectomy patients with refractory diarrhea caused by idiopathic bile acid malabsorption. Aluminum hydroxide or bismuth subsalicylate used intermittently can be helpful, but long-term use should be avoided.

In severe unresponsive cases of diarrhea, alosetron (starting at 1 mg daily), a 5-HT_3 antagonist, slows intestinal transit and relaxes the colon, so it is beneficial for diarrhea and fecal urgency. Alosetron is superior to placebo in diarrhea-predominant IBS, [3] but it is approved by the Food and Drug Administration only for women with severe diarrhea-predominant IBS. Side effects include severe constipation and ischemic colitis, and it is contraindicated in patients with any constipation. Patients who have fecal incontinence may respond to loperamide or biofeedback treatment, depending on the underlying cause.

Simethicone is not usually helpful for bloating. Activated charcoal can reduce flatus after a lactulose challenge in normal persons, but whether it is of benefit in IBS has not been established. α-D-Galactosidase may be helpful in some patients after a vegetable meal to reduce flatus. Treatment of constipation may reduce bloating. Antibiotics such as rifaximin, a nonabsorbed antibiotic, have been reported in a few studies to have some benefit on IBS symptoms.

The probiotic bifidobacterium reduced pain and bloating in one randomized trial. VSL#3 (450 billion lyophilized bacteria per day) has improved bloating but not other symptoms in IBS. The nonabsorbed oral antibiotic rifaximin improves symptoms for up to 10 weeks after its discontinuation. [4]

Tricyclic antidepressants are particularly useful in resistant patients or those with chronic pain because of their anticholinergic effects or central modulation of sensation, or both. Benefits may occur within 3 to 4 weeks even in patients without symptoms of depression. Tricyclic antidepressants should be started at a low dose in the evening (e.g., amitriptyline or desipramine, 10 or 25 mg). If this dose fails, the dose can be titrated slowly upward, although the drugs may worsen constipation. Amitriptyline causes a high incidence of anticholinergic side effects, whereas desipramine causes fewer anticholinergic problems. Other side effects include nausea, weight gain, drowsiness, tremor, postural hypotension, arrhythmias, and rarely cholestasis. Although there is less experience with selective serotonin re-uptake inhibitors (e.g., fluoxetine, citalopram, paroxetine, sertraline) in IBS, these drugs may be useful, especially in constipation-predominant IBS when begun once daily in the morning at full dose (e.g., paroxetine, 20 mg daily [5]); side effects are less than with tricyclic antidepressants but include nausea, diarrhea, and weight loss. If antidepressant therapy is successful, it should usually be continued for 3 to 12 months, and then the dose should be tapered and use of the drug terminated.

Anxiolytics may induce a rebound effect on withdrawal, are potentially habituating, and interact with other drugs and alcohol; currently available benzodiazepines should be avoided in most patients. Leuprolide acetate, a gonadotropin-releasing hormone analogue, initially seemed to improve some symptoms in women with severe functional gastrointestinal complaints, but in clinical practice the drug is rarely used because of its side effects.

Ancillary and Other Therapies

Patients who fail to respond to usual pharmacologic therapy should be encouraged to join a local IBS support group. If referral to a mental health professional is being contemplated, patients should be reassured that this referral is part of a team approach. Relaxation therapy, hypnosis, cognitive behavioral therapy, and psychotherapy seem to be of value, particularly in patients with moderate symptoms who are motivated and can identify a link between emotional difficulties or stressful events and their symptoms. [6] Diarrhea and abdominal pain generally respond better than abdominal distention or constipation. Conversely, patients with chronic, constant pain for many years and those who are resistant to the idea that psychological factors are related to their illness are unlikely to respond.

Prognosis

When a positive diagnosis of IBS has been made, it is rarely altered later. Most patients continue to be intermittently symptomatic. The life expectancy of patients with IBS is no different from that of the background population.

FUNCTIONAL (NONULCER) DYSPEPSIA

Definition

Dyspepsia refers to persistent or recurrent epigastric pain or meal-related upper abdominal discomfort that may be characterized by early satiation or postprandial fullness. Heartburn (typically a burning pain or discomfort that rises up the retrosternum) (Chapter 134) is distinct from dyspepsia. Dyspepsia is not restricted to meal-related pain because patients with peptic ulcer disease often report pain unrelated to meals. With the widespread availability and use of endoscopy, it has become evident that a structural explanation is found in just a minority of patients with new-onset dyspepsia and that most patients have functional (or nonulcer) dyspepsia (see Table 139–1).

Epidemiology

Population-based studies from around the world indicate that the prevalence of dyspepsia is about 25%. In the United States, only one person in four with dyspepsia seeks medical care, however.

Pathobiology

Mucosal Inflammation and Helicobacter pylori

H. pylori infection is the most common cause of histologic gastritis in humans and is causally linked to peptic ulcer disease and gastric cancer (Chapters 141 and 202). Symptoms in patients with functional dyspepsia are indistinguishable from those encountered in patients with peptic ulcer disease. *H. pylori* gastritis is found in 30 to 60% of patients with functional dyspepsia but is also common in totally asymptomatic subjects in the general population. A link between *H. pylori* and functional dyspepsia has been established, but the infection is important only in a small subgroup of infected patients.

Gastric Acid

Basal and peak acid output is normal in patients with functional dyspepsia. Other evidence suggests that the duodenal and sometimes gastric mucosa is more sensitive to acid in patients with functional dyspepsia.

Disturbed Motor Function

Of patients seen at tertiary referral centers with functional dyspepsia, 25 to 40% have delayed gastric emptying of solids, and a similar number have antral hypomotility after meals. The prevalence of gastric motility disturbances in patients with functional dyspepsia seen in primary care is unknown but may be lower. Reflux of bile into the stomach is not more frequent in patients with functional dyspepsia than in healthy controls. Up to 40% of patients with functional dyspepsia may have a stiff fundus that does not relax postprandially and may thereby cause fullness and an inability to finish a normal meal (early satiation).

In patients with otherwise unexplained nausea, slow and rapid sequences of gastric slow waves with either a regular or an irregular rhythm have been observed. Gastric arrhythmias occur in some patients with functional dyspepsia and have also been documented in patients with severe nausea caused by gastroesophageal reflux disease.

Disturbed Sensory Function

Patients with functional dyspepsia have a decreased pain threshold during balloon distention of the stomach. No major differences in sensory thresholds have been observed between *H. pylori*–positive and *H. pylori*–negative patients with functional dyspepsia. Sensory thresholds are lower after intraduodenal lipid, but not after glucose infusion, which may explain why fatty meals induce symptoms in some patients with functional dyspepsia. Lowered duodenal sensory thresholds also occur, as do abnormal rectal and esophageal sensory thresholds in some patients with functional dyspepsia.

Central Nervous System Disturbances

In general, patients with functional dyspepsia who seek medical care are more anxious and depressed than healthy controls and have higher neuroticism and somatization scores. The prolactin response to buspirone, an azaspirone that stimulates central serotoninergic-1α receptors, may be greater in patients with functional dyspepsia than in healthy controls.

Acute stress may result in decreased gastric contractility, but it is not known whether chronic dyspeptic symptoms are explained by these mechanisms. Patients who have functional dyspepsia with or without antral hypomotility demonstrate normal autonomic and humoral responses to acute experimental stressors. The role of major life stresses, such as bereavement or divorce, in the pathogenesis of functional dyspepsia is controversial.

Diet and Environmental Factors

Some patients with functional dyspepsia complain of specific food intolerances, but a convincing relationship between diet and chronic dyspepsia remains to be demonstrated. Coffee may induce symptoms in approximately 50% of patients with functional dyspepsia versus one in five healthy controls, perhaps because coffee acts as a direct irritant, stimulates acid secretion, or precipitates gastroesophageal reflux.

Aspirin and other NSAIDs cause asymptomatic mucosal lesions in 30 to 60% of chronic users and can cause dyspepsia, but symptoms do not correlate with mucosal damage scores. Cyclooxygenase-2–selective NSAIDs also cause dyspepsia. Smoking and alcohol are not important risk factors for functional dyspepsia.

Clinical Manifestations

It has been suggested that patients with functional dyspepsia can be subdivided into those with typical ulcer symptoms, such as epigastric pain related to meals or waking the patient from sleep (ulcer-like dyspepsia), and those with symptoms suggestive of a gut motor disturbance, such as postprandial fullness or early satiation (dysmotility-like dyspepsia). Although this categorization is used in clinical practice, standardized symptom questionnaires have shown considerable overlap among categories. Dyspepsia is frequently associated with minor classic reflux symptoms, in particular, heartburn; if reflux symptoms dominate, the diagnosis is symptomatic gastroesophageal reflux disease until proved otherwise.

Diagnosis

Differential Diagnosis

The major organic causes of dyspepsia are chronic peptic ulcer disease, gastroesophageal reflux (with or without esophagitis), and rarely but importantly, malignancy (Fig. 139–2).

Peptic Ulcer

The most important condition to exclude is peptic ulcer disease because definitive therapy is now available. The type or pattern of symptoms discriminates poorly between peptic ulcer disease and functional dyspepsia. In clinical practice, peptic ulcer disease must be excluded by upper gastrointestinal endoscopy before functional dyspepsia can be diagnosed firmly (Chapter 142).

Gastroesophageal Reflux

Gastroesophageal reflux (Chapter 140) should be strongly suspected in patients with predominant epigastric or retrosternal burning pain or discomfort that radiates up toward the throat and is relieved by antacids or acid-suppressing drugs at least transiently. More than 50% of patients with pathologic gastroesophageal reflux confirmed by esophageal pH testing have no visible esophagitis at endoscopy; these patients should not be misclassified as having functional dyspepsia.

Gastric and Esophageal Cancer

In people younger than 55 years in most Western countries, cancer is a rare cause of dyspepsia; overall, cancer is found in only about 1% of patients with new-onset dyspepsia (Chapters 140 and 202). Nevertheless, a neoplasm must be considered as a possible cause of dyspepsia, although the malignancy is usually advanced and incurable by the time that it causes symptoms.

Biliary Tract Disease

Cholelithiasis causes biliary pain, which is typically severe, constant pain in the epigastrium or right upper quadrant that persists for hours and occurs episodically (Chapter 159). In the absence of characteristic biliary pain, there is no evidence that gallstones are linked to dyspepsia. At ultrasonography, gallstones may be found in 1 to 3% of patients with chronic dyspepsia but are usually incidental. The prevalence of incidental gallstones increases with age; they are three times more prevalent in women. Biliary dyskinesia also causes biliary-type pain and is due to a motility disorder of the sphincter of Oddi. It is typically recognized after cholecystectomy.

Pancreatic Disease

Chronic pancreatitis or pancreatic carcinoma (Chapters 147 and 204) may cause symptoms that are occasionally confused with functional dyspepsia. These patients, however, tend to have severe pain that is persistent and often radiates to the back; they may have a history of risk factors for pancreatitis, such as excess alcohol use.

Drug-Induced Dyspepsia

Drugs that may produce upper abdominal symptoms include NSAIDs, alendronate, orlistat, iron or potassium supplements, digitalis, theophylline, and oral antibiotics, especially erythromycin and ampicillin. Reducing the dose or discontinuing drug therapy generally relieves the dyspepsia.

Other Disorders

Diabetes mellitus can cause postprandial fullness, early satiety, nausea, and vomiting in the presence or absence of gastroparesis (Chapter 247). Diabetic radiculopathy of the thoracic nerve roots can cause upper abdominal pain. Metabolic disturbances (e.g., hypothyroidism, hypercalcemia) can produce upper gastrointestinal distress. Ischemic heart disease is sometimes manifested as upper abdominal pain induced by exertion. Intestinal angina (chronic mesenteric ischemia) should be considered in older patients, particularly smokers; it is typically manifested as postprandial pain that is associated with a fear of eating and significant weight loss (Chapter 146). Colon cancer, gastric lymphoma or sarcoma, and ampullary cancer rarely cause upper abdominal distress that may initially be confused with functional dyspepsia. Infiltrative diseases of the stomach, including eosinophilic gastritis, Crohn's disease, and sarcoidosis, may very rarely cause dyspepsia. Abdominal wall pain can be confused with functional dyspepsia.

Aerophagia

Air swallowing with belching is normal and occurs three to four times per hour. Aerophagia is characterized by excessive unconscious swallowing of air that results in abdominal distention or bloating; patients usually report transient improvement of symptoms after belching. The diagnosis of aerophagia is suggested by a specific history and can be confirmed by observing excessive air swallowing between meals and repetitive belching. Because excessive gas is probably not present, either disturbed upper gastrointestinal tract motility or psychopathology probably explains the symptoms.

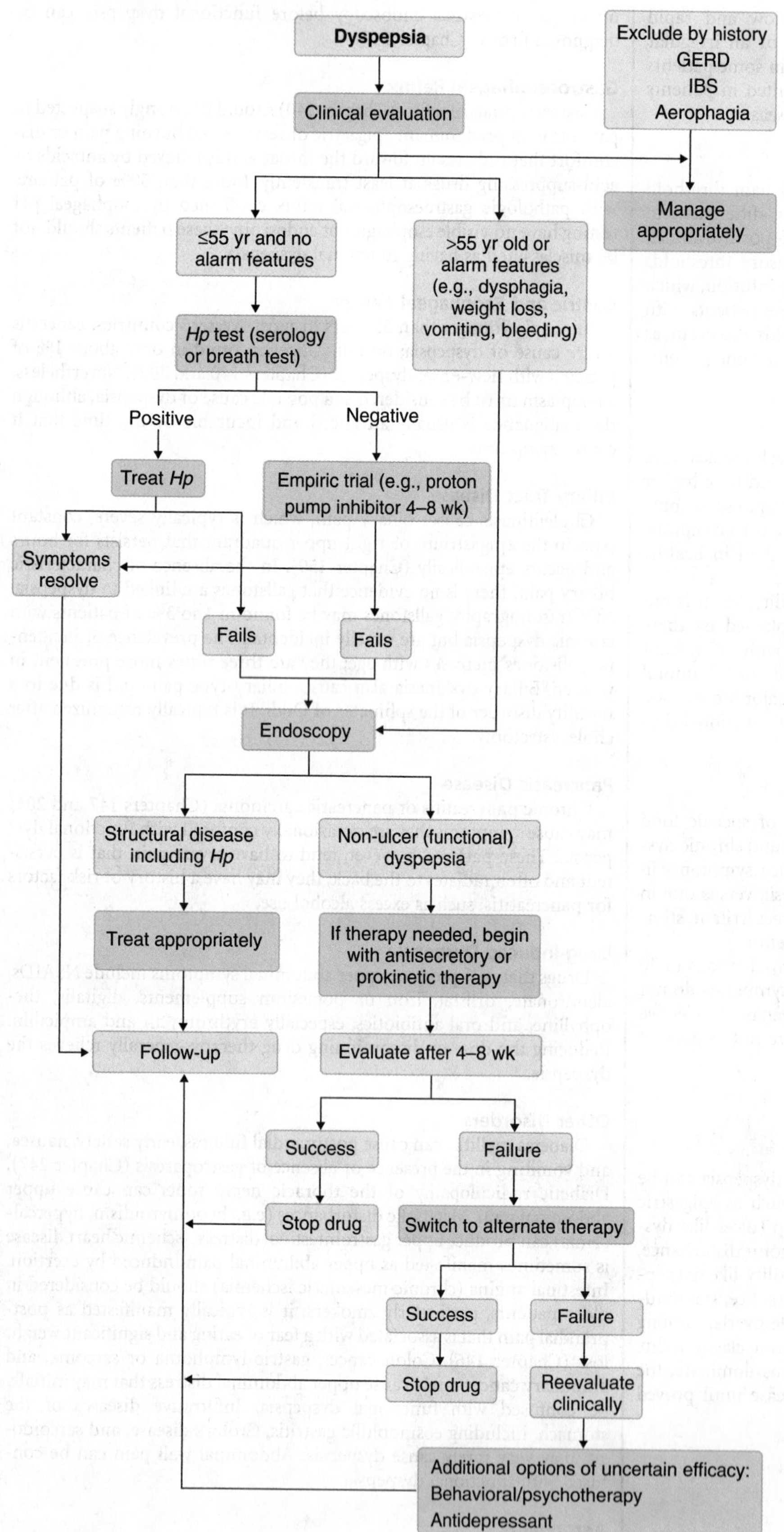

FIGURE 139–2 • Algorithm for the evaluation of dyspepsia. GERD = symptomatic gastroesophageal reflux disease; *Hp* = *Helicobacter pylori;* IBS = irritable bowel syndrome.

Treatment

Rx

General Measures

In patients with documented functional dyspepsia after endoscopy, a positive clinical diagnosis and firm reassurance are the key steps in management. Not all patients want or require medication for functional dyspepsia after a confident diagnosis has been made. A careful explanation of the meaning of the symptoms and their benign nature can have positive therapeutic effects; some patients lose their symptoms spontaneously after a positive diagnosis. It is useful to ask patients with long-standing functional dyspepsia symptoms why they decided to seek care on this occasion; allaying the patient's unwarranted fears is effective therapy. Patients with functional dyspepsia may improve by eating low-fat meals or by ingesting more frequent, but smaller meals throughout the day.

Medical Therapy

There is a considerable response rate to placebo in patients with functional dyspepsia that ranges from 30 to 60%. This placebo response may not reflect a nonspecific effect of treatment but rather, in part, spontaneous regression of the disease. The course of functional dyspepsia is typically characterized by relapsing and remitting symptoms, but over a 1-year period more than 70% continue to be symptomatic.

Eradication of *H. pylori* (Chapter 142) is a standard of care that benefits some infected patients, [7] although many will remain symptomatic despite eradication of infection. Antacids are commonly used by patients with functional dyspepsia, but randomized controlled studies have all failed to show a significant benefit over placebo. The results of controlled trials testing full-dose H_2-receptor antagonists have been conflicting, but a meta-analysis suggested an approximately 20% benefit of H_2-receptor antagonists over placebo. These drugs should be prescribed twice daily (e.g., ranitidine or nizatidine, 150 mg, or famotidine, 20 mg) initially. A meta-analysis concluded that a proton pump inhibitor (e.g., omeprazole, 20 mg/day, or lansoprazole, 30 mg/day) was superior to placebo or an H_2-antagonist in functional dyspepsia, especially in those with epigastric pain.

The dopaminergic receptor blockers metoclopramide and domperidone and the serotonin type 4 receptor agonist cisapride have been used in patients with functional dyspepsia, and evidence from randomized controlled trials has shown that prokinetics are superior to placebo. Cisapride, though efficacious, is available only on a limited-access program and is seldom prescribed because of rare life-threatening arrhythmias. Metoclopramide (5 to 10 mg before meals and at bedtime) can induce serious side effects as a result of its central antidopaminergic effects, including dystonic reactions, drowsiness, and increased prolactin levels. Rarely, tardive dyskinesia may occur, particularly in the elderly, and in some cases it is not reversible. Erythromycin, a motilin agonist, is of no therapeutic value in functional dyspepsia. Tegaserod, a prokinetic, may provide a small benefit, and trials are in progress. Alosetron may also improve symptoms, but its side effect profile restricts its use.

Sucralfate and bismuth subsalicylate may be useful for intermittent dyspepsia but are not clearly superior to placebo. Misoprostol is not efficacious in functional dyspepsia.

Theoretically, anticholinergic agents might be of value in patients with pyloric or antral spasm, but these disturbances have not been documented in functional dyspepsia. Anticholinergic drugs have been evaluated formally in small studies in which dicyclomine was not more efficacious than placebo.

Few formal randomized placebo-controlled trials have investigated the effects of antidepressants in functional dyspepsia, but tricyclics (in low dose) are probably of value in patients with resistant symptoms, even in the absence of depression.

Antinausea Drugs

If nausea is a major complaint, antinausea drugs include antihistamines, phenothiazines (e.g., prochlorperazine), and others with an uncertain mechanism of action (e.g., trimethobenzamide). Benzodiazepines may also help reduce nausea by their sedative effects. The 5-HT_3 receptor antagonist ondansetron and other similar agents are not of established value but may be worth a trial in difficult cases. Combining an antinausea drug with a prokinetic or a low-dose tricyclic antidepressant can be helpful.

Guidelines for Specific Treatment Scenarios

New-Onset (Uninvestigated) Dyspepsia

The medical history is key (see Fig. 139–2). The physician should inquire about typical reflux symptoms; if heartburn or acid regurgitation is the predominant complaint, a diagnosis of gastroesophageal reflux should be made and appropriate treatment instituted. If there is uncertainty, a short trial of high-dose proton pump inhibitor therapy (e.g., omeprazole, 20 mg twice daily for 14 days) has some limited utility as a diagnostic test for distinguishing reflux, in which symptoms are typically abolished, from other causes of upper gastrointestinal symptoms (Chapter 140). Similarly, if bowel dysfunction is linked directly to the epigastric pain or discomfort, a diagnosis of IBS should be considered.

Older patients (>55 years) with new, unexplained dyspepsia and patients with alarm symptoms (e.g., vomiting, bleeding, weight loss, dysphagia) have an increased risk for organic disease and should undergo prompt upper endoscopic evaluation.

In younger patients without alarm symptoms, management depends on the degree of uncertainty that the patient and physician are willing to accept. Use of a noninvasive *H. pylori* test (e.g., breath test or stool antigen test) plus initiation of anti–*H. pylori* treatment in infected subjects is a reasonable initial approach as an alternative to routine endoscopy. This management strategy should relieve symptoms in most patients with peptic ulcer disease and in some with functional dyspepsia (Chapter 141).

In *H. pylori*–negative patients, who are most likely to have functional dyspepsia, the major first-line drug is currently a proton pump inhibitor (e.g., esomeprazole, 40 mg, lansoprazole, 30 mg daily for 4 to 8 weeks). An H_2-blocker (e.g., ranitidine, 150 mg twice daily for 4 to 8 weeks) is an alternative but is less efficacious in uninvestigated dyspepsia. Some clinicians initially prefer to treat ulcer-like dyspepsia with an antisecretory agent and dysmotility-like dyspepsia with a prokinetic agent. Therapy can be switched if there is no benefit after 4 to 8 weeks. Sometimes double-dose proton pump inhibitor therapy is required to relieve symptoms. Patients may be considered for upper endoscopy if they fail to respond within 8 weeks or relapse rapidly, but the yield in this setting remains low.

Refractory Patient with Documented Functional Dyspepsia

Failure to respond to treatment raises the possibility that the diagnosis of functional dyspepsia was incorrect or that the chosen treatment was suboptimal. Simethicone and antispasmodics may be worth a trial but often fail. Another option is to initiate low-dose tricyclic antidepressant treatment. If early satiation or fullness is prominent, drugs that relax the gastric fundus (e.g., sumatriptan, buspirone, tegaserod, or clonidine) may be tried. In patients who need continuous therapy to avoid incapacitating or unremitting symptoms, drug holidays can confirm that the current therapy is still of value.

Aerophagia

Treatment of excessive unconscious air swallowing is difficult. Stress reduction and dietary modifications (avoiding sucking sweets or chewing gum, eating slowly, encouraging small swallows at mealtime, and avoiding diet beverages) may occasionally help. Simethicone and activated charcoal are not of established value. Tranquilizers or prokinetics may sometimes be of benefit. Behavioral therapy can be useful.

Prognosis

A firm diagnosis of functional dyspepsia after endoscopy excludes ulcer or other structural disease, reduces a patient's fears, and may improve the prognosis. Some patients may be symptom-free for years. Patients seen at tertiary centers for functional dyspepsia represent a subgroup with more intractable symptoms, and spontaneous remissions are less common.

NONCARDIAC (FUNCTIONAL) CHEST PAIN

Diagnosis

A third to half of patients arriving at an emergency department with chest pain do not have coronary artery disease. Angina-like chest pain in these patients is most often caused by gastroesophageal reflux and occasionally by motor disorders of the esophagus. Musculoskeletal chest pain and psychiatric disease (e.g., panic attacks) are also important causes to consider (Chapter 48). Microvascular angina explains some cases too, but these conditions can all overlap, thus making management a challenge.

Clinical evaluation should initially be directed at excluding cardiac causes of chest pain (Chapter 48). The history should screen for psychiatric disease and especially panic disorder, which may be manifested as recurrent chest pain. Pain aggravated by movement may be musculoskeletal and can be confirmed by reproducing the patient's typical pain with palpation of the sternum or chest wall.

In patients who do not have cardiac, musculoskeletal, or psychiatric disease, the possibility of esophageal disease must be evaluated (Chapter 140). Upper gastrointestinal endoscopy and ambulatory esophageal pH monitoring are useful in diagnosing reflux. In the remaining patients, esophageal manometry may be considered, but the yield is low. Manometry rules out achalasia (<1% of patients with chest pain) and esophageal spasm (<5% of patients with chest pain). "Nutcracker esophagus" refers to high-amplitude distal contractions (mean, >180 mm Hg) with normal peristalsis. Other less common, nonspecific motor abnormalities include a hypertensive lower esophageal sphincter or exaggerated esophageal body contractions. Although 30% of patients with chest pain have a nonspecific motor abnormality, it rarely coincides with spontaneous chest pain, and the relevance of the manometric disturbances is highly questionable.

Treatment Rx

Treatment relies on reassurance and explanation. A trial of acid suppression with a full-dose proton pump inhibitor (e.g., esomeprazole, 40 mg, lansoprazole, 30 mg daily for 4 to 8 weeks) should be prescribed if there is any suspicion of reflux or if the cause remains unknown, with the dose doubled if no response occurs after 2 weeks (Chapter 140); a meta-analysis has shown that a short trial of a proton pump inhibitor in patients with noncardiac chest pain has a sensitivity and specificity of 80% and 74%, respectively, for abnormal acid reflux. [8] Calcium-channel blockers such as diltiazem (30 to 60 mg four times daily) may be tried for esophageal spasm or in unexplained cases, but their efficacy is questionable; the use of nitrates (short acting and long acting) and anticholinergic agents has been disappointing. The role of sildenafil (50 mg daily) is unclear. Tricyclic antidepressants (starting at a low dose, e.g., imipramine, 25 mg) are of particular value in unexplained noncardiac chest pain, in part because a subset of patients have esophageal hypersensitivity. Behavioral therapy may be useful in patients with and without panic disorder who have unexplained chest pain.

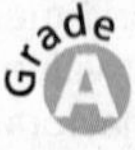

1. Quartero A, Meineche-Schmidt V, Muris J, et al: Bulking agents, antispasmodic and antidepressant medication for the treatment of irritable bowel syndrome. Cochrane Database Syst Rev 2005;2: CD003460.
2. Evans BW, Clark WK, Moore DJ, et al: Tegaserod for the treatment of irritable bowel syndrome. Cochrane Database Syst Rev 2004;1: CD003960.
3. Lembo AJ, Olden KW, Ameen VZ, et al: Effect of alosetron on bowel urgency and global symptoms in women with severe, diarrhea-predominant irritable bowel syndrome: Analysis of two controlled trials. Clin Gastroenterol Hepatol 2004;2:675–682.
4. Pimentel M, Park S, Mirocha J: The effect of a nonabsorbed oral antibiotic (rifaximin) on the symptoms of the irritable bowel syndrome: A randomized trial. Ann Intern Med 2006;145:557–563.
5. Tabas G, Beaves M, Wang J, et al: Paroxetine to treat irritable bowel syndrome not responding to high-fiber diet: A double-blind, placebo-controlled trial. Am J Gastroenterol 2004;99: 914–920.
6. Lackner JM, Mesmer C, Morley S, et al: Psychological treatments for irritable bowel syndrome: A systematic review and meta-analysis. J Consult Clin Psychol 2004;72:1100–1113.
7. Moayyedi P, Soo S, Deeks J, et al: Eradication of *Helicobacter pylori* for non-ulcer dyspepsia. Cochrane Database Syst Rev 2005;1: CD002096.
8. Cremonini F, Wise J, Moayyedi P, et al: Diagnostic and therapeutic use of proton pump inhibitors in non-cardiac chest pain: A meta-analysis. Am J Gastroenterol 2005;100:1226–1232.

SUGGESTED READINGS

Eslick GD, Coulshed DS, Talley NJ: Diagnosis and treatment of noncardiac chest pain. Nat Clin Pract Gastroenterol Hepatol 2005;2:463–472. *Comprehensive clinical review.*

Talley NJ: How to manage the difficult-to-treat dyspeptic patient. Nat Clin Pract Gastroenterol Hepatol 2007;4:35–42. *Comprehensive clinical review.*

Talley NJ, Vakil N, Moayyedi P: AGA Technical Review: Evaluation of dyspepsia 2005. Gastroenterology 2005;129:1756–1780. *Provides official recommendations on management of uninvestigated and nonulcer dyspepsia of the American Gastroenterological Association based on the best evidence.*

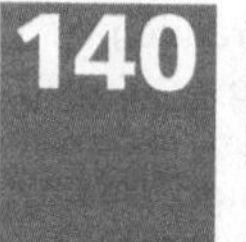

DISEASES OF THE ESOPHAGUS

Roy C. Orlando

Definition

The esophagus is a 22- to 25-cm conduit whose upper third is skeletal muscle and lower two thirds is smooth muscle. Its function is to transport food from the oral cavity to the stomach. When not swallowing, the esophagus is closed at the upper end by the upper esophageal sphincter (UES), or the cricopharyngeus muscle, which creates a high-pressure zone that prevents inspired air from entering the esophagus and esophageal contents from re-entering the oropharynx. The lower esophageal sphincter (LES) creates a high-pressure zone that prevents the gastric contents from entering the esophagus. On swallowing, the swallowing center located in the medulla oblongata coordinates peristalsis in the pharynx and esophagus with relaxation of the UES and LES to enable food to be propelled in a caudad direction to the stomach. The motor signals to the end plates on skeletal muscle from the nucleus ambiguus or to Auerbach's neuronal plexus in smooth muscle from the dorsal motor nucleus of the vagus are carried by vagal postganglionic or preganglionic cholinergic fibers, respectively. Contraction of esophageal muscle is elicited by the release of acetylcholine, and relaxation is induced either by inhibition of the release of acetylcholine (skeletal muscle) or by release of nitric oxide and vasoactive intestinal peptide (smooth muscle). While the esophagus transports food from the mouth to the stomach, it also protects itself from gastric acid reflux injury by a three-tiered system consisting of antireflux barriers (limits reflux frequency), luminal clearance mechanisms (limits duration within the esophagus), and tissue resistance (limits damage on epithelial contact).

Clinical Manifestations

Dysphagia, heartburn, and odynophagia are symptoms with a high degree of specificity for the esophagus (Chapter 134). Chest pain, though common in esophageal disease (Chapter 139), has a far broader differential, including cardiac disease (Chapter 48).

Dysphagia

Dysphagia means difficulty swallowing. When dysphagia arises from disease involving the region of skeletal muscle, it is called *oropharyngeal*

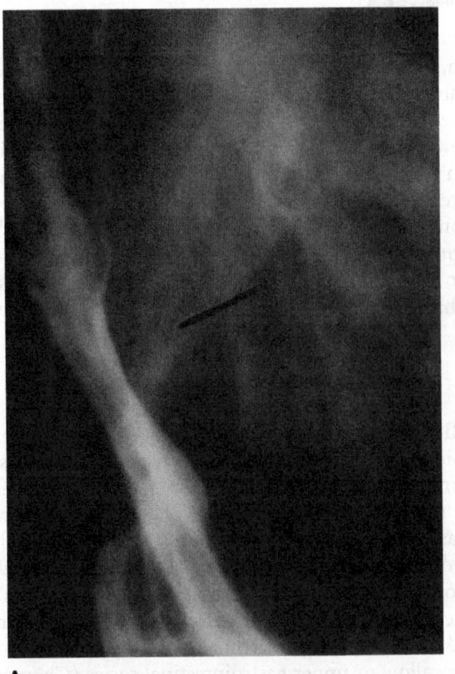
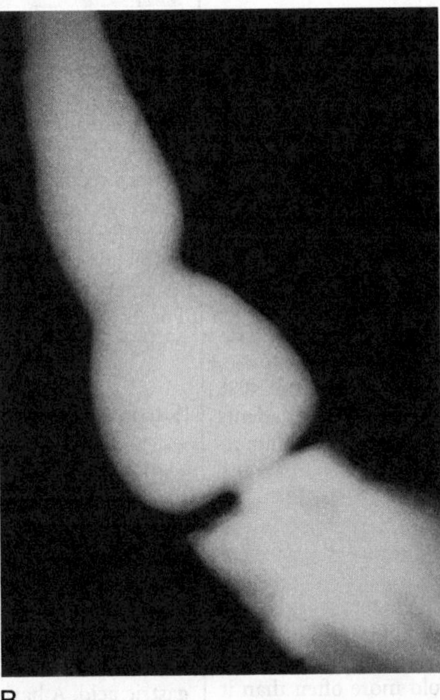
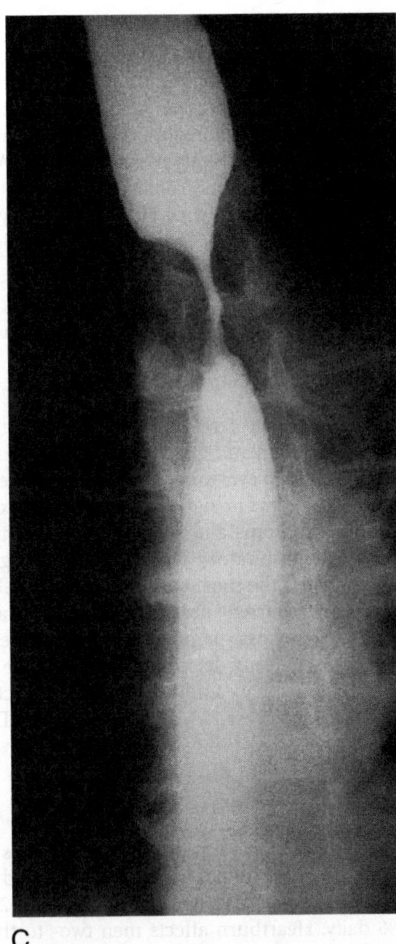

A B C

FIGURE 140–1 • Dysphagia. Barium esophagograms demonstrate three common causes of dysphagia for solids only: peptic stricture **(A)**, Schatzki's ring **(B)**, and malignant stricture **(C)**. A malignant stricture produces rapidly progressive dysphagia for solids in association with both anorexia and weight loss. A peptic stricture occurs in reflux patients and produces slowly progressive dysphagia for solids in the absence of anorexia and weight loss. A Schatzki ring produces either intermittent, nonprogressive dysphagia for solids or acute food impaction in the absence of anorexia or weight loss. (From Feldman M [ed]: Gastroenterology and Hepatology: The Comprehensive Visual Reference. New York, Churchill Livingstone, 1997.)

dysphagia. Oropharyngeal dysphagia is characteristically accompanied by failure to transport a bolus from the mouth to the esophagus, by nasal regurgitation because of lack of occlusion of the nasal air passages by the soft palate, and by coughing with swallowing because of aspiration resulting from failure to elevate the larynx and lower the epiglottis. When dysphagia arises from disease involving the region of smooth muscle, the impairment in bolus transport is perceived substernally and called *esophageal dysphagia.* Oropharyngeal dysphagia but not esophageal dysphagia is accompanied by failure of bolus transport from the mouth to the esophagus, by nasal regurgitation, or by aspiration. Furthermore, esophageal dysphagia can be readily separated into (1) diseases that cause dysphagia for solids only, indicative of a lumen-narrowing (mechanical) lesion such as peptic stricture, cancer, or Schatzki's ring (Fig. 140–1A to C) and (2) diseases that cause dysphagia for liquids as well as solids, indicative of motor dysfunction such as achalasia or diffuse esophageal spasm.

Heartburn

Heartburn is a symptom complex characterized by episodic substernal pain that is worse after meals and on reclining and is relieved, at least temporarily, by antacids. Relief by antacids is especially important because it links the pain with acidity. The quality of the discomfort is often burning, and it commonly radiates toward the mouth. Heartburn is frequently accompanied by complaints of a bitter taste in the mouth (regurgitation) or a welling up in the mouth of a salty tasting (salivary derived) fluid (water brash). When substernal pain relieved by antacids recurs at least once per week over an extended period, the history alone permits the diagnosis of gastroesophageal reflux disease (GERD). Unfortunately, patients often use the term "heartburn" inaccurately, and even "burning" substernal pain lacks specificity for GERD without coincident relief by antacids. As a result, GERD is overdiagnosed, and "treatment failures" often reflect misdiagnoses. Truly *refractory heartburn,* unresponsive to proton pump inhibitors (PPIs), is uncommon when the diagnosis of GERD appropriately requires that substernal pain be "relieved by antacids."

Odynophagia

Odynophagia means painful swallowing and implies an acute and severe form of esophagitis, typically with mucosal ulceration. Odynophagia is experienced substernally as an aching or stabbing pain that is aggravated by the act of swallowing, even swallowing saliva. It is common in esophagitis caused by infection, pills, and radiation but rare in esophagitis caused by reflux.

Noncardiac Chest Pain

Chest pain (Chapter 48), distinctive from heartburn and odynophagia, is common in esophageal disease (Chapter 134). It is termed *atypical* because it has some, but not all, of the characteristics suggestive of angina. For example, esophageal pain, unlike angina, is not brought on by physical exertion but is usually substernal or parasternal; can radiate to the neck, jaw, or arms; may worsen with meals; and may be relieved by nitroglycerin (Chapter 48). Such similarities are not surprising given the overlapping pattern of sensory innervation between the heart and esophagus. When chest pain is accompanied by dysphagia, odynophagia, or heartburn, the origin is probably the esophagus. In the absence of these associated symptoms, patients with chest pain should initially undergo a cardiac evaluation. If cardiac disease is excluded, the patient is said to have *noncardiac chest pain,* whose differential includes but is not limited to GERD and diffuse esophageal spasm.

Esophageal Bleeding

Upper gastrointestinal bleeding may be manifested in many forms, such as hematemesis, melena, coffee-ground emesis, Hemoccult-positive stool, iron deficiency anemia, and hematochezia (Chapter 137). When blood transfusions are required, the most common esophageal causes are ruptured esophageal varices and Mallory-Weiss tears. Less commonly, deep esophageal ulcers from infection with cytomegalovirus (CMV) or human immunodeficiency virus (HIV) may cause significant bleeding. Lower rates of bleeding leading to iron deficiency anemia can be a reflection of GERD.

GASTROESOPHAGEAL REFLUX DISEASE

Definition

Gastroesophageal reflux is a physiologic process that refers to the effortless movement of gastric contents from the stomach to the esophagus. It occurs in everyone, multiple times every day, usually without producing symptoms or signs of damage. Reflux can also be pathologic and produce symptoms and signs of injury to the esophagus, oropharynx, larynx, and respiratory tract. Reflux damage to the esophagus (reflux esophagitis) is the most common form of GERD and is most often recognized by recurrent heartburn. In almost all patients with heartburn, esophageal mucosal pathology is identifiable, although only about 40% have endoscopically detectable erosions. The remaining 60% of patients with heartburn have endoscopically undetectable (microscopic) pathology—termed *nonerosive reflux disease* (NERD).

Epidemiology

GERD is one of the most common diseases in the Western world based on the prevalence of heartburn. In the United States, about 45% of adults have heartburn at least once a month, about 20% once a week, and about 10% daily. Heartburn affects men two- to threefold more often than it affects women and is more common in whites than blacks. Although GERD rarely causes death, it reduces quality of life and has a morbidity rate of 10 to 15% secondary to ulceration, bleeding, stricture, Barrett's esophagus, and adenocarcinoma. The overall risk for esophageal adenocarcinoma in patients with heartburn is very low, with estimates of 1 in 2500 cases per year for those with daily heartburn to 1 in 10,000 cases per year for those with monthly heartburn.

Pathobiology

GERD develops when acidic gastric contents reflux into the esophagus and remain there long enough to overcome the resistance of the esophageal epithelium. Based on 24-hour esophageal pH monitoring, GERD develops in at least two fundamentally different ways: (1) under conditions in which there is prolonged contact of the esophageal epithelium with refluxed gastric acid and (2) under conditions in which the esophageal epithelium is damaged despite a normal duration of contact with refluxed gastric acid. Prolonged acid contact results from defects in the antireflux barriers or luminal clearance mechanisms (or both), with transient LES relaxations accounting for more than 50% of acid reflux events in NERD. These relaxations are non–swallow-induced, reflex relaxations of the LES caused by gastric fundic distention. They are associated with acid reflux because they are twice as long as relaxations with swallowing and, unlike swallow-induced LES relaxations, are accompanied by inhibition of diaphragmatic contraction and unaccompanied by lumen-obliterating esophageal peristalsis. The cause of the increase in the frequency of acid reflux episodes associated with transient relaxations in patients with GERD is unclear but is unrelated to delayed gastric emptying or infection with *Helicobacter pylori.* A diet rich in nonabsorbable carbohydrates may be one possible provocateur. In erosive esophagitis, transient LES relaxations account for less than 50% of acid reflux events, with most occurring across a mechanically weak LES. Whether LES weakness causes erosive esophagitis or is a consequence of it remains unclear because products released during inflammation can impair LES contractility. Similarly, hiatal hernias and impaired peristalsis are common in erosive esophagitis, but whether they are cause or consequence is also unclear because esophagitis can result in both esophageal shortening (by sustained contraction of the longitudinal muscle) and peristaltic dysfunction (by weakening circular muscle contractility). Patients with heartburn despite normal acid contact time presumably have primary defects in tissue resistance, with these defects probably being acquired by dietary indiscretions such as excess exposure to alcoholic, hypertonic, or hot-temperature products.

Clinical Manifestations

Symptoms

Recurrent heartburn, when properly defined (see earlier), is the hallmark of GERD and enables the diagnosis to be made by the history alone. The heartburn associated with GERD typically occurs once or twice per day and lasts from a few minutes to an hour or more if untreated. This pattern recurs, but with considerable variation in frequency and severity. However, neither the frequency, severity, nor duration of heartburn predicts disease severity on endoscopy. GERD can also be associated with dysphagia, an *alarm symptom* because it raises concern for the presence of a peptic stricture or adenocarcinoma arising in Barrett's esophagus. For this reason, dysphagia (Chapter 134) is an indication for early endoscopy.

Signs

The damage in GERD is best assessed by upper endoscopy (Chapter 136) and esophageal biopsy. Endoscopy may reveal friability, erosions, ulcers, strictures, or Barrett's esophagus in a third of subjects. In the other two thirds, endoscopic findings are normal but esophageal biopsy may show basal cell hyperplasia, elongation of the rete pegs, inflammatory cell infiltrates, cell edema, dilated intercellular spaces in squamous epithelium, or any combination of these findings. "Dilated intercellular spaces" is the earliest detectable lesion in NERD and correlates with heartburn because it reflects "leakiness" of the paracellular pathway to refluxed gastric acid. A barium swallow or upper gastrointestinal series (Chapter 135) may also detect ulcers, strictures, and hiatal hernias, but it does not reliably detect inflammation, erosions, or Barrett's esophagus.

Extraesophageal Manifestations

Although GERD is often used synonymously with reflux damage to the esophagus, GERD includes reflux damage to the oropharynx, larynx, and respiratory tract. Consequently, symptoms and signs of GERD can include sore throat (Chapter 455)/pharyngitis (Chapter 455), earache/otitis (Chapter 452), eroded tooth enamel, hoarseness/laryngitis (Chapter 455), bronchitis/chronic cough (Chapter 96), asthma/wheezing (Chapter 87), and aspiration pneumonia (Chapter 97). With the exception of pneumonia, which occurs as a result of gross regurgitation and aspiration of mixed gastric content, damage to the oropharynx, larynx, and airways is mediated by refluxed gastric acid. Asthma (wheezing) and bronchitis (chronic cough) can be triggered either directly by contact of acid with *airway* epithelium (microaspiration) or indirectly through an esophagopulmonary vagal reflex initiated by contact of acid with *esophageal* epithelium. The frequency with which GERD causes, as opposed to being caused by, wheezing/asthma, chronic cough/bronchitis, and hoarseness/laryngitis is unknown.

Associated Conditions

GERD can develop as a consequence of other conditions, such as Zollinger-Ellison syndrome (Chapter 205), scleroderma (Chapter 288), diabetes mellitus (Chapter 247), nasogastric intubation, and pregnancy.

Diagnosis

A history of recurrent heartburn along with a positive response to antacids or acid-suppressing medication is adequate to diagnose GERD. Specific testing is reserved for patients who have (1) GERD plus alarm symptoms of dysphagia, weight loss, or gastrointestinal bleeding; (2) GERD of sufficient chronicity (e.g., 5 years) to raise concern for Barrett's esophagus; and (3) suspected GERD with atypical symptoms, such as chest pain or oropharyngeal, laryngeal, or airway symptoms.

Establishing GERD as a Cause of Nonheartburn Symptoms

Currently, the preferred method for establishing GERD as the cause of symptoms (e.g., chest pain, wheezing) is an *empirical trial of acid suppression* with a PPI (e.g., omeprazole, 20 mg twice daily), which normalizes esophageal acidity in approximately 95% of subjects. In some instances, a bedtime dose of a histamine H_2-receptor antagonist (e.g., ranitidine, 300 mg) is added to reduce the possibility of nocturnal acid breakthrough. The treatment period in which to expect a satisfactory response is 2 to 4 weeks for chest pain and 2 to 3 months for inflammatory disease of the airway. Resolution of the symptoms supports GERD as possibly causal. Confirmation may be obtained by relapse when medication is withdrawn and by a subsequent positive response to re-treatment, as confirmed by documenting control of esophageal acidity on pH monitoring *while undergoing PPI therapy.* Failure of symptoms to improve with PPI therapy is not generally an indication for antireflux surgery (see later) but rather an indication to search for another disease. A rarely used alternative is the *Bernstein test,* in which acid (0.1 N HCl, pH 1.1) or saline (control) is perfused through a catheter positioned in the midesophagus. If symptoms typical of those that occur spontaneously develop with acid but not saline, the test is considered positive for GERD.

Tests for Reflux

Documenting acid reflux is not necessary except when symptoms fail to respond to PPI therapy or when surgery is being considered. *Esophageal pH monitoring,* the "gold standard" for identifying acid reflux, is performed by fixing a small pH probe in the esophagus, 5 cm above the LES, and recording all episodes in which esophageal pH drops to less than 4 over a 24- to 48-hour period. The number and duration of each acidic event, when combined, yield a value for total esophageal acid contact time. Total acid contact times of greater than 5% are abnormal and consistent with a diagnosis of GERD. An event marker activated by the patient also allows symptoms to be related to episodes of esophageal acidity. An *upper gastrointestinal series* (Chapter 135) can detect grossly abnormal reflux by observing movement of barium from the stomach to the esophagus with the patient in the head-down position. It has low sensitivity but, when positive, has high predictive value. The positive predictive value is much lower, however, if reflux is induced by having the subject sip water through a straw in the head-down position. This test is rarely useful for therapeutic decisions.

Tests for Esophageal Injury

See the earlier section Signs.

Tests of Esophageal Motor Function

An upper gastrointestinal series or barium swallow is valuable for identifying gross reflux and marked abnormalities in esophageal anatomy (e.g., hiatal hernia, diverticulum) and peristaltic and sphincter function. More subtle abnormalities, however, require esophageal manometry. Low mean LES pressure (<10 mm Hg) is a specific but insensitive marker of GERD, with 60% of patients having normal values. Currently, the major uses of esophageal manometry in GERD are to (1) position the pH probe for reflux testing, (2) exclude motor disease (achalasia, scleroderma), and (3) quantify peristaltic amplitudes before surgical fundoplication. If contraction amplitudes average less than 30 mm Hg, a partial (Toupet) rather than complete (Nissen) wrap may be preferable to avoid postoperative dysphagia.

Treatment

Rx

Treatment of GERD is primarily medical (Fig. 140–2), the mainstays being lifestyle modifications (Table 140–1) and drug therapy (Table 140–2). The goals of treatment are to relieve symptoms and prevent relapse and complications. All patients should be advised about lifestyle modifications that help reduce symptoms and prevent relapse. Antacids or antacid-alginate combinations are recommended for safe, prompt, inexpensive relief of heartburn. The same agents, however, are poorly suited for regular use because of poor palatability and durability and side effects such as diarrhea, constipation, and possible magnesium or aluminum toxicity in renal patients. Protection against recurrence of heartburn is provided by acid-suppressing medications such as H_2-receptor antagonists and PPIs. H_2-receptor antagonists reduce gastric acid secretion moderately by inhibiting one of three acid-stimulating receptors on the basolateral membrane of the parietal cell. When prescribed twice a day, they can control symptoms in about 50% of GERD patients and heal erosions in about 30%. PPIs irreversibly inhibit the H^+, K^+-ATPase or proton pump, the final common pathway for acid secretion on the apical membrane of the parietal cell. Consequently, PPIs markedly reduce gastric acidity with once-a-day dosing and provide relief of symptoms and healing of lesions in about 80 to 90% of GERD patients. H_2-receptor antagonists (>30 years) and PPIs (≈15 years) have excellent safety profiles. PPI safety beyond 15 years remains unclear because of uncertainty about the long-term risk for chronic gastric hypoacidity and hypergastrinemia. Although vitamin B_{12} levels can be reduced with chronic PPI use, clinically significant vitamin B_{12} deficiency has not been reported, so an increase in vitamin B_{12} intake is not currently recommended.

Early endoscopy is indicated for those with alarm symptoms. Endoscopy is also indicated for patients who fail once-a-day PPI therapy to confirm the diagnosis and assess severity, including the presence of Barrett's esophagus (see later). Testing for *H. pylori* is not recommended because the organism is not etiologic in GERD and, when eradicated, may make treatment more difficult.

Failures with once-a-day PPI therapy are treated with twice-daily PPI therapy with or without H_2-receptor antagonists at bedtime for 6 to 8 weeks, and patients who fail this regimen undergo esophageal pH monitoring *during therapy* to assess for control of esophageal acidity. If the acidity is controlled, the symptoms are not mediated by acid.

Effective therapy is often accompanied by relapse when medication ceases, especially in patients with erosive esophagitis, in whom maintenance therapy is indicated. Patients requiring maintenance therapy should undergo at least one endoscopy procedure to determine whether Barrett's esophagus is present. If endoscopy reveals NERD, no further endoscopy is necessary and treatment is guided by symptoms. If endoscopy reveals erosive esophagitis, treatment to healing should be documented by endoscopy so that Barrett's esophagus can be effectively established or excluded. Once Barrett's esophagus is excluded, endoscopy is unnecessary and treatment is guided by symptoms because subsequent relapse and treatment will rarely result in Barrett's esophagus.

Prognosis

Antacids and acid-suppressing medication effectively control the symptoms of GERD; however, in the absence of adherence to lifestyle modifications or in the presence of advanced disease, relapse is common when medication is stopped.

Complications

The two major complications of GERD are peptic stricture formation and Barrett's esophagus (frequency, 5 to 15%). When endoscopy is performed for heartburn and the diagnosis is NERD, progression to erosive esophagitis is uncommon (≈15%), and complications such as stricture, Barrett's esophagus, and adenocarcinoma are rare. When endoscopy documents erosive esophagitis, the clinical course is more variable and the potential risk for stricture, Barrett's esophagus (see later), and adenocarcinoma is higher. For this reason, repeat endoscopy is desirable to ensure healing without Barrett's esophagus. When healing initially occurs without Barrett's esophagus, it is unlikely to develop in the future irrespective of whether relapse and re-treatment are necessary.

Peptic Stricture

Peptic stricture is a lumen-narrowing lesion that occurs in erosive esophagitis secondary to edema, inflammation, or fibrosis of the distal

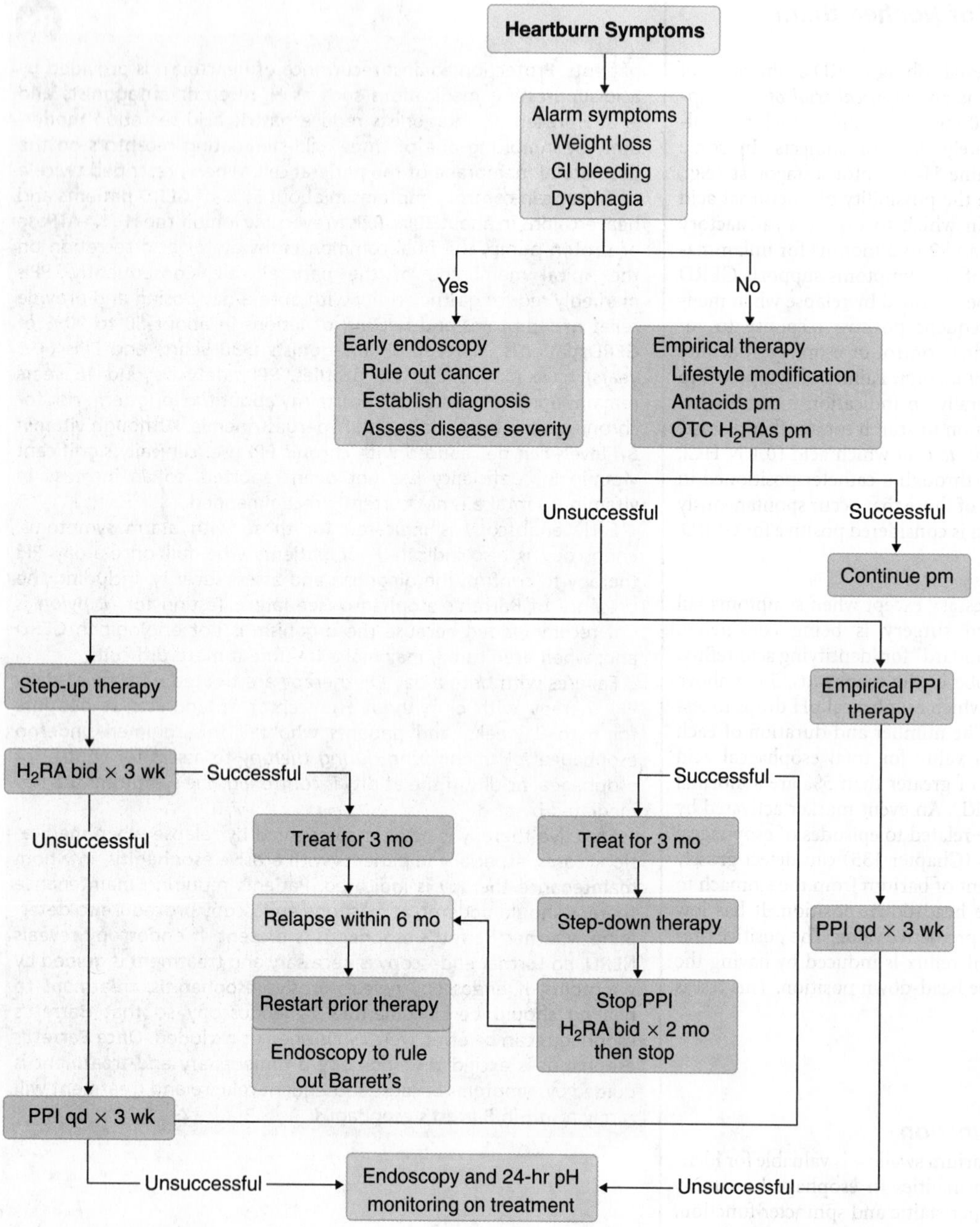

Heartburn Symptoms

Alarm symptoms
Weight loss
GI bleeding
Dysphagia

Yes

Early endoscopy
Rule out cancer
Establish diagnosis
Assess disease severity

No

Empirical therapy
Lifestyle modification
Antacids pm
OTC H_2RAs pm

Unsuccessful

Successful

Continue pm

Step-up therapy

H_2RA bid × 3 wk

Successful

Unsuccessful

Treat for 3 mo

Relapse within 6 mo

Restart prior therapy

Endoscopy to rule out Barrett's

PPI qd × 3 wk

Unsuccessful

Empirical PPI therapy

Successful

Treat for 3 mo

Step-down therapy

Stop PPI
H_2RA bid × 2 mo
then stop

PPI qd × 3 wk

Unsuccessful

Endoscopy and 24-hr pH monitoring on treatment

FIGURE 140–2 • Algorithm for the management of a patient with heartburn. GI = gastrointestinal; OTC H_2RA = over-the-counter H_2-receptor antagonist; PPI = proton pump inhibitor; Rx = treatment. (From Orlando L, Orlando RC: Reflux esophagitis: Evaluation of drug management strategies. Formulary 2002;37:140–146. Reprinted with permission from Formulary. Formulary is a copyrighted publication of Advanstar Communications Inc. All rights reserved.)

TABLE 140–1 LIFESTYLE MODIFICATIONS FOR REFLUX ESOPHAGITIS

Elevate the head of the bed 6 inches
Stop smoking
Stop excessive alcohol consumption
Reduce dietary fat
Reduce meal size
Avoid bedtime snacks
Lose weight (if overweight)
Avoid chocolate, carminatives (spearmint, peppermint), coffee (caffeinated and decaffeinated), tea, cola beverages, tomato juice, citrus fruit juices
Avoid, when possible, anticholinergics, theophylline, diazepam, narcotics, calcium-channel blockers, β-adrenergic agonists (isoproterenol), progesterone (some contraceptives), α-adrenergic antagonists (phentolamine)

end of the esophagus (see Fig. 140–1A). When present, strictures produce dysphagia for solids, a symptom that progresses slowly over a period of months to years. Anorexia and weight loss are absent, which distinguishes dysphagia secondary to stricture from that secondary to cancer. Diagnosis is by barium swallow or upper endoscopy, the latter permitting biopsy to exclude malignancy definitively.

Treatment

Strictures that narrow the esophageal lumen to less than 15 mm often cause dysphagia. When associated with active and marked inflammation of the distal portion of the esophagus, they may respond to medical therapy for GERD alone. However, when strictures are fibrotic, dilation is typically required at various intervals. PPI therapy is useful after dilation to reduce recurrent stricturing and the need for more frequent dilation. Difficult strictures may be dilated by a surgeon under general anesthesia or require partial esophagectomy with esophagogastrostomy and protective fundoplication.

TABLE 140–2 DRUG THERAPY FOR REFLUX ESOPHAGITIS

Agent	Dose
ANTACIDS: LIQUID (TO BUFFER HCl AND INCREASE LESP)	
For example, Mylanta II/Maalox TC (HCl-neutralizing capacity, 25 mEq/5 mL)*	15 mL qid 1 hour after meals and at bedtime or as needed
GAVISCON (TO DECREASE REFLUX VIA A VISCOUS MECHANICAL BARRIER AND BUFFER HCl)	
$Al(OH)_3$, $NaHCO_3$, Mg trisilicate, alginic acid	2–4 tablets qid at bedtime or as needed
H_2-RECEPTOR ANTAGONISTS (TO DECREASE HCl SECRETION)	
Cimetidine (Tagamet)	800 mg bid, 400 mg qid, ≈13 mL bid
Ranitidine (Zantac)	150 mg qid or 10 mL qid; maintenance dose, 150–300 mg bid, 10 mL bid
Famotidine (Pepcid)	20–40 mg bid or 2.5–5 mL bid
Nizatidine (Axid)	150 mg bid
PROKINETICS (TO INCREASE LESP AND INCREASE GASTRIC EMPTYING)	
Bethanechol (Urecholine)	25 mg qid 30 minutes before meals and at bedtime
Metoclopramide (Reglan)	10 mg qid 30 minutes before meals and at bedtime
PROTON PUMP INHIBITORS (TO DECREASE HCl SECRETION AND GASTRIC VOLUME)	
Omeprazole (Prilosec, Zegerid)	20 mg/day; maintenance dose, 20 mg/day
Lansoprazole (Prevacid)	30 mg/day; maintenance dose, 15 mg/day
Pantoprazole (Protonix)	40 mg/day
Rabeprazole (Aciphex)	20 mg/day
Esomeprazole (Nexium)	20–40 mg/day

*Patients with reflux are not generally hypersecretors of gastric acid, so the therapeutic doses of antacids are based on their capacity to buffer (normal) basal HCl secretion rates of approximately 1 to 7 mEq/hr (mean, 2 mEq/hr) and peak meal-stimulated HCl secretion rates of about 10 to 60 mEq/hr (mean, 30 mEq/hr).
LESP = lower esophageal sphincter pressure.

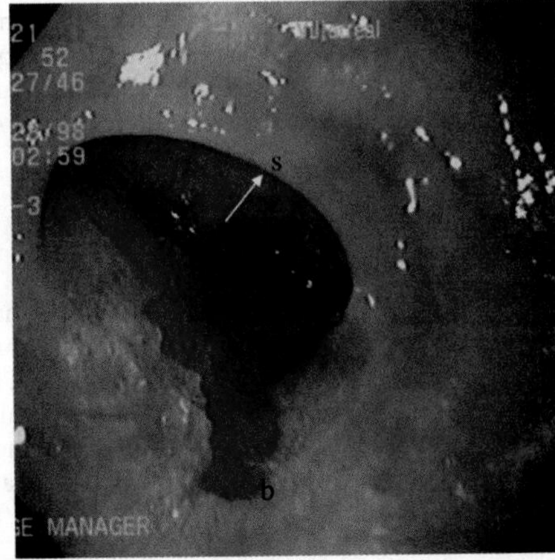

FIGURE 140–3 • Endoscopic view of the distal end of the esophagus in a patient with gastroesophageal reflux disease. A tongue of Barrett's mucosa (b) and a Schatzki ring (s) (arrow) are apparent.

Barrett's Esophagus

Barrett's esophagus is replacement of reflux-damaged squamous epithelium in the distal part of the esophagus by metaplastic, specialized columnar epithelium. It is found in 10 to 15% of patients with GERD, principally in white individuals. Barrett's metaplasia is more acid resistant than squamous epithelium and produces no symptoms. The lesion is suspected on endoscopy by the presence of reddish epithelium extending from the stomach into the tubular lumen of the esophagus (Fig. 140–3). When its length is 3 cm or more, it is called *long-segment Barrett's*, and when the length is less than 3 cm, it is called *short-segment Barrett's*. Confirmation is by biopsy. Barrett's metaplasia is a premalignant lesion that increases the risk for esophageal adenocarcinoma 30- to 125-fold over that of the general population. Factors that increase the risk for malignancy in Barrett's esophagus include white race, male sex, alcohol and tobacco use, obesity, and its length.

When Barrett's esophagus is identified on endoscopy, it generally follows a benign course (life expectancy similar to that of the general population) and remains unchanged for years to decades irrespective of the type or extent of treatment. Nonetheless, the presence of Barrett's esophagus carries up to a 10% lifetime risk for the development of esophageal adenocarcinoma, so periodic (every 2 to 3 years) endoscopy and biopsy are currently recommended for surveillance.

Treatment

Patients with Barrett's esophagus and heartburn or erosive esophagitis are treated like other patients with GERD without Barrett's esophagus. PPI therapy has been reported to reduce cell turnover rates and dysplasia but not the risk for adenocarcinoma. Weight control and cessation of smoking and alcohol are recommended because they are identifiable risk factors for malignancy. Daily aspirin therapy is under investigation for chemoprevention. Esophagectomy to remove all metaplasia is likely to be effective, but the risk is too high (morbidity of 25 to 40% and mortality of 7%) for the relatively low risk of malignancy (0.5% per year). Endoscopic surveillance, though not proved to increase survival, allows detection of phenotypic (dysplasia) and genetic (p53, aneuploidy, increase in G_2 tetraploidy) abnormalities before progression to adenocarcinoma and permits cancer to be detected at a stage (T0 to T2) for potentially curative esophagectomy. Currently, endoscopic surveillance is recommended every 2 to 3 years, with four-quadrant jumbo biopsy specimens obtained every 2 cm throughout the length of Barrett's esophagus. A finding of low-grade dysplasia increases the frequency and intensity of endoscopic surveillance, whereas focal

high-grade dysplasia is probably an indication for endoscopic mucosal resection and diffuse high-grade dysplasia an indication for esophagectomy in good surgical candidates because adenocarcinoma is found in up to a third of diffuse cases and the risk for cancer is approximately 50% over the next 5 years. In poorer surgical candidates, alternatives include endoscopic laser ablation therapy with or without an oral or intravenous photosensitizing agent (e.g., porfimer sodium) immediately or only after adenocarcinoma is confirmed. Laser therapy carries a mortality of about 1% and stricture rates of up to 50%, and many patients have residual islands of Barrett's metaplasia underneath the neosquamous epithelium. After ablative treatment, high-dose PPIs are required to enable replacement of the destroyed tissue by stratified squamous epithelium.

Persistent Reflux

Patients with (refractory) heartburn and abnormal esophageal pH monitoring *while receiving PPI therapy* have "persistent" reflux. Persistent reflux may be due to poor compliance, rapid metabolism or rapidly reversible binding of PPIs to proton pumps, or occasionally, an acid hypersecretory state such as Zollinger-Ellison syndrome (Chapter 250).

Treatment

Rx

Medical Treatment

Persistent reflux with PPI therapy sometimes responds to the addition of high-dose H_2-receptor antagonists (e.g., 300 mg ranitidine three to four times daily), with or without prokinetic therapy (metoclopramide, 10 mg three to four times daily), but the majority require surgical fundoplication for control of pathologic reflux and symptoms.

Surgical Treatment

The primary indications for antireflux surgery in GERD are (1) as an alternative to successful medical maintenance for patients who are good operative risks and (2) as a means of controlling reflux and its attendant risk for aspiration, asthma, and pneumonia. [1] Surgery is not indicated for failure of medical therapy to control "heartburn" or extraesophageal signs and symptoms presumed to be due to acid reflux because failure of high-dose PPI therapy suggests that the symptoms are unrelated to GERD and hence that antireflux surgery will also fail to control the symptoms. When indicated, the operative procedure of choice is laparoscopic Nissen fundoplication, [2] a procedure that can also be performed by open means. It has a success rate (≈85 to 90%) equivalent to that of flexible-dose PPI therapy. Mortality (≈0.2%) and morbidity (2 to 8%) rates are acceptable, and postoperative complications, such as dysphagia and the gas bloating syndrome (inability to belch or vomit), are manageable. Surgery, however, is neither a cure for symptoms because up to 50% of patients may again require medical therapy long-term nor effective in reversing Barrett's esophagus or preventing its progression to esophageal adenocarcinoma. A partial (Belsey, Dor, Toupet) fundoplication is preferred in patients with manometrically defined weak peristaltic amplitudes (<30 mm Hg) to reduce the risk for postoperative dysphagia.

Endoscopic Antireflux Procedures

Three novel endoscopic therapies—Stretta, EndoCinch, and Enteryx procedures—are approved by the U.S. Food and Drug Administration for the treatment of GERD. The Stretta procedure involves thermocoagulation of the LES region, EndoCinch provides suture plication of the gastric cardia, and Enteryx involves injection of a biopolymer into the LES muscle as a bulking agent. All can initially reduce or eliminate reliance on drug therapy in about 30 to 50% of GERD patients, but safety and durability are of major concern and thus none is currently recommended.

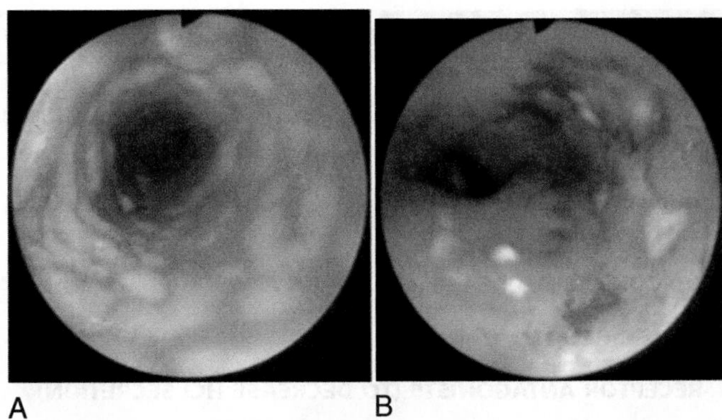

FIGURE 140–4 • Infectious esophagitis in patients with acquired immunodeficiency syndrome. A, Esophageal candidiasis. The multiple small white plaques of *Candida* are seen on the background of abnormally reddened esophageal mucosa. Patients with esophageal candidiasis may also have a smaller number of plaques or a more or less confluent white coating of the mucosa (which must not be confused with a coating of barium if the patient has recently undergone a barium study). **B,** Herpes simplex ulceration of the lower esophagus. Note the multiple shallow ulcers in the lower part of the esophagus. This appearance is not diagnostic of herpes simplex infection because a similar appearance may be seen with other causes of ulceration, including some drugs (such as potassium supplements). The presence of vesicles in the mucosa (not shown here) is virtually diagnostic of herpes simplex. (From Forbes CD, Jackson WF: Color Atlas and Text of Clinical Medicine, 3rd ed. London, Mosby, 2003.)

ESOPHAGITIS

Infectious Esophagitis

Pathobiology

Infectious esophagitis occurs principally, but not exclusively, in immunocompromised patients, usually from cancer chemotherapy, post-transplant antirejection medication, and acquired immunodeficiency syndrome (AIDS) (especially with CD4 counts <200 mm³) (Chapter 416). *Candida albicans* (Chapter 359), herpes simplex virus type 1 (HSV-1) (Chapter 397), and CMV (Chapter 399) are the most common causes, and coinfection with more than one agent may occur. In AIDS, CMV esophagitis may coexist with CMV retinitis or colitis.

Clinical Manifestations

Odynophagia is characteristic and may be severe. Dysphagia, weight loss, and gastrointestinal bleeding are common. Complications are infrequent but may include tracheobronchial fistula, perforation, and hemorrhage. Esophageal candidiasis in AIDS is associated with oral candidiasis (thrush) in only about two thirds of cases, and HSV esophagitis is associated with oral herpetic lesions in about a third of cases. In an immunocompetent host, infectious esophagitis is primarily due to HSV or *Candida.*

Diagnosis

On barium swallow, a "shaggy" mucosa suggests *Candida;* numerous small, volcanic-shaped ulcers suggest HSV; and large, deep linear ulcers suggest CMV (or HIV). Multiple biopsies of ulcerated areas with routine histologic evaluation provide a definitive diagnosis. *Candida* esophagitis is characterized on endoscopy by numerous small white-yellow mucosal plaques containing microorganisms, inflammatory cells, and necrotic mucosa (Fig. 140–4A). Positive brushings and biopsy demonstrate *Candida* pseudohyphae with periodic acid–Schiff reagent or special silver stains. HSV esophagitis on endoscopy begins as numerous vesicles that ulcerate to yield small (<2 cm), shallow, volcano-shaped ulcers (see Fig. 140–4B). A positive biopsy specimen from the ulcer edge demonstrates the characteristic cytopathic effect of HSV within squamous epithelial cells—eosinophilic intranuclear occlusions. CMV esophagitis is characterized by large (>2 cm), deep, often linear ulcers; a positive biopsy specimen from the ulcer base demonstrates the characteristic cytopathic effect of CMV within fibroblasts and endothelial cells—basophilic intranuclear inclusions.

Treatment **Rx**

In non-AIDS patients, *Candida* esophagitis may be treated with oral nystatin, 1 to 3 million units four times a day, or clotrimazole, 100-mg tablets dissolved in the mouth three to five times a day, but patients with AIDS require an azole antifungal such as oral or intravenous fluconazole, 100 to 200 mg/day for 10 to 14 days (Chapter 413). Ketoconazole and itraconazole are also effective but, unlike fluconazole, require normal gastric acidity for absorption. In resistant cases, intravenous caspofungin, 50 mg/day (after a 70-mg loading dose), or low-dose intravenous amphotericin, 0.3 to 0.5 mg/kg/day, for 10 to 14 days is effective. HSV esophagitis is treated with a nucleoside analogue such as acyclovir, 200 to 400 mg orally five times a day or 250 mg/m^2 intravenously every 8 hours for 2 weeks. Valacyclovir and famciclovir are alternatives; for resistant cases, intravenous foscarnet, 60 mg/kg every 8 hours for 2 to 4 weeks, is effective. CMV esophagitis is treated with intravenous ganciclovir, 5 mg/kg every 12 hours for 2 to 4 weeks; for resistant cases, foscarnet is administered intravenously at 60 mg/kg every 8 hours for 2 to 4 weeks. Idiopathic HIV-associated ulcers are treated with prednisone, 40 mg/day, tapering by 10 mg/wk for 1 month; thalidomide, 200 mg/day, may also be effective. Because relapse of all forms of infectious esophagitis is common in immunocompromised patients, maintenance therapy may be required.

Other Causes of Esophagitis

Alkaline Reflux Esophagitis

Alkaline reflux esophagitis is an uncommon and poorly defined clinical entity that develops in the setting of repeated and prolonged contact of the esophageal epithelium with nonacidic gastric or intestinal contents, usually in subjects with a destroyed pylorus after total gastrectomy or a Billroth II gastroenterostomy. Treatment is with bile salt–binding or mucosal-coating agents such as cholestyramine, sucralfate, or colloidal bismuth. Surgical fundoplication (intact stomach) or creation of a Roux-en-Y limb (after gastrectomy) is performed in refractory cases.

Pill-Induced Esophagitis

Pill-induced esophagitis commonly develops in patients, particularly the elderly, who are taking medication improperly (i.e., while supine or with too little liquid). It also occurs in patients with a preexisting abnormality, such as a stricture, diverticulum, or motor disorder. Pills adhere to the esophageal mucosa and cause necrosis and ulceration by the topical release of caustic medication. Among the common offenders are doxycycline, tetracycline, vitamin C, potassium chloride, nonsteroidal anti-inflammatory drugs, quinidine, alendronate and other bisphosphonates (Chapter 27), and iron (Chapter 162). Odynophagia is characteristic and commonly accompanied by dysphagia. Ulceration may lead to hemorrhage, perforation, and stricture. Upper endoscopy is indicated in nonobvious cases to exclude infectious esophagitis. Discontinuation of the offending medication and treatment with sucralfate suspension (1 g orally four times a day for 1 to 2 weeks) or a cocktail (equal parts viscous lidocaine, antacid, and diphenhydramine [Benadryl]) may control the symptoms. Once-a-day PPI therapy is useful to prevent aggravation by reflux. Education about the proper method of taking medication may prevent recurrence.

Radiation Esophagitis

Radiation esophagitis occurs after chest radiation therapy at dose levels that exceed 30 Gy (3000 rad) (Chapter 192). At levels higher than 60 Gy, severe esophagitis and ulceration can develop and lead to hemorrhage, perforation, or fistula. Concomitant chemotherapy with cytotoxic agents (e.g., doxorubicin [Adriamycin]) can potentiate radiation injury. Substernal pain, odynophagia, and dysphagia are typical. Barium swallow and endoscopy can demonstrate the extent and severity of mucosal

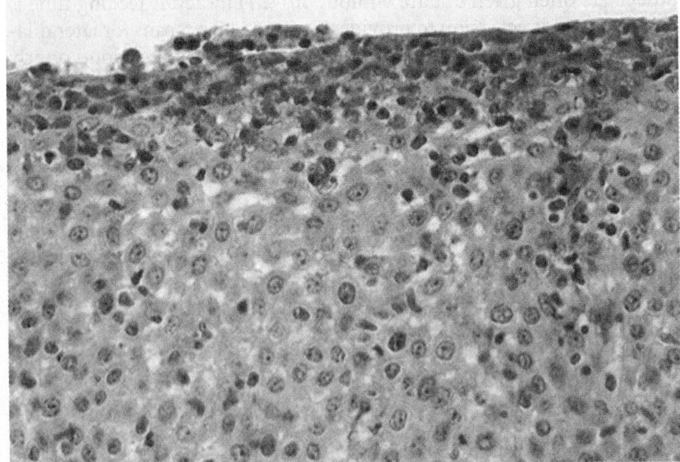

FIGURE 140–5 • Eosinophilic esophagitis. Infiltration of the esophageal epithelium with large numbers of eosinophils, more than 15 to 20 per high-power field, is diagnostic of the condition. (From Castell DO, Richter JE [eds]: The Esophagus, 4th ed. Philadelphia, Lippincott Williams & Wilkins, 2004.)

inflammation, ulceration, and luminal narrowing; endoscopy has the added benefit of biopsy for exclusion of infectious esophagitis. A liquid diet or intravenous fluids plus the treatments described for pill-induced esophagitis are helpful. Strictures may require bougienage for dilation or even esophagectomy with colonic or jejunal interposition.

Eosinophilic Esophagitis

Eosinophilic esophagitis is an uncommon, immunologically mediated entity that is being recognized with increasing frequency in children and adults aged 20 to 40 years. It has a 3 : 1 male-to-female predominance, and half the patients have asthma, skin reactions, and peripheral eosinophilia. The disease is due to food allergy and can be manifested as chest pain or heartburn, but solid food dysphagia and food impaction are characteristic. Endoscopic findings range from grossly normal to a corrugated, inflamed, eroded, or fibrotic esophagus in which a single- or multiple-ringed (feline) esophagus or a stiff, narrowed, noncompliant organ is often produced. Esophageal biopsy is diagnostic with high (>15 to 20 per high-power field) concentrations of mucosal eosinophils (Fig. 140–5). The presence of a dense collagen network within the lamina propria accounts for the rigidity and propensity to fracture (tear) on bougienage. Skin testing and a radioallergosorbent assay (RAST) for allergy should be performed to identify and remove the offending agent or agents—the most common being seafood, nuts, milk, eggs, and soy. Dietary changes or therapy with oral cromolyn (100 to 200 mg four times daily), an H_1-antagonist (e.g., chlorpheniramine, 4 mg four times daily) plus an H_2-antagonist (e.g., cimetidine, 300 mg four times daily), glucocorticoids (topical fluticasone propionate, 220 μg per puff, two puffs swallowed twice to four times daily), or a leukotriene receptor antagonist (montelukast, maintenance dose of 20 to 40 mg/day) may control symptoms, but relapse is common after cessation of therapy. Monoclonal antibodies to interleukin-5 are being investigated as therapy because this cytokine mediates the esophageal eosinophilia.

Caustic Esophagitis

Caustic esophagitis (Chapter 111) occurs from accidental ingestion in children and from suicidal attempts in adults. Among the more common materials ingested are drain cleaners (sodium hydroxide), bleach (sodium hypochlorite), detergents (sodium tripolyphosphates), and disc batteries (sodium hydroxide). Sodium hydroxide (lye) produces liquefaction necrosis on contact with the oropharynx and esophagus and thus has the potential to cause acute ulceration, perforation, and later stricture formation. When perforation is excluded by contrast (diatrizoate [Gastrografin] and, if negative, barium) swallows, endoscopy may be of value to assess the esophageal injury, but passage of the scope beyond an area of severe injury is not recommended to avoid perforation. Emergency esophagogastrectomy is indicated for free perforation and mediastinitis. In the absence of these complications, esophagitis is treated supportively with intravenous fluids and prophylactic antibiotics. Steroids in tapering dosage are often given but are without proven efficacy. A feeding tube is passed under direct vision to provide nutrition and a means for later dilation of a tight stricture. When strictures are complex and respond poorly to dilation, intestinal or colonic interposition should be considered to restore oral intake.

ESOPHAGEAL MOTOR DISORDERS

Esophageal motor disease is characterized by dysphagia for liquids and solids or chest pain (or both). Although the chest pain may mimic cardiac disease (Chapter 48) and be the dominant complaint, careful questioning should also detect dysphagia. Recurrent chest pain without dysphagia is rarely due to esophageal motor disease.

Oropharyngeal Dysphagia

Oropharyngeal dysphagia is due to neuromuscular disorders of the oropharynx and the skeletal muscle portion of the esophagus, including stroke, Parkinson's disease, amyotrophic lateral sclerosis, multiple sclerosis, myasthenia gravis, polymyositis, and myotonic dystrophy. It is characterized by difficulty in bolus transfer from the mouth to the esophagus and by nasal regurgitation or coughing (from aspiration) with swallowing. Oropharyngeal dysphagia commonly occurs amid other signs and symptoms of the underlying neuromuscular disorder. A modified barium swallow with videofluoroscopy is the procedure of choice. The swallows are performed with barium of different consistencies and with the subject swallowing in different head and body positions. Nutritional support via diet, swallow maneuvers, feeding tubes, or percutaneous endoscopic gastrostomy is appropriate, whereas primary therapy is directed at the neuromuscular disorder.

Esophageal Dysphagia

Esophageal dysphagia is due to disease of the smooth muscle–lined portion of the esophagus. The dysphagia is not accompanied by failure of bolus transfer from the mouth to the esophagus, by nasal regurgitation, or by coughing with swallowing, and it characteristically occurs with liquids as well as solids, thus indicating a lack of discrimination for bolus size. Achalasia and diffuse esophageal spasm are primary esophageal motor disorders, whereas scleroderma (Chapter 288) is the most common secondary disorder. Nutcracker esophagus, hypertensive LES, and ineffective peristalsis are best viewed as manometric abnormalities found in association with but not causative of the chest complaints. A barium swallow is valuable as a first test because it provides evidence to support either a motor or mechanical cause of dysphagia. When motor disease is suggested, esophageal manometry is often diagnostic and provides both quantitative and qualitative information about peristaltic and sphincter function.

Achalasia

Epidemiology

Achalasia is the most common primary esophageal motor disorder, with a prevalence of about 10 per 100,000 population. Its etiology is unknown, and it can occur at any age but usually between the ages of 30 and 60 years.

Pathobiology

Achalasia is characterized histopathologically by degeneration of the nerves in Auerbach's plexus, although changes also occur in the vagus nerve and swallowing center. The consequences of neuronal injury are an increase in LES pressure, incomplete LES relaxation with swallowing (achalasia means "failure to relax"), and complete (100%) aperistalsis in the esophageal body. Failure of the LES to relax produces an obstruction at the gastroesophageal junction that leads to esophageal retention. Dilation of the esophageal body occurs as a result of the increase in intraluminal pressure and the presence of weak, aperistaltic contractions.

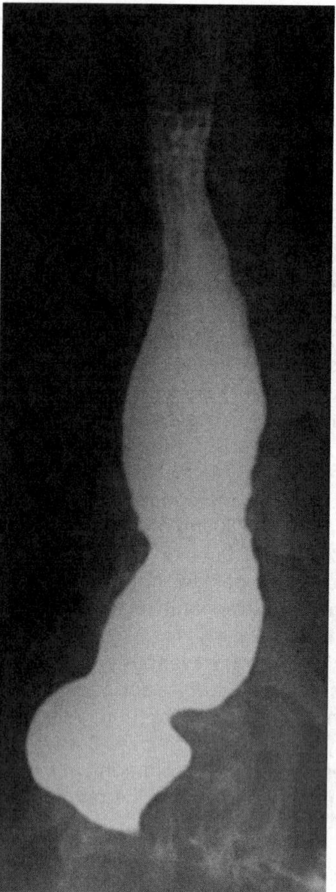

FIGURE 140–6 • Esophagogram of a patient with idiopathic achalasia. Note the dilated esophagus with an air-fluid level and distal tapering providing a "bird's beak" deformity in the area of the lower esophageal sphincter. (From Feldman M, Friedman LS, Sleisenger MH [eds]: Sleisenger and Fordtran's Gastrointestinal and Liver Disease: Pathophysiology, Diagnosis, Management, 7th ed. Philadelphia, Saunders, 2002.)

Clinical Manifestations

Dysphagia for liquids and solids is the primary complaint. Regurgitation is common, and nocturnal cough suggests aspiration on reclining. Atypical chest pain and heartburn occur in about a third of cases secondary to increased intraesophageal pressure and stasis-induced mucosal inflammation, respectively. Weight loss is highly variable and should raise concern about adenocarcinoma of the esophagus or gastric cardia.

Diagnosis

The chest radiograph may show a widened mediastinum, air-fluid level, and absent gastric air bubble. Barium swallow characteristically shows a dilated esophagus, air-fluid level, delayed esophageal emptying, and a smooth, tapered "bird's beak" deformity at the LES (Fig. 140–6). Chagas' disease (Chapter 368) can mimic achalasia by producing megaesophagus, but it also produces megaduodenum and often megaureter and cardiomegaly.

Confirmation is by esophageal manometry, which shows the characteristic incomplete relaxation of the LES with swallows and complete aperistalsis in the esophageal body. LES pressure may or may not be elevated. However, neither radiographic nor manometric criteria can effectively exclude pseudoachalasia, or achalasia secondary to an infiltrating cancer. For this reason, endoscopy is performed to examine the area before treatment; if findings are suspicious but inconclusive, biopsy should be performed, followed by examination of the area by endoscopic ultrasonography or computed tomography (CT).

Treatment

A muscle relaxant such as nifedipine, 10 mg sublingually before meals, may be helpful. More effective treatment requires either endoscopic injection of botulinum toxin into the LES (20 units per quadrant), pneumatic dilation, or surgical Heller myotomy. [3] The benefits of botulinum toxin are relatively short lived (3 to 6 months) when compared with pneumatic dilation, so repeated injections are necessary for the life of the patient. Pneumatic dilation under conscious sedation inflates a balloon (3 to 4 cm in diameter) placed across the LES to rupture its musculature; repeated treatment may be necessary for maximum benefit. A surgical Heller myotomy, which involves direct incision of the LES, is usually performed laparoscopically. Both pneumatic dilation and Heller myotomy provide excellent relief of symptoms for 5 to 10 years in about 85% of subjects. The major risk associated with pneumatic dilation is esophageal perforation (average of ≈3%), and the major side effect of Heller myotomy is reflux esophagitis (≈25%). An antireflux procedure can be combined with a Heller myotomy to reduce the risk for postoperative GERD.

Diffuse Esophageal Spasm

Clinical Manifestations

This uncommon motor disorder is manifested clinically as intermittent chest pain and dysphagia—with chest pain often being the dominant complaint but rarely occurring without dysphagia. Like achalasia, diffuse esophageal spasm is associated with degeneration of the nerves in Auerbach's plexus and, in rare instances, can evolve to achalasia.

Diagnosis

On barium swallow, diffuse esophageal spasm has prominent, spontaneous, nonpropulsive tertiary contractions that can give rise to the appearance of a "corkscrew" esophagus (Fig. 140–7). This appearance, however, is not pathognomonic because it is also observed in asymptomatic elderly patients, hence the term presbyesophagus. On esophageal manometry, more than 30% (but less than 100%) of esophageal contractions are aperistaltic and occasionally repetitive, but manometric findings are not pathognomonic because the diagnosis of diffuse esophageal spasm requires exclusion of diseases that produce similar motor changes, such as diabetes mellitus (Chapter 247), amyloidosis (Chapter 296), scleroderma (Chapter 288), idiopathic pseudo-obstruction, and reflux esophagitis.

Treatment

Therapy is principally supportive and empirical. Recommendations include reassurance of the benign nature of the disease, a trial of smooth muscle relaxants (e.g., isosorbide, 10 mg, nifedipine, 10 mg, or dicyclomine [Bentyl], 20 mg before meals) or a trial of an antidepressant (e.g., amitriptyline, 25 to 50 mg at bedtime, imipramine, 25 to 50 mg at bedtime, and trazodone, 50 mg three times a day). In some instances, relaxation exercises, biofeedback, and psychological counseling are helpful adjuncts to drug therapy.

Scleroderma

The esophagus is the gastrointestinal organ most often affected in scleroderma (Chapter 288), and it results in a characteristic manometric pattern of low LES pressure and weak aperistaltic contractions in the smooth muscle portion of the esophageal body. UES and skeletal muscle–lined upper esophageal contractions are normal. Esophageal involvement in scleroderma results in dysphagia, regurgitation, and heartburn. When dysphagia for solids is prominent, it probably reflects a peptic stricture or adenocarcinoma in Barrett's esophagus. Patients with scleroderma should be treated prophylactically for GERD as recommended earlier.

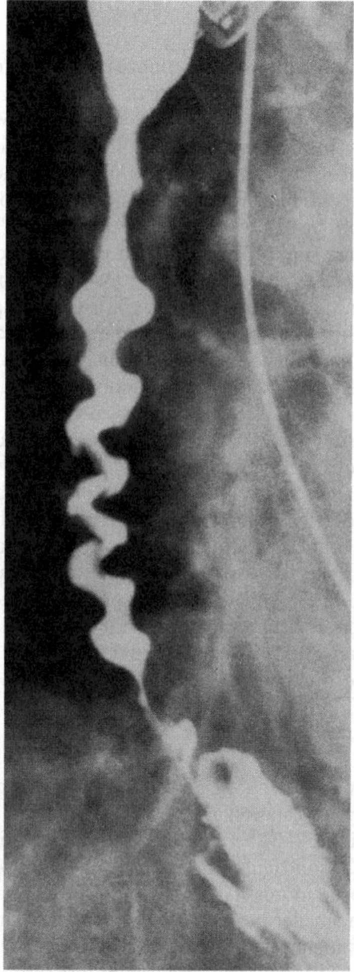

FIGURE 140–7 • Barium esophagogram showing a "corkscrew" esophagus in a patient with diffuse esophageal spasm. The patient had dysphagia, chest pain, and normal endoscopic findings. (From Feldman M [ed]: Gastroenterology and Hepatology: The Comprehensive Visual Reference. New York, Churchill Livingstone, 1997.)

Nutcracker Esophagus

Nutcracker esophagus is a term given to a relatively common manometric pattern found in patients with noncardiac chest pain. This pattern consists of normal peristalsis but with contractions of very high amplitude (average >180 mm Hg). However, a reduction in contraction amplitude by calcium-channel blockers has no consistent effect on chest pain, and chest pain can be relieved by medications (e.g., trazodone) that have no effect on amplitude. Patients with chest pain and nutcracker esophagus commonly exhibit symptoms and signs of depression or anxiety. Treatment of these disorders with (1) amitriptyline (25 to 75 mg at bedtime), imipramine (25 to 50 mg at bedtime), and trazodone (50 mg three times a day) or (2) alprazolam (0.25 to 0.5 mg three times a day) and clonazepam (0.5 to 1 mg twice a day) may relieve the chest pain.

ESOPHAGEAL TUMORS

Epidemiology

Tumors of the esophagus may be benign or malignant. Benign tumors are uncommon and include fibrovascular polyps, leiomyomas, papillomas, lipomas, neurofibromas, and granular cell tumors. When large, benign tumors can cause dysphagia or chest pain from obstruction or stretching. Malignant tumors of the esophagus currently occur at a rate of about 14,000 cases per year in the United States and are divided about equally between squamous cell carcinoma and adenocarcinoma. Rare primary malignancies include leiomyosarcoma, melanoma, lymphoma, and plasmacytoma. Tumors metastatic to the esophagus usually originate from the breast, lung, or skin (melanoma).

Squamous Cell Carcinoma

The incidence of squamous cell carcinoma in the United States is about 2.6 per 100,000, with men having a three- to fourfold higher risk than women and blacks a four- to fivefold higher risk than whites. Regions of high risk also exist in the Transkei of South Africa, China's Linxian and Yangcheng provinces, and Kashmir and Bombay in India. The risk for squamous cell cancer is higher with heavy alcohol and tobacco use, papillomavirus infection, lye ingestion, achalasia, Plummer-Vinson syndrome, tylosis, celiac disease, and radiation exposure. The clinical manifestation is typically rapidly progressive dysphagia for solids, anorexia, and weight loss. Less commonly, squamous cell carcinoma is accompanied by hypercalcemia (pseudohyperparathyroidism), hoarseness (recurrent laryngeal nerve paralysis), or tracheoesophageal fistula. Barium swallow generally reveals a bulky, eroded, partially obstructing esophageal mass that is proved to be squamous cell carcinoma by endoscopic biopsy. Adjacent lymph node invasion is common because the esophagus lacks a serosal layer. Hematogenous metastases usually spread to the liver, lungs, kidney, heart, and bone. Endoscopic ultrasonography or CT, or both, are used for staging. Squamous cell carcinoma is radiosensitive, and chemoradiation therapy, with or without subsequent surgery, can improve the outcome. Nonetheless, late-stage diagnosis is the rule, so the overall 5-year survival rate is only 20 to 30%. Palliation for dysphagia caused by inoperable, obstructing cancers is better with brachytherapy than with endoscopic stenting. [4] Other options include bougienage or tumor ablation by laser, heater probe, or alcohol injection.

Adenocarcinoma

Adenocarcinomas are equally as common as squamous cell cancers but, unlike squamous cancers, arise principally in the distal end of the esophagus (see Fig. 132–7) because the predominant risk for adenocarcinoma is Barrett's esophagus. However, only about 40% of patients with esophageal adenocarcinoma have a history of heartburn, and heartburn occurs in an even smaller percentage of those with Barrett's esophagus. The diagnosis of adenocarcinoma is typically made at endoscopy in a patient with dysphagia, anorexia, and weight loss secondary to a lumen-encroaching lesion. Lymphatic spread is common. Adenocarcinomas are radioinsensitive; although chemoradiation therapy and surgery may improve survival, 5-year survival rates are less than 20%. [5] Palliation is the same as for inoperable squamous cell carcinoma.

STRUCTURAL ABNORMALITIES

Pharyngoesophageal Diverticula

Esophageal diverticula include Zenker's diverticula, midesophageal and epiphrenic diverticula, and intramural pseudodiverticulosis. *Zenker's diverticulum* is an outpouching of pharyngeal mucosa in an area of muscular weakness (Killian's triangle) just proximal to the cricopharyngeus muscle (UES). It is caused by increased hypopharyngeal pressure generated by pharyngeal peristalsis against an incompletely relaxing UES *(cricopharyngeal achalasia)* or the inadequate opening (as a result of inflammation or fibrosis) of a relaxed UES *(cricopharyngeal bar)*. When small, a Zenker diverticulum produces no symptoms, but when large, it leads to dysphagia, regurgitation of undigested food, halitosis, neck pain and swelling, and aspiration. The diagnosis is made by barium swallow (Fig. 140–8), and treatment is cricopharyngeal myotomy, with or without diverticulectomy, or *endoscopic staple-assisted diverticulostomy.*

Midesophageal and epiphrenic diverticula are uncommon and arise from either pulsion, such as an esophageal motor disorder, or traction, such as paraesophageal inflammatory or neoplastic disease. Most are small, wide-mouthed outpouchings and are asymptomatic. When large, they may be associated with dysphagia, regurgitation, aspiration, or chest pain. The diagnosis is made by barium swallow or endoscopy, and treatment is surgical diverticulectomy.

Esophageal intramural pseudodiverticulosis is an uncommon condition noted on barium swallow in which numerous small flask-shaped outpouchings are evident within the esophageal wall. These outpouchings represent dilation of the secretory ducts of the esophageal submucosal glands and arise in the setting of mucosal inflammation or esophageal obstruction. The pseudodiverticula produce no symptoms but occur in the setting of chest pain, dysphagia, heartburn, and odynophagia related to the associated underlying disease. Treatment is directed at the underlying disease.

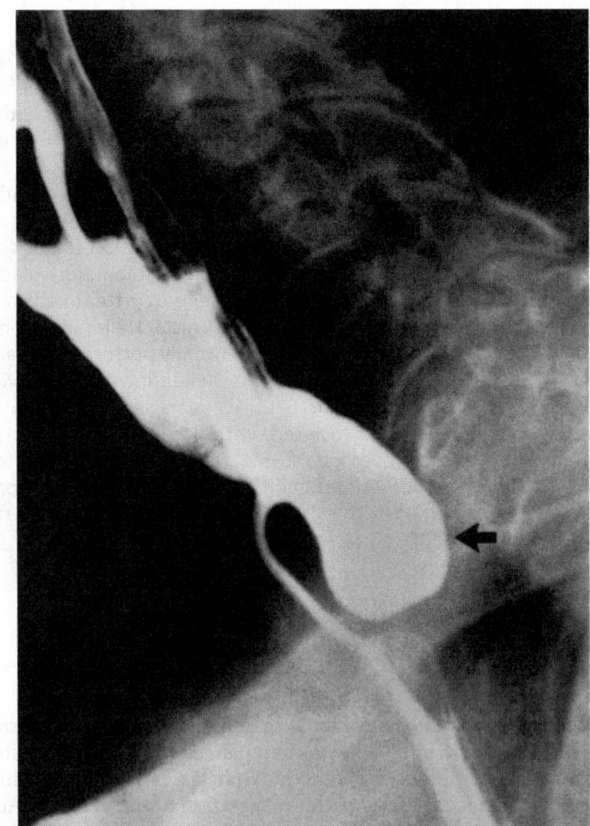

FIGURE 140–8 • Barium esophagogram showing a Zenker diverticulum (arrow). This elderly patient complained of dysphagia, choking with eating, and recurrent pneumonia. (From Feldman M [ed]: Gastroenterology and Hepatology: The Comprehensive Visual Reference. New York, Churchill Livingstone, 1997.)

Esophageal Rings and Webs

The distal end of the esophagus contains two rings, designated the A ring and the B ring, that on barium swallow demarcate the proximal and distal borders of the esophageal vestibule, respectively. The A ring is a broad (4- to 5-mm) band of hypertrophied muscle covered by squamous epithelium. It is rare and usually asymptomatic, but when associated with dysphagia, it can be treated by bougienage or by endoscopic injection with botulinum toxin. The B, or Schatzki, ring, a thin (2-mm) membrane consisting of mucosa and submucosa, is localized to the squamocolumnar junction. It is found in about 15% of barium studies and is often asymptomatic. Schatzki's rings are probably congenital in origin but may extend into the lumen over time secondary to meal-induced (rather than reflux-induced) trauma. When the ring constricts the esophageal lumen to less than 15 mm, dysphagia for solids usually occurs. Diagnosis is by barium swallow (see Fig. 140–1B), often aided by swallowing a marshmallow or barium tablet. When symptomatic, treatment is directed at disrupting the ring either by esophageal bougienage or incision by laser, sphincterotome, or biopsy forceps.

Esophageal webs are thin, fragile membranes of stratified squamous epithelium that occur in the upper and midportion of the esophagus. Unlike rings, these congenital anomalies rarely encircle the lumen but instead protrude, as a shelf, from the anterior wall. Webs are generally asymptomatic and diagnosed incidentally on barium swallow. Upper endoscopy can detect the webs but may rupture them without awareness of their presence. Webs, like rings, can cause dysphagia for solids only and, when symptomatic, are treated by esophageal bougienage. Cervical webs associated with dysphagia and iron deficiency anemia are part of the Plummer-Vinson or Paterson-Kelly syndrome (Chapter 163). This syndrome occurs primarily in women and is associated with an increased risk for sprue and squamous cell carcinoma of the pharynx and esophagus.

Hernias

The two major types are sliding hiatal hernias and paraesophageal hernias. A hiatal hernia is an acquired anomaly in which the esophagogastric junction and stomach project above the diaphragm and into the chest. It is identified in about 15% of upper gastrointestinal series, usually as an incidental finding. Hernias are thought to arise from age-related loss of elasticity of the phrenoesophageal ligament or widening of the right crus of the diaphragm. Hiatal hernias are common in erosive, but not nonerosive forms of GERD. They also occasionally cause gastric erosions (Cameron's ulcers), iron deficiency anemia, and gastrointestinal bleeding as a result of ischemia or mechanical trauma to the herniated gastric mucosa. Treatment is usually medical (acid inhibitors, mucosal-coating agents), but surgical correction is necessary in refractory cases. Paraesophageal hernias are uncommon and result from a defect in the phrenoesophageal ligament. Because the gastroesophageal junction remains fixed, the stomach herniates into the chest and causes close apposition of the gastroesophageal junction and pylorus. Symptoms may be absent, but pain, dysphagia, and bleeding can occur. Surgical repair is generally recommended to prevent incarceration.

MISCELLANEOUS ESOPHAGEAL CONDITIONS

Foreign Bodies

Foreign bodies commonly lodge in the esophagus either at regions of anatomic narrowing (e.g., UES, LES, aorta, or left mainstem bronchus) or at regions of pathology (e.g., stricture, ring). Symptoms include neck pain, chest pain, dysphagia, or odynophagia. Complete obstruction by the object carries a risk for aspiration pneumonia, and delayed relief increases the risk for ulceration, perforation, and stricture.

In the absence of clinical evidence of perforation, foreign bodies are diagnosed and removed by upper endoscopy via a snare, basket, or biopsy forceps. During removal, airway protection is essential. Rigid endoscopy under general anesthesia by an otolaryngologist is an alternative means for the safe retrieval of objects from the hypopharynx or proximal part of the esophagus. Meat impaction in the distal part of the esophagus may respond to smooth muscle relaxation by the administration of 1 mg of intravenous glucagon; ingestion of a papain solution is not recommended because of the potential for coincident damage to the esophageal wall.

Esophageal Trauma

The esophagus, though protected by the bony thorax, is subject to being torn or ruptured by blunt chest trauma (e.g., motor vehicle accident) or a penetrating sharp (e.g., knife) wound. However, most tears and perforations are either iatrogenic and result from esophagogastric diagnostic or therapeutic instrumentation or are caused by abrupt increases in intraluminal pressure during vomiting, retching, and coughing. When increased intraluminal pressure causes a mucosal tear just below or through the esophagogastric junction, it is called a Mallory-Weiss tear (Chapter 140); when it causes complete rupture of the distal end of the esophagus (usually on the left side), the condition is referred to as Boerhaave's syndrome. The consequence of a mucosal tear is gastrointestinal bleeding, which may stop spontaneously or continue with life-threatening hemorrhage (Chapter 137). Cervical rupture is usually confined and leads to a periesophageal abscess. Intrathoracic rupture is accompanied by chest pain, fever, soft tissue emphysema, pleural effusion, pneumothorax, and mediastinitis. Rupture of an intra-abdominal segment leads to peritonitis and sepsis. For tears with bleeding, upper endoscopy is the procedure of choice, both for diagnosis and, when needed, for control of bleeding by epinephrine injection and cautery (Chapters 136 and 137). If endoscopic control fails, emergency angiography with embolization or infusion of vasopressin, exploratory laparotomy to oversew the tear, or balloon tamponade with a Sengstaken-Blakemore or Minnesota tube can be life-saving. For esophageal perforations, diagnosis is by physical examination and chest radiograph to demonstrate extraluminal air, as confirmed by a leak on a diatrizoate swallow. If the diatrizoate swallow is negative, barium may be used. CT can also be helpful. Early recognition (first 24 hours) of an esophageal rupture should prompt primary surgical closure, external drainage, and antibiotics. Later recognition in a clinically stable patient with a walled-off abscess in the neck or mediastinum may be treated medically by nasogastric suction, antibiotics, and parenteral nutrition.

Developmental Anomalies

Congenital anomalies of the esophagus are relatively common and occur in 1 in 3000 to 4500 live births. Such anomalies include esophageal atresia, tracheoesophageal fistulas, strictures, and cysts. Most are diagnosed in infancy or childhood. Small or atypical (H-type) tracheoesophageal fistulas not diagnosed in childhood are manifested as recurrent episodes of aspiration pneumonia and are diagnosed by contrast radiography or by passage of methylene blue from the airway to the esophagus or vice versa. Treatment is surgical.

An aberrant right subclavian artery can be manifested later in life as dysphagia (dysphagia lusoria) arising from vascular compression of the esophagus. The diagnosis is suggested by a barium esophagogram showing a pencil-like indentation near the fourth thoracic vertebra. The diagnosis is confirmed by CT, magnetic resonance imaging, or endoscopic ultrasound. Treatment is often by diet modification, but in refractory cases, surgery is required to reanastomose the artery to the ascending aorta.

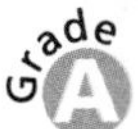

1. Lundell L, Miettinen P, Myrvold HE, et al: Continued (5-year) followup of a randomized clinical study comparing antireflux surgery and omeprazole in gastroesophageal reflux disease. J Am Coll Surg 2001;192:172–179.
2. Mahon D, Rhodes M, Decadt B, et al: Randomized clinical trial of laparoscopic Nissen fundoplication compared with proton-pump inhibitors for treatment of chronic gastro-oesophageal reflux. Br J Surg 2005;92:695–699.
3. Bansal R, Nostrant TT, Scheiman JM, et al: Intrasphincteric botulinum toxin versus pneumatic balloon dilation for treatment of primary achalasia. J Clin Gastroenterol 2003;36:209–214.
4. Homs MYV, Steyerberg EW, Eijkenboom WMH, et al: Single-dose brachytherapy versus metal stent placement for the palliation of dysphagia from oesophageal cancer: Multicentre randomised trial. Lancet 2004;364:1497–1504.
5. Urba SG, Orringer MB, Turrisi A, et al: Randomized trial of preoperative chemoradiation versus surgery alone in patients with locoregional esophageal carcinoma. J Clin Oncol 2001;19:305–313.

SUGGESTED READINGS

Dogan I, Mittal RK: Esophageal motor disorders: Recent advances. Curr Opin Gastroenterol 2006;22:417–422. *Clinical review.*

Kleinberg L, Gibson MK, Forastiere AA: Chemoradiotherapy for localized esophageal cancer: Regimen selection and molecular mechanisms of radiosensitization. Nat Clin Pract Oncol 2007;4:282–294. *Review of treatment options for local esophageal cancer.*

Moayyedi P, Talley NJ: Gastro-oesophageal reflux disease. Lancet 2006;367:2086–2100. *A comprehensive review.*

Rastogi A, Shaarma P: Barrett's esophagus. Endoscopy 2006;38:1065–1069. *Comprehensive review.*

141 ACID PEPTIC DISEASE: EPIDEMIOLOGY AND PATHOBIOLOGY

Ernst J. Kuipers and Martin J. Blaser

Acid peptic diseases can involve the esophagus, stomach, and duodenum. This chapter focuses on gastroduodenal and peptic disease. Acid peptic diseases of the esophagus, in particular gastroesophageal reflux disease, are discussed in Chapter 140, whereas dyspeptic symptoms in patients who have no endoscopic abnormalities, termed *nonulcer dyspepsia*, are discussed in Chapter 139.

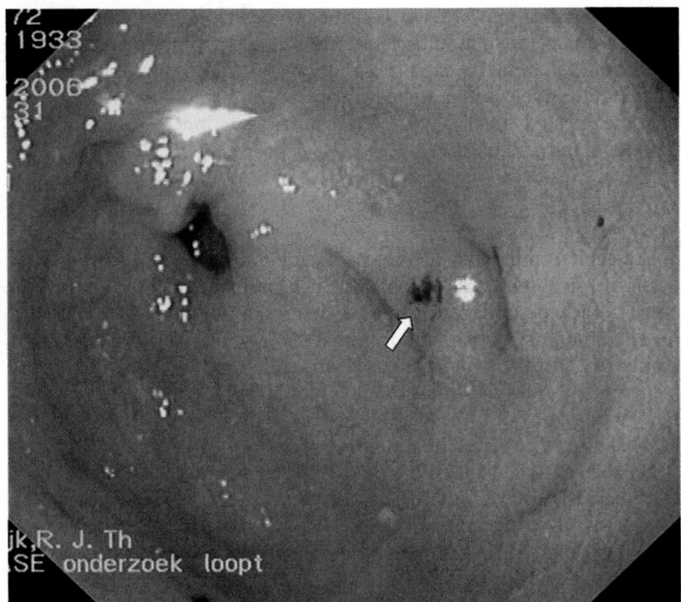

FIGURE 141–1 • Endoscopic view of uncomplicated erosive gastritis. The erosion appears as a small, superficial mucosal break with a black base (arrow).

FIGURE 141–2 • Endoscopic view of an ulcer at the anterior wall of the duodenal bulb. The ulcer has a clean base, with minor signs of recent bleeding at the lower ulcer rim.

Definitions

Gastric and duodenal ulcers usually occur in an area of inflamed mucosa. This inflammation, termed *gastritis, duodenitis, or bulbitis,* sometimes can be recognized during endoscopy by signs of edema, reddening, and swelling of the mucosa, but microscopic evaluation of endoscopic biopsy specimens is required for a definite diagnosis of mucosal inflammation.

Gastritis is usually categorized by endoscopic and histologic criteria, with granulocytes predominating in active gastritis and mononuclear cells in chronic gastritis. Gastritis is also classified by the segment of involved stomach: antral-predominant gastritis, corpus-predominant gastritis, or pangastritis. Finally, the absence or presence of premalignant stages of damage to the mucosa as a result of long-standing inflammation defines the category of nonatrophic or atrophic gastritis, respectively. Endoscopic aspects are usually nonspecific, unless the gastric mucosa has either a typical miniature cobblestone appearance, termed *nodular gastritis* (a lesion found particularly in children colonized by *Helicobacter pylori*), or grossly enlarged folds without evidence of cancer (termed *hypertrophic gastritis*).

A *peptic ulcer* is a mucosal defect that has a diameter of at least 0.5 cm that penetrates the muscularis mucosae. Smaller mucosal defects are called *erosions* (Fig. 141–1). Gastric ulcers are subdivided into proximal ulcers, located in the body of the stomach, and distal ulcers, located in the antrum and angulus of the stomach. Gastric ulcers are mainly located along the lesser curvature, in particular at the transitional zone of corpus to antral-type mucosa. This transitional zone is often in the area of the angulus but may shift proximally. Duodenal ulcers usually are located on the anterior or posterior wall of the duodenal bulb (Fig. 141–2), occasionally at both sites (“kissing” ulcers). Lesions distal to the duodenal bulb are termed *postbulbar ulcers.* Patients who previously underwent a distal gastric resection (Billroth I or II procedure) can develop ulceration at the gastroduodenal anastomosis (anastomotic ulcer). However, ulcers occurring after Billroth II resection are predominantly located in the jejunal mucosa at the junction between the afferent and efferent loops. Other peptic ulcers can occur at sites of metaplastic or heterotopic gastric mucosa, for example, in Meckel’s diverticulum, the rectum, or Barrett’s esophagus. Patients with a large hiatal hernia can develop gastric ulceration, known as *Cameron’s ulcers,* at the level of the herniation.

Epidemiology

The worldwide prevalence of gastritis reflects the prevalence of *H. pylori.* Colonization with this bacterium is virtually always associated with chronic active gastritis, which persists as long as an individual remains colonized and only slowly disappears within 6 to 24 months after *H. pylori* eradication. In developing countries and among first-generation immigrants from these countries to the Western world, the prevalence of *H. pylori* gastritis is very high (often >80%) in all age groups, including children. In Western countries, the prevalence of *H. pylori* gastritis increases with age; it is currently often less than 20% in young adults, but 40 to 60% in elderly persons.

Although peptic ulcer disease is strongly related to *H. pylori* gastritis and duodenitis, the epidemiology of ulcer disease has shown secular variations even at times when *H. pylori* was ubiquitous. The incidence of peptic ulcer disease rose in Western countries steeply in the late 19th and early 20th centuries and has decreased over the past 30 years, yet peptic ulceration remains a common disorder. The decline in incidence, associated with a decrease in hospital admissions and surgery for ulcer disease, is believed mainly to reflect decreasing prevalence of gastric colonization with *H. pylori.* The declining incidence of ulcer disease is also the result of widespread application of eradication therapy, which strongly reduced recurrent ulcers in *H. pylori*-positive patients. Other factors that may have contributed to the decreasing incidence of ulcer disease include the widespread use of acid suppressive medication and the more recent introduction of nonsteroidal anti-inflammatory drugs (NSAIDs) that have lower rates of gastroduodenal complications. Despite these trends, the incidence of hospital admissions for complications of ulcers and mortality from ulcer disease have remained relatively stable over the past decades in both the United States and other countries.

In Western countries, duodenal ulcers occur more frequently than gastric ulcers. The predominant age at which duodenal ulcers occur is between 20 and 50 years, whereas gastric ulcers most commonly occur in patients more than 40 years old. The incidence of gastroduodenal ulcer disease is approximately 1 to 2 per 1000 inhabitants per year. Two thirds of patients with ulcers are male, and the disease is more common in smokers. The risk of recurrent disease after initial healing is high; more than 50% of patients have a recurrent ulcer within 12 months of healing in the absence of treatment. Maintenance acid suppressive therapy reduces this recurrence rate, but only therapeutic measures that remove the underlying cause of the ulcer are able to prevent nearly all ulcer recurrences.

Pathobiology

Helicobacter pylori

Most peptic ulcers are associated with colonization with *H. pylori* (Fig. 141–3). The initial clinical studies into the association between *H. pylori*

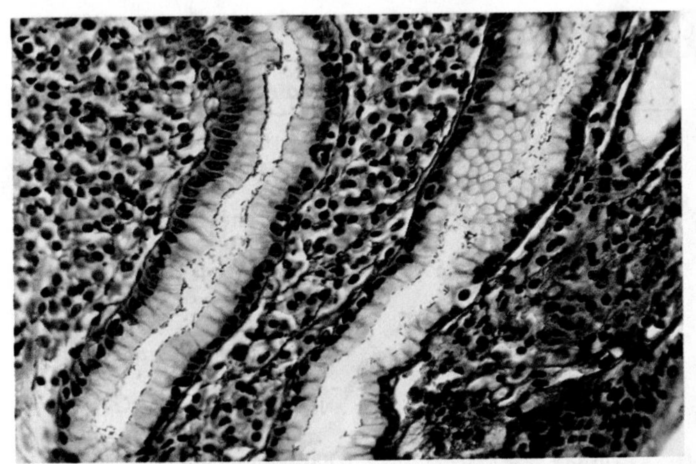

FIGURE 141–3 • Gastric mucosa colonized with *Helicobacter pylori* appearing as curved bacilli on the mucosal surface.

and ulcer disease reported that approximately 85% of patients with gastric ulcer disease and 95% of patients with duodenal ulcer disease were colonized by *H. pylori.* Most persons who are *H. pylori* positive do not have any specific complaints, nor do they develop ulcer disease. The estimated risk for the development of ulcer disease during persistent *H. pylori* colonization is 5 to 15%, that is, three- to eightfold higher than the risk for patients who are *H. pylori* negative. The risk for development of an ulcer in the presence of *H. pylori* is determined by a combination of host- and bacteria-related factors. Host factors include immune response, smoking, and stress. Bacterial factors that increase the risk of ulcer include the following: a high production of cytotoxin, which reflects the presence of the s1m1-type of the *vacA* gene; a high level of cytokine induction, owing to the presence of genes in the *cag* pathogenicity island; and enhanced adherence, resulting from *babA.*

Nonsteroidal Anti-inflammatory Drugs and Aspirin

The other common cause of gastroduodenal ulcer disease is the use of NSAIDs. At least 2 to 4% of the population in many countries use acetylsalicylic acid, acetic acid derivatives (diclofenac, indomethacin, sulindac), or propionic acid derivatives (ibuprofen, ketoprofen, naproxen) on a daily basis. Within 14 days after the start of such treatment, about 5% of patients develop mucosal breaks, that is, erosions and ulcers. In patients who continue therapy for 4 weeks or longer, this proportion increases to 10%. The risk of developing an ulcer during NSAID use is higher in patients who are more than 60 years old, in patients who had a previous ulcer, in patients who use corticosteroids or high-dose NSAIDs, and in patients with major comorbid diseases. In patients who use anticoagulants, such as warfarin, or who have severe comorbid disease, an NSAID-induced ulcer is more likely to lead to life-threatening gastroduodenal hemorrhage.

On the basis of their activities, NSAIDs are divided into cyclooxygenase 1 (COX1) and COX-2 inhibitors (Chapter 27). The COX1 enzyme is involved in the production of prostaglandins, which play a role in normal cell regulation. The COX2 enzyme, which also is involved in the production of prostaglandins, is induced by inflammatory responses. Most NSAIDs have a nonselective COX-inhibitory effect, but selective COX2 inhibitors are associated with fewer gastroduodenal ulcers.

Assessment of NSAID use in an individual patient presenting with ulcer disease can be difficult, both because NSAID use is common and often intermittent and because many different NSAIDs are widely available over the counter in most countries. Nevertheless, because of the strong association of NSAIDs with ulcer disease and the risk for recurrence of ulcers with continued use, it is important that patients with ulcers be thoroughly assessed for the use of NSAIDs. NSAID use is usually evaluated by detailed medical history, focusing not only on current and recent drug use, but also on symptoms of pain, including musculoskeletal complaints. Further information from family members, family practitioners, and pharmacists is sometimes helpful. Urine testing for aspirin and NSAID derivatives is feasible but not commonly used in clinical practice.

Idiopathic or Non–nonsteroidal Anti-inflammatory Drug, non–Helicobacter pylori Ulcer Acid Peptic Disease

H. pylori and NSAID use account in most series for 80 to 95% of cases of gastritis and ulcer disease. The remainder is often referred to as *idiopathic* or *H. pylori–negative, non-NSAID* acid peptic disease. The proportion of ulcer disease that is idiopathic is increasing throughout the world as the prevalence of *H. pylori* decreases. Further, it is likely that some ulcers in *H. pylori*–positive patients were not caused by *H. pylori.* Consistent with this notion is the fact that some of *H. pylori*–positive patients with ulcer disease develop recurrent ulcers after successful bacterial eradication and so presumably had idiopathic ulcer disease. It is not known whether the increased diagnosis of idiopathic ulcer disease is simply proportional to the decreased numbers of *H. pylori*–associated ulcers or whether it reflects a true increase in incidence of idiopathic ulcers.

In patients with idiopathic ulcer disease, specific clues to the underlying cause are often provided by the medical history, including comorbidity and drug use, the endoscopic appearance of the ulcer, and the histologic features of the ulcer's margins and surroundings. In most cases, these initial data can direct further diagnostic studies (Table 141–1).

Malignant Ulcer Disease

Gastroduodenal ulcers can result from underlying malignant disease. In the stomach, these tumors are related to gastric adenocarcinoma and, in rarer cases, to mucosa-associated lymphoid tissue (MALT) lymphomas (Chapter 202). Malignant ulcers in the duodenum may result from primary duodenal carcinomas or from penetrating pancreatic cancers. Duodenal cancers have an association with polyposis syndromes, in particular familial adenomatous polyposis and, to a lesser extent, MYH-associated polyposis and Peutz-Jeghers syndrome (Chapter 203). Both in the stomach and duodenum, ulcer disease also can be caused by metastatic tumors, including cancers of the breast, colon, thyroid, or kidney, or by melanoma, disseminated lymphoma, or Kaposi's sarcoma. Malignant ulcers characteristically are irregular in shape with heaped borders, but they also may be flat or depressed lesions. Current high-resolution and magnification endoscopes allow visualization of the altered mucosal structure surrounding an ulcer, including changes in the microvascular pattern. For a definite diagnosis of malignancy, multiple biopsy specimens are needed, usually from the ulcer margins.

Systemic Inflammatory Disorders

A few gastroduodenal ulcers are caused by systemic inflammatory diseases, in particular, Crohn's disease (Chapter 144). Patients with Crohn's disease affecting the proximal gastrointestinal tract often have multiple ulcers, which are characterized by irregular longitudinal shapes. Ulcers in the duodenum occur atop Kerckring's folds. Patients with gastroduodenal ulcers resulting from Crohn's disease do not invariably have evidence of disease elsewhere in the digestive tract, nor do blood tests suggest an active inflammatory bowel disorder in these patients. The presence of granulomas in biopsy specimens supports a diagnosis of Crohn's disease. However, the absence of granulomas does not exclude Crohn's disease, and these lesions are not specific for Crohn's disease, because they also are associated with *H. pylori* gastritis and other conditions.

Other inflammatory disorders that can cause gastritis or gastroduodenal ulcers include Henoch-Schönlein purpura (Chapter 115), Takayasu's arteritis (Chapter 292), vasculitis (Chapter 291), and sarcoidosis (Chapter 95). Lymphocytic gastroduodenitis, which is strongly associated with celiac disease (Chapter 143), may lead to duodenal ulceration and subsequent stenotic web formation. Ulcer disease may also occur in patients with polycythemia vera (Chapter 168), possibly in relation to reduced mucosal blood flow. Vasculitis underlying ulcer disease should be considered in patients with chronic or recurrent ulceration in whom other causes have been excluded. Lymphocytic phlebitis, which is a rare vasculitic inflammatory disorder affecting the mesenteric veins, may cause gastric ulcer disease. Systemic amyloidosis (Chapter 296) affecting the stomach wall may lead to gastric ulcer disease. Rare cases of duodenal ulceration have been described in the presence of annular pancreas or congenital bands obstructing the descending duodenum.

Hypergastrinemic Syndromes

Peptic ulcers can result from chronic gastric hyperacidity related to hypergastrinemia. The most important hypergastrinemic disorder is the Zollinger-Ellison syndrome (Chapter 250), a condition of marked

TABLE 141–1 DIFFERENTIAL DIAGNOSIS OF PEPTIC ULCER DISEASE

Origin	Condition	Frequency	Diagnostic Test	Findings
Microbes	*Helicobacter pylori*	Very common	*Helicobacter pylori* tests	Bacteria, enzymes, antigens, antibodies
			Histology	Gastritis
	Helicobacter heilmannii	Rare	Histology	Spiral bacteria, gastritis
	Treponema pallidum	Very rare	Serology	Antibodies
	Mycobacterial infection	Very rare	Histology, immune response testing, chest radiograph	Acid-fast bacteria, granuloma, immune response
	Cytomegalovirus, herpes simplex virus type 1	Rare	Histology, serology	Virus inclusions, antibodies
Drug use	Nonsteroidal anti-inflammatory drugs/aspirin	Very common	History, urine test	Nonsteroidal anti-inflammatory drug use
	Bisphosphonates	Rare	History	Bisphosphonate use
	Corticosteroids	Rare	History	Corticosteroid use, comorbidity
	Amphetamines/cocaine	Rare	History, drug testing	Drug use
Malignancy	Gastric cancer	Common	Histology	Malignancy
	Duodenal cancer	Rare	Histology	Malignancy
	Pancreatic cancer	Common	Histology, computed tomography	Malignancy
	Mucosa-associated lymphoid tissue lymphoma	Rare	Histology	Malignancy
	Metastatic cancer	Rare	Histology	Malignancy
Gastritis syndromes	Eosinophilic gastritis	Rare	Histology	Eosinophilic infiltration
	Lymphocytic gastritis	Rare	Histology, celiac disease screening	Lymphocytic infiltration, villous atrophy
Hyperacidic syndromes	Zollinger-Ellison syndrome	Rare	Serum gastrin, secretin test	Extreme hypergastrinemia, positive secretin test
	Antral G-cell hyperfunction	Very rare	Serum gastrin, secretin test	Moderate hypergastrinemia, negative secretin test
	Retained gastric antrum	Very rare	Medical history, gastrin	Billroth II resection, hypergastrinemia
	Systemic mastocytosis	Very rare	Histology of affected sites	Mast cell infiltration
	Chronic myelogenous leukemia	Very rare	Leukemia evaluation	Leukemia
Ischemia	Mesenteric vascular occlusion	Common	Angiography	Vascular disease
	Polycythemia vera	Rare	Blood counts	Polycythemia
Specific ulcer types	Cameron's ulcer	Common	Endoscopy	Ulcer in large hiatus hernia
	Marginal ulcer	Common	Endoscopy	Ulcer at anastomosis
Systemic inflammation	Crohn's disease	Common	Histology, ileocolonoscopy	Inflammation, granulomas
	Vasculitides	Rare	Histology, systemic evaluation	Vasculitis, signs of systemic disease
	Gastric amyloidosis	Very rare	Histology	Amyloid deposition
Other conditions	Stress ulcer	Fairly common in patients in intensive care units	Endoscopy	—
	Radiation therapy/ chemotherapy	Rare	Endoscopy, history	—

hyperacidity leading to severe peptic ulcer disease caused by a gastrin-producing endocrine tumor. These patients usually have multiple, therapy-resistant bulbar and postbulbar duodenal ulcers. The diagnosis can be confirmed by the presence of a high fasting serum gastrin level (usually ≥10-fold increased and >1000 pg/mL). Similar gastrin levels sometimes can be observed in patients treated for chronic ulcer disease with high-dose proton pump inhibitors. For clarification, secretin testing can be performed: in patients with Zollinger-Ellison syndrome, injection of secretin (1 U/kg) leads to a further increase of serum gastrin levels of more than 50%. Imaging techniques, such as computed tomography, magnetic resonance imaging, isotope scanning, endoscopic ultrasonography, videocapsule endoscopy, and double-balloon enteroscopy may be used to detect the primary tumor, which often is located either in the pancreas or in the proximal small bowel. In some patients, Zollinger-Ellison syndrome occurs as part of multiple endocrine neoplasia (Chapter 250), particularly in association with hyperparathyroidism. Other hypergastrinemic hyperacidity syndromes are the retained gastric antrum syndrome (see later) and antral G-cell hyperfunction. In the latter, fasting serum gastrin levels are only modestly increased and do not rise after further injection of secretin, but they respond in an exaggerated way to meals, thereby leading to hyperacidity. When the condition occurs in an *H. pylori*–positive patient, bacterial eradication therapy may be curative. However, some patients with G-cell hyperfunction are *H. pylori* negative.

Ischemia

Stenosis or occlusion of the celiac trunk or the superior mesenteric artery (Chapter 146) also can lead to ulceration in the mucosa of the proximal digestive tract. These ulcers typically occur in elderly patients with risk factors for atherosclerosis, but they also can occur in younger subjects without such risk factors. Ischemic ulcers tend to heal slowly and recur. Pallor of the mucosa, consistent with decreased mucosal blood flow, may be noted at endoscopy. Upper mesenteric ischemia is often associated with upper abdominal pain, which can be elicited by a meal or by physical activity. These symptoms may cause patients to decrease their food intake, thereby leading to weight loss before their clinical presentation. The prevalence of upper mesenteric ischemia with secondary ulcer disease is unknown, in part owing to its variable presentation, often with a gradual history of symptoms, the lack of standardized and reliable diagnostic tests, and the unfamiliarity of clinicians with the condition. Diagnostic evaluation includes a duplex ultrasound scan for vascular flow and conventional or computed tomographic angiography of the affected arteries.

Stress Ulcers

Patients who are stressed by a severe medical condition, such as major trauma, sepsis, extensive burns, head injury, or multiorgan failure, can develop stress ulcers in the stomach or duodenum. Major risk factors for stress ulceration in severely ill patients include mechanical ventilation, coagulopathy, and hypotension, but factors such as hepatic and renal failure and use of ulcerogenic medication may contribute to the development of stress ulcers. Stress ulcers occur independent of *H. pylori* colonization. Ulcers associated with head injury are known as Cushing's ulcers, and ulcers associated with extensive burns are known as Curling's ulcers. Stress ulcers formerly were common in patients in intensive care units, but improvements in overall management, including respiratory and hemodynamic care, acid inhibition, and emphasis on adequate feeding, have reduced the incidence of these ulcers, so they currently affect 1 to 2% of these patients. Stress ulcers may be asymptomatic, but they can also cause complications, especially bleeding.

Other Factors

Cameron's Ulcer

Patients with a large hiatus hernia (Chapter 140) may present with a proximal gastric ulcer, termed *Cameron's ulcer,* at the level of the hiatus, where the stomach is compressed. These ulcers usually are asymptomatic but may cause occult or overt bleeding. During upper gastrointestinal endoscopy, patients with a large hiatus hernia and iron deficiency anemia should be carefully inspected in normal and retroverted position for the presence of Cameron's ulcer.

Anastomotic or Marginal Ulceration

Patients who have undergone partial gastrectomy sometimes later develop recurrent ulcers, often located at the anastomosis or within the jejunum immediately opposite the anastomosis. Ischemia and chronic inflammation resulting from *H. pylori* and biliary reflux may cause such ulcers, as may underlying cancer. If biopsy excludes cancer, treatment should include acid suppression and *H. pylori* eradication, if needed. Ulcer disease can be caused by the retained gastric antrum syndrome, which occurs when the antrum is not completely excised from the detached duodenum and, because it lacks exposure to acid, is not down-regulated by acid but rather continues to secrete gastrin despite normal or even high acid levels. Marginal ulcers also can occur after bariatric Roux-en-Y gastric bypass surgery.

Other Microbes

Colonization with *Helicobacter heilmannii,* formerly known as *Gastrospirillum hominis* and probably a zoonotic organism, often is associated with mild gastritis and sometimes with transient ulcer disease. Ulcer disease also may result from secondary syphilis, mycobacterial infection, infection with herpes simplex virus type 1, and cytomegalovirus infection.

Alcohol

Short-term heavy alcohol use or long-term moderate to heavy alcohol use can lead to signs of acute and chronic gastritis. No evidence indicates that this gastritis is associated with a significant risk for peptic ulceration, although alcohol use may increase the risk of bleeding in patients with peptic ulcer disease.

Hyperhistaminic Syndromes

Similar to the hypergastrinemic syndromes, persistent elevation of histamine also can lead to hyperacidity as a result of chronic stimulation of parietal cells. Elevated histamine levels are observed in two rare syndromes. *Systemic mastocytosis* (Chapter 276) is characterized by proliferation of mast cells in the bone marrow, skin, liver, spleen, and gastrointestinal tract, often associated with both spontaneous and trigger-induced (e.g., alcohol) release of histamine and other vasoactive substances. Patients with systemic mastocytosis often have gastrointestinal symptoms, including pain, diarrhea, and blood loss. Ulceration results from chronic gastric acid hypersecretion. Clues to the diagnosis include symptoms of pruritus, urticaria, or rash. The bone marrow and affected organ mast cell infiltrates carry a specific C-kit mutation and express CD2 and CD25. Histamine hypersecretion leading to peptic ulcer disease also can occur in *chronic myelogenous leukemia* (Chapter 195) with basophilia.

Other Drugs

Treatment with oral bisphosphonates, widely used for osteoporosis (Chapter 264), is complicated by gastric erosions and ulceration in an estimated 3 to 10% of treated patients. The risk for ulcer disease may be synergistically increased by NSAID use but is probably independent of *H. pylori* colonization. Although corticosteroid treatment also can be complicated by peptic ulcer disease, the relative risk is only slightly increased, except in patients who have serious comorbid diseases, use long-term or high-dose therapy, or have had prior ulcers. Other patients who use corticosteroids are not at serious risk for ulcer disease and therefore do not require measures to prevent ulcers.

Persons who use amphetamines and crack cocaine (Chapter 32) more frequently develop ulcer disease, more often with perforation, possibly as a result of vascular insufficiency. Chemotherapy, particularly when selectively given as a high-dose intra-arterial infusion in the celiac system, can be complicated by ulcer disease. Radiation therapy of the upper abdomen is sometimes complicated by chronic ischemic ulceration, especially in long-term follow-up.

SUGGESTED READINGS

Garcia Rodriguez LA, Barreales Tolosa L: Risk of upper gastrointestinal complications among users of traditional NSAIDs and COXIBs in the general population. Gastroenterology 2007;132:498–506. *Large case control study from a health systems database showing that COXIBs are likely safer than NSAIDs.*

Hoffmann KM, Furukawa M, Jensen RT: Duodenal neuroendocrine tumors: Classification, functional syndromes, diagnosis and medical treatment. Best Pract Res Clin Gastroenterol 2005;19:675–697. *A comprehensive review.*

Hung LC, Ching JY, Sung JJ, et al: Long-term outcome of *Helicobacter pylori*-negative idiopathic bleeding ulcers: A prospective cohort study. Gastroenterology 2005;128:1845–1850. *Shows the rising incidence of complicated idiopathic ulcer disease.*

Kusters JG, van Vliet AH, Kuipers EJ: Pathogenesis of *Helicobacter pylori* infection. Clin Microbiol Rev 2006;19:449–490. *Comprehensive review.*

142 ACID PEPTIC DISEASE: CLINICAL MANIFESTATIONS, DIAGNOSIS, TREATMENT, AND PROGNOSIS

Juan-R. Malagelada, Ernst J. Kuipers, and Martin J. Blaser

Clinical Manifestations

The clinical manifestations of acid peptic disease (Table 142–1) do not always predict the various morphologic presentations found at endoscopy. Indeed, gastritis or an ulcer may be silent and recognized only when it presents abruptly with a complication, most commonly perforation or hemorrhage, or incidentally after a diagnostic test is performed for other reasons. Nevertheless, the typical presentation of acid peptic disease is with recurrent episodes of pain. The pain is almost invariably located in the epigastrium and may radiate to the back or, less commonly, to the thorax or other regions of the abdomen (see Table 142–1). Some patients describe the pain as burning or piercing, whereas others describe it as an uncomfortable feeling of emptiness of the stomach, referred to as *painful hunger.* Indeed, the pain may improve with ingestion of food, only to return in the postprandial period. The timing of the pain in relation to meals and the soothing effects of food, however, are quite nonspecific and may also occur in patients with functional dyspepsia without ulcer. Nocturnal epigastric pain that awakens patients several hours after a late meal is more likely to represent ulcer pain.

TABLE 142–1 KEY SYMPTOMS AND SIGNS OF PEPTIC ULCER

UNCOMPLICATED ULCER

- No symptoms ("silent ulcer" up to 40%)
- Epigastric pain
  - Pain may radiate to
    - Back
    - Thorax
    - Rest of abdomen
      - (top most likely, bottom least likely)
  - Pain
    - Nocturnal
    - "Painful hunger"
    - Relieved by food
    - Continuous
      - (top most specific, bottom least specific)
- Nausea
- Vomiting
- Heartburn (mimics or associated with gastroesophageal reflex)

COMPLICATED ULCER

- Acute perforation
  - Severe abdominal pain
  - Shock
  - Abdominal boardlike rigidity
    - (and rebound and other signs of peritoneal irritation)
  - Free intraperitoneal air
- Hemorrhea
  - Hematemesis and/or melena
  - Hemodynamic changes, anemia
  - Previous history of ulcer symptoms (80%)
- Gastric outlet obstruction
  - Satiation, inability to ingest food, eructation
  - Nause, vomiting (and related disturbances)
  - Weight loss

TABLE 142–2 DIAGNOSTIC PATHS AND TOOLS IN ULCER DISEASE

PATH	
PATH 1	**MORPHOLOGIC DIAGNOSIS**
	Gastroduodenoscopy
	Barium contrast (inferior alternative)
	Endoscopic ultrasound (selected cases only)
	Computed tomography (useful in selected cases)
PATH 2	**ETIOLOGIC DIAGNOSIS**
	***HELICOBACTER PYLORI* TESTING**
	Histologic examination of gastric mucosa
	Stool antigen test
	Carbon-13–urea breath test
	Serum antibodies
	ULCER ASSOCIATED WITH NONSTEROIDAL ANTI-INFLAMMATORY DRUG USE
	History of drug ingestion
	Decreased platelet adherence
	Molecular identification (complex, expensive)
	ACID HYPERSECRETORY SYNDROMES
	Serum gastrin elevation
	Gastrin provocative tests (intravenous secretin, meal)
	Gastric analysis

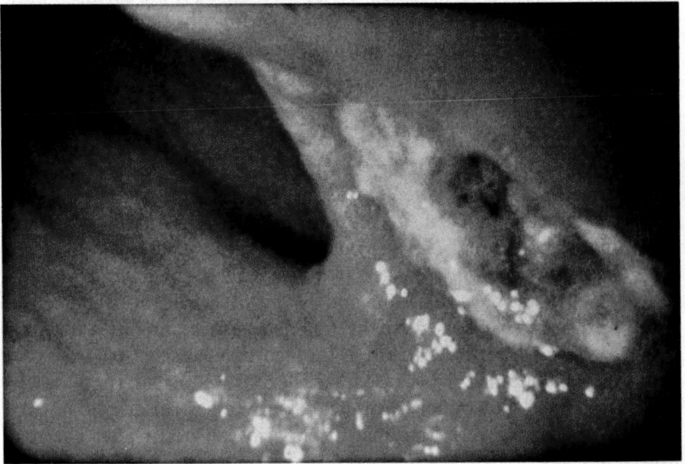

FIGURE 142–1 • Ulcer crater in the gastric wall.

Besides the pain during symptomatic episodes, patients may complain of retrosternal burning (heartburn) or acidic regurgitation into the throat, symptoms reflecting associated gastroesophageal reflux (Chapter 140), which is aggravated by hyperacidity or delayed gastric emptying. Nausea and vomiting may also occur but are quite nonspecific. The presence of significant diarrhea should raise the possibility of Zollinger-Ellison syndrome (Chapter 250), but diarrhea also may result from heavy use of magnesium-containing antacids. In untreated patients, symptoms tend to be intermittent, with flares of daily pain lasting 2 to 8 weeks, separated by prolonged asymptomatic intervals. During periods of remission, patients may feel well and may be able to eat even heavy or spicy meals without apparent discomfort.

Physical Examination

Physical examination is usually unrevealing. If significant bleeding has occurred (Chapter 137), the patient may present with pallor or may even be hypovolemic (Chapter 7). It is always useful to inquire about the characteristics of the stool, because ulcer-related bleeding may manifest not only very obviously in the form of hematemesis but also rather insidiously as melena (black feces). When a patient has acute perforation, severe epigastric and abdominal pain develop, the patient appears distressed. Characteristically, there is intense contracture of the abdominal muscles apparent on palpation, together with rebound and other signs of peritoneal irritation.

Diagnosis

In a patient who presents with symptoms consistent with ulcer disease, the diagnostic process should proceed along two different but complementary paths: confirmation of the anatomic abnormality and investigation of its cause (Table 142–2). In most patients, it is advisable to follow both diagnostic paths simultaneously, but sometimes it is reasonable to skip the anatomic verification as a cost-saving strategy and to proceed to management based on the probable cause.

Anatomic Diagnosis

Endoscopy (Chapter 136) is the primary investigative tool in patients suspected of having acid peptic disease. This technique can detect erosive gastritis (Fig. 141–1) or an ulcer in the gastric wall (see Fig. 142–1) or duodenal bulb (Fig. 141–2). Because of the high prevalence and frequent spontaneous improvement of dyspeptic symptoms, endoscopy usually should not be performed immediately, but rather it should be restricted to selected patients with persistent or recurrent symptoms. However, immediate endoscopy is indicated in patients with alarm symptoms, in particular weight loss, dysphagia, anorexia, considerable vomiting, anemia, or signs of overt bleeding.

Endoscopy has both high sensitivity and high specificity for detection of ulcer disease. The most common locations for a peptic ulcer are the stomach and duodenal bulb, but peptic ulcers may sometimes occur in the esophagus, in the small bowel, and in a Meckel diverticulum lined with heterotopic gastric mucosa. Endoscopic ultrasound also may detect an unsuspected submucosal component or enlarged lymph nodes, such

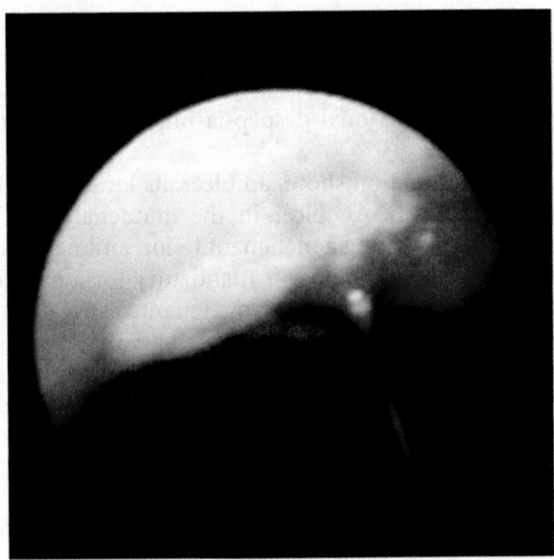

FIGURE 142–2 • Actively bleeding ulcer with a visible blood jet.

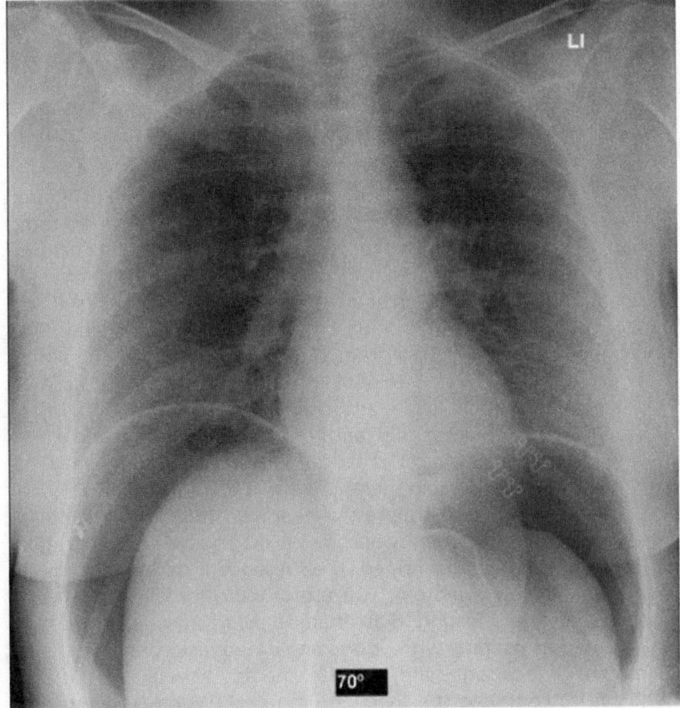

FIGURE 142–3 • Plain abdominal radiograph in a supine patient with a perforated peptic ulcer. The radiograph shows free air under the diaphragm.

as may occur in gastric neoplasia, especially lymphoma and linitis plastica (Chapter 134). Ulcers in the dorsal wall of the duodenal bulb, in particular at the transition from the bulb to the postbulbar descending portion of the duodenum, are most difficult to visualize, and they sometimes require the use of a side-viewing endoscope, particularly when endoscopic treatment is needed. Other regions where gastroduodenal ulcers may be easily missed are the cardia and the gastric angulus. Endoscopy also allows inspection for the following reasons: for ascertaining the presence of concomitant disorders, including esophagitis and duodenitis; for complications, such as bleeding or a visible vessel (see Fig. 142–2); for obtaining biopsy specimens, such as for histologic examination and to assess for *Helicobacter pylori* (Fig. 141–3); and for possible therapeutic interventions.

In rare cases, such as stenosis that blocks the advancing endoscope, conventional barium contrast radiographs (Chapter 135) are indicated. Additional investigations by endosonography or computed tomography are needed when an underlying malignant disease is suspected. The endoscopist should obtain biopsy samples from all ulcers, especially those with a suspicious appearance, to exclude potential underlying malignant diseases.

Etiologic Diagnosis

Diagnosis also must focus on establishing the cause of the ulcer. The first step is to determine whether *H. pylori* is present, since it is the major risk factor for peptic ulcer and can be a contributing factor in ulcers caused by nonsteroidal anti-inflammatory drugs (NSAIDs) and other precipitating causes. The presence of *H. pylori* may be ascertained by four possible approaches.

Testing for Helicobacter pylori

In populations with a high prevalence of *H. pylori*, nearly all patients with peptic ulcer disease are positive for *H. pylori*, so diagnostic testing has little added value, except when antimicrobial susceptibility testing is needed. The prevalence of *H. pylori* remains high in immigrants from developing countries, where most people become *H. pylori* positive in youth. In Western countries, approximately 50% of individuals who are more than 65 years old are colonized with *H. pylori*, but this prevalence is less than 20% in persons who are younger than 30 years old. In these younger persons, the proportion of patients with ulcers who are *H. pylori* negative increases, thus making diagnostic testing for *H. pylori*, followed by targeted therapy in patients who are positive for the bacterium, more attractive than empirical therapy.

Histologic examination of gastric mucosal biopsies, which is the standard procedure when endoscopy is initially performed for diagnosis, is quite sensitive and specific for *H. pylori*. However, the accuracy of this technique may also be affected by sampling error, improper orientation of the specimen, technical issues, and recent therapy with proton pump inhibitors (PPIs).

A second option is *serology*, which is a relatively simple, inexpensive test that has reduced predictive value in areas where the prevalence of *H. pylori* is low. Serology is not helpful to verify whether *H. pylori* has been eradicated with antibiotics because it may take many months or even years for *H. pylori* antibodies to fall to undetectable levels.

A third option is a *stool antigen test*, which is more accurate than serology. This test is capable of detecting *H. pylori* infection in only 1 week after PPIs are discontinued.

Finally, the *carbon-13 (^{13}C)–urea breath test*, which relies on the detection of *H. pylori* urease activity, is a noninvasive and relatively simple test, but it is more expensive than stool or blood testing. Although the test becomes negative as soon as *H. pylori* is eradicated, a minimum interval of 4 to 6 weeks after antibiotic treatment is recommended to reduce false-negative results.

Nonsteroidal Anti-inflammatory Drugs

NSAIDs are usually established as the putative cause of ulcers based on information obtained from the patient. If surreptitious use of NSAIDs is suspected, serum levels may be determined or indirectly assessed by a platelet adherence assay.

Hypersecretory Syndromes

Hypersecretory syndromes not related to *H. pylori* or NSAIDs are rare causes of ulcer disease (Chapter 141) and are diagnosed by special tests (see Table 142–2). Zollinger-Ellison syndrome should be strongly considered and serum gastrin levels determined in patients with multiple ulcers, particularly in atypical locations such as distal to duodenal bulb, and when diarrhea is present, because the latter is uncommon in *H. pylori*–related peptic ulcer disease. Hypergastrinemic syndromes (Zollinger-Ellison syndrome, antral G-cell hyperplasia) are best diagnosed by determination of serum gastrin levels, both basal and after stimulation with intravenous secretin (gastrinoma detection) or a test meal (antral G-cell hyperplasia detection). Measurements of gastrin levels are not routinely recommended but are usually suggested when ulcer disease is associated with refractory symptoms or with hypertrophic gastric folds, to permit earlier detection of small gastrinomas that may still be resectable (Chapter 250).

Gastric analysis, which is performed by placing a nasogastric tube to aspirate gastric juice and to quantify gastric acid output, both basal and after stimulation with subcutaneous pentagastrin, is indicated only in two rare circumstances: patients who have elevated serum gastrin levels suggestive of Zollinger-Ellison syndrome or antral G-cell hyperplasia, but with equivocal responses to standard gastric provocative tests, and patients who have indirect signs of gastric hypersecretion, such as enlarged folds and abundant clear fluid at endoscopy, and normal gastrin levels and negative provocative gastrin tests but who still may be hypersecretors, such as patients with recurrent ulcer disease despite a prior vagotomy with or without an antrectomy. A positive test is a basal acid output greater than 15 mEq/hour or greater than 5 mEq/hour in a postoperative patient.

The diagnosis of Zollinger-Ellison syndrome is best confirmed by gastric analysis showing a basal acid output greater than 15 mEq/hour in conjunction with a fasting serum gastrin level exceeding 1000 pg/mL in the presence of gastric pH less than 2. To skip the cumbersome gastric analysis, a gastric pH determination showing a fasting pH of 2 or less, is adequate. For serum gastrin levels in the range 100 to 1000 pg/mL and intragastric pH greater than 2, an increase in the serum gastrin to more than 200 pg/mL after a secretin stimulation test is suggestive of the diagnosis. An elevated serum gastrin level alone is not sufficient to permit a diagnosis of Zollinger-Ellison syndrome, because serum gastrin levels tend to increase over time with atrophic gastritis and are also increased in patients receiving long-term PPI therapy.

In patients in whom a gastroduodenal ulcer cannot be ascribed to colonization with *H. pylori,* use of NSAIDs, or a hypersecretory syndrome, establishment of a definite etiologic diagnosis may require a more thorough evaluation, starting with a medical history that focuses on the use of other ulcerogenic agents and the presence of symptoms that could suggest an underlying systemic disease. The next, equally important, step is the evaluation of biopsy samples of ulcer borders and of the antrum, corpus, and duodenum. The ulcer specimens may not initially reveal a malignant disease but may provide evidence of other infectious conditions, specific types of gastritis, celiac disease, ischemia, amyloidosis, or a systemic inflammatory condition. These data can be combined with clues provided by the endoscopic evaluation, including the character and location of the ulcer, signs of ischemia, and signs of inflammation at other locations (Chapter 141). Further evaluation should focus on the presence of systemic disorders and may include a chest radiograph, angiography, ileocolonoscopy, and an abdominal computed tomographic scan.

Differential Diagnosis

The differential diagnosis of ulcer-like symptoms includes many disorders of the upper abdominal organs, including malignant diseases of the stomach (Chapter 202), duodenum (Chapter 203), pancreas (Chapter 205), or bile ducts (Chapter 206). The differential diagnosis of upper abdominal symptoms also includes liver and gallstone disease (Chapter 159), pancreatitis (Chapter 147), and motility disorders (Chapter 138). In many patients with upper abdominal dyspeptic complaints, no underlying cause can be identified. In this "nonulcer" or functional dyspepsia group, complaints characteristic of gastroesophageal reflux, ulcer symptoms, or dysmotility symptoms can be prominent (Chapter 138). A few of these patients (generally <5%) benefit from eradication of *H. pylori,* with a slow decrease of dyspeptic complaints over 12 to 24 months, but functional dyspepsia is not a proven or widely accepted indication for treatment of *H. pylori.* If treatment is considered in an individual patient, the patient and the physician should be prepared for persistent symptoms despite eradication of *H. pylori.*

Diagnostic Scenarios: Acute or Initial Clinical Presentation

Younger (<45 years old) patients without alarm symptoms or signs such as anemia, rapid weight loss, or other evidence of serious disease do not necessarily require endoscopy because evidence indicates that malignant gastric disease is unlikely. When a patient who lives in an area of the world with relatively high prevalence of *H. pylori* infection (>10% of the population positive) is seen by a generalist physician, a test and treatment approach can begin with an *H. pylori* stool antigen determination, a urea breath test, or an *H. pylori* serologic examination. If the chosen *H. pylori* test is positive, the patient may be treated with the appropriate *H. pylori* eradication drugs (see later) and observed for 4 to 6 weeks. If the patient was also receiving an NSAID, either orally or parenterally, the same approach will be appropriate, but the NSAID also should be discontinued. If the *H. pylori* test is negative in a person who is taking NSAIDs, these drugs should be discontinued and the patient should be treated with a PPI for 4 to 6 weeks. In patients who are not taking NSAIDs or who do not improve after these drugs are discontinued, endoscopy is indicated to determine whether an ulcer is present.

Conversely, gastroenterologists more commonly proceed directly to endoscopy. If no abnormalities are apparent or the endoscopic study shows gastritis without an overt ulcer, a biopsy should be obtained to ascertain by histologic examination or urease testing whether *H. pylori* is present. If *H. pylori* is found by endoscopic biopsy, the patient could receive eradication treatment because relatively small but consistent (between 5 and 10%) proportions of patients who are positive for *H. pylori* and who have functional dyspepsia improve after eradication of *H. pylori.*

If endoscopic examination shows an ulcer, its location will determine the subsequent approach. An ulcer in the duodenal bulb has only a remote chance of representing a malignant lesion and need not be examined by biopsy. By contrast, biopsy is mandatory for a gastric ulcerative lesion identified at endoscopy, because malignant gastric disease may first appear with similar clinical manifestations and may resemble benign ulcer disease morphologically; even if histologic assessment does not identify a malignant process, repeat endoscopy is recommended about 1 month after therapy to verify complete healing and for biopsy of the scar.

Treatment

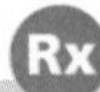

Helicobacter pylori *Infection*

H. pylori–associated ulcers often heal spontaneously but frequently recur. Treatment for 14 days (Table 142–3) has about a 10% advantage over 7-day eradication therapy. [1] Seven-day treatment may be acceptable in regions where local studies have shown that a particular treatment is very effective and is probably the most economical option in countries with low health care costs. After 4 weeks of acid suppressive therapy, more than 80% of ulcers will heal, and this number increases to more than 90% after 8 weeks of therapy. For patients in whom such therapy fails, a 4- to 10-day course of quadruple therapy is advised. This second-line regimen enables eradication of *H. pylori* in an additional 80 to 90% of patients. Resistance of *H. pylori* to metronidazole varies between 10 and 80% throughout the world. Clarithromycin resistance is increasing and is now estimated to be at 5 to 10% in the United States because of widespread use of macrolides as therapy for upper respiratory infections. Resistance to amoxicillin and to tetracycline is rare and is not usually relevant in clinical practice. Sequential therapy may be superior to standard triple therapy. [2]

Continuation of acid suppressive therapy after antibiotic treatment is needed only when symptoms persist and before eradication of *H. pylori* has been confirmed. The subsequent decrease or disappearance of ulcer symptoms is a useful indicator of successful *H. pylori* eradication. Testing to ascertain *H. pylori* status after therapy is indicated in patients with prior complicated ulcer disease or with persistent or recurrent symptoms after therapy, as well as in patients who fail to complete the therapeutic course. When *H. pylori* persists, ulcers recur in 50 to 90% of patients within 12 to 24 months. This rate can be reduced to 20 to 30% with maintenance acid suppression. Ascertainment of therapeutic efficacy must be delayed until at least 1 month after the end of treatment to prevent false-negative results related to the temporary suppression but not eradication of the organism. When repeat endoscopy is needed (e.g., a gastric ulcer that requires repeated histologic examination to exclude underlying malignancy), repeat screening for *H. pylori* can be performed using the gastric biopsy specimens for histologic examination, culture, or urease testing. If no clinical indication exists for repeat endoscopy, then *H. pylori* status can be determined by means of a ^{13}C-urea breath test, stool *H. pylori* antigen, or repeated serology. Serologic determination is based on a more than 40 to 50% decrease in immunoglobulin G antibody levels in the first 6 months after treatment compared with pretreatment in that patient.

Disease Related to Nonsteroidal Anti-inflammatory Drug Use

In patients who are diagnosed with acid peptic disease while they are taking NSAIDs or aspirin, the first step is to stop such therapy. Acid suppression with a PPI (in doses similar to those used for *H. pylori*) leads to healing of 85% of NSAID-induced gastric ulcers and more than 90% of duodenal ulcers within 8 weeks of therapy, whereas acid suppression with an H_2-blocker, equivalent to raniti-

TABLE 142–3 OVERVIEW OF ANTIBIOTICS USED FOR *H. PYLORI* ERADICATION

Drug Class	Drug	Triple Therapy*	Quadruple Therapy†
Acid suppression	Proton pump inhibitor	20–40 mg bid‡	20–40 mg bid‡
Standard antimicrobials	Bismuth compound§	2 tablets bid	2 tablets bid
	Amoxicillin	1 g bid	—
	Metronidazole¶	500 mg bid	500 mg tid
	Clarithromycin	500 mg bid	—
	Tetracycline		500 mg qid
Salvage antimicrobials	Levofloxacin	300 mg bid	—
	Rifabutin	150 mg bid	—
	Furazolidone	100 mg bid	—

*Triple therapy consists of a proton pump inhibitor or bismuth compound, together with two of the listed antibiotics, usually given for 7 to 14 days.
†Quadruple therapy consists of a proton pump inhibitor plus a bismuth compound with two antibiotics as listed given for 4 to 10 days.
‡Proton pump inhibitor dose equivalent to omeprazole 20 mg bid.
§Bismuth subsalicylate or subcitrate.
¶Alternative = tinidazole, 500 mg bid.
bid = twice daily; tid = three times daily.

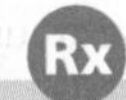

dine, 300 mg twice daily, heals approximately 70% of ulcers within 7 weeks. The mucosal protective drug misoprostol (200 mg twice daily) has a similar effect. Because some patients need to continue the NSAID, a change to a cyclooxygenase 2 inhibitor may be advantageous, but this approach has not been proven. Treatment must be continued for at least 8 weeks, and maintenance therapy is needed in patients who continue NSAID therapy. Gastric ulcers, larger lesions, and recurrent lesions heal more slowly.

Ulcer occurrence during NSAID therapy suggests a causative relationship, but patients also should be tested for *H. pylori.* In patients who are *H. pylori* positive, eradication therapy should be considered, although no clear clinical parameters distinguish between these etiologic factors. In patients who continue to take NSAIDs, *H. pylori* eradication has no benefit above maintenance therapy with a PPI, except in patients who use aspirin, for whom *H. pylori* eradication alone may be curative. Maintenance therapy with H_2-blockers (at a dose equivalent to ranitidine, 300 mg twice daily) reduces duodenal ulcer disease in the first 3 months of NSAID therapy but has no effect on prevention of gastric ulcers. However, stronger acid suppression (equivalent to famotidine, 40 mg twice daily) partially protects against the development of gastric ulcers. Omeprazole, 20 mg once daily, and misoprostol in doses varying between 400 and 800 mg/day also partially protect from both gastric and duodenal ulcers during NSAID use. Patients who require gastroprotection during NSAID use include those who have a prior ulcer, who have severe concomitant disease, who are taking warfarin (Coumadin) or high-dose corticosteroids, or who are elderly (>65 years old).

Prognosis

Four major complications of ulcer disease are intractability, perforation, hemorrhage, and stenosis. Each distinct situation requires specific management approaches.

Intractability

Intractability is a term strictly applied to a patient with a persistent ulcer even after intensive and prolonged PPI therapy. Symptoms may or may not be present. These rare cases may result from poor compliance with recommended treatment, surreptitious use of ulcerogenic drugs, or other diseases (e.g., Crohn's disease, ischemia, bacterial infection with a pathogen other than *H. pylori,* viral infections; Chapter 141). Surgical vagotomy and pyloroplasty can almost always be avoided by recognizing these issues and pursuing these diagnoses.

Other Causes of Acid Peptic Disease

Acid peptic disease related to alcohol or bisphosphonate should be addressed by discontinuing the precipitating agent. Treatment of the Zollinger-Ellison syndrome requires high-dose PPIs and/or surgery (Chapter 141). Crohn's disease (Chapter 144), vasculitis (Chapter 291), sarcoidosis (Chapter 95), celiac disease (Chapter 143), polycythemia vera (Chapter 172), amyloidosis (Chapter 296), and other rare causes of ulcer disease (Chapter 141) should be addressed by treating the underlying condition. Stress ulcers and Cameron's ulcers are treated by potent acid suppression therapy (e.g., omeprazole, 20 mg twice daily).

Perforation

Perforation may manifest as an acute event, whereby gastric contents spill into the peritoneal cavity, or more insidiously by slow penetration of the ulcer into surrounding tissues. Acute free perforation typically causes abrupt and severe abdominal pain associated with abdominal muscular spasm that produces boardlike rigidity of the abdomen and other manifestations of peritoneal irritation. Secondary hemodynamic shock is common. The clinical diagnosis can be confirmed in approximately 80% of patients by a plain abdominal radiograph with the patient standing, sitting up, or lying on the left side (see Fig. 142–3); a computed tomographic scan can be obtained if doubt persists. Leukocytosis develops rapidly, and mild hyperamylasemia may occur. Treatment should begin by correcting hemodynamic, fluid, and electrolyte imbalances. Nasogastric suction is helpful, and prophylactic antibiotics (e.g., amoxicillin-clavulanic acid, 1 g every 8 hours intravenously) are usually administered. Unless a specific contraindication exists, emergency surgery is usually indicated, although more conservative approaches are sometimes appropriate. Given the success in achieving the long-term cure of ulcer disease through the eradication of *H. pylori* and the withdrawal of NSAIDs, suturing of the perforated ulcer may be adequate and may permit the patient to avoid a more radical vagotomy with or without gastric resection.

Hemorrhage

Hemorrhage occurs in about one in six patients with ulcers over the course of their ulcer activity, and ulcers caused by NSAIDs account for a larger proportion of these hemorrhages (Chapter 137). Hemorrhage may manifest either as a serious acute event associated with hemodynamic shock and high mortality or as a slow or intermittent blood loss leading to chronic anemia. Approximately 80% of patients with bleeding ulcers describe a prior history of symptomatic disease, and about 20 to 30% have suffered a previous hemorrhage. Assessment of the magnitude of bleeding is of paramount importance in deciding the need for transfusion and subsequent management. Initial hematocrit levels may be misleading and are likely to fall subsequently because of hemodilution. Rapid bleeding is usually apparent on the basis of clinical signs (pallor, systolic blood pressure <90 mm Hg, pulse >100/minute), and fluids and transfusions are indicated to prevent circulatory collapse (Chapter 137).

Once the patient's hemodynamic status is stabilized, endoscopy should be performed to ascertain the origin of the bleeding, and, it is hoped, to stop it. "Clean base" ulcers carry a significantly lower risk of rebleeding during the succeeding 24 to 72 hours than do oozing ulcers, ulcers with

TABLE 142–5 ROCKALL SCORING SYSTEM FOR THE RISK OF MORTALITY FOLLOWING PEPTIC ULCER BLEEDING

	Score			
Variable	**0**	**1**	**2**	**3**
Age	<60	60–79	80	—
Shock	Not present	Pulse >100	Systolic BP <100 mm Hg	—
Comorbidity	None		Cardiac failure Coronary insufficiency Other serious illness	Renal insufficiency Liver failure Metastatic malignancy
Diagnosis	Mallory-Weiss syndrome or no identifiable cause	Ulcer Varices	Malignancy of proximal digestive tract	—
Endoscopy	No signs of recent bleeding		Bleeding, clot, or visible vessel	—

Data from Rockall TA, Logan RFA, Devlin HB, et al: Risk assessment after acute upper gastrointestinal haemorrhage. Gut 1996;38:316–321.

TABLE 142–4 ENDOSCOPY RESULTS IN PATIENTS WITH BLEEDING ULCERS*

Endoscopy Result	Ulcer Characteristics	Risk of Recurrent Bleeding (%)
Active bleeding	Arterial bleeding	80–90
	Oozing bleeding	10–30
Stigmata of recent bleeding	Nonbleeding visible vessel	50–60
	Adherent clot	25–35
	Flat pigmented spot	0–8
No signs of bleeding	Clean ulcer base	0–12

*The ulcer characteristics determine the risk of recurrent bleeding during follow-up.

a fresh clot, or ulcers with a "visible vessel" (see Fig. 142–2). Meta-analyses suggest that starting intravenous PPIs in the acute phase is associated with reduced rebleeding, less need for blood transfusion and surgical intervention, and lower mortality rates. [4] Other therapies, including tranexamic acid, vasopressin, somatostatin, and octreotide, should be considered experimental.

Ulcer-related bleeding stops spontaneously in about 80% of cases, but approximately 5 to 20% of ulcers may continue to bleed (Table 142–4). Of those ulcers that cease to bleed spontaneously, rebleeding within the first 48 to 72 hours occurs in 20 to 25%. Rebleeding carries a greater risk of mortality than does the initial bleeding, particularly in patients who are more than 55 years old. For persistent or recurrent bleeding, endoscopic intervention is needed, and up to 10% of patients require surgical treatment. Patients with hemodynamic instability, a falling hematocrit, or a need for repeated transfusions are candidates for endoscopic therapy. In patients with a peptic ulcer and active bleeding or a visible vessel, endoscopic therapy is indicated, because this approach may lead to a 75% reduction in episodes of recurrent bleeding and in the need for surgical intervention and also to a 40% reduction in mortality. In patients with an adherent clot, endoscopic removal of the clot and treatment of the underlying lesion are preferred. Endoscopic techniques for hemostasis include the thermal method (thermal or laser coagulation), injection sclerotherapy, and mechanical compression with clips.

The risk for fatal outcome of an upper gastrointestinal hemorrhage can be estimated by means of the Rockall risk score, based on five clinical and endoscopic parameters (Table 142–5). In several studies, mortality in patients with a bleeding peptic ulcer was less than 2% among those with a Rockall score of 2 points or less, 10% in those with 3 to 5 points, and up to 46% in those with 6 points or more. Management of patients who recover after a peptic ulcer hemorrhage is similar to the treatment of patients with ordinary ulcers. Eradication of *H. pylori* provides excellent protection against both recurrence and rebleeding. NSAID-induced ulcers should be managed either by withdrawal of NSAIDs or by the long-term use of adjuvant PPIs.

Stenosis

Gastric outlet obstruction is now a rare complication of ulcer disease because of the early detection and treatment of most ulcers. Most patients who develop clinically relevant gastric outlet obstruction have had an ulcer in the duodenal bulb and/or pyloric channel. Edema and inflammation play an important role, and occasionally a patient with active disease presents with symptoms of outlet obstruction as manifested by nausea, vomiting, and gastric stasis without a tight, chronic stenosis. Management therefore should involve three key steps:

1. Nasogastric tube aspiration and gastric lavage to clean the stomach of retained debris, followed by early endoscopy. This step facilitates accurate diagnosis.
2. Intense antisecretory therapy using intravenous PPIs. Nasogastric suction may need to be maintained for several days if vomiting resumes when the tube is clamped.
3. Treatment of underlying ulcer disease by eradicating *H. pylori* and withdrawing NSAIDs. If the initial treatment resolves the clinical situation and the patient is able to resume eating, it will not be necessary to undertake further specific treatment of the outlet stenosis; however, tight, fibrous scarring may require endoscopic balloon dilation or surgery.

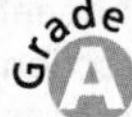

1. Gisbert JP, Pajares JM: Systematic review and meta-analysis: Is 1-week proton pump inhibitor–based triple therapy sufficient to heal peptic ulcer? Aliment Pharmacol Ther 2005;21:795–804.
2. Vaira D, Zullo A, Vakil N, et al: Sequential therapy versus standard triple-drug therapy for *Helicobacter pylori* eradication: A randomized trial. Ann Intern Med 2007;146:556–563.
3. Yeomans ND, Tulassay Z, Juhasz L, et al: A comparison of omeprazole with ranitidine for ulcers associated with non-steroidal anti-inflammatory drugs: Acid Suppression Trial. Ranitidine versus Omeprazole for NSAID-associated Ulcer Treatment (ASTRONAUT) Study Group. N Engl J Med 1998;338:719–726.
4. Leontiadis GI, Sharma VK, Howden CW: Systematic review and meta-analysis: Proton-pump inhibitor treatment for ulcer bleeding reduces transfusion requirements and hospital stay—results from the Cochrane Collaboration. Aliment Pharmacol Ther 2005;22:169–174.

SUGGESTED READINGS

Ford AC, Delaney BC, Forman D, et al: Eradication therapy for peptic ulcer disease in *Helicobacter pylori*–positive patients. Cochrane Database Syst Rev 2006:CD003840. *Meta-analysis of trials concluding that eradication therapy was associated with a decreased risk of recurrent gastrointestinal bleeding.*

Hung LC, Ching JY, Sung JJ, et al: Long-term outcome of *Helicobacter pylori*–negative idiopathic bleeding ulcers: A prospective cohort study. Gastroenterology 2005;128:1845–1850. *The recurrence rate at 1 year was 13%, fivefold higher than for patients with treated HP-positive ulcers.*

Louw JA: Peptic ulcer disease. Curr Opin Gastroenterol 2006;22:607–611. *Comprehensive review.*

APPROACH TO THE PATIENT WITH DIARRHEA AND MALABSORPTION

Carol E. Semrad and Don W. Powell

Definitions

Normal stool frequency ranges from three times a week to three times a day. Although individuals rarely cite increases in frequency alone as the definition of diarrhea, a decrease in stool consistency (increased fluidity) and stools that cause urgency or abdominal discomfort are likely to be termed diarrhea. Consistency is defined as the ratio of fecal water to the water-holding capacity of fecal insoluble solids, which are composed of bacterial mass and dietary fiber. One half of the dry weight of stool is bacteria. Because it is difficult to measure stool consistency and because stool is predominantly (60 to 85%) water, stool weight becomes a reasonable surrogate of consistency.

Physicians often define diarrhea as a physical sign, 24-hour stool excretion by weight or volume, rather than as a symptom. Daily stool weights of children and adults are less than 200 g, and greater stool weights are an objective definition of diarrhea; however, this definition misses 20% of diarrheal symptoms in patients with loose stools less than this daily weight.

Acute diarrheas are those lasting less than 2 to 3 weeks or, rarely, 6 to 8 weeks. The most common cause of acute diarrhea is infection. Chronic diarrheas are those lasting at least 4 weeks, and more usually 6 to 8 weeks or longer. There are three categories of chronic diarrhea: osmotic (malabsorptive) diarrhea, secretory diarrhea, and inflammatory diarrhea.

Epidemiology

Diarrhea is the second leading cause of mortality worldwide and is particularly problematic for children younger than 5 years of age in developing nations. In the United States, the elderly are susceptible to death from diarrheal disease: more than 1600 deaths occur annually among those older than 74 years of age. It is estimated that approximately 5% of the U.S. population suffer from chronic diarrhea and that about 40% of these individuals are older than 60 years of age.

In the United States, the complaint of diarrhea accounts for more than 7 million outpatient visits by 4 million patients per year. The combination of non–food-borne gastroenteritis, food-borne illness, irritable bowel syndrome, chronic diarrhea, and inflammatory bowel diseases accounts for about 250,000 hospital admissions, 2.6 million emergency room visits, and 12.7 million physician visits. Total costs for diarrheal diseases are about $1.2 billion in direct (health care) costs and $5.4 billion in indirect costs (days lost from work).

Pathobiology

Abnormalities of Fluid and Electrolyte Transport

Diarrhea previously was thought to be caused principally by abnormal gastrointestinal motility. It is now clear that most diarrheal conditions are due primarily to alterations of intestinal fluid and electrolyte transport and less to smooth muscle function.

Each 24 hours, 8 to 10 L of fluid enters the duodenum with 800 mEq sodium (Na^+), 700 mEq chloride (Cl^-), and 100 mEq potassium (K^+). The diet supplies 2 L of this fluid; the remainder comes from salivary, stomach, liver, pancreatic, and duodenal secretions. The small intestine normally absorbs 8 to 9 L of this fluid and presents 1.5 L to the colon for absorption. Of the remaining fluid, the colon absorbs all but approximately 100 mL, which contains 3 mEq, 8 mEq, and 2 mEq of Na^+, K^+, and Cl^-, respectively. Diarrhea can result from decreased absorption or increased secretion by either the small intestine or the colon. If deranged electrolyte transport or the presence of nonabsorbable solutes in the intestinal lumen reduced the absorptive capacity of the small intestine by 50%, the volume of fluid presented daily to the normal colon (50% of 10 L, or 5 L) would exceed its maximum daily absorptive capacity of 4 L. Stool excretion of 1000 mL would result, which by definition is diarrhea. Alternatively, if the colon is deranged so that it cannot absorb even the 1.5 L normally presented to it by the small intestine, a stool volume of greater than 200 mL in 24 hours would result, again defined as diarrhea.

At the cellular level, excess intraluminal fluid volumes occur when there is a derangement of electrolyte transport capabilities of the small or large intestine or when osmotic solutes in the bowel lumen create an adverse osmotic gradient that the normal electrolyte absorptive mechanisms cannot overcome. Na^+ transport by the epithelium from lumen to blood (by Na^+-coupled sugar and amino acid transport in the small intestine, by Na^+:H^+ exchange proteins in the small intestine and proximal colon, and by aldosterone-regulated Na^+ channels in the distal colon) creates a favorable osmotic gradient for absorption (Fig. 143–1A and B). Oral rehydration solutions (ORS), which are used extensively to replace diarrheal fluid and electrolyte losses, are effective because they contain Na^+, sugars, and, often, protein (amino acids). If unabsorbable or poorly absorbable solutes (e.g., lactose in lactase-deficient individuals, polyethylene glycol in colon-cleansing solutions, or magnesium [Mg^{2+}] citrate in cathartics) are present in the lumen, the Na^+-absorbing mechanisms are incapable of creating an osmotic gradient favorable for absorption; as a result, fluid remains in the lumen and is the basis of osmotic or malabsorptive diarrhea.

Active Cl^- secretion or inhibited Na^+ absorption also creates an osmotic gradient favorable for the movement of fluids from blood to lumen and is the basis of the secretory diarrheas. Agents that increase enterocyte cyclic adenosine monophosphate (cAMP), cyclic guanosine monophosphate (cGMP), or intracellular ionized calcium (Ca^{2+}), such as cholera toxin, *Escherichia coli* enterotoxins, prostaglandin, and vasoactive intestinal peptide (VIP), all inhibit Na^+ absorption and stimulate Cl^- secretion (Table 143–1; see Fig. 143–1C). Secretion is controlled by neurotransmitters, hormones, and inflammatory mediators (see Fig. 143–1D).

Pathophysiology

To understand the three general categories of diarrhea—malabsorption (osmotic diarrheas), secretory diarrheas, and inflammatory diarrheas—it is necessary to understand how the normal intestine handles fluid and solutes in health and disease. Regardless of whether a subject ingests a hypotonic meal, such as a steak, or a hypertonic meal, such as milk and a doughnut, the volume of the meal is augmented by gastric, pancreatic, biliary, and duodenal secretions. The permeable duodenum then renders the meal approximately isotonic with an electrolyte content similar to that of plasma by the time it reaches the proximal jejunum. As the chyme moves toward the colon, the Na^+ concentration in the luminal fluid remains constant, but Cl^- is reduced to 60 to 70 mmol/L, and bicarbonate (HCO_3^-) is increased to a similar concentration as the result of Cl^- and HCO_3^- transport mechanisms in the enterocyte and HCO_3^- secretion in the ileum (see Figs. 143–1B and 143–1C). In the colon, K^+ is secreted, and the Na^+ transport mechanism of the colonocyte, together with the low epithelial permeability, extract Na^+ and fluid from the stool. As a result, the Na^+ content of stool decreases to 30 to 40 mmol/L; K^+ increases from 5 to 10 mmol/L in the small bowel to 75 to 90 mmol/L; and poorly absorbed divalent cations, such as Mg^{2+} and Ca^{2+}, are concentrated in stool to values of 5 to 100 mmol/L. The anion concentrations in the colon change drastically because bacterial degradation of carbohydrate (i.e., unabsorbed starches, sugars, and fiber) creates short-chain fatty acids that attain concentrations of 80 to 180 mmol/L. At colonic pH, these are present as organic anions, such as acetate, propionate, and butyrate. Depending on the concentrations generated, these fatty acids/anions may decrease stool pH to 4 or lower. The osmolality of the stool is approximately that of plasma (280 to 300 mOsm/kg H_2O) when it is passed.

With ingestion of a poorly absorbable or unabsorbable solute (e.g., Mg^{2+}, polyethylene glycol) or an unabsorbed carbohydrate (e.g., lactulose or, in lactase-deficient individuals, lactose), a considerable proportion of the osmolality of stool results from the nonabsorbed solute. This gap between stool osmolality and the sum of the electrolytes in the stool causes osmotic diarrhea.

Inflammatory diarrheas are characterized by enterocyte damage and death, villus atrophy, and crypt hyperplasia. The enterocytes on rudimentary villi of the small intestine are immature cells with poor disaccharidase and peptide hydrolase activity, reduced or absent Na^+-coupled sugar or amino acid transport mechanisms, and reduced or absent

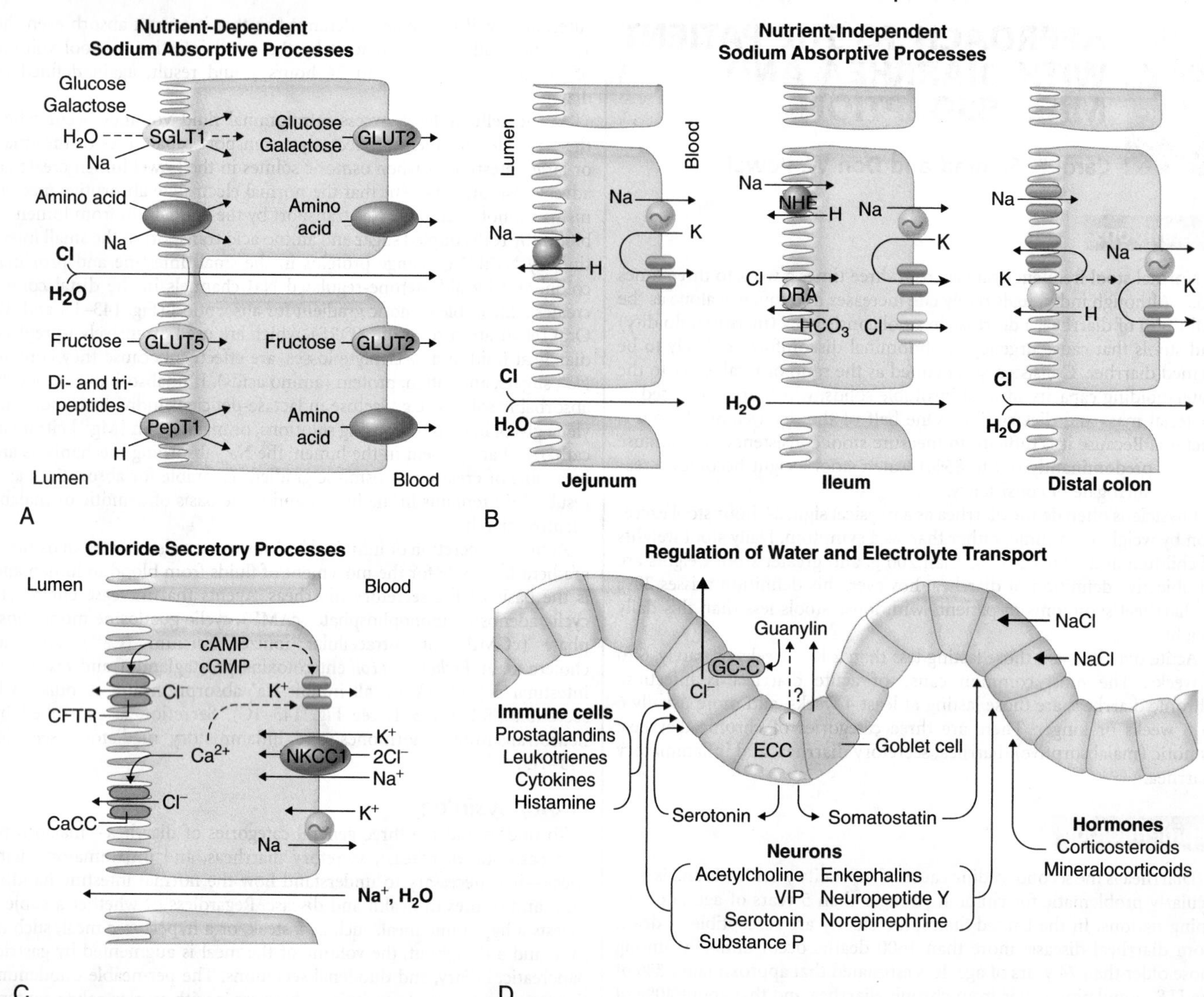

FIGURE 143–1 • Mechanisms of intestinal transport of water and electrolytes. A, Intestinal sodium absorption. Sodium is actively absorbed in villus cells of the small intestine and surface cells of the colon. The sodium-potassium adenosine triphosphatase (Na^+,K^+-ATPase) present on the cell basolateral membrane maintains a low intracellular Na^+ concentration and an electronegative cell interior favoring Na^+ movement across the apical membrane from lumen into cell. In the small intestine, glucose and galactose are taken up with sodium and water at the apical membrane by the sodium-glucose ligand transporter (SGLT1). Several different sodium-dependent amino acid carriers, some with overlapping substrate specificities, transport cationic, anionic, and neutral amino acids into villus cells. Dipeptides and tripeptides are transported by a hydrogen-coupled oligopeptide carrier, PepT1, that is driven by luminal hydrogen ions generated by the epithelial Na^+/H^+ exchanger. Fructose is taken up by the facilitative glucose transporter (GLUT5). **B,** Sodium also is absorbed by nutrient-independent transport processes in the small intestine and colon. The Na^+/H^+ (NHE) and Cl^-/HCO_3^- (DRA) exchangers are inhibited by agents that elevate intracellular cyclic adenosine monophosphate (cAMP), cyclic guanosine monophosphate (cGMP), or calcium. **C,** Chloride secretion by intestinal crypt cells. Chloride can be secreted actively throughout the small intestine and colon. Intracellular mediators of secretion (cAMP, cGMP, Ca^{2+}) open apical Cl^- channels (cystic fibrosis transmembrane conductance regulator [CFTR], calcium-activated chloride channel [CaCC]) and basolateral K^+ channels. Chloride moves from crypt cells into the intestinal lumen, favoring movement of Cl^- from the blood into cells by the Na^+/K^+/$2Cl^-$ cotransporter (NKCC1). Bicarbonate (HCO_3) also may be secreted via the CFTR channel. **D,** Regulation of intestinal water and electrolyte transport. Normally, the intestine is in a net absorptive state under the control of extrinsic adrenergic nerves from the sympathetic nervous system. Guanylin, the natural ligand for the *Escherichia coli* stable-toxin receptor (membrane-bound guanylyl cyclase [GC-C]), may be important in regulating local chloride secretion. The normal tone of the intestine is modified by the enteric nervous system, endocrine and inflammatory cells in the intestinal mucosa, and circulating hormones. The enteric nervous system releases a variety of neurotransmitters, some that stimulate chloride secretion (e.g., vasoactive intestinal peptide [VIP], acetylcholine) and others that promote sodium absorption (e.g., enkephalins, neuropeptide Y). Hormones produced locally from enterochromaffin cells (ECC) in the intestinal epithelium and inflammatory mediators released from immune cells directly affect enterocytes and nearby nerves. Circulating hormones (e.g., aldosterone, glucocorticoids) enhance sodium absorption in the intestine. Glucocorticoids also inhibit release of arachidonic acid and production of prostaglandin by inflammatory cells.

sodium chloride absorptive transporters. Conversely, the hyperplastic crypt cells maintain their ability to secrete Cl^- (and perhaps HCO_3^-). If the inflammation is severe, immune-mediated vascular damage or ulceration allows protein to leak (exudate) from capillaries and lymphatics and contribute to the diarrhea. Activation of lymphocytes, phagocytes, and fibroblasts releases various inflammatory mediators that induce intestinal chloride secretion (see Fig. 143–1D). Interleukin-1 (IL-1) and tumor necrosis factor also are released into the blood, causing fever and malaise.

ACUTE DIARRHEAS

Clinical Manifestations

Approximately 80% of acute diarrheas are due to infections with viruses, bacteria, helminths, and protozoa. The remainder are secondary to the ingestion of medications, poorly absorbed sugars (fructose polymers or sorbitol), fecal impaction, pelvic inflammation (e.g., acute appendicitis [Chapter 145]), or intestinal ischemia (Chapter 146).

TABLE 143–1 AGENTS THAT CAUSE INTESTINAL SECRETION

Laxatives	Phenolphthalein, anthraquinones, bisacodyl, oxyphenisatin, senna, aloe, ricinoleic acid (castor oil), dioctyl sodium sulfosuccinate; endogenous laxatives such as dihydroxy bile acids and long-chain fatty acids
Medications/drugs	Diuretics (furosemide, thiazides); coffee, tea, and cola (caffeine and other methylxanthines); asthma medication (theophylline); thyroid preparations; type II diabetes drug (metformin)
	Cholinergic drugs, glaucoma eye drops, and bladder stimulants (acetylcholine analogues or mimetics); myasthenia gravis medication (cholinesterase inhibitors); cardiac drugs (quinidine and quinine); gout medication (colchicine); antihypertensives (angiotensin-converting enzyme inhibitors); histamine 2 blocker (ranitidine); proton pump inhibitors; antidepressants (selective serotonin reuptake inhibitors); antineoplastic drugs; chenodeoxycholic acid
	Prostaglandins (misoprostol); di-5-aminosalicylic acid (azodisalicylate); gold (also may cause colitis)
	Protease inhibitors
	Human immunodeficiency virus (HIV)
Toxins	Metals (arsenic); plants (e.g., mushroom *Amanita phalloides*); organophosphates (insecticides and nerve poisons); seafood toxins (ciguatera, scombroid poisoning, and paralytic, diarrhetic, or neurotoxic shellfish poisoning); monosodium glutamate
Bacterial enterotoxins	*Vibrio cholerae*, toxigenic *Escherichia coli* (heat-labile and heat-stable toxins), *Campylobacter, Yersinia, Klebsiella, Clostridium difficile, Staphylococcus aureus* (toxic shock syndrome), *Clostridium perfringens, Clostridium botulinum, Bacillus cereus*
Hormone-producing tumors	VIPoma and ganglioneuromas; medullary carcinoma of thyroid (calcitonin and prostaglandins); mastocytosis (histamine); villous adenoma (prostaglandins)
Inflammatory conditions	Allergy and anaphylaxis (histamine, serotonin, platelet-activating factor, prostaglandins); infection (reactive oxygen metabolites, platelet-activating factor, prostaglandins, histamine); idiopathic inflammation; inflammatory bowel disease, celiac disease
	Ischemic colitis

Adapted from Powell DW: Approach to the patient with diarrhea. *In* Yamada T, Alpers DH, Owyang C, et al (eds): Textbook of Gastroenterology, 3rd ed. Philadelphia, Lippincott-Raven, 1999.

TABLE 143–2 EPIDEMIOLOGY OF ACUTE INFECTIOUS DIARRHEA AND INFECTIOUS FOOD-BORNE ILLNESS

Vehicle	Classic Pathogens
Water (including foods washed in such water)	*Vibrio cholerae*, caliciviruses (Norwalk agent), *Giardia, Cryptosporidium*
Food	
Poultry	*Salmonella, Campylobacter, Shigella* species
Beef, unpasteurized fruit juice	Enterohemorrhagic *Escherichia coli*
Pork	Tapeworm
Seafood and shellfish (including raw sushi and gefilte fish)	*V. cholerae, Vibrio parahaemolyticus*, and *Vibrio vulnificus; Salmonella* and *Shigella* species; hepatitis A and B viruses; tapeworm; anisakiasis
Cheese, milk	*Listeria* species
Eggs	*Salmonella* species
Mayonnaise-containing foods and cream pies	Staphylococcal and clostridial food poisonings
Fried rice	*Bacillus cereus*
Fresh berries	*Cyclospora* species
Canned vegetables or fruits	*Clostridium* species
Sprouts	Enterohemorrhagic *E. coli, Salmonella* species
Animal-to-person (pets and livestock)	*Salmonella, Campylobacter, Cryptosporidium*, and *Giardia* species
Person-to-person (including sexual contact)	All enteric bacteria, viruses, and parasites
Daycare center	*Shigella, Campylobacter, Cryptosporidium*, and *Giardia* species; viruses, *Clostridium difficile*
Hospitalization, antibiotics, or chemotherapy	*C. difficile*
Swimming pool	*Giardia* and *Cryptosporidium* species
Foreign travel	*E. coli* of various types; *Salmonella, Shigella, Campylobacter, Giardia*, and *Cryptosporidium* species; *Entamoeba histolytica*

Adapted from Powell DW: Approach to the patient with diarrhea. *In* Yamada T, Alpers DH, Owyang C, et al (eds): Textbook of Gastroenterology, 3rd ed. Philadelphia, Lippincott-Raven, 1999.

Sporadic, Food-Borne, and Water-Borne Infectious Diarrhea

Most infectious diarrheas are acquired through fecal-oral transmission from water, food, or person-to-person contact (Table 143–2). Patients with infectious diarrhea often complain of nausea, vomiting, and abdominal pain and have watery, malabsorptive, or bloody diarrhea and fever (dysentery) (Chapters 325 through 333, 357, 358, 371–373, 377, 378, 402, and 403). As documented using polymerase chain reaction methods of diagnosis, most outbreaks of nonbacterial acute gastroenteritis in the United States and other countries are caused by caliciviruses (Norwalk agent). Rotavirus predominantly causes diarrhea in infants, usually in the winter months, but also may cause nonseasonal acute diarrhea in adults, particularly the elderly. Mechanisms for diarrhea include decreased fluid absorption due to destruction of villus enterocytes and stimulation of fluid secretion by NSP4 rotatoxin and viral activation of the enteric nervous system.

Some of the short-lived watery diarrheas ascribed to "viral gastroenteritis" are likely to be mild, sporadic, food-borne bacterial infections. In addition to enteric infections, certain systemic infections (e.g., hepatitis, listeriosis, legionellosis) and emerging infections (e.g., Hanta virus, severe acute respiratory syndrome [SARS], avian influenza) may cause or manifest with substantial diarrhea.

Food-borne illness affects one in four people in the United States, and the incidence is estimated to be 76 million cases per year, with 325,000 hospitalizations and 5000 deaths annually. The incidence may be underestimated, because most patients present with sporadic diarrhea rather than as part of a clear epidemic, and most endemic diarrheas are not reported. Data suggest that fewer than 11% of these infections are reported to the Centers for Disease Control and Prevention (CDC). Emerging food-borne diseases in the United States include the enteritidis serotype of *Salmonella, Campylobacter jejuni, E. coli* O157:H7, and *Cyclospora* infections. Recent outbreaks of *E. coli* O157:H7 have been associated with petting zoos. Fish can become contaminated in their own environment (especially the filter-feeding bivalve mollusks, such as mussels, clams, oysters, and scallops) or by food handlers. Organisms that are specific for seafood include *Vibrio parahaemolyticus,* which causes either watery or bloody diarrhea, and *Vibrio vulnificus,* which causes watery diarrhea and, especially in patients with liver disease, a fatal septicemia. Ingestion of meat contaminated by anthrax (Chapter 317) causes fever, diffuse abdominal pain, and bloody stool or vomitus. Anthrax invades the intestinal mucosa; the organism, or anthrax toxin, causes inflammation, ulceration, and necrosis. Ascites develops, and death results from blood loss, dehydration and electrolyte imbalance, intestinal perforation, or toxemia.

Food-Borne and Water-Borne Poisonings

Food poisoning occurs with environmental chemicals, such as monosodium glutamate (used in Asian food), heavy metals (arsenic from rat poison), insecticides (organophosphates and carbamates), and natural toxins found in mushrooms and seafood (fin fish or shellfish). Most of these toxins cause varying combinations of gastrointestinal and neurologic symptoms. Arsenic (Chapter 20) also induces cardiovascular collapse at higher, acute doses; one form of mushroom *(Amanita)* poisoning (Chapter 111) can cause acute liver and kidney failure.

Diarrhea and neurologic symptoms (tingling and burning around the mouth, facial flushing, sweating, headache, palpitations, and dizziness) of seafood poisoning may be caused by histamine release from the decaying flesh of blood fish (mahi-mahi, tuna, marlin, or mackerel) after it is caught. This form of seafood poisoning is called scombroid. Plankton, algae, or dinoflagellates ingested by tropical fish (amberjack, snapper, grouper, or barracuda) produce a toxin (ciguatoxin) that causes seafood poisoning called ciguatera. Fish from the Albemarle-Pamlico estuary (eastern United States) ingest toxic dinoflagellates that cause *Pfiesteria piscicida* poisoning. The dinoflagellate toxins cause nausea; vomiting; abdominal pain; diarrhea; neurologic symptoms such as weakness, pruritus, circumoral paresthesias, and temperature reversal (hot drinks taste cold and vice versa); and psychiatric abnormalities and memory loss. Shellfish poisonings are also caused by algae or dinoflagellates ingested by bivalve mollusks; these different toxins can cause predominantly neurologic symptoms (paralytic, neurotoxic, or amnestic shellfish poisonings), which are occasionally severe, or predominantly gastrointestinal symptoms (diarrhetic shellfish poisoning). Puffer fish poisoning (tetrodotoxin) causes neurologic symptoms, respiratory paralysis, and death.

Antibiotic-Associated Diarrheas

Diarrhea occurs in 20% of patients receiving broad-spectrum antibiotics; about 20% of these diarrheas are due to *Clostridium difficile* (Chapter 319). Recently, hypervirulent, fluoroquinolone-resistant strains have emerged, causing an increase in the incidence and severity of *C. difficile* infections, including fulminant *C. difficile* colitis that can lead to colectomy or even death. The A and B toxins produced by *C. difficile* can cause diarrhea. In animal models, IL-8, substance P, and leukotriene B_4 were found to mediate toxin A–stimulated intestinal fluid secretion. *C. difficile* can cause severe diarrhea, pseudomembranous colitis, or toxic megacolon. Patients may have a relapsing course after seemingly successful therapy with metronidazole or vancomycin. Non–*C. difficile* antibiotic-induced diarrhea is generally mild and self-limited, and it usually clears spontaneously or in response to cholestyramine therapy. North American travelers to developing countries and travelers on airplanes and cruise ships where errors in food preparation occur are at high risk for acute infectious diarrhea. Environmental sanitation inspections of cruise ships can decrease diarrheal outbreaks in passengers. Bacterial agents account for 85% of traveler's diarrhea. Enterotoxic *E. coli* is the most common cause. *E. coli* heat-stable toxin binds to guanylate cyclase in the enterocyte brush-border membrane, resulting in elevation of intracellular cGMP. *E. coli* heat-labile toxin, similar to cholera toxin, binds to the monosialoganglioside GM_1 in the brush-border membrane, resulting in the activation of adenylate cyclase and elevation of intracellular cAMP. cAMP and cGMP stimulate intestinal chloride secretion (see Fig. 143–1C) and inhibit nutrient-independent absorption of sodium and chloride (see Fig. 143–1B). Sodium-glucose absorption is not affected; hence, the basis for ORS therapy. Cholera toxin permanently binds to adenylate cyclase (until the natural turnover of the intestinal epithelium, in 5 to 7 days), resulting in persistent secretion and severe diarrhea. Of the 10 to 15 cases of cholera reported in the United States each year, about 60% are travel associated.

Sexually Transmitted and Aids-Related Diarrheas

Men who have sex with men and prostitutes develop infectious diarrhea through the oral-fecal route. The incidence of infectious diarrhea among men who have sex with men ("gay bowel syndrome") has decreased markedly, but the decline has been more than offset by the high incidence and seriousness of enteric infections in patients with acquired immunodeficiency syndrome (AIDS) (Chapter 413). In patients with human immunodeficiency virus (HIV) disease who are receiving highly active antiretroviral therapy, diarrhea is more likely to be due to protease inhibitors than enteric infection.

Daycare Diarrhea

More than 6 million children in the United States attend daycare, and diarrhea from organisms that colonize at a low inoculum dose (e.g., *Shigella, Giardia, Cryptosporidium*) or organisms that are spread easily (e.g., rotavirus, astrovirus, adenovirus) is extremely prevalent in this setting. The secondary attack rate for parents and siblings is 10 to 20%.

Diagnosis

The differential diagnosis of acute watery diarrhea includes food toxins, infections, medications, and diseases (Fig. 143–2; see Table 143–2) (Chapters 326 through 334, 358, 359, 373, 374, 378, 379, 400, 403, and 404). The use of the laboratory to make the diagnosis of infectious diarrhea can be reduced if the evaluation focuses on *Campylobacter, Salmonella, Shigella,* and *C. difficile* and if only liquid stools are cultured. Organisms that can cause diarrhea but are not sought routinely by most clinical microbiology laboratories unless specifically requested include *Yersinia, Plesiomonas,* enterohemorrhagic *E. coli* serotype O157:H7, *Aeromonas, Cryptosporidium, Cyclospora, Microsporidia,* and noncholera *Vibrio.* Parasites such as *Giardia* and *Strongyloides* and enteroadherent bacteria can be difficult to detect in stool but may be diagnosed by intestinal biopsy. Even with the use of all available laboratory techniques, the cause of 20 to 40% of all acute infectious diarrheas remains undiagnosed.

Treatment

Rx

The treatment of diarrhea can be symptomatic (fluid replacement and antidiarrheal agents) or specific (antimicrobial therapy) or both. Because death in acute diarrhea is caused by dehydration, the first task is to assess the degree of dehydration and replace fluid and electrolyte deficits. Severely dehydrated patients should be rehydrated with intravenous Ringer's lactate or saline solution, to which additional K^+ and $NaHCO_3^-$ may be added as necessary. Alert patients should be given ORS, which is equally effective in repairing fluid and electrolyte losses. In mild-to-moderate dehydration, ORS can

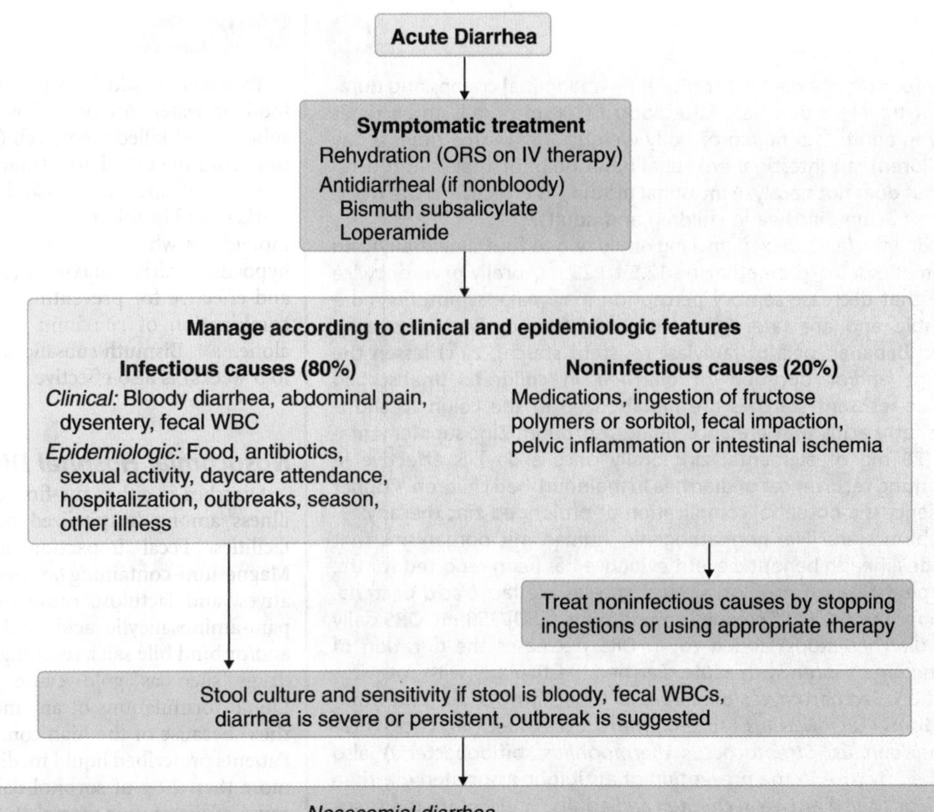

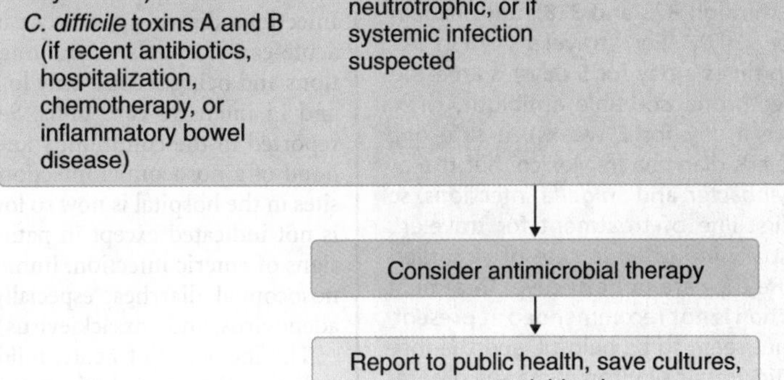

FIGURE 143–2 • Algorithm for the diagnostic approach to acute diarrhea. AIDS = acquired immunodeficiency syndrome; *C. difficile* = *Clostridium difficile;* CMV = cytomegalovirus; *E. coli* = *Escherichia coli;* IV therapy = intravenous rehydration; *M. avium* = *Mycobacterium avium* complex; ORS = oral rehydration solution; WBCs = white blood cells. (Adapted in 2006 with permission from Thielman NM, Guerrant RL: Acute infectious diarrhea. N Engl J Med 2004;350:38–47. Copyright 2004, Massachusetts Medical Society. All rights reserved.)

Rx

be given to infants and children in volumes of 50 to 100 mL/kg over 4 to 6 hours; adults may need to drink 1000 mL/hr. Reduced-osmolarity ORS solutions (Na^+ 75 mmol/L, osmolarity 245 mmol/L versus Na^+ 90 mmol/L, osmolarity 311 mmol/L in standard solutions) are better tolerated and effective in non-cholera diarrhea but may cause hyponatremia in patients with high-volume diarrhea. Glucose-based ORS, although effective in rehydrating the patient, may worsen the diarrhea. In contrast to glucose-based solutions, rice-based ORS decrease diarrhea in cholera victims; rice is digested to many glucose monomers that aid in the absorption of intestinal secretions. These solutions may not decrease stool output in acute diarrheas, but they will effectively rehydrate the patient despite continued diarrhea. After the patient is rehydrated, ORS are given at rates equaling stool loss plus insensible losses until the diarrhea ceases.

Rx

Bismuth subsalicylate (Pepto-Bismol, 525 mg orally every 30 minutes to 1 hour for five doses, may repeat on day 2) is safe and efficacious in bacterial infectious diarrheas. Because of the possibility of worsening the colonization or invasion of infectious organisms by paralyzing intestinal motility, and because of evidence that the use of motility-altering drugs may prolong microorganism excretion time, neither opiates nor anticholinergic drugs are recommended for invasive bacterial infectious diarrheas. However, loperamide (2 mg orally four times a day for 3 to 7 days, maximal dose 16 mg daily) can be useful and safe in acute or traveler's diarrhea, provided that it is not given to patients with dysentery (high fever, with blood or pus in the stool), and especially when administered concomitantly with effective antibiotics. A combination of loperamide (2 mg orally four times a day) plus simethicone (125 mg

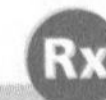

orally four times a day) may reduce the abdominal cramps and duration of traveler's diarrhea. Racecadotril (100 mg orally three times a day in adults, 1.5 mg/kg of body weight orally three times a day in children), an intestinal enkephalinase inhibitor that is antisecretory but does not paralyze intestinal motility, is effective in the treatment of acute diarrhea in children and adults.

Anxiolytics (e.g., diazepam 2 mg orally two to four times daily) and antiemetics (e.g., promethazine 12.5 to 25 mg orally once or twice daily) that decrease sensory perception may make symptoms more tolerable and are safe. Some foods or food-derived substances (green bananas, pectins [amylase-resistant starch], zinc) lessen the amount and/or duration of diarrhea in children. Unabsorbed amylase-resistant starches are metabolized in the colon to short-chain fatty acids that enhance fluid absorption. Zinc supplementation (20 mg of elemental zinc orally once a day) is effective in preventing recurrences of diarrhea in malnourished children. Copper deficiency is a potential complication of prolonged zinc therapy.

Probiotics are live, nonpathogenic, human microorganisms that provide a health benefit. Level 1 evidence has been reported for the therapeutic use of probiotics. Most species are lactic acid bacteria. Lactobacillus GG (10^{10} colony-forming units [CFU]/250 mL ORS daily until diarrhea stops) added to an ORS decreases the duration of diarrhea in children with acute diarrhea, particularly with rotavirus infection. *Saccharomyces boulardii*, lactobacillus GG, [1] and other organisms (*Lactobacillus reuteri, Enterococcus faecium, Lactobacillus acidophilus, Streptococcus thermophilus*, bifidobacteria) also may be effective in the prevention of antibiotic-associated diarrhea and *C. difficile* diarrhea in children and adults. Their role in the treatment of acute infectious and antibiotic-associated diarrheas in adults is less clear. *Saccaromyces boulardii* (500 mg orally two times a day for 30 days) may be effective in preventing recurrent *C. difficile* infection. Some commercially available probiotic preparations contain dead microorganisms and may not be effective.

Certain infectious diarrheas should be treated with antibiotics, including those associated with shigellosis (Chapter 330), cholera (Chapter 325), pseudomembranous enterocolitis (Chapter 319), parasitic infestations (Chapter 371 through 373 and 378), and sexually transmitted diseases (Chapter 307). For traveler's diarrhea, ciprofloxacin (500 mg orally two times a day for 5 days) is an effective treatment. A newly licensed, nonabsorbable antibiotic, rifaximin (200 mg taken orally once a day for 2 weeks), is safe and effective for treatment of traveler's diarrhea in Mexico, but it may not be effective against *Campylobacter* and *Shigella* infections, so fluoroquinolones remain the first line of treatment for traveler's diarrhea. Antibiotics are not usually indicated in case of viral diarrhea or cryptosporidiosis, because they are not effective. Treatment of *E. coli* serotype O157:H7 infection is not recommended at present, because current antibiotics do not seem to be helpful, and the incidence of complications (hemolytic-uremic syndrome) may be greater after antibiotic therapy. Regardless of the cause of infectious diarrhea, patients should be treated if they are immunosuppressed; have valvular, vascular, or orthopedic prostheses; have congenital hemolytic anemias (especially if salmonellosis is involved); or are extremely young or old.

While the clinician is awaiting stool culture results to guide specific therapy (Chapter 309), the fluoroquinolones (e.g., ciprofloxacin 500 mg orally two times a day for 5 days) are the treatment of choice. Trimethoprim-sulfamethoxazole is second-line therapy. If the symptom complex suggests *Campylobacter* infection, azithromycin (500 mg orally one time a day for 3 days) should be added. If *C. difficile* is suspected on an epidemiologic basis, metronidazole (250 mg orally four times a day or 500 mg orally three times a day for 10 days) should be prescribed. Fluoroquinolone-resistant and trimethoprim-sulfamethoxazole–resistant strains of *Shigella, E. coli, Salmonella, Campylobacter*, and *C. difficile* have emerged. Azithromycin, 500 mg orally on day 1 and 250 mg orally one time a day for 4 days, may be an effective alternative treatment for resistant strains of *Shigella* and *Campylobacter* and for traveler's diarrhea acquired in Mexico.

Prevention

Travelers should be vigilant in avoiding ingestion of contaminated food or water. An oral cholera vaccine against recombinant toxin B subunit and killed whole-cell (rBS-WC) is effective in preventing infection from the O1 El Tor strain and partially effective against enterotoxigenic *E. coli* strains. [2] Cholera vaccination is recommended for relief workers and health professionals who work in endemic countries and for individuals who are immunocompromised or have chronic illnesses or hypochlorhydria. Rifaximin (200 mg orally per day for 2 weeks) is safe and effective for preventing traveler's diarrhea in Mexico, [3] and the combination of rifaximin plus loperamide is better than either one alone. [4] Bismuth subsalicylate (525 mg orally four times a day for up to 3 weeks) is also effective.

Nosocomial Hospital Diarrheas

Diarrhea is either the first or the second most common nosocomial illness among hospitalized patients and residents in long-term care facilities. Fecal impaction and medications are common causes. Magnesium-containing laxatives and antacids, sulfate and phosphate laxatives, and lactulose cause osmotic diarrheas. Colchicine, neomycin, para-aminosalicylic acid, and cholestyramine damage the enterocyte and/or bind bile salts, resulting in malabsorption. Radiation therapy and drugs such as gold cause intestinal inflammation and diarrhea. Liquid formulations of any medication can cause diarrhea (elixir diarrhea) because of the high content of sorbitol used to sweeten the elixir. Patients prescribed liquid medications through feeding tubes may receive more than 20 g of sorbitol daily. An important but poorly understood cause of diarrhea is enteral (tube) feeding (Chapter 235), particularly in critically ill patients, who often develop diarrhea. Dysmotility, increased intestinal permeability, and low sodium content in enteral formulas may be contributing factors. The diarrhea often can be managed with pectin or, if there are no contraindications, with loperamide, and diarrhea is not a reason to stop tube feeding unless stool volumes exceed 1 L/day.

Patients in mental institutions and nursing homes have high incidences of nosocomial infectious diarrheas (e.g., hemorrhagic *E. coli, C. difficile*). Infectious diarrhea (mostly caused by *C. difficile*) is also common in acute-care hospitals, accounting for more than 20% of nosocomial infections and being second only to respiratory infections on pediatric wards and in intensive care units. Severe *C. difficile* infection has also been reported in the community and among peripartum women. The likelihood of a nosocomial infection caused by *Salmonella, Shigella*, or parasites in the hospital is now so low that routine evaluation for these agents is not indicated except in patients with neutropenia, HIV infection, or signs of enteric infection. Immunosuppressed patients are susceptible to nosocomial diarrhea, especially viral infections (rotavirus, astrovirus, adenovirus, and coxsackievirus).

The incidence of acute, mild diarrhea with cancer chemotherapy or radiation therapy is high, approaching 100% with some agents, such as amsacrine, azacitidine, cytarabine, dactinomycin, daunorubicin, doxorubicin, floxuridine, 5-fluorouracil, 6-mercaptopurine, methotrexate, plicamycin, and irinotecan (CPT-11). IL-2 therapy, resveratrol, and the combination of 5-fluorouracil plus leucovorin are frequent causes of severe watery diarrhea. Current treatment for chemotherapy-induced and radiation-induced diarrhea is symptomatic and includes loperamide (2 mg orally four times a day) and nonsteroidal anti-inflammatory drugs (NSAIDs) (e.g., naproxen 250 to 500 mg orally twice daily). In patients with severe diarrhea, octreotide may be an effective treatment.

Runner's Diarrhea

Gastrointestinal disturbances including anorexia, heartburn, nausea, vomiting, cramps, urgency, and diarrhea occur in 10 to 25% of persons who exercise vigorously, particularly women marathon runners and triathletes. The pathophysiology in runner's diarrhea is unclear but may involve release of intestinal secretogogues or hormones by ischemia. Loperamide and NSAIDs are taken prophylactically by many runners, but it is not clear whether they are effective.

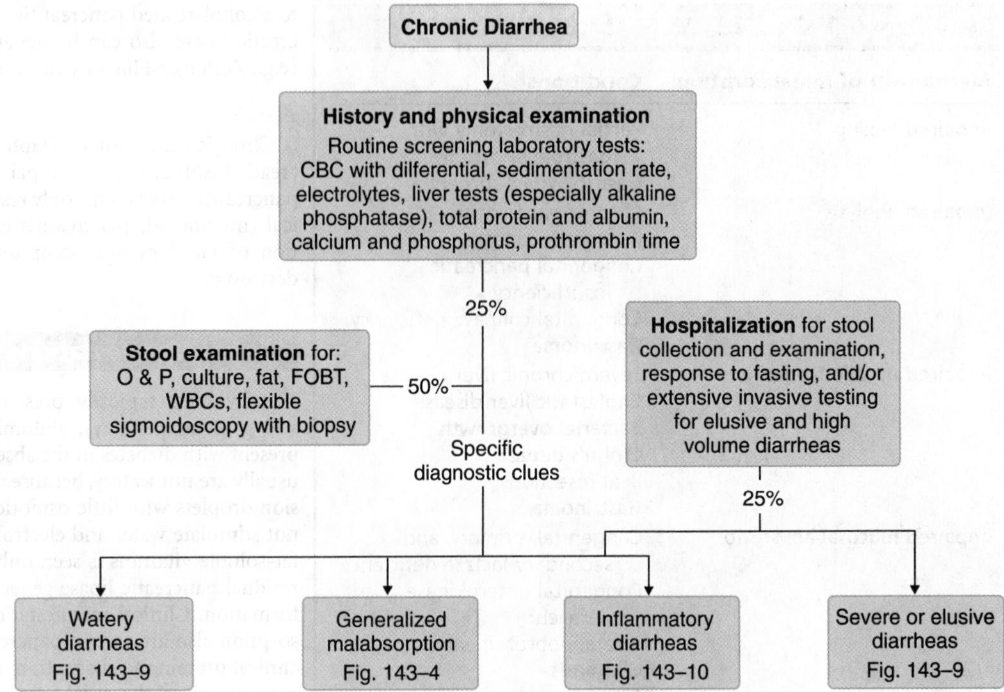

FIGURE 143–3 • Approach to the evaluation of chronic diarrhea. CBC = complete blood count; FOBT = fecal occult blood test; O&P = ova and parasites; WBCs = white blood cells. (Adapted from Powell DW: Approach to the patient with diarrhea. *In* Yamada T, Alpers DH, Owyang C, et al [eds]: Textbook of Gastroenterology, 3rd ed. Philadelphia, Lippincott-Raven, 1999.)

CHRONIC DIARRHEAS

The goal in evaluating a patient with chronic diarrhea is to make a definitive diagnosis as quickly and inexpensively as possible (Fig. 143–3). In 25 to 50% of cases, expert history and physical examination may be sufficient. The addition of stool culture and examination for ova and parasites, determination of stool fat, and flexible sigmoidoscopy with biopsy raises the diagnostic rate to about 75%. The remaining 25% of patients with severe or elusive chronic diarrhea may need extensive testing and perhaps hospitalization.

Prolonged, Persistent, and Protracted Infectious Diarrheas

Stool culture and examination may detect organisms that often cause protracted infectious diarrhea in adults: enteropathogenic (enteroadherent) *E. coli, Giardia, Entamoeba, Cryptosporidium, Aeromonas,* and *Yersinia enterocolitica.* If none of these organisms is found, a therapeutic trial of metronidazole or trimethoprim-sulfamethoxazole may be indicated. Persistent infectious diarrhea lasting longer than 3 to 4 weeks occurs in 3% of returned travelers; if trimethoprim-sulfamethoxazole or the fluoroquinolones have been unsuccessful, tetracycline or metronidazole should be tried.

After documented infectious diarrhea, 25% of patients experience pain, bloating, urgency, a sense of incomplete evacuation, and loose stools for 6 months or longer. This syndrome of infectious diarrhea–induced irritable bowel syndrome, also called Brainerd's diarrhea if it is particularly prolonged and accompanied by severe diarrhea, is initiated by unidentified organisms. Some patients respond to cholestyramine. Celiac disease also may manifest after intestinal infections, so patients should be screened for it in this setting.

Visitors who reside in the tropics for 1 to 3 months may develop tropical sprue (see later discussion). A severe postinfectious diarrhea syndrome (severe protracted diarrhea) may develop in infants and children in developing nations and can occur in milder forms (postenteritis syndrome) in infants and children in developed countries. Malnutrition and death (mortality rate, 50%) can occur with severe disease. Treatment includes dietary lactose exclusion in mild disease or total parenteral nutrition for severely affected patients. Metronidazole, tetracycline, trimethoprim-sulfamethoxazole, folic acid, and zinc therapy also may help.

Malabsorptive Syndromes

Malabsorption is caused by many different diseases, drugs, or nutritional products that impair intraluminal digestion, mucosal absorption, or nutrient delivery to the systemic circulation (Fig. 143–4; Tables 143–3 and 143–4). Dietary fat is the nutrient most difficult to absorb. Fat is predominantly insoluble in the aqueous milieu of the intestine and critically depends on all phases of digestion, absorption, and delivery for its assimilation. Steatorrhea (excess fat in the stool) is the hallmark of malabsorption; a stool test for fat is the best screening test for malabsorption. Malabsorption does not always cause diarrhea. Clinical signs of vitamin or mineral deficiencies may occur in the absence of diarrhea (Table 143–5). A careful history is crucial in guiding further testing to confirm the suspicion of malabsorption and to make a specific diagnosis (see Fig. 143–4). The goals of treatment are to correct or treat the underlying disease and to replenish water, electrolyte, and nutritional losses.

Conditions That Impair Intraluminal Digestion

Most digestion and absorption of nutrients occurs in the small intestine (Fig. 143–5). Pancreatic proteases (trypsinogen, chymotrypsinogen, proelastase, and procarboxypeptidases) are secreted from acinar cells in inactive forms. The cleavage of trypsinogen to trypsin by the duodenal brush-border peptidase enteropeptidase (enterokinase) allows trypsin to cleave the remaining trypsinogen and other proteases to their active form. Neutralization of acid in the small intestinal lumen by bicarbonate secreted from pancreatic duct cells is physiologically important because pancreatic enzyme activity and bile salt micelle formation is optimal at a luminal pH of 6 to 8.

Carbohydrates and most dietary proteins are water soluble and readily digested by pancreatic enzymes. Most dietary lipids (long-chain triglycerides, cholesterol, phosphatidylcholine [lecithin], and fat-soluble vitamins) are water insoluble and must undergo lipolysis and incorporation into mixed micelles before they can be absorbed across the intestinal mucosa. Pancreatic lipase, in the presence of its cofactor, colipase, cleaves long-chain triglycerides into fatty acids and monoglycerides. The products of lipolysis interact with bile salts and phospholipids to form mixed micelles, which also incorporate cholesterol and fat-soluble vitamins (D, A, K, and E) in their hydrophobic centers.

TABLE 143–3 CAUSES OF MALABSORPTION

Mechanism of Malabsorption	Conditions
Impaired mixing	Partial gastrectomy with gastrojejunostomy Gastric bypass surgery
Impaired lipolysis	Chronic pancreatitis Pancreatic cancer Congenital pancreatic insufficiency Congenital colipase deficiency Gastrinoma
Impaired micelle formation	Severe chronic liver disease Cholestatic liver disease Bacterial overgrowth Crohn's disease Ileal resection Gastrinoma
Impaired mucosal absorption	Congenital, primary, and secondary lactase deficiency Congenital enterokinase deficiency Abetalipoproteinemia Giardiasis Celiac disease Tropical sprue Agammaglobulinemia Amyloidosis AIDS-related (infections, enteropathy) Radiation enteritis Graft-versus-host disease Whipple's disease Eosinophilic gastroenteritis Megaloblastic gut Collagenous sprue Ulcerative jejunitis Lymphoma Bacterial overgrowth Short-bowel syndrome Mastocytosis
Impaired nutrient delivery	Congenital intestinal lymphangiectasia Lymphoma Tuberculosis Constrictive pericarditis Severe congestive heart failure
Unknown	Hypoparathyroidism Adrenal insufficiency Hyperthyroidism Carcinoid syndrome

AIDS = acquired immunodeficiency syndrome.

Impaired Mixing

Surgical alterations, such as partial gastrectomy with gastrojejunostomy (a Billroth II anastomosis) or gastrointestinal bypass surgeries for morbid obesity, result in the release of biliary and pancreatic secretions into the intestine at a site remote from the site of entry of gastric contents into the jejunum. This imbalance can result in impaired lipolysis and impaired micelle formation, with subsequent fat malabsorption. Absorption of iron, calcium, and cobalamin is impaired as well. Rapid transit through the jejunum contributes to the malabsorption of nutrients. Individuals with these conditions also have surgical anastomoses that predispose to bacterial overgrowth.

Impaired Lipolysis

A deficiency in pancreatic lipase may be caused by the congenital absence of pancreatic lipase or by destruction of the pancreatic gland due to alcohol-related pancreatitis, cystic fibrosis, or pancreatic cancer. Pancreatic lipase also can be denatured by excess secretion of gastric acid (e.g., Zollinger-Ellison syndrome; Chapter 205).

Chronic Pancreatitis

Chronic pancreatitis (Chapter 147) is the most common cause of pancreatic insufficiency and impaired lipolysis. In the United States, chronic pancreatitis most commonly results from alcohol abuse; in contrast, tropical (nutritional) pancreatitis is most common worldwide. Malabsorption of fat does not occur until more than 90% of the pancreas is destroyed.

Clinical Manifestations

Individuals typically present with bulky, fat-laden stools (usually >30 g of fat per day), abdominal pain, and diabetes, although some present with diabetes in the absence of gastrointestinal symptoms. Stools usually are not watery, because undigested triglycerides form large emulsion droplets with little osmotic force and, in contrast to fatty acids, do not stimulate water and electrolyte secretion in the colon. Deficiency of fat-soluble vitamins is seen only rarely, presumably because gastric and residual pancreatic lipase generates enough fatty acids for some micelle formation. Clinical manifestations of carbohydrate and protein malabsorption also are rare in pancreatic insufficiency. In severe disease, subclinical protein malabsorption, manifested by the presence of undigested meat fibers in the stool, and subclinical carbohydrate malabsorption, manifested by gas-filled, floating stools, can occur. Weight loss, when it occurs, is most often caused by decreased oral intake to avoid abdominal pain or diarrhea and less commonly by malabsorption.

Diagnosis

Between 30 and 40% of individuals with chronic pancreatitis secondary to alcohol abuse have calcifications on abdominal radiographs. A qualitative or quantitative test for fecal fat is positive in individuals whose pancreas is more than 90% destroyed. Noninvasive tests of pancreatic function are not sensitive enough to detect mild to moderate insufficiency, so the secretin stimulation test is preferred (Table 143–6).

Treatment

Rx

Pancreatic enzyme replacement and analgesics are the mainstays of treatment. It is difficult to correct fat malabsorption completely with exogenous pancreatic enzymes because of their inactivation by acid and pepsin in the stomach. Normally, 28,000 U of lipase is present in the duodenal lumen with each meal. A high lipase–containing pancreatic enzyme preparation (25,000 to 40,000 U of lipase in the form of uncoated enzymes or enteric-coated, pH-sensitive microspheres) should be prescribed with each meal. Minimicrosphere preparations (e.g., 20,000 U of lipase taken orally with each meal) may be best tolerated owing to their small capsule size. Pancreatic proteases present in enzyme preparations may reduce abdominal pain by inactivating cholecystokinin (CCK)-releasing factor in the duodenum. Uncoated preparations may be more effective in pain relief, because coated preparations release enzymes predominantly distal to the duodenum. An histamine 2 receptor antagonist (e.g., ranitidine, 150 mg orally taken two times a day) or a proton-pump inhibitor (e.g., Prevacid [lansoprazole], 15 to 30 mg orally once a day) should be added to uncoated pancreatic enzyme replacement therapy in patients with a poor response.

Impaired Micelle Formation

Pathobiology

Bile salt concentrations in the intestinal lumen can fall to less than the critical concentration (2 to 3 mmol/L) needed for micelle formation because of decreased bile salt synthesis (severe liver disease), decreased

TABLE 143–4 DRUGS AND DIETARY PRODUCTS THAT IMPAIR NUTRIENT ABSORPTION

Drug	Mechanism	Nutrient Malabsorbed
Cholestyramine	Bile salt binder	Iron and cobalamin
High fiber, phytates	Chelator	Iron, calcium, magnesium
Tetracycline	Chelator	Calcium
Antacids	Chelator	Calcium, phosphate
Olestra	Nonabsorbable fat (lipophilic)	Fat-soluble vitamins
Orlistat	Lipase inhibitor	Fat, fat-soluble vitamins
Metformin	??	Glucose, cobalamin, folate
Acarbose	Competitive inhibitor of intestinal α-glucosidases	Carbohydrate
Colchicine	?Altered membrane trafficking	Carbohydrate, fat, cobalamin
Neomycin	Inhibitor of protein synthesis, binds bile salts	Carbohydrate, fat, protein
Methotrexate	Villus blunting	Carbohydrate, fat, protein
Phenytoin	Decreases folate absorption	Folate
Sulfasalazine	Inhibits folate hydrolase, ?inhibits folate transporter	Folate

TABLE 143–5 CLINICAL CONSEQUENCES OF MALABSORPTION OF NUTRIENTS, WATER, AND ELECTROLYTES

Nutrient Malabsorbed	Clinical Manifestation
Protein	Wasting, edema
Carbohydrate and fat	Diarrhea, abdominal cramps and bloating, weight loss/growth retardation
Fluid and electrolytes	Diarrhea, dehydration
Iron	Anemia, cheilosis, angular stomatitis
Calcium/vitamin D	Bone pain, fractures, tetany
Magnesium	Paresthesias, tetany
Vitamin B_{12}/folate	Anemia, glositis, cheilosis, paresthesias, ataxia (vitamin B_{12} only)
Vitamin E	Paresthesias, ataxia, retinopathy
Vitamin A	Night blindness, xerophthalmia, hyperkeratosis, diarrhea
Vitamin K	Ecchymoses
Riboflavin	Angular stomatitis, cheilosis
Zinc	Dermatitis, hypogeusia, diarrhea
Selenium	Cardiomyopathy
Essential fatty acids	Dermatitis

bile salt delivery (cholestasis), or removal of luminal bile salts (bacterial overgrowth, terminal ileal disease or resection, cholestyramine therapy, acid hypersecretion). Fat malabsorption resulting from impaired micelle formation is generally not as severe as malabsorption resulting from pancreatic lipase deficiency, presumably because fatty acids and monoglycerides can form lamellar structures, which to a certain extent can be absorbed. Malabsorption of fat-soluble vitamins (D, A, K, and E) may be marked, however, because micelle formation is required for their absorption.

Decreased Bile Salt Synthesis and Delivery

Malabsorption can occur in individuals with cholestatic liver disease or bile duct obstruction. The clinical consequences of malabsorption are seen most often in women with primary biliary cirrhosis because of the prolonged nature of the illness. Although these individuals can present with steatorrhea, bone disease is the most common presentation. Osteoporosis is more common than osteomalacia. The cause of bone disease in these patients is poorly understood and often is not related to vitamin D deficiency. Bone disease is treated with calcium supplements (and vitamin D if a deficiency is documented), weight-bearing exercise, and a bisphosphonate (e.g., alendronate 10 mg orally once daily or 70 mg orally once weekly).

Intestinal Bacterial Overgrowth

In health, only small numbers of lactobacilli, enterococci, gram-positive aerobes, or facultative anaerobes can be cultured from the upper small bowel lumen. Motility and acid are the most important factors in keeping the number of bacteria in the upper small bowel low. Any condition that produces local stasis or recirculation of colonic luminal contents allows development of a predominantly "colonic" flora (coliforms and anaerobes, such as *Bacteroides* and *Clostridium*) in the small intestine (Table 143–7). Anaerobic bacteria cause impaired micelle formation by releasing cholylamidases, which deconjugate bile salts. The unconjugated bile salts, with their higher pK_a, are more likely to be in the protonated form at the normal upper small intestinal pH of 6 to 7 and can be absorbed passively. As a result, the concentration of bile salts decreases in the intestinal lumen and can fall to less than the critical micellar concentration, causing malabsorption of fats and fat-soluble vitamins. Vitamin B_{12} deficiency and carbohydrate malabsorption also can occur with generalized bacterial overgrowth. Anaerobic bacteria ingest vitamin B_{12} and release proteases that degrade brush-border disaccharidases. Lactase is the disaccharidase normally present in lowest abundance and is the first affected. Although anaerobic bacteria use vitamin B_{12}, they synthesize folate. Individuals with bacterial overgrowth usually have low serum vitamin B_{12} levels but normal or high folate levels; this helps distinguish bacterial overgrowth from tropical sprue, in which vitamin B_{12} and folate levels are usually low because of decreased mucosal uptake.

Clinical Manifestations

Individuals with bacterial overgrowth can present with diarrhea, abdominal cramps, gas and bloating, weight loss, and signs and symptoms of vitamin B_{12} and fat-soluble vitamin deficiency. Watery diarrhea occurs because of the osmotic load of unabsorbed carbohydrates and stimulation of colonic secretion by unabsorbed fatty acids.

Diagnosis

The diagnosis of bacterial overgrowth should be considered in the elderly and in individuals with predisposing underlying disorders (see Table 143–7). Bacterial overgrowth may be associated with the irritable bowel syndrome (Chapter 139). The identification of greater than 10^5 CFU/mL in a culture of small intestinal aspirate remains the gold standard in diagnosis. The noninvasive tests with a sensitivity and specificity comparable to intestinal culture are the glucose hydrogen breath test and the ^{14}C- or ^{13}C-D-xylose breath test; in individuals with low vitamin B_{12} levels, a Schilling test before and after antibiotic therapy can be diagnostic (see Table 143–6).

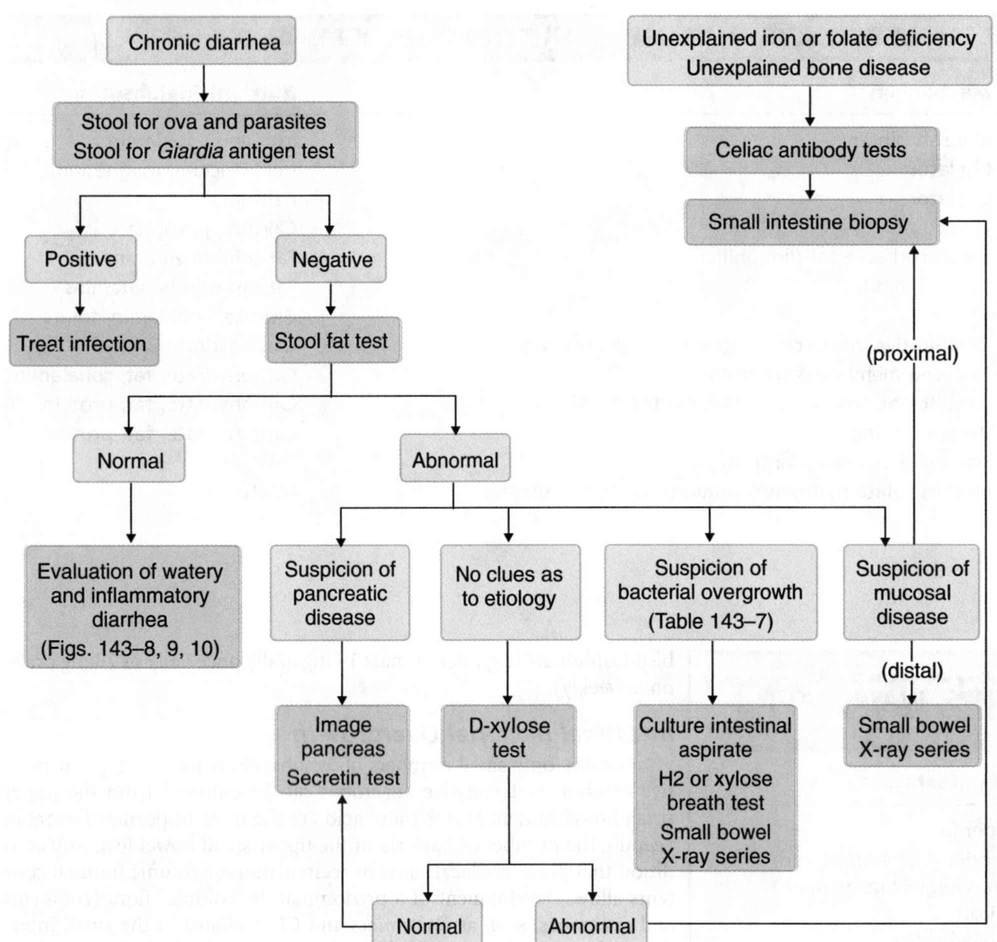

FIGURE 143–4 • Approach to the diagnosis of malabsorption.

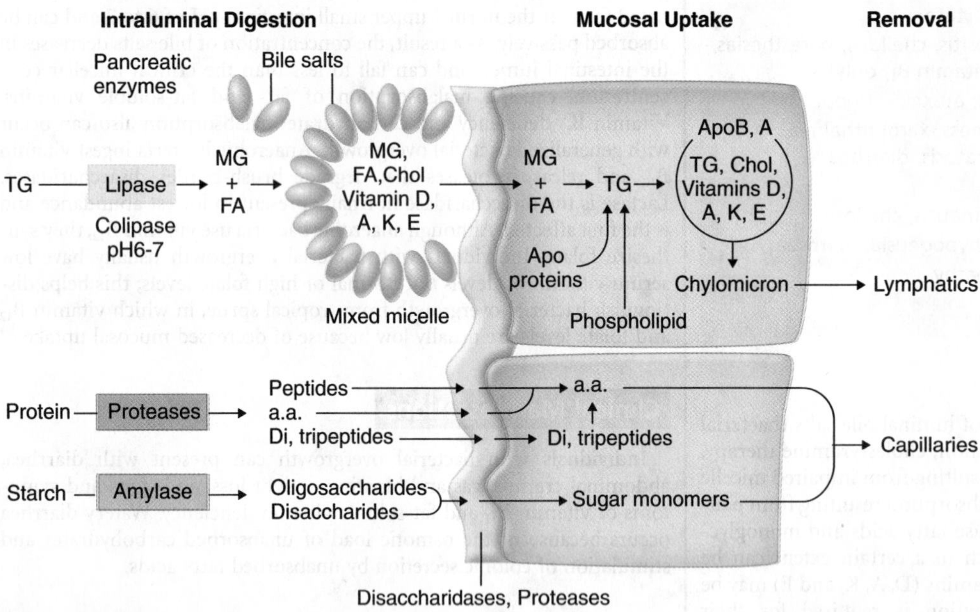

FIGURE 143–5 • Phases of intestinal digestion and absorption of dietary fat, protein, and carbohydrate. a.a. = amino acids; ApoB, A = apolipoproteins B and A; Chol = cholesterol; FA = fatty acids; MG = monoglycerides; TG = triglycerides.

Treatment

Rx

The goals of treatment are to correct the structural or motility defect, if possible; to eradicate offending bacteria, and to provide nutritional support. Acid-reducing agents should be stopped if possible. Treatment with antibiotics should be based on culture results whenever possible; otherwise, empirical treatment is given. Tetracycline (250 to 500 mg orally four times a day) or a broad-spectrum antibiotic against aerobes and enteric anaerobes (ciprofloxacin, 500 mg orally twice a day; amoxicillin/clavulanic acid, 250 to 500 mg orally three times a day; cephalexin, 250 mg orally four times a day with metronidazole, 250 mg three times a day) should be given for 14 days. The nonabsorbable antibiotic rifaximin (400 mg orally three times a day) is also effective, [5] but less so in individuals with an excluded (blind) intestinal loop. Prokinetic agents such as metoclopramide (10 mg orally four times a day) or erythromycin (250 to

TABLE 143–6 TESTS FOR THE EVALUATION OF MALABSORPTION*

Test	Comments
GENERAL TESTS OF ABSORPTION	
Quantitative stool fat test	Gold standard test of fat malabsorption, with which all other tests are compared. Requires ingestion of a high-fat diet (100 g) for 2 days before and during the collection. Stool is collected for 3 days. Normally, <7 g/24 hr is excreted on a high-fat diet. Borderline abnormalities of 8–14 g/24 hr may be seen in secretory or osmotic diarrheas that are not caused by malabsorption. There are false-negative findings if fat intake is inadequate. False-positive results can occur if mineral oil laxatives or rectal suppositories (e.g., cocoa butter) are given to the patient before stool collection.
Qualitative stool fat test	Sudan stain of a stool sample for fat. Many fat droplets per medium-power (40×) field constitute a positive test result. The NMR method determines the percentage of fat in the stool (normal, <20%). The test depends on an adequate fat intake (100 g/day). There is high sensitivity (90%) and specificity (90%) with fat malabsorption of >10 g/24 hr. Sensitivity drops with stool fat in the range of 6–10 g/24 hr.
Acid steatocrit	Reliable screening test for fat malabsorption that is inexpensive and easy to perform. Centrifugation of acidified stool in a hematocrit capillary yields solid, liquid, and fatty layers. Results are expressed as volumetric percentages (lipid phase on solid phase); normal, <10%. High sensitivity (100%) and specificity (95%) compared with the 72-hr stool quantitative fat test. Depends on adequate fat intake (100 g/day).
D-Xylose test	A test of small intestinal mucosal absorption, used to distinguish mucosal malabsorption from malabsorption due to pancreatic insufficiency. An oral dose of D-xylose (25 g/500 mL water) is administered, and D-xylose excretion is measured in a 5-hr urine collection. Normally, >4 g of D-xylose is excreted in the urine over 5 hr. The test also may be positive in bacterial overgrowth owing to metabolism of D-xylose by bacteria in the intestinal lumen. False-positive test results occur with renal failure, ascites, and an incomplete urine collection. Blood levels at 1 and 3 hr improve sensitivity. May be normal with mild or limited mucosal disease.
Hydrogen breath test	Most useful in the diagnosis of lactase deficiency. An oral dose of lactose (1 g/kg body weight) is administered after measurement of basal breath H_2 levels. The sole source of H_2 in the mammal is bacterial fermentation; unabsorbed lactose makes its way to colonic bacteria, resulting in excess breath H_2. A *late peak* (within 3–6 hr) of >20 ppm of exhaled H_2 after lactose ingestion suggests lactose malabsorption. Absorption of other carbohydrates (e.g., sucrose, glucose, fructose) also can be tested.
SPECIFIC TESTS FOR MALABSORPTION	
TESTS FOR PANCREATIC FUNCTION	
Secretin stimulation test	The gold standard test of pancreatic function. Requires duodenal intubation with a double-lumen tube and collection of pancreatic juice in response to IV secretin. Allows measurement of bicarbonate (HCO_3^-) and pancreatic enzymes. A sensitive test of pancreatic function, but labor intensive and invasive.
Fecal elastase-1 test	Stool test for pancreatic function. Equal sensitivity to the secretin stimulation test for the diagnosis of moderate-to-severe pancreatic insufficiency. More specific than the fecal chymotrypsin test. Unreliable with mild insufficiency. False-positive results occur with increased stool volume and intestinal mucosal diseases.
TESTS FOR BACTERIAL OVERGROWTH	
Quantitative culture of small intestinal aspirate	Gold standard test for bacterial overgrowth. Greater than 10^5 colony-forming units (CFU)/mL in the jejunum suggests bacterial overgrowth. Requires special anaerobic sample collection, rapid anaerobic and aerobic plating, and care to avoid oropharyngeal contamination. False-negative results occur with focal jejunal diverticula and when overgrowth is distal to the site aspirated.
Hydrogen breath test	The 50-g glucose breath test has a sensitivity of 90% for growth of 10^5 colonic-type bacteria in the small intestine. If bacterial overgrowth is present, increased H_2 is excreted in the breath. An *early peak* (within 2 hr) of >20 ppm exhaled H_2 suggests bacterial overgrowth. False-negative results occur with non–hydrogen-producing organisms.
^{14}C-D-xylose breath test	This test uses 1 g of carbon 14–labeled D-xylose. It has a sensitivity and specificity >90% for growth of 10^5 colonic-type bacteria in the small intestine. Bacteria metabolize D-xylose with release of $^{14}CO_2$, which is absorbed and exhaled. Non-degraded D-xylose is absorbed in the small bowel and does not reach the colon, yielding a greater specificity than the H_2 breath test. A nonradioactive ^{13}C-D-xylose breath test is suitable for children and pregnant women.
TESTS FOR MUCOSAL DISEASE	
Small-bowel biopsy	Obtained for a specific diagnosis when there is a high index of suspicion for small intestinal disease. Several biopsy specimens (4–5) must be obtained to maximize the diagnostic yield. Distal duodenal biopsy specimens are usually adequate for diagnosis, but occasionally enteroscopy with jejunal biopsy specimens is necessary. Small intestinal biopsy provides a specific diagnosis in some diseases (e.g., intestinal infection, Whipple's disease, abetalipoproteinemia, agammaglobulinemia, lymphangiectasia, lymphoma, amyloidosis). In other conditions, such as celiac disease and tropical sprue, the biopsy specimens show characteristic findings, but the diagnosis is made on improvement after treatment.
Permeability studies	These tests of mucosal integrity are gaining favor as screening tests for small intestinal disease and for monitoring response to treatment. The study is performed by administering an oral dose of nonabsorbable markers (e.g., mannitol/lactulose, lactulose/^{51}Cr-EDTA) and measuring urinary excretion. Currently a research tool.

Continued

TABLE 143–6 TESTS FOR THE EVALUATION OF MALABSORPTION*—cont'd

Test	Comments
TESTS OF ILEAL FUNCTION	
Schilling test	A test of vitamin B_{12} absorption. Performed as part I, followed by parts II, III, and IV if needed Part I: A saturating dose (1 mg IM) of vitamin B_{12} is given, followed by an oral dose of 0.5–2 μg radioactive cyanocobalamin). Urine is collected for 24 hr because of a poorly understood delay in the passage of cobalamins across ileal cells. Part I is abnormal in all individuals with vitamin B_{12} deficiency except those with dietary deficiency and food-cobalamin malabsorption. Part II: The test is repeated with a dose of intrinsic factor. Distinguishes lack of intrinsic factor from other causes of vitamin B_{12} malabsorption. Part III: The test is repeated with pancreatic enzymes. Can be used as a test for pancreatic insufficiency. In such individuals, administration of exogenous enzymes frees cyanocobalamin from R-proteins, reverting the Schilling test to normal. Part IV: The test is repeated with antibiotics. When values for parts I and II are low, bacterial overgrowth can be distinguished from ileal disease by repeating the test after a 5-day course of antibiotics.

*Not all of these tests are readily available. A strong suspicion for any disease may warrant foregoing an extensive work-up and obtaining the test with highest diagnostic yield. In some cases, empirical treatment, such as removing lactose from the diet of an otherwise healthy individual with lactose intolerance, is warranted without any testing.
^{51}Cr-EDTA = chromium 51–labeled ethylenediamine tetraacetic acid; NMR = nuclear magnetic resonance.

TABLE 143–7 ABNORMALITIES CONDUCIVE TO BACTERIAL OVERGROWTH

STRUCTURAL

Surgical
- Afferent loop dysfunction after gastrojejunostomy
- Ileocecal valve resection
- Surgical loops (end-to-side intestinal anastomoses)

Anatomic
- Duodenal and jejunal diverticula
- Obstruction
- Strictures (Crohn's disease, radiation enteritis)
- Adhesions (postsurgical)
- Gastrojejunocolic fistulas

MOTOR

Scleroderma
Diabetes mellitus
Idiopathic pseudo-obstruction

HYPOCHLORHYDRIA

Atrophic gastritis
Proton-pump inhibitors
Acquired immunodeficiency syndrome
Acid-reducing surgery for peptic ulcer disease

MISCELLANEOUS

Immunodeficiency states
Pancreatitis
Cirrhosis
Chronic renal failure

Rx

500 mg orally four times a day) can be tried to treat small bowel motility disorders, but often they are not efficacious. Octreotide (50 μg subcutaneously every day) may improve motility and reduce bacterial overgrowth in individuals with scleroderma. If the structural abnormality or motility disturbance cannot be corrected, the patient is at risk for malnutrition and deficiencies of vitamin B_{12} and fat-soluble vitamins. Cyclic treatment (1 week out of every 4 to 6 weeks) with rotating antibiotics may be required in these patients to prevent recurrent bouts of bacterial overgrowth. If supplemental calories are needed, medium-chain triglycerides should be given, because they are not dependent on micelle formation for their absorption. Monthly treatment with vitamin B_{12} should be considered, along with supplemental vitamins D, A, K, and E and calcium.

Ileal Disease or Resection

Disease of the terminal ileum is most commonly due to Crohn's disease (which also may lead to ileal resection), but it also can be caused by radiation enteritis, tropical sprue, tuberculosis, *Yersinia* infection, or idiopathic bile salt malabsorption. These diseases cause bile salt wasting in the colon.

The clinical consequences of bile salt malabsorption are related directly to the length of the diseased or resected terminal ileum. In an adult, if less than 100 cm of ileum is diseased or resected, watery diarrhea results because of stimulation of colonic fluid secretion by unabsorbed bile salts. Fat absorption remains normal, because increased bile salt synthesis in the liver compensates for bile salt losses and micelle formation is preserved. Bile acid diarrhea responds to cholestyramine (2 to 4 g taken at breakfast, lunch, and dinner). If more than 100 cm of ileum is diseased or resected, bile salt losses (>3 g/day) in the colon exceed the capacity for increased bile salt synthesis in the liver, the bile salt pool shrinks, and micelle formation is impaired. As a result, steatorrhea ensues, and fatty acid–induced intestinal secretion synergizes with the bile acid–induced secretion to cause diarrhea. Treatment is with a low-fat diet, vitamin B_{12} (300 to 1000 μg subcutaneously once every month or 2 mg orally once a day), dietary supplements of calcium (500 mg orally two to three times a day, monitor 24-hour urine calcium for adequacy of dose), and a multiple vitamin-mineral supplement. An antimotility agent should be given for diarrhea. Bile salt binders may worsen diarrhea. Screening for fat-soluble vitamin deficiencies (vitamins A and E, 25-(OH) vitamin D, and prothrombin time) and bone disease (bone densitometry, serum calcium, intact parathyroid hormone, 24-hour urine for calcium) should be done.

Three long-term complications of chronic bile salt wasting and fat malabsorption are renal stones, bone disease (osteoporosis and osteomalacia), and gallstones. Oxalate renal stones occur as a consequence of excess free oxalate absorption in the colon. Free oxalate is generated when unabsorbed fatty acids bind luminal calcium, which is then unavailable for binding oxalate. Renal oxalate stones sometimes can be avoided with a low-fat, low-oxalate diet and calcium supplements. Bone disease is caused by impaired micelle formation with a resulting decrease in absorption of vitamin D; year-round sun exposure reduces this complication. Vitamin D (50,000 U orally one to three times a week) and calcium supplements (500 mg orally two to three times a day) should be given to susceptible individuals, but vitamin D levels and serum and urinary calcium must be monitored for response to treatment, because excess vitamin D can be toxic. The mechanism of gallstone formation in these individuals is unclear; pigmented gallstones are most common.

Conditions That Impair Mucosal Absorption

Pathobiology

Nutrients are absorbed along the entire length of the small intestine, with the exception of iron and folate, which are absorbed predominantly in the duodenum and proximal jejunum, and bile salts and cobalamin, which can be absorbed only in the distal ileum. The efficiency of nutrient uptake at the mucosa is influenced by the number of villus absorptive cells, the presence of functional hydrolases and specific nutrient transport proteins on the brush-border membrane, and transit time. Transit time determines the contact time of luminal contents with the brush-border membrane and influences the efficiency of nutrient uptake across the mucosa.

Fatty Acids

Long-chain fatty acids are transported across the microvillus membrane of villus epithelial cells by the fatty acid transport protein FATP4; are resynthesized into triglycerides; and combine with cholesterol ester, fat-soluble vitamins, phospholipid, and apoproteins to form chylomicrons. The bile salts from mixed micelles remain in the intestinal lumen and are absorbed in the distal ileum by sodium-dependent cotransport.

Oligosaccharides and larger oligopeptides (products of pancreatic enzyme digestion), sucrose and lactose, are hydrolyzed further by enzymes present in the brush-border membrane of villus epithelial cells before they are absorbed. Although only sugar monomers (glucose, galactose, fructose) can be taken up at the apical epithelial cell membrane, dipeptides and tripeptides are readily taken into the cell. Defects in amino acid uptake in Hartnup's disease and cystinuria are characterized by renal and intestinal malabsorption of neutral and basic amino acids. In the intestine, these defects are offset by the absorption of these amino acids as dipeptides and tripeptides.

Vitamins

Water-soluble vitamins are readily absorbed throughout the small intestine. Fat-soluble vitamins, minerals, and cobalamin are more difficult to absorb because of the requirement for micelle formation (vitamins D, A, K, and E), a divalent charge (magnesium, calcium, iron), or selected sites of uptake in the intestine (iron, cobalamin). Calcium is absorbed best in the proximal small intestine by a vitamin D–dependent uptake process. Magnesium from the diet and endogenously secreted magnesium from biliary, gastric, and pancreatic juices are absorbed by the small intestine (throughout its length) by a poorly understood mechanism. Ferrous iron is transported into intestinal epithelial cells by a proton-coupled metal-ion transporter (Nramp2) that has specificity for Fe^{2+} and other divalent cations (Zn^{2+}, Mn^{2+}, Co^{2+}, Cd^{2+}, Cu^{2+}, Ni^{2+}, and Pb^{2+}). The absorption of calcium and nonheme iron is enhanced by solubilization with hydrochloric acid. Intraluminal compounds such as oxalate, phytates, and long-chain fatty acids bind to calcium and magnesium, decreasing their absorption. Individuals with severe mucosal disease or short-bowel syndrome with high fecal fluid outputs lose magnesium and zinc from endogenous secretions.

Mucosal malabsorption can be caused by specific (usually congenital) brush-border enzyme or nutrient transporter deficiencies or by generalized diseases that damage the small intestinal mucosa or result in surgical resection or bypass of small intestine. The nutrients malabsorbed in these general malabsorptive diseases depend on the site of intestinal injury (proximal, distal, or diffuse) and the severity of damage. The main mechanism of malabsorption in these conditions is a decrease in surface area available for absorption. Some conditions (infection, celiac disease, tropical sprue, food allergies, and graft-versus-host disease [GVHD]) are characterized by intestinal inflammation and villus flattening; others are characterized by ulceration (ulcerative jejunitis, NSAIDs diarrhea), infiltration (amyloidosis), or ischemia (radiation enteritis, mesenteric ischemia).

Folates

Folates (Chapters 170 and 237) are both taken in the diet and produced by bacteria in the colon. Deficiency can be caused by poor intake or malabsorption secondary to intestinal disease or drugs. Dietary folates are absorbed in the proximal small intestine. A reduced folate carrier (RFC1), expressed in the small intestine and colon, suggests that folate might be absorbed in the colon and the small intestine.

Cobalamins

The cobalamins (Chapters 170 and 237) are high-molecular-weight, water-soluble molecules that contain a porphyrin-like corrin ring with a cobalt atom in its center. The supplemental form contains a cyanide group attached to the cobalt atom; hence the name cyanocobalamin (vitamin B_{12}). The cobalamins are readily abundant in foods containing animal proteins (e.g., meat, seafood, eggs, milk), so cobalamin deficiency in industrialized countries is rarely due to poor dietary intake but rather reflects the inability to absorb cobalamin. This inability may be caused by a lack of intrinsic factor, consumption of cobalamin by overgrowth of anaerobic bacteria in the small bowel lumen, ileal disease or resection, or defective transcobalamin II. Large amounts of cobalamin are present in the liver (2 to 5 mg), and cobalamin is reabsorbed from bile via the enterohepatic circulation, limiting daily losses to only 0.5 to 1 μg. It usually takes 10 to 12 years for cobalamin deficiency to develop after it is eliminated from the diet, but deficiency can occur more rapidly (2 to 5 years) with malabsorptive syndromes. If lack of gastric acid causes food-cobalamin malabsorption, treatment with oral cyanocobalamin is curative.

Lactase Deficiency

Epidemiology

Acquired lactase deficiency is the most common cause of selective carbohydrate malabsorption. Most individuals, except those of northern European descent, begin to lose lactase activity by the age of 2 years. The prevalence of lactase deficiency is highest (85 to 100%) in Asians, blacks, and Native Americans.

Pathobiology

The persistence/nonpersistence of lactase activity is associated with a single nucleotide polymorphism C/T_{-13910} that is found upstream of the lactase gene on chromosome 2q21-22. Hypolactasia is associated with the C/C_{-13910} genotype in diverse ethnic groups. The mechanism by which this variant downregulates the lactase gene is not known, but functional studies suggest genotype-dependent alterations in levels of messenger RNA.

Clinical Manifestations

Adults with lactase deficiency typically complain of gas, bloating, and diarrhea after the ingestion of milk or dairy products but do not lose weight. Unabsorbed lactose is osmotically active, drawing water followed by ions into the intestinal lumen. On reaching the colon, bacteria metabolize lactose to short-chain fatty acids, carbon dioxide, and hydrogen gas. Short-chain fatty acids are transported with sodium into colonic epithelial cells, facilitating the reabsorption of fluid in the colon. If the colonic capacity for the reabsorption of short-chain fatty acids is exceeded, an osmotic diarrhea results (see later discussion of carbohydrate malabsorption in watery diarrheas).

Diagnosis

The diagnosis of acquired lactase deficiency can be made by empirical treatment with a lactose-free diet, which results in resolution of symptoms; by the hydrogen breath test after oral administration of lactose; or by genetic testing. Many intestinal diseases cause secondary reversible lactase deficiency, including viral gastroenteritis, celiac disease, giardiasis, and bacterial overgrowth.

Congenital Enteropeptidase (Enterokinase) Deficiency

Enteropeptidase is a brush-border protease that cleaves trypsinogen to trypsin, triggering the cascade of pancreatic protease activation in the intestinal lumen. The rare congenital deficiency of enteropeptidase results in inability to activate all pancreatic proteases and leads to severe protein malabsorption. It manifests in infancy as diarrhea, growth retardation, and hypoproteinemic edema.

Abetalipoproteinemia

Formation and exocytosis of chylomicrons at the basolateral membrane of intestinal epithelial cells are necessary for the delivery of lipids to the systemic circulation. One of the proteins required for assembly and secretion of chylomicrons is the microsomal triglyceride transfer protein, which is mutated in individuals with abetalipoproteinemia. Children with this disorder have fat malabsorption and the consequences of vitamin E deficiency (retinopathy and spinocerebellar degeneration). Biochemical tests show low plasma levels of apoprotein B, triglyceride, and cholesterol. Membrane lipid abnormalities result in red blood cell acanthosis (burr cells). Intestinal biopsy is diagnostic; the tissue is characterized by engorgement of epithelial cells with lipid droplets. Calories are provided by treatment with a low-fat diet containing medium-chain triglycerides. Medium-chain fatty acids are easily absorbed and released directly into the portal circulation, bypassing the defect of abetalipoproteinemia. Poor absorption of long-chain fatty acids sometimes can result in essential fatty acid deficiency. High doses of fat-soluble vitamins, especially vitamin E, often are needed. Mutations in the apolipoprotein B gene (hypobetalipoproteinemia) and intracellular retention of chylomicrons (Anderson's disease) cause a similar although less severe clinical syndrome.

Celiac Disease

Definition and Epidemiology

Celiac disease, also called celiac sprue, nontropical sprue, and gluten-sensitive enteropathy, is an inflammatory condition of the small intestine precipitated by the ingestion of wheat, rye, and barley in individuals with certain genetic predispositions. Screening studies for the antigliadin (AGA), antiendomysial (EMA), and anti-tissue transglutaminase (anti-tTG) antibodies that are associated with celiac disease suggest a prevalence in Caucasian populations of about 1%, with the highest prevalence in Northern Ireland. High-risk groups for celiac disease include first-degree relatives and individuals with type I diabetes mellitus, autoimmune thyroid disease, primary biliary cirrhosis, Turner's syndrome, and Down syndrome. About 10% of patients diagnosed with irritable bowel syndrome or with microscopic (lymphocytic) colitis have celiac disease.

Pathobiology

Environmental and genetic factors are important in the development of celiac disease. The alcohol-soluble protein fraction of wheat gluten, the gliadins, and similar prolamins in rye and barley trigger intestinal inflammation in susceptible individuals. Oat grains, which have prolamins rich in glutamine but not proline, are rarely toxic. Gliadins and similar prolamins with high proline content are relatively resistant to digestion by human proteases. A 33-mer peptide that is a natural digestion product of α_2-gliadin may be important in the pathogenesis of celiac disease. This peptide resists terminal digestion by intestinal brush-border proteases and contains three previously identified antigenic epitopes. It also reacts with tissue transglutaminase and stimulates human leukocyte antigen (HLA) DQ2–restricted intestinal T-cell clones from individuals with celiac disease.

Approximately 15% of first-degree relatives of affected individuals are found to have celiac disease. Predisposition to gluten sensitivity has been mapped to the HLA-D region on chromosome 6. More than 90% of individuals with celiac disease have the DQ2 heterodimer encoded by alleles *DQA1*0501* and *DQB1*0201*, compared with 20 to 30% of controls. A smaller celiac group carries HLA DQ8. Genome-wide searches support a strong susceptibility locus for celiac disease in the HLA-D region. Non-HLA loci have been suggested but not yet identified. The DQ2 protein expressed on antigen-presenting cells has positively charged binding pockets; tTG (the autoantigen recognized by EMA) may enhance intestinal inflammation by deamidation of select glutamine residues in gliadin to negatively charged glutamic acid. In the deamidated form, most gliadin peptides have a higher binding affinity for DQ2 and are more potent stimulants of gluten-sensitized T cells. Villous atrophy may be caused by inflammation that is triggered by γ-interferon released from DQ2- or DQ8-restricted CD4 T cells in the lamina propria. Alternatively, intraepithelial lymphocytes may directly kill intestinal epithelial cells under the influence of IL-15 released from stressed enterocytes.

Clinical Manifestations

Celiac disease usually manifests early in life at about 2 years of age (after wheat has been introduced into the diet) or later in the second to fourth decades of life, but it can occur at any age. Breast-feeding and the time of introduction of wheat in the diet (4 to 6 months of age) may lessen the risk or delay the onset of celiac disease in children at risk. About half of adults with celiac disease in the United States present with anemia or osteoporosis without diarrhea or other gastrointestinal symptoms. These individuals most likely have proximal disease that impairs iron, folate, and calcium absorption but an adequate surface area in the remaining intestine for absorption of other nutrients. Other extraintestinal manifestations of celiac disease include rash (dermatitis herpetiformis), neurologic disorders (peripheral neuropathy, ataxia, epilepsy), psychiatric disorders (depression, paranoia), reproductive disorders (infertility, spontaneous abortion), short stature, dental enamel hypoplasia, chronic hepatitis, or cardiomyopathy.

Individuals with significant mucosal involvement present with watery diarrhea, weight loss or growth retardation, and the clinical manifestations of vitamin and mineral deficiencies (see Table 143–5). All nutrients, most notably carbohydrate, fat, protein, electrolytes, fat-soluble vitamins, calcium, magnesium, iron, folate, and zinc, are malabsorbed. Cobalamin deficiency is more common (10% of patients) than previously thought and usually corrects itself on a gluten-free diet. Symptomatic individuals require supplementation of vitamin B_{12}. Diarrhea is caused by many mechanisms, including a decreased surface area for water and electrolyte absorption, the osmotic effect of unabsorbed luminal nutrients, an increased surface area for chloride secretion (crypt hyperplasia), and the stimulation of intestinal fluid secretion by inflammatory mediators and unabsorbed fatty acids. Some individuals have impaired pancreatic enzyme secretion caused by decreased mucosal cholecystokinin release or bacterial overgrowth that may contribute to diarrhea.

Diagnosis

The diagnosis of celiac disease is made by characteristic changes found on a small intestinal biopsy specimen and improvement when a gluten-free diet is instituted (Figs. 143–6 and 143–7). Mucosal flattening may be observed endoscopically as reduced duodenal folds or duodenal scalloping. Characteristic features found on intestinal biopsy include the absence of villi, crypt hyperplasia, increased intraepithelial lymphocytes, and infiltration of the lamina propria with plasma cells and lymphocytes. In some individuals, the only abnormal biopsy finding is increased intraepithelial lymphocytes.

Serologic markers for celiac disease are useful in supporting the diagnosis, in screening first-degree relatives, and in monitoring the response to a gluten-free diet. AGA immunoglobulin A (IgA) and IgG antibodies are sensitive but not specific and should not be used for screening of adults. EMA IgA antibodies, detected by indirect immunofluorescence, are highly sensitive (90%) and specific (90 to 100%) for active celiac disease in skilled laboratory testing. An enzyme-linked immunosorbent assay (ELISA) test to detect antibodies against tTG has equal sensitivity to the EMA test and is less operator dependent. Anti-tTG and EMA IgA antibodies tests are negative in individuals with selective IgA deficiency (present in up to 2.6% of individuals with celiac disease). In these patients, anti-tTG IgG antibodies may be helpful in diagnosis. A new dot blot assay against recombinant human tTG reacts to IgA and IgG antibodies, increasing the specificity to almost 100%. Patients with mild disease may have negative antibody studies. In equivocal cases (negative serology and equivocal biopsy or positive serology and normal biopsy), HLA genotyping is useful to exclude the diagnosis of celiac disease in those who lack the DQ2 or DQ8 gene.

Treatment

Rx

Treatment consists of a lifelong gluten-free diet. Wheat, rye, and barley grains should be excluded from the diet. Rice and corn grains are tolerated. Oats (if not contaminated by wheat grain) are tolerated by most. Early referral to a celiac support group is often helpful in maintaining dietary compliance. Owing to secondary lactase deficiency, a lactose-free diet should be recommended until symptoms improve. All individuals with celiac disease should be screened for vitamin and mineral deficiencies and have bone densitometry performed. Of individuals with celiac disease, 70% have osteopenia. Documented deficiencies of vitamins and minerals should be replenished (Table 143–8), and women of childbearing age should take folic acid supplements.

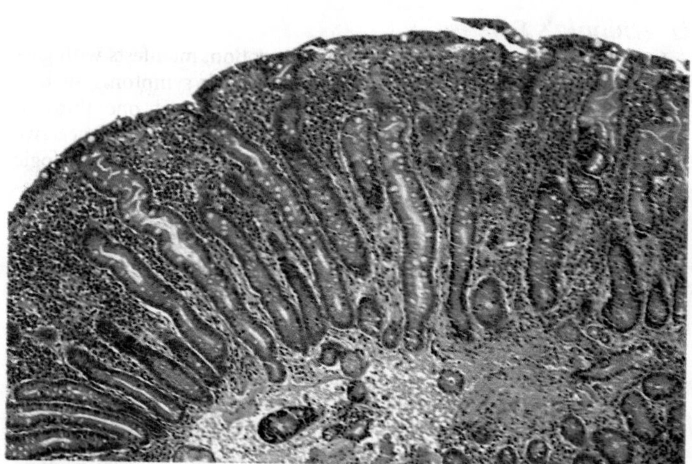

FIGURE 143–6 • Intestinal biopsy appearance of flattened villi, hyperplastic crypts, and increased intraepithelial lymphocytes. (Courtesy of John Hart, MD.)

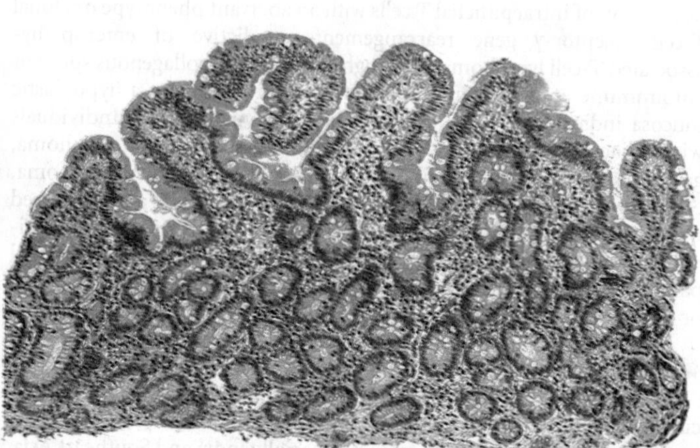

FIGURE 143–7 • Regeneration of villi after initiation of a gluten-free diet. (Courtesy of John Hart, MD.)

TABLE 143–8 VITAMIN AND MINERAL DOSES USED IN THE TREATMENT OF MALABSORPTION

Vitamin	Oral Dose	Parenteral Dose
Vitamin A*	Water-soluble A, 25,000 U/day†	
Vitamin E	Water-soluble E, 400–800 U/day†	
Vitamin D‡	25,000–50,000 U/day	
Vitamin K	5 mg/day	
Folic acid	1 mg/day	
Calcium§	1500–2000 mg elemental calcium/day Calcium citrate, 500 mg calcium/tablet† Calcium carbonate, 500 mg calcium/tablet†	
Magnesium	Liquid magnesium gluconate† 1–3 tbsp (12–36 mEq magnesium) in 1–2 L of ORS or sports drink sipped throughout the day Magnesium chloride hexahydrate† 100–600 mg elemental magnesium/day	2 mL of a 50% solution (8 mEq) both buttocks IM
Zinc	Zinc gluconate† 20–50 mg elemental zinc/day‖	
Iron	150–300 mg elemental iron/day Polysaccharide-iron complex† Iron sulfate or gluconate	Iron sucrose# Sodium ferric gluconate complex# Iron dextran (as calculated for anemia (IV or IM; Chapter 163)¶
B-complex vitamins	1 megadose tablet/day	
Vitamin B_{12}	2 mg/day	1 mg IM or SC/mo**

*Monitor serum vitamin A level to avoid toxicity, especially in patients with hypertriglyceridemia.
†Form best absorbed or with least side effects.
‡Monitor serum calcium and 25-OH vitamin D levels to avoid toxicity.
§Monitor 24-hr urine calcium to assess adequacy of dose.
‖If intestinal output is high, additional zinc should be given. Monitor for copper deficiency with high doses.
¶Parenteral therapy should be given in a supervised outpatient setting because of the risk of fatal reactions.
#Decreased risk of fatal reactions when compared with iron dextran.
**For vitamin B_{12} deficiency, 1 mg IM or SC twice a week for 4 wk, then once a month.
ORS = oral rehydration solution.

Prognosis

Of patients with celiac disease treated with a gluten-free diet, 90% experience symptomatic improvement within 2 weeks. The most common cause of a poor dietary response is continued ingestion of gluten. Other possibilities include a missed diagnosis (intestinal infection, agammaglobulinemia), bacterial overgrowth, pancreatic insufficiency, microscopic colitis, or other food allergies (cow's milk, soy protein). For a small percentage of patients on a strict gluten-free diet, enteropathy persists and no other diagnosis is found; this is so-called refractory sprue. Rarely, collagen deposition is found beneath the surface epithelium (collagenous sprue), or a hypoplastic mucosa shows villus and crypt atrophy. Some patients have antienterocyte antibodies indicative of autoimmune enteritis. Others have ulcerative jejunitis or a monoclonal population of intraepithelial T cells with an aberrant phenotype or clonal T-cell receptor-γ gene rearrangements predictive of enteropathy-associated T-cell lymphoma. Although patients with collagenous sprue or autoimmune enteritis may respond to steroid treatment, a hypoplastic mucosa indicates irreversible (end-stage) intestinal disease. Individuals with celiac disease are at increased risk for intestinal T-cell lymphoma, gastrointestinal tract carcinomas (small bowel adenocarcinoma, esophageal and oropharyngeal squamous carcinomas), and increased mortality; a strict gluten-free diet for life may lessen these risks. Intestinal lymphoma should be suspected in individuals who have abdominal pain, recurrence of symptoms after initial response to a gluten-free diet, or refractory sprue.

Tropical Sprue

Tropical sprue is an inflammatory disease of the small intestine associated with the overgrowth of predominantly coliform bacteria. It occurs in residents or travelers to the tropics, especially India and Southeast Asia. Individuals classically present with diarrhea and megaloblastic anemia secondary to vitamin B_{12} and folate deficiency, but some have anemia only. Intestinal biopsy characteristically shows subtotal and patchy villus atrophy in the proximal and distal small intestine, which may be caused by the effect of bacterial toxins on gut structure or by the secondary effects of vitamin B_{12} deficiency on the gut (megaloblastic gut). Diagnosis is based on history, documentation of vitamin B_{12} and/or folate deficiency, and the presence of an abnormal small intestinal biopsy report. Treatment is a prolonged course of broad-spectrum antibiotics, oral folate, and vitamin B_{12} injections until symptoms resolve. Relapses occur mainly in natives of the tropics.

Infection

Giardia lamblia

Giardia lamblia infection, the most common protozoal infection in the United States, can cause malabsorption in individuals infected with many trophozoites, especially the immunocompromised or IgA-deficient hosts. Malabsorption occurs when many organisms cover the epithelium and cause mucosal inflammation, which results in villus flattening and a decrease in absorptive surface area. Stool for ova and parasites at this stage of infection is often negative because of the attachment of organisms in the proximal small intestine. Diagnosis can be made by a stool antigen-capture ELISA test but may require duodenal aspiration and biopsies.

Human Immunodeficiency Virus

Diarrhea, malabsorption, and wasting are common in individuals with AIDS but are seen less frequently with improved antiretroviral therapy (Chapter 413). Malabsorption is usually due to infection with cryptosporidia, *Mycobacterium avium-intracellulare* complex, *Isospora belli*, or microsporidia. An organism can be identified by stool examination or intestinal biopsy about 50% of the time. AIDS enteropathy (a term used if no organism is identified) also can cause malabsorption. Mechanisms of malabsorption and diarrhea include villus atrophy, increased intestinal permeability, rapid small bowel transit (in patients with protozoal infection), and ultrastructural damage of enterocytes (in AIDS enteropathy). Among individuals with AIDS and diarrhea, results of fecal fat and D-xylose absorption are frequently abnormal. Serum albumin, vitamin B_{12}, and zinc levels are often low. Low serum levels of vitamin B_{12} also have been reported in HIV-infected individuals without AIDS. Vitamin B_{12} deficiency is caused mainly by ileal disease, but low intrinsic factor (IF) and decreased transcobalamin (TC) II may be contributing factors. Management of malabsorption should focus on restoring the immune system by treating the underlying HIV infection with antiviral therapy. If possible, the offending organism should be treated with antibiotics. If the organism cannot be eradicated, chronic diarrhea and malabsorption result; treatment in these cases consists of antimotility agents and a lactose-free, low-fat diet. Pancreatic enzyme replacement therapy can be tried in HIV-infected individuals who are taking highly active antiretroviral therapy or nucleoside analogues and who have fat malabsorption of obscure origin. If supplemental calories are needed, liquid oral supplements that are predigested and high in medium-chain triglycerides (semi-elemental) are tolerated best. Vitamin and mineral deficiencies should be screened for and treated.

Whipple's Disease

Whipple's disease, a rare cause of malabsorption, manifests with gastrointestinal complaints in association with systemic symptoms, such as fever, joint pain, or neurologic manifestations. About one third of patients have cardiac involvement, most commonly culture-negative endocarditis. Occasionally, individuals present with ocular or neurologic disease without gastrointestinal symptoms. Men are affected more commonly than women, particularly white men. The organism responsible for causing Whipple's disease is a gram-positive actinomycete, *Tropheryma whippelii*. The epidemiology and pathogenesis of Whipple's disease are poorly understood. The prevalence of the disease is higher in farmers compared with other workers, which suggests that the organism lives in the soil. Using the polymerase chain reaction, *T. whippelii* has been detected in sewage and in duodenal biopsy specimens, gastric juice, saliva, and stool of individuals without clinical disease. Whether the latter represents a carrier state or the presence of nonpathogenic organisms is not known. Immunologic defects and an association with the HLA-B27 gene may be disease factors. Small intestinal biopsy shows villus blunting and infiltration of the lamina propria with large macrophages that stain positive with the periodic acid–Schiff method and are filled with the organism. It is important to distinguish these macrophages from macrophages infected with *M. avium-intracellulare* complex, which stain positive on acid-fast staining and are found in individuals with AIDS. Treatment is with a prolonged course of broad-spectrum antibiotics (e.g., parenteral penicillin G 1.2 U every day and streptomycin 1.0 g every day for 10 to 14 days, plus 160 mg of trimethoprim and 800 of sulfamethoxazole orally two times a day for 1 year or 160 mg of trimethoprim and 800 of sulfamethoxazole orally two times a day for 1 year). Relapses are common, but initial treatment with parenteral penicillin and streptomycin may lessen the relapse rate.

Graft-versus-Host Disease

Diarrhea occurs frequently after allogeneic bone marrow or stem cell transplantation. Immediately after transplantation, diarrhea is caused by the toxic effects of cytoreductive therapy on the intestinal epithelium. At 20 to 100 days after transplantation, diarrhea is usually due to GVHD or infection. Patients with GVHD present clinically with a skin rash, buccal mucositis, anorexia, nausea, vomiting, abdominal cramps, and diarrhea. The diagnosis of GVHD in the gastrointestinal tract can be made on biopsy of the stomach, small intestine, or colon. In mild cases, the mucosa appears normal on inspection at endoscopy, but apoptosis of gastric gland or crypt cells can be found on biopsy. In severe cases, denudation of the intestinal epithelium results in diarrhea and malabsorption and often requires parenteral nutritional support. Octreotide (50 to 250 μg subcutaneously three times a day) may be helpful in controlling voluminous diarrhea. Treatment of GVHD is with steroids and antithymocyte globulin combined with parenteral nutritional support until intestinal function returns.

Short-Bowel Syndrome

Malabsorption caused by small bowel resection or surgical bypass is called the short-bowel syndrome. The most common causes in the United States are Crohn's disease, radiation enteritis, and mesenteric ischemia, but massive resection due to adhesions, volvulus, or ischemia after intra-abdominal surgery or gastric bypass surgery are increasingly common causes. The severity of malabsorption depends on the site and extent of resection, the capacity for bowel adaptation, and the function of the residual bowel. Adaptive changes to enhance absorption in the remaining bowel include hyperplasia, dilation, and elongation. Mechanisms of malabsorption after small bowel resection include a decreased absorptive surface area, decreased luminal bile salt concentration, rapid transit, and bacterial overgrowth. Limited jejunal resection usually is tolerated best, because bile salt and vitamin B_{12} absorption remain normal. Ileal resection is less well tolerated because of the consequences of bile salt-wasting and the limited capacity of the jejunum to undergo adaptive hyperplasia.

When fewer than 100 cm of jejunum remain, the colon takes on an important role in caloric salvage and fluid reabsorption. Malabsorbed carbohydrates are digested by colonic bacteria to short-chain fatty acids, which are absorbed in the colon. Parenteral nutrition may be avoided by a diet rich in complex carbohydrates, ORS, and an antimotility agent. In comparison, individuals with fewer than 100 cm of jejunum and no colon have high jejunostomy outputs and often require intravenous fluids or parenteral nutrition to survive. These individuals waste sodium, chloride, bicarbonate, magnesium, zinc, and water in their ostomy effluent. Dietary modifications should include a high-salt, nutrient-rich diet given in small meals. An ORS with a sodium concentration greater than 90 mmol/L is absorbed best. Oral vitamin and mineral doses higher than the usual U.S. recommended daily allowances are required (see Table 143–8). Vitamin B_{12} should be given parenterally. Magnesium deficiencies are often difficult to replenish with oral magnesium because of its osmotic effect in the intestinal lumen. A liquid magnesium preparation added to an ORS and sipped throughout the day may minimize magnesium-induced fluid losses. Potent antimotility agents, such as tincture of opium, often are needed to slow transit and maximize contact time for nutrient absorption. High-volume jejunostomy outputs can be lessened by inhibiting endogenous secretions with a proton-pump inhibitor and, in severe cases, octreotide. The benefit of octreotide may be offset by its potential to inhibit intestinal adaptation and impair pancreatic enzyme secretion with doses greater than 300 μg/day. In the most severe cases, supplemental calories must be provided by nocturnal tube feeding or parenteral nutrition. Treatment with growth hormone (0.1 mg/kg/day subcutaneously) with or without glutamine (30 g once a day orally) for 4 weeks may reduce parenteral nutrition requirements in patients who have had massive intestinal resections. 6 A glucagon-like peptide 2 analogue that stimulates adaptive hyperplasia in remnant intestine after resection is in clinical trials. Long-term complications include bone disease, renal stones (oxalate stones if the colon is present, urate stones with a jejunostomy), gallstones, bacterial overgrowth, fat-soluble vitamin deficiencies, essential fatty acid deficiency, and D-lactic acidosis. Small bowel transplantation should be considered for individuals who require parenteral nutrition to survive and then develop liver disease or venous access problems.

Conditions That Impair Nutrient Delivery to the Systemic Circulation

Insoluble lipids (present in chylomicrons) are exocytosed across the basolateral membrane of epithelial cells into the intestinal lymphatics. From there, they enter the mesenteric lymphatics and the general circulation via the thoracic duct. Sugar monomers, amino acids, and medium-chain fatty acids are transported across the basolateral membrane of intestinal epithelial cells into capillaries and into the portal circulation. Sugar monomers are transported across the basolateral membrane by the facilitative glucose transporter isoform (GLUT2) and amino acids by facilitative amino acid carriers (see Fig. 143–1A).

Impaired Lymphatic Drainage

Diseases that cause intestinal lymphatic obstruction, such as primary congenital lymphangiectasia (malunion of intestinal lymphatics), and diseases that result in secondary lymphangiectasia (lymphoma, tuberculosis, Kaposi's sarcoma, retroperitoneal fibrosis, constrictive pericarditis, severe heart failure) result in fat malabsorption. The increased pressure in the intestinal lymphatics leads to leakage and sometimes rupture of lymph into the intestinal lumen, with the loss of lipids, gamma globulins, albumin, and lymphocytes. The diagnosis of lymphangiectasia can be made by intestinal biopsy, but the specific cause may be more difficult to identify. Individuals with lymphangiectasia malabsorb fat and fat-soluble vitamins and have protein loss into the intestinal lumen. The most common presentation is hypoproteinemic edema. Nutritional management includes a low-fat diet and supplementation with medium-chain triglycerides, which are absorbed directly into the portal circulation. Fat-soluble vitamins should be given if deficiencies develop.

WATERY DIARRHEAS

See Figures 143–8 and 143–9 for algorithms concerning evaluation of watery diarrheas.

Ingestion of Nonabsorbable Solutes: Magnesium and Sodium Phosphate/Sulfate Diarrheas

Individuals ingesting significant amounts of Mg^{2+}-based antacids or high-potency multimineral/multivitamin supplements and individuals surreptitiously taking Mg^{2+}-containing laxatives or nonabsorbable anion laxatives, such as Na_2PO_4 (neutral phosphate) or Na_2SO_4 (Glauber's or Carlsbad salt), may develop significant osmotically induced, watery diarrhea.

Carbohydrate Malabsorption

Sorbitol and Fructose Diarrhea

Chewing gum and elixir diarrhea may result from the chronic ingestion of dietetic foods, candy, chewing gum, or medication elixirs that are sweetened with unabsorbable carbohydrates such as sorbitol. Excessive consumption of pears, prunes, peaches, and apple juice, which also contain sorbitol and fructose, can result in diarrhea. Fructose may be malabsorbed if ingested in high concentrations, and an occasional patient may have diarrhea related to ingestion of large volumes of fruit juice or soft drinks that are sweetened with fructose-containing corn syrup.

Rapid Intestinal Transit

Approximately 25% of the normal 200-g carbohydrate diet may be unabsorbed by the normal small intestine. When passed into the colon, it is metabolized to osmotically active short-chain fatty acids by colonic flora. Diets that are high in carbohydrate and low in fat may allow rapid gastric emptying and rapid small intestinal motility, leading to carbohydrate malabsorption and osmotic diarrhea. Rapid orocecal transit time also occurs in thyrotoxicosis. Because carbohydrate is metabolized also to H_2 and CO_2 by colonic bacteria, the symptoms of excess flatus, abdominal bloating, and cramping abdominal pain may be important clues to the diagnosis of carbohydrate malabsorption.

Glucose-Galactose Malabsorption and Disaccharidase Deficiencies

Lactase deficiency and congenital absence of enterocyte brush-border carbohydrate hydrolases and transport proteins may cause diarrheas. Lactase deficiency should be considered in cases of unexplained watery diarrhea, especially if accompanied by abdominal cramps, bloating, and flatus (see earlier discussion). Patients with symptoms on ingestion of mushrooms may have trehalase deficiency.

Prior Surgery: Bile Acid Diarrhea

There are three types of bile acid-induced diarrhea. Type 1 results from severe disease (e.g., Crohn's disease), resection, or bypass of the distal ileum, which allows dihydroxy bile salts to escape absorption (see earlier discussion). Type 2 bile acid diarrhea, or primary bile acid malabsorption, may be congenital or acquired. This form of diarrhea often responds to cholestyramine, 2 to 4 g given orally two to four times daily. Type 3 bile acid diarrhea is caused by measured increases in fecal bile acids in patients with postcholecystectomy diarrhea. It is unclear why interruption of gallbladder storage leads to increased bile acid wastage. Although many patients respond to cholestyramine, some do not. Another cause of type 3 bile acid diarrhea is truncal vagotomy combined with a drainage procedure (postvagotomy diarrhea), after which 20 to 30% of patients develop diarrhea. Many patients do not respond to cholestyramine, but motility-altering drugs such as opiates (e.g., loperamide 2 to 4 mg orally two to four times daily) and anticholinergics (e.g., hyoscyamine sulfate 0.125 to 0.250 mg orally two to four times daily) may be of benefit. Celiac disease also may appear first after gastric surgery or vagotomy.

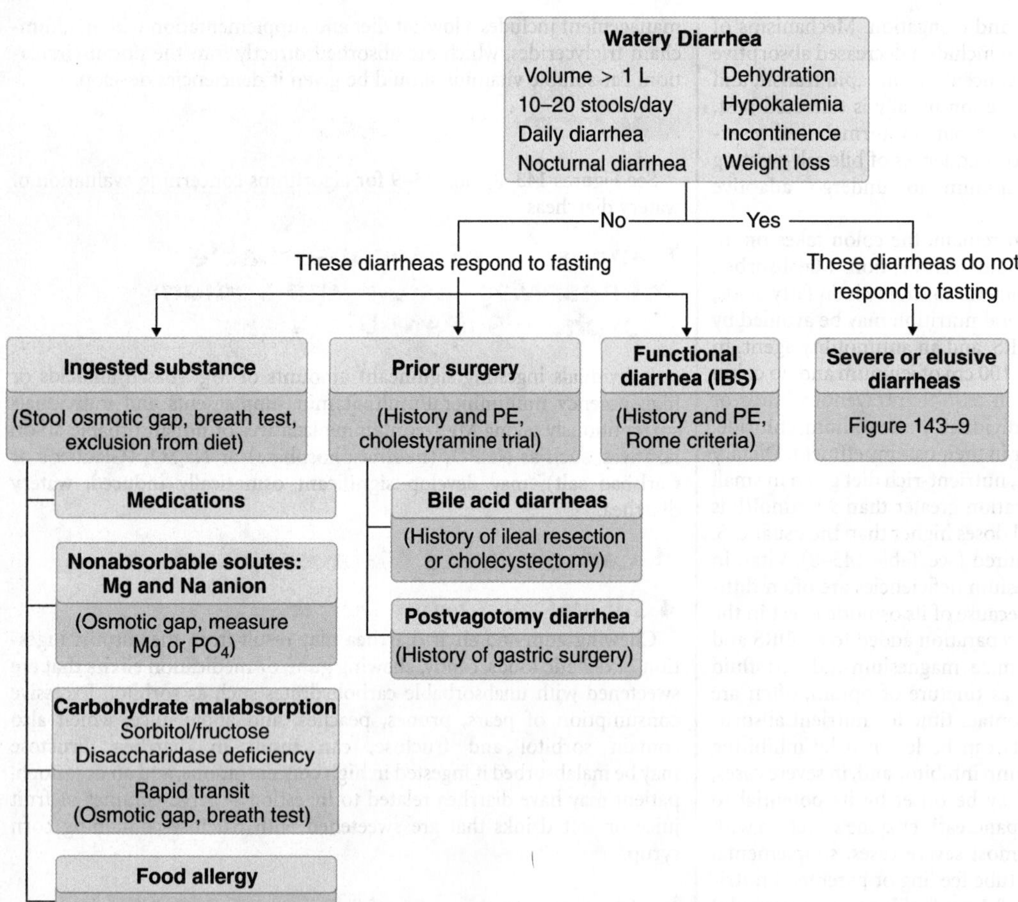

FIGURE 143–8 • Approach to the evaluation of watery diarrheas. IBS = irritable bowel syndrome; PE = physical examination. (Adapted from Powell DW: Approach to the patient with diarrhea. *In* Yamada T, Alpers DH, Owyang C, et al [eds]: Textbook of Gastroenterology, 3rd ed. Philadelphia, Lippincott-Raven, 1999.)

Functional Watery Diarrheas (Irritable Bowel Syndrome)

About 25% of patients with irritable bowel syndrome have a symptom complex of predominantly painless diarrhea (Chapter 139), but many patients are discovered to have other conditions, such as occult lactose intolerance, celiac disease (antibody screening is recommended), collagenous or microscopic/lymphocytic colitis, rapid transit with carbohydrate-wasting diarrhea, malabsorption of fructose or sorbitol, or even primary bile acid malabsorption (type 2). Many of these patients' symptoms begin with an enteric infection (see Prolonged, Persistent, and Protracted Infectious Diarrheas), and many of these patients have an idiopathic bacterial overgrowth syndrome.

TRUE SECRETORY DIARRHEAS

See Figure 143–9.

Endocrine Tumor Diarrheas

Carcinoid Syndrome

Patients with metastatic carcinoid tumors of the gastrointestinal tract or, rarely, primary nonmetastatic carcinoid tumors of the bronchial epithelium may develop a watery diarrhea and cramping abdominal pain in addition to other symptoms (Chapter 251). Because one third of these patients do not have other symptoms at the time the diarrhea begins, carcinoid should be considered in patients with secretory diarrhea.

Gastrinoma

Diarrhea occurs in one third of patients with Zollinger-Ellison syndrome (Chapter 205), may precede the ulcer symptoms, and in about 10% of patients it is the major pathophysiologic manifestation. The diarrhea is caused by high volumes of hydrochloride secretion (which can be reduced by nasogastric aspiration or effective antisecretory therapy) and by maldigestion of fat due to pH inactivation of pancreatic lipase and precipitation of bile acids.

Vipoma or Watery Diarrhea Hypokalemia Achlorhydria Syndrome

Non–beta cell pancreatic adenomas may secrete various peptide secretagogues, including VIP, that produce all of the symptoms of this disease (Chapter 205). Patients with this syndrome have secretory diarrhea, with 70% of patients having more than 3 L of stool per day and almost all having more than 700 mL/day. Stool electrolyte losses account for the dehydration, hypokalemia, and acidosis that give this syndrome its name.

Medullary Carcinoma of the Thyroid

Medullary carcinoma of the thyroid may occur in sporadic form, or it may manifest as part of the multiple endocrine neoplasia type II syndrome with pheochromocytomas and hyperparathyroidism in 25 to 50% of cases (Chapter 250). Watery (secretory) diarrhea is caused by secretion of calcitonin by the tumor; however, these tumors also elaborate other secretogogues, such as prostaglandins, VIP, and serotonin. By the time watery diarrhea occurs, the tumor has metastasized, and this symptom portends a poor prognosis.

Nonendocrine Malignancies

Villous Adenomas

Large (4 to 10 cm) villous adenomas of the rectum or rectosigmoid may cause a secretory form of diarrhea (500 to 3000 mL/24 hours) characterized by hypokalemia, chloride-rich stool, and metabolic alkalosis. Secretogogues such as prostaglandins have been found in the tumor and rectal effluent of patients, and indomethacin administration reduces the diarrhea in some.

Systemic Mastocytosis

The diarrhea of systemic mastocytosis (Chapter 276) may be malabsorptive, secondary to mast cell infiltration of the mucosa with resulting

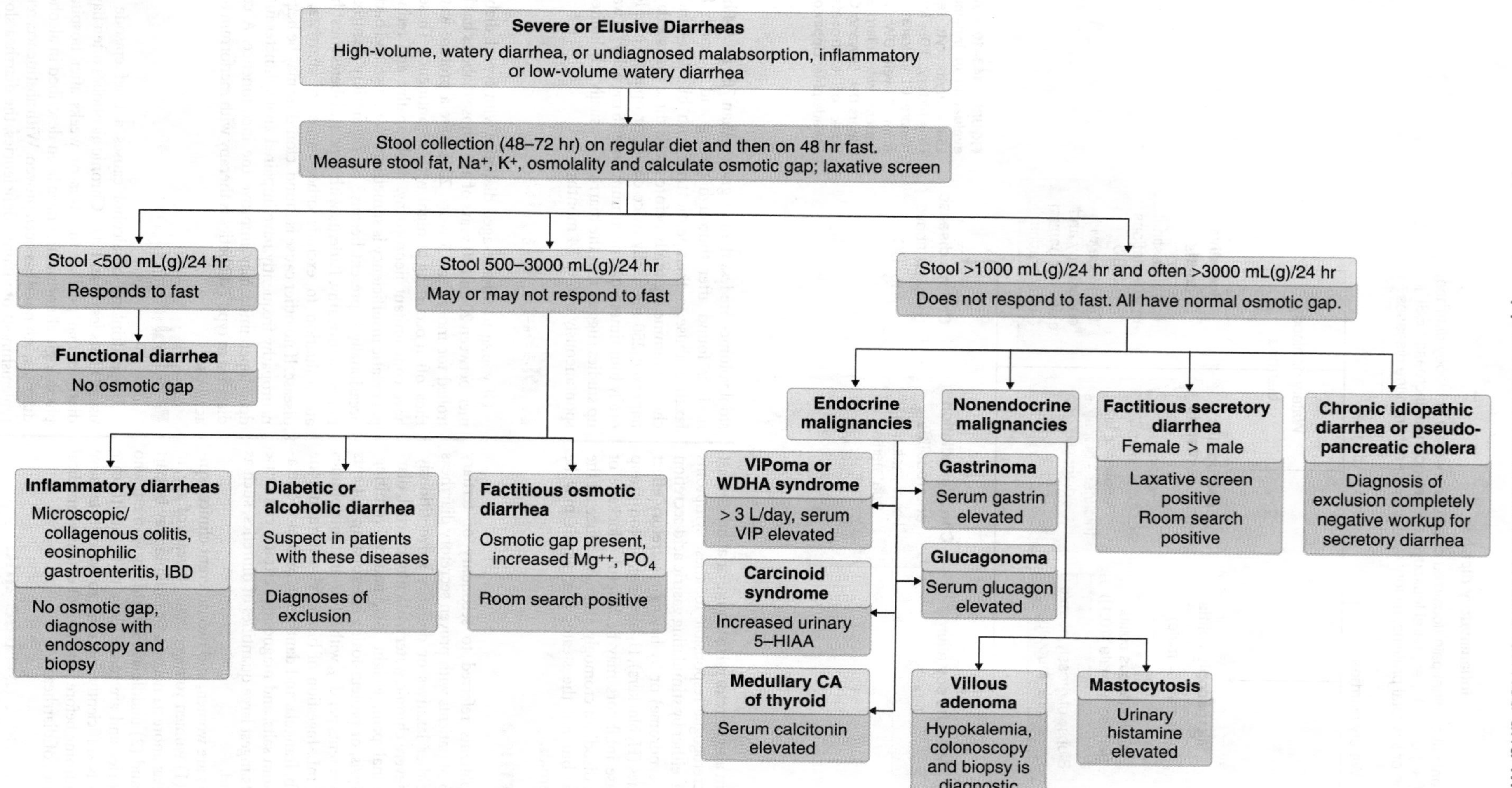

FIGURE 143–9 • Approach to the evaluation of severe or elusive diarrheas. CA = cancer; 5-HIAA = 5-hydroxyindoleacetic acid; IBD = inflammatory bowel disease; VIP = vasoactive intestinal polypeptide; WDHA = watery diarrhea hypokalemia achlorhydria. (Adapted from Powell DW: Approach to the patient with diarrhea. *In* Yamada T, Alpers DH, Owyang C, et al [eds]: Textbook of Gastroenterology, 3rd ed. Philadelphia, Lippincott-Raven, 1999.)

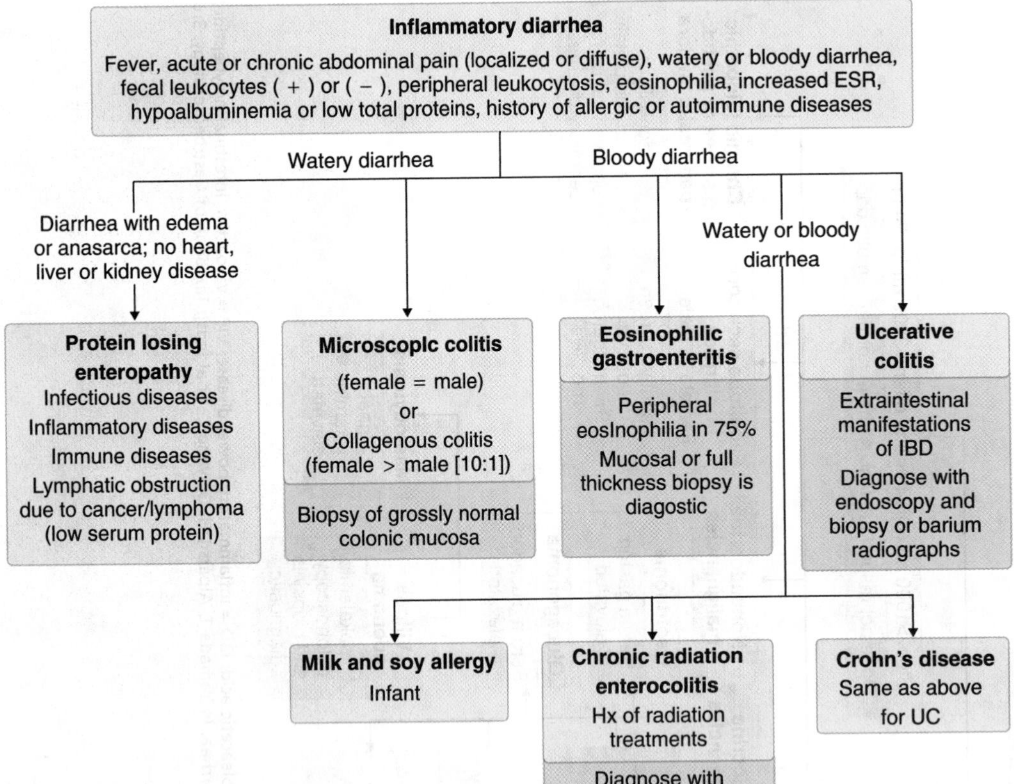

FIGURE 143–10 • Approach to the evaluation of inflammatory diarrheas. ESR = erythrocyte sedimentation rate; Hx = history; IBD = inflammatory bowel disease; UC = ulcerative colitis. (Adapted from Powell DW: Approach to the patient with diarrhea. *In* Yamada T, Alpers DH, Owyang C, et al [eds]: Textbook of Gastroenterology, 3rd ed. Philadelphia, Lippincott-Raven, 1999.)

villous atrophy, or intermittent and secretory. Histamine or another mast cell mediator may be the secretogogue responsible for these symptoms and for the secretory diarrhea, either by stimulating gastric acid secretion (such as in Zollinger-Ellison syndrome) or by having a secretory effect on the intestine. Antihistamines (H_1 blockers), H_2 blockers, proton-pump inhibitors, and cyclooxygenase inhibitors may be helpful. Blockade of mast cell degranulation with disodium cromoglycate may reduce all the symptoms and the diarrhea, but not the steatorrhea, which may be treated better with corticosteroids.

Factitious Diarrhea

Approximately 15% of patients referred to secondary or tertiary centers for diarrhea and 25% of patients with proven secretory diarrheas are found to be ingesting either laxatives or diuretics surreptitiously. These patients present with severe chronic watery, often nocturnal, diarrhea and may have abdominal pain, weight loss, nausea, vomiting, hypokalemic myopathy, acidosis, or protein-losing enteropathy. Patients may have 10 to 20 bowel movements per day, with 24-hour stool volumes in the range of 300 to 3000 mL. Ingestion of bisacodyl, anthraquinone (senna, cascara, aloe, rhubarb, frangula, and danthron), or osmotic laxatives (neutral phosphate, epsom salts, and magnesium citrate) can cause this syndrome. Some patients ingest large quantities of diuretics, such as furosemide or ethacrynic acid.

More than 90% of patients are women, and two different clinical syndromes are most common: (1) women younger than 30 years of age, in whom eating disorders such as anorexia nervosa or bulimia may be part of the psychic abnormality, and (2) middle-aged to elderly women, who have extensive medical histories and are more likely to be health care workers. Factitious diarrhea is sufficiently common to warrant laxative screening to exclude this syndrome before initiation of extensive medical evaluation for the other causes of diarrhea.

Chronic Idiopathic Diarrhea and Pseudopancreatic Cholera Syndrome

Patients in whom extensive evaluation for a cause of secretory diarrhea is negative are said to have either chronic idiopathic diarrhea or pseudopancreatic cholera syndrome, depending on whether the fasting stool volumes are less than or greater than 700 mL/24 hours. If no diagnosis is found after thorough testing and a search for surreptitious laxative abuse, a therapeutic trial with bile salt–binding drugs (e.g., cholestyramine 4 g orally before meals three times a day), NSAIDs (e.g., naproxen 250 mg orally twice daily), or opiates (e.g., loperamide 2 mg orally four times a day, maximum dose 16 mg a day) is warranted. Follow-up studies suggest that the diarrhea is usually self-limited and disappears spontaneously in 6 to 24 months.

Diabetic Diarrhea

Of young to middle-aged diabetics with type 1 diabetes, particularly men between 20 and 40 years of age whose diabetes has been poorly controlled for more than 5 years, 20% have a profuse watery, urgent diarrhea, often occurring at night with incontinence. These patients usually have concomitant neuropathy, nephropathy, and retinopathy. Exocrine pancreatic insufficiency is sometimes the cause, and bacterial overgrowth occasionally is present because of the motility disturbance of the autonomic neuropathy. Patients with type 1 diabetes must have an appropriate evaluation to exclude other causes of diarrhea, especially celiac disease. If no other cause is found, clonidine may be helpful. Patients with neuropathy frequently have impaired anal sphincter function, and high-dose loperamide may improve the incontinence. A common cause of diarrhea in type 2 diabetics is therapy with metformin or, less commonly, acarbose.

Alcoholic Diarrhea

Binge drinking of alcohol causes a brief episode of diarrhea that usually lasts less than 1 day. Chronic alcoholics often have a severe watery diarrhea that persists for days or weeks after hospitalization. Various physiologic abnormalities have been described in alcoholics as a cause of diarrhea, but none has been proven. With abstinence, renourishment, and replenishment of vitamin deficiencies, the diarrhea slowly improves.

INFLAMMATORY DIARRHEAS

See Figure 143–10 for an algorithm for evaluation of inflammatory diarrheas.

Inflammatory Bowel Disease

Patients with Crohn's disease or ulcerative colitis have diarrhea with stool volumes usually less than 1 L/24 hours (Chapter 144). Occasional patients with severe ulcerative colitis have more severe diarrhea, with water and electrolyte secretion in the unaffected small intestine, suggesting the presence of circulating secretogogues originating from the inflamed colon. Pouchitis (inflammation of the ileal reservoir) is a common cause of diarrhea in patients who have ulcerative colitis with an ileoanal anastomosis after colectomy. The cause is unknown. Antibiotic therapy is effective, but relapses are common. A probiotic compound containing lactobacilli, bifidobacteria, and *Streptococcus thermophilus* may be effective at preventing relapses.

Eosinophilic Gastroenteritis

Infiltration of various layers of the gastrointestinal tract with eosinophils is a recognized clinical entity that is accompanied by diarrhea in 30 to 60% of patients. Peripheral eosinophilia is present in 75% of these patients. The disease may involve the entire gastrointestinal tract from esophagus to anus, or it may be isolated to a segment. Abdominal pain, nausea, vomiting, weight loss, steatorrhea, and protein-losing enteropathy are other prominent signs and symptoms of this disease. The cause of eosinophilic gastroenteritis is unknown, but approximately 50% of patients have atopic (allergic) histories, and food allergy is suspected. Corticosteroids (prednisone 20 to 40 mg orally once a day for 7 to 10 days) are the mainstay of therapy; disodium cromoglycate (200 mg orally four times daily) may be useful. Infestation with nematodes must be excluded before this diagnosis is made.

Milk and Soy Protein Intolerance and Food Allergy

Intolerance to cow's milk and soy protein is a well-established cause of enterocolitis in infants (Chapter 274). Approximately 50% of patients who are allergic to one of these proteins are also allergic to the other. The role of food allergy in causing diarrhea in adults is less clear. Commonly suspected allergens include milk, eggs, seafood, nuts, artificial flavors, and food coloring.

Collagenous and Lymphocytic Colitis

These two conditions, collectively known as microscopic colitis, may or may not be the same disease or variants of the same disease. Lymphocytic colitis is equally prevalent in men and women, whereas collagenous colitis occurs 10 times more often in middle-aged or elderly women. These conditions may be associated with autoimmune disease or with NSAID use. There is an increased prevalence (15%) of microscopic colitis among individuals with celiac sprue. These diseases may be categorized as either inflammatory or secretory diarrheas. An epidemiologic relationship to medications such as NSAIDs, H_2-receptor blockers, proton-pump inhibitors, selective serotonin reuptake inhibitors (SSRIs) and others has been reported, and increased luminal prostaglandin levels may cause the diarrhea. Enteric infections, food hypersensitivity, or intraluminal bile has been proposed as a trigger for prostaglandin release from lymphocytes. The disease disappears with fecal stream diversion. Antidiarrheal agents such as loperamide (2 mg orally four times a day) are the mainstay of therapy. Budesonide (9 mg orally once a day), bismuth subsalicylate therapy (eight chewable 262-mg tablets orally once a day), and 5-aminosalicylates (e.g., mesalamine 400 to 800 mg orally three times daily) may be useful. Those with refractory disease may require corticosteroids (e.g., prednisone 40 mg orally once a day).

Protein-Losing Enteropathy

Severe protein loss through the gastrointestinal tract caused by ulceration, obstructed lymphatics, or immune-related vascular injury occurs in a variety of disease states: bacterial or parasitic infection, gastritis, gastric cancer, collagenous colitis, inflammatory bowel disease, congenital intestinal lymphangiectasia, sarcoidosis, lymphoma, mesenteric tuberculosis, Ménétrier's disease, sprue, eosinophilic gastroenteritis, systemic lupus erythematosus, chronic peritoneal dialysis, and food allergies. The condition usually responds to corticosteroids (e.g., prednisone 10 to 60 mg orally once daily) or immunosuppressive therapy (e.g., 6-mercaptopurine in carefully titrated doses).

Radiation Enteritis

Patients receiving pelvic radiation for malignancies of the female urogenital tract or the male prostate may develop chronic radiation enterocolitis 6 to 12 months after total doses of radiation greater than 40 to 60 Gy (Chapters 18 and 145). Symptoms can develop 20 years after treatment, however. In irradiated animal models, early abnormalities include an increase in inflammatory mediators, an increase in cholinergic stimulation of intestinal tissue, and endothelial cell apoptosis that precedes epithelial cell apoptosis. The last finding suggests that vascular injury is the primary event. Vascular endothelial growth factor, basic fibroblast growth factor, and IL-11 protect animal intestine from radiation damage. Diarrhea may be caused by bile acid malabsorption if the ileum is damaged, by bacterial overgrowth if radiation causes small intestinal strictures or bypass, or by radiation-induced chronic inflammation of the small intestine and colon. Rapid transit also may contribute to malabsorption and diarrhea. Treatment is often unsatisfactory. Anti-inflammatory drugs (sulfasalazine, corticosteroids) and antibiotics have been tried with little success. Cholestyramine (4 g orally three times a day) and NSAIDs (e.g., naproxen 250 to 500 mg orally twice daily) may help, as may opiates (loperamide 2 mg orally four times a day or loperamide-*N*-oxide 3 mg orally two times a day).

Miscellaneous Diseases

Although acute mesenteric arterial or venous thrombosis manifests as an acute bloody diarrhea, chronic mesenteric vascular ischemia may manifest as watery diarrhea. Gastrointestinal tuberculosis and histoplasmosis manifest as diarrhea that may be either bloody or watery, as do certain immunologic diseases, such as Behçet's syndrome or Churg-Strauss syndrome. All of these diseases may be misdiagnosed as inflammatory bowel disease. Diarrhea, the hallmark of acute GVHD after allogeneic bone marrow transplantation, manifests with the triad of dermatitis, hepatic cholestasis, and enteritis (see earlier discussion). Neutropenic enterocolitis, an ileocolitis that occurs in neutropenic leukemic patients, sometimes is caused by *C. difficile* infection.

Diagnosis of Chronic Diarrheas

History and Physical Examination

A detailed history, physical examination, and certain screening tests lead to a diagnosis in 75% of patients with watery diarrheas (see Table 143–1 and Figs. 143–3 and 143–8). A history of 10 to 20 bowel movements per day suggests secretory diarrhea (see Fig. 143–9). A history of peptic ulcer should suggest gastrinoma or systemic mastocytosis. Physical examination is helpful only if the thyromegaly of medullary carcinoma, the cutaneous flushing of the neuroendocrine tumors and systemic mastocytosis, the dermatographism of systemic mastocytosis, or the migratory necrolytic erythema of glucagonoma is evident. Scars from previous surgery may suggest postvagotomy diarrhea or terminal ileal resection with bile acid diarrhea. Autonomic dysfunction (e.g., postural hypotension, impotence, gustatory sweating) is almost invariably present in diabetic diarrhea.

Evaluation for malabsorption begins with a careful history of bowel habits, weight loss, travel, food or milk tolerance, underlying gastrointestinal or liver diseases, abdominal surgery, radiation or chemotherapy treatments, family history, and drug and alcohol use. Patients with malabsorption can present with a variety of gastrointestinal or extraintestinal manifestations (see Table 143–5). Significant malabsorption of fat and carbohydrate usually causes chronic diarrhea, abdominal cramps, gas, bloating, and weight loss. Steatorrhea (fat in the stool) manifests as oily, foul-smelling stools that are difficult to flush down the toilet. Stools may be large and bulky (e.g., pancreatic insufficiency) or watery (e.g., bacterial overgrowth, mucosal diseases). Individuals with malabsorption also can present with manifestations of vitamin and mineral deficiencies. Dyspnea can be caused by anemia from iron, folate, or vitamin B_{12} deficiency. Cheilosis, angular stomatitis, or a scaly rash can be caused by many vitamin and mineral deficiencies or essential fatty acid deficiency (see Table 143–5). Dermatitis herpetiformis is a blistering, burning, itchy rash on the extensor surfaces and buttocks that is associated with celiac disease. Manifestations of calcium, magnesium, or vitamin D malabsorption include paresthesias and tetany due to hypocalcemia or hypomagnesemia and bone pain due to osteomalacia or osteoporosis-related fractures. Paresthesias and ataxia are manifestations of cobalamin and vitamin E deficiency.

The important clinical manifestations of inflammatory diarrheas are the signs and symptoms of inflammation and/or the effects of severe chronic protein loss (see Fig. 143–10). Diarrhea in these inflammatory diseases may be meager (e.g., the pseudodiarrhea of proctitis), or it may be fairly severe (e.g., as in GVHD). Systemic manifestations of inflammatory bowel disease include oral aphthous ulcers, polymigratory arthritis, uveitis, erythema nodosum, pyoderma gangrenosum, and the palpable purpura of vasculitis.

Blood Tests

Blood measurements (see Fig. 143–3) of iron, folate, vitamin B_{12}, vitamin D, or prothrombin time (vitamin K) help evaluate malabsorption. Although serum carotene levels may be low simply from poor intake, values lower than 50 µg/dL suggest malabsorption. Peripheral blood findings of leukocytosis, eosinophilia, elevated erythrocyte sedimentation rate, hypoalbuminemia, or low total serum protein suggests an inflammatory diarrhea, whose hallmark is the presence of blood, either gross or occult, and leukocytes in the stool. There are no bedside screening tests to establish the diagnosis in watery diarrheas.

Imaging

Radiographic imaging should be viewed as an adjunct to the diagnosis of diarrheal diseases and not a primary test. Malabsorption may be suggested by a flat plate of the abdomen that shows pancreatic calcification. Some diseases (e.g., previous gastric surgery, gastrocolic fistulas, blind loops from previous intestinal anastomoses, small intestine strictures, multiple jejunal diverticula, abnormal intestinal motility that could lead to bacterial overgrowth) may be shown by computed tomography or magnetic resonance imaging of the abdomen after administration of oral contrast agents or by a traditional upper gastrointestinal radiographic series with small intestine follow-through. Certain diseases may manifest radiographically as uniform thickening of the intestinal folds (e.g., amyloidosis, lymphoma, Whipple's disease); others, such as lymphoma or lymphangiectasia, show uniform or patchy abnormalities. Patients with celiac disease show dilation of the small intestine, with little mucosal abnormality, and segmentation of the barium column as a result of precipitation or flocculation of the barium. Routine contrast radiographs of the gastrointestinal tract usually are not helpful in the diagnosis of watery diarrheas, unless they show a previous vagotomy, extensive small bowel resection or cholecystectomy, the presence of a tumor (carcinoid or villous adenoma), or a bowel filled with fluid (endocrine tumor). Abdominal contrast imaging may show diagnostic evidence of inflammatory bowel disease or changes suggestive of eosinophilic gastroenteritis or radiation enterocolitis. Early or mild gut inflammation may be missed entirely by radiography. Somatostatin receptor scintigraphy with indium 111–labeled octreotide can be useful in localizing gastrinomas, pancreatic endocrine tumors, and carcinoid tumors.

Endoscopy and Biopsy

Upper endoscopy with distal duodenal biopsy should be undertaken if serologic tests for celiac disease are positive or diagnostic clues suggest small bowel mucosal malabsorption. Some patients may have patchy mucosal disease and require enteroscopy with jejunal biopsies for diagnosis. Patients with severe watery or elusive diarrhea should have a flexible sigmoidoscopy or, preferably, a colonoscopy to exclude villous adenomas of the rectosigmoid and biopsy to exclude microscopic or collagenous colitis, mastocytosis, or early inflammatory bowel disease. Colonoscopy and biopsy also may reveal melanosis coli secondary to chronic use of anthracene laxatives. Terminal ileal biopsy may indicate inflammatory bowel disease. Newly developed, longer, flexible push endoscopes and wireless video capsule endoscopy (Chapter 136) are increasingly used to diagnose small bowel diseases.

Other Laboratory Tests

Malabsorption

If chronic diarrhea is the presenting symptom, a stool examination for ova and parasites and a stool antigen-capture ELISA test for *Giardia* should be obtained. A stool test for fat is the best available screening test for malabsorption (see Table 143–6). If the fecal fat test result is negative, selective carbohydrate malabsorption or other causes of diarrhea should be considered. If the fecal fat test result is positive (Fig. 143–11), further testing should be based on clinical suspicion for particular diseases. If pancreatic insufficiency is suspected, imaging studies of the pancreas should be performed. If proximal mucosal damage is suspected, multiple small intestinal biopsy specimens should be obtained. If there are no clues as to the cause of malabsorption, a D-xylose test may help to distinguish mucosal disease from pancreatic insufficiency. The D-xylose test result also can be abnormal in individuals with bacterial overgrowth; if this condition is suspected, culture of an intestinal aspirate or a breath test should be obtained (see Table 143–6). Small bowel contrast imaging is useful in detecting ileal disease and structural abnormalities that predispose to bacterial overgrowth. Some individuals with celiac disease present with selective nutrient deficiencies without diarrhea. In these cases, tTG antibody tests and intestinal biopsy should be performed. If malabsorption is suspected in patients hospitalized for severe diarrhea or malnutrition, a more streamlined evaluation usually includes a stool for culture, ova and parasites, and fat; an abdominal imaging study; and a biopsy of the small intestine.

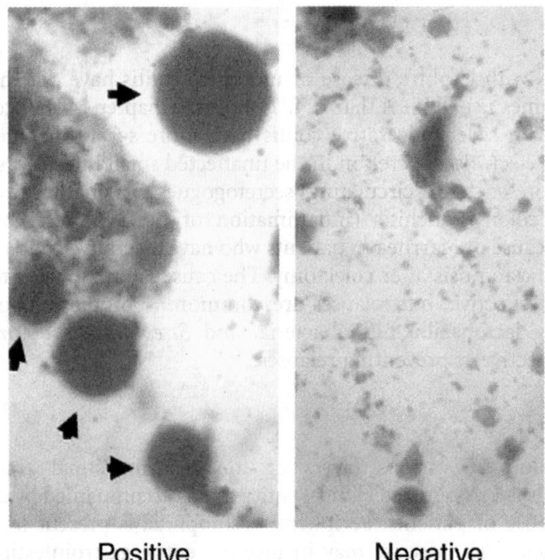

FIGURE 143–11 • Sudan stain of stool for fat. The positive stain (left) shows larger globules of unabsorbed fat (arrows).

Watery Diarrhea

Breath tests to measure the respiratory excretion of labeled CO_2 after oral administration and metabolism of radioactive carbon–labeled substrates, or of H_2 after administration of carbohydrates, can assess fat, carbohydrate, and bile salt malabsorption or bacterial overgrowth (see Table 143–6).

The diagnosis of endocrine tumors, such as carcinoids, gastrinoma, VIPoma, medullary carcinoma of the thyroid, glucagonoma, somatostatinoma, and systemic mastocytosis, is made by showing elevated blood levels of serotonin or urinary 5-hydroxyindoleacetic acid and serum levels for gastrin, VIP, calcitonin, glucagon, somatostatin, histamine, or prostaglandins (Chapter 205). Somatostatin receptor scintigraphy has proved to be sensitive and useful in the diagnosis and evaluation of Zollinger-Ellison syndrome (Chapter 205).

Inflammatory Diarrhea

Video capsule endoscopy (Chapter 136) of the small bowel may detect inflammation not evident by upper or lower endoscopy or conventional barium contrast radiography. Fecal white blood cells can be detected in stool smears with a methylene blue stain. Stool excretion of lactoferrin (a constituent of leukocytes) also may be used as a quantitative index of fecal leukocyte loss. The most sensitive test for certain inflammatory diarrheas is measurement of intestinal protein loss by 24-hour stool excretion or clearance of chromium 51–labeled albumin or α_1-antitrypsin.

Elusive Diarrhea

An important adjunct to diagnosing the cause of diarrhea is to look at the stool. The greasy, bulky stool of steatorrhea and the bloody stool of gut inflammation are distinctive. Patients with steatorrhea sometimes also have severe watery diarrhea, however. Qualitative tests on outpatient spot stool collections and quantitative tests (stool fat, electrolytes, and osmolality) on 48- to 72-hour stool collections can help define the causes of diarrhea, especially severe or elusive diarrheas (see Table 143–6 and Fig. 143–9). Stool collections can be analyzed for appearance, weight, quantitative fecal fat, electrolytes (Na^+, K^+, and, if necessary, Cl^-, PO_4^{2-} and Mg^{2+}), osmolality, fecal pH, and laxative screen. Stool or urine can be analyzed for emetine (a component of ipecac), bisacodyl, castor oil, or anthraquinone. Stool SO_4^{2-}, PO_4^{2-}, and Mg^{2+} analysis detects factitious diarrheas caused by osmotic cathartics.

Carbohydrate malabsorption lowers stool pH because of colonic fermentation of carbohydrate to short-chain fatty acids. Stool pH less than 5.3 usually means pure carbohydrate malabsorption, whereas, in the generalized malabsorptive diseases, stool pH is greater than 5.6 and usually greater than 6.0.

The normal stool osmotic gap, which is the difference between stool osmolality (or 290 mOsm) and twice the stool Na^+ and K^+ concentrations, is 50 to 125. In secretory diarrheas, the solutes causing the movement of water from blood to bowel lumen are the secreted Na^+ and K^+ ions; stool Na^+ concentrations are usually greater than 90 mmol/L, and the osmotic gap is less than 50. In osmotic diarrhea, the ingestion of nonabsorbable (or nonabsorbed) solutes displaces Na^+ from the stool and causes the osmotic gap and the diarrhea (see Pathophysiology); stool Na^+ is less than 60 mmol/L, and the osmotic gap is greater than 125. Stools with Na^+ concentration between 60 and 90 mmol/L and calculated osmotic gaps between 50 and 100 can result from either secretory or malabsorptive abnormalities. Patients with Mg^{2+}-induced diarrhea may be diagnosed by fecal Mg^{2+} values greater than 50 mmol/L. Sodium anion–induced diarrheas mimic secretory diarrhea because the stool Na^+ content is high (>90 mmol/L), and there is no osmotic gap; this diarrhea may be diagnosed by determining stool Cl^- concentration, because these anions displace stool Cl^-, and the resulting stool Cl^- value is usually less than 20 mmol/L.

Treatment of Chronic Diarrheas

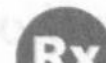

Antidiarrheal Therapy

Antidiarrheal agents are of two types: those that are useful for mild-to-moderate diarrheas and those that are helpful in secretory and other severe diarrheas. The bulk-forming agents (kaolin-pectin, psyllium, and methylcellulose) increase the consistency of stool and have no antisecretory activity. Pectin has been shown to have proabsorptive activity. Other antidiarrheal agents have only mild proabsorptive or antisecretory action, and most have antidiarrheal activity by altering the intestinal motility. Bismuth salicylates, opiates, loperamide, clonidine, phenothiazine, and somatostatin have mild antisecretory activity but also cause dilation of the small intestine and colon and decrease peristalsis. The opiates also increase anal sphincter tone. The therapeutic mechanism of these drugs is to trap fluid within the intestine and put it in contact with the mucosa for a longer period, allowing more complete absorption.

The opiates may be symptomatically useful in mild diarrheas. Paregoric, deodorized tincture of opium, codeine, and diphenoxylate with atropine largely have been supplanted by loperamide. Loperamide does not pass the blood-brain barrier and has a high first-pass metabolism in the liver; it has a high therapeutic-to-toxic ratio and is essentially devoid of addiction potential. It is safe in adults, even in total doses of 24 mg/day. The usual dose is 2 to 4 mg two to four times daily. When opiates are given, stool output is not a reliable gauge for replacing fluid losses, because the antimotility effects of opiates cause fluid to sequester in the bowel lumen (third space). The antimotility effects are a problem in infectious diarrheas, because stasis may enhance bacterial invasion and delay clearance of microorganisms from the bowel, increasing carriage time. Opiates and anticholinergics also are dangerous in severe inflammatory bowel disease, where they may precipitate megacolon. Racecadotril does not seem to affect motility, so it may prove to be a useful, opiate-like antidiarrheal.

The use of drugs with potentially serious side effects can be justified for treatment of severe secretory diarrheas. The somatostatin analogue octreotide has its major antisecretory effect in carcinoid syndrome and in neuroendocrine tumors, because it inhibits hormone secretion by the tumor. Newer, long-acting preparations are now available, easing its use. Octreotide may be of only limited usefulness in short-bowel syndrome and AIDS diarrhea. Agents such as phenothiazine, calcium-channel blockers, or clonidine can have serious side effects but may be tried if octreotide fails. Clonidine can be useful in the diarrhea of diarrhea-predominant irritable bowel syndrome, opiate withdrawal, and, occasionally, in patients with diabetic diarrhea. Serotonin-3 receptor antagonist (alosetron) therapy may be justified for severe diarrhea-predominant irritable bowel syndrome. [7] Indomethacin, a cyclooxygenase blocker that inhibits prostaglandin production, occasionally may be useful in neuroendocrine tumors, irritable bowel syndrome, and food allergy and is most useful in patients with diarrhea caused by acute radiation, AIDS, or villous adenoma of the rectum or colon. Cyclooxygenase blockers may be harmful in inflammatory bowel disease. Glucocorticoids reduce prostaglandin and leukotriene production in inflammatory bowel disease and have a proabsorptive effect on the intestine that is demonstrable by 5 hours after administration. The new anti–tumor necrosis factor antibodies are useful in Crohn's disease and in ulcerative colitis that is unresponsive to conventional therapy (Chapter 144).

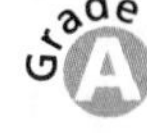

1. McFarland LV: Meta-analysis of probiotics for the prevention of antibiotic associated diarrhea and the treatment of *Clostridium difficile* disease. Am J Gastroenterol 2006;101:812–822.
2. Lucas Me, Dean JL, vonSeidlain, et al: Effectiveness of mass oral cholera vaccination in Beira, Mozambique. N Engl J Med 2005; 32:757–767.
3. Dupont HL, Jiang ZD, Okhuysen PC, et al: A randomized, double-blind, placebo-controlled trial of rifaximin to prevent travelers' diarrhea. Ann Intern Med 2005;142:805–812.
4. Dupont HL, Jiang ZD, Belkind-Gerson J, et al: Treatment of traveler's diarrhea: Randomized trial comparing rifaximin, rifaximin plus loperamide, and loperamide alone. Clin Gastroenterol Hepatol 2007;5:451–456.
5. Di Stefano M, Malservisi S, Veneto G, et al: Rifaximin versus chlortetracycline in the short-term treatment of small intestine bacterial overgrowth. Aliment Pharmacol Ther 2000;14:551–556.
6. Byrne TA, Wilmore DW, Iyer K, et al: Growth hormone, glutamine, and an optimal diet reduces parenteral nutrition in patients with short bowel syndrome: A prospective, randomized, placebo-controlled, double-blind clinical trial. Ann Surg 2005;242:655–661.
7. Chey WD, Chey WY, Heath AT, et al: Long-term safety and efficacy of alosetron in women with severe diarrhea-predominant irritable bowel syndrome. Am J Gastroenterol 2004;99:2195–2203.

SUGGESTED READINGS

Bellemare S, Hartling L, Wiebe N, et al: Oral rehydration versus intravenous therapy for treating dehydration due to gastroenteritis in children: A meta-analysis of randomized controlled trials. BMC Med 2004;2:11–18. *This meta-analysis documents that oral rehydration therapy is as effective as intravenous therapy for treating the dehydration of diarrheal disease in children.*

Camilleri M: Chronic diarrhea: A review on pathophysiology and management for the clinical gastroenterologist. Clin Gastroenterol Hepatol 2004;2:198–206. *An approach to the diagnosis and therapy of chronic diarrhea.*

Elphick HL, Elphick DA, Sanders DS: Small bowel bacterial overgrowth. An under-recognized cause of malnutrition in older adults. Geriatrics 2006;61:21–26. *Overview of symptoms, diagnosis, investigation, and treatment.*

Fedorak RN, Madsen KL: Probiotics and prebiotics in gastrointestinal disorders. Curr Opin Gastroenterol 2004;20:146–155. *Probiotic therapy of gastrointestinal diseases is rapidly moving into the mainstream.*

Jarvela IE: Molecular genetics of adult-type hypolactasia. Ann Med 2005;37: 179–185. *An excellent review of the genes involved in lactase persistence/nonpersistence.*

Kagnoff MF: Celiac disease: Pathogenesis of a model immunogenetic disease. J Clin Invest 2007;117:41–49. *A scientific overview.*

Misiakos EP, Macheras A, Kapetanakis T, et al: Short bowel syndrome: Current medical and surgical trends. J Clin Gastroenterol 2007;41:5–18. *Clinical overview.*

Rostom A, Murray JA, Kagnoff MF: American Gastroenterological Association (AGA) Institute technical review on the diagnosis and management of celiac disease. Gastroenterology 2006;131:1981–2002. *A consensus guideline.*

Thielman NM, Guerrant RL: Acute infectious diarrhea. N Engl J Med 2004;350:38–47. *An up-to-date summary of the diagnostic approach to and antimicrobial therapy for acute infectious diarrhea.*

144 INFLAMMATORY BOWEL DISEASE

William F. Stenson

Definition

Inflammatory bowel diseases (IBDs), including ulcerative colitis and Crohn's disease, are chronic inflammatory diseases of the gastrointestinal tract. They are diagnosed by a set of clinical, endoscopic, and histologic characteristics, but no single finding is absolutely diagnostic for one disease or the other. Moreover, some patients have a clinical picture that falls between the two diseases and are said to have indeterminate colitis.

The inflammatory response in ulcerative colitis is largely confined to the mucosa and submucosa, but in Crohn's disease the inflammation extends through the intestinal wall from mucosa to serosa. Ulcerative colitis is confined to the colon, and colectomy is a curative procedure. Crohn's disease, in contrast, can involve any part of the gastrointestinal tract, although the distal end of the small bowel and the colon are most commonly involved. Resection of the inflamed segment is not curative of Crohn's disease, and inflammation is likely to recur.

Epidemiology

The incidence and prevalence of Crohn's disease and ulcerative colitis vary with geographic location; the highest rates occur in white populations in northern Europe and North America, where the incidence for each disease is about 5 per 100,000 and the prevalence is approximately 50 per 100,000. Rates in central and southern Europe are lower, and in South America, Asia, and Africa they are lower still. Crohn's disease and ulcerative colitis are both more common in Jews than non-Jews. In the United States, the incidence of IBD in the black population has been a fifth to half that in the white population, but in recent years that gap has narrowed. In northern Europe and North America the incidence of ulcerative colitis has leveled off, but that of Crohn's disease is still increasing. For both diseases, the incidence is equal in men and women. The peak age at onset is between 15 and 25 years of age, with a second, lesser peak between 55 and 65 years. Both diseases occur in childhood, although the incidence in children younger than 15 years is low.

The risk for ulcerative colitis is increased in both nonsmokers and former smokers when compared with current smokers. Whether initiation of smoking improves symptoms is unclear, although success has been reported with nicotine patches. In contrast, the incidence of smoking is higher in patients with Crohn's disease than in the general population, and patients who continue to smoke may be less likely to respond to medical therapy.

Pathobiology

Genetics

The most important risk factor for IBD is a positive family history. Approximately 15% of IBD patients have affected first-degree relatives, and the incidence in first-degree relatives is 30 to 100 times that of the general population. The best estimates of the lifetime risk for the development of IBD in first-degree relatives of affected individuals are 3 to 9%. The increased incidence in first-degree relatives contrasts with the absence of an increased incidence in spouses of patients. Dizygotic twins have the same rate of concordance as would be expected for siblings, whereas monozygotic twins have higher rates of concordance for both diseases. Both Crohn's disease and ulcerative colitis are polygenic disorders. The first well-characterized mutations associated with Crohn's disease were in *NOD2*, a gene that codes for a protein that acts as an intracellular receptor for a bacterial product, muramyl dipeptide. Mutations in *NOD2* are seen in about 15% of Crohn's disease patients but are also seen in a smaller percentage of the general population, so mutations in *NOD2* are neither necessary nor sufficient for the development of Crohn's disease.

Pathogenesis

In IBD, the lamina propria is infiltrated with lymphocytes, macrophages, and other cells of the immune system. An intensive search for the antigens that trigger the immune response has yet to identify a specific microbial pathogen. Anticolon antibodies of unclear significance have been identified in the sera of ulcerative colitis patients. IBD may also be related to a failure to suppress (or "downregulate") the normal, finely tuned, low-grade chronic inflammation of the intestinal lamina propria in response to chronic exposure to luminal antigens, particularly commensal bacteria.

Whatever the antigenic trigger, activated lamina propria T cells are involved in the pathogenesis of IBD. In Crohn's disease, the activated lymphocytes appear to be primarily T_H1 lymphocytes that produce interferon-γ (IFN-γ). Pro-inflammatory cytokines, including interleukin-1 (IL-1) and tumor necrosis factor-α (TNF-α), amplify the immune response. Intravenous infusion of antibody to TNF-α is clinically effective in Crohn's disease. Large numbers of neutrophils are attracted by chemotactic agents, including IL-8 and leukotriene B_4, and enter the inflamed mucosa. Epithelial injury in IBD appears to be due to reactive oxygen species from neutrophils and macrophages, as well as cytokines such as TNF-α and IFN-γ.

In mice, colitis develops when the genes for IL-2, IL-10, or transforming growth factor-β_1 are knocked out or when there are certain T-cell receptor mutants, and colitis develops in transgenic rats if the human HLA-B27 gene has been introduced. If the same animals are raised in a germ-free environment, colitis does not develop, thereby suggesting that colitis can be the only manifestation of a variety of abnormalities in systemic immunity and that the colitis is the result of an abnormal immune response to commensal bacteria.

Pathology

Ulcerative colitis and Crohn's disease each have a characteristic pathologic appearance, but in any given case the pathologic picture may not be specific enough to distinguish between them or to differentiate them from other diseases such as infectious colitis or ischemic colitis (Table 144–1). In IBD, pathologic assessment of disease activity may not correlate with clinical and endoscopic assessment.

In ulcerative colitis, inflammation begins in the rectum, extends proximally a certain distance, and then abruptly stops, with a clear demarcation between involved and uninvolved mucosa. In mild disease, there are superficial erosions, whereas in more severe disease, ulcers may be large but superficial and penetrate the muscularis mucosa only in very severe disease. Inflammatory polyps or pseudopolyps may be present. Most of the pathologic findings in ulcerative colitis are limited to the mucosa and submucosa; the muscularis propria is affected only in fulminant disease. Active ulcerative colitis is marked by neutrophils in the mucosa and submucosa and clumps of neutrophils in crypt lumens (crypt abscesses), as well as by mucus depletion, mucosal edema, and vascular congestion with focal hemorrhage. In addition to signs of acute activity, there are also signs of chronicity, with lymphoid aggregates, plasma cells, mast cells, and eosinophils in the lamina propria.

In Crohn's disease, the bowel wall is thickened and stiff. The mesentery, which is thickened, edematous, and contracted, fixes the intestine in one position. Transmural inflammation may cause loops of intestine to be matted together. All layers of the intestine are thickened, and the lumen is narrowed. "Skip lesions" with two involved areas separated by a length of normal intestine suggest Crohn's disease. Colonic inflammation with rectal sparing is more consistent with Crohn's disease than with ulcerative colitis. The earliest lesions of Crohn's disease are aphthous ulcers, which typically occur over Peyer's patches in the small intestine and over lymphoid aggregates in the colon. As the disease progresses, aphthous ulcers enlarge and become stellate or serpiginous. Eventually, the stellate ulcers coalesce to form longitudinal and transverse linear ulcers.

TABLE 144–1 COMPARISON OF ULCERATIVE COLITIS AND CROHN'S DISEASE

Feature	Ulcerative Colitis	Crohn's Disease
PATHOLOGY		
Rectal involvement	Always	Common
Skip lesions	Never	Common
Transmural involvement	Rare	Common
Granulomas	Occasional	Common
Perianal disease	Never	Common
Cobblestone mucosa	Rare	Common
RADIOLOGY		
"Collar button" ulcers	Common	Occasional
Small intestinal involvement	Never	Common
Discontinuous involvement	Never	Common
Fistulas	Never	Common
Strictures	Occasional	Common
ENDOSCOPY		
Aphthous ulcers	Never	Common
Discontinuous involvement	Never	Common
Rectal sparing	Never	Common
Linear or serpiginous ulcers	Never	Common
Ulcers in the terminal ileum	Never	Common

TABLE 144–2 CRITERIA FOR SEVERITY IN INFLAMMATORY BOWEL DISEASE

Mild	Fewer than four bowel movements per day with little or no blood, no fever, and sedimentation rate less than 20 mm/hr
Moderate	Between mild and severe
Severe	Six or more bowel movements per day with blood, fever, anemia, and sedimentation rate greater than 30 mm/hr

The remaining islands of nonulcerated mucosa give a cobblestone appearance. Fissures develop from the base of ulcers and extend down through the muscularis to the serosa. Lymphoid aggregates are found in the submucosa and external to the muscularis propria. Granulomas are common in Crohn's disease but not in ulcerative colitis.

Clinical Manifestations

Ulcerative Colitis

The dominant symptom in ulcerative colitis is diarrhea, which is usually associated with blood in the stool (Table 144–2). Bowel movements are frequent but small in volume as a result of irritability of the inflamed rectum. Urgency and fecal incontinence may limit the patient's ability to function in society. Other symptoms include fever and pain, which may be in either lower quadrant or in the rectum. Systemic features—fever, malaise, and weight loss—are more common if all or most of the colon is involved and may have a greater effect than diarrhea on the patient's ability to function. Some patients, especially elderly persons, complain of constipation rather than diarrhea because rectal spasm prevents the passage of stool. The initial attack of ulcerative colitis may be fulminant with bloody diarrhea, but more commonly the disease begins indolently, with nonbloody diarrhea progressing to bloody diarrhea. Ulcerative colitis may initially be seen with any extent of anatomic involvement, from disease confined to the rectum to pancolitis. Most commonly, ulcerative colitis follows a chronic intermittent course with long periods of quiescence interspersed with acute attacks lasting weeks to months; however, a significant percentage of patients suffer a chronic continuous course.

In ulcerative colitis of mild to moderate severity, there may be tenderness over the affected area of the colon, and rectal examination may reveal tenderness or blood on the glove. In severe disease, the patient is more likely to be febrile and tachycardic.

Anemia and an elevated leukocyte count and erythrocyte sedimentation rate are useful in confirming severe disease and in monitoring the clinical course of a severe exacerbation. Electrolyte disorders, particularly hypokalemia, are seen with severe diarrhea.

Crohn's Disease

Crohn's disease is marked by one of three major patterns: (1) disease in the ileum and cecum (40% of patients), (2) disease confined to the small intestine (30%), and (3) disease confined to the colon (25%). Much less commonly, Crohn's disease involves more proximal parts of the gastrointestinal tract—the mouth, tongue, esophagus, stomach, and duodenum.

The predominant symptoms are diarrhea, abdominal pain, and weight loss; any of these three symptoms may be most prominent in a given individual. The initial manifestation may not be dramatic; patients may complain for months or years of vague abdominal pain and intermittent diarrhea before the diagnosis is considered. Diarrhea occurs in almost all those with Crohn's disease, but the pattern varies with the anatomic location of the disease. In patients with colonic disease, especially with rectal involvement, diarrhea is of small volume and associated with urgency and tenesmus. Inflammation in the rectum causes loss of distensibility; entry of even a small amount of stool into a nondistensible rectum causes an immediate and urgent need to defecate. Prolonged inflammation and scarring in the rectum can leave it so rigid and nondistensible that the patient is incontinent. In disease confined to the small intestine, stools are of larger volume and not associated with urgency or tenesmus. Patients with severe involvement of the terminal ileum and those who have undergone surgical resection of the terminal ileum may have bile salt diarrhea or steatorrhea.

The location and pattern of pain correlate with disease location. In patients with ileal disease, cramping right lower quadrant pain occurs after eating and is related to partial intermittent obstruction of a narrowed intestinal lumen. Abdominal distention, nausea, and vomiting may accompany the pain. Weight loss of some degree, which occurs in most patients with Crohn's disease regardless of the anatomic location, is a product of malabsorption or diminished intake as a result of pain, diarrhea, or anorexia. Fever and chills often accompany disease activity; a low-grade fever may be the patient's first warning sign of a flare. Induction of remission by drugs or surgery is invariably associated with increased energy and a sense of well-being. Crohn's disease, like ulcerative colitis, is a relapsing and remitting disease. About 30% of placebo-treated patients with Crohn's disease of mild to moderate activity go into remission within 4 months. Conversely, of patients in remission and not receiving therapy, about 30% relapse within 1 year and 50% at 2 years.

Physical findings in Crohn's disease vary with the distribution and severity of the disease. Aphthous ulcers of the lips, gingiva, or buccal mucosa are common. The abdomen may be tender, typically over the area of disease activity. Thickened bowel loops, thickened mesentery, or an abscess may cause a mass, often in the right lower quadrant. The presence of perianal disease is suggested by fistulous openings, induration, redness, or tenderness near the anus.

Laboratory findings are largely nonspecific. Anemia may result from chronic disease, blood loss, or nutritional deficiencies of iron, folate, or vitamin B_{12}. A modestly elevated leukocyte count is indicative of active disease, but a marked elevation suggests the presence of an abscess or other suppurative complication. The erythrocyte sedimentation rate has been used to monitor disease activity, and it tends to be higher in colonic disease than in ileal disease. Hypoalbuminemia is an indication of malnutrition. Ileal disease or resection of more than 100 cm of distal ileum results in a diminished serum vitamin B_{12} level because of malabsorption.

Extraintestinal Manifestations

Although IBD primarily involves the bowel, it is also associated with manifestations in other organ systems. The extraintestinal manifestations (e.g., sclerosing cholangitis or ankylosing spondylitis) may be more problematic than the bowel disease. The extraintestinal manifestations can be divided into two major groups: (1) those in which the clinical activity follows the activity of the bowel disease and (2) those in which the clinical activity is unrelated to the activity of the bowel disease.

Arthritis

The most common extraintestinal manifestation of IBD is arthritis, including colitic arthritis and ankylosing spondylitis. Colitic arthritis, a migratory arthritis that affects the knees, hips, ankles, wrists, and elbows, parallels the course of the bowel disease; successful treatment of the intestinal inflammation results in improvement in the arthritis. Ankylosing spondylitis (Chapter 286) is characterized by morning stiffness, low back pain, and a stooped posture; it can be relentlessly progressive and crippling. Patients with ulcerative colitis have a 30-fold increase in the incidence of ankylosing spondylitis in comparison to the general population. Nonsteroidal anti-inflammatory drugs reduce the inflammation and pain but do not halt progression of the disease. Medical treatment of the IBD and colectomy are not helpful in managing ankylosing spondylitis. Sacroiliitis, which is inflammation of the joint between the sacrum and the ilium, occurs in conjunction with ankylosing spondylitis but is more often seen alone. Fifteen percent of patients with ulcerative colitis have radiographs consistent with sacroiliitis, but most patients are asymptomatic.

Hepatic Manifestations

Hepatic complications of IBD include fatty liver, pericholangitis, chronic active hepatitis, and cirrhosis. Biliary tract complications are sclerosing cholangitis (ulcerative colitis) and gallstones (Crohn's disease). Cholesterol gallstones occur in patients with ileal disease or after ileal resection because of malabsorption of bile salts and the resultant decrease in the size of the bile salt pool. Pericholangitis is the most common hepatic complication of IBD, but patients with pericholangitis are usually asymptomatic. Elevations in alkaline phosphatase are seen frequently; elevations in bilirubin are less common.

Sclerosing cholangitis (Chapter 159) is a chronic cholestatic liver disease marked by fibrosing inflammation of the intrahepatic and extrahepatic bile ducts. Even though it occurs in only 1 to 4% of patients with ulcerative colitis and with lower frequency in Crohn's disease, the majority of patients with sclerosing cholangitis have IBD. Colectomy and medical treatment of the bowel disease do not ameliorate the course; sclerosing cholangitis is one of the most common indications for liver transplantation (Chapter 158) in adults.

Dermal Manifestations

The two common dermal complications of IBD are pyoderma gangrenosum and erythema nodosum (Chapter 466). The lesions of pyoderma gangrenosum almost always develop during a bout of acute colitis and generally resolve with control of the colitis by oral or intradermal corticosteroids; in rare cases, colectomy is required. The activity of erythema nodosum, which is seen particularly in association with Crohn's disease in children, follows the activity of the bowel disease.

Ocular Manifestations

Ocular complications of IBD are uveitis and episcleritis (Chapter 449). Local therapy with corticosteroids and agents that dilate the pupil helps prevent scarring and blindness.

Diagnosis

Diagnostic Tests

Radiography

In both ulcerative colitis and Crohn's disease, the radiographic findings may not correlate well with disease activity. The patient's clinical response or endoscopic findings are more useful for this purpose.

Ulcerative Colitis

In early ulcerative colitis, findings on barium enema may be normal, or there may be limited distensibility of the involved segment resulting in a narrowed, shortened, and tubular form of the lumen. The haustral markings disappear, and the normally tortuous appearance of the colon is straightened (Fig. 144–1). Air contrast examination reveals a fine granular appearance of the mucosa with a slightly irregular surface. In more severe disease, the granularity becomes coarser and eventually nodular; ulcers penetrate through the mucosa and can be seen in profile as small collar-button collections of barium extending beyond the colonic lumen.

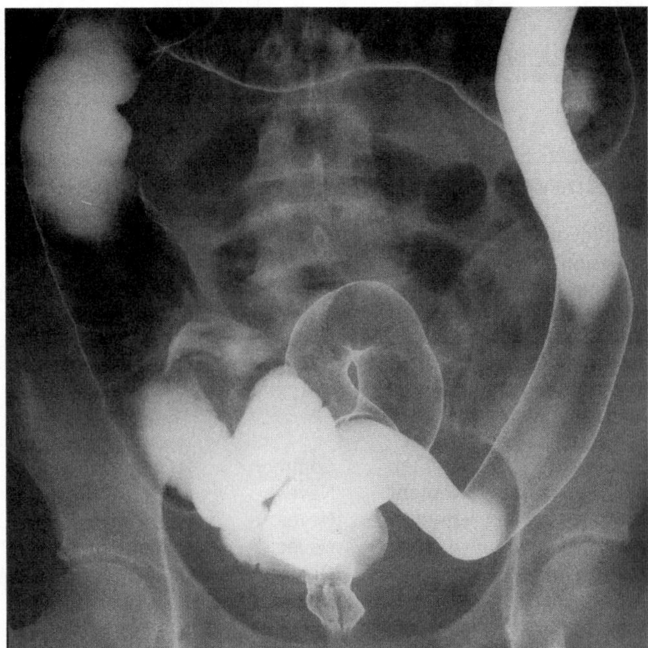

FIGURE 144–1 • Ulcerative colitis. An air contrast barium enema demonstrates luminal narrowing and loss of haustral markings in the sigmoid and descending colon in a patient with ulcerative colitis.

Crohn's Disease

The earliest form of Crohn's disease detectable by air contrast barium enema is marked by the presence of aphthous ulcers, which appear as small discrete collections of barium surrounded by radiolucent halos of inflammatory infiltrate. These small ulcers are usually multiple, and the intervening mucosa is normal. As Crohn's disease becomes more severe, the aphthous ulcers enlarge, deepen, and connect with one another to form linear ulcers; the intervening mucosa develops a nodular appearance on radiographs, a process termed *cobblestoning.* Progressive deepening of ulcers can lead to abscess formation or fistulization. Contrast studies are more likely than endoscopic studies to identify fistulas. Transmural inflammation and fibrosis lead to limited distensibility with decreased luminal diameter and stricture formation. Like fistulas, strictures are more easily appreciated on radiographic studies than by endoscopy. Transmural inflammation and fibrosis result in thickening of the bowel wall with wide gaps between the barium-filled lumens of loops of inflamed small bowel (Fig. 144–2). Small bowel Crohn's disease can be evaluated by small bowel follow-through or by enteroclysis. Computed tomography and ultrasonography are useful in identifying abscesses and other fluid collections and in assessing the thickness of the bowel wall.

Endoscopy

Ulcerative Colitis

The earliest endoscopic manifestations of ulcerative colitis are the development of diffuse erythema and loss of the fine vascular pattern seen in the normal rectal mucosa (Fig. 144–3). Erythema is usually accompanied by mucosal edema, which is manifested endoscopically by blunting of the rectal valves, loss of normal vasculature, and the development of granular-appearing mucosa. Inflammation is associated with the presence of yellowish exudate on the mucosa. The inflamed mucosa bleeds easily if touched with the endoscope; this easy bleeding is termed *friability.* In more severe disease, the mucosa bleeds spontaneously and small ulcerations appear. An important aspect of the endoscopic findings in ulcerative colitis is their distribution: inflammation begins in the rectum, extends proximally a certain distance, and then stops; all the mucosa proximal to that point is normal, and all the mucosa distal to it is abnormal.

Crohn's Disease

The earliest endoscopic manifestation of Crohn's disease is an aphthous ulcer, a small discrete ulcer a few millimeters in diameter sur-

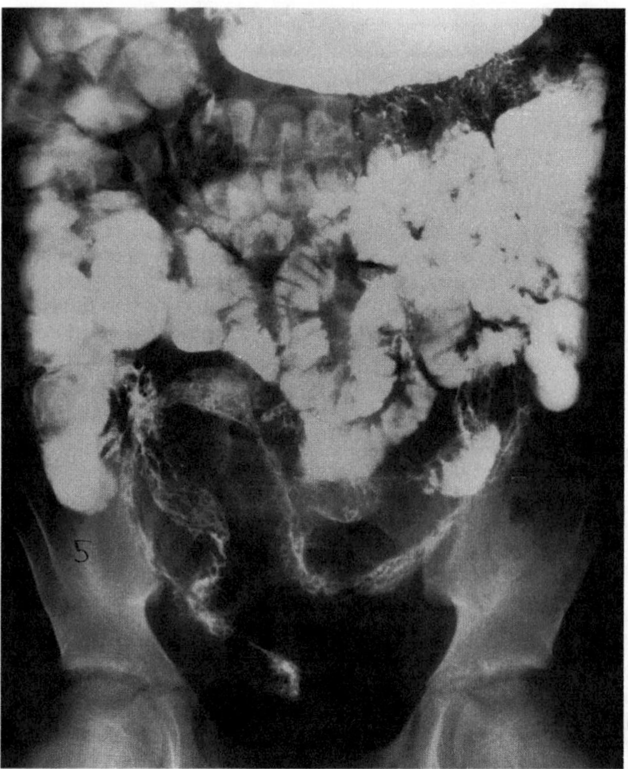

FIGURE 144–2 • Small bowel follow-through in a patient with Crohn's disease of the ileum. Luminal narrowing, mucosal ulceration, and separation of the barium-filled loops because of thickening of the bowel wall are apparent.

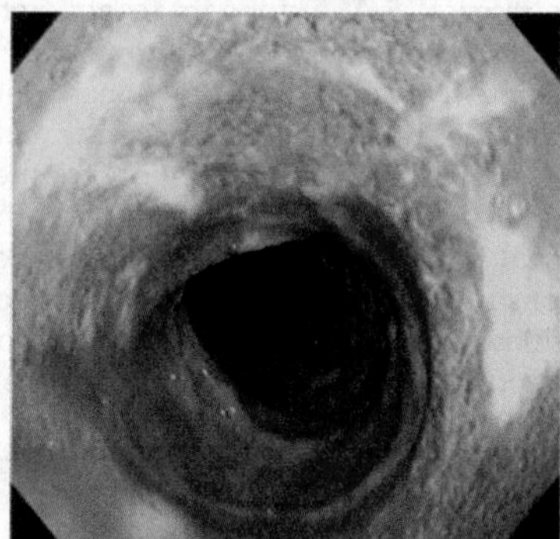

FIGURE 144–3 • Endoscopic view of the colonic mucosa in a patient with idiopathic ulcerative colitis. Friable mucosa, extensive ulceration, and exudates were detected.

rounded by a thin red halo of edematous tissue (Fig. 144–4). Ulcers may be rounded or long and serpiginous. Longitudinal and transverse ulcers may intersect to form a grid with intervening cobblestone-like areas of nonulcerated mucosa (Fig. 144–5). Large, deep, penetrating ulcers can be surrounded by areas of normal-appearing mucosa. The diffuse mucosal irregularities of erythema, edema, and granularity, which are prominent in ulcerative colitis, occur less commonly and later in the course of Crohn's disease. The rectum may or may not be involved in Crohn's disease. Areas of involvement are typically interspersed with normal "skip" areas.

Differential Diagnosis

For many therapeutic decisions it is not particularly important to know whether the patient has ulcerative colitis or Crohn's disease. However, when surgery is contemplated, the distinction is important. For example, colectomy and ileoanal anastomosis could be recommended as a curative procedure if the physician were confident that the patient had ulcerative colitis rather than Crohn's colitis.

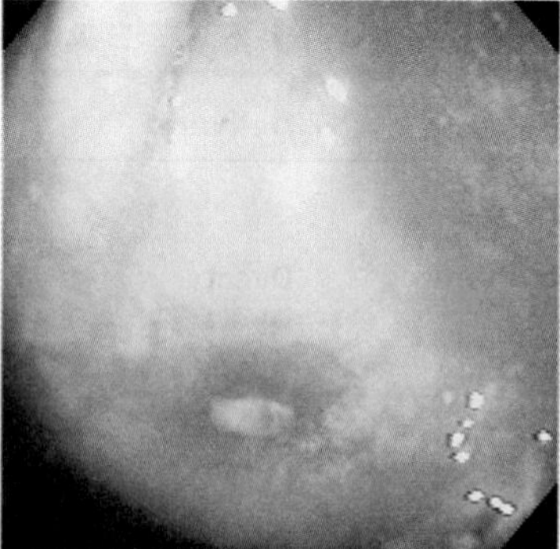

FIGURE 144–4 • A single aphthous ulcer, the earliest endoscopic finding in Crohn's disease.

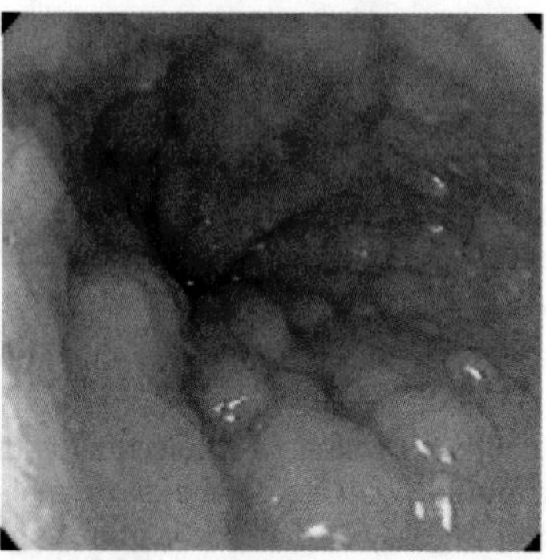

FIGURE 144–5 • Crohn's disease of the colon. Multiple edematous inflammatory polyps give a "cobblestone" appearance to the mucosa. Similar changes may be seen in ulcerative colitis. (From Forbes CD, Jackson WD: Color Atlas and Text of Clinical Medicine, 3rd ed. London, Mosby, 2003.)

Distribution of Inflammation

The anatomic distribution of the inflammatory response may be helpful in distinguishing ulcerative colitis from Crohn's disease. In ulcerative colitis, inflammation is seen in the rectum and extends proximally for some distance; with extensive disease, inflammation extends to the cecum. Although ulcerative colitis does not involve the small intestine, there may be a few centimeters of inflamed mucosa without ulceration in the terminal ileum. If the rectum is spared or if there are areas of uninflamed mucosa (skip areas) between areas of inflamed mucosa, Crohn's colitis is more likely. Not only is ulcerative colitis continuous along the longitudinal axis of the colon, but the degree of inflammation is also consistent and symmetrical circumferentially at any level. In contrast, in Crohn's colitis, deep linear ulcers may be separated by areas of normal mucosa. A major distinguishing mark in favor of Crohn's disease is the presence of transmural inflammatory changes; in ulcerative colitis, inflammation is confined to the mucosa and submucosa. Extensive perianal involvement with fistulas and abscesses point to Crohn's disease. The presence of noncaseating granulomas suggests Crohn's disease, but even in Crohn's disease, most patients have no granulomas on biopsy. Despite all these differences, there is a small but significant number of patients with IBD who cannot be assigned with confidence to one disease category or the other; these patients are considered to have indeterminate colitis.

Infections

Infections with *Shigella, Amoeba, Giardia, Escherichia coli* O157:H7, and *Campylobacter* can be accompanied by bloody diarrhea, cramps, and an endoscopic picture identical to ulcerative colitis (Chapter 305). An important distinction between these infectious diseases (except amebiasis) and IBD is that the diarrhea in infectious diseases tends to be limited to a period of days to a few weeks whereas the diarrhea in IBD is typically of longer duration. Stool cultures for bacterial pathogens and serologic tests for amebiasis help distinguish infectious diarrhea from IBD. In patients with prolonged diarrhea, other protozoal diseases such as giardiasis must be considered. Pseudomembranous colitis is manifested as

TABLE 144–3 PREPARATIONS OF 5-AMINOSALICYLIC ACID

Preparation	Delivery	Distribution	Dose*
TOPICAL			
Mesalamine suppository	Direct	Rectum	500 mg once or twice a day
Mesalamine enema	Direct	Left colon	4 g in 60 mL at bedtime
ORAL			
Sulfasalazine	Bacterial azo reductase	Colon	4–6 g in divided doses
Dipentum	Bacterial azo reductase	Colon	1.5–3.0 g in divided doses
Asacol	Release at pH >7	Distal ileum, colon	2.4–4.8 g in divided doses
Pentasa	Time-release ethyl cellulose microgranules	Ileum, colon	3–4 g in divided doses
Balsalazide	Bacterial azo reductase	Colon	6.75 g in divided doses

*Doses given are for active disease; similar doses can be given for maintenance therapy, although some practitioners use lower doses for maintenance.

profuse watery diarrhea and may last from a few days to months; the presence of small membranous plaques adherent to the mucosa on sigmoidoscopy is pathognomonic. As part of the initial evaluation of patients with acute exacerbations of IBD, it is appropriate to check the stool for *Clostridium difficile* toxin, especially if there has been recent antibiotic exposure.

Other Symptoms

Mild ulcerative colitis, in which rectal bleeding is the primary manifestation, can be confused with hemorrhoids or anal fissures (Chapter 148). The presence of urgency or diarrhea is more consistent with ulcerative colitis. Sigmoidoscopy should easily differentiate ulcerative colitis from these perianal problems.

Collagenous colitis is a chronic inflammatory disease marked pathologically by the presence of thick collagen deposition in the subepithelial layer of the colonic mucosa (Chapter 143). The typical clinical manifestation is chronic watery diarrhea in a middle-aged woman. Endoscopically, the mucosa appears mildly inflamed or, more commonly, absolutely normal; biopsy with histology provides the diagnosis. Ischemic colitis is part of the differential diagnosis of the initial bout of IBD and should be considered in elderly persons or others at particular risk for ischemic disease (Chapter 146). Diverticulitis, which may be difficult to separate from acute Crohn's colitis, tends to be a more acute problem without a chronic inflammatory state (Chapter 145). Intestinal lymphoma can mimic the symptoms of Crohn's disease; in lymphoma, small bowel radiographs may show diffuse involvement with masses in the bowel wall. If Crohn's disease has a long, indolent course with relatively mild symptoms, it may be difficult to differentiate from IBS, and some patients may have both (Chapter 139).

Treatment

Rx

Medical Therapy

Drugs Used for Inflammatory Bowel Disease

General Supportive Therapy

Antidiarrheal agents, usually loperamide or diphenoxylate, are useful in patients with mild IBD to reduce the number of bowel movements and to relieve rectal urgency. Anticholinergics (tincture of belladonna, clidinium, propantheline bromide, and dicyclomine hydrochloride) may reduce cramps, pain, and rectal urgency. An especially effective combination of an antidiarrheal and an antispasmodic is powdered opium (25 mg) and belladonna (15 mg). Antidiarrheal agents and antispasmodics are contraindicated in severe colitis because of the risk of precipitating toxic megacolon. The chronic use of narcotics for pain should not be part of the management of IBD. Sometimes antidepressants can be helpful. Nonsteroidal anti-inflammatory drugs can exacerbate the clinical activity of IBD and should be used cautiously.

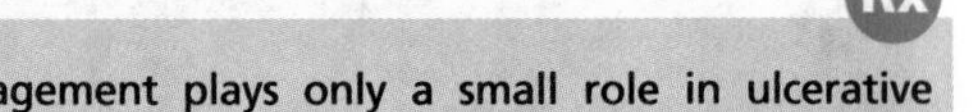

Nutritional management plays only a small role in ulcerative colitis. Patients should avoid specific foods that worsen their symptoms, typically high-fiber foods. Nutritional management plays a much larger role in Crohn's disease, in which many patients have diminished caloric intake and vitamin B_{12}, vitamin D, calcium, magnesium, zinc, and iron may be malabsorbed. Both total parenteral nutrition and elemental enteral diets can decrease intestinal inflammation by reducing the antigen load in the lumen.

Aminosalicylates

Agents that contain 5-aminosalicylic acid (5-ASA) are mainstays of therapy for ulcerative colitis and play a small role in the management of Crohn's disease. 5-ASA appears to act from the luminal surface, so oral formulations are designed to prevent absorption of 5-ASA while making it available in the lumen. In sulfasalazine, olsalazine, and balsalazide, 5-ASA is covalently bound to either another molecule of 5-ASA (olsalazine) or another agent (sulfasalazine and balsalazide); when these covalent bonds are broken by colonic bacteria, 5-ASA is released. In Asacol and Pentasa, the delayed-release or sustained-release 5-ASA is delivered as free 5-ASA to different portions of the gastrointestinal tract (Table 144–3). The efficacy of 5-ASA formulations is highly related to the concentration achieved in the lumen at the site of disease, with this dose-response relationship being seen up to doses of at least 4.8 g of 5-ASA per day, which is 12 tablets of Asacol.

5-ASA is also available as an enema, which reaches the descending colon, and as a suppository, which treats the rectum. The enema and suppository formulations are very effective in treating ulcerative proctitis, both as therapy for active disease and for maintenance of remission, either when used alone or with oral 5-ASA formulations.

Corticosteroids

Oral corticosteroids are effective in mild to moderate ulcerative colitis and Crohn's disease. Parenteral therapy is reserved for moderate to severe disease. The typical initial dose of prednisone is 40 mg/day for moderate to severe disease. The patient takes high doses of corticosteroids until symptoms begin to diminish, after which the dose is gradually reduced. If an inadequate initial dose of prednisone is used because of fear of side effects, the likelihood of a positive response diminishes. In some patients, disease activity flares when the dose of prednisone is reduced to less than a certain level (steroid dependence). For most patients, administration of oral prednisone in a single morning dose is as effective as divided doses. Corticosteroids should not be used in patients with undrained abscesses or when symptoms are due to a stricture or fibrotic process. Maintenance therapy with corticosteroids is ineffective in preventing recurrences in ulcerative colitis or Crohn's disease in remission. The many side effects of corticosteroids (Chapter 33) are the major factor limiting their use in IBD.

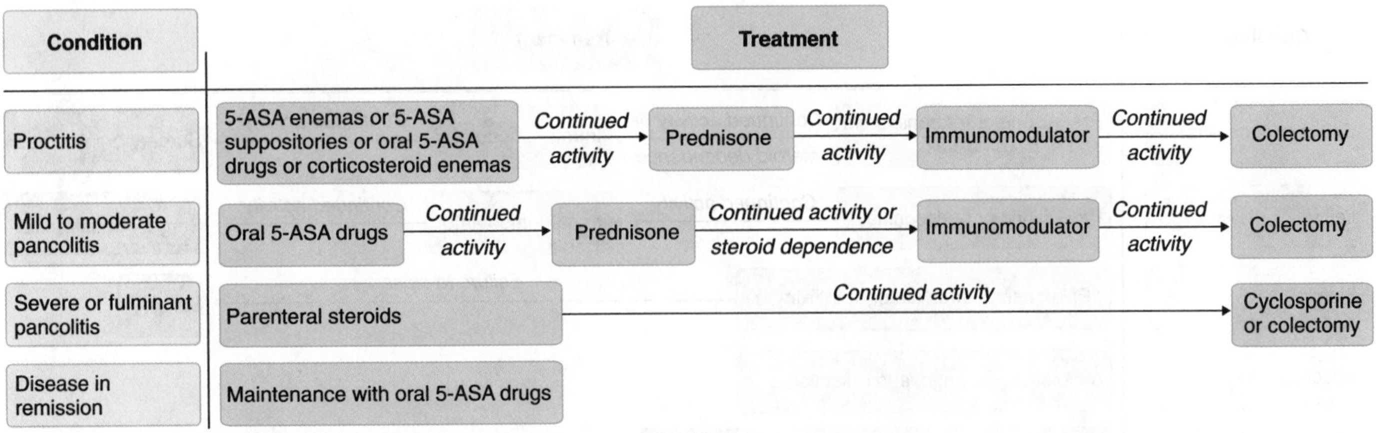

FIGURE 144–6 • Treatment algorithm for ulcerative colitis. ASA = aminosalicylic acid.

Rx

Immunomodulators

Immunomodulator drugs act by blocking lymphocyte proliferation, activation, or effector mechanisms. There is extensive experience with azathioprine and its metabolite 6-mercaptopurine (6-MP) in treating IBD and lesser experience with cyclosporine and methotrexate. Azathioprine and 6-MP are effective in treating active Crohn's disease and in maintaining remission; their role in ulcerative colitis is less clear. Typical initial doses are 1 to 1.5 mg/kg for 6-MP and 2.0 to 2.5 mg/kg for azathioprine. The delay between initiation of therapy and clinical response is typically 3 to 4 months. These drugs are used in patients who have active disease that is unresponsive to corticosteroids (refractory patients) and in corticosteroid-dependent patients. In these patients, 6-MP or azathioprine is added to corticosteroid therapy; after 3 or 4 months, when the 6-MP and azathioprine are likely to have taken effect, the dose of corticosteroids is gradually tapered. Most clinicians maintain patients on 6-MP or azathioprine for several years if remission is induced by these drugs. Some patients are maintained on these drugs indefinitely. The major limiting factor in the use of 6-MP and azathioprine is their toxicity; both commonly cause leukopenia, may cause pancreatitis, and may increase the risk for lymphoma. Methotrexate, given either orally or parenterally, is effective in active Crohn's disease. Cyclosporine, given intravenously, is effective in reducing inflammation in patients with severe ulcerative colitis who are facing colectomy.

Antibiotics

Except in cases of overt sepsis, there is little role for antibiotics in the management of ulcerative colitis. Antibiotics do not affect the remission rate; moreover, the risk of inducing antibiotic-associated pseudomembranous colitis must be considered. Antibiotics play a larger role in Crohn's disease; they are used in management of the suppurative complications, especially abscess formation and perianal disease, although surgical drainage is the primary therapy for abscesses. Metronidazole (10 to 15 mg/kg/day) is effective in perianal Crohn's disease and is as effective as sulfasalazine in Crohn's colitis. The major side effect of metronidazole is peripheral neuropathy, which is dose dependent and generally resolves when use of the drug is discontinued. Ciprofloxacin at 500 mg twice a day for a few weeks is also effective in some patients.

Anti–Tumor Necrosis Factor Antibody

Infliximab, a chimeric mouse-human antibody against TNF-α, is effective in the management of active, moderate to severe Crohn's disease and fistulas associated with Crohn's disease, [1] as well as in patients with refractory ulcerative colitis. [2] The efficacy of infliximab may relate to binding free TNF-α or to lysing lymphocytes and macrophages that have TNF-α bound to their surfaces. Treatment is by intravenous infusion (5 mg/kg), which can be performed every 8 weeks or on an as-needed schedule. About 65% of patients with active Crohn's disease improve, and about a third achieve remission. Long-term response rates, however, are considerably lower. Infliximab is associated with a substantial risk for infection (sepsis, pneumonia, and activation of tuberculosis) and a small but real risk for lymphoma, so it is generally reserved for patients who have failed to respond to azathioprine. Infliximab appears to have a higher rate of efficacy and a lower rate of side effects when it is given with azathioprine rather than as a single agent because azathioprine modulates the intrinsic reaction to the mouse portion of infliximab.

Rx

Medical Management of Ulcerative Colitis (Fig. 144–6)

Proctitis

For active ulcerative proctitis, a relatively effective and rapidly acting approach is nightly administration of 5-ASA retention enemas or suppositories, often supplemented with an oral aminosalicylate. Corticosteroid enemas can also be used. Either 5-ASA suppositories or corticosteroid foam is appropriate for disease involving up to 20 cm of distal colon; 5-ASA or corticosteroid retention enemas can be used for active disease involving up to 60 cm of distal colon. Another approach to proctitis or distal colitis is an oral aminosalicylate, although a response may not be evident for 3 to 4 weeks.

Extensive Colitis

In patients with colitis of mild to moderate activity and extension proximal to the sigmoid colon, the initial drug of choice is an oral aminosalicylate; efficacy increases with increasing doses. Even with more extensive disease, supplementation of oral aminosalicylates with aminosalicylate enemas or suppositories may help reduce the symptoms of urgency that result from rectal involvement. In patients with more active disease (more than five or six bowel movements per day), patients in whom a more rapid response is desired, or those who have not responded to 3 to 4 weeks of aminosalicylates, the treatment of choice is oral prednisone. Patients with severe diarrhea, systemic symptoms, or significant amounts of blood in stool should be started on 40 mg/day; most patients respond to oral corticosteroids within a few days. After the symptoms are controlled, prednisone can be gradually tapered by 5 mg every 1 to 2 weeks. Patients who respond to oral prednisone and can be fully withdrawn from it should be maintained on an aminosalicylate.

For patients who do not respond to corticosteroids (steroid refractory) or who do respond but whose disease flares whenever the corticosteroids are withdrawn (steroid dependent), options include indefinite corticosteroid therapy, an immunomodulator (azathioprine or 6-MP), or colectomy. Continuation of high-dose corticosteroid therapy for too long a time is the most common serious error in the management of ulcerative colitis. If the patient is taking a substantial dose (>15 mg/day of prednisone) for more than 6

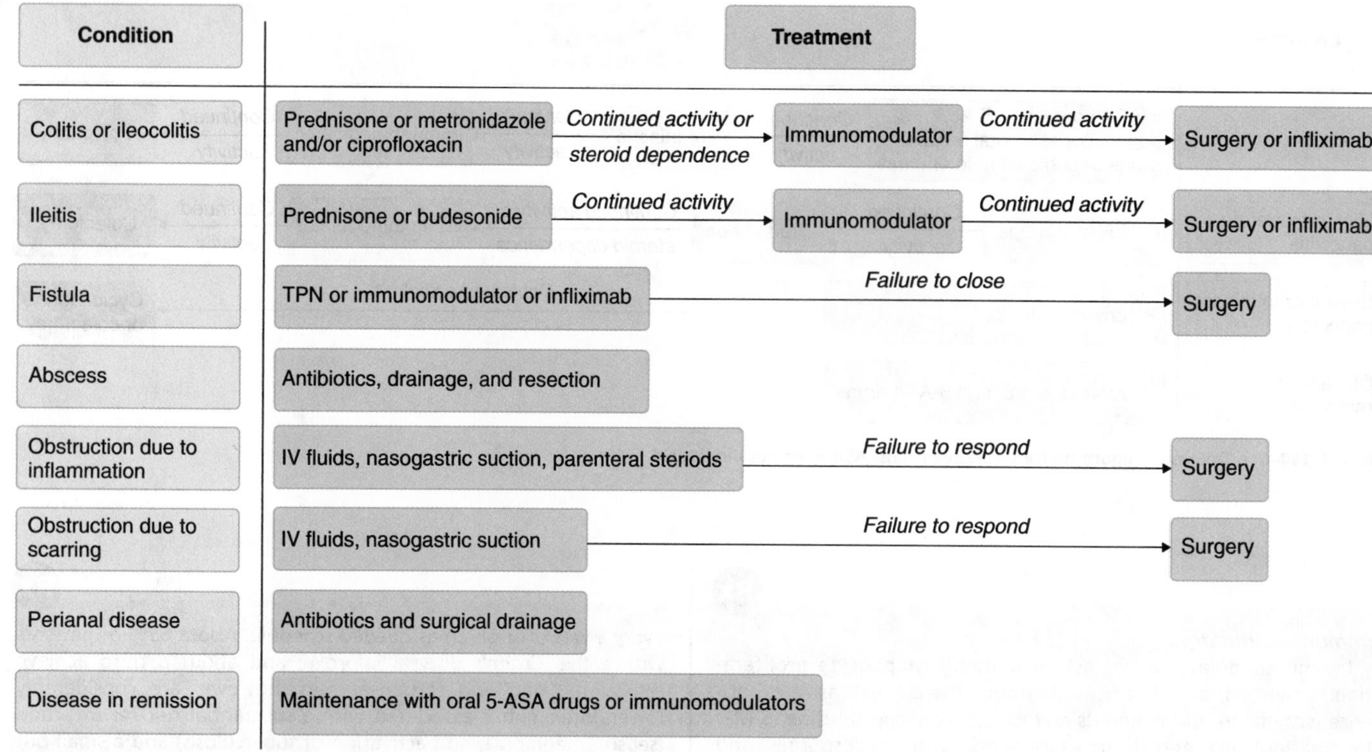

FIGURE 144–7 • Treatment algorithm for Crohn's disease. ASA = aminosalicylic acid; IV = intravenous; TPN = total parenteral nutrition.

months, a trial of an immunomodulator or colectomy should be given serious consideration.

The most common reason for hospitalization is intractable diarrhea, although blood loss is also a frequent problem. Patients with severe active ulcerative colitis should be evaluated for toxic megacolon. Anticholinergics and antidiarrheal agents are contraindicated in patients with severe ulcerative colitis because of the risk of precipitating toxic megacolon. The mainstays of therapy for severe ulcerative colitis are bedrest, rehydration with intravenous fluids, and intravenous corticosteroids (hydrocortisone, 300 mg/day; prednisolone, 60 to 80 mg/day; or methylprednisolone, 48 to 60 mg/day). Total parenteral nutrition may be necessary in the event of malnutrition. Patients with peritoneal signs or signs of systemic infection should be treated with parenteral antibiotics. Patients who do not improve in 7 to 10 days should be considered for either colectomy or a trial of intravenous cyclosporine.

Maintenance Therapy

Aminosalicylates reduce the incidence of recurrence in patients with ulcerative colitis; almost all patients should receive maintenance therapy. The efficacy of sulfasalazine at 3 to 4 g/day is greater than its efficacy at 2 g/day, even though 2 g/day is the usual recommended maintenance dose. Corticosteroids are not effective as maintenance therapy and should not be used. Azothioprine is also an effective maintenance therapy in patients who fail aminosalicylate therapy. [3] Most of the experience with 6-MP as maintenance therapy for ulcerative colitis is in patients whose acute disease has been brought under control with 6-MP; withdrawal of 6-MP from these patients results in a high incidence of exacerbation.

Medical Management of Crohn's Disease (Fig. 144–7)

General Approach

It is difficult to develop generally applicable guidelines for the management of Crohn's disease because of the great variety of anatomic locations, clinical manifestations, and gastrointestinal complications such as fistulas, abscesses, strictures, and perforations. Response to therapy is monitored by empirical clinical assessment directed at the problem that is most troublesome for the patient.

A common problem in the management of Crohn's disease is a marked discrepancy between the severity of the patient's symptoms and the objective signs of disease activity. Patients with severe pain and diarrhea may have minimal findings on endoscopy or radiographic studies. Patients who have undergone ileal resection may have significant diarrhea on the basis of their surgery alone.

Active Disease

For colonic Crohn's disease, either oral corticosteroids (prednisone, 40 mg/day) or antibiotics (metronidazole, 10 to 15 mg/kg/day, and/or ciprofloxacin, 500 mg twice a day) are reasonable first-line therapies. In patients with small bowel Crohn's disease, corticosteroids, either prednisone or budesonide (6 to 9 mg/day), are appropriate. Before corticosteroids are given to a Crohn's disease patient with abdominal pain, fever, and a high leukocyte count, an abdominal computed tomography scan should be obtained to exclude an abscess.

In patients who have been brought into clinical remission with corticosteroids, the rate at which the dose is tapered is arbitrary and has not been defined by controlled trials. Usually the prednisone dose can be tapered from 40 to 20 mg/day relatively rapidly (5 mg/wk) without inducing a flare of disease activity. If the patient has not been taking a 5-ASA preparation, one should be added to increase the likelihood of successful corticosteroid withdrawal. Once the dose of prednisone has reached 20 mg/day, the taper is slowed to 5 mg every 10 to 14 days; if symptoms flare, the dose of prednisone is increased. At this point, the best approach for most patients is a trial of an immunomodulator, either 6-MP or azathioprine; corticosteroid therapy is continued for 3 to 4 months and then tapered gradually. Approximately 60% of corticosteroid-dependent patients are able to withdraw from corticosteroids with this approach; the alternative is surgery if there is a stricture or a focal area of involvement.

Infliximab is typically given in combination with azathioprine or 6-MP to patients who have failed therapy with azathioprine or 6-MP. A novel investigational approach to Crohn's disease is the use of granulocyte-macrophage colony-stimulating factor. The approach to severe Crohn's disease is similar to the approach to

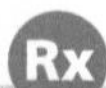

severe ulcerative colitis. The patient is hospitalized, given nothing by mouth, rehydrated with intravenous fluids, and administered parenteral corticosteroids. Patients who respond to parenteral corticosteroids are switched to high-dose oral corticosteroids (prednisone, 40 mg/day), and the dose of prednisone is gradually reduced. Patients with severe Crohn's disease who do not respond to parenteral corticosteroids within a week should be considered for surgery. A course of total parenteral nutrition may be useful as adjunctive therapy.

Maintenance Therapy

Maintenance therapy with aminosalicylates has been recommended for those brought into remission with corticosteroids or by surgery; however, the efficacy of aminosalicylates as maintenance therapy is much less well established in Crohn's disease than in ulcerative colitis. Maintenance with 6-MP or azathioprine is recommended for patients brought into remission with these drugs or who were corticosteroid dependent and then converted to these drugs. [4] There is no role for corticosteroids as maintenance therapy.

Surgical Therapy

Ulcerative Colitis

Twenty percent to 25% of patients with extensive ulcerative colitis eventually undergo colectomy, usually because their disease has not responded adequately to medical therapy. In ulcerative colitis, colectomy is a curative procedure. Emergency colectomy may be required in patients with toxic megacolon or a severe fulminant attack without toxic megacolon. The standard operation for ulcerative colitis is proctocolectomy and Brooke's ileostomy. The most popular alternative operation is proctocolectomy and ileoanal anastomosis; in this procedure a pouch is constructed from the terminal 30 cm of ileum, and the distal end of the pouch is pulled through the anal canal. Ileoanal anastomosis is sometimes complicated by inflammation in the ileal pouch, which can be treated with probiotics. [5] The decision for or against colectomy is influenced by the patient's age, social circumstances, and duration of disease. The risk for the development of malignancy (Chapter 203) enters into the equation when considering colectomy in those with long-standing ulcerative colitis; if the other indications are equivocal, the risk for malignancy may push the balance in favor of colectomy.

Crohn's Disease

Within 10 years of diagnosis, approximately 60% of patients with Crohn's disease undergo surgery for their disease. Because surgical resection is not curative of Crohn's disease and recurrences are likely, the approach is more conservative in terms of the amount of tissue removed. Failure of medical management is a common cause for resection in patients with Crohn's disease, as it is in ulcerative colitis, but complications (e.g., obstruction, fistula, abscess) are often indications for resection in Crohn's disease. Surgery is also performed to allow patients to stop taking medications (usually corticosteroids). For small bowel Crohn's disease, the most common surgical procedure is segmental resection for obstruction or fistula. The incidence of recurrence severe enough to need repeat surgery after ileal or ileocolic resection is about 50% after 10 years and 75% after 15 years. Endoscopic and histologic surgical approaches to Crohn's colitis include segmental resection, subtotal colectomy with ileoproctostomy, and total colectomy with ileostomy. For patients with extensive colonic disease that includes the rectum, the procedure of choice is total proctocolectomy with a Brooke ileostomy. Total colectomy with ileoanal anastomosis is not appropriate in Crohn's colitis because recurrence of Crohn's disease in the ileal segment forming the new pouch would require a repeat operation and loss of a long segment of ileum.

Complications

Ulcerative Colitis

The most severe complication of ulcerative colitis is toxic megacolon, or dilation of the colon to a diameter greater than 6 cm associated with worsening of the patient's clinical condition and the

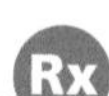

development of fever, tachycardia, and leukocytosis. Physical examination may reveal postural hypotension, tenderness over the distribution of the colon, and absent or hypoactive bowel sounds. Antispasmodics and antidiarrheal agents are likely to initiate or exacerbate toxic megacolon. Medical therapy is designed to reduce the likelihood of perforation and return the colon to normal motor activity as rapidly as possible. The patient is given nothing by mouth and nasogastric suction is begun. Intravenous fluids should be administered to replete water and electrolytes, broad-spectrum antibiotics are given in anticipation of peritonitis resulting from perforation, and parenteral corticosteroids are administered at a dose equivalent to more than 40 mg of prednisone per day. Signs of improvement include a decrease in abdominal girth and the return of bowel sounds. Deterioration is marked by the development of rebound tenderness, increasing abdominal girth, and cardiovascular collapse. If the patient does not begin to show signs of clinical improvement during the first 24 to 48 hours of medical therapy, the risk for perforation increases markedly, and surgical intervention is indicated.

Crohn's Disease

Abscesses and Fistulas

Abscesses and fistulas, which are common complications in Crohn's disease, are products of extension of a mucosal fissure or ulcer through the intestinal wall and into extraintestinal tissue. Leakage of intestinal contents through a fissure into the peritoneal cavity results in an abscess. Extension of the inflammatory process through the wall of adjacent viscera or through the abdominal wall to the exterior results in a fistula. Abscesses occur in 15 to 20% of patients with Crohn's disease and are especially common in the terminal ileum. The typical clinical manifestation of an intra-abdominal abscess is fever, abdominal pain, tenderness, and leukocytosis. Abdominal abscess is most often diagnosed by computed tomography. Broad-spectrum antibiotic therapy, including anaerobic coverage, is indicated. Percutaneous drainage of abscesses in patients with Crohn's disease may improve the clinical picture but does not provide adequate therapy because of persistent communication between the abscess cavity and the intestinal lumen. Resection of the portion of involved intestine containing the communication is usually required for definitive therapy. The prevalence of fistulas is 20 to 40% in Crohn's disease. Most fistulas are enteroenteric or enterocutaneous, with smaller numbers being enterovesical or enterovaginal. Total parenteral nutrition or immunomodulator therapy may induce fistula closure; however, the fistulas often recur after the total parenteral nutrition or immunomodulator therapy is stopped. Surgical treatment includes resection of the segment involved with active disease.

Obstruction

Obstruction is a common complication of Crohn's disease, particularly in the small intestine, and is a leading indication for surgery. Small bowel obstruction in Crohn's disease may be caused by mucosal thickening from acute inflammation, by muscular hyperplasia and scarring as a result of previous inflammation, or by adhesions. Obstruction may also occur because of impaction of a bolus of fibrous food in a stable, long-standing stricture. Obstruction is marked by cramping abdominal pain and diarrhea that worsen after meals and resolve with fasting. Strictures may be evaluated by oral contrast studies, barium enema, or colonoscopy, depending on the anatomic location. Corticosteroids are useful if acute inflammation is an important component of the obstructive process, but not if the obstruction is due to fibrosis. A common error in the management of Crohn's disease is treatment with long courses of corticosteroids in patients who have obstructive symptoms from fixed anatomic lesions. If the obstruction does not resolve with nasogastric suction and corticosteroids, surgery is necessary.

Perianal Disease

Perianal disease is an especially difficult complication of Crohn's disease. A complex of problems is caused by ulcers in the anal canal and the resulting fistulas. The fistulous openings are most commonly

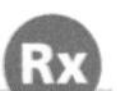

found in the perianal skin but can occur in the groin, the vulva, or the scrotum. Fistulas are accompanied by drainage of serous or mucous material. If the fistula does not drain freely, there is local accumulation of pus (perianal abscess) with redness, pain, and induration. The pain of a perianal abscess is exacerbated by defecation, sitting, or walking. The typical physical manifestation of an abscess is redness with tenderness on digital examination. Adequate evaluation of perianal disease generally requires proctoscopic examination under anesthesia. Computed tomography is useful in defining the presence and extent of perianal abscesses. The goals of therapy for perianal disease are relief of local symptoms and preservation of the sphincter. Limited disease can be approached with sitz baths and metronidazole, but in most cases adequate external drainage is also required. Azathioprine or infliximab may be useful in healing perianal disease, but the disease may reactivate when use of the drug is stopped. Persistent severe perianal Crohn's disease can result in destruction of the anal sphincter and fecal incontinence.

Follow-Up

Colon Cancer, Dysplasia, and Colonoscopic Surveillance

Patients with extensive ulcerative colitis have a markedly increased risk for colon cancer in comparison to the general population beginning 8 to 10 years after diagnosis and increasing with time. The risk for malignancy is also a function of the anatomic extent of the disease; the risk is much greater with pancolitis than with left-sided disease. Patients with long-standing ulcerative colitis are at risk for cancer (Chapter 203) even if their symptoms have been relatively mild; that is, colon cancer is seen in patients whose disease has been quiescent for 10 to 15 years. In ulcerative colitis, colon cancers are frequently submucosal and may be missed at colonoscopy. Colon cancer in patients with ulcerative colitis is associated with dysplastic changes in the mucosa at other sites in the colon. Dysplasia cannot be identified by visual inspection; microscopic examination of biopsy specimens is required. Some practitioners perform surveillance colonoscopy with random biopsies in patients with long-standing ulcerative colitis beginning 8 to 10 years after the onset of disease and repeated every 1 to 2 years. If the specimens show dysplasia, the patient is sent for colectomy. Although it is clear that dysplasia is associated with colon cancer in patients with ulcerative colitis, the utility of surveillance colonoscopy has not been firmly established. The risk for colon cancer in Crohn's colitis is less than in ulcerative colitis but greater than in the general population. The utility of surveillance in Crohn's colitis is unproven.

Pregnancy

Fertility in women with IBD is normal or only minimally impaired, and the incidence of prematurity, stillbirth, and developmental defects in the offspring of women with IBD is similar to that of the general population. The incidence of fetal complications may be somewhat higher in cases in which the mother's disease is clinically active, regardless of drug therapy. Previous proctocolectomy or the presence of an ileostomy is not an impediment to successful completion of a pregnancy. Many women have taken sulfasalazine throughout the course of pregnancy, and there is no evidence of it causing harm to the fetus. Pregnant women have an increased requirement for folic acid, and sulfasalazine interferes with folate absorption. Therefore, women taking sulfasalazine who are pregnant or considering pregnancy should receive folate supplementation (1 mg twice daily) to ensure that the fetus receives amounts adequate for normal development. The use of corticosteroids by pregnant women with IBD is not associated with an increased rate of fetal complications. In general, it appears that the risk to the pregnancy of treatment with sulfasalazine or corticosteroids is less than the risk of allowing disease activity to go untreated. Most of the data on azathioprine and 6-MP in pregnancy come from the transplant literature and involve higher doses than are commonly used for IBD. Reported fetal effects in the transplant population include congenital malformations, immunosuppression, prematurity, and growth retardation; risks in the IBD population are not known. The effects of pregnancy on IBD depend on disease activity. If the patient's disease is inactive at the time of conception, it is likely that it will remain inactive during the course of the pregnancy. If the disease is active at the time of conception, the course is harder to predict. Ulcerative colitis that is active at the time of conception tends to worsen. In two thirds of Crohn's disease cases that are active at conception, the degree of activity remains the same; in the other third, some improve clinically and others deteriorate.

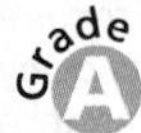

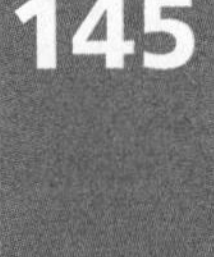

1. Hanauer SB, Feagan BG, Lichtenstein GR, et al: Maintenance infliximab for Crohn's disease: The ACCENT 1 randomized trial. Lancet 2002;359:1541–1549.
2. Lawson MM, Thoas AG, Akobeng AK: Tumour necrosis factor blocking agents for induction of remission in ulcerative colitis. Cochrane Database Syst Rev 2006:CD005112.
3. Timmer A, McDonald JW, MacDonald JK: Azathioprine and 6-mercaptopurine for maintenance of remission in ulcerative colitis. Cochrane Database Syst Rev 2007;CD00478.
4. Hanauer SB, Korelitz BI, Rutgeerts P, et al: Postoperative maintenance of Crohn's disease remission with 6-mercaptopurine, mesalamine, or placebo: A 2-year trial. Gastroenterology 2004; 127:723–729.
5. Gionchetti P, Rizzello F, Venturi A, et al: Oral bacteriotherapy as maintenance treatment in patients with chronic pouchitis: A double-blind placebo controlled trial. Gastroenterology 2000;119: 305–309.

SUGGESTED READINGS

Caprilli R, Viscido A, Latella G: Current management of severe ulcerative colitis. Nat Clin Pract Gastroenterol Hepatol 2007;4:92–101. *Clinical review.*

Gaya DR, Russell RK, Nimmo ER, et al: New genes in inflammatory bowel disease: Lessons for complex diseases? Lancet 2006;367:1271–1284. *A comprehensive review.*

Strober W, Fuss I, Mannon P: The fundamental basis of inflammatory bowel disease. J Clin Invest 2007;117:514–521. *IBD is characterized by an abnormal mucosal immune response facilitated by microbial factors and epithelial cell abnormalities.*

145 INFLAMMATORY AND ANATOMIC DISEASES OF THE INTESTINE, PERITONEUM, MESENTERY, AND OMENTUM

Charlene Prather

APPROACH TO ACUTE ABDOMINAL PAIN

Acute abdominal pain accounts for up to 10% of emergency department visits. Key features in the history and physical examination assist in narrowing the differential diagnosis in a patient with acute abdominal pain (see Table 134–2). Pain characterized by a sudden, intense onset suggests vascular occlusion (Chapter 146). Rupture of a viscous organ (e.g., a perforated duodenal ulcer; Chapters 141 and 142) can also have a similar manifestation. Colicky pain suggests renal calculi (Chapter 127) or small bowel obstruction. Although pain from cholecystitis (Chapter 159) has been referred to "biliary colic," this pain is more commonly steady with a progressive increase in intensity. Disorders with pain that progresses quickly to more severe intensity include acute pancreatitis (Chapter 147), cholecystitis, renal stones, and volvulus. Causes of pain with a more gradual progression include appendicitis, peptic ulcer disease (Chapters 141 and 142), and inflammatory bowel disease (Chapter 144). Acute pain in a patient who lies very still and avoids movement suggests peritonitis and a surgical abdomen. Acute pain in a patient who moves constantly, unable to find a comfortable position, suggests a renal stone, whereas acute pain in a patient who is most comfortable with the torso flexed suggests pancreatic pathology. Pain that increases with leg extension suggests inflammation extending to the iliopsoas muscle, as can be seen in appendicitis, diverticulitis, and abscess formation. Pain that is not localized is seen in mesenteric ischemia, bowel obstruction, obstipation, sickle cell crisis, diabetic ketoacidosis, and gastroparesis.

Physical examination of a patient with acute abdominal pain begins with measurement of vital signs. Tachycardia and hypotension require immediate attention with an assessment for hemorrhage, sepsis, or extreme dehydration. The abdominal examination starts with an explanation to the patient of what to expect. Auscultation for at least 1 minute assesses for the presence or absence of bowel sounds. Absence of bowel sounds may indicate a surgical abdomen, peritonitis, or severe ileus. Hyperperistalsis with rushes suggests bowel obstruction but can also be seen with gastroenteritis. Percussion provides an assessment of bowel gas, ascites, and organomegaly. The least tender part of the abdomen should be palpated first, with progression to the area of suspected greater discomfort last. The area of greatest tenderness and the presence of voluntary or involuntary guarding, rigidity, or rebound should be noted. A rectal examination should be performed in all patients with abdominal pain. The color of stool and the presence of gross or occult blood should be assessed. The rectal examination also provides an evaluation of the presence of fluid in the cul-de-sac. Tenderness on rectal examination can occasionally be seen in diverticulitis, appendicitis, and tubo-ovarian abscess. Pelvic examination in females identifies uterine and tubo-ovarian abnormalities. Females and males should be assessed for hernias. Examination of the male genitalia identifies epididymitis or testicular abnormalities (Chapters 210 and 253). Specific physical examination findings (Tables 145–1 and 145–2) are classically (but not invariably) associated with specific underlying pathology. Laboratory assessment and diagnostic imaging assist in assessing the severity of the underlying malady and help narrow the differential diagnosis.

Appendicitis

Definition and Epidemiology

Acute appendicitis refers to inflammation of the appendix. Appendicitis is the most common acute surgical emergency involving the abdomen. Although appendicitis occurs most commonly in young adults, it can develop at any age. The lifetime prevalence of acute appendicitis is approximately 7%.

Pathobiology

Obstruction of the appendix by a fecalith, which is thought to be the usual inciting event, is found in less than 30% of patients. Other causes of obstruction include ulceration of the appendiceal orifice, lymphoid hyperplasia, tumor (e.g., carcinoid; Chapter 251), inspissation of barium, and ascariasis (Chapter 378). Obstruction blocks the ongoing production of mucus by the appendix, thereby resulting in distention and subsequent mucosal ischemia. This process allows invasion by intraluminal bacteria, infection, and inflammation. Continued obstruction and inflammation can result in perforation, peritonitis, and abscess formation.

Clinical Manifestations

More than 95% of patients with appendicitis have abdominal pain, but only 50 to 60% have the classic symptoms of appendicitis: an acute onset

TABLE 145–1 DIFFERENTIAL DIAGNOSIS OF ACUTE ABDOMINAL PAIN BY LOCATION

Location	Diagnosis
Right upper quadrant	Cholecystitis Choledocholithiasis Duodenal ulcer Fitz-Hugh–Curtis syndrome Hepatic adenoma rupture Right lower lobe pneumonia Pulmonary embolus
Epigastric	Gastric ulcer Gastritis Pancreatitis Esophagitis Myocardial infarction Cholecystitis Choledocholithiasis
Left upper quadrant	Gastritis Peptic ulcer disease Splenic infarct Splenic hematoma Colonic ischemia Left lower lobe pneumonia Pulmonary embolus
Right lower quadrant	Appendicitis Cecal diverticulitis Crohn's disease Ileitis Ovarian cyst Tubal pregnancy Tubo-ovarian abscess
Left lower quadrant	Diverticulitis Inflammatory bowel disease Colonic ischemia Ovarian cyst Tubal pregnancy Tubo-ovarian abscess
Periumbilical	Early appendicitis Small bowel obstruction Pancreatitis Gastroenteritis Abdominal aortic aneurysm

TABLE 145–2 PHYSICAL SIGNS IN PATIENTS WITH ACUTE ABDOMINAL PAIN

Sign	Description	Associated condition
Murphy's sign	Cessation of inspiration during right upper quadrant examination	Acute cholecystitis
McBurney's sign	Tenderness located midway between the anterior superior iliac spine and umbilicus	Acute appendicitis
Cullen's sign	Periumbilical bluish discoloration	Retroperitoneal hemorrhage Pancreatic hemorrhage AAA rupture
Grey Turner's sign	Bluish discoloration of the flanks	Retroperitoneal hemorrhage Pancreatic hemorrhage AAA rupture
Kehr's sign	Severe left shoulder pain	Splenic rupture Ectopic pregnancy rupture
Obturator sign	Pain with flexed right hip rotation	Appendicitis
Psoas sign	Pain when raising a straight leg against resistance	Appendicitis (right side)

AAA = abdominal aortic aneurysm.

TABLE 145–3 DIFFERENTIAL DIAGNOSIS IN SUSPECTED APPENDICITIS

Crohn's ileitis
Mesenteric adenitis
Right-sided colonic diverticulitis
Yersinia, Campylobacter enterocolitis
Meckel's diverticulitis
Tuberculous colitis
Perforated right colon adenocarcinoma
Nephrolithiasis (right sided)
Foreign body perforation (e.g., toothpick bowel perforation)
Right tubo-ovarian abscess
Tubal pregnancy
Ovarian cyst rupture or torsion

of periumbilical pain, often with nausea and vomiting and later localizing to the right lower quadrant. The position of the appendix has important implications for the location of pain, with pain from appendicitis occurring in the suprapubic region or the right upper quadrant. Anorexia is nearly universal, nausea is frequent, but vomiting is uncommon. Acute appendicitis occurs with nonspecific abdominal symptoms and signs in the elderly and the immunosuppressed (e.g., from steroids, organ transplantation, diabetes mellitus). In elderly patients, the diagnosis is unsuspected 25% of the time.

Adults older than 50 years have a perforation rate of greater than 50%, with an intra-abdominal abscess in a third. Signs of perforation include the presence of peritoneal irritation, fever, and increasing abdominal pain.

Diagnosis

A broad differential diagnosis (Table 145–3) may be narrowed by diagnostic testing, which usually includes a complete blood count, serum electrolytes, and tests of renal function, with the addition of amylase and lipase levels when pancreatitis (Chapter 147) is suspected and liver enzymes (aminotransferase levels and alkaline phosphatase) and a bilirubin level when liver or gallbladder conditions are suspected. An elevated white blood cell count, usually in the 12,000 to 18,000/mm^3 range, is common in acute appendicitis but may not be seen early in the course; the presence and degree of elevation are not helpful in identifying complicated appendicitis.

Computed tomography (CT), which is the preferred test [1] to confirm the diagnosis or suggest other causes (Fig. 145–1), has a sensitivity ranging from 88 to 100%, a specificity of 91 to 99%, a positive predictive value of 92 to 98%, and a negative predictive value of 95 to 100%. With a reported overall diagnostic accuracy of 94 to 98% and the ability to detect abscess formation (Fig. 145–2), CT has become the imaging diagnostic modality of choice. Its disadvantages include the need for ionizing radiation (more significant in children and young adults) and intravenous contrast, which entails a risk for adverse reactions, including nephrotoxicity. Ultrasound, though more operator dependent, provides a safe, noninvasive, and relatively inexpensive alternative in relatively thin, younger patients or when gynecologic causes are also included in the differential diagnosis. Plain abdominal radiographs typically provide nonspecific findings, with a calcified fecalith identified in less than 10% of patients; they are not a useful part of the evaluation, which should begin with a CT scan. For nonspecific abdominal pain, watchful waiting is as good as early diagnostic laparoscopy. [2]

Treatment

Rx

When appendicitis is suspected, early surgical consultation is indicated. Treatment of appendicitis is appendectomy, which is increasingly being performed laparoscopically, although 2 days of intravenous antibiotics followed by 10 days of oral antibiotics is a reasonable short-term alternative in the absence of evidence of perforation when surgery cannot be performed safely in the interim. [3] Laparoscopic appendectomy generally takes longer than the open operation but results in faster recovery and a lower rate of wound infection. [4] In the presence of an appendicular abscess, percutaneous ultrasound- or CT-guided drainage may precede surgical intervention.

Preoperative antibiotics (e.g., cefotetan, 2 g intravenously, or cefoxitin, 2 g intravenously, followed by three postoperative doses, or ticarcillin/clavulanic acid) reduce infectious complications in otherwise uncomplicated appendicitis. In the setting of perforation, the duration of antibiotic therapy should be 7 to 10 days with a third-generation cephalosporin or monobactam, plus anaerobic coverage with metronidazole or clindamycin.

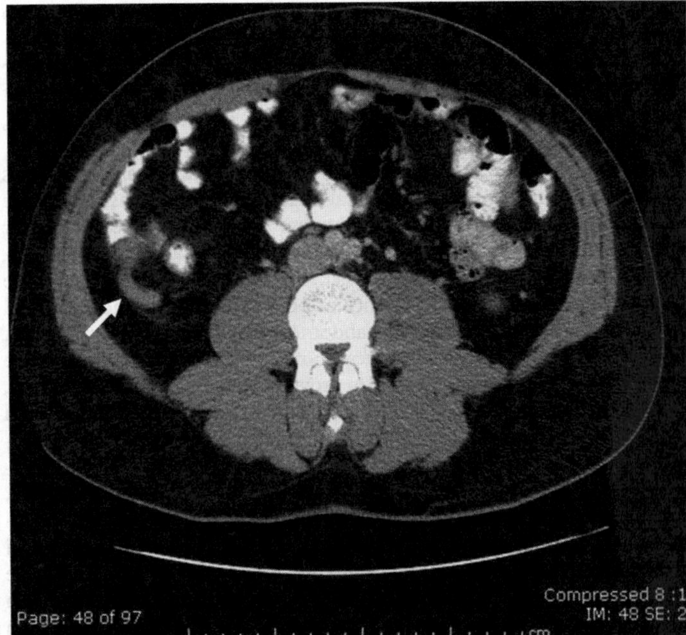

FIGURE 145–1 • Appendicitis. A CT scan shows an edematous appendix with a diameter greater than 1 cm (arrow), consistent with acute, uncomplicated appendicitis.

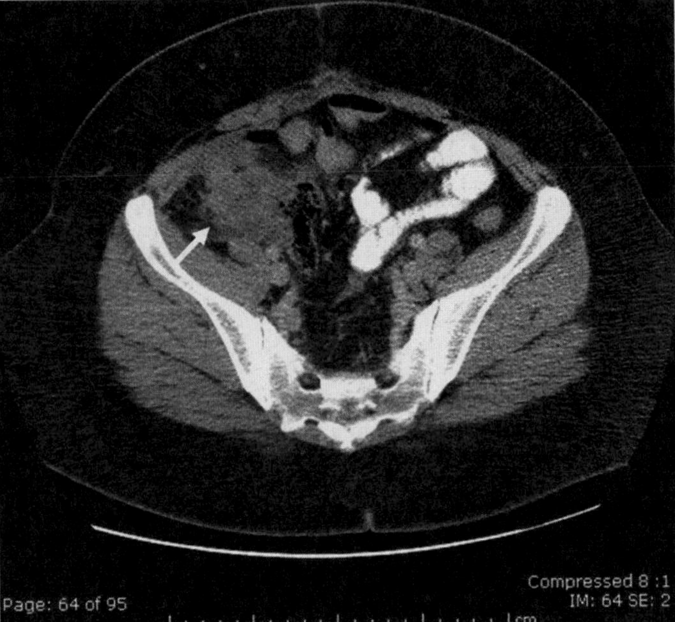

FIGURE 145–2 • Appendicitis. A CT scan shows appendicitis complicated by perforation with abscess formation (arrow).

Section XII Gastroenterology

TABLE 145–4 TERMINOLOGY IN DIVERTICULAR DISEASE

Diverticular disease	The entire spectrum of diverticulosis and its complications
Diverticulosis	The presence of one or more diverticula
Diverticulitis	Inflammation or infection of one or more colonic diverticula
Complicated diverticulitis	Diverticulitis with abscess, fistula formation, free perforation, or obstruction
Painful diverticular disease	Abdominal pain and altered bowel habit in the setting of diverticulosis without another explanation (may be a manifestation of irritable bowel syndrome)
Diverticular bleeding	Acute lower gastrointestinal bleeding from a colonic diverticulum

Prognosis

The frequency of complications associated with perforated appendicitis is greater than 18%, as opposed to a 10% frequency of complications in nonperforated appendicitis. Overall mortality in patients with perforated appendicitis is 3%, but it can be as high as 15% in the elderly.

Diverticulitis of the Colon

Definition

Colonic diverticulosis refers to uncomplicated herniations of the colonic mucosa and submucosa through the muscular layer of the colon. Technically, these lesions are actually pseudodiverticula because all layers of the colon are not involved. Diverticular disease encompasses a spectrum of problems occurring in the setting of diverticulosis, including diverticulitis, painful diverticular disease, and complicated diverticular disease (Table 145–4).

Epidemiology

Although colonic diverticulosis is quite common and affects up to 10% of middle-aged adults and 50 to 80% of those older than 80 years, few people are aware that they have them. Diverticulosis is uncommon in individuals younger than 40 years. Diverticulosis is predominantly a disorder of industrialized or Western populations, where it correlates with low intake of dietary fiber. Obesity appears to be a risk factor for diverticulosis in young males.

Pathobiology

Colonic diverticulosis most commonly occurs at the location where the vasa recta (nutrient artery) penetrates through the muscularis propria. In Western populations, diverticulosis occurs more commonly in the left colon, with the sigmoid colon most frequently involved, perhaps because of the relatively higher pressure present in the lumen of the sigmoid colon. However, in Asian populations, a right-sided distribution is more common.

Diverticulitis is the presence of infection and inflammation of a diverticulum and will develop in 10 to 25% of persons with diverticulosis in their lifetime. Diverticulitis results from inflammation of a colonic diverticulum with subsequent microperforation, which is thought to be caused by the presence of particulate debris within the diverticular sac that compresses or erodes the blood vessel and thereby leads to perforation. Diverticulitis occurs most commonly in the sigmoid colon. Complicated diverticulitis includes abscess formation, free perforation, colonic obstruction, and fistula formation.

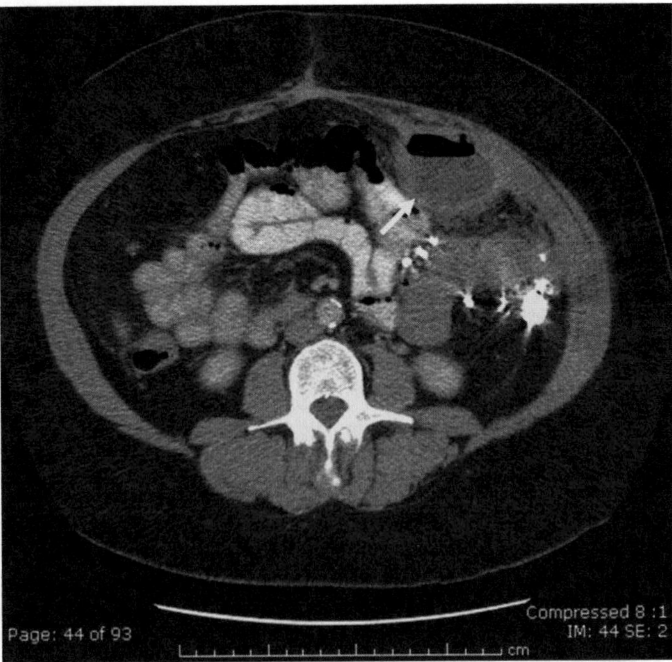

FIGURE 145–3 • Diverticulitis. A CT scan shows perforated diverticulitis with abscess formation (arrow). The abscess is identified as the air-filled collection. Residual contrast remains in the diverticulum.

Clinical Manifestations

Patients with diverticulitis most commonly have anorexia, left lower quadrant pain, and fever. The pain in diverticulitis may radiate to the flank, back, or suprapubic region. Patients may report loose stools or constipation. On physical examination, left lower quadrant tenderness can usually be demonstrated. The examination may also identify the presence of localized guarding and occasionally a tender painful mass. The presence of peritoneal signs (e.g., rebound) suggests a free perforation.

Diverticular bleeding is manifested as painless rectal bleeding, with massive bleeding occurring in 5% of patients with diverticulosis (Chapter 137). Diverticular bleeding is uncommon in the setting of acute diverticulitis.

Diagnosis

Leukocytosis is present in 70 to 80% of patients. When the diverticulitis is adjacent to the bladder, pyuria may occur. Additional associated symptoms include nausea, vomiting, altered bowel pattern, and urinary symptoms. Conditions with findings similar to those of diverticulitis include gastroenteritis, appendicitis, inflammatory bowel disease (Chapter 144), and a perforating colon cancer (Chapter 203).

CT radiography, which reliably identifies the presence and location of inflammation, may show the colonic diverticula, inflammation involving the pericolic fat, and a colonic wall thicker than 4 mm (Fig. 145–3). Barium radiography, which can demonstrate diverticula (Fig. 145–4), will also identify whether the colon connects with the fluid collection in the setting of perforation and abscess formation; it is not recommended in the acute setting because of a higher risk for colonic perforation from contrast or air insufflation. After the acute syndrome has resolved, colonoscopy can also show diverticula (Fig. 145–5) and is essential to exclude malignancy, even in younger patients.

Treatment Rx

Uncomplicated diverticulitis may be treated in the outpatient setting with broad-spectrum antibiotics such as ciprofloxacin and metronidazole for 7 to 10 days (Table 145–5). Patients are started on a clear liquid diet that can be advanced as symptoms resolve. Patients unable to maintain oral intake require hospitalization for hydration and intravenous antibiotics.

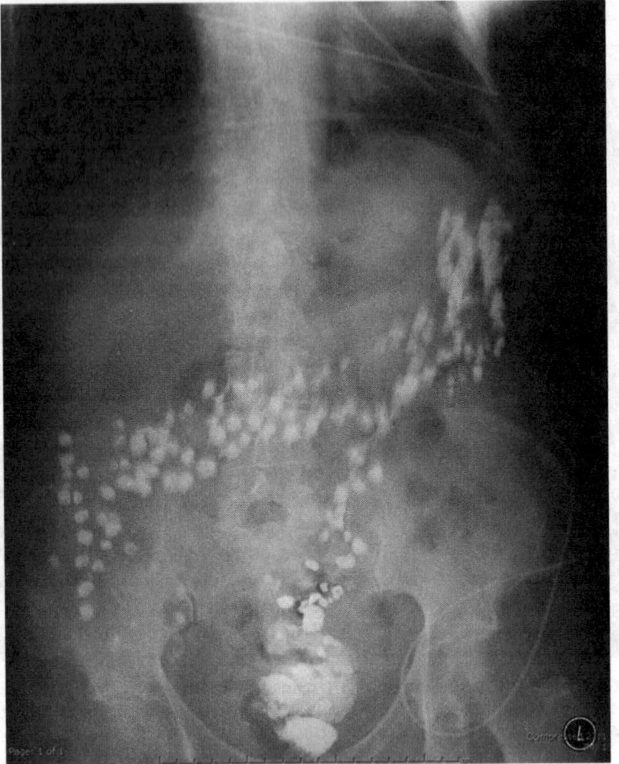

FIGURE 145–4 • Colonic diverticula. An abdominal flat plate shows residual barium in diverticula scattered throughout the colon.

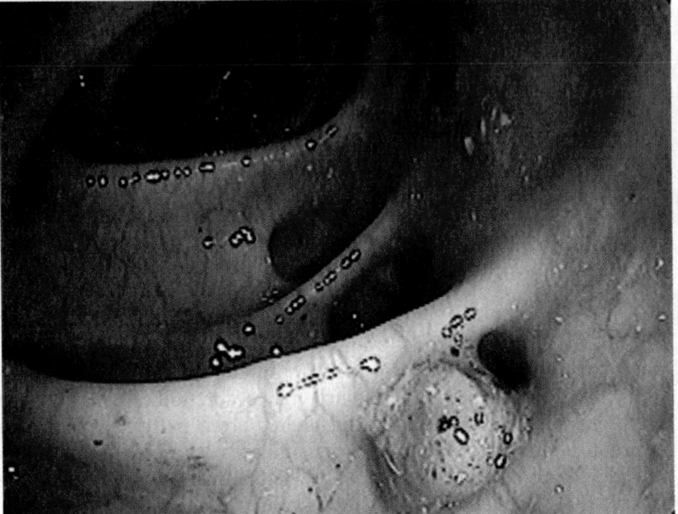

FIGURE 145–5 • Sigmoid diverticula. A colonoscopic photo shows sigmoid diverticula.

Rx

Most patients improve quickly over a period of 2 to 3 days. After recovery, a high-fiber diet is recommended, albeit with little evidence to support its role in preventing further complications. Elective resection carries a mortality rate of 1 to 4%, and expectant management rather than operative treatment is probably associated with less mortality and fewer colostomies, and it is also less expensive.

However, patients younger than 40 years may experience a more aggressive form of the disease, so surgical resection is sometimes recommended after the first episode of diverticulitis. Patients with conditions resulting in immune system compromise may benefit from earlier (after a first episode) surgery because of their reduced

TABLE 145–5 ANTIBIOTIC OPTIONS FOR ACUTE DIVERTICULITIS (GENERALLY FOR 7–10 DAYS)

Ciprofloxacin, 750 mg bid, and metronidazole, 500 mg q6h
Levofloxacin, 750 mg IV q24h, and metronidazole, 500 mg q6h
Trimethoprim/sulfamethoxazole-DS, bid
Piperacillin/tazobactam, 3.375 g q6h
Ampicillin/sulbactam, 3.0 g q6h
Imipenem/cilastatin sodium, 500 mg q6h (reserved for life-threatening infection)

ability to ward off infection and their increased risk for emergency surgery.

Patients with diverticular abscesses are treated by CT-guided drainage and subsequent surgery, usually 6 weeks after successful abscess drainage. Laparoscopic resection, which is increasingly being performed for diverticular disease, results in shorter hospitalization and an early return to full function. Patients with complicated diverticulitis have a mortality of 6.5% and morbidity of 41%; when perforated diverticulitis is excluded, the mortality is less than 2%. Older age, immunosuppressive medications, preexisting medical problems (especially preexisting cardiac and pulmonary disease), and perforated diverticulitis increase postoperative morbidity.

Prevention

A high-fiber diet with avoidance of nuts and seeds has been recommended for patients with diverticulosis, but evidence is inadequate to support or refute this recommendation. Randomized trials show that the combination of fiber and rifaximin (400 mg twice daily for 7 days every month), a poorly absorbable antibiotic, decreases symptoms over a 12-month period. [5] Other medications used to reduce recurrent diverticular symptoms included mesalazine and calcium-channel blockers, although the evidence to support their use is inconclusive. The use of nonsteroidal anti-inflammatory drugs (NSAIDs) increases the risk for diverticular perforation.

Prognosis

The risk for a second attack of diverticulitis is less than 25%. After a second attack of diverticulitis, the risk for subsequent episodes of diverticulitis exceeds 50%, and the risk increases with each subsequent episode. Surgical therapy to remove the segment of colon involved with diverticulosis is often recommended after a second episode of diverticulitis. After elective resection, 25% of patients have persistent symptoms, including altered bowel habits and pain (probably reflecting coexistent irritable bowel syndrome), and 10% have recurrent diverticulitis.

Small Bowel Infections

Small Bowel Bacterial Overgrowth

Definition

The proximal portion of the small bowel normally has relatively few bacteria. An excessive number of bacteria colonize the small bowel (>10^5 organisms/mL) in patients with small bowel bacterial overgrowth. This abnormal colonization includes increased numbers of gram-negative aerobes and anaerobes.

Epidemiology

Bacterial overgrowth is commonly considered in the setting of intestinal dysmotility, such as found in scleroderma or diabetic autonomic neuropathy. In addition, bacterial overgrowth has been reported in patients with acute and chronic pancreatitis, cirrhosis, chronic renal failure, and irritable bowel syndrome and in the elderly, in whom it may be manifested as unexplained weight loss, diarrhea, or vitamin deficiencies (e.g., vitamin B_{12} deficiency). The use of high-dose acid suppression (as with proton pump inhibitors) has also been implicated as increasing the risk for small bowel bacterial overgrowth. Previous gastric resection may predispose to bacterial overgrowth from hypoacidity and intestinal dysmotility. Surgical loss of the ileocecal valve also predisposes to migration of colonic bacteria up into the small intestine. Additionally, bacterial overgrowth occurs in the setting of small bowel strictures and partial bowel obstruction.

Pathobiology

Excess bacteria can deconjugate bile acids, thereby resulting in reduced micelle formation and malabsorption of fat. Small bowel bacterial overgrowth can also cause an osmotic diarrhea from bacterial products or a secretory diarrhea from mucosal damage, including villous atrophy. The excess bacteria in the small bowel consume dietary vitamin B_{12} and thus lead to B_{12} deficiency. The bacteria produce folic acid, levels of which can be elevated in serum. D-Lactate, another byproduct of bacterial overgrowth, can cause a D-lactic acidosis.

Clinical Manifestations

Bacterial overgrowth in the small bowel may be accompanied by chronic diarrhea, bloating, abdominal pain, nausea, malabsorption, macrocytic anemia (vitamin B_{12} deficiency), or steatorrhea.

Diagnosis

Small bowel bacterial overgrowth is difficult to diagnose. The length and relative inaccessibility of the small bowel make culture techniques insensitive, though very specific. A variety of breath tests (see Table 143–7) take advantage of metabolism of the substrate by the bacteria, the production of hydrogen or methane by the bacteria, absorption by the body, and exhalation in breath. The glucose breath test (sensitivity of 67 to 98%, specificity of 77 to 100%) is useful for diagnosing bacterial overgrowth in the proximal portion of the small bowel. The poorly absorbed carbohydrate lactulose provides a more sensitive assessment for more distal bacterial overgrowth but may be falsely positive in patients with rapid small bowel transit or previous resection of the stomach or small bowel. Other substrates sometimes used include fructose and ^{14}C-D-xylose.

Treatment

Rx

A variety of broad-spectrum antibiotics can be used, including doxycycline, amoxicillin–clavulanic acid, ciprofloxacin, norfloxacin, metronidazole, and rifaximin (Table 145–6); a 7- to 14-day duration of therapy is recommended. Nonabsorbable antibiotics (e.g., rifaximin) may reduce systemic side effects. Neomycin is used less commonly because of concern regarding renal toxicity. Patients with intestinal strictures, partial obstruction, and intestinal dysmotility frequently require repeated courses of treatment and, occasionally, chronic suppressive therapy.

TABLE 145–6 ANTIBIOTIC OPTIONS FOR SMALL BOWEL BACTERIAL OVERGROWTH (TYPICALLY FOR 7–10 DAYS)

Doxycycline, 100 mg bid
Amoxicillin–clavulanic acid, 750 mg bid
Ciprofloxacin, 250–500 mg bid
Norfloxacin, 800 mg qd
Metronidazole,* 500 mg tid
Rifaximin, 1200 mg daily

*Limited value as monotherapy.

Whipple's Disease

A rare chronic, relapsing, multisystem condition, Whipple's disease (Chapter 143) is associated with the gastrointestinal manifestations of diarrhea and malabsorption. Thickening of the small bowel is common. Caused by the bacterium *Tropheryma whippelii,* Whipple's disease is diagnosed by upper endoscopy and small bowel biopsy. The small bowel mucosa and submucosa are infiltrated with foamy macrophages and have inclusions that stain positive with periodic acid–Schiff stain. Polymerase chain reaction analysis provides the "gold standard" diagnosis. Treatment includes an induction phase with intravenous penicillin (6 to 24 million U/day) plus streptomycin (1 g/day intramuscularly) or ceftriaxone (2 g/day intravenously) for 10 to 14 days, followed by a year of therapy with oral trimethoprim-sulfamethoxazole (160/800 mg twice daily). Less aggressive antibiotic regimens result in a greater frequency of relapse.

Intestinal Tuberculosis

Mycobacterium tuberculosis (Chapter 345) involving the small intestine is manifested most commonly as abdominal pain, vomiting, and diarrhea. The disease may be subacute with waxing and waning symptoms or be marked by more fulminant sepsis. The intestinal lesions include nodularity, ulcerations, skip lesions, and strictures, features similar to those found in small bowel Crohn's disease. The diagnosis is made by biopsy, stains, and culture. When the small bowel is not accessible endoscopically, exploratory laparotomy for full-thickness biopsy may be required to make the diagnosis. Treatment with conventional antituberculous therapy results in symptomatic improvement.

Histoplasmosis

Histoplasma capsulatum (Chapter 353) typically involves the gastrointestinal tract in the setting of disseminated disease in the immunocompromised, predominately in patients with acquired immunodeficiency syndrome. Gastrointestinal involvement is accompanied by bleeding, obstruction, diarrhea, and malabsorption. Small bowel lesions include ulcerations, polypoid lesions, and masses that simulate carcinoma. The granulomatous changes present on biopsy must be differentiated from Crohn's disease, tuberculosis, and less commonly, sarcoidosis. Treatment is directed at the underlying disseminated infection.

INTESTINAL INVOLVEMENT IN SYSTEMIC DISEASES

Sarcoidosis

Sarcoidosis (Chapter 95) of the gastrointestinal tract is relatively uncommon. Small bowel and colonic involvement has manifestations similar to those of Crohn's disease, with ulceration and non-necrotizing granulomas. Gastrointestinal involvement typically occurs in the setting of other systemic symptoms of sarcoidosis. Patients have abdominal pain, vomiting, diarrhea, or protein-losing enteropathy, or any combination of these findings. Treatment is aimed at the systemic disease.

Neutropenic Enterocolitis

Neutropenic enterocolitis is also referred to as typhlitis. Though originally described in children after induction chemotherapy for acute leukemia, it is an increasingly recognized clinical syndrome in adults as well.

Clinical Manifestations and Diagnosis

The syndrome occurs in neutropenic patients (absolute neutrophil count <500/μL) and consists of right lower quadrant abdominal pain, distention, fever, nausea, vomiting, and diarrhea, which may be bloody. Symptoms typically occur 10 to 14 days after high-dose chemotherapy.

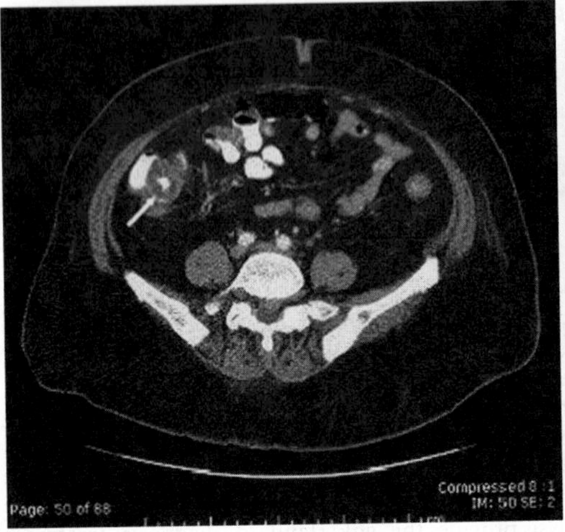

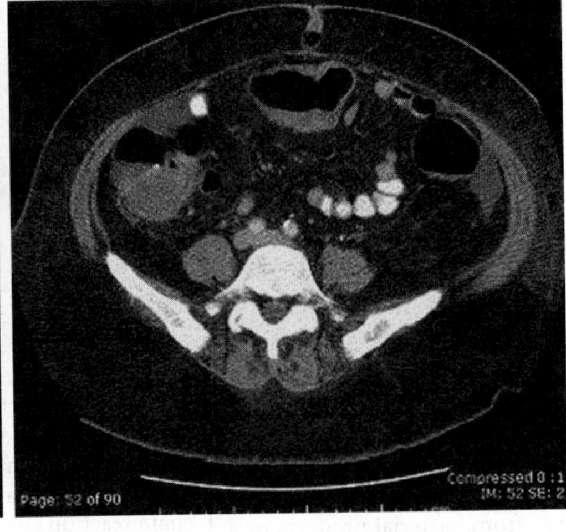

FIGURE 145–6 • CT scans showing neutropenic colitis. The left scan shows a thickened cecal wall (arrow). Eight days latter a follow-up scan showed resolution (right scan).

The clinical findings are nonspecific and overlap with symptoms seen in *Clostridium difficile* colitis (Chapter 319), ischemic colitis (Chapter 146), and colonic pseudo-obstruction (Chapter 138). CT findings include a thickened colonic wall (>4 mm), dilated cecum, and pericecal inflammatory changes (Fig. 145–6).

Treatment

Conservative management includes bowel rest, nasogastric suction when bowel dilation is present, and broad-spectrum antibiotics to cover gram-positive and enteric gram-negative organisms, as well as anaerobes. Recombinant granulocyte colony-stimulating factor has been recommended to correct neutropenia. Lower gastrointestinal bleeding resulting from the colitis with a coexisting coagulopathy necessitates correction of the coagulopathy and blood transfusions. Surgery is indicated in the setting of impending or free perforation, when bleeding cannot be stopped, and for otherwise unexplained clinical deterioration. Symptoms improve rapidly as the neutropenia resolves.

Visceral Angioedema

Visceral angioedema is seen with hereditary and acquired C1 esterase inhibitor deficiency (Chapter 273), hypocomplementemia, drugs (especially angiotensin-converting enzyme inhibitors), or foods or may be idiopathic. Acquired C1 esterase inhibitor deficiency may occur as a paraneoplastic syndrome and is occasionally seen in autoimmune disorders. Angioedema of the gastrointestinal tract is commonly manifested as abdominal pain and distention, nausea, vomiting, and diarrhea. The symptoms may be accompanied by swelling of the mucous membrane, hives, wheezing, or dyspnea. CT findings include thickened, fluid-filled loops of small bowel. Ascites may also be present. The symptoms last 1 to 3 days and may recur periodically. The diagnosis is established by identifying suspect drugs, low serum levels of C4, low C1 esterase quantitative levels, or reduced C1 esterase functional activity.

Systemic Lupus Erythematosus

As a multisystem disease, systemic lupus erythematosus (Chapter 287) frequently affects the gastrointestinal tract. Abdominal pain may be due to serositis, mesenteric ischemia, vasculitis, intestinal dysmotility, angioedema, or pancreatitis. Clinical manifestations include abdominal pain, nausea, vomiting, abdominal bloating, distention, diarrhea, and malabsorption. Small bowel bacterial overgrowth also occurs, presumably secondary to the underlying dysmotility. Treatment consists of management of the underlying systemic disease.

Eosinophilic Gastroenteritis

Eosinophilic gastrointestinal diseases are most commonly recognized in children but can also occur in adults. The disease is characterized by eosinophilic infiltration that can involve the mucosa, submucosa, and muscularis. Any part of the gastrointestinal tract may be affected. Intestinal involvement is manifested as abdominal pain, nausea, vomiting, diarrhea, and occasionally, malabsorption. CT findings include thickened small bowel loops and nodularity of the folds. Peripheral eosinophilia is often present. Treatment of intestinal involvement typically requires the use of systemic steroids, often starting at a dose of 20 to 40 mg of prednisone per day. Up to 90% of patients respond in 1 to 2 weeks and can have the medication tapered, but about 50% of patients may require 5 to 10 mg/day of prednisone long-term.

Radiation Enterocolitis

Patients who receive radiation therapy for intra-abdominal and pelvic neoplasms are at risk for radiation-induced injury.

Epidemiology

The risk for injury varies according to the size of the radiation field and the dose received. Chronic radiation enterocolitis occurs approximately a year after completion of radiation therapy but may develop up to 20 years later. Doses greater than 50 Gy increase the risk for chronic changes, such as the development of obliterative arteritis, intestinal wall fibrosis, and serosal thickening. Other risk factors include older age, previous abdominal surgery, and a larger field of radiation. The quantity of small bowel in the radiation field is a strong predictor of subsequent complications.

Clinical Manifestations and Diagnosis

Symptoms of acute radiation enterocolitis commonly include diarrhea, intestinal bleeding, and fecal incontinence. These symptoms are typically self-limited and resolve within a few months after the completion of radiation treatment.

Symptoms of chronic radiation enterocolitis commonly include abdominal pain and diarrhea. Gastrointestinal bleeding results from vascular ectasia. The bleeding is typically chronic and occult, with the development of iron deficiency anemia, but occasionally it is overt. Complete or partial bowel obstruction from adhesions or strictures, fistulas, small bowel bacterial overgrowth, and malabsorption can also occur.

Diagnostic imaging includes CT radiography or colonoscopy. The finding of a stricture necessitates an evaluation to exclude malignancy.

Prevention and Treatment

Prevention of radiation enteritis includes minimizing the volume of small bowel and colon in the radiation field. Treatment is predominantly supportive. Management of bleeding includes endoscopic ablation of telangiectactic lesions and chronic iron therapy.

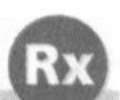

Sucralfate enemas (2 g twice daily) may improve symptoms, but the data are not conclusive.

For acute obstruction, bowel rest and nasogastric suction may allow resolution; surgery is reserved for complete bowel obstruction that does not improve or perforation. Poor wound healing, anastomotic leaks, and fistulas may complicate surgical operations. Patients with diarrhea should be evaluated for small bowel bacterial overgrowth. Cholestyramine, loperamide, and diphenoxylate/atropine provide first-line options for treating diarrhea (Chapter 143), but stronger opiates such as codeine, morphine, or tincture of opium are sometimes required. Caution is necessary when using these agents because of the risk for development of bowel dilation and obstipation.

Intestinal Ulceration

Nonsteroidal Anti-inflammatory Drugs

Small intestinal ulcerations are increasing being recognized with the advent of small bowel capsule endoscopy (Chapter 136). The most common cause of small intestinal ulcers is the use of NSAIDs (Chapter 34). Small bowel and colonic erosions and ulcerations occur in 60 to 70% of long-term users of NSAIDs. Diaphragm-type strictures of the small bowel and, less frequently, the colon also result from chronic NSAID use.

Clinical Manifestations and Diagnosis

Most NSAID-related lesions are asymptomatic, but symptoms suggesting NSAID enteropathy include gastrointestinal bleeding, abdominal pain, iron deficiency anemia, diarrhea, hypoalbuminemia, and obstructive symptoms. Ulceration can be detected by small bowel enteroscopy, small bowel capsule endoscopy, and colonoscopy.

Treatment

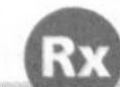

Treatment consists of discontinuing NSAIDs. When obstruction is present and conservative treatment fails, surgical resection may be required.

OTHER INFLAMMATORY CONDITIONS

Ulcerative jejunitis is an uncommon manifestation of celiac disease (Chapter 143). This diagnosis is suspected in patients with persistent symptoms despite a gluten-free diet.

Ulceration of any part of the gastrointestinal tract may occur in *Behçet's disease* (Chapter 291). Symptoms include abdominal pain, diarrhea, and gastrointestinal bleeding. Most patients with gastrointestinal involvement have ileocecal involvement with a single or few ulcers. In the absence of obvious systemic symptoms, Behçet's disease can be difficult to differentiate from Crohn's disease.

Patients with *polyarteritis nodosa* (Chapter 291) may have intermittent or persistent abdominal complications. Gastrointestinal involvement occurs in half or more of patients with polyarteritis nodosa. Most have abdominal pain, nausea, vomiting, melena, hematochezia, diarrhea, and occasionally, constipation; however, severe abdominal pain can also develop as a result of mesenteric vasculitis with gastrointestinal infarction and perforation. These gastrointestinal complications of polyarteritis nodosa result in considerable morbidity and mortality, with a mortality rate of 23% to greater than 60% when the symptoms include an acute abdomen. The diagnosis is typically made by CT radiography and magnetic resonance or CT angiography; less frequently, angiography is required. Although colonoscopy can identify ischemia, its role is limited in the acute setting because of the risk for perforation. Treatment is directed at the systemic disease (Chapter 291).

Henoch-Schönlein purpura (Chapter 291) is an IgA-mediated vasculitis with skin, abdominal, and renal manifestations. Abdominal symptoms include pain, nausea, vomiting, diarrhea, and gastrointestinal bleeding. Small bowel thickening and intussusception can be seen on CT radiography. Upper endoscopy and colonoscopy are not usually necessary diagnostically but can show submucosal hemorrhage, erythema, swelling, and ulcerations. Similar changes are also present in the small intestine as imaged by capsule endoscopy. The disease is often self-limited but may require systemic therapy (Chapter 291).

Peritoneal Disorders

Peritonitis

Definition

The peritoneum is the smooth serous membrane that lines the abdominal and pelvic cavities. The most common clinical disorders of the peritoneum are ascites (Chapter 157) and peritonitis. Peritonitis may be acute or chronic, septic or aseptic, primary or secondary, and localized or diffuse.

Epidemiology and Pathobiology

Acute peritonitis results from acute disruption of the peritoneal cavity with infectious or inflammatory materials. In the setting of perforation of the bowel or an intra-abdominal viscus, the contents themselves may be inflammatory, such as with bile spillage, or may be infectious, such as with contamination from intraluminal contents (e.g., bacteria and fecal material). Aseptic peritonitis results from the introduction of sterile bile, digestive juices, or extrinsic materials (e.g., chemotherapeutic medications) into the peritoneal cavity. Aseptic peritonitis rarely remains that way, with infection typically following in due course. Primary peritonitis refers to spontaneous bacterial peritonitis without an identifiable cause, typically in the setting of chronic liver disease (Chapter 149). Secondary peritonitis results most commonly from a perforated viscus such as the appendix, a diverticulum, peptic ulcer disease, or trauma with secondary spillage of luminal contents into the peritoneum. The most common bacteriology in secondary peritonitis is a mixed flora with *Escherichia coli*, *Streptococcus faecalis*, *Pseudomonas aeruginosa*, *Klebsiella mirabilis*, *Bacteroides fragilis*, *Clostridium* species, and anaerobic streptococci.

Clinical Manifestations

Clinical manifestations of acute diffuse peritonitis typically include the sudden onset of abdominal pain that is usually constant. The pain may be diffuse or referred to the umbilicus or the portion of the abdomen where the inciting event originated. The peritoneal inflammation may subside or localize, thereby resulting in a reduction in pain and improved localization. Additional symptoms include nausea, vomiting, and fever. The development of progressive tachycardia and a falling temperature are grave signs of impending peritoneal shock from bacterial toxemia and septicemia (Chapter 109) (Fig. 145–7).

Additional physical signs (Chapter 134) include a very still patient. Bowel sounds are typically diminished or absent in the setting of peritonitis. Percussion often reveals tympany from the resultant ileus. On palpation, tenderness and rigidity are present. Rebound tenderness, with increasing pain when the examining hand is lifted from the abdomen, is usually present. Increased pain may also be elicited in the affected area on examination of an uninvolved portion of the abdomen. The abdominal muscles may become boardlike with rigidity, although this sign is frequently absent in the elderly and the immunosuppressed.

Diagnosis

Identifying the cause of the peritonitis depends on the age and sex of the patient. In younger patients, appendicitis and a perforated duodenal ulcer (Chapters 141 and 142) are most common. In older patients, perforated diverticula and cancer (Chapter 203) are more common. The use of NSAIDs or aspirin increases the likelihood of a perforated ulcer or diverticula. In young females, tubal pregnancy and a ruptured tubo-ovarian abscess must be considered (Chapters 307 and 323). CT imaging identifies the presence of free air and often is the cause of the intra-abdominal calamity (see Fig. 145–3).

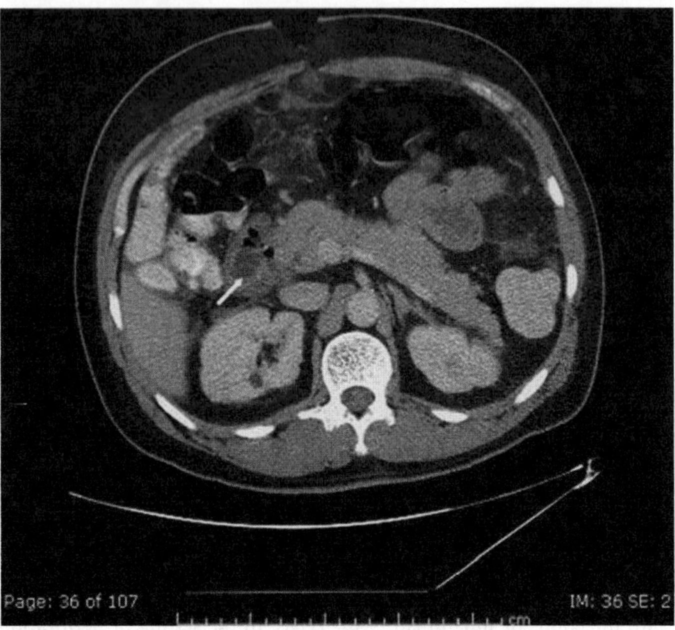

FIGURE 145–7 • CT scan in a patient with peritonitis. Thickening of the duodenal wall (arrow) was identified at surgery as a perforated duodenal ulcer.

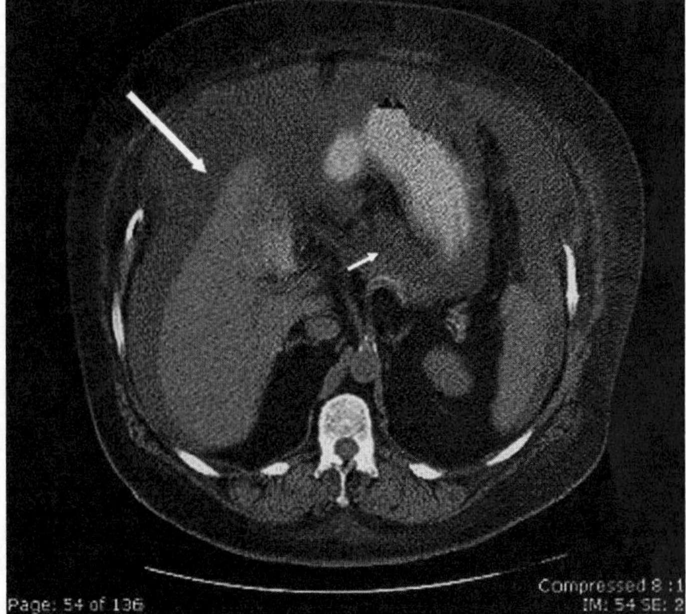

FIGURE 145–8 • Malignant ascites. A CT scan shows ascites (large arrow) and a gastric mass (small arrow).

TABLE 145–7 ANTIBIOTIC OPTIONS FOR INTRA-ABDOMINAL SECONDARY PERITONITIS

Piperacillin/tazobactam, 3.375 g q6h
Ampicillin/sulbactam, 3.0 g q6h
Ciprofloxacin, 400 q12h, and metronidazole, 1 g q12h
Levofloxacin, 750 mg q24h
Cefepime, 2 g q12h, and metronidazole, 1 g q12h
Imipenum/cilastatin sodium, 500 mg q6h

Treatment

Rx

Treatment focuses on resuscitation, control of infection, and laparoscopy. The presence of suspected acute peritonitis necessitates surgical consultation. Correction of volume depletion and electrolyte disturbances with intravenous fluids is the cornerstone of initial management. Blood should be obtained for culture and broad-spectrum antibiotics administered prophylactically to cover gram-negative and anaerobic bacteria (Table 145–7).

Peritoneal Carcinomatosis and Malignant Ascites

Less than 10% of cases of ascites are malignant. Peritoneal carcinomatosis results from the metastatic spread of intra-abdominal malignancy (Table 145–8), usually in the setting of endometrial, colonic, gastric, and pancreatic carcinoma. The manifestation is similar to ascites of other causes (Chapter 149), although the ascites typically occurs rather suddenly in the absence of known portal hypertension, tuberculosis, or right heart failure.

Diagnosis

In the setting of new-onset ascites, diagnostic paracentesis should be performed. Aspirated fluid should be sent for cell count and differential, Gram stain and culture, and measurement of albumin with simultaneous serum albumin measurement. A serum minus ascites albumin value of less than 1.1 g/mL (Chapter 157) supports the diagnosis of malignant ascites but is also seen in pancreatitis, nephrotic syndrome, and peritoneal tuberculosis. In the setting of hepatic metastases, the serum-ascites albumin gradient may be greater than 1.1. Ascitic fluid cytology will identify malignant cells 50 to 60% of the time.

Abnormal ultrasound findings can confirm the presence of ascites, but CT is preferred to help identify the underlying cause (Fig. 145–8). Malignant ascites is frequently loculated, sometimes from previous surgically related adhesions.

TABLE 145–8 CAUSES OF PERITONEAL CARCINOMATOSIS

PRIMARY
Mesothelioma
Sarcoma
SECONDARY INTRA-ABDOMINAL MALIGNANCIES
Gastric adenocarcinoma
Colon adenocarcinoma
Pancreatic adenocarcinoma
Ovarian carcinoma
Neuroendocrine tumors, including carcinoid
Lymphoma
EXTRA-ABDOMINAL MALIGNANCIES
Breast
Melanoma
Lung

Treatment

Treatment of malignant ascites is symptomatic and quite challenging. In general, malignant ascites does not respond to diuretic therapy, except that patients with malignant ascites in the setting of hepatic metastases may respond to spironolactone. Therapeutic paracentesis in the setting of tense ascites improves symptoms, including shortness of breath and abdominal discomfort. Unfortunately, malignant ascites rapidly reaccumulates. The use of intracavitary radioisotopes or chemotherapy has been advocated in some cases for palliation with variable success.

Prognosis

The development of malignant ascites is usually a poor prognostic indicator, with few patients surviving beyond 4 months. An exception is the better prognosis with malignant ascites from ovarian (Chapter 209) or breast cancer (Chapter 208).

Peritoneal Tuberculosis

In the United States, tuberculosis (Chapter 345) is relatively uncommon, although it is increasingly being identified in immigrants. Tuberculous ascites also occurs in cirrhosis and in patients with chronic renal disease who are maintained on peritoneal dialysis.

Peritoneal tuberculosis is accompanied by abdominal swelling, fever, anorexia, and weight loss. The diagnosis should be considered in the setting of refractory ascites. Analysis of ascitic fluid reveals an exudative ascites. The fluid protein is typically greater than 2.5 g/100 mL, with a serum-ascites gradient of less than 1.1 g/mL.

Treatment

Rx

Treatment involves conventional antituberculous therapy (Chapter 345).

Peritonitis Associated with Continuous Ambulatory Peritoneal Dialysis

Patients in whom peritonitis develops while undergoing continuous ambulatory peritoneal dialysis (Chapter 133) have abdominal pain and cloudy peritoneal fluid. Approximately 50% of patients have fever. Nausea and diarrhea may also occur. On physical examination, abdominal pain is usually present.

Diagnosis is based on the peritoneal fluid cell count and differential. Although Gram stain is rarely positive, any organisms that are seen are predictive of subsequent culture results. Peritoneal cultures are positive 90% of the time. Gram-positive organisms predominant, with coagulase-negative staphylococci and *Staphylococcus aureus* most commonly identified. Gram-negative organisms are present about 20% of the time, and 10% of patients have polymicrobial infections. Fungal peritonitis is infrequent and usually due to *Candida* species.

Antibiotic choices for empirical therapy include intraperitoneal cefazolin, cephalothin, and ceftazidime. Aminoglycosides should be used only when residual urine volume is less than 100 mL/day. Once culture results are available, antibiotics are adjusted according to the sensitivity of the organisms.

Miscellaneous Disease of the Mesentery and Omentum

Mesenteric disorders are uncommon. Patients with mesenteric cysts complain of abdominal pain, fever, and emesis. Symptomatic cysts are treated surgically.

Mesenteric panniculitis refers to an inflammatory process of the adipose tissue of the mesentery. A variety of other terms are used, including lipodystrophy, sclerosing lipogranulomatosis, lipogranuloma of the mesentery, and mesenteritis. The disease is manifested as thickening or nodularity of the mesentery with fat necrosis. Mesenteric panniculitis is characterized by a variety of nonspecific abdominal symptoms, including fever, abdominal pain, anorexia, weight loss, and altered bowel habits. The diagnosis is made at laparoscopy. Laboratory studies are rarely helpful, although an elevated erythrocyte sedimentation rate may be seen. Surgical resection is required only when obstruction is present.

ANATOMIC AND MECHANICAL DISORDERS

Groin Hernias

In addition to hiatal hernias (Chapter 140), hernias may occur in the groin as inguinal or femoral hernias or as a result of weakness or abnormalities of other abdominal and pelvic muscles.

Epidemiology

About 3 to 4% of men have groin hernias, and the incidence increases with age. Indirect inguinal hernias, caused by a defect in the abdominal wall, account for about two thirds of hernias. Direct inguinal hernias, which protrude through an area bounded by the rectus abdominis muscle, the inferior upper gastric artery, and the inguinal ligament, account for about 30% of hernias in men and about 2% of hernias in women. Femoral hernias, which pass through an opening associated with the femoral artery and vein, represent about 30% of hernias in women and about 2% in men.

Clinical Manifestations and Diagnosis

Groin hernias may be asymptomatic or be perceived as a mass that enlarges with standing or with increases in intra-abdominal pressure. If a hernia is not readily reducible (i.e., incarcerated), it may be associated with constant discomfort. With strangulation, ischemia or bowel obstruction may occur. The diagnosis is usually readily apparent by palpation of a soft groin mass that becomes larger with standing or with increases in intra-abdominal pressure.

Treatment

Rx

Although femoral hernias should be repaired when first diagnosed because of the risk for strangulation, watchful waiting is an acceptable option for men with minimally symptomatic inguinal hernias. 6 Overall, open repair is preferable to laparoscopic repair. 7

Other Hernias

Incisional hernias develop after 1 to 4% of laparotomy incisions. These hernias may cause chronic abdominal discomfort, especially with maneuvers that increase intra-abdominal pressure. Repair is usually performed with prosthetic mesh.

Colonic Volvulus

Most cases of colonic volvulus involve the sigmoid colon (>90%), with elders at greatest risk. Volvulus can also involve the cecum and transverse colon. Volvulus results in colonic obstruction when the colon twists on its mesentery. Patients with volvulus frequently report a history of chronic constipation or laxative use or have previously been noted to have a dilated colon. A history of psychiatric illness or institutionalization is also associated with an increased risk for the development of volvulus.

Clinical Manifestations

Symptoms of volvulus include the acute development of abdominal distention, nausea, and vomiting, with abdominal pain present initially in about a third of patients. Progressive or severe pain and tenderness suggest developing colonic ischemia and perforation. Much less commonly, patients have an intermittent history of obstructive symptoms and distention suggesting chronic volvulus.

Diagnosis

The diagnosis of volvulus is made by abdominal radiographs, which show a dilated colon that may lack haustral folds and has a "bent inner tube" appearance, with the apex pointing to the right upper quadrant. Cecal volvulus is suspected radiographically when a dilated cecum is located in the epigastrium or left upper quadrant. Small bowel dilation may also be present.

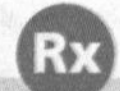

Treatment

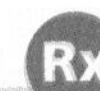

Patients who have suspected colonic volvulus and who exhibit peritoneal signs or have complete obstruction on abdominal radiographs should undergo fluid resuscitation and emergency exploratory laparotomy. In the absence of signs of complete obstruction or impending ischemia and when sigmoid volvulus is suspected, endoscopic sigmoidoscopic examination will document the site of obstruction and may be therapeutic by providing colonic decompression. Endoscopic procedures are generally avoided in patients with suspected cecal volvulus. Water-soluble contrast enema will also confirm the presence and site of obstruction with the classic finding of a "bird's beak" configuration at the obstructed site.

Intussusception

Intussusception results when a segment of intestine is drawn distally into another segment of intestine, thereby resulting in obstruction. Intussusception may occur in the small intestine itself, or the small intestine may intussuscept into the colon. Intussusception occurs most commonly in children, in whom it is seen in the setting of recent viral enteritis (e.g., rotavirus; Chapter 404), cystic fibrosis (Chapter 89), or Meckel's diverticulum. In adults, intussusception is more likely to occur in the setting of small bowel neoplasia (Chapter 203).

Clinical Manifestations

Most patients have symptoms of partial small bowel obstruction—crampy abdominal pain, nausea, vomiting, and occasionally, diarrhea. An abdominal mass may be palpable on examination, and patients may have evidence of occult or overt gastrointestinal bleeding (the passage of "currant jelly" mucus-like stool is described in infants and children).

Diagnosis and Management

The diagnosis is most commonly confirmed by CT radiography, which classically shows a "target" lesion of the small bowel that represents the layers of the small bowel and intussuscepted segment. The finding of intussusception in an adult necessitates abdominal exploration and resection of the intussuscepted segment.

Adhesions

Peritoneal adhesions cause most cases of small bowel obstruction. Adhesions can result from previous laparotomy, with an increased risk for adhesions occurring in patients with intra-abdominal infections, ischemia, and foreign bodies. Symptomatic adhesive bowel obstruction will subsequently develop in 5 to 10% of patients undergoing laparotomy. Adhesive disease may also result in reduced fertility in females. After laparotomy, adhesive-related obstruction can occur at any time from the early postoperative period to many years later.

Clinical Manifestations

Patients have crampy abdominal pain, nausea, vomiting, and increasing abdominal distention. In the setting of complete bowel obstruction, patients no longer pass stool or flatus.

Diagnosis and Treatment

On an upright abdominal radiograph, findings of adhesive-related bowel obstruction include dilated loops of bowel (>6 cm of small bowel) and air-fluid levels, with reduced air distal to the obstruction. Similar findings are present on CT radiography (Fig. 145–9). Limitations of radiographic examination include subtle findings when the obstruction is very proximal in the bowel or the obstruction is only partial. In these settings, small bowel radiographs with water-soluble or barium contrast may be necessary to make the diagnosis.

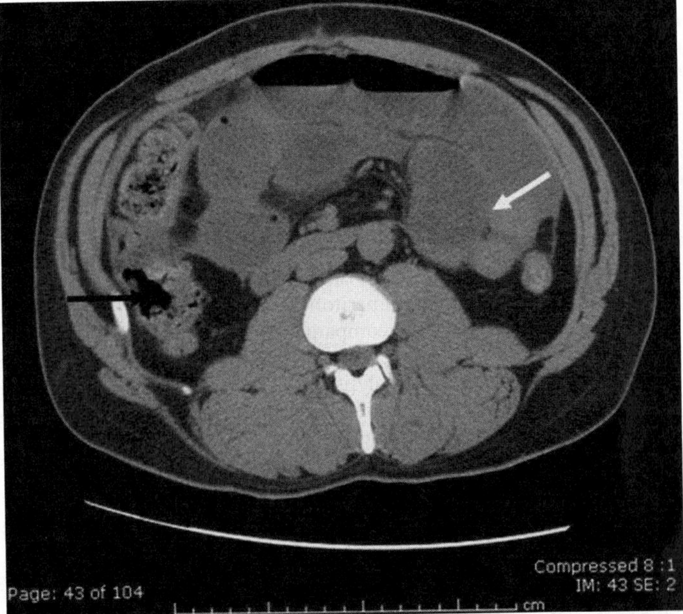

FIGURE 145–9 • Adhesion-related small bowel obstruction. A CT scan shows dilated, fluid-filled small bowel (white arrow) and a nondilated colon (black arrow). At laparotomy, an obstruction secondary to adhesions was found in the midileum.

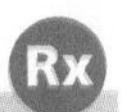

Treatment of complete small bowel obstruction is fluid resuscitation and urgent laparotomy. Nasogastric tube decompression reduces nausea, vomiting, and distention. Nonoperative management may be tried in the setting of partial small bowel obstruction, with surgery reserved for patients whose obstruction fails to resolve. Patients with recurrent small bowel obstruction may benefit from a low-roughage diet to reduce the risk for obstruction from nondigestible food residue in a narrowed lumen.

The presence of chronic or recurrent abdominal pain in the absence of bowel obstruction has often been blamed on adhesions. Unless a clearly identified obstruction is present radiographically, surgical intervention for adhesiolysis is not warranted and does not reliably reduce abdominal pain symptoms. The search continues for intraoperative techniques or substances to reduce the development of adhesions.

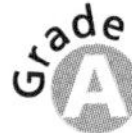

1. Terasawa T, Blackmore C, Bent S, et al: Systematic review: Computed tomography and ultrasonography to detect acute appendicitis in adults and adolescents. Ann Intern Med 2004;141:537–546.
2. Morino M, Pellegrino L, Castagna E, et al: Acute nonspecific abdominal pain: A randomized, controlled trial comparing early laparoscopy versus clinical observation. Ann Surg 2006;244:881–886.
3. Styrud J, Eriksson S, Nilsson I, et al: Appendectomy versus antibiotic treatment in acute appendicitis. A prospective multicenter randomized controlled trial. World J Surg 2006;30:1033–1037.
4. Sauerland S, Lefering R, Neugebauer EAM: Laparoscopic versus open surgery for suspected appendicitis. Cochrane Database Syst Rev 2004;4:CD001546.
5. Latella G, Pimpo MT, Sottili S, et al: Rifaximin improves symptoms of acquired uncomplicated diverticular disease of the colon. Int J Colorectal Dis 2003;18:55–62.
6. Fitzgibbons RJ Jr, Giobbie-Hurder A, Gibbs JO, et al: Watchful waiting vs repair of inguinal hernia in minimally symptomatic men: A randomized clinical trial. JAMA 2006;295:285–292.
7. Neumayer L, Giobbie-Hurder A, Jonasson O, et al: Open mesh versus laparoscopic mesh repair of inguinal hernia. N Engl J Med 2004;350:1819–1827.

SUGGESTED READINGS

Dominguez EP, Sweeney JF, Choi YU: Diagnosis and management of diverticulitis and appendicitis. Gastroenterol Clin North Am 2006;35:367–391. *Comprehensive clinical review.*

Fenollar F, Puechal X, Raoult D: Whipple's disease. N Engl J Med 2007;356:55–66. *Comprehensive review.*

Lee SL, Ho HS: Acute appendicitis: Is there a difference between children and adults? Am Surg 2006;72:409–413. *A useful case review showing that adults had higher "negative" appendectomy rates (19% vs. 10%) and similar perforation rates (about 15%).*

Stollman N, Raskin JB: Diverticular disease of the colon. Lancet 2004; 363:631–639. *Overview of diagnosis and treatment of this common problem, which is symptomatic in 10 to 20% of cases.*

146 VASCULAR DISEASES OF THE GASTROINTESTINAL TRACT

Stephen Crane Hauser

INTESTINAL ISCHEMIA

Intestinal ischemia can occur as a result of a variety of conditions that decrease intestinal blood flow. Both diminished arterial blood flow to the gut and compromised venous circulation from the intestine can cause intestinal or mesenteric ischemia. Several conditions, such as adhesions and malignancy (Chapter 203), may predispose to mesenteric ischemia by secondarily diminishing blood flow via extrinsic compression of otherwise normal intestinal arteries or veins (Table 146–1). These disorders and esophageal varices (Chapters 137 and 157) are discussed elsewhere.

Epidemiology

Intestinal ischemia is responsible for about 1 per 1000 hospital admissions. When considering the diagnosis of intestinal ischemia, it is important to distinguish *primary* (occlusive or nonocclusive) from *secondary* (extrinsic to the blood vessel) mesenteric ischemia, *acute* manifestations from *chronic, arterial* versus *venous,* and *small bowel* versus *colonic* ischemia. Risk factors for intestinal ischemia include age (all the disorders discussed) and conditions that predispose to arterial embolism (e.g., cardiac arrhythmias, heart failure, valvular heart disease, recent myocardial infarction, cardiac catheterization, intracardiac thrombus, atheromatous cholesterol embolism), occlusion of arteries (atherosclerosis, fibromuscular dysplasia, abdominal aortic aneurysm, trauma, vasculitis), low-flow states (sepsis, dialysis, reduced cardiac output, vasoconstrictive drugs), and pathologic thromboses (largely venous; hypercoagulable and hyperviscosity states, trauma, malignancy, inflammation).

Pathobiology

Arterial or venous disease of the esophagus, stomach, duodenum, and rectum is very unusual for anatomic reasons. The esophagus receives its main blood supply segmentally via multiple small vessels from the aorta, right intercostal artery, bronchial arteries, inferior thyroid artery, left gastric artery, short gastric artery, and left phrenic artery. Likewise, the stomach, duodenum, and rectum have numerous arterial input with rich collateralization. Patients who have undergone extensive surgical resection of the esophagus, stomach, or duodenum are at increased risk for ischemia. Vasculitic disorders, which can involve small or large arteries or veins, may affect the esophagus, stomach, duodenum, or rectum.

The arterial supply of blood to the small and large intestine is from the *celiac artery, superior mesenteric artery* (SMA), and *inferior mesenteric artery* (IMA). Collateral vessels, which vary from person to person, may include the meandering mesenteric artery or arc of Riolan at the base of the mesentery (connecting the SMA and IMA), the marginal artery of Drummond along the mesenteric border (connecting the SMA and IMA), the pancreaticoduodenal arcade (connecting the celiac artery and SMA), the arc of Barkow (connecting the celiac artery and SMA), and the arc of Buhler (connecting the celiac artery and SMA). These collaterals can rapidly enlarge in response to localized mesenteric ischemia. During states of low arterial flow, such as in patients with low systemic arterial blood pressure, "watershed" areas such as the splenic flexure, which is furthest away from arterial flow, are more likely to be involved. In contrast, when a major arterial vessel such as the IMA is suddenly occluded, the splenic flexure is less likely to be involved because of collaterals from the SMA circulation.

TABLE 146–1 CONDITIONS PREDISPOSING TO SECONDARY MESENTERIC ISCHEMIA
Adhesions
Herniation
Volvulus
Intussusception
Mesenteric fibrosis
Retroperitoneal fibrosis
Carcinoid syndrome
Malignancy (peritoneal, mesenteric, colonic)
Neurofibromatosis
Amyloidosis
Trauma

Intestinal blood flow, which accounts for approximately 10% of cardiac output, increases to as much as 25% of cardiac output after eating a meal. Blood flow to the intestine is regulated by the sympathetic nervous system and a variety of systemic (angiotensin II, vasopressin) and local (prostaglandins, leukotrienes) humoral factors.

Mesenteric ischemia can occur as a result of decreased *arterial* blood flow, which can be *occlusive* (arterial embolus, arterial thrombus, and vasculitis) or *nonocclusive* (low-flow states). *Venous* obstruction (thrombosis, vasculitis) can also result in mesenteric ischemia.

Whatever the cause of mesenteric ischemia, the gut is able to adapt to as much as a 75% reduction in normal blood flow for as long as 12 hours. Increased flow through available and newly opened collateral vessels and increased oxygen extraction help compensate. However, with a more prolonged and more severe reduction in blood flow, generalized mesenteric arterial vasoconstriction often develops and can become irreversible, even with correction of the original underlying condition (i.e., relief of focal arterial obstruction or resolution of a low-flow state). Hypoxia and reperfusion injury via oxygen radicals, reduced endothelial synthesis of nitric oxide, and an enhanced cellular inflammatory response cause microvascular and end-organ damage. Initially, the end-organ damage is primarily mucosal, but damage can rapidly progress to transmural necrosis (gangrene). Some ischemic segments of bowel will heal with fibrosis (strictures).

Clinical Manifestations

Symptoms of intestinal ischemia at initial evaluation may be acute (sudden, lasting hours), subacute (days), or chronic (intermittent, occurring over a period of weeks to months). With acute and many subacute manifestations, abdominal pain (see Table 134–2) is often the cardinal symptom. Usually the pain is severe, persistent, and poorly localized. Initially, the pain is typically more severe than the findings on abdominal palpation (i.e., pain out of proportion to tenderness). With or without pain, other initial features may include fever, altered mental status, abdominal distention, difficulty eating, nausea, vomiting, and diarrhea. With small bowel ischemia, overt gastrointestinal bleeding (Chapter 137) is a late and ominous finding that often suggests small bowel infarction.

Findings on physical examination can include hypotension, tachycardia, abdominal distention, initially increased and later decreased bowel sounds, and nonspecific diffuse abdominal tenderness, often mild at first. Over time, peritoneal signs with localized to generalized abdominal tenderness, rebound, and rigidity may become manifest. Occult gastrointestinal bleeding can be an early finding.

Diagnosis

Even as the diagnostic evaluation is begun, appropriate attention must be directed to emergency therapy, including fluid resuscitation, antibiotics, and invasive therapy (Fig. 146–1).

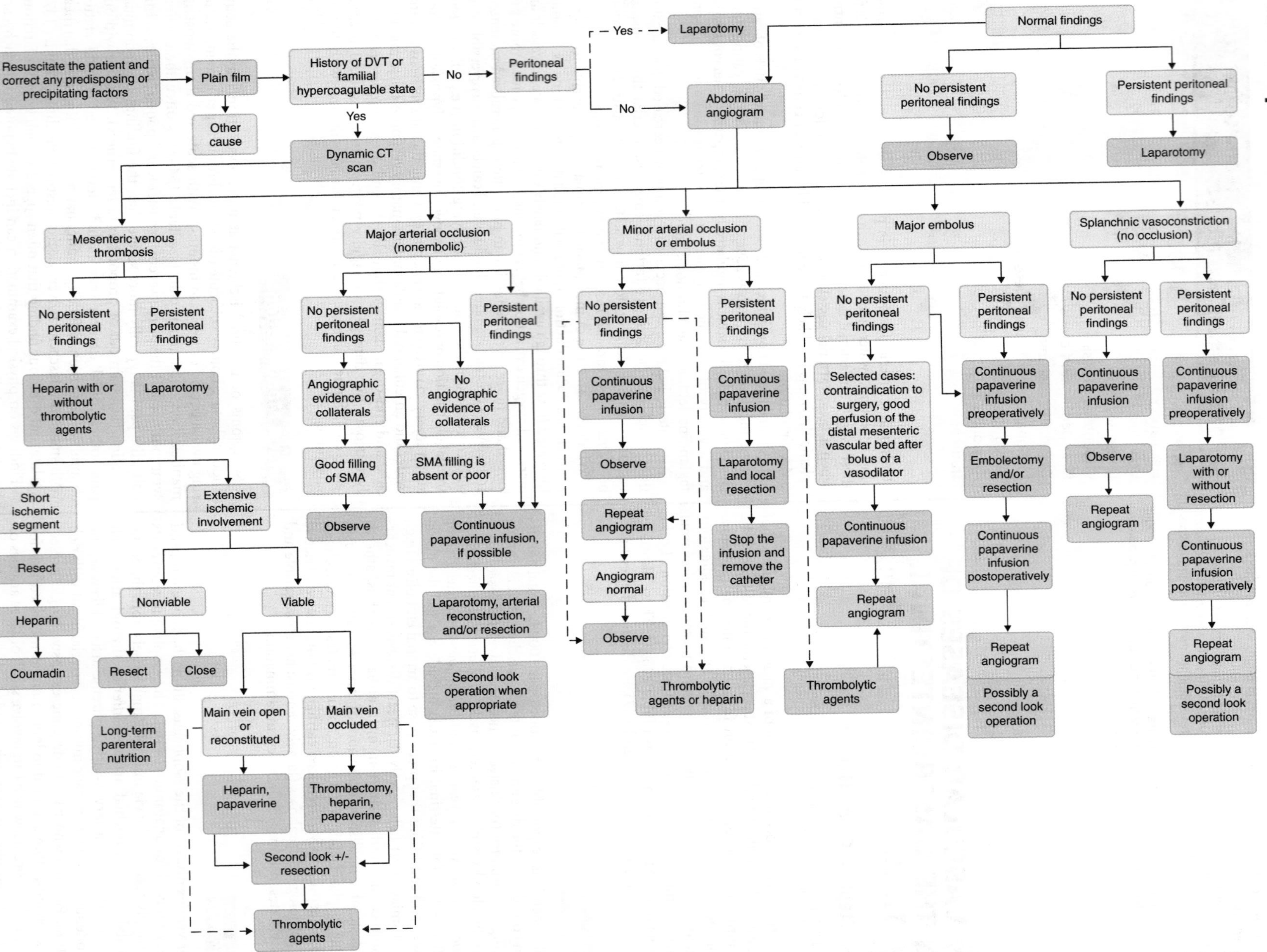

FIGURE 146–1 • Algorithm for managing patients with suspected acute mesenteric ischemia: diagnosis and management. Solid lines indicate an accepted management plan; dashed lines indicate an alternative management plan. CT = computed tomography; DVT = deep venous thrombosis; SMA = superior mesenteric artery. (From American Gastroenterological Association Medical Position Statement: Guidelines on intestinal ischemia. Gastroenterology 2000;118:951–953 [corrected algorithm in Gastroenterology 2000;119:281].)

Initial Diagnostic Evaluation

The initial laboratory findings in patients with an acute onset of bowel ischemia can be entirely normal. Nonspecific abnormalities such as leukocytosis with a left shift and hemoconcentration may be seen. Elevated serum levels of amylase, lactate, aminotransferases, lactate dehydrogenase, creatine kinase, and phosphate often portend more advanced (necrotic) small bowel ischemia, but these findings lack sensitivity as well as specificity.

Noninvasive Imaging

The presence or absence of radiographic features suggestive of ischemia in patients with acute-onset mesenteric ischemia varies and depends on the duration and extent of ischemia. Plain abdominal radiographs are useful in helping exclude secondary causes of mesenteric ischemia, as well as other causes of acute abdominal pain, nausea, vomiting, or distention, such as obstruction and perforation. Radiographic findings such as "thumbprinting" (caused by submucosal hemorrhage), an ileus pattern, formless loops of small bowel, or with more advanced disease, pneumatosis intestinalis or portal venous gas (often a sign of transmural necrosis or gangrene) may on occasion be seen. Contrast-enhanced abdominal/pelvic computed tomography (CT) is also helpful to exclude alternative diagnoses. CT may demonstrate entirely *normal* findings in acute mesenteric ischemia, or findings such as segmental bowel wall thickening, submucosal hemorrhage, mesenteric stranding, mesenteric venous thrombosis, pneumatosis, and portal venous gas may be present (Fig. 146–2). Subacute manifestations of bowel ischemia may be due to a wide variety of causes, including mesenteric venous thrombosis, which is best diagnosed by CT scan. However, the time needed to obtain a CT scan should not delay resuscitation or arteriography in very ill patients with suspected acute-onset ischemia.

Treatment

Rx

Acutely ill patients require prompt, definitive diagnosis and treatment, which usually requires selective mesenteric angiography (Fig. 146–3). If transmural intestinal necrosis (gangrene) is suspected from peritoneal signs, pneumatosis, or portal venous gas on imaging procedures, emergency laparotomy is indicated. The presence of predisposing conditions (e.g., arrhythmias, systemic hypotension) and their extraintestinal manifestations (e.g., heart failure, sepsis, respiratory insufficiency, acute renal failure, anemia) dictate the initial therapy: volume replacement, optimization of cardiac output, management of respiratory function, avoidance of splanchnic vasoconstrictors such as digoxin, and administration of broad-spectrum antibiotics (e.g., meropenem, imipenem/cilastatin, metronidazole and a third-generation cephalosporin, ciprofloxacin and metronidazole, or piperacillin/tazobactam) to cover aerobic gram-negative and anaerobic organisms and to prevent sepsis secondary to translocation of bacteria across ischemic gut mucosa.

Prognosis

Acute primary arterial mesenteric ischemia involving the small bowel is an urgent condition that if unidentified or untreated can result in death within hours. Mortality rates may be as high as 70% but are much lower with early diagnosis and prompt therapy. Overall, colonic ischemia has a much better prognosis than small bowel ischemia does. Mesenteric venous thrombosis also has a much better prognosis than acute primary arterial mesenteric ischemia of the small intestine does.

Specific Ischemic Bowel Syndromes

Superior Mesenteric Embolism

Embolization to the intestine via the SMA (*SMA embolus*) accounts for 5% of peripheral emboli and nearly 50% of cases of primary noncolonic mesenteric ischemia. Emboli most commonly originate from the heart, with an aortic origin being less common (Table 146–2), and tend to obstruct beyond the origin of the SMA.

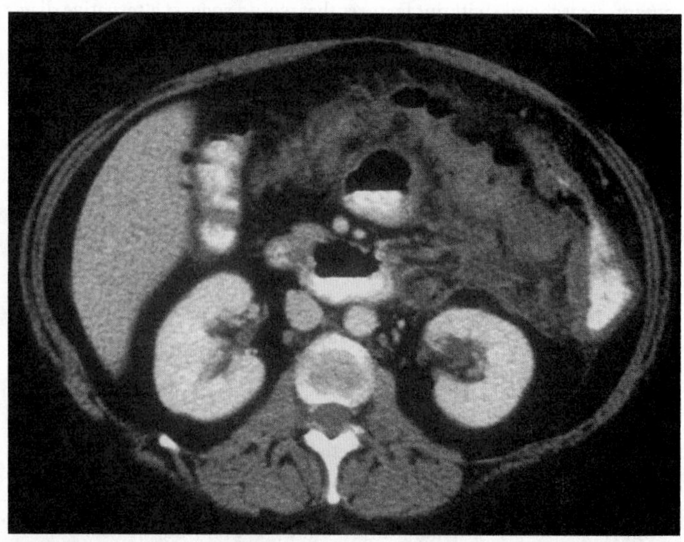

FIGURE 146–2 • Computed tomography of the abdomen in a patient with ischemic colitis as a result of superior mesenteric vein thrombosis. A segmental area of the transverse colon demonstrates a thick wall, as well as considerable fluid and soft tissue stranding in the adjacent mesentery. (From Johnson CL, Schmit GD [eds]: Mayo Clinic Gastrointestinal Imaging Review. Boca Raton, FL, Mayo Clinic Scientific Press, Taylor and Francis Group, 2005. By permission of the Mayo Foundation for Medical Education and Research. All rights reserved.)

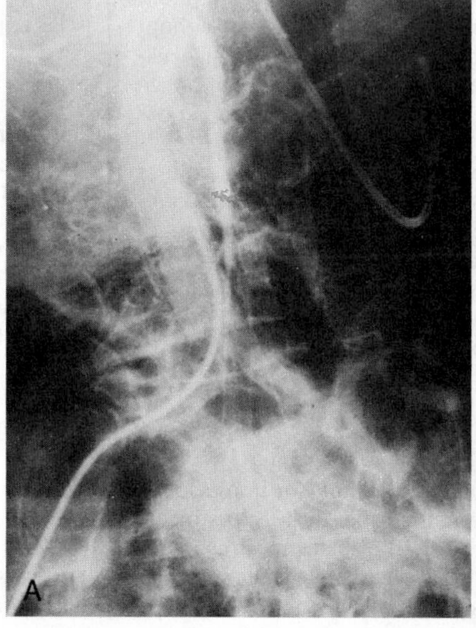

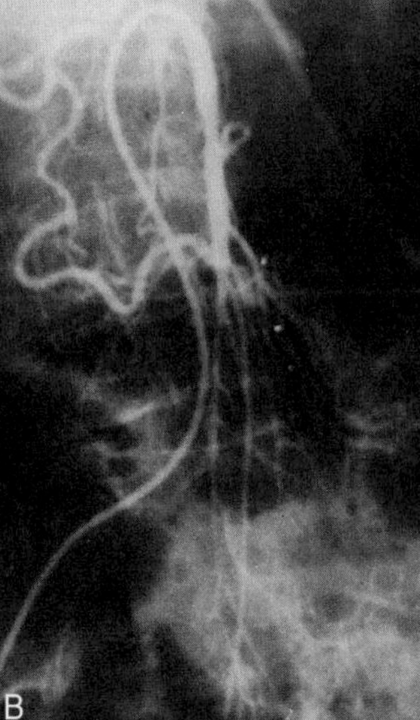

FIGURE 146–3 • Selected films from superior mesenteric angiography. A, Diffuse vasoconstriction characteristic of nonocclusive mesenteric ischemia. **B,** Intra-arterial infusion of papaverine (30 to 60 mg/hr) resulted in vasodilation.

TABLE 146–2 CONDITIONS ASSOCIATED WITH EMBOLIZATION TO THE GASTROINTESTINAL TRACT

Cardiac arrhythmias
Valvular heart disease
Heart failure
Myocardial infarction
Intracardiac thrombus
Cardiac catheterization
Cardioversion
Atherosclerosis of the aorta

Clinical Manifestations and Diagnosis

Patients who are evaluated early in the course of their illness may have entirely normal CT scans, or the CT findings may be consistent with mesenteric ischemia without features that would suggest alternative diagnoses (e.g., perforation, obstruction). At the present time, CT angiography (CTA), magnetic resonance angiography (MRA), and Doppler ultrasound (US) are not sensitive enough to diagnose embolic disease reliably in the mesenteric arterial vasculature. Selective mesenteric angiography is the diagnostic test of choice for acute mesenteric arterial embolization, which usually involves the vascular territory of the SMA.

Treatment

Select patients with acute onset of a partial or small SMA branch occlusion may be candidates for thrombolytic therapy (e.g., streptokinase, urokinase, tissue plasminogen activator) infused via an arterial catheter directly into the vicinity of the embolus; such therapy can lyse the embolus and resolve symptoms such as abdominal pain. Because segmental arterial embolic occlusion of a small portion of the SMA vascular bed results in widespread splanchnic visceral arterial vasoconstriction, which may persist even after the original inciting event (i.e., an embolus) is rectified, infusion of a vasodilator such as papaverine (often given as a 60-mg bolus, followed by a continuous infusion of 30 to 60 mg/hr for 12 to 48 hours) via an arterial catheter reverses this reflex vasoconstriction and improves the outcome, including mortality rates. The same scenario occurs with other arterial occlusive lesions (SMA thrombi), arterial nonocclusive disease (nonocclusive mesenteric ischemia), and disorders associated with mesenteric venous occlusion.

Patients initially seen later in the course of their acute embolic illness with peritoneal signs require laparotomy, with or without resection and with or without embolectomy, which is usually performed during surgical exploration. A second-look operation 24 hours after embolectomy to make sure that all necrotic tissue has been resected may be necessary.

Any patient in whom SMA embolization is diagnosed requires preoperative systemic anticoagulation (e.g., intravenous heparin) to prevent propagation of clot around the embolus and to guard against further embolization to the intestine or other organs (i.e., brain, coronary arteries, kidneys, extremities). Anticoagulation is usually discontinued before surgery and is often resumed 24 to 48 hours postoperatively, depending on the operative findings.

Superior Mesenteric Thrombosis

Thrombosis of the SMA *(SMA thrombus)* accounts for nearly 15% of cases of primary noncolonic mesenteric ischemia. Risk factors include older age, atherosclerosis (e.g., hypertension, diabetes mellitus, hyperlipidemia, smoking history), low-flow states, hypercoagulable states, and less often, vasculitis and aortic or mesenteric aneurysms.

Clinical Manifestations and Diagnosis

Nearly a third of these patients have a history of symptomatic chronic mesenteric ischemia (see later) antedating their acute manifestation of SMA thrombosis. Proximal mesenteric arterial occlusions are well recognized by CTA, MRA, and Doppler US, but similar abnormalities are common in asymptomatic elderly persons. Similar to acute SMA embolism, the diagnosis is confirmed by selective mesenteric angiography, with intra-arterial infusion of a vasodilator used to reverse reflex-generalized vasoconstriction.

Treatment

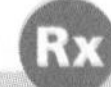

Although thrombolytic therapy has been helpful in a few case reports, surgical thrombectomy or bypass grafting, with or without bowel resection, is the most common therapeutic approach. Because many of these thrombi occur near the origin of the SMA, angioplasty may be therapeutic in very select cases, but the risk for reocclusion is high. Similar to acute SMA embolism, anticoagulation (intravenous heparin) is important preoperatively and at some point postoperatively in the acute state, as is administration of broad-spectrum antibiotics (see earlier).

Acute Nonocclusive, Noncolonic Primary Arterial Ischemia

Nonocclusive mesenteric ischemia, which accounts for about 20% of cases of primary noncolonic mesenteric ischemia, is caused by low arterial blood flow to the intestine. Risk factors include advanced age, decreased systolic blood pressure (e.g., cardiac arrhythmia, heart failure, myocardial infarction, shock, sepsis, burns, pancreatitis, hemorrhage, multiple organ failure, dialysis, perioperative states), vasospasm (e.g., digoxin, vasopressin, amphetamines, cocaine), and atherosclerotic disease.

Clinical Manifestations and Diagnosis

The clinical findings are generally indistinguishable from those of embolic or thrombotic vascular disease, except that the symptoms may be less acute. As a result, patients may initially be seen without acute abdominal pain but rather with more nonspecific symptoms such as distention, nausea, fever, altered mental status, and borderline or low systolic blood pressure. Selected mesenteric angiography establishes the diagnosis (lack of embolus or thrombus, alternating areas of vessel spasm and dilation, vascular pruning and spasm).

Treatment

The best specific treatment is prolonged intra-arterial instillation of a vasodilator (e.g., papaverine, often given as a 60-mg bolus, followed by a continuous infusion of 30 to 60 mg/hr) to reverse the vasospasm. Avoidance of vasospastic medications and optimization of cardiac output, blood volume, and blood pressure are crucial. Anticoagulation is not generally necessary, but broad-spectrum antibiotics (similar to those recommended earlier) should be given to cover aerobic gram-negative and anaerobic organisms. Although many of these patients have serious conditions that predispose them to low-flow states and their ultimate prognosis is dependent on the outcomes of these serious conditions, diagnosis and treatment of acute nonocclusive mesenteric ischemia with therapeutic angiography can be life-saving.

Mesenteric Venous Thrombosis

Occlusive disease of the mesenteric venous circulation *(mesenteric venous thrombosis)* usually involves the superior mesenteric vein (SMV)

TABLE 146–3 RISK FACTORS FOR MESENTERIC VENOUS THROMBOSIS

Hypercoagulable and hyperviscosity states
Protein S deficiency
Protein C deficiency
Antithrombin III deficiency
Factor V Leiden mutation
Hyperfibrinogenemia
Antiphospholipid syndrome
Primary myeloproliferative syndrome
Sickle cell disease
Estrogen or progesterone
Intra-abdominal infections and inflammation
Appendicitis
Diverticulitis
Crohn's disease
Abscess
Pancreatitis
Cholecystitis
Pyelophlebitis
Neonatal omphalitis
Portal hypertension
Variceal sclerotherapy
Malignancy
Trauma
Vasculitis

and may be accompanied by symptoms that are acute in onset (hours to days) or subacute (weeks to months).

Epidemiology and Pathobiology

Thrombosis of the SMV accounts for about 10% of cases of primary noncolonic mesenteric ischemia. Colonic involvement with ischemic colitis is much less common. In contrast to arterial occlusive disease, risk factors and causes for SMV thrombosis are more numerous and diverse. Individuals with a personal or family history of a hypercoagulable state or deep venous thrombosis are at increased risk for SMV thrombosis. Hypercoagulable states, hyperviscosity syndromes, portal hypertension, intra-abdominal infections (e.g., pyelophlebitis, diverticulitis, appendicitis) or inflammation (e.g., Crohn's disease, pancreatitis), malignancy, vasculitis, and trauma may all cause thrombosis of the SMV (Table 146–3).

Clinical Manifestations

Symptoms in acute-onset cases are similar to those of acute occlusive and nonocclusive arterial mesenteric ischemia—abdominal pain, anorexia, nausea, vomiting, abdominal fullness, diarrhea, and constipation—but tend to persist over a longer period. Some patients may have bacteremia, especially with *Bacteroides.* Gastrointestinal hemorrhage, if present, is often indicative of infarction. However, many patients with SMV thrombosis experience more vague symptomatic abdominal pain, nausea, distention, or diarrhea over a period of weeks to months (subacute).

Diagnosis

Abdominal/pelvic contrast-enhanced CT, which is the preferred diagnostic test, usually (>90% sensitivity) demonstrates thrombosis of the SMV with or without portal vein or splenic vein thrombosis. By definition, chronic mesenteric venous thrombosis is asymptomatic and usually detected as an incidental CT finding in patients with portal hypertension, pancreatitis (acute or chronic), or malignancy. The presence of abundant collateral vessels suggests chronic or sometimes subacute mesenteric venous obstruction.

Small bowel radiography may demonstrate segmental bowel wall thickening and separation of bowel loops. Selective mesenteric angiography is not generally necessary.

Treatment

Therapy for acute-onset cases may include laparotomy with or without bowel resection when infarction is suspected, fluid resuscitation, broad-spectrum antibiotics (similar to those recommended earlier to cover aerobic gram-negative and anaerobic organisms), avoidance of vasoconstrictors, and anticoagulation (e.g., intravenous heparin) in the absence of gastrointestinal bleeding. Selected patients may be candidates for thrombolytic therapy (e.g., streptokinase, urokinase, tissue plasminogen activator), followed by anticoagulation. Underlying conditions such as hypercoagulable states, portal hypertension, intra-abdominal infections, intra-abdominal inflammation, and malignancy require concomitant diagnosis and therapy. The indications for anticoagulation in the chronic setting are uncertain, and it is generally avoided in patients who have portal hypertension but do not have symptoms related to their mesenteric venous thrombosis.

Chronic Mesenteric Ischemia

Chronic atherosclerotic stenosis of the visceral arteries is the cause of most cases of chronic mesenteric ischemia, sometimes called *intestinal angina.*

Epidemiology and Pathobiology

Risk factors for chronic mesenteric ischemia are principally older age and the risk factors for atherosclerosis. Rarely, vasculitis or an aortic aneurysm can be manifested as chronic mesenteric ischemia. Atherosclerotic stenoses usually involve the origins of two or all of the three major visceral arteries supplying the intestine. However, many age-matched patients also harbor atherosclerotic lesions and do not have symptoms of chronic mesenteric ischemia.

Clinical Manifestations

Patients typically complain of episodic ischemic abdominal pain. The pain is usually upper or midabdominal, typically begins 15 to 30 minutes after a meal, lasts 1 to 3 hours, and progresses in severity over time, as well as occurs after smaller meals and more frequently after meals. Patients may lose weight as a result of fear of eating (sitophobia). Nausea, vomiting, bloating, diarrhea, and constipation can also occur. Malabsorption with steatorrhea, otherwise unexplained gastroduodenal ulcerations, and small bowel biopsy findings of villous atrophy, nonspecific surface cell flattening, and chronic inflammation may be seen in some patients. More than half of patients will have a bruit on abdominal examination. In some patients with episodic symptoms, acute thrombotic mesenteric ischemia will suddenly develop.

Diagnosis and Treatment

Atherosclerotic lesions can usually be identified by Doppler US because they are proximal in these vessels and demonstrate increased flow velocity through areas of marked stenosis. MRA is also useful to screen for arterial stenoses consistent with chronic mesenteric ischemia in symptomatic patients, but neither technique is adequately sensitive to exclude the diagnosis of chronic mesenteric ischemia when the pretest probability is high. Thus, selective mesenteric angiography is important to ensure that the anatomic findings are consistent with the diagnosis. Patients must be evaluated thoroughly to exclude other causes of abdominal pain (i.e., gastric cancer, gastroparesis, gastric volvulus, partial small bowel obstruction, small bowel bacterial overgrowth states, pancreatic cancer, biliary disease, paraesophageal hernias). For symptomatic patients with appropriate findings on angiography and no other causes of symptoms, surgical reconstruction provides better long-term outcomes than angioplasty and stenting do.

TABLE 146–4 MEDICATIONS AND DRUGS ASSOCIATED WITH ISCHEMIC COLITIS

Digitalis
Vasopressin
Pseudoephedrine
Amphetamines
Cocaine
Ergot
Sumatriptan
Gold
Danazol
Estrogens
Progestins
Alosetron
Psychotropics
Nonsteroidal anti-inflammatory drugs
Various enemas

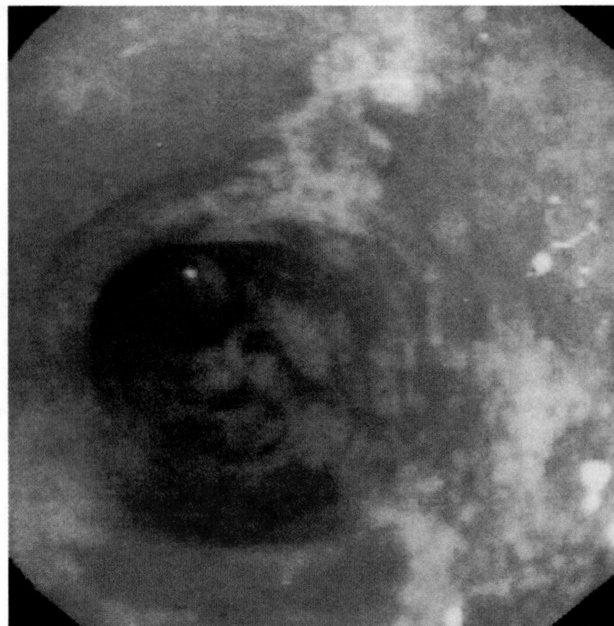

FIGURE 146–4 • Endoscopy of the splenic flexure of the colon in a patient with ischemic colitis. Note the shallow, irregular, exudative ulceration with interspersed erythema. (From Emory TS, Carpenter HA, Gostout CJ, Sobin LH [eds]: Atlas of Gastrointestinal Endoscopy and Endoscopic Biopsies. Washington, DC, Armed Forces Institute of Pathology, American Registry of Pathology, 2000.)

Ischemic Colitis

Epidemiology and Pathobiology

Ischemic colitis, which is the single most common cause of mesenteric ischemia, accounts for nearly 50% of all cases and for almost 1 in 2000 hospital admissions. Many cases are acute and self-limited and occur in persons older than 60 years without any apparent cause; these cases are probably due to transient nonocclusive hypoperfusion involving a segment of the colon. It is controversial whether subtle hypercoagulable states contribute to the pathogenesis of idiopathic cases. Atherosclerotic or thrombotic occlusion of the IMA or its branches and low-flow states are recognizable causes of ischemic colitis. Less common causes include hypercoagulable states (especially in younger persons), iatrogenic ligation of the IMA (e.g., with aortic surgery), embolism, vasculitis, and any cause of colonic obstruction, including malignancy, stricture, and fecalith, that can produce localized compression of the vasculature with an upstream segment of ischemia. Other unusual associations include long-distance running (dehydration, mechanical trauma to the vasculature, generally involving the cecum) and intra-abdominal infections or inflammatory disease. A variety of medications, illicit drugs, and chemicals can also result in a chemical picture identical or similar to ischemic colitis (Table 146–4), sometimes probably secondary to vasoconstriction that can affect other parts of the gastrointestinal tract, liver, and other organ systems (e.g., cocaine, amphetamines, pseudoephedrine) and sometimes as a result of a chemical effect (e.g., sodium polystyrene with sorbitol enemas).

Clinical Manifestations

The clinical manifestation of ischemic colitis is acute and, in most patients, includes abdominal pain (mostly left lower quadrant), often with urgency, diarrhea, and passage of bright red blood per rectum. Anorexia, nausea, vomiting, abdominal distention, and passage of maroon material per rectum may also occur. Although the blood loss is not usually enough to require transfusion, some patients may be orthostatic because of loss of blood and fluid. Fever, tachycardia, abdominal tenderness over the affected portion of colon, and distention may be found on physical examination.

Diagnosis

Laboratory findings range from normal to nonspecific findings such as leukocytosis and hemoconcentration to those found in persons with bowel necrosis (see earlier). Evaluation of patients younger than 50 years should include tests for thrombophilic disorders (Chapter 182).

Plain radiographs of the abdomen may reveal "thumbprinting" or may be normal. Similar to small bowel ischemia, CT scanning can be useful to help exclude other disorders, especially in more symptomatic and sicker patients; the findings may be consistent with segmental colonic edema and inflammation, with or without adjacent pericolonic inflammatory stranding. These radiographic features are consistent with ischemic colitis in an appropriate clinical setting but are nonspecific and may be seen in patients with other disorders such as acute diverticulitis (Chapter 145), infectious colitis (Chapter 143), and inflammatory bowel disease (Chapter 144). The diagnosis is best made by colonoscopy, which should provide endoscopic and histologic findings consistent with acute ischemic colitis: segmental patchy ulceration, edema, erythema, and submucosal bluish purple hemorrhagic nodules (Fig. 146–4).

Typically, visceral angiography is not required because most patients with ischemic colitis have self-limited involvement of the left colon or distal transverse colon/splenic flexure with sparing of the rectum, and findings on urgent angiography in these patients are usually normal. However, about 10% of patients with acute ischemic colitis have predominantly right-sided involvement of the cecum, ascending colon, hepatic flexure, and proximal transverse colon. Because the arterial supply to the right colon is via the ileocolic branch of the SMA, there may be concomitant distal ileal ischemia; these patients more often have ischemia secondary to low-flow states or embolization and are at risk for small bowel necrosis.

Differential Diagnosis

Gastrointestinal infections, such as with *Escherichia coli* O157:H7, *Clostridium difficile,* and cytomegalovirus, can mimic ischemic colitis clinically and even histologically. Acute-onset inflammatory bowel disease involving the colon can also be difficult to distinguish from ischemic colitis. However, patients with subacute or chronic pain, diarrhea, obstructive symptoms, weight loss, or bleeding may be thought to have complicated diverticular disease, Crohn's disease, or malignancy with stricture, and chronic ischemic stricture of the colon may not be correctly diagnosed until after surgery is performed.

Stool culture can exclude infection, especially with *E. coli* O157:H7, *C. difficile,* and parasites. In immunocompromised patients, colonic biopsy can be performed to diagnose cytomegalovirus infection.

Treatment

Rx

Patients with right-sided ischemic colitis require visceral angiography not only for diagnosis but also for intra-arterial administration of vasodilators (e.g., papaverine as a 60-mg intravenous bolus followed by an infusion of 30 to 60 mg/hr). Some patients may require urgent surgery. The clinical course in patients with right-sided ischemic colitis may be subacute, with a mortality rate as high as 50% or greater.

In contrast, left-sided acute ischemic colitis, which accounts for most cases, tends to resolve within hours to a few days with supportive therapy, including volume replacement, correction of any low-flow state, broad-spectrum antibiotics (similar to those recommended earlier for patients with small bowel ischemia), avoidance of vasoconstrictive medications, and rarely, blood transfusion; surgery is required only in patients with signs and symptoms of transmural necrosis, perforation, or massive bleeding. Occasional patients with acute-onset left-sided ischemic colitis have persistent or recurrent symptoms of pain, diarrhea, bleeding, sepsis, or stricture formation that develop over a period of weeks to months and may require segmental surgical resection.

VASCULITIS

Many vasculitic syndromes can involve the gastrointestinal tract. Usually, but not always, other organ systems are also involved.

Large and Medium Vessel Vasculitis

Takayasu's arteritis (Chapters 78 and 291) and *giant cell arteritis* (Chapter 292), which affect large to medium-sized muscular arteries, rarely involve the gastrointestinal tract. Takayasu's arteritis has rarely been associated with inflammatory bowel disease.

Medium to Small Vessel Vasculitis

Polyarteritis nodosa (Chapter 291) is characterized by segmental microaneurysms typically involving small and medium-sized arteries. The small bowel is involved more commonly than the large bowel. Many patients will have abdominal pain, fever, hypertension, and multiple organ involvement. Gastrointestinal bleeding or perforation will develop in some patients. The gallbladder, spleen, pancreas, and liver may also be involved. Nearly half of patients with polyarteritis nodosa are infected with hepatitis B virus.

Both *Wegener's granulomatosis* (Chapter 291) and *Churg-Strauss syndrome* (Chapter 291) affect small and medium-sized arteries. Although gastrointestinal involvement is not common in Wegener's granulomatosis with granulomatous inflammation, in up to a third of patients with Churg-Strauss syndrome, abdominal pain or gastrointestinal bleeding may develop as a result of ischemia. Mesenteric venous involvement can also occur with Churg-Strauss syndrome.

Thromboangiitis obliterans (Buerger's disease; Chapter 80) involves small and medium-sized arteries and can cause multiple distal occlusions of the mesenteric arterial circulation. Patients with *Behçet's disease* (Chapter 291) often have lymphocytic inflammation of small and medium-sized arteries, as well as veins. Like Crohn's disease, the ileocecal region is frequently involved with ulceration. Abdominal pain, diarrhea, gastrointestinal bleeding, and perforation may occur.

Small Vessel Vasculitis

Small vessel involvement with IgA immune complex deposition in blood vessel walls is typical in *Henoch-Schönlein purpura* (Chapter 291). These patients usually have palpable purpura, arthritis, and abdominal pain, as well as gastrointestinal bleeding. *Hypersensitivity vasculitis* (Chapter 291), which affects small arterioles, venules, and capillaries, is related to a variety of drugs, infections, and chemicals; on occasion there may be gastrointestinal involvement. *Cryoglobulinemia* (Chapter 198) with immune complex involvement of small blood vessels can sometimes involve the gastrointestinal tract. These patients are often infected with hepatitis C virus.

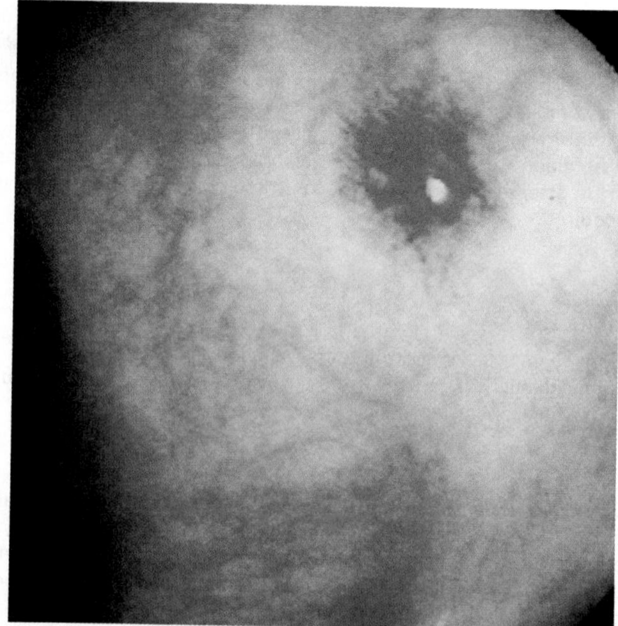

FIGURE 146–5 • Endoscopy of the sigmoid colon in a patient with angiectasia. The lesion is discrete and contains a tight, radiating cluster of ectatic mucosal vessels. (From Emory TS, Carpenter HA, Gostout CJ, Sobin LH [eds]: Atlas of Gastrointestinal Endoscopy and Endoscopic Biopsies. Washington, DC, Armed Forces Institute of Pathology, American Registry of Pathology, 2000.)

HEMORRHAGIC VASCULAR DISORDERS

Angiodysplasia

Definition and Epidemiology

Angiodysplasia or vascular ectasia is a thin-walled, dilated, punctate red vascular structure in the mucosa or submucosa of the bowel; it typically involves adjacent venules, capillaries, and arterioles. Angiodysplasia is found in the colon, especially the right colon, in up to 1% of persons and is also found in the stomach and small bowel but rarely in the esophagus. Angiodysplastic lesions may be single or multiple, and they increase in frequency with age. Some data suggest associations with chronic renal failure (Chapter 131), von Willebrand's disease (Chapter 180), and aortic stenosis (Chapter 75); whether correction of these associated disorders diminishes future gastrointestinal hemorrhage from angiodysplasia is uncertain.

Clinical Manifestations

Clinically, these lesions can produce painless bleeding, which may be occult and manifested only by guaiac-positive stools or iron deficiency anemia, or the bleeding may be overt, with hematochezia, maroon stools, melena, and hematemesis.

Diagnosis

Endoscopic procedures most often make the diagnosis of bleeding secondary to angiodysplasia (Fig. 146–5). In some patients, endoscopic procedures may need to be repeated, especially in volume-depleted patients and after the administration of narcotics. Small bowel angiodysplasia, beyond the reach of both a colonoscope from below and an extended-length endoscope from above, may be the cause of major bleeding (Chapter 137) and require video capsule endoscopy (Chapter 136) for diagnosis.

Treatment

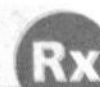

Electrocoagulation laser therapy or argon plasma coagulation can be accomplished during endoscopy. When very active bleeding makes urgent colonoscopy technically difficult, visceral angiography can be diagnostic and also permit embolization of bleeding lesions or intra-arterial infusion of a vasoconstrictor. Rarely, bowel resection is required.

Prognosis

More than 90% of gastrointestinal angiodysplasias never bleed. If found incidentally in patients without a history of bleeding, they should not be treated.

Dieulafoy's Lesion

Dieulafoy's lesion is an unusually large submucosal artery typically found in the proximal portion of the stomach within 6 cm of the gastroesophageal junction. Similar lesions may also occur in the rectum, colon, small bowel, and far less often, the esophagus. Dieulafoy's lesion is manifested clinically as sudden, massive bleeding, which may be recurrent.

Diagnosis and Treatment

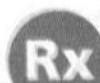

Urgent endoscopy is required to identify what is usually a very small vascular protuberance (Fig. 146–6) but can rapidly become inapparent once the acute bleeding stops. Ulceration is not seen, and repeat endoscopic procedures during active bleeding may be required to make the diagnosis. Sometimes the diagnosis requires angiography during a bleeding episode. Endoscopic injection and electrocoagulation therapy are generally effective, but endoscopic band therapy and hemoclips may also be used, and surgery is sometimes required.

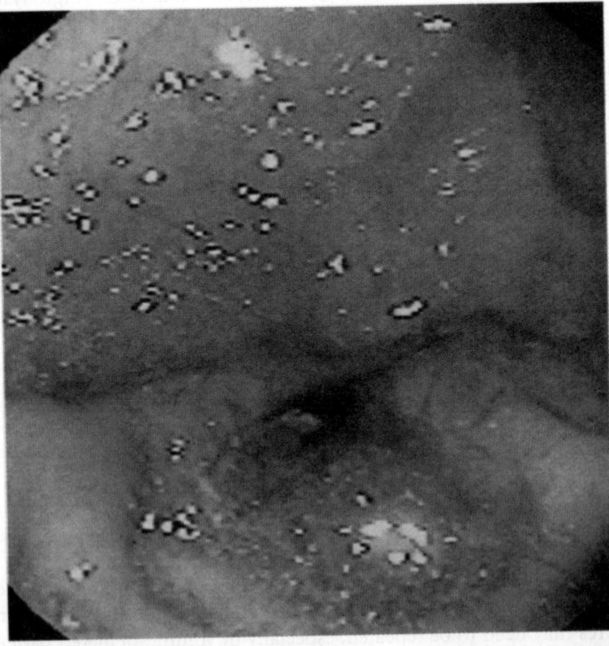

FIGURE 146–6 • Endoscopy of the stomach in a patient with a Dieulafoy lesion. Note the visible vessel manifested as a pale protuberance surrounded by a clot with adjacent normal-appearing mucosa. (From Emory TS, Carpenter HA, Gostout CJ, Sobin LH [eds]: Atlas of Gastrointestinal Endoscopy and Endoscopic Biopsies. Washington, DC, Armed Forces Institute of Pathology, American Registry of Pathology, 2000.)

Other Ectasias

Telangiectases are similar to angiodysplasias but occur in all the layers of the bowel wall, are usually congenital, and often occur in other organ systems. *Hereditary hemorrhagic telangiectasia* (Osler-Weber-Rendu disease; Chapter 179) is an autosomal dominant disorder with telangiectases involving the lips; mucous membranes, especially in the mouth and nose; gastrointestinal tract, especially the stomach and small bowel; liver; lung; retina; and central nervous system. Patients with *Turner's syndrome* (Chapter 255), *scleroderma* (Chapter 288), and the *CREST syndrome* (Chapter 288) (calcinosis, Raynaud's phenomenon, esophageal dysmotility, sclerodactyly, telangiectasia) may also have gastrointestinal tract telangiectases.

Vascular ectasias involving venules and capillaries can also be seen in the small bowel *(congestive enteropathy)*, in the colon *(congestive colopathy)*, and more commonly, in the stomach *(congestive gastropathy)* in patients with portal hypertension (Chapter 157). In contrast to angiodysplasias, these lesions tend to be more diffuse, appear as multiple, fine punctate red spots or as a mosaic pattern similar to the gastritis of *Helicobacter pylori*, and are more often found in the proximal than the distal part of the stomach. Therapies that decrease portal hypertension can reduce or eliminate these lesions and bleeding from them.

Gastric antral vascular ectasia (GAVE), or watermelon stomach, also involves venules and capillaries with thrombosis as well as ectasia. Erythematous streaks similar to the stripes on a watermelon are typically seen in the antrum radiating toward the pylorus. Patients usually have occult bleeding and less often melena. GAVE is associated with connective tissue diseases (e.g., systemic lupus erythematosus [Chapter 287], mixed connective tissue disease [Chapter 288], scleroderma [Chapter 288]), pernicious anemia (Chapter 170), and portal hypertension (Chapter 157). However, unlike congestive gastropathy, treatment of portal hypertension does not eliminate GAVE or bleeding from it. Argon plasma coagulation is the usual therapy if iron replacement alone is not effective. Antrectomy is rarely needed.

Neoplastic Vascular Lesions

Hemangiomas are uncommon, usually benign vascular tumors that can be found throughout the gastrointestinal tract, often in the rectum or colon. They may be single or multiple, bluish purple, sessile or polypoid. In some persons these lesions are multiple and associated with skin lesions, such as the *blue rubber bleb nevus syndrome* with purple-blue cutaneous hemangiomas or the *Klippel-Trenaunay* syndrome with port-wine–colored cutaneous hemangiomas, hemihypertrophy, and varicose veins. Rare vascular malignant neoplasms of the gastrointestinal tract include *angiosarcomas* and *hemangioendotheliomas.*

Miscellaneous Vascular Disorders

Aortoenteric fistulas, which most commonly occur after surgery for an aortic aneurysm (Chapter 78), may be related to infection of the graft and can result in torrential gastrointestinal bleeding. Many of these fistulas communicate with the duodenum. Evaluation of bleeding in persons who have previously undergone abdominal aortic surgery should include urgent extended-length upper endoscopy to document a fistula or diagnose another definitive source of the bleeding. Angiography and radiographic tests (CT, magnetic resonance imaging [MRI]) are helpful only if the findings are abnormal (i.e., there is evidence of a fistula) because of their poor sensitivity for the presence of aortoenteric fistulas. If no clear alternative source for the bleeding can readily be found, explorative surgery is indicated.

Celiac artery compression syndrome (median arcuate ligament syndrome) is a very rare pseudo-ischemic syndrome. Patients are often young and healthy and have postprandial upper abdominal pain, most likely caused by extrinsic compression of the celiac axis by the median arcuate ligament of the diaphragm. Sitophobia can result in considerable weight loss, and there may be a loud systolic bruit in the epigastric region on physical examination. Visceral angiography supports the diagnosis, but bruits and celiac axis compression may occur without symptoms. Surgical therapy is indicated after other possible causes of the patient's symptoms have been excluded.

Bowel as well as large vessel rupture can occur as a complication of *Ehlers-Danlos syndrome type IV* (Chapter 281). Similar vascular catastrophes with gastrointestinal or intraperitoneal hemorrhage can occur in patients with *pseudoxanthoma elasticum type I* (Chapter 281) or with *visceral artery aneurysms* (secondary to atherosclerosis, fibrodysplasia, portal hypertension, pregnancy, pancreatitis, vasculitis, or trauma).

HEPATIC AND SPLENIC VASCULAR DISEASE

Budd-Chiari Syndrome

Budd-Chiari syndrome can occur as a result of any process that interferes with the normal flow of blood out of the liver, including constrictive pericarditis (Chapter 77) and veno-occlusive disease (Chapter 153). Hepatic vein thrombosis, which is the main cause of Budd-Chiari syndrome, may involve one, two, or all three of the major hepatic veins, with or without partial or complete occlusion of the inferior vena cava. Often, Budd-Chiari syndrome is due to a hypercoagulable state (Chapter 182), such as a chronic myeloproliferative disorder (e.g., polycythemia vera [Chapter 172], essential thrombocythemia [Chapter 177], myeloid metaplasia [Chapter 177]) or other hypercoagulable condition (e.g., factor V [Leiden] gene mutation, antiphospholipid antibody syndrome, antithrombin III deficiency). Malignancies (direct compression or invasion of hepatic veins, hypercoagulable state), infections (liver abscess), pregnancy, and membranous obstruction (webs) of the inferior vena cava are also associated with Budd-Chiari syndrome.

Clinical Manifestations

The syndrome is usually subacute, occurs over a period of weeks to months, and is characterized by the insidious onset of upper abdominal pain, hepatomegaly, and ascites. Fulminant or acute manifestations consisting of encephalopathy, jaundice, ascites, and liver failure are rare.

Diagnosis

Liver function testing usually reveals mild nonspecific elevations in serum aspartate and alanine aminotransferase levels. Doppler US of the liver is the initial diagnostic test of choice, but the absence of hepatic venous flow or venous thrombosis (or both) is also readily apparent with contrast-enhanced CT scanning or MRI. Hepatic venography can confirm the diagnosis (Fig. 146–7) and, with imaging of the inferior vena cava, as well as selective venous pressure measurements, can help guide therapy.

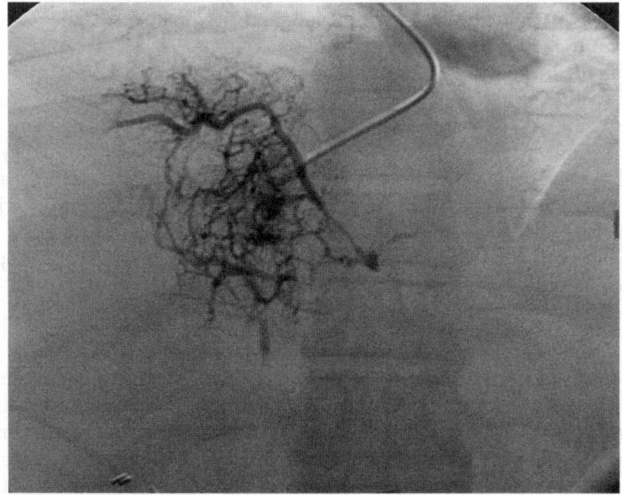

FIGURE 146–7 • Budd-Chiari syndrome. A hepatic vein contrast study depicts the "spider web" pattern of venovenous collaterals attempting to bypass a thrombosed hepatic vein. (Courtesy of Patrick Kamath.)

Treatment

Therapy includes diagnosis and treatment of underlying conditions, anticoagulation (intravenous heparin; see Table 81–4) to prevent the propagation of thrombi, and treatment of the ascites (e.g., diuretics; Chapter 157). To decompress the congested liver, most patients require interventional radiologic procedures, such as angioplasty, stenting, or transjugular intrahepatic portosystemic shunts, to restore hepatic venous flow. Surgical procedures such as surgical shunts to drain the portal or mesenteric venous system into the inferior vena cava can also decompress the liver. Liver transplantation (Chapter 158) should be considered for patients with fulminant liver failure or cirrhosis, or both. Many but not all patients with Budd-Chiari syndrome require lifelong warfarin anticoagulation (Chapter 35), even after liver transplantation.

Portal Vein Thrombosis

In adults, cirrhosis, hypercoagulable states, inflammatory disorders (e.g., pancreatitis, Crohn's disease), and medical procedures (e.g., splenectomy, liver transplantation, transjugular intrahepatic portosystemic shunt) are most often the cause of portal vein thrombosis. Clinical manifestations include portal hypertension with variceal bleeding and ascites. Abdominal pain may indicate extension of the thrombus into the SMV with intestinal ischemia. The diagnosis is confirmed by Doppler US or MRA. Endoscopy for the diagnosis and treatment of varices (Chapter 136), with or without pharmacologic treatment of the portal hypertension (e.g., β-blockade with propranolol; Chapter 157), is often beneficial. Surgical shunts are rarely necessary.

Splenic Vein Thrombosis

Splenic vein thrombosis is usually secondary to malignancy (e.g., pancreatic cancer), pancreatitis, or trauma. In many of these patients, isolated gastric varices develop and are difficult to treat by therapeutic endoscopy. Liver function and portal pressure are normal. Most patients with splenic vein thrombosis have splenomegaly (Chapter 174). Doppler US, MRI, and CT assist in making the diagnosis. Patients with symptomatic isolated splenic vein thrombosis are best treated by splenectomy.

Hepatic and Splenic Arterial Disease

Hepatic arterial disease may be nonocclusive or occlusive. Nonocclusive disease, termed *ischemic hepatitis,* occurs when arterial blood flow to the liver is insufficient, usually because of cardiogenic hypotension, volume depletion, or sepsis. Typically, serum aminotransferase rises acutely to levels greater than 1000 U/L. With restoration of adequate hepatic arterial blood flow, serum aminotransferase levels eventually fall back to their baseline by about 40 to 60% per day. Hepatic artery thrombosis is extremely rare except in a post–liver transplantation (Chapter 158) patient, in whom it may be manifested as mild abnormalities in liver function test results, bile duct injury (e.g., biliary stricture, cholangitis, liver abscess), or liver failure. Doppler US and angiography will confirm the diagnosis, and these patients often require biliary stents, drainage of abscesses, surgical reconstruction of the hepatic artery, or retransplantation of the liver.

The splenic artery or hepatic artery may be predisposed to the development of aneurysmal dilation, usually secondary to atherosclerosis, trauma, infection, or vasculitis. Common clinical manifestations include abdominal pain and intra-abdominal hemorrhage. Hemobilia may occur with hepatic artery aneurysms. Angiography is usually required to make the diagnosis. Symptomatic as well as sizable (variably defined, usually 1 cm or greater for a hepatic aneurysm and 2 cm or greater for a splenic artery aneurysm) aneurysms require surgery.

Fistulas from the hepatic artery to the portal vein can occur as a result of trauma, malignancy, or the inherited disorder hereditary hemorrhagic telangiectasia. The resultant portal hypertension may cause abdominal pain, ascites, and gastrointestinal bleeding, and involvement of the hepatic artery may result in biliary strictures and hepatobiliary infection. Radiographic embolization of these fistulas, surgery, or liver transplantation may be required.

SUGGESTED READINGS

Alva S, Abir F, Longo WE: Colorectal manifestations of collagen vascular disease. Am J Surg 2005;189:685–693. *Emphasizes the value of conservative, nonoperative therapies.*

Condat B, Valla D: Nonmalignant portal vein thrombosis in adults. Nat Clin Pract Gastroenterol Hepatol 2006;3:505–515. *Clinical review.*

Hirsch AT, Haskal ZJ, Hertzer NR, et al: ACC/AHA 2005 Practice Guidelines for the management of patients with peripheral arterial disease (lower extremity, renal, mesenteric, and abdominal aortic). Circulation 2006;113:e463–e654. *Consensus guidelines.*

Sreenarasimhaiah J: Diagnosis and management of ischemic colitis. Curr Gastroenterol Rep 2005;7:421–426. *A clinical review.*

Yasuharu H: Acute mesenteric ischemia: The challenge of gastroenterology. Surg Today 2005;35:185–195. *A succinct review of the pathophysiology, clinical manifestations, diagnosis, and management of acute mesenteric ischemia.*

147 PANCREATITIS

Chung Owyang

ACUTE PANCREATITIS

Definition

Acute pancreatitis, which is an inflammatory disease of the pancreas, is characterized by a discrete episode of abdominal pain and elevated serum amylase and lipase levels. In contrast to chronic pancreatitis, which is characterized by changes in pancreatic structure and by persistence of dysfunction even after the precipitating cause has been corrected, acute pancreatitis is distinguished by complete restitution of the pancreas both morphologically and functionally after the derangements that precipitated the attack have been corrected.

Epidemiology

The incidence of acute pancreatitis ranges from 1 to 5 per 10,000 per year. Among the many causes of acute pancreatitis (Fig. 147–1), alcoholism and biliary tract disease are most frequent and account for more than 70% of cases. Rare causes are responsible for about 10% of cases, but in the remainder, the cause remains unknown.

Specific Causes

Alcohol

Alcohol-induced acute pancreatitis usually occurs in patients who consume large quantities of alcohol for 5 to 10 years before the first attack (Chapter 31). However, a recent study has indicated that an increased risk for alcoholic pancreatitis may occur with as little as 25 g (or two drinks) per day. In individuals who use large amounts of alcohol, acute pancreatitis develops in only 5 to 10%. A polymorphism in the detoxifying enzyme uridine 5-diphosphate (UDP) glucuronyl transferase (UGT1A7*3) confers an increased risk for alcoholic pancreatitis. Environmental factors or cofactors such as smoking and consumption of a high-fat diet may also affect a person's susceptibility to the disease.

Several mechanisms may contribute to the development of alcoholic pancreatitis, including abnormal sphincter of Oddi spasm in the presence of stimulated pancreatic secretion, obstruction of small ductules by proteinaceous plugs, and direct toxic effects of alcohol metabolic byproducts. Alcohol may also change the amounts of potentially damaging proteases in pancreatic secretions. Increased amounts of lysosomal enzymes and an increased trypsinogen–pancreatic trypsin ratio have been reported in the pancreatic juice of alcoholic patients.

Gallstones

The frequency of acute pancreatitis is inversely proportional to the size of gallstones (Chapter 159). Persistence of stones in the bile duct or ampulla is associated with more severe disease. An impacted gallstone may permit reflux of bile into the pancreatic duct or occlude the duct's orifice.

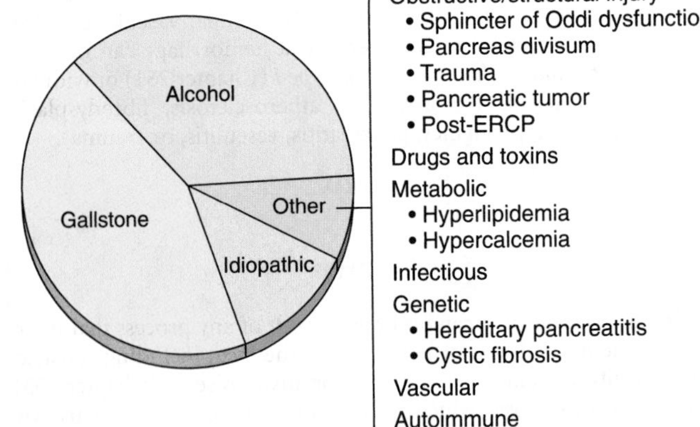

FIGURE 147–1 • Factors associated with acute pancreatitis. ERCP = endoscopic retrograde cholangiopancreatography.

Microlithiasis (crystals in bile) may cause recurrent pancreatitis, although the precise mechanism remains unknown. Microlithiasis is common after prolonged fasting, total parenteral nutrition (Chapter 236), rapid weight loss, and the use of drugs such as octreotide or ceftriaxone. Microlithiasis may be identified by the presence of sludge by ultrasonography (US) or the presence of birefringent cholesterol crystals in bile; the diagnosis should be considered in patients who have recurrent bouts of apparently idiopathic pancreatitis.

Pancreatic Obstruction

Obstruction of pancreatic secretion is a less common cause of acute pancreatitis. Sphincter of Oddi dysfunction is associated with increases in sphincter pressure caused by increased smooth muscle tone or fibrotic stricturing. Pancreas divisum results from failure of the ventral and dorsal ducts to join during fetal development; the small accessory duct of Santorini and minor papillae may produce high outflow resistance. Sphincter of Oddi dysfunction or pancreas divisum has been reported in more than 25% of patients with idiopathic pancreatitis in some series, although whether this association is causal or coincidental is difficult to determine. Pancreatitis has been reported in up to 10% of patients with pancreatic cancer (Chapter 204), but it is usually mild. Older patients with unexplained pancreatitis should undergo careful evaluation to exclude a minute pancreatic cancer amenable to resection.

Drugs and Toxins

Toxins and drugs that have been implicated in acute pancreatitis include insecticides, methanol, organophosphates, and the venom of a scorpion found in the West Indies. Some of these agents cause pancreatitis by overstimulation of the pancreas via cholinergic pathways. The most prominent family of drugs causing pancreatitis are immunosuppressants, including azathioprine and its major metabolite (6-mercaptopurine), cyclosporine, and tacrolimus. Drugs used to treat acquired immunodeficiency syndrome (AIDS), such as trimethoprim-sulfamethoxazole, pentamidine, and 2′,3′-dideoxyinosine (ddI), may cause severe pancreatitis. Furosemide, thiazide diuretics, angiotensin-converting enzyme inhibitors, sulfasalazine, and oral 5-aminosalicylic acid appear to be rare causes of pancreatitis. Therapy with estrogens is associated with a dose-dependent increase in triglyceride levels and with pancreatitis. Tetracycline has been linked to pancreatitis, usually in patients with fatty liver. Other drugs such as corticosteroids, methyldopa, procainamide, nitrofurantoin, metronidazole, and interleukin-2 (IL-2) have also been implicated, but their causal relationship is less certain.

Metabolic Factors

Attacks of acute pancreatitis are associated with hypertriglyceridemia, including familial forms (Chapter 217). Serum triglyceride levels higher than 1000 mg/dL may precipitate attacks of acute pancreatitis, and lowering serum triglyceride levels to less than 200 mg/dL can prevent pancreatitis. It is currently believed that pancreatitis occurs as a result of the harmful effects of fatty acids released into the pancreatic circulation or parenchyma by the action of pancreatic lipase. Hypercalcemia secondary to hyperparathyroidism, immobilization, multiple myeloma, or total parenteral nutrition has been linked to hyperamylasemia but probably causes pancreatitis infrequently.

Genetic Factors

In patients with a family history of pancreatitis, the possibility of familial pancreatitis should be considered. This autosomal dominant disorder has a penetrance of about 80%. The majority of patients have their first symptoms before reaching 20 years of age, with attacks frequently precipitated by alcohol, high fat intake, or emotional disturbances. Patients with this disorder also have a higher risk for pancreatic cancer. The most common genetic defect is an arginine-histidine substitution (R122H) at 7q35, the site of the trypsinogen gene, that results in resistance to trypsin hydrolysis, but other mutations involving the trypsinogen gene can also predispose to pancreatitis. Sporadic genetic mutations occur, and up to 11% of mutation-positive individuals may be silent carriers.

Mutation in the pancreatic trypsin inhibitor gene (serine protease inhibitor, kazal type 1; *SPINK1*) may also predispose to pancreatitis. Loss of function of the inhibitor gene may impair inhibition of activated trypsin within acinar cells. The relatively common *SPINK1* missense mutation in codon N34S is probably a disease modifier rather than a cause of pancreatitis because the prevalence of the N34S *SPINK1* gene mutation (≈2%) is far greater than the prevalence of pancreatitis (0.006%) and the pancreatitis phenotype is no different with either a homozygous or heterozygous N34S *SPINK1* gene mutation. However, specific *SPINK1* mutations combined with other inherited mutations, such as mutations of the calcium-sensing receptor gene, may cause pancreatitis.

Mutations in the cystic fibrosis transmembrane regulator (CFTR; Chapter 89) can cause pancreatitis. Classically, cystic fibrosis results in pulmonary disease and pancreatic insufficiency in 20% of patients, but rarely pancreatitis. Recently, a second phenotype, including recurrent acute pancreatitis and early-onset chronic pancreatitis, has been identified in heterozygotic patients without pulmonary disease.

Trauma and Iatrogenic Factors

Most cases of trauma-induced pancreatitis occur as a result of blunt rather than penetrating injury. Postoperative pancreatitis is most frequently associated with procedures that involve manipulation of the pancreas or the periampullary region, or both. Reduced vascular perfusion (e.g., shock), as may occur when surgical procedures are associated with hypotension or hypoperfusion, can also precipitate acute pancreatitis. Hyperamylasemia and abdominal pain are common after endoscopic retrograde cholangiopancreatography (ERCP) (Chapter 136), but evidence of significant pancreatitis occurs in less than 5% of patients undergoing ERCP.

Miscellaneous and Idiopathic Factors

Other unusual causes of pancreatitis include autoimmune diseases, renal and cardiac transplantation, and infections with mumps (Chapter 392) and coxsackieviruses (Chapter 402). Cytomegalovirus infection (Chapter 399) can cause acute inflammation of the pancreas in patients with AIDS (Chapter 412). Although about 20% of patients are still classified as having unexplained pancreatitis, the wider use of sphincter of Oddi manometry, biliary crystal analysis, and genetic testing should reduce this percentage in the future.

Pathobiology

Pathologically, two morphologic classifications are recognized: acute interstitial pancreatitis and acute hemorrhagic pancreatitis. The latter type is associated with much higher morbidity and mortality.

The precise mechanisms responsible for acute pancreatitis are not well understood. However, the fundamental mechanism for transformation of the initial injury into pancreatitis appears to be intracellular activation of digestive enzymes and autodigestion. The complex cascade of cellular events leading to acute pancreatitis begins in the pancreatic acinar cells. Intracellular conversion of pancreatic zymogens into active enzymes most likely involves several pathways, including (1) cleavage of trypsinogen to trypsin by the lysosomal hydrolase cathepsin B, (2) disruption of intracellular Ca^{2+} signaling, and (3) trypsinogen autoactivation. In experimental models, hyperstimulation of the pancreas may result in the fusion of lysosome and zymogens within large vacuoles, followed by activation of enzymes and acute intracellular injury. Cathepsin B is a lysosomal enzyme capable of activating trypsinogen to trypsin. Trypsin then catalyzes the conversion of many proenzymes into active forms, which in turn are responsible for the major systemic complications of acute pancreatitis. Intracellular Ca^{2+} may also play an important role in the initiation of acute pancreatitis. A rise in intracellular Ca^{2+} and disruption of acinar cell Ca^{2+} signaling occur in pancreatitis that is induced by cerulean hyperstimulation and by pancreatic duct obstruction; this rise is associated with vacuolization of acinar cells and autoactivation of trypsinogen mediated by the translocation of vacuolar adenosine triphosphatase to membrane compartments in the acinar cell and the resulting acidification of intracellular compartments.

The pancreas has several safety mechanisms to cope with the problem of autoactivation of zymogens. One mechanism is the pancreatic secretory trypsin inhibitor (PSTI), which is found in secretory granules. PSTI binds with the active site of trypsin in a ratio of 1 : 1 and inhibits trypsin activity. When more than 10% of the trypsinogen is activated, this inhibitory mechanism becomes ineffective. Thus, any disorders or agents that adversely affect or overwhelm this protective mechanism can cause pancreatitis.

During pancreatitis, inflammatory mediators, including cytokines (such as tumor necrosis factor-α and platelet-activating factor) and chemokines (such as IL-6), are generated and released. These agents stimulate the recruitment of inflammatory cells, enhance the activation and adherence of inflammatory cells to the vascular wall, or cause direct cell injury. Generation of pro-inflammatory mediators can lead to the systemic inflammatory response syndrome (SIRS; Chapters 107 and 109). Marked leukocyte activation can result in distant organ injury and the development of multisystem organ failure. SIRS and pancreatic infection are the two major causes of death from acute pancreatitis.

Clinical Manifestations

The typical symptoms of acute pancreatitis are abdominal pain, nausea, and vomiting. Pain usually develops first and remains constant, without the waxing and waning pattern typical of intestinal or renal colic (Chapter 134 and see Table 134–2). The pain is frequently located in the epigastrium with radiation to the midback region; it typically lasts for hours to days and is not relieved by vomiting. Abdominal findings vary with the severity of the attack, from minimal local tenderness to marked generalized rebound tenderness, guarding, and abdominal distention. Bowel sounds are frequently diminished or absent because of intestinal ileus. Jaundice can occur even without stone-induced pancreatitis as a result of compression of the common bile duct by the edematous pancreas. With severe attacks, hypotension, tachypnea, tachycardia, and hyperthermia may be noted. Fever is usually less than 38.5° C. Examination of the skin may reveal tender areas of induration and erythema resulting from subcutaneous fat necrosis. In severe necrotizing pancreatitis, large ecchymoses may occasionally appear in the flanks (Grey Turner's sign) or the umbilical area (Cullen's sign); these ecchymoses are caused by blood dissecting from the retroperitoneally located pancreas along the fascial planes.

Diagnosis

Laboratory Findings

Serum Amylase

The diagnosis of acute pancreatitis is based on clinical findings and supported by an elevation in serum amylase and lipase. Most, but not all patients with acute pancreatitis have hyperamylasemia. Typically, the serum amylase level rises rapidly over the initial 2 to 12 hours of an attack and then slowly declines to its normal values over the next 3 to 5 days. The magnitude of hyperamylasemia has no prognostic value. Hyperamylasemia is not specific to pancreatitis, but marked elevations in serum amylase (more than three times the upper limit of normal) support the diagnosis of pancreatitis in a patient with severe abdominal pain. Apart from acute pancreatitis, modest hyperamylasemia may result from small bowel obstruction, perforation, or infarction; a perforated duodenal ulcer; or liberation of amylase into the circulation from nongastrointestinal sources such as the lung, fallopian tubes, and salivary glands

TABLE 147–1 CAUSES OF INCREASED SERUM AMYLASE AND LIPASE LEVELS

	Amylase	Lipase
Pancreatitis	↑	↑
Intestinal injury/obstruction	↑	↑
Biliary stone	↑	↑
Tubo-ovarian disease	↑	Normal
Renal failure	↑	↑
Macroamylasemia	↑	Normal
Parotitis	↑	Normal

(Table 147–1). Alternatively, hyperamylasemia may result from release of amylase from certain tumors or be caused by reduced renal clearance of amylase secondary to renal failure. Pancreatic hyperamylasemia can occur after ERCP or after passage of common duct stones, even in the absence of pancreatitis. Macroamylasemia, an unusual but not rare condition, can occasionally cause isolated elevation of the serum amylase level. In this condition, amylase is bound to an abnormal serum protein; the complex is not cleared by the kidney and results in hyperamylasemia. Macroamylasemia should be suspected when hyperamylasemia is associated with low urinary amylase levels. Hypertriglyceridemia may spuriously depress serum amylase measurements; diluting the serum unmasks the increased serum amylase level.

Amylase activity in blood is composed of isoenzymes from both the pancreas and salivary glands. Pancreatic isoamylase normally accounts for approximately 40% of total serum amylase activity. In acute pancreatitis, serum pancreatic isoamylase increases substantially. Unfortunately, such increases can also occur in conditions other than acute pancreatitis, including intestinal injury and renal insufficiency, thereby rendering its measurement nonspecific.

Serum Lipase

During acute pancreatitis, serum lipase levels increase in parallel with serum amylase levels. The lipase level remains elevated longer and thus may help diagnose pancreatitis after an attack has passed. Additionally, lipase levels are normal in patients with macroamylasemia and parotitis. Though not entirely specific for pancreatitis, serum lipase has supplanted amylase as the single test of choice for the diagnosis of pancreatitis.

Other Blood Tests

Routine laboratory tests in patients with moderate to severe acute pancreatitis usually reveal leukocytosis. Transient mild hyperglycemia is common and occurs when excess glucagon is released from alpha cells of the islets of Langerhans. Hypocalcemia is generally caused by extravasation of nonionized, albumin-bound calcium from inflamed retroperitoneal and, at times, peritoneal surfaces; this form of hypocalcemia is common, usually causes no symptoms, and requires no treatment. In necrotizing pancreatitis, hypocalcemia can be more severe because of loss of ionized calcium within areas of fat necrosis in the pancreas and peripancreatic tissue. Hyperbilirubinemia and elevations in serum aminotransferase and alkaline phosphatase levels are seen in up to 50% of patients as a result of either compression of the common bile duct by the inflamed pancreas or the nonobstructive cholestasis that accompanies severe illness. In the presence of pancreatitis, an increase in liver enzyme values, especially alanine aminotransferase to more than three times normal, suggests a biliary cause. Hypoalbuminemia may occur as a result of extravasation of albumin from inflamed retroperitoneal and peritoneal surfaces. The serum triglyceride level should be measured in all patients because of its etiologic implications and to interpret unexpectedly normal serum amylase levels. Serum triglyceride levels less than 500 mg/dL are unlikely to be a cause of pancreatitis. For example, most individuals who abuse alcohol have moderate, but transient elevations in triglyceride levels, probably as an epiphenomenon but not as the cause of pancreatitis.

Urine Tests

The urinary amylase–to–creatinine clearance ratio increases from 3% to approximately 10% in acute pancreatitis. Even moderate renal insufficiency interferes with the accuracy and specificity of this test. Excretion of urinary amylase is not increased in patients with macroamylasemia. Thus, other than to diagnose macroamylasemia, urinary amylase and the amylase–to–creatinine clearance ratio are not used clinically.

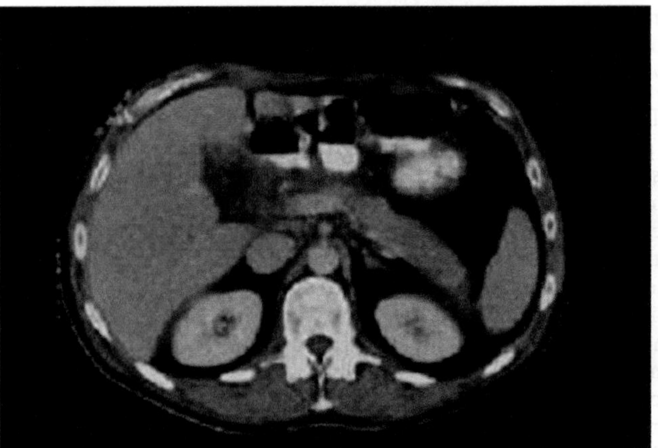

FIGURE 147–2 • Typical computed tomography scan in a patient with acute non-necrotizing pancreatitis. After intravenous contrast injection, the normally enhancing pancreatic parenchyma can be seen separately from the nonenhancing peripancreatic fluid that surrounds the pancreatic tail. (Courtesy of Poonputt Chotiprasidhi.)

Imaging

Chest and Abdominal Radiographs

Standard and upright chest and abdominal radiographs should be obtained in patients suspected of having acute pancreatitis. Chest radiographs may show pleural effusions and basilar atelectasis. Bilateral pulmonary opacification with a normal-sized heart is the hallmark of adult respiratory distress syndrome (ARDS; Chapter 105). Abdominal radiographs should be obtained to exclude nonpancreatic diseases such as intestinal perforation. Intestinal gas patterns may indicate ileus, which may sometimes appear as an isolated dilated loop of small bowel overlying the pancreas (a sentinel loop) or dilation of the transverse colon with abrupt termination of the gas column at the splenic flexure (colon cutoff sign) when the inflammatory process affects the phrenicocolic ligament.

Ultrasound and Computed Tomography

US and computed tomography (CT) play important roles in the diagnosis and management of acute pancreatitis. US is the single best noninvasive test for detecting cholelithiasis (Chapters 134 and 135), although it is less reliable for direct visualization of a bile duct stone. An inflamed pancreas may appear hypoechoic on US because of edema in the parenchyma. However, visualization of the pancreas is limited by intestinal gas or adipose tissue in 30 to 40% of patients.

CT is the primary modality for evaluating the extent and local complications of pancreatitis. Pancreatic inflammation may be seen as pancreatic enlargement, inhomogeneity of the pancreatic parenchyma, or fluid infiltrating the peripancreatic fat in 90% of patients (Fig. 147–2). Dynamic CT during bolus administration of intravenous contrast is useful to evaluate the severity of pancreatitis because it can demonstrate the poor pancreatic perfusion that is suggestive of pancreatic necrosis (Fig. 147–3). The CT finding of necrosis identifies patients who are at higher risk for pancreatic infection and death (Table 147–2).

Magnetic Resonance Imaging and Endoscopic Retrograde Cholangiopancreatography

Magnetic resonance imaging (MRI) is probably equivalent to CT for imaging an acutely inflamed pancreas. MRI is better than CT for distinguishing between an uncomplicated pseudocyst and one that contains necrotic debris. Though more expensive and less accessible, MRI is preferred in patients who are pregnant or have contrast allergies. In patients with suspected biliary pancreatitis, magnetic resonance cholangiopancreatography (MRCP) may identify more than 90% of bile duct stones.

ERCP is not useful for establishing the diagnosis of acute pancreatitis, but it is very useful to diagnose and treat persistent bile duct stones in acute pancreatitis. It should also be used in the investigation of patients with unexplained recurrent pancreatitis. It is especially useful for the diagnosis of mild chronic pancreatitis, pancreas divisum, or sphincter of Oddi disease. However, it should be noted that pancreatitis occurs in about 5% of patients undergoing ERCP. This risk for pancreatitis increases significantly in female patients with normal serum bilirubin, patients suspected of sphincter of Oddi dysfunction, and those with a previous history of post-ERCP pancreatitis. In fact, patients with the lowest probability of harboring truly obstructive pathology are at the highest risk for the development of pancreatitis after ERCP, even if the procedure is performed for diagnosis alone. Because new techniques such as MRCP and endoscopic ultrasound (EUS) have accuracy rates rivaling that of ERCP, they may be preferable to ERCP for patients with equivocal evidence of biliary obstruction, especially those at high risk for post-ERCP pancreatitis.

Differential Diagnosis

Acute pancreatitis must be distinguished from a number of conditions that cause upper abdominal pain, nausea, and vomiting (see Table 134–1)—especially a perforated viscus, bowel obstruction, mesenteric ischemia, and cholecystitis (Chapters 145, 146, and 159). Each of these processes can be marked by elevated serum amylase/lipase levels and be difficult to distinguish from acute pancreatitis. Features that favor the diagnosis of acute pancreatitis include greater than a one- to two-fold elevation in the serum amylase level, CT evidence of pancreatic inflammation, lack of free air on an abdominal plain radiograph or CT scan, and improvement with nonoperative treatment. If doubt persists and clinical deterioration continues, surgical intervention may be necessary to establish the diagnosis.

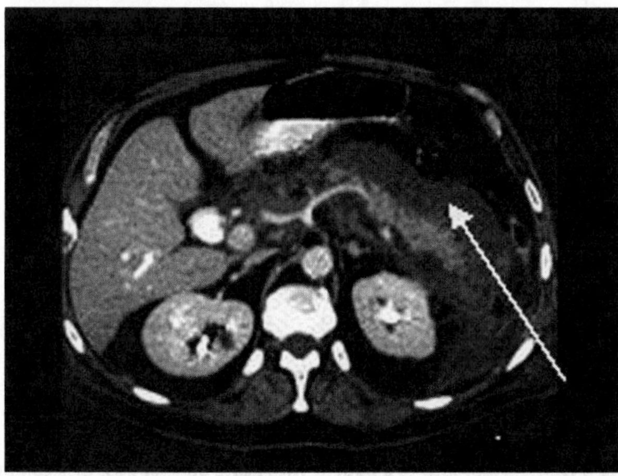

FIGURE 147–3 • Typical computed tomography scan in a patient with necrotizing pancreatitis. Peripancreatic and retroperitoneal edema, as well as large nonenhancing areas of necrosis (arrow), are visible in the body and tail of the pancreas. This degree of necrosis is classified as grade D (see Table 147–2).

Evaluation of Severity

Among the 200,000 patients admitted to hospitals each year in the United States with acute pancreatitis, approximately 20% have severe acute pancreatitis. In contrast to mild acute pancreatitis, which has a mortality rate of less than 1%, the death rate for severe acute pancreatitis is much higher: 10% with sterile pancreatitis and 25% with infected pancreatic necrosis. Thus it is important to establish the severity of acute pancreatitis to predict the patient's course and anticipate complications. Prognostic information from specific laboratory tests, clinical and physiologic assessment, and CT should guide the use of prophylactic antibiotics, urgent bile duct imaging, and early ERCP.

Laboratory Tests

Routine blood tests such as serum amylase/lipase or white blood cell counts provide little prognostic information, whereas markers such as serum or urinary trypsinogen activation peptide (TAP) and C-reactive protein may help separate mild pancreatitis from severe pancreatitis. The TAP assay, which is an indirect measure of the amount of active trypsin, appears to discriminate between mild and severe disease. Urinary TAP can accurately predict the severity of acute pancreatitis 24 hours after onset and may be used as a single marker to assess severity in clinical practice. Neutrophil-specific elastase and IL-6 are released from inflammatory cells and are elevated in blood during the first 12 hours of acute pancreatitis; their elevation correlates with the severity of pancreatitis. C-reactive protein is induced by IL-6 and is a later marker to distinguish patients with severe disease on the second hospital day. A peak of more than 210 mg/L on days 2 to 4 or more than 120 mg/L at the end of the first week may be as predictive as the multiple factor scoring system (see the next section).

Clinical and Physiologic Evaluation

A number of scoring systems can predict the morbidity and mortality of acute pancreatitis. Ranson's criteria, which are the most well known (see Table 147–2), include 11 characteristics. The five that are assessed at admission reflect the intensity of the inflammatory response, whereas the six evaluated during the initial 48 hours reflect serious complications, including fluid shifts, cardiovascular instability, and end-organ failure. In general, patients with fewer than two criteria have less than 1% mortality. Conversely, patients with more than six positive criteria have an increased likelihood of pancreatic necrosis and infection, as well as a

TABLE 147–2 PROGNOSTIC CRITERIA FOR ACUTE PANCREATITIS

Ranson's Criteria*	Simplified Glasgow Criteria†	CT Criteria‡
On admission	Within 48 hr of admission	A. Normal
Age >55 yr	Age >55 yr	B. Enlargement
WBC >16,000/μL	WBC >15,000/μL	C. Pancreatic inflammation
AST >250 U/L	LDH >600 U/L	D. Single fluid collection
LDH >350 U/L	Glucose >180 mg/dL	E. Multiple fluid collection
Within 48 hr after admission	Albumin <3.2 g/dL	
Glucose >200 mg/dL	Ca^{2+} <8 mg/dL	
HCT decrease by >10%	Arterial Po_2 <60 mm Hg	
BUN increase by >5 mg/dL	BUN >45 mg/dL	
Ca^{2+} <8 mg/dL		
Arterial Po_2 <60 mm Hg		
Base deficit >4 mEq/L		
Fluid sequestration >6 L		

AST = aspartate aminotransferase; BUN = blood urea nitrogen; Ca^{2+} = serum calcium level; HCT = hematocrit; WBC = white blood count.
*Three or more Ranson's criteria predict a complicated clinical course. Ranson JH, Rifkind KM, Turner JW: Prognostic signs and nonoperative peritoneal lavage in acute pancreatitis. Surg Gynecol Obstet 1976;143:209–219.
†Blamey SL, Imrie CW, O'Neill J, et al: Prognostic factors in acute pancreatitis. Gut 1984;25:1340–1346.
‡Grades A and B represent very mild disease with essentially no risk for infection or death. Grade C represents moderately severe disease with a minimal likelihood of infection and essentially no risk of mortality. Grades D and E represent severe pancreatitis with an infection rate of 30 to 50% and a mortality rate of 15%. Balthazar EJ, Robinson DL, Megibow AJ, et al: Acute pancreatitis: Value of CT in establishing prognosis. Radiology 1990;174:331–336.

higher mortality rate. The Glasgow system, which can be calculated anytime within the first 48 hours of hospitalization, measures only eight parameters (see Table 147–2) but appears to have prognostic accuracy similar to that of Ranson's criteria. The Acute Physiology and Chronic Health Evaluation (APACHE) II system uses 14 routinely measured parameters to produce a numerical score based on a patient's deviation from the normal range; however, it is more complex and difficult to use outside an intensive care unit.

Both standard CT and contrast-enhanced CT provide useful prognostic information. The CT severity index (see Table 147–2) correlates with the Ranson criteria for assessing severity. Contrast-enhanced CT can be used to evaluate the presence and extent of pancreatic necrosis, which correlates well with morbidity and mortality. In non-necrotizing acute pancreatitis, infection is very rare and mortality is less than 1% (see Fig. 147–2). Conversely, necrotizing pancreatitis (see Fig. 147–3) is associated with a 30 to 50% rate of infection, and mortality ranges between 10 and 30%.

The Atlanta classification categorizes acute pancreatitis as mild or severe. Pancreatitis without parenchymal necrosis on CT scan is termed interstitial or edematous pancreatitis and is usually mild. Patients have severe acute pancreatitis if they have any of four criteria: (1) organ failure with one or more of the following: shock (systolic blood pressure <90 mm Hg), pulmonary insufficiency (Pao_2 <60 mm Hg), renal failure (serum creatinine >2 mg/dL after hydration), or gastrointestinal tract bleeding (>500 mL in 24 hours); (2) local complications such as necrosis, pseudocyst, or abscess; (3) at least three of Ranson's criteria; or (4) at least eight of the APACHE II criteria.

Treatment

Rx

Because there is no proven therapy that directly affects pancreatic inflammation, the main treatment goal for acute pancreatitis is to provide supportive care, including fluid resuscitation, maintenance of optimal fluid balance, and close monitoring for signs of local and systemic complications (Fig. 147–4). More than 80% of patients with acute pancreatitis have mild disease with no complications. Nasogastric suction is not necessary in mild pancreatitis, but it is recommended in the presence of vomiting and ileus. Patients with mild acute pancreatitis can generally begin oral feeding within a few days of the onset of pain. Three randomized control trials have demonstrated that enteral feeding is not only safe and feasible but also associated with fewer infectious complications and lower cost than parenteral nutrition is. [1] Nasogastric feeding is as safe as nasojejunal feeding, even with severe pancreatitis. [2] Parenteral nutrition is reserved for patients who cannot tolerate enteral feeding or in whom an adequate infusion rate cannot be reached within 2 to 4 days.

Patients should receive sufficient analgesic medication for pain control. Abdominal pain may be treated with 50 to 100 mg of meperidine every 4 hours as needed. More severe pain requires hydromorphone (Dilaudid, 2 to 4 mg every 4 hours as needed), which has a longer half-life than meperidine and may be given parenterally by a patient-controlled anesthesia pump. Prophylactic antibiotic therapy is not indicated in patients with uncomplicated acute pancreatitis. Severe intravascular volume contraction and hypovolemia, which can be caused by exudation of fluid into the inflamed peripancreatic retroperitoneum, as well as by gastrointestinal fluid loss from vomiting and nasogastric suction, should be corrected promptly. Patients who are still hypotensive after adequate volume replacement require placement of central lines to allow more precise assessment and management of fluid and electrolyte requirements. Patients with severe necrotizing pancreatitis frequently have a high cardiac index and low peripheral vascular resistance typical of SIRS. Most patients with gallstone pancreatitis have a mild episode, do well, and can undergo cholecystectomy during the same admission. A meta-analysis of four randomized controlled trials showed that patients with severe acute pancreatitis who demonstrate evidence of acute cholangitis or progressive jaundice benefit from early ERCP for bile duct clearance. [3] The role of

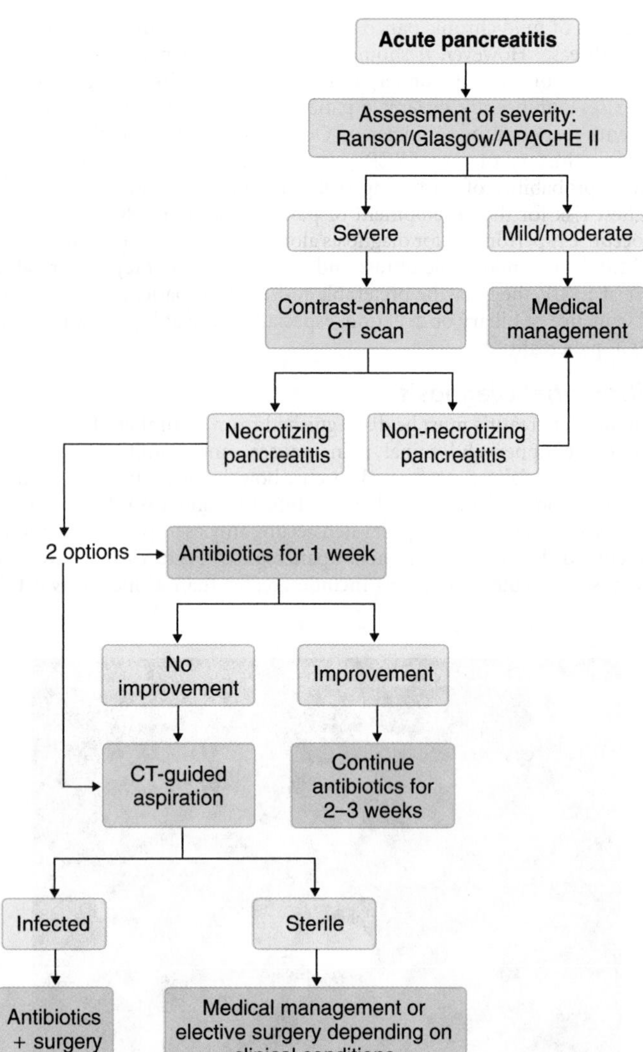

FIGURE 147–4 • Approach to a patient with acute pancreatitis. CT = computed tomography.

Rx

early ERCP in patients without biliary obstruction or cholangitis is unclear.

The major indication for early surgical intervention is diagnostic uncertainty in the presence of an acute abdomen. Intestinal perforation or necrosis, which sometimes mimic hemorrhagic acute pancreatitis, can be confirmed and corrected only when laparotomy is performed. Infected necrosis (see later) also requires urgent intervention. Surgical débridement plus drainage is usually necessary.

Hypertriglyceridemia may cause 1 to 4% of cases of acute pancreatitis. Every attempt should be made to lower serum triglyceride levels to less than 200 mg/dL, usually with a statin but with other medications as needed (Chapter 217).

Complications

In patients who show evidence of smoldering persistent pancreatitis, every effort should be made to exclude infected pancreatic necrosis, an impacted gallstone in the duodenal ampulla, and a pseudocyst. If US does not demonstrate a pseudocyst or an enlarged pancreas, a CT scan is indicated. CT will often reveal structural abnormalities such as a pseudocyst, pancreatic necrosis, or dilated ducts that may have escaped detection.

Local Complications

Infected pancreatic necrosis should be suspected in patients who have moderate to severe acute pancreatitis and worsening of symp-

Rx

toms after initial improvement or in those in whom new fever (especially >38.5° C), marked leukocytosis, positive blood cultures or, other evidence of sepsis develops (see Fig. 147–4). If necrotic pancreatitis is suspected, an emergency abdominal CT scan with intravenous contrast enhancement should be performed. Pancreatic or peripancreatic infection, usually occurring at least 10 days after the onset of pancreatitis, develops in 40 to 70% of patients with pancreatic necrosis and is the leading cause of morbidity and mortality in patients with severe acute pancreatitis. A meta-analysis of eight randomized trials showed that prophylactic broad-spectrum antibiotics that penetrate pancreatic tissue reduce mortality in patients with severe acute pancreatitis. [4] If fever or leukocytosis persists or develops later than 7 to 10 days after diagnosis without an obvious source of infection, fine-needle aspiration of the necrotic area should be performed to exclude infection. The demonstration of polymorphonuclear cells and bacteria is highly suggestive of infected pancreatic necrosis and should lead to urgent surgical intervention because the mortality in conservatively treated patients with infected pancreatic necrosis is greater than 60%. Antibiotic therapy should be initiated or continued to cover gram-negative enteric and anaerobic organisms; antibiotics with high penetration into pancreatic tissue include imipenem-cilastatin, fluoroquinolones, and metronidazole. Standard regimens include imipenem, 500 mg intravenously three times daily, or pefloxacin, 400 mg intravenously twice daily, and/or metronidazole, 500 mg three times daily for 10 to 14 days. [5]

Management of clinically sterile pancreatic necrosis remains controversial; the necrotic tissue may resolve or gradually evolve into a pseudocyst or a region of organized pancreatic necrosis. In patients with persistent necrosis, 40% or more become infected during their course; others may experience persistent organ failure despite prolonged supportive care. Careful clinical monitoring and repeated dynamic CT scans are recommended to monitor the progression of necrotizing pancreatitis. If the condition deteriorates, surgery should be contemplated.

Pancreatic pseudocysts occur in 10 to 20% of cases of acute pancreatitis. The diagnosis is most easily made by abdominal US or CT scan. Smaller cysts tend to disappear without specific treatment. Cysts that have been present for more than 6 weeks and are larger than 5 cm in diameter usually require treatment. The presence of severe pain, rapid expansion, or complications such as bleeding, leakage, or rupture may accelerate the need to intervene. Internal surgical drainage into the stomach or small intestine remains the most widely used treatment, but endoscopic or percutaneous drainage can be an attractive nonsurgical option.

Acute pancreatitis can cause true pancreatic ascites, defined by the presence of large amounts of fluid that is rich in pancreatic amylase and protein and that results from a communication between the pancreatic duct or a pseudocyst and the peritoneal cavity (Chapters 149 and 157). The site of ductal disruption is usually identified by ERCP. Acute pancreatitis may infrequently cause bleeding or thrombosis of peripancreatic vessels. Arterial hemorrhage occurs when a pseudocyst erodes into a pancreatic artery and transforms the pseudocyst cavity into a pseudoaneurysm. The diagnosis is made by CT scan and angiography; the bleeding artery can often be treated by embolization, but surgical intervention is sometimes required. The most common venous complication of pancreatitis is occlusion of the splenic vein, which may result in splenomegaly and gastric varices.

Systemic Complications

The two most important systemic complications of acute pancreatitis are renal and respiratory failure. Renal failure generally occurs as a result of hypovolemia and decreased renal perfusion (Chapter 121). Prevention and treatment of pancreatitis-associated renal failure depend, to a large extent, on correction of fluid and electrolyte abnormalities. Mild and transient respiratory failure is believed to be the result of infradiaphragmatic inflammation, splinting of respiration, and atelectasis. Arterial hypoxemia with an arterial PO_2 less than 70 mm Hg is often associated with mild respiratory alkalosis and is frequently noted in patients with severe acute pancreatitis; it is usually detected within the first 2 or 3 days of an attack. Hypoalbuminemia and fluid overload are probably important contributory factors. In most cases, the respiratory failure generally improves as the acute phase of pancreatitis ends. Some patients, however, progress to a more severe form of respiratory failure that resembles ARDS (Chapter 105). This poor prognostic sign is frequently associated with a complicated clinical course or death (or both). Pancreatitis-associated ARDS results from injury to the alveolar membrane or degradation of surfactant by circulating enzymes, such as phospholipase, that may be released from the inflamed pancreas. Treatment is mainly supportive because specific therapy for pancreatitis-associated ARDS has not been defined.

Surgical Therapy

Infected pancreatic necrosis should be treated by surgical débridement. Outcomes are better if surgery is delayed until the necrosis has organized for at least 12 days and usually for about 4 weeks after the onset of pancreatitis, [6] when separation of tissue planes is easier and pancreatectomy can be avoided. In general, surgery is not indicated for patients with sterile necrosis unless clinical deterioration continues despite optimal medical care. In patients who are poor surgical candidates, minimal-access necrosectomy (débridement) by either CT-guided percutaneous or endoscopic routes has shown encouraging results.

Prognosis

The natural history of pancreatitis is unpredictable and depends on the cause. In gallstone pancreatitis, cholecystectomy will prevent further attacks. Hyperparathyroidism, hyperlipidemia, and implicated drugs may cause or contribute to pancreatitis; elimination of these precipitants should prevent reoccurrence. With the exception of alcoholic pancreatitis, progression from acute to chronic pancreatitis is rare. In most cases of alcoholic pancreatitis, structural and functional abnormalities have generally already occurred, so pancreatic structure and function may continue to deteriorate despite alcohol abstinence, albeit at a slower pace. Nevertheless, alcohol abstinence will decrease the risk for future episodes of acute pancreatitis.

CHRONIC PANCREATITIS

Definition

Chronic pancreatitis is an inflammatory disease of the pancreas characterized by the presence of permanent and progressive morphologic or functional damage to the pancreas. Many patients have intermittent flares of acute pancreatitis. Sometimes, clinical distinction between acute recurrent pancreatitis, with restoration of normal pancreatic function and structure between attacks, and chronic pancreatitis may be difficult without structural or functional studies of the pancreas.

Epidemiology

The prevalence of chronic pancreatitis in autopsy series is 0.04 to 5.0%, although it may be much higher in alcoholics. Chronic pancreatitis can be subdivided into calcifying pancreatitis and obstructive pancreatitis. Chronic calcifying pancreatitis is characterized by an irregular distribution of fibrosis and calcification within the pancreas, with varying degrees of obstruction of the primary and secondary pancreatic ducts. It is by far the most common form of chronic pancreatitis and may be associated with chronic alcoholic pancreatitis, tropical pancreatitis (see the next section), hereditary pancreatitis, pancreatitis secondary to hypercalcemia or hyperlipidemia, and idiopathic pancreatitis. Chronic obstructive pancreatitis is characterized by dilation of the ductal system, diffuse atrophy of the acinar parenchyma, and uniform fibrosis. It may be caused by pancreatic tumors, duct strictures, and possibly, pancreas divisum. In contrast to other forms of chronic pancreatitis, intraductal plugs or stones are rare or absent, and both structural and functional changes may improve when the obstruction is relieved.

Specific Causes

In the United States, alcohol consumption is by far the principal cause of chronic pancreatitis; it accounts for approximately 70% of all cases. In contrast to acute pancreatitis, gallstones do not cause chronic pancreatitis. Malnutrition-induced (tropical) pancreatitis is the most prevalent form of chronic pancreatitis in developing Asian and African countries. Consumption of cassava, a plant indigenous to these regions, may contribute to pancreatic injury by increasing serum thiocyanate levels, which subsequently increase cellular free radical production. Ingestion of a diet deficient in micronutrients and antioxidants then exposes the pancreas to injury by unopposed free radicals. In a minority of cases, chronic pancreatitis results from trauma or from prolonged metabolic disturbances such as hypercalcemia and hypertriglyceridemia. In rare instances, pancreatitis can be inherited as an autosomal dominant disease and be manifested as acute or chronic pancreatitis with prominent pancreatolithiasis.

About 4 to 6% of patients with chronic pancreatitis have *autoimmune pancreatitis* associated with hypergammaglobulinemia, histologic evidence of lymphoplasmacytic infiltration, frequent coexistence of other autoimmune diseases, and a favorable response to steroid therapy. This disease typically occurs in older male patients who have painless jaundice and weight loss but not the typical severe abdominal pain of pancreatitis. Diabetes is common in patients with autoimmune pancreatitis (42 to 76%). Up to 50% of patients may have other autoimmune diseases such as Sjögren's syndrome, primary sclerosing cholangitis, inflammatory bowel disease, and retroperitoneal fibrosis. Most patients have normal or only mildly elevated levels of serum amylase and lipase with a cholestatic profile on liver function tests. IgG4, a subtype of IgG, may distinguish autoimmune pancreatitis from other pancreatic disorders with a sensitivity of 95% and a specificity of 97%. On CT scan, most patients have a diffusely enlarged pancreas without peripancreatic fat, phlegmonous changes, or pseudocysts. The hallmark findings on ERCP are diffuse or segmental irregular narrowing of the main pancreatic duct.

Recent data indicate an increased incidence of heterozygotic mutations in the cystic fibrosis gene *(CFTR)* in patients with idiopathic chronic pancreatitis. In contrast to cystic fibrosis, which is usually accompanied by painless pancreatic insufficiency, these patients experience recurrent pancreatitis despite normal sweat test results and pulmonary function.

Approximately 20% of cases of chronic pancreatitis are idiopathic. A bimodal age distribution in adolescents and the elderly suggests that there may be two distinct pathophysiologic causes.

Pathobiology

The pathophysiologic mechanism responsible for chronic pancreatitis is unclear. Theories include stone and ductal obstruction, necrosis-fibrosis, toxic-metabolic, and oxidative stress. The stone and ductal obstruction theory stems from the observation that obstruction causes an increase in the basal secretion of pancreatic proteins and a decrease in trypsin inhibitor in experimental animal models. The proteins in pancreatic juice precipitate as protein plugs and block small ductules in a random fashion, thereby activating pancreatic enzymes that result in episodes of acute pancreatitis. In time, calcium is complexed to the protein plugs, which results in further structural deterioration of the pancreatic ducts and acinar tissue, infiltration of inflammatory cells, and eventual acinar atrophy and fibrosis of exocrine tissue. Lack of normal secretion of specific proteins that inhibit calcium carbonate stone formation has been proposed as a cause of stone formation and chronic pancreatitis. Though widely espoused, the stone and duct obstruction theory fails to explain why protein plugs are not found in all cases of chronic pancreatitis, especially in the early stages of disease. The necrosis-fibrosis hypothesis proposes that the inflammation and scarring from bouts of acute pancreatitis cause obstruction and stasis within the duct with the subsequent formation of stones. Chronic pancreatitis may require "two hits," including the early formation of protein plugs and postnecrotic fibrosis, to result in ductular obstruction. The toxic-metabolic theory proposes that alcohol produces an accumulation of cytoplasmic lipid within the acinar cells, thereby leading to fatty degeneration, cellular necrosis, and eventually fibrosis. The oxidative stress theory suggests that the fundamental cause of pancreatic disease is overactivity of hepatic mixed-function oxidases, which can produce reactive molecules that induce oxidative damage. The pancreas is exposed to this "oxidative stress" through the systemic circulation or through reflux of bile into the pancreatic duct, and the result is recurrent inflammation and tissue damage. All four proposed models of chronic pancreatitis have scientific merit, but it is unlikely that all cases of chronic pancreatitis can be explained by a single theory.

Clinical Manifestations

Abdominal pain (see Table 134–2), which is the major symptom of chronic pancreatitis, occurs in about 80% of patients. Pain may be intermittent or chronic, and it may continue, diminish, or disappear completely over time. Pain may actually improve as the severity of pancreatitis worsens. In about 15% of patients, chronic pancreatitis is relatively painless. Possible causes of pain include inflammation of the pancreas, increased intrapancreatic pressure, neural inflammation, and extrapancreatic causes such as stenosis of the common bile duct and duodenum.

Weight loss occurs in more than 50% of patients. Initially, the major cause of weight loss is decreased caloric intake because of fear of aggravating the abdominal pain. In advanced chronic pancreatitis, weight loss is usually due to pancreatic insufficiency with malabsorption or uncontrolled diabetes.

Diarrhea and steatorrhea secondary to inadequate digestion of fats occur when pancreatic lipase is reduced to less than 10% of normal levels, a reduction that indicates extensive structural damage (Chapter 143). Amylase deficiency results in diminished carbohydrate digestion and leads to osmotic diarrhea. Maldigestion of proteins is caused by deficiency of protease. Even though maldigestion affects all nutrients, the most clinically significant problem concerns maldigestion of fat and fat-soluble vitamins (A, D, E, and K).

Although glucose intolerance is common early in the course of chronic pancreatitis, clinical diabetes (Chapter 247) occurs relatively late in the disease. Ketoacidosis and diabetic neuropathy are relatively uncommon in this form of diabetes. Management of pancreatic diabetes is often difficult because the loss of both insulin and glucagon makes for a brittle form of diabetes. Insulin requirements are generally lower than for most patients with genetic diabetes because insulin receptors are not down-regulated and insulin antibodies are not initially present.

Diagnosis

If chronic pancreatitis is suspected, imaging techniques such as US and CT scan may reveal diagnostic information in approximately 70 to 90% of cases. If these tests are equivocal or negative, ERCP should be performed to visualize abnormalities of the pancreatic duct that may not be visible by imaging techniques. Less invasive EUS or MRCP can substitute for ERCP. If findings on ultrasound, CT, and ERCP or EUS are normal, a secretin/cholecystokinin stimulation test, which may disclose evidence of mild chronic pancreatitis, may be useful, especially with small duct disease.

Structural Studies

Demonstration of diffuse, speckled calcification of the pancreas on a plain film of the abdomen is diagnostic of chronic pancreatitis, but the sensitivity of this finding is only 30 to 40%. US has a sensitivity of about 70% and a specificity of 90%, and the finding of chronic pancreatitis on US generally requires no confirmatory testing. Findings associated with mild chronic pancreatitis include an irregular contour of the gland, a reduction in echogenicity or echogenic foci in the parenchyma, and mild dilation of the duct. Calcification and dilation of the main pancreatic duct are suggestive of more severe chronic pancreatitis. CT is more sensitive than US but has comparable specificity. The most common diagnostic findings of chronic pancreatitis on CT include ductal dilation, calcifications, and cystic lesions. Other findings include enlargement or atrophy of the pancreas and heterogeneous density of the parenchyma.

ERCP is commonly considered to be the most sensitive (≈90%) and specific (≈100%) diagnostic test for chronic pancreatitis. In minimal chronic pancreatitis, the branches and fine ducts show dilation and irregularity. Moderate pancreatitis is characterized by the additional finding of dilation, tortuosity, and stenosis of the main pancreatic duct. Advanced pancreatitis is defined by marked dilation of the main duct with total loss of the normal, tapered appearance; the secondary ducts are similarly dilated and blunted. ERCP should be reserved for patients in whom the diagnosis cannot be clearly established by other imaging techniques or those who have recurrent acute pancreatitis without an obvious cause.

MRCP with or without stimulation of secretin is a useful alternative to ERCP when ERCP is contraindicated or not feasible because of technical difficulties. This imaging technique allows visualization of pancreatic ductal anatomy, peripancreatic fluid collections, and the pancreatic parenchyma. Although the quality, sensitivity, and specificity of MRCP currently vary greatly among centers, MRCP may replace ERCP in this setting as these technical limitations are overcome.

EUS has equivalent sensitivity and specificity as ERCP without the risk of inducing pancreatitis. EUS-guided fine-needle aspiration can differentiate chronic pancreatitis from malignancy. As with ERCP, EUS should be used only when less invasive procedures fail to substantiate the diagnosis of chronic pancreatitis.

Assessment of Pancreatic Exocrine Function

The simplest way to assess pancreatic exocrine function is quantitative 72-hour fecal fat measurement. Increased fat in stool (>7 g/day) occurs if exocrine secretion is reduced by more than 90%, but the test is neither sensitive nor specific (Chapter 143). Among the pancreatic function tests, the secretin or cholecystokinin stimulation test with simultaneous collection of pancreatic secretions through a catheter positioned in the distal duodenum is most sensitive (sensitivity ≈90 to 95%). The collected fluid is assayed for bicarbonate (secretin stimulation) or lipase and trypsin. However, this test is time consuming (2 hours) and not widely available.

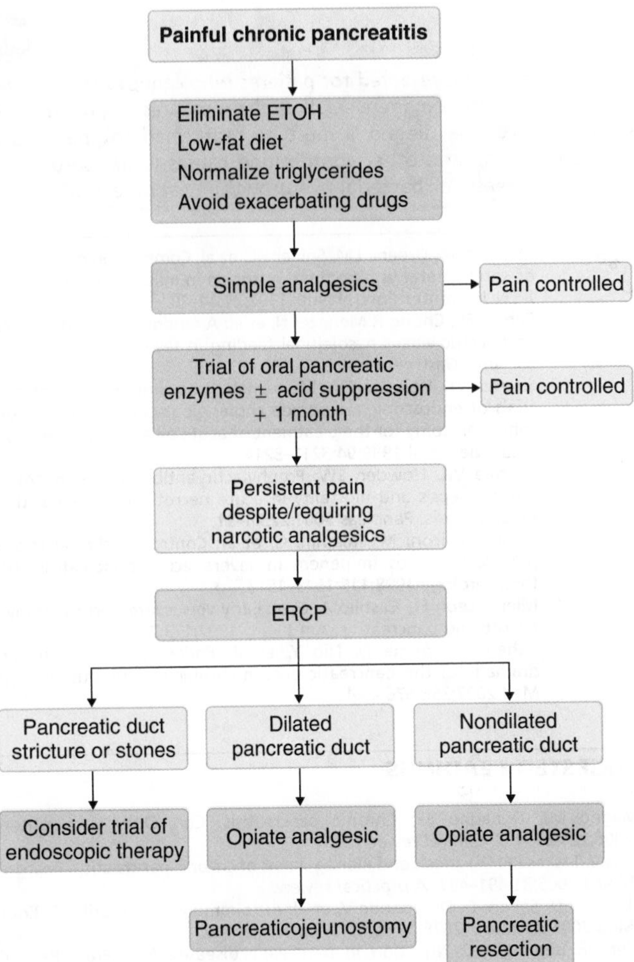

FIGURE 147–5 • Approach to a patient with chronic painful pancreatitis. ERCP = endoscopic retrograde cholangiopancreatography; ETOH = alcohol.

Treatment Rx

Medical treatment is aimed mainly at control of pain and correction of malabsorption with adequate enzyme replacement. Most patients with autoimmune chronic pancreatitis respond dramatically to steroids with resolution of clinical symptoms and imaging abnormalities within 4 weeks. Prednisolone is usually initiated at 30 to 40 mg/day for 1 to 2 months and tapered by 5 mg every 2 to 4 weeks. In some patients, a maintenance dose of 5 to 10 mg/day of prednisolone may be needed to prevent relapse.

Pain Control

Pain control (Fig. 147–5) includes avoidance of alcohol or the elimination of other offending agents (or both), use of analgesics, and celiac plexus block. Elevated (>500 mg/dL) triglyceride levels should generally be reduced beginning with a statin (e.g., atorvastatin starting at 10 to 20 mg/day), and implicated drugs, such as azathioprine, should be discontinued. It makes sense to eliminate these precipitants as possible causes of ongoing inflammation and pain. An initial trial of acetaminophen or nonsteroidal anti-inflammatory drugs (e.g., ibuprofen, 400 mg every 4 to 6 hours) is preferable, but patients may require opiate analgesics (e.g., hydrocodone, 10 mg every 6 hours as needed) (Chapter 28). Concerns about addiction should not interfere with the goal of pain relief; a strong patient-physician relationship may prevent abuse of prescribed narcotics. Percutaneous radiologically or sonographically guided celiac plexus block can control pain from pancreatic cancer (Chapter 204), but the procedure's occasional benefits almost never persist for more than a few months in patients with chronic pancreatitis.

Oral pancreatic enzymes (25,000 to 30,000 units of lipase per meal) that are not enteric coated provide more protease activity in the proximal duodenum than do enteric-coated preparations and can reduce pain in a subset of patients with chronic pancreatitis, perhaps because the administration of trypsin or chymotrypsin can inhibit the intrinsic secretion of cholecystokinin and pancreatic enzymes. The greatest success (70%) is in patients with small duct disease rather than large duct disease (25%).

The somatostatin analogue octreotide inhibits pancreatic secretion and has visceral analgesic effects. Clinical trials are under way to ascertain the utility of this drug in patients with painful chronic pancreatitis. Octreotide may also have a role in the management of refractory pancreatic fistulas or pseudocysts.

Endoscopic therapy can control pain in some patients who have a prominent stricture in the proximal pancreatic duct. In most cases, dilation is followed by stent placement across the stricture. Pain improves in 55 to 100% of selected patients with an isolated proximal stricture during 2 to 69 months of follow-up.

If all measures fail to relieve pain, surgery, which is superior to endoscopic drainage, 7 should be considered. Patients with ductal dilation have a 60% chance of obtaining pain relief if they undergo either partial resection with pancreaticojejunostomy or lateral pancreaticojejunostomy (modified Puestow procedure). In patients with ductal obstruction and dilation, the modified Puestow pancreaticojejunostomy relieves pain in about 60% of patients with morbidity less than 5% and mortality less than 2%. For patients with moderate to severe parenchymal disease and no ductal dilation, partial pancreatic resection can reduce pain in about 50% of cases.

Management of Pancreatic Insufficiency

Pancreatic steatorrhea should be treated with pancreatic enzyme replacement. At least 25,000 to 30,000 units of lipase per meal is necessary to provide adequate lipolysis, so patients must take 2 to 10 pills with each meal, depending on the preparation. Most patients achieve satisfactory nutritional status with this regimen and become relatively asymptomatic. A reduction in dietary fat can also help alleviate symptoms. In some patients, the use of enteric-coated preparations may be necessary because their gastric acid can destroy pancreatic enzymes; H_2-receptor antagonists or proton pump

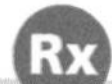

inhibitors should be reserved for patients who cannot achieve adequate relief by other maneuvers. If all the measures just mentioned are ineffective, the diagnosis must be reaffirmed (by pancreatic function testing), and other contributing causes (celiac sprue, terminal ileal disease, or bacterial overgrowth) must be excluded.

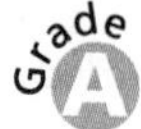

1. McClave SA, Greene LM, Snider HL, et al: Comparison of the safety of early enteral vs parenteral nutrition in mild acute pancreatitis. JPEN J Parenter Enteral Nutr 1997;21:14–20.
2. Eatock FC, Chong P, Menezes N, et al: A randomized study of early nasogastric versus nasojejunal feeding in severe acute pancreatitis. Am J Gastroenterol 2005;100:432–439.
3. Sharma VK, Howden CW: Meta-analysis of randomized controlled trials of endoscopic retrograde cholangiography and endoscopic sphincterotomy for the treatment of acute biliary pancreatitis. Am J Gastroenterol 1999;94:3211–3214.
4. Sharma VK, Howden SW: Prophylactic antibiotic administration reduces sepsis and mortality in acute necrotizing pancreatitis: A meta-analysis. Pancreas 2001;22:28–31.
5. Bassi C, Falconi M, Talamini G, et al: Controlled clinical trial of pefloxacin versus imipenem in severe acute pancreatitis. Gastroenterology 1998;115:1513–1517.
6. Mier J, Leon EL, Castillo A, et al: Early versus late necrosectomy in necrotizing pancreatitis. Am J Surg 1997;173:71–75.
7. Cahen D, Gouma D, Nio Y, et al: Endoscopic versus surgical drainage of the pancreatic duct in chronic pancreatitis. N Engl J Med 2007;356:676–684.

SUGGESTED READINGS

DiMagno MJ, Dimagno EP: Chronic pancreatitis. Curr Opin Gastroenterol 2006;22:487–497. *Clinical review.*

Gupta V, Toskes PP: Diagnosis and management of chronic pancreatitis. Postgrad Med J 2005;81:491–497. *A practical review.*

Finkelberg D, Sahani D, Deshpande V, et al: Autoimmune pancreatitis. N Engl J Med 2006;355:2670–2676. *A comprehensive review.*

Meier RF, Beglinger C: Nutrition in pancreatic diseases. Best Pract Res Clin Gastroenterol 2006;20:507–529. *Review of the role of nutritional support in pancreatic diseases.*

Pandol SJ, Saluja AK, Imrie CW, et al: Acute pancreatitis: Bench to bedside. Gastroenterology 2007;132:1127–1151. *Review of the basic science of pancreatitis.*

Whitcomb DC: Value of genetic testing in the management of pancreatitis. Gut 2004;53:1710–1717. *Describes both benefits and risks.*

Whitcomb DC: Acute pancreatitis. N Engl J Med 2006;354:2142–2150. *A case-based review.*

148 DISEASES OF THE RECTUM AND ANUS

Heidi Nelson

Pathobiology

The anal canal is a 2- to 4-cm-long muscular cuff (Fig. 148–1). It is distinctly different from the rectum, but some of its components, such as the mucosal lining, are essentially a continuance of rectal structures, and they work together to regulate defecation. The internal sphincter, which is an involuntary muscle innervated by the autonomic nervous system, must relax for rectal emptying. The external sphincter, which is a voluntary skeletal muscle innervated by the internal pudendal nerve, can contract for a short period to delay rectal emptying.

The anal canal transitions from rectal columnar epithelium and sensory responses to distention to perianal skin with squamous epithelium and responses to thermal and traumatic cutaneous stimuli. The dentate line represents the transition point between these two types of lining. For diagnostic purposes, this transition is important because ulcerative colitis, adenocarcinomas, and internal hemorrhoids occur cephalad to the dentate line whereas squamous cell carcinomas, hidradenitis suppurativa, and external hemorrhoids occur caudad to this line. For treatment purposes, simple procedures (hemorrhoidal ligation) can be performed cephalad to the dentate without the need for anesthesia.

Diagnosis

For acute problems, the history should focus on the duration, intensity, and character of symptoms. For chronic and recurring problems, the possibility of underlying inflammatory bowel disease (Chapter 144) or cancer (Chapter 203) should be considered, and diagnostic tests should be ordered accordingly. The anus can be examined with the patient lying in the left lateral decubitus position or lying prone in the jackknife position. Gentle retraction of the buttocks allows for inspection followed by palpation of the anal canal to assess for skin conditions, sphincter strength, and the presence of masses or inflammation. A rigid proctoscope or anoscope best visualizes the anal canal and distal part of the rectum. Flexible sigmoidoscopy or colonoscopy best evaluates the proximal portion of the bowel (complete evaluation is particularly indicated for bleeding or changes in bowel habits).

HEMORRHOIDS

Pathobiology

The normal anal canal contains cushions typically located in the left lateral, right anterior, and right posterior positions within the canal. Anal cushions are discrete areas of thickened submucosa containing blood vessels, smooth muscle, and elastic and connective tissues. Repetitive downward pressure gradually exaggerates the cushion and produces a hemorrhoid.

Clinical Manifestations

Internal hemorrhoids originate above the dentate line and therefore rarely cause pain; they are typically associated with symptoms of bleeding or prolapse. In contrast, external hemorrhoids originate distal to the dentate line and are typically manifested as swellings and problems with hygiene. Thrombosis of the underlying vessels can cause severe anal pain (Fig. 148–2).

Diagnosis and Treatment

Anoscopy and inspection with straining give the best assessment of the location and extent of prolapse. The severity of the symptoms dictates the management (Table 148–1). Dietary fiber, [1] stool softeners (e.g., docusate sodium [Colace], 100 mg once daily), sitz baths, and excision can ameliorate symptoms. For fourth-degree prolapse of internal hemorrhoids, urgent hemorrhoidectomy, preferably with conventional surgery rather than a staple procedure, [2] may be required to prevent tissue necrosis.

ANAL FISSURES

Pathobiology

Anal fissures are among the most common causes of anal pain (see Fig. 148–2). An initiating event, such as strain from constipation, probably produces a small tear in the anal lining. Local anal pain from the tear generates spasm of the underlying internal sphincter muscle, and this hypertonia reduces blood flow, thereby causing mucosal ischemia. Anal fissures typically occur as linear ulcers just inside the anal verge, most commonly with a posterior commissure.

Clinical Manifestations and Diagnosis

The classic symptoms of pain and bleeding on defecation may be severe and have an acute onset, or they may be insidious and chronic. The diagnosis can be confirmed by gentle retraction near the anal verge to expose and visualize the ulcer. Acute ulcers tend to be red with rough edges, whereas chronic fissures tend to be white and show exposed internal sphincter fibers; they are also likely to be associated with a sentinel tag externally and a hypertrophied anal papilla internally. The resting

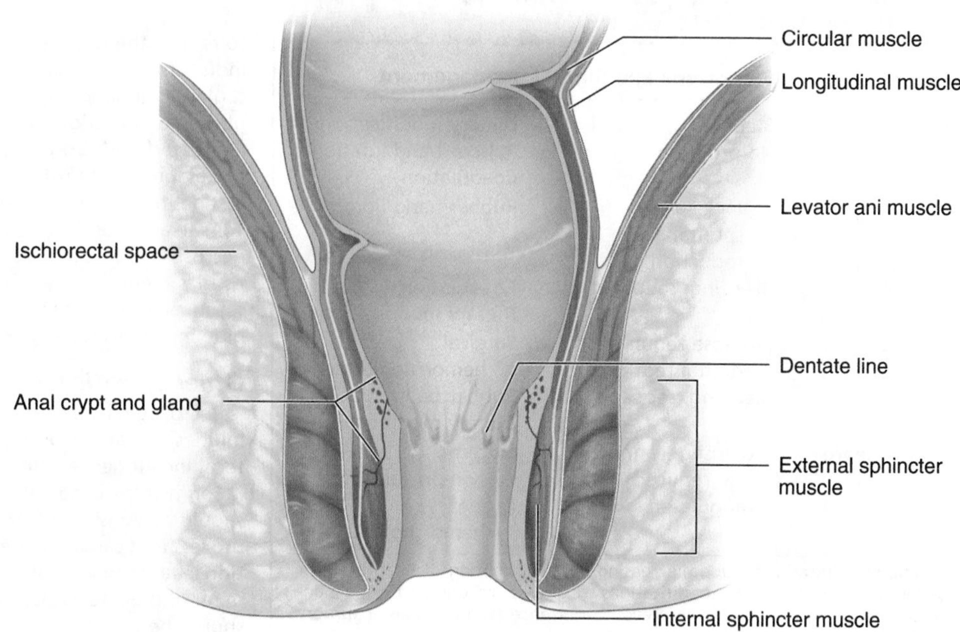

FIGURE 148–1 • Anorectal anatomy. (By permission of Mayo Foundation.)

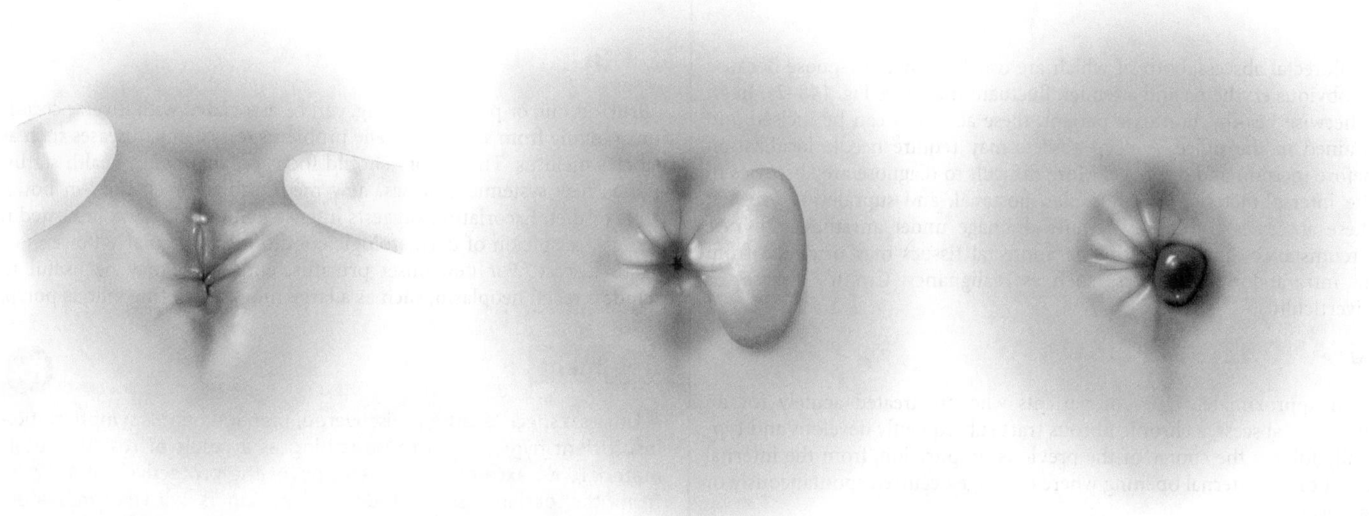

FIGURE 148–2 • Causes of anal pain. (By permission of Mayo Foundation.)

tone of the anal sphincter is typically quite tense and the pain so severe that digital and anoscopic examinations cannot be performed. When fissures are multiple, have an unusual appearance, or are located laterally, colorectal cancer (Chapter 203), Crohn's disease (Chapter 144), or sexually transmitted diseases should be considered.

Treatment

Rx

Medical management of acute and chronic anal fissures starts with short-term measures such as sitz baths and the topical applications of anesthetics (e.g., 2% lidocaine hydrochloride jelly USP topically applied to the perianal skin) and stool softeners (e.g., Colace, 100 mg once daily) for patients with hard constipated stools. Long-term preventive measures include modifications of diet and bowel habits, as well as the use of bulking agents (e.g., Konsyl, 6 g once to three times daily; Citrucel, 9 g once to three times daily; or Metamucil, 3.4 g once to four times daily), to provide more consistency and regularity. The internal sphincter can be relaxed by nitric oxide donors (e.g., either 0.2% nitroglycerin twice daily or isosorbide-dinitrate, 2.5 mg three times daily as topical therapy for 4 to 8 weeks). Approximately 70% heal and require no further management.

An alternative to topical medical therapy is injection of a single dose of botulinum toxin A into the internal sphincter; 2 to 3 months of sphincter relaxation promotes healing. Patients who fail medical therapy can be treated surgically with a lateral internal sphincterotomy. 3

ANORECTAL ABSCESS

An anorectal abscess should always be considered in patients with acute anal pain because a delay in diagnosis can lead to necrotizing infections, particularly in an immunocompromised host. Most anorectal infections arise from an obstructed crypt and an infected gland (see Fig. 148–1). The infection can be manifested as a superficial perianal or

TABLE 148–1 INTERNAL HEMORRHOIDS: GRADING AND MANAGEMENT

Grade	Symptoms and Signs	Management
First degree	Bleeding No prolapse	Dietary modifications* Rubber band ligation Coagulation
Second degree	Prolapse with spontaneous reduction	Rubber band ligation
	Bleeding, seepage	Coagulation Dietary modifications
Third degree	Prolapse requiring digital reduction	Surgical hemorrhoidectomy
	Bleeding, seepage	Rubber band ligation Dietary modifications
Fourth degree	Prolapsed, cannot be reduced	Surgical hemorrhoidectomy
	Strangulated	Urgent hemorrhoidectomy

*Dietary modifications include increasing the consumption of fiber, bran, or psyllium and water. Dietary modifications are always appropriate for the management of hemorrhoids and to prevent recurrence after banding or surgery (or both).

From Nelson H, Dozois RR: Anus. *In* Townsend CM (ed): Sabiston Textbook of Surgery, 16th ed. Philadelphia, Saunders, 2001, p 979.

ischiorectal abscess, both of which are usually easy to diagnose because of obvious erythema and a tender, fluctuant mass (see Fig. 148–2). In an otherwise healthy, nontoxic patient, these abscesses can be incised and drained in the office. A deep abscess may require needle localization before incision and drainage. More difficult to diagnose are abscesses in the intersphincteric, intermuscular, postanal, and supralevator spaces; these abscesses commonly require drainage under anesthesia. In rare circumstances, an abscess in the anorectal tissues may originate from an intra-abdominal process such as malignancy, Crohn's disease, or diverticulitis.

ANORECTAL FISTULA

In approximately 30% of patients who are treated acutely for an anorectal abscess, a chronic fibrous tract subsequently develops and typically follows the course of the previous suppuration, from the internal crypt to the external opening where drainage occurred spontaneously or surgically.

Diagnosis

Although it is typically easy to identify the external opening of an anorectal fistula (also called fistula in ano), it may be difficult to visualize the internal opening. Sometimes a fibrous tract can be palpated or located via a probe in the office, but other fistulas can be delineated only in the operating room. For anterior fistulas in which the external opening is close to the anus, the internal opening is typically in a straight radial line toward the anus. For posterior fistulas, or those with a horseshoe-type or long tract, the opening is generally in the posterior midline.

Pretreatment diagnostic imaging with contrast-enhanced endosonography [4] or digital subtraction magnetic resonance fistulography is highly accurate at differentiating simple versus complex tracts and can help reduce rates of recurrent fistulas.

Treatment

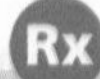

Treatment is indicated to manage symptoms of purulent or feculent drainage and to prevent the recurrent infections that occur whenever the tract becomes occluded and fecal material accumulates. Trans-sphincteric fistulas are often managed with conservative approaches, including fibrin glue injections and island flap anoplasty to reduce the risk for permanent fecal incontinence from surgically induced sphincter damage. [5] For simple fistulas arising from cryptoglandular sources, treatment is fistulotomy, seton placement, or fibrin glue injection. For complex or refractory anal fistulas or those associated with an internal opening proximal to the dentate line, the diagnosis of Crohn's disease must be entertained; the gastrointestinal tract should be evaluated and treated accordingly (Chapter 144). In addition to specific treatment of Crohn's disease (e.g., tumor necrosis factor-α monoclonal antibodies [6]), complex or refractory fistulas generally require treatment with surgical drainage and seton placement for control of suppuration, antibiotics, or fibrin glue injections (or any combination of these measures).

Other Specific Causes of Fistulas

Rectovaginal or anovaginal fistulas often occur after childbirth injuries and are associated with sphincter damage and symptoms of fecal incontinence. Surgical repair is required.

For fistulas distal to the dentate line, hidradenitis suppurativa should be considered. This condition is a chronic inflammatory skin process that can affect perianal tissues, with apocrine gland obstruction leading to local abscesses and sinuses. In addition to acute treatment of the infection, preventive measures such as frequent hygiene should be instituted.

On rare occasion, neglected rectal cancers are manifested as perianal fistulas. Alternatively, cancers can develop in chronic fistula tracts.

PRURITUS ANI

Pruritus ani, or perianal itching, can be associated with diverse conditions ranging from simple hygiene problems to systemic diseases such as diabetes mellitus. The history should focus on changes in health status, such as new systemic illnesses, new medications, or changes in bowel habits or diet. Excoriation suggests intense itching. Biopsy is indicated if there is a suspicion of dermatologic conditions, particularly Bowen's or Paget's disease. For new-onset pruritus, endoscopy may be useful to exclude a rectal neoplasm, such as a large mucus-secreting villous polyp.

Treatment

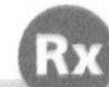

Unless a specific cause is discovered, management is symptomatic. Insufficient hygiene can cause itching as a result of residual fecal material, but excessive hygiene removes the protective natural oils from the perianal skin. Optimal cleansing is with warm water without soap, followed by gentle drying, preferably with warm air rather than abrasive towels. Cornstarch or talc powder may be applied to maintain moisture-free perianal conditions.

Stool bulking agents (see earlier) and modifications in diets may be required to improve daily bowel function. If food diaries suggest that certain foods (e.g., citrus fruits and juices, cola, coffee, tea, alcoholic beverages, nuts, popcorn, and milk) are associated with pruritus, reduction or elimination of them may alleviate the symptoms.

SEXUALLY TRANSMITTED DISEASES

Sexually transmitted diseases involve the rectum and anus primarily in persons who practice anal intercourse. Nonviral sexually transmitted diseases (Chapter 307) may produce pruritus, bloody or mucopurulent rectal discharge, pain, diarrhea, and fever. Etiologic agents include *Neisseria gonorrhoeae* (Chapter 322), *Treponema pallidum* (Chapter 340), *Chlamydia* (Chapter 339), *Shigella* (Chapter 330), *Campylobacter* (Chapter 326), and *Haemophilus ducreyi* (Chapter 324). Endoscopic evaluation and cultures of stool or anorectal swabs facilitate diagnosis and treatment based on the causative agent.

Viral sexually transmitted diseases are most typically manifested as pain, discharge, or bleeding (or any combination), with physical features characteristic of the specific causative agents. Herpes simplex, which causes vesicles or ulcers (or both), can be diagnosed by culture and treated with acyclovir. Human papillomavirus 6 (HPV-6) and HPV-11 are commonly associated with benign warts or condylomata acuminata. HPV-16 and HPV-18 are more often associated with dysplasia and malignancy. Condylomata may be small and external only, or they may be extensive, coalescing, and internal (Fig. 148-3). Medical management includes podophyllin (0.5% self-applied sequentially for 3 days) and imiquimod (5% cream applied nightly, three times per week for 6 weeks). Surgical therapies include excision, removal by laser, and cauterization; excised specimens should be examined histologically to exclude malignancy. The lesions of molluscum contagiosum are painless, round, and umbilicated. Human immunodeficiency virus (HIV) infections involving the anus can be associated with painful anal ulcers or with lower gastrointestinal symptoms such as bleeding, proctalgia, and diarrhea.

Parasitic sexually transmitted diseases are accompanied by systemic symptoms such as abdominal cramping, fever, and bloody diarrhea. Common agents include *Entamoeba histolytica* (Chapter 373), *Giardia lamblia* (Chapter 372), and *Isospora belli* (Chapter 413).

Evolving evidence now links sexually transmitted diseases of the anus and rectum to premalignant and malignant conditions of the same organs (see later). Anal intraepithelial neoplasia is a precursor to squamous cell cancer of the anus, much like the biology described for cervical intraepithelial neoplasia. The frequency of anal intraepithelial neoplasia and squamous cell carcinoma of the anus is increasing, specifically in patients with long-standing HIV infection. Screening programs for "at-risk" individuals with chronic HIV and HPV infection make use of cytologic investigations.

FECAL INCONTINENCE

Fecal incontinence is an inability of the sphincter complex to contract sufficiently to control the release of gas, stool, or diarrhea. In patients with symptoms of leakage or incontinence, evaluation should focus on testing the pressure, nerve, and anatomic profiles of the anal sphincter muscles (Fig. 148–4). Diet and bulking agents (see earlier) may improve

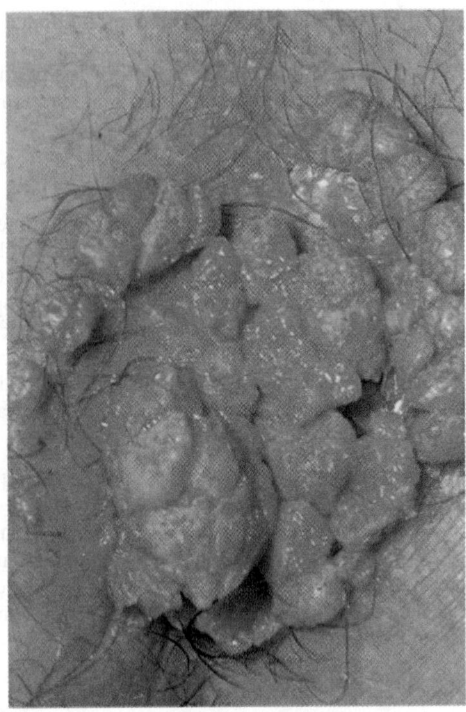

FIGURE 148–3 • Perianal condylomata resulting from human papillomavirus infection. They are usually sexually transmitted and are most common in homosexual men. (From Forbes CD, Jackson WF: Color Atlas and Text of Clinical Medicine, 3rd ed. London, Mosby, 2003.)

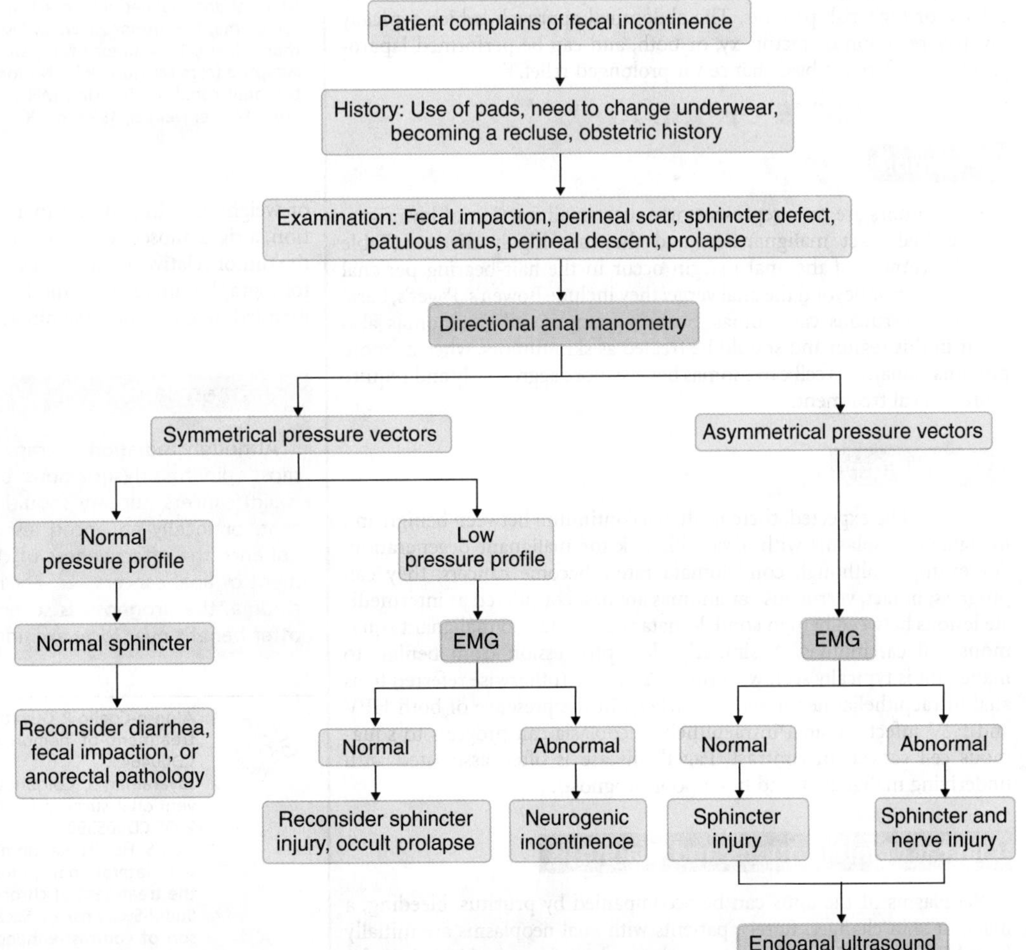

FIGURE 148–4 • Algorithm for the investigation of fecal incontinence. EMG = electromyogram. (From Sagar PM, Pemberton JH: Anorectal and pelvic floor function: Relevance to continence, incontinence, and constipation. Gastroenterol Clin North Am 1996;25:163–182.)

the consistency and regularity of bowel function. In difficult or extreme cases of diarrhea, constipating medications such as loperamide (Imodium; 2 mg as needed, not to exceed eight tablets per day) may be required. If constipation is complicating the ability to control bowel evacuation, laxatives or enemas may be helpful.

SOLITARY RECTAL ULCER SYNDROME

Solitary rectal ulcer syndrome is a benign, but oftentimes disabling condition in which excessive straining at defecation results in focal mucosal changes with pain, bleeding, and mucous discharge. Occult prolapse or internal intussusception may be implicated. Endoscopy typically discloses a raised erythematous patch with or without frank ulceration, and biopsy confirms a solitary rectal ulcer or colitis cystica profunda. Exclusion of malignancy is essential. Symptomatic relief may be achieved by optimizing bowel consistency and regularity with daily evacuation, as well as by correcting pelvic floor disorders.

DESCENDING PERINEUM SYNDROME

Descending perineum syndrome is a pelvic floor disorder in which the patient senses an inability to completely evacuate the rectum at defecation. On examination, the perineum can be seen to protrude below the level of the ischial tuberosities. Symptomatic treatment is similar to that described for solitary rectal ulcer syndrome.

RECTAL PROLAPSE

Rectal prolapse or intussusception of the rectum may be occult, partial (mucosal only), or complete (i.e., procidentia or full-thickness protrusion beyond the anus). It tends to occur more often in women, in patients with straining conditions, or in patients with chronic mental conditions. The patient typically describes a rectal bulge while straining, and this sign may be reproduced during the examination to determine the degree and extent of prolapse, which may be a few to several centimeters in length.

Full-thickness rectal prolapse should be surgically corrected with a perineal or abdominal procedure. Patients recover more rapidly after a perineal approach, but its higher recurrence rate makes it best suited for frail, elderly, or high-risk patients. The abdominal approach, which typically involves resection or rectopexy, or both, and can be performed laparoscopically, offers the best chance for prolonged relief.

NEOPLASMS OF THE ANUS

Definition

Anal tumors are rare, representing only a small fraction of lower gastrointestinal tract malignancies, and they are highly diverse (Table 148–2). Tumors of the anal margin occur in the hair-bearing perianal skin, outside or beyond the anal verge; they include Bowen's, Paget's, basal cell, and verrucous carcinomas. Some squamous cell carcinomas also occur in this region and should be treated as skin tumors, whereas more proximal squamous cell carcinomas behave more aggressively and require more radical treatment.

TABLE 148–2 SUMMARY OF THERAPIES FOR ANAL NEOPLASMS

Bowen's disease (intraepithelial squamous cell carcinoma)
Accurate lesion mapping
Wide local excision with flap repair as indicated
Exclude the presence of a locally invasive component and underlying gynecologic malignancy
Paget's disease (intraepithelial adenocarcinoma)
Accurate lesion mapping
Wide local excision with flap repair as indicated
Exclude any underlying malignancy
APR and chemoradiation therapy if invasive adenocarcinoma is present
Basal cell and anal margin squamous cell carcinoma
Local excision with clear margins
Radiation therapy or chemotherapy for poor-prognosis lesions or recurrence as indicated
Verrucous carcinoma
Wide local excision; APR if very extensive
Combined-modality therapy if transformation to SCC has occurred
Epidermoid cancer
Combined-modality, external beam radiation therapy plus 5-FU and mitomycin
Local excision if favorable T1
APR if incontinent, local treatment failure, or recurrence after combined chemoradiation therapy
Triple-modality therapy for bulky T3 and T4 lesions (role of APR is controversial)
Adenocarcinoma
APR with 5-FU and radiation therapy as indicated, based on stage
Melanoma
APR or local excision (controversial) if potentially curable

APR = abdominal perineal resection; 5-FU = 5-fluorouracil; SCC = squamous cell carcinoma; T1 = tumor 2.0 cm or less in greatest dimension; T3 = tumor greater than 5.0 cm; T4 = tumor of any size that invades adjacent organs.
Adapted from McMurrick PJ, Nelson H, Goldberg RM, Haddock MG: Cancer of the anal canal. *In* Torosian MH (ed): Integrated Cancer Management. New York, Marcel Dekker, 1999, p 200. Courtesy of Marcel Dekker, Inc.

Pathobiology

As would be expected, there is often a continuum between benign and malignant neoplasms with a variable risk for malignant degeneration. For example, although condylomata rarely become cancers, they can progress; in fact, verrucous carcinomas are best considered as intermediate lesions between benign condylomata acuminata and malignant squamous cell carcinomas. A similarly slow progression from benign to malignant is typically seen with Bowen's disease (otherwise referred to as anal intraepithelial neoplasia, see earlier). In the presence of both HPV and HIV infection, anal intraepithelial neoplasia can progress to squamous cell cancer. In contrast, Paget's disease is often associated with underlying malignancy and has a poor prognosis.

Clinical Manifestations and Diagnosis

Neoplasms of the anus can be accompanied by pruritus, bleeding, a mass, or skin changes. Rarely, patients with anal neoplasms are initially found to have systemic symptoms such as enlarged inguinal lymph nodes or weight loss. In addition to a complete history and physical examination, a rigid anoscope or proctoscope can define the size and location of the tumor relative to the anal canal, rectum, and perianal skin. Computed tomographic imaging of the lungs, liver, and pelvis is typically recommended to assess for disseminated disease.

Treatment and Prognosis

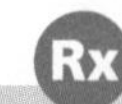

Although radiation therapy plus chemotherapy is standard for most epidermoid (squamous, basaloid, cloacogenic, or mucoepidermoid) cancers, surgery should be considered for refractory, recurrent, or locally advanced lesions. Intracavitary hyperthermia may enhance the effectiveness of chemoradiation therapy in the treatment of anal cancers. 7 For melanoma and anal canal adenocarcinoma, the prognosis is so poor that aggressive surgery may not offer benefit over local excision.

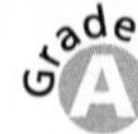

1. Alonso-Coello P, Guyatt G, Heels-Ansdell D, et al: Laxatives for the treatment of hemorrhoids. Cochrane Database Syst Rev 2005: CD004649.
2. Jayaraman S, Colquhoun PH, Malthaner RA: Stapled versus conventional surgery for hemorrhoids. Cochrane Database Syst Rev 2006:CD005393.
3. Ho KS, Ho YH: Randomized clinical trial comparing oral nifedipine with lateral anal sphincterotomy and tailored sphincterotomy in the treatment of chronic anal fissure. Br J Surg 2005;95:403–408.
4. Sudol-Swopinska I, Szczepkowski M, Panorska AK, et al: Comparison of contrast-enhanced with non-contrast endosonography in the diagnostics of anal fistulas. Eur Radiol 2004;14:2236–2241.

5. Ho KS, Ho YH: Controlled, randomized trial of island flap anoplasty for treatment of trans-sphincteric fistula-in-ano: Early results. Tech Coloproctol 2005;9:166–168.
6. Sand BE, Anderson FH, Bernstein CN, et al: Infliximab maintenance therapy for fistulizing Crohn's disease. N Engl J Med 2004;350: 876–885.
7. Kouloulias V, Plataniotis G, Kouvaris J, et al: Chemoradiotherapy combined with intracavitary hyperthermia for anal cancer. Am J Clin Oncol 2005;28:91–99.

SUGGESTED READINGS

Abbasakoor F, Boulos PB: Anal intraepithelial neoplasia. Br J Surg 2005; 92:277–290. *A comprehensive review of evolving diagnostic and treatment issues pertinent to anal intraepithelial neoplasia.*

Cummings BJ: Current managemnt of anal canal cancer. Semin Oncol 2005;32:S123–128. *Comprehensive review.*

Kaidar-Person O, Person B, Wexner SD: Hemorrhoidal disease: A comprehensive review. J Am Coll Surg 2007;204:102–117. *Comprehensive review.*

Nelson R: Operative procedures for fissure in ano. Cochrane Database Syst Rev 2005;2:CD002199. *An evidence-based review of best data on five different surgical approaches to chronic anal fissures.*

Sagap I, Remzi FH: Controversies in the treatment of common anal problems. World J Gastroenterol 2006;12:3146–3154. *Clinical review.*

Wald A: Fecal incontinence in adults. N Engl J Med 2007;356:1648–1655. *Clinical review.*

Zuccati G, Lotti T, Mastrolorenzo A, et al: Pruritus ani. Dermatol Ther 2005;18:355–362. *Clinical review.*

Section XIII

Diseases of the Liver, Gallbladder, and Bile Ducts

149 APPROACH TO THE PATIENT WITH LIVER DISEASE

Nora V. Bergasa

Identification of a chief complaint, a complete medical history, and a thorough physical examination form the basis for the approach to a patient with liver disease. Identification of risk factors for liver disease is particularly important.

Patients with liver disease may have subtle symptoms, recognition of which will alert the clinician to hepatic pathology. Other times, the quality of life of patients may be markedly impaired. Often, however, the first suggestion of liver disease is from laboratory data obtained as part of routine health maintenance, for nonspecific symptoms, or for other medical reasons.

The range of liver injury varies from inflammation to fibrosis and cirrhosis. Liver failure, which is characterized by impaired function, can be acute and fulminant (Chapter 158), but most liver conditions that lead to long-term complications tend to be chronic and progress slowly, so accurate diagnosis may provide an opportunity for successful treatment.

SYMPTOMS AND SIGNS OF LIVER DISEASE

Jaundice

Classically recognized as a sign of liver disease, jaundice may be identified by the patient and hence be part of the chief complaint as "yellow eyes" (Fig. 149–1). In general, jaundice is a good indication that some aspect of bilirubin metabolism is altered (e.g., bilirubin availability, uptake, conjugation, or excretion; Chapter 150).

Fatigue

Lack of energy or fatigue, which may be the most common symptom of liver disease, is sometimes associated with acute liver injury (e.g., acute viral hepatitis; Chapter 151) or a chronic condition (e.g., primary biliary cirrhosis [Chapter 159] and chronic hepatitis C infection [Chapter 152]). The pathogenesis of fatigue in liver disease is unknown, and it does not appear to be related to abnormal musculoskeletal function or neurologic impairment. Fatigue has been associated with poor-quality sleep and with depression, perhaps via the opioid and serotoninergic systems. When fatigue is prominent, conditions other than liver disease, including hypothyroidism (Chapter 244), anemia (Chapter 162), and depression (Chapter 420), should be excluded.

Pruritus

Pruritus, or itching (Chapter 462), can be a manifestation of liver disease, particularly diseases characterized by cholestasis (i.e., impaired secretion of bile; Chapters 157 and 159), presumably because of the accumulation of substances that are normally excreted in bile and that as a result of cholestasis accumulate in tissues. However, the nature of the pruritogen or pruritogens is unknown, and there is no specific evidence indicating a role of bile acids in this symptom. It has been hypothesized that the pruritus of cholestasis is mediated, at least in part, by increased opioidergic neurotransmission; amelioration of the pruritus by opiate antagonists (e.g., naloxone, 0.4 mg by intravenous push, followed by a continuous infusion of 0.02 μg/kg/min) supports this hypothesis. It is important to appreciate that pruritus and fatigue can precede the diagnosis of liver disease by years.

Poor Appetite and Weight Loss

Poor appetite may accompany the onset of acute liver disease. Patients with advanced liver disease may also have chronic poor appetite, weight loss, or muscle wasting. In advanced liver disease, weight loss may not be a reliable indicator of liver disease because fluid retention may compensate for the lost dry weight.

Abdominal Pain

Patients with liver disease can report more abdominal pain than other individuals do, and the pain is worse after meals. Biliary colic and acute cholecystitis must also be considered in patients with liver disease because the prevalence of gallstones is increased in patients with cirrhosis.

Alterations in the Senses of Taste and Smell

Taste abnormalities (e.g., hypogeusia and dysgeusia; Chapter 453) are recognized complications of liver disease. Smokers with acute hepatitis B and perhaps other acute liver diseases may lose interest in cigarettes because of a perverted sense of taste from liver inflammation. Impaired gustatory function with decreased sensitivity to or recognition of bitter, salt, sweet, and sour taste has been reported in patients with cirrhosis. Serum concentrations of certain elements, including magnesium, zinc, and vitamin A, are decreased in some patients with liver disease and an altered sense of taste. A central mediation of taste abnormalities in patients with liver disease has been proposed. Hyposmia can be associated with cirrhosis and may resolve after liver transplantation.

Personality Changes and Sleep Disturbances

One of the most dramatic manifestations of decompensated liver disease is hepatic encephalopathy (Chapter 157), which is characterized by inhibitory neurotransmission. Its manifestation can be subtle or florid. Reversal of the sleep pattern is well recognized, with patients reporting both insomnia and an inability to stay awake during the day. Family members may report confusion, cognitive deficiencies, and changes in personality, including combativeness.

Dyspnea

Decreased exercise tolerance and shortness of breath in patients with liver disease may be caused by the hepatopulmonary syndrome (Chapter 157), portopulmonary hypertension (Chapters 67 and 157), and cardiomyopathy (Chapter 59), the latter traditionally associated with alcohol abuse and recently also being recognized as a complication of chronic hepatitis C infection. Dyspnea can also result from impaired diaphragmatic excursion secondary to ascites.

Bleeding

A history of hematemesis, melena, or hematochezia may identify patients with portal hypertension (Chapter 157).

Stool Characteristics

Jaundice associated with acholic (e.g., pale) stools, which result from decreased bile pigments in feces, suggests biliary obstruction. In liver diseases characterized by profound cholestasis, the critical micellar concentration of bile acids is decreased in the small intestine; hence, diarrhea (Chapter 143) from fat malabsorption and, in some cases, from maldigestion may ensue. Diarrhea is also a cardinal manifestation of inflammatory bowel disease (Chapter 144), which can be associated with primary sclerosing cholangitis (Chapter 159) and cholestasis.

Vision Disturbances

Deficiency of vitamin A is usually manifested as impaired visual adaptation to darkness, of which patients may not be aware. Patients with liver disease may be deficient in vitamin A because of malabsorption and decreased availability of retinol binding protein. In addition, there may be impaired release of vitamin A from liver stores.

Bone Pain and Fractures

Pain in the long bones (e.g., tibia) and joints, sometimes associated with clubbing, is suggestive of hypertrophic osteoarthropathy (Chapter 189), a complication of cirrhosis. A dramatic manifestation of liver disease of the cholestatic type can be bone fractures from osteopenia (Chapter 264), the etiology of which is uncertain but may relate to osteomalacia (Chapter 265) from decreased bowel absorption of vitamin D.

Pain

Peripheral neuropathy (Chapter 446) manifested by localized neurologic deficits and pain can be a symptom in patients with liver disease secondary to cholestasis, primarily in children. Xanthomatous neuropathy can be caused by lipid deposition on peripheral nerves in patients with hyperlipidemia as a result of profound cholestasis.

Hyperpigmentation

Hyperpigmentation (Chapter 467) is a complication of liver disease, mostly of the cholestatic type. Its pathogenesis is unknown, but increased availability of α-melanocyte–stimulating hormone has been proposed as a contributing factor.

Chills and Rigors

Chills and rigors are manifestations of infection. Examples that can complicate the course of liver disease are spontaneous bacterial peritonitis (Chapter 157) in patients with ascites, an infected biliary tree in patients with primary sclerosing cholangitis (Chapter 159), and pneumonia (Chapter 97) or meningitis (Chapter 437) in an immunocompromised patient with alcoholic liver disease.

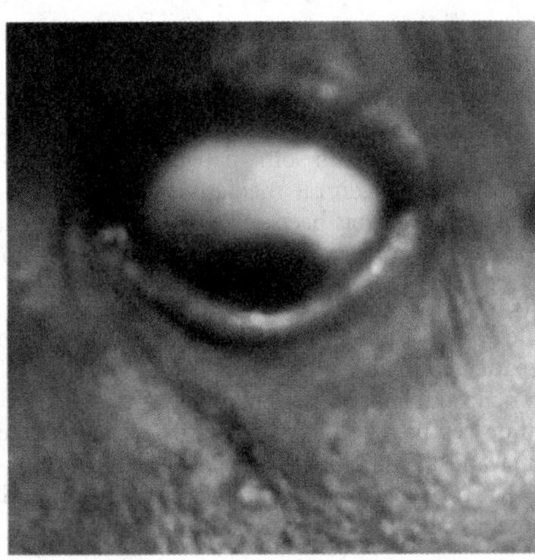

FIGURE 149–1 • Scleral icterus in a patient with biliary cirrhosis.

Dark Urine

Dark brown urine suggests bilirubinuria, which is a reflection of hyperbilirubinemia. This finding can precede jaundice.

Sexual Dysfunction and Disinterest

Decreased libido and impotence (Chapter 253) are manifestations of cirrhosis in men. Decreased serum levels of testosterone and increased serum levels of gonadotropins are known complications of alcoholic cirrhosis. Hypogonadism may also result from the toxic effect of alcohol and its metabolites on the gonads and from the systemic effect of estrogens on the hypothalamic-pituitary-gonadal axis. In women, the most relevant factors in lack of interest in sexual activities have been reported to be depression and fatigue.

Muscle Cramps

Mostly nocturnal, muscle cramps affecting the calves, toes, and fingers can complicate cirrhosis of the liver and have a marked negative impact on quality of life. The pathogenesis is unknown.

IDENTIFICATION OF RISK FACTORS FOR LIVER DISEASE

Activities that involve contact with blood and body fluids are risks for acquiring viral hepatitis (Chapter 151). In the United States, individuals are at risk for contracting viral hepatitis (e.g., hepatitis C and B and delta hepatitis) from transfusion of blood, especially before 1992, and other blood products (e.g., clotting factors), especially before 1987, intravenous injection of illicit drugs (Chapter 32), and chronic hemodialysis. Body piercings and tattoos with contaminated tools and certain sexual behavior (e.g., multiple sexual partners) are risk factors for viral hepatitis.

Alcohol abuse is an important cause of cirrhosis of the liver (Chapter 156), and many medications or dietary supplements, by prescription or over the counter, can cause liver disease (Chapter 153). The drinking of "bush tea" in some Caribbean islands (e.g., Jamaica) can be associated with veno-occlusive disease, which can present dramatically as ascites and hepatic insufficiency. Hepatic vascular thrombosis (Chapter 146) and hepatic adenomas are complications of estrogens and anabolic steroids. Malignant tumors of the liver (Chapter 206) have been associated with exposure to certain compounds used in industry (e.g., vinyl chloride, inorganic arsenicals) and to aflatoxin B_1, which can result from the ingestion of food products (e.g., grains) contaminated with the mold *Aspergillus flavus.* Travel to endemic areas may expose individuals to infectious diseases that may involve the liver, including leptospirosis, malaria, Q fever, amebiasis, echinococcosis, and schistosomiasis (Chapter 155).

RECOGNIZING HEPATIC MANIFESTATIONS OF COMORBID CONDITIONS

Systemic disorders can cause clinical or subclinical involvement of the liver. Jaundice can be seen in patients with decompensated right heart failure (Chapter 57) and in patients with sepsis (Chapter 109). Obesity can be associated with abnormal serum liver profile, as can diabetes mellitus (Chapter 248). Patients with amyloidosis may have their liver infiltrated with amyloid, manifested as hepatomegaly, and disseminated tuberculosis and fungemia may involve the liver. Patients with renal insufficiency from polycystic kidney disease (Chapter 128) may have liver cysts as part of the syndrome. Stauffer's syndrome, characterized by hepatomegaly and cholestasis in the absence of liver metastasis, can be a manifestation of renal cell carcinoma (Chapter 207); the syndrome resolves when the tumor is resected. Cystic fibrosis (Chapter 89) can be associated with cholestasis. Hypothyroidism and hyperthyroidism (Chapter 244) can be accompanied by increased serum aminotransferase levels; Basedowiana-Haban cirrhosis, characterized by hepatomegaly and episodes of jaundice, was originally described in patients with thyrotoxicosis. An increase in thyroid-binding globulin, not hyperthyroidism itself, appears to be the most common cause of increased total levels of thyroxine in patients with liver disease; determination of free thyroxin levels is necessary to confirm true hyperthyroidism.

PAST MEDICAL AND SURGICAL HISTORY

A history of jaundice or abnormal serum liver profile may suggest prior hepatitis or the passage of a gallstone. A history of gallbladder surgery, including laparoscopic cholecystectomy, in a patient with cholestasis should trigger a search for postsurgical biliary strictures (Chapter 159), which must be repaired to prevent biliary cirrhosis. Biliary strictures can also be a complication of chronic pancreatitis (Chapter 147).

FAMILY HISTORY

A history of liver disease in family members is relevant for the diagnosis of hereditary liver diseases (Chapter 154), including primary hemochromatosis (Chapter 231), α_1-antitrypsin deficiency (Chapter 154), and Wilson's disease (Chapter 230). A history of viral hepatitis B in the mother may suggest perinatally acquired hepatitis in the patient.

REVIEW OF SYSTEMS

A florid manifestation of hemochromatosis (Chapter 231) may include arthralgias, glucose intolerance, hypogonadism, and cardiomyopathy. Psychiatric and neurologic alterations may suggest Wilson's disease (Chapter 230). Classically, emphysema and liver disease suggest α_1-antitrypsin deficiency (Chapter 154), although liver disease may occur without pulmonary complications in this condition. Easy bruising in a patient with infiltrative liver disease suggests amyloidosis (Chapter 296). A patient with "red eyes," silvery skin nodules, and pulmonary complaints should be evaluated for possible sarcoidosis (Chapter 95). Dyspnea may suggest hepatopulmonary syndrome. The CREST syndrome (*c*alcinosis, *R*aynaud's phenomenon, *e*sophageal dysmotility, *s*clerodactyly, and *t*elangiectasia) (Chapter 288) can be associated with primary biliary cirrhosis.

THE PHYSICAL EXAMINATION

Signs of liver disease may be overt, subtle, or absent. Fever in a patient with liver disease should trigger the exclusion of infections, including bacterial peritonitis in patients with ascites and cholangitis in patients with biliary obstruction. In patients with decompensated liver disease, blood pressure tends to be lower than average because of systemic arterial vasodilation.

Fetor Hepaticus

A sweet odor emanating from the breath can be perceived in patients with advanced liver disease, including those with extensive portosystemic shunting.

The Skin, Mucous Membranes, and Nails

Scleral icterus may be subtle or obvious. A yellow discoloration of the skin and mucous membranes defines jaundice, which may be secondary to biliary tract obstruction, acute hepatitis, hepatocellular failure, or excess bilirubin production from hemolysis (Chapter 164). Kayser-Fleischer rings (see Fig. 230–11), a brown rim on the periphery of the cornea secondary to copper accumulation in Descemet's membrane, is a classic finding of Wilson's disease (Chapter 230) that is often seen only by slit lamp examination. In prolonged cholestasis not related to Wilson's disease, Kayser-Fleischer rings may also be seen.

In advanced liver disease, the skin is warm from a hyperdynamic circulation. Spider telangiectases (see Fig. 134–4), which are characterized by vascular arborizations that blanch on pressure, are found on the face, upper part of the back, thorax, and upper part of the arms. The pathogenesis of spider angiomas is thought to be a systemic excess of estrogen combined with portosystemic shunting from cirrhosis. Skin hyperpigmentation is common in patients with cholestasis and especially in those with primary biliary cirrhosis, who may display what has been named the "butterfly sign," an area of relative hypopigmentation between the scapulae as compared with the surrounding skin. A gray to brown discoloration of the skin and mucous membranes from the accumulation of hemosiderin and hemofuscin (gray hue) and melanin (brown hue) suggests hereditary hemochromatosis (Chapter 231). Xanthomatosis, which is accumulation of lipids in the skin, is a manifestation of hyperlipidemia in cholestasis (e.g., primary biliary cirrhosis). It is associated with xanthomas on the palms, soles, trunk, and flexor surfaces; tuberous xanthomas over the joints; and xanthelasmas on the eyelids and under the eyes. Lichen planus (Chapter 464) is also associated with primary biliary cirrhosis. "Paper money" skin, characterized by telangiectases on the cheeks, can be a sign of cirrhosis. Purpura (Chapter 465) is a manifestation of vasculitis, which can be associated with chronic hepatitis C and B infections. Telangiectases on mucous membranes (e.g., lips) suggest CREST syndrome (Chapter 288) or hereditary hemorrhagic telangiectasia (Chapter 179), in which vascular malformations can occur in the liver. The distribution of body hair in men with cirrhosis is in a feminine pattern. Excoriations and prurigo nodularis (Fig. 149–2) result from chronic scratching in patients who suffer from pruritus. Nails can display white horizontal (Muehrcke's) lines (Chapter 467), indicative of hypoalbuminemia. Azure lunulae (sky blue moon) of the nails and a green hue on the skin from the accumulation of copper are described in Wilson's disease (Chapter 230).

Parotid Glands, Breasts, and Genitalia

Parotid gland enlargement (Chapter 451) can be detected in 20% of patients with cirrhosis secondary to alcohol abuse. Testicular atrophy and feminization, including gynecomastia, which is a classic finding in men with cirrhosis, may result from increased peripheral conversion of androgens; tender gynecomastia is also a side effect of spironolactone, a diuretic used to treat ascites.

Cardiovascular System

Heart failure from any cause (Chapter 57) may result in hepatomegaly; clues include cardiomegaly, cardiac gallops, and distended neck veins. Constrictive pericarditis (Chapter 77) is classically manifested as distended neck veins, a pericardial knock, hepatomegaly, and ascites. Pulmonary hypertension associated with portal hypertension or liver disease (i.e., portopulmonary hypertension) is suggested by an accentuated pulmonary component of the second heart sound or the presence of a systolic murmur consistent with tricuspid insufficiency, or both (Chapter 48). Pounding pulses are characteristic of patients with decompensated liver disease and are caused by systemic vasodilation and increased cardiac output (Chapter 157).

Respiratory System

Decreased breath sounds at the lung bases, usually at the right base, suggest hydrothorax in a patient with decompensated liver disease and, usually, ascites. Hepatopulmonary syndrome, which is associated with intrapulmonary vascular dilation, is characterized by orthodeoxia (i.e., arterial deoxygenation when moving from the supine to the upright position) and platypnea (i.e., dyspnea on moving from the supine to the upright position) (Chapter 157). These phenomena result from an increase in intrapulmonary shunting of blood to the lower lobes.

Abdomen

Dilated veins on the abdominal wall may be a sign of intrahepatic portal hypertension. This phenomenon results from recanalization of the paraumbilical or umbilical veins in an effort to decompress the portal system. Dilated veins are classically described as emerging from the umbilicus, a finding known as "caput medusae." When compressed, the veins fill up from the umbilicus. Dilated abdominal veins can also be seen high up in the abdomen, not emanating from the umbilicus.

In patients with liver disease, abdominal auscultation may reveal a venous hum suggestive of portal hypertension. A bruit over the liver area, in synchrony with the pulse, suggests a vascular tumor with arterial blood supply (e.g., hepatocellular carcinoma) or florid alcoholic hepatitis. A hepatic friction rub has been described in tumors eroding the liver capsule, hepatic syphilis, and liver abscesses.

A distended abdomen with bulging flanks suggests ascites (Fig. 149–3), which is a defining complication in the natural history of liver disease because of its correlation with increased morbidity and mortality (Chapter 157). The detection of shifting dullness, which suggests ascites, results from movement of fluid to the most dependent portion of the abdomen. The subject is examined in the supine position, and the abdomen is percussed from the midline toward the right or left flanks. A change from a tympanic sound to a dull sound indicates a change from air to fluid, and the location of that change identifies the surface of the fluid pool. The examiner should percuss beyond the point at which dullness is elicited and ask the subject to turn toward the examiner without moving the hand so that the hand is then at the highest point. With the subject on the side, the examiner percusses again; if the sound is resonant, the presence of ascites is supported. This maneuver should be performed on the right side and again on the left side for confirmation. A fluid wave can be felt by placing the medial border of one hand on the abdomen and tapping the right or left lateral abdominal walls; the resulting wave will be felt by the first hand. Abdominal tenderness in a patient with ascites suggests peritonitis (e.g., spontaneous bacterial peritonitis), which is an ominous complication of liver disease.

The liver is dull to percussion. To feel the liver, the abdomen is examined with the patient in the supine position, arms parallel to the sides of the body, and the knees bent to relax the abdominal muscles. It is useful to start palpating from the right lower quadrant of the abdomen toward the rib cage so that the liver edge is encountered on the way up. The liver

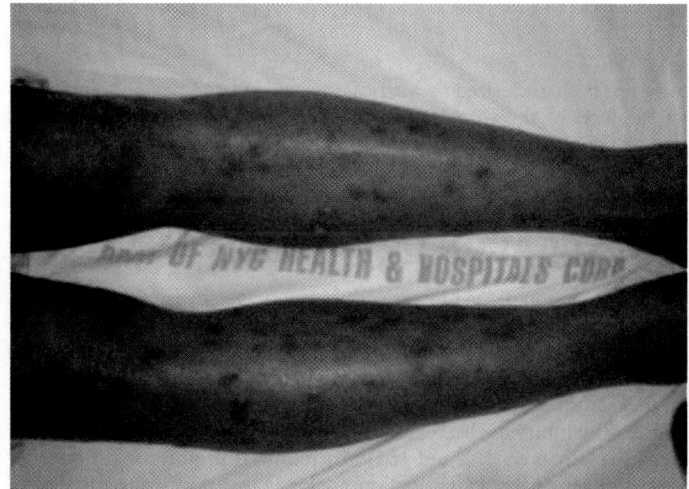

FIGURE 149–2 • Prurigo nodularis on the skin of the patient whose sclera is depicted in Figure 149–1 secondary to chronic scratching to relieve the pruritus of cholestasis.

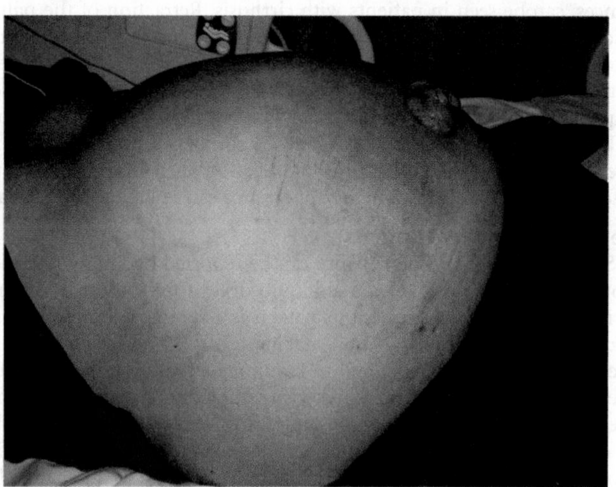

FIGURE 149–3 • Marked ascites and an umbilical hernia, which had ruptured a few days before the photograph, in a patient with cirrhosis and portal hypertension secondary to hepatitis C.

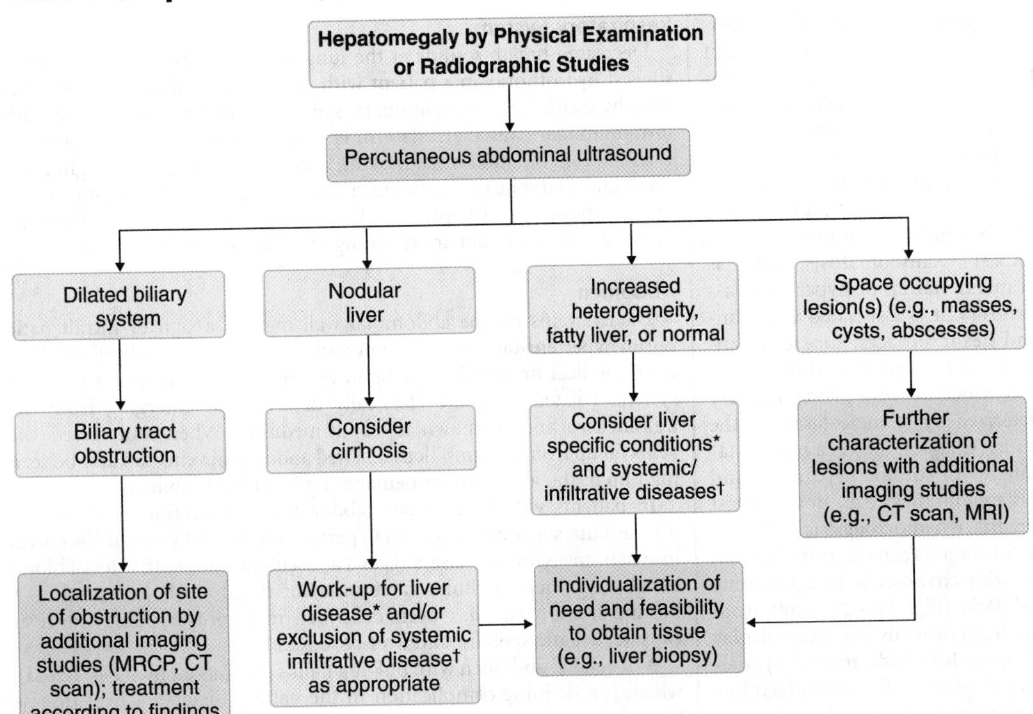

FIGURE 149–4 • A diagnostic approach to hepatomegaly. *Conditions to be excluded include viral hepatitis, alcohol- and drug-induced liver disease, steatohepatitis, autoimmune liver diseases, and metabolic disorders including hemochromatosis, Wilson's disease, and α_1-antitrypsin deficiency. †Systemic and infiltrative diseases include amyloidosis, lymphoma, sarcoidosis, and infectious processes such as disseminated tuberculosis and fungemia. CT = computed tomography; MRCP = magnetic resonance cholangiopancreatography; MRI = magnetic resonance imaging.

edge is smooth and sometimes slightly tender when palpated. In general, a liver that is felt up to 2 cm below the right costal margin is considered normal. A normal-sized liver can be displaced downward by emphysematous lungs. In thin subjects, the liver edge can be felt on deep inspiration, even in the absence of hepatic pathology. Hepatomegaly may indicate cirrhosis, infiltrative disease, or space-occupying lesions (e.g., tumors) (Fig. 149–4). A liver with a firm or hard consistency is consistent with cirrhosis. The liver can extend across the midline, and the left lobe can be felt in the epigastrium. When the presence or absence of hepatomegaly is uncertain, the scratch test, which is conducted by placing the bell of the stethoscope on the right upper quadrant over the rib cage and scratching the surface of the abdominal wall from the midabdomen towards the liver, may demonstrate amplification of the sound of the scratch on an area under which the liver lies. In the presence of ascites, the liver edge can be made to bounce by exerting quick pressure with the fingertips below the rib cage. Splenomegaly (Chapter 174) suggests portal hypertension (Chapter 157).

Extremities

Red palms (Fig. 149–5), especially on the thenar and hypothenar eminences, can be seen in patients with cirrhosis. Retraction of the palmar fascia with subsequent contracture of the palms and fingers is known as Dupuytren's contracture, a condition that is more prevalent in patients with liver disease. Acquired finger clubbing (see Fig. 48–10) can be seen in patients with cirrhosis and in those with hepatopulmonary syndrome.

Lower extremity edema (see Fig. 48–7) complicates fluid retention in liver disease. The edema is usually pitting, but when chronic or complicated by venous insufficiency, the appearance can resemble elephantiasis.

Neuropsychiatric Alterations

Subtle alterations in personality can be reported by family members. Constructional apraxia (e.g., inability to draw a five-pointed star or to write legibly) in a fully conscious patient is a typical finding of hepatic encephalopathy. The Reitan trail-making test can be used to assess the presence of encephalopathy and to monitor its evolution in response to therapy. The test, which measures visual motor integration and motor speed, is performed by asking the subject to connect in sequence a series of numbers from 1 to 25 randomly printed on a page. The baseline time is recorded, and change to more rapid completion is interpreted as improvement. Asterixis, a sign of encephalopathy, can be appreciated by having the patient extend the arms, with the palms down, and then dorsiflex the wrists while separating the fingers for at least 15 seconds; a positive test is characterized by a series of extension and flexion movements at the level of the wrist. Electromyography of the contracted muscles reveals lapses of electrical input that coincide with asterixis. Tremors (Chapter 434) can also be noted.

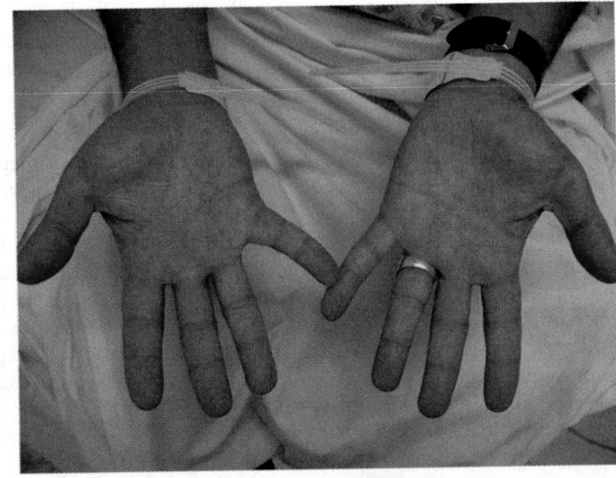

FIGURE 149–5 • Palmar erythema in a patient with cirrhosis.

GENERAL COMMENTS ON THE INVESTIGATION OF LIVER DISEASE

An impression of liver disease can be confirmed by laboratory or radiographic tests (or both), all of which should be analyzed in concert. A liver profile suggestive of cholestasis (Chapter 150) of any cause is characterized by an increase in the serum activity of alkaline phosphatase and, in the majority of cases, γ-glutamyl transpeptidase. Aminotransferases are released by injury to the hepatocytes, such as occurs in acute or chronic hepatitis (Chapters 151 and 152). A prolonged prothrombin time suggests synthetic hepatic dysfunction, as does a decreased concentration of serum albumin (Chapter 150). A complete blood count may reveal pancytopenia as a result of bone marrow suppression and hypersplenism, which is caused by portal hypertension (Chapter 157). Jaundice in the absence of urobilinogen in urine indicates unconjugated hyperbilirubinemia (e.g., from hemolysis; Chapter 164). Microscopic hematuria and proteinuria suggest glomerulopathies (e.g., associated with cryoglobulinemia or deposition of immune complexes, most commonly IgA; Chapter 122). An alkaline urine pH suggests renal tubular acidosis (Chapter 123), which can complicate Wilson's disease and, in the partial form, primary biliary cirrhosis. Renal insufficiency, oliguria, and a marked reduction in urine sodium (Chapter 117) are consistent with hepatorenal syndrome (Chapter 157), a dreaded complication of liver disease.

Exclusion of biliary obstruction by percutaneous ultrasound is a defining point in the investigation of an abnormal liver profile in the presence or absence of hepatomegaly (Chapter 135). A sonographic study of the liver can also provide some suggestion of the presence or absence of parenchymal liver disease (e.g., increased echogenicity, nodularity) and an opportunity to identify space-occupying lesions, including tumors and cysts. Inclusion of Doppler studies during the sonographic examination provides information on the patency of relevant blood vessels and the direction and characteristics of blood flow.

LIVER BIOPSY

Examination of liver histology provides the opportunity to diagnose or confirm a particular disease, determine the degree of liver injury (e.g., the presence of cirrhosis), and assess response to treatment. The decision to perform a liver biopsy must be individualized by weighing the risks versus the benefits. Liver fibrosis is associated with a decrease in tissue elasticity. An evolving noninvasive method to assess liver fibrosis is transient elastography. This technique uses ultrasound and low-frequency elastic waves and allows for the measure of the waves' propagation velocity, which increases as tissue elasticity decreases.

Exclusion of congenital liver diseases (e.g., primary hemochromatosis, Wilson's disease, α_1-antitrypsin deficiency) in patients in whom an acquired disease (e.g., viral hepatitis) has been diagnosed is always prudent because missing such diagnoses has dire consequences. By the same reasoning, a patient in whom a congenital or autoimmune disease is diagnosed should be evaluated to exclude any acquired diseases (e.g., viral hepatitis).

SUGGESTED READINGS

Blei AT: Portal hypertension and its complications. Curr Opin Gastroenterol 2007;23:275–282. *A clinical overview.*

Brienza N, Dalfino L, Cinnella G, et al: Jaundice in critical illness: Promoting factors of a concealed reality. Intensive Care Med 2006;32:267–274. *Jaundice is common in critically ill patients and those with shock, sepsis, and mechanical ventilation.*

Cardenas A, Arroyo V: Refractory ascites. Dig Dis 2005;23:30–38. *The pathophysiology, clinical features, and treatment of refractory ascites in cirrhosis.*

150 APPROACH TO THE PATIENT WITH JAUNDICE OR ABNORMAL LIVER TEST RESULTS

Paul D. Berk and Kevin M. Korenblat

Definition

Jaundice, from the French *jaune* (yellow), is the yellow-orange discoloration of the skin, conjunctivae, and mucous membranes that results from elevated concentrations of bilirubin in plasma. Mild hyperbilirubinemia may be clinically undetectable, but jaundice becomes evident at plasma bilirubin concentrations of 3 to 4 mg/dL, depending on the patient's normal pigmentation, the conditions of observation, and the bilirubin fraction that is elevated. Optimal interpretation of an elevated plasma bilirubin concentration is based on an appreciation of its sources and disposition.

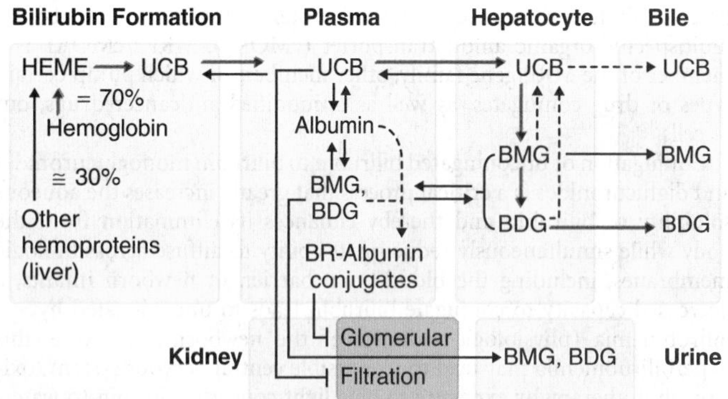

FIGURE 150–1 • Overview of bilirubin metabolism. Unconjugated bilirubin (UCB) formed from the breakdown of heme from hemoglobin and other hemoproteins is transported in plasma reversibly bound to albumin and converted in the liver to bilirubin monoglucuronide (BMG) and diglucuronide (BDG), the latter being the predominant form secreted in bile. BMG and BDG together usually account for less than 5% of normal serum bilirubin. In patients with hepatobiliary disease, BMG and BDG accumulate in plasma and appear in urine. Bilirubin glucuronides in plasma also react nonenzymatically with albumin and possibly other serum proteins to form protein conjugates, which do not appear in urine and have a plasma half-life similar to that of albumin.

Bilirubin Metabolism

Bilirubin Production

Bilirubin is the degradation product of the heme moiety of hemoproteins, a class of proteins involved in the transport or metabolism of oxygen (Fig. 150–1). Normal adults produce about 4 mg of bilirubin per kilogram of body weight per day. Between 70 and 90% of bilirubin is derived from the hemoglobin of erythrocytes that are sequestered and destroyed by mononuclear phagocytic cells of the reticuloendothelial system, principally in the spleen, liver, and bone marrow. The remainder results primarily from the turnover of nonhemoglobin hemoproteins such as myoglobin, the P-450 cytochromes, catalase, and peroxidase, principally in the liver; a minor fraction reflects ineffective erythropoiesis, which is the premature destruction of newly formed erythrocytes within the bone marrow.

The two-step conversion of heme to bilirubin begins with opening of the heme molecule at its α-bridge carbon by the microsomal enzyme *heme oxygenase*, a process that results in the formation of equimolar quantities of carbon monoxide and the green tetrapyrrole biliverdin. This nontoxic, water-soluble pigment is the main excretory product of heme in birds, reptiles, and amphibians. However, biliverdin cannot cross the placenta. Accordingly, reduction of biliverdin to bilirubin in mammals by a second enzyme, *biliverdin reductase*, allows its transplacental removal from the fetus to the maternal circulation. The unconjugated bilirubin produced in the periphery is transported to the liver in plasma. Because of its insolubility in aqueous media, it is kept in solution by tight, but reversible binding to albumin. A number of compounds, including sulfonamides, furosemide, and radiographic contrast agents, competitively displace bilirubin from its binding sites on albumin, a phenomenon that is of little clinical significance except in neonates, in whom the resulting increased concentration of unbound bilirubin raises the risk for kernicterus.

Disposition of Bilirubin by the Liver

Excretion of bilirubin from the body is a major function of the liver (see Fig. 150–1), where specialized microanatomy enhances the extraction of tightly protein-bound compounds from the circulation. Hepatic translocation of bilirubin from blood to bile involves four distinct steps: (1) uptake of unconjugated bilirubin, principally by an incompletely characterized, facilitated transport process and, to a lesser extent, by diffusion; (2) intracellular binding, mainly to various cytosolic proteins of the glutathione-*S*-transferase family; (3) conversion of unconjugated bilirubin to bilirubin monoglucuronides and diglucuronides by a specific uridine diphosphate (UDP)-glucuronosyltransferase isoform designated UGT1A1 encoded by the *UGT1* gene complex; and (4) transfer of bilirubin monoglucuronides and diglucuronides into bile by a canalicular membrane adenosine triphosphate (ATP)-dependent transporter designated multidrug resistance–associated protein 2 (MRP2) or canalicular multispecific organic anion transporter (cMOAT). MRP2/cMOAT is a member of the MRP gene family, other members of which pump certain types of drug conjugates, as well as unmodified anticancer drugs, out of cells.

Conjugation of unconjugated bilirubin to bilirubin monoglucuronides and diglucuronides is a critical process that greatly increases the aqueous solubility of bilirubin and thereby enhances its elimination from the body while simultaneously reducing its ability to diffuse across biologic membranes, including the blood-brain barrier. In newborn infants, a decreased capacity to conjugate bilirubin leads to unconjugated hyperbilirubinemia (physiologic jaundice of the newborn). If severe, this hyperbilirubinemia may lead to irreversible central nervous system toxicity. Phototherapy by exposure to blue light converts bilirubin to water-soluble photo-isomers that are readily excreted in bile, thereby protecting the central nervous system from bilirubin toxicity. Gilbert's syndrome and Crigler-Najjar syndrome types 1 and 2, which result from genetic defects in bilirubin conjugation, are characterized by unconjugated hyperbilirubinemia; in contrast, Dubin-Johnson syndrome, which results from inheritable defects in MRP2/cMOAT (see later), is characterized by conjugated or mixed hyperbilirubinemia.

Bilirubin in Plasma

The total plasma bilirubin concentration in normal adults is less than 1 to 1.5 mg/dL, depending on the measurement method used. Modern analytic techniques show that normal plasma contains principally unconjugated bilirubin, with only traces of conjugates. Clinical laboratories typically quantify plasma bilirubin by a reaction in which bilirubin is cleaved by a diazo reagent, such as diazotized sulfanilic acid, to azodipyrroles, which are readily quantitated spectrophotometrically. Bilirubin conjugates react rapidly ("prompt" or "direct"-reacting bilirubin). Unconjugated bilirubin reacts slowly because the site of attack by the diazo reagent is protected by internal hydrogen bonding. Accordingly, accurate measurement of the total plasma bilirubin concentration requires the addition of an accelerator, such as ethanol or urea, to disrupt this internal hydrogen bonding and to ensure complete reaction of any unconjugated bilirubin. The "indirect"-reacting bilirubin is calculated by subtracting the direct-reacting bilirubin from the total. Even though physicians traditionally equate the direct-reacting fraction of bilirubin in plasma with conjugated bilirubin and the indirect fraction with unconjugated bilirubin, this approach is, at best, a rough approximation. Although 10 to 20% of bilirubin in normal plasma gives a prompt (direct) diazo reaction, this percentage is an artifact of the kinetics of the diazo reaction inasmuch as more than 95% of the total bilirubin in normal plasma is unconjugated. Consequently, unqualified interpretation of the direct and indirect fractions as reflecting conjugated and unconjugated bilirubin, respectively, may lead to diagnostic errors, particularly in the diagnosis of isolated, hereditary hyperbilirubinemia.

Interpretation of Clinical Measurements of the Plasma Bilirubin Concentration

At virtually any total bilirubin concentration, a direct-reacting fraction of less than 15% of total bilirubin can be considered as essentially being all unconjugated. When the direct-reacting fraction is greater than 15%, a simple dipstick test for bilirubinuria may clarify the situation. Unconjugated bilirubin is not excreted in urine regardless of the height of its plasma concentration because its binding to albumin is too tight for effective glomerular filtration and it is not secreted by the tubules. The canalicular transport mechanism for excretion of bilirubin conjugates is especially sensitive to injury. Accordingly, in hepatocellular disease, as well as with either cholestasis or mechanical bile duct obstruction, bilirubin conjugates within the hepatocyte or biliary tract may reflux into the blood stream and result in a mixed or, less often, a purely conjugated hyperbilirubinemia. Conjugated bilirubin, which is normally loosely bound to albumin, is readily filtered at the glomerulus; even modest degrees of conjugated hyperbilirubinemia result in bilirubinuria, which is *always* a pathologic finding. With prolonged conjugated hyperbilirubinemia, some of the conjugated bilirubin binds *covalently* to albumin and produces what is designated the delta (δ) bilirubin fraction. Although δ-bilirubin gives a direct diazo reaction, it is not filterable by the glomerulus and does not appear in urine; it disappears slowly from plasma, with the 14- to 21-day half-life of the albumin to which it is bound. δ-Bilirubin accounts for the sometimes slow rate at which conjugated (direct) hyperbilirubinemia resolves as hepatitis improves or biliary obstruction is relieved. Although δ-bilirubin is not easily measured, its presence can be inferred when an elevated direct-reacting bilirubin persists after bilirubinuria resolves.

Bilirubin in Bile

Normal bile contains an average of less than 5% unconjugated bilirubin, 7% bilirubin monoconjugates, and 90% bilirubin diconjugates. The proportion of monoconjugates increases with either an increased bilirubin load (hemolysis) or reduced bilirubin conjugating capacity (e.g., Crigler-Najjar syndrome type 1).

Posthepatic Aspects of Bilirubin Disposition

Unconjugated bilirubin ordinarily does not reach the gut except in neonates or, by ill-defined alternative pathways, in the presence of severe unconjugated hyperbilirubinemia (e.g., Crigler-Najjar syndrome type 1). In these circumstances, unconjugated bilirubin is reabsorbed from the gut, thereby amplifying the hyperbilirubinemia. After canalicular secretion, conjugated bilirubin traverses the biliary tree, reaches the duodenum, and passes down the gastrointestinal tract without reabsorption by either the gallbladder or intestinal mucosa. Although some bilirubin reaches the feces, most is converted to urobilinogen and to related compounds by bacteria within the ileum and colon, where the urobilinogen is reabsorbed, returns to the liver through the portal circulation, and is re-excreted into bile in a process of enterohepatic recirculation. Any urobilinogen that is not taken up by the liver reaches the systemic circulation, from which it is cleared by the kidneys. Normal urine urobilinogen excretion is 4 mg/day or less. With hemolysis, which increases the load of bilirubin entering the gut and therefore the amount of urobilinogen formed and reabsorbed, or with liver disease, which decreases the hepatic extraction of bilirubin, plasma urobilinogen levels rise, and more urobilinogen is excreted in urine. Severe cholestasis, bile duct obstruction, or broad-spectrum antibiotics that reduce or eliminate the bacterial conversion of bilirubin to urobilinogen markedly decrease the formation and urinary excretion of urobilinogen.

Differential Diagnosis of Hyperbilirubinemia and Jaundice

Hyperbilirubinemia and jaundice (Fig. 150–2) may result from isolated disorders of bilirubin metabolism, liver disease, or obstruction of the biliary tract. Jaundice represents the most visible sign of hepatobiliary disease of many causes (Table 150–1).

DISORDERS OF BILIRUBIN METABOLISM

Pure hyperbilirubinemia may result either from extrahepatic factors or from inherited or acquired defects in specific aspects of hepatic bilirubin disposition.

Unconjugated Hyperbilirubinemia

The plasma unconjugated bilirubin concentration ([UCB]) is determined by a balance between the bilirubin production rate (BRP) and hepatic bilirubin clearance (C_{BR}) according to the relationship

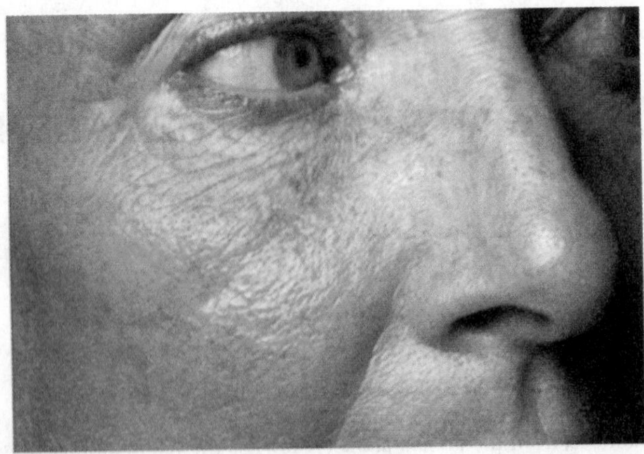

FIGURE 150–2 • Severe cholestatic jaundice in a patient with primary biliary cirrhosis. The high level of conjugated bilirubin, maintained over a long period, gives a characteristic dark brown-orange pigmentation to the skin and sclerae. Large xanthelasmas and corneal arcus usually develop in patients with primary biliary cirrhosis as a consequence of disordered lipid metabolism. (From Forbes CD, Jackson WF: Color Atlas and Text of Clinical Medicine, 3rd ed. London, Mosby, 2003.)

TABLE 150–1 DIFFERENTIAL DIAGNOSIS OF HYPERBILIRUBINEMIA AND JAUNDICE

ISOLATED DISORDERS OF BILIRUBIN METABOLISM

Unconjugated hyperbilirubinemia
- Increased bilirubin production
  - *Examples:* hemolysis, ineffective erythropoiesis, blood transfusion, resorption of hematomas
- Decreased hepatocellular uptake
  - *Examples:* drugs (e.g., rifampin)
- Decreased conjugation
  - *Examples:* Gilbert's and Crigler-Najjar syndromes, physiologic jaundice of the newborn, breast milk jaundice, HIV protease inhibitors

Conjugated or mixed hyperbilirubinemia
- Decreased canalicular transport: Dubin-Johnson syndrome
- Mechanism uncertain: Rotor's syndrome

LIVER DISEASE

Acute or chronic hepatocellular dysfunction
- Acute or subacute hepatocellular injury
  - *Examples:* viral hepatitis A, B, C, hepatotoxins (e.g., ethanol, acetaminophen, mushroom *[Amanita phalloides]* poisoning), drugs (e.g., isoniazid, α-methyldopa), metabolic diseases (e.g., Wilson's disease, Reye's syndrome), pregnancy related (e.g., acute fatty liver of pregnancy, preeclampsia), hepatic ischemia (e.g., hypotension, postoperative, hepatic artery thrombosis)
- Chronic hepatocellular disease
  - *Examples:* hepatitis B and C, hepatotoxins (e.g., ethanol, vinyl chloride, vitamin A), autoimmune hepatitis, metabolic disease (Wilson's disease, hemochromatosis, α_1-antitrypsin deficiency)

Hepatic disorders with prominent cholestasis
- Familial cholestatic disorders
- Single-gene disorders
  - *Examples:* benign recurrent intrahepatic cholestasis, progressive familial intrahepatic cholestasis types 1–3
- Familial cholestatic disorders of unknown pathogenesis
  - *Examples:* Aagenaes' syndrome, Navajo neurohepatopathy, North American Indian cholestasis
- Diffuse infiltrative disorders
  - *Examples:* granulomatous diseases (e.g., mycobacterial and fungal infections, sarcoidosis, lymphoma, drugs, Wegener's granulomatosis), amyloidosis, infiltrative malignancies
- Inflammation of intrahepatic bile ductules and/or portal tracts
  - *Examples:* primary biliary cirrhosis, liver allograft rejection, graft-versus-host disease, drugs (e.g., chlorpromazine, erythromycin)
- Miscellaneous conditions
  - *Examples:* uncommon manifestations of viral or alcoholic hepatitis, intrahepatic cholestasis of pregnancy, contraceptive jaundice, estrogens, anabolic steroids, postoperative cholestasis, total parenteral nutrition, bacterial infections, drugs

OBSTRUCTION OF BILE DUCTS

Choledocholithiasis
- *Examp les:* cholesterol gallstones, pigment gallstones

Diseases of the bile ducts
- Inflammation/infection
  - *Examples:* primary sclerosing cholangitis, AIDS cholangiopathy, hepatic arterial chemotherapy, postsurgical strictures
- Neoplasms (e.g., cholangiocarcinoma)

Extrinsic compression of the biliary tree
- Neoplasms
  - *Examples:* pancreatic carcinoma, metastatic lymphadenopathy, hepatoma
- Pancreatitis with or without pseudocyst formation
- Vascular enlargement (e.g., aneurysm, cavernous transformation of the portal vein)

AIDS = acquired immunodeficiency syndrome; HIV = human immunodeficiency virus.

$$[UCB] \approx BRP/C_{BR} \quad (1)$$

C_{BR} is analogous to creatinine clearance in the test of kidney function; it is a measure of the rate at which bilirubin is extracted from plasma, and it is a true quantitative test of liver function. Although BRP and C_{BR} are not easily quantified, investigative measurements have yielded useful pathophysiologic insights. Equation 1 indicates that [UCB] increases linearly with an increase in BRP or hyperbolically with a decrease in C_{BR}, thereby providing a basis for classifying unconjugated hyperbilirubinemias according to their pathogenesis.

Increased Bilirubin Production

Increased production of bilirubin and subsequent unconjugated hyperbilirubinemia can be caused by hemolysis, accelerated destruction of transfused erythrocytes, resorption of hematomas, or ineffective erythropoiesis (e.g., lead poisoning, megaloblastic anemias related to deficiency of either folic acid or vitamin B_{12}, sideroblastic anemia, congenital erythropoietic porphyria, or myeloproliferative or myelodysplastic diseases). In these settings, other liver tests are typically normal and the hyperbilirubinemia is modest, rarely exceeding 4 mg/dL; higher values imply concomitant hepatic dysfunction. However, after brisk blood transfusion or resorption of massive hematomas caused by trauma, the increased bilirubin load may be transiently sufficient to lead to frank jaundice. The causes of hemolysis are numerous (Chapters 164 to 167). Besides specific blood disorders, mild hemolysis accompanies many acquired diseases. In the setting of systemic disease, which may include a degree of hepatic dysfunction, hemolysis may produce a component of conjugated hyperbilirubinemia in addition to an elevated unconjugated bilirubin concentration. Prolonged hemolysis may lead to the formation of bilirubin gallstones, which may cause cholecystitis, obstruction, or any other biliary tract consequence of calculous disease (Chapter 159).

Decreased Hepatic Bilirubin Clearance

Decreased Bilirubin Uptake

Several drugs (e.g., rifampin, flavaspidic acid, novobiocin, and various cholecystographic contrast agents) competitively inhibit the hepatocellular uptake of bilirubin. The resulting unconjugated hyperbilirubinemia resolves with cessation of the medication. Decreased hepatic bilirubin uptake is also believed to contribute to the unconjugated hyperbilirubinemia of Gilbert's syndrome, although the principal molecular basis for this syndrome is a reduction in the conjugation of bilirubin.

Impaired Bilirubin Conjugation

The most frequent cause of decreased bilirubin clearance is a decrease in bilirubin conjugating activity. Bilirubin conjugation with glucuronic acid is catalyzed by a specific UDP-glucuronosyltransferase that is designated UGT1A1 and encoded by the *UGT1* gene complex. The *UGT1A1* gene is assembled by alternative splicing of a bilirubin-specific variant of exon 1, designated exon A_1, with four common exons (exons 2 to 5) that encode the shared carboxyl-terminal end of all *UGT1*-encoded proteins. Its promoter region normally contains an $A(TA)_6TAA$ TATA box–like construct.

Genetic Disorders of Bilirubin Conjugation

The hereditary hyperbilirubinemias (Table 150–2) are a group of five syndromes in which hyperbilirubinemia occurs as an isolated biochemical abnormality without evidence of either hepatocellular necrosis or cholestasis. The molecular defects have been identified in all but Rotor's syndrome.

Crigler-Najjar syndrome types 1 and 2 and *Gilbert's syndrome* are hereditary forms of unconjugated hyperbilirubinemia that result from mutations in *UGT1A1.* In Crigler-Najjar type 1, essentially no functional enzyme activity is present, whereas patients with Crigler-Najjar type 2 have up to 10% of normal and patients with Gilbert's syndrome have 10 to 33% of normal activity, which leads to bilirubin concentrations of 18 to 45, 6 to 25, and 1.5 to 4 mg/dL, respectively (see Table 150–2). Because total UGT1A1 enzymatic activity must be reduced to less than 50% of normal to produce unconjugated hyperbilirubinemia, phenotypic expression of mutations in this enzyme requires either homozygosity or double heterozygosity. Thus, despite earlier reports to the contrary, each of these disorders is inherited as an autosomal recessive trait. Patients with types 1 and 2 Crigler-Najjar syndrome are either homozygotes or double heterozygotes for structural mutations within the coding region. In Western countries, patients with Gilbert's syndrome are typically homozygous for an $A(TA)_7TAA$ promoter mutation. Structural

TABLE 150–2 PRINCIPAL FEATURES OF HEREDITARY DISORDERS OF BILIRUBIN METABOLISM

Feature	Crigler-Najjar Syndrome TYPE I	Crigler-Najjar Syndrome TYPE II	Gilbert's Syndrome	Dubin-Johnson Syndrome	Rotor's Syndrome
Incidence	Very rare	Uncommon	Up to 12% of the population	Uncommon	Rare
Total serum bilirubin (mg/dL)	18–45 (usually >20), unconjugated	6–25 (usually ≤20), unconjugated	Typically ≤4 in the absence of fasting or hemolysis; mostly unconjugated	Typically 2–5, less often ≤25; about 60% direct reacting	Usually 3–7, occasionally ≤20; about 60% direct reacting
Defect(s) in bilirubin metabolism	Bilirubin UDPGT activity markedly reduced: trace to absent	Bilirubin UDPGT activity reduced: ≤10% of normal	Bilirubin UDPGT activity typically reduced to 10–33% of normal; reduced bilirubin uptake in some cases; mild hemolysis in up to 50% of patients	Impaired canalicular secretion of conjugated bilirubin because of MRP2/cMOAT mutation	Impaired hepatic secretion or storage of conjugated bilirubin; molecular defect not known
Routine liver tests	Normal	Normal	Normal	Normal	Normal
Serum bile acids	Normal	Normal	Normal	Usually normal	Normal
Plasma sulfobromophthalein removal (% retention of a 5-mg/kg dose at 45 min)*	Normal	Normal	Usually normal (<5%); mild 45-min retention (<15%) in some patients	Slow initial decline in plasma concentration (retention ≤20% at 45 min) with secondary rise at 90–120 min	Very slow initial decline in plasma concentration (45-min retention = 30–45%) without secondary rise
Oral cholecystography	Normal	Normal	Normal	Faint or nonvisualization of the gallbladder	Usually normal
Pharmacologic responses/ special features	No response to phenobarbital	Phenobarbital reduces bilirubin by ≤75%	Phenobarbital reduces bilirubin, often to normal	Increased bilirubin concentration with estrogens; diagnostic urine coproporphyrin isomer pattern (total is normal, with isomer I increased to ≤80% of total)	Characteristic urine coproporphyrin excretion pattern (total is increased ≥2.5-fold in ≈65% of cases, but isomer I always <80% of total)
Major clinical features	Kernicterus in infancy if untreated; may occur later despite therapy	Rare late-onset kernicterus with fasting	None	Occasional hepatosplenomegaly	None
Hepatic morphology/ histology	Normal	Normal	Normal; occasionally increased lipofuscin pigment	Liver grossly black; coarse, dark centrilobular pigment	Normal
Bile bilirubin fractions†	>90% unconjugated	Largest fraction (mean 57%) is monoconjugates	Mainly diconjugates, but monoconjugates are increased (mean 23%)	Mixed conjugates, reported increase in diconjugates	Increased conjugates
Inheritance (all autosomal)	Recessive	Recessive	Promoter mutation is recessive; missense mutation often dominant	Recessive; rare kindred appears dominant	Recessive
Diagnosis	Clinical and laboratory findings; lack of response to phenobarbital	Clinical and laboratory findings; response to phenobarbital	Clinical and laboratory findings; promoter genotyping; liver biopsy rarely necessary	Clinical and laboratory findings; liver biopsy unnecessary if coproporphyrin studies available; BSP disappearance	Clinical and laboratory findings; urine coproporphyrin analysis; BSP disappearance
Treatment	Phototherapy or tin protoporphyrin as short-term therapy; liver transplantation definitive	Consider phenobarbital if baseline bilirubin ≥8 mg/dL	None necessary	Avoid estrogens; no other therapy necessary	No treatment necessary

*Sulfobromophthalein studies may be useful in distinguishing the Dubin-Johnson and Rotor syndromes if coproporphyrin isomer studies are not available.
†Bilirubin in normal bile: less than 5% is unconjugated bilirubin, with an average of 7% bilirubin monoconjugates and 90% bilirubin diconjugates.
BSP = sulfobromophthalein; cMOAT = canalicular multispecific organic anion transporter; MRP2 = multidrug resistance–associated protein 2; UDPGT = uridine diphosphate glucuronosyltransferase.

mutations causing modest reductions in UGT1A1 enzymatic activity have been reported in some Japanese patients with Gilbert's syndrome.

Crigler-Najjar syndrome type 1 is characterized by striking unconjugated hyperbilirubinemia that appears in the neonatal period, persists for life, and is unresponsive to phenobarbital. The majority of patients (type 1A) exhibit defects in glucuronide conjugation of a spectrum of substrates in addition to bilirubin as a result of mutations in one of the common exons (2 to 5) of the *UGT1* complex. In a smaller subset (type 1B), a mutation in the bilirubin-specific exon A1 limits the defect to bilirubin conjugation. More than 30 structurally diverse *UGT1A1* mutations can cause type 1 Crigler-Najjar syndrome; their common feature is that they all encode proteins with absent or, at most, traces of enzymatic activity. Before the availability of phototherapy, most patients with Crigler-Najjar type 1 died of bilirubin encephalopathy (kernicterus) in infancy or early childhood. Optimal treatment for a neurologically intact patient includes (1) about 12 hr/day of phototherapy from birth throughout childhood, perhaps supplemented by exchange transfusion in the neonatal period; (2) use of tin-protoporphyrin to blunt transient episodes of increased hyperbilirubinemia; and (3) early liver transplantation, before the onset of brain damage. Transplantation with isolated allogeneic hepatocytes is being evaluated as an experimental therapeutic approach.

Bilirubin concentrations are typically lower in type 2 Crigler-Najjar syndrome, and plasma bilirubin levels can be reduced to 3 to 5 mg/dL by phenobarbital. At least 10 different mutations in *UGT1A1* have been associated with Crigler-Najjar type 2; all encode a bilirubin-UDP-glucuronosyltransferase with markedly reduced but detectable enzymatic activity. Though uncommon in Crigler-Najjar type 2, kernicterus has occurred at all ages and is typically associated with factors that temporarily raise the plasma bilirubin concentration above baseline (e.g., fasting, intercurrent illness). For this reason, phenobarbital therapy is often recommended; a single bedtime dose usually maintains clinically safe plasma bilirubin concentrations.

Gilbert's syndrome is the most common of the hereditary hyperbilirubinemias, with a genotypic prevalence of up to 12% and a phenotypic prevalence of up to 7%. Its high prevalence may explain the frequent appearance of mild unconjugated hyperbilirubinemia in liver transplant recipients. Plasma bilirubin concentrations are most often less than 3 mg/dL, although both higher and lower values are frequent, with increases of two- to three-fold commonly occurring with fasting and intercurrent illness. The phenotypic distinction between mild Gilbert's syndrome and a normal state is often blurred. Phenobarbital normalizes both the bilirubin concentration and C_{BR}. Oxidative drug metabolism and the disposition of most xenobiotics that are metabolized by glucuronidation appear to be normal in Gilbert's syndrome. A critical exception is the antitumor agent irinotecan (CPT-11), whose active metabolite (SN-38) is glucuronidated specifically by UGT1A1. In patients with Gilbert's syndrome, CPT-11 can cause intractable diarrhea, myelosuppression, and other serious toxicities. Unconjugated hyperbilirubinemia related to selective inhibition of UGT1A1 also occurs with several human immunodeficiency virus (HIV) protease inhibitors (e.g., indinavir). Abnormal disposition of menthol, estradiol benzoate, acetaminophen, tolbutamide, rifamycin SV, and other agents has not been associated with significant complications, but prudence should be exercised in prescribing agents that are metabolized by glucuronidation to patients with Gilbert's syndrome.

Unconjugated Hyperbilirubinemia in the Newborn Period

Mild unconjugated hyperbilirubinemia develops in most neonates between days 2 and 5 after birth because of hepatic immaturity and low levels of UGT1A1. Peak bilirubin levels are typically less than 5 to 10 mg/dL, and levels return to normal within 2 weeks as mechanisms of bilirubin disposition mature. Prematurity, with hemolysis or hepatic immaturity, is associated with higher bilirubin levels that may require phototherapy. The progestational steroid 3α,20β-pregnanediol and certain fatty acids found in the breast milk (but not serum) of some mothers inhibit bilirubin conjugation and can cause excessive neonatal hyperbilirubinemia *(breast milk jaundice)*. By comparison, *transient familial neonatal hyperbilirubinemia* (Lucey-Driscoll syndrome) is caused by a UGT1A1 inhibitor that is found in maternal serum.

Acquired Conjugation Defects

A modest reduction in bilirubin conjugating capacity occurs in patients with advanced hepatitis or cirrhosis (Chapters 157 and 158). However, in this setting, conjugation is better preserved than other aspects of bilirubin disposition, such as canalicular excretion. Pharmacologic and metabolic perturbations may also lead to acquired reductions in bilirubin conjugation. Various drugs (e.g., pregnanediol, novobiocin, chloramphenicol, gentamicin, and several HIV protease inhibitors) may cause unconjugated hyperbilirubinemia by inhibiting UGT1A1. In all settings in which UGT1A1 inhibitors cause unconjugated hyperbilirubinemia, the hyperbilirubinemia is greater in patients with underlying Gilbert's syndrome.

Conjugated or Mixed Hyperbilirubinemia

Two phenotypically similar, but mechanistically distinct inherited disorders, Dubin-Johnson syndrome and Rotor's syndrome, are characterized by conjugated or mixed hyperbilirubinemia with normal values for other standard liver tests (see Table 150–2). Dubin-Johnson syndrome results from any of several mutations in the gene encoding the ATP-dependent canalicular organic anion transporter MRP2/cMOAT (see Fig. 150-1). The molecular defect in Rotor's syndrome remains unknown, although some data suggest that it is precanalicular. Despite the conjugated hyperbilirubinemia, patients with these syndromes are not cholestatic and can be distinguished noninvasively by analysis of urine coproporphyrins (see Table 150–2), so liver biopsy is not required. Both syndromes carry a benign prognosis without specific therapy.

LIVER AND BILIARY TRACT DISEASE

Jaundice is a common sign of generalized hepatobiliary dysfunction, both acute and chronic. Icteric hepatobiliary disease is readily distinguished from the isolated disorders of bilirubin metabolism because the increase in plasma bilirubin concentration occurs in association with abnormalities in other standard liver tests. Liver diseases can be categorized as those in which the primary injury results from inflammation and hepatocellular necrosis versus those in which the central feature is inhibition of bile flow (cholestasis) and retention of bile constituents, some of which (e.g., bile acids) may be toxic. Although an accurate classification into one of these two broad categories is possible in most patients on the basis of clinical findings and standard biochemical studies (see later), further classification of patients with a predominantly cholestatic picture into those with decreased hepatocellular bile secretion and those with mechanical obstruction of the biliary tree may be more difficult. These diagnostically challenging conditions include several familial cholestatic syndromes; infiltrative disorders, particularly those involving the intrahepatic biliary tree; certain other inflammatory or neoplastic conditions; and drug reactions (see Table 150–1 and Chapters 151 to 157).

Familial Cholestasis Syndromes

Benign recurrent intrahepatic cholestasis is a rare, autosomal recessive disorder characterized by recurrent attacks of malaise, pruritus, and jaundice beginning in either childhood or adulthood and varying in duration from weeks to months. Intervals between attacks may vary from months to years. This benign disorder does not progress to chronic liver disease or cirrhosis, and there is complete resolution between episodes; treatment during the cholestatic episodes is symptomatic. The familial intrahepatic cholestasis 1 *(FIC1)* gene, which is mutated in this condition, encodes a protein that transports aminophospholipids from the outer to the inner leaflet of various cell membranes. The gene is expressed strongly in the small intestine but only weakly in the liver. *Progressive familial intrahepatic cholestasis* describes three phenotypically related syndromes of cholestasis during infancy and end-stage liver disease during childhood. In contrast to the selective bilirubin transport defect in Dubin-Johnson syndrome, the conjugated hyperbilirubinemia in these syndromes is caused by generalized bile secretory failure.

Postoperative Jaundice

This multifactorial syndrome can be caused by increased bilirubin production (e.g., breakdown of transfused erythrocytes, resorption of hematomas), by decreased hepatic clearance (e.g., bacteremia, endotoxemia, parenteral nutrition, perioperative hypoxia), or by both. Hyperbilirubinemia, which is the main biochemical feature, is often accompanied by a several-fold increase in levels of alkaline phosphatase, γ-glutamyl transpeptidase (GGT), or both. Aminotransferases are, at most, minimally elevated, and synthetic function is typically normal. The differential diagnosis includes biliary obstruction (Chapter 159) or hepatocellular injury related to shock, anesthetic injury (Chapter 153), or post-transfusion hepatitis (Chapter 151). Postoperative jaundice per se is not a threat to the patient, and it usually resolves in parallel with the patient's overall condition.

Jaundice in Pregnancy

Jaundice in pregnancy (Chapter 259) may result from any liver disease that also affects nonpregnant women or from conditions unique to pregnancy. The unique conditions include a generally modest and self-limited elevation in aminotransferase and bilirubin levels during the first trimester, often in patients with hyperemesis gravidarum; intrahepatic cholestasis of pregnancy, which occurs during the second and third trimesters and resolves spontaneously after delivery; or acute fatty liver or the HELLP syndrome (*h*emolysis, *e*levated *l*iver enzymes, and *l*ow *p*latelets) in association with preeclampsia in the third trimester (Chapters 154, 181, and 259). Acute fatty liver may resemble fulminant hepatic failure, with early delivery being a prerequisite to maternal recovery; a defect in the oxidation of fatty acids is found in some infants born after these pregnancies.

Diagnostic Tools for the Evaluation of Liver Disease

Accurate diagnosis and the distinction between acute and chronic disease are often dependent on appropriate selection and interpretation of a spectrum of laboratory and imaging studies.

Tests used for the initial evaluation of liver disease fall into two categories: (1) tests that indicate injury, such as release of intracellular enzymes, and (2) tests that measure, or at least reflect, actual function. Tests that reflect injury do not measure liver function and should not be called liver function tests.

The important functions of the liver include clearance, biotransformation and detoxification of potentially toxic metabolites and exogenous compounds, synthesis and export of various plasma proteins, and a critical integrative role in the intermediary metabolism of carbohydrates, amino acids, and lipids (Chapter 149). In specific diseases, some of these functions may be markedly compromised, whereas others are little affected. Liver tests must be chosen with care and interpreted within the total clinical context. In specific situations, serial determinations are often helpful to assess the course of disease or the effects of therapy.

Serum Enzyme Tests

The levels of hepatic enzymes found in plasma are a measure of hepatocyte turnover or injury. Enzymes released during normal hepatocyte turnover are believed to be the basis for normal circulating levels. Cell injury and cell death activate phospholipases that create holes in the plasma membrane, thereby increasing the release of intracellular contents.

Aminotransferases

The aminotransferases (formerly called transaminases) catalyze transfer of the α-amino group of aspartate (aspartate aminotransferase [AST]) or alanine (alanine aminotransferase [ALT]) to the α-keto group of ketoglutarate. Serum levels are normally 40 IU/L or less (see Appendix) but can exceed 1000 IU/L in acute hepatocyte injury, such as from viral infection (Chapter 151) or toxins (Chapter 153). ALT is a purely cytosolic enzyme. Distinct isoforms of AST are present in the cytosol and mitochondria. Expression of the mitochondrial isoform and its physiologic export from the hepatocyte are upregulated by ethanol. Circulating levels of AST and ALT are elevated in most hepatic diseases, and the degree of aminotransferase activity found in plasma roughly reflects the current activity of the disease process. There are, however, critical exceptions. In even the most severe cases of alcoholic hepatitis, aminotransferase levels of 200 to 300 IU/L or greater are uncommon (Chapter 156). By contrast, aminotransferase activity of 1000 IU/L or greater is often present in even mild acute viral hepatitis (Chapter 151) or shortly after acute biliary obstruction, such as during passage of a gallstone (Chapter 159). Conversely, aminotransferase levels may decline during the course of massive hepatic necrosis because the liver injury is so extensive that little enzyme activity remains (Chapter 158).

Aminotransferase levels are useful in several distinct ways. First, they provide a relatively specific screening test for hepatobiliary disease. Although AST levels may be increased with disease of other organs (notably myocardial and skeletal muscle), values equal to or greater than 10 times the upper limit of normal almost invariably indicate hepatobiliary pathology. Moreover, in the total clinical context, the source of increased aminotransferase activity is usually obvious. Aminotransferase levels are also used to monitor the activity of acute or chronic parenchymal liver disease and its response to therapy. However, levels in a given patient may correlate poorly with severity of the disease as assessed by liver biopsy, particularly in chronic hepatitis C (Chapter 152). Aminotransferases are also often normal in advanced cirrhosis (Chapter 157), in which they are of limited prognostic value. Finally, aminotransferase levels may provide diagnostic clues. AST levels 15 or more times normal are unusual in *chronic* bile duct obstruction without cholangitis, and AST levels 6 or more times normal are uncommon in alcoholic liver disease in the absence of other causes. In most liver diseases, the ratio of AST to ALT is usually 1 or less. However, ratios are typically 2 or higher in alcoholic fatty liver and alcoholic hepatitis (Chapters 156 and 157) as a result of increased synthesis and secretion of mitochondrial AST into plasma and selective loss of ALT activity because of the pyridoxine deficiency commonly seen in alcoholism. An elevated AST/ALT ratio also occurs in fulminant hepatitis related to Wilson's disease (Chapter 230).

Alkaline Phosphatase

Alkaline phosphatases are widely distributed enzymes (e.g., liver, bile ducts, intestine, bone, kidney, placenta, and leukocytes) that catalyze the release of orthophosphate from ester substrates at an alkaline pH. The normal activity level in adult serum is highly dependent on the measurement method, age, and sex. Two methods in current use have upper limits of normal in adults of 85 and 110 IU/L (see Appendix). Higher levels are normal in children and in pregnancy. Results must always be compared with the appropriate normal range. In bone, alkaline phosphatase participates in the deposition of hydroxyapatite in osteoid. In other sites, including the liver, phosphatase activity may facilitate movement of molecules across cell membranes. Serum alkaline phosphatase activity usually reflects the hepatic and bone isozymes principally, but the intestinal form may account for 20 to 60% of the total after a fatty meal. There is a substantial placental contribution to the alkaline phosphatase level late in pregnancy; the *Regan isozyme,* a variant that appears identical to the placental form, is associated with hepatoma, lung cancer, and other tumors (Chapter 206).

Elevations in serum alkaline phosphatase activity in cholestatic hepatobiliary disease result from two distinct mechanisms: increased synthesis and secretion of the enzyme and solubilization from the apical (canalicular) surface of hepatocytes and the luminal surface of biliary epithelial cells by the increased local concentrations of bile acids that occur with cholestasis. Serum alkaline phosphatase activity may also be increased in bone disorders (e.g., Paget's disease [Chapter 268], osteomalacia [Chapter 265], bone metastases [Chapters 201, 208, and 211]), during rapid bone growth in children, in the later stages of pregnancy, with chronic renal failure (Chapter 131), and occasionally, in the presence of malignancy not involving bones or the liver. The source is often obvious, but when it is not, methods such as heat stability and electrophoretic separation can distinguish hepatobiliary alkaline phosphatase from other forms. A simpler alternative is to measure serum levels of GGT or 5′-nucleotidase (5-NT), which tend to parallel levels of alkaline phosphatase in hepatobiliary disease but are not usually increased in bone disease. With a serum half-life of approximately 1 week, serum alkaline phosphatase levels may remain elevated for days to weeks after resolution of the biliary obstruction. This delay may be especially misleading when it is accompanied by prolonged direct-reacting hyperbilirubinemia because of delayed clearance of δ-bilirubin.

Modest increases in serum alkaline phosphatase activity (three times normal or less) occur in many hepatic parenchymal disorders, including hepatitis and cirrhosis. In the absence of bone disease, larger increases (3 to 10 times normal) generally indicate obstruction of bile flow. Although the highest levels usually reflect obstruction of the common bile duct, major elevations also occur with intrahepatic cholestasis and with infiltrative or mass lesions (primary or metastatic cancer, lymphoma, leukemia, sarcoidosis, or infection with *Mycobacterium avium-intracellulare*). A normal serum bilirubin level in the setting of chronic elevation of the alkaline phosphatase level can occur early in primary biliary cirrhosis (Chapter 157), but this combination also suggests localized infiltrative disease or obstruction of a portion of the biliary tree related to other localized lesions, such as stricture or tumor (Chapter 159). Alkaline phosphatase is a relatively sensitive screening test for primary or metastatic tumors of the liver, but up to a third of patients with isolated elevations in hepatobiliary alkaline phosphatase have no detectable liver or biliary disease.

Other Hepatic Enzymes

5′-NT is a plasma membrane enzyme that cleaves orthophosphate from the 5′ position on the pentose sugar of adenosine or inosine phosphate. *Leucine aminopeptidase (LAP)* is a ubiquitous cellular peptidase. The serum levels of both usually increase in cholestasis. Accordingly, their major use is to confirm whether an elevated serum alkaline phosphatase level is hepatic in origin. Both enzymes may be increased in the latter stages of a healthy pregnancy.

GGT is present in many tissues. Its serum activity increases in hepatobiliary disease but also after myocardial infarction; in neuromuscular diseases, pancreatic disease (even in the absence of biliary obstruction), pulmonary disease, and diabetes; and during the ingestion of ethanol and other inducers of microsomal enzymes. Nevertheless, because serum GGT levels are generally normal in bone disease, the enzyme may be helpful in confirming the hepatic origin of alkaline phosphatase. Measurement of GGT has been proposed as a sensitive screening test for hepatobiliary disease and for monitoring abstinence from ethanol. Because of its low specificity, many persons who test positive have no identifiable liver disease on further study. GGT offers no clear advantage over LAP or 5′-NT for identifying the source of increased serum alkaline phosphatase activity except in pregnancy. Serum GGT levels may be normal despite elevated hepatobiliary alkaline phosphatase levels in certain rare disorders, including benign recurrent intrahepatic cholestasis and progressive familial intrahepatic cholestasis types 1 and 2 (see earlier and Chapter 154).

Lactate dehydrogenase levels are often elevated in liver disease but are not usually helpful diagnostically because this enzyme is also found in most other body tissues.

Tests Based on Clearance of Metabolites and Drugs

A major function of the liver is to remove various metabolites and toxins from blood. In liver disease, clearance of such molecules may be impaired because of loss of parenchymal cells, diminished bile secretion, biliary obstruction, decreased cellular uptake or metabolism, or reduced or heterogeneous hepatic blood flow. When a metabolite is produced at a relatively constant rate (e.g., bilirubin), its serum level can be a sensitive indicator of liver function. The rate of removal of certain exogenous drugs and dyes from plasma can be similarly interpreted.

Bilirubin

The differential diagnosis of hyperbilirubinemia (see earlier) includes generalized liver disease, inherited disorders of bilirubin metabolism (e.g., Gilbert's and Crigler-Najjar syndromes), and nonhepatic conditions (e.g., hemolysis). Higher bilirubin levels correlate with a poorer prognosis in alcoholic hepatitis (Chapter 156), primary biliary cirrhosis (Chapter 157), and fulminant hepatic failure (Chapter 158).

Ammonia

Ammonia, a byproduct of amino acid metabolism, is removed from blood by the liver, converted to urea in the Krebs-Henseleit cycle, and excreted by the kidneys (Chapters 116 and 226). In the setting of portosystemic shunting or severe hepatic dysfunction (e.g., fulminant hepatic failure), ammonia levels rise. Measurements of blood ammonia are principally used to confirm a diagnosis of hepatic encephalopathy and to monitor the success of therapy, but the correlation of ammonia levels with the degree of encephalopathy is only approximate (Chapter 158). Correlations may be somewhat better if the measurement is made rapidly on an iced arterial blood sample. Elevated ammonia levels also occur when ammonia production is increased by intestinal flora (e.g., after a high-protein meal or gastrointestinal bleeding), by the kidney (in response to metabolic alkalosis or hypokalemia), or in rare genetic diseases that affect the pathway of urea synthesis (Chapter 226).

Drug Clearance

The rate of hepatic clearance of compounds such as sulfobromophthalein, lidocaine, and aminopyrine from the circulation can be measured chemically or with radiolabeled tracers. Although such tests can quantify hepatic function, they are rarely used in clinical practice.

Tests Reflecting Hepatic Synthetic Function

Coagulation Tests (Chapters 35, 178, and 181)

Prothrombin Time

The prothrombin time (PT) reflects the plasma concentrations of both extrinsic and common pathway factors, that is, factors VII, X, and V, prothrombin, and fibrinogen. A prolonged PT most often results from vitamin K deficiency, liver disease, or both. Vitamin K, a fat-soluble vitamin, is found in many foods and is also synthesized by gut bacteria (Chapter 178). Vitamin K deficiency can be caused by poor dietary intake and malabsorptive states, including the fat malabsorption that results from cholestasis, and it also occurs with antibiotic suppression of gut flora, particularly in patients who receive inadequate vitamin K replacement.

The half-lives of clotting factors are typically less than 1 day. Factor VII, which has the shortest half-life, is usually the earliest and most severely depressed during periods of defective hepatic synthesis. Because the PT is dependent on the level of factor VII, it responds rapidly with changes in hepatic synthetic function; it is useful for monitoring the course of acute liver diseases, with a significant or growing prolongation of the PT possibly indicating a poor prognosis (Chapter 151). An abnormal PT that is due solely to vitamin K deficiency generally becomes normal within 24 to 48 hours after parenteral repletion. However, if decreased synthesis of clotting factors reflects hepatocyte dysfunction, there may be little or no response to vitamin K. Finally, prolongation of the PT may also reflect disseminated intravascular coagulation (Chapter 181), which should always be considered in the context of both acute liver failure and end-stage chronic liver disease.

Partial Thromboplastin Time

This test reflects both the intrinsic and common pathway factors, that is, all of the classic clotting factors except factor VII, and is therefore complementary to the PT. It is especially useful in detecting circulating anticoagulants (Chapter 181) but adds little to the PT in evaluating hepatic synthetic function.

Albumin

Albumin is produced solely by the liver. Its plasma concentration reflects a balance between its synthetic rate of about 100 to 200 mg/kg/day and its plasma half-life of about 21 days. The synthetic rate is affected by the patient's nutritional state, thyroid and glucocorticoid hormone levels, plasma colloid osmotic pressure, exposure to hepatotoxins (e.g., alcohol), and presence of systemic disorders or liver disease (or both). Many conditions increase albumin loss and shorten its plasma half-life, including nephrotic syndrome (Chapter 122), protein-losing enteropathy (Chapter 143), severe burns (Chapter 113), exfoliative dermatitis, and major gastrointestinal bleeding (Chapter 137). In cirrhosis with ascites (Chapter 157), hypoalbuminemia indicates diminished synthesis or redistribution into ascitic fluid. Thus, a reduced serum albumin concentration can be considered an indicator of decreased hepatic synthetic function only when these factors are not involved.

Examination of Urine and Stool

Bilirubinuria always indicates a pathologic increase in plasma conjugated bilirubin levels and is frequently seen with plasma conjugated bilirubin concentrations of 2 to 3 mg/dL; it often appears before the onset of clinical jaundice and persists after the jaundice has resolved. Quantification of urobilinogen in urine or feces is of limited clinical value. By contrast, stool culture or examination for ova and parasites may provide important information in selected patients. Testing of stool for occult blood may lead to discovery of a gastrointestinal lesion related to hepatobiliary disease (e.g., tumors metastatic to the liver, ulcerative colitis associated with sclerosing cholangitis) or may explain the onset or worsening of hepatic encephalopathy.

Hematologic Tests for Liver Disease

In moderate to severe acute liver disease, mild anemia may reflect low-grade hemolysis or marrow depression; modest leukopenia, often with atypical lymphocytes, and mild thrombocytopenia are also common. Bone marrow suppression may be caused by ethanol or drugs, and aplastic anemia may sometimes complicate acute viral hepatitis (Chapters 151 and 171). Zieve's syndrome (hemolytic anemia and hypertriglyceridemia) is a rare, but well-characterized complication of alcoholic liver disease (Chapters 156 and 157). Coagulopathy frequently complicates both acute and chronic liver failure as a result of depressed hepatic synthesis of clotting factors or disseminated intravascular coagulation, or both (Chapters 180 and 181).

Chronic liver disease, especially if cholestatic, may be accompanied by target cells in the peripheral blood smear. Target cells are erythrocytes with an expanded cell membrane that reflects abnormalities in serum lipids. Spur cells (acanthocytes), most often found in advanced alcoholic cirrhosis, reflect a still greater increase in membrane cholesterol. Red blood cells, white blood cells, and platelets may all be decreased in the presence of portal hypertension related to hypersplenism (Chapters 157 and 174).

Tests for Specific Liver Diseases

Patients with findings of acute or chronic parenchymal liver disease are most likely to fall into one of three categories: viral or toxic hepatitis, including alcoholic liver disease; autoimmune liver disease; or an inherited metabolic disorder (Chapters 151 to 154, 156, and 397, 399, and 400). Specific tests for viral antigens, nucleic acids, and antibodies are available for the conventional hepatitis viruses (Chapter 151), as well as for Epstein-Barr virus (Chapter 400), cytomegalovirus (Chapter 399), and herpesviruses (Chapter 397), which are well-established but less common causes of liver disease. The major autoimmune diseases of the liver include primary biliary cirrhosis (Chapter 157), autoimmune hepatitis (Chapter 152), and various overlap syndromes. The starting point for establishing a specific diagnosis within this category is a search for specific autoantibodies in serum, including antimitochondrial antibodies against epitopes of the pyruvate dehydrogenase complex, which are virtually diagnostic of primary biliary cirrhosis (Chapter 157), and antinuclear, anti–smooth muscle, and anti–liver microsomal antibodies, which suggest a diagnosis of one of the subtypes of autoimmune hepatitis (Chapters 152, 157, and 159). The most prevalent of the hereditary metabolic disorders affecting the liver include hemochromatosis (Chapter 231), α_1-antitrypsin deficiency (Chapter 154), and Wilson's disease (Chapter 230).

Liver Biopsy

Liver biopsy can be of great help in the diagnosis of diffuse or localized parenchymal diseases, including chronic hepatitis, cirrhosis, and primary or metastatic malignancy in the liver. The value of liver biopsy in acute hepatitis or acute cholestatic jaundice may be primarily prognostic because the histologic changes in these settings may be nonspecific. However, toxic hepatitis (Chapter 153) related to certain medications may display diagnostic features. Liver biopsy for assessment of diffuse disease can be performed percutaneously after localization of the liver by physical examination or ultrasonographic visualization. When specific lesions such as tumors must be sampled, the biopsy can be guided by ultrasonographic or radiographic imaging or performed under direct visualization during laparoscopy or laparotomy. Relative or absolute contraindications include coagulopathy, high-grade biliary obstruction, biliary sepsis, ascites, and right pleural disease. Although liver biopsy remains the standard for assessment of hepatic histology in diffuse disease (Chapter 149), the procedure's invasiveness and concern for sampling error have generated interest in noninvasive measures of hepatic fibrosis. Transient elastography uses ultrasound to assess tissue stiffness as a measure of hepatic fibrosis. Commercially available biomarker panels have also been developed to provide a noninvasive assessment of hepatic fibrosis by blood testing alone. These panels typically include standard laboratory measures of hepatic injury (GGT, total bilirubin) and other serum markers (e.g., haptoglobin, hyaluronic acid, apolipoprotein A-I). However, the ability of currently available noninvasive markers to assess the extent of hepatic fibrosis across the clinically relevant histologic spectrum remains to be established.

APPROACH TO A PATIENT WITH JAUNDICE OR ABNORMAL LIVER TEST RESULTS

History, Physical Examination, and Initial Laboratory Studies

Patients with liver disease may have jaundice or other signs or symptoms, or the disease may be detected in an asymptomatic patient by the finding of abnormal liver test results during routine evaluation. Regardless of how the patient comes to medical attention, the diagnostic approach (Fig. 150–3) begins with a careful history and physical examination (Chapter 149), as well as screening laboratory studies (complete blood cell count; measurement of plasma bilirubin concentration; assay of ALT, AST, and alkaline phosphatase levels; and PT) to formulate an initial differential diagnosis. The ability to distinguish expeditiously between liver disease and extrahepatic biliary tract obstruction is the major goal of the initial evaluation, in part because the latter may call for prompt surgical intervention. Appropriate selection of second-level laboratory tests and imaging studies leads to a definitive diagnosis in most patients. Care in selecting tests, particularly imaging studies, can both maximize the likelihood of making a correct diagnosis and protect the patient from unnecessary discomfort, risk, and expense.

If the patient is asymptomatic and hepatic test results other than bilirubin are normal, hemolysis or an isolated disorder of bilirubin metabolism should be considered. If signs, symptoms, or laboratory abnormalities indicate hepatobiliary disease, certain patterns of findings can help distinguish intrinsic liver disease from biliary obstruction (Table 150–3). Pain in the right upper quadrant accompanied by a predominant increase in serum alkaline phosphatase activity suggests biliary obstruction (Chapter 159), as does a history of previous biliary surgery, right upper quadrant scars, or an abdominal mass. Fever and rigors, indicative of cholangitis, strengthen this conclusion. The incidence of gallstone disease

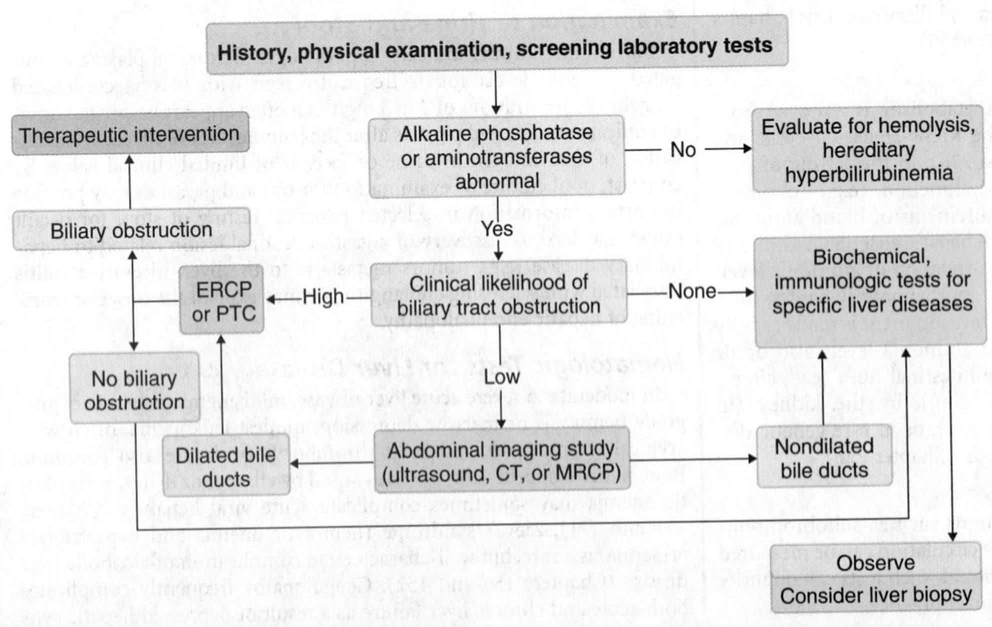

FIGURE 150–3 • Diagnostic algorithm for the evaluation of hyperbilirubinemia and other liver test abnormalities and/or signs and symptoms suggestive of liver disease. CT = computed tomography; ERCP = endoscopic retrograde cholangiopancreatography; MRCP = magnetic resonance cholangiopancreatography; PTC = percutaneous transhepatic cholangiogram. (Modified from Lidofsky SD, Scharschmidt BF: Jaundice. *In* Feldman M, Scharschmidt BF, Sleisenger MH [eds]: Gastrointestinal and Liver Disease, 6th ed. Philadelphia, Saunders, 1998, p 227.)

TABLE 150–3 OBSTRUCTIVE JAUNDICE VERSUS CHOLESTATIC LIVER DISEASE

Feature	Suggests Obstructive Jaundice	Suggests Parenchymal Liver Disease
History	Abdominal pain Fever, rigors Previous biliary surgery Older age Acholic stools	Anorexia, malaise, myalgias, suggestive of a viral prodrome Known infectious exposure Receipt of blood products, use of intravenous drugs Exposure to a known hepatotoxin Family history of jaundice
Physical examination	High fever Abdominal tenderness Palpable abdominal mass Abdominal scar	Ascites Other stigmata of liver disease (e.g., prominent abdominal veins, gynecomastia, spider angiomas, asterixis, encephalopathy, Kayser-Fleischer rings)
Laboratory studies	Predominant elevation of serum bilirubin and alkaline phosphatase Prothrombin time that is normal or normalizes with vitamin K administration Elevated serum amylase	Predominant elevation of serum aminotransferases Prolonged prothrombin time that does not correct with vitamin K administration Blood tests indicative of specific liver disease

and malignant neoplasm increases with age, although risk factors such as obesity or recent extensive diet-induced weight loss increase the risk for gallstones. Other risk factors (e.g., hepatitis exposure, transfusions, intravenous drug use, alcohol use, certain medications, and a family history of genetic diseases) and a predominant elevation in serum aminotransferase levels favor a diagnosis of parenchymal liver disease. Physical evidence of cirrhosis (e.g., spider angiomas, gynecomastia, ascites, splenomegaly) supports the diagnosis of chronic parenchymal disease.

Despite the general validity of these patterns, many exceptions exist. In particular, parenchymal disorders with prominent cholestasis may mimic biliary obstruction. Both alkaline phosphatase and GGT are usually elevated in patients with cholestasis; the combination of an elevated alkaline phosphatase and normal GGT level suggests that the alkaline phosphatase is from bone. Conversely, an isolated elevation in GGT may result from certain drugs (e.g., diphenylhydantoin) or alcohol even in the absence of liver disease. Because of the risk for life-threatening infection in the setting of unrelieved biliary tract obstruction, this possibility must always be considered and excluded if an alternative diagnosis is not definitely established.

Imaging Studies

If extrahepatic obstruction is suspected, it should be possible to determine its site and nature in virtually all patients (see Fig. 150–3). A reasonable initial step is the use of a noninvasive study such as ultrasonography (US) or computed tomography (CT) to determine whether the intrahepatic or extrahepatic biliary system (or both) is dilated, which implies mechanical obstruction. Because of its lesser expense, lack of radiation exposure, portability, and convenience, US is often the procedure of choice and is substantially better than CT for detecting gallstones. CT may be preferred when better anatomic definition and information about the general level of obstruction are desired. Still more precise resolution may be obtained with magnetic resonance cholangiopancreatography (MRCP). Each of these techniques can fail to identify dilated ducts, particularly in patients with cirrhosis or primary sclerosing cholangitis. Conversely, a modest degree of ductal dilation is common in a patient after previous cholecystectomy and does not necessarily signify current obstruction. US has the disadvantage of being highly operator dependent, whereas optimal CT imaging requires the use of intravenous contrast agents that may be nephrotoxic.

If dilated ducts are found, the biliary tree should be examined by endoscopic retrograde cholangiopancreatography (ERCP) or percutaneous transhepatic cholangiography (PTC) (Chapter 136). ERCP involves positioning an endoscope in the duodenum, inserting a catheter through the ampulla of Vater, and injecting contrast medium into the distal common bile duct or pancreatic duct, or both. PTC involves percutaneous passage of a needle through the hepatic parenchyma into a peripheral bile duct, followed by injection of contrast medium into the biliary tree through the peripheral duct. The choice of procedure is based on the suspected site of obstruction (proximal vs. distal); the presence of coagulopathy or a history of previous gastroduodenal surgery, which might preclude PTC or ERCP, respectively; the probable need for a therapeutic procedure (e.g., stent placement or endoscopic sphincterotomy); and the skills of available staff. Endoscopic ultrasound (EUS) is a complementary approach that permits internal ultrasonographic analysis of the pancreas, extrahepatic bile ducts, and regional lymph nodes and blood vessels. EUS combined with fine-needle aspiration permits tissue sampling of abnormalities in areas such as the bile ducts and pancreas, which have typically been difficult to sample percutaneously.

Selection of Imaging Tests

If the likelihood of obstruction is negligible on the basis of the clinical findings and laboratory test results, no imaging studies are required. Conversely, if obstruction is considered very likely, direct cholangiography by ERCP or PTC, which offer therapeutic as well as diagnostic capabilities, may be an appropriate initial choice. If obstruction is considered possible but not highly likely, noninvasive imaging with US, CT, or even MRCP is a reasonable first study. Individual radiology suites have different levels of expertise for these procedures, and the local radiology staff may be quite helpful in recommending the best procedure for a given patient.

APPROACH TO AN ASYMPTOMATIC PATIENT WITH ABNORMAL LIVER TEST RESULTS

An apparently healthy patient with an isolated abnormality in aminotransferase or alkaline phosphatase levels requires careful evaluation to identify any underlying disease while avoiding unneeded testing. Often, no significant disease is found despite extensive evaluation. Common causes of abnormal enzyme test results include obesity, alcohol consumption, chronic hepatitis C, steatohepatitis, bone disease, and muscle injury.

Asymptomatic Aminotransferase Elevation

Epidemiologic data suggest that up to 25% of asymptomatic adult Americans have a mild to moderate elevation in aminotransferase levels. The incidental discovery of such abnormalities is currently the most frequent means by which liver disease is first recognized. Whereas up to a third of such patients have no elevation on subsequent testing, many others prove to have steatohepatitis (Chapter 156) or chronic hepatitis C (Chapter 152) (Fig. 150–4). Further evaluation is generally indicated only in patients with persistent abnormalities. Initial screening should include a careful history of exposure to hepatotoxins (alcohol, prescription drugs, over-the-counter medications, herbs, chemicals, and occupational exposure). If the abnormal test result was an AST determination, a hepatic origin for the enzyme elevation should be confirmed with an ALT determination. If the ALT level is normal, a muscle source is likely. If the ALT level is abnormal, the patient should be screened serologically for hepatitis B and C; young women should also be screened for markers of

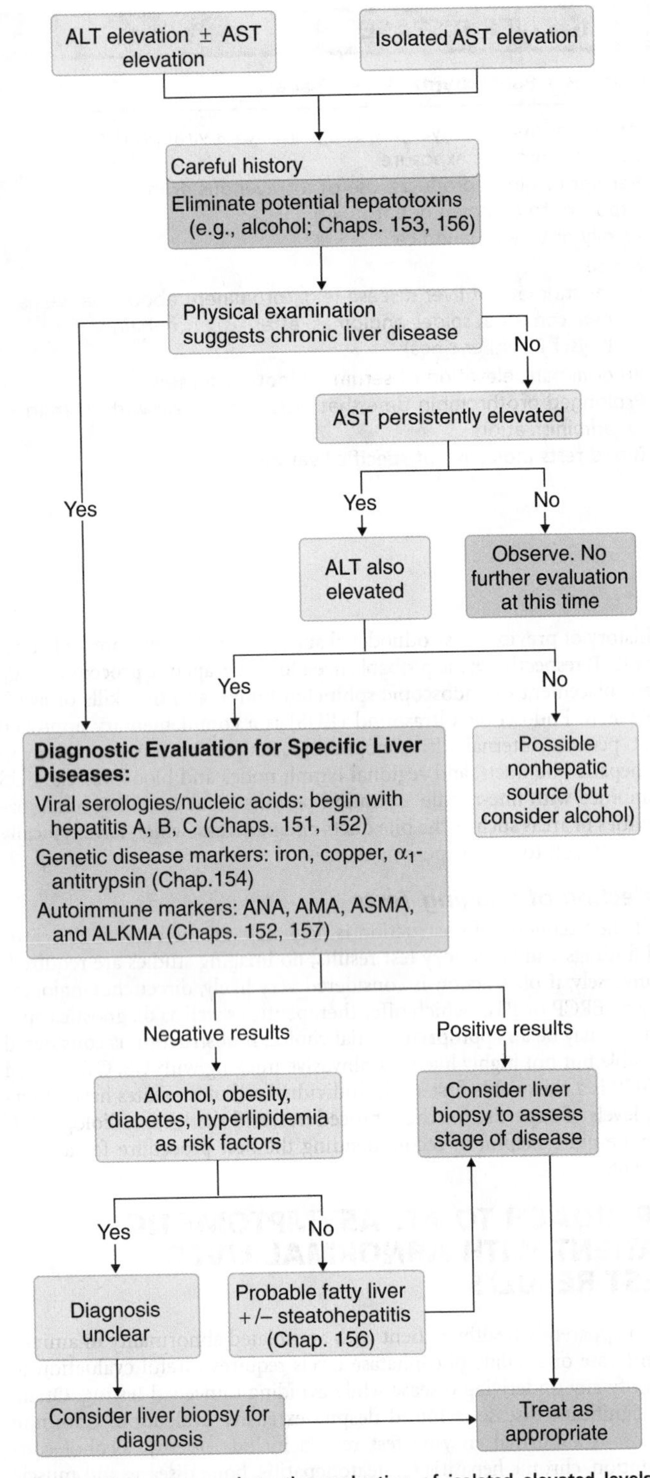

FIGURE 150–4 • Approach to the evaluation of isolated elevated levels of serum alanine aminotransferase (ALT) or aspartate aminotransferase (AST), or both, in an asymptomatic patient. ALKMA = anti-liver/kidney microsomal antibody; AMA = antimitochondrial antibody; ANA = antinuclear antibody; ASMA = anti–smooth muscle antibody.

autoimmune liver disease. Older persons should be screened for hemochromatosis with an iron and transferrin level (Chapter 231), whereas younger persons should be screened with ceruloplasmin and urine copper for Wilson's disease (Chapter 230). If these tests are negative, screening for α_1-antitrypsin deficiency is indicated (Chapters 88 and 154). Malaria (Chapter 366), schistosomiasis (Chapter 376), and other parasitic diseases should be considered in appropriate settings. A substantial fraction of patients prove to have fatty liver, with or without nonalcoholic steatonecrosis (Chapter 156). AST abnormalities caused by alcohol-induced steatosis should become normal with several weeks of abstinence. If the abnormalities persist for 6 to 12 months without an apparent cause, liver biopsy should be considered.

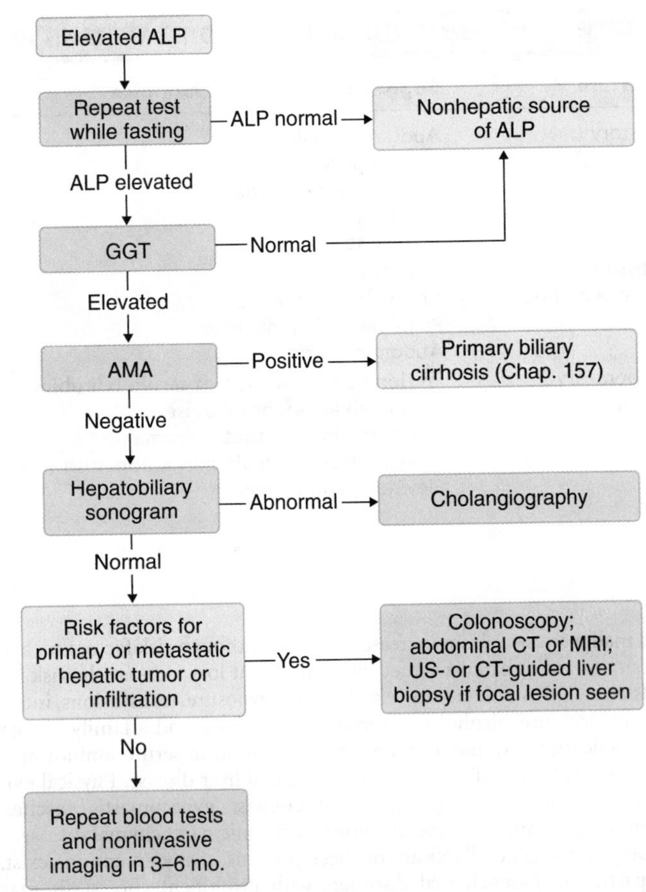

FIGURE 150–5 • Approach to an asymptomatic patient with isolated elevated levels of serum alkaline phosphatase (ALP). AMA = antimitochondrial antibody; CT = computed tomography; GGT = γ-glutamyl transpeptidase; MRI = magnetic resonance imaging; US = ultrasonography.

Asymptomatic Alkaline Phosphatase Elevation (Fig. 150–5)

Many patients with isolated elevation of the alkaline phosphatase level have nonhepatic causes such as pregnancy or bone disease. The origin of an elevated alkaline phosphatase level should be confirmed with a fasting sample because intestinal alkaline phosphatase may be elevated after a meal. A hepatic source is highly likely if the serum GGT level is also abnormal. Women should be screened with an antimitochondrial antibody test; a positive result suggests primary biliary cirrhosis (Chapter 157). A careful history (Chapter 149) identifies patients at risk for intrahepatic cholestasis related to drugs or toxins. Essentially all other patients with persistently abnormal alkaline phosphatase levels should undergo hepatobiliary sonography or other noninvasive imaging test. Demonstration of dilated intrahepatic or extrahepatic bile ducts should prompt direct visualization of the biliary tract by ERCP or PTC (Chapters 136 and 159). Evidence of an intrahepatic mass should prompt thorough evaluation for possible malignancy (Chapters 159 and 206). Because colon cancer often metastasizes to the liver, colonoscopy may be useful in appropriate cases (Chapter 203). Infiltrative diseases, including schistosomiasis and granulomatous hepatitis (Chapter 154), should be considered. Liver biopsy may be useful in patients whose abnormalities persist without an apparent cause.

SUGGESTED READINGS

Bosma PJ: Inherited disorders of bilirubin metabolism. J Hepatol 2003;38:107–117. *A thorough review.*

Giannini EG, Testa R, Savarino V: Liver enzyme alteration: A guide for clinicians. Can Med Assoc J 2005;172:367–379. *A practical approach to a common clinical problem.*

Hussain SM, Semelka RC: Hepatic imaging: Comparison of modalities. Radiol Clin North Am 2005;43:929–947. *Review of ultrasound, CT, MRI, and PET.*

Korenblat K, Berk PD: Hyperbilirubinemia in the setting of anti-viral therapy. Clin Gastroenterol Hepatol 2005;3:303–310. *Reviews a new and increasingly common diagnostic problem.*

Watkins PB, Kaplowitz N, Slattery JT, et al: Aminotransferase elevations in healthy adults receiving 4 grams of acetaminophen daily: A randomized controlled trial. JAMA 2006;296:87–93. *Emphasizes that high-dose acetaminophen use is a common cause of ALT elevations.*

151 ACUTE VIRAL HEPATITIS

Jay H. Hoofnagle

Definition

Acute viral hepatitis is a distinct clinical syndrome that can be caused by five separate, unrelated viruses. Clinically, acute viral hepatitis is marked by symptoms of malaise, nausea, poor appetite, vague abdominal pain, and jaundice; biochemically, by abrupt increases in serum bilirubin and aminotransferase levels; serologically, by the appearance of a hepatitis viral genome in the liver and serum followed by antibodies to viral antigens; and histologically, by varying degrees of hepatocellular necrosis and inflammation. Acute viral hepatitis is typically self-limited and resolves completely without residual liver injury or viral replication. A proportion of some forms of hepatitis, however, can result in persistent infection with chronic liver injury. The clinical manifestations of the five forms of viral hepatitis are quite similar, and the diseases can be distinguished only by serologic assays.

The five known causes of acute hepatitis are the hepatitis A (HAV), B (HBV), C (HCV), D or delta (HDV), and E (HEV) viruses (Table 151–1). All except HBV are RNA viruses. Hepatitis A and E are forms of *infectious* hepatitis; they are spread largely by the fecal-oral route, are associated with poor sanitary conditions, are highly contagious, occur in outbreaks as well as sporadically, and cause self-limited hepatitis only. Hepatitis B, C, and D are forms of *serum* hepatitis, are spread largely by parenteral routes and less commonly by intimate or sexual exposure, and are not highly contagious but instead occur sporadically and rarely cause outbreaks. They are capable of leading to chronic hepatitis and, ultimately, to cirrhosis and hepatocellular carcinoma. Cases of an acute viral hepatitis–like syndrome that cannot be identified as being due to a known hepatitis virus occur and are termed acute *non-A, non-B, non-C, non-D, non-E (non-A–E) hepatitis* or *acute hepatitis of unknown cause.* Despite many attempts, the viral etiology of non-A–E hepatitis remains unproven.

Epidemiology

Acute viral hepatitis is a common disease that affects 0.5 to 1% of persons in the United States each year. The annual incidence of acute hepatitis has been decreasing steadily since 1990, largely because of the use of hepatitis A and B vaccines and decreases in high-risk behaviors. In recent population-based surveys, viral causes of acute hepatitis were HAV in 37%, HBV in 45%, and HCV in 18% of cases. Hepatitis D is rare in the United States (<1% of acute cases), and most reported cases of hepatitis E have been imported. In up to 3% of cases, the cause of hepatitis cannot be ascertained even after extensive testing. In clinical practice, other nonviral forms of acute hepatitis must be considered, especially mononucleosis (Chapter 400); secondary syphilis (Chapter 340); drug-induced liver disease (Chapter 153); acute cholecystitis (or acute biliary obstruction; Chapter 159); Wilson's disease (Chapter 230); and various forms of ischemic, malignant, or toxic hepatic injury (Chapters 146 and 154 to 157).

Pathobiology

The pathogenesis of the liver injury in viral hepatitis is not well understood. None of the five agents seems to be directly cytopathic, at least at levels of replication found during typical acute and chronic hepatitis. The timing and histologic appearance of hepatocyte injury in viral hepatitis suggest that immune responses, particularly cytotoxic T-cell responses to viral antigens expressed on hepatocyte cell membranes, may be the major effectors of injury. Other pro-inflammatory cytokines, natural killer cell activity, and antibody-dependent cellular cytotoxicity may also play modulating roles in cell injury and inflammation during acute hepatitis virus infection. Recovery from hepatitis virus infection is usually accompanied by the appearance of rising titers of antibody against envelope antigens, such as anti-HAV, anti-HBs, anti-HCV-E1 and anti-HCV-E2, and anti-HEV; these antibodies may provide at least partial immunity to reinfection.

Clinical Manifestations

The course of acute hepatitis is highly variable and ranges in severity from a transient, asymptomatic infection to severe or fulminant disease. The disease may be self-limited and resolve, run a relapsing course, or lead to chronic infection. In a typical, clinically apparent course of acute resolving viral hepatitis (Fig. 151–1), the *incubation period* varies from 2 to 20 weeks, largely on the basis of the viral etiology and exposure dose. During this phase, virus becomes detectable in blood, but serum aminotransferase and bilirubin levels are normal, and antibody is not detected.

The *preicteric phase* of illness is marked by the onset of nonspecific symptoms such as fatigue, nausea, poor appetite, and vague right upper quadrant pain. Viral-specific antibody first appears during this phase. The preicteric phase typically lasts 3 to 10 days, but this phase may last longer and even constitute the entire course of illness in patients with subclinical or anicteric forms of acute hepatitis. Viral titers are generally highest at this point, and serum aminotransferase levels start to increase.

The onset of dark urine marks the *icteric phase* of illness, during which jaundice appears and symptoms of fatigue and nausea worsen. Typically, acute viral hepatitis is rarely diagnosed correctly before the onset of jaundice. If jaundice is severe, stool color lightens, and pruritus may appear. Anorexia, dysgeusia, and weight loss may also occur. Physical examination usually shows jaundice and hepatic tenderness. In more severe cases, hepatomegaly and splenomegaly may be present. Serum bilirubin levels (total and direct) rise, and aminotransferase levels are generally greater than 10 times the upper limit of normal, at least at the onset. During the icteric, symptomatic phase, levels of hepatitis virus begin to decrease in serum and liver.

The duration of clinical illness is variable; it typically lasts 1 to 3 weeks. Recovery is first manifested by return of appetite and is accompanied by resolution of the serum bilirubin and aminotransferase elevations and clearance of virus. *Convalescence* can be prolonged, however, before full energy and stamina return. Neutralizing antibodies usually appear during the icteric phase and rise to high levels during convalescence.

Complications of acute viral hepatitis include chronic infection, fulminant hepatic failure, relapsing or cholestatic hepatitis, and extrahepatic syndromes. Chronic hepatitis (Chapter 152), generally defined as at least 6 months of illness, eventuates in approximately 2 to 7% of adults

TABLE 151–1 FIVE CAUSES OF ACUTE VIRAL HEPATITIS

Hepatitis Virus	Size (nm)	Genome	Spread	Incubation Period (Days)	Fatality Rate	Chronic Rate	Antibody
A	27	RNA	Fecal-oral	15–45, mean of 25	1%	None	Anti-HAV
B	45	DNA	Parenteral Sexual	30–180, mean of 75	1%	2–7%	Anti-HBs Anti-HBc Anti-HBe
C	60	RNA	Parenteral	15–150, mean of 50	<0.1%	50–85%	Anti-HCV
D (delta)	40	RNA	Parenteral Sexual	30–150	2–10%	2–7% 50%	Anti-HDV
E	32	RNA	Fecal-oral	30–60	1%	None	Anti-HEV

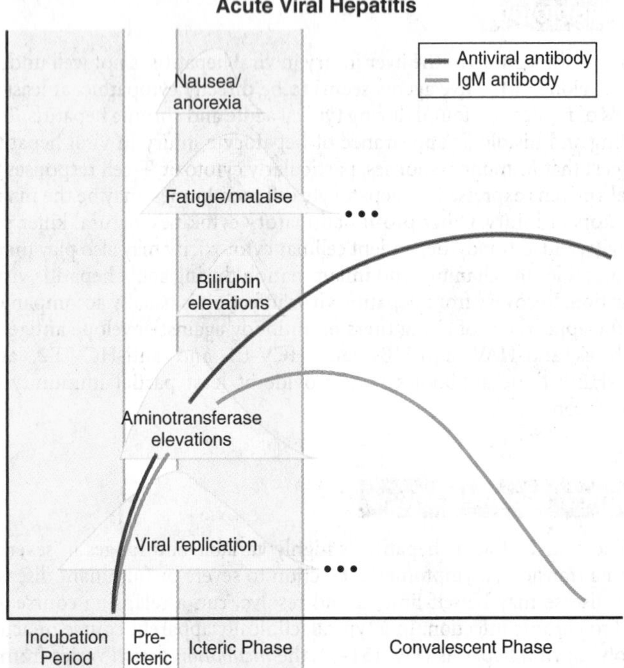

FIGURE 151–1 • Typical course of acute viral hepatitis.

with hepatitis B and 50 to 85% of adults with hepatitis C. Hepatitis B, C, and D are said to be chronic if viremia persists for more than 6 months but can be suspected if viremia persists for 3 months after the onset of symptoms.

Acute liver failure or fulminant hepatitis occurs in 1 to 2% of patients with symptomatic acute hepatitis, perhaps most commonly with hepatitis B and D and least commonly with hepatitis C. The disease is called *fulminant* if hepatic encephalopathy appears; however, the initial symptoms (changes in personality, aggressive behavior, or abnormal sleep patterns) may be subtle or misunderstood. The most reliable prognostic factor in acute hepatic failure is the degree of prolongation of the prothrombin time; other signs of poor prognosis are persistently worsening jaundice, ascites, and decreases in liver size. Serum aminotransferase levels and viral titers have little prognostic value and often decrease with worsening hepatic failure.

In a proportion of patients with acute hepatitis, a cholestatic pattern of illness consisting of prolonged and fluctuating jaundice and pruritus develops. Patients may have one or more clinical relapses and may feel relatively good despite marked jaundice. Cholestatic hepatitis is generally benign and ultimately resolves.

In 10 to 20% of patients with acute hepatitis, a serum sickness–like syndrome marked by variable combinations of rash, hives, arthralgias, and fever develops during the preicteric phase. This immune complex–like syndrome is often mistakenly attributed to other illnesses until the onset of jaundice, at which time the fever, hives, and arthralgias quickly resolve. Other extrahepatic manifestations of acute hepatitis are uncommon but include severe headaches, encephalitis, aseptic meningitis, seizures, acute ascending flaccid paralysis, nephrotic syndrome, and seronegative arthritis.

Diagnosis

Serologic tests are adequate for the diagnosis of acute viral hepatitis (see later), so liver biopsy is not recommended unless the diagnosis remains unclear and a therapeutic decision is needed. If biopsy is required, the liver histology in acute viral hepatitis is characterized by widespread parenchymal inflammation and spotty necrosis. Inflammatory cells are predominantly lymphocytes, macrophages, and histiocytes. Fibrosis is absent. Immunohistochemical stains for hepatitis antigens are generally negative during the acute disease, and there are no reliably distinctive features that separate the five viral forms of acute hepatitis from each other.

Treatment

Rx

Though not proven to be effective in prospective controlled trials, recent uncontrolled studies suggest that antiviral therapies may be effective in acute hepatitis B and C (see later). However, several recommendations are applicable to all patients with acute hepatitis. Bedrest and sensible nutrition are appropriate for patients who are symptomatic and jaundiced. Alcohol should be avoided until convalescence. Sexual contacts should be limited until partners receive prophylaxis. In hepatitis A, all household contacts should be given immune globulin, and initiation of HAV vaccination is appropriate. In hepatitis B, family members should be vaccinated, and hepatitis B immune globulin (HBIG) should also be given to recent sexual contacts. Patients in whom any signs of fulminant hepatic failure develop (prolongation of the prothrombin time, personality changes, confusion) should be considered for antiviral therapy and be evaluated quickly for possible liver transplantation (Chapter 158). The success of transplantation for severe, acute viral hepatitis often depends on early referral and careful attention to all details of clinical management in the context of an experienced team of physicians. Follow-up of acute hepatitis should be adequate to show that resolution has occurred, particularly for patients with hepatitis C. Finally and importantly, all cases of acute hepatitis should be reported to the local or state health department as soon as possible after diagnosis.

HEPATITIS A

Epidemiology

Hepatitis A is highly contagious and is spread largely by the fecal-oral route, especially when sanitary conditions are poor. Hepatitis A has been decreasing in frequency in the United States but is still an important cause of acute liver disease worldwide. Acute hepatitis A can occur in sporadic as well as epidemic forms. Investigation of the source of hepatitis A cases reveals that most are due to direct person-to-person exposure and, to a lesser extent, to direct fecal contamination of food or water. Consumption of shellfish from contaminated waterways is a well-known, but quite uncommon source of hepatitis A. Rare instances of spread of hepatitis A from blood transfusions and pooled plasma products have been described. High-risk groups for acquiring hepatitis A include travelers to developing areas of the world, children in daycare centers (and secondarily their parents), men who have sex with men, injection drug users, hemophiliacs given plasma products, and persons in institutions.

Pathobiology

HAV is a small RNA virus that belongs to the family Picornaviridae (genus Hepatovirus). The viral genome is 7.5 kilobases (kb) in length and has a single, large open reading frame that encodes a polyprotein with structural and nonstructural components. The virus replicates largely in the liver and is assembled in the hepatocyte cytoplasm as a 27-nm particle with a single RNA genome and an outer capsid protein (HAVAg). The virus is secreted into bile and, to a lesser extent, serum. The highest titers of HAV are found in stool (10^6 to 10^{10} genomes per gram) during the incubation period and early symptomatic phase of illness.

Clinical Manifestations

The clinical course of typical acute hepatitis A (Fig. 151–2) begins with an incubation period that is usually 15 to 45 days (mean of 25). Jaundice occurs in 70% of adults infected with HAV but in smaller proportions of children. Antibody to HAV (anti-HAV), which develops in all patients infected with the virus, is first detectable shortly before the onset of symptoms, then rises to high titer and persists for life. In contrast, IgM-specific anti-HAV arises early in the disease and persists for only 4 to 12 months. Severe and fulminant cases of hepatitis A can occur, particularly in the elderly and in patients with preexisting chronic liver disease. Hepatitis A is the most common cause of relapsing cholestatic hepatitis.

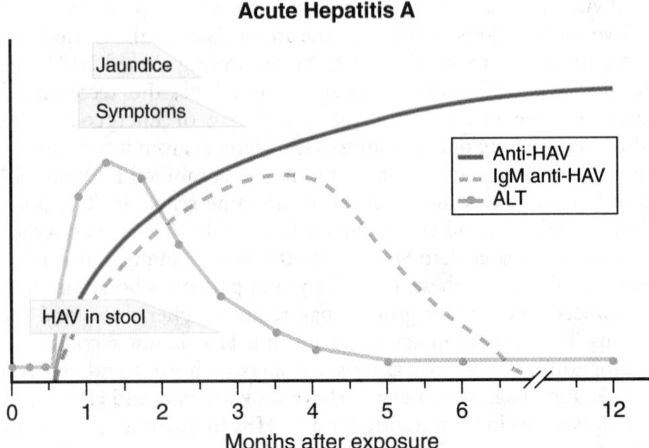

FIGURE 151–2 • Serologic course of acute hepatitis A. ALT = alanine aminotransferase; HAV = hepatitis A virus.

Diagnosis

The diagnosis of acute hepatitis A is made by detection of IgM anti-HAV in the serum of a patient with the clinical and biochemical features of acute hepatitis. Testing for total anti-HAV is not helpful in diagnosis but is a means of assessing immunity to hepatitis A.

Prevention

A safe and effective HAV vaccine is available and recommended for all children 1 year of age and older and persons at increased risk of acquiring hepatitis A, including travelers to endemic areas of the world, men who have sex with men, and illicit drug users. HAV vaccine is also recommended for all patients with chronic liver disease and recipients of pooled plasma products, such as hemophiliacs.

Two formulations of HAV vaccine are available in the United States; both consist of inactivated hepatitis A antigen purified from cell culture. Havrix (GlaxoSmithKline, Philadelphia) is recommended as two injections 6 to 12 months apart in an adult dose of 1440 enzyme-linked immunosorbent assay (ELISA) units (1.0 mL) and a pediatric (2 to 18 years of age) dose of 720 ELISA units (0.5 mL). Vaqta (Merck, West Point, PA) is recommended as two injections 6 to 18 months apart in an adult dose of 50 U (1.0 mL) and a pediatric dose (1 to 18 years) of 25 U (0.5 mL). A combination HAV and HBV vaccine (Twinrix; GlaxoSmithKline) is also available; it is recommended for adults who require vaccination against both forms of hepatitis and is given in a three-injection schedule at 0, 1, and 6 months. HAV vaccines have an excellent safety record, with serious complications occurring in less than 0.1% of recipients. Seroconversion rates after HAV vaccine are greater than 95% but are lower in patients with chronic liver disease, human immunodeficiency virus (HIV) infection, and other immune-compromised conditions. Nevertheless, neither follow-up testing for anti-HAV nor late booster inoculations are currently recommended. Prevaccination serologic testing for anti-HAV is not recommended except perhaps for adults born in endemic countries and for older (>50 years of age) U.S.-born adults.

Postexposure prophylaxis with immune globulin still is recommended for household and intimate contacts of persons with acute hepatitis A. The dose is 2 mL in adults and 0.02 mL/kg in children, given intramuscularly within 2 weeks of exposure. Concurrent HAV vaccination is appropriate.

Treatment

No specific therapies have been shown to shorten or ameliorate the course of illness in hepatitis A. An important element of management should be prophylaxis for contacts. Persons with fulminant hepatitis should be referred early for possible liver transplantation (Chapter 158).

Prognosis

Acute hepatitis A is invariably a self-limited infection. The virus can persist for months, but it does not lead to a chronic infection, chronic hepatitis, or cirrhosis.

HEPATITIS B

Epidemiology

Hepatitis B is spread predominantly by the parenteral route or by intimate personal contact. It is endemic in many areas of the world, such as Southeast Asia, China, Micronesia, and sub-Saharan Africa. Lesser rates occur in the Indian subcontinent and Middle East. In the United States, hepatitis B is the most common cause of acute hepatitis, and chronic infection affects approximately 0.5% of the population. Investigations of the source of hepatitis B reveal that most adult cases are due to sexual or parenteral contact. Hepatitis B is common in injection drug users, heterosexuals with multiple sexual partners, and men who have sex with men. Blood transfusion and plasma products are now rarely infectious for hepatitis B because of the institution of routine screening of blood donations for hepatitis B surface antigen (HBsAg) and antibody to hepatitis B core antigen (HBcAg), anti-HBc. Maternal-infant spread of hepatitis B is another important mode of transmission not only in endemic areas of the world but also in the United States among immigrants from these endemic areas. Routine screening of pregnant women and prophylaxis of newborns are now recommended. Intrafamilial spread of hepatitis B can also occur, although the mode of spread in this situation is not well defined. Unfortunately, lack of attention to universal precautions and aseptic technique, especially the cleaning of shared medical devices, remains an important root cause of small outbreaks and sporadic cases of acute hepatitis B.

Pathobiology

HBV is a double-shelled, enveloped DNA virus belonging to the family Hepadnaviridae (genus Orthohepadnavirus). The viral genome consists of partially double-stranded DNA, is 3.2 kb in length, and possesses four partially overlapping open reading frames that encode the genes for HBsAg (*S* gene), HBcAg (*C* gene), HBV polymerase (*P* gene), and a small protein that seems to have transactivating functions (*X* gene, HBxAg). The *S* gene has three start codons and is capable of producing three different sizes of HBsAg (small, medium, and large *S*). The *C* gene has two start codons and can produce two antigenically distinct products: HBcAg, which is retained in hepatocytes until assembled and incorporated into HBV virions, and hepatitis B e antigen (HBeAg), which is secreted into serum as a small soluble protein. The virus infects only humans and higher apes and replicates predominantly in hepatocytes and perhaps to a lesser extent in stem cells in the pancreas, bone marrow, and spleen. During acute and chronic infection, patients with hepatitis B have large amounts of HBsAg in serum, most in the form of incomplete 20-nm virus-like spherical and tubular particles. The intact virion is a double-shelled particle with an envelope of HBsAg, an inner nucleocapsid of HBcAg, and an active polymerase enzyme that is linked to a single molecule of double-stranded HBV DNA. Persons who produce large amounts of HBV in serum also typically produce HBeAg, thus making HBeAg a surrogate marker for high levels of viral replication.

Clinical Manifestations

The typical course of acute, self-limited hepatitis B (Fig. 151–3) begins with an incubation period of 30 to 150 days (mean of 75). During the incubation period, HBsAg, HBeAg, and HBV DNA become detectable in serum and rise to high titer, with the virus reaching titers of 10^8 to 10^{11} virions/mL. By the onset of symptoms, anti-HBc arises and serum aminotransferase levels are elevated. Jaundice appears in a third of adults with hepatitis B and lesser percentages of children. Generally, HBV DNA and HBeAg begin to fall at the onset of illness and may be undetectable at the time of peak clinical illness. HBsAg becomes undetectable and anti-HBs arises during recovery, several weeks to months after loss of HBsAg. Anti-HBs is a long-lasting antibody and is associated with immunity.

Diagnosis

The diagnosis of acute hepatitis B can be made on the basis of finding HBsAg in the serum of a patient with the clinical and biochemical features of acute hepatitis. HBsAg may also be present as a result of chronic hepatitis B or the carrier state, however, and a patient with acute hepatitis and HBsAg in serum may actually have chronic hepatitis and a superimposed form of acute injury, such as acute hepatitis A or D or drug-induced liver disease. For this reason, testing for IgM anti-HBc is helpful because this antibody arises early and is lost within 6 to 12 months of the onset of illness. Testing for HBeAg, anti-HBe, HBV DNA, and anti-HBs is not generally helpful in the diagnosis of hepatitis B but may be valuable in assessing prognosis. Persons who remain HBV DNA or HBeAg positive (or both) 6 weeks after the onset of symptoms are likely to be developing chronic hepatitis B. Loss of HBeAg or HBV DNA is a favorable serologic finding. Similarly, loss of HBsAg plus the development of anti-HBs denotes recovery.

Hepatitis B is also an important cause of fulminant hepatitis. Factors associated with severe outcomes of acute hepatitis B include advanced age, female sex, and perhaps some strains of virus. There are variants of HBV that lack the ability to produce HBeAg because of a mutation in the precore region of the viral genome. These precore or HBeAg-negative mutants are associated with atypical forms of acute and chronic hepatitis B. Several clusters of severe or fulminant hepatitis B have been associated with infection with the HBeAg-negative forms of virus.

Prevention

Vaccination against HBV is recommended for all newborns, children, and adolescents, as well as adults at risk for acquiring HBV, including health care and public safety workers with exposure to blood, injection drug users, men who have sex with men, persons at risk for sexually transmitted infections, persons traveling internationally to endemic regions, and individuals with close contact with patients who have chronic hepatitis B. Two formulations of HBV vaccine are available in the United States; both are made from recombinant techniques using cloned HBV *S* gene expressed in *Saccharomyces cerevisiae.* For adults, the recommended regimen is three injections of 1.0 mL (20 µg of Energix-B [GlaxoSmithKline] or 10 µg of Recombivax HB [Merck]) given intramuscularly in the deltoid muscle at 0, 1, and 6 months. A combined HAV and HBV vaccine (GlaxoSmithKline) is given at the same schedule. The dose in newborns, children, and adolescents is less (Table 151–2). The seroconversion rate is greater than 90% in healthy, young adults, but it may be lower in smokers, the obese, the elderly, and patients who are immunocompromised; these latter groups may require higher doses and more injections. Prevaccination screening for anti-HBs is not recommended except for adults in high-risk groups (e.g., persons born in endemic countries, injection drug users, men who have sex with men, and HIV-infected persons). Postvaccination testing for anti-HBs to document seroconversion is not recommended routinely except for persons whose subsequent clinical management depends on knowledge of their immune status, particularly health care and public safety workers. At present, booster doses are not recommended but they may be appropriate for high-risk individuals if titers of anti-HBs fall below what is considered protective (10 IU/mL).

Postexposure prophylaxis with HBIG is recommended at birth for infants born to infected mothers and for patients with percutaneous exposure to a patient with hepatitis B. A single dose of HBIG (0.5 mL in newborns of infected mothers, 0.06 mL/kg in other settings and in adults) should be given as soon as possible after exposure, and HBV vaccination should be started immediately. HBIG is unlikely to provide benefit if the time since exposure is longer than 14 days; vaccine alone can be used in these circumstances. For patients with sexual or household contact with a patient who has chronic hepatitis B, vaccination alone is appropriate; HBIG is recommended in addition for sexual exposure to a patient with acute hepatitis B.

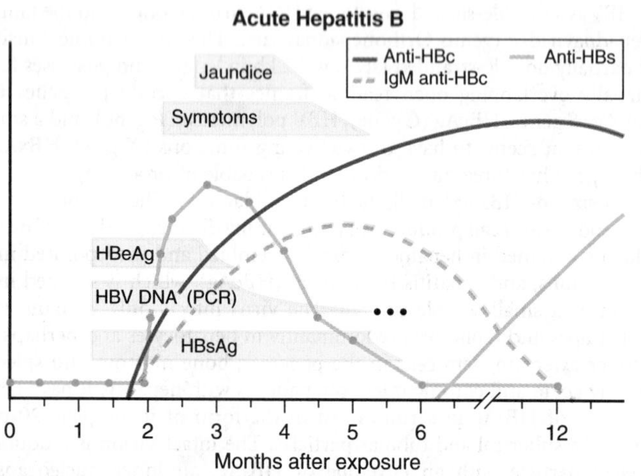

FIGURE 151–3 • Serologic course of acute hepatitis B. HBc = hepatitis B core; HBeAg = hepatitis B e antigen; HBs = hepatitis B surface; HBsAg = hepatitis B surface antigen; HBV = hepatitis B virus; PCR = polymerase chain reaction.

Treatment

The use of antiviral therapy for acute hepatitis B is controversial. Interferon alfa and lamivudine are established therapies for chronic hepatitis B (Chapter 152), but they have not been adequately evaluated for acute infection. In a small study, interferon alfa did not decrease the rate of chronicity or speed recovery. Uncontrolled observations using lamivudine in patients with fulminant and severe hepatitis B, however, suggest that this therapy may ameliorate the course of infection. Because of the safety of lamivudine therapy and the unpredictable and potentially serious outcome of severe cases of acute hepatitis B, therapy with lamivudine (100 mg daily until the disease has resolved and HBsAg has become negative) is prudent for patients with symptoms or signs of fulminant liver disease (rising prothrombin time, severe jaundice), particularly if high levels of HBV DNA are present. Management of acute hepatitis B should also focus on avoidance of further hepatic injury and prophylaxis of contacts. The patient should be monitored by repeat testing for HBsAg and alanine aminotransferase levels 3 to 6 months later to determine whether chronic hepatitis B has developed (Chapter 152).

TABLE 151–2 HEPATITIS B VIRUS VACCINATION RECOMMENDATIONS

Group	No. Doses	Schedule (mo)	Recombivax HB	Energix-B
Infants	3	0, 1, and 6	5 µg (0.5 mL)	10 µg (0.5 mL)
Infants born to HBsAg-positive mothers	3	0*, 1, and 6	5 µg (0.5 mL)	10 µg (0.5 mL)
Children (1–10 yr)	3	0, 1, and 6	5 µg (0.5 mL)	10 µg (0.5 mL)
Adolescents (11–19 yr)†	3	0, 1, and 6	5 µg (0.5 mL)	10 µg (1 mL)
Adults	3	0, 1, and 6	10 µg (1 mL)	20 µg (1 mL)
Adults on dialysis‡	4	0, 1, 2, and 6	40 µg (1 mL)	40 µg (2 mL)

*Hepatitis B immune globulin and initial vaccination should be given within 12 hours of birth.
†Adolescents aged 11 to 15 years can receive an alternative regimen of two doses of 10 µg (1 mL) at 0 and 4 to 6 months.
‡Recombivax HB is available in a dialysis formulation of 40 µg/mL; Energix-B must be given as two 1-mL injections to achieve a dose of 40 µg.
HBsAg = hepatitis B surface antigen.

Prognosis

Chronic hepatitis B (Chapter 152) develops in 2 to 7% of adults infected with HBV, more commonly in men and in immunosuppressed individuals. The risk for chronic infection also correlates with age: it occurs in 90% of newborns infected with HBV, in approximately 30% of infants, but in less than 10% of adults. Chronic hepatitis B is still the third or fourth most common cause of cirrhosis (Chapter 157) in the United States and is an important cause of liver cancer (Chapter 206).

HEPATITIS C

Epidemiology

Hepatitis C is spread predominantly by the parenteral route. At highest risk are injection drug users and persons with multiple parenteral exposures. Sexual transmission of hepatitis C occurs but is not common. Prospective follow-up of spouses and sexual partners of patients with chronic hepatitis C shows the risk for sexual transmission to be low (<1% per year of exposure). Maternal-infant spread occurs in approximately 5% of cases, usually to infants whose mothers have high levels of HCV RNA in serum and a protracted delivery or early rupture of membranes. Other potential sources of HCV are needlestick accidents and either contamination or inadequate sterilization of reusable needles and syringes. Unfortunately, outbreaks of hepatitis C in health care settings continue to be identified from reuse of syringes and other failures in appropriate aseptic technique. Since the introduction of routine screening of blood for anti-HCV, post-transfusion hepatitis C has become rare. Inactivation procedures performed on plasma products have made transmission of HCV from clotting factor concentrates uncommon. There remain, however, many persons with chronic hepatitis C who were infected with this virus by these means in the past. Current studies of acute hepatitis C indicate that more than 60% of cases are attributable to injection drug use; 15 to 20% to sexual exposure (usually involving multiple sexual partners); and only a small proportion to maternal-infant spread, needlestick accidents, and iatrogenic causes. Approximately 10% of cases are not associated with any history of potential exposure and remain unexplained.

Pathobiology

HCV is an RNA virus that belongs to the family Flaviviridae (genus Hepacivirus). HCV was originally identified by molecular techniques, and the virus has not been well visualized. HCV probably circulates as a double-shelled enveloped virus, 50 to 60 nm in diameter. The genome is a positively stranded RNA molecule; it is approximately 9.6 kb in length and contains a single open reading frame that encodes a large polyprotein that is post-translationally modified into three structural and several nonstructural polypeptides. The structural proteins include two highly variable envelope antigens (E1 and E2) and a relatively conserved nucleocapsid protein (C). HCV replicates largely in the liver and is detectable in serum in titers of 10^5 to 10^7 virions/mL during acute and chronic infection.

Clinical Manifestations

The clinical course of acute hepatitis C (Fig. 151–4) begins with an incubation period that ranges from 15 to 120 days (mean of 50). During the incubation period, often within 1 to 2 weeks of exposure, HCV RNA can be detected by sensitive assays such as reverse transcriptase polymerase chain reaction (PCR). HCV RNA persists until well into the clinical course of disease. Antibody to HCV (anti-HCV) arises late in the course of acute hepatitis C and may not be present at the time of onset of symptoms and serum aminotransferase elevations. If the hepatitis is self-limited, HCV RNA soon becomes undetectable in serum; in this situation, titers of anti-HCV are generally modest and may eventually fall to undetectable levels as well.

Diagnosis

Diagnosis of acute hepatitis C is generally based on detection of anti-HCV in serum in a patient with the clinical and biochemical features of acute hepatitis. In some patients, however, detectable levels of anti-HCV

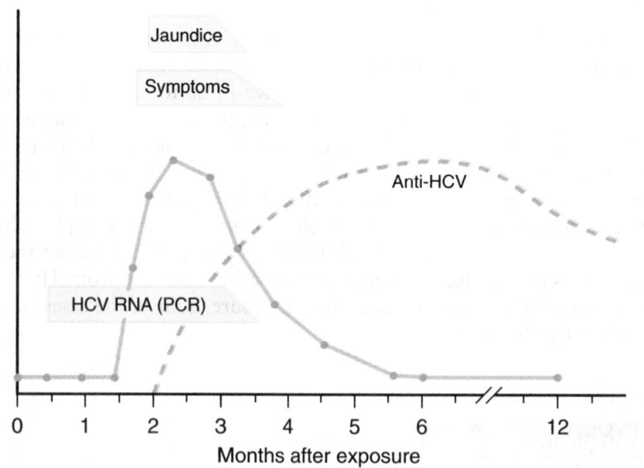

FIGURE 151–4 • Serologic course of acute hepatitis C. HCV = hepatitis C virus; PCR = polymerase chain reaction.

do not develop until weeks or months after the onset of illness, so retesting for anti-HCV during convalescence or direct tests for HCV RNA are necessary to exclude the diagnosis of acute hepatitis C in a patient who tests negative for all serologic markers. Several commercial tests for HCV RNA are now licensed and are reliable in detecting HCV RNA at levels greater than 100 copies/mL. Tests that quantify the HCV RNA level are also available, but measuring viral levels is not clinically useful in diagnosis or monitoring of acute hepatitis C.

Prevention

At present, there are no means of prevention of hepatitis C other than avoidance of high-risk behaviors and appropriate use of universal precautions. Injection drug use is currently the most common cause of newly acquired cases of hepatitis C. In this regard, needle exchange programs and education regarding the risks of drug use, including intranasal cocaine, and the risk of transmission from shared injection equipment are important.

Accidental needlestick exposure is perhaps the most frequent issue in prevention of transmission. At present, neither immune globulin nor preemptive therapy with antiviral agents or interferon is recommended in this situation. Monitoring by means of aminotransferase levels, HCV RNA, and anti-HCV testing (at baseline and 1 and 6 months after exposure) is appropriate. This approach allows for early intervention and treatment.

Treatment

Rx

Therapy with peginterferon alfa and ribavirin has been shown to be beneficial in chronic hepatitis C (Chapter 152); such therapy leads to sustained clearance of virus and resolution of disease in slightly more than 50% of cases. The role of therapy during acute infection is still unresolved. Because 50 to 85% of patients with acute disease progress to chronic infection, the issue of early therapy often arises. Several studies have now documented that more than 90% of patients with acute hepatitis C treated with peginterferon with or without ribavirin for 24 weeks experience resolution of disease and sustained loss of HCV RNA.  Importantly, initiation of therapy can be delayed for 2 to 3 months after the onset of infection without a decrease in the high response rate. For these reasons, patients with acute hepatitis C should be treated only if HCV RNA remains detectable for 2 to 3 months after the onset of infection. An appropriate regimen is either peginterferon alfa-2a (180 μg) or alfa-2b (1.5 μg/kg) once weekly for 24 weeks in combination with ribavirin (1000 mg/day if body weight <70 and 1200 mg if >70 kg). The possible roles of HCV genotyping in guiding therapy and limiting therapy to 12 to 16 weeks in patients who become HCV RNA negative within 4 weeks of starting therapy are currently under investigation (Chapter 152).

Prognosis

The major complication of acute hepatitis C is the development of chronic hepatitis. The clinical course depicted in Figure 151–4 is not typical because hepatitis C does not resolve in 50 to 85% of cases but rather progresses to chronic infection (Chapter 152). In this situation, HCV RNA remains detectable, and aminotransferase levels generally remain elevated, though often in a fluctuating pattern. In some instances, aminotransferase levels become normal despite persistence of viremia. Other complications include the development of immune complex phenomena and cryoglobulinemia, although these complications are more typical of chronic disease. Fulminant hepatitis resulting from HCV is rare; in several large surveys of acute liver failure, none of the cases could be attributed to HCV.

HEPATITIS D

Epidemiology

Hepatitis D is linked to hepatitis B, and consequently its epidemiology is similar. HDV can be spread by the parenteral route and sexually. Persons at greatest risk are chronic carriers of hepatitis B and persons who have repeated parenteral exposures. In the United States and western Europe, delta hepatitis is most common in injection drug users and, before routine screening of blood donations, recipients of blood products, including persons with hemophilia and thalassemia. Delta hepatitis is endemic in the Amazon basin and central Africa and is common in some European and Mediterranean countries, including southern Italy, Greece, and eastern Europe.

Pathobiology

The hepatitis delta virus is a unique RNA virus that requires HBV for replication. The viral genome is a short, 1.7-kb circular single-stranded molecule of RNA that has a single open reading frame and a highly conserved nontranslated region that resembles the self-replicating element of viroids. The single open reading frame encodes delta antigen, and RNA editing can vary the size of the molecule to produce either a small (195 amino acids) or large (214 amino acids) delta antigen. The small delta antigen promotes the replication of HDV RNA; the large delta antigen promotes viral assembly and secretion into serum as the mature 36-nm delta viral particle.

Clinical Manifestations

Delta hepatitis occurs in two clinical patterns, termed *coinfection* and *superinfection*. Delta coinfection is the simultaneous occurrence of acute HDV and acute HBV infection. It resembles acute hepatitis B but may manifest a second elevation in aminotransferase levels associated with the period of delta virus replication. The diagnosis of acute delta coinfection can be made in a patient with clinical features of acute hepatitis who has HBsAg, anti-HDV, and IgM anti-HBc in serum. Immunoassays for anti-HDV are commercially available and reliable, although antibody may appear late during the illness. In patients suspected of having delta hepatitis, repeat testing for anti-HDV during convalescence is appropriate.

Diagnosis

Acute delta superinfection is the occurrence of acute HDV infection in a person with chronic hepatitis B or the HBsAg carrier state. The diagnosis of acute delta superinfection can be made in a patient with clinical features of acute hepatitis who has HBsAg and anti-HDV but no IgM anti-HBc in serum. Superinfection with HDV is more frequent than coinfection and is far more likely to lead to chronic delta hepatitis. Other tests that are helpful in making the diagnosis of ongoing HDV infection are serum HDV RNA (detectable by PCR) and HDV antigen (detectable by immunoblot); both of these tests are currently research assays and not standardized. Delta antigen can also be detected readily in liver biopsy specimens with immunohistochemical stains.

Prevention

Delta hepatitis can be prevented by preventing hepatitis B. The severity of delta hepatitis is another compelling rationale for routine hepatitis B vaccination in areas of the world where delta hepatitis is endemic. There are no means of prevention of delta hepatitis in a person who is already an HBsAg carrier; in this situation, avoidance of further exposure is important.

Treatment

No specific therapies are available for acute delta hepatitis. Lamivudine and other anti-HBV agents are ineffective against HDV replication. Most cases of acute coinfection resolve; patients with superinfection should be treated when it is clear that chronic delta hepatitis has supervened.

Prognosis

Delta hepatitis tends to be more severe than hepatitis B alone and is more likely to lead to fulminant hepatitis and to cause severe chronic hepatitis and ultimately cirrhosis.

HEPATITIS E

Epidemiology

Hepatitis E is responsible for epidemic and endemic forms of non-A, non-B hepatitis that occur in lesser developed areas of the world. Large outbreaks have been described from India, Pakistan, China, northern and central Africa, and Central America. In studies from India and Egypt, hepatitis E has accounted for a high proportion of cases of sporadic acute hepatitis. In the United States and western Europe, hepatitis E is rare, with most cases being imported or caused by zoonotic spread from swine or rats that harbor a similar virus. HEV is spread by the fecal-oral route, and most cases can be traced to exposure to contaminated water under poor hygienic conditions. Hepatitis E seems to be less contagious than hepatitis A, the other form of infectious hepatitis, and secondary cases are rare.

Pathobiology

HEV is a small nonenveloped, single-stranded RNA virus that is currently unclassified. The viral genome is 7.5 kb in length and encodes three open reading frames, the first (ORF1) for the nonstructural proteins responsible for viral replication, the second (ORF2) for the capsid protein (HEV antigen), and the third (ORF3) for a short protein of unknown function. The virus and HEV antigen can be detected in hepatocytes during acute infection. The highest levels of virus are detectable in stool during the incubation period of the disease. Viruses similar to HEV are found in other species, and strains found in domesticated swine may be infectious in humans.

Clinical Manifestations

The clinical course of hepatitis E resembles that of other forms of hepatitis. The incubation period is 15 to 60 days (mean of 35). The disease is frequently cholestatic, with prominence of bilirubin and alkaline phosphatase elevations. Hepatitis E also tends to be more severe than other forms of epidemic jaundice, with a fatality rate of 1 to 2% and a particularly high rate of acute liver failure in pregnant women. HEV virions and antigen can be detected in stool and liver during the incubation period and early symptomatic phase, but these tests are not practical means for diagnosis. ELISAs for IgM and IgG antibody to HEV (anti-HEV) have been developed and are reactive in at least 90% of patients at the onset of clinical illness. These tests are neither generally available nor standardized, however. In addition, anti-HEV is found in 1 to 2% of the normal population, which may represent resolved subclinical cases of hepatitis E acquired during travel or as a result of exposure to livestock or other infected animals.

Diagnosis

The diagnosis of hepatitis E should be considered in a patient with acute hepatitis who has recently traveled to an endemic area, particularly if tests for other forms of hepatitis are nonreactive. The finding of anti-HEV, particularly of the IgM subclass, is sufficient to make the diagnosis in this situation. Hepatitis E is rare in the United States and Western world, however, so testing for anti-HEV is rarely necessary.

Prevention and Treatment

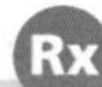

There are no known means of prevention or treatment of hepatitis E. Immune globulin, even when prepared from the plasma of populations with a high rate of hepatitis E, does not seem to be effective. No specific means of treatment have been evaluated.

Travelers to areas of the world (particularly pregnant women) where hepatitis E is endemic should be cautioned regarding drinking water and uncooked food. Recombinant vaccines against HEV have been developed and shown to be effective in animal models of hepatitis E. Efficacy trials of an HEV vaccine are now under way in endemic areas.

DIFFERENTIAL DIAGNOSIS

The diagnostic approach to a patient with the clinical features of acute hepatitis (Table 151–3) begins with a careful history for risk factors and possible exposure; for medication use, including herbal and over-the-counter drugs; and for alcohol use. The onset and progression of symptoms may give clues to other causes of liver disease, such as alcohol or gallstones. Biochemical laboratory tests, including serum bilirubin, alanine and aspartate aminotransferase, alkaline phosphatase, lactate dehydrogenase, albumin, complete blood cell counts, and prothrombin time, are valuable in defining whether the clinical picture is typical of acute hepatitis (high aminotransferases, normal or modest elevations in alkaline phosphatase and lactate dehydrogenase) or resembles that of obstructive jaundice or alcoholic liver disease. In atypical cases, testing for antinuclear antibodies to evaluate for autoimmune hepatitis and a Venereal Disease Research Laboratory test to exclude secondary syphilis (Chapter 340) are needed. The presence of fever and atypical lymphocytosis should suggest mononucleosis (Chapter 400). The presence of hemolysis should suggest Wilson's disease (Chapter 230). Serologic tests that are helpful in all cases of acute hepatitis include IgM anti-HAV, HBsAg or IgM anti-HBc (or both), and anti-HCV. Follow-up testing for anti-HDV or anti-HCV can be useful in making the diagnosis of delta hepatitis (in a patient with HBsAg) or hepatitis C (in a patient initially testing negative for all viral antibodies).

TABLE 151–3 SEROLOGIC DIAGNOSIS OF ACUTE HEPATITIS

Diagnosis	Screening Assays	Supplemental Assays
Hepatitis A	IgM anti-HAV	None needed
Hepatitis B	HBsAg, IgM anti-HBc	HBeAg, anti-HBe, HBV DNA
Hepatitis C	Anti-HCV by EIA	HCV RNA by PCR; anti-HCV by Immunoblot
Hepatitis D	HBsAg	Anti-HDV
Hepatitis E	History	Anti-HEV
Mononucleosis	History, white blood cell differential counts	Heterophile antibody
Drug-induced hepatitis	History	

EIA = enzyme immunoassay; PCR = polymerase chain reaction.

HEPATITIS NON-A–E

Epidemiology and Pathobiology

Cases of acute hepatitis that appear to be viral in etiology but cannot be attributed to any known virus are called *hepatitis non-A–E.* Various candidate viruses have been reported in association with this disease, including paramyxoviruses, togaviruses, and flaviviruses (GBV-C, hepatitis G, and TT virus), but none has been clearly linked to this disease. In serologic surveys of cases of acute hepatitis in Western countries, 2 to 20% of cases cannot be attributed to any of the five known hepatitis viruses. Animal inoculation and tissue culture studies in search of the agent of hepatitis non-A–E have been unrevealing.

Clinical Manifestations

The clinical features of non-A–E hepatitis are similar to the features of known forms of acute hepatitis. Most cases of non-A–E hepatitis have no clear source of exposure. Cases are rare after blood transfusion and are no more common than in control, nontransfused subjects. The absence of typical risk factors for viral hepatitis suggests that some cases of non-A–E hepatitis may be due to nonviral causes, such as an autoimmune process, environmental exposure, or drugs.

Diagnosis

Non-A–E hepatitis is a diagnosis of exclusion that is usually made on the basis of occurrence of acute hepatitis in a patient without anti-HAV, HBsAg, anti-HBc, HCV RNA, or anti-HCV and without any other known cause of acute hepatic injury. Testing of serum during convalescence is helpful in excluding hepatitis C with delayed seroconversion. Tests for anti-HEV are not generally necessary unless there is a history of travel to an endemic area or exposure to swine. The most important diagnoses to exclude are infectious mononucleosis and the nonviral causes of an acute hepatitis–like syndrome, most particularly drugs, over-the-counter medications, herbal preparations, toxins, alcoholic liver injury, acute cholecystitis, autoimmune hepatitis, and Wilson's disease. A careful history of exposure to drugs and toxins, abdominal ultrasonography to exclude gallstone disease, and tests for antinuclear antibodies and ceruloplasmin (and urine copper if necessary) are helpful in fully defining a case of non-A–E hepatitis.

Treatment

There are no means of either treatment or prevention of non-A–E hepatitis. A viral etiology of this syndrome is being investigated, particularly in the situation of acute liver failure and aplastic anemia.

Prognosis

The syndrome of non-A–E hepatitis has been particularly associated with the complications of acute liver failure and aplastic anemia. Hepatitis non-A–E is a more common cause of fulminant hepatic failure than hepatitis A or B combined is and often accounts for 30 to 40% of cases. Chronic hepatitis develops in approximately a third of patients with non-A–E hepatitis, and cirrhosis ultimately develops in a small percentage.

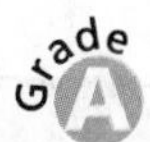

1. Jeckel E, Cornberg M, Wedemeyer H, et al: Treatment of acute hepatitis C with interferon alfa-2b. N Engl J Med 2001;345:1452–1457.

SUGGESTED READINGS

Ganem D, Prince AM: Hepatitis B virus infection—natural history and clinical consequences. N Engl J Med 2004;350:1118–1129. *A comprehensive review.*

Hoofnagle JH: Course and outcome of hepatitis C. Hepatology 2002;36(5 Suppl. 1):S21–S29. *Emphasizes good short-term outcome but a higher rate of chronic manifestations.*

Mast EE, Margolis HS, Fiore AE, et al: A comprehensive immunization strategy to eliminate transmission of hepatitis B virus infection in the United States:

Recommendations of the Advisory Committee on Immunization Practices (ACIP) part 1: Immunization of infants, children, and adolescents. MMWR Recomm Rep 2005;54(RR-16);1–31. *Current status of hepatitis B in the United States and recommendations for and prevention of acute and chronic infection.*

Prevention of hepatitis A through active or passive immunization: Recommendations of the Advisory Committee on Immunization Practices (ACIP). MMWR Recomm Rep 2006;55(RR07):1–23. *Recommendations for hepatitis A vaccination and use of immune globulin and rationale for each.*

Shrestha M, Scott R, Joshi D, et al: Safety and efficacy of a recombinant hepatitis E vaccine. N Engl J Med 2007;356:895–903. *In a high-risk population, the rHEV vaccine was effective.*

Vinholt Schiodt F, Davern TJ, Obaid Shakil A, et al: Viral hepatitis–related acute liver failure. Am J Gastroenterol 2003;98:448–453. *Viral hepatitis now accounts for only an eighth of all cases of acute liver failure in the United States; hepatitis B carries a worse prognosis than hepatitis A does.*

Wasley A, Samandari T, Bell BP: Incidence of hepatitis A in the United States in the era of vaccination. JAMA 2005;294:194–201. *Documents the decline in hepatitis A in the United States as a result of HAV vaccination strategies.*

152 CHRONIC HEPATITIS

Jay H. Hoofnagle

Definition

Chronic hepatitis comprises several diseases that are marked by chronic necro-inflammatory injury to the liver. The disease is defined as chronic if there is evidence of ongoing injury for 6 months or longer. The various forms of chronic hepatitis have similar clinical manifestations and outcomes, and each can lead to cirrhosis and end-stage liver disease (Table 152–1). The most common forms are chronic hepatitis B and C and autoimmune hepatitis. Drug-induced (Chapter 153) or metabolic (Chapter 154) liver diseases, alcoholic steatohepatitis (Chapter 156), and nonalcoholic steatohepatitis (Chapter 156) can also cause chronic necro-inflammatory lesions of the liver. Despite extensive testing, some cases cannot be attributed to any known cause.

Epidemiology

The incidence and prevalence of chronic hepatitis in the general U.S. population have not been well defined. In population-based surveys, 2.3% of Americans have elevations in serum alanine aminotransferase (ALT) levels, 0.2% are seropositive for hepatitis B surface antigen (HBsAg), and 1.6% are reactive for antibody to hepatitis C virus (anti-HCV). Not all ALT elevations are due to chronic hepatitis, however, and not all HBsAg-positive or anti-HCV–positive individuals have active liver disease. A fair estimate is that chronic hepatitis affects 2% of the population, but these diseases tend to occur mostly in high-risk groups rather than the general population. For hepatitis B, high-risk groups include recent immigrants from endemic areas of the world (Africa, eastern Europe, Southeast Asia), persons with multiple sexual partners, men who have sex with men, injection drug users, recipients of blood or blood products before 1987, hemophiliacs, oncology and renal dialysis patients, and health care workers. For hepatitis C, high-risk groups include recipients of blood or blood products before 1992, hemophiliacs who received blood products before 1986, injection drug users, renal dialysis patients, health care workers, and persons with multiple sexual partners. Chronic hepatitis B and C probably cause 10,000 to 12,000 deaths yearly, and about another 2000 patients with these diseases undergo liver transplantation annually for end-stage liver failure.

TABLE 152–1 MAJOR CAUSES OF CHRONIC HEPATITIS

Chronic hepatitis B
Chronic hepatitis D
Chronic hepatitis C
Autoimmune hepatitis
Drug-induced chronic hepatitis
Wilson's disease
Cryptogenic hepatitis (non-A–E hepatitis)

Clinical Manifestations

The clinical symptoms of chronic hepatitis are typically nonspecific, intermittent, and mild; a large proportion of patients have no symptoms of liver disease. The most common symptom is fatigue, which may be intermittent. Some patients have sleep disorders or difficulty concentrating. Right upper quadrant pain, if present, is usually mild, intermittent, and aching in character. In many cases, the diagnosis of chronic hepatitis is made in a person without any symptoms after liver test abnormalities are identified when blood is drawn for a routine health evaluation, during assessment for an unrelated health problem, or at the time of voluntary blood donation (Chapter 150). Symptoms of advanced disease or an acute exacerbation include nausea, poor appetite, weight loss, muscle weakness, itching, dark urine, and jaundice. When cirrhosis is present, weakness, weight loss, abdominal swelling, edema, ready bruisability, gastrointestinal bleeding, and hepatic encephalopathy with mental confusion may arise.

The clinical signs of liver disease in patients with chronic hepatitis are also usually minimal. The most common finding is liver tenderness. In patients with severe or advanced disease, other findings may include a firm liver or enlargement of the spleen, spider angiomas (see Fig. 134–4), and palmar erythema (see Fig. 149–5). When cirrhosis is present, signs may include muscle wasting, ascites (see Fig. 149–3), edema, skin excoriations (see Fig. 149–2) or bruises, and hepatic fetor.

Diagnosis

Although symptoms and signs are not particularly useful in identifying chronic hepatitis, biochemical and hematologic blood test results are reliable. Most typical are elevations in ALT and aspartate aminotransferase (AST) levels with little or no elevation in the alkaline phosphatase level. The elevations are usually in the range of one to five times the upper limit of normal, and the ALT level is generally higher than the AST level, unless cirrhosis is present. Serum aminotransferase levels can be normal when the disease is mild or inactive but can also be markedly elevated in the range typical of acute hepatitis (10 to 25 times the upper limit of normal) during acute exacerbations. Although there may be major discrepancies between the height of the liver enzyme elevations and histologic estimates of activity as shown by liver biopsy, monitoring of these values over time generally provides a reasonable estimate of the severity of disease and likelihood of progression.

In general, alkaline phosphatase and γ-glutamyl transpeptidase elevations are minimal in chronic hepatitis, unless cirrhosis is present. Creatine kinase and lactate dehydrogenase levels are normal. Serum bilirubin and albumin levels and the prothrombin time are normal in patients with chronic hepatitis, unless the disease is severe or advanced. Any elevation in serum direct bilirubin or decrease in albumin should be considered evidence of serious disease activity or injury. Serum immunoglobulin levels are mildly elevated or normal in chronic viral hepatitis but may be strikingly elevated in chronic autoimmune hepatitis. Blood counts are normal in chronic hepatitis, unless cirrhosis or portal hypertension is present with associated decreases in the white blood cell and platelet counts. Serial determinations of platelet counts may provide the earliest clinical evidence of progression of chronic hepatitis to advanced fibrosis and cirrhosis. Blood tests results that suggest the presence of advanced fibrosis are low platelet counts (below 160,000), AST levels higher than ALT levels, elevations in serum bilirubin, decreases in serum albumin, prolongation of the prothrombin time, elevations in α-fetoprotein levels, and the presence of rheumatoid factor or high globulin levels.

Imaging

Imaging with ultrasound can be performed to define hepatic texture and size, determine the presence of hepatic masses, assess the gallbladder and intrahepatic bile ducts, define the size of the spleen, and determine the presence of collateral vessels and portal venous flow. Computed tomography and magnetic resonance imaging of the liver are less helpful unless a mass or other abnormality is found by ultrasound. More recently, hepatic elastography has been used to assess hepatic stiffness as a marker for liver fibrosis. Though still experimental, preliminary results suggest that elastography may be a reliable, noninvasive means of detecting worsening of hepatic fibrosis and cirrhosis.

Histologic Analysis

Hepatic histologic characteristics include spotty hepatocellular necrosis, chronic inflammatory cell infiltration in the portal areas, and variable degrees of fibrosis. The hepatocellular necrosis is typically eosinophilic degeneration or ballooning degeneration. The necrosis is spotty throughout the parenchyma, but activity is usually greater in the periportal area; the pattern is termed piecemeal necrosis or interface hepatitis. The hepatocellular necrosis seems to be mediated largely by apoptosis in association with cytotoxic lymphocytes. Chronic inflammatory cells ($CD4^+$ and $CD8^+$ lymphocytes and plasma cells, histiocytes, and macrophages) are found in the areas of necrosis and in sinusoids but most prominently in the portal areas. Fibrosis occurs insidiously during the course of chronic hepatitis and typically begins in the periportal regions. Ultimately, bands of fibrosis can link up adjacent portal areas or portal and central areas (bridging fibrosis), distort the hepatic architecture, and lead to cirrhosis and portal hypertension.

Hepatic histologic analysis is useful for grading the severity of necroinflammation and for staging the degree of fibrosis in chronic hepatitis and is generally obtained to confirm the diagnosis made through the patient's history, physical examination, and blood test results. Hepatic histologic evaluation may help confirm the diagnosis of autoimmune hepatitis and clarify the role of α_1-antitrypsin deficiency or Wilson's disease. Most importantly, liver histologic analysis can exclude other diagnoses that can mimic chronic hepatitis clinically or cause similar patterns of elevated liver enzyme levels, including fatty liver, alcoholic liver disease, steatohepatitis (Chapter 156), drug-induced liver disease (Chapter 153), sclerosing cholangitis (Chapter 159), iron overload (Chapter 231), and veno-occlusive disease.

The grade of chronic hepatitis refers to the activity of the disease in terms of necrosis and inflammation; the grade of disease fluctuates and is reversible. The stage of disease refers to how advanced the fibrosis process is and whether cirrhosis is present; stages of disease have previously been considered irreversible, but it is now clear that successful treatment of chronic hepatitis caused by hepatitis B, hepatitis C, or autoimmune processes can result in reversal of hepatic fibrosis. The most commonly used system of grading and staging is the histology activity index, in which the combined scores for periportal necrosis and inflammation (0 to 10), lobular necrosis and inflammation (0 to 4), and portal inflammation (0 to 4) define the grade or activity of disease. Disease stage is defined by scores between 0 and 4 for fibrosis, with 4 indicating cirrhosis. A modification of the histology activity index system scores fibrosis from 0 to 6 (Ishak score), with stages 3 and 4 indicating bridging hepatic fibrosis and stages 5 and 6 representing incomplete and established cirrhosis. The Metavir system, which is used widely in Europe, grades activity on a 4-point scale (A0, A1, A2, A3) and fibrosis (F0, F1, F2, F3, F4) on a 5-point scale.

Differential Diagnosis

Chronic hepatitis can be caused by several diseases that are similar clinically but respond differently to therapy and must be managed individually. Patients with suspected chronic hepatitis should be evaluated carefully for fatty liver, alcohol- (Chapter 156) or drug-induced (Chapter 153) liver disease, and metabolic liver diseases (Chapter 154), not only because these conditions mimic disorders that cause chronic hepatitis but also because they can coexist with the disorders that cause chronic hepatitis. After taking a history designed to elucidate risk factors for viral hepatitis, specific and appropriate serologic tests (Table 152–2) can be used to make the diagnosis. Liver biopsy with special stains can be performed to confirm the diagnosis, assess the activity and severity of injury, and stage the disease.

Treatment

Rx

A treatment strategy should arise from careful consideration of the diagnosis and the grade and stage of disease (see later). With advances currently being made in antiviral and immunomodulatory therapeutics, it is anticipated that the considerable progress made in treating these diseases will continue in the future.

CHRONIC HEPATITIS B

Pathobiology

Chronic hepatitis B is caused by infection with the hepatitis B virus (HBV), a DNA virus belonging to the family Hepadnaviridae (Chapter 151). The diagnosis of chronic hepatitis B is generally suspected on the basis of HBsAg in the serum of a patient with chronic hepatitis and confirmed by the finding of HBV DNA in serum or hepatitis B core antigen (HBcAg) in the liver. Most patients with chronic hepatitis B also have hepatitis B e antigen (HBeAg) in serum as a result of high levels of viral replication. Some patients have active liver disease with HBsAg and high levels of HBV DNA but no HBeAg in serum. These patients usually harbor a mutant HBV that replicates efficiently and is pathogenic but does not produce HBeAg.

Liver injury and the pathogenesis of chronic hepatitis B are believed to be immunologically mediated, so the severity and course of disease do not correlate well with the level of virus in serum or with antigen expression in the liver. Antigen-specific cytotoxic T cells are believed to mediate the cellular injury in hepatitis B and account for ultimate viral clearance. Specific cytokines produced by cytotoxic and other T cells also have

TABLE 152–2 DIFFERENTIAL DIAGNOSIS OF CHRONIC HEPATITIS

Diagnosis	Screening Tests	Confirmatory Tests (Serum or Liver)	Comments
Chronic hepatitis B	HBsAg	HBV DNA, HBeAg, or HBcAg in liver	
Chronic hepatitis C	Anti-HCV	HCV RNA (using PCR)	Immunoblot for anti-HCV can be used to confirm antibody reactivity
Chronic hepatitis D	Anti-HDV	HDV RNA or HDV antigen in the liver	
Autoimmune hepatitis	ANA (anti-LKM1)	Exclusion of other causes and patterns of clinical disease	Suggested by raised IgG levels and by response to corticosteroid therapy
Drug-induced liver disease	History	Rechallenge, if necessary, is considered safe	Medications most suspected include isoniazid, NSAIDs, methyldopa, nitrofurantoin
Wilson's disease	Ceruloplasmin	Urine and hepatic copper concentration	Suggested by hemolysis or severe chronic hepatitis in a child or adolescent
Cryptogenic	Exclusion of other causes		Major differential is with autoimmune hepatitis and drug-induced liver disease

ANA = antinuclear antibody; anti-LKM1 = liver-kidney microsomal 1 antibody; HBcAg = hepatitis B core antigen; HBeAg = hepatitis B e antigen; HBsAg = hepatitis B surface antigen; HBV = hepatitis B virus; HCV = hepatitis C virus; HDV = hepatitis D virus; IgG = immunoglobulin G; NSAIDs = nonsteroidal anti-inflammatory drugs.

antiviral effects on hepatocytes that contribute to viral clearance without cell death. The progression of acute to chronic hepatitis B is attributed to lack of a vigorous cytotoxic T-cell response to hepatitis B antigens. Similarly, spontaneous seroconversion from HBeAg to anti-HBe during chronic hepatitis B may be immunologically mediated, as suggested from the transient flare of disease that often immediately precedes clearance of HBeAg. Some HBV strains may be more pathogenic and more likely to lead to chronic infection because they are less immunogenic or more resistant to T-cell attack. Seroconversion may be due to spontaneous mutations in the predominant HBV species to forms that produce HBsAg without HBeAg (e-negative mutant) and that are less efficient in replication and less pathogenic.

Epidemiology

There are at least six different genotypes of HBV, the most common being A, B, C, and D. The genotypes of HBV have distinct geographic variation in frequency and, in the United States, vary in prevalence by risk group. Genotype A is found largely in Western countries and is the most common genotype identified in men who have sex with men. Genotype D is most frequent in Mediterranean and eastern European countries and is common in injection drug users in the United States. Genotypes B and C are the major genotypes of China and Southeast Asia. Genotyping tests using line probe hybridization assays are available and generally accurate. There may be minor differences in the natural history of hepatitis B related to genotypes, with genotype C being associated with a greater likelihood of cirrhosis and hepatocellular carcinoma. More importantly, there may be genotypic differences in response to interferon-based therapy.

Clinical Manifestations

In the typical course of hepatitis B, HBsAg, HBeAg, and HBV DNA become detectable in serum during the incubation period and gradually rise in titer (Fig. 152–1). Symptoms appear 30 to 152 days after exposure (mean incubation period, 75 days), usually at the time of peak viral levels. Symptoms are mild and nonspecific, and jaundice is rare. The appearance of jaundice during the course of acute infection is highly predictive of eventual recovery.

In chronic hepatitis, serum ALT levels decrease after the acute phase of infection but persist at levels between 1 and 10 times the upper limit of normal. HBsAg, HBeAg, and HBV DNA persist, generally at high levels; the finding of HBeAg more than 2 months after the onset of symptoms indicates evolution to chronicity. Levels of HBV DNA are generally in the range of 10^7 to 10^{11} genome copies/mL.

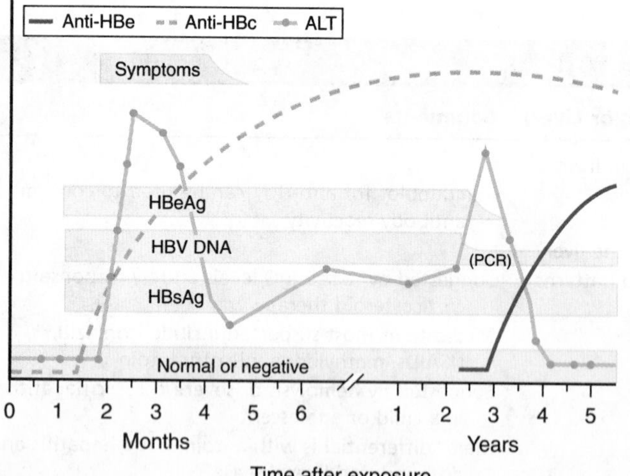

FIGURE 152–1 • Typical serologic course of chronic hepatitis B. ALT = alanine aminotransferase; HBc = hepatitis B core antigen; HBeAg, HBe = hepatitis B e antigen; HBsAg = hepatitis B surface antigen; HBV = hepatitis B virus; PCR = polymerase chain reaction.

The subsequent course of chronic hepatitis B is highly variable. Some patients continue to have active viral replication with high levels of HBV DNA and HBeAg in serum and progressive liver injury; cirrhosis and end-stage liver disease may soon develop. In other patients, the disease is more indolent and insidiously leads to cirrhosis in decades. In a large proportion of patients, however, the outcome is more benign; the disease eventually goes into remission spontaneously, symptoms (if present) resolve, serum aminotransferase levels decrease to the normal range, and liver histologic characteristics improve. Remission is often preceded by a transient flare of disease and can be precipitous; it coincides with a major decrease in the level of HBV DNA and seroconversion from HBeAg to anti-HBe. HBsAg persists in serum at levels lower than before this seroconversion, and HBV DNA can be detected at low levels (generally $<10^5$ genome copies/mL) if sensitive techniques such as polymerase chain reaction (PCR) are used.

With the decrease in viral levels and loss of HBeAg, the disease seems to go into remission, thus suggesting that there has been a transition from chronic hepatitis B to an "inactive" carrier state with no symptoms, normal serum aminotransferase levels, and inactive liver disease indicated by biopsy findings. Loss of HBeAg is not always followed by permanent resolution of disease, however. In some patients, reactivation occurs with reappearance of HBeAg; in others, an HBV mutant develops and replicates efficiently but cannot produce HBeAg. These patients with HBeAg-negative chronic hepatitis B can have severe disease and often experience multiple clinical relapses.

Extrahepatic manifestations of chronic hepatitis B include mucocutaneous vasculitis, glomerulonephritis, and polyarteritis nodosa. The glomerulonephritis of hepatitis B occurs more commonly in children than adults and is usually characterized by nephrotic syndrome with little decrease in renal function. Polyarteritis nodosa (Chapter 291) occurs primarily in adults and is marked by a sudden, severe onset of hypertension, renal disease, and systemic vasculitis with arteritis in vessels of the kidney, gallbladder, intestine, or brain.

Diagnosis

There are two general forms of chronic hepatitis B: typical, HBeAg-positive chronic hepatitis B, in which there is HBsAg, HBeAg, and high levels of HBV DNA in serum, and the less common HBeAg-negative form, in which there is HBsAg and anti-HBe without HBeAg in serum. Patients with HBeAg-negative chronic hepatitis B often have moderate or fluctuating levels of HBV DNA in serum. These forms of chronic hepatitis B should be distinguished from the inactive (which has been inappropriately referred to as healthy) HBsAg carrier state, in which HBsAg persists in serum without active liver disease and minimal or no detectable viral replication (Table 152–3); in the inactive carrier state, HBV DNA is not detectable in serum with conventional hybridization assays sensitive to levels of 10^6 viral copies/mL. Testing for HBV DNA by the more sensitive PCR assays generally shows low levels of viral genome (almost always $<10^4$ viral copies/mL) in the serum of patients with the inactive carrier state.

Treatment

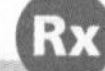

Nonspecific recommendations for the management of chronic hepatitis B include vaccination of all household and sexual contacts. Patients should be counseled on the modes of transmission of hepatitis B and means of prevention of spread. Vaccination against hepatitis A is also recommended. Patients with hepatitis B should be advised to abstain from alcohol and to avoid all but the most necessary use of immunosuppressive medications. Severe flares of hepatitis B and even deaths have followed short courses of corticosteroids or cancer chemotherapy. If corticosteroids or chemotherapy is required for other conditions, prophylaxis against reactivation should be given (see later).

Medical Therapy

The conventional treatment of chronic hepatitis B is a course of standard or pegylated interferon alfa (peginterferon). Because of its

TABLE 152–3 THREE FORMS OF CHRONIC HEPATITIS B VIRUS INFECTION

Pattern	HBsAg	HBeAg	HBV DNA* (Titer)	HBcAg in Liver	Chronic Hepatitis
Typical chronic hepatitis B	Positive	Positive	Positive, 10^7–10^{11}	Positive (nuclear)	Active
HBeAg-negative chronic hepatitis B	Positive	Negative	Positive, 10^5–10^9	Positive (cytoplasmic)	Active (relapsing)
Inactive HBsAg carrier state	Positive	Negative	Positive, 10^1–10^5	Negative	Inactive

*Positive or negative result by hybridization techniques (sensitive to a titer of 10^6 genome-equivalents/mL). Titers less than 10^6 genome-equivalents/mL generally require polymerase chain reaction assays for detection.
HBcAg = hepatitis B core antigen; HBeAg = hepatitis B e antigen; HBsAg = hepatitis B surface antigen; HBV = hepatitis B virus.

TABLE 152–4 RESPONSE RATES TO 48 WEEKS OF THERAPY FOR CHRONIC HEPATITIS B*

Antiviral Agent	Loss of HBsAg	Loss of HBeAg	Loss of HBV DNA (by PCR)	Normal ALT Levels	Improved Histology
HBeAg-POSITIVE CHRONIC HEPATITIS B					
Peginterferon†	3.0%	34%	14%	41%	38%
Lamivudine	1.1%	20%	36%	60%	62%
Adefovir	<1%	24%	21%	48%	53%
Entecavir	1.7%	22%	67%	68%	72%
Placebo	<1%	11%	<1%	16%	25%
HBeAg-NEGATIVE CHRONIC HEPATITIS B					
Peginterferon†	4.0%	NA	19%	59%	48%
Lamivudine	<1%	NA	72%	71%	61%
Adefovir	<1%	NA	51%	72%	64%
Entecavir	<1%	NA	90%	78%	70%
Placebo	<1%	NA	<1%	29%	33%

*Summarized from six recent randomized controlled trials.
†Results were measured at the end of 48 weeks of therapy and while still on treatment, with the exception of results for peginterferon, which were measured 24 weeks after stopping treatment.
ALT = alanine aminotransferase; HBeAg = hepatitis B e antigen; HBsAg = hepatitis B surface antigen; HBV = hepatitis B virus; NA = not applicable; PCR = polymerase chain reaction.

Rx

ease of administration and better efficacy, peginterferon has largely replaced standard interferon. Peginterferon is given by subcutaneous injection in doses of 180 μg (peginterferon alfa-2a) or 1.5 μg/kg body weight (alfa-2b) weekly for 24 to 48 weeks, a regimen that results in clearance of HBeAg in about a third and clearance of HBsAg in up to 5% of patients (Table 152–4). The combination of other antiviral agents with peginterferon does not appear to increase the sustained response rate.

Therapy with peginterferon is indicated for patients who have chronic hepatitis B with HBsAg, HBeAg, and HBV DNA in serum and elevations in serum aminotransferase levels. Therapy with peginterferon is contraindicated in patients with advanced cirrhosis, in solid organ transplant recipients, in immunosuppressed patients, and in patients with other serious major illnesses. Peginterferon therapy is not recommended for patients with normal or near-normal serum aminotransferase levels (even if high levels of HBV DNA are present), largely because it is usually ineffective in this situation. The major factors associated with a higher likelihood of response to peginterferon are initial high levels of serum aminotransferase (elevated more than five-fold), lower levels of HBV DNA (less than 10^7 genome copies/mL), HBV genotypes A and B (vs. C and D), and absence of immunosuppression. The potential benefits and risks of interferon therapy should be discussed thoroughly before treatment. The major side effects of interferon include fatigue, muscle aches, fever, depression, and irritability; uncommon severe side effects include suicide, psychosis, renal and cardiac failure, bacterial infections, and induction of autoimmune disorders (see the discussion of treatment of chronic hepatitis C).

Rx

With initiation of treatment, levels of HBV DNA usually decrease. In patients with a beneficial response (as defined by loss of HBeAg with treatment), the disease may flare transiently with elevations in serum ALT to levels two to three times baseline after 2 to 3 months of therapy, coinciding with a precipitous fall in HBV DNA levels and loss of HBeAg. Serum aminotransferase levels decrease to normal, and a proportion of patients lose HBsAg, often many months to several years after loss of HBeAg. Reactivation of disease with rises in aminotransferase levels and reappearance of HBeAg and high levels of HBV DNA occurs rarely. Nonresponders to peginterferon therapy, who remain HBeAg positive, may have improvements in serum aminotransferase levels and disease activity, but over time these improvements are generally lost. Such patients should be considered for maintenance therapy with oral antiviral agents.

Several oral nucleoside and nucleotide analogues, including lamivudine, adefovir dipivoxil, tenofovir disoproxil fumarate, entecavir, clevudine (L-FMAU), emtricitabine (FTC), and telbivudine (L-thymidine), have been shown to have potent effects against HBV in vitro and in vivo. Four of these agents (lamivudine, telbivudine, adefovir, and entecavir) are currently approved for use in the United States (see Table 152–4), and several others are likely to be approved in the near future.

Lamivudine is a negative enantiomer of a 3′ sulfated cytidine analogue and has major activity against HBV and human immunodeficiency virus (HIV). Lamivudine is recommended at a dose of 100 mg/day for 1 year. Initiation of therapy is followed rapidly by marked falls in HBV DNA by 4 to 6 $\log_{10}$ units to levels less than 10^5 viral copies/mL within the first 3 to 6 months of starting therapy.

Rx

Prolonged therapy (≥1 year) is associated with loss of HBeAg in up to a third of patients. With loss of HBeAg and the development of anti-HBe, lamivudine therapy can be stopped; relapses are uncommon when seroconversion occurs. Most patients remain HBeAg positive, however, despite improvements in HBV DNA and aminotransferase levels. In patients with HBeAg-negative chronic hepatitis B, lamivudine is associated with a higher rate of response, with improvements in ALT levels and liver histology in two thirds of patients. However, relapse is almost invariable in HBeAg-negative chronic hepatitis B once lamivudine therapy is discontinued. Lamivudine is well tolerated; in randomized trials, side effects were no more common with lamivudine than with placebo. The lack of side effects with lamivudine and the improvements in HBV DNA and serum aminotransferase levels that occur with therapy support the use of lamivudine as maintenance, long-term therapy for hepatitis B with the goal of long-term suppression of HBV replication. [1] Instances of long-term biochemical and histologic improvement have been reported in chronic hepatitis B with continuous lamivudine therapy. However, long-term therapy is associated with development of viral resistance in a high proportion of patients. Lamivudine resistance is marked by a rise in HBV DNA toward baseline levels, followed by elevations in serum aminotransferase levels. Most patients with viral resistance harbor an HBV mutant with amino acid changes in the conserved region of the polymerase gene (*YMDD* mutates to either *YIDD* or *YVDD*). Typically, patients with *YMDD* mutations have lower levels of HBV DNA and serum aminotransferase levels than were present before therapy, thus suggesting that the mutant HBV is less efficient in replication and less pathogenic than the wild-type virus. Lamivudine resistance develops in 20 to 25% of patients in each year of therapy, so after 4 to 5 years of treatment, more than two thirds of patients have HBV mutants.

Telbivudine, the L-enantiomer of deoxythymidine, is a potent and specific inhibitor of HBV replication in vitro and in vivo. In preliminary studies in patients with HBeAg-positive chronic hepatitis B, a 1-year course of telbivudine resulted in a 10^6 $\log_{10}$ decrease in HBV DNA levels and loss of HBeAg in 28% of patients. Adefovir dipivoxil is a nucleotide analogue (bis-POM-PMEA) that acts as a prodrug of adefovir with enhanced oral availability. Adefovir has activity in vitro and in vivo against both wild-type and lamivudine-resistant HBV strains. Monotherapy with adefovir dipivoxil (given in a dose of 10 mg daily) leads to marked decreases in HBV DNA levels (by 3 to 4 $\log_{10}$ units) and subsequent improvements in serum aminotransferase levels and hepatic histology in approximately half of patients (see Table 152–4). Even higher rates of response are reported in HBeAg-negative chronic hepatitis B. However, discontinuation of therapy is usually followed by relapse and return of disease activity, particularly in HBeAg-negative patients. Long-term trials of adefovir dipivoxil therapy are now under way; studies of treatment for up to 4 years show that clinical and genetic evidence of viral resistance occurs slowly (0% at 1, 3% at 2, 11% at 3, and 18% at 4 years). [2,3] The safety of 10 mg of adefovir daily has been shown in randomized trials in which side effects were no more common with adefovir than with placebo. Higher doses of adefovir are associated with the development of renal toxicity (renal tubular acidosis) after 6 to 12 months of treatment. For these reasons, the dose of adefovir should be kept to 10 mg daily or less, and patients should be monitored for increases in serum creatinine; any elevation of greater than 0.5 mg/dL above baseline levels should lead to an immediate modification of the dose or temporary withholding of therapy. The safety of adefovir dipivoxil in patients with preexisting renal disease has not been shown. Thus, adefovir dipivoxil monotherapy is a practical approach to long-term therapy for both HBeAg-positive and HBeAg-negative disease and can be used in cases of lamivudine resistance.

Entecavir, a recently approved oral nucleoside analogue therapy for chronic hepatitis B, appears to be the most potent. Entecavir is a guanosine analogue with activity against wild-type HBV in cell culture, but somewhat less activity against lamivudine-resistant strains. Studies in humans at doses of 0.5 mg daily show that therapy is followed by a rapid decrease in HBV DNA levels averaging 10^5 to 10^7 $\log_{10}$ declines within 6 to 12 months. Entecavir is well tolerated and associated with a high rate of response as assessed by loss of detectable HBV DNA, normalization of aminotransferase levels, and improvement in liver histology (see Table 152–4). Unfortunately, entecavir, like lamivudine and adefovir, leads to loss of HBeAg in only 20 to 25% of patients, and relapse is frequent once treatment with the drug is stopped. [4] Thus, long-term therapy is required for continued suppression of HBV and improvement in liver disease. Importantly, entecavir has been associated with a very low rate of antiviral resistance: in preliminary reports, no resistance was detected after 1 to 2 years of treatment except in patients with preexisting lamivudine resistance. Although entecavir is effective against lamivudine-resistant HBV strains, higher doses (1 mg daily) are recommended and response rates are lower than in patients without resistance. These findings lend support to the recommendation to avoid the use of long-term lamivudine monotherapy in HBeAg-positive chronic hepatitis B. The safety and continued efficacy of long-term entecavir therapy are still under evaluation.

There are no clear guidelines for the use of antiviral therapy for hepatitis B. Peginterferon is effective in approximately a third of patients with HBeAg-positive chronic hepatitis B, but it is expensive and poorly tolerated. Lamivudine, telbivudine, adefovir, and entecavir are easy to administer and have minimal side effects, but they are less likely to lead to sustained loss of HBeAg or HBsAg (see Table 152–4). Furthermore, the decision of whether to stop or continue therapy after 1 to 2 years is often difficult. Withdrawal of therapy with nucleoside or nucleotide analogues usually results in a rapid return of HBV DNA levels toward baseline, and this return of viral replication can be associated with a transient exacerbation of disease, which in some instances can be severe or even fatal and ultimately reverse any benefit of years of treatment. Management of lamivudine resistance is particularly challenging; it is often appropriate to stop therapy when resistance develops.

At present, monotherapy with nucleoside or nucleotide analogues should be limited to patients who have moderate to severe chronic hepatitis B as shown by liver biopsy histology or by clinical features. Selected patients with HBeAg-positive chronic hepatitis B should be treated first with peginterferon, with the oral antiviral agents reserved for those who fail to respond to or cannot tolerate a course of peginterferon. When using nucleoside or nucleotide therapy for hepatitis B, the need for long-term treatment should be expected. The benefits of long-term therapy with the oral antiviral agents in patients with advanced fibrosis and cirrhosis have been shown dramatically in studies of lamivudine therapy in which it was demonstrated that long-term suppression of viral replication can decrease the rate of hepatic decompensation and hepatocellular carcinoma and improve survival. The benefits of long-term therapy in patients with less-advanced stages of chronic hepatitis B have not been proved, although marked improvements in biochemical test results and liver histology have been shown in selected patients. The choice of oral antiviral agent should be based on the response rate and likelihood of resistance. Patients with lamivudine resistance should be reevaluated for the necessity of therapy and perhaps are best switched to adefovir dipivoxil therapy (discontinuing lamivudine). Combinations of antiviral agents have been proposed as being effective in preventing antiviral resistance, but the added benefit of combination therapy over monotherapy for hepatitis B has yet to be demonstrated in clinical trials. [5]

The oral antiviral agents should not be used in patients with mild or minimal disease despite the presence of HBeAg or high levels of HBV DNA (or both). An exception to this caution is a patient with chronic hepatitis B or an inactive carrier state who requires therapy with a pulse or short course of immunosuppression or corticosteroids, as with cyclic cancer chemotherapy or bone marrow transplantation. The use of lamivudine in this situation is directed at preventing reactivation of hepatitis, which can be severe and even life-threatening. These patients should be treated for the duration of immunosuppressive therapy. Recommendations regarding indications and regimens and the duration of therapy will change as more effective combination antiviral therapies are developed.

CHRONIC HEPATITIS D

Epidemiology and Pathobiology

Hepatitis D is caused by combined infection with hepatitis B and the hepatitis D virus (HDV), a defective RNA virus that replicates and spreads efficiently only in the presence of HBsAg (Chapter 151). Hepatitis D is the least common form of chronic viral hepatitis but is also the most severe. On average, cirrhosis develops in 70% of patients with chronic hepatitis D, generally at a younger age than in patients with hepatitis B alone.

Diagnosis

The diagnosis of chronic hepatitis D is usually made on the basis of finding antibody to HDV (anti-HDV) in a patient with chronic hepatitis and HBsAg in serum. The diagnosis can be confirmed by identification of HDV antigen in liver or by detection of HDV RNA in serum, a research test not generally available. Most patients with chronic hepatitis D have HBsAg without serologic markers of active viral replication (i.e., they have a negative result for HBeAg and either low levels [$<10^5$ viral copies/mL] or no detectable HBV DNA). Delta hepatitis should be considered in all patients with HBsAg in serum and active liver disease, particularly those who have low levels or no detectable HBV DNA in serum. Replication of HDV seems to suppress replication of HBV.

Treatment

Rx

Therapy for hepatitis D is difficult. A prolonged course of high doses of interferon alfa (5 to 10 million U/day or three times weekly) results in improvements in serum aminotransferase levels and liver histology in approximately a third of patients. With the exception of patients who become HBsAg negative during treatment, however, most patients have a relapse when therapy is stopped. Trials of long-term therapy with peginterferon are currently under way. Neither corticosteroids nor lamivudine or adefovir is helpful. General management recommendations for hepatitis D are the same as for hepatitis B.

CHRONIC HEPATITIS C

Epidemiology

Hepatitis C is spread largely by the parenteral route, most commonly as a result of injection drug use or receipt of blood transfusions before the introduction of routine screening of blood for anti-HCV (in 1992) or receipt of plasma products before the introduction of inactivation procedures (in 1986). Hepatitis C also occurs after accidental needlesticks and is an occupational hazard for health care workers. In 10 to 30% of patients, a parenteral source of infection cannot be identified, even after careful questioning. These sporadic cases of hepatitis C are probably related to sexual contact or "inapparent" parenteral spread. Sexual spread of hepatitis C can occur, but the risk is low, and sexual transmission has been described primarily in individuals with multiple partners and in patients after exposure to acute rather than chronic hepatitis C. Maternal-infant spread of HCV occurs in approximately 5% of infants of mothers with chronic hepatitis C. Neither breast-feeding nor the type of delivery correlates with transmission, but transmission is more frequent in newborns of women with prolonged labor, early rupture of membranes, and invasive fetal monitoring. Coinfection with HIV in the mother may also increase the risk for transmission of HCV.

Pathobiology

Chronic hepatitis C is caused by infection with HCV, an RNA virus classified in the genus Hepacivirus, family Flaviviridae (Chapter 151). HCV has marked genetic heterogeneity, with nucleotide variability between different isolates ranging from 1 to 50%. Phylogenetic analysis indicates that there are at least six different genotypes of HCV (differing by 30 to 50% in sequence) and more than 90 subtypes (differing by 15 to 30%). Different isolates of a single genotype can vary by 5 to 15%, and virions isolated from a single individual often differ by 1 to 5%, a phenomenon that is termed quasispecies diversity and that may account for the propensity of this virus to lead to chronic infection. The most common genotypes in the United States are 1a and 1b (approximately 75%), 2a and 2b (approximately 15%), and 3a (approximately 7%). Genotype 4 typically occurs in Africa and the Middle East and is uncommon in the United States. Genotype 5 is rare outside South Africa, and genotype 6 is rare outside Southeast Asia. Infections with different genotypes do not differ in clinical expression or disease severity, but responses to interferon-based therapies depend on the genotype of the infection.

The pathogenesis of viral persistence and the cause of hepatic injury in chronic HCV infection are unknown, but cytotoxic T-lymphocyte–mediated responses are probably important. In general, the degree of liver injury does not correlate with the level or genotype of virus but tends to increase with the duration of infection. Nevertheless, some individuals remain infected with HCV for decades yet have minimal changes on liver biopsy. Alcohol ingestion and other causes of liver injury (e.g., iron overload, nonalcoholic steatohepatitis, or concurrent hepatitis virus infection) may augment the liver injury in chronic HCV infection.

Clinical Manifestations

In the typical course of chronic hepatitis C (Fig. 152–2), HCV RNA becomes detectable soon after exposure and remains present throughout the course of the acute illness and thereafter. Approximately a third of patients experience symptoms during the acute episode, and a similar percentage are jaundiced. Aminotransferase levels vary widely but after the acute episode are usually less than 10 times the upper limit of normal. In about a third of infected individuals, serum aminotransferase levels decrease and remain in the normal range despite persistence of HCV RNA. These individuals nevertheless have chronic hepatitis on liver biopsy. Anti-HCV rises after the onset of ALT elevations and symptoms, and it generally persists at high titer. Anti-HCV may not become detectable in patients who have renal failure, are immunosuppressed, or have hypogammaglobulinemia or agammaglobulinemia.

Natural History

The natural history of hepatitis C is highly variable. A small proportion of patients have severe and progressive disease, and cirrhosis and end-stage liver disease develop within a few years; other patients have a benign outcome. In patients monitored from the time of acute infection (e.g., after blood transfusion or receipt of contaminated blood products), chronic infection arises in approximately 55 to 85%, but cirrhosis develops in only 5 to 20% within the first 20 years. In these patients there is little or no increase in hepatitis C–related mortality during the first 2 decades of infection. When patients with established chronic hepatitis C are monitored prospectively, cirrhosis develops in 30 to 50% and mor-

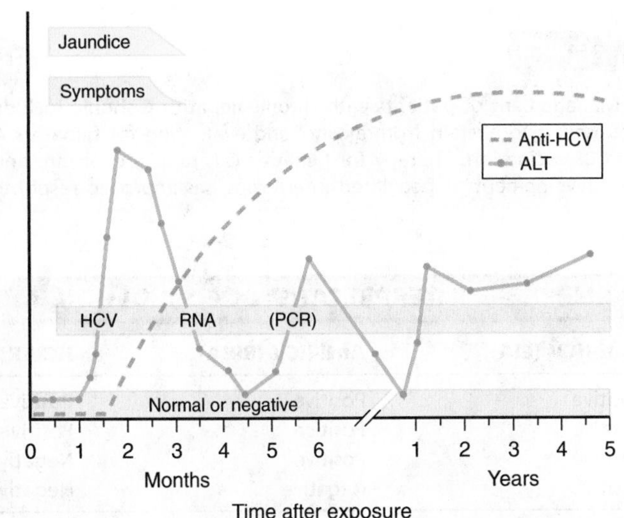

FIGURE 152–2 • Typical serologic course of chronic hepatitis C. ALT = alanine aminotransferase; HCV = hepatitis C virus; PCR = polymerase chain reaction.

bidity and mortality rates are substantial, with the development of end-stage liver disease or hepatocellular carcinoma, particularly in patients with cirrhosis or severe fibrosis indicated on initial liver biopsy. At the time of diagnosis, the average patient probably has had the infection for 15 to 25 years (dating the onset from the time of presumed exposure).

Factors associated with a risk for development of cirrhosis in patients with chronic hepatitis C include age, male sex, alcohol use, and coinfection with other hepatitis viruses or HIV. Factors associated with an increased rate of development of hepatocellular carcinoma are cirrhosis or advanced fibrosis on liver biopsy, age, male sex, and alcohol abuse. In some retrospective studies, treatment with interferon alfa, even without a sustained virologic response, has been associated with a lower rate of development of liver cancer. Obesity, diabetes, and steatosis on liver biopsy have been associated with more advanced disease in some studies, but it remains unclear whether these factors are the result rather than the cause of the worse disease. Viral genotype and high virus levels have not been linked to an increased rate of cirrhosis or liver cancer.

Extrahepatic manifestations of chronic hepatitis C include cryoglobulinemia (Chapter 198), glomerulonephritis (Chapter 122), mucocutaneous vasculitis (Chapter 291), sicca syndrome (Chapter 289), non-Hodgkin's B-cell lymphoma (Chapter 196), porphyria cutanea tarda (Chapter 229), lichen planus (Chapter 464), and perhaps fibromyalgia (Chapter 295). Cryoglobulinemia, which is the most common and well-defined complication of hepatitis C, occurs in approximately 1% of adults with this infection. Typical manifestations are fatigue, myalgias, arthralgias, rash (purpura, hives, and leukocytoclastic vasculitis), neuropathy, and renal disease (glomerulonephritis). Laboratory testing reveals high levels of rheumatoid factor and cryoglobulins containing anti-HCV and HCV RNA, with low levels of complement. Cryoglobulinemia can be severe and lead to end-stage renal disease or severe neuropathies. Long-term cryoglobulinemia has been linked to B-cell lymphomas.

Diagnosis

The diagnosis of chronic hepatitis C is usually based on detection of anti-HCV in a patient with serum aminotransferase elevations or a risk factor for hepatitis C (Table 152–5). The typical test for anti-HCV is an enzyme immunoassay, which can occasionally yield a false-positive result. A recombinant immunoblot assay can be used to confirm anti-HCV reactivity. The diagnosis of hepatitis C is confirmed more aptly, however, by a qualitative, sensitive assay for HCV RNA in serum, such as reverse transcriptase PCR. If anti-HCV is present without HCV RNA, recovery from hepatitis C rather than persistent infection has probably occurred. Several commercial assays are available to quantify HCV RNA levels in serum, but these tests have been difficult to standardize. Most patients with chronic hepatitis C have 10^5 to 10^7 IU of HCV RNA in serum, and levels are usually stable over time. HCV RNA levels should be measured before and during therapy, but otherwise there is little clinical value in monitoring levels of HCV RNA.

Treatment

Rx

Management of patients with chronic hepatitis C should include counseling to abstain from alcohol and evaluation for hepatitis A and B vaccination. Therapy for hepatitis C is rapidly evolving, and the development of pegylated interferons has improved response rates to a 48-week course of the combination of peginterferon and ribavirin to 54 to 56%. [6]

Combination Therapy

With combination therapy, HCV RNA levels typically decrease rapidly on starting treatment and, in responders, become undetectable within 1 to 3 months (Fig. 152–3). Serum aminotransferase levels become normal in most patients with a virologic response. In patients who relapse, HCV RNA and elevations in serum ALT levels reappear soon after therapy is stopped. In nonresponders, ALT levels may decrease and become normal, but HCV RNA remains detectable. The presence or absence of HCV RNA during therapy is the most accurate means of assessing response, and the most accurate end point in defining a beneficial response to treatment is absence of detectable HCV RNA (by a reliable and sensitive PCR technique) for at least 6 months after stopping therapy. A 6-month, post-treatment sustained virologic response is highly predictive of long-term remission and resolution of the liver disease and probably indicates eradication of the infection and cure of the disease.

The major pretreatment factor associated with a beneficial response to combination therapy is the viral genotype, which determines the optimal recommendations for dose and duration of therapy. In patients with genotypes 2 and 3, sustained response rates are 70 to 80%, and these rates can be achieved by a 24-week course of therapy with a lower dose of ribavirin (800 mg daily). In contrast, in patients with genotype 1, sustained response rates are higher with a 48-week course of therapy (40 to 45%) than with a 24-week course, and optimal response rates require a full dose of ribavirin (1000 to 1200 mg daily). In patients with genotype 1 infection, other pretreatment factors that are associated with a higher likelihood of response are low levels of HCV RNA (below 800,000 IU/mL), lack of severe hepatic fibrosis or cirrhosis, young age, female sex, and non–African American race. These factors have minimal effects on response rates in patients with HCV genotypes 2 and 3.

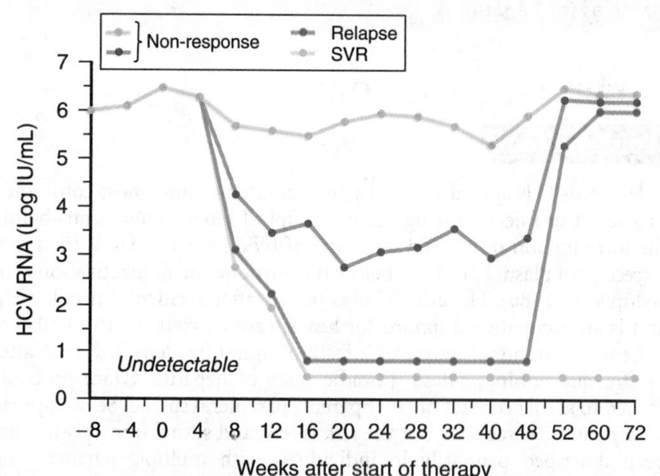

FIGURE 152–3 • Virologic responses to treatment of chronic hepatitis C for 48 weeks. HCV = hepatitis C virus; SVR = sustained virologic response.

TABLE 152–5 INTERPRETATION OF SEROLOGIC MARKERS FOR HEPATITIS C

Anti-HCV (EIA)	Anti-HCV (RIBA)	HCV RNA (PCR)	ALT	Interpretation
Positive	Positive	Positive	Elevated	Acute or chronic hepatitis C
Positive	Positive	Positive	Normal	Chronic hepatitis C
Positive	Positive	Negative	Normal	Resolved hepatitis C
Positive	Negative	Negative	Normal	False-positive EIA assay result

ALT = alanine aminotransferase; Anti-HCV = antibody to hepatitis C virus; EIA = enzyme immunoassay; HCV RNA = hepatitis C viral RNA; PCR = polymerase chain reaction; RIBA = recombinant immunoblot assay.

Rx

Response rates to combination therapy are lower in African American patients (25 to 30%) than in white patients (45 to 55%) with HCV genotype 1 infection for reasons that are unclear. Response rates are also lower in patients with cirrhosis. However, these negative predictive factors should not be used to deny or exclude patients from treatment; indeed, patients with advanced fibrosis and cirrhosis are the most likely to benefit from a sustained virologic response. Patients with genotype 1 infection can be assessed for the likelihood of response during therapy to allow for early discontinuation in those who are unlikely to have a sustained response. The conventional approach is to test for HCV RNA after 24 weeks of combination therapy and discontinue treatment in patients who are still reactive. An alternative approach is to measure HCV RNA levels at the start of therapy and again after 12 weeks. Patients who fail to have a 2-$\log_{10}$ decrease in HCV RNA levels (or to become negative) are unlikely to have a sustained virologic response (<2% likelihood). This early stopping rule can be helpful in limiting the expense and side effects of treatment in patients who are unlikely to have a sustained response to a full 48-week course of treatment. This approach is not necessary in patients with genotypes 2 or 3.

At present, therapy is recommended for patients with chronic hepatitis C and HCV RNA in serum, raised serum aminotransferase levels, chronic hepatitis of at least moderate severity on a liver biopsy specimen (presence of fibrosis or moderate degrees of inflammation and necrosis), and no contraindications to treatment. Contraindications to combination therapy with peginterferon and ribavirin are decompensated liver disease, renal failure, severe immunosuppression, solid organ transplantation, cytopenia, severe psychiatric disease, and active substance abuse. Ribavirin therapy is contraindicated in patients with hemolysis, anemia, significant coronary or cerebrovascular disease, or renal insufficiency. Because ribavirin is teratogenic, it is essential that adequate contraception be practiced during therapy in men and women and for at least 6 months thereafter. Patients with genotype 1 should receive a 48-week course of peginterferon (1.5 μg/kg of alfa-2b or 180 μg of alfa-2a) weekly in combination with ribavirin at a dose of 1000 mg if body weight is less than 75 kg and 1200 mg if body weight is greater than 75 kg. Patients with genotype 2 or 3 should receive a 24-week course of peginterferon (at the same dose as for genotype 1 patients) and ribavirin at a dose of 800 mg/day. The side effects of interferon and ribavirin must be reviewed carefully before starting therapy. Interferon induces an influenza-like syndrome with the first several doses. Thereafter, the major side effects are fatigue, malaise, depression, difficulty concentrating, bone marrow suppression, and in rare instances, bacterial infections or induction of autoimmune disease. Side effects of ribavirin include a dose-related hemolysis that usually results in a 5 to 15% decrease in hemoglobin level, mild itching, and nasal congestion. Dose modification is frequently required during therapy. Ribavirin should be decreased in 200-mg increments for side effects of anemia and hemolysis. In the event of interferon side effects, peginterferon should be decreased stepwise, from 180 to 135 to 90 μg/wk for peginterferon alfa-2a and from 1.5 to 1.0 to 0.5 μg/kg/wk for peginterferon alfa-2b.

Even with combination therapy, the overall sustained virologic response rate to interferon treatment in hepatitis C is only 50%, and many patients find the therapy difficult to tolerate. At present there are no satisfactory therapies for patients who have contraindications to therapy or who are nonresponders. For patients with decompensated liver disease secondary to hepatitis C, liver transplantation (Chapter 158) is indicated. The use of long-term peginterferon with and without ribavirin in nonresponder patients with the goal of suppression rather than eradication of HCV is undergoing evaluation in randomized controlled trials and cannot be recommended at present. Patients who relapse after a conventional course of peginterferon and ribavirin may achieve a sustained response with retreatment for a longer duration or with higher doses of either drug, but the overall efficacy and safety of this approach have not been proved. Several HCV protease, helicase, and polymerase inhibitors are in early clinical trials for chronic hepatitis C.

AUTOIMMUNE HEPATITIS

Definition

Autoimmune hepatitis is a chronic inflammatory disorder of the liver of unknown cause. It is characterized by presence of autoantibodies, high levels of serum immunoglobulins, and frequent association with other autoimmune diseases.

Epidemiology

The disease is more common in women than men and typically has its onset either in childhood and young adulthood (between the ages of 15 and 25) or around the time of menopause (between the ages of 45 and 60). Two types of autoimmune hepatitis have been described: type 1 (or classic) and type 2. Both forms have similar clinical and serum biochemical features. Type 2 autoimmune hepatitis is found largely in Europe and typically affects young women or girls.

Autoimmune hepatitis is one of the three major autoimmune liver diseases, along with primary biliary cirrhosis and primary sclerosing cholangitis (Chapters 157 and 159). Also within this group of autoimmune liver diseases are variant forms of autoimmune hepatitis, which have been termed overlap syndromes because they share features of autoimmune hepatitis and another type of chronic liver disease, and outlier syndromes, which have features of autoimmune hepatitis but do not meet the criteria established by the International Autoimmune Hepatitis Group.

Pathobiology

The pathogenesis of autoimmune hepatitis is not known, but it is believed to be caused by autoimmune reactions against normal hepatocytes. The disease seems to occur in genetically predisposed individuals on exposure to as yet unidentified noxious environmental agents that trigger an autoimmune process directed at liver antigens. In patients with autoimmune hepatitis, primary associations are seen with the human leukocyte antigen (HLA) class I B8 and class II DR3 and DR52a loci. In Asians, autoimmune hepatitis is associated with HLA-DR4, an association that is less common in Western patients.

Clinical Manifestations

Autoimmune hepatitis is a heterogeneous disease with a wide spectrum of clinical features. It tends to be more severe and florid in onset than chronic hepatitis B or C. Autoimmune hepatitis is usually progressive and leads to end-stage liver disease if not treated with immunosuppression. In some patients it is detected before the onset of symptoms and jaundice if elevated serum aminotransferase levels are found on a routine health evaluation. More typically, patients are first seen because of jaundice and fatigue. Abnormalities in routine liver test results are also similar to the abnormalities found in other forms of chronic hepatitis with elevations in serum aminotransferase levels. Elevations in bilirubin or alkaline phosphatase indicate more severe or advanced disease. Perhaps most characteristic of autoimmune hepatitis are striking elevations in serum gamma globulin and, specifically, immunoglobulin G (IgG), accompanied by autoantibodies directed at non–organ-specific cellular constituents.

Diagnosis

The presence of serum autoantibodies is the basis for diagnosis of the two types of autoimmune hepatitis: type 1 (classic) autoimmune hepatitis is characterized by the detection of antinuclear (ANA), anti–smooth muscle (SMA), antiactin, and antiasialoglycoprotein receptor antibodies. Type 2 autoimmune hepatitis is characterized by the detection of anti–liver-kidney microsomal 1 antibodies (anti-LKM1) and anti–liver cytosol 1 antibodies and the absence of ANA or SMA. To meet criteria for the diagnosis of autoimmune hepatitis, these antibodies should be present in titers of at least 1:80 in adults and 1:20 in children.

Liver biopsy specimens in patients with autoimmune hepatitis show features characteristic of chronic hepatitis (as described earlier). Plasma cell infiltrates, which are rare in other forms of chronic hepatitis, are characteristic of autoimmune hepatitis.

Treatment

Rx

Most typical of autoimmune hepatitis is a rapid clinical response to corticosteroid therapy in terms of resolution of clinical symptoms and improvement in serum aminotransferase and serum bilirubin elevations. In typical cases, prednisone should be initiated at a dose of 20 to 30 mg/day. Higher doses of prednisone may be needed in patients with more severe disease. A biochemical response with a decrease in serum aminotransferase levels to the normal or near-normal range should occur within 1 to 3 months. A lack of biochemical or clinical response should lead to reevaluation of the diagnosis. To prevent the side effects of long-term prednisone therapy, azathioprine, 50 to 100 mg, can be combined with prednisone starting at the same time or added later. In the typical patient, prednisone can be tapered slowly to a maintenance regimen of 5 to 10 mg/day combined with azathioprine, 50 to 150 mg/day. In some patients, azathioprine alone, at a dose of 2 mg/kg body weight per day, can be used instead of prednisone as maintenance therapy. The long-term side effects of azathioprine (immune suppression, bone marrow suppression, and risk of cancer) need to be considered. Corticosteroid or immunosuppressive therapy is usually continued indefinitely. In patients with long-term remission (3 years or more), attempts can be made to withdraw therapy, but these patients should be monitored carefully thereafter because severe and even fatal flares of disease can occur weeks to months after stopping prednisone.

Prognosis

The prognosis in this disease is generally related to the histologic stage of disease at the time of diagnosis and initiation of therapy, but patients whose disease responds to immunosuppressive therapy can do well for many years. Patients with autoimmune hepatitis that progresses to end-stage liver disease have excellent survival rates after liver transplantation (Chapter 158).

CRYPTOGENIC CHRONIC LIVER DISEASE

The term cryptogenic chronic liver disease is normally reserved for patients with chronic hepatitis or cirrhosis of unknown cause. Cryptogenic hepatitis is a diagnosis of exclusion and should be made only after hepatitis B, C, and D, autoimmune hepatitis, and other causes of a chronic hepatitis–like syndrome are excluded (see Table 152–1). It is most important to exclude drug-induced (Chapter 153) and inherited metabolic liver diseases (Chapter 154) such as Wilson's disease (by serum ceruloplasmin and, if necessary, urine and liver copper concentrations) and α_1-antitrypsin deficiency (by serum levels of α_1-antitrypsin and phenotyping). Diseases that can resemble chronic hepatitis on blood tests but are readily excluded by liver biopsy histologic findings include alcoholic liver disease, fatty liver, nonalcoholic steatohepatitis (Chapter 156), hemochromatosis (Chapter 231), primary biliary cirrhosis (Chapter 159), and sclerosing cholangitis (Chapter 159). Cryptogenic cirrhosis may represent the end stage of any of these diseases, but particularly nonalcoholic steatohepatitis, which in its later stages may be associated with little or no fat and loss of the other usual characteristics of the disease.

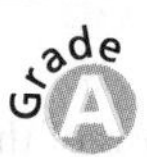

1. Liaw Y-F, Sung JJY, Chow WC, et al: Lamivudine for patients with chronic hepatitis B and advanced disease. N Engl J Med 2004;351:1521–1531.
2. Marcellin P, Chang T-T, Lim SG, et al: for the Adefovir Dipivoxil 437 Study Group: Adefovir dipivoxil for the treatment of hepatitis B e antigen–positive chronic hepatitis B. N Engl J Med 2003; 348:808–816.
3. Hadziyannis SJ, Tassopoulos NC, Heathcote EJ, et al: for the Adefovir Dipivoxil 438 Study Group: Adefovir dipivoxil for the treatment of hepatitis B e antigen–negative chronic hepatitis B. N Engl J Med 2003;348:800–807.
4. Chang T-T, Gish RG, de Man R, et al: for the Entecavir BEHoLD A1463022 Study Group: A randomized comparison of entecavir to lamivudine for treatment of HBeAg–positive chronic hepatitis B in nucleoside-naïve patients. N Engl J Med 2006;354:1001–1010.
5. Lau GKK, Piratvisuth T, Luo KX, et al: Peginterferon alfa-2a, lamivudine and the combination for HBeAg-positive chronic hepatitis B. N Engl J Med 2005;352:2682–2695.
6. Hadziyannis SJ, Sett H Jr, Morgan TR, et al: Peginterferon-alpha2a and ribavirin combination therapy in chronic hepatitis C: A randomized study of treatment duration and ribavirin dose. Ann Intern Med 2004;140:346–355.

SUGGESTED READINGS

Armstong GL, Wasley A, Simard EP, et al: The prevalence of hepatitis C virus infection in the United States, 1999 through 2002. Ann Intern Med 2006; 144:705–715. *Most recent data on the frequency of anti-HCV and HCV RNA in the general U.S. population and specific rates in minority cohorts.*

Ganem D, Prince AM: Hepatitis B virus infection—natural history and clinical consequences. N Engl J Med 2004;350:1118–1129. *Summary of natural history, immunopathogenesis, and treatment.*

Hoofnagle J, Seeff L: Peginterferon and ribavirin for chronic hepatitis C. N Engl J Med 2006;355:2444–2451. *A case-based review.*

Krawitt EL: Autoimmune hepatitis. N Engl J Med 2006;354:54–66. *Summary of pathogenesis, natural history, and therapy.*

153 TOXIN- AND DRUG-INDUCED LIVER DISEASE

William M. Lee

Definition

Toxin-induced and drug-induced hepatotoxicity, defined as any degree of liver injury caused by a drug or a toxic substance, is a frequent cause of acute liver injury and accounts for more than 50% of all cases of acute liver failure with hepatic encephalopathy in the United States. Hepatotoxicity has been described with many drugs (see Table 27–5), although the number of cases is low given the number of prescriptions written.

Epidemiology

Few data are available on the epidemiology of toxic and drug-induced liver disease. The exact number of drug-induced liver injuries per year in the United States is unknown, but European data on adverse drug reactions report about 22 cases of drug-induced liver disease per 1 million people per year. In developing parts of the world, drug-induced liver disease is much less common and related to fewer drugs. It is estimated that less than 10% of actual cases are reported, so a true estimate of the incidence of toxic and drug-induced liver disease may be impossible to obtain.

Pathobiology

The liver, which is situated between the absorptive surface of the gastrointestinal tract and the targets of drugs throughout the body, is central to the metabolism of foreign substances. Most drugs and xenobiotics cross the intestinal brush border because they are lipophilic. *Biotransformation* is the process by which lipophilic therapeutic agents are rendered more hydrophilic by the liver, thereby resulting in drug excretion in urine or bile. In most instances, biotransformation changes a nonpolar to a polar compound through several steps. Foremost are oxidative pathways (e.g., hydroxylation) mediated by the cytochromes (CYPs) P-450 (Chapter 27). The next step is typically esterification to form sulfates and glucuronides, a process that results in the addition of highly polar groups to the hydroxyl group. These two enzymatic steps are referred to as *phase I* (CYP oxidation) and *phase II* (esterification). Other important metabolic pathways involve glutathione-*S*-transferase, acetylating enzymes, and alcohol dehydrogenase, but the principal metabolic pathways for most pharmacologic agents involve CYPs and subsequent esterification.

Pathogenesis

The exact details of the pathogenesis of liver injury are unclear for most drugs. A single drug may cause toxic effects in several ways. An oversimplified approach suggests that high-energy unstable metabolites of the parent drug, the result of CYP activation, bind to cell proteins or DNA and disrupt cell function. Perhaps the best example is acetaminophen. Though used universally for non-narcotic pain relief, acetaminophen taken in large quantities causes profound centrilobular necrosis. The metabolic pathway of acetaminophen involves phase I and phase II reactions, glutathione detoxification, and the formation of reactive intermediates (Fig. 153–1). Glucuronidation and sulfation occur as the initial detoxifying step because the parent compound contains a hydroxyl group. Glucuronidation and sulfation capacity greatly exceeds daily needs, so even patients with far-advanced liver disease continue to have adequate glucuronidation capacity, which explains why no obvious enhancement of toxicity is observed when cirrhotic patients take acetaminophen.

Genetics

Enzyme Polymorphism

Although acetaminophen is a dose-related toxin, the rarity of idiosyncratic drug toxicity (1 in 10,000 patients) suggests the importance of environmental and host factors (Table 153–1). Genetically variant CYP isoenzymes may partially explain the observed individual variation in response to drugs. An example is debrisoquine, an antihypertensive drug marketed in Europe that is hydroxylated by CYP2D6, an isoform that is totally absent in 5% of normal individuals. Lack of CYP2D6 greatly prolongs the half-life of the parent compound in affected individuals. Another example is the phenomenon of fast versus slow acetylation, which affects whole races and has been implicated in variation in the metabolism of isoniazid. Most known genetic variants that occur relatively frequently, however, cannot explain the formation of a toxic intermediate in only a rare individual.

Most drugs are small organic compounds, unlikely to evoke an immune response. Although some toxic drug reactions are associated with an obvious allergic response, most are not. Nevertheless, immune mechanisms not associated with systemic allergic IgE reactions or skin hypersensitivity might be involved. Studies suggest that the products of cytochrome P-450 metabolism, the highly reactive intermediates that are formed within the microsomes, covalently bind to the enzyme itself to form a drug-hapten adduct that disables the enzyme and injures the cell. Haptenization then evokes an immune response directed against the newly formed antigen or neoantigen. P-450s have been shown to traffic to the plasma membrane, thereby allowing the drug–P-450 adduct to become the target of a subsequent cytolytic attack. Whether these adducts or smaller peptides processed and presented by the major histocompatibility complex class I and class II schemes are the targets is unclear. The association among neoantigens, autoantibodies, and hepatotoxic drugs implicates an immunologic mechanism.

Regardless of whether an individual drug causes significant cell necrosis, the P-450–drug adducts can evoke the immune response. Any subsequent P-450–drug adduct present on the hepatocyte surface would evoke a further response. Responses may be antibody mediated or occur as a result of direct cytolytic attack by primed T cells.

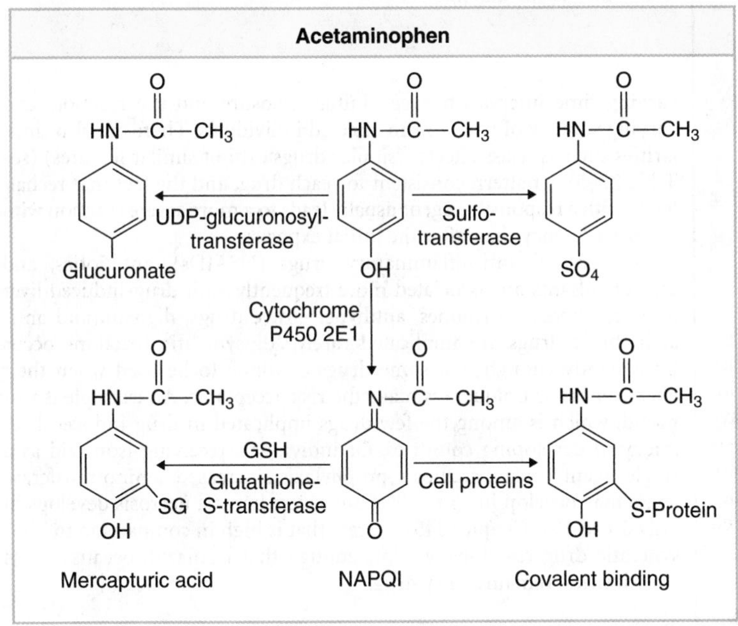

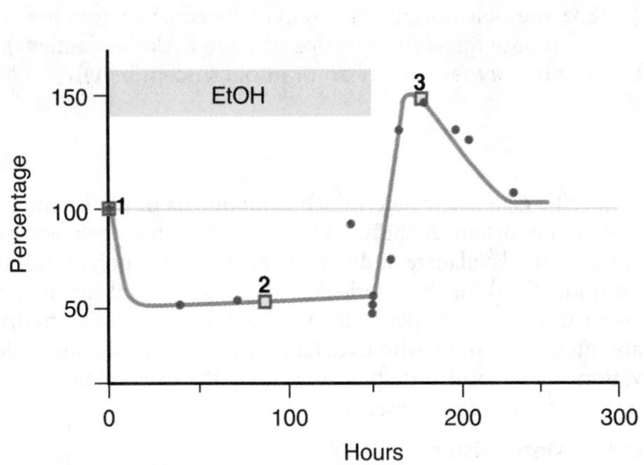

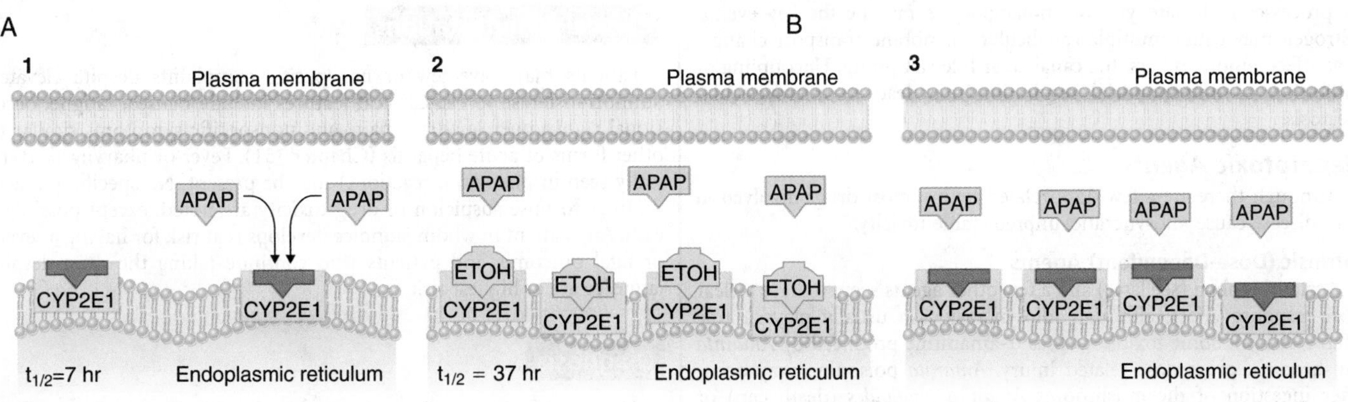

FIGURE 153–1 • Acetaminophen metabolism. Although acetaminophen is metabolized largely by sulfation or glucuronidation under normal conditions, exceeding the recommended doses increases the proportion metabolized by cytochrome P-450 2E1, which leads to the highly reactive intermediate *N*-aminoparaquinoneamine (NAPQI) (**A**). This compound leads to liver injury unless scavenging by glutathione yields the inert, water-soluble mercapturic acid. The presence of alcohol (EtOH), which competes for cytochrome P-450 2E1, not only inhibits NAPQI formation but also induces the enzyme so that its half-life is slowed and more enzyme is present (**B** and **C**). After cessation of alcohol, NAPQI formation is enhanced by the presence of the induced enzyme and the lack of competition from alcohol. Toxicity is a dynamic process and may be most pronounced in the 24 hours after cessation of alcohol. (Adapted from Thummel KE, Slattery JT, Ro H, et al: Ethanol exposure and acetaminophen hepatotoxicity: Inhibition and induction of hepatotoxic metabolite formation. Clin Pharmacol Ther 2000;67:5991–5999.)

TABLE 153–1 FACTORS THAT MAY INFLUENCE THE METABOLIC FATE OF DRUGS

Factor	Description
Age	The elderly seem to be affected more often. Adults are more susceptible than children in some instances (acetaminophen, halothane, isoniazid), less susceptible in others (aspirin, valproic acid)
Alcohol, acute and chronic	Induction of CYP2E1 affects drugs metabolized by this pathway, including acetaminophen and isoniazid
Gender	Females are affected more often, but the mechanism is unknown
Pregnancy	Effects of drugs in pregnancy have been poorly studied
Preexisting liver disease	Hepatic disease may *protect* against idiosyncratic reactions and may *enhance* toxicity in dose-dependent hepatotoxins (e.g., acetaminophen)
Renal disease	Slowed disappearance of the parent compound yields higher concentrations and affects P-450 (e.g., enhancement of tetracycline toxicity in renal disease)
Certain foods	Grapefruit has an unknown substance that interferes with the metabolism of some drugs
Concomitant drugs	Drug-drug interactions are common causes of adverse effects (e.g., valproate and chlorpromazine together lead to enhanced cholestasis)
Genetic factors	Enzyme polymorphisms (e.g., enhanced phenytoin liver disease in patients with defective epoxide hydrolase activity), HLA phenotypes (e.g., nitrofurantoin susceptibility)

TABLE 153–2 DRUGS/TOXINS IN WHICH A DOSE-RESPONSE EFFECT IS OBSERVED

Drug	Response
Acetaminophen	Total dose, single vs. multiple time points
Amiodarone	Total dose over time
Bromfenac	Toxicity occurs only after extended use
Cocaine	Dose-related vascular collapse
Cyclophosphamide	Dose related, worse with previous ALT elevations
Cyclosporine	Cholestasis with toxic blood levels, CYP3A phenotype
Methotrexate	Aminotransferase/fibrosis; single dose/total dose
Niacin	Large doses yield vascular collapse
Oral contraceptives	Prolonged use yields hepatic adenomas
Tetracycline	Total dose, renal dysfunction
Toxins (yellow phosphorus, carbon tetrachloride, *Amanita* toxin, bacterial toxins)	Total dose

ALT = alanine aminotransferase.

Specific genetically determined components of the immune response may be important. A specific HLA haplotype has been associated with amoxicillin-clavulanate–induced hepatitis, and polymorphisms have been identified for the interleukin-10 promoter and for tumor necrosis factor-α. For every patient with a severe injury secondary to drugs, there are often many more who have had asymptomatic aminotransferase elevations that subsided despite continuing the drug—sometimes referred to as an adaptive response.

Other Mechanisms

In drug-induced cholestasis, disruption of specific transport proteins or processes in hepatocytes or cholangiocytes may be the key events. Estrogen may cause multiple canalicular membrane transport changes that affect, among others, the canalicular bile salt pump. Uncoupling or inhibition of mitochondrial respiration may lead to microvesicular steatosis.

Hepatotoxic Agents

Although there are a few dose-related toxins, most drugs involved in liver disease cause idiosyncratic, unpredictable toxicity.

Intrinsic (Dose-Dependent) Agents

Acetaminophen (see later) and a few other agents seem to have a clear dose-response effect, although idiosyncrasy also usually plays a role (Table 153–2). Some toxins, such as α-amanitine produced by *Amanita* mushrooms, cause dose-related injury. *Amanita* poisoning may occur after ingestion of the mushrooms *Amanita phalloides* (death cap) or *Amanita virosa* (deadly agaric). The dose-dependent toxic effect on the liver is attributed to amatoxin, an ingredient of the mushrooms that further enhances the toxic effect by its enterohepatic recirculation characteristics; the toxic effect is exerted on each cycle of the recirculation through the liver.

Idiosyncratic Reactions

Most drug reactions occur in 1 in 1000 to 1 in 200,000 patients. Characteristics of these idiosyncratic reactions include infrequent occurrence, varying time intervals between initial exposure and the reaction, and varying severity of reactions in affected individuals. There are also similarities such as "class effects" (similar drugs exhibit similar features) (see Table 27–5), a pattern consistent for each drug, and the fact that rechallenge with a responsible agent usually leads to a more severe reaction with a shorter latency than after the initial exposure.

Nonsteroidal anti-inflammatory drugs (NSAIDs), antibiotics, and anticonvulsants are associated more frequently with drug-induced liver disease, whereas hormones, antihypertensive drugs, digoxin, and antiarrhythmic drugs are implicated rarely. Idiosyncratic reactions occur infrequently enough that some drugs continue to be used when their effectiveness or uniqueness make the risk acceptable. An example is isoniazid, which is among the few drugs implicated in drug-induced liver injury in developing countries. Of individuals receiving isoniazid as a single agent for tuberculosis prophylaxis, increased aminotransferase levels may develop in 15 to 20%, but severe hepatic necrosis develops in only 0.1 to 1% (Chapter 345)—a rate that is high in comparison to idiosyncratic drug reactions, yet low enough that isoniazid, because of its effectiveness, remains a key drug.

Clinical Manifestations

Patients may have few or nonspecific complaints despite elevated aminotransferase levels. Clinical features include nausea, fatigue, occasional right upper quadrant pain, and nonspecific symptoms similar to other forms of acute hepatitis (Chapter 151). Fever or pharyngitis (typically seen in phenytoin reactions) may be present. No specific physical findings to raise suspicion of drug toxicity are noted, except possibly a rash. Any patient in whom jaundice develops is at risk for having a severe or fatal outcome, and patients who continue taking the drug despite jaundice are at highest risk.

Diagnosis

Abnormal aminotransferase levels with the use of a new drug should raise suspicion of a drug-induced reaction and prompt immediate discontinuation of the drug rather than waiting for further diagnostic tests to confirm or exclude the diagnosis. Rapid discontinuation of medication at the first sign of liver disease can prevent most fatal liver injuries.

Evaluation of a patient with a suspected drug reaction is directed toward establishing the time line for all drugs or herbs that the patient may have taken. Responsible drugs would usually have been started between 5 and 90 days before the onset of symptoms. Evidence of viral hepatitis (Chapter 151), gallstones (Chapter 159), alcoholic liver disease (Chapter 156), pregnancy (Chapter 259), severe right heart failure (Chapter 57), or a period of hypotension (Chapter 107) points to these specific causes. Less commonly, cytomegalovirus (Chapter 399), Epstein-Barr virus (Chapter 400), or herpesviruses (Chapter 397) can cause hepatic injury, primarily in immunosuppressed individuals. If all these causes can be excluded, if the temporal relationship fits, and if the patient begins to improve after withdrawal of the drug, the diagnosis is more secure. Liver biopsy is of limited value because the histologic picture of most cases of drug-induced liver injury is not different from that of viral hepatitis. Nevertheless, an occasional liver biopsy specimen in a puzzling case shows eosinophils or granulomas consistent with a drug reaction.

Types of Drug Reactions

Although most liver injury involves direct hepatocyte necrosis/apoptosis (hepatocellular injury), some drugs primarily injure bile ducts or canaliculi and cause cholestasis without significant damage to hepatocytes. Other drugs affect sinusoidal cells or present a particular pattern of liver injury affecting multiple cell types (mixed type). Another approach to drug reactions emphasizes the histologic changes involved and the cell type (Table 153–3 and Fig. 153–2).

Hepatocellular Reactions

Hepatocellular reactions are the most common type of drug-induced liver disease and account for 90% of cases (Table 153–4). They are characterized by a pattern of serum liver test results that reflect hepatocellular injury (Chapter 150). Usually, improvement is quick after discontinuation of the drug (1 to 2 months), and fulminant, acute liver failure with hepatic encephalopathy develops in only a few patients.

Histologic findings include necrosis and cellular infiltration. The necrosis may be zonal (e.g., induced by acetaminophen or carbon tetrachloride) or diffuse (e.g., induced by halothane), and the inflammatory response consists of lymphocytes or eosinophils. Massive necrosis may cause acute liver failure and death.

Acetaminophen toxicity is the most common form of acute liver failure observed in the United States and has been the best understood example of direct hepatocyte toxicity. The incidence of acetaminophen poisoning varies widely throughout the world, but it is becoming more frequent and widespread. Liver injury occurs predictably after an intentional suicidal overdose (Chapter 111); it also occurs when acetaminophen is used in excessive doses or sometimes even in therapeutic doses for pain relief. Enhanced toxicity occurs when patients are fasting or are chronic alcohol users because of enzyme induction and depletion of glutathione by alcohol and fasting; by comparison, acute alcohol intake may protect against acetaminophen toxicity during the period of alcohol ingestion. Thereafter, a rebound increase in available CYP2E1 results in increased toxicity in the 12 hours after ingestion because of enzyme induction (see Fig. 153–1). Patients with an unintentional acetaminophen overdose may fare worse than suicidal patients because the former seek treatment later in their course, even though suicidal patients take larger doses. The better outcome after an acute overdose may be explained by earlier medical attention and the use of *N*-acetylcysteine, an effective antidote. Nevertheless, a fifth of acetaminophen suicidal attempts are associated with severe liver injury and the potential for a fatal outcome.

The extremely elevated aminotransferase values (often >6000 IU/L and sometimes as high as 30,000 IU/L) observed in suicidal and unintentional acetaminophen ingestion help distinguish these cases from viral hepatitis or other drug injury. The antidote *N*-acetylcysteine (Chapter 111) may be given by nasogastric tube on admission and for the ensuing 72 hours to provide glutathione substrate. The standard treatment is intravenous *N*-acetylcysteine beginning at a dose of 140 mg/kg in 300 mL of 5% dextrose given over a period of 1 hour, followed by a dose of 70 mg/kg in 5% dextrose given over 1-hour period every 4 hours for 48 hours. A loading dose of 140 mg/kg can be given orally, followed by 70 mg/kg every 4 hours for 17 doses (72 hours). Expected survival rates are greater than 80%, although liver transplantation is occasionally required.

TABLE 153–3 TYPES OF TOXIC AND DRUG REACTIONS

Autoimmune *(attack on cell surface markers)*
Lovastatin, methyldopa, nitrofurantoin
Cholestatic *(attack on bile ducts)*
Anabolic steroids, carbamazepine, chlorpromazine, estrogen, erythromycin
Fibrosis *(activation of stellate cells leads to fibrosis)*
Methotrexate, vitamin A excess
Granulomatous *(macrophage stimulation)*
Allopurinol, diltiazem, nitrofurantoin, quinidine, sulfa drugs
Hepatocellular *(damage to smooth endoplasmic reticulum and immune cell surface)*
Acetaminophen, *Amanita* poisoning, diclofenac, isoniazid, lovastatin, nefazodone, trazodone, venlafaxine
Immunoallergic *(cytotoxic cell attack on surface determinants)*
Halothane, phenytoin, sulfamethoxazole
Mixed *(see above)*
Amoxicillin-clavulanate, carbamazepine, cyclosporine, herbs, methimazole
Oncogenic *(hepatic adenoma formation)*
Oral contraceptives, androgenic agents
Steatohepatitis *(mitochondrial dysfunction: β-oxidation and respiratory chain)*
Amiodarone, perhexiline maleate, tamoxifen
Vascular collapse *(ischemic damage)*
Cocaine, ecstasy, nicotinic acid
Veno-occlusive disease *(endotheliitis of sinusoidal endothelial cells)*
Busulfan, cytoxan

Cholestatic Reactions

Cholestatic reactions have been described for many drugs. Cholestasis is defined best as failure of bile to reach the duodenum, and common symptoms are jaundice and pruritus. *Pure cholestasis* with no signs of hepatocellular necrosis is seen almost exclusively in patients taking oral contraceptives, anabolic steroids, or sex hormone antagonists such as tamoxifen. Acute *cholestatic hepatitis* is histologically characterized by cholestasis (dilated canaliculi, brown granules in the cytoplasm of hepatocytes), some degree of liver cell necrosis and bile duct injury, and inflammatory infiltration by polymorphonuclear leukocytes. Drugs that cause this type of reaction include carbamazepine, trimethoprim-sulfamethoxazole, and captopril.

Generally, drug-induced cholestasis requires a longer time to resolve than hepatocellular drug reactions do. In some cases, segments of the intrahepatic biliary tree may be destroyed progressively, the so-called *vanishing bile duct syndrome* that occurs after a protracted course (>6 months) of drug-induced cholestasis. The result is a state of chronic cholestasis that resembles primary biliary cirrhosis (Chapter 159). Approximately 30 drugs have been implicated in the vanishing bile duct syndrome, including chlorpromazine and ajmaline. A sclerosing cholangitis–like syndrome with jaundice caused by intrahepatic and extrahepatic strictures in the bile ducts is sometimes observed in patients receiving intra-arterial floxuridine chemotherapy for hepatic metastases of colorectal cancer.

Immunoallergic Reactions

Drugs may also be associated with definite allergic reactions. A combined toxic/immunologic mechanism is involved in the liver injury caused by halothane, a fluorinated hydrocarbon anesthetic that causes severe, often fatal liver injury after multiple exposures (Chapter 458). Other fluorinated hydrocarbons, including isoflurane and desflurane, occasionally result in the same response. Although halothane has never been withdrawn, its use has been limited by the advent of safer agents. Hypersensitivity reactions, such as fever, eosinophilia, and rash, are common. Halothane may induce fever, eosinophilia, and antimitochondrial antibodies. Direct cytotoxicity and immune-mediated toxicity are observed, consistent with the clinical observation that severe halothane toxicity occurs with repeated exposure. Although evidence of injury can usually be identified within 1 week of the first exposure, the interval to toxicity is shortened and the damage is more severe with each successive exposure, as befits an immune reaction.

Phenytoin (Chapter 426) induces the simultaneous onset of fever, rash, lymphadenopathy, and eosinophilia. The mechanisms responsible for the combined allergic and hepatotoxic reaction are unknown, but the slow resolution of the illness suggests that the allergen remains on the surface of the hepatocyte for weeks or months. A concurrent mononucleosis-like picture is frequently confused with a viral illness or streptococcal pharyn-

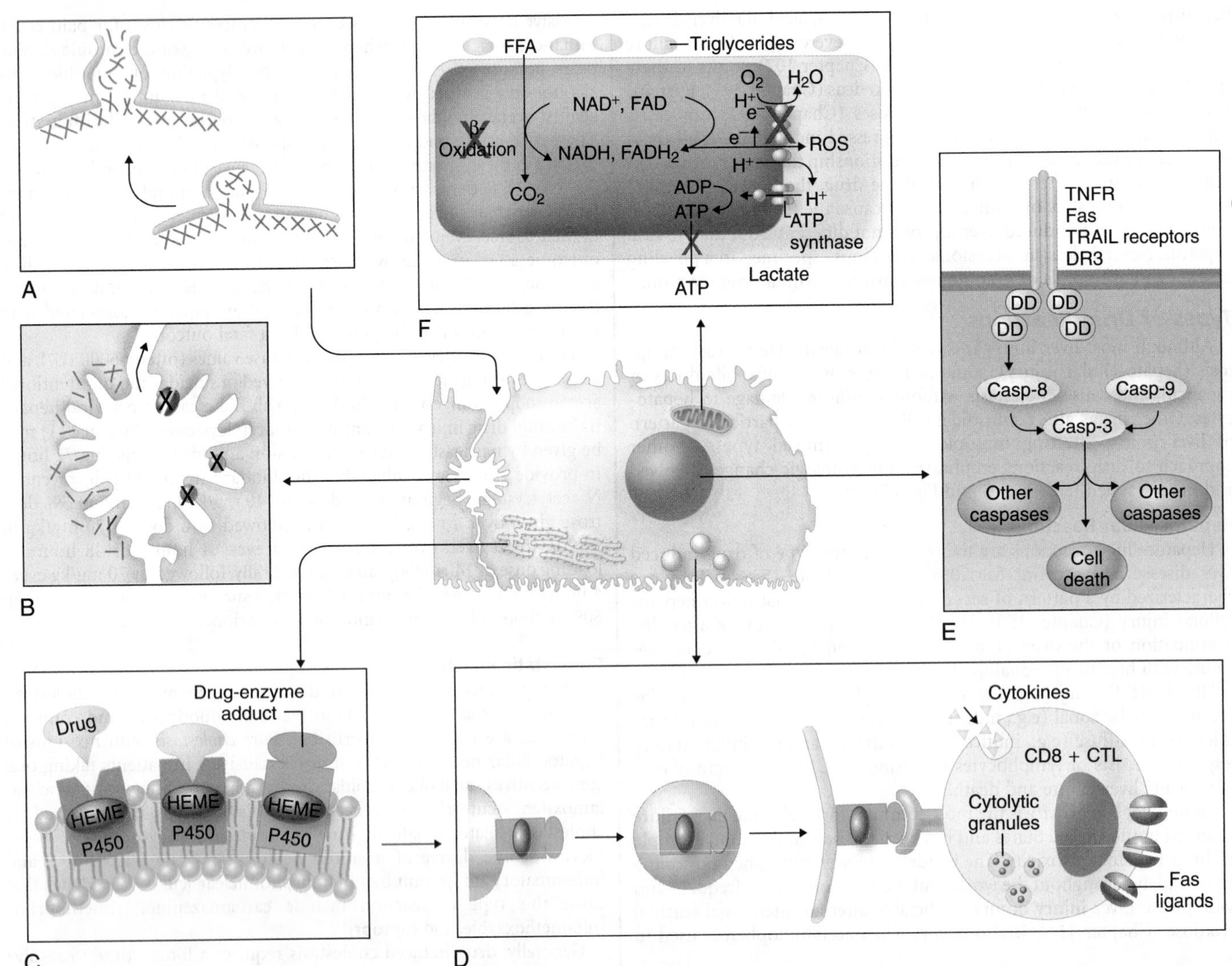

FIGURE 153–2 • Mechanisms of liver injury. Each form of liver injury targets specific organelles, although multiple organelles may be affected. The hepatocyte in the center may be affected in at least six ways. **A,** Disruption of intracellular calcium leads to actin fibril disassembly at the hepatocyte surface, which results in blebbing of the cell membrane and subsequent rupture and cell lysis. **B,** In cholestatic diseases, disruption of actin filaments may occur with the loss of villus processes. Interference with ion pumps limits the excretion of bilirubin and other organic compounds. **C,** Most hepatocellular reactions involve the cytochrome P-450 system. The high-energy reaction involved may lead to binding of drug to enzyme and create a new adduct. **D,** Enzyme-drug adducts may traffic to the cell surface and serve as target immunogens for cytolytic attack by T cells. **E,** Activation of apoptotic pathways results in cell death. **F,** Inhibition of β-oxidation or respiration in mitochondria results in microvesicular fat accumulation and lactic acidosis, a pattern characteristic of a variety of agents, including nucleoside analogues, tetracycline, and aspirin. ATP = adenosine triphosphate; FAD = flavin adenine dinucleotide; FFA = free fatty acid; NAD = nicotinamide adenine dinucleotide; ROS = reactive oxygen species; TNFR = tumor necrosis factor receptor. (**A,** Adapted from Farrell GC: Drug-Induced Liver Disease. Edinburgh, Churchill Livingstone, 1994, p 44. **B,** Adapted from Trauner M, Meier PJ, Boyer J: Mechanisms of disease: Molecular pathogenesis of cholestasis. N Engl J Med 1998;339:1217–1227. **C,** Aadapted from Watkins Zimmerman HJ: Hepatotoxicity, 2nd ed. Philadelphia, Lippincott Williams & Wilkins, 2000. **D,** From Robin M-A, Le Roy M, Descatoire V, Pessayre D: Plasma membrane cytochromes P450 as neoantigens and autoimmune targets in drug-induced hepatitis. J Hepatol 1997;26(Suppl. 1):23–30. **E,** From Reed JC: Apoptosis-regulating proteins as targets for drug discovery. Trends Mol Med 2001;7:314–319. **F,** Adapted from Pessayre D: Personal communication.)

gitis. If use of phenytoin is not discontinued promptly despite signs of hepatitis, a severe Stevens-Johnson drug eruption (Chapters 465 and 466) and prolonged fever may result. As with any therapeutic agent, rapid recognition of the presence of a toxic drug reaction and immediate discontinuation of the compound are key to limiting hepatic damage. Systemic features of an allergic reaction may not be obvious, even when eosinophilia or granulomas are present on liver biopsy.

Steatohepatitis

Steatosis in the liver (Chapter 156) can be present in a microvesicular or macrovesicular pattern. Macrovesicular steatosis, the most common form, is histologically characterized by a single vacuole of fat filling up the hepatocyte and displacing the nucleus to the cell's periphery. Macrovesicular steatosis is typically caused by alcohol, diabetes, or obesity. Sometimes drugs such as corticosteroids or methotrexate may cause these hepatic changes. Amiodarone (Chapters 63 and 64) has been associated with a picture resembling alcoholic hepatitis, occasionally with progression to cirrhosis. The pathophysiology involves accumulation of phospholipids in the liver, eyes, thyroid, and skin. Treatment is primarily withdrawal of the drug and observation, although the half-life of amiodarone is prolonged. Tamoxifen, which has been used in long-term regimens for the prevention of recurrent breast cancer (Chapter 208), has also been associated with a steatohepatitis picture evolving to cirrhosis.

In microvesicular steatosis, hepatocytes contain numerous small fat vesicles that do not displace the nucleus. Valproic acid, an anticonvulsant (Chapter 426), causes hepatotoxicity, either as microvesicular fat deposition resembling Reye's syndrome or in a more chronic indolent fashion associated with macrovesicular fat accumulation. Toxicity is more severe and frequent in children. These lesions are associated with disruption of mitochondrial DNA, with resulting anaerobic metabolism that leads to lactic acidosis in the most severe cases. Macrovesicular and microvesicular lesions may be observed concomitantly in some patients, and the microvesicular lesions are associated more often with a poor prognosis. Hepatocellular necrosis may also be present. Acute fatty liver of pregnancy (Chapter 154) and Reye's syndrome are two examples of severe liver diseases caused by microvesicular steatosis.

Drugs involved in microvesicular steatosis include valproate, tetracycline, and fialuridine. Aspirin use in children has been associated with Reye's syndrome, but the incidence of Reye's syndrome has decreased dramatically since warnings were issued concerning aspirin use in children.

TABLE 153–4 SCORING SYSTEM FOR ASSESSING CAUSALITY FOR HEPATOCELLULAR TYPES OF REACTIONS

TEMPORAL RELATIONSHIP OF START OF DRUG TO START OF ILLNESS	
Initial treatment: 5–90 days; subsequent treatment course: 1–15 days	+2
Initial treatment: <5 or >90 days; subsequent treatment course: >15 days	+1
From cessation of drug: ≤15 days*	+1
COURSE	
ALT decreases ≥50% from peak within 8 days	+3
ALT decreases ≥50% from peak within 30 days	+2
If the drug is continued, inconclusive	0
RISK FACTORS	
Alcohol†	+1
No alcohol†	0
Age ≥55 years	+1
Age <55 years	0
CONCOMITANT DRUG	
Concomitant drug with suggestive time of onset	−1
Concomitant drug known to be a hepatotoxin with suggestive time of onset	−2
Concomitant drug with further evidence of involvement (rechallenge)	−3
NUMBER OF NONDRUG CAUSES	
Hepatitis A, B, or C; biliary obstruction; alcoholism (AST ≥2 × ALT); recent hypotension; CMV, EBV, or HSV infection excluded	
All excluded	+2
4–5 causes excluded	+1
<4 causes excluded	−2
Nondrug cause highly probable	−3
PREVIOUS INFORMATION ON HEPATOTOXICITY OF THE DRUG IN QUESTION	
Package insert mentions	+2
Published case reports but not on package label	+1
Reaction unknown	0
RECHALLENGE	
Positive (ALT doubles with drug alone)‡	+2
Compatible (ALT doubles, compounding features)‡	+1
Negative (increase in ALT but ≤2 × ULN)‡	−2
Not done	0

Highly probable (score >8), *probable* (score 6–8), *possible* (score 3–5), *unlikely* (score 1–2), or *excluded* (score ≤0).

For cholestatic reactions: *≤30 days; †alcohol or pregnancy; ‡read alkaline phosphatase (or total bilirubin) instead of ALT.

ALT = alanine aminotransferase; AP = alkaline phosphatase; AST = aspartate aminotransferase; CMV = cytomegalovirus; EBV = Epstein-Barr virus; HSV = herpes simplex virus; TB = total bilirubin; ULN = upper limits of normal.

Adapted from Danan G, Benichou C: Causality assessment of adverse reactions to drugs: I. A novel method based on the conclusions of international consensus meetings: Application to drug-induced liver injuries. J Clin Epidemiol 1993;46:1323–1330; and Benichou C, Danan G, Flahault A: Causality assessment of adverse reactions to drugs: II. An original model for validation of drug causality assessment methods: Case reports with positive rechallenge. J Clin Epidemiol 1993;46:1331–1336.

Effects of Sex Steroids

Anabolic steroids, such as methyltestosterone, may cause cholestasis. Androgens may cause peliosis hepatis and benign or malignant tumors. Oral contraceptives (Chapter 257) may cause cholestasis, hepatic adenomas, or Budd-Chiari syndrome (hepatic vein thrombosis). Antiandrogens used to treat prostate cancer (Chapter 211), such as flutamide and nilutamide, and antipituitary drugs, such as cyproterone acetate, have also been associated with severe hepatocellular injury.

Other Drug Reactions

Other less severe drug reactions involving the liver include granulomatous reactions, fibrosis, ischemic injury, and chronic autoimmune liver injury (see Table 153–3). The type of reaction observed can be helpful in determining the probable agent because most drugs have a specific injury profile.

A pattern of veno-occlusive disease with obliteration of small intrahepatic veins, sinusoidal congestion, and necrosis is observed frequently in bone marrow transplant patients (Chapter 184) who receive chemotherapy with cyclophosphamide (Cytoxan) or busulfan. Symptoms, including rapidly accumulating ascites, painful hepatomegaly, and jaundice, develop soon after the chemotherapeutic regimen has begun. Rarely, herbal medicines (Chapter 36) such as pyrrolizidine alkaloids (*Crotalaria* and *Senecio* found in Jamaican bush tea) may cause veno-occlusive disease.

Toxins are associated with direct injury to hepatocytes in a dose-dependent fashion. Organic solvents such as carbon tetrachloride and trichloroethylene (Chapter 111) cause centrilobular injury. Yellow phosphorus, found in firecrackers and rat poisons, is a rare cause of liver injury either from accidental or from intentional exposure. Symptoms from poisoning are similar to those of any other types of hepatitis.

Mushroom poisoning (Chapter 111), which follows the ingestion of *A. phalloides* and related species, typically occurs in amateur mushroom fanciers in a dose-related fashion. The associated muscarinic effects, including severe diarrhea, vomiting, and profuse sweating, predominate in the first hours after ingestion. Hepatic failure follows if antidotes (see later) are not given. The overall prognosis for spontaneous recovery is poor; liver transplantation may be life-saving.

Differential Diagnosis

The differential diagnosis of toxic and drug-induced liver injury includes almost the entire spectrum of liver diseases. Because the clinical picture of drug-induced liver injury ranges from pure hepatocellular to pure cholestatic variants, a high index of suspicion must be maintained, even when toxic or drug-induced liver injury is not obvious initially.

For dose-dependent hepatotoxins, the diagnosis may be easier to establish than for idiosyncratic drug reactions. Serum levels of acetaminophen, a thorough history, and characteristic biochemical abnormalities (high aminotransferase levels) usually reveal an acetaminophen overdose, whereas a diagnosis of *Amanita* poisoning depends on the history, symptoms of gastroenteritis (muscarinic reaction), and positive mushroom identification.

For idiosyncratic drug reactions, the diagnosis is sometimes more difficult to establish. A standardized reporting form called the *RUCAM* (*R*oussel *U*claf *c*ausality *a*ssessment *m*ethod; see Table 153–4) developed by an international panel provides a worthwhile causality assessment scoring system. These guidelines outline the steps that an experienced clinician might use to assess the likelihood of drug reactions. Causality assessment methods typically include the temporal relationship, course after cessation of the drug, risk factors, concomitant drugs, a search for nondrug causes (viral hepatitis), previous information concerning the drug, and response to rechallenge, which is not usually attempted.

Treatment

Prompt discontinuation of a suspected drug is mandatory. Available antidotes should be used for acetaminophen (*N*-acetylcysteine) and *Amanita* poisoning (penicillin, given intravenously at 300,000 to 1 million U/kg/day, and thioctic acid, 5 to 100 mg every 6 hours intravenously, have been recommended, but there are no controlled trials). General supportive therapy ranges from intravenous fluid replacement to intensive monitoring and treatment of patients with hepatic encephalopathy secondary to acute liver failure (Chapter

158). Liver transplantation (Chapter 158) is performed in more than 50% of patients with idiosyncratic drug-induced acute liver failure because the survival rate in this setting without transplantation is less than 20%.

Future Directions

Research in *pharmacogenomics* may allow the patient's own genetic information to guide individualized drug therapy and monitoring of idiosyncratic drug reactions. The genetic information would probably concentrate initially on enzymes with variant alleles associated with poor metabolism, such as CYP1A2 or CYP2C19 for isoniazid, CYP2C9 for piroxicam, or CYP2D6 for nortriptyline. Better postmarketing surveillance of all drugs to identify those whose hepatotoxicity was not previously appreciated should be a high priority.

Prevention

It is wise to defer embracing new drugs during their first year of introduction, particularly if they show no unique advantages over accepted formulations. Physicians must strive to instill in their patients a healthy level of alertness with regard to drug-induced liver injury, particularly for agents with known hepatotoxicity. Monitoring of aminotransferase levels on a monthly basis is suggested for known hepatotoxins such as isoniazid or diclofenac, but it is unlikely to be cost-effective when an adverse reaction occurs less frequently, such as in only 1 in 50,000 patients. Because many drug reactions develop within days, monitoring provides no guarantee. Most fatal drug reactions could be prevented if the offending agent were withdrawn immediately, at the first sign of illness.

SUGGESTED READINGS

Arunded C, Lewis JH: Drug-induced liver disease in 2006. Curr Opin Gastroenterol 2007;23:244–254. *A practical update of the literature.*

Bjornsson E, Jerlstad P, Bergqvist A, et al: Fulminant drug-induced hepatic failure leading to death or liver transplantation in Sweden. Scand J Gastroenterol 2005;40:1095–1101. *A comprehensive study.*

Larson AM, Fontana RJ, Davern TJ, et al: Acetaminophen-induced acute liver failure: Results of a United States multicenter, prospective study. Hepatology 2005;42:1364–1372. *Overview of acetaminophen poisoning in the United States based on 275 cases.*

Lee WM: Medical progress: Drug-induced hepatotoxicity. N Engl J Med 2003; 349:474–485. *Review of hepatotoxicity, specific drugs involved, and the role of the FDA in monitoring drug toxicity.*

154 INHERITED AND METABOLIC HEPATIC DISORDERS

Kris V. Kowdley

INHERITED LIVER DISORDERS

Inherited Liver Disorders in Which the Metabolic Disorder Is Localized to the Liver (Table 154–1)

Wilson's Disease

Definition

In Wilson's disease, a disorder of copper metabolism leads to progressive accumulation of copper in the liver and various other tissues with eventual tissue toxicity and end-organ damage. Copper accumulates within the liver because of failure to excrete copper in bile, which is the major method of elimination of copper from the body.

TABLE 154–1 INHERITED AND METABOLIC DISORDERS OF THE LIVER

Inherited liver disorders in which the metabolic disorder is localized to the liver
Wilson's disease
α_1-Antitrypsin deficiency
Glycogen storage disease types I and IV
Amyloidosis, including familial amyloidotic polyneuropathy
Inherited disorders in which the metabolic disorder is extrahepatic
Hereditary hemochromatosis
Erythropoietic protoporphyria
Gaucher's disease
Inherited diseases in which the metabolic disorder is systemic but liver involvement is a major component
Cystic fibrosis
Miscellaneous
Liver disease associated with pregnancy
Liver disease associated with total parenteral nutrition

Epidemiology and Pathobiology

The Wilson disease gene, *ATP7B*, is on chromosome 13 and encodes an intracellular P-type adenosine triphosphatase located within the Golgi complex in hepatocytes. The frequency of *ATP7B* mutations ranges from 1 in 90 to 1 in 150, and estimates of the prevalence of Wilson's disease are between 1 in 30,000 and 1 in 60,000. More than 200 mutations of the *ATP7B* gene, including deletions, insertions, and missense or nonsense mutations, can cause phenotypic Wilson's disease, and the phenotypic pattern may vary among different genotypes. The usual presumed mode of inheritance is autosomal recessive, but some mutations may be present in heterozygous or homozygous forms, whereas others may be compound heterozygous forms.

Pathophysiology

Loss or deficiency of functional ATP7B results in reduced vesicular secretion of copper into bile and impaired incorporation of copper into ceruloplasmin. Consequently, copper accumulates in hepatocytes and extrahepatic sites, particularly in the central nervous system, kidneys, endocrine organs, heart, and musculoskeletal system. Over time, copper accumulation in the liver leads to chronic liver injury. Acute release of copper from the liver may result in a characteristic syndrome of acute fulminate liver failure (Chapter 158), Coombs-negative hemolytic anemia, and a Fanconi syndrome type of renal tubular defect (Chapter 123).

Clinical Manifestations

The clinical features of Wilson's disease are varied and may include liver disease, neurologic or psychiatric abnormalities, renal disease, osteoporosis, osteoarthritis, chondrocalcinosis, cardiac disease, hemolytic anemia, and endocrine abnormalities such as infertility, amenorrhea, and hypoparathyroidism. The age at diagnosis ranges from 5 years to older than 80 years, with the diagnosis made in about 50% of patients by 15 years of age.

Most patients with Wilson's disease demonstrate evidence of liver disease that may range from nonspecific changes such as microvesicular and macrovesicular steatosis to chronic active hepatitis, fibrosis, fulminant hepatitis, and cirrhosis with portal hypertension. Chronic hepatitis, the most common manifestation of hepatic Wilson's disease, may be difficult to differentiate from chronic hepatitis of other causes (Chapter 152), so Wilson's disease should be included in the differential diagnosis of any patient with chronic liver disease. Fulminant hepatitis is frequently associated with Coombs-negative hemolytic anemia, as well as with low serum alkaline phosphatase and uric acid levels. Liver cancer is uncommon in patients with Wilson's disease.

Neuropsychiatric symptoms of Wilson's disease generally occur in the second decade of life and follow signs of liver disease. Motor disorders are typically observed and may include tremors, dysarthria, micrographia, drooling, and pseudobulbar palsy; dysphagia may result in weight loss. Psychiatric symptoms may range from anxiety to personality disorders to frank psychosis.

Diagnosis

The diagnosis of Wilson's disease requires a high level of clinical suspicion, usually because of the presence of hemolytic anemia or neurologic or neuropsychiatric disease in addition to the liver disease. The initial diagnostic test is the serum ceruloplasmin level, which is generally less than 20 mg/dL. Hypoproteinemia may result in reduced serum ceruloplasmin levels in the absence of Wilson's disease. Conversely, ceruloplasmin is an acute phase reactant that may be falsely elevated into the normal range in patients with Wilson's disease. Although the total serum copper level is low in parallel with the low ceruloplasmin level, the free serum copper level is elevated (>25 μg/dL). Similarly, urinary copper excretion usually exceeds 100 μg/24 hr in symptomatic patients, but it can be normal in asymptomatic individuals.

A decreased serum ceruloplasmin level should raise suspicion for Wilson's disease but does not confirm the diagnosis. Liver biopsy to measure the hepatic copper concentration and measurement of total urinary copper excretion over a 24-hour period are considered confirmatory tests for the diagnosis of Wilson's disease. Hepatic copper concentrations greater than 250 μg/g dry weight (normal, <35 μg/g) are often found in untreated patients with Wilson's disease, but the hepatic copper concentration may also be elevated into the range associated with Wilson's disease in patients with chronic cholestatic disorders because copper is normally excreted through bile.

Treatment

Rx

Medical treatment is based on copper chelating agents, which bind copper and allow it to be excreted in urine. Trientine at a dose of 1.0 to 1.2 g/day has largely replaced D-penicillamine at a dose of 1.0 to 1.5 g/day as the initial copper chelator of choice because it is less toxic. Chelators are indicated in patients with evidence of significantly increased copper stores (i.e., ≥250 μg/g); lifelong therapy is frequently needed to achieve negative copper balance and to remove excess copper from parenchymal tissues. Zinc acetate at a dose of 50 mg three times daily is an alternative treatment option for patients in whom Wilson's disease is diagnosed early in the course of the disease, before the development of significant end-organ damage, or as maintenance therapy after negative copper balance has been achieved and storage sites have been depleted, as evidenced by a reduction in urinary copper excretion (i.e., <500 mg/24 hr) after initial cupruresis. Zinc inhibits the intentional absorption of copper via induction of metallothionein in the intestine. New agents being tested include ammonium tetrathiomolybdate, particularly for neurologic Wilson's disease.

Liver transplantation is indicated for fulminant hepatic failure, liver dysfunction unresponsive to chelation, or noncompliance with chelation therapy. Liver transplantation is curative in Wilson's disease because the primary site of the metabolic defect is in the liver. As serum ceruloplasmin and copper levels return to normal after liver transplantation, neuropsychiatric symptoms may improve, although this possibility is not a primary indication for liver transplantation.

α_1-Antitrypsin Deficiency

Definition and Epidemiology

α_1-Antitrypsin deficiency (Chapter 88) is an autosomal recessive disorder with a prevalence of 1 in 1550 to 2800 among populations of northern European descent. It has been estimated that approximately 116 million individuals carry the trait and that 1.1 million have clinically significant α_1-antitrypsin deficiency.

Pathobiology

α_1-Antitrypsin, a 52-kD glycoprotein, is secreted into blood by hepatocytes, phagocytes, and epithelial cells in the lungs. The protein is an inhibitor of serine proteases, primarily human neutrophil elastase. Absent or severely reduced α_1-antitrypsin levels may result in emphysema as a result of degradation of connective tissue. The associated liver disease is a consequence of progressive accumulation of deformed, aggregated polymers of α_1-antitrypsin in the endoplasmic reticulum of hepatocytes, as seen by periodic acid–Schiff staining of histologic specimens.

The more than 75 structural variants of α_1-antitrypsin can be classified by their migration velocity on starch gel electrophoresis as F (fast), M (medium), S (slow), or Z (very slow). The most common phenotypes associated with normal α_1-antitrypsin levels (85 to 215 mg/dL) are the M1 to M4 variants. The Z variant is the most common deficiency variant; patients homozygous for this mutation (designated PiZZ) have only 15% normal α_1-antitrypsin levels with an increased risk for lung or liver disease. The S variant is also a common "deficient" variant with α_1-antitrypsin levels less than 80 mg/dL. Null or QO variants have undetectable plasma levels of α_1-antitrypsin and an increased risk for emphysema but not liver disease.

Clinical Manifestations

α_1-Antitrypsin deficiency is the most common cause of inherited liver disease in neonates and children. In the newborn, liver disease may initially be manifested as jaundice at 4 to 8 weeks of age. Many such patients will have spontaneous resolution of jaundice and cholestasis and become asymptomatic by 1 year of age. Patients with persistent symptoms may demonstrate any feature of chronic liver disease or bleeding, including chronic active hepatitis, cryptogenic cirrhosis, or portal hypertension. The odds ratio for liver disease and hepatocellular carcinoma in adult homozygotes has been estimated to be 8.3 to 18.3 and 5.0, respectively.

Diagnosis

α_1-Antitrypsin deficiency should be included in the differential diagnosis of any patient with unexplained chronic liver disease or hepatocellular carcinoma. The key initial diagnostic test is a low serum α_1-antitrypsin level (<85 mg/dL), although the value may be increased into the normal range as an acute phase reactant or be decreased because of hypoproteinemia in patients with other causes of liver dysfunction. Confirmation of the diagnosis requires demonstration of an abnormal α_1-antitrypsin phenotype (such as PiZZ) and evidence of periodic acid–Schiff–positive, diastase-resistant globules on liver biopsy.

Treatment

Rx

No specific medical therapy is available for the liver disease of α_1-antitrypsin deficiency. Because it is now believed that phenotypic expression of α_1-antitrypsin deficiency requires both increased accumulation and decreased degradation of the abnormal protein, patients should avoid alcohol or other hepatotoxins that may reduce clearance of the abnormal protein. Treatment is otherwise aimed at management of the complications of chronic liver disease. Liver transplantation (Chapter 158) should be offered to patients with decompensated liver disease. α_1-Antitrypsin deficiency is the most common inherited liver disease for which liver transplantation is performed in children.

Glycogen Storage Diseases

The hepatic glycogen storage diseases (Chapter 219) include a rare group of inherited enzymatic disorders in which the metabolism of glycogen to glucose is impaired. Consequently, excess glycogen accumulates in the liver, heart, muscle, kidney, and other organs, where it leads to organ dysfunction. The three major glycogen storage diseases that lead to liver disease are types I, III, and IV, each of which is inherited in an autosomal recessive pattern and is associated with specific enzymatic deficiencies.

Type I (Von Gierke's Disease)

Definition and Pathobiology

This disorder (Chapter 219) results from a deficiency in glucose-6-phosphatase, an enzyme expressed in the hepatic microsomal system and also in the renal tubular epithelium, pancreas, and intestine. Loss-of-function mutations in the gene encoding glucose-6-phosphatase reduce the activity of this enzyme, thereby resulting in accumulation of glycogen in multiple organs.

Clinical Manifestations

The disease may be manifested in infancy and rarely in adulthood with hypoglycemia, lactic acidosis, hyperlipidemia, and hyperuricemia. Clinical features include failure to thrive, growth retardation, and hypoglycemic seizures. Hepatomegaly, elevated serum bilirubin levels, and abnormal serum aminotransferase levels may be observed as a result of increased glycogen deposition. Children may be disposed to the development of hepatocellular adenomas with a high risk for subsequent malignant transformation. Other complications include renal disease, renal stones, and osteoporosis. The diagnosis is confirmed by demonstrating decreased or absent activity of glucose-6-phosphatase.

Treatment

Rx

Treatment is aimed at preventing hypoglycemia with multiple daytime carbohydrate feedings and enteral glucose administration. Diagnosis early in life can prevent irreversible complications and preserve growth and development. Liver transplantation, which has been performed in patients with progressive liver disease or neoplasms, corrects the underlying metabolic defect.

Type III

Type III glycogen storage disease is caused by a deficiency in amylo-1,6-glucosidase, an enzyme responsible for structural modification of glycogen. In contrast to other forms of glycogen storage disease, the phenotypic manifestations are less severe because of the availability of alternative methods of gluconeogenesis. However, significant end-organ damage may develop in the liver, musculoskeletal system, and heart. Medical management should focus on dietary protein intake as a source of gluconeogenic amino acids. There are anecdotal reports of successful liver transplantation for type III glycogen storage disease.

Type IV (Andersen's Disease)

Glycogen storage disease type IV (Chapter 219) is related to deficiency in another structural enzyme, α-1,4-α-1,6-glucosyltransferase, which results in accumulation of glycogen molecules similar to amylopectin. Type IV glycogen storage disease may be complicated by advanced liver disease, neurologic disease, cardiomyopathy, and skeletal muscle abnormalities. Liver transplantation is indicated for decompensated liver disease, but cardiac complications may reduce survival after liver transplantation.

Amyloidosis

Definition

Amyloidosis describes abnormal deposition of the fibrillar amyloid protein in various tissues (Chapter 296).

Clinical Manifestations

Amyloidosis may result in nonspecific signs and symptoms, but typical findings include macroglossia, heart failure, arrhythmias, hepatosplenomegaly, carpal tunnel syndrome, peripheral neuropathy, renal failure, and nephrotic-range proteinuria. Liver involvement occurs in about 60% of patients with systemic amyloidosis. Hepatic amyloidosis may be accompanied by abdominal pain and is commonly associated with a palpable, firm, and enlarged liver. Decompensated liver disease characterized by severe cholestasis and massive hepatic amyloid deposition is an uncommon late complication.

Diagnosis

Laboratory tests typically reveal an elevated serum alkaline phosphatase level (86%), hypoalbuminemia, proteinuria, and a monoclonal protein spike in serum or urine (89%). The diagnosis of amyloidosis is confirmed by demonstration of apple-green birefringence on polarization microscopy after Congo red staining of the affected tissue.

Treatment

For patients with secondary or AA amyloidosis, treatment of the primary disorder is indicated. For primary or AL amyloidosis, no treatment is curative, but melphalan, colchicine, and corticosteroids can improve survival (Chapter 296). Liver transplantation can be successful in patients with acute liver failure secondary to amyloidosis.

Familial Amyloidotic Polyneuropathy

Definition and Pathobiology

Familial amyloidotic polyneuropathy is a unique form of hereditary amyloidosis associated with the accumulation of amyloidogenic transthyretin (TTR, the most common type), gelsolin, or apolipoprotein A-I. It is an autosomal dominant disorder with variable penetrance, even in patients with the same mutation in the *TTR* gene. TTR is primarily synthesized in the liver and is bound to thyroxine or to a retinol binding protein in plasma. More than 100 mutations in the gene encoding TTR, which is located at 18q12.1, can create an abnormally folded TTR, thereby resulting in accumulation of fibrillar amyloid deposits.

Clinical Manifestations

The clinical manifestations, which are related to deposition of abnormal amyloid fibril in various parenchymal tissues, include sensorimotor and autonomic polyneuropathy, ocular disease, cerebral angiopathy, gastrointestinal dysmotility, cardiomyopathy, renal dysfunction, and hematologic sequelae.

Treatment

Familial amyloidotic polyneuropathy may be fatal. However, liver transplantation can correct the underlying metabolic defect and may prevent progressive neuromuscular disease, with reported overall survival rates of 82% at 1 year and 60% at 5 years. Therefore, liver transplantation has been recommended early in the course of disease, before the development of neurologic, cardiac, renal, or gastrointestinal disease.

Inherited Disorders in Which the Metabolic Disorder Is Extrahepatic

Hereditary Hemochromatosis

Definition

Hemochromatosis (Chapter 231) is a syndrome of end-organ damage caused by excessive deposition of iron in various tissues. At the present time, four types of primary iron overload disorders have been described, including HLA-linked hereditary hemochromatosis, one of the most common genetic disorders in the white population.

Pathobiology

HLA-linked hereditary hemochromatosis, or HFE-associated hemochromatosis (type 1), is the most common form. The normal HFE protein is a transmembrane protein localized to the basolateral aspect of the villus cell in the small intestine. HFE binds transferrin and appears to play a role in internalization of the transferrin–transferrin receptor complex. The *C282Y*-mutated HFE protein is trapped intracellularly and thus does not bind transferrin. Furthermore, hepatic release of hepcidin, a circulating peptide that has antimicrobial properties and inhibits iron absorption in the duodenum, appears to be inappropriately low in type 1 hereditary hemochromatosis. However, despite these observations, it remains unclear how the mutant HFE protein disrupts normal regulation of iron metabolism.

The other types of hereditary hemochromatosis are distinctly uncommon. Juvenile hemochromatosis, called type 2 hereditary hemochromatosis, may be associated with mutations in the hemojuvelin gene (*HJV*), which is located on chromosome 1 and encodes a glycosylphosphatidylinositol-linked membrane protein, or with mutations in *HAMP*, a gene located on chromosome 19 that encodes hepcidin. Type 3 hereditary hemochromatosis is associated with mutations in transferrin receptor 2 (TFR2), which is highly expressed in hepatocytes and thought to play a role in signaling the liver regarding body iron stores. Type 4 hereditary hemochromatosis is an autosomal dominant condition associated with mutations in ferroportin, a protein thought to be responsible for transporting iron out of cells.

Clinical Manifestations

Type 1 hereditary hemochromatosis is generally associated with the development of symptoms in middle age. Although men and women may inherit the mutation equally, phenotypic expression is milder in women and occurs later in their life. The clinical manifestation of type 1 hereditary hemochromatosis reflects the sequelae of iron deposition in multiple organs, including the liver, heart, pancreas, skin, joints, and anterior pituitary. The resulting classic complications may include cirrhosis and hepatocellular carcinoma, diabetes mellitus, cardiomyopathy, hyperpigmentation or "bronzing" of the skin, arthropathy of the metacarpophalangeal joints, and hypogonadotropic hypogonadism. However, most patients may be asymptomatic or have nonspecific symptoms such as weakness, lethargy, arthralgias, and abdominal pain. It should be emphasized that hepatic iron overload is also seen in alcoholic liver disease, which sometimes causes confusion between these two diagnoses. The development of cirrhosis is associated with an increased risk for hepatocellular carcinoma and reduced life expectancy.

Type II hereditary hemochromatosis is associated with severe phenotypic expression in the second and third decades of life. Men and women are affected equally, and cardiac manifestations predominate. Clinical features of iron overload associated with *TFR2* mutations (type II hereditary hemochromatosis) are similar to those of HFE-associated hereditary hemochromatosis. The pattern of hepatic iron deposition and clinical features in type IV hereditary hemochromatosis are different from other forms of hereditary hemochromatosis. This disorder is characterized by hepatic iron deposition predominantly in reticuloendothelial cells, frequently normal serum transferrin iron saturation, and increased serum ferritin levels.

Diagnosis

Appropriate evaluation of suspected hereditary hemochromatosis should include a complete medical history, family history, and physical examination. The initial screening test is measurement of the serum transferrin iron saturation percentage; if the saturation is 45% or greater, a repeat fasting measurement should be obtained along with a serum ferritin level. If the repeat serum transferrin iron saturation is 45% or higher, *HFE* gene testing is appropriate, especially if the serum ferritin level is elevated (>200 ng/mL in women and >300 ng/mL in men). The majority of white patients (>85%) with typical phenotypic hereditary hemochromatosis are homozygous for the *C282Y* mutation. Compound heterozygosity for the *C282Y* and *H63D* mutations is found in approximately 5% of patients who have clinical evidence of hereditary hemochromatosis, although the severity of iron loading is less in these patients. In individuals heterozygous for the *C282Y* mutation, iron overload typically does not develop except in the presence of another disorder such as chronic hepatitis C infection or alcoholic liver disease. Therefore, only the *C282Y* homozygous and *C282Y/H63D* compound heterozygous genotypes are currently considered diagnostic of type 1 hereditary hemochromatosis. Patients with suspected hereditary hemochromatosis based on elevated serum transferrin iron saturation who have either of these two mutation patterns can be confirmed to have hereditary hemochromatosis.

The diagnosis of hereditary hemochromatosis by phenotypic criteria is problematic in the setting of advanced liver disease. Serum iron studies may lack specificity for iron overload in this population because serum transferrin is frequently low as a result of decreased hepatic function and because it is a negative acute phase reactant. Furthermore, many patients with alcohol- or hepatitis C–related end-stage liver disease have hepatic iron overload despite the absence of *HFE* mutations.

Liver biopsy, previously considered to be the "gold standard" for the diagnosis of hereditary hemochromatosis, shows increased stainable iron in hepatocytes and bile duct cells with a paucity of iron in Kupffer cells and a hepatic iron concentration usually greater than 4000 μg/g dry weight. Liver biopsy remains important to identify possible cirrhosis in patients who are homozygous for *C282Y* or are *C282Y/H63D* compound heterozygotes if liver enzymes are elevated or if the serum ferritin level is 1000 ng/mL or greater. Liver biopsy should also be considered both to clarify the diagnosis and to exclude cirrhosis in patients who have elevated serum transferrin iron saturation and ferritin levels but are neither homozygous *C282Y* nor *C282Y/H63D* compound heterozygotes. Noninvasive measurement of hepatic iron content with magnetic resonance imaging and susceptometry for estimation of iron content and fibrosis may substitute for liver biopsy in the future.

Treatment

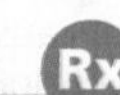

Iron reduction therapy by phlebotomy, which is the mainstay of treatment, is safe, easy, and inexpensive and should not be delayed until the development of symptoms. Weekly phlebotomy of 500 mL of whole blood is generally well tolerated. Phlebotomy is continued until iron depletion is confirmed by mild anemia and a ferritin concentration lower than 50 ng/mL, a process that may take up to 2 years. Maintenance phlebotomy is then continued throughout the patient's life, typically via removal of 1 to 2 units of blood three to four times a year to maintain a serum ferritin level of less than 50 ng/mL. Patients should likewise be counseled to avoid vitamin C supplements, which can increase the absorption of iron. Phlebotomy should also be offered to patients with evidence of cirrhosis because it probably improves quality of life and may decrease complications of portal hypertension. Fatigue, elevated liver enzymes, and hepatomegaly may improve after phlebotomy is undertaken. Cardiac function may improve if treatment is begun before the development of dilated cardiomyopathy. However, joint symptoms may not respond to therapy.

Although HFE-associated hereditary hemochromatosis is an uncommon indication for liver transplantation (Chapter 158), liver transplantation is the only effective treatment for patients with decompensated cirrhosis or hepatocellular carcinoma. However, survival after liver transplantation is adversely affected by the risk for cardiac and infectious complications.

Erythropoietic Protoporphyria

Definition and Pathobiology

The porphyrias (Chapter 229) are characterized by genetic or acquired abnormalities in enzymes involved in heme biosynthesis. A deficiency in ferrochelatase, which is responsible for the final step in heme synthesis, results in erythropoietic or erythrohepatic protoporphyria. Erythrohepatic protoporphyria has an autosomal dominant pattern of inheritance with variable penetrance. In a subset of patients, protoporphyrin accumulates in hepatocytes and bile duct cells after biliary canalicular excretion is overwhelmed by the excess protoporphyrin produced in the bone marrow.

Clinical Manifestations

The most common symptom is photosensitivity secondary to accumulation of protoporphyrin in skin and associated vasculature, a process that can lead to pruritus and an acute cutaneous erythematous reaction (see Fig. 465–11). Occasionally, burning and itching can occur in the absence of skin damage or may be associated with petechiae and purpuric lesions. Continued sun exposure leads to the formation of bullous skin lesions, cholestasis, and nodular cirrhosis. Pigmented gallstones can form as a consequence of hemolysis.

Diagnosis

Liver disease should be suspected in patients with elevated serum liver enzymes and markedly high erythrocyte protoporphyrin levels (<1500 μg/dL). Liver biopsy may reveal increased deposition of protoporphyrin.

Treatment

Therapies used to treat this disorder include high-dose oral β-carotene supplementation, erythrocyte transfusion, intravenous heme administration, oral charcoal, oral cholestyramine, or oral chenodeoxycholic acid. Progressive liver disease, cirrhosis, and hepatic failure may require liver transplantation, which has been reported to have good outcomes, although great care must be taken to avoid cholestasis, such as from the formation of biliary strictures, because the ferrochelatase deficiency is unchanged and the excess production of protoporphyrin in bone marrow and elevated levels of protoporphyrin in erythrocytes and feces persist after liver replacement.

Inherited Diseases with a Systemic Metabolic Disorder and Significant Liver Involvement

Cystic Fibrosis

Definition and Epidemiology

Cystic fibrosis (Chapter 89) is a relatively common genetic disease in white individuals, with an incidence of 1 in 3000 newborns. The disease, which is inherited in an autosomal recessive pattern, is the result of a mutation in the gene on chromosome 7 that encodes the cystic fibrosis transmembrane regulator (CFTR) and regulates an apical cyclic adenosine monophosphate–dependent chloride channel that is ubiquitous in cells lining the epithelia of various tissues, including the bronchial tree, pancreatic ducts, bile ducts, sweat ducts, intestinal tract, and vas deferens. A large number of mutations result in variable penetrance and expressivity. The prevalence of cystic fibrosis–associated liver disease ranges from a low of 2% to a high of 68% in children and adolescents. However, it is likely that the prevalence of liver disease is increasing, given the improvements in management and longer life expectancy. Liver disease is now the second leading cause of death in patients with cystic fibrosis.

Pathobiology

The pathophysiology of liver disease is related to the lack of CFTR in bile duct epithelial cells, which results in obstruction of bile ducts by inspissated bile with a high protein content. Consequently, intrahepatic cholestasis and extrahepatic bile duct obstruction lead to jaundice and cirrhosis. The histologic features are consistent with a biliary tract disease and may be evidenced by periductular inflammation in addition to focal or diffuse biliary cirrhosis. Liver disease is associated with a history of meconium ileus and pancreatic insufficiency.

Clinical Manifestation and Diagnosis

Cystic fibrosis–associated liver disease may become apparent within the first decade of life, but the prevalence of liver disease increases over time into the teenage years and early adulthood. Ultimately, liver disease develops in up to 40% of patients, and advanced liver disease may develop in 2 to 8%. Once cirrhosis is established, portal hypertension and its complications may ensue, including hepatosplenomegaly, ascites, variceal bleeding, and liver failure. The presence of portal hypertension is a marker for worse prognosis, with a mean survival of 4.5 years after diagnosis.

Treatment

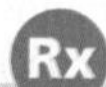

Treatment should focus on nutrition, especially fat-soluble vitamins, essential fatty acids, and mineral deficiencies, as in patients with pancreatic insufficiency of other causes (Chapter 147). High-dose ursodeoxycholic acid (20 to 30 mg/kg/day) appears to improve biochemical parameters but has not been shown to improve clinical outcomes.

Liver transplantation has been used successfully to treat advanced liver disease. Candidates for liver-only transplantation should have stable lung function with a forced vital capacity of 75% of the predicted value or greater and a forced expiratory volume in 1 second of 70% or greater. Outcome after liver transplantation in patients with cystic fibrosis is comparable to other indications, with long-term survival rates of up to 75%. Combined lung-liver or heart-lung-liver transplantation should be considered in patients with severe pulmonary disease, hypercapnia, recurrent lung infections, colonization with multidrug-resistant organisms, diminished pulmonary reserve, hepatopulmonary syndrome, or severe pulmonary hypertension. A transjugular intrahepatic portosystemic shunt or a surgical portosystemic shunt can be used to manage severe variceal hemorrhage in patients with otherwise compensated liver disease or those who are not candidates for liver transplantation.

NONINHERITED METABOLIC HEPATIC DISORDERS

Liver Diseases of Pregnancy

Liver diseases unique to pregnancy include hyperemesis gravidarum, intrahepatic cholestasis of pregnancy, HELLP syndrome (*h*emolysis, *e*levated *l*iver enzymes, and *l*ow *p*latelet count), and acute fatty liver of pregnancy (Table 154–2).

Hyperemesis Gravidarum

The symptoms of this condition, the pathogenesis of which is unknown, include severe nausea and vomiting in the first trimester and rarely after 20 weeks of gestation. The incidence is 0.35 to 0.8%. Up to 50% of patients have abnormal liver enzymes, although the degree of elevation is mild to moderate. Treatment is supportive with hydration and antiemetics.

Intrahepatic Cholestasis of Pregnancy

Intrahepatic cholestasis is generally observed in the second trimester of pregnancy. The etiopathology is likely to be due to increased sensitivity to the cholestatic effects of estrogen in a genetically predisposed individual. Mutations in the gene encoding a biliary canalicular phospholipid transporter may account for some cases.

Clinical Manifestations and Diagnosis

The clinical features, which include severe pruritus and jaundice in the mother, may result in prematurity and an increased risk for fetal demise. Elevated serum bile acid levels are the hallmark of the diagnosis; increased serum bilirubin and aminotransferase levels are frequent. Jaundice develops in a large proportion of patients a few weeks after the onset of itching. Liver biopsy may reveal primarily a cholestatic reaction with bile plugs in zone 3 and a paucity of periportal inflammation or necrosis. However, liver biopsy is not usually needed for diagnosis.

TABLE 154–2 LIVER DISEASES UNIQUE TO PREGNANCY

	Trimester of Onset	Symptoms	Laboratory Abnormalities	Recurrence with Future Pregnancies
Hyperemesis gravidarum	1	Nausea, vomiting	Mild to moderate elevation in AST/ALT, occasionally hyperbilirubinemia	
Cholestasis	2, 3	Pruritus, jaundice	Bile acids >8 μM, elevated AST/ALT and bilirubin in more severe cases	Common
Acute fatty liver	3	Nausea, vomiting, abdominal pain	Elevated AST/ALT (100–1000 U/L), bilirubin >5 mg/dL, prolonged prothrombin time*	Rare
HELLP syndrome	2, 3, or postpartum	Abdominal pain, nausea, vomiting	Elevated AST/ALT (60–1500 U/L), platelets <100,000/mm^3, LDH >600 U/L, hemolytic anemia	3–25%

*Useful diagnostic distinction from HELLP syndrome in which the prothrombin time, partial thromboplastin time, and fibrinogen are usually normal.
ALT = alanine aminotransferase; AST = aspartate aminotransferase; HELLP = hemolysis, elevated liver enzymes, and low platelet count; LDH = lactate dehydrogenase.

Treatment

Rx

Symptoms may be treated with antihistamines or cholestyramine, but severe disease may require early delivery. The syndrome may recur with future pregnancies.

HELLP Syndrome

HELLP syndrome is most commonly observed in the third trimester of pregnancy. It is usually diagnosed at 32 to 34 weeks' gestation. Associated conditions include preeclampsia, which is diagnosed by the triad of hypertension, proteinuria, and edema.

Clinical Manifestations and Prognosis

Patients may have no symptoms or may report nonspecific abdominal pain. Aminotransferase levels may exceed 1000 U/L. Coagulopathy may be present if the hemolysis is severe and associated with disseminated intravascular coagulation. The peripheral blood smear reveals schistocytes and burr cells, although the period of active hemolysis may be transient. Serum haptoglobin should be measured if the peripheral smear is not consistent with hemolysis. Thrombocytopenia with a platelet count lower than 100,000 is typical, but low platelet counts are not pathognomonic for HELLP syndrome because thrombocytopenia is present in up to 8% of pregnant women.

Histopathologic analysis of liver tissue may demonstrate periportal hemorrhage and fibrin deposition. The differential diagnosis includes hemolytic-uremic syndrome (Chapter 179), thrombocytopenic purpura (Chapter 179), acute viral hepatitis (Chapter 151), and acute fatty liver of pregnancy.

The most serious complication of HELLP syndrome is the development of hepatic infarction, which may be accompanied by subcapsular hematoma or intraperitoneal hemorrhage. Clues to this complication include an acute onset of severe abdominal pain, fever, and a marked elevation in aminotransferase levels (>5000 U/L). Immediate surgical intervention may be required in such cases, and the risk for mortality is increased.

Treatment

Treatment of HELLP syndrome is primarily early delivery, which generally resolves the abnormalities. If the fetus has not yet reached 37 weeks' gestation, corticosteroids can be given to promote fetal lung development and may help stabilize the syndrome itself. [1]

Acute Fatty Liver of Pregnancy

Acute fatty liver of pregnancy is a rare complication, usually seen in the last trimester, with an incidence of 1 in 13,000 to 16,000. Primigravidas account for up to 70% of cases, and the average maternal age is the middle of the second decade. The etiology of acute fatty liver of pregnancy is unknown.

Clinical Manifestations and Diagnosis

Patients may be asymptomatic or may have right upper quadrant or epigastric pain that may mimic acute cholecystitis or reflux esophagitis. The disease may progress rapidly within days to acute liver failure with hepatic encephalopathy, ascites, edema, and renal insufficiency. Preeclampsia is present in more than 50% of patients.

Marked jaundice and hyperbilirubinemia are common, and the serum bilirubin level may rise to greater than 40 mg/dL. Extrahepatic complications include gastrointestinal bleeding and renal dysfunction, which may require dialysis. Pancreatitis may develop in up to 30% of patients, and severe hypoglycemia may be seen in 25 to 50%.

Liver biopsy, which confirms the diagnosis, reveals vacuolization of hepatocytes and pallor in the central zone regions; microvascular steatosis is characteristic. Fresh-frozen tissue should be used to stain for fat.

Treatment

Acute fatty liver of pregnancy should be considered a medical and obstetric emergency. Patients should be promptly admitted to a liver failure unit; urgent liver transplantation may be needed. Mortality rates may be up to 15% even with early delivery, and fetal demise is common.

Liver Disease with Parenteral Nutrition

Liver disease may develop in up 40% of adult patients who receive chronic nutritional supplementation with long-term total parenteral nutrition (TPN; Chapter 236) for intestinal failure. The liver disease associated with TPN is quite variable and may include fatty infiltration (steatosis), biliary calculous disease (microlithiasis and macrolithiasis), and intrahepatic cholestasis with variable degrees of fibrosis. Fortunately, progressive liver disease with cirrhosis and its attendant complications are uncommon. Parenteral carbohydrates, which are converted to triglycerides, presumably contribute to the hepatic steatosis. Increased administration of lipid emulsions and possibly deficiencies of certain choline or other nutrients may also contribute to the steatosis. Other contributing factors include reduced bile flow, decreased intestinal secretion of gastrointestinal hormones, and cholestasis. A short residual functional small bowel may contribute to impaired enterohepatic circulation of bile salts.

Prevention and Treatment

Strategies to reduce the likelihood and severity of hepatic involvement associated with the use of TPN include attention to adequate vitamin supplementation, administration of adequate choline, [2] balancing the lipid and carbohydrate content of TPN solutions, [3] and the use of enteral nutrition whenever possible. Ursodeoxycholic acid therapy may be helpful to avoid cholestasis and promote bile flow.

Grade A

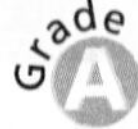

1. Magann EF, Bass D, Chauhan SP, et al: Antepartum corticosteroids: Disease stabilization in patients with the syndrome of hemolysis, elevated liver enzymes, and low platelets (HELLP). Am J Obstet Gynecol 1994;171:1148–1153.
2. Buchmiller CE, Kleiman-Wexler RL, Ephgrave KS, et al: Liver dysfunction and energy source: Results of a randomized clinical trial. JPEN J Parenter Enteral Nutr 1993;17:301–306.
3. Buchman AL, Ament ME, Sohel M, et al: Choline deficiency causes reversible hepatic abnormalities in patients receiving parenteral nutrition: Proof of a human choline requirement: A placebo-controlled trial. JPEN J Parenter Enteral Nutr 2001;25:260–268.

SUGGESTED READINGS

Alexander J, Kowdley KV: Hereditary hemochromatosis: Genetics, pathogenesis, and clinical management. Ann Hepatol 2005;4:240–247. *Review of clinical aspects with a suggested approach to management.*

Ando Y, Nakamura M, Araki S: Transthyretin-related familial amyloidotic polyneuropathy. Arch Neurol 2005;62:1057–1062. *Emphasizes the molecular genetics, with a suggested diagnostic algorithm.*

Brewer GJ, Askari FK: Wilson's disease: Clinical management and therapy. J Hepatol 2005;42:S13–S21. *Review of clinical manifestations and treatment options.*

Brigman C, Feranchak A: Liver involvement in cystic fibrosis. Curr Treat Options Gastroenterol 2006;9:484–496. *Practical recommendations.*

Kelly DA: Intestinal failure–associated liver disease: What do we know today? Gastroenterology 2006;130:S70–S77. *A comprehensive review.*

Park MA, Mueller PS, Kyle RA, et al: Primary (AL) hepatic amyloidosis: Clinical features and natural history in 98 patients. Medicine (Baltimore) 2003; 82:291–298. *A comprehensive treatise describing one of the largest cohorts with this condition.*

Perlmutter DH: Alpha-1-antitrypsin deficiency: Diagnosis and treatment. Clin Liver Dis 2004;8:839–859. *Review of basic science, diagnostic testing, and management.*

Pietrangelo A: Hereditary hemochromatosis—a new look at an old disease. N Engl J Med 2004;350:2383–2397. *State-of-the-art review with a particular focus on newer forms of hereditary hemochromatosis.*

155 BACTERIAL, PARASITIC, FUNGAL, AND GRANULOMATOUS LIVER DISEASES

Brent A. Neuschwander-Tetri

Epidemiology

Infection of the liver by nonviral pathogens accounts for a large burden of human disease worldwide. In developed countries, where chronic viral hepatitis (Chapter 152) is the most common form of infectious disease of the liver, diagnosis and treatment of nonviral infections of the liver continue to be a significant clinical challenge. In less-developed regions, amebae, other protozoa, and helminths such as *Schistosoma* are enormous public health problems. Up to 10% of the world's population is colonized with *Entamoeba histolytica* or schistosomal species, thus underscoring the need for effective treatment and public health measures.

Diagnosis

Nonviral infections of the liver often result in an indolent course of fever, right upper quadrant abdominal pain, and malaise. In this setting, routine testing of blood, determination of liver enzymes, and abdominal imaging may lead to a general diagnosis of nonviral liver infection. Serologic testing and aspirates of focal lesions identified within the liver lead to a specific diagnosis and guide appropriate therapy. A common difficulty in establishing a specific diagnosis in developed countries is distinguishing between amebic liver abscess and bacterial (pyogenic) liver abscess. Other nonviral infectious diseases and granulomatous liver diseases often present an additional diagnostic challenge.

BACTERIAL INFECTIONS OF THE LIVER

Bacterial (Pyogenic) Abscess

Definition

A *bacterial,* or *pyogenic,* liver abscess is a focal accumulation of purulent necro-inflammatory debris within the liver parenchyma caused by single or multiple bacterial pathogens.

Epidemiology

Because bacterial liver abscesses are the result of diverse infections such as biliary tract infections (Chapter 159), intra-abdominal infections (e.g., diverticulitis and appendicitis, Chapter 145), extra-abdominal infections (e.g., bacterial endocarditis, Chapter 76), or infections of the oral cavity, their incidence shows no major gender, ethnic, or geographic influence. The typical age of patients is 50 to 70 years, an age when diverticulitis and biliary tract occlusion by stones or malignancy are more prevalent.

Pathobiology

Bacterial liver abscesses most commonly develop as a result of seeding of the liver through an infected biliary tract (cholangitis) or bacteremia (Table 155–1). Bacteremia of portal blood flow is caused by focal infections in regions drained by the mesenteric circulation. Appendicitis and diverticulitis are the two most common infections associated with liver abscesses. Inflammatory bowel disease, especially Crohn's disease (Chapter 144), is a major risk factor because of the compromised mucosal barrier separating enteric bacteria from the circulation. Cirrhosis (Chapter 157) is also a risk factor for liver abscess formation, probably because of impaired clearance of transient portal bacteremia by the cirrhotic liver. Systemic bacteremia caused by untreated infections of the oral cavity or bacterial endocarditis likewise predisposes to the development of bacterial liver abscesses. Less common causes include blunt or penetrating trauma to the liver and extension of an adjacent abscess into the liver parenchyma. Penetrating trauma may be obvious, as in the case

TABLE 155–1 CONDITIONS THAT PREDISPOSE TO BACTERIAL LIVER ABSCESSES

MAJOR
Bacterial cholangitis (typically caused by biliary tract manipulation, duct obstruction by stones, malignancy, *Ascaris lumbricoides*)
Diverticulitis
Appendicitis
Alcoholism
Diabetes
LESS COMMON
Inflammatory bowel disease
Peptic ulcer
Cirrhosis
Necrotizing pancreatitis
Omphalitis
Bacterial endocarditis
Pneumonia
Pelvic inflammatory disease
Hemorrhoidal abscess
Poor oral hygiene
Iatrogenic bacteremia (line sepsis)
Penetrating liver trauma
Liver necrosis (blunt trauma, sickle crisis)
Tumor necrosis within the liver
Neutrophil defects (chronic granulomatous disease, leukemia)
Hemochromatosis (*Yersinia enterocolitica*)

of a knife wound, or less obvious, such as penetration of an ingested toothpick or fish bone from the duodenum into the liver. Bacterial liver abscesses are multifocal in about 50% of patients.

The organisms responsible for bacterial liver abscesses reflect the underlying source of bacteremia. Colonic flora such as *Escherichia coli, Klebsiella pneumoniae,* and viridans streptococci are common pathogens when primary colonic infections such as diverticulitis, appendicitis, and inflammatory bowel disease are the predisposing processes. Such abscesses are typically polymicrobial and may involve coexisting enteric anaerobes such as *Bacteroides* species. Abscesses in the setting of endocarditis are generally monomicrobial and are due to organisms such as *Staphylococcus aureus.*

Clinical Manifestations

The symptoms of a bacterial liver abscess are nonspecific. Fever, malaise, loss of appetite, and weight loss are the most common. Surprisingly, fever is absent in 5 to 20% of patients. Right upper quadrant abdominal pain is helpful in leading to an appropriate evaluation, but it is present in less than half the patients. Jaundice is even less common unless the underlying infection is cholangitis secondary to biliary obstruction. About a third of patients have nausea and vomiting.

Diagnosis

Identifying the presence of a liver abscess as a cause of nonspecific constitutional symptoms requires a high index of suspicion. Physical examination reveals right upper quadrant abdominal tenderness and hepatomegaly in 50% of patients. Laboratory testing typically reveals a leukocytosis. Blood cultures may be negative. Liver enzymes are usually normal to mildly elevated unless biliary obstruction is present, in which case alkaline phosphatase can be substantially elevated. The chest radiograph may identify an elevated right hemidiaphragm. Imaging of the abdomen by ultrasonography (US) or computed tomography (CT) with intravenous contrast (Fig. 155–1) identifies single or multiple abscesses within the liver. CT has somewhat better sensitivity, and both US and CT are superior to technetium-labeled sulfur colloid scanning.

The greatest challenge facing a clinician in the management of a liver abscess is distinguishing a bacterial abscess from an amebic abscess (Table 155–2) and an echinococcal cyst. In the absence of fever and leukocytosis, a noninvasive approach for obtaining imaging studies plus serologic tests for *Entamoeba histolytica* and *Echinococcus granulosus* is reasonable. If these tests are negative, if fever and leukocytosis are present, or if a focal lesion is suspected of being a bacterial abscess, US- or CT-guided needle aspiration with Gram stain and culture of the aspirate is indicated.

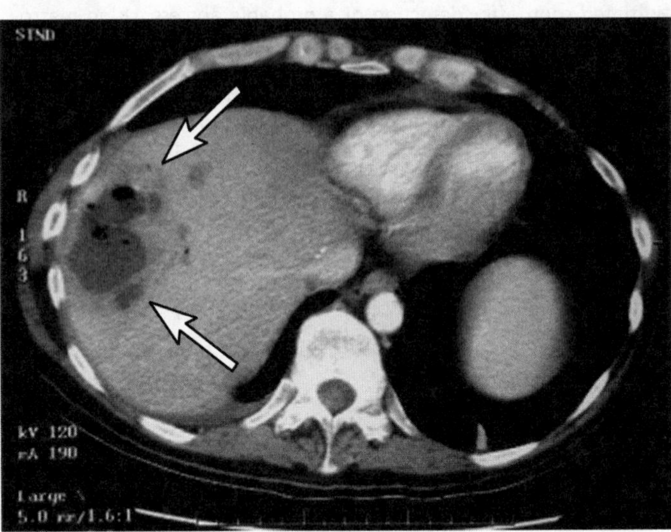

FIGURE 155–1 • Bacterial abscess. An abdominal computed tomography scan obtained after intravenous contrast administration demonstrates an irregular hypodense area containing gas bubbles in the right lobe of the liver (arrows). Aspiration revealed purulent material from which *Klebsiella pneumoniae* organisms were cultured.

TABLE 155–2 DISTINGUISHING FEATURES OF BACTERIAL AND AMEBIC ABSCESSES OF THE LIVER

	Bacterial Liver Abscess	Amebic Liver Abscess
Demographics	Age: 50–70 yr Equal gender ratio	Age: 20–40 yr Strong male preponderance (>10:1)
Major risk factors	Recent bacterial infection, especially intra-abdominal Biliary obstruction/manipulation Diabetes mellitus	Travel to or living in an endemic area (even in the remote past)
Symptoms	Right upper quadrant abdominal pain, fever, chills, rigors, weakness, malaise, anorexia, weight loss, diarrhea, cough, pleuritic chest pain	Acute manifestation: high fever, chills, abdominal pain, sepsis Subacute manifestation: weight loss; fever and abdominal pain less common Typically no symptoms of enteric colonization or colitis
Signs	Tender hepatomegaly, abdominal mass, jaundice	Variable right upper quadrant abdominal tenderness
Laboratory testing	Leukocytosis, anemia, elevated liver enzymes (alkaline phosphatase more than aminotransferases), elevated bilirubin, hypoalbuminemia Blood cultures positive in 50–60%	Positive amebic serology (70–95%) Variable leukocytosis and anemia No eosinophilia Alkaline phosphatase elevated but aminotransferases usually normal
Imaging	Abscesses are multifocal in 50% Usually right lobe Irregular margins	Typically single abscess in 80% Usually right lobe Round or oval, can be septated Wall enhancement on computed tomography scan with intravenous contrast
Aspirate	Purulent Organisms on Gram stain Culture positive in 80% with proper handling	Variable consistency and color Sterile Trophozoites rarely visualized

Treatment

Rx

Once a bacterial abscess of the liver is suspected, treatment with antibiotics should also be initiated. In the setting of a known predisposing infection such as *S. aureus* endocarditis, antibiotic therapy can be tailored immediately to the probable organism. In most circumstances, however, empirical therapy (e.g., ceftriaxone, 2 g intravenously every 24 hours, and metronidazole, 500 mg every 8 hours, until adequate drainage is achieved and the patient is stable, at which time oral antibiotics should be continued for a total of 4 to 6 weeks) directed at enteric flora, including anaerobes, should be initiated soon after detection of a probable abscess. Using metronidazole to treat possible anaerobic coinfection offers the additional advantage of effectively treating *E. histolytica* when an amebic abscess has not been excluded. Delays in initiating therapy while arranging for aspiration and culture should be avoided.

Most bacterial abscesses of the liver should be treated with percutaneous drainage as well as antibiotics, but small abscesses in patients who are not severely ill can be successfully managed with antibiotics alone. Multiple large abscesses and abscesses not responding to percutaneous drainage may require surgical drainage. Effective drainage of an obstructed biliary tract, either endoscopically or percutaneously, is also necessary when cholangitis has led to liver abscess formation.

Prognosis

Bacterial abscesses respond well to drainage and appropriate antibiotic therapy. However, if appropriate diagnostic testing does not lead to effective treatment in timely fashion, death from sepsis is the most likely outcome.

Other Bacterial Liver Infections

Listeria monocytogenes (Chapter 316) infection commonly involves the liver in neonates and occasionally gives rise to a clinical picture of acute hepatitis in adults. Preexisting liver disease is a major risk factor for liver involvement; it is manifested as elevations in liver enzymes and is diagnosed by positive blood cultures.

Yersinia enterocolitica (Chapter 333) infection may cause multiple liver abscesses when active enteric infection, usually manifested as terminal ileitis, develops in patients with underlying cirrhosis, diabetes, or hemochromatosis. If abscesses are large, drainage and antibiotics are indicated. *Salmonella typhi* and *Salmonella paratyphi* infections (Chapter 329) can be associated with aminotransferase elevations that range from mild to severe, sometimes mimicking viral hepatitis. Jaundice is occasionally seen.

Legionnaires' disease (Chapter 335) causes mild elevations in aminotransferase and alkaline phosphatase levels in more than half the cases. Direct liver infection can be seen on liver biopsy, but biopsy is rarely indicated because the hepatic abnormalities gradually improve with appropriate antibiotic treatment.

Ehrlichiosis (Chapter 348) usually causes aminotransferase elevations that range from mild to severe, even to levels suggesting acute viral hepatitis. Alkaline phosphatase and bilirubin elevations are less common, although severe cholestasis has been reported. The presence of fever, neutropenia, and thrombocytopenia suggest the diagnosis. Improvement is seen after treatment with doxycycline.

Q fever (Chapter 348) can cause granulomatous hepatitis, but acute infection is commonly associated with mild elevations in aminotransferase and alkaline phosphatase levels. Q fever should be suspected in individuals with exposure to cattle, sheep, goats, unprocessed milk, or raw goat cheese.

Tularemia (Chapter 332) is commonly associated with mild to moderate elevations in aminotransferase levels. In severe disease, markedly elevated aminotransferase levels, jaundice, hepatomegaly, and ascites may develop.

Gonococcal infections (Chapter 322) frequently cause elevations in liver enzymes, most commonly alkaline phosphatase. Jaundice is occasionally seen. Although these abnormalities may represent nothing more than the response of the liver to systemic infection, they may also be a manifestation of infection of the liver capsule (perihepatitis, or Fitz-Hugh–Curtis syndrome), which reflects intra-abdominal spread of pelvic gonococcal infection in women. Gonococcal perihepatitis is accompanied by sudden right upper quadrant pain and liver tenderness. Although cholecystitis is often a consideration, coexisting arthritis, pericarditis, or myocarditis may suggest gonococcal disease, which is confirmed by vaginal swabs. A history of previous gonococcal infection, sometimes years earlier, is often elicited.

Spirochete and Rickettsial Infections

Syphilis (Chapter 340) most commonly involves the liver in the secondary stage. It is manifested as tender hepatomegaly with enzyme elevations in a predominantly cholestatic pattern. The abnormalities gradually improve over a period of weeks after effective therapy.

Leptospirosis (Chapter 344) is associated with a range of abnormalities from minor enzyme elevations to severe jaundice, with the latter occurring in the severe form of leptospirosis known as Weil's disease. Liver failure is not a manifestation of the infection, and the hepatic abnormalities gradually resolve after the infection subsides.

Lyme disease, caused by tick-transmitted *Borrelia burgdorferi* (Chapter 342), is sometimes associated with mild aminotransferase elevations, usually only during the early phase of the infection. Infections by the *Borrelia* species responsible for relapsing fever (Chapter 343) commonly involve the liver. In severe forms, the liver infection is manifested as tender hepatosplenomegaly, jaundice, and even hepatic failure. The diagnosis is established by manual examination of the peripheral blood smear.

Rocky Mountain spotted fever, caused by *Rickettsia rickettsii* (Chapter 348), is generally accompanied by mild to moderate aminotransferase elevations. Rarely, infection leads to marked vasculitic involvement of the liver with jaundice, as well as increased mortality.

Mycobacterial Infections

See information on granulomatous liver disease later.

Hepatic Manifestations of Systemic Bacterial Infections

Abnormalities in liver function can develop in the setting of systemic bacterial infection, even without direct involvement of the liver. The most common clinical problem is cholestasis of sepsis (Chapter 150). Bacterial endotoxins exert an inhibitory effect on hepatocellular bilirubin secretion, thereby leading to conjugated hyperbilirubinemia. Total bilirubin levels from 10 mg/dL to as high as 30 mg/dL can occur. Alkaline phosphatase can also become elevated, but aminotransferase levels typically remain normal or only mildly elevated. The most commonly implicated organisms are *Streptococcus pneumoniae* (Chapter 311) and enteric gram-positive and gram-negative bacteria. Jaundice is a common manifestation of *S. aureus* infections, such as toxic shock syndrome (Chapter 310), and is an occasional manifestation of gangrene caused by *Clostridium perfringens* (Chapter 319). The keys to diagnosing cholestasis of sepsis are recognizing the underlying infection, excluding biliary tract obstruction by imaging, and observing gradual resolution after appropriate antibiotic therapy. The possibility of a cholestatic drug reaction must also be considered (Chapter 150) in this setting, and the use of potentially offending drugs should be discontinued if the diagnosis is uncertain.

PARASITIC PROTOZOAL AND HELMINTHIC INFECTIONS OF THE LIVER

Amebic Liver Abscess

Definition

An amebic liver abscess (Chapter 373) is a focal accumulation of fluid and proteinaceous debris within the liver parenchyma surrounded by a rim of granulomatous inflammation caused by invading *E. histolytica* trophozoites.

Epidemiology

Amebic infection is second only to malaria as a protozoan cause of death. Ingestion of amebic cysts with subsequent colonization of the gastrointestinal tract may occur years before the development of a liver abscess. Persons at highest risk live in or have a history of travel to an endemic area. Colonic infection and liver abscess are much more common in men than women. Alcohol abuse is a significant risk factor, and persons at higher risk include men who have sex with men, immunosuppressed individuals, and institutionalized, mentally retarded persons.

Pathobiology

Humans are the principal host of *E. histolytica,* a motile nonflagellated protozoan parasite. Shedding of cysts in stool from colonized individuals and ingestion of fecally contaminated food or water by susceptible hosts perpetuates the organism's life cycle. Cysts mature into motile trophozoites in the intestinal lumen, and the trophozoites are responsible for human disease. In only a minority of infected individuals does amebic colitis develop, and the development of colitis is not necessary for the development of a liver abscess. Invasion of trophozoites through the colonic mucosa into the portal circulation, with or without clinically evident colitis, can lead to liver abscess formation.

Clinical Manifestations

Amebic liver abscesses can have either an acute clinical picture or a more indolent course. Patients with symptoms of less than 10 to 14 days' duration typically have high temperatures, chills, abdominal tenderness, leukocytosis, relatively low alkaline phosphatase but higher aspartate aminotransferase levels, and a higher chance of multifocal disease in the liver. Patients with indolent symptoms, ranging from 2 weeks to 6 months in duration, are more likely to have a solitary abscess, higher alkaline phosphatase levels, and anemia; fever and abdominal pain are less common, and leukocytosis is not generally present. Untreated amebic abscesses can spontaneously rupture into the peritoneal cavity or erode into the pleural or pericardial spaces.

Diagnosis

Most patients have a history of previous travel to endemic areas ranging from weeks to decades before the onset of symptoms. The physician should have a low threshold for obtaining abdominal US, CT, or magnetic resonance imaging in patients who have unexplained fever. Serologic testing, which has greater than 94% sensitivity and specificity, plays an important role in diagnosing amebic abscess. However, serologic testing is less useful for residents or migrants from endemic regions because of a high prevalence of preexisting seropositivity. Eosinophilia is not a feature.

Stool should be evaluated for *E. histolytica* with commercially available tests that specifically detect antigens of this *Entamoeba* species. Even with such highly sensitive stool tests, however, colonization with *E. histolytica* is often missed. Routine microscopic stool evaluation for ova and parasites lacks adequate sensitivity and specificity and is not recommended.

Aspiration may be needed to exclude a primary bacterial abscess or secondary bacterial infection of an amebic abscess. The aspirate is variable in appearance and viscosity, ranging from thin yellow fluid to thick brown fluid.

Treatment and Prevention

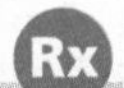

The cornerstone of treatment is oral or parenteral metronidazole (500 to 750 mg orally three times daily or a 15-mg/kg loading dose followed by 7.5 mg/kg every 6 hours intravenously). The recommended duration of treatment is 5 to 10 days, and most patients improve clinically within 3 days. The related nitroimidazole tinidazole, 2 g daily for 3 days, is also effective. At some point during treatment, intestinal cysts must be eradicated by the administration of a luminal agent such as iodoquinol, 650 mg three times daily for 20 days, to prevent continued colonization and possible recurrence of the abscess. Failure to obtain a clinical response within 3 to 5 days should prompt percutaneous cyst drainage to exclude secondary bacterial infection and prevent rupture of large abscesses. Abscesses typically require 6 months to 2 years to resolve fully, and interim imaging in a clinically improved patient may lead to unwarranted concern and unnecessary procedures. Abscesses that erode into adjacent tissue spaces respond equally well to treatment, and no further intervention is generally needed unless organ function is compromised.

Prevention of infection requires boiling of water used for drinking and preparing food. Iodine treatment can be ineffective. Prophylactic antibiotic use during travel to endemic areas is not recommended. Household contacts of infected individuals should undergo stool antigen tests to detect colonization.

Prognosis

With appropriate antibiotic therapy, amebic liver abscesses resolve fully without sequelae. If diagnosis and appropriate treatment are delayed, amebic liver abscesses may rupture or become secondarily infected. Mortality rates can reach 13% without treatment; overall mortality is highest in patients seen acutely with high fever and abdominal pain.

Other Protozoal Liver Diseases

The key features of the other major protozoal diseases affecting the liver are shown in Table 155–3.

Helminthic Liver Diseases

Echinococcosis (Chapter 375)

Hepatic infection with *E. granulosus* is sometimes called hydatid disease because of the watery cysts that characterize the infection. The liver cysts may be septated or multiple, and they grow at an average rate of 1 to 5 cm/yr. Because of this slow growth, the diagnosis may be delayed for months to years after the initial infection. Infection occurs worldwide. Canids such as dogs and wolves are the primary hosts and serve as reservoirs for the 5-mm-long intestinal tapeworms that shed *Echinococcus* eggs in the feces. Humans become accidental secondary hosts by ingesting food or water that is fecally contaminated with eggs. Because sheep and other livestock are the usual secondary hosts, human contact with canids such as sheepdogs, which are in frequent contact with livestock, is a major risk for infection. The initial infection is asymptomatic, but growing hydatid cysts may cause abdominal pain, nausea, hepatomegaly, or a palpable mass. Liver enzymes are generally normal or nearly normal, and eosinophilia is not reliably present. Cysts may rupture or become secondarily infected with bacteria. Intra-abdominal rupture can cause pruritus and anaphylaxis. The diagnosis is suggested by the presence of septated liver cysts or cysts that have adjacent daughter cysts. Serologic tests can be helpful but lack sufficient sensitivity to exclude the diagnosis. Fine-needle aspiration under US guidance can establish the diagnosis, but anthelmintic therapy should be initiated before aspiration to prevent complications. Treatment is challenging and usually relies on a combination of a skilled surgical approach and anthelmintic therapy (3 or more months of albendazole, 400 mg twice daily with food for 4 weeks, followed by a 2-week rest period).

Hepatic infection with *Echinococcus multilocularis* is becoming a growing concern because of its expanding distribution in the Northern Hemisphere and its resistance to treatment. Foxes typically serve as the primary host, and rodents are the secondary host. The associated disease, alveolar echinococcosis, is an insidiously progressive disease that is typically asymptomatic for a decade or more and then appears as tumor-like masses of small (<1 to 30 mm) vesicles, primarily in the liver. Radical surgical excision and prolonged anthelmintic therapy (cycles of albendazole, 400 mg twice daily with food for 4 weeks, followed by a 2-week rest period, for at least several years) are the best options, although the disease is usually managed and not cured.

Schistosomiasis (Chapter 376)

Although primary schistosomiasis does not occur in the United States, the enormous burden of infection with this parasite (5% of the world's population) makes it a major international public health issue and cause of disease in immigrants. Worms lodge in the tributaries of the portal vasculature, where they induce a granulomatous and fibrotic reaction. The end result is presinusoidal portal hypertension, marked splenomegaly,

TABLE 155–3 PARASITIC INFECTIONS INVOLVING THE LIVER

	Characteristics	Risk Factors and Endemic Areas	Major Hepatic Manifestations	Diagnosis	Treatment
MAJOR PROTOZOA					
Entamoeba histolytica	Ingested cysts develop into invasive trophozoites that colonize the colon and occasionally spread to the liver by the portal blood	Male gender; Mexico, regions of Central and South America, India, and regions of Africa	Amebic liver abscesses develop as a tissue response to trophozoite invasion with acute and chronic manifestations (see text)	Imaging, serology, stool antigen test (microscopic evaluation of stool has a poor yield)	Metronidazole, 500–750 mg PO tid × 5–10 days, or tinidazole, 2 g daily × 3 days; iodoquinol, 650 mg tid × 20 days, also needed to eradicate intestinal colonization
OTHER PROTOZOA					
Cryptosporidium sp and Microsporidia	Ingested cysts develop into trophozoites in intestinal mucosa	AIDS; worldwide distribution	Biliary tract infection with obstruction and cholangitis	See Chapter 371	See Chapter 371
Toxoplasma gondii	Ingestion of oocysts in contaminated soil or water or in infected meat; systemic spread of tachyzoites in the circulation	Worldwide distribution	Immunocompetent: asymptomatic or hepatomegaly and mild enzyme elevations Immunocompromised: occasional overt hepatitis	See Chapter 370	See Chapter 370
Leishmania sp	Sand fly bite transmits promastigotes; proliferation in the reticuloendothelial system	Worldwide distribution	Hepatosplenomegaly months to years after infection	See Chapter 369	See Chapter 369
Plasmodium sp	Mosquito (*Anopheles*) bite transmits sporozoites	Exposure to anopheline mosquito bites in multiple regions throughout the world	Proliferation in hepatocytes causes hepatomegaly, enzyme elevations, and jaundice	See Chapter 375	See Chapter 375
Babesia microti	Tick bite transmits the agent, which parasitizes erythrocytes	Asplenia is a risk for fatal hepatic failure, especially bovine babesiosis (Europe)	Mild liver enzyme elevations	See Chapter 374	See Chapter 374
MAJOR HELMINTHS					
Schistosoma sp	Cercaria in fresh water penetrate the skin, travel by the circulation to portal vein radicals	Contact with fresh water in regions of Africa, Asia, South America, and the Caribbean	Progressive presinusoidal blood flow obstruction, periportal fibrosis, portal hypertension, varices, ascites, splenomegaly	Rectal biopsy, liver biopsy	Praziquantel or oxamniquine, see Chapter 376
Echinococcus granulosus	Eggs of small (3–7 mm) tapeworms in stool of canid hosts; ingested eggs produce larval oncospheres that migrate to the liver and form cysts in sheep, humans, and other intermediate hosts	Ingestion of food or water contaminated by dog or other canid feces; worldwide distribution, found especially in areas where dogs are in contact with livestock	Initial infection asymptomatic; liver cysts increase in diameter by 1–5 cm yearly and cause variable abdominal pain, hepatomegaly, and variable eosinophilia; occasional cyst rupture, secondary bacterial infection	See Chapter 375	See Chapter 375

Echinococcus multilocularis	Eggs of small tapeworms in stool of foxes; ingested eggs produce oncospheres in the liver of rodents, humans, and other intermediate hosts	Endemic in Northern Hemisphere; human exposure increasing with growing fox populations	Metacestodes colonize the liver as a tumor-like mass of small vesicles	See Chapter 375	See Chapter 375
Fasciola sp	Leaf-shaped flukes up to 13 × 30 mm derived from ingested cysts; the fluke excysts in the duodenum, migrates directly across the bowel wall into the peritoneal cavity, and burrows directly into the liver (or occasionally out to the skin)	Consumption of freshwater or aquatic plants contaminated by colonized livestock; worldwide distribution	Acute: fever, abdominal pain, eosinophilia Chronic: symptomatic biliary obstruction, variable eosinophilia	Serology, stool examination	Triclabendazole, 10 mg/kg once or twice
Opisthorchis (Clonorchis) sinensis	Flukes of 8–25 mm derived from ingested cysts; the fluke excysts in the duodenum and migrates into the bile ducts	Consumption of raw, pickled, dried, smoked, or salted freshwater fish or crayfish originating from East Asia or, in the case of *Opisthorchis felineus*, Russia and eastern Europe	Acute: typically asymptomatic Chronic: abdominal pain, fever, anorexia, tender hepatomegaly, sometimes eosinophilia Late sequelae: intermittent biliary obstruction, cholelithiasis, cholecystitis, cholangitis, secondary bacterial abscesses, cholangiocarcinoma	Stool examination	Praziquantel, 25 mg/kg q8h ×3 doses
Toxocara sp	Nematode infection disseminates to cause visceral larva migrans after ingestion of soil contaminated with dog or cat feces	Consumption of food contaminated with soil containing eggs; distributed throughout the United States, highest prevalence in southeastern United States	Often an asymptomatic cause of eosinophilia (exclude *Trichinella, Strongyloides,* filaria, hookworm, schistosomiasis); hepatomegaly is common, but nonhepatic manifestations dominate the clinical picture	See Chapter 378	See Chapter 378
OTHER HELMINTHS					
Ascaris lumbricoides	Ingested eggs develop into larvae that migrate to the lungs and are coughed and swallowed; develop into roundworms 15–30 mm long in the small intestine	Consumption of fecally contaminated food or water; 20% of the world's population is colonized	Colonization is typically asymptomatic with eosinophilia; biliary migration of worms can cause symptomatic biliary obstruction, cholangitis, cholecystitis, and secondary bacterial liver abscess	Stool examination	Albendazole, 400 mg once
Capillaria hepatica	Ingested eggs develop into larvae in the intestinal mucosa; larvae migrate to the liver by portal blood flow and develop into short-lived roundworms	Consumption of food contaminated with rodent feces; human infection is rare	Fever, eosinophilia, and hepatomegaly; subsequent foci of liver fibrosis, granulomas, and calcification in involved areas	Stool and tissue examination	Mebendazole, 200 mg bid ×20 days
Strongyloides stercoralis	Ingested eggs develop into 1.5-to 2.5-mm nematodes that invade the hepatic vasculature, lymphatics, and biliary tract	Consumption of food contaminated with soil containing eggs in warm, moist climates	Hepatic disease in the setting of immunosuppression: jaundice, abdominal pain; eosinophilia is uncommon	Serology and stool examination	Ivermectin, 200 μg/kg/day ×2 days, *or* albendazole, 400 mg/day ×7 days

ascites, and gastroesophageal varices. In the late phase of the disease, the diagnosis is established by examination of a rectal biopsy specimen for eggs. Liver biopsy can also be helpful. Infection is treated with antischistosomal agents; decompression of portal hypertension may be needed to prevent recurrent variceal hemorrhage in selected patients.

Other Helminthic Liver Diseases

For other helminthic infections (see Table 155–3), a careful history of travel and dietary habits may identify important risk factors.

FUNGAL DISEASES OF THE LIVER

Candidiasis (Chapter 359)

Hepatic infection with *Candida albicans* is seen primarily in patients with severe, prolonged neutropenia. Unexplained fever, often already treated with broad-spectrum antibiotics and even amphotericin, is invariably present. Liver enzymes may be elevated in a cholestatic pattern, and contrast-enhanced CT scanning may identify focal low-density areas in the liver parenchyma. The diagnosis is confirmed by identification of fungal elements on liver biopsy or by culture of liver biopsy specimens. However, the sensitivity of these diagnostic tests is poor, especially if the patient has already received amphotericin. Eradication of hepatic candidal infection is difficult and may require prolonged administration of amphotericin even after reconstitution of the immune system.

Other Fungal Diseases

Clinically significant hepatic involvement by other fungal pathogens is unusual and typically manifested as hepatic granulomas in immunocompromised hosts (Table 155–4).

GRANULOMATOUS DISEASES OF THE LIVER

In patients with abnormal aminotransferase or alkaline phosphatase levels, granulomas are frequently found on liver biopsy. The recommended evaluation to establish an underlying cause depends on the patient's clinical status, coexisting diseases, and exposure history. The evaluation of an asymptomatic patient is usually limited, whereas a patient with constitutional symptoms or signs should be more extensively evaluated with cultures, serologic testing, and imaging as indicated by the travel history, immunologic competence, and other risk factors (see Table 155–4).

Definition

Granulomas are focal aggregates of epithelioid cells, macrophages, and other inflammatory cells (Fig. 155–2). The macrophages of granulomas may coalesce to form multinucleated giant cells. Central necrosis, or caseation, may also develop, especially in tuberculous granulomas (Fig. 155–3). *Granulomatous hepatitis* is a poorly defined term that is generally used to describe an illness characterized by cholestatic liver enzyme abnormalities and granulomatous inflammatory changes as the predominant histologic manifestation.

Epidemiology

Up to 10% of liver biopsy specimens show granulomas, either as an incidental finding or as part of the primary process. Sarcoidosis (Chapter 95) accounts for up to a third of cases, and about two thirds of patients with sarcoidosis have hepatic granulomas, but rarely in the absence of pulmonary involvement.

Pathobiology

Granuloma formation is the response of the immune system to the presence of foreign substances that are nondigestable by the enzymes of inflammatory cells and macrophages. Such substances are typically derived from infectious organisms (e.g., mycobacteria and schistosomes) or from injected or ingested material (e.g., talc and mineral oil). The

TABLE 155–4 CAUSES OF GRANULOMATOUS LIVER DISEASE

Underlying Disease Process	Factors and Coexisting Conditions That Suggest the Diagnosis
Sarcoidosis	Evidence of pulmonary sarcoidosis, African American ancestry, elevated angiotensin-converting enzyme level
Primary biliary cirrhosis	Female, positive antimitochondrial antibody, elevated IgM
Other immunologic disorders (Wegener's granulomatosis, chronic granulomatous disease, temporal arteritis, polymyalgia rheumatica, Crohn's disease, ulcerative colitis, idiopathic hypogammaglobulinemia, allergic granulomatosis, erythema nodosum, systemic lupus erythematosus, AIDS)	Specific serologic findings, previous established diagnosis
Malignancy (Hodgkin's lymphoma, non-Hodgkin's lymphoma, carcinoma)	Adenopathy, known primary disease
Mycobacterium tuberculosis	Fever, active pulmonary or miliary tuberculosis, caseating granulomas on biopsy
Other mycobacteria (*Mycobacterium leprae*, atypical, bacille Calmette-Guérin)	Exposure history, HIV infection
Other bacterial infections (syphilis, Q fever, brucellosis, Whipple's disease, tularemia, yersiniosis, melioidosis, listeriosis, nocardiosis, actinomycosis, typhoid fever, cat-scratch disease, psittacosis, ehrlichiosis, Lyme disease)	Fever, specific risk factors for unusual infections
Parasitic infections (schistosomiasis, fascioliasis, toxocariasis, capillariasis, strongyloidiasis, amebiasis, toxoplasmosis, malaria, leishmaniasis)	Travel to endemic regions, positive serologic testing
Fungal infections (histoplasmosis, candidiasis, cryptococcosis, coccidioidomycosis, blastomycosis, aspergillosis, mucormycosis)	Fever, immunocompromised
Viral infections (cytomegalovirus, Epstein-Barr virus, influenza B, coxsackievirus)	Characteristic clinical illness, positive serology for acute or recent exposure
Drug reactions (allopurinol, carbamazepine, hydralazine, penicillins, phenylbutazone, procainamide, quinidine, sulfonamides)	Previous or ongoing exposure to the suspected drug
Toxins (beryllium, copper sulfate, Thorotrast)	Previous exposure history
Foreign body reactions (talc, mineral oil)	Talc: history of intravenous drug use, birefringent crystals in granulomas

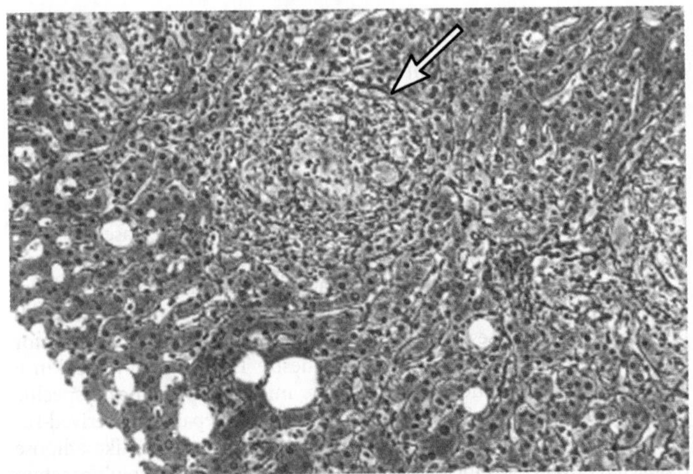

FIGURE 155–2 • Sarcoidosis. Well-defined non-necrotizing granulomas (e.g., arrow) are seen in the liver of a 48-year-old man with unexplained fevers (original magnification, ×20). (Courtesy of E. M. Brunt.)

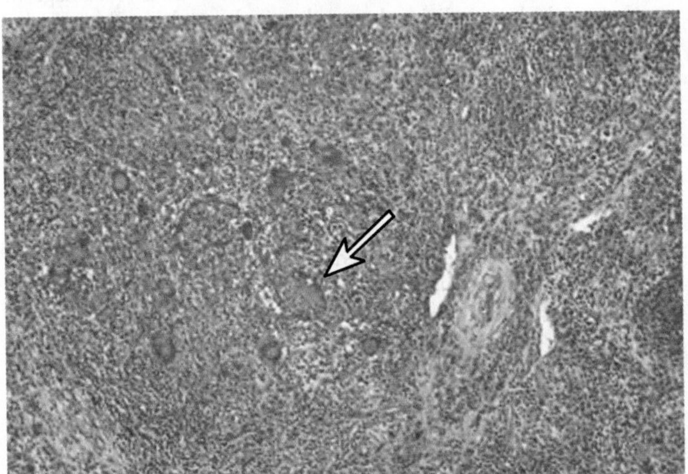

FIGURE 155–3 • Tuberculous granuloma. A large necrotizing hepatic granuloma from a patient with active *Mycobacterium tuberculosis* infection fills this entire field. Several focal aggregates of histiocytes are present (e.g., arrow). Although tissue sections did not reveal organisms by acid-fast staining, culture of the tissue confirmed the diagnosis (original magnification, ×20). (Courtesy of E. M. Brunt.)

response may also be elicited by hypersensitivity reactions to drugs and toxins. The antigenic stimulus in sarcoidosis remains uncertain. Sometimes the collagen deposition in and around a granuloma forms a fibrin ring, which is a characteristic finding in brucellosis (Chapter 331). Lipogranulomas are associated with hepatic steatosis (Chapter 156) and may be due to ingestion by macrophages of large, unmetabolizable lipid droplets that originate in hepatocytes.

Clinical Manifestations

Hepatic granulomas are typically asymptomatic. Constitutional symptoms such as fever, weight loss, anorexia, and night sweats are more often manifestations of an underlying disease process rather than the liver involvement itself. Laboratory evaluation most commonly reveals liver enzyme elevations in a cholestatic pattern, with alkaline phosphatase levels being higher than aminotransferases. Jaundice occasionally develops in severe granulomatous hepatitis. Imaging of the liver may reveal hepatomegaly. Focal lesions on imaging studies are unusual but can be seen with coalescence of sarcoid granulomas or extensive mycobacterial granulomas in an immunocompromised host.

Diagnosis

Incidentally encountered granulomas require minimal further evaluation. Tuberculosis should be excluded, and sarcoidosis should be considered. The antimitochondrial antibody titer should be measured to identify primary biliary cirrhosis (Chapter 159). Granulomas discovered during the evaluation of systemic illness or unexplained liver enzyme elevations require more extensive diagnostic testing, often guided by the exposure history (see Table 155–4). The use of potentially causative drugs should be stopped if possible (see Table 155–4). Certain pathologic features, often revealed by additional staining such as Gomori methenamine silver stain for fungal elements or acid-fast staining for mycobacteria, can point to specific underlying processes.

Treatment

Treatment of granulomatous liver disease depends on the underlying cause and clinical status of the patient. Granulomas associated with sarcoidosis do not require treatment unless they are accompanied by significant constitutional symptoms or severe cholestasis, in which case corticosteroid therapy may be indicated (Chapter 95).

Prognosis

Incidental hepatic granulomas in the absence of sarcoidosis, primary biliary cirrhosis, or other specific underlying causes do not cause progressive liver disease. Sarcoidosis is usually an asymptomatic manifestation of the primary disease, but it can occasionally progress to biliary cirrhosis with portal hypertension, ascites, and variceal hemorrhage.

SUGGESTED READINGS

Dourakis SP, Saramandou R, Alexopoulou A, et al: Hepatic granulomas: A 6-year experience in a single center in Greece. Eur J Gastroenterol Hepatol 2007; 19:101–104. *Of 66 cases, primary biliary cirrhosis, overlap syndrome, and autoimmune hepatitis were the most common causes, followed by sarcoidosis.*

Elzi L, Laifer G, Sendi P, et al: Low sensitivity of ultrasonography for the early diagnosis of amebic liver abscess. Am J Med 2004;117:519–522. *The sensitivity of ultrasound was 92% for pyogenic liver abscess but only 58% for amebic liver abscess.*

Jepsen P, Vilstrup H, Schonheyder HC, et al: A nationwide study of the incidence and 30-day mortality rate of pyogenic liver abscess in Denmark, 1977–2002. Aliment Pharmacol Ther 2005;21:1185–1188. *Mortality has declined to about 10%.*

Karagiannidis A, Karavalaki M, Koulaouzidis A: Hepatic sarcoidosis. Ann Hepatol 2006;5:251–256. *Review of diagnosis and treatment of hepatic sarcoidosis.*

Kibiki GS, Drenth JP, Nagengast FM: Hepatosplenic schistosomiasis: A review. East Afr Med J 2004;81:480–485. *Review of liver disease caused by schistosomiasis.*

Kurland JE, Brann OS: Pyogenic and amebic liver abscesses. Curr Gastroenterol Rep 2004;6:273–279. *Concise review of bacterial and amebic liver abscesses.*

McManus DP, Zhang W, Li J, Bartley PB: Echinococcosis. Lancet 2003;362: 1295–1304. *Concise review of echinococcosis.*

Stanley SL Jr: Amoebiasis. Lancet 2003;361:1025–1034. *Excellent review of the pathobiology of amebiasis and the distinction between* E. histolytica *and* E. dispar.

156 ALCOHOLIC AND NONALCOHOLIC STEATOHEPATITIS

Anna Mae Diehl

Definition

Steatohepatitis is an intermediate stage in the spectrum of fatty liver disease, an entity that ranges from relatively clinically benign steatosis to cirrhosis. Alcoholic steatohepatitis develops in some individuals who consume alcohol habitually. Nonalcoholic steatohepatitis (NASH) shows the same histopathology but occurs in the absence of excess alcohol consumption. NASH is strongly associated with the metabolic syndrome, an insulin-resistant state that is common in individuals with truncal obesity (Chapter 239), type 2 diabetes mellitus (Chapter 248), and dyslipidemia (high triglyceride and low high-density lipoprotein levels; Chapter 217). Though strongly associated with obesity, NASH has also been demonstrated in about 3% of lean individuals, including those with generalized lipodystrophy. In addition, certain drugs can cause steatohepatitis (see later).

Epidemiology

The true incidence and prevalence of alcoholic steatohepatitis and NASH are unknown because no currently available noninvasive test can reliably distinguish steatohepatitis from simple fatty liver (steatosis). Moreover, estimates of the prevalence of fatty liver disease vary according to the sensitivity of various diagnostic tests.

Population-based surveys of adults 18 years or older with abdominal ultrasonography have demonstrated fatty liver disease (at least steatosis) in about 20% of the adult populations of Japan, Western Europe, and the United States. However, when screening is performed with very sensitive imaging modalities such as magnetic resonance imaging (MRI), the overall prevalence of hepatic steatosis is considerably higher (≈34%) in the general adult population older than 18 years. MRI screening also demonstrates racial differences in the prevalence of fatty liver: almost 50% of Hispanic Americans, about a third of whites, and almost 25% of African Americans have fatty livers. However, 80% or so of individuals with hepatic steatosis by MRI have normal serum aminotransferase levels, thus indicating that blood tests are the least sensitive tool for diagnosing the condition. Not surprisingly, the reported prevalence of fatty liver disease falls to 5 to 8% if elevations in serum aminotransferase levels are used for screening. Nevertheless, despite the limited utility of serum aminotransferase levels for diagnosing fatty liver disease, there is now overwhelming consensus that this condition is the main cause of elevated liver enzymes in the Western world.

Most individuals with fatty liver disease deny excessive alcohol consumption but are likely to fulfill the criteria for metabolic syndrome, which suggests that nonalcoholic (rather than alcohol-induced) fatty liver disease is the most common chronic liver disease in these populations. However, because neither abdominal imaging tests nor blood tests reliably differentiate steatosis from more advanced stages of fatty liver disease (e.g., steatohepatitis and cirrhosis) and because liver biopsy studies show that steatohepatitis or cirrhosis sometimes occurs in individuals with normal serum aminotransferase levels, the true prevalence of steatohepatitis (as opposed to simple steatosis) remains unknown.

Liver biopsy studies of selected patient populations suggest that steatosis is probably twice as common as steatohepatitis and that at least 10% of patients with steatohepatitis progress to cirrhosis over time. Thus, in the adult U.S. population, in which the prevalence of fatty liver is approximately 34%, the prevalence of steatohepatitis and cirrhosis is estimated to be about 17% and 2%, respectively. The validity of these crude estimates is supported by a recent study in Olmsted County, Minnesota, where the prevalence of cirrhosis related to nonalcoholic fatty liver disease was reported to be 5% of the adult population.

Pathobiology

In the early stages of fatty liver disease, fat accumulates within hepatocytes when mechanisms that promote lipid removal (by oxidation or export) cannot keep pace with mechanisms that promote lipid import or biosynthesis. Although alcohol consumption has long been known to promote lipid biosynthesis while inhibiting lipid export, it has been appreciated only recently that the molecular mechanisms involved are very similar to those that promote steatosis in nonalcoholic fatty liver disease.

Three of the best-characterized factors that modulate the evolution of fatty liver disease are fatty acids, tumor necrosis factor-α (TNF-α), and adiponectin. Fatty acids routinely traffic between the liver and adipose tissue. Fat and the liver are also important sources of TNF-α and adiponectin. Adiponectin generally reduces lipid accumulation within hepatocytes by inhibiting fatty acid import and increasing fatty acid oxidation and export. It is also a potent insulin-sensitizing agent. TNF-α antagonizes the actions of adiponectin and thereby promotes hepatocyte steatosis and insulin resistance.

Situations that increase TNF-α relative to adiponectin promote hepatic steatosis and insulin resistance. TNF-α increases mitochondrial generation of reactive oxygen species, which have been shown to induce cellular insulin resistance. TNF-α also promotes hepatocyte apoptosis and recruits inflammatory cells to the liver. Hence, protracted exposure to TNF-α generates oxidative and apoptotic stress that sometimes overwhelms antioxidant and antiapoptotic defenses and leads to steatohepatitis. Studies in mouse models of NASH, as well as mice with ethanol-induced steatohepatitis, show that overproduction of TNF-α relative to adiponectin causes steatohepatitis and that treatments that inhibit TNF-α or that increase adiponectin improve steatohepatitis. In addition, studies in humans with NASH demonstrate that the relative risk for the development of steatohepatitis correlates with increases in TNF-α or decreases in adiponectin levels.

The simple accumulation of fatty acids within hepatocytes induces signaling in hepatocytes to activate kinases such as inhibitor κ kinase-β (IKK-β); these kinases then activate the nuclear transcription factor NFκB, which drives hepatocytes to synthesize TNF-α and interleukin-6 (IL-6). In addition, studies in transgenic mice with hepatocyte-specific overexpression of IKK-β have demonstrated that hepatocyte-derived IL-6 is responsible for systemic insulin resistance. Therefore, like adipose tissue, fatty livers (specifically, fatty hepatocytes) also make soluble factors that circulate to distant tissues and contribute to systemic insulin resistance (i.e., the metabolic syndrome).

Alcohol-induced steatohepatitis, as well as possibly NASH, can clearly develop in nonobese individuals. The mechanism of liver damage in nonobese and obese individuals may be similar and involve excessive exposure of hepatocytes to fatty acids, fatty acid–inducible inflammatory mediators (i.e., TNF-α), and reactive oxygen species. Intestinal microflora help regulate intestinal uptake of diet-derived lipids, in addition to hepatic fatty acid synthesis, so the gut bacteria of some nonobese individuals might promote excessive hepatic accumulation of fatty acids, as well as exposure to other bacterial factors (e.g., lipopolysaccharide or other Toll-like receptor agonists) that trigger hepatic TNF production.

The role of intestinal flora in the pathogenesis of fatty liver disease has been particularly well demonstrated for alcohol-induced liver disease. Experimental animals housed under germ-free conditions or treated with poorly absorbed oral antibiotics are protected from alcohol-induced hepatotoxicity. Products from intestinal bacteria are thought to injure the liver by increasing hepatic production of TNF-α and reactive oxygen species because mice that are genetically deficient in either TNF-α or certain enzyme systems that generate reactive oxygen species are also protected from the early stages of alcoholic liver damage.

It is generally believed that progression from fatty liver disease to cirrhosis is predominately dictated by the severity of oxidant stress and the consequent necro-inflammation that occurs in individuals with steatohepatitis. However, findings in animal models of steatohepatitis cast some doubt on this assumption because mice in which severe steatohepatitis develops do not uniformly progress to cirrhosis. In fact, progression to cirrhosis is also poorly predicted by the gravity of the injurious insult in human fatty liver disease. For example, although there is no doubt that alcohol is hepatotoxic, most lifelong heavy drinkers do not become cirrhotic. Similarly, although obesity clearly increases exposure to fat-derived inflammatory mediators and is an independent risk factor for progression of alcoholic fatty liver disease to cirrhosis, some morbidly obese individuals have normal livers at the time of gastric bypass surgery. Individuals in whom just steatosis develops despite constant bombardment with inflammatory factors might be better at repairing their liver damage without the development of fibrosis than those in whom steatohepatitis or cirrhosis develops. In this regard, leptin, angiotensin, and norepinephrine promote the proliferation of hepatic stellate cells, upregulate their expression of profibrogenic cytokines such as transforming growth factor-β, and induce collagen gene expression. Conversely, adiponectin appears to inhibit the activation of hepatic stellate cells and decrease liver fibrosis. Consistent with these pathophysiologic findings is the clinical observation that angiotensin is an independent risk factor for advanced liver fibrosis in nonalcoholic fatty liver disease and the suggestion, in a small open-label trial, that angiotensin receptor blockade might decrease liver fibrosis and slow disease progression in patients with NASH and arterial hypertension.

Clinical Manifestations

Fatty liver (steatosis) without steatohepatitis is relatively asymptomatic, and individuals with alcoholic steatohepatitis or NASH may be entirely asymptomatic as well, although vague constitutional complaints such as malaise and weakness are common. Careful physical examination detects hepatomegaly in almost 75% of patients with steatohepatitis. When sufficient fibrosis has developed to cause portal hypertension, patients may have splenomegaly, spider telangiectases, palmar erythema, gynecomastia, ascites, lower extremity edema, portal hypertensive bleeding, or hepatic encephalopathy. Severe steatohepatitis can also lead to jaundice, coagulopathy, and fever.

Classically, severe alcoholic steatohepatitis (formerly called "alcoholic hepatitis") is characterized by the sudden development of tender hepatomegaly, jaundice, and fever in an individual who has been drinking heavily. Often, the illness is associated with a flulike prodrome that includes malaise, anorexia, and weakness. These symptoms sometimes prompt reduced alcohol ingestion, which in turn may precipitate alcohol withdrawal (Chapter 31). Some individuals require hospitalization because of decompensated liver disease or associated conditions such as alcohol withdrawal, gastrointestinal bleeding, infection, or pancreatitis. Although most people gradually recover during early abstinence, others deteriorate despite abstinence and aggressive management of their associated problems.

Diagnosis

The diagnosis of alcoholic steatohepatitis and NASH requires a combination of noninvasive and invasive tests because no single test is perfectly sensitive or specific. Patients generally have elevated alanine and aspartate aminotransferase levels that are detected incidentally on blood tests, as well as elevated γ-glutamyl transpeptidase levels, but some simply have hepatomegaly or the incidental finding of a fatty liver on abdominal imaging studies. Steatosis, steatohepatitis, and even cirrhosis may occur without elevations in aminotransferase levels, so patients are occasionally first seen with hypersplenism, gastrointestinal bleeding, or encephalopathy.

History

Risk factors for viral hepatitis (Chapter 151) should be sought. Although the rare hepatitis C genotype 3 may cause steatosis, a diagnosis of chronic hepatitis B or C (Chapter 152) generally excludes alcoholic steatohepatitis and NASH; however, these diseases may coexist.

Information about lifetime alcohol consumption should be obtained. More than 60 g/day in men or 20 g/day in women increases the risk for alcoholic steatohepatitis, and lower levels may potentiate liver damage in cases of NASH. A history of exposure to any drugs that have been associated with NASH (Table 156–1) should be elicited. Obesity, type 2 diabetes, other insulin resistance syndromes (e.g., lipodystrophy, dyslipidemia, polycystic ovary syndrome), and other rarer inherited conditions have also been associated with NASH.

The history and physical examination should also include a thorough search for clues to other types of chronic liver disease, including autoimmune hepatitis (Chapter 152), hemochromatosis (Chapters 154 and 231), α_1-antitrypsin deficiency (Chapter 154), Wilson's disease (Chapters 154 and 230), primary biliary cirrhosis (Chapter 159), and primary sclerosing cholangitis (Chapter 159).

The severity of any underlying liver damage is assessed by evidence of cirrhosis (Chapter 157), such as jaundice, dark urine, acholic stools, pruritus, gastrointestinal bleeding, ascites or lower extremity edema, personality changes, insomnia, decreased memory or ability to concentrate, asterixis, lethargy, confusion, or coma.

Laboratory Findings

In steatohepatitis, serum alanine aminotransferase, aspartate aminotransferase, and γ-glutamyl transpeptidase values are generally increased less than 4-fold; elevations greater than 10-fold are very unusual and suggest either an alternative diagnosis or superimposed drug- or virus-induced liver injury. The liver enzyme values correlate poorly with the severity of the underlying liver disease and cannot predict which patients have steatosis rather than steatohepatitis, with or without cirrhosis. The aspartate aminotransferase value tends to be at least twice the alanine aminotransferase value in many patients with alcoholic steatohepatitis, whereas this pattern of liver enzyme values generally does not occur until cirrhosis develops in patients with NASH. γ-Glutamyl transpeptidase elevations are common in both alcoholic steatohepatitis and NASH, and increased γ-glutamyl transpeptidase values may be a sensitive marker of insulin resistance. Some patients with alcoholic steatohepatitis or NASH also have accompanying minor (generally, 1.5- to 2-fold) elevations in serum alkaline phosphatase values. Greater increases in alkaline phosphatase values should prompt suspicion of associated biliary tract disease or a hepatic infiltrative process (Chapters 154 and 159). Levels of bilirubin, albumin, and ammonia, the prothrombin time, and the platelet count help estimate the severity of liver disease.

Hyperglycemia and dyslipidemia (increased total and low-density lipoprotein levels, decreased high-density lipoprotein levels, and hypertriglyceridemia) are associated with alcoholic steatohepatitis and NASH. Classically, patients with alcoholic steatohepatitis and NASH test negative for autoantibodies and have normal values for viral markers, the α_1-antitrypsin phenotype, transferrin saturation, and ceruloplasmin. However, autoantibody titers are elevated in some patients with biopsy-proven NASH, thus demonstrating the difficulty of differentiating the

TABLE 156–1 POTENTIAL CAUSES OF NONALCOHOLIC STEATOHEPATITIS

DRUGS
Cytotoxic/cytostatic drugs
L-Asparaginase
Azacitidine
Azaserine
Azauridine
Bleomycin
Methotrexate
Antibiotics
Puromycin
Tetracycline
Other causes
Amiodarone
Coumadin
Dichloroethylene
Ethionine
Ethyl bromide
Estrogens
Flectol H
Glucocorticoids
Hydrazine
Hypoglycin
Orotate
Perhexiline maleate
Safrole
Total parenteral nutrition
INHERITED AND ACQUIRED METABOLIC CONDITIONS
Inborn errors of metabolism
Abetalipoproteinemia
Congenital generalized lipodystrophy
Familial hepatosteatosis
Galactosemia
Glycogen storage disease
Hereditary fructose intolerance
Homocystinuria
Prader-Willi syndrome
Refsum's syndrome
Shwachman's syndrome
Systemic carnitine deficiency
Tyrosinemia
Weber-Christian syndrome
Wilson's disease
Acquired metabolic disorders
Diabetes mellitus, type 2
Lipodystrophy—drug induced
Inflammatory bowel disease
Jejunoileal bypass
Kwashiorkor and marasmus
Obesity

two conditions without liver biopsy. Similarly, some patients with alcoholic steatohepatitis are chronically infected with hepatitis C or hepatitis B virus, and the predominant cause of liver damage cannot be determined without examining liver histology. Finally, hyperferritinemia and increased transferrin saturation have been noted in many individuals with NASH, even in the absence of detectable mutations in the *HFe* gene, and most of these patients do not exhibit significant iron accumulation on subsequent liver biopsy.

Serum concentrations of TNF-α, IL-1α, IL-6, and IL-8 are increased in most patients with severe alcoholic steatohepatitis, and the greatest mortality rates occur in those with the highest cytokine levels. Similarly, serum cytokines gradually decline during recovery.

Imaging

Abdominal ultrasonography is the most common imaging test used to screen for hepatic steatosis, but a fatty liver on an ultrasonogram has a positive predictive value of only 77% and a negative predictive value of only 67% when compared with liver biopsy. Computed tomography is less sensitive than ultrasonography. Abdominal MRI provides the most reliable noninvasive approach for detecting and quantifying hepatic steatosis, but its expense limits its usefulness in routine practice. Most importantly, none of these imaging modalities can distinguish simple steatosis from steatohepatitis nor identify cirrhosis until hepatic fibrosis has caused overt portal hypertension.

Liver Biopsy

Liver biopsy is the "gold standard" for confirming the clinical suspicion of alcoholic steatohepatitis and NASH, particularly in patients who have physical findings or blood test results that suggest the presence of more than one type of liver disease. Biopsy is also the most sensitive means for staging fatty liver disease because histology distinguishes steatohepatitis from steatosis and permits the identification of hepatic fibrosis long before overt sequelae of portal hypertension develop.

Histologically, steatohepatitis is characterized by the presence of steatosis and foci of hepatocellular ballooning (Fig. 156–1). The latter are dying hepatocytes that sometimes contain Mallory bodies, which are ropelike condensations of ubiquitinated cytokeratins. Patchy infiltration of inflammatory cells within the hepatic parenchyma is common but not necessary to establish the diagnosis of steatohepatitis. Fibrosis (accumulation of type 1 collagen) is seen at diagnosis in more than 60% of cases. Collagen deposition around individual hepatocytes (pericellular fibrosis), along hepatic sinusoids (sinusoidal fibrosis), and around terminal hepatic venules (perivenular fibrosis) is typical and helps distinguish steatohepatitis from other types of chronic hepatitis in which the fibrosis is more localized to periportal areas. Like patients with other types of chronic hepatitis, bridging hepatic fibrosis may develop in patients with steatohepatitis, and they are at risk of progressing to cirrhosis. Nevertheless, biopsy is an imperfect test with sampling error; for example, two consecutive biopsy passes in patients with fatty liver disease can show discordant findings 40% of the time. Despite its limitations, whenever a definitive diagnosis will influence management, liver biopsy is indicated in patients older than 45 years and those who are obese or diabetic because of the risk for liver-related morbidity and mortality.

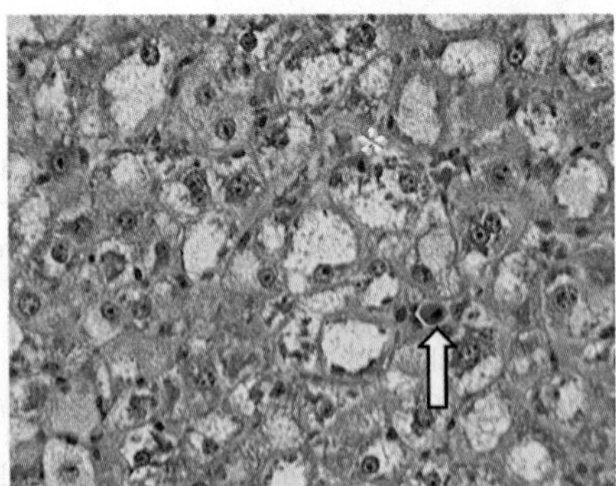

FIGURE 156–1 • Histology typical of steatohepatitis. The hepatocytes have accumulated lipid droplets. Small foci of inflammatory cells are apparent, and a few ballooned hepatocytes contain Mallory bodies. Dead (apoptotic) hepatocytes (*arrow*) are noted.

Prevention

Secondary Prevention

In individuals in whom alcoholic or nonalcoholic fatty liver disease has already developed, situations that increase hepatic oxidative stress promote progression from steatosis to steatohepatitis. Such patients should discontinue alcohol consumption and consider supplemental antioxidants or treatments that inhibit endogenous factors that promote TNF-α production; however, the data for such interventions are currently limited to small, mostly uncontrolled studies in patients and experimental animal models.

Primary Prevention

Abstinence from alcohol is the primary prevention for alcoholic steatohepatitis. In humans with fatty livers, diet modification and exercise to improve insulin resistance may reduce the fatty liver state that is the substrate for NASH.

Treatment (Table 156–2)

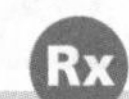

Alcoholic Steatohepatitis

In humans hospitalized with severe alcoholic steatohepatitis (Chapter 157), prospective, randomized, placebo-controlled trials have demonstrated the efficacy of corticosteroids [1,2] and pentoxifylline. [3] Both agents are known to inhibit either the production or the activities of pro-inflammatory cytokines, and each reduces acute liver-related mortality by about 50%. Patients with severe alcoholic steatohepatitis should be treated with corticosteroids (40 mg prednisolone orally every day for 4 weeks) or pentoxifylline (400 mg orally three times a day for 4 weeks) if they have no contraindications; maintenance therapy is not recommended. All patients with alcoholic steatohepatitis are strongly urged to discontinue alcohol consumption, and referral to alcohol rehabilitation services may improve long-term success (Chapter 31). Actively drinking individuals with alcoholic steatohepatitis are advised to take supplemental B vitamins and eat a nutritious diet.

Nonalcoholic Steatohepatitis

The goals for treating NASH are to reduce hepatic exposure to fatty acids and TNF-α while increasing adiponectin activity, thereby improving both fatty liver disease and insulin resistance. In obese individuals, lifestyle modifications that gradually reduce adiposity, such as calorie-restricted diets and increased physical activity, achieve these objectives and also improve the histologic features of steatohepatitis. Similar benefits have been observed in morbidly obese patients with NASH who lose weight after gastric bypass surgery. Several small studies of insulin-sensitizing agents (e.g., the biguanide metformin and the thiazolidinediones troglitazone, rosiglitazone, and pioglitazone) have also demonstrated improvements in steatohepatitis and associated fibrosis. Each of these agents has anti-inflammatory actions that reduce TNF-α and increase adiponectin activity. Pioglitazone, a thiazolidinedione that activates the peroxisome proliferator–activating receptor-γ (PPAR-γ), a factor that inhibits the activation of hepatic stellate cells, has shown encouraging short-term metabolic and histologic benefits. [4] Additional, randomized controlled trials of biguanides and thiazolidinediones are in progress. Three small studies of the TNF antagonist pentoxifylline have also shown efficacy in patients with NASH. Antioxidants such as vitamin E, silymarin, betaine, and *S*-adenosylmethionine reduce TNF-α activity and are predicted to improve NASH. Ursodeoxycholic acid is not beneficial, and trials of vitamins C and E have demonstrated inconsistent benefits. Pilot studies of the antioxidants betaine and *S*-adenosylmethionine suggest that these agents may have efficacy. Orlistat, a drug that decreases absorption of dietary lipids, reduces hepatic exposure to fatty acids and has seemed to improve NASH in several small, uncontrolled studies. Other lipid-lowering agents, such as fibrates (which reduce hypertriglyceridemia) and statins (which decrease low-density lipoprotein cholesterol levels) also appear to have some benefits.

TABLE 156–2 APPROACH TO TREATMENT

Mild–Moderate*	**Severe†**		
ALCOHOLIC STEATOHEPATITIS			
Discontinue alcohol	Discontinue alcohol		
Nutritious diet	Enteral or parenteral nutrition		
	Treat alcoholic steatohepatitis		
	Prednisolone (40 mg/day PO)‡ or		
	Pentoxifylline (400 mg PO tid)		
	Treat comorbid conditions		
Body Mass Index <27		**Body Mass Index >27**	
No Diabetes	**Diabetes**	**No Diabetes**	**Diabetes**
NONALCOHOLIC STEATOHEPATITIS			
Vitamin E	Metformin or thiazolidinedione Vitamin E	Diet/exercise Vitamin E	Diet/exercise Metformin or thiazolidinedione Vitamin E

*4.6 × (Patient's prothrombin time – Control prothrombin time) + Bilirubin (mg/dL) ≤ 32.
†4.6 × (Patient's prothrombin time – Control prothrombin time) + Bilirubin (mg/dL) > 32.
‡Contraindicated in patients with active, systemic infection.

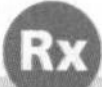

Hence, despite the dearth of prospective controlled treatment trials for NASH, evidence from many small studies suggests that most, if not all of the therapies that improve metabolic syndrome (Chapter 248) also improve NASH. Moreover, treatment with all of these agents appears to be generally safe for patients with fatty liver disease. For patients with NASH but no other clinical manifestations of metabolic syndrome, it is still reasonable to suggest dietary modification and exercise because even very minor reductions in body weight (i.e., about 10 to 20%) improve insulin sensitivity. By comparison, rapid, extreme weight loss may accelerate the progression of NASH to cirrhosis and also increases the risk for gallstone disease.

Prognosis

Among patients hospitalized because of severe alcoholic steatohepatitis, cirrhosis develops in up to 50% within 5 years, an outcome that is more common in patients who have severe liver damage by histology, patients who continue drinking alcohol, and women. Emerging data suggest that cirrhosis will develop in 10 to 50% of patients with steatohepatitis. Factors strongly associated with disease progression include age (older than 40 or 50 years), increased body mass index, and diabetes. Cirrhosis can also develop in relatively asymptomatic individuals with alcoholic steatohepatitis or NASH in whom the hepatic fibrosis evolves gradually over a period of 1 to 2 decades and may not be recognized until an overt manifestation of portal hypertension such as hypersplenism or ascites develops. Advanced fibrosis or cirrhosis develops in about 10 to 50% of patients with alcoholic steatohepatitis within 5 to 10 years. The natural history of patients with cirrhosis is similar, regardless of whether the cirrhosis resulted from alcoholic steatohepatitis or NASH (Chapter 157). Alcohol abuse accelerates the rate of hepatic decompensation and doubles the risk for liver-related mortality in patients with cirrhosis.

Once a diagnosis of cirrhosis has been established, patients should be monitored carefully for the appearance of varices, ascites, encephalopathy, or liver tumors and then treated accordingly. General treatments to prevent or palliate the complications of cirrhosis (Chapter 157) are effective in patients with alcoholic steatohepatitis and NASH.

Presently, 13% of cases of hepatocellular carcinoma in the United States are related to NASH, and this percentage is predicted to increase in parallel with the rising incidence of NASH in the general adult population. Regular screening by abdominal ultrasonography and serum tests for α-fetoprotein improve the early detection of hepatocellular carcinoma.

Ultimately, liver transplantation (Chapter 158) improves the survival of patients who have decompensated cirrhosis or small hepatocellular carcinomas confined to the liver. Most transplant centers do not recommend transplantation for patients with alcoholic liver disease unless they have demonstrated at least 6 months of abstinence from alcohol. However, in sober patients who undergo liver transplantation for alcoholic liver disease, post-transplant survival is outstanding, with 5-year survival rates approaching 85%.

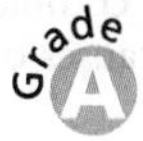

1. Carithers RL, Herlong HF, Diehl AM, et al: Methylprednisolone therapy in patients with severe alcoholic hepatitis: A randomized multicenter trial. Ann Intern Med 1989;110:685–690.
2. Ramond MJ, Poynard T, Rueff B, et al: A randomized trial of prednisolone in patients with severe alcoholic hepatitis. N Engl J Med 1992;326:507–512.
3. Akrividis E, Botla R, Briggs W, et al: Pentoxifylline improves short-term survival in severe acute alcoholic hepatitis: A double-blind, placebo-controlled trial. Gastroenterology 2000;119:1637–1648.
4. Belfort R, Harrison S, Brown K, et al: A placebo-controlled trial of pioglitazone in subjects with nonalcoholic steatohepatitis. N Engl J Med 2006;355:2297–2307.

SUGGESTED READINGS

Adams LA, Angulo P: Recent concepts in non-alcoholic fatty liver disease. Diabet Med 2005;22:1129–1133. *Comprehensive overview of pathobiology and treatment.*

Adams LA, Lymp JF, St Sauver J, et al: The natural history of nonalcoholic fatty liver disease: A population-based cohort study. Gastroenterology 2005;129:113–121. *Epidemiologic evidence that NAFLD progresses to cirrhosis and reduces life expectancy.*

Browning JD, Szczepaniak LS, Dobbins R, et al: Prevalence of hepatic steatosis in an urban population in the United States: Impact of ethnicity. Hepatology 2004;40:1387–1395. *Sensitive imaging techniques demonstrated the prevalence of hepatic steatosis in various ethnic subgroups in the United States.*

Furuya CK Jr, de Oliveira CP, de Melle ES, et al: Effects of bariatric surgery on nonalcoholic fatty liver disease: Preliminary findings after 2 years. J Gastroenterol Hepatol 2007;22:510–514. *Documents benefit on measures of NAFLD.*

Hamaguchi M, Kojima T, Takeda N, et al: The metabolic syndrome as a predictor of nonalcoholic fatty liver disease. Ann Intern Med 2005;143:722–728. *Patients with the metabolic syndrome were more likely to develop NASH and less likely to have NASH regress.*

McCullough AJ: The clinical features, diagnosis and natural history of nonalcoholic fatty liver disease. Clin Liver Dis 2004;8:521–533. *Contemporary practical review of this disease.*

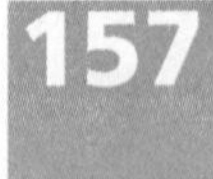

CIRRHOSIS AND ITS SEQUELAE

Guadalupe Garcia-Tsao

Definition

Cirrhosis, which can be the final stage of any chronic liver disease, is a diffuse process characterized by fibrosis and conversion of normal architecture to structurally abnormal nodules (Fig. 157–1). These "regenerative" nodules lack normal lobular organization and are surrounded by fibrous tissue. The process involves the whole liver and is essentially irreversible. Although cirrhosis is histologically an "all or nothing" diagnosis, clinically it can be classified by its status as compensated or decompensated. Decompensated cirrhosis is defined by the presence of ascites, variceal bleeding, encephalopathy, or jaundice, which are complications that result from the main consequences of cirrhosis: portal hypertension and liver insufficiency.

Epidemiology

Because many patients with cirrhosis are asymptomatic until decompensation occurs, it is very difficult to assess the real prevalence and incidence of cirrhosis in the general population. The prevalence of chronic liver disease/cirrhosis worldwide is estimated to be 100 (range, 25 to 400) per 100,000 subjects, but it varies widely by country and by region.

Cirrhosis is an important cause of morbidity and mortality worldwide and in the United States. According to the World Health Organization, about 800,000 people die of cirrhosis annually. In the United States, cirrhosis accounts for about 27,000 deaths each year, or a death rate of 9.4 per 100,000, which makes it the 12th leading cause of death overall. Importantly, chronic liver disease and cirrhosis are the seventh leading cause of death in the United States in individuals between 25 and 64 years of age, with a death rate of 19.9 per 100,000. Because chronic liver disease affects people in their most productive years of life, it has a significant impact on the economy as a result of premature death, illness, and disability.

Any chronic liver disease can lead to cirrhosis (Table 157–1). Chronic viral hepatitis C and alcoholic liver disease are the most common causes of cirrhosis, followed by nonalcoholic fatty liver disease and chronic hepatitis B (Chapters 152 and 156). However, the many other causes of cirrhosis include cholestatic and autoimmune liver diseases such as primary biliary cirrhosis, primary sclerosing cholangitis (Chapter 159), autoimmune hepatitis (Chapter 152), and metabolic diseases such as hemochromatosis, Wilson's disease, and α_1-antitrypsin deficiency (Chapter 154). When all the causes have been investigated and excluded, cirrhosis is considered "cryptogenic." Many cases of cryptogenic cirrhosis are now thought to be due to nonalcoholic fatty liver disease (Chapter 156).

It is important to mention that although the entity termed "primary biliary *cirrhosis*" assumes the presence of cirrhosis, this term is actually misleading. Primary biliary cirrhosis (Chapter 159) is an immune-mediated cholestatic chronic liver disease that is characterized by progressive destruction of intrahepatic bile ducts and progresses over time from an initial stage in which fibrosis is minimal (stage 1) to a final stage in which there is well-established cirrhosis (stage 4).

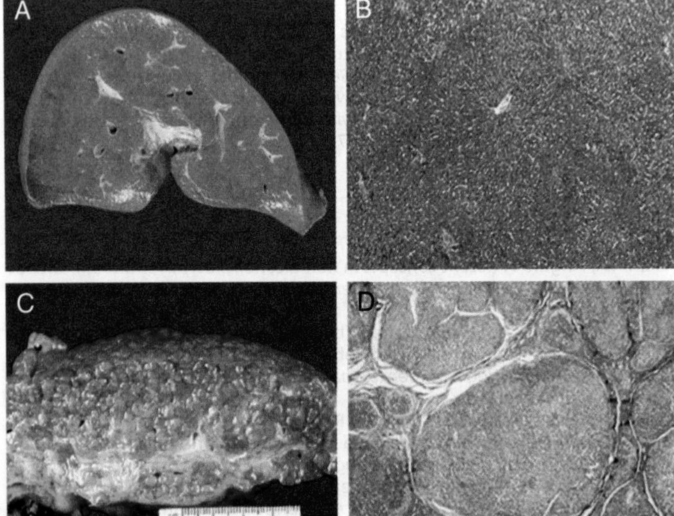

FIGURE 157–1 • Gross and microscopic images of a normal and cirrhotic liver. A, Gross image of a normal liver with a smooth surface and homogeneous texture. **B,** Microscopically, liver sinusoids are organized and vascular structures are normally distributed. **C,** Gross image of a cirrhotic liver. The liver has an orange-tawny color with an irregular surface and a nodular texture. **D,** Microscopically, the architecture is disorganized and there are regenerative nodules surrounded by fibrous tissue.

Pathobiology

Liver Fibrosis/Cirrhosis

The key pathogenic feature underlying liver fibrosis and cirrhosis is activation of hepatic stellate cells. Hepatic stellate cells, which are known as Ito cells or perisinusoidal cells, are located in the space of Disse between hepatocytes and sinusoidal endothelial cells. Normally, hepatic stellate cells are quiescent and serve as the main storage site for retinoids (vitamin A). In response to injury, hepatic stellate cells become activated, as a result of which they lose their vitamin A deposits, proliferate, develop a prominent rough endoplasmic reticulum, and secrete extracellular matrix (collagen types I and III, sulfated proteoglycans, and glycoproteins). Additionally, they become contractile hepatic myofibroblasts.

Unlike other capillaries, normal hepatic sinusoids lack a basement membrane. The sinusoidal endothelial cells themselves contain large fenestrae (100 to 200 nm in diameter) that allow the passage of large molecules with molecular weights up to 250,000. Collagen deposition in the space of Disse, as occurs in cirrhosis, leads to defenestration of the sinusoidal endothelial cells ("capillarization" of the sinusoids), thereby altering exchange between plasma and hepatocytes and resulting in a

TABLE 157–1 CAUSES OF CIRRHOSIS

MAIN FACTORS CAUSING CIRRHOSIS
Chronic hepatitis C
Alcoholic liver disease
Nonalcoholic fatty liver disease
Chronic hepatitis B
OTHER CAUSES OF CIRRHOSIS (<2% OF ALL CASES)
Cholestatic and autoimmune liver diseases
Primary biliary cirrhosis
Primary sclerosing cholangitis
Autoimmune hepatitis
Intrahepatic or extrahepatic biliary obstruction
Mechanical obstruction
Biliary atresia
Cystic fibrosis
Metabolic disorders
Hemochromatosis
Wilson's disease
α_1-Antitrypsin deficiency
Glycogen storage diseases
Abetalipoproteinemia
Porphyria
Hepatic venous outflow obstruction
Budd-Chiari syndrome
Veno-occlusive disease
Right-sided heart failure
Drugs and toxins
Intestinal bypass
Indian childhood cirrhosis

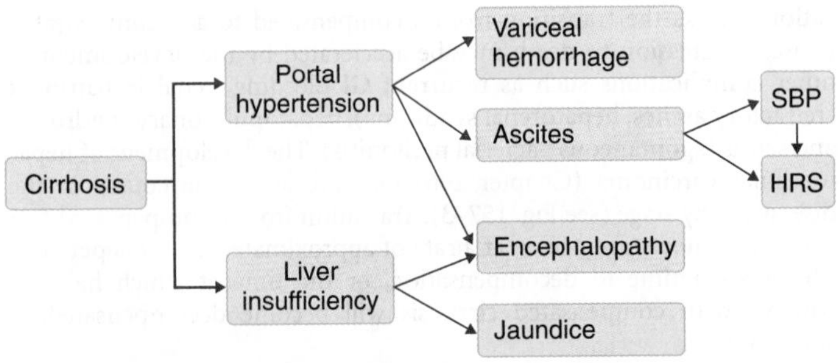

FIGURE 157–2 • Complications of cirrhosis result from portal hypertension or liver insufficiency. Varices and variceal hemorrhage are a direct consequence of portal hypertension. Ascites results from sinusoidal portal hypertension and can be complicated by infection (spontaneous bacterial peritonitis [SBP]) or renal dysfunction (hepatorenal syndrome [HRS]). Hepatic encephalopathy results from portosystemic shunting (i.e., portal hypertension) and liver insufficiency. Jaundice results solely from liver insufficiency.

decreased sinusoidal diameter that is further exacerbated by the contraction of stellate cells.

Complications of Cirrhosis

The two main consequences of cirrhosis are portal hypertension, with the accompanying hyperdynamic circulatory state, and liver insufficiency (Fig. 157–2). The development of varices and ascites is a direct consequence of portal hypertension and the hyperdynamic circulatory state, whereas jaundice occurs as a result of an inability of the liver to excrete bilirubin (i.e., liver insufficiency). Encephalopathy is the result of both portal hypertension and liver insufficiency. Ascites, in turn, can become complicated by infection, which is called spontaneous bacterial peritonitis, and by functional renal failure, which is called hepatorenal syndrome.

Portal Hypertension and the Hyperdynamic Circulatory State

In cirrhosis, portal hypertension results from both an increase in resistance to portal flow and an increase in portal venous inflow. The initial mechanism is increased sinusoidal vascular resistance secondary to (1) deposition of fibrous tissue and subsequent compression by regenerative nodules (fixed component) and (2) active vasoconstriction (functional component), which is amenable to the action of vasodilators such as nitroprusside and is caused by a deficiency in intrahepatic nitric oxide (NO), as well as enhanced activity of vasoconstrictors.

Early in the portal hypertensive process, the spleen grows and sequesters platelets and other formed blood cells, thereby leading to hypersplenism. In addition, vessels that normally drain into the portal system, such as the coronary vein, reverse their flow and shunt blood away from the portal system to the systemic circulation. These portosystemic collaterals are insufficient to decompress the portal venous system and offer additional resistance to portal flow. As collaterals develop, an increase in portal blood inflow maintains the portal hypertensive state as a result of splanchnic vasodilation, which in turn is secondary to increased production of NO. Thus, the paradox in portal hypertension is that a deficiency of NO in the intrahepatic vasculature leads to vasoconstriction and increased resistance whereas overproduction of NO in the extrahepatic circulation leads to vasodilation and increased flow.

In addition to splanchnic vasodilation, there is systemic vasodilation, which by causing a decreased *effective* arterial blood volume, leads to activation of neurohumoral systems, retention of sodium, expansion of plasma volume, and development of a hyperdynamic circulatory state. This hyperdynamic circulatory state maintains the portal hypertension, thereby leading to the formation and growth of varices, and plays an important role in the development of all other complications of cirrhosis.

Varices and Variceal Hemorrhage

The complication of cirrhosis that results most directly from portal hypertension is the development of portal-systemic collaterals, the most relevant of which are those that form through dilation of the coronary and gastric veins and constitute gastroesophageal varices. The initial formation of esophageal collaterals depends on a threshold portal pressure, which is a hepatic venous pressure gradient of 10 to 12 mm Hg, below which varices do not develop.

Development of a hyperdynamic circulatory state leads to further dilation and growth of varices and eventually to their rupture and variceal hemorrhage, one of the most dreaded complications of portal hypertension. Tension in a varix determines variceal rupture and is directly proportional to variceal diameter and intravariceal pressure and inversely proportional to variceal wall thickness.

Ascites and Hepatorenal Syndrome

Ascites in cirrhosis is secondary to sinusoidal hypertension and retention of sodium. Cirrhosis leads to sinusoidal hypertension by blocking hepatic venous outflow both anatomically by fibrosis and regenerative nodules and functionally by increased postsinusoidal vascular tone. Similar to the formation of esophageal varices, a threshold hepatic venous pressure gradient of 12 mm Hg is needed for the formation of ascites. In addition, retention of sodium replenishes the intravascular volume and allows the continuous formation of ascites. Retention of sodium results from vasodilation that is mostly due to an increase in NO production; NO inhibition in experimental animals increases urinary sodium excretion and lowers plasma aldosterone levels. With progression of cirrhosis and portal hypertension, vasodilation is more pronounced, thereby leading to further activation of the renin-angiotensin-aldosterone and sympathetic nervous systems and resulting in further sodium retention (refractory ascites), water retention (hyponatremia), and renal vasoconstriction (hepatorenal syndrome).

Spontaneous Bacterial Peritonitis

Spontaneous bacterial peritonitis, which is an infection of ascitic fluid, occurs in the absence of perforation of a hollow viscus or an intra-abdominal inflammatory focus such as an abscess, acute pancreatitis, or cholecystitis. Bacterial translocation, or the migration of bacteria from the intestinal lumen to mesenteric lymph nodes and other extraintestinal sites, is the main mechanism implicated in spontaneous bacterial peritonitis. Impaired local and systemic immune defenses are a major element in promoting bacterial translocation and, together with shunting of blood away from the hepatic Kupffer cells through portosystemic collaterals, allow a transient bacteremia to become more prolonged, thereby colonizing ascitic fluid. Spontaneous bacterial peritonitis occurs in patients with reduced ascites defense mechanisms, such as a low complement level in ascitic fluid. Another factor that promotes bacterial translocation in cirrhosis is bacterial overgrowth attributed to a decrease in small bowel motility and intestinal transit time. Infections, particularly from gram-negative bacteria, can precipitate renal dysfunction through worsening of the hyperdynamic circulatory state.

Encephalopathy

Ammonia, a toxin normally removed by the liver, plays a key role in the pathogenesis of hepatic encephalopathy. In cirrhosis, ammonia accumulates in the systemic circulation because of shunting of blood through portosystemic collaterals and decreased liver metabolism (i.e., liver insufficiency). The presence of large amounts of ammonia in the brain damages supporting brain cells or astrocytes and leads to structural changes characteristic of hepatic encephalopathy (Alzheimer's type II astrocytosis). Ammonia results in upregulation of astrocytic peripheral-type benzodiazepine receptors, the most potent stimulants of neurosteroid production. Neurosteroids are the major modulators of γ-aminobutyric acid, which results in cortical depression and hepatic encephalopathy. Other toxins, such as manganese, also accumulate in the brain, particularly the globus pallidus, where they lead to impaired motor function.

Jaundice

Jaundice (Chapters 149 and 150) in cirrhosis is a reflection of the inability of the liver to excrete bilirubin and is therefore the result of liver insufficiency. However, in cholestatic diseases leading to cirrhosis (e.g., primary biliary cirrhosis, primary sclerosing cholangitis, vanishing bile duct syndrome), jaundice is more likely due to biliary damage than liver insufficiency. Other indicators of liver insufficiency, such as the prothrombin time or the presence of encephalopathy, help determine the most likely contributor to hyperbilirubinemia (Chapter 150).

Cardiopulmonary Complications

The hyperdynamic circulatory state eventually results in high-output heart failure with decreased peripheral utilization of oxygen, a complication that has been referred to as cirrhotic cardiomyopathy. Vasodilation at the level of the pulmonary circulation leads to arterial hypoxemia, the hallmark of hepatopulmonary syndrome. Normal pulmonary capillaries are 8 μm in diameter, and red blood cells (slightly <8 μm) pass through them one cell at a time, thereby facilitating oxygenation. In hepatopulmonary syndrome, the pulmonary capillaries are dilated up to 500 μm, so passage of red cells through the pulmonary capillaries may be many cells thick. As a result, a large number of red cells are not oxygenated, which causes the equivalent of a right-to-left shunt.

Conversely, portopulmonary hypertension occurs when the pulmonary bed is exposed to vasoconstrictive substances that may be produced in the splanchnic circulation and bypass metabolism by the liver; the initial result is reversible pulmonary hypertension. However, because these factors result in endothelial proliferation, vasoconstriction, in situ thrombosis, and obliteration of vessels, irreversible pulmonary hypertension ensues.

Clinical Manifestations

The clinical manifestations of cirrhosis range widely, depending on the stage of cirrhosis, from an asymptomatic patient with no signs of chronic liver disease to a patient who is confused and jaundiced and has severe muscle wasting and ascites. The natural history of cirrhosis is characterized by an initial phase, termed "compensated" cirrhosis, followed by a rapidly progressive phase marked by the development of complications of portal hypertension or liver dysfunction (or both), termed "decompensated" cirrhosis (Fig. 157–3). In the compensated phase, portal pressure may be normal or below the threshold level identified for the development of varices or ascites. As the disease progresses, portal pressure increases and liver function decreases, thereby resulting in the development of ascites, portal hypertensive gastrointestinal (GI) bleeding, encephalopathy, and jaundice. The development of any of these complications marks the transition from a compensated to a decompensated phase. Progression to death may be accelerated by the development of other complications such as recurrent GI bleeding, renal impairment (refractory ascites, hepatorenal syndrome), hepatopulmonary syndrome, and sepsis (spontaneous bacterial peritonitis). The development of hepatocellular carcinoma (Chapter 206) may accelerate the course of the disease at any stage (see Fig. 157–3). Transition from a compensated to a decompensated stage occurs at a rate of approximately 5 to 7% per year. The median time to decompensation, or the time at which half the patients with compensated cirrhosis will become decompensated, is about 6 years.

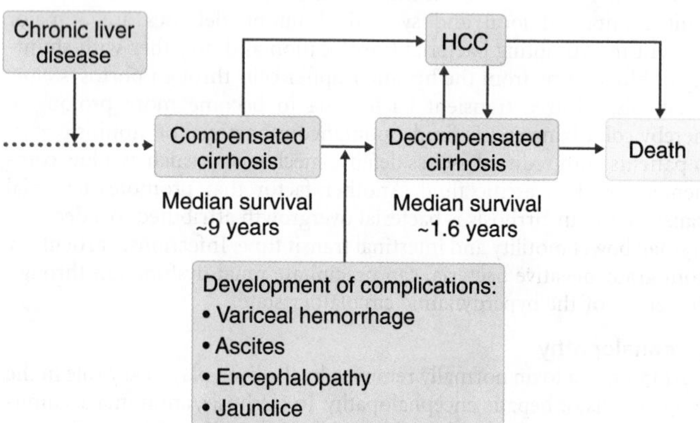

FIGURE 157–3 • Natural history of cirrhosis. Any chronic liver disease will lead to cirrhosis. Initially, cirrhosis will be compensated (median survival, 9 years), but once complications (ascites, variceal hemorrhage, encephalopathy, jaundice) develop, it becomes decompensated (median survival, 1.6 years). Hepatocellular carcinoma (HCC) can develop at any stage and precipitate decompensation and death.

Compensated Cirrhosis

In this stage, cirrhosis is mostly asymptomatic and is diagnosed either (1) when a liver biopsy is performed during the evaluation of chronic liver disease or (2) fortuitously during routine physical examination, biochemical testing, imaging for other reasons, or abdominal surgery. Nonspecific fatigue, decreased libido, or sleep disturbances may be the only complaints.

About 40% of patients with compensated cirrhosis have esophageal varices. Nonbleeding gastroesophageal varices are asymptomatic, and their presence (without bleeding) does not denote decompensation.

Decompensated Cirrhosis

At this stage there are signs of decompensation: ascites, variceal hemorrhage, jaundice, hepatic encephalopathy, or any combination of these findings. Ascites, which is the most frequent sign of decompensation, is present in 80% of patients with decompensated cirrhosis.

Variceal Hemorrhage

Gastroesophageal varices are present in approximately 50% of patients with newly diagnosed cirrhosis. The prevalence of varices correlates with the severity of liver disease and ranges from 40% in Child A cirrhotic patients (Table 157–2) to 85% in Child C cirrhotic patients.

Both the development of varices and the growth of small varices occur at a rate of 7 to 8% per year. The incidence of a first variceal hemorrhage in patients with small varices is about 5% per year, whereas medium and large varices bleed at a rate of approximately 15% per year. Large varices, severe liver disease, and red wale markings on varices are independent predictors of variceal hemorrhage. Bleeding from gastroesophageal varices can be manifested as overt hematemesis or melena, or both (Chapter 137).

Ascites and Hepatorenal Syndrome

Ascites (Chapter 145) is the most common cause of decompensation in cirrhosis and occurs at a rate of 7 to 10% per year. The most frequent symptoms associated with ascites are increased abdominal girth, which is often described by the patient as tightness of the belt or garments around the waist, and recent weight gain. When present in small to moderate amounts, ascites can be identified on examination by bulging flanks, flank dullness, and shifting dullness (Chapter 149).

TABLE 157–2 THE TWO MOST COMMONLY USED SCORING SYSTEMS IN CIRRHOSIS

1. Child-Pugh-Turcotte (CPT) score (range, 5–15)

	Points Ascribed		
Parameters	**1**	**2**	**3**
Ascites	None	Grade 1–2 (or easy to treat)	Grade 3–4 (or refractory)
Hepatic encephalopathy	None	Grade 1–2 (or induced by a precipitant)	Grade 3–4 (or spontaneous)
Bilirubin (mg/dL)	<2	2–3	>3
Albumin (g/dL)	>3.5	2.8–3.5	<2.8
Prothrombin time (seconds > control) or INR	<4 <1.7	4–6 1.7–2.3	>6 >2.3

CPT classification: Child A: score of 5–6; Child B: score of 7–9; Child C: score of 10–15

2. Model of End-Stage Liver Disease (MELD) score (range, 6–40):

[0.957 × LN (creatinine in mg/dL) + 0.378 × LN (bilirubin in mg/dL) + 1.12 × LN (INR) + 0.643] × 10

INR = international normalized ratio; LN = natural logarithm.

Hepatorenal syndrome is divided into two types based on clinical characteristics and prognosis. Type 1 hepatorenal syndrome is rapidly progressive renal failure in which a doubling of serum creatinine (or halving of creatinine clearance) occurs within a 2-week period. Type 2 hepatorenal syndrome is more slowly progressive and associated with ascites that is refractory to diuretics. Patients with hepatorenal syndrome usually have tense ascites that responds poorly to diuretics, but no specific symptoms or signs typify this entity.

Spontaneous Bacterial Peritonitis

About a third of cirrhotic patients are admitted for or acquire bacterial infections during hospitalization, the most common being spontaneous bacterial peritonitis. The two most important predictors of the development of bacterial infection are the severity of liver disease and admission for GI hemorrhage. The most frequent clinical manifestations of spontaneous bacterial peritonitis are fever, jaundice, and abdominal pain. On physical examination there is typically abdominal tenderness, with or without rebound tenderness, or ileus (or both). However, patients with spontaneous bacterial peritonitis may have just encephalopathy or evidence of shock. Up to a third of patients may be entirely asymptomatic.

Hepatic Encephalopathy

Hepatic encephalopathy, which is the neuropsychiatric manifestation of cirrhosis, occurs at a rate of approximately 2 to 3% per year. Hepatic encephalopathy associated with cirrhosis is of gradual onset and rarely fatal. Clinically, it is characterized by alterations in consciousness and behavior ranging from inversion of the sleep/wake pattern and forgetfulness (stage 1); to confusion, bizarre behavior, and disorientation (stage 2); to lethargy and profound disorientation (stage 3); to coma (stage 4) (Chapter 158). On physical examination, early stages may demonstrate only a distal tremor, but the hallmark of hepatic encephalopathy is the presence of asterixis (Chapter 149). Additionally, patients with hepatic encephalopathy may have sweet-smelling breath, a characteristic termed *fetor hepaticus*.

Pulmonary Complications

Hepatopulmonary syndrome is associated with exertional dyspnea, which can lead to extreme debilitation. Clubbing of the fingers, cyanosis, and vascular spiders may be seen on physical examination. Hepatopulmonary syndrome is present in approximately 5 to 10% of patients awaiting liver transplantation.

Portopulmonary hypertension is manifested as exertional dyspnea, syncope, and chest pain. On examination, an accentuated second sound and right ventricular heave are prominent (Chapter 67).

Diagnosis

The diagnosis of cirrhosis should be considered in any patient with chronic liver disease. In asymptomatic patients with *compensated cirrhosis*, typical signs of cirrhosis may not be present, and the diagnosis may often require histologic confirmation by liver biopsy, which is the "gold standard" for the diagnosis of cirrhosis. In patients with symptoms or signs of chronic liver disease, however, the presence of cirrhosis can frequently be confirmed noninvasively by imaging studies without the need for liver biopsy.

Physical Examination

On physical examination, stigmata of cirrhosis consist of muscle atrophy, mainly involving the bitemporal muscle regions and the thenar and hypothenar eminences; spider angiomas, mostly on the trunk, face, and upper limbs; and palmar erythema involving the thenar and the hypothenar eminences and the tips of the fingers. Although muscular atrophy is a marker of liver insufficiency, spider angiomas and palmar erythema are markers of vasodilation and a hyperdynamic circulation. Males may have hair loss on the chest and abdomen, gynecomastia, and testicular atrophy. Petechiae and ecchymoses may be present as a result of thrombocytopenia or a prolonged prothrombin time. Dupuytren's contracture, which is a thickening of the palmar fascia, occurs mostly in alcoholic cirrhosis. A pathognomonic feature of cirrhosis is the finding on abdominal examination of a small right liver lobe, with a span of less than 7 cm on percussion, and a palpable left lobe that is nodular with increased consistency. Splenomegaly may also be present and is indicative of portal hypertension. Collateral circulation on the abdominal wall (caput medusae) may also develop as a consequence of portal hypertension. Absence of any of the aforementioned physical findings does not exclude cirrhosis.

Laboratory Tests

Laboratory test results suggestive of cirrhosis include even subtle abnormalities in serum levels of albumin or bilirubin or elevation of the international normalized ratio. The most sensitive and specific laboratory finding suggestive of cirrhosis in the setting of chronic liver disease is a low platelet count (<150,000/mm^3), which occurs as a result of portal hypertension and hypersplenism. Other serum markers that are often abnormal include levels of aspartate and alanine aminotransferase, alkaline phosphatase, γ-glutamyl transpeptidase, hyaluronic acid, α_2-macroglobulin, haptoglobin, and apolipoprotein A. Although attempts have been made to use such markers to predict the presence of cirrhosis, none have sufficient sensitivity and specificity to be useful clinically.

Imaging Studies

Confirmatory imaging tests include computed tomography, ultrasound, and magnetic resonance imaging. Findings consistent with cirrhosis include a nodular contour of the liver, a small liver with or without hypertrophy of the left/caudate lobe, splenomegaly, and in particular, identification of intra-abdominal collateral vessels indicative of portal hypertension. On a liver-spleen scan, findings consistent with cirrhosis are heterogeneous colloid uptake by a small liver, splenomegaly, and colloid shift to the bone marrow. Typical findings on any of these imaging studies together with a compatible clinical picture are indicative of the presence of cirrhosis; a liver biopsy is not required unless the degree of inflammation or other features require investigation.

In *decompensated cirrhosis*, detection of ascites, variceal bleeding, or encephalopathy in the setting of chronic liver disease essentially establishes the diagnosis of cirrhosis; a liver biopsy is not necessary to establish the diagnosis. Patients with decompensated cirrhosis often exhibit malnutrition, more severe muscle wasting, more numerous vascular spiders, and hypotension and tachycardia as a result of the hyperdynamic circulatory state.

Portal Pressure Measurements

Direct measurements of portal pressure involve catheterization of the portal vein, are cumbersome, and may be associated with complications. Hepatic vein catheterization with measurement of wedged and free pressure is the simplest, safest, most reproducible, and most widely used method to indirectly measure portal pressure. Portal pressure measurements are expressed as the hepatic venous pressure gradient: the gradient between wedged hepatic venous pressure, which is a measure of sinusoidal pressure, and free hepatic or inferior vena cava pressure, which is used as an internal zero reference point. In a patient with clinical evidence of portal hypertension (e.g., varices), the hepatic venous pressure gradient is useful in the differential diagnosis of the cause of portal hypertension: it will be normal in prehepatic causes of portal hypertension, such as portal vein thrombosis (Chapter 158), and in intrahepatic but presinusoidal causes, such as schistosomiasis (Chapter 376), but will be abnormal in sinusoidal causes of portal hypertension, such as cirrhosis, and in postsinusoidal causes, such as veno-occlusive disease. Not unexpectedly, the hepatic venous pressure gradient predicts the development of complications of portal hypertension, and its reduction on pharmacologic therapy predicts a favorable outcome in patients with cirrhosis.

Complications of Cirrhosis

Varices and Variceal Hemorrhage

Upper GI endoscopy (Chapters 136 and 137) remains the main method for diagnosing varices and variceal hemorrhage. Varices are classified as small (straight, minimally elevated veins above the esophageal mucosal surface), medium (tortuous veins occupying less than a third of the esophageal lumen), or large (occupying more than a third of the esophageal lumen). The diagnosis of variceal hemorrhage is made when diagnostic esophagogastroduodenoscopy shows one of the following: active bleeding from a varix, a "white nipple" overlying a varix, clots overlying a varix, or varices with no other potential source of bleeding.

Ascites

The most common cause of ascites is cirrhosis, which accounts for 80% of cases; peritoneal malignancy (e.g., peritoneal metastases from GI tumors or ovarian cancer; Chapter 145), heart failure (Chapter 57), and peritoneal tuberculosis (Chapters 145, 155, and 345) account for another 15% of cases. The initial, most cost-effective, and least invasive method to confirm the presence of ascites is abdominal ultrasonography.

Diagnostic paracentesis is a safe procedure that should be performed in every patient with new-onset ascites, even in those with coagulopathy. Ultrasound guidance should be used in patients in whom percussion cannot locate the ascites or in whom a first paracentesis attempt does not yield fluid. The fluid in a patient with new-onset ascites should always be evaluated for albumin (with simultaneous estimation of serum albumin), total protein, polymorphonuclear (PMN) blood cell count, bacteriologic cultures, and cytology. The PMN cell count and bacteriologic culture are useful to exclude infection (spontaneous or secondary bacterial peritonitis), and cytologic evaluation is needed if peritoneal carcinomatosis is suspected. Depending on the clinical setting, additional tests can be performed on the fluid: glucose and lactate dehydrogenase levels (if secondary bacterial peritonitis is suspected), smear and culture for acid-fast bacilli (if peritoneal tuberculosis is suspected), and an amylase level (if pancreatic ascites is suspected).

The serum-ascites albumin gradient and ascites protein levels are useful in the differential diagnosis of ascites (Table 157–3). The serum-ascites albumin gradient correlates with sinusoidal pressure and will therefore be elevated (>1.1 g/dL) in patients in whom the source of ascites is the hepatic sinusoid (e.g., cirrhosis or cardiac ascites). Protein levels in ascitic fluid are an indirect marker of the integrity of the hepatic sinusoids: normal sinusoids are permeable structures that "leak" protein, whereas sinusoids in cirrhosis are "capillarized" and do not leak as much protein. The three main causes of ascites—cirrhosis, peritoneal malignancy or tuberculosis, and heart failure—can easily be distinguished by combining the results of both the serum-ascites albumin gradient and ascites total protein content. Cirrhotic ascites typically has a high serum-ascites albumin gradient and low protein, cardiac ascites has a high serum-ascites albumin gradient and high protein, and ascites secondary to peritoneal malignancy typically has a low serum-ascites albumin gradient and high protein.

Hepatorenal Syndrome

Hepatorenal syndrome represents the extreme of the spectrum of abnormalities that lead to cirrhotic ascites and is characterized by maximal peripheral vasodilation as well as maximal activation of hormones that cause the retention of sodium and water and vasoconstriction of renal arteries. Ascites unresponsive to diuretics is universal, and dilutional hyponatremia is almost always present.

Hepatorenal syndrome, which is a diagnosis of exclusion, should be made only after discontinuing diuretics, expanding intravascular volume with albumin, and excluding or treating any condition that leads to worsening of the hemodynamic status of the cirrhotic patient. The differential diagnosis includes conditions that worsen vasodilation, such as sepsis, the use of vasodilators, and large-volume paracentesis not accompanied by albumin infusion; conditions that decrease effective arterial blood volume, such as fluid losses through overdiuresis or diarrhea (often induced by overdoses of lactulose); conditions that induce renal vasoconstriction, such as nonsteroidal anti-inflammatory drugs; and nephrotoxic insults, such as from aminoglycosides.

Spontaneous Bacterial Peritonitis

A high index of suspicion and early diagnosis are key in the management of spontaneous bacterial peritonitis. Diagnostic paracentesis should be performed in any patient with symptoms or signs of spontaneous bacterial peritonitis, including unexplained encephalopathy and renal dysfunction. Because spontaneous bacterial peritonitis is often asymptomatic and frequently community acquired, diagnostic paracentesis should be performed when any cirrhotic patient is admitted to the hospital, regardless of the cause for admission.

The diagnosis of spontaneous bacterial peritonitis is established by an ascitic fluid PMN count greater than 250/mm^3. Bacteria can be isolated from ascitic fluid in only 40 to 50% of cases, even with sensitive methods such as inoculation directly into a blood culture bottle. Spontaneous bacterial peritonitis is mostly a monobacterial infection, usually with gram-negative enteric organisms. Anaerobes and fungi very rarely cause spontaneous bacterial peritonitis; their presence, as well as a polymicrobial infection, should raise suspicion of secondary bacterial peritonitis.

Hepatic Encephalopathy

The diagnosis of hepatic encephalopathy is clinical and based on the history and physical examination showing alterations in consciousness and behavior, as well as the presence of asterixis. Ammonia levels are unreliable, and there is poor correlation between the stage of hepatic encephalopathy and ammonia blood levels. Therefore, measurements of ammonia are not useful. Psychometric tests and an electroencephalogram are typically used in research but are not useful for clinical diagnosis. Minimal hepatic encephalopathy, formerly called "subclinical" hepatic encephalopathy, which occurs in about 30 to 70% of patients who have cirrhosis without overt hepatic encephalopathy, is detected by psychometric and neuropsychological testing of attention (e.g., number connection test, digit symbol test) and psychomotor function (e.g., grooved pegboard) alone. However, screening of cirrhotic patients for asymptomatic hepatic encephalopathy is not recommended because diagnostic tests are not standardized and the benefits of treatment are unknown.

Hepatopulmonary Syndrome and Portopulmonary Hypertension

The diagnostic criteria for hepatopulmonary syndrome are arterial hypoxemia with a $Pa{O_2}$ less than 80 mm Hg or an alveolar arterial oxygen gradient greater than 15 mm Hg, along with evidence of pulmonary vascular shunting on contrast echocardiography (Chapter 53) or a ^{99m}Tc-labeled macroaggregated albumin scan demonstrating abnormal shunting of radioactivity to the brain. Portopulmonary hypertension is diagnosed by the presence of mean pulmonary arterial pressure higher than 25 mm Hg on right heart catheterization, provided that pulmonary capillary wedge pressure is less than 15 mm Hg.

TABLE 157–3 USING THE SERUM-ASCITES ALBUMIN GRADIENT AND THE ASCITES TOTAL PROTEIN LEVEL TO DIAGNOSE THE CAUSE OF ASCITES

Condition	Serum-Ascites Albumin Gradient*	Ascites Total Protein Level†
Cirrhosis	High	Low
Malignant ascites	Low	High
Cardiac ascites	High	High

*High is greater than 1.1 g/dL; low is less than 1.1 g/dL.
†High is greater than 2.5 g/dL; low is less than 2.5 g/dL.

Treatment

Rx

Treatment of cirrhosis should ideally be aimed at interrupting or reversing fibrosis. However, antifibrotic drugs have not been shown to reverse fibrosis consistently or improve outcomes in cirrhotic patients. Treatment of compensated cirrhosis is currently directed at preventing the development of decompensation by (1) treating the underlying liver disease (e.g., antiviral therapy for hepatitis C or B) to reduce fibrosis and prevent decompensation; (2) avoiding factors that could worsen liver disease, such as alcohol and hepatotoxic drugs; and (3) screening for varices (to prevent variceal hemorrhage) and for hepatocellular carcinoma (to treat at an early stage) (Fig. 157–4). Treatment of decompensated cirrhosis is directed toward specific decompensating events.

Varices and Variceal Bleeding

Reducing portal pressure decreases the risk for the development of varices and variceal hemorrhage, as well as the risk for ascites and death. Nonselective β-adrenergic blockers (propranolol, nadolol) reduce portal pressure by producing splanchnic vasoconstriction and decreasing portal venous inflow. In patients with cirrhosis and medium/large varices that have never bled, nonselective β-blockers significantly reduce the risk for first variceal hemorrhage, and their use in this setting is considered the standard of care. [1] Propranolol should be initiated at a dose of 20 mg orally twice a day, whereas nadolol should be initiated at a dose of 20 mg orally every day. The dose should be titrated to produce a resting heart rate of about 55 to 60 beats per minute. In patients who cannot tolerate or have contraindications to β-blockers, particularly those with large

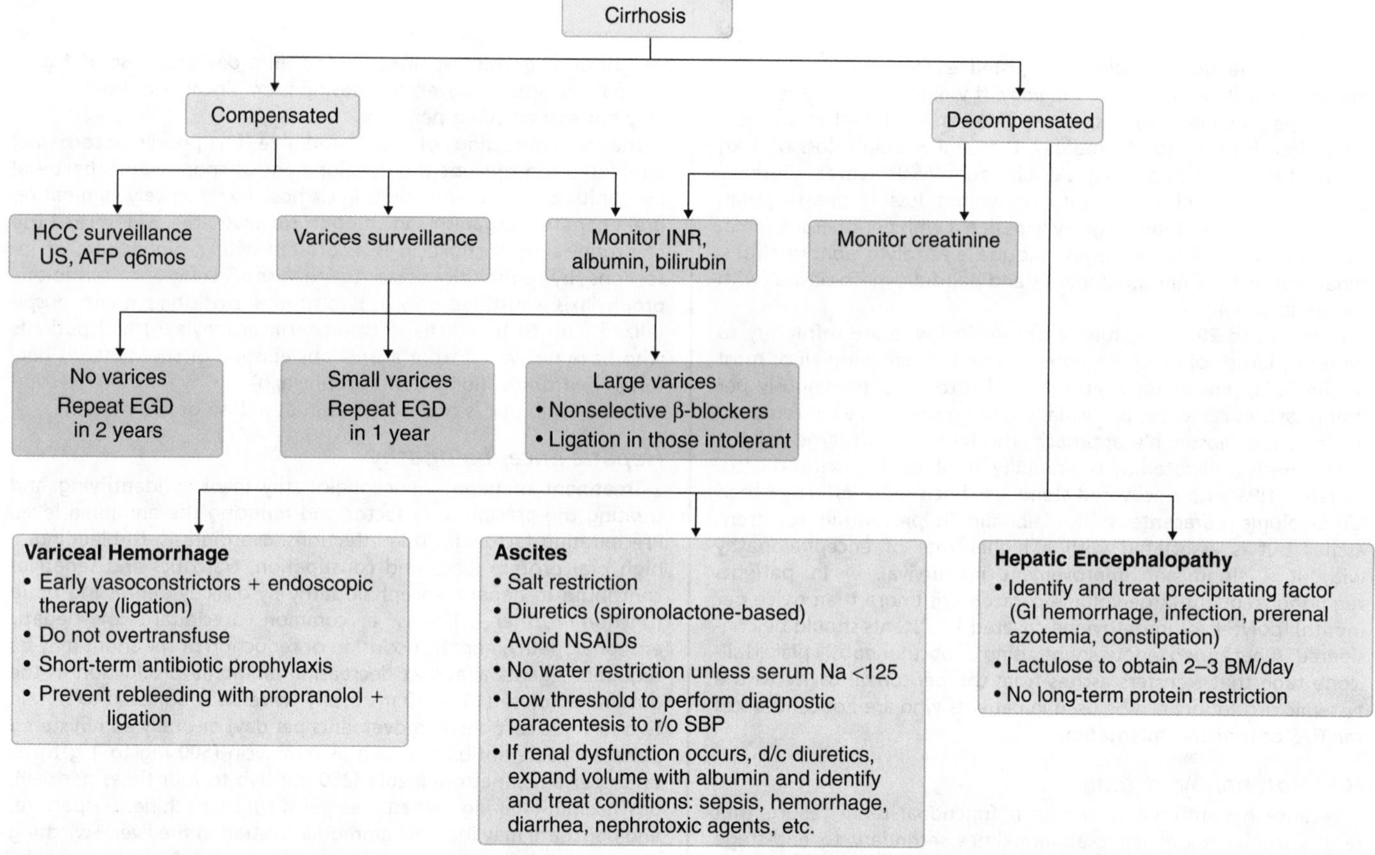

FIGURE 157–4 • Summary of the management of compensated and decompensated cirrhosis. AFP = α-fetoprotein; BM = bowel movement; EGD = esophagogastroduodenoscopy; GI = gastrointestinal; HCC = hepatocellular carcinoma; INR = international normalized ratio; Na = sodium; NSAIDs = nonsteroidal anti-inflammatory drugs; SBP = spontaneous bacterial peritonitis; US = ultrasound.

Rx

varices with red wale marks, endoscopic variceal ligation is indicated. Ligation is a local therapy that aims to obliterate varices by placement of rubber rings on variceal columns. In patients with no varices, nonselective β-blockers do not prevent the development of varices and are associated with more side effects. 2 In patients with small varices, data are insufficient to recommend therapy with nonselective β-blockers. Endoscopy should be repeated every 2 to 3 years in patients with no varices, every 1 to 2 years in patients with small varices, and sooner in patients with decompensated disease so that effective therapy can be instituted before the varices grow in size and bleed.

Patients with cirrhosis and variceal hemorrhage require resuscitation in an intensive care unit. However, overtransfusion and volume overexpansion should be avoided because they can precipitate rebleeding. Prophylactic antibiotics should be used in this setting not only to prevent bacterial infections but also to decrease rebleeding 3 and death. The recommended antibiotic is oral norfloxacin at a dose of 400 mg twice daily for 5 to 7 days, although ciprofloxacin (orally at a dose of 500 mg twice daily or intravenously at a dose of 400 mg twice daily) for 5 to 7 days is a reasonable alternative.

The most effective specific therapy for the control of active variceal hemorrhage is the combination of a vasoconstrictor with endoscopic therapy. Safe vasoconstrictors include terlipressin, somatostatin, and the somatostatin analogues octreotide and vapreotide; they can be initiated at admission to the hospital and continued for 2 to 5 days. The vasoconstrictor currently available in the United States is octreotide, which is used as a 50-μg bolus followed by an infusion at 50 μg/hr.

After control of hemorrhage, the 1-year recurrence of hemorrhage without treatment is very high at about 60%. Therefore, therapy to prevent rebleeding should be instituted before the patient is discharged. The lowest rebleeding rates (about 10%) are observed in patients who achieve a significant reduction in the hepatic venous pressure gradient with pharmacologic therapy (β-blockers, at the same dose recommended for prevention of first hemorrhage, with or without isosorbide mononitrate at stepwise dosing starting at 20 mg/day and increased as tolerated up to 40 mg twice a day); however, because hepatic venous pressure gradient measurements are not widely used, the next best results (rebleeding rates of 14 to 23%) are obtained with the combination of nonselective β-blockers (propranolol or nadolol) and endoscopic variceal ligation. 4 The dose of β-blockers should be the maximal dose tolerated, and endoscopic variceal ligation should be repeated every 2 to 4 weeks until the varices are obliterated.

Shunt therapy should be used in patients whose variceal bleeding has persisted or recurred despite combined pharmacologic and endoscopic therapy. Shunt therapy is most commonly accomplished with a transjugular intrahepatic portosystemic shunt (TIPS) to connect the portal vein to the hepatic vein, bypass the liver, and normalize portal pressure; however, TIPS can also cause complications or worsen hepatic encephalopathy and liver failure. Moreover, TIPS stents can occlude, but newer polytetrafluoroethylene-covered stents are associated with lower occlusion rates and lower rates of hepatic encephalopathy. 5

Ascites

Salt restriction and diuretics constitute the mainstay of management of ascites. Dietary sodium intake should be restricted to 2 g/day. A more restrictive diet is not recommended and may compromise nutritional status. Fluid restriction is not required unless the serum sodium concentration is below 125 mEq/L.

Spironolactone, which is more effective than loop diuretics, should be started at a dose of 100 mg/day (once a day in the

Rx

morning). The dose should be adjusted every 3 to 4 days to a maximal effective dose of 400 mg/day. If weight loss is inadequate or if hyperkalemia develops, furosemide can be added at an escalated dose from 40 to 160 mg/day. The goal is weight loss of 1 kg in the first week and 2 kg/wk subsequently. However, diuretics should be reduced if the rate of weight loss is greater than 0.5 kg/day or more than 1 kg/day in patients with peripheral edema. Side effects of diuretic therapy include electrolyte abnormalities, renal dysfunction, encephalopathy, and painful gynecomastia (with spironolactone).

In the 10 to 20% of patients with ascites who are refractory to diuretics, large-volume paracentesis, aimed at removing all or most of the fluid, plus albumin at a dose of 6 to 8 g intravenously per liter of ascites removed, particularly when more than 5 L is removed at once, is a reasonable approach. The frequency of large-volume paracentesis is dictated by the rapidity at which the ascites reaccumulates. TIPS with uncovered stents has been more effective than large-volume paracentesis plus albumin in preventing recurrent ascites but is associated with a higher rate of encephalopathy without a significant improvement in survival. [6] In patients requiring frequent large-volume paracentesis (more than twice per month), polytetrafluoroethylene-covered TIPS stents should be considered. A peritoneovenous shunt, using a subcutaneously placed silicone tube that transfers ascites from the peritoneal cavity to the systemic circulation, can be used in patients who are not candidates for TIPS or liver transplantation.

Hepatorenal Syndrome

Because hepatorenal syndrome is functional renal failure that results from hemodynamic abnormalities secondary to end-stage liver disease and severe portal hypertension, the mainstay of therapy is liver transplantation (Chapter 158). Therapies that have been used to "bridge" a patient to transplantation include vasoconstrictors plus albumin, TIPS, and extracorporeal albumin dialysis, which is an experimental hemofiltration dialysis method that uses an albumin dialysate. Evidence for the use of these treatments is not strong, and randomized trials will be necessary to determine the best therapeutic strategy for hepatorenal syndrome. The largest experience is with the combination of potent vasoconstrictors (terlipressin, octreotide plus midodrine, noradrenaline), which act by ameliorating the vasodilatory state of advanced cirrhosis, plus intravenous albumin (25 to 50 g/day), which acts by expanding arterial blood volume. The most investigated drug is terlipressin, used at a dose 0.5 to 2.0 mg intravenously every 4 to 6 hours. Because terlipressin is not yet available in the United States, the most used combination is octreotide (100 to 200 μg subcutaneously three times a day) plus midodrine (7.5 to 12.5 mg orally three times a day), with the dose adjusted to obtain an increase of at least 15 mm Hg in mean arterial pressure. Improvements may become clinically noticeable at day 7.

Spontaneous Bacterial Peritonitis

Empirical antibiotic therapy with an intravenous third-generation cephalosporin (e.g., cefotaxime, 2 g intravenously every 12 hours, or ceftriaxone, 1 to 2 g intravenously every 24 hours) or amoxicillin–clavulanic acid (1 g/0.5 g intravenously every 8 hours) should be initiated as soon as the diagnosis is established and before culture results are available; the minimal duration of therapy should be 5 days. Aminoglycosides should be avoided because of the high incidence of renal toxicity in cirrhotic patients. Repeat diagnostic paracentesis should be performed 2 days after starting antibiotics, by which time the number of PMN neutrophils in ascitic fluid should have decreased by more than 25% from baseline. Lack of response should prompt further investigations to exclude secondary peritonitis. The renal dysfunction associated with spontaneous bacterial peritonitis can be prevented by the intravenous administration of albumin, particularly in patients who have any evidence of renal dysfunction (blood urea nitrogen >30 mg/dL and/or creatinine >1 mg/dL) or serum bilirubin greater than 4 mg/dL at the time of diagnosis. Albumin has been used at a dose of 1.5 g/kg of body weight at diagnosis, repeated on the third day at a dose of 1 g/kg of body weight. However, this dosing is empirical and should probably not exceed 100 g per dose.

The administration of nonabsorbable (or poorly absorbable) antibiotics can prevent the development of spontaneous bacterial peritonitis and other infections in cirrhosis by selectively eliminating gram-negative organisms in the gut. However, the widespread use of prophylactic norfloxacin is associated with a higher rate of infections by antibiotic-resistant organisms. Long-term antibiotic prophylaxis is justified only in two groups: cirrhotic patients hospitalized with GI hemorrhage (short-term prophylaxis) and patients who have recovered from a previous episode of spontaneous bacterial peritonitis (long-term prophylaxis), in whom the recommended antibiotic is oral norfloxacin at a dose of 400 mg/day.

Hepatic Encephalopathy

Treatment of hepatic encephalopathy involves identifying and treating the precipitating factor and reducing the ammonia level. Precipitating factors include infections, overdiuresis, GI bleeding, a high oral protein load, and constipation. Narcotics and sedatives contribute to hepatic encephalopathy by directly depressing brain function further. TIPS is a common precipitant of hepatic encephalopathy; hepatic occlusion or reduction of the shunt may be required. Agents aimed at decreasing ammonia production in the gut are lactulose (15 to 30 mL orally twice daily adjusted to obtain two to three soft bowel movements per day) or orally administered nonabsorbable antibiotics such as neomycin (500 mg to 1 g three times per day), metronidazole (250 mg two to four times per day), or rifaximin (400 mg three times per day). L-Ornithine, L-aspartate, and benzoate may increase ammonia fixation in the liver. Switching dietary protein from an animal source to a vegetable source may be beneficial, but protein restriction is not necessary and should not be used long-term. [7]

Pulmonary Complications

Hepatopulmonary syndrome rarely resolves spontaneously, and medical therapy is disappointing. TIPS is not generally recommended. The only viable treatment is liver transplantation (Chapter 158).

By comparison, portopulmonary hypertension is not an indication for liver transplantation. In fact, a mean pulmonary arterial pressure higher than 50 mm Hg is an absolute contraindication to liver transplantation.

Surgical Therapy

Liver Transplantation

Orthotopic liver transplantation (Chapter 158), which is the definitive therapy for cirrhosis, is indicated when the risk of dying from liver disease is greater than the risk of dying from transplantation, as determined by a Child-Pugh score of 7 or higher (see Table 157–2) or a Model for End-Stage Liver Disease (MELD) score of 15 or higher. MELD (see Table 158–4), which is a mathematical model that estimates the risk for 3-month mortality, is used to determine the priority for liver transplantation. The number of available deceased donor organs is lower than the number of patients awaiting liver transplantation; as a result, 15 to 20% of patients awaiting liver transplantation in the United States die before an organ becomes available.

Primary Prevention

Treatment of the underlying liver disease, before the development of cirrhosis, is a primary prevention strategy. Because the major causes of cirrhosis are related to lifestyle choices such as injection drug use (Chapter 32), alcohol consumption (Chapter 31), and unprotected sex, primary prevention programs that focus on encouraging alcohol abstinence, reducing high-risk behavior for hepatitis virus infection, and vaccinating for hepatitis B are even better prevention strategies.

Prognosis

The outcome of cirrhosis depends on the patient's stage. Patients with compensated cirrhosis die of liver disease only after transition to a decompensated stage. The 10-year survival rate of patients who remain in a compensated stage is approximately 90%, whereas their likelihood of decompensation is 50% at 10 years. Inception cohort studies of patients with compensated cirrhosis show a median survival of all patients, including those in whom decompensation develops over time, of about 10 years, whereas the median survival after decompensation is around 2 years.

Four clinical stages of cirrhosis have recently been identified, each with a different prognosis. In stage 1, or patients without varices or ascites, mortality is about 1% per year. Stage 2 patients, or those with varices but without ascites or bleeding, have a mortality rate of about 4% per year. Stage 3 patients have ascites with or without esophageal varices that have never bled; their mortality rate while remaining in this stage is 20% per year. Stage 4 patients, or those with portal hypertensive GI bleeding with or without ascites, have a 1-year mortality rate of 57%, with nearly half of these deaths occurring within 6 weeks after the initial episode of bleeding. Stages 1 and 2 correspond to compensated cirrhosis, whereas stages 3 and 4 are decompensated cirrhosis. Hepatocellular carcinoma develops at a fairly constant rate of 3% per year and is associated with a worse outcome at whatever stage it develops.

Predictors of survival are different in compensated and decompensated patients, with parameters of portal hypertension (varices, splenomegaly, platelet count, gamma globulin) assuming greater importance in compensated patients, whereas renal dysfunction, bleeding, and hepatocellular carcinoma are important predictive factors in patients with decompensated cirrhosis. In clinical practice, the Child-Pugh score is applicable to all cirrhotic patients, and the MELD score is used in decompensated patients to determine priority for liver transplantation.

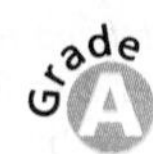

1. D'Amico G, Pagliaro L, Bosch J: Pharmacological treatment of portal hypertension: An evidence-based approach. Semin Liver Dis 1999;19:475–505.
2. Groszmann RJ, Garcia-Tsao G, Bosch J, et al: for the Portal Hypertension Collaborative Group: Beta-blockers to prevent gastroesophageal varices in patients with cirrhosis. N Engl J Med 2005;353:2254–2261.
3. Hou MC, Lin HC, Liu TT, et al: Antibiotic prophylaxis after endoscopic therapy prevents rebleeding in acute variceal hemorrhage: A randomized trial. Hepatology 2004;39:746–753.
4. De la Pena J, Brullet E, Sanchez-Hernandez E, et al: Variceal ligation plus nadolol compared with ligation for prophylaxis of variceal rebleeding: A multicenter trial. Hepatology 2005;41:572–578.
5. Bureau C, Garcia-Pagan JC, Otal P, et al: Improved clinical outcome using polytetrafluoroethylene-coated stents for TIPS: Results of a randomized study. Gastroenterology 2004;126:469–475.
6. D'Amico G, Luca A, Morabito A, et al: Uncovered transjugular intrahepatic portosystemic shunt for refractory ascites: A meta-analysis. Gastroenterology 2005;129:1282–1293.
7. Cordoba J, Lopez-Hellin J, Planas M, et al: Normal protein diet for episodic hepatic encephalopathy: Results of a randomized study. J Hepatol 2004;41:38–43.

SUGGESTED READINGS

D'Amico G, Garcia-Tsao G, Pagliaro L: Natural history and prognostic indicators of survival in cirrhosis. A systematic review of 118 studies. J Hepatol 2006; 44:217–231. *A comprehensive overview.*

Garcia-Pagan JC, Bosch J: Endoscopic band ligation in the treatment of portal hypertension. Nat Clin Pract Gastroenterol Hepatol 2005;2:526–535. *Review of its role for primary and secondary prophylaxis in the context of other therapies for varices.*

Garcia-Tsao G: Bacterial infections in cirrhosis: Treatment and prophylaxis. J Hepatol 2005;42(Suppl.):S85–S92. *Overview of antibiotic treatment of the acute episode, as well as primary and secondary prophylaxis.*

Gines P, Cardenas A, Arroyo V, et al: Management of cirrhosis and ascites. N Engl J Med 2004;350:1646–1654. *The pathogenesis and management of ascites and its complications, especially refractory ascites and hepatorenal syndrome.*

Hoeper MM, Krowka MJ, Strassburg CP: Portopulmonary hypertension and hepatopulmonary syndrome. Lancet 2004;363:1461–1468. *Review of the pathogenesis, clinical features, diagnosis, and management.*

Shawcross D, Jalan R: Dispelling myths in the treatment of hepatic encephalopathy. Lancet 2005;365:431–433. *Overview of data suggesting lack of benefit from reducing dietary protein or intestinal bacteria.*

158 HEPATIC FAILURE AND LIVER TRANSPLANTATION

Emmet B. Keeffe

Liver transplantation is the treatment of choice for patients with severe liver failure, end-stage liver disease, and certain metabolic liver diseases for which no alternative therapies are available. More than 6000 liver transplantations are performed in the United States annually, with a waiting list that has grown to approximately 18,000 patients. With modern immunosuppressive drug regimens, technical advances, and improved perioperative care, the current 1-year survival rate after liver transplantation is 85 to 90%, except in cases of hepatic malignancies, for which it is 72% (Table 158–1). Many studies show that liver transplantation significantly improves the physical, cognitive, and psychological functioning of the recipient. In recent years, the disparity between a limited supply of cadaver donor organs and much greater need for liver transplantation has resulted in an unacceptable number of deaths of patients listed for transplantation and created a mandate to optimize the selection of patients and timing of transplantation.

INDICATIONS AND SELECTION CRITERIA FOR LIVER TRANSPLANTATION

The indications and contraindications for liver transplantation, the most appropriate candidates to receive a transplant, and the organ allocation scheme continue to evolve. The diseases for which liver transplantation is performed in adults includes cirrhosis with end-stage liver disease, acute liver failure, hepatic malignancies (particularly hepatocellular carcinoma), and metabolic diseases in which the inborn error of metabolism resides in the hepatocytes (e.g., hemochromatosis, α_1-antitrypsin deficiency, Wilson's disease). The most common indications for liver transplantation are chronic hepatitis C and alcoholic liver disease in adults (together accounting for approximately 50% of transplantations), and biliary atresia and α_1-antitrypsin deficiency in children.

General selection criteria that should be considered in the referral of patients for liver transplantation include (1) the absence of alternative forms of therapy that may reverse liver failure and defer the need for liver transplantation, (2) the absence of any absolute contraindication to transplantation (discussed later), (3) expected compliance with longitudinal follow-up care, and (4) the ability to provide for the financial costs of liver transplantation and follow-up care, including medications that may be expensive. Insurance coverage for transplantation is typically determined before referral by a financial counselor at the transplantation center.

Referral for Liver Transplantation

Patients with chronic (Table 158–2) or acute (Table 158–3) liver disease should be referred when hepatic decompensation first develops or the presence of hepatocellular carcinoma is first detected. The greatest like-

TABLE 158–1 KAPLAN-MEIER PATIENT SURVIVAL RATES FOR LIVER TRANSPLANTATION PERFORMED FROM 1997–2004

	Kaplan-Meier Survival Rate (%)		
Diagnosis	**1-Year**	**3-Year**	**5-Year**
Acute hepatic necrosis	82	73	70
Cholestatic cirrhosis	90	85	80
Noncholestatic cirrhosis	86	76	69
Other liver disease	80	72	64
Metabolic disease	90	85	81
Malignant neoplasm	86	70	58
Benign neoplasm	86	82	71

From The Organ Procurement and Transplantation Network. Available at: *http://www.unos.org→Data→View* data reports→National Data→Survival/Liver/Patient→Survival by recipient diagnosis category. Accessed January 13, 2007.

TABLE 158–2 BIOCHEMICAL AND CLINICAL INDICATIONS FOR LIVER TRANSPLANTATION IN CHRONIC LIVER DISEASE

CHOLESTATIC LIVER DISEASE
Bilirubin >10 mg/dL
Intractable pruritus
Progressive cholestatic bone disease
Recurrent bacterial cholangitis
HEPATOCELLULAR LIVER DISEASE
Serum albumin <3 g/dL
Prothrombin time >3 sec above control
BOTH CHOLESTATIC AND HEPATOCELLULAR LIVER DISEASES
Recurrent or severe hepatic encephalopathy
Refractory ascites
Spontaneous bacterial peritonitis
Recurrent portal hypertensive bleeding
Severe chronic fatigue and weakness
Progressive malnutrition
Development of hepatorenal syndrome
Detection of small hepatocellular carcinoma

INR = international normalized ratio.
From Keeffe EB: Selection of patients for liver transplantation. *In* Maddrey WC, Sorrell MF, Schiff ER (eds): Transplantation of the Liver, 3rd ed. Philadelphia, Lippincott Williams & Wilkins, 2001, pp. 5–34, with permission.

TABLE 158–3 KING'S COLLEGE CRITERIA FOR LIVER TRANSPLANTATION IN FULMINANT HEPATIC FAILURE

PATIENTS TAKING ACETAMINOPHEN
pH <7.3, or prothrombin time >6.5 (INR) and serum creatinine >3.4 mg/dL
PATIENTS NOT TAKING ACETAMINOPHEN
Prothrombin time >6.5 (INR) *or* any three of the following:
1. Age <10 or >40 yr
2. Etiology: non-A, non-B hepatitis; halothane hepatitis; idiosyncratic drug reaction
3. Duration of jaundice before encephalopathy >7 days
4. Prothrombin time >3.5 (INR)
5. Serum bilirubin >17.6 mg/dL

INR = international normalized ratio.
Adapted from O'Grady JG, Alexander GJ, Hayllar KM, Williams R: Early indicators of prognosis in fulminant hepatic failure. Gastroenterology 1989;97:439–445.

lihood of survival and return to an excellent quality of life occurs in patients who undergo liver transplantation before the onset of multiorgan failure. Meticulous attention to medical management of the complications of cirrhosis, such as avoidance of excessive diuretic therapy or aminoglycosides to protect renal function in patients with ascites or spontaneous bacterial peritonitis, is critically important. Blood loss in patients with gastrointestinal bleeding should be judiciously replaced with blood products to avoid fluid overload and pulmonary edema.

For long-term management in patients with chronic liver disease who may ultimately become candidates for transplantation, nonsurgical interventions, such as transjugular intrahepatic portosystemic shunt (TIPS) for refractory portal hypertensive bleeding and endoscopic or radiologic approaches to dominant biliary strictures in patients with primary sclerosing cholangitis, are preferable to abdominal procedures that can cause adhesions. Patients with cirrhosis (Chapter 157) should undergo surveillance for hepatocellular carcinoma with ultrasound or computed tomography and α-fetoprotein testing every 6 months to facilitate early diagnosis of lesions, when they are small and amenable to treatment with modalities such as resection or liver transplantation.

Chronic Liver Disease

Although the survival of patients with compensated cirrhosis is good (approximately 90% at 5 years), the development of decompensation with ascites, portal hypertensive bleeding, or encephalopathy implies a lower 5-year survival rate of about 50%. A patient with a Child-Turcotte-Pugh (CTP) score of 5 or 6 (Child's class A cirrhosis; see Table 157–2) without a history of portal hypertensive bleeding or spontaneous bacterial peritonitis is likely to remain stable for a considerable period and does not require listing for transplantation. Criteria for listing should be clinical decompensation and/or biochemical deterioration of synthetic function that yields a CTP score of 7 or greater (Child's class B or C), or the development of a small hepatocellular carcinoma.

Liver transplantation for hepatocellular carcinoma (Chapter 206) is reserved for selected patients who have advanced cirrhosis, who do not have the hepatic reserve to undergo resection, and who have no evidence of extrahepatic tumor after thorough evaluation. Risks for recurrent hepatocellular carcinoma after transplantation include advanced disease (stage 3 or greater) as defined by lymph node involvement, gross vascular invasion by imaging studies, tumor burden (single lesion >5 cm, or two or more lesions >3 cm), and/or involvement of more than one lobe. In low-risk patients with stage 1 or 2 disease (single lesion of 5 cm, or two or three lesions of ≤3 cm), the actuarial survival rate is about 75% at 4 years, whereas the survival in patients with higher risk is about 50% at 4 years.

Acute Liver Failure

Liver transplantation is a major advance in the management of severe acute liver failure. *Fulminant hepatic failure* refers to the presence of acute liver failure with superimposed hepatic encephalopathy developing within 2 to 8 weeks after the onset of illness in a patient without preexisting liver disease. *Subfulminant hepatic failure* (or *late-onset hepatic failure*) is applied to a syndrome that develops more slowly, after 2 to 8 weeks up to 3 to 6 months. The selection of patients with acute liver failure who are likely to die and therefore would benefit from liver transplantation is challenging but can be predicted by certain biochemical and clinical features, the most popular of which were established at King's College Hospital in London (see Table 158–3).

Aggressive supportive care is necessary in patients with fulminant hepatic failure to prevent and treat bleeding, infection, cerebral edema, renal failure, and respiratory failure. These complications are the main reasons why transplantation may not be possible and may also contribute to postoperative morbidity and mortality.

Potential alternative treatment strategies for fulminant hepatic failure include extracorporeal liver assist devices, hepatocyte transplantation, and heterotopic auxiliary liver transplantation. The goals of these therapies are to prevent irreversible brain damage, provide time for possible hepatic regeneration and recovery of acceptable function, and stabilize patients who do not recover until liver transplantation can be performed. Clinical experience with hepatic support devices, primarily using either porcine or human hepatocytes, is encouraging but limited to ongoing trials. Hepatocyte transplantation and heterotopic liver transplantation have a number of technical problems that limit their application.

Patients with fulminant hepatic failure should be treated in an intensive care unit, with the patient's head elevated at 20 to 30 degrees. Although lactulose is the cornerstone of treatment of chronic hepatic encephalopathy, it is less effective in patients with acute encephalopathy, and the role of antibiotics such as neomycin is unknown. However, a trial of lactulose, 30 mL two to four times daily, adjusted to achieve two to three loose bowel movements daily, is worthwhile, and the drug may need to be administrated by nasogastric tube or by rectal enema. Factors precipitating hepatic encephalopathy, such as gastrointestinal bleeding, hypokalemia, or sepsis, should be identified and treated.

Cerebral edema is frequently manifested by hypertension, bradycardia, and neurologic findings such as decerebrate posturing or abnormal pupillary reflexes. These findings may occur late; therefore, monitoring of intracranial pressure (ICP) with institution of therapy to maintain ICP at less than 20 mm Hg is preferred. ICP may be monitored with either a subdural or an epidural transducer, and the risk of hemorrhage as a complication of placement is outweighed by the benefit of monitoring and early intervention.

Initial treatment of increased ICP is with mannitol (0.5 to 1 g/kg by intravenous infusion over 5 minutes). Repeated doses of mannitol may be required to treat recurrent increases in ICP. Mannitol can be given only if the serum osmolality is less than 320 mOsm/L. Caution is advised in patients with renal failure, and mannitol may need to be administered in combination with hemodialysis or continuous arteriovenous hemofiltration. Other useful therapies include disturbing the patient as little as possible, controlling agitation, and administering moderate hyperventilation to a partial carbon dioxide pressure of 25 to 30 mm Hg. A persistent ICP greater than 40 mm Hg that is refractory to treatment precludes liver transplantation.

Listing for Liver Transplantation

Before final selection and listing for liver transplantation, prospective candidates with acute or chronic liver disease undergo a pretransplantation evaluation to define the current status of systemic diseases and to determine whether any absolute or relative contraindications are present. Routine evaluation includes blood bank and hematologic studies, complete liver and kidney chemistry profiles, viral serology assays (hepatitis A, B, and C viruses; human immunodeficiency virus [HIV]; cytomegalovirus [CMV]), chest radiography, and abdominal computed tomography or Doppler ultrasound studies of the hepatic vasculature. Additional routine tests include skin testing for tuberculosis, creatinine clearance, electrocardiogram, and, in the presence of lung disease, pulmonary function testing. Patients who are at risk for coronary artery disease undergo cardiology consultation and, if indicated, stress testing, cardiac catheterization, or both. Cancer screening, depending on age and gender, includes Papanicolaou smear, mammogram, occult fecal blood testing, and lower gastrointestinal endoscopy. Consultations with a social worker, financial counselor, and psychiatrist are routinely performed at the transplantation center.

Patients are generally assigned to one of four categories by the liver transplantation center selection committee: (1) suitable and ready, with listing for transplantation; (2) suitable but too well, with placement on inactive status and continued follow-up with the referring physician; (3) potentially reversible relative contraindication, with treatment and recategorization at a later date; and (4) absolute contraindication, with denial of transplantation. Patients who are approved for liver transplantation are then listed for a donor organ with the United Network for Organ Sharing (UNOS), and final approval by the insurance carrier or third party payer is sought.

Allocation of Donor Organs

In the current UNOS system, patients with fulminant liver failure receive the first priority for available organs. The Model for End-Stage Liver Disease (MELD), which is an accurate indicator of chronic liver disease severity, is used to allocate organs to patients with end-stage liver disease (Table 158–4). The MELD score is calculated using three biochemical variables (serum bilirubin, serum creatinine, and the international normalized ratio of prothrombin time), which are readily available, reproducible, and objective. Although initially developed to predict survival after the TIPS procedure, MELD has been validated as an accurate predictor of short-term mortality in patients with advanced liver disease independent of etiology or the presence of clinical complications of cirrhosis.

TABLE 158–4 RELATIONSHIP BETWEEN MELD SCORE AND 3-MONTH MORTALITY IN HOSPITALIZED CIRRHOTIC PATIENTS

MELD Score	No. Deaths/Total No. of Patients	Mortality Rate (%)
≤9	6/148	4
10–19	28/103	27
20–29	16/21	76
30–39	5/6	83
≥40	4/4	100

MELD = Model for End-Stage Liver Disease.
Adapted from Wiesner RH, McDiarmid SV, Kamath PS, et al: MELD and PELD: Application of survival models to liver allocation. Liver Transpl 2001;7:567–580.

Contraindications to Liver Transplantation

Absolute Contraindications

The list of absolute contraindications to transplantation is short: advanced cardiopulmonary disease, active untreated sepsis, extrahepatic malignancy, anatomic abnormality precluding transplantation, active alcohol or substance abuse, and documented poor compliance with medical care. In addition, patients should not undergo liver transplantation if they have compensated cirrhosis (Child's class A; see Chapter 157) and no history of portal hypertensive bleeding. Patients are not candidates for liver transplantation if they have poor ventricular function or severe valvar heart disease. Coronary artery disease, if anatomically reversible by angioplasty or bypass surgery, is not a contraindication to listing if left ventricular function is adequate.

Half of all liver transplantation candidates have abnormal arterial oxygenation, but only patients with advanced chronic obstructive pulmonary disease or pulmonary fibrosis are precluded from liver transplantation. Previous tuberculosis is not a contraindication to liver transplantation. Active tuberculosis should be treated for at least 2 to 3 weeks and preferably for several months before liver transplantation and for up to 1 year afterward. Hepatopulmonary syndrome (Chapter 157), which is diagnosed on the basis of the triad of chronic liver disease with portal hypertension, intrapulmonary vascular dilation with right-to-left shunting, and arterial hypoxemia, may be reversed by liver transplantation. In contrast, portopulmonary hypertension is associated with high operative mortality; for example, patients with a mean pulmonary artery pressure of 50 mm Hg or greater have a postoperative mortality rate that approaches 100%. Conversely, patients with mean pulmonary artery pressures lower than 35 mm Hg do not have increased perioperative mortality.

Active untreated infection should be controlled before proceeding with liver transplantation. In the setting of spontaneous bacterial peritonitis, most programs defer transplantation until antibiotic treatment has been administered for 48 hours and resolution of infection is documented on repeat paracentesis. Sepsis and pneumonia remain absolute contraindications to liver transplantation. Serious chronic infections such as osteomyelitis, chronic fungal diseases, and abscesses preclude transplantation unless they can be treated effectively. Selected HIV-positive patients are currently undergoing liver transplantation in a few centers in the United States to determine whether the benefits outweigh the risks.

Liver transplantation is not performed in the presence of extrahepatic malignancy, except perhaps for patients with isolated liver metastases from slow-growing neuroendocrine tumors (Chapter 205), such as gastrinoma, insulinomas, glucagonomas, somatostatinomas, and carcinoid tumors. The results of liver transplantation are so poor with cholangiocarcinoma (Chapter 159) that most centers consider this diagnosis to be an absolute contraindication, although a few centers have demonstrated acceptable tumor-free survival rates when liver transplantation is combined with adjuvant chemotherapy and radiation in highly selected patients.

Most programs accept patients with alcoholic liver disease as candidates for liver transplantation only after proven alcohol abstinence for at least 6 months and completion of an inpatient or outpatient rehabilitation program. Isolated portal vein thrombosis, previously considered an absolute contraindication, is only a relative problem in light of novel reconstructive innovations, including thrombectomy or jump grafts.

Relative Contraindications

Patient selection should be based on an assessment of biologic age and absence of major systemic illnesses rather than an arbitrary chronologic age cutoff. Patients undergoing evaluation for liver transplantation may have the hepatorenal syndrome, chronic renal failure, or reversible acute renal failure that may be related to intercurrent events such as spontaneous bacterial peritonitis, gastrointestinal bleeding, or excessive diuresis; however, these conditions are not contraindications to transplantation. Chronic renal failure secondary to intrinsic kidney disease is not a contraindication to liver transplantation but necessitates consideration for dual transplantation of liver and kidney. Transient deterioration in renal function due to an acute injury usually is not a problem unless it is complicated by the development of hepatorenal syndrome, which is reversible only if urgent liver transplantation can be performed.

THE TRANSPLANTATION PROCEDURE

Donors and recipients are matched according to blood type and body size. In general, organs are transplanted into recipients in keeping with standard ABO compatibility rules. Most surgeons believe that a satisfactory size match exists if the donor's and recipient's body weights are within 20% of one another. The donor organ is harvested according to standard protocols to ensure that the physiologic condition of the donor is close to normal when the organ is removed and to limit warm ischemia time. The cold ischemia time while the organ is in a preservation solution is also kept as short as possible—the usual goal is less than 12 hours—to minimize the risk of delayed graft function or nonfunction.

The recipient undergoes bilateral subcostal incision with upper midline extension. The standard hepatectomy includes removal of both the vena cava and the liver, often with use of a pump-driven venovenous bypass to return the inferior vena cava and portal venous flow to the heart through the axillary vein. A popular alternative method is to preserve the retrohepatic vena cava during hepatectomy. After hepatectomy, the donor liver is put in place, with repair of the inferior vena cava if it was interrupted, portal reperfusion, hepatic arterial reconstruction, and, finally, duct-to-duct reconstruction of the common bile duct. A Roux-en-Y choledochojejunostomy is used when a duct-to-duct anastomosis is not suitable, such as in patients who have primary sclerosing cholangitis, in whom the diseased common bile duct is removed in its entirety.

Evolving Approaches to Liver Transplantation

The growing discrepancy between the number of available organs and the need for transplantation has led to increasing application of novel approaches to liver replacement, including deceased donor split-liver transplantation and adult living donor liver transplantation. Xenotransplantation and hepatocyte transplantation are future hopes.

Split-liver transplantation allows two liver transplants from a single deceased donor liver, usually a right lobe implanted into an adult recipient and left lobe or left lateral segment implanted into a pediatric recipient. This technique has the potential to provide grafts to the majority of listed pediatric patients and to decrease substantially the waiting time for adult patients.

Living donor liver transplantation uses the left lateral segment for adult-to-child donation, with a very low risk to the adult donor, who usually is a parent. Good results also have been achieved in recent years with elective adult-to-adult living donor liver transplantation grafting the right lobe (segments 5 to 8), which represents 60 to 65% of the liver, into the recipient. This operation has also been applied to urgent cases with good outcomes. Patients with small hepatocellular carcinomas and those with primary sclerosing cholangitis at risk for cholangiocarcinoma are excellent candidates for a timely living donor liver transplantation. Unfortunately, adult-to-adult living donor liver transplantation is just a partial solution to the donor shortage for adult liver transplantation, because only about 15% of potential donors are satisfactory candidates after complete evaluation. The morbidity and mortality rates for the donor average 15% and 0.5%, respectively, making the operation formidable and necessitating careful informed consent from the donor.

POST-TRANSPLANTATION MANAGEMENT

Allograft dysfunction is the most important complication after liver transplantation. Liver biopsy is critical in differentiating the various causes of dysfunction, because many of them share similar but nonspecific clinical and biochemical presentations. Diagnostic evaluations may also include a cholangiogram and duplex ultrasound of the vessels supplying the liver.

Standard Medical Therapies

In general, all patients receive corticosteroids in large intravenous doses during the operation. Steroid doses are rapidly reduced over 5 days and can be discontinued by 3 to 12 months after transplantation in many patients, depending on the underlying disease and the presence or absence of rejection. Either cyclosporine or tacrolimus is initiated at the time of liver transplantation and is used long-term in most patients to prevent acute and chronic allograft rejection. In recent years, a paradigm shift in the use of immunosuppression has taken place, with movement away from triple therapy (prednisone, a calcineurin agent [cyclosporine or tacrolimus], and azathioprine or mycophenolate mofetil) to early withdrawal of corticosteroids (from 14 days to 3 months after transplantation) followed by use of a calcineurin agent alone. In patients with renal dysfunction, calcineurin-sparing regimens using mycophenolate mofetil with lower doses of a calcineurin agent or sirolimus alone are used. Calcineurin-sparing regimens reduce the incidence of late renal failure, which approaches 15 to 20% by 20 years after transplantation. Immunosuppressive drugs are typically titrated to therapeutic or slightly subtherapeutic blood levels, but different drug strategies are used in different centers. Other routine medications after liver transplantation include those used for preemptive prevention of viral and fungal infection (see later discussion).

Early Complications after Liver Transplantation

Problems that may occur in the first few days after liver transplantation include hepatic artery thrombosis, portal vein thrombosis, primary graft nonfunction, and hyperacute rejection. Hepatic artery thrombosis, which occurs in about 2 to 8% of adults and in 3 to 20% of children who undergo liver transplantation, is more common among patients who receive sirolimus. Hepatic artery thrombosis typically manifests early after transplantation as fulminant liver failure; occasionally, it occurs 1 to 2 months after transplantation and manifests with stenosis or intimal hyperplasia with eventual rearterialization from collaterals. Early hepatic artery thrombosis is first treated by immediate revascularization via thrombectomy or use of a surgical conduit, but it often requires urgent retransplantation. Hepatic artery stenosis without thrombosis is usually associated with multiple ischemic biliary strictures and manifests somewhat later. Retransplantation is indicated if biliary sepsis or graft failure develops.

Portal vein thrombosis complicates only 1 to 3% of liver transplantation cases. Early acute portal vein thrombosis leads to fulminant liver failure and requires immediate revascularization or urgent retransplantation. Conversely, late portal vein thrombosis manifests as portal hypertension.

Primary graft nonfunction, or delayed ischemia-reperfusion injury, is the most common cause of graft loss within the early postoperative period after a technically successful liver transplantation. The clinical presentation resembles that of fulminant liver failure, with persistent or new hepatic encephalopathy and elevated serum aminotransferase levels (>2500 IU/L).

Initial poor graft function is characteristic of a marginally functioning graft that typically recovers adequate function days to weeks after transplantation. This syndrome has a milder clinical presentation than primary nonfunction, and serum aminotransferases are usually less than 2500 IU/L. Treatment is largely supportive, and most grafts eventually recover.

Acute and Chronic Allograft Rejection

The most common cause of allograft dysfunction after the first postoperative week is acute cellular rejection, which occurs overall in one half to two thirds of cases and is seen between the fifth day and 3 weeks after transplantation. The incidence of acute rejection with the use of low-dose prednisone, tacrolimus, and mycophenolate mofetil is 25 to 30%. An acute rejection episode occurring beyond 6 weeks after transplantation should raise suspicion for a subtherapeutic immunosuppressive regimen or for noncompliance with the medical regimen. The patient is usually asymptomatic and presents with increases in serum bilirubin, alkaline phosphatase, and γ-glutamyltransferase in the early post-transplantation course and with predominant elevations in the serum aminotransferases if acute rejection occurs several weeks after transplantation. However, recipients may also present with fever, malaise, abdominal pain, or portal hypertensive changes such as ascites. Histologic examination reveals a mixed portal or periportal inflammatory infiltrate (with neutrophils, eosinophils, plasma cells, and lymphocytes) leading to destructive suppurative cholangitis and endotheliitis. Treatment, which reverses 65 to 85% of episodes, consists of high-dose intravenous corticosteroids, usually 1 g of methylprednisolone, followed by oral prednisone with a rapid taper over 7 days.

Chronic ductopenic rejection now occurs in 2 to 3% of patients, most commonly between 6 weeks and 6 months after transplantation. Cholestatic enzymes, such as alkaline phosphatase and γ-glutamyltransferase, gradually increase for weeks to months before the onset of jaundice that signals the late stage of chronic ductopenic rejection. Histologic evaluation reveals sparse lymphocytic portal inflammation but progressive loss of interlobular and septal bile ducts in at least half of the portal tracts—a condition known as vanishing bile duct syndrome. Approximately 10 to 20% of retransplantations are done because of chronic ductopenic rejection.

Biliary Complications after Liver Transplantation

The biliary tree has very poor regenerative and reparative capacity when damaged and is the most common site for technical complications after transplantation. Biliary complications occur in 10 to 25% of all recipients, with more than two thirds of cases diagnosed within 1 month and 80% within 6 months after transplantation. Causes of biliary complications include technical factors, preservation injury, hepatic artery thrombosis, immunologic factors, and infection, particularly with CMV. Bile leaks and strictures are the most common presentations of biliary complications in the first 3 months postoperatively.

Choledochocholedochostomy and choledochojejunostomy are the two methods of primary biliary reconstruction in liver transplantation. The more commonly performed choledochocholedochostomy, or duct-to-duct anastomosis, preserves the sphincter of Oddi and endoscopic access to the biliary tree after transplantation. Choledochojejunostomy, or Roux-en-Y anastomosis, is used for retransplantation, for transplantation of small liver grafts, and in patients with intrinsic disease of the extrahepatic bile ducts, such as primary sclerosing cholangitis.

Bile leakage occurs in up to 25% of all recipients and can be diagnosed by cholangiogram or biliary scintigraphy if the leak is sufficiently large. Patients may present with fever, abdominal pain, peritonitis, hypotension, or sepsis with biloma. For patients who suffer from bile leak after T-tube removal, endoscopic placement of a nasobiliary drain or internal plastic stent allows the leakage to heal as the bile flows preferentially through the ampulla. Surgical creation or revision of choledochojejunostomy should be performed only after failure of endoscopic or radiologic interventions.

Anastomotic biliary stricture, which affects 4 to 10% of all recipients, occurs within the first 6 months after transplantation. Clinical presentation is typical of cholangitis but may be asymptomatic, with only elevation of cholestatic enzymes (predominantly alkaline phosphatase and γ-glutamyltransferase). Balloon dilation or stenting endoscopically or radiologically should be attempted before resorting to surgery. Nonanastomotic biliary strictures, affecting up to 20% of all recipients, occur within the first 4 months after transplantation. The biliary strictures are usually multiple and may be associated with extrahepatic and intrahepatic bile leaks. Management of these strictures depends on their number, location, and severity, as well as liver function. Diffuse strictures in the setting of bile leakage and biloma indicate the need for retransplantation. Focal intrahepatic strictures may benefit from repeated sessions of balloon dilation and stenting performed endoscopically or radiologically.

Infections

Most infections occur within the first 2 months after transplantation, while recipients are receiving a high-dose induction immunosuppressive regimen. Bacteria and fungi cause more than 90% of infections during this period. Pneumonia, urinary infection, intra-abdominal and hepatic abscesses, peritonitis, wound infection, and line sepsis are the most common infections. *Candida albicans* is the most common infecting fungal agent in the immediate post-transplantation period. Other frequently seen fungi include *Aspergillus fumigatus* and non-*albicans Candida* species. Despite its nephrotoxicity, amphotericin B is the treatment of choice for invasive fungal infections. Oral fluconazole, 100 mg daily, prevents most fungal infections and is the standard antifungal prophylaxis used for the first 6 weeks after transplantation.

The routine use of trimethoprim-sulfamethoxazole prophylaxis, one single-strength tablet (80/400) three times weekly, has made infection with *Pneumocystis jiroveci* (formerly *P. carinii*) rare in liver transplant recipients. Inhalational pentamidine, 300 mg every 4 weeks, and oral dapsone, 50 mg daily, are alternative prophylactic regimens for patients who are allergic to sulfa. Prophylaxis lasts for 1 year after transplantation but should be extended for an extra year if the patient received additional high-dose immunosuppressants (e.g., steroid boluses, muromonab-CD3, increased tacrolimus) during the first year after transplantation.

CMV infection and disease are less common than in the past but remain a risk after liver transplantation. Prophylaxis with acyclovir, ganciclovir, or valganciclovir is effective and reduces mortality; [1] oral valganciclovir (900 mg daily) is most commonly used for the first 3 months after transplantation. Prophylaxis with oral acyclovir (200 mg daily) or valganciclovir is also a useful preventive strategy against the reactivation of oral or genital herpes simplex virus in the first 3 months after transplantation. Reactivation of varicella zoster virus may manifest as localized dermatomal vesicles or, in patients who were seronegative before transplantation, as cutaneous and visceral dissemination; treatment is with high-dose acyclovir (800 mg five times daily for 7 to 10 days).

By 6 months after liver transplantation, recipients who have normal allograft function and are receiving standard doses of immunosuppressive drugs share the same risks as immunocompetent hosts for community-acquired infections and are not at increased risk for opportunistic infections. Conversely, recipients who have been receiving high-dose immunosuppressive drug regimens for antirejection therapy continue to be at high risk for life-threatening opportunistic infections.

Long-Term Follow-up

Long-term management after liver transplantation requires continuing communication and cooperation between the transplantation center and the primary care physician. Patients require careful routine medical management, screening for malignancy, and immunization updates and boosters.

Hypertension

Hypertension (Chapter 66) occurs among 30 to 90% of all liver transplant recipients and is related to cyclosporine and tacrolimus, which cause vasoconstriction in the systemic and renal vasculature, and corticosteroids, which result in sodium retention, increased plasma volume, and weight gain. Management of hypertension in these patients follows a stepwise approach. Dietary sodium restriction, resumption of physical activity, and weight reduction are the first steps. Because of the pathophysiology of vasoconstriction, calcium-channel blockers are the drugs of first choice. The preferred calcium-channel blockers belong to the dihydropyridine class, such as nifedipine. Verapamil, diltiazem, and nicardipine are also effective, but they increase the drug levels of cyclosporine and tacrolimus. Second-line antihypertensive agents include diuretics, β-blockers, and α-adrenergic blockers. Angiotensin-converting enzyme inhibitors should be used with caution because they can aggravate hyperkalemia and, in rare instances, exacerbate leukopenia. Hypertension may improve with time as corticosteroids are discontinued and the dose of cyclosporine or tacrolimus is lowered.

Diabetes Mellitus

Diabetes mellitus (Chapter 248) develops in more than one third of liver recipients after transplantation, with the majority of cases being insulin-dependent. The pathogenesis is multifactorial, including genetic predisposition and use of tacrolimus, cyclosporine, and corticosteroids. Steroid tapering is the key to management of early post-transplantation hyperglycemia. Management is otherwise similar to that for the nontransplanted population.

Hyperlipidemia

Hyperlipidemia (Chapter 217) develops in approximately one fourth of all liver transplant recipients. The management of hyperlipidemia includes appropriate dietary restrictions of fat and carbohydrate, weight reduction, regular exercise, and smoking cessation. The preferred medication for patients with resistant hyperlipidemia is 3-hydroxy-3-methylglutaryl coenzyme A (HMG-CoA) reductase inhibitors.

Bone Mineral Density

Bone mineral density decreases during the first few months after transplantation but eventually regains its preoperative level. Fractures most frequently involve trabecular bones such as the vertebrae and the ribs. *Osteonecrosis* or *avascular necrosis* of the hips and, less often, the knees and the humerus bones, may occur. Contributing risk factors to bone disease include preexisting osteopenia, prolonged bed rest, malnutrition, corticosteroids, cyclosporine, tacrolimus, furosemide, and the original diagnosis of primary biliary cirrhosis or primary sclerosing cholangitis with associated metabolic osteodystrophy. Management includes regular exercise and pharmacologic therapies such as calcium supplementation, vitamin D derivatives, and bisphosphonates (Chapter 264).

Cancer

Skin cancer (Chapter 214) is the most common malignancy occurring in the setting of solid-organ transplantation and immunosuppression. Squamous cell carcinoma is more common than basal cell carcinoma or malignant melanoma in this population, and some recipients develop hundreds of squamous cell carcinomas. Patients should seek medical attention if they have a skin growth that bleeds or crusts, increases in size or thickness, or changes in color or texture. Sunscreen with a sun protection factor of at least 15 is recommended. Patients should undergo at least annual skin examinations depending on their previous history of skin cancers.

Colon cancer (Chapter 203) is a common de novo neoplasia after transplantation. Colonoscopic surveillance with multiple biopsies every 6 months for the first 2 years after transplantation, followed by annual examinations, has been recommended for high-risk patients with ulcerative colitis.

If not given before liver transplantation, hepatitis A, hepatitis B, and pneumococcal vaccines (Chapter 16) should be given. Other immunizations include influenza vaccine annually and tetanus toxoid booster every 5 years. Vaccines based on live or attenuated microorganisms should be avoided, including those for measles, mumps, rubella, chickenpox, polio, and bacille Calmette-Guérin (BCG).

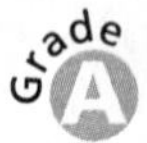

1. Hodson EM, Jones CA, Webster AC, et al: Antiviral medications to prevent cytomegalovirus disease and early death in recipients of solid-organ transplants: a systematic review of randomised controlled trials. Lancet 2005;365:2105–2115.

SUGGESTED READINGS

Burroughs AK, Sabin CA, Rolles K, et al: Three-month and 12-month mortality after first liver transplant in adults in Europe: Predictive models for outcome. Lancet 2006;367:225-232. *The 3-month and 12-month mortality models can compare outcomes both within and between centers.*

Carithers RL Jr, Murray KF: AASLD Practice guidelines: Evaluation of the patient for liver transplantation. Hepatology 2005;41:1407–1432. *A consensus statement on the selection of patients for liver transplantation from the American Association for the Study of Liver Diseases.*

Clavien PA, Petrowsky H, De Oliveira ML, et al: Strategies for safer liver surgery and partial liver transplantation. N Engl J Med 2007;356:1545–1559. *A scholarly overview.*

Larson AM, Curtis JR: Integrating palliative care for liver transplant candidates: "Too well for transplant, too sick for life." JAMA 2006;295:2168–2176. *A case-based perspective.*

Shawcross D, Jalan R: Dispelling myths in the treatment of hepatic encephalopathy. Lancet 2005;365:431–433. *Overview of data suggesting lack of benefit from reducing dietary protein or intestinal bacteria.*

159 DISEASES OF THE GALLBLADDER AND BILE DUCTS

Nezam H. Afdhal

THE BILIARY SYSTEM

Definition

The biliary tract consists of the intrahepatic biliary canaliculus; the small, medium, and large intrahepatic bile ducts; the common bile duct; the gallbladder; the cystic duct; and the ampulla of Vater. The primary functions of the biliary system are secretion and storage of bile salts that solubilize intestinal lipids, excretion of cholesterol to maintain cholesterol homeostasis, excretion of excess bilirubin, and excretion of organic ions, including drug metabolites.

CHOLESTASIS

Pathobiology

Cholestasis is the systemic retention of biliary constituents as a result of failure of formation and flow of bile (Table 159–1). In the liver, hepatocytes are organized into cribriform, anastomosing plates along the sinusoids. At the apical pole, between adjacent hepatocytes, is the 1- to 2-μM biliary canaliculus or space. Each hepatocyte can have multiple canaliculi (up to three), which are characterized by microvilli that protrude into the canalicular lumen.

Bile consists of water, electrolytes, and organic solutes (Table 159–2). It is continuously modified both by the cholangiocytes that line the bile ducts and by the gallbladder mucosa, and therefore gallbladder bile is markedly different from hepatic bile. The gallbladder mucosa absorbs water and concentrates bile, so the total lipid content of gallbladder bile is much higher than that of hepatic bile (10 vs. 3 g/dL, respectively).

TABLE 159–1 CAUSES OF CHOLESTASIS

Extrahepatic	Intrahepatic
Choledocholithiasis	Viral hepatitis
Bile duct stricture	Alcoholic hepatitis
Cholangiocarcinoma	Drug induced
Pancreatic carcinoma	Ductopenia syndromes
Chronic pancreatitis	Primary biliary cirrhosis
Papillary stenosis	Benign recurrent intrahepatic cholestasis
Ampullary cancer	Byler's disease
Primary sclerosing cholangitis	Primary sclerosing cholangitis
Choledochal cysts	Alagille's syndrome
Parasites (e.g., *Ascaris, Clonorchis*)	Sarcoid
Acquired immunodeficiency syndrome cholangiography	Lymphoma
Biliary atresia	Postoperative
Portal lymphadenopathy	Total parenteral nutrition
Mirrizzi's syndrome	α_1-Antitrypsin deficiency

TABLE 159–2 CONSTITUENTS OF HUMAN CANALICULAR BILE

Bile salts, 12 g/L	Cholates, 35%
Glycine conjugates, 75%	Chenodeoxycholates, 35%
Taurine conjugates, 24.8%	Deoxycholates, 25%
Free bile acids, 0.2%	Lithocholates, 1%
	Miscellaneous, 40%
Phospholipids, 5 g/L	Phosphatidylcholine, 96%
	Phosphatidylethanolamine, 3%
Cholesterol, 1 g/L	Free, unesterified, 99%
Bilirubin, 0.2 g/L	Diglucuronide, 80%
	Monoglucuronide, 18%
	Unconjugated, 2%
Proteins, 2 g/L	Albumin, 50%
	Immunoglobulins, 23%
	Calcium binding protein/anionic peptide fraction, 17%
	Serum proteins, 9%
	Canalicular proteins, 1%
Electrolytes	Sodium, 150 mEq/L
	Magnesium, 2 mEq/L
	Calcium, 3 mEq/L
	Potassium, 5 mEq/L
	Chloride, 110 mEq/L
	Bicarbonate, 30 mEq/L

The major primary bile acids are cholic and chenodeoxycholic acid. The secondary bile acids, lithocholic and deoxycholic acids, which are derived from the intestinal breakdown of primary bile acids, are more hydrophobic, increase in cholestasis, and can be toxic to hepatocytes. Amidation with glycine or taurine results in the formation of bile salts that are preferentially secreted into bile. Bile salts are amphophilic detergent-like molecules synthesized from cholesterol via a pathway dependent on either 7α-hydroxylase or sterol 27-hydroxylase. Bile salt synthesis accounts for approximately 50% of the liver metabolism of cholesterol. Bile salts are secreted into the canalicular space by an energy-dependent bile salt export pump (Fig. 159–1). In the canalicular membrane, bile salts exist as simple (bile salt only) or mixed (with phosphatidylcholine and cholesterol) micelles and are transported into the gallbladder. A fatty meal results in contraction of the gallbladder with expulsion of bile salts into the duodenum, where they form micelles with intraluminal fat. About 95% of bile acids are absorbed by a sodium-dependent bile acid transporter in the terminal ileum. The total bile acid pool is circulated four to six times per day, and the volume of biliary secretion is approximately 1 L/day. The major phospholipid in bile is phosphatidylcholine, also called lecithin. Phosphatidylcholine in bile is derived from newly synthesized hepatic phosphatidylcholine, which is then transported through the hepatocyte by a phosphatidylcholine transfer protein and delivered to the multidrug resistance receptor 3 (MDR3), a phosphatidylcholine-specific transporter for final secretion into bile (see Fig. 159–1). All biliary lipids, including cholesterol, are secreted in a controlled manner by adenosine triphosphate (ATP) binding cassette transporters (Table 159–3).

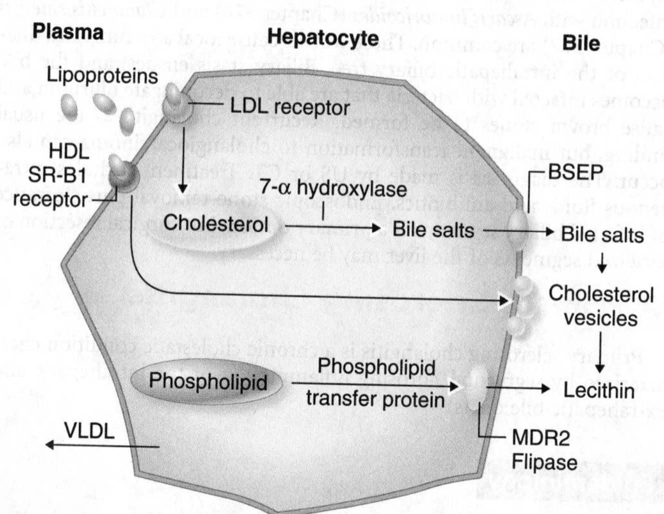

FIGURE 159–1 • Schematic diagram of the metabolism of phospholipid and cholesterol by the hepatocyte. BSEP = bile salt export pump; HDL = high-density lipoprotein; LDL = low-density lipoprotein; MDR2 = multidrug resistant receptor 2, a phospholipid lipase highly selective for phosphatidylcholine or lecithin; VLDL = very low density lipoprotein.

Clinical Manifestations

The clinical manifestations depend on the location and cause of the obstructive process and the degree to which an associated increase in proinflammatory cytokines decreases bile salt synthesis and secretion. *Intrahepatic cholestasis* is usually the result of either hepatocellular dysfunction (Chapter 149) or injury to the small and medium bile ducts secondary to viruses (Chapters 151 and 152), alcohol (Chapters 156 and 157), or drugs (Chapter 153).

Bile salt retention can lead to an excess of hydrophobic bile salts, such as deoxycholate, which are hepatotoxic. These retained bile salts can overflow out of the liver and lead to increased levels of bile salts in serum and the skin; the result is pruritus. Excess cholesterol is deposited in all tissues, particularly as tendinous xanthomas and periorbital xanthelasmas, but clinically significant atherosclerosis is uncommon.

In cholestasis, concentrations of intestinal bile salts are inadequate to solubilize dietary lipids; the result is the excretion of excess nonabsorbed fat. Long-chain dietary fats also irritate the colonic mucosa. Steatorrhea, which is characterized by greasy, foul-smelling diarrhea, develops (Chapter 143). Steatorrhea is suggested by the presence of stainable fat in stool (see Fig. 143–11) and confirmed by quantitative analysis of a 32-hour stool collection (see Table 143–6).

Because malabsorption of the fat-soluble vitamins A, D, E, and K can result in deficiency syndromes, fat-soluble vitamins and essential fatty acids should be given as dietary supplements. The combination of osteomalacia and osteoporosis is a serious consequence of cholestasis and chronic liver disease.

Diagnosis

In pure cholestasis, alkaline phosphatase and γ-glutamyltransferase levels are elevated significantly, whereas aminotransferase levels are normal or only mildly increased (Chapter 150). Bilirubin may be elevated but can be normal even in severe intrahepatic cholestasis until the very late stages of disease. Dilation of the intrahepatic ducts on ultrasonography (US) suggests *extrahepatic obstructive cholestasis.*

Treatment

Rx

Therapy should attempt to remove the cause of cholestasis, such as bypassing an obstructing pancreatic cancer (Chapter 204) with surgery or a stent. In the progressive cholestasis of intrahepatic biliary disease (e.g., primary biliary cirrhosis [PBC]), liver transplantation (Chapter 158) may be the only recourse.

Bile acid binders or sequestrants, such as cholestyramine, can lower the bile acid concentration but are associated with bloating and constipation (Table 159–4). Replacement of hydrophobic bile salts with hydrophilic bile salts, such as ursodeoxycholic acid (UDCA), treats all forms of intrahepatic cholestasis and the associated pruritus. The sensorineural pathway can also be blocked by using opioid antagonists such as naloxone and naltrexone, but care must be taken to avoid the risk for opioid withdrawal syndrome. Hepatic

TABLE 159–3 CANALICULAR ATP-BINDING CASSETTE TRANSPORTERS FOR PRIMARY BILIARY CONSTITUENTS

Transporter Name	Gene Code	Substrate	Associated Hereditary Disease
FIC1	*ATP8B1*	?	Byler's disease, PFIC type 1
BSEP	*ABCB11*	Bile salts	PFIC type 2
MDR3	*ABCB4*	Phosphatidylcholine	PFIC type 3
MDR1	*ABCB1*	Amphipathic drugs	
MRP2 (cMOAT)	*ABCC2*	Anionic neutral drugs	Dubin-Johnson syndrome
ABCG5/ABCG8	*ABCG5/8*	Cholesterol	Sitosterolemia

ATP = adenosine triphosphate; BSEP = bile salt export pump; cMOAT = canalicular multispecific organic anion transporter; MDR = multidrug-resistant receptor; MRP2 = multidrug resistance–associated protein 2; PFIC = progressive familial intrahepatic cholestasis.

TABLE 159–4 CLINICAL FEATURES OF AND THERAPY FOR CHOLESTASIS

Clinical Syndrome	Treatment
Pruritus	Bile salt binders (e.g., cholestyramine), ursodeoxycholic acid, rifampicin, naltrexone, carbinoids, phenobarbital
Hypercholesterolemia	Bile salt binders (e.g., cholestyramine) Statins—poor effect
Malabsorption	Medium-chain triglycerides, fat-soluble vitamins (A, D, E, K), essential fatty acids
Osteopenia	Calcium, vitamin D, bisphosphonates

Rx

enzyme inducers such as phenobarbital and rifampicin have also been successfully used for pruritus. Rifampicin may induce drug-metabolizing transporters, thereby resulting in increased excretion of pruritogens but with a risk of hepatotoxicity. In some cases of intractable pruritus, marijuana or its synthetic form Marinol has been useful in controlling symptoms. Finally, for situations such as the intractable pruritus of biliary cirrhosis, liver transplantation is the only option.

Supplementation with calcium, 1500 mg daily, plus vitamin D is essential. If bone density scans show osteopenia, therapy with bisphosphonates should be instituted (Chapter 264).

BILIARY TRACT DISEASES

Lesions of the intrahepatic and extrahepatic biliary tree, including the ampulla of Vater, are rare.

Biliary Atresia

Biliary atresia is a fibro-obliterative process that affects the perinatal bile ducts from the hilar bifurcation to the duodenum in 1 in every 13,000 live births in the United States. Associated genetic abnormalities in 25% of cases include polysplenia, anomalies of the portal vein and hepatic artery, abdominal situs inversus, intestinal malrotation, and cardiovascular and urinary tract anomalies. The clinical findings consist of jaundice with acholic stools persisting for 2 weeks after birth. The diagnosis can be suspected by endoscopic retrograde cholangiopancreatography (ERCP) or magnetic resonance cholangiopancreatography (MRCP) but is usually confirmed by laparotomy. Surgical correction by portoenterostomy should be performed within the first 60 days of life. About 80% of children grow normally through the first years of life, but subsequent stenosis of the anastomosis with progressive biliary cirrhosis and liver failure is common and an indication for liver transplantation.

Choledochal Cysts

Choledochal cysts are congenital ductal ectasias involving either a segment or the entirety of the biliary tree. The incidence is 1 per 13,000 live births in the United States but is 13 times higher in Japan and Asia. Female gender carries a four-fold greater prevalence, and there is an association of cysts with an abnormal pancreatic ductal junction and congenital hepatic fibrosis. The usual clinical manifestation is a right upper quadrant mass, jaundice, and pain. Acute pancreatitis, cholangitis, variceal hemorrhage, and cyst rupture are alternative findings. The diagnosis is usually made by imaging studies, including US, computed tomography (CT), MRCP, and ERCP. Therapy is generally surgical excision of the cyst with a Roux-en-Y hepaticojejunostomy because of the high (3 to 26%) incidence of malignant transformation of the cysts into cholangiocarcinoma. When there is extensive intrahepatic ductal dilation (Caroli's disease), recurrent cholangitis and intrahepatic stones are common, and liver transplantation is the optimal therapy.

TABLE 159–5 DISEASES ASSOCIATED WITH SCLEROSING CHOLANGITIS

Primary Sclerosing Cholangitis	Secondary Sclerosing Cholangitis
Ulcerative colitis	Choledocholithiasis
Crohn's colitis or ileocolitis	Infections in immunocompromised patients (*Cryptosporidium*, *Trichosporon*, cytomegalovirus, *Cryptococcus*, visceral protothecosis)
Type 1 autoimmune hepatitis	HTLV-1–associated myelopathy
	Ischemic injury to the hepatic artery or arterioles
	Trauma
	Neoplasia
	Toxic injury
	Floxuridine (hepatic artery injection)
	Formalin injection of echinococcal cysts
	Congenital abnormalities
	Celiac sprue

HTLV = human T-cell lymphotropic virus.

Oriental Cholangiohepatitis

Recurrent cholangitis with hepatolithiasis is endemic in East Asia, especially in Taiwan where the incidence is as high as 13% in areas where infection with *Ascaris lumbricoides* (Chapter 378) and *Clonorchis sinensis* (Chapter 377) are common. These worms cause local strictures and dilation of the intrahepatic biliary tree. Biliary stasis ensues, and the bile becomes infected with bacteria that are able to deconjugate bilirubin and cause brown stones to be formed. Recurrent cholangitis is the usual finding, but malignant transformation to cholangiocarcinoma can also occur. The diagnosis is made by US or CT. Treatment includes intravenous fluids and antibiotics. Endoscopic stone removal plus clearance of infected biliary segments is a primary option, but surgical resection of localized segments of the liver may be necessary.

Primary Sclerosing Cholangitis

Primary sclerosing cholangitis is a chronic cholestatic condition characterized by segmental fibrosing inflammation of the intrahepatic and extrahepatic bile ducts.

Epidemiology

The prevalence of primary sclerosing cholangitis is 1 to 6 cases per 100,000 in the U.S. population, with a male-to-female ratio of 2.3:1. The mean age at diagnosis is 32 to 40 years of age, but children can be affected.

Pathobiology

The etiology remains unknown, but primary sclerosing cholangitis is thought to be a primary autoimmune disease. The disease is progressive, with obliteration of small, medium, and large bile ducts leading to three distinct clinical syndromes: (1) cholestasis with eventual biliary cirrhosis, (2) recurrent cholangitis and large duct strictures, and (3) cholangiocarcinoma. The multiple causes of secondary sclerosing cholangitis can be accompanied by symptoms and signs that are indistinguishable from the primary form (Table 159–5).

Primary sclerosing cholangitis is associated with both ulcerative colitis and Crohn's disease of the colon (Chapter 144). Between 70 and 90% of patients with primary sclerosing cholangitis have clinical or microscopic colitis, and between 1.3 and 13% of patients with colitis have primary sclerosing cholangitis. Inflammatory bowel disease usually precedes primary sclerosing cholangitis, but in some cases the colitis is asymptomatic and discovered only by subsequent colonoscopy and biopsy. There is also a crossover syndrome between primary sclerosing cholangitis and primary autoimmune hepatitis (Chapter 152).

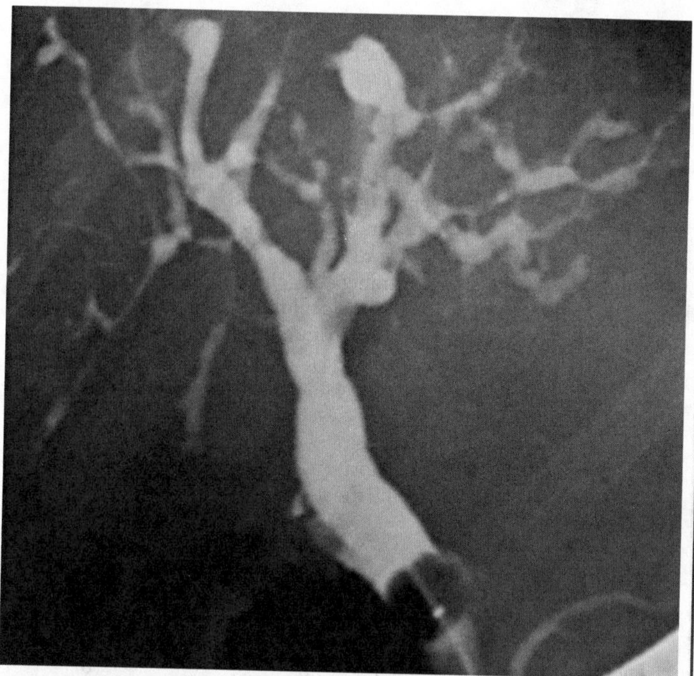

FIGURE 159–2 • Endoscopic retrograde cholangiopancreatography for primary sclerosing cholangitis with contrast injected through a balloon catheter (seen in the lower common duct). The intrahepatic ducts are mainly affected and show diminished arborization (pruning); diffuse segmental strictures alternating with normal-caliber or mildly dilated duct segments (cholangiectases) have resulted in a beaded appearance. (From Mahadevan U, Bass NM: Sclerosing cholangitis and recurrent pyogenic cholangitis. *In* Feldman M, Friedman LS, Sleisenger MH [eds]: Gastrointestinal and Liver Disease: Pathophysiology/Diagnosis/Management, 7th ed. Philadelphia, Saunders, 2002, p 1137.)

Clinical Manifestations

The most common laboratory finding is an elevated alkaline phosphatase level, which is present in 90% of patients, and mildly elevated aminotransferase levels. The bilirubin level is initially normal in 60% of patients but increases over time and is an important prognostic factor. Autoantibodies, including antinuclear antibodies and anti–smooth muscle antibodies, are seen in 22% of patients, but a positive antimitochondrial antibody (AMA) is rare and suggests PBC. Perinuclear antineutrophilic cytoplasmic antibody (pANCA) is positive in 90% of patients with primary sclerosing cholangitis and colitis, but pANCA is nonspecific and is also found in ulcerative colitis and in autoimmune hepatitis without primary sclerosing cholangitis.

Diagnosis

The diagnosis is based on pathologic and radiologic findings, and all patients should undergo both liver biopsy and cholangiography. Large duct disease, which is diagnosed most frequently by ERCP or MRCP, includes strictures, beading, and dilation (Fig. 159–2). Liver biopsy shows an obliterative cholangitis with inflammation and characteristic periductular onion ring fibrosis (Fig. 159–3). As the disease progresses, ductopenia and secondary biliary cirrhosis predominate. In stage I, inflammation is confined to the portal tracts; in stage II, there is hepatitis and portal fibrosis; in stage III, bridging fibrosis appears; and stage IV is characterized by biliary cirrhosis and regenerative nodules. Associated conditions include pancreatitis (15% of patients), perihepatic lymphadenopathy, and cholangiocarcinoma (27 to 41% of patients at autopsy or transplantation).

Treatment

Rx

No treatment slows disease progression. Medical therapy includes treatment of cholangitis and endoscopic therapy for large strictures via balloon dilation and stent insertion. Surgery is avoided, if possible, because it increases the risk for recurrent cholangitis. Immuno-

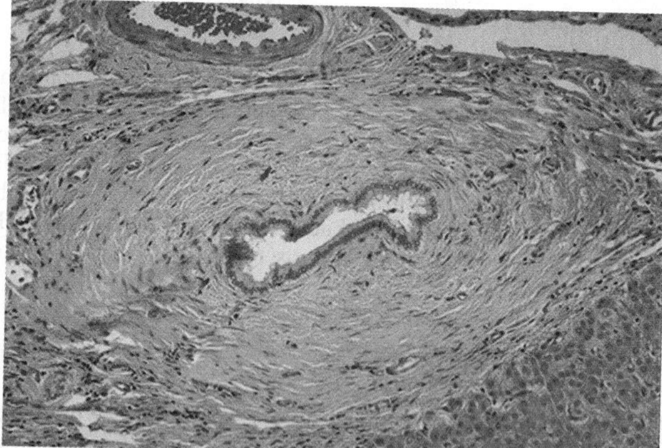

FIGURE 159–3 • Microscopically, this bile duct in a case of sclerosing cholangitis is surrounded by marked collagenous connective tissue deposition. (Reproduced from http://library.med.utah.edu/WebPath/GUIDE/INTRO.html with permission.)

Rx

suppressive therapy is not effective. In randomized trials, UDCA (15 mg/kg/day) has improved bilirubin, alkaline phosphatase, and albumin levels but has not provided any definite benefit on survival or time to liver decompensation. Higher doses (20 mg/kg) are often used because some preliminary reports have suggested a better biochemical response to these doses. 1

Liver transplantation (Chapter 158), which is the only potentially curative therapy, provides an actuarial survival rate of 83% at 1 year and 73% at 5 years. All patients with primary sclerosing cholangitis who undergo transplantation should be screened periodically for colon carcinoma because they have chronic colitis (Chapter 144). Recurrent primary sclerosing cholangitis after transplantation is rare and difficult to distinguish from other causes of bile duct injury. If small (<1 cm), incidental cholangiocarcinomas are found at transplantation, survival is not affected, but larger cholangiocarcinomas (>2 cm) detected in the pretransplant evaluation by CT or magnetic resonance imaging are a contraindication to liver transplantation.

Patients with primary sclerosing cholangitis should be screened for possible cholangiocarcinoma by cholangiography of strictures every 6 to 12 months with brushings and biopsies. If cholangiocarcinoma is detected, patients should be offered surgical resection or radiotherapy (Chapter 206).

Prognosis

The natural history is variable. Some patients have severe recurrent cholangitis, whereas others progress to biliary cirrhosis. The median survival to death or transplantation is approximately 12 years, with a range of up to 21 years. Actuarial survival is greater for asymptomatic patients (10-year survival rate of 80%) than for symptomatic patients (10-year survival rate of 50%).

Primary Biliary Cirrhosis

Definition

PBC is a slowly progressive obliterative autoimmune cholangiopathy involving the small and medium-sized bile ducts. It leads to ductopenia, progressive fibrosis, cholestasis, and liver failure.

Epidemiology

PBC is predominantly a disease of women (95% of cases) between the ages of 20 and 60. The age- and gender-adjusted prevalence has been estimated at 65 and 12 per 100,000 persons, respectively, for women and men. The incidence of the disease may be increasing, and a U.S. study estimated it at 2.7 per 100,00 person years or 4.5 and 0.7 for women and men, respectively.

Pathobiology

PBC is thought to be an autoimmune disorder, but the mechanism of progressive destruction of the small interlobular ducts is unknown. The disease is slowly progressive and can eventually lead to biliary cirrhosis with portal hypertension and liver failure. The classic histologic finding is the presence of noncaseating granulomas associated with small bile ducts and an overall paucity of bile ducts in the portal tracts. The presence of significant bridging fibrosis or cirrhosis carries a worse prognosis.

Clinical Manifestations

Almost 60% of patients with PBC are asymptomatic at the time of initial diagnosis. The most common symptoms are fatigue (50%) and pruritus (30%). Fatigue is unrelated to the degree of underlying liver injury or cholestasis and can be extremely debilitating. Pruritus is often first noticed in pregnancy but persists after delivery, and many patients are initially referred for dermatologic evaluation.

In addition to the features of cholestasis, multiple clinical syndromes are associated with PBC and are suggestive of an autoimmune origin. Autoimmune thyroid dysfunction (Chapter 244), sicca syndrome (Chapter 289), Raynaud's phenomenon (Chapter 288), and celiac disease (Chapter 143) have all been associated with PBC. Metabolic bone disease can be particularly troublesome because of the long duration of cholestasis; bone density studies are mandatory every 2 years to guide and monitor therapy.

Diagnosis

The most common biochemical abnormality is an elevation in serum alkaline phosphatase, which should be confirmed by an elevated γ-glutamyl transpeptidase and indicates cholestasis. The bilirubin level is not elevated until late in the course of disease, and most of the elevation is usually of conjugated bilirubin. US should be performed to image the biliary tree and confirm the absence of extrahepatic disease. AMA, which has a sensitivity and specificity higher than 95% when the titer is greater than 1:40, can be positive before there is any clinical or biochemical evidence of PBC. Total immunoglobulins are generally normal, but the IgM fraction can be elevated. Liver biopsy is performed to stage the disease and occasionally to confirm the diagnosis, particularly in AMA-negative patients.

Treatment

Rx

UDCA therapy reduces intracellular hydrophobic bile acids and may have a cytoprotective effect on cell membranes. Randomized trials show a significant increase in survival after up to 4 years of therapy with UDCA (12 to 15 mg/kg), [2] as judged by time to liver transplantation. The greatest benefit is seen in patients with the most severe disease. Serum bilirubin, alkaline phosphatase, and cholesterol levels improve with UDCA therapy, but treatment does not benefit the fatigue and has a variable effect on pruritus. Side effects are rare, the most common being diarrhea.

There is no definite benefit to steroids, colchicine, or azathioprine. Low-dose methotrexate (2.5 mg three times per week) has been tried, but data are insufficient to support its routine use at this time. PBC is a common indication for liver transplantation (Chapter 158), but there is considerable debate regarding the timing of transplantation.

Prognosis

PBC is a progressive disease, with up to two thirds of asymptomatic patients becoming symptomatic in 2 to 4 years. Median survival is 9.3 years from diagnosis, and the most reliable determinants of prognosis are the height of the serum bilirubin level and the Mayo risk score, a composite score that predicts clinical outcomes and is calculated as R = 0.871 log(e) (bilirubin in mg/dL) + 2.53 log(e) (albumin in g/dL) + 0.039 (age in years) + 2.38 log(e) (prothrombin time in seconds) + 0.859 (edema score of 0, 0.5, or 1). Liver failure develops in 26% of patients by 10 years after diagnosis.

Vanishing Bile Duct Syndromes

Vanishing bile duct syndromes are characterized by a paucity of intrahepatic bile ducts and by eventual cholestasis and biliary cirrhosis. Causes include PBC, primary sclerosing cholangitis, autoimmune hepatitis (Chapter 152), graft-versus-host disease, chronic liver allograft rejection (Chapter 158), ischemia, intrahepatic chemotherapy, drug toxicity (e.g., ampicillin, amoxicillin, flucloxacillin, erythromycin, tetracycline, doxycycline, cotrimoxazole), human immunodeficiency virus infection (Chapter 413), sarcoidosis (Chapter 95), idiopathic or paraneoplastic bile duct paucity, and histiocytosis. Almost all these conditions are accompanied by chronic cholestasis and elevated alkaline phosphatase levels. Treatment is for the complications of cholestasis, and UDCA (15 mg/kg) is given to increase bile flow. Most of these conditions are slowly progressive and result in biliary cirrhosis, which ultimately requires liver transplantation.

GALLSTONE DISEASE

Definition

There are three different types of gallstones: cholesterol gallstones, mixed gallstones, and pigment stones, which can be further divided into black and brown stones. Cholesterol and mixed stones account for 80% of gallstone disease in the United States. Cholesterol stones contain more than 70% cholesterol, whereas mixed stones also contain significant amounts of pigments such as bilirubin. Black pigment stones, which are generally associated with hemolytic diseases, contain calcium salts, bilirubin, and proteins. Brown pigment stones are more common in Asia, where they are associated with intrahepatic cholangitis and infection; in the United States, brown stones are seen after cholecystectomy, especially when manifested as choledocholithiasis.

Epidemiology

Approximately 30 million people in the United States have gallstones, and the estimated annual cost of gallstone disease is $15 billion. In Europe, large ultrasound studies in subjects between 30 and 65 years of age have shown gallstones in 18.8% of women and 9.5% of men. In a study in which 1930 subjects were monitored for 10 years, the cumulative incidence of new stones was 4.6%.

Age is a major risk factor for gallstone disease (Table 159–6); less than 2% of cholecystectomies for gallstones are performed in children, usually because of hemolytic diseases. However, the increased prevalence of obesity in children may result in an earlier incidence of gallstone disease.

The age-adjusted female-to-male ratio for gallstone disease is 2.9 between the ages of 30 and 39 years, but it decreases to 1.2 between the ages of 50 and 59 years. Women with gallstone disease also appear to be

TABLE 159–6 RISK FACTORS FOR GALLSTONE DISEASE
Age
Female gender
Parity
Obesity
Rapid weight loss
Hypertriglyceridemia
Genetic (e.g., Pima Indians, Chileans)
Medications: estrogen, clofibrate, ceftriaxone, Sandostatin
Terminal ileal resection
Gallbladder hypomotility: pregnancy, diabetes, after vagotomy
Somatostatinoma
Total parenteral nutrition
Spinal cord injury

more likely than men to undergo cholecystectomy. Pregnancy appears to be the major risk factor for the increased prevalence of gallstones in younger women, with a prevalence of 1.3% in nulliparous women versus 13% in multiparous women. Estrogen use is also associated with a higher risk for symptomatic gallstones and cholecystectomy: a relative risk of 2.1 to 3.7 versus no estrogen use. The mechanisms of increased risk include activation of estrogen α-receptor–mediated hepatic cholesterol secretion, a progesterone-induced reduction in gallbladder contraction, and a pregnancy-induced alteration in hydrophobic/hydrophilic bile salt balance.

Obesity increases the risk for gallstones as a result of enhanced cholesterol absorption, synthesis, and secretion. The risk is higher in women and in the morbidly obese, but rapid weight reduction by very low calorie diets is also associated with gallstones. Diets high in polyunsaturated and monounsaturated fats may reduce the risk for gallstone disease.

Pathobiology

Gallstone disease is predominantly an inability to maintain free cholesterol in solution in bile. As canalicular bile passes down the bile duct system, cholangiocytes maintain bile flow and volume by secreting chloride, bicarbonate, and water into bile. In cystic fibrosis (Chapter 89), defects in the cystic fibrosis transmembrane conductance regulator, which in the liver is found only on cholangiocytes, reduces choleresis and results in the formation of mucous plugs with subsequent focal biliary cirrhosis and gallstone disease.

The gallbladder, which acts as the final storage reservoir for bile, concentrates bile by removing water and thereby increasing the lipid concentration from 3 g/dL in hepatic bile to 10 g/dL in gallbladder bile. Bile salt concentrations can be as high as 300 mM and would digest the biliary epithelium if the gallbladder did not secrete mucin for protection. The gallbladder mucosa also secretes hydrogen ions to prevent calcium salt deposition and maintain a bile pH of about 6.5. A normal gallbladder ejects 10 to 20% of its contents in response to duodenal-gallbladder enteric nervous stimulation. Postprandially, duodenal lipids cause about a 70% contraction of the gallbladder mediated by both the enteric nervous system and cholecystokinin. Impaired contractility is one of the critical steps in the pathogenesis of gallstones.

Genetics

Family history studies have shown that gallstones are twice as common in first-degree relatives of gallstone patients as in age- and sex-matched control subjects. In the United States, descendants of the original Amerindians have a markedly increased prevalence of gallstones, with the highest rates in female Pima Indians older than 25 years, who have a 75% prevalence of cholesterol gallstones. Amerindians in South America and Mexico also have a very high prevalence of gallstones, and these populations have the highest rate of complications of gallstone disease, such as gallbladder cancer, in the world. South Americans of Hispanic origin have much lower rates of gallstone disease.

No specific gallstone genes have been found in humans, but lithogenic genes, including the bile salt export pump gene, have been described in gallstone-susceptible mice. Human gallstone disease is probably a combination of complex multigene susceptibility and environmental factors.

Cholesterol Gallstones

Cholesterol gallstones contain 50 to 90% cholesterol and are the most common form of stones in countries with a Western diet that is high in protein and fat. Cholesterol is an intensely hydrophobic molecule that can remain soluble in aqueous solution only as saturated micelles and vesicles in conjunction with bile salts and lecithin. Cholesterol in gallbladder bile is found in multiple phases; in the presence of cholesterol supersaturation, unstable cholesterol vesicles nucleate to form cholesterol crystals (Fig. 159–4). Nucleation is promoted by a variety of factors, including proteins and lipids.

Increased biliary secretion of cholesterol results in cholesterol supersaturation of bile. The result is excess secretion of mucus into the gallbladder, formation of a gel layer, and stasis, which causes cholesterol to nucleate and cholesterol crystals to be deposited.

Cholesterol monohydrate crystals are only several hundred micrometers in size and should easily be expelled through the cystic duct. However, the mucous sludge containing calcium salts, bilirubin, mucin, and crystals is not easily expelled by contraction of the gallbladder. Biliary sludge, also known as microlithiasis, can be seen as an echogenic, freely mobile mass in the gallbladder on US. Biliary sludge can cause the symptoms of gallstone disease, including cholecystitis, cholangitis, and pancreatitis.

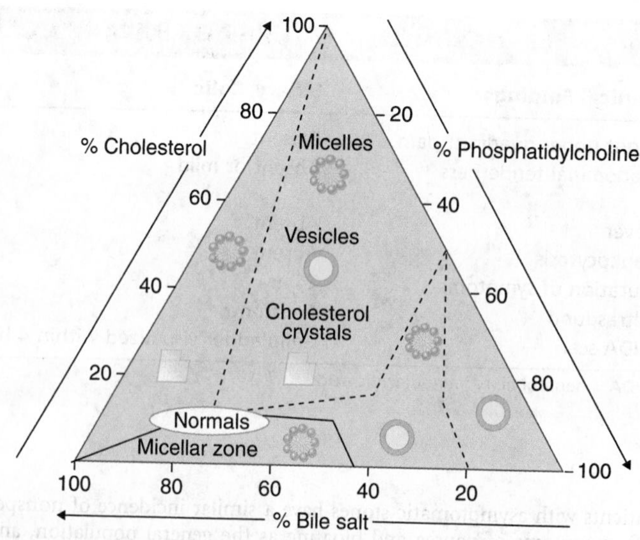

FIGURE 159–4 • Equilibrium phase diagram for a lithogenic model bile system with a total lipid content of 10 g/dL.

Biliary sludge can resolve, persist, or progress to stones when its crystals grow to form plates, in part because of an impairment in gallbladder contractility. Cholesterol supersaturation of bile is associated with increased absorption of cholesterol by the gallbladder smooth muscle, a process that impairs smooth muscle contractility and reduces the response of the gallbladder to cholecystokinin.

Pigment Gallstones

Black pigment stones contain 10 to 90% calcium bilirubinate in combination with a variety of other calcium salts, such as hydroxyapatite and carbonate. These stones are common in India (40%) but rare in Minnesota (5%). Older age is associated with a higher incidence of pigment stones, as are total parenteral nutrition and hemolytic diseases.

Brown pigment stones represent 30% of gallstones in Japan and up to 90% of gallstones in rural China. They are related to low-calorie, high-vegetable diets, occur in both the biliary tract and the liver, and have a strong association with recurrent pyogenic cholangitis and cholangiohepatitis. In the United States, these stones are seen as postcholecystectomy cholelithiasis, presumably secondary to stasis and infection. Bacterial enzymes deconjugate bilirubin from its glucuronide and hydrolyze phospholipids, thereby leading to precipitation of calcium, bilirubin, and free fatty acids. These stones, which are often soft and easy to crush endoscopically, are commonly treated by endoscopic extraction.

Clinical Manifestations

The symptoms caused by gallstones are often nonspecific and include nausea, bloating, and right upper quadrant pain. Biliary pain, which is described as an intermittent right upper quadrant or epigastric pain occurring 15 to 30 minutes after a meal, often with radiation to the back, is unpredictable, severe, and usually constant rather than a true colic. The pain persists for 3 to 4 hours and may be associated with nausea and vomiting. In uncomplicated cholecystitis, fever and leukocytosis are absent, the pain can usually be adequately treated with a single dose of narcotic analgesics or nonsteroidal anti-inflammatory agents (NSAIDs), and the pain generally subsides within 6 hours. Attacks of colic may be separated by days or months.

Diagnosis

Asymptomatic Gallstones

Asymptomatic gallstones, which are frequently diagnosed by US performed for other indications, account for about 85% of gallstones.

TABLE 159–7 CLINICAL FEATURES OF BILIARY COLIC COMPARED WITH ACUTE CHOLECYSTITIS

Clinical Findings	Biliary Colic	Acute Cholecystitis
Right upper quadrant pain	Present	Present
Abdominal tenderness	Absent or mild	Moderate to severe, especially over the liver and/or gallbladder (Murphy's sign)
Fever	Absent	Usually present
Leukocytosis	Absent	Usually >11,000/μL
Duration of symptoms	<4 hr	>6 hr
Ultrasound	Gallstones	Gallstones, thickening of the gallbladder wall
HIDA scan	Gallbladder visualized within 4 hr	No filling of the gallbladder

HIDA = hepatobiliary iminodiacetic acid.

Patients with asymptomatic stones have a similar incidence of nonspecific symptoms of nausea and bloating as the general population, and complications of gallstone disease rarely develop. Biliary colic, however, is more predictive of gallstones, and it is an indicator of increased risk for cholecystitis or other complications. Because the current standard of care is to treat only symptomatic stones, it is critically important to determine whether any symptoms are related to gallbladder stones.

Among patients with asymptomatic stones, biliary colic develops in about 2 to 3% annually. In the absence of antecedent symptoms, complications of gallstone disease, such as acute cholecystitis, develop at a rate of less than 1% per year. As a result, the recommendation is to reserve cholecystectomy until after biliary colic develops, with prophylactic or incidental cholecystectomy recommended only for Amerindians, transplant recipients, or patients with sickle cell anemia, morbid obesity, an anomalous pancreatic ductal junction, a porcelain gallbladder, or gallbladder polyps larger than 1 cm (see Cholecystectomy).

Acute Calculous Cholecystitis

Acute cholecystitis, which is the most common serious complication of gallstone disease, can lead to a variety of complications, including perforation of the gallbladder, peritonitis, fistula into the intestine or duodenum with gallstone ileus or obstruction, and abscesses in the liver or abdominal cavity. Acute cholecystitis is caused by obstruction of the cystic duct, and the ensuing increased intraluminal pressure can lead to vascular compromise of the gallbladder. *Salmonella* and other less common microorganisms such as *Vibrio cholerae*, *Leptospira*, and *Listeria* can cause primary cholecystitis. Clinical differentiation of biliary colic from acute cholecystitis is difficult but can usually be made from clinical and radiologic findings (Table 159–7).

Blood Tests

In uncomplicated acute cholecystitis, laboratory testing usually shows leukocytosis but otherwise is not very helpful. Elevated liver enzyme levels, hyperbilirubinemia, and elevated amylase or lipase levels are not common in cholecystitis and suggest other complications of gallstone disease, such as cholangitis or pancreatitis. When acute cholecystitis is accompanied by an inflammatory mass, the gallbladder can compress the common duct and lead to bile duct obstruction (Mirrizzi's syndrome).

Imaging Studies

Right upper quadrant US noninvasively diagnoses gallstones in 95% of patients with cholecystitis (Fig. 159–5). US can also exclude common bile duct obstruction and may occasionally show bile duct stones. In cholecystitis, the gallbladder wall may be thickened, and free pericholecystic fluid may be present. Murphy's sign is also useful and can be elicited by the ultrasonographer or on physical examination. Gentle pressure is placed by the probe or hand at the border of the rectus sheath in the right upper quadrant, and the patient is asked to inspire. The gallbladder moves down with inspiration onto the examiner's hand or ultrasound probe, and the patient complains of pain when the inflamed gallbladder comes into contact with the examining hand. US can also exclude gangrenous cholecystitis with free air in the gallbladder wall, perforation, and abscess. The most specific test for acute cholecystitis is a technetium-labeled hepatobiliary iminodiacetic acid (HIDA) scan. Intravenously,

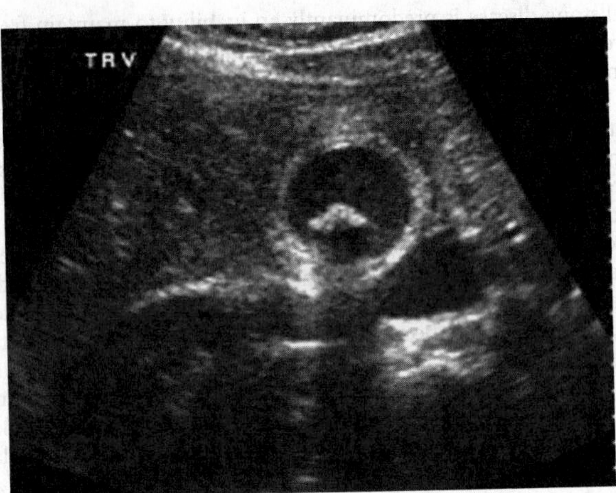

FIGURE 159–5 • Ultrasound showing a gallstone.

HIDA is normally taken up by the liver, excreted into the biliary tract, and concentrated in the gallbladder. When a stone obstructs the cystic duct, the gallbladder fails to fill with HIDA; the sensitivity of HIDA scan is 95%, but the specificity varies markedly and can be as poor as 50% in critically ill or jaundiced patients.

Treatment Rx

Medical Stabilization of Acute Cholecystitis

Treatment of uncomplicated acute cholecystitis is intravenous fluids, antibiotics for 7 to 10 days, and bowel rest. Antibiotic choices include ampicillin (2 g intravenously every 6 hours) and an aminoglycoside (gentamicin, 5.1 mg/kg every 24 hours), but cephalosporins (ceftriaxone, 1 to 2 g once daily) and ampicillin-sulbactam (1.5 to 3 g every 6 hours) can also be used. Broader coverage should be used in immunosuppressed patients, including the addition of metronidazole (500 mg every 8 hours), piperacillin-tazobactam (3.375 g every 6 hours), and levofloxacin (500 mg to 1 g once daily). Early cholecystectomy (at the time of first admission) is generally recommended. 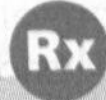

Cholecystectomy

Indications for cholecystectomy include biliary colic, acute and chronic cholecystitis, and acalculous cholecystitis. Diabetic patients may have fewer symptoms because of their neuropathy, so their cholecystitis may more frequently be complicated by gangrene and perforation; however, prophylactic cholecystectomy is not recommended in patients with diabetes.

Laparoscopic cholecystectomy has now all but replaced conventional open cholecystectomy as the procedure of choice for gallstones. Advantages of laparoscopic cholecystectomy include less pain, early discharge (usually 1 day after the procedure), fewer

Rx

wound infections, earlier return to work, and lower cost. A planned laparoscopic approach is changed to open cholecystectomy in only 3% of cases, usually because of difficulty identifying critical anatomic structures such as the cystic or common bile ducts.

Operative cholangiography can be performed during laparoscopic cholecystectomy, and bile duct stones can be removed concurrently or subsequently by ERCP. The incidence of unsuspected, retained common bile duct stones after laparoscopic cholecystectomy is about 2.3%.

The most serious complication of laparoscopic cholecystectomy is bile duct injury, which now occurs in 0.25% of cases, is more common when the indication for surgery is acute cholecystitis, and is less common after a surgeon has performed more than 25 laparoscopic surgeries. Bile duct injuries include cystic duct leak, laceration of the duct, complete transection of the duct, and thermal injuries to the duct. Early recognition permits primary open bile duct repair. Leakage from the cystic duct is usually recognized as jaundice, fever, and abdominal pain several days after the procedure; it can be treated successfully by ERCP with insertion of an endoscopic stent or by sphincterotomy.

Gallstone Dissolution Therapies

In patients who have relative or absolute contraindications to laparoscopic cholecystectomy, such as concomitant advanced cardiopulmonary or liver disease, a combination of chenodeoxycholic acid (10 mg/kg/day) with UDCA (7 to 15 mg/kg/day) or UDCA alone (15 mg/kg/day) can dissolve multiple small (<5 mm) stones in up to 60% of patients with a functioning gallbladder. If CT shows the stones to be calcified, the efficacy is lower, and complete dissolution occurs in only about 10% of patients. Gallstones generally dissolve at a rate of 1 mm/mo. After dissolution, gallstones recur at a rate of 10% per year for 5 years, but recurrence is unusual after that time. Continuous therapy may be necessary, thereby making this therapy unattractive except in selected patients in whom cholecystectomy cannot be performed safely.

Extracorporeal shock wave lithotripsy, which uses a focused ultrasound beam, can fragment larger stones. The fragmented stones can be passed through the cystic duct and expelled into the common bile duct. The fragments that remain behind in the gallbladder should be treated with UDCA for dissolution. Gallstones disappear in more than 50% of patients, but they recur in 50% of successfully treated patients, particularly those with multiple stones and poorly functioning gallbladders.

Topical dissolution therapy involves the insertion of a catheter into the gallbladder under ultrasound guidance; stones are dissolved with methyl terbutyl ether or ethyl propionate. The technique is still experimental but may soon be ready for widespread testing.

Choledocholithiasis

Common bile duct stones can descend from the gallbladder or arise de novo in a tortuous, dilated common bile duct as a result of infection and biliary stasis (usually cholesterol stones), or they can occur in a postcholecystectomy patient (usually brown stones), in whom they are frequently missed at surgery (2% of cholecystectomies). The clinical findings are cholangitis, pancreatitis, or biliary obstruction; large, obstructing stones can cause jaundice.

Acute bacterial cholangitis, which is most frequently caused by common duct stones that obstruct the common bile duct and raise intrabiliary pressure, is a medical emergency. The bile in these patients is generally infected with *Escherichia coli*, *Bacteroides*, *Klebsiella*, or *Clostridium* species, and the increase in pressure results in transient bacteremia.

Diagnosis

Patients with bacterial cholangitis have Charcot's triad of jaundice, abdominal pain, and fever with rigors. Severe renal dysfunction and disseminated intravascular coagulation can complicate severe cholangitis. Aminotransferase, bilirubin, and alkaline phosphatase levels are usually increased. The diagnosis of common bile duct stones can be made with US, which generally shows dilated bile ducts and occasionally identifies a stone. MRCP can identify 95% of stones larger than 1 cm (Fig. 159–6). ERCP remains the "gold standard" for the diagnosis and treatment of common bile duct stones. If cholangitis is suspected, ERCP should be performed.

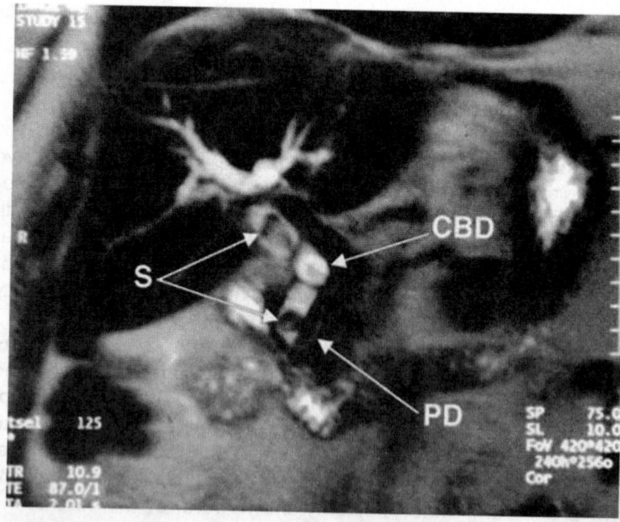

FIGURE 159–6 • Magnetic resonance cholangiopancreatogram of a dilated biliary tract. The common bile duct (CBD), pancreatic duct (PD), and two large common duct stones (S) are shown.

Treatment

Rx

Endoscopic therapy includes sphincterotomy and stone extraction with a balloon or basket. Small (<2 cm) stones can be removed easily, whereas larger stones may be crushed with mechanical or US lithotriptors before removal. Fluids and antibiotics with broad gram-negative coverage (e.g., ceftriaxone, 1 to 2 g once daily; ampicillin-sulbactam, 1.5 to 3 g every 6 hours; piperacillin-tazobactam, 3.375 g every 6 hours; levofloxacin, 500 mg to 1 g once daily) are recommended for bacterial cholangitis. In an acutely ill patient, initial decompression of a pus-filled common bile duct with a stent may be the first line of treatment, followed subsequently by definitive endoscopic or surgical therapy. After successful endoscopic therapy, laparoscopic cholecystectomy should be performed routinely because of the high risk for recurrent biliary events. 

In certain situations, such as after Roux-en-Y choledochojejunostomy, ERCP may not be possible. Alternative approaches include radiologic percutaneous transhepatic cholangiography (PTC) or open exploration of the common bile duct. At PTC, the radiologist can decompress the bile ducts with catheters or stents, and stones can subsequently be removed through the fistula tract by direct cholangiography.

Unusual Complications of Gallstone Disease

Gallstone pancreatitis (Chapter 147) is more common in patients with multiple small stones; it has also been associated with microlithiasis and biliary sludge. Patients have acute epigastric pain radiating into the back, hyperamylasemia, and an imaging study that demonstrates an edematous or necrotic pancreas. Concomitant cholangitis or jaundice can rarely be seen if the stone is obstructive. Clinical features that suggest gallstone pancreatitis include elevated aspartate aminotransferase and alkaline phosphatase levels. Early ERCP with sphincterotomy plus stone extraction within 24 hours of suspected acute gallstone pancreatitis reduces morbidity and mortality, but in 50% of cases the stones are not visible or have passed by the time of ERCP. After successful treatment of common duct

stones, patients who still have a gallbladder should have it removed electively.

Vascular compromise to the gallbladder and the presence of gas-forming bacteria, which are more common in patients who have diabetes or are immunocompromised, can cause *gangrenous or emphysematous cholecystitis*. Clinically, patients are usually very ill with a high temperature, features of systemic sepsis, and obtundation. US may show air in the gallbladder or gallbladder wall; perforation of the gallbladder with peritonitis may then occur. Emergency cholecystectomy is required.

If a fistula develops from the gallbladder to the duodenum, stomach, or colon, a large gallstone can pass through the fistula and into the bowel. If obstruction occurs at the duodenum or the ileocecal valve, *gallstone ileus* occurs with symptoms and signs of intestinal obstruction. A plain abdominal radiograph shows bowel obstruction with free air in the gallbladder or biliary tract. Treatment is generally cholecystectomy and removal of the obstructing gallstone.

Prevention

UDCA, 600 mg at night, markedly reduces gallstone formation in patients on low-fat, low-calorie diets. Primary prevention of cholesterol gallstones is based on dietary alteration to avoid cholesterol supersaturation (i.e., a diet rich in whole grains and roughage and low in cholesterol and saturated fats). Secondary prevention includes using bile acid therapy with UDCA to reduce cholesterol supersaturation, improving gallbladder motility with cholecystokinin analogues, and reducing mucin secretion with aspirin and NSAIDs. All these strategies have been used effectively in high-risk groups, such as patients on low-calorie diets or patients maintained on total parenteral nutrition. [5]

Prognosis

Overall, the prognosis of gallstone disease is excellent for younger and otherwise healthy patients. However, with the aging population, there is a higher prevalence of complicated gallstone disease with common duct stones, cholangitis, and pancreatitis, each of which is associated with substantial morbidity and mortality.

ACUTE ACALCULOUS CHOLECYSTITIS

Epidemiology and Pathobiology

Acalculous cholecystitis is inflammation of the gallbladder or the presence of gallbladder-related symptoms in the absence of stones. Acute acalculous cholecystitis accounts for 2 to 17% of all cholecystectomies. Ischemia, infections, chemical injury by biliary contents, and obstruction of the cystic duct have all been implicated as causes (Table 159–8).

TABLE 159–8 RISK FACTORS AND PRIMARY ORGANISMS ASSOCIATED WITH ACALCULOUS CHOLECYSTITIS

RISK FACTORS
Fasting
Total parenteral nutrition
Septicemia, biliary infections
Major trauma
Burns
Major nonbiliary surgery
Childbirth
Multiple blood transfusions
Mechanical ventilation
Opiates
Immunosuppression—chemotherapy, human immunodeficiency virus infection, transplantation
Diabetes
Ischemic heart disease
Malignancy
ORGANISMS IMPLICATED AS A PRIMARY CAUSE
Salmonella typhi
Vibrio cholera
Staphylococcus
Leptospira
Listeria
Pneumocystis carinii
Mycobacterium sp
Cytomegalovirus
Candida
Ascaris
Echinococcus

Clinical Manifestations

Primary infections may be manifested as acute cholecystitis with unexplained fever, right upper quadrant pain, or clinical deterioration postoperatively or after transplantation, trauma to the abdomen, chemotherapy, or total parenteral nutrition. Pain, fever, leukocytosis, and abnormal liver enzyme test results are common.

Diagnosis

The diagnosis is confirmed by US showing a distended gallbladder, often with a thin wall, pericholecystic fluid, or a positive Murphy sign (see earlier text) in the absence of gallstones. Sludge may be present. Intraluminal gas or bubbles, the so-called champagne sign, indicates emphysematous cholecystitis.

Treatment

Rx

Treatment includes intravenous fluids, antibiotics as for gallstone disease, and general supportive measures. Because gangrene and perforation are more common in acalculous than calculous cholecystitis, urgent cholecystectomy is recommended. Postcholecystectomy complications such as leaks, abscess, and wound infection are also more common and reflect the underlying multisystemic problems. In severely ill patients in whom cholecystectomy is contraindicated, radiologic decompression of the gallbladder via percutaneous cholecystostomy can be performed. The overall mortality associated with acute acalculous cholecystitis is 5 to 20%.

CHRONIC ACALCULOUS CHOLECYSTITIS

Chronic acalculous cholecystitis is a poorly understood clinical syndrome in which patients have symptoms of biliary colic in the absence of gallstones. The gallbladder may be normal or show changes of chronic inflammation. Cholesterolosis may also be present, with deposits of cholesterol in the mucosa and muscle layers of the gallbladder. Affected patients, who are often young and female, have abdominal pain and nonspecific symptoms such as nausea and intolerance of fatty food. Biliary dyskinesia may be diagnosed by food-cholecystokinin–stimulated US or a HIDA scan. In 80 to 90% of patients with abnormal stimulated motility, symptoms are relieved by cholecystectomy.

GALLBLADDER CANCER

Gallbladder cancer constitutes 0.76 to 1.2% of all cancers and is the most common biliary cancer, with about 7200 new cases reported in the United States each year. The highest incidence occurs in Amerindians, particularly in Chile, Mexico, and Colombia. Gallbladder cancer is a disease of the elderly and is more common in women than men. There is a strong association with cholelithiasis, chronic cholecystitis, and inflammation; 90% of patients with gallbladder cancer have concomitant stones. Patients who have a porcelain gallbladder, defined as calcification of the gallbladder wall, have a 25% risk for the development of gallbladder cancer, and patients with an anomalous pancreatic ductal junction in which the pancreatic duct drains into the lower common bile duct instead of the ampulla have an increased risk for gallbladder cancer. Both these lesions are indications for prophylactic cholecystectomy.

About 90% of gallbladder cancers are adenocarcinomas; the remainder are squamous cell or other cancers. Gallbladder cancer spreads locally, with invasion of the liver, and to the local lymph nodes and peritoneal cavity. About 90% of patients have symptoms and signs suggestive of cholecystitis. Surgery, which is the only therapeutic option, can be curative when the tumor is confined to the gallbladder. Adjuvant radiation therapy and chemotherapy have not been shown to be effective. The median survival for all patients with gallbladder cancer is 3 months, with a 1-year survival rate of 14% and a 5-year survival rate of 5%.

DISORDERS OF THE AMPULLA OF VATER

The ampulla of Vater is the final sphincter that controls entry of bile into the duodenum. Hormonal control of the sphincter is mediated by cholecystokinin, which causes the gallbladder to contract and the ampulla to relax. The most common disorder of the ampulla is stenosis or dysfunction after cholecystectomy, the so-called sphincter of Oddi dysfunction.

Sphincter of Oddi Dysfunction or Biliary Dyskinesia

In true sphincter stenosis, the sphincter is narrowed by inflammation and fibrosis secondary to pancreatitis, passage of a gallstone through the papilla, intraoperative trauma, infection, or adenomas. Sphincter stenosis can be manifested as abdominal pain and pancreatitis. The common bile duct is often dilated above the stenosis, and treatment is a large sphincterotomy performed at ERCP.

In sphincter of Oddi dyskinesia, a functional disorder of the sphincter leads to intermittent biliary obstruction. Most patients have undergone cholecystectomy and are being evaluated for recurrent biliary pain or, less frequently, pancreatitis. The diagnosis is usually made by ERCP, which can demonstrate delayed excretion of contrast. In patients who have pain associated with abnormal aminotransferases on two or more occasions, a dilated common bile duct, and delayed drainage of contrast, sphincterotomy is recommended. Patients without all three of these criteria are usually given a trial of relaxants, such as nitrates or calcium-channel blockers.

Ampullary Tumors

Adenocarcinoma of the ampulla has an incidence of three per million. Adenomas appear as protruding ampullary lesions, may grow either inside the ampulla or into the duodenum, and can transform into adenocarcinomas (Fig. 159–7). The cancer tends to be locally invasive. Ampullary adenomas are associated with familial polyposis coli (Chapter 203) and the *FAP* gene: almost 80% of patients with the *FAP* gene have adenomas of the ampulla, and their risk for ampullary cancer is 100-fold that of the normal population.

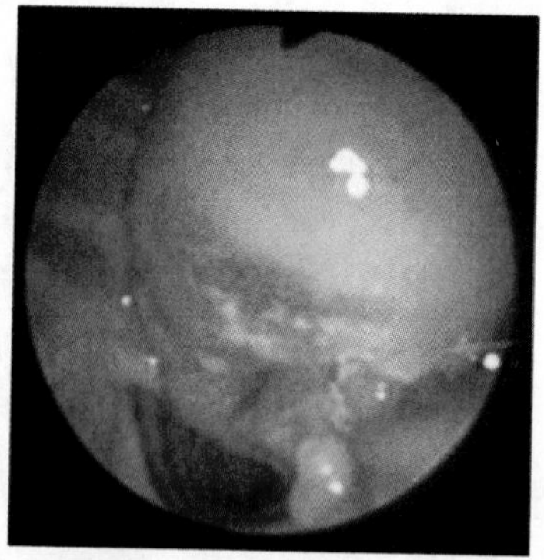

FIGURE 159–7 • Carcinoma of the ampulla of Vater. The carcinoma is seen toward the bottom of the picture. The bulging swelling above is the grossly dilated common bile duct, which is obstructed by the carcinoma. (From Forbes CD, Jackson WF: Color Atlas and Text of Clinical Medicine, 3rd ed. London, Mosby, 2003.)

The average age at diagnosis is 50 years, with a peak at 70 years; there is no gender predilection. About 80% of patients have jaundice, which is usually progressive and associated with abdominal pain and weight loss. Liver enzymes are generally abnormal, and the diagnosis is suggested by US or CT findings of dilated biliary and pancreatic ducts all the way to the ampulla. Confirmation is by endoscopy with biopsy and brushings. Staging of the tumor, particularly for lesions growing into the ampulla, can best be performed by endoscopic US. Adenomas and small cancers can be removed by endoscopic ampullectomy. The standard recommended curative operation is pancreaticoduodenectomy (the Whipple procedure), which provides a 25 to 55% 5-year survival rate, depending on the extent of the tumor. Adjuvant chemotherapy and radiation therapy have no proven benefit in the treatment of ampullary lesions.

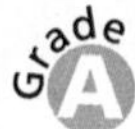

1. Lindor KD: Ursodiol for primary sclerosing cholangitis. Mayo Primary Sclerosing Cholangitis–Ursodeoxycholic Acid Study group. N Engl J Med 1997;336:691–695.
2. Goulis J, Leandro G, Burroughs AK: Randomised controlled trials of ursodeoxycholic-acid therapy for primary biliary cirrhosis: A meta-analysis. Lancet 1999;354:1053.
3. Lo C, Liu C, Lai E, et al: Early versus delayed laparoscopic cholecystectomy for treatment of acute cholecystitis. Ann Surg 1996;223;37–42.
4. Boerma D, Rauws EA, Keulemans YC, et al: Wait-and-see policy or laparoscopic cholecystectomy after endoscopic sphincterotomy for bile-duct stones: A randomised trial. Lancet 2002;360:761–765.
5. Shiffman ML, Kaplan GD, Brinkman-Kaplan V, et al: Prevention of gallstone formation with ursodeoxycholic acid in patients participating in a very low calorie diet program. Ann Intern Med 1995;122:899–905.

SUGGESTED READINGS

Bergasa NV: The pruritus of cholestasis. J Hepatol 2005;43:1078–1088. *Extensive review of the pathophysiology of pruritus in liver disease and its treatment.*

Byrnes V, Afdhal NH: Cholangiocarcinoma of the hepatic hilum (Klatskin tumor). Curr Treat Options Gastroenterol 2002;6:87–94. *A complete review of treatment options for cholangiocarcinoma.*

Hawn MT: Gallbladder and biliary tract disease in the intensive care unit. Semin Gastrointest Dis 2003;14:28–33. *A lucid overview.*

Maggs JR, Chapman RW: Sclerosing cholangitis. Curr Opin Gastroenterol 2007;23:310–316. *A practical overview.*

Portincasa P, Moschetta A, Palasciano G: Cholesterol gallstone disease. Lancet 2006;368:230–239. *A clinical overview.*

Section XIV

Hematologic Diseases

160 HEMATOPOIESIS AND HEMATOPOIETIC GROWTH FACTORS

Peter J. Quesenberry

The production of hematopoietic and lymphoid cells is complex but tightly regulated. The system is exquisitely responsive to functional needs. Red blood cell (erythroid) production changes with tissue oxygen levels; neutrophil and monocyte production responds to noxious foreign stimuli, especially bacterial infection; and platelet levels respond to blood loss, tissue damage, and platelet deficiency.

Lymphohematopoietic cells, which are produced by a small number of marrow cells termed stem cells, proliferate, differentiate, and self-renew. Stem cells respond to inductive stimuli and differentiate to progenitor cells (Table 160–1) that are progressively restricted in their potential for proliferation, differentiation, and self-renewal but that have increasing functional characteristics as defined by their specific lineages (Fig. 160–1). An alternative cell cycle model postulates that stem cells may represent phenotypic shifts in a reversible continuum and that differentiation comes from different phenotypes in the continuum (Fig. 160–2).

In either model, differentiation results in the cell lineages recognizable by standard Wright-Giemsa stains as erythroid, granulocytic, monocytic, lymphoid, and megakaryocytic. These events occur continuously with a large turnover of differentiated cells, as illustrated by the blood lifespan of human erythrocytes (120 days), platelets (10 days), and granulocytes (9 hours). The lifespans of lymphocytes (T and B cells) vary tremendously from hours to years. The production of different types of blood cells occurs predominantly in the bone marrow, but the spleen, lymph nodes, and accessory lymphoid tissues are also ongoing sites of lymphoid cell production; under stress, myeloid cell production also occurs at these sites. The end cells produced in the marrow are released into the blood stream under various stimuli and circulate in the blood. With the exception of erythrocytes and platelets, these cells emigrate to tissues where they have variable lifespans: days for granulocytes and weeks to years for monocytes, macrophages, and lymphocytes.

LYMPHOHEMATOPOIESIS

The classically recognizable differentiated marrow lineages represent the end stages of a carefully orchestrated production system. Progenitors and possibly stem cells (the continuum model) feed into the various blast compartments (myeloblast, proerythroblast, lymphoblast, and megakaryoblast), which in turn feed into lineages that show increasingly differentiated characteristics while losing proliferative potency. Myeloblasts become promyelocytes, which then differentiate into myelocytes, the stage at which neutrophilic (Fig. 160–3), eosinophilic, and basophilic lineages are distinguished. Erythrocyte and platelet lineages result in anucleate functional cells, whereas B, T, and NK lymphocyte lineages give rise to a variety of effector cell populations. This system is an irreversible in-out production system, with final demise of end cells occurring in the blood stream (platelets and red cells) or tissues (all others).

STEM CELL ONTOGENY

Early multipotent stem cells are present in the yolk sac and in mesenchymal tissues. These stem cells subsequently traffic predominantly to the liver (and, to a lesser extent, to the kidney), followed by the establishment of marrow as the major site of active hematopoiesis. The earlier in ontogeny that stem cells are harvested, the greater their proliferative potential, as illustrated by the proliferative and growth potential of fetal liver and cord blood cells in clinical transplantation.

The hematopoietic cell in both murine and human species has been characterized in regard to its surface proteins and physical, metabolic, and cell cycle characteristics; these characteristics have been used physically to purify stem cells (Fig. 160–4). Early stem cells differentially express more than 2000 nonredundant genes involved with energy metabolism, signaling pathways, cell cycle regulation, chromatin, the translational apparatus, DNA metabolism, transcription factors, surface proteins, cytoskeleton, the mitochondrial apparatus, and membrane trafficking. Early stem cells do not express many differentiated cell functions, but they do express functions involving movement and membrane deformation, probably as part of their homing function. Recent work indicates a high degree of functional plasticity with cell cycle transit and reversible fluctuations of cell surface–based markers such as CD34. The most primitive marrow stem cells are either slowly cycling or intermittently entering the cell cycle, and their phenotype changes reversibly with cell cycle. Traditionally, primitive stem cells have been thought to give rise to committed progenitors (the hierarchical model, Fig. 160–5; see also Fig. 160–1), but recent data suggest that there may be a continuum whereby stem cells convert to progenitor cells and then back to stem cells (see Fig. 160–2); if so, progenitor cells might not be a discrete class of cells. Some cells may divide to give rise to two stem cells, and some divide into two differentiating cells, but the most common outcome is probably an asymmetrical stem cell division in which the stem cell divides and gives rise to another stem cell and a differentiating cell. Apoptosis presumably also modifies the system.

Lymphohematopoietic Stem Cell (Classic System)

The existence of a stem cell common to all lymphoid and myeloid lineages was established by studies in mice in which the infusion of a single cytogenetically or retrovirally marked stem cell gave rise to all cell lineages, which then persisted over time. Sustained in vivo engraftment is the "gold standard" for the true stem cell, although different subpopulations may show different engraftment kinetics, ranging from weeks to more than a year in the mouse. The engrafting cell, which is quiescent or dormant but slowly cycling over time, appears to have high p170 pump activity (stains low for rhodamine, a p170-pumped dye). The existence of a similar multipotent stem cell in humans was inferred from studies of marrow and blood cells from patients with chronic myelogenous leukemia, in whom all lineages were marked with the Philadelphia chromosome, and from glucose-6-phosphate dehydrogenase studies of patients with myeloproliferative disorders.

There is not an in vivo engraftment assay in humans, but in vitro assays appear to measure relatively primitive multilineage cells and have been proposed as true surrogates for the long-term renewable lymphohematopoietic stem cell. The colony-forming unit–blast (an assay in which marrow cells give rise to small colonies of primitive blast cells), with extensive proliferative and differentiative potential, may in fact be a good surrogate, but few laboratories have mastered this technique, so it is not generally applicable. The high proliferative potential colony-forming cell, an assay in which marrow cells proliferate in the presence of combinations of growth factors to give rise to large (>0.5 mm) colonies in vitro, also appears to be a reasonable surrogate and is probably the best generally available. The stroma-based assays, long-term culture-initiating cell (LTC-IC) and cobblestone-forming assays, are of interest but appear to monitor both primitive and more differentiated cells and are difficult to reproduce. These assays, in which marrow cells grow on an adherent stromal layer, remain interesting research areas without practical applications, although the LTC-IC extended (a 60+-day assay) may come closer to mirroring the real stem cell.

Regulation and Cytokines

By both in vitro and in vivo assays, a large number of cytokines have been characterized and shown to affect lymphohematopoiesis. Regulation of lymphohematopoiesis is based on a large number of circulating and membrane-based cytokines as well as integrin modulation and antigen presentation to B and T cells. More than 70 cytokines maintain, stimulate, or inhibit various aspects of lymphohematopoiesis (Table 160–2).

Cytokines exert a wide variety of actions on diverse types of cells both within and outside specific differentiation lineages, but many cytokines have predominant or primary actions, especially when they are evaluated after in vivo administration (Table 160–3; see also Table 160–2). Erythropoietin (erythroid), macrophage colony-stimulating factor (M-CSF), and granulocyte colony-stimulating factor (G-CSF) are cytokines with a relatively high degree of specificity. Most cytokines, however, have multiple actions. Examples include interleukin (IL)–6, which acts on primitive stem cells as well as lymphoid, granulocyte, megakaryocyte, and macrophage lineages, and IL-3, which has an impact on virtually all lineages. IL-1 induces many other cytokines and illustrates the difficulty in ascertaining primary or secondary effects, especially with the potential for paracrine or autocrine loops.

Most cells produce multiple cytokines, which can be differentially induced by various stimuli, including other cytokines, such as IL-1. The

TABLE 160–1 STEM AND PROGENITOR CELLS (HIERARCHICAL MODEL)

Characteristic	Stem Cell	Progenitor Cell
Proliferative potential	Tremendous	More limited
Renewal	On a population basis	Probably none
Potential for differentiation	All lymphohematopoietic lineages	Restricted
Differentiated characteristics	Minimal—lineage negative	Progressively increases
Functional characteristics	Rapid directed motility and expression of proteopodia; homing	Less defined
Cycle status	Dormant (either slowly cycling or intermittently entering and exiting cycle)	Cycling
Cytokine responsiveness	Large number of cytokines needed for expression of phenotype	Restricted
Cell of origin	Unknown	Stem cell
Stains with rhodamine and Hoechst dyes (partial measure of p170 pump activity)	Active p170 pump—stains dimly	Less active p170 pump—rhodamine "bright"
Produces long-term hematopoiesis after in vivo transplantation	Defines cells	Limited to none
Adheres to marrow stroma	Yes	No or limited

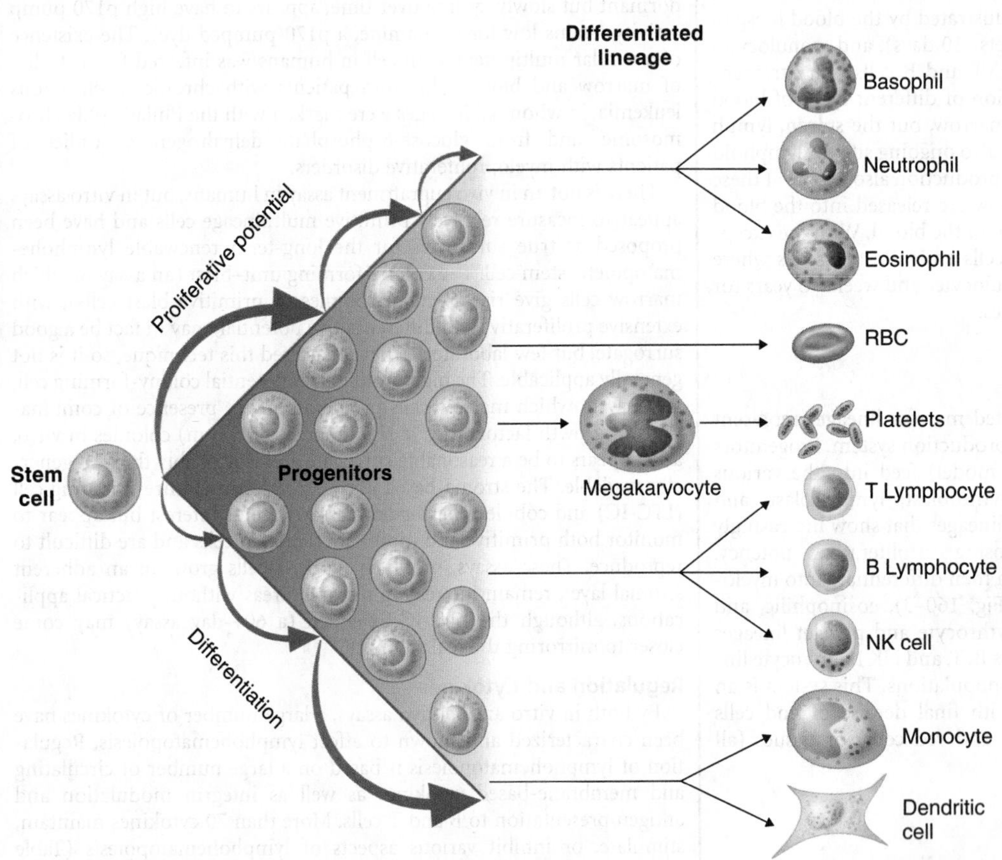

FIGURE 160–1 • Hierarchical model of lymphohematopoiesis. NK = natural killer; RBC = red blood cell.

suggestion that "everything makes everything" is perhaps too drastic but also not too far off target. The key is differential production in response to different stimuli and probably in local production. Monocytes, T lymphocytes, endothelial cells, fibroblasts, and "marrow stromal" cells are important sources of lymphohematopoietic cytokines. Erythropoietin is an exception to the general rule because it is largely produced in the kidney in response to hypoxia, although it can also be produced by the liver. Stimuli that induce white blood cell formation are, in general, related to exposure to foreign or noxious agents, whereas platelet production occurs in response to hemorrhage, anemia, and thrombocytopenia.

Perhaps the best way to define the cytokine responsiveness of a particular cell class is to characterize its cytokine receptor expression. Each cytokine has its private receptor, but different cytokines may share class-specific signal transducers. Many receptors dimerize on cytokine binding and then activate tyrosine kinase, thereby promoting phosphorylation of intracellular proteins; other receptors do not have intrinsic enzymatic activity but induce protein phosphorylation through associated nonreceptor-type tyrosine kinase activities, such as JAK2, Fes, and Lyn. Receptors are expressed in low numbers and do not exceed a few hundred per cell. The multipotent repopulating stem cell possesses receptors for most cytokines, but more mature cells have a more restricted distribution of receptors.

Two major receptor families have been described. First, the hematopoietic receptor family includes IL-2, IL-3, IL-4, IL-5, IL-6, IL-7, IL-9, IL-13, IL-15, oncostatin M, leukemia inhibitory factor, ciliary neurotrophic factor, G-CSF, granulocyte-macrophage colony-stimulating factor

(GM-CSF), and erythropoietin. The extracellular binding domains of these receptors contain four conserved cysteine residues and a WS-X-WS motif (X is a variable nonconserved amino acid). Some also have an immunoglobulin-like structure. Receptors for GM-CSF, IL-3, and IL-5 each contain specific low-affinity α chains, but a high-affinity β chain is shared by all three receptors. The common β chain plays a role in the competitive binding of these ligands. Second, the tyrosine kinase receptor family includes receptors for Flt3 ligand, steel factor (c-*kit* ligand), colony-stimulating factor 1, and thrombopoietin. These receptors have an immunoglobulin-like structure and 10 conserved cysteines in the extracellular domain, with tyrosine kinase activity in the cytoplasmic domain. Receptors not fitting into these families include those for IL-1, IL-8, transforming growth factor-β, and the chemokine receptors.

Signaling through these receptors activates transcription factors that then may direct differentiation toward specific lineages. For example, GATA-1 and FOG promote erythroid and megakaryocyte differentiation, whereas SCL, AML1, and GATA-2 regulate primitive stem cell differentiation. A sequential pathway determining myeloid and lymphoid development appears to work through Jagged-based signaling to Notch, then activating PU.1; PU.1 and GATA-1 then signal development of myeloid differentiation. Conversely, low PU.1 levels in concert with Ikarios expression signal lymphoid differentiation. Physical combinations of various transcription factors appear critical for mediating these effects and may be inhibiting or stimulating.

Adhesion molecules function both to bind cells or extracellular matrix and as signaling molecules. Steel factor, IL-3, and GM-CSF activate very late antigens 4 and 5, which are adhesion molecules expressed on $CD34^+$ cells. This activation results in promotion of the ability of very late antigens 4 and 5 to bind fibronectin. Other adhesion proteins important in hematopoiesis include stroma-derived growth factor 1, CD84, and CD44. Stromal or microenvironmental cells are major regulators of hematopoiesis, both by positioning stem-progenitor cells and by signaling with secreted and membrane-based cytokines. Homing studies indicate that long-term repopulating lymphohematopoietic stem cells move closely adjacent to osteogenic surfaces; others have suggested that bone cells are major stem cell regulators.

These regulatory influences affect hematopoietic lineages in a variety of ways. An important effect of erythropoietin on erythrocyte progenitors and precursors is to prevent apoptosis and thus maintain the viability of these cells. Cell cycle transit and the induction of proliferation are major effects of many of the early-acting cytokines, such as steel factor, and all lineages exhibit cytokine-modulated differentiation. Erythropoietin induces erythroid hemoglobinization, G-CSF causes the acquisition of myeloid enzymes in granulocytes, and thrombopoietin induces the expression of platelet-specific proteins. Thus, differentiation is a general feature, although whether this is specifically cytokine-mediated induction from a multipotent cell or simply a manifestation of survival of cells with a genetic probability of differentiation into a specific lineage remains an area of controversy. Regulatory influences also affect the function of many end cells, such as granulocytes, monocytes, T cells, B cells, NK cells,

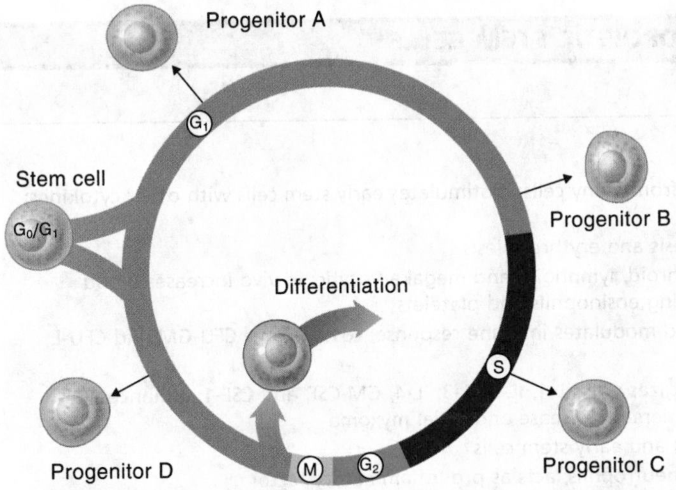

FIGURE 160–2 • Cell cycle–based model of stem cell regulation.

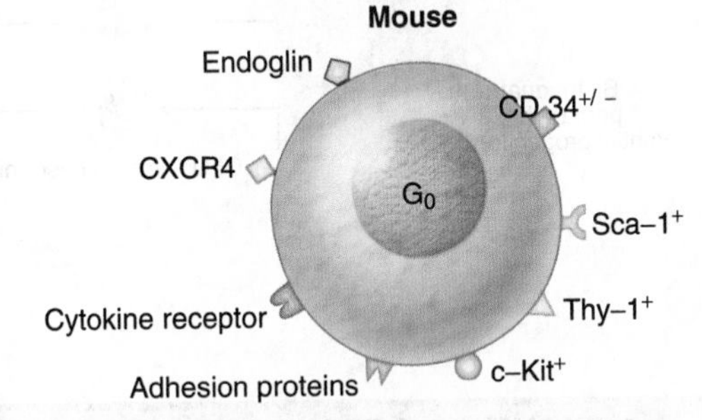

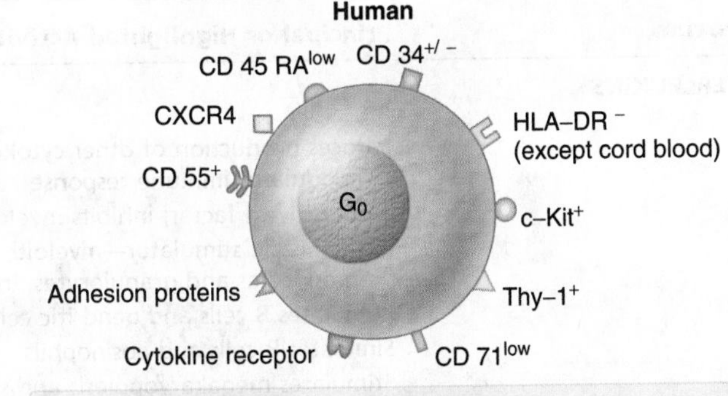

FIGURE 160–4 • Characteristics of the lymphohematopoietic stem cell.

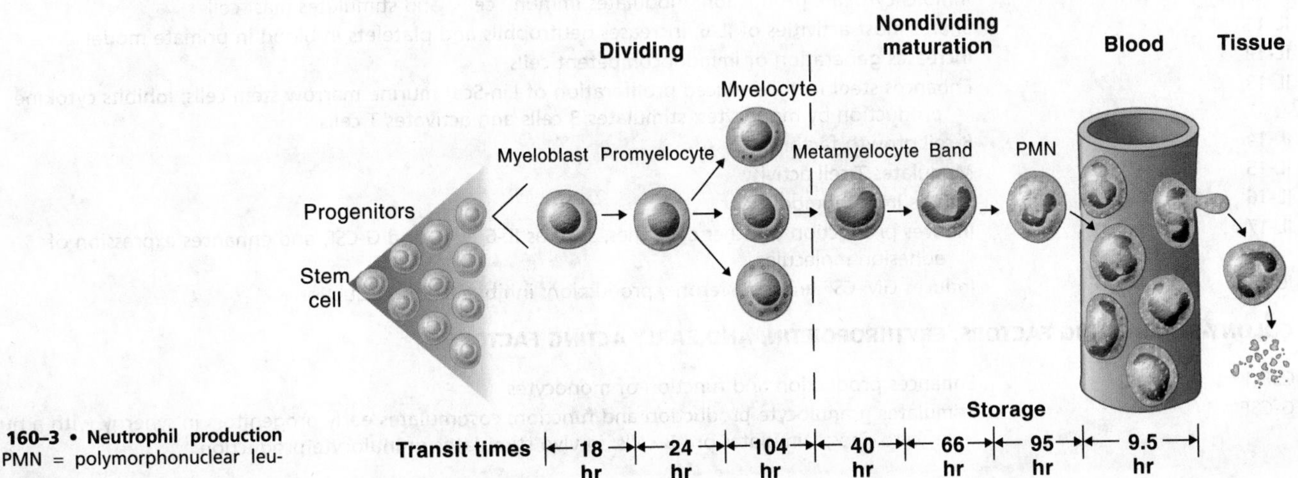

FIGURE 160–3 • Neutrophil production system. PMN = polymorphonuclear leukocyte.

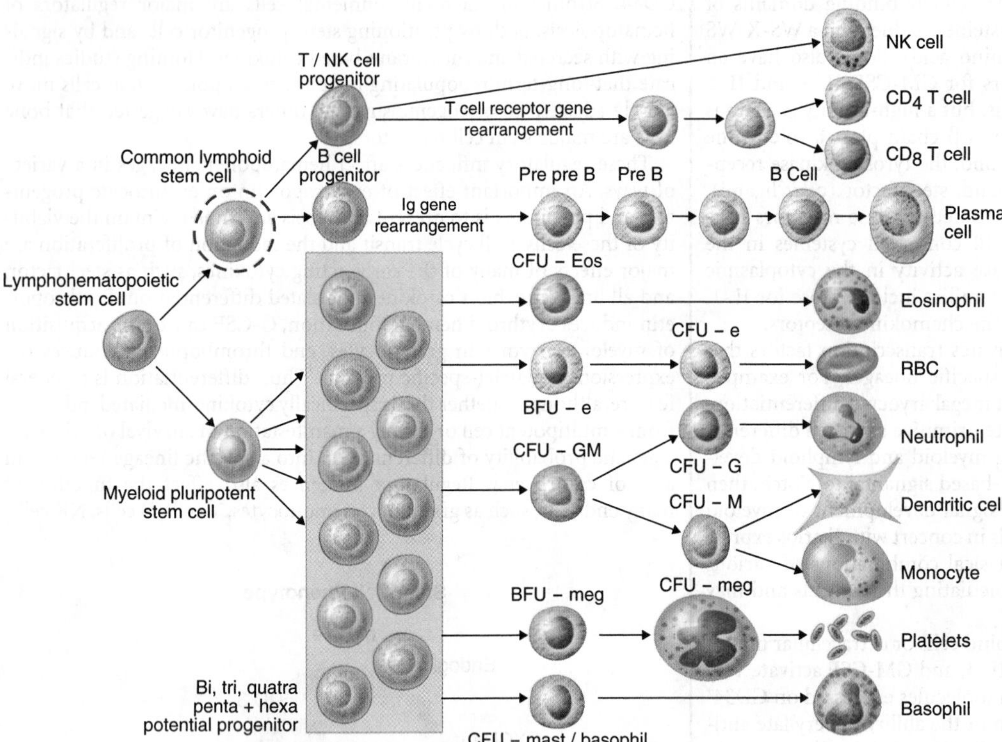

FIGURE 160–5 • Hierarchical model of stem cell regulation.

TABLE 160–2 CYTOKINES ACTIVE ON LYMPHOHEMATOPOIETIC STEM CELLS

Cytokine	Principal or Highlighted Activity
INTERLEUKINS	
IL-1	Induces production of other cytokines from many cells; costimulates early stem cells with other cytokines; modulates immune response
IL-2	T-cell growth factor; inhibits myelopoiesis and erythropoiesis
IL-3	Multilineage stimulator—myeloid, erythroid, lymphoid, and megakaryocytic; in vivo increases blood monocytes and granulocytes, including eosinophils and platelets
IL-4	Stimulates B cells and dendritic cells and modulates immune response; costimulates CFU-GM and CFU-E
IL-5	Simulates B cells and eosinophils
IL-6	Stimulates megakaryopoiesis and synergizes with IL-1, IL-2, IL-3, IL-4, GM-CSF, and CSF-1; enhances plasma cell proliferation; role in Castleman's disease and atrial myxoma
IL-7	Stimulates pre-B cells (with steel factor) and early stem cells
IL-8	Stimulates production and function of neutrophils; acts as pro-inflammatory factor
IL-9	Costimulates CFU-GM and CFU-Mix; stimulates BFU-E with erythropoietin; enhances T-cell production and, with IL-3, mast cell production
IL-10	Inhibits cytokine production, modulates immune cells, and stimulates mast cells
IL-11	Shares most activities of IL-6; increases neutrophils and platelets in blood in primate model
IL-12	Increases generation of immunocompetent cells
IL-13	Enhances steel factor–induced proliferation of $Lin^{-}Sca^{+}$ murine marrow stem cells; inhibits cytokine production by monocytes; stimulates B cells and activates T cells
IL-14	B-cell growth factor
IL-15	Modulates T-cell activity
IL-16	Acts as immunomodulator
IL-17	Induces production of other cytokines, such as IL-6, IL-8, and G-CSF, and enhances expression of adhesion molecules
IL-18	Induces GM-CSF and interferon-γ production; inhibits IL-10 production
COLONY-STIMULATING FACTORS, ERYTHROPOIETIN, AND EARLY-ACTING FACTORS	
CSF-1	Enhances production and function of monocytes
G-CSF	Stimulates granulocyte production and function; costimulates early progenitors in synergy with a number of cytokines; stimulates pre-B cells; in vivo stimulate granulocyte production

TABLE 160–2 CYTOKINES ACTIVE ON LYMPHOHEMATOPOIETIC STEM CELLS—cont'd

Cytokine	Principal or Highlighted Activity
GM-CSF	Stimulates GM-CFC and production of monocytes, granulocytes, eosinophils, and basophils; synergizes with IL-4 to produce dendritic cells; costimulates many types of progenitors, including early multipotent stem cells
Erythropoietin	Stimulates erythrocyte production in vitro and in vivo; costimulates BFU-E and CFU-Meg and stimulates CFU-E
Flt3 ligand	Costimulates multipotential stem cells, especially with thrombopoietin and steel factor; stimulates generation of dendritic cells
Steel factor	Similar to Flt3; enhances generation of mast cells
Thrombopoietin, c-Mpl ligand	Major regulator of proliferation and differentiation of megakaryocytes; costimulates multipotential stem cells in combination with steel factor and IL-11; promotes erythropoiesis in synergy with erythropoietin
CYTOKINE INHIBITORY FACTORS AND OTHERS	
MIP-1α	Inhibits early multipotent colony formation but stimulates that of committed precursors
TGF-β	Suppresses early multipotent progenitors but stimulates later progenitors
MCAF, platelet factor 4, H-ferritin	Similar to TGF-β
TNF-α	Similar to TGF-β, but a more pronounced effect on BFU-E and CFU-E
Activin	Enhances IL-3 and erythropoietin-stimulated BFU-E and CFU-E; inhibits IL-3–stimulated CFU-GM
Inhibin	Inhibits CFU-Mix, CFU-GM, and BFU-E
Interferons α, β, and γ	Coinhibits CFU-Mix, CFU-GM, and BFU-E; inhibits production of cytokines; immune modulator
Prostaglandin E_2	Suppresses CFU-M with less or no activity on CFU-GM and CFU-G; enhances BFU-E indirectly through $CD8^+$ lymphocytes
Glu-Glu-Asp-Asp-Lys (pentapeptide)	Inhibits CFU-S proliferation and CFU-GM
N-Acetyl-Ser-Asp-Lys-Pro (tetrapeptide)	Inhibits CFU-S and other progenitors' entry into cell cycle
Leukemia inhibitory factor	Inhibits GM-CSF–stimulated CFU-GM and G-CSF–stimulated CFU-G
Insulin-like growth factor 2	Stimulates erythroid and granulocyte progenitors
Hepatocyte growth factor (scatter factor)	Synergistic activity on progenitors
Basic fibroblast growth factor	Acts in concert with other cytokines on early multipotential and megakaryocyte progenitors
Platelet-derived growth factor	Stimulates erythroid and granulocyte progenitors

BFU-E = blast-forming unit–erythroid; CFU-E = colony-forming unit–erythroid; CFU-G = colony-forming unit–granulocyte; CFU-GM = colony-forming unit–granulocyte-macrophage; CFU-M = colony-forming unit–macrophage; CFU-Meg = colony-forming unit–megakaryocytes; CFU-Mix = colony-forming unit–mixed lineages; CFU-S = colony-forming unit–spleen; CSF-1 = colony-stimulating factor 1; G-CSF = granulocyte colony-stimulating factor; GM-CFC = granulocyte-macrophage colony-forming cell; GM-CSF = granulocyte-macrophage colony-stimulating factor; MCAF = monocyte chemotactic and activating factor; MIP-1α = macrophage inflammatory protein 1α; TGF-β = transforming growth factor-β; TNF-α = tumor necrosis factor-α.

TABLE 160–3 CHARACTERISTICS OF LYMPHOHEMATOPOIETIC CYTOKINES

- Are glycoproteins
- Act on cell surface receptors
- Initiate complex second messenger and transcriptional and post-transcriptional regulation
- May act on stem cells, progenitor cells, and differentiated cells of the same lineage
- May act on multiple different lineages (e.g., erythroid, granulocyte, and lymphoid)
- Stimulate or inhibit proliferation, apoptosis, differentiation, or function
- Usually act on neoplastic counterpart of normal target cell

and dendritic cells. These data are consistent with either a hierarchical or a continuum model of hematopoiesis.

Stem Cell Plasticity: Functional and Hierarchical

Studies indicate that bone marrow–derived hematopoietic stem cells have much greater potential than previously realized. Marrow cells are capable of giving rise to cardiac myocytes, keratinocytes, pneumocytes, hepatocytes, neural cells, skeletal muscle, and a variety of mesenchymal cells including cartilage, fat, and bone. Several murine studies have shown quantitatively significant replacement of cardiac and hepatic cells in models of cardiac ischemia and liver failure. More important, improved cardiac and hepatic function was also seen. In one intriguing study, a single purified marrow hematopoietic stem cell was shown by limiting dilution techniques to give rise to hematopoietic cells and to a wide variety of nonhematopoietic cells; such cells might possibly be used to restore tissue in various disease states. Other studies have suggested that muscle, neural, or hepatic cells could give rise to hematopoietic cells.

Another form of hematopoietic plasticity is functional plasticity tied to the cell cycle. Continuing studies have indicated that all stem cells continuously or intermittently enter the cell cycle; during cell cycle transit, the stem cell phenotype continually and reversibly changes. These data suggest that a primitive stem cell and a progenitor may present a phenotypic continuum rather than being part of a hierarchy and, in fact, that there may not be a discrete population of hematopoietic progenitors.

Mobilization of Stem-Progenitor Cells

Engraftable, long-term repopulating stem cells and their progenitors are easily mobilized into the peripheral blood by a number of cytokines, including G-CSF, steel factor, Flt3, IL-11, IL-12, IL-3, IL-8, IL-7, macrophage inflammatory protein 1β, and erythropoietin. In addition, previous exposure to cyclophosphamide or other cytotoxic agents also mobilizes stem cells, presumably through the actions of cytokines. Pretreatment with cyclophosphamide followed by treatment with steel factor and G-CSF may be the most potent regimen for mobilizing stem-progenitor cells. In general, mobilized stem-progenitor cells appear to restore hematopoiesis more rapidly than unstimulated marrow does, although marrow that has been primed with in vivo cytokines may be equivalent to mobilized peripheral blood cells for rapid engraftment. Whether these mobilized stem cells have the same long-term repopulation capacity as that of marrow cells remains to be established.

Stem-Progenitor Cell Expansion

The ability to expand lymphohematopoietic stem cells in vitro has immediate implications for strategies of repetitive transplantation, immunotherapy, and gene therapy. A large number of studies have established that exposure of marrow cells to a variety of cytokines in liquid culture leads to differentiation and progenitor cell expansion. These cells can also be effective in transplantation, but as yet no study has established expansion of long-term engraftable stem cells, and studies have shown that cytokine stimulation of marrow stem cells can lead to fluctuations in engraftment phenotype that are reversible and correlate with the phase of the cell cycle.

Historic dogma had contended incorrectly that marrow transplant recipients needed to be treated with cytotoxic agents, usually irradiation or cytotoxic drugs, to open space in the marrow for stem cells to engraft. In fact, marrow stem cells engraft quantitatively in nontreated hosts, and the final ratio of donor to host cells after transplantation appears to be determined simply by the ratio of donor to host stem cells (Chapter 184). Homing to marrow appears complete within several hours, and engrafted stem cells rapidly enter the cell cycle after intravenous infusion (within 12 hours). They move to the bone surface, giving rise to both hematopoietic and bone cells. The blood stream clears quickly of stem cells, and there appears to be virtually no primary thymic engraftment, although secondary engraftment of the thymus occurs later. These observations form the basis of the current minitransplant approaches, although additional steps are necessary in the allogeneic setting to ensure engraftment and to avoid graft-versus-host disease.

DISEASES OF STEM CELLS AND CYTOKINES

Stem Cell Diseases (Table 160–4)

Acute (Chapter 194) and chronic (Chapter 195) myelogenous leukemia and polycythemia vera (Chapter 172) are neoplastic diseases of the myeloid multilineage pluripotent stem cell. Paroxysmal nocturnal hemoglobinuria (Chapter 164), a disease that is due to *PIGA* mutations with missing cellular glycosylphosphatidylinositol anchors, is a clonal disease at the pluripotent (including lymphoid) cell level. Cyclic neutropenia (Chapter 173), which is manifested by 21-day cycles of neutropenia and is due to mutations in the elastase 2 gene, is also a disease of pluripotent stem cells, with cycling also occurring in the red cell and platelet lineages. Severe chronic neutropenia (Kostmann's syndrome; Chapter 173) also usually is associated with mutations in the elastase 2 gene and shows a high predilection for evolution to acute myelocytic leukemia when it is treated with G-CSF.

The deficiency states, such as aplastic anemia (Chapter 171), are the other broad category of stem cell diseases. The idiopathic variety is usually due to an immune attack against the stem cell, but drug-induced, virus-induced, or genetic causes may be related to death or deficiency of the pluripotent stem cell, independent of any immune cause. In Fanconi's anemia (Chapter 171), an inherited aplastic anemia with a high risk for subsequent development of solid tumors or acute myelocytic leukemia, a failure to form monoubiquinated FANCD2 leads to defective DNA repair and fewer progenitor cells.

Dyskeratosis congenita (Chapter 171) is X-linked and may represent a mutation of the *DKC1* gene, which codes for the nuclear protein dyskerin. Progenitors are reduced, and marrow failure (aplastic anemia) occurs in 50% of cases. In congenital amegakaryocytic thrombocytopenia, aplastic anemia due to mutations in *MPL*, the thrombopoietin receptor, develops in about 45% of patients in the first year of life. Other X-linked thrombocytopenia syndromes are due to mutations of *GATA1* or in the Wiskott-Aldrich syndrome gene. Trisomy 21 can lead to leukemia, myelodysplasia, or aplastic anemia. Multilineage or unilineage marrow failure can be due to viral infections, such as parvovirus (B19) and dengue fever.

TABLE 160–4 STEM CELL DISEASES

Disease	Mechanism
CLONAL STEM CELL NEOPLASMS	
Acute myelogenous leukemia	Many specific chromosome abnormalities
Chronic myelogenous leukemia	9 : 22 translocation
Polycythemia vera	JAK2
Primary thrombocytosis	Unknown
Myelofibrosis, myeloid metaplasia	A stem cell malignancy with secondary fibrosis
Myelodysplasia	Many chromosome abnormalities; when secondary to myelotoxic chemotherapy, abnormalities on chromosomes 5 and 7
Paroxysmal nocturnal hemoglobinuria	Defective glycosylphosphatidylinositol-anchored membrane proteins and mutation in *PIGA* gene
Cyclic neutropenia	Mutations in elastase 2 gene
Kostmann's syndrome	In most, a mutation in elastase 2 gene
FAILURE OF PLURIPOTENT MARROW STEM CELLS	
Aplastic anemia	Deficient multipotent stem cell due to immune attack against stem cells; telomerase mutations are common
Fanconi's anemia	Genetic lesion with failure to form monoubiquinated FANCD2 and defects in DNA repair
Dyskeratosis congenita	Mutations in *DKC1* gene with decreased progenitors
Congenital megakaryocyte thrombocytopenia	Mutations in thrombopoietin receptor (*MPL*) cause aplastic anemia in about 50% by 1 year of age
Trisomy 21 (Down syndrome) and a variety of familial aplastic anemias	Variety of genetic lesions
Viral infections—hepatitis, parvovirus, cytomegalovirus, or dengue	Direct effect on the stem cell
Toxicity from irradiation or chemotherapy	Direct effect on the stem cell

TABLE 160–5 CYTOKINE DISORDERS AFFECTING HEMATOPOIESIS

Cytokine or Receptor	Mechanism	Hematology	Disease
Erythropoietin	Decreased production	Anemia	Renal failure
	Increased levels by tumor production	Polycythemia	Large uterine fibroids, cerebellar hemangioblastomas, hepatocellular or renal carcinoma
	Increased production due to tissue (renal) hypoxia	Polycythemia	Cyanotic heart disease, pulmonary disease, sleep apnea, pickwickian syndrome, high altitude, carbon monoxide from smoking, high-affinity hemoglobin, methemoglobinemia, and ischemic kidney
	Increased response to erythropoietin, sometimes with mutations of the erythropoietin receptor	Polycythemia	Primary familial or congenital polycythemia; Chuvash polycythemia
IL-7 receptor α chain	Deficiency due to mutation	T-cell disease deficiency	Severe combined immunodeficiency
γ chain of IL-2, IL-4, IL-7, IL-9, IL-15, and IL-21 receptors	Deficiency due to mutation	Defect in development of T cells and NK cells	X-linked immunodeficiency
IL-7	Excess production	Eosinophilia	Parasitic diseases, collagen vascular diseases, allergies
IL-6	Excess production	Leukocytosis, malaise	Castleman's disease, atrial myxoma, inflammation, or infection
	Increased production by marrow cells	Increased growth of myeloma cells	Multiple myeloma
IL-1 and TNF-β	Increased production by malignant cell or normal cell	Hypercalcemia	Multiple myeloma, carcinoma
G-CSF	Tumor production	Granulocytosis	Carcinomas (lung)

G-CSF = granulocyte colony-stimulating factor; TNF-β = tumor necrosis factor-β.

Cytokine Disorders (Table 160–5)

A number of disorders are associated with abnormal levels of hematopoietic cytokines or specific responses to these cytokines. Renal disease, perhaps the only true hematopoietic cytokine deficiency, is caused by decreased erythropoietin levels and is corrected by treatment with erythropoietin. Increases in IL-6 play a role in the systemic anemia associated with Castleman's disease, atrial myxoma, and inflammation or infection (Chapter 169). The anemia of chronic disease has been associated with increased serum levels of IL-1, IL-6, IL-10, tumor necrosis factor, and interferon-α.

Inappropriate overproduction of erythropoietin by the ischemic kidney, renal tumors, hepatocellular carcinoma, cerebellar hemangioblastoma, and large uterine fibroids may cause polycythemia. Appropriate production of high levels of erythropoietin and resultant polycythemia are seen in response to hypoxic stimuli in patients with cyanotic heart disease, pulmonary disease, sleep apnea, the pickwickian syndrome, residence at high altitude, high levels of carbon monoxide from smoking, high oxygen affinity hemoglobins, or congenital methemoglobinemia. Primary familial or congenital polycythemias are associated with an increased response to erythropoietin, in some cases due to mutations of the erythropoietin receptor.

Several immune deficiency syndromes relate to impaired cytokine signaling. IL-7 receptor α-chain deficiency is one of several causes of severe combined immunodeficiency in which peripheral T cells are markedly decreased and normal numbers of B cells are present. A defect in the development of T cells and NK cells due to mutation of the common γ chain of IL-2, IL-4, IL-7, IL-9, IL-15, and IL-21 receptors is manifested as X-linked immunodeficiency.

STEM CELL AND CYTOKINE THERAPIES

Stem Cell Therapies

Stem cell transplantation (Chapter 184) has been successfully used to cure marrow deficiency states (e.g., aplastic anemia), genetic marrow diseases (hemoglobinopathies, enzymopathies), osteopetrosis, and a variety of predominantly marrow or lymphoid malignant neoplasms. Marrow cells were the initial source of stem cells for transplantation, but pheresis of peripheral blood stem cells has supplemented marrow in autologous transplantation, and its use in allogeneic transplantation is still being evaluated. Fetal liver has been used as a source of stem cells, and umbilical cord blood is becoming a major source of cells, especially for unrelated pediatric transplantation.

Cytokines in Therapy

The only cytokine deficiency that clearly causes a clinical disorder is the deficiency of erythropoietin in patients with renal failure (Chapters 131 and 169). Administration of erythropoietin corrects this anemia. Erythropoietin is also approved for treatment of the anemia of malignancy, but in trials in which patients with breast cancer and head and neck cancer were treated with erythropoietin, outcomes worsened because of more progressive cancer. 1,2 Erythropoietin should be used in cancer patients only in clinical trials addressing the role of erythropoietin. If it is used in select cancer patients, a detailed discussion with the patient about these trials should occur before treatment.

Unfortunately, the results of cytokine therapy for other diseases (despite approval by the Food and Drug Administration) are equivocal at best. A major emphasis has been placed on the use of G-CSF and GM-CSF (Table 160–6) to expedite marrow recovery after cytotoxic therapy for cancer. Although the use of G-CSF or GM-CSF allows higher doses of chemotherapy to be administered, cancer control and survival are not improved. 3 Neither G-CSF nor GM-CSF has proved effective in active infection, presumably because endogenous levels of G-CSF are already high in neutropenic and infected patients.

GM-CSF has been combined with cytosine arabinoside as an effective therapy for myelodysplasia (Chapter 193). G-CSF, frequently in the context of recovery from cyclophosphamide treatment, helps mobilize stem cells. It also appears effective in certain severe chronic neutropenic states, including Kostmann's neutropenia and cyclic neutropenia (Chapter 173). Evolution to leukemia in patients with Kostmann's neutropenia, however, is a concern. The malignant counterparts of the marrow cells usually retain the cytokine responsiveness of normal cells,

TABLE 160–6 G-CSF AND GM-CSF USE IN CLINICAL THERAPY

	Established Benefit	
Condition	**G-CSF**	**GM-CSF**
Chronic neutropenia (cyclic, idiopathic, and Kostmann's)	Yes	No
Cancer chemotherapy–induced neutropenia	Uncertain	Uncertain
Stem cell mobilization	Yes	Yes
Active infection	No	No
Other inflammatory conditions	No	No
Drug-induced (not chemotherapy) neutropenia	No	No

G-CSF = granulocyte colony-stimulating factor; GM-CSF = granulocyte-macrophage colony-stimulating factor.

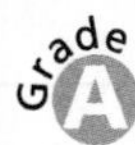

Section XIV Hematology

and many neoplastic cells proliferate in response to cytokines. G-CSF and GM-CSF also stimulate a wide variety of nonhematopoietic cells and, not surprisingly, have a wide variety of side effects, including bone pain, fever, chills, pleural and pulmonary effusions or infiltrates, vasculitis, splenic enlargement, proteinuria, and rashes, including neutrophilic dermatitis (Sweet's syndrome). Thrombopoietin and IL-11 can stimulate platelet production, but their clinical usefulness is not documented.

Grade A

1. Henke M, Laszig R, Rube C, et al: Erythropoietin to treat head and neck cancer patients with anaemia undergoing radiotherapy: Randomised, double-blind, placebo-controlled trial. Lancet 2003;362:1255–1260.
2. Leyland-Jones B, Semiglazov V, Pawlicki M, et al: Maintaining normal hemoglobin levels with epoetin alfa in mainly nonanemic patients with metastatic breast cancer receiving first-line chemotherapy: A survival study. J Clin Oncol 2005;23:5960–5972.
3. Lyman GH, Kuderer NM, Djulbegovic B: Prophylactic granulocyte colony-stimulating factor in patients receiving dose-intensive cancer chemotherapy: A meta-analysis. Am J Med 2002;112:406.

SUGGESTED READINGS

Burns CE, Zon LI: Homing sweet homing: Odyssey of hematopoietic stem cells. Immunity 2006;25:859–862. *Overview of the migration of nascent hematopoietic stem cells.*

Jelkmann W: Erythropoietin after a century of research: Younger than ever. Eur J Haematol 2007;78:183–205. *A comprehensive review.*

Quesenberry PJ, Colvin GA, Abedi M, et al: The stem cell continuum. Ann N Y Acad Sci 2005;1044:228–235. *Describes the potential of cells at various stages of differentiation.*

161 THE PERIPHERAL BLOOD SMEAR

James R. Newland

Wright-Giemsa–stained peripheral blood is examined for its formed elements: red blood cells (RBCs), white blood cells (WBCs), and platelets. A careful review of the peripheral smear is useful when a patient has an abnormal WBC count or platelet count with or without anemia, has a report of "atypical" WBCs, or is suspected of having a condition for which the smear is especially useful. Even in other circumstances, it is important for the physician to have an understanding of the morphologic characteristics that underlie the report of an automated complete blood count so that the likelihood of reaching the correct diagnosis is enhanced (Table 161–1).

TABLE 161–1 EXAMPLES OF WHEN REVIEW OF THE PERIPHERAL BLOOD SMEAR CAN AID IN DIAGNOSIS

Diagnosis	Peripheral Blood Smear Clue
Pernicious anemia	Hypersegmented neutrophils
Acute leukemia	Blasts, Auer rods
Disseminated intravascular coagulation	Fragmented erythrocytes
Myelofibrosis/marrow replacement	Teardrop-shaped erythrocytes, nucleated erythrocytes
Malaria, babesiosis	Characteristic erythrocyte inclusions
Fungal/bacterial infections	Granulocytes with cytoplasmic organisms
Viral infections	Reactive lymphocytes
Lead poisoning	Basophilic stippling of erythrocytes

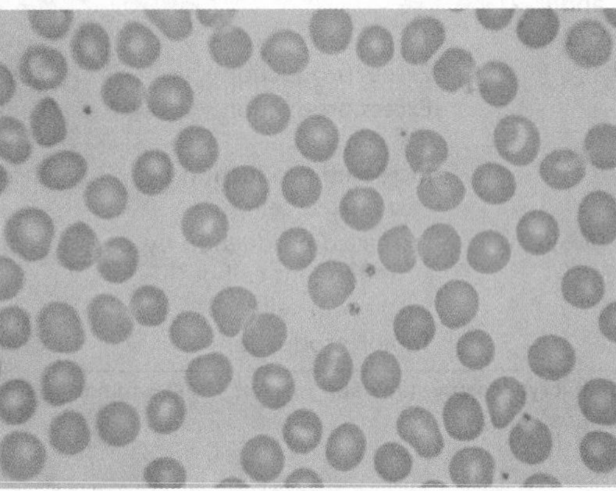

FIGURE 161–1 • Normal peripheral blood smear. These normal red cells are biconcave discs. Central pallor is less than a third the diameter of the cell. There are also scattered normal platelets (×1000).

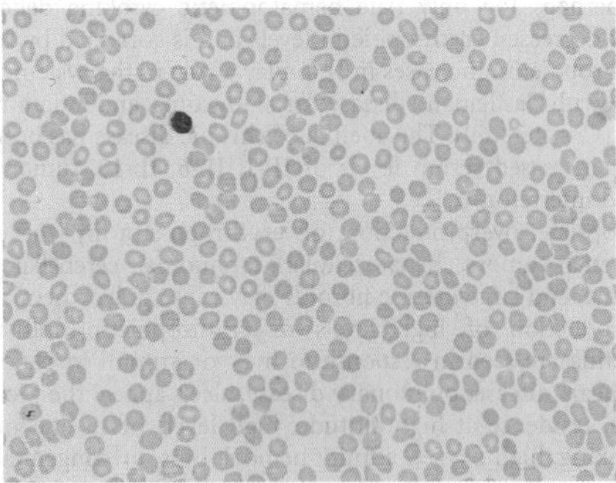

FIGURE 161–2 • Normal peripheral blood smear. The red cell diameter is about the same size as the nucleus of the small lymphocyte (×400).

DISORDERS OF RED BLOOD CELLS

Size and Color of Red Blood Cells

RBCs are normally biconcave discs measuring about 7 μm in diameter (Fig. 161–1), or about the same as the nucleus of a small lymphocyte (Figs. 161–2). The central pallor of the concavity in a normochromic RBC is about a third of the cell's diameter, and the remaining cytoplasm has a homogeneous pinkish color. The diameter of RBCs is proportional to mean corpuscular volume.

Excessive numbers of RBCs of various size on a peripheral smear is termed *anisocytosis*. If RBCs are smaller than the normal range, the term is *microcytosis* (Fig. 161–3). Microcytosis (Chapter 163) occurs in iron

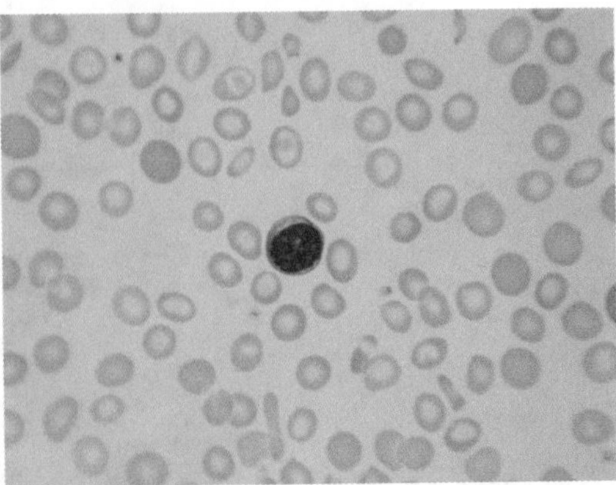

FIGURE 161–3 • Microcytic red cells from a case of thalassemia minor. The red cell diameter is smaller than that of the nucleus of the small lymphocyte (×1000).

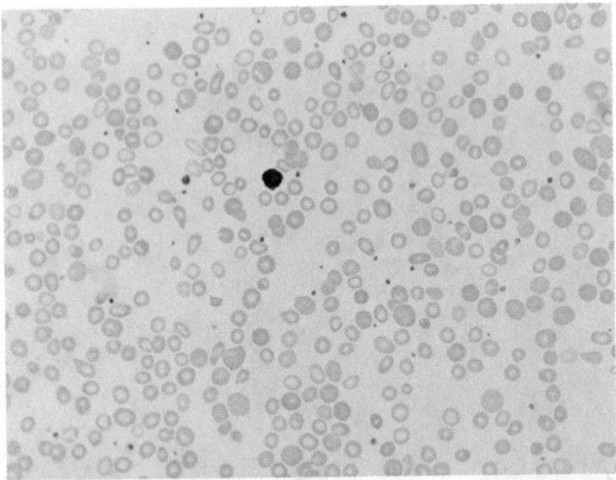

FIGURE 161–4 • Microcytic, hypochromic anemia. The red cell diameter is smaller than that of the nucleus of the small lymphocyte, and the central pallor is greater than a third the diameter of the red cells (×400).

deficiency anemia (Chapter 163), some cases of anemia of chronic disease (Chapter 163), α- and β-thalassemia (Chapter 166), the sideroblastic anemias (Chapter 163), and vitamin B_6 deficiency (Chapter 169).

Hypochromia, in contrast to normochromia, denotes a central pallor greater than a third the diameter of the RBC. This finding appears in iron deficiency anemia (Chapter 163), some cases of anemia of chronic disease (Chapter 163), and the thalassemias (Chapter 166). Hypochromic, microcytic red cells indicate more advanced iron deficiency anemia (Fig. 161–4).

Larger than normal RBCs, or "macrocytosis," occur in folate and vitamin B_{12} deficiencies (Chapter 170), liver disease, some myelodysplastic disorders (Chapter 193), and conditions with reticulocytosis (Fig. 161–5). In more severe instances of folate and vitamin B_{12} deficiency, macrocytic RBCs may have an oval shape called "macro-ovalocytosis." Reticulocytes, which are RBCs that have just been released from the bone marrow, retain RNA for about 48 hours and are also slightly larger than normal-sized RBCs. Polychromasia, which is evidenced by increased numbers of bluish tinged RBCs, occurs in any condition with an outpouring of reticulocytes from the marrow (Fig. 161–6).

Shapes of Red Blood Cells

"Poikilocytosis" denotes a peripheral smear with RBCs of various shape. Spherocytic RBCs, which lack central pallor (Fig. 161–7), appear when antibody coats the RBC surface (Chapter 164) and in congenital spherocytosis (Chapter 165), a heterogeneous condition with cytoskeletal defects in RBCs. The target or Mexican hat cell, which has a central bull's-eye of hemoglobin surrounded by an area of pallor (Fig 161–8), is typical of liver disease, hemoglobinopathies (Chapter 168), and sometimes iron deficiency anemia.

Sickle cells (Chapter 167) have a crescentic shape with pointed ends as a result of distortion by elongated curvilinear tactoids of hemoglobin S within their cytoplasm (Fig 161–9). This irreversible change is regularly observed in the homozygous SS state. Sickled red cells may be seen in

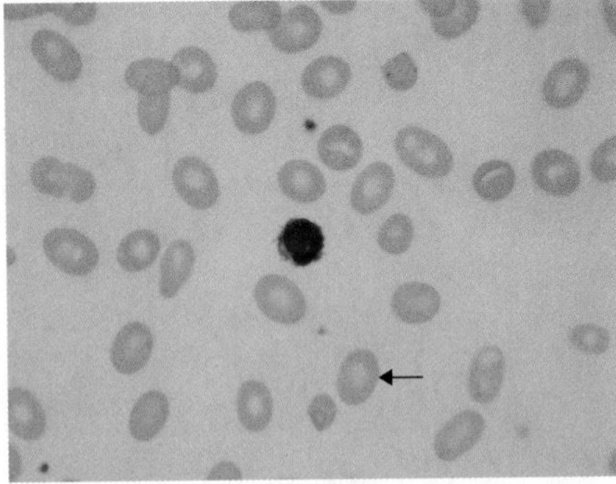

FIGURE 161–5 • Macrocytic anemia. Here the red cell diameter is greater than that of the nucleus of the small lymphocyte (×1000). A macro-ovalocyte is indicated by the arrow.

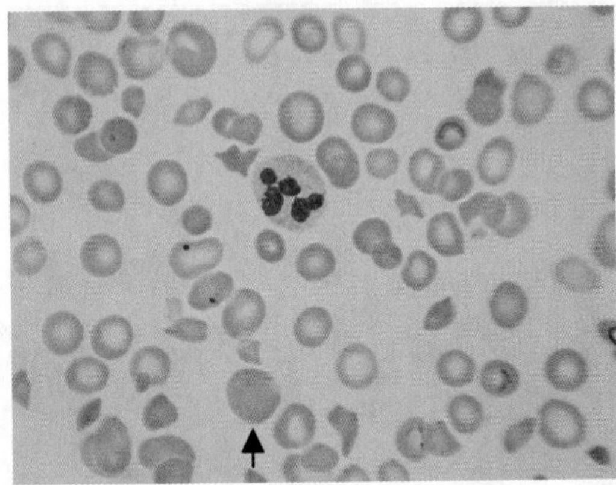

FIGURE 161–6 • Polychromasia. A polychromatic red cell is indicated by the arrow. Also present are two red cells with small, round, blue Howell-Jolly bodies (×1000).

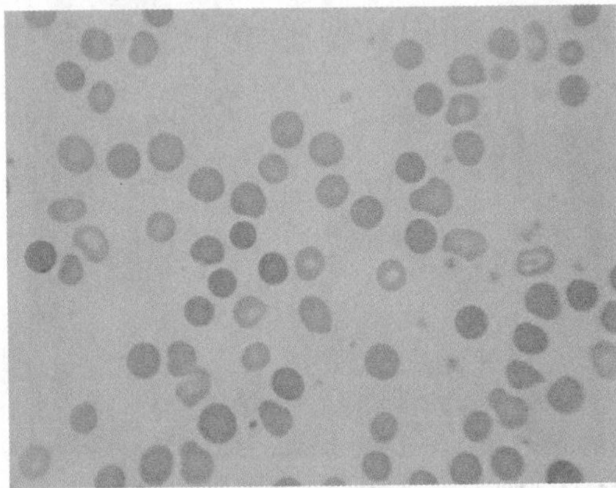

FIGURE 161–7 • Congenital spherocytosis. These red cells lack central pallor because of their more spherical shape (×1000).

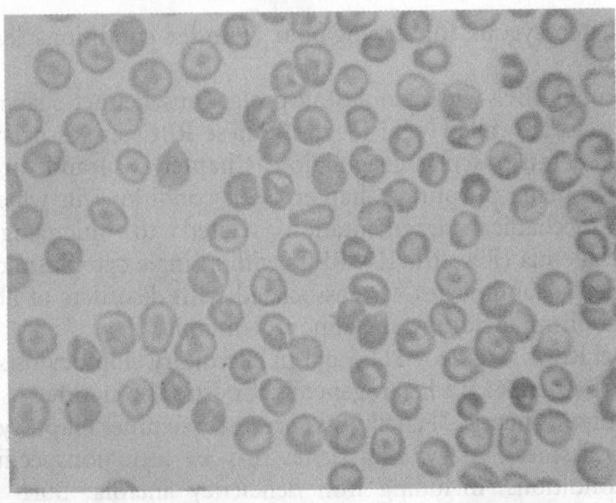

FIGURE 161–8 • Target cells. These cells have a central knob of hemoglobin surrounded by an area of pallor and then a peripheral area of hemoglobin (×1000).

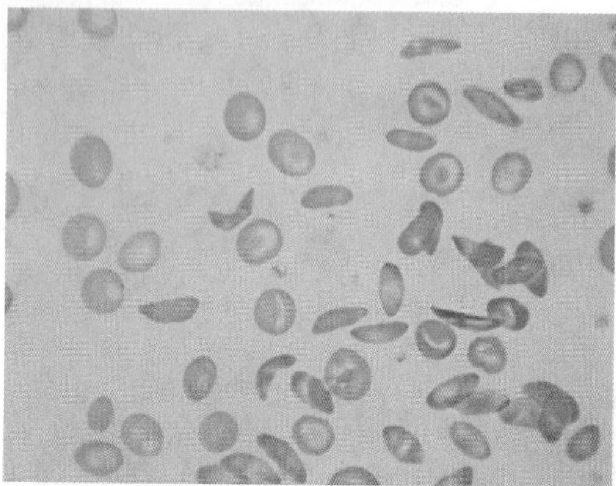

FIGURE 161–9 • Sickle cells. These sickle-shaped cells give sickle cell anemia its name (×1000).

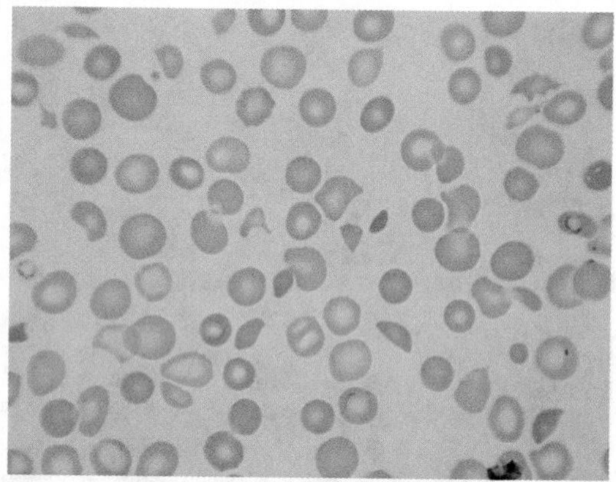

FIGURE 161–10 • Disseminated intravascular coagulation. Fragmented red cells with helmet shapes, cytoplasmic projections, and burrs are present (×1000).

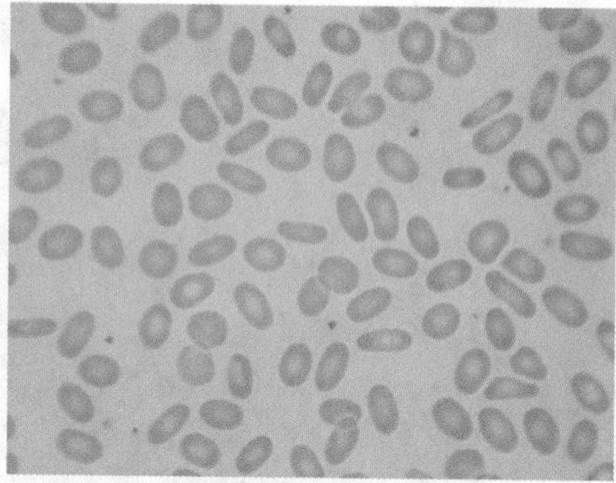

FIGURE 161–11 • Elliptocytosis. Elliptocytes (ovalocytes) are seen in a patient with hereditary elliptocytosis (×1000).

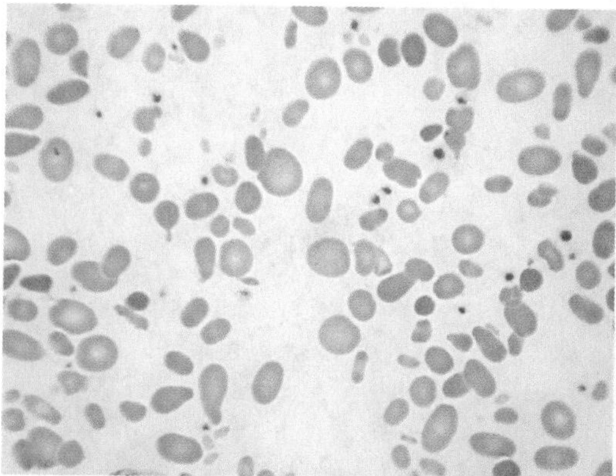

FIGURE 161–12 • Hereditary pyropoikilocytosis. This congenital condition of the red cell cytoskeleton results in various sizes and shapes of red cell fragments, including microspherocytes. The peripheral smear from a burn patient would be similar (×1000).

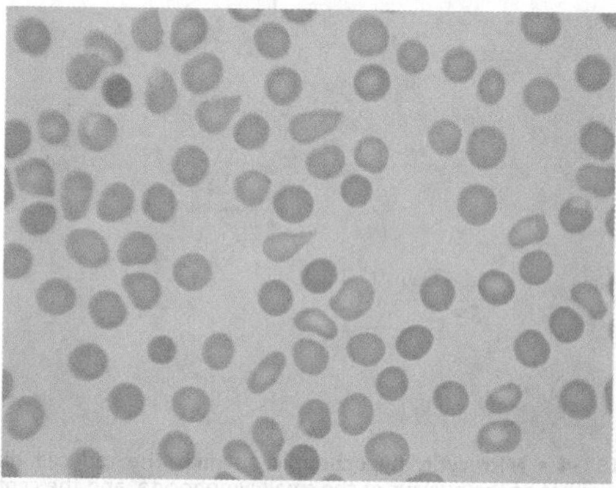

FIGURE 161–13 • Teardrop red blood cells. A teardrop-shaped red cell (dacryocyte) is present in the center of the photo (×1000).

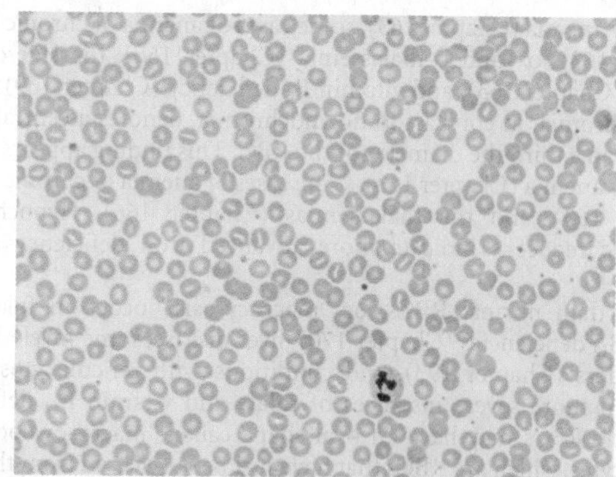

FIGURE 161–14 • Stomatocyte. Red cells with mouth-shaped central pallor ("stomatocyte") are seen scattered throughout this smear (×400).

patients heterozygous for hemoglobin S under conditions leading to hypoxia.

Fragmented RBCs with cytoplasmic projections, helmet-shaped forms, and burr cells are called "schistocytes." These RBCs are associated with disseminated intravascular coagulation (Chapter 181) and thrombotic thrombocytopenia purpura (Chapter 179), conditions in which RBCs undergo mechanical fragmentation related to microangiopathic hemolytic anemia (Fig. 161–10). RBCs with a single cytoplasmic projection, termed "acanthocytes," are associated with disorders of abnormal lipid metabolism, including abetalipoproteinemia.

Elliptical RBCs (Fig. 161–11) occur in hereditary elliptocytosis (ovalocytosis) (Chapter 165), a heterogeneous condition sometimes associated with hemolytic anemia. "Pencil poikilocytosis" signifies elliptocytosis on a peripheral smear. A few elliptocytes may be seen nonspecifically in various conditions, including iron deficiency anemia. Burn patients (Chapter 113) may exhibit RBCs in markedly varying size, including microspherocytes and irregular RBC fragments related to thermal damage. A similar appearance is seen in a congenital cytoskeletal RBC defect named "pyropoikilocytosis" (Fig. 161–12).

Teardrop RBCs (Fig. 161–13) have a pointed end resembling a tear, hence the other term, "dacryocyte." When an RBC must course through a particularly narrowed lumen of a vessel, it may assume this shape. These teardrop forms occur in myelofibrosis (Chapter 177), myelophthisic states secondary to bone marrow replacement by tumor or granulomas, and megaloblastic anemia (Chapter 170). An RBC with central pallor in the shape of a mouth, termed a "stomatocyte," is associated with liver disease but can also appear as a genetic condition (Fig. 161–14).

Inclusions in Red Blood Cells

A usually single, 1- to 2-μm nuclear fragment retained within the red cell, termed a Howell-Jolly body (see Fig. 161–6), is seen most frequently

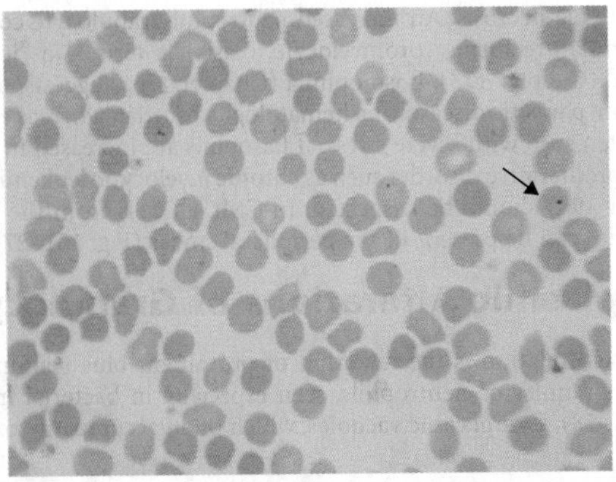

FIGURE 161–15 • Pappenheimer body. Pappenheimer bodies are the small, rounded inclusions present in the red cell at the arrow (×1000).

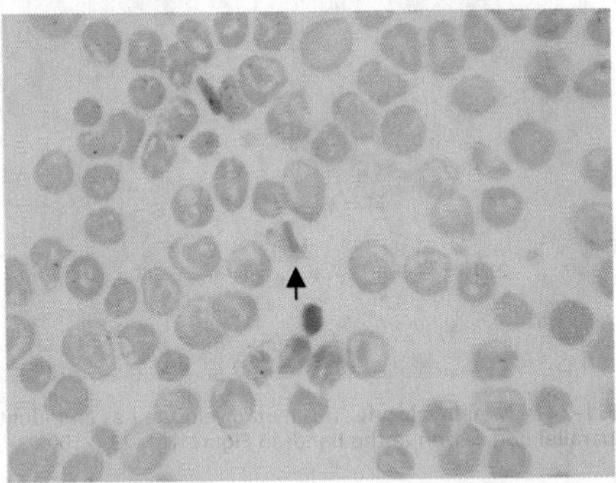

FIGURE 161–16 • Homozygous hemoglobin C. A hemoglobin C crystal is present within the red cell at the arrow in this case of hemoglobin C (×1000).

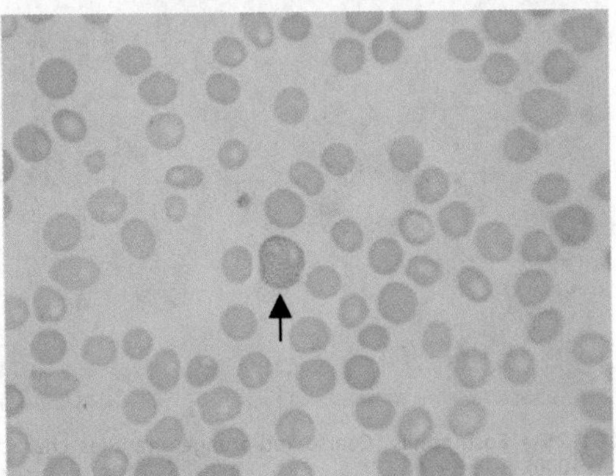

FIGURE 161–17 • Basophilic stippling. Fine basophilic stippling is seen within the red cell at the arrow (×1000).

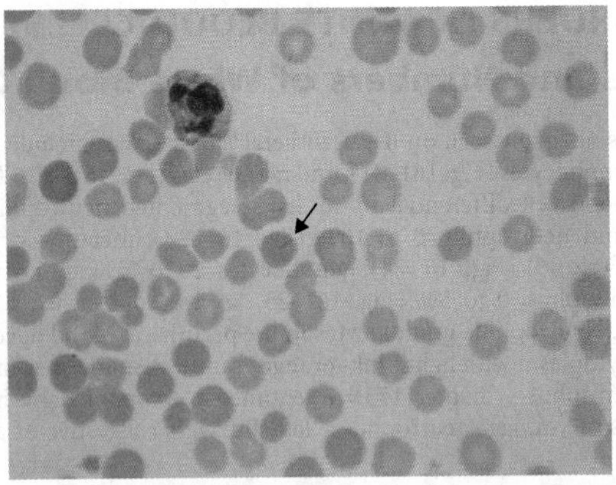

FIGURE 161–18 • Red blood cell inclusion. A red cell containing a bacterium is seen at the arrow (×1000).

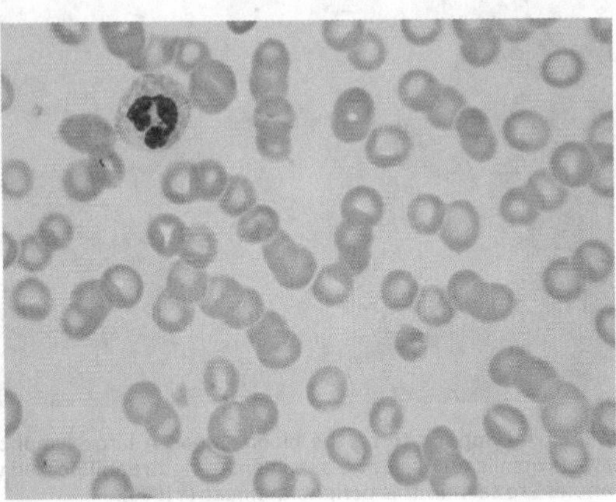

FIGURE 161–19 • Rouleaux formation. Red cells stacked like coins is called rouleaux formation and is often related to a monoclonal gammopathy (×1000).

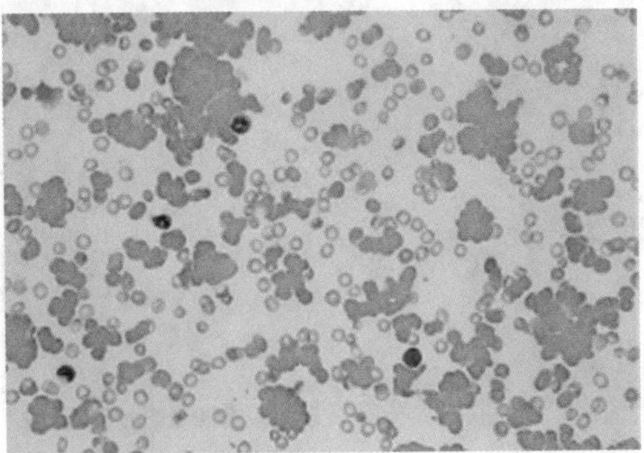

FIGURE 161–20 • Clumps of red blood cells. Large amorphous aggregates (agglutination) of red blood cells as seen in *Mycoplasma pneumoniae* (×100). (Courtesy of Jean Schafer.)

in patients with an absent or nonfunctional spleen. Small, rounded iron inclusions, termed Pappenheimer bodies (Fig. 161–15), occur in patients with sideroblastic anemia (Chapter 163). On an iron stain, these inclusions are termed "siderotic granules." Hemoglobin C crystals are hexagonally shaped rods that occur in the red cell cytoplasm of patients with homozygous hemoglobin C (Chapter 167; Fig. 161–16). These crystals may also be extracellular.

Basophilic stippling, which is the appearance of regularly spaced fine to coarse blue-staining dots of RNA in RBC cytoplasm (Fig. 161–17), is sometimes associated with lead poisoning (Chapter 20) (the stippling tends to be coarse), severe anemia, and β-thalassemia (Chapter 166). Parasites residing within the cytoplasm of the red cell include malarial organisms (Chapter 366 and Fig. 366–1) and babesiosis (Chapters 374). On rare occasion, bacteria may be seen in the RBC with or without the help of a Gram stain (Fig. 161–18).

Other Red Blood Cell Conditions

Nucleated RBCs in the peripheral smear suggest increased production of RBCs or infiltration of the bone marrow. Nucleated RBCs in combination with increased numbers of immature granulocytes, a "leukoerythroblastic reaction," suggests marrow replacement or infiltration as a result of metastatic tumor to the bone marrow, leukemia (Chapter 194), a myeloproliferative disorder (Chapter 177), or hemolytic anemia (Chapter 165).

RBCs clumped as stacks of coins, called rouleaux formation (Fig. 161–19), suggest a monoclonal gammopathy as seen in multiple myeloma (Chapter 198). Clusters of red cells in clumps are seen in the presence of a cold agglutinin (Chapter 164; Fig. 161–20).

DISORDERS OF WHITE BLOOD CELLS

Types and Numbers of White Blood Cells

WBCs normally seen on the peripheral blood smear include granulocytes, lymphocytes (Fig. 161–21), and monocytes (Fig. 161–22). A normal white blood cell differential in adults is segmented neutrophils, 50 to 70%; band neutrophils, 0 to 10% (Fig. 161–23); metamyelocyte neutrophils, 0 to 1% (Fig. 161–24); lymphocytes, 20 to 40%; monocytes, 0 to 7%; eosinophils, 0 to 5% (Fig. 161–25); and basophils, 0 to 1% (Fig. 161–26). Neutrophilic granulocytes in the peripheral blood have a finely dotted cytoplasm with light pink–orange granules. An increase in peripheral neutrophils (Chapter 173), oftentimes accompanied by increased numbers of younger neutrophils ("left shift"), is suggestive of an infection or tissue necrosis. An increased neutrophil granulocyte count with more immature forms (promyelocyte, blasts) is termed a "leukemoid reaction" (Chapter 173). Eosinophilia (Chapter 176) suggests an allergic condition, parasitic disease, or a hematologic disorder, whereas eosinopenia is often seen with severe stress. If basophils are increased in number, a myeloproliferative disorder such as chronic myelocytic leukemia (CML) (Chapter 195) should be suspected. In CML all cells from the granulocytic series can be present in the peripheral smear (Fig. 161–27).

Cytoplasmic Alterations of Granulocytes

Toxic granulation is the retention of prominent blue staining in the primary granules of neutrophils, seen especially in bacterial infections (Fig. 161–28). Cytoplasmic vacuoles, which often accompany toxic gran-

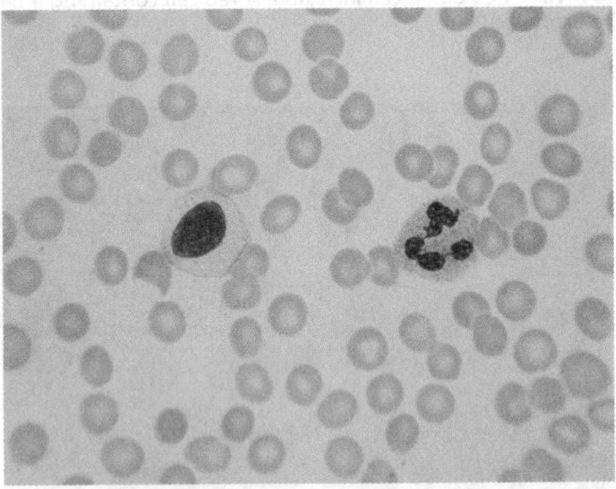

FIGURE 161–21 • Lymphocyte on the blood smear. A large lymphocyte with cytoplasmic azurophilic granules and a segmented neutrophil packed with pink-orange granules are seen in this peripheral smear (×1000).

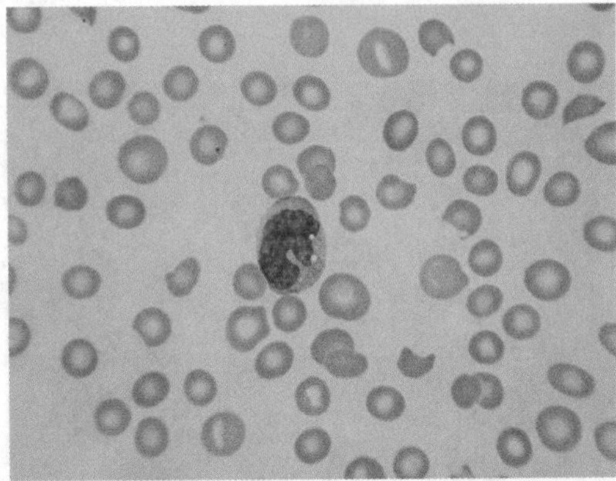

FIGURE 161–22 • Monocyte on the blood smear. This normal monocyte has a "dirty gray" cytoplasm with vacuoles and a cerebriform nucleus (×1000).

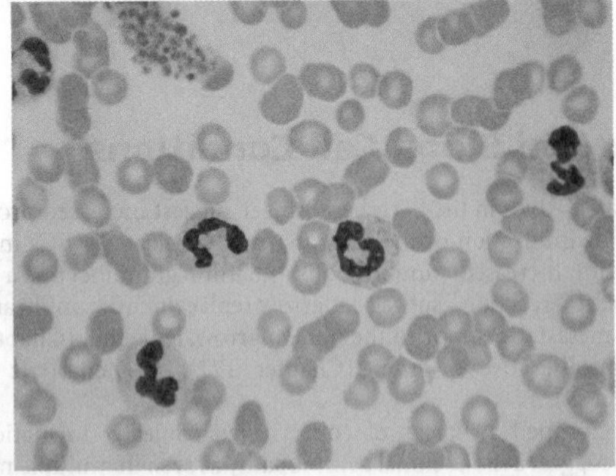

FIGURE 161–23 • Band neutrophil. There are two definite band neutrophils in the center of this photomicrograph.

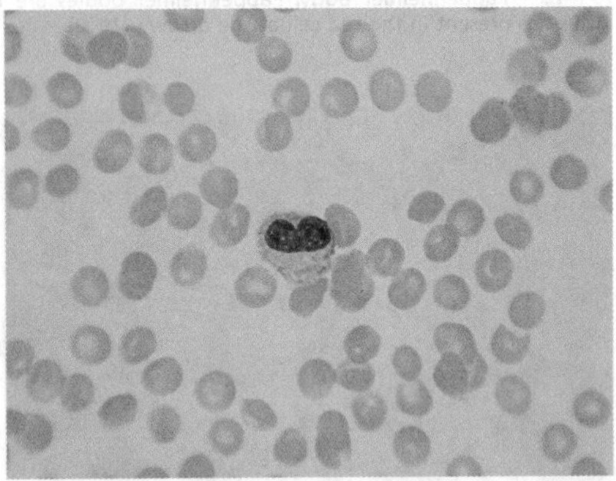

FIGURE 161–24 • Metamyelocyte. This metamyelocyte has an indentation but lacks the parallel edges seen in the bands in Figure 161–23 (×1000).

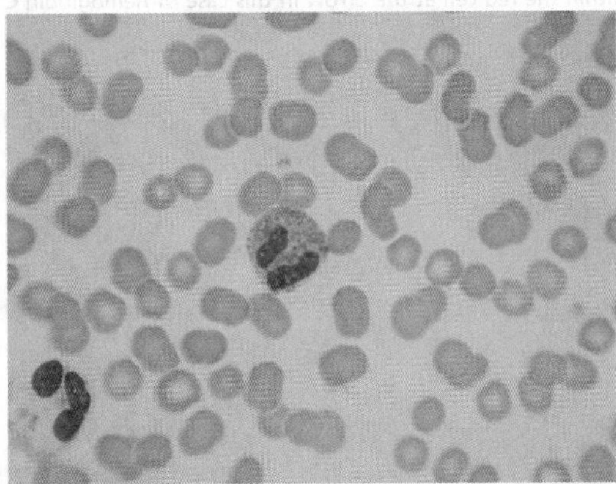

FIGURE 161–25 • Eosinophils. Coarse red-orange granules characterize the eosinophil (×1000).

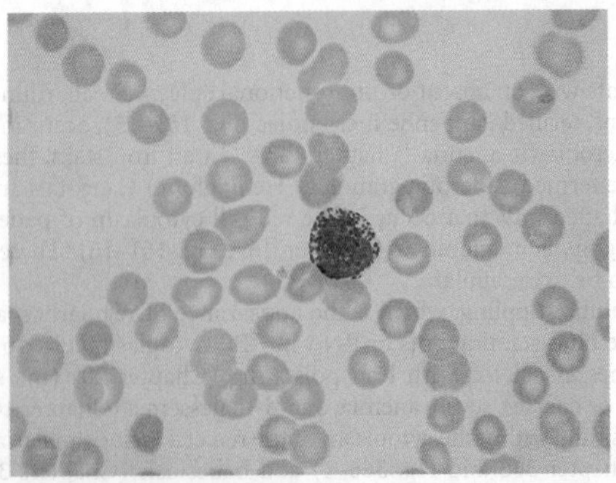

FIGURE 161–26 • Basophils. The basophil has basophilic granules in the cytoplasm and overlying the nucleus (×1000).

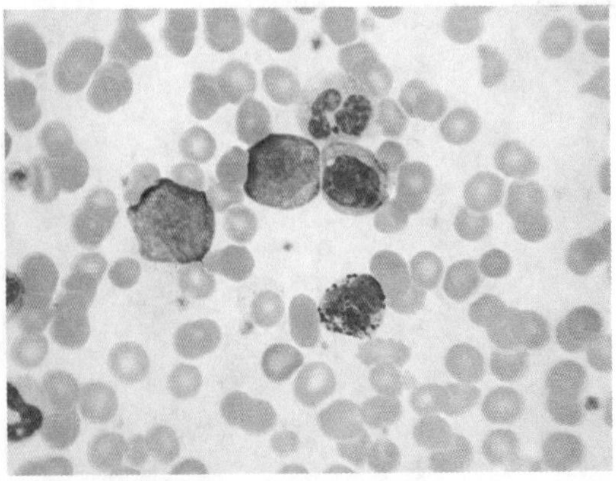

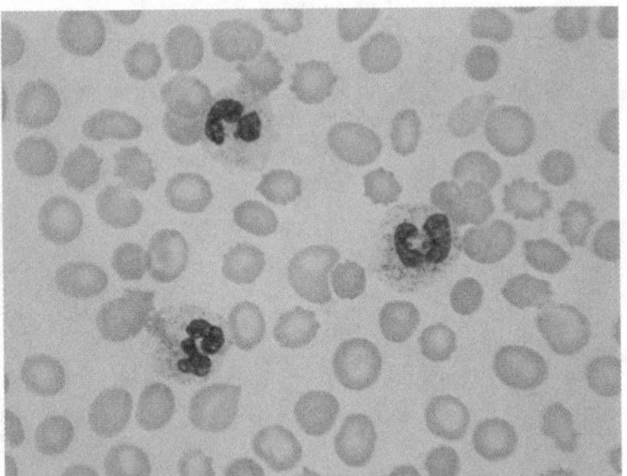

FIGURE 161–27 • Chronic myelogenous leukemia. In this view there are myeloblasts, a myelocyte, a basophil, and a segmented neutrophil (×1000).

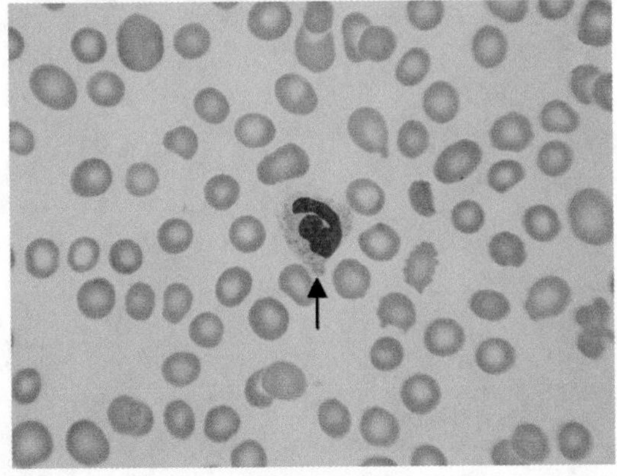

FIGURE 161–28 • Toxic granulation. Cytoplasmic vacuoles and toxic granulation are present in these neutrophils from a patient with infection (×1000).

FIGURE 161–29 • Döhle bodies. A Döhle body is present in the peripheral cytoplasm as indicated by the arrow (×1000).

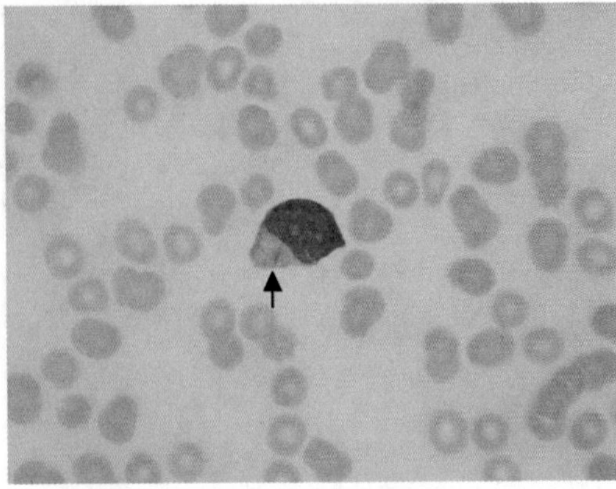

FIGURE 161–30 • Auer rod. Note the Auer rod indicated by the arrow in this blast from a case of acute myelogenous leukemia (×1000).

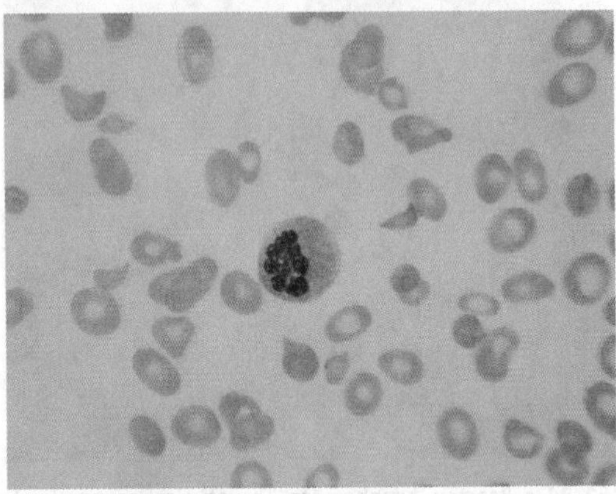

FIGURE 161–31 • Hypersegmented neutrophils. A hypersegmented neutrophil (more than five segments) in a patient with megaloblastic anemia is seen in this photomicrograph (×1000).

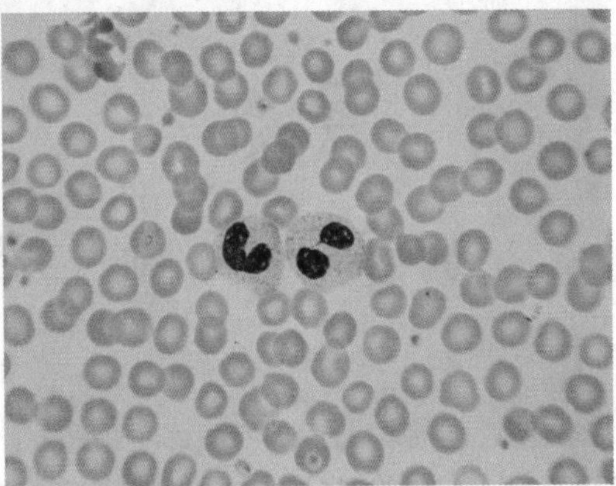

FIGURE 161–32 • Pelger-Huët anomaly. The "band" neutrophil on the left has hyperclumped chromatin giving it a peanut shell appearance, whereas the one on the right has nuclear segments suggesting pince-nez spectacles (×1000).

ulations in infections, indicate intracytoplasmic sites of bacterial destruction (see Fig. 161–28). In more severe infections, the Döhle body, a bluish smudge within the cytoplasm consisting of light blue fragments of RNA (Fig. 161–29), can also be seen. Neutrophil hypogranularity may accompany severe infections but is also a feature of myelodysplasia (Chapter 193) and CML (Chapter 195). On occasion, a bacterium or yeast is found within a granulocyte and suggests septicemia. The presence of Auer rods (Fig. 161–30) in even one peripheral granulocyte demands further evaluation for acute myelogenous leukemia (Chapter 194).

Nuclear Alterations of Granulocytes

Six or more distinct segmented lobes in a mature neutrophil (Fig. 161–31) is classically associated with vitamin B_{12} and folate deficiencies (Chapter 170). Hyposegmentation typifies the Pelger-Huët anomaly (Fig. 161–32), which can accompany myelodysplastic syndrome (Chapter 193), acute myelogenous leukemia (Chapter 194), or the accelerated phase of CML (Chapter 195).

Monocytes

The abundant gray-blue cytoplasm of monocytes contains vacuoles and very fine, barely discernible granules (see Fig. 161–22). An increased number of peripheral monocytes is seen in chronic inflammatory reactions, recovery from cell injury, nonhematopoietic malignancies, and some hematopoietic malignancies (Chapter 173).

Lymphocytes

Lymphocytes vary from small (see Fig. 161–3) with minimal cytoplasm to medium and large with larger nuclei (Fig. 161–33). Occasionally, reddish granules are seen in the cytoplasm. Reactive (atypical) lympho-

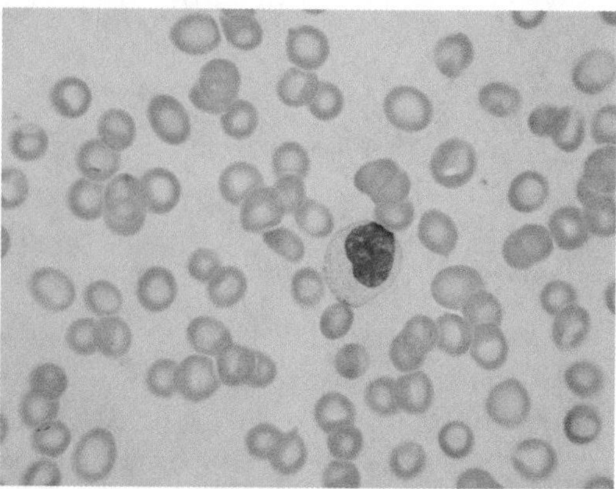

FIGURE 161–33 • Large lymphocyte.

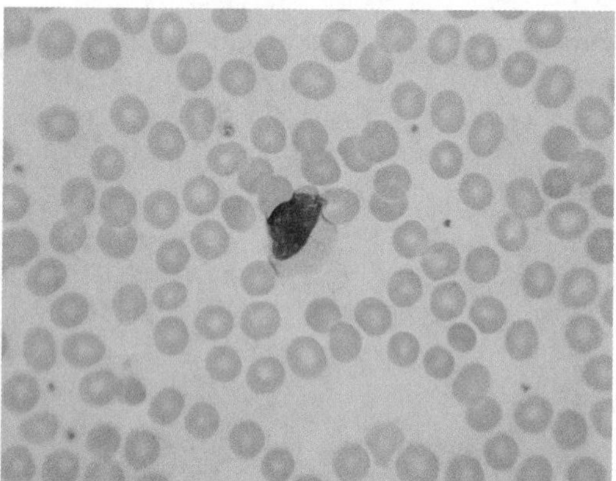

FIGURE 161–34 • Reactive lymphocytes. This atypical or reactive lymphocyte has a bluish cytoplasm that is indented by adjacent red cells (×1000).

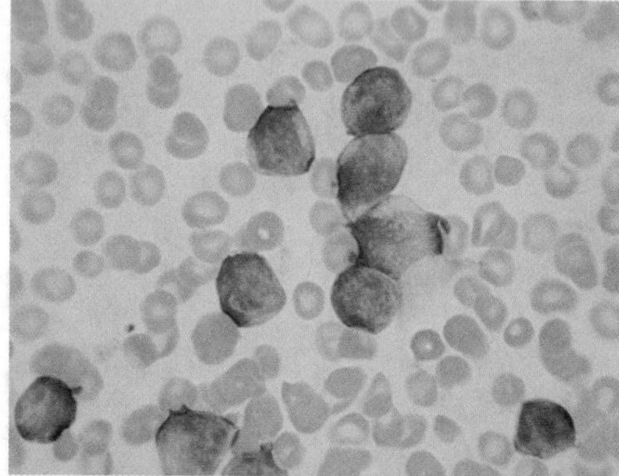

FIGURE 161–35 • Acute lymphocytic leukemia. Multiple blasts are present in this view. Platelets are decreased in number (×1000).

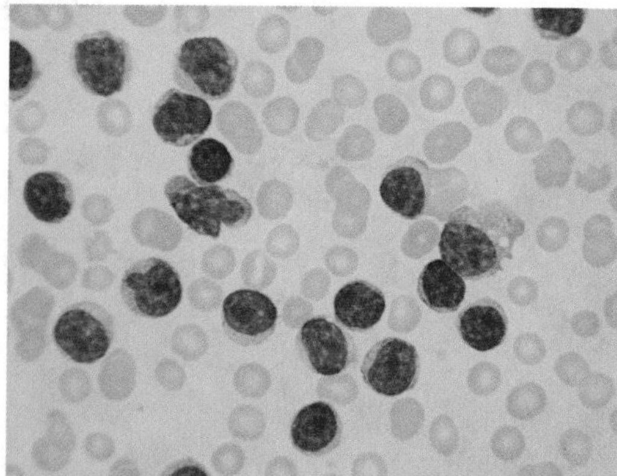

FIGURE 161–36 • Chronic lymphocytic leukemia. Large numbers of rather monotonous small lymphocytes in a case of chronic lymphocytic leukemia are seen in this photomicrograph (×1000).

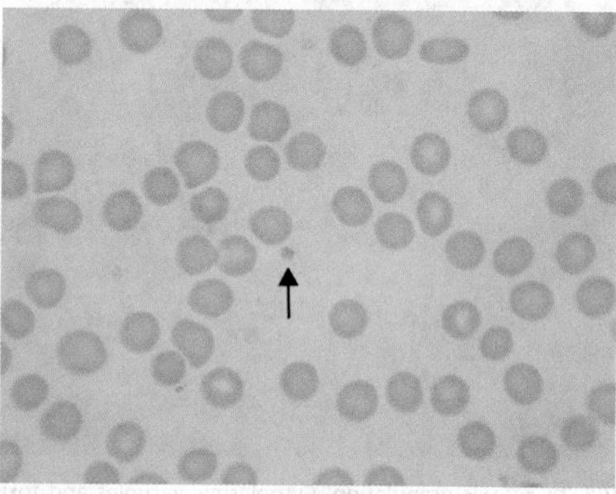

FIGURE 161–37 • Normal platelet indicated by the arrow. Platelets are granular, although this is not apparent in this view (×1000).

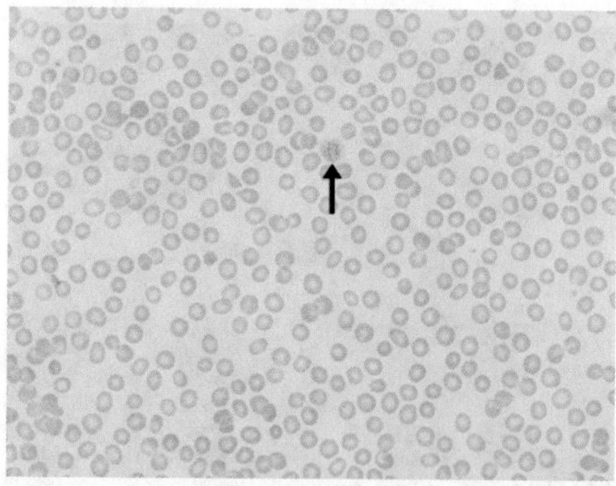

FIGURE 161–38 • Giant platelets. They are as large as or larger than the diameter of a normal red cell as shown by the arrow. Giant platelets indicate increased platelet turnover (×1000).

cytes, which occur in a variety of disorders, including infectious mononucleosis (Fig. 161–34; Chapter 400), have abundant cytoplasm that may have prominent blue shading and vacuoles; on occasion, reactive lymphocytes may closely resemble monocytes. Lymphocytosis is also typical of acute lymphocytic leukemia (Chapter 194) (Fig. 161–35), chronic lymphocytic leukemia (Chapter 195) (Fig. 161–36), and lymphoma (Chapter 196).

Platelets

Platelets are 2 to 4 μm in size and normally stain bluish with a granular appearance (Fig. 161–37). When there is increased turnover of platelets, giant platelets appear (Fig. 161–38). Increased platelet counts occur after acute hemorrhage, during hemolysis, in neoplastic states, and in the myeloproliferative disorders, including essential thrombocythemia (Chapter 177). Thrombocytopenia is seen with the immune thrombocytopenias (Chapter 179), hypersplenism (Chapter 174), drugs and toxins, and hemopoietic malignancies.

Rarely, true thrombocytopenia can be masked by fragments of leukocytes in patients with acute leukemia. An incorrectly low automated platelet count can be recognized by discovery of platelet clumping—a phenomenon occasionally seen in blood collected in ethylenediaminetetraacetic acid (EDTA).

SUGGESTED READINGS

Bain BJ: Diagnosis from the peripheral blood smear. N Engl J Med 2005;353:498–507. *Highlights the broad range of disorders that can be diagnosed from the peripheral blood smear.*

Hernandez AM: Peripheral blood manifestations of lymphoma and solid tumors. Clin Lab Med 2002;22:215–252. *A wide variety of underlying tumors can be suspected by the peripheral blood smear.*

Kroft SH: Infectious diseases manifested in the peripheral blood. Clin Lab Med 2002;22:253–277. *Review of peripheral blood findings in a broad spectrum of infectious diseases.*

162 APPROACH TO THE ANEMIAS

Kenneth S. Zuckerman

Definition

Anemia is defined as a reduction in the number of circulating erythrocytes. It is a common manifestation of primary bone marrow disorders (resulting in impaired production of erythrocytes), primary abnormalities of erythrocytes (resulting in an increased rate of destruction), immunologic disorders, nutritional deficiencies, and a broad spectrum of systemic diseases that secondarily result in anemia. Any condition that can impair the production or increase the rate of destruction or loss of erythrocytes can result in anemia if the bone marrow is unable to compensate for the rate of loss of red blood cells (RBCs). At least some degree of anemia is detectable in 20 to 40% of hospitalized patients.

Pathobiology

Electronic, automated blood cell counters provide a considerable amount of information that is useful in determining the severity, pathophysiology, and etiology of anemia (Table 162–1). The hemoglobin (Hgb), measured in grams per deciliter, represents the total amount of hemoglobin in all the erythrocytes in 100 mL of blood. The hematocrit (Hct) is the percentage of the total blood volume that is composed of erythrocytes. The mean corpuscular or cell volume (MCV) is measured directly on automated cell counters but can be calculated as MCV (μm^3 or fL) = Hct (%) × 10/RBC count (× 10^6/μL of whole blood). The mean cell hemoglobin (MCH) is calculated by automated cell counters as MCH (pg) = Hgb (g/dL) × 10/RBC (× 10^6/μL). The mean cell hemoglobin concentration (MCHC) is calculated by automated cell counters as MCHC = Hgb (g/dL) × 100/Hct (%). MCH and MCHC are of limited value because of relatively poor sensitivity for any individual disorders, whereas MCV is extremely useful in classification and determination of the cause of anemia. The RBC distribution width (RDW/CV) is a ratio of the width of the RBC size distribution curve at 1 SD from the mean size divided by the MCV. Because this value is a ratio with the MCV as the denominator, it tends to magnify any variation in cell size in patients with microcytosis but is relatively insensitive to mild or early macrocytosis. A less frequently used value, RDW/SD, is the width of the RBC size distribution curve that encompasses 80% of the erythrocytes in the measured population. This latter measurement is particularly sensitive even to small populations of microcytic or macrocytic RBCs. In addition to these standard measurements, automated absolute reticulocyte counts per microliter of blood or evaluations of new methylene blue–stained peripheral blood smears for the percentage of positive-staining erythrocytes (reticulocytes) give a measure of the number of newly released (generally 1- to 2-day-old) erythrocytes. These newly formed erythrocytes still contain residual ribosomal RNA, which can easily be recognized on supravital staining with new methylene blue. Because ribosomal RNA is lost from the cell within the first 1 to 2 days in circulation and erythrocytes in blood survive an average of about 120 days, reticulocytes account for about 1 to 2% of all erythrocytes in the circulation; a normal, nonanemic adult has 40,000 to 100,000 reticulocytes per microliter of blood. Automated blood cell counters also provide the total white blood cell (WBC) count, the WBC differential count, and the platelet count. All of this information is useful in assessing the mechanism of anemia.

Pathogenesis

Normal Erythropoiesis

A circulating erythrocyte under normal conditions has an average lifespan of approximately 120 days. It is a non-nucleated, nondividing cell in which more than 90% of the protein content is the oxygen-carrying molecule hemoglobin. The erythrocyte's sole responsibility is to deliver oxygen to the tissues of the body. The primary consequence of anemia is tissue hypoxia. Erythropoiesis is driven by a feedback loop. Oxygen-sensing cells, which are thought to be located near the tip of the juxtamedullary region of the cortical labyrinths of the kidney, respond to local tissue hypoxia by increasing production of erythropoietin (EPO), the primary regulatory hormone for erythropoiesis. A small proportion (no more than 10%) of EPO production occurs outside the kidney, primarily in the liver. EPO plays little, if any role in maintaining or producing early hematopoietic precursors or even the earliest detectable erythroid progenitor cells, known as *burst forming units–erythroid* (BFU-E); however, EPO is essential for the maturation of BFU-E to late erythroid progenitor cells, known as *colony-forming units–erythroid* (CFU-E), and to proerythroblasts in the bone marrow. The main mechanism of action of EPO is to prevent apoptosis, also called *programmed cell death*, of erythroid precursor cells and to permit their proliferation and maturation. When erythroid precursor cells mature to the level of proerythroblasts, further maturation to normoblasts, reticulocytes, and mature erythrocytes no longer requires the presence of EPO. Under normal circumstances, RBC mass is maintained at a nearly constant level by means of the EPO feedback loop's ability to match new erythrocyte production with the rate of natural senescence and loss of RBCs. Although total absence of EPO in the circulation never or almost never occurs, severe depression of circulating EPO levels results in near cessation of erythrocyte production.

Hypoxia, as sensed in the kidney, results in increased production of EPO, which leads to increased erythrocyte production by the bone marrow. When the local tissue hypoxia is due to a reduction in the number of circulating erythrocytes, the amount of hemoglobin, and the

TABLE 162–1 NORMAL VALUES FOR RED BLOOD CELL MEASUREMENTS

Measurement	Unit	Normal Range (Approximate)*
Hemoglobin	g/dL	Males: 13.5–17.5 Females: 12–16
Hematocrit	%	Males: 40–52 Females: 36–48
Red blood cell (RBC) count	×10^6/μL of blood	Males: 4.5–6.0 Females: 4.0–5.4
Mean cell volume (MCV)	fL	81–99
Mean cell hemoglobin (MCH)	pg	30–34
Mean cell hemoglobin concentration (MCHC)	g/dL	30–36
Red blood cell size distribution width		
RDW-CV	%	12–14
RDW-SD	fL	37–47
Reticulocyte count (absolute number)	No./μL of blood	40,000–100,000
Reticulocyte percentage	% of RBCs	0.5–1.5

*Actual normal ranges for many of these values may vary slightly, depending on factors such as the location and type of laboratory instruments used, altitude above sea level, and patient age.

consequent decreased total body oxygen-carrying capacity, the increased EPO produced by the kidney stimulates the bone marrow to produce increased numbers of erythrocytes to compensate for the existing deficiency of RBCs. When an increase in EPO levels in the circulation occurs in response to an acute onset of anemia, new proerythroblasts and normoblasts appear in the bone marrow within 2 to 4 days, and new reticulocytes begin to appear in the peripheral blood within 3 to 7 days. Reestablishment of normal numbers of circulating erythrocytes and normal tissue oxygenation results in reduced production of EPO and a reduced rate of production of erythrocytes back to the normal basal level that is required to maintain a stable, normal number of erythrocytes in blood. When hypoxia is caused by a decreased ambient oxygen concentration, impaired delivery of oxygen through the lungs and to hemoglobin molecules in erythrocytes, venous to arterial shunting of blood, hemoglobin mutants with increased oxygen affinity and decreased ability to release oxygen to tissues, or localized renal disease that the renal sensor cannot distinguish from generalized hypoxemia, the increase in EPO results in increased erythropoiesis, erythrocytosis, and secondary polycythemia.

Pathogenesis of Anemias

The basic mechanisms of anemia can be divided into conditions that result in accelerated destruction or loss of RBCs and conditions in which the primary abnormality is impaired ability of the bone marrow to produce sufficient numbers of erythrocytes to replace the erythrocytes that are lost. Although this classification makes it easier to understand the pathophysiology of anemia and to determine the proper diagnostic studies to perform, more than one mechanism may occur simultaneously in many patients.

Anemias Caused by Impaired Production of Erythrocytes by Bone Marrow

If there is a reduced erythrocyte mass secondary to impaired production of erythroid precursors and mature RBCs by the bone marrow, the number of reticulocytes in circulating blood and the number of normoblasts in bone marrow would be lower than would be appropriate in the presence of the existing degree of anemia. A wide variety of conditions can be responsible for impaired erythropoiesis (Table 162–2).

Erythropoietin Deficiency

Insufficient production of EPO results in failure of an otherwise normal bone marrow to produce the required number of erythrocytes despite the production of normal numbers of other hematopoietic cells such as neutrophils and platelets. The prototype for impaired EPO production is renal failure (with particularly severe EPO deficiency after bilateral nephrectomy), in which only low levels of EPO, generally less than 10% of normal, are produced (Chapter 131). The small amount of EPO produced by patients after nephrectomy is derived from the liver and is sufficient to generate only a small portion of the required numbers of erythrocytes. Patients with chronic renal failure and particularly patients who have undergone bilateral nephrectomy have severe anemia, with hemoglobin values less than 5g/dL in the absence of exogenous EPO therapy or RBC transfusions. Rare patients with autoantibodies against EPO have extremely low to undetectable circulating EPO levels and severe anemia with pure RBC aplasia in the bone marrow. Patients with infectious or inflammatory diseases or cancer can also have anemia that is associated with inappropriately low levels of EPO for the degree of anemia; in these circumstances, cytokines such as interleukin-1 (IL-1), IL-6, or tumor necrosis factor-α may be responsible, at least in part, for the impaired EPO production.

Quantitative Deficiency of Hematopoietic Stem Cells and/or Committed Erythroid Progenitor Cells

A second mechanism of anemia caused by reduced production of cells by the bone marrow is deficiency of hematopoietic stem cells or committed erythroid progenitor cells, or both. Any condition that is characterized by a deficiency of hematopoietic stem cells or committed erythroid precursor cells also results in anemia. Even if EPO production is appropriately increased for the degree of anemia, anemia results if the target marrow precursor cells are deficient in number. In almost all such cases, the defect is a more generalized bone marrow abnormality that results in reduced production of all lineages of bone marrow–derived cells, particularly erythrocytes, granulocytes, and platelets. Idiopathic bone marrow failure, commonly called *aplastic anemia*, is the prototype of these disorders (Chapter 171). Bone marrow aplasia or hypoplasia may also occur as a result of toxic substances such as benzene; cancer chemotherapeutic agents; other pharmacologic agents such as chloramphenicol or gold salts; ionizing radiation; or certain viral infections such as with Epstein-Barr virus, human immunodeficiency virus (HIV), hepatitis (non-A, non-B, non-C) virus, or dengue virus. Other conditions, such as bone marrow fibrosis (myelofibrosis; Chapter 177) or extensive replacement of bone marrow by neoplastic cells, can also result in deficiencies of hematopoietic stem and progenitor cells or impaired ability of these cells to proliferate and differentiate into mature hematopoietic cells. Patients with severe malnutrition (Chapter 234), including anorexia nervosa, may likewise have bone marrow hypoplasia. In addition, a few patients with myelodysplasia (Chapter 193) or paroxysmal nocturnal hemoglobinuria have significant bone marrow hypoplasia. Selective anemia is also seen in pure RBC aplasia; this disorder usually has an immunologic basis, with selective immune-mediated destruction of erythroid progenitor cells and absence or near absence of detectable nucleated erythroid precursors in bone marrow despite elevated levels of circulating EPO. Viral infection, particularly with parvovirus B19, which selectively infects committed erythroid progenitor cells, can also cause transient or prolonged pure RBC aplasia because of the cytotoxic effect of this virus on the infected erythroid precursor cells.

TABLE 162–2 PATHOPHYSIOLOGIC CLASSIFICATION OF ANEMIAS CAUSED BY IMPAIRED PRODUCTION OF ERYTHROCYTES BY BONE MARROW

Erythropoietin (EPO) deficiency (normocytic anemias)
- Renal insufficiency (worse after bilateral nephrectomy)
- Pure red cell aplasia as a result of anti-EPO antibodies (extremely rare)
- Anemia of inflammation (an inappropriately low EPO level is a partial contributing factor)

Quantitative deficiency of hematopoietic/erythroid progenitor cells (normocytic anemias)
- Idiopathic bone marrow aplasia/hypoplasia
- Secondary bone marrow aplasia/hypoplasia (drugs, toxins, infections, radiation, malnutrition)
- Myelofibrosis (primary or secondary)
- Bone marrow replacement by neoplastic cells (myelophthisis)
- Myelodysplasia (minority of myelodysplasia patients)
- Paroxysmal nocturnal hemoglobinuria (10-15% of PNH patients)
- Pure red cell aplasia (antierythroid precursor cell antibodies, parvovirus B19 infection)

Impaired DNA synthesis and erythroid precursor cell division (macrocytic/megaloblastic anemias)
- Cobalamin (vitamin B_{12}) deficiency
- Folate deficiency
- Myelodysplasia
- Cancer chemotherapeutic drugs and some immunosuppressive and antimicrobial drugs

Impaired heme synthesis in differentiating erythroid cells (microcytic anemias)
- Iron deficiency
- Anemia of inflammation
- Sideroblastic anemias (particularly hereditary forms)

Impaired globin synthesis in differentiating erythroid cells (microcytic anemias)
- Thalassemias

Impaired Ability of Erythroid Progenitors to Respond to Erythropoietin

A third general mechanism responsible for reduced erythrocyte production by the bone marrow is impaired responsiveness of erythroid precursors to appropriate circulating EPO concentrations. This category covers a broad range of disorders, including intrinsic erythrocyte abnormalities, exogenous inhibitory effects, and nutritional deficiencies. No mutations or abnormalities of EPO receptors or EPO-related signal transduction pathways in erythroid precursors have been identified as causes of anemia thus far. There are many potential ways to categorize this large, diverse group of anemias. One method is to divide these conditions pathophysiologically into conditions in which there is impaired DNA synthesis and cell division and conditions in which there is impaired synthesis of hemoglobin.

Disorders Characterized by Impaired DNA Synthesis: Megaloblastic Anemias

Impaired DNA synthesis and the resulting impaired cell division by erythroid precursors result in RBC macrocytosis (increased MCV) and variable degrees of anemia (Chapter 170). These abnormalities may occur whenever there is a significant deficiency of key substrates in the DNA synthetic pathways, as caused by deficiencies in cobalamin (vitamin B_{12}) and folate. Folate deficiency may frequently be due to insufficient dietary intake but may also be due to diffuse intestinal disorders and drugs that interfere with folate metabolism, such as ethanol, sulfonamides or sulfa-related drugs, trimethoprim, methotrexate, anticonvulsants, and possibly oral contraceptives. Folate deficiency may occur in individuals with an increased requirement for folate, such as patients with chronic hemolytic anemia, pregnant women, and children. In addition, severe alcoholics, patients with general malnutrition from any cause, and patients with certain unconventional dietary habits are susceptible to the development of folate deficiency. A severely folate-deficient diet results in clinically significant folate deficiency within about 6 weeks. Cobalamin deficiency almost never occurs because of lack of dietary cobalamin intake; instead, it is most often due to impaired absorption of cobalamin as a result of a lack of intrinsic factor, gastric atrophy, and abnormalities of cobalamin absorption in the terminal ileum. Because of substantial stores and low daily requirements for cobalamin in normal individuals, deficiency of cobalamin usually takes at least 3 to 5 years to become manifest. In patients with myelodysplasia, one of the mechanisms of anemia and other hematopoietic cell deficiencies can be a moderately severe to severe impairment in DNA synthesis, with the development of megaloblastosis and macrocytosis. A broad range of cancer chemotherapeutic agents impair DNA synthesis in the short term, and some cause stem cell damage that can result in long-term adverse effects on DNA synthesis, which may result in mild to moderate anemia or may be manifested only by an increased MCV. In association with the reduced DNA synthesis and delays in or decreased number of cell divisions in megaloblastic anemias, there is generally intramedullary death of hematopoietic precursors, predominantly by apoptosis, and reduced numbers of mature erythrocytes and sometimes granulocytes and platelets released into blood. This condition of hypercellular bone marrow combined with the death of precursors before full maturation of hematopoietic cells is called *ineffective hematopoiesis* or, in the case of RBCs alone, ineffective erythropoiesis.

Impaired Hemoglobin Synthesis: Disorders Characterized by Diminished Heme Synthesis

Impaired hemoglobin synthesis occurs with disorders in which there is reduced production of either heme or globin and, when sufficiently severe, results in microcytic anemias (decreased MCV; Chapter 163). Most or all of the rare disorders collectively called *hereditary sideroblastic anemias* seem to be due to mutations in the coding regions of genes for the erythroid-specific forms of heme synthetic pathway enzymes or erythroid-specific promoters (especially 5-aminolevulinate synthase, hydroxymethylbilane synthase, and possibly ferrochelatase); the result is reduced heme synthesis in erythroid cells. Iron is required for the final stage of synthesis of heme, and iron deficiency impairs heme synthesis and results in anemia. Although iron deficiency anemia is classically associated with microcytosis, most patients with mild iron deficiency anemia actually have normocytic erythrocytes. Over time, iron-deficient patients commonly have a progressive decrease in MCV within the normal range, and microcytosis occurs generally in the most severe 20 to 30% of cases. In patients with acute or chronic infectious or inflammatory diseases or with cancer, the responsiveness of erythroid precursors to endogenous and exogenous EPO may be impaired. The mechanisms responsible for this impaired responsiveness to EPO are not understood completely, but most recent evidence indicates that induction of hepcidin by inflammatory cytokines leads to impaired iron accessibility for erythropoiesis. One of the hallmarks of anemia of inflammation is impaired transfer of iron into developing erythroid cells, which leads to a functional iron deficiency in normoblasts even when iron stores in bone marrow and the rest of the body are adequate. The result is impaired heme synthesis and a mild to moderate normocytic or microcytic anemia. In many of the circumstances in which anemia of inflammation occurs, there may be concomitant iron deficiency.

Impaired Hemoglobin Synthesis: Disorders Characterized by Impaired Globin Synthesis—Thalassemias

Impaired synthesis of α-globin chains in α-thalassemias or β-globin chains in β-thalassemias results in unbalanced synthesis of globin chains and a reduction in the number of hemoglobin $\alpha2/\beta2$ tetramers (Chapter 166). Because of the reduced numbers of hemoglobin tetramer molecules in each cell, thalassemia patients have a microcytic anemia. The unpaired excess β-chains in the erythrocytes of patients with α-thalassemia and the unpaired excess α-chains in patients with β-thalassemia tend to aggregate, precipitate, and form insoluble cytoplasmic inclusion bodies that result in oxidative damage to the membranes of developing normoblasts and death of a large proportion of these developing erythroid cells within the marrow, thereby leading to anemia secondary to ineffective erythropoiesis. The normoblasts that do survive produce erythrocytes that contain similar inclusions (Heinz bodies), which leads to premature destruction of these cells in the spleen and liver and results in a hemolytic component of the anemia. The overall degree of anemia is related to the severity of the defect in globin synthesis, so patients who have deletion of only one of their four α-globin genes generally have microcytosis but no anemia, patients with deletion of two α-globin genes have microcytosis and mild anemia, and patients who are heterozygous for β-thalassemia have microcytosis and mild anemia.

Ineffective Erythropoiesis

Ineffective erythropoiesis is defined as anemia with increased numbers of erythroid precursor cells in bone marrow but decreased numbers of mature circulating erythrocytes being released from bone marrow. In ineffective erythropoiesis, there are inappropriately low numbers of reticulocytes in blood. This condition is usually caused by defects in the maturing proerythroblasts and normoblasts in bone marrow and results in their premature death within the bone marrow, usually by apoptosis. The most common causes of anemia secondary to ineffective erythropoiesis are myelodysplasia, megaloblastic anemias, and thalassemias.

Anemias Caused by Accelerated Destruction, Consumption, or Loss of Circulating Erythrocytes

Any intrinsic defects in erythrocytes or extrinsic conditions that cause erythrocytes to be damaged intravascularly, removed from the circulation prematurely by the spleen or liver, or lost through bleeding result in increased EPO production, increased numbers of maturing erythroid precursors in bone marrow, and release of increased numbers of newly formed reticulocytes into blood. In a patient with normal bone marrow, accelerated loss of circulating erythrocytes is always associated with increased erythropoiesis, which can be judged by the presence of an increased reticulocyte count. An increased reticulocyte count implies that there is at least a mildly increased rate of loss or destruction of erythrocytes. If the bone marrow is able to keep up with the increased demand for replacement erythrocytes, the patient will not have a decreased RBC mass. Anemia occurs only if the rate of production of erythrocytes by bone marrow is unable to compensate completely for the loss or destruction of RBCs. Although chronic hemolysis or blood loss is associated with compensatory increased erythropoiesis (assuming no additional abnormalities in the bone marrow, kidney, or required nutrients), signs of compensatory increased erythropoiesis do not appear until several days after acute hemolysis or blood loss.

Hemolytic Anemias Caused by Intrinsic Red Blood Cell Membrane Defects

Abnormalities in RBC membrane proteins and lipids lead to deformed erythrocytes, which are prone to be removed prematurely from the circulation, primarily by the filtering functions of the spleen (Chapter 165). The most common membrane protein abnormalities involve spectrin, ankyrin, band 3 protein, and protein 4.1 and lead to the RBC membranopathies known as *hereditary spherocytosis, hereditary elliptocytosis,* and *hereditary pyropoikilocytosis.* In each of these disorders, the decreased deformability of RBCs results in their premature clearance from blood, primarily in the spleen. Abnormalities in the lipid bilayer of the erythrocyte membrane lead to bizarrely shaped RBCs that have poor deformability and cytoplasmic projections that result in an increased rate of destruction of erythrocytes, primarily in the spleen. One abnormality of the lipid bilayer is acanthocytosis or spur cell anemia, which may be caused by hereditary lipoprotein defects such as abetalipoproteinemia, cholesterol metabolism abnormalities that occur in patients with severe liver disease, or the McLeod phenotype of severely deficient Kell blood group antigen on erythrocytes. Stomatocytes or xerocytes result from an imbalance in the size of the outer and inner portions of the membrane lipid bilayer and dehydration of erythrocytes; abnormalities in membrane phospholipids or absence of Rh antigens on the surface of RBCs (Rh null phenotype) result in these morphologic abnormalities, which may lead to mild hemolysis. In paroxysmal nocturnal hemoglobinuria, a defect in a crucial membrane-anchoring molecule (glycosylphosphatidylinositol) that is responsible for anchoring many cell surface proteins results in the absence of at least three surface proteins essential for the prevention of complement-mediated cell damage and lysis. Absence or a significant reduction in decay accelerating factor (DAF, CD55), membrane inhibitor of reactive lysis (MIRL, CD59), and C8-binding protein results in variably increased susceptibility of these defective cells to lysis by complement.

Hemolytic Anemias Caused by Intrinsic Red Blood Cell Enzymopathies

RBC enzymopathies (Chapter 165) that may lead to hemolytic anemia generally fall into two groups. Defects in enzymes in the hexose monophosphate shunt (e.g., glucose-6-phosphate dehydrogenase) or enzymes responsible for maintaining reduced glutathione (e.g., γ-glutamylcysteine synthetase) to prevent oxidative injury to RBCs most frequently tend to be associated with episodic hemolysis during times of physiologic stress, such as surgery, infections, or oxidants in foods or pharmacologic agents. The oxidant damage causes Heinz body formation. In contrast, deficiencies of enzymes in the Embden-Meyerhof pathway (e.g., pyruvate kinase and glucose phosphate isomerase) or enzymes responsible for supporting nucleotide metabolism (e.g., adenosine deaminase and pyrimidine 5′-nucleotidase) tend to cause chronic hemolytic anemias, presumably as a result of adenosine phosphate deficiency, which leads to impaired homeostasis of water, sodium, potassium, and calcium. Because erythrocytes are unable to synthesize new proteins, older erythrocytes are most likely to have the lowest levels of enzymes that are susceptible to intracellular degradation and are the most likely to be removed from the circulation.

Hemolytic Anemias Caused by Hemoglobin Variants with Reduced Solubility or Protein Instability

More than 100 different structural variants of hemoglobin exhibit either reduced solubility (e.g., hemoglobins S, C, O Arab, and D Los Angeles) or a higher susceptibility than normal to oxidation of amino acids within the globin chains (e.g., hemoglobins Zurich, Köln, Hammersmith, and Gun Hill) (Chapter 168). The less soluble and more unstable hemoglobins tend to form abnormal hemoglobin polymers or crystals, precipitate, and form cytoplasmic Heinz bodies, which then become attached to the cell membrane and decrease erythrocyte deformability; the result is membrane damage, followed by sequestration and destruction of erythrocytes in the spleen.

Hemolytic Anemias Caused by Abnormalities Extrinsic to the Red Blood Cell

Erythrocytes can be sequestered or destroyed prematurely as a result of other conditions that secondarily cause damage to otherwise normal RBCs. In autoimmune hemolytic anemia, antibodies form against RBC membrane antigens (most commonly Rh-D antigen for so-called warm IgG antibodies and I or i antigen for so-called cold, complement-fixing IgM antibodies) (Chapter 164). These antibody-coated erythrocytes are recognized by Fc or complement receptors on macrophages in the spleen (especially IgG) or liver (especially C3 complement). IgG-coated RBCs usually undergo repeated partial phagocytosis with progressive loss of RBC membrane until the cells that survive and reenter the circulation are spherocytes, which have decreased deformability and are eventually sequestered and permanently removed from the circulation. A long list of drugs can result in hemolysis via similar mechanisms by causing antierythrocyte antibodies or by causing antidrug antibodies that lead to subsequent immune complex deposition on erythrocytes, which also results in hemolysis by similar mechanisms. Alloimmune hemolysis may result from transfusion of blood with "minor" blood group mismatches into recipients previously sensitized to those antigens by prior transfusions or pregnancies (or both). Severe acute intravascular hemolysis (Chapter 164) can occur from transfusion of ABO-incompatible blood and less commonly from transfusion of blood that has Rh or so-called minor blood group antigen mismatches. Microangiopathic hemolysis with fragmented erythrocytes, intravascular release of hemoglobin and other erythrocyte contents, and intravascular and splenic destruction of RBCs occur in the presence of fibrin deposition in small arterioles, in conditions such as thrombotic thrombocytopenic purpura and disseminated intravascular coagulation, and in the presence of diffuse small vessel vasculitis, eclampsia, or malignant hypertension. Prosthetic heart valves or arterial grafts with roughened endothelial surfaces can also cause mechanical fragmentation of erythrocytes. Trauma (e.g., march hemoglobinuria), thermal injury from severe burns, and osmotic lysis secondary to freshwater drowning or mistaken intravenous infusion of high volumes of hypotonic fluids are additional causes of mechanical damage to otherwise normal erythrocytes. Certain infections, such as malaria, bartonellosis, and babesiosis, can cause direct intravascular destruction of infected erythrocytes, and clostridial sepsis can result in the release of toxins that directly damage RBC membrane phospholipids and massive intravascular lysis of RBCs. Certain snake and spider venoms can cause hemolysis (i.e., cobra venom via phospholipases that destroy the erythrocyte membrane and pit viper and brown recluse spider venoms via induction of disseminated intravascular coagulation). Finally, many drugs and ingested toxins, including nitrofurantoin, phenazopyridine, sulfones, amyl nitrite, naphthalene mothballs, paraquat, and hydrogen peroxide, can cause direct oxidative damage to erythrocytes. Several cancer chemotherapeutic agents probably also cause oxidant or membrane damage (or both), which can result in anemia within a few days after drug administration.

Blood Loss

Although anemia is obvious with acute blood loss, it may be much more difficult to document slow, chronic blood loss, in which case the bone marrow is almost always able to compensate until the patient becomes iron deficient. The gastrointestinal tract is a major site of chronic blood loss (Chapter 137). Malignancies, gastritis, peptic ulcer disease, inflammatory bowel disease, diverticulitis, proctitis, hemorrhoidal bleeding, angiodysplasia, arteriovenous malformations, and hereditary hemorrhagic telangiectasia (Osler-Weber-Rendu syndrome) are among the major causes of chronic or intermittent gastrointestinal blood loss. Chronic excessive menstrual blood loss, chronic urinary tract bleeding, and recurrent epistaxis can also lead to iron deficiency and anemia. In addition, because of the substantial consumption of maternal iron by the developing fetus, multiple pregnancies may contribute to the development of iron deficiency and anemia. Patients with chronic intravascular hemolysis (e.g., paroxysmal nocturnal hemoglobinuria, malaria, or traumatic hemolysis from a prosthetic cardiac valve) lose hemoglobin in urine and may become iron deficient and anemic. The blood drawn from and lost by a hospitalized patient can also contribute to an otherwise unexplained recent anemia, especially in patients who are unable to mount an erythropoietic response.

Dilutional Pseudoanemia

Certain conditions lead to an expansion of plasma volume, which results in decreased hemoglobin, hematocrit, and RBC count without any decrease in the patient's total RBC mass. The chronic intravascular volume expansion that occurs in pregnancy can reduce the hemoglobin concentration to 10 g/dL. Acute volume overload can also cause a dilutional decrease in the concentration of RBCs, which resolves after equilibration and diuresis occur. Certain medications, particularly some cytokines such as IL-2 and granulocyte-macrophage colony-stimulating factor, may likewise cause acute dilutional pseudoanemia.

Clinical Manifestations

There are three main types of clinical manifestations of anemia. In anemia that has developed rapidly, symptoms related to hypotension may develop as a result of loss of blood volume. In chronic and acute anemias, tissue and organ hypoxia is a major source of symptoms, although eventually orthostatic and nonorthostatic hypotension and tachycardia may occur secondary to chronically decreased blood volume. In hemolytic anemias, the toxicity of products of lysed erythrocytes may also cause specific clinical findings. The signs and symptoms of anemia can vary widely from patient to patient with the same degree and tempo of anemia. The major factors that determine the specific response of each individual to anemia include the severity of the anemia, the rapidity of onset of the anemia, the age of the patient, the patient's overall physical condition, and comorbid events or disorders. Mild anemia is often associated with no clinical symptoms and may be discovered only when a complete blood cell count is performed for another reason. The earliest clinical symptoms of mild to moderate anemia tend to be a sense of fatigue, generalized weakness, and loss of stamina, followed by tachycardia and exertional dyspnea. In young, healthy patients, these symptoms are not frequently noticed until the hemoglobin level decreases to less than 7 or 8 g/dL. In elderly patients and those with cardiovascular or pulmonary disease, symptoms may occur with even modest degrees of anemia and hemoglobin levels of 9 to 11 g/dL. Modest increases in the hemoglobin level can sometimes result in an improved quality of life, even though symptoms may not be obvious before correction of the anemia.

Physiologic Compensatory Mechanisms

The five main physiologic compensatory responses to anemia vary in prominence, depending on rapidity of onset and duration of the anemia and the condition of the patient. First, in acute-onset anemia with severe loss of intravascular volume, peripheral vasoconstriction and central vasodilation preserve blood flow to vital organs. Second, over time and with increasingly severe anemia, systemic small vessel vasodilation results in increased blood flow to ensure better tissue oxygenation. These vascular compensations lead to decreased systemic vascular resistance, increased cardiac output, and tachycardia, which result in a higher rate of delivery of oxygen-bearing erythrocytes to tissues. Third, an increased level of 2,3-diphosphoglycerate accumulates in RBCs and interacts with hemoglobin molecules to cause a rightward shift of the hemoglobin oxygen dissociation curve, which in turn enhances the release of oxygen to tissues at any given partial pressure of oxygen. Fourth, in chronic anemias there is a compensatory increase in plasma volume that maintains total blood volume and enhances tissue perfusion. The fifth compensatory response in otherwise normal individuals is stimulation of EPO production, which in turn stimulates new erythrocyte production. The latter occurs if the stem cells and erythroid precursors are normal, the erythroid precursors are able to respond normally to EPO, and the developing normoblasts are normal.

Clinical Manifestations of Chronic Anemia

Weakness, fatigue, lethargy, decreased stamina, palpitations, dyspnea on exertion, and orthostatic light-headedness are common symptoms in patients with chronic anemia, although the compensatory mechanisms described earlier may prevent these symptoms from being manifested in patients with mild or moderate anemia. Occasional patients with slowly developing or long-standing anemia may report being asymptomatic with hemoglobin levels of 5 or 6 g/dL, although virtually all such patients notice a distinct improvement in their performance status after correction of the anemia. As is true of acute anemias, comorbid conditions, particularly with impaired blood supply or oxygenation of specific organs, may result in symptoms and signs secondary to organ-specific dysfunction. Anemic patients with previous myocardial dysfunction may have more pronounced edema, dyspnea, orthopnea, tachycardia, fatigue, and loss of stamina. In patients with coronary artery disease, anemia may result in the onset or worsening of angina or may precipitate myocardial infarction. New or worsening claudication may develop in anemic patients with significant peripheral arterial disease. Anemic patients with cerebrovascular disease may experience decreased cognition and more frequent or severe transient ischemic attacks or strokes.

In patients who are anemic without an immediately obvious cause, careful probing of the patient's past medical and family history is essential. In particular, it is important to obtain the results of previous blood cell counts to determine whether the anemia is of recent or even lifelong duration. A careful, in-depth discussion of the personal and family history can be helpful, particularly if positive for anemia, splenectomy, cholecystectomy, gallstones, or jaundice at birth or later in life. The new mutation rate for congenital/hereditary hemolytic anemias is sufficiently high, however, that lack of a family history should not deter one from a search for these conditions if the remainder of the clinical picture is compatible with a congenital hemolytic anemia. Mild hereditary and congenital hemolytic anemias sometimes escape detection until patients are elderly or a second event compromises the ability of the patient's bone marrow to compensate for the chronic, excessive rate of destruction of erythrocytes. In some patients, past treatment may have been inappropriate or ineffective because of inadequate evaluation and incorrect diagnosis.

The most prominent general physical examination findings that may occur in patients with significant anemia include pallor of the skin, especially under the nails, and mucosal surfaces (Fig. 162–1), orthostatic hypotension, resting or orthostatic tachycardia, a systolic ejection murmur, increased prominence of the cardiac apical impulse, bounding pulses, and a wide pulse pressure. The presence of splenomegaly or a history of previous splenectomy raises the possibility of chronic hemolytic anemia. A right upper quadrant surgical scar or a history of gallstones or cholecystectomy (or both) should also raise the possibility of a chronic hemolytic state with the formation of bilirubin-containing gallstones.

General Clinical Manifestations of Acute Development of Anemia from Blood Loss or Hemolysis

In a patient with severe acute hemolysis or blood loss, prominent early symptoms include resting or orthostatic hypotension from a decrease in total blood volume, along with subsequent light-headedness or syncope, exertional or resting tachycardia (or both) and palpitations, diaphoresis, anxiety, agitation, generalized severe weakness and lethargy, and possibly decreased mental function. All of the physical examination findings described earlier for chronic anemias tend to be more pronounced with anemias of rapid onset that also are complicated by acute loss of intravascular blood volume. Depending on the severity of the anemia and blood volume depletion, comorbid conditions, age, and overall health, there may also be signs of oxygen deprivation in one or multiple organ systems. Loss of 25 to 35% of total blood volume in 12 to 24 hours cannot be ameliorated by the normal compensatory mechanisms, and loss of more than 40% of blood volume in 12 hours leads to profound symptoms resulting more from intravascular volume depletion than from anemia.

Diseases of Other Body Systems That Can Cause or Be Associated with Anemia

A broad spectrum of disorders of other organ systems can give rise to anemia. Any chronic infection, chronic inflammatory disease, or malignant disease can result in anemia of inflammation (Chapter 169). Recently, it has been recognized that conditions such as heart failure and diabetes mellitus, which may not have been considered to be inflammatory disorders in the past, are associated with sufficiently increased levels of mediators of inflammation to induce anemia of inflammation. In addition, elderly patients with anemia have been found to have elevated levels of circulating inflammatory cytokines, even in the absence of clinical evidence of inflammatory disease. Thus, what has been called anemia of chronic disease in the past is now more accurately designated as anemia of inflammation or, in some cases, as anemia of chronic inflammation. Autoimmune hemolytic anemia may develop in patients with lymphoproliferative and rheumatologic diseases. Moderate to severe renal insufficiency can cause anemia secondary to impaired EPO production. Any cause of marked splenomegaly, including myeloprolifera-

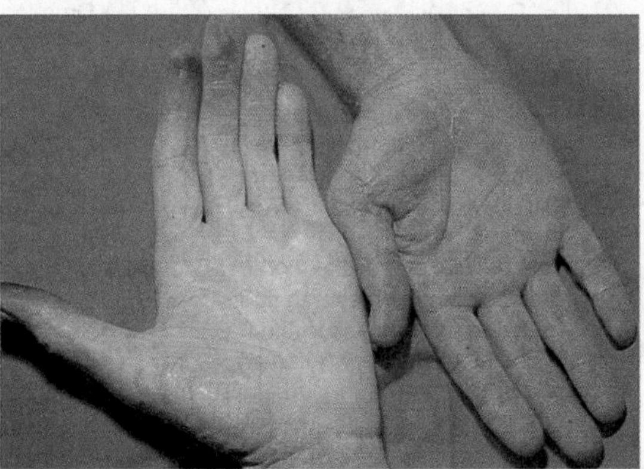

FIGURE 162–1 • Chronic anemia. Pallor of the hand in anemia is obvious in this patient, especially when compared with the physician's hand on the right. The patient's hemoglobin concentration was 7 g/dL. The hand also shows that the patient was a heavy smoker. His anemia resulted from chronic blood loss from a carcinoma in the esophagus, a site where the risk for carcinoma is increased in smokers. (From Forbes CD, Jackson WF: Color Atlas and Text of Clinical Medicine, 3rd ed. London, Mosby, 2003.)

tive and lymphoproliferative disorders, certain chronic infectious diseases (e.g., malaria, tuberculosis), portal vein thrombosis, or portal hypertension, may cause excessive RBC sequestration and destruction. Gastritis, peptic ulcer disease, gastrointestinal angiodysplasia, and hereditary hemorrhagic telangiectasia are frequently associated with chronic blood loss that leads to iron deficiency and anemia. Iron deficiency can also be caused by removal or significant dysfunction (e.g., Whipple's disease, Crohn's disease) of the duodenum, which is the major site of iron absorption. Anti–gastric parietal cell antibodies, gastric achlorhydria, previous gastrectomy, intestinal bacterial overgrowth, or dysfunction (e.g., inflammatory bowel disease) or surgical removal of the terminal ileum can result in cobalamin deficiency and anemia. Gastroduodenal bypass surgery for the treatment of obesity frequently causes chronic iron deficiency as a result of loss of duodenal absorption of iron, as well as chronic vitamin B_{12} deficiency as a result of loss of intrinsic factor. Patients with hypopituitarism or hypothyroidism may have a mild macrocytic anemia. Severe alcoholics may be susceptible to folate deficiency from poor dietary intake, iron deficiency from chronic gastric blood loss, or toxic suppression of bone marrow resulting in decreased erythropoiesis. Patients with severe liver disease often have shortened RBC survival secondary to splenomegaly caused by portal hypertension or secondary to excess deposition of unesterified cholesterol on erythrocyte membranes and the resulting formation of acanthocytes and schistocytes, which are cleared from the blood prematurely. Anemia is a common manifestation of HIV infection and may be multifactorial, including contributions from cytokine-mediated anemia of inflammation, relative EPO deficiency, malnutrition, myelodysplastic changes in bone marrow, bone marrow fibrosis and necrosis, immune-mediated hemolysis, and drug-induced (e.g., zidovudine) myelosuppression.

Diagnosis

Laboratory Evaluation

The initial diagnostic evaluation (Fig. 162–2) of anemia is based on using readily available information, including a careful in-depth evaluation of the patient's past medical and family history (Table 162–3), physical examination (splenomegaly is the most important physical finding in an anemic patient), complete blood cell count, reticulocyte count, and microscopic evaluation of the peripheral blood smear (Table 162–4). More specialized laboratory tests are indicated only after these screening studies have been obtained. In a patient with anemia, the first distinction

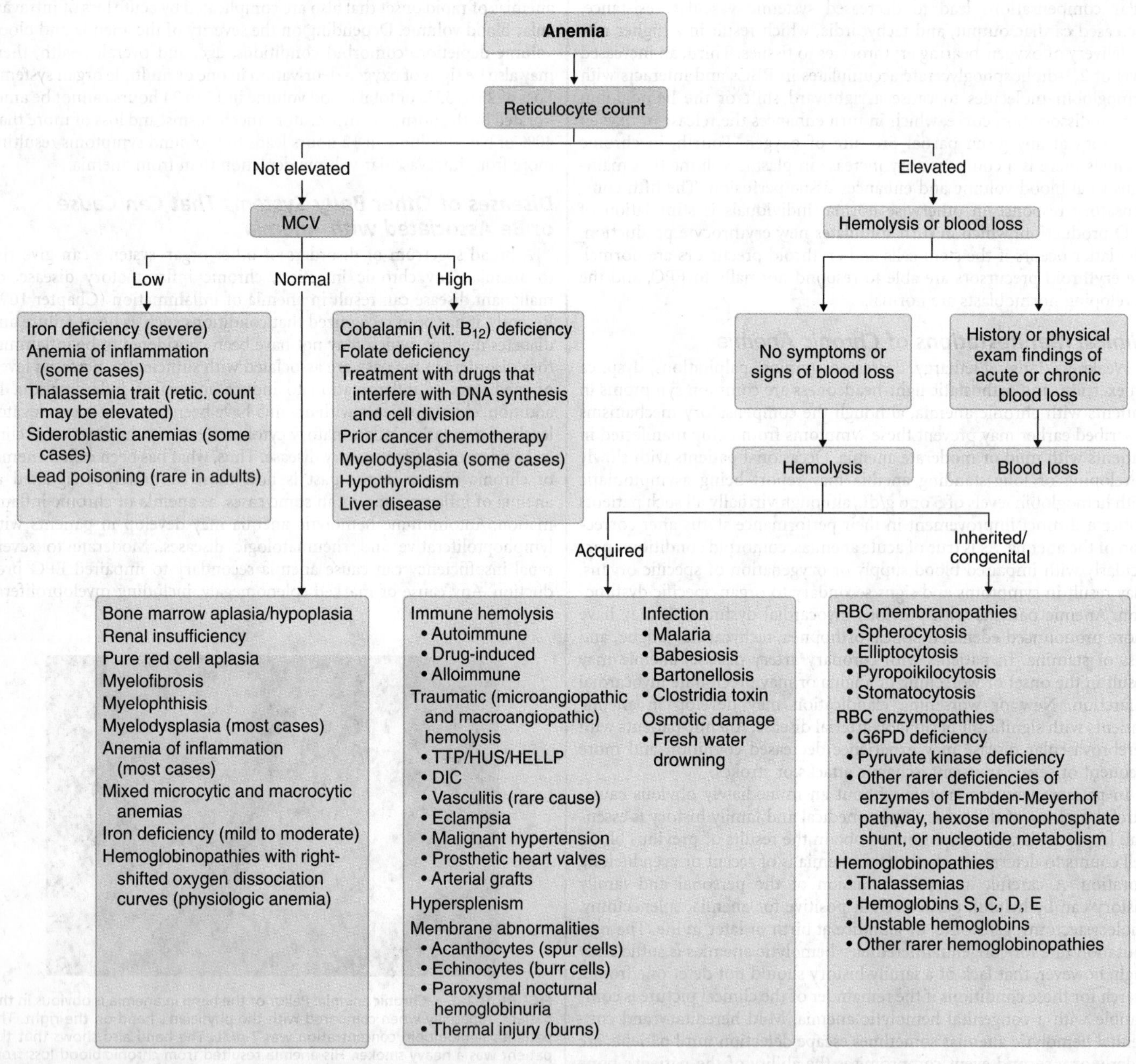

FIGURE 162–2 • Algorithm for the diagnosis of anemias. DIC = disseminated intravascular coagulation; G6PD = glucose-6-phosphate dehydrogenase; HELLP = *h*emolysis, *e*levated *l*iver (function tests), *l*ow *p*latelets; HUS = hemolytic uremic syndrome; MCV = mean corpuscular volume; RBC = red blood cell; TTP = thrombotic thrombocytopenic purpura.

TABLE 162–3 USE OF THE PERSONAL AND FAMILY MEDICAL HISTORY IN DIAGNOSIS OF ANEMIAS

History: Signs and Symptoms	Possible Etiology of Anemia
Known normal complete blood cell count in the past	Probably not a hereditary/congenital disorder
Anemia known since childhood	Inherited/congenital hemolytic anemia or (less likely) bone marrow hypoplasia
Splenectomy, gallstones, and/or jaundice	Chronic hemolytic anemia, liver disease
Family history of splenectomy, gallstones, and/or jaundice	Hereditary hemolytic anemia (RBC enzyme or membrane disorder, thalassemia, or hemoglobinopathy)
Poor or unconventional diet, malnutrition, or severe alcoholism	Bone marrow hypoplasia, folate deficiency
Paresthesias, foot numbness, loss of balance, altered mental status	Cobalamin (vitamin B_{12}) deficiency
Gastrectomy, surgical removal of the ileum, chronic malabsorption disorder	Cobalamin (vitamin B_{12}) deficiency
Chronic gastritis, peptic ulcer disease, chronic use of ASA or NSAIDs, recurrent epistaxis or rectal bleeding, melena, menorrhagia, metrorrhagia, multiple pregnancies, duodenal surgery, gastrectomy	Iron deficiency
Chronic rheumatologic, immunologic, infectious, or neoplastic disease	Anemia of inflammation, autoimmune hemolytic anemia
Decreased urine output	Anemia secondary to renal insufficiency
Dark urine	Hemolytic anemia (intravascular hemolysis)
Recent onset of infections, mucosal and skin bleeding, easy bruising, oral ulcerations	Bone marrow aplasia/hypoplasia, acute leukemia, myelodysplasia, myelophthisis
Occupational/environmental toxin exposure (benzene, ionizing radiation, lead)	Bone marrow aplasia/hypoplasia, acute leukemia, myelodysplasia, lead poisoning
Drug/medication exposure:	
Penicillin, cephalosporin, procainamide, quinidine, quinine, sulfonamide	Drug-induced immune hemolytic anemia
Fava beans, dapsone, naphthalene	Oxidant-induced hemolysis (G6PD deficient)
Cancer chemotherapeutic drugs (recent use)	Bone marrow aplasia/hypoplasia, oxidant damage, fluid retention/dilutional anemia, megaloblastic anemia
Cancer chemotherapeutic drugs (past use)	Bone marrow hypoplasia, myelodysplasia, acute myeloid leukemia
Chloramphenicol, gold salts, sulfonamides, anti-inflammatory drugs	Bone marrow aplasia/hypoplasia
Ethanol, chloramphenicol	Acute reversible bone marrow toxicity
Methotrexate, azathioprine, pyrimethamine, trimethoprim, zidovudine, sulfa drugs, hydroxyurea, antimetabolites	Bone marrow aplasia/hypoplasia, megaloblastic anemia

ASA = acetylsalicylic acid (aspirin); G6PD = glucose-6-phosphate dehydrogenase; NSAIDs = nonsteroidal anti-inflammatory drugs; RBC = red blood cell.

TABLE 162–4 RED BLOOD CELL MORPHOLOGIC ABNORMALITIES AS CLUES TO THE DIAGNOSIS OF ANEMIAS

Red Blood Cell Morphology	Representative Causes of Anemia
Microcytosis	Iron deficiency, anemia of inflammation, thalassemia, and rarely, lead poisoning, vitamin B_6 deficiency, or hereditary sideroblastic anemias
Macrocytosis	Polychromatophilia (reticulocytes), vitamin B_{12} (cobalamin) or folate deficiency, myelodysplasia, use of drugs that inhibit DNA synthesis
Basophilic stippling	Hemolysis, lead poisoning, thalassemia
Target cells	Thalassemia; hemoglobins C, D, E, and S; liver disease; abetalipoproteinemia
Microspherocytes	Autoimmune hemolytic anemia, alloimmune hemolysis, hereditary spherocytosis, some cases of Heinz body hemolytic anemias
Schistocytes and fragmented RBCs	Thrombotic thrombocytopenic purpura, disseminated intravascular coagulation, vasculitis, malignant hypertension, eclampsia, traumatic hemolysis secondary to a prosthetic heart valve or damaged vascular graft, thermal injury (burns), post-splenectomy status
Teardrop cells	Myelofibrosis, myelophthisis (bone marrow infiltration by neoplastic cells)
Sickle cells	Hemoglobin SS, SC, or S–β-thalassemia
Acanthocytes (spur cells)	Severe liver disease, malnutrition, McLeod blood group phenotype
Echinocytes (burr cells)	Renal failure, hemolysis from malnutrition with hypomagnesemia and hypophosphatemia, pyruvate kinase deficiency, common in vitro artifact
Stomatocytes	Alcoholism, hereditary stomatocytosis
"Bite" cells or "blister" cells	Glucose-6-phosphate dehydrogenase deficiency, other oxidant-induced hemolysis, unstable hemoglobins
Howell-Jolly bodies	Post-splenectomy status, hyposplenism
Intraerythrocytic parasitic or bacterial inclusions	Malaria (parasites), babesiosis (parasites), bartonellosis (gram-negative coccobacilli)
Agglutinated RBCs	Cold agglutinin disease, in vitro artifact
Rouleaux formation	Multiple myeloma, monoclonal gammopathy of undetermined significance

to be made is whether the primary cause of the anemia is failure of the bone marrow to produce sufficient numbers of erythrocytes or accelerated loss or destruction of erythrocytes. A single test, the reticulocyte count, often provides the answer to this question. An elevated absolute reticulocyte count in an anemic patient indicates that the bone marrow is responding to the requirement for new erythrocyte production to replace prematurely destroyed or lost erythrocytes as a result of hemolysis or blood loss. A reticulocyte count that is below normal or below the level expected for the degree of anemia indicates an inability of the bone marrow to maintain the rate of production of RBCs required to compensate for those lost or destroyed and is the primary cause or a major contributing factor of the anemia.

Microscopic examination of the morphology of RBCs in a peripheral blood smear is an essential part of the evaluation of defective production and excessive destruction of RBCs (see Fig. 161–1). In a patient with an elevated reticulocyte count, specific morphologic changes in the RBCs observed on microscopic examination often make the diagnosis readily apparent or reduce the list of possible diagnoses considerably. The finding of sickle cells should lead to hemoglobin electrophoresis, which confirms the type of sickling disorder (see Fig. 161–9). A predominant finding of spherocytes means that the patient almost certainly has autoimmune or alloimmune hemolysis or hereditary spherocytosis (Fig. 162–3). The evaluation includes a careful past medical and family history (for the duration of anemia; medications; history of blood transfusions; anemia in other family members; and history of splenectomy, cholecystectomy, gallstones, and jaundice in the patient and family members). Examination of the patient (for splenomegaly, jaundice, or signs of autoimmune disorders) may be helpful.

Laboratory studies play a crucial role in diagnosis of the specific cause of anemia. The direct antiglobulin (Coombs) test or more sensitive tests of antierythrocyte antibodies help diagnose autoimmune hemolytic anemia, and the indirect antiglobulin test helps diagnose alloimmune hemolysis. Elevated levels of total and particularly indirect hyperbilirubinemia support a general diagnosis of hemolysis. Microcytic RBCs in a patient without an elevated reticulocyte count suggest iron deficiency (see Fig. 161–4), anemia of inflammation, or thalassemia trait (or in more severe cases, homozygous β-thalassemia or hemoglobin H disease) as the most likely cause. Sideroblastic anemia with or without myelodysplasia and lead poisoning are rare causes of microcytic anemia in adults. In microcytic anemia, helpful clues include the duration and severity of the anemia; previous menstrual and pregnancy history in women; dietary history; occupational history; history of gastric, duodenal, or ileal surgery; history of gastrointestinal, upper respiratory, or urinary tract bleeding; history of chronic infections or autoimmune or inflammatory disorders; response to previous therapy for anemia; and family history of anemia. A low or low normal RBC count and normal RDW favor anemia of inflammation, an elevated RDW favors iron deficiency, and a high normal or elevated RBC count and normal RDW favor thalassemia. Serum iron, iron-binding capacity, and particularly ferritin levels can often distinguish between anemia of inflammation and iron deficiency anemia (Table 162–5); in patients with anemia of inflammation, an elevated serum soluble transferrin receptor level favors the associated presence of iron deficiency. Determination of marrow iron stores on bone marrow aspiration or biopsy, the "gold standard" for determining iron stores for several decades, is rarely required for this purpose now.

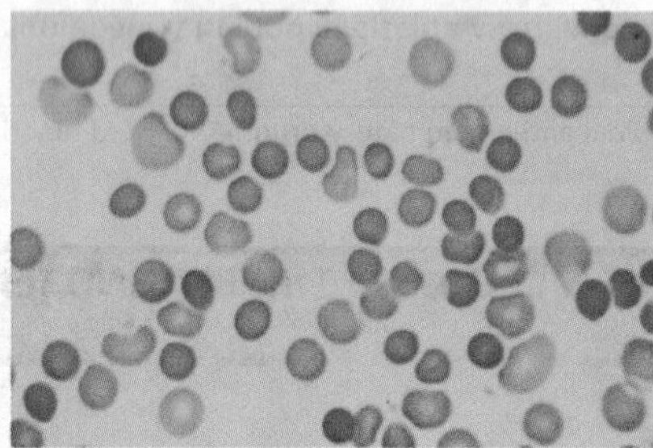

FIGURE 162–3 • Hereditary spherocytosis. A peripheral blood smear shows a predominance of microspherocytes (small, densely staining red blood cells with loss of the central areas of pallor) alongside larger, grayish, "polychromatic" cells that usually represent reticulocytes.

The diagnosis of myelodysplasia requires microscopic examination of bone marrow cell morphology, and diagnosis of sideroblastic anemia (see Fig. 163–5) also requires Prussian blue staining (for detection of iron) of normoblasts in the bone marrow (Table 162–6). If microcytosis and mild anemia with substantial numbers of target cells are present, thalassemia trait is the most likely diagnosis. β-Thalassemia heterozygotes can almost always be distinguished from α-thalassemia heterozygotes on the basis of an elevated hemoglobin A_2 level, as measured by chromatography (estimates of hemoglobin A_2 levels on starch gel electrophoresis are much less accurate). More sophisticated tests, including direct sequencing of the β-globin gene, may be needed to determine the specific type of β-thalassemia. α-Thalassemia can be diagnosed definitively only with globin chain synthesis studies, Southern blotting, polymerase chain reaction, or α-globin gene sequencing; however, a normal hemoglobin A_2 level in a patient with microcytosis, target cells, and no or mild anemia strongly suggests a one- or two-gene deletion α-thalassemia trait.

Differential Diagnosis

Patients often have multiple potential causes of anemia. A patient with a rheumatologic or lymphoproliferative disease may have anemia of inflammation but may also have a marked change in the severity of the anemia because of the development of autoimmune hemolysis. A patient with chronic hemolytic anemia, such as sickle cell disease, thalassemia, or hereditary spherocytosis, may become deficient in folate or infected with parvovirus B19, which prevents the bone marrow from continuing to overproduce erythrocytes and leads to a decreased number of reticulocytes and a resulting marked increase in the severity of the anemia. If the entire clinical picture cannot be explained by a single cause, the physician must search for secondary factors that may be important contributing components to the patient's anemia.

TABLE 162–5 LABORATORY TESTS TO DISTINGUISH IRON DEFICIENCY ANEMIA FROM ANEMIA OF (CHRONIC) INFLAMMATION (ACI OR AI)

Measurement	Units	Normal Values	Iron Deficiency	ACI/AI	ACI/AI + Iron Deficiency
Serum iron	µg/dL	50–150	↓	Low normal–↓	↓
Serum total iron-binding capacity	µg/dL	250–400	↑	Low normal–↓	Low normal–↓
Transferrin saturation	%	20–50	↓	Normal–↓	Low normal–↓
Serum ferritin	µg/L	20–350	↓	Normal–↑	Normal–↓
Serum soluble transferrin receptor	nM	9–28	↑	Normal	↑
Bone marrow iron stores	0–4+	2–3+	↓	Normal	↓
Iron-containing normoblasts in bone marrow	%	20–80%	↓	↓	↓

TABLE 162–6 SELECTED LABORATORY STUDIES THAT ARE USEFUL IN THE DIAGNOSIS OF ANEMIAS

If This Is Considered to Be a Possible Cause of a Patient's Anemia	These Are Potentially Useful Diagnostic Laboratory Tests
HYPOPROLIFERATIVE ANEMIAS	
Bone marrow aplasia/hypoplasia or myelophthisis	Platelet count, white blood cell count with differential, bone marrow aspirate and biopsy
Myelodysplasia	Bone marrow aspirate and biopsy (including Prussian blue stain of iron), karyotype analysis
Acute leukemia	Bone marrow aspirate and biopsy, flow cytometry, immunohistochemical staining, karyotype analysis
Myelofibrosis	Bone marrow biopsy with stains for collagen (trichrome stain) and reticulin (silver stain)
Iron deficiency	Serum iron, TIBC, ferritin, soluble transferrin receptor (± bone marrow iron stain)
Anemia of inflammation	Serum iron, TIBC, ferritin, soluble transferrin receptor (± bone marrow iron stain)
Folate deficiency	Red blood cell folate level, serum folate level, bone marrow aspirate
Vitamin B_{12} (cobalamin) deficiency	Serum vitamin B_{12} level, urine (± serum) methylmalonic acid level, bone marrow aspirate, Schilling tests
HEMOLYTIC ANEMIAS	
General measures of hemolysis (intravascular [I] and extravascular [E])	Reduction in serum haptoglobin (I > E), presence of urine hemoglobin (I) and/or urine hemosiderin (I), increased serum LDH (I > E) and serum unconjugated bilirubin (I > E)
Thalassemias	Hemoglobin A_2 level, globin DNA analysis (Southern blotting, polymerase chain reaction, sequencing), globin chain synthesis ratios, hemoglobin electrophoresis (looking for mutated globins with altered electrophoretic mobility, which result in a thalassemia phenotype)
Sickle cell disorders	Hemoglobin electrophoresis
Autoimmune hemolysis	Direct antiglobulin (Coombs) test, quantitation of red blood cell surface antibodies, cold agglutinin titer
Alloimmune hemolysis	Direct and indirect antiglobulin (Coombs) test with specificity analysis of eluted antibodies
Traumatic (microangiopathic or macroangiopathic) hemolysis	History and physical examination findings of hypertension, pregnancy, prosthetic heart valves or vascular grafts, systemic vasculitis, neurologic changes, fever; schistocytes, anemia, and destructive thrombocytopenia; BUN and creatinine; urinalysis; DIC panel; von Willebrand factor multimers, ADAMTS13
Hereditary spherocytosis, elliptocytosis, pyropoikilocytosis, and stomatocytosis	Primarily morphologic diagnoses; specific mutations detected by sequencing spectrin, ankyrin, band 3, or protein 4.1 DNA
Red blood cell enzymopathies	G6PD assay (1-2 months after acute hemolysis), Heinz body preparation, specific enzyme assays
Unstable hemoglobins	Heat/isopropanol denaturation tests, hemoglobin electrophoresis
Paroxysmal nocturnal hemoglobinuria	Acid hemolysis (Ham) or sucrose hemolysis test, flow cytometry analysis of GPI-anchored cell surface proteins (e.g., CD55, CD59)

BUN = blood urea nitrogen; DIC = disseminated intravascular coagulation; G6PD = glucose-6-phosphate dehydrogenase; GPI = glycosylphosphatidylinositol; TIBC = total iron-binding capacity.

SUGGESTED READINGS

Denny SD, Kuchibhatla MN, Cohen HJ: Impact of anemia on mortality, cognition, and function in community-dwelling elderly. Am J Med 2006;119:327–334. *Anemia is an independent predictor of functional and cognitive impairment, as well as subsequent mortality.*

Marks PW, Glader B: Approach to anemia in the adult and child. *In* Hoffman R, Benz EJ Jr, Shattil SJ, et al (eds): Hematology: Basic Principles and Practice. Philadelphia, Churchill Livingstone, 2005, pp 455–463. *Excellent diagnostic approaches to anemia in both children and adults.*

Schechter GP: Differential diagnosis of anemia. *In* Young NS, Gerson SL, High KA (eds): Clinical Hematology. Philadelphia, Mosby, 2006, pp 1037–1048. *Concise discussion of the pathophysiology of anemia and superb algorithms for diagnostic approaches to various types of anemia.*

Tefferi A: Anemia in adults: A contemporary approach to diagnosis. Mayo Clin Proc 2003;78:1274–1280. *An excellent approach using traditional and more recently available tools for diagnosing the cause of anemia.*

Valeri CR, Dennis RC, Ragno G, et al: Limitations of the hematocrit level to assess the need for red blood cell transfusion in hypovolemic anemic patients. Transfusion 2006;46:365–371. *In hypovolemic patients, the measured hematocrit overestimates the "true" hematocrit after volume repletion by 4 to 5 "points."*

163 MICROCYTIC AND HYPOCHROMIC ANEMIAS

Gordon D. Ginder

The oxygen-carrying hemoglobin molecule executes the principal function of the mature erythrocyte. The hemoglobin content of erythrocytes is determined by the coordinated production of globin protein, the heme porphyrin ring, and the availability of iron. A deficiency in any of these three critical components of hemoglobin results in hypochromic and/or microcytic anemia. Microcytic anemia is typically reported initially by automated red blood cell (RBC) indices. Hypochromic microcytic anemia can be confirmed on the peripheral blood smear (Fig. 163–1). Disorders of globin protein production typically produce microcytosis but not hypochromia and are discussed elsewhere (Chapter 166).

IRON DEFICIENCY ANEMIA

Epidemiology

Iron deficiency is by far the most common cause of anemia worldwide and is among the most frequently encountered medical problems seen by primary care physicians in the United States. It is estimated that between 2 and 5% of adolescent females in the United States have iron deficiency sufficient to cause anemia. Elsewhere, the prevalence of iron deficiency–induced anemia is much higher, with estimates of up to 10% of the world population, or more than 500 million people, being affected. The prevalence rates are especially high in developing countries where dietary insufficiency and intestinal parasites are prevalent.

Pathobiology

The majority of the approximately 4 g of iron in the adult human body is incorporated into hemoglobin (approximately 2100 mg) in erythrocytes, or myoglobin (approximately 300 mg) in muscle. The remainder is chiefly present as storage iron in the liver (1000 mg) and in the reticuloendothelial macrophages of bone marrow and spleen (600 mg) (Fig. 163–2). Only a small amount of iron (3 to 7 mg) is freely circulating in plasma bound to transferrin, but this pool is kinetically very active, turning over every 3 to 4 hours. Because of the potent conservatory mechanisms of iron recycling through the reticuloendothelial macrophage system, only an average of about 1 to 2 mg of iron is normally lost per day, largely through mucosal sloughing, desquamation, and, in females of reproductive age, menstruation.

The ability of iron to donate or accept electrons readily through conversion between ferrous (Fe^{2+}) and ferric (Fe^{3+}) states makes it a critical component of the hemoglobin and myoglobin porphyrin rings that transport oxygen, as well as cytochromes and various other vital enzymes. Free iron is extremely toxic due to its capacity to catalyze the formation of free radicals, which lead to cellular damage. Therefore, the majority of body iron that is not stably incorporated into porphyrin rings is associated with proteins. Transferrin is the major protein associated with circulating plasma iron, and ferritin is the major protein associated with stored intracellular iron, both in the cytoplasm and in mitochondria.

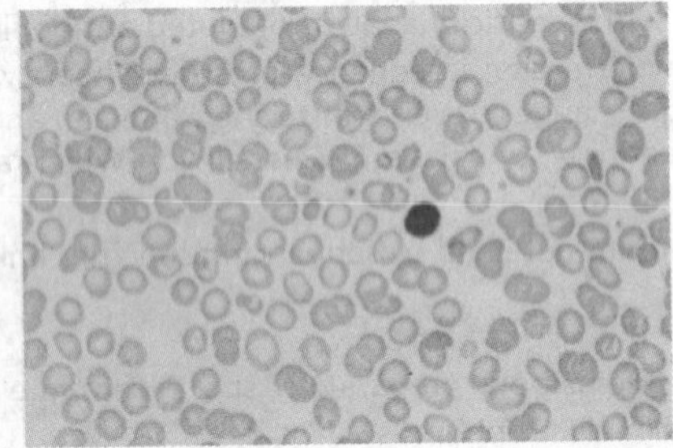

FIGURE 163–1 • Iron deficiency anemia. Many of these red blood cells are microcytic (smaller than the nucleus of the normal lymphocyte near the center of the field) and hypochromic (with central areas of pallor that exceed half of the diameter of the cells).

Because the normal rate of iron loss is low, only about 1 to 2 mg of dietary iron intake is needed to maintain homeostasis. The average daily Western diet contains about 20 mg of iron, and the efficiency of absorption of iron in the duodenum is usually sufficient to maintain the necessary amount of iron intake required for homeostatic balance.

Control of iron absorption by the duodenal crypt cells is critical because of the lack of any regulated mechanism for iron excretion. As a result, excessive iron intake can lead to deleterious iron overload with concomitant organ damage (Chapter 231). Non-heme dietary iron is dissolved in part by the low pH of the stomach effluent. After reduction to the ferrous state by ferroreductase, iron is transferred across the apical crypt cell membrane by the divalent metal transporter-1 (DMT1). Several levels of regulation are involved in iron absorption by the intestine. One of these is modulated by dietary intake such that, after a large influx of dietary iron, the duodenal absorptive capacity is diminished. A second regulatory mechanism modulates iron absorption capacity based on total body iron stores. Finally, the so-called erythropoietic regulator modulates the capacity for enterocyte absorption based on the requirements for iron needed for erythropoiesis. A paradoxical increase in iron absorption through this mechanism occurs in certain types of anemia characterized by intravascular and intramedullary destruction of erythroid cells: sideroblastic anemia, the thalassemias (Chapter 166), and congenital dyserythropoietic anemias.

Once inside the intestinal absorbing cell, iron is stored in complex with ferritin. Circulating plasma iron is complexed with the iron transport protein, transferrin. The transferrin iron complex is then taken up by erythroid precursors via the transferrin receptor. The high density of transferrin receptors on erythroid precursors insures the preferential uptake of iron by these cells and explains why erythropoiesis proceeds normally until a critical deficiency of transferrin-bound iron, reflecting a depletion of total body iron, is present. The levels of transferrin, transferrin receptor, ferritin, and other proteins important in iron metabolism are regulated by the iron regulatory proteins, IRP-1 and IRP-2.

Hepcidin, a 25-amino-acid peptide originally isolated as an antimicrobial substance found in both serum and urine, is believed to be a central regulator of iron homeostasis through its effects on intestinal absorption, macrophage recycling of iron from senescent RBCs, and iron mobilization from hepatic stores. Thus, hepcidin affects all major sites of iron uptake and storage. Hepcidin is produced in the liver and acts as a negative regulator of iron absorption by the intestine and iron release from storage in macrophages and hepatocytes. It is believed that hepcidin binds to ferroportin, the major iron transporter in the membranes of the enterocyte, macrophage, and hepatocyte, causing its internalization and degradation. This process blocks transport of iron across the membrane of the basolateral crypt cell, thereby preventing its incorporation into transferrin-

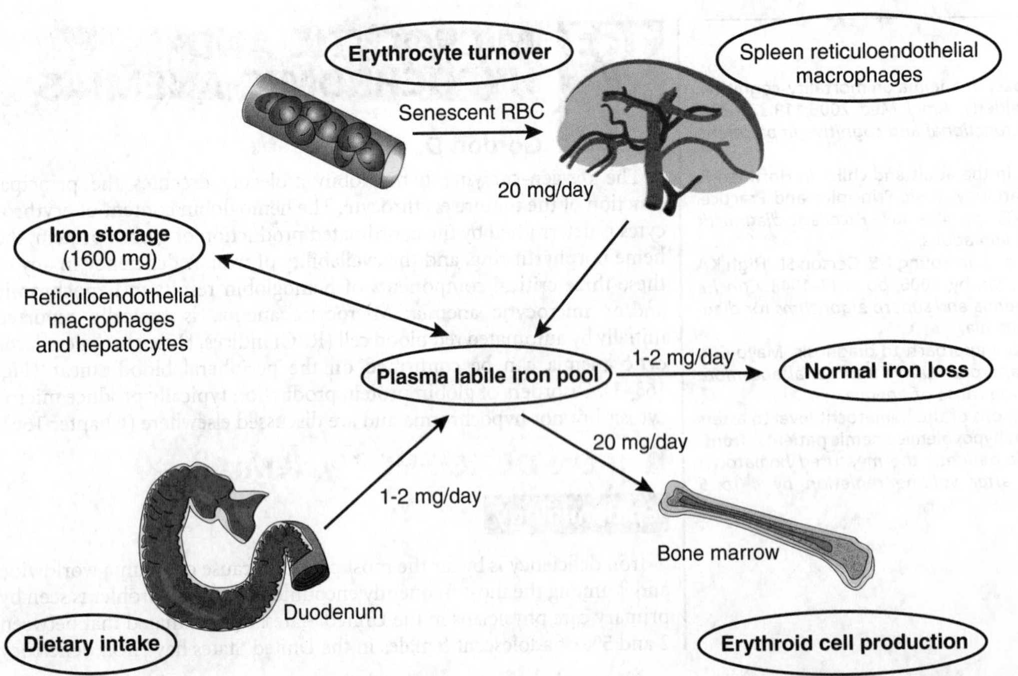

FIGURE 163–2 • Iron homeostasis in normal humans. RBC = red blood cells.

bound plasma iron. Likewise, loss of ferroportin function results in a block in the major export pathway of iron stores from macrophages and hepatocytes. Hepcidin production is upregulated by iron and downregulated by hypoxia, consistent with its homeostatic role. Because hepcidin is also upregulated by inflammatory cytokines, it is believed to play an important role in the paradoxical lack of transferrin-bound iron available for erythropoiesis in the face of adequate or even excess iron stores found in the anemia of chronic inflammation (Chapter 169).

Blood Loss

Iron deficiency anemia results from an imbalance between available body iron for hemoglobin production and the minimal requirements needed to sustain normal hemoglobin production during erythropoiesis (see Fig. 163–2). Because of the combined effectiveness of dietary absorption and retention of iron under normal circumstances, this mismatch is most often due to blood loss. Gastrointestinal (GI) blood loss is the most common type of blood loss leading to iron deficiency (Chapter 137). In developed countries, the blood loss is usually secondary to benign or neoplastic lesions of the GI tract (Chapter 203). Chronic ingestion of drugs that cause GI mucosal damage is another frequent cause of blood loss (Chapter 141): the most common offending agents are alcohol and salicylates or other nonsteroidal anti-inflammatory agents. In developing countries, helminthic infections, including hookworm (Chapter 378) and schistosomiasis (Chapter 376), are among the most common causes of GI blood loss.

Genitourinary (GU) tract blood loss resulting in iron deficiency is most common in menstruating women. Less common are urinary tract malignancies (Chapter 207) and hemoglobinuria due to intravascular hemolysis (Chapter 164). Respiratory tract blood loss is far less common as a cause of iron deficiency.

Reproduction and Growth

Although in most cases an increased iron requirement is due to blood loss, there are also other causes of increased iron needs: rapid growth in infancy and adolescence, and both pregnancy and lactation in adulthood. It is estimated that the increased iron requirements during pregnancy, if not met with supplemental iron, may result in a deficiency equivalent to a cumulative blood loss of up to 1500 mL.

Inadequate Iron Intake

The other major cause of iron deficiency is inadequate iron intake. Because normally only about 1 to 2 mg per day of dietary iron intake is required to maintain homeostasis, only diets lacking this amount fail to provide adequate iron. The average Western meal contains about 6 mg of iron, and normal intestinal absorption mechanisms are highly efficient, so dietary insufficiency is not a common cause of iron deficiency. Certain diets that lack iron or contain large quantities of phytates from cereals or tannate from tea, both of which inhibit intestinal iron absorption, may result in inadequate iron absorption. Although iron is usually readily absorbed, primarily in the duodenum, pathologic states that can impair the process include generalized intestinal malabsorption (Chapter 143), atrophic gastritis (Chapter 141) with achlorhydria, and extensive gastric surgery. In contrast, chronic use of histamine 2 (H_2) receptor blockers or proton-pump inhibitors does not appear to be sufficient to cause iron deficiency. In the United States, celiac disease (Chapter 143) is an increasingly common cause of iron deficiency, and anemia can be the presenting manifestation of the disease.

Clinical Manifestations

Because of physiologic compensatory mechanisms, patients with mild iron deficiency anemia may be asymptomatic. Iron deficiency in these patients may be recognized during the evaluation of an underlying disease process or as part of routine laboratory studies. The findings of microcytosis and hypochromia occur only after the hematocrit has fallen to approximately 30%, so neither finding may be present in early stages.

The anemia of iron deficiency, like other anemias, manifests with nonspecific symptoms such as weakness, pallor, dizziness, decreased exercise tolerance, or irritability. Because iron is a critical component of the porphyrin complex in muscle as well as many essential metabolic enzymes, its deficiency affects other organ systems besides the erythron. As a result, the degree of fatigue and weakness in iron deficiency may be out of proportion to the hemoglobin level. Rare patients, most frequently elderly women, may have dysphagia due to an esophageal stricture or web (Plummer-Vinson syndrome). A clinical manifestation unique to iron

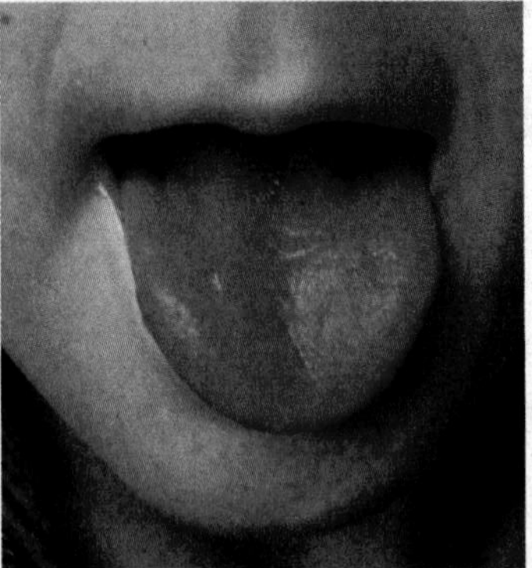

FIGURE 163–3 • Clinical symptoms of iron deficiency anemia. Iron deficiency anemia commonly leads to pallor of the face, lips, and tongue and, if chronic, to atrophic glossitis and angular stomatitis. All of these symptoms are seen in this young woman whose iron deficiency anemia resulted from excessive menstrual bleeding. The anemia responded to oral iron supplementation. (From Forbes CD, Jackson WF: Color Atlas and Text of Clinical Medicine, 3rd ed., London, Mosby, 2003, with permission.)

deficiency is pica, which is an unusual craving for certain non-nutritional substances. Pica may be manifested as a craving for ice (pagophagia), or less commonly for clay (geophagia) or starch (amylophagia); pagophagia is believed to be the most specific to iron deficiency.

Physical findings that may be associated with the iron-deficient state include glossitis and angular stomatitis (Fig. 163–3). Other less common but highly specific abnormal findings in iron deficiency are spooning of the fingernails (koilonychia) and blue-tinged sclerae.

Diagnosis

The diagnosis of iron deficiency anemia is made by laboratory testing. Because microcytic hypochromic RBCs are a sine qua non of this type of anemia, the initial screening tests consist of determination of hemoglobin levels, mean corpuscular volume, erythrocyte hemoglobin content, and reticulocyte count. In experienced hands, the peripheral blood smear (Chapter 161) is an excellent indicator of iron deficiency anemia. In iron deficiency anemia, most erythrocytes are smaller in diameter than the nucleus of a typical lymphocyte, and the area of central pallor is greater than 50% of the total diameter of the erythrocyte (see Fig. 163–1). Another feature is the variability of size of the erythrocytes, a finding that is in contrast to other conditions that give rise to microcytosis; the calculated variability in RBC volume (the so-called RBC volume distribution width, or RDW), is elevated early in iron deficiency anemia.

The definitive diagnosis of iron deficiency anemia is made by tests that measure total body iron stores, because absence of mobilizable iron stores is unique to this microcytic hypochromic anemia. Transferrin levels and transferrin-bound iron are not reliable indicators of iron deficiency because the tests are also abnormal in the anemia of chronic disease, despite adequate total body iron stores.

The serum ferritin level is the most reliable, noninvasive, and cost-effective indicator that is routinely available in most clinical laboratories (Table 163–1). In a large study of 259 anemic patients, a serum ferritin level of less than 18 μg/L was diagnostic of iron deficiency with greater than 95% specificity and a 55% sensitivity. At a level of 45 μg/L, the sensitivity rises to approximately 70%, and a serum ferritin level higher than 100 μg/L in populations with a less than 40% prevalence of iron deficiency excludes a diagnosis of iron deficiency with more than 90% sensitivity. Although some recent studies have questioned the accuracy of routine determination of stainable marrow iron, this test is still generally considered to be the gold standard of available tests for iron deficiency. However, determination of total bone marrow iron stores is rarely necessary to make a diagnosis of iron deficiency anemia except when there is some other complicating process.

One such setting in which serum ferritin levels can be spuriously elevated is chronic inflammation or chronic disease. The soluble serum transferrin receptor (StFR) level is an excellent measure of total erythroid precursor mass. The StFR is aberrantly elevated in the presence of iron deficiency, so it is considered a useful test for the latter. A number of studies have demonstrated the utility of the StFR/ferritin ratio in distinguishing iron deficiency from the anemia of chronic disease. However, the lack of reliable standards has prevented this assay from becoming a routinely available test in clinical practice.

TABLE 163-1 LABORATORY FINDINGS FOR IRON STUDIES IN MICROCYTIC HYPOCHROMIC ANEMIAS

Anemia	Serum Iron	Total Iron Binding Capacity (TIBC)	Percent Transferrin Saturation	Serum Ferritin	Serum Transferrin Receptor (sTfR)	Marrow RE Iron	Marrow Ringed Sideroblasts
Iron deficiency anemia	Low	High	0–15	Low (<30 μ/L)	High	Absent	Absent
Anemia of chronic disease	Low	Normal or low	5–15	Normal or high	Normal	Normal or high	Absent
Sideroblastic anemia	High	Normal	60–90	High	Normal or high	High	Present

RE = reticuloendothelial.

Treatment

Rx

The treatment of iron deficiency anemia is replenishment of body iron stores. However, the underlying cause should always be investigated before treatment is begun, because in many cases it is a correctable and potentially fatal GI lesion (Chapters 137 and 203).

Oral Administration

The preferred route of iron administration is oral. Oral iron is most readily absorbed in the absence of food, especially in the setting of decreased stomach acid production due to atrophic gastritis, gastric surgery, or chronic suppression of gastric acid with an H_2 antagonist or proton-pump inhibitor. The major obstacle to oral iron replacement is unacceptable side effects, chiefly epigastric discomfort or nausea, although diarrhea or constipation also occurs in some patients. Reducing the dose often eliminates nausea and epigastric discomfort. Despite the development of a number of orally effective iron-containing compounds, the original salt, ferrous sulfate (325 mg three times daily), remains the most useful. Although some newer oral iron preparations, such as ferrous gluconate (300 mg two or three times daily) or ferrous fumarate (325 mg two or three times daily) may induce less GI side effects per milligram of iron, they are also less well absorbed, so there is no net advantage to these costlier formulations except for patients who cannot tolerate ferrous sulfate. Given both the low toxicity and the low cost of oral iron replacement, a therapeutic trial is a complementary means for confirming a diagnosis of iron deficiency anemia.

Parenteral Administration

In situations in which primary blood loss is uncontrollable, iron cannot be absorbed due to severe malabsorption, or oral iron is not tolerated despite concerted efforts to minimize side effects, parenteral iron is an effective alternative treatment. Intramuscular dosing is limited to 100 mg per injection, so intravenous (IV) administration of iron is recommended. Sodium ferric gluconate (given intravenously as a 125-mg dose over 10 minutes) is the preferred form of parenteral iron for routine use due to the low incidence of adverse reactions. A multi-institutional, double-blind, randomized, placebo-controlled trial of more than 2500 patients showed similar adverse events in patients receiving sodium ferric gluconate versus placebo, and only one life-threatening complication occurred, compared with 23 such events among 3768 patients treated with iron dextran in a historical control arm. [1] One limitation of serum ferric gluconate is that the maximum dose that can be delivered in a single injection is approximately 125 mg, and a total dose of 500 to 2000 mg is usually required for adequate repletion. Although iron dextran can be used to deliver very large doses of iron in a single IV injection, it is currently reserved for situations in which rapid iron replacement is required, because of the life-threatening anaphylactic and delayed adverse reactions that occur in 0.6% and 2.5% of cases, respectively. If iron dextran is to be given intravenously, premedication with diphenhydramine and a slow test dose injection of 30 to 40 mg diluted in normal saline is recommended.

The response to iron repletion therapy is usually quite rapid, with elimination of symptoms within a few days. Increased reticulocytosis usually begins within 4 to 5 days, and the hemoglobin level often rises within 1 week and reaches a normal level after 6 weeks of therapy if adequate iron replacement is achieved. The goal of therapy, which is to reach a serum ferritin level of greater than 50 mg/L, usually takes 4 to 6 months. Therapy must be continued after adequate replacement is achieved if the underlying cause of iron deficiency is not reversible. Because of the avidity of transferrin receptor–rich erythroid precursors for transferrin-bound iron, the serum ferritin level usually will not rise until hemoglobin levels reach normal. An incomplete response, as determined by failure to normalize the hemoglobin level, usually means either that iron replacement has not been adequate or that another condition, such as anemia of chronic disease, is coexistent.

Prognosis

In most cases, iron deficiency anemia can be corrected rapidly by either oral or parenteral replacement, but the long-term prognosis ultimately depends on the clinical course of the underlying cause. It is critical that the patient undergo a full evaluation to determine the underlying cause of the iron deficiency, especially because an occult GI lesion, often malignant, may be present, particularly in patients older than 50 years of age (Chapter 203).

ANEMIA OF CHRONIC DISEASE AND INFLAMMATION

Definition

Anemia of chronic disease refers to anemia that occurs in the setting of a chronic disease state, usually one associated with elevated levels of inflammatory cytokines. Because of this tight association, more recently the condition has also been referred to as anemia of inflammation. Although anemia of chronic inflammation is usually manifested as a normochromic normocytic process (Chapter 169), between 20 and 50% of cases are associated with microcytic RBC indices. The anemia is usually mild to moderate, and it may not be symptomatic.

Epidemiology

Anemia of chronic inflammation is a common cause of anemia, believed to be second only to iron deficiency in incidence. It is the most common type of anemia encountered among hospitalized patients. A wide spectrum of underlying diseases includes acute and chronic infections, autoimmune-associated diseases, cancers, and chronic kidney diseases.

Pathobiology

The underlying mechanisms of anemia of chronic inflammation are all believed to result from the effects of abnormal levels of inflammatory cytokines, and three major mechanisms are believed to account for this type of anemia. The first is dysregulated iron homeostasis, manifested by low serum iron (hypoferremia) in the presence of normal or elevated serum ferritin levels and abundant reticuloendothelial macrophage iron stores. The functional consequence is a limitation of iron for erythroid progenitor cells and resultant restriction of erythropoiesis. Proinflammatory stimuli, including lipopolysaccharides, interferon-γ, and tumor necrosis factor-α (TNF-α), upregulate DMT1, which increases iron uptake by the reticuloendothelial cells. At the same time, these stimuli cause downregulation of expression of ferroportin, which is the protein required for release of ferrous iron from storage cells and for transport of dietary iron from duodenal enterocytes into the circulation.

Because hepcidin is an iron-regulated, acute phase–reactant peptide that blocks both iron uptake in the gut and iron release from hepatocytes and macrophage storage, its upregulation by lipopolysaccharides, interleukin-6 (IL-6), and possibly IL-1 (indirectly through induction of IL-6) results in anemia. Also, patients with hepatic adenomas that secrete high levels of hepcidin have iron-refractory anemia in the presence of normal or elevated ferritin and macrophage iron stores, despite the absence of elevated inflammatory cytokine levels. Elevated urinary hepcidin concentrations correlate with ferritin levels in patients with anemia of inflammation, iron overload, and iron deficiency.

Another pathophysiologic feature of anemia of chronic inflammation is inhibition of erythroid progenitor expansion. Interferon-γ is the most potent inhibitory factor of erythropoiesis, but similar inhibition is believed to be mediated by IL-1, TNF-α, interferon-α, and interferon-β. These mediators of inflammation act to increase erythroid progenitor apoptosis, downregulate erythropoietin receptors, and antagonize pro-hematopoietic factors. The action of erythropoietin appears to be directly antagonized by these pro-inflammatory cytokines, which would explain why responsiveness to erythropoietin appears to be inversely related to the severity of the underlying chronic inflammation and the levels of interferon-γ and TNF-α. Finally, increased erythrophagocytosis in the presence of inflammation results in a modest shortening of RBC half-life.

Clinical Manifestations

The clinical manifestations in patients with anemia of chronic inflammation are usually dominated by the underlying disease process. The anemia in this condition is usually mild, with hemoglobin levels in the range of 8 to 10 g/dL. However, supervening blood loss, absolute iron deficiency, or other aggravating factors can produce life-threatening anemia. Even mild to moderate anemia contributes to the debilitating effects of the underlying disease on performance status and quality of life. Moreover, the presence of anemia is associated with poorer overall prognosis in many of the frequently associated underlying chronic diseases, although correction of anemia as yet has not been directly demonstrated to improve survival.

Diagnosis

The clinical diagnosis of anemia of chronic disease presenting with microcytic hypochromic RBC indices is one of exclusion, based on low serum iron in the presence of normal or increased total body iron stores (see Table 163–1). Serum ferritin is the best single laboratory marker for assessing iron storage, and it is almost invariably normal or elevated in anemia of chronic disease. If both the serum iron and the transferrin saturation are reduced, reflecting dysregulation of iron homeostasis, the diagnosis of anemia of chronic disease can be made in the appropriate clinical setting after exclusion of other causes of anemia, such as coexistent blood loss, thalassemia (Chapter 166), and drug-induced suppression of erythropoiesis. In the presence of inflammation, however, up to 30% of patients with true iron deficiency have serum ferritin levels greater than 100 μg/L, potentially obscuring the diagnosis of iron deficiency. Assays for StFR are useful to diagnose iron deficiency in the presence of the inflammation associated with anemia of chronic disease, but problems with standardization have limited this test's availability in clinical practice. Examination of the bone marrow for reticuloendothelial macrophage iron stores (hemosiderin) and erythroblasts containing iron granules (sideroblasts) can provide definitive evidence of absent iron stores in the setting of anemia of chronic inflammation. A low serum erythropoietin level is also useful in supporting a diagnosis of anemia of chronic inflammation, but only when the hemoglobin level is less than 10 g/dL.

Treatment

Treatment of the Underlying Disease

The most effective treatment for anemia of chronic disease is successful treatment of the underlying inflammatory disease process, whether it be an acute or chronic infection, treatable cancer, renal failure, or rheumatoid arthritis. Even if definitive treatment is not possible, quality of life and perhaps prognosis can improve if symptomatic anemia is treated directly. Unfortunately, anemia of chronic inflammation remains undertreated, even in developed countries, as illustrated by a study of 200,000 patients, in which 23% of patients with chronic renal failure had a hematocrit lower than 30, and only 30% of them were receiving treatment for their anemia.

Blood Transfusion

Blood transfusion (Chapter 183) offers immediate resolution of anemia but it is indicated chiefly in situations in which anemia is life-threatening or imposes serious limitations on the patient's function. These situations almost always involve supervening blood loss or some other acute process that compounds the anemia of chronic disease. Transfusion is not recommended for long-term treatment of mild or moderate anemia of chronic inflammation because of the secondary risks, which include iron overload, human leukocyte antigen (HLA) sensitization in potential renal transplantation, and other side effects of transfusion.

Intravenous Iron Therapy

If iron replacement is needed in anemia of chronic inflammation, parenteral iron administration is usually required to replenish stores because of the block in intestinal absorption. In hemodialysis patients receiving erythropoietin therapy, IV iron therapy improves anemia; however, when IV iron replacement raises the transferrin saturation to greater than 20%, there appears to be an increased risk of developing bacteremia, thereby underscoring the complex relationship between iron homeostasis and immunity.

Erythropoietin therapy is currently approved for use in patients with chronic kidney disease with HIV infection, and in patients with cancer who are undergoing myelosuppressive treatment. Patients with demonstrated iron deficiency should receive supplemental iron with IV iron gluconate (see earlier discussion) while being treated with erythropoietin.

In patients with cancer and anemia of chronic inflammation, erythropoietin therapy improves quality of life and performance status. [2] However, erythropoietin receptors are present in many types of cancer cells, including those from the head and neck, breast, ovary, prostate, and kidney. Some studies of patients with breast cancer and head and neck cancers have suggested adverse clinical outcomes with erythropoietin therapy, [3] but a meta-analysis involving 3287 patients [4] failed to show any adverse effect of erythropoietin therapy on clinical outcomes. Given its benefits in cancer patients with symptomatic anemia, erythropoietin is recommended for such patients.

Prognosis

The overall prognosis in anemia of chronic inflammation is determined almost exclusively by the course of the underlying disease. It is well established that the degree of anemia correlates well with the severity of the underlying disease process and therefore with the concomitant levels of inflammatory cytokines. In the absence of a supervening process, the anemia of chronic inflammation is not life-threatening, and, as yet, treatment of the anemia per se has not been proven to affect overall survival.

SIDEROBLASTIC ANEMIAS

Definition

This heterogeneous group of anemias is distinguished by the characteristic finding of excessive mitochondrial iron in erythroblasts, as manifested by iron-laden, ringed sideroblasts in the bone marrow in the presence of moderate to severe anemia. These disorders result from mitochondrial defects either in the biosynthesis of the heme porphyrin ring or in the metabolism of iron. Both hereditary and acquired types of sideroblastic anemia have been described. Although often characterized by microcytic and sometimes hypochromic anemia, these disorders can manifest with normochromic normocytic RBCs; if the anemia is associated with myelodysplasia, macrocytic RBC indices may be present.

Epidemiology

Although acquired sideroblastic anemias are relatively rare, they are much more prevalent than hereditary forms. The true incidence of acquired sideroblastic anemia is not well established, in part due to the heterogeneity of causes and clinical presentations. Hereditary X-linked sideroblastic anemias usually manifest in childhood or early adulthood.

Pathobiology

Genetics

The pathophysiologic mechanisms of hereditary sideroblastic anemias are much better understood than those of the more common idiopathic acquired variety. Two main forms of X-linked hereditary sideroblastic anemia have been characterized, and both result from defects in the heme synthesis pathway (Fig. 163–4). The first type is caused by mutations in the gene coding for erythroid-specific δ-aminolevulinic acid synthase, known as ALAS-2, on the X chromosome. These mutations may affect the affinity of the enzyme for pyridoxal phosphate or its structural stability, catalytic site, or susceptibility to mitochondrial proteases. In those cases in which the affinity of ALAS-2 for pyridoxal phosphate is altered, pyridoxine supplementation can ameliorate the associated anemia. The other major group of X-linked sideroblastic anemias results from defects in the adenosine triphosphate (ATP) binding cassette (ABC) protein known as hABC7. The hABC7 protein is believed to be involved in iron-sulfur [FeS] cluster formation. Because [FeS] cluster–associated proteins include ferrochelatase and the cytosolic IRP-1, defects in hABC7 are believed to result in defective iron metabolism or inadequate incorporation of iron into the heme porphyrin ring by ferrochelatase. This type of X-linked sideroblastic anemia is associated with ataxia.

In addition to the two X-linked causes, both autosomal dominant and recessive forms of hereditary sideroblastic anemia have been described. However, the exact mechanisms involved in these disorders are not known.

Other types of hereditary sideroblastic anemia are believed to result from mutations in the mitochondrial genome rather than in nuclear genes. The inheritance of these disorders is complex, owing to the exclusively maternal inheritance pattern of mitochondria, because the ovum is the only source of embryonic mitochondria.

Exposure to Drugs or Toxins

The most common form of acquired sideroblastic anemia results from nutritional deficiency or exposure to exogenous drugs or toxins, especially alcohol. Although sideroblastic anemia is not a common finding in alcoholism, the high incidence of alcohol abuse in Western cultures accounts for its frequency as a cause. Alcohol directly inhibits erythropoiesis, but sideroblastic anemia is usually seen only in the setting of concurrent alcoholism and nutritional deficiencies. Other well-documented drug exposures associated with sideroblastic anemia include isoniazid, chloramphenicol, and cycloserine. Sideroblastic anemia also has been attributed to lead exposure (Chapter 20), but there are limited primary data to support this association. Deficiency of pyridoxine causes sideroblastic anemia in animals and may also occur in the setting of alcoholism in humans, although ethanol is believed to be an antagonist of the interaction of pyridoxal phosphate with 5-aminolevulinic acid as a

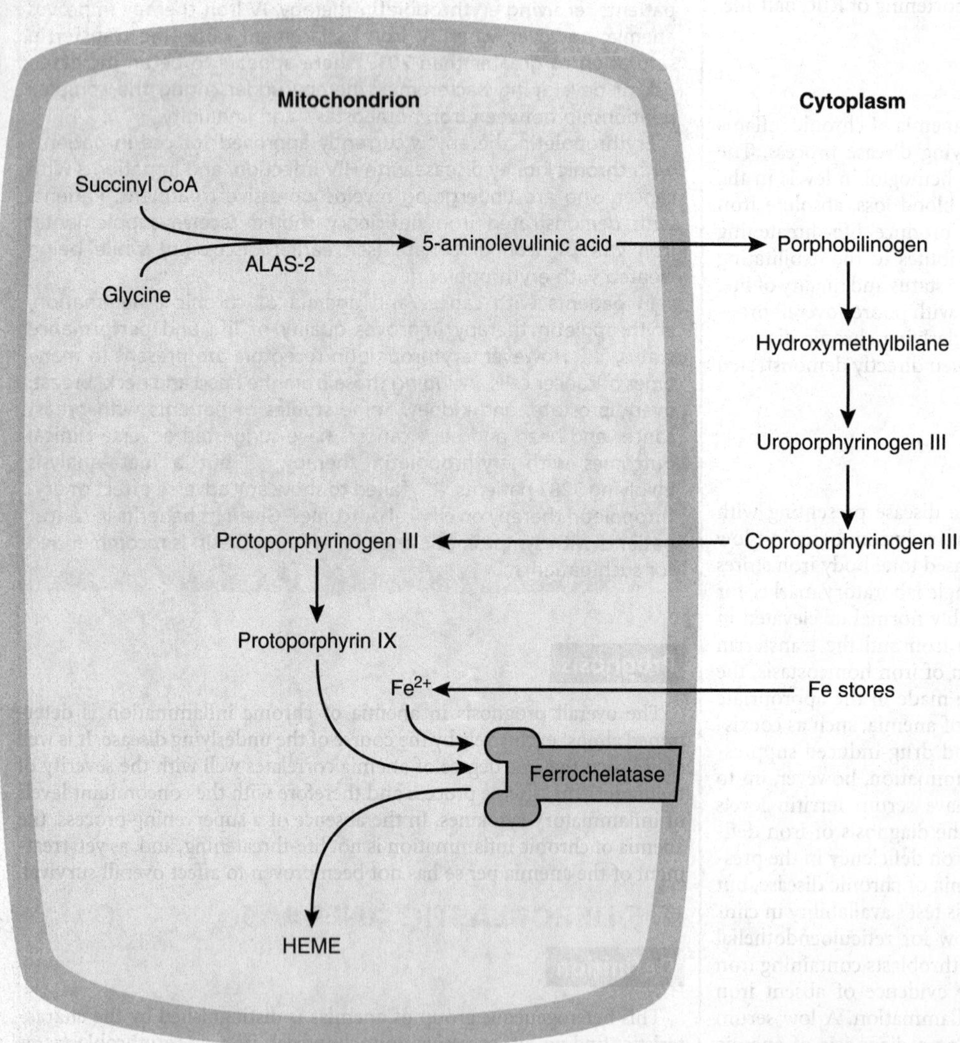

FIGURE 163–4 • The heme synthetic pathway. ALAS-2 = δ-aminolevulinic acid synthase; CoA = coenzyme A.

cofactor in the first step of heme biosynthesis. Copper deficiency, although rare, has also been associated with sideroblastic anemia, usually in the setting of an overdose of bivalent cation chelators, such as penicillamine or trientine, used to treat the copper overloading found in Wilson's disease (Chapter 230).

Idiopathic Forms

The other major cause of acquired sideroblastic anemia is idiopathic in association with myelodysplastic syndromes (Chapter 193). Refractory anemia with ringed sideroblasts is characterized by abnormalities in all three hematopoietic cell lineages in addition to the presence of ringed sideroblasts.

A second form, known as pure sideroblastic anemia, is less frequently associated with cytogenetic abnormalities, is characterized by dysplasia only in erythroid progenitors, and lacks cytopenias other than anemia. The prognosis in this type of acquired idiopathic sideroblastic anemia is much better than that in refractory anemia with ringed sideroblasts, in part because of a very low incidence (<10%) of evolution to acute leukemia.

Because of the important differences in prognosis, it is imperative to evaluate cytogenetics and marrow morphology at the time of diagnosis. Recent evidence suggests that mitochondrial DNA mutations and attendant mitochondrial cytopathies account for many, if not all, cases.

Clinical Manifestations

Because of the heterogeneous nature of the sideroblastic anemias, many of the clinical manifestations vary according to the underlying pathophysiologic cause. The anemia is usually moderate to severe, with hemoglobin levels in the range of 4 to 10 g/L. The peripheral blood smear frequently reveals hypochromia, often with basophilic stippling. Microcytosis is often seen in hereditary forms, but normochromic, normocytic or even macrocytic RBCs may be seen, especially in the setting of myelodysplasia or in a rare X-linked hereditary form known as Pearson's syndrome.

Diagnosis

The most useful diagnostic laboratory test for sideroblastic anemia is bone marrow morphology with Prussian blue iron staining, which reveals abnormally large and numerous bluish-green siderosomes within at least 15% of erythroblasts, giving the characteristic appearance of ringed sideroblasts (Fig. 163–5). These ringed sideroblasts distinguish this disorder from iron deficiency anemia and anemia of chronic inflammation. Bone marrow findings in idiopathic acquired sideroblastic anemias include dyspoietic features of erythroid and/or myeloid and megakaryotic cell lineages.

Iron studies usually reveal normal iron stores or evidence of iron overload, which is caused by the ineffective erythropoiesis found in sideroblastic anemia as well as the transfusion therapy often required for its treatment. Iron deficiency can occur coincident with sideroblastic anemia, complicating the diagnosis due to the lack of characteristic ringed sideroblasts, particularly in myelodysplastic syndromes in which thrombocytopenia leads to GI blood loss. In cases in which coexisting iron deficiency is suspected, a repeat bone marrow examination after iron repletion fails to correct the anemia will reveal the diagnostic ringed sideroblasts.

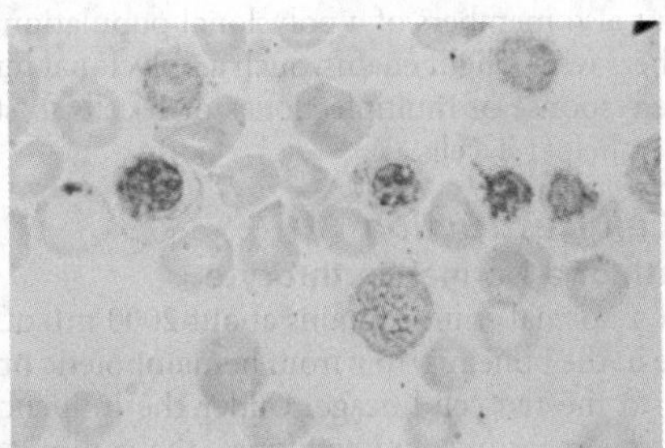

FIGURE 163–5 • Sideroblastic anemia. Prussian blue iron stain of the bone marrow shows ringed sideroblasts, which are nucleated red blood cell precursors with perinuclear rings of iron-laden mitochondria.

Treatment

Rx

Treatment of Underlying Disease

Most forms of sideroblastic anemia lack a specific therapy aimed at the underlying mechanism. Exceptions are those forms caused by alcohol or other drugs, for which removal of the offending agent usually results in resolution, or at least improvement, of the anemia. Abstinence from alcohol usually reverses the abnormalities in heme biosynthesis in 1 to 2 weeks, as evidenced by disappearance of ringed sideroblasts in the marrow.

Pyridoxine markedly improves the relatively rare cases of nutritional deficiency, which are usually associated with alcoholism, and some forms of X-linked hereditary sideroblastic anemias in which the binding of pyridoxine by ALAS-2 is defective. Because of its low toxicity in moderate doses, a trial of pyridoxine, 100 to 200 mg/day orally for up to 3 months, is worthwhile in all patients. In responsive cases, reticulocytosis occurs within 2 to 3 weeks, and the hemoglobin level improves over several months. High-dose pyridoxine has been shown to overcome the defect in ALAS-2 activity in some patients with X-linked sideroblastic anemia, but prolonged high-dose therapy can be associated with peripheral neuropathy.

Transfusion

The mainstay of therapy for most severe sideroblastic anemias remains RBC transfusions. Because of the risks of long-term transfusion therapy, treatment should be aimed at achieving normal performance status rather than a specific target hemoglobin level. Iron stores should be monitored regularly, and iron chelation with desferrioxamine should be used in the setting of iron overload.

Erythropoietin

Therapy with erythropoietin, with or without granulocyte colony-stimulating factors (G-CSF), benefits a small percentage of patients with acquired sideroblastic anemia due to myelodysplasia. A meta-analysis of 17 studies in which 205 patients were treated with erythropoietin showed an overall response rate of only 16%. However, patients with a diagnosis other than refractory anemia with ringed sideroblasts who were not transfusion dependent had response rates greater than 50%, whereas none of the patients who had refractory anemia with ringed sideroblasts and a serum erythropoietin level greater than 200 U/L responded. Studies using a combination of erythropoietin and G-CSF showed somewhat higher response rates, although none of these studies were large or randomized. Allogeneic bone marrow transplantation (Chapter 184) benefits patients whose myelodysplasias (Chapter 193) have a high risk of evolving into acute leukemia.

Prognosis

As with the underlying pathophysiology, the prognosis in sideroblastic anemias is highly variable. Secondary acquired forms of the disease due to alcohol or toxins respond well to withdrawal of the offending agent, with rapid and often complete normalization of erythropoiesis. The pure sideroblastic anemia variant of myelodysplasia-associated sideroblastic anemia usually can be managed well for many years with transfusion and, if necessary, concordant iron chelation therapy. Other myelodysplasia-related sideroblastic anemias generally have a poor prognosis because of the coexistent prevalence of pancytopenia and the relatively high incidence of progression to acute leukemia.

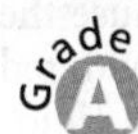

1. Michael B, Coyne DW, Fishbane S, et al: Sodium ferric gluconate complex in hemodialysis patients: Adverse reactions compared to placebo and iron dextran. Kidney Int 2002;61:1830–1839.
2. Witzig TE, Silberstein PT, Loprinzi CL, et al: Phase III, randomized, double-blind study of epoetin alfa compared with placebo in anemic patients receiving chemotherapy. J Clin Oncol 2005;23:2606–2617.
3. Henke M, Laszig R, Rube C, et al: Erythropoietin to treat head and neck cancer patients with anaemia undergoing radiotherapy: Randomised, double-blind, placebo-controlled trial. Lancet 2003;362:1255–1260.
4. Bohlius J, Langensiepen S, Schwarzer G, et al: Recombinant human erythropoietin and overall survival in cancer patients: Results of a comprehensive meta-analysis. Natl Cancer Inst 2005;97:489–498.

SUGGESTED READINGS

Beyan C, Kaptan K, Ifran A: Predictive value of discrimination indices in differential diagnosis of iron deficiency anemia and beta-thalassemia trait. Eur J Haematol 2007;78:524–526. *The RBC level is often diagnostic, but total body iron status and hemoglobin A(2) levels confirm diagnosis.*

Bridges KR, Alcindor T: Sideroblastic anemias. Br J Haematol 2002;116:733–743. *A comprehensive review.*

Cook JD: Diagnosis and management of iron-deficiency anaemia. Best Pract Res Clin Haematol 2005;18:319–332. *Review of practical clinical aspects of iron deficiency anemia.*

Fleming RE, Bacon BR: Orchestration of iron homeostasis. N Engl J Med 2005;352:1741–1744. *A concise review of iron metabolism and its disorders.*

Weiss G, Goodnough LT: Anemia of chronic disease. N Engl J Med 2005;352: 1011–1023. *A comprehensive review.*

164 AUTOIMMUNE AND INTRAVASCULAR HEMOLYTIC ANEMIAS

Robert S. Schwartz

Definition

The immune-mediated hemolytic anemias comprise a group of disorders in which antibodies, complement, and macrophages, usually acting in concert, send the patient's red blood cells to a premature demise. In the most common type of this class of hemolytic anemia, the antibodies bind to native constituents of the membrane of the patient's own red blood cells. For this reason, the antibodies qualify as autoantibodies, and the diseases that they cause fall under the rubric of autoimmune hemolytic anemia.

There are, in addition, less common types of immune-mediated hemolytic anemia. Some drugs elicit antidrug antibodies that can cause hemolytic anemia if the drug plants itself in the erythrocyte membrane, thereby making the red cell a target of the antibodies. A high titer of IgM antierythrocyte autoantibodies that bind to red blood cells at cold temperatures is the distinguishing serologic feature of cold agglutinin disease. In paroxysmal cold hemoglobinuria, an IgG antibody binds to the erythrocyte at cold temperatures, thereby setting the stage for complement-mediated hemolysis at warm temperatures. Paroxysmal nocturnal hemoglobinuria (PNH), a disease in which complement also mediates hemolysis, arises from a somatic mutation in a hematopoietic stem cell that renders erythrocytes susceptible to complement-mediated lysis in the absence of antibody. The hemolytic transfusion reaction (Chapter 183) is another disorder with complement-mediated destruction of erythrocytes, but in such cases alloantibodies in the recipient against red cell antigens of the donor trigger lysis of the transfused cells.

AUTOIMMUNE HEMOLYTIC ANEMIAS

Autoimmune Hemolytic Anemia Associated with IgG Autoantibodies

Epidemiology

Autoimmune hemolytic anemia associated with IgG autoantibodies accounts for about 75% of cases of autoimmune hemolytic anemia. Generally referred to simply as autoimmune hemolytic anemia, it has also been called warm antibody autoimmune hemolytic anemia because the IgG anti–red blood cell autoantibodies in this disorder react best with red cells at 37° C. Autoimmune hemolytic anemia can be primary (idiopathic) or occur in association with another disease (secondary autoimmune hemolytic anemia).

Autoimmune hemolytic anemia is uncommon. The estimated overall (not age-adjusted) annual incidence is about 1 case per 100,000 in the population; after the age of 60, the annual incidence reaches 10 per 100,000. The disorder occurs in children and adults, but most patients are older than 40 years. About 65% of patients with primary autoimmune hemolytic anemia are women, and almost all cases that complicate systemic lupus erythematosus (Chapter 287) occur in women.

Pathobiology

Red Cell Antibodies

IgG anti–red cell autoantibodies mediate the destruction of red blood cells outside the circulating blood in a process called extravascular hemolysis. By contrast, when lytic components of the complement system enter the mechanism, destruction of red cells occurs directly within the circulating blood (intravascular hemolysis). The participation of lytic complement components in IgG-mediated autoimmune hemolytic anemia is, however, rare.

Molecular Structure of IgG Anti–Red Cell Autoantibodies

IgG antibodies consist of two identical heavy chains and two identical light chains (Fig. 164–1A); both kinds of chains contain variable and constant regions (Chapter 42). The variable regions form the antigen-binding pocket of the molecule and are held together by the first domains of the constant (Fc) regions of the heavy and light chains. The affinity of an antierythrocyte antibody is a measure of how tightly its antigen-binding pocket fits the red cell antigen, whereas avidity is a measure of the binding strength of a population of anti–red cell antibodies. Each IgG molecule has two identical antigen-binding sites, thus making it bivalent with respect to an antigen. Disulfide bonds hold the constant regions of the heavy and light chains together and give the molecule its characteristic Y shape.

Mechanism of Immunoglobulin Variation

Linear arrays of genes in germline DNA code for the variable and constant regions of the heavy and light chains. There are three types of heavy chain variable region genes, termed V, D, and J, and two kinds of light chain variable region genes, V and J. During its maturation in bone marrow, the B lymphocyte randomly rearranges these germline genes by means of a cut-and-paste mechanism to form a somatic combination of VDJ genes for the heavy chain variable region and VJ genes for the light chain variable region. Because there are almost 290 germline variable region genes, the mechanism of random recombination has the potential to create an astronomical number of distinctive antibodies. Recombination of immunoglobulin V genes accounts for the production of an antibody with a structurally unique antigen-binding pocket by each newly formed B-cell clone and is the basis of the polyclonal population of antibodies that appears in response to an immunogenic stimulus. In a mature B cell, the nascent antibody moves from the Golgi apparatus to the surface, where it serves as a transmembrane receptor for antigens. The B cell secretes the antibody only later, when it differentiates into a plasma cell.

The Constant Region of Immunoglobulins

After joining the VDJ and VJ cassettes that encode the V regions of the heavy and light chains, the B cell aligns them with one of several constant region genes that specify the effector functions of immunoglobulins. There are only two variants of the constant region of light chains: χ and λ. By contrast, the nine heavy chain constant region genes—M, D, G3, G1, A1, G2, G4, E1, and A2 (the order on chromosome 14q32)—allow nine types of heavy chains: μ (IgM), δ (IgD), $\gamma 3$ (IgG3), $\gamma 1$ (IgG1), $\alpha 1$ (IgA1), $\gamma 2$ (IgG2), $\gamma 4$ (IgG4), $\varepsilon 1$ (IgE1), or $\alpha 2$ (IgA2). These various constant regions determine the isotype of the antibody.

Initially, B cells produce IgM antibodies, but later in the immune response an isotype switch from IgM to IgG, IgA, or IgE occurs under the influence of T cells ($CD4^+$ helper T cells). This switch is the signature of an immune response that is driven by antigen-activated helper T cells. In a given case of autoimmune hemolytic anemia, the autoantibodies are not only IgG but also members of a polyclonal population, some with χ light chains, others with λ light chains. Such a polyclonal mixture is characteristic of the response of multiple clones of B cells to stimulation by antigen-activated helper T cells.

Red Blood Cell Destruction

Birth and Death of a Normal Erythrocyte

The blood of a normal adult contains about 2000 mL of erythrocytes. These cells arise in the bone marrow from hematopoietic precursors with a commitment to the red cell lineage. Under the influence of erythropoietin, other growth factors, and cytokines, the committed precursors differentiate, synthesize hemoglobin, and emerge from the marrow 3 days after their debut as proerythroblasts (Chapter 160). The earliest red cells in the blood are reticulocytes. These immature cells lose the blue-

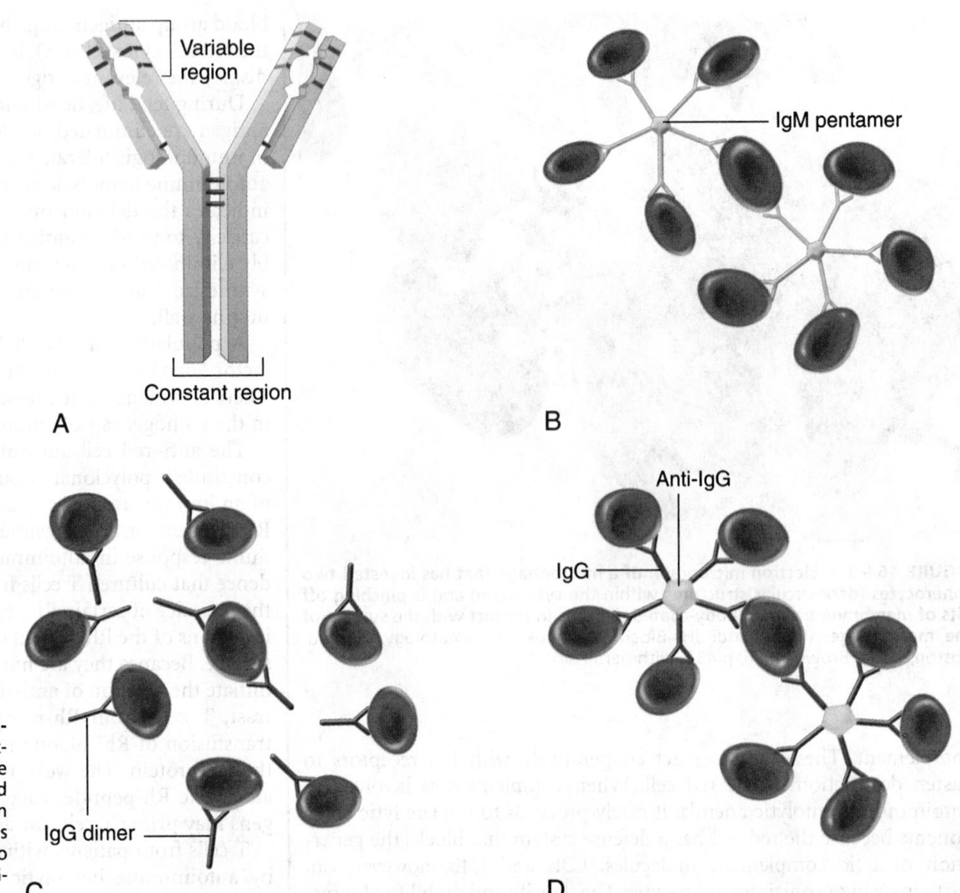

FIGURE 164–1 • IgG anti–red cell autoantibodies. A, Structure of an IgG molecule demonstrating its variable and constant regions and the heavy and light chains. B, Agglutination of red cells by pentameric IgM antibodies, which can join the cells into a lattice. C, Coating of red cells by IgG antibodies. The antibodies are unable to agglutinate the cells. D, Agglutination of IgG-coated red cells by an anti-IgG antibody.

staining remnants of cytoplasmic RNA and ribosomes in a little more than a day to become mature oxygen-transporting erythrocytes. The red cell's biconcave shape, the lack of a nucleus, and the lipid bilayer arrangement of its membrane give the cell the flexibility it needs to complete a traversal of over 100 miles through the circulatory system during its lifespan of 4 months.

Normally, production and destruction of erythrocytes are matched. To maintain the steady state, the marrow of a 70-kg adult produces about 25 mL of red blood cells (2×10^{11} erythrocytes) daily. About 1% of the circulating red cells die every day, mainly because worn-out adenosine triphosphate–fueled pumps cannot prevent water overload in the cell. The result is transformation of red cell discs into spheres. Spherocytes constitute 1% of the erythrocytes in blood, a figure equal to the proportion of reticulocytes in blood. In sinusoids of the spleen, lymph nodes, and liver, where blood flow is sluggish, macrophages ingest spherocytes and break down the hemoglobin that they carry into bilirubin and amino acids. Enzymes in the liver add glucuronide moieties to the bilirubin, thereby converting it from an insoluble form termed unconjugated or indirect-reacting bilirubin to a soluble form termed conjugated or direct-reacting bilirubin.

Dead erythrocytes release about 6 to 7 g of hemoglobin daily, most of it within macrophages. About 10% of dying spherocytes empty hemoglobin directly into the blood stream, where it binds to haptoglobin. Hepatocytes take up the hemoglobin-haptoglobin complexes, cleave globin from heme, and break it down into its constituent amino acids. If massive intravascular hemolysis overwhelms the haptoglobin disposal mechanism, the unbound (free) hemoglobin appears in urine. Renal tubular cells can convert hemoglobin into bile pigments, but they retain most of the heme iron. Tubular cells in urine that contain excess iron stain with Prussian blue, and together with cola-colored urine (hemoglobinuria), the blue renal tubular cells are characteristic of chronic (or massive) intravascular hemolysis. Table 164–1 lists causes of black or brown urine.

The Role of Macrophages in Red Blood Cell Destruction

IgG anti–red cell autoantibodies are opsonins; when bound to autoantigens on red cell membranes, they instigate phagocytosis of the cells by macrophages. Using its Fcγ receptors, the macrophage can ingest the entire IgG-coated erythrocyte or can transform it into a spherocyte by nibbling away its surface (Fig. 164–2). These antibody-coated spherocytes cannot resist osmotic forces; ultimately, they surrender to macrophages, especially in the splenic sinusoids where blood flows sluggishly.

The Fcγ receptors of macrophages bind to structures in the constant regions of all four subclasses of IgG, thereby bringing antibody-coated erythrocytes into a fatal embrace with the macrophage. Macrophages display three types of Fcγ receptors: FcγI, FcγII, and FcγIII. FcγI reacts avidly with IgG1 and IgG3, and it may follow FcγII and FcγIII in the sequence of events that culminate in phagocytosis of an antibody-coated red cell. Polymorphisms of the FcγII receptor genes affect the efficiency of the interaction of the receptor with IgG2; one variant interacts with high efficiency, the other only weakly.

The Fc (constant) region of IgG has a binding site for C1q, the first component of the complement system, and macrophages display receptors (CR1 receptors) for the later-acting C3b and C4b components of

TABLE 164–1 CAUSES OF BLACK OR DARK BROWN URINE

Hemoglobinuria
Intravascular hemolysis
Myoglobinuria (from rhabdomyolysis, Chapter 114)
Ischemic muscle damage
Crush injury
March myoglobinuria
Drugs (see Table 27–5)
Porphyria cutanea tarda (Chapter 229)
Melanin (metastatic malignant melanoma)
Alkaptonuria (Chapter 224)
Methemoglobinuria

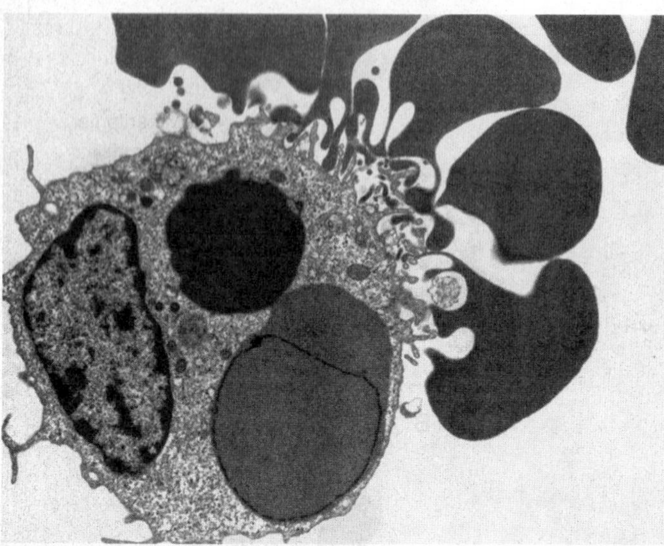

FIGURE 164–2 • Electron micrograph of a macrophage that has ingested two spherocytes (dark circular structures within the cytoplasm) and is pinching off bits of membrane from antibody-coated red cells in contact with the surface of the macrophage. (From Jandl JH: Blood. Textbook of Hematology, 2nd ed. Boston, Little, Brown, 1996, p 432, with permission.)

complement. These receptors act cooperatively with Fcγ receptors to hasten destruction of the red cell. When complement is involved in autoimmune hemolytic anemia, it rarely proceeds to the late lytic components because the red cell has a defense system that blocks the generation of lytic complement molecules. C3b and C4b, however, can participate in opsonizing erythrocytes. The density and mobility of target antigens on the erythrocyte membrane are also important because binding of C1q to the constant region of the antibody requires two closely adjacent Fcγ structures on the membrane.

The Hemolytic Rate

The rate of hemolysis in autoimmune hemolytic anemia depends on the amount of autoantibody on the red cell surface, the affinity and avidity of autoantibodies for the red cell autoantigen, and the number of macrophages in the environment of the antibody-coated erythrocyte. The amount and distribution of antigenic sites on the red cell surface influence the avidity of the polyclonal population of antierythrocyte autoantibodies. Populations of autoantibodies with high avidity cause a higher rate of red cell destruction than do populations with low avidity. Free (monomeric) IgG competes with the interaction of antibody-coated red cells with the Fc receptors of macrophages, but the concentration of IgG in plasma has only a minor influence on the hemolytic rate. The importance of the subclasses of IgG is unclear, but IgG3 antibodies seem more potent than IgG1 antibodies in promoting phagocytosis. The IgG subclass is also important for complement fixation. The order of potency is IgG1 > IgG3 > IgG2 > IgG4.

The degree of anemia depends not only on the rate of red cell destruction but also on the ability of marrow to increase erythrocyte production. With an adequate supply of nutrients and growth factors, bone marrow can overcome a hemolytic rate of about three times normal; anemia does not appear until the half-life of the red cell population drops to about 10 days (the half-life of a population of normal red cells is about 30 days as measured with ^{51}Cr-labeled red cells). A half-life of 5 or 6 days is not unusual in autoimmune hemolytic anemia. The marrow can compensate for accelerated red cell destruction by increasing the number of red cell precursors by up to 10 times the normal number (erythroid hyperplasia), accelerating the release of reticulocytes, and in some cases, allowing nucleated red cells to enter the blood.

Causes of Autoimmune Hemolytic Anemia

The cause of autoimmune hemolytic anemia is unknown. In about a third of cases, the autoantibodies have specificity for an antigen in the Rh system. In another third, the antibodies target proteins in membrane glycoproteins (glycophorins) of the red cell; in other cases, the antibodies have specificity for antigens in the Kell or Duffy blood group system (very rarely for ABO antigens) or for structures in the membrane that are not blood group antigens (e.g., band 3, an anchor point in the membrane for the red cell cytoskeleton). In all these cases the patient's own erythrocytes display the relevant antigen.

During fetal life, developing lymphocytes that come into contact with antigen are eliminated or silenced. This effect is one of the mechanisms of immunologic tolerance of endogenous antigens. The extreme rarity of autoimmune hemolytic anemia secondary to anti-A or anti-B antibodies indicates the deletion from the immune repertoire of B cells with the capacity to produce anti-A or anti-B antibodies. Such clones are probably eliminated or inactivated early in ontogeny because the embryo can synthesize A and B substances within 5 weeks of its implantation in the uterine wall.

A population of $CD4^+/CD25^+$ T cells that express the transcription factor Foxp3 restrains immune responses against autoantigens in adults. There is evidence that a deficiency of these regulatory T cells plays a role in the pathogenesis of autoimmune hemolytic anemia.

The anti–red cell autoantibodies in autoimmune hemolytic anemia constitute a polyclonal population of IgG antibodies—a typical feature of an immune response to an exogenous antigen. That the patient's own Rh antigens or an exogenous cross-reactive antigen drives the autoimmune response in autoimmune hemolytic anemia is supported by evidence that cultured T cells from patients with the disorder proliferate in the presence of certain Rh peptides. These self-stimulatory peptides occur in regions of the Rh protein that are not normally exposed on the red cell surface. Because they are hidden, the antigens may not have been able to initiate the deletion of anti-self T cells with receptors for self-Rh. By contrast, T cells from Rh-negative persons who were alloimmunized by transfusion of Rh^+ blood respond to Rh peptides in exposed regions of the Rh protein. The weak response of T cells from normal subjects to allogeneic Rh peptides suggests that cross-reactive environmental antigens may prime T cells for an anti-Rh response.

T cells from patients with chronic lymphocytic leukemia complicated by autoimmune hemolytic anemia also respond in vitro to self Rh proteins. Notably, the leukemic B cells from these patients are highly effective in presenting Rh protein to T cells. In some cases of chronic lymphocytic leukemia with autoimmune hemolytic anemia, the leukemic cells display surface immunoglobulins with light chain isotypes that differ from those of the patient's anti–red cell autoantibodies, thus indicating that the source of the autoantibodies in these patients is not the leukemic clone.

Drug-Induced Immune Hemolytic Anemia

Many drugs or their metabolites have the potential to elicit antidrug antibodies. Drugs that form covalent bonds with proteins in the red cell membrane can bind antidrug antibodies to the red cell surface, thereby causing a positive direct antiglobulin test and, in some cases, initiating antibody-mediated destruction of red cells. Some drugs, such as the cephalosporins, can bind to red cell membranes and take up IgG nonspecifically from plasma. In these cases there is no antidrug antibody.

The diagnosis of drug-induced, immune-mediated hemolytic anemia should come to mind if the patient has a history of receiving or taking a medication, there is acute complement-mediated hemolysis, only complement components are detectable on the red cell surface, or the patient's serum reacts with red cells in the presence of the suspected drug. Some drugs can induce true autoantibodies against red cells. Fludarabine, a purine nucleoside analogue used in the treatment of chronic lymphocytic leukemia, and interferon-α have this property. The cause of this type of drug-induced autoimmune hemolytic anemia is unknown, and there is no certain way of distinguishing it from primary autoimmune hemolytic anemia. Resolution of the hemolytic anemia after discontinuation of the suspected drug is not a constant feature of the phenomenon.

Clinical Manifestations

Autoimmune hemolytic anemia usually unfolds insidiously, but in some cases it begins abruptly with overt symptoms of severe anemia. When the disease is secondary to chronic lymphocytic leukemia (Chapter 195), systemic lupus erythematosus (Chapter 287), or some other disorder, the primary condition generally brings the patient to the physician first.

The symptoms are nonspecific and varied. They depend on the age of the patient; the presence of comorbid conditions, especially atherosclerotic cardiovascular disease; whether the autoimmune process is primary or a complication of another disorder; and the degree of anemia. In primary autoimmune hemolytic anemia, symptoms of anemia predominate; asthenia and easy fatigue are typical. Dyspnea suggests coexisting heart disease, and angina or myocardial infarction can occur in patients with severe anemia and coronary artery disease.

Diagnosis

History

The history can provide clues that help differentiate among the many causes of hemolytic anemia (Table 164–2) and is key to the diagnosis of drug-induced hemolytic anemia. It is essential to question the patient about drugs, both prescribed and over-the-counter medications, because drug-induced hemolytic anemia can be confused with autoimmune hemolytic anemia and management of the two conditions differs. It is also important to inquire about comorbid conditions; for example, symptoms of cardiovascular disease will influence management.

Autoimmune hemolytic anemia is a well-recognized complication of chronic lymphocytic leukemia (Chapter 195) and non-Hodgkin's B-cell lymphomas (Chapter 196). It can also occur occasionally in ulcerative colitis (Chapter 144), rheumatoid arthritis (Chapter 285), and various carcinomas (Chapter 189). Autoimmune hemolytic anemia occurs in about 10% of cases of systemic lupus erythematosus (Chapter 287); it may be the initial clinical manifestation of the disease or occur later. It may also complicate the antiphospholipid antibody syndrome; such cases constitute an unusual subset of systemic lupus erythematosus. In most diseases with autoimmune hemolytic anemia as a secondary feature, the primary disorder will be at the center of the clinical problem.

Physical Examination

There are no specific findings on physical examination. Nevertheless, the combination of pallor, jaundice, and a palpable spleen (Chapter 174) strongly point to hemolytic anemia, but not necessarily to autoimmune hemolytic anemia. Pallor is often difficult to gauge; examination of the palmar creases, the buccal mucosa, and the subconjunctival membranes, including side-by side comparison of the examiner's nail beds with the patient's, can be revealing. More than half the patients have a palpable spleen, but the frequency of this finding depends on the skill of the examiner. The tip of the spleen rarely descends more than 6 cm below the costal margin except in the presence of a lymphoma or chronic lymphocytic leukemia. Hepatomegaly is also frequent; a firm, nontender edge is easily palpable in about 50% of patients.

The examiner should search for an underlying disease because of differences between primary and secondary autoimmune hemolytic anemia in management and prognosis. The malar rash of systemic lupus erythematosus and the enlarged lymph nodes of a lymphoma or chronic lymphocytic leukemia should not be overlooked. A very large spleen should raise the possibility of coexisting lymphoma or chronic lymphocytic leukemia.

Laboratory Findings

Anemia

Examination of the blood smear will reveal the attempt of marrow to compensate for accelerated hemolysis and the effects of the interaction between antibody-coated red cells and macrophages. Two populations are evident: large, blue-tinged red cells, which correspond to reticulocytes, and small, dark red spherocytes (Fig. 164–3). Such a dimorphic population is characteristic of hemolytic anemia but is not diagnostic of any particular type of hemolytic anemia.

Automated instruments that directly measure hemoglobin, red cell numbers, and red cell volume (mean corpuscular volume [MCV]) have virtually displaced microscopy in routine practice. The instruments reveal abnormal populations of red cells with histograms of the red cell volume distribution and calculate the red cell distribution width (RDW), a reflection of the variation in red cell size (anisocytosis). They also count reticulocytes by means of a fluorescent dye that binds to RNA or supravital stains. The combination of a high MCV (because of reticulocytosis), a high RDW (because of the dimorphic population of reticulocytes and spherocytes), and a high reticulocyte count points to hemolytic anemia. In rare cases, the reticulocyte count is unexpectedly low, probably because the autoantibody destroys reticulocytes before they leave the bone marrow.

TABLE 164–2 DIFFERENTIAL DIAGNOSIS OF HEMOLYTIC ANEMIA

HEREDITARY HEMOLYTIC ANEMIA

The thalassemias
- β-Thalassemia
- α-Thalassemia
- Combined thalassemia and hemoglobinopathy

The hemoglobinopathies
- Sickle cell disease (hemoglobin S)
- Hemoglobin C disease
- Hemoglobin E disease
- Combined hemoglobinopathies (hemoglobin SC disease)

Defects of the red cell membrane
- Hereditary spherocytosis
- Hereditary elliptocytosis
- Acanthocytosis

Deficiencies in red cell enzymes
- Glucose-6-phosphate dehydrogenase deficiency
- Pyruvate kinase deficiency
- Defects of the Embden-Meyerhof pathway

ACQUIRED HEMOLYTIC ANEMIA

Immune-mediated hemolytic anemia
- Autoimmune hemolytic anemia
- Cold agglutinin disease
- Paroxysmal nocturnal hemoglobinuria
- Paroxysmal cold hemoglobinuria
- Drug-induced immunohemolytic anemia
- Hemolytic transfusion reaction
- Hemolytic disease of the newborn secondary to maternal alloantibodies
- Systemic lupus erythematosus

Microangiopathic hemolytic anemia (Fig. 164–4)
- Disseminated intravascular coagulation
- Thrombotic thrombocytopenic purpura
- Hemolytic-uremic syndrome
- Infections (e.g., *Clostridium*, malaria, babesiosis, *Bartonella*)
- Deficiency of factor H
- Giant hemangioma
- Disseminated carcinomatosis
- Chemotherapy (e.g., mitomycin C)
- Solid organ transplantation
- Bone marrow transplantation
- Malignant hypertension
- Scleroderma
- Eclampsia, preeclampsia, HELLP syndrome (*h*emolysis, *e*levated *l*iver enzymes, *l*ow *p*latelet count)
- Prosthetic materials
  - Heart valves
  - Ventricular or atrial septal patches
  - Left ventricular assist devices
  - Vascular grafts
  - Transjugular intrahepatic portosystemic shunts
- Physical or chemical injuries
  - Trauma to small vessels (e.g., exercise related)
  - Burn related
  - Venoms
  - Bacterial infection (e.g., *Clostridium*)
  - Copper
  - Freshwater near-drowning

Other Blood Cells

The white blood cell count is often moderately elevated, a reflection of a stressed bone marrow with severe hemolytic anemia. In uncomplicated cases, platelet counts are normal or occasionally increased slightly. Platelet counts may be low in systemic lupus erythematosus or in Evans' syndrome, a rare combination of autoimmune hemolytic anemia and immune thrombocytopenia (Chapter 179).

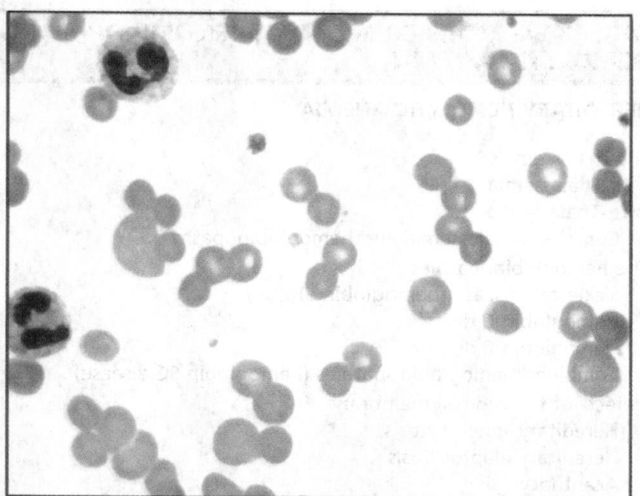

FIGURE 164–3 • Representative peripheral blood smear in a patient with autoimmune hemolytic anemia. (Courtesy of Thomas K. Chacko.)

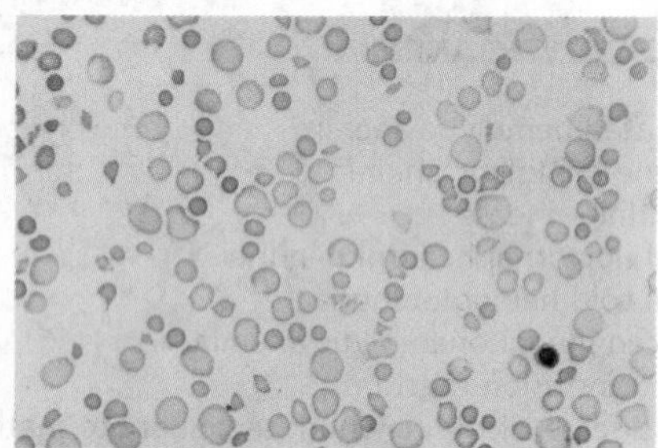

FIGURE 164–4 • Microangiopathic hemolytic anemia. A peripheral smear shows fragmental red blood cells or schistocytes in a variety of shapes and sizes.

Bone Marrow

The characteristic finding in bone marrow is erythroid hyperplasia. However, examination of marrow is needed only if there are unexpected findings or suspicion of a lymphoma.

Biochemical Signs of Increased Destruction of Erythrocytes

Elevated serum levels of prehepatic (indirect) bilirubin and lactate dehydrogenase (LDH) and a reduced serum haptoglobin concentration are signs of hemolytic anemia. The indirect bilirubin in hemolytic anemia does not usually exceed 4.0 mg/dL unless there is coexisting liver disease. Serum LDH can be useful, especially in cases with intravascular hemolysis, but neither LDH nor the haptoglobin level is specific for hemolytic anemia. Moreover, the presence of inflammation may negate the value of measuring haptoglobin, which is an acute phase protein. Oral contraceptives, estrogen replacement therapy, and tamoxifen all affect haptoglobin levels. Laboratory signs of intravascular destruction of red blood cells (hemoglobinemia, hemoglobinuria, and hemosiderinuria; see later) are unusual in autoimmune hemolytic anemia.

The Antiglobulin (Coombs) Test

The antiglobulin test is key to the diagnosis of autoimmune hemolytic anemia and central to an understanding of the antibody-mediated mechanism of destruction of red blood cells in this disorder (see Fig. 164–1B to D).

The terms complete and incomplete antibodies refer to the ability (or inability) of antibodies to cross-link adjacent red cells, thereby building the lattice needed for macroscopic clumping of red cells. The strong negative charge of red blood cells suspended in saline keeps them apart, even if they have a coating of antibodies—the average distance between cells is 24 nm. IgM antibodies, being pentamers, are efficient agglutinins; with five antigen-binding sites, they can bridge this distance. In contrast, bivalent IgG antibodies often cannot cause clumping of saline-suspended erythrocytes.

In 1945, Robin Coombs showed that animal (rabbit) antibodies against human IgG agglutinated Rh^+ red blood cells that were coated with "incomplete" anti-Rh antibodies. The test that revealed antibody-coated red blood cells was named the direct antiglobulin test, and its first clinical application was for the diagnosis of hemolytic disease of the newborn secondary to anti-Rh antibodies. The indirect antiglobulin test was devised to seek the presence of incomplete anti-Rh antibodies in maternal serum. In this procedure, serum suspected of harboring anti-Rh antibodies is incubated with Rh^+ red blood cells, which are then subjected to the direct antiglobulin test. As presently used, the standard antiglobulin reagent contains antibodies against all four classes of IgG and components of complement (usually C3 and C4). The Coombs test has become central to the diagnosis of autoimmune hemolytic anemia, and with few exceptions, a positive direct antiglobulin test leads to the diagnosis of antibody-mediated hemolytic anemia.

Nevertheless, a positive antiglobulin test requires cautious interpretation when there are no other features of autoimmune hemolytic anemia. False-positive test results are not unusual. The reported incidence of positive antiglobulin tests in normal blood donors and general populations of hospitalized patients varies widely—from 1 in 100 to 1 in 15,000. Differences in the technique used in performing the test account for this variation. The most common reason for a false-positive direct antiglobulin test is low-avidity adherence of nonspecific IgG to red cells. In rare cases, however, the result is not a false-positive but a harbinger of the development of autoimmune hemolytic anemia. False-negative tests are usually due to low-affinity autoantibodies that spontaneously elute from the red cell in vitro or amounts of erythrocyte-coating antibodies that are below the limit of detection by the antiglobulin test. The distinction between a true-positive and a false-positive direct antiglobulin test can be made by eluting the antibody from the red cells and testing its ability to bind to normal red cells. In a false-positive reaction, the eluted antibody does not bind to normal red cells, whereas binding occurs in a true-positive test.

Treatment

Rx

There are no prospective controlled trials of the treatment of autoimmune hemolytic anemia. A corticosteroid, usually prednisone, is the standard initial treatment. Splenectomy is indicated in patients who fail to attain or sustain a remission. If splenectomy does not cause improvement, one or more immunosuppressive agents can be tried. Red cell transfusions should never be withheld from symptomatic patients.

Initial Medical Therapy

Corticosteroids

In the initial management of the disease, the standard of practice is administration of prednisone in a dose of 1.0 to 1.5 mg/kg/day. The duration of treatment at this dose is an unsettled question, but a response, manifested by a rise in the hematocrit and a fall in the reticulocyte count, is usually evident within 3 to 4 weeks. A patient who fails to improve within this time is unlikely to respond to further treatment with prednisone. In a patient who does respond, slow reduction of the dose of prednisone is essential to avoid a relapse. The usual tapering schedule is a weekly reduction of the initial dose by 10 mg/day to a dose of 30 mg/day, followed by a weekly reduction of 5 mg/day to 15 mg/day. Thereafter, slow, cautious tapering over a period of at least 4 months is the rule. A rise in the reticulocyte count or a fall in the hematocrit should prompt an increase in the dose, usually to the previous level.

About 25% of patients treated with corticosteroids in the manner described enter a stable, complete remission; half the patients require continuous, low-dose prednisone; and the remaining 25% respond only transiently or not at all or are unable to tolerate continuous corticosteroid treatment. There is no reliable evidence that alternate-day maintenance treatment is superior to daily treatment, but some patients tolerate this schedule better than daily prednisone. Very high doses of intravenous methylprednisolone have been advocated for stubborn cases, but such treatment is risky and should be considered experimental.

Transfusion

Red blood cell transfusions (Chapter 183) are indicated in patients with disabling symptoms of anemia: marked fatigue, reduced exer-

Rx

cise tolerance, or an inability to work. These symptoms often develop when the hemoglobin concentration falls below 10 g/dL, but the decision to administer red cell transfusions should not depend primarily on laboratory tests—the patient's clinical status is the dominant factor. Some patients can tolerate a stable hemoglobin level as low as 8 g/dL; however, symptoms of coronary artery disease or heart failure may force the decision to transfuse before the hemoglobin level falls below 10 g/dL. Regardless of the patient's clinical status, rapid transfusion of large volumes of red cells can have serious adverse consequences. The blood should be administered at a rate that does not exceed 1 mL/kg/hr.

The risk of reactions to blood transfusions (Chapter 183) in autoimmune hemolytic anemia is ever present because of destruction of transfused blood by the patient's autoantibody. This hazard is increased if the patient also has alloantibodies that were induced by pregnancy or previous transfusions. For these reasons, the blood bank should be alerted to the diagnosis and to whether the patient was ever pregnant or ever had transfusions.

It is important for the managing physician to understand that no patient with symptomatic autoimmune hemolytic anemia should be denied blood transfusions because of an "incompatible crossmatch." The patient's positive antiglobulin test always interferes with compatibility testing. Communication and cooperation between the patient's physician and specialists in transfusion medicine (Chapter 183) are essential in reducing the risk of transfusion in patients with autoimmune hemolytic anemia.

Surgical Therapy

Splenectomy

Because the spleen is the major site of red cell destruction in autoimmune hemolytic anemia, splenectomy should be considered for patients who have not responded to corticosteroids or who have maintained a stable, but corticosteroid-dependent remission. A complete, durable remission follows splenectomy in half to two thirds of cases. Attempts to predict responsiveness to splenectomy with measurement of splenic sequestration of ^{51}Cr-labeled erythrocytes are not reliable. The only way of knowing the effectiveness of splenectomy in a given patient is to perform the procedure. Laparoscopic splenectomy, a safe method of removing the organ, is now the preferred surgical technique.

A major risk of splenectomy is post-splenectomy sepsis secondary to encapsulated bacteria, particularly pneumococci and especially in children. Splenectomy also increases susceptibility to babesiosis, ehrlichiosis, and malaria. Preoperative immunization with polyvalent pneumococcal and *Haemophilus influenzae* vaccines reduces the risk for post-splenectomy sepsis. In children, a prophylactic antibiotic, generally penicillin or amoxicillin, is essential after splenectomy. The usual dose of penicillin for prophylaxis is 250 mg twice daily for 2 to 3 years after splenectomy (or at least until the age of 5). Although evidence for the effectiveness of (or need for) prophylactic antibiotics in splenectomized adults is inconclusive, it is reasonable to give adults prophylactic penicillin, 250 mg twice daily for 1 year after splenectomy. Penicillin-resistant pneumococci have emerged in some parts of the United States; in those areas of the country a macrolide should be used. Education of the patient concerning the risk for serious infection after splenectomy is also important.

A rise in the platelet count occurs after splenectomy in almost all patients. The increase rarely exceeds 500,000/μL and usually subsides within 3 to 5 months. The low risk for thromboembolism in post-splenectomy thrombocytosis argues against the need for routine antithrombotic prophylaxis.

Other Medical Treatments

Rituximab

Rituximab is a chimeric monoclonal antibody with high affinity for the CD20 antigen on the surface of normal and malignant B lymphocytes. The antibody consists of murine light chain and heavy chain variable region sequences and human constant region sequences. The limited data on its use in autoimmune hemolytic anemia are encouraging. The antibody is usually given at a dose of 375 mg/m^2 by intravenous infusion once weekly for four or eight doses, but it may be continued weekly or biweekly if necessary. Rituximab rapidly depletes the circulation and lymphoid tissue of B cells; it can cause allergic reactions and increase the risk for infection.

Immunosuppressive Drugs and Other Agents

Immunosuppressive drugs other than corticosteroids can be useful in stubborn cases of autoimmune hemolytic anemia, but no trials have compared the efficacy of these drugs head-to-head. The choice usually depends on safety and familiarity with the agent. Azathioprine has the least short-term and long-term toxicity; cyclosporine is nephrotoxic; and cyclophosphamide damages the bone marrow, ovaries, and bladder, and it impairs spermatogenesis. In general, these drugs should be administered only by specialists and reserved for refractory cases: patients who have failed to respond to splenectomy or who, because of comorbidity, are not suitable candidates for splenectomy.

A variety of other treatments have been used in stubborn cases of autoimmune hemolytic anemia, including plasma exchange, vinca alkaloids, danazol (a synthetic androgen), and intravenous IgG. None of these forms of therapy are reliably effective.

Autoimmune Hemolytic Anemia Associated with IgM Antibodies: Cold Agglutinin Disease

Definition and Epidemiology

Of the two types of cold agglutinin disease, the acute form occurs as a complication of an infectious disease, usually caused by *Mycoplasma pneumoniae* (Chapter 338) or Epstein-Barr virus (infectious mononucleosis [Chapter 400]). The onset in these cases is abrupt and generally makes its appearance during recovery from the infection. The acute disease, which almost always affects young adults, is rare and self-limited and seldom requires treatment. The usual type of cold agglutinin disease is a chronic disorder of older patients, many of whom have a B-cell lymphoma (Chapter 196), chronic lymphocytic leukemia (Chapter 195), or Waldenström's macroglobulinemia (Chapter 198). In these cases the cold agglutinin is a monoclonal IgM, in contrast to the polyclonal IgM cold agglutinins of postinfectious cold agglutinin disease.

Pathobiology

Cold Agglutinins

Cold agglutinins are IgM autoantibodies that react with erythrocytes at temperatures below 37° C. Normal serum contains low titers of cold agglutinins, usually not detectable in a dilution higher than 1:10, but in chronic cold agglutinin disease the titer of the cold agglutinin can exceed 1:10^5. The temperature at which cold agglutinins react with red cells in vitro—the thermal amplitude of the antibodies—varies considerably, but in almost all cases the red cells agglutinate readily at 4° C and quickly disaggregate at 37° C. The temperature-dependent reversibility of the reaction is a manifestation of the weak affinity of cold agglutinins for red cell antigens.

Most cold agglutinins react with polysaccharides on the red cell surface. The principal targets are the i antigen (a straight-chain paragloboside) and the I antigen (a branched paragloboside with the same composition as the i antigen). Less common are the Pr glycoproteins and sialylated polysaccharides. The erythrocytes of almost all adults are I$^+$ and lack the i antigen. The i antigen is characteristic of the red cells of newborns because the enzyme that converts i to I becomes active only after birth. Cold agglutinins associated with *M. pneumoniae* infection have anti-I specificity, whereas cold agglutinins related to infectious mononucleosis have anti-i specificity. In chronic cold agglutinin disease, the cold agglutinins are almost always monoclonal IgM, χ anti-I antibodies with a heavy chain segment that is encoded by the VH4-34 gene. The shape of the antigen-binding surface of this heavy chain favors binding to polysaccharides. Curiously, about 10% of B cells from normal subjects have rearranged the VH-34 gene segment; these cells are probably the source of the cold agglutinins in normal serum. Anti-Pr cold agglutinins tend to have a similar χ light chain variable region; presumably, the binding surface of this light chain promotes attachment of the agglutinins to red cell glycoproteins.

Erythrocyte Destruction in Cold Agglutinin Disease

The basis of red cell destruction in cold agglutinin disease is the ability of IgM antibodies to fix complement readily. Unlike IgG antibodies, each IgM molecule has two binding sites for C1q. An inhibitor on the red cell surface (the membrane inhibitor of reactive lysis) stops the complement cascade before lytic components can be activated, with fragments termed C3b and C4b left behind. This step prepares the red cell for engulfment by phagocytic cells with CR1 receptors for C3b and C4b. If such coated red cells escape into the circulation, enzymes degrade the C3b and C4b fragments to harmless peptides (C3dg and C4d).

In the hands and feet, blood cools sufficiently to allow cold agglutinins to bind red cells. During this fraction of a second, the adherent IgM attracts C1q, which initiates the generation of C3b and C4b on the erythrocyte's surface. On entering the warmer visceral circulation, the red cell releases the cold agglutinin, but the remaining C3 fragments, by engaging the CR1 of macrophages, enable phagocytosis of the red cell. The efficiency of this process depends on the amount of cold agglutinin on the red cell surface, the ability of the cold agglutinin to activate the complement pathway, and its thermal amplitude. An antibody that binds only at very low temperatures causes little harm, whereas an antibody that binds at a temperature close to 37° C can cause severe hemolytic anemia. These variables account for the widely different degrees of severity of cold agglutinin disease.

Clinical Manifestations

Most cases of chronic cold agglutinin disease occur between the ages of 50 and 70. The main symptoms are due to anemia, which may worsen in cold weather. The anemia is not generally severe and can remain static without treatment for many months because of the action of an inhibitor of C3b in serum.

In a patient with high-affinity cold agglutinins, exposure to cold can precipitate an attack of acrocyanosis as a result of massive agglutination of red cells in the capillary circulation, intravascular hemolysis with hemoglobinuria, and rarely, acute renal failure. The acrocyanosis is not Raynaud's phenomenon (white, blue, and red digits caused by vasospasm [Chapter 80]) nor the vasculitis of cryoglobulinemia (Chapter 198). Enlargement of the spleen is uncommon unless there is an associated B-cell neoplasm.

Diagnosis

Agglutination of the patient's red cells at room temperature or, more often, on chilling the blood is distinctive. Characteristically, the agglutination disappears on warming the blood to 37° C. Hemagglutination causes rouleaux formation in the blood smear and may interfere with automated blood counts. Spherocytosis is not prominent; the reticulocyte count is proportional to the degree of anemia.

The titer of cold agglutinins is often 1:10^5 or higher, and the direct antiglobulin test is positive if the cold agglutinin has a high thermal amplitude. In the presence of a B-cell lymphoma, a monoclonal IgM-χ cold agglutinin may be detectable in serum by electrophoresis or immunofixation.

Treatment

Rx

Cold agglutinin disease, whether postinfectious or chronic, often requires no treatment. Postinfectious cold agglutinin disease is self-limited and generally of mild degree. Because chronic cold agglutinin disease is frequently a stable condition, its management requires mainly avoidance of the cold. Safe transfusion is possible; there is no agreement concerning the need for transfusion with warmed blood.

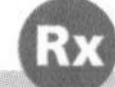

Prednisone, usually in a dose of 1.0 to 1.5 mg/kg/day for 3 to 6 weeks, can be tried, but it is rarely effective. The use of immunosuppressive drugs such as azathioprine or cyclophosphamide is not recommended. Splenectomy generally fails to induce a remission because the liver is a major site of destruction of C3b-coated red cells. Rituximab (375 mg/m^2 by intravenous infusion once weekly for four or eight doses) has been used successfully in some cases. In patients with chronic cold agglutinin disease and a B-cell neoplasm, treatment should be directed against the tumor.

Paroxysmal Cold Hemoglobinuria

Definition

Paroxysmal cold hemoglobinuria is a rare form of immune-mediated hemolytic anemia in which an IgG autoantibody binds to red cells at low temperatures and brings with it C1q. The antibody dissociates from red cells at 37° C, but C1q remains on the membrane; at the warmer temperature it triggers progression of the complement cascade to its lytic components. The result is intravascular hemolysis.

Pathobiology

An unsolved problem is how the lytic components of complement are generated on the red cell surface in paroxysmal cold hemoglobinuria but not in cold agglutinin disease. The antibody is named for Donath and Landsteiner, who in 1904 described it in a patient with tertiary syphilis. With the waning of late syphilis in modern times, the Donath-Landsteiner antibody is encountered most often during convalescence from a viral infection, usually a childhood exanthem.

The Donath-Landsteiner autoantibody has no clinical effects unless the patient is exposed to the cold. With cold exposure, even of only an arm or a leg, intravascular hemolysis begins soon after return to a warm temperature. Chills, fever, back pain, abdominal cramps, and hemoglobinuria are typical. Urticaria is common, acute renal failure is rare, and anemia is an inevitable consequence of severe intravascular hemolysis. The attack is self-limited, lasting only 1 or 2 days.

Diagnosis

A positive Donath-Landsteiner test is diagnostic, but the test is relatively insensitive. The procedure should demonstrate hemolysis in the test tube when the patient's blood is chilled and then warmed to 37° C. Addition of normal serum as a source of complement is often necessary to bring out the hemolytic phase of the reaction.

Treatment

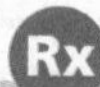

Treatment is generally unnecessary, and spontaneous recovery should be expected within weeks or a few months.

Paroxysmal Nocturnal Hemoglobinuria

Definition

PNH is an acquired form of hemolytic anemia in which a somatic mutation in a hematopoietic stem cell renders erythrocytes susceptible to the lytic components of complement, thereby causing intravascular hemolysis in the absence of an anti–red blood cell antibody.

Epidemiology

PNH can occur at any age, but usually between the ages of 10 and 50. At the time of diagnosis, the median age is about 40 years; median survival from diagnosis is approximately 10 years. It is a rare disorder with an estimated prevalence in the population of 1 in 10^5 to 1 in 10^6. There is no sex preference, and a family history of the disorder is unusual.

Pathobiology

Genetics

PNH is due to a somatic mutation that causes a defect in the red cell membrane. The disease begins in a single hematopoietic stem cell when the *pig-a* gene on the short arm of the active X chromosome acquires a mutation. The *pig-a* gene encodes PIG-A, an enzyme that is essential for the synthesis of glycosylphosphatidylinositol (GPI). This lipid in the red cell membrane forms a peptide link with the C-terminal amino acid of numerous proteins, thereby anchoring them to the membrane.

Because the mutation occurs in a hematopoietic stem cell, blood cells of all lineages are deficient in PIG-A. Almost 150 different mutations of *pig-a* have been identified. Most of them completely inactivate PIG-A and cause total loss of GPI in the descendents of the carrier stem cell; other mutations only partially disable the synthesis of GPI. Red cells with complete deficiency of GPI are termed PNH III erythrocytes, and those with partial deficiency are called PNH II erythrocytes. The coexistence of PNH III and PNH II red cells in the same patient is indicative of the presence of at least two mutant clones. The simultaneous presence of normal and mutant clones results in two (or more) populations of blood cells in the patient: one is normal, whereas the other carries the mutation. In effect, a patient with PNH is a hematopoietic chimera.

Functional Consequences of Deficiency of Glycosylphosphatidylinositol

The membrane inhibitor of reactive hemolysis (CD59, or protectin) is one of the many proteins that GPI anchors to the red cell. It prevents polymerization of C9, the final step in assembly of the membrane attack complex that begins with cleavage of C5 to C5b. If unimpeded by C59, polymers of C9 drill holes in the red cell membrane and cause lysis of the red cell, which releases its hemoglobin into the circulation. The deficiency of CD59 in PNH allows unimpeded assembly of the membrane attack complex on the erythrocyte surface, thereby initiating intravascular hemolysis. A variety of nonspecific factors, such a reduction in the pH of blood, can activate complement. The morning hemoglobinuria of PNH is probably the result of acidification of blood during sleep.

Clinical Manifestations

Classically, a patient with PNH arises in the morning and passes urine the color of a cola beverage. During the ensuing hours, the color of urine gradually returns to the usual shade of yellow. In all cases, these paroxysms of hemoglobinuria occur on a background of chronic, low-grade intravascular hemolysis, the cause of the constant hemosiderinuria in PNH. About a third of cases evolve into a picture of aplastic anemia (Chapter 171); transformation to acute myelogenous leukemia is a rare event. Abdominal pain, dysphagia, and erectile dysfunction are additional clinical features. The basis of these symptoms is probably scavenging by free plasma hemoglobin of nitric oxide, which has an important role in regulating vasomotor tone and relaxing smooth muscle. A feared complication that occurs in about a third of cases is venous thrombosis, which often causes Budd-Chiari syndrome (Chapter 146) by obstructing the hepatic veins. Splenomegaly is uncommon; hepatomegaly and ascites point to hepatic vein thrombosis. Petechiae and susceptibility to infection are indications of bone marrow failure. Hemosiderinuria, a constant finding, is the result of chronic intravascular hemolysis. Subtle or overt signs of bone marrow damage (leukopenia and thrombocytopenia) are frequent.

The extent of red cell destruction in PNH depends on the number of PNH red cells in blood, the level of GPI on the red cell membrane (PNH III cells are devoid of GPI), and activation of complement. The anemia is often aggravated by iron deficiency, which is caused by the constant hemosiderinuria. The reason for the tendency to thrombosis is unclear; hypercoagulability from the release of prothrombotic materials in red cell and platelet membranes (which are also abnormal in PNH) and impaired fibrinolysis have been implicated. Nitric oxide scavenging by free plasma hemoglobin may damage endothelial cells and cause aggregation of platelets.

Paroxysmal Nocturnal Anemia and Aplastic Anemia

Signs of bone marrow damage are detectable in almost all patients with the clinical picture of PNH. Injury to the marrow plays a key role in the development of PNH, and in some patients the disease evolves into a picture of aplastic anemia (Chapter 171). Conversely, patients with aplastic anemia often have PNH red cells in their blood. Moreover, small numbers of hematopoietic precursor cells bearing the *pig-a* mutation occur in normal people, but the mutant precursor clones do not expand, and the few PNH descendents of these cells have no clinical consequences. In the presence of bone marrow damage, however, clones bearing the mutation have a growth advantage, perhaps because cells lacking GPI-anchored proteins resist the injury that damaged the marrow and expand to the point of clinical significance. A second mutation could also give a mutant clone a growth advantage, and chromosomal abnormalities have been reported in PNH.

Diagnosis

Often, the clinical picture is virtually diagnostic. The diagnosis can be established accurately by demonstrating, through the use of flow cytometry, a deficiency of CD59 on erythrocytes. A promising sensitive test for CD59 entails the use of aerolysin, a bacterial toxin that binds to the GPI anchor. When tagged with a fluorescent dye for use in flow cytometry, aerolysin can detect small numbers of GPI-deficient cells in blood. Flow cytometry can also measure the proportions of PNH III and PNH II red cells in blood, thereby providing information on the severity of the disease. Laboratory tests that depend on the sensitivity of PNH red cells to complement, such as the Ham acidification test, are insensitive and have largely been abandoned.

Treatment

Rx

A humanized monoclonal antibody (eculizumab) against C5, a complement component essential for formation of the membrane attack complex, was found to reduce signs of intravascular hemolysis and the requirement for transfusions in patients with PNH. [1] In a randomized trial, the dose of the antibody was 600 mg every week for 4 weeks, followed 1 week later by a 900-mg dose and then by 900 mg every other week through week 26. Oral iron can correct the iron deficiency (treatment with iron does not exacerbate the hemolysis), and warfarin can prevent thrombosis in patients with a history of a thrombotic event. Transfusions are helpful in supportive care. Aplastic anemia has been treated successfully with immunosuppressive agents (antithymocyte globulin, usually in a dose of 1.5 mg/kg daily for 7 to 14 days) or cyclosporine (3 to 5 mg/kg for at least 3 months). Bone marrow transplantation is risky but can be curative.

Hemolytic Transfusion Reactions

Definition

Of the various types of acute transfusion reactions (Chapter 183), acute hemolytic transfusion reaction is the most dangerous. Redundant blood bank systems of crosschecks, automated blood typing and crossmatching, and computer-based techniques of patient identification have reduced the risk of a hemolytic transfusion reaction, but the possibility of this complication is ever present.

Epidemiology and Pathobiology

Fatal hemolytic transfusion reactions are rare—about 16 for every 10 million red cell transfusions. The cause of hemolytic transfusion reactions is intravascular lysis of the donor's red cells by antibodies (alloantibodies or isoantibodies) in the recipient that bind to one or more blood group antigens on the transfused cells. The recipient's isoantibodies can be natural anti-A or anti-B antibodies, or they can be induced by previous transfusions or pregnancy. Whether IgM or IgG, the isoantibodies trigger the assembly of lytic complement components on the surface of the donor's red cell. The rapid formation of large amounts of C3a and C5a fragments causes hypotension and bronchial and smooth muscle spasm. Renal failure is a consequence of severe, prolonged hypotension;

TABLE 164–3 EXTRAVASCULAR AND INTRAVASCULAR HEMOLYSIS

Condition	Diagnostic Finding	Red Cell Morphology	Other Findings	Treatment
Autoimmune hemolytic anemia	Positive antiglobulin test	Spherocytosis	Splenomegaly	Chapter 164
Drug-induced hemolytic anemia	Drug-dependent antibody	Spherocytosis	History of drug ingestion	Chapter 164
Cold agglutinin disease	Cold agglutinins	Normal	Acrocyanosis	Chapter 164
Paroxysmal nocturnal hemoglobinuria	Lack of CD59	Normal	Hemoglobinuria, hemosiderinuria	Chapter 164
Paroxysmal cold hemoglobinuria	Donath-Landsteiner antibody	Normal	Cold-dependent hemoglobinuria	Chapter 164
Prosthetic heart valve	Heart murmur	Schistocytosis	Hemosiderinuria	Iron, folic acid, and vitamin B_{12}. Valve replacement for severe hemolysis; Chapter 75
Thrombotic thrombocytopenic purpura	Intravascular hemolysis + thrombocytopenia	Schistocytosis	Renal failure, autoantibody against ADAMTS-13	Chapter 177
Hemolytic-uremic syndrome	Intravascular hemolysis + thrombocytopenia	Schistocytosis	Renal failure, *Shigella* toxin	Chapter 177
HELLP syndrome	Pregnancy	Schistocytosis	Coagulopathy	Chapter 154
Arteriovenous malformations (Kasabach-Merritt syndrome)	Large cavernous hemangioma	Schistocytosis	Thrombocytopenia	Chapter 177
Postperfusion syndrome	Cardiopulmonary Bypass surgery	Ghost erythrocytes	Complement activation	Chapter 74
March hemoglobinuria	History of jogging	No consistent abnormality	Hematuria, hemoglobinuria	Symptomatic
Oxidative hemolysis	Drugs	Heinz bodies	G6PD deficiency	Avoid responsible drug (Chapter 27)
Chemical-induced hemolysis	Strong oxidizing chemicals (e.g., sodium chlorate)	Microspherocytes	Hemoglobinuria, methemoglobinemia, renal failure	Plasma exchange, dialysis
Burns	Severe burn	Spherocytes, schistocytes	Hemoglobinuria	Treatment of burn (Chapter 113)
Malaria	*Plasmodium falciparum* infection	Red cell sporozoites	Hemoglobinuria	Chapter 366
Babesiosis	Tick bite	Intracellular protozoa	Splenectomy scar	Chapter 374
Clostridium perfringens	*C. perfringens* bacteremia	Spherocytosis	Intravascular hemolysis	Chapter 319

G6PD = glucose-6-phosphate dehydrogenase; HELLP = *h*emolysis, *e*levated *l*iver enzymes, *l*ow *p*latelet count.

the main renal lesion is renal cortical ischemia secondary to shunting of blood away from the kidneys. Hemoglobin itself is not nephrotoxic.

Clinical Manifestations

The signs and symptoms of a hemolytic transfusion reaction are nonspecific and include fever, back pain, urticaria, dyspnea, hypotension, and evidence of disseminated intravascular coagulation. These nonspecific signs appear and worsen during administration of the transfusion.

Treatment

Rx

Immediate steps must be taken to stop the transfusion, submit the transfused blood and a sample of the patient's blood to the blood bank, and order tests of plasma and urine for free hemoglobin. Hydration is necessary to ward off renal failure; intravenous fluid, usually normal saline, should be started at once together with a diuretic (usually furosemide) in amounts to keep urine flow at a rate of at least 100 mL/hr. A nephrologist should be consulted without delay if these measures are ineffective, if hypotension persists, or if renal failure worsens.

OTHER CAUSES OF INTRAVASCULAR HEMOLYSIS

Conditions in which vascular abnormalities, toxins, infections, or drugs damage red blood cells and cause them to lose pieces of membrane and ultimately fragment into hemoglobin-containing bits should be considered in the differential diagnosis of intravascular hemolysis (Table 164–3; see also Table 164–2). Most of these conditions are readily apparent from the history and physical examination. Treatment focuses on the underlying cause of the hemolysis (see Table 164–3).

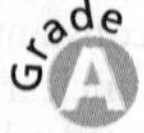

1. Hillmen P, Young NS, Schubert J, et al: The complement inhibitor Eculizumab in paroxysmal nocturnal hemoglobinuria. N Engl J Med 2006;355:1233–1243.

SUGGESTED READINGS

Bain BJ: Diagnosis from the blood smear. N Engl J Med 2005;353:498–507. *Excellent photomicrographs of blood smears in various forms of hemolytic anemia.*

Jiang H, Chess L: Regulation of immune responses by T cells. New Engl J Med 2006;54:1166–1176. *Review of regulatory T cells and autoimmunity.*

Johnson ST, Fueger JT, Gottschall JL: One center's experience: The serology and drugs associated with drug-induced immune hemolytic anemia—a new paradigm. Transfusion 2007;47:697–702. *Drug-induced causes are common, with cephalosporins, penicillins, and NSAIDs now more frequent than quinine or quinidine.*

King KE, Ness PM: Treatment of autoimmune hemolytic anemia. Semin Hematol 2005;42:131–136. *An overview of treatment.*

Parker C, Omine M, Richards S, et al: Diagnosis and management of paroxysmal nocturnal hemoglobinuria. Blood 2005;106:3699–3709. *An authoritative review.*

Petz LD: A physician's guide to transfusion in autoimmune haemolytic anemia. Br J Haematol 2004;124:712–716. *Good advice on the difficult problem of transfusion therapy in patients with autoimmune hemolytic anemia.*

Schollkopf C, Kjeldsen L, Bjerrum OW, et al: Rituximab in chronic cold agglutinin disease: A prospective study of 20 patients. Leuk Lymphoma 2006;47:253–260. *A phase II trial in which 45% of patients responded to rituximab.*

Wheeler CA, Calhoun L, Blackall DP: Warm reactive autoantibodies: Clinical and serologic correlations. Am J Clin Pathol 2004;122:680–685. *The serology of autoimmune hemolytic anemia.*

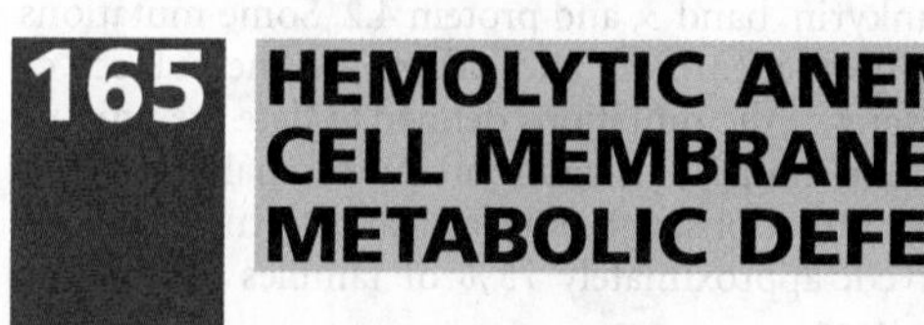

165 HEMOLYTIC ANEMIAS: RED CELL MEMBRANE AND METABOLIC DEFECTS

David E. Golan

NORMAL RED CELL MEMBRANE

Structure

Membrane Lipids

The red cell membrane, which was the first biologic membrane to be characterized biochemically, consists of an asymmetrically organized lipid bilayer in which some membrane proteins are embedded and to which other membrane proteins are attached. The lipids consist principally of a mixture of phospholipids and unesterified cholesterol in an approximately 1:1 molar ratio. The cholesterol is randomly distributed between the inner and outer leaflets of the bilayer, but the phospholipids are asymmetrically arranged such that the amino phospholipids (phosphatidylserine and phosphatidylethanolamine) and phosphatidylinositols are localized mainly in the inner leaflet, whereas the choline phospholipids (phosphatidylcholine and sphingomyelin) are mainly in the outer leaflet. This phospholipid asymmetry is maintained by the action of a selective amino phospholipid translocase, or flippase, that uses the energy of adenosine triphosphate (ATP) hydrolysis to translocate phosphatidylserine and phosphatidylethanolamine vectorially from the outer to the inner bilayer leaflet. The action of the translocase is functionally important because exposure of phosphatidylserine and phosphatidylethanolamine at the outer surface of the circulating red cell not only activates the coagulation pathways but also promotes mononuclear phagocyte adhesion, which leads to hemolysis. Red cell membrane lipids appear to exchange freely with those in plasma lipoproteins.

Membrane Proteins

Like membrane phospholipids, red cell membrane proteins are asymmetrically arranged to optimize membrane structure and function (Fig. 165–1). The major integral membrane proteins, which penetrate or span the lipid bilayer and are commonly decorated with carbohydrate on their extracellular surfaces, include functionally important transport proteins, such as band 3 (the anion exchange protein), and proteins that carry cell surface antigens, such as the glycophorins. The major peripheral membrane proteins, which do not penetrate the lipid bilayer but are instead attached to the intracellular surface of the bilayer by virtue of binding interactions with one or more integral proteins, include structural proteins, such as spectrin and actin, and some glycolytic enzymes, such as glyceraldehyde-3-phosphate dehydrogenase.

The structural proteins are organized into a dense, two-dimensional fibrous meshwork that laminates the inner membrane surface but does not extend into the cytoplasm of the cell. The principal components of this meshwork are spectrin, actin, and protein 4.1. Spectrin is a long, flexible, rod-shaped heterodimer consisting of an α chain and a β chain that associate stably with one another. In turn, these heterodimers associate with one another to form spectrin heterotetramers (and a few higher order oligomers) at the "head" (self-association) end of the heterodimers and with short filaments of actin at the "tail" end of the heterodimers.

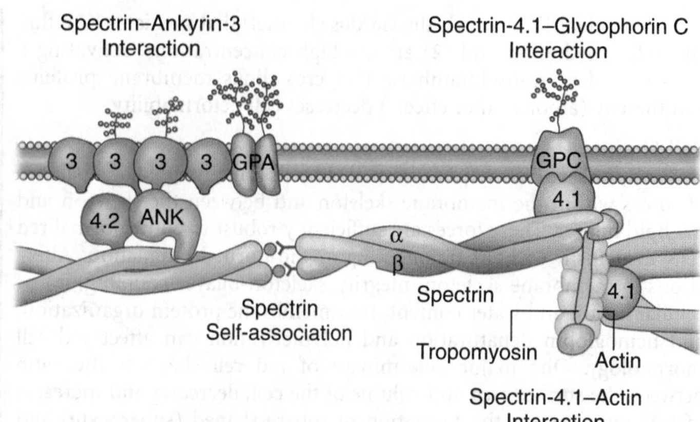

FIGURE 165–1 • Molecular binding interactions among the major proteins of the red cell membrane. 3 = band 3; 4.1 = protein 4.1; 4.2 = protein 4.2; ANK = ankyrin; GP = glycophorin.

The spectrin-actin binding interaction is strengthened by protein 4.1, which binds to both actin and the spectrin β chain. Because each actin filament can accommodate the binding of about six spectrin heterodimers (this assembly is sometimes called the junctional complex), the spectrin–actin–protein 4.1 complex can extend as a two-dimensional "membrane skeleton" around the entire inner membrane surface.

The membrane skeleton is coupled to the overlying lipid bilayer by the action of several "linking" proteins. The most important linking action is provided by ankyrin, which binds to the spectrin β chain near the self-association site and to the cytoplasmic domain of the integral protein band 3. Protein 4.2 may play a role in strengthening the spectrin-ankyrin interaction. Other linking mechanisms, the importance of which was demonstrated by the existence of intact (albeit abnormal) red cells in mammalian species that are completely lacking in band 3 protein, include the binding interaction between protein 4.1 and glycophorin C and the interaction between skeletal proteins (especially spectrin) and inner leaflet membrane lipids.

Function

Membrane Strength and Deformability

The exquisite mechanical coupling between the membrane skeleton and the overlying lipid bilayer confers on the normal red cell its remarkable properties of strength and deformability. On release from the bone marrow, mature red cells must withstand the high pressure and shear forces in the heart and large arteries and also traverse the small-diameter microcirculatory vessels for 120 days. The ability of the skeleton-bilayer couple to withstand high shear and to deform readily allows normal red cells to perform these tasks. Abnormal red cells with defective membrane skeletons or defective coupling between the skeleton and the overlying bilayer fragment spontaneously in the circulation, which leads to the clinical picture of nonimmune hemolytic anemia.

Cation and Volume Homeostasis

The red cell uses protein pumps and channels in its lipid bilayer membrane to control intracellular concentrations of sodium, potassium, and calcium ions and thereby to regulate cell volume. Normal intracellular concentrations of Na^+, K^+, and Ca^{2+} are about 10 mmol/L, 100 mmol/L, and 100 nmol/L, respectively. The physiologically most important pumps include the ATP-dependent Na^+-K^+ exchanger, which uses the energy provided by ATP hydrolysis to pump Na^+ outward against its concentration gradient and K^+ inward against its concentration gradient, and the ATP-dependent Ca^{2+} pump, which pumps Ca^{2+} outward against its concentration gradient. The activities of these pumps counteract the small passive leaks of Na^+, K^+, and Ca^{2+} down their concentration gradients through the relatively impermeable lipid bilayer. Pathologic increases in the passive leak rates of these three cations—or decreases in the activities of these two pumps—can have deleterious effects. A net gain of intracellular cations obligates net water entry and causes cells to swell, whereas a net loss of intracellular cations dehydrates cells. The free flow of water molecules in both directions across the lipid bilayer is mediated by the aquaporin-1 water channel protein. A pathologic increase in intracellular Ca^{2+} concentration can be especially harmful by (1) activating a

Ca^{2+}-dependent K^+ channel (the Gardos channel) that mediates K^+ efflux and cell dehydration and (2) at very high concentrations, activating a Ca^{2+}-dependent transglutaminase that cross-links membrane proteins and thereby (among other effects) decreases cell deformability.

Cell Shape

The biconcave disc shape of normal red cells is maintained by a balance of forces within the membrane skeleton and between the skeleton and the lipid bilayer. These forces are sufficiently robust to allow normal red cells to deform without fragmenting in the normal circulation. Alterations in membrane skeleton integrity, skeleton-bilayer coupling, intracellular cation and water content, transmembrane protein organization, and hemoglobin denaturation and polymerization can affect red cell morphology. One major determinant of red cell shape is the ratio between the surface area and volume of the cell; decreases and increases in this ratio lead to the formation of sphere-shaped (spherocyte) and cup- (stomatocyte) or target-shaped red cells, respectively. Irreversible shape change can also be mediated by permanent deformation of the membrane skeleton; orderly plastic deformation causes the formation of elliptical or oval red cells (elliptocytes or ovalocytes), whereas random membrane injury with denatured hemoglobin precipitation on the skeleton and oxidative cross-linking of proteins leads to the formation of spiculated (echinocyte), irreversibly sickled, and other abnormal red cell forms.

Anion Exchange

The red cell membrane plays an important physiologic role in carbon dioxide (CO_2) transport. CO_2 handling is facilitated by red cell enzyme-mediated conversion of this molecule to bicarbonate (HCO_3^-) in the tissues and back to CO_2 for excretion in the lungs. To increase the HCO_3^--carrying capacity of the blood, some of the HCO_3^- is carried in the plasma. Movement of HCO_3^- in and out of red cells is facilitated by the presence of about 1 million anion exchanger molecules (band 3 proteins) in each red cell membrane. Band 3 mediates the passive bidirectional exchange of HCO_3^- for Cl^-; no energy is required for this process. Band 3 therefore serves at least two important roles in red cell membrane structure and function: coupling the membrane skeleton to the overlying lipid bilayer and mediating anion exchange across the membrane.

Interactions with the Spleen: Red Cell Senescence

Most normal red cells are removed from the circulation by the spleen after a 120-day lifespan. The fenestrations between splenic cords and sinuses provide mechanical stress as red cells squeeze through these openings, whereas the low-oxygen, low-glucose, low-pH environment of the splenic cords places metabolic stress on the cells. The spleen uses two major mechanisms to sequester and remove aged red cells. First, as red cells become less deformable with age, they are less able to traverse the splenic fenestrations. Second, as red cells age, their membranes are progressively decorated with autoantibodies or complement proteins that bind to receptors on mononuclear phagocytes in the spleen; these autoantibodies may be directed against clustered or proteolytically altered band 3 at the red cell surface.

RED CELL MEMBRANE DISORDERS

Hereditary Spherocytosis

Epidemiology

The incidence of hereditary spherocytosis is between 1:2000 and 1:5000 among northern European people, although the disease can occur in any population.

Pathobiology

Etiology

Hereditary spherocytosis is an inherited hemolytic anemia caused by a defect in one of the proteins that couples the red cell membrane skeleton to the overlying lipid bilayer. These proteins include spectrin (either the α or the β chain), ankyrin, band 3, and protein 4.2. Some mutations in these proteins have been identified, and others are the subject of current investigation. Many of the mutations defined to date are unique, thus indicating that no one mutation is common. Autosomal dominant, autosomal recessive, new mutations, and nonclassical patterns of inheritance have been observed; approximately 75% of families exhibit the autosomal dominant pattern.

Pathogenesis

Molecular defects in spectrin, ankyrin, band 3, and protein 4.2 lead to spectrin deficiency as the "final common pathway" that characterizes all red cells with hereditary spherocytosis. This molecular phenotype results either from a primary deficiency of spectrin or, more commonly, from a deficiency of one of the proteins that allows spectrin to bind with high affinity to the overlying lipid bilayer. Spectrin deficiency appears to cause the spherocytic cellular phenotype by weakening "vertical" interactions between the membrane skeleton and the bilayer and thereby leading to "unsupported" areas of lipid that are spontaneously lost as red cells traverse the circulation. Spherocytic red cells are less able than normal cells to squeeze through the fenestrations between splenic cords and sinuses, and the increased metabolic stress placed on the cells in the environment of the cords leads to further membrane loss. Although some hyperchromic microspherocytes eventually escape back into the peripheral circulation, many of these cells are hemolyzed in the spleen (Fig. 165–2).

The discovery that spectrin deficiency is the sine qua non of hereditary spherocytic red cells led some to hypothesize that primary defects in spectrin would be found in most cases of hereditary spherocytosis. Surprisingly, mutations in α-spectrin (autosomal recessive hereditary spherocytosis) and β-spectrin (autosomal dominant hereditary spherocytosis) are each present in only about 10% of patients with hereditary spherocytosis. Instead, mutations in ankyrin (autosomal dominant and recessive hereditary spherocytosis; about 40 to 50% of cases) and band 3 (autosomal dominant hereditary spherocytosis; about 20% of cases) are much more common. Mutations in protein 4.2 (autosomal recessive

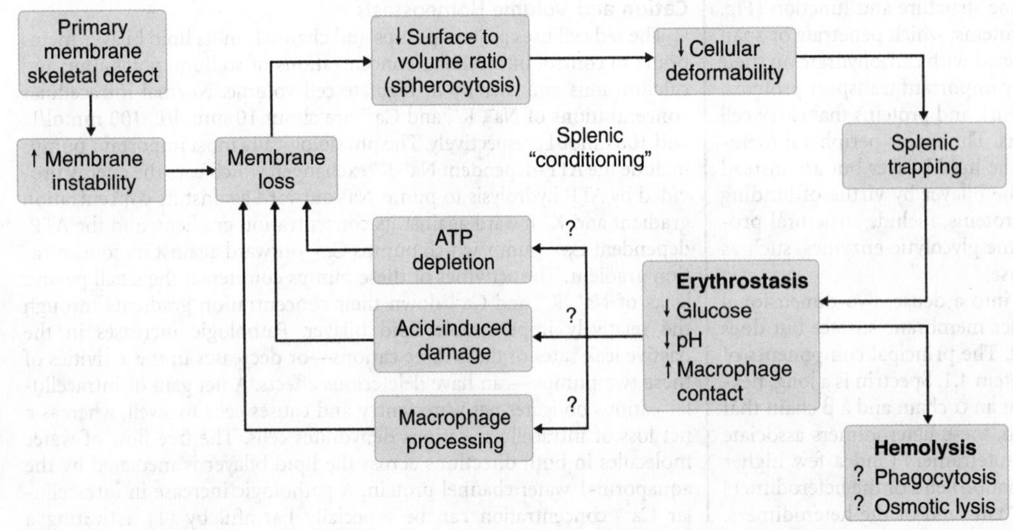

FIGURE 165–2 • Model of the pathophysiologic mechanism of spherocytosis and hemolysis in hereditary spherocytosis. ATP = adenosine triphospate.

hereditary spherocytosis) are relatively rare except in Japan, where a number of families have been described. The severity of hemolysis correlates with the cellular spectrin content in spherocytic red cells, providing strong evidence in support of the pathogenetic mechanisms described before.

Clinical Manifestations

Symptoms and Signs

The clinical manifestations of hereditary spherocytosis can vary from a clinically insignificant hemolytic state that is fully compensated by increased marrow erythropoiesis to a life-threatening hemolytic state that is dependent on red cell transfusion. This variation in clinical phenotype is a reflection of the variation in the molecular consequences of the mutations in spectrin, ankyrin, band 3, or protein 4.2, all of which result in weakened interaction between the membrane skeleton and the overlying lipid bilayer. In general, an autosomal recessive inheritance pattern is associated with clinically more severe disease, whereas an autosomal dominant pattern is associated with a milder phenotype.

Although all cases of hereditary spherocytosis are present from birth, the diagnosis can be made at any age. Clinical manifestations common in hereditary spherocytosis include jaundice and splenomegaly (Table 165–1). Approximately 50% of neonates experience marked jaundice that may require exchange transfusion, and some infants may require periodic red cell transfusions to maintain an adequate hematocrit. The potential for erythropoietin therapy to obviate the need for red cell transfusions in neonates and infants with hereditary spherocytosis is under investigation.

By several months of age, most patients with hereditary spherocytosis achieve a partially compensated hemolytic state characterized by mild to moderate anemia (hemoglobin concentration, 9 to 11.5 g/dL), intermittent jaundice (exacerbated by viral infection), and splenomegaly. Even in patients with fully compensated hemolysis, states associated with splenic enlargement or increased splenic blood flow (e.g., infectious mononucleosis and, occasionally, intense physical activity) may provoke severe hemolysis and anemia. Previously compensated elderly patients with hereditary spherocytosis may experience more severe anemia with aging because of a decline in compensatory bone marrow activity.

Complications

Common clinical complications of hereditary spherocytosis include occasional crises and the formation of bilirubinate gallstones. Hemolytic crisis appears to be caused by the increased activity of the mononuclear phagocyte (reticuloendothelial) system associated with many infections; such crises are typified by a small decrease in the hematocrit that is not clinically significant. Aplastic crisis is most often associated with parvovirus B19 infection (Chapter 394); such crises may be clinically severe and require prompt red cell transfusion. Fortunately, infection with parvovirus B19 generally produces lifelong immunity, so most patients are subjected to no more than one such crisis in a lifetime. Megaloblastic crisis is caused by a relative lack of folic acid in the diet; because of the increased need for this vitamin during pregnancy, such crises are more common in pregnant women. The increased generation of bilirubin associated with ongoing hemolysis leads to the formation of bilirubinate gallstones in most untreated teenagers and adults with hereditary spherocytosis. The incidence of this complication increases from about 5% in children 0 to 10 years old to about 45% in patients aged 11 to 50 years and about 65% in older patients. Because a large fraction of bilirubinate gallstones are not radiopaque, abdominal ultrasonography is the most reliable imaging method to detect these stones.

Relatively rare clinical complications of hereditary spherocytosis in adults include gout, rashes and ulcers of the lower extremities, and extramedullary hematopoietic tumors of the thorax. The gout and lower extremity complications usually disappear after splenectomy (see later), but the tumors commonly undergo fatty change after splenectomy and therefore persist on routine chest film. Several families with hereditary spherocytosis and either spinocerebellar degeneration or cardiomyopathy have been described, perhaps suggesting a common genetic basis for these disorders in these families.

TABLE 165–1 HEREDITARY SPHEROCYTOSIS

Clinical Manifestations	Laboratory Features
Common manifestations	Anemia, reticulocytosis
Splenomegaly	Spherocytosis on blood smear
Gallstones	Elevated MCHC
Intermittent jaundice from hemolysis or biliary obstruction	Increased osmotic fragility (especially on incubated osmotic fragility test)
Aplastic crises	Negative result of direct antiglobulin (Coombs) test
Good response to splenectomy	Decrease in red cell membrane proteins:
Rare manifestations	Spectrin and/or
Leg ulcers	Ankyrin and/or
Gout	Band 3 and/or
Spinal cord dysfunction	Protein 4.2
Extramedullary hematopoietic tumors of the thorax	
Cardiomyopathy	

MCHC = mean cell hemoglobin concentration.

Diagnosis

Laboratory features common to all cases of hereditary spherocytosis include an elevated reticulocyte count and the presence of spherocytes on the blood smear (see Fig. 161–7). Patients with mild disease may not be anemic or manifest hyperbilirubinemia, although many patients with hereditary spherocytosis do exhibit mild to moderate anemia and an elevated indirect bilirubin level. The laboratory test most commonly used to confirm the presence of spherocytosis is the osmotic fragility test, which measures the ability of red cells to withstand swelling in solutions of decreasing osmotic strength. Because spherocytes have a decreased ratio of surface area to volume, these cells are less able to swell in a hypotonic environment than normal discocytes are. Thus, populations of red cells containing a significant proportion of spherocytes exhibit increased osmotic fragility compared with normal red cell populations. In some cases of mild hereditary spherocytosis, however, neither striking spherocytosis on the blood smear nor an abnormal finding on the osmotic fragility test is apparent. The most reliable test in this situation is the incubated osmotic fragility test, in which red cells are metabolically stressed by incubation in the absence of glucose for 24 hours. Whereas normal red cells can withstand this treatment without significant membrane damage, hereditary spherocytic red cells shed bilayer lipids under these conditions and become less able to remain intact in a hypotonic environment. Finally, because hereditary spherocytic red cells tend to be dehydrated, an elevated mean cell hemoglobin concentration (MCHC) can be a helpful clue in the diagnosis of hereditary spherocytosis; even in patients with hereditary spherocytosis but no increase in MCHC, the presence of a subpopulation of dehydrated cells can usually be observed by use of laboratory instruments that provide a histogram of MCHC values. Biochemical quantification of spectrin, ankyrin, band 3, and protein 4.2, which could theoretically yield the most specific test for hereditary spherocytosis, is available only in research laboratories.

Differential Diagnosis

The differential diagnosis of spherocytosis includes a number of clinical entities (Table 165–2), but the most common other clinical state characterized by spherocytosis—autoimmune hemolytic anemia—can be readily distinguished from hereditary spherocytosis by the direct antiglobulin (Coombs) test.

Treatment

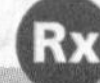

Most hematologists recommend splenectomy for children with severe hereditary spherocytosis (hemoglobin concentration, <8 g/dL; reticulocyte count, >10%) and for children with moderate disease (hemoglobin concentration, 8 to 11 g/dL; reticulocyte count, 8 to

TABLE 165–2 DISEASES CHARACTERIZED BY PROMINENT SPHEROCYTOSIS ON THE BLOOD SMEAR

COMMON
Hereditary spherocytosis
Autoimmune hemolytic anemia (warm antibody type)
ABO incompatibility (neonates)
UNCOMMON TO RARE
Hemolytic transfusion reaction
Clostridial sepsis
Severe burn
Spider, bee, and snake venom
Acute red cell oxidant injury
Severe hypophosphatemia
Bartonellosis

Rx

10%) if the degree of anemia compromises physical activity. In adults with moderate hereditary spherocytosis, additional indications for splenectomy include a degree of anemia that compromises oxygen delivery to vital organs, the development of extramedullary hematopoietic tumors, and the occurrence of bilirubinate gallstones, which could predispose to cholecystitis and biliary obstruction. Splenectomy is generally deferred in patients with mild hereditary spherocytosis (hemoglobin concentration, >11 g/dL; reticulocyte count, <8%).

Several European groups have advocated the use of subtotal splenectomy as a compromise operation that ameliorates most of the extravascular hemolysis associated with splenic function while retaining some immune and phagocytic activity of the normal spleen. In 40 children treated with this operation, the success rate in relieving hemolysis during a 1- to 14-year follow-up period was adequate (although less than that achieved with total splenectomy), and the rate of complications has been low; however, data are currently too limited for this procedure to be recommended in the general hereditary spherocytosis population.

All patients undergoing splenectomy should receive polyvalent pneumococcal vaccine, preferably several weeks before the operation; children should also receive meningococcal and *Haemophilus influenzae* B vaccines. In the first several years after splenectomy, many patients are treated with prophylactic oral penicillin to protect against pneumococcal sepsis, although the emergence of penicillin-resistant pneumococci may force a change in this practice in the coming years. All patients with hereditary spherocytosis should be given 1 mg of folate as a daily supplement (patients with moderate to severe disease may require 5 mg daily) to prevent megaloblastic crisis.

After splenectomy, the blood smear in patients with hereditary spherocytosis acquires several characteristic alterations. Howell-Jolly bodies, acanthocytes, target cells, and siderocytes normally mark red cells for removal by the spleen, but such cells now remain in the circulation. Although spherocytes are still present, the microspherocytes formed by splenic conditioning disappear. Failure of splenectomy to ameliorate the degree of hemolysis in hereditary spherocytosis, either immediately after the operation or many years later, is often due to an accessory spleen. The presence of this structure, which is found in about 15 to 20% of patients with hereditary spherocytosis, can be revealed by the disappearance of Howell-Jolly bodies from the blood smear or by laboratory abnormalities associated with hemolysis, such as an increased reticulocyte count. The radionuclide liver-spleen scan can be a useful imaging modality in searching for an accessory spleen.

Prognosis

Because red cell destruction in the spleen is the primary mechanism by which abnormal hereditary spherocytic red cells are prematurely removed from the circulation, splenectomy is highly effective in restoring a normal hematocrit and a nearly normal reticulocyte count (1 to 3%) to almost all patients with hereditary spherocytosis. In patients with the most severe form of the disease, a mild anemia may remain after splenectomy; however, this anemia represents a state of compensated hemolysis rather than the transfusion dependence that characterizes such patients before splenectomy. In all patients with hereditary spherocytosis, the benefits of splenectomy must be weighed against its risks. The major risks include bacterial sepsis, often caused by pneumococcal, meningococcal, or *H. influenzae* B bacteria, and mesenteric or portal venous occlusion. The risk of post-splenectomy sepsis is so great in children younger than 3 to 5 years that splenectomy should be avoided in such patients even with the necessity of transfusion dependence. One series of 226 adult patients with hereditary spherocytosis estimated the lifetime risk of fulminant post-splenectomy sepsis to be about 2%. After splenectomy, a small but significant increase in the risk of ischemic heart disease has also been reported.

Hereditary Elliptocytosis

Epidemiology

The incidence of mild hereditary elliptocytosis is about 1:2500 among northern Europeans and as common as 1:150 in some areas of Africa, although the disease can occur in any population. Hereditary pyropoikilocytosis and spherocytic hereditary elliptocytosis are considerably more rare. Southeast Asian ovalocytosis (SAO) is caused by a specific deletion in band 3 that allows the mutant protein to form linear aggregates in the plane of the lipid bilayer. The incidence of this autosomal dominant disorder is as common as 1:3 among some lowland aboriginal populations of Indonesia, Malaysia, Melanesia, and the Philippines, although SAO is rare in other areas of the world.

Pathobiology

Hereditary elliptocytosis comprises a family of inherited hemolytic anemias caused primarily by defects in one or more of the proteins that make up the two-dimensional membrane skeletal network. The four clinical phenotypes of hereditary elliptocytosis appear to be caused by different sets of molecular defects. Mild hereditary elliptocytosis and hereditary pyropoikilocytosis arise most often from α- and β-spectrin chain defects that affect the ability of spectrin heterodimers to self-associate and from protein 4.1 defects that affect the strength of binding in the ternary spectrin–actin–protein 4.1 complex. Spherocytic hereditary elliptocytosis can be caused by defects in the β chain of spectrin that may affect spectrin-ankyrin binding as well as spectrin self-association; other mutations are the subject of current investigation. In general, mild hereditary elliptocytosis and spherocytic hereditary elliptocytosis are inherited as autosomal dominant traits, and hereditary pyropoikilocytosis is inherited in an autosomal recessive pattern.

Pathogenesis

In mild hereditary elliptocytosis, a molecular defect near the "head" region of the spectrin heterodimer (i.e., a mutation near the aminocarboxy terminus of α-spectrin or the aminocarboxy terminus of β-spectrin) leads to weakening of the "horizontal" interactions that give the red cell membrane skeleton its properties of strength and deformability. Heterozygous deficiency of protein 4.1—or a mutation that prevents formation of the spectrin–actin–protein 4.1 ternary complex at the "tail" region of the spectrin heterodimer—has a similar mechanical effect. In both cases, red cells are released from the bone marrow with a normal discocytic shape, but the membrane skeletons (and consequently the red cells themselves) undergo plastic deformation to a permanent elliptocytic shape as the cells traverse the microcirculation. Because the vertical interactions that couple the membrane skeleton to the overlying lipid bilayer remain intact in these cells, membrane loss does not occur, and the cells may have a relatively normal lifetime in the circulation. Hereditary pyropoikilocytosis, in contrast, results from either a homozygous or a compound heterozygous defect in spectrin (typically, α-spectrin) or protein 4.1. In addition to the defects described before, coinheritance of an α-spectrin mutation with the spectrin α^{LELY} polymorphism can cause the hereditary pyropoikilocytosis phenotype. In spectrin α^{LELY}, α-spectrin mRNA splicing is altered such that the resulting protein chains lose the ability to pair with β-spectrin. Because α-spectrin is synthesized in excess of β-spectrin in normal erythropoiesis, the spectrin α^{LELY} polymorphism is silent by itself. When paired in *trans* with an α-spectrin coding region mutation, however, the polymorphism causes the majority of spectrin heterodimers at the membrane to carry the coding region (functional) defect, which leads to the much more severe hereditary pyropoikilocytosis phenotype.

In spherocytic hereditary elliptocytosis, the molecular defect in the spectrin β chain appears to affect both horizontal interactions at the spectrin self-association site and vertical interactions at the spectrin-ankyrin binding site. This combined defect results in features of both hereditary elliptocytosis (because of the horizontal interaction defect) and hereditary spherocytosis (because of the vertical interaction defect). The linear aggregates of mutant band 3 protein in SAO red cells are thought to cause extreme rigidification of the membrane by preventing the local expansions and contractions of the membrane skeletal network that are responsible for membrane deformability. Membrane rigidity or reduced lateral mobility of the aggregated band 3 protein is likely to be the mechanism by which SAO red cells resist invasion by malaria parasites, which accounts for the high prevalence of this variant in certain areas of Southeast Asia. Interestingly, unlike the nondeformable spherocytes found in hereditary spherocytosis and autoimmune hemolytic anemia, the rigid SAO red cells are not removed prematurely from the circulation. The mechanisms by which SAO cells survive normally in the circulation remain to be elucidated. The SAO mutation must have some deleterious effect on red cell membrane structure and function, however, because the homozygous state appears to be lethal.

Diagnosis

The majority of individuals with mild hereditary elliptocytosis are heterozygous carriers of a dominantly inherited molecular and cellular defect that is clinically insignificant. These individuals have no anemia, little or no hemolysis (reticulocyte count, 1 to 3%), and no splenomegaly. Diagnosis is based on a prominent elliptocytosis (often greater than 40%) on the blood smear (see Fig. 161–11), a normal finding on the osmotic fragility test, and a positive family pedigree. Individuals who inherit a mild α-spectrin defect in *trans* with spectrin α^{LELY} may exhibit mild chronic hemolysis and some fragmented red cells on the blood smear. Mild hereditary elliptocytosis can be associated with significant hemolysis in patients in whom splenic enlargement develops from, for example, viral infection or portal hypertension. Neonates with mild hereditary elliptocytosis often exhibit a syndrome, called transient infantile poikilocytosis, characterized by a moderately severe hemolytic anemia for the initial 6 to 12 months of life. The increased hemolysis in the neonatal and early infant period appears to result from the increase in intracellular 2,3-diphosphoglycerate (2,3-DPG) concentration that is present in fetal red cells. Elevated levels of this normal metabolite weaken the ternary spectrin–actin–protein 4.1 binding interaction and thereby exacerbate the spectrin self-association defect caused by the mild hereditary elliptocytosis mutation. As fetal red cells are lost from the circulation, the intracellular 2,3-DPG concentration falls and the clinical condition spontaneously reverts to that of mild hereditary elliptocytosis.

Hereditary pyropoikilocytosis is a recessively inherited disorder that is clinically manifested by a severe (sometimes life-threatening) hemolytic anemia in which the blood smear contains bizarre poikilocytes and red cell fragments. The mean cell volume is markedly decreased (45 to 75 fL), and because spectrin deficiency and spherocytosis are often secondary consequences of the combined molecular defects, osmotic fragility is increased. The name is derived from the property of hereditary pyropoikilocytosis red cells to fragment at 45° to 46° C rather than the normal 49° C; this abnormal heat sensitivity is most often due to a lowering of the temperature at which the mutant spectrin chains denature.

Differential Diagnosis

As implied by the name, spherocytic hereditary elliptocytosis has clinical and diagnostic features of both hereditary spherocytosis and mild hereditary elliptocytosis. Patients manifest mild to moderate hemolytic anemia with splenomegaly and intermittent jaundice, the blood smear contains rounded elliptocytes and sometimes spherocytes, and osmotic fragility is increased. In contrast, individuals with the SAO mutation are clinically normal, with little or no anemia or hemolysis; the blood smear shows characteristic rounded elliptocytes that often exhibit a transverse bar dividing the central clear area.

Treatment

Spherocytic hereditary elliptocytosis should be treated like hereditary spherocytosis, with the considerations for and against splenectomy as noted. Virtually all patients with hereditary pyropoikilocytosis require splenectomy, which ameliorates but does not completely cure the hemolytic anemia. As in treatment of patients with moderate to severe hereditary spherocytosis, it is important to defer splenectomy until 3 to 5 years of age if possible, especially because of the possibility that a severe poikilocytic anemia in the neonatal and infant period could represent transient infantile poikilocytosis rather than true hereditary pyropoikilocytosis.

Prognosis

Mild hereditary elliptocytosis and SAO are clinically insignificant variants that require no treatment and have no effect on lifespan (other than the beneficial protection against malaria afforded to individuals with SAO).

Hereditary Defects in Membrane Permeability

Hereditary Xerocytosis

The hallmark of this rare autosomal dominant disorder is an alteration in red cell membrane cation permeability that leads to a net loss of intracellular cations and water and to cell dehydration. The molecular defect responsible for this phenotype remains to be elucidated, although the gene for a subset of xerocytosis has been mapped to the long arm of chromosome 16. The dehydrated red cells appear on the blood smear as target cells or spiculated acanthocytes, and the increased MCHC leads to relatively nondeformable cells that can be sequestered and removed by the spleen. The differential diagnosis of dehydrated red cells also includes the much more common sickle cell syndromes, hereditary spherocytosis, and hemoglobin C disease. Splenectomy is relatively contraindicated in patients with hereditary xerocytosis because of the high risk of postprocedure thrombosis in these patients.

Hereditary Stomatocytosis

This rare autosomal dominant disorder appears to be due to an inherited defect in Na^+ permeability that leads to a net influx of Na^+ and water and to cell swelling. Several molecular defects are probably responsible for this phenotype because some families with this disorder experience severe hemolytic anemia whereas others have clinically mild disease. The swollen red cells appear on the blood smear to have a mouth-like invagination in the membrane and are therefore called stomatocytes. The differential diagnosis of stomatocytosis also includes the much more common acquired effects of acute alcoholism or liver disease. Patients with the severe form of hereditary stomatocytosis often respond well to splenectomy, but some patients have developed hypercoagulability and catastrophic thrombosis after splenectomy.

NORMAL RED CELL METABOLISM

Glycolysis

Normal mature red cells have lost the cellular machinery responsible for oxidative phosphorylation, and the metabolism in these cells is almost entirely anaerobic. The major red cell energy source is glucose, which is metabolized primarily by the glycolytic pathway (also called the Embden-Meyerhof pathway) and secondarily by the pentose phosphate pathway (also called the hexose monophosphate shunt) (Fig. 165–3). The glycolytic pathway converts 90 to 95% of the metabolized glucose in red cells

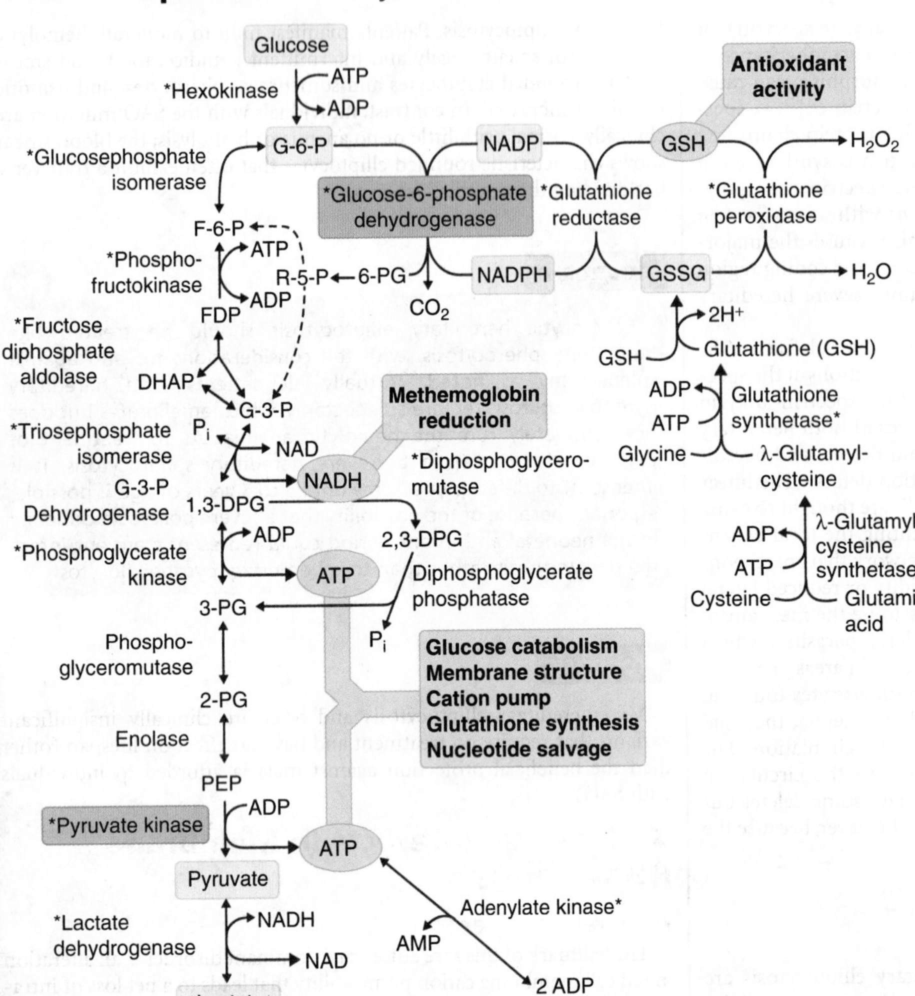

FIGURE 165–3 • Biochemical glycolysis, pentose phosphate, and glutathione pathways in human red cell metabolism. Asterisks denote enzymes that have been shown to be deficient in hereditary metabolic defects. ADP = adenosine diphosphate; AMP = adenosine monophosphate; ATP = adenosine triphosphate; DHAP = dihydroxyacetone phosphate; 1,3-DPG = 1,3-diphosphoglycerate; 2,3-DPG = 2,3-diphosphoglycerate; F-6-P = fructose-6-phosphate; FDP = fructose-1,6-diphosphate; G-3-P = glyceraldehyde-3-phosphate; G-6-P = glucose-6-phosphate; GSH = reduced glutathione; GSSG = oxidized glutathione; NAD = nicotinamide adenine dinucleotide; NADH = reduced NAD; NADP = nicotinamide adenine dinucleotide phosphate; NADPH = reduced NADP; PEP = phosphoenolpyruvate; 2-PG = 2-phosphoglycerate; 3-PG = 3-phosphoglycerate; 6-PG = 6-phosphogluconate; P_i = phosphate; R-5-P = ribulose-5-phosphate. (Modified from Valentine WN: Hemolytic anemia and inborn errors of metabolism. Blood 1979;54:549.)

to lactate, in the process generating 2 mol of ATP per mole of glucose consumed. Although this rate of ATP generation is inefficient compared with that provided in other cells by the tricarboxylic acid cycle, it is sufficient in normal red cells to renew 150 to 200% of the total red cell ATP per hour. ATP is an essential energy source that is used to maintain homeostasis in red cells by cation pumps and channels, by protein kinases, and by enzymes that regulate glycolysis, glutathione synthesis, and nucleotide salvage. Two important metabolic cofactors generated in the glycolytic pathway are reduced nicotinamide adenine dinucleotide (NADH) and 2,3-DPG. NADH is an essential cofactor for the enzyme methemoglobin reductase, which maintains heme iron in the ferrous (Fe^{2+}) state that is necessary for the ligation of molecular oxygen by hemoglobin. 2,3-DPG, generated by the Rapoport-Luebering shunt, regulates the affinity of hemoglobin for oxygen and thereby increases oxygen delivery to tissues.

Pentose Phosphate Pathway and Glutathione Metabolism

The pentose phosphate pathway handles 5 to 10% of metabolized glucose in normal red cells, in the process generating 2 mol of reduced nicotinamide adenine dinucleotide phosphate (NADPH) for each mole of glucose metabolized. NADPH is an essential cofactor for the enzyme glutathione reductase, which maintains glutathione in the reduced state necessary for detoxification of toxic oxygen products such as superoxide anion (O_2^-), hydrogen peroxide (H_2O_2), and hydroxyl radical (·OH). Normal red cells are continually subjected to these products as a result of intracellular heme oxidation. In addition, certain drugs can markedly enhance oxidant generation by red cells, and many infections can induce oxidant generation by phagocytic cells in the circulation. In the absence of reduced glutathione, toxic oxygen products can damage red cell lipids and proteins and result in hemolysis. Under conditions of oxidative stress, the pentose phosphate pathway can increase in activity to use 50% or more of the available glucose. This increase in activity is stimulated by NADP and inhibited by NADPH, thereby tightly coupling intracellular antioxidant supply and demand.

Glutathione is a tripeptide that is synthesized by mature red cells in relatively high amounts (2 mmol/L steady-state concentration) from the amino acids cysteine, glutamic acid, and glycine. Two enzymes catalyze this synthetic pathway, and two other enzymes couple glutathione metabolism to NADPH oxidation (see Fig. 165–3).

■ RED CELL METABOLISM DISORDERS

■ Defects in the Pentose Phosphate Pathway and Glutathione Metabolism

■ *Glucose-6-Phosphate Dehydrogenase Deficiency*

Epidemiology

Glucose-6-phosphate dehydrogenase (G6PD) deficiency, which is by far the most common enzyme defect associated with hereditary hemolytic anemia, affects hundreds of millions of individuals from all races around the world. More than 300 molecular G6PD variants have been described. The most common normal variants of the enzyme are called $G6PD^B$ or Gd^B, found in 99% of whites and about 70% of blacks, and Gd^{A+}, found in about 20% of blacks. The most common abnormal variants of the enzyme are called Gd^{A-}, found in about 10% of American blacks and a number of black African populations, and Gd^{Med}, found in Mediterranean (Arabs, Greeks, Italians, Sephardic Jews, and others), Indian, and Southeast Asian populations. Both Gd^{A-} and Gd^{Med} represent mutant enzymes that differ from the respective normal variants by a

TABLE 165–3 COMMON FORMS OF ABNORMAL GLUCOSE-6-PHOSPHATE DEHYDROGENASE

Feature	Gd^{A-}	Gd^{Med}
Frequency	Common in African populations	Common in Mediterranean populations
Chronic hemolysis	None	None
Degree of acute hemolysis	Moderate	Severe
Abnormal G6PD activity	Old red cells	All red cells
Hemolysis with		
Drugs	Unusual	Common
Infection	Common	Common
Need for transfusions	Rare	Sometimes

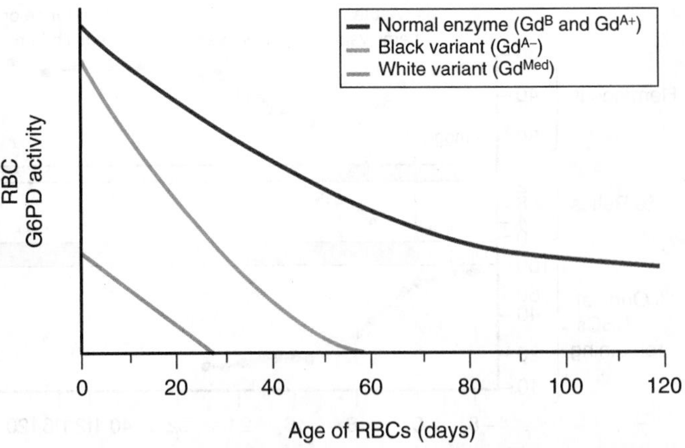

FIGURE 165–4 • Decline in red cell G6PD activity as a function of cell age. Shown are curves for the normal Gd^B and Gd^{A+} enzymes and for the unstable Gd^{A-} and Gd^{Med} variants. Note that although the activity of the normal enzyme declines as red cells age, even the oldest cells have a sufficient level of activity to provide protection against oxidative damage and hemolysis. In contrast, few Gd^{Med} red cells have sufficient enzyme activity to prevent such damage, whereas a substantial fraction of young Gd^{A-} red cells are so protected. Under oxidative stress, then, nearly all Gd^{Med} cells but only the oldest Gd^{A-} cells are susceptible to hemolysis. Assuming a normally functioning bone marrow, individuals with Gd^{A-} red cells can compensate by increasing the reticulocyte count and thereby populating the red cell pool with younger cells. In this way, G6PD screening assays may be falsely negative in Gd^{A-} males immediately after a hemolytic episode. G6PD = glucose-6-phosphate dehydrogenase; RBC = red blood cell. (Modified from Lux SE: Hemolytic anemias. Metabolic defects. *In* Beck WS [ed]: Hematology, 4th ed. Cambridge, MA, MIT Press, 1985, p 223.)

single amino acid. The prevalence of G6PD deficiency in African black, Mediterranean, Indian, and Southeast Asian populations is thought to derive from the relative protection afforded G6PD-deficient individuals against *Plasmodium falciparum* malaria. Although the electrophoretic mobilities of the Gd^B and Gd^{Med} enzymes are identical, and those of the Gd^{A+} and Gd^{A-} isoforms are also identical, the overall catalytic activity of each abnormal variant is markedly less than that of the corresponding normal variant (see later).

Because the G6PD gene is located on the X chromosome, the inheritance pattern of G6PD deficiency is sex linked. Thus, whereas males have either a normal or an abnormal G6PD variant, females can exhibit either homozygous or heterozygous G6PD deficiency. Although relatively rare, homozygous G6PD deficiency in females is phenotypically identical to hemizygous deficiency in males. Even in female heterozygotes, each individual red cell is either normal or abnormal (i.e., there is no intermediate state) because only one X chromosome is active in each somatic cell (according to the Lyon hypothesis). The overall effect of G6PD deficiency in female heterozygotes may be mild, moderate, or severe, depending on the proportion of red cells in which the abnormal G6PD enzyme is expressed.

Pathobiology

The primary metabolic consequence of G6PD deficiency is the diminished ability of the variant enzyme to generate sufficient NADPH to keep up with the requirement for reduced glutathione in a red cell population stressed by oxidizing agents. Depletion of cellular glutathione allows toxic oxygen products to damage red cell macromolecules, including hemoglobin, band 3, spectrin, membrane lipids, and other molecules. Oxidation of the heme iron of hemoglobin generates methemoglobin, which is incapable of ligating molecular oxygen. Oxidative denaturation of the globin chain produces intracellular hemoglobin precipitates called Heinz bodies that localize to the inner surface of the red cell membrane, probably through specific binding interactions between denatured hemoglobin and the cytoplasmic domain of band 3. Heinz bodies cause further oxidative damage to the membrane, manifested by clustering of band 3 proteins into large aggregates, which can be recognized by low-affinity autoantibodies and thereby targeted for removal by the mononuclear phagocyte system, and by increasing membrane cation permeability, which is accompanied by changes in cell hydration and deformability. Oxidative cross-linking of spectrin is likely to contribute to the decreased deformability of oxidatively stressed G6PD-deficient red cells, and peroxidation of membrane lipids may be a major contributing factor in the intravascular hemolysis that accompanies acute hemolytic episodes.

Normal and abnormal G6PD variants differ in both the stability and the catalytic activity of the various enzymes (Table 165–3). Normal Gd^B and Gd^{A+} enzymes are slowly degraded during the lifetime of a normal red cell in vivo, such that intracellular G6PD activity falls to half its original value in about 60 days. This slow decline in enzyme activity over time is clinically inconsequential because even the oldest normal red cells in the circulation retain sufficient G6PD activity to maintain intracellular reduced glutathione levels and to withstand nearly all oxidant stresses (Fig. 165–4). The catalytic activity of the Gd^{A-} variant is only mildly reduced compared with the normal enzyme; the major defect in Gd^{A-} red cells is the more rapid degradation of Gd^{A-} in comparison with the normal enzyme, such that G6PD activity falls to half its original value in only 13 days. Thus, young Gd^{A-} red cells are capable of withstanding oxidant stresses, whereas old Gd^{A-} red cells are not. This cellular heterogeneity allows a substantial fraction of Gd^{A-} red cells to survive even severe oxidant stress, and the acute hemolytic episode is therefore self-limited and usually not life-threatening. In contrast, both the catalytic activity and the stability of Gd^{Med} are much less than those of either the normal enzymes or Gd^{A-}; this feature renders nearly all Gd^{Med} red cells susceptible to oxidant-induced hemolysis and results in potentially life-threatening acute hemolytic episodes. Chronic ongoing hemolysis is not observed even in Gd^{Med} red cells in vivo, thus suggesting that endogenous oxidant generation must be low in the absence of oxidant stresses, such as drugs and infections.

In a Gd^{A-} individual treated with an oxidant drug, the acute hemolytic episode occurs immediately after initiation of drug therapy and is indicated by progressive anemia, hemoglobinuria, and reticulocytosis (Fig. 165–5); during this phase, the older red cells with low G6PD activity are hemolyzing. Despite continuation of the offending drug, however, the hemolysis spontaneously abates, red cell survival improves, and the hematocrit increases; during this phase, the bone marrow is compensating for the acute hemolytic episode by increasing its production of young Gd^{A-} red cells, which have sufficient G6PD activity to withstand the ongoing oxidant stress. Although the individual now appears to be resistant to drug-induced hemolysis, this "resistance" actually results from increased bone marrow erythropoiesis, which compensates for the ongoing hemolysis. The individual's continuing vulnerability to the effects of the drug is unmasked by withdrawal of the drug for several months to allow the rate of red cell production by the bone marrow to fall to its original value; during this phase, the older red cells are again allowed to survive, and the red cell population is again rendered sensitive to drug-induced hemolysis.

Clinical Manifestations

Except in a few rare cases (see later), the clinical manifestations of G6PD deficiency occur only under conditions of oxidant stress. In the

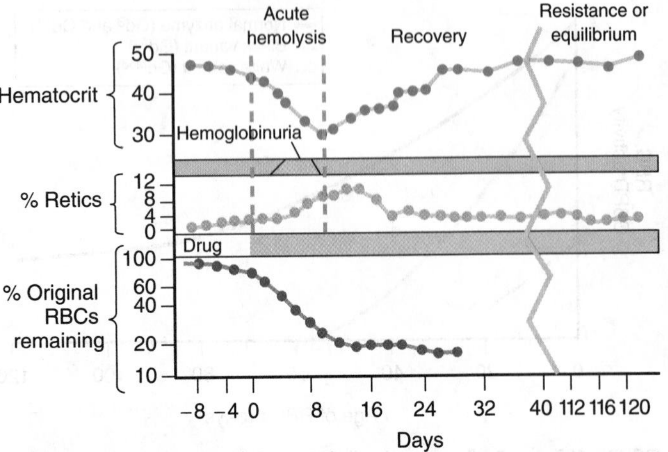

FIGURE 165–5 • Time course of primaquine-induced hemolysis in an individual with Gd^{A-} G6PD deficiency. Drug was administered from day 0 through day 120. Note that hemolytic anemia, hemoglobinuria, and reticulocytosis develop shortly after the drug is started but that red cell survival stabilizes and hemolysis abates shortly thereafter because of repopulation of the red cell pool with young cells that have sufficient G6PD activity to protect against oxidative damage and hemolysis. G6PD = glucose-6-phosphate dehydrogenase; RBC = red blood cell. (Modified from Alving AS: Bull World Health Organ 1960;22:621.)

absence of such stress, individuals with the Gd^{A-} and Gd^{Med} variants have a normal blood smear and no hemolysis. In the presence of such stress, individuals with G6PD deficiency manifest hemolysis that can range from a chronic low-level hemolytic state, with a modest (3 to 4 g/dL) decrease in hemoglobin concentration and a modest increase in the reticulocyte count, to an acute episode of intravascular hemolysis characterized by anemia, hemoglobinemia, hemoglobinuria, hyperbilirubinemia, and jaundice. Severe hemolytic episodes can lead to symptoms of acute anemia such as chest pain, dyspnea, palpitations, dizziness, and headache; to acute abdominal and back pain; and to hemoglobin-induced renal tubular necrosis and renal failure. Changes in the blood smear include the appearance of Heinz bodies (visualized with supravital stains), bite cells (cells with small localized membrane invaginations, probably caused by splenic removal of Heinz bodies at the invagination sites), and blister cells (cells with a hemoglobin-free area adjacent to the membrane).

Hemolysis in the setting of G6PD deficiency is most often caused by acute infection, in which oxidant molecules are liberated in large amounts by granulocytes and mononuclear phagocytes. Oxidant drugs represent the other major category of oxidant stress that can lead to acute or chronic hemolysis (Table 165–4). Ingestion of fava beans (Italian broad beans) can also cause acute hemolysis in some patients with Gd^{Med}, probably because of the high levels of oxidant pyrimidine analogues in the beans. Many neonates with G6PD deficiency manifest jaundice at 1 to 4 days of age; although this complication can occasionally require exchange transfusion, it is usually managed successfully with phototherapy. A few rare patients with extremely unstable or low-activity G6PD variants have chronic ongoing hemolysis in the absence of oxidant stress.

Diagnosis

The most widely used screening tests for G6PD deficiency rely on a change in NADPH-induced dye decolorization or in methylene blue–mediated methemoglobin reduction to detect a decrease in enzyme activity. These tests suffer from low sensitivity, however, because 30 to 40% of the cells in the sample must be deficient for the abnormal state to be detected and most if not all of the deficient cells may be hemolyzed (especially in Gd^{A-} individuals) after an acute oxidant stress. More sensitive than these screening tests is the specific enzyme assay, which relies on a direct measurement of NADPH generation; however, even this assay requires that 20 to 30% of the cells be deficient to yield an abnormal result, although careful comparison between the activity of G6PD and that of other age-dependent enzymes in the sample may allow the diagnosis to be made immediately after an acute hemolytic episode. The most sensitive functional test for G6PD deficiency is the G6PD-tetrazolium cytochemical test, which requires that only 1 to 5% of the cells be deficient to discriminate an abnormal result; this test is capable not only of making the diagnosis after a hemolytic episode but also of detecting the enzyme deficiency in female heterozygotes. Increasingly, molecular diagnostic techniques are used to detect common mutations (e.g., mutations coding for Gd^{Med} or Gd^{A-} at the genomic or cDNA level).

TABLE 165–4 DRUGS THAT COMMONLY CAUSE HEMOLYSIS IN GLUCOSE-6-PHOSPHATE DEHYDROGENASE DEFICIENCY*

SULFONAMIDES AND SULFONES
Sulfisoxazole (Gantrisin)
Trimethoprim-sulfamethoxazole (Bactrim, Septra)
Salicylazosulfapyridine (Azulfidine, sulfasalazine)
Sulfanilamide
Sulfapyridine
Sulfadimidine
Sulfacetamide (Albucid)
Diaminodiphenylsulfone (Dapsone)†
Sulfoxone†
Glucosulfone sodium (Promin)
OTHER ANTIBACTERIALS
Nitrofurans
Nitrofurantoin (Furadantin)
Nitrofurazone (Furacin)
Furazolidone
Chloramphenicol
p-Aminosalicylic acid
Nalidixic acid‡
ANTIMALARIALS
Primaquine§
Pamaquine**
Mepacrine (quinacrine HCl)
ANTHELMINTICS
β-Naphthol
Stibophen
Niridazole
ANALGESICS‡‡
Acetylsalicylic acid (aspirin) (can give moderate doses)
Acetophenetidin (phenacetin)
MISCELLANEOUS
Probenecid
Vitamin K analogues (1 mg phytonadione can be given to infants)
Dimercaprol (BAL)
Methylene blue
Toluidine blue
Naphthalene (mothballs)†
Phenazopyridine (Pyridium)
Fava beans
Quinine

*Persons with all forms of G6PD deficiency should avoid the drugs listed in bold print; G6PD-deficient persons of Mediterranean, Middle Eastern, and Asian origin should avoid the drugs listed in bold and plain print.
†These drugs or chemicals may cause hemolysis in normal persons if they are given in large doses.
‡This drug applies only to individuals with Gd^{A-}.
§Persons with Gd^{A-} may take this drug at reduced dosage (15 mg/day or 45 mg twice weekly) under surveillance.
**Chloroquine may be used under surveillance (instead of pamaquine) when it is required for prophylaxis or treatment of malaria in susceptible individuals.
‡‡Acetaminophen (paracetamol) is a safe alternative.
Modified from WHO Working Group: Glucose-6-phosphate dehydrogenase deficiency. Bull World Health Organ 1989;67:601–611.

Treatment

Rx

Because all but a few rare individuals with G6PD deficiency are hematologically normal in the absence of an exogenous oxidant stress, no treatment is required for the deficiency itself. Mild to moderate episodes of acute hemolysis can often be managed by removal of the offending drug or by treatment of the concurrent infection. Severe hemolytic episodes in individuals with Gd^{Med} and other unstable G6PD variants may require red cell transfusions to alleviate the signs and symptoms of acute anemia as well as measures designed to protect against the potential renal complications of hemoglobinuria.

Defects in Glutathione Metabolism

Deficiencies in all of the enzymes responsible for glutathione synthesis and metabolism have been described (see Fig. 165–3). Red cells deficient in either γ-glutamylcysteine synthetase or glutathione synthetase, the two enzymes that catalyze glutathione synthesis, have abnormally low levels of glutathione and are sensitive to drug- and infection-induced oxidant hemolysis. Deficiencies of these two enzymes are rare, and the clinical syndromes are similar to G6PD deficiency. Inherited defects in glutathione reductase are also rare; the clinical consequence of this deficiency is uncertain, however, because no case of glutathione reductase–associated hemolysis has been carefully documented. Deficiencies in glutathione peroxidase are relatively common, but this disorder appears not to be associated with hemolytic anemia by virtue of the ability of glutathione to reduce hydrogen peroxide by a nonenzymatic as well as by an enzymatic route.

Defects in Glycolysis

Pyruvate Kinase Deficiency

Epidemiology

Pyruvate kinase deficiency, which is the most common hereditary defect in the glycolytic pathway, affects hundreds to thousands of individuals worldwide.

Pathobiology

The disease is inherited in an autosomal recessive pattern. Homozygotes manifest clinically significant hemolytic anemia, whereas heterozygote carriers are phenotypically normal.

Pathogenesis

Hemolysis in pyruvate kinase deficiency is thought to result from an intracellular deficiency of ATP, which leads to alterations in many of the biochemical pathways responsible for cellular homeostasis (see Fig. 165–3). These inherent biochemical abnormalities are magnified in the stressful environment of the splenic cords. Depending on the level of residual enzyme activity, the degree of hemolysis can range from mild (compensated hemolysis without anemia) to severe (red cell transfusion dependent). One factor that may mitigate the deleterious effects of pyruvate kinase deficiency on ATP generation is the two- to three-fold increase in 2,3-DPG that results from the distal block in the glycolytic pathway (see later).

Clinical Manifestations

Pyruvate kinase deficiency, unlike G6PD deficiency, results in a chronic hemolytic anemia that is not affected by drugs or other oxidant-producing states. Splenomegaly is a common feature of the disorder, probably because the ATP-deficient red cells are not capable of rapidly traversing the splenic fenestrations. The clinical sequelae of hemolytic anemia in pyruvate kinase deficiency are often milder than those seen in other conditions with the same degree of anemia, perhaps because the elevated levels of 2,3-DPG in pyruvate kinase–deficient red cells permit more efficient delivery of oxygen to the tissues for the same concentration of hemoglobin in the blood.

Diagnosis

Pyruvate kinase deficiency is diagnosed by spectrophotometric assays of enzyme activity, by measurements of enzyme substrate and product concentrations in the affected red cells, and by molecular diagnostic detection of specific mutations at the genomic or cDNA level. Measurement of red cell ATP content is not a reliable method for determination of pyruvate kinase activity, perhaps because the most severely affected cells with the lowest ATP content are quickly removed from the circulation and because the young reticulocytes that remain in the circulation have a high ATP content. Similarly, the morphology of pyruvate kinase–deficient red cells is often relatively normal in the presence of a functioning spleen.

Treatment

Splenectomy ameliorates the hemolysis in moderate to severe pyruvate kinase deficiency, although the improvement may not be as marked as that seen in diseases such as hereditary spherocytosis. After splenectomy, a "paradoxical reticulocytosis" often occurs (sometimes with a reticulocyte count of 50 to 70%) despite an improvement in the anemia. This striking finding is thought to be due to improved survival of the pyruvate kinase–deficient reticulocytes, which must depend on mitochondrial oxidative phosphorylation for ATP generation and are therefore susceptible to accelerated splenic "conditioning" (see Fig. 165–2) and extravascular hemolysis in the hypoxic environment of the splenic cords.

Other Defects in Glycolysis

Although abnormalities in most of the other enzymes in the glycolytic pathway have been described (see Fig. 165–3), the incidence of these deficiencies is so rare that together they affect only 5 to 10% of the number of individuals with pyruvate kinase deficiency. Like pyruvate kinase deficiency, most of these defects have an autosomal recessive inheritance pattern; the only exception is phosphoglycerate kinase deficiency because the gene coding for this enzyme is located on the X chromosome. The pathogenesis, clinical manifestations, diagnosis, and treatment of these deficiencies are generally similar to those described for pyruvate kinase deficiency.

Defects in Red Cell Nucleotide Metabolism

Two rare defects in red cell nucleotide metabolism can cause chronic hereditary hemolytic anemia. Pyrimidine-5′-nucleotidase deficiency is inherited in an autosomal recessive pattern. Lack of this enzyme prevents red cell precursor cells from degrading pyrimidine nucleotides to cytidine and uridine, which allows the intracellular accumulation of partially degraded RNA that appears in the mature red cells as basophilic stippling. (This mechanism may also explain the basophilic stippling seen in lead poisoning because the same enzyme is also inhibited by lead.) Although splenomegaly is common in this disorder, splenectomy is of little benefit, thus indicating that the mechanism of hemolysis may be fundamentally different from that involved in the other hereditary anemias discussed in this chapter. Overproduction of adenosine deaminase also causes chronic hemolytic anemia, apparently by depleting the intracellular pool of adenine to the point that ATP synthesis is affected; the molecular mechanism responsible for overexpression of this apparently normal protein remains to be elucidated.

SUGGESTED READINGS

Beutler E, Vulliamy TJ: Hematologically important mutations: Glucose-6-phosphate dehydrogenase. Blood Cells Mol Dis 2002;28:93–103. *Reviews the genetic bases of G6PD deficiency.*

Bolton-Maggs PHB, Stevens RF, Dodd NJ, et al: Guidelines for the diagnosis and management of hereditary spherocytosis. Br J Haematol 2004;126:455–474. *Reviews the diagnosis and current management of hereditary spherocytosis.*

Delaunay J: The hereditary stomatocytoses: Genetic disorders of the red cell membrane permeability to monovalent cations. Semin Hematol 2004; 41:165–172. *Reviews the pathophysiology of hereditary xerocytosis and hereditary stomatocytosis.*

Delaunay J: The molecular basis of hereditary red cell membrane disorders. Blood Rev 2007;21:1–20. *Reviews the genetic basis of disorders of red cell mechanics.*

Gallagher PG: Hereditary elliptocytosis: Spectrin and protein 4.1R. Semin Hematol 2004;41:142–164. *Reviews the pathophysiology of hereditary elliptocytosis.*

Gallagher PG: Red cell membrane disorders. Hematology Am Soc Hematol Educ Program 2005;13–18. *Discusses management considerations, including the risks and benefits of splenectomy.*

166 HEMOGLOBINOPATHIES: THE THALASSEMIAS

Griffin P. Rodgers

Definition

The thalassemia syndromes are a heterogeneous group of inherited anemias characterized by defects in the synthesis of one or more globin chain subunits of the adult hemoglobin tetramer (HbA). Patients with β-thalassemia have a decrease in β-chain production relative to α-chain production; the converse is the case in α-thalassemia. The clinical syndromes associated with thalassemia arise from the combined effects of inadequate hemoglobin production and unbalanced accumulation of globin subunits. The former causes hypochromia and microcytosis; the latter leads to ineffective erythropoiesis and hemolytic anemia. Clinical manifestations are diverse and range from asymptomatic hypochromia and microcytosis to profound anemia leading to death in utero or in early childhood if untreated. This clinical heterogeneity reflects the variable severity of the primary biosynthetic defect and coinherited modulating factors, such as accelerated synthesis of fetal hemoglobin subunits, the overall effectiveness of a wide range of cellular and circulatory adaptive factors, and perhaps not yet appreciated environmental factors. These disorders differ from the hemoglobinopathies that result from mutations in the coding sequences of the α-globin or β-globin genes; these mutations alter protein structure and lead to other disease manifestations (e.g., HbS in sickle cell disease) (Chapters 167 and 168). These disorders are not mutually exclusive in that some mutations (e.g., HbE and Hb Constant Spring) alter the structure of a globin chain and the rate at which it is produced. Table 166–1 presents a clinical classification and distinguishing characteristics of specific thalassemia syndromes.

Pathobiology

Genetics

Many structural genes encode for the globin polypeptides in maturing human erythroid cells. Normal functional hemoglobin consists of a tetramer of two α-like and two β-like globin polypeptide chains. Two clusters of closely linked genes encode the globin chains. The non-α (β-like) genes reside on chromosome 11 and include the two adult genes, δ

TABLE 166–1 CLINICAL CLASSIFICATION OF THALASSEMIAS

Classification	Genotypes	Clinical Severity*	Treatment
α-THALASSEMIA SYNDROMES†			
$α^+$-Carrier (silent)	–α/αα	Silent	None
α-Thalassemia trait	–α/–α; —/αα	Mild	None
HbH disease	–α/—	Mild-moderate; hemolytic anemia	Folic acid; avoidance of oxidant drugs; transfusion support and splenectomy, as indicated
Hydrops fetalis	—/—	Lethal	Early referral to high-risk obstetric service
Hb Constant Spring genotypes	$αα^{cs}/αα$	Silent-mild	None
β-THALASSEMIA SYNDROMES‡			
β-Thalassemia minor (trait)	$β/β^+$	Silent	None
β-Thalassemia intermedia	$β/β^0$ $β^+/β^+$; $β^+/β^0 = β^+$ HbE/$β^0$	Moderate-severe	Folic acid; periodic blood transfusion support and/or splenectomy, as indicated
β-Thalassemia major	$β^0/β^0 = β^0$	Severe	Early referral for hematopoietic stem cell transplantation, if feasible; regular blood transfusions and iron chelation therapy; splenectomy, as indicated
COMPLEX β-THALASSEMIA SYNDROMES			
Coinherited β-thalassemia‡	Various combinations of α- and β-thalassemia syndromes		
Hereditary persistence of fetal Hb	Various point mutations or deletions in or around γ-globin gene	Mild-moderate	Folic acid; periodic blood transfusion support and/or splenectomy, as indicated
γ-Thalassemia	Deletion of ≥1 γ-genes		
δ-Thalassemia	Deletion of ≥1 δ-genes		
γδβ-Thalassemia	Complex deletions of ≥1 γ-, δ-, β-genes in tandem		

Hb = hemoglobin.
**Silent* = normal or minimally abnormal hematology values; *mild* = hemoglobin level normal or slightly reduced with disproportionate microcytic hypochromic indices; *moderate* = hemolytic anemia, icterus, splenomegaly, although no regular transfusion requirement; *severe* = profound anemia with transfusion dependency, extramedullary hematopoiesis, growth retardation, bone abnormalities, hemosiderosis; *lethal* = death in utero from anemic congestive heart failure.
†The α-thalassemia syndromes usually result from deletions in one or more α-genes, indicated by the minus sign, or from mutations in the coding sequence (e.g., α-Constant Spring, $α^{cs}$).
‡The β-thalassemia syndromes are typically the consequence of mutations that lead to a *decreased* level of normal β-chain production ($β^+$) or *absence* of β-chain production ($β^0$). Various combinations of these mutations give rise to syndromes of increasing severity.

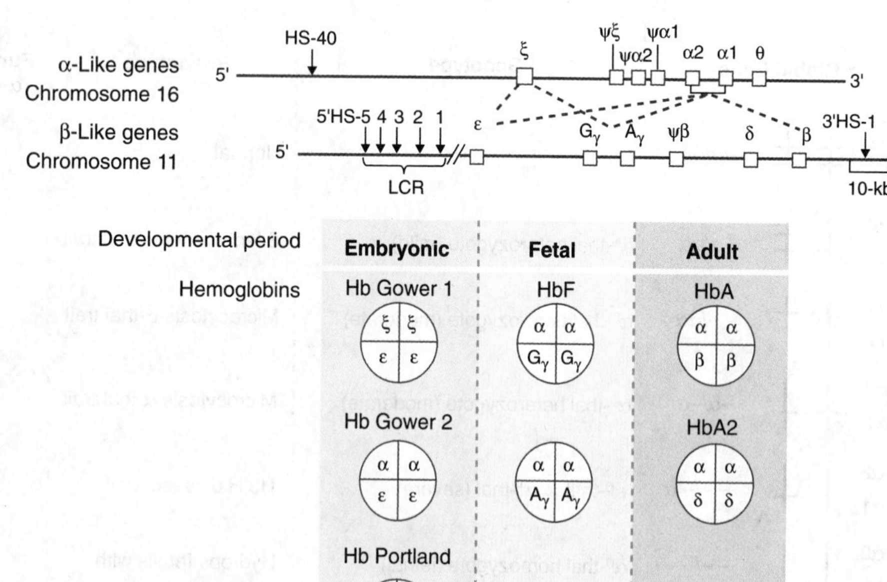

FIGURE 166–1 • Organization and expression of the human globin genes. The human globin genes consist of two clusters of closely linked genes on two separate chromosomes encoding the globin chains. The genes are arranged with the same transcriptional orientation from 5′ to 3′ as the order in which they are sequentially expressed during development. The α- and β-globin gene clusters also contain several pseudogenes, indicated by the ψ prefix. Upstream (5′) of these clusters are major transcriptional control elements, HS-40 → (α) and LCR → (β), that are crucial for high-level expression in a developmentally specific manner. Hb = hemoglobin.

and β, the two similar fetal genes (differing by one amino acid, alanine or glycine) Aγ and Gγ, and the single embryonic ε-gene. On chromosome 16 are found the α-like genes, including the duplicated and almost identically functional α-genes ($\alpha_2\alpha_1$), which are present in the fetal and adult stages of erythropoiesis, and the embryonic ζ-gene. A θ-gene downstream from the α_1-gene has been shown to be a pseudogene incapable of producing normal messenger RNA (mRNA). High-level tissue and developmentally specific globin gene expression is governed in large part by novel upstream regulatory elements designated HS-40 and LCR for the α-globin and β-globin clusters, respectively. As the descriptors of these genes imply, several distinct hemoglobin species are present during the transition from intrauterine to adult life (Fig. 166–1).

On a smaller scale, individual α-like and β-like globin genes share many general features. Each gene consists of three coding sequences (exons) interrupted by two intervening sequences (introns). As with other eukaryotic genes, globin genes have short segments of 5′ and 3′ untranslated regions, appropriate recognition sequences at the intron/exon junctions to facilitate normal splicing, and polyadenylation sequences in the 3′ untranslated regions. In the 5′ promoter region are three elements crucial for normal globin gene expression: the ATA, CCAAT, and CACCC boxes. Enhancers and silencing elements also have been recognized in these 5′ and 3′ flanking sequences. Mutations (or deletions) in any of these important elements in the promoters, enhancers, or intron-exon junctions lead to a decrease in overall gene transcription.

These mutations or deletions in and around the α-globin and β-globin genes or in the α-HS-40 or β-LCR may lead to disease manifestations ranging from inconsequential laboratory findings (microcytosis and hypochromia in α-thalassemia, β-thalassemia trait) to events incompatible with normal intrauterine growth and development (hydrops fetalis) (Fig. 166–2; see Table 166–1).

Molecular Defects

α-Thalassemia syndromes have been classified by defects resulting in severe (α-thalassemia type 1) and mild (α-thalassemia type 2) forms (Fig. 166–3). This nomenclature gradually is being replaced to reflect the current classification scheme of the β-thalassemias into two groups: α^0-thalassemias and α^+-thalassemias. In the α^0-thalassemias, production of α-globin chains by the affected chromosome is completely abolished, whereas the α^+-thalassemias are defined by a variable amount of globin chain production resulting from the remaining α-globin genes on the chromosome. The α^0-thalassemias usually result from deletion of the α_2-globin and α_1-globin genes in cis (i.e., on the same chromosome), deletion of the entire cluster together with the main regulatory sequence

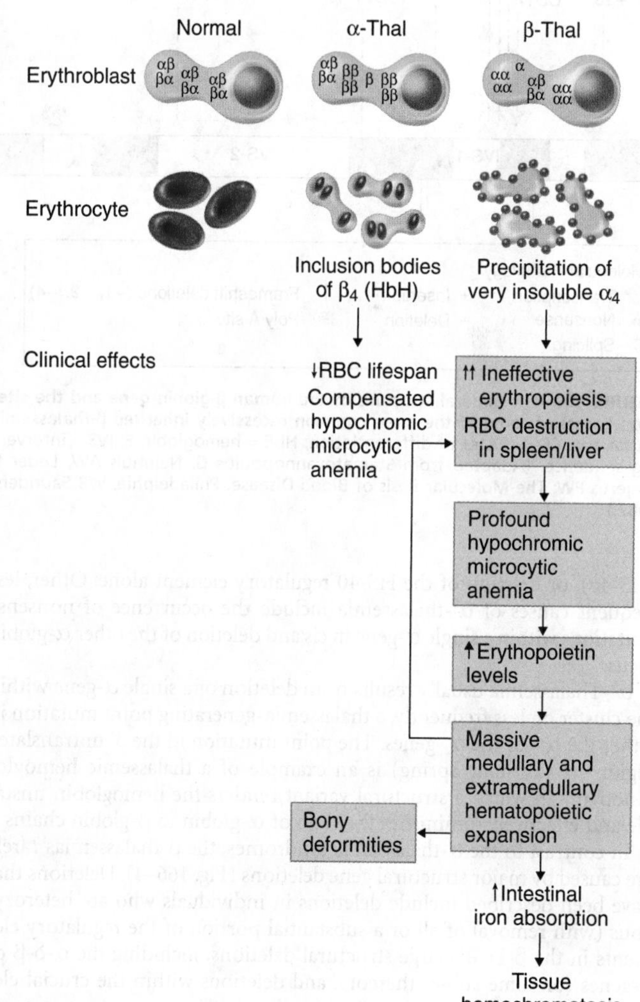

FIGURE 166–2 • α- and β-thalassemia. Schematic representation of the pathophysiology of the clinically significant α- and β-thalassemia (Thal) syndromes. RBC = red blood cell.

α-Globin Gene		Genotype	Phenotype	No. of Functional α-Genes
α2 α1	αα/αα	Normal	Normal	4
α2 α1	–α/αα	α⁺-thal heterozygote (mild)	Silent carrier α-thal trait	3
α2 α1	– –/αα	α⁰-thal heterozygote (moderate)	Microcytosis α-thal trait	2
α2 α1	–α/–α	α⁺-thal heterozygote (moderate)	Microcytosis α-thal trait	2
α2 α1	– –/– α	α⁰-thal × α⁺-thal (severe)	Hb H disease	1
α2 α1	– –/– –	α⁰-thal homozygote (lethal)	Hydrops fetalis with Hb Bart's	0

FIGURE 166–3 • The genetic bases of the more common forms of α-thalassemia. The hematologic and clinical severity is directly proportional to the number of deleted α-globin genes, as indicated. (Adapted from Gelehrter TD, Collins FS: Principles of Medical Genetics. Baltimore, Williams & Wilkins, 1990.)

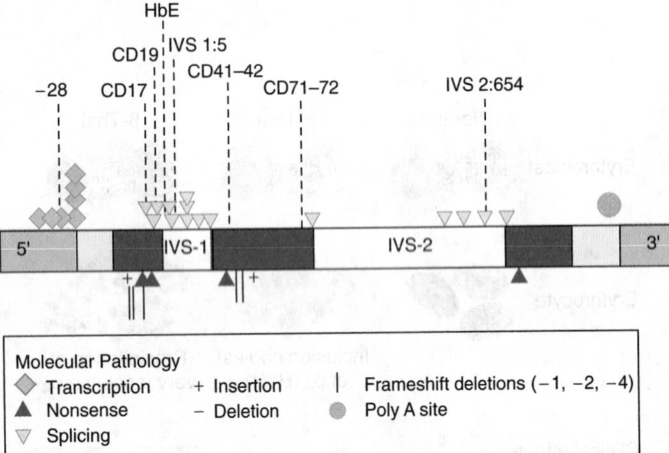

FIGURE 166–4 • General structure of the human β-globin gene and the sites (and bases) of some of the more common recessively inherited β-thalassemia mutations. CD = cluster of differentiation; HbE = hemoglobin E; IVS = intervening sequence. (Adapted from Stamatoyannopoulos G, Neinhuis AW, Leder P, Majerus PW: The Molecular Basis of Blood Disease. Philadelphia, WB Saunders, 1987.)

(HS-40), or deletion of the HS-40 regulatory element alone. Other, less frequent causes of α⁰-thalassemia include the occurrence of nonsense mutations within a single α-gene in cis and deletion of the other α-globin locus.

α⁺-Thalassemia usually results from deletion of a single α-gene within the cluster or, less frequently, a thalassemia-generating point mutation in either the α_1- or the α_2-genes. The point mutation in the 3′ untranslated region (α Constant Spring) is an example of a thalassemic hemoglobinopathy in which a structural variant renders the hemoglobin unstable and effectively diminishes the ratio of α-globin to β-globin chains.

In contrast to the α-thalassemia syndromes, the β-thalassemias rarely are caused by major structural gene deletions (Fig. 166–4). Deletions that have been described include deletions in individuals who are heterozygous (with removal of all or a substantial portion of the regulatory elements in the β-LCR); large structural deletions, including the α-δ-β or β-genes (or some subset thereof); and deletions within the crucial elements in the β-promoter described previously. The most common cause of β-thalassemia is the so-called nondeletional variant, which affects gene function in many ways, including abnormalities in transcription, RNA processing, or RNA translation of the β-globin gene.

Despite the large number of these mutations—more than 200 β-thalassemia alleles have been characterized—probably only 20 β-thalassemic alleles account for more than 80% of the β-thalassemia mutations. *Transcriptional mutants* result from mutations either in the promoter of regulatory elements, usually between position –101 and position –28, or in the 5′ untranslated regions, especially in the region of the canonical CAP site. An example of such a transcriptional mutant is the –28 point mutation, which is common in American and African blacks and Southeast Asians and gives rise to a β⁺-phenotype. *RNA processing abnormalities,* perhaps the most common of all mutations thus characterized, occur near splice junctions next to the consensus splice site (e.g., the intervening sequence [IVS] 1:5 mutation common in Mediterranean populations, Northern Europeans, and Algerians), in cryptic splice sites in introns (e.g., IVS 2:654 producing β⁰-thalassemia or β⁺-thalassemia in Chinese, Southeast Asians, and Japanese), or in cryptic splice sites in exons (e.g., codon 19 in Southeast Asians). A mutation in codon 26 (GTA→GTG) results in HbE, which is prevalent among Southeast Asians; this mutation gives rise to a quantitative reduction in normal β-globin gene mRNA because of activation of a cryptic splice donor site and to a qualitative abnormality of the β-globin chain because of substitution of a lysine for the normal glutamic acid (Chapter 167). The third major category of mutations results in *RNA translation abnormalities.* These mutations produce a β⁰-thalassemia phenotype and include abnormalities in the initiation (ATG) codon; production of nonsense codons (codon 39 in Mediterranean populations); or frame-shift mutations such as the codon 41/42 mutations common in Chinese, Southeast Asian, and Asian Indian populations or the codon 71/72 mutations in Chinese populations.

Pathophysiology

Patients with α-thalassemia have a decrease in α-globin chain production relative to β-globin chain, with the formation of β_4 (HbH) inclusion bodies. Red blood cells bearing these inclusion bodies are removed rapidly from the circulation by the reticuloendothelial system, shortening their survival. The resulting mild anemia is compensated partially by an increase in red blood cell production.

In contrast, patients with β-thalassemia have a decrease in β-globin chain production relative to α-globin chain production, which leads to an excess of α-globin chains. Although this decrease in β-synthesis is compensated slightly by the γ-globin and δ-globin chains, the combined β-globin, δ-globin, and γ-globin chains are insufficient to match the number of α-globin chains present. Unbound α-globin chains are extremely insoluble and precipitate in red blood cell precursors and their progeny, a process leading to defective erythroid maturation (ineffective erythropoiesis). The α-chain monomers form hemichromes that bind and modify red blood cell membrane proteins including protein bands 3 and 4.1, ankyrin, and spectrin; they also lead to the externalization of phosphatidylserine, which may activate the coagulation system. The few cells that do emerge into the peripheral circulation are removed rapidly in the spleen and liver. Progressive splenomegaly occurs in an attempt to entrap these abnormal red blood cells and further exacerbates the anemia through hemodilution. The resulting profound anemia increases circulating levels of erythropoietin and causes a massive expansion of medullary and extramedullary hematopoietic tissue. This expansion leads to skeletal abnormalities and various growth and metabolic derangements. The expanded erythroid marrow induces signals that increase intestinal iron absorption. Recent studies in animal models have identified ferroportin (Fpn) and hepcidin (Hepc) as critical proteins in the mechanisms by which iron is regulated with respect to absorption and movement throughout the body. This process, along with the iatrogenic iron overload (secondary to long-term transfusion therapy), leads to tissue hemochromatosis and its attendant complications.

Clinical Manifestations

α-Thalassemias

Deletion of one or both α-globin genes on chromosome 16 is the most common mutation of the human genome. The α-globin gene cluster is a dynamic locus in which tandemly duplicated long blocks of nucleotide sequences promote nonhomologous recombination between chromosomes during meiosis. The α-thalassemia syndromes result predominately from deletions of one or more of the four genes coding for the α-chain, although nondeletional forms also have been described. These disorders have their highest prevalence among Africans and their descendants (30%), in whom a single α-gene or two α-genes in trans (i.e., on opposite chromosomes) may be deleted. In contrast, in Southeast Asian populations, where the prevalence may reach 40%, more typically two α-genes in cis may be deleted, although single α-gene deletions also are seen (see Fig. 166–3).

The clinical spectrum of the α-thalassemia syndromes is related directly to the number of functioning α-globin genes. Accordingly, deletions of one (αα/–α) or two (–α/–α, —/αα) α-globin genes, which occur frequently in many parts of the world, are virtually asymptomatic. Correct diagnosis of these genotypes allows for the identification of couples at risk for pregnancies with homozygous fetuses (see later discussion). In addition, proper recognition of these syndromes provides a molecular basis for microcytosis and hypochromia (and possibly mild anemia) and averts the injudicious and often extended use of iron supplementation for the erroneous diagnosis of iron deficiency (Chapter 163). HbH disease, which is caused by deletions of three genes (—/–α), is manifested as a moderately severe anemia with splenomegaly and a hypochromic, microcytic blood film appearance (see Table 166–1). HbH ($β_4$) is demonstrable by special staining of the red blood cell and by hemoglobin electrophoresis. In most cases, the hemolytic anemia in HbH disease is compensated partially, with an average hemoglobin value of 8 to 10 g/dL, and long-term transfusion therapy may not be required. However, HbH is prone to precipitation in red blood cells during oxidative stress and under conditions of increased temperature, and consequently the hemolytic anemia may be exacerbated in these patients by agents known to induce oxidant injury or in the presence of infection. Accordingly, the same drugs that induce hemolysis in patients who are deficient in glucose-6-phosphate dehydrogenase (Chapter 164), especially the sulfonamides, should be avoided in susceptible patients with HbH disease.

In its most severe form, in which all four genes are deleted, α-thalassemia is incompatible with life, and the fetus is stillborn or critically ill with hydrops fetalis. Occasionally, fetuses have survived after treatment with intrauterine transfusions and postnatal stem cell transplantation, or, more recently, intrauterine stem cell transplantation. Reports also indicate that mothers carrying affected fetuses have a high incidence of pregnancy-induced hypertension (75%), seizures, postpartum hemorrhage (10%), and other peripartum complications. Accordingly, every effort should be made to identify these women (typically Asians or Asian-Americans) during the early course of their pregnancy for appropriate referral.

β-Thalassemias

The β-thalassemia syndromes represent the classic molecular paradigm in which disparate defects in a eukaryotic structural gene can culminate in decreased to absent (β) polypeptide chain production. This diverse group of disorders for the most part results from single nucleotide changes in or around either or both of the two β-globin genes. Some of the molecular mechanisms accounting for the thalassemic phenotype include nonsense, frame-shift, splicing, and polyadenylation mutations, insertions, and deletions (see Fig. 166–4). These alterations give rise to significant changes in the level of gene transcription that lead to absent ($β^0$) or markedly diminished ($β^+$) amounts of β-globin gene mRNA (see Table 166–1). In addition, long deletions lead to more complex forms of β-thalassemia syndromes, such as β-thalassemia or hereditary persistence of fetal hemoglobin. These large deletions in the β-globin cluster occur less commonly than in the α-globin cluster.

The condition is ubiquitous but is especially common in Mediterranean, Asian, and African populations (and their American descendants), in whom the high gene frequency has been thought to reflect geographic areas with a high prevalence of malaria. Within a given ethnic group, relatively few genotypes account for most cases, each of which now has been defined by DNA analysis. At a lower level of resolution, the pattern of DNA resolved on gel electrophoresis after restriction enzyme digestion has been used to define certain haplotypes or restriction fragment length polymorphisms. Specific β-globin cluster haplotypes are linked genetically to certain of these thalassemic mutations, and haplotype analysis has been used to define mutation prevalence in various populations and to assess population migration.

The clinical spectrum of disease severity in the β-thalassemia syndromes is related directly to the quantitative effect of individual mutations on β-globin synthesis. Although β-thalassemia trait is asymptomatic, disease occurs in homozygotes or compound heterozygotes such as patients with β-thalassemia/HbE (see Table 166–1). In these latter instances, reduced or absent β-globin synthesis results in the accumulation of free α-globin chains that precipitate during early erythroblast development because of their relative insolubility. These inclusions lead to ineffective erythropoiesis in the bone marrow and enhanced peripheral destruction of the erythrocytes that emerge from the bone marrow. The associated pathophysiologic changes resulting from the subsequent anemia include splenomegaly, which may lead to hypersplenism; osteoporosis and other skeletal and soft tissue changes associated with an expanded bone marrow; and iron overload resulting from a combination of enhanced gastrointestinal iron absorption and red blood cell transfusions. The liver, heart, pancreas, pituitary, and other endocrine organs are the major sites of excessive iron deposition, which ultimately leads to damage and failure of these organs.

Diagnosis

Historically, the diagnosis of β-thalassemia and α-thalassemia has relied heavily on clinical and hematologic features (Fig. 166–5). Often, patients were referred for evaluation of anemia or microcytosis or both, or in the context of neonatal or population screening. The discovery of low mean corpuscular volume and hemoglobin on automated complete blood counts has increased the number of these referrals. In the presence of normal iron status, increased levels of HbA_2 (as high as 4 to 6%) and/or HbF (5 to 20%) on quantitative hemoglobin analysis support the diagnosis. Differentiation between iron deficiency anemia and β-thalassemia or α-thalassemia trait can be difficult in practice if no reciprocal increases in levels of HbA_2 and/or HbF are present. In the presence of concomitant iron deficiency, HbA_2 levels in individuals with β-thalassemia may fall into the normal range. In these instances, the demonstration of a modified ratio of β-globin to α-globin synthetic chain, usually using tritium (^3H)-labeled leucine to analyze globin chain production in reticulocytes, is required for a conclusive diagnosis.

In the contemporary era of DNA technology, reference laboratories can swiftly clone and directly sequence the α-globin or β-globin genes or perform other techniques of DNA analysis for patients with suspected

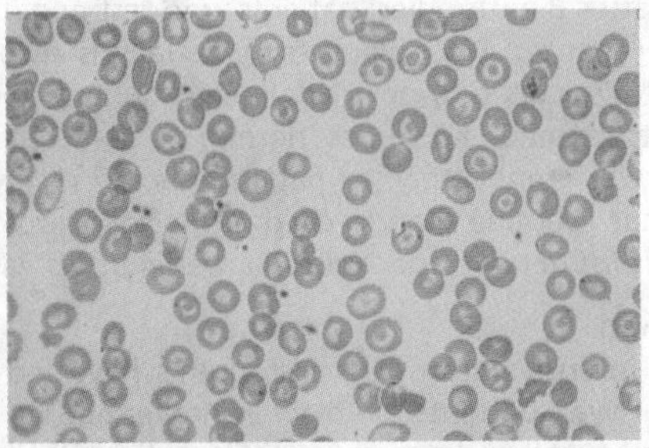

FIGURE 166–5 • **Thalassemia minor.** Smear shows hypochromic red blood cells with many target cells.

thalassemia syndromes. This approach, which has revolutionized prenatal diagnosis of the severe thalassemia syndromes, can be performed at 14 weeks' gestation on amniotic fluid cells and at 10 weeks if chorionic villus sampling is performed. These procedures carry a risk of miscarriage of 1% and 5%, respectively.

A hydrops fetalis (—/—) genotype can be shown by the complete absence of α-globin genes in the DNA on use of α-globin–specific probes. For β-thalassemia mutations, antenatal diagnosis can be made by polymerase chain reaction (PCR) gene amplification of white blood cell–derived DNA and hybridization with a panel of DNA probes specific for common mutations within the patient's ethnic group. If the diagnosis is suspected but the likely mutations are unknown, other DNA-based methods to diagnose and differentiate the thalassemia syndromes include single-strand conformation polymorphism, denaturing gradient electrophoresis, heteroduplex analysis, and direct DNA sequencing of PCR products. These methods all use to great advantage an initial step of PCR gene amplification.

Treatment

α-Thalassemia

Some deletions of one ($\alpha\alpha$/–α) or two (–α/–α, —/$\alpha\alpha$) α-globin genes are asymptomatic, and no therapy is indicated. For HbH disease (three-gene deletion, —/–α), folic acid, 1 mg orally, should be administered daily to compensate for folate loss from accelerated red blood cell turnover. Splenectomy may be indicated for progressive anemia and often is associated with a mean rise in hemoglobin of 2 to 3 g/dL.

β-Thalassemia

Despite an almost comprehensive understanding of the molecular and cellular pathogenesis of the β-thalassemia syndromes, a widely available curative form of treatment for homozygotes remains elusive. Nonetheless, dramatic improvement in life expectancy and morbidity has been observed since the 1980s, primarily because of aggressive transfusion support and the institution of effective iron chelation therapy in these regularly transfused patients. Except for curative allogeneic bone marrow transplantation (Chapter 184), therapy is considered symptomatic and supportive. Treatment of compound heterozygotes for HbS is discussed in Chapter 167.

Transfusion

As treatment of severe β-thalassemia has improved, so have morbidity and median survival. Nontransfused patients in the 1920s had a median survival time of 2 years. Transfusion therapy aimed at maintenance of a hemoglobin concentration of 11 to 13 g/dL (with pretransfusion level >10 g/dL) has been shown to extend average survival into the second decade and to minimize the bony abnormalities and improve sexual development. Transfusion support usually is initiated when the hemoglobin level decreases to less than 7 g/dL and remains there in the absence of infection or blood loss. To minimize febrile reactions and avoid prejudicing the potential future application of bone marrow transplantation (see later discussion), leukocyte-poor red blood cells should be administered (Chapter 183). An accurate record of the date and amount of blood administered, along with pretransfusion and post-transfusion hemoglobin levels and the occurrence of any transfusion reactions, facilitates optimal therapy. Patients should be tested for the presence of hepatitis B antibodies; patients who test negative should be immunized (Chapter 16). Splenectomy usually is recommended in children (6 to 7 years old) or in adolescents when their transfusion requirements exceed 1.5 times normal (e.g., >200 mL/kg/year). Before elective splenectomy, all patients should receive polyvalent pneumococcal vaccine, and children also should be given *Haemophilus influenzae* and *Neisseria meningitidis* vaccines.

Iron Chelation

Although intensive transfusion programs have led to markedly improved survival, patients die from iron overload unless chelation therapy is instituted and maintained (Chapter 231). Historically, this therapy involved subcutaneous deferoxamine, a parenterally administered iron chelator, given as a 12- to 24-hour infusion 5 or 6 days a week. Now, however, treatment in the United States can also be achieved with oral deferasirox (20 to 30 mg/kg/day), which is roughly comparable to deferoxamine in removing excess iron. [1] Because of its relatively long half-life, deferasirox can be administered once daily. It has an acceptable side-effect profile; the most common side effects are gastrointestinal or relate to iron deprivation.

Chelation therapy should be individualized according to age, risks, compliance history, and other factors. Patients with high liver iron concentrations (>6000 μg per gram of dry tissue) and patients with evidence of cardiac involvement (i.e., heart failure, arrhythmias) require more intensive therapy and should be referred to specialized medical centers caring for large numbers of patients who require long-term transfusion support. Periodic assessment of the effectiveness of chelation therapy should include an estimate of iron burden (e.g., serum iron, total iron-binding capacity, ferritin) and an estimate of liver iron concentration by the judicious use of percutaneous liver biopsy or, ideally, by validated noninvasive testing. At present, the options include superconducting quantum interference device (SQUID) susceptometry or, potentially, magnetic resonance susceptometry. A yearly cardiac evaluation should be done to detect clinical evidence of cardiac disease and should include a complete history and physical examination, electrocardiogram, echocardiogram, and chest radiograph. A Holter monitor should be used for any patient who complains of palpitations or who is noted on physical examination to have an irregular heartbeat. Potential iron-induced damage to the endocrine glands should be evaluated by glucose tolerance testing, thyroid function tests, and cortisol determinations. Hormone replacement therapy is dictated by the results of basal and/or provocative endocrine function studies.

Another alternative, not currently approved by the U.S. Food and Drug Administration, is deferiprone. At a mean dose of 92 mg/kg/day, it has been shown to be more promising than deferoxamine in reducing myocardial iron overload in beta-thalassemia major. [2]

Stem Cell Transplantation and Experimental Therapies

Allogeneic bone marrow transplantation (Chapter 184) is increasingly effective for patients with homozygous β-thalassemia. Among good-risk children (defined by good compliance with chelation and the absence of hepatomegaly and portal fibrosis), the 3-year event-free survival rate is 95%. Older patients and those exhibiting one or more risk factors have rejection-free survival rates of less than 75%. Currently, bone marrow transplantation can be recommended as a reasonable option only for selected good-risk pediatric candidates who have a human leukocyte antigen (HLA)-matched donor. There has also been increased interest in the application of low-intensity conditioning regimens (nonmyeloablative, minitransplants) for older patients with compatible donors, in whom high doses of conditioning radiation and chemotherapy lead to unacceptable morbidity and mortality.

One alternative form of therapy involves the manipulation of globin gene expression with drugs such as 5-azacytidine, hydroxyurea, erythropoietin, or butyrate analogues. The rationale for these trials is that these agents are known to stimulate fetal hemoglobin synthesis and that γ-globin chain augmentation may compensate for the reduced β-chain synthesis, normalizing the ratio of α-chain to non–α-chain; the result could be decreased transfusion requirements, decreased extramedullary hematopoiesis, and reduced iron overload. Although some patients have responded impressively to these therapies, the overall low response rate and the requirement for frequent parenteral administration have tempered enthusiasm for this approach. Nonetheless, these initial successes have led investigators to examine the efficacy of related classes of orally administered agents to stimulate HbF production.

Finally, gene therapy has been directed at replacing or compensating for the defective β-globin alleles, especially in view of the comparative ease of obtaining hematopoietic stem cells. Although this approach remains theoretically attractive, methodologic and logistic hurdles persist.

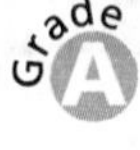

1. Cappellini MD, Cohen A, Piga A, et al: A phase 3 study of deferasirox (ICL670), a once-daily oral iron chelator, in patients with beta-thalassemia. Blood 2006;107:3455–3462.
2. Pennell DJ, Berdoukas V, Karagiorga M, et al: Randomized controlled trial of deferiprone or deferoxamine in beta-thalassemia major patients with asymptomatic myocardial siderosis. Blood 2006;107:3738–3744.

SUGGESTED READINGS

Birgens H, Ljung R: The thalassaemia syndromes. Scand J Clin Lab Invest 2007;67:11–25. *Overview of the biologic and clinical aspects of thalassemia.*

Hahalis G, Alexopoulos D, Kremastinos DT, et al: Heart failure in beta-thalassemia syndromes: A decade of progress. Am J Med 2005;118:957–967. *By increasing the proportion of patients receiving optimal chelation, survival in β-thalassemia major has improved and may improve further.*

Neufeld EJ: Oral chelators deferasirox and deferiprone for transfusional iron overload in thalassemia major: new data, new questions. Blood 2006;107:3436–3441. *Review of oral chelators.*

Rund D, Rachmilewitz E: Beta-Thalassemia. N Engl J Med 2005:1135–1146. *Update on pathophysiology, diagnosis, and treatment.*

Vichinsky EP, MacKlin EA, Waye JS, et al: Changes in the epidemiology of thalassemia in North America: A new minority disease. Pediatrics 2005;116:e818–e825. *Asian patients now account for >50% of the thalassemia population in the United States.*

167 SICKLE CELL DISEASE AND ASSOCIATED HEMOGLOBINOPATHIES

Martin H. Steinberg

SICKLE CELL DISEASE

Definition

Sickle cell disease, caused by a mutation in the β-globin gene (*HBB*) is a group of chronic hemolytic anemias, all characterized by vasculopathy, vaso-occlusive disease, widespread acute and chronic organ damage, and a reduced lifespan.

Epidemiology

The prevalences of the various forms of sickle cell disease and of the sickle cell trait, which is not truly a form of sickle cell disease, vary in the United States and worldwide (Table 167–1; Fig. 167–1). The sickle hemoglobin mutation became prominent in equatorial Africa, the Middle East, and India several thousand years ago, when deforestation, agriculture, and stagnant pooling of water permitted *Plasmodium falciparum* to become endemic. Carriers of the sickle hemoglobin gene were more likely to survive to reproductive age and had a selective advantage where falciparum malaria was present. At least five distinct origins of this identical mutation can be distinguished by the accompanying haplotype of the β-globin gene-like cluster. Voluntary and forced population shifts, predominantly the Atlantic slave trade of the 17th through 19th centuries, spread this mutation to the Americas, throughout the Mediterranean basin, and eastward to the Indian subcontinent. In some sites in Africa, half the population carries the sickle hemoglobin gene.

Pathobiology

Globin, the protein portion of hemoglobin, harbors the porphyrin heme ring and permits the molecule to operate efficiently in oxygen transport and its other physiologic functions (Fig. 167–2). Mutations can alter the primary amino acid sequence of the globin polypeptide, sometimes resulting in clinically significant diseases called hemoglobinopathies, including sickle cell disease. Sickle hemoglobin (HbS; $\alpha_2\beta_2^S$) is caused by an adenine (A) to thymidine (T) substitution (GAG→GTG) in codon 6 of the β-globin gene, resulting in replacement of the normal glutamic acid residue by a valine (Glu6Val). HbS polymerizes when it is deoxygenated, a property only of hemoglobin variants that have the β Glu6Val substitution. Critical amounts of HbS polymer within sickle erythrocytes cause cellular injury and lead to the phenotype of sickle cell disease, which is recognized by hemolytic anemia and vaso-occlusion. Other common hemoglobin variants, such as HbE and HbC, are clinically recognizable. More than 1000 hemoglobin mutations are known, and occasionally they can affect the stability and function of hemoglobin and cause hemolytic anemia (Chapter 168), disordered oxygen transport (Chapter 172), or methemoglobinemia (Chapter 168). However, most globin mutations are clinically insignificant. Thalassemias (Chapter 166) are also caused by mutations in globin genes, but these mutations affect globin gene expression so that synthesis of a globin chain is reduced or absent, although the structure of any globin produced is normal.

In sickle cell disease, erythrocytes are heterogeneous as a result of membrane damage and the cellular distribution of fetal hemoglobin (HbF). HbF concentrations vary among patients with sickle cell anemia and among erythrocytes of each individual. Because HbF inhibits HbS polymerization (see later discussion), its concentration within each cell and its distribution among all cells influence cell heterogeneity.

Sickle cell anemia is noteworthy for its clinical heterogeneity. Any patient can have almost all known disease complications; some have almost none but die suddenly; some skip one or more phases of the disease but suffer intensely from others. Thus, this prototypical single-gene, mendelian disorder behaves clinically as a multigenic trait with exceptional phenotypic variability. Understanding the vascular and inflammatory components of the disease provides many loci where the disease phenotype can be influenced by modifying genes. These genes potentially affect the pathogenesis of sickle cell anemia by modulating inflammation, oxidant injury, nitric oxide (NO) biology, vasoregulation, cell-cell interaction, blood coagulation, and hemostasis. Polymorphisms have been noted in candidate genes that affect these functions, and some may be prognostically useful. The sickle mutation is found on several different haplotypes of the β-globin gene-like cluster, reflecting different origins of the mutation in Africa and the Middle East. The Senegal haplotype is often associated with higher HbF levels than other haplotypes and with a more benign clinical course. Conversely, the Bantu haplotype may be associated with more disease complications.

Cation homeostasis is impaired in some sickle cells. A reduced capacity of sickle cells to maintain normal potassium (K^+) gradients is mediated by activation of the Gardos and K^+/Cl^- cotransport channels. As a result, sickle erythrocytes vary in their density and deformability. Irreversibly sickled cells (ISCs; Fig. 167–3) always appear deformed because of permanent membrane damage, even though they may not contain HbS polymer. In some dense cells, the mean corpuscular hemoglobin concentration reaches 50 g/dL (normal, 27 to 38 g/dL) and HbS polymer is always present. Individuals with the highest numbers of ISCs and dense cells have the most hemolysis and anemia but not necessarily the highest incidence of vaso-occlusive events.

Hemolysis is mainly extravascular due to erythrophagocytosis by reticuloendothelial cells that recognize the damaged sickle erythrocyte. In some patients, intravascular destruction of sickle erythrocytes liberates excessive amounts of hemoglobin into the circulation, thereby depleting haptoglobin and scavenging NO. This process promotes a vasoconstrictive, proinflammatory phenotype that triggers vaso-occlusive complications (Fig. 167–4). Certain complications of sickle disease, such as pulmonary hypertension, priapism, leg ulcer, and stroke, are closely linked to the intensity of hemolysis, whereas other complications, such as painful episodes, acute chest syndrome, and osteonecrosis, are linked to high blood viscosity and the interactions among sickle cells, leukocytes, and the endothelium.

Vaso-occlusive events probably depend on features intrinsic to the sickle erythrocyte, such as polymer content and the degree of cellular damage, interacting with factors in the cell's environment, such as endothelial injury, vascular tone, and other blood cells. In the first hours of a painful episode, the number of dense cells falls; it rises again as pain resolves. These observations suggest the possibility that more deformable, more adherent, and fewer dense cells might initiate vaso-occlusion, whereas dense cells become sequestered or destroyed in the microvasculature. Endothelial cells are responsive to many biologic modifiers that can be generated during sickle vaso-occlusive episodes and infection. Their activation and damage may be provoked by adherent sickle cells and shear stresses that cause release of oxidant radicals, expression of

TABLE 167–1 GENETIC AND LABORATORY FEATURES OF COMMON SICKLE HEMOGLOBINOPATHIES*

Genotype	Genetics	Prevalence among African Americans†	Hematocrit (%)	MCV (fl)	HbS (%)	HbA_2 (%)	HbF (%)	Severity‡
Sickle cell anemia (HbSS)	Homozygous, HbS	1:600	18–28	85–95	>85	2–3	2–15	4
HbSS-α-thalassemia	Homozygous, HbS α-thalassemia	30% of HbSS patients	25–33	70–85	>85	4–6	2–15	4
HbSC disease (HbSC)	Compound heterozygous HbS, HbC	1:800	28–40	70–85	50	2–3	1–8	2
HbS–β^0-thalassemia (HbS–β^0-Thal)	Compound heterozygous HbS, β^0-thalassemia	1:1600	20–30	65–75	>85	4–6	5–15	4
HbS–β^+-thalassemia (HbS–β^+-Thal)	Compound heterozygous HbS, β^+-thalassemia	1:1600	30–40	60–70	70–95	4–6	2–10	1–3
HbSE disease (HbSE)	Compound heterozygous HbS, HbE	Rare§	30–45	70–80	60	2–3	1	1
HbS-HPFH	Compound heterozygous HbS and gene deletion HPFH	Rare	38–45	70–80	70	2	20–30	0
Sickle cell trait (HbAS)¶	Heterozygous HbS	1:12	38–50	80–90	35–40	2–3	<1	0
Normal (HbAA)	Homozygous HbA	—	38–50	80–90	0	2–3	<1	—

Hb = hemoglobin; HPFH = hereditary persistence of HbF; MCV = mean corpuscular volume.
*Many other abnormal globin genes can be found as compound heterozygotes with the HbS gene. The most common of these are α-thalassemia, HbD, HbO^{Arabia}, $HbG^{Philadelphia}$, HPFH, Hb Hope, and Hb Lepore. Average ranges of laboratory values are shown, but these can vary according to patient age.
†These figures differ depending on the prevalence of the involved genes in the population studied. In West and Central Africa, where the disease is most common, approximately 2% of all newborns have sickle cell disease. The prevalence of the HbC trait in African Americans is 3%, and that of the β-thalassemia trait is 1%. About 30% of African Americans carry an α-thalassemia gene, which can alter the phenotype of sickle cell disease by causing microcytosis, reduced cell density, and less hemolysis.
‡Vaso-occulsive severity of disease compared with sickle cell anemia, clinically the most severe genotype. This is a qualitative ranking of the clinical vaso-occlusive severity of each genotype; within each genotype, there is great clinical heterogeneity.
§Although this combination is still a rare genotype, the rising Asian population in the United States (HbE is a Southeastern Asian gene) will make it more frequent with time. With few cases reported compared with the other genotypes, the phenotype of HbSE disease is not totally defined. It may resemble HbS–β^+ thalassemia with symptoms appearing mainly in adults.
¶Sickle cell trait should not be classified as a form of sickle cell disease. About 8% of African Americans are carriers of HbS and are hematologically normal with a normal lifespan. The few abnormalities traceable to the presence of HbS include hyposthenuria, increased risk of urinary tract infection during pregnancy, hematuria, and the rare medullary carcinoma of the kidney.

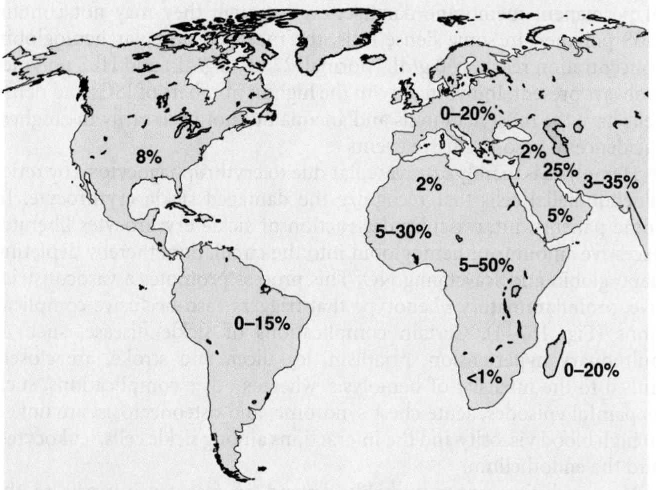

FIGURE 167–1 • Worldwide prevalence of the sickle cell trait. Shown are the percentages of individuals with sickle cell trait in regions of the world where the hemoglobin S (HbS) gene is often present. In each geographic area, the prevalence of sickle cell trait can vary markedly according to racial or ethnic group, historical migration patterns, and even from village to village. Not shown is the high concentration of the HbS gene in areas of Europe such as London, Manchester, and Paris, where migrants from Africa or Afro-Caribbean populations have settled.

endothelin, and disturbed NO balance. Cellular damage enables adhesive interactions among sickle cells, endothelial cells, and leukocytes. Reperfusion injury can also induce endothelial activation. The association of sickle and endothelial cells by a variety of adhesion molecules and their ligands may sufficiently delay cellular passage so that HbS polymerization, cell sickling, and vaso-occlusion happen before transit through the microvasculature is complete. Reticulocytes that are prematurely released from bone marrow display adhesive ligands that facilitate erythrocyte-endothelial interactions. Individuals with the greatest amount of hemolysis have the highest reticulocyte counts, and these adherent cells provide another link of hemolysis with vaso-occlusion. Neutrophils, which are modulators of inflammation and tissue damage, are increased in patients who have the acute chest syndrome, priapism, or stroke and are a risk factor for survival.

Clinical Manifestations

The clinical phenotype of sickle cell disease can be a result of many different genotypes, but most patients have either sickle cell anemia, HbSC disease, or HbS–β-thalassemia (see Table 167–1). Although hemolytic anemia and vaso-occlusive events are found in all genotypes, genotypes with higher cellular concentration of HbS are clinically more severe. Within milliseconds to seconds after HbS deoxygenation, depending on the intracellular concentration of HbS, HbS polymer appears in the sickle erythrocyte. In sickle cell trait (i.e., the heterozygote carriage of the HbS mutation), each cell contains only 30 to 40% HbS, so polymer is not found under most conditions (see Fig. 167–3). Therefore, carriers have few complications and a normal lifespan.

The features of sickle cell anemia change as life advances (Table 167–2). The switch from HbF to HbS underlies the clinical shift in life's first

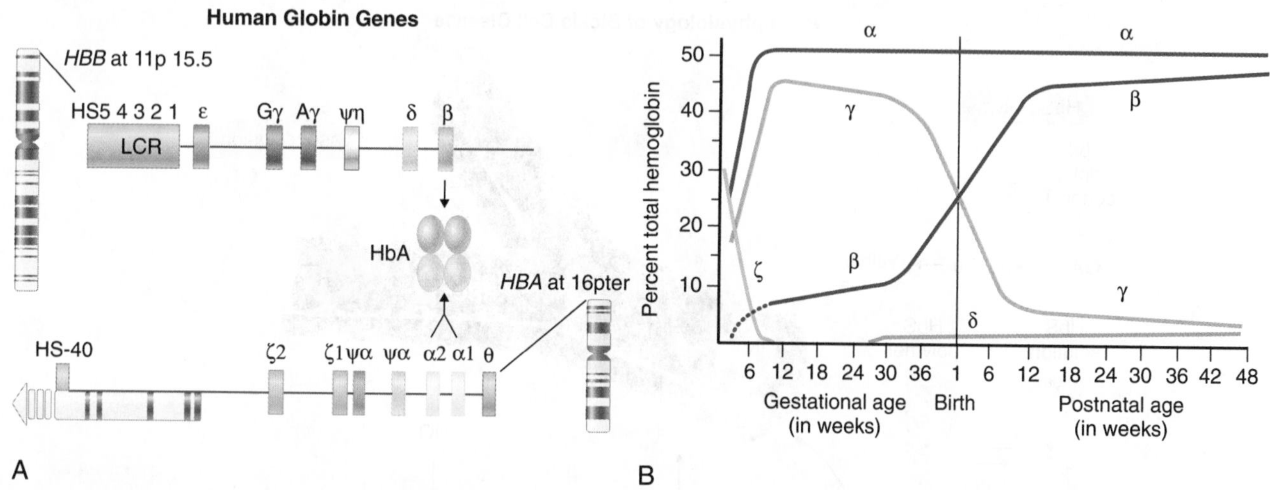

FIGURE 167–2 • Human globin genes. A, The β-like globin gene cluster on chromosome 11 is shown above, and the α-like globin gene cluster below. Two β-globin chains and two α-globin chains combine to form the normal hemoglobin A (HbA) tetramer, represented between the globin genes. Each globin chain contains one heme group, and oxygen transport takes place sequentially at the four iron-containing heme groups. Fetal hemoglobin (HbF) is composed of two α- and two γ-globin chains; the minor hemoglobin of adults, HbA_2, contains two α- and two δ-globin chains. Normally present at a level of only 2 to 3%, HbA_2 concentration is increased to 4 to 6% in most carriers of β-thalassemia. The ζ *(HBZ)* and ε *(HBE1)* genes are normally expressed only in the embryo. The 5′ ψα gene has recently been found to be expressed at a very low level and is now called the μ-globin gene *(HBM)*. The θ-globin gene *(HBQ1)* is also expressed at low levels. Neither the θ nor the μ gene has been found in a functional hemoglobin. Any of the globin chains participating in hemoglobin formation may have a mutation altering its amino acid sequence. HbS, HbE, and HbC mutations affect the β-globin gene *(HBB)*. Other mutations can affect the α- *(HBA1, HBA2)*, γ- *(HBG1, HBG2)*, and δ-globin *(HBD)* genes. LCR = locus control region. **B,** Expression of globin genes during development. α-Chains are expressed throughout gestation and adult life, fetal γ-globin chains are expressed predominantly in utero, and the β- and δ-globin genes are expressed mainly postnatally. This switching of gene expression patterns accounts for the different hemoglobins present in the embryo, fetus, and adult. It also accounts for the observation that disorders of α-globin can affect both fetus and adult, whereas β-globin chain diseases usually are not clinically apparent in the first months of life, when HbF levels are still high.

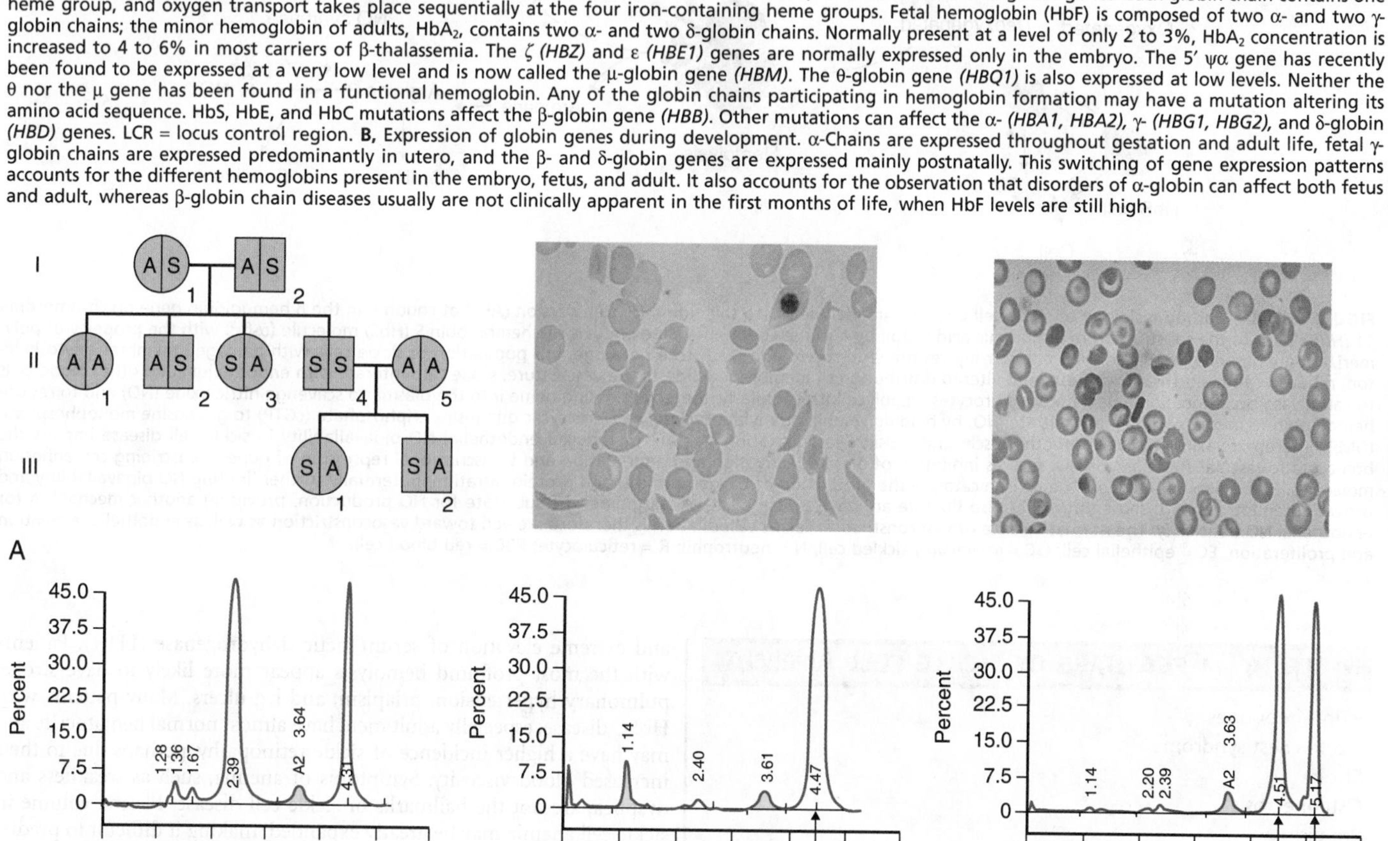

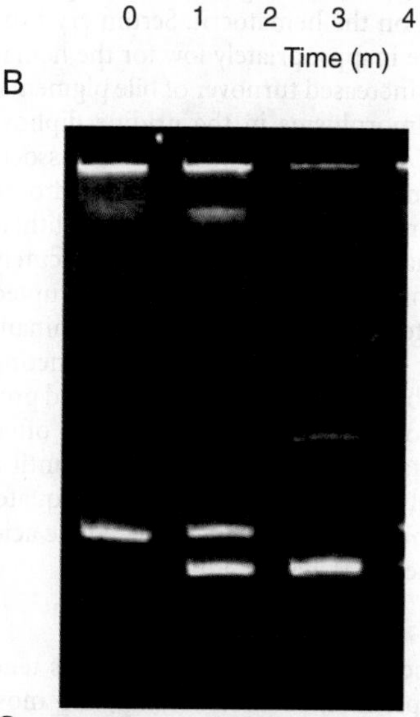

FIGURE 167–3 • Diagnosis of sickle cell disease. A, A prototypical family structure in which both parents (I) have sickle cell trait and each offspring (II) has a 25% chance of having sickle cell anemia (SS). Each child of an affected parent (III) will have sickle cell trait (SA) if the other parent has a normal hemoglobin (AA) genotype. The center and right blood films are from patients with sickle cell anemia and HbSC disease, respectively. Note the irreversibly sickled cells (ISCs) in the former and the hemoglobin C (HbC) crystal and target cells in the latter. **B,** High-performance liquid chromatography (HPLC) profiles from patients with sickle cell trait (left), sickle cell anemia (center), and HbSC disease (right). **C,** Amplification refractory mutation system (ARMS)-based separation of the β-globin genes from a normal subject (AA), a carrier of sickle cell trait (AS), and a patient with sickle cell anemia (SS).

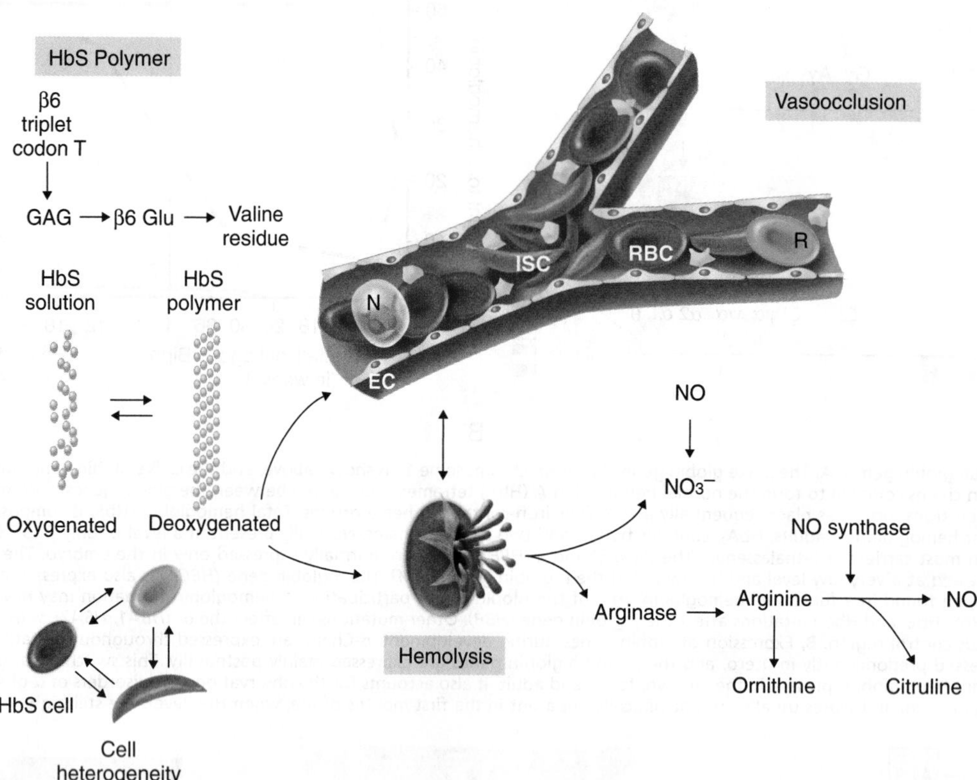

FIGURE 167–4 • Pathophysiology of sickle cell disease. An adenine (A) to thymidine (T) transversion (A6T) at codon 6 in the β hemoglobin gene on chromosome 11 *(HBB)* leads to the substitution of a glutamic acid codon by a valine codon. β^6 valine endows the hemoglobin S (HbS) molecule ($\alpha_2\beta_2{}^S$) with the property of polymerization when deoxygenated. HbS polymer injures the erythrocyte and leads to a heterogenous population of sickle cells with damaged membrane cytoskeleton, reduced cation and water content, and altered distribution of membrane lipids. In the vasculature, sickle cells interact with endothelium and other blood cells to cause vaso-occlusion. Some damaged erythrocytes hemolyze intravascularly, thereby releasing heme into the plasma to scavenge nitric oxide (NO) and to reduce hemoglobin to methemoglobin and nitrate. NO, by binding soluble guanylate cyclase, converts cyclic guanosine triphosphate (cGTP) to guanosine monophosphate (GMP), thereby relaxing vascular smooth muscle and causing vasodilatation. A state of reduced endothelial NO bioavailability in sickle cell disease impairs the homeostatic vascular functions of NO, such as inhibition of platelet activation and aggregation and transcriptional repression of genes transcribing cell adhesion molecules. Hemoglobin, heme, and heme iron catalyze the production of oxygen radicals and protein nitration, potentially further limiting NO bioavailability and activating endothelium. Lysed erythrocytes also liberate arginase, which destroys L-arginine, the substrate for NO production, providing another mechanism for endothelial NO deficiency. The normal balance of vasoconstriction versus vasodilation is therefore skewed toward vasoconstriction as well as endothelial activation and proliferation. EC = epithelial cell; ISC = irreversibly sickled cell; N = neutrophil; R = reticulocyte; RBC = red blood cell.

TABLE 167–2 FEATURES OF SICKLE CELL ANEMIA

Painful episodes
Acute chest syndrome
Stroke
Osteonecrosis
Priapism
Proliferative retinopathy
Splenic infarction and sequestration
Leg ulcers
Gallstones
Aplastic crisis
Osteopenia—bone marrow hyperplasia
Nutritional deficiencies—folic acid, zinc, calories
Pneumococcal disease and sepsis
Placental insufficiency

decade. This time is typified by acute problems: high risks of severe life-threatening infection, acute chest syndrome, splenic sequestration, and stroke. Chronic organ damage (renal failure, pulmonary hypertension, and late effects of previous cerebrovascular disease) becomes paramount in adults.

Most patients with sickle cell anemia have moderate anemia with a hematocrit between 25 and 30%. Some patients appear to have more severe hemolysis, with hematocrit less than 20%, marked reticulocytosis, and extreme elevation of serum lactic dehydrogenase (LDH). Patients with the most profound hemolysis appear more likely to have stroke, pulmonary hypertension, priapism, and leg ulcers. Many patients with HbSC disease, especially adult men, have almost normal hematocrits and may have a higher incidence of sickle retinopathy, perhaps due to their increased blood viscosity. Symptoms of anemia, such as weakness and dyspnea, are not the hallmarks of sickle cell disease. Plasma volume in sickle cell anemia may be greatly expanded, making it difficult to predict the red blood cell (RBC) mass based on the hematocrit. Serum erythropoietin levels in sickle cell anemia are inappropriately low for the hematocrit. A consequence of hemolysis is increased turnover of bile pigments, regulated in part by promoter poylmorphisms in the uridine diphosphate-glucuronosyltransferase 1A *(UGT1A)* gene, which is also associated with unconjugated hyperbilirubinemia and Gilbert syndrome (Chapter 150). As a result, more than half of all adults have cholelithiasis (Chapter 159). Hemolytic anemia places patients at risk for acutely developing severe anemia when erythropoiesis is temporarily interrupted by B19 parvovirus infection (Chapter 394), which is the predominant cause of the aplastic crisis. Aplastic crisis is typified by a plummeting hematocrit, reticulocytopenia, and a bone marrow without erythroid precursors. It is a transient process, most common in children, and often requires blood transfusion to maintain circulatory competence until a spontaneous recovery follows. Rarely, if a patient's diet is inadequate, hemolysis-induced accelerated turnover of erythrocytes causes folic acid deficiency and megaloblastic and anemia (Chapter 170).

First 20 Years

Although any complication can occur at any age, certain events tend predominate in different age groups. In life's first decades, the most common sickle cell disease-related clinical events are painful episodes, acute chest syndrome, and stroke. Delayed growth and sexual development, more severe in patients with sickle cell anemia than in those with HbSC disease, become major issues of concern to the adolescent, but sexual maturation is eventually achieved.

Psychosocial problems are common in adolescents with sickle cell disease. Difficulties with medical staff often begin in adolescence and frequently center on issues of pain management and inpatient stay.

The Painful Episode

Pain, presumed to be caused by sickle vaso-occlusion, often starts in young children as the hand-foot syndrome: painful swelling of the hands and feet caused by inflammation of the metacarpal and metatarsal periosteum. Acute painful episodes are the most commonly encountered vaso-occlusive events in patients of all ages, but what triggers an acute painful episode is usually unknown. Commonly, painful episodes begin with little warning; some patients, however, may sense one in the offing. These episodes, which last from hours to many days, may wax and wane in intensity and migrate from site to site. No useful laboratory test can tell if a vaso-occlusive pain episode is occurring, and the history remains the best clue. Sickle cell pain is described as worse than postoperative or traumatic pain. Some women describe the pain of childbirth as paling in comparison with the pain experienced during painful episodes. These agonizing attacks of acute pain must be separated from chronic pain perhaps caused by osteoporosis of the spine, pain associated with osteonecrosis of the hips and shoulders, neuropathic pain, iatrogenic pain, and the milder aches, pains, and soreness that are frequently present between severe episodes.

Patients vary greatly in the number, severity, and frequency of their painful episodes. Painful episodes are often stereotypical, affecting individuals in the same manner from episode to episode. Patients usually know whether the pain they are experiencing is different from their typical painful episode, and the wise physician should heed a patient's advice about the need for hospitalization or the likelihood that the pain has an alternative explanation.

About 40% of patients do not have pain requiring a hospital visit in a given year, whereas 3% have more than six painful episodes per year. Having more than three pain episodes requiring hospitalization per year is associated with increased mortality among patients aged 20 years and older.

HbF levels are inversely related to the frequency of painful episodes. Concurrent α-thalassemia may increase the pain rate because of its effect on the hematocrit. The day-to-day management of sickle cell disease often equates with the management of acute and chronic pain. Because patients manage many painful events at home, hospital visits underestimate the frequency of pain.

The pain accompanying acute chest syndrome, acute cholecystitis, splenic sequestration crisis, splenic infarction, or right upper quadrant syndrome may sometimes be mistaken for uncomplicated pain episodes. Acute painful episodes often herald the acute chest syndrome, and occasionally pain episodes end with multiorgan failure. Unexplained death can occur during acute painful episodes, perhaps as a result of an arrhythmia secondary to unrecognizable myocardial damage or perhaps as a sequela of pulmonary hypertension. Currently, it is not possible to foretell whether a "usual" pain episode will have an unexpected mortal outcome or presage acute chest syndrome, but the presence of atypically severe pain or an uncommonly high leukocyte count or low hematocrit should be cause for extra scrutiny.

Stroke

A major complication of sickle cell anemia in early life is stroke caused by stenosis and occlusion of large vessels (Chapter 431). Sickle erythrocytes and anemia-related high blood flow velocity lead to vascular damage. Hemorrhagic stroke is often caused by rupture of aneurysms. Moya Moya disease, a proliferation of small vessels found in sickle cell patients with stenotic lesions, may also cause hemorrhage in adults (Chapter 431). Hemorrhagic stroke is associated with a mortality rate of more than 20%. Stroke is most common among patients with sickle cell anemia, with much lower rates among those with HbSC disease or HbS–β^+-thalassemia. Beyond age 1 year, the incidence of stroke in sickle cell anemia is approximately 0.5 events per 100 patient-years until age 40 years. The risk of having a first stroke is 11% by age 20 years, 15% by age 30 years, and 24% by age 45 years. Severe anemia, acute chest syndrome, and elevated systolic blood pressure are associated with ischemic strokes, whereas an elevated leukocyte count is a risk factor for hemorrhagic stroke. α-Thalassemia may protect patients with sickle cell anemia from stroke, perhaps because these patients have less hemolysis and a higher hematocrit. Subclinical neurologic events and silent cerebral infarction are even more common than stroke. The aberrant behavior of some sickle cell patients is most likely a result of otherwise silent cerebral infarction with deteriorating neurocognitive function.

Acute Chest Syndrome

Acute chest syndrome, characterized by fever, chest pain, wheezing, cough, hypoxia, and a new lung infiltrate, is a sometimes lethal complication that affects more than half of all patients with sickle cell anemia. It is the second most common reason for hospitalization and is a frequent cause of death in adults. The syndrome is more frequent in children, in whom its course is often mild, than in adults, in whom it tends to be more severe.

Commonly, acute chest syndrome develops after several days in individuals hospitalized for an acute painful episode (see earlier discussion). Acute chest syndrome also often occurs postoperatively, even when patients are properly prepared with blood transfusion. Other causes include rib infarction with atelectasis and regional hypoxia; fat emboli from the bone marrow (Chapter 99); infection with chlamydia, B19 parvovirus, or other viral agents; microvascular or large vessel in situ thrombosis; thromboembolic disease; and vascular injury and inflammation. Fat embolism can be identified by finding lipid within pulmonary macrophages obtained by bronchopulmonary lavage, but this nonstandardized test is not recommended.

In most cases of acute chest syndrome, a cause cannot be found early enough to guide treatment. Elevated concentrations of phospholipase A_2 have been found in patients with sickle cell disease in association with acute chest syndrome and may predict its occurrence.

Acute Anemia

Acute anemia can result from sequestration of blood in the spleen or liver, an aplastic crisis caused by parvovirus B19 infection (Chapter 394), or a severe vaso-occlusive event, such as acute chest syndrome or multiorgan failure. Transfusion may be needed. Megaloblastic arrest of erythropoiesis is uncommon if the diet is adequate in folic acid.

Infection

Because patients with sickle cell anemia are hyposplenic early in life and functionally asplenic later, they are susceptible to infection with encapsulated bacteria. Persistent gross splenomegaly but not normal splenic function is common in patients with sickle cell disease in Africa and is related to endemic malaria. Splenomegaly and splenic function often persist in patients with HbSC disease; hence, the reduced incidence of infection but risk of splenic sequestration and infarction in adults. Prevention of mortality from pneumococcal infection is the basis for screening of newborns for sickle cell disease and the use of prophylactic oral penicillin in affected individuals. Pneumococcal vaccine (Chapter 16) is also recommended.

Age 20 to 40 Years

Pregnancy

There is no absolute contraindication to pregnancy for patients with sickle cell anemia, and fertility is probably normal. All approved methods of contraception can be used satisfactorily.

Modern medical management generally achieves good results of pregnancy, but the rates of pyelonephritis, pregnancy-induced hypertension (Chapter 259), and cesarean section are increased, and babies are more likely to have low birth weight. Some obstetricians believe that blood transfusions should be used routinely, but limited data suggest that, with good prenatal care, transfusions do not improve the outcome.

Osteonecrosis and Bone Diseases

Osteonecrosis of the hip and shoulder joints (Chapter 269) affects about half of all patients with sickle cell anemia or HbSC disease. Its onset is insidious but progressive, and most patients with early-stage disease progress to collapse of the femoral head within 2 years. Osteonecrosis of the hip usually manifests with pain in and around the affected joint, or at times with spasm of the surrounding muscles. Patients with higher hematocrits and with sickle cell anemia–α-thalassemia have the highest prevalence of osteonecrosis. Osteonecrosis can be detected very early by magnetic resonance imaging, but only more advanced disease is visible on plain radiographs.

Osteomyelitis (Chapter 293) is often difficult to distinguish from bone infarction. Osteomyelitis is usually caused by staphylococcal infection, but salmonella infection (Chapter 329) is a particular cause of sickle cell osteomyelitis.

Leg Ulcers

About 5 to 10% of patients with sickle cell anemia older than 10 years of age develop leg ulcers, but leg ulcers are rare in HbSC disease or HbS–β^+-thalassemia and in children before age 10 years. In the tropics, leg ulcers are more common. Small and superficial ulcers leg ulcers heal spontaneously with rest and careful local hygiene. Control of local inflammation and infection remains the mainstay of treatment. Dressing the ulcer with an Unna boot protects the involved area and is a reasonable method of conservative management. Deep, large, painful ulcers may require large doses of narcotic analgesics, prolonged bed rest, transfusion, and even surgery.

Priapism

Priapism, a prolonged undesirable painful erection, may be seen in 40% of men with sickle cell anemia. Priapism in sickle cell anemia is usually bicorporeal, with only the corpora cavernosa affected. Venous outflow is obstructed rather than arterial flow increased. In bicorporeal priapism, the glans remains soft and urination is normal. Recurrent, self-limited attacks of priapism can last for several hours with tolerable discomfort. These episodes have been termed stuttering priapism and usually have a nocturnal onset. Erectile function is usually preserved between attacks. Major episodes of priapism often, but not always, follow a history of stuttering attacks, last for days, and can be excruciatingly painful; they often end in impotency. Priapism is a notable example of sickle vasculopathy and may be triggered by hemolysis. Affected patients have a higher incidence of stroke, pulmonary hypertension, renal failure, leg ulcers, and premature death than individuals without priapism.

Digestive Diseases

Sickle hepatopathy, hepatic crisis, and right upper quadrant syndrome are terms applied to sickle cell–associated liver disease. Liver disease may be related to intrahepatic and extrahepatic cholestasis, viral hepatitis (Chapter 152), cirrhosis, hypoxia, infarction, erythrocyte sequestration, iron overload (Chapter 154), or drug reactions (Chapter 153). Differentiation among these potential causes can be difficult. Increased bilirubin levels (Chapter 150) are often the result of unconjugated bilirubinemia and are a manifestation of hemolytic anemia.

Gallstones

Cholelithiasis (Chapter 159), a consequence of the accelerated bile pigment turnover typical of hemolytic anemia, can appear in the first decade of life, and more than half of all adults are affected. Depending on the degree of calcification, pigmented gallstones may be either radiopaque or radiolucent. Ultrasonography is the preferred means of detection, and laparoscopic cholecystectomy is the preferred method of dealing with symptomatic stones. Documented episodes of acute cholecystitis and typical obstructive jaundice are much less frequent than the presence of stones. If stones are asymptomatic or symptoms and laboratory findings suggesting cholecystitis are equivocal, careful observation may be the best course.

Beyond the Fifth Decade

Pulmonary Hypertension

Pulmonary hypertension (Chapter 67), defined by a regurgitant pulmonary jet velocity of more than 2.5 m/sec by echocardiography (Chapter 53), is found in 30 to 40% of adult patients with sickle cell anemia. It is also seen in children and in patients with HbSC disease. The higher frequency of pulmonary vasculopathy at autopsy confirms that it is often asymptomatic or unrecognized. Possible causes include decreased availability of NO owing to hemolysis, chronic hypoxemia, recurrent acute chest syndrome, in situ thrombosis, and asplenia.

Pulmonary hypertension occurs primarily in patients older than 35 years of age. Half of the patients with a regurgitant pulmonary jet velocity of more than 2.5 m/sec die within 2 years after diagnosis, but the reasons for this high mortality rate are unclear. Patients with sickle cell anemia should be screened for the presence of pulmonary hypertension because of this prognostic importance.

Nephropathy

Hyposthenuria is present in almost all patients with sickle cell anemia and even in most carriers of sickle cell trait (Table 167–3). Clinically, the loss of urine concentrating ability is not important unless access to fluid is restricted. Isosthenuria, distal renal tubular acidosis, and impaired potassium excretion are signs of medullary dysfunction.

TABLE 167–3 RENAL ABNORMALITIES IN SICKLE CELL DISEASE*

DISTAL NEPHRON
Impaired urine concentrating ability
Impaired urine acidification—incomplete renal tubular acidosis
Impaired K^+ excretion
HEMATURIA
PAPILLARY NECROSIS
PROXIMAL TUBULE
Increased phosphate reabsorption
Increased β_2-microglobulin reabsorption
Increased uric acid secretion
Increased creatinine secretion
HEMODYNAMIC CHANGES
Increased glomerular filtration rate
Increased renal plasma flow
Decreased filtration fraction
GLOMERULAR ABNORMALITIES
Proteinuria
Nephrotic syndrome with focal glomerular sclerosis
Chronic renal failure

*In carriers of sickle cell trait, the distal nephron can be affected, about 5% of patients develop hematuria, and papillary necrosis rarely occurs. Medullary carcinoma is a rare tumor found in patients with sickle cell trait.

Glomerular hyperfiltration, increased creatinine secretion, and a very low serum creatinine are characteristic of young patients with sickle cell anemia, so renal dysfunction can be present even with normal serum creatinine values. Glomerulopathy begins very early in life, but an increasing prevalence of renal failure is a hallmark of an aging population of sickle cell anemia patients. About 4% of patients with sickle cell anemia and 2% of those with HbSC develop renal failure, at median ages of 23 and 50 years, respectively. Among sickle cell patients, 60% of those older than 40 years of age have proteinuria, and 30% have renal insufficiency. Nephrotic syndrome is found in 40% of adults, with creatinine levels greater than 1.5 mg/dL. Survival time for patients with sickle cell anemia after the diagnosis of sickle renal failure is 4 years, even with dialysis.

Eye Disease

Proliferative sickle retinopathy is present in fewer than 20% of patients with sickle cell anemia but in more than 40% of those with HbSC disease by the third decade of life. Vitreal hemorrhage and retinal detachment can occasionally lead to visual loss, but proliferative lesions may regress spontaneously. Screening for proliferative retinopathy using fluorescence angiography is commonly recommended to guide possible laser photocoagulation.

Cardiovascular Complications

The heart is usually enlarged, with a hyperactive precordium and systolic ejection murmurs. Myocardial infarction is rare and suggests small vessel disease. Sudden unexpected and unexplained death (Chapter 62) is common in adults, most likely due to arrhythmias, but screening is not recommended currently.

Patients with sickle cell anemia usually have blood pressures that are in the normal range but are inappropriately high compared with controls who have similar levels of anemia. "Relative" hypertension in sickle cell anemia might reflect endothelial cell damage and NO scavenging. Survival is decreased and the risk of stroke is increased as blood pressure rises. Treatment goals of 120/80 mm Hg or less are generally the same as for other patients (Chapter 66).

Diagnosis

Normocytic or microcytic anemia with reticulocytosis, increased levels of lactate dehydrogenase and aspartate aminotransferase, and a compatible clinical history should suggest the presence of sickle cell disease. Nevertheless, because of the multiple genotypes and considerable clinical heterogeneity of each genotype, milder cases may not be diagnosed for many years.

The Blood

In sickle cell anemia, the erythrocytes are normocytic or macrocytic depending on the reticulocyte count. Microcytosis in a suspected case of sickle cell anemia can be seen very early in life, when iron deficiency has developed, or when β-thalassemia or α-thalassemia is present. Sickled cells are usually present in sickle cell anemia and in HbS–β^0-thalassemia but are less common in other forms of sickle cell disease. In HbSC disease, target cells are prominent and HbC crystalizes in some cells (see Fig. 167–3A). ISCs remain relatively constant over time, although their percentage may rise early during a painful episode. Finding ISCs has no value for establishing whether a patient is experiencing a vaso-occlusive episode.

Hemoglobin Composition of the Blood

After 1 year of age, hemoglobin fractions are sufficiently stable to be relied on for diagnosis, but the high HbF concentrations of early infancy often make the results of hemoglobin analysis at that time difficult to interpret. In patients with sickle cell anemia, except in infancy, HbS almost always forms more than 80% of the hemolysate. HbS is best detected by high-performance liquid chromatography (HPLC), which is also the method of choice for quantitation of the hemoglobin fractions in newborns and adults (see Fig. 167–3B), or by isoelectric focusing that provides qualitative information. HPLC provides excellent resolution of hemoglobin fractions, gives quantitative results, and is automated. DNA-based methods of detecting HbS are specific but usually are not needed for uncomplicated cases. Nevertheless, they are necessary for antenatal diagnosis and, sometimes, for genetic counseling (see Fig. 167–3C).

Family Studies

The *HBB* gene on chromosome 11 (see Fig. 167–2) is inherited as a codominant trait, implying that both normal and mutant alleles are expressed and are easily detectable. However, the sickle cell phenotype (see Table 167–1) is present only in homozygotes for HbS and in certain compound heterozygotes. Family studies (see Fig. 167–3) can suggest a patient's hemoglobin genotype.

TABLE 167–4 HYDROXYUREA TREATMENT IN SICKLE CELL ANEMIA*

INDICATIONS
Adults, adolescents, and some children with frequent pain episodes, history of acute chest syndrome, or other severe vaso-occlusive complications. Severe symptomatic anemia.
BASELINE EVALUATION
Blood counts, RBC indices, HbF level, serum chemistries, pregnancy test, willingness to adhere to all recommendations for treatment, not receiving chronic RBC transfusions.
INITIATION OF TREATMENT
Hydroxyurea 10–15 mg/kg/day or, for adults, 500 mg every morning for 6–8 wk.
CONTINUATION OF TREATMENT
If counts are acceptable by CBC every 2 wk (granulocytes, ≥2000/mm^3; platelets, ≥80,000/mm^3), escalate dose to 1500 mg every morning in increments of 200 to 500 mg every 6–8 wk. When a stable nontoxic dose of hydroxyurea is reached, CBC may be done at 4- to 8-wk intervals. Most good responses require 1000 to 2000 mg/day.
GOALS OF TREATMENT
Less pain, increase in HbF (usually measured every 6–8 wk) or MCV, increased hematocrit if severely anemic, acceptable toxicity. Failure of HbF to increase may be due to biologic inability to respond to treatment or, more often, to poor compliance with treatment. If compliance is documented, the dose can be increased cautiously to 2000–2500 mg/day (maximum dose, 30 mg/kg).

*Special caution should be exercised in patients with compromised renal or hepatic function and in those patients who are habituated to narcotics. Contraception should be practiced by both men and women. Without chronic RBC transfusions or an intercurrent illness suppressing erythropoiesis, a trial period of 6 to 12 months is probably adequate.
CBC = complete blood count; HbF = fetal hemoglobin; MCV = mean corpuscular volume; RBC = red blood cell.

Prevention and Treatment

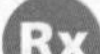

Primary Prevention

In populations with a high prevalence of the HbS gene, heterozygote detection is simple, but there is little benefit of a broad screening effort to detect carriers. A preferred approach consists of educational programs about sickle cell disease, followed by counseling for couples who are planning families. These couples are offered the choice of testing, after which the risks of having affected fetuses can be discussed and the availability of antenatal diagnosis by chorionic villus sampling or amniocentesis presented.

General Measures

Sickle cell disease is a chronic disorder, for which good nutrition and timely immunizations are critical. Work should be encouraged.

Older children do not routinely need continued antibiotic prophylaxis. Neonatal screening to detect newborns with sickle cell disease allows early administration of prophylactic penicillin, which reduces the incidence of and mortality from pneumococcal bacteremia in children younger than 5 years of age who have sickle cell anemia. [1]

Because of increased rates of RBC production and inadequate nutrition, folic acid, 1 mg daily, is generally recommended but may not be necessary with a good dietary intake. There is no evidence that high concentrations of inhaled oxygen are of preventive value.

Hydroxyurea

Hydroxyurea, the sole drug approved by the U.S. Food and Drug Administration for treatment of sickle cell anemia, increases HbF in these patients, because its cytotoxicity causes erythroid regeneration and perhaps because its metabolism leads to NO-related increases in soluble guanylate cyclase, with a subsequent increase in cyclic guanosine monophosphate (cGMP) that augments γ-globin gene expression. In a multicenter trial in adults with sickle cell anemia, hydroxyurea reduced the incidence of pain and acute chest syndrome by almost 50%, with little risk during more than 9 years of observation. In follow-up studies, cumulative mortality was reduced almost 40%, and the favorable result was related to the ability of the drug to increase HbF and reduce painful episodes and the acute chest syndrome. [2] Children have a more robust HbF response to hydroxyurea than adults do. Cancer and leukemia have been reported in patients with sickle cell disease treated with hydroxyurea, but whether the incidence is higher than in the general population is not known. Hydroxyurea should be used in all adults with appropriate indications (Table 167–4). However, only a fraction of patients who might benefit from this treatment receive it. The clinical benefits of hydroxyurea in HbSC disease are just beginning to be studied.

Red Blood Cell Transfusion

Acute transfusions of packed red blood cells can be life-saving, and chronic transfusions reduce the incidence and severity of most complications of sickle cell disease. However, repeated transfusions

produce iron overload, alloimmunization, loss of venous access, and viral infection. Whether exchange transfusion is preferable to simple transfusion in the acute chest syndrome, stroke, or other acute complications has not been tested in clinical trials. For severe symptomatic anemia or stroke prophylaxis, simple transfusions are preferred.

Treatment of Common Complications

Painful Crisis

A decision as to whether hospitalization is needed can be made after an assessment of the duration and severity of the pain and the response to treatment. Associated factors such as excessive tachycardia, hypotension, fever greater than 101° F, marked leukocytosis, a fall in the hematocrit and platelet count, hypoxia, or a new infiltrate on chest radiography should prompt admission.

Physical examination is usually not helpful, but sometimes there is localized swelling and pain over an involved bone. Low-grade fever and a mild increase in leukocytosis can accompany uncomplicated painful episodes, but higher temperature elevations may point to infection or extensive tissue damage.

The cornerstones of pain management (Chapter 28) are fluid replacement and opioid analgesics (Table 167–5). Because almost every patient is hyposthenuric, urinary output in patients with sickle cell anemia may exceed 2 L/day, making them susceptible to dehydration. Pain is often accompanied by reduced fluid intake and increased water losses, so increased fluid intake is essential. Administration of 5% dextrose in water and 0.25 to 0.5 normal saline should be used for initial fluid replacement. Although needs vary and hydration should be monitored closely to avoid iatrogenic heart failure or electrolyte imbalance, the daily fluid intake should be approximately 3 to 5 L for adults and 100 to 150 mL/kg for children. Oxygen should be reserved for patients who are hypoxic or have acute respiratory distress. Infection should always be considered and treated early if present, although bacterial infections are uncommon.

Pain management (Chapter 28) is complicated by the influence of learned pain behavior, pain memories, and pain therapy–induced pain. Management proves extremely difficult in perhaps 10% of all patients, and often enormous doses of opioids are required for relief.

TABLE 167–5 ANALGESIC MANAGEMENT OF THE ACUTE PAINFUL EPISODE (UNCOMPLICATED BY ACUTE CHEST SYNDROME, SEQUESTRATION SYNDROMES, OR PRIAPISM)*

ASSESSMENT
Use an available pain measurement instrument and repeat frequently as the benchmark for titrating the dose of analgesics (see Chapter 28)
TREATMENT
NONSTEROIDAL ANTI-INFLAMMATORY DRUGS FOR MILD TO MODERATE PAIN†
Aspirin
Acetaminophen
Ibuprofen
Ketorolac
ORAL OPIOIDS FOR MODERATE TO SEVERE PAIN‡
Codeine
Oxycodone
Methadone
Morphine
Hydromorphone
PARENTERAL OPIOIDS FOR SEVERE PAIN§
Morphine
Hydromorphone
Fentanyl
TRANSCUTANEOUS OPIOIDS FOR SEVERE PAIN
Fentanyl

*Analgesic management presupposes that other treatments, such as hydration, oxygen, and antimicrobial agents, are used if needed. The key to successful pain management is individualized treatment and dosing, taking into account prior pain management and prior use of opioids. Patient-controlled analgesia and a scheduled regimen of drug dosing are preferable, and PRN analgesics should be avoided. Frequent reassessment of the effects of treatment is paramount so that opioid doses can be titrated for pain relief and tapered when relief is obtained. Meperidine should be avoided, because its metabolites (e.g., normeperidine) can cause central nervous system excitation.
†May cause renal dysfunction (see Chapter 34).
‡Can cause impaired ventilation (see Table 28–2).
§Commonly impairs ventilation (see Table 28–2).

Stroke

After initial stabilization and transfusion, chronic RBC transfusion reduces the chance of recurrent ischemic stroke. However, it is not known how long chronic transfusions should continue. In practice, transfusions are often stopped after children make the transition from pediatric to adult care. Long-term management of hemorrhagic stroke is unclear, and whether transfusion reduces recurrence is unknown. Increased intracranial flow velocity, measurable only in children, increases the risk of stroke, but its sensitivity is only 10%, with a far from perfect specificity. Children found to be at risk for stroke by transcranial Doppler flow velocities should be started on chronic transfusions, but it is unclear whether or when such transfusions may be discontinued. 3 Emerging work suggests that stroke may also be predicted by polymorphisms in selected genes.

Acute Chest Syndrome

Routine treatments for acute chest syndrome initially include bronchodilators (e.g., albuterol nebulizer 0.25 mL in 2.5 mL normal saline; or albuterol measured-dose inhaler during the acute episode), incentive spirometry, empiric antimicrobial agents as used for community-acquired pneumonia (e.g., ceftriaxone or azithromycin or levofloxacin for 5 to 7 days [see Chapter 97]), and supplemental oxygen when hypoxia is noted by continuous or frequent monitoring of blood oxygen saturation. Opioid analgesics (e.g., morphine [see Table 28–2]) are often needed, but their dose should be titrated carefully to avoid respiratory depression and worsening of hypoxia.

Blood transfusion is the cornerstone of treatment when a patient becomes hypoxic, develops respiratory distress, has a clinically significant fall in the hematocrit and platelet count or increase in leukocyte count, or shows any sign of multiorgan failure, such as impaired mentation, rhabdomyolysis, renal failure, or liver failure. Both simple transfusion and exchange transfusions appear to reverse many adverse findings of the acute chest syndrome, but controlled studies have never tested the superiority of either method. Although the death rate in acute chest syndrome is less than 10%, a few patients have a rapidly deteriorating course with sudden development of the acute respiratory distress syndrome (ARDS; see Chapter 105), as manifested by increased oxygen requirements, extensive pulmonary opacification, and multiorgan failure. Excessive hydration and fat emboli are potential contributing causes. Successful management of the severe acute chest syndrome and ARDS requires close coordination among physicians and nurses. Some patients have repeated episodes of severe acute chest syndrome, and chronic transfusion can reduce the recurrence rate. Hydroxyurea also reduces the rate of acute chest syndrome by about 50%.

Osteonecrosis and Bone Disease

Treatment with reduced weight bearing, nonsteroidal anti-inflammatory drugs (NSAIDs), and physical therapy is the mainstay of conservative management but does not retard progression of osteonecrosis and bone disease. Total hip arthroplasty can be very successful, but about one third of prostheses fail within 4 to 5 years.

Rx

Core decompression for osteonecrosis of the femoral head is being studied as an alternative treatment.

Diffuse osteoporosis (Chapter 264) is usually present, and osteomalacia (Chapter 265) due to vitamin D deficiency is common in both children and adults. If vitamin D deficiency is present, treatment with calcium (1000 mg PO daily) and vitamin D (50,000 IU PO every week for 2 months, then 50,000 IU PO every other week) is reasonable.

Priapism

Conservative treatment of priapism includes analgesics (see Tables 167–5 and Table 28–2), hydration, and transfusions. Aspiration and irrigation of the corporeal bodies should be performed within a 12-hour window from the onset of erection if the episode differs from prior episodes of stuttering priapism. Operative treatment, which should be considered after 24 to 48 hours of priapism, includes the creation of shunts between the corpora cavernosa and spongiosum. For a typical episode of low-flow priapism, a Winter shunt between the glans penis and corpora cavernosa should be performed within 24 to 48 hours. Oral or intracavernous administration of α-adrenergic agonists such as pseudoephedrine may help reverse priapism and is being studied.

Pulmonary Hypertension

The NO precursor, L-arginine, can acutely reverse sickle cell pulmonary hypertension. For symptomatic individuals, transfusions, sildenafil, bosentan, and epoprostenol have all been used, but controlled trials reporting their effectiveness in sickle cell patients have not been conducted. It is unknown how asymptomatic pulmonary hypertension should be managed.

Renal Disease

In a small randomized trial, 6 months' treatment with 25 mg/day of captopril caused a 37% reduction in microalbuminuria, compared with a 17% increase in placebo-treated patients; such treatment would be reasonable in patients with known microalbuminuria, but whether screening or long-term treatment is worthwhile is unknown. NSAIDs reduce the glomerular filtration rate in sickle cell anemia and should be avoided in older individuals with creatinine levels of 1.2 mg/dL or higher. Dialysis and renal transplantation are used in end-stage sickle cell nephropathy, but with outcomes less favorable than in other types of renal failure.

Surgery and Anesthesia

Preoperative blood transfusion should be used for all surgeries requiring general anesthesia and selected other surgeries. Simple transfusion to a hematocrit of about 30% before surgery is as effective in preventing postoperative complications as exchange transfusion and causes fewer transfusion-related complications. 4

Implantable infusion ports and catheters have higher risks of complications in sickle cell anemia, including thrombosis of large veins and bacteremia. Low-dose warfarin may retard thrombosis of these devices.

Red Blood Cell Transfusion and Chelation Therapy

Anemia alone is seldom an indication for transfusion. With aging and the onset of renal failure, anemia worsens and can become symptomatic. Transfusion may become necessary, although judicious use of erythropoietin (e.g., darbepoetin, 0.45 µg/kg every 2 weeks, increased as needed) can often restore the hematocrit to pre–renal failure levels.

It is advised that patients undergo erythrocyte phenotyping to determine their RBC antigens before embarking on a transfusion program. Otherwise, alloimmunization occurs in about one quarter of frequently transfused patients. In the presence of multiple alloantibodies, it may be difficult to find compatible blood.

With repeated transfusion, iron overload inevitably develops and can result in heart and liver failure and many other complications (Chapters 59, 154, and 231). Serum ferritin is an inaccurate means of estimating the iron burden. Liver biopsy is the most accurate means of determining tissue iron concentration and the response to chelation, but magnetic resonance imaging is a reasonable alternative.

Chelation of excessive iron can be achieved using parenteral desferrioxamine, usually starting with 25 to 30 mg/kg given subcutaneously five times per week in 8- to 12-hour infusions, with the dose not to exceed 50 mg/kg in adults (Chapter 231). Because of its expense and difficulty of administration, this treatment is used in fewer than half of eligible patients. Side effects include skin reactions, ototoxicity, retinal toxicity, bone and growth abnormalities, and *Yersinia* infection resulting from the sudden mobilization of iron. The effectiveness of desferrioxamine is impaired by the failure of patients, especially adolescents and teenagers, to comply with treatment. Deferasirox (20 mg/kg orally daily) is as efficacious as desferrioxamine and is easier to administer. Increases in serum creatinine and proteinuria occur in about 40% of patients. Another oral chelator, deferiprone, is less potent than desferrioxamine but is useful instead of or in addition to it; it is approved for use in more than 40 countries but is not available in the United States. Side effects requiring discontinuation of deferiprone, seen in 5 to 10% of patients, include agranulocytosis, neutropenia, arthropathy, and gastrointestinal symptoms.

Stem Cell Transplantation

Successful stem cell transplantation (Chapter 184) can cure sickle cell anemia, but only about 10% of patients have suitable donors. Stem cell transplantation carries a 5 to 10% mortality rate, and patients older than 16 years of age have more toxicity, are less likely to engraft, and have a higher peritransplantation mortality rate during myeloablative conditioning regimens for transplantation. Reduced-intensity conditioning with the hope of establishing stable mixed chimerism for older patients who might benefit from transplantation is in development. Transplantation is best done under the aegis of ongoing clinical trials and only for those patients with multiple episodes of acute chest syndrome or severe painful episodes but otherwise good renal and liver function.

Future Directions

Experimental treatments to induce higher levels of HbF more consistently and to reduce HbS polymer with drugs that may remodel chromosomal structure (e.g., short-chain fatty acids and their derivatives) or affect hypomethylation of the HbF gene promoters (e.g., decitabine) are undergoing clinical trials. By preventing the leak of potassium and water from the sickle cell, other agents in clinical trials, such as clotrimazole derivatives and magnesium (which are inhibitors of the Gardos channel and the K^+/Cl^- cotransport channel, respectively), may prevent dehydration of RBCs, reduce cell density, and retard polymer formation by reducing the concentration of HbS. In areas where malaria is endemic, malaria prophylaxis reduces episodes of malaria and increases mean hemoglobin levels 5; whether such therapy can be effectively disseminated is less clear. Agents that improve the bioavailability of NO, such as arginine, nitrite, and sildenafil, may also be useful. Gene therapy is the ultimate hope.

Prognosis

Average life expectancy for patients with sickle cell anemia in the United States is between 50 and 60 years; patients with HbSC disease typically live 60 to 70 years. Patients with HbS–β^0-thalassemia are likely to have a life expectancy similar to those with sickle cell anemia, and the lifespan for patients with the HbS–β^+ form may resemble that of patients with HbSC disease. Death is often caused by infection, and another 20% of deaths are related to organ failure. However, death in adults often is unexpected, happening in the midst of an acute event such as a pain crisis, and occurring within the first 24 hours of hospitalization. In areas of the developing world without access to modern medical care, death in childhood is usual.

OTHER HEMOGLOBINOPATHIES

Hemoglobinopathies other than those associated with HbS, HbE, and HbC rarely cause clinically recognizable disorders. HbC (Glu6Lys) and HbE (Glu26Lys) are common β-globin variants. As with HbS, their high gene frequencies are a result of the positive selective pressure of endemic falciparum malaria. HbC is present in about 2% of African Americans, and HbE is seen in Southeast Asians where, in some areas, the gene frequency may reach 50%. Heterozygotes with either mutation are asymptomatic, although the blood of HbC trait carriers contains target cells and HbE carriers may have very mild anemia and microcytosis. Even homozygotes for HbC and HbE have virtually no clinical disease, only mild hematologic abnormalities such as microcytosis, target cells, and mild anemia. Compound heterozygotes for HbE and β-thalassemia usually have the phenotype of transfusion-dependent β-thalassemia, although genotype-phenotype correlations are difficult to make because of the likelihood that other genes affect the expression of disease.

Rare hemoglobinopathies may change the affinity of hemoglobin for oxygen, render it susceptible to oxidation, or cause molecular instability. Amino acid substitutions involving heme-binding residues may lead to irreversible iron oxidation, methemoglobinemia, and cyanosis (Chapter 168). Patients with these conditions have congenital pseudocyanosis but are usually asymptomatic and need no treatment.

Substitutions at contacts between globin subunits may alter the affinity of hemoglobin for oxygen. When hemoglobin-oxygen affinity is increased, less oxygen is available in tissues, erythropoietin production is enhanced, and erythrocytosis results (Chapter 172). Usually, no treatment is required because the erythrocytosis is mild. Hemoglobin-oxygen affinity may also be reduced by some mutations, resulting in anemia or cyanosis. Hemoglobin instability, produced by several molecular mechanisms (including introduction of proline residues into the alpha helix, substitutions near the heme ring, and deletion or addition of amino acids), often causes loss of heme from the molecule and hemolytic anemia. Hb Koln is the most frequent example of this class of hemoglobinopathy, but more than 200 unstable variants have been described. Sometimes, oxidant drugs provoke increased hemolysis. Splenectomy is sometimes effective treatment if anemia is severe.

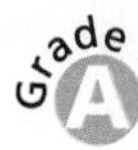

1. Gaston MH, Verter J, Woods G, et al: Prophylaxis with oral penicillin in children with sickle cell anemia. N Engl J Med 1986;314:1593–1599.
2. Steinberg MH, Barton F, Castro O, et al: Effect of hydroxyurea on mortality and morbidity in adult sickle cell anemia: Risks and benefits up to 9 years of treatment. JAMA 2003;289:1645–1651.
3. Adams RJ, Brambilla D: Discontinuing prophylactic transfusions used to prevent stroke in sickle cell disease. N Engl J Med 2005;353:2769–2778.
4. Vichinsky EP, Haberkern CM, Neumayr L, et al: A comparison of conservative and aggressive transfusion regimens in the perioperative management of sickle cell disease. N Engl J Med 1995;333:206–213.
5. Oniyangi O, Omari AA: Malaria chemoprophylaxis in sickle cell disease. Cochrane Database Syst Rev 2006;4:CD003489.

SUGGESTED READINGS

Atkins RC, Walters MC: Haematopoietic cell transplantation in the treatment of sickle cell disease. Expert Opin Biol Ther 2003;3:1215–1224. *Stem cell transplantation can "cure" sickle cell anemia: Is the cure worth the "price"?*

Howard J, Davies SC: Sickle cell disease in North Europe. Scand J Clin Lab Invest 2007;67:27–38. *A practical overview.*

Kato GJ, Gladwin MT, Steinberg MH: Deconstructing sickle cell disease: Reappraisal of the role of hemolysis in the development of clinical subphenotypes. Blood Rev 2007;21:37–47. *A review of the effect of hemolysis on nitric oxide dysregulation.*

Machado RF, Anthi A, Steinberg MH, et al: N-terminal pro-brain natriuretic peptide levels and risk of death in sickle cell disease. JAMA 2006;296:310–318. *Elevated levels of NT-proBNP were associated with pulmonary hypertension and mortality.*

Machado RF, Martyr S, Kato GJ, et al: Sildenafil therapy in patients with sickle cell disease and pulmonary hypertension. Br J Haematol 2005;130:445–453. *By increasing bioavailable NO, this phosphodiesterase 5 inhibitor may reduce pulmonary artery pressure.*

Steinberg MH: Predicting clinical severity in sickle cell anaemia. Br J Haematol 2005;129:465–481. *The phenotype of sickle cell anemia is likely to be affected by the interactions of many modifying genes.*

168 METHEMOGLOBINEMIAS AND UNSTABLE HEMOGLOBINS

Ronald L. Nagel

METHEMOGLOBINEMIA

Definition

Methemoglobinemia, which arises from a nonfunctional hemoglobin containing oxidized Fe^{3+}, results in reduced O_2 supply to tissues and hence cyanosis. It can develop by four mechanisms: (1) a deficiency of the methemoglobin reductase enzyme, (2) a genetic mutation resulting in an abnormal cytochrome b_5 reductase (b5R), (3) toxin-induced oxidation of hemoglobin, or (4) hemoglobin M disease (Table 168–1).

Pathobiology

Methemoglobin results from the continuous deoxygenation of hemoglobin, but endogenous hemoglobin reductase enzymes routinely lower the methemoglobin level to maintain a very low steady-state blood level of 1% or less of total hemoglobin. Increased levels of methemoglobin above this steady state, termed *methemoglobinemia,* result from either enhanced methemoglobin production or decreased methemoglobin reduction (Fig. 168–1). Heme iron is oxidized from the ferrous (Fe^{2+}) to the ferric (Fe^{3+}) state. The ferric hemes of methemoglobinemia cannot bind O_2, and the O_2 affinity of the ferrous hemes in the hemoglobin tetramer is increased. As a result, the O_2 dissociation curve (Fig. 168–2) is shifted to the *left* and O_2 delivery is *reduced,* thereby leading to hypoxia.

Congenital Methemoglobinemias

Epidemiology

The most common cause of congenital methemoglobinemia is deficiency of the *b5R enzyme.* Inherited in an autosomal recessive pattern, type I b5R deficiency is found worldwide but is endemic in Athabascan and Navajo native Americans and in Yakutsk natives of Siberia. In other ethnic groups the defect occurs sporadically.

About 10 to 15% of cases of *enzymopenic congenital methemoglobinemia* are type II, caused by a general deficiency of b5R in all cell types. Type II b5R deficiency is found sporadically worldwide.

Pathobiology

Reduction of methemoglobin back to hemoglobin is catalyzed by the reduced form of nicotinamide adenine dinucleotide (NADH) b5R. Electrons are transferred from NADH (generated by glyceraldehyde-3-phosphate in the glycolytic pathway) to an enzyme, NADH b5R, and then to cytochrome b_5 (see Fig. 168–1). In hemoglobin-containing red blood cells (RBCs), cytochrome b_5 transfers electrons directly to methemoglobin to convert it to hemoglobin. In nucleated cells and reticulocytes, cytochrome b_5 transfers electrons to stearyl–coenzyme A desaturase.

The b5R enzyme is constitutively expressed and is the product of a single gene that produces multiple transcripts. In type I deficiency, the

TABLE 168–1 TYPES OF METHEMOGLOBINEMIA

Acquired methemoglobinemia
Medications/chemicals, especially in heterozygotes for congenital methemoglobinemia
Congenital methemoglobinemia
Autosomal recessive; clinical disease in homozygotes or compound heterozygotes
Cytochrome b_5 reductase deficiency
Cytochrome b_5 deficiency
Autosomal dominant
Hemoglobin M disease

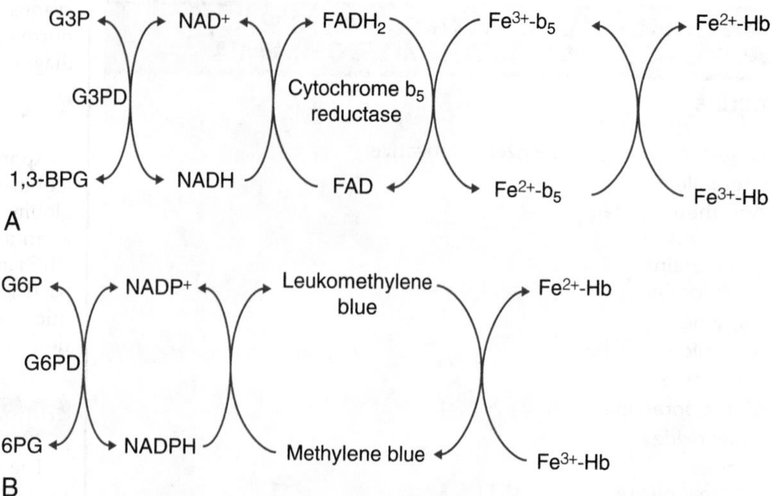

FIGURE 168–1 • Reduction of methemoglobin. A, Reduced nicotinamide adenine dinucleotide (NADH)-dependent methemoglobin reduction. NADH is generated during glycolysis in the reaction mediated by glucose-3-phosphate dehydrogenase (G3PD). Transfer of a pair of electrons from NADH to the flavin adenine dinucleotide (FAD) prosthetic group of cytochrome b_5 reductase reduces it to $FADH_2$. Two molecules of ferric (Fe^{3+}) cytochrome b_5 are then sequentially bound and reduced to form ferrous (Fe^{2+}) cytochrome b_5. An ionic complex between ferrous (Fe^{2+}) cytochrome b_5 and a ferric (Fe^{3+}) subunit of a hemoglobin (methemoglobin) tetramer is formed, and an electron is transferred between the two hemes to create ferrous (Fe^{2+}) hemoglobin. 1,3-BPG = 1,3-biphosphonate glyceraldehyde; G3P = glyceraldehyde-3-phosphate; Hb = hemoglobin. **B,** NADPH-dependent methemoglobin reduction. NADPH methemoglobin reduction can be activated by exogenously administered methylene blue. G6P = glucose-6-phosphate; G6PD = glucose-6-phosphate dehydrogenase; 6PG = 6-phosphogluconate. (From Gregg XT, Prchal JT: Red cell enzymopathies. *In* Hoffman R, Benz E, Shattil S, et al [eds]: Hematology: Basic Principles and Practice, 4th ed. Philadelphia, Saunders, 2005, p 654.)

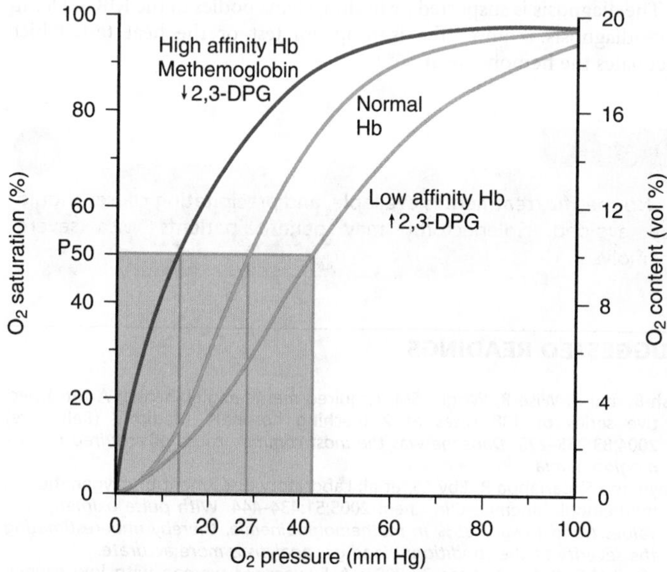

FIGURE 168–2 • Hemoglobin (Hb) oxygen dissociation curve. A left-shifted curve is characteristic of mutant Hb with increased oxygen affinity or decreased 2,3-bisphosphoglycerate (formerly called 2,3-diphosphoglycerate [2,3-DPG]) levels and low oxygen half saturation value (P_{50}), whereas a right-shifted curve is characteristic of mutant Hb with decreased oxygen affinity or increased 2,3-DPG levels and increased P_{50}. The normal P_{50} value is 27 mm Hg.

abnormal, unstable gene product is generated at a normal rate. Hence, only mature RBCs, which cannot synthesize proteins, are affected.

By contrast, type II deficiency results when mutations reduce production of the enzyme or the enzyme has decreased enzymatic activity. In this form, b5R deficiency is generalized to all cells.

Clinical Manifestations

Methemoglobinemia is manifested as cyanosis when it accounts for about 10 to 15% of hemoglobin, or about 1.5 g/dL. Patients who are *homozygotes* or *compound heterozygotes* for type I b5R deficiency have methemoglobin concentrations of 10 to 35% under baseline conditions. Symptoms of headache and easy fatigability are sometimes reported, but patients are typically asymptomatic despite cyanosis, even with methemoglobin levels of 40%. Life expectancy is normal, and women have normal pregnancies. Compensatory polycythemia typically does not occur. However, oxidizing drugs and other toxic chemicals (Table 168–2) may greatly enhance the normal spontaneous rate of production of methemoglobin. If as a result methemoglobin level exceeds 70% of total hemoglobin, vascular collapse results and leads to coma and death.

In heterozygotes, b5R activity of the RBC is approximately 50% of normal. This level is usually adequate to maintain normal methemoglobin levels, but if *oxidant stress* from medications or chemicals (see Table 168–2) exceeds the capacity of RBCs to reduce methemoglobin, cyanosis develops, with tachycardia and dyspnea occurring acutely if methemoglobin levels are 20% or higher. The classic clinical manifestation of shortness of breath and cyanosis often suggests pulmonary embolism. Common precipitants include benzocaine 20% spray, commonly used in transesophageal echocardiography and gastroenterologic endoscopy, with which the incidence of methemoglobinemia is less than 2 per 1000 patients. Sprays should be limited to 1 second. A similar syndrome has been reported with Chinese herbal medicine, with methemoglobin levels reaching as high as 65 to 70%. Inhaled nitrites can also cause life-threatening methemoglobinemia. Methemoglobinemia is seen in some patients who receive primaquine or dapsone for malaria.

Amniotic cells contain easily measurable b5R activity, so prenatal diagnosis should be made available to all families with type II b5R deficiency. Nevertheless, high enough exposure to offending drugs and chemicals can produce methemoglobinemia, even in persons without discernible enzymatic deficiencies.

In type II b5R deficiency, the main symptoms are cyanosis, mental retardation, and severe developmental delay. Life expectancy is reduced because of these neurologic complications, although their pathophysiologic basis remains unexplained.

Diagnosis

Methemoglobinemia should be suspected when a cyanotic patient has a normal Po_2 on blood gas analysis. The blood is a dark red or chocolate color, which does not change with exposure to oxygen. Laboratory methods for assessing oxygenation status typically involve pulse oximetry to measure O_2 saturation (So_2) and blood gas instruments that calculate the estimated So_2 from empirical equations using pH and Po_2 values. In most patients the results from these two methods will be virtually identical. In patients with methemoglobinemia, however, So_2 via pulse oximetry, which is calculated from the pH and Po_2, is often inaccurate because the algorithms used assume normal O_2 affinity, normal 2,3-diphosphoglycerate concentrations, and no hemoglobinopathies. CO oximeter reports should include the dyshemoglobin fractions in addition to the oxyhemoglobin fraction. In patients with an increased methemoglobin fraction, pulse oximeter values trend toward 85%, thus underestimating the actual So_2. Hemoglobin M variants may yield normal methemoglobin and increased carboxyhemoglobin or sulfhemoglobin fractions measured by CO oximetry.

Differentiation of methemoglobinemia from the more rare sulfhemoglobinemia of cyanide poisoning (Chapter 111) can be made by special laboratory testing of the absorption spectrum of the patient's hemoglobin. Hereditary forms of methemoglobinemia are diagnosed by pedigree analysis. Incubation of blood with methylene blue rapidly reduces methemoglobin caused by enzymatic deficiencies, but not that caused by hemoglobin M (see later).

TABLE 168–2 DRUGS AND CHEMICALS ASSOCIATED WITH METHEMOGLOBINEMIA

DRUGS
Acetaminophen (nitrobenzene derivative)
Acetanilide
Anesthetics (local)
Benzocaine
Lidocaine
Prilocaine
Dapsone
Flutamide
Ifosfamide
Metoclopramide
Nitric oxide
Nitrites
Amyl nitrite
Isobutyl nitrite
Nitroglycerin
Sodium nitrite
Nitrofurantoin
Phenacetin
Phenazopyridine
Primaquine
Sulfamethoxazole
CHEMICALS
Aniline dyes
Nitrates (bacterial conversion to nitrites)
Nitrobenzenes/nitrobenzoates
Nitroethane (nail polish remover)
Paraquat/monolinuron

Treatment

Rx

Precipitating drugs and chemicals must be discontinued. No specific therapy is required in asymptomatic patients. For toxic causes and patients with type I b5R deficiency, treatment with 1% methylene blue, 1 to 2 mg/kg intravenously over a 5-minute period, rapidly reduces methemoglobinemia and can be life-saving; the dose may be repeated in 1 hour if needed. Large cumulative doses (>7 mg/kg) can cause dyspnea, chest pain, and hemolysis. Patients with glucose-6-phosphate dehydrogenase deficiency (Chapter 165) should not receive methylene blue but can receive oral ascorbic acid (300 to 1000 mg/day in divided doses). For severe methemoglobinemia, hyperbaric oxygen and exchange transfusion can be used. If the source of toxicity can be eliminated, methemoglobin levels will return to normal.

For cosmetic purposes, patients with homozygous or compound heterozygous b5R deficiency can be treated with methylene blue, 100 to 300 mg/day orally, or ascorbic acid, 300 to 1000 mg/day orally in divided doses. Riboflavin (20 to 30 mg/day) may also be effective.

For type II b5R deficiency, treatment is the same as for type I. However, the treatment is effective only for cosmetic purposes because it has no effect on neurologic complications.

Methemoglobinemia from M Forms of Hemoglobin

Hemoglobin M mutations, which carry an amino acid substitution in or near the heme pocket, create the propensity to form methemoglobin instead of oxyhemoglobin in the presence of molecular O_2. Hemoglobin M mutations are usually caused by substitution of tyrosine for either the proximal or distal histidine residue that binds to the iron atom of heme. These amino acid substitutions stabilize iron in the oxidized form, thus making it resistant to reduction by endogenous enzyme mechanisms or reducing agents (e.g., methylene blue). In affected patients, asymptomatic cyanosis has been present since birth or infancy. RBC morphology is normal, and specialized laboratory testing may be required to make the diagnosis. No therapy is beneficial.

UNSTABLE HEMOGLOBINS

Approximately 100 different globin mutations cause unstable hemoglobins by interfering with the binding of heme, the structure of hemoglobin, or hemoglobin hydrophobic interactions. Mutations are inherited as an autosomal dominant phenotype. Hemoglobin precipitates within RBCs are visualized microscopically as Heinz bodies. Rigid hemoglobin particles interfere with the plasticity of RBCs and create a block in the microcirculation, especially in the spleen, thereby leading to sequestration of RBCs.

Clinical Manifestations and Diagnosis

The spleen of affected patients is typically enlarged. Fever and many oxidant drugs, such as sulfonamides, exacerbate hemolysis and can precipitate an acute hemolytic crisis. Severe hemolysis may be associated with intravascular hemolysis and hemoglobinuria.

The diagnosis is suspected by finding Heinz bodies in the RBCs. Definitive diagnosis requires the isopropanol test or the heat test, which incubates the hemolysate at 50° C.

Treatment

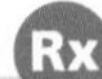

No specific treatment is available, and precipitating causes should be avoided. Splenectomy may benefit patients with severe hemolysis.

SUGGESTED READINGS

Ash-Bernal R, Wise R, Wright SM: Acquired methemoglobinemia: A retrospective series of 138 cases at 2 teaching hospitals. Medicine (Baltimore) 2004;83:265–273. *Dapsone was the most common cause of acquired methemoglobinemia.*

Haymond S, Cariappa R, Eby CS, et al: Laboratory assessment of oxygenation in methemoglobinemia. Clin Chem 2005;51:434–444. *With pulse oximetry, Po_2 values trend toward 85% in methemoglobinemia, thereby underestimating the severity of the condition; blood gas analysis is more accurate.*

Hurford WE, Kratz A: Case 23-2004: A 50-year-old woman with low oxygen saturation. N Engl J Med 2004;351:380–387. *Review of congenital methemoglobinemia.*

Percy MJ, McFerran NV, Lappin TR: Disorders of oxidised haemoglobin. Blood Rev 2005;19:61–68. *A clinical overview of methemoglobinemia.*

Umbreit J: Methemoglobin—it's not just blue: A concise review. Am J Hematol 2007;82:134–144. *Overview of biology and pathophysiology.*

169 NONHEMOLYTIC NORMOCHROMIC, NORMOCYTIC ANEMIAS

Ayalew Tefferi

Definition

For practical purposes, it is reasonable to define "normocytic" anemia strictly as a mean corpuscular volume (MCV) reading that lies within the normal reference range (approximately 80 to 100 fL) (Chapter 162) and then consider seven broad categories of diseases that can be accompanied by normocytic anemia (Table 169–1). Nonhemolytic normochromic, normocytic anemia includes the categories that are not related to either hemolysis or nutrient deficiency.

TABLE 169–1 OPERATIONAL CLASSIFICATION OF NORMOCYTIC ANEMIA

Anemia of inflammation (a.k.a. anemia of chronic disease)
Anemia of renal insufficiency (Chapter 131)
Acute blood loss
Nutrient-deficient anemia
Iron deficiency anemia (Chapter 163)
Megaloblastic anemia from vitamin B_{12} or folate deficiency (Chapter 170)
Anemia associated with primary bone marrow failure (Chapter 171)
Aplastic anemia
Pure red cell aplasia
Drug- or virus-induced suppression of erythropoiesis
Anemia associated with ineffective clonal erythropoiesis
Myelodysplastic syndrome (Chapter 193)
Myeloproliferative disorders (Chapter 177)
Anemia associated with an infiltrative process in the bone marrow
Leukemia (Chapter 194)
Lymphoma (Chapters 196 and 197)
Multiple myeloma (Chapter 198)
Metastatic cancer (Chapter 189)
Myelofibrosis (Chapter 177)
Hemolytic anemia (Chapters 164 and 165)

Epidemiology

Anemia is an often under-recognized, but frequent problem in elderly patients and contributes to increased mortality from cardiovascular and neurologic complications, poor health, fatigue, and a decline in activity levels. In a U.S. national survey, anemia, as defined by a hemoglobin level lower than 13 g/dL in men or 12 g/dL in women, was documented in approximately 11.0% of men and 10.2% of women 65 years or older, although the degree of anemia was usually mild. Either anemia of inflammation (serum iron <60 µg/dL without evidence of iron deficiency) or renal insufficiency accounted for a third of the cases, but oftentimes the cause of anemia was uncertain. There is a statistically significant decrease in hemoglobin level among men starting at a creatinine clearance of 70 mL/min or less and among women starting at 50 mL/min or less (approximately a 1- to 1.5-g/dL drop in hemoglobin level as creatinine clearance decreases to <30 mL/min). Overall, it is estimated that 800,000 elderly persons in the United States have chronic renal insufficiency–associated anemia. In another systematic survey of patients with rheumatoid arthritis, 30 to 60% had anemia of inflammation.

Pathobiology

Impaired erythropoiesis (Chapter 160) can result from either a stem/progenitor cell defect or intrinsic/extrinsic causes of ineffective production of erythrocytes. Examples of the former include aplastic anemia and pure red blood cell aplasia (Chapter 171). Ineffective erythropoiesis accompanies chronic myeloid malignancies (e.g., myelodysplastic syndrome, myeloproliferative disorders; Chapter 177), as well as certain nutrient deficiencies (e.g., vitamin B_{12} and folate; Chapter 170). In addition, optimal red blood cell production is affected when the bone marrow space is compromised by infiltration with either neoplastic (e.g., metastatic cancer [Chapter 189], acute leukemia [Chapter 194], lymphoma [Chapters 196 and 197], multiple myeloma [Chapter 198]) or non-neoplastic processes (e.g., infectious granulomas, myelofibrosis with myeloid metaplasia). However, adequate bone marrow cell reserve and space do not necessarily ensure effective erythropoiesis, which requires response to both positive (e.g., erythropoietin, insulin-like growth factor [IGF-1], stem cell factor [SCF], granulocyte colony-stimulating factor [G-CSF], granulocyte-macrophage colony-stimulating factor [GM-CSF], interleukin-3 [IL-3] and other interleukins) and negative (uremic toxins) cytokine/hormone stimulation.

Anemia of Renal Insufficiency

Erythropoietin, the major growth and development factor for erythrocytes, provides proliferative, differentiation, and survival signals to erythroid progenitors; it acts mostly at the colony-forming unit—erythroid (CFU-E) and, to a much lesser extent, at the burst-forming unit—erythroid (BFU-E) stages of erythroid development. The erythropoietin receptor is mainly expressed by CFU-E cells and early pronormoblasts and transduces signaling through the JAK2-STAT (Janus kinase 2–signal transducers and activators of transcription) pathway. The primary and secondary sites of erythropoietin production are the kidney and liver, respectively. In the kidney, tissue oxygen pressure determines the production of erythropoietin by the juxtamedullary region (peritubular interstitial cells) through hypoxic activation of erythropoietin gene transcription mediated by the transcription factor hypoxia-inducible factor 1 (HIF-1). The mechanism of anemia in renal insufficiency is linked to the decline in erythropoietin production by the diseased kidney, as well as a blunted erythroid progenitor cell response to erythropoietin in the presence of uremia.

Anemia of Chronic Inflammation

Anemia of inflammation accompanies a heterogenous group of disorders, such as acute and chronic infections, autoimmune disorders, chronic inflammatory conditions, and cancer. Often, multiple factors contribute to the anemia, including medications for the underlying disease, as well as both iatrogenic and occult blood loss. Anemia of inflammation is currently believed to constitute a cytokine-mediated impairment of erythropoiesis in which iron homeostasis, erythroid proliferation, and both the production of and sensitivity to erythropoiesis are variably affected. Cytokines that are implicated include IL-1α, IL-1β, IL-6, transforming growth factor β (TGF-β), and tumor necrosis factor α (TNF-α). The key pathologic mechanism in anemia of inflammation is considered to be the preferential sequestration of iron in macrophages, thereby restricting the access of erythroid progenitors to iron. Such impaired release of iron from macrophages might be the result of decreased expression of ferroportin (a membrane molecule that exports iron out of macrophages and enterocytes), possibly mediated by hepcidin, a liver-derived peptide that is a major regulator of the intestinal absorption of iron and recycling of iron from macrophages. The increased production of hepcidin in anemia of inflammation is believed to be mediated by inflammatory cytokines, including IL-6, and might involve several other proteins, such as the hemochromatosis gene product (HFE), transferrin receptor 2, and hemojuvelin (Chapter 231).

Diagnosis

In patients with "normocytic" anemia, the wide range of the normal interval for MCV (80 to 100 fL) means that a patient-specific microcytic or macrocytic process might be spuriously termed normocytic if the individual's baseline MCV is not known. In iron deficiency, for example, anemia antedates microcytosis (Chapter 163). Key clues from the history include bleeding, pica, malnutrition, and substance abuse. Causes of both microcytic and macrocytic anemia, especially readily treatable ones, must be included in the differential diagnosis of normocytic anemia (e.g., iron, vitamin B_{12}, and folate deficiency anemias) (Fig. 169–1). It is clinically prudent always to start with a review of the present and past serum creatinine levels and exclude the possibility of hemolysis because such cases lend themselves to specific and usually effective therapy. Additional guidance toward a specific diagnosis (Table 169–2) is obtained from careful review of the red blood cell indices, the complete blood count, and the peripheral blood smear (Chapter 161; Fig. 169–2).

Differential Diagnosis

The differential diagnosis of a normocytic anemia that is not linked to bleeding, nutrient deficiency, renal insufficiency, or hemolysis is either anemia of inflammation or a primary bone marrow disorder. Anemia of inflammation is a diagnosis of exclusion, without any specific diagnostic markers.

TABLE 169–2 CLUES FROM THE COMPLETE BLOOD COUNT AND PERIPHERAL BLOOD SMEAR IN THE DIFFERENTIAL DIAGNOSIS OF NORMOCYTIC ANEMIA

Differential Diagnosis	Complete Blood Count Clues	Peripheral Blood Smear Clues
Bleeding	Usually unremarkable	Polychromasia
Nutrient-deficient anemia	Increased RDW	Anisocytosis Dimorphic erythrocytes
Anemia of renal insufficiency	Normal RDW	Usually unremarkable
Hemolysis	Normal or elevated RDW Thrombocytosis	Polychromasia Spherocytes Schistocytes Bite cells
Anemia of chronic disease	Normal RDW	Unremarkable
A primary marrow disorder	Increased RDW Other cytopenias Monocytosis Leukocytosis Thrombocytosis Abnormal differential	Dimorphic erythrocytes (MDS) Pseudo–Pelger-Huët anomaly (MDS) Oval macrocytes (MDS) Myelophthisis* (myelofibrosis, metastatic cancer) Rouleaux formation (multiple myeloma) Blasts (acute leukemia, chronic myeloid disorder)

MDS = myelodysplastic syndrome; RDW = red cell distribution width.
*Myelophthisis implies the presence of nucleated red blood cells, immature myeloid cells, and tear drop–shaped erythrocytes.

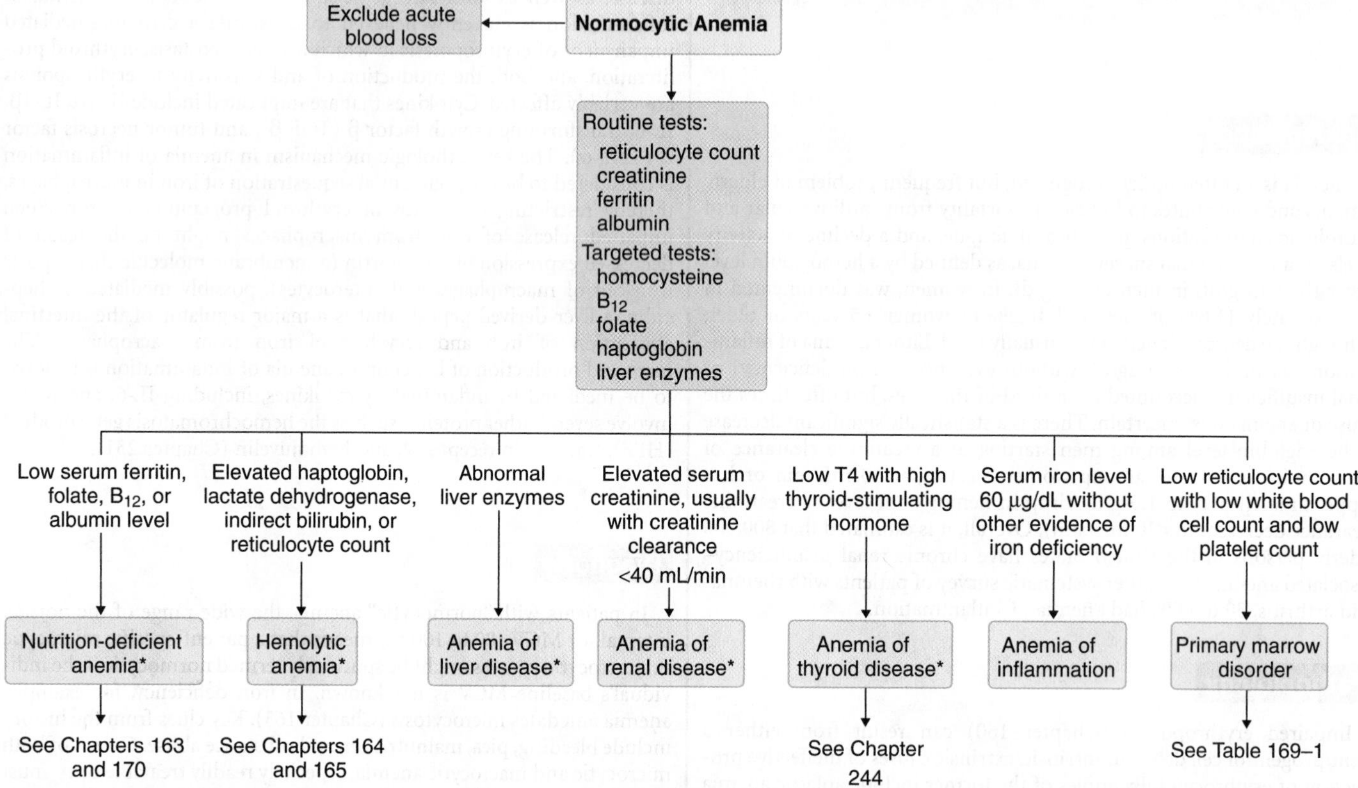

FIGURE 169–1 • Diagnostic algorithm for normocytic anemias. *Anemias associated with vitamin B_{12} or folate deficiency or with thyroid or liver disease will typically be macrocytic or megaloblastic (Chapter 170), and iron deficiency anemia will be microcytic (Chapter 163) as it becomes more severe. T4 = levothyroxine.

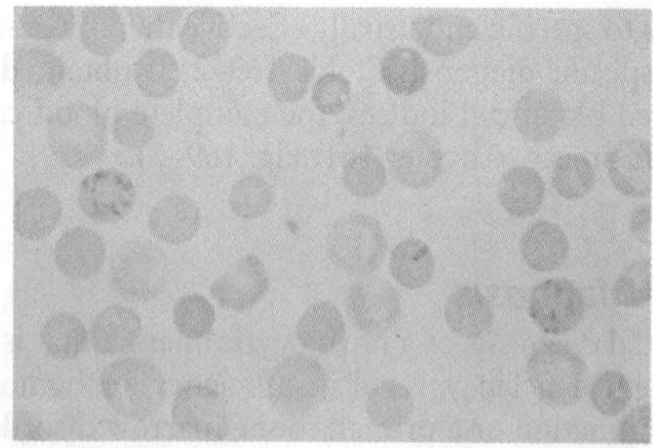

FIGURE 169–2 • Reticulocytes. Special supravital (methylene blue) staining of the blood smear reveals dark purple reticulin, which represents residual RNA in immature red blood cells.

Treatment

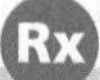

The goal of anemia-directed therapy in patients with either renal insufficiency or inflammation is to improve the hemoglobin level, reduce the need for blood transfusion, and improve quality of life. Interestingly, data suggest that survival might also be improved in anemic patients with heart failure, but higher target hemoglobin levels increase adverse effects and death in patients with chronic kidney disease. 1,2

Three forms of recombinant erythropoietin are available: epoetin alfa (human recombinant erythropoietin), epoetin beta (NeoRecormon, which differs from epoetin alfa in terms of glycosylation and

Rx

sialic acid content), and a longer-acting derivative of epoetin alfa (darbepoetin). All three products have amino acid sequences identical to those of endogenous human erythropoietin but differ from it as well as from each other in terms of glycosylation and the sialic acid content of the glycoprotein. All three brands of recombinant erythropoietin are safe and effective for treating anemia in patients with either renal insufficiency or chronic inflammation, but only the two types of epoetin alpha are available in the United States. The subcutaneous and intravenous routes of drug administration are roughly equivalent, and once-weekly subcutaneous administration of 10,000 U of any of these three erythropoietin preparations appears to be adequate. 3 Some data suggest that concomitant administration of intravenous iron (Chapter 163) is of incremental benefit even with adequate bone marrow stores. However, iron therapy is currently considered only if patients do not show the expected increase in their hemoglobin level after an adequate trial of erythropoietin therapy by itself. Erythropoietin therapy benefits both critically 4 and chronically ill patients with anemia of inflammation caused by rheumatoid arthritis, Crohn's disease, and cancer. Currently, such therapy is formally approved by the Food and Drug Administration only for patients with either human immunodeficiency virus infection or cancer undergoing myelosuppressive therapy. In general, higher doses of erythropoietin (e.g., 40,000 U subcutaneously weekly) are used in the setting of anemia of inflammation.

Treatment with recombinant erythropoietin is generally safe, and untoward drug effects are very rare. One rare complication (fewer than 200 cases reported) is pure red cell aplasia (Chapter 171) caused by neutralizing anti-erythropoietin antibodies, which are usually seen in patients with renal insufficiency. This complication may be more common with a formulation of epoetin alfa (Eprex) that is marketed only outside the United States. Pure red cell aplasia caused by erythropoietin usually responds to immunosuppressive therapy with corticosteroids or cyclosporine with no recurrence. Other side effects of erythropoietin therapy include a rise in blood pressure, reactions at the injection site, and very rarely, seizures.

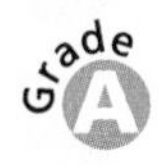

1. Singh AK, Szczech L, Tang KL, et al: Correction of anemia with epoetin alfa in chronic kidney disease. N Engl J Med 2006;355: 2085–2098. *A higher target hemoglobin was associated with an increased risk of adverse events.*
2. Phrommintikul A, Haas SJ, Elsik M, et al: Mortality and target haemoglobin concentrations in anaemic patients with chronic kidney disease treated with erythropoietin: A meta-analysis. Lancet 2007;369:381–388. *Notes an increased risk of death in patients treated with a higher hemoglobin target.*
3. Locatelli F, Baldamus CA, Villa G, et al: Once-weekly compared with three-times-weekly subcutaneous epoetin beta: Results from a randomized, multicenter, therapeutic-equivalence study. Am J Kidney Dis 2002;40:119–125.
4. Corwin HL, Gettinger A, Pearl RG, et al: Efficacy of recombinant human erythropoietin in critically ill patients: A randomized controlled trial. JAMA 2002;288:2827–2835.

SUGGESTED READINGS

Ferrucci L, Guralnik JM, Bandinelli S, et al: Unexplained anaemia in older persons is characterised by low erythropoietin and low levels of pro-inflammatory markers. Br J Haematol 2007;136:849–855. *Unexplained anemia is associated with a reduced kidney EPO response, low levels of pro-inflammatory markers, and low lymphocyte counts.*

Means RT Jr.: Hepcidin and anaemia. Blood Rev 2004;18:219–225. *This acute phase protein may be pathogenic in anemia of chronic disease.*

Verhelst D, Rossert J, Casadevall N, et al: Treatment of erythropoietin-induced pure red cell aplasia: A retrospective study. Lancet 2004;363:1768–1771. *Review of this rare condition.*

Weiss G, Goodnough LT: Anemia of chronic disease. N Engl J Med 2005; 352:1011–1023. *A comprehensive review.*

170 MEGALOBLASTIC ANEMIAS

Aśok C. Antony

Definition

Megaloblastic anemias, a group of disorders characterized by a distinct morphologic pattern in hematopoietic cells, are commonly due to deficiency of vitamin B_{12} (cobalamin) or folates. Folates and cobalamin are both required to sustain one-carbon metabolism, which involves the transfer of one-carbon groups such as methyl-, formyl-, methylene-, forminyl-, and formimino- in reactions essential for pyrimidine and purine biosynthesis, including the synthesis of three of the four nucleotides of DNA. Thus, a deficiency in cobalamin or folate results in the common biochemical feature of a defect in DNA synthesis, with lesser alterations in RNA and protein synthesis, that leads to a state of unbalanced cell growth and impaired cell division. In contrast to a normal population of cells, the majority of megaloblastic cells are not resting but rather are vainly engaged in attempting to double their DNA, with frequent arrest in the S phase and lesser arrest in other phases of the cell cycle; as a result, an increased percentage of these cells have DNA values between 2N and 4N because of delayed cell division. This increased DNA content in megaloblastic cells is morphologically expressed as larger than normal "immature" nuclei with finely particulate chromatin, whereas the relatively unimpaired RNA and protein synthesis results in large cells with greater "mature" cytoplasm and cell volume. The microscopic appearance of this nuclear-cytoplasmic asynchrony (or dissociation) is morphologically described as megaloblastic. Megaloblastic hematopoiesis is commonly manifested as anemia, the most easily recognized manifestation of a more global defect in DNA synthesis that affects all proliferating cells. Because correct vitamin replacement is curative, precise diagnosis of the deficient vitamin is essential. In the case of cobalamin, knowledge of the causes of the deficiency (Table 170–1) dictates the dose and duration of replacement therapy.

Epidemiology

Cobalamin

Nutrition

Cobalamin is a pink, water-soluble vitamin with a complex structure that generally resembles the heme molecule but with cobalt replacing iron in the center of the pyrrole ring. The recommended daily allowance of cobalamin is 2.4 µg for men and nonpregnant women, 2.6 µg for pregnant women, 2.8 µg for lactating women, and between 1.5 and 2 µg for children 9 to 18 years old. Cobalamin is produced in nature only by microorganisms, and humans receive cobalamin solely from the diet. Meat from parenchymal organs is richest in cobalamin (>10 µg per 100 g wet weight); fish and animal muscle, milk products, and egg yolk have 1 to 10 µg per 100 g wet weight. An average nonvegetarian Western diet with abundant meat, milk and dairy products, and eggs contains 5 to 7 µg/day of cobalamin, which adequately sustains normal cobalamin equilibrium. For vegetarians, consumption of eggs, milk, and dairy products provides most of the cobalamin. Other sources include contamination of plants by cobalamin-producing bacteria that grow in the roots and nodules of legumes, manure that is rich in cobalamin and used for fertilization, microscopic insects that infest plants, and *nori* (dried seaweed) and *tempeh* (fermented soybean cake) used in Asian cuisine.

Vegetarian diets that provide less than 0.5 µg of cobalamin daily cannot sustain adequate cobalamin balance. In addition to vegan diets, both lactovegetarian and lacto-ovovegetarian diets (in ascending order of cobalamin content) are generally insufficient to prevent cobalamin deficiency. These individuals have increased blood levels of homocysteine and methylmalonic acid (MMA), which is strongly suggestive biochemical evidence of cobalamin deficiency (with or without folate deficiency). Furthermore, the normalization of sensitive electroencephalographic, evoked potential, and electrophysiologic markers of cognitive ability by cobalamin treatment in otherwise apparently asymptomatic individuals with subclinical cobalamin deficiency indicates that these individuals can benefit from prophylactic cobalamin replacement. Poverty-imposed

TABLE 170–1 ETIOPATHOPHYSIOLOGIC CLASSIFICATION OF COBALAMIN AND FOLATE DEFICIENCIES

I. Cobalamin deficiency
  A. Nutritional cobalamin deficiency *(insufficient cobalamin intake)*—vegetarians, poverty-imposed near-vegetarians, breast-fed infants of mothers with pernicious anemia
  B. Abnormal intragastric events *(inadequate proteolysis of food cobalamin)*—atrophic gastritis, partial gastritis with hypochlorhydria, proton pump inhibitors, H_2 blockers
  C. Loss/atrophy of gastric oxyntic mucosa *(deficient intrinsic factor molecules)*—total or partial gastrectomy, adult and juvenile pernicious anemia, caustic destruction (lye)
  D. Abnormal events in the small bowel lumen
    1. Inadequate pancreatic protease *(R factor–cobalamin not degraded, cobalamin not transferred to intrinsic factor)*
      a. Insufficient pancreatic protease—pancreatic insufficiency
      b. Inactivation of pancreatic protease—Zollinger-Ellison syndrome
    2. Usurping of luminal cobalamin *(inadequate binding of cobalamin to intrinsic factor)*
      a. By bacteria—stasis syndromes (blind loops, pouches of diverticulosis, strictures, fistulas, anastomosis), impaired bowel motility (scleroderma), hypogammaglobulinemia
      b. By *Diphyllobothrium latum* (fish tapeworm)
  E. Disorders of ileal mucosa/intrinsic factor-cobalamin receptors *(intrinsic factor–cobalamin not bound to intrinsic factor–cobalamin receptors)*
    1. Diminished or absent intrinsic factor–cobalamin receptors—ileal bypass/resection/fistula
    2. Abnormal mucosal architecture/function—tropical/nontropical sprue, Crohn's disease, tuberculous ileitis, infiltration by lymphomas, amyloidosis
    3. Intrinsic factor/post–intrinsic factor–cobalamin receptor defects—Imerslund-Gräsbeck syndrome, hereditary megaloblastic anemia, TCII deficiency
    4. Drug-effects—metformin, cholestyramine, colchicine, neomycin
  F. Disorders of plasma cobalamin transport *(TCII-cobalamin not delivered to TCII receptors)*—congenital TCII deficiency, defective binding of TCII-cobalamin to TCII receptors (rare)
  G. Metabolic disorders *(cobalamin not used by cell)*
    1. Inborn enzyme errors (rare)
    2. Acquired disorders: *(cobalamin functionally inactivated by irreversible oxidation)*—nitrous oxide (N_2O) inhalation

II. Folate deficiency
  A. Nutritional causes
    1. Decrease dietary intake—poverty and famine, institutionalized individuals (psychiatric/nursing homes)/chronic debilitating disease, prolonged feeding of infants with goat's milk, special slimming diets or food fads *(folate-rich foods not consumed)*, cultural/ethnic cooking techniques *(food folate destroyed)*
    2. Decreased diet and increased requirements
      a. Physiologic: pregnancy and lactation, prematurity, hyperemesis gravidarum, infancy
      b. Pathologic
        (1) *Intrinsic hematologic diseases* involving hemolysis with compensatory erythropoiesis, abnormal hematopoiesis, or bone marrow infiltration with malignant disease
        (2) *Dermatologic disease*—psoriasis
  B. Folate malabsorption
    1. With normal intestinal mucosa
      a. Some drugs (controversial)
      b. Congenital folate malabsorption (rare)
    2. With mucosal abnormalities—tropical and nontropical sprue, regional enteritis
  C. Defective cellular folate uptake—infantile cerebral folate deficiency *(antifolate receptor antibodies)* (rare)
  D. Inadequate cellular utilization
    1. Folate antagonists (methotrexate)
    2. Hereditary enzyme deficiencies involving folate
  E. Drugs (multiple effects on folate metabolism)—alcohol, sulfasalazine, triamterene, pyrimethamine, trimethoprim-sulfamethoxazole, diphenylhydantoin, barbiturates

III. Miscellaneous megaloblastic anemias not caused by cobalamin or folate deficiency
  A. Congenital disorders of DNA synthesis
    1. Orotic aciduria
    2. Lesch-Nyhan syndrome
    3. Congenital dyserythropoietic anemia
  B. Acquired disorders of DNA synthesis
    1. Deficiency—thiamine-responsive megaloblastic anemia (DIDMOAD syndrome)
    2. Malignancy—erythroleukemia
      a. Refractory sideroblastic anemias (?pyridoxine responsive)
      b. All antineoplastic drugs that inhibit DNA synthesis *(including antinucleosides used against HIV and other viruses)*
    3. Toxic—alcohol

DIDMOAD = diabetes insipidus, diabetes mellitus, optic atrophy, deafness; HIV = human immunodeficiency virus; TCII = transcobalamin II.

near-vegetarians who consume meat infrequently have a cobalamin status that is only marginally better than that of lacto-ovovegetarians. Because vegetarians have a lifelong low cobalamin status, superimposition of additional conditions that perturb either absorption or metabolism of cobalamin can easily tip them into frank cobalamin deficiency far earlier than nonvegetarians who have substantially greater preexistent stores.

Cobalamin is stored exceptionally well in tissues. Of the total body content of 2 to 5 mg in adults, half is in the liver. With a daily loss of 1 μg, dietary cobalamin deficiency can take up to 5 to 10 years to become apparent. However, it takes about 3 to 4 years to deplete cobalamin stores if dietary cobalamin is abruptly malabsorbed, thereby interfering with an efficient enterohepatic circulation that accounts for the turnover of 5 to 10 μg of cobalamin per day and reabsorption of 75% of the cobalamin secreted into bile. Cobalamin is stable and resists high-temperature cooking processes. A pH greater than 12 (during food processing) or high doses of ascorbic acid (vitamin C) convert cobalamin to inactive analogues.

Worldwide, the most common cause of cobalamin deficiency in all age groups is nutritional deficiency. In affluent countries, however, inadequate absorption of adequate dietary cobalamin is the more common cause.

The incidence of pernicious anemia is approximately 25 new cases per year per 100,000 persons older than 40 years, and the average age at onset is about 60 years. In one study, up to 1.9% of free-living individuals older than 60 years in southern California had undiagnosed pernicious anemia with minimal clinical manifestations of cobalamin deficiency. The prevalence was 2.7% in women and 1.4% in men, but 4.3% of African American women and 4.0% of white women had pernicious anemia. However, pernicious anemia is found in persons of all ages, race, and ethnic origin. About 30% of patients have a positive family history, and there is an association with other autoimmune diseases (i.e., polyglandular autoimmune syndrome, Graves' disease [Chapter 244], Hashimoto's thyroiditis [Chapter 244], vitiligo [Chapter 467], Addison's disease [Chapter 250], idiopathic hypoparathyroidism [Chapter 266], primary ovarian failure [Chapter 255], myasthenia gravis [Chapter 448], type 1 diabetes [Chapter 247], and adult hypogammaglobulinemia [Chapter 271]).

Folates

Nutrition

Folates are synthesized by microorganisms and plants. Rich food sources include green leafy vegetables (spinach, lettuce, broccoli), beans, fruit (bananas, melons, lemons), yeast, mushrooms, and animal protein (liver, kidney). The recommended daily allowance of folate is 400 μg for adult men and nonpregnant women, 600 μg for pregnant women, 500 μg for lactating women, and 300 to 400 μg for children 9 to 18 years of age. A balanced Western diet can prevent folate deficiency, but the net dietary intake of folate in many developing countries is often insufficient to sustain folate balance. For example, in rural areas of northern India, estimates of folate intake are often less than half of optimum.

Folates are susceptible to breakdown during prolonged cooking (for >15 minutes), which is common in many cultures; for example, many ethnic cooking techniques involve prolonged boiling of lentils or beans or frying foods in an open pan—methods that destroy 50 to 95% of folate. Eating fresh raw or stir-fried vegetables or salads that are rich in folate is not common in many cultures. Finally, processing food with additives such as nitrites destroys folate, but adding ascorbic acid before processing preserves the folate.

Folate deficiency can arise from decreased supply (reduced intake, absorption, transport, or utilization) or increased requirements (from metabolic consumption, destruction, or excretion). The same individual may have multiple causes for folate deficiency, but specific tests to define each mechanism are not available clinically. Folate deficiency varies among different populations, and nutritional deficiency is the most common cause worldwide in all age groups. With food folate fortification programs, folate deficiency has been dramatically reduced in the United States; nevertheless, folate deficiency may be present in 5 to 10% of the elderly (>70 years of age).

Pathobiology

Cobalamin

Normal Physiology

Absorption and Transport

Cobalamin in food is usually in coenzyme form (as deoxyadenosylcobalamin and methylcobalamin) and bound to proteins (Fig. 170–1). In the stomach, peptic digestion at low pH is a prerequisite for release of cobalamin from food protein. Once released by proteolysis, cobalamin preferentially binds with a high-affinity cobalamin-binding protein called R protein, which is secreted in salivary and gastric juice. These cobalamin–R protein complexes along with unbound intrinsic factor, which is produced by gastric parietal cells, pass into the second part of the duodenum, where pancreatic proteases degrade the R protein to which cobalamin is bound, thereby allowing transfer of cobalamin to intrinsic factor.

The stable intrinsic factor–cobalamin complex then passes through the jejunum to the ileum, where it binds to membrane-associated intrinsic factor–cobalamin receptors on the microvilli of ileal mucosal cells. Within enterocytes, cobalamin is transferred to transcobalamin II, which efficiently delivers cobalamin to transcobalamin II receptors found on cell surfaces. Another protein, transcobalamin I, which binds 75% of serum cobalamin but does not participate in transport, appears to be a storage protein for cobalamin in blood. A third quantitatively minor protein, transcobalamin III, binds a wide spectrum of cobalamin analogues that are rapidly cleared by the liver into bile for fecal excretion.

Cellular Processing

More than 95% of intracellular cobalamin is bound to two intracellular enzymes, methylmalonyl–coenzyme (CoA) mutase and methionine synthase. In mitochondria, deoxyadenosylcobalamin is a coenzyme for methylmalonyl-CoA mutase, which converts the products of propionate metabolism methylmalonyl-CoA to succinyl-CoA, a form that is easily metabolized. In the cytoplasm, methylcobalamin is a coenzyme for methionine synthase, which catalyzes the transfer of methyl groups from methylcobalamin to homocysteine to form methionine. The methyl group of 5-methyltetrahydrofolate (methyl-THF) is donated to regenerate methylcobalamin, thereby forming the THF that is essential to sustain one-carbon metabolism. The methionine so formed can be adenylated to *S*-adenosylmethionine, which donates its methyl group in a critical series of biologic methylation reactions involving more than 80 proteins, phospholipids, neurotransmitters, RNA, and DNA.

Pathogenesis of Cobalamin Deficiency

Nutritional Cobalamin Deficiency

Vegetarianism and poverty-imposed near-vegetarianism, which is especially common in developing countries, are important causes of nutritional cobalamin deficiency.

Inadequate Dissociation of Cobalamin from Food Protein

Dietary cobalamin requires proteolytic digestion of food by gastric acid and pepsin. Thus, failure to release cobalamin from food protein can lead to cobalamin deficiency despite the presence of intrinsic factor.

Absent Secretion

Deficiency of intrinsic factor as a result of gastric parietal cell atrophy is associated with insufficient HCl secretion and can be caused by (1) total or partial gastrectomy, (2) autoimmune destruction (chronic atrophic gastritis) as found as in classic pernicious anemia, or (3) destruction of gastric mucosa by caustic (lye) ingestion.

Total gastrectomy invariably leads to cobalamin deficiency in 2 to 10 years, thus warranting prophylactic cobalamin (and iron) replacement. After partial gastrectomy, up to a third of patients may have multifactorial cobalamin deficiency from decreased secretion of intrinsic factor, hypochlorhydria, or intestinal bacterial overgrowth of cobalamin-consuming organisms. Morbidly obese patients who have undergone gastric bypass surgery have more malabsorption of cobalamin from food than do those treated by vertical banded gastroplasty. Malabsorption of cobalamin can also occur with the long-term use of H_2 blockers or proton pump inhibitors.

In *pernicious anemia,* the primary event is autoimmune destruction and atrophy of the gastric parietal cell mucosa, thereby leading to the absence of intrinsic factor and HCl, which causes severe cobalamin malabsorption and deficiency. The autoimmune gastritis that eventually leads to chronic atrophic gastritis involves the gastric fundus and body. Intrinsic factor antibodies are found in the serum of 60% and in the gastric juice of 75% of patients with pernicious anemia. Type I anti–intrinsic factor antibodies prevent binding of cobalamin to intrinsic factor, whereas type II anti–intrinsic factor antibodies prevent binding of intrinsic factor–cobalamin complexes to ileal intrinsic factor–cobalamin receptors and can interfere with tests for cobalamin absorption. About 96% of African American women with pernicious anemia have high titers of blocking anti–intrinsic factor antibodies but lack anti–parietal cell antibodies. Juvenile pernicious anemia is manifested in the second decade, often in conjunction with endocrinopathies; recently, mutations in intrinsic factor resulting in qualitative abnormalities and cobalamin deficiency have been described.

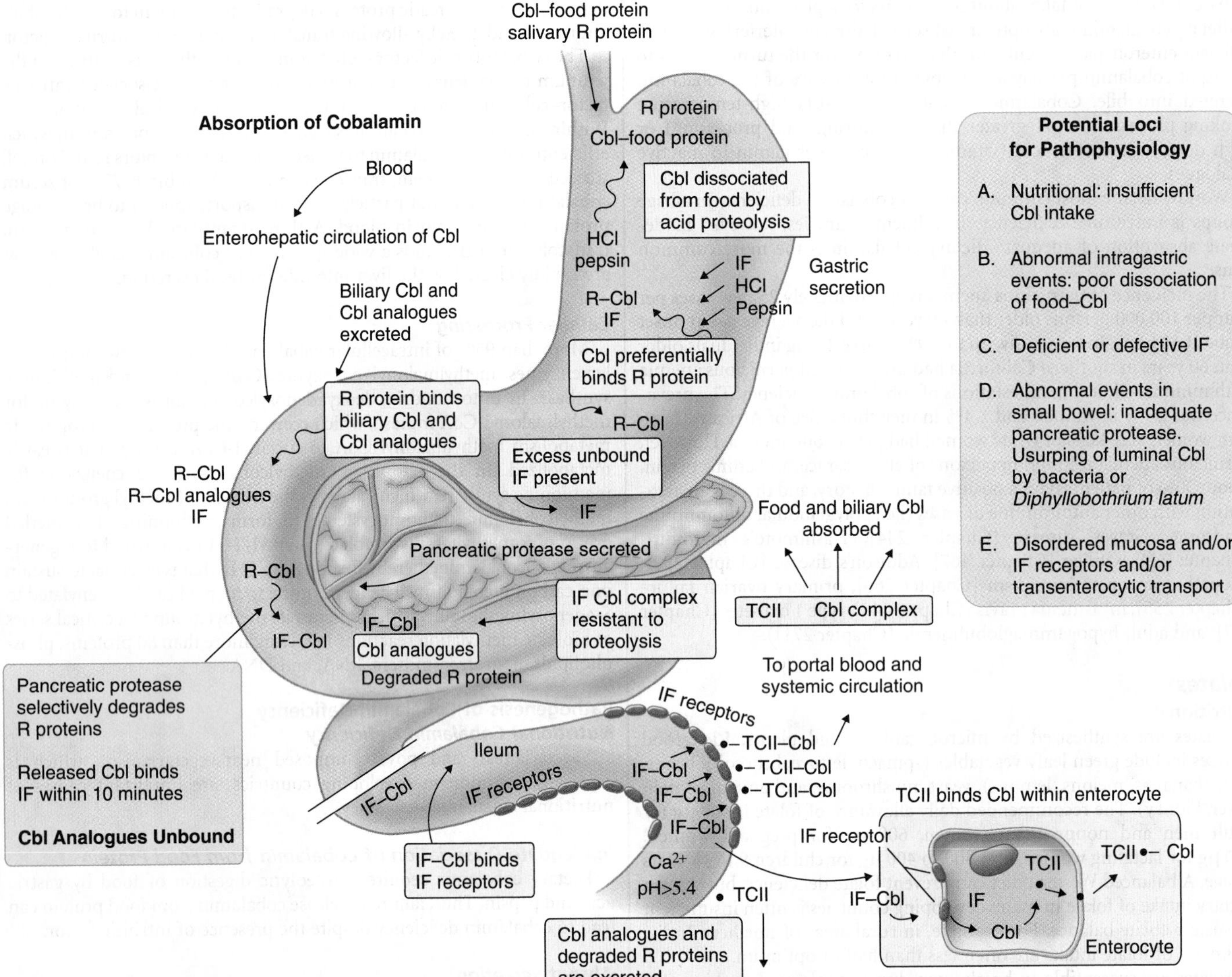

FIGURE 170–1 • Components and mechanism of cobalamin absorption with an indication of the locus for malabsorption. See text for details. IF = intrinsic factor; TCII = transcobalamin II. (From Antony AC: Megaloblastic anemias. *In* Hoffman R, Benz EJ Jr, Shattil SJ, et al [eds]: Hematology: Basic Principles and Practice, 4th ed. Philadelphia, Churchill Livingstone, 2005, pp 519–556.)

Abnormal Events Precluding Absorption of Cobalamin

Pancreatic insufficiency (Chapter 147) with a deficiency of pancreatic protease will fail to break down the R proteins to which cobalamin is preferentially bound in the stomach, thereby precluding transfer of cobalamin to intrinsic factor. However, with the widespread early use of pancreatic replacement, frank cobalamin deficiency is now uncommon. Endogenous pancreatic protease can be inactivated by massive gastric hypersecretion arising from a gastrinoma in Zollinger-Ellison syndrome (Chapters 141, 142, and 205), where the low pH of the luminal contents in the ileum can also preclude binding of the intrinsic factor–cobalamin complex with intrinsic factor–cobalamin receptors, a process that requires a pH higher than 5.4.

Bacterial overgrowth in the small bowel (Chapter 143) (arising from stasis, impaired motility, and hypogammaglobulinemia) favors colonization by bacteria, which can then usurp free cobalamin before it can bind to intrinsic factor; this problem can be reversed by a short course of antibiotic therapy. Individuals heavily infested with the fish tapeworm *Diphyllobothrium latum* (by consuming raw or partially cooked freshwater fish from lakes in Russia, Japan, Switzerland, Germany, and the United States) can become cobalamin deficient when these 10-m-long adult worms in the jejunum avidly usurp cobalamin. After the worms have been expelled (praziquantel, 10 to 20 mg/kg, single dose orally), cobalamin replenishment is curative.

Disorders of the Intrinsic Factor Receptors or Mucosa

Because the distal ileum has the greatest density of intrinsic factor–cobalamin receptors, removal, bypass, or dysfunction of only 1 to 2 ft of terminal ileum can result in cobalamin malabsorption. Among drugs, biguanides (i.e., metformin) decrease intrinsic factor and acid secretion and can inhibit transenterocytic transport of cobalamin in up to a third of patients, which can be avoided by intake of calcium (1.2 g/day). Other drugs (extended-release potassium chloride, cholestyramine, colchicine, and neomycin) can also impair transepithelial transport of cobalamin and interfere with the Schilling test.

Acquired Cobalamin Deficiency

Nitrous oxide (N_2O) irreversibly inactivates cobalamin and results in a state of functional intracellular cobalamin deficiency, which can be bypassed by administration of 5-formyl-THF (leucovorin). Although N_2O exposure during prolonged surgery can induce megaloblastosis, especially in those with marginal or low cobalamin stores, chronic intermittent (surreptitious, accidental, or occupational) exposure leads more frequently to a neuromyelopathic manifestation.

Folates

Normal Physiology

Absorption and Transport

In general, only half the folate in food, which is mainly in polyglutamylated form, is nutritionally available (bioavailable), whereas 85% of folic acid that is added to food or ingested as a supplement is bioavailable. The small intestine can absorb folic acid unchanged, but food folate polyglutamates must be hydrolyzed to monoglutamate by folate polyglutamate hydrolase at the brush border before transport into enterocytes, where it is reduced to THF and methylated before release into plasma as methyl-THF. The normal serum folate level is maintained by dietary folate intake and by an efficient enterohepatic circulation.

From plasma, there is rapid uptake of folate (methyl-THF and folic acid) into tissues by two physiologic transport processes for cellular entry. The reduced-folate carrier is a low-affinity, but high-capacity system that can mediate the uptake of physiologic methyl-THF and pharmacologic folates (methotrexate and folinic acid) into a variety of cells. In addition, membrane-associated folate receptors can also bind and take up methyl-THF and folic acid with high affinity at concentrations found in serum. The relative density of these two pathways on cells generally determines the route of entry of folates and antifolates into normal and malignant cells. Finally, physiologic transplacental folate transport involves capture of maternal folate by placental folate receptors, followed by displacement of this pool by dietary folates, a process that leads to transfer to the fetal circulation along a downhill concentration gradient. Passive diffusion also operates to transport folate across biologic membranes at supra-physiologic folate concentrations.

The acquired transport resistance in patients with relapsed acute lymphocytic leukemia is associated with decreased reduced-folate carrier expression. Antibodies to folate receptors in mothers and infants have been linked to recurrent neural tube defects and infantile cerebral folate deficiency, respectively.

Cellular Retention and Excretion

Polyglutamylation of folate is the major factor for intracellular retention. After glomerular filtration, folate receptors on the brush border membranes on proximal renal tubular cells bind luminal folate and transport it back into blood.

Intracellular Metabolism and Cobalamin-Folate Interactions

After cellular uptake, methyl-THF must first be converted to THF via methionine synthase. Only then can the THF be polyglutamated by folate polyglutamate synthase, which allows it to play a central role in one-carbon metabolism. THF can be converted to 10-formyl-THF, which can be used for de novo biosynthesis of purines, and to methylene-THF, which can be used for the synthesis of thymidylate.

The central role of methylene-THF is that it can be used either in the thymidylate cycle via thymidylate synthase for the synthesis of thymidine and DNA or in the methylation cycle via methionine synthase, but only after its conversion to methyl-THF by methylene-THF reductase. Inactivation of methionine synthase during cobalamin deficiency results in accumulation of the substrate methyl-THF, which cannot be polyglutamylated and thus leaks out of the cell, thereby resulting in an intracellular THF deficiency and reduction of one-carbon metabolism. This process explains why cobalamin deficiency responds to replacement with folic acid, which can be converted to THF via dihydrofolate reductase, or to replacement with 5-formyl-THF (folinic acid), which bypasses methionine synthase and can be converted to methylene-THF or 10-formyl-THF via intermediates.

Pathogenesis of Folate Deficiency

Nutritional Causes (Decreased Intake or Increased Requirements)

With an abrupt reduction in folate consumption, body stores of folate are adequate for approximately 4 months; however, these stores are depleted even faster in individuals who are chronically in negative folate balance and who often have multiple nutritional deficiencies (and diseases) that tip them into frank folate deficiency. Children and women in developing countries are at particular risk, but even the elderly in developed countries are at risk if their diet is poor because of physical disabilities or social isolation. A seasonal reduction in folate-rich food, poverty, cultural or ethnic diets that are intrinsically poor in folates, cooking techniques that destroy food folate, and the anorexia that accompanies chronic illnesses are among the myriad of reasons for folate deficiency, especially in developing countries.

Patients with hematologic diseases involving increased intrinsic cell proliferation or with compensatory erythropoiesis in response to chronic peripheral red blood cell destruction are at risk. Folate deficiency in the face of chronic hemolysis can lead to an acute reticulocytopenic aplastic crisis, an unexpected increase in transfusional requirements, or a fall in platelets. Exfoliative skin diseases (Chapter 464) also cause folate deficiency when there is a combination of increased demand from excess loss of skin cells.

Pregnancy and Infancy

Pregnancy with poor folate intake is a very common cause of megaloblastic anemia in developing countries because pregnancy and lactation require additional folate for growth of the fetus and maternal tissues. Transplacental maternal to fetal folate transport relies on provision of adequate dietary folate. However, mothers with short intervals between consecutive pregnancies, with twin pregnancies, or with hyperemesis gravidarum are unable to maintain adequate folate stores, thereby leading to premature, low-birthweight infants and other predominantly midline developmental abnormalities in the fetus.

Tropical and Nontropical (Celiac) Sprue

With the development of intestinal mucosal abnormalities, patients are at increased risk for folate malabsorption. In tropical sprue (Chapter 143), for example, a dramatic response to folate can cure about 60% of patients of their sprue in the first year. In the short term, malabsorption leads to folate deficiency, but later in the chronic phase of the disease (longer than 3 years), malabsorption of cobalamin also develops. In addition, iron deficiency (Chapter 163), pellagra, and beriberi (Chapter 237) may coexist in these patients.

Drugs

Excess alcohol consumption at the expense of a balanced diet may be the most common cause of folate deficiency in the United States. Inhibition of dihydrofolate reductase by *trimethoprim* and *pyrimethamine* or *methotrexate* can be acutely reversed by the administration of 5-formyl-THF (folinic acid). *Sulfasalazine* induces megaloblastosis in two thirds of subjects taking full doses (>2 g/day) by decreasing the breakdown of folate polyglutamates to monoglutamates before absorption or by inducing Heinz body hemolytic anemia, which leads to increased requirements. *Oral contraceptives* may increase folate catabolism, whereas *anticonvulsants* can reduce absorption and induce microsomal liver enzymes. *Antineoplastics* and *antiretroviral antinucleosides* (azidothymidine) induce megaloblastosis by perturbing DNA synthesis.

Cellular Consequences of Perturbed One-Carbon Metabolism

In either cobalamin or folate deficiency, a net decrease in methylene-THF interrupts the reaction mediated by thymidylate synthase, which converts deoxyuridine monophosphate (dUMP) to deoxythymidine monophosphate (dTMP). Because of decreased dTMP (and eventually deoxythymidine triphosphate [dTTP]), dUMP is converted to deoxyuridine triphosphate (dUTP), which is then misincorporated into DNA by DNA polymerase. An editorial enzyme, DNA uracil glycosylase, recognizes this misincorporation and excises dUTP; however, with persistently low dTTP, the DNA strand is not repaired. Repetition of this cycle results in repeated DNA strand breaks and, ultimately, fragmentation of DNA, which then leaks out of the cell. Defective DNA synthesis also leads to additional epigenetic changes, such as altered sensitivity of folate-sensitive fragile sites, acetylation and methylation of histones, and numerous chromosomal abnormalities, that cause progressive nuclear-cytoplasmic asynchrony as a cobalamin- or folate-deficient cell divides, thereby resulting in classic megaloblastic changes in all proliferating cells (hematopoietic cells and epithelial cells in the gastrointestinal tract, cervix, vagina, and uterus).

Clinical Manifestations

The finding of macrocytosis on a routine complete blood count may be the first clinical manifestation. In other patients, the findings may be dominated by the condition that caused the deficiency of cobalamin or folate, such as malabsorption, alcoholism, or malnutrition (see Table 170–1).

The clinical manifestations of folate deficiency may involve the hematologic (pancytopenia with megaloblastic marrow), cardiopulmonary (secondary to anemia), gastrointestinal (megaloblastosis with or without malabsorption), dermatologic (hyperpigmentation of the skin and premature graying), genital (megaloblastosis of the cervical epithelium), infertility (sterility), and psychiatric (with primarily a flat affect) systems. If patients have additional neurologic findings, other diseases that predispose to folate deficiency (alcoholism with thiamine deficiency) or associated cobalamin deficiency must be considered. Because megaloblastosis secondary to either folate or cobalamin deficiency results in functional folate deficiency, the hematologic manifestations of both deficiencies, including pancytopenia with megaloblastic bone marrow, are indistinguishable (see later). However, only cobalamin deficiency results in a patchy demyelination process, which is expressed clinically as cerebral abnormalities and subacute combined degeneration of the spinal cord (Chapter 443). This widespread demyelination begins in the dorsal columns in the thoracic segments of the spinal cord and then spreads contiguously to involve the corticospinal tracts and later the spinothalamic and spinocerebellar tracts. Hematologic manifestations, neurologic manifestations, or both may dominate the clinical picture.

Megaloblastosis can lead to atrophy of epithelial cells lining the gastrointestinal lumen and functional defects (failure of secretion of intrinsic factor and malabsorption of cobalamin and folate). This vicious cycle, whereby megaloblastosis begets more megaloblastosis, can be interrupted only by specific therapy with cobalamin or folate.

In folate deficiency there is increased susceptibility to carcinogenesis and neural tube defects. Moreover, with chronic hyperhomocysteinemia associated with severe cobalamin or folate deficiency (or both), there may be additional clinical manifestations that stem from the fact that homocysteine is a continuous, progressive risk factor for occlusive vascular diseases such as myocardial infarction (Chapter 72), stroke (Chapter 431), vascular disease in end-stage renal failure (Chapter 131), thromboangiitis obliterans (Chapter 79), aortic atherosclerosis (Chapter 78), arterial and venous thromboembolism (Chapters 81 and 182), and placental abruption or infarction. For example, in western India, about 75% of ambulatory subjects have hyperhomocysteinemia consistent with nutritional deficiency of cobalamin alone or with folate and/or pyridoxine deficiency.

Diagnosis

Diagnostic Approach to the Patient

The general approach to a patient with megaloblastic anemia is first to *recognize* that megaloblastic anemia is present; then to *distinguish* whether folate, cobalamin, or combined folate and cobalamin deficiencies have led to the anemia; and finally to diagnose the *underlying disease* and *mechanism* causing the deficiency (see Table 170–1 and Fig. 170–2). Deficiencies of cobalamin and folate are but two of the causes of macrocytosis, although they become increasingly more likely as MCV increases (Table 170–2).

TABLE 170–2 CAUSES OF MACROCYTOSIS BY LEVEL OF MEAN CORPUSCULAR VOLUME

CATEGORY 1: MACROCYTOSIS WITH MCV >110 fL*
Megaloblastic anemia caused by folate or cobalamin deficiency
Megaloblastic anemia caused by drug-induced disorders of DNA synthesis (antineoplastic chemotherapy, immunosuppressive agents, antiretroviral agents)
Myelodysplastic syndromes (especially the 5q– syndrome)
Erythroleukemia (rare)
Inherited disorders affecting DNA synthesis (pediatric age group)
CATEGORY 2: MACROCYTOSIS WITH MCV <110 fL*
Reticulocytosis† secondary to the broad categories of acute blood loss *or* hemolysis
Post-splenectomy status
Hepatic disease with or without alcoholism
Aplastic/hypoplastic anemia, myelophthisic anemia, multiple myeloma
Myeloproliferative disease
Hypothyroidism
Smoking, chronic lung disease

*This table is only a rough guide because there are several exceptions. For example, early stages of diseases in category 1 can be accompanied by smaller rises in MCV to less than 110 fL, whereas some diseases in category 2 such as hemolysis, alcoholism, hepatic disease, or myeloproliferative disease may be associated with folate deficiency and megaloblastic anemia. Furthermore, a combination of causes in category 2 such as hepatic disease or alcoholism (or both) with acute bleeding can result in an MCV greater than 110 fL.
†Marked reticulocytosis could result in an MCV greater than 110.
Note: Cold agglutinins may result in an abnormal high MCV from adherent cells being counted as single cells. Severe hyperglycemia or leukocytosis can also lead to spuriously raised MCV.
MCV = mean corpuscular volume.

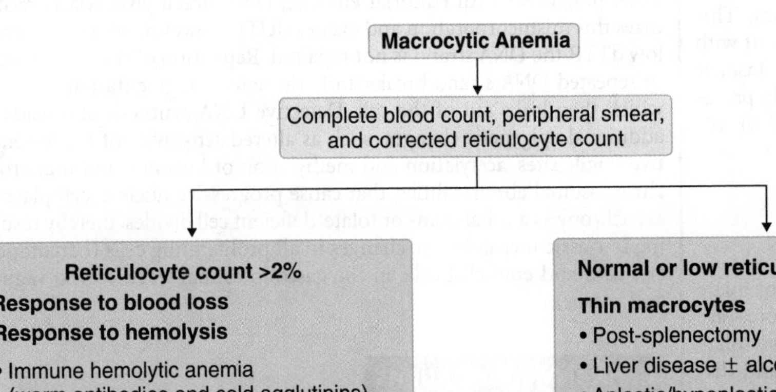

FIGURE 170–2 • Algorithm for evaluation of a patient with macrocytosis.

The underlying condition that predisposed to the development of folate deficiency usually began within the previous 6 months and will often dominate the overall clinical picture. Alcoholism can be identified as the basis for folate deficiency from the history and physical examination, but associated thiamine deficiency may result in a more complex manifestation (e.g., heart failure from cardiovascular disease ["wet beriberi"] and peripheral neuropathy ["dry beriberi"] with Wernicke-Korsakoff syndrome [Chapters 237 and 443]). By contrast, cobalamin deficiency takes several years to become clinically manifested. Therefore, the underlying condition is more chronic and symptoms develop more insidiously, so specific tests will often be required to define the cause.

History and Physical Examination

The dietary history may be revealing (food faddism, vegetarianism, alcohol intake), whereas the medical or family history may uncover blood diseases, gluten sensitivity, autoimmune diseases, epilepsy treated with an anticonvulsant, use of offending drugs, previous hemolytic anemia, a past surgical history (e.g., gastrectomy, fistula, or bowel resection), accidental or surreptitious inhalation of nitrous oxide, or a travel history suggestive of tropical sprue.

Physical examination of cobalamin-deficient vegetarians or those with pernicious anemia may reveal well-nourished individuals. By contrast, patients with folate deficiency are poorly nourished and may have other stigmata of multiple deficiencies from malabsorption (Chapter 143). Associated deficiency of vitamins A, D, and K or protein-calorie malnutrition, or both, may give rise to angular cheilosis, bleeding mucous membranes, dermatitis, osteomalacia, and chronic infections. Varying degrees of pallor with lemon-tint icterus (a combination of pallor and icterus best observed in fair-skinned individuals) are common features of megaloblastosis. The skin may reveal either a diffuse brownish pigmentation or abnormal blotchy tanning. Premature graying is observed in both light- and dark-haired individuals.

Examination of the mouth may reveal glossitis with a smooth (depapillated), beefy red tongue and occasional ulceration of the lateral surface. Thyromegaly may be observed in the neck if there is associated autoimmune disease, but it also raises suspicion for macrocytosis related to hypothyroidism (see later). The characteristic findings of cardiovascular failure from severe anemia may be accompanied by mild splenomegaly and extramedullary hematopoiesis.

In prolonged cobalamin deficiency, neurologic examination will reveal evidence of involvement of the posterior and pyramidal spinocerebellar and spinothalamic tracts. Posterior column dysfunction results in loss of position sense in the index toes (before great toe involvement) (Chapter 443) and loss of the ability to discern vibration of a high-pitched (256 cps) tuning fork. Diminished vibratory sensation and proprioception of the lower extremities are the most common early objective signs. Neuropathic involvement of the legs precedes the arms. Upper motor neuron signs may be modulated by the subsequent involvement of peripheral nerves. A positive Romberg sign and a Lhermitte sign may be elicited. Loss of sphincter and bowel control or involvement of cranial nerves, such as optic neuritis, may accompanied by other dysfunction of the cerebral cortex, including dementia, psychoses, and disturbances of mood. Folate deficiency in adults does not give rise to significant neurologic findings. Thus, the coexistence of folate deficiency with neurologic disease should prompt investigations to exclude cobalamin and other nutrient deficiencies arising from dietary insufficiency or malabsorption.

Nutritional cobalamin deficiency in developing countries can be manifested as florid pancytopenia, mild hepatosplenomegaly, fever, and thrombocytopenia, with the neuropsychiatric syndrome developing as a later manifestation. However, cobalamin-related neurologic disease has also been found in patients with only mild to moderate anemia secondary to cobalamin deficiency in both developing and developed countries. Between 25 and 50% of patients who have neuropsychiatric abnormalities attributable to cobalamin deficiency can have a normal hematocrit and MCV if they have adequate folate stores to protect them from hematologic abnormalities. In fact, in the United States there is often an inverse correlation between the hematocrit and neurologic disease in cobalamin deficiency—most subjects have mild neurologic deficits, and 25% have only moderate deficits with paresthesias or ataxia as the initial symptoms.

Laboratory Tests

Megaloblastosis

To establish the diagnosis of megaloblastosis, the evaluation begins with a complete blood count, MCV (which often reveals a steady increase over a period of several months or years), peripheral smear, and reticulocyte count (see Fig. 170–2). Classic megaloblastosis from cobalamin or folate deficiency may be accompanied by a hemoglobin level of less than 5 g/dL. Neutropenia and thrombocytopenia occur less commonly than anemia and are not usually severe. Occasionally, however, neutrophil counts less than 1000/μL and platelet counts less than 50,000/μL can be seen. Additional abnormalities supporting intramedullary hemolysis include elevated levels of serum lactate dehydrogenase and bilirubin, as well as decreased serum haptoglobin levels.

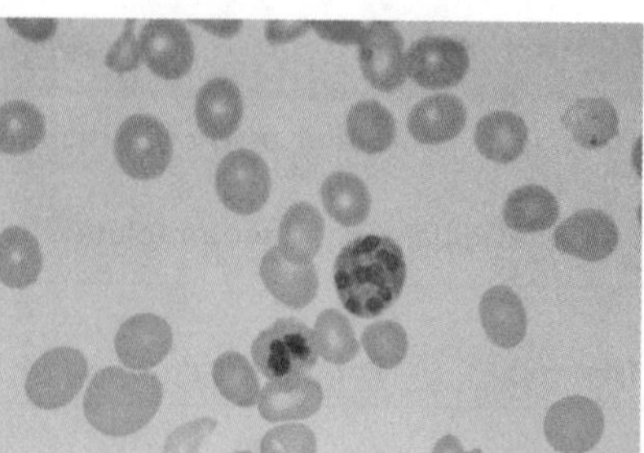

FIGURE 170–3 • Megaloblastic anemia. The peripheral blood has oval macrocytes (large red blood cells) and marked neutrophil hypersegmentation.

Megaloblastic anemia can be masked when there is a coexisting condition that neutralizes the tendency to generate large cells, such as with iron deficiency (Chapter 163) or thalassemia (Chapter 166). In these situations, giant myelocytes and metamyelocytes in bone marrow and hypersegmented neutrophils in bone marrow and peripheral blood (Fig. 170–3) are important clues to a masked megaloblastosis. This problem is clinically relevant because appropriate replacement with cobalamin or folate will elicit a maximal hematologic response only when any associated iron deficiency is corrected. Conversely, if combined iron and cobalamin deficiency (after gastrectomy) or iron and folate deficiency (pregnancy) is treated with iron alone, megaloblastosis will be unmasked. Thus, the diagnosis of megaloblastic anemia should not be excluded until bone marrow aspirates have been examined and the presence of bone marrow iron is established.

Cobalamin and Folate Levels

Laboratory evaluation of suspected cobalamin or folate deficiency begins with measurement of the serum levels of these vitamins and then progresses to confirmatory tests (Table 170–3). Use of clinical information will improve the pretest probability of serum cobalamin and folate levels. Moreover, without detailed clinical information, the combined results of serum cobalamin, folate, and metabolite test results are not sufficiently unambiguous to diagnose and distinguish cobalamin deficiency from combined cobalamin plus folate deficiency.

Serum Cobalamin Levels

A low serum cobalamin level (<200 pg/mL) is a valuable (albeit relatively insensitive) indicator of cobalamin deficiency when compared with metabolite levels. Serum cobalamin is less than 300 pg/mL in 99% of patients with clinical hematologic or neurologic manifestations of cobalamin deficiency, whereas a cobalamin level greater than 300 pg/mL suggests folate deficiency or another cause of macrocytosis (see later) or neurologic disease.

About 90% of older patients with serum cobalamin levels less than 200 pg/mL show evidence of true tissue cobalamin deficiency, but individuals with neuropsychiatric disorders attributed to cobalamin deficiency may not have anemia and may have normal or minimally depressed cobalamin levels. Indeed, mild and usually subclinical cobalamin deficiency has been recognized in up to a quarter of free-living elderly (75 to 80 years of age). The serum cobalamin concentration is falsely low in the absence of true cobalamin deficiency in patients with folate deficiency (in a third of patients), pregnancy, multiple myeloma, transcobalamin I deficiency, or megadose vitamin C therapy or when the serum contains other radioisotopes (e.g., ^{99m}Tc, ^{67}Ga, or ^{125}I) from organ scanning.

A falsely raised cobalamin level in the presence of a true cobalamin deficiency will lead to clinical manifestations if uncorrected. Examples include an artificial increase in transcobalamin I and II, which can occur with myeloproliferative states, hepatomas, and fibrolamellar hepatic tumors; when transcobalamin II–producing macrophages are activated in autoimmune diseases, monoblastic leukemias, and lymphomas; and on release of cobalamin from hepatocytes during active liver disease in

TABLE 170–3 STEPWISE APPROACH TO THE DIAGNOSIS OF COBALAMIN AND FOLATE DEFICIENCY

Megaloblastic anemia *or* neurologic-psychiatric manifestations consistent with cobalamin deficiency
plus
Test results on serum cobalamin and serum folate

Cobalamin* (pg/mL)	Folate† (ng/mL)	Provisional Diagnosis	Proceed With Metabolites?‡
>300	>4	Cobalamin/folate deficiency is unlikely	No
<200	>4	*Consistent* with cobalamin deficiency	No
200–300	>4	*Rule out* cobalamin deficiency	Yes
>300	<2	*Consistent* with folate deficiency	No
<200	<2	*Consistent* with combined cobalamin *plus* folate deficiency or with isolated folate deficiency	
>300	2–4	*Consistent* with folate deficiency or with an anemia unrelated to vitamin deficiency	Yes

TEST RESULTS ON METABOLITES: SERUM METHYLMALONIC ACID AND TOTAL HOMOCYSTEINE

Methylmalonic Acid (Normal = 70–270 nM)	Total Homocysteine (Normal = 5–14 μM)	Diagnosis
Increased	Increased	Cobalamin deficiency confirmed; folate deficiency still possible (i.e., combined cobalamin plus folate deficiency possible)
Normal	Increased	Folate deficiency is likely; <5% may have cobalamin deficiency
Normal	Normal	Cobalamin and folate deficiencies are excluded

*Serum cobalamin levels: abnormally low, less than 200 pg/mL; clinically relevant low-normal range, 200 to 300 pg/mL.
†Serum folate levels: abnormally low, less than 2 ng/mL; clinically relevant low-normal range, 2 to 4 ng/mL.
‡Any frozen-over sample from serum folate/cobalamin determination can be subjected to metabolite tests.

cobalamin-deficient patients. Studies suggest that approximately 10% of the U.S. population, especially the elderly, have true cobalamin deficiency manifested by low or low-normal serum cobalamin levels, as well as elevated levels of serum methylmalonic acid (MMA) and homocysteine that fall to normal with cobalamin therapy.

Serum Folate Levels

When combined with a clinical picture of megaloblastic anemia and additional results of cobalamin levels, serum folate is the cheapest and most useful initial biochemical test to diagnose folate deficiency. Although red blood cell folate levels by microbiologic assay correlate well with hepatic folate stores, they are not widely available, and the newer radioisotopic or colorimetric assays are too unreliable for routine clinical use.

The serum folate level is highly sensitive to the intake of a single folate-rich meal; nutritional folate deficiency first leads to a decline in the serum folate level below normal (<2 ng/mL) in about 3 weeks; thus, it is a sensitive indicator of negative folate balance. If the serum folate level is borderline or normal and the patient has megaloblastic anemia with vitamin B_{12} levels higher than 300 pg/mL, metabolite tests or a therapeutic trial may be necessary to exclude underlying folate deficiency. However, isolated reduction of serum folate in the absence of megaloblastosis (i.e., a false-positive result) occurs in a third of hospitalized patients with anorexia and is likewise seen with acute alcohol consumption, normal pregnancy, and the use of anticonvulsants; because these groups are also at high risk for folate deficiency, additional testing with metabolites or modified therapeutic trials (discussed later) may be required. Conversely, in 25 to 50% of alcoholic abusers (Chapter 31) with folate deficiency, serum folate levels may be low normal or borderline low.

Metabolite Levels

The normal value for serum homocysteine is 5.1 to 13.9 μM, and that for MMA is 73 to 271 nM; these values rise proportionate to the severity of deficiency. Although serum MMA and homocysteine tests are the "gold standard" for the diagnosis of cobalamin deficiency, they are too expensive for initial use. Serum MMA levels are elevated in more than 95% of patients with clinically confirmed cobalamin deficiency (with median values of 3500 nM). Serum homocysteine concentrations are elevated in both cobalamin deficiency (median values of 70 μM) and folate deficiency (median values of 50 μM). Both homocysteine and MMA rise with dehydration or renal failure. Propionic acid, derived from anaerobic fecal bacterial metabolism, can also contribute to MMA values, which can be lowered by metronidazole. Thus, although these metabolites can help distinguish between isolated cobalamin or folate deficiency, an increase in both metabolites cannot differentiate between isolated cobalamin deficiency and combined cobalamin plus folate deficiency. The abnormally high metabolites will return to normal in a week when replaced with the appropriate (deficient) vitamin.

Clinicians can use serum MMA and homocysteine to assist in the diagnosis in patients with (1) borderline cobalamin and folate levels; (2) existing conditions known to perturb folate/cobalamin tests, thereby leading to difficulties in interpreting test results; (3) low levels of both cobalamin and folate, where a high MMA level is useful to confirm cobalamin deficiency (rather than attributing the condition to folate deficiency alone); and (4) low serum cobalamin levels when there is an alternative explanation for the syndrome that led to obtaining a cobalamin level (e.g., a diabetic or alcoholic patient with peripheral neuropathy or an alcoholic patient with a high MCV and a low cobalamin level without anemia). In the context of diagnosing a subclinical deficiency of cobalamin (or folate) based on increased serum MMA or homocysteine (or both) despite normal serum cobalamin (or folate) levels, positive attribution can be made confidently only after demonstrated reversal of laboratory values following treatment with cobalamin (and/or folate).

Peripheral Smear

In peripheral blood, the earliest manifestation of megaloblastosis is an increase in MCV with macro-ovalocytes (up to 14 μm). Nuclear hypersegmentation of neutrophils, diagnosed if greater than 5% of polymorphonuclear leukocytes have five lobes or a single cell has six lobes on the smear (Fig. 170–3), strongly suggests megaloblastosis when associated with macro-ovalocytosis. Macro-ovalocytes (MCV >100 fL) have decreased central pallor, which normally occupies a third of the normal red blood cell. Although macro-ovalocytes and hypersegmented polymorphonuclear neutrophils are the hallmarks of megaloblastosis, macrocytosis is not present in nearly 50% of cases. Moreover, neutrophil hypersegmentation is not sensitive for the diagnosis of *mild* cobalamin deficiency. Furthermore, thin macrocytes that have an increase in central pallor can be found in conditions in which there is reticulocytosis: liver disease, aplastic anemia, myelodysplastic syndromes, multiple myeloma, hypoxemia, and tobacco smoking (see Table 170–3; also see later).

Bone Marrow Examination

In florid hematologic disease with or without neurologic disease suggestive of cobalamin or folate deficiency, identification of nucleated red cells with megaloblastic changes in the peripheral smear—which reflects the morphology in the bone marrow—can clinch the diagnosis of megaloblastosis. If not found, a bone marrow aspirate can be invaluable in assisting in the rapid diagnosis of megaloblastosis (within an hour). However, in the outpatient setting when there is less urgency to make the diagnosis because the anemia is mild to moderate and the patient has a suggestive peripheral smear or when the manifestation is primarily neuropsychiatric, a good case could be made to initiate the sequence of diagnostic tests without bone marrow aspiration by proceeding with measurement of serum levels of vitamins or metabolites (see Table 170–2 and Fig. 170–2).

In a bone marrow aspirate (Fig. 170–4), which is better than biopsy for observing megaloblastosis, the cells are actually proliferating very slowly despite what looks like exuberant cell proliferation with numerous mitotic figures. In early cobalamin or folate deficiency, normoblasts may dominate the marrow, with only few megaloblasts seen, but the full spectrum of megaloblastic hematopoiesis is observed in florid deficiency and is accompanied by varying degrees of pancytopenia. In contrast to the normally dense chromatin of comparable normoblasts, megaloblastic erythroid precursors have an open, finely stippled, reticular, sievelike pattern. The orthochromatic megaloblast, with its hemoglobinized cytoplasm, continues to retain its large sievelike immature nucleus, in sharp contrast to the clumped chromatin of orthochromatic normoblasts. The majority of megaloblastic cells (80 to 90%) die in the bone marrow and are scavenged by macrophages in a process called ineffective erythropoiesis or intramedullary hemolysis. There is an absolute increase in leukopoiesis, with megaloblastic cells also having a sievelike chromatin. Giant (20 to 30 μm) metamyelocytes and "band" forms are pathognomonic for megaloblastosis. Hypersegmented polymorphonuclear leukocytes may be seen in the marrow and peripheral blood. Megakaryocytes may be normal or increased in number and can exhibit complex hypersegmentation with liberation of fragments of cytoplasm and giant platelets into the circulation. The net output of platelets is decreased in severe megaloblastosis.

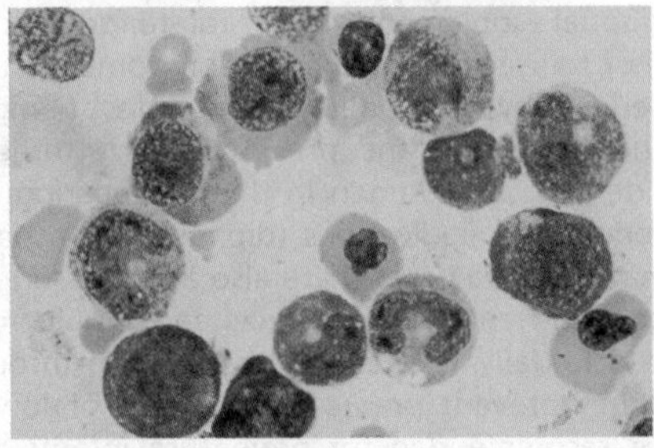

FIGURE 170–4 • Megaloblastic anemia. A bone marrow aspirate shows red blood cell precursors that are giant megaloblasts with nuclear-cytoplasmic dissociation (nuclear maturation lagging behind cytoplasmic maturation). Megaloblastic changes in the leukocyte series are shown by the "giant metamyelocyte."

Determining the Cause of the Vitamin Deficiency

By the time that the megaloblastic state is established, the cause of the folate deficiency is usually clear from the history, physical examination, and clinical setting. With rare exception, adults with cobalamin deficiency have either cobalamin malabsorption (pernicious anemia, malabsorption of cobalamin from food, bacterial overgrowth, or ileal malabsorption) or, in the case of vegetarians, dietary cobalamin insufficiency. All these conditions can be treated similarly with either monthly parenteral cobalamin or daily oral cobalamin. However, it is important to try to determine the underlying mechanism of the cobalamin deficiency because identifying the basis for malabsorption can point to whether additional diagnostic tests (e.g., intestinal biopsy, examination of stool for malabsorption or *D. latum* infestation) and specific therapy (e.g., gluten-free diet, folate, antibiotics, or anthelmintics) are indicated. This evaluation, in turn, indicates whether cobalamin replacement should be lifelong. A positive test result for serum anti–intrinsic factor antibodies confirms pernicious anemia (about 60% of cases); for the remaining 40%, the Schilling test can identify the locus of malabsorption. If a Schilling test cannot be performed, cobalamin deficiency should be treated based on its severity (see later).

The Schilling Test

The Schilling test evaluates the locus and etiology of cobalamin malabsorption (Table 170–4). If the blood contains an excess of cobalamin (Cbl) (from a diagnostic "flushing" injection of cobalamin), greater than 8% of orally administered radiolabeled CN-[^{57}Co]Cbl will be excreted in urine within 24 hours (stage I test). If there is a decrease in endogenous intrinsic factor, as in pernicious anemia, less than 8% will ultimately be excreted; however, if intrinsic factor is given together with CN-[^{57}Co]Cbl, this abnormality will be corrected (stage II test). If usurping of radiolabeled cobalamin by bacterial overgrowth is suspected, previous therapy

TABLE 170–4 INTERPRETATION OF THE SCHILLING TEST

	Material Administered				
Condition	**CN-[^{57}Co]Cbl Plus H_2O—Stage I Test**	**CN-[^{57}Co]Cbl Plus IF—Stage II Test**	**CN-[^{57}Co]Cbl After 7–10 Days of Antibiotics—Stage III Test**	**CN-[^{57}Co]Cbl Plus Pancreatic Extract**	**CN-[^{57}Co]Cbl—Food Cbl Absorption Test (Research Tool)**
Normal	N*†				
Lack of IF	Low*	N			
Usurping of Cbl by bacteria	Low	Low	N		
Pancreatic insufficiency	Low	Low	Low	N	
Lack/bypass of ileal IF-Cbl receptors/ defective transenterocytic Cbl transport	Low	Low	Low	Low	
Inadequate dissociation of food Cbl	N				Low†

*"N" means that the results indicate normal absorption; "low" means that the results indicate less than normal absorption. Cbl = cobalamin; IF = intrinsic factor.
†Patients with food Cbl malabsorption can normally absorb crystallizing CN-[^{57}Co]Cbl but cannot absorb CN-[^{57}Co]Cbl that is bound to food protein.

with either amoxicillin-clavulanate (875 mg twice daily), cephalexin (250 mg four times daily) plus metronidazole (250 mg three times daily), or norfloxacin (800 mg daily) for 7 to 10 days will correct cobalamin malabsorption (stage III test). However, antibiotics will not correct cobalamin malabsorption caused by fish tapeworm infestation or defects involving a net deficiency of intrinsic factor–cobalamin receptors, such as ileal resection, fistulas, diseases of the ileal mucosa, and transcobalamin II deficiency (see Fig. 170–1 and Table 170–1).

The most common cause of an abnormal Schilling test result is incomplete collection of urine, but renal impairment and drugs that interfere with cobalamin absorption must be also considered. Waiting at least 4 months after the administration of other radioactive agents will avoid potential interference with the test result. The Schilling test is never an emergency and should be delayed until after therapy has been given for at least 2 months to reverse any functional cobalamin malabsorption arising from megaloblastosis of intestinal cells.

Treatment

Rx

If the patient is decompensated or decompensation is imminent, after blood is drawn for determination of serum folate and cobalamin levels (and enough for metabolite levels if indicated later) and bone marrow aspiration is performed if needed to confirm megaloblastosis, the patient should be transfused slowly with 1 U of packed red cells and diuretics administered if necessary, and both cobalamin and folate should be started at full doses. *If the patient is moderately symptomatic,* transfusions should be avoided because patients are likely to have a dramatic improvement in well-being within 2 to 3 days of appropriate vitamin replacement, even before hematologic improvement. *If the patient is well compensated or is in the ambulatory setting,* or both, the orderly sequence of diagnostic tests (see Fig. 170–2 and Table 170–3) should precede therapy. Resumption of normal hematopoiesis can lead to an acute reduction in the serum potassium level (1- to 2-mEq/dL drop in 48 hours), which can precipitate potentially fatal arrhythmias; supplemental potassium should be administered *before* therapy is initiated if patients have borderline or low potassium levels, and the potassium level should be monitored carefully, with subsequent replacement therapy given to maintain a normal serum level.

Drug Dosage

Therapy with full doses of parenteral cobalamin (1 mg/day) and oral folate (folic acid) (1 to 5 mg) before knowledge of the type of vitamin deficiency is established should be reserved for severely ill patients. An aggressive scheme to replace cobalamin rapidly is 1 mg of intramuscular cyanocobalamin per day (week 1), 1 mg twice weekly (week 2), 1 mg/wk for 4 weeks, and then 1 mg/mo for life. Because 1 to 2% of an oral dose is absorbed by passive diffusion, even in patients with malabsorption of physiologic cobalamin for any reason, an equally good alternative approach to parenteral maintenance therapy with monthly cobalamin injections is to administer 2-mg cobalamin tablets orally daily after rapidly replenishing cobalamin parenterally. [1] The oral approach is generally preferred by patients and is especially recommended for patients with disorders of hemostasis. In patients with malabsorption of food-bound cobalamin, cobalamin doses of 1 mg/day are required. If there is a question of adherence to a daily cobalamin regimen, the serum cobalamin level can be rechecked periodically. For patients with nutritional cobalamin deficiency without absorptive problems, smaller oral cobalamin doses of 5 to 10 μg, as found in conventional multivitamin tablets, taken for a lifetime of vegetarianism is adequate after repletion of cobalamin stores, either by intramuscular injections or by 2 mg/day of oral cobalamin for at least 3 months.

Oral folate (folic acid) at doses of 1 to 5 mg/day results in adequate absorption despite intestinal malabsorption of physiologic food folate. Therapy should be continued until complete hematologic recovery is documented, and the subsequent duration of therapy is dictated by the etiology.

Folinic acid is of value to bypass the block of dihydrofolate reductase by methotrexate and trimethoprim-sulfamethoxazole. Congenital folate malabsorption arising from inadequate folate

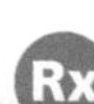

transport across the gastrointestinal tract and blood-brain barrier responds to parenteral leucovorin in high doses.

Modified Therapeutic Trials

Failure to respond to a modified therapeutic trial (1 mg of folic acid orally for 10 days and 1 mg of cobalamin intramuscularly or subcutaneously daily for 10 days) can confirm the clinical suspicion that the patient does not have deficiency of either vitamin. Such a trial is appropriate when there is a clinical suspicion that the underlying disease is *not* due to a vitamin deficiency despite clinical, morphologic, and/or biochemical abnormalities. Examples include a megaloblastic bone marrow that could be secondary to chemotherapy, myelodysplastic syndromes, or acute myeloid leukemia or patients with pregnancy, acquired immunodeficiency syndrome, or alcoholism, when the anemia is likely to be multifactorial. After all such negative trials, bone marrow evaluation is indicated to identify another primary hematologic disease.

Prophylaxis with Cobalamin or Folate

Prophylaxis with cobalamin must be given to infants of cobalamin-deficient mothers, as well as to patients who have undergone total gastrectomy. For vegetarians, prophylaxis with cobalamin, 5- to 10-μg tablets per day orally, should suffice. In malabsorption of cobalamin from food secondary to an inability to cleave food cobalamin by acid and pepsin and in patients maintained on long-term therapy (>5 years) with H_2 blockers or proton pump inhibitors, replacement therapy should be with 1 mg tablets orally each day. In all other conditions involving any abnormality of cobalamin absorption, oral administration of cobalamin tablets containing 2000 μg/day is sufficient to meet daily needs.

Periconceptional supplementation of folate for all normal women (with 400 μg of folic acid per day) and for women who have previously delivered a baby with a neural tube defect (4 mg of folic acid per day) is now standard and prevents nearly three quarters of neural tube defects. [2] Women in the childbearing age who are taking anticonvulsant medications (diphenylhydantoin, phenobarbital, carbamazepine, valproate) are also at increased risk for delivery of babies with neural tube defects and should routinely take 1 mg of folic acid daily. Folate supplementation throughout pregnancy also helps prevent premature delivery of low-birthweight infants and is recommended for premature infants and lactating mothers. Folic acid supplements (1 mg orally daily) are taken by patients with hemolysis or myeloproliferative diseases and reduce the toxicity of methotrexate in patients with rheumatoid arthritis and psoriasis. Individuals in whom cobalamin deficiency develops while undergoing long-term folate replacement will have a pure neurologic syndrome.

In the United States, the mandatory fortification of rice, flour, pasta, macaroni, bread, and cake at 140 μg of folic acid per 100 g of food ensures that women of childbearing age have an increase in folic acid intake of 100 μg/day (≈25% of the recommended daily intake). Follow-up studies indicate a nearly two-fold increase in serum folate values and a reduced incidence of neural tube defects. Unfortunately, most developing countries have not yet instituted comprehensive programs to protect their women from having babies with neural tube defects.

Prognosis

Megaloblastic hematopoiesis reverts to normal rapidly (within 12 hours) and resolves by 48 hours; the only persisting clue may be giant metamyelocytes in bone marrow and hypersegmented neutrophils in blood for up to 14 days. Thus, a single nutritious hospital meal could mask megaloblastosis if the diagnostic bone marrow test is performed later.

The general response to cobalamin replacement is a dramatic improvement in well-being, with alertness, a good appetite, and resolution of a sore tongue. The accelerated hematopoiesis can also increase the serum urate level (peaks by day 4) and precipitate an attack of gout, but prophylactic therapy is not generally advised. The reticulocyte count peaks by days 5 to 8, followed by a rise in the red cell count, hemoglobin level, and hematocrit. By the end of the first week, the white blood cell count rises, sometimes with a transient left shift, as does the platelet count; both normalize by approximately 2 months.

On cobalamin replacement, the degree of reversal of neurologic damage is generally inversely related to the extent of disease and the duration of signs and symptoms. Most neurologic abnormalities improve in up to 90% of patients with documented subacute combined degeneration, and most signs and symptoms of less than 3 months' duration are reversible. With signs and symptoms of longer duration, there is invariably some residual neurologic dysfunction. The maximal response often takes up to 6 months, but recovery beyond 12 months is unusual.

If there is clear evidence for megaloblastic anemia from cobalamin or folate deficiency but there is no response to treatment, the patient may have a combined deficiency that is being treated with only one vitamin. Incorrect treatment of cobalamin deficiency with folate does not improve the neuropsychiatric abnormalities, which will actually continue to progress; hematologic improvements, however, often occur. Alternatively, there may be associated iron deficiency or hypothyroidism that needs replacement or another hemoglobinopathy (such as sickle cell disease or thalassemia) that limits the normalization of hemoglobin values.

In patients with pernicious anemia, subsequent iron deficiency anemia (Chapter 163), osteoporosis (Chapter 264) with fractures of the proximal end of the femur and vertebrae, gastric cancer (Chapter 202), and cancer of the buccal cavity and pharynx can develop. Some experts recommend periodic endoscopic surveillance.

MACROCYTOSIS AND EVALUATION OF MACROCYTIC ANEMIA

The descriptive term *macrocytosis* is used when macrocytes are identified on the peripheral smear and red cell MCV is elevated. Macrocytic anemia describes a macrocytosis associated with a reduction in the hemoglobin concentration. Macrocytic anemias in which the MCV is greater than 110 fL and accompanied by a reduction in central pallor to less than a third of the cell are for the most part induced by an intrinsic interference with DNA synthesis that leads to megaloblastic anemia (see Table 170–2). However, other conditions increase red cell volume but not to an MCV greater than 110 fL.

The first challenge in evaluating a patient with macrocytic anemia (see Fig. 170–2) is to distinguish whether the MCV is increased as a result of reticulocytosis (because reticulocytes are 20% larger than mature red cells) or whether the red cells are morphologically abnormal as a result of either a nonmegaloblastic or megaloblastic anemia. Polychromatophilia of red cells on a routine hematoxylin-eosin–stained peripheral smear implies a high reticulocyte count and suggests either acute blood loss or hemolysis. The reticulocyte count must be corrected to account for premature release of reticulocytes from the bone marrow, a process that is common during intense erythroid hyperplasia. Such prematurely released "shift" reticulocytes are even larger than circulating reticulocytes and may be accompanied by thrombocytosis and leukocytosis during acute blood loss or peripheral hemolysis. If there is no blood loss in a patient with reticulocytosis, evidence for hemolysis followed by specific tests to define the cause of hemolysis should be dictated by the clinical findings (Chapter 164).

A normal or low corrected reticulocyte count could accompany thin macrocytes, which are defined as cells with an increased cell surface but without an increase in volume. The morphology of these thin macrocytes is the result of factors that influence the lipid composition of the erythrocyte membrane. Whereas the target cells that are found in hepatic disease are one form of thin macrocytes, other examples of thin macrocytes can be identified on the peripheral smear as red cells that have an enlarged central pallor that occupies more than a third of the cell. Thin macrocytes are also found in the post-splenectomy state because normal reticulocytes undergo a form of "remodeling" with a loss of membrane lipids during their maturation in the spleen; when this function is lost in the post-splenectomy state, these reticulocytes will mature into thin macrocytes that contain an increase in membrane lipid.

A low reticulocyte count with macro-ovalocytes suggests an underlying megaloblastic anemia that may be associated with teardrop-shaped erythrocytes, anisocytosis, and hypersegmented polymorphonuclear cells with mild leukopenia and thrombocytopenia. Whereas the patient's history can point to a drug-induced cause for perturbed DNA synthesis as a side effect of antineoplastic, immunosuppressive, or antiretroviral therapy, further evaluation of serum folate and cobalamin may also lead to the diagnosis of cobalamin or folate deficiency.

The frequency with which a high MCV is found depends on the patient population studied. Thus, in a U.S. hospital, up to two thirds of cases of macrocytosis (MCV ≥100) can be due to drug therapy (chemotherapy, antiretroviral therapy) or alcoholism and liver disease. By contrast, in a developing country such as India, where a substantial percentage of the population is vegetarian, the major cause would be nutritional deficiency of cobalamin or folate, or both, with an associated iron deficiency possibly resulting in a dimorphic anemia: large red cell distribution width from a mix of macrocytic and microcytic cells.

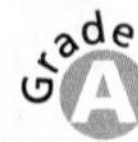

1. Vidal-Alaball J, Butler CC, Cannings-John R, et al: Oral vitamin B12 versus intramuscular vitamin B12 for vitamin B12 deficiency. Cochrane Database Syst Rev 2005;3:CD004655.
2. Berry RJ, Li Z, Erickson JD, et al: Preventing neural-tube defects with folic acid in China. N Engl J Med 1999;341:1485–1490.

SUGGESTED READINGS

Andrès A, Loukili NH, Noel E, et al: Vitamin B_{12} (cobalamin) deficiency in elderly patients. CMAJ 2004;171:251–259. *An excellent review.*

Antony AC: Vegetarianism and vitamin B-12 (cobalamin) deficiency. Am J Clin Nutr 2003;78:3–6. *Emphasizes the equivalence between vegetarianism and poverty-imposed near-vegetarianism.*

Carmel R, Green R, Rosenblatt DS, et al: Update on cobalamin, folate, and homocysteine. Hematology (Am Soc Hematol Educ Program). 2003;62–81. *Discussion of clinical issues related to folate and cobalamin, hyperhomocysteinemia, polymorphisms, and congenital diseases.*

Cherian A, Seena S, Bullock RK, et al: Incidence of neural tube defects in the least-developed area of India: A population-based study. Lancet 2005; 366:930–931. *Highlights the challenge of reducing neural tube defects and neurocristopathies by periconceptional folate supplementation in developing countries.*

Ramaekers VT, Rothenberg SP, Sequeira JM, et al: Autoantibodies to folate receptors in the cerebral folate deficiency syndrome. N Engl J Med 2005; 352:1985–1991. *Identification of a new autoimmune syndrome that may be responsible for preventing folate uptake in the brain in infancy.*

Stabler SP, Allen RH: Vitamin B_{12} deficiency as a worldwide problem. Annu Rev Nutr 2004;24:299–326. *Summary of the problem.*

Wickramasinghe SN: Diagnosis of megaloblastic anaemias. Blood Rev 2006;20: 299–318. *A practical review.*

171 APLASTIC ANEMIA AND RELATED DISORDERS

Hugo Castro-Malaspina and Richard J. O'Reilly

APLASTIC ANEMIA

Definition

Aplastic anemia is a disorder of hematopoiesis characterized by pancytopenia and a marked reduction or depletion of erythroid, granulocytic, and megakaryocytic cells in bone marrow. Hematopoiesis (Chapter 160) is markedly decreased as shown by the near absence of myeloid elements and by the absence or low numbers of CD34 and colony-forming cells in bone marrow. In aplastic anemia, hematopoietic stem cells are unable to proliferate, differentiate, or give rise to mature blood cells and their precursors. In most cases, this failure of stem cells seems to result from an immune mechanism.

Epidemiology

The incidence of aplastic anemia in Western countries is about two new cases per 1 million persons per year. The incidence is higher in Asia, with almost four new cases per 1 million persons per year in Bangkok and rural Thailand. The disease occurs at all ages but is more common in young adults aged 15 to 30 years and in persons older than 60. The incidence is similar in males and females.

TABLE 171–1 CAUSES OF APLASTIC ANEMIA

ACQUIRED
Drugs: antimetabolites, antimitotic agents, chloramphenicol, phenylbutazone, sulfonamides
Radiation
Chemicals: benzene, solvents, insecticides
Viruses: non-A, non-B, non-C hepatitis, Epstein-Barr virus
Paroxysmal nocturnal hemoglobinuria
Miscellaneous: pregnancy, connective tissue disorders
HEREDITARY
Fanconi anemia
Dyskeratosis congenita
Schwachman syndrome
IDIOPATHIC: 50–65% OF CASES

TABLE 171–2 DRUGS ASSOCIATED WITH APLASTIC ANEMIA

Antineoplastic drugs
Antimetabolites: fluorouracil, mercaptopurine, methotrexate
Alkylating agents: busulfan, cyclophosphamide, nitrogen mustard melphalan
Cytotoxic antibiotics: daunorubicin, doxorubicin, mitoxantrone
Sulfonamides and derivatives
Antibacterials: sulfonamides
Diuretics: acetazolamide, chlorothiazide, furosemide
Hypoglycemics: chlorpropamide, tolbutamide
Other antimicrobial drugs
Antibacterials: chloramphenicol, dapsone, β-lactam antibiotics
Antifungals: amphotericin, flucytosine
Antiprotozoals: quinacrine, chloroquine, pyrimethamine, mepacrine
Anti-inflamatory drugs: phenylbutazone, oxyphenbutazone, indomethacin, ibuprofen, naproxen, sulindac
Antiarthritic drugs: gold salts, colchicine
Anticonvulsant drugs: carbamazepine, hydantoins, ethosuximide, primidone
Analgesic drugs: phenacetin, salicylamide, aspirin
Antiarrhythmic drugs: quinidine, tocainide
Antithyroid drugs: carbimazole, methimazole, methylthiouracil, potassium perchlorate, propylthiouracil, sodium thiocyanate
Antihypertensive drugs: captopril, enalapril, methyldopa
Antihistamine drugs: chlorpheniramine, pyrilamine, tripelennamine
Sedatives: chlordiazepoxide, chlorpromazine, lithium, meprobamate
Antiplatelet drugs: ticlopidine

Etiology

Aplastic anemia may occur as the result of inherited abnormalities, such as Fanconi's anemia, but most cases are acquired. Causative factors include drugs, viruses, organic compounds, and radiation (Table 171–1). For more than 50% of patients, however, no cause can be determined. Even when a well-defined association exists between an exposure and the subsequent development of aplastic anemia (e.g., chloramphenicol), it remains unclear why the disease develops in only a small proportion of exposed individuals. Furthermore, the mechanisms by which certain agents or classes of agents (e.g., viruses, drugs) contribute to the pathogenesis of aplastic anemia are still poorly understood.

Drugs

Population-based studies have demonstrated an association between certain drugs and aplastic anemia. Drug-induced aplastic anemia is most commonly caused by anticonvulsants, antibacterial agents, antidiabetic drugs, diuretics, sulfonamides, antimetabolites, antimitotic agents, and synthetic antithyroid drugs (Table 171–2). Many other drugs have been linked to aplastic anemia, but the current data are less convincing. For antineoplastic drugs, antimetabolites, and sulfonamides, the myelotoxicity is dose dependent. For the other agents, however, particularly chloramphenicol, phenylbutazone, oxyphenbutazone, indomethacin, and gold salts, aplasias are idiosyncratic and not dose related. The mechanisms contributing to aplasia are unclear. For example, chloramphenicol can induce a dose-related reversible suppression of erythropoiesis during treatment or an idiosyncratic dose-independent marrow aplasia that develops many weeks or months after cessation of therapy.

Radiation

Acute exposure to total body irradiation causes a dose-related transient marrow suppression that is reversible at low doses but permanent and life-threatening at high doses (Chapter 18). Total body irradiation exceeding 700 to 1000 cGy can induce persistent aplasia by eradicating hematopoietic cells, depending on the radiation energy and dose rate. At a dose exceeding 4000 cGy, the marrow microenvironment in sites of irradiation does not support hematopoiesis. Chronic exposure to low-dose and extensive localized radiation may cause late permanent marrow failure; for example, patients irradiated for ankylosing spondylitis (Chapter 286) have a higher incidence of aplastic anemia. However, the incidence of aplastic anemia has not been increased in long-term survivors of the atomic bombings in Hiroshima and Nagasaki.

Benzene and Insecticides

Benzene, which was the first organic solvent linked to aplastic anemia, has a dose-dependent marrow-suppressive effect. Chronic exposure has been associated with the development of aplastic anemia and leukemias. Benzene and related aryl hydrocarbons may generate catabolites that are directly toxic to stem cells, and they may also induce the formation of haptens that may stimulate immune responses.

Viruses

The most common viral infection associated with aplastic anemia is viral hepatitis (Chapters 151 and 152), with approximately 1 to 5% of cases of aplastic anemia following overt hepatitis. Even though hepatitis A, B, C, and G viruses have been implicated in aplastic anemia in a small number of cases, most cases are not related to these viruses. Although hepatitis viruses may induce lytic infection of primitive hematopoietic stem cells, the remission of aplasia induced by immunosuppressive therapy in a proportion of cases of posthepatitic aplasia has suggested that the immune responses induced by infection may play a central role.

Parvovirus B19, the etiologic agent of exanthema subitum, can cause transient erythroid aplasia in patients with underlying spherocytic anemia and hemoglobinopathy. This virus infects and lyses erythroid progenitor cells. Persistent infection results from an inability to mount an adequate antibody response. Epstein-Barr virus–induced infectious mononucleosis (Chapter 400) is rarely associated with aplastic anemia, and blood counts usually recover spontaneously in most patients. Cytomegalovirus (CMV) infections in newborns and immunocompromised individuals commonly cause neutropenia or thrombocytopenia, or both (Chapter 399). CMV has also been associated with marrow failure, particularly in recipients of marrow transplants. Evidence suggests that certain strains of CMV may infect the bone marrow's stromal cells, which support hematopoietic cell growth, thereby inducing secondary aplasia. Human immunodeficiency virus (Chapter 416) can also suppress erythropoiesis.

Pregnancy

Case reports have documented that aplastic anemia develops during pregnancy in some women. The aplasia has resolved with natural or premature termination of pregnancy in some cases but has recurred with a subsequent pregnancy. The pathogenesis and causal relationship between pregnancy and aplastic anemia remain unknown.

Paroxysmal Nocturnal Hemoglobinuria

Paroxysmal nocturnal hemoglobinuria (PNH) (Chapter 164) is a clonal disease caused by acquired mutations in the *PIGA* gene, which results in partial or complete inability to construct a glycosyl phosphatidylinositol (GPI) anchor for the attachment of membrane proteins such as CD55, CD59, and others. Aplastic anemia can be the initial hematologic manifestation of PNH. Conversely, PNH can develop in patients with aplastic anemia months to years after immunosuppressive therapy. This clinical observation and laboratory studies have shown that a PNH clone can expand in a marrow that is depleted of normal stem cells. A history of thrombosis plus evidence of hemolysis in a patient with an aplastic anemia picture suggests PNH. However, the diagnosis may be difficult to make because the proportion of PNH cells in blood may be too small to be detected by the Ham test; flow cytometric studies using antibodies against cell surface proteins such as CD55 and CD59, which are lacking in PNH, are helpful in establishing the diagnosis.

Other Acquired Causes

Eosinophilic fasciitis (Chapter 447), a rare connective tissue disease characterized by painful swelling and induration of the skin and subcutaneous tissue, has been associated with aplastic anemia. Suppression of marrow function in this condition is thought to be antibody mediated. A similar mechanism has been implicated in the rare case reports of patients with systemic lupus erythematosus (SLE) (Chapter 287) in whom spontaneous aplastic anemia develops. However, patients with SLE and other autoimmune diseases are often treated with anti-inflammatory drugs and gold salts, both of which have been linked to aplastic anemia; as a consequence, the independent role of SLE in the pathogenesis of secondary aplasia is uncertain. In recipients of allogeneic stem cell transplants (Chapter 184), graft-versus-host disease (GvHD) may cause severe marrow suppression. Aplasia has also been documented in rare patients with congenital or acquired immunodeficiency (Chapter 271) and in recipients of organ allografts who have been engrafted with HLA-mismatched T cells derived from nonirradiated blood products or allografts. Certain disorders of the immune system, including thymoma, X-linked lymphoproliferative disorder, and T gamma lymphocyte proliferation, have also been associated with marrow failure. In addition, aplastic anemia may, in rare instances, precede acute leukemia. The hypocellular variant of myelodysplastic syndrome (Chapter 193) may be manifested by clinical and pathologic features that are difficult to distinguish from aplastic anemia.

Pathobiology

The observation that 40 to 50% of syngeneic transplants for aplastic anemia can achieve hematologic reconstitution without pretransplant immunosuppression is consistent with an isolated stem cell defect. Conversely, the fact that the other 50 to 60% of recipients of syngeneic grafts fail to engraft but can achieve hematologic reconstitution if adequate immunosuppression is given before a second transplant strongly suggests that an immune mechanism contributes to the disease. This suggestion is further supported by documentation of autologous recovery in patients who receive allogeneic marrow transplants after immunosuppressive conditioning or antithymocyte globulin (ATG) or cyclosporine (or both). Moreover, the observation that approximately 25% of patients with aplastic anemia are cured by immunosuppressive therapy suggests that in some patients, the disease is due to an isolated reversible immune defect that induces a quantitative deficiency of healthy hematopoietic stem cells. Conversely, the observation that 20 to 30% of patients with aplastic anemia who achieve partial or, less commonly, complete reconstitution of hematopoiesis after treatment with ATG or cyclosporine (or both) contract a clonal disease, either PNH (10 to 13%) or a myelodysplastic syndrome (10 to 15%), months to years after completion of immunosuppressive therapy suggests that aplastic anemia develops in these patients as a manifestation of an immune response directed against preexisting abnormal hematopoietic stem cells or that these abnormal hematopoietic stem cells preferentially recover after immunosuppressive therapy.

In vitro studies have confirmed that the pancytopenia in acquired aplastic anemia results from a quantitative deficiency of hematopoietic stem cells, as documented by colony-forming cell assays, long-term marrow cultures, and quantification of marrow cells expressing CD34 antigen. This stem cell deficiency is due to the cytotoxic or suppressive effect of the patient's own T cells, but the nature of the antigen or antigens causing this pathologic immune response and the intimate mechanisms triggering this abnormal response are not known. In vitro studies have also demonstrated that oligoclonal populations of activated cytotoxic T cells derived from the blood and marrow of a significant proportion of patients with aplastic anemia cause a Fas-mediated death of stem cells and that they overproduce T helper type 1 (T_H1)-associated cytokines, specifically interferon-γ and tumor necrosis factor-β, that suppress hematopoietic progenitors. In patients who respond to immunosuppressive therapy, these colony-inhibiting and interferon γ–producing T cells are no longer detected in the marrow. T cells from patients with aplastic anemia kill hematopoietic stem cells in an HLA-DR–restricted manner, via Fas ligand. The most primitive hematopoietic stem cells express little or no HLA-DR or Fas and can therefore escape the cytolytic effect of T cells and then repopulate the marrow after immunosuppressive therapy. As in other autoimmune diseases, certain histocompatibility genotypes, especially within the HLA-DR2 locus, are associated with a predisposition to acquired aplastic anemia. Moreover, polymorphisms of the interferon-γ and transforming growth factor-β_1 genes are associated with an increased risk for acquired aplastic anemia.

Clinical Manifestations

The most common initial symptoms of aplastic anemia are caused by anemia and thrombocytopenia: progressive weakness, fatigue, headaches, dyspnea on exertion, petechia, ecchymoses, epistaxis, metrorrhagia, and gum bleeding. Even when the neutropenia is very severe, infection is rarely an initial symptom. The most frequent physical findings are cutaneous and conjunctival pallor and hemorrhages (petechiae, ecchymoses, and gum bleeding). If the anemia is severe, the patient may be tachycardic and have cardiac murmurs associated with high-flow states. Hepatosplenomegaly and lymphadenopathy are notably absent.

Diagnosis

Diagnostic Evaluation

The diagnosis of aplastic anemia should be considered if a pancytopenic patient has a normochromic, normocytic (or slightly macrocytic), and aregenerative anemia; thrombocytopenia with normal-sized platelets; neutropenia; and no abnormal cells in the leukocyte differential. The absolute reticulocyte count is low because the anemia is secondary to reduced or absent red cell production. Confirmation of the diagnosis requires morphologic and cytogenetic evaluation of the bone marrow.

Bone marrow typically shows numerous spicules with empty fatty spaces and a few hematopoietic cells (Fig. 171–1). The hypocellularity is due to a marked decrease in megakaryocytes and granulocytic and erythroid cells. Lymphocytes, plasma cells, and mast cells are relatively increased and, in severe cases, constitute more than 65% of the cells. Although erythroid cells may exhibit megaloblastic changes, the morphology of marrow elements is generally normal. The presence of overt dysplasia favors the diagnosis of hypocellular myelodysplasia (Chapter 193). Sometimes the cellularity may appear normal because of isolated foci (hot spots) of hematopoiesis. The marrow biopsy allows better assessment of cellularity and permits evaluation for the presence of tumor cells, hairy cells, and fibrosis. Cytogenetic studies are important to distinguish aplastic anemia from myelodysplasia: the presence of clonal chromosomal abnormalities favors myelodysplasia, but a normal karyotype does not exclude it.

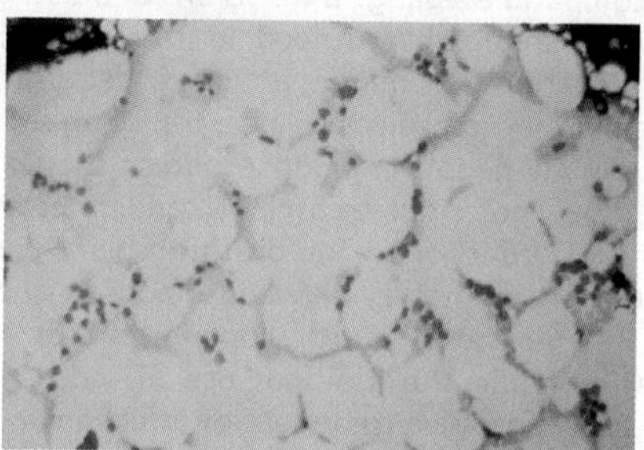

FIGURE 171–1 • **Aplastic anemia.** A bone marrow biopsy specimen shows a virtually empty marrow. (Courtesy of Andrew Schafer, MD.)

Lactate dehydrogenase levels, serum haptoglobin levels, and flow cytometric analysis of peripheral blood cells with antibodies against GPI-linked proteins are useful to establish or exclude the diagnosis of PNH (Chapter 164). In younger patients, cytogenetic studies of marrow cells in the presence or absence of diepoxybutane should be performed because patients with Fanconi's anemia may not have a family history or other clinical findings of the disease.

Differential Diagnosis

Patients with *hypocellular myelodysplastic syndrome* (Chapter 193) also have pancytopenia and hypocellular bone marrow. However, review of blood smears may show the presence of immature granulocytes or nucleated red cells. The few myeloid elements in the marrow have dysplastic changes, and the marrow karyotype may show a clonal abnormality. The differential diagnosis may be difficult when the dysplastic changes are subtle and there are no chromosomal abnormalities. *Hypocellular acute leukemia* (Chapter 194) can be misdiagnosed as aplastic anemia when the few mononuclear cells present in bone marrow are not identified as blasts. Although *hairy cell leukemia* (Chapter 195) is usually manifested as splenomegaly and hypercellular marrow, it occasionally occurs without these features; the diagnosis is established by recognizing the few hairy cells by their typical morphology, as well as by their cytochemical and phenotypic characteristics.

Determination of Severity

Aplastic anemia can be categorized as moderate, severe, or very severe based on the degree of pancytopenia. Severe aplastic anemia is defined by two or more of the following criteria: neutrophils less than 500/mL, platelets less than 20,000/mL, and reticulocytes less than 20,000/mL; these patients have an 80% risk for death by 2 years after diagnosis if treated with supportive care alone. The very severe form meets the aforementioned criteria and in addition has a neutrophil count of less than 200/mL; this very severe form has the worst prognosis, with a lower response rate and poorer survival rate after immunosuppressive therapy. Patients with less profound cytopenia (neutrophils >500/mL, platelets >20,000/mL, and reticulocytes >20,000/mL) are classified as having a moderate form of aplastic anemia.

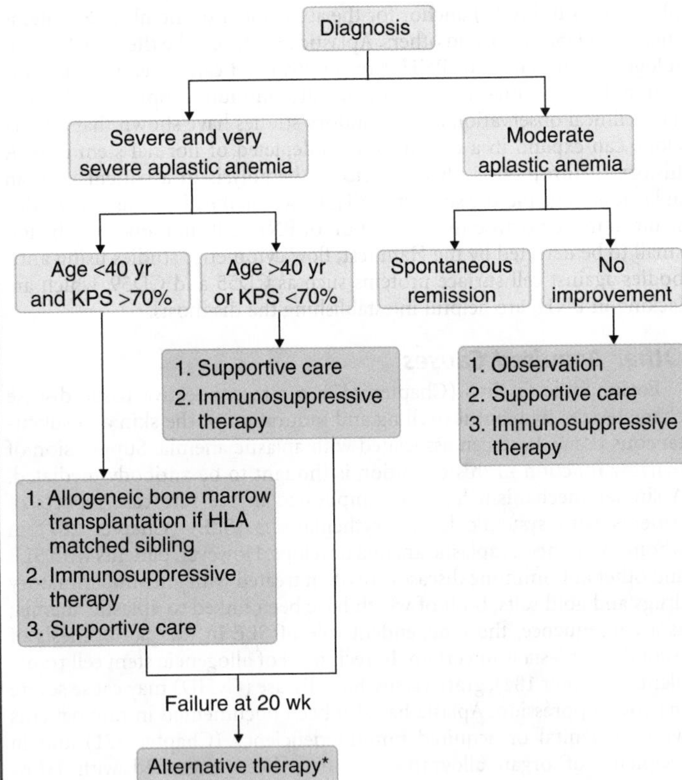

FIGURE 171–2 • Management of aplastic anemia. HLA = human leukocyte antigen; KPS = Karnofsky performance status score. *Alternative therapy includes a second course of immunosuppressive therapy and allogeneic stem cell transplantation from an HLA-matched sibling for older patients and stem cell transplantation from an unrelated donor or a partially matched related donor for younger and older patients who are refractory to immunosuppressive therapies and are also severely thrombocytopenic and refractory to platelet transfusions.

Treatment

Rx

Prompt and aggressive treatment is indicated for most patients (Fig. 171–2). If a specific cause is suspected, withdrawal of the etiologic agent is the most direct approach to treatment. Discontinuation of the suspected drug, thymectomy in patients with thymoma (Chapter 448), and delivery or therapeutic abortion in pregnancy-associated aplastic anemia may result in recovery of blood counts. Aplastic anemia that develops after hepatitis B may resolve if the virus is cleared with antiviral therapy (Chapter 152). Unfortunately, however, remissions are observed in only a small proportion of patients.

Once the diagnosis of aplastic anemia is established, family HLA typing should be performed as soon as possible, particularly in younger patients (<50 years) because these individuals are most likely to benefit from stem cell transplantation from a histocompatible sibling (Chapter 184). Transplantation is a curative treatment, but it is associated with an early mortality risk ranging from 10% in children and young adults to more than 20% in older patients. Transplantation is the preferred therapy in children who have a histocompatible sibling. Transfusions of blood products from family members should be avoided in transplant candidates to prevent sensitization to minor antigens because sensitization increases the risk for graft rejection after transplantation. Whenever possible, only CMV-negative blood products should be given to CMV-seronegative potential transplant candidates to reduce the incidence of CMV infection in the post-transplant period. At diagnosis and during the interval between diagnosis and response to immunosuppressive therapy and allogeneic transplantation, supportive care, including the judicious use of red cell and platelet transfusions and aggressive treatment of infections with parenteral antimicrobial agents, is essential in the treatment of patients with aplastic anemia.

Rx

Immunosuppression is the most common therapy used for aplastic anemia because only 25 to 30% of patients have a histocompatible sibling. In older adult patients, the choice between immunosuppression and allogeneic stem cell transplantation is sometimes difficult because of differences in short- and long-term complications. Immunosuppression has a low early mortality rate (<10%), but it is not curative and carries a 30 to 50% risk for relapse and a 20 to 30% probability of development of a myelodysplastic syndrome or PNH.

Immunosuppressive Therapy

ATG (40 mg/kg/day for 4 days) alone or in combination with cyclosporine (10 mg/kg/day divided into two doses, with dose adjustments as needed to maintain levels of 200 to 400 µg/mL for 3 to 6 months and then tapered over a period of 3 months) is the treatment of choice for aplastic patients who lack a histocompatible sibling or are older than 40 years. Prospective trials have demonstrated that ATG in combination with cyclosporine induces a higher response rate (60 to 80% vs. 40 to 60%) and a more rapid response (median of 60 days vs. 80 days) than ATG alone does, but rates of relapse, development of secondary clonal disease, and survival are similar. [1] Combined ATG plus cyclosporine is recommended for patients with the severe and very severe forms of aplastic anemia, whereas ATG alone is often used for patients with moderate aplastic anemia.

The exact mechanism for the response to immunosuppressive therapy in patients with aplastic anemia is unclear. The licensed ATG preparations contain purified and concentrated IgG from hyperimmune sera derived from horses or rabbits immunized with human thymocytes or thoracic duct lymphocytes. These antibodies may delete an abnormal clone of T cells. Cyclosporine induces immuno-

Rx

suppression by inhibiting the first phase of T-cell activation. Response to immunosuppressive therapy is slow and progressive and may not be detected until 12 weeks after administration. Response rates and post-treatment survival correlate with severity of the disease; patients with very severe forms have a lower response rate.

Of the 60 to 80% of patients responding to immunosuppression, about 20 to 30% achieve a complete and durable recovery of blood counts. The other 50 to 70% achieve a partial response and become transfusion independent with platelet counts exceeding 20,000/mL and neutrophil counts exceeding 500/mL. About 10 to 40% of responders to immunosuppressive therapy require chronic immunosuppression with cyclosporine therapy to maintain adequate blood counts.

Of the 20 to 40% of patients who fail to respond to an initial course of combined immunosuppressive therapy with ATG and cyclosporine, about 75% may respond to second course of immunosuppression with rabbit ATG and cyclosporine. Similarly, 30 to 50% of patients who initially respond to immunosuppressive therapy later relapse, particularly if they have achieved only a partial response. Retreatment with a second course of immunosuppressive therapy can induce a second response in more than 50 to 75% of patients.

Overall, the quality of the initial response is a strong predictor of ultimate outcome. Of patients who achieve a complete remission, 90% survive event free. In contrast, only 50 to 60% of patients who have partial responses or relapse survive 5 years.

Major long-term complications of immunosuppressive therapy include the development of overt myelodysplastic syndrome or PNH in 20 to 30% of patients many months to years after therapy; both are markedly more frequent in patients who achieve only a partial response. ATG is associated with a higher incidence of secondary solid tumors, similar to what is observed in patients who have aplastic anemia and are prepared for allogeneic stem cell transplantation with radiation-containing regimens. Whether there is an increase in the incidence of solid tumors in patients treated with more intensive immunosuppression remains to be determined.

High-dose cyclophosphamide (50 mg/kg/day for 4 days) has also been used successfully to treat patients with aplastic anemia who lack a suitable donor, but experience with this approach is limited. In a prospective randomized trial, a standard course of ATG plus cyclosporine was better than cyclophosphamide plus cyclosporine, which caused more toxicity, fungal infections, and deaths. Although very high-dose corticosteroids (10 to 20 mg/kg) can induce responses in a small proportion of patients with aplastic anemia, corticosteroids are no longer used as single agents because of their side effects and the better response rates achieved with ATG and cyclosporine. Treatment with androgens is not beneficial in aplastic anemia.

Allogeneic Hematopoietic Stem Cell Transplantation

Hematopoietic stem cell transplantation from an HLA-compatible sibling is curative in patients with aplastic anemia (Chapter 184). Unfortunately, this approach is applicable only to a minority of patients because the proportion who have an HLA-matched sibling is on the order of 25 to 30%. Current survival rates are about 70 to 90%.

The preparative regimen that is currently considered the standard of care for allogeneic transplantation in patients with aplastic anemia consists of pretransplant immunosuppression with high-dose cyclophosphamide and ATG, followed by post-transplant immunosuppression with cyclosporine and methotrexate as prophylaxis against GvHD. Marrow transplants from HLA-matched siblings administered with this regimen are associated with a low (<5%) incidence of graft failure and a 30 to 50% incidence of grade III/IV acute GvHD; the long-term survival rate is up to 90% at 2 years after transplantation.

Marrow or peripheral blood stem cell transplants from a related single HLA allele–mismatched donor or from an HLA-matched unrelated donor are an accepted form of therapy for aplastic anemia when patients have no histocompatible siblings, have failed immunosuppressive therapy, and are refractory to platelet transfusions. Transplants from such donors are associated with a higher incidence of acute and chronic GvHD, as well as a high incidence of transplant-related complications. As a result, the usually reported survival rates (30 to 50%) have not been as good as those achieved after HLA-matched sibling transplants. Nevertheless, these survival rates are superior to those seen in otherwise refractory patients maintained on supportive therapy. The outcome of unrelated donor transplants has improved as a result of the use of less toxic preparative regimens and better selection of donors by high-resolution DNA-based HLA typing.

Supportive Therapy

Red cell and platelet transfusions should be used with caution because of short- and long-term complications. The risk of bleeding should be carefully assessed, and platelet transfusions should be given only when the platelet count is less than 10,000/mL or if there is active bleeding with a higher platelet count (Chapter 183). Pooled-donor platelets are generally used until sensitization occurs. Ideally, single-donor platelets should be used from the beginning to minimize the risk for sensitization, but in practice this alternative is difficult to implement. Refractoriness to platelet transfusions is a major problem with long-term transfusion support; such patients may require HLA-compatible platelet transfusions. Menstruating patients should be placed on a regimen of suppressive doses of birth control pills to avoid severe blood loss.

Packed red cells should also be transfused when the hemoglobin concentration is less than 7 g/dL. Younger patients may tolerate lower values, whereas a higher threshold may be clinically indicated in older patients. To reduce sensitization, packed red cells should be filtered to remove leukocytes and platelets. Chronic administration of red cell transfusions results in secondary hemochromatosis because each unit has approximately 200 to 250 mg of iron. Serum ferritin values should be monitored, and chelation therapy with deferoxamine should be given to treat iron overload (Chapter 231).

Patients with aplastic anemia in whom sepsis or other severe bacterial or fungal infections develop require intensive treatment with parenteral antibacterial and antifungal agents (Chapter 303). Leukocyte transfusions are indicated only in severely neutropenic (<200/mL) patients who have documented fungal or bacterial infections that are caused by organisms resistant to first-line antifungal or antibacterial therapy. Prophylactic use of antibiotics in afebrile neutropenic patients has no benefit and increases the emergence of resistant strains.

A common drawback to immunosuppressive treatment is that recovery of blood counts does not occur until 12 to 16 weeks after ATG treatment. The resulting significant early mortality is usually due to infections. Hematopoietic growth factors, particularly granulocyte colony-stimulating factor (G-CSF), may stimulate more rapid correction of severe neutropenia. However, when patients with aplastic anemia have been maintained on long-term G-CSF, the long-term incidence of myelodysplastic syndromes with clonal chromosomal abnormalities is increased.

When used as first-line therapy, recombinant hematopoietic growth factors improve blood counts, particularly the neutrophil count, in only a small proportion of patients. Unfortunately, these increments are entirely dependent on the presence of residual hematopoietic progenitors, so patients with very severe neutropenia (<200/mL) rarely respond to growth factors. In patients who do respond, blood counts drop to pretreatment values after discontinuation of growth factor administration.

Prognosis

The pancytopenia of aplastic anemia is progressive and life-threatening. The prognosis at diagnosis is closely correlated with the severity of neutropenia. The risk for infection (mainly bacterial and fungal) and associated mortality is high in patients with very severe aplastic anemia.

HLA-matched related bone marrow transplantation is curative in 80 to 90% of patients, but it carries a substantial risk for early morbidity and mortality (Chapter 184). Furthermore, a proportion of long-term survivors may have chronic GvHD. In contrast, immunosuppressive therapy has fewer early risks and can induce at least partial remission in 60 to 80% of patients. However, it is not curative, so a large proportion of patients may relapse and secondary clonal diseases can develop. The success of allogeneic bone marrow transplantation correlates with age and degree of matching. The upper age limit for marrow transplantation continues to increase as better approaches are developed to prevent or treat transplant-related complications. However, allogeneic bone marrow transplantation should be used as first-line of therapy only in younger patients. There is no consensus regarding the definition of a younger patient, but it is well accepted that patients who are younger than 20 years and who have an HLA-matched sibling should undergo allogeneic stem cell transplantation. It is also well accepted that patients older than 50 years should be treated with immunosuppressive therapy. Patients who do not respond to immunosuppression can be maintained with supportive therapy, but their prognosis is poor. Transplants from partially matched family members or matched unrelated donors are an increasingly effective option for these patients. However, at this time, the higher rates of transplant-associated morbidity and mortality with such grafts continue to argue against their use in the front-line management of severe aplastic anemia.

FANCONI'S ANEMIA AND OTHER CONGENITAL CYTOPENIA

Fanconi's anemia is an autosomal recessive disorder characterized by progressive pancytopenia, diverse congenital abnormalities, enhanced chromosomal fragility or cellular hypersensitivity to mutagenic chemicals, and an increased predisposition to acute myelogenous leukemia and epithelial cancers, particularly of the head and neck and genitourinary system. Cells from patients with Fanconi's anemia are uniquely hypersensitive to the clastogenic effect of DNA cross-linking agents such as diepoxybutane and cyclophosphamide; the increased chromosomal breakage resulting from exposure to diepoxybutane establishes the diagnosis. At least 12 complementation groups are now recognized within the spectrum of Fanconi's anemia. The genes affected by mutations corresponding to 11 of these complementation groups (FANC A, B, C, D1, D2, E, F, G, J, L, and M) have been mapped and cloned, and their respective coded proteins have been characterized. It is now recognized that in response to DNA damage and during the S phase of the normal cell cycle, a complex of eight of these gene products (FANC A, B, C, E, G, L, and M) is formed and catalyzes the monoubiquitination of another Fanconi's anemia protein, FANC D2. After monoubiquitination, FANC D2 relocalizes from a soluble nuclear compartment to foci on the chromatin, where it promotes the loading and colocalization of FANC D1 (now recognized to be identical to BRCA2) to form stable complexes of FANC D1 and D2, as well as BRCA1, on damaged chromatin. Current studies suggest that these complexes may stabilize broken replication forks and thereby foster efficient homologous recombination through the DNA repair protein RAD51. Another protein in this chromatin-bound complex, BRCA1, also contributes to DNA repair, and mutations in an associated helicase, BACH1, have recently been proposed as the basis for FANC J. Defects in any of the Fanconi anemia–associated genes forming the initial seven protein complexes or in the later proteins in this pathway will result in chromosome instability and enhanced sensitivity to DNA breakage induced by alkylating agents—the distinctive diagnostic feature of Fanconi's anemia.

The mechanisms whereby these gene mutations induce aplasia are still unclear. However, the limitations to efficient DNA repair associated with these defects may limit the ultimate replicative potential of hematopoietic stem cells, thereby predisposing them to depletion or malignant transformation. Specific mutations within the common variant of Fanconi's anemia, type C, are associated with earlier onset of severe aplasia. In addition, Fanconi type G and specific mutations of type A are associated with a particularly high risk for secondary myelodysplasia and acute myelogenous leukemia.

Clinical Manifestations

The most widely recognized features include short stature, cafe au lait spots, kidney and urinary tract abnormalities, microphthalmos, mental retardation, and skeletal abnormalities, most often affecting the thumb and radius. However, many patients with Fanconi's anemia have no morphologic abnormalities, with anemia or progressive aplasia being the only manifestation of disease.

Diagnosis

Patients with Fanconi's anemia are now most commonly detected early in life in families of known predisposition, at which time they may have normal hematologic indices, mild anemia, or neutropenia. The diagnosis is generally obvious from the pancytopenia and typical associated features.

Treatment

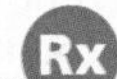

Initially, up to 75% of patients with moderate to severe Fanconi's anemia may attain improved hemoglobin levels when treated with androgens, with or without corticosteroids. However, long-term androgen use in these patients is associated with significant complications, including hepatocellular carcinoma. Prompt improvements in neutrophil counts have also been observed with G-CSF or granulocyte-macrophage colony-stimulating factor (GM-CSF), and daily to three times–weekly doses of these cytokines can sustain neutrophil counts for many months. However, once pancytopenia develops, these cytokines are rarely effective.

Currently, allogeneic hematopoietic cell transplantation (Chapter 184) is the only curative treatment of Fanconi's anemia. It is the treatment of choice for patients with HLA-matched related donors, in whom long-term survival rates are 70 to 90%. Transplants of T cell–depleted hematopoietic progenitor cell grafts from partially matched related and unrelated donors administered after conditioning based on the immunosuppressive activity of the antimetabolite fludarabine have resulted in extended disease-free survival rates of 75 to 82%.

Although a hematopoietic stem cell graft can cure aplasia and prevent the subsequent development of myelodysplastic syndrome or acute myelocytic leukemia, the increased risk for solid tumors remains. Indeed, squamous cell carcinoma of the head and neck has developed in more than 25% of patients with Fanconi's anemia after successful stem cell transplantation. A high proportion of these tumors are associated with the human papillomavirus (Chapter 396), so trials are under way to test whether vaccination of the donor before transplantation and the host after transplantation can reduce this risk. The possibility of gene therapy for Fanconi's anemia is also being explored.

DYSKERATOSIS CONGENITA

Aplastic anemia also develops in a majority of patients with dyskeratosis congenita, a rare genetic disorder clinically characterized by the triad of skin hyperpigmentation, dystrophic nails, and oral leukoplakia.

Pathobiology

Autosomal dominant as well as autosomal and X-linked recessive forms are recognized. The X-linked form is ascribed to mutations in the *DKCI* gene encoding dyskerin, a protein contributing to telomere maintenance and the function of ribosomes. The autosomal dominant form is due to mutations in the RNA component of telomerase. These mutations result in deficiencies in the activity of telomerase, which catalyzes repair of telomeres at the end of chromosomes in germ cells and stem cells of different lineages after each cell division. Such deficiencies may result in an abnormal and progressive shortening of telomeres, thereby limiting the progenitor cell's ultimate proliferative potential. In patients with dyskeratosis congenita, the degree of shortening is directly correlated with the severity of clinical manifestations. The autosomal dominant form is characterized by the phenomenon of "disease anticipation," in which the severity of clinical manifestations increases and occurs earlier in successive generations. Average age-adjusted telomere lengths are also shorter in children of affected probands.

Clinical Manifestations

The typical pancytopenia, skin pigmentation, dystrophic nails, and oral leukoplakia are often associated with short stature; structural abnormalities of the gastrointestinal, genitourinary, and pulmonary systems; and a predisposition to myelodysplastic syndrome, acute myelocytic leukemia, and epithelial malignancies. The diagnosis is usually clear from the characteristic clinical findings.

Treatment

Rx

The cytopenia in dyskeratosis congenita can be treated for varying periods with androgens, erythropoietin, G-CSF or GM-CSF, and transfusion support. However, progressive aplasia commonly requires hematopoietic cell transplantation from a normal HLA-compatible related or unrelated allogeneic donor, which can provide full and durable reconstitution of normal hematopoiesis.

SCHWACHMAN-DIAMOND SYNDROME

Schwachman-Diamond syndrome is a rare autosomal recessive disorder characterized by exocrine pancreatic insufficiency, short stature, and neutropenia. More than 36% of cases progress to aplastic anemia, myelodysplasia, or overt acute myelocytic leukemia by the age of 30 years. In most (80%) but not all cases, the disease has been ascribed to mutations in the Schwachman-Bodian-Diamond gene, which is located on 7q11 and produces a protein that is concentrated in pseudopods and may contribute to normal chemotaxis. Most patients have significant neutropenia and defective chemotaxis of phagocytes. Treatment with G-CSF (5 µg/kg/day subcutaneously) corrects the neutropenia in most patients, and long-term treatment must be continued. For patients in whom aplastic anemia, myelodysplastic syndrome, or acute myelocytic leukemia develops, the only curative option is hematopoietic cell transplantation from a normal HLA-compatible allogeneic donor. Recent results of marrow and cord blood transplants, mostly from unrelated donors, indicate an extended disease-free survival rate of 64%.

PURE RED CELL APLASIA

Pure red cell aplasias (PRCAs) are rare disorders that selectively affect the growth and differentiation of erythroid precursors in bone marrow. Affected patients have varying degrees of anemia. Myeloid, megakaryocytic, and lymphoid lineages appear normal. Several distinctive forms of red cell aplasia are recognized, including a congenital form, Blackfan-Diamond anemia, which is usually diagnosed at or shortly after birth, and acquired forms, which may have their onset at any time but are generally first detected in older children and adults.

Blackfan-Diamond Anemia

Blackfan-Diamond anemia is a rare form of hypoplastic anemia characterized by intrinsic abnormalities in erythroid progenitor differentiation that result in varying degrees of normochromic or macrocytic anemia, elevated levels of red cell adenosine deaminase and hemoglobin F, and either absence or severely reduced erythroid elements in the marrow. A family history consistent with an autosomal dominant disorder is detected in 10 to 20% of cases.

Pathobiology

Approximately 25% of all patients, particularly those with the autosomal dominant form, have mutations involving a gene termed *DBA1* or *RPS19*, which is located on chromosome 19q13.2 and encodes the ribosomal protein S19. Mutations in another as yet uncloned gene, termed *DBA2* and mapped to 8p23-22, have been implicated in an additional 35% of patients. An etiologic role for *RPS19* mutations is suggested because transduction of $CD34^+$ marrow progenitor cells from these patients with a retroviral vector encoding a normal gene for the S19 protein increases the formation of normal erythroid colonies in vitro by over three-fold.

Clinical Manifestations

This disorder is also associated with craniofacial dysmorphologies, malformations of the thumb or upper limbs, atrial or ventricular septal defects of the heart, and abnormalities of the urogenital system.

Diagnosis

The diagnosis is usually obvious from the characteristic clinical manifestations.

Treatment

The severity of anemia is variable. Approximately 80% of affected patients achieve partial or full remission when treated with low-dose steroids (prednisone, 2 mg/kg/day until hemoglobin increases to 10 g/dL, followed by a slow taper to alternate-day doses needed to sustain the hemoglobin level), and about 15% sustain remission off steroids. The survival rate at age 40 is 100% for patients achieving a sustained remission and 75% for those who can be maintained on steroids. However, for patients with severe or steroid-refractory anemia, only 57% survive to age 40. In phase II trials, 15 to 30% of such patients have achieved partial or complete remissions when treated with interleukin-3 (5 to 10 µg/kg/day subcutaneously) or with the prolactin-inducing drug metoclopramide (10 mg orally three times per day for 4 months). In contrast, erythropoietin is ineffective. In approximately 2% of patients leukemia ultimately develops. Stem cell transplantation from an HLA-matched sibling administered after myeloablative and immunosuppressive conditioning can reconstitute normal donor-derived hematopoiesis and provide about a 75% disease-free survival rate at 3 to 5 years after transplantation. Unfortunately, the disease-free survival rate after transplants from unrelated or HLA-disparate related donors is still poor and ranges from 17 to 39%.

Acquired Forms

Definition and Epidemiology

Acquired PRCA may develop for unknown reasons, but more commonly it develops in association with specific types of malignancy, infection, or drugs. Most commonly, acquired PRCA develops as a complication of a neoplastic process such as a thymoma (Chapter 448), B- or T-cell chronic lymphocytic leukemia (Chapter 195), non-Hodgkin's lymphoma (Chapter 196), or an autoimmune disorder such as rheumatoid arthritis (Chapter 285) or SLE (Chapter 287).

Pathobiology

When PRCA is a complication of lymphoreticular malignancies or chronic Epstein-Barr virus infection, interferon γ-secreting T cells that inhibit erythroid colony growth in vitro can often be isolated from blood or marrow. In patients with B-cell chronic lymphocytic leukemia or autoimmune diseases in whom PRCA develops, antibodies that suppress erythropoiesis have often been identified. In rare instances, these antibodies have been shown to neutralize erythropoietin.

The emergence of T or B cells that are active against erythroid progenitors has also been hypothesized to play an etiologic role in the development of PRCA in patients treated with specific drugs such as phenytoin, chlorpropamide, isoniazid, and azathioprine. However, certain agents, such as chloramphenicol and the antibiotic linezolid, may induce a dose-dependent selective inhibition of red cell production.

Acquired PRCA may also result from a lytic infection of erythroid progenitors by human parvovirus B19, the etiologic agent of fifth disease. Erythroid cells are selectively targeted by virtue of their expression of globoside, the blood group P antigen that is expressed on a proportion of erythroid colony-forming units and all more differentiated erythroid elements. Such infections probably occur in normal individuals, but anemia is not observed because of the rapidity of the immune response and the regrowth of normal erythroid elements. However, in patients with spherocytosis or sickle cell anemia, whose erythroid cell production is already stressed by chronic hemolysis, red cell aplastic crises may develop. Similarly, acquired PRCA may develop after parvovirus B19 infection in patients with acquired immunodeficiency syndrome (AIDS) as a result of impairment in viral clearance ascribable to their immunodeficiency.

Acquired PRCA may also be the first manifestation of a myelodysplastic syndrome (Chapter 193); in this case it is a clonal disorder of erythropoiesis rather than a sequela of a secondary immune response. Consistent with this hypothesis is the low rate of response to immunosuppressive therapy in these patients.

Treatment Rx

Treatment of acquired PRCA is usually suggested by the disorder co-associated with its development. Removal of a thymoma, treatment of an underlying malignancy, or cessation of an instigating drug may induce remission. For patients with autoimmune forms, treatment with prednisone (2 mg/kg/day with a slow taper after remission) generally improves erythropoiesis. Refractory patients may also respond to prednisone combined with cyclosporine (10 mg/kg/day divided into two doses, with dose adjustments to maintain levels of 200 to 400 μg/mL for 3 to 6 months, followed by a taper over a 3-month period) or low-dose cyclophosphamide (2 to 3 mg/kg/day until remission or 3 to 4 months). Studies indicate that the CD20-specific monoclonal antibody rituximab can induce durable remissions in patients whose PRCA is refractory to these agents. In contrast, for patients with parvovirus B19 infection–induced aplasia, brief treatment with high doses of intravenous immunoglobulin (400 mg/kg/day every 3 to 4 weeks) alone usually fosters rapid recovery of normal erythropoiesis by providing significant doses of parvovirus-specific antibody and thereby hastening viral clearance. For patients with AIDS, chronic parvoviremia may necessitate repeated doses of immunoglobulin.

MYELOPHTHISIC ANEMIAS

Deposition of fibrous tissue in bone marrow (myelofibrosis) generally causes leukoerythroblastosis in the peripheral blood (immature granulocytes, nucleated red cells, and teardrop-shaped red cells). This process can occur as a primary hematologic disease, called *myelofibrosis with myeloid metaplasia* (Chapter 177), or as a secondary process, called *myelophthisis,* which is often associated with anemia. Myelophthisis represents a reaction of the marrow tissue to invading tumor cells, infectious agents (particularly mycobacteria or fungi), lipid storage diseases (notably Gaucher's disease [Chapter 223]), or other granulomatous diseases such as sarcoidosis (Chapter 95). Tumors associated with myelophthisis are of both hematopoietic (acute leukemias, chronic myeloproliferative disorders, hairy cell leukemia, Hodgkin's disease, non-Hodgkin's lymphomas, multiple myeloma) and epithelial (breast, lung, prostate, and stomach adenocarcinomas) origin. Myelophthisis can also occur as a result of osteopetrosis (Chapter 269), a congenital disease characterized by failure of osteoclasts to remodel bone, thereby resulting in obliteration of the marrow space with bone and fibrous tissue. Marrow fibrosis results from an overproduction of collagen by marrow stromal cells as a consequence of abnormal concentrations of cytokines produced by tumor cells or inflammatory cells that control collagen metabolism.

The blood smear in myelophthisis is characterized by a normocytic, normochromic anemia with low reticulocyte counts, teardrop-shaped red cells, and circulating erythroblasts. Platelet counts are usually decreased, whereas the granulocyte count, which includes immature forms, is normal or increased. The marrow fibrosis is often associated with extramedullary hematopoiesis and sometimes hepatosplenomegaly. Marrow often cannot be aspirated (dry tap), but biopsy reveals fibrosis. The primary process is generally apparent, but it is extremely important to exclude an infectious cause. Therapy is aimed at the primary cause; infections can be successfully treated, whereas metastatic marrow disease is more difficult to treat.

FUTURE DIRECTIONS

Identification of the genes responsible for dyskeratosis congenita, Fanconi's anemia, and an increasing fraction of Diamond-Blackfan anemia cases permits antenatal screening in affected families, in vitro selection of unaffected conceptuses, and potential gene replacement therapy for affected individuals. The introduction of T cell–depleted transplants and novel nonmyeloablative preparative regimens has improved the results of allogeneic marrow transplants, reduced the risk for transplant-associated mortality, and fostered increasingly effective transplant strategies for patients who lack an HLA-matched sibling donor.

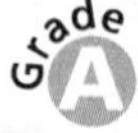

1. Frickhofen N, Heimpel H, Kaltwasser JP, et al: Antithymocyte globulin with or without cyclosporin A: 11-year follow-up of a randomized trial comparing treatments of aplastic anemia. Blood 2003;101:1236–1242.

SUGGESTED READINGS

Brodsky RA, Jones RJ: Aplastic anemia. Lancet 2005;365:1647–1652. *A comprehensive review.*

Federman N, Sakamoto KM: The genetic basis of bone marrow failure syndromes in children. Mol Genet Metab 2005;86:100–109. *A useful review of current information regarding the genetics of congenital aplasia.*

Kahl C, Leisenring W, Deeg HJ, et al: Cyclophosphamide and antithymocyte globulin as a conditioning regimen for allogeneic marrow transplantation in patients with aplastic anaemia: A long-term follow-up. Br J Haematol 2005;130:747–751. *Long term evaluation of a large series.*

Lipton JM, Aatsidaftos E, Zyskind I, Vlachos A: Improving clinical care and elucidating the pathophysiology of Diamond Blackfan anemia: An update from the Diamond Blackfan anemia registry. Pediatr Blood Cancer 2006;46:558–564. *Review of diagnosis, management, and outcomes in the North American registry.*

Yamaguchi H, Calado RT, Ly H, et al: Mutations in TERT, the gene for telomerase reverse transcriptase, in aplastic anemia. N Engl J Med 2005;352:1413–1424. *Mutations were found in 7 unrelated patients among 124 with aplastic anemia.*

Young NS, Brown KE: Parvovirus B19. N Engl J Med 2004;350:586–597. *Overview of the many clinical manifestations, including transient aplastic crisis.*

Young NS, Calado RT, Scheinberg P: Current concepts in the pathophysiology and treatment of aplastic anemia. Blood 2006;108:2509–2519. *An excellent review.*

172 POLYCYTHEMIAS

Ayalew Tefferi

Definition

The word *polycythemia* is derived from the Greek and literally translates as "too many blood cells." However, in conventional terminology, polycythemia refers to either a real (true polycythemia) or spurious (apparent polycythemia) perception of an increase in red blood cell mass. True polycythemia may represent either a clonal myeloproliferative disorder (polycythemia vera) or a nonclonal increase in red blood cell mass that is often mediated by erythropoietin (secondary polycythemia). Apparent polycythemia results from either a decrease in plasma volume (relative polycythemia) or a misperception of what constitutes the upper limit of normal values for either hemoglobin or hematocrit (Fig. 172–1). Occasionally, a true increase in red blood cell mass may be masked by a normal-appearing hematocrit because of a concomitant increase in plasma volume, often accompanied by marked splenomegaly (inapparent polycythemia).

APPARENT POLYCYTHEMIA

Most conditions that cause acute depletion of plasma volume (i.e., relative polycythemia) are clinically obvious (e.g., severe dehydration, diarrhea, vomiting, use of diuretics, capillary leak syndrome, severe burns) and do not require diagnostic confirmation with the use of specialized tests. Conversely, the existence of chronic contraction of the plasma volume, such as postulated for both Gaisböck's syndrome (relative polycythemia associated with hypertension and nephropathy) and stress polycythemia (relative polycythemia associated with emotional stress), is controversial. Accurate reference to the race- and sex-adjusted normal laboratory values should minimize the inappropriate use of the term apparent polycythemia in physiologically normal persons with hemat-

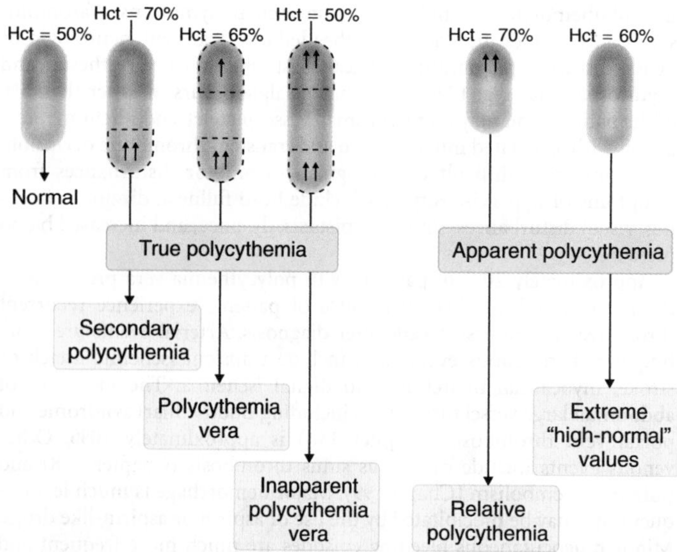

FIGURE 172–1 • Clonal and nonclonal causes of polycythemia. True polycythemia denotes an increase in red cell mass (denoted in blue). Apparent polycythemia is not associated with increased red cell mass and can be caused by contracted plasma volume (denoted in red). Hct = hematocrit.

ocrit values that lie in the upper percentiles of the normal distribution. In such instances, the performance of costly diagnostic tests, including the measurement of red blood cell mass, is unwarranted.

SECONDARY POLYCYTHEMIA

Definition

Secondary polycythemia is classified as acquired or congenital (Table 172–1). In each instance, the serum erythropoietin level is helpful in the differential diagnosis. Erythropoietin is a 35-kD glycosylated protein that is synthesized in response to hypoxia, mainly by the peritubular capillary endothelial cells of the renal cortex by means of an intricate oxygen-sensing mechanism. Erythropoietin acts at both the late burst-forming unit erythroid and colony-forming unit erythroid levels of erythropoiesis (Chapter 160). Stimulants of physiologic erythropoietin production include both anemia and hypoxia. However, secondary polycythemia may or may not be associated with increased production of erythropoietin, and certain cases may not even be mediated by erythropoietin.

Pathobiology

Acquired secondary polycythemia is usually associated with increased erythropoietin production that is either hypoxia driven or hypoxia independent. In the former instance, the hypoxic stimulus is usually central, with cardiopulmonary conditions most responsible. Other causes of central hypoxia include high-altitude (Chapter 94) habitat and carbon monoxide poisoning (Chapter 94). Hypoxia in peripheral tissues is exemplified by the acquired polycythemia associated with renal artery stenosis (Chapter 126). In both central and peripheral hypoxia-driven secondary polycythemia, the serum erythropoietin level, although initially elevated, may fall within the normal reference range after the hemoglobin level has stabilized at a higher level. By contrast, in erythropoietin-mediated but hypoxia-independent secondary polycythemia, the serum erythropoietin level often remains elevated despite the rise in hemoglobin level. Thus, hypoxia-independent elevation of erythropoietin with an elevated hemoglobin level is also associated with malignant or benign tumors of the liver (Chapter 206), kidney (Chapter 207), uterus, and cerebellum (see Table 172–1). Exogenous administration of drugs such as androgen preparations or erythropoietin itself also causes acquired secondary polycythemia.

Congenital polycythemia can be associated with increased, normal, or decreased serum erythropoietin levels. For example, the serum erythropoietin level is usually increased or normal in the autosomal dominant, high–oxygen affinity hemoglobinopathies (e.g., hemoglobin Chesapeake, hemoglobin Heathrow), the autosomal recessive red cell enzymopathy, 2,3-diphosphoglycerate mutase deficiency (Chapter 164), and the autosomal recessive Chuvash polycythemia that is endemic in Russia and is associated with a von Hippel–Lindau (*VHL*) (Chapter 444) gene mutation.

TABLE 172–1 CLASSIFICATION OF "POLYCYTHEMIA"

1. APPARENT POLYCYTHEMIA

a. Relative polycythemia
b. Extreme "high normal" values

2. TRUE POLYCYTHEMIA

a. Polycythemia vera
b. Secondary polycythemia
 i. Congenital
  1. Associated with high or normal serum erythropoietin level
   (a) Chuvash and other polycythemias associated with von Hippel–Lindau (*VHL*) gene mutation (autosomal recessive)
   (b) High–oxygen affinity hemoglobinopathy (autosomal dominant)
   (c) 2,3-Diphosphoglycerate mutase deficiency (autosomal recessive)
   (d) Pathogenetically undefined cases
  2. Associated with low serum erythropoietin level
   (a) Activating mutation of the erythropoietin receptor (autosomal dominant)
 ii. Acquired
  1. Erythropoietin mediated
   (a) Hypoxia-driven
    (i) Central hypoxic process
     1. Chronic lung disease
     2. Right-to-left cardiopulmonary vascular shunts
     3. High-altitude habitat
     4. Carbon monoxide poisoning
     5. Smoker's polycythemia (chronic carbon monoxide exposure)
     6. Hypoventilation syndromes including sleep apnea
    (ii) Peripheral hypoxic process
     1. Localized
     2. Renal artery stenosis
   (b) Hypoxia-independent (pathologic erythropoietin production)
    (i) Malignant tumors
     1. Hepatocellular carcinoma
     2. Renal cell cancer
     3. Cerebellar hemangioblastoma
     4. Parathyroid carcinoma
    (ii) Nonmalignant conditions
     1. Uterine leiomyomas
     2. Renal cysts (polycystic kidney disease)
     3. Pheochromocytoma
     4. Meningioma
  2. Drug associated
   (a) Erythropoietin doping
   (b) Treatment with androgen preparations
  3. Unknown mechanisms
   (a) Post–renal transplant erythrocytosis

Conversely, the serum erythropoietin level is low in patients with an activating mutation of the erythropoietin receptor gene that results in a C-terminal truncated receptor that is more efficient in signal transduction, possibly because of defective recruitment of regulatory phosphatases.

Finally, in the absence of an identifiable cause, true polycythemia has been termed *idiopathic erythrocytosis.* However, substantial numbers of patients with the latter entity may have early polycythemia vera, congenital polycythemia, or occult secondary polycythemia.

Diagnosis

The serum erythropoietin level does not reliably differentiate among the different causes of secondary polycythemia. If family history suggests a congenital cause, it is essential to measure P_{50} (oxygen pressure at 50%

hemoglobin-oxygen saturation). A low P_{50} value is consistent with either a high–oxygen affinity hemoglobinopathy or a 2,3-diphosphoglycerate mutase deficiency (Chapter 164). A normal P_{50} value in the presence of congenital polycythemia warrants consideration of other causes, such as Chuvash polycythemia or a mutation in the erythropoietin receptor (see earlier).

In acquired secondary polycythemia, initial laboratory tests should include the measurement of arterial hemoglobin-oxygen saturation. In the absence of a central hypoxic state, renal vascular studies should be performed to exclude the possibility of renal artery stenosis (Chapter 126). Evaluation for possible tumors of the kidney (Chapter 207), liver (Chapter 206), and central nervous system (Chapter 199) may be considered when the aforementioned studies are unrevealing or the serum erythropoietin level is persistently elevated. For suspected erythropoietin doping, immunoblotting techniques can differentiate endogenous erythropoietin from exogenously administered recombinant erythropoietin.

Treatment

Rx

Both the frequency and severity of thrombotic and nonthrombotic complications of polycythemia are significantly less in secondary polycythemia than in polycythemia vera. Therefore, if prophylactic phlebotomy is ever recommended, it is reserved for a higher target hematocrit level (≥60%) in secondary polycythemia than in polycythemia vera (40 to 45%). Angiotensin-converting enzyme inhibitors (e.g., enalapril 2.5 to 10 mg/day for 8 weeks) and angiotensin II receptor blockers (e.g., losartan 50 mg/day for 14 weeks) can significantly reduce hematocrit levels in secondary polycythemia that is associated with either renal transplantation or chronic obstructive lung disease by inducing apoptosis in erythroid precursor cells. [1]

POLYCYTHEMIA VERA

Definition

Polycythemia vera is currently classified with both essential thrombocythemia and myelofibrosis with myeloid metaplasia as the third *BCR/ABL*-negative, classic myeloproliferative disorder (Chapter 177). Accordingly, polycythemia vera is a clonal stem cell disease with growth factor–independent erythroid proliferation that results not only in increased red blood cell mass, but also in thrombocytosis and leukocytosis in a substantial number of patients.

Epidemiology

Population-based epidemiologic studies suggest a stable prevalence of polycythemia vera at approximately 2.3 per 100,000 population. A higher incidence has been suggested in persons of Ashkenazi Jewish ancestry, but no known environmental exposures have been implicated. Median age at diagnosis is approximately 60 years, with a slight male preponderance. Approximately 7% of cases are diagnosed in patients less than 40 years old, and rare cases have occurred in children.

Pathobiology

Polycythemia vera is a clonal stem cell disease that is not only erythropoietin independent but also hypersensitive to insulin-like growth factor-I, interleukin-3, granulocyte-monocyte colony-stimulating factor, stem cell factor, and thrombopoietin. All these abnormalities may be related to an activating mutation of the *JAK2* kinase gene that has recently been described in 65 to 97% of patients with polycythemia vera. The $JAK2^{V617F}$ mutation occurs within the autoinhibitory JH2 domain (pseudokinase domain) of the gene, so the oncogenic mechanism is thought to involve dysregulation of the kinase activity that resides in the catalytically intact JH1 domain. In mice, this mutant allele induces hypersensitivity to erythropoietin and, as a result, erythrocytosis.

Clinical Manifestations

More and more cases of polycythemia vera are diagnosed at an asymptomatic stage based on routine blood counts. When symptoms are present (Table 172–2), they fall into three major categories: vasomotor, thrombohemorrhagic, and other nonvascular symptoms. Vasomotor symptoms include headache, lightheadedness, transient neurologic or ocular disturbances, tinnitus, atypical chest discomfort, paresthesias, and erythromelalgia (Fig. 172–2). Erythromelalgia occurs in fewer than 5% of the patients and may represent small vessel platelet-endothelium interaction with associated inflammation and transient thrombotic occlusion. It is sometimes difficult to distinguish vasomotor disturbances from symptoms of hyperviscosity that include head fullness, dizziness, flushing, visual disturbances, tinnitus, epistaxis, dyspnea, and increased blood pressure.

Approximately 20% of patients with polycythemia vera present with thrombosis, and another 20 to 30% of patients experience recurrent thrombosis in the first decade after diagnosis. Arterial events are more frequent than venous events and include transient ischemic attack or stroke, myocardial infarction, and digital ischemia. The incidence of abdominal large vessel thrombosis including Budd-Chiari syndrome and portal vein thrombosis (Chapter 146) is approximately 10%. Other venous events include cavernous sinus thrombosis (Chapter 438) and pulmonary embolism (Chapter 99). Major hemorrhage is much less frequent but may be precipitated by the use of aspirin or aspirin-like drugs. Minor mucocutaneous bleeding episodes are much more frequent and include epistaxis, gingival bleeding, and ecchymoses.

Nonvascular symptoms include pruritus and hypercatabolic symptoms. Pruritus (Chapter 461), which is often exacerbated by water contact (aquagenic), occurs in more than 50% of patients with polycythemia vera and may be sufficiently severe to prevent patients from taking daily showers. Hypercatabolic symptoms include weight loss, fatigue, diaphoresis, and night sweats. Patients may present with peptic ulcer symptoms or toe or joint pain secondary to gouty arthritis (Chapter 294).

A patient with untreated polycythemia vera may display plethora or ruddiness (a red and congested facial complexion), palmar erythema, and sausage-shaped distention of retinal veins. Palpable splenomegaly (Chapter 174) occurs in approximately 70% of patients and may be associated with early satiety. Laboratory findings may include leukocytosis (20 to 43%), thrombocytosis (48 to 63%), microcytosis (50 to 80%), and increased serum levels of uric acid, lactate dehydrogenase (a general indicator of high cell turnover), vitamin B_{12}, and vitamin B_{12} binding capacity. The leukocyte alkaline phosphatase score is often elevated.

TABLE 172–2 POLYCYTHEMIA VERA–RELATED CLINICAL AND LABORATORY FEATURES

Persistent leukocytosis
Persistent thrombocytosis
Microcytosis secondary to iron deficiency
Increased leukocyte alkaline phosphatase
Splenomegaly
Generalized pruritus (usually after bathing)
Unusual thrombosis (e.g., Budd-Chiari syndrome)
Erythromelalgia (acral dysesthesia and erythema; see Fig. 172–2)

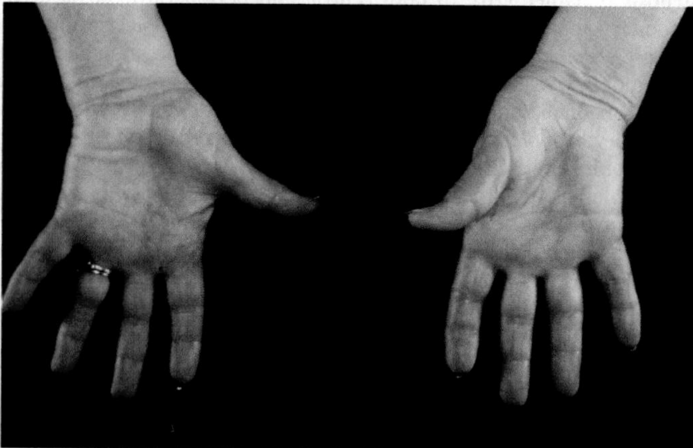

FIGURE 172–2 • Erythromelalgia refers to a painful red discoloration of the hands or toes (Chapter 80).

Section XIV Hematology

Diagnosis

The diagnostic possibility of polycythemia vera (Fig. 172–3) may be entertained only if (1) the hemoglobin and hematocrit levels are greater than the 95th percentile of the normal distribution adjusted for sex and race, (2) the hemoglobin level is documented to be greater than a historical baseline for the individual patient, or (3) polycythemia vera–related features (see Table 172–2) are present. If any of these conditions is present, a serum erythropoietin level should be obtained. In the absence of all three criteria, a follow-up blood test in 3 months should be adequate. A rare exception is the patient with suspected polycythemia vera who presents with a normal or even low hemoglobin or hematocrit after bleeding from a peptic ulcer.

A low serum erythropoietin level is highly suggestive of polycythemia vera. This diagnosis is unlikely in the presence of an increased serum erythropoietin level, but a normal serum erythropoietin level does not exclude polycythemia vera. A bone marrow examination is indicated if the serum erythropoietin level is low. In contrast, if the serum erythropoietin level is normal, a bone marrow examination is recommended only if either the leukocyte alkaline phosphatase score is elevated or the patient manifests a characteristic clinical feature of polycythemia vera (see Table 172–2).

Histologic features of the bone marrow that are characteristic of polycythemia vera include both numeric and morphologic abnormalities of megakaryocytes, including cluster formation, increased reticulin fibrosis, and bone marrow hypercellularity. However, the utility of bone marrow histology in the diagnosis of polycythemia vera is not universally appreciated, so concomitant screening for the *JAK2*^{V617F} mutation is recommended (see Fig. 172–3). At present, however, screening for the *JAK2*^{V617F} mutation cannot substitute for bone marrow histology because the specific mutation is not detected in all patients. Nevertheless, if an asymptomatic patient with polycythemia of no apparent cause has a normal serum erythropoietin level and no characteristic features of polycythemia vera, the *JAK2*^{V617F} screening can help the clinician to decide whether to obtain a bone marrow biopsy.

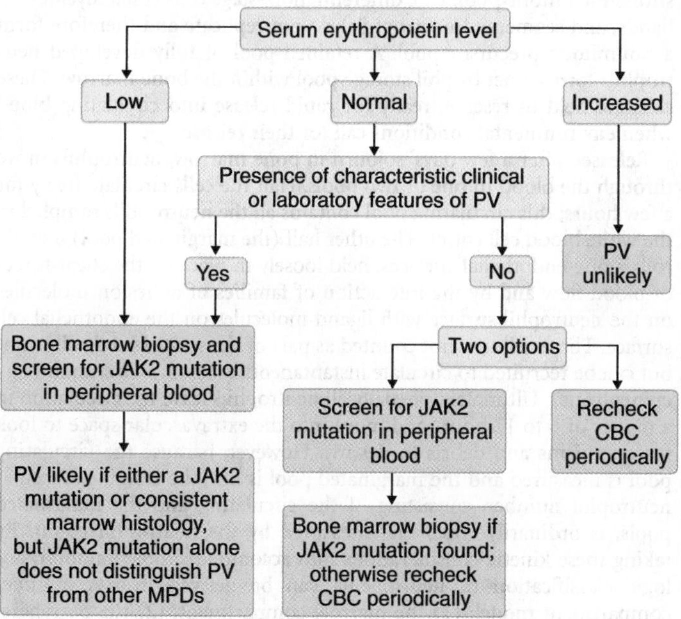

FIGURE 172–3 • A diagnostic algorithm for polycythemia vera (PV) that incorporates mutation screening for *JAK2*^{V617F}. A normal erythropoietin level is 536 μ/L. "Periodically" is usually interpreted clinically as approximately every 6 months. (See Table 172–2 for features related to polycythemia vera, including increased leukocyte alkaline phosphatase [LAP] score, thrombocytosis, leukocytosis, splenomegaly, thrombosis, pruritus, and erythromelalgia.) CBC = complete blood count; JAK = Janus kinase; MPD = myeloproliferative disorder.

Treatment

Treatment of polycythemia vera is primarily directed at preventing thrombotic complications. The mainstays of therapy in polycythemia vera are phlebotomy and aspirin. Phlebotomy is used to achieve a goal of keeping the hematocrit lower than 45% in white men and 42% in women and African American men. These levels reduce blood hyperviscosity, improve cerebral blood flow, and lower the rate of thrombotic complications. The current consensus is to supplement phlebotomy with hydroxyurea only in patients who are at high risk for thrombosis (Tables 172–3 and 172–4). Low-dose (81 mg/day) aspirin therapy has additional antithrombotic value without an increased risk of major hemorrhage. 2 Aspirin therapy is also effective in controlling microvascular symptoms such as headaches and erythromelalgia. Whether any therapy modifies the risk of transformation into myelofibrosis with myeloid metaplasia is not clearly ascertained.

The addition of oral chlorambucil or intravenous radioactive phosphorus (P-32) to phlebotomy significantly reduces the rate of early thrombotic complications but also significantly lessens survival because of an increased incidence of therapy-related acute leukemia. In patients with polycythemia vera who are at high risk for thrombosis (see Table 172–3), hydroxyurea appears to lower the risk of thrombosis compared with phlebotomy alone, with a lower risk of acute leukemia compared with either chlorambucil or radioactive phosphorus, but these data are not from randomized trials. Pipobroman (not available in the United States) is as effective as hydroxyurea in the treatment of polycythemia vera without being more or less leukemogenic. In nonrandomized settings, both busulfan and interferon alfa have also shown activity against

TABLE 172–3 RISK STRATIFICATION IN POLYCYTHEMIA VERA

LOW RISK

Age <60 yr, *and*
No history of thrombosis, *and*
Platelet count <1.5 million/μL, and
Absence of cardiovascular risk factors

INTERMEDIATE RISK

Neither low-risk nor high-risk

HIGH RISK

Age ≥60 years, or
A history of thrombosis

TABLE 172–4 TREATMENT ALGORITHM IN POLYCYTHEMIA VERA

Risk Category	Age <60 Yr	Age ≥60 Yr	Women of Childbearing Age
Low risk	Phlebotomy and low-dose aspirin	Not applicable	Phlebotomy and low-dose aspirin
Indeterminate risk	Phlebotomy and low-dose aspirin*	Not applicable	Phlebotomy and low-dose aspirin*
High risk	Phlebotomy and low-dose aspirin and hydroxyurea	Phlebotomy and low-dose aspirin and hydroxyurea	Phlebotomy and low-dose aspirin and Interferon alfa†

*The possibility of clinically significant acquired von Willebrand's syndrome must be excluded in the presence of a platelet count >1 million/μL before aspirin is given.
†Based on anecdotal evidence of safety.

polycythemia vera, but they have not been compared rigorously with hydroxyurea. Anagrelide has been used to treat polycythemia vera, both in the presence and the absence of associated thrombocytosis, without any evidence of additional advantage over hydroxyurea. Finally, paroxetine, a selective serotonin reuptake inhibitor, is used to treat polycythemia vera–associated pruritus.

Future Directions

Studies are currently ongoing to define the precise pathogenetic role of $JAK2^{V617F}$ in polycythemia vera and to design new therapies based on these discoveries.

Prognosis

Life expectancy in polycythemia vera exceeds 10 years but is worse than in the sex- and age-matched control population, owing to premature death from fatal thrombohemorrhagic complications and to transformation into myelofibrosis with myeloid metaplasia (Chapter 183) and acute myeloid leukemia (Chapter 194). Age older than 60 years, a white blood cell count above 15,000/mm³, and history of thrombosis are considered adverse risk factors for thrombotic complications (see Table 172–3). The estimated rates of recurrent thrombosis in low- and high-risk patients are approximately 5 and 30%, respectively. The incidences of myelofibrosis with myeloid metaplasia and acute myeloid leukemia in the first decade of the disease are approximately 10 and 5%, respectively. More patients experience disease transformation in the second decade of the disease.

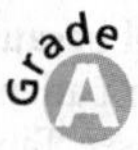

1. Yildiz A, Cine N, Akkaya V, et al: Comparison of the effects of enalapril and losartan on posttransplantation erythrocytosis in renal transplant recipients: Prospective randomized study. Transplantation 2001;72:542–544.
2. Landolfi R, Marchioli R, Kutti J, et al: Efficacy and safety of low-dose aspirin in polycythemia vera. N Engl J Med 2004;350:114–124.

SUGGESTED READINGS

Campbell PJ, Green AR: The myeloproliferative disorders. N Engl J Med 2006;355:2452–2466. *An excellent review.*

Gordeuk VR, Stockton DW, Prchal JT: Congenital polycythemias/erythrocytoses. Haematologica 2005;90:109–116. *A detailed review of the different causes of secondary polycythemia, with emphasis on congenital causes.*

Landolfi R, Di Gennaro L, Barbui T, et al: Leukocytosis as a major thrombotic risk factor in patients with polycythemia vera. Blood 2007;109:2446–2452. *A WBC >15,000 is associated with increased risk of thrombosis (HR 1.71).*

Schafer AI: Molecular basis of the diagnosis and treatment of polycythemia vera and essential thrombocythemia. Blood 2006;107:4214–4222. *A comprehensive review.*

Scott LM, Tong W, Levine RL, et al: JAK2 exon 12 mutations in polycythemia vera and idiopathic erythrocytosis. N Engl J Med 2007;356:459–468. *Four somatic gain-of-function mutations in JAK2 are described.*

Sirhan S, Fairbanks VF, Tefferi A: Red cell mass and plasma volume measurements in polycythemia. Cancer 2005;104:213–215. *The first systematic study demonstrating the suboptimal diagnostic accuracy of red cell mass measurement in polycythemia vera.*

173 LEUKOPENIA AND LEUKOCYTOSIS

Grover C. Bagby, Jr.

The normal peripheral white blood cell count ranges from 5.0 to 10.0×10^9/L, and a low total white blood cell count ($<4.5 \times 10^9$/L) is known as *leukopenia*. When leukopenia is discovered, a most important first step is to determine which type of white blood cell is at low levels. Circulating leukocytes consist of heterogeneous cell types (neutrophils, monocytes, basophils, eosinophils, B lymphocytes, T lymphocytes, and natural killer cells), each of which serves a unique purpose and represents a different fractional component of the total body leukocyte population. Therefore, patients may be either severely neutropenic or lymphocytopenic despite having total white blood cell counts that fall within the normal range. Consequently, in a number of clinical settings (e.g., patients with an acute infection or those with recurrent infections), differential white blood cell counts are important to obtain even in the absence of leukopenia.

NEUTROPENIA

Definition

The clinical consequences of prolonged phagocyte dysfunction can be life-threatening. Fortunately, acquired and inherited phagocyte dysfunction syndromes are rare. However, a reduction in the number of circulating phagocytes is more common in clinical practice, the most life-threatening instances of which result from bone marrow failure. Neutropenia is said to exist when a patient's peripheral *neutrophil* count is less than 2.0×10^9/L. Because the normal range in Yemenite Jews and black individuals is somewhat lower, neutropenia in these populations is defined as counts less than 1.5×10^9/L. The role of the neutrophil in phagocytic defense of the host is generally met if the neutrophil count is higher than 1.0×10^9/L. If the neutrophil count drops further, particularly below 0.5×10^9/L, the threat of recurrent, severe, life-threatening, and difficult-to-treat infections increases enormously.

Pathobiology

Categorizing the causes of neutropenia requires an understanding of normal neutrophil kinetics. Neutrophils arise from a pool of marrow precursor cells through serial divisions and synchronous maturation steps (Fig. 173–1). The rate of neutrophil production is high: more than 10^{11} cells per day. In the bone marrow, neutrophil precursors that retain replicative potential (myeloblasts, promyelocytes, and myelocytes) constitute the mitotic pool. Late differentiation–stage cells (metamyelocytes, bands, and segmented neutrophils) do not replicate and therefore form a nonmitotic precursor pool. A retained pool of fully developed neutrophils forms a neutrophil storage pool within the bone marrow. These cells are held in reserve, ready for rapid release into circulating blood when environmental conditions call for their release.

Released after a few days' sojourn in bone marrow, neutrophils move through the blood in one of two pools. Half the cells circulate freely for a few hours; this circulating pool contains all the neutrophils sampled in the white blood cell count. The other half (the marginated pool) literally rolls along endothelial surfaces, held loosely in place by the shear forces of blood flow and by the interaction of families of adhesion molecules on the neutrophil surface with ligand molecules on the endothelial cell surface. These cells are not counted as part of the white blood cell count but can be recruited to circulate instantaneously by various stimuli (e.g., epinephrine). Ultimately, virtually all neutrophils leave the circulation in a matter of 6 to 12 hours and move into the extravascular space to look for organisms and debris to destroy. However, because the circulating pool is measured and the marginated pool is not, the true intravascular neutrophil number, consisting of the circulating and the marginated pools, is ordinarily twice that measured by the neutrophil count. By taking these kinetic considerations into account, a simple pathophysiologic classification of neutropenia can be derived from the three-compartment model: (1) the marrow compartment, (2) the peripheral blood compartment, (3) the extravascular compartment, or (4) combinations of these three (Fig. 173–2).

Abnormalities in the Marrow Compartment

Bone marrow defects (failure to produce and release neutrophils at a normal rate) account for the majority of neutropenia in clinical practice. Failure of the marrow compartment can occur as a result of direct injury to either hematopoietic progenitors and stem cells or cells in the hematopoietic microenvironment. With both types of injury, the marrow usually contains fewer than normal numbers of hematopoietic cells, or maturation defects of hematopoietic cells result in normal or increased numbers of morphologically abnormal hematopoietic cells. In either case, neutropenia of this type frequently occurs along with abnormalities in the number of platelets and red blood cells.

Marrow injury can occur as a consequence of a variety of diseases, but drug-induced injury is most common (Table 173–1). Antineoplastic, certain antiviral, and some immunosuppressive agents are generally designed to inflict injury on a nonmyeloid cell population (e.g., neoplastic cells); myelosuppressive toxicity is the rule but is generally predictable because its intensity varies directly with the dose. Drugs that are not

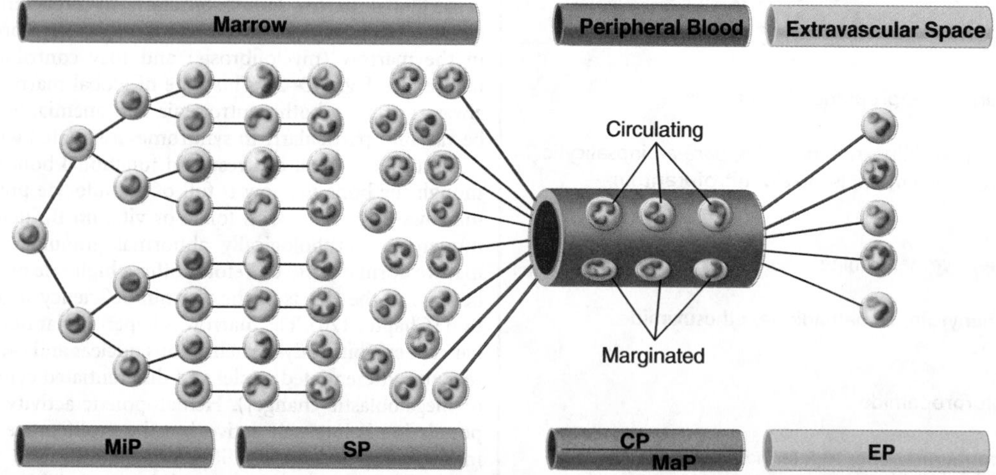

FIGURE 173–1 • Production and distribution of neutrophils involve three compartments: marrow, peripheral blood, and the extravascular space. Unlike red blood cells, phagocytes are destined to function primarily in the extravascular space. The critical issue for clinicians to consider is whether delivery of phagocytes to this extracellular space is adequate. Stem cells, committed progenitor cells, and morphologically recognizable bone marrow precursor cells proliferate and mature; they differentiate under the influence of a variety of humoral regulatory factors that govern the production of neutrophils (granulocyte colony-stimulating factor), monocytes (macrophage colony-stimulating factor), and eosinophils (interleukin-5). These replicative responses occur in the mitotic pool (MiP). Once more differentiated cells reach the intermediate maturation stage known as the metamyelocyte, they stop replicating but continue differentiating into bands and segmented neutrophils. These cells, though capable of leaving the marrow when needed (e.g., in the setting of an acute bacterial infection), spend up to 5 days in the marrow in the storage pool (SP). The neutrophils then enter the blood stream. Half of these circulating cells adhere to endothelial cells and compose the marginated pool (MaP). The nonmarginated cells make up the circulating pool (CP). After their very brief sojourn in peripheral blood, the neutrophils invade the extravascular compartments of most organs, where they are used as defenders or garbage disposal devices (a process that involves both destruction of the offending organism and self-destruction), or they die within 1 to 2 days. EP = extravascular pool.

Marrow

ABNORMALITIES IN THE BONE MARROW COMPARTMENT

1. Bone marrow injury
   - A. Drugs
     - Cytotoxic and noncytotoxic agents
   - B. Radiation
   - C. Chemicals
     - Benzene, DDT, dinitrophenol, arsenic, bismuth, nitrous oxide
   - D. Certain congenital and hereditary neutropenias
   - E. Immunologically mediated (largely seen in patients with rheumatic disorders)
     - Cytotoxic T cell–mediated (T)
     - Antibody-mediated (Ab)
     - Mechanisms that require both T and Ab
   - F. Infection
     - Viral (hepatitis, parvovirus, AIDS)
     - Bacterial (*Mycobacterium tuberculosis, Mycobacterium kansasii*)
   - G. Bone marrow replacement (infiltrative diseases)
     - Malignancies (lung, breast, prostate, stomach, lymphomas, and lymphoid leukemias)
     - Fibrosis
     - Agnogenic myeloid metaplasia
     - Long-standing polycythemia vera
     - Chronic myelogenous leukemia
     - Radiation injury
     - Injury from chronic cytotoxic drug therapy
     - Acute megakaryocytic leukemia
   - H. Inherited neutropenia syndromes (precursor cell apoptosis)
     - Cyclic neutropenia
     - Severe congenital neutropenia
     - Shwachman-Diamond syndrome
     - Myelokathexis
2. Maturation defects
   - A. Acquired
     - Folic acid deficiency
     - Vitamin B_{12} deficiency
   - B. Neoplastic and other clonal disorders
     - Acute nonlymphocytic leukemia
     - Myelodysplastic syndromes
     - Paroxysmal nocturnal hemoglobinuria

Peripheral Blood

ABNORMALITIES IN THE PERIPHERAL BLOOD COMPARTMENT

1. Shift of neutrophils from the circulating to the marginated pool (known as pseudoneutropenia)
   - A. Hereditary or constitutional benign pseudoneutropenia
   - B. Acquired
     - Acute: Severe bacterial infection, frequently associated with endotoxemia
     - Chronic: Protein-calorie malnutrition, malaria
2. Intravascular sequestration
   - A. In lung (complement-mediated leukoagglutination)
   - B. In spleen (hypersplenism)

Extravascular

ABNORMALITIES IN THE EXTRAVASCULAR COMPARTMENT

1. Increased utilization
   - A. Severe bacterial, fungal, viral, or rickettsial infection
   - B. Anaphylaxis

FIGURE 173–2 • Causes of neutropenia arranged according to the compartment with which the pathophysiologically relevant mechanism is linked. One should begin the diagnostic approach to a neutropenic patient by seeking to identify the pathophysiologically relevant compartment. Management of a neutropenic patient whose neutrophil production is reduced is entirely different from that of a neutropenic patient whose production is normal and in whom the rate of delivery to the extravascular compartment is normal or appropriately increased in the context of acute infections. AIDS = acquired immunodeficiency syndrome.

TABLE 173–1 DRUGS THAT CAUSE NEUTROPENIA

Antiarrhythmics
Tocainide, procainamide, propranolol, quinidine
Antibiotics
Chloramphenicol, penicillins, sulfonamides, *para*-aminosalicylic acid, rifampin, vancomycin, isoniazid, nitrofurantoin, ganciclovir
Antimalarials
Dapsone, quinine, pyrimethamine
Anticonvulsants
Phenytoin, mephenytoin, trimethadione, ethosuximide, carbamazepine
Hypoglycemic agents
Tolbutamide, chlorpropamide
Antihistamines
Cimetidine, brompheniramine, tripelennamine
Antihypertensives
Methyldopa, captopril
Anti-inflammatory agents
Aminopyrine, phenylbutazone, gold salts, ibuprofen, indomethacin
Antithyroid agents
Propylthiouracil, methimazole, thiouracil
Diuretics
Acetazolamide, hydrochlorothiazide, chlorthalidone
Phenothiazines
Chlorpromazine, promazine, prochlorperazine
Immunosuppressive agents
Antimetabolites
Cytotoxic agents
Alkylating agents, antimetabolites, anthracyclines, vinca alkaloids, cisplatin, hydroxyurea, dactinomycin
Other agents
Recombinant interferons, allopurinol, ethanol, levamisole, penicillamine, zidovudine, streptokinase, carbamazepine, clozapine

usually myelosuppressive and that are well tolerated in the majority of patients can sometimes induce either marrow injury or peripheral neutrophil destruction. These idiosyncratic drug-induced reactions can result from direct drug-mediated cytotoxicity or from an immune mechanism in which (1) neutrophils are destroyed in extramedullary sites as a result of antineutrophil antibodies (e.g., the penicillins) or (2) the marrow compartment is injured (e.g., procainamide, chloramphenicol, dapsone, tocainide).

Radiation (Chapter 18) may result in acute self-limited bone marrow injury and chronic marrow failure. Chronic radiation-induced injury can also result in the later development of myelodysplasia and nonlymphocytic leukemia, both of which may be accompanied by neutropenia. In addition, benzene toxicity can result in acute or chronic neutropenia and, like radiation-induced marrow failure, is associated with a high risk for acute nonlymphocytic leukemia.

Immune-mediated bone marrow failure can be mediated by autoantibodies or, more often, by T lymphocytes that inhibit the growth of bone marrow precursor cells. Apart from those with acquired aplastic anemia (often immunologically mediated; see Chapter 171), most patients with immune-mediated leukopenia have concurrent rheumatic or autoimmune diseases, which are especially likely if the neutropenia is "isolated" (i.e., the only severe hematologic defect in patients who otherwise have normal red blood cell and platelet counts). Infection of the marrow per se is unusual and most often does not result in neutropenia; some exceptions include mycobacterial infections (especially those caused by *Mycobacterium tuberculosis* and *Mycobacterium kansasii;* see Chapters 345 and 346) and certain viral infections.

Bone marrow invasion by abnormal cells can result in neutropenia. Carcinoma of the lung (Chapter 201), breast (Chapter 208), prostate (Chapter 211), and stomach (Chapter 202), as well as malignant hematopoietic disorders, can occupy enough of the medullary space to cause global marrow failure. Similarly, in certain myeloproliferative diseases and leukemias, bone marrow fibroblasts can proliferate significantly in the marrow (myelofibrosis) and may contribute to bone marrow failure (see Fig. 173–2). This type of global marrow dysfunction nearly always results in both neutropenia and anemia, but platelet counts can be variable, particularly in syndromes associated with myelofibrosis.

Maturation arrest can result in functional bone marrow failure even though the bone marrow is full of granulocyte precursors. In the bone marrows of patients with folate or vitamin B_{12} deficiency, for example, numerous morphologically abnormal granulocyte precursors fail to mature normally and therefore suffer a high rate of intramedullary death because of the effects of the vitamin deficiency state on nuclear replication (Chapter 170). The marrow is hypercellular but is packed with peculiar cells exhibiting dys-synchronous nuclear and cytoplasmic maturation (e.g., undifferentiated nuclei and differentiated cytoplasm [the hallmark of megaloblastic change]). Hematopoietic activity in the primitive cell population is intensely active, but the proliferative activity is ineffective in delivering terminally differentiated cells into the blood stream—a process known as *ineffective hematopoiesis.* Certain congenital neutropenias also represent maturation abnormalities, as do the acute nonlymphocytic leukemias, myelodysplastic syndromes, and paroxysmal nocturnal hemoglobinuria.

Abnormalities in the Peripheral Blood Compartment

Perturbations of the peripheral blood compartment result from shifts from the marginated to the circulating pool and vice versa (see Figs. 173–1 and 173–2). In one syndrome, pseudoneutropenia, neutrophil production and utilization are normal, but the size of the marginated pool is increased and the circulating pool is decreased. Because these marginated cells, while hidden from the blood cell counting machine, maintain their capacity to migrate to sites of infection, patients with pseudoneutropenia are not at increased risk for infection unless an abnormality in neutrophil function coexists. Acquired pseudoneutropenia often occurs as an acute or subacute response to systemic infection; it is generally associated with acute changes in other compartments (Fig. 173–3) and resolves when the infection is appropriately treated or spontaneously abates. Finally, a truly artifactual type of pseudoneutropenia can be seen as a result of clumping of neutrophils induced by ethylenediaminetetraacetic acid (EDTA; the anticoagulant in the complete blood count tube), which can be eliminated by adding kanamycin to the sample.

Demands of the Vascular Compartment

Neutrophils and their precursors respond to a number of environmental cues in a highly regulated fashion. The most frequent of these cues evolve in response to infection. These responses are governed by a variety of hematopoietic growth factors, adhesion molecules, and interleukins, including two granulopoietic factors, granulocyte-macrophage colony-stimulating factor (GM-CSF) and granulocyte colony-stimulating factor (G-CSF), and an important chemokine, interleukin-8 (IL-8). These factors, along with IL-1 and tumor necrosis factor-α, cytokines that induce the synthesis and release of granulopoietic factors and adhesion molecules on both neutrophils and endothelial cells, account for (1) a prompt increase in the rate of production of neutrophils in the mitotic compartment, a response mediated by a complex network of cellular and humoral regulatory interactions; (2) early release of neutrophils from the marrow storage pool to the peripheral blood pool; (3) an increase in the rate of neutrophil egress from the peripheral blood pool to the invaded tissue or tissues; and (4) increased phagocytic and bactericidal activity of the neutrophils. Rarely, increased demand for neutrophils in the extravascular compartment can lead to transient neutropenia, especially in patients with severe acute infections (see Fig. 173–3). In such cases, the immediate demand for neutrophils in the zone of infection calls forth such a substantial release response that the marrow storage pool is used up before it can be restored by increased proliferative activity of the granulocyte progenitor cells. This kind of neutropenia is not uncommon in cases of *Salmonella* typhoid fever (Chapter 329), in which leukopenia is common in the acute phase. In such cases, the infected tissue serves as a sink for neutrophils for a brief period (sometimes up to 5 to 6 days). Ultimately, even under these conditions the neutrophil count generally rises well above normal within a few days because the bone marrow is highly effective in responding to infectious events, so the demand for neutrophils almost never exceeds the capacity of the mitotic pool to supply them if the bone marrow is completely normal. In contrast, neutrophil

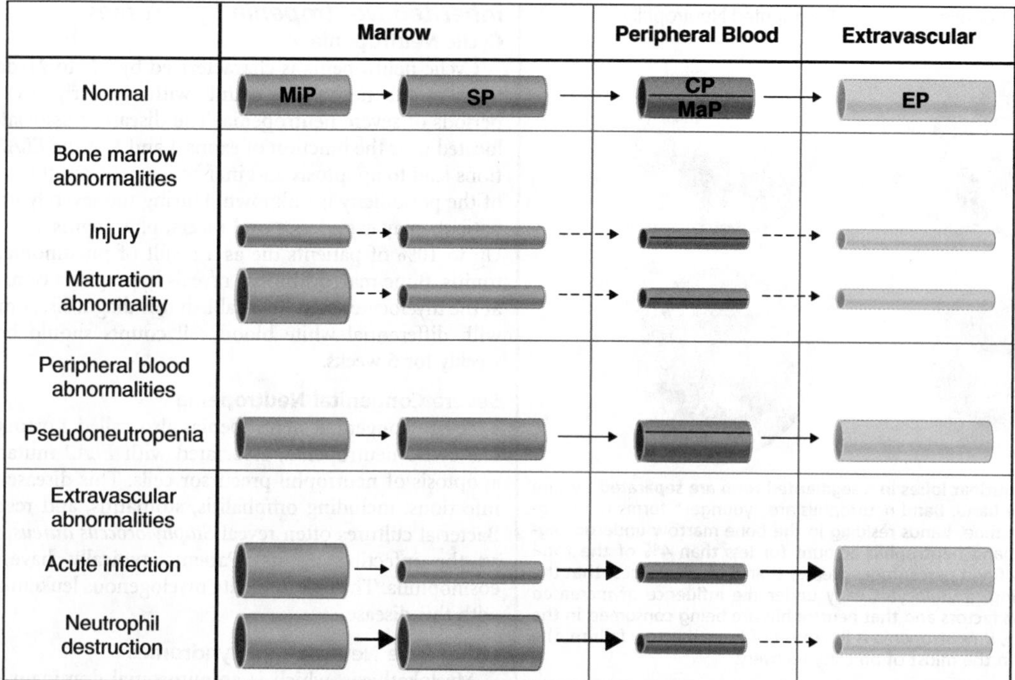

FIGURE 173–3 • Pathophysiologic mechanisms of neutropenia. The size of a given compartment is represented by the size of the corresponding cylindrical pool. The relative number of cells leaving one compartment and headed for the next (highly variable from case to case) is represented by the size of the arrow between those compartments. Flow between compartments is unidirectional. CP = circulating pool; EP = extravascular pool; MaP = marginated pool; MiP = mitotic pool; SP = storage pool. Notice that in every case the circulating neutrophil pool is small but the size of the other pools is variable. In marrow injury, there is a global decline in the size of all pools. A maturation abnormality (e.g., deficiency of folic acid or vitamin B_{12}), however, is characterized by an increase in the number of precursor cells that do not mature, which results in an absolute decrease in mature neutrophils in the marrow, blood, and tissues. Pseudoneutropenia is characterized by movement of circulating neutrophils to the marginated pool, but because delivery of cells to the extravascular space is usually normal, such patients are not at increased risk for infections. In patients who have acute infections, the demand for neutrophils in the infected extravascular site can result in a transient loss of storage pool neutrophils before the hypercellular (but as yet immature) mitotic compartments can renew the storage pool. This kind of neutropenia is very transient and occurs most often in cases of overwhelming infection, although certain organisms (e.g., *Salmonella typhosa*) seem to induce this type of response more than others do. Excessive destruction of neutrophils can also result in neutropenia, but this is not particularly common, except in cases of human immunodeficiency virus infection.

consumption in patients with autoimmune neutropenia and hypersplenism can, indeed, outstrip the capacity of the bone marrow to keep up with the losses.

Clinical Manifestations

Neutropenia can occur as a manifestation of a wide variety of systemic diseases (see Fig. 173–2), the manifestations of which may dominate the clinical picture. Many neutropenic patients remain asymptomatic, most often those whose neutrophil count exceeds 1.0×10^9/L or those whose neutropenia is acute or of brief duration. When symptoms do occur, they generally result from recurrent, often severe bacterial infections because of the pivotal importance of the neutrophil in defense of the host against microorganisms (Chapter 175).

This risk for bacterial infection increases slightly as the peripheral neutrophil count falls below 1.0×10^9/L, but it is substantially increased at levels below 0.5×10^9/L. The degree to which monocytosis compensates for neutropenia may modify the risk. Some patients with severe congenital neutropenia have such substantial compensatory monocytosis that their clinical course is very mild. Because of the capacity of the extra monocytes to "cover" for neutrophil deficiencies, such rare patients have few bacterial infections. The lungs, genitourinary system, gut, oropharynx, and skin are the most frequent sources of infection in neutropenic patients. The infecting organisms are the "usual suspects" for the given anatomic site, with the caveat that for patients who have recurrent infections and require prolonged and recurrent antibacterial therapy, unusual (often hospital-acquired) organisms can colonize and subsequently cause infection. Consequently, the antibiotic history of infected neutropenic patients is important to obtain.

One must look carefully for infections in neutropenic patients because the usual signs and symptoms of infection are often diminished or absent as a result of the reduction in cells that mediate much of the inflammatory responses to infection. Thus, neutropenic patients with severe bilateral bacterial pneumonia may initially be seen with minimal infiltrates demonstrable on chest imaging (sometimes no infiltrates can be seen at all until after about 3 or 4 days of full-blown symptoms) and can have benign-looking, nonpurulent sputum, patients with pyelonephritis may not exhibit much pyuria, patients with bacterial pharyngitis may not have purulence in their oropharynx, and patients with severe bacterial infection of the skin may have only mild erythroderma rather than furunculosis. In a neutropenic patient, infections that in an otherwise normal individual might have been well localized quickly become disseminated. Therefore, not only does an infected neutropenic patient represent a diagnostic problem, but in addition, because any given infection is more likely to be widespread at the time of diagnosis, these patients are often gravely ill at the time that they are initially seen by their caregivers.

Diagnosis

The diagnostic evaluation of neutropenia is influenced by its severity and the clinical setting in which it occurs. The assessment of patients with neutrophil counts of less than 0.5 to 1.0×10^9/L must proceed briskly. A patient with fever, sepsis, or both in whom neutropenia is discovered for the first time presents a particularly difficult problem. In such patients, it is impossible to determine immediately whether the neutropenia antedated the sepsis, a situation with both prognostic and therapeutic implications, or whether the neutropenia is merely a short-lived response to the infection itself (see Fig. 173–3). Examination of the peripheral blood smear and differential white blood cell count can be helpful in such cases. An increase in the fraction of circulating band neutrophil forms to levels above 20% suggests that marrow granulopoietic activity is responding appropriately (Fig. 173–4). Although the clinical context is more important to consider than this single data point, colloquially known as "bandemia," it is nonetheless a data point more compatible with the notion that the bone marrow of the patient is in the midst of recovering from injury or that the neutropenia is derived from a transient shift to the marginated pool or to the extravascular compartment.

The diagnostic evaluation of neutropenia must first address the question of severity and then whether the patient has fever, sepsis, or both. A patient with sepsis and severe neutropenia should be treated promptly

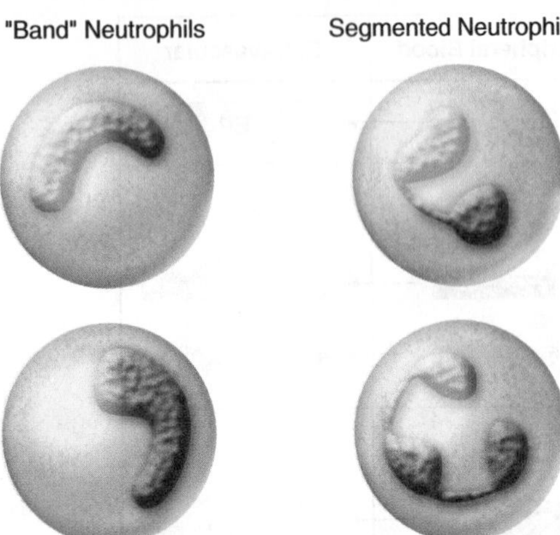

FIGURE 173–4 • The nuclear lobes in a segmented form are separated by fine filaments absent in the band. Band neutrophils are "younger" forms than segmented neutrophils. In time, bands residing in the bone marrow undergo segmentation. Normally, band neutrophils account for less than 4% of the total circulating neutrophils. Band percentages greater than 6 to 7% suggest that the storage pool is releasing granulocytes early under the influence of increased levels of granulopoietic factors and that neutrophils are being consumed in the periphery. Alternatively, if neutropenia is the result of bone marrow failure, the bone marrow may be in the midst of an early recovery.

with intravenous antibiotics after obtaining blood for appropriate cultures but without waiting for the results of those cultures. Once these important initial questions are answered, the remainder of the diagnostic evaluation can proceed (Fig. 173–5): (1) identifying any potential drugs and toxins to which the patient might have been exposed (see Table 173–1); (2) determining, if possible, the chronicity of the neutropenia (e.g., seeking evidence about whether the patient ever had a normal white blood cell count and when); (3) ascertaining whether there have been recurrent infections; (4) identifying any underlying systemic disease that might be causative; and (5) examining the blood counts and blood and bone marrow morphology (marrow examination is virtually always warranted unless a diagnosis is clear from simple blood tests, e.g., serum folate, homocysteine, methylmalonate, or vitamin B_{12} levels) to determine the most likely pathophysiologic explanation. In some cases, specialized bone marrow studies (e.g., progenitor cell colony assays before and after removing T lymphocytes from the sample) are warranted even with a clear diagnosis. Felty's syndrome, for example, a well-recognized syndrome of neutropenia in patients with rheumatoid arthritis (Chapter 285), is caused by one of two pathophysiologic mechanisms. One is mediated by antineutrophil antibodies, the other by T lymphocyte–mediated bone marrow failure. Each mechanism has a distinctly different therapeutic implication.

After the severity of the neutropenia is quantified, careful examination of the peripheral blood counts and blood smear is in order (see Fig. 173–5). Patients with selective neutropenia are approached differently from those with additional deficiencies of platelets and red blood cells, although drugs or toxins may be involved in either category. Potentially offending drugs should obviously be discontinued if such a maneuver is possible based on the nature of the disease for which the agent was prescribed and the availability of alternative drugs. Patients with selective neutropenia but with no drug or toxin exposure, no history of recurrent sepsis, and no underlying chronic inflammatory or autoimmune disease may have stable and benign neutropenia; this category includes some cases of familial and congenital neutropenia and pseudoneutropenia. Any patient with selective neutropenia and a history of sepsis and all patients with known toxin exposure should undergo bone marrow examination to assess (1) the cellularity of each compartment (storage and mitotic pools), (2) the distribution of differentiation stages found in each pool, and (3) whether any morphologic abnormality (e.g., acute leukemia or myelodysplasia) exists in the hematopoietic cells.

In patients with pancytopenia or bicytopenia, bone marrow aspiration plus biopsy is absolutely required. The only exception to this rule would be patients with unambiguous evidence of vitamin B_{12} or folate deficiency (Chapter 170).

Inherited Neutropenia Syndromes

Cyclic Neutropenia

Cyclic neutropenia is characterized by 14- to 21-day periodic oscillations of the neutrophil count, with regularly occurring 3- to 5-day periods of severe neutropenia. The disease is associated with mutations located near the junction of exons 4 and 5 of the *ELA2* gene; these mutations lead to apoptosis and ineffective neutrophil production. The cause of the periodicity is unknown. During the severely neutropenic periods, patients may experience oral ulcers, pharyngitis, and lymphadenopathy. Up to 10% of patients die as a result of pneumonia, cellulitis, or peritonitis. Bone marrow biopsy reveals hyperplasia or arrest of cell division at the myelocyte stage. To establish this diagnosis, complete blood counts with differential white blood cell counts should be performed twice weekly for 6 weeks.

Severe Congenital Neutropenia

Severe congenital neutropenia, also called Kostmann's syndrome, is, like cyclic neutropenia, associated with *ELA2* mutations that result in apoptosis of neutrophil precursor cells. This disease is accompanied by infections, including omphalitis, stomatitis, and respiratory infections. Bacterial cultures often reveal *Staphylococcus aureus* and *Escherichia coli* as the infecting agents. Patients typically have monocytosis and eosinophilia. The risk for acute myelogenous leukemia is high in patients with this disease.

Other Rare Neutropenia Syndromes

Myelokathexis, which is an autosomal dominant disorder caused by truncating mutations of the chemokine receptor CXCR4, is associated with hypersegmentation of neutrophils in the marrow and peripheral blood. In light of the characteristic bone marrow hypercellularity, apoptosis of well-differentiated neutrophil precursors in the marrow is thought to result because abnormalities in the proper release of neutrophils from marrow lead to severe neutropenia and recurrent infections.

The Shwachman-Diamond syndrome is an autosomal recessive disease caused by mutations of a gene *(SDBS)* that encodes a protein involved in ribosome biosynthesis. The disease is associated with neutropenia, pancreatic insufficiency, short stature, and skeletal abnormalities. Like all of the inherited neutropenia syndromes just mentioned, bone marrow myeloid precursor cells are apoptotic. Similar to severe congenital neutropenia, the disease is associated with a high risk for acute leukemia.

Treatment

Treatments Specifically Designed to Increase the Neutrophil Count

Immunosuppressive therapy (e.g., glucocorticoids, antithymocyte globulin, cyclosporine) very commonly elicits favorable responses in patients with marrow failure mediated by cytotoxic T lymphocytes or antineutrophil antibodies. Splenectomy is rarely helpful in the management of neutropenic patients, even those with Felty's syndrome; it is now reserved for patients with unambiguous hypersplenism in whom bone marrow function is normal.

Recombinant Human Granulopoietic Factors

GM-CSF and G-CSF (either native G-CSF or the pegylated long-acting form) can increase the neutrophil count in selected neutropenic patients. As a general rule, patients with drug-induced neutropenia (e.g., after cancer chemotherapy) recover more rapidly if they receive either GM-CSF or G-CSF. These agents are indicated in the settings of (1) bone marrow transplantation; (2) management of patients with inherited neutropenic syndromes, including cyclic neutropenia; (3) induction of stem cell mobilization from marrow to peripheral blood in preparation for transplantation; and (4) combined therapy with erythropoietin for selected patients with myelodysplastic syndromes. Additional potential roles of these agents in clinical practice are unclear. Large clinical studies indicate that G-CSF hastens neutrophil recovery in patients receiving cytotoxic therapy but does not reduce the rate of hospitalization for febrile episodes, prolong survival, reduce culture-positive infections, or reduce the cost of supportive care, whether given preemptively or to treat neutropenic fever. [1] In addition, there is no evidence

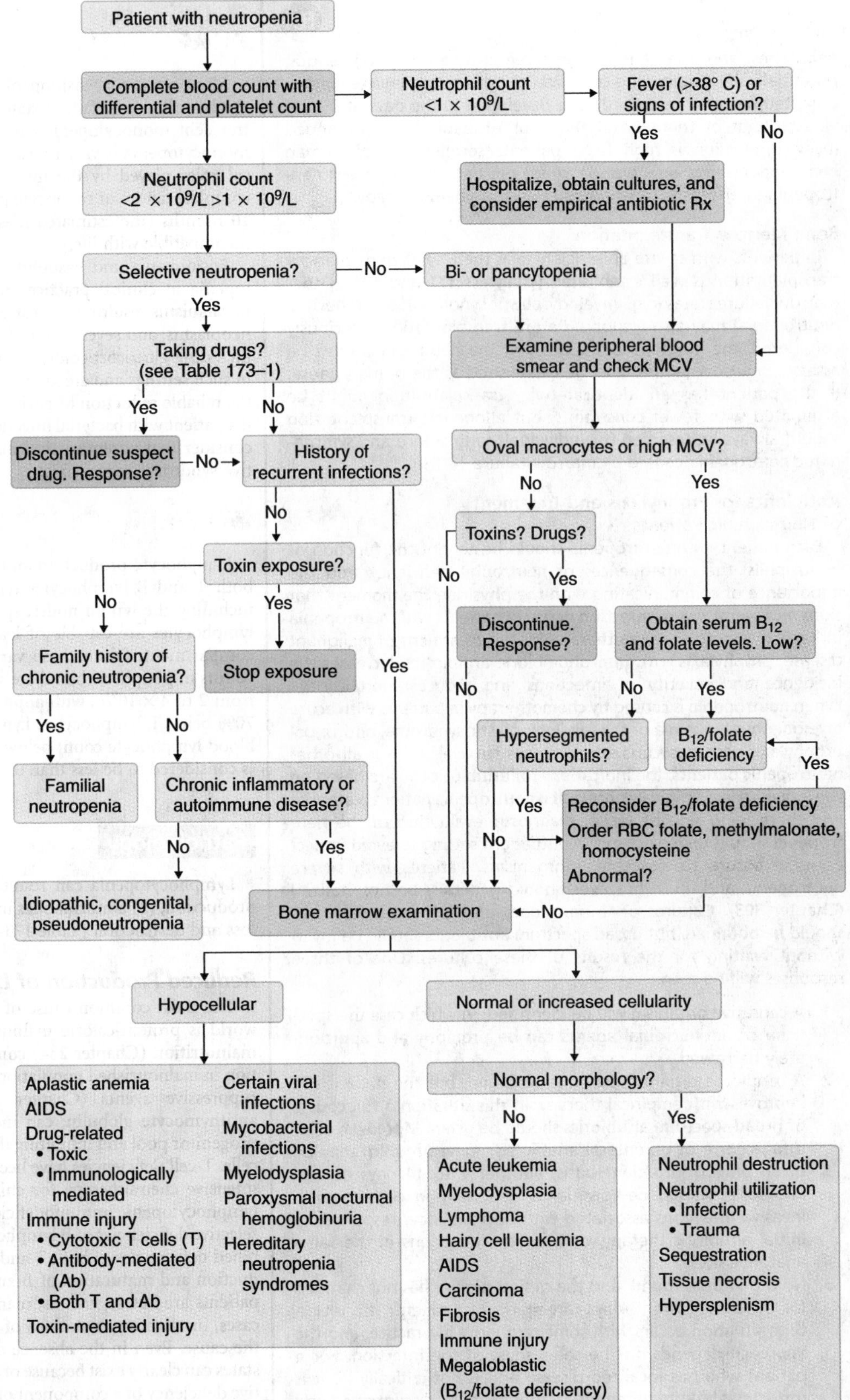

FIGURE 173–5 • Practical algorithm for the evaluation of patients with neutropenia. The fundamental diagnostic principle is that for patients with severe neutropenia or for those with bicytopenia or pancytopenia, bone marrow examination will probably be necessary unless the following diagnoses are made: (1) a nutritional (folate or vitamin B_{12}) deficiency or (2) drug- or toxin-induced neutropenia in a patient whose neutropenia resolves after discontinuation of the offending agent. AIDS = acquired immunodeficiency syndrome; MCV = mean corpuscular volume; RBC = red blood cell.

Rx

that these recombinant growth factors reduce mortality in nonneutropenic patients with nosocomial pneumonia in the intensive care unit. 2 In view of their attendant costs, routine use of G-CSF or GM-CSF to prevent infection in neutropenic cancer patients cannot be encouraged outside the setting of well-designed controlled clinical trials. For nontransplant patients not participating in such studies, it seems most rational to use these granulopoietic factors in patients undergoing cytotoxic chemotherapy only if the dose intensity of the chemotherapeutic agents has a demonstrated impact on overall survival (e.g., Hodgkin's disease, germ cell

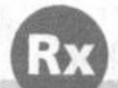

neoplasms) *and* one of following three criteria apply: (1) serious, potentially life-threatening complications of neutropenia (e.g., documented bacterial infection) have developed in the patient in previous rounds of therapy; (2) the prior probability for prolonged myelosuppression is high (e.g., patients seropositive for human immunodeficiency virus type 1); or (3) the patient's persistent neutropenia interferes with scheduled doses of chemotherapy.

Bone Marrow Transplantation

In patients with severe aplastic anemia, the role of bone marrow transplantation is well established (Chapters 171 and 184). Other marrow failure states (e.g., myelodysplastic syndromes and inherited neutropenia) may also respond. Before transplantation is seriously considered, the duration and severity of the neutropenia must be assessed; marrow failure must be established as the primary cause. If the patient has an identical twin, transplantation might be attempted with fewer constraints, but allogeneic transplantation should always be reserved for individuals with severe and symptomatic neutropenia caused by marrow failure.

Antibiotics for Prophylaxis and Treatment of Neutropenic Patients

Each patient with neutropenia should be taught the function of neutrophils, the consequences of neutrophil deficiency, and the importance of communicating with the physician the moment that signs and symptoms of infection occur. In patients with neutropenia induced by cytotoxic chemotherapy for the treatment of malignant disease, prophylaxis with fluoroquinolone antibiotics decreases the incidence and severity of infections and reduces mortality. [3] When neutropenia is caused by chemotherapy in patients with acute myelogenous leukemia or the myelodysplastic syndrome, antifungal prophylaxis with posaconazole improves survival. [4] For all other neutropenic patients, the indications for antibiotic use are based on the individualized clinical context. If a neutropenic patient is afebrile and there is no sign of sepsis, diagnostic evaluation of the neutropenia should take place in the outpatient setting to avoid unnecessary exposure to nosocomial organisms. Patients with severe neutropenia and fever, however, should generally be hospitalized (Chapter 303). Cultures of urine, blood, and other relevant sites should be obtained, but broad-spectrum antibiotics should be given without waiting for the results of these cultures. One of three responses will be seen:

1. A causative organism will be identified, in which case the spectrum of antimicrobial agents can be promptly and appropriately narrowed.
2. A candidate organism will not be found, but the patient still improves with empirical therapy. In this situation a full course of broad-spectrum antibiotics should be given. Moreover, after a full course of parenteral antibiotics, some of which may be given on an outpatient basis, another 7 to 14 days of oral antibiotics should be considered, especially in patients with invasive infections associated with necrosis, slow responses to initial antibiotic therapy, or recurrent infections in the same anatomic site.
3. No organism is found, and the clinical picture has not changed for the better after 3 days of empirical treatment. This unsettling situation occurs with some regularity in practice, and the approach depends on the seriousness of the infection. For a patient who has localized disease and is not critically ill, it is sometimes helpful for empirical therapy to be discontinued and for repeat cultures to be obtained. If the patient is critically ill, however, antibiotics should be discontinued only if other antibiotics are substituted. Among the antibiotics to consider under these circumstances are antiviral and antifungal agents. Antifungal agents should be added to the therapeutic regimen for patients with acute leukemia, diabetes, dysphagia or esophagitis, endophthalmitis, or defective cell-mediated immunity (including those receiving immunosuppressive therapy) and for those who have received prolonged treatment with broad-spectrum antibacterial agents in the recent past.

DEFICIENCIES OF OTHER CIRCULATING PHAGOCYTES

Monocytopenia, eosinopenia, and basophilopenia are seen in most of the bone marrow failure states associated with neutropenia. Although transient monocytopenia can result from hemodialysis, stable isolated monocytopenia is very unusual. In view of the heterogeneous and critical roles played by the monocyte-macrophage in normal physiology, complete failure of monocyte production for a period of more than 9 to 10 months (the estimated lifespan of tissue macrophages) is probably incompatible with life.

Eosinopenia and basophilopenia are more common than monocytopenia in clinical practice and most often represent redistributional mechanisms resulting from stress, including acute infections, widespread neoplasms, and severe injury (e.g., burns). A variety of humoral factors, including glucocorticoids, prostaglandins, and epinephrine, are released in such settings and are known to induce eosinopenia. In fact, because of the reliable reduction of peripheral eosinophils during infectious events, if a patient with bacterial infection does not have eosinopenia, one should consider that adrenocortical insufficiency or a primary myeloproliferative syndrome may coexist.

LYMPHOCYTOPENIA

Lymphocyte production and traffic are difficult to assess because (1) both T and B lymphocytes replicate in heterogeneous anatomic sites, including the lymph nodes, spleen, tonsils, and bone marrow, and (2) lymphocytes are capable of leaving and then later re-entering a given compartment. Given these variables, it is surprising that lymphocyte counts in peripheral blood are so tightly regulated; normal counts range from 2 to 4×10^9/L, with approximately 20% being B lymphocytes and 70% being T lymphocytes. Lymphocytopenia is defined as a peripheral blood lymphocyte count below 1.5×10^9/L, but severe lymphocytopenia is considered to be less than 0.7×10^9/L.

Pathobiology

Lymphocytopenia can result from (1) abnormalities in lymphocyte production, (2) abnormalities in lymphocyte traffic, and (3) lymphocyte loss and destruction (Table 173–2).

Reduced Production of Lymphocytes

The most common cause of reduced lymphocyte production in the world is protein-calorie malnutrition. Immune paresis resulting from malnutrition (Chapter 234) contributes to the high incidence of infection in malnourished populations. Radiation (Chapter 18) and immunosuppressive agents (Chapter 33), including alkylating agents and antithymocyte globulin, can induce lymphocytopenia by injuring the progenitor pool and inhibiting the replication of more well differentiated cells. T-cell deficiencies have been found in some long-term survivors of intensive chemotherapy for childhood cancer. A variety of congenital lymphocytopenic immunodeficiency states exist, some of which result in selective deficiencies of B lymphocytes, some of T cells, and some of combined deficiencies of both T and B cells. The mechanisms by which production and maturation of B and T lymphocytes are impaired in these patients are heterogeneous; many remain ill defined, although in some cases, inactivating mutations of receptors for lymphopoietic factors are the cause. Even in the absence of lymphocytopenia, immunodeficiency states can clearly exist because of abnormal lymphocyte function or selective deficiency of a component of the circulating lymphocyte population.

Certain viruses are capable of inducing lymphocytopenia; some of these agents infect lymphoid cells and cause their destruction. Such viruses include measles, polio, varicella-zoster, and human immunodeficiency virus. Human immunodeficiency virus does not frequently cause lymphocytopenia, but it infects the helper ($CD4^+$) subset of T lymphocytes and destroys them, a process that results in a marked decline in the absolute numbers of helper T cells in the peripheral circulation (Chapter 416). Patients with untreated Hodgkin's disease occasionally have lymphocytopenia, especially during the late stages of the disease or in instances associated with the least favorable histologic subtypes (Chapter 197).

TABLE 173–2 CAUSES OF LYMPHOCYTOPENIA

ABNORMALITIES IN LYMPHOCYTE PRODUCTION

Protein-calorie malnutrition
Radiation
Immunosuppressive therapeutic agents
  Glucocorticosteroids
  Cyclosporine
Congenital immunodeficiency states
  Wiskott-Aldrich syndrome
  Nezelof's syndrome
  Adenosine deaminase deficiency
Viral infections
Hodgkin's disease
Multiple myeloma
Widespread granulomatous infection (mycobacterial, fungal)
Cytotoxic chemotherapy
Direct dose-related effects (e.g., fludarabine)
Long-term effects (e.g., cyclophosphamide)
Idiosyncratic drug reactions (e.g., quinine)

ALTERATIONS IN LYMPHOCYTE TRAFFIC

Acute bacterial/fungal infection
Surgery
Trauma
Hemorrhage
Glucocorticosteroid therapy
Viral infection
Widespread granulomatous infection
Hodgkin's disease

LYMPHOCYTE DESTRUCTION OR LOSS

Viral infection (e.g., human immunodeficiency virus, severe acute respiratory syndrome [SARS])
Antibody-mediated lymphocyte destruction (e.g., systemic lupus erythematosus)
Protein-losing enteropathy
Chronic right ventricular failure
Thoracic duct drainage or rupture
Extracorporeal circulation
Graft-versus-host disease

Alterations in Lymphocytic Traffic

Traffic redistribution is common and most frequently represents transient responses to a variety of stressful events, including bacterial infections, surgery, trauma, and hemorrhage. These responses are probably mediated by high levels of endogenous glucocorticoids that induce rapid declines in circulating levels of B and T lymphocytes. In hospitalized patients with lymphocytopenia, glucocorticosteroid therapy (Chapter 33) is the third most common cause, after acute bacterial or fungal infections and surgery. The lymphocytopenic response to this type of steroid results from a self-limited shift of lymphocytes away from the peripheral blood compartment. Lymphocyte values generally return to normal within 24 to 48 hours. For this reason, the transient declines induced by endogenous steroid production are not associated with functional immunologic deficiency. Certain viruses can also bind to lymphocyte populations and cause their departure from the blood compartment into other sites. Given the rapid onset of disease in patients with severe acute respiratory syndrome (SARS; Chapter 97), this mechanism may also account for the prevalence of lymphocytopenia in such patients.

More persistent lymphocytopenia has been described in patients with widespread granulomatous disease, a phenomenon that is probably multifactorial and derived from both inhibition of production and alterations in traffic. Patients with these disorders are often difficult to treat. In daily practice, establishing a cause-and-effect relationship between the infection and lymphocytopenia can be difficult when one considers that the reverse might just as easily be true; consider, for example, the frequency of mycobacterial infection in patients with the acquired immunodeficiency syndrome.

Increased Destruction of Lymphocytes

Viral infections or antilymphocyte antibodies, especially in patients with underlying autoimmune or rheumatic diseases, increase lymphocyte destruction. Loss of viable lymphocytes can also occur as a result of structural defects in sites of high-density lymphocyte traffic (e.g., via thoracic duct fistulas). In such patients, both T cells and B cells decline in the peripheral blood. Loss of lymphocytes from intestinal lymphatics can occur in cases of protein-losing enteropathy, severe heart failure, or primary diseases of the gut or intestinal lymphatics (see Table 173–2).

Clinical Manifestations

There are no specific clinical manifestations of lymphocytopenia per se. Whether the patient exhibits signs of immunologic deficiency depends on the pathophysiology of the disorder, the duration of the disease, the type of lymphocytes affected, the intactness of nodal tissues, and the degree to which cellular or humoral immunity is functionally perturbed.

Diagnosis

Unless the clinical setting is clearly one in which transient lymphocytopenia is likely, the approach to diagnosis should involve comprehensive assessment of the integrity of the immune apparatus. Specifically, the subsets of lymphocytes remaining in the circulating blood should be quantified, including B cells, helper-inducer T cells ($CD4^+$), and cytotoxic-suppressor T cells ($CD8^+$). In addition, quantitative immunoglobulin levels in serum should be measured and a series of skin tests should be performed to detect deficiencies of cell-mediated immunity.

Treatment

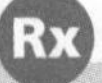

Because lymphocytopenia ordinarily represents a response to an underlying disease, primary attention must be paid to establishing the nature of that disease and instituting therapy for it. Patients whose lymphocytopenia is accompanied by hypogammaglobulinemia may benefit significantly from the administration of intravenous immunoglobulin, which often reduces the incidence of infectious events. Treatment of severe deficiencies of cell-mediated immunity remains experimental. Responses have been described with transplantation of allogeneic bone marrow, fetal liver, or thymic epithelial cells. Treatment with IL-7 can hasten immune recovery in nonhuman primates rendered neutropenic by radiation and antithymocyte globulin, so IL-7 and other lymphopoietic factors may have future roles that parallel the role of granulopoietic factors.

LEUKOCYTOSIS AND LEUKEMOID REACTIONS

Circulating leukocytes consist of neutrophils, monocytes, eosinophils, basophils, and lymphocytes (T cells, B cells, and natural killer cells). Any one or all of these cell types can increase to abnormal levels in peripheral blood in response to various stimuli. Each type of leukocyte is produced in the bone marrow (and in the case of lymphocytes, in lymph nodes, the spleen, and the thymus as well) in response to specific growth factors and, in the case of some lymphocytes, in response to antigenic stimuli. The term *leukocytosis* is used to describe a total leukocyte count above 11.0×10^9/L; it is a common and diagnostically important finding in clinical practice. Once leukocytosis is discovered, it is essential to examine the differential white blood cell count so that one can determine which white blood cell types are increased. The terms *neutrophilia* (neutrophilic leukocytosis), *monocytosis, lymphocytosis, eosinophilia,* and *basophilia* suggest specific sets of diagnostic considerations.

Leukocytosis is a common finding in acutely ill patients. When the leukocyte count exceeds 25 to 30 × 10^9/L, the condition is sometimes termed a *leukemoid reaction.* Leukemoid reactions generally reflect the response of healthy bone marrow to cytokines released by auxiliary cells (lymphocytes, macrophages, and stromal cells) exposed to infection or trauma. Leukemoid reactions are not synonymous with *leukoerythroblastosis,* which indicates the presence of immature white blood cells *and* nucleated red blood cells in the peripheral blood, irrespective of the total leukocyte count. Leukoerythroblastosis is less common than leukemoid reactions but frequently, especially in adult patients, reflects serious marrow dysfunction (Table 173–3). Consequently, the finding of leukoerythroblastosis represents a clear indication to perform bone marrow aspiration and biopsy, unless the clinical setting is specifically an acute severe hemolytic anemia, sepsis in a patient with hyposplenism, or acute massive trauma with multiple fractures.

TABLE 173–3 CAUSES OF LEUKOERYTHROBLASTOSIS

NORMAL BONE MARROW
Severe acute hemolytic anemia
Acute infection in hyposplenic patients
ABNORMAL BONE MARROW
Marrow infiltration
Metastatic malignancy (e.g., carcinoma of the lung, breast, prostate, or stomach)
Hematologic malignancies
Acute leukemia
Multiple myeloma
Chronic myeloproliferative diseases (e.g., myeloid metaplasia or chronic myelogenous leukemia)
Lymphoma
Granulomatous diseases
Mycobacterial infection
Fungal diseases
OTHER DISORDERS
Osteopetrosis
Gaucher's disease
Amyloidosis
Paget's disease of bone
Severe tissue hypoxia
Multiple fractures

Neutrophilia

Pathobiology

The number of neutrophil precursors in the marrow mitotic pool (Fig. 173–6) is largely influenced by the hematopoietic growth factors, the most neutrophil lineage specific of which is the granulopoietic factor G-CSF. G-CSF not only functions to stimulate the growth and differentiation of granulocyte progenitor cells but also functionally activates neutrophils by enhancing their capacity to kill ingested organisms. The same holds true for macrophage colony-stimulating factor (M-CSF, which activates mononuclear phagocytes) and IL-5 (the growth factor that activates eosinophils).

The marrow storage pool can provide the periphery with neutrophils for about 5 days in the steady state, even if it received no input from the mitotic pool. Neutrophils are released from the storage pool into the circulating pool in response to a variety of physiologic stresses, including endogenous glucocorticoids (see Fig. 173–6B). Neutrophilia can result from a shift of neutrophils from the marginated to the circulating pool, termed *demargination* (see Fig. 173–6C). This response is rapid and can be induced by injections of epinephrine and glucocorticosteroids. In patients with acute inflammatory illnesses, storage pool release and demargination usually occur together (see Fig. 173–6D).

Neutrophilic leukocytosis is the most common type of leukocytosis in clinical practice. It evolves in response to the release of factors that govern the production and traffic of this cell type, including G-CSF, and factors that augment the mitotic activity of G-CSF, including IL-3, Steel factor, and GM-CSF. These and additional less well defined granulopoietic factors are produced by a network of auxiliary cells in the bone marrow, including mononuclear phagocytes, microvascular endothelial cells, fibroblasts, and lymphocytes. These growth factor–producing cells respond to acute inflammatory events by augmenting production of the critically important colony-stimulating factors. The colony-stimulating factors stimulate replication of granulopoietic progenitor cells, which leads to expansion of the neutrophil storage pool and subsequent neutrophilia (see Fig. 173–6E). In response to the infection and the induced cytokines and adhesion molecules, the transit time of neutrophils in the mitotic and postmitotic pools in the bone marrow is shorter than in the uninfected state, and immature neutrophils (bands and metamyelocytes) are released from the storage pool. This new high level of production persists until the inflammatory process resolves.

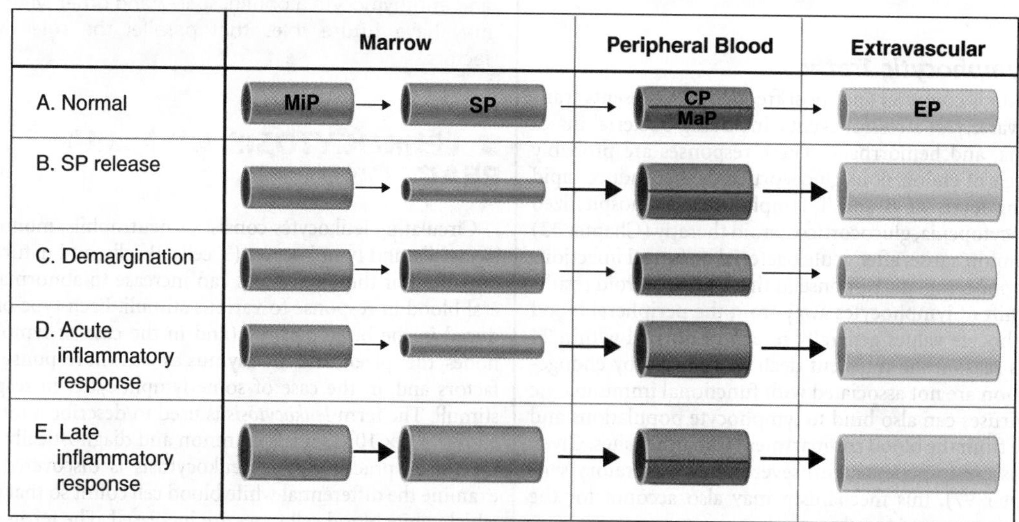

FIGURE 173–6 • Pathophysiologic mechanisms of neutrophilia. A, In this figure, the size of a given compartment is represented by the relative size of the cylinder-shaped "pool." The absolute number of cells leaving one pool for the next is represented by the size of the arrows between the pools. CP = circulating granulocyte pool; EP = extravascular pool; MaP = marginated pool; MiP = mitotic pool of neutrophil precursor cells; SP = neutrophil storage pool. Notice that the circulating neutrophil pool is large (necessarily true for patients with neutrophilic leukocytosis) but the size of the other pools is variable. **B,** A variety of stresses, such as infection, can result in the release of storage pool granulocytes, probably mediated through the actions of glucocorticosteroids or the granulopoietic factors granulocyte colony-stimulating factor and granulocyte-macrophage colony-stimulating factor. **C,** The circulating granulocyte pool can also increase in size because of a shift of neutrophils from the marginated to the circulating pool. The demargination response can be regularly elicited by the administration of epinephrine. This is a response that also occurs in infections, but not generally without other dynamic alterations in other pools. **D,** In most bacterial infections and other inflammatory processes, the demand for neutrophils in the infected extravascular site results in the simultaneous release of storage pool neutrophils and demargination. **E,** Later in the inflammatory response, after the hematopoietic growth factors released in response to the inflammatory stimulus have induced a few days of proliferation in the mitotic pool, the content of neutrophils in all pools increases and delivery to the tissues is maximized.

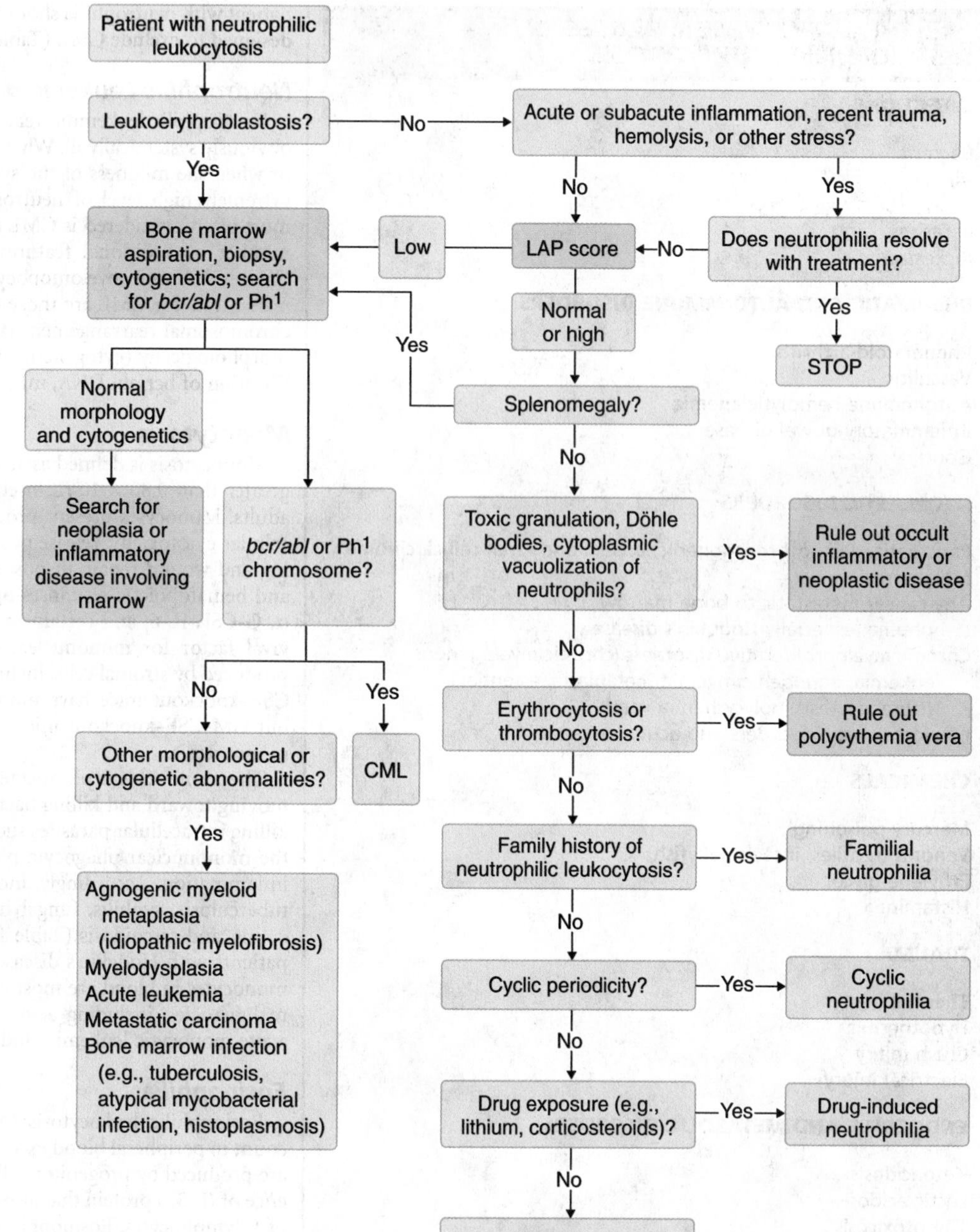

FIGURE 173–7 • Evaluation of patients with neutrophilic leukocytosis. *bcr/abl* = translocation of the *c-abl* gene from chromosome 9 to the *bcr* gene on chromosome 22q; CML = chronic myelogenous leukemia; LAP = leukocyte alkaline phosphatase; Ph[1] = Philadelphia chromosome.

Diagnosis

Neutrophilia (neutrophil counts >7.5 × 10^9/L), a common finding in clinical practice, usually reflects the inflammatory response to acute or subacute infections (Fig. 173–7; Table 173–4), so it should trigger a diagnostic search for its cause. Such searches generally involve a careful history and physical examination and just a few inexpensive laboratory tests (the nature of which depends on the findings on physical examination) because in most cases the cause will become apparent and usually proves to be an active infectious process.

When neutrophilia occurs in the absence of evidence of acute inflammation or illness, three explanations should be considered: (1) chemical effects, including agents such as glucocorticoids, lithium chloride, and epinephrine; (2) malignant tumors, in which cancer cells may inappropriately express certain of the genes encoding granulopoietic factors (e.g., G-CSF or IL-5); and (3) chronic myeloproliferative disorders, including chronic myelogenous leukemia (CML), agnogenic myeloid metaplasia, essential thrombocytosis, and polycythemia vera.

Neutrophil morphology can lead to early diagnosis. Toxic granulation of neutrophils (Fig. 161–29), Döhle bodies (Fig. 161–30), and vacuoles in the neutrophil cytoplasm suggest that overt or subclinical inflammation, toxin exposure, trauma, or neoplasia exists. Because glucocorticoids induce prompt eosinopenia and basophilopenia, these cells are almost universally absent in the blood of an acutely injured or infected patient. Thus, the presence of eosinophils should indicate that (1) the acutely ill patient may have concomitant adrenocortical insufficiency (Chapter 245), (2) the neutrophilia derives from the inappropriate production of GM-CSF or IL-5 (e.g., by malignant cells), or (3) the neutrophilia is one manifestation of a hematopoietic neoplasm (a chronic myeloproliferative disorder, myelodysplastic syndrome, lymphoma, or acute nonlymphocytic leukemia associated with eosinophilia).

The diagnostic approach to patients with neutrophilia (see Fig. 173–7) leads quickly to the performance of bone marrow aspiration and biopsy for patients with leukoerythroblastosis. In patients without leukoerythroblastosis, neutrophilic leukocytosis usually results from acute toxic, inflammatory, or traumatic stress, and it is generally best to observe the course of neutrophilia to determine its degree of linkage with the underlying disease. If the underlying disease resolves and the neutrophilia does not, other, less common explanations must be pursued.

Leukocyte alkaline phosphatase (LAP) is an enzyme found in neutrophils. When neutrophilia represents a reaction to an acute illness, LAP levels usually increase substantially. In patients with CML (Chapter 195), however, the LAP score is markedly decreased. A low LAP level in a

TABLE 173–4 COMMON CAUSES OF NEUTROPHILIC LEUKOCYTOSIS
INFECTIONS
Bacteria
Viruses
Fungi
Parasites
Rickettsia
RHEUMATIC AND AUTOIMMUNE DISORDERS
Rheumatoid arthritis
Vasculitis
Autoimmune hemolytic anemia
Inflammatory bowel disease
Gout
NEOPLASTIC DISORDERS
Pancreatic, gastric, bronchogenic, breast, and renal cell carcinoma
Melanoma
Any cancer metastatic to bone marrow
Lymphoma, especially Hodgkin's disease
Chronic myeloproliferative disorders (chronic myelogenous leukemia, agnogenic myeloid metaplasia, essential thrombocytosis, polycythemia vera)
Myelodysplastic disorders and acute leukemia
CHEMICALS
Mercury poisoning
Venoms (reptiles, insects, jellyfish)
Ethylene glycol
Histamine
TRAUMA
Thermal injury
Hypothermia
Crush injury
Electrical injury
ENDOCRINE AND METABOLIC DISORDERS
Ketoacidosis
Lactic acidosis
Thyrotoxicosis
HEMATOLOGIC DISORDERS (NON-NEOPLASTIC)
Acute hemolytic anemias and transfusion reactions
Post-splenectomy status
Recovery from marrow failure
OTHER DISORDERS
Tissue necrosis
Pregnancy
Eclampsia
Exfoliative dermatitis
Hypoxia
DRUGS
Corticosteroids
Lithium
Epinephrine
Granulocyte colony-stimulating factor
Granulocyte-macrophage colony-stimulating factor

patient with neutrophilia should therefore lead to a diagnostic evaluation designed to exclude CML (Table 173–5).

Neutrophilic Leukemoid Reactions

Neutrophilic leukemoid reactions generally occur in patients who are obviously systemically ill. When the neutrophil count exceeds 80×10^9/L or when the mildness of the systemic illness seems discordant with the extremely high level of neutrophils in peripheral blood, the diagnosis most often considered is CML or chronic myelomonocytic leukemia. A number of additional features distinguish leukemoid reactions from CML and chronic myelomonocytic leukemia (see Table 173–5). The diagnostic tests for CML are those designed to identify the classic balanced chromosomal rearrangement (a chromosome 9;22 translocation) either morphologically (cytogenetic analysis) or by molecular methods (identification of bcr/abl DNA, mRNA, or protein).

Monocytosis

Monocytosis is defined as absolute peripheral blood monocyte counts greater than 0.80×10^9/L in children and greater than 0.50×10^9/L in adults. Monocytes present processed antigens to lymphocytes, mediate cellular cytotoxicity, release procoagulants, participate in bone remodeling and wound repair, dispose of damaged cells, and regulate immune and hematopoietic responses by producing IL-1, tumor necrosis factor-α, G-CSF, IL-6, and certain interferons. The most specific growth/survival factor for mononuclear phagocytes is M-CSF (see Fig. 173–7) produced by stromal cells, including endothelial cells and fibroblasts. M-CSF–knockout mice have monocytopenia and macrophage deficiency, but GM-CSF–knockout mice do not. The cytokine IL-13 also induces monocytosis.

The mononuclear phagocyte is more sluggish than the neutrophil in moving toward and killing bacteria but is as effective, if not more so, in killing intracellular parasites such as fungi, yeast, and viruses. In addition, the mononuclear phagocyte participates in all types of granulomatous inflammation. Accordingly, monocytosis is often seen in patients with tuberculosis, syphilis, fungal infections, ulcerative and granulomatous colitis, and sarcoidosis (Table 173–6). Mild monocytosis is common in patients with Hodgkin's disease and a variety of cancers. High levels of monocytes in blood are most often seen in patients with hematopoietic malignancies, including acute and chronic myelomonocytic leukemia, acute monocytic leukemia, and the juvenile type of CML.

Eosinophilia

Eosinophilic leukocytosis (eosinophilia) exists when the eosinophil count in peripheral blood exceeds 0.4×10^9/L (Chapter 176). Eosinophils are produced by progenitor cells in the marrow, largely under the influence of IL-5, a protein that also stimulates the growth and differentiation of B lymphocytes. Eosinophils not only function as phagocytes but also play an extraordinarily important role in modulating the potentially toxic effects of mast cell degranulation in hypersensitivity reactions.

Lymphocytosis

Lymphocytosis (Table 173–7) is defined as a lymphocyte count in excess of 5.0×10^9/L. Atypical lymphocytosis is present when atypical lymphocytes account for more than 20% of the total peripheral blood lymphocyte population. A number of humoral factors induce the growth of T lymphocytes (IL-2, IL-3, IL-7, IL-15), natural killer cells (IL-2, IL-12, IL-1), and B lymphocytes (IL-10, IL-6, IL-5, IL-4, IL-7, IL-13, IL-14, IL-15).

Diagnosis

Mild to moderate lymphocytosis (lymphocyte counts $<12 \times 10^9$/L) is most commonly caused by viral infections, including infectious mononucleosis and viral hepatitis. Careful examination of peripheral blood lymphocyte morphology can help distinguish between these two disorders. In cases of infectious mononucleosis, many of the lymphocytes are large, with abundant cytoplasm and a "ballerina skirt"–like cytoplasmic border; these are the characteristic "atypical" lymphocytes that exceed 20% of the total lymphocyte population during the course of this disease (Fig. 173–8). Interestingly, whereas the B lymphocyte is the target of the causative Epstein-Barr virus, the majority of cells in the peripheral blood of patients with this disease are T lymphocytes. This proliferation of T lymphocytes in response to Epstein-Barr virus infection of B cells plays

TABLE 173–5 DISTINCTIONS BETWEEN NEUTROPHILIC LEUKEMOID REACTIONS AND CHRONIC MYELOGENOUS LEUKEMIA

Finding/Result	Leukemoid Reaction	CML
Presence of fever or other manifestations of acute or subacute inflammation	Usual*	Infrequent†
Splenomegaly	Rare	Frequent
Natural course of neutrophilia	Resolution linked with abatement of the underlying disease	Progressive slow increase over time
Peripheral blood basophilia	Rare‡	Common
LAP score	High	Low§
Philadelphia chromosome	Absent	Frequent (>85%)
bcr/abl translocation	Absent	Frequent (>90%)

*Exceptions include patients with leukemoid reactions associated with certain cancers.
†Infections can also develop in patients with CML. The time to evaluate this possibility is when the inflammatory process resolves and the neutrophilia does not.
‡Patients with acute allergic reactions and patients with parasitic diseases are exceptions to this rule.
§LAP scores can be normal in some CML patients, particularly after splenectomy.
CML = chronic myelogenous leukemia; LAP = leukocyte alkaline phosphatase.

TABLE 173–6 CAUSES OF MONOCYTOSIS

INFECTIONS

Tuberculosis
Brucellosis
Endocarditis
Typhoid and paratyphoid
Syphilis
Fungal
Recovery from acute infections
Protozoal
Viral (e.g., varicella, dengue)

NEOPLASTIC DISEASES

Hodgkin's disease
Carcinoma (many varieties)
Acute and chronic myelomonocytic leukemia
Juvenile chronic myelomonocytic leukemia
Acute monocytic leukemia
Myelodysplasia
Myeloma and Waldenström's macroglobulinemia
Chronic lymphocytic leukemia (rare)

GASTROINTESTINAL DISORDERS

Ulcerative colitis
Granulomatous colitis
Cirrhosis
Sarcoidosis
Drug reactions
Recovery from marrow suppression
Congenital neutropenia

TABLE 173–7 CAUSES OF LYMPHOCYTOSIS

HIGH (>15 × 10^9/L)

Infectious mononucleosis
Pertussis
Acute infectious lymphocytosis
Chronic lymphocytic leukemia and variants thereof
Acute lymphocytic leukemia

MODERATE (<15 × 10^9/L)

Many viral infections
Infectious mononucleosis
Measles
Varicella
Hepatitis
Coxsackievirus
Adenovirus
Mumps
Cytomegalovirus
Human immunodeficiency virus type 1 (acute lymphadenopathy)
Other infectious diseases
Toxoplasmosis
Brucellosis
Tuberculosis
Typhoid fever
Syphilis (secondary)
Neoplastic disorders
Carcinoma
Hodgkin's disease
Acute lymphocytic leukemia (early)
Chronic lymphocytic leukemia
Thymoma
Sjögren's syndrome
Graves' diseases
Drug reactions (e.g., tetracycline)

a role in eradicating the infected B-cell population. This response is a critical one in view of the oncogenic potential of this virus.

Acute bacterial infections rarely cause lymphocytosis. One exception is pertussis (seen almost exclusively in children), in which profound lymphocytosis (up to 60 × 10^9/L) is sometimes seen. It has been known for 30 years that specific soluble factors derived from the causative organism *Bordetella pertussis* induce lymphocytosis in experimental animals. Perhaps with the exception of patients with early chronic lymphocytic leukemia, most patients with lymphocytosis and especially those with substantial lymphocytosis (>12 to 15 × 10^9/L) have overt signs of an underlying illness involving anatomic sites other than the lymphohematopoietic system. The diagnostic approach depends simply on establishing a tissue diagnosis to exclude malignant disease in patients who do not have clear-cut evidence of one of the more benign disorders. Bone marrow aspiration and biopsy are required when lymphocytosis coexists with leukoerythroblastosis, peripheral lymphocytes are immature (lymphoblasts), and the lymphocytosis is persistent in a patient who has no evidence of acute or subacute infection.

Immunophenotyping by flow cytometric analysis ("lymphocyte markers") should be performed with monoclonal antibodies to definitive integral membrane proteins. Not only will such studies provide evidence for or against dominance of one lymphocyte type and differentiation stage, but analysis of immunoglobulin light chain types can also determine whether B lymphocytes in the circulation are all members of a single (and therefore probable neoplastic) clone.

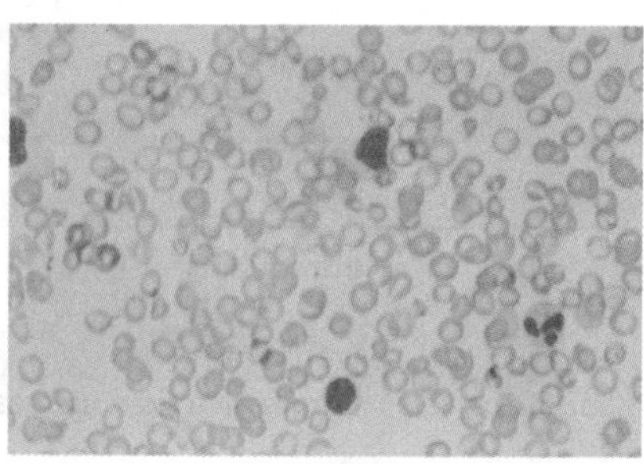

FIGURE 173–8 • Infectious mononucleosis. A peripheral smear shows pleomorphic, atypical (or "reactive") lymphocytes.

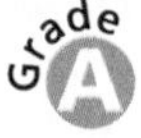

1. Rusthoven J, Bramwell V, Stephenson B, et al: Use of granulocyte colony-stimulating factor (G-CSF) in patients receiving myelosuppressive chemotherapy for the treatment of cancer. Cancer Care Ontario Practice Guideline Initiative CPG 12-2, 2002 (http://www.ccopebc.ca/guidelines/sys/cpg12_f.html).
2. Root RK, Lodato RF, Cade JF, et al: Multicenter, double-blind, placebo-controlled study of the use of filgrastim in patients hospitalized with pneumonia and severe sepsis. Crit Care Med 2003;31:635–637.
3. Gafter-Gvili A, Fraser A, Paul M, et al: Meta-analysis: Antibiotic prophylaxis reduces mortality in neutropenic patients. Ann Intern Med 2005;142:979–995.
4. Cornely OA, Maertens J, Winston DJ, et al: Posaconazole vs. fluconazole or itraconazole prophylaxis in patients with neutropenia. N Engl J Med 2007;356:348–359.

SUGGESTED READINGS

Klastersky J, Paesmans M, Georgala A, et al: Outpatient oral antibiotics for febrile neutropenic cancer patients using a score predictive for complications. J Clin Oncol 2006;24:4129–4134. *An oral regimen followed by early discharge may be an effective strategy in selected patients.*

Paul M, Yahav D, Fraser A, et al: Empirical antibiotic monotherapy for febrile neutropenia: Systematic review and meta-analysis of randomized controlled trials. J Antimicrob Chemother 2006;57:176–189. *Ceftazidime, piperacillin /tazobactam, imipenem/cilastatin and meropenem were suitable monotherapy, but cefepime increased mortality.*

Smith TJ, Khatcheressian J, Lyman GH, et al: 2006 update of recommendations for the use of white blood cell growth factors: an evidence-based clinical practice guideline. J Clin Oncol 2006;24:3187–3205. *Primary prophylaxis is indicated in high-risk patients.*

Welte K, Zeidler C, Dale DC: Severe congenital neutropenia. Semin Hematol 2006;43:189–195. *A comprehensive review.*

174 APPROACH TO THE PATIENT WITH LYMPHADENOPATHY AND SPLENOMEGALY

James O. Armitage

LYMPHADENOPATHY

Physiology and Anatomy

Lymph nodes are found throughout the body along the course of lymphatics, strategically located to allow filtering of lymphatic fluid and interdiction of microorganisms and abnormal proteins. Lymphatic fluid enters the node in afferent lymphatic vessels that empty into the subcapsular sinus. The fluid then transverses the node and exits in a single efferent lymphatic vessel. In doing so, the lymph and its contents are exposed to immunologically active cells throughout the node. Lymph nodes are populated predominantly by macrophages, dendritic cells, B lymphocytes, and T lymphocytes. B lymphocytes are located primarily in the follicles and perifollicular areas, whereas T lymphocytes are found principally in the interfollicular or paracortical areas of the lymph node. These cells function together to provide antigen processing, antigen presentation, antigen recognition, and proliferation of effector B and T lymphocytes as part of the normal immune response to microorganisms or foreign proteins.

Because the normal immune response leads to proliferation and expansion of one or more of the cellular components of lymph nodes, it also often leads to significant lymph node enlargement. In young children, who are continuously undergoing exposure to new antigens, palpable lymphadenopathy is the rule. In fact, the absence of palpable lymphadenopathy would be considered abnormal. In adults, lymph nodes larger than 1 to 2 cm in diameter are generally considered abnormal. However, lymph nodes 1 to 2 cm in diameter in the groin are sufficiently common to often be considered "normal."

Lymphoid proliferation is a normal response to exposure to foreign antigens. The location of the enlarged lymph nodes will often reflect the site of invasion. For example, cervical lymphadenopathy would be typical in a patient with pharyngitis. Generalized immune proliferation and lymphadenopathy can occur with a systemic disorder of the immune system, disseminated infection, or disseminated neoplasia. Malignancies of the immune system might be manifested as localized or disseminated lymphadenopathy.

Differential Diagnosis

The differential diagnosis of lymphadenopathy (Table 174–1) is vast, with the underlying causes responsible for either proliferation of immunologically active cells or infiltration of the lymph node by foreign cells or substances. In practice, the cause of enlarged lymph nodes is often not certain even in retrospect; in such cases, unrecognized infectious processes are generally blamed.

Infections by bacteria, mycobacteria, fungi, chlamydiae, parasites, and viruses are the major causes of lymph node enlargement. Lymph nodes in the drainage area of essentially all pyogenic infections can enlarge. In certain infections such as bubonic plague caused by *Yersinia pestis*, dramatic regional lymph node enlargement with fluctuant lymph nodes (i.e., buboes) can be a hallmark of the disease (Chapter 333). Other bacterial infections have lymph node enlargement as a prominent feature (e.g., cat-scratch disease, Chapter 336) and can mimic lymphoproliferative disorders. Mediastinal lymphadenopathy is seen in inhalational anthrax (Chapter 317). In some parts of the world, cervical lymphadenopathy is a sufficiently frequent manifestation of tuberculosis to lead to the institution of antituberculous therapy rather than biopsy. Disseminated

TABLE 174–1 CAUSES OF LYMPHADENOPATHY
Infection Bacterial (e.g., all pyogenic bacteria, cat-scratch disease, syphilis, tularemia) Mycobacterial (e.g., tuberculosis, leprosy) Fungal (e.g., histoplasmosis, coccidioidomycosis) Chlamydial (e.g., lymphogranuloma venereum) Parasitic (e.g., toxoplasmosis, trypanosomiasis, filariasis) Viral (e.g., Epstein-Barr virus, cytomegalovirus, rubella, hepatitis, human immunodeficiency virus)
Benign disorder of the immune system (e.g., rheumatoid arthritis, systemic lupus erythematosus, serum sickness, drug reactions such as to phenytoin, Castleman's disease, sinus histiocytosis with massive lymphadenopathy, Langerhans cell histiocytosis, Kawasaki's syndrome, Kimura's disease)
Malignant disorders of the immune system (e.g., chronic and acute myeloid and lymphoid leukemia, non-Hodgkin's lymphoma, Hodgkin's disease, angioimmunoblastic-like T-cell lymphoma, Waldenström's macroglobulinemia, multiple myeloma with amyloidosis, malignant histiocytosis)
Other malignancies (e.g., breast carcinoma, lung carcinoma, melanoma, head and neck cancer, gastrointestinal malignancies, germ cell tumors, Kaposi's sarcoma)
Storage diseases (e.g., Gaucher's disease, Niemann-Pick disease)
Endocrinopathies (e.g., hyperthyroidism, adrenal insufficiency, thyroiditis)
Miscellaneous (e.g., sarcoidosis, amyloidosis, dermatopathic lymphadenitis)

TABLE 174–2 MOST FREQUENT CAUSES OF LYMPHADENOPATHY IN ADULTS IN THE UNITED STATES

Unexplained
Infection
In drainage area of infection (e.g., cervical adenopathy with pharyngitis)
Disseminated (e.g., mononucleosis, human immunodeficiency virus infection)
Immune disorders (e.g., rheumatoid arthritis)
Neoplasms
Immune system malignancies (e.g., leukemia and lymphomas)
Metastatic carcinoma or sarcoma

lymphadenopathy can be seen in cases of infection by a variety of organisms, such as *Toxoplasma,* Epstein-Barr virus (i.e., infectious mononucleosis), cytomegalovirus, and human immunodeficiency virus.

A variety of nonmalignant disorders of the immune system can lead to localized or disseminated lymphadenopathy. Autoimmune diseases such as rheumatoid arthritis (Chapter 285) and systemic lupus erythematosus (Chapter 287) often have accompanying lymphadenopathy, which can pose a diagnostic challenge because of the increased incidence of lymphoma in patients with these disorders. In the lymphadenopathy that occurs as a reaction to drugs such as phenytoin, lymph node biopsy findings can sometimes be confused with those of lymphoma. Benign proliferative diseases of the immune system that can also be confused with lymphoma include Castleman's disease (Chapter 196; angiofollicular lymph node hyperplasia), sinus histiocytosis with massive lymphadenopathy, and disorders seen more frequently in Asia, such as Kawasaki syndrome (Chapter 465) and Kimura's disease.

All of the cells in the immune system can become malignant. Several of these malignancies are typically manifested as lymphadenopathy, and it can be seen in all. Lymphadenopathy as the initial manifestation is the rule for Hodgkin's disease and non-Hodgkin's lymphoma and is common in Waldenström's macroglobulinemia and B-cell chronic lymphocytic leukemia, but it is only occasionally seen in the myeloid leukemias (Chapters 194 through 198). Malignancies of all organ systems can metastasize to the lymph nodes and cause lymphadenopathy, which is usually seen in the drainage area of the primary tumor, for example, axillary lymph nodes in patients with breast cancer, hilar and mediastinal lymph nodes in patients with lung cancer, and cervical lymph nodes in patients with head and neck cancer. However, widespread lymphadenopathy can also occur with many solid tumors.

Other disorders that can have lymphadenopathy as an initial finding include storage diseases such as Gaucher's disease (Chapter 223), endocrinopathies such as hyperthyroidism (Chapter 244), sarcoidosis (Chapter 95), and dermatopathic lymphadenitis. Amyloidosis (Chapter 296) can cause lymphadenopathy in patients with multiple myeloma, hereditary amyloidosis, or amyloidosis associated with chronic inflammatory states.

Among patients with lymphadenopathy actually seen in practices in the United States, diagnoses will not be determined in a high proportion (Table 174–2). In such cases, the lymphadenopathy will usually be blamed on infection. When the lymphadenopathy is in the drainage site of a known infection (e.g., cervical lymphadenopathy in a patient with pharyngitis) or the patient has a known infection associated with lymphadenopathy (e.g., infectious mononucleosis; Chapter 400), this infectious assumption is usually correct. Alternatively, if a patient has an immunologic disorder that is known to cause lymphadenopathy, such as rheumatoid arthritis, this disorder is usually an acceptable explanation; however, progressive lymphadenopathy in such patients should trigger a biopsy because these patients are at increased risk for lymphoma. Localized, progressive lymphadenopathy, particularly when associated with fever, sweats, or weight loss, requires biopsy to exclude lymphoma.

Lymph Node Evaluation

Evaluation of a patient with lymphadenopathy includes a careful history, a thorough physical examination, laboratory tests, and sometimes imaging studies to determine the extent and character of the lymphadenopathy. The age of the patient and any associated systemic symptoms might be important hints in the evaluation (Table 174–3). Cervical lymphadenopathy in a child would be much less worrisome than equally prominent lymphadenopathy in a 60-year-old adult. The occurrence of fever, sweats, or weight loss raises the possibility of a malignancy of the immune system. The explanation for the lymphadenopathy might become apparent by identification of a site of infection, a particular medication, a travel history, or a previous malignancy.

TABLE 174–3 FACTORS TO CONSIDER IN THE DIAGNOSIS OF LYMPHADENOPATHY

Associated systemic symptoms
Patient's age
History of infection, trauma, medications, travel experience, previous malignancy, etc.
Location: cervical, supraclavicular, epitrochlear, axillary, intrathoracic (hilar vs. mediastinal), intra-abdominal (retroperitoneal vs. mesenteric vs. other), iliac, inguinal, femoral
Localized vs. disseminated
Tenderness/inflammation
Size
Consistency

TABLE 174–4 METHODS OF LYMPH NODE EVALUATION

Physical examination
Imaging
Chest radiography
Lymphangiography
Ultrasonography
Computed tomography
Magnetic resonance imaging
Positron emission tomography
Sampling
Needle aspiration
Cutting needle biopsy
Excisional biopsy

Physical examination allows the identification of localized versus widespread lymphadenopathy. The particular sites of involvement can be important hints to the diagnosis inasmuch as infections and carcinomas are likely to cause lymphadenopathy in the lymphatic drainage of the site of the disorder. In general, lymph nodes that are tender are more likely to be due to an infectious process, whereas painless adenopathy raises concern for malignancy. Lymph node consistency can also aid in the diagnosis: typically, lymph nodes containing metastatic carcinoma are rock hard, lymph nodes containing lymphoma are firm and rubbery, and lymph nodes enlarged in response to an infectious process are soft.

The larger the lymph node, the more likely that a serious underlying cause exists; lymph nodes greater than 3 to 4 cm in diameter in an adult are very worrisome. Physical examination to assess lymph node size is only marginally accurate and reproducible, although it is by far the most widely used method. More precise methods are available with various imaging techniques.

Imaging

Imaging studies, including routine radiographs or computed tomography (CT), ultrasonography, lymphangiography, magnetic resonance imaging, gallium scans, and positron emission tomography, are the only methods that can be used to assess the extent of lymphadenopathy in the chest and abdomen (Table 174–4). Chest radiographs provide the most economical and easiest method to assess mediastinal and hilar lymphadenopathy but are not as accurate as CT of the chest. Although the technique is no longer widely available, lymphangiography provides an

TABLE 174–5 AN APPROACH TO A PATIENT WITH LYMPHADENOPATHY

Does the patient have a known illness that causes lymphadenopathy? Treat and monitor for resolution.
Is there an obvious infection to explain the lymphadenopathy (e.g., infectious mononucleosis)? Treat and monitor for resolution.
Are the nodes very large and/or very firm and thus suggestive of malignancy? Perform a biopsy.
Is the patient very concerned about malignancy and unable to be reassured that malignancy is unlikely? Perform a biopsy.
If none of the preceding is true, perform a complete blood cell count and, if unrevealing, monitor for a predetermined period (usually 2 to 8 weeks). If the nodes do not regress or if they increase in size, perform a biopsy.

extremely accurate assessment of the lower abdominal lymph nodes and, because of retained contrast material, allows repeat examinations and assessment of response to therapy. CT and ultrasonography are the most useful modalities for assessing abdominal and retroperitoneal lymphadenopathy. In most patients, CT is probably the most accurate approach, but ultrasonography has the advantage of being less expensive and not requiring radiation exposure. Magnetic resonance imaging and positron emission tomography are not first-line studies for the assessment of lymphadenopathy. Positron emission tomography is frequently positive in patients with Hodgkin's disease and aggressive non-Hodgkin's lymphomas and can be used to assess the presence of active lymphoma in patients with lymphadenopathy and a proven diagnosis; they are especially useful for re-evaluating patients after therapy because lymph nodes do not always regress to normal size after treatment, particularly those in the mediastinum and retroperitoneum.

Interventional Evaluation

Lymph node aspiration or biopsy is often necessary for an accurate diagnosis of the cause of the lymphadenopathy. Fine-needle aspiration is currently popular and is often an accurate means of diagnosing infection or carcinoma involving a lymph node. Although lymphomas can occasionally be diagnosed with this approach, it is inappropriate as an initial diagnostic maneuver for lymphoma. Cutting needle biopsy will occasionally provide sufficient material for an unequivocal diagnosis and subtyping of the lymphoma. However, excisional biopsy, which is most likely to provide the pathologist with adequate material to perform histologic, immunologic, and genetic studies, is the approach most likely to yield the correct diagnosis.

An Approach to the Patient with Lymphadenopathy

Patients with lymphadenopathy (Table 174–5) come to medical attention in several ways. Perhaps the most common is a patient who has felt a lymph node in the neck, axilla, or groin and then seeks a physician's opinion. Lymphadenopathy might also come to medical attention as an unexpected finding on routine physical examination or as part of evaluation for another complaint. Finally, patients might be found to have unexpected lymphadenopathy on imaging studies of the chest or abdomen. When the nodes are multiple or larger than 2 to 3 cm, biopsy via mediastinoscopy, a paramediastinal incision, laparoscopy, or laparotomy is often required for diagnosis.

The approach to a patient complaining of newly discovered lymphadenopathy in the neck, axilla, or groin depends on the size, consistency, and number of enlarged lymph nodes and the patient's general health. In most cases, very large or very firm lymph nodes in the presence of systemic symptoms such as unexplained fever, sweats, or weight loss should lead to lymph node biopsy. Patients who have enlarged lymph nodes in the drainage area of a previously treated malignancy (e.g., neck nodes in a patient with a history of head and neck cancer) might be best approached by lymph node aspiration. Carcinoma can often be diagnosed in this manner, although it is a poor approach for the diagnosis of lymphoid malignancies. For the cervical lymph nodes, excisional biopsy should be delayed in a patient who has head and neck cancer (Chapter 200) as a diagnostic consideration. These patients should initially undergo careful ear, nose, and throat examinations to avoid performing a biopsy that can complicate the patient's subsequent therapy.

For the most common situation, in which a lymph node is soft and not larger than 2 to 3 cm and the patient has no obvious systemic illness, observation for a brief period is usually the best approach. Performance of a complete blood cell count and examination of a peripheral smear can be helpful in recognizing a systemic illness (e.g., infectious mononucleosis) (see Fig. 161–35). These patients are often also given antibiotics. If the lymph node does not regress over the course of a few weeks or if it grows in size, a biopsy should be performed.

Part of the care of such patients involves the art of medicine and responsiveness to the patient's particular needs. For example, biopsy might be performed more quickly in a patient who is very anxious about malignancy or who needs a definitive diagnosis expeditiously.

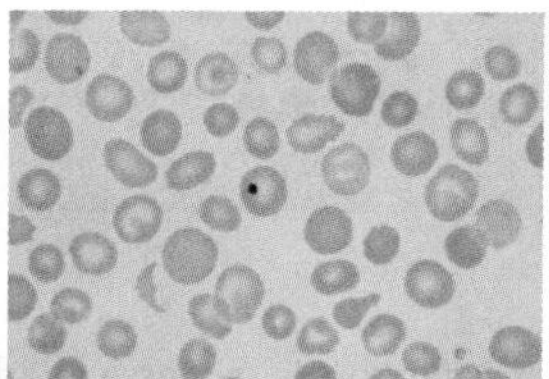

FIGURE 174–1 • A Howell-Jolly body in an erythrocyte, evidence of splenectomy or a nonfunctional spleen.

SPLENOMEGALY

Definition

The spleen is the largest lymphatic organ in the body and is sometimes approached clinically as though it were a very large lymph node. However, although it also participates in the primary immune response to invading microorganisms and foreign proteins, the spleen has many other functions. It functions as a filter for the blood and is responsible for removing senescent red blood cells from the circulation, as well as blood cells and other cells coated with immunoglobulins. Blood enters the spleen, filters through the splenic cords, and is exposed to immunologically active cells in the spleen.

The splenic red pulp occupies more than half the volume of the spleen and is the site where senescent red cells are identified and destroyed and red blood cell inclusions are removed by a process known as *pitting.* In the absence of splenic function, basophilic inclusions known as *Howell-Jolly bodies* are seen in circulating red blood cells. The presence of Howell-Jolly bodies (Fig. 174–1) in peripheral blood indicates that the patient has undergone splenectomy or has a process that has rendered the spleen nonfunctional (e.g., sickle cell disease with repeated splenic infarcts and chronic graft-versus-host disease).

The white pulp of the spleen contains macrophages, B lymphocytes, and T lymphocytes; participates in the recognition of microorganisms and foreign proteins; and is involved in the primary immune response. Absence of this splenic function makes individuals particularly sensitive to certain infections, including sepsis with encapsulated organisms such as *Streptococcus pneumoniae.* The risk for overwhelming sepsis is related to the age at the time of splenectomy or other cause of loss of splenic function. Children and young adults are at highest risk. If possible, all patients should undergo vaccination against *S. pneumoniae* (Chapter 16) before splenectomy. Some physicians have patients take oral penicillin (penicillin VK, 250 mg twice daily) indefinitely if splenectomy has been performed in childhood or adolescence.

Pathobiology

As with lymphadenopathy, the conditions associated with splenomegaly are extremely numerous (Table 174–6). Certain bacterial infections such as endocarditis (Chapter 76), brucellosis (Chapter 331), and typhoid fever (Chapter 329) have splenomegaly as a frequent manifestation. Disseminated tuberculosis (Chapter 345) is often associated with splenomegaly, and splenomegaly can also be seen in cases of disseminated histoplasmosis (Chapter 353) and toxoplasmosis (Chapter

TABLE 174–6 CAUSES OF SPLENOMEGALY

Infection
- Bacterial (e.g., endocarditis, brucellosis, syphilis, typhoid, pyogenic abscess)
- Mycobacterial (e.g., tuberculosis)
- Fungal (e.g., histoplasmosis, toxoplasmosis)
- Parasitic (e.g., malaria, leishmaniasis)
- Rickettsial (e.g., Rocky Mountain spotted fever)
- Viral (e.g., Epstein-Barr virus, cytomegalovirus, human immunodeficiency virus, hepatitis)

Benign disorders of the immune system (e.g., rheumatoid arthritis with Felty's syndrome, systemic lupus erythematosus, drug reactions such as to phenytoin, Langerhans cell histiocytosis, serum sickness)

Malignant disorders of the immune system (e.g., acute or chronic myeloid or lymphoid leukemia, non-Hodgkin's lymphoma, Hodgkin's disease, Waldenström's macroglobulinemia, malignant histiocytosis)

Other malignancies (e.g., melanoma, sarcoma)

Congestive splenomegaly (e.g., portal hypertension secondary to liver disease, splenic or portal vein thrombosis)

Hematologic disorders (e.g., autoimmune hemolytic anemia, hereditary spherocytosis, thalassemia major, hemoglobinopathies, elliptocytosis, megaloblastic anemia, extramedullary hematopoiesis)

Storage diseases (e.g., Gaucher's disease)

Endocrinopathies (e.g., hyperthyroidism)

Miscellaneous (e.g., sarcoidosis, amyloidosis, tropical splenomegaly, cysts)

370). Splenomegaly is an almost constant accompaniment of malaria (Chapter 366). Rickettsial disorders such as Rocky Mountain spotted fever are frequently associated with splenomegaly. A wide variety of viral infections typically cause splenomegaly, including infectious mononucleosis associated with Epstein-Barr virus (Chapter 400) and viral hepatitis (Chapter 151). Splenomegaly can accompany human immunodeficiency virus infection. Splenic abscesses, which are usually the result of hematogenous spread of pyogenic organisms, represent an unusual and difficult-to-diagnose cause of splenomegaly.

Splenomegaly is also seen in a variety of benign disorders of the immune system, including rheumatoid arthritis (Chapter 285), in which some patients will have Felty's syndrome and accompanying granulocytopenia. Splenomegaly is frequently detected in patients with systemic lupus erythematosus (Chapter 287), certain drug reactions, and serum sickness.

Malignancies of the immune system and nonimmune organs can also lead to splenomegaly. Splenomegaly is usually seen in patients with chronic myeloid leukemia and is frequent in chronic lymphoid leukemia (Chapter 195). It can develop in patients with acute myeloid or lymphoid leukemia, non-Hodgkin's lymphoma, Hodgkin's disease, and Waldenström's macroglobulinemia (Chapters 196 to 198) but is rare in multiple myeloma (Chapter 198). The condition previously known as angioimmunoblastic lymphadenopathy, which is now usually thought to represent a T-cell lymphoma, often has splenomegaly as one manifestation. Isolated splenomegaly (i.e., without any enlarged lymph nodes) is characteristic of certain immune system malignancies, including hairy cell leukemia (Chapter 195), the prolymphocytic variant of chronic lymphocytic leukemia (Chapter 195), and splenic marginal zone lymphoma (Chapter 197). Metastasis of carcinomas and sarcomas to the spleen is unusual except for malignant melanoma; even with melanoma, however, palpable splenomegaly is an unusual finding.

Splenomegaly can develop as a result of increased pressure in the splenic circulation, especially in patients with portal hypertension caused by a variety of hepatic disorders, including alcoholic cirrhosis (Chapter 157). However, it also can be due to splenic or portal vein thrombosis.

Hematologic disorders that can lead to palpable splenomegaly include autoimmune hemolytic anemia, hereditary spherocytosis, and a number of other anemias (Chapters 164, 165, and 167). In cases of idiopathic myelofibrosis, the spleen is frequently a site of extramedullary hematopoiesis (Chapter 177).

A variety of less common conditions can lead to splenomegaly. The storage disorder Gaucher's disease (Chapter 223) is usually manifested as splenomegaly. Splenomegaly can be seen in endocrinopathies such as hyperthyroidism (Chapter 244). Sarcoidosis (Chapter 95) and amyloidosis (Chapter 296) can be manifested as splenomegaly. *Tropical splenomegaly* is a term used to describe the palpable spleens found in patients who live in tropical areas and might have numerous causes.

TABLE 174–7 METHODS FOR EVALUATING THE SPLEEN

Physical examination

Imaging
- Ultrasonography
- Computed tomography
- Liver-spleen scanning
- Positron emission tomography

Biopsy
- Needle aspiration
- Splenectomy
  - Laparotomy (total or partial splenectomy)
  - Laparoscopy

Diagnosis

Evaluation of Splenic Size and Function

Physical Examination

The ability to perform an accurate physical examination and determine the presence of an enlarged spleen (Table 174–7) is an important skill, but it is not easily learned. Physical examination of the spleen can be performed with the patient supine or in the right lateral decubitus position. Inspection, percussion, auscultation, and palpation can all be important in accurate assessment. It is rare to have a spleen so large that it is visible and can be seen to move with respiration. However, in patients with such a condition, it is possible to miss the splenomegaly by failing to start palpation sufficiently low to find the edge. Occasionally, percussion of the left upper quadrant will help identify an area of dullness that moves with respiration and can lead to the identification of splenomegaly. Splenic size is generally recorded as the number of centimeters that the spleen descends below the left costal margin in the midclavicular line on inspiration. Although auscultation is not usually a regular part of splenic examination, the existence of a splenic rub on inspiration can lead to the diagnosis of splenic infarction. The left kidney is sometimes confused with the spleen on physical examination, but its failure to move with respiration in the manner typical for the spleen will usually allow distinction.

Laboratory Evaluation

Laboratory studies are frequently valuable in assessing splenic function. In patients with an absent or nonfunctional spleen, Howell-Jolly bodies will be seen in circulating red blood cells (see Fig. 174–1). Splenic hyperfunction (a condition often referred to as *hypersplenism*) is associated with cytopenias: the spleen is the normal reservoir for a significant proportion of platelets, and this reservoir function can lead to thrombocytopenia in patients with splenomegaly. Patients with autoimmune hemolytic anemia usually have palpable splenomegaly, but patients with idiopathic (immune) thrombocytopenic purpura usually do not.

The spleen can be imaged with ultrasonography, CT, traditional radionuclide scans, and positron emission tomography (Fig. 174–2). Ultrasonography can provide accurate determination of splenic size and is easy to repeat. CT will frequently give a better view of the consistency of the spleen and can identify splenic tumors or abscesses that would otherwise be missed. Positron emission tomography can aid in evaluating focal lesions in the spleen. The technetium-labeled liver-spleen scan can be important in identifying liver disease as the cause of splenomegaly; in patients with cryptogenic cirrhosis who are found to have thrombocytopenia, a technetium liver-spleen scan that shows higher activity in the spleen than in the liver might be the initial hint of liver disease.

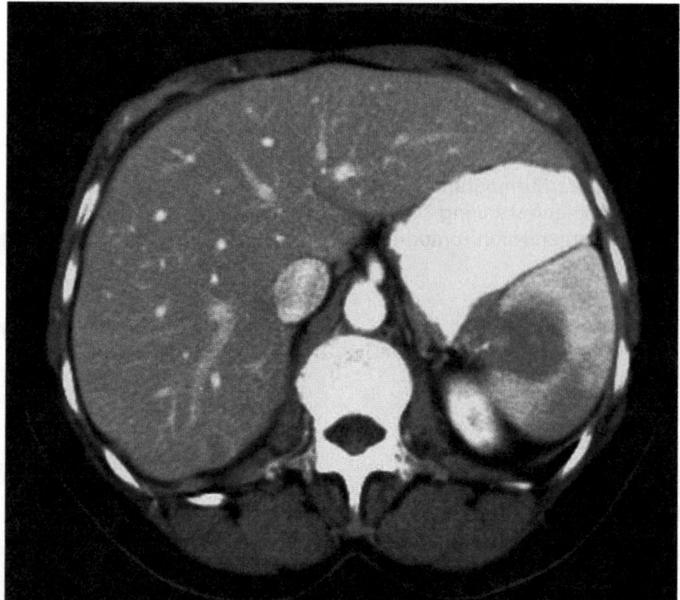

FIGURE 174–2 • Enlarged spleen with metastatic adenocarcinoma.

Because of the spleen's location and its propensity to bleed, needle aspiration or cutting needle biopsy of the spleen is rarely performed. In general, splenic "biopsy" involves splenectomy, which can be performed at the time of laparotomy or via laparoscopy. However, performing splenectomy laparoscopically usually leads to maceration of the organ and can reduce the diagnostic information. In very young children, in whom splenectomy causes a high risk for serious infections such as pneumococcal septicemia, partial splenectomy can sometimes be performed. Patients who undergo splenectomy at the time of splenic trauma and rupture can have seeding of splenic cells to other sites in the abdomen. Some patients have additional small or accessory spleens. Persistent, functional splenic tissue can be the explanation for recurrent immune thrombocytopenia after splenectomy and might be recognized by the absence of Howell-Jolly bodies in circulating red blood cells.

An Approach to the Patient with Splenomegaly

Patients with splenomegaly (Table 174–8) may come to medical attention for a variety of reasons. Patients may complain of left upper quadrant pain or fullness or early satiety. A splenic infarct, which is typically manifested as left upper quadrant pain that sometimes radiates to the left shoulder, can be the first clue to the existence of an enlarged spleen. Rarely, splenomegaly can initially be manifested by the catastrophic symptoms of splenic rupture. Some patients are found to have splenomegaly as a result of evaluation for unexplained cytopenia. Splenomegaly can be discovered incidentally on physical examination. In recent years, splenomegaly has been frequently discovered on imaging studies of the abdomen performed for other purposes.

The presence of a palpable spleen on physical examination is almost always abnormal. The one exception to this rule is a palpable spleen tip in a slender, young woman. In general, the presence of a palpable spleen should be considered a serious finding, and an explanation should be sought. It is less clear whether the same rules would apply to borderline splenomegaly discovered incidentally on routine imaging studies.

The approach to a patient with an enlarged spleen should focus initially on excluding a systemic illness that could explain the splenomegaly. Infectious mononucleosis, leukemia or lymphoma, rheumatoid arthritis, sarcoidosis, cirrhosis of the liver, malaria, and a host of other illnesses would be accepted as a reasonable explanation for the splenomegaly. The systemic condition should be treated and then the spleen should be re-evaluated. If the systemic illness can be treated successfully, the spleen should regress to normal size over time.

Patients with no obvious explanation for an enlarged spleen present a difficult diagnostic problem. Careful follow-up of these patients sometimes reveals occult liver disease or an autoimmune process that initially defied diagnosis. Concerns about malignancy, particularly in patients with systemic symptoms such as fever, sweats, or weight loss or in patients

TABLE 174–8 AN APPROACH TO A PATIENT WITH SPLENOMEGALY

Does the patient have a known illness that causes splenomegaly (e.g., infectious mononucleosis)? Treat and monitor for resolution.
Search for an occult infection (e.g., infectious endocarditis), hematologic disorder (e.g., hereditary spherocytosis), occult liver disease (e.g., cryptogenic cirrhosis), autoimmune disease (e.g., systemic lupus erythematosus), or storage disease (e.g., Gaucher's disease). If found, manage appropriately.
If systemic symptoms are present and suggest malignancy and/or focal replacement of the spleen is seen on imaging studies and no other site is available for biopsy, splenectomy is indicated.
If none of the above is true, monitor closely and repeat studies until the splenomegaly resolves or a diagnosis becomes apparent.

in whom imaging studies show a focal abnormality, are sometimes indications for splenectomy. However, in the absence of such findings, it is generally preferable to monitor patients closely with repeated attempts to establish the diagnosis by approaches other than splenectomy. It is particularly important to avoid splenectomy in a patient with occult liver disease and portal hypertension.

Splenectomy was once performed routinely as part of the staging evaluation for Hodgkin's disease or other lymphomas (Chapters 196 and 197). Today, this procedure is rarely needed to choose the correct therapy, and it should generally be avoided. Splenectomy can be an effective therapy for immune thrombocytopenic purpura (Chapter 179) and autoimmune hemolytic anemia (Chapter 164) and can occasionally be an appropriate therapy to relieve cytopenia in other conditions such as advanced myelofibrosis (Chapter 177).

SUGGESTED READINGS

Casaccia M, Torelli P, Squarcia S, et al: The Italian Registry of Laparoscopic Surgery of the Spleen (IRLSS): A retrospective review of 379 patients undergoing laparoscopic splenectomy. Chir Ital 2006;58:697–707. *A safe procedure for diagnosis and therapy.*

Habermann TM, Steensma DP: Lymphadenopathy. Mayo Clin Proc 2000;75: 723–732. *A comprehensive review.*

Petroianu A: Drug-induced splenic enlargement. Expert Opin Drug Saf 2007;6:199–206. *An increasingly common cause, via hemolysis or portal vein occlusion.*

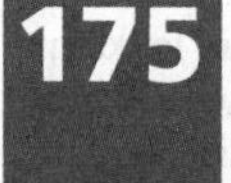

175 DISORDERS OF PHAGOCYTE FUNCTION

Michael Glogauer

Neutrophils and monocyte-macrophages are the key phagocytes of the innate immune system. Their principal innate immune role is to recognize and eliminate microorganisms that make their way past primary physical barriers, such as the epithelium and body secretions that protect the external and lining surfaces of the body. Phagocytes identify foreign invaders through a series of pattern recognition receptors, the majority of which belong to the Toll-like receptor family. Whereas macrophages carry out sentinel duty looking for microbes in healthy tissue and act as a bridge between the innate and adaptive immune systems, neutrophils appear only in infected or damaged tissue after being recruited by inflammatory mediators released from activated macrophages and endothelial cells or by chemical signals released by invading microorganisms themselves (Table 175–1). After accumulation of these key immune cells at sites of infection, the microbes are eliminated through the process of phagocytosis, which is defined as the engulfment, internalization, and degradation of extracellular material.

NEUTROPHILS

Neutrophils develop in the bone marrow from myeloid precursors, migrate into the circulation, and if required, make their way into infected or damaged tissue (Fig. 175–1; also see Fig. 173–1). Their travels are essentially one-way trips because once they leave a compartment, they do not return. After release from the bone marrow compartment, a mature neutrophil has a blood half-life of about 10 hours and may survive up to an additional 48 hours within infected or damaged tissue.

The Bone Marrow Compartment: The Site of Granulopoiesis

Neutrophils are the most abundant white blood cell and account for up to 70% of circulating leukocytes. Although they normally number about 3 to 5 × 10^6 cells per milliliter of blood, neutrophil numbers can increase rapidly by as much as 5- to 10-fold during periods of acute infection. Because these cells have a very short half-life in blood, the bone marrow compartment provides a steady supply of mature neutrophils with the capability to upregulate cell production rapidly during times of infection. Neutrophils originate in the bone marrow from a common population of hematopoietic stem cells through a 10- to 14-day process of proliferation, differentiation, and maturation.

TABLE 175–1 PRIMARY IMMUNE ROLES OF MONOCYTE-MACROPHAGES AND NEUTROPHILS

MONONUCLEAR PHAGOCYTE FUNCTIONS
Elimination of invading pathogens
Elimination of cellular debris from sites of tissue damage and the blood stream
Wound healing-remodeling of normal tissue
Amplification of the innate immune response: release of immune regulators
Bridge to the adaptive immune system: presentation of antigens to lymphocytes
NEUTROPHILS
Elimination of invading pathogens

Steps in Granulopoiesis

The stages of neutrophil granulopoiesis (Fig. 175–2) are divided and identified by the major transitions from the pluripotent stem cell to the mature neutrophil. The *myeloblast* is the first recognizable progenitor cell committed to granulopoiesis. This proliferating cell is characterized by its large nucleus and agranular cytoplasm. The *promyelocyte* follows and displays the initial development of primary granules. *Myelocytes* occupy the next stage of neutrophil maturation and are characterized by development of the first specific or "secondary" (peroxidase negative) granules. *Metamyelocytes,* which follow myelocytes, are incapable of further mitosis and are readily identifiable by their now numerous cytoplasmic granules. The functional maturation of metamyelocytes results in the development of *band* cells, which are usually slightly larger than mature neutrophils and have a 15-μm diameter, a "horseshoe"-shaped nucleus, and a moderate to abundant supply of specific granules. Band cells can be found in the circulation during periods of acute infection. The final mature *neutrophil,* which is released into the circulation, has a diameter of approximately 10 μm with a characteristic nucleus that is segmented and multilobed and occupies about 20% of the cell's volume; the remaining cytoplasm is taken up by granules.

Laboratory Evaluation of Granulopoiesis

Defects in granulopoiesis are manifested clinically as low circulating levels of neutrophils (neutropenia; Chapter 173). Verification of the stage at which neutrophil developmental arrest occurs can be determined by a bone marrow biopsy to assess the cellularity and characteristics of the neutrophil precursors present in the marrow space.

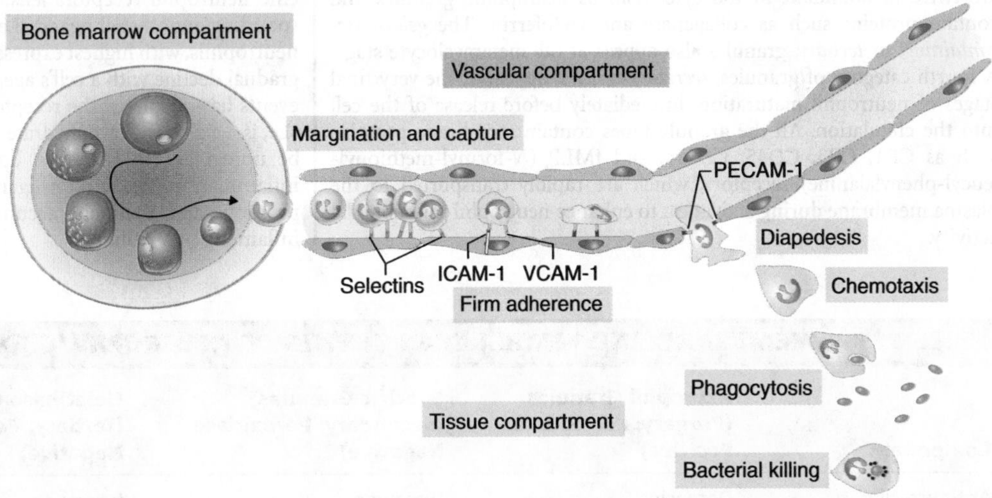

FIGURE 175–1 • Life cycle of the neutrophil. The three major neutrophilic compartments and the various steps involved in recruiting neutrophils to sites of infection are shown. ICAM = intercellular adhesion molecule; PECAM = platelet endothelial cell adhesion molecule; VCAM = vascular cell adhesion molecule.

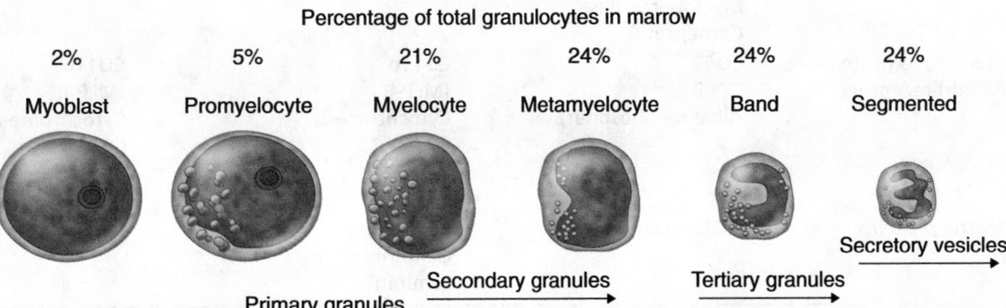

FIGURE 175–2 • Cellular stages of granulopoiesis in bone marrow.

Regulation of Granulopoiesis

Granulopoiesis is driven by hematopoietic growth factors. These factors, which are synthesized by a variety of cells, including fibroblasts and endothelial cells, are known to work together with other regulatory molecules, such as cytokines, to regulate hematopoiesis. Hematopoietic growth factors such as *interleukin-3* (IL-3), *granulocyte-macrophage colony-stimulating factor* (GM-CSF), and *granulocyte colony-stimulating factor* (G-CSF) bind to their target cells through specific receptors and are critical for the hematopoietic system to respond rapidly to infection or inflammation by dramatically increasing the production of leukocytes.

Granulocyte Colony-Stimulating Factor

G-CSF is a potent cytokine that influences the proliferation, survival, maturation, and functional activation of cells from the neutrophil-granulocyte lineage. Although G-CSF is not essential for neutrophil differentiation during steady-state granulopoiesis in the bone marrow, without it the pool of mature neutrophils is significantly reduced because of increased apoptosis of neutrophil precursors. In normal individuals, circulating levels of G-CSF are very low (<100 pg/mL). However, in conditions of stress, G-CSF levels can rise to 20 times baseline levels, thereby resulting in a rapid increase in circulating neutrophils. Some studies have shown that G-CSF regulates this increased granulopoiesis by increasing the mitotic pool at the promyelocyte and myelocyte stages, whereas other studies suggest that G-CSF affects granulopoiesis by shortening neutrophil transit time in bone marrow.

Neutrophil Granules

One of the major mechanisms used by neutrophils to eliminate bacteria is a remarkable arsenal of antimicrobial proteins that are packed into cytoplasmic granules (Table 175–2). These antimicrobial proteins are securely contained within their respective granules and are released only when granules fuse with phagosomes or directly with the plasma membrane. Granulogenesis begins between the myeloblast and promyelocyte stages of neutrophil development and continues throughout the differentiation and maturation process of the cell. *Azurophilic* granules, which make up 30% of granules in a mature neutrophil (≈1500 total), are the first to appear at the promyelocyte stage; they contain hydrolytic enzymes, microbicidal peptides, and myeloperoxidase. The *secondary*, or specific, granules appear later, beginning at the metamyelocyte stage; they are twice as abundant in the cytoplasm as azurophilic granules and contain proteins such as collagenase and lactoferrin. The *gelatinase-containing*, or *tertiary*, granules also appear at the metamyelocyte stage. A fourth category of granules, *secretory vesicles*, appear at the very final stages of neutrophil maturation, immediately before release of the cell into the circulation. All the granule types contain membrane proteins such as CR1, CR3, CD45, CD11c, and fMLP (*N*-formyl-methionyl-leucyl-phenylalanine) receptors, which are rapidly transported to the plasma membrane during activation to enhance neutrophil microbicidal activity.

Laboratory Evaluation of Granule Content

A number of clinical conditions result from specific defects in granule development and formation. Initial assessment for granule defects can be made by microscopic evaluation of a peripheral blood smear. Examples of obvious clinical diagnoses made with the peripheral smear include specific granule deficiency, which is characterized by bilobed nuclei in more than 80% of the neutrophils and a significant decrease in cytoplasmic granularity. Abnormally large cytoplasmic granules are seen in individuals with Chédiak-Higashi syndrome.

The Vascular Compartment

Mature neutrophils are released from the postmitotic bone marrow compartment into the circulation, where they have an approximate lifespan of 8 to 12 hours and either circulate within the center of the blood vessel or attach to its endothelial lining, a process termed margination. Marginalized neutrophils on the vessel walls are able to detach and reenter the circulation when required. For example, corticosteroids and epinephrine induce a rapid increase in circulating neutrophils by releasing neutrophils from the marginalized pool. Neutrophils circulate until they are recruited to a site of infection. The initial phase of recruitment involves changes in the endothelial cell surface receptors lining the capillary beds closest to the site of infection or tissue damage. These critical changes in endothelial cells are mediated by immune regulators released by tissue macrophages, which initially detect the tissue damage or bacterial invasion. Emigration of circulating neutrophils from the vasculature to the site of infection or tissue damage requires three steps (see Fig. 175–1): capture and margination, firm adhesion to the endothelial wall, and diapedesis.

Margination and Capture

The marginated pool of neutrophils consists of neutrophils transiently retained against the walls of pulmonary capillaries and postcapillary venules. In the 20-μm diameter of a postcapillary venule, the smaller and faster circulating red blood cells displace the slower-moving and larger neutrophils, which move to the vessel margins, where a low-affinity molecular interaction occurs between surface adhesion molecules of the neutrophil and the endothelial cells. This interaction results in neutrophil rolling and capture along the vessel walls, an event that requires the specific neutrophil receptors *leukocyte selectin* (L-selectin) and the corresponding endothelial ligand sLe. L-selectin is constitutively expressed in neutrophils, with highest expression in young circulating neutrophils and gradual decline with a cell's age, probably because previous margination events have depleted the receptor. The endothelial ligand for L-selectin, sLe, is a sialylated carbohydrate linked to a mucin-like molecule that can be upregulated by bacterial lipopolysaccharide or other mediators of inflammation. The selectin-ligand interactions are reversible and serve to promote and maintain accumulation of circulating neutrophils on inflamed endothelium.

TABLE 175–2 MEMBRANE AND MATRIX COMPONENTS OF NEUTROPHILIC GRANULES

Component	Azurophil Granules (Primary; Peroxidase Positive)	Specific Granules (Secondary; Peroxidase Negative)	Gelatinase Granules (Tertiary; Peroxidase Negative)	Secretory Vesicles
Antimicrobial proteins	Defensins Lysozyme Elastase Myeloperoxidase Cathepsin G	Lysozyme Lactoferrin	Lysozyme	
Membrane proteins and receptors	CD63 CD68 Alkaline phosphatase	CD11b fMLP-R Cytochrome b_{558} CR3	CD11b fMLP-R Cytochrome b_{558} CR3 CD45	CD11b fMLP-R Cytochrome b_{558} CR1 CD14 CD16
Matrix proteins	β-Glucuronidase	Collagenase Gelatinase Laminin	Gelatinase	Albumin

Modified from Edwards SW: Biochemistry and Physiology of the Neutrophil. Cambridge, Cambridge University Press, 2005, p 55.

Adherence to the Endothelial Wall

Low-affinity, selectin-mediated transient interactions must be replaced by high-affinity, adhesive contacts between neutrophils and endothelial cells. During an acute inflammatory event, mediators derived from bacteria, damaged host cells, complement activation, or other immune cells are released from the site of infection and diffuse to the capillary beds, where they induce an immediate and transient vascular response that results in vascular leakage, which further encourages neutrophil margination. Endothelial cells adjacent to the site of inflammation, as well as the activated neutrophils that are bound to them, express integrin receptors that lead to high-affinity attachments between the neutrophils and endothelial cells. These high-affinity connections occur between neutrophil β2 *integrins* and their endothelial counterparts, the intercellular adhesion molecules (ICAMs). Integrins, which are a receptor family of heterodimeric transmembrane glycoproteins made up of an α- and β-subunit, are integral for cell adhesion. Neutrophil β2 integrins consist of three different α-subunits (CD11a, CD11b, and CD11c) that bind to a common β-subunit (CD18). The cytoplasmic tails of these transmembrane receptors possess phosphorylation sites for attachment of signal transduction and cytoskeletal proteins. The neutrophil integrins that mediate this adhesion step are *macrophage antigen-1* (Mac-1; CD11b/CD18) and *lymphocyte-associated function antigen-1* (LFA-1; CD11a/CD18). The receptors are stored in the neutrophil granule compartments to facilitate quick transfer to the plasma membrane during cell stimulation. The integrins bind to endothelial ICAM-1 and ICAM-2 and *vascular cell adhesion molecule-1* (VCAM-1), which are upregulated on the endothelial cell membranes when a cell is exposed to inflammatory cytokines. L-selectin receptors on neutrophils are concentrated on microvillus projections of the cell membrane, whereas the integrins are restricted to the body of the neutrophil. As a result, soon after initial contact during rolling interactions, the projections retract, thereby allowing integrins to interact with their ligands.

Diapedesis

Firm adherence through the L-selectin and integrin receptors facilitates transendothelial migration, or diapedesis, which marks the "point of no return" in the process of neutrophil recruitment to the site of injury. Unlike rolling and firm adhesion, which require heterophilic interactions between one class of molecules on the neutrophil and another class of molecules on the endothelial cell, diapedesis involves homophilic interactions between the same class of molecules on both cells—the *platelet–endothelial cell adhesion molecule-1* (PECAM-1 or CD31). PECAM-1 is expressed evenly on the surface of neutrophils and concentrated at endothelial cell junctions. Once firmly bound to the endothelial cell surface, neutrophils migrate between the closest tricellular endothelial cell junctions through interactions with PECAM-1 receptors. The neutrophil has now entered the tissue compartment, where it is primed for its final critical role in the elimination of microorganisms and cellular debris.

Laboratory Evaluation of Margination and Firm Adhesion

A defect in neutrophil margination or adhesion to the endothelial lining of the vascular compartment results in neutrophilia (elevated circulating neutrophil levels). This condition is usually associated with leukocyte adhesion deficiency (LAD), which is the result of a lack of CD11/CD18 receptor surface expression in peripheral blood neutrophils. If LAD is suspected, surface expression of these receptors can be measured with a flow cytometer and specific antibodies to CD11, CD18, or CD15 receptors.

The Tissue Compartment

Chemotaxis

Chemotaxis is the directed movement of cells up a chemical concentration gradient of a *chemoattractant*. Chemoattractants are soluble proteins or peptides, including bacterial products, complement factors, and chemokines produced by both inflammatory and noninflammatory cells, that are released from damaged or infected tissue. A concentration difference of 1% at the opposite ends of the neutrophil is sufficient to activate neutrophil chemotaxis. Once a chemoattractant binds to its corresponding neutrophil membrane receptor, a series of cytoplasmic signaling pathways lead to activation of the neutrophil cytoskeleton. This activation results in the neutrophil assuming a polarized state characterized by an actin-rich leading lamella or pseudopod that drives cell motility.

Directional cell crawling, the intrinsic basis of chemotaxis, can be broken down into smaller processes, including extension of the cell membrane, adhesion to the tissue matrix, and contraction of the cell body in an organized and reversible manner. The actin-dependent protrusion of the leading edge, which is a sheetlike structure rich in actin filaments, is critical for normal neutrophil motility. The actin filaments within these lamellar regions are assembled into highly organized structures that push the membrane forward. These structures are formed by different collections of actin-binding proteins under the regulation of specific signal transduction cascades linking chemotactic receptors with cell movement. Defects in actin assembly also result in defects in chemotaxis and recurrent infections.

Actin Assembly Biology

Actin filaments are polar structures, with each end differing in its equilibrium-binding constant for actin monomers (Fig. 175–3). Filaments grow at the high-affinity or barbed end, whereas depolymerization occurs at the low-affinity or pointed end. This difference, generated by the ability of actin to bind and hydrolyze adenosine triphosphate, provides a physical polarity that regulatory proteins use to drive filament dynamics with high temporal and spatial precision. Three classes of proteins regulate the availability of high-affinity actin filament ends: filament-nucleating proteins (e.g., ARP2/3 de novo nucleation), filament-capping proteins (e.g., gelsolin), and filament-severing proteins (e.g., cofilin). Actin-nucleating factors bind actin monomers under conditions otherwise unfavorable for assembly and generate a new filament with a free high-affinity end available for assembly. Actin filament-capping proteins bind to the high-affinity filament end and regulate the addition of monomers by their presence or absence at the end of the filament. Actin-binding proteins are regulated by various second messengers, including calcium. On stimulation, localized changes in the intracellular Ca^{2+} concentration lead to the rapid initiation of actin assembly and disassembly. The changes in actin filament length and the extent of cross-linkage between the filaments may account for the directional extension of actin-rich lamellae and contraction of the tail-like uropod at the other end of the cell. Movement in the neutrophil is therefore the result of lamellar protrusions resulting from the growth of actin filaments. Actin-rich lamellae will continue to be maintained as long as the neutrophil detects the chemoattractant gradient.

Laboratory Evaluation of Chemotaxis

A defect in neutrophil chemotaxis can be measured in the laboratory with a Boyden chamber, which uses a porous membrane to separate isolated neutrophils from a chemoattractant. A chemical gradient develops across the porous membrane and activates the neutrophils to crawl through the membrane toward the compartment containing the chemoattractant. Defects in chemotaxis can be determined by a lack of neutrophil transmigration through the membrane as compared with control neutrophils from a healthy donor.

Phagocytosis

Phagocytosis is the process whereby neutrophils engulf and internalize invading pathogens into membrane compartments called phagosomes. Bacterial targets are "highlighted" or opsonized by antibodies (IgG) or products from the classical complement pathway that coat the target and serve to mediate phagocytic adhesion. Neutrophilic phagocytosis involves two separate classes of receptors: *Fcγ receptors* (CD32 and CD16) for antibody-coated targets and *complement receptors* (CR1 and CR3) for complement-coated targets. CD32 and CR3 are functional receptors directly involved in neutrophilic phagocytosis, whereas CD16 and CR1 are coreceptors that assist their mate in completing binding and internalization. Activation of Fcγ receptors brings about phosphorylation of their cytoplasmic *immunoreceptor tyrosine-based activation motifs* (ITAMs) via activation of *Src family kinases;* the result is transduction of signals that induce extension of pseudopods, including signaling to the small Rho family of small guanosine triphosphatases (GTPases). These GTPases are responsible for the assembly of actin filaments, thereby leading to remodeling of the plasma membrane and the formation of actin-rich pseudopods, which are essential for the ingestion of particles and formation of phagosomes.

Laboratory Evaluation of Phagocytosis

Neutrophils can be incubated with fluorescently labeled bacteria after opsonization with serum from either the patient or a control. Phagocytosis is assessed by flow cytometry, which measures the increase in neutrophilic fluorescence after uptake of the fluorescently tagged bacteria.

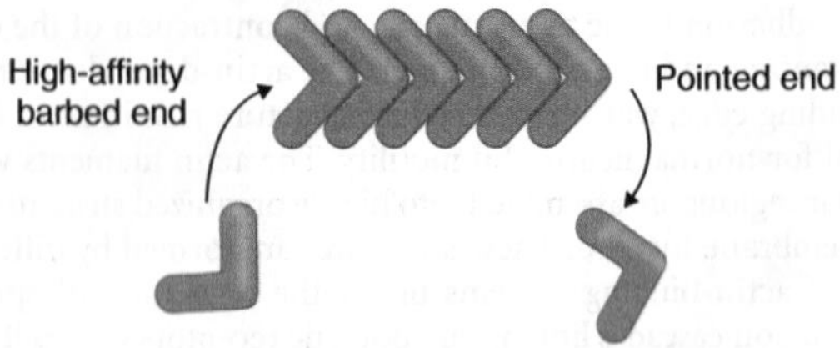

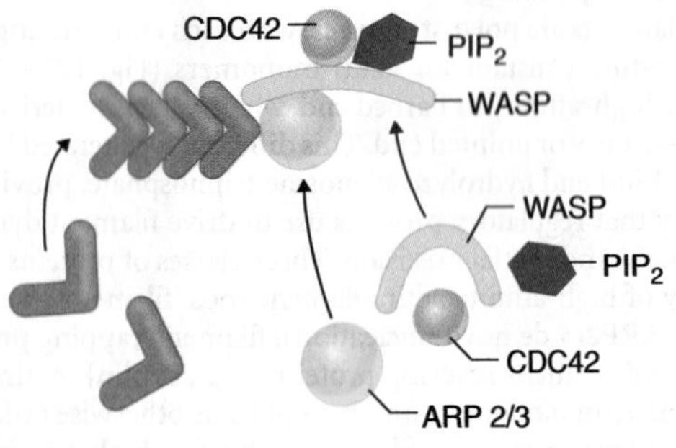

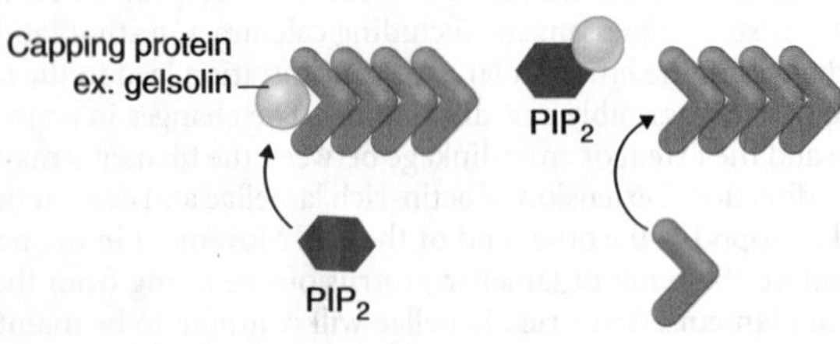

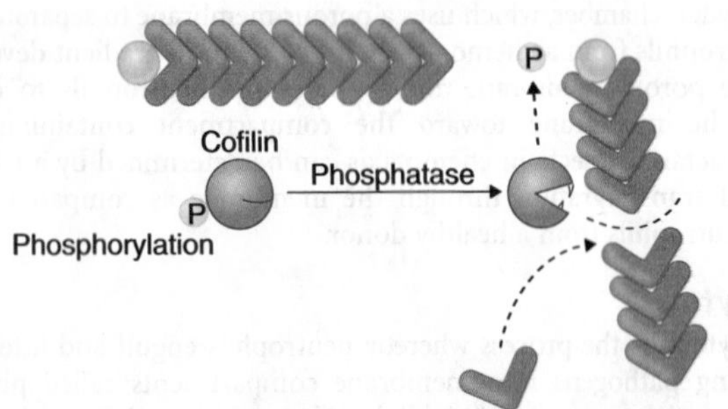

FIGURE 175–3 • Regulation of actin assembly through the generation of free barbed ends by actin-binding proteins. A, The components below join together to form a nucleation complex (above). **B,** PIP_2 binds the capping protein, leading to its removal from the high-affinity end, allowing for addition and filament growth. **C,** A phosphatase removes the (p) from cofilin, thereby allowing it to sever the actin filament and leaving a free high affinity end. PIP_2 = phosphatidylinositol 4,5-biphosphate; WASP = Wiskott-Aldrich syndrome protein.

Bacterial Killing

Phagocytes use two potent mechanisms for killing bacteria within the membrane-bound phagosome. The first involves fusion of the previously described storage granules with the phagosome to deliver microbicidal and lytic enzymes into the membrane compartment that contains the ingested microorganisms. The second mechanism uses a multiprotein enzyme complex to generate microbicidal oxidants via partial reduction of oxygen. The multiprotein enzyme complex known as reduced nicotinamide adenine dinucleotide phosphate (NADPH) oxidase generates oxidants by means of oxygen consumption, hence the term respiratory burst.

TABLE 175–3 SYMPTOMS SUGGESTIVE OF A PHAGOCYTIC DISORDER

Recurrent infections that fail to resolve with conventional treatment
Recurrent infections of unusual severity
Recurrent infections in the lung, liver, or bone
Normally nonpathogenic bacteria or fungi identified in cultures from the infection sites
Aphthous ulcers
Severe periodontal diseases, including gingivitis
Lymphadenopathy or hepatosplenomegaly
Severe recurrent cutaneous infections with *Staphylococcus aureus*
Recurrent mycobacterial infections

Components of the NADPH Oxidase Complex

The NADPH enzyme system is made up of four essential polypeptide subunits that are denoted by their molecular weight (kD) and the superscript phox, which denotes phagocyte oxidase. Within the cytoplasmic membrane, the subunits $p22^{phox}$ and $gp91^{phox}$ bind the electron-carrying components of the oxidase (NADPH, a flavin adenine dinucleotide, and two nonidentical hemes) and form the cytochrome b_{558} redox center of the oxidase complex. Cellular activation by inflammatory mediators results in the addition of two cytosolic components, $p47^{phox}$ and $p67^{phox}$, to the complex along with the Rac small GTPase.

Product of the NADPH Oxidase Complex

The membrane-bound electron transport chain NADPH oxidase catalyzes the reduction of molecular oxygen to superoxide (O_2^-). The superoxide generated by this process is in turn catalytically converted to hydrogen peroxide and serves as a cosubstrate for myeloperoxidase to oxidize halides and produce hypochlorous acid (HOCl), a very potent antimicrobial agent. These oxidants are able to kill bacteria within the phagosomes by oxidizing their cellular constituents.

Laboratory Evaluation of the Respiratory Burst and Bacterial Killing

Flow cytometry, a rapid and effective method for quantitatively assessing the respiratory burst, measures the fluorescence generated by cytoplasmic fluorescent probes such as dihydrorhodamine, which is converted to rhodamine by H_2O_2. The nitroblue tetrazolium test is still used for rapid assessment of the respiratory burst when flow cytometry is not available.

Bacterial killing assays using a patient's neutrophils with either the patient's or control serum and bacteria such as *Staphylococcus aureus* or *Escherichia coli* are a definitive method to determine whether a given patient's neutrophils has an intracellular killing defect. Neutrophils from a healthy control subject phagocytose and kill approximately 95% of the bacteria within 2 hours. In assays in which an intracellular killing defect is present, neutrophils kill less than 10% of bacteria over a 2-hour period. It is necessary to confirm that there is no phagocytic defect before performing the bacterial killing assay to be sure that any defect in bacterial killing is not due to an internalization defect.

Clinical Manifestations of Phagocytic Defects

In addition to fever and recurrent infections, the most common findings in patients with phagocytic defects are oral infections resulting in gingival inflammation, periodontal bone loss, mobile/loose teeth, and premature loss of teeth (Table 175–3). An oral examination should be performed at the initial evaluation, followed by a full dental examination, depending on the findings. The history and laboratory tests can differentiate among the various clinical causes of disordered phagocytosis (Table 175–4).

DEFECTS IN LEUKOCYTE ADHESION

A defect in neutrophil adhesion to the endothelial lining leads to neutrophilia—an accumulation of neutrophils in the circulation, with very few neutrophils at sites of infection. Defects in neutrophil adhesion can either be induced by drugs or be due to a genetic defect. Drugs such as corticosteroids and epinephrine result in a transient leukocyte adhesive

TABLE 175–4 DISORDERS OF PHAGOCYTIC FUNCTION

Disorder	Etiology	Impaired Function	Clinical Consequence
DEGRANULATION ABNORMALITIES			
Chédiak-Higashi syndrome	Autosomal recessive; disordered coalescence of lysosomal granules. Responsible gene found at 1q42-45. The encoded protein (LYST) has structural features homologous to a vacuolar sorting protein	Decreased neutrophilic chemotaxis, degranulation, and bactericidal activity; platelet storage pool defect; impaired NK function; failure to disperse melanosomes	Neutropenia, recurrent pyogenic infections, propensity for the development of marked hepatosplenomegaly in the accelerated phase, partial albinism
Specific granule deficiency	Autosomal recessive; abnormal regulation of various myeloid granule genes by a transacting factor	Impaired chemotaxis and bactericidal activity; bilobed nuclei in neutrophils; reduced content of neutrophil defensins, gelatinase, collagenase, vitamin B_{12}–binding protein, and lactoferrin	Recurrent infections, especially sinopulmonary and skin infections
ADHESION ABNORMALITIES			
Leukocyte adhesion deficiency type 1	Autosomal recessive; absence of CD11/CD18 surface adhesive glycoprotein (β2-integrins) on leukocyte membranes, most commonly arising from failure to express CD18 mRNA	Decreased binding of C3bi to neutrophils and impaired adhesion to ICAM-1 and ICAM-2	Neutrophilia, recurrent bacterial infection associated with lack of pus formation
Leukocyte adhesion deficiency type 2	Autosomal recessive; absence of neutrophil sialyl-Lewis^{X}	Decreased adhesion to activated endothelium expressing ELAM	Neutrophilia, recurrent bacterial infection without pus
Neutrophil actin dysfunction	Altered polymerization of neutrophil cytoplasmic actin, perhaps arising from the presence of an inhibitor to F-actin formation	Impaired neutrophil adhesion, chemotaxis, and bacterial killing	Neutrophilia, recurrent bacterial infections without pus
DISORDERS OF CELL CHEMOTAXIS			
HYPERACTIVE CHEMOTAXIS			
Familial Mediterranean fever (FMF)	Autosomal recessive gene responsible for FMF on chromosome 16, which encodes for a protein called "pyrin"; pyrin may modify neutrophil activation	Excessive accumulation of neutrophils at inflamed sites	Recurrent fever, peritonitis, pleuritis, arthritis, amyloidosis
DEPRESSED CHEMOTAXIS			
Intrinsic defects of the neutrophil, e.g., leukocyte adhesion deficiency, Chédiak-Higashi syndrome, specific granule deficiency, neutrophil actin dysfunction, neonatal neutrophils	In the neonatal neutrophil there is diminished ability to express β2-integrins and a qualitative impairment in β2-integrin function	Diminished chemotaxis	Propensity for the development of pyogenic infections
Direct inhibition of neutrophil mobility, e.g., drugs	Ethanol, glucocorticoids, cyclic AMP	Impaired locomotion and ingestion, impaired adherence	Possible causes of frequent infections; neutrophilia seen with epinephrine is the result of cyclic AMP release from the endothelium
Immune complexes	Bind to Fc receptors on neutrophils in patients with rheumatoid arthritis, systemic lupus erythematosus, and other inflammatory states	Impaired chemotaxis	Recurrent pyogenic infections

Continued

TABLE 175–4 DISORDERS OF PHAGOCYTIC FUNCTION—cont'd

Disorder	Etiology	Impaired Function	Clinical Consequence
Hyperimmunoglogulin E syndrome	Autosomal dominant; variable expression of a soluble inhibitor from mononuclear cells affecting neutrophil chemotaxis; high levels of antistaphylococcal IgE	Impaired chemotaxis, impaired IgG opsonization of *Staphylococcus aureus*	Recurrent skin and sinopulmonary infections
DEFECTS OF MICROBICIDAL ACTIVITY			
Chronic granulomatous disease (CGD)	X-linked and autosomal recessive; failure to express functional gp91^{phox} (in the phagocyte membrane) and p22^{phox} (autosomal recessive). Other autosomal recessive forms of CGD arise from failure to express protein p47^{phox} or p67^{phox}	Failure to activate neutrophil respiratory burst leading to failure to kill catalase-positive microbes	Recurrent pyogenic infections with catalase-positive microorganisms
G6PD deficiency	Less than 5% of normal activity of G6PD	Failure to activate NADPH-dependent oxidase	Infections with catalase-positive microorganisms
Myeloperoxidase deficiency	Autosomal recessive; failure to process modified precursor protein arising from missense mutation	H_2O_2-dependent antimicrobial activity not potentiated by myeloperoxidase	None
Deficiencies of glutathione reductase and glutathione synthetase	Failure to detoxify H_2O_2	Excessive formation of H_2O_2	Minimal problems with recurrent pyogenic infections
IMPAIRED MACROPHAGE FUNCTION			
Defects in the interferon-γ–IL-12 axis	Interferon-γ receptor ligand-binding chain, interferon-γ receptor signaling chain, IL-12 receptor β_1 chain, IL-12 p40 deficiency; the interferon-γ receptor abnormalities may be autosomal dominant or recessive; the IL-12 receptor and IL-12 abnormalities are autosomal recessives	Impaired killing of microorganisms. Fatal BCG infection secondary either to an inability to produce IL-12 by dendritic cells and macrophages or to depressed bactericidal activity of macrophages lacking normal function of the interferon receptor	Infection with atypical mycobacteria, *Salmonella*, and *Listeria*

AMP = adenosine monophosphate; BCG = bacille Calmette-Guérin; ELAM = endothelial leukocyte adhesion molecule; G6PD = glucose-6-phosphate dehydrogenase; ICAM = intracellular adhesion molecule; IL-12 = interleukin-12; NADPH = nicotinamide adenine dinucleotide phosphate; NK = natural killer; phox = phagocyte oxidase.
Modified from Boxer LA: Quantitative abnormalities of granulocytes. *In* Beutler E, Lichtman MA, Coller BS, et al (eds): Williams Hematology, 6th ed. New York, McGraw-Hill, 2001, p 836.

defect that results in an apparent dramatic increase in circulating neutrophils because of release of the marginated neutrophil pool. The major genetic disease that results in an adhesion deficiency is termed *leukocyte adhesion deficiency.*

Leukocyte Adhesion Deficiency

LAD-I

Pathobiology

LAD-I is an autosomal recessive inherited disorder in which patients have a mutation in the gene encoding CD18. The result is a deficiency of β2 integrin receptors, which are required for neutrophil migration from the vasculature into the tissues, thereby impairing the binding of neutrophils to C3bi and endothelial ICAM-1 and ICAM-2.

Clinical Manifestations and Diagnosis

Patients have soft tissue bacterial and fungal infections, delayed wound healing, impaired pus formation, and severe destructive periodontitis with rapid tooth loss. This condition is also characterized by delayed separation of the umbilical cord. Patients usually die during childhood. Flow cytometry is used to measure CD11/CD18 surface expression levels on neutrophils.

Treatment

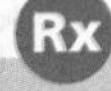

Treatment is mainly supportive with prophylactic antibiotics in patients with recurrent infections. In severe cases, bone marrow transplantation is the treatment of choice.

LAD-II

LAD-II, a variant of LAD-I, is associated with neutrophilia, the Bombay (hh) blood phenotype, dwarfism, and mental retardation. This disorder is due to a mutation in the guanosine diphosphate–fucose transporter gene, which results in impaired expression of CD15s and other selectin ligands. Symptoms are similar to those of LAD-I, and the diagnosis is confirmed by flow cytometry for CD15s.

DEFECTS IN NEUTROPHILIC CHEMOTAXIS

After phagocytes enter the tissue compartment from the vascular pool, they migrate up the concentration gradients of various chemoattractants to the site of focal infection. A number of chemotactic defects result in severe recurrent infections.

Hyperimmunoglobin E

Pathobiology

Hyperimmunoglobin E, also referred to as Job's syndrome, is an autosomal dominant neutrophilic disorder characterized by recurrent skin abscesses, pneumonia, and periodontal diseases.

Clinical Manifestations

After birth, patients usually have moderate to severe dermatitis, eczematous skin eruptions, nonerythematous abscesses, pneumatoceles, and severe osteoporosis that can result in bone fractures. The organisms most commonly present at infected sites are *S. aureus, Haemophilus influenzae, E. coli,* and *Candida albicans.*

Diagnosis

Patients have elevated IgE levels and eosinophilia. The defect in neutrophilic chemotaxis is less severe than that in Chédiak-Higashi syndrome.

Treatment

Treatment is prophylactic antibiotics and aggressive treatment of infections. In severe cases, bone marrow transplantation may be considered.

Familial Mediterranean Fever

Pathobiology

Familial Mediterranean fever (Chapter 297), also known as recurrent polyserositis, is an autosomal recessive inflammatory disease that is widespread among people of Mediterranean descent, including Arabs, Armenians, and Sephardic Jews. The genetic defect is a missense mutation in the *MEFV* gene, which encodes the protein pyrin. Pyrin is believed to be a transcription factor involved in downregulating inflammation, possibly through an effect on chemotaxis in neutrophils and monocytes. The *MEFV* mutation results in a hyperinflammatory response characterized by abundant neutrophilic infiltration into the peritoneal, pleural, and joint spaces.

Clinical Manifestations

The most common findings include acute, self-limited attacks of fever accompanied by pleuritis, peritonitis, arthritis, pericarditis, and erythematous skin lesions. Although first attacks may be observed during infancy, clinical disease commonly occurs in childhood or adolescence.

Diagnosis

Leukocytosis has been observed during attacks, but the leukocyte count is normal between episodes. Genetic testing is available for the most common mutations. This disease can be fatal if renal failure develops as a result of amyloidosis (Chapter 296), which occurs in up to 25% of those affected.

Treatment

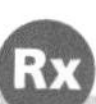

The hyperinflammatory attacks can be reduced significantly with 0.6 mg of prophylactic colchicine orally two or three times daily.

Prognosis

The prognosis is generally good for the majority of affected individuals maintained with colchicine.

DISORDERS OF NEUTROPHILIC DEGRANULATION

Granules supply key membrane proteins, including receptors required for phagocytosis. Granule-related defects result in profound defects in bacterial killing.

Chédiak-Higashi Syndrome

Pathobiology

Chédiak-Higashi syndrome is a rare autosomal recessive disorder of the *LYST* gene, which encodes a protein responsible for lysosomal trafficking. Defective targeting of granules to the membrane results in large cytoplasmic granules that are unable to target to the plasma membrane in neutrophils, monocytes, and lymphocytes.

Clinical Manifestations

Symptoms are recurrent bacterial infections of the skin, mouth, and respiratory tract; partial albinism; and mild bleeding disorders as a result of a deficiency in serotonin- and adenosine phosphate–containing granules in platelets. Defects in myelopoiesis result in neutropenia and peripheral neuropathy. Death usually occurs by 7 years of age because of infection. Advanced disease is characterized by lymphocytic tissue infiltrates and pancytopenia.

Diagnosis

Giant cytoplasmic granules are seen in the peripheral blood smear. Neutrophil function testing shows defects in chemotaxis and bacterial killing.

Treatment

Prophylactic antibiotics should be used to prevent infections. Bone marrow transplantation from an HLA-matched donor may be successful if performed before the disease becomes advanced.

Specific Granule Deficiency

Specific granule deficiency is an autosomal recessive disorder that is manifested during infancy as the recurrent appearance of deep and superficial skin infections, respiratory infections, and abscesses. Azurophilic granules in neutrophils lack defensins, gelatinase, cytochrome *b,* and vitamin B_{12}. Neutrophils are morphologically altered and have a bilobed rather than a trilobed nucleus. This disorder is characterized by impaired neutrophil chemotaxis, reduced respiratory burst, and a defect in bacterial killing. Infections are commonly caused by *S. aureus, Pseudomonas aeruginosa,* and *C. albicans.* Aggressive treatment of infections is required.

DISORDERS OF OXYGEN-DEPENDENT BACTERIAL KILLING

A genetic defect in any component of the respiratory burst results in delayed or ineffective bacterial killing.

Section XIV Hematology

Chronic Granulomatous Disease

Pathobiology

Chronic granulomatous disease is a genetic disease that occurs in about 1 in 200,000 live births. Neutrophils and macrophages cannot generate superoxide and are therefore unable to kill catalase-positive organisms. This condition results from mutations in one of the four structural genes of the NADPH oxidase complex. The most common genetic defect occurs in the 91-kD component of cytochrome b_{558}, which is coded on the X chromosome. The other mutations are autosomal recessive and have been detected in the 22-, 47-, and 67-kD structural proteins.

Clinical Manifestations

Children are prone to infections or granulomatous lesions in the lungs, skin, and liver. *S. aureus* is the most common organism, but other organisms include *Serratia marcescens, Burkholderia cepacia, Aspergillus* species, and *Nocardia* species. Staphylococcal liver abscesses are pathognomonic of chronic granulomatous disease.

Diagnosis

Flow cytometry is used to measure the increase in fluorescence generated when dihydrorhodamine is converted to rhodamine by H_2O_2.

Treatment

Rx

Abscesses can be removed by surgery. Trimethoprim-sulfamethoxazole prophylaxis (5 mg/kg/day divided into two equal doses) and antifungal prophylaxis with itraconazole (100 mg/day for <50 kg, 200 mg/day for >50 kg) have been shown to reduce the frequency of infections in these patients. Interferon gamma (50 µg/m² subcutaneously three times per week) prophylaxis is now considered "standard of care" in many centers. Bone marrow transplantation can also be considered for patients with refractory infections.

Myeloperoxidase Deficiency

Myeloperoxidase deficiency is a relatively common disorder (1 in 4000) in which the enzyme for conversion of neutrophilic hydrogen peroxide to HOCl is absent. This deficiency is not associated with increased susceptibility to infections, probably because of the accumulation of hydrogen peroxide, which is also bactericidal. Myeloperoxidase deficiency is usually asymptomatic, although patients with diabetes mellitus may occasionally experience candidal infections. The diagnosis is made by observation of a negative peroxidase stain of the peripheral blood smear. Symptomatic patients may be treated with prophylactic antibiotics.

Glutathione Synthetase Deficiency

Glutathione, which is a potent antioxidant found in granulocytes, is required for a normal respiratory burst and bacterial killing. Patients with glutathione synthetase deficiency typically have recurrent otitis and hemolytic anemia. The diagnosis is confirmed by verifying low or no glutathione synthetase in red blood cells.

Severe Glucose-6-Phosphate Dehydrogenase Deficiency

Glucose-6-phosphate dehydrogenase (G6PD) deficiency is an X-linked disorder. White individuals with a severe reduction in G6PD activity are subject to recurrent infections, whereas Asians or blacks with similarly reduced G6PD levels are not. G6PD is crucial for regulating the availability of NADPH for the respiratory burst. G6PD deficiency results in recurrent bacterial infections, hemolysis, recurrent bouts of severe anemia, and jaundice. The diagnosis can be made with flow cytometry to assess the respiratory burst, as well as demonstration of the absence of G6PD in all blood cells.

MACROPHAGE-RELATED ABNORMALITIES

Accumulation of monocytes/macrophages at sites of infection occurs after the major influx of neutrophils. Macrophages have a critical role in antigen presentation to lymphocytes, thereby activating the adaptive arm of the immune system. A critical defect in macrophage signaling results in susceptibility to mycobacterial infection.

Interferon-γ Receptor 1 Defects

When macrophages phagocytose mycobacteria, they produce IL-12, which in turn stimulates T cells to produce interferon-γ (IFN-γ). IFN-γ is critical to the killing of mycobacteria and other intracellular bacteria. Patients with recurrent and severe mycobacterial infections who are not infected with human immunodeficiency virus should be assessed for abnormalities in pathways that lead to the generation and utilization of IFN-γ.

Pathobiology

Patients with autosomal recessive mutations in the IFN-γ receptors typically have a complete loss of function of the IFN-γ receptors. Autosomal dominant mutations in the IFN-γ receptors result in normal ligand binding but defective intracellular signal transduction because of a cytoplasmically truncated form of the receptor.

Clinical Manifestations

Recessive mutations are typically manifested as severe disseminated infections and poor formation of granulomas. Multifocal mycobacterial osteomyelitis is pathognomonic of an autosomal dominant mutation in the IFN-γ receptor.

Diagnosis

Flow cytometry confirms the absence of membrane expression of IFN-γ receptor 1 in the autosomal recessive form and up to 10-fold higher membrane expression levels of the cytoplasmically truncated receptor in the autosomal dominant form.

Treatment

Rx

For patients with autosomal dominant mutations, subcutaneous IFN-γ is effective. For autosomal recessive patients completely lacking IFN-γ receptor function, bone marrow transplantation should be considered. Long-term antibiotic prophylaxis against mycobacterial infections with azithromycin or clarithromycin is recommended.

ASSESSING PHAGOCYTE FUNCTION: MAKING THE DIAGNOSIS

If a phagocyte functional disorder may be the underlying cause of recurrent infections in a patient, a complete blood count (CBC) and peripheral smear guide subsequent definitive testing (Fig. 175–4). Cultures from infected areas allow antimicrobial targeting and also provide critical diagnostic information. If the defect is a result of abnormal neutrophil development and maturation, the CBC will show neutropenia; a bone marrow biopsy might be required. Repeated CBC (twice per week for 6 weeks) is indicated if cyclic neutropenia is suspected because of a periodicity of the infections.

If the CBC reveals neutrophilia, a defect in the recruitment of neutrophils into tissues is suggested. An assessment of the receptors required for transmigration by flow cytometry and specific antibodies to the surface receptors is indicated.

If circulating levels of phagocytes are normal yet the patient is experiencing recurrent infections, a phagocytic defect within the infected tissue is likely. Laboratory testing to evaluate chemotaxis, phagocytosis, and bacterial killing is indicated.

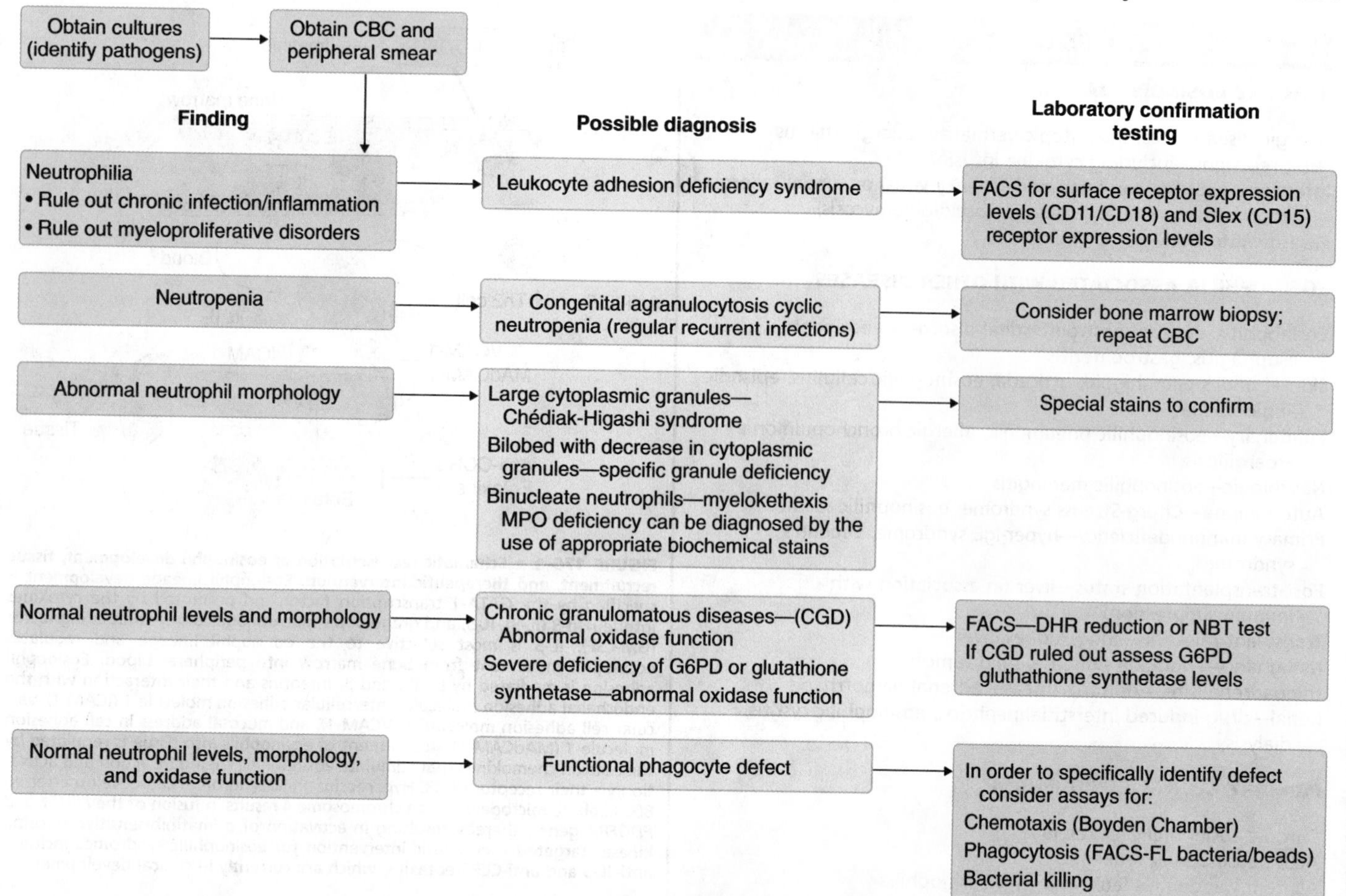

FIGURE 175–4 • Approach to diagnosing a suspected phagocytic defect. CBC = complete blood count; DHR = dihydrorhodamine; FACS = flow cytometry; FL = fluorescent; G6PD = glucose-6-phosphate dehydrogenase; MPO = myeloperoxidase; NBT = nitroblue tetrazolium.

SUGGESTED READINGS

Dinauer MC: Chronic granulomatous disease and other disorders of phagocyte function. Am Soc Hematol Educ Program 2005;89–95. *A practical review.*

El-Shanti H, Majeed HA, El-Khateeb M: Familial mediterranean fever in Arabs. Lancet 2006;367:1016–1024. *A clinical and molecular review.*

Long SS: Periodic fever. Adv Exp Med Biol 2005;568:101–115. *A scientific review.*

Onen F: Familial Mediterranean fever. Rheumatol Int 2006;26:489–496. *A clinical update.*

Rosenzweig SD, Holland SM: Phagocyte immunodeficiencies and their infections. J Allergy Clin Immunol 2004;113:620–626. *A comprehensive review.*

176 EOSINOPHILIC SYNDROMES

Marc E. Rothenberg

Definition

Eosinophilic syndromes are a heterogeneous group of disorders that involve eosinophilia, which is defined as the accumulation of eosinophils in peripheral blood or tissues, or both. Circulating eosinophils normally account for only 1 to 3% of peripheral blood leukocytes, and the upper limit of the normal range is 350 cells/mm^3 of blood. Eosinophilia occurs in a variety of disorders (Table 176–1) and is usually arbitrarily classified according to the degree of blood eosinophilia: mild (351 to 1500 cells/mm^3), moderate (>1500 to 5000 cells/mm^3), or severe (>5000 cells/mm^3). Tissue eosinophilic disorders, such as eosinophil-associated gastrointestinal disorders and eosinophilic fasciitis, are not necessarily associated with blood eosinophilia, so their diagnosis is based on the microscopic identification of eosinophil-rich inflammatory infiltrates associated with tissue damage.

Historically, hypereosinophilic syndromes were generally classified as idiopathic and were defined by (1) the presence of eosinophilia (>1500 cells/mm^3 for at least 6 months) that remained unexplained despite a comprehensive evaluation for known causes of eosinophilia (such as drug reactions and infections) and (2) evidence of organ dysfunction directly attributable to the eosinophilia. Now, however, it is known that in some patients a chromosome 4 microdeletion results in the generation of an activated tyrosine kinase (FIP1L1–platelet-derived growth factor receptor α [PDGFRA]) that causes a clonal hematologic disorder now better classified as chronic eosinophilic leukemia. Identification of FIP1L1-PDGFRA–positive disease has important therapeutic implications because PDGFRA-associated disease can be treated with imatinib, a tyrosine kinase inhibitor.

Epidemiology

The most common cause of eosinophilia worldwide is helminth infections, which affect hundreds of millions of people worldwide. The most frequent cause in industrialized nations is atopic disease, which affects 10 to 30% of the population (Chapter 270). Hypereosinophilic disorders such as FIP1L1-PDGFRA–associated disease and Churg-Strauss syndrome (Chapter 291) are very rare. For example, Churg-Strauss syndrome affects 4 to 6 cases per million per year, whereas true idiopathic hypereosinophilic syndromes may affect only 4000 to 5000 people worldwide. Other syndromes such as eosinophil-associated gastrointestinal disorders are more common, with an incidence of approximately 1 in 10,000 children.

TABLE 176–1 CAUSES OF EOSINOPHILIA

REACTIVE EOSINOPHILIA
Allergic diseases—asthma, atopic dermatitis, allergic rhinitis
Drug reactions—including cytokine infusions
Infection—viral (human immunodeficiency virus) or fungal (allergic bronchopulmonary aspergillosis, coccidioidomycosis)
Parasitic infection—mostly helminths
EOSINOPHILIA ASSOCIATED WITH OTHER DISEASES
Eosinophil-associated gastrointestinal disorders—eosinophilic esophagitis, gastroenteritis
Skin—bullous pemphigoid, urticaria, eosinophilic cellulitis, episodic angioedema
Pulmonary—eosinophilic pneumonia, allergic bronchopulmonary aspergillosis
Neurologic—eosinophilic meningitis
Autoimmune—Churg-Strauss syndrome, eosinophilic fasciitis
Primary immunodeficiency—hyper-IgE syndrome, Omenn's syndrome
Post-transplantation status—liver (in association with immunosuppression)
Transplant rejection—lung, kidney, liver
Malignancy—Hodgkin's disease, solid tumors
Hypoadrenalism—Addison's disease, adrenal hemorrhage
Renal—drug-induced interstitial nephritis, eosinophilic cystitis, dialysis
PRIMARY CLONAL EOSINOPHILIA
Chronic eosinophilic leukemia
Acute eosinophilic leukemia
Acute myelogenous leukemia with eosinophilia
Acute lymphoblastic leukemia with eosinophilia
Myeloblastic disorders with eosinophilia
Myeloproliferative disorders with eosinophilia
Systemic mastocytosis with eosinophilia
FIP1L1-PDGFRA fusion gene–positive disease
IDIOPATHIC HYPEREOSINOPHILIA

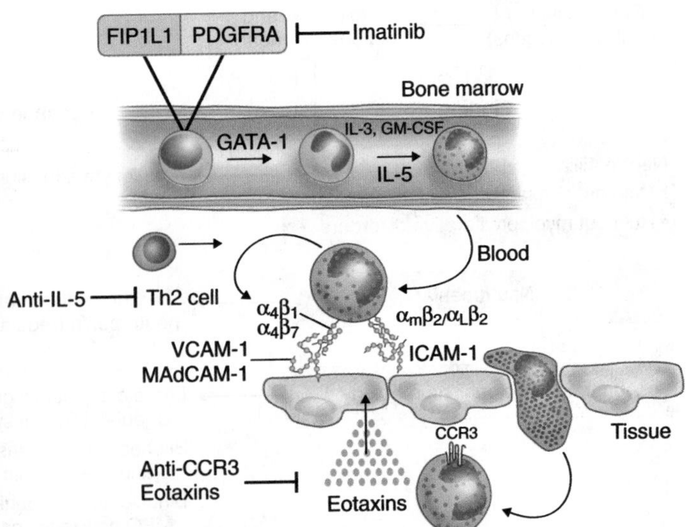

FIGURE 176–1 • Schematic representation of eosinophil development, tissue recruitment, and therapeutic intervention. Eosinophil lineage development is specified by the GATA-1 transcription factor and promoted by the cytokines interleukin-3 (IL-3), IL-5, and granulocyte-macrophage colony-stimulating factor (GM-CSF). IL-5 is most selective to the eosinophil lineage and regulates eosinophil movement from bone marrow into peripheral blood. Eosinophil adhesion is mediated by β_1, β_2, and β_7 integrins and their interaction with the endothelial adhesion molecules intercellular adhesion molecule 1 (ICAM-1), vascular cell adhesion molecule 1 (VCAM-1), and mucosal address in cell adhesion molecule 1 (MAdCAM-1). Recruitment of eosinophils into tissue is regulated by the eotaxin chemokines that stimulate eosinophilic chemoattraction and activation via their receptor CCR3. Hypereosinophilic syndromes can develop after an 800-kilobase microdeletion on chromosome 4 results in fusion of the *FIP1L1* and *PDGFRA* genes, thereby resulting in activation of a imatinib-sensitive tyrosine kinase. Targeted therapeutic intervention for eosinophilic syndromes includes anti–IL-5 and anti-CCR3/eotaxins, which are currently in clinical development.

Pathobiology

Eosinophils are produced in the bone marrow from pluripotential stem cells under regulation of the transcription factor GATA-1 and the cytokines interleukin-3 (IL-3), IL-5, and granulocyte-macrophage colony-stimulating factor (GM-CSF) (Fig. 176–1). Eosinophils are under the regulation of helper type 2 T cells (T_H2) that secrete IL-4, IL-5, and IL-13. Notably, IL-5 is a cytokine that specifically regulates the selective differentiation of eosinophils, their release from bone marrow into the peripheral circulation, and their survival. A humanized anti–IL-5 drug markedly lowers circulating eosinophilia and reduces tissue eosinophilia more modestly. Early studies in patients with asthma have shown that anti–IL-5 therapy does not appear to improve airway function but improves markers of lung remodeling (associated with decreases in transforming growth factor β_1 [TGF-β_1] levels); humanized anti–IL-5 therapy is currently in clinical testing for a variety of indications, including hypereosinophilic syndromes. IL-4 and IL-13 induce eosinophil recruitment and survival, expression of critical adhesion molecules on the endothelium that bind to the β_1 and β_2 integrins on eosinophils (such as intercellular adhesion molecule 1 [ICAM-1] and vascular cell adhesion molecule 1 [VCAM-1]), and eosinophil-active chemokines such as the eotaxins. The eotaxins are three structurally related eosinophil chemoattractant and activating proteins that signal exclusively through the eosinophil-selective receptor CCR3. In addition to regulating the baseline homing of eosinophils into various tissues, such as the gastrointestinal tract, wherein most eosinophils reside, the eotaxins are induced by T_H2-associated inflammatory triggers (e.g., IL-13) and thereby promote tissue accumulation of eosinophils. Humanized antibodies against the eotaxins and small-molecule inhibitors against CCR3 are promising new approaches for treating eosinophilic disorders that are in clinical development.

Eosinophil granules contain a crystalloid core composed of major basic protein (MBP-1 and MBP-2), as well as a matrix composed of eosinophil cationic protein (ECP), eosinophil-derived neurotoxin (EDN), and eosinophil peroxidase (EPO). MBP, EPO, and ECP have cytotoxic effects on a variety of tissues in concentrations similar to those found in biologic fluids from patients with eosinophilia. Additionally, ECP and EDN belong to the ribonuclease A superfamily and possess antiviral and ribonuclease activity. ECP can insert voltage-insensitive, ion-nonselective toxic pores into the membranes of target cells, and these pores may facilitate the entry of other toxic molecules. MBP directly increases smooth muscle reactivity by causing dysfunction of vagal muscarinic M_2 receptors, and this process has been postulated to contribute to the airway hyperresponsiveness associated with asthma. MBP also triggers degranulation of mast cells and basophils. Triggering of eosinophils by engagement of receptors for cytokines, immunoglobulins, and complement can lead to the generation of a wide range of inflammatory cytokines, including IL-1, IL-3, IL-4, IL-5, IL-13, GM-CSF, TGF-α/β, tumor necrosis factor α (TNF-α), RANTES, macrophage inflammatory protein 1α (MIP-1α), and the eotaxins, thus indicating that eosinophils have the potential to modulate multiple aspects of the immune response. Additionally, eosinophils can directly activate T cells by antigen presentation. Further eosinophil-mediated damage is caused by toxic hydrogen peroxide and halide acids generated by EPO and by superoxide generated by the respiratory burst oxidase enzyme pathway in eosinophils. Eosinophils also generate large amounts of cysteinyl leukotriene C_4 (LTC_4), which is metabolized to LTD_4 and LTE_4. These three lipid mediators increase vascular permeability and mucus secretion and are potent stimulators of smooth muscle contraction. Finally, bipyramidal Charcot-Leyden crystals are derived from a nongranule lysophospholipase in eosinophils and are frequently found in sputum, feces, and tissues infiltrated by eosinophils.

Clinical Manifestations

Hypereosinophilia is often recognized on a routine blood count in a patient who is asymptomatic or being evaluated for unrelated or nonspecific signs or symptoms. On other occasions, the possibility of eosinophilia may be specifically investigated in a patient with gastrointestinal or respiratory symptoms because helminthic disease or allergic causes are suspected. The clinical signs and symptoms of hypereosinophilic syndromes are heterogeneous because of the diversity of the causes and potential organ involvement. Common signs and symptoms include dermatitis, heart failure, neuropathy, and abdominal pain. One of the most serious complications of hypereosinophilia is cardiac disease secondary to endomyocardial thrombus formation and restrictive fibrosis (Chapter 59). Mitral and tricuspid valve regurgitation may result from progressive fibrotic damage to the chordae tendineae, and resultant heart failure can develop from valvar insufficiency and endomyocardial fibrosis. Cardiac involvement can occur in association with eosinophilia from diverse causes, including parasitic infections. Hypereosinophilic syndromes can result in cerebral emboli from cardiac disease, diffuse encephalopathy, and peripheral neuropathy.

Diagnosis

Differential Diagnosis

The differential diagnosis of eosinophilia includes reactive eosinophilia, eosinophilia associated with other primary disorders, and eosinophilia associated with clonal hematopoiesis (see Table 176–1). Evaluation of patients is based on their history and clinical characteristics (Fig. 176–2). The initial goal is to determine whether the eosinophilia is secondary to a reactive cause (i.e., in response to another primary trigger such as allergy, infection, solid tumor, vasculitis). If reactive causes are not identified, further evaluation should determine whether the eosinophilia is secondary to a clonal hematologic disorder. If no evidence of clonality is determined, the patient is considered to have an idiopathic hypereosinophilic syndrome.

The differential diagnosis of eosinophilia requires a review of the patient's history, which may reveal wheezing (Chapter 83), rhinitis (Chapter 272), or eczema (indicating atopic causes); travel to areas where helminth infections (e.g., schistosomiasis [Chapter 376]) are endemic; the presence of a pet dog (indicating possible infection with *Toxocara canis* [Chapter 378]); symptoms of cancer; or drug ingestion (indicating a possible hypersensitivity reaction [Chapter 275]). Eosinophilia caused by drugs (Chapter 275) is usually benign but can sometimes be accompanied by tissue damage, as in hypersensitivity pneumonitis (Chapter 92). In most cases, the eosinophilia resolves when use of the drug ceases, but in some cases, such as eosinophilia-myalgia syndrome secondary to the ingestion of contaminated L-tryptophan, the disease can persist despite withdrawal of the drug.

The presence of abnormal morphologic features of eosinophils, an increase in immature and dysplastic cells in the bone marrow or blood, elevated levels of vitamin B_{12}, and splenomegaly raises suspicion of a clonal hypereosinophilic syndrome. In such cases, evidence of clonality (e.g., by analysis of X chromosome inactivation patterns in female patients), an elevated level of mast cell tryptase (elevated in myelodysplastic variants of hypereosinophilic syndrome), the presence of aberrant lymphocyte phenotypes (elevated in lymphocytic variants of hypereosinophilic syndrome), abnormal cytogenetics, and the possible presence of specific fusion genes such as *FIP1L1-PDGFRA* should be investigated.

Other eosinophilic syndromes such as Churg-Strauss syndrome (Chapter 291) should be considered in patients with a history of worsening asthma, sinus disease, neuropathy, or blood eosinophilia and the presence of abnormal laboratory findings associated with autoimmunity, such as an elevated erythrocyte sedimentation rate, C-reactive protein, and antineutrophil cytoplasmic antibodies.

An accumulation of eosinophils that is limited to specific organs is characteristic of particular diseases, such as eosinophilic cellulitis (Wells' syndrome), eosinophilic pneumonias (e.g., Löffler's syndrome [Chapter 59]), and eosinophilic fasciitis (Shulman's syndrome).

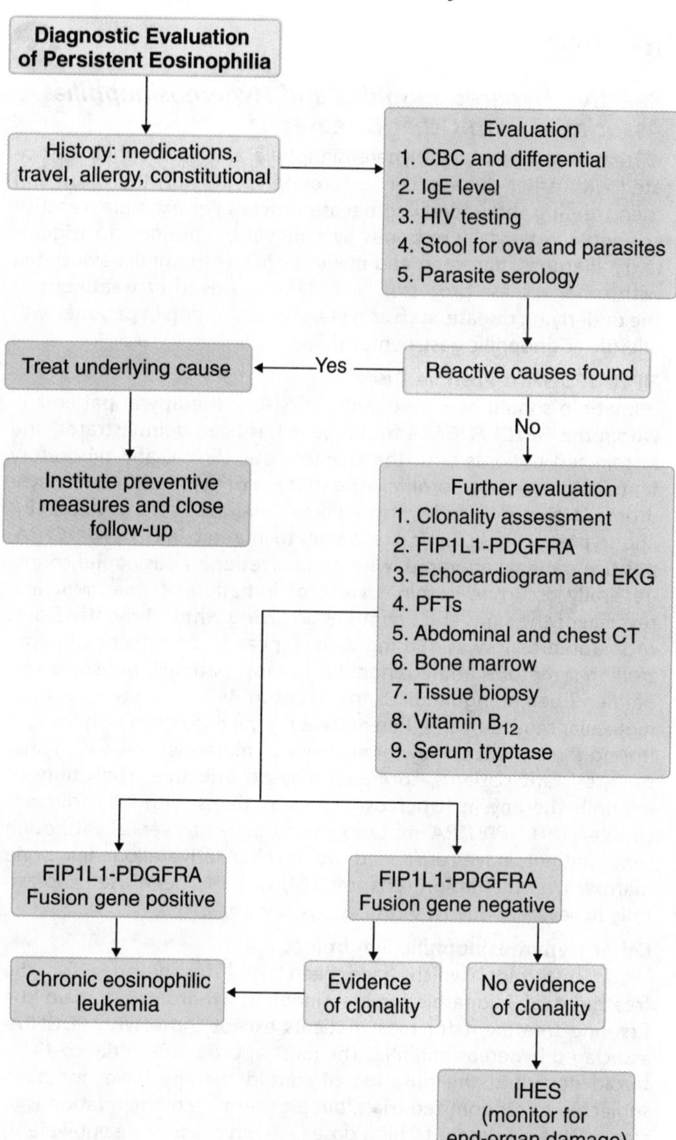

FIGURE 176–2 • Diagnostic evaluation of persistent eosinophilia. CBC = complete blood count; CT = computed tomography; ECG = electrocardiogram; IgE = immunoglobulin E; IHES = idiopathic hypereosinophilic syndrome; HIV = human immunodeficiency virus; PDGFRA = platelet-derived growth factor α; PFTs = pulmonary function tests.

Diagnostic Evaluation

Diagnostic studies that should be performed in patients with moderate to severe eosinophilia and considered in patients with persistent mild eosinophilia include morphologic examination of a blood smear, human immunodeficiency virus (HIV) screen, serial stool examinations for ova and parasites, parasite serology, and plasma immunoglobulin E (IgE) level. Parasitic infections that cause eosinophilia are usually limited to helminthic parasites, with the exception of two enteric protozoans, *Isospora belli* (Chapter 374) and *Dientamoeba fragilis* (Chapter 374). *Strongyloides stercoralis* (Chapter 378) infection is important to diagnose because it can cause disseminated fatal disease in immunosuppressed patients; detection of such infection often requires serologic testing. Other infections to consider include trichinosis (Chapter 378), *T. canis* infection (Chapter 378), and HIV infection (Chapter 407).

Patients with sustained hypereosinophilia should be monitored closely for the subsequent development of cardiac disease. A pathologically similar disease, Löffler's endomyocarditis (Chapter 59), has been noted in tropical regions, where antecedent parasite-elicited eosinophilia may be responsible for the cardiac damage.

Treatment

Rx

Reactive Hypereosinophilia and Hypereosinophilia Associated with Other Diseases

Treatment of reactive hypereosinophilia and eosinophilia associated with other diseases centers around identifying the cause and then treating the underlying disease process. For example, reactive eosinophilia typically responds by removal of the inciting triggers (e.g., allergens, parasites, and medications). Eosinophilia associated with other disease processes typically improves after treatment of the underlying disease, such as dietary manipulation in patients with allergic eosinophilic gastroenteritis.

FIP1L1/PDGFRA-Positive Disease

Imatinib should be considered as first-line therapy in patients in whom the *FIP1L1-PDGFRA* fusion gene has been demonstrated and in selected patients with the characteristic clinical and laboratory features of this myeloproliferative subtype of hypereosinophilic syndrome (e.g., male gender, tissue fibrosis, elevated serum vitamin B_{12} and tryptase levels). Clinical responses to imatinib in *FIP1L1/PDGFRA*-positive patients are rapid, with normalization of eosinophil counts generally occurring within 1 week of initiation of treatment and reversal of the signs and symptoms occurring within 1 month. Doses of imatinib as low as 100 mg daily appear to be effective in controlling symptoms and eosinophilia in most patients, but some recommend beginning imatinib treatment at 400 mg daily to achieve molecular remission and then decreasing the dose slowly while monitoring the patient closely for evidence of molecular relapse. In imatinib-resistant patients, sorafenib may be effective. The utility of imatinib therapy in hypereosinophilic patients without a demonstrable *FIP1L1-PDGFRA* mutation remains controversial, although some patients have responded. Nonmyeloablative allogeneic bone marrow transplantation (Chapter 184) has also been used successfully in several patients with hypereosinophilia.

Other Hypereosinophilic Syndromes

Corticosteroids, which have been used for decades for the treatment of idiopathic hypereosinophilic syndromes, remain the first-line treatment for most patients except those with PDGFRA-associated hypereosinophilia. The most appropriate initial corticosteroid dose and the duration of steroid therapy have not been subjected to randomized trials, but a general recommendation is to start with a moderate to high dose (≥40 mg prednisone equivalent) and taper very slowly while monitoring the eosinophil count closely. With this approach, most but not all patients will respond initially, and some will be able to be maintained on low doses of corticosteroids for prolonged periods. Of the cytotoxic therapies that have been used for steroid-refractory hypereosinophilia, hydroxyurea has been the most extensively studied at doses of 1 to 3 g/day. Vincristine at a dose of 1 to 2 mg intravenously can rapidly lower eosinophilia in patients with extremely high eosinophil counts (>100,000/mm^3) and may be useful for the treatment of children whose aggressive disease is unresponsive to other therapies. In patients who have corticosteroid-refractory hypereosinophilic syndromes or in whom intolerable side effects of steroid treatment develop, immunomodulatory agents that are sometimes helpful include interferon alfa, cyclosporine, and alemtuzumab. Responses can often be achieved with relatively low doses of interferon alfa (1 to 2 × 10^6 U/day) and may persist for prolonged periods. Because the effects of interferon alfa on eosinophil numbers in peripheral blood may not become evident for several weeks, escalation to an effective dose may require several months. Rarely, patients have remained in remission for extended periods after cessation of interferon alfa therapy, thus suggesting that interferon alfa may be curative in a small subset of individuals. Low-dose (500 mg daily) hydroxyurea appears to act synergistically with interferon alfa to lower the eosinophil count without increasing side effects. Monoclonal anti–IL-5 antibody therapy (e.g., mepolizumab at monthly intravenous doses of 750 mg) for hypereosinophilia has a number of unique advantages related to the specificity of IL-5 for the eosinophil lineage. The safety and efficacy of anti–IL-5 therapy as a steroid-sparing agent in hypereosinophilia are currently being assessed in a large, double-blind, placebo-controlled study.

Future Directions

Treatments on the horizon for hypereosinophilic disorders include targeted therapy against the eotaxin chemokines and their receptor CCR3.

Prognosis

The prognosis of hypereosinophilic syndromes depends on the primary cause. Whereas *FIP1L1-PDGFRA* positive disease and other forms of clonal disorders have a poor prognosis (25 to 50% 5-year mortality if responsiveness to therapeutic intervention is not achieved), the prognosis of hypereosinophilia from reactive and other causes is usually better.

SUGGESTED READINGS

Klion AD, Bochner BS, Gleich GJ, et al: Approaches to the treatment of hypereosinophilic syndrome: A workshop summary report. J Allergy Clin Immunol 2006;117:1292–1302.

Pardanani A, Brockman SR, Paternoster SF, et al: FIP1L1-PDGFRA fusion: Prevalence and clinicopathologic correlates in 89 consecutive patients with moderate to severe eosinophilia. Blood 2004;104:3038–3045. *The prevalence of the FIP1L1-PDGFRA mutation in primary eosinophilia was 14%.*

Sade K, Mysels A, Levo Y, et al: Eosinophilia: A study of 100 hospitalized patients. Eur J Intern Med 2007;18:196–201. *Common causes were asthma or atopic disease (13%), eosinophilic pneumonia (10%), cancer (10%), infections (10%), and drug reactions (6%), but 34% were of unknown cause.*

Shorr AF, Scoville SL, Cersovsky SB, et al: Acute eosinophilic pneumonia among US military personnel deployed in or near Iraq. JAMA 2004;292:2997–3005. *Occurring in 1 per 10,000, the cause is unknown; most responded to corticosteroids.*

Tefferi A: Blood eosinophilia: A new paradigm in disease classification, diagnosis, and treatment. Mayo Clin Proc 2005;80:75–83. *A clinical review.*

177 MYELOPROLIFERATIVE DISORDERS: ESSENTIAL THROMBOCYTHEMIA AND PRIMARY MYELOFIBROSIS

Ayalew Tefferi

Definition

Essential thrombocythemia and primary myelofibrosis (formerly called myelofibrosis with myeloid metaplasia) are currently classified with polycythemia vera (Chapter 172) as the classic *BCR/ABL*-negative myeloproliferative disorders. These clinicopathologic entities have biologic and phenotypic similarity to other chronic myeloid diseases, including chronic myeloid leukemia (CML; Chapter 195), myelodysplastic syndrome (Chapter 193), and other atypical myeloproliferative disorders (Table 177–1). X-linked glucose-6-phosphate dehydrogenase cell assays initially established the stem cell–derived, clonal (neoplastic) nature of trilineage myeloproliferation in most chronic myeloid disorders, including both essential thrombocythemia and primary myelofibrosis. Current diagnosis is therefore based on a constellation of clinical findings, bone marrow histology, cytogenetics, and most recently, mutation screening for $JAK2^{V617F}$ based on the demonstration of this specific mutation in the majority of patients with polycythemia vera (Chapter 172) and half of those with either essential thrombocythemia or primary myelofibrosis.

Epidemiology

The myeloproliferative disorders are rare, with an approximate annual incidence of 0.2 to 2.5, 0.8 to 2.8, and 0.4 to 1.3 per 100,000 for essential thrombocythemia, polycythemia vera, and myeloid metaplasia, respectively. The median age at initial evaluation across the three disorders is similar (55 to 65 years), with a slight male preponderance (1.2:1) in polycythemia vera and myeloid metaplasia and a female preponderance (2:1) in essential thrombocythemia. All three disorders have infrequently been

TABLE 177–1 APPROACH TO THE CLASSIFICATION OF CHRONIC MYELOID DISORDERS

Myelodysplastic syndrome
Myeloproliferative disorders
- Classic myeloproliferative disorders
  - Molecularly defined
    - Chronic myeloid leukemia (*BCR/ABL*-positive)
  - Clinicopathologically assigned (*BCR/ABL*-negative and frequently associated with *JAK2*^{V617F} mutation)
    - Essential thrombocythemia
    - Polycythemia vera
    - Primary myelofibrosis
- Atypical myeloproliferative disorders
  - Molecularly defined
    - *PDGFRA*-rearranged eosinophilic/mast cell disorders (e.g., *FIP1L1-PDGFRA*)
    - *PDGFRB*-rearranged eosinophilic disorders (e.g., *TEL/ETV6-PDGFRB*)
    - Systemic mastocytosis associated with *c-kit* mutation (e.g., *c-kit*^{D816V})
    - *8p11* Myeloproliferative syndrome (e.g., *ZNF198/FIM/RAMP-FGFR1*)
  - Clinicopathologically assigned (infrequently associated with *JAK2*^{V617F} mutation)
    - Chronic neutrophilic leukemia
    - Chronic eosinophilic leukemia, molecularly not defined
    - Hypereosinophilic syndrome
    - Chronic basophilic leukemia
    - Chronic myelomonocytic leukemia
    - Juvenile myelomonocytic leukemia (associated with recurrent mutations of RAS signaling pathway molecules, including *PTPN11* and *NF1*)
    - Systemic mastocytosis, molecularly not defined
    - Unclassified myeloproliferative disorder

RAS = renin-angiotensin system.
With permission from Tefferi A, Gilliland DG: Classification of chronic myeloid disorders: From Dameshek towards a semi-molecular system. Best Pract Res Clin Haematol 2006;19:365–385.

described in children. No convincing evidence links specific environmental exposures to these diseases.

Pathobiology

Clonal myeloproliferation involving granulocytes, monocytes, erythroid cells, platelets, and sometimes even lymphocytes has been demonstrated in most patients with myeloproliferative disorders, including essential thrombocythemia and primary myelofibrosis, by X chromosome–linked DNA or gene product analysis, as well as other molecular clonality assays. Cytogenetic studies have been of limited value because such abnormalities occur in less than 5% of patients with essential thrombocythemia and in approximately 50% of those with primary myelofibrosis and are nonspecific in both instances. An acquired point mutation involving an auto-inhibitory domain of the JAK2 kinase (JAK2^{V617F}) occurs in about 25 to 60% of patients who have essential thrombocythemia and 35 to 60% of those who have primary myelofibrosis.

Clonal myeloproliferation in primary myelofibrosis associated with an intense bone marrow stromal reaction that consists of excess deposition of extracellular matrix proteins, including collagen, angiogenesis (new blood vessel formation), and osteosclerosis (osteoblast proliferation and new bone formation). Observations from experimental myelofibrosis in mice and the finding that bone marrow fibroblasts in myeloid metaplasia are polyclonal form the basis for the current assumption that the bone marrow stromal changes in myeloid metaplasia represent a reactive process that is mediated by cytokines such as basic fibroblast growth factor, vascular endothelial growth factor, transforming growth factor-β, and tumor necrosis factor-α; such cytokines are furnished by the clonal proliferation of megakaryocytes, monocytes, and/or histiocytes.

TABLE 177–2 CAUSES OF THROMBOCYTOSIS (PLATELET COUNT >500,000/μL OR HIGHER) IN UNSELECTED COHORTS OF CONSECUTIVE PATIENTS (APPROXIMATE PERCENTAGES)

Condition	Adults, >500,000/μL	>1,000,000/μL
Infection	22%	31%
Rebound thrombocytosis	19%	3%
Tissue damage (surgery)	18%	14%
Chronic inflammation	13%	9%
Malignancy	6%	14%
Renal disorders	5%	<1%
Hemolytic anemia	4%	<1%
Post-splenectomy status	2%	19%
Blood loss	NS	6%
Primary thrombocythemia	3%	14%

From Tefferi A, Gilliland DG: Classification of chronic myeloid disorders: From Dameshek towards a semi-molecular system. Best Pract Res Clin Haematol 2006;19:365–385.

ESSENTIAL THROMBOCYTHEMIA

Clinical Manifestations

Approximately 50% of patients with essential thrombocythemia may be asymptomatic at initial evaluation. Vasomotor disturbances (headaches, lightheadedness, visual symptoms, palpitations, atypical chest pain, erythromelalgia, distal paresthesia) are the most frequent symptoms and occur in 25 to 50% of patients. It is believed that these symptoms, especially erythromelalgia (see Fig. 177–2), are the result of small vessel platelet-endothelium interaction with associated inflammation and transient thrombotic occlusion. The life-threatening complications of essential thrombocythemia are thrombosis, hemorrhage, and transformation into either primary myelofibrosis or acute myeloid leukemia (Chapter 194).

Arterial thrombosis (e.g., cerebrovascular or cardiovascular ischemia or infarcts, digital gangrene) is more frequent than venous thrombosis (pulmonary embolism, Budd-Chiari syndrome, portal vein thrombosis, deep vein thrombosis) in both essential thrombocythemia and polycythemia vera. The upper gastrointestinal system is the usual site of hemorrhage in essential thrombocythemia, and the risk for this complication is enhanced by the use of nonsteroidal anti-inflammatory drugs (NSAIDs). Increased mucocutaneous bleeding is frequent and may be related to an acquired von Willebrand (vW) defect (Chapter 180). More than a third of women with essential thrombocythemia may have a first trimester spontaneous miscarriage, which may be unrelated to the platelet count or use of aspirin. Complications late in pregnancy are unusual and appear not to be reduced by prophylactic platelet apheresis during delivery.

Major thrombosis or hemorrhage is noted at initial evaluation in 11 to 25% and 2 to 5% of patients, respectively; subsequent events during the first decade of the disease occur in 11 to 22% and 1 to 7%, respectively. The overall incidence of superficial or deep thrombosis in essential thrombocythemia is 20 to 40%, but major thrombosis (stroke, myocardial infarction, deep vein thrombosis, pulmonary embolism, digital arterial occlusion) occurs in only 10 to 20% of patients. Leukemic transformation is rare (<5%) during the first 10 years but may be higher thereafter.

Physical examination is often unremarkable, but approximately 25% of patients have palpable splenomegaly at diagnosis.

Diagnosis

In routine clinical practice, more than 80% of cases of thrombocytosis are considered reactive and are not associated with a clonal hematologic disorder (Table 177–2). It is important to distinguish reactive thrombocytosis from essential thrombocythemia (Fig. 177–1) because

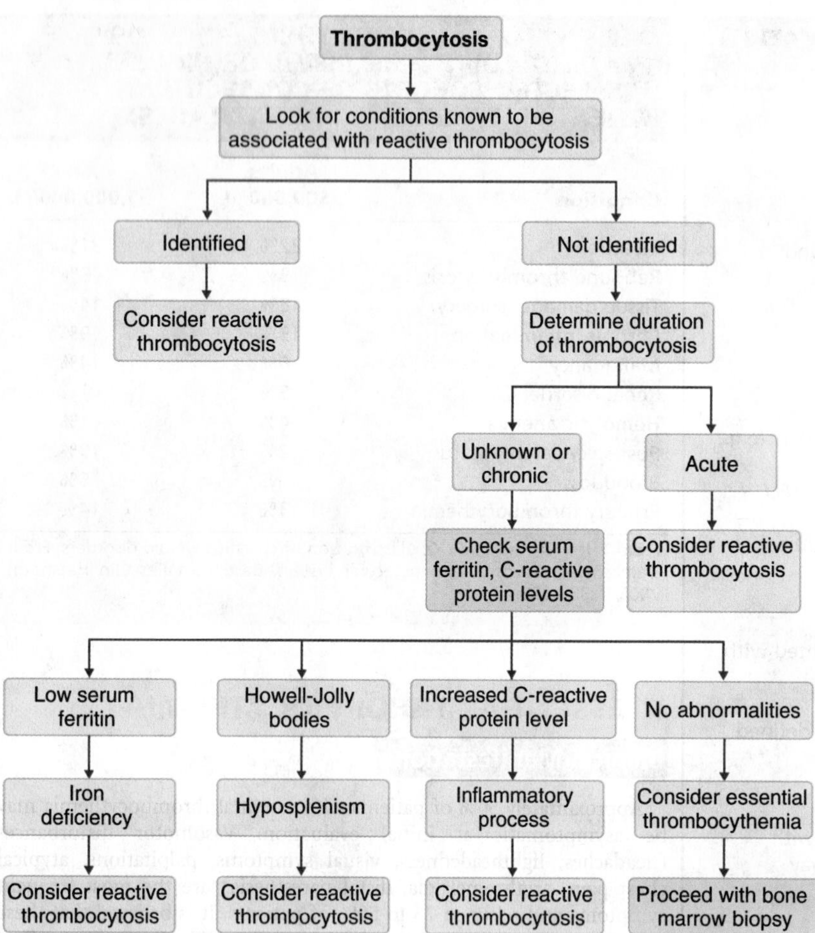

FIGURE 177–1 • Diagnostic evaluation of thrombocytosis in routine clinical practice.

there is an increased risk for thrombosis associated with essential thrombocythemia but not with reactive thrombocytosis. The degree of thrombocytosis, platelet morphology, and platelet function tests are neither specific nor sensitive enough to distinguish essential from reactive thrombocytosis.

However, serum levels of both ferritin and C-reactive protein may help address the possibility of iron deficiency anemia (Chapter 163) and occult inflammatory process, respectively, as causes of possible reactive thrombocytosis. Uncomplicated essential thrombocythemia is characterized by normal C-reactive protein levels. A normal serum ferritin level excludes iron deficiency–associated reactive thrombocytosis, but a low level does not exclude the possibility of essential thrombocythemia. Howell-Jolly bodies on the peripheral blood smear suggest surgical or functional hyposplenism as a cause of reactive thrombocytosis (Fig. 177–2). Serum thrombopoietin levels are not generally helpful in distinguishing essential thrombocythemia from either reactive thrombocytosis or other causes of primary thrombocytosis.

The peripheral smear in essential thrombocythemia is often unremarkable except for the abundance of platelets. However, some patients may display morphologic pleomorphism as well as giant platelets. Primary thrombocytosis may be ascribed to essential thrombocythemia only when bone marrow morphologic and cytogenetic findings do not suggest another chronic myeloid disorder. Bone marrow histology in essential thrombocythemia often reveals abnormal clusters of megakaryocytes (Fig. 177–3) that may or may not be accompanied by either increased overall cellularity or mild reticulin fibrosis.

A Philadelphia chromosome (or its molecular equivalent, *BCR/ABL*) establishes CML as the diagnosis and excludes essential thrombocythemia. A trilineage dysplasia suggests myelodysplastic syndrome, and intense marrow cellularity with florid atypical megakaryocytic hyperplasia suggests "cellular phase" myeloid metaplasia. Mutation screening for $JAK2^{V617F}$ is appropriate when one suspects the diagnosis of a myeloproliferative disorder in general and essential thrombocythemia in particular (Fig. 177–4).

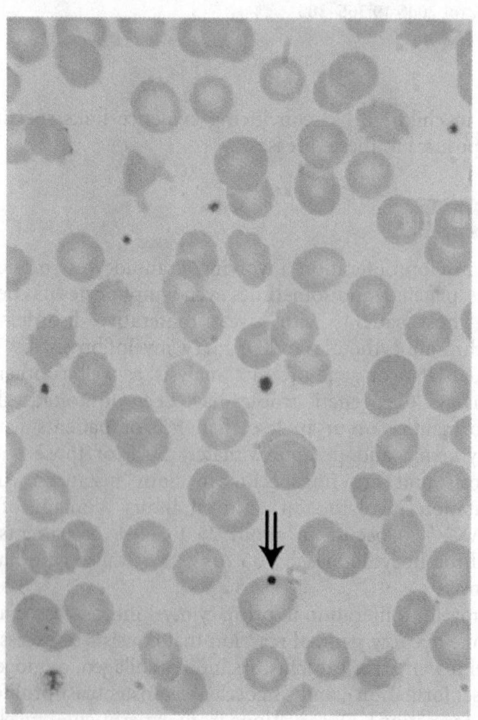

FIGURE 177–2 • Peripheral smear showing Howell-Jolly bodies (arrow) in red blood cells, a finding typical of surgical or functional hyposplenism.

Treatment

Rx

The key guide to long-term management of essential thrombocythemia is the patient's risk for thrombosis based on a history of previous thrombosis and age older than 60 years (Table 177–3). Cytoreductive (platelet-lowering) therapy reduces the risk for thrombosis in high-risk patients, in whom the platelet count may need to be reduced to less than 400,000/μL. In other patients, the use of platelet-lowering agents is not supported. Only hydroxyurea (Table 177–4) has been shown prospectively to reduce the risk for thrombosis in patients with essential thrombocythemia, and in a randomized trial it was also superior to anagrelide. [1] In high-risk women who are or wish to be pregnant, cytoreductive therapy with interferon alfa has been safe and effective in anecdotal reports.

Acute thrombosis in patients with essential thrombocythemia requires an immediate reduction of the platelet count to less than 400,000/μL. If the platelet count is higher than 800,000/μL, platelet apheresis is indicated, usually combined with hydroxyurea. Systemic anticoagulation with full-dose heparin followed by warfarin (with an international normalized ratio goal of 2 to 2.5) should also be started, and warfarin may be switched to low-dose aspirin after 6 months of treatment if the thrombocytosis has been adequately controlled.

In general, the use of aspirin or other NSAIDs is discouraged in patients with platelet counts greater than 1 million/μL because of the danger of bleeding from acquired vW disease (Chapter 180). However, low-dose aspirin (81 to 325 mg/day) is currently recommended as a supplement to cytoreductive therapy in high-risk patients, as well as an optional consideration in most patients with essential thrombocythemia in the absence of risk factors for bleeding such as acquired vW disease and a history of upper gastrointestinal bleeding.

Rx

For vasomotor disturbances, low-dose aspirin (one baby aspirin, 81 mg/day) is effective. If aspirin is not adequate, platelet-lowering (cytoreductive) therapy, including hydroxyurea (starting dose of 500 mg/day twice a day), may be indicated, with the goal being a platelet count that relieves symptoms.

Prognosis

In patients with essential thrombocythemia, life expectancy in the first decade of the disease may not be significantly different from that of the age- and sex-matched control population, in part because the risk for early leukemic transformation is well below 5%. The subsequent risk for leukemia is thought to be higher, however, and natural history studies suggest worse survival than in age-matched control subjects after the first decade of the disease.

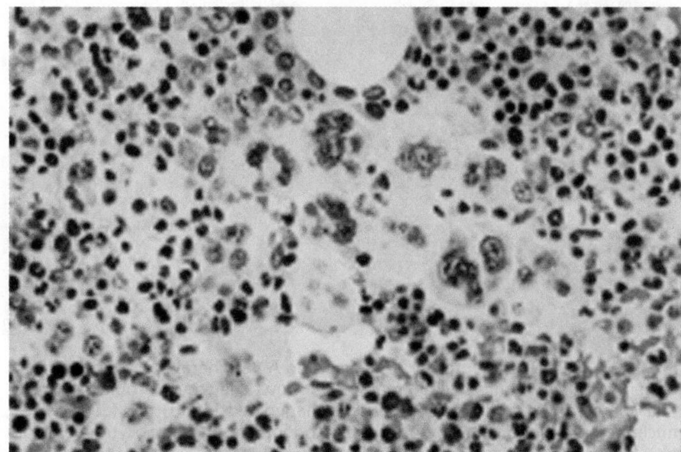

FIGURE 177–3 • Myeloproliferative disorder. Bone marrow shows megakaryocytic clusters seen in essential thrombocythemia and other conditions associated with clonal thrombocytosis.

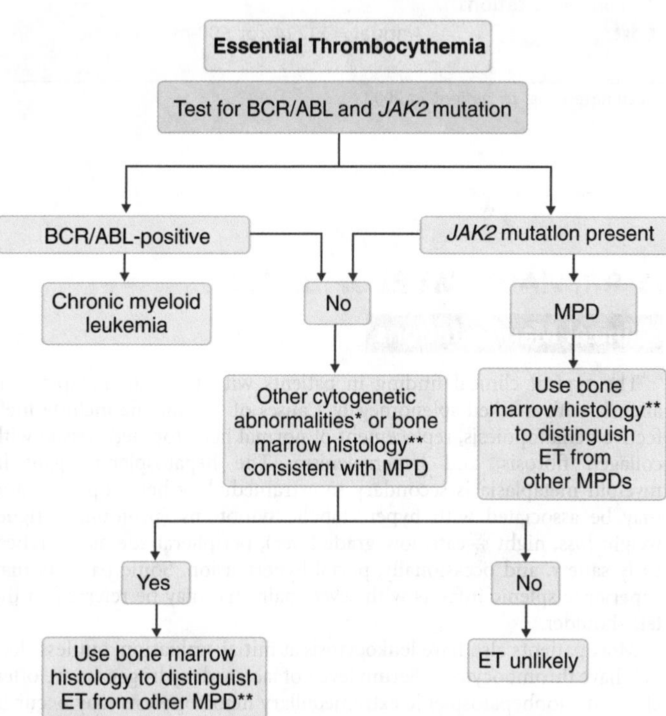

FIGURE 177–4 • Diagnostic algorithm for essential thrombocythemia (i.e., clinically not consistent with reactive thrombocytosis; see Table 177–2). ET = essential thrombocythemia; FISH = fluorescence in situ hybridization; *JAK2* = Janus kinase 2; MPD = myeloproliferative disorder. *Cytogenetic abnormalities include those of chromosomes 8 and 9. **Bone marrow histology abnormalities include megakaryocyte clustering and giant megakaryocytes. (From Tefferi A, Sirhan S, Lasho TL, et al: Concomitant neutrophil *JAK2*^{V617F} mutation screening and *PRV-1* expression analysis in myeloproliferative disorders and secondary polycythemia. Br J Haematol 2005;131:166–171, with permission.)

TABLE 177–3 TREATMENT OF ESSENTIAL THROMBOCYTHEMIA BASED ON THE RISK FOR THROMBOSIS

Risk category	Low risk*	High risk†	Indeterminate risk‡ + Cardiovascular risk factors + Extreme thrombocytosis
Cytoreductive therapy	No	Yes, and current treatment of choice is hydroxyurea	No Sometimes
Aspirin therapy	Optional but recommended in the absence of contraindications	Yes	Yes No

*Age younger than 60 years *and* no history of thrombosis, extreme thrombocytosis (platelet count ≥1 to 1.5 million/μL), or cardiovascular risk factors (smoking, hyperlipidemia).
†Age 60 years or older *or* a history of thrombosis.
‡Neither low risk nor high risk.

TABLE 177–4 CLINICAL PROPERTIES OF PLATELET-LOWERING AGENTS

Drug (Class)	Hydroxyurea (Myelosuppressive)	Anagrelide (Platelet Specific)	Interferon Alfa (Myelosuppressive)
Mechanism of action	Antimetabolite	Unknown	Biologic agent
Pharmacology	Half-life ≅5 hr, renal excretion	Half-life ≅1.5 hr, renal excretion	Kidney is main site of metabolism
Starting dose	500 mg PO bid	0.5 mg PO tid	5 million U SC 3×/wk
Onset of action	≅3–5 days	≅6–10 days	1–3 weeks
Frequent side effects	Leukopenia, oral ulcers, anemia, hyperpigmentation, nail discoloration, xeroderma	Headache, palpitations, diarrhea, fluid retention, anemia	Flulike syndrome, fatigue, anorexia, weight loss, lack of ambition, alopecia
Infrequent side effects	Leg ulcers, nausea, diarrhea, alopecia, skin atrophy	Arrhythmias, lightheadedness, nausea	Confusion, depression, autoimmune thyroiditis, myalgia, arthritis
Rare side effects	Fever, cystitis, platelet oscillations	Cardiomyopathy	Pruritus, hyperlipidemia, transaminasemia
Absolute contraindications	Pregnancy	Pregnancy	
Relative contraindications		Congestive heart failure	
Cost*	Annual = $1714 for 500-mg dose tid	Annual = $8500 for 0.5-mg dose qid	Annual = $10,500 for 3 million U 5 days/wk

*Estimated cost to patient in 2003.

PRIMARY MYELOFIBROSIS

Clinical Manifestations

The typical clinical finding in patients with myeloid metaplasia is anemia with marked splenomegaly. Causes of the anemia include ineffective hematopoiesis, replacement of normal hematopoietic tissue with collagen fibrosis, and hypersplenism. The hepatosplenomegaly in myeloid metaplasia is secondary to extramedullary hematopoiesis and may be associated with hypercatabolic symptoms (profound fatigue, weight loss, night sweats, low-grade fever), peripheral edema, diarrhea, early satiety, and occasionally, portal hypertension. Some patients may experience splenic infarcts with severe pain that may be referred to the left shoulder.

Most patients also have leukocytosis at initial evaluation, but less than half have thrombocytosis. Serum levels of lactate dehydrogenase are often elevated. Nonhepatosplenic extramedullary hematopoiesis may occur in the lymph nodes, pleura (effusion), peritoneum (ascites), lung (interstitial process), and paraspinal and epidural spaces (spinal cord and nerve root compression).

Diagnosis

The diagnosis of primary myelofibrosis is actively considered when anemia or splenomegaly is accompanied by a "myelophthisic" blood picture consisting of immature granulocytes, nucleated red cells, and teardrop-shaped red blood cells (dacryocytes) on the peripheral blood smear (Fig. 177–5). However, myelophthisis may also be associated with other bone marrow–infiltrating processes, including metastatic cancer, Hodgkin's disease (Chapter 194), and multiple myeloma (Chapter 198). Therefore, bone marrow biopsy is essential for further clarification of the diagnosis.

The bone marrow in patients with primary myelofibrosis is not easily aspirated (dry tap). The usual findings in the core biopsy include atypical megakaryocyte hyperplasia, collagen fibrosis, osteosclerosis, and intrasinusoidal hematopoiesis (Fig. 177–6). The degree of fibrosis may be better estimated by the use of either a reticulin (silver impregnation) or trichrome stain. Occasionally, the degree of bone marrow fibrosis may be minimal ("cellular phase" myeloid metaplasia). Bone marrow fibrosis may also be associated with other hematologic and nonhematologic conditions (Table 177–5).

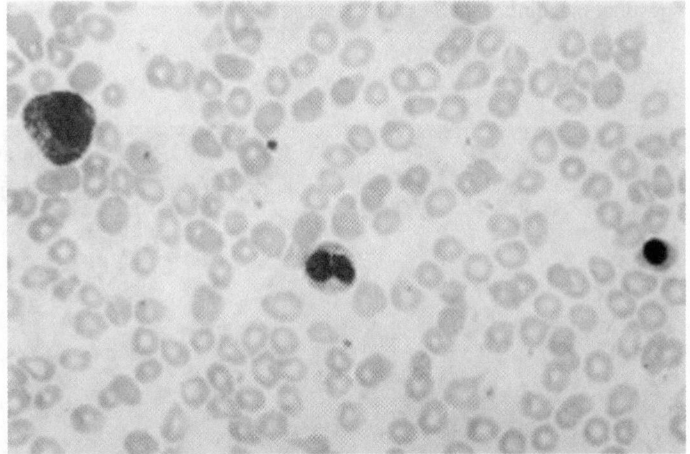

FIGURE 177–5 • Myeloproliferative disorder. A peripheral blood smear from a patient with agnogenic myeloid metaplasia shows a leukoerythroblastic picture. The characteristic findings are teardrop-shaped red blood cells (dacryocytes), nucleated red blood cells (erythroblasts), and immature granulocyte precursors.

The bone marrow morphologic features of myeloid metaplasia may sometimes be difficult to distinguish from those of both myelodysplastic syndrome with fibrosis (Chapter 193) and acute myelofibrosis. Acute myelofibrosis is characterized by severe constitutional symptoms, a nonpalpable spleen, pancytopenia, and the presence of circulating blasts. Some cases of acute myelofibrosis are classifiable as acute megakaryoblastic leukemia (Chapter 194). When compared with myeloid metaplasia, both myelodysplastic syndrome with fibrosis and acute myelofibrosis are associated with lower survival rates and may require more aggressive treatment.

Cytogenetic studies are most important in excluding any atypical forms of CML that may be accompanied by substantial bone marrow fibrosis. At diagnosis, approximately a third of patients with myeloid metaplasia display karyotypic abnormalities, including del(13q), del(20q), trisomy 8, and abnormalities of chromosomes 1 and 7. However, none of these cytogenetic markers carries diagnostic specificity.

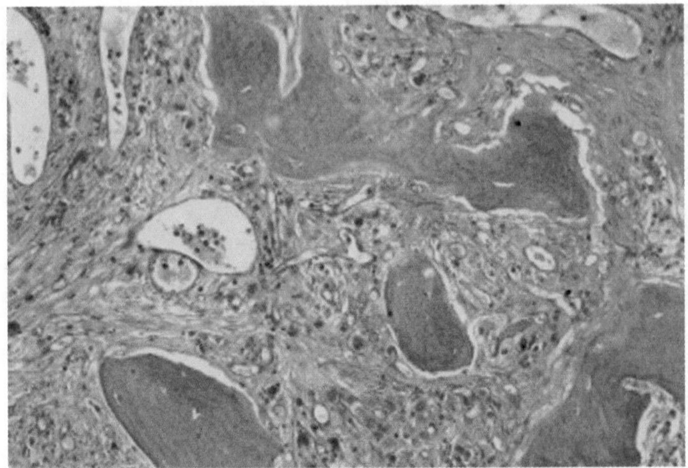

FIGURE 177–6 • A bone marrow biopsy specimen from a patient with primary myelofibrosis shows reticulin fibrosis, osteosclerosis, and intrasinusoidal hematopoiesis.

TABLE 177–5 CAUSES OF BONE MARROW FIBROSIS

MYELOID DISORDERS
Primary myelofibrosis
Metastatic cancer
Chronic myeloid leukemia
Myelodysplastic syndrome
Atypical myeloid disorder
Acute megakaryocytic leukemia
Other acute myeloid leukemias
Gray platelet syndrome
LYMPHOID DISORDERS
Hairy cell leukemia
Multiple myeloma
Lymphoma
NONHEMATOLOGIC DISORDERS
Connective tissue disorder
Infections (tuberculosis, kala-azar)
Vitamin D deficiency rickets
Renal osteodystrophy

Treatment

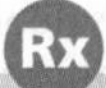

Conventional Medical Therapy

Conventional therapy for primary myelofibrosis is largely palliative and has not been shown to improve survival. Anemia is often treated with an androgen preparation (oral fluoxymesterone, 20 mg/day), with or without the addition of corticosteroids (oral prednisone, 30 mg/day). Response occurs in less than a third of patients and lasts for less than a year. Before instituting androgen therapy, the possibility of occult prostate cancer (Chapter 211) should be excluded. Furthermore, female patients should be warned about possible virilizing side effects, and all patients should be periodically monitored by serum liver chemistry assays.

Alternative treatments of anemia include subcutaneous erythropoietin (40,000 U weekly), thalidomide (50 mg/day), and danazol (400 mg/day). Overall response rates with each of these drugs range from 10 to 30%. Complete disclosure of drug side effects is important, including neuropathy with thalidomide and liver function test abnormalities with danazol.

Hydroxyurea (starting dose, 500 mg two times a day) remains the drug of choice for the control of leukocytosis, thrombocytosis, or organomegaly. Hydroxyurea-refractory splenomegaly, if symptomatic, may require surgical removal. Other indications for splenectomy include disabling constitutional symptoms associated with marked splenomegaly, symptomatic portal hypertension, and the need for frequent red cell transfusions. Approximately a fourth of patients with transfusion-requiring anemia may derive durable benefit from splenectomy. However, the perioperative mortality rate may be as high as 9%, and overall survival may not be affected (median post-splenectomy survival is approximately 2 years).

After splenectomy, acute leukemia, marked hepatomegaly, and extreme thrombocytosis may develop in approximately 16, 16, and 22% of surgical survivors, respectively, with the latter being significantly associated with perioperative thrombosis. Therefore, prophylactic hydroxyurea is strongly advised to prevent the post-splenectomy elevation in platelet count. In poor surgical candidates with symptomatic splenomegaly, palliative splenic irradiation is reasonable (approximately 300 cGy given in 10 fractions). Splenic irradiation may also be used in the management of splenic infarcts that are refractory to opiate analgesics. Treatment of nonsplenic extramedullary hematopoiesis requires low doses of involved field irradiation (100 to 150 cGy) given in multiple fractions.

Investigational Therapy

Allogeneic hematopoietic stem cell transplantation has provided durable disease remission in approximately a third of patients with primary myelofibrosis who have undergone such treatment. However, the substantial mortality and morbidity (approximately 50%) associated with the procedure currently limit it to poor-risk young patients. Lenalidomide, an immunomodulatory analogue of thalidomide, has therapeutic activity in primary myelofibrosis, and additional studies are ongoing.

Future Directions

In essential thrombocythemia, the most important goal may be the identification of patients who are at risk for either thrombohemorrhagic complications or clonal evolution to guide selection for specific treatment. In primary myelofibrosis, the immediate goal is to identify the causal genetic mutation. The spectacular benefits of imatinib mesylate in CML (Chapter 195) suggest that targeted therapy with small molecules may provide great benefit in chronic myeloproliferative disorders.

Prognosis

The most frequent disease-related causes of death in patients with primary myelofibrosis are infection and leukemic transformation. The latter occurs in approximately 20% of patients over the first 10 years. The presence of anemia (hemoglobin level less than 10 g/dL), thrombocytopenia (platelet count less than 100,000/µL), extreme ranges of white blood cell count (leukocytes either below 4000 or above 30,000/µL), circulating myeloblasts, unfavorable cytogenetic abnormalities (i.e., clones other than 13q– and 20q–), severe constitutional symptoms, or advanced age is predictive of poor survival. A simple complete blood count–based prognostic scoring system (Table 177–6) reliably discriminates low-risk (median survival >10 years), intermediate-risk (median survival of 5 to 10 years), and high-risk disease (median survival <5 years). On the other hand, the degree of either hepatosplenomegaly or bone marrow fibrosis may not affect survival.

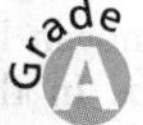

1. Harrison CN, Campbell PJ, Buck G, et al: Hydroxyurea compared with anagrelide in high-risk essential thrombocythemia. N Engl J Med 2005;353:33–45.

Section XIV Hematology

TABLE 177–6 USING THE COMPLETE BLOOD COUNT FOR RISK STRATIFICATION IN PATIENTS WITH PRIMARY MYELOFIBROSIS

Risk category	Low risk	High risk	Intermediate risk
Properties	**All of the following:** Hemoglobin ≥10 g/dL Platelet count ≥100,000/µL WBC ≥4000 and <30,000/µL	**2 or 3 of the following:** Hemoglobin <10 g/dL Platelet count <100,000/µL WBC <4,000 or ≥30,000/µL	Neither low nor high risk
Median survival	More than 10 yr	Less than 5 yr	5–10 yr

WBC = white blood cell count.

SUGGESTED READINGS

Campbell P, Green A: The myeloproliferative disorders. N Engl J Med 2006;355:2452–2466. *A clinical overview.*

Cervantes F: Modern management of myelofibrosis. Br J Haematol 2005;128: 583–592. *A comprehensive summary.*

Schafer AI: Molecular basis of the diagnosis and treatment of polycythemia vera and essential thrombocythemia. Blood 2006;107:4214–4222. *A comprehensive review.*

Tefferi A, Cortes J, Verstovsek S, et al: Lenalidomide therapy in myelofibrosis with myeloid metaplasia. Blood 2006;108:1158–1164. *Suggests efficacy in a subset of patients.*

Tefferi A, Huang J, Schwager S, et al: Validation and comparison of contemporary prognostic models in primary myelofibrosis: Analysis based on 334 patients from a single institution. Cancer 2007;109:2083–2088. *Hemoglobin level and platelet, leukocyte, and monocyte counts were predictive.*

Wolanskyj AP, Schwager SM, McClure RF, et al: Essential thrombocythemia beyond the first decade: Life expectancy, long-term complication rates, and prognostic factors. Mayo Clin Proc 2006;81:159–166. *Life expectancy is significantly reduced, and leukocytosis is an independent risk factor.*

178 APPROACH TO THE PATIENT WITH BLEEDING AND THROMBOSIS

Andrew I. Schafer

MECHANISMS OF HEMOSTASIS AND THROMBOSIS

The major components of coagulation are (1) platelets and (2) soluble plasma clotting factors (proteins) that generate fibrin. The coagulation system is normally maintained in a quiescent state by the actions of a continuous monolayer of endothelial cells that line the intimal surface of the vasculature throughout the circulatory tree. At a site of vascular damage, the antithrombotic properties of endothelium are lost, and thrombogenic constituents of the subendothelial vessel wall become exposed to circulating blood. The result is rapid formation of a hemostatic clot that consists of platelets and fibrin and is localized to the area of vascular injury. Activation of platelets and formation of fibrin occur essentially simultaneously and interdependently to effect hemostasis. Subsequently, vascular repair is accomplished by thrombolysis and recanalization of the occluded site.

Platelet activation at a site of vascular damage is initiated by the process of adhesion to the de-endothelialized intimal surface (platelet–vessel wall interaction). Platelet adhesion is mediated by von Willebrand's factor, which anchors circulating platelets to the vessel wall by binding to its platelet receptors located in membrane glycoprotein Ib. Adherent platelets undergo the "release reaction," during which they discharge constituents of their storage granules, including adenosine diphosphate (ADP), and synthesize thromboxane A_2 from arachidonic acid by means of the aspirin-inhibitable cyclooxygenase reaction. ADP, thromboxane A_2, and other components of the release reaction act in concert to recruit and activate additional platelets from the circulation to the site of vascular injury. These activated platelets expose binding sites for fibrinogen by forming the surface membrane glycoprotein IIb/IIIa complex. In the process of platelet aggregation (platelet–platelet interactions), fibrinogen

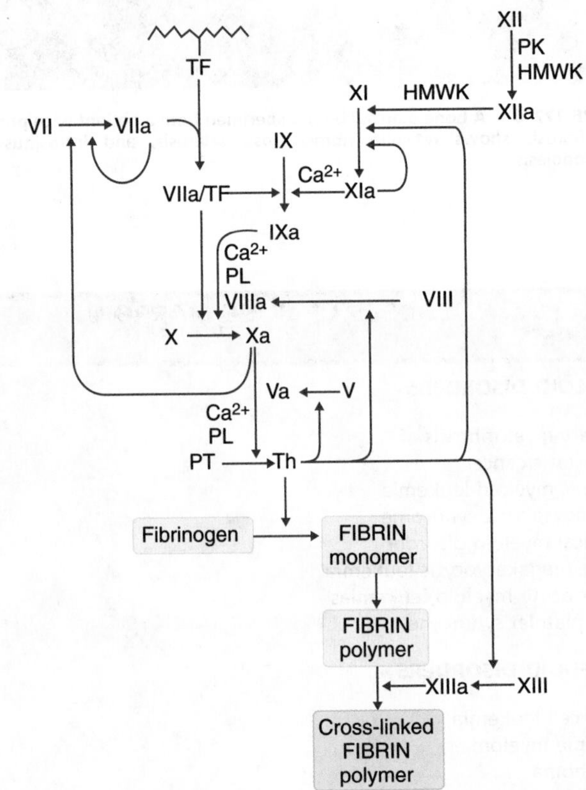

FIGURE 178–1 • The coagulation cascade. This scheme emphasizes understanding of (1) the importance of the tissue factor pathway in initiating clotting in vivo, (2) the interactions among pathways, and (3) the pivotal role of thrombin in sustaining the cascade by feedback activation of coagulation factors. HMWK = high-molecular-weight kininogen; PK = prekallikrein; PL = phospholipid; PT = prothrombin; TF = tissue factor; Th = thrombin. (From Schafer AI: Coagulation cascade: An overview. *In* Loscalzo J, Schafer AI [eds]: Thrombosis and Hemorrhage. Cambridge, MA, Blackwell Scientific Publications, 1994, pp 3–12.)

(or von Willebrand's factor under conditions of high shear stress) mediates the formation of an occlusive platelet plug.

Fibrin, which anchors the hemostatic platelet plug, is formed from soluble plasma fibrinogen by the action of the potent protease enzyme, thrombin (Fig. 178–1). The fibrin mesh is stabilized by covalent cross-linking mediated by factor XIII. Thrombin is formed from its inactive (zymogen) plasma precursor, prothrombin, by the action of activated factor X (Xa) and its cofactor, factor Va. This sequence of reactions classically has been referred to as the *common pathway* of coagulation. Factor X can be activated by either the tissue factor *(extrinsic) pathway* or the contact activation *(intrinsic) pathway* of coagulation. The former, which is now considered to be the major physiologic pathway of coagulation activation, is initiated by the complex of tissue factor and factor VIIa. The latter involves a series (or cascade) of zymogen–protease reactions that are initiated by factor XII, high-molecular-weight kininogen, and prekallikrein. Activated factor XII (XIIa) converts factor XI to XIa, which in turn activates factor IX to IXa. Factor IXa is the enzyme that converts factor X to Xa, a reaction that requires factor VIIIa as a cofactor.

Intact, normal endothelium promotes blood fluidity by inhibiting platelet activation. It likewise plays a crucial role in preventing fibrin accumulation. Among the physiologic antithrombotic systems that produce this latter effect are (1) antithrombin III, (2) protein C and protein S, (3) tissue factor pathway inhibitor (TFPI), and (4) the fibrinolytic system. Antithrombin is the major protease inhibitor of the coagulation system: it inactivates thrombin and other activated coagulation factors. Heparin functions as an anticoagulant by binding to antithrombin and greatly accelerating these reactions. Heparin and heparin sulfate proteoglycans are naturally present on endothelial cells, so antithrombin inactivation of thrombin and other coagulation proteases most likely occurs physiologically on vascular surfaces rather than in fluid plasma. Activated protein C, with its cofactor, protein S, functions as a natural anticoagulant by destroying factors Va and VIIIa, two essential cofactors of the coagulation cascade. Thrombin itself is the activator of protein C, and this reaction occurs rapidly only on the surfaces of intact vascular endothelial cells where thrombin binds to the glycosaminoglycan thrombomodulin. TFPI is a plasma protease inhibitor that specifically quenches tissue factor–induced coagulation. Finally, what little fibrin can be produced, despite these potent physiologic antithrombotic mechanisms, is digested rapidly by the endogenous fibrinolytic system. Fibrinolysis is mediated by the protease plasmin, which is generated from plasminogen in plasma by the action of endothelium-derived plasminogen activators.

EVALUATION OF THE PATIENT WITH A POSSIBLE BLEEDING DISORDER

History and Physical Examination

A thorough history is paramount in evaluating a patient for a possible systemic bleeding disorder. Not only should the patient be asked about spontaneous bleeding episodes in the past, but also responses to specific hemostatic challenges should be recorded. A bleeding tendency may be suspected if a patient previously experienced excessive hemorrhage after surgery or trauma, including commonly encountered events such as circumcision, tonsillectomy, labor and delivery, menses, dental procedures, vaccinations, and injections. Conversely, a history of normal blood clotting after specific challenges in the recent past is at least as important to note, because it may reflect a better test of systemic hemostasis than any laboratory measurement could provide.

In a patient with a history of excessive or unexplained bleeding, the initial problem is to determine whether the cause is a systemic coagulopathy or an anatomic or mechanical problem. This situation is encountered most frequently in patients with excessive postoperative bleeding. A history of prior bleeding suggests a coagulopathy, as does the finding of bleeding from multiple sites. However, even diffuse bleeding may arise from anatomic rather than hemostatic abnormalities (e.g., recurrent mucosal hemorrhage in patients with hereditary hemorrhagic telangiectasia). Conversely, a single episode of bleeding from an isolated site may be the initial manifestation of a systemic coagulopathy.

The history must include a survey of coexisting systemic diseases and drug ingestions that could affect hemostasis. Renal failure and the myeloproliferative disorders are associated with impaired platelet–vessel wall interactions and qualitative platelet abnormalities; connective tissue diseases and lymphomas are associated with thrombocytopenia; and liver disease causes a complex coagulopathy. Ingestion of aspirin and other nonsteroidal anti-inflammatory drugs (NSAIDs) that cause nonselective inhibition of cyclooxygenase leads to platelet dysfunction; these drugs often are contained in over-the-counter preparations that patients may neglect to report without specific questioning. Other drugs, such as antibiotics, also may be associated with a bleeding tendency by causing abnormal platelet function or thrombocytopenia. Finally, it is important to elicit a family history of bleeding problems. Although a positive history provides a clue to a possible inherited coagulopathy, a negative history does not exclude a familial cause; for example, 20% of patients with classic hemophilia have a completely negative family history of bleeding.

Patterns of clinical bleeding, as revealed by the history and physical examination, may be characteristic of certain types of coagulopathy (Table 178–1). In general, patients with thrombocytopenia or qualitative platelet or vascular disorders present with bleeding from superficial sites in the skin and mucous membranes; these may involve petechiae, which are pinpoint cutaneous hemorrhages that appear particularly over dependent extremities (characteristic of severe thrombocytopenia), ecchymoses (common bruises), purpura, gastrointestinal and genitourinary tract bleeding, epistaxis, and hemoptysis. In these disorders, bleeding from these sites tends to occur spontaneously or immediately after trauma. In contrast, patients with inherited or acquired coagulation factor deficiencies, such as hemophilia or therapeutic anticoagulation, tend to bleed from deeper tissue sites (e.g., hemarthroses, deep hematomas, retroperitoneal hemorrhage) and in a delayed manner after trauma.

Laboratory Testing

Four simple screening tests are used in the initial evaluation of patients with a suspected coagulopathy: (1) platelet count, (2) bleeding time, (3) prothrombin time (PT), and (4) activated partial thromboplastin time (aPTT). Thrombocytopenia, reported by electronic particle counting, should be verified by examination of the peripheral smear. Pseudothrombocytopenia, a laboratory artifact of ex vivo platelet clumping, may be caused by the ethylenediamine tetraacetic acid (EDTA) anticoagulant used in tubes for blood cell counts, by other anticoagulants, or by cold agglutinins acting at room temperature; it should be suspected whenever a very low platelet count is reported in a patient who does not exhibit any clinical bleeding. Pseudothrombocytopenia is indicated by the finding of platelet clumps on the peripheral smear, and the diagnosis is supported by the finding of simultaneously normal platelet counts in blood samples obtained by fingerstick, in tubes containing other anticoagulants, or in a tube maintained at 37° C before platelet counting. Examination of the blood smear in patients with thrombocytopenia also can reveal clues to the cause, such as fragmented red blood cells in thrombotic thrombocytopenic purpura.

The bleeding time has been a widely used clinical screening test for disorders of platelet–vessel wall interactions. It measures the time to cessation of bleeding after a standardized incision over the volar aspect of the forearm, now most commonly performed by disposable automated devices. The bleeding time is prolonged in thrombocytopenia, qualitative platelet abnormalities, defects in platelet–vessel wall interactions (e.g.,

TABLE 178–1 CHARACTERISTIC PATTERNS OF BLEEDING IN SYSTEMIC DISORDERS OF HEMOSTASIS

Type of Disorder	Sites of Bleeding: General	Skin	Mucous Membranes	Others	Onset of Bleeding	Clinical Examples
Platelet-vascular disorders	Superficial surfaces	Petechiae, ecchymoses	Common: oral, nasal, gastrointestinal, genitourinary	Rare	Spontaneous or immediately after trauma	Thrombocytopenia, functional platelet disorder, vascular fragility, disseminated intravascular coagulation, liver disease
Coagulation factor deficiency	Deep tissues	Hematomas	Rare	Common: joint, muscle, retroperitoneal	Delayed after trauma	Inherited coagulation factor deficiency, acquired inhibitor, anticoagulation, disseminated intravascular coagulation, liver disease

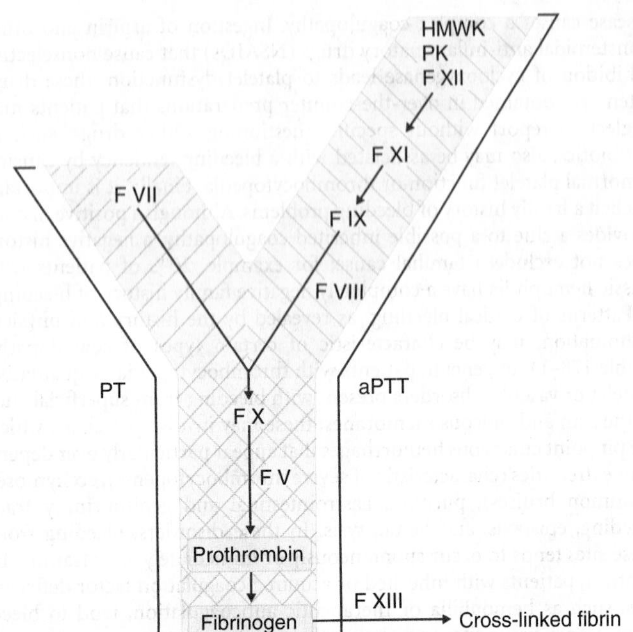

FIGURE 178–2 • The classic coagulation cascade. The prothrombin time (PT) measures the integrity of the extrinsic and common pathways, whereas the activated partial thromboplastin time (aPTT) measures the integrity of the intrinsic and common pathways. Factor (F) XIII deficiency is not detected by PT or aPTT. HMWK = high-molecular-weight kininogen; PK = prekallikrein.

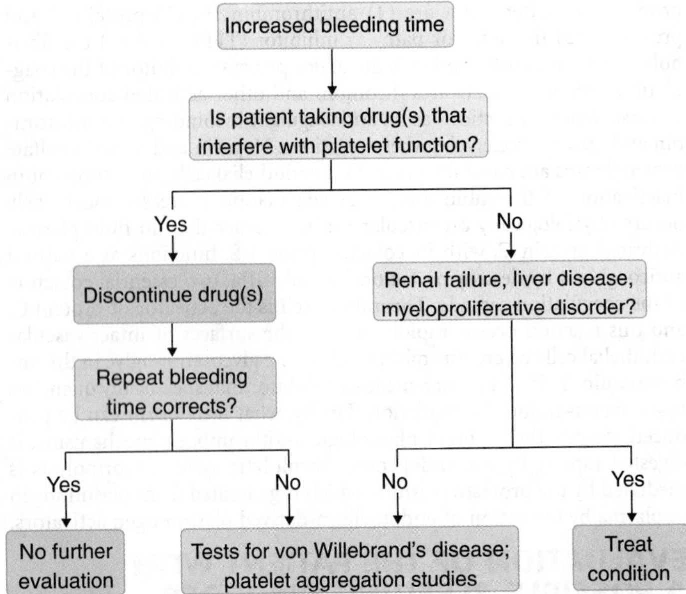

FIGURE 178–3 • Algorithm for diagnostic decisions in evaluating patients with a prolonged bleeding time (unless tests for von Willebrand's disease preceded the bleeding time). The scheme assumes that the platelet count is normal because thrombocytopenia itself can prolong the bleeding time.

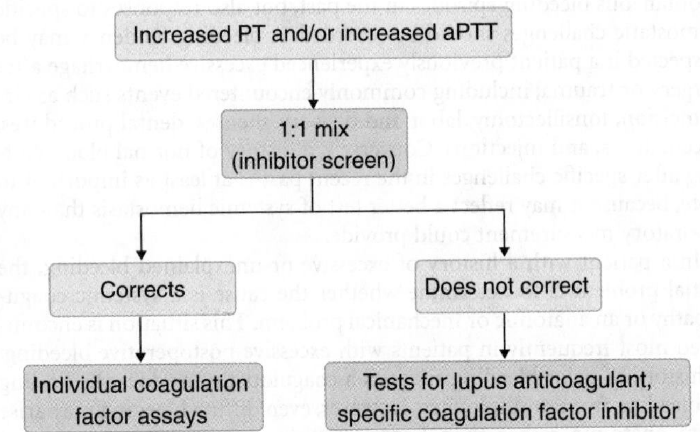

FIGURE 178–4 • Approach to evaluating patients with prolonged prothrombin time (PT) or activated partial thromboplastin time (aPTT).

von Willebrand's disease), and primary vascular disorders. The bleeding time usually is not prolonged in patients with coagulation factor deficiencies. The test is prone to problems of reproducibility, sensitivity, and specificity. Therefore, because von Willebrand's disease is the most common cause of abnormal platelet–vessel wall interactions, some experts now recommend replacing the bleeding time with specific tests for von Willebrand's disease in the initial evaluation of patients with a suspected coagulopathy (Chapter 180).

The PT measures the integrity of the extrinsic and common pathways of coagulation (factors VII, X, and V; prothrombin; and fibrinogen) (Fig. 178–2). The aPTT measures the integrity of the intrinsic and common pathways of coagulation (high-molecular-weight kininogen; prekallikrein; factors XII, XI, IX, VIII, X, and V; prothrombin; and fibrinogen). The sensitivity of the PT and aPTT in detecting coagulation factor deficiencies may vary with the reagents used to perform these tests, and each laboratory must determine its own reference standards.

With a few notable exceptions, as follows, normal results for all four of the screening tests of hemostasis essentially exclude any clinically significant systemic coagulopathy. Patients with factor XIII deficiency may have a serious bleeding diathesis but normal screening tests; specific tests for factor XIII deficiency should be performed if this disease is suspected. The PT and aPTT detect only the more severe deficiencies of coagulation factors, usually at levels of less than 30% of normal; specific factor levels should be determined if a mild coagulation factor deficiency is suspected. Patients with von Willebrand's disease sometimes have normal bleeding times and usually do not have sufficiently reduced levels of factor VIII to affect the aPTT. Rare disorders of fibrinolysis also may be associated with normal screening tests, necessitating more specialized tests when indicated. Abnormalities in the screening tests of hemostasis may be pursued by more specialized tests to establish a specific diagnosis (Chapters 179 through 182).

A prolonged bleeding time in the absence of thrombocytopenia initially should be approached by determining whether the patient is taking any drugs that might interfere with platelet function (e.g., aspirin, other NSAIDs) or has a coexisting disease that might explain the finding (e.g., renal failure) (Fig. 178–3). If these conditions are not found or if the bleeding time fails to correct after discontinuation of any potentially offending drugs, further specialized testing may include platelet aggregation studies to identify specific qualitative abnormalities of platelet function and specific assays to exclude one of the types of von Willebrand's disease.

The finding of a prolonged PT and/or aPTT indicates either a deficiency of one or more coagulation factors or the presence of an inhibitor, usually an antibody, directed at one or more components of the coagulation system (Fig. 178–4). These two possibilities can be distinguished by performing an inhibitor screen, which involves a 1:1 mix of the patient's plasma and normal plasma. The premise of the test is that even if a patient's plasma is completely deficient (0% level) in a certain factor, mixing it 1:1 with normal plasma (100% level) should bring the concentration of the factor to 50% in the mixture; as noted earlier, this is sufficient to correct the prolonged PT or aPTT. If correction occurs with the inhibitor screen, individual coagulation factor levels should be assayed for a specific deficiency state. If the 1:1 mix fails to correct the prolonged PT and/or aPTT, an inhibitor is likely to be present and interfering with coagulation in both the patient's and the normal plasma. Specific assays should be then performed to determine whether there is a true inhibitor against a coagulation factor (e.g., factor VIII antibody) or whether the inhibitor is a lupus anticoagulant.

EVALUATION OF THE ASYMPTOMATIC PATIENT WITH ABNORMAL COAGULATION TESTS

In asymptomatic individuals who are discovered incidentally to have abnormalities in screening laboratory tests of hemostasis, the first critical question is whether the findings are clinically relevant. Patients with inherited deficiencies of one of the contact activation coagulation factors (factor XII, high-molecular-weight kininogen, prekallikrein) characteristically have a markedly prolonged aPTT, yet they do not have a clinical bleeding tendency. Likewise, patients with lupus anticoagulants typically have prolongation of the aPTT and sometimes the PT; they more often have thrombotic rather than bleeding complications. In patients with heparin-induced thrombocytopenia, a marked decrease in the platelet count sometimes is associated with arterial and venous thrombosis. It is crucial to view the clinical setting, history, physical examination, and screening laboratory tests as complementary facets of the approach to patients with suspected coagulopathies.

EVALUATION OF THE PREOPERATIVE PATIENT

Routine screening of all preoperative patients with a platelet count, bleeding time, PT, and aPTT is not only uninformative but may be counterproductive if follow-up testing causes unnecessary expense and delays in surgery (Chapter 457). Preoperative bleeding time, PT, and aPTT do not predict surgical bleeding risk in patients who are not found to be at increased risk on clinical grounds, so a thorough clinical assessment should guide the need for obtaining these preoperative screening tests. Laboratory testing and possibly further specialized tests of coagulation are indicated for patients whose bleeding histories are suspicious for a hemostatic abnormality. Preoperative screening tests of coagulation probably also are warranted for patients who cannot cooperate with an adequate clinical assessment and for those who are to undergo procedures in which even minimal postoperative hemorrhage could be hazardous.

EVALUATION OF THE PATIENT WITH A POSSIBLE HYPERCOAGULABLE STATE

Many (possibly most) patients with venous thromboembolism have an inherited basis for hypercoagulability (Chapter 182). Most patients with inherited hypercoagulable states (or thrombophilia) present with their initial episode of venous thromboembolism in early adulthood, but thrombotic manifestations may begin at any time from early childhood to old age. Patients typically have deep vein thrombosis of the lower extremities or pulmonary embolism, but other unusual sites of venous thrombosis may be involved. Arterial thrombosis is unusual in patients with inherited hypercoagulable states. Arterial thrombosis that occurs prematurely or in the absence of apparent risk factors should trigger a different line of investigation, possibly including evaluation for vasculitis, myeloproliferative disorders, hyperhomocysteinemia, antiphospholipid syndrome, and potential sources of systemic embolization.

The primary or hereditary hypercoagulable states (see Table 182–1) result from specific mutations or polymorphisms that lead to decreased levels of physiologic antithrombotic proteins or increased levels of procoagulant proteins. The hereditary form of heterozygous hyperhomocysteinemia, which often manifests in adulthood with venous or arterial thrombosis, is caused by discrete mutations in the enzymes that mediate homocysteine metabolism. In contrast, the secondary or acquired hypercoagulable states (see Fig. 182–2) are a heterogeneous group of disorders that predispose to thrombosis by complex mechanisms. Venous thrombosis often is precipitated by the combination of a hypercoagulable genotype and an acquired prothrombotic, hypercoagulable state, such as pregnancy, immobilization, or the postoperative state. Certain clinical characteristics suggest the presence of an inherited hypercoagulable state (Table 178–2). Patients with recurrent thrombosis should be tested for these disorders and, in most cases, committed to lifelong prophylactic anticoagulation. It is not clear whether it is essential to order these tests after a single episode of venous thromboembolism. Even if not maintained on long-term anticoagulation, patients with diagnosed primary hypercoagulable states should receive prophylactic anticoagulation during situations that pose a high risk for thrombosis, such as the peripartum period. There is no simple screening test for primary hypercoagulable states, and the timing of obtaining these tests is crucial to avoid erroneous diagnoses. Acute thrombosis itself can cause transient decreases in the levels of antithrombin, protein C, and protein S. Heparin therapy can cause a decrease in plasma antithrombin activity. Warfarin therapy lowers the functional levels of protein C and protein S. Inherited deficiency states can be diagnosed spuriously under these conditions.

Patients who present with venous thromboembolism probably have an increased risk of harboring an occult malignancy (Chapter 189). This association is increased further in patients who have recurrent and idiopathic thrombosis. Evaluation for occult malignancy in these patients need not be exhaustive, however. It can be limited to a thorough history, physical examination, routine complete blood cell count and chemistries, test of fecal occult blood, urinalysis, mammogram (in women), and chest radiograph; further testing should be guided by any abnormalities found in this initial evaluation.

In addition to classic deep vein thrombosis and pulmonary embolism, certain characteristic types of thrombosis may provide important clues to the etiology and trigger specific evaluation. Migratory, superficial thrombophlebitis (Trousseau's syndrome) or nonbacterial thrombotic endocarditis suggests the presence of an occult malignancy (Chapter 189). Hepatic vein thrombosis (Budd-Chiari syndrome; Chapter 146) or portal vein thrombosis may indicate a myeloproliferative disorder (Chapter 177) or paroxysmal nocturnal hemoglobinuria (Chapter 164). Warfarin-induced skin necrosis strongly suggests an underlying protein C or protein S deficiency. Recurrent, spontaneous miscarriages are associated with the antiphospholipid syndrome (Chapter 259).

TABLE 178–2 CLINICAL CHARACTERISTICS OF PATIENTS WITH INHERITED HYPERCOAGULABLE STATES

Venous thromboembolism (>90% of cases)
Deep vein thrombosis of lower limbs (common)
Pulmonary embolism (common)
Superficial thrombophlebitis
Mesenteric vein thrombosis (rare but characteristic)
Cerebral vein thrombosis (rare but characteristic)
Frequent family history of thrombosis*
First thrombosis usually at young age (<40 yr)*
Frequent recurrences*
Neonatal purpura fulminans (homozygous protein C and protein S deficiency)

*All of these features are less evident in patients with activated protein C resistance, who appear to be less severely affected clinically.
From De Stefano V, Finazzi G, Manucci PM: Inherited thrombophilia: Pathogenesis, clinical syndromes, and management. Blood 1996;87:3531–3544.

SUGGESTED READINGS

Key NS: Inhibitors in congenital coagulation disorders. Br J Haematol 2004;127:379–391. *Comprehensive review of the immunobiology, laboratory evaluation, and management in patients with coagulation factor inhibitors.*

Mathew P: Current opinion on inhibitor treatment options. Semin Hematol 2006;43(2 Suppl 4):S8–13. *A clinical review.*

Pruthi RK: A practical approach to genetic testing for von Willebrand disease. Mayo Clin Proc 2006;81:679–691. *A guide to judicious use of genetic testing.*

Tripodi A: A review of the clinical and diagnostic utility of laboratory tests for the detection of congenital thrombophilia. Semin Thromb Hemost 2005;31:25–32. *How laboratory testing for inherited hypercoagulable states should be linked to treatment and prevention.*

179 HEMORRHAGIC DISORDERS: ABNORMALITIES OF PLATELET AND VASCULAR FUNCTION

Robert McMillan

Definition

Hemostasis, which is the body's response to vascular damage, includes several sequential processes: adhesion of platelets to the site of injury, platelet activation and aggregation, formation of a platelet plug, and development of a localized clot (Fig. 179–1). Maintaining a balance between normal blood flow and the need to form thrombi only when

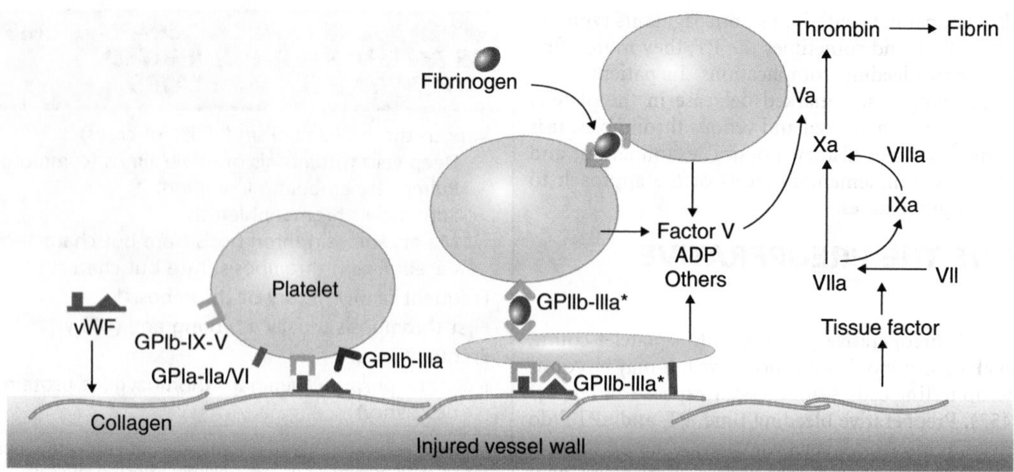

FIGURE 179–1 • Hemostasis. The resting platelet has several surface glycoprotein complexes, including GPIb-IX-V, GPIIb-IIIa, and GPIa-IIa/VI. After vascular injury, the extracellular matrix is exposed, and platelets are temporarily tethered to collagen-bound von Willebrand factor (vWF) via the platelet surface glycoprotein GPIb-IX-V complex. This reaction, as well as exposure of platelets to collagen and subsequently thrombin, activates platelets, thereby resulting in (1) conversion of the platelet surface GPIIb-IIIa complex into its active conformation (GPIIb-IIIa*) and causing irreversible binding of platelets to vWF; (2) secretion of a variety of factors from the platelet granules, including adenosine diphosphate (ADP; causing further activation) and factor V, which is converted to the active form Va, which then binds to the platelet's surface and serves as a reaction site for coagulation); and (3) recruitment of additional platelets to the site of injury via fibrinogen bridging between the activated GPIIb-IIIa complexes on adjacent platelets to form a platelet plug. Simultaneously, tissue factor released from the site of injury activates factor VII to VIIa, which with the aid of factors IXa and VIIIa, converts factor X to Xa, thereby resulting in the production of thrombin and the formation of fibrin, which stabilizes the platelet plug.

necessary requires tightly controlled collaboration among platelets, the coagulation system, and the endothelial surface of blood vessels.

Pathobiology

The physiologic trigger for hemostasis after vascular injury is loss of the endothelial cell barrier that separates flowing blood from the extracellular matrix. The platelet response to vascular injury can be arbitrarily divided into three closely integrated phases: adhesion, activation, and aggregation. The initial step in platelet adhesion is binding of the platelet surface receptor glycoprotein (GP) Ib-IX-V to von Willebrand factor (vWF). Although some vWF is normally present in the subendothelial space, the majority is due to binding of circulating plasma vWF to one of the subendothelial collagens, usually type I or III, after the injury. This initial interaction between GPIb-IX-V and vWF is transient and reversible. Platelets are temporarily tethered but can move slowly along the damaged vascular surface and are eventually released unless platelet activation occurs. Other interactions may also contribute to the adhesion process (e.g., binding of the platelet collagen receptor GPIa-IIa/GPVI to subendothelial collagen fibrils), but only under low-shear situations that might be seen in areas of slow blood flow, such as in capillaries.

Subsequent platelet plug formation depends on platelet activation, which may be due to a variety of stimuli, including the adhesion interaction between vWF and platelet GPIb-IX-V, agonists released from platelets on activation (adenosine diphosphate [ADP], epinephrine), thrombin produced during coagulation, or factors exposed or generated at the site of vascular injury (collagen, thromboxane A_2). Platelet activation converts the platelet surface GPIIb-IIIa complex from an inactive to an active conformation, thereby resulting in irreversible platelet adhesion to collagen-bound plasma vWF and recruitment of additional platelets to the site of injury by aggregation via fibrinogen bridging between GPIIb-IIIa complexes on adjacent platelets.

Concurrently, tissue factor from the site of injury triggers the coagulation system and results in the formation of factor Xa, and activated platelets release factor V, which binds to anionic lipids on the platelet surface and is activated to factor Va. The factor Va on the platelet surface provides an assembly site for the prothrombinase complex (factor Xa and prothrombin), thereby allowing efficient generation of local thrombin and the formation of fibrin at the site of the vascular injury.

Control mechanisms to limit thrombosis to the site of injury include modulators of platelet and vascular reactivity (nitric oxide, prostacyclin) and coagulation inhibitors (antithrombin III, protein C and protein S, tissue factor pathway inhibitor). In addition, procoagulants are diluted and removed from the site of injury by flowing blood, and activated coagulation factors are removed by the reticuloendothelial system. Eventually, the process of fibrinolysis removes the fibrin clot.

Platelets

Platelet Production and Kinetics

Platelets are small, anucleated blood cells whose primary function is to "survey" the integrity of the vascular system. They are produced in the bone marrow from megakaryocytes, which are large, polyploid cells derived from hematopoietic stem cells under the control of a variety of stimulators, most notably thrombopoietin (Chapter 160). After stem cells commit to the megakaryocyte lineage, they become progressively larger through a series of endomitotic divisions that result in cellular chromosomal content ranging from 2n to 64n and form cytoplasmic demarcation membranes. Two types of cytoplasmic storage granules also develop in these cells and release their contents during platelet activation: (1) α-granules, which contain adhesive proteins (fibrinogen, fibronectin, thrombospondin, and vWF), procoagulants (factor V, platelet factor 4 [PF4]), growth factors, adhesion proteins (P-selectin), and enzymes (plasminogen), and (2) dense granules, which contain ADP, adenosine triphosphate (ATP), serotonin, and other factors. Fully mature megakaryocytes develop cytoplasmic extensions through the endothelial barrier into the sinusoidal lumen of the bone marrow, where the platelets are released into the circulation.

Thrombopoietin is the most important platelet growth factor, although stem cell factor, interleukin-3 (IL-3), IL-6, and IL-11 also contribute. Thrombopoietin is produced primarily in the liver and binds to the c-mpl receptor, which is present on both megakaryocytes and platelets. The production of thrombopoietin is thought to remain relatively constant, whereas the quantity of unbound thrombopoietin, available to stimulate platelet production, increases as the number of megakaryocytes and platelets diminish and decreases as they increase. Bone marrow responds to a need for more platelets in two ways: committing a larger number of stem cells to the megakaryocytic lineage and increasing the average number of endomitotic cycles per megakaryocyte so that they become larger. It is estimated that each megakaryocyte produces 1000 to 3000 platelets, depending on its size.

The normal platelet lifespan ranges from 7 to 10 days, and about a third of the circulating platelets are present in the spleen in a freely exchangeable pool. In patients with splenomegaly, up to 90% of the platelets may be in the splenic pool, thereby resulting in peripheral thrombocytopenia despite a normal total platelet mass. The near linear decline of radiolabeled platelets in normal individuals suggests that most platelets are removed from the blood stream by senescence rather than by utilization. In individuals with thrombocytopenia secondary to decreased platelet production, the elimination profile is curvilinear, thus indicating that a minimum number of platelets, estimated at about 7000/μL, is needed to maintain vascular integrity.

Platelet-associated bleeding symptoms can arise from either decreased platelet numbers (thrombocytopenia) or qualitative platelet abnormalities, which may be inherited or acquired. Less commonly, pathologic thrombosis can occur as a result of uncontrolled activation of platelets.

THROMBOCYTOPENIA

Thrombocytopenia may be due to either increased platelet destruction or utilization, abnormal platelet distribution (an enlarged splenic pool), or decreased platelet production (Table 179–1). Assuming normal platelet function, the symptoms and signs expected with various platelet counts are as follows: greater than 50,000/μL, no symptoms or signs, although patients may bleed longer with major trauma; 25,000 to 50,000/μL, petechiae and bruising with minor trauma; 10,000 to 25,000/μL, spontaneous petechiae and bruising greater on the lower extremities and menorrhagia; less than 10,000/μL, prominent bruising, mucosal bleeding (epistaxis, gum bleeding, gastrointestinal [GI] or genitourinary [GU] bleeding), and a risk for central nervous system (CNS) bleeding.

Patients with thrombocytopenia generally have a history of easy bruising and varying degrees of mucosal bleeding (e.g., gum bleeding, epistaxis, GU or GI bleeding), depending on the severity of the thrombocytopenia; CNS bleeding is rare but often lethal. Deep muscular bleeding, hemarthroses, or retroperitoneal bleeding suggests a coagulation factor disorder (Chapter 180). Special attention should be directed to the onset, duration, and severity of bleeding symptoms because this information will help direct subsequent therapy. The patient should specifically be asked about a history of anemia; recent infection or transfusion of blood products; and possible exposure to human immunodeficiency virus (HIV), hepatitis, or drugs associated with thrombocytopenia, particularly quinine, quinidine, sulfa drugs, and heparin. Onset at a young age or a family history of thrombocytopenia suggests congenital or inherited thrombocytopenia. Thrombocytopenia in a patient in an intensive care unit is commonly due to either bacterial sepsis or heparin-induced thrombocytopenia (HIT). Physical findings of fever, adenopathy, or splenomegaly suggest infection, collagen vascular disease, or a primary hematologic or oncologic illness.

All patients should have a complete blood count (CBC), and the peripheral blood smear (Chapter 161) should be carefully examined for other cytopenias, abnormal white blood cells, cellular inclusions, schistocytes or nucleated red cells, abnormally large or small platelets, or aggregated platelets. The latter finding suggests pseudothrombocytopenia, which most commonly is due to ethylenediaminetetraacetic acid (EDTA)-dependent platelet antibodies and can be diagnosed by repeating the platelet count with citrate or ammonium oxalate as the anticoagulant instead of EDTA. Other studies that may be indicated, depending on the clinical findings and the CBC, include antinuclear antibody, HIV or hepatitis studies, cultures, coagulation studies, and bone marrow aspiration and biopsy. A bleeding time and platelet aggregation studies are helpful in evaluating patients suspected of having qualitative platelet defects.

TABLE 179–1 CAUSES OF THROMBOCYTOPENIA

INCREASED PLATELET DESTRUCTION OR UTILIZATION
Immune destruction
Autoantibodies: ITP, disease-associated IT (collagen disease, lymphoproliferative disorders)
Alloantibodies: post-transfusion purpura, neonatal purpura
Drug-induced IT: quinidine, quinine, sulfonamides, gold, etc.
Acute ITP
Infection—HIV, hepatitis, cytomegalovirus, Epstein-Barr virus
Nonimmune destruction or platelet removal
Infection (bacterial, viral, malarial)
Thrombotic thrombocytopenic purpura/hemolytic-uremic syndrome
Disseminated intravascular coagulation
Hemangiomas
Platelet loss (massive bleeding)
Platelet redistribution (enlarged splenic pool)
Congestive splenomegaly
Other (non-Hodgkin's lymphoma, Gaucher's disease, etc.)
DECREASED PLATELET PRODUCTION
Myeloproliferative disorders (acute or chronic leukemias, multiple myeloma, myelofibrosis)
Lymphoproliferative disorders (non-Hodgkin's lymphoma, CLL)
Aplasia or hypoplasia (idiopathic, drug induced, radiation)
Ineffective hematopoiesis (myelodysplasia, vitamin B_{12} or folate deficiency)
Myelophthisis (prostate, lung, breast, gastrointestinal cancers)
Drugs (chemotherapy, thiazides, alcohol, etc.)
Congenital/hereditary disorders

CLL = chronic lymphocytic leukemia; HIV = human immunodeficiency virus; IT = immune thrombocytopenia; ITP = immune thrombocytopenic purpura.

Immune Thrombocytopenias

Chronic Immune Thrombocytopenic Purpura

Definition

Chronic immune thrombocytopenic purpura (ITP) is an autoimmune disorder manifested by immune-mediated thrombocytopenia. The diagnosis is one of exclusion and is based on American Society of Hematology guidelines (Table 179–2).

Pathobiology

The primary disturbance leading to an immune response against platelet autoantigens is unknown. T and B lymphocytes, reactive with platelet autoantigens, have been detected in the blood and spleen of patients with ITP, and autoantibody production by cells from the spleen, blood, and bone marrow has been shown. There is skewed cytokine production compatible with the activation of T-helper (T_H) T_H0/T_H1 cells (increased IL-2 and interferon-γ with reduced IL-10), and a reduced T_H2 response has been described. Antibody-coated platelets may be destroyed by either phagocytosis or complement-induced lysis. Platelet survival studies show reduced intravascular survival, but either normal or reduced platelet turnover has been demonstrated in about 75% of patients with ITP, thus suggesting either inhibition of platelet production or intramedullary platelet destruction. In vitro studies showing reduced production and maturation of megakaryocytes in the presence of ITP plasma provide evidence for autoantibody-induced suppression of megakaryocytopoiesis. Cytotoxic T lymphocyte–induced platelet lysis may also play a role in pathogenesis.

TABLE 179–2 AMERICAN SOCIETY OF HEMATOLOGY CRITERIA FOR THE DIAGNOSIS OF CHRONIC IMMUNE THROMBOCYTOPENIC PURPURA: DIAGNOSIS OF EXCLUSION

History compatible with the diagnosis of chronic ITP
Normal physical examination findings except for signs of thrombocytopenia (petechiae, purpura, or mucosal bleeding); no adenopathy or splenomegaly
Complete blood count showing isolated thrombocytopenia with large platelets but no anemia unless bleeding or immune hemolysis is present
Bone marrow examination showing normal or increased numbers of megakaryocytes (not required for diagnosis unless unusual manifestation or age >60 yr)
No clinical or laboratory evidence for other causes of thrombocytopenia

Helicobacter pylori Infection

Studies from Italy and Japan report an increased incidence of *H. pylori* infection in patients with ITP and partial or complete remission in many patients after its eradication. A prospective study in the United States showed neither an increased incidence of ITP with *H. pylori* nor a platelet response after its treatment. At present, no definitive recommendation can be made about whether routine *H. pylori* testing or treatment, or both, are indicated in ITP.

Clinical Manifestations

On initial evaluation, patients may be asymptomatic, with moderate thrombocytopenia discovered during a routine blood count. More commonly, patients note increasing petechiae and ecchymoses. In more severe cases there is evidence of mucosal bleeding (epistaxis, gum bleeding, GI or GU bleeding), and CNS bleeding may develop in the most severely affected, usually with platelet counts below 5000/µL. Lymphadenopathy or splenomegaly suggests another diagnosis.

Diagnosis

The diagnosis is one of exclusion (see Table 179–2). The symptoms and physical examination findings reflect the degree of thrombocytopenia (petechiae, purpura, or mucosal bleeding), and other causes of thrombocytopenia must be excluded. A careful history is important to exclude drugs that cause thrombocytopenia, familial thrombocytopenia, post-transfusion purpura, or disorders associated with secondary immune thrombocytopenia. The CBC is normal except for thrombocytopenia, although anemia can be seen if excessive bleeding or associated autoimmune hemolytic anemia (Evans syndrome, Chapter 164) has occurred. The peripheral blood smear is normal except for a decreased number of platelets, many of which are enlarged. Bone marrow examination is not required for diagnosis if the findings are typical, although it is recommended in patients whose clinical or CBC findings suggest another disorder or in patients older than 60 years to exclude myelodysplasia; when performed, it shows normal or increased numbers of megakaryocytes and is otherwise normal.

The utility of measuring antiplatelet antibodies remains controversial. With the use of antigen-specific assays, autoantibodies against one or more platelet surface glycoproteins, including GPIIb-IIIa, GPIb-IX, and GPIa-IIa, can be detected with a sensitivity of 49 to 66% and a specificity of 78 to 93% when patients with ITP are compared with healthy subjects or patients with nonimmune thrombocytopenia. A positive antigen-specific assay provides strong evidence for the diagnosis of ITP, but a negative assay does not exclude it. The frequency of a positive assay and the degree of positivity increase with increasing severity of the disease. Unfortunately, antigen-specific assays are not readily available and, though helpful in the diagnosis, are not necessary. Platelet-associated immunoglobulin assays lack specificity and cannot be recommended.

Differential Diagnosis

Because an ITP-like syndrome can be seen in patients with HIV or hepatitis C infection, appropriate testing is indicated in at-risk individuals. Secondary ITP may be induced by drugs or occur in patients with collagen vascular disease (Chapters 285 and 287), lymphoproliferative disorders (Chapters 196 and 197), immune thyroid disease (Chapter 244), or common variable hypogammaglobulinemia (Chapter 271). The presence of these disorders is usually suggested by a careful history, physical examination, and CBC findings; the diagnosis can be confirmed by appropriate laboratory and radiologic studies.

Treatment

Treatment includes two phases, emergency therapy and long-term therapy, but oftentimes both treatments must be used concurrently. Table 179–3 lists the treatments used for ITP with doses, expected response times, and common side effects; Figure 179–2 shows a treatment algorithm.

TABLE 179–3 TREATMENTS USED FOR ADULT CHRONIC IMMUNE THROMBOCYTOPENIC PURPURA

Therapy	Dose	Response Time	Common Side Effects
IVIG	1 g/kg IV qd × 2–3 days	5–7 days	Headache, aseptic meningitis, fluid overload
Anti-D	50–75 µg/kg IV	5–7 days	Infusional symptoms: fever, chills, hemolysis, renal failure, DIC
Prednisone	1.0 mg/kg PO qd	1–4 weeks	Hypokalemia, gastric upset, sodium and fluid retention, hyperglycemia, hypertension, myopathy, osteoporosis, infection risk, psychosis
Dexamethasone	40 mg PO qd × 4 days q4wk	1–4 weeks	Same as for prednisone
Splenectomy	—	1–3 weeks	Usual postoperative complications, overwhelming bacterial sepsis (rare)
Rituximab	375 mg/m² IV qwk × 4	3–4 weeks	Infusional symptoms: fever, chills, headache, bronchospasm. Severe B cell reduction and potential for infection
Danazol	200 mg PO qid	3–6 months	Fluid retention, seborrhea, hirsutism, amenorrhea, acne, headache, liver toxicity, thrombocytopenia
Colchicine	0.6 mg PO bid	4–8 weeks	Diarrhea (may limit therapy), nausea, vomiting
Dapsone	75–100 mg PO qd	4–8 weeks	Hemolysis, agranulocytosis, aplastic anemia, exfoliative dermatitis, toxic hepatitis, cholestatic jaundice, peripheral neuropathy
Cyclophosphamide	150 mg PO qd	6–8 weeks	Cytopenias, hemorrhagic cystitis, GI symptoms, sterility, secondary malignancies*
Azathioprine	150 mg PO qd	2–10 months	Cytopenias, GI symptoms, secondary malignancies*
Cyclosporine	1.25–2.5 mg/kg PO bid	Variable	Renal insufficiency, hepatotoxicity, hypertension, tremor, hirsutism, gum hyperplasia, hypomagnesemia, secondary malignancies*
Mycophenolate mofetil	0.5–1.0 g PO bid	3–4 weeks	Diarrhea, leukopenia, headache, secondary malignancies*
High-dose cyclophosphamide	1.0–1.5 g/m² IV q4wk	1–4 weeks	Cytopenias, hemorrhagic cystitis, GI symptoms, alopecia, sterility, myocardiopathy, secondary malignancies*
Combination chemotherapy	See below†	1–4 weeks	Cytopenias, hemorrhagic cystitis, alopecia, dermatitis, anaphylaxis, GI symptoms, sterility, myocardiopathy, mucositis, secondary malignancies*

*Lymphoproliferative disorders or acute leukemia has occurred in patients with other disorders who were receiving these drugs.
†Several combinations have been used.
DIC = disseminated intravascular coagulation; GI = gastrointestinal; IVIG = intravenous immune globulin.

Section XIV Hematology

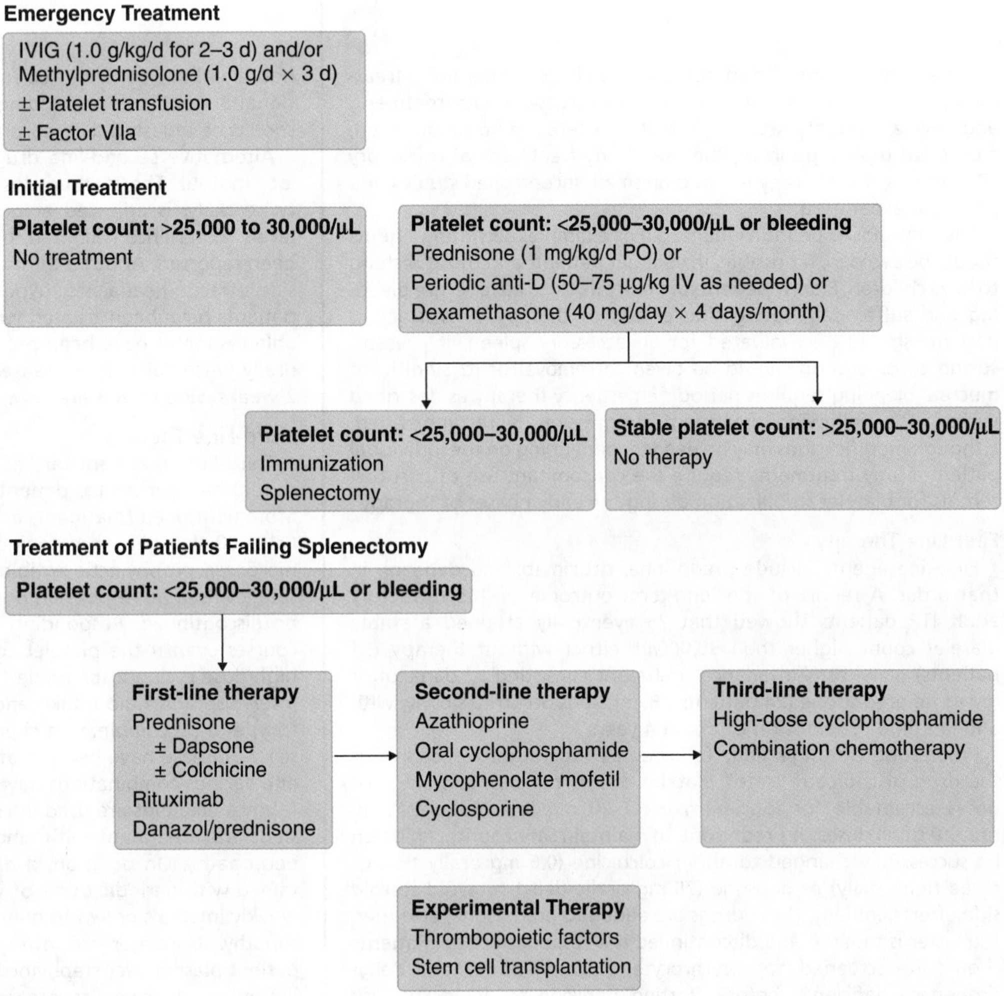

Emergency Treatment

IVIG (1.0 g/kg/d for 2–3 d) and/or Methylprednisolone (1.0 g/d × 3 d)
± Platelet transfusion
± Factor VIIa

Initial Treatment

Platelet count: >25,000 to 30,000/μL
No treatment

Platelet count: <25,000–30,000/μL or bleeding
Prednisone (1 mg/kg/d PO) or
Periodic anti-D (50–75 μg/kg IV as needed) or
Dexamethasone (40 mg/day × 4 days/month)

Platelet count: <25,000–30,000/μL
Immunization
Splenectomy

Stable platelet count: >25,000–30,000/μL
No therapy

Treatment of Patients Failing Splenectomy

Platelet count: <25,000–30,000/μL or bleeding

First-line therapy
Prednisone
± Dapsone
± Colchicine
Rituximab
Danazol/prednisone

Second-line therapy
Azathioprine
Oral cyclophosphamide
Mycophenolate mofetil
Cyclosporine

Third-line therapy
High-dose cyclophosphamide
Combination chemotherapy

Experimental Therapy
Thrombopoietic factors
Stem cell transplantation

FIGURE 179–2 • Treatment of adult chronic immune thrombocytopenic purpura. IVIG = intravenous immune globulin.

Section XIV Hematology

Rx

Emergency Treatment

Hospitalization should be strongly considered in patients with significant mucosal bleeding or extremely low platelet counts (<5000/μL). Treatment should be started immediately. A rapid, though temporary increase in the platelet count can usually be achieved with one of the following: intravenous gamma globulin (IVIG, 1.0 g/kg/day intravenously [IV] for 2 to 3 days); methylprednisolone (1.0 g/day IV for 3 days), or a combination of both. Platelet transfusions are indicated in all patients who are actively bleeding. Recombinant factor VIIa (35 to 100 μg/kg IV) has been reported as useful in unresponsive patients with uncontrolled bleeding.

Long-Term Treatment

Initial Therapy

On diagnosis, patients with platelet counts less than 25,000 to 30,000/μL should be treated with the aim of obtaining a stable, safe platelet count (>25,000 to 30,000/μL) off treatment. Recent evidence shows that if the platelet count can be supported at this level for a period of months, some adult patients with ITP will achieve a stable remission without splenectomy. Prednisone (1 mg/kg/day) should be administered, and if a response occurs, the dose should be slowly tapered with the aim of maintaining safe platelet counts at doses causing tolerable side effects (<10 to 15 mg/day). Some physicians prefer pulsed dexamethasone (40 mg/day on 4 days per month for four to six courses) as an alternative to prednisone. In Rh^+ patients who either do not respond to corticosteroids or cannot be tapered to safe doses, anti-D (50 to 75 μg/kg IV) should be given whenever the platelet count falls below 25,000 to 30,000/μL. Treatment with corticosteroids or anti-D should be continued for up to 6 to 12 months if possible, with the aim of eventually discontinuing treatment. Failure to show any response to corticosteroids, anti-D, or IVIG should prompt reconsideration of the diagnosis, and bone marrow examination should be performed if not previously done.

Splenectomy is indicated if (1) safe platelet counts cannot be achieved, (2) a stable remission with safe platelet counts while off therapy has not occurred in 6 to 12 months, (3) drug toxicity is severe, or (4) this treatment approach becomes too burdensome for the patient. If splenectomy is indicated, pneumococcal, *Haemophilus influenzae,* and meningococcal immunizations are advised at least 2 weeks before surgery. If possible, the platelet count should be boosted before surgery with either IVIG, anti-D, or corticosteroids. Prophylactic platelet transfusions are not indicated, although platelets should be available at the time of surgery. About 75 to 85% of patients respond initially to splenectomy; of these, 10 to 20% relapse over the next 5 to 10 years. Laparoscopic and conventional transabdominal approaches give comparable results, although the former hastens recovery. In view of the small, but finite risk for overwhelming sepsis after splenectomy, febrile illnesses demand careful evaluation, and prophylactic antibiotics should be given for any illness with a temperature of 101° F or higher until sepsis can be ruled out.

Treatment of Patients Refractory to Splenectomy

Refractory patients are defined as those who have undergone splenectomy but have postoperative thrombocytopenia that requires additional treatment. In general, sedentary patients with stable platelet counts greater than 25,000 to 30,000/μL require no treatment, but patients with an active lifestyle may require higher counts. Treatment is necessary for those with lower platelet counts or active bleeding.

Rx

Refractory patients often respond slowly to subsequent treatment, have significant morbidity from the disease and its treatment, and have a mortality rate of 10 to 16%. There are no randomized, controlled trials supporting the use of any treatment of refractory ITP patients, and therapy is based on small uncontrolled studies and physician experience.

Therapy should be individualized. For example, alkylating agents should be avoided, if possible, in younger patients and those wishing to have children. Elderly patients are more likely to have severe bleeding and suffer debilitating side effects of therapy. All refractory patients should be evaluated for an accessory spleen; if present, strong consideration should be given to removal or it. Significant mucosal bleeding requires periodic emergency therapy as described earlier. The following treatment progression is recommended, although modifications may be needed, depending on the individual patient. Many treatments require the concomitant use of corticosteroids for platelet stabilization during the early phases of therapy.

First-Line Therapy

First-line agents include prednisone, rituximab, and danazol, in that order. A report of the long-term outcome of 105 refractory adult ITP patients showed that 75 eventually attained a stable platelet count higher than 30,000/μL either without therapy (51 patients) or with maintenance treatment consisting of danazol or low-dose prednisone (24 patients). Remissions occurred slowly, with a mean time to remission of about 4 years.

Prednisone (1.0 mg/kg/day followed by tapering if responsive) is the drug of choice if "safe" platelet counts can be maintained at doses acceptable for long-term use (≤10 mg/day). Patients who require small doses of prednisone to maintain safe counts can often be successfully changed to either colchicine (0.6 mg orally two or three times daily) or dapsone (75 mg orally daily) to avoid steroid side effects. Initially, these drugs are added to prednisone, and then the latter is tapered and discontinued if a response occurs. Patients should be screened for erythrocyte glucose-6-phosphate dehydrogenase deficiency before starting dapsone to avoid the risk for hemolysis. Some physicians prefer pulsed dexamethasone (40 mg/day for 4 days every 4 weeks for four to six cycles) instead of prednisone. Patients respond more quickly, but side effects are more prominent.

Rituximab (375 mg/m² IV every week for four courses) is indicated in patients who fail corticosteroids. A stable long-term complete or partial remission is seen in about 20% of treated patients and occurs within 4 to 8 weeks after the first infusion. Patients who relapse may respond to subsequent courses.

If there is no response to rituximab, danazol is given initially at a dose of 200 mg four times daily with full-dose prednisone (1 mg/kg/day). Treatment with danazol should be continued for 3 to 6 months because responses occur slowly. If a response is obtained, prednisone should be tapered and stopped, if possible. Danazol, at full doses, should be continued for at least 1 year and then tapered slowly by 50 mg/day every 4 months. Liver function should be monitored monthly. Danazol maintenance therapy, with or without low-dose prednisone, may be required by some patients.

Second-Line Therapy

Azathioprine or cyclophosphamide is generally recommended when there is no response to prednisone, rituximab, or danazol. Responses to cyclophosphamide occur faster, but serious side effects are more common. For these reasons, drug selection depends on the urgency of the clinical situation because overall response rates are similar (20 to 40%). In the event of a relapse in a patient responding to either agent, the long-term risks (e.g., myelodysplasia, secondary malignancy) should be weighed against the potential benefits of continued therapy. The initial dose of azathioprine is 150 mg/day orally, which is adjusted with the aim of maintaining mild neutropenia. Responses to this agent occur slowly, sometimes requiring 3 to 6 months. Treatment should be continued at full doses for 12 to 18 months in responding patients and then tapered gradually and stopped. Cyclophosphamide is started at 150 mg/day orally and the dose adjusted to maintain mild neutropenia. Responses are noted within 8 to 12 weeks, and full doses are indicated for an additional 3 months in responding patients. At least 2 quarts of liquid should be ingested daily to prevent hemorrhagic cystitis.

Alternative second-line drugs are cyclosporine and mycophenolate mofetil. The starting dose of cyclosporine, 1.25 to 2.5 mg/kg twice daily, is adjusted according to cyclosporine and creatinine levels. Experience is limited, but response rates of 25 to 30% have been reported. About a third of patients stop treatment because of side effects (headaches, hypertension, and myalgias). Only a few patients have been treated with mycophenolate mofetil, and variable responses have been reported. Treatment is begun at 500 mg orally twice daily and increased to 1000 mg orally twice daily after 2 weeks. Side effects are few.

Third-Line Therapy

Third-line treatments are associated with severe side effects and should be reserved for patients who have failed to respond to the aforementioned treatments and have extremely low platelet counts (<10,000/μL) or life-threatening symptoms. Should severe neutropenia occur, prophylactic antibiotics are indicated until counts reach safe levels. If no response is noted after two courses, therapy should be discontinued. Responding patients should receive three to six courses even if the platelet count normalizes. Options include (1) high-dose cyclophosphamide (1.0 to 1.5 g/m² IV infused at 4-week intervals; high fluid intake and frequent blood counts are mandatory) and (2) combination chemotherapy. Only a few patients with severe disease have been treated with combination chemotherapy, and various combinations have been used.

Vinca alkaloids are used infrequently because responses are transient and treatment with vincristine is complicated by peripheral neuropathy. On occasion, a patient's platelet count can be maintained with periodic doses of vinblastine (5 to 10 mg IV infused at weekly intervals or less frequently), which is less likely to cause neuropathy. Responses are infrequently noted with the perfusion of patient plasma over staphylococcal protein A columns, but its use is limited by occasional severe side effects.

Experimental Therapy

In preliminary studies, agents that activate the thrombopoietin receptor have stimulated an increase in the platelet counts of both healthy subjects and some patients with ITP. In an ongoing study using AMG 531 (mean dose/week of 3.4 μg/kg subcutaneously), 29 of 36 ITP patients (30 patients were refractory to splenectomy) had a protocol-defined response (doubling of the platelet count and an increase to ≥50,000/μL), with a mean platelet count of 100,000/μL in weeks 1–24 and 131,000/μL in weeks 25–48. The only adverse events were bone pain (1 patient) and increased marrow reticulum (1 patient). A second experimental agent, eltrombopag (30, 50, or 75 mg/kg PO), resulted in a dose-dependent increase in the platelet count and an 80% response rate at the 75 mg/day dose; headache was the only adverse event and was not dose-related. Clinical trials are continuing, and the role of these agents in ITP therapy remains to be determined.

Autologous stem cell transplantation (Chapter 184) has been used in a small number of patients with refractory ITP, and stable remissions have been reported in about half the patients. However, this treatment is expensive and carries a high rate of morbidity and potential mortality, so it must be performed at centers with the necessary experience and should be considered only in patients who have failed all other treatments.

Disease-Associated Immune Thrombocytopenia

Autoimmune thrombocytopenia, though associated with a variety of diseases, is most commonly seen in patients with collagen vascular or lymphoproliferative disorders. In some patients, thrombocytopenia is a major symptomatic feature, whereas in others, symptoms and signs of the primary disease dominate.

Collagen Vascular Disease

Thrombocytopenia is noted in 14 to 26% of patients with systemic lupus erythematosus (Chapter 287) and is seen much less frequently with other collagen vascular diseases. Clinical features related to thrombocytopenia are similar to those in chronic ITP and mirror the platelet level. Splenomegaly and mild adenopathy are not unusual. Laboratory findings show increased numbers of megakaryocytes in the bone marrow and, if performed, shortened platelet survival. Autoantibodies, similar to those seen in chronic ITP, are common. Because patients with collagen vascular disorders produce a variety of autoantibodies, it seems likely that thrombocytopenia is another manifestation of their altered immune system. Therapy is similar to that for chronic ITP, although the response to splenectomy varies in different series. Danazol is particularly useful both before and after splenectomy, and intermittent pulsed cyclophosphamide has been helpful in individuals unresponsive to other treatments.

Lymphoproliferative Disorders

A low platelet count is commonly seen in patients with lymphoproliferative disorders. In most cases it is due to decreased platelet production because of marrow infiltration or the effects of treatment. However, immune thrombocytopenia is sometimes noted, particularly in individuals with chronic lymphocytic leukemia (Chapter 195) or indolent non-Hodgkin's lymphoma (Chapter 196). Symptoms and signs reflect the severity of both the primary disease and the degree of thrombocytopenia. Adenopathy or splenomegaly, or both, are common. Bone marrow examination shows adequate or increased numbers of megakaryocytes, as well as findings of the primary disease. Platelet-associated and plasma autoantibodies against platelet surface glycoproteins are demonstrable in many patients. In some individuals, the thrombocytopenia responds to the treatment used for the primary disease; otherwise, therapy is similar to that for chronic ITP.

Alloimmune Thrombocytopenia

Post-transfusion Purpura

This rare disorder almost always occurs in women and appears about 7 to 10 days after transfusion. There is usually a history of either a previous transfusion or pregnancy, and most cases occur in multiparous women after their first blood transfusion.

Pathobiology

Alloantibodies react with epitopes on one of three plasma membrane glycoproteins: GPIIIa (Pl^{A1}, Pl^{A2}, and Pen^{a}), GPIIb (Bak^{a} and Bak^{b}), or GPIa (Br^{a}). The patient's platelets invariably lack the alloantigen. The alloantibodies are easily detected by a variety of assays, which are available only in specialized laboratories. The most commonly involved antigen is Pl^{A1}.

Three explanations have been offered to explain alloantibody-induced destruction of autologous platelets that lack the alloantigen: (1) after lysis of the transfused platelets, platelet-specific alloantigen persists in the circulation and forms immune complexes with the alloantibody, which then bind to autologous platelets; (2) the platelet-specific alloantigen released on platelet lysis binds to autologous platelets, which are then destroyed by alloantibody; or (3) an autoantibody that reacts with the patient's platelets is produced in addition to the alloantibody.

Clinical Manifestations and Diagnosis

Post-transfusion purpura is associated with rapidly developing purpura and frequent mucosal bleeding. About 10% of reported cases also have intracranial hemorrhage.

Thrombocytopenia is usually severe (<10,000/μL) but self-limited, lasting 2 to 6 weeks if untreated. Physical findings are those due to thrombocytopenia.

Treatment

Rx

Left untreated, patients recover spontaneously within 6 weeks. However, because intracranial hemorrhage occurs in up to 10% of untreated patients, therapy should be given to all patients. IVIG (1 g/kg/day for 2 to 3 days) has become the treatment of choice. Plasma exchange (1.0 to 1.5 plasma volumes daily for 3 to 4 days), which can normalize the platelet count within a few days, is reserved for patients who fail to respond to IVIG. Although most patients receive corticosteroids, their benefit remains uncertain. Platelet transfusions are not usually helpful and may be associated with severe febrile reactions; however, in the setting of severe bleeding, platelet transfusions should not be withheld. If available, single-donor platelets compatible with the offending antibody (usually PL^{A1} negative) should be used.

Drug-Induced Immune Thrombocytopenia

Definition

The list of drugs that cause immune thrombocytopenia is extremely large, but most cases are caused by a few drugs. In an older review of 357 cases, 70% were due to eight drugs: quinidine, quinine, gold salts, sulfonamides, sulfonamide derivatives, chlorothiazide, chloroquine, and rifampicin. In recent years it has become apparent that platelet GPIIb-IIIa antagonists (abciximab, eptifibatide, and tirofiban), used in the treatment of acute coronary syndrome (Chapter 71) or as an adjunct for management after coronary angioplasty (Chapter 73), can also cause platelet destruction. A complete database of drugs associated with immune thrombocytopenia can be found at the website http://moon.ouhsc.edu/jgeorge/DITP.html. HIT is discussed separately (see later).

Pathobiology

Because of their molecular weight, the drugs most likely function as a hapten bound to a carrier protein, which induces antibody against either a neoantigen generated by a drug-induced structural change in the carrier protein or an antigen consisting of the drug and a portion of the carrier protein. Although only a few drugs have been studied (e.g., quinine, quinidine, sulfa drugs), antigens that have been defined involve the major platelet surface glycoproteins GPIb-IX or GPIIb-IIIa (or both). Some patients have multiple antibodies against different epitopes on the same glycoprotein, whereas others have antibodies against one or more of the glycoproteins. Interestingly, the antibodies are often highly drug specific and do not cross-react with drugs of similar structure. For example, quinidine antibodies do not bind to quinine. In view of the rapid onset of thrombocytopenia within the first 24 hours with GPIIb-IIIa inhibitors, patients are thought to have preexisting autoantibodies to GPIIb-IIIa that bind to epitopes exposed after drug-induced conformational changes in GPIIb-IIIa.

Clinical Manifestations

The clinical picture of most cases of drug-induced immune thrombocytopenia is similar. The onset of thrombocytopenia is sudden, with petechiae, ecchymoses, and frequently mucosal bleeding noted; blood-filled blisters in the mouth are common. Other symptoms may include nausea, vomiting, fever, or a rash. In a study of 247 patients, 23 had major bleeding, 68 had overt but minor bleeding, and 96 had minimal bleeding or purpura alone. Two patients died of bleeding (both while taking quinine).

Diagnosis

A complete drug history must be obtained that includes not only prescription drugs but also quinine-containing drinks and over-the-counter drugs. The clinical history should document that thrombocytopenia occurred after starting the drug (the median time in one large study was 14 days, although it may be noted within the first few hours with GPIIb-IIIa inhibitors). The physical findings are those associated with thrombocytopenia unless other diseases are present. Routine laboratory findings generally show severe isolated thrombocytopenia (although some drugs can cause leukopenia) with adequate or increased numbers of megakaryocytes.

Normalization of the platelet count should usually be noted after stopping the drug, typically within 7 to 10 days, although thrombocytopenia may persist for up to 3 to 4 weeks. In patients with thrombocytopenia secondary to gold therapy, reduced counts may persist for months, presumably because of slow excretion of this agent. Although drug-dependent antibodies are detectible with a variety of methods (e.g., flow cytometry and antigen-specific assays), these tests are not readily available, and diagnosis and treatment must be based on clinical judgment. Rechallenge with the drug is the surest way to confirm the diagnosis, but the risk to the patient rarely warrants this approach.

Treatment

Rx

Therapy consists of stopping use of the offending drug. In patients with severe thrombocytopenia or significant mucosal bleeding, consideration should be given to platelet transfusion and possibly to IVIG (1 g/kg/day for 2 days) or corticosteroids (methylprednisolone, 1.0 g/day IV for 3 days), or to both. Patients receiving GPIIb-IIIa antagonists should have their platelet counts monitored within the first 4 hours and at 24 hours. If thrombocytopenia (<100,000/μL) develops, the GPIIb-IIIa antagonist and any other possible causative medications, such as heparin, should be discontinued. Depending on the degree of thrombocytopenia, consideration should be given to stopping antiplatelet agents such as aspirin or clopidogrel, although the high risk for acute coronary artery or in-stent thrombosis must be considered (Chapter 73). Platelet transfusion may be required for severe thrombocytopenia. The platelet count usually returns to normal within the first few days but may take up to 2 weeks.

Heparin-Induced Thrombocytopenia (HIT)

HIT (Chapter 35), which is a relatively common prothrombotic disorder caused by an immunoglobulin G (IgG) antibody against heparin-PF4 complexes, results in mild to moderate thrombocytopenia, as well as activation of platelets and possibly endothelial cells, at times leading to debilitating or fatal venous or arterial thrombosis, or both. Unlike other drug-induced antiplatelet antibodies, thrombosis is the most feared complication; severe thrombocytopenia or significant bleeding rarely occurs. The frequency of HIT varies widely, depending on the type of heparin (bovine > porcine > low-molecular-weight heparin) and the patient population (surgical > medical > obstetric) (Chapter 35).

Pathobiology

HIT is due to the formation of an IgG antibody against a neoantigen on PF4 created by the binding of heparin to this cationic platelet α-granular protein. Antibody binding to PF4-heparin forms an immune complex that binds to the platelet membrane FcγRII receptor, thereby leading to platelet activation, thrombocytopenia, and in some cases, thrombosis. The immune complexes also bind to sulfated glycosaminoglycans on endothelial cells, which may also contribute to thrombus formation.

Clinical Manifestations

HIT occurs most commonly in postoperative patients receiving prophylactic heparin therapy. It usually develops 5 to 10 days after starting heparin, although the onset may occur within hours in patients who have received heparin in the previous 3 to 4 months. Thrombosis generally occurs during the first week after the onset of thrombocytopenia. Venous thrombosis and pulmonary embolism are the most common events; arterial thrombosis is less frequent but may result in limb ischemia (often requiring amputation), myocardial infarction, or cerebrovascular accidents. Intracardiac thrombosis and microvascular thrombosis have also been described.

Diagnosis

Platelet counts in high-risk patients (e.g., postoperative patients receiving unfractionated heparin) should be obtained every other day from day 4 to day 10. In medical or obstetric patients or those receiving low-molecular-weight heparin, less frequent counts are required. If there has been previous exposure to any type of heparin, a count should be obtained in the first 24 hours.

The diagnosis of HIT is based on clinical findings and requires (1) a platelet count of less than 150,000/μL or a decrease in the platelet count of more than 50% of the pretreatment peak count occurring at the appropriate time (5 to 10 days after starting heparin) and (2) the absence of other causes of thrombocytopenia. The median platelet count nadir is 50,000 to 60,000/μL, and counts below 20,000/μL are uncommon. In some patients, normal platelet counts are present despite the 50% decrease. Patients who satisfy these criteria for HIT but have no clinically evident thrombosis should have a sonogram of the lower extremities because clinically silent deep venous thrombosis is often noted and, if present, will influence therapy. In many patients the diagnosis of HIT is difficult because postoperative complications or other conditions such as infection, postpump thrombocytopenia, or venous thrombosis for other reasons may provide alternative explanations for the clinical findings.

To support the diagnosis of HIT, heparin-induced platelet aggregation in the presence of the patient's plasma is highly specific if positive but lacks sensitivity. Platelet activation assays, such as the serotonin release assay, are both sensitive and specific but technically demanding and not readily available. The most commonly used assays that are commercially available are enzyme-linked immunosorbent assays (ELISAs) for antibodies against the PF4-heparin complex. These assays are easily performed in a clinical laboratory and have high sensitivity, but clinically insignificant positive results are common (10 to 15% in medical patients, >20% in surgical patients, and up to 50% in patients undergoing cardiopulmonary bypass surgery). Therefore, the initial diagnosis of HIT should be based on clinical findings, and if the clinical criteria are met, treatment should be started while awaiting laboratory test results. When the clinical findings are unclear, the results of both an antigen and activation assay may help confirm or exclude the diagnosis. The diagnosis of HIT is unlikely if either the serotonin release assay or ELISA is negative for antibody.

Treatment

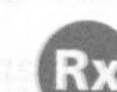

Because HIT occurs much less commonly in patients receiving low-molecular-weight heparin, these agents should be used preferentially when possible (Chapter 35). When HIT is diagnosed, heparin should be discontinued immediately, including heparin line flushes and, if possible, removal of heparin-impregnated catheters. Alternative anticoagulation should be started in all patients, even without evidence of ongoing thrombosis, because thrombosis may develop within several days after stopping heparin in up to 50% of patients whose only initial manifestation of HIT is thrombocytopenia. Low-molecular-weight heparin is contraindicated in patients with HIT because most heparin antibodies cross-react with these agents. Alternatives include lepirudin, argatroban, and fondaparinux. Lepirudin and argatroban have resulted in improved outcomes in large studies of patients with HIT when compared with historic controls and are approved for use in HIT, whereas fondaparinux (7.5 mg daily subcutaneously) has been helpful in case reports but is not approved for this indication.

Lepirudin is a recombinant form of the direct thrombin inhibitor hirudin and acts by interfering with the active site of thrombin. The initial dose is 0.4 mg/kg by IV bolus, followed by a continuous infusion at 0.15 mg/kg/hr, which is adjusted to a dose that results in an activated partial thromboplastin time (aPTT) 1.5 to 2.5 times the patient's baseline aPTT. Because the drug is excreted by the kidney, dose adjustment or substitution of another agent is required in patients with renal insufficiency. Lepirudin is preferred in patients with hepatobiliary disease because argatroban is excreted by the liver. Side effects include bleeding (up to 18%) and the development of non-neutralizing antihirudin antibodies, which may affect drug clearance. There is no antidote for lepirudin.

Argatroban is a synthetic direct thrombin inhibitor derived from L-arginine that also interferes with the active site of thrombin. The initial dose is 2 μg/kg/min IV adjusted to an aPTT of 1.5 to 3.0 times the baseline value. Argatroban is cleared by the liver, so dose adjust-

Rx

ment or substitution of another agent may be required in patients with hepatobiliary disease. In patients with renal insufficiency, argatroban is the preferred agent. As with lepirudin, the major side effect is bleeding (up to 7%), and there is no antidote.

For HIT patients who manifest only thrombocytopenia, direct thrombin inhibitor treatment should continue until the platelet count has returned to normal, which generally occurs within a week, although some investigators recommend therapy for up to a month even after the platelet count normalizes. For patients who require long-term anticoagulation because of thrombotic complications from HIT or for other indications, warfarin is the drug of choice. However, it should be emphasized that warfarin should never be started until adequate anticoagulation has been achieved with a direct thrombin inhibitor and the platelet count has returned to normal. Warfarin causes a rapid decrease in the natural anticoagulant protein C, and this decrease may trigger microvascular thrombosis, which can be devastating. Once started, warfarin and the direct thrombin inhibitor should be given concurrently for at least 5 days. Because both lepirudin and argatroban affect the international normalized ratio, it must be checked after stopping these agents to determine whether adequate anticoagulation has been achieved with warfarin. For HIT-associated thrombosis, warfarin should be continued for at least 3 to 4 months. Because of the increase in severe bleeding in some clinical trials, thrombolytic agents should not be used concurrently with direct thrombin inhibitors.

Even if treated with thrombin inhibitors, HIT is a serious disorder. It carries a substantial risk for mortality (≈15%) and severe morbidity (amputation, ≈2%; new thromboses, ≈8%).

Acute Immune Thrombocytopenic Purpura

Acute ITP is a transient, mostly postinfectious disorder characterized by increased platelet destruction that occurs almost exclusively in children with a peak age between 2 and 5 years and no sex predilection. Chronic ITP, defined as immune thrombocytopenia persisting for more than 6 months, occurs in 10 to 15% of children initially thought to have acute ITP, and its frequency increases with the age of the child. Chronic ITP in children is an autoimmune disease comparable to adult ITP.

Viral Infection

Thrombocytopenia associated with some viral infections, such as rubella (Chapter 391), mumps (Chapter 392), infectious mononucleosis (Chapter 400), and cytomegalovirus (Chapter 399), appears to be primarily of immune origin and closely mimics acute ITP. Symptoms of the primary viral disease are usually well established (7 to 10 days) before the onset of thrombocytopenia, which is often acute and severe with symptoms of generalized purpura and severe mucosal bleeding; rarely, deaths have been reported. Splenomegaly may be noted, particularly in patients with infectious mononucleosis or cytomegalovirus infection. Bone marrow examination shows increased megakaryocytes in most patients, although reduced or absent megakaryocytes have occasionally been reported. The thrombocytopenia generally remits spontaneously within 2 to 4 weeks, but in occasional individuals it may persist for months before remitting. Patients with severe thrombocytopenia or active bleeding may require emergency treatment with platelet transfusions combined with either IVIG (1 g/kg/day IV for 1 to 3 days), anti-D (50 to 75 µg/kg IV), or methylprednisolone (1.0 g/day IV for 1 to 3 days). Rarely, when severe thrombocytopenia with uncontrolled bleeding occurs, splenectomy has been used successfully.

Thrombocytopenia Associated with the Human Immunodeficiency Virus

Pathobiology

In HIV disease, thrombocytopenia is due to both immune-mediated platelet destruction (manifested by shortened platelet survival and increases in platelet-associated IgG, platelet-associated IgM, platelet-associated C3, and circulating immune complexes [Chapter 416]) and decreased platelet production, probably secondary to infection of megakaryocytes, which show ultrastructural alterations and the presence of HIV-1 RNA.

Clinical Manifestations

The thrombocytopenia associated with HIV infection may be clinically indistinguishable from chronic ITP. Patients may be asymptomatic or demonstrate petechiae or bruising; severe mucosal bleeding is unusual. Unlike chronic ITP, adenopathy and splenomegaly may be present. Bone marrow examination shows normal or increased numbers of megakaryocytes. Other symptoms related to HIV infection or to associated complications may be present. Thrombocytopenia may occur before or at any time during HIV infection, although the incidence increases as the disease progresses.

Treatment

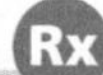

If the patient is not yet receiving highly active antiretroviral therapy, it should be started. Antiretroviral therapy is aimed at improving platelet production, and this effect may take several weeks.

Because thrombocytopenia is partially due to platelet destruction, patients who are actively bleeding should receive IVIG (1 g/kg/day for 1 to 2 days) or anti-D (50 to 75 µg/kg IV) with platelet transfusions, as described for chronic ITP. Patients whose low platelet counts do not require emergency therapy should receive a trial of prednisone (1 mg/kg/day with tapering if responsive). About 60 to 80% of patients respond to prednisone, but most relapse on tapering the drug. Although short courses appear to be safe, prednisone is not recommended for long-term use because of its immunosuppressive properties. IVIG or anti-D therapy at the aforementioned doses may be used chronically to maintain the platelet count, but these alternatives are inconvenient and expensive. Patients who continue to have symptomatic thrombocytopenia after an adequate trial of antiretroviral therapy should undergo splenectomy, which results in stable complete or partial remissions in 60 to 80% of patients. In patients who fail splenectomy, variable success has been reported with several agents, including dapsone, danazol, vincristine, and interferon alfa.

Platelet Destruction Caused by Nonimmune Disorders

Thrombotic Thrombocytopenic Purpura

Thrombotic thrombocytopenic purpura (TTP) is a life-threatening disorder characterized by platelet aggregation and thrombosis in the microvasculature; it results in thrombocytopenia, hemolytic anemia, organ ischemia, and unless treated, a mortality rate higher than 90%. Hemolytic-uremic syndrome (HUS) is a clinically similar disorder that primarily affects children and is marked by a predominance of renal failure. Clinically similar syndromes have been reported with disseminated malignancies (Chapter 189), stem cell transplantation (Chapter 184), pregnancy (Chapter 259), and a variety of drugs, including mitomycin C, ticlopidine, clopidogrel, cyclosporine, and quinine.

Pathobiology

In the early 1980s, unusually large vWF multimers, similar in size to those produced by endothelial cells in culture, were noted in the plasma of patients with TTP. It was postulated that these multimers were responsible for in vivo platelet clumping in small blood vessels and that patients with TTP lacked the depolymerase responsible for controlling multimer size. In the mid-1990s, a plasma protease that specifically cleaves vWF multimers at the peptide bond Tyr842-Met843, the site previously shown to be cleaved during physiologic vWF processing, was isolated. This protease was subsequently cloned, identified as a member of the ADAMTS family of metalloproteases, and designated ADAMTS-13. Subsequent studies showed that histamine-stimulated, cultured endothelial cells secrete extremely large vWF multimers that remain linked to the endothelial cells and, when perfused with platelets, form "beads-on-a-string" structures. Perfusion with normal plasma or purified ADAMTS-13 results in rapid detachment of the adherent platelets, thus suggesting that ADAMTS-13 regulates the in vivo size of vWF multimers and prevents platelet adherence.

Several ADAMTS-13 assays have been developed, most of which are based on the degradation of large vWF multimers into smaller multimers by a patient's plasma. Inhibitors of ADAMTS-13 are measured by preincubating the patient's plasma with pooled normal plasma and then measuring the residual vWF-cleaving activity of normal plasma. Interlaboratory agreement is good in samples with severe ADAMTS-13 deficiency and high-titer inhibitors but less good in samples with mild or moderately reduced ADAMTS-13 or low-titer inhibitors.

Hereditary TTP is caused by homozygous or double-heterozygous gene mutations that result in a severe deficiency of ADAMTS-13. After the discovery of ADAMTS-13, two large series reported that almost all patients with acquired TTP had severe vWF-cleaving protease deficiency, most often associated with an IgG inhibitor. It was concluded that autoantibody-induced ADAMTS-13 deficiency explained the pathogenesis of the disease. However, subsequent studies have shown that ADAMTS-13 activity can be severely deficient in asymptomatic patients and that patients with the characteristic syndrome of TTP can have normal or nearly normal ADAMTS-13 activity. At present, it must be concluded that deficient ADAMTS-13 is one important factor in many patients with acquired TTP but that other, as yet undefined factors must be involved in other patients with this syndrome.

Clinical Manifestations

The classic TTP "pentad" of signs and symptoms includes (1) thrombocytopenia, which is usually moderate or severe with an associated increase in bone marrow megakaryocytes; (2) microangiopathic hemolytic anemia with a blood smear showing schistocytes (Fig. 161–10; similar to what is seen with disseminated intravascular coagulation), as well as an extremely high serum lactic dehydrogenase (LDH) level; (3) renal insufficiency, which is generally mild with moderate increases in serum creatinine and urine protein levels; (4) fever; and (5) neurologic abnormalities, which range from mild headache and disorientation to severe symptoms such as hemiparesis, seizures, focal neurologic deficits, coma, and death. Symptoms vary among patients, and any of the common symptoms can dominate the clinical course. About a third of patients with acquired TTP will have a relapse after an initial response to treatment, especially during the first year. The relapse rate appears to be higher in patients with severe ADAMTS-13 deficiency. Patients with hereditary TTP show an age-dependent clustering of the onset of the disease, with the initial manifestation occurring either before 5 years of age or between the ages of 20 and 41, although some patients in whom TTP is diagnosed during family studies remain asymptomatic.

Diagnosis

Because of the high fatality rate in untreated TTP patients, the diagnosis is urgent but may be difficult if the patient does not have the complete pentad of symptoms. The presence of hemolytic anemia with schistocytes, thrombocytopenia, and a markedly increased LDH that is unexplained by another condition allows a tentative diagnosis. It is better to err on the side of treatment rather than awaiting additional symptoms, which may be lethal. Assays for ADAMTS-13 and inhibitors may be clinically helpful but are not readily available on an urgent basis.

Treatment

Rx

Acquired Thrombotic Thrombocytopenic Purpura

In patients with acute acquired TTP, plasma exchange with fresh-frozen plasma should be started immediately. [1] If there is a delay in arranging for plasma exchange, patients should be transfused with fresh-frozen plasma alone until plasma exchange can be instituted. If the patient is clinically stable and does not have significant neurologic symptoms, a daily single-volume plasma exchange is sufficient. If the clinical situation deteriorates, a daily double-volume plasma exchange is indicated. Cryosupernatant can also be used as the replacement fluid. When the patient shows objective signs of improvement, as indicated by improvement in CNS function, rising platelet counts, and falling LDH levels, the intensity and frequency of plasma exchange can be tapered. Microangiopathy may persist for weeks to months. Corticosteroids (prednisone, 2 mg/kg/day with tapering if responsive) are used by some physicians, either alone in mild cases or in addition to plasma exchange in more severe cases.

In refractory patients, a variety of immunosuppressants (vincristine, azathioprine, cyclophosphamide) have been used with varied success. Splenectomy is effective in some patients, although it is best performed in remission. Recently, there have been several case reports of patients with relapsing TTP who have had successful responses to the anti-CD20 monoclonal antibody rituximab (375 mg/m^2/wk IV for four to eight doses), although long-term follow-up is not available.

Hereditary Thrombotic Thrombocytopenic Purpura

Patients with hereditary TTP as a result of ADAMTS-13 gene defects should receive an infusion of fresh-frozen plasma every 2 to 3 weeks to prevent relapse.

Hemolytic-Uremic Syndrome

Pathobiology

Patients with HUS do not have reduced ADAMTS-13 levels. Children with HUS after infection with *Escherichia coli* (Chapter 327) are thought to have endothelial damage secondary to Shiga toxins elaborated by the bacteria. Familial HUS accounts for 5 to 10% of cases. Some of these patients have been found to have a deficiency or an abnormal form of complement factor H.

Clinical Manifestations

HUS is seen most commonly in children, predominantly after a GI infection with *E. coli* (Chapter 327), usually serotype O157 : H7, associated with severe bloody diarrhea. HUS is also seen in adults, often in association with exposure to various drugs (e.g., mitomycin C, ticlopidine, cyclosporine, tacrolimus, quinine, combination chemotherapy), during the postpartum period, with immunosuppression, or after bone marrow (Chapter 184) or organ transplantation. Renal dysfunction is the dominant feature and frequently requires dialysis. Neurologic symptoms are generally less prominent. With the exception of the rare familial type, HUS almost always occurs as a single episode.

Diagnosis

Proteinuria, hematuria, and elevated blood urea nitrogen and creatinine levels reflect the degree of renal failure. Additional laboratory findings may include microangiopathic hemolytic anemia, thrombocytopenia, and an elevated LDH level, but these findings are less prominent than in TTP. If performed, ADAMTS-13 assays are negative.

Treatment

Rx

Children with HUS as a result of *E. coli* infection are generally treated with supportive therapy and renal dialysis as needed; plasma infusion or exchange does not improve the clinical outcome. Some physicians use supportive therapy only and avoid antibiotic therapy for fear that it will result in an increase in toxin production, but comparative studies have not substantiated this fear. The outcome of HUS in other clinical situations is usually either self-limited or determined by the associated disease.

Disseminated Intravascular Coagulation

A wide variety of clinical disorders, including infection, burns, trauma, and malignancies, may introduce procoagulants into the circulation that overcome control mechanisms and thereby result in the widespread generation of thrombin, intravascular coagulation, and multiorgan dysfunction. Thrombocytopenia is due to platelet utilization during this process. This entity is discussed in detail in Chapter 181.

Other Infections

Thrombocytopenia is commonly seen in individuals with gram-positive or gram-negative infections. The incidence of thrombocytopenia ranges from 46 to 77% in patients with positive blood cultures and up to 90% in patients with septic shock (Chapter 109). Platelet counts are usually in the 30,000 to 70,000/μL range, although more severe thrombocytopenia may be seen. The relative role of disseminated intravascular coagulation (Chapter 181) and the immune system in producing thrombocytopenia is unknown. A similar syndrome is associated with malarial infection (Chapter 366). Treatment of the thrombocytopenia consists of therapy for the primary infection. In the rare event of severe thrombocytopenia or mucosal bleeding, platelet transfusions and specific treatment of disseminated intravascular coagulation are indicated.

Kasabach-Merritt Syndrome

Patients with Kasabach-Merritt syndrome have giant cavernous angiomas, and the condition is usually diagnosed at a young age, although thrombocytopenia may be first noted in adulthood. Patients have a pathologically distinctive vascular tumor that may infiltrate progressively and require intensive treatment. Thrombocytopenia is often associated with low fibrinogen, consistent with platelet consumption and intravascular coagulation within the tumor. Laboratory studies show thrombocytopenia, red cell fragmentation, and findings consistent with disseminated intravascular coagulation. Eradication of the lesion by surgery, embolization, or radiation therapy can be curative. The coagulopathy may be improved with the use of an anticoagulant such as heparin or an antifibrinolytic drug such as aminocaproic acid, which may help eliminate the vascular lesion by promoting local thrombosis. Shrinkage of the hemangiomas may occur after glucocorticoid or interferon treatment or may occur spontaneously. A similar syndrome can rarely occur with aortic aneurysms.

Massive Transfusion

Thrombocytopenia will develop in patients requiring massive transfusion (Chapter 183), defined as 10 or more units of red cells within a 24-hour period. The degree of thrombocytopenia parallels the number of red cell units transfused. In one study, the platelet count after 15 or more red cell units ranged from 47,000 to 100,000/μL and after 20 red cell units ranged from 25,000 to 61,000/μL. The cause of the thrombocytopenia is a combination of the loss of platelets from bleeding and replacement with red cell units that have no functioning platelets because of storage at cold temperatures. Platelet transfusions may be given but are rarely required.

Platelet Redistribution (Enlarged Splenic Pool)

Patients with an enlarged spleen (Chapter 174) have an increase in their splenic platelet pool and a corresponding decrease in their peripheral platelet count. This phenomenon is most commonly seen in congestive splenomegaly associated with chronic liver disease but may also occur in other disorders characterized by a large spleen such as Gaucher's disease, lymphoma, myelofibrosis, and Felty's syndrome (Chapter 285). Platelet counts of less than 30,000 to 40,000/μL are unusual, and therapy is rarely required. Mild anemia or leukopenia may also be seen.

Thrombocytopenia Caused by Decreased Platelet Production

Disorders that cause thrombocytopenia as a result of decreased platelet production (Table 179–1) can usually be suspected from the history and physical examination, blood counts, and the blood smear and can confirmed by bone marrow aspiration and biopsy. In most cases the low platelet count is due to either bone marrow infiltration (e.g., leukemia [Chapter 194], multiple myeloma [Chapter 198], lymphoproliferative disorders [Chapters 196 and 197], myelofibrosis [Chapter 177], or solid tumor), abnormally functioning marrow (e.g., aplastic anemia [Chapter 171], myelodysplasia [Chapter 193], or megaloblastic anemia [Chapter 170]), an inherited or congenital disorder (May-Hegglin anomaly, Wiskott-Aldrich syndrome, or familial thrombocytopenia), or less commonly, marrow suppression as a result of drugs, radiation therapy (Chapter 18), or the excessive use of alcohol (Chapter 31). In most cases, therapy involves either stopping use of the offending drug or treating the primary disorder.

Congenital or Inherited Platelet Disorders

These disorders are rare but in some cases may be associated with isolated thrombocytopenia in an asymptomatic patient and be confused with a common platelet disorder, such as chronic ITP, and result in inappropriate treatment with splenectomy, immunosuppressive agents, or both. The following findings suggest a congenital or hereditary platelet disorder: (1) onset at birth; (2) a family history of thrombocytopenia; (3) specific diagnostic features on the blood film, such as abnormally large or small platelets, absence of α-granules (gray platelets), or abnormal blood cell inclusions; (4) associated clinical features such as orthopedic abnormalities (e.g., absent radii), mental retardation, renal failure, cataracts, high-tone hearing loss, or the development of leukemia; (5) a long history of stable thrombocytopenia; (6) bleeding out of proportion to the platelet count; and (7) lack of a platelet response after therapy in a patient suspected of having ITP.

Amegakaryocytic Thrombocytopenias

Congenital amegakaryocytic thrombocytopenias are manifested as severe thrombocytopenia during the first month of life. This condition is often confused with neonatal alloimmune thrombocytopenia, except that patients fail to improve. Bone marrow examination demonstrates reduced or absent megakaryocytes. The defect has been shown, in most cases, to be due to a mutation of the thrombopoietin receptor c-mpl; in the absence of this receptor, megakaryocytes do not proliferate normally. A substantial proportion of these patients have orthopedic or neurologic abnormalities, and many progress to aplastic anemia within a few years. Allogeneic stem cell transplantation is the only curative therapy. Platelet transfusion is indicated for significant bleeding. The syndrome of thrombocytopenia and absent radii (TAR syndrome) is often associated with less severe thrombocytopenia after the first year of life, so platelet transfusions are no longer required.

Wiskott-Aldrich Syndrome

Patients with Wiskott-Aldrich syndrome (Chapter 271) usually have significant thrombocytopenia with small platelets noted on the peripheral smear. The risk for hemorrhage in some patients is out of proportion to the platelet count, possibly because the platelet mass is low as a result of the small platelets. These patients also have a congenital immunodeficiency, including an inability to produce antipolysaccharide antibodies, that results in the frequent occurrence of pneumococcal sepsis. Eczema is commonly seen. This disorder is unusual in that the thrombocytopenia responds to splenectomy, possibly because of removal of a site of destruction of the defective platelets. The lifetime risk for lymphoma is approximately 10%. Allogeneic transplantation is indicated for severe disease. In patients who are not transplantation candidates, splenectomy can be helpful. However, in view of the associated immunodeficiency, presplenectomy vaccinations should be performed (see the section on chronic ITP), and prophylactic antibiotics are indicated after splenectomy.

MYH9-Related Diseases

These diseases include the May-Hegglin, Fechtner, Sebastian, and Epstein syndromes, all of which involve mutations of the gene coding for myosin IIA. Patients have varying degrees of thrombocytopenia with extremely large platelets. Platelet function is generally preserved, and patients are frequently asymptomatic. Associated clinical features may include leukocyte inclusions, renal failure, hearing loss, and cataracts. Therapy is not usually required.

Other Inherited Thrombocytopenias

Many families have been reported with isolated thrombocytopenia, typically with an autosomal dominant inheritance pattern. The diagnosis is made in most of these patients as adults, and they have only minimal symptoms with moderate thrombocytopenia, normal platelet morphology, and normal bone marrow findings. Recognition of these patients is important because their condition is often misdiagnosed as chronic ITP and in some cases they have undergone splenectomy or received immunosuppressive therapy without benefit. Treatment is not usually required.

QUALITATIVE PLATELET DISORDERS

Inherited Disorders

Bernard-Soulier Syndrome

This autosomal recessive disorder is manifested early in life by purpura and bleeding out of proportion to the platelet count. The platelets show abnormal adhesion to vascular subendothelium because of the absence or dysfunctional expression of the platelet GPIb-IX-V complex. Laboratory studies show a prolonged bleeding time, isolated moderate thrombocytopenia, and extremely large platelets that aggregate normally to ADP, epinephrine, and collagen but do not aggregate to ristocetin. Genetic mutations have been associated with GPIbα, GPIbβ, and GPIX, but not with GPV.

Glanzmann's Thrombasthenia

This bleeding disorder, also with autosomal recessive inheritance, develops in early childhood and causes severe purpura and mucosal bleeding. Bleeding tends to decrease in older patients. Laboratory studies show a prolonged bleeding time, a normal platelet count, and abnormal platelet aggregation to a variety of agonists (including ADP, epinephrine, thrombin, and collagen), but normal aggregation to ristocetin. The interaction of platelets with subendothelium shows normal adhesion but no aggregation. Patients have either a marked reduction, dysfunction, or absence of the platelet surface GPIIb-IIIa complex.

Gray Platelet Syndrome

Patients with gray platelet syndrome have a mild to moderate bleeding diathesis manifested by varying degrees of purpura and mucosal bleeding, although some patients remain asymptomatic. Bleeding is thought to be due to the lack of α-granule proteins, such as vWF, fibronectin, and thrombospondin. Laboratory studies show a prolonged bleeding time and usually moderate thrombocytopenia. Platelets and megakaryocytes appear gray on peripheral blood smear because of the absence of α-granules. Aggregation studies show decreased aggregation to threshold concentrations of collagen and thrombin.

Storage Pool Deficiency

Patients with storage pool deficiency have a variable bleeding disorder of autosomal dominant inheritance caused by a deficiency of dense bodies in megakaryocytes and circulating platelets. The dense bodies serve as a storage pool for ATP, ADP, serotonin, calcium, and pyrophosphate, which are secreted on platelet activation. It is postulated that the reduced release of ADP may result in decreased GPIIb-IIIa–dependent aggregation. Patients have various degrees of purpura and mucosal bleeding. Laboratory studies show a prolonged bleeding time with normal platelet counts and morphology. Platelet aggregation studies characteristically demonstrate an absence of the secondary wave after ADP, epinephrine, and low concentrations of thrombin; aggregation to collagen is markedly impaired. When measured, there is an increased platelet ATP/ADP ratio. The absence of platelet dense bodies can be documented by the use of mepacrine dye.

Treatment Rx

In patients with severe bleeding, platelet transfusion (Chapter 183) with HLA-matched platelets is indicated, if possible, to reduce alloantibody formation against HLA antigens. In some patients, transfusion-induced antibodies develop against the deficient platelet glycoprotein (e.g., GPIIb-IIIa in Glanzmann's thrombasthenia, GPIb-IX-V in Bernard-Soulier syndrome), which makes transfusion difficult. Other agents that have been used include desmopressin, ε-aminocaproic acid (especially for mouth or nose bleeding), hormonal therapy to lessen menses, and recombinant factor VIIa. Allogeneic stem cell transplantation may be indicated in patients with severe Glanzmann's thrombasthenia or Bernard-Soulier syndrome if a suitable match is available.

Acquired Disorders

Renal Disease

Bleeding is often a problem in patients with renal failure. The bleeding pattern, which is characteristic of a deficiency of primary hemostasis, is manifested primarily as purpura, epistaxis, and GI bleeding. Acute GI bleeding often occurs from ulcers or erosions in the upper GI tract. Platelet counts are generally normal, but the bleeding time is prolonged and correlates to some degree with the severity of bleeding. Platelet aggregation study results vary widely and are not useful in the diagnosis. The bleeding tendency of patients with renal failure is usually controlled by dialysis. The specific toxins involved have not been clearly defined, and the mechanisms are probably complex.

Treatment Rx

Correction of the anemia of renal failure with either red cell transfusions or erythropoietin (Chapters 131 and 169) normalizes the bleeding time and lessens the bleeding tendency. Because complete correction of the anemia may lead to complications such as hypertension, the target hematocrit should range from 27 to 32%. Other agents that are useful include desmopressin and estrogens. Desmopressin may be given intravenously (0.3 to 0.4 μg/kg), with improvement in the bleeding time within 1 hour and persisting for up to 8 hours. The drug can also be given subcutaneously at the same dose or intranasally (2 μg/kg). Tachyphylaxis limits the frequency of administration. Conjugated estrogens are also useful. Intravenous infusion (Premarin, 0.6 mg/kg IV) daily for 4 to 5 days improves the bleeding time within the first 6 to 8 hours, and this effect persists for up to 2 weeks. Oral conjugated estrogens (e.g., Premarin, 50 mg/day) or transdermal 17β-estradiol (50 to 100 μg/day) are also effective.

Liver Disease

Patients with liver failure (Chapter 158) have a high risk for bleeding because of a combination of factors, including hypersplenism with associated thrombocytopenia; anatomic abnormalities, including esophageal varices and gastritis; and abnormalities of the coagulation system as a result of impaired synthesis of coagulation factors, abnormal fibrinogens, and disseminated intravascular coagulation. The bleeding time may be prolonged, but there are no characteristic platelet aggregation findings. As in renal insufficiency, anemia may contribute to the platelet dysfunction. Therapy is difficult because of the complexity of the situation and must be individualized according to the factors involved.

Drug-Induced Bleeding

Many drugs are known to interfere with platelet function, including aspirin, nonsteroidal anti-inflammatory drugs, antiplatelet agents such as diclopidine and clopidogrel, and a variety of antibiotics. Bleeding is not usually severe and rarely requires therapy unless the drugs are given to patients who already have significant thrombocytopenia from other causes or have dysfunctional platelets.

VASCULAR PURPURAS

Senile Purpura (Purpura Simplex)

This condition (Chapter 23) is manifested as bruising, usually over the exposed skin of the arms and legs, and is noted most frequently in older patients or in association with corticosteroid therapy. It is thought to be caused by lack of capillary support because of alterations in connective tissue.

Scurvy

Patients with scurvy (Chapter 237) have defective collagen synthesis as a result of vitamin C deficiency. Scurvy is uncommon but may be seen in persons following dietary fads, those in extreme poverty, or individuals who have psychiatric problems or are socially isolated. Clinical findings include follicular hyperkeratosis, perifollicular bruising, and abnormal hair growth resulting in corkscrew hairs. Scurvy is cured by the administration of vitamin C.

Infection-Related Purpura

A wide variety of bacterial (*Neisseria meningitidis* [Chapter 321], *Haemophilus influenzae* [Chapter 323], *Streptococcus pneumoniae* [Chapter 312], etc.) viral (coxsackievirus [Chapter 402], rubella [Chapter 391], measles [Chapter 390], hepatitis A and B [Chapter 151], etc.), rickettsial (Rocky Mountain spotted fever; Chapter 348), and fungal infections (*Candida;* Chapter 359) can be associated with purpura. Mechanisms include vascular invasion, septic emboli, immune complex vasculitis, or less commonly, thrombocytopenia. Treatment is directed at the primary illness.

Ehlers-Danlos Syndrome

Excessive bleeding as a result of vascular defects has been noted in Ehlers-Danlos syndrome (Chapter 281). Patients are characterized clinically by lax skin, hypermobile joints, and delayed wound healing with prominent scarring. Easy bruising is a common finding, and in some subtypes of the syndrome, bleeding manifestations may be severe and at times fatal (e.g., spontaneous rupture of arteries, veins, or viscera). The diagnosis is based on clinical findings. Laboratory tests are not usually helpful, and the bleeding time is generally normal.

Dysproteinemias

Palpable petechiae and purpura are noted in Waldenström's macroglobulinemia, amyloidosis, benign polyclonal hypergammaglobulinemia, cryoglobulinemia, and cryofibrinogenemia (Chapter 198). Treatment depends on the primary diagnosis.

Hereditary Hemorrhagic Telangiectasia (Osler-Weber-Rendu Syndrome)

This autosomal dominant disorder is characterized by telangiectasia involving the skin, mucous membranes, and solid organs, as well as by large arteriovenous malformations that can involve the lung, liver, and brain. Mutations involve either of two proteins, endoglin or activin receptor–like kinase, both of which are associated with the signal transduction mechanisms of transforming growth factor-β, a potent angiogenic factor.

The vascular lesions usually appear during the second or third decades and almost always by the age of 40. The lesions are red spots that blanch on pressure and occur most commonly on the face, lips, nares, fingers, tongue, and oral mucosa (Fig. 179–3). Epistaxis is the most common symptom (90%), but painless upper or lower GI bleeding (50%) and hematuria (15%) are also seen. Arteriovenous fistulas in the lung may result in clubbing, hypoxemia, right-to-left shunting, and pulmonary hypertension. Fistulas in the liver can cause cirrhosis or high-output heart failure. Neurologic symptoms are most frequently due to paradoxical or septic emboli.

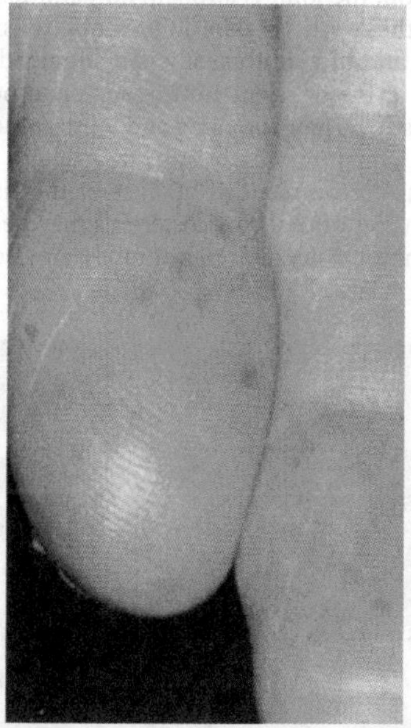

FIGURE 179–3 • Hereditary hemorrhagic telangiectasia. Patients commonly have lesions on or close to mucous membranes, but telangiectases may occur anywhere on the body, as in this patient whose fingers were affected. The lesions are dilated capillaries, and they blanch if pressure is applied with a glass slide. (From Forbes CD, Jackson WF: Color Atlas and Text of Clinical Medicine, 3rd ed. London, Mosby, 2003.)

Treatment

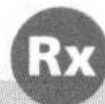

Treatment is primarily supportive. Patients with GI bleeding should receive supplemental iron and folate; red blood cell transfusions and parenteral iron may be required in some patients. Other agents such as desmopressin, danazol, and aminocaproic acid have been used with varied success. Embolization of arteriovenous fistulas may be required. Estrogen or progesterone treatment had been advised, but no benefit could be demonstrated in a placebo-controlled randomized trial.

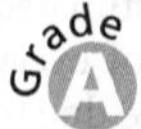

1. Rock GA, Shumak KH, Buskard NA, et al: Comparison of plasma exchange with plasma infusion in the treatment of thrombotic thrombocytopenic purpura. Canadian Apheresis Study Group. N Engl J Med 1991;325:393–397.

SUGGESTED READINGS

Arnold DM, Dentali F, Crowther MA, et al: Systematic review: Efficacy and safety of rituximab for adults with idiopathic thrombocytopenic purpura. Ann Intern Med 2007;146:25–33. *Rituximab is effective in >60% of patients, but was associated with significant risk of adverse events.*

Arepally GM, Ortel TL: Heparin-induced thrombocytopenia. N Engl J Med 2006:355:809–817. *A clinical review.*

Bussel JB, Kuter DJ, George JN, et al: AMG 531, a thrombopoiesis-stimulating protein, for chronic ITP. N Engl J Med 2006;355:1672–1681. *AMG 531 caused no major adverse effects and increased platelet counts.*

Drachman JG: Inherited thrombocytopenia: When a low platelet count does not mean ITP. Blood 2004;103:390–398. *A comprehensive review.*

George JN: Thrombotic thrombocytopenic purpura. N Engl J Med 2006:354: 1927–1935. *A case-based review.*

Moake JI: Thrombotic microangiopathies. N Engl J Med 2002;347:589–600. *Overview comparing and contrasting TTP and HUS.*

Nurden AT: Qualitative disorders of platelets and megakaryocytes. J Thromb Haemost 2005;3:1773–1782. *A detailed overview.*

180 HEMORRHAGIC DISORDERS: COAGULATION FACTOR DEFICIENCIES

Craig M. Kessler

COAGULATION DEFICIENCIES

Severe coagulation deficiencies, or coagulopathies, typically are characterized by the development of excessive bleeding or bruising that is unprovoked or, more commonly, is precipitated by trivial incidental or surgical trauma. Frequently, these hemorrhagic events result in life- and limb-threatening complications. Moderate and mild coagulopathies may remain clinically silent until they are detected serendipitously on routine laboratory screening assays for global coagulation (e.g., prothrombin time [PT] or activated partial thromboplastin time [aPTT]) or when these assays are ordered to evaluate the cause of abnormal bleeding or easy bruisability. Much of the morbidity of coagulopathies can be minimized or avoided altogether by advanced awareness and prophylactic replacement of the deficient clotting factor proteins. In contrast to the lifelong clinical manifestations of hereditary or congenital coagulopathies, acquired deficiencies usually appear acutely in previously asymptomatic individuals, may not be suspected immediately on examination, and may remit spontaneously or after eradication of an inciting disease state or the withdrawal of an offending medication. Acquired coagulation disorders often are associated with more severe bleeding than are those derived from congenital causes. Coagulopathies predominantly result from inadequate biosynthesis of coagulation factor proteins or from direct or indirect inhibition of activated clotting factor proteins by acquired antibodies or anticoagulant medications; however, qualitative defects, either congenital or acquired, also can result in bleeding.

Hereditary Hemophilias

Definition

The hemophilias include hemophilia A, caused by a deficiency of clotting protein factor VIII (antihemophilic factor), and hemophilia B, caused by a deficiency of factor IX (also called antihemophilic factor B, plasma thromboplastin component, or Christmas factor, named after an individual with the disease). A deficiency of either of these two intrinsic coagulation pathway components results in inefficient and inadequate generation of thrombin.

Epidemiology

The sex-linked recessive disorders of hemophilia A and B are estimated to occur, respectively, in approximately 1 of every 5000 and 1 of every 30,000 male births. The higher incidence of hemophilia A may be due to the greater amount of DNA "at risk" for mutation in the factor VIII gene (186,000 base pairs) compared with the factor IX gene (34,000 base pairs). Hemophilia A and B are observed throughout all races and ethnic groups, and more than 25,000 individuals in the United States are recognized to have one of the hemophilias. Although carrier testing, genetic counseling, and prenatal diagnosis are widely available in the United States through the network of federally funded Hemophilia Treatment Centers, fecundity rates remain high, and few confirmed carriers elect to terminate their pregnancies even if an affected fetus is detected in utero. These decisions probably are influenced by the wide availability of efficacious and safe commercial coagulation factor replacement concentrates and by the prospect that gene therapy may eventually cure the hemophilias. The advent of highly active antiretroviral therapy (Chapter 412), biological response modifiers such as pegylated interferon-α, and liver transplantation (Chapter 158) has prolonged the survival of hemophiliacs with acquired immunodeficiency syndrome (AIDS) and chronic hepatitis. A substantial proportion (30%) of cases of hemophilia result from unanticipated new, spontaneous mutations. Overall, the hemophilias are much more common than the autosomal recessive coagulation disorders, which often affect progeny from consanguineous relationships and require the inheritance of two defective alleles for the bleeding manifestations to become evident.

Pathobiology

Genetics

As with other sex-linked recessive diseases, the genes for factor VIII and factor IX are located on the long arm of the X chromosome. Males with a defective allele on their single X chromosome do not transmit this gene to their sons, but all of their daughters become obligate carriers. Female carriers transmit the coagulation disorder to half of their sons, and half of their daughters become carriers. Female carriers can manifest hemophilia-like symptoms if the alleles on the X chromosome are unequally inactivated (lyonization); the defective hemophilic allele is expressed in preference to the normal allele, and a phenotypic hemophiliac is produced. Female hemophilia can arise as the result of mating between a hemophilic male and a female carrier (homozygous for the defective factor VIII or IX gene) or in carrier females who have the 45 XO karyotype (Turner's syndrome) and are hemizygous for the defective hemophilia gene.

No single mutation is responsible for the hemophilias, and many missense and nonsense point mutations, deletions, and inversions have been described. Severe molecular defects predominate, with 40 to 50% of all cases of severe hemophilia A evolving from a unique inversion of intron 22 (the largest of the factor VIII introns). This inversion results from the recombination and translocation of DNA within intron 22 of the factor VIII gene, with areas of extragenic but homologous "nonfunctional" DNA located at a distance from intron 22. Other, less commonly encountered severe molecular defects include large gene deletions (5 to 10% of cases) and nonsense mutations (10 to 15% of cases). The encoded proteins resulting from these mutations are defective and do not express any factor VIII activity. Mild and moderate hemophilia A commonly are associated with point mutations and deletions. In contrast, factor IX mutations are more diverse, and severe hemophilia B more likely is caused by large deletions. Hemophilia B also may result from mutations that alter the γ-glutamyl residues of the factor IX protein, which normally become carboxylated through a vitamin K–dependent process and then assemble on a phospholipid surface for eventual activation. Mutated clotting factor genes responsible for the hemophilias may code for the production of defective nonfunctional proteins that circulate in the plasma and can be detected by immunoassays. Designated *cross-reacting material,* these proteins have no clinical relevance except that individuals without cross-reacting material may be more susceptible to alloantibody inhibitor formation.

Clinical Manifestations

The clinical pictures of hemophilia A and hemophilia B are indistinguishable from each other, with their clinical severity corresponding inversely to the circulating levels of plasma coagulant factor VIII or IX activity. Individuals with less than 1% of normal factor VIII or IX activity have severe disease characterized by frequent spontaneous bleeding events in joints (hemarthrosis) and soft tissues and by profuse hemorrhage with trauma or surgery. Spontaneous bleeds are uncommon with mild deficiencies (>5% normal activity); however, excessive bleeding still can occur with trauma or surgery. A moderate clinical course is associated with factor VIII or IX levels between 1 and 5%. Approximately 60% of all cases of hemophilia A are clinically severe, whereas only 20 to 45% of cases of hemophilia B are severe.

Severe hemophilia typically is suspected and diagnosed during infancy in the absence of a family history. Although the trauma of uncomplicated childbirth (vaginal or cesarean section) rarely produces intracranial hemorrhage, prolonged labor, forceps delivery, and the use of vacuum extraction are major risk factors. Circumcision within days after birth is accompanied by excessive bleeding in fewer than half of severely affected boys. The first spontaneous hemarthrosis in severely affected hemophiliacs usually occurs between 12 and 18 months of age, when ambulation begins, and in moderately affected individuals it occurs at about 2 to 5 years of age. The knees are the most prominent sites of spontaneous bleeds, followed by the elbows, ankles, shoulders, and hips; wrists are less commonly involved.

Acute hemarthroses (Fig. 180–1) originate from the subsynovial venous plexus underlying the joint capsule and produce a tingling or burning sensation, followed by the onset of intense pain and swelling. On physical examination, the joint is swollen, hot, and tender to palpation, with erythema of the overlying skin. Joint mobility is compromised by pain and stiffness, and the joint usually is maintained in a flexed position. Replacement of the deficient clotting factor to normal hemostatic levels rapidly reverses the pain. Swelling and joint immobility improve as the intra-articular hematoma resolves. Intra-articular needle aspiration of fresh blood is not recommended because of the risk of introducing infection. Short courses of oral corticosteroids may be helpful to reduce the acute joint symptoms in children but rarely are used in adults.

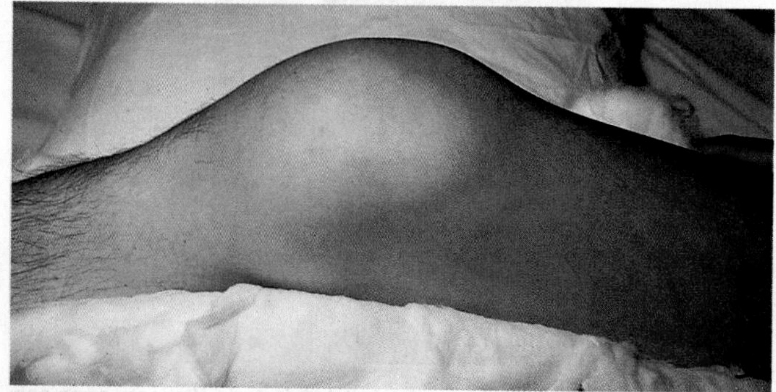

FIGURE 180–1 • Acute hemarthrosis of the knee is a common complication of hemophilia. It may be confused with acute infection unless the patient's coagulation disorder is known, because the knee is hot, red, swollen, and painful. (From Forbes CD, Jackson WF: Color Atlas and Text of Clinical Medicine, 3rd ed. London, Mosby, 2003, with permission.)

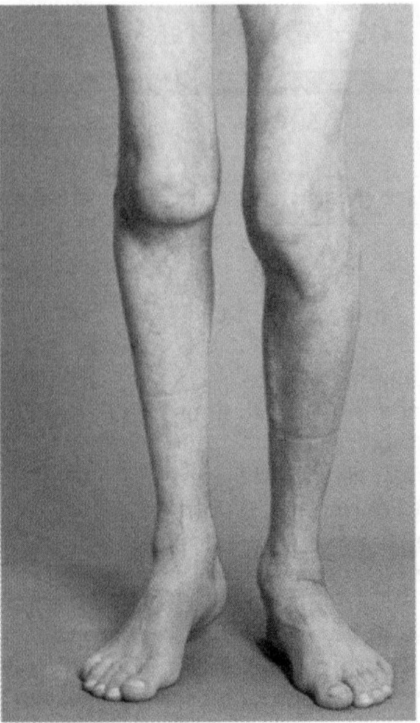

FIGURE 180–2 • Severe chronic arthritis in hemophilia. The knee is the most commonly affected joint. Both knees are severely deranged in this patient. Note that he is unable to stand with both feet flat on the floor. (From Forbes CD, Jackson WF: Color Atlas and Text of Clinical Medicine, 3rd ed. London, Mosby, 2003, with permission.)

Recurrent or untreated bleeds result in chronic synovial hypertrophy and eventually damage to the underlying cartilage, with subsequent subchondral bone cyst formation, bony erosion, and flexion contractures. The intra-articular iron deposited in hemarthroses may activate oncogenes, which subsequently stimulate synovial proliferation. Abnormal mechanical forces from weight bearing can produce subluxation, misalignment, loss of mobility, and permanent deformities of the lower extremities (Fig. 180–2). These changes are accompanied by chronic pain, swelling, and arthritis. Plain radiographs and clinical examination of chronic hemarthroses often underestimate the extent of bone and joint damage; serial magnetic resonance imaging (MRI) appears to be the most sensitive and specific means of detecting and monitoring early and progressive disease.

Intramuscular hematomas account for about 30% of hemophilia-related bleeding events and are rarely life-threatening. They usually are precipitated by physical or iatrogenic trauma (i.e., after intramuscular injection of vaccines or medications) and can compromise sensory and motor function and arterial circulation if they entrap and compress vital structures in closed fascial compartments. Retroperitoneal hematomas may be confused clinically with appendicitis or hip bleeds. Unless these bleeding episodes are treated immediately and aggressively, permanent anatomic deformities, such as flexion contractures and pseudotumors (expanding hematomas that erode and destroy adjacent skeletal structures), may occur. Bleeding from mucous membranes is very common and may be exaggerated by the degradation of fibrin clots by proteolytic enzymes contained in secretions. Bleeding involving the tongue or the retropharyngeal space can rapidly produce life-threatening compromise of the airways. Gastrointestinal hemorrhages typically originate from anatomic lesions proximal to the ligament of Treitz and can be exacerbated by esophageal varices secondary to cirrhosis and portal hypertension or by the use of nonsteroidal anti-inflammatory drugs (NSAIDs) for the treatment of hemarthroses. Spontaneous bleeding in the genitourinary tract secondary to hemophilia is a diagnosis of exclusion after renal stones and infection are ruled out. Ureteral blood clots produce renal colic, which may be confused with nephrolithiasis and may be worsened by the use of antifibrinolytic agents. Ninety percent of hemophiliacs experience at least one episode of gross hematuria or hemospermia.

Intracranial bleeds occur in 10% of patients, usually are induced by trauma, and are fatal in 30% of the cases. The risk of development of an intracranial hemorrhage is approximately 2% per year. Neuromuscular defects, seizure disorders, and intellectual deficits may ensue.

Diagnosis

The diagnosis of hemophilia in infancy is confirmed by detection of significantly reduced factor VIII or IX activities in the plasma of male babies born into families known to be affected by hemophilia or of male children who present with excessive bruising or bleeding at the time of circumcision, when intramuscular injections of immunizing vaccinations are administered, or after trauma during the toddler years. Hemarthrosis, the most common cause of morbidity in severe hemophilia, is not prevalent in pretoddler years. The diagnosis of mild hemophilia B in the neonate may be confounded by the fact that factor IX activity may be decreased substantially in normal infants owing to reduced hepatic synthesis of vitamin K–dependent proteins by an immature liver. Newborns without hemophilia have reduced levels of factor IX (to approximately 40% of normal), and there is a gradual rise during the first year of life into the low-normal adult range. Prematurity is associated with even lower factor IX levels due to the immaturity of the liver. Evaluation of suspected hemophilia in a female should exclude von Willebrand's disease (vWD) and its variants (e.g., type 2 Normandy), as well as the rare occurrence of a normal male karyotype associated with testicular feminization. Molecular genetic testing may be useful to confirm suspected hemophilia in any patient with low circulating levels of factor VIII or factor IX.

Treatment

Rx

Reversal and prevention of acute bleeding events in hemophilia A and B are based on replacement of the missing or deficient clotting factor protein to restore adequate hemostasis (Table 180–1). The morbidity, mortality, and overall cost of care for individuals with hemophilia are reduced significantly if care is provided by comprehensive hemophilia centers, where the multispecialty expertise, specialized coagulation laboratory, and diagnostic capabilities exist to coordinate and monitor specific patient needs.

Replacement guidelines (Table 180–2) are intended to achieve plasma levels of factor VIII and IX activity of 25 to 30% for minor spontaneous or traumatic bleeds (e.g., hemarthroses, persistent hematuria), at least 50% clotting factor activity for the treatment or prevention of severe bleeds (e.g., major dental surgery, maintenance replacement therapy after major surgery or trauma), and 80 to 100% activity for any life-threatening or limb-threatening hemorrhagic event (e.g., major surgery, trauma). After major trauma or if visceral or intracranial bleeding is suspected, replacement therapy adequate to achieve 100% clotting factor activity should be administered before diagnostic procedures are initiated. Although replacement dosing is often empiric, plasma factor VIII activity increases about 2% (0.02 IU/mL) for each unit of factor VIII administered per kilogram of body weight, , and factor IX activity increases about 1% (0.01 IU/mL) for each unit of factor IX administered per kilogram of body weight. The initial dose of factor IX diffuses into the extravascular space and binds to endothelial cell surfaces to a much greater degree than is observed with factor VIII. A 70-kg individual with severe hemophilia A or B (factor VIII or IX activity <1% of normal) who requires replacement to 100% activity for major surgery initially should receive 3500 IU of factor VIII or 7000 IU of factor IX concentrate. The circulating kinetics of factors VIII and IX require subsequent dosing every 8 to 12 hours and every 18 to 24 hours, respectively, and dosing should be individualized according to the peak recovery increment within 15 to 30 minutes after bolus infusion as well as trough activity levels. The frequency of repeat dosing also is determined by the rapidity of pain relief, recovery of joint function, and resolution of active bleeding. Replacement usually is maintained for 10 to 14 days after major surgery to allow for proper wound healing. Bolus dosing typically results in wide fluctuations in clotting factor activity levels and requires frequent laboratory monitoring to avoid suboptimal troughs. Continuous infusion regimens, consisting of 1 to 2 IU of factor VIII or IX concentrate per kilogram per hour after a bolus dose, maintain a plateau level without the necessity for frequent laboratory testing and reduce total concentrate consumption by 30 to 75% in surgical settings.

TABLE 180–1 FDA-APPROVED CLOTTING FACTOR CONCENTRATES FOR HEMOPHILIA A AND B AVAILABLE IN THE UNITED STATES

Virucidal Technique	Type/Name of Product (Manufacturer)	Specific Activity (IU/mg Protein Discounting Albumin)
ULTRAPURE RECOMBINANT FACTOR VIII		
First generation: Immunoaffinity; ion exchange chromatography	Recombinate (Baxter); synthesized in CHO cell lines	>4000
Second generation: Albumin-free final formulation; solvent detergent viral attenuation (TNBP/Triton X100); ion exchange chromatography; nanofiltration	Refacto (Wyeth); B-domain–deleted molecule; synthesized in CHO cell lines; sucrose added as stabilizer	11,200–15,000
Second generation: Albumin-free final formulation; immunoaffinity and ion exchange chromatography; solvent detergent viral attenuation (TNBP/polysorbate 80); ultrafiltration	Kogenate FS (Bayer, Inc.), Helixate FS (Bayer, Inc. for ZLB Behring, Inc.); both synthesized in baby hamster kidney cell lines; sucrose added as a stabilizer	>4000
Third generation: No human or animal protein used in the culture medium or manufacturing process; immunoaffinity and ion exchange chromatography; solvent detergent viral attenuation (TNBP/polysorbate 80)	Advate (Baxter); synthesized in CHO cell lines; trehalose added as a stabilizer	>4000–10,000
ULTRAPURE HUMAN PLASMA–DERIVED FACTOR VIII		
Immunoaffinity chromatography and pasteurization (60° C, 10 hr)	Monoclate P (ZLB Behring, Inc.)	>3000
Immunoaffinity chromatography, solvent detergent (TNBP/Octoxynol 9)	Hemofil M (Baxter), Monarc M (Baxter, distributed by the American Red Cross, which also provides the donor plasma)	>3000
INTERMEDIATE-PURITY AND HIGH-PURITY HUMAN PLASMA–DERIVED FACTOR VIII		
Affinity chromatography, solvent detergent (TNBP and polysorbate 80), and terminal dry heating (80° C, 72 hr)	Alphanate SD (Grifols, Inc.); contains functional vWF protein	50–100 (>400 when corrected for vWF protein content)
Solvent detergent; terminal dry heating (80° C, 72 hr)	Koate-DVI (Bayer, Inc.); contains functional vWF protein	50–100
Pasteurization (heating in solution, 60° C, 10 hr)	Humate-P (ZLB-Behring, Inc.); used predominantly for von Willebrand's disease	1–10
INTERMEDIATE-PURITY PORCINE PLASMA–DERIVED FACTOR VIII		
(TNBP/polysorbate 80)	Hyate-C (Ibsen/Biomeasure, Inc.); porcine plasma–derived factor VIII used for patients with alloantibody or autoantibody factor VIII inhibitor	>50 (available in limited quantities)
ULTRAPURE RECOMBINANT FACTOR IX		
Affinity chromatography and ultrafiltration	BeneFix (Wyeth); CHO cell lines maintained in fetal calf serum-free medium	>200 (albumin free)
VERY HIGHLY PURIFIED PLASMA-DERIVED FACTOR IX		
Dual-affinity chromatography, solvent detergent (TNBP/polysorbate 80), and nanofiltration (viral filter)	AlphaNine SD (Grifols, Inc.)	>200
Monoclonal antibody immunoaffinity chromatography, solvent detergent (sodium thiocyanate), and ultrafiltration	Mononine (ZLB-Behring, Inc.)	>160 (albumin free)
LOW-PURITY PLASMA-DERIVED FACTOR IX COMPLEX CONCENTRATES		
Solvent detergent (TNBP/polysorbate 80)	Profilnine SD (Grifols, Inc.)	<50
Vapor heat (10 hr, 60° C, 1190 mbar pressure plus 1 hr 80° C, 1375 mbar)	Bebulin VH (Baxter)	<50
ACTIVATED PLASMA–DERIVED FACTOR IX COMPLEX CONCENTRATE (RESERVED PRIMARILY FOR PATIENTS WITH ALLOANTIBODY AND AUTOANTIBODY FACTOR VIII AND IX INHIBITOR)		
Vapor heat (10 hr, 60° C, 1190 mbar plus 1 hr, 80° C, 1375 mbar)	FEIBA VH (Baxter)	<50

TABLE 180–1 FDA-APPROVED CLOTTING FACTOR CONCENTRATES FOR HEMOPHILIA A AND B AVAILABLE IN THE UNITED STATES—cont'd

Virucidal Technique	Type/Name of Product (Manufacturer)	Specific Activity (IU/mg Protein Discounting Albumin)
RECOMBINANT FACTOR VIIa (INDICATED FOR PATIENTS WITH ALLOANTIBODY AND AUTOANTIBODY FACTOR VIII AND IX INHIBITOR)		
Affinity chromatography; solvent detergent (TNBP/polysorbate 80)	NovoSeven (Novo Nordisk, Inc.); synthesized in baby hamster kidney cells; solvent (bovine calf serum used in culture medium); albumin-free formulation	50,000 IU/mg

Baxter = Baxter/Immuno, Inc.; CHO = Chinese hamster ovary; FDA = U.S. Food and Drug Administration; TNBP = tri(*n*-butyl)phosphate; vWF = von Willebrand's factor; Wyeth = Wyeth-Ayerst/Genetics Institute.

TABLE 180–2 FDA-APPROVED COAGULATION PROTEINS AND REPLACEMENT THERAPIES AVAILABLE IN THE UNITED STATES

Coagulation Protein Deficiency	Inheritance Pattern	Prevalence	Minimum Hemostatic Level	Replacement Sources
Factor I (fibrinogen):			50–100 mg/dL	Cryoprecipitate/FFP
Afibrinogenemia	Autosomal recessive	Rare (<300 families)		
Dysfibrogenemia	Autosomal dominant or recessive	Rare (>300 variants)		
Factor II (prothrombin)	Autosomal dominant or recessive	Rare (25 kindreds)	30% of normal	FFP, factor IX complex concentrates
Factor V (labile factor)	Autosomal recessive	1 per 1 million births	25% of normal	FFP
Factor VII	Autosomal recessive	1 per 500,000 births	25% of normal	Recombinant factor VIIa (20–30 μg/kg), FFP, factor IX complex concentrates
Factor VIII (antihemophilic factor)	X-linked recessive	1 per 5000 male births	80–100% for surgery/life-threatening bleeds, 50% for serious bleeds, 25–30% for minor bleeds	Factor VIII concentrates (see Table 180–1)
von Willebrand's disease:			>50% vWF antigen and ristocetin cofactor activity	DDAVP for mild to moderate disease (except type 2B; variable response to 2A); cryoprecipitate and FFP (not preferred except in emergencies); factor VIII concentrates, viral attenuated, intermediate purity (preferred for disease unresponsive to DDAVP and for type 3) (see Table 180–1)
Type 1 and 2 variants	Usually autosomal dominant	1% prevalence		
Type 3	Autosomal recessive	1 per 1 million births		
Factor IX (Christmas factor)	X-linked recessive	1 per 30,000 male births	25–50% of normal, depending on extent of bleeding and surgery	Factor IX concentrates; FFP not preferred except in dire emergencies (see Table 180–1)
Factor X (Stuart-Prower factor)	Autosomal recessive	1 per 500,000 births	10–25% of normal	FFP or factor IX complex concentrates
Factor XI (hemophilia C)	Autosomal dominant; severe type is recessive	4% Ashkenazi Jews; 1 per 1 million general population	20–40% of normal	FFP or factor XI concentrate
Factor XII (Hageman factor), prekallikrein, high-molecular-weight kininogen	Autosomal recessive	Not available	No treatment necessary	—
Factor XIII (fibrin stabilizing factor)	Autosomal recessive	1 per 3 million births	5% of normal	FFP, cryoprecipitate, or viral-attenuated factor XIII concentrate

DDAVP = desmopressin; FDA = U.S. Food and Drug Administration; FFP = fresh-frozen plasma; vWF = von Willebrand's factor.

Rx

Because of the potential thrombogenicity associated with repeated administration of prothrombin complex concentrates for replacement of factor IX deficiency, high-purity, plasma-derived, or genetically engineered factor IX concentrates, which lack activated vitamin K–dependent clotting factors, are preferred therapies in hemophilia B.

Cryoprecipitate (the precipitate remaining after fresh-frozen plasma [FFP] is thawed at 4° C) and FFP contain factor VIII, but factor IX is contained only in FFP. However, they are not the optimal replacement products for either hemophilia A or hemophilia B because of their potential to transmit blood-borne pathogens. Plasma-derived clotting factor concentrates are manufactured from the plasma donations pooled from thousands of individual donors and are subjected to various types of viral inactivation techniques. Only lipid-enveloped viruses are susceptible to these procedures, which increases the risk that these products can transmit viruses such as parvovirus B19, hepatitis A, and prions, which have been implicated in variant Creutzfeldt-Jakob disease (vCJD) (Chapter 442). The safety of these products has been enhanced by deferring the inclusion of first-time donor plasma collections from the plasma pool and by implementing more rigorous and specific viral surveillance of "minipools" (16 individual plasma donors) prior to manufacture. Nucleic acid amplification testing is used to detect hepatitis C, West Nile virus, and human immunodeficiency virus (HIV), and polymerase chain reaction (PCR) testing is used to detect parvovirus B19. Hepatitis B surface antigen is also measured. No assay is available to detect vCJD in plasma.

All clotting factor concentrates available in the United States (see Table 180–1), whether plasma derived or genetically engineered, are equally efficacious and are considered extremely safe; none has ever been implicated in the transmission of blood-borne viral pathogens or prions. Newer recombinant factor VIII and IX concentrates are manufactured free of added human or animal proteins in the culture medium or in the final formulation, to eliminate the theoretical risks of transmission of prions or murine viruses.

Hemarthroses

The moderate or severe levels of pain that accompany acute hemarthroses respond to immediate analgesic relief, temporary immobilization, restraint from weight bearing, and clotting factor replacement. Narcotic analgesics, such as codeine (30 to 60 mg up to four times daily) or synthetic derivatives of codeine, should be prescribed alone or combined with doses of acetaminophen that are low enough (<10 g) to avoid hepatic toxicity in patients with chronic hepatitis. Although these medications do not possess significant anti-inflammatory activity, they are preferable to NSAIDs or aspirin, which can exacerbate bleeding complications through their antiplatelet aggregatory effects. Despite its possible arterial hypercoagulable side effects when used in high doses, the cyclooxygenase 2 inhibitor, celecoxib, when used judiciously (100 to 200 mg once or twice daily in patients without sulfonamide allergy, a dose that does not antagonize platelet function in vitro), often provides safe and effective pain relief for the chronic arthritis produced by recurrent hemarthroses. Alternative approaches to analgesia include acupuncture, transdermal nerve stimulation, and hypnosis (Chapter 36); these modalities may reduce narcotic consumption.

Strategies intended to prevent end-stage joint destruction should be initiated at an early age. Synovectomy through open surgery or arthroscopy removes the inflamed tissue and should result in substantially decreased pain and recurrent bleeding. Nonsurgical synovectomy (synoviorthosis), which involves the intra-articular administration of a radioisotope, is particularly useful for high-risk patients and for patients with alloantibody inhibitors against factor VIII or factor IX. Neither synovectomy nor synoviorthosis reverses joint damage, but both procedures may delay its progression. Non–weight-bearing exercises, such as swimming and isometrics, are important to periarticular muscle development and maintenance of joint stability for ambulation. Intractable pain and severe joint destruction secondary to repeated hemorrhage require prosthetic replacement. Chronic ankle pain responds best to open surgical or arthroscopic fixation and fusion (arthrodesis).

Rx

The ultimate strategy to minimize or eliminate progressive joint destruction by recurrent hemarthroses is predicated on the concept of primary prophylaxis—the scheduled administration of clotting factor concentrates two (for factor IX products) or three (for factor VIII replacement) times weekly at doses adequate to maintain trough clotting factor activity levels greater than 1% to 2% of normal. The first and only prospective, randomized clinical trial of primary prophylaxis in young children with severe hemophilia A compared a regimen of every-other-day infusions of factor VIII at 25 IU/kg to prevent hemorrhage (primary prophylaxis) with intensive therapy using more than 3 infusions, totaling more than 80 IU/kg of factor VIII, at the time of each acute joint hemorrhage (on-demand therapy) to minimize joint damage, reverse bleeding, and relieve acute pain. Primary prophylaxis reduced the total number of total bleeds and hemarthroses by up to 90% compared with intensive on-demand therapy. [1] Long-term compliance with primary prophylaxis prevented the development or progression of bone and cartilage damage, as observed by serial MRI studies, and preserved overall joint function. An alternative and potentially more cost-effective approach to primary prophylaxis individualizes the dose of factor VIII replacement therapy and dosing intervals based on the variability of the individual's bleeding pattern. One schema initiates primary prophylaxis with factor VIII at 50 IU/kg weekly and escalates to 30 IU/kg twice weekly if the frequency of bleeding is unacceptable (i.e., four joint/soft tissue bleeds) or if a target joint develops (three bleeds into a single joint over a consecutive 3-month period). If breakthrough bleeding continues, a third escalation dose to 25 IU/kg every other day can be implemented. Primary prophylaxis is facilitated by the placement of a central venous access device.

As obligate recipients of clotting factor replacement products, virtually all hemophiliacs treated before 1985, when techniques for elimination of lipid-enveloped viruses were introduced, have been exposed to hepatitis C virus (HCV), often with multiple genotypes (Chapter 151). Hepatitis G, observed in 15% to 25% of hemophiliacs, is susceptible to current viral attenuation procedures. Hepatitis B virus, also lipid enveloped, is a rare problem for hemophiliacs now because vaccination at an early age is the standard of care. Hepatitis A virus is not lipid coated and was transmitted to a small but significant number of patients through solvent detergent–treated factor VIII and factor IX concentrates in the past; hepatitis A vaccination now should eliminate this risk. Parvovirus B19 seroprevalence approaches 80% in older adult hemophiliacs exposed to plasma-derived products. Hepatitis A and parvovirus B19 have unclear long-term clinical consequences. Nevertheless, their transmission in plasma-derived concentrates symbolizes the vulnerability of hemophiliacs to blood-borne pathogens that escape viral attenuation processes. Cadaver and living-donor liver transplantation (Chapter 158) has improved the survival of hemophiliacs with chronic hepatitis-induced liver failure and cured the coagulopathy, suggesting that the liver is the predominant source of normal synthesis of factors VIII and IX. Liver transplantation may be performed successfully in HIV/HCV-coinfected individuals who have an undetectable HIV viral titer while receiving highly active antiretroviral therapy.

Ancillary and Other Therapies

Ancillary treatment strategies for hemophilias include the use of antifibrinolytic agents, such as ε-aminocaproic acid (1 to 2 g PO up to four times daily) or tranexamic acid (3 or 4 g PO daily in divided doses), to minimize mucous membrane bleeding and the application of fibrin glues to bleeding sites. Desmopressin (DDAVP [Stimate] may be administered by nasal insufflation 2 hours before a scheduled surgical procedure (one spray per nostril, to provide a total dose of 300 μg; or, in patients weighing less than 50 kg, 150 μg administered as a single spray); or DDAVP may be administered intravenously (dissolved in 50 mL normal saline) over 20 minutes at a dose of 0.3 μg/kg. DDAVP is useful in patients with mild hemophilia A, inasmuch as an adequate incremental rise in factor VIII activity can circumvent the use of clotting factor concentrates. Repeated administration of DDAVP (intravenously or by intranasal spray) can be complicated by tachyphylaxis, hyponatremic seizures, and angina.

Rx

Alloantibody Inhibitors to Factors VIII and IX

Alloantibodies usually are detected in childhood after a median of 9 to 12 consecutive days of exposure to clotting factor. These inhibitors occur with an increased incidence in sibships; they are more common in individuals with large, multidomain factor VIII and factor IX gene deletions; and they manifest a racial predilection. The incidence of factor VIII alloantibodies is 24 to 52%, with an increased frequency in blacks and Hispanics. Factor IX alloantibodies are observed with a 1.5% to 3% incidence and predominate among Scandinavians. Patients with factor IX inhibitor seem to be susceptible to anaphylaxis and the development of nephrotic syndrome with subsequent exposure to sources of factor IX.

Alloantibody inhibitors arise predominantly in individuals with severe congenital deficiencies of factor VIII or IX, and they are suspected when replacement therapy does not provide the usual immediate relief in bleeding symptoms. These immunoglobulin G (IgG) antibodies, usually IgG4 subclass, completely neutralize clotting factor activity; no or reduced increments in factor VIII or IX levels are observed after the administration of bolus doses of concentrate. These inhibitors are time and temperature dependent. The strength of the inhibitor is quantitated in Bethesda units (BU); 1 BU is defined arbitrarily as the amount of inhibitor that neutralizes 50% of the specific clotting factor activity in normal plasma. Patients with high-titer inhibitor, or "high responders," have greater than 5 BU, and an anamnestic antibody enhancement usually develops 5 to 7 days after subsequent exposure to the antigenic clotting factor protein. Patients with low-titer inhibitor (i.e., ≤5 BU) are "low responders" and do not manifest anamnesis. Low-titer inhibitors, in contrast to the high-titer situation, can be overwhelmed easily by large amounts of human factor VIII or factor IX concentrate, usually three to four times the usual dose.

Treatment of patients with high-titer inhibitors against factor VIII or factor IX is complicated by the observation that no single approach is uniformly successful. Bypassing agents are available to treat bleeding episodes (see Table 180–1); specifically, the activated prothrombin complex concentrate FEIBA VH (50 to 100 IU/kg every 8 hours) and recombinant factor VIIa (rFVIIa; 90 μ/kg every 3 hours) may be administered as indicated until bleeding is controlled. In congenital hemophilia A patients with inhibitors, one dose of FEIBA VH or two doses of rFVIIa controlled hemarthrosis episodes 81 and 79% of the time, respectively, in patients with congenital hemophilia A and alloantibody inhibitors. 1 The activated and unactivated prothrombin complex concentrates contain activated vitamin K–dependent clotting factors that "bypass" the intrinsic pathway inhibitor. As a result, repeated administration over a short time frame is complicated by potential thrombogenicity, and the aPTT and clotting factor assays are useless monitors of adequate hemostasis. The availability of porcine plasma–derived factor VIII concentrate is severely limited, but at doses between 50 and 100 U/kg it has an 80% excellent or good response rate. Factor VIII activity can be measured after its administration and provides objective laboratory evidence of hemostasis. This product is nonthrombogenic, but anamnestic immune responses can result in increased antibody titers against porcine and human factor VIII. A recombinant form of porcine factor VIII concentrate is currently in clinical trials and may supplant the plasma formulation in the future. Recombinant factor VIIa is an additional effective therapy in patients with high-titer inhibitors, particularly those who have factor IX alloantibodies and who experience anaphylactic reactions or the nephrotic syndrome after exposure to factor IX–containing replacement products or FFP.

Immune tolerance induction regimens are often useful to eradicate alloantibody inhibitors. Consisting of daily administration of factor VIII or IX concentrates, this regimen is essentially a desensitization process with a 68% success rate. Young age, low-titer inhibitor, and immediate initiation after detection of the inhibitor increase the likelihood of success. After tolerance has been achieved, maintenance prophylaxis with factor VIII or IX concentrate administered two to three times weekly (20 to 30 IU/kg) is necessary.

Prevention

Carrier Detection and Prenatal Diagnosis

Carrier detection and prenatal diagnosis have become technically feasible, very sensitive, and widely available, but their application is influenced by ethical, cultural, religious, economic, educational, and personal considerations. For instance, carrier detection is particularly useful to identify women who themselves may be at risk for hemorrhagic complications during the delivery process, and it can identify male offspring who will be particularly vulnerable to develop intracerebral bleeds at birth. Alternatively, these techniques can provide important information for making difficult reproductive decisions. Patients may decide to accept the 50% likelihood that any male child of a confirmed carrier of hemophilia A or B will be affected; to abstain from pregnancy and/or to adopt; to determine the sex of the fetus and terminate pregnancy if an affected male child is identified; or to embark on in vitro fertilization with subsequent uterine transfer of only harvested female embryos (as confirmed by fluorescent in situ hybridization) or genetically unaffected male and female embryos (as determined by PCR-based techniques for specific hemophilia gene mutations). Genetic counseling and testing have not resulted in increased rates of termination of pregnancy for hemophilia in developed countries, where the availability of safe and effective replacement products is ubiquitous and offers the potential of an almost normal lifespan with greatly reduced disability. In economically developing nations with limited health resources, however, hemophiliacs do not receive timely or adequate treatment and often die in childhood.

The phenotypic identification of obligate female carriers of hemophilia, who are related to affected males, can be accomplished with 90% accuracy by measuring low levels of factor IX activity or relatively low factor VIII coagulant activity compared with levels of von Willebrand's factor antigen (vWF : Ag). Coagulation activity assays used for the phenotypic identification of carriers or affected males lose their sensitivity when large populations are screened for random mutations and cannot be applied easily to fetal blood specimens or amniotic fluid, which are usually contaminated by thromboplastic materials that provide spuriously high clotting factor activity results. In addition, in the case of hemophilia B, the presence of cross-reactive factor IX antigen may confound the ability to predict carrier status or fetal involvement. Genotypic analysis for specific mutations is the most accurate and reliable means of prenatal detection and carrier testing for the hemophilias. More than 150 heterogeneous point mutations of the factor VIII gene (comprising 186 kb with 26 exons) have been associated with development of hemophilia A, necessitating linkage analysis employing DNA polymorphic markers in assays based on restriction fragment length polymorphism. Increased accuracy is achieved if the specific gene defect is known and genetic material is available from the propositus and the carrier. PCR amplification of DNA and denaturing gradient gel electrophoresis analysis are useful for detection of the intron 22 inversion, which is associated with half of the cases of severe hemophilia A. The molecular basis of hemophilia B is even more heterogeneous than that of hemophilia A, with several hundred causative mutations, predominantly single nucleotide polymorphisms with ethnic variation but no frequent mutation type, reported in this considerably smaller gene comprising 34 kb, 8 exons, and 7 introns. A listing of the mutations that have been characterized to cause the hemophilias can be accessed via the Human Gene Mutation Database *(www.hgmd.org)*, through HAMSTeRS (The Haemophilia A Mutation, Structure, Test, and Resource Site) at *http://europium.csc.mrc.ac.uk*, and the Haemophilia B Mutation Database at *www.kcl.ac.uk/ip/petergreen/haemBdatabase.html* (all accessed August 24, 2006).

Prognosis

The life expectancy of severe hemophiliacs approaches 65 years when HIV-related issues are excluded. The age-matched death rate of hemophiliacs who are HIV seropositive is 5 times greater than that of the normal population, 33 times greater for hemophiliacs with frank AIDS, and 2.4 times greater for those coinfected with hepatitis C. HIV is currently responsible for more than 55% of all hemophilia-related deaths. In contrast, the lifetime risk of intracranial hemorrhage is 2 to 8%. Approximately one third of all hemophiliacs between the ages of 21 and 60 years are HIV infected, with infection more common among those with hemophilia A. The availability of anti-HIV protease inhibitors (Chapter 412) has prolonged the HIV disease-free survival time of infected hemophiliacs. Those coinfected with hepatitis C have a poorer prognosis, however, despite the initiation of pegylated interferon-α and ribavirin therapy (Chapter 152). The progression of hepatitis C can be exacerbated by alcohol and by hepatotoxic medications prescribed for prophylaxis of opportunistic infections and chronic pain (e.g., large doses of acetaminophen). Life expectancy is related to the severity of hemophilia, with the mortality rate of severely affected patients being four to six times greater than that of patients with mild deficiencies. With timely treatment, there is no increased mortality associated with the presence of alloantibody inhibitors. Problems with growth and development are exaggerated in HIV-infected boys, with increased cortical atrophy on magnetic resonance imaging (15% in HIV-positive vs. 6.5% in HIV-negative boys) and delayed growth velocity in adolescence. IQ does not seem to be affected by either HIV or hemophilia.

Future Directions

Gene Therapy for Hemophilia A and B

The hereditary hemophilias are model diseases for gene therapy, because they are caused by specific, well-defined gene mutations; a small incremental rise in clotting factor synthesis can lead to substantially improved treatment and quality of life; and inadvertent overexpression by successful gene transfer would not be detrimental. Successful gene transfer techniques have been developed to provide long-term therapeutic benefits in hemophilic mice and dog models, but not thus far in humans, probably because current gene delivery systems and their viral vectors have induced antibodies that suppress long-term expression of clotting factor activity.

Acquired Hemophilias

Epidemiology and Pathobiology

Autoantibody inhibitors can occur spontaneously in individuals with previously normal hemostasis (nonhemophiliacs). Although approximately 50% of patients have no obvious underlying cause, the remainder of cases are associated with autoimmune diseases, lymphoproliferative disorders, idiosyncratic drug associations, and pregnancy.

Clinical Manifestations and Diagnosis

Patients typically have massive hemorrhagic events, usually much more severe than events produced by alloantibodies in patients with congenital hemophilia. The laboratory expression of autoantibodies is similar to that of alloantibodies, except that clotting factor activity is not completely neutralized. Residual clotting factor activities between 3% and 20% of normal frequently are observed in patients with autoantibodies.

Treatment

Rx

The same principles of replacement therapy for alloantibodies also apply to these acquired autoantibody inhibitors. Porcine factor VIII concentrate is particularly useful in acquired hemophilia A, because little cross-reactivity usually occurs even with extremely high titers of anti–human factor VIII antibodies. Because of its limited availability, clinical studies are underway with genetically engineered forms of this protein. Immunosuppressive therapy with corticosteroids (prednisone, 1 mg/kg PO daily for 3 weeks) or cytotoxic agents (such as cyclophosphamide, 150 mg daily PO or 500 to 750 mg/m^2 IV bolus every 3 to 4 weeks, with dose titration or delays depending on the development of cytopenias), is typically required to suppress the inhibitor and is usually continued until the autoantibody inhibitor has disappeared. Whether addition of cytotoxic agents improves outcome at 2 years, however, is unclear. Administration of anti-CD20 antibody (rituximab, 375 mg/m^2 IV weekly for 4 weeks) appears promising for the long-term eradication of autoantibody inhibitors, although no randomized controlled studies have been performed. There are also anecdotal cases of successful rituximab eradication of alloantibody inhibitors. High-dose intravenous gamma globulin may be a useful adjunctive therapy. Immune tolerance induction regimens that combine alkylating agents, daily administration of clotting factor concentrate, and high-dose corticosteroids have been successful in eradicating autoantibody inhibitors. If inhibitor-related hemorrhage is refractory to administration of the bypassing clotting factor agents, the initiation of intense extracorporeal plasmapheresis over a staphylococcal protein A column may remove enough neutralizing IgG alloantibody or autoantibody to facilitate successful hemostasis after replacement therapy.

Prognosis

Several large series of patients with acquired hemophilia have revealed a substantial mortality rate, ranging from 15 to 25%, which is considerably higher than that observed with alloantibody factor VIII inhibitors. A large meta-analysis indicated that overall survival in acquired hemophilia was influenced primarily by achievement of a complete remission; age younger than 65 years at diagnosis; and related diseases (malignancy versus postpartum versus others). Fifteen percent of the deaths were associated with sepsis, and 71% of these patients had developed cyclophosphamide-induced neutropenia. Hemorrhagic complications, which were the primary cause of death, could be reduced if the inhibitor could be eradicated. Of note, complete remission was observed in 89% of cyclophosphamide-treated individuals, compared with 70% of those treated with corticosteroids alone and 41% of those who received no treatment.

Hereditary von Willebrand's Disease

Definition

The most common bleeding disorder is vWD, an autosomal dominantly inherited hemorrhagic disease that affects both sexes, with a prevalence of 1 to 3% of the population and no ethnic predominance. Homozygous patients are rare and carry a recessive mutant gene.

Pathobiology

Normal vWF is a large, multimeric glycoprotein product of the vWF gene, located on chromosome 12. The protein consists of 220,000-D monomeric subunits, and the fully processed protein may reach a total molecular weight of 20 million D, with its platelet agglutination properties mediated predominantly by the highest-molecular-weight multimers. The phenotypic classification of vWD recognizes three major types of the disease based on the multimeric structure and function of the vWF protein (Table 180–3).

Type 1 vWD accounts for 75 to 80% of patients and is inherited predominantly via an autosomal dominant mode; a qualitative defect is present in which the vWF structure is normal but vWF:Ag and activity are reduced. Defects in synthesis or secretion from the endothelial cell or megakaryocyte or increased intravascular clearance, probably independent of proteolysis by the metalloprotease ADAMTS-13 (a disintegrin and metalloprotease with thrombospondin, also known as von Willebrand factor cleaving protease), induce the type 1 vWD phenotype. However, several vWF gene mutations produce increased intracellular retention (i.e., decreased secretion) or enhanced plasma clearance without altering the structure of vWF.

Type 2 vWD includes approximately 20% of vWD patients, is inherited in either a dominant or a recessive pattern, and is characterized by qualitative and quantitative abnormalities in the vWF protein. Further subclassification is based on multimeric structure and responses in the ristocetin-induced platelet aggregation (RIPA) assay. Defects in vWF multimeric assembly and/or enhanced ADAMTS-13–mediated proteolytic degradation of vWF account for many of these qualitatively abnormal molecules. Up to 30 variants have been described, each with unique aberrations in vWF multimer structure. In type 2A, the most common variant, there is loss of the largest and intermediate-sized multimers, whereas type 2B lacks only the largest vWF multimers. The multimeric patterns in type 2A may result from defective synthesis of the vWF protein or increased susceptibility of vWF to proteolysis in vivo. In type 2B, the highest-molecular-weight multimers of vWF are adsorbed preferentially and with abnormally high affinity to the glycoprotein Ib receptor binding site on the platelet membrane surface. Alternatively, a structural defect in the glycoprotein Ib platelet receptor binding site for

TABLE 180–3 PATTERNS OF VON WILLEBRAND'S DISEASE

Type	vWF:AG/vWF:RCOF	RIPA	RIPA–Low Dose	Multimeric Pattern
1 (classic)	↓/↓	±↓	Absent	Uniform ↓ in all multimers
2 (variant)				
2A	↓/↓↓↓	↓↓	Absent	↓ in large and intermediate multimers
2B	±↓/±↓	Normal	Increased	↓ in large multimers
2N (Normandy)	Normal/normal	Normal	↓	Normal
Platelet type	±↓/±↓	±↑	Increased with cryoprecipitate	↓in large multimers
3 (Homozygote or compound heterozygote)	Absent/absent	Absent	Absent	Absent

↓, reduced; ±↓, more or less reduced; ↓↓↓, greatly reduced; RIPA = ristocetin-induced platelet aggregation; vWF:Ag = von Willebrand's factor antigen; vWF:RCoF = von Willebrand's factor ristocetin cofactor activity.

vWF can produce a multimeric pattern similar to that of type 2B by virtue of its preferential adsorption of the highest-molecular-weight multimers from normal vWF in the circulation. This latter variant is designated *platelet-type pseudo-vWD.* Type 2N (Normandy) is an unusual variant that resembles hemophilia A, although it is inherited in an autosomal dominant pattern. The defective vWF protein is normal from functional and multimeric perspectives but lacks an intact binding site for factor VIII. Unbound factor VIII is cleared from the circulation with a short half-life.

Type 3 vWD is an exceedingly rare variant that occurs in 1 of every 1 million individuals. It is characterized by almost complete absence of circulating vWF.

Clinical Manifestations

Most patients with vWD have mild disease that may go undiagnosed until trauma or surgery occurs. Symptomatic individuals manifest easy bruisability and mucosal surface bleeding, including epistaxis and gastrointestinal hemorrhage. Menorrhagia affects 50 to 75% of affected women and may be the initial symptom. These symptoms are consistent with platelet-based defects and reflect the crucial role of vWF protein in mediating platelet-platelet and platelet–subendothelial matrix interactions in the process of vascular plug formation and primary hemostasis. The use of aspirin or NSAIDs with anti–platelet aggregation effects may exacerbate the symptoms. Deep subcutaneous and intramuscular bleeds, hemarthroses, and intracranial hemorrhages are unusual in vWD except in the rare type 3 variant. The factor VIII deficiency is caused by to the absence of vWF protein, which normally complexes with factor VIII, delivers it to sites of ongoing coagulation, and prevents its clearance from the circulation.

Diagnosis

Because the physical examination usually reveals nonspecific evidence of easy bruising and bleeding, the diagnosis of vWD depends in large part on laboratory findings that measure the bleeding time, factor VIII activity, vWF:Ag level, and vWF activity or ristocetin cofactor activity (vWF:RCoF).

The bleeding time in patients with vWD is variably prolonged and may be influenced by the thrombocytopenia associated with vWD type 2B. The test is labor intensive and performer dependent. Although it is used to diagnose vWD, it is less useful as a predictor of adequate hemostasis after replacement therapy. The platelet function analyzer (PFA-100; Dade-Behring, Liederbach, Germany) provides a global perspective of vWF and platelet function and may substitute for bleeding time in the diagnosis of vWD; however, both bleeding time and the PFA-100 results are relatively insensitive for the diagnosis of vWD, particularly in the absence of other, more specific assays and a significant medical history, and they do not always correlate with bleeding propensity after replacement therapy. The aPTT is also variably prolonged because of concurrent factor VIII deficiency, but a normal aPTT does not exclude the diagnosis of vWD.

The vWF activity assay or vWF:RCoF is the most specific and sensitive test for vWF function but may be only slightly decreased in mild vWD. The vWF:Ag assay measures the immunologic expression of vWF and usually is performed via electroimmunoassay or enzyme-linked immunosorbent assay (ELISA). It is reduced slightly in mild vWD and its variants and is virtually absent in type 3. Because these assays are sensitive to the molecular mass of vWF, vWF:RCoF activity is discordantly low as a result of a low-normal or slightly reduced vWF:Ag level in the type 2 variants of vWD. Both vWF:RCoF and vWF:Ag are acute phase reactants; they are increased by exercise, stress, pregnancy, oral contraceptives, and liver disease and are decreased with hypothyroidism and in the presence of blood group O. vWD subtypes can be analyzed by in vitro platelet aggregation assays in which the patient's platelet-rich plasma is activated by the addition of standard and low concentrations of ristocetin or cryoprecipitate. Types 1 and 3 vWF show mild or marked hyporesponsiveness to the standard concentration of ristocetin, whereas type 2B shows hyperaggregation with half-standard concentrations of ristocetin. Platelet-type pseudo-vWD can be differentiated from type 2B by observing spontaneous platelet agglutination after the addition of cryoprecipitate.

Gene-based assays are the most specific means of diagnosing vWF variants via restriction enzyme mapping of the vWF gene. These assays are available predominantly through research laboratories and should be obtained if the routine laboratory tests for vWF activity are equivocal. Type 3 vWF exhibits large deletions, whereas the other types are caused by variable point mutation defects. Type 2N has defects in the functional domain coding for vWF binding to factor VIII.

Treatment

The goals of therapy for vWD consist of correcting the deficiencies in vWF protein activity to greater than 50% of normal and in factor VIII activity to levels appropriate for the clinical situation. Although cryoprecipitate is licensed by the U.S. Food and Drug Administration (FDA) for prophylaxis or treatment of vWD-related bleeding complications, the lack of viral safety relegates its use exclusively to emergency circumstances when no other options are readily available. Replacement therapy with viral-attenuated, intermediate-purity or high-purity factor VIII concentrates containing an incomplete complement of high-molecular-weight multimers of vWF (e.g., Humate-P, Koate-DVI, Alphanate SD) is preferred and should be reserved for patients with type 1 and 2A variants unresponsive to DDAVP and for those with type 2B and type 3 diseases. These products also are indicated for the 2N variant and provide a source of normal vWF to complex with the normal intrinsic factor VIII. Dosing of these concentrates for vWD is calculated according to ristocetin cofactor units. On-demand IV bolus administration (60 RCoF U/kg) and continuous infusion regimens have been used successfully. An ultra-high-purity, plasma-derived vWF concentrate, which is virtually devoid of FVIII:C, is available in France and corrects deficient vWF:Ag and vWF:RCoF activity as efficiently as do products that contain FVIII:C; however, there is a 6- to 10-hour delay in the recovery of endogenous FVIII:C activity levels to adequate hemostatic ranges. This product has limited value to treat acute severe bleeds or to provide hemostasis for emergent surgery in patients

Rx

with type 3 vWD, who require concurrent additional therapy with sources of factor VIII:C. The proportion of high-molecular-weight multimers, which are restored after the administration of these replacement products, is variable and correlates poorly with clinical efficacy. Excellent to good hemostatic responses are achieved in more than 90% of surgeries and bleeding episodes after administration of one or two doses of any of these products.

Any of these plasma-derived concentrates may precipitate thrombotic complications or exacerbate the thrombocytopenia in patients with vWD variant 2B or platelet-type pseudo-vWD. These individuals should receive transfusions with normal platelets that possess glycoprotein Ib/IX complexes with normal vWF affinity. Otherwise, DDAVP (0.3 μg/kg in 50 mL of normal saline infused over 20 minutes or intranasally at 150 μg per nostril for adults) is the recommended treatment and eliminates potential exposure to blood-borne pathogens.

The adjunctive use of antifibrinolytic agents, such as ε-aminocaproic acid (1 to 2 g PO up to four times daily) or tranexamic acid (3 or 4 grams PO daily in divided doses), is helpful after DDAVP therapy for bleeds. These agents should not be used routinely for renal bleeds or menorrhagia.

The following important caveats for vWD treatment should be considered: (1) A prolonged bleeding time does not need to be normalized to achieve adequate hemostasis after replacement therapy. Correction of vWF and factor VIII activity suffices and correlates closely with the clinical risk of bleeding. (2) DDAVP administration should be avoided in most individuals with type 2B variant vWD. Their thrombocytopenia may worsen, because DDAVP induces the release of abnormal vWF into the circulation, with additional in vivo platelet agglutination/aggregation. (3) Individuals with variant type 2N may not manifest a sustained factor VIII response to DDAVP, because the vWF released cannot complex with the simultaneously released factor VIII and prevent its clearance from the circulation. (4) Individuals who respond adequately to intravenously administered DDAVP may not respond adequately to the intranasal DDAVP preparation. Ideally, patients should be tested for their responses *before* treatment is needed for surgery. (5) Pregnant women with type 2B variant vWD may experience an exacerbation of thrombocytopenia as pregnancy progresses. Levels of the abnormal vWF increase as estrogen levels increase. (6) Free water intake, whether intravenous or by mouth, should be severely restricted for 4 to 6 hours after DDAVP administration to minimize the risk of hyponatremia and seizures. (7) vWD is associated clinically with Osler-Weber-Rendu syndrome (hereditary hemorrhagic telangiectasia), so gastrointestinal bleeding may occur. (8) Replacement therapy in type 3 vWD occasionally may precipitate the formation of alloantibody inhibitors that neutralize vWF activity. Recombinant factor VIIa concentrate is an effective alternative replacement product for vWF patients with alloantibody inhibitor.

Prognosis

In Western countries, the mortality rate for vWD approaches zero because of the ability to diagnose the disease and to treat it safely and effectively with a variety of replacement products.

Acquired von Willebrand's Disease

Acquired vWD is a rare condition that usually occurs as a complication of autoimmune, myeloproliferative, or lymphoproliferative disorders. The acquired vWD associated with neuroblastoma is secondary to proteolysis of vWF by tumor-secreted hyaluronidase. Abnormal vWF multimeric composition is a hallmark of these syndromes. vWF replacement regimens in this condition are similar to those for congenital vWD, but responses are unpredictable. In some patients with refractory bleeding, intravenous gamma globulin (IVIG, 1 g/kg), recombinant activated factor VII concentrate (90 μg/kg), plasmapheresis with albumin exchange, corticosteroids (1 mg/kg/day), alkylating agents, and rituximab (375 mg/m^2 weekly for 4 doses) have been initiated to enhance recovery of adequate hemostasis.

Factor XI Deficiency (Hemophilia C)

Epidemiology

Factor XI deficiency occurs at a prevalence of 1 per 1 million in the general population and 1 per 500 births in Ashkenazi Jewish families. Factor XI is the only component of the contact phase system (factor XII, prekallikrein, and high-molecular-weight kininogen) of the intrinsic pathway of coagulation that is associated with excessive bleeding complications when a deficient state exists.

Pathobiology

Factor XI deficiency is predominantly an autosomal recessive trait, although some mutations may have a dominant transmission pattern. The factor XI gene *(FXI)* is located on chromosome 4, and the Glu117stop mutation in *FXI* is the most common cause of factor XI deficiency, secondary to poor secretion/stability of the truncated protein or decreased levels of messenger RNA. To date, 65 mutations of *FXI* have been identified in factor XI–deficient patients (see *www.FactorXI.org*), but close correlation between hemorrhagic phenotype and genotype is lacking. In Ashkenazi Jewish individuals, two predominant gene mutations occur with equal frequency and are designated type II (a stop codon in exon 5) and type III (a single base defect in exon 9). The most severe clinical disease is observed in patients homozygous for type II, who usually have less than 1% factor XI activity. Homozygous type III individuals also manifest severe symptoms, but typically less severe than those of type II patients, and have slightly higher factor XI levels of about 10 to 20%. Compound heterozygotes, type II/III, make up the bulk of factor XI–deficient patients; they have clinically mild disease, with factor XI levels between 30 and 50%. Genotypic identification of affected patients is determined practically by measuring factor XI levels rather than by defining the specific gene defect.

Clinical Manifestations

The clinical bleeding tendencies in factor XI deficiency are less severe than those observed in severe hemophilia A or B and are not correlated with the extent of the deficiency. Most individuals with less than 20% of normal factor XI activity experience excessive bleeding after trauma or surgery; however, a few do not bleed. In contrast, bleeding has been observed in approximately 35 to 50% of mildly affected patients with factor XI levels between 20 and 50% of normal. Spontaneous hemorrhagic episodes, hemarthroses, and intramuscular and intracerebral bleeds are unusual; traumatic and surgical bleeds typically involve the mucous membranes. Patients undergoing tonsillectomy, prostatectomy, or dental extraction are at highest risk for bleeding unless replacement therapy is administered. Women may experience significant menorrhagia. Patients with mild factor XI deficiency and coincident mild vWD have an increased risk of bleeding.

Diagnosis

Factor XI deficiency is diagnosed in the laboratory by a prolonged aPTT, normal PT, and decreased factor XI activity ascertained in a specific quantitative clotting assay (normal range, 60 to 130%).

Treatment

FFP remains the mainstay for factor XI replacement (15 to 20 mL/kg); however, it is not viral inactivated. A minimum factor XI level of 40% is essential for major bleeds and major surgery. A viral-inactivated factor XI concentrate is not available in the United States, but such products have been used in Europe for more than 15 years (Factor XI, Bio Products Laboratory, Elstree, United Kingdom; Hemoleven, LFB, Les Ulis, France). Hypercoagulability

Rx

(e.g., fatal disseminated intravascular coagulation, myocardial infarction, acute cerebrovascular events) occurs in approximately 10% of patients, particularly in older individuals with preexisting cardiovascular disease and malignancy. Replacement dosing levels should never exceed 70% factor XI activity. Repeat dosing with FFP or factor XI concentrate should be in the context of the long (60- to 80-hour) biologic half-life of factor XI in vivo.

The decision to treat heterozygotes with factor XI at levels greater than 20% is empiric and should be based on the individual's prior history of bleeding after trauma or surgery. Alternatively, the family medical history of previous bleeding complications can be considered. For symptomatic patients, the preoperative or post-trauma use of FFP and pooled plasma products can be minimized or avoided by administering DDAVP, 0.3 μg/kg intravenously. Because hemorrhagic complications originate most commonly from mucosal membrane surfaces, antifibrinolytic agents such as ε-aminocaproic acid or tranexamic acid are frequently helpful as adjunctive therapy.

Alloantibody inhibitors, which neutralize the hemostatic effects of exogenously administered factor XI replacement, can develop in patients who have factor XI levels lower than 1 IU/dL and who have been exposed to plasma or factor XI concentrate. Recombinant factor VIIa can prevent bleeding during or after surgery in these patients.

Contact Activation Factors

Although factor XI is important for activating factor IX in the intrinsic pathway generation of thrombin, it is only one of the four components of the contact phase of coagulation. Deficiencies in any of the other three factors (factor XII, prekallikrein, and high-molecular-weight kininogen) produce in vitro laboratory abnormalities.

Patients have no clinical bleeding. Counterintuitively, 8 to 10% of individuals with severe factor XII deficiency (<1% activity) have experienced premature venous thromboembolic events, occasionally fatal in nature. This finding has led to speculation that factor XII deficiency may lead to hypercoagulability through defective participation of the contact phase proteins in the activation of fibrinolysis.

Autoantibody inhibitors and antiphospholipid antibodies have been associated with decreased levels of factor XII. No clinical sequelae have been associated.

Diagnosis

Deficiencies of each of these factors prolong the aPTT, which may normalize after prolonged incubation of the patient's plasma at 37° C with a negatively charged activator of the aPTT assay (i.e., kaolin or Celite). Specific assays are also available to quantitate each of the contact factors.

Treatment

Rx

No therapy is indicated. Routine anticoagulation regimens are used to treat the thrombogenic events (Chapter 178).

Factor XIII (Fibrin-Stabilizing Factor) Deficiency

Factor XIII is a transglutaminase that is activated by thrombin and subsequently cross-links fibrin to protect it from lysis by plasmin. It also is involved in wound healing and tissue repair and seems to be crucial for maintaining a viable pregnancy. Homozygous severe deficiency states are rare and are inherited in an autosomal recessive manner with a prevalence of 1 per 3 million births. Consanguinity is common.

Clinical Manifestations

Typically, patients are first seen shortly after birth with persistent bleeding around the umbilical stump. Intracranial bleeding events, usually precipitated by minimal trauma, occur commonly enough in infants to justify initiation of a primary prophylaxis regimen of replacement therapy. Delayed bleeding after surgery and trauma is the hallmark of the disease; however, easy bruisability, poor wound healing with defective scar formation and dehiscence, and hemarthroses are characteristic. Spontaneous abortions are increased in severely affected women.

Diagnosis

The diagnosis usually is suspected on clinical grounds, inasmuch as factor XIII deficiency is not detected by the conventional screening coagulation assays (i.e., the aPTT or the PT). Most laboratories use a rapid screening assay that assesses the ability of a fibrin clot to remain intact with incubation in 5 mol/L of urea or 1% monochloroacetic acid. With factor XIII levels less than 1% of normal, the clot dissolves within 2 to 3 hours.

Treatment

Rx

Replacement therapy for prophylaxis or treatment of acute bleeds can be accomplished by administering cryoprecipitate, FFP, or, preferably, plasma-derived factor XIII concentrate (Fibrogammin P, which is pasteurized for viral safety and is available in the United States via compassionate investigational new drug [IND] use through ZLB-Behring, Inc., Marburg, Germany, and King of Prussia, PA). Clinical studies are in progress to evaluate a placentally derived product. Normal hemostasis is achieved with a factor XIII level of only 5% of normal. The circulating half-life of factor XIII is 10 days, so prophylactic replacement can be scheduled every 3 to 4 weeks. Acquired alloantibody inhibitors can develop in severely affected individuals. Autoantibodies also occur, usually in association with systemic lupus erythematosus (SLE).

Dysfibrinogenemia and Afibrinogenemia

Approximately 300 abnormal fibrinogens have been described, but few cause symptoms. Abnormal fibrinogens are rare, autosomally inherited proteins. Their characterization has provided valuable information on the structure and function of fibrinogen and better understanding of wound healing and fibrinolysis.

Clinical Manifestations

More than 50% of the dysfibrinogenemias are asymptomatic, 25% are associated with a mild hemorrhagic tendency (commonly caused by defective release of fibrinopeptide A), and 20% predispose individuals to thrombophilia (usually caused by impaired fibrinolysis). Concurrent bleeding and thrombosis also may occur. The prevalence of dysfibrinogenemia in patients with a history of thromboembolic episodes approaches 0.8%, typically occurring in late adolescence and early adulthood. Women experience a high incidence of pregnancy-related complications, such as spontaneous abortion and postpartum thromboembolic events. Thrombin times and reptilase times (plasma-based clotting times with substitution of reptilase snake venom for thrombin) are not helpful in predicting whether an abnormal fibrinogen will be prothrombotic, prohemorrhagic, or asymptomatic, but clinical history, fibrinopeptide release studies, and fibrin polymerization studies may be useful. Clinically insignificant dysfibrinogenemias may be acquired in association with hepatocellular carcinoma.

In contrast to the hepatic synthesis of a qualitatively abnormal protein in dysfibrinogenemia, congenital afibrinogenemia, an autosomal recessive disorder, represents the markedly deficient production of a normal protein. Severe life-threatening hemorrhagic complications can occur at any site, beginning at birth with umbilical bleeding. Intracranial hemorrhage is a frequent cause of death. Poor wound healing is characteristic. All coagulation-based assays that depend on the detection of a fibrin clot end point are markedly prolonged. Afibrinogenemia is usually detectable by specific functional or immunologic assays. Platelet dysfunction may accompany afibrinogenemia and exacerbate bleeding.

Diagnosis

Abnormalities usually are detected incidentally when routine coagulation screening assays reveal decreased fibrinogen concentrations and prolonged thrombin clotting times. On further evaluation, discordance between functional and immunologic fibrinogen levels (>50 mg/dL more antigenic than functional) is observed; clotting times using snake venom (reptilase or ancrod) are variably prolonged.

Treatment

Deficiencies of fibrinogen may be corrected by the administration of FFP or cryoprecipitate; however, viral safety remains an issue. Viral-attenuated (pasteurized), plasma-derived fibrinogen concentrates (not available in the United States but licensed in France, Japan, Scotland, and China) or solvent detergent—or psoralen-treated FFP (when licensed by the FDA) will be preferable alternatives. The replacement goal is 100 mg/dL of fibrinogen. With a circulating biologic half-life of at least 96 hours, treatment every 3 to 4 days is adequate. Primary prophylaxis regimens may be useful in afibrinogenemia; on-demand or prophylactic replacement for trauma or surgery is recommended for prohemorrhagic dysfibrinogenemias. Individuals with thrombophilic manifestations should receive anticoagulation indefinitely.

Deficiency of Factor V (Proaccelerin, Labile Factor)

Factor V is a component of the prothrombinase complex that assembles factors Va and Xa on the phospholipid membrane of the platelet for prothrombin (factor II) activation to thrombin.

Congenital Factor V Deficiency

Deficiency of factor V is a rare, autosomal recessive disorder (1 per 1 million births). The factor V Leiden protein, which is responsible for resistance to activated protein C and thrombophilia, does not affect factor V coagulant activity (Chapter 182). The severity of the plasma factor V reduction correlates less well with the risk of clinical bleeding than does the platelet factor V content in the α-granule. This observation illustrates the crucial role of the platelet in promoting adequate hemostasis at bleeding sites and explains why transfusions of normal platelets may be preferred over FFP for the treatment of hemorrhagic episodes secondary to congenital or acquired factor V deficiency. Hemostasis can be maintained without correcting plasma factor V activity (>25% of normal).

Combined Deficiencies of Factors V and VIII

Factors V and VIII are structurally homologous proteins, and combined deficiencies of these factors occur as an autosomal recessive disorder with a prevalence of 1 per 100,000 births among Jews of Sephardic origin. The severity of bleeding is determined by the levels of these factors, which usually range from 5% to 30% of normal. Replacement therapy should be aimed at normalizing both clotting protein activities.

Acquired Factor V Deficiency

Acquired factor V deficiency has been described in individuals exposed to bovine factor V, which contaminates the thrombin preparations used topically to control bleeding during cardiovascular surgery. This abnormality probably represents the development of anti–bovine factor V antibodies that cross-react with the human factor V protein. Profuse bleeding accompanies this complication.

Deficiencies of Vitamin K–Dependent Coagulation

Deficiencies of Factors II, VII, and X

Pathobiology and Clinical Manifestations

Congenital deficiencies of factors II, VII, and X are rare, autosomally inherited disorders. Heterozygotes (with factor levels approximately 20% of normal) are typically asymptomatic except in the immediate newborn period, when physiologic vitamin K deficiency exacerbates the underlying clotting factor deficiency. Homozygotes with clotting factor levels lower than 10% of normal manifest variable symptoms. As with other coagulopathies, these deficiencies usually are suspected after the onset of neonatal umbilical stump bleeding. Thereafter, unless replacement or prophylactic therapy is provided, these patients are subject to mucosal bleeding from epistaxis, menorrhagia, and dental extractions; to hemarthroses and intramuscular hematomas; and to bleeding after surgery or trauma.

The genetic factor II variant resulting from a glycine-to-alanine (G-to-A) mutation at nucleoside 20210 is associated with elevated prothrombin levels and an increased risk of venous and arterial thrombosis (Chapter 182). The PT and aPTT are not affected.

Acquired factor VII deficiency has been associated with Dubin-Johnson and Gilbert syndromes (Chapter 150).

Acquired factor IX deficiency has been associated with Gaucher's disease, because factor IX binds to glucocerebroside (Chapter 223). Factor IX deficiency also may accompany Noonan's syndrome, an autosomal dominant disease complex characterized by congenital heart disease, abnormal facies, and excessive bleeding or bruising.

Diagnosis

In the coagulation laboratory, factor VII deficiency is associated with a prolonged PT and a normal aPTT. This pattern localizes the deficiency to the extrinsic pathway. In contrast, deficiencies of factors II and X prolong the PT and the aPTT, with the defects localized to the common pathway of coagulation. A Russel viper venom–based clotting assay can differentiate between these two deficiencies, because, as a direct activator of factor X, the assay is prolonged with factor X but not factor II deficiency. Mixing patient plasma with normal plasma shows correction of these assays, and specific clotting assays using plasma that is deficient in the coagulation protein to be studied confirm the diagnosis.

Treatment

Replacement therapy is indicated for acute symptomatic bleeds and for prophylaxis before surgery. In addition to FFP, which has the potential to transmit blood-borne viruses, factor IX complex concentrates can be administered to achieve hemostatic levels of any of these vitamin K–dependent factors (25 to 30% of normal).

Bleeding complications caused by acquired IgG autoantibodies directed against any coagulation factor protein may be reversed rapidly, albeit temporarily, by extracorporeal immunoadsorption over a Sepharose-bound polyclonal antihuman IgG or staphylococcal A column with concomitant replacement therapy and initiation of immunosuppression.

Factor Deficiency in Amyloidosis

Acquired severe deficiency of factor X, often accompanied by deficiencies of other vitamin K–dependent factors, occasionally occurs in individuals with systemic amyloidosis (Chapter 296). Because amyloid fibrils in the reticuloendothelial system bind endogenous and exogenous sources of factor X, replacement therapy with FFP or factor IX complex concentrates, even in large quantities, may not always be sufficient. Recombinant factor VIIa concentrate has been used to reverse acute bleeding. Splenectomy may ameliorate recurrent bleeding complications.

Other Acquired Coagulation Deficiencies

Lupus Anticoagulants and the Antiphospholipid Syndrome

Epidemiology

The lupus anticoagulant may be discovered incidentally when routine coagulation assays reveal prolongations in the PT, the aPTT, or both; when young women experience recurrent spontaneous miscarriages or pregnancy-related thromboembolic events; when young women and elderly men are detected with cerebral arterial thromboses; when patients are affected by SLE (20 to 40%; see Chapter 287) or other autoimmune diseases or lymphoproliferative malignancies; and when patients have been receiving long-term therapy with psychotropic medications (e.g., chlorpromazine; see Chapter 420). Lupus anticoagulant also can occur with the active opportunistic infections and malignancies associated with AIDS.

Pathobiology

The lupus anticoagulant is the functional expression of an IgG or IgM antiphospholipid autoantibody, which prolongs coagulation in in vitro assays but typically does not produce bleeding complications in vivo. The immunologic expression of the antiphospholipid autoantibodies can be measured by anticardiolipin antibody ELISA. The antiphospholipid antibodies are not directed specifically against the anionic phospholipids that function as templates for activation of the prothrombinase complex but in actuality appear to interact with plasma proteins (β_2-glycoprotein I or apolipoprotein H), which in turn bind to anionic phospholipids. β_2-Glycoprotein I modulates the normal coagulation process by binding to phospholipid membranes; there is impaired thrombin generation in a β_2-glycoprotein I knockout mice model. However, when so-called antiphospholipid antibodies complex with β_2-glycoprotein in vivo, the modulatory function for β_2-glycoprotein I is negated, thereby resulting in increased risks for recurrent venous thromboembolism, fetal wastage, and arterial thrombotic episodes, including stroke. There is evidence that the antiphospholipid antibodies inhibit protein C activation, interfere with antithrombin III activity, disrupt the annexin V "shield," and interfere with normal fibrinolysis. All of these phenomena are prothrombotic events.

Clinical Manifestations

The lupus anticoagulant can precipitate clinical bleeding complications when antiphospholipid/anticardiolipin antibodies complex with factor II (prothrombin) and produce an acquired prothrombin deficiency, probably because of accelerated clearance of lupus anticoagulant-prothrombin complexes from the circulation. Bleeding tendencies also arise when the lupus anticoagulant targets platelet membranes and produces quantitative and/or qualitative platelet abnormalities.

Nonpregnant individuals with thrombotic manifestations of lupus anticoagulant or antiphospholipid antibody have a 50% risk of experiencing recurrent events over a 5-year period. Typically, recurrent hypercoagulable episodes occur in a pattern consistent with the initial findings (i.e., venous recurrence follows an initial deep venous thrombosis).

Diagnosis

The in vitro anticoagulant properties of the antiphospholipid antibodies are detected when mixing studies of the patient's plasma with normal plasma reveal immediate inhibition of the aPTT or the PT at baseline with no additional prolongation after a 2-hour incubation (in contrast to the findings with factor VIII autoantibody). Confirmatory assays include the kaolin clotting time (the most sensitive test), the dilute Russell's viper venom time, the dilute tissue thromboplastin inhibition assay, the textarin:ecarin venom clotting time ratio, and the platelet neutralization assay. All of these laboratory tests depend on the presence of phospholipid; antiphospholipid antibodies block the binding of coagulation factors and the modulators of coagulation (protein S and activated protein C) to their phospholipid assembly surface template.

Treatment

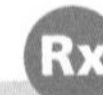

The approach to the management of lupus anticoagulant or antiphospholipid antibody varies according to the severity of symptoms and the clinical circumstances. In the setting of idiopathic fetal loss, there is a 15 to 20% association with the antiphospholipid syndrome, with 75% of the pregnancy losses occurring in the first trimester. Treatment with low-dose unfractionated heparin (5000 U subcutaneously every 8 hours) and daily aspirin (81 mg) has resulted in 80% fetal survival. The use of corticosteroids is controversial and is not recommended because of attendant diabetes and hypertension. Supplemental calcium and vitamin D (Chapter 264) should be administered to minimize the risks of osteoporosis from prolonged heparin use. Clinical trials with preparations of low-molecular-weight heparin (LMWH) and immunosuppressive agents such as intravenous gamma globulin are in progress. An FDA-mandated advisory suggested that the use of LMWHs may be associated with a low incidence of teratogenicity and possibly with thrombogenicity; although these complications have not been observed in meta-analyses of LMWH in pregnancy; controlled studies are needed to confirm any potential risk.

Individuals who experienced venous thromboembolism associated with antiphospholipid antibodies should be treated for at least 6 months with oral anticoagulation with warfarin to maintain a target international normalized ratio (INR) of 2.0 to 3.0. For patients with recurrent noncardioembolic stroke and antiphospholipid antibodies, oral anticoagulation with warfarin at a target INR of 2.0 to 3.0 is preferred, rather than use of antiplatelet agents.

The nonvirilizing androgen preparations danazol and stanozolol may be helpful in raising depressed factor II levels into the hemostatic range. Asymptomatic individuals may benefit from prophylactic aspirin therapy 81 mg/day, which has a favorable risk-to-benefit profile.

Coagulopathies Secondary to Anticoagulation

The most common acquired clinical coagulopathies occur secondary to anticoagulation with warfarin and other coumarin analogues and to the use of heparin.

Warfarin

Vitamin K–dependent clotting factors II, VII, IX, and X are functionally defective after warfarin use because post-translational carboxylation of their γ-glutamyl residues cannot be accomplished. The risks for life-threatening bleeding increase proportionally with the intensity of anticoagulation and INRs rising to greater than 6.0. Warfarin effects can be exaggerated by potentiating medications, excessive ethanol use, and simultaneous dietary vitamin K deficiency. Bleeding may be severe or occult and may unmask the presence of pathologic lesions, such as gastrointestinal or genitourinary carcinomas.

Treatment

For acute and profuse bleeding events caused by warfarin with any INR, vitamin K_1, 1 to 5 mg, should be administered subcutaneously or intravenously in conjunction with FFP (10 to 20 mL/kg) or small amounts of factor IX complex concentrate (25 to 50 IU/kg). Recombinant factor VIIa concentrate (20 to 30 μg/kg) also has been reported to be a useful salvage therapy to reverse refractory hemorrhage caused by overanticoagulation with warfarin. For minor bleeding or markedly increased INRs without bleeding, warfarin should be withheld for 1 to 2 days and vitamin K_1 administered (1 to 2 mg subcutaneously or intravenously). A single dose of oral vitamin K_1 (1 mg) also has been used successfully in this scenario, but the INR may not correct significantly for about 48 hours. Administration of FFP may be considered for INRs greater than 9.0 to facilitate reduction of the INR and to minimize potential bleeding in high-risk patients. These maneuvers allow for easy reinitiation of warfarin with appropriate dose adjustment. The frequency of major

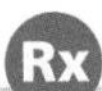

hemorrhage, the mortality rate, and the incidence of recurrent thromboembolic complications all are reduced greatly when anticoagulated patients receiving long-term warfarin therapy are managed in anticoagulation clinics.

Heparin

Heparin anticoagulation also can induce life-threatening hemorrhagic complications. The aPTT and thrombin times are prolonged even with minimal amounts of heparin in the circulation or with contaminating indwelling catheters from which blood specimens are obtained. The reptilase time can be used to distinguish heparin from other causes of thrombin time prolongation (e.g., fibrin degradation products, abnormal fibrinogens). The PT may be prolonged in the presence of large concentrations of heparin. Heparin functions as a circulating inhibitor, so that mixing studies of patient plasma with normal plasma do not result in correction of the aPTT. LMWH preparations do not affect the aPTT but may affect the thrombin time, depending on the thrombin concentration used in the assay (Chapter 35). The anticoagulant properties of LMWHs can be monitored by the anti-factor Xa assay.

Treatment

Acute and profuse bleeding episodes secondary to heparin can be reversed by administration of protamine sulfate (1 mg/100 U of residual heparin). Overdosing with protamine sulfate can produce its own coagulopathy. Otherwise, the circulating survival time of standard heparin in plasma is short enough (2 to 4 hours) to allow the anticoagulant state to dissipate on its own. The half-life of LMWH is longer, but bleeding is uncommon unless the patient has renal dysfunction. The anticoagulation effects of LMWH may be reversed with protamine sulfate, although the response can be marginal and unpredictable. Recombinant factor VIIa (30 to 90 μg/kg) has been used anecdotally to reverse refractory bleeding associated with LMWH.

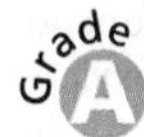

1. Manco-Johnson MJ, Abshire TC, Brown D, et al: Initial results of a randomized, prospective trial of prophylaxis to prevent joint disease in young children with factor VIII (FVIII) deficiency. Blood 2005;106:Abstract 3.
2. Astermark J, Donfield A, DiMichele DM, et al: A randomized comparison of bypassing agents in hemophilia complicated by an inhibitor. Blood 2007;109:546–551.

SUGGESTED READINGS

Ansel J, Hirsh J, Poller L, et al: The pharmacology and management of vitamin K antagonists. The seventh ACCP conference on antithrombotic and thrombolytic therapy. Chest 2004;126:204S–233S. *Approaches to the reversal of anticoagulation-related bleeding complications.*

Armout J, Jankowski M: Understanding the antiphospholipid syndrome and its treatment. Current Hematol Rep 2005;4:385–390. *Concise review of clinical, immunological, and diagnostic issues of the antiphospholipid antibody syndrome and the lupus anticoagulant.*

Collins PW, Hirsch S, Baglin TP, et al: Acquired haemophilia A in the UK: A two year national surveillance study by UK Haemophilia Centre Doctors' Organisation. Blood 2007;109:1870–1877. *No difference in outcomes between treatment with steroids and cytotoxics vs. steroids alone.*

Feldman BM, Pai M, Rivard GE, et al: Tailored prophylaxis in severe hemophilia A: Interim results from the first 5 years of the Canadian Hemophilia Primary Prophylaxis Study. J Thromb Haemost 2006;4:1228–1236. *An individualized approach provides good outcomes and requires less factor infusion than traditional prophylaxis.*

Kessler CM: New perspectives in hemophilia treatment. Hematology Am Soc Hematol Educ Program 2005;429–435. *Review of all aspects of care, with a comprehensive list of available replacement products.*

Mannucci PM: Treatment of von Willebrand's disease. N Engl J Med 2004;351:683–694. *Overview of pathophysiology, diagnosis, and treatment.*

White CC, Kempton CL, Grimsley A, et al: Cellular immune responses in hemophilia: Why do inhibitors develop in some, but not all hemophiliacs? J Thromb Haemostas 2005;3:1676–1681. *Discussion of the genetics, clinical manifestations, diagnosis, and treatment of alloantibodies in hemophilia.*

181 HEMORRHAGIC DISORDERS: DISSEMINATED INTRAVASCULAR COAGULATION, LIVER FAILURE, AND VITAMIN K DEFICIENCY

Andrew I. Schafer

DISSEMINATED INTRAVASCULAR COAGULATION

Definition

Disseminated intravascular coagulation (DIC), also referred to as *consumptive coagulopathy* or *defibrination,* is caused by a wide variety of serious disorders (Table 181–1). In most patients, the underlying process dominates the clinical picture, but in some cases (e.g., occult malignancy, envenomation), DIC may be the initial or predominant manifestation of the disorder.

Pathobiology

DIC is primarily a thrombotic process, although its clinical manifestation may be widespread hemorrhage in acute, fulminant cases. The basic pathophysiology (Fig. 181–1), regardless of cause, is entry into the circulation of procoagulant substances that trigger systemic activation of the

TABLE 181–1 MAJOR CAUSES OF DISSEMINATED INTRAVASCULAR COAGULATION

Infections
Gram-negative bacterial sepsis
Other bacteria, fungi, viruses, Rocky Mountain spotted fever, malaria
Immunologic reactions
Transfusion reactions
Transplant rejection
Obstetric complications
Amniotic fluid embolism
Retained dead fetus
Abruptio placentae
Toxemia, preeclampsia
Septic abortion
Malignancies
Pancreatic carcinoma
Adenocarcinomas
Acute promyelocytic leukemia
Other neoplasms
Liver failure
Acute pancreatitis
Envenomation
Respiratory distress syndrome
Trauma, shock
Brain injury
Crush injury
Burns
Hypothermia/hyperthermia
Fat embolism
Hypoxia, ischemia
Surgery
Vascular disorders
Giant hemangioma (Kasabach-Merritt syndrome)
Aortic aneurysm
Vascular tumors

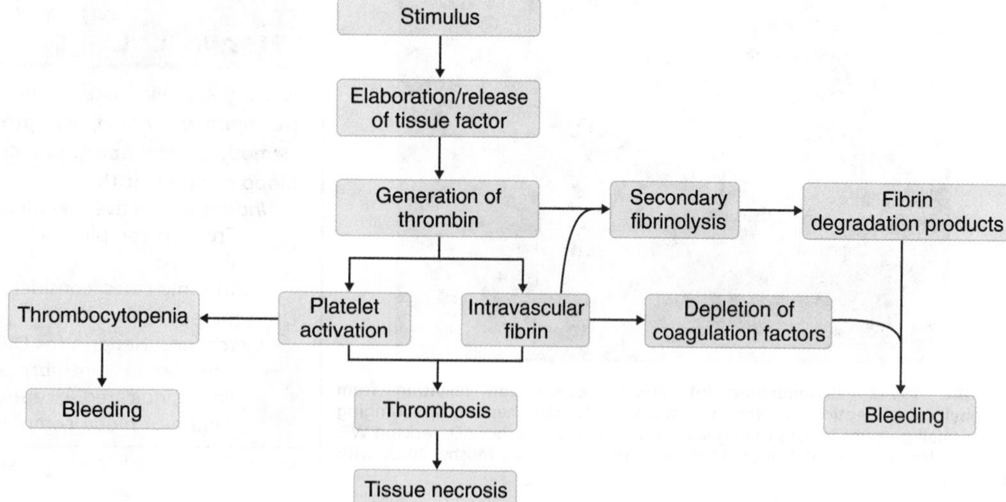

FIGURE 181–1 • Pathophysiology of bleeding, thrombosis, and ischemic manifestations in patients with disseminated intravascular coagulation.

coagulation system and platelets and subsequent disseminated deposition of fibrin-platelet thrombi. In most cases the procoagulant stimulus is tissue factor, a lipoprotein that is not normally exposed to blood. In DIC, tissue factor gains access to blood by tissue injury, its elaboration by malignant cells, or its expression on the surface of monocytes and endothelial cells by inflammatory mediators. Components of the inflammatory response and the coagulation system are mutually activated in some forms of DIC, such as sepsis. Tissue factor triggers generation of the coagulation protease thrombin, which induces fibrin formation and platelet activation. In some specific cases of DIC, procoagulants other than tissue factor (e.g., a cysteine protease or mucin in certain malignancies) and proteases other than thrombin (e.g., trypsin in pancreatitis, exogenous proteins in envenomation) provide the procoagulant stimulus.

In acute, uncompensated DIC, coagulation factors are consumed at a rate in excess of the capacity of the liver to synthesize them, and platelets are consumed in excess of the capacity of bone marrow megakaryocytes to release them. The resulting laboratory manifestations are a prolonged prothrombin time (PT) and activated partial thromboplastin time (aPTT) and thrombocytopenia. Increased fibrin formation in DIC stimulates the process of secondary fibrinolysis, in which plasminogen activators generate plasmin to digest fibrin (and fibrinogen) into fibrin(ogen) degradation products (FDPs). FDPs are potent circulating anticoagulants that further contribute to the bleeding manifestations of DIC. Intravascular fibrin deposition can cause fragmentation of red blood cells and lead to the appearance of schistocytes in blood smears; however, frank hemolytic anemia is unusual in DIC. Microvascular thrombosis in DIC can compromise the blood supply to some organs and lead to multiorgan failure, particularly when accompanied by systemic hemodynamic and metabolic derangements.

Underlying Causes

DIC always has an underlying cause that generally must be identified and eliminated if the coagulopathy is to be treated successfully. The development of DIC in many of these disorders is associated with an unfavorable outcome. Infection is the most common cause of DIC. The syndrome is particularly associated with gram-negative or gram-positive sepsis (Chapter 109), although it can be triggered by a variety of other bacterial, fungal, viral, rickettsial, and protozoal microorganisms. The placenta and uterine contents are rich sources of tissue factor and other procoagulants that are normally excluded from the maternal circulation; a spectrum of clinical manifestations of DIC may accompany obstetric complications, especially in the third trimester. These syndromes range from acute, fulminant, and often fatal DIC in amniotic fluid embolism to chronic or subacute DIC with a retained dead fetus. Other obstetric problems associated with DIC include abruptio placentae, toxemia, and septic abortion. Chronic forms of DIC accompany a variety of malignancies, particularly pancreatic cancer (Chapter 204) and mucin-secreting adenocarcinomas of the gastrointestinal tract (Chapter 203), in which thrombotic rather than bleeding manifestations predominate. Treatment with all-*trans*-retinoic acid has greatly reduced the incidence of severe DIC in patients with acute promyelocytic leukemia (Chapter 194). It is not known whether liver failure (Chapter 158) can cause DIC or whether its coexistence merely exacerbates intravascular coagulation because of impaired clearance of activated clotting factors, plasmin, and FDPs. Snake venom contains a variety of substances that can affect coagulation and endothelial permeability. Bites from rattlesnakes and other vipers can induce profound DIC by introduction of these exogenous toxins and release of endogenous tissue factor via tissue necrosis. The likelihood and degree of DIC caused by trauma, surgery, and shock (Chapter 107) are related to the extent of tissue damage and the organs involved; the brain is a particularly rich source of tissue factor, so traumatic brain injury (Chapter 422) can precipitate acute DIC. Large aortic aneurysms (Chapter 78), giant hemangiomas (Chapter 179), and other vascular malformations can cause subclinical or clinical DIC that is initiated locally in the abnormal vasculature but can "spill" into the systemic circulation.

Clinical Manifestations

The clinical manifestations of DIC are determined by the nature, intensity, and duration of the underlying stimulus. The coexistence of liver disease enhances DIC of any etiology. Low-grade DIC is often asymptomatic and diagnosed only by laboratory abnormalities. Thrombotic complications of DIC occur most often with chronic underlying diseases, as exemplified by Trousseau's syndrome in cancer (Chapter 189). Gangrene of the digits or extremities, hemorrhagic necrosis of the skin (Fig. 181–2), or purpura fulminans may also be manifestations of DIC. Bleeding is the most common clinical finding in acute, uncompensated DIC. Bleeding can be limited to sites of intervention or anatomic abnormalities, but it tends to be generalized in more severe cases, including widespread ecchymoses and diffuse oozing from mucosal surfaces and orifices.

Diagnosis

The laboratory diagnosis of severe, acute DIC is not usually difficult. Consumption and inhibition of the function of clotting factors cause prolongation of the PT, aPTT, and thrombin time. Consumption of platelets causes thrombocytopenia. Secondary fibrinolysis generates increased titers of FDPs, which can be measured by latex agglutination or D-dimer assays. Some schistocytes may be seen in the peripheral blood smear, but this finding is neither sensitive nor specific for DIC. Chronic or compensated forms of DIC are more difficult to diagnose, with highly variable patterns of abnormalities in "DIC screen" coagulation tests. Increased FDPs and a prolonged PT are generally more sensitive measures than abnormalities of the aPTT and platelet count are. Overcompensated synthesis of consumed clotting factors and platelets in some chronic forms of DIC may actually cause shortening of the PT and aPTT or thrombocytosis (or both), even though elevated levels of FDPs indicate secondary fibrinolysis in such cases.

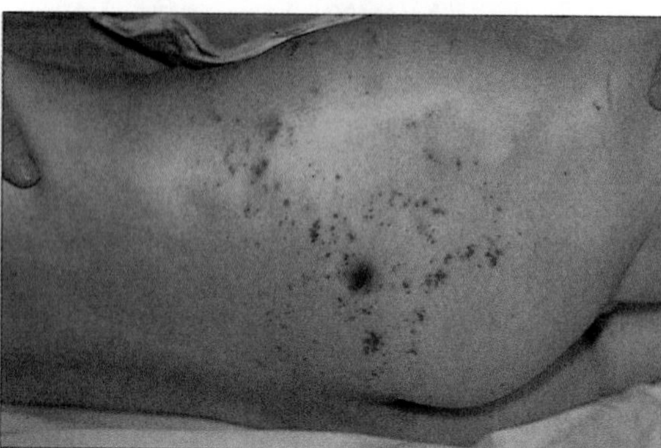

FIGURE 181–2 • Disseminated intravascular coagulation resulting from staphylococcal septicemia. Note the characteristic skin hemorrhage ranging from small purpuric lesions to larger ecchymoses. (From Forbes CD, Jackson WF: Color Atlas and Text of Clinical Medicine, 3rd ed. London, Mosby, 2003, with permission.)

The most difficult differential diagnosis of DIC occurs in patients who have coexisting liver disease. The coagulopathy of liver failure is often indistinguishable from that of DIC, partly because advanced hepatic dysfunction is accompanied by a state of DIC. In liver failure, the combination of decreased synthesis of clotting factors, impaired clearance of activated clotting factors, secondary fibrinolysis, and thrombocytopenia from portal hypertension and hypersplenism may make the coagulopathy practically impossible to differentiate from DIC. In thrombotic microangiopathies, including thrombotic thrombocytopenic purpura and hemolytic-uremic syndrome, platelet consumption and thrombocytopenia are not accompanied by activation of clotting factors or secondary fibrinolysis; the PT, aPTT, thrombin time, and FDPs are generally normal in these disorders. Schistocytes, often with frank hemolysis, are much more prominent in the peripheral smear in thrombotic thrombocytopenic purpura and hemolytic-uremic syndrome (Chapter 179) than in DIC.

Primary fibrinolysis is disputed as a distinct entity. Some patients with a serious clinical bleeding diathesis, however, have laboratory evidence of predominantly fibrinolysis, including high levels of FDPs (D-dimers) and severe hypofibrinogenemia, with relatively little consumption of coagulation factors and normal or near-normal platelet counts. These unusual findings, which approximate the findings expected with fibrinolytic therapy, are encountered occasionally, particularly in patients with prostate cancer.

Treatment

Rx

Successful treatment of DIC (Table 181–2) requires that the underlying cause be identified and eliminated. All other therapies, including hemodynamic support, replacement of coagulation factors and platelets, and pharmacologic inhibitors of coagulation and fibrinolysis, are just temporizing measures. In many patients with asymptomatic, self-limited DIC who have only laboratory manifestations of the coagulopathy, no treatment may be necessary. In patients with DIC who are actively bleeding or who are at high risk for bleeding, the blood component treatments of choice are transfusions of platelets to improve the thrombocytopenia and fresh-frozen plasma to replace all consumed coagulation factors and correct the prolonged PT and aPTT. Large volumes of plasma (e.g., 6 U/24 hr) may be required to ameliorate bleeding in severe cases. In some patients who have particularly profound hypofibrinogenemia, the additional transfusion of cryoprecipitate, a plasma concentrate that is enriched in fibrinogen, may be useful. The theoretical concern that these blood products may "fuel the fire" and exacerbate the DIC has not been supported by clinical experience. Infusion of antithrombin III concentrate may be considered as an adjunctive measure in selected cases, particularly in DIC associated with sepsis.

The use of pharmacologic inhibitors of coagulation and fibrinolysis in DIC is controversial. Heparin is of theoretical benefit because it blocks thrombin activity and quenches intravascular coagulation and the resultant secondary fibrinolysis. In practice, heparin might exacerbate the bleeding tendency in acute DIC. Heparin is usually reserved for special forms of DIC, including those manifested by thrombosis or acrocyanosis and forms that accompany cancer, vascular malformations, retained dead fetus, and possibly acute promyelocytic leukemia. Antifibrinolytic agents, including ε-aminocaproic acid and tranexamic acid, are generally contraindicated in DIC. By blocking the secondary fibrinolytic response to DIC, these drugs cause unopposed fibrin deposition and may precipitate thrombosis. Antifibrinolytic agents may be effective in decreasing life-threatening bleeding in DIC, however, particularly in extreme cases in which aggressive blood component replacement fails to control the hemorrhage; in such situations, simultaneous infusion of low doses of heparin may reduce the risk for thrombosis.

A 96-hour infusion of recombinant human activated protein C (rhAPC), which has both anticoagulant and anti-inflammatory properties, significantly reduces mortality in patients with severe sepsis [1] and should be urgently considered in cases of sepsis related to DIC. However, it does not benefit septic patients with a low risk of death. [2] Because of the increased risk for intracerebral hemorrhage with severe thrombocytopenia, rhAPC must be used cautiously in patients with DIC and in conjunction with platelet transfusion if the platelet count is less than 30,000/mm^3. Although recombinant tissue factor pathway inhibitor and antithrombin III concentrates may have some efficacy in improving laboratory and clinical parameters of DIC, the overall survival benefit with these agents in patients with DIC has yet to be demonstrated.

TABLE 181–2 TREATMENT OF DISSEMINATED INTRAVASCULAR COAGULATION

Identify and eliminate the underlying cause
No treatment if mild, asymptomatic, and self-limited
Hemodynamic support, as indicated, in severe cases
Blood component therapy
Indications: active bleeding or high risk for bleeding
Fresh-frozen plasma
Platelets
In some cases, consider cryoprecipitate, antithrombin III
Drug therapy
Indications: Heparin for DIC manifested by thrombosis or acrocyanosis; antifibrinolytic agents generally contraindicated except with life-threatening bleeding and failure of blood component therapy

DIC = disseminated intravascular coagulation.

LIVER FAILURE

Bleeding complications in patients with advanced liver disease (Chapters 157 and 158) can be severe and even fatal and directly account for about 20% of the deaths associated with hepatic failure. The extent of the bleeding tendency depends on the severity and type of liver disease involved. About a third of deaths in patients undergoing liver transplantation are attributable to perioperative hemorrhage.

Pathobiology

The pathophysiology of bleeding in liver failure is complex and multifactorial. Anatomic abnormalities resulting from portal hypertension are frequently the major cause of gastrointestinal bleeding in patients with liver disease. Upper gastrointestinal bleeding can be caused by esophageal varices or hemorrhagic gastritis (congestive gastropathy), whereas lower gastrointestinal bleeding, though seldom life-threatening, can be due to hemorrhoids.

TABLE 181–3 COAGULATION ABNORMALITIES IN LIVER DISEASE

ABNORMALITIES IN COAGULATION
Decreased synthesis of coagulation factors
Impaired vitamin K–dependent γ-carboxylation
Dysfibrinogenemia
Disseminated intravascular coagulation
Increased fibrinolytic activity
ABNORMALITIES IN PLATELETS
Thrombocytopenia (hypersplenism)
Abnormal platelet function

The complexity of the systemic coagulopathy of liver failure is not surprising inasmuch as the liver is the principal organ site for the synthesis of coagulation and fibrinolytic factors and their protein inhibitors (Table 181–3). Hepatocytes produce all of the clotting factors except von Willebrand factor, and advanced parenchymal liver disease results in impaired synthesis of these proteins (Chapter 180). Liver disease can also cause impairment in vitamin K–dependent γ-carboxylation of the procoagulant factors II, VII, IX, and X, as well as the anticoagulant proteins C and S. Functional abnormalities of fibrinogen, termed *dysfibrinogenemias,* are frequently found in various forms of liver disease, particularly in hepatomas. Most forms of advanced liver disease are accompanied by some degree of DIC caused by impaired synthesis of inhibitors of blood coagulation and defective hepatocellular clearance of activated coagulation factors. DIC is an especially important potential complication of LeVeen shunts used to treat intractable ascites because this procedure introduces procoagulant-rich ascitic fluid into the systemic circulation. In many of these cases, shunt ligation is required to terminate the DIC. DIC and bleeding risk are exacerbated by the enhanced fibrinolytic activity of liver disease caused by increased levels of tissue plasminogen activator accompanied by decreased synthesis of inhibitors of plasminogen activator and plasmin.

Quantitative and qualitative abnormalities of platelets also contribute to the bleeding diathesis of liver failure. Congestive splenomegaly secondary to portal hypertension causes increased pooling of platelets in the spleen (hypersplenism). The resultant thrombocytopenia, the degree of which generally correlates with spleen size, rarely causes a reduction in the platelet count to less than 50,000/mm^3. In alcoholic patients, suppression of bone marrow thrombopoiesis by the acute toxic effects of alcohol or folate deficiency may contribute to the thrombocytopenia. Qualitative platelet abnormalities have also been described in patients with liver disease.

Liver transplantation (Chapter 158) poses special problems to the coagulation system. During the anhepatic stage of surgery, which lasts about 2 hours, the complete cessation of synthesis of coagulation factors causes further prolongation of the PT and aPTT. Release of tissue plasminogen activator from the newly grafted liver leads to increased fibrinolysis and transient exacerbation of bleeding risk in the postoperative period.

Clinical Manifestations

The most common hemorrhagic complication of liver disease is gastrointestinal bleeding, which is usually caused by anatomic abnormalities and exacerbated by the systemic coagulopathy of liver failure. Bleeding from other mucosal sites, extensive ecchymoses, or more serious hemorrhage into the retroperitoneum or central nervous system generally indicates more significant derangements of the coagulation system.

The severe coagulopathy in patients with liver disease makes liver biopsy a potentially hazardous procedure. The PT and platelet count are the best guides to bleeding risk. In general, liver biopsy can be performed safely if the PT and aPTT do not exceed 1.5 times control and the platelet count is greater than 50,000/mm^3. Fresh-frozen plasma (see Treatment) can be infused to correct the prolonged PT and aPTT. Bleeding time is not a reliable predictor of bleeding risk after biopsy.

Diagnosis

Although the PT and aPTT are often prolonged in patients with advanced liver disease, the former tends to be a more sensitive assay early in the course; a disproportionate prolongation of the aPTT should raise suspicion of a coexisting coagulation abnormality, such as a lupus anticoagulant or clotting factor inhibitor. A prolonged PT is also a useful prognostic indicator of poor outcome in patients with cirrhosis, acute acetaminophen hepatotoxicity, and acute viral hepatitis; in the latter, it is a better index of prognosis than serum albumin or transaminases are. A disproportionate prolongation of the thrombin time should suggest the presence of dysfibrinogenemia. Hypersplenism (Chapter 174), possibly associated with nutritional folate deficiency or the acute toxic effects of alcohol on bone marrow, often causes mild to moderate thrombocytopenia in patients with liver disease; however, consideration should be given to other coexisting causes of thrombocytopenia if the platelet count is significantly less than 50,000/mm^3.

The coagulopathy of liver failure is often indistinguishable from that of DIC, in part because some degree of DIC is a necessary accompaniment of advanced liver disease. In general, patients with DIC have more marked decreases in levels of factor VIII and increases in titers of FDPs, however, particularly D-dimers, than do patients with liver failure.

Treatment

Therapy for the coagulopathy of liver disease may be directed at preventing the hemorrhagic complications of invasive procedures or treating active bleeding. The most effective treatment is blood component therapy with fresh-frozen plasma (which contains all the coagulation factors) and platelet transfusions (Chapter 183). Some patients require large volumes of fresh-frozen plasma (15 to 20 mL/kg) to lower the prolonged PT; rarely, plasmapheresis with plasma exchange is required to avoid fluid overload in these situations. Because of the short half-lives of some clotting factors, fresh-frozen plasma may have to be administered every 8 to 12 hours to maintain acceptable coagulation test parameters. In some patients, especially those with cholestasis, parenteral administration of vitamin K can at least partially reverse the coagulation abnormalities; however, in patients with advanced hepatocellular failure, vitamin K is largely ineffective. Prothrombin complex concentrates are relatively contraindicated in patients with liver failure, as in those with DIC, because of the risk of thrombotic complications. Because of immediate pooling of transfused platelets in the enlarged spleens of patients with hypersplenism, a higher than calculated dose of platelet concentrates is usually required to increase circulating platelet counts significantly.

The use of recombinant activated factor VII (rhVIIa) reduces bleeding complications, particularly upper gastrointestinal bleeding, in some patients with advanced liver disease. However, the routine use of rfVIIa in this setting cannot currently be justified in the absence of controlled clinical trials and Food and Drug Administration approval. Desmopressin (DDAVP), which can shorten the bleeding time of patients with cirrhosis, may be considered as ancillary therapy in patients undergoing invasive procedures.

VITAMIN K DEFICIENCY

Vitamin K is required for γ-carboxylation of glutamic acid residues of the procoagulant factors II (prothrombin), VII, IX, and X and the anticoagulant factors protein C and protein S. This post-translational modification normally renders these proteins functionally active in coagulation. The PT is more sensitive than the aPTT in detecting vitamin K deficiency states because factor VII, the only vitamin K–dependent factor that is in the extrinsic pathway of coagulation, is the most labile of these proteins.

The two major sources of vitamin K are dietary intake and synthesis by the bacterial flora of the intestine. In the absence of malabsorption, nutritional deficiency alone rarely causes clinically significant vitamin K deficiency. This condition can arise, however, when eradication of gut flora is combined with inadequate dietary intake. This situation typically occurs in critically ill patients in intensive care units who have no oral intake and are receiving broad-spectrum antibiotics for prolonged periods. Vitamin K deficiency can also develop in patients receiving total parenteral nutrition unless the infusions are supplemented with vitamin K.

Vitamin K is absorbed predominantly in the ileum and requires the presence of bile salts. Clinically significant vitamin K deficiency occurs with malabsorption of fat-soluble vitamins secondary to obstructive jaundice (Chapter 159) or with malabsorption caused by intrinsic small bowel diseases, including celiac sprue, short-bowel syndrome, and inflammatory bowel disease (Chapters 143 and 144).

Warfarin (Chapter 35) acts as an anticoagulant by competitive antagonism of vitamin K. Rare cases of hereditary deficiency of the vitamin K–dependent coagulation factors may cause a lifelong bleeding tendency.

Correction of vitamin K deficiency, when clinically significant, can be achieved with oral supplementation, unless malabsorption is present. In the latter case, parenteral vitamin K (10 mg subcutaneously daily) should be administered. Emergency treatment of bleeding caused by vitamin K deficiency is transfusion of fresh-frozen plasma.

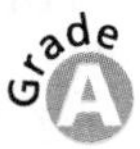

1. Bernard GR, Vincent JL, Laterre PF, et al: Efficacy and safety of recombinant human activated protein C for severe sepsis. N Engl J Med 2001;344:699–709.
2. Abraham E, Laterre PF, Garg R: Drotrecogin alfa (activated) for adults with severe sepsis and a low risk of death. N Engl J Med 2005;353:1332–1341.

SUGGESTED READINGS

Laposata M, Van Cott EM, Lev MH: Case records of the Massachusetts General Hospital. Case 1-2007. A 40-year-old woman with epistaxis, hematemesis, and altered mental status. N Engl J Med 2007;356:174–182. *A discussion of warfarin poisoning.*

Levi M: Current understanding of disseminated intravascular coagulation. Br J Haematol 2004;124:567–576. *Comprehensive review emphasizing the pathophysiology of DIC.*

Mercer KW, Gail Macik B, Williams ME: Hematologic disorders in critically ill patients. Semin Respir Crit Care Med 2006;27:286–296. *Systematic review of coagulation problems encountered in the intensive care unit, including thrombocytopenia, DIC, and vitamin K deficiency.*

Silva MA, Muralidharan V, Mirza DF: The management of coagulopathy and blood loss in liver surgery. Semin Hematol 2004;41:132–139. *Review of the risk factors for and prevention of perioperative hemorrhage.*

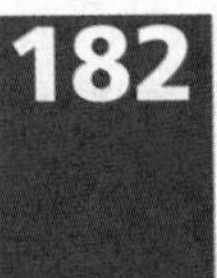

THROMBOTIC DISORDERS: HYPERCOAGULABLE STATES

Andrew I. Schafer

The *hypercoagulable states,* also referred to as *thrombophilias,* encompass a group of inherited or acquired conditions that cause a pathologic thrombotic tendency or risk for thrombosis.

The primary hypercoagulable states are caused by quantitative or qualitative abnormalities in specific coagulation proteins that induce a prothrombotic state. Most of these disorders involve inherited mutations that lead to either (1) deficiency of a physiologic antithrombotic factor or (2) increased level of a prothrombotic factor (Table 182–1). Particularly when combined with other prothrombotic mutations (multigene interactions), these primary hypercoagulable states are associated with a lifelong predisposition to thrombosis. The trigger for a discrete, clinical thrombotic event is often the development of one of the acquired, secondary hypercoagulable states superimposed on an inherited state of hypercoagulability. The secondary hypercoagulable states, a diverse group of mostly acquired conditions (see Fig. 182–2), cause a thrombotic tendency by complex, often multifactorial mechanisms.

TABLE 182–1 PRIMARY HYPERCOAGULABLE STATES

DEFICIENCY OF ANTITHROMBOTIC FACTORS
Antithrombin (III) deficiency
Protein C deficiency
Protein S deficiency
INCREASED PROTHROMBOTIC FACTORS
Factor Va (activated protein C resistance; factor V Leiden)
Prothrombin (prothrombin G20210A mutation)
Factors VII, XI, IX, VIII; von Willebrand's factor; fibrinogen

PRIMARY HYPERCOAGULABLE STATES

Antithrombin III Deficiency

Epidemiology and Pathobiology

Inherited quantitative or qualitative deficiency of antithrombin III leads to increased fibrin accumulation and a lifelong propensity to thrombosis (Chapter 178). Antithrombin is the major physiologic inhibitor of thrombin and other activated coagulation factors; therefore, its deficiency leads to unregulated protease activity and fibrin formation.

The frequency of asymptomatic heterozygous antithrombin deficiency in the general population may be 1 in 350. Most of these individuals have clinically silent mutations and never have thrombotic manifestations. The frequency of symptomatic antithrombin deficiency in the general population has been estimated to be between 1 in 2000 and 1 in 5000. Among all patients seen with venous thromboembolism, antithrombin deficiency is detected in only about 1%, but it is found in approximately 2.5% of selected patients with recurrent thrombosis or onset of thrombosis at a younger age (<45 years old).

Patients with type I antithrombin deficiency have proportionately reduced plasma levels of antigenic and functional antithrombin that result from a quantitative deficiency of the normal protein. Impaired synthesis, defective secretion, or instability of antithrombin in type I antithrombin-deficient individuals is caused by major gene deletions, single nucleotide changes, or short insertions or deletions in the antithrombin gene. Patients with type II antithrombin deficiency have normal or nearly normal plasma antigen accompanied by low activity levels, characteristics indicative of a functionally defective molecule. Type II deficiency is usually caused by specific point mutations leading to single amino acid substitutions that produce a dysfunctional protein. More than 250 different mutations causing type I or type II antithrombin deficiency have been recognized to date.

The pattern of inheritance of antithrombin deficiency is autosomal dominant. Most affected individuals are heterozygotes whose antithrombin levels are typically about 40 to 60% of normal. These individuals may have the full clinical manifestations of hypercoagulability. Rare homozygous antithrombin-deficient patients generally have type II deficiency with reduced heparin affinity, a variant that is associated with a low risk for thrombosis in its heterozygous form; other forms of homozygous antithrombin deficiency are probably incompatible with life.

Protein C Deficiency

Protein C deficiency leads to unregulated fibrin generation because of impaired inactivation of factors VIIIa and Va, two essential cofactors in the coagulation cascade.

Epidemiology

The prevalence of heterozygous protein C deficiency in the general population is about 1 per 200 to 500. Protein C deficiency is found in 3 to 4% of all patients with venous thromboembolism.

Pathobiology

As with antithrombin deficiency, two general forms of protein C deficiency are recognized: type I, in which quantitative deficiency of the protein is associated with a proportionate decrease in protein C antigen and activity, and type II, in which qualitative defects in protein C are associated with disproportionately reduced protein C activity relative to antigen. More than 160 mutations are known to cause protein C deficiency. In the more common type I deficiency, frameshift, nonsense, or missense mutations cause premature termination of synthesis or loss of protein C stability. In type II deficiency, different mutations can cause abnormalities in protein C activation or function. The mode of inheritance of protein C deficiency is autosomal dominant. As in antithrombin deficiency, most affected individuals are heterozygotes.

Protein S Deficiency

Protein S is the principal cofactor of activated protein C (APC), and its deficiency mimics that of protein C in causing loss of regulation of fibrin generation by impaired inactivation of factors VIIIa and Va.

Epidemiology

The prevalence of protein S deficiency in the general population is unknown. Its frequency in all patients evaluated for venous thromboembolism (2 to 3%) is comparable, however, to that of protein C deficiency.

Pathobiology

Protein S circulates in plasma partly in complex with C4b binding protein; only free protein S, which normally constitutes about 35 to 40% of total protein S, can function as a cofactor of APC. As in antithrombin and protein C deficiencies, quantitative (type I) and qualitative (type II) forms of inherited protein S deficiency are known. In addition, type III protein S deficiency is characterized by normal plasma levels of total protein S but low levels of free protein S.

Relatively few specific mutations of the protein S gene have been described to date. Most involve frameshift, nonsense, or missense point mutations.

Activated Protein C Resistance (Factor V Leiden)

Epidemiology

The factor V Leiden mutation is remarkably frequent (3 to 7%) in healthy white populations but is far less prevalent in certain black and Asian populations. In various studies, APC resistance was found in a wide range of frequencies (10 to 64%) in patients with venous thromboembolism.

Pathobiology

Most subjects with functional APC resistance have a single, specific point mutation in the gene for factor V, which is a critical target of the physiologic anticoagulant action of APC. In this mutation, termed *factor V Leiden,* guanine is replaced with adenine at nucleotide 1691 (G1691A), which leads to the amino acid substitution of Arg504 by Gln and renders factor Va incapable of being inactivated by APC. Heterozygosity for the autosomally transmitted factor V Leiden mutation increases the risk for thrombosis by a factor of 5 to 10, whereas homozygosity increases the risk by a factor of 50 to 100.

Prothrombin Gene Mutation

The substitution of G for A at nucleotide 20210 of the prothrombin gene has been associated with elevated plasma levels of prothrombin and an increased risk for venous thrombosis. The allele frequency for this gain-of-function mutation is 1 to 6% in white populations, but it is much less prevalent in other racial groups. The prothrombin G20210A mutation is found in 6 to 8% of all patients with venous thromboembolism.

Other Primary Hypercoagulable States

Elevated levels of factor VIII coagulant activity are a significant risk factor for venous thrombosis, and family studies suggest that high factor VIII levels are often genetically determined. Increased levels of factors VII, IX, and XI, fibrinogen, von Willebrand's factor, and thrombin-activatable fibrinolysis inhibitor, as well as very low levels of tissue factor pathway inhibitor, may also confer increased risk. Many other inherited abnormalities of specific physiologic antithrombotic systems may be associated with a thrombotic tendency. Most of these conditions are limited to case reports or family studies, their molecular genetic bases are less well defined, and their prevalence rates are unknown, but are probably much lower than those of the disorders described earlier. The other primary hypercoagulable states include heparin cofactor II deficiency, dysfunctional thrombomodulin, and many fibrinolytic disorders that lead to impaired fibrin degradation, including hypoplasminogenemia, dysplasminogenemia, plasminogen activator deficiency, and certain dysfibrinogenemias that cause a thrombotic rather than a bleeding diathesis.

Clinical Manifestations

The primary hypercoagulable states are associated with predominantly venous thromboembolic complications (Chapter 81). Deep venous thrombosis of the lower extremities and pulmonary embolism are the most frequent clinical manifestations. More unusual sites of venous thrombosis include superficial thrombophlebitis and mesenteric and cerebral venous thrombosis (see Table 178–2). Arterial thrombosis involving the coronary, cerebrovascular, and peripheral circulations is not linked to any of the primary hypercoagulable states, although some reports have described their occurrence with protein S deficiency and homozygous antithrombin deficiency. Venous thrombosis can also result in arterial occlusion by paradoxical embolism across a patent foramen ovale.

The initial episode of venous thromboembolism can occur at any age in patients with primary hypercoagulable states, but it typically takes place in early adulthood. Positive family histories of thrombosis can frequently be elicited. The risk for thrombosis varies among the individual primary hypercoagulable states and is highest in patients with deficiencies of antithrombotic factors (see Table 182–1); it is markedly increased with the coexistence of multiple prothrombotic mutations. Patients with homozygous deficiency states tend to have more severe thrombotic complications. A peculiar manifestation of homozygous protein C or protein S deficiency is neonatal purpura fulminans. This serious, sometimes fatal syndrome is caused by ischemic necrosis secondary to widespread thrombosis of small cutaneous and subcutaneous vessels. Fatal purpura fulminans associated with a bleeding diathesis has also been described in a patient with an acquired IgG inhibitor of protein C. Warfarin-induced skin necrosis (Chapter 35 and see Fig. 182–1) may infrequently complicate the initiation of oral anticoagulant therapy in patients with heterozygous protein C or protein S deficiency. Because both these proteins depend on vitamin K for normal function, their plasma levels in patients with inherited deficiency states may drop to nearly zero within a few days of starting therapy with warfarin, a vitamin K antagonist, and lead to a transient prothrombotic imbalance and skin necrosis caused by dermal vascular thrombosis. Nevertheless, oral anticoagulation provides effective long-term antithrombotic prophylaxis in these individuals.

In most patients with primary hypercoagulable states, discrete clinical thrombotic complications seem to be precipitated by acquired prothrombotic events (e.g., pregnancy, use of oral contraceptives, surgery, trauma, immobilization), many of which are the secondary hypercoagulable states discussed subsequently. In particular, thrombosis complicates pregnancy, especially during the puerperium, in about 30 to 60% of women with antithrombin deficiency, 10 to 20% with protein C or protein S deficiency, and almost 30% with APC resistance, unless prophylactic anticoagulation is administered during this period.

Diagnosis

Laboratory diagnosis (Chapter 178) of the primary hypercoagulable states requires testing for each of the disorders individually because no general screening test is available to determine whether a patient may have such a condition. At this time, functional, immunologic, or DNA-based assays are available to test for antithrombin deficiency, protein C deficiency, protein S deficiency, APC resistance (factor V Leiden), and the prothrombin G20210A mutation.

A reasonable diagnostic approach at this time is to screen at least all "strongly thrombophilic" patients after an initial episode of venous thromboembolism: individuals with (1) a documented event before 50 years of age, (2) a positive family history, (3) massive or submassive pulmonary embolism, or (4) spontaneous thrombosis at an unusual site (e.g., intra-abdominal or cerebral). Although indefinite anticoagulation is recommended for patients who have had two or more venous thromboembolic events, regardless of whether a primary hypercoagulable state is found, testing these individuals for thrombophilia may also be useful to guide family screening strategies. Individuals with arterial thrombosis generally should not be tested for any of these disorders because primary hypercoagulable states (see Table 182–1) are not clearly associated with an increased risk for arterial thrombosis. In contrast, some of the secondary hypercoagulable states, including hyperhomocysteinemia and the antiphospholipid syndrome (see later), are associated with an increased risk for arterial thrombosis.

In general, testing for primary hypercoagulable states is not recommended immediately after a major thrombotic event, but rather in clinically stable patients at least 2 weeks after completing oral anticoagulation following a thrombotic episode. Active thrombosis may transiently consume and deplete some of the proteins in plasma and lead to the erroneous diagnosis of inherited antithrombin, protein C, or protein S deficiency. In addition to acute thrombosis, pregnancy, estrogen use, liver disease, and disseminated intravascular coagulation (DIC) may cause acquired deficiencies of antithrombin, protein C, or protein S. Anticoagulation may also interfere with some of the functional tests for primary hypercoagulable states. Heparin treatment can cause a decline in antithrombin levels to the deficiency range even in normal individuals. In contrast, warfarin can elevate antithrombin levels into the normal range in patients who do have an inherited deficiency state. Warfarin therapy also reduces the functional levels and, less prominently, the immunologic levels of protein C and protein S, thereby potentially leading to a misdiagnosis of inherited deficiency. When testing is indicated in patients in whom interruption of prophylactic oral anticoagulation is considered to be too risky, protein C and protein S levels can be determined after warfarin therapy has been discontinued under heparin coverage for at least 2 weeks.

Functional assays are the best screening tests for antithrombin, protein C, and protein S deficiencies because these assays detect both quantitative and qualitative defects; antigenic (immunologic) assays detect only quantitative deficiencies of these proteins. Functional coagulation assays for protein C and protein S may yield spuriously low values, however, if APC resistance is present. APC resistance can be diagnosed by the newer high-sensitivity and high-specificity coagulation assays or by DNA analysis of peripheral blood mononuclear cells for the factor V Leiden mutation.

Treatment

Rx

The initial treatment of acute venous thrombosis or pulmonary embolism in patients with primary hypercoagulable states is not different from that in patients without genetic defects (Chapters 35 and 81). As in patients without known thrombophilia, thrombolytic therapy should be considered after massive venous thrombosis or pulmonary embolism. Acute management is initiated with at least 5 days of unfractionated or low-molecular-weight heparin. Oral anticoagulation with warfarin can be started on the first day of heparin use and continued for at least 6 months in patients with venous thromboembolism in the absence of triggering factors (e.g., postoperative state), with regulation of the dose to maintain an international normalized ratio (INR) of the prothrombin time between 2.0 and 3.0. 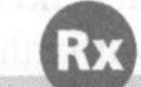

Continuing oral anticoagulant prophylaxis beyond the initial 6 to 12 months after an acute episode of venous thromboembolism must be weighed against continued exposure of the individual patient to the significant risk for bleeding complications. Patients with primary hypercoagulable states who have had two or more thrombotic events should receive indefinite or lifelong prophylactic anticoagulation with warfarin (Chapter 81). Indefinite or lifelong anticoagulation is probably indicated for individuals with recurrent thrombosis even in the absence of identifiable primary hypercoagulable states.

TABLE 182–2 LONG-TERM MANAGEMENT OF PATIENTS WITH PRIMARY HYPERCOAGULABLE STATES

Risk Classification	Management
High risk ≥2 spontaneous thromboses 1 spontaneous life-threatening thrombosis 1 spontaneous thrombosis at an unusual site (e.g., mesenteric, cerebral venous) 1 spontaneous thrombosis in the presence of antiphospholipid syndrome, antithrombin deficiency, or more than a single hypercoagulable state	Indefinite anticoagulation or lifelong chronic anticoagulation
Moderate risk 1 thrombosis with an acquired prothrombotic stimulus	Vigorous prophylaxis during high-risk situations
Asymptomatic	

Modified from Bauer K: Approach to thrombosis. *In* Loscalzo J, Schafer AI (eds): Thrombosis and Hemorrhage, 3rd ed. Philadelphia, Lippincott Williams & Wilkins, 2003, pp 330–342.

Rx

The decision to continue prophylactic oral anticoagulation beyond the initial period after the first episode of thrombosis is more difficult (Table 182–2). After a single episode of thrombosis, patients with inherited hypercoagulable states should probably receive indefinite or lifelong anticoagulation if their initial episodes were life-threatening or occurred in unusual sites (e.g., mesenteric, cerebral venous thrombosis) or if they have more than one prothrombotic genetic abnormality (Chapter 81). Some authorities also recommend indefinite or lifelong anticoagulation after an initial venous thromboembolic event in patients whose risk of recurrence likewise appears to be increased: those with isolated heterozygous deficiencies of antithrombin, protein C, or protein S or patients with homozygous factor V Leiden. In the absence of these characteristics, particularly if the initial episode was precipitated by a transient acquired prothrombotic situation (e.g., pregnancy, postoperative state, immobilization), it is reasonable at this time to discontinue warfarin therapy after 6 to 12 months and administer subsequent prophylactic anticoagulation only during high-risk periods.

Asymptomatic individuals with known thrombophilia who have not had previous thrombotic complications do not require prophylactic anticoagulation except during periods of high risk for thrombosis. Because about half of the first-degree relatives of a patient with a primary hypercoagulable state should be affected, these individuals should be counseled about the implications of making a diagnosis.

Management of pregnancy in women with primary hypercoagulable states requires special consideration because of the high risk for thrombosis, particularly during the puerperium. Women with thrombophilia who have previously had thrombosis—and probably also asymptomatic women with thrombophilia—should receive prophylactic anticoagulation throughout pregnancy and for 4 to 6 weeks postpartum, a particularly high-risk period. Coumarin derivatives cross the placenta and have the potential to cause both bleeding and teratogenic effects in the fetus; therefore, oral anticoagulants should not be used during pregnancy. Heparin does not cross the placenta and does not cause these fetal complications.

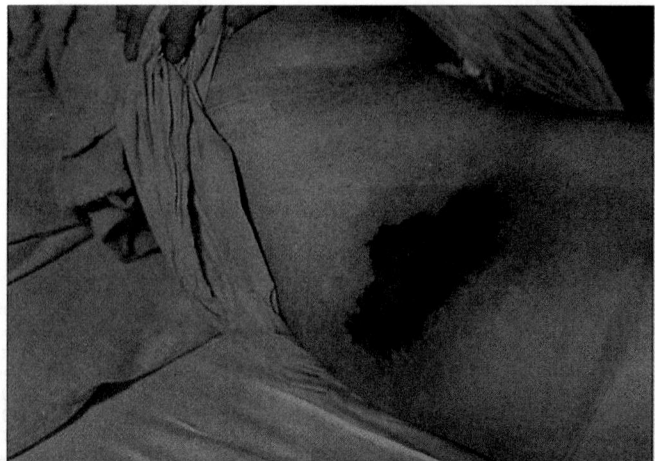

FIGURE 182–1 • Acute skin necrosis in a patient with protein C deficiency who was treated with heparin and warfarin for deep vein thrombosis that occurred after elective hip surgery. Warfarin treatment was withdrawn and anticoagulation continued with heparin. Skin grafting of the affected area was required. (From Forbes CD, Jackson WF: Color Atlas and Text of Clinical Medicine, 3rd ed. London, Mosby, 2003.)

Rx

Therefore, either unfractionated heparin or fixed-dose, low-molecular-weight heparin is the anticoagulant of choice during pregnancy. Neither warfarin nor heparin induces an anticoagulant effect in a breast-fed infant when the drug is given to a nursing mother, so either can be given safely when indicated in the postpartum period.

Because warfarin-induced skin necrosis (Fig. 182–1) is a rare problem, screening of all patients for inherited protein C or protein S deficiency, conditions that are known to predispose to this complication, is not indicated before starting warfarin therapy. Most cases can be avoided by not initiating warfarin therapy with high loading doses and by concomitant coverage with heparin. When the complication does occur, as manifested by painful red and subsequently dark, necrotic skin lesions within a few days of starting warfarin, such therapy must be discontinued immediately, vitamin K administered, and heparin started (Chapter 35). The use of fresh-frozen plasma or purified protein C concentrate to normalize protein C levels rapidly can improve results. Despite this rare complication, warfarin is an effective, long-term prophylactic anticoagulant in patients with inherited protein C or protein S deficiency.

Antithrombin III concentrate purified from normal human plasma may be a useful adjunct to anticoagulation in "heparin-resistant" patients, who represent unusual cases of type II antithrombin deficiency, and in antithrombin-deficient patients with recurrent thrombosis despite adequate anticoagulation. Infusion of antithrombin concentrate can also be considered in some perioperative or obstetric settings in which anticoagulation poses an unacceptable bleeding risk.

SECONDARY HYPERCOAGULABLE STATES

Definition

The secondary hypercoagulable states (Fig. 182–2) are diverse, mostly acquired disorders that predispose patients to thrombosis by complex, multifactorial pathophysiologic mechanisms. Many of these conditions also represent the acquired precipitating stimuli for clinical thrombotic events in individuals with a genetic predisposition (primary hypercoagulable states). Although each disorder causes thrombosis primarily through abnormalities in blood flow (rheology), the composition of blood (coagulation factors and platelet function), or the vessel wall, multiple overlapping mechanisms are operative in many of them.

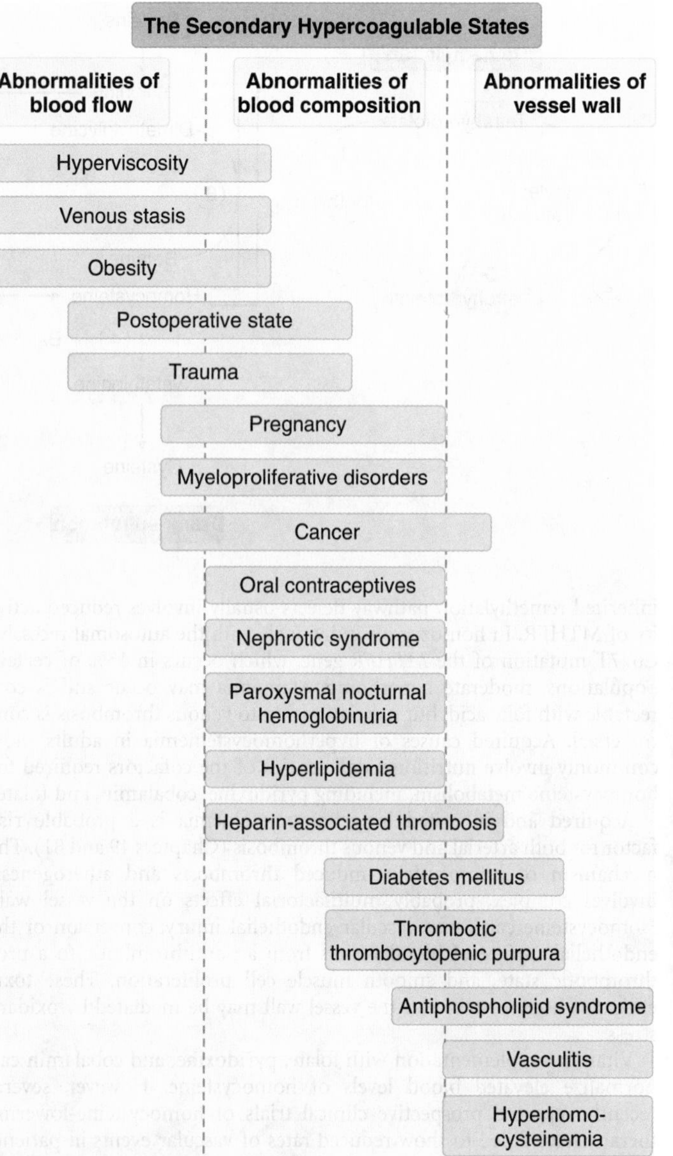

FIGURE 182–2 • Secondary hypercoagulable states. The pathophysiologic basis of thrombotic risk in these diverse disorders is complex and multifactorial. Predominant mechanisms of thrombosis for the different secondary hypercoagulable states shown are based on Virchow's triad of thrombogenesis: abnormalities in blood flow, abnormalities in blood composition, and abnormalities of the vessel wall. (Modified from Schafer AI: The primary and secondary hypercoagulable states. *In* Schafer AI [ed]: Molecular Mechanisms of Hypercoagulable States. New York, Chapman & Hall, 1997, p 16.)

Hyperhomocysteinemia

Hyperhomocysteinemia is an elevated blood level of homocysteine, a sulfhydryl amino acid derived from methionine by a transmethylation pathway (Fig. 182–3). Homocysteine is remethylated to methionine or catabolized to cystathionine. The major remethylation pathway requires folate and cobalamin (vitamin B_{12}) and involves the action of methylenetetrahydrofolate reductase (MTHFR); a minor remethylation pathway is mediated by betaine-homocysteine methyltransferase. Alternatively, homocysteine is converted to cystathionine in a trans-sulfuration pathway catalyzed by cystathionine β-synthase (CBS), with pyridoxine used as a cofactor.

Homozygous CBS deficiency states that lead to severe hyperhomocysteinemia (homocystinuria) (Chapter 228) cause premature arterial atherosclerotic disease and venous thromboembolism, as well as mental retardation, neurologic defects, lens ectopy, and skeletal abnormalities. By comparison, adults with heterozygous CBS deficiency, with resultant mild to moderate hyperhomocysteinemia, may have only venous or arterial thrombotic manifestations. Hyperhomocysteinemia resulting from

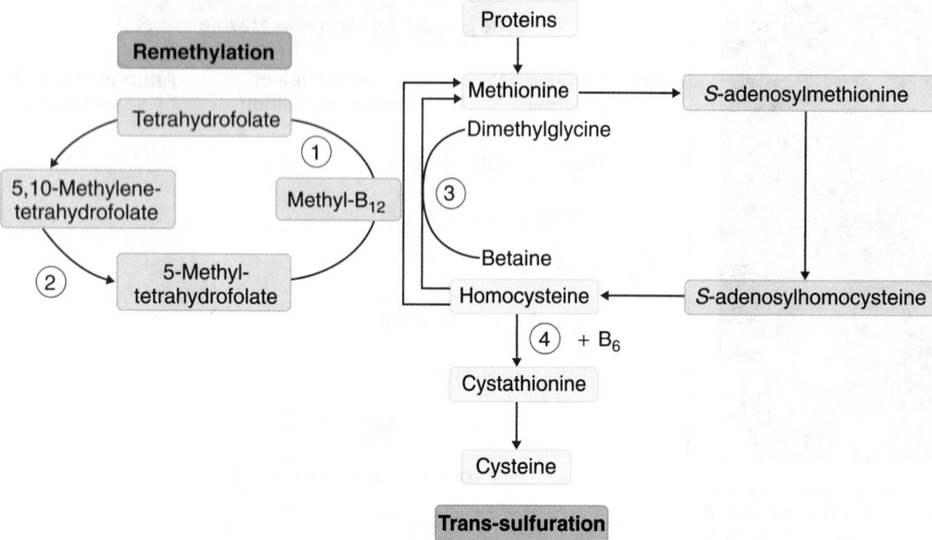

FIGURE 182-3 • Intracellular metabolism of homocysteine occurs through remethylation to methionine or trans-sulfuration to cysteine. Numbered circles indicate the principal enzymes involved: (1) methionine synthase; (2) 5,10-methylenetetrahydrofolate reductase; (3) betaine-homocysteine methyltransferase; (4) cystathionine β-synthase. (Modified from De Stefano V, Finazzi G, Mannucci PM: Inherited thrombophilia: Pathogenesis, clinical syndromes, and management. Blood 1996;87:3531–3544.)

inherited remethylation pathway defects usually involves reduced activity of MTHFR. In homozygous individuals with the autosomal recessive C677T mutation of the *MTHFR* gene, which occurs in 15% of certain populations, moderate hyperhomocysteinemia may occur and is correctable with folic acid, but its relationship to venous thrombosis is controversial. Acquired causes of hyperhomocysteinemia in adults most commonly involve nutritional deficiencies of the cofactors required for homocysteine metabolism, including pyridoxine, cobalamin, and folate.

Acquired and inherited hyperhomocysteinemia is a probable risk factor for both arterial and venous thrombosis (Chapters 49 and 81). The mechanism of homocysteine-induced thrombosis and atherogenesis involves complex, probably multifactorial effects on the vessel wall. Homocysteine can cause vascular endothelial injury, conversion of the endothelial surface of blood vessels from an antithrombotic to a prothrombotic state, and smooth muscle cell proliferation. These toxic effects of homocysteine on the vessel wall may be mediated by oxidant stress.

Vitamin supplementation with folate, pyridoxine, and cobalamin can normalize elevated blood levels of homocysteine. However, several recently reported prospective clinical trials of homocysteine-lowering therapy have failed to show reduced rates of vascular events in patients with established vascular disease. It remains to be determined whether this disappointing lack of clinical benefit with homocysteine-lowering vitamin therapy indicates that homocysteine is not a direct atherogenic factor, or that vitamin therapy in this setting might have other, offsetting deleterious effects, or that possibly other mechanisms are operative.

Malignancy

Multiple abnormalities of hemostasis are involved in the hypercoagulable state in cancer patients, many of which initiate a systemic process of chronic DIC (Chapters 181 and 189). The thrombotic tendency of patients with cancer may also be related to mechanical factors, such as immobility, indwelling central venous catheters, or a bulky tumor mass compressing vessels, and to comorbid conditions, such as sepsis, surgery, liver dysfunction secondary to metastases, and the prothrombotic effects of certain antineoplastic agents.

The incidence of thrombotic complications in cancer patients depends in part on the type of malignancy. Hypercoagulability seems to be most prominent in patients with pancreatic cancer (Chapter 204), adenocarcinoma of the gastrointestinal tract (Chapters 202 and 203) or lung (Chapter 201), and ovarian cancer (Chapter 209). The presence of underlying malignancy compounds the independent risk for thrombosis in the postoperative state. Thrombosis most commonly occurs in patients with established or concurrently diagnosed malignancy (Chapters 81 and 189).

The most frequent thrombotic manifestations in patients with neoplasms are deep vein thrombosis and pulmonary embolism, but more unusual and distinctive thrombotic complications are also found. Trousseau's syndrome, characterized by migratory superficial thrombophlebitis of the upper or lower extremities, is strongly linked to cancer. Nonbacterial thrombotic endocarditis involves fibrin-platelet vegetations on heart valves, which produce clinical manifestations by systemic embolization (Chapter 59). Of patients with nonbacterial thrombotic endocarditis, 75% have underlying malignancies at autopsy. Trousseau's syndrome and nonbacterial thrombotic endocarditis are highly associated with adenocarcinomas. The occurrence of either syndrome in patients without known cancer demands a more vigorous search for occult malignancy than in patients with deep vein thrombosis or pulmonary embolism. Thrombotic microangiopathy (Chapter 189), characterized by hemolysis with red blood cell fragmentation, thrombocytopenia, and microvascular thrombosis with involvement of target organs, occurs in about 5% of patients with metastatic carcinomas, most commonly those with gastric (Chapter 202), lung (Chapter 201), and breast (Chapter 208) primary sites.

Treatment

Rx

Treatment of acute venous thromboembolism in cancer patients should be initiated as in other patients, but subsequent prophylactic anticoagulation should be continued while active malignancy is present. Anticoagulation can be difficult in many cancer patients; these patients may be resistant to warfarin prophylaxis. Anticoagulation can also be complicated by bleeding into tumors. Long-term treatment of cancer patients with low-molecular-weight heparin after venous thromboembolism (Chapter 35) reduces recurrences and possibly decreases bleeding complications when compared with treatment with warfarin. 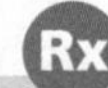

Myeloproliferative Disorders and Paroxysmal Nocturnal Hemoglobinuria

Thrombosis and, apparently paradoxically, bleeding are major causes of morbidity and mortality in patients with myeloproliferative disorders (Chapters 172 and 177) and the related stem cell disorder paroxysmal nocturnal hemoglobinuria (Chapter 164). In uncontrolled polycythemia vera (Chapter 172), increased whole blood viscosity contributes to the thrombotic tendency. Thrombocytosis, abnormal platelet function, and other less well understood factors are also probably involved in the hemostatic defect of the myeloproliferative disorders and paroxysmal nocturnal hemoglobinuria.

In addition to deep vein thrombosis and pulmonary embolism, some distinctive thrombotic manifestations are seen. Hepatic vein thrombosis (Budd-Chiari syndrome) and portal and other intra-abdominal venous thromboses (Chapter 146) are associated with myeloproliferative disorders and paroxysmal nocturnal hemoglobinuria (Chapter 164) and may be the initial manifestations of the disease. Myeloproliferative disorders, particularly polycythemia vera (Chapter 172) and essential thrombocythemia (Chapter 177), may cause erythromelalgia (see Fig. 172–2), a syndrome of microvascular thrombosis manifested by intense pain accompanied by warmth, duskiness, and mottled erythema, sometimes resembling livedo reticularis, in a patchy distribution in the extremities, most prominently in the feet; digital microvascular ischemia progressing to vascular insufficiency and gangrene may ensue (Chapter 80). A wide spectrum of neurologic manifestations may be caused by cerebrovascular ischemia, especially in patients with essential thrombocythemia.

Treatment

Treatment of venous thromboembolism in patients with the myeloproliferative disorders and paroxysmal nocturnal hemoglobinuria should be initiated as in patients without these hematologic disorders. In patients with thrombosis associated with polycythemia vera, the hematocrit should be maintained in the normal range with phlebotomies or chemotherapy, or with both (Chapter 172). Low-dose aspirin (100 mg daily) can prevent thrombotic complications without increasing the incidence of major bleeding in patients with polycythemia vera who have no contraindications to such treatment. 3 In patients with essential thrombocythemia, cytoreduction of the elevated platelet count should be achieved with chemotherapy (Chapter 177).

Antiphospholipid Syndrome

Antiphospholipid syndrome is characterized by venous and arterial thrombosis, recurrent spontaneous abortions (which may also be due to thrombosis), thrombocytopenia, and a variety of neuropsychiatric manifestations. The syndrome is associated with a heterogeneous group of autoantibodies that bind to anionic phospholipid-protein complexes, a protein cofactor of which is β_2-glycoprotein I. Patients with this syndrome have any combination of positive tests to detect different plasma antiphospholipid-protein antibodies (e.g., anticardiolipin antibodies) and/or phospholipid-based clotting tests (lupus anticoagulants) (Chapter 287). The predominant prothrombotic effects of these antibodies are probably directed to the vessel wall.

Deep vein thrombosis and pulmonary embolism are the most frequent venous thrombotic events in these patients. Cerebrovascular events are the most common arterial thrombotic complications and are manifested as stroke, transient ischemic attacks (Chapter 431), multi-infarct dementia (Chapters 26 and 425), or retinal artery occlusion (Fig. 449–20). Peripheral and intra-abdominal vascular occlusion is encountered more rarely. About a third of these patients have nonbacterial heart valve vegetations (Libman-Sacks endocarditis). The most prominent obstetric complications are recurrent spontaneous abortions and fetal growth retardation, which are probably due to thrombosis of placental vessels. Patients are occasionally seen with "catastrophic" antiphospholipid syndrome involving a series of acute and sometimes fatal vascular occlusive events, or "thrombotic storm." Thrombotic complications are limited largely to patients with primary antiphospholipid syndrome or patients in whom the antibodies are associated with collagen vascular disease, not with drugs or infections.

Treatment

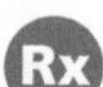

Acute management of thrombosis in these patients is essentially the same as in other individuals. Monitoring of heparin anticoagulation is difficult in patients with a lupus anticoagulant because they already have a prolonged activated partial thromboplastin time at baseline; the use of low-molecular-weight heparin, which does not require monitoring, can circumvent this problem. Warfarin is effective in preventing recurrent thrombosis but usually requires prolonged or indefinite therapy with doses to achieve an INR of 2.0 to 3.0. 4 No established treatment of women with antiphospholipid syndrome has been shown to prevent recurrent fetal loss. Treatment with prednisone and aspirin during pregnancy is not effective in promoting live birth and may increase the risk for prematurity.

Pregnancy, Oral Contraceptives, and Hormone Replacement Therapy

The pathophysiology of hypercoagulability associated with pregnancy (Chapter 259) involves a progressive state of DIC throughout the course of pregnancy. Activation of the coagulation system is initiated locally in the uteroplacental circulation, where the placenta is the source of increased thrombin generation. Platelet activation and increased platelet turnover also occur during normal pregnancy, and about 8% of healthy women have mild thrombocytopenia at term. Simultaneously, the fibrinolytic system is progressively blunted throughout pregnancy because of the action of placental plasminogen activator inhibitor type 2. The net effect of these coagulation changes is creation of a state of hypercoagulability that makes pregnant women vulnerable to thrombosis, particularly in the puerperium. These systemic alterations are compounded by prothrombotic mechanical and rheologic factors in pregnancy, including venous stasis in the legs caused by the gravid uterus, pelvic vein injury during labor, and the trauma of cesarean section. Oral contraceptives induce a prothrombotic state by increasing procoagulant effects and decreasing physiologic anticoagulant effects. The use of oral contraceptives is associated with an increased risk for venous thrombosis, myocardial infarction, stroke, and peripheral arterial disease, particularly during the first year of use (Chapter 262). Unexpectedly, third-generation oral contraceptives, which contain less estrogen and a different progestin, double the risk for venous thromboembolism in comparison to second-generation preparations. Postmenopausal hormone replacement increases the risk for deep venous thromboembolism by a factor of 2 to 3.5, at least during the first year. Hormone replacement therapy has no beneficial and possibly even a detrimental effect on the risk for arterial disease (Chapter 262).

Deep vein thrombosis and pulmonary embolism are the most common thrombotic complications of pregnancy and the use of oral contraceptives or hormone replacement therapy. Coexisting primary hypercoagulable states are an additive risk factor in all of these settings. In the absence of a clear family history of venous thromboembolism, there is little justification, however, to screen for prothrombotic mutations with pregnancy or before starting hormone replacement therapy or oral contraceptives. Increasing age, increasing parity, cesarean delivery, prolonged bedrest or immobilization, obesity, and previous thromboembolism are additional prothrombotic risk factors in pregnant women. Most thrombotic events associated with pregnancy occur in the peripartum period, especially after delivery. Special considerations for anticoagulation in the setting of pregnancy are noted in the section on treatment of primary hypercoagulable states.

Postoperative State, Immobilization, and Trauma

Postoperative thrombosis (Chapter 459) is caused by a combination of local mechanical factors, including decreased venous blood flow in the lower extremities, and systemic changes in coagulation (Chapter 81). The level of risk for postoperative thrombosis depends largely on the type of surgery performed. It is probably compounded by coexisting risk factors, such as an underlying inherited primary hypercoagulable state or malignancy, advanced age, and prolonged procedures. Postoperative deep vein thrombosis and pulmonary embolism, the most common thrombotic complications, are often asymptomatic but detectable by noninvasive studies. The incidence of deep vein thrombosis after general surgical procedures is about 20 to 25%, with almost 2% of these patients having clinically significant pulmonary embolism. The risk for deep vein thrombosis after hip surgery and knee reconstruction ranges from 45 to 70% without prophylaxis, and clinically significant pulmonary embolism occurs in 20% of patients undergoing hip surgery. Postoperative thrombosis risk after urologic and gynecologic surgery more closely approximates that found after general surgery. Although the process of thrombosis generally begins intraoperatively or within a few days of surgery, the risk for this complication can be protracted beyond the time of discharge from the hospital, particularly in hip replacement patients.

Patients who are bedridden or experiencing prolonged air travel are at increased risk for venous thromboembolism. Venous thromboembolism is also one of the most common causes of morbidity and mortality in survivors of major trauma, and asymptomatic deep vein thrombosis of the lower extremities has been detected by venography in more than 50% of hospitalized trauma patients (Chapter 113). The risk for venous thrombosis after trauma is increased by advanced age, need for surgery or transfusions, and the presence of lower extremity fractures or spinal cord injury.

Mechanical methods of prophylaxis against venous thromboembolism should be considered in high-risk postoperative patients and bedridden patients with medical conditions, either in combination with anticoagulant prophylaxis or instead of it in patients who have an unusually high risk for bleeding with anticoagulation. Such methods include graduated compression stockings, intermittent pneumatic compression devices, and venous foot pumps. For long-distance travelers with thrombophilia, either properly fitted below-knee graduated compression stockings or a single prophylactic dose of low-molecular-weight heparin injected before departure is recommended in addition to general measures such as avoidance of dehydration and frequent stretching of calf muscles.

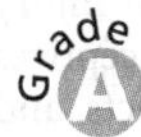

1. Kearon C, Ginsberg JS, Kovacs MJ, et al: Comparison of low-intensity warfarin therapy with conventional-intensity warfarin therapy for long-term prevention of recurrent venous thromboembolism. N Engl J Med 2003;349:631–639.
2. Lee AY, Levine MN, Baker RI, et al: Low-molecular-weight heparin versus a coumarin for the prevention of recurrent venous thromboembolism in patients with cancer. N Engl J Med 2003; 349:146–153.
3. Landolfi R, Marchioli R, Kutti J, et al: Efficacy and safety of low-dose aspirin in polycythemia vera. N Engl J Med 2004;350:114–124.
4. Crowther MA, Ginsberg JS, Julian J, et al: A comparison of two intensities of warfarin for the prevention of recurrent thrombosis in patients with the antiphospholipid antibody syndrome. N Engl J Med 2003;349:1133–1138.

SUGGESTED READINGS

Büller HR, Agnelli G, Hull RD, et al: Antithrombotic therapy for venous thromboembolic disease: The Seventh ACCP Conference on Antithrombotic and Thrombolytic Therapy. Chest 2004;126:401S–428S. *Updated, comprehensive guidelines with graded, evidence-based recommendations.*

De Stefano V, Rossi E, Za T, Leone G: Prophylaxis and treatment of venous thromboembolism in individuals with inherited thrombophilia. Semin Thromb Hemost 2006;32:767–780. *Concise review of how thrombophilias guide anticoagulation strategies.*

Giannakopoulos B, Passam F, Rahgozar S, et al: Current concepts on the pathogenesis of the antiphospholipid syndrome. Blood 2007;109:422–430. *An excellent review.*

Lim W, Crowther MA, Eikelboom JW: Management of antiphospholipid antibody syndrome: A systematic review. JAMA 2006;295:1050–1057. *A comprehensive review.*

Merriman L, Greaves M: Testing for thrombophilia: An evidence-based approach. Postgrad Med 2006;82:699–704. *Critical review of the benefits and pitfalls of testing for acquired and inherited hypercoagulable states in cases of venous thromboembolism.*

Walker ID: Exogenous sex hormones and thrombophilia. Obstet Gynecol Clin North Am 2006;33:467–479. *Discussion of risk of thrombosis with the use of oral contraceptives and postmenopausal hormone replacement in women with thrombophilia.*

183 TRANSFUSION MEDICINE

Lawrence T. Goodnough

DEVELOPMENT OF TRANSFUSION MEDICINE

Issues in blood transfusion and blood conservation include the safety of blood, the formation of guidelines and consensus statements on the use of blood components and products, new strategies in blood conservation, emerging alternatives to blood transfusion, and issues related to informed consent for transfusion. The broad-based constituency of transfusion medicine includes blood collection facilities, hospital-based transfusion services, research laboratories, and the commercial sector.

The Transfusion Medicine Specialist

Medical management of the blood bank addresses issues related to blood inventory and safety, as well as oversight of laboratory policies and procedures (Fig. 183–1). Management of the transfusion service includes the coordination of blood transfusion and blood conservation activities, in addition to serving as a consultant to clinicians managing patients undergoing massive transfusion, apheresis, or transplantation or having problems such as difficulty finding compatible blood products. Finally, the transfusion medicine specialist supervises quality assurance to satisfy regulatory and accreditation requirements.

TRANSFUSION

Worldwide, more than 75 million units of whole blood are estimated to be donated every year. In the United States, the yearly transfusion of more than 13 million units corresponds to transfusion of 1 unit of blood every 0.39 second.

Blood Availability

Blood centers must be able to supply blood in response to acute crises. Sporadic shortages of blood and blood products (e.g., packed red cells, platelet products, albumin, intravenous immunoglobulin, and clotting factor concentrates) are potentially life-threatening. Such shortages have been attributed to disruptions in production, increasingly strict criteria

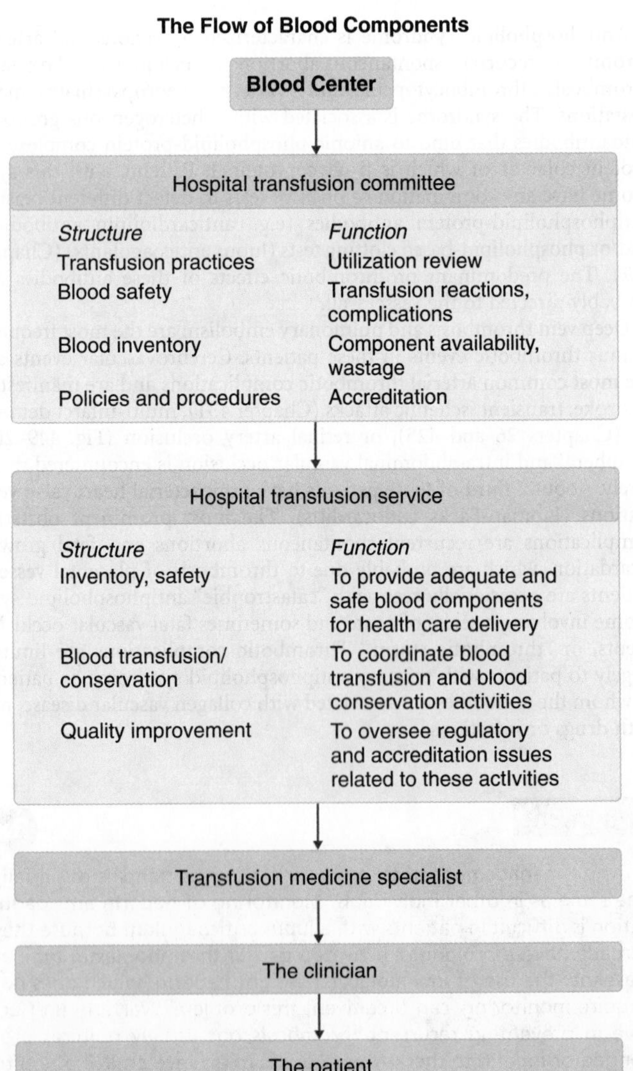

FIGURE 183–1 • A hospital's transfusion committee and transfusion service help clinicians manage the availability, safety, and use of blood products. (From Goodnough LT: What is a transfusion medicine specialist? Transfusion 1999;39:1031–1033. Reprinted with permission.)

for accepting donors, product recalls, increased use (including off-label), and possibly supply disruptions because of stockpiling or other market issues.

In an attempt to anticipate and manage such shortages better, the United Kingdom uses web-based submission of data and instant graphic feedback from 54% of hospitals served by the National Blood Service to track 1.44 million red cell units per year. In the United States, the Department of Health and Human Services monitors three sentinel community blood services and 26 sentinel hospital transfusion services, which account for about 10% of the U.S. inventory of red blood cells and platelets.

In the United States, blood transfusion and collection activities peaked in 1986 and then declined until 1994. However, blood transfusions and collections increased 8.0% in 1997, 10.2% in 1999, and an estimated 4% to 5% annually thereafter.

Within the American Red Cross, which supplies about half of all blood products in the United States, a 3- to 4-day supply of red blood cell products is typical, but some independent centers have higher reserves. Use of frozen red cells as a hedge against inventory shortages has generally not been practical because the shelf-life of thawed units is only 24 hours, but an automated, functionally closed system for the glycerolization and deglycerolization processes allows for a 2-week post-thaw shelf life. With the availability of such a system, many blood centers and transfusion services can expand their available red cell inventory for reserves. After disasters, human or natural, on-hand blood supplies are adequate in the short term and can be rapidly mobilized over great distances. Because of the need to maintain reserves, collections of blood routinely surpass transfusions—by 13 million units in 2000 and 15 million units in 2001.

Red Blood Cell Transfusion

Whole Blood

A unit of blood is collected as a donation of 450 mL ± 10% into a citrate anticoagulant that also contains phosphate and dextrose. The red cell and hemoglobin (Hgb) content is variable and dependent on the donor's hematocrit and the precise volume bled.

Whole blood is stored at 4 ± 2° C to diminish red cell utilization of adenosine triphosphate and to preserve their viability, which should be at least 70% at the end of a shell life of 35 days. After 10 days of storage, all predonation 2,3-diphosphoglycerate is lost, but up to 50% is regenerated within 8 hours after transfusion.

In Western countries, however, whole blood is rarely used because within a few hours or days, some coagulation factors (especially factors V and VIII) and platelets decrease in quantity or lose viability. After a 7-day hold at 4° C, factor VIII levels will have fallen to 0.32 ± 0.09 IU/mL, and there is a lesser fall in factor V levels to 0.78 ± 0.15 IU/mL. At 4° C, platelets undergo a shape change from discoid to spherical that is irreversible after 8 hours, and their in vivo survival is reduced to 2 days.

There are no absolute indications for the transfusion of whole blood and little good clinical trial evidence to compare the effectiveness of whole blood with red cell concentrates. However, some physicians continue to use whole blood for selected indications, such as large-volume transfusion in children or exchange transfusion in neonates, in whom there is a need for both red cells and expansion of plasma volume, and the supply of coagulation factors may offset the development of a dilutional coagulopathy.

Red Cell Components

Red cells are provided in various formats that differ with respect to the presence of additive solutions and the extent to which white cells are removed. Solutions that contain combinations of saline, adenine, phosphate, bicarbonate, glucose, and mannitol provide better red cell viability during storage and allow up to a 42-day shelf life. Red cells and red cells in additive solution can be used interchangeably, with the exception that red cells in additive solution are not recommended for exchange or massive transfusion in neonates.

Red cells should not be taken out of refrigeration until the time of the transfusion because of a risk for bacterial proliferation within the pack at room temperature. Red cells that have been out of refrigeration for 30 minutes or longer cannot be returned to stock and, if still required, should be transfused immediately. A unit of red cells should be infused over a maximum period of 4 hours.

Irradiated Cellular Blood Components

Gamma-irradiated cellular blood components are used to prevent the occurrence of transfusion-associated graft-versus-host disease (see later).

Leukocyte-Reduced Blood Components

Blood components are depleted of leukocytes by means of filtration. A leukocyte-reduced component is defined as one with less than 5×10^6 residual white cells per liter, and 100% of tested units should meet this standard. Leukocyte removal should be performed while the cells are still intact by filtering the blood as soon as possible after collection.

Leukocyte reduction reduces the incidence of human leukocyte antigen (HLA) alloimmunization in multitransfused recipients, but immunization rates of 10 to 25% are still seen in women who have already been exposed to HLA alloantigens in pregnancy. However, leukocyte reduction has less impact on refractoriness to random platelet donations because of the importance of nonimmune factors in the poor response to transfused platelets.

Leukocyte reduction also lowers the risk for nonhemolytic febrile reactions after the transfusion of red cells or platelets. Several, but not all studies suggest a beneficial impact of leukocyte reduction on the rate of postoperative infections. The impact of leukocyte reduction on the incidence of transfusion-associated graft-versus-host disease is unknown.

Preventing Transmission of Cytomegalovirus

A small number of studies of prestorage leukocyte reduction have suggested its efficacy in preventing transfusion-transmitted cytomegalovirus (CMV) infection (Chapter 399), which occurs in 4% of cases, even with seronegative components. Prestorage leukocyte depletion reduces the infection rate to less than 1%, thus suggesting that this technology may prove to be at least equivalent to serologic testing for CMV antibodies for the prevention of CMV transmission, but CMV testing of leukocyte-reduced components continues to be performed by most transfusion services. Indications for CMV-seronegative components include transfusion in pregnancy, intrauterine transfusions, transfusions to neonates less than 37 weeks' gestation, transfusions to CMV-seronegative patients who are potential or actual recipients of allogeneic bone marrow/peripheral blood progenitor transplants when the donor is also CMV seronegative, and patients infected with human immunodeficiency virus (HIV).

Immunomodulatory Effects

Previous transfusion has an immunomodulatory benefit for the survival of renal allografts, even with the use of potent immunosuppressive drugs (Chapter 133), although the exact mechanism of this benefit remains unknown. Retrospective studies suggest an adverse effect of transfusion on the rate of recurrent cancers, particularly colorectal cancer.

Typing and Crossmatching

Blood and blood components for transfusion should, in most cases, be the same blood type as the patient. Obtaining an accurate ABO/Rh grouping for a patient is the most significant serologic test performed before transfusion. When type-specific blood and components are unavailable or emergency circumstances do not allow their identification or use, type O-negative red cells should be used unless the recipient is blood group AB, in which case options include A, B, or O red cells. Group O is the only choice for group O recipients and is the alternative choice for both group A and group B.

Red cell antigens other than ABO and D are not routinely considered when selecting *donor* blood products for transfusion unless clinically significant, unexpected red cell antibodies are determined to be present by an antibody screen or have previously been identified. Red cell alloantibodies are produced by exposure to foreign red cell antigens via previous transfusion or pregnancy, or both. For an antibody to be considered clinically significant, it must be associated with a hemolytic transfusion reaction or decreased survival of transfused incompatible red cells. Most of the clinically significant antibodies are optimally reactive at 37° C or are detected by the antiglobulin test. If an antibody screen is negative in the *recipient,* the probability is greater than 99% that an ABO and Rh crossmatch will also be compatible. If no clinically significant, unexpected antibodies are detected and there is no record of previous detection of such antibodies, only serologic testing to detect ABO incompatibility is required (i.e., antiglobulin testing is not required when the crossmatch is performed).

Indications for Red Blood Cell Transfusion

If a transfusion is appropriate, a benefit should occur. In a large study of Jehovah's Witnesses, the risk for death was higher in surgical patients with cardiovascular disease than in those without. A follow-up analysis of a subset of these patients reported that the odds of death in patients with a postoperative Hgb level of less than 7 g/dL increased 2.5 times for each gram decrease in the Hgb level; although no deaths occurred in 98 patients with postoperative levels of 7.1 to 8.0 g/dL, 34.4% of 32 patients with postoperative levels of 4.1 to 5.0 g/dL died. These data suggest that in surgery-induced anemia, survival in patients at risk is improved if blood transfusion is administered to maintain the Hgb concentration at greater than 7 g/dL. In a large, retrospective study of elderly patients who underwent surgical repair of hip fractures, the use of perioperative transfusion in patients with Hgb levels as low as 8.0 g/dL did not appear to influence 30- or 90-day mortality.

In a multi-institutional study, 418 critical care patients received red cell transfusions when the Hgb level dropped below 7.0 g/dL and had their Hgb levels maintained between 7.0 and 9.0 g/dL, whereas another 420 patients received transfusions when the Hgb level declined below 10.0 g/dL and had their Hgb levels maintained between 10.0 and 12.0 g/dL. Thirty-day mortality rates were not significantly different in the two groups (18.7 vs. 23.3%, $P = .11$), thus suggesting that a transfusion threshold as low as 7.0 g/dL may be as safe as a higher transfusion threshold of 10.0 g/dL in critically ill patients. [1] A follow-up analysis found that the more restrictive strategy of red blood cell transfusion also appeared to be safe in most patients with cardiovascular disease.

A retrospective study analyzed the relationships among anemia, blood transfusion, and mortality in nearly 80,000 patients older than 65 years hospitalized for acute myocardial infarction. Anemia, defined as a hematocrit below 39%, was present on hospital admission in 44% of patients and was 33% or less in 10% of patients; blood transfusion in patients with hematocrit levels lower than 33% at admission was associated with a significantly lower 30-day mortality. On the basis of this study, transfusion to maintain hematocrit levels above 33% has been recommended in patients with acute myocardial infarction. In patients with heart failure, transfusion to maintain an Hgb level above 10 g/dL appears to improve outcomes.

Guideline

Guidelines from several professional groups recommend that blood not be transfused prophylactically in patients without risk factors until the Hgb level is 6.0 to 8.0 g/dL; an Hgb threshold of 8.0 g/dL seems appropriate in surgical patients with no risk factors for ischemia, whereas a threshold of 10 to 11 g/dL can be justified for patients who are considered to be at risk: those with myocardial ischemia or infarction, heart failure, chronic lung disease, or chronic kidney disease. With substantial improvements in blood safety, the concern now is that some patients may be at risk for undertransfusion.

Platelet Transfusion

The use of intensive chemotherapy regimens and bone marrow/stem cell transplantation has increased the demand for platelet products, particularly in patients with severe thrombocytopenia or bleeding complications. The use of apheresis platelet transfusions (i.e., a platelet unit collected from a dedicated donor via an apheresis procedure) has increased substantially, driven by the need for platelet inventories to support cardiac surgery, oncology, and stem cell transplantation programs. Emerging issues in platelet transfusion therapy include (1) re-evaluation of the platelet threshold for prophylactic transfusion and (2) modification of the dose of platelet transfusions.

Threshold for Platelet Transfusion

The appropriate threshold for platelet transfusion depends on the clinical situation (Fig. 183–2). Prospective, randomized studies indicate that a platelet transfusion threshold of 10,000 cells/μL is as safe and effective as higher thresholds in patients undergoing chemotherapy or stem cell transplantation. [2-4]

For consumptive thrombocytopenias such as disseminated intravascular coagulation (DIC) (Chapter 181), platelet therapy is supportive but not effective until the underlying cause is treated. Platelet transfusions are generally not indicated in patients with idiopathic thrombocytopenic purpura or the thrombotic microangiopathies (thrombotic thrombocytopenic purpura and hemolytic-uremic syndrome [Chapter 179]).

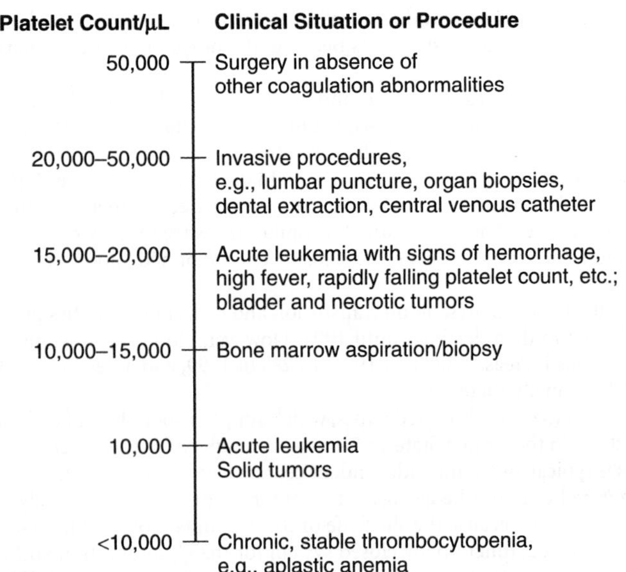

FIGURE 183–2 • Threshold for providing platelet transfusions in thrombocytopenic patients.

Platelet Dose

Standards of the American Association of Blood Banks require that 75% of apheresis products (i.e., platelet apheresis units) contain more than 3×10^{11} platelets and that 75% of platelet concentrates contain more than 5.5×10^{10} platelets; however, no consensus exists for a standardized platelet dose, and clinical trials have used a broad range of platelet doses. Leukoreduction of apheresis platelets results in an approximately 20% loss of platelets. In general, higher platelet doses result in greater incremental increases in the platelet count and prolonged time to the next transfusion, but the estimated platelet half-life is similar and there are no other differences in patients' outcomes.

Mathematical modeling suggests that low-dose platelet therapy (i.e., <1 platelet unit) may be more beneficial in thrombocytopenic patients who are receiving prophylactic platelet transfusions. The fixed platelet requirement for hemostasis is estimated to be 7100/μL^3/day, and platelet needs above this threshold are mainly a result of platelet consumption. For patients who become thrombocytopenic as a result of myeloablative therapy, platelet survival decreases with increasing severity of thrombocytopenia: platelet survival is 5 to 7 days in patients with platelet counts in the normal range, but only 1 to 2 days in patients with platelet counts of 10,000 to 20,000 cells/μL—levels at which most thrombocytopenic patients are maintained to prevent hemorrhage. One mathematical model predicted that low-dose platelet therapy allows a 22% decrease in the need for platelets while maintaining a platelet threshold greater than 10,000 cells/μL, even with a shorter transfusion-free interval and a greater daily relative risk of receiving additional transfusions.

Blood Safety (Table 183–1)

Errors in Transfusion Medicine

The mistransfusion rate (blood transfused to other than the intended recipient) is about 1 in 14,000 to 28,000 units. About two thirds of the errors occur in the clinical arena (incorrect identification of the recipient to the blood unit, phlebotomy errors, failure to recognize a transfusion reaction) and about a third in the laboratory. Half of mistransfusions are ABO incompatible, and about 10% are fatal. The frequency of death as a result of ABO error can therefore be estimated to be approximately 1 per 600,000 blood units, a risk that is higher than the risk of transmitting HIV or hepatitis C virus.

Transfusion Reactions

Acute Hemolytic Transfusion Reaction

An acute hemolytic transfusion reaction is most commonly defined as hemolysis of donor red cells within 25 hours of transfusion by preformed alloantibodies in the recipient's circulation. Life-threatening acute hemolytic transfusion reactions are most commonly due to ABO-incompatible blood being transfused to a recipient with naturally occurring

TABLE 183–1 TRANSFUSION-ASSOCIATED ADVERSE REACTIONS

	Risk per Unit Infused
ABO incompatible blood transfusions	1 in 30,000 to 60,000
Symptoms	40%
Fatalities	1 in 600,000
Delayed serologic reactions	1 in 1600
Delayed hemolytic reactions	1 in 6700
Transfusion-related acute lung injury	1 in 8,000
Graft-versus-host disease	Rare
Fluid overload	Underestimated
Febrile, nonhemolytic transfusion reactions	
Red blood cells (non–leukocyte reduced/leukocyte reduced)	1 in 200/1 in 300
Platelets (non–leukocyte reduced/leukocyte reduced)	1 in 5–20/1 in 25–50
Allergic reactions	1 in 30–100
Anaphylactic reactions	1 in 150,000
Iron overload	After 80–100 U
Post-transfusion purpura	Rare
Immunosuppressive effects	Unknown

ABO alloantibodies (anti-A, anti-B, anti-A, B). Clerical errors (mislabeling blood or misidentification of patients) account for 80% of such reactions.

Signs and symptoms of an acute intravascular hemolytic transfusion reaction may develop when as little as 10 to 15 mL of ABO-incompatible blood has been infused. Fever, which is the most common initial manifestation, is frequently accompanied by chills. The patient may have complaints such as a general sense of anxiety or uneasiness or may complain of pain at the infusion site or in the back or chest (or both). The most serious sequela is acute renal failure. In an unconscious or anesthetized patient, diffuse bleeding at the surgical site may be the first indication of intravascular hemolysis and may be accompanied by hemoglobinuria and hypotension.

Treatment begins with immediate cessation of the transfusion. The risk for renal failure may be reduced by the administration of crystalloid fluids, including sodium bicarbonate (250 to 500 mg intravenously over a 1- to 4-hour period), to maintain urine pH at 7.0 and by diuresis with 20% mannitol (100 mL/m^2 in 30 to 60 minutes, followed by 30 mL/m^2/hr for 12 hours) or furosemide (40 to 120 mg intravenously).

Febrile Nonhemolytic Transfusion Reactions

Febrile nonhemolytic transfusion reactions are common and estimated to occur in 0.5% of all red cell transfusions and up to 30% of platelet transfusions. A febrile transfusion reaction is defined as a rise in temperature of greater than 1° C, which may be accompanied by chills or rigor, or both.

These reactions are thought to be due to a reaction of HLA or leukocyte-specific antigens (or both) on transfused lymphocytes, granulocytes, or platelets in the donor unit with antibodies in previously alloimmunized recipients. Multiply transfused individuals and multiparous women are most likely to experience this type of transfusion reaction. Febrile nonhemolytic transfusion reactions, especially those associated with platelet transfusions, may be caused by the infusion of biologic response modifiers, such as cytokines, that have accumulated in the platelet concentrate during storage.

Symptoms may occur during the transfusion or not be manifested until 1 to 2 hours after its completion. The diagnosis of a febrile nonhemolytic transfusion reaction is generally made by excluding other causes of fever (e.g., bacterial contamination of blood, acute hemolytic transfusion reaction).

Febrile nonhemolytic transfusion reactions in susceptible populations can often be prevented by administering antipyretics before transfusion of blood components. Prestorage leukocyte reduction is recommended to prevent reactions that occur as a result of the accumulation of cytokines during storage.

Allergic Reactions

Allergic reactions can be mild, moderate, or life-threatening in severity and are associated with the amount of plasma transfused. From 1 to 5% of all blood transfusion recipients experience mild allergic reactions.

Anaphylactic transfusion reactions are sometimes associated with antibodies to IgA, which are common in the population and have an incidence of approximately 1 in 700 individuals. However, the incidence of anaphylactic transfusion reactions is much lower, 1 in 20,000 to 50,000.

Urticarial reactions are not well understood but are believed to be an interaction between antibodies in the recipient's plasma and plasma proteins in donor blood. There is not usually a specific identifiable antigen to which the patient is reacting.

Symptoms are generally mild and include localized urticaria, erythema, and itching. However, anaphylactic or anaphylactoid reactions, which can occur after the transfusion of only a few milliliters of blood or plasma, include skin flushing, nausea, abdominal cramps, vomiting, diarrhea, laryngeal edema, hypotension, shock, cardiac arrhythmia, cardiac arrest, and loss of consciousness. Fever is notably absent. In some instances there may be symptoms indicative of airway involvement, such as hoarseness, wheezing, dyspnea, and substernal pain. Management begins with discontinuation of the transfusion. Treatment is diphenhydramine (25 to 50 mg intravenously), but more severe episodes may require aggressive therapy (Chapters 273 and 274).

Patients who experience recurrent allergic or urticarial reactions can be pretreated with antihistamines before transfusion. Washed red blood cells may be indicated for patients who experience repeated severe urticarial reactions.

Bacterial Contamination

Bacterial contamination may be introduced into a unit of blood through skin contaminants during venipuncture or from donors with asymptomatic bacteremia. Multiplication of bacteria may occur in blood and blood components stored at refrigerated temperatures but is more likely to occur in blood components stored at room temperature.

Bacterial contamination of red cells is most often due to *Yersinia enterocolitica,* followed by *Serratia liquefaciens,* whereas platelets are most often contaminated with *Staphylococcus* and Enterobacteriaceae. The incidence of bacterial contamination of red cells has been estimated to be 1 in 60,000 with an overall fatality rate of 1 in 1,000,000. The incidence of bacterial contamination of platelets was estimated to be 1 in 5000 before the initiation of bacterial detection systems in 2004, but it is much lower now.

Recipients of units with low bacterial counts may have relatively mild symptoms such as fever and chills, but transfusion of units with high bacterial counts may result in severe or fatal reactions. Clinically, the patient may experience high fever, shock, hemoglobinuria, renal failure, and DIC. The blood transfusion must be stopped immediately, the patient's and any untransfused blood must be cultured, and broad-spectrum antibiotics (Chapter 109) should be started.

Circulatory Overload

Acute pulmonary edema, caused by the inability of the circulatory system to handle an increased fluid volume, can occur in any patient who is transfused too rapidly. Although the true frequency of this type of transfusion reaction is unknown, it is believed to be a common occurrence. Susceptible populations are primarily the very young, the elderly, and patients with a small total blood volume or cardiopulmonary disease. Treatment is the same as for heart failure (Chapter 58).

Delayed Reactions

A delayed hemolytic transfusion reaction generally occurs 3 to 7 days after transfusion of the implicated unit. Hemolysis is usually extravascular, and red cells are destroyed in the recipient's circulation by antibody produced as a result of an immune response induced by the transfusion. These reactions are most commonly due to an anamnestic response (secondary exposure to a red cell antigen) in a patient who had a negative antibody screen despite a low level of antibody as a result of previous exposure, either through pregnancy or transfusion, to a foreign red cell antigen. Exposure to the same antigen a second time may cause IgG antibody to reappear within hours or days of the transfusion. This subsequent exposure to the antigen produces an anamnestic antibody response resulting in increased production of IgG antibodies that are capable of reacting with any transfused cells present.

In most cases, anamnestic production of antibody does not result in acute hemolysis, but red cell destruction does occur between 3 days and 2 weeks after the transfusion. Patients are generally asymptomatic, and hemolysis may be noted only by a more rapid decline than usual in the patient's Hgb or absence of the expected rise in Hgb. Fever, the most common initial symptom, may occasionally be noted, along with jaundice; renal failure is rare. Prednisone (1 to 2 mg/kg/day) is indicated for more severe reactions.

Transfusion-Associated Graft-versus-Host Disease

Transfusion-associated graft-versus-host disease results from the transfusion of immunologically competent lymphocytes into an immunologically incompetent host. The risk for an individual depends on whether the recipient is immunocompromised (and the degree to which the recipient is immunocompromised), the degree of HLA similarity between the transfusion donor and recipient, and the number of transfused T lymphocytes capable of multiplying and engrafting. The engrafted lymphocytes mount an immunologic response against the recipient's tissue, thereby resulting in pancytopenia with bleeding and infectious complications. Symptoms usually appear within 12 days of transfusion. Transfusion-associated graft-versus-host disease is rare, but it is fatal in approximately 90% of affected patients.

Transfusion-Related Acute Lung Injury

Transfusion-related acute lung injury (TRALI; Chapter 94) is an acute respiratory distress syndrome (Chapter 105) that occurs within 4 hours after transfusion and is characterized by dyspnea and hypoxia secondary to noncardiogenic pulmonary edema. Although the actual incidence is almost certainly underreported, the estimated frequency is approximately 1 in 8000 transfusions. In approximately 50% of cases, blood donor antibodies with HLA or neutrophil antigenic specificity can be shown to react with the recipient's leukocytes, thereby leading to increased permeability of the pulmonary microcirculation.

Most recently, reactive lipid products from donor blood cell membranes that arise during the storage of blood products have been implicated in the pathophysiology of TRALI. Such substances are capable of neutrophil priming, with subsequent damage to the pulmonary-capillary endothelium of the recipient, particularly in patients who receive massive transfusions in defined clinical settings such as cardiac surgery or trauma or in patients receiving chemotherapy for malignancy. In each of these settings, the true incidence of TRALI may be underreported because the findings may be blamed on the underlying disease process or the surgical procedure. As in other causes of acute respiratory distress syndrome (Chapter 105), therapy is supportive, and 90% of patients recover.

Transmission of Viral Pathogens

The implementation of nucleic acid testing of multiple minipools (donation samples/test well) from blood donations has markedly reduced transmission of HIV and hepatitis C virus during the infectious window period. Current estimates of the risk per unit of blood in the post–nucleic acid testing era are 1 in 1.4 to 2.4 million for HIV and 1 in 872,000 to 1.7 million for hepatitis C virus (Fig. 183–3).

Only 43% of the World Health Organization's 191 member states test blood for HIV, hepatitis C virus, and hepatitis B virus, so at least 13 million units of blood donated every year are not tested for these transmissible viruses. In the poorest countries, access to safe blood is financially prohibitive because testing costs between $40 and $50 per blood donation. Every year, unsafe transfusions are estimated to account for 8 to 16 million hepatitis B infections, 2.3 to 4.7 million hepatitis C infections, and 80,000 to 160,000 HIV infections.

EMERGING TECHNOLOGIES

Stimulants of red blood cell production, including recombinant human erythropoietin, modified erythropoietin molecules, erythropoietin receptor agonists, and artificial oxygen carriers, can decrease the need for chronic red cell transfusion. It is important that oversight of these biotechnology products and other specialized blood products (such as solvent/detergent-treated plasma, leukoreduced blood products, irradiated blood components, and CMV-negative blood components) now included be placed under the auspices of standing hospital medical committees, such as a transfusion medicine committee. Otherwise, promotion of such products by the commercial sector directly to consumers

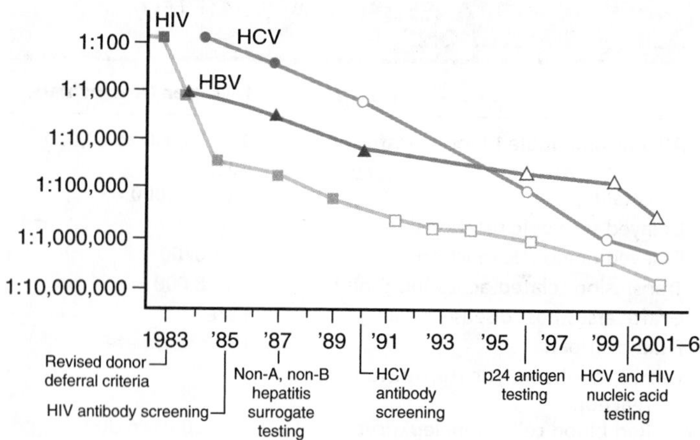

FIGURE 183–3 • Decline in transmission of human Immunodeficiency virus (HIV), hepatitis B virus (HBV), and hepatitis C virus (HCV) through transfusion of blood or blood components. Data were derived from studies sponsored by the National Heart, Lung and Blood Institute. Estimates are approximately 1 in 200,000 for HBV and about 1 in 2,000,000 each for HCV and HIV. (Adapted with permission from Busch MP, Kleinman SH, Nemo GJ: Current and emerging infectious risks of blood transfusions. JAMA 2003;289:959–962.)

could undermine both institutional oversight and evidence-based rationale for their use.

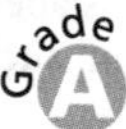

1. Herbert PC, Wells G, Blajchman MA, et al: A multicenter, randomized, controlled clinical trial of transfusion requirements in critical care. N Engl J Med 1999;340:409–417.
2. Rebulla P, Finazzi G, Marangoni F, et al: The threshold for prophylactic platelet transfusions in adults with acute myeloid leukemia. N Engl J Med 1997;337:1870–1875.
3. Norol F, Bierling P, Roudot-Thoraval F, et al: Platelet transfusion: A dose-response study. Blood 1998;92:1448–1453.
4. Diedrich B, Remberger M, Shanwell A, et al: A prospective randomized trial of a prophylactic platelet transfusion trigger of 10×10^9 per L versus 30×10^9 per L in allogeneic hematopoietic progenitor cell transplant recipients. Transfusion 2005;45:1064–1072.

SUGGESTED READINGS

Gajic O, Moore SB: Transfusion-related acute lung injury. Mayo Clin Proc 2005;80:766–770. *A clinical review.*

Goodnough L: Current issues in transfusion medicine. Clin Adv Hematol Oncol 2005;3:614–616. *A practical overview.*

Greinacher A, Warkentin TE: Transfusion medicine in the era of genomics and proteomics. Transfus Med Rev 2005;19:288–294. *An agenda for improvement.*

Spiess BD: Red cell transfusions and guidelines: A work in progress. Hematol Oncol Clin North Am 2007;21:185–200. *Reviews emerging risks.*

Vincent JL, Piagnerelli M: Transfusion in the intensive care unit. Crit Care Med 2006;34(5 Suppl.):S96–S101. *Overview of benefits and risks.*

184 HEMATOPOIETIC STEM CELL TRANSPLANTATION

Julie M. Vose and Steven Z. Pavletic

Hematopoietic stem cell transplantation is the process of collection and infusion of hematopoietic stem cells obtained from bone marrow (bone marrow transplantation [BMT]) or peripheral blood (blood stem cell transplantation). High-dose chemotherapy followed by subsequent BMT or peripheral blood progenitor (stem cell) transplantation is increasingly being used for the treatment of many hematologic, immunologic, and neoplastic diseases. Hematopoietic stem cells can be obtained directly from bone marrow by multiple aspirations from the pelvic bones while the patient is under general anesthesia (BMT). Alternatively, hematopoietic stem cells can be obtained from peripheral blood after stimulation with hematopoietic growth factors, such as granulocyte colony-stimulating factor (G-CSF), followed by leukapheresis (peripheral blood stem cell transplantation). The subsequent availability of hematopoietic stem cell transplantation permits the administration of supralethal chemotherapy or radiotherapy to patients with malignancies in an attempt to increase the destruction of malignant cells. Additionally, the healthy transplanted cells may reconstitute the patient's immune system to provide an antitumor effect or, in the case of BMT for congenital diseases, provide cells that are no longer deficient in certain vital components.

ALLOGENEIC AND SYNGENEIC TRANSPLANTATION

Allogeneic BMT or peripheral blood transplantation involves the transfer of stem cells from a donor to another person. Syngeneic transplantation, which occurs in about 1% of transplant procedures, is the special rare case of a donor and a recipient who are genetically identical twins. Allogeneic transplants are usually considered for patients no older than 55 to 60 years, but older patients are occasionally treated. Results tend to be poorer in older patients because of the increasing incidence of graft-versus-host disease (GVHD) with age. The decision in any patient must take into account all factors, including not only chronologic age but also the physiologic age of the patient. The donor and recipient must be matched for human leukocyte antigens (HLA); the most important gene pairs include HLA-A, HLA-B, HLA-C, and HLA-DR loci, all of which are closely linked on chromosome 6 and inherited in haplotypes. The chance of having an HLA match from a sibling is 1 in 4; however, as a result of the relatively small size of families in the United States, only about 30% of patients have an HLA-matched sibling. For patients who lack an HLA-identical sibling donor, there are other possible solutions: identify an unrelated but closely HLA-matched person through the National Marrow Donor Program (NMDP), use a partially matched related donor, or identify one or more cord blood units from a cord blood bank. The genes encoding HLA antigens are numerous, and the odds that any two unrelated individuals are HLA-identical for main loci are less than 1 in 10,000. About 4 million volunteer donors have been HLA-typed through the NMDP registry, however, and a donor can be found for about 50% of patients for whom a search is initiated. About 4 months is usually required to locate an unrelated donor, a waiting time that may be too long for some patients with rapidly progressive malignancies. Allogeneic partially matched sibling or placental/umbilical cord blood is an alternative source of stem cells. Umbilical cord blood stem cells are already stored in cord blood banks, and no additional harvest procedures are needed. Because of the unique immature biology of umbilical cord blood stem cells, these transplants are associated with less GVHD; consequently, the HLA-matching requirements are less strict. However, cord blood cells need to be partially matched to the recipient, as well as to each other if more than 1 U is given. The small volume of cord blood stem cells often makes these transplants unsuitable for adult recipients. The time to engraftment and immune reconstitution may also be different for this type of transplant.

When an adequate donor has been identified, the patient is prepared for the allogeneic or syngeneic transplant with high doses of chemotherapy, alone or combined with radiation therapy. This treatment is designed to destroy any remaining malignant cells, provide sufficient immunosuppression to allow engraftment of the new cells, and clear the marrow space for engraftment of the new cells. The preparative agents must have few toxicities at doses that are much greater than their hematologic effects. High doses of anthracyclines are often impractical because of their cardiac toxicities (Chapter 192). Most regimens consist of total body irradiation combined with alkylating agents, etoposide, or cytarabine.

An integral component of the regimens for allogeneic transplantation is immunosuppression to prevent GVHD and graft rejection. Because the recipient's immune system is ablated with high-dose chemotherapy and radiation therapy, graft rejection is a rare event. Drugs that are used most commonly to prevent GVHD include tacrolimus, mycophenolate mofetil, rapamycin, and the combination of cyclosporine and methotrexate. For allogeneic hematopoietic stem cell transplantation, prophylactic immunosuppression is not lifelong; when immunologic tolerance is established, immunosuppressive agents can be discontinued. Another approach to prevent GVHD is to deplete the donor's T cells from the graft; the disadvantage of this approach is that it is associated with increased rates of disease relapse and infection, and overall survival also does not seem to be improved. To accelerate engraftment, hematopoietic growth factors, such as G-CSF, are administered after transplantation until the neutrophil count recovers. Allogeneic transplantation regimens also include prophylactic antiviral drugs (acyclovir, ganciclovir), antifungal drugs (fluconazole), broad-spectrum antibiotics (cephalosporins, fluoroquinolones), and anti-*Pneumocystis* drugs (trimethoprim-sulfamethoxazole, dapsone, pentamidine).

Leukemias (Chapters 194 and 195) that relapse after allogeneic stem cell transplantation can sometimes be controlled by further infusions of lymphocytes from the same allogeneic donor. The donor T lymphocytes destroy leukemia cells by an immune mechanism called the *graft-versus-leukemia effect.* For solid tumors, a graft-versus-tumor effect can sometimes be demonstrated. These observations have led to the development of a new approach to allogeneic stem cell transplantation: nonmyeloablative transplantation regimens based on the philosophy that allogeneic stem cell transplantation is a form of immunotherapy by which the donor lymphocytes eradicate the malignant disease, with high-dose chemotherapy and irradiation not being necessary for success.

AUTOLOGOUS BONE MARROW TRANSPLANTATION

In autologous BMT, the patient's own hematopoietic cells are infused to reestablish bone marrow function after the administration of high-dose chemotherapy and radiation therapy. These reinfused hematopoietic cells can come from the patient's bone marrow or peripheral blood, or both. Because a major limitation to the use of allogeneic BMT is that only a few patients have an HLA-matched sibling donor, the use of autologous hematopoietic cells greatly increases the number of patients eligible for transplantation. Autologous transplantation can also be used safely in older patients because of the absence of GVHD, which is a major concern with older patients. A disadvantage of autologous hematopoietic cell transplantation is the risk of contaminating the graft with viable tumor cells. Although patients undergoing autologous transplantation have higher relapse rates than do patients undergoing allogeneic transplantation, the lower rate of other complications with autologous transplantation seems to translate into similar long-term outcomes (Table 184–1). A variety of methods have been developed to decrease the contamination of autologous grafts with tumor cells (graft "purging"), but no prospective data have yet confirmed that these interventions are beneficial because most relapses originate from incompletely eradicated disease in the host.

INDICATIONS FOR TRANSPLANTATION

For many diseases, hematopoietic stem cell transplantation is now part of standard therapy (Table 184–2). More than 17,000 allogeneic and autologous transplants are performed per year for various diseases in the United States (Fig. 184–1).

Lymphoproliferative Malignancies

Non-Hodgkin's Lymphoma

Autologous transplantation has been used for the treatment of intermediate-grade and high-grade non-Hodgkin's lymphoma (Chapter 196). Patients with relapsed disease seem to benefit most from this therapy if they undergo transplantation when they still have chemotherapy-sensitive disease. Patients who have high-risk characteristics and undergo transplantation as part of their planned therapy early in the course of

TABLE 184–1 COMPARISON OF ALLOGENEIC AND AUTOLOGOUS TRANSPLANTATION

Feature	Allogeneic	Autologous
Upper age limits	55–60	Physiologic status limits
Availability	40–60% of patients	Only limitation may be the ability to collect enough stem cells
Main cause of failure	Graft-versus-host disease Infections	Disease relapse

TABLE 184–2 RESULTS OF STANDARD-OF-CARE ALLOGENEIC OR AUTOLOGOUS STEM CELL TRANSPLANTATION IN SPECIFIC DISEASES*

	Three-Year Survival (%)	
	Allogeneic	**Autologous**
HEMATOLOGIC MALIGNANCIES		
Acute myelogenous leukemia	41–61	37–62
Chronic myelogenous leukemia	52–71	NU
Myelodysplastic syndrome	33–78	NU
Acute lymphocytic leukemia	42–62	10–51
Chronic lymphocytic leukemia	50	83
Hodgkin's disease	NU	58–82
Follicular lymphoma	60	67–85
Diffuse large cell lymphoma	23–33	41–66
Multiple myeloma	48–52	54–63
Neuroblastoma	NU	41–53
NONMALIGNANT CONDITIONS		
Aplastic anemia	33–82	NA
Fanconi's anemia	16–81	NA

*Information based on the Center for International Bone Marrow Transplant Research report for patients who underwent transplantation between 1996 and 2001. Results are typically better in patients younger than 20 years, patients in earlier stages of the disease, and recipients of HLA-identical sibling transplants.

NA = not applicable; NU = not routinely used.

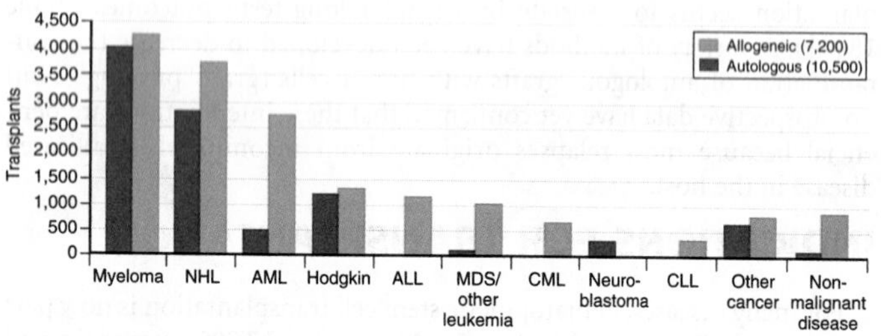

FIGURE 184–1 • Indications for blood and marrow transplantation in North America. ALL = acute lymphocytic leukemia; AML = acute myelogenous leukemia; CLL = chronic lymphocytic leukemia; CML = chronic myelogenous leukemia; MDS = myelodysplastic syndrome. (Information reprinted with permission of the Center for International Bone Marrow Transplant Research [CIBMTR], 2003.)

disease in first partial or complete response may have a better outcome than similar patients treated with conventional therapy. [1] The use of high-dose chemotherapy and radiation therapy and autologous transplantation in patients with indolent disease is associated with a failure-free survival rate of 40 to 60% at a median follow-up of 3 years; because late relapses are common, much longer follow-up is necessary to assess the long-term results of this treatment.

Hodgkin's Disease

High-dose chemotherapy followed by autologous hematopoietic stem cell transplantation has been widely accepted for patients with relapsed Hodgkin's disease (Chapter 197). Allogeneic transplantation has not been used as extensively because of increased morbidity and mortality. The outcome is poorer in patients who have received multiple chemotherapy regimens than in patients who have undergone less pretreatment. Autologous transplantation performed in first remission is being evaluated in patients with B symptoms, disseminated disease with bone marrow or pulmonary involvement, and other high-risk features.

Multiple Myeloma

Autologous and allogeneic transplant procedures have been performed successfully in patients with multiple myeloma (Chapter 198). The major concern with conventional myeloablative allogeneic transplantation has been its high mortality rate. With improvements in supportive care, however, the transplant-related mortality associated with autografts for multiple myeloma has been reduced to 1%, and a randomized trial has confirmed better survival after autologous stem cell transplantation than after conventional chemotherapy. [2] Autologous transplantation for multiple myeloma is more successful in patients who undergo less pretreatment and have a smaller tumor burden. Multiple myeloma is now the most common indication for autologous stem cell transplantation in North America.

Acute Lymphoblastic Leukemia

The results of conventional induction and consolidation chemotherapy for acute lymphoblastic leukemia (ALL) in children are excellent except in a few clinical circumstances, such as ALL associated with the Philadelphia chromosome (Chapter 194). The use of transplantation for ALL in children is generally reserved for these high-risk patients and those who relapse after initial therapy. In adults, the indications for transplantation are similar, although a much higher percentage of adults fail after initial therapy.

Chronic Lymphocytic Leukemia

Selected younger patients with B-cell chronic lymphocytic leukemia (B-CLL) that is refractory or has relapsed more than once might benefit by transplantation from a related or unrelated donor; durable disease-free survival rates are 40 to 60% (Chapter 195). Because the allogeneic graft-versus-leukemia effect seems to be especially important against B-CLL, this disease has become one of the most popular indications for nonmyeloablative allogeneic transplantation. Autologous transplantation also yields high rates of remission in pretreated B-CLL patients, but relapse rates are high and eventual survival may not be improved.

Myeloproliferative Malignancies

Acute Myelogenous Leukemia

Because patients with good-risk or average-risk acute myelogenous leukemia (AML) can be cured with conventional chemotherapy, most centers use transplantation only for (1) relapsed AML in adults or (2) as part of the initial therapy in patients with known poor prognostic characteristics, such as certain high-risk chromosomal abnormalities, including complex abnormalities or deletions of chromosomes (Chapter 194). Most studies show a decreased relapse rate with allogeneic transplantation, but long-term overall survival is not as improved because of the morbidity and mortality related to the transplantation itself.

Myelodysplastic Syndromes

Myelodysplastic syndromes in young, otherwise healthy patients are best treated with an allogeneic transplant from an HLA-identical sibling donor (Chapter 193). Most patients with myelodysplastic syndromes are elderly, which often precludes use of this successful therapy.

Chronic Myelogenous Leukemia

Allogeneic transplantation from an HLA-matched sibling donor produces long-term disease-free survival in 55 to 75% of patients with Philadelphia chromosome–positive chronic myelogenous leukemia (CML) (Chapter 195). The results seem to be better when the patients are younger, undergo transplantation within the first year of diagnosis, have received hydroxyurea rather than busulfan, and have not received extensive interferon. When an HLA-matched related donor is not available, the use of alternative donors can yield a cure in about 50% patients with chronic phase CML. However, the development of effective and nontoxic tyrosine kinase inhibitors for the treatment of *BCR-ABL*–positive CML is tempering enthusiasm for allogeneic transplantation in patients with CML.

Solid Tumors

Breast Cancer

The use of high-dose chemotherapy for the treatment of metastatic breast cancer can result in a higher complete response rate than with conventional treatment (Chapter 208). The reported disease-free survival rate in chemotherapy-sensitive stage IV breast cancer is only 10 to 25%, however, and no overall survival benefit has yet been shown in several randomized trials. [3] As a result, transplantation has lost favor in this condition.

Other Solid Tumors

High-dose chemotherapy plus transplantation has had success in the treatment of some chemotherapy-sensitive solid tumors, including testicular cancer (Chapter 210), ovarian carcinoma (Chapter 209), and childhood tumors such as neuroblastoma and Wilms' tumor. Other solid tumors that are refractory to chemotherapy, such as melanoma or many gastrointestinal malignancies, are poor targets for this therapy. Limited reports of a high rate of regression of metastatic renal carcinoma (Chapter 207) after nonmyeloablative allogeneic peripheral blood stem cell transplantation holds promise for wider use of allogeneic stem cell transplantation for solid tumors.

Nonmalignant Conditions

Immunodeficiency Disorders

Disorders such as Wiskott-Aldrich syndrome or severe combined immunodeficiency syndrome have been treated successfully with HLA-matched sibling transplants or transplants from alternative donors (Chapter 271).

Genetic Disorders

Genetic disorders such as osteopetrosis (Chapter 269), Gaucher's disease (Chapter 223), and Hurler's syndrome (Chapter 281) can be treated successfully with an allogeneic transplant. Other indications for allogeneic transplantation include hemoglobinopathies, such as sickle cell anemia (Chapter 167) and thalassemia (Chapter 166), and acquired blood disorders such as paroxysmal nocturnal hemoglobinuria (Chapter 164). The transplant must be performed before the onset of secondary organ failure.

Aplastic Anemia

Allogeneic transplantation can lead to long-term disease-free survival in more than 50% of patients with severe aplastic anemia (Chapter 171). When compared with standard immunosuppressive therapy, allogeneic transplantation is more likely to produce a complete and durable reversal of the hematologic abnormalities. For patients with less severe aplastic anemia, patients older than 40 years, and those without a matched sibling donor, a trial of immunosuppression therapy is usually appropriate before consideration of allogeneic transplantation.

Autoimmune Disease

Autologous stem cell transplantation to engraft a tolerant immune system has had promising results in selected patients with systemic lupus erythematosus, rheumatoid arthritis, scleroderma, and multiple sclerosis. Randomized prospective trials comparing conventional treatments are currently being planned.

Cardiac Disease

Much attention has focused on the possible use of autologous bone marrow–derived or circulating peripheral blood stem cells to promote recovery of myocardial function after acute myocardial infarction. To date, infusion of such cells, usually directly into the relevant coronary artery after successful percutaneous coronary intervention (Chapter 73), has shown promising results in improving regional but not necessarily global myocardial function. Further research will be required to define the appropriate clinical role for such approaches.

COMPLICATIONS

Infections

Infections are a major cause of morbidity and mortality after hematopoietic stem cell transplantation, especially allogeneic transplantation, because of prolonged immunosuppression for the prevention or treatment of GVHD (Chapter 303). Bacterial infections are frequently related to central venous catheters. Among fungal infections, *Aspergillus* infections typically occur in patients receiving prolonged therapy with high-dose steroids for the treatment of GVHD. Viral infections include reactivation cytomegalovirus (Chapter 399), human herpesvirus 6, and Epstein-Barr virus infection (Chapter 400). These patients are also susceptible to seasonal respiratory viruses. Prophylactic use of granulocyte colony-stimulating factor and granulocyte-macrophage colony-stimulating factor reduces infections but does not improve survival. [4]

At 1 year after allogeneic or autologous transplantation, patients should receive the following vaccinations: diphtheria, tetanus, *Haemophilus influenzae* type b, hepatitis B virus, 23-valent pneumococcal polysaccharide, hepatitis A virus, seasonal influenza virus, inactivated poliovirus, and only in areas of outbreaks, meningococcal vaccine (Chapter 16). Live vaccines against measles, mumps, and rubella should not be administered until 2 years after transplantation and only in the absence of chronic GVHD and immunosuppressive therapy. Family members may receive routine vaccines, including influenza virus vaccine, but patients should avoid contact with a child who has received oral poliovirus vaccine for about 1 month after vaccination. Despite these recommendations, vaccines may not always induce protective immunity in an immunodeficient patient who has chronic GVHD or is taking immunosuppressive drugs.

Cardiac Toxicity

Most transplant centers screen potential patients for underlying cardiac abnormalities that would place them at potential increased risk during the procedure. Nevertheless, a few patients experience cardiotoxicity, either acutely during the transplant procedure or at a later time, that is manifested as arrhythmias, heart failure, or ischemia as a result of the large volumes of fluids administered during the procedure or the added physiologic stress. Pericardial effusion can develop in patients who have disease near the pericardium or are receiving radiation therapy in that area (Chapter 77). An idiosyncratic cardiomyopathy can occur after high doses of cyclophosphamide (Chapters 59 and 192). Viral cardiomyopathies can also develop.

Pulmonary Toxicities

Pulmonary toxicities include infections from bacterial, fungal, or viral sources during the transplantation. In addition, in patients receiving certain chemotherapy agents, such as carmustine, chemotherapy-induced lung damage (Chapters 92 and 192) may develop but can usually be treated with steroids. Patients undergoing allogeneic transplantation are at increased risk for pneumonitis caused by cytomegalovirus and fungal infections, for adult respiratory distress syndrome, and for interstitial pneumonia of unknown etiology. Chronic GVHD can also be manifested in the lung as bronchiolitis obliterans with or without obstructive pneumonia.

Liver Toxicity

The most frequent liver complication associated with transplantation is veno-occlusive disease of the liver (Chapter 153). Symptoms associated with this complication include jaundice, tender hepatomegaly, ascites, and weight gain. Progressive hepatic failure and multiorgan system failure can develop. Predisposing factors seem to be previous hepatic injury, the use of estrogens, and perhaps the use of HLA-mismatched donors.

Renal Toxicity

Acute renal failure requiring dialysis occurs infrequently during the transplant procedure. The judicious use of nephrotoxic agents can decrease the incidence of this complication. Idiopathic or cyclosporine-induced hemolytic-uremic syndrome (Chapter 179) can be a serious complication after allogeneic stem cell transplantation, with a high risk for end-stage renal disease or death.

Graft-versus-Host Disease

In the allogeneic transplant setting, acute GVHD is manifested by symptoms in the skin, gastrointestinal tract, and liver within the first 100 days after transplantation. The skin manifestations range from a maculopapular rash to generalized erythroderma or desquamation. The severity of liver disease is scored on the basis of the bilirubin, and the severity of the gastrointestinal disease is graded by the quantity of diarrhea per day. Patients who receive transplants from unrelated donors are at increased risk, and the incidence and severity of GVHD rise with the age of the patient. Other risk factors include a female donor (particularly a multiparous donor), advanced age, and cytomegalovirus seropositivity of the donor or patient. Prophylaxis with cyclosporine or tacrolimus, with or without methotrexate, corticosteroids, or mycophenolate mofetil, reduces the incidence and severity. Treatment of acute GVHD includes high-dose corticosteroids, antithymocyte globulin, or various monoclonal antibodies.

Chronic GVHD occurs more than 100 days after transplantation and is most likely to develop in older patients who also had acute GVHD. Symptoms include the sicca syndrome, chronic sinusitis, rashes, scleroderma-like skin thickening, diarrhea, wasting syndrome, and liver abnormalities. Patients are also at greatly increased risk for infectious complications resulting from either the GVHD itself or the treatment for it. Adverse prognostic factors for survival include thrombocytopenia, progressive clinical manifestations, involvement of more than 50% of the skin, poor performance status, and elevated bilirubin. Treatment of chronic GVHD includes corticosteroids, cyclosporine, tacrolimus, mycophenolate mofetil, thalidomide, ultraviolet light, and other immunosuppressive agents.

Graft Rejection

Graft rejection occurs when immunologically competent cells of host origin destroy the transplanted cells of donor origin. This complication is rare after fully matched, related donor transplantation and occurs more commonly in patients who receive transplants from alternative donors or T cell–depleted transplants. Graft rejection is less likely in nontransfused patients with aplastic anemia.

LATE COMPLICATIONS

As the number of long-term survivors after transplantation increases, complications that develop years later are beginning to be recognized.

Secondary Malignancies

One complication of the chemotherapy or radiation therapy (or both) used to treat malignancy is the development of a secondary malignancy. There have been several reports of the development of secondary AML or myelodysplastic syndrome after autologous transplantation. Some studies have suggested that total body irradiation may increase the risk for these complications. After allogeneic transplantation, the overall incidence of secondary malignancies is 2.2% at 10 years and 6.7% at 15 years after transplantation. Within the first 1 to 2 years, the most common malignancies are Epstein-Barr virus–related lymphoproliferative disorders; solid tumors are more likely to occur more than 3 years after transplantation. Risk factors include the use of antithymocyte globulin to treat GVHD, the use of a T-cell-depleted graft, HLA incompatibility, and perhaps total body irradiation.

Infertility and Hypogonadism

The risk of gonadal failure is likely to be lower with the increased use of nonmyeloablative preparative regimens. The use of total body irradiation is almost always associated with sterility, but successful pregnancies have occurred in some patients after other regimens. Gynecomastia (sometimes tender) occasionally occurs in males. To address all the complexities of functional castration from high-dose therapy, a reproductive endocrinologist should be consulted before transplantation in patients for whom future fertility is an issue.

Endocrine Dysfunction

Iatrogenic Cushing's syndrome is commonly due to long-term steroid therapy in patients with chronic GVHD (Chapters 33 and 245). Particularly disabling are consequences such as steroid-induced myopathy, avascular necrosis of the hip, and osteoporosis. Because many patients are taking steroids for many months, tapering can be associated with malaise, nausea, hypotension, and musculoskeletal pains. In these situations, slower tapering over a period of several months or reintroduction of physiologic replacement doses (e.g., 7.5 to 10 mg/day of prednisone) is appropriate. Hypothyroidism (Chapter 244) is typically related to the use of total body irradiation or local irradiation of the head and neck for lymphoma or other cancer. Osteoporosis (Chapter 264) occurs in 50 to 60% of patients after hematopoietic stem cell transplantation. The major contributing causes include hypogonadism, secondary hyperparathyroidism caused by low serum calcium, and post-transplant steroid therapy. Bone mineral density should be evaluated before and after transplantation; osteopenia should be treated as appropriate with bisphosphonates, calcium, vitamin D, estrogen, and testosterone.

Other Complications

The long-term incidence of cataracts is about 20 to 50%; the risk is related to the use of total body irradiation and corticosteroids (Chapter 449). About 50% of patients with cataracts require surgical therapy. Alopecia is typically reversible, but in rare cases it may be irreversible, especially after the use of busulfan-containing preparative regimens.

FUTURE DIRECTIONS

The safety and efficacy of transplantation may be improved by the use of hematopoietic cytokines to stimulate immunologic reconstitution, ex vivo expansion of progenitors, genetic modulation of cells, improved supportive care for transplant patients, better prophylaxis against GVHD, better HLA typing, and newer anticancer agents. Whether stem cells can be infused to improve the function of adult organs is an area of active investigation.

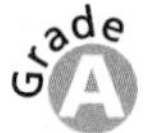

1. Milpied N, Deconinck E, Gaillard F, et al: Initial treatment of aggressive lymphoma with high-dose chemotherapy and autologous stem-cell support. N Engl J Med 2004;350:1287–1295.
2. Attal M, Harousseau JL, Stoppa AM, et al: A prospective, randomized trial of autologous bone marrow transplantation and chemotherapy in multiple myeloma. N Engl J Med 1996;335:91–97.
3. Farquhar C, Marjoribanks J, Basser R, et al: High dose chemotherapy and autologous bone marrow or stem cell transplantation versus conventional chemotherapy for women with metastatic breast cancer. Cochrane Database Syst Rev 2006;4:CD003142.
4. Dekker A, Bulley S, Beyene J, et al: Meta-analysis of randomized controlled trials of prophylactic granulocyte colony-stimulating factor and granulocyte-macrophage colony-stimulating factor after autologous and allogeneic stem cell transplantation. J Clin Oncol 2006;24:5207–5217.

SUGGESTED READINGS

Copelan EA: Hematopoietic stem-cell transplantation. N Engl J Med 2006;354: 1813–1826. *A comprehensive review.*

de Witte T, Oosterveld M, Muus P: Autologous and allogeneic stem cell transplantation for myelodysplastic syndrome. Blood Rev 2007;21:49–59. *A clinical review.*

Horwitz ME, Sullivan KM: Chronic graft-versus-host disease. Blood Rev 2006;20:15–27. *A clinical review.*

Ljungman P, Urbano-Ispizua A, Cavazzana-Calvo M, et al: Allogeneic and autologous transplantation for haematological diseases, solid tumours and immune disorders: Definitions and current practice in Europe. Bone Marrow Transplant 2006;37:439–447. *A comprehensive overview.*

Parimon T, Au DH, Martin PJ, et al: A risk score for mortality after allogeneic hematopoietic cell transplantation. Ann Intern Med 2006;144:407–414. *A 50-point pretransplantation score predicted risk of death within 2 years.*

Rizzo JD, Wingard JR, Tichelli A, et al: Recommended screening and preventive practices for long-term survivors after hematopoietic cell transplantation: Joint recommendations of the European Group for Blood and Marrow Transplantation, the Center for International Blood and Marrow Transplant Research, and the American Society of Blood and Marrow Transplantation. Biol Blood Marrow Transplant 2006;12:138–151. *Consensus recommendations.*

Section XV

Oncology

185 EPIDEMIOLOGY OF CANCER

Michael J. Thun

EPIDEMIOLOGY

Prevalence

Collectively, all cancers combined account for about 23% of deaths in the United States, thereby placing cancer second only to heart disease as a cause of death. Although the age-standardized death rate from all cancers combined decreased by more than 13% in the United States from 1991 to 2004, the number of people in whom cancer is diagnosed has continued to increase because of growth and aging of the population, improved detection of certain cancers, and the long-term consequences of cigarette smoking in women. In contrast, the number of Americans dying from cancer has decreased since 2002 because of the large decrease in death rates. Worldwide, approximately 7 million deaths from cancer occurred in the year 2000, evenly divided between developed and developing countries. The number of cancer deaths in economically developing countries will soon surpass that in developed countries because of the global dissemination of Western patterns of tobacco use and diet, as well as growth and aging of the population.

The magnitude of suffering and death from cancer continues to be enormous. Fortunately, there has been progress on several fronts. Research has identified the causes of many types of cancer, as well as basic mechanisms that drive carcinogenesis (Chapter 191). Various control measures have reduced exposure to tobacco (Chapter 30) and occupational carcinogens (Chapter 17) in most industrialized countries. Advances in early detection and treatment (Chapter 192) have improved survival. However, an estimated 75 to 80% of cancer cases and deaths in the United States could, in principle, be prevented, even without further improvements in treatment.

Incidence

Measures of Occurrence and Survival

Incidence and Death Rates

Cancer *incidence* and *death rates* are usually expressed per 100,000 people per year and are age-standardized to allow valid comparisons across populations of different size and age structure. Conventionally, comparisons of rates within the United States are standardized to the age distribution of the U.S. population (currently the year 2000 age standard), whereas international comparisons are based on the world population standard in 1960. In the United States, cancer incidence rates are measured in special population-based tumor registries that now encompass 92% of the population. Temporal trends in cancer incidence have been monitored since 1973 in 10% of the population by the National Cancer Institute (NCI) Surveillance, Epidemiology, and End Results (SEER) program. Deaths from cancer have been tabulated nationally in U.S. vital statistics since 1930. Mortality rates are based on the underlying cause of death as coded from death certificates using systematic nosologic rules. Validation studies have documented that despite the well-known limitations of death certificates, there is greater than 90% agreement between the clinical diagnosis and the underlying cause of death coded systematically from death certificates for the 17 cancer sites that represent over two thirds of cancers in the United States.

Relative Survival

Survival in patients with cancer is usually expressed as *relative survival*, which compares the percentage of cancer patients alive after a designated period (often 5 years) with the corresponding percentage in a population without cancer but of similar age, race, and sex. A relative survival of 100% signifies that cancer patients have the same survival as people without cancer. Survival has been monitored by NCI SEER registries since 1975.

Cumulative Incidence

The terms *cumulative incidence* and *cumulative risk* describe the average probability of development or death from disease (all cancers or a specific type of cancer) over a defined period. Cumulative risk over a 1-year period is the same as the annual incidence or death rate. For longer periods, cumulative risk increases with the duration of observation and age. The lifetime risk of cancer being diagnosed has increased with improvements in life expectancy such that invasive cancer will be diagnosed in slightly less than one in every two men and more than one in every three women during their lifetime. Except for nonmelanoma skin cancer, prostate cancer ranks first in lifetime risk among men (17.1%) and breast cancer ranks first among women (12.7%).

Geographic Variation

Cancer occurs in all countries of the world, although the types of cancer that predominate in different countries vary widely. For several cancers, such as malignancies of the esophagus, skin, ovary, and prostate, the cumulative risk by age 74 is at least 200 times higher in regions with the highest risk than in those with the lowest risk (Table 185–1). Even for all sites combined, the cumulative incidence is almost 10 times higher in African American men than men in parts of India; these large variations in overall cancer risk indicate that geographic variability does not simply represent substitution of one form of cancer for another. Although some of the geographic variation reflects incomplete diagnoses in developing countries, much of it is real. The regional cancer registries that provide these data are maintained by the International Agency for Research on Cancer (IARC), which makes special effort to improve the completeness of registration.

The reasons for this geographic variation are better understood for cancers caused by infectious agents and tobacco use than by other factors. For example, the high incidence of liver cancer (Chapter 206) in parts of Asia and sub-Saharan Africa closely parallels the geographic patterns of *hepatitis B virus (HBV)* infection in childhood, just as mortality from stomach (Chapter 202) and cervical (Chapter 209) cancer correlates closely with the prevalence of infection with pathogenic strains of *Helicobacter pylori* and *human papillomavirus (HPV)*, respectively. The incidence of oropharyngeal (Chapter 200) cancer is high throughout much of the Indian subcontinent and Southeast Asia because of oral use of tobacco mixed with betel nut, just as the incidence of lung cancer (Chapter 201) is highest in countries with a prolonged history of widespread cigarette smoking. In contrast, it is not fully understood why esophageal cancer (Chapter 140) occurs with extraordinary frequency in countries surrounding the Caspian Sea, although the combination of severe nutritional deficiency and the practice of swallowing the charred residue from opium pipes has been proposed. Nor is it clear why ovarian cancer (Chapter 209) is more common in certain European countries or exactly how dietary consumption of salted fish may interact with Epstein-Barr virus (EBV) infections and genetic susceptibility to cause nasopharyngeal cancer (Chapter 200) in southern China and Eskimos in Alaska and Greenland.

Temporal Variation

Temporal variations in the incidence or death rates from certain cancers further illustrate the importance of potentially modifiable "environmental" factors on the burden of disease. For example, the large changes in mortality from stomach and lung cancer in the United States (Fig. 185–1A and B) reflect changes in external exposure rather than inherited genetic susceptibility. Cancers of the stomach and uterus (principally the uterine cervix) were the most common fatal cancers in the United States in 1930 but decreased dramatically by 2003, the most recent year for which mortality data are available. In contrast, cancer of the lung and bronchus was uncommon in 1930 but had become the leading fatal cancer in both men and women in the United States by 1987. The global decrease in stomach cancer (Chapter 202) was an unexpected consequence of changes in food preservation and reduced prevalence of *H. pylori* infection. The advent of refrigeration increased the availability of fresh vegetables and fruit and decreased reliance on salted, smoked, and pickled foods, whereas improvements in sanitation and housing and widespread antibiotic use decreased the prevalence of chronic infection with *H. pylori*. Progress in reducing the incidence and death rate from cervical cancer (Chapter 209) is largely attributable to the introduction of Papanicolaou testing and early removal of premalignant and cancerous lesions. The increase and subsequent decrease in lung cancer (Chapter 201) mortality in men in the United States reflect the rise and partial decline of cigarette smoking. The epidemic of lung cancer in women lags behind that in men by approximately 25 years because of later uptake of smoking.

TABLE 185–1 COMPARISON OF THE CUMULATIVE INCIDENCE* OF SELECTED CANCERS IN COUNTRIES AT HIGHEST AND LOWEST RISK

Site or Origin of Cancer	High Incidence Area	Sex	Cumulative Incidence,* % in High-Incidence Area	Ratio of Highest to Lowest Cumulative Incidence*	Low-Incidence Area
Esophagus	China, Cixian	M	20.4	253	Kuwait, Kuwaitis
Melanoma	Australia, Queensland	M	5.3	236	Kuwait
Ovary	Iceland	F	1.8	217	China, Hong Kong
Prostate	USA, African Americans	M	22.4	204	China, Quidong County
Nasopharynx	China, Hong Kong	M	2.2	171	Belgium, Limburg
Penis	Uganda	M	0.5	121	Israel
Stomach	China, Changle	M	17.8	99	Thailand, Songkhla
Colon	Japan, Hiroshima	M	7.1	86	India, Karunagappally
Liver	Thailand, Khon Kaen	M	10.5	80	Canada, Yukon
Corpus uteri	USA, Hawaii	F	3.1	66	Oman, Omani
Cervix uteri	Zimbabwe, Harave	F	6.6	48	China, Jiashan
Lung and bronchus	Canada, Northwest Territory	M	11.4	39	Mali
Rectum	Japan, Hiroshima	M	2.9	35	Kuwait, Non-Kuwaitis
Pharynx	France, Somme	M	0.4	32	Czech Republic
Larynx	Spain, Zaragoza	M	2.2	27	China, Jiashan
Bladder	Italy, Genoa	M	4.9	18	India, Trivandrum
Non-Hodgkin's lymphoma	USA, San Francisco	M	2.2	12	Mali, Bamako
Pancreas	USA, African Americans	M	1.5	12	Thailand, Songkhla
Breast	Uruguay, Montevideo	F	12.4	11	China, Jiashan
All sites	USA, African Americans	M	45.9	4.8	India, Trivandrum
All sites	Switzerland, Geneva	F	33.8	4.5	India, Karunagappally

*Cumulative incidence (risk) of cancer being diagnosed by the age of 75 years, in the absence of other causes of death, based on age-specific rates, 1993 to 1997.
M = male; F = female.
From: Parkin DM, Whelan SL, Ferlay J, et al (eds): Cancer Incidence in Five Continents, vol VIII, IARC Scientific Publications No. 155. Lyon, International Agency for Research on Cancer, 2002.

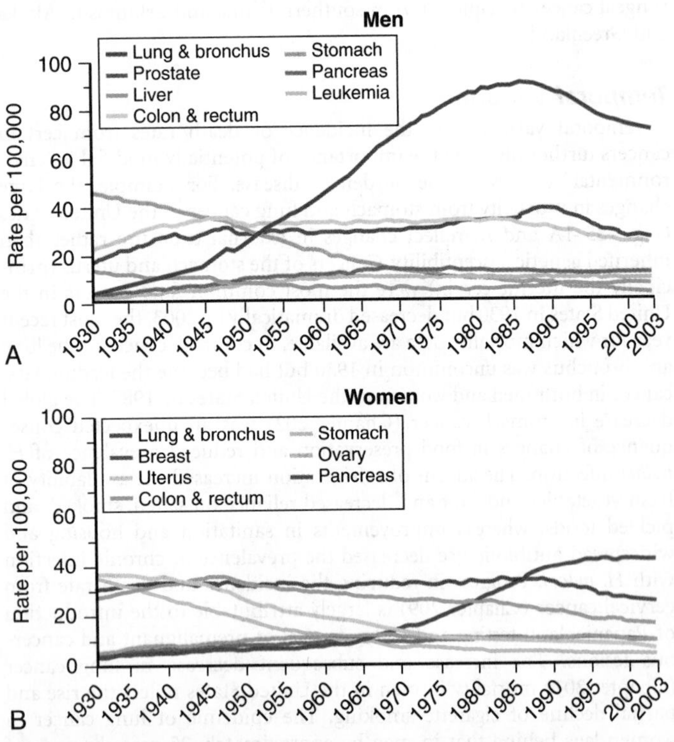

FIGURE 185–1 • Cancer mortality rates. A, Temporal trends in cancer mortality rates, United States, 1930 to 2003, men. **B,** Temporal trends in cancer mortality rates, United States, 1930 to 2003, women.

Screening

Trends in cancer incidence rates are more difficult to interpret than trends in mortality, especially for sites that are detectable by screening. The introduction of a new screening test can create the appearance of a sudden increase in cancer incidence, especially when the test detects prevalent but undiagnosed tumors that would otherwise be missed. For example, a sudden increase in the incidence of prostate cancer (Chapter 211) in the United States occurred with the introduction of prostate-specific antigen (PSA) screening in the late 1980s (Fig. 185–2). The upward trend reversed after 1992 because of saturation of screening among older men. The upward trend in reported incidence has since returned to the more gradual increase that prevailed before the introduction of PSA testing.

The introduction of new screening tests also complicates the interpretation of temporal trends in *relative survival* among patients with cancer (Table 185–2). Screening tests detect cancer earlier, before the tumor would otherwise have been diagnosed, thus creating an apparent lengthening of survival that exaggerates actual progress. This so-called lead-time bias can be difficult to separate completely from improvements in relative survival for sites that are commonly diagnosed by screening, such as breast and prostate cancer, even in analyses that stratify for stage at diagnosis. New screening tests can also alter the mix of cancers being diagnosed by increasing the detection of indolent tumors that may not be life-threatening. Advances in the molecular characterization of tumors may ultimately resolve this problem by providing more homogeneous groupings of tumors in which to measure relative survival.

Demographic Factors

Age

The incidence of most cancers increases exponentially with age from 10 to 84 years (Fig. 185–3). This age-related increase is consistent with the multistage nature of carcinogenesis and reflects the time required for

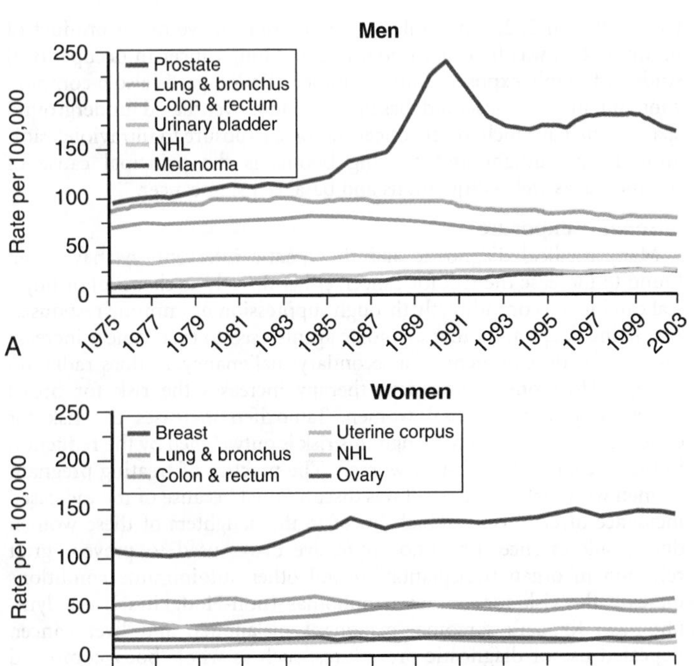

FIGURE 185–2 • Cancer incidence rates. A, Temporal trends in cancer incidence rates adjusted for delayed reporting, Surveillance, Epidemiology, and End Results (SEER), 1975 to 2003, men. **B,** Temporal trends in cancer incidence rates adjusted for delayed reporting, SEER, 1975 to 2003, women.

TABLE 185–2 RELATIVE SURVIVAL* (%) FOR SELECTED CANCER SITES DURING THREE TIME PERIODS, UNITED STATES, SEER

Site	1975–1977	1984–1986	1996–2002
All sites	50	53	66
Breast (female)	75	79	89
Colon	51	59	65
Leukemia	35	42	49
Lung and bronchus	13	13	16
Melanoma of the skin	82	86	92
Non-Hodgkin's lymphoma	48	53	63
Ovary	37	40	45†
Pancreas	2	3	5
Prostate	69	76	100
Rectum	49	57	66
Urinary bladder	73	78	82

*Five-year relative survival rates based on follow-up of patients through 2003.
†Recent changes in the classification of ovarian cancer have affected 1996 to 2002 survival rates.
From Surveillance, Epidemiology and End Results Program (SEER), 1975–2003, Division of Cancer Control and Population Sciences, National Cancer Institute, 2006.

a single cell line to accumulate all the mutations or epigenetic events (or both) needed for malignant transformation (Chapter 187). Age is a stronger predictor of the risk for cancer than any other factor is. Three quarters (76%) of all cancers occur in the approximately 19% of the U.S. population 55 years or older. The apparent decrease in the incidence of cancer after 85 years of age reflects incomplete diagnosis of cancer in the elderly, as well as the fact that generations born before 1920 preceded the peak of cigarette smoking.

Age affects the types of cancer that occur, as well as their frequency. In the United States, the five most common fatal cancers before age 20 are acute lymphocytic leukemia and cancer of the brain and other nervous system, bones and joints, endocrine system, and soft tissues. In women aged 20 to 59 years, breast cancer is the most common fatal cancer. At age 60 and older, the four most common cancers are lung and bronchus

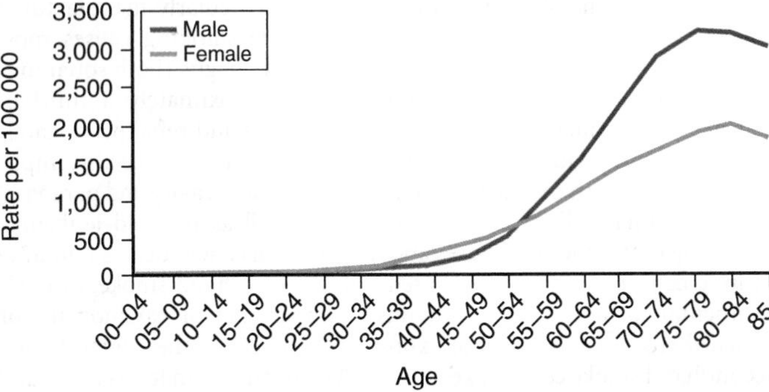

FIGURE 185–3 • Age- and sex-specific incidence rates for all cancer combined in the nine Surveillance, Epidemiology and End Results (SEER) areas, 2003.

(Chapters 201), breast (Chapter 208), prostate (Chapter 211), and colon and rectum cancer (Chapter 203).

Sex

For most cancers that affect both sexes, the incidence rate is higher in men than women, with the exceptions being cancers of the thyroid, gallbladder, and anus. The male excess for cancers of the oropharynx, esophagus, larynx, lung, pancreas, and kidney can be attributed to higher tobacco or alcohol use, or both. For other sites, such as brain, hematopoietic, and childhood cancers, however, the reasons are unclear.

Socioeconomic Status, Race, and Ethnicity

African Americans experience disproportionately high incidence and death rates from most cancers. Racial disparities in death rates are largest for cancers of the prostate, stomach, larynx (men), myeloma, and uterine cervix. Relatively few studies have attempted to separate the impact of biologic differences associated with race from factors related to poverty and its effects on education, risk factors, and access to high-quality care for prevention, early detection, and treatment. Accumulating data suggest that socioeconomic factors account for most of these disparities (Chapter 5). For example, black women have the highest death rate from breast cancer among all racial or ethnic groups in the United States. Although the incidence rate is reportedly higher in white than in black women, this lower incidence rate reflects underdiagnosis of breast cancer in black women. Survival among women with breast cancer is lower in black than in white women in the general population, but it is similar in military hospitals where both races have equal access to care. Relative survival is lower in African Americans than in whites for many other cancers, including prostate, uterine cervix and corpus, colon, and rectum cancer.

Other ethnic groups in the United States also have distinctive cancer patterns. Relative to whites, age-adjusted incidence and mortality rates among Hispanics are higher for gallbladder, stomach, and cervical cancer; those among American Indians are higher for cancer of the gallbladder, stomach, and cervix; rates in Japanese Americans are higher for stomach and liver cancer; those in Chinese Americans are higher for nasopharynx, liver, and stomach cancer; Native Hawaiians have higher death rates from breast, esophagus, liver, pancreas, lung, and cervical cancer; and Filipino Americans have a lower risk of most cancers except for cancers of the stomach, liver, oral cavity, and esophagus. Many of these ethnic differences are known to reflect differences in the use of tobacco, dietary habits, infectious exposure, or medical care. Research is needed to identify practical interventions to reduce these disparities.

Causes of Cancer

Whereas infectious diseases are defined by exposure to a specific microorganism, chronic diseases such as cancer may have multiple causes, none of which need be necessary or sufficient for the disease to occur. For instance, tobacco smoking is the major cause of lung cancer, but it is neither necessary nor sufficient for the disease to occur. Approximately 10 to 15% of lung cancers occur in people who have never smoked actively, and in only about 20% of long-term cigarette smokers does lung cancer develop.

Tobacco

Exposure to tobacco (Chapter 30) is the single largest cause of cancer in the United States. Tobacco smoke contains more than 4000 chemicals, at least 50 of which are known to be carcinogenic in humans or animals, or both. All forms of tobacco cause cancer, parti-cularly manufactured cigarettes. In industrialized countries, cigarette smoking causes most cancers of the lung, oropharynx, larynx, and esophagus (both squamous cell carcinoma and adenocarcinoma) and approximately a third of cancers of the pancreas, kidney (adenocarcinoma and renal pelvis carcinoma), urinary bladder, and uterine cervix. Recent evidence also implicates smoking with cancer of the nasopharynx, nasal cavity and paranasal sinuses, stomach, liver, and colorectum, as well as myeloid leukemia. Active cigarette smoking causes about 30% of all cancer deaths and 87% of lung cancer deaths in the United States. Secondhand smoke, or environmental tobacco smoke, contains a similar mix of carcinogens for which there is no safe level of exposure. Each year in the United States, secondhand smoke causes an estimated 3000 deaths from lung cancer and 30,000 to 40,000 deaths from heart disease.

Diet, Obesity, Physical Inactivity

For the majority of Americans who do not use tobacco, the most important modifiable determinants of the risk for cancer are dietary patterns, physical inactivity, and obesity. Approximately a third of cancer deaths in the United States are attributed to nutritional factors. Obesity, physical inactivity, and an excess of caloric intake over energy expenditure are known to increase the risk for several types of cancer. Obesity (Chapter 239) is causally related to cancer of the endometrium, kidney, breast (in postmenopausal but not premenopausal women), esophagus, colon (especially in men), and gallbladder (particularly in women). More limited evidence suggests that obesity may also increase the risk for cancer of the liver, pancreas, and stomach, as well as some hematopoietic cancers. Excessive alcohol consumption (Chapter 31) is an established cause of cancer of the oropharynx, larynx, esophagus, and liver; even moderate drinking increases the risk for breast cancer. The importance of other specific components of diet to the risk for cancer in Western populations is more controversial. The strongest evidence pertains to increased risk for colon cancer in people who have inadequate intake of folic acid or excessive consumption of red or processed meat.

Infectious Agents

It is estimated that about 17% of cancer cases worldwide are attributable to infectious agents. This percentage is higher in economically developing (26%) than in developed countries (7.2%). Viruses known to cause cancer in humans include *HPV* (Chapter 396), *HBV* (Chapter 152), *hepatitis C virus* (HCV) (Chapter 152), *EBV* (Chapter 400), *human immunodeficiency virus (HIV)* (Chapter 416), and *human herpesvirus 8* (Chapter 397). Viruses increase the risk for cancer through a variety of mechanisms, including direct effects on DNA, promotion of tumor development by means of chronic inflammation *(HPV, HBV, HCV)*, or suppression of specific elements of the immune system (e.g., *HIV*) (Chapter 187).

H. pylori, which is the only bacterial infection known to cause cancer, is a gram-negative, spiral bacteria that colonizes the mucous layer of the stomach. Chronic inflammation caused by strains of *H. pylori* that express the CagA (a 128-kD cytotoxin-associated gene—A positive) protein promotes the development of gastric ulcers, gastric carcinoma, and mucosa-associated lymphoid tissue (MALT) lymphoma of the stomach (Chapter 202). Parasitic infections known to increase the risk for cancer include *Schistosoma haematobium* (Chapters 207 and 377) (bladder cancer) and liver flukes such as *Clonorchis sinensis* (Chapter 378) and *Opisthorchis viverrini* (Chapter 378) (biliary tract cancer, Chapter 206).

Ionizing Radiation

Ionizing radiation (Chapter 18) from x-rays, gamma radiation, and other sources is one of the most extensively studied human carcinogens. Leukemia and cancer of the thyroid and female breast are most strongly associated with radiation, although cancer of the lung, esophagus, stomach, colon, and bladder and myeloma are also promoted. The risk for development of cancer from ionizing radiation depends not only on cumulative exposure but also on the intensity, rate, and nature of the exposure, as well as on the age at which it occurs. Childhood exposure from medical treatments or fallout from atomic bombs or nuclear accidents principally increases the risk for leukemia and thyroid cancer. Girls exposed to radiation during adolescence and young adulthood are more susceptible to breast cancer from this exposure than are women exposed later in life. Radioactive isotopes such as iodine 131, radium (224, 226, 236), and phosphorus 32 concentrate in the thyroid, bone, and bone marrow, respectively, and deliver high localized doses to radiosensitive tissues. Radon 222, a naturally occurring radioactive decay product of uranium 238, was first discovered to cause lung cancer in occupational studies of highly exposed uranium miners. Radon gas is also a common contaminant of household basements and unventilated underground spaces, albeit at much lower concentrations. Exposure to ultraviolet radiation from sunlight and tanning booths is the principal cause of melanoma, as well as squamous and basal cell skin cancer.

Iatrogenic Exposure

Many medical diagnostic and therapeutic interventions have been found to increase the risk for cancer, either directly as chemical or physical carcinogens or indirectly through suppression of immune responses. Alkylating drugs and other cytotoxic agents used to treat cancer increase the risk for development of a secondary malignancy, as does radiation therapy. Hormone replacement therapy increases the risk for breast cancer in postmenopausal women. Tamoxifen increases the risk for endometrial cancer, even though this risk is outweighed by the reduction in breast cancer in high-risk women. The practice of treating pregnant women with diethylstilbestrol was discontinued because of the increased incidence of clear cell vaginal cancer in the daughters of these women during adolescence. Immunosuppressive drugs used to prevent graft rejection in organ transplantation and other autoimmune conditions increase the risk for certain lymphomas (non-Hodgkin's B-cell lymphomas), Kaposi's sarcoma, malignant melanoma, and liver cancer. Repeated use of diagnostic procedures, such as whole body computed tomography, results in substantial radiation exposure, although the potential long-term consequences receive surprisingly little attention.

Occupational and Environmental Carcinogens

Occupationally exposed workers (Chapter 17) have unfortunately served as the sentinel for many of the recognized industrial carcinogens, especially in workplaces where prolonged, heavy exposure caused unusual clusters of rare cancers. For example, clusters of scrotal cancer in London chimney sweeps, osteosarcoma of the jaw in watch dial painters exposed to radium, mesothelioma in asbestos workers, and angiosarcoma of the liver in chemical workers exposed to vinyl chloride monomer attest to the carcinogenicity of coal tar, radium, asbestos, and vinyl chloride monomer. In other instances, increases in the risk for common cancers have been sufficiently large to be detected in epidemiologic studies of several thousand workers. Examples include arsenic, asbestos, beryllium, bis (chloromethyl) ether, cadmium, chromium (hexavalent), coal tar, coke oven emissions, nickel, polycyclic aromatic hydrocarbons, and radon.

What Constitutes "Proof" of Causation?

There has been vigorous philosophic and scientific debate over what constitutes "proof" of causation in scientific studies. When policy decisions relate to exposures judged to be harmful, epidemiologic evidence alone is often considered sufficient to justify protective intervention. It is unethical to propose randomized clinical trials to confirm that smoking causes lung cancer, that ionizing radiation causes leukemia, or that HPV causes cervical cancer. Moreover, in these examples, the observational evidence is so strong that the epidemiologic evidence itself is virtually incontrovertible. In other instances, especially when the exposure of interest is difficult to measure and the observed association is weaker, judgments about causality must be based on the weight of the evidence with consideration of all potentially relevant information from observational, clinical, experimental, and basic studies.

The inference that an association is causal is supported when a number of the following apply:

1. The association is strong (higher relative risk being more likely to indicate cause).
2. The risk increases or decreases with exposure in a dose-response gradient.
3. Consistent findings are seen in multiple studies with different investigators, study populations, and designs.
4. The exposure or cause precedes disease onset.
5. It is biologically plausible that the exposure could cause the disease.
6. The association is specific between the exposure and a single disease.
7. The epidemiologic findings fit coherently with information from other types of research and other epidemiologic studies.

Reviews and listings of substances known or suspected to cause cancer in humans are maintained by the National Toxicology Program (NTP)

TABLE 185–3 SELECTED KNOWN CAUSES OF CANCER AND THE ASSOCIATED CANCER SITES*

Cause	Associated cancer sites
TOBACCO	
Active smoking	Lip, oral cavity, nasal cavities, sinus, pharynx, larynx, lung, esophagus, pancreas, liver, stomach, bladder, kidney, cervix, acute myeloid leukemia
Environmental tobacco smoke	Lung
Spit tobacco (snuff, chewing)	Oral cavity, pancreas
NUTRITION, OBESITY, PHYSICAL INACTIVITY, AND FOOD CONTAMINANTS	
Aflatoxins	Liver
Alcohol	Mouth, pharynx, larynx, esophagus, breast,† liver†
Chinese salted fish†	Nasopharynx
Obesity	Postmenopausal breast, endometrium, colon, kidney, gallbladder
Physical inactivity	Colon, breast
MEDICAL	
CHEMOTHERAPY	
Chlorambucil	Acute nonlymphocytic leukemia
Cyclophosphamide	Bladder, leukemia
Melphalan	Acute nonlymphocytic leukemia
Methyl-CCNU	Leukemia
Myleran	Leukemia
Thiotepa	Leukemia
RADIOTHERAPY (see Ionizing Radiation)	
HORMONES	
Diethylstilbestrol	Breast, endometrium, cervix, vagina, testicles
Estrogen, steroidal	Endometrium, breast
Tamoxifen	Endometrium (reduces breast cancer risk)
OTHER DRUGS	
Analgesic mixtures containing phenacetin	Kidney, bladder
Azathioprine	Non-Hodgkin's lymphoma, skin, liver, mesenchyma
Chlornaphazine†	Bladder
Cyclosporine	Lymphoma, skin
Methoxsalen with ultraviolet A therapy (PUVA)	Skin
INFECTIOUS AGENTS	
VIRUS	
Epstein-Barr virus	Non-Hodgkin's lymphoma (Burkitt's lymphoma), Hodgkin's lymphoma, nasopharynx
Hepatitis B	Liver
Hepatitis C	Liver
Human immunodeficiency virus	Kaposi's sarcoma, Hodgkin's lymphoma, non-Hodgkin's lymphoma
Human papillomavirus	Cervix
Human herpesvirus 8	Kaposi's sarcoma, lymphoma
Human T-cell lymphotrophic virus	Leukemia
BACTERIA	
Helicobacter pylori	Stomach
PARASITES	
Liver flukes (*Clonorchis sinensis* and *Opisthorchis viverrini*)	Bile duct, liver
Schistosoma haematobium	Bladder
RADIATION	
NONIONIZING RADIATION	
Broad-spectrum solar ultraviolet radiation	Skin
Sunlamps or sunbeds	Skin, eye
IONIZING RADIATION	
X-radiation and gamma radiation	Leukemia, thyroid, breast, lung
Radium	Bone sarcoma
Radon	Lung
Thorium dioxide	Liver, leukemia, bone
Neutrons	Leukemia, thyroid, breast, lung

Continued

TABLE 185–3 SELECTED KNOWN CAUSES OF CANCER AND THE ASSOCIATED CANCER SITES*—cont'd

OCCUPATION AND ENVIRONMENTAL CHEMICALS	
4-Aminobiphenyl	Bladder
Arsenic compounds, inorganic	Skin, lung, digestive tract, liver, bladder, kidney, lymphatic and hematopoietic systems
Asbestos	Respiratory tract, pleural and peritoneal mesothelioma
Benzene	Acute myeloid leukemia
Benzidine and dyes	Bladder
Beryllium and beryllium compounds	Lung
1,3-Butadiene	Lymphatic, hematopoietic systems
Cadmium and cadmium compounds	Lung, prostate, kidney, bladder
Bis(chloromethyl) ether and technical-grade chloromethyl methyl ether	Lung
Chromium hexavalent compounds	Lung, sinonasal cavity
Coal tar and coal tar pitch	Skin, scrotum, lung, bladder, kidney, digestive tract, leukemia
Coke oven emissions	Skin, respiratory tract, kidney, bladder
Dioxin	Lung, non-Hodgkin's lymphoma
Erionite	Mesothelioma, lung
Ethylene oxide	Leukemia, stomach
Formaldehyde†	Nasopharynx
Mineral oils (untreated and mildly treated)	Skin, gastrointestinal tract, sinonasal, scrotum, bladder
Mustard gas	Respiratory tract
2-Napthylamine	Bladder
Nickel compounds	Lung, nasal
Silica, crystalline	Lung
Soot	Scrotum, skin, lung, prostate, bladder, hematopoietic and lymphatic systems
Strong inorganic acid mists containing sulfuric acid	Larynx, lung
Vinyl chloride	Liver, brain, lung, lymphatic and hematopoietic systems
Wood dust	Nasal cavity, paranasal sinus

*Modified from lists compiled by the International Agency for Research on Cancer (IARC) and the National Toxicology Program (NTP).
†Classified as carcinogenic by the IARC but not by the NTP.

and by the IARC, a branch of the World Health Organization (Table 185–3). The IARC evaluations classify exposures into one of four categories: (1) "sufficient evidence" of carcinogenicity in humans (in the working group's opinion, chance, bias, and confounding can be excluded with reasonable confidence), (2) "limited evidence" of carcinogenicity (the agent has been associated with increased risk for human cancer, but chance, bias, and confounding cannot be ruled out with reasonable confidence), (3) "inadequate evidence" of carcinogenicity (available studies are of insufficient quality, consistency, or statistical power to permit a conclusion regarding the carcinogenicity of the agent, or no data on carcinogenicity in humans are available), and (4) "evidence suggesting lack of carcinogenic activity" (several adequate studies of use or exposure are mutually consistent in not showing an increased risk for specified cancer sites, conditions, and levels of exposure). The NTP uses only two categories, "known to be a human carcinogen" and "reasonably anticipated to be a human carcinogen."

FUTURE DIRECTIONS

An exciting frontier in cancer epidemiology involves efforts to integrate insights from molecular biology and genetics into large-scale population studies to examine how the interaction of inherited genetic susceptibility (nature) with exposure after conception (nurture) influences an individual's risk for the development of cancer. It is hoped that such studies will identify modifiable, intermediate factors that influence the development or progression of cancer, just as cardiovascular research has identified lipid abnormalities and hypertension as therapeutic targets for the prevention of heart disease.

SUGGESTED READINGS

International Agency for Research on Cancer website. Accessed February 26, 2007. http://www.iarc.fr. *Listing of numerous resources available through the branch of the World Health Organization that deals with cancer.*

Jemal A, Siegel R, Ward E, et al: Cancer statistics, 2007. CA Cancer J Clin 2007;57:43–66. *Documents a drop in cancer-related mortality in 2004, the second consecutive year.*

National Toxicology Program website. Department of Health and Human Services. Accessed February 26, 2007. http://ntp-server.niehs.nih.gov/. *Website lists substances that are known or "reasonably anticipated to be" human carcinogens.*

186 GENETICS OF CANCER

Raju S. K. Chaganti

Cancer is a multistep process, the earliest step of which in some cases is an inherited mutation, followed by one or more somatic mutations in the target cell. Each cancer ultimately traces back to a single transformed normal cell and hence is clonal in nature. This chapter examines the role of genetics in the natural history and clinical implications of cancer.

CANCER AS AN INHERITED DISEASE

The aggregation of cancer in a family can be due to genetic or nongenetic causes, the former through mendelian (single-gene mutation; Chapter 39) or nonmendelian (polygenic or multifactorial; Chapter 37) inheritance of genes that predispose to cancer and the latter related to common exposure to carcinogenic agents (Chapter 187), lifestyle, or simply coincidence. The modern understanding of familial aggregation of cancer has required increasingly sophisticated epidemiologic and statistical methods in combination with genetic concepts and methods.

Although mendelian inheritance accounts for a small minority of all cancers, mutations that predispose to cancer have provided some of the most penetrating insights into the understanding of the genetic basis of normal as well as abnormal development; these mutations manifest the classical recessive or dominant modes of inheritance (Table 186–1). Nonmendelian inheritance, which also plays a major role in the overall incidence of cancer, has been more difficult to characterize. In addition, the interaction of mutated genes with the environment adds another level of complexity in deciphering the role of genetics of cancer in individuals as well as in families.

Some of the best known dominantly inherited syndromes are retinoblastoma, the hereditary breast cancer syndromes (Chapter 208), hereditary gastrointestinal malignancies (Chapter 203), and the endocrine tumor syndromes (Chapter 250). In many of the dominant syndromes, a defect in a tumor suppressor gene is generally inherited as a germline mutation from one parent; a subsequent acquired (somatic) mutation in the second copy of the gene from the other parent leads to complete loss of function and the development of cancer. In others, a gain-of-function mutation leads to formation of an oncogene, which promotes cancer even when only one copy of the gene is affected. Likewise, the so-called chromosome breakage (Bloom's syndrome [Chapter 38], ataxia telangiectasia [Chapter 271], Fanconi's anemia [Chapter 171]) and DNA repair disorders (xeroderma pigmentosum) illustrate recessively inherited cancer syndromes.

Hereditary retinoblastoma, which is a paradigm of a rare cancer syndrome, accounts for only 1% of pediatric cancers, although it is the most common eye cancer in children. It may be unilateral or bilateral, with bilateral tumors arising at a median age of 8 months whereas unilateral tumors arise at a median age of 2 years. Bilateral tumors are generally hereditary, although only 10% of patients present with a positive family history. Epidemiologic features of this disease suggested the "two-hit" hypothesis, which was validated upon cloning the gene and showing that the hereditary form represents a germline (present in one copy of the gene in all somatic cells of the gene carrier) mutation in the retinoblastoma gene as well as a second mutation, deletion, or other genetic event in the other copy of the retinoblastoma gene occurring in the target retinal cells and leading to suppression of the gene's function. In contrast, nonhereditary tumors arise when both mutations occur in the target cells, thus also fulfilling the criteria for the two-hit model. Functional characterization of the retinoblastoma gene showed that it regulates a key checkpoint in mitotic cell cycle progression from the G_1 to S phase. Mutational inactivation of the gene eliminates the checkpoint, thereby leading to abnormal cell cycle progression and uncontrolled mitotic proliferation. The recognition that loss of function of a key regulatory gene leads to the development of a tumor by abrogating the normal control of a key cell function led to the concept that such genes represent tumor suppressor genes, of which the retinoblastoma gene was the first to be discovered.

Another cell cycle checkpoint regulator, which functions as a potent tumor suppressor when functionally inactivated, is the *TP53* (p53) gene. The p53 protein is a transcription factor that regulates a number of growth regulatory genes, mediates apoptosis, and modulates cellular response to DNA damaging agents. In recognition of its multiple cellular regulatory functions, it is sometimes called the cell's gatekeeper. Germline mutations of the *TP53* gene underlie the Li-Fraumeni syndrome (Chapter 187), which is characterized by bone or soft tissue sarcomas, as well as multiple other cancer types. Several other dominantly inherited cancer syndromes, such as hereditary breast cancer syndromes and hereditary gastrointestinal malignancies, are caused by dysfunction of tumor suppressor genes.

CANCER AS A SOMATIC CELL DISEASE

Chromosomal Changes

Cytogenetic studies of various leukemias established four cardinal attributes of genetic change in cancer: (1) specific or nonrandom chromosomal changes may characterize individual cancer types; (2) tumor genomes are genetically unstable and subject to continuing change, a feature now recognized as genomic instability; (3) all cells in a given tumor trace back to a single progenitor cell and therefore are clonal; and (4) tumor progression is often associated with additional specific or nonrandom chromosomal changes, presumably "selected" from the genomic instability, in subpopulations of tumor cells that lead clonal diversity and evolution. Chromosomal changes are of many types, the most common being gain of an entire chromosome (aneuploidy) or a region of it (duplication), loss of an entire chromosome (monosomy) or a region of it (deletion), translocation or inversion (rearrangement), and amplification (Fig. 186–1).

Thousands of human tumors belonging to all five cancer lineages (hematopoietic, epithelial, mesenchymal, neuronal, germ cell) have been investigated for their chromosomal changes using molecular cytogenetic methods. These studies generally confirmed the principles of chromosomal change deduced from studies of leukemia. In addition, detailed cytogenetic characterization showed that all tumors display all the types of aberrations illustrated in Figure 186–1, and hematopoietic and mesenchymal tumors tend to exhibit specific translocations that are associated with specific histologies.

Oncogenes

Early in the 20th century, Peyton Rous showed that infection of chickens with a transforming retroviral sequence, termed the viral oncogene (v-*onc* gene), transduced and activated by mutation its normal cellular counterpart (c-*onc* gene) and caused the development of sarcomas. This particular c-*onc* gene was thus named c-*src* (sarcoma). Over the years, more than 30 isolated retroviruses have been shown to cause acute transformation in eukaryotic, although not human, cells. In humans, c-*onc* genes (homologous to *ras*), which are members of the so-called *ras* family of c-*onc* genes, cause bladder, lung, colon, and other cancers. Other transforming genes that are neither members of the *ras* family nor homologous with transforming sequences in retroviruses include multiple receptor tyrosine kinases, growth factors, and transcription factors. All these genes are now generically referred to as oncogenes. Oncogenes as a class tend to be highly conserved and, in their normal state, regulate development, growth, and other important cell functions.

A reciprocal translocation between two nonhomologous chromosomes leads to exchange of chromosomal segments following breakage and healing of the broken ends (see Fig. 186–1). In cancer-causing translocations, genes situated at the breakpoints are subject to either juxtaposition to other key genes with subsequent deregulation or the formation of fusion genes that generate abnormal proteins. For example, the Ph chromosome translocation, which involves the *ABL* oncogene on chromosome 9 (at 9q34) and the *BCR* gene (at 22q11), leads to the generation of one of two fusion genes that code for an 210-kD protein (p210) in chronic myelogenous leukemia (Chapter 195) or a 190-kD (p190) protein in acute lymphoblastic leukemia (Chapter 194) (Fig. 186–2). Another example is Burkitt's lymphoma, in which breakpoints in a translocation affecting chromosomes 8 and 14, with breaks at bands 8q24 and 14q32, cause *MYC* (a homologue of the avian myelomatosis retroviral oncogene) situated at 8q24 to rearrange with *IGH* (immunoglobulin heavy chain gene) at 14q32, thereby leading to the generation of a hybrid *IGH*:*MYC* transcriptional unit. The protein-coding region *MYC* remains intact but is brought under the transcriptional control of the *IGH* gene, thereby leading to deregulated expression of *MYC*, which then sets the stage for neoplastic transformation. This general pattern of translocations is common in lymphomas, where a variety of oncogenes are deregulated by juxtaposition with IG or TCR (T-cell receptor) antigen loci, the latter constitutively active in immune cells. Specific translocations also characterize sarcomas (Chapters 212 and 213), all of which generate fusion proteins involving oncogenes.

Finally, amplification of an oncogene to form multiple copies of itself can lead to overexpression of the gene product. This frequent, tumor-specific mechanism is associated with aggressive behavior or poor outcome. Thus, the *MYC* family of oncogenes (*MYC, MYCL, MYCN*) is amplified in small cell lung cancer, *MYCN* in neuroblastoma, *ERBB1* (estrogen growth factor receptor) in glioblastoma, and *ERBB2 (HER2), MYC,* and *CCND1* (cyclin D1) in breast cancer (Chapter 208).

Epigenetics

The traditional view of gene function is based on the concept that both parental (paternal and maternal) alleles of a gene are equivalent. Genomic imprinting is an epigenetic modification that occurs in only one parental allele of the gene in germline or somatic cells and that leads to differential expression of the two parental alleles in an individual cell or all of its

TABLE 186–1 SYNDROMES OF INHERITED CANCER PREDISPOSITION IN CLINICAL ONCOLOGY SYNDROME

Syndrome	Mode of Inheritance	Gene(s)
HEREDITARY BREAST CANCER SYDROMES		
Hereditary breast and ovarian cancer syndrome	Dominant	*BRCA1* *BRCA2*
Li-Fraumeni syndrome	Dominant	*TP53*
Cowden's syndrome	Dominant	*PTEN*
Bannayan-Riley-Ruvalcaba syndrome	Dominant	*PTEN*
HEREDITARY GASTROINTESTINAL MALIGNANCIES		
Hereditary nonpolyposis colon cancer	Dominant	*MLH1* *MLH2* *MSH6*
Familial polyposis	Dominant	*APC*
Hereditary gastric cancer	Dominant	*CDH1*
Juvenile polyposis		*SMAD4/DPC4* *BMPR1A*
Peutz-Jeghers syndrome	Dominant	*STK11*
Hereditary melanoma–pancreatic cancer syndrome	Dominant	*CDKN2A*
Hereditary pancreatitis	Dominant	*PRSS1*
Turcot's syndrome	Dominant	*APC* *MLH1* *PMS2*
Familial gastrointestinal stromal tumor	Dominant	*KIT*
GENODERMATOSES WITH CANCER PREDISPOSITION		
Melanoma syndromes	Dominant	*CDKN2A* *CDK4* *CMM*
Basal cell cancer, Gorlin's syndrome	Dominant	*PTCH*
Cowden's syndrome	Dominant	*PTEN*
Neurofibromatosis 1	Dominant	*NF1*
Neurofibromatosis 2	Dominant	*NF2*
Tuberous sclerosis	Dominant	*TSC1* *TSC2*
Carney's complex	Dominant	*PRKAR1A*
Muir-Torre syndrome	Dominant	*MLH1* *MSH2*
Xeroderma pigmentosum	Recessive	*XPA,B,C,D,E,F,G* *POLH*
Rothmund-Thomson syndrome	Recessive	*RECOL4*
LEUKEMIA/LYMPHOMA PREDISPOSITION SYNDROMES		
Bloom's syndrome	Recessive	*BLM*
Fanconi's anemia	Recessive	*FANCA,B,C* *FANCA,*D_2 *FANCE,F,G* *FANCL*
Ataxia-telangiectasia	Recessive	*ATM*
Shwachman-Diamond syndrome	Recessive	*SBDS*
Nijmegen breakage syndrome	Recessive	*NBS1*
Canale-Smith syndrome	Dominant	*FAS* *FASL*
Wiskott-Aldrich syndrome	X-linked recessive	*WAS*
Common variable immune deficiency	Recessive	
Severe combined immune deficiency	X-linked recessive Recessive	*IL2RG* *ADA* *JAK3* *RAG1* *RAG2* *IL7R* *CD45* *Artemis*
X-linked lymphoproliferative syndrome	X-linked recessive	*SH2D1A*
GENITOURINARY CANCER PREDISPOSITION SYNDROMES		
Hereditary prostate cancer	Dominant	*HPC1* *HPCX* *HPC2/ELAC2* *PCAP* *PCBC* *PRCA*
Simpson-Golabi-Behmel syndrome	X-linked recessive	*GPC3*
von Hippel–Lindau syndrome	Dominant	*VHL*
Beckwith-Wiedemann syndrome	Dominant	*CDKN1C* *NSD1*
Wilms' tumor syndrome	Dominant	*WT1*
Wilms' tumor, aniridia, genitourinary abnormalities, mental retardation (WAGR) syndrome	Dominant	*WT1*
Birt-Hogg-Dubé syndrome	Dominant	*FLCL*
Papillary renal cancer syndrome	Dominant	*MET,PRCC*
Constitutional t(3;8) translocation	Dominant	*TRCB*
Hereditary bladder cancer	Sporadic	
Hereditary testicular cancer	Possibly X-linked	
Rhabdoid predisposition syndrome	Dominant	*SNF5INI1*
CENTRAL NERVOUS SYSTEM/VASCULAR CANCER PREDISPOSITION SYNDROMES		
Hereditary paraganglioma	Dominant	*SDHD* *SDHC* *SDHB*
Retinoblastoma	Dominant	*RB1*
Rhabdoid predisposition syndrome	Dominant	*SNF5/INI1*
SARCOMA/BONE CANCER PREDISPOSITION SYNDROMES		
Multiple exostoses	Dominant	*EXT1* *EXT2*
Leiomyoma/renal cancer syndrome	Dominant	*FH*
Carney's complex	Dominant	*PRKAR1A*
Werner's syndrome	Recessive	*WRN*

TABLE 186–1 SYNDROMES OF INHERITED CANCER PREDISPOSITION IN CLINICAL ONCOLOGY SYNDROME—cont'd

Syndrome	Mode of Inheritance	Gene(s)
ENDOCRINE CANCER PREDISPOSITION SYNDROMES		
Multiple endocrine neoplasia 1	Dominant	*MEN1*
Multiple endocrine neoplasia 2	Dominant	*RET*
Familial papillary thyroid cancer	Dominant	Multiple loci

Modified from Garber JE, Offit K: Hereditary cancer predisposition syndromes. J Clin Oncol 2005;23:276–292.

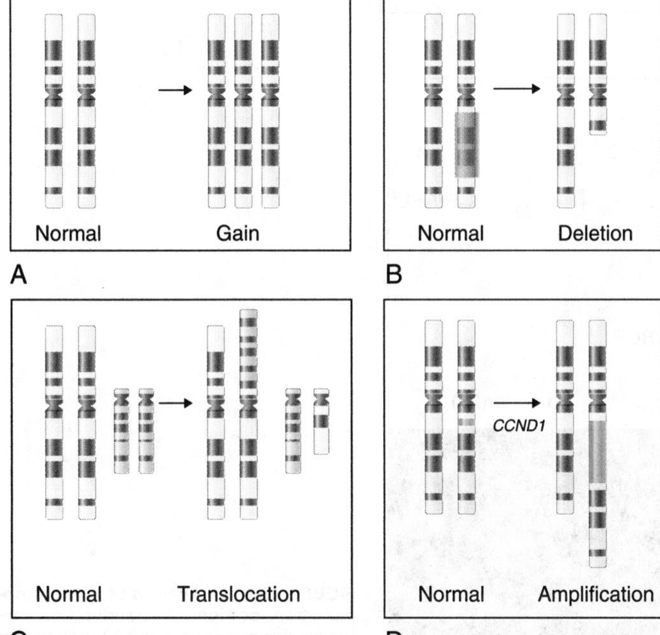

FIGURE 186–1 • Common cytogenetic changes in cancer. The chromosome (at metaphase) is traditionally distinguished by its short and long arms separated by a centromere. Stylized bands (dark and light stripes along the length of the chromosome) produced by special treatments are also shown. The abnormality (right) and the corresponding normal image of the chromosome are illustrated in each panel. **A,** Gain of a chromosome leading to aneuploidy. **B,** Deletion of a chromosomal segment from one of the two homologues. **C,** Translocation showing exchange of segments between nonhomologous chromosomes. **D,** Amplification, with an increase in a region of a chromosome by replicating many times in place.

progeny. Loss of imprinting may activate a normally inactive growth-enhancing gene or inactivate a tumor suppressor gene. Genomic imprinting is normally maintained by methylation of cytosine within DNA sequences that are rich in CpG dinucleotides (CpG islands). Loss of imprinting, which is detectable as abnormal methylation of CpG islands, is found in many types of tumors and affects many genes (e.g., *APC, CDKN2A, MLH1, RASFA1, MGMT*).

Genetic Counseling

Risk assessment based on testing for the mutation status of the relevant gene in a family is an integral component of management of affected and at-risk individuals in a family (Chapter 38). In the communication of genetic risk information to a patient or family, the provider must be equipped to deal with the medical, psychological, and social consequences in all their complexity. Furthermore, as ability to identify individuals at risk increases, especially at early ages, the responsibility to institute effective surveillance and prevention strategies also increases.

Genetic Testing for Diagnosis and Prognosis

Cytogenetic chromosomal analysis or fluorescence in situ hybridization is now routine for all newly diagnosed leukemias (Chapters 194 and 195) because both good and bad prognostic cytogenetic markers have been identified. Cytogenetic analysis is equally important in the differential diagnosis of lymphomas, sarcomas, and other tumors and in the prognostic evaluation of neuroblastoma and metastatic breast cancer. In addition, cytogenetic analysis after chemotherapy or stem cell transplantation can assess residual tumor burden and engraftment. Prognostic markers include the *EGFR* gene in lung cancer (Chapter 201) and the *IGHV* mutation in chronic lymphocytic leukemia (Chapter 195). Molecular methods such as the polymerase chain reaction also provide increasing precision to detect chromosomal translocations and other abnormalities in treated patients to detect minimal residual disease.

GENETICS IN CANCER THERAPY

The greatest hope for therapy is that when a causal mutation or other genetic aberration for any cancer is discovered, it should be possible either to replace a defective gene with a normal one by genetic or cellular engineering or to develop drugs that block the action of an aberrant gene. In the latter area, the growth factor gene *ERBB2 (HER2)* is amplified and the HER2 protein encoded by it is overexpressed in a proportion of metastatic breast cancers with poor prognosis (Chapter 208). The drug trastuzumab, an antibody against HER2, specifically blocks the overexpressed protein in HER2-positive breast cancers and is a highly effective therapy. The normal *ABL* gene encodes a protein tyrosine kinase, the Abl tyrosine kinase, whereas the *BCR-ABL* fusion gene in chronic myelogenous leukemia (Chapter 195) encodes the aberrant Bcr-Abl tyrosine kinase. Inhibitors of Bcr-Abl tyrosine kinase, such as imatinib mesylate, are highly effective in this otherwise refractory leukemia as well as in gastrointestinal stromal tumors (Chapter 202). Another kinase inhibitor, sunitinib, was introduced as a potential drug for kidney cancer, with promising results. Given the current pace of research, more genetically based targeted therapeutic agents can be expected in the near future.

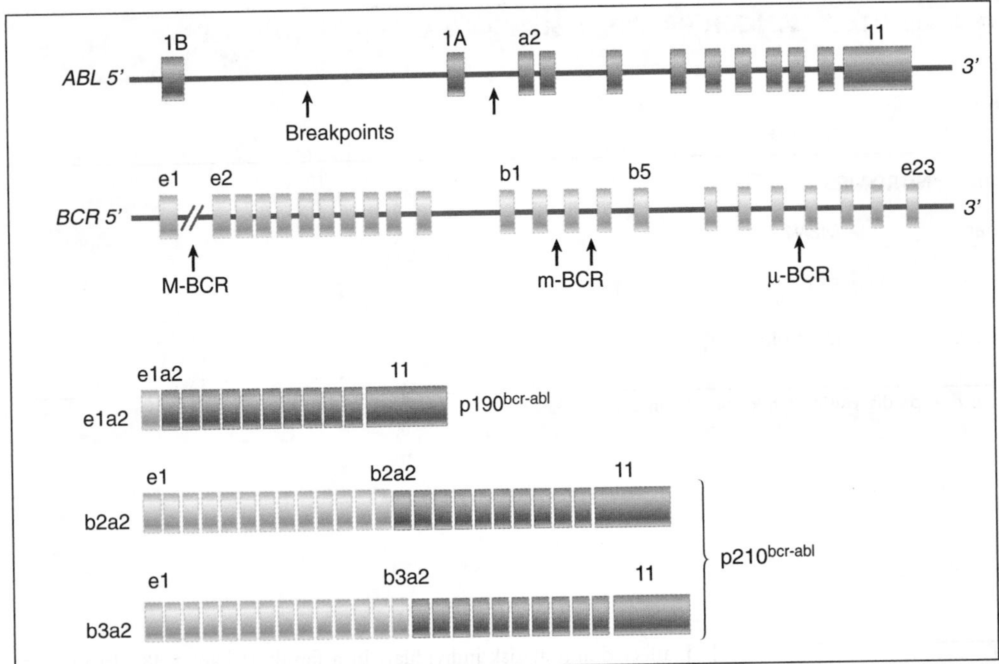

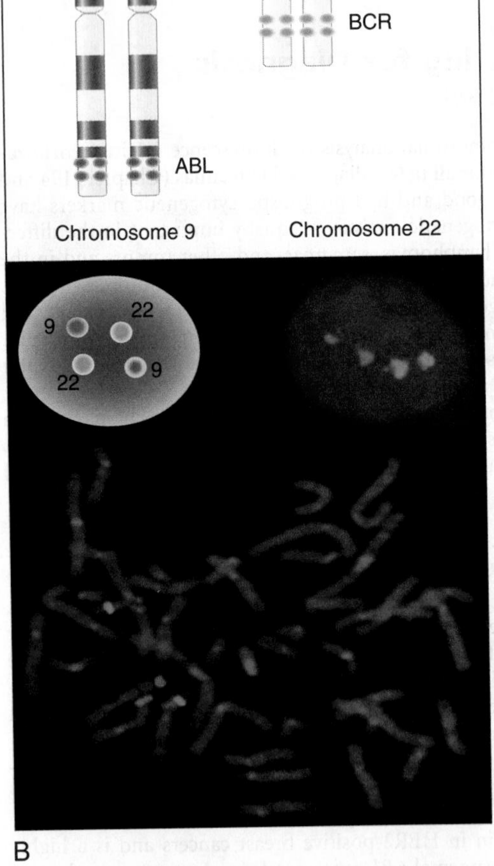

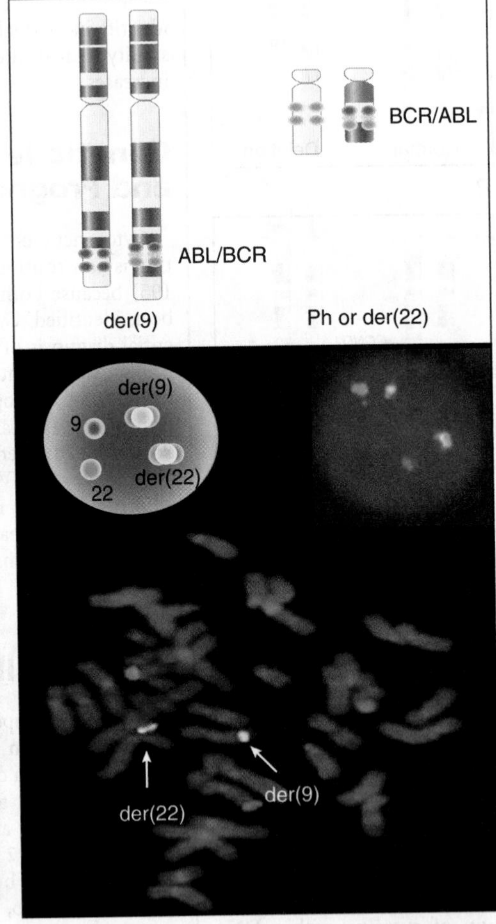

FIGURE 186–2 • Analysis of a chromosomal translocation. A translocation between chromosomes 9 and 22 with breaks through the *ABL* (chromosome 9) and *BCR* (chromosome 22) genes results in abnormal expression of the *ABL* gene and development of chronic myelogenous leukemia (CML). **A,** The molecular structure of *ABL* and *BCR* genes, the breakpoints in the genes, and the P190 and P210 proteins encoded by the fusion genes. **B,** Cytogenetic depiction of the translocation. Top, The normal and translocated chromosome illustrated in a cartoon form. Bottom, Fluorescence in situ images of the translocation. Left, A normal metaphase and interphase showing two red *(ABL)* and two green *(BCR)* signals. Right, A tumor metaphase and interphase showing one red *(ABL),* one green *(BCR),* and two fusion red-green signals.

SUGGESTED READINGS

Chen HY, Yu SL, Chen CH, et al: A five-gene signature and clinical outcome in non-small-cell lung cancer. N Engl J Med 2007;356:11–20. *Associated with relapse-free and overall survival.*

Garber JE, Offit K: Hereditary cancer predisposition syndromes. J Clin Oncol 2005;23:276–292. *A comprehensive overview.*

Hitchins MP, Wong JJ, Suthers G, et al: Inheritance of a cancer-associated MLH1 germ-line epimutation. N Engl J Med 2007;356:697–705. *Demonstrates transgenerational epigenetic inheritance.*

Holleman A, Cheok MH, den Boer ML, et al: Gene-expression patterns in drug-resistant acute lymphoblastic leukemia cells and response to treatment. N Engl J Med 2004;351:533–542. *A relatively small number of genes determine sensitivity and resistance to four drugs used in this disease.*

Quackenbush J: Microarray analysis and tumor classification. N Engl J Med 2006;354:2463–2472. *An excellent review of recent advances in tumor classification using high-throughput genome analysis methods.*

Tomlinson SA, Rhodes DR, Perner S, et al: Recurrent fusion of TMPRSS and ETS transcription factor genes in prostate cancer. Science 2005;310:644–648. *Example of advanced methods of detection of chromosome translocations based on gene expression profiles.*

187 BIOLOGY OF CANCER

Jeffrey A. Moscow and Kenneth H. Cowan

GENETIC CANCER BIOLOGY

Cancer is an acquired genetic disease (Chapter 186). Spontaneous genetic changes overwhelm the mechanisms that maintain normal cellular homeostasis, disrupt the normal tight control of cell division and death, and result in the malignant phenotype.

The genetic damage that results in cancer can occur in several ways: translocations of genes can juxtapose two genes in ways that cause dysregulation of their function; mutations can activate cancer-causing genes or deactivate cancer-preventing genes; and epigenetic modifications of proteins that associate with DNA can alter the expression of critical genes (Chapter 186). Sometimes, the first step is the mutation of genes that normally prevent mutations in other genes—cells then quickly gain additional mutations that, through a morbid natural selection, ultimately produce the mutant clone that gives rise to a malignancy.

The very processes that generate malignant transformations also present obstacles to their treatment. The genetic plasticity that can manufacture cancer-causing mutations can also generate mutations that result in resistance to anticancer drugs.

Tumor formation after malignant transformation requires changes in cell biology that, in the processes of invasion and metastases, favor propagation of the malignant cells. Because individual cells, like organisms, are programmed to die, cancer cells must learn to evade the intricate systems of apoptosis that ensure cell death. Cancer cells must also enable the formation of new blood vessels to provide nutrition for the growing mass and develop strategies to escape the immune surveillance that suppresses tumor formation. These processes that give rise to malignant tumors can again raise barriers to successful therapies; for example, cells with impaired apoptosis may be resistant to anticancer drugs that kill cells through activation of apoptosis. However, the distinctive biology of malignancies can also provide opportunities for directed therapies.

Specific Mutations, Targeted Therapies

All cancer cells contain some genomic damage. In most cases, several abnormalities must occur, but sometimes even a single mutation appears sufficient to produce malignant transformation. The latter examples demonstrate clearly that cancer is a genetic disease of dysregulated growth, and they demonstrate that identification of a genetic cause can lead to a specific targeted therapy aimed at the product of the damaged gene.

In the case of acute promyelocytic leukemia (APL; Chapter 194), the characteristic t(15;17) translocation is the only identified genetic lesion. This genetic mishap splices the retinoic acid receptor *(RAR)* gene to another gene called *PML*, and the resulting hybrid RAR-PML protein does not function properly. In normal cells, RAR binds to its ligand, vitamin A, which causes the RAR to disassociate with a complex of proteins that repress transcription of certain genes and recruit a different complex of proteins that activate transcription of those genes. In APL, the hybrid RAR-PML protein has lost the capacity to activate gene transcription in response to normal levels of vitamin A. However, the functional defect of the RAR-PML hybrid protein product can be overcome with pharmacologic doses of a vitamin A analogue, all-*trans*-retinoic acid (ATRA). The addition of ATRA to chemotherapy for APL doubles disease-free survival, from approximately 40% to approximately 80%.

Cancers driven by single mutations appear to be restricted to specific tissue types. The t(15;17) creates malignancy in promyelocytes, but this translocation does not lead to cancer when it occurs in other tissues. Similarly, the accidental genetic recombination that creates the BCR/ABL hybrid protein results in malignant transformation of myeloid cells (Chapters 186 and 195), but this genetic alteration is found only in a limited number of nonhematologic tissues (Chapter 202). Thus, genetic alterations that lead to malignant transformation are also dependent on the cellular context in which they occur.

The Multistage Evolution of Malignancy

Most cancers do not have a single cause but rather are the products of a progression of genetic lesions that can be years in the making, as evidenced by their multiple and complex genetic alterations. The classical model of two stages of cancer development, initiation and promotion, has been replaced by a more dynamic and multistep model in which accumulated genetic damage leads to dysregulation of cell division and the disarming of the mechanisms of cell death.

Often the first step in the creation of a tumor is the development of genomic instability. During each cell division, some 3 billion nucleotide pairs must be faithfully copied to produce exact replicas in each daughter cell. The process of cancer can begin with alterations in any one of a number of factors that influence the accuracy of this process of genetic replication. Two major mechanisms create this acquired genetic damage: spontaneous mutations can disable the machinery that edits DNA replication and removes damaged genes, or, more frequently, cells are exposed to carcinogens that directly damage DNA, and the imprecise repair of damaged DNA results in an increase in spontaneous mutations.

The evidence for the loss of genomic integrity in cancer is exemplified by studies that examine the stability of DNA sequences scattered throughout the genome, that is, microsatellite repeats. These sequences have no apparent role in gene expression or regulation, but they can be viewed as a bellwether for the fidelity of genomic replication. In most tumors, the increase in microsatellite instability, or an increase in the variation of the length of these DNA sequences in tumor tissue versus normal tissues, demonstrates the loss of the ability to replicate the genome faithfully in malignant cells.

Heritable conditions that impair the proteins that ensure genomic fidelity cause a predisposition to a variety of types of cancer. For example, defects in genes that repair DNA damage (Table 187–1) cause disorders such as xeroderma pigmentosum (Chapter 462) and ataxia-telangiectasia (Chapter 271) and are associated with an increased risk of cancer. The colon cancer predisposition syndrome, hereditary nonpolyposis colon cancer (Chapter 203), is caused by inherited defects in a number of related genes that repair DNA mismatches (*MSH2, MSH6, MLH1,* and *PMS2*).

Carcinogens are substances that create genomic alterations. As cancer is a genetic disease, carcinogens are genomic toxins that damage DNA and create mutations. The DNA damage from cigarette smoke (Chapter 30) results from exposure to dangerous hydrocarbon products that bind DNA and disrupt faithful replication. Ultraviolet irradiation causes characteristic DNA damage in the skin that can lead to melanoma and other skin cancers (Chapter 214). Ionizing radiation (Chapter 18) from diagnostic and therapeutic radiation can also cause cancer.

TABLE 187–1 GENOMIC INSTABILITY GENES ASSOCIATED WITH INCREASED HEREDITARY CANCER RISK

Genes	Syndrome	Hereditary Tumor Types
MUTYH	Attenuated polyposis	Colon
ATM	Ataxia-telangiectasia	Leukemias, lymphomas, brain
BLM	Bloom's	Leukemias, lymphomas, skin
BRCA1, BRCA2	Hereditary breast cancer	Breast, ovary
FANCA, FANCC, FANCD2, FANCE, FANCF, FANCG	Fanconi's anemia A, C, D2, E, F, and G	Leukemias
NBS1	Nijmegen breakage	Lymphomas, brain
MSH2, MLH1, MSH6, PMS2	Hereditary nonpolyposis colon cancer	Colon
XPA, XPC, ERCC2, ERCC3, ERCC4, ERCC5, DDB2	Xeroderma pigmentosum	Skin

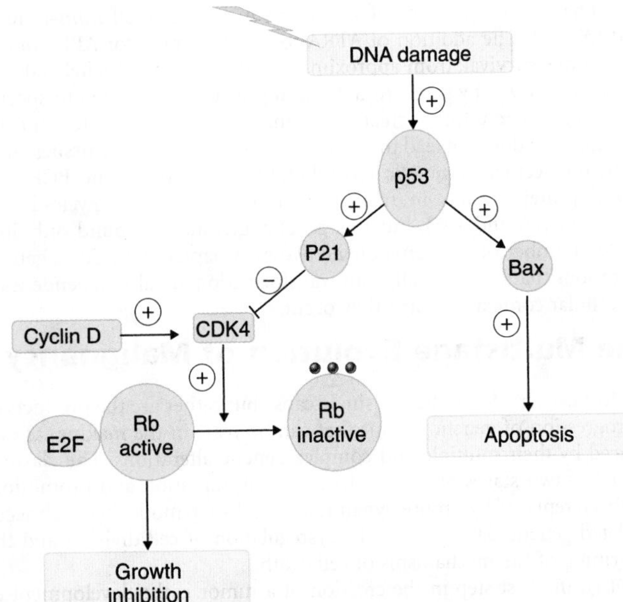

FIGURE 187–1 • P53 and DNA damage response. Following DNA damage, p53 expression induces the cyclin kinase inhibitor p21, resulting in cell cycle arrest, and bax, which induces apoptosis. Rb, retinoblastoma.

One key regulator of genomic integrity is the p53 protein, the product of a tumor suppressor gene that is commonly referred to as the "guardian of the genome." The p53 protein can sense DNA damage and direct the cell either to cell cycle arrest by increased expression of the cyclin kinase inhibitor p21 (Fig. 187–1), which provides the cell with the opportunity to repair genetic damage prior to cell division, or down the path of programmed cell death (apoptosis) by increased expression of bax, a proapoptotic protein. Inactivating mutations in p53 are among the most common abnormalities observed in cancer, emphasizing the critical role of unrepaired genetic damage in the etiology of cancer. Individuals with inherited mutations of the p53 gene have the Li-Fraumeni syndrome (Chapter 186), with increased susceptibility to specific types of cancer. The retinoblastoma (RB) gene is another tumor suppressor gene whose normal function is to regulate cell growth (see Fig. 187–1). Mutations in a number of other tumor suppressor genes are also associated with specific cancer syndromes (Table 187–2).

The relative impact of heritable predispositions and environmental exposures depends on the frequency of the genetic abnormality and its penetrance. Mutations in the breast cancer susceptibility genes *BRCA1* and *BRCA2* (Chapter 208) are rare, so relatively few women inherit abnormal copies of these gene alleles from their parents, and only approximately 10% of breast cancers can be attributed to *BRCA1* and *BRCA2* mutations. The mechanisms involved in carcinogenesis induced by *BRCA1* and *BRCA2* mutations are not clear. *BRCA1* is involved in the regulation of gene expression, whereas both *BRCA1* and *BRCA2* associate with many intracellular proteins that are involved in DNA repair, including rad50, rad51, ATM, and p53 (Fig. 187–2). Cells defective in *BRCA1* or *BRCA2* display defects both in the response to DNA and in DNA repair.

The penetrance of BRCA1 is high, so that an affected woman has a 60 to 85% lifetime risk for breast cancer. By comparison, other cancer susceptibility genes are both more common and less penetrant, and the interactions among these genes are complex. For example, studies in monozygotic twins estimate that inherited genes may account for almost a third of breast, colorectal, and prostate cancers, with the remaining attributable risk thought to be environmental.

DNA damage, whether from heritable conditions, from unfortunate somatic mutations in the DNA repair mechanisms themselves, or from carcinogen exposure, increases the rate of spontaneous mutations in cells and sets the stage for the natural selection of malignant clones. Although mutations of most of the approximately 25,000 genes in the genome do not result in malignancy, mutations or other disruptions of a few critical genes, which confer a selective proliferative or survival advantage, are frequently altered in many types of cancers.

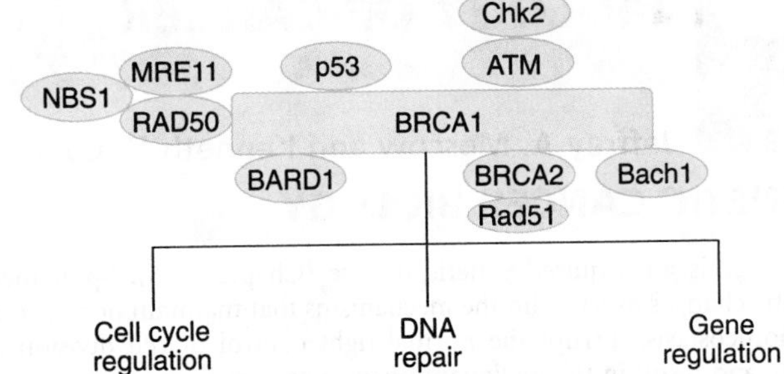

FIGURE 187–2 • Protein interactions with BRCA1 and BRCA2. BRCA1 and BRCA2 act as molecular scaffolds and promote assembly of protein complexes involved in cell cycle regulation in response to DNA damage as well as DNA repair.

TABLE 187–2 TUMOR SUPPRESSOR GENES ASSOCIATED WITH INCREASED HEREDITARY CANCER RISK

Genes	Syndrome	Hereditary Tumor Types
P53	Li-Fraumeni	Breast, sarcoma, adrenal, brain,
APC	Familial adenomatous polyposis	Colon, thyroid, stomach, intestine
CDHI	Familial gastric carcinoma	Stomach
VHL	von Hippel–Lindau	Kidney
WT1	Familial Wilms' tumor	Wilms'
PTEN	Cowden's	Hamartoma, glioma, uterus
CDKN2A	Familial malignant melanoma	Melanoma, pancreas
CDK4	Familial malignant melanoma	Melanoma
RB1	Hereditary retinoblastoma	Eye
NF1	Neurofibromatosis	Neurofibroma
MEN1	Multiple endocrine neoplasia type 1	Parathyroid, pituitary, islet cell,
NF2	Neurofibromatosis	Meningioma, acoustic neuromas

Disease of the Messenger Proteins

In health, cells respond to external stimuli with complex and redundant protein networks that interact with external stimuli and transmit appropriate signals to the nucleus. The proteins involved in signal transduction include cell surface receptors, second messenger systems, and multiple transcription factors that directly regulate gene expression. Each of these elements of the signal transduction network is controlled by multiple proteins that tightly regulate the activation state of each element of the network. Disruption of any of the genes that encode the proteins involved in signal transduction—proteins that relay the external stimulus to the nucleus—occurs frequently in cancer.

Cell surface receptors for external stimuli involve families of receptor tyrosine kinases, proteins that become activated after binding to specific ligands, often as a result of homodimerization or heterodimerization and subsequent phosphorylation of cytoplasmic proteins. For example, the epidermal growth factor (ERBB) family receptor kinases are often amplified or found activated by mutations in breast, ovary, gastric, and lung cancers. Identification of genetic abnormalities in cancer cells has provided valuable targets for selective therapies. Thus, trastuzumab, a monoclonal antibody directed against the ERBB2/Her2neu protein, which is amplified and overexpressed in 25% of breast cancers, has proved to be very useful in improving disease-free survival and overall survival when given in combination with chemotherapy (Chapter 208). Erlotinib, an inhibitor of ERBB1 (epidermal growth factor [EGF]) receptor, may be effective in treatment of lung cancers that contain mutations in the ERBB1 (EGF) receptor (Chapter 201).

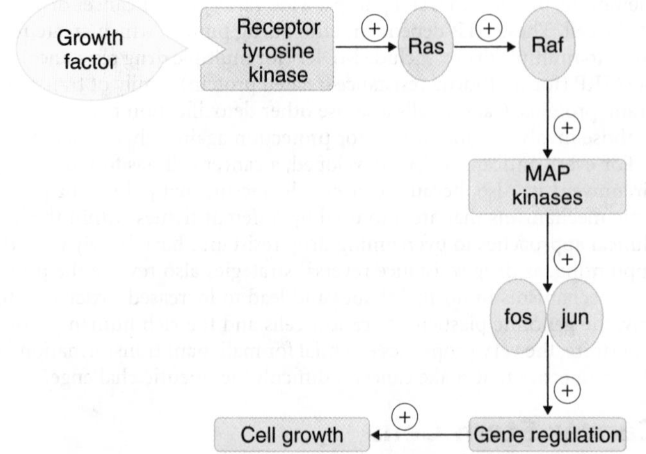

FIGURE 187–3 • Growth factor–mediated signal transduction. Upon binding to specific receptor ligands, receptor tyrosine kinases activate downstream signal transduction cascades that result in changes in gene expression and enhanced cell growth. Alterations in various steps in the signal transduction cascade are frequently observed in cancer. MAP, mitogen-activated protein.

Unregulated growth can also result from mutations that affect downstream signal transduction networks (Fig. 187–3). Receptor tyrosine kinases transmit their signals through biochemical pathways and ultimately drive gene transcription. In some pathways, receptor tyrosine kinases activate Ras proteins, which act as second messengers that amplify and direct signals from receptor tyrosine kinases to other intracellular proteins, which then ultimately generate the cellular response to the stimulus. Ras proteins are guanosine triphosphate binding proteins that sit in the cell membrane, and their activation is tightly regulated in normal cells. Ras mutations, which are frequently found in cancer, typically result in the Ras protein being stuck in the "on," or activated, position; instead of switching on and off in response to a stimulus, activated (mutated) Ras provides a constant, unregulated stimulus to downstream proteins, which in turn creates a cascading effect that stimulates cell growth. Although mutations in other genes are also commonly found in tumors that harbor Ras mutations, mutation of Ras alone has been shown to transform normal cells into malignant cells. Activating mutations of Ras family proteins can frequently be found in melanoma, myeloid leukemias, and cancers of the colon, pancreas, and lung. Genetic abnormalities are also frequently found in the other signaling pathways that transmit signals from receptor tyrosine kinases, including the PIP3/PDK1/Akt pathway, as well as in the nonreceptor tyrosine kinases signaling pathways, including the Jak/STAT and the c-Src pathways.

Disruption of the genes that encode the proteins that regulate gene transcription, which are the downstream targets of signal transduction cascades, can also create malignancy. For example, amplification of the Myc family of transcription factors is frequently observed in neuroblastoma and in cancers of the lung, bladder, breast, stomach, and colon. Certain acute leukemias (Chapter 194) arise when the normal gene recombination process that produces diverse immune responses goes awry and an immunoglobulin or T-cell receptor locus is accidentally spliced onto a gene encoding a transcription factor, resulting in loss of regulation of the transcription factor activity. Several pathognomonic oncogenic chromosomal translocations commonly found in sarcomas also involve genes for transcription factors; for example, the t(11;22) of Ewing's sarcoma (Chapter 212) creates the Fli1-EWS hybrid transcription factor, and the characteristic t(2;13) of alveolar rhabdomyosarcoma creates the hybrid Pax3/FKHR DNA binding protein.

Suppression of Tumor Suppressors

Normal cells contain proteins that prevent malignant transformation. Inactivation of the tumor suppressor genes that encode these proteins also leads to cancer. Because a loss of function is required for a malignant effect, both copies of the tumor suppressor gene must be affected. In almost all cases, patients have a physical loss of one copy of a gene and an acquired mutation of the other. The spontaneous deletion of genetic material, called loss of heterozygosity, is a frequently observed genetic abnormality in tumors.

Some familial cancer predisposition syndromes are based on the inheritance of one damaged copy of a tumor suppressor gene (Chapter 186). Hereditary retinoblastoma, which results from inheritance of a mutated RB gene, and the Li-Fraumeni syndrome (Chapter 186), which results from inheritance of a mutant p53 gene, predispose affected individuals to cancers. Both the RB and p53 proteins play critical roles in regulating the progression of proliferating cells through the cell cycle, and the loss of this checkpoint regulation can contribute to uncontrolled cell growth and cancer.

The importance of the p53 and RB signaling pathways in tumor suppression is further revealed by the mechanism by which infection with the human papillomavirus (HPV; Chapter 396) in cervical epithelial cells leads to cervical cancer (Chapter 209). HPV proteins E6 and E7 inactivate p53 and RB proteins, respectively, thereby creating a virally induced premalignant state in which the machinery that prevents damaged cells from proliferating has been turned off. For this reason, vaccination against certain HPV serotypes holds the promise of preventing most cases of cervical cancer.

DISTINCTIVE CANCER BIOLOGY

Cancer cells do not behave like normal cells. The alterations in the regulation of cell growth, differentiation, and death that give rise to cancer also produce common abnormal biologic characteristics, which are shared by tumors that arise from different cells of origin. These common features conspire to allow the transformed cell to grow into a tumor.

Normal cells are programmed to differentiate and ultimately to die, and this programming is regulated through enzymatic pathways that lead to terminal differentiation, senescence, or apoptosis. Cancer cells evade the mechanisms that are designed to steer cells toward terminal differentiation and senescence by altering the function of telomerase. As primitive cells divide and differentiate, the ends of chromosomes, called telomeres, progressively shorten and ultimately lead to a growth arrest that is termed replicative senescence. An enzyme called telomerase adds length back to the telomeres and reverses the process of replicative senescence. Telomerase is usually expressed at significant levels only in stem cells. However, telomerase is highly expressed in most malignant tissues, demonstrating a common alteration of cell biology that is necessary for creation and maintenance of the malignant phenotype.

In addition to bypassing senescence, cancer cells disable the pathways that lead to apoptosis. Because apoptosis is literally a life-and-death decision for the cell, it must be tightly controlled by intricate pathways of regulatory proteins. Apoptosis can be triggered through either external or internal pathways that converge to activate a family of enzymes, called caspases, that systematically degrade cellular proteins and DNA in a characteristic pattern resulting in cell death. Cancer cells contain many common aberrations in the machinery that regulates apoptosis, including increased activity of antiapoptotic proteins, such as Bcl-2 and Mcl-1, or increased levels of inhibitors of apoptosis, such as the protein survivin, which inhibits caspase activity.

Epigenetic changes in gene expression are also hallmarks of malignancy (Chapter 186). In normal cells, gene expression is controlled by epigenetic processes that limit the physical accessibility of genes to transcription factors. Gene expression can be silenced by processes that methylate specific DNA sequences on chromosomes, called CpG islands. In cancer, tumor suppressor genes are frequently found to be abnormally methylated, leading to a loss of their expression and function. The drug 5-azacytidine and the newer agent decitabine reverse methylation and have activity in the myelodysplastic syndrome (Chapter 193) and leukemia. However, drug resistance genes may also be methylated, and strategies to reverse global methylation may have uncertain effects on cellular sensitivity to chemotherapy. Gene expression is also controlled by histone acetylases, which influence how tightly genomic DNA is spooled around large complex nuclear proteins called histones and alter the interaction of chromatin proteins with DNA. A novel group of drugs called histone deacetylase inhibitors, such as suberoylanilide hydroxamic acid and depsipeptide, are currently under development as novel anticancer agents.

Cancer cells also demonstrate characteristic alterations in glucose metabolism, known as the Warburg effect. Malignant cells tend preferentially to shunt glucose into the glycolytic pathway, taking up excessive amounts of glucose and metabolizing glucose into lactate instead of channeling glucose into the typical aerobic pathway that more efficiently captures energy and creates the end products of carbon dioxide and water. This disruption of normal cellular energy metabolism is thought to be due to dysregulation of a gene that is also involved in the regulation of apoptosis, Akt, and its downstream effectors. This abnormal metabolism of glucose in cancer cells is also the principle behind the use of positron emission tomographic scans to image tumors. Inherited inactivating mutations of the phosphatase and tensin homologue (PTEN), which inactivates Akt, are also responsible for Cowden's syndrome (Chapter 186), in which the susceptibility to breast and thyroid cancers is increased.

Normal cells have tightly regulated mechanisms to degrade and recycle proteins by attaching one or more ubiquitin molecules to a protein. Ubiquitinylation can serve as a signal that a protein should be trafficked to and degraded by lysosomes or the proteasome. Ubiquitinylation plays an important role in the regulation of receptor tyrosine kinases, in cell cycle progression, and in repair of DNA damage. This regulatory mechanism is altered in many types of cancer. The first anticancer drug targeted at this abnormality in cancer cells is bortezomib, which inhibits proteasome activity and is effective in the treatment of multiple myeloma (Chapter 198).

Because tumors must find mechanisms to feed themselves as they grow, the malignant transformation must include the ability to stimulate new blood vessel formation, or angiogenesis. Malignant cells have in common the ability to stimulate the formation of endothelial cells and the breakdown of extracellular membranes, often by secreting vasculature endothelial growth factor (VEGF). The resulting tumor vasculature, although functional, does not have the vessel architecture or endothelial wall characteristics of a normal vascular bed. The realization that tumor cells have unique angiogenesis has led to the novel therapeutic approach of targeting tumor vessel formation, and not the malignant cell itself, such as with the monoclonal anti-VEGF antibody bevacizumab in metastatic colorectal cancer (Chapter 203).

Tumors also develop strategies to evade immune surveillance. The T cells and natural killer cells of the immune system play a role in protecting the host against malignancy, just as they also protect against infectious agents. Tumors can grow unimpeded after malignant cells have been selected with properties that disarm the host's immune response to tumors; these mechanisms include down-regulation of costimulatory and major histocompatibility complex molecules, as well as secretion of cytokines that inhibit the immune system, such as transforming growth factor β, interleukin-10, and signal transducer and activator of transcription 3 (STAT3). The development of therapies designed to harness the immune system for cancer treatment, including tumor antigen vaccines, has been hindered by properties that allow tumors to escape immune destruction.

Drug Resistance

Genomic instability sets the stage for the natural selection of cells with acquired genetic alterations that permit dysregulated growth. The same genetic plasticity also allows cancer cells access to the repertoire of the human genome and its capability to express and mutate any of its genes—sometimes resulting in resistance to anticancer therapy.

Cancer cells can specifically alter the target to become resistant. In the case of imatinib mesylate, the targeted therapy for chronic myeloid leukemia (Chapter 195), cells can become resistant by mutating the binding site of the drug to the already mutant BCR/ABL protein. Cancer cellular resistance to older targeted drugs such as methotrexate, which targets the enzyme dihydrofolate reductase, can be mediated by multiple steps in the folate metabolic pathway.

Cancer cells can also reach into their genomes and call upon more general mechanisms of protection from stress. Normal cells can upregulate genes to protect against environmental toxins. In cancer, malignant cells use the same proteins to evade chemotherapy. For example, when exposed to lipid-soluble anticancer drugs that diffuse through the cell membrane, cancer cells respond by increasing the expression of cell membrane proteins that can pump a wide variety of anticancer drugs out of the cell. These ATP-dependent efflux drug pumps, which create resistance to multiple drugs, include MDR1 (for multiple drug resistance) and the MRP (for multidrug resistance–related protein) family of transmembrane proteins. Cancer cells also use other detoxification pathways, such as those involving glutathione, for protection against chemotherapy.

For every anticancer drug developed, a cancer cell has found a way to circumvent it. Also, because cancer cells recruit many different physiologic mechanisms that are also used by different tissues within the host, clinical approaches to overcoming drug resistance have largely been disappointing, as drug resistance reversal strategies also reverse the protective mechanisms in normal tissues and lead to increased toxicity. In this way, the genomic plasticity of cancer cells and the rich human genomic repertoire, the very properties essential for malignant transformation, are also properties that make cancer a difficult therapeutic challenge.

Cancer Stem Cells

Tissues are composed of a vast majority of cells that are irreversibly committed toward terminal differentiation. Hidden within tissues are also a very small minority of primitive, seemingly nondescript cells that are capable of repopulating the tissue with new cells and have the potential for self-renewal, that is, the ability to divide without differentiating. Cells that possess both the ability to produce the different, specialized cells of a tissue and the additional capacity for self-renewal are called stem cells (Chapter 160). For example, a very small population of hematopoietic stem cells in the bone marrow gives rise to more committed erythroid, myeloid, and lymphocytic lineage progenitor cells that ultimately undergo terminal differentiation to produce the formed elements in blood and have the ability to repopulate the marrow, such as in a stem cell transplantation (Chapter 184).

The view of cancer as a homogeneous mass of clonally derived malignant cells has been replaced by a view that cancer cell division is organized more like a tissue in that most of the cells of a tumor do not have the capacity for self-renewal but rather are the progeny of a minute population of cancer stem cells. In hematopoietic malignancies and other tumors, flow cytometric techniques have demonstrated small, unique populations of cancer cells within tumors that have the ability to re-form the tumor, whereas the vast majority of cells in a malignancy do not have this potential.

This concept of cancer, in which tumors contain small numbers of malignant stem cells and a vast majority of malignant but biologically differentiated cells, has enormous consequences for the study and treatment of cancer. Most important, all previous studies that have examined the overall expression of genes in a malignancy may not reveal critical and unique characteristics of the cancer stem cells from which the tumor has arisen. The pattern of treatment response followed by treatment relapse may be due not only to the acquisition of drug resistance but also to a failure of the therapy to treat the distinctive biology of the cancer stem cell. Isolation and characterization of cancer stem cells derived from different malignancies may reveal new cancer stem cell–specific targets that distinguish them from both their malignant progeny and normal stem cells. Specific therapeutics aimed at cancer stem cells hold the potential for markedly improving cancer therapy.

SUGGESTED READINGS

Beyer M, Schultze JL: Regulatory T cells in cancer. Blood 2006;108:804–811. *Review of antitumor immunity.*

Clarke MF, Fuller M: Stem cells and cancer: Two faces of eve. Cell 2006;124:1111–1115. *Reviews regulatory pathways in cancer stem cells.*

Jordan CT, Guzman ML, Noble M: Cancer stem cells. N Engl J Med 2006;355:1253–1261. *An excellent review.*

Thompson JE, Thompson CB: Putting the rap on Akt. J Clin Oncol 2004;22:4217–4226. *Review of molecular mechanisms underlying altered glucose metabolism in cancer.*

Vogelstein B, Kinzler KW: Cancer genes and the pathways they control. Nat Med 2004;10:789–799. *A review of cancer genetics and hereditary cancer predisposition.*

188 ENDOCRINE MANIFESTATIONS OF TUMORS: "ECTOPIC" HORMONE PRODUCTION

Robert F. Gagel

It is now commonly accepted that genetic abnormalities cause disordered cell growth that leads to transformation of the phenotype. A corollary of this fundamental tenet is that changes in a handful of important cellular genes can result in altered expression of other genes and thereby lead to the production of cellular proteins not normally expressed in the differentiated cell type (Chapter 186). Among the more interesting and clinically relevant types of abnormal protein are those associated with "ectopic" hormone syndromes, a small but clinically important group of disorders.

There are several patterns of "ectopic" hormone production. The most common is the production of small polypeptide hormones by tumors derived from a specific class of neuroendocrine cells. These neuroendocrine cells are widely dispersed throughout the lung, gastrointestinal tract, pancreas, thyroid gland, adrenal medulla, breast, prostate, and skin; they share several common cytologic and biochemical characteristics (amine precursor uptake and decarboxylation [APUD]), are often derived from the neural crest, and normally produce both biogenic amines and small polypeptide hormones. The list of hormones produced by tumors derived from members of this group of neuroendocrine cells includes adrenocorticotropic hormone (corticotropin, ACTH), calcitonin, vasoactive intestinal peptide, growth hormone–releasing hormone (GHRH), corticotropin-releasing hormone (CRH), somatostatin, and other small peptides. A second group of tumors, generally derived from squamous epithelium, produce parathyroid hormone–related protein (PTHrP) and vasopressin.

Current evidence suggests that aberrant hormone production is due to reversion to an earlier state of differentiation and an earlier developmental pattern of transcription factor expression. Expression of human achaete-scute homologue (hASH), a helix-loop-helix transcription factor, is necessary for differentiation of pulmonary neuroendocrine cells, the cell type involved in small cell carcinoma of the lung, but it is not expressed in normal differentiated cells. Recent studies have shown that a negative regulator of hASH, hairy enhancer of split-1 (HES-1), is expressed at low levels in small cell carcinoma of the lung and that overexpression of this gene in these cancers and in other neuroendocrine carcinoma cell lines returns the cell to a more differentiated phenotype. These results suggest that a perturbation in a normal differentiation factor is involved not only in development of the transformed phenotype but also in aberrant expression of several small polypeptide hormones.

In a second common hormonal syndrome, hypercalcemia caused by ectopic production of PTHrP, activation of the *ras*–mitogen-activated protein (MAP) kinase signaling pathway, through mutation, appears to be responsible for PTHrP production by squamous epithelium. For example, normal fibroblasts can be stimulated to overexpress PTHrP by combined expression of an activated *ras* gene and a mutated tumor suppressor gene, *p53*. In this example, a combinatorial effect of common genetic changes in human cancer apparently results in abnormal expression of this hypercalcemic peptide.

The clinical syndromes associated with "ectopic" hormone production are important because they are often difficult diagnostic dilemmas, they are a major cause of morbidity and death in cancer patients, and their therapy can be challenging (Table 188–1). Management of these clinical syndromes is often difficult because of the necessity to treat both the cancer and the syndrome caused by excessive hormone production.

HUMORAL HYPERCALCEMIA OF MALIGNANCY

Hypercalcemia (Chapter 266) is one of the most common hormonal syndromes associated with cancer and one of the most difficult to manage. It is the final common manifestation for several different pathophysiologic processes, so each patient must be approached in an organized manner to facilitate correct diagnosis and treatment.

TABLE 188–1 SOME CLINICAL SYNDROMES OF ECTOPIC HORMONE PRODUCTION

- Humoral hypercalcemia
  - Parathyroid hormone–related protein
    - Squamous cell carcinoma
    - Breast cancer
    - Neuroendocrine tumors
    - Renal cell cancer
    - Melanoma
    - Prostate cancer
  - Increased calcitriol
    - Lymphoma
    - Benign conditions: sarcoid, berylliosis, tuberculosis, fungal infections
- Corticotropin
  - Proopiomelanocortin
    - Small cell lung cancer
    - Pulmonary carcinoid
    - Medullary thyroid cancer
    - Islet cell tumor
    - Pheochromocytoma
    - Ganglioneuroma
  - Corticotropin-releasing hormone
    - Medullary thyroid cancer
    - Paraganglioma
    - Prostate cancer
    - Islet cell tumors
- Human chorionic gonadotropin
  - Choriocarcinoma
  - Testicular embryonal cell carcinoma
  - Seminoma
- Hypoglycemia
  - Insulinoma
  - Sarcomas or large retroperitoneal tumors
- Inappropriate antidiuretic hormone secretion
  - Small cell lung cancer
  - Squamous cell head and neck cancer
- Erythropoietin
  - Renal cell cancer
  - Hepatoma
  - Pheochromocytoma
  - Benign conditions: cerebellar hemangioblastoma, uterine fibroids

Pathobiology

Parathyroid Hormone–Related Protein

PTHrP is normally involved in chondrocytic and dermatologic differentiation. Eight of the first 16 amino acids of PTHrP are homologous with parathyroid hormone (PTH), and both peptides exert their various effects through interaction with the osteoblast PTH receptor. Activation of this receptor increases the expression of an osteoblast-specific cell surface protein, RANK ligand (RANKL). Interaction of RANKL with the RANK receptor on undifferentiated osteoclasts causes increased osteoclast differentiation, bone resorption, and hypercalcemia. Ectopic production of PTHrP by a wide variety of tumors is one of the most common causes of hypercalcemia associated with malignancy.

Increased Production of Calcitriol

Increased production of calcitriol occurs in a high percentage of patients with lymphoma (Chapters 196 and 197). There is compelling evidence for increased expression of 1α-hydroxylase by lymphomatous tissue. Other granulomatous conditions such as sarcoid (Chapter 95), berylliosis (Chapter 93), and tuberculous (Chapter 345) or fungal infection may also cause this clinical syndrome.

Bone Metastasis

Bone metastasis (Chapter 212) should always be considered in the differential diagnosis of hypercalcemia in a cancer patient. Bone metastases are frequently associated with local production of cytokines, PTHrP, or other substances that cause increased bone resorption. Indeed, the distinction between humoral hypercalcemia of malignancy and localized osteolysis has become blurred because of evidence that tumors such as breast carcinoma (Chapter 208) or myeloma (Chapter 198) cause localized osteolysis by local production and secretion of PTHrP in addition to RANKL. In breast carcinoma there is considerable evidence supporting a local regulatory loop between transforming growth factor β (TGF-β) and PTHrP production. TGF-β is a normal component of bone matrix. Local PTHrP production by breast carcinoma cells can stimulate osteoclastic bone resorption and release of TGF-β. The release of TGF-β in turn stimulates greater PTHrP production, thereby accelerating the osteolytic process. Other activators of bone resorption, including tumor necrosis factor, lymphotoxin, interleukin-1 (IL-1), and IL-6, can be produced by other tumors that metastasize to (renal cell carcinoma) or reside in (myeloma) bone.

Clinical Manifestations

The clinical syndrome associated with elevated levels of parathyroid hormone–related protein is nearly identical to that observed with hyperparathyroidism and includes increased osteoclast-mediated bone resorption, as well as an increase in renal tubular calcium resorption and a decrease in renal phosphorus resorption. The only significant clinical difference between PTHrP- and PTH-mediated hypercalcemia is the finding of increased serum calcitriol (1,25-dihydroxycholecalciferol) levels in hyperparathyroidism and low or normal values in PTHrP-mediated hypercalcemia, presumably because of the inhibitory effects of cancer on the enzyme that produces calcitriol, 1α-hydroxylase. PTHrP production is most commonly associated with squamous cell carcinoma (Chapter 201), although production has been observed in other types of cancer, including breast (Chapter 208), neuroendocrine (Chapter 205), renal (Chapter 207), skin (Chapter 214), and prostate cancer (Chapter 211).

Other clinical features of patients with increased production of calcitriol include a suppressed intact serum PTH (iPTH) level (Fig. 188–1), an increased or normal serum phosphorus level, hypercalciuria, and no evidence of bone metastasis. An elevated serum calcitriol concentration is found in approximately half of hypercalcemic cancer patients.

Diagnosis

Measurement of iPTH provides a useful starting point for diagnosis (see Fig. 188–1). An elevated PTH level in the context of hypercalcemia should prompt further evaluation for parathyroid disease (Chapter 266). However, in the majority of cancer patients with hypercalcemia, the iPTH value will be suppressed, thus indicating that the malignancy is generating the hypercalcemia. Several different clinical syndromes have been elucidated.

Treatment

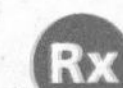

Management of hypercalcemia should focus initially on reversing dehydration and increasing urine calcium excretion by infusion of normal saline solution at rates of 100 to 300 mL/hr, depending on cardiac status. A patient with a serum calcium concentration greater than 13 mg/dL (3.25 mM/L), altered mental status, or renal dysfunction should also be treated with bisphosphonate (intravenous pamidronate, 60 to 90 mg/4 hr, or intravenous zoledronate, 4 mg over a 15-minute period), glucocorticoids (40 to 60 mg/day prednisone or methylprednisolone), gallium nitrate (200 mg/m^2/day, infused for 7 days), or salmon calcitonin (100 to 200 U intravenously or subcutaneously every 6 to 12 hours) alone or in combination. PTHrP-mediated or localized osteolysis is most responsive to bisphosphonates or gallium nitrate; vitamin D–mediated hypercalcemia is most responsive to glucocorticoid therapy (Chapter 266). Use of high-dose intravenous bisphosphonates for extended periods has been associated with osteonecrosis of the jaw, a condition in which the mandibular or maxillary bone becomes devascularized, thereby leading to loss of the overlying mucosa and exposed bone. This condition has developed in approximately 1 to 2% of patients with breast cancer and 2 to 3% with myeloma who received monthly intravenous pamidronate or zoledronate. Replacement of the devascularized and sclerotic bone occurs slowly—some patients have had exposed bone for 3 to 5 years. Because many of the cases have been associated with dental procedures, such as removal of a tooth or tooth implantation, or with poorly fitting dentures, patients starting intravenous bisphosphonate therapy should undergo a dental examination and have any dental issues addressed before initiation of therapy. The benefits of intravenous bisphosphonates in the context of bone metastasis or myeloma are substantial, and their continued use seems appropriate; however, trials are ongoing to address the question of whether less intensive therapy involving the use of bone turnover markers to indicate suppression of bone resorption will provide the beneficial effect of an intravenous bisphosphonate without the toxicity.

Long-term management is focused on treatment of the underlying malignancy. Average survival in a patient with PTHrP-mediated hypercalcemia is less than 3 months, in part related to the underlying malignancy. Long-term therapy for PTHrP-mediated hypercalcemia, like that associated with parathyroid carcinoma, is difficult:

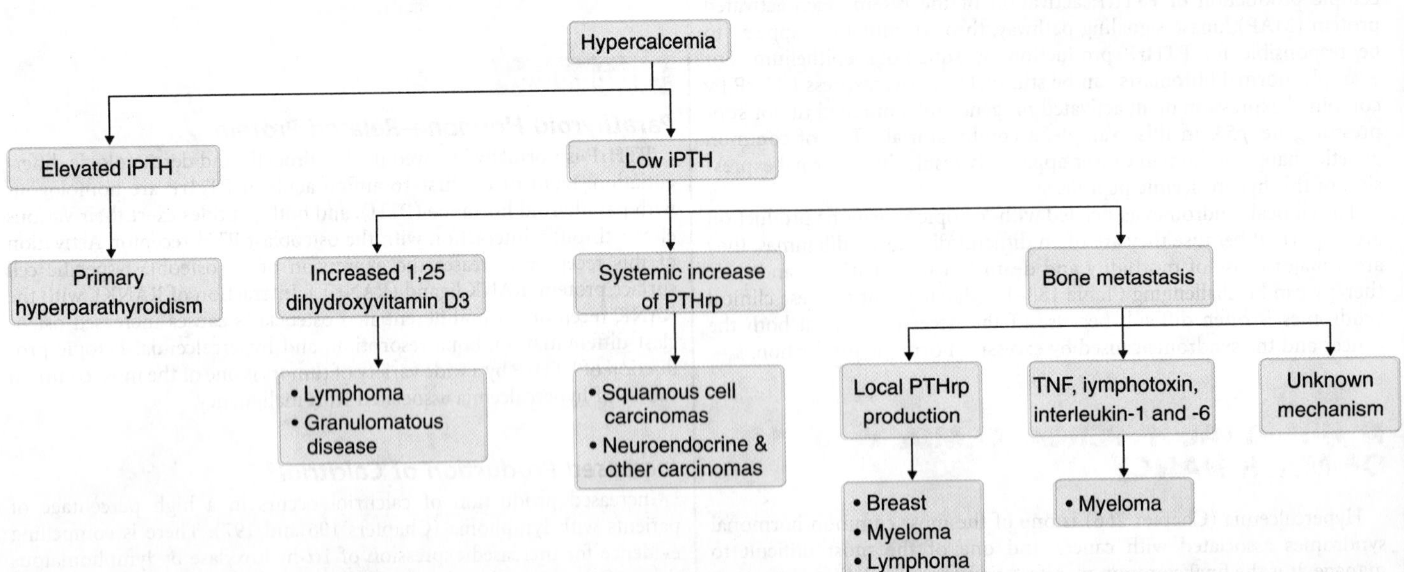

FIGURE 188–1 • Strategy for evaluation of hypercalcemia in the context of malignancy based on measurement of intact parathyroid hormone (iPTH). PTHrp = parathyroid hormone–related protein; TNF = tumor necrosis factor.

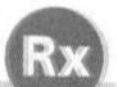

patients tend to become less responsive to the effects of bisphosphonate or salmon calcitonin therapy over time and may experience renal toxicity from gallium nitrate therapy when it is used for extended periods.

Identification of the aforementioned RANKL/RANK receptor system has led to the identification of osteoprotegerin, a soluble receptor produced by osteoblasts that binds to RANKL, thereby preventing activation of the RANK receptor. The effect of osteoprotegerin has been mimicked by the development of a monoclonal antibody that binds RANKL and prevents activation of the RANK receptor. This agent shows promise and is in phase III trials.

ECTOPIC ADRENOCORTICOTROPIC HORMONE SECRETION

Pathobiology

Inappropriate secretion of ACTH is a rare, but important cause of morbidity and mortality in cancer patients. It can be caused by two different mechanisms: expression of the proopiomelanocortin (POMC) gene by a tumor or ectopic expression of CRH. In cell types that express the POMC gene, post-translational processing of this gene product can proceed down one of several mutually exclusive pathways and result in expression of β-lipotropin, γ-lipotropin, and β-endorphin or big melanocyte-stimulating hormone and ACTH. Although POMC expression by malignant tumors is relatively common, the enzymes necessary to cleave ACTH from the precursor are found less frequently outside the pituitary gland. ACTH production occurs in a broad spectrum of tumors, but it is most commonly associated with small cell carcinoma of the lung (Chapter 201) or more classic neuroendocrine tumors such as pulmonary carcinoid (Chapter 251), medullary thyroid carcinoma (Chapter 244), islet cell adenoma or carcinoma (Chapter 249), pheochromocytoma (Chapter 246), and occasional neural tumors such as ganglioneuroma. Ectopic ACTH production causes adrenal cortical hyperplasia and excessive cortisol production (Chapter 245).

Clinical Manifestations

Ectopic production of CRH causes a clinical syndrome characterized by pituitary corticotrope hyperplasia and laboratory results that mimic those of pituitary Cushing's disease (Chapter 245). Diagnosis requires a high index of suspicion, combined with either measurement of CRH in blood or identification of a neoplasm outside the pituitary. Some neoplasms produce both ACTH and CRH. Tumors reported to produce CRH include medullary thyroid carcinoma, paraganglioma, prostate cancer, and islet cell neoplasms.

Hypercorticism associated with ectopic ACTH syndrome may be manifested as classic features of Cushing's syndrome, such as easy bruisability, centripetal obesity, muscle wasting, hypertension, diabetes, and metabolic alkalosis. In other patients, particularly those with rapidly growing small cell carcinoma of the lung, the clinical picture may be dominated by profound hypokalemic metabolic alkalosis and hypertension without the other clinical findings of Cushing's syndrome.

Diagnosis

Evaluation of Cushing's syndrome (Chapter 245) is based on the plasma ACTH measurement in a patient with suggestive clinical and laboratory features (Fig. 188–2). The finding of a marked elevation in the plasma ACTH concentration (>100 pg/mL) should prompt a search for an ectopic source of ACTH. In a patient with a plasma ACTH value greater than 10 pg/mL but less than 100 pg/mL, a more detailed evaluation is appropriate. Differentiation between a pituitary and an ectopic source may require stimulation of ACTH secretion by CRH combined with measurement of ACTH in blood from the pituitary venous drainage (inferior petrosal sinus sampling). Lack of an increase in the inferior petrosal sinus ACTH concentration (more than three times the peripheral ACTH concentration) after peripheral CRH stimulation should prompt a search for an ectopic source. In patients who have an increased (more than three times the peripheral level) inferior petrosal sinus ACTH level after CRH, a pituitary source is likely. Ectopic CRH can yield confusing results and may not be diagnosed unless the clinician considers the possibility and measures plasma CRH or looks for an ectopic source.

Other approaches have also been applied to the diagnosis of ectopic ACTH syndrome. For example, ACTH production from an ectopic source is not generally suppressed by high-dose dexamethasone. In a patient with an ACTH concentration greater than 10 pg/mL, administration of a single 8-mg oral dose of dexamethasone at 11:00 PM, followed by measurement of the serum cortisol level at 8:00 AM, can differentiate between a pituitary and an ectopic source. The serum cortisol level in pituitary Cushing's syndrome will generally be suppressed 50% after dexamethasone, whereas levels in ectopic ACTH are not usually suppressed. However, false-positive or false-negative results occur with each of these testing procedures, thus making the differential diagnosis of Cushing's syndrome among the most challenging in medicine.

Treatment

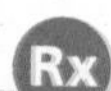

Hypercortisolism associated with ectopic ACTH can be managed by removal of the ACTH- or CRH-producing tumor or by inhibition of cortisol synthesis with metyrapone (1 to 4 g/day orally), aminoglutethimide (250 mg orally four times per day with upward titration), or ketoconazole (200 to 400 mg twice a day orally). Parenteral etomidate, used for sedation and induction of anesthesia, rapidly inhibits cortisol synthesis at subhypnotic concentrations. It is titrated from 0.3 to 4 mg/kg/hr to normalize serum cortisol measurements and has been used to rapidly reverse hypercorticism in a small number of patients. Replacement glucocorticoid therapy is needed to prevent adrenal insufficiency in patients receiving inhibitors of cortisol synthesis. If surgical removal of an ACTH- or CRH-producing tumor is not possible and inhibition of cortisol synthesis is inadequate, bilateral adrenalectomy (with replacement glucocorticoid and mineralocorticoid therapy) may be required. In patients with a rapidly progressive small cell carcinoma of the lung and ectopic ACTH syndrome, the oncologic imperative to initiate immediate cytotoxic therapy must be counterbalanced by the desire to normalize cell-mediated immunity by normalizing cortisol secretion, hypokalemia, and metabolic alkalosis. Cytotoxic chemotherapy should generally be delayed, if possible, until the serum cortisol level is normalized because of the high rate of infection that often causes death in neutropenic patients with hypercortisolism. If oncologic therapy is initiated, prophylactic therapy for pulmonary *Pneumocystis carinii* (Chapter 362) and fungal infections should be considered.

HUMAN CHORIONIC GONADOTROPIN PRODUCTION

Pathobiology

Two different genes encode the α- and β-subunits of human chorionic gonadotropin (HCG). The β-subunit is common to all of the pituitary glycoprotein hormones (luteinizing hormone, follicle-stimulating hormone, thyroid-stimulating hormone [TSH], and HCG), whereas each of these hormones has a unique β-subunit gene. Inappropriate production of the α-subunit occurs in a variety of pituitary and nonpituitary tumors and does not cause any discernible clinical syndrome. The β-subunit confers biologic specificity. Production of intact HCG occurs commonly in trophoblastic tumors (choriocarcinoma, testicular embryonal carcinoma, and seminoma; Chapter 210) and less commonly in other tumors such as those of the lung and pancreas.

Clinical Manifestations and Diagnosis

Clinical syndromes associated with production of HCG include precocious puberty, gynecomastia, and hyperthyroidism. Hyperthyroidism results from the low-affinity interaction of HCG with the TSH receptor

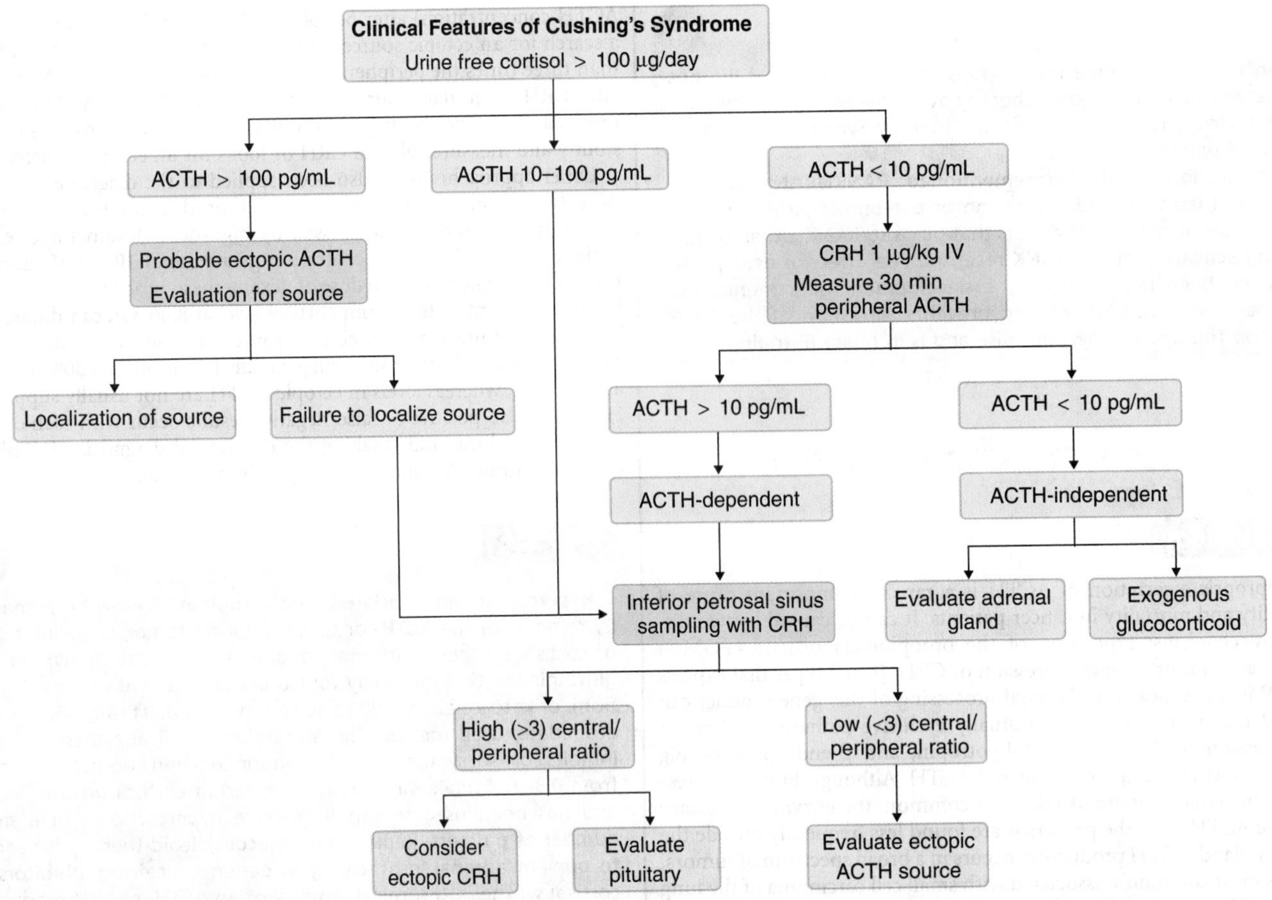

Clinical Features of Cushing's Syndrome
Urine free cortisol > 100 μg/day

ACTH > 100 pg/mL → Probable ectopic ACTH / Evaluation for source → Localization of source; Failure to localize source → Inferior petrosal sinus sampling with CRH

ACTH 10–100 pg/mL → Inferior petrosal sinus sampling with CRH

ACTH < 10 pg/mL → CRH 1 μg/kg IV / Measure 30 min peripheral ACTH → ACTH > 10 pg/mL → ACTH-dependent → Inferior petrosal sinus sampling with CRH; ACTH < 10 pg/mL → ACTH-independent → Evaluate adrenal gland; Exogenous glucocorticoid

Inferior petrosal sinus sampling with CRH → High (>3) central/peripheral ratio → Consider ectopic CRH; Evaluate pituitary

Inferior petrosal sinus sampling with CRH → Low (<3) central/peripheral ratio → Evaluate ectopic ACTH source

FIGURE 188–2 • Evaluation strategy for a patient with Cushing's syndrome and suspected ectopic adrenocorticotropic hormone (ACTH) production. In patients with a plasma ACTH concentration greater than 100 pg/mL, an ectopic ACTH source should be considered, although some patients with pituitary Cushing's disease may have values in this range. In patients with a plasma ACTH concentration between 10 and 100 pg/mL, inferior petrosal sinus sampling (IPSS) for ACTH should be performed after peripheral corticotropin-releasing hormone (CRH) injection (Chapter 245) to separate a pituitary (high central-peripheral ACTH ratio) from an ectopic ACTH (low central-peripheral ACTH ratio) source. In patients with a low basal peripheral ACTH value (<10 pg/mL), a low-dose CRH test (1 μg/kg) should be performed, followed by IPPS in individuals whose plasma ACTH concentration rises to greater than 10 pg/mL.

when β-HCG is present in high concentrations. β-HCG concentrations that are several orders of magnitude higher than normal interact with the TSH receptor and increase the production of thyroid hormone, thereby suppressing endogenous TSH production below normal.

Treatment

Therapy for precocious puberty and gynecomastia is directed toward removal or treatment of the underlying tumor. Hyperthyroidism is treated by inhibition of thyroid hormone synthesis, usually with thionamide therapy, followed by therapy for the underlying tumor. Treatment of hyperthyroidism by surgical removal of the thyroid gland or ablation with radioactive iodine is rarely required because the hyperthyroidism resolves rapidly after treatment of the underlying tumor.

HYPOGLYCEMIA ASSOCIATED WITH CANCER

Pathobiology

Tumor-associated hypoglycemia is a rare, but important cause of morbidity in cancer patients. Three different clinical syndromes cause most cancer-related hypoglycemia. The first is production of insulin by an islet tumor. Although primary insulinomas are rare, dedifferentiation and bulky hepatic metastasis of an islet cell carcinoma may be associated with excessive insulin production (Chapter 249). A second cause of hypoglycemia, insufficient gluconeogenesis to maintain the plasma glucose concentration in the fasting state, is caused by nearly complete replacement of the liver by metastatic tumor. A third cause of hypoglycemia is increased concentrations of insulin-like growth factor type II (IGF-II), a ligand that activates the insulin receptor in large abdominal tumors, most commonly fibrosarcoma, hemangiopericytoma, or hepatoma. This increase appears to be due to the failure to form normal IGF binding protein 3 (IGFBP-3) and the acid-labile subunit (ALS) complex that normally binds IGF-II; the result is an increase in free IGF-II concentrations. It is usually possible to differentiate among these causes by measurement of serum insulin, C-peptide, proinsulin, IGF-I, IGF-II, and ALS levels during a controlled fast that causes hypoglycemia (Chapter 249).

Clinical Manifestations, Diagnosis, and Treatment

In all three types of hypoglycemia, the patient is at greatest risk for symptoms during periods of fasting, most commonly during sleeping hours. Therapy should focus on surgical excision, when possible, or antineoplastic therapy directed at the tumor. Initial therapy for hypoglycemia is focused on frequent meals, and patients may occasionally be maintained symptom free if awakened for one or more snacks during sleeping hours. If the tumor progresses or the patient's caloric intake is inadequate, additional measures may be required. In patients in whom hepatic replacement by tumor is evident, a continuous infusion of 20% dextrose through a central line may be required, especially during sleeping hours. In patients with insulin-producing or large retroperitoneal tumors, glucagon infusion (0.5 to 2 mg/hr) stimulates hepatic gluconeogenesis and prevents hypoglycemia, although in rare patients a rash associated with glucagonoma may develop. An increase in glucose concentration after a single injection of glucagon (1 mg) should be documented before initiating therapy. In patients with large retroperitoneal tumors, treatment with growth hormone (3 to 6 μg/kg subcuta-

Rx

neously) or glucocorticoids (20 to 40 mg/day) may reverse the hypoglycemia, possibly by facilitating IGFBP-3/ALS complex formation, thereby reducing free serum IGF-II levels. Growth hormone doses as high as 2600 μg/day have been administered in this condition, although long-term treatment with this dose may cause acromegalic side effects. Somatostatin analogues (octreotide or lanreotide) are not generally effective for normalizing the plasma glucose level in patients with islet cell tumors; diazoxide (3 to 8 mg/kg/day in two or three divided doses) may be effective, but problems with fluid retention frequently preclude its long-term use.

SYNDROME OF INAPPROPRIATE ANTIDIURETIC HORMONE SECRETION

Pathobiology

Ectopic production of vasopressin by head and neck tumors (3%), small cell carcinoma of the lung (15%), and other lung carcinomas (1%) causes a clinical syndrome characterized by hyponatremia, hypo-osmolality, excessive urine sodium excretion, an inappropriately high urine osmolality for the low serum osmolality, and normal function of the kidneys, adrenal glands, and thyroid (Chapter 243). Other malignant neoplasms (primary brain tumors; hematologic neoplasms; skin tumors; gastrointestinal, gynecologic, breast, and prostate cancers; and sarcomas) are rare causes of this clinical syndrome.

Clinical Manifestations and Diagnosis

In most cases the hyponatremia is asymptomatic, although altered mental status and seizures may develop when the serum sodium concentration falls below 120 mEq/L. Hyponatremic women of reproductive age may experience profound cerebral degeneration.

Treatment

Rx

Fluid restriction may be effective for short-term management but is difficult to maintain over long periods. Hypertonic fluids can be given with great caution to symptomatic patients (Chapter 117); the serum sodium concentration should be monitored to prevent more than a 12-mEq/day increase. Treatment with 150 to 300 mg/day demeclocycline can block the effects of vasopressin on the kidney and is an effective long-term therapy in patients with cancer. Oral tolvaptan [1] and intravenous conivaptan [2] are vasopressin receptor antagonists that are effective treatments for hyponatremia and are approved in an intravenous form as an effective inpatient treatment of trials, and other members of this class are being developed.

RARE ECTOPIC HORMONE SYNDROMES

Oncogenic Osteomalacia

A clinical syndrome characterized by profound hypophosphatemia, muscle weakness, and osteomalacia (Chapter 265) can be produced by mesenchymal tumors (osteoblastoma, giant cell osteosarcoma, hemangiocytoma, and rarely, prostate and lung carcinoma). Recent studies have shown that fibroblast growth factor 23 (FGF-23), mutated in autosomal dominant hypophosphatemic rickets (Chapter 265), is overexpressed in neoplasms causing this disorder. Therapy is directed toward correction of hypophosphatemia with either oral or intravenous supplementation and vitamin D treatment. Surgical removal of the tumor is curative. Identification of FGF-23 overexpression as a cause may lead to the development of specific antagonists.

Hematologic Syndromes

The kidney is the primary site of erythropoietin production, and therefore the relatively common erythropoietin production by benign or malignant renal tumors is not an "ectopic" hormone syndrome. Production of erythropoietin by cerebellar hemangioblastoma (Chapter 199), uterine fibroids (Chapter 256), pheochromocytomas (Chapter 246), and ovarian (Chapter 209) and hepatic tumors (Chapter 206) is generally considered "ectopic." Patients with excessive erythropoietin production may or may not have polycythemia (Chapter 172). Other ectopic syndromes, less well defined, include production of thrombopoietin, leukopoietin, or colony-stimulating factor by some tumors. These conditions are treated by removal of the tumor or by appropriate chemotherapy.

Hypertension

Renal (Wilms' tumor, renal cell carcinoma, or hemangiopericytoma), lung (small cell carcinoma of the lung, adenocarcinoma), hepatic, pancreatic, and ovarian carcinomas may produce renin. The clinical findings in these patients can include hypertension, hypokalemia, and evidence of increased aldosterone production. Therapy with aldosterone antagonists or angiotensin-converting enzyme inhibitors may be effective.

Growth Hormone and Prolactin Production

Rare examples of growth hormone production have been identified in lung and gastric adenocarcinoma. Ectopic production of GHRH has been documented for islet cell tumors (Chapter 249), bronchogenic carcinoids (Chapter 251), and small cell carcinoma of the lung (Chapter 201). Increased prolactin production is a rare phenomenon associated with lymphomas and cancer of the lung, colon, kidney, and oral cavity. Hyperprolactinemia produces galactorrhea and amenorrhea in women and hypogonadism and gynecomastia in men. Treatment with dopamine agonists (bromocriptine, quinagolide, or cabergoline), effective in pituitary prolactinoma (Chapter 242), should be tried but is most commonly ineffective.

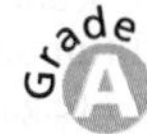

1. Schrier RW, Gross P, Gheorghiade M, et al: Tolvaptan, a selective oral vasopressin V2-receptor antagonist, for hyponatremia. N Engl J Med 2006;355:2099–2112.
2. Ghali JK, Koren MJ, Taylor JR, et al: Efficacy and safety of oral conivaptan: A V1A/V2 vasopressin receptor antagonist, assessed in a randomized, placebo-controlled trial in patients with euvolemic or hypervolemic hyponatremia. J Clin Endocrinol Metab 2006; 91:2145–2152.

SUGGESTED READINGS

Body JJ: Bisphosphonates for malignancy-related bone disease: Current status, future developments. Support Care Cancer 2006;14:408–418. *Review of the use of bisphosphonates in reducing skeletal complications in patients with bone metastases.*

Stewart AF: Hypercalcemia associated with cancer. N Engl J Med 2005; 352:373–379. *An overview of causes and treatment of hypercalcemia associated with malignancy.*

Vu L, Theodore PR: Localization of a corticotropin-secreting tumor by thoracoscopic pulmonary venous sampling. N Engl J Med 2005;353:851–852. *Case report describing novel approach to localizing ACTH-secreting tumor.*

189 PARANEOPLASTIC SYNDROMES AND OTHER NON-NEOPLASTIC EFFECTS OF CANCER

Hope S. Rugo

Definition

The direct clinical manifestations of cancer are usually due to local effects of tumor growth, either in the primary site or at a distant site, or are nonspecific such as anorexia, malaise, weight loss, night sweats, and fever. The term *paraneoplasia*, which means "alongside cancer," has been commonly used to denote remote effects that cannot be attributed either to direct invasion or to distant metastases.

Epidemiology

These syndromes may be the first sign of a malignancy and may affect up to 15% of patients with cancer. However, if patients with cachexia are excluded, the incidence probably drops to only a few percent.

Paraneoplastic syndromes are important clinically for a number of reasons. First, they may be the initial presenting sign or symptom of an underlying malignancy. Up to two thirds of paraneoplastic syndromes arise before an associated malignancy is diagnosed. In some cases, the paraneoplastic syndrome may be associated with relatively small tumors; recognition of these associations may lead to earlier diagnosis and better therapy. Second, one of the hallmarks in defining a paraneoplastic syndrome is that the course of the syndrome generally parallels the course of the tumor. Therefore, effective treatment of the underlying malignancy is often accompanied by improvement or resolution of the syndrome. Conversely, recurrence of the cancer may be heralded by return of systemic symptoms. One exception is the neurologic paraneoplastic syndromes, in which damage to structures within the nervous system may not be reversible. Third, the clinical manifestations of the paraneoplastic syndrome (or the toxic effects of electrolyte disturbances) may constitute a more urgent hazard to life or have a greater impact on quality of life than the underlying cancer.

Pathobiology

Paraneoplastic syndromes may be caused by a variety of mechanisms; the endocrine (Chapter 188) and neurologic syndromes are the best understood. Possible etiologies include (1) secretion of proteins that are not associated with the normal tissue equivalent of the cancer (e.g., ectopic endocrine syndromes, local destruction of tissues by tumor-secreted cytokines), (2) antibodies that are directed against aberrantly expressed antigens on the tumor cell that cross-react with antigens that are normally expressed on other tissues (e.g., neurologic syndromes), and (3) effects related to unknown mechanisms, such as unidentified tumor products or circulating immune complexes stimulated by the tumor (e.g., osteoarthropathy associated with bronchogenic carcinoma; Chapter 201). Clinical findings may resemble those of primary metabolic, hematologic, dermatologic, or neuromuscular disorders or be specific to a cancer-related syndrome. Even such nonspecific symptoms as fever and weight loss are truly paraneoplastic and are due to the production of specific factors (e.g., tumor necrosis factor) by tumor cells or by normal cells in response to the tumor (see later).

Diagnosis

In a patient who presents with symptoms or signs of a paraneoplastic syndrome, the screening evaluation (Table 189–1) should focus on the most common associated malignancies. If the initial evaluation is unrevealing, a repeated evaluation should be considered after several months. If the relationship between the syndrome and malignancy is less clear or less frequently observed, the evaluation should be focused on the patient's individual risks and symptoms.

The most common cancer associated with paraneoplastic syndromes is small cell cancer of the lung (Chapter 201), probably because of its neuroectodermal origin. Other neoplasms commonly associated with paraneoplastic syndrome include carcinomas of the breast (Chapter 208), ovary (Chapter 209), other adenocarcinomas, lymphoproliferative diseases (especially Hodgkin's disease; Chapter 197), and thymoma (Chapter 448).

TABLE 189–1 EVALUATION AND DIAGNOSIS OF PARANEOPLASTIC SYNDROMES

Characterize abnormality; obtain laboratory studies and biopsy as necessary.
Carefully elicit any additional symptoms and signs.
Eliminate common causes.
If there is no obvious etiology, consider a paraneoplastic syndrome.
If findings are consistent with a known syndrome, screen for underlying malignancy.
If signs and symptoms are consistent with a known paraneoplastic syndrome, undertake a search for an unknown primary cancer or recurrence or progression of a known primary tumor.
Screening should include a careful physical examination including breast, gynecologic, and prostate evaluations; basic hematology, chemistry, and urine studies; chest radiograph; and mammogram. Computed tomography of the abdomen and pelvis is indicated if there are any suspicious symptoms, signs, or laboratory abnormalities. Antibody testing for paraneoplastic neurologic syndromes and/or skin biopsy should be performed as indicated.
Consider treatment of cancer and/or appropriate palliative treatment including immunosuppressive therapy for paraneoplastic symptoms when possible.

NEUROLOGIC PARANEOPLASTIC SYNDROMES

Pathobiology

Research over the past four decades has helped to elucidate the underlying mechanisms of neurologic syndromes associated with cancer; increasing evidence suggests that most effects are autoimmune in origin (Table 189–2). Tumors express antigens that are normally isolated to the nervous system and are found on neurons, referred to as "onconeuronal antigens." Antineuronal antibodies that are produced against the new tumor cell antigen circulate in serum and spinal fluid and, at least in some patients, cause damage at the primary site of normal antigen expression. Pathologically, perivascular and interstitial lymphocytic infiltrates are found in the affected area of the brain. Indirect immunofluorescence of serum detects antibodies reactive with neurons.

It is unclear what susceptibility factors lead to development of a neurologic paraneoplastic syndrome. In addition to direct antibody-mediated damage, there is evidence that cell-mediated autoimmune mechanisms may contribute. The finding of $CD8^+$ T lymphocytes infiltrating neurologic tissue in postmortem studies of patients with neurologic paraneoplastic syndromes, combined with data that patients with antibodies (with or without neurologic paraneoplastic syndromes) may have longer survival rates than otherwise similar patients without circulating antibodies, suggests that $CD8^+$ T lymphocytes play a beneficial role in tumor-directed immune responses. This immune response may be mediated by aberrant expression of native antigens.

Clinical Manifestations

Neurologic paraneoplastic syndromes may involve the brain, cranial nerves, spinal cord, dorsal root ganglia, peripheral nerves, neuromuscular junction, muscle, or multiple levels of the nervous system. Perhaps because of cross-reactivity of antibodies, it is not uncommon for patients to develop more than one paraneoplastic syndrome, making the diagnosis of a particular syndrome more difficult. Therapy includes treatment of the underlying tumor as well as immunosuppressive therapy with or without plasmapheresis, although this approach usually results in only modest, if any, improvement of the neurologic deficit.

The differential diagnosis of neurologic paraneoplastic syndromes includes idiopathic presentations of the same syndrome, side effects of chemotherapy (Chapter 192) and radiation therapy (Chapter 18; Table 189–3), infections (usually associated with lymphoproliferative diseases), vascular disease (including infarction and hemorrhage), and metabolic and nutritional abnormalities (including hormonal paraneoplastic syndromes).

Diagnosis

A patient presenting with neurologic complaints regardless of a prior diagnosis of malignancy should undergo a standard evaluation for diseases such as a primary central nervous system (CNS) malignancy, a metastatic malignancy, bleeding, vascular events, and infection. Generally, this evaluation includes a careful history regarding onset, associated

TABLE 189–2 SOME PARANEOPLASTIC NEUROLOGIC SYNDROMES, ASSOCIATED ANTIBODIES, AND MALIGNANCIES

Neurologic Syndrome	Clinical Presentation	Antibody	Associated Malignancy
Lambert-Eaton myasthenic syndrome	See text	Anti-VGCC	SCLC (>80%)
Paraneoplastic encephalomyelitis/ subacute sensory neuropathy	See text	Anti-Hu Anti-amphiphysin Anti-Ma Anti-Trk (sensory)	SCLC (75–80%), neuroblastoma SCLC, breast Various carcinomas Lymphoma
Paraneoplastic cerebellar degeneration	See text	Anti-Yo Anti-Ri Anti-Hu Anti-Tr, Anti-GluR Anti-Ma	Breast, ovarian, and other gynecologic malignancies Breast (50%) SCLC Hodgkin's lymphoma Various carcinomas
Limbic encephalopathy	Subacute amnestic syndrome, affective disorder, seizures. DDX: Herpes encephalitis. Improvement common with treatment of underlying tumor; immunosuppression is of unclear benefit	Anti-Hu, antiamphiphysin, others Anti-Ta	SCLC Testicular, breast
Opsoclonus/myoclonus	Saccadic eye movements with ataxia and myoclonus. Majority occur in children with neuroblastomas. Pathology reveals diffuse dropout of Purkinje cells. Treatment of underlying tumor may improve symptoms; ACTH, steroids, and IVIG may also benefit	Anti-Ri Anti-Hu Antiamphiphysin Anti-Ta	Breast (70%), ovarian SCLC, neuroblastoma (50%) SCLC Testicular
Stiff-person syndrome	Progressive muscle stiffness and rigidity, with intermittent and painful muscle spasms. EMG: continuous firing of motor unit potentials. Treat with muscle relaxants; may improve with cancer therapy	Antiamphiphysin Anti-GAD	Breast, SCLC Breast
Neuromyotonia	Diffuse muscle stiffness and cramps; may be associated with myasthenia gravis. Responds to treatment of tumor and immunosuppression	Anti-VGCC	Thymoma
VISUAL SYNDROMES			
CAR	Gradual to acute and progressive visual loss	Antiretinal, antirecoverin	SCLC
MAR	Reports of response to immunosuppressive therapy, and plasmapheresis	Antibipolar cell	Melanoma
Bilateral diffuse melanocytic proliferation		?	Gynecologic malignancy
SYNDROMES WITH NO ASSOCIATED ANTIBODY IDENTIFIED			
Demyelinating neuropathies (including CDP, mononeuritis multiplex)	Sensory more common than motor or both. May improve with treatment of paraprotein, plasmapheresis	IgM paraprotein may cross-react with MAG, cryoglobulins	Plasma cell and lymphoproliferative neoplasms, osteosclerotic myeloma, POEMS, amyloid, SCLC, other carcinomas
Necrotizing myelopathy	Symptoms associated with specific levels of spinal cord dysfunction. Rapid deterioration and death		Variety of carcinomas and lymphomas
Motor neuron disease	Similar to ALS with progressive weakness; may improve with plasmapheresis and treatment of paraproteinemia		Plasma cell and lymphoproliferative neoplasms
Polymyositis/dermatomyositis	Unclear relationship to cancer, higher risk with dermatomyositis. May improve with treatment of cancer, otherwise treat as idiopathic		Variety of carcinomas

ACTH = adrenocorticotropic hormone; ALS = amyotrophic lateral sclerosis; amphiphysin = synaptic vesicle–associated protein; CAR = carcinoma-associated retinopathy; CDP = chronic demyelinating polyneuropathy; DDX = differential diagnosis; EMG = electromyogram; GAD = glutamic acid decarboxylase; IgM = immunoglobulin M; IVIG = intravenous immunoglobulin; MAG = myelin-associated glycoprotein; MAR = melanoma-associated retinopathy; POEMS = polyneuropathy, organomegaly, endocrinopathy, monoclonal protein, and skin changes associated with osteosclerotic myeloma; SCLC = small cell lung cancer; VGCC = voltage-gated calcium channel.

TABLE 189–3 NEUROLOGIC COMPLICATIONS OF THERAPEUTIC RADIATION

Latency Period (Time following Radiation)	Site of Injury	Clinical Findings
Immediate	Brain	Acute encephalopathy (self-limited)
Early (1–4 mo)	Brain	Somnolence syndrome (steroid responsive) Focal neurologic signs
	Spinal cord	Lhermitte's sign (shocklike sensation down the spine when bending the neck so that the chin meets the chest)
Delayed (months to years)	Brain	Cognitive dysfunction Focal neurologic signs
	Spinal cord	Transverse myelopathy
	Peripheral nerves	Peripheral neuropathy, decreased Function
Secondary effects at other organ sites (years)	CNS including nerve sheaths	Secondary malignancy
	Arteries	Premature atherosclerosis Telangiectasias (increased risk for hemorrhage)
	Thyroid or parathyroid	Hypothyroid or hypoparathyroid (hyperthyroidism or hyperparathyroidism may be an early symptom)

CNS = central nervous system.

symptoms, and other general medical conditions, as well as a careful physical and neurologic examination. Studies should include an initial contrast-enhanced magnetic resonance imaging (MRI) scan and examination of the cerebrospinal fluid (CSF) for protein and cells if the MRI is normal or showed leptomeningeal enhancement. If the evaluation does not reveal evidence of primary CNS disease, a body positron emission tomography or computed tomography scan along with standard laboratory testing may be useful to screen for undetected malignancies.

In addition, serum testing for antibodies associated with specific neurologic syndromes (see later) should be performed. However, a high degree of specificity of an antibody for a particular syndrome does not prove that the antibody is pathogenic. Finding a circulating antibody is useful but not diagnostic of any particular syndrome; patients can have circulating antibodies without the associated clinical syndrome, and the majority of lung cancers as well as many breast and gynecologic malignancies express neuronal antigens. Diagnosis of a neurologic paraneoplastic syndrome should instigate a reasonable search for the commonly associated malignancy (see Table 189–1).

Lambert-Eaton Myasthenic Syndrome—Anti-VGCC Antibodies

Definition and Epidemiology

The Lambert-Eaton myasthenic syndrome is one of the first recognized and most common neurologic paraneoplastic syndromes, and it is one of the only syndromes with direct evidence to support the role of autoantibodies in producing clinical disease. This disorder affects 1 to 2% of patients with small cell cancer of the lung, and two thirds of the cases are associated with an underlying malignancy.

Pathobiology

Lambert-Eaton myasthenic syndrome is associated with a defect in the release of neurotransmitters (acetylcholine) from the presynaptic neurons at the neuromuscular junction and other sites. Acetylcholine release is mediated by P-type voltage-gated calcium channels (VGCCs); antibodies to VGCC are found in the serum of more than 85% of patients with Lambert-Eaton myasthenic syndrome.

Clinical Manifestations and Diagnosis

Clinically, patients present with proximal lower limb weakness, with improvement in strength after several seconds of sustained voluntary contraction (Chapter 448). Autonomic symptoms, including dry mouth, ptosis, and impotence, are also common. Patients may also have associated CNS dysfunction, such as encephalomyelitis, cerebellar dysfunction, and peripheral neuropathy resulting from cross-reactivity or the presence of combinations of antibodies. The diagnosis is made by an electromyogram, which shows *increased* muscle action potential with repeated nerve stimulation greater than 10 Hz (the opposite of myasthenia gravis; Chapter 448).

Treatment

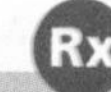

Treatment consists of a combination of plasmapheresis, intravenous immunoglobulin (IVIG) to bind circulating antibodies, and immunosuppression (to remove antibodies and suppress their production), as well as treatment of the underlying malignancy (Chapter 192). Pharmacologic facilitation of neuromuscular transmission with pyridostigmine, 3,4-diaminopyridine, and guanidine may be useful.

Paraneoplastic Encephalomyelitis/ Subacute Sensory Neuropathy— Anti-Hu Antibodies

This heterogeneous group of disorders can affect the cerebral hemispheres, limbic system, cerebellum, brain stem, spinal cord, dorsal root, and autonomic ganglia.

Pathobiology

About 75 to 80% of paraneoplastic encephalomyelitis/subacute sensory neuropathy (Chapter 446) is associated with small cell lung cancer (Chapter 201), with a variety of other neoplasms representing the remainder. The majority of patients have circulating antineuronal anti-Hu autoantibodies; a small number have either no antibodies or antibodies to other proteins. One report found evidence of impairment of the Trk-neurotrophin receptor by the serum of a patient with subacute sensory neuropathy, suggesting production of anti-Trk autoantibodies. Although neuronal loss is accompanied by perivascular and leptomeningeal infiltration of lymphocytes, the pathogenesis of this syndrome is unknown.

Clinical Manifestations

The most common manifestations are related to subacute sensory neuropathy, with patchy or asymmetric numbness, burning or aching paresthesias, and sensory ataxia with loss of proprioception and vibration sense. Patients may also present primarily with subacute cerebellar degeneration or brain stem encephalitis, and nearly all patients have evidence of multifocal involvement of the CNS and dorsal root ganglia.

Diagnosis

The diagnosis is made on clinical grounds and is aided by finding circulating antibody in serum. MRI scans are usually normal, and the CSF can show elevated protein levels with a lymphocytosis. The usual course is deterioration over weeks to months, with stabilization at a level of severe neurologic disability.

Treatment

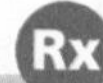

Treatment has been largely unsuccessful, but a small number of patients have improved with immunosuppressive therapy including prednisone and IVIG.

Paraneoplastic Cerebellar Degeneration—Anti-Yo Antibodies

Paraneoplastic cerebellar degeneration is usually the initial manifestation of cancer. About 90% of patients have breast cancer, ovarian or other gynecologic tumors, small cell lung cancer, or Hodgkin's disease.

Pathobiology

Patients with paraneoplastic cerebellar degeneration and carcinomas of the breast or ovary or other gynecologic cancers have been found to have high titers of an anti–Purkinje cell antibody, anti-Yo, in the serum and CSF, but other antibodies that react against Purkinje cell antigens can also be found (see Table 189–2). Autopsy reveals nearly complete loss of cerebellar Purkinje cells, with occasional inflammatory infiltrates.

Clinical Manifestations and Diagnosis

Symptoms are often abrupt in onset and include dysarthria, ataxia, and oculomotor dysfunction. Syndromes such as paraneoplastic encephalomyelitis or Lambert-Eaton myasthenic syndrome may be superimposed. The diagnosis is based on clinical signs and may be aided by the presence of circulating antibody; however, anti-Yo antibodies are also found in patients who have a variety of cerebellar disorders but no evidence of cancer even on follow-up. CSF may reveal a pleocytosis and an elevated protein level or may be normal. MRI scans may show diffuse cerebellar atrophy, but they are often normal.

Treatment

Treatment of the underlying malignancy occasionally results in significant improvement of cerebellar function. Rarely, responses have been seen to immunosuppressive therapy.

Neurologic Complications of Therapeutic Radiation

Although improvements in technique have significantly reduced the neurologic complications of radiation therapy, profound side effects can still occur and may be seen more frequently as patients with advanced cancers enjoy longer survival owing to improved systemic treatment (Table 189–3). Complications may be acute or delayed, and delayed reactions can be seen within 1 to 4 months or up to months to years after completion of treatment. The risk of any reaction is related to the total dose, the extent of the radiation field, the dose of radiation per fraction, and the length of time over which the radiation was given. Lowering the dose per fraction and extending the duration of treatment decrease both short- and long-term risks, but variations in susceptibility among individuals are not well understood. Treatment is generally supportive, except for the somnolence syndrome, which may respond to corticosteroids. Rarely, radiation-induced tumors, including meningiomas or gliomas, may occur many years after successful cranial irradiation.

DERMATOLOGIC PARANEOPLASTIC SYNDROMES

Clinical Manifestations and Diagnosis

Recognition of cutaneous manifestations of malignancy can be critical for the early diagnosis and successful treatment of malignancy, but some abnormalities are seen only with advanced, incurable disease. Cutaneous manifestations include direct involvement of the skin with tumor as well as the remote effects of cancer.

Benign skin changes may be the only sign of genetic syndromes that predispose to an increased risk for malignancy over a lifetime (Table 189–4). Recognition of these syndromes is critical for screening, early diagnosis, and genetic counseling of affected family members.

Associations between cutaneous syndromes and underlying malignancies may be difficult to confirm. Generally, and unlike the situation in neurologic paraneoplastic syndromes, the skin condition and cancer should follow a parallel course, and the two diagnoses should be made at about the same time (Table 189–5). Some skin lesions are almost always associated with malignancy. Others, however, are nonspecific and are

TABLE 189–4 GENETIC SYNDROMES WITH CUTANEOUS MANIFESTATIONS ASSOCIATED WITH AN INCREASED RISK OF SYSTEMIC CANCERS

Genetic Syndrome	Skin Lesion	Associated Cancers	Risk
Torre's	Multiple sebaceous gland tumors, basal cell cancers	GI and GU cancers	High
Gardner's	Multiple epidermal/sebaceous cysts of face and scalp, desmoid tumors of skin, osteomas of face and head, GI polyps	GI cancers	High
Cowden's	Multiple hamartomas of skin, mucous membranes (trichilemmomas), lipomas	Breast, thyroid cancers	High
MEN 2B	Multiple papular mucosal neuromas on lips, oropharynx, conjunctiva	Medullary carcinoma of thyroid, pheochromocytoma	High
Ataxia-telangiectasia	Telangiectasias over face, conjunctiva	Lymphomas	Medium
Neurofibromatosis	Café au lait spots, axillary freckles, neurofibromas	Neurofibrosarcoma, pheochromocytoma, acoustic neuromas	Low
Peutz-Jeghers	Pigmented macules on the lips, oral mucosa, hands, feet; hamartomatous GI polyps	GI, pancreas, ovary, testes	Low
Basal cell carcinoma nevus	Multiple basal cell cancers	Medulloblastoma, fibrosarcoma	Low
Bloom's	Telangiectatic redness of skin in photoexposed areas, stunted growth	Lymphomas, leukemias	Medium

GI = gastrointestinal; GU = genitourinary; MEN = multiple endocrine neoplasia.

TABLE 189–5 EXAMPLES OF CUTANEOUS AND RHEUMATOLOGIC LESIONS ASSOCIATED WITH MALIGNANT DISEASE

Syndrome	Clinical Presentation	Associated Malignancy	Association/Risk
CUTANEOUS			
Acanthosis nigricans	Velvety, verrucous, brown hyperpigmentation involving body folds and mucosal membranes	Gastric cancer (also endocrinopathies)	High
Acquired hypertrichosis lanuginosa (malignant down)	Long, fine, nonpigmented lanugo hairs on face, trunk, limbs, axillae	Carcinomas of the lung, colon, breast, uterus, bladder, and lymphoma (also seen with AIDS, anorexia, thyrotoxicosis, porphyria, medications)	Moderate to high
Acquired tylosis	Hyperkeratosis of palms	Lung cancer	Likely low
Bazex's syndrome	Acral hyperkeratotic papulosquamous lesions, onychodystrophy	Squamous cell carcinomas of the oropharynx, larynx, bronchi, esophagus	High
Extramammary Paget's	Nonhealing superficial dermatitis	Genitourinary and rectal cancers	Moderate to high
Sign of Leser-Trélat	Diffuse eruption of seborrheic keratoses	Gastrointestinal cancers (also seen with aging)	Likely moderate
Tripe palms	Thickened, velvety palms	Lung and gastric cancers (almost always seen with acanthosis nigricans)	High
Necrolytic migratory erythema	Circinate erosive erythematous rash, stomatitis	Glucagonoma	Likely moderate
Erythema gyratum repens	Concentric rings on trunk and proximal extremities; may have pruritus	Carcinomas of the lung, esophagus, and breast	High
Erythroderma	Diffuse erythema	Lymphoma	Low to moderate
Paraneoplastic pemphigus (PNP)	Painful erythematous lesions with blistering; mucous membrane ulcerations	Lymphoma	High
Sweet's syndrome	Red nodules or plaques, fever, dermal neutrophilic infiltrates	Acute myelogenous leukemia (also seen with infection)	Moderate
Pruritus	Excoriations, pruritus occurs on extremities, upper trunk, extensor surfaces	Lymphoma and myeloproliferative disease	Low
CUTANEOUS WITH ARTHRITIS OR MYOPATHY			
Amyloidosis	Waxy papules and nodules, occasionally with associated symmetrical arthritis; renal insufficiency	Multiple myeloma	Moderate
Palmar fasciitis-polyarthritis	Thickening of the palmar fascia; inflammatory distal symmetrical arthritis	Ovarian cancer	Low
Panniculitis-arthritis	Erythematous subcutaneous tender nodules; inflammatory monoarticular or polyarticular arthritis	Cancer of the pancreas (also pancreatitis)	Low
Eosinophilic fasciitis	Edema, thickening of the dermis and fascia associated with joint contractures	Breast cancer, myeloproliferative disease, lymphoproliferative disease	Low
Dermatomyositis/polymyositis	Heliotrope rash (erythema in periorbital area); Gottron's papules (erythematous papules over phalangeal joints); proximal myopathy	Various tumors, primarily adenocarcinomas	Low to moderate, more with dermatomyositis

TABLE 189–5 EXAMPLES OF CUTANEOUS AND RHEUMATOLOGIC LESIONS ASSOCIATED WITH MALIGNANT DISEASE—cont'd

Syndrome	Clinical Presentation	Associated Malignancy	Association/Risk
ARTICULAR			
Digital clubbing	Loss of nail bed angle	Lung cancer (also seen with benign cardiopulmonary disorders)	Low
Hypertrophic pulmonary osteoarthropathy	Periostosis of long bones; pain and swelling in distal joints	Lung cancer	High
Carcinoma polyarthropathy	Sudden onset of seronegative arthritis at a late age	Cancers of the breast and lung	Low to moderate
Gout	Classical acute painful gouty arthritis	Acute leukemias, lymphomas associated with rapid tumor cell turnover and tumor lysis	Low
VASCULAR			
Leukocytoclastic vasculitis	Palpable purpura, urticaria, maculopapular rash with or without arthritis	Myeloproliferative and lymphoproliferative diseases, myelodysplasia; rarely with adenocarcinoma and melanoma	Low to moderate
Polyarteritis nodosa	Cutaneous and/or mesenteric vasculitis; fever, myalgia; arthritis; mononeuritis multiplex	Hairy cell leukemia	Low
Raynaud's syndrome	Classic Raynaud's with progression to digital necrosis or gangrene common	Lymphoma, leukemia, myeloma, and cancers of the lung, ovary, small bowel, breast, pancreas, kidney	Low to moderate in patients older than 50 years
Erythromelalgia	Painful, erythematous digits, relieved by aspirin	Myeloproliferative disease	Moderate to high

most commonly seen with nonmalignant conditions, making it difficult or impossible to connect the skin disease with the underlying malignancy. In addition, biopsies of the skin lesion are usually nonspecific, with features identical to those when the same lesion is seen with a nonmalignant condition. The formation of tumor-related autoantibodies has been rarely associated with dermatologic paraneoplastic syndromes, although inflammatory cell infiltration may be seen.

The finding of a new skin lesion that is almost always associated with an underlying malignancy (e.g., Bazex's syndrome, erythema gyratum repens) should prompt a directed evaluation for that tumor. In contrast, diagnosis of a common problem that is only occasionally associated with cancer (e.g., pruritus, dermatomyositis) should prompt a careful physical examination and routine cancer screening as well as continued awareness of this possible association over time. The etiology of most dermatologic paraneoplastic syndromes is not well understood. The diagnosis of a paraneoplastic dermatologic syndrome is based on characteristic clinical and pathologic findings, including deposition of immunoglobulin G (IgG) and C3 at the basement membrane of affected skin in a variety of syndromes and the finding of an underlying malignancy.

Specific Syndromes

Acanthosis Nigricans

One of the most well-known paraneoplastic syndromes is acanthosis nigricans, whose pathogenesis is unclear. The tumor may produce factors that activate insulin-like growth factors or the insulin receptor in skin. Many tumors are known to produce transforming growth factor α (TGF-α), which might activate epidermal growth factor receptors in skin to cause hyperpigmentation and thickening.

Clinical Manifestations and Diagnosis

The skin lesions (Fig. 189–1) arise as velvety, verrucous hyperpigmentation of the neck, axilla, groin, and mucosal membranes, including the lips, periocular area, and anus. Although this lesion clearly occurs as a benign entity associated with obesity and endocrinopathy, its appearance in older adults, especially when it includes mucosal lesions, has been

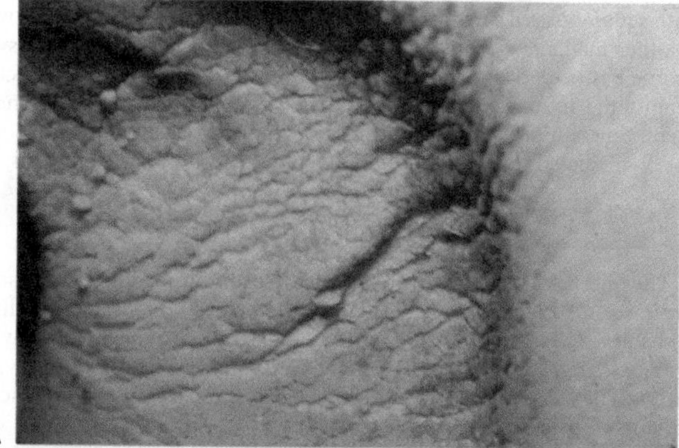

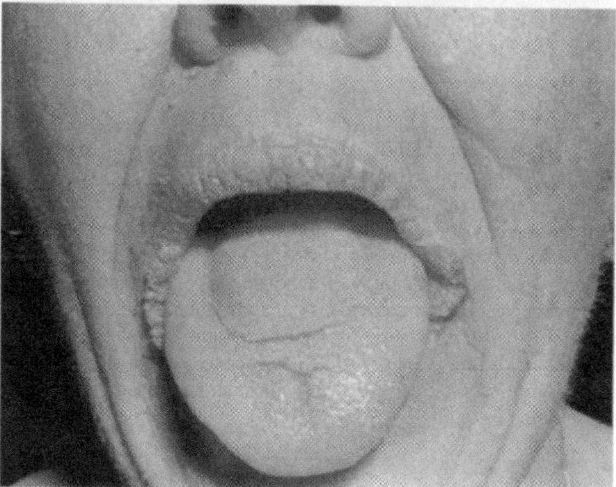

FIGURE 189–1 • Acanthosis nigricans. A, Paraneoplastic acanthosis nigricans with a velvety hyperpigmented rash in the axilla in a patient with gastric cancer. **B,** Acanthosis nigricans of the oral mucosa. This pattern of involvement is almost always associated with cancer. (Courtesy Dr. Timothy Berger.)

highly associated with malignancies of the gastrointestinal tract as well as other adenocarcinomas. The lesions often regress with successful treatment of the underlying tumor.

Paraneoplastic Pemphigus

This syndrome is manifested by ulcerative and blistering mucocutaneous lesions with acantholysis; it is primarily associated with lymphoma (Chapters 196 and 197), other lymphoproliferative diseases, and thymic cancers. Patients have high titers of autoantibodies that react against tumor antigens and cross-react with antigens at the epidermal cell junction, including the plakin family of desmosomal proteins and desmogleins; indirect immunofluorescent staining shows IgG and C3 deposition on the surface of keratinocytes and on the basement membrane zone. Antibody titers may correlate with the severity of the skin disease and its response to therapy.

Diagnosis

The diagnosis of paraneoplastic pemphigus should include finding specific major criteria including a polymorphic cutaneous eruption, concurrent internal neoplasia, and a specific immunoprecipitation pattern on testing of serum. Minor criteria include histologic evidence of acantholysis, intercellular and basement membrane staining with antibodies to IgG and C3 on direct immunofluorescence, and staining of rat urothelium with antibodies to desmoplakin on indirect immunofluorescence. The development of paraneoplastic pemphigus in patients with lymphoma (Chapters 196 and 197), chronic lymphocytic leukemia (Chapter 195), Castleman's disease (Chapter 196), and, less commonly, other malignancies is associated with a very poor prognosis and is often associated with pulmonary involvement.

Bazex's Syndrome

Bazex's syndrome is a papulosquamous eruption that is also termed acrokeratosis paraneoplasia owing to the characteristic location of the hyperkeratotic lesions on the palms and soles. It is seen in association with squamous cell carcinoma of the head and neck (Chapter 200) as well as other malignancies involving the oropharynx or larynx. Bazex's syndrome has been postulated to be caused by antibodies that are directed against the tumor but that cross-react with keratinocyte or basement membrane antigens, similar to those in paraneoplastic pemphigus, or a T-cell–mediated immune response to epidermal tumor-like antigens.

Clinical Manifestations and Diagnosis

The findings are similar in appearance to psoriatic plaques but are seen in unexpected locations including the ears, nails, node, fingers, palms, and soles. These lesions can predate the diagnosis of malignancy by as long as 1 year, and they may progress in parallel with the underlying tumor. The main differential diagnosis involves exclusion of benign acral variants of psoriasis.

RHEUMATOLOGIC PARANEOPLASTIC SYNDROMES

Definition and Epidemiology

A wide variety of rheumatologic paraneoplastic syndromes have been associated with underlying malignancies, but almost all of these syndromes are identical to their benign counterparts (see Table 189–5). The rheumatologic paraneoplastic syndromes can be classified as cutaneous with arthritis, articular, or vasculitic. Paraneoplastic rheumatologic syndromes may either coincide with the diagnosis of malignancy or precede it by several years. An increased risk of subsequent malignancy may exist in patients with a variety of rheumatologic diseases. For example, Sjögren's syndrome (Chapter 289) is associated with a slightly increased risk of lymphoproliferative disease, although the cause of this relationship remains unclear.

Clinical Manifestations

In contrast to the nonparaneoplastic rheumatologic syndromes, rheumatologic paraneoplastic syndromes are associated with rapid onset, late age at onset (older than 50 years), negative serologies, and effusions characterized by the absence of inflammatory markers. Considerable overlap exists among the rheumatologic, dermatologic, and neurologic paraneoplastic syndromes.

Diagnosis

In general, when a rheumatologic paraneoplastic syndrome is suspected, screening should include a physical examination, laboratory tests, and standard radiographic tests, such as a mammogram.

POEMS Syndrome

Osteosclerotic myeloma (Chapter 198) associated with the POEMS syndrome (*p*olyneuropathy, *o*rganomegaly, *e*ndocrinopathy, *m*onoclonal protein, and skin changes suggestive of *s*cleroderma) is a rare condition that has features of all three of the paraneoplastic syndromes owing to the effects of a circulating paraprotein. It is likely that other factors also play a role in the pathogenesis of POEMS syndrome, including production of high levels of vascular endothelial growth factor and inflammatory cytokines.

Hypertrophic Osteoarthropathy

One of the more common and specific paraneoplastic syndromes is hypertrophic osteoarthropathy, which arises as an oligoarthritis or polyarthritis of the distal joints with clubbing, tender periostitis of the distal long bones, and noninflammatory synovial effusions. Hypertrophic osteoarthropathy may affect up to 10% of patients with adenocarcinoma of the lung. It is also seen with a variety of other pulmonary malignancies, including metastases to the lung. The etiology is unknown. Laboratory studies may reveal an elevation in the erythrocyte sedimentation rate; bone radiographs show linear ossification of the distal long bones separated by a radiolucent zone from the underlying cortex (Fig. 189–2). Treatment is symptomatic with anti-inflammatory agents; treatment of the underlying tumor may also improve symptoms.

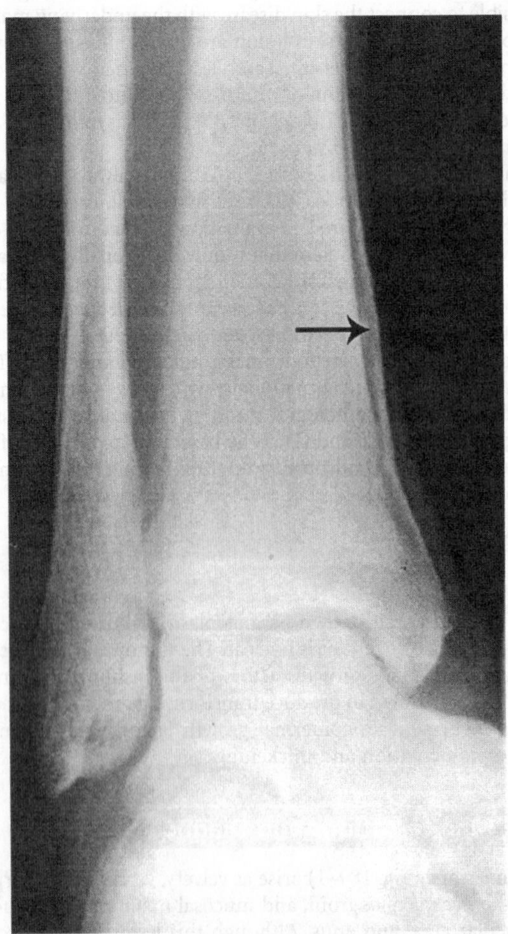

FIGURE 189–2 • Hypertrophic pulmonary osteoarthropathy characterized by periosteal elevation of the tibia (arrow). (Courtesy Dr. Lynne S. Steinbach.)

Dermatomyositis/Polymyositis

Dermatomyositis/polymyositis has been reported to be associated with an underlying malignancy in less than 10% to as high as 60% of cases (Chapter 290). Dermatomyositis has been more closely associated with malignancy than has polymyositis. Studies of patients with dermatomyositis suggest a two- to four-fold increased risk of malignancies, including cancer of the lung, ovaries, breast, gastrointestinal tract, and testes. The true incidence of malignancy in patients diagnosed with dermatomyositis is probably in the range 10 to 15%. Although the etiology is unknown, autoantibodies to muscle have been described in patients with dermatomyositis. These antibodies have not been well characterized and do not appear to be directly related to tumor antigens. The diagnosis of malignancy is usually made within 1 year preceding or following the diagnosis of dermatomyositis; a longer duration of dermatomyositis substantially decreases the risk of association.

Hematologic Paraneoplastic Syndromes

Routine blood testing may identify a hematologic paraneoplastic syndrome as well as the underlying malignancy. Hematologic paraneoplastic syndromes may involve all three cell lines.

Red Cells

The most prevalent and commonly recognized paraneoplastic syndrome, seen with many cancers, is a normochromic, normocytic anemia associated with a low reticulocyte count (Chapter 169). This hypoproductive anemia, generally termed *anemia of chronic disease,* must be differentiated from anemia as a result of side effects of treatment or direct tumor infiltration of the bone marrow. It is associated with inappropriately low erythropoietin levels as well as the inability to reuse iron. Cytokines including interleukin-1 (IL-1), tumor necrosis factor (TNF), and TGF-β released by the tumor or local inflammatory cells mediate this disorder, which may be effectively treated with weekly subcutaneous injections of erythropoietin at a dose of 40,000 units or darbepoetin at a dose of 200 μg every 2 weeks. Adequate iron intake must be ensured. The rare syndrome of pure red cell aplasia (Chapter 171) is associated with cancer of the thymus gland (thymoma; Chapter 448) and is thought to be due to an autoimmune mechanism. Bone marrow examination shows an absence of red cell precursors.

Paraneoplastic anemia can also be caused by hemolytic anemia (Chapter 164) related to warm- or cold-reacting antibodies in the setting of B-cell malignancies, especially chronic lymphocytic leukemia (Chapter 195) and lymphoma (Chapters 196 and 197). Treatment is directed toward the underlying lymphoproliferative disease but may also include splenectomy for warm antibody hemolysis; cold-reacting hemolysis may require plasmapheresis. Microangiopathic hemolytic anemia (Chapter 164) with thrombocytopenia may occur with mucinous adenocarcinomas or after specific types of chemotherapy. Erythrocytosis is an uncommon paraneoplastic syndrome that is associated with tumors that produce erythropoietin, including renal cell cancer, hepatocellular carcinoma, and posterior fossa tumors (e.g., cerebellar hemangioblastoma) (Chapters 172 and 188).

White Cells

Leukocytosis (Chapter 173) is common in advanced cancer. Although infection and myeloproliferative disease must be excluded, the leukocytosis is generally caused by cytokines that are probably produced by the tumor itself, including granulocyte stimulating factor and granulocyte-macrophage stimulating factor. Although paraneoplastic leukocytosis requires no specific treatment, it may represent a poor prognostic sign. Eosinophilia (Chapter 176) is often seen with lymphoproliferative diseases.

Platelets

Paraneoplastic thrombocytosis, which is a relatively common laboratory finding, is caused by tumors that produce stimulatory cytokines (IL-6, thrombopoietin); platelet counts generally do not exceed 1 million. The thrombocytosis does not require specific treatment. Iron deficiency, especially caused by gastrointestinal blood loss, should be excluded. Thrombocytopenia is uncommon except when it is associated with microangiopathic hemolytic anemia, disseminated intravascular coagulopathy (DIC), or marrow infiltration.

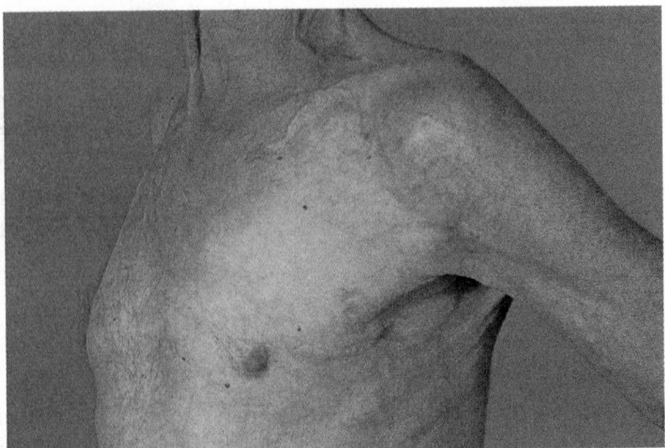

FIGURE 189–3 • Thrombophlebitis in superficial or deep veins is relatively common in many forms of malignant disease, but it is particularly associated with carcinoma of the pancreas and sometimes is the presenting feature. In this patient, thrombosis in the veins of the upper arm is associated with an extensive collateral circulation in the superficial veins around the shoulder. Recurrent episodes of thrombophlebitis may precede the diagnosis of carcinoma by many months, and their occurrence in an otherwise apparently fit patient should lead to a search for underlying malignancy, especially in the pancreas. (From Forbes CD, Jackson WF: Color Atlas and Text of Clinical Medicine, 3rd ed. London, Mosby, 2003.)

Thrombosis

Epidemiology

The best known and one of the first described hematologic paraneoplastic syndromes is Trousseau's syndrome, or the association of venous or arterial thrombosis with malignancy (Fig. 189–3). Although thrombosis frequently complicates progressive cancer, it may also be the first sign of cancer. Deep venous thrombosis may herald an underlying malignancy in approximately 10% of patients, particularly in patients who present with an initial episode without other obvious risk factors, in the setting of recurrent thrombosis despite adequate doses of warfarin (warfarin resistance), or when the thrombosis occurs in usual sites (e.g., subclavian vein, Budd-Chiari syndrome, portal vein thrombosis).

Pathobiology

Paraneoplastic thrombosis is most commonly associated with adenocarcinomas, particularly of the stomach, breast, and ovary. The etiology of malignant thrombosis is complex, and it may be due to release of procoagulant mediators (e.g., sialic residues of tumor-secreted mucin) directly by tumor cells or to tumor-mediated endothelial damage. The thrombosis can be associated with low-grade DIC (Chapter 181) and abnormal platelet activation. As with other hematologic paraneoplastic syndromes, cytokines play a role in the systemic activation of coagulation. Other factors that contribute to a high risk of thrombosis in patients with known malignancy include the procoagulant effects of chemotherapy, indwelling catheters, and immobility.

Diagnosis

The evaluation of patients with a malignancy-associated thrombosis should include laboratory testing for DIC as well as a careful assessment of bleeding risk at sites of tumor, such as metastases to the nervous system or involvement of the gastrointestinal tract. It is important to exclude inherited clotting disorders, especially in younger patients who present with a deep venous thrombosis without known underlying cause (Chapters 81 and 182).

Treatment

Rx

Treatment for thrombosis without evidence of DIC should include initial standard anticoagulation with heparin. Chronic treatment with low-molecular-weight heparin may be better than warfarin for

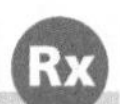

preventing recurrent thromboembolism without increasing the risk of bleeding. 1 Venous interruption (Chapters 81 and 99) is associated with significant complications and should be reserved for patients without other treatment options. Successful treatment of the underlying malignancy is the most effective way to reduce the risk of thrombosis.

Hemorrhagic Paraneoplastic Syndromes

DIC caused by activation of the hemostatic system with consumption of coagulation factors and platelets can result in both thrombosis and hemorrhage. Acute DIC can be seen with a variety of malignancies. Essentially all patients with acute promyelocytic leukemia (Chapter 194) either present with acute DIC and associated hemorrhage or develop it during treatment. Procoagulant material released from the leukemia cells activates the fibrinolytic pathway; treatment with all-*trans*-retinoic acid and low-dose heparin has significantly reduced the complications of hemorrhage with this leukemia.

Other causes of malignancy-associated bleeding disorders include paraproteins that interfere with fibrin polymerization, amyloid deposits associated with monoclonal gammopathies such as multiple myeloma (Chapters 198 and 296), and, rarely, acquired von Willebrand disease associated with lymphoproliferative and myeloproliferative disorders (Chapter 180). Increased fibrinolysis may be seen in patients with advanced prostate cancer (Chapter 211).

RENAL PARANEOPLASTIC SYNDROMES

Renal involvement in the setting of malignancy may be due to direct tumor infiltration of the renal parenchyma or, less commonly, to a paraneoplastic syndrome. Paraneoplastic syndromes involving the kidney may be caused by tumor-related hormone production (Chapter 188), may directly involve the glomerulus or the microvasculature, may be related to proteins produced by the tumor (e.g., amyloid, paraproteins), or may be caused by electrolyte disorders (hyponatremia, hyperuricemia).

Glomerulonephritis

The renal paraneoplastic syndrome most clearly linked to malignancy is membranous glomerulonephritis, which is characterized by nephrotic range proteinuria, edema, hypoalbuminemia, microscopic hematuria, hypertension, and increased risk of thrombosis (Chapter 122). Associated cancers include adenocarcinomas of the lung (Chapter 201), breast (Chapter 208), and stomach (Chapter 202), as well as others. The pathology is related to thickening of the glomerular basement membrane from subepithelial deposition of tumor antigen that has reacted with circulating immunoglobulins (IgG) and complement. Other glomerular lesions include minimal change nephropathy complicating lymphoproliferative disorders, in particular Hodgkin's disease (Chapter 197); rapidly progressive glomerulonephritis associated with lymphoplasmacytic diseases; and other glomerulopathies (including nephrotic syndrome and minimal change disease) associated with a variety of malignant diseases.

It may be very difficult to differentiate a renal paraneoplastic syndrome from a benign disorder of the kidney; a biopsy demonstrating immune complex deposition as well as a parallel course with an underlying malignancy can help make the diagnosis.

Microvascular Disease

Renal microvascular involvement is uncommon and may be due to vasculitis or microangiopathy. Vasculitis may be caused by cryoglobulinemia in patients with hepatitis C–related hepatocellular carcinoma (Chapter 206) or rarely in patients with IgA monoclonal gammopathy in association with cancer of the lung. Thrombotic microangiopathy (hemolytic-uremic syndrome) or thrombotic thrombocytopenic microangiopathy (Chapter 179) is most commonly a complication of chemotherapy (Chapter 192), including mitomycin-C, cisplatin, and others, but it may also be seen in association with a variety of adenocarcinomas as well as with promyelocytic leukemia. The etiology is unknown; the underlying malignancy should be treated, if possible, and plasma exchange may be indicated.

HEPATOPATHY

Paraneoplastic hepatopathy is an uncommon disorder characterized by hepatic dysfunction with elevated liver enzymes and abnormal synthetic function with fever and weight loss. This syndrome has been associated with nonmetastatic renal cell cancer (Chapter 207) and is probably due to either autoimmune effects or direct toxicity from tumor-related products. This unusual syndrome resolves with resection of the tumor.

FEVER AND CACHEXIA

Fever (Chapters 302 and 303), night sweats, and cachexia are nonspecific symptoms that, when paraneoplastic, often suggest the diagnosis of an underlying malignancy. Cytokines clearly play a pathogenetic role in inducing both fever and cachexia. TNF-α (previously known as cachectin), interleukins (including IL-1 and IL-6), and interferon-γ are produced directly by the tumor or by normal host cells, such as macrophages, in response to inflammation and result in a catabolic state. Cytokines may produce fever directly by acting at the hypothalamic thermoregulatory center (Chapters 302 and 303). In addition to the burden of tumor and the production of cytokines, cachexia may be caused or worsened by the side effects of cancer treatment, by intestinal blockage or malabsorption caused by tumor infiltration, and by depression.

Fever is generally cyclic and may be associated with drenching night sweats. Symptoms resolve with treatment of the underlying tumor, and return of fever usually heralds relapse. When treatment of the tumor is not possible or is ineffective, nonsteroidal anti-inflammatory agents or steroids given around the clock significantly improve quality of life. Although fever is most commonly seen in association with lymphoproliferative disease (Chapters 196 and 197), renal cell carcinoma (Chapter 207), and leukemias (Chapters 194 and 195), it may also occur with other cancers.

Cachexia, or the cancer wasting syndrome, is probably the single most common paraneoplastic syndrome, eventually affecting up to 80% of patients with cancer. This syndrome is characterized by anorexia, muscle wasting, loss of subcutaneous fat, and fatigue. It appears to be caused by a combination of protein wasting, malabsorption, immune dysregulation, and increased glucose turnover in the setting of tumor-induced increased energy expenditure. Successful treatment of the underlying tumor reverses the process, but, in many cases, no treatment is successful. Megestrol acetate given in high concentrations in liquid form (400 to 800 mg/day) can significantly improve appetite and result in weight gain, as can dronabinol (Marinol; 2.5 to 5 mg three times a day). Corticosteroids may also help. Although agents that block TNF production are theoretically attractive to treat cancer-related cachexia, there is also concern that such agents may block cytokines that may inhibit tumor growth. In addition, preclinical data suggest that antibodies to parathyroid hormone–related protein may block the production of inflammatory cytokines in cancer; whether this effect is of clinical value remains a research question.

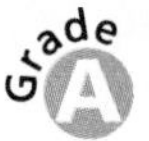

1. Lee AY, Levine MN, Baker RI, et al: Low-molecular-weight heparin versus coumarin for the prevention of recurrent venous thromboembolism in patients with cancer. N Engl J Med 2003;349:146–153.

SUGGESTED READINGS

Blom JW, Doggen CJM, Osanto S, et al: Malignancies, prothrombotic mutations, and the risk of venous thrombosis. JAMA 2005;293:715–722. *The overall risk of venous thrombosis was increased seven-fold in patients with a malignancy.*

Dalmau J, Gonzalez RG, Lerwill MF: Case records of the Massachusetts General Hospital. Case 4-2007. A 56-year-old women with rapidly progressive vertigo and ataxia. N Engl J Med 2007;356:612–620. *Case of cerebellar degeneration due to Anti-Yo antibodies in breast cancer, with a useful general discussion.*

Dropcho EJ: Immunotherapy for paraneoplastic neurologic disorders. Expert Opin Biol Ther 2005;5:1339–1348. *A summary of current understanding of clinical immunology, immunologic therapies, and clinical outcomes.*

Muscaritoli M, Bossola M, Aversa Z, et al: Prevention and treatment of cancer cachexia: New insights into an old problem. Eur J Cancer 2006;42:31–41. *A thorough review of the potential mechanisms and treatment of this common complication of malignancy.*

Sommer C, Weishaupt A, Brinkhoff J, et al: Paraneoplastic stiff-person syndrome: Passive transfer to rats by means of IgG antibodies to amphiphysin. Lancet 2005;365:1406–1411. *Suggests a direct pathogenic role.*

Stone SP, Buescher LS: Life-threatening paraneoplastic cutaneous syndromes. Clin Dermatol 2005;23:301–306. *A brief description of the most common serious syndromes.*

190 CANCER BIOMARKERS

Anna D. Barker

USE OF BIOMARKERS

Cancer biomarkers, which are used in many aspects of the management of cancer patients and in drug development, represent a major strategic platform for the development of personalized medicine. Although it is likely that new cancer biomarkers will emerge from high-throughput genomics and proteomics, only a few biomarkers are currently approved by the Food and Drug Administration (FDA).

Biomarkers, which are indicators of normal and disease-related processes or pharmacologic responses to therapy, range from proteins, genes, or other biomolecules to multimolecule complexes such as gene expression profiles. Most currently validated biomarkers (Table 190–1) are cell surface antigens that are not cancer specific, but the several exceptions provide proof of concept for the ultimate usefulness of biomarkers in cancer diagnosis and treatment. Biomarkers have historically been measured primarily in serum but are now increasingly being measured in tissue. They are clinically useful for diagnosis, selection of treatment, monitoring during and after treatment, and assessment of prognosis. They are also used investigationally for drug development and to identify and stratify cohorts in clinical trials.

TYPES OF CANCER BIOMARKERS

Currently, the most clinically useful cancer biomarkers are those that correlate with risks and clinical outcomes, especially measures of progression (e.g., recurrence or metastasis). Many biomarkers of cancer progression are cellular proteins, such as carcinoembryonic antigen (CEA), α-fetoprotein (AFP), prostate-specific antigen (PSA), and CA-125. These *risk biomarkers,* which are frequently used for screening to describe the likelihood that cancer is present or will progress, may measure genetic predisposition, pharmacogenomic parameters, and previous disease or precursor lesions. *Drug effect biomarkers,* which correlate with biologic or clinical effects, are often measures of reduced expression or activity of a molecular target in a mechanism-based therapy. *Cellular, histopathologic,* and *imaging biomarkers* reflect biologic alterations that occur during cancer progression, including histologic changes measured by imaging and immunohistochemical techniques, or biomarkers such as altered differentiation, gene expression, or gene mutations. Increasingly, *pharmacodynamic* and *pharmacogenomic biomarkers* are being used to measure drug effects and predict drug-specific toxicities. Criteria for validating biomarkers include standardization and validation of their assays, as well as validation by correlation with disease and outcomes.

CANCER BIOMARKERS AND CLINICAL CARE

Breast Cancer (Chapter 208)

Screening

No biomarkers are currently effective in screening for breast cancer.

Selecting Therapy and Monitoring Therapeutic Response

Rx

Three tissue-based tumor biomarkers are routinely assayed in all newly diagnosed breast cancers—estrogen receptor (ER), progesterone receptor (PR), and HER-2/neu (c-ErbB-2). Both ER and PR, used to identify patients for hormone therapy, are nuclear hormone receptors. ER is found in 50 to 70% of invasive breast cancers; approximately 50 to 60% of ER-positive patients and 70 to 80% of patients who are positive for both ER and PR respond to hormone therapy. HER-2/neu, which belongs to the superfamily of receptor tyrosine kinases, is assayed primarily to identify patients who will benefit from treatment with trastuzumab (Herceptin), an antibody inhibitor of HER-2/neu. 1 Overexpression of HER-2/neu has also been investigated as a predictor of resistance to hormonal therapy, but evidence does not yet support routine use for this indication. Although CA 15-3 and CA 27-29 are approved by the FDA for monitoring in breast cancer, they are not specific for breast cancer and are of little value in patient management.

Prognosis

Urokinase-type plasminogen activator (uPA) and plasminogen activator inhibitor type 1 (PAI-1) are tissue-based proteins that are also validated for clinical use as tumor biomarkers in breast cancer. To date their use has been limited by the assays' requirements for fresh tissue. Both uPA and PAI-1 are strong prognostic factors in breast cancer independent of nodal metastases, tumor size, and hormone receptor status. Combined measurements of both proteins are used as a prognostic factor in node-negative breast cancer patients. Patients with low levels of both uPA and PAI-1 have a low risk for relapse and are unlikely to benefit from adju-

TABLE 190–1 ROLE OF BIOMARKERS IN SPECIFIC CANCERS

Breast Cancer	Colorectal Cancer	Hepatocellular Cancer	Lymphoma	Ovarian Cancer	Prostate Cancer
ER/PR Response to hormone therapy Prognostic biomarker	**CEA** Cancer recurrence, metastasis Selection for adjuvant chemotherapy	**AFP** Detection and diagnosis Treatment monitoring (elevated before therapy) Prognosis	**LDH** Prognostic factor—identify probable responders to standard therapy	**CA-125** Recurrence, selection for chemotherapy	**PSA levels (PSA-DT, %fPSA, PSA-V) and nomogram with other factors (e.g., DRE, Gleason score)**
HER-2/neu Response to trastuzumab (metastatic and adjuvant settings) and anthracycline-based therapy Prognostic with other factors	**CA 19-9, CA-242** Recurrence		**β_2-Microglobulin** Prognostic for patients with newly diagnosed lymphoma Treatment monitoring		Detection Recurrence Selection for therapy Treatment monitoring

AFP = α-fetoprotein; CA = cancer antigen; CEA = carcinoembryonic antigen; %fPSA = percent free (unconjugated) PSA; LDH = lactate dehydrogenase; PSA = prostate-specific antigen; PSA-DT = PSA doubling time; PSA-V = PSA velocity.

vant chemotherapy, whereas patients with high levels of one or both of these proteins have a higher risk for relapse and are likely to benefit from adjuvant chemotherapy.

Biomarkers in Development

CA 15-3/BR 27.29 (MUC1) mucin, a membrane-bound glycoprotein that is overexpressed and aberrantly glycosylated in breast cancers, detects metastases in approximately 70% of cases before clinical symptoms appear (Table 190–2). CEA may detect asymptomatic metastatic disease even when MUC1 does not. However, treatment of progressive disease based on these serum biomarkers has not been shown to increase survival. In the future, gene expression profiles may identify patients who are likely to respond to therapy.

Colorectal Cancer (Chapter 203)

Screening

CEA, which is a 200-kD glycoprotein biomarker found in many types of cells, may be increased in colon and other cancers (e.g., pancreatic, stomach, lung, thyroid, and ovarian cancer) and a range of benign conditions, including infection, inflammatory bowel disease, pancreatitis, cirrhosis, and some benign tumors. In adults, normal blood levels of CEA are less than 2.5 ng/mL in nonsmokers and less than 5.0 ng/mL in smokers. Blood levels are typically 10 ng/mL or less in benign disease. The most common cancers with elevated CEA levels are those of the colon and rectum, and CEA is the only tumor biomarker widely accepted for clinical use in these cancers. Although levels greater than 20 ng/mL are indicative of metastatic disease before therapy, the sensitivity and specificity of CEA are not sufficiently robust for screening.

Prognosis

In colorectal cancer, CEA is a useful tool for estimating prognosis, monitoring patients for recurrent disease, and assessing the success of treatment of metastatic disease. In patients with newly diagnosed cancer, high preoperative levels are associated with aggressive disease and recurrence. Serial monitoring of CEA levels every 2 to 3 months for 2 years or longer is widely accepted as a validated biomarker for surveillance and detection of recurrent disease in patients with stage II and III disease. However, there is no consensus on the definition of clinically significant increases in CEA. Current criteria range from a 30% or greater increase substantiated by two measurements within a month to an increase of 15 to 20% sustained over three successive measurements. Because CEA elevation is not seen in 20 to 30% of recurrences, even with distant metastases, CEA should not be the only method to monitor for recurrence.

Monitoring Therapeutic Response

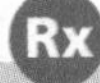

Measurements of CEA at 2- to 3-month intervals may lead to early detection of treatment failure, with the potential to change treatment and reduce side effects and treatment costs. In metastatic colorectal cancer, elevation of CEA levels above baseline in serial measurements strongly suggests treatment failure and progressive disease.

Biomarkers in Development

Serum proteins being evaluated as biomarkers for colorectal cancer include CA-242 antigen, CA 19-9 antigen, tissue inhibitor of metalloproteinases type 1 (TIMP-1), and soluble urokinase plasminogen activator receptor (suPAR). In preliminary studies, TIMP-1 was found to detect early- and late-stage colorectal cancer with high specificity and sensitivity.

Fecal DNA-based biomarkers with high sensitivity and specificity show promise in screening for colorectal cancer. These biomarkers are combinations of mutated tumor suppressor genes, oncogenes, and indicators of microsatellite instability that are prevalent in colorectal cancer. Patients with locally advanced stage II/III colorectal cancer with aneuploidy and mutated K-*ras*, *p53*, and adenomatosis polyposis coli (APC) show aggressive tumor growth and reduced survival.

Hepatocellular Carcinoma (Chapter 206)

Screening

AFP, a 70-kD glycoprotein normally produced during gestation, is highly elevated in the serum of newborns and decreases during the first year of life to 0 to 20 μg/L. Although AFP is not specific for hepatocellular cancer, it is currently used in conjunction with ultrasound for the diagnosis of hepatocellular cancer in high-risk patients with cirrhosis or chronic hepatitis B or C, for monitoring of patients with hepatocellular cancer to detect recurrences after liver transplantation or tumor resection, for monitoring response after chemotherapy, and for prognosis. About 20 to 40% of adults with hepatitis or liver cirrhosis have AFP levels higher than 10 μg/L, levels of 10 to 1000 μg/L have been associated with benign disease, and patients with hepatocellular cancer may have levels up to 10×10^6 μg/L. When used in conjunction with ultrasound, AFP levels of 400 to 500 μg/L are currently used to distinguish malignant from benign disease; at these levels, AFP has greater than 90% specificity for detecting hepatocellular cancer, although sensitivity (20 to 40%) and positive predictive value (5 to 15%) are low. Serial measurements of AFP are recommended; if inflammation can be excluded as a cause, serial rises are considered suggestive of hepatocellular cancer.

Prognosis

Preoperative AFP values higher than 20 μg/L are associated with poor outcomes; survival of patients with AFP levels higher than 10,000 μg/L at diagnosis is significantly shorter than when the AFP level is less than 200 μg/L.

Monitoring Therapeutic Response

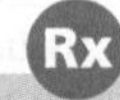

Effective chemotherapy for hepatocellular cancer can result in dramatic decreases in serum AFP, and some patients return to normal levels. Decreases in AFP appear to reflect tumor regression more consistently than do changes in tumor size or volume as measured by computed tomography. Progressive disease is seen in patients with continued increases in AFP.

Biomarkers in Development

The most promising serum biomarkers for detecting hepatocellular cancer include des-γ-carboxyprothrombin, human hepatocyte growth factor, and insulin-like growth factor type I (IGF-I). Several laboratories have recently reported that glypican-3 (GPC3), which is expressed by a large percentage of hepatocellular cancers, is undetectable in normal hepatocytes and nonmalignant liver disease, thus suggesting that serum GPC3 may be useful as a serologic test for diagnosis. Because elevated GPC3 does not correlate with elevated AFP but at least one of these two markers is elevated in a large majority of patients with hepatocellular cancer, simultaneous measurement of both biomarkers may be worthwhile.

Lymphoma

Screening

The most important serum markers for the diagnosis, staging, and therapeutic monitoring of non-Hodgkin's lymphoma (Chapter 196) are β_2-microglobulin, lactate dehydrogenase (LDH), and CA-125, but no traditional tumor biomarkers have been validated for clinical use in management of the various types of lymphoma.

Prognosis

In non-Hodgkin's lymphoma, high LDH levels are associated with a poor prognosis.

Monitoring Therapeutic Response

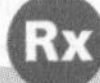

Elevation of LDH levels over time suggests treatment failure and can guide the selection of more aggressive therapy, especially in clinical trials.

TABLE 190–2 BIOMARKERS IN DEVELOPMENT

Breast Cancer	Colorectal Cancer	Hepatocellular Cancer	Lymphoma	Ovarian Cancer	Prostate Cancer
CA 15-3/BR 27.29 (glycoprotein encoded by MUC1) Recurrence, metastasis in symptomatic patients	**Fecal DNA molecular markers** *APC, p53, KRAS, BAT26,* combinations Microsatellite instability Hypermethylation Early disease detection	**DCP** Cancer detection Prognostic factor for portal venous invasion	**DNA microarray (diffuse large B-cell lymphoma)** Identify probable responders to chemotherapy	**Osteopontin** Detection Adjunct to CA-25 in detection of recurrence	**PSMA** Recurrence, metastasis
CEA Recurrence, metastasis (combination with other factors) Monitoring therapy in advanced disease	**TIMP-1** Detection (early- and late-stage disease with high specificity and sensitivity) Predictive of response to adjuvant therapy	**GPC3 (alone and in combination with AFP)** Detection (high specificity, sensitivity to differentiate HCC from other disorders)		***BRCA1/BRCA2*** Disease risk (germline mutations)	**GSTP1 (hypermethylation)** Detection (*GSTP1* is the most frequently inactivated gene in prostate cancer)
21-Gene expression profile (OncotypeDX) Predictive biomarker for response to therapy (locally advanced disease)	***UGT1A* gene polymorphisms** Identify potential toxicity of irinotecan in affected patients	**Human hepatocyte growth factor/IGF-I** Detection (in combination with other factors)		**Prostasin** Detection (alone and in combination with CA-125)	**PCA3** Detection (prostate-specific gene overexpressed in cancers)
uPA, PAI-1 Identification of patients (lymph node negative) likely to benefit from adjuvant chemotherapy Prognostic in advanced disease	**TS, DD, TP levels** Selection of patients likely to respond to 5-fluorouracil			**HER-2/*neu*** Prognostic (identification of patients with aggressive disease)	**hK-2** Detection (in combination with PSA)
Circulating tumor cells Prognostic Monitoring treatment				**Proteome** Cancer detection (development phase)	**Telomerase** Detection, disease risk
Abnormal FNA (or NAF or ductal lavage) Detection/risk					**PTEN loss** Detection, disease risk
BRCA1/BRCA2 Disease risk					**PSCA** Detection, disease risk (highly expressed in cancers vs. other genitourinary tissue)

AFP = α-fetoprotein; BR = breast antigen; *BRCA1/BRCA2* = breast cancer gene 1/2; CA = cancer antigen; CEA = carcinoembryonic antigen; DCP = des-γ-carboxyprothrombin (precursor of prothrombin); DD = dihydropyrimidine dehydrogenase; FNA = fine-needle aspiration; GPC3 = glypican-3 (oncofetal antigen); GSTP1 = glutathione-*S*-transferase P1; HCC = hepatocellular carcinoma; HER-2/neu = human epidermal growth factor receptor-2; hK-2 = human kallikrein-2 (protease); IGF-I = insulin-like growth factor type I; NAF = nipple aspirate fluid; PAI-1 = plasminogen activator inhibitor-1; *PCA3* = prostate cancer gene 3 (also called *DD3*); PSCA = prostate stem cell antigen; PSMA = prostate-specific membrane antigen; PTEN = phosphate and tensin homologue; TIMP-1 = tissue inhibitor of metalloproteinases type 1; TP = thymidine phosphorylase; TS = thymidylate synthase; UGT1A1 = UDP glycosyltransferase 1A1; uPA = urokinase plasminogen activator.

Biomarkers in Development

New lymphoma subtypes with unique molecular gene expression profiles correlate with specific genetic abnormalities and prognosis. DNA microarray expression analysis has defined molecularly distinct diseases within the diffuse large B-cell lymphoma classification. The germinal center B-cell–like and the activated B-cell–like subgroups differ in the expression of more than 1000 genes and have markedly different clinical outcomes. The genes identified as consistently abnormal in microarray profiles might provide clues for identifying proteins that can be used as future biomarkers.

Ovarian Cancer (Chapter 209)

Screening

Serum CA-125, a mucin with a large glycosylated extracellular domain, is the only tumor biomarker currently accepted for clinical use in ovarian cancer. CA-125 is used for detection in high-risk women, for diagnosis (distinguishing malignant from benign pelvic lesions), for post-treatment monitoring of patients for recurrence, and potentially for monitoring response to chemotherapy. CA-125 has insufficient sensitivity and specificity for screening asymptomatic women at normal risk for ovarian cancer; however, annual CA-125 measurements along with pelvic and ultrasound examinations have been recommended for high-risk women (i.e., women with potential hereditary disease, who have a lifetime risk of 40%).

CA-125 is more useful for diagnosis than for screening. Overall, 80% of women with ovarian cancer have CA-125 levels higher than 35 U/mL. CA-125 is recommended in postmenopausal women to distinguish malignant and benign disease (specificity of 75 to 94%, sensitivity of 71 to 78%, and positive predictive value as high as 95%). For example, in more than 90% of postmenopausal women who have a pelvic mass and elevated CA-125 level (>65 U/mL), ovarian cancer will be diagnosed. Conversely, because a variety of benign conditions can result in elevated CA-125 levels in younger women, the probability of ovarian cancer is much lower (15 to 40%) in younger women with a pelvic mass and elevated CA-125. Attempts to improve the performance of CA-125 assays have focused on increasing the specificity of CA-125 by measuring just the peptide moiety (MUC16) and using CA-125 within panels of biomarkers.

Monitoring Therapeutic Response

CA-125 is also used to monitor patients after treatment. CA-125 levels higher than 35 U/mL after treatment indicate residual disease, whereas elevated, rising, or doubling levels over limited time frames predict relapse (>85% accuracy). Current practice calls for measuring CA-125 at 2-to 4-month intervals for 2 years after treatment and then less frequently thereafter.

The rate of decrease in CA-125 levels appears to correlate with response to treatment. For example, when pretreatment CA-125 levels are two or more times the upper limit of the laboratory reference range, response has been defined as a 50% or greater reduction in CA-125 levels that is maintained for 28 or more days. However, CA-125 is of little value in the detection of microscopic disease because of the fact that only significant disease is associated with elevated CA-125.

Prognosis

Preoperative CA-125 levels higher than 65 U/mL correlate with a significantly lower 5-year survival rate and a 6.37-fold increased risk for death when compared with lower levels. Persistent CA-125 elevations indicate a poor prognosis. A CA-125 half-life of less than 20 days correlates with a 50% prolongation in survival, and normalization of CA-125 levels within three cycles of treatment also correlates with improved survival. CA-125 is not elevated in patients with serous or mucinous epithelial ovarian tumors, which have low malignant potential and are usually cured by surgery.

Biomarkers in Development

Three biomarkers, osteopontin, prostasin, and HER-2/neu, may all become of value for ovarian cancer. Osteopontin is upregulated in ovarian cancer, with higher expression in invasive cancer. Though potentially less sensitive than CA-125, osteopontin levels rise earlier than CA-125 in 90% of patients in whom recurrent disease develops, thus indicating that it may be a clinically useful adjunct to CA-125. Prostasin has also been detected at higher levels in ovarian cancer: mean serum levels are 13.7 μg/mL in ovarian cancer versus 7.5 μg/mL in controls. In patients with nonmucinous ovarian cancer, the combination of prostasin and CA-125 has 94% specificity and 92% sensitivity for detecting ovarian cancer. Amplification and overexpression of HER-2/neu in ovarian cancer has been correlated with aggressive disease, advanced clinical stages, and poor outcome. Individuals bearing germline *BRCA1*/*BRCA2* mutations also have an increased risk for the development of ovarian cancer.

Prostate Cancer (Chapter 211)

Screening/Detection

PSA, a 33-kD androgen-regulated glycoprotein, is the only tumor biomarker widely accepted for clinical use in prostate cancer. Serum PSA-based biomarkers are used for early detection and diagnosis, for post-treatment monitoring for recurrent disease, and for determining prognosis. Most PSA is made in epithelial cells in the transition zone of the prostate, so levels increase with age as a result of increases in prostate volume. Though controversial, PSA screening for prostate cancer has become standard clinical practice, and such screening clearly detects more prostate cancer than digital rectal examination does. Although elevated serum PSA is specific for prostatic disease, it is not cancer specific because levels are increased in conditions such as benign prostatic hyperplasia (Chapter 130), prostatitis, and prostate trauma. Levels higher than 4 ng/mL are usually considered abnormal in men 50 to 70 years old.

The lack of specificity of PSA for organ-confined prostate cancer remains controversial because at levels greater than 4 ng/mL, nearly 50% of men with the disease would be considered normal based on their PSA levels. Conversely, a large number of men with elevated PSA levels are subjected to needless biopsies. Although the extent of overtreatment because of elevated PSA has not been quantified, the side effects of overtreatment can include impotence and incontinence. One approach to the PSA screening question is to recommend screening for organ-confined disease only in men who have sufficient life expectancy to benefit from intervention.

Because of lack of specificity, total serum PSA is not generally used alone. Other PSA-derived biomarkers currently include percent free PSA, also known as free (unconjugated) PSA, PSA velocity, and PSA doubling time. Total serum PSA contains 5 to 30% free PSA with the remainder bound to serum protease inhibitors. Lower percent free PSA values are seen in men with prostate cancer than in men with benign disease. PSA velocity, which reflects the expected enhanced growth rate of cancer as compared with benign disease, is calculated from at least three PSA measurements during a 2-year period. However, this potentially promising approach has not been widely adopted because of the high variability in PSA levels over time.

Prognosis

PSA doubling time is used primarily to assess prostate cancer growth, with shorter doubling times associated with more aggressive disease. After successful surgery, PSA should decrease to undetectable levels, and a rising PSA thereafter is a biochemical sign of recurrence. However, a rising PSA level usually precedes clinical progression by many years, and not all patients will need treatment in their lifetime. PSA doubling time in combination with time to biochemical recurrence and the Gleason score can estimate the risk for progression and need for further treatment in such patients.

Monitoring Therapeutic Response

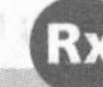

Nomograms incorporating PSA, PSA-derived biomarkers, Gleason scores, and other variables are increasingly being used to individualize therapy and predict outcome in patients with prostate cancer. Although elevated or rising PSA levels after surgery indicate that the tumor has spread systemically, treatment for men with disseminated disease remains inadequate.

Cancer Biomarkers in Development

A number of serum and tissue biomarkers are being evaluated, including human kallikrein-2 (hK-2), IGF, IGF binding protein-3, *PCA3* gene, α-methylacyl-CoA racemase, glutathione *S*-transferase-π, DNA hypermethylation, telomerase, circulating prostate cells, PTEN loss, cyclin-dependent kinase inhibitor, Ki-67, prostate stem cell antigen, and prostate-specific membrane antigen. Some of these markers have high specificity for prostate cancer and have already shown promise. For example, hK-2, which is 80% homologous with PSA, may enhance specificity for detection of prostate cancer in combination with PSA.

Future Directions

Postgenomics technologies increasingly demonstrate that cancer is a remarkably heterogeneous disease at the molecular level. Biomarkers carry the best hope of identifying not only which patients are at highest risk but also how to target therapy, perhaps even directly at the biomarkers or associated proteins.

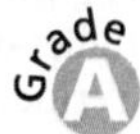

1. Romond EH, Perez EA, Bryant J, et al: Trastuzumab plus adjuvant chemotherapy for operable HER2-positive breast cancer. N Engl J Med 2005;353:1673–1684.

SUGGESTED READINGS

Chun FK, Karakiewicz PI, Huland H, et al: Role of nomograms for prostate cancer in 2007. World J Surg 2007; epub ahead of print. *Review of nomograms for pedicting disease and its prognosis.*

Diamandis EP, Sturgeon C, Hoffman B: The National Academy of Clinical Biochemistry Laboratory Medicine Practice Guidelines. Tumor Markers (Draft Guidelines), 2005. Available at http://www.nacb.org/lmpg/tumor_lmpg_draft.stm. *Consensus guidelines.*

Duffy MJ: Predictive markers in breast and other cancers: A review. Clin Chem 2005;51:494–503. *Critical review of clinical biomarkers in breast and other tissues, including discussion of biomarkers derived from microarray and proteomic analysis.*

Duffy MJ, Ging P: Guidelines for the use of tumor biomarkers. Produced on behalf of the Association of Clinical Biochemists in Ireland (ACBI), 3rd ed, 2005. Available at http://www.acbi.ie/tm%20booklet%203rd%20edition%202005.pdf. *Consensus guidelines.*

McShane LM, Altman DG, Sauerbrei W, et al: Reporting recommendations for tumor marker prognostic studies. Nat Clin Pract Oncol 2005;2:416–422 Available at http://www.nature.com/npcponc/index.html. *Describes criteria for reporting biomarker evaluations.*

Quackenbush J: Microarray analysis and tumor classification. N Engl J Med 2006;354:2463–2472. *A comprehensive review.*

191 CANCER PREVENTION

Scott M. Lippman and Waun Ki Hong

Recent estimates indicate that annual cancer deaths number 6.2 million worldwide and will grow to more than 10 million by 2025. An estimated 1,372,910 new cancer cases and 570,280 cancer deaths occurred in the United States alone in 2005. More than half these cases or deaths involved cancer of the lung, breast, prostate, and colon and rectum. Besides mortality, cancer causes substantial anguish, economic hardship, and morbidity from the disease, as well as from treatment. Cancer therapy has had limited success in reducing the suffering and mortality from many common cancers, so prevention is a high public health priority for improving the control of cancer and its consequences.

EPIDEMIOLOGY OF CAUSES OF CANCER

Tobacco

Tobacco use (Chapter 30) is estimated to cause 30% of the cancer deaths in the United States and is the greatest preventable cause of morbidity and mortality from cancer. Tobacco smoking is associated with more than a two-fold increased risk for lung (Chapter 201), head and neck (Chapter 200), esophagus (Chapter 140), bladder (Chapter 207), kidney (Chapter 207), and pancreas cancer (Chapter 204); moderately increased risk for leukemia (Chapter 195) and colon (Chapter 203), stomach (Chapter 202), and cervical (Chapter 209) cancer; and probably an increased risk for prostate and liver cancer. There is a clear dose-response relationship of the intensity (number of cigarettes per day) and duration of smoking with cancer. The prevalence of smoking in the U.S. population is 24% overall and is higher in younger people and those with less education and lower incomes. Environmental (passive) tobacco smoke has been declared a human carcinogen by the U.S. Environmental Protection Agency.

Quitting smoking can reduce cancer risk; for example, it can reduce the risk for lung cancer by 30 to 50% (at 10 years after quitting) and the risk for oral and esophageal cancer by 50% (at 5 years after quitting). Community-based smoking cessation interventions produce similar quit rates in heavy smokers and significantly increased quit rates in light to moderate smokers when compared with quit rates in control communities. In other trials, rates of cessation for short durations (6 to 12 months) are nearly two-fold higher with nicotine replacement therapy products (patch, gum, nasal spray, inhaler, or lozenge) than with placebo or no intervention. Antidepressant therapy (e.g., bupropion) and smoking cessation counseling alone, even if brief, can also increase smoking cessation rates. In a large, randomized trial, a strong physician message plus 12 group sessions and nicotine gum for 10 weeks reduced all-cause mortality by 15% in the intervention group at 14.5 years. [1] Public education and health policies to discourage smoking (e.g., increasing tobacco excise taxes and legislating clean indoor air) can help in controlling tobacco use.

Alcohol

Alcohol (Chapter 31) is strongly associated with a risk for squamous cell carcinoma of the oral cavity (Chapter 451), pharynx (Chapter 200), larynx (Chapter 200), and esophagus (Chapter 140), as well as hepatocellular carcinoma (Chapter 206). Alcohol is also associated with colorectal (Chapter 203), ovarian (Chapter 209), pancreatic (Chapter 204), and breast cancer (Chapter 208). The risk for breast cancer increases at a relatively low level of alcohol consumption.

Diet

The influence of diet (Chapter 232) on the risk for cancer is extremely complex. Epidemiologic studies have suggested that reduced dietary fat is associated with a reduced risk for breast cancer or that diets high in fruits and vegetables or fiber are independently associated with a reduced risk for colorectal neoplasia. However, randomized trials of dietary interventions have not yielded positive results.

Overweight

By some estimates, obesity or being overweight is second only to smoking as the largest avoidable cause of cancer mortality in the United States. Although the true impact of obesity on cancer is under debate, it has been estimated that this risk factor contributes to one in seven cancer deaths in men and to one in five in women in the United States. Obesity is associated with an increased risk for breast, colorectal, renal cell, esophageal, endometrial, liver, gallbladder, pancreas, and aggressive prostate cancer. Nearly two thirds of U.S. adults meet the definition of obesity or being overweight (body mass index of 25 or greater). Obesity probably promotes tumorigenesis through mechanisms involving insulin resistance, steroid hormones, and inflammation. Obesity has a strong inverse association with physical activity (Chapter 14), which is associated with a moderate protective effect against colon cancer and a small protective effect against breast and possibly endometrial cancer.

Infection

Infections are a major cause of cancer worldwide, especially in developing countries, and cause about 1.6 million cancers annually. Cancer-causing infections include hepatitis B and C (Chapter 152) for hepatocellular cancer, certain human papillomaviruses (HPVs) (Chapter 396) for cervical cancer, Epstein-Barr virus (Chapter 400) for Burkitt's lymphoma (Chapter 196) and nasopharyngeal cancer, human herpesvirus-8 for Kaposi's sarcoma, human immunodeficiency virus serotype 1 for non-Hodgkin's lymphoma, human T-cell leukemia virus type I for T-cell leukemia, *Schistosoma haematobium* (Chapter 376) for urinary bladder cancer, *Clonorchis sinensis* and *Opisthorchis viverrini* for liver cholangiocarcinoma, and *Helicobacter pylori* for gastric adenocarcinoma. Vaccines, antibiotics and other treatments, and environmental control of parasites to control infectious diseases can be effective in preventing cancer. Vaccinating children against hepatitis B virus and treating chronic hepatitis B have been shown to reduce the incidence of liver cancer. A randomized trial of a vaccine targeting HPV-16 reduced the incidence of both HPV-16 infection and HPV-16–related cervical intraepithelial neoplasia. [2] Another, more recent randomized trial in women aged 16 to 26 years and not previously infected with HPV-16 and HPV-18 found that a vaccine against HPV-16 and HPV-18 (associated with 70% of cervical cancers) prevented high-grade precancer and carcinoma in situ of the cervix (versus placebo). The FDA recently approved an HPV vaccine (Chapter 16) for girls and women 9 to 26 years old to reduce their risk of cervical cancer, adenocarcinoma in situ, and high-grade precancer, as well as vulvar and vaginal precancer. This vaccine may reduce the incidence of cervical cancer and the 290,000 deaths that it causes worldwide each year. Evidence is inconclusive regarding whether antibiotic treatment of the bacterium *H. pylori* may prevent gastric carcinogenesis; anti–gastric cancer vaccines targeting *H. pylori* are also under development. These approaches have major public health implications because *H. pylori* is the principal cause of gastric cancer, which is the fourth most common cancer and second most common cause of cancer death in the world. An estimated 50% of the world's population harbored *H. pylori* and more than 335,000 deaths resulted from *H. pylori*–associated gastric cancer in 2000.

Chronic inflammation not linked to specific infections (e.g., the chronic inflammatory bowel diseases ulcerative colitis and Crohn's disease [Chapter 144]) is also associated with increased cancer risk.

BIOLOGY OF CANCER PREVENTION

Pathobiology

Neoplasia is both a multistep process, driven by genetic instability and involving accumulated genetic and epigenetic alterations, and a multifocal process involving multiple genetically independent or related clones. These processes result in several key biologic characteristics that promote cancer, including the evasion of apoptosis, strong replicative potential, and sustained angiogenesis, which are frequently present in both cancer and precancer, or intraepithelial neoplasia. The U.S. Food and Drug Administration (FDA) has approved several treatments of intraepithelial neoplasia, including oral tamoxifen for breast ductal carcinoma in situ and atypical ductal hyperplasia (Chapter 208), oral porfimer (Photofrin) with photodynamic therapy for high-grade esophageal dysplasia (Chapter 140), celecoxib for familial adenomatous polyposis (Chapter 203), instillation therapy with bacillus Calmette-Guérin or valrubicin for bladder dysplasia (Chapter 207), and topical treatment with 5-fluorouracil, diclofenac sodium, or aminolevulinic acid with photodynamic therapy for actinic keratosis (Chapter 214).

Genetics

Cancer genetics (Chapter 186) is intrinsic to assessment of cancer risk and prevention. Genetic testing for highly penetrant mutations (e.g., in people with a strong family cancer history) can benefit individuals in whom such mutations are detected (e.g., they can undergo risk-reducing surgery to prevent primary or second primary cancers), as well as their family members, who should be screened for the presence of such mutations.

BRCA1 and *BRCA2* mutations associated with breast cancer risk are two of the best-studied, highly penetrant germline mutations (Chapter 186). The prevalence of germline *BRCA1* or *BRCA2* mutations in the general population is 0.1 to 0.2%, and carriers of either mutation have lifetime risks of 50 to 85% for breast cancer (Chapter 208) and 15 to 45% for ovarian cancer (Chapter 209). Prophylactic bilateral mastectomy reduces the risk for breast cancer in carriers of *BRCA* mutations by over 95%, whereas prophylactic bilateral salpingo-oophorectomy reduces the risk for ovarian cancer by over 95% and for breast cancer by over 50%, with the breast risk reduction probably being a result of eliminating estrogen produced by the ovaries.

Germline mutations in the mismatch repair genes *MLH1, MSH2,* and *MSH6* are associated with hereditary nonpolyposis colorectal cancer (HNPCC), and germline *APC* mutations are associated with familial adenomatous polyposis and colorectal cancer (Chapter 203). *MLH1, MSH2,* and *MSH6* mutations have a general population prevalence similar to that of *BRCA* mutations and confer a lifetime risk of 80% for colorectal cancer in men and 40 to 60% for colorectal cancer or endometrial cancer in women. Colorectal cancer can be prevented by colonoscopic screening followed by partial or total colectomy (e.g., when large adenomas are detected), and endometrial cancer can be prevented by prophylactic hysterectomy (e.g., in younger mutation carriers who decide not to have more children). Germline *APC* mutations, which can be associated with hundreds to thousands of adenomatous polyps in early childhood, carry a nearly 100% risk for colorectal cancer.

SCREENING AND PREVENTION

Breast cancer screening with breast self-examination does not decrease mortality, but mammography, either alone or with clinical breast examination, every 1 to 2 years decreases mortality in average-risk women older than 50 years (Chapters 13 and 208). No randomized trials have evaluated the Pap smear, but a number of cohort and case-control studies indicate that it can reduce mortality (Chapters 13 and 209). Randomized trials of screening for lung cancer with chest radiography alone or with sputum cytology found no reduction in lung cancer mortality; studies of screening with spiral computed tomography are in progress. Periodic visual screening of the oral cavity can reduce mortality from oral cancer in high-risk individuals. [3] Screening with prostate-specific antigen (PSA) and digital rectal examination is common in the United States, where such screening enhances the detection of early prostate cancer but has not yet been proved to reduce mortality from prostate cancer.

Randomized studies have shown that colorectal screening by testing stool for the presence of hemoglobin, either annually or biennially in people aged 50 to 80 years, can reduce mortality from colorectal cancer by about a third. [4] Regular screening of people older than 50 years by sigmoidoscopy may further reduce colorectal cancer mortality. Little is known about the value of screening with digital rectal examination or barium enema. Colorectal screening with colonoscopy is widely used and is the only technique that offers screening, diagnostic, and therapeutic management of the entire colon-rectum in one procedure. Although no randomized trials have been conducted, the use of colonoscopy is supported by data showing a 76 to 90% reduction in the incidence of colorectal cancer at an average of 5.9 years after complete colonoscopy and polypectomy (vs. three nonconcurrent control groups). Despite its proven efficacy, colorectal screening is greatly underused, and strategies involving public education and other approaches to make these screening tests more acceptable and readily available are being studied.

CHEMOPREVENTION

Chemoprevention is the use of pharmacologic interventions to prevent or treat intraepithelial neoplasia or reduce the risk for cancer, or both. Although high-dose isotretinoin is too toxic for long-term use, a randomized trial provided proof of principle by showing that it prevented second primary cancers in patients after definitive treatment of a first head or neck cancer. A subsequent trial of low-dose isotretinoin unfortunately did not reduce second primary cancers, recurrences, or mortality. Several major chemoprevention trials are summarized in Table 191–1.

Despite consistent data suggesting that β-carotene is associated with a lower risk for lung cancer, β-carotene supplements alone or combined with retinyl palmitate increased rates of cancer in randomized trials involving patients at high risk for lung cancer. [5] In randomized trials of persons at average or below average risk for cancer (e.g., nonsmokers), β-carotene had neither benefit nor harm. By comparison, the combination of β-carotene, vitamin E, and selenium significantly reduced the incidence of gastric cancer and all cancers, as well as mortality from cancer in a randomized trial in Linxian, China, possibly because of restoration of healthy nutrient levels in an undernourished population. [6]

For women at a higher than average risk for breast cancer, the selective estrogen receptor modulator (SERM) tamoxifen (20 mg/day) reduces the incidence of invasive and noninvasive breast cancer by 50% in one study and by 32% in another. This reduction in risk was limited to estrogen receptor–positive tumors. Tamoxifen also reduced the risk for osteoporotic fractures but increased the risk for endometrial cancer, thromboembolism, and cataracts. There was no effect on cardiovascular disease or mental function. The U.S. FDA approved tamoxifen

TABLE 191–1 SELECTED MAJOR PLACEBO-CONTROLLED, RANDOMIZED, CONTROLLED PREVENTION TRIALS

Intervention	Cohort	N	Results
HPV-16 vaccine	16–23-Year-old women	2,392	Reduced HPV-16 infection and HPV-16–related CIN*
HPV-16, HPV-18 vaccine	16–26-Year-old women	12,167	Reduced CIN/CCIS*
Tamoxifen	High-risk women	13,388	Reduced breast cancer*
Tamoxifen	High-risk women	7,410	Reduced breast cancer*
Raloxifene/tamoxifen	High-risk women	19,747	Equivalent breast cancer rates
Finasteride	≥55-Year-old men	18,882	Reduced overall PC,* increased HG PC*
Aspirin	Previous adenoma	1,121	
81 mg/day			Reduced adenomas*
325 mg/day			Reduced adenomas
Aspirin (325 mg/day)	Previous CRC	635	Reduced adenomas*
Aspirin (100 mg every other day)	≥45-Year-old women	39,876	Negative (CRC, other cancers)
Rofecoxib	Previous adenoma	2,586	Reduced adenomas*
Celecoxib (200/400 mg bid)	Previous adenoma (high risk)	2,035	Reduced adenomas*
Celecoxib (400 mg/day)	Previous adenoma	1,561	Reduced adenomas but increased cardiovascular events
Calcium	Previous adenoma	913	Reduced adenomas*
LD isotretinoin	Previous stage I/II HNC	1,190	Negative
LD isotretinoin	Previous stage I NSCLC	1,166	Negative

*Statistically significant.
CCIS = cervical carcinoma in situ; CIN = cervical intraepithelial neoplasia; CRC = colorectal cancer; HG = high grade; HPV = human papillomavirus; HNC = head and neck cancer; LD = low dose; NSCLC = non–small cell lung cancer; PC = prostate cancer.

(20 mg/day for 5 years) to reduce the risk for breast cancer in women with a 5-year predicted risk of at least 1.66% (Chapter 208). The FDA has also approved tamoxifen to reduce the risk for a second, contralateral breast cancer or invasive tumor in women with ductal carcinoma in situ. Another SERM, raloxifene at 60 mg/day, is equally good for reducing the incidence of invasive breast cancer but with lower rates of uterine cancer, thromboembolic events, and cataracts. 7

Other promising drugs to prevent breast cancer include the aromatase inhibitors, which are currently being tested in large randomized trials. Combination oral contraceptives containing estrogen and progesterone reduce the risk for endometrial and ovarian cancer by 50%. However, the adverse effects of this therapy—heart disease, stroke, and venous thromboembolism—make it unattractive (Chapter 262).

Finasteride (5 mg/day), which inhibits 5α-reductase, the enzyme that converts testosterone to the more potent androgen dihydrotestosterone, reduced the 7-year cumulative incidence of prostate cancer by 25% and reduced symptoms of benign prostatic hypertrophy in men older than 55 years with a normal digital rectal examination and PSA level, but it also increased the rate of sexual dysfunction and high-grade prostate cancer. A randomized trial of selenium and vitamin E to prevent prostate cancer is ongoing in the United States.

In randomized trials, aspirin significantly (but modestly) reduced recurrent adenomas of the colon. The selective cyclooxygenase-2 inhibitors rofecoxib and celecoxib significantly reduce adenomas but also significantly increase adverse cardiovascular events. 8 No randomized study, however, has shown a reduction in colorectal cancer.

Calcium modestly reduced the risk for sporadic adenomas in two randomized trials but did not reduce colorectal cancer in a large-scale trial of calcium plus vitamin D. The incidence of colorectal cancer was also reduced by 37% in a randomized trial of combined estrogen and progestin therapy, but at the expense of an absolute increase in adverse cardiovascular outcomes.

FUTURE DIRECTIONS

Virtual colonoscopy, assays for genetic and epigenetic alterations (e.g., in stool and sputum), serum proteomics, molecular imaging, and other new approaches promise to improve screening for cancer and intraepithelial neoplasia in many sites. Cancer risk–reducing surgical procedures (e.g., colonoscopy and polypectomy for patients with sporadic adenoma and HNPCC; prophylactic bilateral salpingo-oophorectomy for *BRCA* mutation carriers) are becoming increasingly practical options for high-risk patients. The major direction of chemoprevention is molecularly targeted drug development, especially for high-risk intraepithelial neoplasia such as familial adenomatous polyposis and oral intraepithelial neoplasia with allelic imbalance.

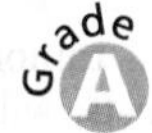

1. Anthonisen NR, Skeans MA, Wise RA, et al: The effects of smoking cessation intervention on 14.5-year mortality. Ann Intern Med 2005;142:233–239.
2. Koutsky LA, Ault KA, Wheeler CM, et al: A controlled trial of a human papillomavirus type 16 vaccine. N Engl J Med 2002;347: 1645–1651.
3. Sankaranarayanan R, Ramadas K, Thomas G, et al: Effect of screening on oral cancer mortality in Kerala, India: A cluster-randomised controlled trial. Lancet 2005;365:1927–1933.
4. Mandel JS, Bond JH, Church TR, et al: Reducing mortality from colorectal cancer by screening for fecal occult blood. Minnesota Colon Cancer Control Study. N Engl J Med 1993;328:1365–1371. Erratum in N Engl J Med 1993;329:672.
5. The ATBC Study Group: Incidence of cancer and mortality following α-tocopherol and β-carotene supplementation. A postintervention follow-up. JAMA 2003;290:476–485.
6. Blot WJ, Li JY, Taylor PR, et al: Nutrition intervention trials in Linxian, China: Supplementation with specific vitamin/mineral combinations, cancer incidence, and disease-specific mortality in the general population. J Natl Cancer Inst 1993;85:1483–1492.
7. Vogel VG, Costantino JP, Wickerham DL, et al: Effects of tamoxifen vs raloxifene on the risk of developing invasive breast cancer and other disease outcomes: The NSABP Study of Tamoxifen and Raloxifene (STAR) P-2 trial. JAMA 2006;295:2727–2741.
8. Bertagnolli MM, Eagle CJ, Zauber AG, et al: Celecoxib for the prevention of sporadic colorectal adenomas. N Engl J Med 2006; 355:873–884.

SUGGESTED READINGS

Chan AT, Giovannucci EL, Meyerhardt JA, et al: Long-term use of aspirin and nonsteroidal anti-inflammatory drugs and risk of colorectal cancer. JAMA 2005;294:914–923. *Data suggesting that high-dose aspirin can reduce colorectal cancer risk, with a discussion on different doses and their effects.*
Dale KM, Coleman CI, Henyan NN, et al: Statins and cancer risk: A meta-analysis. JAMA 2006;295:74–80. *No evidence of reduction of cancer risk.*
Garber JE, Offit K: Hereditary cancer predisposition syndromes. J Clin Oncol 2005;23:276–292. *Comprehensive summary of the prevalence, penetrance, clinical and molecular features, and medical management of the major inherited cancer syndromes.*
Khuri FR, Lee JJ, Lippman SM, et al: Randomized phase III trial of low-dose isotretinoin for prevention of second primary tumors in stage I and II head

and neck cancer patients. J Natl Cancer Inst 2006;98:441–450. *Therapy using tolerable doses was not effective.*

Lippman SM, Lee JJ: Reducing the "risk" of chemoprevention: Defining and targeting high risk—2005 AACR Cancer Research and Prevention Foundation Award Lecture. Cancer Res 2006;66:2893–2903. *Discusses the complex risk-benefit issues of cancer chemoprevention.*

Walter LC, Lewis CL, Barton MB: Screening for colorectal, breast, and cervical cancer in the elderly: A review of the evidence. Am J Med 2005;118: 1078–1086. *No evidence of one age at which potential benefits of screening suddenly cease or potential harms suddenly become substantial for everyone.*

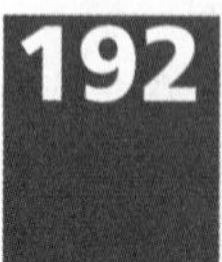

192 PRINCIPLES OF CANCER THERAPY

Michael C. Perry

Diagnosis

Approach to the Patient with Cancer

Few diagnoses produce such emotional responses as "cancer" or "leukemia," and the first moments after those words are uttered often produce a storm of feelings that limit useful discussion. When the time is right, however, the physician must discuss the diagnosis, its implications, and, so far as he or she understands them, the therapeutic alternatives. It is best if other family members or close friends are also in the consulting room, both for emotional support and for another "set of ears." It is often useful to ask "what do you understand about your diagnosis?"

If the physician is not current with the latest treatments, advance reading, for example from the National Cancer Institute's Physician Data Query, will make the interview more meaningful. Prompt referral to a specialist, whether surgical oncologist, radiation oncologist, or medical oncologist, is imperative. The generalist should not be a therapeutic nihilist unless he or she is intimately involved in the field and knows of all current therapies and clinical trials.

The consulting medical oncologist, often advised by a local tumor board comprised of medical, surgical, and radiation oncologists, will usually outline the prognosis and alternatives: standard therapy, possible clinical trials, a second opinion, or no treatment. Many oncologists actively participate in clinical trials and may have investigational drugs available or may suggest referral to a tertiary cancer center as appropriate.

Diagnostic Procedures

In most settings, a lesion has been found on physical examination or by radiographic studies, and a subsequent biopsy has confirmed the diagnosis. It is critical that the biopsy be representative of the entire tumor and that appropriate investigations (e.g., special stains, flow cytometry, cytogenetics, hormone assays) be performed before treatment is initiated. If there is a question as to whether the lesion is benign or malignant or as to its proper classification, consideration should be given to additional biopsies, and consultation with a reference pathologist may be indicated. There is seldom a need for such rapid therapy that appropriate pretreatment evaluations cannot be performed. For many tumor sites, such as the colon (Chapter 203), there is one predominant histology; in others, for example the lung (Chapter 201), the distinction between small cell lung cancer and non–small cell lung cancers is critical for treatment. For breast cancer (Chapter 208), the treating physician is interested in a variety of factors, such as histology, tumor grade, the presence or absence of estrogen and progesterone receptors, and the presence of ERBB2 (Her-2/neu) overexpression.

Staging

After a diagnosis has been established, staging is next. The American Joint Committee on Cancer (AJCC) staging system is considered the standard in the United States and is based on the T (tumor), N (node), and M (metastases) system. The approach to staging depends on the type of cancer but commonly includes plain films, such as chest radiographs, computed tomographic (CT) scans, magnetic resonance (MR) imaging scans, radionuclide scans, and, increasingly, positron emission tomography (PET) scans. These studies are typically supplemented by routine hematologic and chemistry profiles, tumor markers, and, in some cases, bone marrow aspiration and biopsies.

Treatment

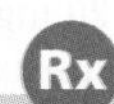

Development of a Treatment Plan

For cancers amenable to surgery, resection is usually the best alternative if the patient is a suitable candidate for anesthesia (Chapter 457) and otherwise is in acceptable condition in terms of concomitant or comorbid illnesses. A joint discussion among the internist, oncologist, surgeon, and anesthesiologist is often very useful in this regard. Determination of the patient's performance score (Table 192–1) is a simple means of assessing functional status. If life expectancy is limited or the patient is not a good candidate for

TABLE 192–1 KARNOFSKY AND ZUBROD PERFORMANCE SCORE SCALES

KARNOFSKY PERFORMANCE STATUS SCALE

Value	Level of Functional Capacity
100	Normal, no complaints, no evidence of disease
90	Able to carry on normal activity, minor signs or symptoms of disease
80	Normal activity with effort, some signs or symptoms of disease
70	Cares for self, unable to carry on normal activity or to do active work
60	Requires occasional assistance but is able to care for most needs
50	Requires considerable assistance and frequent medical care
40	Disabled, requires special care and assistance
30	Severely disabled, hospitalization is indicated although death is not imminent
20	Hospitalization is necessary, very sick, active supportive treatment necessary
10	Moribund, fatal processes progressing rapidly
0	Dead

EASTERN COOPERATIVE ONCOLOGY GROUP (ECOG, ZUBROD) PERFORMANCE SCALE

Performance Status	Definition
0	Asymptomatic
1	Symptomatic; fully ambulatory
2	Symptomatic; in bed <50% of day
3	Symptomatic; in bed >50% of day
4	Bedridden

Rx

surgery, radiation therapy is usually considered as the next "local therapy," with chemotherapy reserved for patients whose disease is too extensive or metastatic. The increasing effectiveness of chemotherapy has resulted in its incorporation into therapy earlier, often as part of an "organ-sparing" approach. The ideal discussion with the patient should include a multidisciplinary approach, with clarification of diagnosis, prognosis, treatment goals, alternatives, side effects, and risks and benefits.

Surgical Therapy

Surgery is used to biopsy a suspected lesion, to remove the primary tumor, to bypass obstructions, and to provide palliation. A preoperative discussion may establish the need for placement of a venous access device at the time of surgery, thus eliminating a second procedure.

Surgery remains the most common method to cure localized cancers, such as breast cancer (Chapter 208), colorectal cancer (Chapter 203), and lung cancer (Chapter 201), but it is limited by the location of the tumor, its extension, and distant metastases. Even if a tumor cannot be removed, a biopsy provides confirmation of the diagnosis. Occasionally, an obstructing lesion can be bypassed to provide palliation.

Surgical staging also establishes the extent of the disease. For ovarian cancer (Chapter 209) surgical "debulking" aims to remove all visible disease, leaving minimal residual disease, to enhance chemotherapy.

In rare circumstances when the primary tumor is controlled, removal of a single metastasis ("metastastectomy") can result in long-term survival; an example is resection of a single liver metastasis found at the time of colectomy for colorectal cancer. A variety of surgical techniques, such as radiofrequency ablation or cryoablation, can treat hepatic metastases in carefully selected patients. "Adjuvant" chemotherapy is often given after surgery in this situation to treat microscopic metastases.

Reconstruction after a disfiguring procedure is critical to long-term physical and emotional functioning. Examples include post-mastectomy breast reconstruction (Chapter 208) and plastic surgery procedures to correct deformities after head and neck surgery (Chapter 200).

Radiation Therapy

Ionizing radiation (Chapter 18) can be delivered using high-energy rays, known as teletherapy, via a linear accelerator; by brachytherapy, through the application of radioactive implants, seeds, wires, or plaques; and intravenously by using radioisotopes. Radiation interacts with molecular oxygen, inducing the formation of superoxide, hydrogen peroxide, or hydroxyl radicals that damage DNA, leading to cell death. Like chemotherapy, radiation therapy is most effective against rapidly dividing cells.

As "local therapies," both surgery and radiation therapy are limited in their effectiveness by inapparent extension of disease, the location of tumors next to normal structures that must be preserved, and the presence of distant metastases. Normal tissue tolerance, which varies among the various organs and tissues, often prevents the use of doses that could uniformly eradicate cancers. Radiation therapy is also limited by tumor hypoxia: large, bulky tumors are frequently relatively "radioresistant," whereas well-oxygenated tumors can be more effectively treated at lower doses.

Radiation therapy can be used as the primary treatment, as part of multimodality therapy, in the adjuvant setting, and for palliation. As a single modality, radiation therapy can be curative for early-stage malignancies such as laryngeal cancer (Chapter 200), cervical cancer (Chapter 209), and prostate cancer (Chapter 211). Breast-conserving surgery (Chapter 208) requires the use of radiation to treat the remaining breast. Partial irradiation techniques using three-dimensional planning with external beam radiation or with a balloon catheter have recently been developed and used for selected patients with appropriately placed breast cancers. For localized prostate cancer (Chapter 211), implanted radioactive seeds of gold or palladium offer an alternative to surgery or external beam radiation therapy, again in carefully selected patients.

Rx

It is important to note that the combination of chemotherapy and radiation therapy may result in synergistic toxicities, such as esophagitis (Chapter 140) in the treatment of lung cancer (Chapter 201) or mucositis in the treatment of head and neck cancer (Chapter 200).

Newer techniques, such as intensity-modulated radiation therapy, permit more exact tailoring of the dose to the target and therefore reduce damage to surrounding normal tissues. Stereotactic radiation therapy or "gamma knife" techniques allow treatment of primary or metastatic brain tumors (Chapter 199) of up to 3 cm with pinpoint accuracy, thereby minimizing damage to normal brain.

Low- to moderate-dose palliative radiation is used to ameliorate symptomatic cancer when cure is no longer the goal. For instance, radiotherapy can improve brain metastases (Chapter 199); relieve pain from bone lesions (Chapter 212); relieve obstructing lesions; and sometimes relieve hemoptysis caused by a lung cancer (Chapter 201) or bleeding from a gynecologic malignancy (Chapter 209). Bone-seeking radioisotopes such as samarium or strontium may relieve pain from bone metastases in prostate cancer (Chapter 211) or breast cancer (Chapter 208).

Systemic Therapy

Chemotherapy

Pharmacogenomics, the study of inherited differences in interindividual drug disposition and effects, is becoming important in cancer therapy because genetic polymorphisms in drug-metabolizing enzymes are often responsible for the variations in efficacy and toxicity observed with many chemotherapeutic agents. Drugs potentially affected by polymorphisms identified to date include the thiopurines, 5-fluorouracil, irinotecan, and the platinum agents. In patients who are heterozygous or homozygous for metabolizing enzymes, toxicity can be dramatically enhanced.

Currently available tests do not reliably permit assessment of the likelihood of response to therapy, so treatment is largely empirical and based on predictive factors from the tumor itself. Gene expression microarrays currently under development may predict responses reliably in the future.

Assessing Treatment

Assessment of the response to therapy depends largely on tumor size, determined either by direct measurement or from diagnostic imaging studies. The categories of response are complete response, with total absence of the tumor and correction of tumor-associated changes; partial response, defined as greater than 50% reduction of tumor size; stable disease, defined as greater than 25% but less than 50% reduction in tumor size; and progressive disease, characterized by either tumor growth or the development of new tumors. Leukemias can be assessed by bone marrow aspirates, and multiple myeloma is typically assessed by measurement of monoclonal proteins, peripheral blood counts, and percentages of malignant plasma cells in bone marrow samples, as well as radiographs of bone lesions.

Chemotherapy is now used in a variety of settings without, before, with, and after surgery and radiation therapy (Table 192–2). Considerable experimental evidence suggests that cancers are most sensitive to chemotherapy during the early stages of growth, as a result of the high growth fraction and shorter cell cycle times, so that a given dose of drug will exert a greater therapeutic effect against a rapidly growing tumor than against a larger, quiescent tumor.

Neoadjuvant Chemotherapy

Neoadjuvant therapy, also called primary or induction chemotherapy, is used before surgery or radiation therapy to decrease the size of locally advanced cancers, thereby permitting better surgical resection, and to eradicate undetectable metastases. It also affords an opportunity to evaluate the effectiveness of treatment by histologic analysis of resected tissue. This approach is most often used for locally advanced breast cancer (Chapter 208), although other primary tumors can be targeted. Disadvantages result from the initially incomplete pathologic staging and the possibility that ineffective chemotherapy will permit the tumor to grow beyond the point of resection.

TABLE 192–2 EXAMPLES OF TIMING OF CHEMOTHERAPY

Adjuvant Therapy	Neoadjuvant Therapy	Organ-Sparing Therapy	Combination Chemotherapy
Stage I and II breast cancer	Stage III breast cancer	Anal cancer	Metastatic solid tumors*
Stage III colorectal cancer		Larynx cancer	Hematologic malignancies
Stage III melanoma		Esophageal cancer	
Stage I–III lung cancer			

*Usually palliative.

Rx

Organ-sparing therapy is the use of chemotherapy, radiation therapy, or both to permit salvage of organs that otherwise would have been surgically removed if cure were the intended result. This technique is often effective in patients with cancers of the larynx (Chapter 200), esophagus (Chapter 140), bladder (Chapter 207), and anus (Chapter 203).

Adjuvant Therapy

Adjuvant chemotherapy is the use of chemotherapy in patients in whom the primary tumor and all evidence of cancer (e.g., regional lymph nodes), have been surgically removed or treated definitively with radiation but the risk of recurrence is thought to be high because of the presence of involved lymph nodes or certain morphologic or biologic characteristics of the cancer. Common examples include cancers of the breast (Chapter 208) and colon (Chapter 203). The typical end points of clinical chemotherapy, such as shrinkage of measurable tumor on serial radiographic studies, are not available in this situation; instead, relapse-free survival and overall survival are the principal measures of treatment effect. For an individual patient receiving adjuvant therapy, there is no means to determine whether the toxicity and expense of the therapy were beneficial or necessary, so decisions are generally based on evidence from clinical trials.

Adjuvant therapy has been used in a wide variety of tumors with variable success. In the cases of breast cancer (Chapter 208) and colon cancer (Chapter 203), the number of lives saved by the use of adjuvant therapy is significant because of the large number of affected patients, despite the modest absolute differences seen between treated and control patients with current treatment programs. Resectable lung cancer (Chapter 201) has recently been added to this list.

Palliative Chemotherapy

Chemotherapy rarely cures cancers that remain after surgical or radiation treatment or that recur after such therapy. Pancreatic cancer (Chapter 204) is perhaps the best example of this scenario, because few patients are deemed eligible for surgery, and most have recurrent cancer after surgery. Most adult patients with recurrent or metastatic disease are considered for palliative therapy if there is no realistic chance of cure, but the potential for prolongation of useful life and/or relief of tumor-related symptoms makes such therapy reasonable.

Combination Chemotherapy

Virtually all the curative chemotherapy regimens developed for hematologic malignancies or solid tumors use combinations of active agents. Combination chemotherapy is also usually superior to the use of single agents in adjuvant and neoadjuvant therapy. The improved results achieved by combination chemotherapy can be explained in several ways. Resistance to any given single agent is almost always present at diagnosis, even in clinically responsive tumors. Tumors that are initially "sensitive" to chemotherapy rapidly acquire resistance to single agents, either as a result of selection of a preexisting clone of resistant tumor cells or because of an increased rate of mutation leading to drug resistance. Combination chemotherapy theoretically addresses both phenomena by providing a broader range of coverage against initially resistant clones of cells and preventing or slowing the development of resistant clones.

TABLE 192–3 HORMONAL THERAPY

Corticosteroids
- Prednisone
- Dexamethasone (Decadron)

Androgens
- Halotestin

Estrogens
- Diethylstilbestrol (DES)

Antiandrogens
- Bicalutamide (Casodex)
- Flutamide (Eulexin)
- Nilutamide (Nilandron)

Antiestrogens
- Tamoxifen (Nolvadex)
- Toremifene (Fareston)

Progestational agents
- Medroxyprogesterone acetate (Megace)

Luteinizing hormone–releasing hormone analogues
- Leuprolide (Lupron)
- Goserelin (Zoladex)

Aromatase inhibitors
- Anastrazole (Arimidex)
- Exemestane (Aromasin)
- Letrozole (Femara)

Estrogen receptor antagonist
- Fulvestrant (Faslodex)

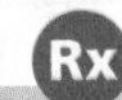

Combination chemotherapy follows a set of principles. All drugs must be active against the tumor. All drugs must be given at an optimal dose and schedule. The drugs should have different mechanisms of antitumor activity as well as differing toxicity profiles, and the drugs should be given at consistent intervals for the shortest possible treatment time.

Hormonal Therapy

Endocrine or hormonal therapy for cancer, the earliest form of systemic therapy, is almost entirely limited to breast cancer (Table 192–3) and prostate cancer (Chapter 211). Many premenopausal breast cancers are thought to be under the influence of estrogens, and hormonal deprivation (ablation) may produce long-term responses in properly selected patients (those with estrogen and/or progesterone receptor positivity who have predominantly soft tissue or bone disease). This hormonal ablation may take the form of surgical removal of the ovaries, ablative radiation therapy, or the use of luteinizing hormone–releasing hormone (LHRH) antagonists. The antiestrogen, tamoxifen, is effective against breast cancer, and it may decrease the incidence of contralateral breast cancers in both premenopausal and postmenopausal women with breast cancer. It also has an estrogen-like activity that is responsible for an increased rate of endometrial cancers. Somewhat paradoxically, postmenopausal women who are candidates for hormonal therapy may also respond to tamoxifen.

TABLE 192–4 IMMUNOTHERAPY

Interferon-alfa (Intron A, Roferon)
Interleukin-2 (Proleukin)

Aromatase Inhibitors

Patients who have experienced a prolonged objective response or stable disease with hormonal therapy may be candidates for second, third-, or fourth-line hormonal therapy. However, such responses tend to become less frequent and shorter, and many patients eventually need chemotherapy. Recently, aromatase inhibitors (e.g., anastrazole, letrozole, exemestane), which decrease the conversion of metabolites in fat and muscle into estrogen, have been found to be more effective than tamoxifen as first-line therapy in both the adjuvant and metastatic settings, although the optimal schedule for tamoxifen and the aromatase inhibitors in the adjuvant setting is still under study (Chapter 208).

Prostate cancer is androgen dependent, and androgen deprivation though castration or antiandrogens can produce meaningful responses. Estrogen therapy now is used infrequently because of its cardiovascular side effects and the availability of better alternatives. Once prostate cancer becomes androgen independent, second-line hormonal therapy rarely produces useful responses.

Corticosteroids

The corticosteroids, typically prednisone or dexamethasone, are widely used in the treatment of hematologic and oncologic cancers. In Hodgkin's disease (Chapter 197), the non-Hodgkin's lymphomas (Chapter 196), and multiple myeloma (Chapter 198), corticosteroids have antitumor activity. In solid tumors, they are used as antiemetics, rarely for the treatment of hypercalcemia of cancer (Chapter 266), and for symptomatic relief of cerebral edema in cases of central nervous system metastases (Chapter 199) or as an adjunct to radiation therapy for spinal cord metastases. Medroxyprogesterone acetate (Megace) is often used in an attempt to relieve anorexia, which is common among cancer patients.

Immunotherapy

Two cancers that are characterized by often unpredictable clinical behavior, melanoma (Chapter 214) and renal cell carcinoma (Chapter 207), are treated with interferon or interleukin-2 or both (Table 192–4). Dramatic responses are uncommon, and immunotherapy is only a minor component of cancer therapy.

Molecularly Targeted Agents

Targeted agents (Table 192–5) are drugs directed at a specific molecular point, such as a protein tyrosine kinase, or at the presence of a specific antigen on a tumor cell. Tyrosine kinase inhibitors include imatinib and erlotinib. The current best example of the success of tyrosine kinase inhibitor therapy is the dramatic response of chronic myelogenous leukemia (CML; see Chapter 195) to imatinib (Gleevec). Imatinib also has activity against gastrointestinal stromal cell tumors (Chapter 202).

Erlotinib, directed against the epidermal growth factor receptor (EGFR), has antitumor effects in patients whose non–small cell lung cancers (Chapter 201) have EGFR mutations. Current research aims to identify the specific types of mutations so that patients can be prospectively selected for therapy, analogous to the measurement of estrogen receptors to select breast cancer patients for hormonal therapy.

The vascular endothelial growth factor receptor (VEGFR) inhibits the formation of new blood vessels that are critical for tumor growth. Anti-VEGFR agents, such as the monoclonal antibody bevacizumab, prevent VEGF from inducing its signal in endothelial cells, thereby preventing their division. Bevacizumab has antitumor effects in metastatic colorectal cancer, non–small cell lung cancer, and breast cancer. Thalidomide inhibits angiogenesis through an unknown mechanism and is used against multiple myeloma (Chapter 198).

TABLE 192–5 MOLECULARLY TARGETED AGENTS AND MONOCLONAL ANTIBODIES

MOLECULARLY TARGETED AGENTS
Imatinib (Gleevec)
Erlotinib (Tarceva) EGFR TKI
Antiangiogenesis agents
Bevacizumab (Avastin) VEGF inhibitor
Thalidomide (Thalomid)
Lenalidomide (Revlimid)
Multikinase inhibitor
Sorafenib (Nexavar)
Scinitinib (Sutent)
Bortezomib (Velcade)-proteasome inhibitor
MONOCLONAL ANTIBODIES
Trastuzumab (Herceptin)
Rituximab (Rituxan)
Gemtuzumab ozogamicin (Mylotarg)
Alemtuzumab (CamPath)
Cetuximab, C-225 (Erbitux)
Tositumomab Iodine 131 (Bexxar)
Ibritumomab tiuxetan Y 90 (Zevalin)

EGFR = epidermal growth factor receptor; VEGF = vascular endothelial growth factor.

Bortezomib (Velcade), a unique drug, is a reversible inhibitor of the proteasome pathway that normally regulates the intracellular concentration of specific proteins, thus controlling homeostasis. It has been effective in the treatment of refractory multiple myeloma (Chapter 198) and non-Hodgkin's lymphomas (Chapter 196).

The development of monoclonal antibodies directed against antigens found on cancer cells represents an additional treatment modality, often complementary to conventional chemotherapy. Examples include alemtuzumab, cetuximab, rituximab, and trastuzumab. Trastuzumab has recently been shown to add significantly to disease-free survival time in patients positive for ERBB2 who receive adjuvant therapy for early-stage breast cancer (Chapter 208). These monoclonal antibodies can be used alone ("naked") or, in some cases, labeled with a radioactive molecule to enhance cell killing. This radioimmunoconjugate approach has been most effective in the treatment of non-Hodgkin's lymphomas (Chapter 196) and chronic lymphocytic leukemia (Chapter 195). The effectiveness of monoclonal antibodies is limited by changes in the antigenic composition of neoplastic cells, called "antigenic drift."

Bone Marrow/Stem Cell Transplantation

Because the major dose-limiting toxicity of most chemotherapeutic agents is myelosuppression, approaches have been developed to harvest the pluripotent stem cells found in bone marrow, peripheral blood, or, less often, cord blood before marrow-damaging chemotherapy, so that the stem cells can be reinfused later (Chapter 184). This technique is most effective for acute leukemias (Chapter 194), relapsed lymphomas (Chapter 196), and germ cell tumors (Chapter 210). The effectiveness of this approach is limited more by inability to eradicate cancer cells than by the inability to achieve engraftment. Transplants may be syngeneic (from identical twin), autologous (from self), allogeneic (from a matched donor, such as a sibling or parent), or from matched unrelated donors (MUD). Nonablative hematopoietic transplants that do not completely abolish myelopoiesis reduce toxicity and allow treatment of older and medically infirm patients.

Individual Agents

A general list of the currently most commonly used chemotherapeutic agents (Table 192–6) can help in understanding the key issues

Text continued on p. 1386.

TABLE 192–6 CHEMOTHERAPEUTIC AGENTS

Agent	Class	Action	Excretion	Unique Side Effects	Drug Interactions	Indications
ALKYLATING AGENTS						
Busulfan (Myleran)	Bifunctional alkylating agent	Interacts with thiol groups of proteins and nucleic acids, forming DNA cross-links; cell cycle nonspecific	Metabolized in liver, excreted by kidneys	Hepatotoxicity (veno-occlusive disease), pulmonary fibrosis, cataracts, skin darkening (pseudo-Addison's syndrome)	None	Chronic granulocytic leukemia, preparative regimens for stem cell transplantation
Carboplatin (Paraplatin)	Platinum coordination compound	Produces interstrand DNA cross-links, similar to those with bifunctional alkylating agents; cell cycle nonspecific	Renal	Nephrotoxicity, ototoxicity, neuropathy, hypomagnesemia, hypersensitivity reactions, hepatotoxicity	Avoid other nephrotoxic or ototoxic drugs	Ovarian cancer, testicular cancer, lung cancer, head and neck cancer, breast cancer
Carmustine (BCNU, BiCNU)	Nitrosourea	Alkylates DNA and RNA; cell cycle nonspecific	Hepatic biotransformation, renal excretion	Delayed and cumulative myelosuppression, pulmonary toxicity (dose-related), hepatotoxicity, nephrotoxicity, cutaneous toxicity	None	Brain tumors, Hodgkin's and non-Hodgkin's lymphomas, myeloma
Chlorambucil (Leukeran)	Bifunctional alkylating agent	Formation of interstrand DNA cross-links with resultant inactivation of DNA; cell cycle nonspecific	Hepatic biotransformation, renal excretion	Hepatotoxicity, pulmonary toxicity	None	CLL, Waldenström's macroglobulinemia, Hodgkin's and non-Hodgkin's lymphomas, myeloproliferative disorders, ovarian cancer
Cisplatin (Platinol)	Platinum coordination compound	Produces interstrand DNA cross-links similar to bifunctional alkylating agents; cell cycle nonspecific	Renal	Nephrotoxicity, ototoxicity, neuropathy, hypomagnesemia, hypersensitivity reactions, hemolytic anemia, SIADH	Avoid other nephrotoxic or ototoxic drugs	Testicular cancer, other germ cell tumors, ovarian cancer, bladder cancer, prostate cancer, lung cancer, sarcomas, cervical cancer, endometrial cancer, gastric cancer, breast cancer, adrenal cancer, head and neck cancer
Cyclophosphamide (Cytoxan, Neosar)	Alkylating agent of the nitrogen mustard type	Cross-linking of DNA and RNA, inhibits protein synthesis; cell cycle nonspecific	Hepatic biotransformation with renal excretion	Hemorrhagic cystitis, SIADH	Phenobarbital increases rate of metabolism and leukopenia; cyclophosphamide potentiates the effects of succinylcholine and may increase oral anticoagulant activity	Breast cancer, ovarian cancer, Hodgkin's and non-Hodgkin's lymphomas, leukemias, neuroblastoma, retinoblastoma, other sarcomas, bladder cancer, lung cancer, cervical cancer, endometrial cancer, prostate cancer, osteogenic sarcoma, Wilms' tumor

Dacarbazine (DTIC-Dome)	Nonclassic alkylating agent	Inhibits DNA and RNA synthesis via formation of carbonium ions; cell cycle nonspecific	Hepatic biotransformation, renal excretion	Pain on injection, flulike syndrome, hepatic veno-occlusive disease, photosensitivity	Heparin, lidocaine, hydrocortisone, phenytoin, phenobarbital, interleukin-2	Melanoma, Hodgkin's disease, sarcomas
Ifosfamide (Ifex)	Alkylating agent of the nitrogen mustard type	Alkylated metabolites interact with DNA; cell cycle nonspecific	Hepatic biotransformation, renal elimination	Hemorrhagic cystitis, nephrotoxicity, CNS toxicity	None	Germ cell tumors, sarcomas, non-Hodgkin's lymphomas, cervical cancer, Ewing's sarcoma, lung cancer
Lomustine (CCNU, CeeNU)	Nitrosourea	Alkylates DNA and RNA, inhibits DNA synthesis; cell cycle nonspecific	Hepatic biotransformation, renal excretion	Delayed and cumulative myelosuppression, pulmonary toxicity (dose-related), hepatotoxicity, nephrotoxicity	Cimetidine enhances toxicity	Brain tumors, Hodgkin's disease, multiple myeloma, GI cancers
Mechlorethamine, nitrogen mustard (Mustargen)	Bifunctional alkylating agent	Cross-links strands of DNA and RNA, inhibits protein synthesis; cell cycle nonspecific	Rapidly deactivated in body fluids and tissues	Extravasation	None	Hodgkin's disease, intracavitary treatment of effusions; topically for mycosis fungoides
Melphalan (Alkeran)	Alkylating agent of nitrogen mustard type	Forms interstrand, intrastrand, or DNA protein cross-links; cell cycle nonspecific	Deactivated in body fluids and tissues, renal elimination 50%	Pulmonary toxicity	Cimetidine decreases oral bioavailability; cyclosporine enhances risk of renal toxicity	Multiple myeloma, breast cancer, ovarian cancer, rhabdomyosarcoma, bone marrow ablation for stem cell transplantation
Mitomycin (Mutamycin)	Antitumor antibiotic	Acts as a bifunctional alkylating agent, inhibiting DNA synthesis; cell cycle nonspecific, but most active in G and S phases	Hepatic biotransformation, renal elimination	Cumulative myelosuppression, extravasation, renal toxicity, pulmonary toxicity, cardiac toxicity, hemolytic-uremic syndrome	Prior treatment with vinca alkaloids may predispose to pulmonary toxicity; if used with doxorubicin, may potentiate cardiotoxicity	Gastric cancer, pancreatic cancer, anal cancer, lung cancer, head and neck cancer, cervical cancer
Oxaliplatin (Eloxatin)	Platinum coordination compound	Produces interstrand DNA cross-links similar to bifunctional alkylating agents; cell cycle nonspecific	Renal	Nephrotoxicity, neurotoxicity (worse with cold), allergic reactions	Avoid other nephrotoxic drugs, incompatible with 5-fluorouracil	Colorectal cancer
Procarbazine (Matulane)	Nonclassic alkylating agent and an MAO inhibitor	Unknown; metabolism produces highly active free radicals that may alkylate and methylate DNA; cell cycle specific, S phase	Renal 70% after hepatic biotransformation	Disulfiram (Antabuse)–like side effects with alcohol ingestion; patients should avoid foods containing tyramine due to the drug's MAO inhibitory effects; central and peripheral neurotoxicity, hepatotoxicity, pulmonary toxicity	>100, including alcohol, antihistamines, anticoagulants, anticonvulsants, hypoglycemics, certain antihypertensives, caffeine-containing preparations, narcotics,	Hodgkin's disease, brain tumors

Continued

TABLE 192–6 CHEMOTHERAPEUTIC AGENTS—cont'd

Agent	Class	Action	Excretion	Unique Side Effects	Drug Interactions	Indications
					methyldopa, metrizamide, sympathomimetics, tyramine or other high pressor amine-containing foods	
Streptozocin (Zanosar)	Nitrosourea	Inhibits DNA synthesis	Renal	Cumulative, dose-related renal toxicity, hepatotoxicity, glucose intolerance	None	Islet cell carcinoma of the pancreas, carcinoid tumors
Temozolomide (Temodar)	Nonclassic alkylating agent	Inhibits DNA and RNA synthesis via formation of carbonium ions; cell cycle nonspecific	Hepatic biotransformation, renal excretion	Photosensitivity	None	Melanoma, brain tumors
DIFFERENTIATING AGENTS						
All-*Trans* retinoic acid (TRA)	Retinoid	Induces differentiation and/or inhibition of clonogenicity	Conjugation to glucuronic acid with subsequent biliary excretion and enterohepatic circulation	Mucocutaneous toxicity, ocular toxicity, musculoskeletal toxicity, neurologic toxicity, hepatotoxicity, lipid toxicity	None	Acute progranulocytic leukemia
Arsenic trioxide (Trisenox)	Natural product	Induces differentiation of acute progranulocytic leukemia cells	Hepatic metabolism, excreted in urine	Prolonged QT interval, acute progranulocytic leukemia differentiation syndrome, leukocytosis, peripheral neuropathy	Medications that increase the QT interval, such as antiarrhythmics and amphotericin	Acute progranulocytic leukemia
ENZYMES						
Asparaginase (Elspar)	Enzyme	Hydrolyzes 1-asparaginine to aspartic acid and ammonia, resulting in a cellular deficiency of 1-asparaginine; sensitive tumor cells lack asparagine synthetase; interferes with protein, DNA, and RNA synthesis; cell cycle specific for G1 phase of cell division	Metabolized in liver	Hypersensitivity reactions, inhibitory effects on protein synthesis with resultant decreases in hepatic synthesis of coagulation factors, pancreatitis, hyperglycemia, CNS depression, hepatotoxicity	Abolishes effects of methotrexate on malignant cells; concurrent vincristine may enhance the hyperglycemic effects of asparaginase and may increase risk of neuropathy	Acute lymphoblastic leukemia
ANTIMETABOLITES						
5-Azacitidine (Vidaza)	Antimetabolite, a pyrimidine nucleoside analogue of cytidine	Causes hypomethylation of DNA and direct cytotoxicity on abnormal hematopoietic cells	Hepatic metabolism, excreted in urine	Renal toxicity, low serum bicarbonate levels	None	Myelodysplasia

Capecitabine (Xeloda)	Antimetabolite of the pyrimidine analogue type	Fluoropyrimidine carbamate prodrug form of 5-fluorouracil; given orally; inactive as itself; inhibits DNA and RNA synthesis; cell cycle specific, S phase	Hepatic catabolism	Hand and foot syndrome, angina	Warfarin potentiation, phenytoin, antacids, leucovorin, thymidine	Breast cancer, colorectal cancer
Cladribine (Leustatin), 2-chloro-2-deoxy-D-adenosine	Antimetabolite	Purine nucleoside analogue, inhibits both DNA synthesis and repair	Uncertain	Bone marrow suppression, fever, paralysis, and/or acute renal failure when used at very high doses for bone marrow transplantation	None known	Hairy cell leukemia
Cytarabine (Cytosar-U, Tarabine PFS)	Antimetabolite	Activated to cytarabine triphosphate in tissues, inhibits DNA synthesis; cell cycle specific, S phase	Deaminated in blood and tissues	Pancreatitis; with high doses, cerebral dysfunction, GI damage, hepatotoxicity, pulmonary edema, corneal damage, "Ara-C syndrome"	With high-dose cyclophosphamide, may increase cardiotoxicity	Acute granulocytic leukemia and its variants, non-Hodgkin's lymphoma, myelodysplasia*
Fludarabine phosphate (Fludara)	Antimetabolite of the purine type	2-Fluoro-ara-ATP inhibits DNA synthesis by inhibition of ribonucleotide reductase and the DNA polymerases; cell cycle specific, S phase	Renal	Neurologic, pulmonary toxicity	None	CLL
Fluorouracil (5-FU, Adrucil)	Antimetabolite of the pyrimidine analogue type	Inhibits DNA and RNA synthesis; cell cycle specific, S phase	Respiratory, small renal elimination	Cerebellar ataxia, myocardial ischemia	None	Breast cancer, GI cancers, head and neck cancer, bladder cancer, ovarian cancer, endometrial cancer, effusions
Floxuridine (FUDR)	Antimetabolite of the pyrimidine analogue type	Inhibits DNA and RNA synthesis; cell cycle specific, S phase	Respiratory, small renal elimination	Cerebellar ataxia, myocardial ischemia, hepatotoxicity	Leucovorin enhances activity and toxicity; thymidine rescues toxic effects	Intra-arterial therapy for hepatic malignancies
Hydroxyurea (Hydrea)	Antimetabolite	Inhibits ribonucleotide reductase, causing inhibition of DNA synthesis; cell cycle specific, S phase	Renal after hepatic biotrans-formation	Megaloblastosis	May enhance the effects of anti-HIV drugs	Myeloproliferative disorders, ovarian cancer, head and neck cancer, cervical cancer (with radiation therapy)
Mercaptopurine (Purinethol, 6-MP)	Antimetabolite of the purine analogue type	Inhibits DNA synthesis; cell cycle specific, S phase	Metabolic alteration by xanthine oxidase, renal excretion	Hepatotoxicity, skin rashes	Dose must be reduced when used with allopurinol; concomitant methotrexate enhances bioavailability of 6-MP; inhibits Coumadin effects	Acute lymphoblastic leukemia

Continued

TABLE 192–6 CHEMOTHERAPEUTIC AGENTS—cont'd

Agent	Class	Action	Excretion	Unique Side Effects	Drug Interactions	Indications
Methotrexate (Folex, Mexate)	Antimetabolite of the folic acid analogue type	Inhibits DNA, RNA, thymidylate, and protein synthesis as a result of binding to dihydrofolate reductase; cell cycle specific, S phase	Renal	Hepatotoxicity, lung disease; in high doses, acute renal failure, acute neurologic dysfunction; avoid use with ascites, pleural effusions	Salicylates, NSAIDs, folic acid–containing vitamins, oral nonabsorbable broad- spectrum antibiotics, trimethoprim/ sulfamethoxazole, other nephrotoxic drugs	Breast cancer, head and neck cancer, choriocarcinoma, acute lymphoblastic leukemia, non-Hodgkin's lymphomas, osteosarcoma, intrathecal treatment of meningeal leukemia, bladder cancer, lung cancer
Pemetrexed (Alimta)	Antimetabolite of the folic acid analogue type	Inhibits thymidylate synthetase, dihydrofolate reductase, and de novo purine synthesis; cell cycle specific, S phase	Renal, after hepatic metabolism	Must be given with folic acid and vitamin B_{12}; avoid use with ascites, pleural effusions	Salicylates, NSAIDs	Mesothelioma, breast cancer, lung cancer
Pentostatin (Nipent)	Purine antagonist	Inhibits adenosine deaminase; also inhibits RNA synthesis	Renal	Fever, fatigue, rash, pain, hepatotoxicity, chronic immunosuppression	Enhances the effects of vidarabine, a purine nucleoside with antiviral activity; must not be given with fludarabine because of fatal pulmonary toxicity	Hairy cell leukemia, CLL
Thioguanine (6-TG, Tabloid)	Antimetabolite of purine antagonist type	Purine antagonist; cell cycle specific, S phase	Hepatic transformation, renal excretion	Hepatotoxicity	None	Acute lymphocytic and granulocytic leukemia
NONCOVALENT DNA-BINDING DRUGS						
Bleomycin (Blenoxane)	Antitumor antibiotic	Inhibition of DNA synthesis; most effective in G2 phase of cell division	Renal	Dose-related pulmonary fibrosis, hypersensitivity reactions, skin and mucocutaneous toxicity, including Raynaud's phenomenon (in combination with other agents), fever, chills; usually considered nonmyelosuppressive	Cisplatin may decrease renal clearance; high oxygen concentrations may enhance pulmonary toxicity, even after therapy	Testicular cancer and other germ cell tumors; Hodgkin's and non-Hodgkin's lymphomas; mycosis fungoides; squamous cell carcinomas of the head and neck, cervix, and vulva; pleural effusions
Daunorubicin (Cerubidine)	Antitumor antibiotic	Binds to DNA by intercalation between base pairs and inhibits DNA and RNA synthesis by template disordering and steric obstruction; most active in S phase but not cell cycle phase specific	Hepatic biotrans-formation with 40% biliary excretion	Dose-related cardiotoxicity, extravasation, red urine	None	Acute granulocytic leukemia and its variants, acute lymphoblastic leukemia

Doxorubicin (Adriamycin, Rubex)	Antitumor antibiotic	Binds to DNA by intercalation between base pairs and inhibits DNA and RNA synthesis by template disordering and steric obstruction; cell cycle specific, S phase	Hepatic biotransformation with 50% biliary excretion	Dose-related cardiotoxicity, extravasation, red urine	None	Acute granulocytic leukemia and its variants, acute lymphoblastic leukemia, breast cancer, bladder cancer, ovarian cancer, thyroid cancer, lung cancer, Hodgkin's and non-Hodgkin's lymphomas, sarcomas, gastric cancer, multiple myeloma, endometrial cancer, bladder cancer, prostate cancer, Wilms' tumor, neuroblastoma
Idarubicin (Idamycin)	Anthracycline glycoside	Intercalates DNA and inhibits DNA synthesis, interacts with RNA polymerases, and inhibits topoisomerase II	Hepatic biotransformation, biliary	Dose-related cardiotoxicity, extravasation	None	Acute granulocytic leukemia and its variants
Mitoxantrone (Novantrone)	Antitumor antibiotic	Binds to DNA by intercalation between base pairs and a nonintercalative electrostatic interaction, resulting in inhibition of DNA and RNA synthesis; not cell cycle specific, but most active in late S phase	Hepatic biotransformation with biliary/fecal excretion	Dose-related cardiotoxicity, extravasation, blue-green urine	None	Prostate cancer, acute myelogenous leukemia and its variants, breast cancer, non-Hodgkin's lymphomas
INHIBITORS OF CHROMATIN FUNCTION						
Docetaxel (Taxotere)	Mitotic spindle poison	Unique mitotic spindle inhibitor; cell cycle specific, M phase	Hepatic metabolism, biliary	Hypersensitivity reactions, fluid retention syndrome, nail discoloration, neuropathy, arthralgias	Inhibitors or activators of the liver cytochrome P-450 CYP34A enzyme system may affect metabolism	Breast cancer, prostate cancer, lung cancer, ovarian cancer, esophageal cancer, gastric cancer, head and neck cancer, bladder cancer
Etoposide (VP-16, VePesid)	Epipodophyllotoxin	Inhibits DNA synthesis; cell cycle dependent and phase specific, with maximum effect in S and G2 phases	Hepatic biotransformation, then renal elimination	Allergic reactions, hepatotoxicity, CNS toxicity, hypotension	None	Testicular cancer, lung cancer, Hodgkin's and non-Hodgkin's lymphomas, choriocarcinoma, Ewing's sarcoma, acute granulocytic leukemia
Irinotecan (Camptosar)	Topoisomerase I inhibitor	Binds to the topoisomerase I–DNA complex and prevents relegation of these single-strand breaks	Metabolized in the liver	Early and late diarrhea may be severe	None	Colorectal cancer, small cell lung cancer

Continued

TABLE 192–6 CHEMOTHERAPEUTIC AGENTS—cont'd

Agent	Class	Action	Excretion	Unique Side Effects	Drug Interactions	Indications
Paclitaxel (Taxol)	Mitotic spindle poison	Unique mitotic spindle inhibitor; cell cycle specific, M phase	Hepatic metabolism, biliary	Hypersensitivity reactions, neuropathy, arthralgias, cardiotoxicity	Enhanced myelosuppression with doxorubicin	Lung cancer, ovarian cancer, breast cancer, esophageal cancer, gastric cancer, head and neck cancer
Paclitaxel protein-bound particles (Abraxane)	Mitotic spindle poison	Unique mitotic spindle inhibitor; cell cycle specific, M phase	Hepatic metabolism, biliary	Hypersensitivity reactions, neuropathy, arthralgias/myalgias, cardiotoxicity	Enhanced myelosuppression with doxorubicin	Metastatic breast cancer
Topotecan (Hycamtin)	Topoisomerase I inhibitor	Binds to the topoisomerase I–DNA complex and prevents relegation of these single-strand breaks	Excreted unchanged in urine	—	None	Relapsed ovarian cancer, small cell lung cancer
Vinblastine (Velban)	Vinca alkaloid	Blocks mitosis by arresting cells in metaphase; cell cycle specific, M phase	Biliary/fecal	Extravasation, neurotoxicity	None	Testicular cancer, breast cancer, choriocarcinoma, Hodgkin's and non-Hodgkin's lymphomas, Kaposi's sarcoma, bladder cancer, neuroblastoma, renal carcinoma
Vincristine (Oncovin)	Vinca alkaloid	Blocks mitosis by arresting cells in metaphase; cell cycle specific, M phase	Biliary/fecal	Extravasation, neurotoxicity, constipation, SIADH	Concurrent use with 1-asparaginase may increase neurotoxicity	Acute lymphocytic leukemia, neuroblastoma, Wilms' tumor, Hodgkin's and non-Hodgkin's lymphomas, rhabdomyosarcoma, Ewing's sarcoma, breast cancer, small cell lung cancer, multiple myeloma
Vinorelbine (Navelbine)	Vinca alkaloid	Inhibits tubulin polymerization, disrupting formation of microtubule assembly during mitosis; cell cycle specific, M phase	Biliary/fecal	Extravasation, neurotoxicity, constipation, SIADH	Drugs metabolized by liver P-450 system, phenytoin	Non–small cell lung cancer, breast cancer, non-Hodgkin's lymphomas
HORMONAL AGENTS						
Anastrozole (Arimidex)	Nonsteroidal aromatase inhibitor	Inhibits the synthesis of estrogens by inhibiting the conversion of adrenal estrogens to estrogens	Metabolized in the liver	Hot flashes, arthralgias	None	Adjuvant and metastatic breast cancer in postmenopausal women
Bicalutamide (Casodex)	Nonsteroidal antiandrogen	Binds to androgen receptors in prostate	Hepatic metabolism	Worsening bone pain, gynecomastia, hot flashes	None	Prostate cancer (usually in conjunction with LHRH antagonist)
Dexamethasone (Decadron)	Corticosteroid	Multiple	Renal excretion of inactive metabolites	Cushingoid appearance, hyperglycemia, fluid retention, osteoporosis,	Efficacy impaired by phenytoin	Acute lymphoblastic leukemia, Hodgkin's and non-Hodgkin's

				muscular weakness, peptic ulcer disease, cataracts, psychosis, aseptic necrosis		lymphomas, CLL, multiple myeloma, Waldenström's macroglobulinemia, for treatment of cerebral edema, hypercalcemia, lymphangitic metastases, and as an antiemetic
Diethylstilbestrol (DES)	Estrogen	Stimulation of autocrine growth factors	Renal	Feminization in men, fluid retention, thromboembolic phenomena, induction of endometrial cancer	None	Breast cancer, prostate cancer
Estradiol	Estrogen	Stimulation of autocrine growth factors	Renal	Feminization in men, fluid retention, thromboembolic phenomena, induction of endometrial cancer	None	Breast cancer, prostate cancer
Estramustine (Emcyt)	Phosphorylated combination of estradiol and nitrogen mustard	Inhibits microtubule structure and function; cell cycle specific, M-phase	Biliary/fecal	Feminization, fluid retention	None	Prostate cancer
Estrogens (Conjugated or esterified)	Estrogen	Stimulation of autocrine growth factors, inhibition of pituitary secretion of LH, resulting in decreased serum testosterone concentration	Primarily renal	Feminization in men, fluid retention, thromboembolic phenomena, induction of endometrial cancer	None	Breast cancer, prostate cancer
Exemestane (Aromasin)	Steroidal aromatase inhibitor	Permanently binds to and irreversibly inhibits aromatase, inhibits the synthesis of estrogens by inhibiting the conversion of adrenal estrogens to estrogens	Metabolized in the liver	Hot flashes, arthralgias	None	Metastatic breast cancer in postmenopausal women
Fluoxymesterone (Halotestin)	Androgen	Suppresses GnRh, LH, and FSH through a negative feedback mechanism involving the hypothalamus and anterior pituitary	Renal	Masculinization in women, hepatotoxicity	May increase anticoagulant effects of Coumadin; decreased blood glucose, resulting in potential for hypoglycemia in diabetics	Breast cancer
Flutamide (Eulexin)	Antiandrogen	Inhibition of androgen uptake and/or inhibition of nuclear binding of androgen in target tissues; its interference with testosterone at the cellular level complements the "medical castration" produced by LHRH analogues	Renal	Worsening bone pain, hot flashes, gynecomastia	None	Prostate cancer (usually in conjunction with LHRH antagonist)

Continued

TABLE 192–6 CHEMOTHERAPEUTIC AGENTS—cont'd

Agent	Class	Action	Excretion	Unique Side Effects	Drug Interactions	Indications
Fulvestrant (Faslodex)	Estrogen receptor antagonist	Competitively binds to the estrogen receptor and down-regulates the estrogen receptor protein in breast cancer cells	Cleared by hepatobiliary route	Arthralgias	None	Recurrent breast cancer in postmenopausal women
Goserelin (Zoladex)	Synthetic decapeptide analogue of LHRH	Suppresses pituitary gonadotrophins, with fall of serum testosterone into castrate range	Metabolism	Worsening bone pain, hot flashes	None	Breast cancer, prostate cancer
Letrozole (Femara)	Nonsteroidal competitive inhibitor of aromatase	Inhibits synthesis of estrogens by inhibiting the conversion of adrenal estrogens to estrogens	Metabolized in the liver	Hot flashes, arthralgias	None	Adjuvant and metastatic breast cancer in postmenopausal women
Leuprolide (Lupron, Lupron Depot)	Synthetic LHRH analogue	Suppresses secretion of GnRh, with a resultant fall in testosterone secretion, producing a "medical castration"	Metabolized in liver	Increased bone pain, hot flashes, thromboembolic phenomena	None	Prostatic cancer, breast cancer
Medroxyprogesterone (Provera, Depo-Provera)	Progestational drug	Inhibition of pituitary gonadotropin production with resultant decrease in estrogen secretion	Renal	Weight gain, thromboembolic phenomena, fetal hazard	None	Breast cancer, endometrial cancer
Megestrol acetate (Megace)	Progestational drug	Inhibition of pituitary gonadotrophin production, with resultant decrease in estrogen secretion	Renal	Weight gain, thromboembolic phenomena, fetal hazard	None	Breast cancer, endometrial cancer
Nilutamide (Nilandron)	Nonsteroidal antiandrogen	Binds to androgen receptors in prostate, inhibiting androgen uptake and binding in the nucleus	Hepatic metabolism	Worsening bone pain, gynecomastia, hot flashes, visual disturbances, interstitial pneumonitis	Increased warfarin effect; inhibits liver cytochrome P-450 system; increased risk of alcohol intolerance	Prostate cancer (usually in conjunction with LHRH antagonist)
Octreotide (Sandostatin)	Synthetic octapeptide analogue of somatostatin	Suppresses secretion of serotonin and GI peptides; blocks carcinoid flush, decreases serum 5-HIAA, and controls other symptoms associated with the carcinoid syndrome	Renal	Hyper/hypoglycemia, hepatic dysfunction	None	Palliative treatment of carcinoid tumors and vasoactive intestinal peptide tumors (VIPomas)
Prednisone (Deltasone)	Corticosteroid	Multiple	Renal excretion of inactive metabolites	Cushingoid appearance, hyperglycemia, fluid retention, osteoporosis, muscular weakness, peptic ulcer disease, cataracts, psychosis, aseptic necrosis	Efficacy impaired by phenytoin	Acute lymphoblastic leukemia, Hodgkin's Hodgkin's and non-lymphomas, CLL, multiple myeloma, Waldenström's macroglobulinemia, for treatment of cerebral edema, hypercalcemia, lymphangitic metastases,

Tamoxifen (Nolvadex)	Nonsteroidal antiestrogen	Competes with estradiol for estrogen receptor protein	In feces, mainly as conjugates	Hot flashes, nausea/vomiting, vaginal bleeding or discharge, hypercalcemia, visual disturbances, thrombocytopenia, endometrial cancer, rare liver dysfunction	When used with coumarin anticoagulants a significant increase in anticoagulant effect may be seen	Adjuvant and metastatic breast cancer
BIOLOGIC RESPONSE MODIFIERS						
Aldesleukin (Human Recombinant IL-2, Proleukin)	Lymphokine	Supports T-cell proliferation, augments natural killer cytotoxicity, induces lymphokine-activated killer (LAK) cell development, and participates in the activation of monocytes and B cells	Renal	Cardiovascular toxicity, nephrotoxicity, pulmonary toxicity, GI toxicity, endocrine toxicity, dermatologic complications, CNS toxicity, hematologic toxicity, fever and chills, infection, capillary leak syndrome	May potentiate effects of psychotropics, nephrotoxic drugs, and antihypertensive agents; corticosteroids may reduce effectiveness	Renal cancer, melanoma
Erythropoietin (Aranesp, Epogen, Procrit)†	Hematopoietic growth factor	Stimulates division and differentiation of committed erythroid progenitors in the bone marrow	Metabolized in liver	Headache, hypertension, possible seizures, allergic reactions	None	Correction of anemia in chronic renal failure, azathioprine-treated HIV infection, myelodysplasia, multiple myeloma, chemotherapy-induced anemia
Filgrastim (G-CSF, Neupogen)	Class II hematopoietic growth factor (acts on progenitor cells capable of forming only one differentiated cell type, the neutrophil)	CSFs bind to specific cell surface receptors and stimulate proliferation and differentiation	Metabolized in liver	Pain at site of subcutaneous injection, allergic reactions, arthralgias, bone pain	None	Decreases the incidence of infection after myelosuppressive chemotherapy, enhances myeloid engraftment after bone marrow transplantation, enhances peripheral progenitor cell yield
Interferon-α (Intron-A, Roferon)‡	Interferon	Antiviral, antiproliferative, and immunomodulatory properties	Renal	Fever, flulike symptoms, cardiotoxicity, neurotoxicity	None	Hairy cell leukemia, Kaposi's sarcoma, renal cancer, non-Hodgkin's lymphoma
Sargramostim (GM-CSF, Leukine, Prokine)	Class I hematopoietic growth factor (stimulates formation of granulocytes and macrophages and is not lineage specific)	CSFs bind to specific cell surface receptors and stimulate proliferation and differentiation	Metabolized in liver	Fever, capillary leak syndrome, pain at site of subcutaneous injection, allergic reactions, arthralgias, bone pain	None	Decreases the incidence of infection after myelosuppressive chemotherapy, enhances myeloid engraftment after bone marrow transplantation, enhances peripheral progenitor cell yield

Continued

TABLE 192–6 CHEMOTHERAPEUTIC AGENTS—cont'd

Agent	Class	Action	Excretion	Unique Side Effects	Drug Interactions	Indications
TARGETED AGENTS						
Alemtuzumab (Campath)	Humanized monoclonal antibody	Targets CD52 antigen present on the surface of most normal lymphocytes and malignant B and T lymphocytes	Metabolism unclear	Hypersensitivity reactions, immunosuppressive	None	Relapsed B-cell CLL, T-cell prolymphocytic leukemia
Bevacizumab (Avastin)	Recombinant humanized monoclonal antibody to VEGF; inhibits angiogenesis	Binds to all human forms of VEGF, preventing it from binding to its receptors, reducing blood vessel formation	Metabolized	Hemorrhage, hypertension, proteinuria, thrombophlebitis	SN-38 metabolite of irinotecan is higher with concurrent use	Metastatic colorectal cancer, lung cancer, breast cancer
Bortezomib (Velcade)	Targeted agent	A reversible inhibitor of the 26S proteasome; inhibits the breakdown of ubiquinated intracellular proteins and disrupts the ubiquitin–proteasome pathway, eventually leading to apoptosis	Undergoes oxidative metabolism via cytochrome P-450 enzymes	Myelosuppression, peripheral neuropathy, asthenia, hypotension	Unknown	Relapsed multiple myeloma
Cetuximab (Erbitux)	Chimeric monoclonal antibody targeted against EGFR	Blocks growth factor from binding to EGFR, preventing cell signaling by tyrosine kinase phosphorylation	Metabolized	Hypersensitivity reactions, rash, diarrhea	None	Metastatic colorectal cancer
Erlotinib (Tarceva)	Targeted agent	Inhibits the tyrosine kinase domain of the EGFR	Metabolized	Rash, diarrhea, interstitial lung disease	CYP3A4 induces and inhibitors may alter metabolism	Second- or third-line non–small cell lung cancer
Gemtuzumab ozogamicin (Mylotarg)	Monoclonal antibody conjugated to a cytotoxic antibody, calicheamicin	Antibody binds to the CD33 antigen found on leukemia cells; when inside the cell, calicheamicin binds to DNA, causing double-strand breaks and cell death	Calicheamicin is metabolized to many metabolites	Hypersensitivity reactions, prolonged myelosuppression	None	Relapsed myeloid leukemia in patients >60 yr

Imatinib (Gleevec)	Targeted agent; signal transduction inhibitor	Inhibits BCR-ABL tyrosine kinase	Hepatic metabolism, excreted in feces	Myelosuppression, hypophosphatemia, fluid retention	Drugs inhibiting/ stimulating liver microsomal CYP3A4 enzyme	Chronic myelogenous leukemia, gastrointestinal stromal tumors (GIST)
Lenalidomide (Revlimid, CC-5013)	Targeted agent	Induces apoptosis	Renal excretion	Neutropenia, thrombocytopenia, diarrhea, pruritus, rash, fatigue, leg cramps	Other myelosuppressive agents	Myelodysplasia, myeloma§
Nexavar (Sorafenib, BAY 43-9006)	Targeted agent	Multikinase inhibitor, inhibits RAF kinase, VEGF, and PDGF receptors	Hepatic	Rash, hand and foot syndrome, fatigue, diarrhea, hair loss	CYP2C9 inducers, UGT1A1 pathway excreted agents (irinotecan)	Renal cell carcinoma
Rituximab (Rituxan)	Chimeric anti-CD20 antibody	Targets CD20 antigen expressed on lymphocytes	Metabolized	Hypersensitivity reactions, lymphopenia	None	Relapsed low grade non-Hodgkin's lymphomas
Thalidomide (Thalomid)	Immunomodulatory agent antigenic agent	Inhibits TNF-α, may inhibit angiogenesis through inhibition of bFGF and VEGF	Nonenzymatic hydrolysis	Teratogenicity, sedation, constipation, peripheral neuropathy, rash	Sedation enhanced with alcohol, other sedatives	Multiple myeloma
Trastuzumab (Herceptin)	Recombinant humanized monoclonal antibody against Her-2/neu	Down regulates expression of ERBB2 pathways	Metabolized	Hypersensitivity reactions	Increased risk of cardiotoxicity when used with anthracyclines or taxanes	Metastatic or adjuvant Her-2/neu-positive breast cancer
DRUGS TO OFFSET SIDE EFFECTS OF CHEMOTHERAPY						
Leucovorin (Folinic Acid, Citrovorum Factor, Wellcovorin)	Water-soluble folate vitamin	Increases general body pool of reduced folates	Metabolized in liver	None	In large amounts may counteract action of anticonvulsives	Prophylaxis and treatment of hematopoietic side effects of folic acid antagonists
Mesna (Mesnex)	Synthetic sulfhydryl compound	Only metabolite, mesna disulfide, reacts chemically with urotoxic ifosfamide metabolites, resulting in their detoxification	Renal	Bad taste, diarrhea	None	Prophylaxis of cyclophosphamide/ ifosfamide-induced hemorrhagic cystitis

*Note: An intrathecal formulation, DepoCyt, is used for the treatment of carcinomatous meningitis.
†Note: Dosing differs among agents.
‡Note: Dosages differ between brands.
§Note: An analogue of thalidomide, a severe human teratogen. Restricted prescribing.
ATP = adenosine triphosphate; bFGF, basic fibroblast growth factor; CLL = chronic lymphocytic leukemia; CNS = central nervous system; CSF = colony-stimulating factor; EGFR = epidermal growth factor receptor; ERBB2 = Her-2/neu; FSH = follicle-stimulating hormone; G-CSF = granulocyte-colony stimulating factor; GM-CSF = granulocyte-monocyte colony stimulating factor; GI = gastrointestinal; GnRh = gonadotrophin-releasing hormone; 5-HIAA = 5-hydroxyindolacetic acid; HIV = human immunodeficiency virus; LH = luteinizing hormone; LHRH = luteinizing hormone–releasing hormone; MAO = monoamine oxidase; NSAIDs = nonsteroidal anti-inflammatory drugs; PDGF = platelet-derived growth factor; SIADH = syndrome of inappropriate secretion of antidiuretic hormone; TNF = tumor necrosis factor-α; VEGF = vascular endothelial growth factor.

each raises. In all cases, the most current information from the manufacturer should be sought before therapy is initiated. The number of new drugs continues to increase, and some older drugs, now less commonly used, have been omitted.

The administration of chemotherapy is best done by specifically trained individuals because of the dual risks of hypersensitivity reactions and extravasation. No doses or schedules are suggested, because these agents are often used in combination, and the doses must be reduced in many cases. End-organ function also affects dosing. The administration of chemotherapy during pregnancy (Chapter 258) is an especially difficult circumstance and requires a particularly high level of expertise.

Unless otherwise specified, all chemotherapeutic agents are capable of producing some degree of nausea/vomiting, myelosuppression, alopecia, mucositis, and/or diarrhea after treatment. Most agents are also teratogenic, mutagenic, and carcinogenic, so these toxicities are not repeated for each agent. Drugs used routinely to offset agent-specific toxicities are also included in Table 192–6.

Management of Complications

Supportive Care

Nutrition is always a concern for patients newly diagnosed with cancer, even if they have not experienced weight loss. In fact, significant weight loss is an adverse prognostic factor for several cancers, especially lung cancer. Patients are often concerned with whether their diet could have contributed to the development of the cancer (Chapter 185) and whether diet can influence the results of therapy. In most settings, neither of these scenarios is the case. Malnourished patients should be evaluated by a dietitian to determine whether they are ingesting sufficient calories and to suggest dietary supplements (Chapters 235 and 237). Some patients, such as those with head and neck cancers (Chapter 200) or esophageal cancers (Chapter 140), may require parenteral nutrition through a percutaneous endoscopic gastrostomy (PEG) tube. Total parenteral nutrition (Chapter 236) is rarely indicated, is not particularly helpful, and is likely to produce an ethical dilemma when therapy has failed and a decision to discontinue it is discussed. Corticosteroids increase appetite but have many undesirable side effects. Megestrol acetate (Megace) at a dose of 800 mg daily improves appetite and allows weight gain in many patients; it is expensive, although the suspension is less expensive than the tablets. The synthetic cannabinoid dronabinol (Marinol) stimulates appetite and reduces nausea in some patients, but it can produce dysphoria, particularly in older patients. A multiple vitamin with zinc may help with abnormal taste and provide trace minerals. Larger than recommended doses of vitamins are not helpful and may be toxic. It is always useful to inquire what over-the-counter and "alternative" medications (Chapter 36) are being contemplated or used by the patient.

Symptom Management

Symptom management is key to successful treatment and a patient's quality of life. Pain control (Chapter 28) can be accomplished with a variety of analgesics, both non-narcotic and narcotic. Oncologists use a 10-point scale for evaluating pain control (Fig. 192–1), and start with nonsteroidal analgesics (NSAIDs) such as aspirin and acetaminophen, progressing through ibuprofen and related drugs, through combinations of NSAIDs and narcotics to stronger narcotics. Newer narcotics are available in both short-duration and long-duration forms, with patches that last 72 hours, which are ideal for patients who have severe pain and are unable to take oral medication. Oral transmucosal fentanyl is more effective than standard release morphine in this setting. [1] Oral mucositis, a common complication of intensive therapy for hematologic malignancies, may be treated with local measures or, potentially, with recombinant human keratinocyte growth factor. [2,3] Oral anti-*Candida* drugs that are absorbed or partially absorbed from the gastrointestinal tract can help prevent oral candidiasis. [4]

Many patients still fear chemotherapy because of the risk of nausea and vomiting. New antiemetics, used in combination, have

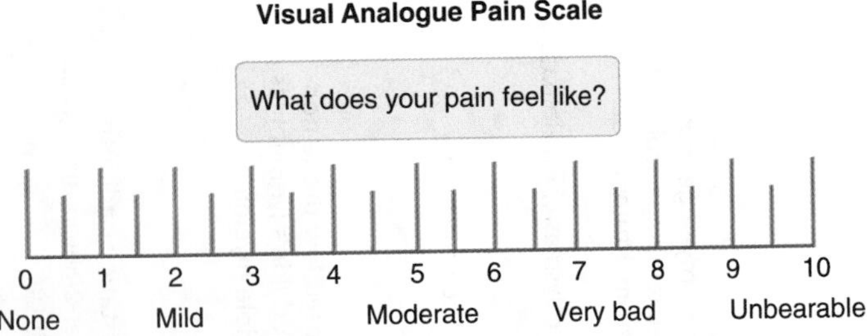

FIGURE 192–1 • Grading pain in cancer patients.

made this side effect much less common. Chemotherapeutic drugs can be ranked according to their probability of causing nausea and vomiting, with prophylactic treatment given accordingly. The availability of the serotonin 5-hydroxytryptamine type 3 (5-HT3) receptor antagonists (dolasetron, granisetron, ondansetron) has dramatically improved the rate of complete control of nausea and vomiting. Although prochlorperazine may be adequate for mildly emetogenic chemotherapy, more emetogenic regimens require combination therapy with a corticosteroid (usually dexamethasone), a 5-HT3 antagonist, and a benzodiazepine (e.g., lorazepam). A newer antiemetic, aprepitant, is particularly useful for the treatment of delayed nausea and vomiting. Treating patients before the development of nausea and vomiting is much more effective and helps patients adhere to their treatment schedule.

Growth factors, such as granulocyte-colony stimulating factor (G-CSF) and granulocyte-monocyte colony stimulating factor (GM-CSF), permit more rapid recovery of white blood cell nadirs, thus permitting chemotherapy to be given on schedule, without reducing doses in many cases. However, such therapy does not reduce hospitalizations or improve survival. [5] It is possible to determine which individuals are at greatest risk for febrile neutropenia (Chapter 173) and treat them in advance, [6,7] based on published guidelines. Anemia induced by chemotherapy can be alleviated, and the need for transfusions and quality of life improved, by the use of either erythropoietin (Procrit) or darbepoetin (Aranesp).

The bisphosphonates (Chapter 264), pamidronate (Aredia) or zoledronate (Zometa), are very effective, not only to treat tumor-induced hypercalcemia, but also to reduce pathologic fractures in bones with metastatic lesions, particularly from breast cancer (Chapter 208) or prostate cancer (Chapter 211) and myeloma (Chapter 198). They are also used to treat osteoporosis caused by chemotherapy-induced premature menopause in young women with breast cancer.

Hematologic malignancies and chemosensitive solid tumors should be treated with prophylactic allopurinol to prevent gout and renal colic from hyperuricemia. The effects of the acute tumor lysis syndrome (hyperuricemia, hyperphosphatemia, hypocalcemia, and hyperkalemia) may be minimized by the use of allopurinol, vigorous hydration, and careful assessment of serum electrolytes.

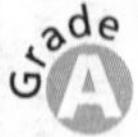

1. Zeppetella G, Ribeiro MD: Opioids for the management of breakthrough (episodic) pain in cancer patients. Cochrane Database Syst Rev 2006;1:CD004311.
2. Spielberger R, Stiff P, Bensinger W, et al: Palifermin for oral mucositis after intensive therapy for hematologic cancers. N Engl J Med 2004;351:2590–2598.
3. Worthington HV, Clarkson JE, Eden OB: Interventions for preventing oral mucositis for patients with cancer receiving treatment. Cochrane Database Syst Rev 2006;2:CD000978.
4. Clarkson J, Worthington H, Eden O: Interventions for preventing oral candidiasis for patients with cancer receiving treatment. Cochrane Database Syst Rev 2007;CD003807.
5. Rusthoven J, Bramwell V, Stephenson B, et al: Use of granulocyte colony-stimulating factor (G-CSF) in patients receiving myelosuppressive chemotherapy for the treatment of cancer. Cancer Care Ontario Practice Guideline Initiative CPG 12-2, 2002. Available at:

www.ccopebc.ca/guidelines/sys/cpg12_f.html (accessed August 25, 2006).
6. Bucaneve G, Micozzi A, Menichetti F, et al: Levofloxacin to prevent bacterial infection in patients with cancer and neutropenia. N Engl J Med 2005;353:977–987.
7. Cullen M, Steven N, Billingham L, et al: Antibacterial prophylaxis after chemotherapy for solid tumors and lymphomas. N Engl J Med 2005;353:988–998.

SUGGESTED READINGS

Aapro MS, Cameron DA, Pettengell R, et al: EORTC guidelines for the use of granulocyte-colony stimulating factor to reduce the incidence of chemotherapy-induced febrile neutropenia in adult patients with lymphomas and solid tumours. Eur J Cancer 2006;42:2433–2453. *Consensus guidelines.*

Halfdanarson TR, Hogan WJ, Moynihan TJ: Oncologic emergencies: Diagnosis and treatment. Mayo Clin Proc 2006;81:835–848. *Comprehensive review.*

Kris MG, Hesketh PJ, Somerfield MR, et al: American Society of Clinical Oncology guideline for antiemetics in oncology: Update 2006. J Clin Oncol 2006;24:2932–2947. *Recommendations based on emetic risk.*

National Cancer Institute's Patient Data Query (PDQ): Current version of therapy for cancers and hematologic malignancies, updated every three months. Available at: *www.cancer.gov* (accessed August 25, 2006). *Addresses common management issues.*

Smith TJ, Khatcheressian J, Lyman GH, et al: 2006 update of recommendations for the use for white blood cell growth factors: an evidence-based clinical practice guideline. J Clin Oncol 2006;24:3187–3205. *Primary prophylaxis is recommended when the risk of febrile neutropenia exceeds 20%.*

Soares HP, Kumar A, Daniels S, et al: Evaluation of new treatments in radiation oncology: Are they better than standard treatments? JAMA 2005;293:970–978. *A comprehensive overview.*

Spinazze S, Schrijvers D: Metabolic emergencies. Crit Rev Oncol Hematol 2006;58:79–89. *An overview of diagnosis and therapy.*

193 MYELODYSPLASTIC SYNDROME

D. Gary Gilliland and Alan F. List

Definition

Myelodysplastic syndrome (MDS) refers to a heterogeneous group of acquired bone marrow disorders characterized by dysplastic growth of hematopoietic progenitors, a hypercellular bone marrow with peripheral cytopenia, and a propensity to progress to acute myelogenous leukemia (AML; Chapter 194).

Epidemiology

Although rare kindreds have an inherited predisposition to develop MDS, most cases are sporadic. In most instances, the etiology of de novo MDS is unknown, although exposure to chemical solvents, including benzene, and exposure to pesticides have been identified as risk factors. De novo MDS occurs only rarely in young patients, but therapy-related MDS and AML (t-MDS/AML) is increasingly recognized as a potentially fatal complication of chemotherapy or radiation therapy, or both, for other malignancies. De novo MDS is rare, occurring at a frequency of approximately 1 per 100,000 per year in the general population. However, the incidence increases dramatically with age, with an incidence of 25 to 50 per 100,000 per year in populations older than 60 years. In this age group, the incidence approximates that of other common hematologic malignancies, such as chronic lymphocytic leukemia and multiple myeloma. As longevity increases in developed countries, the prevalence of MDS will increase. Similarly, with advances in technology that include the use of stem cell support and hematopoietic growth factors, the intensity and duration of treatment for cancer have increased dramatically; to the extent that these therapeutic maneuvers are successful in eradicating the underlying disease, the incidence of t-MDS/AML is likely to increase.

The treatment of Hodgkin's disease (Chapter 197) and non-Hodgkin's lymphoma (Chapter 196) is an example of the problem. Autologous stem cell transplantation (Chapter 184) has proved to be a significant advance in the treatment of Hodgkin's disease and non-Hodgkin's lymphoma, with cure rates approaching 40 to 50% in subgroups of patients in whom the expected survival had been lower than 20%. The counterpoint to the success of intensive therapy has been an increased risk of t-MDS/AML in this population. Because autologous stem cell transplantation is a relatively new procedure and follow-up is not sufficiently long, the exact incidence of secondary t-MDS/AML in this population is not known. However, reported actuarial incidences of t-MDS/AML in patients undergoing autologous stem cell transplantation for Hodgkin's disease and non-Hodgkin's lymphoma range from 4 to 25%.

Pathobiology

Genetics

Clonality

MDS is a clonal disorder with an acquired somatic mutation that affects an early hematopoietic progenitor and gives rise to clonally derived neutrophils, red cells, and platelets. There is no convincing evidence for clonal involvement of B and T cells.

Cytogenetic Abnormalities

Identification of mutant genes in MDS has been difficult, in part because MDS is characterized by loss of genetic material, in contrast to the balanced reciprocal chromosomal translocations typical of de novo AML. Consistent loss of genetic material has led to the hypothesis that MDS is caused by homozygous loss of genes with tumor suppressor activity. The most common cytogenetic abnormalities in MDS are deletions of the long arm of chromosomes 5, 7, and 20. 5q- is present in approximately 15% of de novo MDS and 50% of t-MDS, and abnormalities of 5q or 7, or both, are present in 70% of t-MDS. It has been hypothesized that tumor suppressor genes reside in these loci in which one allele is deleted and that there is concomitant loss of function of the residual allele through point mutation or epigenetic influences. Despite significant progress in identifying the critically deleted regions on chromosomes 5 and 7, genes meeting criteria for classical tumor suppressors associated with 5q-, 7q-, or 20q- have not yet been identified. There is evidence that MDS may be associated with loss of a single allele, or haploinsufficiency, of the *AML1* gene (see later discussion), suggesting that loss of a single copy of a critical gene or genes located on 5q, 7q, or 20q may be sufficient for MDS.

Rare but recurring chromosomal translocations are also associated with MDS. For example, the *MLL (HRX)* gene localized to chromosome 11q23 has been implicated in the pathogenesis of de novo AML and in t-MDS/AML. The t(11;16)(q23;p13) is exclusively associated with t-MDS/AML and results in fusion of *MLL* to the transcriptional coactivator *CBP* (cyclic AMP response element binding protein [CREB] binding protein).

The t(3;21)(q22;q22) translocation, which is associated with some cases of t-MDS/AML as well as with chronic myelogenous leukemia (CML) in blast crisis, results in fusion of *AML1* with one of several fusion partners on chromosome 3, including *EAP, EVI1,* and *MDS1. AML1,* which is also involved in the t(8;21) translocation in de novo AML, contains a highly conserved DNA binding domain that regulates expression of myeloid-specific genes, including myeloperoxidase and neutrophil elastase. It has been suggested that the t(3;21) and t(8;21) fusions disrupt *AML1* function and thereby inhibit early myeloid differentiation.

t(5;12)(q33;p13) is a rare recurring translocation associated with chronic myelomonocytic leukemia (CMML). The consequence of the translocation is fusion of the tyrosine kinase domain of the platelet-derived growth factor-β receptor (PDGFRβ) to a member of the ETS family of transcription factors, TEL. Fusion of TEL to PDGFRβ constitutively activates the tyrosine kinase domain of PDGFRβ, leading to abnormal myeloid proliferation. It has subsequently been demonstrated that a spectrum of chromosomal translocations associated with a CMML phenotype all result in constitutive activation of a tyrosine kinase, including the TEl/ABL, HIP1/PDGFβR, RAP5E/PDGFβR, TEL/JAK2, and H4/PDGFβR fusions.

Many of the chromosomal translocations associated with AML have also been observed in MDS, including the t(15;17), t(8;21), and inv(16) giving rise to the PML/RARa, AML1/ETO, and CBFβ/SMMHC fusions, respectively, suggesting that MDS and AML are a continuum of the same disease.

Point Mutations

Activating mutations that confer transforming potential to the *RAS* gene family occur in 5 to 15% of patients with MDS and are associated with progression to AML. Mutations are rare in *p53*, in the macrophage colony-stimulating factor receptor gene *(M-CSFR)*, and in the neurofibromatosis gene *NF1*, which acts in the *RAS* signal transduction pathway. However, some patients with MDS harbor mutations in the hematopoietic receptor tyrosine kinase FLT3, resulting in constitutive activation of FLT3. FLT3 and RAS may therefore be therapeutic targets of FLT3 and farnesyl transferase inhibitors, respectively.

Loss-of-function point mutations may occur in hematopoietic transcription factors in MDS, including the *AML1 (RUNX1)* gene. *AML1* is required for normal hematopoietic development; thus, loss-of-function mutations associated with inherited forms of MDS, such as the FPD/AML syndrome (familial platelet disorder with propensity to develop AML), and sporadic cases of MDS would be expected to impair hematopoiesis.

Cell Culture Analysis

Hematopoietic progenitors from patients with MDS grow poorly in culture, although poor growth can be partially overcome by addition of exogenous growth factors such as granulocyte-macrophage colony-stimulating factor. There are functional defects in neutrophils (decreased phagocytosis, chemotaxis, microbicidal activity), red cells (ringed sideroblasts with defective iron processing, qualitative defects in red cell glycolytic enzymes), and platelets (defects in aggregation and morphology). Most patients have normal T- and B-cell numbers and normal levels of immunoglobulins and hence are not particularly susceptible to opportunistic infections unless they have been treated with immunosuppressive agents.

Clinical Manifestations

The clinical presentation of MDS is frequently related to cytopenia in one or more hematopoietic cell lineages, with neutropenia occurring in 24 to 39% of patients, anemia in 45 to 93%, and thrombocytopenia in 28 to 45% in various series. In the geriatric population, patients may present with symptoms related to comorbid illnesses. For example, a patient with coronary artery disease may present with mild anemia associated with an increase in the frequency and duration of angina. Other common presenting symptoms include easy bruising, epistaxis or petechiae, and signs and symptoms of infection. Because infection may itself suppress myelopoiesis, any patient with a mild cytopenia (Chapter 173) in the setting of infection should have follow-up blood cell counts to determine whether the cytopenia persists after the infection has resolved. This evaluation is particularly important because MDS confers not only a quantitative defect in the production of myeloid lineage cells but also a qualitative defect in function of those cells. Therefore, a patient with a mild leukopenia may have MDS and be highly susceptible to bacterial infections owing to abnormal neutrophil function. Patients with MDS usually have normal number and function of T and B cells and rarely present with evidence of opportunistic infections. Infections related to opportunistic pathogens are usually seen only in MDS patients who have been heavily treated with antibacterial antibiotics for extended periods of time or who have received marrow suppressive therapy for MDS.

The clinical course of MDS is characterized by inexorably progressive pancytopenia. Although the rate of decline of peripheral blood cell counts is highly variable and may affect one hematopoietic lineage more than another, a clinically significant improvement in blood cell counts rarely, if ever, occurs during the course of MDS. The clinical problems encountered during the course of MDS depend in part on comorbid illness and the extent to which each of the hematopoietic lineages is involved. For example, although it is relatively easy to provide red cell transfusion therapy for patients with isolated macrocytic anemia as the primary manifestation of MDS, anemia may be a significant and life-threatening problem in an elderly MDS patient with coexistent severe coronary artery disease. Similarly, an elderly MDS patient with diabetes may encounter little difficulty with anemia or thrombocytopenia but may have recurrent life-threatening infections requiring frequent hospitalization from persistent neutropenia in the setting of diabetes. Because de novo MDS occurs most commonly in elderly persons, about 30% of patients die of underlying medical conditions unrelated to MDS. About 40% of patients die of complications of marrow failure, such as infection or bleeding, and about 30% die of transformation to acute leukemia.

Diagnosis

Examination of the peripheral blood smear is often helpful in establishing the diagnosis of MDS. Granulocytes are poorly granulated and may be hyposegmented and display the Pelger-Huët anomaly (see Fig. 161–33). Red cells are usually hypochromic with polychromasia. Other abnormalities in red cell morphology can include teardrop-shaped cells, especially in the subset of MDS patients with bone marrow fibrosis, as well as red cell fragments and nucleated cells. Mild macrocytosis is a hallmark of MDS, with mean corpuscular volume (MCV) in the range 100 to 110 μm^3. MCVs outside this range make a diagnosis of MDS less likely. Platelets may be large, and megakaryocyte fragments may be present.

A bone marrow aspirate and biopsy are required to provide a definitive diagnosis. Evidence of dysmyelopoiesis can include abnormal granules, such as large primary granules or decreased numbers of granules, the presence of bizarre nuclear forms in myeloid lineage cells, the Pelger-Huët anomaly, and Auer rods (see Fig. 161–31). Signs of dyserythropoiesis may include multinuclear forms, nuclear fragments, megaloblastic changes, nuclear-cytoplasmic dyssynchrony, and ringed sideroblasts. Finally, dysplasia affecting megakaryocyte lineage cells can include bizarre nuclear figures, decreased ploidy, separated nuclei (so-called pawn ball nuclei), and micro-megakaryocytes. The percentage of myeloblasts may be increased and is used as part of the classification of MDS. The bone marrow cellularity is usually normal or increased despite the fact that most patients present with peripheral blood cytopenia.

Characteristic cytogenetic abnormalities are another helpful clue in the diagnosis of MDS, although normal cytogenetics do not exclude the diagnosis. Most cytogenetic abnormalities in MDS are characterized by loss of genetic material through deletions. Nonrandom chromosomal abnormalities associated with MDS include 5q-, which occurs in approximately 15% of de novo MDS and 50% of secondary MDS; monosomy 7; trisomy 8; 21q-; 17q-; and 20q-. As many as 80% of patients have detectable chromosomal abnormalities.

Differential Diagnosis

A diagnosis of MDS requires the exclusion of other disorders that may cause peripheral cytopenias (Table 193–1). The evaluation of a patient with unexplained cytopenia (Chapters 171 and 173) should always include exclusion of congenital disorders associated with cytopenia, vitamin deficiencies, and toxic drugs. Whenever possible, patients should discontinue any medications that can cause cytopenia for at least 6 to 8 weeks. A careful physical examination should search for evidence of hypersplenism (Chapter 174), with attention to various potential underlying causes, such as myelofibrosis, hepatic cirrhosis, and other hematologic disorders (e.g., hairy cell leukemia or primary splenic lymphoma). Alcoholic patients may present with a combination of vitamin deficiency, alcoholic myelosuppression, and hypersplenism that may resemble MDS (Chapter 157). Some physicians incorporate testing for autoimmune diseases, such as antinuclear antibody tests, in the evaluation of cytopenia, although it is rare that cytopenia is the only presenting finding for autoimmune disorders (Chapters 171 and 173). When the initial physical examination, laboratory evaluation, and removal of potentially causative drugs fail to disclose a cause for a cytopenia, bone marrow aspiration and biopsy with cytogenetic analysis should be performed to address the possibility that the patient may have MDS or another cause of the cytopenia, such as aplastic anemia, leukemia, or marrow infiltration by malignant cells.

MDS is currently classified by a scheme developed by the World Health Organization (Table 193–2). Although these categories carry prognostic information, the International Prognostic Scoring System (IPSS) provides the most reliable estimates of survival and likelihood of progression to AML.

Treatment

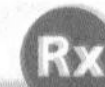

Supportive care may include transfusion of red cells (Chapter 183) with chelation therapy to prevent iron overload, prevention and treatment of infection, and transfusion of platelets for clinically significant bleeding. Pyridoxine, a cofactor in heme biosynthesis, is nontoxic and is often given for 3 months in patients with anemia from MDS; responses are rare. There is no clear role for corticosteroids, androgens, or other vitamins in the therapy of MDS, despite anecdotal reports of response.

Hematopoietic Growth Factors

There is no known survival benefit from administration of any hematopoietic growth factor either alone or in combination. About 15 to 30% of patients respond to recombinant human erythropoietin (rhuEPO), which is most effective when pretreatment serum EPO levels are less than 200 U/mL, the transfusion requirement is low (less than 2 U/month), and blasts represent less than 10% of bone marrow cells. For patients who are refractory to rhuEPO monotherapy, dose escalation or coadministration of granulocyte colony-stimulating factor (G-CSF), or both, may elicit a response. G-CSF given alone almost invariably results in hematologic responses and may be of value in management of infections that complicate moderate to severe neutropenia. Darbepoetin alfa, a hypersialylated erythropoietic stimulating protein with a long half-life, may be as effective as rhuEPO and permit less frequent dosing.

Hematopoietic Stem Cell Transplantation

(Chapter 184)

Related or unrelated donor hematopoietic stem cell transplantation (HSCT) remains the only known cure for MDS and should be considered the treatment of choice for patients who meet age and donor criteria. Disease-free survivals can exceed 15 years. Allogeneic HSCT, especially including experimental nonmyeloablative HSCT, is being used in older (age 55 to 66 years) patients; as a result, as many as 50% of patients with MDS may be candidates for HSCT, usually without prior chemotherapy. Age younger than 40 years and a short duration of disease before transplantation are favorable prognostic indicators.

Overall long-term survival after HSCT is about 46%, and patients who have refractory anemia and receive transplants with fully matched related donors have as high as 75% long-term, disease-free survival. Even in patients 55 to 66 years old, overall 3-year, disease-free survival is greater than 53%. The risk of relapse is higher in patients with worse IPSS scores (see later text).

Epigenetic Therapy

5-Azacytidine, which interferes with DNA methylation, prolongs median time to progression to AML and median survival [1]; it is approved by the U.S. Food and Drug Administration (FDA) for treatment of all subtypes of MDS. Decitabine, another methyltransferase inhibitor with activity in MDS, is under review for approval by the FDA.

Drugs with Antiangiogenic Activity

Oral lenalidomide, a 4-aminoglutaramide analogue of thalidomide with putative anti-angiogenic activity, provides about a 60% response rate in erythropoietin-unresponsive MDS patients, with most patients no longer requiring transfusions. [2] Response rates are highest in patients with chromosomal deletions of 5q31.1 (83%), compared with 56% in patients with normal karyotype and only 12% in patients with other karyotypic abnormalities. As a result, lenalidomide is approved by the FDA for treatment of transfusion-dependent MDS with 5q deletion. Other angiogenic drugs with modest activity in MDS include arsenic trioxide and vascular endothelial growth factor receptor inhibitors, such as bevacizumab; these agents are under active investigation.

TABLE 193–1 DIFFERENTIAL DIAGNOSIS OF MYELODYSPLASTIC SYNDROME

CONGENITAL DISORDERS

Hereditary sideroblastic anemia
Fanconi's anemia
Diamond-Blackfan syndrome
Kostmann's syndrome
Shwachman's syndrome
Down syndrome

VITAMIN DEFICIENCY

B_{12}, folate, or iron deficiency

DRUG TOXICITY

Marrow suppression from oral or parenteral medications
Toxins
Chemotherapy and/or radiation therapy
Alcohol

ANEMIA OF CHRONIC DISEASE

Renal failure
Chronic infection, including tuberculosis
Rheumatologic disorders

VIRAL MARROW SUPPRESSION

Including Epstein-Barr virus, parvovirus B19, human immunodeficiency virus, and others

MARROW INFILTRATION

Acute and chronic leukemias
Metastatic solid tumor infiltration

PAROXYSMAL NOCTURNAL HEMOGLOBINURIA
HYPERSPLENISM

TABLE 193–2 WORLD HEALTH ORGANIZATION CLASSIFICATION OF MYELODYSPLASTIC SYNDROME

Category	Peripheral Blood	Bone Marrow
1a. RA without dysplasia	Blasts <1%; monocytes <1000/mm^3	Blasts <5%; ringed sideroblasts <15%
1b. RA with dysplasia	Same + dysgranulocytes and/or giant platelets	Same + dysgranulocytes and/or dysmegakaryocytes
2a. RARS without dysplasia	Blasts <1%; monocytes <1000/mm^3	Blasts <5%; ≥15% ringed sideroblasts
2b. RARS with dysplasia	Same + dysgranulocytes and/or giant platelets	Same + dysgranulocytes and/or dysmegakaryocytes
3a. RAEB-I	Blasts 1–4%; monocytes <1000/mm^3	Blasts 5–10%
3b. RAEB-II	Blasts 5–19%; monocytes <1000/mm^3	Blasts 11–19%

RA = refractory anemia; RAEB = refractory anemia with excess blasts; RARS = refractory anemia with ringed sideroblasts.

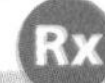

Conventional Chemotherapy

Remission rates for MDS or secondary AML (evolving from MDS) range from 18 to 44% with standard antileukemia regimens; treatment-related deaths occur in as many as half of patients. Treatment with fludarabine 30 mg/m^2, cytarabine 2 g/m^2 daily for 5 days, and G-CSF has provided complete response rates comparable to those for induction chemotherapy for de novo AML. However, duration of remission is brief, and it is not yet clear whether intensive chemotherapy prolongs survival. Intensive chemotherapy, with or without growth factor support, can be recommended only under the auspices of a clinical trial.

Immunosuppressive Therapy

Several clinical observations have suggested a link between MDS and aplastic anemia (Chapter 171), which often responds to immunosuppressive therapy with antithymocyte globulin (ATG) or cyclosporin A, or both. Several phase II trials have suggested that ATG or cyclosporin A is well tolerated and effective in some patients with MDS, but treatment should be undertaken only in the context of a clinical trial.

Signal Transduction Inhibitors

RAS inhibition using farnesyl transferase inhibitors and FLT3 inhibition using small molecule ATP analogues, such as tipifarnib and lonafarnib, are being tested in clinical trials but are not FDA approved for this indication. In MDS patients who progress to CMML and have activating alleles of the PDGFRβ, imatinib is effective.

Prognosis

Median survival has historically ranged from 0.4 years in high-risk patients to 5.7 years in low-risk patients. In the 1990s, a prognostic score based on the presence of peripheral cytopenias, bone marrow blasts, and karyotype correlated well with overall survival and likelihood of progression to AML. It still is potentially useful for guiding therapy but is no longer likely to be accurate in the era of azacitidine and lenalidomide.

Future Directions

The remarkable efficacy of lenalidomide, particularly in patients with 5q deletions, may provide new insights into the pathophysiology of MDS.

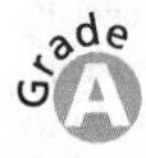

1. Silverman LR, Demakos EP, Peterson BL, et al: Randomized controlled trial of azacitidine in patients with the myelodysplastic syndrome: A study of the cancer and leukemia group B. J Clin Oncol 2002;20:2429–2440.
2. List A, Kurtin S, Roe DJ, et al: Efficacy of lenalidomide in myelodysplastic syndromes. N Engl J Med 2005;352:549–557.

SUGGESTED READINGS

Bowen DT: Treatment strategies and issues in low/intermediate-1-risk myelodysplastic syndrome (MDS) patients. Semin Oncol 2005;32:S16–S23. *Approach to treatment in different subgroups.*

de Witte T, Oosterveld M, Muus P: Autologous and allogeneic stem cell transplantation for myelodysplastic syndrome. Blood Rev 2007;21:49–59. *A clinical review.*

Hofmann WK, Koeffler HP: Myelodysplastic syndrome. Annu Rev Med 2005; 56:1–16. *A comprehensive review.*

List A, Dewald G, Bennett J, et al: Lenalidomide in the myelodysplastic syndrome with chromosome 5q deletion. N Engl J Med 2006;355:1456–1465. *Lenalidomide can reduce transfusion requirements and reverse cytologic and cytogenetic abnormalities.*

Mano H: DNA micro-array analysis of myelodysplastic syndrome. Leuk Lymphoma 2006;47:9–14. *The course of MDS consists of distinct stages, each with its own "molecular signature."*

Steensma DP, Bennett JM: The myelodysplastic syndromes: Diagnosis and treatment. Mayo Clin Proc 2006;81:104–130. *A comprehensive review.*

194 THE ACUTE LEUKEMIAS

Frederick R. Appelbaum

Definition

Normal hematopoiesis (Chapter 160) requires tightly regulated proliferation and differentiation of pluripotent hematopoietic stem cells that become mature peripheral blood cells. Acute leukemia is the result of a malignant event or events occurring in an early hematopoietic precursor. Instead of proliferating and differentiating normally, the affected cell gives rise to progeny that fail to differentiate but continue to proliferate in an uncontrolled fashion. As a result, immature myeloid cells in acute myeloid leukemia (AML), or lymphoid cells in acute lymphoblastic leukemia ALL)—often called blasts—rapidly accumulate and progressively replace the bone marrow, diminishing the production of normal red cells, white cells, and platelets. This loss of normal marrow function in turn gives rise to the common clinical complications of leukemia: anemia, infection, and bleeding. With time, the leukemic blasts pour out into the blood stream and eventually occupy the lymph nodes, spleen, and other vital organs. If untreated, acute leukemia is rapidly fatal; most patients die within several months after diagnosis. With appropriate therapy, however, the natural history of acute leukemia can be markedly altered, and many patients can be cured.

Epidemiology

Incidence

About 35,000 new cases of leukemia are diagnosed in the United States each year, at a rate of about 8.5 cases per 100,000 persons; this rate has remained consistent for the past 3 decades. Approximately 34% of these cases are AML, 28% are chronic lymphocytic leukemia (CLL), 13% are chronic myeloid leukemia (CML), 11% are ALL, and the remainder are all others. The leukemias account for about 3% of all cancers in the United States. The impact of leukemia is heightened because of the young age of some patients. For example, with a maximum incidence between ages 2 and 10 years, ALL is the most common cancer and the second leading cause of death in children younger than 15 years of age. In contrast, the incidence of AML gradually increases with age, without an early peak. The median age at diagnosis of AML is about 60 years.

Determinants

In most cases, acute leukemia develops for no known reason, but sometimes a possible cause can be identified.

Radiation

Ionizing radiation (Chapter 18) is leukemogenic. ALL, AML, and CML are all increased in incidence among patients given radiation therapy for ankylosing spondylitis and among survivors of the atomic bomb blasts at Hiroshima and Nagasaki. The magnitude of the risk depends on the dose of radiation, its distribution in time, and the age of the individual. Greater risk results from higher-dose radiation delivered over shorter periods to younger patients. In areas of high natural background radiation (often from radon), chromosomal aberrations have been reported to be more frequent, but an increase in acute leukemia has not been consistently found. Concern has been raised about the possible leukemogenic effects of extremely low-frequency nonionizing electromagnetic fields emitted by electrical installations. If such an effect exists at all, its magnitude is small.

Oncogenic Viruses

The search for a viral cause of leukemia has been intensely pursued, but only two clear associations have been found. Human T-cell lymphotropic virus type I (HTLV-I), an enveloped, single-stranded RNA virus, is considered to be the causative agent of adult T-cell leukemia (ATL) (Chapter 195). This distinct form of leukemia is found within geographic clusters in southwestern Japan, the Caribbean basin, and Africa. The virus can be spread vertically from mother to fetus or horizontally by sexual contact or through blood products. The cumulative lifetime risk of developing ATL is estimated to be 3% among individuals infected with

HTLV-I. Although previously rare in the United States, HTLV-I seropositivity has been found with increasing frequency among patients undergoing frequent transfusions and intravenous drug users. Screening of blood products for antibodies to HTLV-I is routine practice in blood banks in the United States. Epstein-Barr virus (Chapter 401), the DNA virus that causes infectious mononucleosis, is associated with Burkitt's lymphoma (Chapter 196) and its leukemic counterpart, mature B-cell ALL.

Chemicals and Drugs

Heavy occupational exposure to benzene and benzene-containing compounds such as kerosene and carbon tetrachloride may lead to marrow damage, which can take the form of aplastic anemia, myelodysplasia, or AML. A link between leukemia and tobacco use has recently been reported.

With increasing use of chemotherapy to treat other malignancies, the incidence of AML secondary to prior chemotherapy has increased and may represent 6 to 10% of all cases. Prior exposure to alkylating agents such as melphalan and the nitrosoureas is associated with an increased risk of secondary AML, often first manifested as a myelodysplastic syndrome (Chapter 193), frequently with abnormalities of chromosomes 5, 7, and 8, but with no distinct morphologic features. These secondary AMLs typically develop 4 to 6 years after exposure to alkylating agents, and their incidence may be increased with greater intensity and duration of drug exposure. Prolonged exposure to epipodophyllotoxins (teniposide or etoposide) has also been identified as a risk factor for the development of AML. The secondary leukemias associated with epipodophyllotoxin exposure tend to have a shorter latency period (1 to 2 years), lack a myelodysplastic phase, have a monocytic morphology, and involve abnormalities of the long arm of chromosome 11 (band q23) or chromosome 21 (band q22). Recently, an association between the development of acute promyelocytic leukemia (APL) and prior treatment for psoriasis with bimolane, a dioxopiperazine derivative, has been reported.

Pathobiology

Genetics

If leukemia develops before 10 years of age in a patient with an identical twin, the unaffected twin has a 20% chance of subsequently developing leukemia. Several syndromes with somatic cell chromosome aneuploidy (Chapter 39), including trisomy 21 (Down), trisomy 13 (Patau), and XXY (Klinefelter; Chapters 39 and 252) are associated with an increased incidence of AML. Other inherited mutations, for example, a mutation at 21q22, have been associated with a high incidence of AML in rare families. Several autosomal recessive disorders associated with chromosomal instability are prone to terminate in acute leukemia, including Bloom's syndrome, Fanconi's anemia (Chapter 171), and ataxia-telangiectasia (Chapter 271).

Clonality and Cell of Origin

The acute leukemias are clonal disorders, and all leukemic cells in a given patient are descended from a common progenitor. The clonal nature of acute leukemia suggests that there are leukemic stem cells capable of both self-renewal and proliferation. Recent studies suggest that the leukemic stem cells in AML are rare among the leukemic mass, with a frequency of 0.2 to 10×10^6, and are within the primitive $CD34^{++}$ $CD38^-$ fraction. Less is known about the ALL stem cell.

Classification

The acute leukemias can be classified in a number of ways, including morphology, cytochemistry, cell surface markers, cytoplasmic markers, cytogenetics, and oncogene expression. For more than three decades the French-American-British (FAB) system, which relies on morphology, was the principal method of classification (Table 194–1). The more recent World Health Organization classification includes molecular and clinical features as well as morphologic features (Table 194–2).

Morphology

Leukemic cells in AML are typically 12 to 20 nm in diameter, with discrete nuclear chromatin, multiple nucleoli, and cytoplasm that usually contains azurophilic granules. Auer rods, which are slender, fusiform cytoplasmic inclusions that stain red with Wright-Giemsa stain, are virtually pathognomonic of AML. The FAB system divides AML into eight subtypes based on morphology: M0, M1, M2, and M3 reflect increasing degrees of differentiation of myeloid leukemic cells; M4 and M5 leukemias have features of the monocytic lineage; M6 has features of the erythroid cell lineage; and M7 is acute megakaryocytic leukemia.

The leukemic cells in ALL tend to be smaller than AML blasts and relatively devoid of granules. ALL can be divided, by FAB criteria, into L1, L2, and L3 subgroups. L1 blasts are uniform in size, with homogeneous nuclear chromatin, indistinct nucleoli, and scanty cytoplasm with few, if any, granules. L2 blasts are larger and more variable in size and may have nucleoli. L3 blasts are distinct, with prominent nucleoli and deeply basophilic cytoplasm with vacuoles.

Cell Surface Markers

Monoclonal antibodies reactive with cell surface antigens have been used to classify acute leukemias. Antibodies that react with antigens found on normal immature myeloid cells, including CD13, CD14, CD33, and CD34, also react with blast cells from most patients with AML. Exceptions are the M6 and M7 variants, which have antigens restricted to the red cell and the platelet lineage, respectively. Myeloid leukemia blasts also express human leukocyte antigen (HLA)-DR antigens but usually lack T-cell, B-cell, and other lymphoid antigens. In 10 to 20% of patients, however, otherwise typical AML blasts also express antigens usually restricted to B- or T-cell lineage. Expression of lymphoid antigens by AML cells does not change either the natural history or the therapeutic response of these leukemias.

Approximately 75% of cases of ALL express B-lineage antigens and can be further divided into four categories. The most immature group, pro-B ALL, expresses CD19 but not other B-lineage antigens and represents about 10% of cases of ALL. Approximately 50 to 60% of cases of ALL express the common ALL antigen (CALLA, or CD10), which is a glycoprotein that is also found occasionally on normal early lymphocytes and other nonhematopoietic tissues. CALLA-positive ALL is thought to represent an early pre–B-cell differentiation state. Approximately 10% of cases of ALL have intracytoplasmic immunoglobulin and are termed pre–B-cell ALL. B-cell ALL is signified by the presence of immunoglobulin on the cell surface and accounts for fewer than 5% of cases of ALL. In general, the best therapeutic outcomes among B-cell ALL types are with early pre–B-cell (CALLA positive) ALL. Among the 25% of cases of ALL that express T-lineage antigens, fewer than half are so-called pre–T-cell types that express CD3 with either CD4 and CD8 or neither CD4 nor CD8; the majority of cases, termed T-cell ALL, express CD3 and either CD4 or CD8. The prognosis for T-cell ALL is superior to that for pre–T-cell ALL. In about 25% of patients with ALL, the leukemic cells also express myeloid antigens. The presence of such antigens defines a group of patients who historically had a somewhat worse prognosis; with current, more aggressive regimens, however, the impact of myeloid antigen expression has disappeared.

Occasional cases of acute leukemia lack evidence of lineage commitment and are termed acute undifferentiated leukemia. Other cases display characteristics of both myeloid and lymphoid commitment. In some of these cases, single neoplastic cells express features of both lineages (biphenotypic), whereas in other cases two distinct subpopulations of leukemia cells can be found, one expressing myeloid and the other lymphoid features (bilineal). In general, the prognosis for patients with truly undifferentiated, biphenotypic or bilineal acute leukemia is poor whether they are treated as myeloid or lymphoid malignancies.

Cytogenetics and Molecular Biology

In most cases of acute leukemia, an abnormality in chromosome number or structure is found. These abnormalities are clonal, involving all of the malignant cells in a given patient; they are acquired and are not found in the normal cells of the patient; and they are referred to as "nonrandom," because specific abnormalities are found in multiple cases of AML and are associated with distinct morphologic or clinical subtypes of the disease. These abnormalities may be simply the gain or loss of whole chromosomes, but more often they include chromosomal translocations, deletions, or inversions. When patients with acute leukemia and a chromosomal abnormality receive treatment and enter into complete remission (CR), the chromosomal abnormality disappears; when relapse occurs, the abnormality reappears. In many cases, these abnormalities have provided clues into the pathobiology of acute leukemia.

TABLE 194–1 FRENCH-AMERICAN-BRITISH (FAB) CLASSIFICATION OF ACUTE LEUKEMIAS

		Histochemistry				
Subtype	**Morphology**	**Myeloperoxidase**	**Nonspecific Esterase**	**PAS**	**Monoclonal Reactivity**	**Cytogenetic Abnormalities**
M0—Acute undifferentiated leukemia	Uniform, very undifferentiated	–	–	–	For subtypes M0–M5b, approximately 90% react with at	Various
M1—Acute myeloid leukemia with minimal differentiation	Very undifferentiated, few azurophilic granules	+/–	+/–	–	least one of the following antimyeloid antibodies: anti-CD13	Various
M2—Acute myeloid leukemia with differentiation	Granulated blasts predominate; Auer rods may be seen	+++	+/–	+	anti-CD14 anti-CD33 anti-CD34	Various, including t(8;21)
M3—Acute promyelocytic leukemia	Hypergranular promyelocytes	+++	+	+		t(15;17)
M4—Acute myelomonocytic leukemia	Both monoblasts and myeloblasts are present	++	+++	++		Various, including inv/del (16)
M4E	Like M4 but with eosinophils					
M5—Acute monocytic leukemia	Monoblasts predominate					
M5a M5b	Type a, >80% monoblasts; type b, >20% promonocytes	+/–	+++	++		Various, including abnormalities of 11q23
M6—Acute erythroleukemia	Erythroblasts and megaloblastic red cell precursors seen	–	–	++	Antiglycopherin, antispectrin	Various
M7—Acute megakaryocytic leukemia	Undifferentiated blasts	–	+/–	+	CD41, CD61	Various
L1—Acute lymphoid leukemia, childhood variant	Small, uniform blasts, nucleoli indistinct	–	–	+++	65% react with anti-CD10 (anti-CALLA); 20% react with anti-CD5, -CD3, or -CD2 (anti-T cell)	Various including t(9;22), t(4;11), and t(1;9)
L2—Acute lymphoid leukemia, adult variant	Larger, more irregular nucleoli present	–	–	++		
L3—Burkitt-like acute lymphoid leukemia	Large with strongly basophilic cytoplasm and vacuoles	–	–	–	Anti-surface immunoglobulin, anti-CD19, anti-CD20	t(8;14)

PAS = periodic acid–Schiff.

The most common cytogenetic abnormalities seen in AML can be categorized according to their underlying biology and prognostic significance. The translocation t(8;21) and the inversion inv(16) result in abnormalities of a transcription factor made up of core binding factor-α (CBF-α) and CBF-β. The t(8;21) results in fusion of the CBF, a subunit on chromosome 21, with the *ETO* gene on chromosome 8, whereas inv(16) results in the fusion of the CBF subunit on the q arm of chromosome 16 with the *MYH11* gene on the p arm. Both of these "core binding factor" AMLs are characterized by a high complete response rate and relatively favorable long-term survival. An additional translocation with a favorable prognosis, t(15;17), involves two genes, *PML* and *RAR-α* (a gene encoding the a retinoic acid receptor), and is invariably associated with APL, the M3 subtype of AML. Translocations involving the *MLL* gene, located at chromosome band 11q23, carry an intermediate prognosis. MLL is perhaps the most promiscuous oncogene partner in oncology, with more than 30 fusion partners identified. Trisomy 8 is among the most common nonrandom cytogenetic abnormalities seen in AML; it accounts for 9% of cases and carries an intermediate prognosis. Trisomies of chromosome 21, chromosome 11, and other chromosomes are also sometimes seen. Deletions of part or all of chromosomes 5 or 7 each account for 6% to 8% of cases of AML. These abnormalities are seen with greater frequency in older patients and in patients with AML secondary to myelodysplasia or prior exposure to alkylating agents, and they are associated with an unfavorable prognosis.

In addition to the abnormalities detectable by routine cytogenetic analysis, other mutations exist in the malignant cells in substantial proportions of AML cases. Many of these involve signal transduction pathways. Activating mutations in the FLT3 receptor have been found in 20

TABLE 194–2 WORLD HEALTH ORGANIZATION CLASSIFICATION OF ACUTE LEUKEMIAS

ACUTE MYELOID LEUKEMIA (AML)
AMLs with recurrent cytogenetic translocations
AML with t(8;21)(q22;q22), AML1 (CBF-α)/ETO
Acute promyelocytic leukemia (AML with t[15;17][q22;q11-12] and variants, PML/RAR-α)
AML with abnormal bone marrow eosinophils (inv[16][p13q22] or t[16;16][p13;q11], CBF-β/MYH11X)
AML with 11q23 (MLL) abnormalities
AML with multilineage dysplasia
With prior myelodysplastic syndrome
Without prior myelodysplastic syndrome
AML and myelodysplastic syndromes, therapy-related
Alkylating agent–related
Epipodophyllotoxin-related (some may be lymphoid)
Other types
AML not otherwise categorized
AML minimally differentiated (FAB M0)
AML without maturation (FAB M1)
AML with maturation (FAB M2)
Acute myelomonocytic leukemia (FAB M4)
Acute monocytic leukemia (FAB M5)
Acute erythroid leukemia (FAB M6)
Acute megakaryocytic leukemia (FAB M7)
Acute basophilic leukemia
ACUTE PANMYELOSIS WITH MYELOFIBROSIS
ACUTE BIPHENOTYPIC LEUKEMIAS
ACUTE LYMPHOID LEUKEMIAS
Precursor B-cell acute lymphoblastic leukemia (cytogenetic subgroups)
t (9;22) (a34;q11); *BCR/ABL*
t(v;11q23); *MLL* rearranged
t(1;19)(q23;p13) *E2A/PBX1*
t(12;21)(p12;q22) *ETV/CBF-α*
PRECURSOR T-CELL ACUTE LYMPHOBLASTIC LEUKEMIA
BURKITT-LIKE LEUKEMIA

FAB = French-American-British classification (see Table 194–1).

to 40% of cases of AML. These mutations may be internal tandem repeats (15 to 30%) or point mutations (5 to 10%), and they tend to be associated with a poorer overall response to therapy. Mutations in FMS, which, like FLT3, is a receptor tyrosine kinase, are seen in 10 to 20% of cases of AML, and mutations in HRAS, KRAS2, or NRAS1, which are cellular proteins involved with signal transduction, are seen in 15 to 20% of AML cases. *CEBPA* is a gene encoding a leucine zipper transcription factor involved in myeloid differentiation. Recent reports indicate that the gene is mutated in 4 to 15% of cases of AML and may be associated with a more favorable outcome. All of these mutations have become of interest not only for their prognostic importance, but also because they may serve as targets for new therapies.

The most common cytogenetic abnormality seen in adults with ALL is the Philadelphia (Ph) chromosome [t(9;22)], a translocation that results in fusion of the *BCR* gene on chromosome 22 to the *ABL* tyrosine kinase gene on chromosome 9. This translocation results in the constitutive activation of *ABL*, but the precise mechanism by which this activity leads to leukemia is unclear. The *BCR/ABL* fusion is associated with both ALL and CML (Chapter 195), with a minor difference in the breakpoint of *BCR* distinguishing the two. A slightly smaller 190-kD protein is usually found in ALL, whereas a larger 210-kD protein is characteristic of CML. The frequency of t(9;22) increases with age: it is found in approximately 5% of childhood cases, 25% of adults, and 50% of adults older than 50 years of age. ALL with t(9;22) has a poor prognosis when treated with conventional chemotherapy. The most common translocation seen in childhood ALL is t(12;21), which involves the genes *TEL* and *AML1*. Like the AML-associated t(8;21) and inv(16), t(12;21) is thought to result in abnormal DNA transcription by interfering with the normal function of CBF. The t(12;21) is difficult to diagnose by routine cytogenetics, but by molecular studies it has been shown to account for 25% of childhood ALL and 4% of adult ALL. Other abnormalities sometimes seen in B-cell ALL include t(8;14) and t(8;22), which result in translocation of the *MYC* gene on chromosome 8 and immunoglobulin enhancer response genes on chromosomes 14 or 22, as well as abnormalities involving 11q23. T-cell ALLs are frequently associated with abnormalities of chromosome 7 or 14 at the sites of T-cell receptor enhancer genes on these chromosomes. The leukemia cells in about 20% of patients with ALL have a propensity to gain chromosomes, sometimes reaching an average of 50 to 60 chromosomes per cell. Patients with such hyperdiploid leukemias tend to respond well to chemotherapy.

Clinical Manifestations

The signs and symptoms of acute leukemia are usually rapid in onset, developing over a few weeks to at most a few months, and result from decreased normal marrow function and invasion of normal organs by leukemic blasts. Anemia is present at diagnosis in most patients and causes fatigue, pallor, headache, and, in predisposed patients, angina or heart failure. Thrombocytopenia is usually present, and approximately one third of patients have clinically evident bleeding at diagnosis, usually in the form of petechiae, ecchymoses, bleeding gums, epistaxis, or hemorrhage. Most patients with acute leukemia are significantly granulocytopenic at diagnosis. As a result, approximately one third of patients with AML and slightly fewer patients with ALL have significant or life-threatening infections when initially seen, most of which are bacterial in origin.

In addition to suppressing normal marrow function, leukemic cells can infiltrate normal organs. In general, ALL tends to infiltrate normal organs more often than AML does. Enlargement of lymph nodes, liver, and spleen is common at diagnosis. Bone pain, thought to result from leukemic infiltration of the periosteum or expansion of the medullary cavity, is a common complaint, particularly in children with ALL. Leukemic cells sometimes infiltrate the skin and result in a raised, non-pruritic rash, a condition termed leukemia cutis. Leukemic cells may infiltrate the leptomeninges and cause leukemic meningitis, typically manifested by headache and nausea. As the disease progresses, central nervous system (CNS) palsies and seizures may develop. Although fewer than 5% of patients have CNS involvement at diagnosis, the CNS is a frequent site of relapse, particularly with ALL; because of the so-called blood-brain barrier, the CNS requires special therapy. Testicular involvement is also seen in ALL, and the testicles are a frequent site of relapse. In AML, collections of leukemic blast cells, often referred to as chloromas or myeloblastomas, can occur in virtually any soft tissue and appear as rubbery, fast-growing masses.

Certain clinical manifestations are unique to specific subtypes of leukemia. Patients with APL of the M3 type commonly have subclinical or clinically evident disseminated intravascular coagulation (DIC) (Chapter 181) caused by tissue thromboplastins that are present in the leukemic cells and released as these cells die. Acute monocytic or myelomonocytic leukemias are the forms of AML most likely to have extramedullary involvement. M6 leukemia often has a long prodromal phase. Patients with T-cell ALL frequently have mediastinal masses.

Diagnosis

Abnormalities in peripheral blood counts are usually the initial laboratory evidence of acute leukemia. Anemia is present in most patients. Most are also at least mildly thrombocytopenic, and up to one fourth have severe thrombocytopenia (platelets <20,000/μL). Although most patients are granulocytopenic at diagnosis, the total peripheral white cell count is more variable; approximately 25% of patients have very high white cell counts (>50,000/μL), approximately 50% have white cell counts between 5000 and 50,000/μL, and about 25% have a low white cell count (<5000/μL). In most cases, blasts are present in the peripheral blood, although in some patients the percentage of blasts is quite low or absent.

The diagnosis of acute leukemia is typically established by marrow aspiration and biopsy, usually from the posterior iliac crest. Marrow aspirates and biopsy specimens are usually hypercellular and contain 20 to

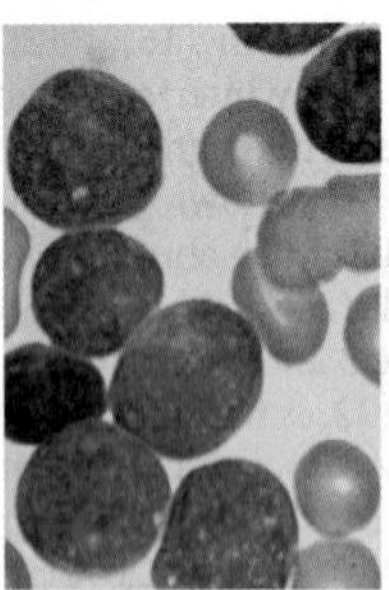
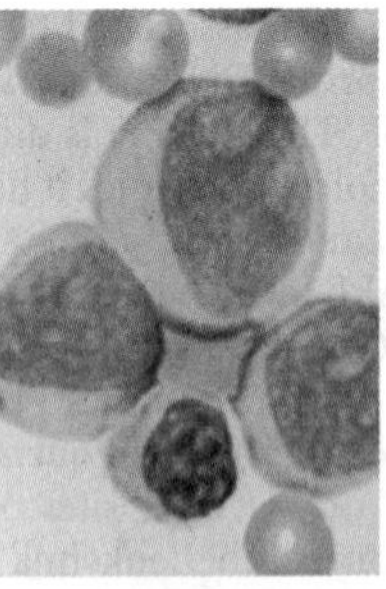

FIGURE 194–1 • Acute leukemia. Left, Acute lymphoblastic leukemia (ALL). Right, Acute myeloid leukemia (AML). Lymphoblasts in ALL are smaller, with a higher ratio of nuclear to cytoplasmic material and less distinct nucleoli than in the myeloblasts in AML. The nucleoli in the myeloblasts are clear and "punched out."

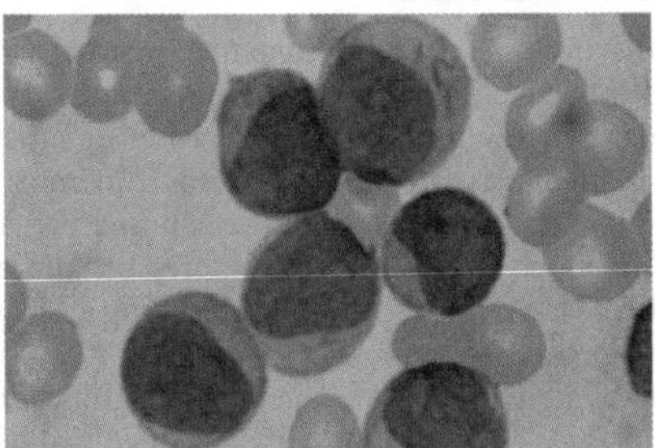

FIGURE 194–2 • Acute myeloid leukemia. The myeloblasts in the smear show Auer rods as cytoplasmic inclusions.

100% blast cells, which largely replace the normal marrow (Figs. 194–1 and 194–2). Occasionally, in addition to the blast cell infiltrate, other findings are present, such as marrow fibrosis (especially with M7 AML) or bone marrow necrosis.

The prothrombin and partial thromboplastin times are sometimes elevated. In APL, reduced fibrinogen and evidence of DIC are also often seen. Other laboratory abnormalities frequently present are hyperuricemia, especially in ALL, and increased serum lactate dehydrogenase. In cases of high cell turnover and cell death (e.g., L3 ALL), evidence of tumor lysis syndrome may be noted at diagnosis, including hypocalcemia, hyperkalemia, hyperphosphatemia, hyperuricemia, and renal insufficiency. This syndrome, which is more commonly seen shortly after therapy is begun, can be rapidly fatal if untreated.

Differential Diagnosis

The diagnosis of acute leukemia is usually straightforward but can occasionally be difficult. Both leukemia and aplastic anemia (Chapter 171) can be manifested by peripheral pancytopenia, but the finding of a hypoplastic marrow without blasts usually distinguishes aplastic anemia. Occasionally, a patient has a hypocellular marrow and a clonal cytogenetic abnormality, which establishes the diagnosis of myelodysplasia or hypocellular leukemia. A number of processes other than leukemia can lead to the appearance of immature cells in the peripheral blood. Although other small round cell neoplasms can infiltrate the marrow and sometimes mimic leukemia, immunologic markers are effective in differentiating the two. Leukemoid reactions to infections such as tuberculosis can result in the outpouring of large numbers of young myeloid cells, but the proportion of blasts in marrow or peripheral blood almost never reaches 20% in a leukemoid reaction (Chapter 173). Infectious mononucleosis (Chapter 400) and other viral illnesses can sometimes resemble ALL, particularly if large numbers of atypical lymphocytes are present in the peripheral blood and if the disease is accompanied by immune thrombocytopenia or hemolytic anemia.

Treatment

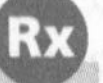

With the development of effective programs of combination chemotherapy and advances in hematopoietic stem cell transplantation, many patients with acute leukemia can be cured. These therapeutic measures are complex and are therefore best carried out at centers with appropriate support services and experience in treating leukemia. Because leukemia is a rapidly progressive disease, specific antileukemic therapy should be started as soon after diagnosis as possible, usually within 48 hours. The goal of initial chemotherapy is to induce a CR with restoration of normal marrow function. In general, induction chemotherapy is intensive and is accompanied by significant toxicities. Therefore, patients should be stabilized to the extent possible before specific antileukemic therapy is begun.

Preparing the Patient for Therapy

Severe bleeding usually results from thrombocytopenia, which can be reversed with platelet transfusions (Chapter 183). Once thrombocytopenic bleeding is stopped, continued prophylactic transfusions of platelets may be warranted to maintain the platelet count higher than 10,000 to 20,000/μL. Occasionally, patients also have evidence of DIC, usually associated with the diagnosis of M3 AML. If active bleeding is due to DIC (Chapter 181), low doses of heparin (50 U/kg) given intravenously every 6 hours can be of benefit. Platelets and fresh-frozen plasma (or cryoprecipitate) should be transfused to maintain the platelet count higher than 50,000/μL and the fibrinogen level greater than 100 mg/dL until the DIC abates. Whether heparin should be given prophylactically to patients with laboratory evidence of DIC but no active bleeding is an often debated but unsettled question.

Patients with fever and granulocytopenia should have blood cultures obtained; while awaiting culture results, infection should be assumed and broad-spectrum antibiotics begun empirically (Chapters 173 and 304). It is preferable to bring an infection under control before starting initial chemotherapy if the patient has an adequate granulocyte count. However, patients often have infection but essentially no granulocytes; in this situation, delaying chemotherapy is unlikely to be of benefit.

Patients with very high blast counts (>100,000/μL) may have symptoms attributable to the effects of masses of these immature cells on blood flow. The leukostasis may evolve into vascular injury and local hemorrhage. If this situation occurs in the CNS, the outcome can be fatal. Leukapheresis, immediate whole-brain irradiation (600 cGy in one dose), and administration of hydroxyurea (3 g/m^2 given orally for 2 or 3 days) can usually prevent this complication.

Before treatment, management in all patients should be aimed at preventing the tumor lysis syndrome. Patients should be hydrated, have their urine alkalinized with acetazolamide (500 mg/day), and be given allopurinol 100 to 200 mg orally three times per day before chemotherapy is initiated. Patients with very high white cell counts may have uremia and anuria secondary to greatly increased serum uric acid levels, with subsequent intratubular crystallization, even before starting therapy. Hyperuricemia usually responds rapidly to rasburicase 0.20 mg/kg/day intravenously, over 30 minutes.

The diagnosis of leukemia usually comes as a profound psychological shock to the patient and family. Therefore, in addition to stabilizing the patient hematologically and metabolically, it is worthwhile having at least one formalized conference, in which the patient and the family are advised about the meaning of the diagnosis of leukemia and the consequences of therapy, before treatment is initiated.

Treatment of Acute Lymphoblastic Leukemia

After the patient's condition has been stabilized, antileukemic therapy should be started as soon as possible. Treatment of newly diagnosed ALL can be divided into three phases: remission induction, postremission therapy, and CNS prophylaxis.

Remission Induction

The initial goal of treatment is to induce CR, defined as the reduction of leukemic blasts to undetectable levels and restoration of normal marrow function. A number of different chemotherapeutic combinations can be used to induce remission; all include vincristine and prednisone, and most add L-asparaginase and daunorubicin, administered over a period of 3 to 4 weeks. With such regimens, CR is achieved in 90% of children and 80 to 90% of adults (Table 194–3).

TABLE 194–3 COMMON REGIMENS FOR COMMON FORMS OF ACUTE LEUKEMIA

I. MANAGEMENT OF NEWLY DIAGNOSED ACUTE MYELOID LEUKEMIA

A. Induction—Daunorubicin 45–60 mg/m²/day for 3 days (or idarubicin 10–12 mg/m²/day for 3 days) and cytarabine 200 mg/day for 7 days

B. Postremission
1. Favorable risk—Cytarabine, 3 g/m² over 3 hours every 12 hours on days 1, 3, and 5 every month for 4 months
2. Intermediate risk—As for favorable risk; or, if HLA-matched sibling exists, allogeneic hematopoietic cell transplantation; or, if no matched sibling exists, two courses of cytarabine followed by autologous transplantation
3. Unfavorable risk—If HLA-matched related or unrelated donor is available, proceed to allogeneic transplantation; if not, treat as for intermediate risk

II. MANAGEMENT OF NEWLY DIAGNOSED ACUTE PROMYELOCYTIC LEUKEMIA

A. Induction—ATRA 45 mg/m²/day until complete remission plus daunomycin 45–60 mg/m²/day for 3 days and cytarabine 200 mg/m²/day for 7 days

B. Consolidation—ATRA 45 mg/m²/day for 7 days and daunomycin 50 mg/m²/day for 3 days; repeat course 1 month later

C. Maintenance—ATRA 45 mg/m²/day for 15 days every 3 months plus 6-MP 100 mg/m²/day and MTX 10 mg/m² per week for 2 years

III. MANAGEMENT OF NEWLY DIAGNOSED ADULT PH-NEGATIVE ACUTE LYMPHOID LEUKEMIA

A. Induction (and courses 3, 5, 7)—Cyclophosphamide 300 mg/m² over 3 hours every 12 hours for 6 doses on days 1, 2, 3; doxorubicin 50 mg/m² on day 4; vincristine 2 mg/day on days 4 and 11; and dexamethasone 40 mg/day on days 1 through 4 and days 11 through 14

B. Consolidation (courses 2, 4, 6, 8)—MTX (200 mg/m² over 2 hours followed by 800 mg/m² over 22 hours on day 1) and high-dose cytarabine (3 g/m² over 2 hours every 12 hours for 4 doses on days 2 and 3)

C. Four intrathecal treatments of MTX 12 mg alternating with cytarabine 100 mg are given during the first four courses of systemic therapy.

ATRA = all-*trans*-retinoic acid; HLA = human leukocyte antigen; 6-MP, 6-mercaptopurine; MTX = methotrexate; Ph = Philadelphia chromosome [t(9;22)].

Because vincristine, prednisone, and L-asparaginase are relatively nontoxic to normal marrow precursors, the disease often enters CR after a relatively brief period of myelosuppression. Failure to achieve CR is usually due to either resistance of the leukemic cells to the drugs used or progressive infection. These two complications occur with approximately equal frequency.

Postremission Chemotherapy

If no further therapy is given after induction of CR, relapse occurs in almost all cases, usually within several months. Chemotherapy after CR can be given in a variety of combinations, dosages, and schedules. The term *consolidation chemotherapy* refers to short courses of further chemotherapy given at doses similar to those used for initial induction (requiring rehospitalization). Attempts are usually made to select different drugs for consolidation than were used to induce the initial remission. In the case of ALL, such drugs include high-dose methotrexate, cyclophosphamide, and cytarabine, among others. Maintenance involves the administration of low-dose chemotherapy on a daily or weekly outpatient basis for long periods. The most commonly used maintenance regimen in ALL combines daily 6-mercaptopurine and weekly or biweekly methotrexate. The optimal duration of maintenance chemotherapy is unknown, but maintenance is usually given for 2 to 3 years. Optimal chemotherapy for ALL requires both consolidation and maintenance chemotherapy.

Central Nervous System Prophylaxis

Most chemotherapeutic agents, when given intravenously or orally, do not penetrate the CNS well. However, systemic chemotherapy with high-dose methotrexate (e.g., 200 mg/m² intravenously over 2 hours followed by 800 mg/m² over 22 hours) and cytarabine (e.g., 3 g/m² over 2 hours every 12 hours for 4 doses) can achieve therapeutic drug levels within the CNS. Alternatives are intrathecal methotrexate, intrathecal methotrexate combined with 2400 cGy radiation to the cranium, or 2400 cGy to the craniospinal axis.

Burkitt-like ALL

Burkitt-like ALL (also termed FAB L3 or mature B-cell ALL) is characterized by the presence of monoclonal surface immunoglobulin, cytogenetics showing t(8;14), and the constitutive expression of the *MYC* oncogene. Burkitt-like ALL, which accounts for 3 to 5% of adult cases of ALL, responds well to regimens that incorporate short, intensive courses of high-dose methotrexate (1.5 g/m² over 24 hours with leucovorin), cytarabine (3 g/m² over 2 hours every 12 hours for 4 doses), and cyclophosphamide (200 mg/m²/day for 5 days); this regimen yields high rates of complete response and cures about 50% of patients. Preliminary results suggest that the addition of rituximab may further improve outcomes.

Philadelphia Chromosome–Positive ALL

Approximately 5% of pediatric cases and 25% of adult cases of ALL have cytogenetics showing t(9;22), the Ph chromosome. Historically, such patients had CR rates slightly lower than seen in Ph-negative ALL, but had markedly reduced remission durations, averaging less than a year, and few if any such patients were cured with conventional chemotherapy. Therefore, the general recommendation has been that such patients should receive an allogeneic transplant from a matched sibling or a matched unrelated donor while in first remission, if possible. With this approach, approximately 50% of patients can be cured. More recently, the addition of the tyrosine kinase inhibitor, imatinib mesylate, to conventional chemotherapeutic regimens has increased complete response rates to be as good as are seen in Ph-negative ALL, but the impact of the addition of imatinib mesylate on the duration of remission is not yet known. The general recommendation remains in favor of transplantation during first remission for this high-risk group of patients.

Prognosis after Initial Chemotherapy

A number of factors are predictive of outcome in ALL, the most important of which are younger age, a lower white cell count at diagnosis, and favorable cytogenetics. With currently available treatment regimens, 50 to 70% of children and 25 to 45% of adults who initially achieve CR maintain that state for more than 5 years, and these patients are probably cured of their disease.

Treatment of Relapsed ALL

Most relapses occur within 2 years after diagnosis, and most occur in the marrow. Occasionally, relapse is initially found in an extramedullary site such as the CNS or testes. Extramedullary relapse is usually followed shortly by systemic (marrow) relapse and should be considered part of a systemic recurrence. With the use of chemotherapeutic regimens similar to those used for initial induction, 50 to 70% of patients achieve at least a short-lived second remission. A small percentage of patients for whom the initial remission was longer than 2 years may be cured with salvage chemotherapy. If the CNS or testes is the initial site of the relapse, specific therapy to that site is also required, along with systemic retreatment. Because the prognosis of relapsed leukemia treated with

Rx

chemotherapy is so poor, marrow transplantation is usually recommended in this setting.

Hematopoietic Stem Cell Transplantation

The use of high-dose chemoradiotherapy followed by hematopoietic stem cell transplantation (Chapter 184) from an HLA-identical sibling can cure 20 to 40% of patients with ALL who fail to achieve an initial remission or who have a relapse after an initial CR and 50 to 60% of patients who undergo transplantation during first remission. Although there is still considerable debate, several recent studies have reported improved survival for adults with high-risk or standard-risk ALL who receive a stem cell transplant during first remission rather than being treated with standard chemotherapy. [1] The major limitations of transplantation are graft-versus-host disease, interstitial pneumonia, and recurrence of disease. If an HLA-identical sibling is not available, alternative sources are marrow from a partially matched family member, marrow or stored cord blood from an HLA-matched unrelated donor, and autologous marrow that has been removed during remission, treated in vitro to remove contaminating tumor cells, and subsequently stored. The outcome of transplantation of either autologous marrow or alternative sources of marrow has not been as favorable as that using marrow from matched family member donors.

Treatment of Acute Myeloid Leukemia

Remission Induction

Treatment with a combination of an anthracycline (daunomycin 45 to 60 mg/m^2/day for 3 days or idarubicin 12 mg/m^2/day for 3 days) and cytarabine (100 to 200 mg/m^2/day for 7 days) leads to CR in 60 to 80% of patients with AML. Profound myelosuppression always follows when these agents are used at doses capable of achieving CR. Failure to achieve CR is usually due to either drug resistance or fatal complications of myelosuppression.

Postremission Therapy

Intensive consolidation chemotherapy with repeated courses of daunomycin and cytarabine at doses similar to those used for induction, high-dose cytarabine (1 to 3 g/m^2/day for 3 to 6 days), or other agents prolongs the average remission duration and improves the chances for long-term disease-free survival. The best results reported to date with chemotherapy have generally been with repeated cycles of high-dose cytarabine. [2] Unlike the situation with ALL, low-dose maintenance therapy is of limited benefit after intensive consolidation treatment. In AML, leukemic recurrence occurs less often in the CNS (~10% of cases), most commonly in patients with the M4 or M5 variant. There is no evidence that CNS prophylaxis improves survival in AML.

Prognosis of Acute Myeloid Leukemia after Initial Chemotherapy

Among patients in whom CR is achieved, 20 to 40% remain alive in continuous CR for more than 5 years, suggesting probable cure. As with ALL, younger patients and those with a low white cell count at diagnosis have a more favorable outcome. Patients whose disease is characterized by certain chromosomal abnormalities, particularly t(8;21), t(15;17), and inv(16), do somewhat better, whereas those with 5q-, −7, 11q23, inv(3), or t(6;9) do worse. Patients who have a preleukemic phase before their condition evolves into acute leukemia and those whose leukemia is secondary to prior exposure to alkylating agents or radiation respond poorly to chemotherapy. Expression of the multidrug resistance gene 1 *(MDR1)* is also associated with a worse outcome.

Treatment of Recurrent Acute Myeloid Leukemia

Patients whose AML recurs after initial chemotherapy can achieve a second remission in about 50% of cases after retreatment with daunomycin-cytarabine or high-dose cytarabine. The likelihood of achieving a second remission is predicted by the duration of first remission: 70% in patients whose first remission persisted beyond 2 years, compared with less than 15% in those whose first remission lasted less than 6 months. Older patients may benefit from gemtuzumab ozogamicin (9 mg/m^2 on days 1 and 15), a form of antibody-targeted chemotherapy. Second remissions tend to be short lived, however, and few patients in whom relapse occurs after first-line chemotherapy are cured by salvage chemotherapy.

Treatment of Acute Promyelocytic Leukemia

CR can be induced in at least 90% of patients with APL by using all-*trans*-retinoic acid (ATRA; 45 mg/m^2/day until CR) in combination with an anthracycline. Patients treated with ATRA usually have their coagulation disorders corrected within several days. A unique toxicity of ATRA in the treatment of APL is the development of hyperleukocytosis accompanied by respiratory distress and pulmonary infiltrates. The syndrome responds to temporary discontinuation of ATRA and the addition of corticosteroids. By combining ATRA with anthracyclines for induction and consolidation, then using ATRA as maintenance therapy, approximately 70% of patients can be cured. [3] Patients with higher white cell counts at diagnosis do worse. Arsenic trioxide (0.15 mg/kg/day until CR) is effective in patients with recurrent APL and is being studied as part of the primary treatment.

Hematopoietic Stem Cell Transplantation

For patients with AML in whom an initial remission cannot be achieved or for those who have a relapse after chemotherapy, stem cell transplantation (Chapter 184) from an HLA-identical sibling offers the best chance for cure. Fifteen percent of patients with end-stage disease can be saved by this treatment. If the procedure is applied earlier, the outcome is better: approximately 30% of patients who undergo stem cell transplantation at first relapse or second remission are cured, and 50 to 60% of patients are cured if stem cell transplantation is performed during first remission. A large number of studies have prospectively compared the outcome of allogeneic stem cell transplantation with that of chemotherapy in patients with AML in first remission. The trends in all of these studies have been toward higher treatment-related mortality but improved disease-free survival time with allogeneic transplantation. Less difference has been seen in overall survival. Currently, allogeneic stem cell transplantation is the treatment of choice for patients with AML who have an initial relapse, and it should be strongly considered for patients with high- or intermediate-risk disease during first remission. The major limitations to allogeneic stem cell transplantation are lack of a matched sibling donor, graft-versus-host disease, interstitial pneumonia, and disease recurrence. Because transplant-related toxicities increase with patient age, most centers limit stem cell transplantation to those 55 years of age or younger. However, recent studies of reduced-intensity or nonmyeloablative allogeneic transplantation have shown encouraging results in patients with AML in remission at ages up to 70 years. Allogeneic transplantation using matched unrelated donors gives results not too dissimilar from those with matched siblings, although with a higher incidence of complications. Autologous stem cell transplantation offers an alternative for patients without matched siblings to serve as donors. In randomized trials, the use of autologous BMT after consolidation chemotherapy significantly prolonged the duration of disease-free survival for patients with AML in first remission but was not of benefit if used as a substitute for intensive consolidation.

Treatment of AML in Older Patients

The benefits of intensive consolidation chemotherapy in younger patients do not translate to patients older than 60 years of age, in part because older patients are less able to tolerate therapy, but also because AML in older patients is more often associated with unfavorable cytogenetics (particularly abnormalities of chromosomes 5 and 7) and more often over expresses p-glycoprotein, thereby resulting in the multidrug resistance phenotype. Accordingly, long-term survival rates of only 5 to 10% are seen with chemotherapy in patients older than 60 years of age. Intensive chemotherapy can cause more harm than good in older patients with poor performance status, and such patients may be candidates for supportive care only or for alternative therapies currently under study (e.g., tipifarnib). Otherwise healthy older individuals should be offered intensive chemotherapy.

Management of Complications

Treatment of acute leukemia, especially AML, is accompanied by a number of complications, the two most serious and frequent being infection and bleeding. During the granulocytopenic period that follows induction and consolidation chemotherapy, most patients become febrile, and in approximately 50% of cases a bacterial infection can be documented. The most commonly isolated organisms vary somewhat from medical center to medical center, but gram-positive organisms such as *Staphylococcus epidermidis* and gram-negative enteric organisms such as *Pseudomonas aeruginosa, Escherichia coli,* and *Klebsiella/Aerobacter* are the most commonly isolated bacteria. Even if no cause for fever is found, bacterial infection should be assumed, and, in general, all patients with fever and neutropenia should begin receiving broad-spectrum antibiotics (Chapters 173 and 304). Commonly used antibiotic approaches include monotherapy with imipenem or a combination of an antipseudomonal penicillin and a third-generation cephalosporin. Once begun, antibiotic use should be continued until patients recover their granulocyte count, even if they become afebrile first. If documented bacterial infection persists despite appropriate antibiotics, the physician should consider removal of indwelling catheters.

Frequently, patients taking broad-spectrum antibiotics become afebrile for a time, only to have a second fever develop. Such patients should be carefully reassessed with a high index of suspicion for fungal infection. Granulocytopenic patients who remain febrile for more than 1 week while taking broad-spectrum antibiotics should be treated empirically with amphotericin or voriconazole for presumed fungal infection. The prophylactic use of fluconazole can reduce the incidence of invasive candidal infections.

In addition to being granulocytopenic, patients undergoing induction chemotherapy for leukemia have deficient cellular and humoral immunity, at least temporarily, and therefore are subject to infections common in other immunodeficiency states, including *Pneumocystis jiroveci* (formerly *P. carinii*) infection (PCP) and a variety of viral infections. PCP can be prevented by prophylactic use of trimethoprim-sulfamethoxazole. Cytomegalovirus (CMV) infection can be prevented in a CMV-seronegative patient by the sole use of CMV-seronegative blood products (Chapter 399). Herpes simplex (Chapter 397) can often complicate existing mucositis and can be prevented with prophylactic acyclovir. Acyclovir is also useful for the treatment of disseminated varicella-zoster virus infection (Chapter 398).

Myeloid growth factors (granulocyte or granulocyte-macrophage colony-stimulating factor; Chapter 160), if given shortly after the completion of chemotherapy, shorten the period of severe myelosuppression by, on average, approximately 4 days. In most studies, this accelerated recovery has resulted in fewer days with fever and less use of antibiotics, but it has not improved the complete response rate or altered survival.

The platelet count that signals a need for platelet transfusion has been the subject of recent debate. Traditionally, platelet transfusions from random donors were used to maintain platelet counts greater than 20,000/μL, but more recently it has been demonstrated that lowering this threshold to 10,000/μL is safe in patients with no active bleeding. In 30% to 50% of cases, patients eventually become alloimmunized and require the use of HLA-matched platelets (Chapter 183). Occasionally, cells (presumably T cells) within the blood product can engraft in an immunosuppressed leukemic patient and cause a graft-versus-host reaction. Transfusion-induced graft-versus-host disease is manifested as a rash, low-grade fever, elevated values in liver function tests, and decreasing blood counts. This syndrome can be prevented by irradiating all blood products with at least 1500 cGy before transfusion.

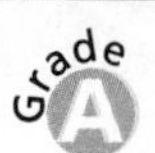

1. Thiebaut A, Vernant JP, Degos L, et al: Adult acute lymphocytic leukemia study testing chemotherapy and autologous and allogeneic transplantation: A follow-up report of the French protocol LALA 87 (review). Hematol Oncol Clin North Am 2000;14:1353–1366.
2. Mayer RJ, Davis RB, Schiffer CA, et al: Intensive post-remission chemotherapy in adults with acute myeloid leukemia. N Engl J Med 1994;331:891–903.
3. Tallman MS, Andersen JW, Schiffer CA, et al: All-trans retinoic acid in acute promyelocytic leukemia: Long-term outcome and prognostic factor analysis from the North American Intergroup protocol. Blood 2002;100:4298–4302.

SUGGESTED READINGS

Estey E, Döhner H: Acute myeloid leukemia. Lancet 2006;368:1894–1907. *A clinical overview.*

O'Donnell MR, Appelbaum FR, Baer JC, et al: Acute myeloid leukemia. NCCN Practice Guidelines in Oncology, vol 2. National Comprehensive Cancer Network. 2005. Available at: www.nccn.org/professionals/physician_gls/PDF/aml.pdf (accessed August 25, 2006). *A practical approach to therapy.*

Pui CH, Evans WE: Treatment of acute lymphoblastic leukemia. N Engl J Med 2006;354:166–178. *A clinical overview.*

Tallman MS, Gilliland DG, Rowe JM: Drug therapy for acute myeloid leukemia. Blood 2005;106:1154–1163. *A comprehensive overview.*

Talpaz M, Shah NP, Kantarjian H, et al: Dasatinib in imatinib-resistant Philadelphia chromosome-positive leukemias. N Engl J Med 2006;354:2531–2541. *Dasatinib induces hematologic and cytogenetic responses in patients with CML or Ph-positive ALL.*

195 THE CHRONIC LEUKEMIAS

Hagop Kantarjian and Susan O'Brien

CHRONIC MYELOGENOUS LEUKEMIA

Definition

Chronic myelogenous leukemia (CML), also called chronic myeloid leukemia, chronic myelocytic leukemia, and chronic granulocytic leukemia, is a clonal myeloproliferative disorder of the primitive hematopoietic stem cell that is characterized by overproduction of cells of the myeloid series, which results in marked splenomegaly and leukocytosis. Basophilia and thrombocytosis are common. A characteristic cytogenetic abnormality, the Philadelphia (Ph) chromosome, is present in the bone marrow cells in more than 90% of cases. Most patients (85 to 90%) present in the chronic phase. Eventually, if poorly controlled, CML evolves into the accelerated and blastic phases.

Epidemiology

CML constitutes one fifth of all cases of leukemia in the United States. It is diagnosed in 1 or 2 persons per 100,000 per year and has a slight male preponderance. This incidence of 5000 to 7000 cases annually has not changed significantly in the past few decades. The incidence of CML increases with age; the median age at diagnosis is 45 to 55 years. Ph-positive CML is uncommon in children and adolescents. No familial association of CML has been noted; for example, the risk is not increased in monozygotic twins or in relatives of patients with CML. Because of the availability of effective therapy, the prevalence of CML is predicted to increase gradually, from 15,000 to 20,000 cases up to as many as 100,000 to 150,000 cases in the United States.

Often, no etiologic agent is incriminated in CML. Exposure to ionizing radiation (e.g., in survivors of the atomic bomb explosions in Japan in 1945, via radiation treatment of ankylosing spondylitis of cervical cancer) has increased the risk of CML; the peak incidence occurs 5 to 12 years after exposure and is dose related. No increase in the risk of CML has been demonstrated among individuals working in the nuclear industry. Radiologists working without adequate protection before 1940 were more likely to develop myeloid leukemia, but no such association has been found in recent studies. Benzene exposure increases the risk of acute myelogenous leukemia (AML) but not of CML. CML is not a frequent secondary leukemia after treatment of other cancers with radiation or alkylating agents or both.

Pathobiology

Molecular Pathogenesis

The Ph chromosome abnormality, present in more than 90% of patients with typical CML (Fig. 195–1), results from a balanced translocation of genetic material between the long arms of chromosomes 9 and 22: t(9;22)(q34;q11.2). The breakpoint at band q34 of chromosome 9

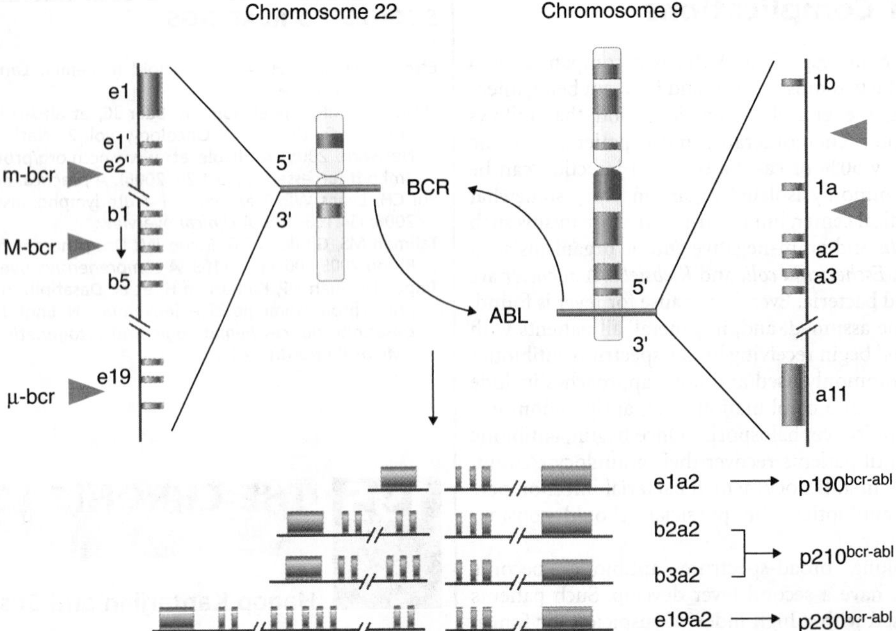

FIGURE 195–1 • The Philadelphia chromosome. Originally described as a shortened long arm of chromosome 22, the Philadelphia chromosome (Ph) was later found to be the result of a balanced translocation of genetic material between the long arms of chromosomes 9 and 22, t(9;22)(q34;q11.2). This results in the juxtaposition of *ABL* to *BCR*, producing a hybrid *BCR-ABL* oncogene. Depending on the breakpoint on BCR, three oncoproteins may be produced: (1) $p210^{BCR-ABL}$, which is associated with 98% or more of the cases of Ph-positive chronic myelogenous leukemia (CML); (2) $p190^{BCR-ABL}$, which is associated with 60 to 80% of cases of Ph-positive acute lymphocytic leukemia (ALL; the other 20 to 40% of cases are $p210^{BCR-ABL}$); and (3) $p230^{BCR-ABL}$, which is associated with rare cases of Ph-positive CML. The dysregulated expression of *BCR-ABL*, through phosphorylation of substrate proteins, triggers the abnormal signal transduction of multiple downstream events, some of them thought to cause excessive proliferation, reduced apoptosis, abnormal cytoskeletal regulation and cytoadhesion, and other events contributing to the growth advantage of CML cells.

results in translocation of the cellular oncogene, *ABL1* (previously *c-ABL*), to a region on chromosome 22 coding for the major breakpoint cluster region *(BCR)*. *ABL1* is a homologue of *v-ABL*, the Abelson virus that causes leukemia in mice. This translocation allows juxtaposition of a 5′ portion of a BCR and 3′ position of ABL; the two genetic sequences produce a new hybrid oncogene *(BCR-ABL)*, which codes for a novel BCR-ABL oncoprotein of molecular weight 210 kD ($p210^{BCR-ABL}$). The $p210^{BCR-ABL}$ oncoprotein results in uncontrolled kinase activity of BCR-ABL, which triggers the excessive proliferation and reduced apoptosis of CML cells, thereby giving CML cells a growth advantage over normal cells and suppressing normal hematopoiesis. Although in most cases 100% of the metaphases on cytogenetic analysis show BCR-ABL, some normal stem cells emerge on long-term bone marrow culture and after treatment with interferon-α (IFN-α), imatinib, high-dose chemotherapy, and autologous stem cell transplantation.

The constitutive activation of BCR-ABL results in autophosphorylation and activation of multiple downstream pathways that affect gene transcription, apoptosis, cytoskeletal organization, cytoadhesions, and degradation of inhibitory proteins. The signal transduction pathways implicated involve RAS, mitogen-activated-protein (MAP) kinases, signal transducers and activators of transcription (STAT), phosphatidyl inositol 3-kinase (PI3K), MYC, and others. Many of these interactions are mediated through tyrosine phosphorylation and require binding of the BCR-ABL to adapter proteins such as GRB-2, CRK, CRK-like protein (CRKL) and SCR-homology containing proteins (SHC). Although imatinib has been extremely successful at targeting BCR-ABL, understanding of the pathophysiology of the downstream events of BCR-ABL is important for future development of agents that may target these events.

In Ph-positive acute lymphocytic leukemia (ALL), the breakpoint in BCR is proximal, in the minor *BCR* region, resulting in a smaller BCR gene apposing ABL; the resulting fusion gene, messenger RNA, and BCR-ABL oncoprotein ($p190^{BCR-ABL}$) are of smaller sizes. A third, rare, mu (µ) BCR breakpoint distal to the major *BCR* region produces a $p230^{BCR-ABL}$ hybrid oncoprotein, which is associated with a more indolent CML course.

What induces this molecular rearrangement is unknown. Molecular techniques that amplify detection of *BCR-ABL* have demonstrated its presence in the marrow cells of 25 to 30% of healthy volunteers and 5% of infants, but not in cord blood. Because clinical CML develops in only 1 to 2 of 100,000 individuals (i.e., 1 to 2 per 25,000 to 30,000 individuals who express *BCR-ABL* in their bone marrow), immune regulatory processes or additional molecular events presumably contribute to the development of CML.

BCR-ABL is found only in hematopoietic cells and has its origin close to the pluripotent stem cell. For example, the Ph chromosome occurs in erythroid, myeloid, monocytic, and megakaryocytic cells, less commonly in B lymphocytes, rarely in T lymphocytes, and not at all in marrow fibroblasts. The fusion *BCR-ABL* gene and the p210 protein can be found in cases of typical morphologic CML in which no cytogenetic abnormality occurs or in which changes other than the typical t(9;22)(q34;q11.2) are identified. These patients have a survival rate and a response to therapy similar to those of patients with Ph-positive CML. Patients with atypical CML (usually older and more frequently exhibiting anemia, thrombocytopenia, monocytosis, and dysplasia) who are Ph-negative and *BCR-ABL* negative have a worse prognosis than those with either Ph-positive or Ph-negative *BCR-ABL*-positive CML; they resemble more closely patients with myelodysplastic syndrome (MDS; see Chapter 193). Thus, three groups of patients with CML can be identified: (1) those who are positive for Ph and *BCR-ABL*, (2) those who are Ph-negative but *BCR-ABL* positive, and (3) those who are negative for Ph and *BCR-ABL*. *PDGFB* (previous *SIS*), which codes for platelet derived growth factor (PDGF) and is the homologue of the simian sarcoma virus, is also translocated from chromosome 22 to chromosome 9 in CML, but it is distant from the breakpoint and is not expressed.

Clinical Manifestations

About 40 to 50% of patients diagnosed with CML are asymptomatic until the disease is found on routine physical examinations or blood tests. In these patients, the white blood cell (WBC) count may be relatively low at diagnosis. The degree of leukocytosis correlates with tumor burden as defined by spleen size.

The symptoms of CML, when present, are due to anemia and splenomegaly: fatigue, weight loss, malaise, easy satiety, and left upper quadrant fullness or pain (Table 195–1). Rarely, bleeding (associated with

TABLE 195–1 CLINICAL AND LABORATORY FEATURES OF PH-POSITIVE CHRONIC MYELOGENOUS LEUKEMIA IN NEWLY DIAGNOSED PATIENTS REFERRED TO M. D. ANDERSON CANCER CENTER FROM 1980 TO 2005 (N = 1809)

Parameter	Percentage
Age ≥60 yr	26
Female	40
Splenomegaly	36
Hepatomegaly	8
Lymphadenopathy	6
Other extramedullary disease	7
Hemoglobin <10 g/dL	12
Platelets	
>450,000/µL	34
<100,000/µL	4
WBC ≥50,000/µL	43
Marrow	
≥5% blasts	7
≥5% basophils	14
Peripheral smear	
≥3% blasts	12
≥7% basophils	15
Cytogenetic clonal evolution other than the Ph chromosome	9

Ph = Philadelphia chromosome; WBC = white blood cells.

a low platelet count and/or platelet dysfunction) or thrombosis (associated with thrombocytosis and/or marked leukocytosis) occur. Other rare presentations include gouty arthritis (from elevated uric acid levels), priapism (usually with marked leukocytosis or thrombocytosis), retinal hemorrhages, and upper gastrointestinal ulceration and bleeding (from elevated histamine levels due to basophilia). Headaches, bone pain, arthralgias, pain from splenic infarction, and fever are uncommon in the chronic phase but more frequent as CML progresses. Leukostatic symptoms, such as dyspnea, drowsiness, loss of coordination, or confusion, which are due to sludging in the pulmonary or cerebral vessels, are uncommon in the chronic phase despite WBC counts exceeding 50,000 cells/µL, but these symptoms appear more frequently in the accelerated or blastic phases.

Splenomegaly, the most consistent physical sign in CML, occurs in 50 to 60% of cases. Hepatomegaly is less common (10 to 20%) and usually minor (1 to 3 cm below the right costal margin). Lymphadenopathy is uncommon, as is infiltration of skin or other tissues. If present, these findings suggest Ph-negative CML or the accelerated or blastic phase of CML.

Diagnosis

The diagnosis of typical CML is not difficult. Patients with untreated CML usually have leukocytosis ranging from 10,000 to 500,000/µL. The predominant cells are neutrophils, with a left shift extending to blast cells. Basophils and eosinophils are commonly increased. Monocytes may be slightly increased in some cases that overlap with chronic myelomonocytic leukemia (CMML; see later discussion). Thrombocytosis is common, whereas thrombocytopenia is rare and, if present, suggests a worse prognosis. A hemoglobin level of less than 11 g/dL is present in one third of patients. Biochemical abnormalities in CML include a low leukocyte alkaline phosphatase (LAP) score. A low LAP score also occurs in some patients with agnogenic myeloid metaplasia. Serum levels of vitamin B_{12}, lactate dehydrogenase, uric acid, and lysozyme are often increased. Some patients demonstrate a cyclic oscillation of the WBC count. The presence of unexplained myeloid leukocytosis (Fig. 195–2) with splenomegaly should lead to a bone marrow examination and cytogenetic analysis.

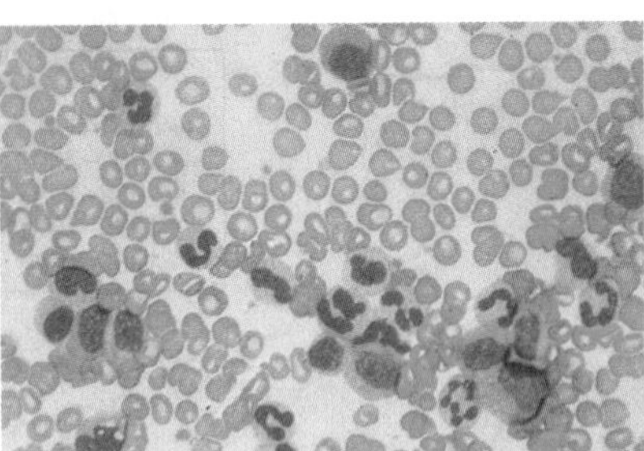

FIGURE 195–2 • Chronic myelogenous leukemia, chronic phase. Peripheral smear shows leukocytosis, with representation by the entire spectrum of leukocyte differentiation, ranging from myeloblasts to mature neutrophils. (Courtesy of Andrew Schafer, MD.)

Bone Marrow

The bone marrow is hypercellular with marked myeloid hyperplasia and, at times, evidence of increased reticulin or collagen fibrosis. The myeloid/erythroid ratio is 15:1 to 20:1. About 15% of patients have 5% or more blast cells in the peripheral blood or bone marrow at diagnosis.

Cytogenetics

The presence of the t(9;22)(q34;q11.2) abnormality establishes the diagnosis of CML. If the Ph chromosome is not found in a patient with suspected CML, molecular studies for the presence of the hybrid *BCR-ABL* gene should be performed. About 25 to 30% of patients with a typical morphologic picture of CML who are Ph-negative have *BCR-ABL* rearrangement. The Ph chromosome is usually present in 100% of metaphases, often as the sole abnormality. Between 10 and 15% of patients have additional chromosomal changes (loss of the Y chromosome, trisomy 8, an additional loss of material from 22q, or double Ph). Some patients have complex chromosomal changes involving chromosome 9 or chromosome 22 (Ph-variants; three-way translocations).

Differential Diagnosis

CML must be differentiated from leukemoid reactions (Chapter 173), which usually produce WBC counts lower than 50,000/µL, toxic granulocytic vacuolation, Döhle bodies in the granulocytes, absence of basophilia, a normal or increased LAP level, and a clinical history and physical examination suggesting the origin of the leukemoid reaction. Corticosteroids can rarely cause extreme neutrophilia with a left shift, but this abnormality is self-limited and of short duration.

CML may be more difficult to differentiate from other myelodysplastic or myeloproliferative syndromes (Chapters 172, 177, and 193). Patients with agnogenic myeloid metaplasia with or without myelofibrosis frequently have splenomegaly, neutrophilia, and thrombocytosis. Polycythemia rubra vera with associated iron deficiency, which causes normal hemoglobin and hematocrit values, can manifest with leukocytosis and thrombocytosis. Such patients usually have a normal or increased LAP score, a WBC count less than 25,000/µL, and no Ph chromosome.

The greatest diagnostic difficulty lies with patients who have splenomegaly and leukocytosis but do not have the Ph chromosome. In some, the *BCR-ABL* hybrid gene can be demonstrated despite a normal or atypical cytogenetic pattern. Patients who are Ph-negative and *BCR-ABL* negative are considered to have Ph-negative CML or CMML (see later discussion). Rarely, patients have myeloid hyperplasia, which involves almost exclusively the neutrophil, eosinophil, or basophilic cell lineage. These patients are described as having chronic neutrophilic, eosinophilic, or basophilic leukemia and do not have evidence of the Ph chromosome or the *BCR-ABL* gene. Isolated megakaryocytic hyperplasia can give rise to idiopathic thrombocythemia (Chapter 177) with marked thrombocytosis and splenomegaly. Some patients who present with clinical characteristics of essential thrombocythemia (with marked thrombocytosis but without leukocytosis) have CML; cytogenetic and molecular studies showing the Ph chromosome or the *BCR-ABL* rearrangement, or both, lead to the appropriate diagnosis and treatment.

Clinical Course

Evolution of Chronic Myelogenous Leukemia: Accelerated and Blastic Phases

More than 90% of patients present with CML in the benign or chronic phase, which becomes asymptomatic once controlled. Death rarely occurs during chronic phase CML.

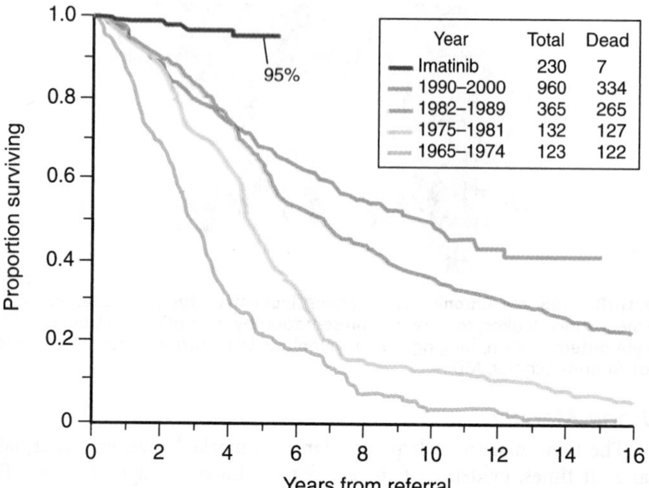

FIGURE 195–3 • Survival of patients with Ph-positive chronic myelogenous leukemia in chronic phase. (M. D. Anderson data; 1810 patients from 1965 to 2005.)

When poorly controlled, CML evolves into an accelerated phase, usually defined by the presence of 15% or more blasts, 30% or more blasts + promyelocytes, 20% or more basophils, thrombocytopenia less than 100,000/μL unrelated to therapy, or cytogenetic clonal evolution. About 5 to 10% of patients present in the accelerated phase. The accelerated phase is also characterized by worsening anemia; increasing splenomegaly or hepatomegaly; infiltration of nodes, skin, bones, or other tissues; increasing peripheral blasts or basophils; or fever, malaise, and weight loss. In accelerated phase CML, bone marrow studies may show dysplastic changes, increased percentages of blasts and basophils, myelofibrosis, and chromosomal abnormalities in addition to the Ph chromosome (clonal evolution).

Before the era of imatinib therapy, the risk of developing accelerated or blastic phase in CML was 10% per year in the first 2 years after diagnosis, then 15 to 20% per year thereafter, unless therapies such as IFN-α or allogeneic stem cell transplantation were used. With imatinib, the annual incidence of progression of CML from chronic to accelerated-blastic phases has been 2% in the first 5 years of observation (Fig. 195–3). Before imatinib therapy, the median survival of accelerated phase CML was 18 months or less, but now survival has increased to 4 years or more.

The blastic phase of CML is diagnosed when 30% or more blast cells are present in the bone marrow and/or peripheral blood, or in the presence of extramedullary blastic disease (Table 195–2). Most patients develop accelerated phase features prior to blastic, but 20% of patients evolve quickly into a blastic phase without warning. Most patients in accelerated or blastic phase have additional chromosomal abnormalities (clonal evolution), such as duplication of the Ph chromosome, trisomy of chromosome 8, or development of an isochromosome 17. Extramedullary blastic phase of CML can occur in the spleen, lymph nodes, skin, meninges (especially in lymphoid blastic phase), bone, and other sites; extramedullary transformation is usually followed shortly by evidence of marrow involvement. Blastic phase CML is associated with a very poor median survival time of 5 months. About 25% develop a lymphoid blastic phase; their response rate to anti-ALL–like chemotherapy and imatinib is about 60%, and their median survival time is about 1 year.

BCR-ABL–Negative Chronic Myelogenous Leukemia

Ph-negative and *BCR-ABL*-negative CML often appear to overlap clinically with CMML in their behavior, progress, and response to therapy and to resemble the myelodysplastic syndromes (Chapter 193) more than Ph-positive CML. A male preponderance and older age are noted; splenomegaly is common (60 to 70%). The WBC count is usually in the range of 25,000 to 100,000/μL. Anemia, thrombocytopenia, and monocytosis are more common than in Ph-positive CML, whereas eosinophilia and basophilia are less common. The median survival time is 18 to 24 months; patients die of infection, bleeding, or transformation to acute leukemia.

TABLE 195–2 FEATURES AND DEFINITIONS OF ACCELERATED AND BLASTIC PHASE CHRONIC MYELOGENOUS LEUKEMIA

ACCELERATED PHASE CHRONIC MYELOGENOUS LEUKEMIA
Commonly used criteria
Marrow or peripheral blasts: 10% or more
Marrow or peripheral basophils and eosinophils: 20% or more
Frequent Pelger-Huët–like neutrophils, nucleated red cells, or megakaryocytic nuclear fragments
Increased marrow reticulin or collagen fibrosis
Leukocytosis (>50,000/μL), anemia (hematocrit <25%), or thrombocytopenia (<100,000/μL) not responsive to antileukemic therapy
Progressive splenomegaly unresponsive to therapy
Unexplained fever or bone pain
Requirement of increased doses of medication
Documented extramedullary leukemia
Chromosomal abnormality in addition to the Ph chromosome (excludes loss of chromosome Y, Ph variants, constitutional abnormalities)
Criteria used in recent studies of accelerated phase CML
Percent blasts: 15% or more
Percent basophils: 20% or more
Percent blasts + promyelocytes: 30% or more
Thrombocytopenia <100,000 μL not related to therapy
Chromosomal abnormality in addition to the Ph chromosome (excludes loss of chromosome Y, Ph variants, constitutional abnormalities)
BLASTIC PHASE CHRONIC MYELOGENOUS LEUKEMIA
Marrow or peripheral blasts: 30% or more
Extramedullary hematopoiesis with immature blasts

CML = chronic myelogenous leukemia; Ph = Philadelphia chromosome.

Treatment

Treatment decisions in CML are based on the patient's age, the availability of a donor, the phase of CML, and the patient's or physician's preferences or experience. Definitive therapy is divided into transplantation and nontransplantation alternatives.

Nontransplantation Therapies

Imatinib Mesylate

Since its discovery in 1999, imatinib mesylate has become standard therapy for CML. Imatinib is a 2-phenylaminopyrimidine derivative that binds to the canonical adenosine triphosphate (ATP) lining the groove between the N and C lobes of the ABL kinase domain, thus blocking the phosphorylation of tyrosine residues on substrate protein. Blocking of ATP binding inactivates the ABL kinase, because it cannot transfer phosphate to its substrate. By inhibiting phosphorylation, imatinib prevents activation of signal transduction pathways that induce the leukemic transformation processes that cause CML (Fig. 195–4). Imatinib inhibits several tyrosine kinases, including $p210^{BCR\text{-}ABL}$, $p190^{BCR\text{-}ABL}$, v-ABL, c-ABL, c-Kit, and PDGF-receptor.

In a randomized trial of 1106 patients with newly diagnosed CML, imatinib 400 mg orally daily provided significantly higher rates of major cytogenetic response (87% versus 35%) and complete cytogenetic response (76% versus 14%), as well as lower rates of progression (8% versus 26%) and transformation (3% versus 9%) after 12 months of therapy, compared with the prior standard nontransplantation therapy (a combination of IFN-α plus cytosine arabinoside). 1, 2 The longer-term follow-up results continue to demonstrate outstanding outcomes with imatinib therapy (Table 195–3; see Fig. 195–3): with a median follow-up time of 5 years, the complete cytogenetic response rate is 84%, the annual rate of pro-

Rx

gression to accelerated-blastic phase is only 7%, and the estimated 5-year survival rate is 89%. 3

Imatinib has a 5% or lower rate of serious side effects, including nausea, vomiting, diarrhea, skin rashes, muscle cramps, bone aches, periorbital or leg edema, weight gain, and, rarely, hepatic, renal, or cardiopulmonary dysfunction; most of these are manageable with dose reductions or treatment interruptions. Drug-related myelosuppression occurs in 10 to 20% of patients with newly diagnosed CML and is manageable with brief treatment interruptions or dose modifications or both, or with growth factors (erythropoietin for anemia, granulocyte colony-stimulating factor [G-CSF] for neutropenia). Hypophosphatemia associated with altered bone metabolism can occur, and the serum phosphate level should be monitored. Chromosomal abnormalities may appear in the Ph-negative diploid cells in 5 to 10% or responding patients, probably due to unmasking of a fragile stem cell prone to development of CML or to chromosomal instability; such changes disappear spontaneously in 70% of cases and rarely evolve into a myelodysplastic syndrome or acute myeloid leukemia, probably as part of the natural course of CML.

Transplantation Therapies

Allogeneic Stem Cell Transplantation

Allogeneic stem cell transplantation, a potentially curative therapy in selected patients with CML, is most effective during the chronic phase, when it is associated with a 20-year survival rate of 40 to 50%. Transplant-related mortality ranges from 5 to 50%, depending on the patient's age, whether the donor is related or unrelated, the degree of matching, and other, less important factors, such as positivity for cytomegalovirus, preparative and post-transplantation regimens, and institutional expertise. Disease-free survival rates with related allogeneic stem cell transplantation are 40 to 80% in chronic phase, 15 to 40% in accelerated phase, and 5 to 20% in blastic phase. In chronic phase CML, patients younger than 30 to 40 years of age have disease-free survival rates of 60 to 80%, compared with only 30 to 40% for patients older than 50 years of age. A major limitation of allogeneic stem cell transplantation is the availability of related donors. Human leukocyte antigen (HLA)-compatible unrelated donors can be found for 50% of patients; the median time from initiation of the donor search to transplantation is 3 to 6 months.

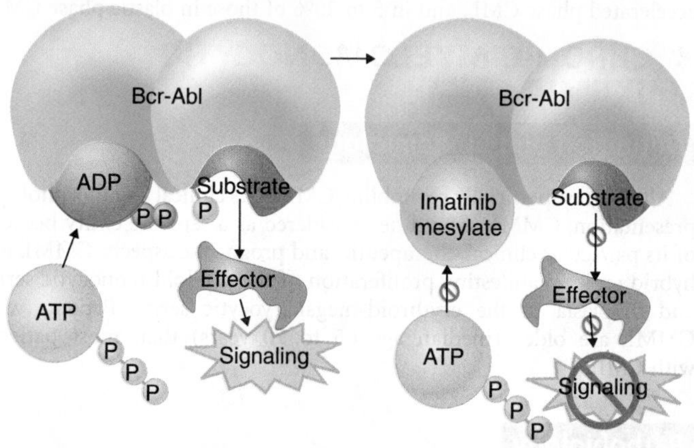

FIGURE 195–4 • Mechanism of action of imatinib. By occupying the ATP binding pocket of the ABL kinase domain, imatinib prevents substrate phosphorylation and downstream activation of signals, thus inhibiting the leukemogenic effects of BCR-ABL on cells in chronic myelogenous leukemia. ADP = adenosine diphosphate; ATP = adenosine triphosphate; P = phosphate group.

Nonmyeloablative preparative regimens have expanded the indications for allogeneic stem cell transplantation to older patients and have reduced transplantation-related mortality and complications (Chapter 184). Early results show acceptable degrees of engraftment, less mortality and organ damage, more persistent residual disease, and perhaps similar degrees of graft-versus-host disease. Patients whose CML recurs after allogeneic stem cell transplantation may respond to donor lymphocyte infusions, imatinib, IFN-α, or a second allogeneic transplant.

Initial Choice of Therapy in Chronic Myelogenous Leukemia

Most patients with CML (80% or more) are not candidates for allogeneic stem cell transplantation owing to age restrictions, comorbid conditions, or donor availability; imatinib is then clearly the treatment of choice. Patients who are transplantation candidates face the difficult decision of choosing between two effective but vastly different treatment options: allogeneic stem cell transplantation or imatinib therapy. The advantages of stem cell transplantation are its proven track record, with an estimated cure rate of 40% at 20 years. However, it is associated with a 1-year mortality rate of 5 to 40%, and with morbidities including cataracts, infertility, second cancers (5 to 10%), immune-mediated complications, and chronic graft-versus-host disease. Delaying allogeneic stem cell transplantation beyond the first 1 to 3 years after diagnosis may be associated with worse results and with occasional sudden CML blastic transformation, which may not be salvageable. The major disadvantages of imatinib therapy are the short current follow-up of its results (maximum of 6 to 7 years), the low rate of eradication of molecular disease, and the present need for indefinite therapy. It has a low rate of serious, often transient side effects, although drug-induced hypophosphatemia may be associated with impaired bone remodeling.

Initial choice of therapy in younger patients with a related matched donor is still a subject of controversy, However, many investigators and physicians now believe that most patients with CML should receive initial imatinib therapy and be considered for allogeneic stem cell transplantation only if imatinib therapy fails. Alternatively, a more potent tyrosine kinase inhibitor may be tried if imatinib resistance is seen. For example, nilotinib (AMN107), a selective BCR-ABL tyrosine kinase inhibitor, is 20 to 50 times more potent than imatinib, and dasatinib (BMS-354825), a dual SRC/ABL inhibitor, is 300 times more potent than imatinib. In phase I and II studies, both agents have been associated with complete hematologic response rates of 70 to 80% and cytogenetic response rates of 40 to

TABLE 195–3 EARLY RESULTS OF IMATINIB MESYLATE THERAPY IN CHRONIC MYELOGENOUS LEUKEMIA

Phase	% Cytogenetic Response		Estimated Survival
	Complete (Ph 0%)	Major (Ph <35%)	
Blastic	7	10–20	10–15% at 4 yr
Accelerated	20–40	40–60	40–50% at 4 yr
Chronic, after failure of IFN-α	55–63	60–80	80–85% at 4 yr
Chronic, newly diagnosed	65–85	80–90	90–95% at 4–5 yr

IFN-α = interferon-α; Ph = Philadelphia chromosome.

50% in chronic phase CML, and with encouraging results in accelerated-blastic phase CML in patients for whom imatinib therapy has failed.

Treatment of Accelerated and Blastic Phase Chronic Myelogenous Leukemia

Response rates to combination chemotherapy are 20% in nonlymphoid blastic phase CML and 60% in lymphoid blastic phase CML. Median survival times are 3 to 6 months and 9 to 12 months, respectively. The addition of imatinib to chemotherapy has improved the response rates and prolonged the median survival time in CML blastic phase from 3 to 5 months to 6 to 10 months.

Allogeneic stem cell transplantation is presently the only curative therapy for accelerated and blastic phase CML: overall cure rates are in the ranges of 5 to 20%, and 15 to 40%, respectively, and patients with cytogenetic clonal evolution as the only accelerated phase criterion have a long-term event-free survival rate of about 60%. Otherwise, imatinib, the only approved treatment for accelerated or blastic phase CML, provides hematologic responses in 80% of patients and an estimated 4-year survival rate of 40 to 55% in accelerated phase CML, but only a 40% response rate and a median survival of 7 months in blastic phase CML. Patients in accelerated or blastic phases should be encouraged to participate in investigational strategies to improve their prognosis. Combinations of imatinib with chemotherapy may improve results in CML-transformation, as may the new tyrosine kinase inhibitors.

Special Therapeutic Considerations

Patients with severe leukocytosis and leukostatic manifestations may benefit from initial leukapheresis. Severe thrombocytosis uncontrolled with anti-CML measures may respond to anagrelide, thio-TEPA, IFN-α, and leukapheresis. CML during pregnancy may be controlled with pheresis in the first trimester and then with hydroxyurea until delivery. Use of IFN-α during pregnancy has been reported to be safe anecdotally. There is little experience with the use of imatinib during pregnancy. Splenectomy is useful as a palliative measure in patients with massive painful splenomegaly, hypersplenism, or thrombocytopenia.

Follow-up

Monitoring Response to Therapy in CML

With improved therapy, the incidences of complete cytogenetic response and minimal residual disease have increased. This has required the development of new techniques to measure these responses more accurately (rather than relying on only 20 metaphases by cytogenetic analysis), with less tedious and painful procedures (peripheral blood rather than marrow studies), and with techniques that can measure minimal (molecular) disease below the level of detection by routine cytogenetic studies. Fluorescent in situ hybridization (FISH) studies with improved probes can measure 200 interphase cells, can be done using peripheral blood, and have false-positive rates of less than 2% or 3%. Quantitative polymerase chain reaction (QPCR) studies usually measure the ratio of the abnormal message BCR-ABL to a normal message ABL. A BCR-ABL/ABL ratio of less than 0.05 to 0.1%, about a 3-log reduction of disease, has been associated with a very low risk of CML relapse on imatinib therapy. This is now referred to as a major molecular response. A negative QPCR analysis (i.e., undetectable BCR-ABL levels, usually less than 10^{-5} to 10^{-6}) may be very dependent on the technique used and could be referred to as a complete molecular response.

In monitoring the response to imatinib-based therapies, patients require a bone marrow analysis before therapy (to determine the percentages of blasts and basophils and clonal evolution) and once a year (again to look for chromosomal abnormalities in both Ph-positive and Ph-negative cells). Monitoring can then continue with peripheral blood FISH studies every 3 to 4 months until Ph-positive cells are less than 5%, at which time monitoring can be continued with either FISH or QPCR studies. The frequency of monitoring depends on the treatment plan and is more frequent in younger patients, less frequent in very old patients. "Resistance" to imatinib therapy can be defined as persistent 100% Ph-positivity after 6 months of therapy, Ph-positivity of more than 35% after 12 to 18 months of therapy, or cytogenetic or hematologic relapse. A positive QPCR in a patient in complete cytogenetic response is not, at present, an indication of imatinib resistance or for change of therapy.

Future Directions

New tyrosine kinase inhibitors may soon be approved for first-line or salvage strategies, either alone or in combinations with existing therapies or novel agents. Immunotherapeutic strategies, including vaccines, may improve eradication of minimal residual disease, thereby potentially obviating the need for indefinite therapy with imatinib. Further understanding of the pathophysiology and events downstream of BCR-ABL may help in a rational development of new strategies that could target these events. Such strategies may include inhibitors of pathways involving Raf, protein farnesylation, mTOR, JAK/STAT, proteasome, MEK/MAPK, PI3K/AKT, or others.

Prognosis

Imatinib therapy has revolutionized the treatment of CML. In cases of newly diagnosed CML, imatinib therapy is associated with an estimated 5-year survival rate greater than 90%. If this favorable trend continues with longer follow-up, the median survival time in CML may exceed 20 years. During the first 5 years of follow-up, the annual mortality has been about 2%. Many previously well-established poor prognostic factors in CML have lost much of their importance since the advent of imatinib therapy. With allogeneic stem cell transplantation, cures are expected in 40 to 80% of patients in chronic phase CML, in 15 to 40% of those in accelerated phase CML, and in 5 to 20% of those in blastic phase CML.

CHRONIC MYELOMONOCYTIC LEUKEMIA

Definition and Epidemiology

Although superficially resembling CML in its clinical and morphologic presentation, CMML should be considered as a separate entity because of its particular clinical, therapeutic, and prognostic aspects. CMML is a hybrid entity manifesting proliferation of the myeloid monocytic series and dysplasia of the erythroid-megakaryocytic series. Patients with CMML are older (median age 65 to 70 years) than most patients with CML.

Pathobiology

The cytogenetic findings in patients with CMML are normal or involve an additional chromosome 8 or findings other than the Ph chromosome. Patients with CMML have *RAS* mutations in 40 to 60% of cases.

Clinical Manifestations and Diagnosis

Patients often present with symptoms related to anemia and thrombocytopenia (fatigue, bleeding). Other typical features include splenomegaly, leukocytosis, and monocytosis. Organ infiltration (lymph nodes, skin, liver) is less common. Basophilia and thrombocytosis are not presenting features.

Treatment and Prognosis

Allogeneic stem cell transplantation (Chapter 184), which is the only curative modality, should be considered as front-line therapy in candidate patients. Other therapies include hydroxyurea to control leukocytosis; erythropoietin to improve anemia; azacitidine or decitabine (both approved by the U.S. Food and Drug Administration [FDA] for the treatment of CMML); topotecan and cytarabine, or other anti-AML (Chapter 194) intensive regimens for CMML transformation; splenectomy for symptomatic splenomegaly and/or hypersplenism; and investigational agents.

Poor prognostic factors include the presence of anemia (hemoglobin <10 g/dL), thrombocytopenia, and more than 5% blasts. Median survival time is 12 to 18 months.

HAIRY CELL LEUKEMIA

Definition and Epidemiology

Hairy cell leukemia (HCL) is an uncommon and indolent B-cell leukemia (1 to 2% of all leukemias). The median age at diagnosis is 50 years, and there is a 4:1 male preponderance.

Pathobiology

The cell of origin of HCL is the B lymphocyte, as documented by the demonstration of heavy- and light-chain immunoglobulin gene rearrangements. Hairy cells express CD19, CD20, CD11C, CD103, FMC7, and CD22, but not CD21, CD5, CD10, or CD23. The cells demonstrate a κ or λ light-chain phenotype excess. The cells also express CD25 (TAC), the low-affinity interleukin-2 (IL-2) receptor. High levels of soluble IL-2 receptor (>5 times normal) are present in the sera of almost all patients with HCL, with extremely high levels being noted in many cases. A number of different cytogenetic abnormalities have been reported in HCL, but none appears to be consistently present, and all have been described in other hematologic malignancies. Immune dysfunction is wide-ranging in HCL. Monocytopenia is universal; B and T lymphocytes are decreased in number; the CD4/CD8 (T-helper/T-suppressor) ratio is often inverted; and skin test reactivity to recall antigens is impaired, as is antibody-dependent cellular cytotoxicity. Humoral immunity is relatively preserved, with normal immunoglobulin levels. Marrow failure in HCL may be due in part to inhibitory factors (e.g., tumor necrosis factor) produced by the leukemic infiltrate; the pancytopenia is often more marked than would be anticipated from the degree of leukemic infiltration.

Clinical Manifestations

The majority of patients present with pancytopenia and splenomegaly. Patients may also have fatigue, fever, weight loss, and infection secondary to granulocytopenia or monocytopenia. Leukocytosis is uncommon, and lymphadenopathy is rare. Anemia is present in up to 85% of patients, whereas leukopenia and thrombocytopenia are present in 60 to 75%. The cytopenias are caused by a combination of bone marrow failure due to leukemic infiltration and hypersplenism. Patients may experience repeated infections and, rarely, a systemic vasculitis resembling polyarteritis nodosa. Although bacterial infections occur as expected with neutropenia, patients with HCL have a predilection to develop tuberculosis, atypical mycobacterial infections, and fungal infections, perhaps related to the severe monocytopenia that is characteristic of this disorder.

Diagnosis

In conjunction with the described clinical features, careful examination of the peripheral blood smear may demonstrate the occasional typical cells with cytoplasmic projections, giving rise to the name *hairy cell leukemia* (Fig. 195–5). The hairy cells are 10 to 15 mm in diameter, with pale blue cytoplasm, a nucleus with a loose chromatin structure, and one or two indistinct nucleoli. Bone marrow aspiration is often inadequate owing to increased deposition of reticulin, collagen, and fibrin; bone marrow biopsy is usually necessary. Bone marrow involvement is interstitial or patchy, and the infiltrate is characterized by widely spaced nuclei due to the abundant cytoplasm, giving rise to the commonly described "fried egg" appearance.

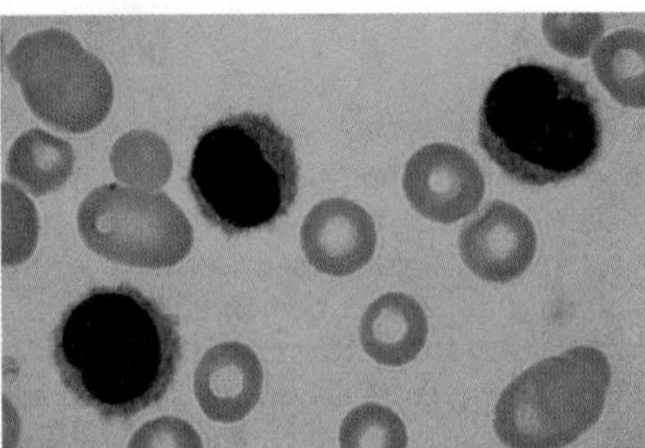

FIGURE 195–5 • Hairy cell leukemia. Peripheral smear shows hairy cells with blue-gray cytoplasm; fine, hairlike projections (resembling ruffles); and oval or slightly indented nuclei with loose chromatin and indistinct nucleoli. (Courtesy of Andrew Schafer, MD.)

Hairy cells exhibit a strong acid phosphatase (isoenzyme 5) cytochemical reaction in 95% of cases, a reaction that is resistant to the inhibitory effect of tartaric acid (TRAP). Other lymphoproliferative diseases are rarely TRAP positive. Electron microscopy clearly demonstrates the microvillar projections. Often, ribosomal-lamellar complexes, which are characteristic but not diagnostic of HCL, can be identified. The peroxidase stain is negative, and lysozyme activity is absent in hairy cells, thereby differentiating these cells from monocytes.

Differential Diagnosis

The differential diagnosis must distinguish HCL from lymphoma (Chapter 196) or CLL, which can manifest with predominant splenomegaly and minimal lymphadenopathy. Some patients with a myelodysplastic syndrome (Chapter 193) or a myeloproliferative syndrome (Chapter 177) have splenomegaly and pancytopenia with only a few atypical cells. Patients with other diseases, such as systemic lupus erythematosus (Chapter 287) and other autoimmune diseases, B-cell and T-cell prolymphocytic leukemias (Chapter 194), infiltrative splenomegaly (Chapter 174), or tuberculosis (Chapter 345), may have splenomegaly and cytopenia, but these diagnoses can usually be made by history, physical examination, and appropriate blood and bone marrow tests. Splenomegaly, cytopenia, and nonaspirable marrow in a middle-aged man should create a high index of suspicion for HCL. Splenectomy and lymph node biopsy are sometimes necessary to establish the diagnosis in difficult cases. Cases of HCL variant manifest with higher WBC counts, are TRAP negative, have prominent nucleoli, and are only occasionally positive for antibodies against CD25. HCL variant responds less well to the agents that usually are effective in the management of typical HCL.

Treatment

A small proportion (<5%) of patients with HCL do not require therapy. These patients have mild cytopenias, are not transfusion dependent, have no history of infections, and have a low level of marrow infiltration by hairy cells.

2-Chlorodeoxyadenosine (cladribine), an adenosine analogue that is resistant to deamination by adenosine deaminase, produces complete remission in more than 80% of HCL patients after a single course of 0.1 mg/kg/day for 7 days given by continuous intravenous infusion, and it is now the recommended first-line therapy. Remissions are durable, and patients who relapse can often attain a second remission after retreatment with cladribine. The drug is well tolerated, with a low infection rate. Despite long-lasting suppression of $CD4^+$ lymphocyte counts, there does not appear to be an increase in late opportunistic infections or second malignancies.

Deoxycoformycin (pentostatin; 4 mg/m^2 weekly or every 2 weeks for up to 6 months), an adenosine deaminase inhibitor, produces complete remission in 50 to 60% of patients and partial remission in 40%. The response to treatment is rapid, and the drug is active in patients previously treated with IFN. Toxicity includes nausea and vomiting, infection, renal and hepatic dysfunction, conjunctivitis, and photosensitivity, albeit mild in most cases.

Human leukocyte interferon (HuIFN) or r-IFN-α, rapidly improves granulocyte, platelet, and hemoglobin levels (1 to 3 months); reduces spleen size; and decreases marrow infiltration. Peripheral

Rx

blood cell counts return to normal in 80% of cases, but complete remission is uncommon. In addition, when treatment is discontinued, relapse occurs within 1 to 2 years.

An immunotoxin, LMV2, composed of the Fc portion of the anti-TAC antibody linked to a *Pseudomonas* exotoxin, is effective in patients with refractory HCL. Rituximab also has activity in patients with relapsed HCL. Splenectomy is recommended mainly for patients with splenic infarcts or massive splenomegaly.

Prognosis

More than 85 to 90% of patients treated with 2-cladribine or pentostatin are projected to be alive at 10 years.

CHRONIC LYMPHOCYTIC LEUKEMIA

Definition

Chronic lymphocytic leukemia (CLL) is a neoplasm characterized by accumulation of monoclonal lymphocytes of B-cell origin. The cells accumulate in the bone marrow, lymph nodes, liver, spleen, and occasionally other organs.

Epidemiology

CLL is the most common leukemia (one third of all cases) in the Western world and is twice as common as CML. The disease occurs rarely in those younger than 30 years of age; most patients with CLL are older than 60 years. CLL increases in incidence exponentially with time; by age 80, the incidence rate is 20 cases per 100,000 persons per year. The male/female ratio is approximately 2:1. Asians in Japan and China have a CLL incidence only 10% of that in the United States and other Western countries. Intermediate incidence rates are seen in persons of Hispanic origin.

The cause of CLL is unknown. Ionizing radiation and viruses have not been associated with CLL, although recently hepatitis C infection has been associated with splenic lymphoma with villous lymphocytes (another indolent B-cell disorder). Familial clustering in CLL is more common than in other leukemias; first-degree relatives of patients have a two- to four-fold higher risk and develop CLL at a younger age, compared with the general population (anticipation). Farmers have a higher incidence of CLL than do those in other occupations, raising the question of the possible etiologic role of herbicides or pesticides. No definite leukemogenic role of chemicals, including benzene, has been established for CLL.

Pathobiology

Leukemia cells in CLL are homogeneous and have an appearance of normal mature lymphocytes. However, clonality can be documented by the presence of immunoglobulin gene rearrangements and the restriction to either κ or λ light chains on the cell surface. The cells express low-intensity monoclonal surface immunoglobulin (SmIg, usually immunoglobulin M [IgM] ± IgD) as well as the pan–B-cell antigens CD19, CD20, CD23, and CD24 in almost all cases and CD21 (which includes the receptor for the Epstein-Barr virus and the C3D component of complement) in more than 75% of cases. Almost all cells exhibit Ia antigen, receptors for the Fc fragment of IgG, and spontaneously form rosettes with mouse erythrocytes. In addition to B-cell antigens, CLL cells express CD5 (Leu 1, T1, and T101), a pan–T-cell antigen. Other T-cell antigens are absent. CD25 (TAC, IL-2 receptor) antigen is positive in about 25% of cases. T-cell function is invariably abnormal in CLL. T cells are increased in number at diagnosis, and the CD4/CD8 ratio is often inverted, owing to a relatively greater increase in $CD8^+$ cells. The CD4/CD8 ratio declines as the disease progresses and after therapy. The T cells have a blunted response to T-cell mitogens and decreased delayed hypersensitivity reactions to recall antigens. However, these T-cell functions may be impaired by factors produced by the CLL cells, because purified T cells have a normal response to T-cell mitogens.

Genetics

Standard cytogenetic analysis identifies abnormalities in 40 to 50% of cases of CLL, but CLL cells have low mitotic activity. By FISH, the likelihood of detecting abnormalities increases to 80%. A 13q deletion is the most common abnormality; other abnormalities include 11q deletion (15 to 20%), trisomy 12 (15 to 20%), and 17p deletion (5 to 10%). The 17p deletion increases in frequency as the disease progresses, recurs after therapy, and is associated with a very poor prognosis. The 11q deletion also is associated with a poorer prognosis, whereas 13q deletion, if present as the sole abnormality, is associated with a favorable prognosis.

Clinical Manifestations

Most patients with CLL are asymptomatic, and the disease is diagnosed when absolute lymphocytosis is noted in the peripheral blood (see Fig. 195–5) during evaluation for other illnesses or when the patient undergoes a routine physical examination. Symptoms such as fatigue, lethargy, loss of appetite, weight loss, and reduced exercise tolerance are nonspecific. Many patients have enlarged lymph nodes. B symptoms (fever, night sweats, weight loss) are rarely present initially, and their presence in later stages of the disease suggests transformation to large cell lymphoma. The most common infections are sinopulmonary. As the disease progresses, the frequency of neutropenia, T-cell deficiency, and hypogammaglobulinemia increases, resulting in infections with gram-negative bacteria, fungi, and viruses such as herpes zoster and herpes simplex.

The major physical findings relate to infiltration of the reticuloendothelial system. Lymphadenopathy with discrete, rubbery, mobile lymph nodes is present in two thirds of patients at diagnosis. Later, as the lymph nodes enlarge, they can become matted. Enlargement of the liver or spleen is less common at diagnosis (approximately 10% and 40% of cases, respectively) but occurs more frequently with progression. Organ failure resulting from infiltration with CLL is uncommon. Infiltration of the central nervous system in CLL is rare, and central nervous system symptoms are more likely to be caused by opportunistic infections, such as cryptococcosis or listeriosis.

Diagnosis

CLL is characterized by absolute lymphocyte counts ranging from 5000 to 600,000/μL in the peripheral blood. Even with markedly elevated WBC counts, hyperviscosity symptoms rarely occur, probably because of the small size and pliability of the cells. Anemia (hemoglobin <11 g/dL) is present in 15 to 20% of patients at diagnosis, and thrombocytopenia (platelet count <100,000/μL) in 10%. However, bone marrow replacement and hypersplenism, which are seen with progressive disease, increase the frequency of anemia and thrombocytopenia. The anemia is usually normochromic and normocytic, and the reticulocyte count is normal unless the patient has autoimmune hemolytic anemia (Chapter 164), which usually results from the development of a warm-reacting IgG antibody. The diagnosis of autoimmune hemolytic anemia, which occurs in 10% of cases, is confirmed by a positive direct Coombs' test (80 to 90% of cases), reticulocytosis, a low serum haptoglobulin concentration, and an elevated unconjugated serum bilirubin level. In such patients, reactive erythroid hyperplasia as a response to the hemolysis may be masked in the bone marrow by the marked lymphocytic infiltration. Cold agglutinin hemolysis occurs rarely in CLL. Autoimmune thrombocytopenia (immune thrombocytopenic purpura [ITP; see Chapter 179]) can be diagnosed in some cases by a positive test for platelet antibodies. The antibodies causing the red cell and platelet destruction are not produced by the CLL cells, and the mechanisms for the autoimmune diseases are not known. Pure red cell aplasia (Chapter 171) is an additional underappreciated cause of anemia in CLL.

The lymphocytes in CLL are indistinguishable on light or electron microscopy from normal small B lymphocytes (Fig. 195–6). On bone marrow aspiration, the proportion of lymphocytes is greater than 30% and may be up to 100%. Four patterns of lymphocyte infiltration on bone marrow biopsy occur: nodular (15%), interstitial (30%), mixed nodular and interstitial (30%), and diffuse (35%). Most early-stage cases have one of the first three patterns; diffuse histology is common in advanced-stage disease and becomes more prominent as the disease evolves. A diffuse histologic pattern confers a poor prognosis regardless of the stage of disease.

Differential Diagnosis

The many diseases that can cause lymphocytosis, such as pertussis (Chapter 334), cytomegalovirus (Chapter 399), Epstein-Barr virus mononucleosis (Chapter 400), tuberculosis (Chapter 345), toxoplasmosis (Chapter 370), chronic inflammatory disorders, and autoimmune syndromes, are seldom confused with B-cell CLL, largely because the lymphocytosis in these conditions is usually less than 15,000/μL and is not sustained. If doubt persists, immunophenotypic or molecular studies can distinguish the monoclonal lymphocytosis in CLL from the T-cell or polyclonal B-cell proliferation in the other disorders.

Other Chronic Lymphocytic Leukemias

The more difficult differential diagnosis is from other lymphoproliferative disorders, such as prolymphocytic leukemia (PLL), splenic lymphoma with villous lymphocytes, HCL, the leukemic phase of mantle cell lymphoma, and Waldenström's macroglobulinemia. Whereas certain clinical features are more common in some of these disorders (e.g., marked splenomegaly with minimal or no lymphadenopathy in PLL, splenic lymphoma and HCL versus extensive lymphadenopathy with or without splenomegaly in CLL), none of these clinical features is specific. The differential diagnosis therefore depends largely on histopathologic and, more specifically, immunophenotypic features (Table 195–4).

Prolymphocytic Leukemia

PLL is an uncommon disease (<5% of the incidence of CLL), and its characteristics of massive splenomegaly, minimal lymphadenopathy, and markedly elevated WBC count (often >100,000/μL), with 10 to 90% of the cells being prolymphocytes, distinguish this disease from typical B-cell CLL. Prolymphocytes are larger cells that have a distinct nucleolus and express FMC-7. The male/female ratio is 4:1, and the median age at diagnosis is 70 years. Survival is shorter than in CLL (median 3 years), and response to therapies usually applied in CLL is poor. A monoclonal spike, typically IgG or IgA, is present in one third of cases. The immunoglobulin on the surface of the cells is occasionally IgG or IgA, not IgM ± IgD, as in CLL. Several karyotypic abnormalities have been reported in PLL, including t(11;14) (q13;q32). Deletions of 11q3, 23, and 17p are more common in B-cell PLL than in CLL. Abnormalities in the *TP53* oncogene are found in 75% of cases B-cell PLL. One fifth of PLL cases express a T-cell phenotype.

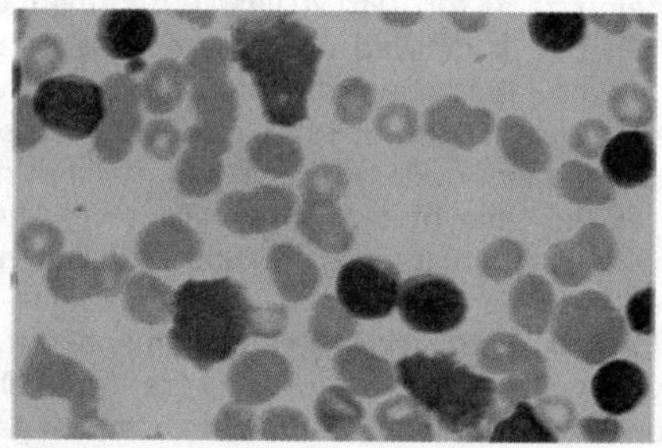

FIGURE 195–6 • Chronic lymphocytic leukemia. Peripheral smear shows that the predominant leukocytes are "normal," mature-appearing lymphocytes, with occasional "smudge" cells. (Courtesy of Andrew Schafer, MD.)

Small Lymphocytic Lymphoma

Small lymphocytic lymphoma (SLL) shares histopathologic and immunophenotypic features with CLL, differing only in the lack of lymphocytosis in the peripheral blood. The bone marrow in SLL may or may not have more than 30% lymphocytes. LFA-1 adhesion protein is much more commonly expressed on SLL cells than on CLL cells. Occasionally, other lymphomas, such as follicular and mantle cell lymphomas (Chapter 196), manifest a leukemic phase on initial presentation. Follicular lymphoma cells are often cleaved on light microscopy, have bright staining for SmIg, and are FMC-7 and CD10 positive. Lymph node biopsy should be performed to identify these cases with greater precision. The presence of lymphoma cells in the blood in follicular lymphoma is more common with advanced disease. Follicular lymphoma can usually be identified by the presence of the translocation t(14;18) and consequent *BCL2* rearrangement, both of which are rare in CLL. The WBC count in Waldenström's macroglobulinemia (Chapter 198) is usually much lower than in CLL (<10,000/μL), and many patients are leukopenic. The cells have a plasmacytoid appearance, CD38 and PCA-1 positivity, and more SmIg and cytoplasmic Ig. A monoclonal IgM plasma peak is present in almost all cases of Waldenström's macroglobulinemia but is uncommon in CLL.

T-Cell Leukemias

The predominant clinical manifestation of Sézary's syndrome (a CD4$^+$ T-cell malignant disorder related to mycosis fungoides) is chronic exfoliative erythroderma with a low number of circulating monoclonal T cells. The clinical and laboratory differential diagnosis from CLL is not difficult. Other T-cell malignant disorders with peripheral blood involvement are adult T-cell leukemia-lymphoma and large granular lymphocytosis (LGL), also referred to as large granular lymphoproliferative disorder, T-cell lymphocytosis with neutropenia, or T-gamma lymphocytosis syndrome. Adult T-cell leukemia-lymphoma is associated with a

TABLE 195–4 DIFFERENTIAL DIAGNOSIS OF INDOLENT LYMPHOPROLIFERATIVE DISORDERS

Disease	Lymphadenopathy (%)	Splenomegaly (%)	Cell of Origin (B/T)	Positive Markers* SmIg	CD5	CD19, CD20 (%)	Other
Chronic lymphocytic leukemia (CLL)	75	50	B (20:1)	Weak	>90%	≥90	Mouse red blood cell receptors
Prolymphocytic leukemia (PLL)	33	95	B (4:1)	Bright	T-cell PLL	75	FMC-7
Hairy cell leukemia	<10	80	B (T rare)	Bright	—	>90	CD25, CD11C, CD103
Lymphoma (leukemic phase)	90	90	B (T rare)	Bright	Some	>90	CD10
Splenic lymphoma with villous lymphocytes	10	80	B	Bright	20%	>90	FMC-7, CD22
Waldenström's macroglobulinemia	33	33	All B	Weak	Some	Many	CD38, PCA-1
Large granular lymphocytosis	10	10	All T	Absent	—	—	CD2, CD3, CD8

*CD2 = pan–T cell; CD3 = pan–mature T cell; CD5 = pan–T cell, B-cell CLL; CD8 = T cell (suppressor cytotoxic); CD10 = early B cell; CD11C = hairy cell, activated T cell, NK cell; CD19 = early pan–B cell; CD20 = pan–B cell; CD25 = low-affinity interleukin-2 receptor; CD38 = activated B cell, thymocyte, plasma cell; FMC-7 = PLL, hairy cell leukemia; PCA-1 = plasma cell; SmIg = monoclonal surface immunoglobulin.

TABLE 195–5 RAI AND BINET STAGING SYSTEMS IN CHRONIC LYMPHOCYTIC LEUKEMIA

Stage	Lymphocytosis	Lymphadenopathy	Hepatomegaly or Splenomegaly	Hemoglobin (g/dL)	Platelets ×10³/mL
RAI STAGING SYSTEM					
0	+	–	–	≥11	≥100
I	+	+	–	≥11	≥100
II	+	±	+	≥11	≥100
III	+	±	±	<11	≥100
IV	+	±	±	Any	<100
BINET STAGING SYSTEM					
A	+	±	± (<3 lymphatic groups* positive)	≥10	≥100
B	+	±	± (≥3 lymphatic groups* positive)	≥10	≥100
C	+	±	±	<10†	<100†

*The three lymphatic groups are (1) cervical, axillary, and inguinal nodes; (2) liver; and (3) spleen. Each group is considered one group whether unilateral or bilateral.
†The criterion is hemoglobin <10 g/dL and/or platelets <100 × 10³/mL.

retrovirus (human T-cell leukemia-lymphoma virus [HTLV-I]) and is common in Japan and the Caribbean. It is frequently manifested by lytic bone lesions and hypercalcemia. In T-large granular lymphoproliferative disorders, the absolute lymphocyte count is usually low (<5000/μL), with a CD2⁺, CD3⁺, CD8⁺, and CD16⁺ (T-suppressor) phenotype (T-gamma cells). These patients often have splenomegaly, neutropenia, and rheumatoid arthritis–like symptoms. A subset, called *natural killer* (NK) *cell LGL*, has an NK cell phenotype (CD16⁻) and no molecular evidence of T-cell receptor rearrangement. The lymphocytes have abundant cytoplasm with azurophilic granules. In most patients, a benign course is noted, although repeated infections can occur.

Staging and Prognostic Factors

The natural history of CLL is heterogeneous, with survival times ranging from 2 to 20 years after diagnosis. Either of two validated clinical staging systems can be used. The Rai staging system (1975) defines five stages and is most frequently used in the United States, whereas the Binet system (1981) defines three stages and is most frequently used in Europe (Table 195–5). Patients with anemia and thrombocytopenia (Rai stages III and IV, Binet C) have the worst prognosis; patients with lymphocytosis alone (Rai 0, some Binet A patients) have an excellent prognosis. A group of patients with a lymphocyte count of less than 30,000/μL, hemoglobin greater than 13 g/dL, platelet count greater than 100,000/μL, fewer than three involved node areas, and lymphocyte doubling time of greater than 12 months has been described as having "smoldering" CLL, with survival equal to that of an age- and sex-matched population. Patients tend to progress through stages, with many patients developing more sites of involvement with time and eventually experiencing marrow failure, but anemia and thrombocytopenia can develop abruptly even without antibody-mediated destruction or markedly increased tumor burden.

Other adverse factors include a diffuse pattern of lymphocytic infiltration observed on bone marrow biopsy; molecular abnormalities, including deletion of 11q or 17p; advanced age; male sex; elevated serum levels of thymidine kinase, β_2-microglobulin, and soluble CD23; rapid lymphocyte doubling time; an increased proportion of large or atypical lymphocytes in the peripheral blood; and lack of somatic mutation of the VH gene within the B-CLL cell, often manifested by the presence of the ZAP-70 protein.

Treatment

Rx

The major therapeutic questions for CLL are when to treat and which therapeutic regimen to use. Patients with CLL are usually older, and the prognosis of the disease is variable (with some early-stage cases being stable for 10 to 20 years). Treatment of early-stage CLL (Rai 0, Binet A) is delayed until the disease progresses. Early treatment with alkylating agents does not prolong survival and may be associated with a heightened risk of developing second malignant tumors. Treatment of Rai stages III and IV (Binet stage C) is recommended at the time of diagnosis because of the morbidities associated with cytopenias and the poor survival time of these patients (median 3 years). Treatment of intermediate-stage disease (Rai stages I and II, Binet stage B) is recommended if symptomatic disease (fever, sweats, weight loss, severe fatigue), or massive lymphadenopathy, with or without hepatosplenomegaly, is present.

Medical Therapy

Chemotherapy

Fludarabine monophosphate (25 mg/m²/day for 5 days every 4 weeks), an adenosine analogue, is approved by the FDA for treatment of relapsed CLL, with overall response rates of 50 to 60%. The dose-limiting toxicity is myelosuppression. When used in conjunction with steroids, the treatment may be complicated by infections with organisms usually associated with immunodeficiency syndromes involving T lymphocytes (e.g., those caused by *Pneumocystis jiroveci* [PCP] or herpes viruses). In a large randomized trial of initial therapy of CLL, fludarabine resulted in higher overall and complete remission rates, longer durations of remission, and improved response rates on crossover, but no survival advantage compared with chlorambucil, 4 the prior standard therapy. This finding was probably related both to the crossover design of the study, in which patients who failed one treatment received the other, and to the low rates of complete response. Fludarabine combined with cyclophosphamide can provide responses in 86 to 100% of previously untreated patients, with complete responses in 35 to 47%, rates that were substantially better than with fludarabine alone in two randomized trials. 5 Cladribine is less effective and more toxic than fludarabine, and pentostatin has not been as widely studied in CLL as in HCL.

The COP regimen (cyclophosphamide, 100 to 300 mg/m²/day given orally on days 1 through 5; vincristine [Oncovin], 2 mg given intravenously on day 1; and prednisone, 100 mg given orally on days 1 through 5) does not have any advantage over chlorambucil alone, usually given as 0.1 to 0.2 mg/kg/day for 3 to 6 weeks until the desired effect is obtained or until thrombocytopenia or neutropenia develops; the dose is then adjusted for maintenance and is continued for 6 to 12 months. Regimens using cyclophosphamide,

TABLE 195–6 **DEFINITION OF REMISSION IN CHRONIC LYMPHOCYTIC LEUKEMIA (CLL): COMPARISON OF THE INTERNATIONAL WORKSHOP IN CLL (IWCLL) AND THE NATIONAL CANCER INSTITUTE WORKING GROUP (NCI-WG) CRITERIA**

	Complete Remission		Partial Remission	
Criteria	**IWCLL**	**NCI-WG**	**IWCLL**	**NCI-WG**
Physical examination				
Nodes	None	None	Shift to a lower Binet stage (e.g., C → A or B, B → A)	≥50% decrease
Liver/spleen	Not palpable	Not palpable		≥50% decrease
Symptoms	None	None		N/A
Peripheral blood				
Neutrophils	≥1500/mL	≥1500/mL		≥1500/mL or ≥50% increase from baseline
Platelets	>100,000/mL	>100,000/mL		100,000/mL or ≥50% increase from baseline
Hemoglobin	Not specified	>11 g/dL		>11 g/dL or >50% increase from baseline
Lymphocytes	<4000/mL	≤4000/mL		>50% decrease
Bone marrow	Normal aspirate and biopsy*			N/A
Lymphocytes		<30%		N/A

*Nodules or focal aggregates of lymphocytes are compatible with complete remission in IWCLL, not NCI-WG.

Rx

doxorubicin, and prednisone with vincristine (CHOP) or without vincristine (CAP) have produced response rates of 50 to 70% in previously untreated patients with Binet stage C disease and are well tolerated in CLL despite the advanced age of most patients; however, they do not prolong survival when compared with chlorambucil or fludarabine.

After therapy, many patients remain stable for months to years before progressive disease indicates the need for further treatment. The goal of treatment is to achieve a complete response (Table 195–6).

Monoclonal Antibodies

Rituximab, a monoclonal antibody targeting the CD20 antigen, is associated with response rates of about 50% when given at the standard dose (375 mg/m^2 weekly for 4 weeks) as initial therapy for CLL, and significantly lower rates when it is used in the salvage setting, but complete responses are rare in either setting. The major benefit of this antibody appears to be its use in combination with chemotherapy. The combination of fludarabine with rituximab appears better than fludarabine alone, [6] and a three-drug regimen of fludarabine, cyclophosphamide, and rituximab appears to produce the best and most durable complete remission rates (70%) when used as first-line therapy.

Alemtuzumab (CamPath-1H; 30 mg IV three times a week for 4 to 12 weeks), a monoclonal antibody that binds to the CD52 antigen, is approved for the treatment of fludarabine-refractory CLL. One third of such patients can achieve a remission.

Stem Cell Transplantation

Autologous stem cell transplantation has no proven benefit in terms of survival or long-term disease control in CLL. Data on allogeneic stem cell transplantation are limited to young patients with refractory disease, in whom a long-term control rate of 40 to 55% has been reported. Nonmyeloablative stem cell transplantation, which works mainly by its graft-versus-leukemia effect, has been used in older patients with CLL with some success.

Radiation Therapy

In CLL, radiation therapy is used in a palliative mode to shrink unsightly or painfully enlarged nodal masses or an enlarged spleen.

Autoimmune and Infectious Manifestations

Autoimmune hemolytic anemia and immune-mediated thrombocytopenia do not correlate closely with the activity of CLL. Prednisone (60 to 100 mg/day) is indicated as treatment for autoimmune hemolytic anemia (Chapter 164) and for some cases of immune-mediated thrombocytopenia (ITP; Chapter 179) in CLL. If there is no response in 3 to 4 weeks, the treatment has failed, and the dose should then be tapered over 1 to 2 weeks. If a response is obtained, the dose is reduced by 25% each week over 4 weeks. Patients for whom corticosteroids fail often respond to low-dose cyclosporin given orally at 100 mg three times daily. Other therapeutic options include splenectomy, intravenous immunoglobulin, and rituximab.

Intravenous immunoglobulin (400 mg/kg every 3 to 4 weeks) significantly decreases the incidence of infections in patients with recurrent infections and hypogammaglobulinemia. However, the cost of this therapy is substantial.

Prognosis

Approximately one third of patients who present with early-stage CLL never require therapy and have the same survival of age-matched controls. Frequent characteristics of such patients include WBC less than 30,000/μL, hemoglobin greater than 13 g/dL, nondiffuse pattern on bone marrow biopsy, and slow lymphocyte doubling time.

A poor response to therapy is an adverse factor in all phases of the disease. As CLL progresses, the development of a prolymphocytic transformation (10% of cases) or transformation to large cell lymphoma portends a median survival time of less than 6 months. Other factors that may suggest transformation are the development of B-symptoms or a markedly elevated lactate dehydrogenase (LDH) level. A high incidence of second malignant tumors (10 to 20% of patients) either precedes or follows the diagnosis of CLL, with the roles of therapy versus impaired immune surveillance as causative factors being unclear. Skin cancer, including melanoma, as well as colorectal and lung cancers, are common. CLL tends to develop in older people; in indolent cases, death often occurs from other intercurrent illnesses seen in this age group. Patients younger than 60 years of age and patients with progressive disease almost all die as a result of CLL, primarily from infections. Gram-positive organisms usually cause nonfatal infections early in CLL, but most deaths due to infection are associated with gram-negative bacterial or fungal infections. Infection with other opportunistic organisms, such as *Mycobacterium tuberculosis*, herpesvirus, and *P. jiroveci*, may also be fatal.

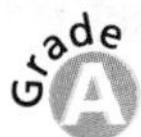

1. O'Brien SG, Guilhot F, Larson RA, et al: Imatinib compared with interferon and low-dose cytarabine for newly diagnosed chronic-phase chronic myeloid leukemia. N Engl J Med 2003;348:994–1004.
2. Hughes T, Kaeda J, Branford S, et al: Frequency of major molecular responses to imatinib or interferon alfa plus cytarabine in newly diagnosed chronic myeloid leukemia. N Engl J Med 2003;349: 1423–1432.
3. Druker B, Guilhot F, O'Brien S, et al: Five-year follow-up of patients receiving imatinib for chronic myeloid leukemia. N Engl J Med 2006;355:2408–2417.
4. Rai KR, Peterson BL, Appelbaum FR, et al: Fludarabine compared with chlorambucil as primary therapy for chronic lymphocytic leukemia. N Engl J Med 2000;343:1750–1757.
5. Eichhorst BF, Busch R, Hopfinger G, et al: Fludarabine plus cyclophosphamide versus fludarabine alone in first-line therapy of younger patients with chronic lymphocytic leukemia. Blood 2006;107:885–891.
6. Byrd JC, Peterson BL, Morrison VA, et al: Randomized phase 2 study of fludarabine with concurrent versus sequential treatment with rituximab in symptomatic, untreated patients with B-cell chronic lymphocytic leukemia: Results from Cancer and Leukemia Group B 9712 (CALGB 9712). Blood 2003;101:6–14.

SUGGESTED READINGS

Baccarani M, Saglio G, Goldman J, et al: Evolving concepts in the management of chronic myeloid leukemia: Recommendations from an expert panel on behalf of the European Leukemianet. Blood 2006;108:1809–1820. *Consensus guidelines.*

Chiorazzi N, Rai KR, Ferrarini M: Chronic lymphocytic leukemia. N Engl J Med 2005;352:804–815. *A comprehensive review.*

Mauro MJ, Maziarz RT: Stem cell transplantation in patients with chronic myelogenous leukemia: When should it be used? Mayo Clin Proc 2006; 81:404–416. *Suggests a limited role in the imatinib era.*

Shanafelt TD, Byrd JC, Call TG, et al: Initial management of newly diagnosed, early-stage chronic lymphocytic leukemia. Ann Intern Med 2006;145:435–447. *A clinical overview.*

Talpaz M, Shah NP, Kantarjian H, et al: Dasatinib in imatinib-resistant Philadelphia chromosome-positive leukemias. N Engl J Med 2006;354:2531–2541. *Dasatinib induces hematologic and cytogenetic responses in patients with CML or Ph-positive ALL.*

Yee KW, O'Brien SM: Chronic lymphocytic leukemia: Diagnosis and treatment. Mayo Clin Proc 2006;81:1105–1129. *A clinical review.*

196 NON-HODGKIN'S LYMPHOMAS

Philip J. Bierman, Nancy Harris, and James O. Armitage

Definition

Lymphomas are solid tumors of the immune system. Rapidly increasing knowledge of the biology of the immune system has led to corresponding increases in the understanding of these malignancies. In addition to better systems of classification and clinical evaluation, this new knowledge has led to the development of new therapies. Beneficial treatment is available for essentially every patient with non-Hodgkin's lymphoma, and many patients can be cured.

Epidemiology

In the United States, about 55,000 new cases of non-Hodgkin's lymphoma are diagnosed annually, and about 20,000 people are estimated to die each year of this disease. Non-Hodgkin's lymphomas account for about 4% of new cancers in the United States and result in about 4% of cancer deaths. The U.S. lifetime risk of developing non-Hodgkin's lymphoma is 2.18% (1 in 46) for men and 1.80% (1 in 56) for women. In 2002, the U.S. age-adjusted incidence rate for non-Hodgkin's lymphoma was about 23.2 per 100,000 for men and 16.3 per 100,000 in women. The incidence rate increases dramatically with age and is higher in whites than in other ethnic groups (Figs. 196–1 and 196–2).

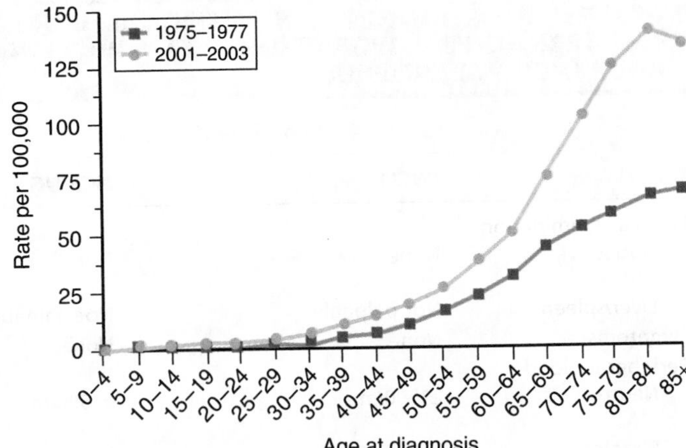

FIGURE 196–1 • Non-Hodgkin's lymphoma incidence by age in men. (From the Surveillance, Epidemiology, and End Results Program of the National Cancer Institute. *In* Ries LAG, Harkins D, Krapcho M, et al: SEER Cancer Statistics Review, 1975–2003. Bethesda, MD, National Cancer Institute, http://seer.cancer.gov/csr/1975_2003/, based on November 2005 SEER data submission, posted to the SEER website 2006.)

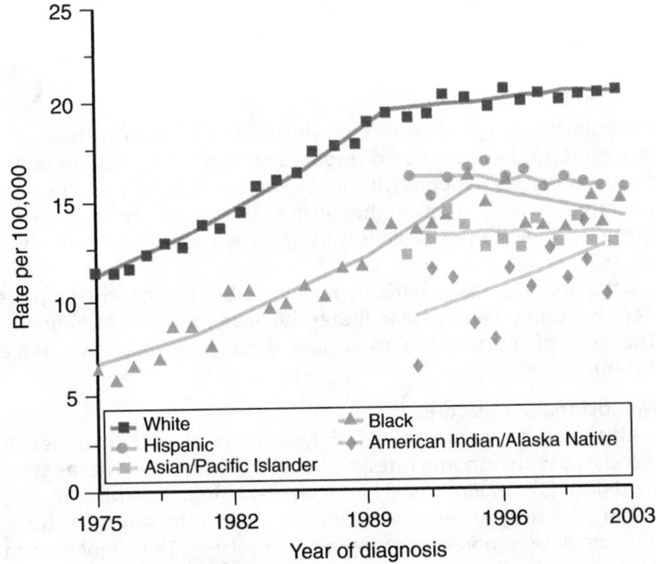

FIGURE 196–2 • Non-Hodgkin's lymphoma incidence, both genders. (From the Surveillance, Epidemiology, and End Results Program of the National Cancer Institute. *In* Ries LAG, Harkins D, Krapcho M, et al: SEER Cancer Statistics Review, 1975–2003. Bethesda, MD, National Cancer Institute, http://seer.cancer.gov/csr/1975_2003/, based on November 2005 SEER data submission, posted to the SEER website 2006.)

Geographic differences in the incidence of non-Hodgkin's lymphomas vary as much as five-fold. The highest rates are seen in the United States, Europe, and Australia, whereas lower rates are seen in Asia. Even more striking are geographic differences in the incidence of certain types of non-Hodgkin's lymphomas, such as Burkitt's lymphoma, follicular lymphoma, extranodal natural killer (NK)/T-cell nasal lymphoma, and adult T-cell leukemia/lymphoma (see later discussion).

Between 1950 and the early 1990s, the incidence rate for non-Hodgkin's lymphomas in the U.S. increased by about 3 to 4% yearly, but it has declined slightly since the mid-1990s (see Fig. 196–2). Increases have occurred among both men and women in all parts of the world. This increase in incidence is partially related to the aging population (see Fig. 196–1) and to the acquired immunodeficiency syndrome (AIDS) epidemic (Chapter 416); occupational and environmental exposures (e.g., farm chemicals) may also explain some of the increase. Finally, some of the increase may be explained by improvements in the ability of pathologists to diagnose lymphoma and by improvements in imaging techniques.

TABLE 196–1 FACTORS ASSOCIATED WITH THE DEVELOPMENT OF NON-HODGKIN'S LYMPHOMA

IMMUNE ABNORMALITIES
Inherited disorders
Severe combined immunodeficiency disease
Common variable immunodeficiency disease
Wiskott-Aldrich syndrome
Ataxia-telangiectasia
X-linked lymphoproliferative disorder
Acquired disorders
Solid organ transplantation
Acquired immunodeficiency syndrome
Methotrexate therapy for autoimmune disorders
Rheumatoid arthritis
Sjögren's syndrome
Hashimoto's thyroiditis
Infectious agents
Epstein-Barr virus
Human T-cell lymphotropic virus type I
Human herpesvirus 8
Hepatitis C virus
Helicobacter pylori
Borrelia burgdorferi
Chlamydia psittaci
Campylobacter jejuni
Occupational and environmental exposure
Herbicides
Organic solvents
Hair dyes
Ultraviolet light
Diet
Smoking

Pathobiology

For most cases of non-Hodgkin's lymphoma, the etiology is unknown, although genetic, environmental, and infectious agents have been implicated (Table 196–1).

Genetic Factors

Familial clusters have been described, and there is a slightly higher risk of non-Hodgkin's lymphoma among siblings and first-degree relatives of patients with lymphoma or other hematologic malignancies. Polymorphisms of tumor necrosis factor (308G→A) and interleukin (IL)-10 (3575 T→A) are associated with the development of diffuse large B-cell lymphoma.

Immune System Abnormalities

Several inherited disorders increase the risk of developing non-Hodgkin's lymphoma as much as 250-fold (see Table 196–1). In some of these conditions, the lymphoma may be related to the Epstein-Barr virus (EBV) (Chapter 400). For example, patients with the X-linked lymphoproliferative disorder have mutations in the *SH2D1A* gene, which encodes proteins that regulate host immune response against EBV-infected cells; they may develop fatal infectious mononucleosis or non-Hodgkin's lymphoma after primary exposure to EBV virus. Acquired immunodeficiency states are also associated with an increased risk of non-Hodgkin's lymphoma. For example, post-transplantation lymphoproliferative disorders occur in as many as 20% of patients who have received solid organ transplants, related to the proliferation of B lymphocytes that have been transformed by EBV immunosuppressive therapy. The risk of non-Hodgkin's lymphoma is also increased more than 100-fold in patients infected with the human immunodeficiency virus (HIV); almost all central nervous system (CNS) lymphomas and approximately 50% of other lymphomas in patients with AIDS are related to EBV (Chapter 415). Some studies have shown a two-fold increase in the incidence of non-Hodgkin's lymphomas among patients with rheumatoid arthritis (Chapter 285), and the risk of marginal zone lymphomas is increased approximately 30- to 40-fold in patients with Sjögren's syndrome (Chapter 289). Increases in the incidence of thyroid lymphoma are seen in patients with Hashimoto's thyroiditis (Chapter 244). Enteropathy-type T-cell lymphomas are associated with celiac disease (Chapter 143).

Infectious Agents

EBV is associated with the majority of post-transplantation lymphoproliferative disorders and many AIDS-associated lymphomas. This viral genome is detectable in more than 95% of cases of endemic Burkitt's lymphoma and in approximately 40% of cases of sporadic Burkitt's lymphoma and AIDS-associated lymphomas.

The human T-cell lymphotropic virus type I (HTLV-I; Chapter 401) is detectable in virtually all cases of adult T-cell leukemia/lymphoma. The risk of lymphoma is approximately 3% in patients infected with HTLV-I; in endemic areas, up to 50% of all non-Hodgkin's lymphomas may be related to HTLV-I. Reports of an association of Simian virus 40 with non-Hodgkin's lymphoma have not been supported by further research.

Human herpesvirus 8 (HHV-8, Kaposi's sarcoma–associated herpesvirus; Chapters 397 and 415), which is associated with expansion of the B-cell population, is also associated with primary effusion lymphoma (see later discussion) in immunocompromised patients and with multicentric Castleman's disease. Patients with primary effusion lymphoma are often coinfected with EBV.

Epidemiologic evidence has linked hepatitis C virus (Chapter 152) to lymphoplasmacytic lymphoma and splenic marginal zone lymphoma. Chronic antigenic stimulation from this virus may lead to the emergence of malignant B-cell clones.

Helicobacter pylori is associated with gastric lymphoma (see Chapter 202) of extranodal marginal zone/mucosa-associated lymphoid tissue (MALT). Colonized patients develop gastritis (Chapter 141) from chronic antigenic stimulation that is mediated by T cells, which respond to *H. pylori*–specific antigens; malignant B-cell clones emerge. *Borrelia burgdorferi* (Chapter 342) has been associated with marginal zone B-cell lymphoma of the skin. Evidence also links *Chlamydia psittaci* (Chapter 339) with ocular adnexal lymphomas and *Campylobacter jejuni* with immunoproliferative small intestinal disease (Chapter 326).

Environmental and Occupational Exposure

Agricultural chemicals have been associated with an increased risk of developing non-Hodgkin's lymphomas, and the strongest associations have been described with phenoxy herbicides such as 2,4-dichlorophenoxyacetic acid (2,4-D), which was also a component of Agent Orange (Chapter 17). An increased risk has also been associated with ionizing radiation (Chapter 18), organic solvents, hair dyes, and nitrates in drinking water, although contradictory results have been reported. Some studies have also linked non-Hodgkin's lymphomas to high-fat diets and ultraviolet radiation (Chapter 185). The risk of non-Hodgkin's lymphomas is increased approximately 20-fold after treatment for Hodgkin's disease (Chapter 197). Heavy smokers (Chapter 30) have an increased risk of developing follicular lymphoma.

Pathology

Non-Hodgkin's lymphomas are derived from cells of the immune system at varying stages of differentiation. In some cases, the cell of origin is directly linked to the morphology, immunophenotype, and clinical behavior of the lymphoma (Fig. 196–3 and Table 196–2).

The transformation of cells from the normal immune system into malignant lymphoma reflects the acquisition of specific genetic abnormalities. In many cases, cytogenetic studies can identify chromosomal translocations that underlie the development or progression of the lymphoma. In most cases of non-Hodgkin's lymphoma, the activation of proto-oncogenes is the major abnormality, but occasionally chromosomal translocations can lead to fusion genes that code for chimeric proteins. In addition, some cases are associated with deletion of tumor suppressor genes. Specific genetic abnormalities are associated with some specific subtypes of non-Hodgkin's lymphoma (Table 196–3).

Classification

The recognition of the Reed-Sternberg cell approximately 100 years ago made it possible to define Hodgkin's disease (Chapter 197) as a distinct entity, whereas other lymphomas were included under the heading of "non-Hodgkin's lymphomas." In the 1990s, a classification system

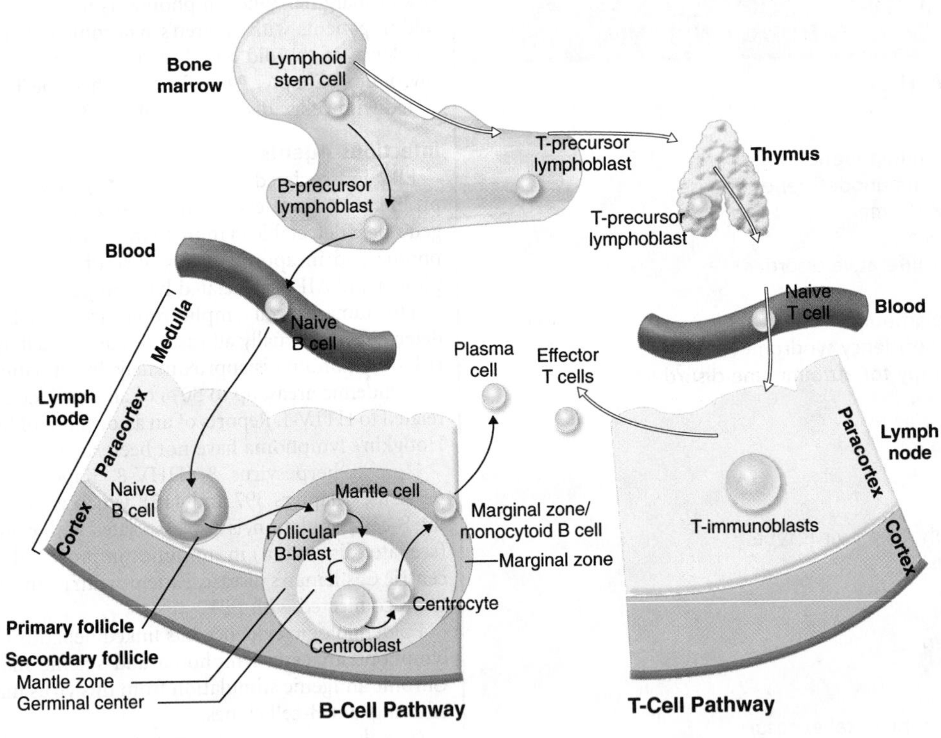

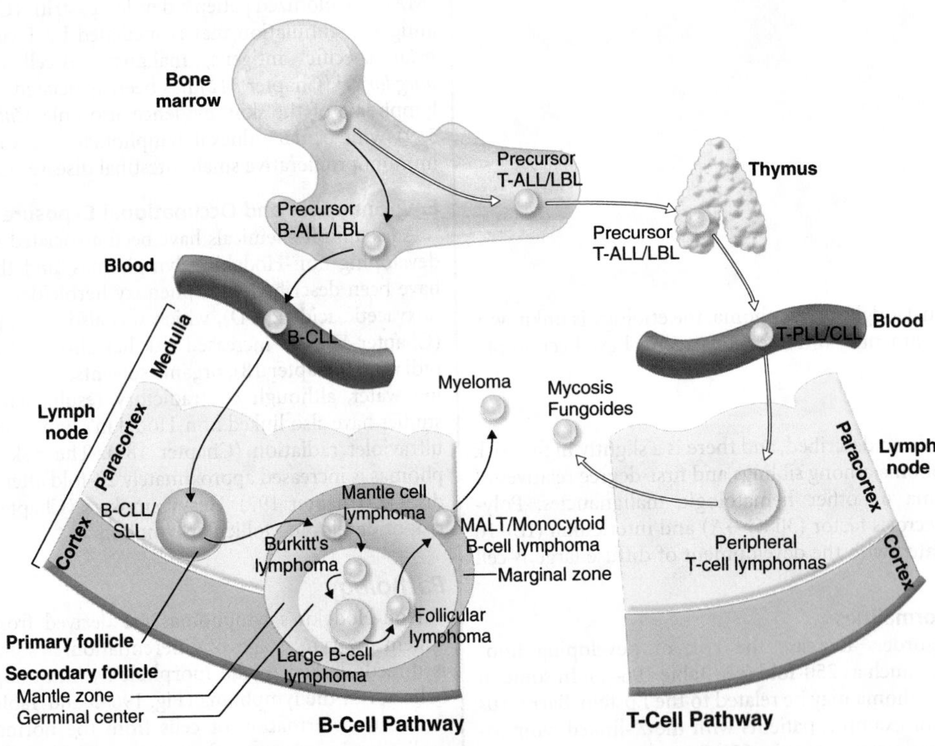

FIGURE 196–3 • Postulated normal counterparts of currently recognized B- and T-cell malignancies. A, Schema of normal B- and T-cell differentiation. Bone marrow–derived lymphoid stem cells differentiate into committed B-cell precursors or into T-cell precursors that undergo further maturation in the thymus. These B- and T-cell precursors mature into naive B or T cells that circulate to lymph nodes. After antigen exposure, normal B blasts proliferate and undergo further differentiation in the germinal center of the secondary follicle. The germinal center is surrounded by a mantle zone and a marginal zone. Antigen-specific B cells generated in the germinal center leave the follicle and reappear in the marginal zone. Thereafter, immunoglobulin-producing plasma cells accumulate in the lymph node medulla and subsequently exit to the periphery. Antigen-dependent T-cell proliferation occurs in the lymph node paracortex. After antigen exposure, mature T cells become immunoblasts and, subsequently, antigen-specific effector T cells that exit to the periphery. The postulated normal counterparts of many currently recognized T- and B-cell neoplasms are shown. **B,** T- and B-cell malignancies derived from the postulated normal counterparts shown in **A.** MALT = mucosa-associated lymphoid tissue.

TABLE 196–2 TYPICAL IMMUNOPHENOTYPES OF COMMON HON-HODGKIN'S LYMPHOMAS

Lymphoma	CD20	CD3	CD10	CD5	CD23	Other
Small lymphocytic	+	–	–	+	+	
Lymphoplasmacytic	+	–	–	–	–	Cytoplasmic Ig+
Extranodal marginal zone MALT	+	–	–	–	–	
Nodal marginal zone	+	–	–	–	–	
Follicular	+	–	+			
Mantle cell	+	–	–	+	–	Cyclin D1+
Diffuse large B cell	+	–				
Mediastinal large B cell	+	–				
Burkitt's	+	–	+	–		TdT–
Precursor T lymphoblastic	–	+/–				TdT+, CD1a +/–, CD7+
Anaplastic large T cell	–	+/–				CD30+, CD15–, EMA+, ALK+
Peripheral T cell	–	+/–				Other pan-T variable

ALK = anaplastic lymphoma kinase; EMA = epithelial membrane antigen; MALT = mucosa-associated lymphoid tissue; TdT = terminal deoxynucleotidyl transferase.

TABLE 196–3 CHROMOSOMAL TRANSLOCATIONS CHARACTERISTIC OF NON-HODGKIN'S LYMPHOMA (NHL)

NHL Subtype	Translocation	Genes Involved	Frequency (%)
Diffuse large B-cell	t(3q27)	BCL6	35
	t(14;18)(q32;q21)	IgH, BCL2	15–20
	t(18;14)(q24;q32)	MYC (c-Myc), IgH	<5
Burkitt's	t(8;14)(q24;q32)	MYC, IgH	100% have one of these, most commonly t(8;14)
	t(8;22)(q24;q11)	MYC, IgL	
	t(2;8)(p12;q24)	IgK, MYC	
Follicular	t(14;18)(q32;q21)	IgH, BCL2	~90
Mantle cell	t(11;14)(q13;q32)	BCL1, IgH	>90
ALCL	t(2;5)(p23;q35)	ALK, NPM	>80 of ALK+ ALCLs
MALT	t(11;18)(q21;q21)	API2, MALT1	35
	t(14;18)(q21;q32)	IgH, MALT1	20
	t(1;14)(p22;q32)	BCL10, IgH	10

ALCL = anaplastic large cell lymphoma; ALK = anaplastic lymphoma kinase; MALT = mucosa-associated lymphoid tissue.

incorporating morphologic, immunologic, genetic, and clinical information (the Revised European-American Lymphoma Classification, or REAL) was developed to identify distinct clinicopathologic subgroups representing diseases that can be recognized by clinicians. This system was subsequently adopted as the World Health Organization (WHO) classification of lymphomas in 2001 (Table 196–4).

The WHO classification divides lymphomas on the basis of B-cell or T/NK-cell origin and whether they are derived from primitive precursor cells or from more mature "peripheral" cells. Specific clinical and pathologic entities are recognized within each of these groupings. In the United States and Europe, 85 to 90% of non-Hodgkin's lymphomas are B cell in origin.

The most frequent type is diffuse large B-cell lymphoma, which represents 31% of all non-Hodgkin's lymphomas worldwide. The next most frequent type is follicular lymphoma, which represents 22% of cases; follicular lymphoma is relatively more frequent in North America and Western Europe and less frequent in Asia. Less common types, each representing between 5% and 10% of all non-Hodgkin's lymphomas, are the extranodal marginal zone/MALT lymphomas, the peripheral T-cell lymphomas, small lymphocytic lymphoma, and mantle cell lymphoma. Rarer types, each of which constitutes more than 1% of cases, include mediastinal large B-cell lymphoma, anaplastic large T-cell lymphoma, and lymphoblastic lymphoma. Other groups such as Burkitt's lymphoma, adult T-cell leukemia/lymphoma, and rare types of T-cell lymphomas each represent less than 1% of non-Hodgkin's lymphomas seen in the United States.

The non-Hodgkin's lymphomas recognized in the WHO classification have clinically distinctive characteristics (Table 196–5), such that an experienced hematopathologist can accurately classify 85% of patients by WHO criteria when adequate material is available. Some diagnoses, such as follicular lymphoma, can be made with a high degree of accuracy without immunologic or genetic studies. The diagnosis of T-cell lymphomas cannot be made accurately without immunophenotyping. Cytogenetic studies and molecular genetic studies can help resolve difficult differential diagnoses. For example, the presence of a t(8;14) translocation would support the diagnosis of a Burkitt's lymphoma, whereas a t(11;14) with cyclin D1 overexpression can confirm the diagnosis of mantle cell lymphoma (see Tables 196–2 and 196–3).

Recently the use of complementary DNA (cDNA) microarrays has allowed the identification of distinct subsets of patients with diffuse large B-cell lymphoma. Patients with histologically identical lymphomas can be divided into those with tumor gene expression patterns resembling normal germinal center B cells and those whose tumors resemble activated post–germinal center B cells.

Clinical Manifestations

The most common presentation of non-Hodgkin's lymphoma is lymphadenopathy (Fig. 196–4; Chapter 174). In many cases, patients notice cervical, axillary, or inguinal adenopathy and seek a physician's advice. In general, lymph nodes containing lymphoma are firm, nontender, and not associated with a regional infection. However, patients are frequently treated with a course of antibiotics before a biopsy is performed to confirm the diagnosis of lymphoma. In other patients, lymphadenopathy occurring in sites such as the mediastinum or retroperitoneum causes

TABLE 196–4 WORLD HEALTH ORGANIZATION CLASSIFICATION OF NON-HODGKIN'S LYMPHOMA

B-CELL LYMPHOMAS

Precursor B-cell lymphoma
- Precursor B-lymphoblastic lymphoma/leukemia

Mature B-cell lymphomas
- Chronic lymphocytic leukemia/small lymphocytic lymphoma
- Lymphoplasmacytic lymphoma
- Splenic marginal zone lymphoma
- Extranodal marginal zone B-cell lymphoma of mucosa-associated lymphoid tissue (MALT-lymphoma)
- Nodal marginal zone B-cell lymphoma
- Follicular lymphoma
- Mantle cell lymphoma
- Diffuse large B-cell lymphoma
- Mediastinal (thymic) large B-cell lymphoma
- Intravascular large B-cell lymphoma
- Primary effusion lymphoma
- Burkitt's lymphoma/leukemia

T/NK-CELL LYMPHOMAS

Precursor T-cell lymphoma
- Precursor T-cell lymphoblastic leukemia/lymphoma
- Blastic NK cell lymphoma

Mature T/NK cell lymphoma
- Adult T-cell leukemia/lymphoma
- Extranodal NK/T cell lymphoma, nasal type
- Enteropathy-type T-cell lymphoma
- Hepatosplenic T-cell lymphoma
- Subcutaneous panniculitis-like T-cell lymphoma
- Mycosis fungoides
- Sézary syndrome
- Primary cutaneous anaplastic large cell lymphoma
- Peripheral T-cell lymphoma, unspecified
- Angioimmunoblastic T-cell lymphoma
- Anaplastic large cell lymphoma

NK = natural killer.
Adapted from Jaffe ES, Harris NL, Stein H, Vardiman JW (eds): World Health Organization Classification of Tumours: Pathology and Genetics. Tumours of Haematopoietic and Lymphoid Tissues. Lyon, IARC Press, 2001.

symptoms that bring the patient to the physician. Chest pain, cough, superior vena cava syndrome, abdominal pain, back pain, spinal cord compression, and symptoms of renal insufficiency associated with ureteral compression are characteristic.

Non-Hodgkin's lymphomas are often associated with systemic symptoms that may lead to the diagnosis. The most obvious symptoms are fevers, night sweats, and unexplained weight loss. Any of these symptoms without an obvious cause should lead a physician to consider the diagnosis of lymphoma. Other, less characteristic symptoms include fatigue, which is frequently present at the time of diagnosis of lymphoma if the patient is questioned carefully, and pruritus.

Non-Hodgkin's lymphomas can involve essentially any organ in the body, and malfunction of that organ can cause symptoms that lead to the diagnosis. Examples include neurologic symptoms with primary brain lymphoma (Chapter 199), shortness of breath with MALT lymphomas in the lung, epigastric pain and vomiting with gastric MALT or diffuse large B-cell lymphomas (Chapter 202), bowel obstruction with small bowel lymphomas (Chapter 203), testicular masses with diffuse large B-cell lymphoma (Chapter 210), and skin lesions with cutaneous lymphomas (Chapter 466). Many lymphomas involve the bone marrow and can occasionally cause extensive myelophthisis (Chapter 171) and bone marrow failure; these patients can present with infections, bleeding, and anemia.

Non-Hodgkin's lymphomas can also manifest with a variety of immunologic abnormalities. For example, autoimmune hemolytic anemia (Chapter 164) and immune thrombocytopenia (Chapter 179) can be the presenting manifestations of non-Hodgkin's lymphoma, especially small lymphocytic lymphoma/chronic lymphocytic leukemia but also other subtypes, including diffuse large B-cell lymphoma. Peripheral neuropathies (Chapter 446), often associated with overproduction of a monoclonal protein, can be seen in a variety of subtypes but are most characteristic of lymphoplasmacytic lymphoma and are also sometimes seen with POEMS syndrome (*p*olyneuropathy, *o*rganomegaly, *e*ndocrinopathy, *M* protein, *s*kin changes) associated with Castleman's disease (Chapters 189 and 446). Paraneoplastic neurologic complications of non-Hodgkin's lymphoma include demyelinating polyneuropathy, Guillain-Barré syndrome, autonomic dysfunction, and peripheral neuropathy. Paraneoplastic syndromes (Chapter 189) associated with non-Hodgkin's lymphoma can affect the skin (e.g., pemphigus), kidney (e.g., glomerulonephritis), and miscellaneous organ systems (e.g., vasculitis, dermatomyositis, and cholestatic jaundice).

The differential diagnosis in patients who are found to have non-Hodgkin's lymphoma is broad. Any cause of lymphadenopathy or splenomegaly can potentially be confused with non-Hodgkin's lymphoma (Chapter 174). However, this confusion is resolved by appropriate biopsy. It is extremely important to recognize that the diagnosis of non-Hodgkin's lymphoma must be considered in patients with compatible clinical presentations and then confirmed by means of an adequate biopsy that is read by an experienced hematopathologist. The diagnosis should never be inferred, and patients should not be treated until the diagnosis is confirmed by biopsy.

Diagnosis

Each new patient with a non-Hodgkin's lymphoma should be thoroughly evaluated in a systematic manner (Table 196–6). Because subtle pathologic distinctions may alter therapy, the most important issue in managing non-Hodgkin's lymphoma is to establish an accurate diagnosis. Core needle biopsies can occasionally be used for a primary diagnosis if the specimen is handled properly. Fine-needle aspirates should not be used to diagnose lymphoma, and they preclude accurate diagnosis of the specific subtype of non-Hodgkin's lymphoma. In most cases, an excisional biopsy is necessary for the initial diagnosis; another biopsy should be performed if sufficient material is not obtained. Review by an experienced hematopathologist is essential.

Staging

After diagnosis, a meticulous staging evaluation is necessary to estimate prognosis and to determine therapy. Staging requires a careful history and physical examination; a complete blood count; renal and hepatic function tests; a serum lactate dehydrogenase (LDH) level; computed tomographic (CT) scans of the chest, abdomen, and pelvis; and a bone marrow biopsy. Positron-emission tomographic (PET) scans can be helpful to identify initial sites of involvement and, after treatment, to distinguish persisting lymphoma from residual fibrosis in masses seen on CT. The most common staging system is the Ann Arbor classification, which separates patients into four stages based on anatomic sites of disease (Table 196–7). In addition, each stage is subdivided into A (without defined general symptoms) and B (unexplained weight loss of more than 10% in the previous 6 months, unexplained temperature greater than 38° C, or night sweats) categories. Known sites of disease can be reexamined later to evaluate the response to therapy.

Treatment Rx

Lymphomas may behave in an indolent or an aggressive manner. The behavior of many of these neoplasms is distinctive, but within each category the behavior is frequently influenced by sites of disease, bulk of tumor, and the performance status of the patient. Some lymphomas can be managed, at least initially, with observation, whereas other situations, such as spinal cord compression (Chapter 199), are medical emergencies. It is important to consider three questions before starting therapy: (1) Does treatment have curative potential? (2) Can treatment prolong survival? (3) Will treatment alleviate symptoms?

Surgical excision is sometimes curative for patients with localized MALT lymphoma. Sometimes, resection of colon and small bowel

TABLE 196–5 PRESENTING CLINICAL CHARACTERISTICS OF THE MOST COMMON SUBTYPES OF NON-HODGKIN'S LYMPHOMAS

Type of Lymphoma	Median Age (yr)	% Male	Ann Arbor Stage (%) 1	2	3	4	B Symptoms (%)	Bone Marrow Involved (%)	IPI Score (%) 0/1	2/3	4/5	5-Year Survival (%)
B-CELL LYMPHOMAS												
Small lymphocytic	65	53	4	5	8	83	33	72	23	64	13	51
Lymphoplasmacytic	63	53	7	13	7	73	13	73	16	69	15	59
Extranodal marginal zone MALT	60	48	39	28	2	31	19	14	44	48	8	74
Nodal marginal zone	58	42	13	13	34	40	37	32	60	27	13	57
Follicular	59	42	18	15	16	51	28	42	45	48	7	72
Mantle cell	63	74	13	7	9	71	28	64	23	54	23	27
Diffuse large B cell	64	55	25	29	13	33	33	16	35	46	19	46
Mediastinal large B cell	37	34	10	56	3	31	38	3	52	37	11	50
Burkitt's	31	89	37	25	0	38	22	33	57	29	14	44
PRECURSOR B/T-CELL LYMPHOMAS												
Precursor T-lymphoblastic	28	64	0	11	14	75	21	50	33	41	26	26
T-CELL LYMPHOMAS												
Anaplastic large T cell	34	69	19	32	10	39	53	13	61	18	21	77
Peripheral T cell	61	55	8	12	15	65	50	36	17	52	31	25

B symptoms = fevers, night sweats, and weight loss; IPI = International Prognostic Index (see Table 196–9); MALT = mucosa-associated lymphoid tissue.
Adapted from Armitage JO, Weisenburger DD, for the Non-Hodgkin's Lymphoma Classification Project: New approach to classifying non-Hodgkin's lymphomas: Clinical features of the major histologic subtypes. J Clin Oncol 1998;16:2780–2795.

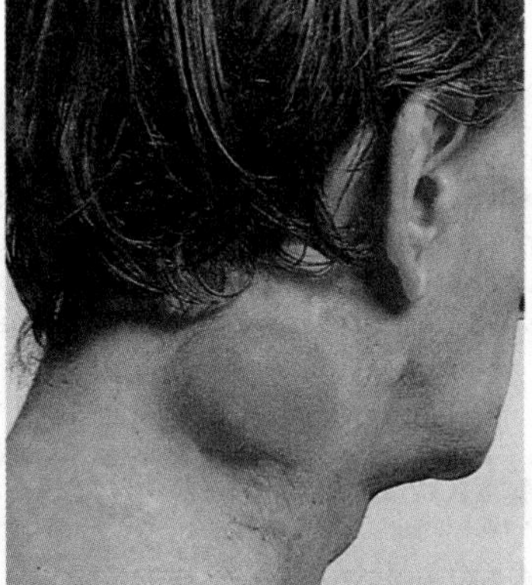

FIGURE 196–4 • Non-Hodgkin's lymphoma. Despite the redness of the skin over the enlarged lymph node in this patient, the lesion was completely painless. (From Forbes CD, Jackson WF: Color Atlas and Text of Clinical Medicine, 3rd ed. London, Mosby, 2003, with permission.)

lymphoma is appropriate to avoid the potential complications of perforation and hemorrhage with the initiation of chemotherapy. Splenectomy can improve cytopenias and is sometimes used as palliative therapy for symptomatic splenomegaly. Otherwise, surgery has little role in the treatment of non-Hodgkin's lymphoma.

Radiotherapy is frequently used alone or in combination with chemotherapy for localized disease and is sometimes used after chemotherapy to consolidate treatment of bulky disease. Radiation therapy is also used as palliative therapy to treat symptomatic sites of relapse.

Most patients require chemotherapy, which may consist of single agents or combinations of drugs (Table 196–8). Three monoclonal antibodies (rituximab, ^{131}I-tositumomab, and ^{90}Y-ibritumomab) are approved in the United States for the treatment of follicular non-Hodgkin's lymphoma; these agents are also active for more aggressive histologic subtypes. In addition, one antibody (alemtuzumab) is approved for use in small lymphocytic lymphoma.

TABLE 196–6 TYPICAL EVALUATION OF A PATIENT NEWLY DIAGNOSED WITH NON-HODGKIN'S LYMPHOMA

1. Biopsy to establish diagnosis
2. Careful history and physical examination
3. Laboratory evaluation
   A. Complete blood count
   B. Chemistry screen including lactate dehydrogenase and β_2-microglobulin levels
4. Imaging studies
   A. Chest radiograph
   B. Computed tomographic scan of chest, abdomen, and pelvis
   C. Positron-emission tomographic scan (consider for patients with diffuse large B-cell lymphoma and other aggressive histologic subtypes)
5. Further biopsies
   A. Bone marrow
   B. Any other suspicious site if the results of the biopsy would change therapy

SPECIFIC TYPES OF NON-HODGKIN'S LYMPHOMAS

Precursor T-Cell and B-Cell Lymphomas

These tumors are nodal or other solid tissue infiltrates of cells that are morphologically and immunophenotypically identical to the immature cells seen in B-cell or T-cell acute lymphoblastic leukemia (Chapter 194). Patients who have predominantly nodal disease with minimal or no involvement of the bone marrow are frequently classified as having *lymphoblastic lymphoma,* whereas those with more than 25% neoplastic cells in the marrow are classified as having *lymphoblastic leukemia.* These distinctions are arbitrary and reflect the stage of disease rather than different diagnoses. These neoplasms are more common in children than in adults.

B-cell precursor lymphomas frequently manifest as solid tumors with involvement of the skin and bones, whereas T-cell neoplasms typically manifest as a mediastinal mass in a young male. Involvement of the CNS is common. Approximately 90% of patients who present with lymphoblastic lymphoma have a T-cell phenotype, whereas about 85% of patients who present with acute lymphoblastic leukemia have a B-cell precursor phenotype. Adverse prognostic characteristics include CNS involvement, stage IV disease, and an elevated LDH level.

TABLE 196–7 STAGING OF NON-HODGKIN'S LYMPHOMA

Stage	Description
I	Involvement of a single lymph node region (I) or a single extralymphatic organ or site (I_E)
II	Involvement of 2 or more lymph node regions on the same side of the diaphragm (II) or localized involvement of extralymphatic organ or site and 1 or more lymph node regions on the same side of the diaphragm (II_E)
III	Involvement of lymph node regions on both sides of the diaphragm (III), which may also be accompanied by localized involvement of extralymphatic organ or site (III_E) or by involvement of spleen (III_S), or both (III_{SE})
IV	Diffuse or disseminated involvement of 1 or more extralymphatic organs or tissues with or without associated lymph node enlargement
A	no "B" symptoms
B	unexplained weight loss ≥10% of body weight in prior 6 months, unexplained fever >38° C, or night sweats

Adapted from Carbone PP, Kaplan HS, Musshoff K, et al: Report of the Committee on Hodgkin's Disease Staging Classification. Cancer Res 1971;31:1860–1861.

Treatment — Rx

Patients with either T-cell lymphoblastic lymphoma or precursor B-cell lymphoblastic lymphoma are typically treated with regimens modeled after ones used for acute lymphoblastic leukemia (Chapter 194). These regimens frequently contain cytarabine and high-dose methotrexate, and they often include maintenance therapy. CNS prophylaxis with intrathecal chemotherapy, high-dose methotrexate, or cranial irradiation is also a component of these regimens.

Mature B-Cell Lymphomas

Small Lymphocytic Lymphoma/Chronic Lymphocytic Leukemia

Small lymphocytic lymphoma is defined as a lymph node or other tissue infiltrate that is morphologically and immunophenotypically identical to chronic lymphocytic leukemia. Patients are frequently asymptomatic, and the diagnosis is often made when blood counts are performed for other reasons. Patients frequently have lymphadenopathy or splenomegaly. Fatigue is common. Hypogammaglobulinemia can occur and lead to an increased susceptibility to infection.

In addition to advanced stage and systemic symptoms, a poorer prognosis is associated with expression of high levels of CD38 and ZAP-70 on the tumor cells, lymphomas without rearranged immunoglobulin heavy chain genes, and genetic abnormalities such as del(17p) and del(11q). Approximately 2 to 3% of patients exhibit transformation to diffuse large B-cell lymphoma (Richter's syndrome), which is associated with a poor prognosis.

The median survival time is more than 10 years for patients without adverse characteristics, and these patients can often be managed with observation. Therapy is necessary for patients who have rapidly progressive or symptomatic lymphadenopathy and for those who develop cytopenias.

Treatment — Rx

Management must be individualized, because therapy is not curative, and patients are often elderly. Fludarabine in combination with cyclophosphamide and rituximab (see Table 196–8) is a frequent regimen used in the United States for relatively young, fit patients. Single-agent fludarabine plus rituximab is more commonly used in elderly patients. Fludarabine is more effective than chlorambucil,

TABLE 196–8 COMBINATION CHEMOTHERAPY REGIMENS FOR NON-HODGKIN'S LYMPHOMA

Regimen	Dose (mg/m²)	Days of Administration	Frequency
CHOP-R			Every 21 d
Cyclophosphamide	750 IV	1	
Doxorubicin	50 IV	1	
Vincristine*	1.4 IV	1	
Prednisone, fixed dose	100 PO	1–5	
Rituximab	375 IV	1	
CVP-R			Every 21 d
Cyclophosphamide	1000 mg/m² IV	1	
Vincristine	1.4 mg/m² IV*	1	
Prednisone, fixed dose	100 mg PO	1–5	
Rituximab	375 mg/m² IV	1	
FCR			Every 28 d
Fludarabine	25 mg/m² IV	1–3	
Cyclophosphamide	250 mg/m² IV	1–3	
Rituximab	375 mg/m²	1	

*Vincristine dose often capped at 2 mg total.

Section XV Oncology

Rx

but chlorambucil is administered orally, has few side effects, and is still sometimes used in older patients. Alemtuzumab, a monoclonal antibody directed against the CD52 antigen, is sometimes effective after other treatments have failed. Allogeneic hematopoietic stem cell transplantation may be curative, but few patients are candidates for this approach.

Patients may develop autoimmune thrombocytopenia (Chapter 179), autoimmune neutropenia (Chapter 173), and red blood cell aplasia (Chapter 171). These autoimmune disorders may respond to treatment with steroids, intravenous immune globulin, or splenectomy as used in patients without underlying lymphoma.

Extranodal Marginal Zone Lymphoma of Mucosa-Associated Lymphoid Tissue (MALT Lymphoma)

MALT lymphomas are indolent tumors that originate in association with epithelial cells and are seen most commonly in the gastrointestinal tract, salivary glands, breast, thyroid, orbit, conjunctiva, skin, and lung. The majority of cases are stage I or II at diagnosis, although in some series as many as 30% disseminate to bone marrow or other sites. These lymphomas tend to remain localized for extended periods. Local treatment with surgery or radiotherapy cures a high proportion of localized neoplasms. Disseminated disease is treated similarly to follicular lymphoma (see later discussion).

Gastric MALT lymphomas are usually associated with infection by *H. pylori.* Eradication of *H. pylori* with antibiotics leads to complete regression in more than 50% of gastric MALT lymphomas, although polymerase chain reaction analysis demonstrates minimal residual disease in many of the patients, and the long-term outcome of this approach is unknown. The likelihood of response to antibiotic therapy is less if invasion is deeper, lymph node metastases are found, or the t(11;18) chromosomal translocation is present. Patients may have tumors in more than one extranodal site, and these locations can sometimes be successfully treated with local therapy. Asymptomatic patients can be monitored closely without antilymphoma therapy until symptoms progress. Gastric MALT lymphoma that does not respond to antibiotics can be treated with radiation, rituximab as a single agent (similar to its use in follicular lymphoma), or several traditional combination chemotherapy regimens (see Table 196–8).

Follicular Lymphoma

Follicular lymphoma comprises the majority of indolent or "low-grade" lymphomas in the United States. Follicular lymphoma is divided into three grades based on the proportion of large transformed cells (centroblasts).

Patients with follicular lymphoma are frequently asymptomatic. The most common presenting complaint is painless lymphadenopathy. Some patients have cough or dyspnea related to pulmonary or mediastinal involvement or have pleural effusions. Other patients have symptoms of abdominal pain or fullness related to subdiaphragmatic or splenic disease. A minority of patients have systemic symptoms of fevers, night sweats, or weight loss.

The clinical behavior and treatment of follicular lymphoma grade 1 and follicular lymphoma grade 2 are the same and are discussed in this section. Grade 3 follicular lymphoma may have a more aggressive clinical course and is frequently treated similarly to diffuse large B-cell lymphoma (see later discussion).

Treatment

Rx

Localized Disease

Approximately 5 to 15% of patients have localized disease (stage I or minimal stage II disease) at diagnosis. These lymphomas are usually treated with involved-field radiation, and most series report 10-year disease-free survival rates of approximately 50% and overall survival rates of 60 to 70%. Some retrospective series have reported improved outcomes when chemotherapy is combined with radiation.

Rx

Advanced Disease

Most patients with follicular lymphoma have extensive disease at diagnosis. The median survival time of these patients is 8 to 10 years. Although spontaneous regression has been described, 30 to 50% of patients experience transformation to a more aggressive histology—usually diffuse large B-cell lymphoma. Transformation is frequently associated with new systemic symptoms and rapidly progressive lymphadenopathy, typically follows an aggressive clinical course, and has a poor prognosis.

Asymptomatic patients, especially elderly patients and those with other medical illnesses, can frequently be managed with a "watch and wait" approach. Prospective trials have demonstrated that this approach does not influence overall survival, and patients can sometimes be observed for long periods before treatment is required.

Most patients with follicular lymphoma eventually require treatment because of systemic symptoms, symptomatic or progressive lymphadenopathy, splenomegaly, effusions, or cytopenias. In elderly patients, those who are poor candidates for intensive chemotherapy regimens, and those who want to avoid the side effects (e.g., alopecia) of standard chemotherapy regimens, single-agent rituximab at a dose of 375 mg/m^2 intravenously given weekly for four consecutive weeks yields an objective response rate of well over 50%. The median duration of response is approximately 1 to 2 years for patients who receive no more therapy, but response can be extended with ongoing administration of rituximab once every 2 months or with the initial four doses repeated every 6 months. When rituximab is combined with standard chemotherapy regimens such as CVP (cyclophosphamide, vincristine, and prednisone) or CHOP (cyclophosphamide, doxorubicin, vincristine, prednisone) (see Table 196–8), the response rate, duration of response, and probably survival are increased compared with the use of the chemotherapy regimen alone. [1] Fludarabine, used alone or in combination with mitoxantrone is also effective. One study of ^{131}I-tositumomab radioimmunotherapy appeared to produce prolonged benefit. [2] Interferon-α may be beneficial when combined with initial chemotherapy, but is rarely used for primary treatment of follicular lymphoma in the United States because of its side effects. One study from Europe showed an improvement in failure-free survival with the use of autologous bone marrow transplantation in patients who achieved an initial remission.

Salvage Therapy

Most patients respond to initial chemotherapy, and initial responses typically persist for 1 to 3 years. However, follicular lymphoma eventually progresses in most patients with advanced-stage disease. Patients who have a relapse usually respond to additional therapy, often with the same agents, although the duration of response becomes progressively shorter with repeated courses of therapy. Approximately 50 to 60% of patients with relapsed follicular lymphoma respond to rituximab, and maintenance therapy prolongs remission in responding patients; however, fewer than 10% attain a complete response. Some patients who do not respond to rituximab respond to the radiolabeled antibodies tositumomab or ibritumomab or to interferon-α. Radiation therapy may also be useful for patients with a localized site of symptomatic disease.

Prolonged remissions have been observed after autologous hematopoietic stem cell transplantation. Allogeneic hematopoietic stem cell transplantation may cure some patients with relapsed follicular lymphoma, although the transplant-related mortality rate is high.

Mantle Cell Lymphoma

Mantle cell lymphoma is a B-cell neoplasm composed of small lymphoid cells that may resemble small lymphocytic lymphoma or follicular lymphoma. It is most common in elderly patients and is usually at an advanced stage at the time of diagnosis. Male patients are more frequently affected, and extranodal disease, especially involvement of the bone marrow, Waldeyer's ring, and the gastrointestinal tract, is common. Mantle cell lymphoma is the most common cause of multiple lymphomatous polyposis, and the gastrointestinal tract should be evaluated with endoscopy during the initial evaluation.

Some patients present with involvement of the peripheral blood as well as the bone marrow, a clinical picture that resembles chronic lymphocytic leukemia (Chapter 195). The lymphocytes in both disorders are CD5 positive, but the t(11:14) and overexpression of cyclin D1 seen in mantle cell lymphoma usually allows an accurate diagnosis.

Mantle cell lymphoma has a poor prognosis, with a median survival time of 3 to 4 years. Although there is some evidence that prognosis may be improved with aggressive chemotherapy, mantle cell lymphoma is usually not curable with standard chemotherapy regimens. Autologous hematopoietic stem cell transplantation for patients in their first remission may improve survival, but randomized trials have not been performed. Allogeneic transplantation can be curative but is associated with considerable morbidity and mortality.

Diffuse Large B-Cell Lymphoma

These tumors are the most common type of non-Hodgkin's lymphoma, but their morphology and genetic features are heterogeneous. Signs and symptoms are similar to those of other subtypes, although patients are more likely to be symptomatic with B symptoms or symptoms from the local tumor than are patients with follicular lymphoma.

Treatment

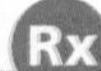

Localized Disease

As many as 30% of patients with diffuse large B-cell lymphoma have stage I or minimal stage II disease. These patients may occasionally be cured with radiation therapy alone, but initial treatment with chemotherapy is more effective. Although one study in France suggested that a very intensive chemotherapy regimen alone might be better than CHOP plus radiation, [3] most patients in the United States receive CHOP plus rituximab (see Table 196–8), followed by consolidative radiation therapy. It remains unclear whether any other regimen is superior to CHOP plus rituximab. Although the necessity of consolidative radiotherapy after CHOP plus rituximab has not been tested, this combination is still widely used.

Advanced Disease

More than 30 prospective randomized trials have compared aggressive combination chemotherapy regimens for diffuse large B-cell lymphoma, and dozens of combination chemotherapy regimens can cure this disease. Most regimens are combinations of an alkylating agent, anthracycline, vinca alkaloid, and corticosteroid, but others contain agents such as bleomycin, methotrexate, cytarabine, and etoposide. All of these regimens yield complete response rates of 60 to 80%, and long-term disease-free survival is seen in 50% to 65% of those who attain a complete response. The combination of CHOP with rituximab (R-CHOP) is generally considered to be the gold standard for treatment of adults of all ages with advanced-stage diffuse large B-cell lymphoma in the United States. Among patients older than 60 years of age, 75% achieve a complete response, with a 5-year event-free survival rate of 47% and a 5-year overall survival rate of 58% [4]; these results are markedly better than with CHOP alone.

The use of hematopoietic growth factors permits the administration of higher doses of chemotherapeutic drugs and allows chemotherapy cycles to be administered at shorter intervals, although a clear benefit from this approach remains uncertain. Several prospective trials have examined the role of high-dose chemotherapy followed by autologous hematopoietic stem cell transplantation as consolidation therapy after initial chemotherapy for patients with adverse prognostic characteristics. Although results vary, some of the trials have shown benefits for autologous transplantation in first remission, and many investigators recommend early transplantation for selected patients. [5]

Salvage Therapy

A variety of chemotherapy regimens have been developed for patients who relapse after attaining a remission with initial chemotherapy. These regimens commonly contain agents such as cisplatin, cytarabine, etoposide, carboplatin, and ifosfamide. Response rates exceeding 50% can be observed with these combinations, although no more than 10 to 15% of patients achieve long-term disease-free survival. High-dose therapy followed by autologous hematopoietic stem cell transplantation has become accepted therapy for patients with relapsed diffuse large B-cell lymphoma; approximately 40% of these patients attain long-term disease-free survival with transplantation if they are still responsive to conventional salvage chemotherapy.

Mediastinal Large B-Cell Lymphoma

Primary mediastinal large B-cell lymphoma originates in the thymus and is most common in young women. This entity is distinguished by the presence of a mediastinal mass, which usually causes symptoms of cough, chest pain, or superior vena cava syndrome. Genetic studies have shown that some patients with this lymphoma have gene expression patterns that are distinct from those of other diffuse large B-cell lymphomas and are similar to that seen in classic Hodgkin's disease.

Disease is confined to the chest and neck in most cases. A very large mass (>10 cm) or the existence of a malignant pleural effusion is associated with worse prognosis. The management of patients with mediastinal large B-cell lymphoma involves initial chemotherapy with regimens used for diffuse large B-cell lymphoma, followed, in some cases, by consolidative radiotherapy, and the prognosis is similar to that of other patients with diffuse large B-cell lymphoma. Relapses often occur in extranodal sites such as the CNS, lungs, gastrointestinal tract, liver, ovaries, and kidneys.

Burkitt's Lymphoma

Burkitt's lymphoma is a highly aggressive B-cell lymphoma that is more common in children and immunosuppressed individuals than in healthy adults. Widespread extranodal involvement is common. The endemic form of Burkitt's lymphoma is seen most frequently in children who reside in equatorial Africa. Involvement of bones of the jaw is common in this form. The sporadic form of Burkitt's lymphoma is seen most commonly in children in the United States. Males are more frequently affected. Both children and adults frequently have bulky abdominal disease, sometimes with involvement of the kidneys, ovaries, and breasts. Bone marrow involvement is seen in about one third of cases.

Tumors may progress extremely rapidly, so therapy should be started as soon as possible. Tumor lysis syndrome may occur because of the frequent presence of bulky disease, the high rate of tumor proliferation, and the extreme sensitivity of the tumor to chemotherapy. Patients are usually treated with specialized high-intensity regimens including rituximab of relatively short duration. CNS prophylaxis with intrathecal chemotherapy or high-dose methotrexate is required. Cure rates well in excess of 50% are typical.

Rare Types of B-Cell Lymphoma

Several rare types of lymphoma have distinct clinical features.

Lymphoplasmacytic lymphoma is an indolent lymphoma that frequently involves the bone marrow, peripheral blood, and spleen. Patients frequently have an immunoglobulin M paraprotein (and therefore could be called Waldenström's macroglobulinemia) that may lead to symptoms of hyperviscosity, autoimmune phenomena, or neuropathies (Chapter 198). Plasmapheresis can reduce symptoms of hyperviscosity. Chemotherapy with alkylating agents, combination chemotherapy, or fludarabine may be used. Rituximab is also effective.

Splenic marginal zone lymphoma is an indolent lymphoma that usually manifests with splenomegaly and lymphocytosis. A monoclonal gammopathy is frequently seen. Peripheral lymphadenopathy is unusual. Anemia and thrombocytopenia may respond to splenectomy. Chemotherapy with single agents or anthracycline-based combinations may be useful, and responses to interferon have been described. This lymphoma appears to be particularly responsive to rituximab.

Nodal marginal zone B-cell lymphoma is an indolent disorder that is usually associated with generalized lymphadenopathy. The clinical course and prognosis are similar to those of follicular lymphoma, and it is usually treated in a similar manner.

Intravascular large B-cell lymphoma is an aggressive lymphoma caused by cells that infiltrate the lumina of small blood vessels. Widespread extranodal involvement is common. Focal neurologic deficits and mental status changes are frequent. Most cases are diagnosed at autopsy, although durable responses to combination chemotherapy have been described.

Primary effusion lymphoma is associated with HHV-8 and is seen in HIV-infected and other immunosuppressed patients. Effusions occur in serous body cavities; peripheral lymphadenopathy is not seen. Prognosis is poor despite chemotherapy.

Small intestinal immunoproliferative disease, a disorder most frequently seen in the Middle East, begins as a polyclonal process and can progress to a large B-cell lymphoma. The process is often associated with *Campylobacter jejuni* infection. Early in the disease, patients may respond to antibiotics, and frank lymphoma can respond to combination chemotherapy regimens.

Mature T-Cell Lymphomas

Mycosis Fungoides

Mycosis fungoides (often referred to as cutaneous T-cell lymphoma) is an indolent malignancy that is most common in middle-aged and older adults. The clinical course usually progresses slowly from isolated patches or plaques, to thickened widespread plaques, and then to multiple cutaneous tumors that may ulcerate (Chapter 464). A subset of patients present with generalized erythroderma and circulating tumor cells, a presentation that is called Sézary syndrome. Lymph node and visceral involvement may occur late in the course of the disease.

Treatment Rx

Cutaneous radiotherapy may be curative for patients with limited-stage patch or plaque disease. Patients with early stage (<10% body surface area) disease are frequently treated with skin-directed therapy that may include ultraviolet radiation, topical steroids, or topical nitrogen mustard.

Patients with more advanced disease frequently benefit from total skin electron beam therapy or extracorporeal photopheresis. Medical treatments include interferon-α, retinoids, monoclonal antibodies, the fusion toxin denileukin diftitox, and traditional cytotoxic chemotherapeutic agents; however, these treatments are usually only palliative. Results with autologous hematopoietic stem cell transplantation are usually poor, although allogeneic stem cell transplantation has yielded promising results in some cases.

Adult T-Cell Lymphoma/Leukemia

Adult T-cell lymphoma/leukemia, which is associated with HTLV-I infection (Chapter 401), is most commonly seen in southern Japan and the Caribbean. Most infected patients are asymptomatic, and the lifetime risk of developing adult T-cell lymphoma/leukemia is approximately 3%.

Patients may have acute leukemia, aggressive lymphoma, or an indolent lymphoproliferative disease. Patients with aggressive disease present with generalized lymphadenopathy, hepatosplenomegaly, cutaneous infiltration, and hypercalcemia. Many patients have characteristic circulating tumor cells with a "flower" or "clover leaf" nucleus.

Patients with indolent disease can sometimes be monitored without therapy. Aggressive disease is usually treated with combination chemotherapy, but there is no consensus on the best regimen. The 5-year survival rate historically has been less than 10%, although recent trials have reported better outcomes.

CD30-Positive Cutaneous Lymphoproliferative Disorders

These disorders represent a spectrum of diseases that may have an identical histologic appearance and overlapping clinical manifestations. Treatment decisions must often be based on the clinical behavior of the lesions. These lymphomas express CD30 but do not express the anaplastic lymphoma kinase (ALK) protein (see later discussion).

Lymphomatoid papulosis is a "histologically malignant" clonal disorder consisting of erythematous or skin-colored papules that frequently undergo spontaneous ulceration and necrosis over a period of weeks. The prognosis is excellent, although patients may eventually develop lymphoma.

Primary cutaneous anaplastic large cell lymphoma occurs most commonly in older men and also undergoes frequent spontaneous regression. The 5-year survival rate is greater than 90%. Treatment usually consists of local measures (surgery or radiation), although chemotherapy may be required.

Primary Systemic Anaplastic Large Cell Lymphoma

Anaplastic large cell lymphoma (ALCL) is a $CD30^+$, aggressive T-cell non-Hodgkin's lymphoma that is seen most frequently in young males. B-cell lymphomas with similar morphology can occur, but they have clinical features identical to other diffuse large B-cell lymphomas and are not considered part of this disease. A morphologically similar but biologically unrelated and clinically distinct neoplasm, primary cutaneous ALCL, occurs predominantly in older adults and represents part of the spectrum of cutaneous $CD30^+$ lymphoproliferative disorders (see earlier discussion) Primary systemic ALCL frequently has a t(2;5) chromosomal translocation leading to overexpression of ALK, a protein not normally detectable in lymphoid cells.

Patients usually have lymphadenopathy, and involvement of the skin, bone, and gastrointestinal tract may be observed. Patients are usually treated with chemotherapy regimens such as CHOP. Patients whose tumors express ALK have an excellent outcome, and 5-year survival rates of 70 to 90% have been observed. ALK-negative ALCL is more common in older patients and is associated with an inferior response rate and shorter survival times. Autologous hematopoietic stem cell transplantation may be curative for patients who relapse.

Other Peripheral T-Cell Lymphomas

The largest group of patients with peripheral T-cell lymphomas are defined in the WHO classification as having "peripheral T-cell lymphoma, unspecified." These patients have signs and symptoms that are similar to those of patients with aggressive B-cell lymphomas, although systemic symptoms (fevers, night sweats, and weight loss) and extranodal involvement are frequent. The diagnosis of peripheral T-cell lymphoma requires immunophenotyping to demonstrate the T-cell origin. Patients are generally treated with the same regimens used for diffuse large B-cell lymphomas (e.g., CHOP), although the outcome is substantially worse (see Table 196–5). Patients who relapse after complete remission can sometimes be cured with autologous hematopoietic stem cell transplantation.

Unusual Subtypes of T-Cell Lymphoma

As with B-cell lymphomas, rare types of T-cell lymphoma also occur.

Angioimmunoblastic T-cell lymphoma is associated with generalized lymphadenopathy, fever, weight loss, skin rash, and polyclonal hypergammaglobulinemia. Results of therapy are similar to those for peripheral T-cell lymphoma, unspecified.

Extranodal NK/T-cell lymphoma usually occurs in extranodal sites, especially the nose, palate, and nasopharynx. Involvement of the nose and face leads to the syndrome that was previously called lethal midline granuloma. This disorder is unusual in the United States, but it is frequent in Southeast Asia and Peru. The prognosis is extremely poor, although patients with localized disease can sometimes be cured with aggressive combination radiotherapy and chemotherapy.

Hepatosplenic T-cell lymphoma is characterized by sinusoidal infiltration of the spleen, liver, and bone marrow, which leads to hepatosplenomegaly, systemic symptoms, and cytopenias. Lymphadenopathy is unusual. Patients are typically young males, and this disease can occur in allograft recipients and in the setting of immune dysfunction. The prognosis is poor, and remissions are rarely observed with chemotherapy.

Enteropathy-type T-cell lymphoma is usually seen in patients with gluten-sensitive enteropathy (Chapter 143). Patients typically present with abdominal pain and diarrhea, and sometimes with bowel perforation. Treatment of celiac disease with a gluten-free diet appears to reduce the risk of lymphoma. The prognosis in these often undernourished patients is poor.

Subcutaneous panniculitis-like T-cell lymphoma manifests with multiple subcutaneous nodules and is often misdiagnosed as panniculitis.

Patients with disseminated disease can have a syndrome consisting of fevers, weight loss, hepatosplenomegaly, pancytopenia, and phagocytosis of blood cells (hemophagocytic syndrome). Patients sometimes respond to combination chemotherapy regimens used for diffuse large B-cell lymphoma, interferon, and radiotherapy, but long-term disease-free survival is unusual.

SPECIAL CLINICAL SITUATIONS

The diagnosis and management of patients with the various types of non-Hodgkin's lymphoma can be profoundly influenced by the site of origin of the lymphoma or by certain clinical characteristics of the patients. Examples of the latter include pregnant patients with lymphoma, elderly patients with lymphoma, and lymphoma occurring in patients who are severely immunosuppressed.

Specific Primary Sites of Diffuse Large B-Cell Lymphoma

Approximately 30% of diffuse large B-cell lymphomas originate in extranodal sites. Presentation in certain extranodal sites is associated with unique clinical behaviors that may necessitate diagnostic studies or additional therapy beyond what is used for patients with nodal presentations.

Patients with primary CNS lymphoma (Chapter 199) commonly have ocular involvement, and all patients with this diagnosis should have a slit-lamp examination. Surgical resection of primary CNS lymphoma is not beneficial, and the only role for surgery is diagnosis. Primary lymphomas of the CNS are very sensitive to corticosteroids, but the best results have been observed with chemotherapy regimens that use high-dose methotrexate, alone or in combination with other agents such as cytarabine. By comparison, conventional chemotherapy regimens, such as CHOP, are of little benefit. Whole brain irradiation is also effective therapy, although the incidence of leukoencephalopathy is extremely high, especially in elderly patients. Radiation therapy is frequently reserved for relapse rather than being used as adjunctive treatment with primary chemotherapy.

Treatment of primary testicular lymphoma (Chapter 210) usually consists of orchiectomy followed by combination chemotherapy. Relapse in the contralateral testicle is common, and most oncologists recommend adjuvant radiation to the scrotum. CNS involvement is common, and prophylactic intrathecal chemotherapy is usually recommended. Late relapses occur frequently.

Diffuse large B-cell lymphoma of the stomach and gastrointestinal tract is treated differently from gastric MALT lymphoma even if a history of prior MALT lymphoma exists. Patients can be cured with surgery and adjunctive radiation or chemotherapy, although surgery is rarely performed for gastric lymphomas because of the morbidity associated with gastric resection. Patients should be treated with chemotherapy regimens used for other patients with diffuse large B-cell lymphoma. Radiation therapy is sometimes used after chemotherapy, although the role of combined modality treatment is not defined.

Lymphoma in Immunocompromised Patients and Post-transplantation Lymphoproliferative Disorders

Non-Hodgkin's lymphoma is an AIDS-defining illness in HIV-infected individuals (Chapter 407), and the risk of developing a non-Hodgkin's lymphoma is increased more than 150-fold after the diagnosis of another AIDS-defining illness. Most cases are diffuse large B-cell lymphomas or Burkitt's lymphomas. AIDS-associated lymphomas behave aggressively and frequently involve the CNS and other unusual sites, such as the gastrointestinal tract, anus, rectum, skin, and soft tissue (Chapter 416). Factors associated with poor survival include low CD4 counts, poor performance status, older age, and advanced stage. The prognosis of these lymphomas is poor, with median survival times of approximately 6 months in the absence of concomitant aggressive therapy for HIV. If chemotherapy is given in association with highly active antiretroviral agents to patients with a good performance status, the likelihood of controlling the lymphoma is similar to that in patients without HIV infection. Intrathecal prophylaxis is generally recommended because of a higher risk of CNS involvement.

The risk of developing a non-Hodgkin's lymphoma is also markedly increased in patients who have received a solid organ transplant. The histologic appearance of these lymphomas is variable, but they frequently resemble aggressive lymphomas in nonimmunocompromised patients. Similar disorders can be seen in patients who are treated with methotrexate for autoimmune disorders and in recipients of allogeneic hematopoietic stem cell transplants, especially if the transplants are T-cell depleted. These post-transplantation lymphoproliferative disorders, which may develop within weeks after surgery, are more common in those patients who have received more aggressive immunosuppression after transplantation. Involvement of extranodal sites is common, and lymphoma frequently involves the transplanted organ. Post-transplantation lymphoproliferative disorders may respond to reduction or withdrawal of immunosuppression. Some investigators have advocated the use of acyclovir or ganciclovir, because these lymphomas are usually related to EBV, but this practice is controversial. Other patients require treatment with combination chemotherapy regimens. High response rates are also seen with rituximab.

Non-Hodgkin's Lymphoma in Elderly Patients

More than 50% of patients who develop non-Hodgkin's lymphomas are older than 60 years of age, and the prognosis is generally worse for elderly patients. These poorer outcomes are related to increased toxicity of drug therapy, lower remission rates, increased rates of relapse, and higher death rates from cardiovascular disease and causes other than the lymphoma itself. Older patients are more likely to have other adverse prognostic characteristics (Table 196–9), which also contribute to poorer outcomes.

Several chemotherapy regimens have been developed specifically for elderly patients (i.e., older than 65 to 70 years), but it is unclear whether they yield better outcomes. The practice of arbitrary dose reductions based solely on age should be discouraged if patients have a good performance status and no comorbid illnesses.

Non-Hodgkin's Lymphoma and Pregnancy

Non-Hodgkin's lymphoma in pregnancy involves major clinical and ethical issues, and a multidisciplinary approach is needed (Chapter 258). Although chest radiographs are generally considered to be safe, ultrasound examination is usually used instead of computed tomography for staging in the abdomen and pelvis.

Treatment can occasionally be delayed until after delivery; however, most women have a tumor that is potentially curable, and treatment delays may decrease the chance for cure. Other patients have conditions such as superior vena cava syndrome that require immediate treatment. After the first trimester, full-dose standard therapy such as CHOP may be used; several studies indicate high probabilities of cure without adverse long-term physical or intellectual deficits for the child. Although it is reasonable to offer therapeutic abortion for women in the first trimester, chemotherapy may also be successful in this situation.

DISEASES SOMETIMES CONFUSED WITH LYMPHOMA

The most common atypical lymphoid proliferations that can be confused with lymphoma are florid reactions to immune stimulation. Follicular hyperplasia with diffuse proliferation of B cells and T cells can be seen in a variety of autoimmune diseases (e.g., Sjögren's syndrome, systemic lupus erythematosus, rheumatoid arthritis) and infectious processes (e.g., EBV, cytomegalovirus, cat-scratch disease) (Chapter 174). If the definitive diagnosis of lymphoma cannot be made even after immunologic and molecular studies, the patient should be closely observed. The clinical course or subsequent biopsies can usually resolve the confusion.

TABLE 196–9 THE INTERNATIONAL PROGNOSTIC INDEX

Category	International Prognostic Index Score (No. of Risk Factors)	Complete Response Rate (%)	5-Yr Relapse-Free Survival (%)	5-Yr Overall Survival (%)
ALL PATIENTS*				
Low	0 or 1	87	70	73
Low intermediate	2	67	50	51
High intermediate	3	55	49	43
High	4 or 5	44	40	26
AGE-ADJUSTED INDEX, PATIENTS ≤60 YR†				
Low	0	92	86	83
Low intermediate	1	78	66	69
High intermediate	2	57	53	46
High	3	46	58	32

*Adverse factors for all patients: age >60 yr, ↑LDH, performance status 2–4, >1 extranodal site, Ann Arbor stage III or IV.
†Adverse factors for patients ≤60 yr: ↑LDH, performance status 2–4, Ann Arbor stage III or IV.
LDH = lactate dehydrogenase.
Adapted from Shipp M, Harrington D, Anderson J, et al: A predictive model for aggressive non-Hodgkin's lymphoma. N Engl J Med 1993;329:987–994.

Several rare lymphoproliferative disorders other than lymphoma have distinctive clinical courses.

Castleman's disease, or angiofollicular lymph node hyperplasia, usually appears with a hyaline vascular pattern of lymphoid proliferation, but a subset of patients have hyperplastic lymphoid follicles and sheets of plasma cells. Patients with Castleman's disease often present with a localized lymphoid mass, but some patients have a systemic illness with fevers, night sweats, weight loss, and fatigue. Frequently, the systemic symptoms of Castleman's disease are related to excessive production of IL-6. Castleman's disease in HIV-infected patients is frequently associated with HHV-8. Patients with disseminated and plasma cell–rich forms of Castleman's disease may occasionally progress to lymphoma. Patients with localized Castleman's disease can be treated with surgical removal or radiotherapy. Patients with systemic disease may respond to treatment with high-dose corticosteroids. Patients with overexpression of IL-6 frequently benefit from treatment with an anti-IL6 antibody. If other treatments fail, patients sometimes benefit from combination chemotherapy regimens or autologous or allogeneic hemopoietic stem cell transplantation, or both.

Sinus histiocytosis with massive lymphadenopathy, also known as *Rosai-Dorfman disease,* manifests as bulky lymphadenopathy in children and young adults. Extranodal sites such as the skin, upper airways, gastrointestinal tract, and CNS can be involved. There is a characteristic pattern of lymphoid proliferation with a thick fibrous capsule, distention of lymphoid sinuses, accumulation of plasma cells, and proliferation of large, often atypical, histiocytes. The disease is usually self-limited, but it has been associated with autoimmune hemolytic anemia.

Kikuchi's disease (histiocytic necrotizing lymphadenitis) is a disease of unknown origin that most commonly affects young women. Symptoms most commonly consist of painless cervical lymphadenopathy that is often accompanied by fever, flulike symptoms, and rash. Treatment is symptomatic, and symptoms usually resolve within weeks or months. Lymph node biopsies reveal foci of necrotic histiocytes.

Prognosis

Within each category of non-Hodgkin's lymphoma, the prognosis may vary according to factors related to the patient and the tumor. The International Prognostic Index, which has become the most widely used means to evaluate prognosis for non-Hodgkin's lymphoma (see Table 196–9), incorporates five factors (age, performance status, LDH level, number of extranodal sites of disease, and stage) to determine the probability of attaining a complete remission with chemotherapy and the probability of survival. The index is used primarily for diffuse large B-cell lymphomas, but it is also useful for peripheral T-cell lymphomas and follicular lymphomas.

Other factors that influence prognosis include the bulk of the tumor, cytogenetics, the cellular proliferation rate, the β_2-microglobulin level, BCL2 protein expression, and *P53* gene mutations. Gene expression profiles identified with cDNA or oligonucleotide microarrays have the potential to identify patterns that could be better predictors of prognosis than currently used clinical prognostic factors. For example, patients whose diffuse large B-cell lymphoma has a gene expression pattern similar to that of normal germinal center B cells have a better prognosis than patients whose tumor expresses genes similar to activated B cells.

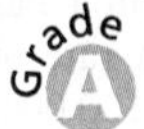

1. Marcus R, Imrie K, Belch A, et al: CVP chemotherapy plus rituximab compared with CVP as first line treatment for advanced follicular lymphoma. Blood 2005;105:1417–1423.
2. Kaminski MS, Tuck M, Estes J, et al: ^{131}I-Tositumomab therapy as initial treatment for follicular lymphoma. N Engl J Med 2005;352:441–449.
3. Reyes F, Lepage E, Ganem G, et al: ACVBP versus CHOP plus radiotherapy for localized aggressive lymphoma. N Engl J Med 2005;352:1197–1205.
4. Feugier P, Van Hoof A, Sebban C, et al: Long-term results of the R-CHOP study in the treatment of elderly patients with diffuse large B-cell lymphoma: A study by the Groupe d'Etude des Lymphomes de l'Adulte. J Clin Oncol 2005;23:4117–4126.
5. Milpied N, Deconinck E, Gaillard F, et al: Initial treatment of aggressive lymphoma with high-dose chemotherapy and autologous stem-cell support. N Engl J Med 2004;350:1287–1295.

SUGGESTED READINGS

Armitage JO, Bierman PJ, Bociek RG, Vose JM: Lymphoma 2006: Classification and Treatment. Oncology 2006;3:231–239. *An overview of recent advances in the classification, staging, and therapy of major subtypes of non-Hodgkin's lymphoma.*

Bachelor T, Loeffler JS: Primary CNS lymphoma. J Clin Oncol 2006;24:1281–1288. *Overview of diagnosis and therapy for this difficult condition, which is increasing in incidence even in patients not known to be immunosuppressed.*

Farinha P, Gascoyne RD: *Helicobacter pylori* and MALT lymphoma. Gastroenterology 2005;128:1579–1605. *Review of molecular pathogenesis.*

Hummel M, Bentink S, Berger H, et al: A biologic definition of Burkitt's lymphoma from transcriptional and genomic profiling. N Engl J Med 2006;354:2419–2430. *A molecular definition that clarifies and extends the WHO criteria.*

Rizvi MA, Evens AM: T-cell non-Hodgkin lymphoma. Blood 2006;107:1255–1264. *A comprehensive review.*

Savage KJ, Monti S, Kutok JL, et al: The molecular signature of mediastinal large B-cell lymphoma differs from that of other diffuse large B-cell lymphomas and shares features with classical Hodgkin lymphoma. Blood 2003;102:3871–3879. *The gene expression of mediastinal large B-cell lymphoma is similar to that of Hodgkin's disease.*

Thorley-Lawson DA, Gross A: Persistence of the Epstein-Barr virus and the origins of associated lymphomas. N Engl J Med 2004;350:1328–1337. *Overview of the pathophysiology and its clinical relevance.*

197 HODGKIN'S LYMPHOMA

Joseph M. Connors

Definition

Hodgkin's lymphoma, formerly called Hodgkin's disease, is one of the B-cell lymphomas. It has a characteristic neoplastic cell, the Reed-Sternberg cell, a distinct natural history, and most importantly, an excellent response to treatment, with the large majority of patients being cured. Its management, which requires careful multidisciplinary cooperation, serves as a paradigm for the successful application of modern oncologic concepts. Highly effective chemotherapy is the cornerstone of treatment. Carefully selected patients may require the addition of radiation or, if the lymphoma recurs after primary treatment, high-dose chemoradiation therapy and autologous hematologic stem cell transplantation (HDC/HSCT). The current challenge to clinicians managing this neoplasm is not only to cure it but also to do so with the least burden of long-term toxicity.

Epidemiology

The incidence of Hodgkin's lymphoma varies substantially around the world. The highest rates occur in the United States, Canada, Switzerland, and northern Europe. Intermediate rates are seen in southern and eastern Europe and low rates in eastern Asia. No clear explanation for this variation in incidence has been found. Postulated reasons include differences in the age at onset or genotype of any associated Epstein-Barr virus (EBV) infection, crowding during childhood as a result of lower socioeconomic status predisposing to passage of an as yet undiscovered infectious vector, or intrinsic genetic differences in susceptibility.

Approximately 20,000 new cases are seen annually in North America and Europe. The age-adjusted incidence of Hodgkin's lymphoma has declined modestly but significantly over the past 20 years at a rate of approximately 0.9% per year and is now approximately 2.7 per 100,000. Age-adjusted annual mortality is 0.5 per 100,000. Hodgkin's lymphoma occurs slightly more often in men and is seen more frequently in whites than African-Americans and much less frequently in Asian populations. Much of the difference in incidence between whites and blacks in North America can be attributed to the higher incidence seen in higher socioeconomic classes. The cumulative lifetime risk for development of Hodgkin's lymphoma is approximately 1 in 250 to 1 in 300 in North America.

The incidence of Hodgkin's lymphoma rises from a very low level in childhood to a plateau in early adulthood and then remains stable. In the Western world, only about 5% of cases occur in persons younger than 15 years and 5% in persons older than 70 years. In contrast, however, the age distribution in the Indian subcontinent is strongly shifted into childhood.

Pathobiology

The cause of Hodgkin's lymphoma remains unclear. Hodgkin's lymphoma is not associated with exposure to radiation, chemicals, biocidal agents, working in health care–related professions, or previous tonsillectomy. The leading suspect remains EBV based on much suggestive evidence but no definitive proof.

Epstein-Barr Virus

EBV is a large B-lymphocyte tropic herpesvirus (Chapter 400). Approximately 90% of the general population acquires infection with EBV by early adulthood. In the developing world, this infection usually occurs in childhood, but in developed countries, infection is often delayed into the teens, when it is associated with the syndrome of infectious mononucleosis in up to 30% of new cases. A history of infectious mononucleosis increases the likelihood for subsequent Hodgkin's lymphoma three-fold. Antibodies to the viral capsid antigen reach higher levels in patients with Hodgkin's lymphoma than in controls, and these higher levels appear several years before the neoplasm. In situ hybridization studies have demonstrated that the Reed-Sternberg cells in approximately 50% of cases of Hodgkin's lymphoma contain EBV-encoded small RNA (EBER), and in these cases virtually all the Reed-Sternberg cells are positive for the virus. The EBV genome is amplified 50-fold or more in Reed-Sternberg cells and is monoclonal in an individual patient's Reed-Sternberg cells. In some populations, virtually all cases of Hodgkin's lymphoma occur in EBV-positive individuals, but up to 50% of patients in developed countries do not have EBV in their Reed-Sternberg cells. Thus, although EBV may play an important role in the development of Hodgkin's lymphoma, that role is neither straightforward nor universal.

Genetic Factors

Circumstantial evidence for a genetic contribution to the etiology of Hodgkin's lymphoma comes from studies showing that Hodgkin's lymphoma is almost 100-fold more likely to develop in the monozygotic twin of an affected individual than in a dizygotic twin. First-degree relatives of individuals with the disease have up to a five-fold increased risk for development of the lymphoma. Perhaps genetically predisposed individuals react differently to EBV, thereby increasing the chance that a lymphoid neoplasm will develop.

Polymerase chain reaction–based genotypic analysis has demonstrated the clonal derivation of Reed-Sternberg cells, including identical *p53* mutations from multiple Reed-Sternberg cells extracted from a single biopsy specimen, thereby unequivocally establishing clonality. The presence of clonal immunoglobulin gene rearrangements from multiple cells in the same biopsy specimen also confirms a B-cell origin. Only a few rare cases with a T-cell genotype have been reported but are obviously exceptional. The presence of clonal somatic mutations provides proof of the germinal center origin of the neoplastic cells. Finally, identification of cells with identical immunoglobulin gene rearrangements both at diagnosis and at relapse verify that the B-cell clonality of the disease is preserved over time.

Despite their B-cell origin, the neoplastic cells of Hodgkin's lymphoma are incapable of making intact antibodies, perhaps because they lack the ability to make the transcription factors necessary to activate the immunoglobulin promoter. B cells that are incapable of manufacturing antibody should undergo apoptosis, but the Hodgkin/Reed-Sternberg cells avoid this self-destruction. The observation that the anti-apoptotic nuclear transcription factor NFκB is constitutively activated in these cells may provide an explanation.

Classic cytogenetics has been unrevealing in Hodgkin's lymphoma. Aneuploidy and hyperploidy consistent with the multinucleated nature of Hodgkin's/Reed-Sternberg cells are frequent, but no consistent translocations have been detected.

Clinical Manifestations

Hodgkin's lymphoma is usually manifested as lymphadenopathy (Chapter 174), typically in the cervical, axillary, or mediastinal areas, and only about 10% of the time as nodal disease below the diaphragm. Although peripherally located nodes seldom reach large size, very large mediastinal masses or, less often, retroperitoneal masses can develop with only modest symptoms. Lymph node involvement in Hodgkin's lymphoma is usually painless, but an occasional patient notes discomfort in involved nodal sites immediately after drinking alcohol.

Approximately 25% of patients with Hodgkin's lymphoma have constitutional symptoms. The classic B symptoms, significant weight loss (>10% of baseline), night sweats, or persistent fever, usually signal widespread or locally extensive disease and imply a need for systemic treatment. Generalized pruritus, occasionally severe, can antedate the diagnosis of Hodgkin's lymphoma by up to several years. Some patients have symptoms suggestive of a growing mass lesion, such as cough or stridor as a result of tracheobronchial compression from mediastinal disease or bone pain secondary to metastatic involvement. Because Hodgkin's lymphoma can involve the bone marrow extensively, an occasional patient has symptomatic anemia or incidentally noted pancytopenia. Paraneoplastic neurologic or endocrine syndromes have been reported with Hodgkin's lymphoma but are rare.

Diagnosis

The diagnosis of Hodgkin's lymphoma is based on recognition of Reed-Sternberg cells (Fig. 197–1) or Hodgkin's cells (or both) in an appropriate cellular background in tissue sections from a lymph node or extralymphatic organ, such as bone marrow, lung, or bone. Fine-needle

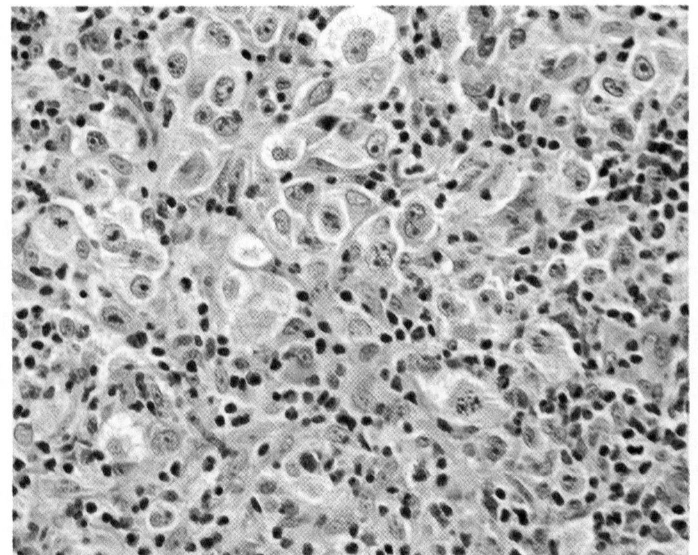

FIGURE 197–1 • Nodular sclerosing Hodgkin's lymphoma. This figure shows a typical case of classic nodular sclerosing Hodgkin's lymphoma with many lacunar cells, occasional diagnostic Reed-Sternberg cells, and the characteristic background of lymphocytes and eosinophils. (Photomicrograph courtesy of Randy D. Gascoyne, MD, British Columbia Cancer Agency.)

TABLE 197–1 WORLD HEALTH ORGANIZATION CLASSIFICATION OF HODGKIN'S LYMPHOMA SUBTYPES

Subtype Name	Frequency (%)*
Classic Hodgkin's lymphoma	
Nodular sclerosis	65
Lymphocyte rich	3
Mixed cellularity	12
Lymphocyte depleted	2
Nodular lymphocyte-predominant Hodgkin's lymphoma	6
Hodgkin's lymphoma, not otherwise classifiable	12

*Frequency based on all new cases (N = 302) seen in British Columbia since January 1998 when the category of lymphocyte-rich classic Hodgkin's lymphoma became well established.

aspiration biopsy is not adequate for the diagnosis of Hodgkin's lymphoma. Open biopsy and standard histochemical staining are required to establish the diagnosis unequivocally and to determine the histologic subtype. Immunohistochemical studies can prove helpful in difficult cases or to distinguish special subtypes such as lymphocyte-rich classic Hodgkin's lymphoma and the nodular lymphocyte-predominant type. In classic Hodgkin's lymphoma, scattered large Reed-Sternberg cells are either multinucleated or have a large polyploid nucleus. Variations include mononuclear cells that are similar to the usual polylobated or multinuclear cells but have only one large nucleus with a prominent nucleolus, as well as lacunar cells, which are Reed-Sternberg variants with abundant cytoplasm that has retracted as an artifact of formalin fixation. The infrequent Reed-Sternberg cells are usually present in a background mixture of polyclonal lymphocytes, eosinophils, neutrophils, plasma cells, fibroblasts, and histiocytes. Occasionally, granulomas form with a prominent histiocytic component.

Hodgkin's lymphoma can typically be classified into one of five well-described subtypes (Table 197–1). Reproducibility of the distinctions among these subtypes has been confirmed in the current widely accepted World Health Organization classification of lymphoid neoplasms. With addition of the new category of lymphocyte-rich classic Hodgkin's lymphoma, this newest classification scheme permits confident identification of nodular lymphocyte-predominant Hodgkin's lymphoma as a separate entity. The most common subtype is nodular sclerosing, which has characteristic course bands of sclerosis surrounding nodules composed of typical Reed-Sternberg cells in the usual background mixture of reactive and inflammatory cells.

The immunophenotype of the neoplastic cells in Hodgkin's lymphoma can help identify the specific subtype. Typically, the Hodgkin/Reed-Sternberg cells stain positively for CD30 (80 to 100% of cases), CD15 (75 to 85% of cases), and B-cell–specific activating protein (BSAP), which is the product of the *PAX5* gene (>90% of cases). However, often only a minority of the malignant cells stain positively for the CD15 and BSAP markers. CD20, a generally reliable marker of B-cell lineage, is positive in about 40% of cases of classic Hodgkin's lymphoma, but usually only a minority of cells are positive, and the staining can be weak. In contrast, nodular lymphocyte-predominant Hodgkin's lymphoma almost always stains strongly positive for CD20 and for the specialized B-cell markers CD79a and CD45, but it is negative for CD30 and CD15. Nodularity signals the diagnosis of nodular lymphocyte-predominant Hodgkin's lymphoma. Finally, anaplastic large cell lymphoma (Chapter 196) is reliably negative for CD15, CD20, and CD79a but frequently positive for anaplastic lymphoma kinase (ALK).

Differential Diagnosis

Depending on the site of occurrence and associated symptoms, the differential diagnosis of Hodgkin's lymphoma includes non-Hodgkin's lymphoma (Chapter 196), germ cell tumors (Chapter 210), thymoma (Chapter 448), sarcoidosis (Chapter 95), and tuberculosis (Chapter 345). However, the specific diagnosis is readily determined by obtaining an adequate biopsy specimen for review by an experienced hematopathologist. Proceeding to such a biopsy early in the assessment of patients with lymphadenopathy (Chapter 174), especially of the mediastinum, often saves time and spares the patient needless testing and delay in diagnosis.

With the widespread availability of computed tomography (CT) and appropriate biopsy procedures to investigate enlarged central thoracic or intra-abdominal lymph nodes, the diagnosis of Hodgkin's lymphoma seldom presents difficulty. The immunophenotype can also help distinguish Hodgkin's lymphoma from other diseases. For example, T cell–rich B-cell lymphoma (Chapter 196) is distinguished from classic Hodgkin's lymphoma by being CD30 and CD15 negative but positive for CD20 and CD45. However, T cell–rich B-cell lymphoma (Chapter 196) can be very difficult to distinguish from nodular lymphocyte-predominant Hodgkin's lymphoma because both are negative for CD30 and CD15 but positive for CD45. This distinction is best made by focusing on the histologic pattern of the neoplastic cells. In fact, the combination of appropriate immunohistopathologic evaluation by an expert hematopathologist and clinical assessment has virtually eliminated difficulties with the differential diagnosis. Problems mostly arise when inadequate or improperly processed material is all that is available for diagnosis.

Staging

Physical Examination

Given its tendency to spread in an orderly fashion, usually from initially involved lymph nodes, the stage of Hodgkin's lymphoma can be established by using readily available imaging and laboratory tests (Fig. 197–2 and Table 197–2). The evaluation should start with a careful history to search for the presence of localizing signs, such as bone pain, or the constitutional symptoms of fever, weight loss, or night sweats. The history may also reveal comorbid conditions that may affect the safe delivery of planned treatment. The physical examination may identify lymphadenopathy or organomegaly.

Laboratory Testing

Laboratory testing should include blood cell counts and the erythrocyte sedimentation rate, assessment of liver and renal function, serologic testing for hepatitis B and hepatitis C if liver enzyme abnormalities are detected, human immunodeficiency virus (HIV) antibody testing if the history indicates an increased risk or if the sites of disease are unusual, an albumin level, and serum protein electrophoresis. Bone marrow aspiration and biopsy are most useful for the minority of patients with constitutional (B) symptoms or those with lower than normal peripheral blood counts at diagnosis.

Imaging

Imaging techniques to evaluate Hodgkin's lymphoma continue to evolve (Fig. 197–3). All patients should undergo contrast-enhanced CT scanning of the thorax, abdomen, and pelvis with slices at intervals of 1 cm or less. Magnetic resonance imaging is occasionally useful when the extent of bone or soft tissue involvement must be determined precisely or for a patient with an absolute contraindication to the use of intravenous contrast agents. Gallium scanning adds little to what can be

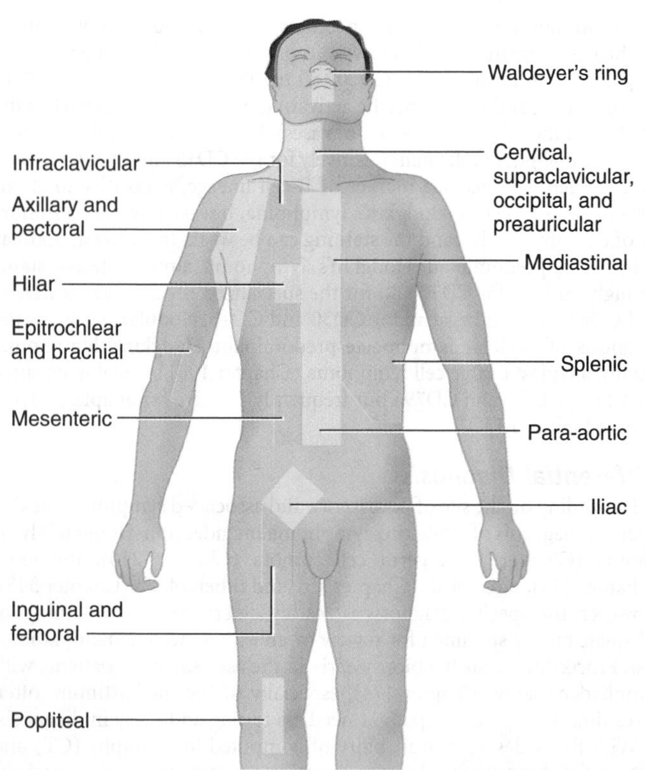

FIGURE 197–2 • Anatomic definition of lymph node regions for staging of Hodgkin's disease. (From Kaplan HS, Rosenberg SA: The treatment of Hodgkin's disease. Med Clin North Am 1966;50:1591–1610.)

TABLE 197–2 TESTS REQUIRED FOR STAGING OF HODGKIN'S LYMPHOMA

Complete history to search for B symptoms (fever, weight loss, night sweats) or other symptomatic problems suggesting more advanced disease

Physical examination for lymphadenopathy or organomegaly

Complete blood count plus erythrocyte sedimentation rate

Serum creatinine, alkaline phosphatase, lactate dehydrogenase, bilirubin, and protein electrophoresis (including albumin level)

Chest radiograph, posteroanterior and lateral views

Computed tomography scan of the neck, thorax, abdomen, and pelvis

Certain tests are required only for specific manifestations

Manifestation/Condition	Test
B symptoms or WBC count <4.0 × 10^9/L, Hgb <120 g/L (women) or 130 g/L (men), or platelets <125 × 10^9/L	Bone marrow biopsy and aspiration
Stage IA or IIA disease with upper cervical lymph node involvement (supra-hyoid)	ENT examination

ENT = ear, nose, and throat; Hgb = hemoglobin; WBC = white blood cell.

learned with CT scanning and is prone to false-negative and false-positive results.

Positron Emission Tomography

Positron emission tomography (PET) is more sensitive and specific than CT or gallium scanning both for staging and for assessment of residual masses after treatment. However, it has not been proved that the addition of PET to standard staging imaging tests for Hodgkin's lymphoma will actually improve outcome, so whether PET could replace other studies is not clear. The greatest usefulness of PET presently appears to be the assessment of residual masses during or after planned treatment so that the minority of patients who should receive altered or additional therapy can be identified.

TABLE 197–3 MODIFIED ANN ARBOR STAGING SYSTEM FOR HODGKIN'S LYMPHOMA

Stage	Involvement
I	Single lymph node region (I) or one extralymphatic site (I_E)
II	Two or more lymph node regions, same side of the diaphragm (II), or local extralymphatic extension plus one or more lymph node regions, same side of the diaphragm (II_E)
III	Lymph node regions on both sides of the diaphragm (III); may be accompanied by local extralymphatic extension (III_E)
IV	Diffuse involvement of one or more extralymphatic organs or sites
A	No "B" symptoms
B	Presence of at least one of the following: Unexplained weight loss >10% of baseline during 6 months before staging Recurrent unexplained fever >38° C Recurrent night sweats

The Ann Arbor staging system with the Cotswold modification (Table 197–3) categorizes patients into four stages. The first three indicate the expanding extent of lymph node disease (see Fig. 197–2): stage I, a single nodal area; stage II, two or more nodal areas but still on one side of the diaphragm; and stage III, nodal disease on both sides of the diaphragm. The spleen and the lymphoid tissue of Waldeyer's ring each count as nodal sites in this system. Stage IV is reserved for extranodal disease, which for all practical purposes is disease in the bone marrow, lung, bone, or liver. Hodgkin's lymphoma at any other extranodal site should prompt questioning of the diagnosis or a search for HIV infection.

Bulky disease is defined as the presence of any tumor mass with the largest diameter greater than 10 cm or a mediastinal mass with a transverse diameter exceeding a third of the largest transverse transthoracic diameter. Now that CT scanning is widely available, use of the mediastinal mass ratio is obsolete, and the term *bulky* is best assigned to tumors exceeding 10 cm in largest single diameter.

The E lesion designation identifies patients whose limited extranodal extension of Hodgkin's lymphoma could be included in a reasonable involved field of irradiation. After staging, patients are further subdivided into those with or without fever, night sweats, or weight loss (B symptoms).

Treatment

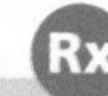

Over the past 50 years, Hodgkin's lymphoma has been transformed from a nearly uniformly fatal illness to one that is usually cured. This remarkable success has provided a paradigm on which much of modern oncologic treatment is based. The principles underlying combined-modality treatment and multiagent chemotherapy, the mainstays of today's successful treatment of many malignancies, were first demonstrated to be effective with Hodgkin's lymphoma. The essential involvement of a multidisciplinary team, including pathologists, experts in diagnostic imaging, medical and radiation oncologists, nurses, and support staff, has served as a model for all cancer. The necessity to balance greater efficacy of initial treatment, which often requires an increase in intensity and therefore toxicity, against troublesome and occasionally fatal late complications has encouraged a long-term perspective.

From a practical therapeutic viewpoint, patients with stage III or IV disease, bulky disease, or B symptoms are defined as having advanced disease, whereas patients without these characteristics have limited-stage disease. In Europe, patients with limited disease are further subdivided into those with favorable and unfavorable outcomes, but cure rates exceed 90 to 95% for all patients with non-bulky stage IA or IIA (limited) disease. However, for patients with advanced-stage disease, independent predictors of progression include gender, age, stage, hemoglobin level, white blood cell count, lymphocyte count, and serum albumin level (Table 197–4). For the 80% of patients with no more than three factors, the likelihood

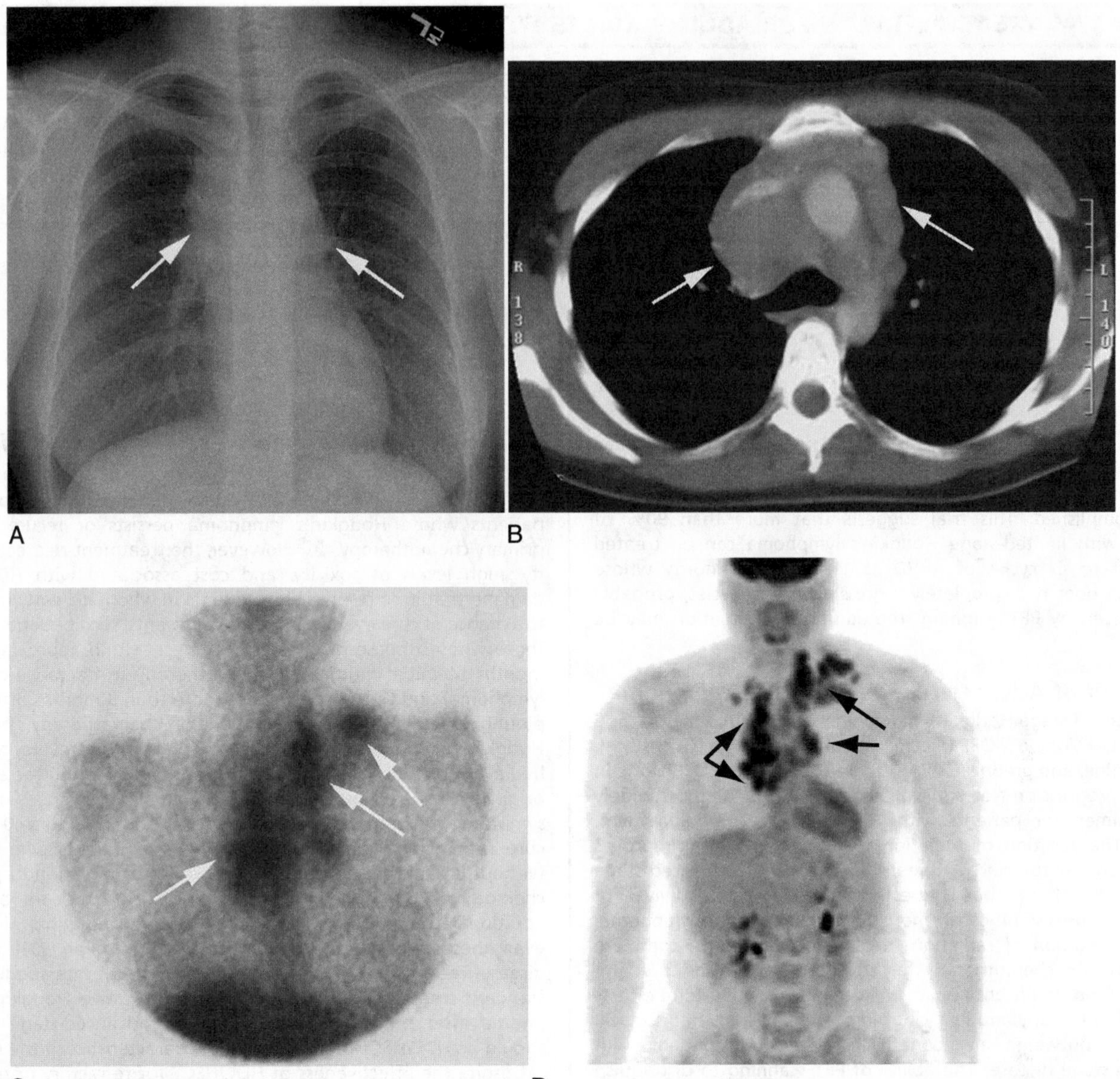

FIGURE 197–3 • Imaging of Hodgkin's lymphoma. Bulky Hodgkin's disease as seen on chest radiograph **(A)**, computed tomography (CT) of the chest **(B)**, gallium scan **(C)**, and positron emission tomography (PET) **(D)**. The arrows indicate sites of disease. Note that the PET and CT scans provide more detailed information than the chest radiograph and gallium scan.

TABLE 197–4 RATES OF PROGRESSION IN 5 YEARS IN PATIENTS WITH ADVANCED-STAGE HODGKIN'S LYMPHOMA

Number of Factors*	Frequency (%)	Percentage with Progression-Free Survival at 5 Years
0–3	81	70
4–7	19	47

*Male sex, age older than 45 years, stage IV, hemoglobin level less than 10.5 g/dL, white blood cell count greater than 15,000/mL, lymphocyte count less than 600/mL or less than 8% of the white cell count, or serum albumin less than 4 g/dL.

Rx

of progression-free survival is 70%. For the 20% who have four or more factors, the progression-free survival rate falls to less than 50%. A straightforward plan of treatment for the 90% of patients in whom Hodgkin's lymphoma is diagnosed between the ages of 16 and 70 can be based on clinical stage, the presence of B symptoms, and bulk of the largest tumor mass (Table 197–5).

Rx

Treatment of Limited-Stage Hodgkin's Lymphoma

Most of the 35% of patients with Hodgkin's lymphoma initially seen with-limited stage disease can be cured regardless of the site of occurrence, the presence of disease above or below the diaphragm, or the histologic subtype. The greatest challenge is to achieve this goal with the least toxicity and cost.

Two cycles of ABVD (Adriamycin [doxorubicin], bleomycin, vinblastine, and dacarbazine) chemotherapy followed by involved-field irradiation cures nearly 95% of patients with limited-stage disease and nearly completely eliminates the risk for infertility, premature menopause, and leukemia and minimizes cardiopulmonary toxicity. 1,2 The chemotherapy in the combined-modality treatment of limited-stage Hodgkin's lymphoma eradicates subclinical disease and allows smaller fields of irradiation to be used. However, a substantial proportion of the excess, long-term mortality in patients with limited-stage Hodgkin's lymphoma is due to cardiovascular disease and second neoplasms that are closely related to the use of irradiation. In a randomized trial that compared four to six cycles of ABVD chemotherapy alone versus irradiation, either alone or augmented with two cycles of ABVD chemotherapy, the strategy of chemotherapy alone proved equivalent to irradiation-based treatment in terms of event-free and overall survival, although the irradiation-based

TABLE 197–5 TREATMENT PLAN FOR ADULT PATIENTS WITH HODGKIN'S LYMPHOMA

Stage	Prognostic Category	Treatment
IA or IIA, no bulky disease*	≤3 adverse factors†	ABVD‡ × 4 if CR after 2 cycles or ABVD × 2 + IRRT
IB, IIB, or any stage III or IV, but no bulky disease	≤3 adverse factors	ABVD‡ until 2 cycles past CR (minimum 6, maximum 8)
Bulky disease, any stage	≥4 adverse factors	Stanford V‡ or BEACOPP‡ ABVD × 6 + IRRT

*Bulky refers to disease with the largest diameter of any single mass equal to or greater than 10 cm.
†See Table 197–4.
‡See text for drugs in each regimen. Optimal dosing must be individualized.
CR = complete response; IRRT = involved-region radiation therapy.

approach did produce a modest improvement in progression-free survival. [3] Longer follow-up will be necessary to see whether the goal of a reduction in cardiovascular events and second neoplasms was accomplished. This trial suggests that more than 90% of patients with limited-stage Hodgkin's lymphoma can be treated with four to six cycles of ABVD alone; for the minority whose lymphoma does not completely regress after two cycles, probably best assessed by PET scanning, the addition of radiation may be optimal.

Treatment of Advanced-Stage Hodgkin's Lymphoma

In advanced-stage Hodgkin's lymphoma (stages IIIA, IIIB, IVA, and IVB), both ABVD and MOPP (mechlorethamine, Oncovin [vincristine], procarbazine, and prednisone)/ABVD are superior to MOPP alone in terms of progression-free survival. Today, ABVD is the most widely used regimen for patients with advanced-stage Hodgkin's lymphoma. The addition of radiation therapy significantly improves progression-free survival at 10 years in patients with advanced-stage Hodgkin's lymphoma, but it does not improve overall survival [4] because it causes significantly more deaths unrelated to lymphoma. Even the addition of radiation therapy for patients in complete remission after chemotherapy for advanced-stage Hodgkin's lymphoma has no significant impact. [5] The adverse long-term effects of radiation therapy and its lack of improvement in overall survival appear to outweigh any benefits for the usual patient with advanced-stage disease. The ability of PET scanning to distinguish between residual fibrosis and persistent lymphoma may provide a mechanism to identify selected patients who might benefit from localized radiation therapy.

Recently devised regimens for patients with advanced Hodgkin's lymphoma are the Stanford V regimen (doxorubicin, vinblastine, mechlorethamine, etoposide, vincristine, bleomycin, and prednisone) and escalated BEACOPP (bleomycin, etoposide, doxorubicin, cyclophosphamide, vincristine, prednisone, and procarbazine) (see Table 197–5). As originally described, both include postchemotherapy irradiation to sites of initial or residual tumor bulk (≥5 cm). In phase II testing, the Stanford V regimen provided 91% freedom from progression at 8 years with an overall survival rate of 95%; fertility was maintained. BEACOPP plus radiation therapy provides better progression-free and overall survival at a median follow-up of 6.9 years than COPP/ABVD plus radiation therapy despite a higher rate of hematologic toxicity and infertility. [6]

About 50% of patients who are not cured by primary chemotherapy can be effectively treated with HDC/HSCT (Chapter 184). For the 80% of patients with zero to three adverse prognostic factors, who have a 70% chance of cure with primary chemotherapy, the most widely used approach is to start with ABVD. For the 30% of these low-risk patients in whom progressive lymphoma develops despite primary treatment, HDC/HSCT (Chapter 184) should be offered. Such a strategy confines the high cost and toxicity of intensified treatment to the minority of patients whose disease demands it. Conversely, for the 20% of high-risk patients who have four or more adverse factors and less than a 50% likelihood of cure with primary chemotherapy, more intense initial treatment with the Stanford V or BEACOPP protocol is reasonable.

Management of Refractory or Relapsed Hodgkin's Lymphoma

HDC/HSCT has become the established treatment for most patients whose Hodgkin's lymphoma persists or recurs despite primary chemotherapy. [7] However, the treatment-related mortality, high levels of toxicity, and cost associated with HDC/HSCT demand that it be reserved for patients in whom it clearly increases the chance of cure over alternative treatments; such patients include those whose disease progresses during or within approximately 3 months of initial multiagent chemotherapy (refractory Hodgkin's lymphoma) and those who relapse more than 3 months after completing a full course of multiagent chemotherapy (relapsed Hodgkin's lymphoma). For relapsed lymphoma, controversy remains, however, for two special subgroups: patients who relapse solely in originally involved but unirradiated lymph nodes and without B symptoms or extranodal disease, who may obtain up to a 40 to 50% cure rate with wide-field irradiation, and patients who relapse without B symptoms more than 1 year after completion of primary chemotherapy, who may achieve up to a 30 to 40% cure rate with additional chemotherapy with or without irradiation. However, even these two subgroups may achieve up to an 80% 10-year disease-free survival rate after HDC/HSCT. Thus, data suggest that standard treatment for patients with progressive Hodgkin's lymphoma after primary chemotherapy for advanced-stage disease should be HDC/HSCT regardless of the characteristics of the relapse.

Despite the effectiveness of HDC/HSCT for refractory or relapsed Hodgkin's lymphoma, randomized trials of HDC/HSCT for patients with adverse prognostic factors in complete or partial remission after primary chemotherapy for advanced Hodgkin's lymphoma failed to show a difference in outcome. [8] Based on present evidence, HDC/HSCT should be reserved for patients who have progressive lymphoma after primary chemotherapy.

Management of Complications

Follow-up and Late Complications of Treatment

Most adult patients with Hodgkin's lymphoma are cured and experience minimal long-term toxicity from their treatment. However, the risk for certain predictable and occasional rare and less predictable late effects warrants careful but not intrusive follow-up and selective intervention (Table 197–6). First, at the conclusion of treatment a thorough reassessment of the initial sites of lymphoma should be completed to provide post-treatment baseline measurements. Patients should be seen by a specialist knowledgeable in the management of lymphoma, preferably about every 3 months for 2 years, then every 6 months for 3 years, then annually. Patients should be strongly encouraged to refrain from smoking, to perform careful breast and skin examinations on a regular basis, and to undergo regular immunizations for influenza annually, pneumococcus at diagnosis and 5 years after treatment, and diphtheria and tetanus every 10 years (Chapter 16). Patients who have received radiation to the head or neck area should follow a vigorous program of dental prophylaxis in anticipation of the deleterious effect of reduced saliva production and have their thyroid-stimulating hormone level checked annually in recognition of about a 50% risk for eventual hypothyroidism.

TABLE 197–6 MONITORING AFTER SUCCESSFUL PRIMARY TREATMENT OF HODGKIN'S LYMPHOMA

Risk/Problem	Incidence/Response
Relapse	Ten percent to 30% of patients relapse. Careful attention should be directed to lymph node sites, especially if previously involved with disease and not treated with radiation. New persistent focal symptoms such as bone pain should be investigated with appropriate laboratory and imaging studies.
Dental caries	Neck or oropharyngeal irradiation may cause decreased salivation. Patients should have regular dental care and should make their dentist aware of the previous irradiation.
Hypothyroidism	After external beam thyroid irradiation at doses sufficient to cure Hodgkin's lymphoma, at least 50% of patients eventually become hypothyroid. All patients who have been exposed to neck irradiation should have an annual TSH level determined. Patients whose TSH level becomes elevated should be treated with lifelong thyroxine replacement in doses sufficient to suppress TSH levels to low normal (Chapter 244).
Infertility	ABVD is not known to cause permanent gonadal toxicity, although temporary oligospermia or irregular menses may persist for 1 to 2 years after treatment. Direct or scatter radiation to gonadal tissue may cause infertility, amenorrhea, or premature menopause, but this adverse event seldom occurs with the current fields used for the treatment of Hodgkin's lymphoma. In general, women who continue menstruating are fertile, but men require semen analysis to provide a specific answer.
Secondary neoplasms	Though uncommon, certain secondary neoplasms occur with increased frequency in patients who have been treated for Hodgkin's lymphoma: acute myelogenous leukemia; thyroid, breast, lung, cervical, and upper gastrointestinal carcinoma; and melanoma. It is appropriate to "be vigilant" for these neoplasms for the remainder of the patient's life because they may have a lengthy induction period.

ABVD = Adriamycin, bleomycin, vinblastine, and dacarbazine; TSH = thyroid-stimulating hormone.

Special Problems in the Management of Hodgkin's Lymphoma

Hodgkin's Lymphoma during Pregnancy

Between 0.5 and 1.0% of cases of Hodgkin's lymphoma occur coincident with pregnancy (Chapter 258). When the lymphoma is discovered during pregnancy, it is almost always possible to control the lymphoma and allow the pregnancy to go to full term.

Standard staging tests (see Table 197–2) should be completed, except that imaging requiring radiation must be minimized. For example, abdominal ultrasonography can identify bulky retroperitoneal disease, and a single posteroanterior radiograph of the chest, with proper shielding, can identify bulky mediastinal disease.

More than 50% of patients can continue the pregnancy to term without any treatment of the lymphoma. If symptomatic or progressive disease develops, systemic chemotherapy can be given in the second and third trimester with very small risk of injuring the fetus. An alternative is intermittent single-agent vinblastine, given in the lowest dose that can control symptoms until delivery, followed by a full course of six to eight cycles of multiagent chemotherapy after delivery.

Hodgkin's Lymphoma and Acquired Immunodeficiency Syndrome

In patients with HIV infection, the incidence of Hodgkin's lymphoma is increased as much as 5- to 10-fold, and the lymphoma is manifested differently and pursues a more aggressive natural history (Chapter 416). Hodgkin's lymphoma in HIV-positive individuals is almost always associated with EBV within Hodgkin's/Reed-Sternberg cells. The histology is much more likely to be mixed cellularity or lymphocyte depleted. The disease most commonly develops in extranodal sites, especially the bone marrow. More than 80% of patients have advanced-stage disease, and most patients have B symptoms.

Patients are prone to opportunistic infections, and the interaction of chemotherapeutic agents with other medications may compromise the patient's ability to tolerate treatment. The best approach is a combination of vigorous supportive care with antiviral and antifungal agents, neutrophil-stimulating growth factors, and their usual highly active antiretroviral agents (Chapter 412) along with standard multiagent chemotherapy. With appropriate supportive care, regimens such as ABVD [9] and EBVP (epirubicin, bleomycin, vinblastine, and prednisone) can be delivered. However, worse than normal toxicity must be anticipated, and cure rates are much lower than in the non–HIV-infected population. Median survival is typically 1 to 2 years.

Rx

Hodgkin's Lymphoma in the Elderly

Elderly patients with Hodgkin's lymphoma have a worse outcome. For example, the 5-year overall survival rate falls from 80% in patients younger than 65 years to less than 50% in patients older than 65. Explanations include more advanced stage at diagnosis, comorbid diseases, delay in diagnosis, incomplete staging, inadequate adherence to treatment protocols, and failure to maintain full dose intensity.

Of note is that elderly patients achieve outcomes equivalent to those of younger patients when they receive similar doses of chemotherapy. The best approach for elderly patients is to attempt to treat them in a manner similar to younger patients, with the addition of neutrophil growth factors if necessary to enable safe delivery of full doses. For patients with preexisting pulmonary or cardiac disease, it might be necessary to reduce or eliminate bleomycin or doxorubicin, respectively.

Future Directions

The ability to profile multigene expression patterns and identify genetic polymorphisms associated with specific malignancies may provide better insight into the molecular genesis of Hodgkin's and other lymphomas.

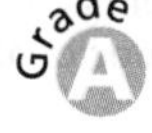

1. Engert A, Schiller P, Josting A, et al: Involved-field radiotherapy is equally effective and less toxic compared with extended-field radiotherapy after four cycles of chemotherapy in patients with early-stage unfavorable Hodgkin's lymphoma: Results of the HD8 trials of the German Hodgkin's Lymphoma Study Group. J Clin Oncol 2003;21:3601–3608.
2. Bonadonna G, Bonfante V, Viviani S, et al: ABVD plus subtotal nodal versus involved-field radiotherapy in early-stage Hodgkin's disease: Long-term results. J Clin Oncol 2004;22:2835–2841.
3. Meyer RM, Gospodarowicz MK, Connors JM, et al: Randomized comparison of ABVD chemotherapy with a strategy that includes radiation therapy in patients with limited-stage Hodgkin's lymphoma: National Cancer Institute of Canada Clinical Trials Group and the Eastern Cooperative Oncology Group. J Clin Oncol 2005;23:4634–4642.
4. Loeffler M, Brosteanu O, Hasenclever D, et al: Meta-analysis of chemotherapy versus combined modality treatment trials in Hodgkin's disease. International Database on Hodgkin's Disease Overview Study Group. J Clin Oncol 1998;16:818–829.
5. Ferme C, Sebban C, Hennequin C, et al: Comparison of chemotherapy to radiotherapy as consolidation of complete or good partial response after six cycles of chemotherapy for patients with advanced Hodgkin's disease: Results of the Groupe d'Etudes des Lymphomes de l'Adulte H89 trial. Blood 2000;95:2246–2252.

6. Diehl V, Franklin J, Pfreundschuh M, et al: Standard and increased-dose BEACOPP chemotherapy compared with COPP-ABVD for advanced Hodgkin's disease. N Engl J Med 2003;348:2386–2395.
7. Schmitz N, Pfistner B, Sextro M, et al: Aggressive conventional chemotherapy compared with high-dose chemotherapy with autologous haemopoietic stem-cell transplantation for relapsed chemosensitive Hodgkin's disease: A randomised trial. Lancet 2002;359:2065–2071.
8. Federico M, Bellei M, Brice P, et al: High-dose therapy and autologous stem-cell transplantation versus conventional therapy for patients with advanced Hodgkin's lymphoma responding to front-line therapy. J Clin Oncol. 2003;21:2320–2325.
9. Levine AM, Li P, Cheung T, et al: Chemotherapy consisting of doxorubicin, bleomycin, vinblastine, and dacarbazine with granulocyte-colony-stimulating factor in HIV-infected patients with newly diagnosed Hodgkin's disease: A prospective, multi-institutional AIDS clinical trials group study (ACTG 149). J Acquir Immune Defic Syndr 2000;24:444–450.

SUGGESTED READINGS

Ansell SM, Armitage JO: Management of Hodgkin lymphoma. Mayo Clin Proc 2006;81:419–426. *A practical overview.*

Connors JM: State-of-the-art therapeutics: Hodgkin's lymphoma. J Clin Oncol 2005;23:6400–6408. *Up-to-date review of the current state-of-the-art of treatment of Hodgkin's lymphoma.*

Re D, Kuppers R, Diehl V: Molecular pathogenesis of Hodgkin's lymphoma. J Clin Oncol 2005;23:6379–6386. *Concise but comprehensive review of new insights into the basic molecular biology and etiology of Hodgkin's lymphoma.*

Swerdlow AJ, Higgins CD, Smith P, et al: Myocardial infarction mortality risk after treatment for Hodgkin disease: A collaborative British cohort study. J Natl Cancer Inst 2007;99:206–214. *Increase in risk of death due to MI in survivors of Hodgkin's lymphoma (SMR 2.5).*

198 PLASMA CELL DISORDERS

S. Vincent Rajkumar and Robert A. Kyle

Definition

Plasma cell disorders are neoplastic or potentially neoplastic diseases associated with the proliferation of a single clone of immunoglobulin-secreting plasma cells (Table 198–1). They are characterized by the secretion of electrophoretically and immunologically homogeneous (monoclonal) proteins that represent intact or incomplete immunoglobulin molecules. Monoclonal proteins are commonly referred to as M proteins, myeloma proteins, or paraproteins.

Syndromes associated with plasma cell disorders and monoclonal proteins include monoclonal gammopathy of undetermined significance (MGUS), multiple myeloma, Waldenström's macroglobulinemia, cryoglobulinemia, and primary amyloidosis (see Table 198–1). Occasionally, free hemoglobin-haptoglobin complexes resulting from hemolysis, large amounts of transferrin in patients with iron deficiency anemia, or increased levels of fibrinogen may simulate the presence of a monoclonal protein in serum.

Serum Immunoglobulins

Intact immunoglobulins consist of two heavy (H) polypeptide chains of the same class and subclass and two light (L) polypeptide chains of the same type (Chapter 42). The heavy polypeptide chains are designated by Greek letters: γ in immunoglobulin G (IgG), α in immunoglobulin A (IgA), μ in immunoglobulin M (IgM), δ in immunoglobulin D (IgD), and ε in immunoglobulin E (IgE). IgG includes the subclasses IgG1, IgG2, IgG3, and IgG4; IgA includes the subclasses IgA1 and IgA2; and no subclasses have been recognized for IgM, IgD, or IgE. The light chain types are kappa (κ) and lambda (λ). Both heavy chains and light chains have "constant" and "variable" regions with respect to the amino acid sequence. The class specificity of each immunoglobulin is defined by a series of antigenic determinants on the constant regions of the heavy chains (γ, α, μ, δ, and ε) and the two major classes of light chains (κ and λ). The amino acid sequence in the variable regions of the immunoglobulin molecule corresponds to the active antigen-combining site of the antibody, whereas the constant regions convey other biologic properties (Chapter 42).

TABLE 198–1 CLASSIFICATION OF PLASMA CELL PROLIFERATIVE DISORDERS

I. Monoclonal gammopathies of undetermined significance (MGUS)
   A. Benign (IgG, IgA, IgD, IgM, and rarely, free light chains)
   B. Associated neoplasms or other diseases not known to produce monoclonal proteins
   C. Biclonal gammopathies
   D. Idiopathic Bence Jones proteinuria
II. Malignant monoclonal gammopathies
   A. Multiple myeloma (IgG, IgA, IgD, IgE, and free light chains)
      1. Overt multiple myeloma
      2. Smoldering multiple myeloma
      3. Plasma cell leukemia
      4. Nonsecretory myeloma
      5. IgD myeloma
      6. Osteosclerotic myeloma (POEMS syndrome)
      7. Solitary plasmacytoma of bone
      8. Extramedullary plasmacytoma
   B. Waldenström's macroglobulinemia
      1. Other lymphoproliferative diseases
III. Heavy chain diseases (HCDs)
   A. γ-HCD
   B. α-HCD
   C. μ-HCD
IV. Cryoglobulinemia
V. Primary amyloidosis (AL)

Ig = immunoglobulin; POEMS = polyneuropathy, organomegaly, endocrinopathy, M protein, and skin changes.
Modified from Kyle RA: Classification and diagnosis of monoclonal gammopathies. *In* Rose NR, Friedman H, Fahey JL (eds): Manual of Clinical Laboratory Immunology, 3rd ed. Washington, DC, American Society for Microbiology, 1986, p 152, with permission of the American Society for Microbiology (ASM Press).

In the majority of plasma cell disorders, intact immunoglobulin molecules are secreted as M proteins. In some patients, however, heavy chain expression is completely lost, and only monoclonal light chains (Bence Jones proteins) are secreted. Even less frequently, only heavy chains are secreted (heavy chain diseases [HCDs]).

Serum protein electrophoresis detects M protein as a narrow peak (like a church spire) on the densitometer tracing or as a dense, discrete band on agarose gel (Fig. 198–1). Monoclonal light chains (Bence Jones proteinemia) are rarely seen on agarose gel electrophoresis. In the HCDs, the M component is not usually apparent.

Immunofixation should be performed when a peak or band is first seen on protein electrophoresis to identify the heavy and light chain type of the M protein. It should also be performed when multiple myeloma or related disorders are suspected despite normal findings on protein electrophoresis. Immunofixation is especially useful for finding a small M protein in primary amyloidosis, solitary plasmacytoma, or extramedullary plasmacytoma or after successful treatment of multiple myeloma or macroglobulinemia..

An M protein can be present when the total protein concentration, β- and γ-globulin levels, and quantitative immunoglobulin values are all within normal limits. A small M protein can be concealed in the normal β or γ areas and may be overlooked. In 5% of sera with a monoclonal peak, there is an additional M protein of a different immunoglobulin class; this condition is designated a biclonal (double) gammopathy.

In some patients, the M protein has specificity to one of various antigens. Examples include actin, dextran, antistreptolysin O, antinuclear antibody, riboflavin, von Willebrand's factor, thyroglobulin, insulin, double-stranded DNA, and apolipoprotein. Binding of calcium by an M protein may produce hypercalcemia without symptomatic or pathologic consequences. M proteins have also been found to bind to copper and to phosphate.

Monoclonal proteins must be distinguished from an excess of polyclonal immunoglobulins (one or more heavy chain types and both κ and

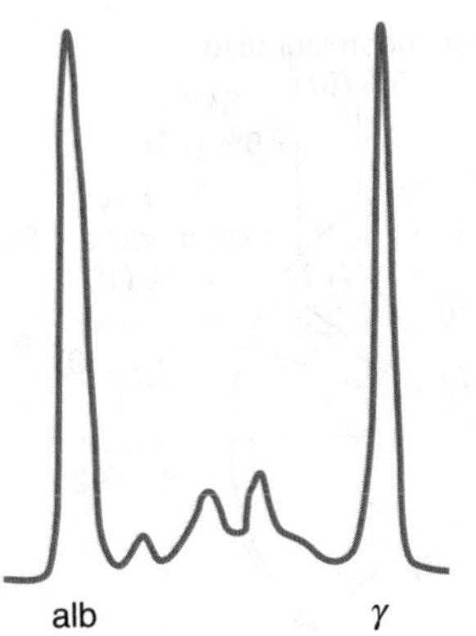

A

B

FIGURE 198–1 • Serum protein electrophoresis showing a monoclonal (M) protein. A, Monoclonal pattern of serum protein as traced by a densitometer after electrophoresis on agarose gel: tall, narrow-based peak of γ mobility. **B,** Monoclonal pattern from electrophoresis of serum on agarose gel (anode on the left): dense, localized band representing monoclonal protein of γ mobility. (From Kyle RA, Katzmann JA: Immunochemical characterization of immunoglobulins. *In* Rose NR, Conway de Macario E, Folds JD, et al [eds]: Manual of Clinical Laboratory Immunology, 5th ed. Washington, DC, ASM Press, 1997, p 156, with permission of the American Society for Microbiology.)

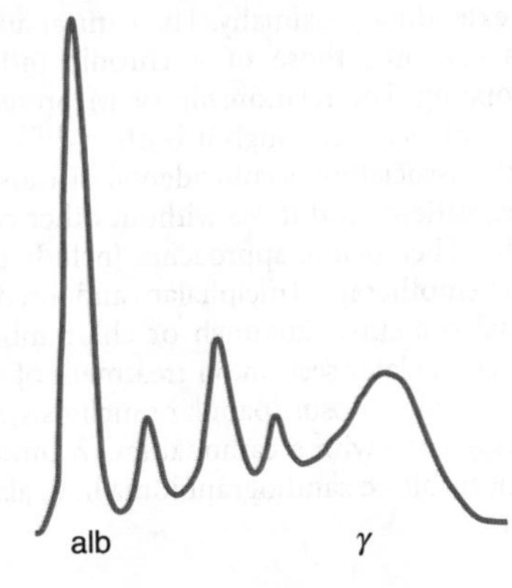

A

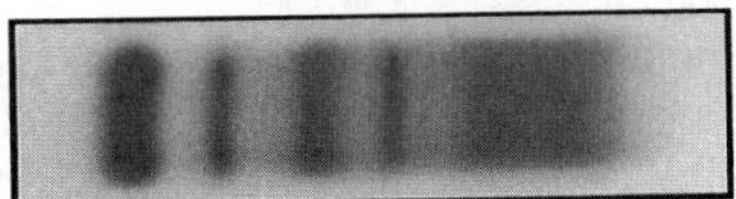

B

FIGURE 198–2 • Serom protein electrophoresis showing increased polyclonal immunoglobulins. A, Polyclonal pattern from a densitometer tracing of agarose gel: broad-based peak of γ mobility. **B,** Polyclonal pattern from electrophoresis of agarose gel (anode on the left). The band at the right is broad and extends throughout the γ area. (From Kyle RA, Katzmann JA: Immunochemical characterization of immunoglobulins. *In* Rose NR, Conway de Macario E, Folds JD, et al [eds]: Manual of Clinical Laboratory Immunology, 5th ed. Washington, DC, ASM Press, 1997, p 156, with permission of the American Society for Microbiology.)

λ light chains, usually limited to the γ region [Fig. 198–2]), which produce a broad-based peak or broad band. This finding is associated with a reactive or inflammatory process.

Serum Free Light Chains

The serum free light chain assay measures the level of free κ and λ immunoglobulin light chains (i.e., light chains that are not bound to intact immunoglobulin). An abnormal κ/λ free light chain ratio (normal range, 0.26 to 1.65) indicates an excess of one light chain type versus the other and is interpreted as representing a monoclonal elevation of the corresponding light chain type.

Analysis of Urine

Dipstick tests are insensitive to Bence Jones protein (monoclonal light chain in urine). Sulfosalicylic acid or Exton reagent is better than dipstick testing, but immunofixation of an adequately concentrated 24-hour urine specimen is recommended to detect Bence Jones protein. Bence Jones protein can be quantified according to the size of the monoclonal spike on urine protein electrophoresis and the amount of total protein in a 24-hour specimen.

MONOCLONAL GAMMOPATHY OF UNDETERMINED SIGNIFICANCE

Definition

MGUS (formerly called benign monoclonal gammopathy) denotes the presence of an M protein in persons without evidence of multiple myeloma, macroglobulinemia, amyloidosis, or other related diseases. At diagnosis it is not known whether the process that produces the M protein will remain stable or progress to symptomatic disease. MGUS is defined by a serum M protein concentration lower than 3 g/dL, less than 10% plasma cells in the bone marrow, and absence of lytic bone lesions, anemia, hypercalcemia, and renal insufficiency that can be attributed to a plasma cell disorder.

Epidemiology

More than 50% of patients with serum M protein have an initial clinical diagnosis of MGUS (Fig. 198–3). The prevalence of MGUS increases with age, from approximately 1% in patients 50 to 60 years old to greater than 5% in those older than 70 years. The age-adjusted prevalence is higher in males than in females and is twice as high in patients of African descent as in patients of European descent.

Pathobiology

MGUS represents a limited, initially nonmalignant expansion of monoclonal plasma cells. The etiology of MGUS is unknown. It is hypothesized that infection, inflammation, or other antigenic stimuli in concert with the development of primary translocations involving the immunoglobulin heavy chain locus on chromosome 14q32 may be the initiating pathogenetic events in more than 50% of patients with MGUS. The most common primary translocations that have been identified thus far are t11;14 (which results in upregulation of the cyclin D1 oncogene), t4;14 (upregulation of the *MMSET* and *FGFR3* oncogenes), and t14;16 (upregulation of the C-*maf* oncogene).

Clinical Manifestations

MGUS is asymptomatic and usually diagnosed incidentally on laboratory testing. Patients with MGUS progress to multiple myeloma or related malignancy at a rate of approximately 1% per year. The interval from the time of recognition of the M protein to the diagnosis of serious disease ranges from 1 to 32 years (median, 10.6 years), and the relative risk versus a control population is 25.0 for progression to multiple myeloma, 2.4 for the development of IgM lymphoma, 8.4 for primary amyloidosis, 46 for Waldenström's macroglobulinemia, 8.5 for plasmacytoma, but 0.9 for chronic lymphocytic leukemia. In a small percentage of patients, the M protein level increases to greater than 3 g/dL or the percentage of plasma cells in bone marrow increases to more than 10% without progression to overt myeloma or a related disorder.

Diagnosis

MGUS is differentiated from multiple myeloma and smoldering multiple myeloma by the size of the M protein, the bone marrow plasma cell percentage, and the presence or absence of anemia, renal failure, hypercalcemia, or lytic bone lesions (Table 198–2). Because anemia and renal

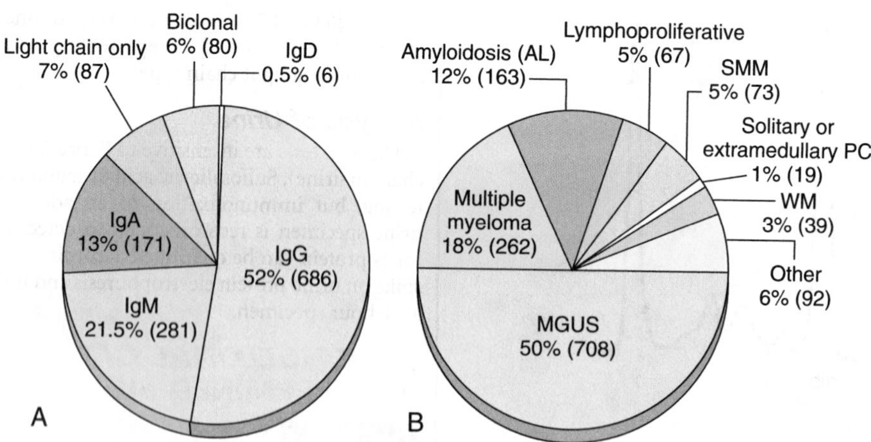

FIGURE 198–3 • Monoclonal gammopathy. A, Distribution of serum monoclonal proteins in 1311 patients seen at the Mayo Clinic during 2004. **B,** Diagnoses in 1423 cases of monoclonal gammopathy seen at the Mayo Clinic during 2004. Ig = immunoglobulin; MGUS = monoclonal gammopathy of undetermined significance; PC = plasmacytoma; SMM = smoldering multiple myeloma; WM = Waldenström's macroglobulinemia.

TABLE 198–2 CRITERIA FOR THE DIAGNOSIS OF MONOCLONAL GAMMOPATHY OF UNDETERMINED SIGNIFICANCE, SMOLDERING MULTIPLE MYELOMA, AND MULTIPLE MYELOMA

Monoclonal gammopathy of undetermined significance	Serum monoclonal protein <3 g/dL *and* bone marrow plasma cells <10% *and* absence of anemia, renal failure, hypercalcemia, and lytic bone lesions
Smoldering multiple myeloma	Serum monoclonal protein ≥3 g/dL *and/or* bone marrow plasma cells ≥10% *and* absence of anemia, renal failure, hypercalcemia, and lytic bone lesions
Multiple myeloma	Presence of serum or urine monoclonal protein, bone marrow plasmacytosis, *and* anemia, renal failure, hypercalcemia, or lytic bone lesions. Patients with primary systemic amyloidosis and ≥30% bone marrow plasma cells are considered to have both multiple myeloma and amyloidosis

From Rajkumar SV, Dispenzieri A, Fonseca R, et al: Thalidomide for previously untreated indolent or smoldering multiple myeloma. Leukemia 2001;15:1274–1276, with permission of Nature Publishing Group.

insufficiency are relatively common in the elderly population with MGUS, the cause of these conditions should be carefully investigated with adequate laboratory studies. For example, in a patient with anemia, tests to exclude iron, vitamin B_{12}, or folate deficiency must be performed. In certain instances, such as unexplained renal failure, a renal biopsy may be needed. Only patients with strong evidence of end-organ damage thought to be directly related to a plasma cell disorder can be considered to have myeloma or related malignancy.

Levels of the immunoglobulin classes other than M protein (i.e., the normal polyclonal or background immunoglobulins) are generally reduced in multiple myeloma or Waldenström's macroglobulinemia, but a reduction also occurs in almost 40% of patients with MGUS. The presence of osteolytic lesions strongly suggests multiple myeloma, but metastatic carcinoma may produce lytic lesions, as well as plasmacytosis, and may be associated with an unrelated monoclonal gammopathy.

Association with Other Diseases

Monoclonal gammopathy may be seen after liver, bone marrow, or kidney transplantation. M protein is found in 3 to 4% of patients with a diffuse lymphoproliferative process but in less than 1% of those with a follicular lymphoma. IgM monoclonal gammopathies are more common than IgG or IgA in lymphoproliferative diseases. M proteins occur in the sera of some patients with chronic lymphocytic leukemia (Chapter 195) but have no recognizable effect on the clinical course. M proteins are also detected in some patients with other leukemias, but no more often than in the normal population.

Approximately 5% of patients with sensorimotor peripheral neuropathy of unknown cause (Chapter 446) have an associated monoclonal gammopathy. In half of such patients, the M protein binds to myelin-associated glycoprotein. These patients have a slowly progressive sensory more than motor neuropathy, beginning in the distal ends of the extremities and extending proximally. The clinical and electrodiagnostic manifestations resemble those of a chronic inflammatory demyelinating polyneuropathy. The relationship of M protein to the peripheral neuropathy is not clear. Although it is often difficult to determine clinically whether the association is coincidental or causal, causality is more likely in younger patients and those without other conditions known to cause neuropathy. Therapeutic approaches include plasmapheresis and, occasionally, chemotherapy (melphalan and prednisone for IgG and IgA monoclonal proteins, rituximab or chlorambucil for IgM monoclonal proteins; see the later section on treatment of multiple myeloma).

Lichen myxedematosus (papular mucinosis, scleromyxedema [Chapter 465]) is associated with a cathodal IgG λ protein. Pyoderma gangrenosum and necrobiotic xanthogranuloma have also been associated with an M protein.

Prevention and Treatment

Rx

No treatment is necessary for MGUS. The M protein level in serum and urine should be measured serially, together with periodic reevaluation of clinical and other laboratory findings, to determine whether multiple myeloma or another related disorder is present. In general, if the serum M protein value is less than 2 g/dL, electrophoresis should be repeated at 6 months; if it is stable, it should be rechecked annually. If the serum M protein value is greater than 2.0 g/dL without evidence of myeloma or related disorders, electrophoresis should be repeated in 3 months; if it is stable, the test should be repeated annually.

Prognosis

Differentiation of a patient with MGUS in whom the disorder remains stable from one in whom multiple myeloma, macroglobulinemia, or a related disorder eventually develops may be difficult when the M protein is first recognized. The size of the M protein at diagnosis of MGUS is the most important predictive factor for progression, but patients with IgM and IgA M proteins or an abnormal serum free light chain ratio also have an increased risk of progression (Table 198–3).

TABLE 198–3 RISK OF PROGRESSION OF MONOCLONAL GAMMOPATHY OF UNDETERMINED SIGNIFICANCE TO MYELOMA OR RELATED DISORDERS

Risk Group	Relative Risk	Cumulative Absolute Risk of Progression at 20 Years*	Cumulative Absolute Risk of Progression at 20 Years Accounting for Death as a Competing Risk†
Low risk: serum M protein <1.5 g/dL, IgG subtype, normal free light chain ratio (0.26–1.65)	1	5%	2%
Low–intermediate risk: any 1 factor abnormal	5.4	21%	10%
High–intermediate risk: any 2 factors abnormal	10.1	37%	18%
High risk: all 3 factors abnormal	20.8	58%	27%

*Estimates in this column represent the risk of progression assuming that patients do not die of other causes during this period.
†Estimates in this column represent the risk of progression calculated by using a model that accounts for the fact that patients can die of unrelated causes during this time.
Ig = immunoglobulin.
Adapted from Rajkumar SV, Kyle RA, Therneu TM, et al: Serum free light chain ratio is an independent risk factor for progression in monoclonal gammopathy of undetermined significance (MGUS) Blood 2005;106:812–817. © The American Society of Hematology.

BICLONAL GAMMOPATHIES

Biclonal gammopathies occur in at least 5% of patients with clonal gammopathies. Biclonal gammopathy of undetermined significance accounts for about two thirds of such patients. The remainder have multiple myeloma, macroglobulinemia, or other lymphoproliferative diseases. Rarely, triclonal gammopathies may also occur.

IDIOPATHIC BENCE JONES PROTEINURIA

Bence Jones proteinuria is a recognized feature of multiple myeloma, primary amyloidosis, Waldenström's macroglobulinemia, and other malignant lymphoproliferative disorders. An apparently benign, idiopathic Bence Jones proteinuria, analogous to MGUS, may also occur, with the proteinuria persisting for more than 20 years in the absence of multiple myeloma or related disorders.

MULTIPLE MYELOMA

Definition

Multiple myeloma is characterized by the neoplastic proliferation of a single clone of plasma cells engaged in the production of a monoclonal immunoglobulin. This clone of plasma cells proliferates in bone marrow and frequently invades the adjacent bone to produce extensive skeletal destruction that results in bone pain and fractures. The diagnosis of myeloma requires 10% or more plasma cells on bone marrow examination, M protein in serum or urine (except in the case of nonsecretory myeloma), and evidence of hypercalcemia, renal insufficiency, anemia, or bone lesions thought to be related to the plasma cell proliferative disorder. Patients with multiple myeloma must be differentiated from those with MGUS and smoldering multiple myeloma (see Table 198–2).

Epidemiology

Multiple myeloma accounts for 1% of all malignant disease and slightly more than 10% of hematologic malignancies in the United States. The annual incidence of multiple myeloma is 4 per 100,000. An apparent increased incidence in recent years is probably related to increased availability and use of medical facilities, especially for older persons. Multiple myeloma occurs in all races and all geographic locations. Its incidence in blacks is almost twice that in whites. Multiple myeloma is slightly more common in men than in women. The median age of patients at the time of diagnosis is about 65 years; only 2% of patients are younger than 40.

Pathobiology

The cause of multiple myeloma is unclear. Exposure to radiation, benzene, and other organic solvents, herbicides, and insecticides may play a role. Multiple myeloma has been reported in familial clusters of two or more first-degree relatives and in identical twins.

In most cases, the plasma cells in myeloma are cytoplasmic Ig^+, $CD38^+$, $CD138^+$, and PCA-1^+; only a minority express CD10 and HLA-DR, and 20% express CD20. However, the nature of the clonogenic cells in myeloma is still unknown. Circulating clonogenic premyeloma cells or long-lived plasma cells may, by means of adhesion molecules, home to the marrow where they find an appropriate microenvironment (cytokine network) to differentiate and expand further. T cells may play an important role. In patients with multiple myeloma, $CD4^+$ T cells are often reduced. Levels of interleukin-6 (IL-6) are higher in patients with progressive myeloma than in those with MGUS. Macrophage inflammatory protein-α, IL-1β, and tumor necrosis factor-α (TNF-α), each of which has bone-resorbing activity, are overproduced in patients with multiple myeloma.

The lytic bone lesions, osteopenia, hypercalcemia, and pathologic fractures in patients with myeloma are a result of abnormal osteoclast activity induced by the neoplastic plasma cells and inhibition of osteoblast differentiation. Osteoclasts are activated by stimulation of the transmembrane receptor RANK (receptor activator of nuclear factor κB), which belongs to the TNF receptor superfamily. The ligand for this receptor (RANKL) also has a decoy receptor, osteoprotegerin (OPG). Stimulation of RANK is controlled by the ratio of RANKL to OPG. The cytokines secreted by myeloma cells, such as macrophage inflammatory protein-α, IL-6, IL-1β, and TNF-α, increase the RANKL/OPG ratio, thereby inducing osteoclast activation (Chapter 188).

Cytogenetic Abnormalities

Conventional cytogenetic studies show an abnormal karyotype in less than 40% of patients with myeloma. However, fluorescent in situ hybridization (FISH) with chromosome-specific probes reveals chromosome abnormalities in almost 100% of patients. Primary translocations involving the immunoglobulin heavy chain loci (chromosome 14q32), which represent early events originating at the MGUS stage, are seen in up to 70% of patients with multiple myeloma. Other cytogenetic abnormalities, such as activating mutations of N- and K-*ras*, inactivating mutations of *p53*, and dysregulation of c-*myc*, are late events that occur during the course of symptomatic myeloma. Complete or partial deletions of chromosome 13 can occur at the MGUS stage, but these deletions in myeloma (15% of patients by conventional cytogenetic studies and 50% by FISH studies) carry an adverse prognosis. Flow cytometry studies have shown aneuploidy in about 80% of patients, hyperdiploidy in 70%, and hypodiploidy in the remaining 10%.

Clinical Manifestations

History

Bone pain, particularly in the back or chest and less often in the extremities, is present at the time of diagnosis in more than two thirds of

TABLE 198–4 CLINICAL MANIFESTATIONS OF MULTIPLE MYELOMA

Skeletal involvement: pain, reduced height, pathologic fractures, hypercalcemia
Anemia: mainly caused by decreased erythropoiesis; produces weakness and fatigue
Renal insufficiency: mainly caused by "myeloma kidney" from light chains or hypercalcemia, rarely from amyloidosis
Recurrent infections: respiratory and urinary tract infections or septicemia caused by gram-positive or gram-negative organisms
Bleeding diathesis: from thrombocytopenia or coating of platelets with M protein
Amyloidosis: develops in 10%
Extramedullary plasmacytomas: occur late in the disease
Cryoglobulinemia type I: rarely symptomatic

patients (Table 198–4). The pain is usually induced by movement and does not occur at night except with change of position. The patient's height may be reduced by several inches because of vertebral collapse. Weakness and fatigue are common and are often associated with anemia. Fever is rare and, when present, is generally from an infection; in some patients the infection itself is the initial feature. Other symptoms may result from renal insufficiency (Chapters 121 and 131), hypercalcemia (Chapter 266), nephrotic syndrome (Chapter 122), a radiculopathy (Chapter 423), or amyloidosis (see Organ Involvement, later).

Physical Examination

Pallor is the most frequent physical finding. The liver is palpable in about 5% of patients and the spleen in 1%. Tenderness may be noted at sites of bone involvement. Radiculopathy may be caused by spinal compression fractures. Occasionally, extramedullary plasmacytomas may appear.

Diagnosis

Laboratory Findings

A normocytic, normochromic anemia (Chapter 169) is present initially in approximately 75% of patients but eventually occurs in nearly every patient with multiple myeloma. Serum protein electrophoresis shows an M protein in 80% of patients, hypogammaglobulinemia in almost 10%, and no apparent abnormality in the remainder. With serum immunofixation, 93% of patients have detectable M protein. The type of M protein is IgG in 52%, IgA in 21%, light chain only (Bence Jones proteinemia) in 16%, IgD in 2%, and biclonal gammopathy in 2%; 7% have no serum M protein at diagnosis. Immunofixation of urine reveals an M protein in approximately 75% of patients. The light chain type is kappa in 65% of cases and lambda in 35%. At the time of diagnosis, 97% of patients with multiple myeloma have an M protein in serum or urine by immunofixation; the remainder are considered to have nonsecretory myeloma.

In the bone marrow, plasma cells account for greater than 10% of all nucleated cells in 96% of patients (Fig. 198–4). In 4% of patients, bone marrow examination shows less than 10% plasma cells, even though the patient otherwise meets the criteria for myeloma, because bone marrow involvement in myeloma may be focal rather than diffuse, and thus repeated bone marrow examinations may be required. Identification of a monoclonal immunoglobulin in the cytoplasm of plasma cells by immunoperoxidase staining is helpful for differentiating monoclonal plasma cell proliferation in multiple myeloma from reactive plasmacytosis related to connective tissue disease, metastatic carcinoma, liver disease, and infections.

Radiologic Findings

Conventional radiographs reveal abnormalities consisting of punched-out lytic lesions (Fig. 198–5), osteoporosis, or fractures in nearly 80% of patients. The vertebrae, skull, thoracic cage, pelvis, and proximal ends of the humerus and femur are the most frequent sites of involvement. Technetium-99m bone scanning is inferior to conventional radiography and should not be used. Computed tomography or magnetic resonance imaging is helpful in patients who have skeletal pain but no abnormality on radiographs.

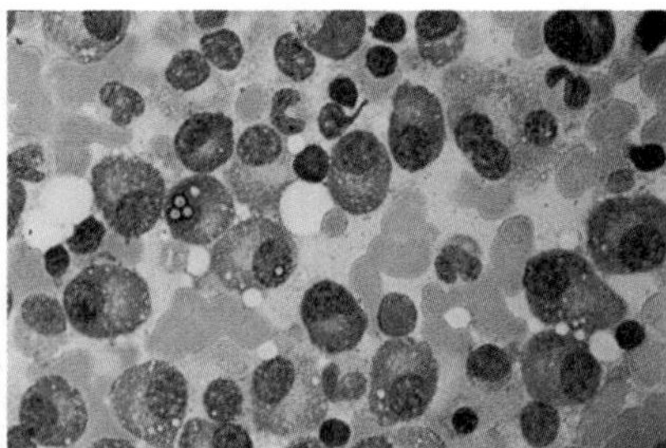

FIGURE 198–4 • Multiple myeloma. A bone marrow aspirate shows a predominance of plasma cells.

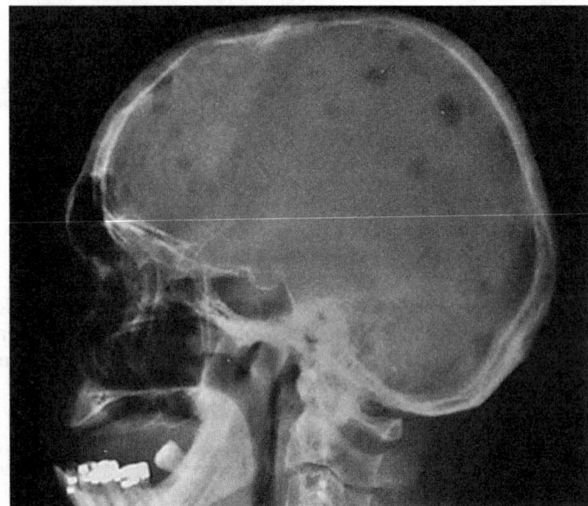

FIGURE 198–5 • Skull radiograph showing multiple lytic lesions.

Organ Involvement

Renal

Bence Jones proteinuria is detected by immunofixation in 75%. The serum creatinine value is increased initially in almost half of patients and is greater than 2 mg/dL in 20%.

The two major causes of renal insufficiency are light chain cast nephropathy ("myeloma kidney") and hypercalcemia. Myeloma kidney is characterized by the presence of large, waxy, laminated casts in the distal and collecting tubules. The casts are composed mainly of precipitated monoclonal light chains. The extent of cast formation correlates directly with the amount of free urinary light chain and with the severity of renal insufficiency. Dehydration may precipitate acute renal failure.

Hypercalcemia, which is present in 15 to 20% of patients initially, is a major and treatable cause of renal insufficiency. It results from destruction of bone. Hyperuricemia may contribute to renal failure. Amyloidosis occurs in nearly 10% of patients and may produce nephrotic syndrome (Chapter 122), renal insufficiency (Chapter 121), or both. Acquired Fanconi's syndrome (Chapter 119), characterized by proximal tubular dysfunction, results in glycosuria, phosphaturia, and aminoaciduria. Deposition of monoclonal light chains in the renal glomerulus (light chain deposition disease) may also produce renal insufficiency and nephrotic syndrome.

Neurologic

Radiculopathy (Chapter 423), the single most frequent neurologic complication, usually occurs in the thoracic or lumbosacral area and results from compression of the nerve by the vertebral lesion or by the collapsed bone itself. Compression of the spinal cord occurs in up to 10% of patients. Peripheral neuropathy (Chapter 446) is uncommon in multiple myeloma and, when present, is generally caused by amyloidosis. Rarely, myeloma cells diffusely infiltrate the meninges. Intracranial plasmacytomas almost always represent extensions of myelomatous lesions of the skull.

Other Systemic Involvement

Hepatomegaly from plasma cell infiltration is uncommon. Plasmacytomas of the ribs are common and arise either as expanding bone lesions or as soft tissue masses. The incidence of infections is increased in patients with multiple myeloma. *Streptococcus pneumoniae* and *Staphylococcus aureus* have been the most frequent pathogens, but gram-negative organisms now account for more than half of all infections. The propensity for infection results from impairment of the antibody response, deficiency of normal immunoglobulins, and neutropenia (Chapters 173 and 303). Bleeding from coating of the platelets by M protein may occur. Occasionally, a tendency to thrombosis is present.

Prevention and Treatment

Patients with MGUS or smoldering multiple myeloma should not be treated, but an increasing level of M protein in serum or urine suggests that therapy will be needed in the near future. Indications for therapy (Fig. 198–6) include significant anemia, hypercalcemia, or renal insufficiency; the occurrence of lytic bone lesions; and the finding of extramedullary plasmacytomas. If there is doubt in the physician's mind, it is usually better to withhold therapy and re-evaluate the patient in 2 or 3 months.

Radiation Therapy

Palliative radiation in a dose of 20 to 30 Gy should be limited to patients who have multiple myeloma with disabling pain and a well-defined focal process that has not responded to chemotherapy and to patients with spinal cord compression from a plasmacytoma. Analgesics in combination with chemotherapy can usually control the pain.

Autologous Stem Cell Transplantation

In the approximately 50% of patients with newly diagnosed multiple myeloma who are considered candidates for the procedure based on good performance status, no or limited comorbid conditions, and younger physiologic age (<65 to 70 years), autologous peripheral blood stem cell transplantation (Chapter 184) with high-dose chemotherapy improves overall survival in comparison to conventional chemotherapy. [1,2] Currently, it is not possible to eradicate myeloma cells completely with conditioning regimens, and reinfused autologous stem cells are usually contaminated by myeloma cells or their precursors. As a result, autologous transplantation is not curative, but it prolongs event-free and overall survival.

Initial therapy typically consists of pulsed dexamethasone (40 mg daily on days 1 to 4, 9 to 12, and 17 to 20 every 28 days) plus thalidomide (200 mg daily) for approximately 4 months to reduce the number of tumor cells in the bone marrow and peripheral blood. Toxicities include a high risk for deep vein thrombosis; clinical trials are now testing the use of lenalidomide instead of thalidomide. After induction therapy, peripheral blood stem cells adequate for

Newly Diagnosed Myeloma
Symptomatic myeloma: Therapy is indicated
Smoldering multiple myeloma: No therapy except in approved clinical trials investigating novel therapy
Not a transplant candidate
Transplant candidate
Chemotherapy with melphalan plus prednisone until plateau (minimum 12 months): consider melphalan, prednisone, thalidomide for patients 65–75 years of age; alternative is investigational therapy in an approved clinical trial. If rapid tumor reduction is needed, consider alternative regimen (e.g., thalidomide plus dexamethasone)
Induction therapy ×4 cycles with thalidomide plus dexamethasone: alternative is investigational regimen in an approved clinical trial (e.g., lenalidomide plus dexamethasone)
Peripheral blood stem cell harvest (preferably adequate for 2 transplants)
Early autologous transplant (melphalan 200 mg/m²)
Conventional therapy (e.g., continue induction therapy at reduced doses or use melphalan plus prednisone until plateau; stem cell transplant at time of relapse)
Complete response or very good partial response (>90% reduction in monoclonal protein levels): observe and/or consider maintenance therapy in a clinical trial
Complete response or very good partial response is not achieved: consider second (tandem) autologous transplant

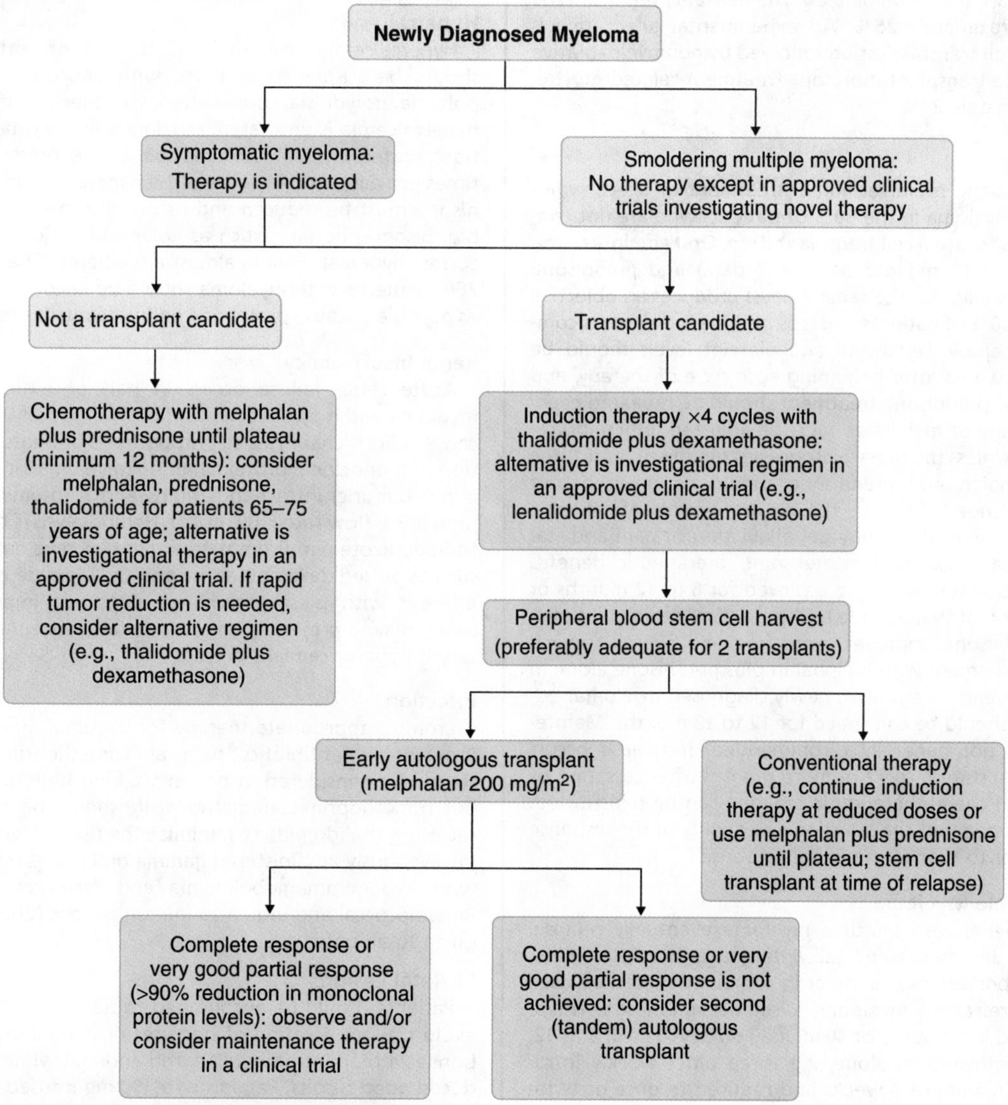

FIGURE 198–6 • Approach to newly diagnosed multiple myeloma.

Rx

two stem cell transplants are collected with the use of granulocyte colony-stimulating factor to aid in mobilization. Autologous stem cell transplantation (Chapter 184) is performed with melphalan, 200 mg/m^2, as the conditioning regimen, followed by infusion of the peripheral blood stem cells. Patients who do not achieve a complete or nearly complete response with the first autologous transplantation are considered for a second autologous transplantation. 3

An alternative approach in patients with newly diagnosed disease is to cryopreserve stem cells for future use after initial therapy. Patients then continue initial therapy or conventional chemotherapy, such as melphalan and prednisone, until a plateau phase is reached, followed by observation until relapse or progression, at which point stem cell transplantation is considered. Data from randomized trials comparing early versus delayed transplantation indicate no significant difference in survival between the two strategies. The choice between the two options is based on patients' preferences and other clinical conditions, but early transplantation is often preferred because its mortality is low (<1%) and it avoids the inconvenience, cost, and potential side effects of prolonged chemotherapy.

Allogeneic Bone Marrow Transplantation

Ninety to 95% of patients with multiple myeloma cannot undergo allogeneic bone marrow transplantation because of their age, lack of an HLA-matched sibling donor, or inadequate renal, pulmonary, or cardiac function (Chapter 184). Although a complete response occurs in 40% of patients, most have a relapse; in long-term follow-up there is no apparent survival plateau. The mortality rate from the procedure is approximately 25%. An experimental alternative is autologous stem cell transplantation followed by nonmyeloablative ("mini") allogeneic transplantation, but treatment-related mortality is still approximately 20%.

Chemotherapy

Chemotherapy is the preferred initial treatment of overt, symptomatic multiple myeloma in the 50% of patients who are not considered candidates for stem cell transplantation. Oral administration of melphalan (8 to 10 mg per day for 7 days) and prednisone (20 mg three times daily for the same 7 days) produces an objective response in 50 to 60% of patients and is as good as intravenous combination chemotherapy. Leukocyte and platelet levels should be measured every 3 weeks after beginning each cycle of therapy, and the melphalan and prednisone treatment should be repeated every 6 weeks. The dosage of melphalan must be adjusted until midcycle cytopenia occurs. Unless the disease progresses rapidly, at least three courses of melphalan and prednisone should be given before therapy is discontinued. Because the natural course of multiple myeloma is progression of the disease, alleviation of pain and stabilization of disease usually indicate some therapeutic benefit. Objective improvement may not be achieved for 6 to 12 months or longer. The addition of thalidomide to the standard regimen of melphalan plus prednisone improves event-free and overall survival compared with treatment with melphalan plus prednisone alone in patients 65 to 75 years of age with newly diagnosed myeloma. 4

Chemotherapy should be continued for 12 to 18 months. Maintenance therapy is not generally recommended. If relapse occurs during the plateau state 6 to 12 or more months after cessation of therapy, the initial chemotherapeutic regimen can be reinstituted. Most patients respond, but the duration and quality of the response are usually inferior to that of the initial response.

Refractory Multiple Myeloma

Almost all patients with multiple myeloma eventually relapse. High-dose pulse dexamethasone, alkylating agents, thalidomide, lenalidomide, or bortezomib, alone or in combination, can be used to treat relapsed refractory myeloma. Pulsed dexamethasone is typically administered in a dosage of 40 mg/day on days 1 to 4, 9 to 12, and 17 to 20. Methylprednisolone, 2 g three times weekly intravenously for a minimum of 4 weeks and reduced to once or twice weekly if there is a response, is helpful for patients with pancytopenia and may be associated with fewer side effects than is the case with dexamethasone.

Thalidomide (50 to 200 mg orally daily) produces an objective response, with a median duration of about 1 year, in about a third of patients with refractory myeloma. Side effects are sedation, constipation, peripheral neuropathy, rash, bradycardia, and thrombotic events. The addition of dexamethasone to thalidomide increases the response rate to approximately 50%, and combinations of thalidomide, dexamethasone, and alkylating agents produce response rates exceeding 70% in patients with relapsed refractory disease.

The thalidomide analogue lenalidomide appears to be well tolerated and produces objective benefit in approximately 40% of patients with relapsed refractory myeloma as a single agent and in 60% of patients in combination with dexamethasone. The starting dose is 25 mg orally on days 1 to 21 every 28 days. Lenalidomide has significantly fewer nonhematologic toxicities than thalidomide does; myelosuppression is the most common adverse event.

Bortezomib, an inhibitor of the ubiquitin-proteasome pathway, acts through multiple mechanisms to arrest tumor growth, tumor spread, and angiogenesis. It produces objective responses in about a third of patients with refractory myeloma. As with thalidomide and lenalidomide, bortezomib can also be combined with dexamethasone to increase response rates. 5 The starting dose is 1.3 mg/m^2 administered intravenously on days 1, 4, 8, and 11 every 21 days. The most common adverse events are gastrointestinal side effects, fatigue, and neuropathy.

Management of Complications

Hypercalcemia

Hypercalcemia, present in 15 to 20% of patients at diagnosis, should be suspected in those with anorexia, nausea, vomiting, polyuria, polydipsia, constipation, weakness, confusion, or stupor. If hypercalcemia is untreated, renal insufficiency may develop. Hydration, preferably with isotonic saline plus prednisone (25 mg four times per day), usually relieves the hypercalcemia. The dose of prednisone must be reduced and its use discontinued as soon as possible. Bisphosphonates such as zoledronic acid or pamidronate will correct hypercalcemia in almost all patients (Chapters 188, 263, and 266). Patients with myeloma should be encouraged to be as active as possible because prolonged bedrest contributes to hypercalcemia.

Renal Insufficiency

Acute renal failure occurs in half of patients with multiple myeloma and may develop insidiously or rapidly. The most common cause is light chain cast nephropathy in patients with excess excretion of monoclonal protein in urine (myeloma kidney). If the patient is not oliguric, intravenous fluids and furosemide can maintain a high urine flow rate (100 mL/hr). Hemodialysis is necessary for symptomatic azotemia. Prompt treatment of myeloma with a regimen such as pulsed dexamethasone and thalidomide is essential. Plasmapheresis with plasma exchange does not improve outcomes in patients who present with acute renal failure. Allopurinol is necessary if hyperuricemia is present.

Infection

Prompt, appropriate therapy for bacterial infections is necessary. Prophylactic antibiotics such as trimethoprim-sulfamethoxazole should be considered in patients taking high-dose corticosteroids, but trimethoprim-sulfamethoxazole should be avoided in patients receiving thalidomide to minimize the risk for serious skin reactions. Intravenously administered gamma globulin is reserved for patients with hypogammaglobulinemia and recurrent severe infections. Pneumococcal and influenza immunizations (Chapter 16) should be given to all patients.

Skeletal Lesions

Patients should be encouraged to be as active as possible but to avoid trauma. Fixation of fractures or impending fractures of long bones with an intramedullary rod and methylmethacrylate has produced good results. Pamidronate (90 mg infused intravenously over a 4-hour period every 4 weeks) or zoledronic acid (4 mg intra-

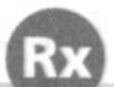

venously over at least a 15-minute period) reduces the incidence of bone pain, pathologic fractures, and spinal cord compression; such prophylaxis is now routinely recommended for all patients with myeloma bone disease.

Spinal cord compression from an extramedullary plasmacytoma (Chapter 423) should be suspected in patients who have severe back pain, weakness or paresthesias of the lower extremities, or bladder or bowel dysfunction. Magnetic resonance imaging, computed tomography, or myelography must be performed immediately. Initial treatment is with dexamethasone and radiation therapy. If the neurologic deficit increases, surgical decompression is necessary.

Miscellaneous Complications

Symptomatic hyperviscosity (see later) is less common than in Waldenström's macroglobulinemia. Anemia that is persistent despite adequate treatment of underlying myeloma often responds to erythropoietin.

Prognosis

Multiple myeloma has a progressive course, and the median survival is approximately 3 years, but survival varies widely according to clinical stage and other characteristics (Table 198–5). In some patients, an acute or aggressive terminal phase is characterized by rapid tumor growth, pancytopenia, soft tissue subcutaneous masses, decreased M protein levels, and fever; survival in this subset is generally only a few months.

Future Directions

Future efforts must be directed toward identifying new active agents and developing effective combinations of active drugs. Studies are under way to improve the conditioning regimen used in autologous stem cell transplantation and to better integrate novel therapies with stem cell transplantation. Immunotherapy using dendritic cell vaccination with the myeloma cell idiotype as a tumor-specific antigen and monoclonal antibody therapy are also under investigation.

TABLE 198–5 STAGING AND PROGNOSTIC FACTORS IN MULTIPLE MYELOMA

	Median Survival
I. INTERNATIONAL STAGING SYSTEM (SERUM β_2-MICROGLOBULIN AND ALBUMIN)	
Stage I (serum β_2-microglobulin <3.5 mg/L and serum albumin ≥3.5 g/dL)	62 months
Stage II (neither stage I or III)	44 months
Stage III (serum β_2-microglobulin ≥5.5 mg/L)	29 months
II. RISK STRATIFICATION	
High-risk myeloma (any of the following)	24–36 months
Karyotyping: deletion 13 or hypodiploidy	
Molecular genetics: t4;14, t14;16, deletion 17p	
Plasma cell labeling index >3%	
III. OTHER ADVERSE PROGNOSTIC FACTORS	
Elevated lactate dehydrogenase level	
Poor performance status	
Increased circulating plasma cells	
Plasmablastic morphology	
High C-reactive protein level	

VARIANT FORMS OF MULTIPLE MYELOMA (See Table 198–1)

Smoldering Multiple Myeloma

Smoldering (asymptomatic) multiple myeloma is defined by the presence of an M protein level greater than 3 g/dL in serum or 10% or more plasma cells in bone marrow in the absence of anemia, renal insufficiency, hypercalcemia, or skeletal lesions. Often, a small amount of M protein is found in urine, and the concentration of normal immunoglobulins in serum is decreased. The plasma cell labeling index is typically low. Biologically, patients with smoldering multiple myeloma are similar to those with MGUS but carry a much higher risk for progression to myeloma or related malignancy. As a result, patients must be observed more closely, but smoldering multiple myeloma should not be treated unless progression to symptomatic multiple myeloma occurs.

Plasma Cell Leukemia

Patients with plasma cell leukemia have more than 20% plasma cells in the peripheral blood and an absolute plasma cell count of 2000/μL or greater. Plasma cell leukemia is classified as primary when it is diagnosed in the leukemic phase (60%) or as secondary when there is leukemic transformation of a previously recognized multiple myeloma (40%). Patients with primary plasma cell leukemia are younger and have a greater incidence of hepatosplenomegaly and lymphadenopathy, a higher platelet count, fewer bone lesions, a smaller serum M protein component, and longer survival (median, 6.8 vs. 1.3 months) than do patients with secondary plasma cell leukemia. Treatment of plasma cell leukemia is unsatisfactory, but partial responses occur with regimens such as thalidomide plus dexamethasone or alkylating agents. Autologous stem cell transplantation after myeloablative therapy is beneficial for some patients. Secondary plasma cell leukemia rarely responds to chemotherapy because the patients have already received chemotherapy and are resistant.

Nonsecretory Myeloma

Patients with nonsecretory myeloma have no M protein in either serum or urine and account for only 3% of cases of myeloma. To make the diagnosis, the clonal nature of bone marrow plasma cells should be established by immunoperoxidase, immunofluorescence, or flow cytometric methods. Responses to therapy and survival rates in patients with nonsecretory myeloma are similar to those in patients with a serum or urinary M component, but renal involvement is less. The serum free light chain assay is abnormal in more than 60% of patients and can be used to monitor the response to therapy.

Immunoglobulin D Myeloma

The M protein is smaller in IgD myeloma than in IgG or IgA myeloma, and Bence Jones proteinuria of the λ type is more common. Amyloidosis and extramedullary plasmacytomas are more frequent with IgD myeloma. Survival is generally believed to be shorter than with other myeloma types, but IgD myeloma is often not diagnosed until later in its course.

Osteosclerotic Myeloma (POEMS Syndrome)

This syndrome is characterized by *p*olyneuropathy, *o*rganomegaly, *e*ndocrinopathy, *M* protein, and *s*kin changes (POEMS). The major clinical features are a chronic inflammatory-demyelinating polyneuropathy with predominantly motor disability and sclerotic skeletal lesions. Except for the presence of papilledema, the cranial nerves are not involved. The autonomic nervous system is intact. Hepatomegaly occurs in almost 50% of patients, but splenomegaly and lymphadenopathy occur in a minority. Hyperpigmentation and hypertrichosis are often evident. Gynecomastia and atrophic testes may be seen, as well as clubbing of the fingers and toes. In contrast to findings in multiple myeloma, the hemoglobin level is usually normal or increased, and thrombocytosis is common. The bone marrow usually contains less than 5% plasma cells, and hypercalcemia and renal insufficiency rarely occur. Most patients have a λ protein. Evidence of Castleman's disease (Chapter 196) may be found. The diagnosis is confirmed by identification of monoclonal plasma cells obtained at biopsy of an osteosclerotic lesion.

If the lesions are in a limited area, radiation therapy produces substantial improvement of the neuropathy in more than 50% of patients. If the patient has widespread osteosclerotic lesions, treatment is with autologous stem cell transplantation or other systemic therapy similar to that used for myeloma.

Solitary Plasmacytoma (Solitary Myeloma) of Bone

Diagnosis of this disease is based on histologic evidence of a tumor consisting of monoclonal plasma cells identical to those in multiple myeloma. In addition, complete skeletal radiographs must show no other lesions of myeloma, and the bone marrow aspirate must contain no evidence of multiple myeloma. An M protein may be present in serum or urine at diagnosis, but persistence of the M protein after radiation therapy is associated with an increased risk for progression to multiple myeloma. Magnetic resonance imaging of the spine and pelvis is helpful for detecting marrow involvement. Treatment consists of radiation in the range of 40 to 50 Gy. Almost 50% of patients who have a solitary plasmacytoma are alive at 10 years, and disease-free survival rates at 10 years range from 15 to 25%. Progression to myeloma, when it occurs, usually takes place within 3 years, but patients must be monitored on an indefinite basis. There is no convincing evidence that adjuvant chemotherapy decreases the rate of conversion to multiple myeloma.

Extramedullary Plasmacytoma

Extramedullary plasmacytomas outside the bone marrow are most commonly (80%) found in the upper respiratory tract, especially in the nasal cavity and sinuses, nasopharynx, and larynx. Extramedullary plasmacytomas may also occur in the gastrointestinal tract, central nervous system, urinary bladder, thyroid, breast, testes, parotid gland, or lymph nodes. The diagnosis is based on detection of a plasma cell tumor in an extramedullary site and the absence of multiple myeloma on bone marrow examination, radiography, and appropriate studies of blood and urine. Treatment consists of tumoricidal irradiation. The plasmacytoma may recur locally, metastasize to regional nodes, or rarely, develop into multiple myeloma.

WALDENSTRÖM'S MACROGLOBULINEMIA (PRIMARY MACROGLOBULINEMIA)

Definition

Waldenström's macroglobulinemia is the result of uncontrolled proliferation of lymphocytes and plasma cells in which an IgM M protein is produced. The cause is unknown; familial clusters have been reported. The median age of patients at the time of diagnosis is about 65 years, and approximately 60% are male. The diagnostic criteria require IgM monoclonal gammopathy (regardless of the size of the M protein), 10% or greater bone marrow infiltration (usually intertrabecular) by small lymphocytes that exhibit plasmacytoid or plasma cell differentiation, and a typical immunophenotype (e.g., surface IgM^+, $CD5^{+/-}$, $CD10^-$, $CD19^+$, $CD20^+$, $CD23^-$) that would satisfactorily exclude other lymphoproliferative disorders, including chronic lymphocytic leukemia and mantle cell lymphoma.

Clinical Manifestations

Weakness, fatigue, and bleeding (especially oozing from the oronasal area) are common initial symptoms. Blurred or impaired vision, dyspnea, loss of weight, neurologic symptoms, recurrent infections, and heart failure may occur. In contrast to multiple myeloma, lytic bone lesions, renal insufficiency, and amyloidosis are rare. Physical findings include pallor, hepatosplenomegaly, and lymphadenopathy. Retinal hemorrhages, exudates, and venous congestion with vascular segmentation ("sausage" formation) may occur. Sensorimotor peripheral neuropathy is common. Pulmonary involvement is manifested by diffuse pulmonary infiltrates and isolated masses. Pleural effusion may occur. Diarrhea and steatorrhea are uncommon.

Laboratory Evaluation

Almost all patients have moderate to severe normocytic, normochromic anemia. Coombs-positive hemolytic anemia is uncommon. The serum cholesterol value is often low. The serum electrophoretic pattern is characterized by a tall, narrow peak or dense band and is usually of γ mobility. Low-molecular-weight IgM (7S) is present and may account for a significant part of the increased IgM level. A monoclonal light chain is detected in the urine of 80% of patients, but the amount of urinary protein is generally modest.

The bone marrow aspirate is often hypocellular, but the biopsy is hypercellular and extensively infiltrated with lymphoid cells and plasma cells. The number of mast cells is frequently increased. Rouleaux formation is prominent (see Fig. 161–19), and the sedimentation rate is markedly increased unless gelation of the plasma occurs. About 10% of macroglobulins have cryoproperties.

Diagnosis

The lymphoplasmacytic cells express CD19, CD20, and CD22, whereas expression of CD5 and CD10 occurs in a minority. The combination of typical symptoms and physical findings, the presence of an IgM M protein, and 10% or greater lymphoplasmacytic infiltration of the bone marrow provide the diagnosis. Asymptomatic patients are considered to have smoldering Waldenström's macroglobulinemia. Multiple myeloma, chronic lymphocytic leukemia, and MGUS of the IgM type must be excluded.

Patients meeting the diagnostic criteria for Waldenström's macroglobulinemia but who have less than 3 g/dL IgM protein at diagnosis have sometimes been classified as having "lymphoplasmacytic lymphoma with an IgM M protein" (Chapter 196). However, except for hyperviscosity, the clinical picture, therapy, and prognosis for these patients are no different from that of patients with an IgM level of 3 g/dL or greater, and hence these patients are also considered to have Waldenström's macroglobulinemia by the current definition.

Prevention and Treatment

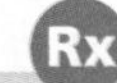

Patients should not be treated unless they have anemia; constitutional symptoms such as weakness, fatigue, night sweats, or weight loss; hyperviscosity; or significant hepatosplenomegaly or lymphadenopathy. Rituximab, a chimeric anti-CD20 monoclonal antibody, produces a response in at least 50% of untreated patients. Chlorambucil is an alternative, especially for elderly patients; it is usually given orally in a dosage of 6 to 8 mg/day and is reduced when the leukocyte or platelet value decreases. Patients should be treated until the disease has reached a plateau state, at which time the treatment can be discontinued and the patients observed closely. Another choice for initial therapy is a purine nucleoside analogue, either fludarabine or 2-chlorodeoxyadenosine.

Chemotherapy should be reinstituted when the disease relapses. Agents used as initial therapy can be used alone or in combination at the time of relapse. Other options include combinations of alkylating agents, autologous stem cell transplantation, and interferon α-2.

Erythropoietin or transfusions of packed red blood cells should be given for symptomatic anemia. Spuriously low hemoglobin and hematocrit levels may occur because of the increased plasma volume from the large amount of M protein. Consequently, transfusions should not be given solely on the basis of the hemoglobin or hematocrit value. Symptomatic hyperviscosity should be treated by plasmapheresis. The median survival of patients with macroglobulinemia is 5 years.

HYPERVISCOSITY SYNDROME

Hyperviscosity syndrome occurs in patients with Waldenström's macroglobulinemia who have high levels of serum M protein (>5 g/dL) and occasionally in those with myeloma, especially of the IgA type. Chronic nasal bleeding and oozing from the gums are frequent, but postsurgical or gastrointestinal bleeding may also occur. Retinal hemorrhages are common, and papilledema may be seen. The patient occasionally complains of blurring or loss of vision. Dizziness, headache, vertigo, nystagmus, decreased hearing, ataxia, paresthesias, diplopia, somnolence, and coma may occur. Hyperviscosity can precipitate or exacerbate heart failure. Most patients have symptoms when the relative viscosity is greater than 4 cP, but the relationship between serum viscosity and clinical manifestations is not precise. Patients with symptomatic hyperviscosity should be treated with plasmapheresis and with chemotherapy to treat the underlying malignancy. Plasma exchange of 3 to 4 L with albumin should be performed daily until the patient is asymptomatic.

HEAVY CHAIN DISEASES

The HCDs are characterized by the presence of an M protein consisting of a portion of the immunoglobulin heavy chain in serum or urine, or both. These heavy chains are devoid of light chains and represent a lymphoplasma cell proliferative process. There are three major types: γ-HCD, α-HCD, and μ-HCD.

γ-HCD

The abnormal protein consists of monoclonal γ chains with significant deletions of amino acids, including the C_{H1} domain of the constant region. The median age of patients is approximately 60 years, although the condition has been noted in persons younger than 20. Patients with γ-HCD often initially have a lymphoma-like illness, but the clinical findings are diverse and range from an aggressive lymphoproliferative process to an asymptomatic state. Hepatosplenomegaly and lymphadenopathy occur in about 60% of patients. Anemia is found in approximately 80% initially and in nearly all eventually. A few patients have had a Coombs-positive hemolytic anemia. The electrophoretic pattern often shows a broad-based band more suggestive of a polyclonal increase than an M protein. The urinary protein value ranges from trace to 20 g/day, but it is usually less than 1 g/day.

The number of lymphocytes, plasma cells, or plasmacytoid lymphocytes in the bone marrow and lymph nodes is increased. The histologic pattern varies, with generalized or localized lymphoma or myeloma usually included, but in some cases there is no evidence of a lymphoplasmacytic proliferative process.

Treatment is indicated only for symptomatic patients and consists of chemotherapy with melphalan plus prednisone or regimens used to treat non-Hodgkin's lymphoma, such as cyclophosphamide, vincristine, and prednisone (Chapter 196). The prognosis of γ-HCD is variable and ranges from a rapidly progressive downhill course of a few weeks' duration to the asymptomatic presence of a stable monoclonal heavy chain in serum or urine.

α-HCD

α-HCD is the most common form of HCD and occurs in patients from the Mediterranean region or Middle East, generally in the second or third decade of life. About 60% are men. Most commonly the gastrointestinal tract is involved, and severe malabsorption with diarrhea, steatorrhea, and loss of weight is noted (Chapter 143). Plasma cell infiltration of the jejunal mucosa is the most frequent pathologic feature. Immunoproliferative small intestinal disease is restricted to patients with small intestinal lesions who have the same pathologic features as those of α-HCD, but these patients do not synthesize α heavy chains.

The serum protein electrophoretic pattern is normal in half the cases, and in the remainder an unimpressive broad band may appear in the α_2 or β regions. The diagnosis depends on identification of a monoclonal α heavy chain on immunofixation. The amount of α heavy chain in urine is small.

In the absence of therapy, α-HCD is typically progressive and fatal. The usual treatment is administration of antibiotics such as tetracyclines and eradication of any concurrent parasitic infection. Patients who do not respond adequately to antibiotics are treated with chemotherapy similar to that used to treat non-Hodgkin's lymphoma, for example, the cyclophosphamide, hydroxydaunomycin, Oncovin (vincristine), and prednisone (CHOP) regimen (Chapter 196).

μ-HCD

This disease is characterized by the demonstration of a monoclonal μ-chain fragment in serum. The patient may have chronic lymphocytic leukemia or lymphoma, but it is likely that the clinical spectrum will broaden when more cases are recognized.

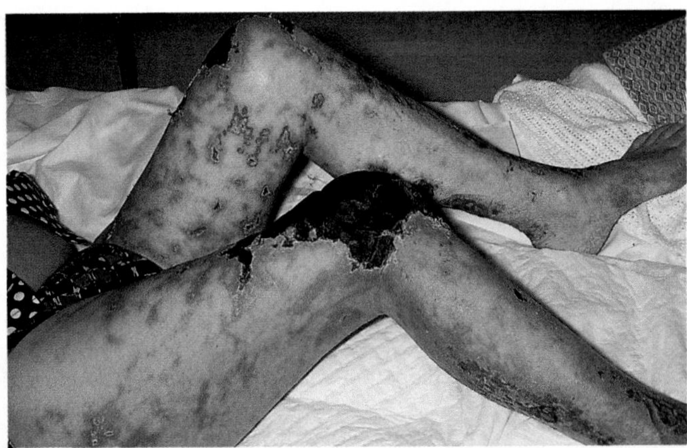

FIGURE 198–7 • Skin infarction in cryoglobulinemia. The skin has a reticulated pattern as a result of leakage of red blood cells from damaged skin capillaries. Necrosis and ulceration have occurred in peripheral sites because of vessel blockage. This patient eventually required plastic surgery. (From Forbes CD, Jackson WF: Color Atlas and Text of Clinical Medicine, 3rd ed. London, Mosby, 2003.)

The serum protein electrophoretic pattern is usually normal except for hypogammaglobulinemia. Bence Jones proteinuria has been found in two thirds of cases. Lymphocytes, plasma cells, and lymphoplasmacytoid cells are increased in the bone marrow. Vacuolization of the plasma cells is common and should suggest the possibility of HCD. The course of μ-HCD is variable, and survival ranges from a few months to many years. Treatment is with corticosteroids and alkylating agents.

CRYOGLOBULINEMIA

Cryoglobulins are proteins that precipitate when cooled and dissolve when heated. They are designated as idiopathic or essential when they are not associated with any recognizable disease. Cryoglobulins are classified into three types: type I (monoclonal), type II (mixed monoclonal plus polyclonal), and type III (polyclonal).

Type I Cryoglobulinemia

Type I (monoclonal) cryoglobulinemia is most commonly of the IgM or IgG class, but IgA and Bence Jones cryoglobulins have been reported. Most patients, even with large amounts of type I cryoglobulin, are completely asymptomatic from this source. Others with monoclonal cryoglobulins in the range of 1 to 2 g/dL may have pain, purpura, Raynaud's phenomenon, cyanosis, and even ulceration and sloughing of skin and subcutaneous tissue (Fig. 198–7) on exposure to cold because their cryoglobulins precipitate at relatively high temperatures. Type I cryoglobulins are associated with macroglobulinemia, multiple myeloma, or MGUS. Therapy for patients with type I cryoglobulinemia and significant symptoms is similar to that for Waldenström's macroglobulinemia for the IgM type and multiple myeloma for the non-IgM type.

Type II Cryoglobulinemia

Type II (mixed) cryoglobulinemia typically consists of an IgM M protein and polyclonal IgG, although monoclonal IgG or monoclonal IgA may also be seen with polyclonal IgM. Serum protein electrophoresis generally shows a normal pattern or a diffuse, polyclonal hypergammaglobulinemic pattern. The quantity of mixed cryoglobulin is usually less than 0.2 g/dL. Hepatic dysfunction and serologic evidence of infection with hepatitis C virus (Chapter 152) are common, and hepatitis C is thought to be the cause of most cases of type II cryoglobulinemia. Vasculitis, glomerulonephritis, lymphoproliferative disease, and chronic infectious processes have also been associated with the disease.

Most clinical manifestations are related to the development of vasculitis and include purpura, polyarthralgias, and neuropathy. Involvement of the joints is symmetrical, but joint deformities rarely develop. Raynaud's phenomenon, necrosis of the skin, and neurologic involvement may be present. In almost 80% of renal biopsy specimens, glomerular damage can be identified. Nephrotic syndrome may result, but severe renal insufficiency is uncommon.

TABLE 198–6 CLINICAL CLASSIFICATION OF AMYLOIDOSIS

Amyloid Type	Classification	Major Protein Component
AL	Primary	κ or λ light chain
AA	Secondary	Protein A
AL	Localized	κ or λ light chain
ATTR	Familial	
	Neurologic	Transthyretin mutant (prealbumin)
	Cardiopathic	Transthyretin mutant (prealbumin)
	Nephropathic	
	Familial	
	Mediterranean fever	Protein A
	Fibrinogen α chain	
	Lysozyme	
	Apolipoprotein A-I	
	Senile systemic amyloidosis	Normal transthyretin (prealbumin)
β2M	Long-term dialysis	β_2-Microglobulin

Early administration of corticosteroids is the most frequent therapy. Treatment should also target underlying hepatitis C infection with interferon α-2 or ribavirin (Chapter 152). Agents such as cyclophosphamide, chlorambucil, azathioprine, or rituximab are used if there is no response. Plasmapheresis is helpful in the acute management of symptoms by removing circulating immune complexes.

Type III Cryoglobulinemia

Type III (polyclonal) cryoglobulinemia does not have a monoclonal component and is not associated with a clonal plasma cell proliferative disorder. Type III cryoglobulins are found in many patients with infections or inflammatory diseases and are usually of no clinical significance unless associated with hepatitis C infection.

PRIMARY AMYLOIDOSIS (Chapter 296)

Definition

The term *amyloid* refers to a fibrillar proteinaceous material that consists of rigid, linear, nonbranching fibrils 7.5 to 10 nm in width and aggregated in a β-pleated sheet conformation. When stained with Congo red, amyloid produces a characteristic apple-green birefringence under polarized light. Clinically, there are several types of amyloidosis, with classification based on the major protein component of the amyloid (Table 198–6). The type of amyloid cannot be differentiated by organ distribution or by electron microscopy. The amyloid fibrils in primary amyloidosis (also called light chain amyloidosis or AL amyloidosis) consist of the variable portion of a monoclonal light chain or, in rare instances, the intact light chain. The light chain class is more frequently λ than κ (2:1), with a predominance of the λ_{VI} subclass. Primary amyloidosis is a systemic disease and its diagnosis requires documentation of positive amyloid staining on a tissue biopsy specimen plus evidence that the amyloid is the result of a clonal plasma cell proliferative disorder (Table 198–7). Patients with amyloidosis may have aberrant de novo synthesis or abnormal proteolytic processing of light chains. The catabolism, or breakdown, of amyloid fibrils is an important, but poorly understood factor in the pathogenesis of primary amyloidosis.

Clinical Manifestations

The median age at diagnosis is 65 years, and only 1% of patients are younger than 40. Two thirds are male. Weakness or fatigue and loss of weight are the most frequent symptoms. Dyspnea, pedal edema, paresthesias, light-headedness, and syncope are frequent in patients with heart failure or peripheral neuropathy. Hoarseness or change of voice, as well as jaw claudication, may occur.

The liver is palpable in a fourth of patients, but splenomegaly occurs in only 5%. Macroglossia is present in 10%. Purpura often involves the neck, face, and eyes. Ankle edema is common.

Almost a third of patients have nephrotic syndrome. Carpal tunnel syndrome (about 20%), heart failure (15 to 20%), peripheral neuropathy (15 to 20%), and orthostatic hypotension (about 10%) are other major syndromes initially seen. The presence of one of these syndromes and an M protein in serum or urine is a strong indication of amyloidosis, for which appropriate biopsy specimens must be taken for diagnosis.

TABLE 198–7 DIAGNOSIS OF PRIMARY AMYLOIDOSIS*

I. Evidence of an amyloid-related systemic syndrome—positive amyloid staining by Congo red in one or more of the following sites:
   1. Fat aspirate
   2. Bone marrow biopsy specimen
   3. Organ biopsy specimen (such as kidney, liver, heart, gastrointestinal tract, sural nerve)

II. Evidence that amyloid is light chain related by one or more of the following methods:
   1. Immunoperoxidase staining of amyloid tissue showing positive light chain staining
   2. Presence of serum or urine monoclonal protein (or both)
   3. Presence of monoclonal plasma cells in a bone marrow specimen

*Both I and II must be present for the diagnosis of primary amyloidosis.

Diagnosis

In patients with suspected primary amyloidosis, the initial diagnostic procedure should be abdominal fat aspiration, which is positive in 75% of patients. Bone marrow aspiration and biopsy should be performed to determine the degree of plasmacytosis; amyloid staining of the bone marrow is positive in more than 50% of patients. Either abdominal fat or bone marrow biopsy results are positive in 90%; if both are negative, options include rectal biopsy or biopsy of a suspected organ (see Table 198–7).

Specific antisera are helpful for identifying the type of systemic amyloidosis. Antiserum to amyloid P component, which reacts with all amyloid types, should be used to demonstrate the presence of amyloid.

Anemia is not a prominent feature, but when present, it is usually due to renal insufficiency, multiple myeloma, or gastrointestinal bleeding. Thrombocytosis occurs in 10% of patients. Proteinuria is present initially in 80%, and the serum creatinine level is greater than 2 mg/dL in 20%. The serum alkaline phosphatase level may be increased. Hyperbilirubinemia is infrequent, but when present, it is an ominous sign. Hypoalbuminemia and increased cholesterol and triglyceride levels are common in patients with nephrotic syndrome. The factor X level is decreased in more than 10% of patients but is rarely the cause of bleeding. The prothrombin time is increased in about 15% of patients, and the thrombin time is prolonged in 60%.

A serum M protein is found in about 50% of patients on electrophoresis, but it is modest in size (median, 1.4 g/dL). Hypogammaglobulinemia is present in about 20%. Immunofixation reveals an M protein in serum or urine in almost 90% of patients at diagnosis.

Bone marrow plasma cells are generally only modestly increased, with a median value of 7%. Less than 20% of patients have more than 20% plasma cells in the marrow. Radiographs of the bones are normal unless the patient has multiple myeloma.

Organ System Involvement

Cardiac and Circulatory

Heart failure is present in approximately 20% of patients at diagnosis and develops during the course of the disease in an additional 10% (Chapters 57 and 59). The electrocardiogram frequently shows either low voltage in the limb leads or features consistent with an anteroseptal infarction (loss of anterior forces), but there is no evidence of myocardial infarction at autopsy. Atrial fibrillation, atrial or junctional tachycardia, ventricular premature complexes, and heart block are common electrocardiographic features.

Echocardiography (Chapter 53) is valuable for evaluation of amyloid heart disease. Increased thickness of the ventricular wall and septum correlates with an increased prevalence of heart failure. Early cardiac amyloidosis is characterized by abnormal relaxation, whereas advanced involvement is characterized by restrictive hemodynamics. Intermittent claudication of the lower extremities, the upper extremities, or the jaw may be a prominent feature.

Other Organs

Nephrotic syndrome is present in more than 25% of patients at the time of diagnosis (Chapter 122). The degree of proteinuria does not correlate well with the extent of amyloid deposition in the kidney. Gross hematuria is rare. Sensorimotor peripheral neuropathy (Chapter 446) characterized by dysesthetic numbness involving the lower extremities is present in about 15% of patients at diagnosis. Autonomic dysfunction (Chapter 445) may be a prominent feature and is usually manifested as orthostatic hypotension, diarrhea, or impotence. Amyloidosis can involve the periarticular structures and produce the shoulder pad syndrome. Rarely, osteolytic lesions from amyloid may occur. Pseudohypertrophy of skeletal muscles from amyloid deposition may be impressive. Petechiae, ecchymoses, papules, plaques, nodules, tumors, bullous lesions, thickening of the skin, and dystrophy of the nails may occur.

Prevention and Treatment

Rx

Treatment of amyloidosis is not satisfactory. Standard therapy consists of melphalan (0.22 mg/kg) plus dexamethasone (40 mg) given orally on days 1 to 4 every 28 days for nine cycles.

Encouraging results have been reported with high-dose intravenous melphalan (140 to 200 mg/m^2) followed by autologous peripheral blood stem cell transplantation. This approach should be considered in selected patients who have no significant cardiac involvement and three or fewer involved organs. Other treatments depend on the type and extent of organ involvement (Chapters 58, 59, 122, 427, and 445).

Prognosis

Currently, the median survival of patients with amyloidosis is approximately 18 months. Survival is only 4 months after the onset of heart failure. Patients with just peripheral neuropathy have a median survival of 2 years.

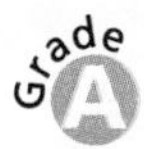

1. Attal M, Harousseau JL, Stoppa AM, et al: A prospective, randomized trial of autologous bone marrow transplantation and chemotherapy in multiple myeloma. N Engl J Med 1996;335:91–97.
2. Child JA, Morgan GJ, Davies FE, et al: High-dose chemotherapy with hematopoietic stem-cell rescue for multiple myeloma. N Engl J Med 2003;348:1875–1883.
3. Attal M, Harousseau JL, Facon T, et al: Single versus double autologous stem-cell transplantation for multiple myeloma. N Engl J Med 2003;349:2495–2502.
4. Palumbo A, Bringhen S, Caravita T, et al: Oral melphalan and prednisone chemotherapy plus thalidomide compared with melphalan and prednisone alone in elderly patients with multiple myeloma: Randomised controlled trial. Lancet 2006;367:825–831.
5. Richardson PG, Sonneveld P, Schuster MW, et al: Bortezomib or high-dose dexamethasone for relapsed multiple myeloma. N Engl J Med 2005;352:2487–2498.

SUGGESTED READINGS

Barlogie B, Tricot G, Anaissie E, et al: Thalidomide and hematopoietic-cell transplantation for multiple myeloma. N Engl J Med 2006;354:1021–1030. *Thalidomide increased complete responses but did not affect overall survival in patients having stem cell transplants.*

Blade J: Monoclonal gammopathy of undetermined significance. N Engl J Med 2006;355:2765–2770. *A clinical review.*

Dimopoulos MA, Anagnostopoulos A: Waldenström's macroglobulinemia. Best Pract Res Clin Haematol 2005;18:747–765. *Review of the disease, including complications and management.*

Hideshima T, Bergsagel PL, Kuehl WM, et al: Advances in biology of multiple myeloma: Clinical applications. Blood 2004;104:607–618. *Excellent review of recent advances in myeloma biology.*

Lacy MQ, Dispenzieri A, Gertz MA, et al: Mayo Clinic consensus statement for the use of bisphosphonates in multiple myeloma. Mayo Clin Proc 2006;81:1047–1053. *Recommendations with an emphasis on safety concerns (osteonecrosis of the jaw).*

Sirohi B, Powles R: Multiple myeloma. Lancet 2004;363:875–887. *Review of the disease, including complications and management.*

199 TUMORS OF THE CENTRAL NERVOUS SYSTEM AND INTRACRANIAL HYPERTENSION AND HYPOTENSION

Lisa M. DeAngelis

INTRACRANIAL TUMORS

General Approach to Brain Tumors

Epidemiology

About 17,000 new primary brain tumors and nervous system cancers are diagnosed annually in the United States, making central nervous system (CNS) tumors more than twice as common as Hodgkin's disease and approximately one third as common as melanoma. In contrast, intracranial metastases are five times more common than primary brain tumors. More than 120 types of primary brain tumors arise from the different cells that comprise the CNS (Table 199–1). In addition to classifying tumors by their cell of origin, in clinical practice it is often useful to classify a tumor by its intracranial site as well, such as pineal region tumors or pituitary and suprasellar tumors.

Pathobiology

In contrast to tumors arising elsewhere in the body, there is little distinction between benign and malignant tumors when they occur in the brain. The growth of brain tumors is restricted to the CNS; they rarely, if ever, metastasize to other organs. In the CNS, a malignant tumor is characterized by aggressive pathologic features, including local tissue invasion, neovascularity, regional necrosis, and cytologic atypia. These features confer a growth advantage to malignant cells and lead to rapid expansion and, frequently, to early regrowth after treatment. Tumors lacking these aggressive histologic features are preferably classified as low-grade rather than benign. Many low-grade tumors continue to grow within the CNS, causing progressive neurologic disability, and some may acquire a more malignant phenotype over time. The low-grade tumors that transform into high-grade neoplasms are primarily the intra-axial tumors that cannot be cured by resection because of their diffuse infiltration of brain. Almost all truly benign CNS tumors are extra-axial tumors, such as meningiomas and acoustic neuromas, that can be cured with complete surgical resection.

Clinical Manifestations

A patient with a brain tumor can present with one or both of two types of symptoms and signs. *Generalized symptoms,* which typically reflect the increased intracranial pressure (ICP) that often accompanies cerebral tumors, include headaches, lethargy, personality change, nausea, and vomiting. *Lateralizing symptoms,* which reflect the specific location of the tumor, include hemiparesis, hemisensory deficits, aphasia, visual field impairment, and seizures (Table 199–2).

Most patients have symptoms that progress over a week to a few months. A sudden intensification of symptoms may precipitate the

TABLE 199–1 WORLD HEALTH ORGANIZATION CLASSIFICATION OF BRAIN TUMORS*

TUMORS OF NEUROEPITHELIAL TISSUE

- Astrocytic tumors
  - Astrocytoma
  - Anaplastic (malignant) astrocytoma
  - Glioblastoma multiforme
  - Pilocytic astrocytoma
  - Pleomorphic xanthoastrocytoma
  - Subependymal giant cell astrocytoma
- Oligodendroglial tumors
  - Oligodendroglioma
  - Anaplastic (malignant) oligodendroglioma
- Ependymal tumors
  - Ependymoma
  - Anaplastic (malignant) ependymoma
  - Myxopapillary ependymoma (spinal tumor)
  - Subependymoma
- Mixed gliomas
  - Oligoastrocytoma
  - Anaplastic (malignant) oligoastrocytoma
- Choroid plexus
  - Choroid plexus papilloma
  - Choroid plexus carcinoma
- Neuronal and mixed neuronal-glial tumors
  - Gangliocytoma
  - Dysembryoplastic neuroepithelial tumor
  - Ganglioglioma
  - Anaplastic (malignant) ganglioglioma
  - Central neurocytoma
- Pineal parenchymal tumors
  - Pineocytoma
  - Pineoblastoma
- Embryonal tumors
  - Medulloblastoma
  - Primitive neuroectodermal tumor

TUMORS OF CRANIAL AND SPINAL NERVES

- Schwannoma
- Neurofibroma

TUMORS OF MENINGES

- Meningioma
- Hemangiopericytoma
- Hemangioblastoma

PRIMARY CENTRAL NERVOUS SYSTEM LYMPHOMAS

GERM CELL TUMORS

- Germinoma
- Embryonal carcinoma
- Yolk sac tumor (endodermal sinus tumor)
- Choriocarcinoma
- Teratoma
- Mixed germ cell tumors

CYSTS AND TUMOR-LIKE LESIONS

- Rathke cleft cyst
- Epidermoid cyst
- Dermoid cyst
- Colloid cyst of the third ventricle

TUMORS OF THE SELLAR REGION

- Pituitary adenoma
- Pituitary carcinoma
- Craniopharyngioma

METASTATIC TUMORS

*Abridged and modified from World Health Organization classification.

TABLE 199–2 FOCAL CLINICAL MANIFESTATIONS OF BRAIN TUMORS

- Frontal lobe
  - Generalized seizures
  - Focal motor seizures (contralateral)
  - Expressive aphasia (dominant side)
  - Behavioral changes
  - Dementia
  - Gait disorders, incontinence
  - Hemiparesis
- Basal ganglia
  - Hemiparesis (contralateral)
  - Movement disorders (rare)
- Parietal lobe
  - Receptive aphasia (dominant side)
  - Spatial disorientation (nondominant side)
  - Cortical sensory dysfunction (contralateral)
  - Hemianopia (contralateral)
  - Agnosias
- Occipital lobe
  - Hemianopia (contralateral)
  - Visual disturbances (unformed)
- Temporal lobe
  - Complex partial (psychomotor) seizures
  - Generalized seizures
  - Behavioral changes
  - Olfactory and complex visual auras
  - Language disorder (dominant side)
  - Visual field defect
- Corpus callosum
  - Dementia (anterior)
  - Memory loss (posterior)
  - Behavioral changes
  - Asymptomatic (middle)
- Thalamus
  - Sensory loss (contralateral)
  - Behavioral changes
  - Language disorder (dominant side)
- Midbrain/pineal
  - Paresis of vertical eye movement
  - Pupillary abnormalities
  - Precocious puberty (boys)
- Sella/optic nerve/pituitary
  - Endocrinopathy
  - Bitemporal hemianopia
  - Monocular visual defects
  - Ophthalmoplegia (cavernous sinus)
- Pons/medulla
  - Cranial nerve dysfunction
  - Ataxia, nystagmus
  - Weakness, sensory loss
  - Spasticity
- Cerebellopontine angle
  - Deafness (ipsilateral)
  - Loss of facial sensation (ipsilateral)
  - Facial weakness (ipsilateral)
  - Ataxia
- Cerebellum
  - Ataxia (ipsilateral)
  - Nystagmus

patient's initial visit to the physician; however, a careful history usually reveals symptoms that predated the acute deterioration and slowly worsened over time. Two exceptions are the new appearance of a seizure in a previously asymptomatic individual (Chapter 426) and sudden hemorrhage into a tumor.

Symptoms of brain tumors can be produced by tumor invading brain parenchyma, tumor and edema compressing brain tissue, cerebrospinal fluid (CSF) obstruction caused directly by the tumor or by a shift of brain tissue, and herniation. Invasion and compression typically produce focal symptoms, many of which can be relieved if the compression is reduced. Obstruction of CSF flow and herniation are frequently a consequence of elevated ICP and typically produce generalized symptoms of headache, nausea, and vomiting, but they can also cause false localizing signs, such as an abducens nerve palsy, as a result of diffuse increased ICP.

Headache (Chapter 421) is a presenting symptom of approximately 35% of brain tumors. It is more common in younger than older patients, and more common in patients who have rapidly growing tumors than in those whose tumors have evolved slowly (Fig. 199–1). Mental and cognitive abnormalities (Chapters 424 and 425) may be a reflection of local tumor (e.g., aphasia, alexia, agnosia) or of general impairment (e.g., lethargy, confusion, word finding difficulty, apathy). Seizures affect approximately one third of patients with brain tumors, and they are especially common as the presenting and only symptom of a low-grade tumor. The seizures, which are focal because they originate at the site of the tumor, may remain restricted (e.g., focal motor seizures), or they may generalize secondarily, producing loss of consciousness (Chapter 426), sometimes so quickly that the focal signature is missed by the patient or even an observant witness.

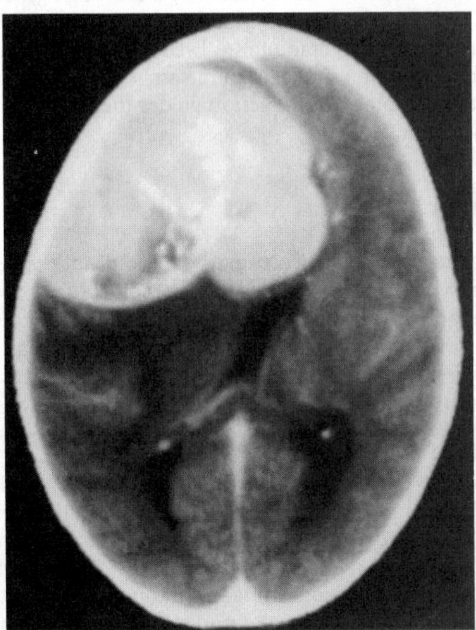

FIGURE 199–1 • Meningioma. Computed tomography scan with contrast of a meningioma in a patient who presented with mild cognitive deficits, illustrative of the size a slow-growing tumor can attain in the brain. The tumor was completely resected.

Diagnosis

Imaging

Magnetic resonance imaging (MRI) is far superior to computed tomography (CT) scans and should be used in all cases of suspected intracranial tumor (Chapter 419). MRI should be performed both without and with intravenous gadolinium. A well-performed MRI scan identifies any intracranial tumor, and normal MRI results effectively exclude a neoplasm. The MRI of some extra-axial tumors (e.g., acoustic neuromas, meningiomas) is so characteristic that histologic confirmation is not required (Table 199–3). A non–contrast-enhancing infiltrative lesion that is visible primarily on T2 or fluid-attenuated inversion recovery (FLAIR) images is most consistent with a low-grade glioma (Fig. 199–2), whereas a contrast-enhancing lesion with an area of central necrosis and surrounding edema is most likely to be a glioblastoma or possibly a brain metastasis. Although these diagnoses must be confirmed histologically, the preoperative diagnostic possibilities affect the choice of surgical procedure and the surgical approach to the lesion.

Magnetic resonance (MR) perfusion imaging after rapid infusion of gadolinium can measure the relative cerebral blood volume and neovascularity associated with a tumor; high perfusion is associated with higher grade of malignancy. This technique can help estimate the tumor's grade preoperatively and guide the planning of treatment.

Magnetic resonance spectroscopy (MRS) noninvasively assesses tissue composition (Chapter 419). High-grade primary brain tumors are asso-

TABLE 199–3 MAGNETIC RESONANCE IMAGING OF COMMON BRAIN TUMORS

Tumor Type	Noncontrast T1	Contrast T1	T2
Malignant glioma	↓ density	+	↑ density
Low-grade glioma	↓ density	–	↑ density
Primary central nervous system lymphoma	↑ density	+	↑ density
Meningioma	Iso to ↑	+	Iso to ↓
Acoustic neuroma	↓ to Iso	+	Iso to ↑
Metastases	↑ to ↓	+	Variable, ↑ to ↓

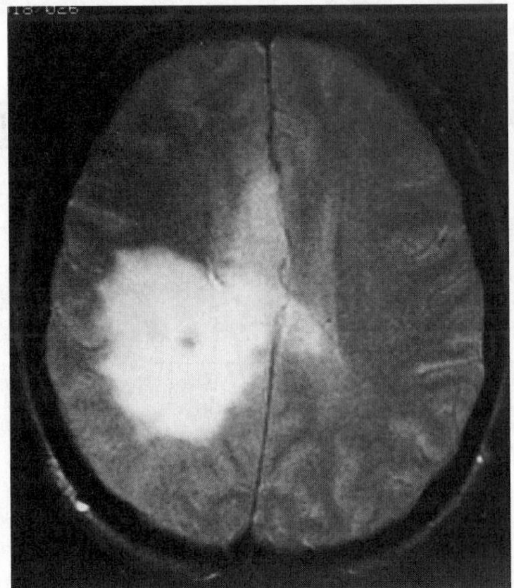

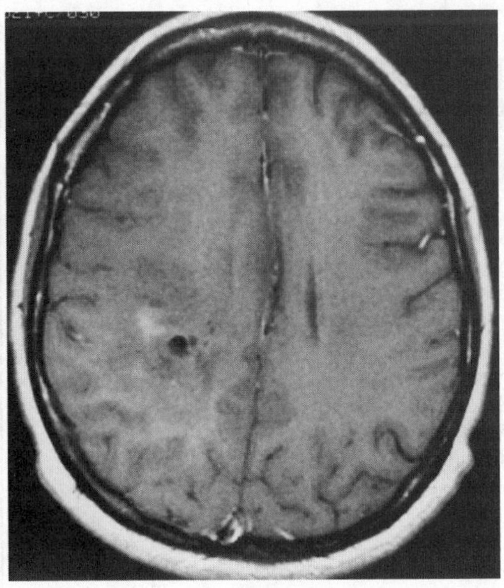

FIGURE 199–2 • Glioma. Magnetic resonance imaging (MRI) scan of a low-grade glioma. **Left,** T2-weighted image; **right,** T1-weighted image, gadolinium contrast with minimum enhancement. The images are typical of this tumor, which is being detected with increasing frequency by MRI in seizure patients. Many are invisible on computed tomography scans.

ciated with a decrease in *N*-acetylaspartate (NAA) and an increase in choline (Cho). More malignant tumors are associated with a greater Cho/NAA ratio and frequently contain areas with elevation of lactate and lipid.

Surgical resection is a major objective in the treatment of almost every kind of brain tumor, but resection must be balanced against possible damage to adjacent normal brain. The development of functional MRI (fMRI), which measures cerebral blood flow when areas of cortex are activated, has greatly enhanced the ability to localize critical neurologic functions and their relationship to the tumor preoperatively (Chapter 419). When the fMR image is fused with the anatomic MR image, critical functions can be identified in relationship to the patient's tumor, and a more safe and complete resection may be planned.

On positron-emission tomography (PET), high-grade tumors are usually hypermetabolic, whereas low-grade tumors are hypometabolic (Chapter 419). New technologies using ^{11}C-methionine PET may differentiate low- from high-grade gliomas much more efficiently than deoxyglucose PET does.

CT scanning, without and with intravenous contrast, should be used only for patients who cannot undergo MRI. A CT scan, even with contrast, may miss low-grade tumors and tumors in the posterior fossa.

Currently, angiography has no role in the diagnosis of intracranial tumors. However, angiographic embolization is occasionally useful preoperatively to reduce the vascularity of some meningiomas, thereby making a complete resection safer and more feasible.

Other Tests

Electroencephalography (EEG) is rarely needed in the diagnosis or management of brain tumors. An EEG can occasionally be useful in a patient who has prolonged or unexplained stupor and in whom nonconvulsive status epilepticus is a consideration. Intraoperative monitoring is also frequently used to help guide resection of epileptogenic cortex adjacent to or within brain tumor tissue.

CSF analysis has little role in the diagnosis of most intracranial neoplasms. In primary CNS lymphoma (PCNSL), the diagnosis may be established on CSF cytologic examination in about 15% of patients. Rarely, a lumbar puncture is required to exclude inflammatory conditions or other processes that may be confused with a primary brain tumor. Lumbar puncture must be avoided in patients with cerebellar tumors, because the release of pressure through the spinal needle may result in herniation of the cerebellar tonsils through the foramen magnum.

Differential Diagnosis

Patients who present with symptoms of raised ICP or the new onset of central neurologic symptoms such as hemiparesis or seizure should be hospitalized and evaluated rapidly. Prompt neuroimaging discloses a mass, and the radiographic features narrow the differential diagnosis (Table 199–4). Extra-axial tumors, such as a meningioma or acoustic neuroma, can be confused with a dural metastasis. Low-grade intra-axial tumors, which are nonenhancing on MRI, have been confused with infections such as herpes encephalitis when they involve the temporal lobe. Contrast-enhancing intra-axial tumors can be confused with a stroke (Chapters 431 and 432), brain abscess (Chapter 438), or focal plaque of demyelination (Chapter 436). Subacute infarction can show brisk contrast enhancement, usually in a gyral pattern, unlike brain tumors, in which enhancement is primarily in the white matter; occasionally, however, the two are indistinguishable radiographically. Brain abscesses typically have a thinner enhancing wall than a malignant tumor, but they sometimes appear similar on MRI. Despite careful evaluation, patients thought to have a malignant glioma occasionally are found at surgery to have a brain abscess. A single large plaque of demyelination can also be confused radiographically with a brain tumor, and sometimes the diagnosis can be established only by biopsy.

When MRI suggests a primary brain tumor, there is no need for an extensive systemic search for a possible source of metastasis. Brain metastases are more common than primary brain tumors, but most occur in patients with known cancer, typically with active systemic disease. If an obvious systemic cancer is not revealed by a thorough general examination, chest radiograph, routine blood tests, and urinalysis, then the patient should proceed to craniotomy. Even if a brain metastasis is found at surgery, resection of a single brain metastasis is the appropriate treatment, and the pathology of the lesion guides the subsequent search for the primary tumor.

Treatment

Rx

The treatment for all brain tumors can be divided into two main categories: symptomatic and definitive (Table 199–5). Symptomatic treatment addresses the associated problems, such as cerebral edema, seizures, and thromboembolic disease, which can contribute substantially to clinical symptoms. Definitive treatment addresses the tumor itself.

Symptomatic Treatment

Symptomatic management includes the use of corticosteroids, anticonvulsants, and prophylaxis for deep vein thrombosis (DVT; Chapter 81). Corticosteroids decrease the vasogenic edema that surrounds primary and metastatic brain tumors. Blood vessels associated with tumor formation are leaky and do not share the normal morphologic and physiologic features that form the blood-brain barrier; corticosteroids effectively reconstitute the blood-brain barrier by decreasing the abnormal permeability of these neovessels. Clinical improvement may begin within minutes, and frequently patients are dramatically improved within 24 to 48 hours.

Dexamethasone is the most commonly used glucocorticoid, because it has the least mineralocorticoid activity. The usual start-

TABLE 199–4 DIFFERENTIAL DIAGNOSIS OF INTRACRANIAL TUMORS

Infection
Brain abscess
Bacterial
Fungal
Parasitic (e.g., cysticercosis)
Herpes encephalitis
Vascular disease
Stroke
Intracranial hemorrhage
Inflammatory conditions
Granuloma (sarcoid)
Multiple sclerosis: single large lesion
Vascular malformations
Cavernous angiomas
Venous angiomas
Congenital abnormalities
Cortical dysplasia
Heterotopia

TABLE 199–5 TREATMENT FOR BRAIN TUMORS

SYMPTOMATIC
Glucocorticoids
Anticonvulsants
DVT prophylaxis and treatment
DEFINITIVE
Surgery
Goal is gross total excision
Radiotherapy
Standard external beam
Fractionated
Usually focal
Stereotactic radiosurgery
Chemotherapy
Limited by intrinsic drug resistance and blood-brain barrier

DVT = deep vein thrombosis.

Section XV Oncology

Rx

ing dose is 12 to 16 mg/day, but this can be adjusted up or down to find the lowest possible dose that alleviates neurologic symptoms. After definitive treatment is instituted, many patients can be tapered off their corticosteroid completely. Chronic high-dose corticosteroid therapy is associated with substantial side effects (Chapter 33). Patients who will be taking glucocorticoids for 6 weeks or longer should receive prophylaxis against *Pneumocystis jiroveci* (formerly *P. carinii;* Chapter 362).

Anticonvulsants are administered to any patient who has had a seizure, but prophylactic anticonvulsants should not be prescribed for patients who have never had a seizure, except that they may be useful in the perioperative period. 1,2

DVT, which occurs in about 25% of patients with brain tumors, can occur early in the illness or at any time during treatment. All patients undergoing neurosurgery should have pneumatic compression boots in the postoperative period to reduce the incidence of DVT. Prophylactic anticoagulants have also been used successfully in the immediate postoperative period without increasing postoperative hemorrhage. Appropriately regulated anticoagulation (Chapters 35 and 81) is the optimal therapy for DVT and is not associated with an increased risk of intracerebral hemorrhage in patients with intracranial tumors. Inferior vena cava filters can be used for patients who have DVTs or pulmonary emboli and who cannot be fully anticoagulated.

Definitive Treatment

Surgery

Complete excision is the goal for a primary brain tumor. Surgical excision can often be accomplished for primary extra-axial tumors, such as meningiomas and acoustic neuromas. However, meningiomas often occur in intracranial locations that make resection impossible. Tumors of the skull base are particularly difficult to remove, and partial resection for decompression is often performed to preserve neurologic function. The safe boundaries for resecting cortical lesions while preserving function can often be elucidated by preoperative fMRI and intraoperative cortical mapping. However, lesions involving many critical structures, such as the brain stem or thalamus, cannot be excised safely.

Lesions that cannot be resected are still amenable to biopsy for diagnostic purposes. In particular, the use of stereotactic biopsy has made it feasible to reach lesions in almost any area of the brain with minimal morbidity. The risks of stereotactic biopsy include (1) inadequate tissue sample to make a diagnosis, (2) a tissue sample that does not accurately reflect the most malignant grade of the tumor, and (3) a procedure-related complication, such as hemorrhage. Hemorrhage that causes neurologic impairment occurs in only 2% of stereotactic biopsies, typically in patients with glioblastoma multiforme.

Complete excision can cure extra-axial primary brain tumors, and it is associated with prolonged survival and better neurologic outcome even in patients with primary intra-axial tumors. Gross total excision, as measured by postoperative neuroimaging, is associated with prolonged survival in patients with malignant gliomas and probably in those with low-grade gliomas as well. However, most low-grade gliomas are not amenable to gross total excision, and usually only partial excision is feasible. Macroscopic tumor can frequently be removed completely in patients with high-grade gliomas, but there is always remaining microscopic disease that infiltrates surrounding brain.

Some tumors, such as brain stem gliomas, are in such critical locations that not even biopsy is attempted. Their characteristic radiographic appearance permits diagnosis and initiation of medical treatment.

Radiation Therapy

A course of external beam radiation therapy is delivered in small daily fractions to a total cumulative dose usually between 45 and 60 Gy. Dividing the treatment into small daily fractions permits sublethal repair in normal tissues and markedly reduces neurologic toxicity associated with cerebral radiation. External beam irradiation, which is the most effective nonsurgical treatment for brain tumors, doubles median survival time of patients with malignant primary brain tumors or metastatic lesions. It can also be useful for recurrent meningiomas and acoustic neuromas. However, it only rarely cures any of these lesions, and most patients develop recurrent disease despite maximal radiation therapy.

Rx

Stereotactic radiosurgery has been developed to deliver high fractions of focused radiation therapy that spare normal surrounding tissue. The technique is limited to tumors that are 3 cm in diameter or smaller and is less useful for malignant gliomas because of their infiltrative nature.

The neurologic complications of radiation therapy, which are usually observed in patients months to years after completion of treatment, include radionecrosis, dementia, and leukoencephalopathy. The incidence is reported as less than 5%, and most patients die of their brain tumor before the delayed consequences of treatment can be observed. However, in long-term survivors (e.g., patients with low-grade glioma or primary CNS lymphoma, children with medulloblastoma) the late consequences of radiation therapy are important. Dementia accompanying radiation-induced leukoencephalopathy can progress and result in severe neurologic impairment. Radionecrosis can mimic recurrent tumor with a large contrast-enhancing lesion on MRI. Corticosteroids can reduce the edema and sometimes are sufficient to treat small areas of radionecrosis. However, if the lesion is sufficiently large, resection may be required to decompress the mass and reduce the steroid requirements.

Chemotherapy

Chemotherapy for brain tumors has usually been disappointing because of the intrinsic resistance of these tumors to most conventional agents. Carboplatin and cisplatin (Chapter 192) are active agents against medulloblastoma, even when the tumor is disseminated in the CSF. Temozolomide (150 to 200 mg/m^2 for 5 days every 4 weeks) is active in all gliomas, and high-dose methotrexate (3 to 8 g/m^2 for 3 to 12 months) is effective for primary CNS lymphoma. For patients with glioblastoma, polymers impregnated with carmustine (BCNU) and placed in a resection cavity offer modest benefit when compared with no chemotherapy, but they are associated with local tissue injury and edema.

SPECIFIC TYPES OF BRAIN TUMORS

Primary Extra-axial Tumors

The most common primary extra-axial tumors are meningiomas, pituitary adenomas, and acoustic neuromas. These tumors arise within the intracranial cavity but are not tumors of brain tissue. Almost all are benign; because the brain is rarely invaded, complete excision often enables cure with full recovery of neurologic function. These tumors produce neurologic symptoms and signs by compressing the underlying brain; however, edema of the underlying brain is infrequent, so glucocorticoids have a limited role.

Meningiomas

Epidemiology

Meningiomas are usually benign. Between 5 and 10% of meningiomas are atypical or malignant variants with a more aggressive course. Meningiomas are more common in women, may be multiple in about 10% of patients with sporadic meningioma, and are occasionally part of a familial syndrome. They occur with increased frequency in patients with neurofibromatosis type 2 (Chapter 444).

Diagnosis

Meningiomas grow slowly and produce symptoms that are insidious in onset and typically slowly progressive. Tumors can reach a consider-

Section XV Oncology

able size, but they grow so slowly that the brain accommodates to the progressive compression. Meningiomas typically occur in specific locations: over the convexity, along the falx and parasagittal area, the olfactory groove, base of the skull near the sphenoid bone, cavernous sinus, cerebellopontine angle, and foramen magnum. Cortical and parasagittal tumors typically manifest with seizures or progressive hemiparesis. Tumors in the anterior cranial fossa can cause slowly progressive changes in personality and cognition. Meningiomas at the base of the skull manifest with cranial neuropathies and gait difficulties when there is brain stem compression. Frequently, tumors are completely asymptomatic and are identified on neuroimaging done for another purpose, such as head trauma.

On MRI, meningiomas have a characteristic appearance consisting of a diffusely enhancing, dural-based lesion that is associated with a thin enhancing dural tail extending from the tumor; often the radiographic features are so characteristic that surgery is performed for therapeutic purposes only. The radiographic differential diagnosis includes the less common *hemangiopericytoma* and *dural metastasis.* Most meningiomas are not accompanied by significant edema, but marked edema is seen with high-grade malignant lesions or the secretory variant.

If small meningiomas are discovered in the absence of clinical symptoms or the symptoms are minor, lesions may be monitored with serial images, because growth can be so slow.

Treatment

Rx

If treatment is indicated, complete resection is often curative, but even completely resected benign tumors may recur (as many as 20% in some series), so radiologic follow-up is essential. Tumors at the base of the skull often cannot be resected completely and tend to recur despite successive attempts at surgical resection. Radiation therapy can sometimes slow progression and is essential for the treatment of malignant meningiomas. No effective chemotherapy has yet been identified.

Acoustic Neuromas

Acoustic neuromas (Chapter 454), better called vestibular schwannomas, are benign tumors that arise from the eighth cranial nerve. Acoustic neuromas are twice as common in women as in men; the peak age is between 40 and 60 years. Sporadic vestibular schwannomas are unilateral; bilateral acoustic neuromas are pathognomonic of neurofibromatosis type 2 (Chapter 444).

Acoustic neuromas usually arise from the vestibular portion of the nerve and typically manifest with unilateral hearing loss, sometimes preceded or accompanied by tinnitus and a sensation of dizziness or unsteadiness but not true vertigo. The slow, progressive enlargement of the tumor produces ipsilateral facial numbness or weakness by compressing the fifth or seventh cranial nerve, respectively. Tumors originate within the internal auditory meatus but grow out of the acoustic canal and into the cerebellopontine angle, where they can compress the brainstem and cause ataxia and ipsilateral cerebellar signs. Cranial MRI with gadolinium delineates even small acoustic neuromas with ease.

Treatment is often surgical; stereotactic radiosurgery may be an alternative for lesions smaller than 3 cm. It is preferable to treat the tumors when they are small, to preserve facial nerve function and hearing.

Pituitary Adenomas

Pituitary adenomas (Chapter 242) can be classified according to their size as microadenomas (<1 cm in diameter) or macroadenomas; by the presence or absence of endocrine function; and by the endocrinologic syndromes or neurologic syndromes caused by tumor compression. Microadenomas typically manifest with endocrine symptoms such as amenorrhea, galactorrhea, infertility, and sexual dysfunction (all related to prolactin-secreting tumors); acromegaly (related to growth hormone hypersecretion); Cushing's syndrome (related to adrenocorticotropic hormone–producing tumors), and hyperthyroidism (related to thyroid-stimulating hormone–producing tumors). As pituitary tumors enlarge and become macroadenomas, they compress the surrounding neural structures, including the optic chiasm and optic nerves, typically causing bitemporal hemianopia and occasionally causing unilateral visual loss. Macroadenomas are frequently nonsecreting but destroy pituitary tissue, causing panhypopituitarism. Rarely, pituitary tumors manifest with the abrupt onset of headache, ophthalmoplegia, unilateral blindness, and even a depressed level of alertness or coma—a syndrome of *pituitary apoplexy* caused by hemorrhage or infarction.

Cranial MRI, particularly with coronal images and gadolinium administration, can completely outline the pituitary tumor and surrounding neural structures. All macroadenomas and some microadenomas can be treated with transsphenoidal pituitary surgery, which is associated with minimal morbidity. Occasionally, residual or recurrent tumor necessitates radiation therapy. Some hormone-secreting tumors, particularly prolactinomas or growth hormone–secreting tumors, can be treated medically with cabergoline or octreotide, respectively (Chapter 242). These medications not only correct the hormonal excess but also shrink the tumor; they must be taken for life.

Other tumors in the pituitary and suprasellar region include craniopharyngiomas, suprasellar epidermoid cysts, Rathke cleft cysts, germinomas (discussed later), and lymphocytic hypophysitis, which is a benign inflammatory condition that usually manifests with diabetes insipidus (Chapter 243). MRI frequently differentiates these conditions, which are usually suprasellar and erode into the pituitary fossa only secondarily. Some of these lesions also have characteristic radiographic features. These lesions are benign. Except for hypophysitis, which resolves completely with corticosteroid treatment (e.g., methylprednisolone 120 mg daily for 2 weeks and then tapered for one additional week), complete surgical excision is the curative therapy.

Other Extra-axial Tumors

Pineal region tumors all have a characteristic clinical presentation that includes Parinaud's syndrome, which consists of paresis of upward gaze, poor pupillary reaction to light with brisk reaction on accommodation, impairment of convergence, and convergence–retraction nystagmus. Some of these lesions may also cause hydrocephalus and symptoms of increased ICP. Pineal region tumors include pineal parenchymal tumors, such as pineocytomas and the more aggressive pineoblastomas, and germ cell tumors, including germinomas and nongerminomatous germ cell tumors. Germinomas can be completely cured with focal radiation therapy, whereas nongerminomatous germ cell tumors are more aggressive and frequently relapse despite chemotherapy plus cranial irradiation.

Chordomas are rare tumors of residual notochordal tissue. They usually occur at the base of the skull, are locally invasive, and are characterized by multiple recurrences despite surgery and radiation therapy.

Lipomas are benign tumors that can occur in midline structures, particularly near the corpus callosum. They can be cured by complete removal.

Arachnoid cysts are not tumors per se but can manifest with headaches, seizures, or focal neurologic symptoms if they become large enough to compress underlying brain tissue. Many are completely asymptomatic and are found incidentally on neuroimaging. Only symptomatic cysts require removal.

Primary Intra-axial Tumors

Most primary intra-axial brain tumors are gliomas, including the astrocytomas, oligodendrogliomas, and ependymomas. Less common are medulloblastomas, other rare neuroectodermal tumors, and primary CNS lymphomas. All of these tumors have a tendency to invade brain tissue, and none can be completely excised surgically.

Gliomas

Definition

Astrocytomas, which are the most common glioma, are classified into one of four World Health Organization (WHO) categories: grade I is the pilocytic astrocytoma, grade II is the fibrillary astrocytoma, grade III is the anaplastic astrocytoma, and grade IV is the glioblastoma multiforme. Pilocytic astrocytomas (grade I) are extremely low-grade focal tumors that are more common in children and may be associated with neurofibromatosis type 1; they are often cured by complete surgical excision. Astrocytomas, anaplastic astrocytomas, and glioblastomas are diffuse tumors that tend to infiltrate widely into brain; even grade II tumors progress over time, and the majority acquire the histologic features and growth patterns of grade III and IV tumors.

Epidemiology

Gliomas occur at any age, but the peak age is 20 to 30 years for an astrocytoma, 40 years for anaplastic astrocytoma, and 55 to 60 years for glioblastoma. Age is the single most important prognostic factor: younger patients live substantially longer than older patients. Histology is also critical: patients with glioblastoma do significantly worse than patients with lower-grade lesions. Performance status, duration of symptoms, and whether a complete resection has been achieved are also strong predictors of improved outcome and prolonged survival. For all grades of glioma, men are more frequently affected than women, and whites significantly more frequently than blacks. Gliomas are typically single lesions, but multifocal disease is seen in approximately 5% of patients with high-grade tumors. A variant of gliomas, called *gliomatosis cerebri,* causes widespread infiltration of the entire brain; most patients have relatively low-grade pathology on biopsy, but focal regions of high-grade transformation can exist.

Pathobiology

At least 95% of gliomas are sporadic, and only 5% occur in patients with a family history of brain tumor. Furthermore, patients with a familial history of glioma usually do not fall into a well-recognized hereditary syndrome. However, neurofibromatosis 1 (von Recklinghausen's disease; Chapter 444) is associated with an increased incidence of gliomas particularly in the optic pathway, hypothalamus, and brain stem. Gliomas also occur with increased frequency in Turcott's syndrome, in which colorectal neoplasms are seen in association with a variety of CNS tumors.

Clinical Manifestations and Diagnosis

Patients with gliomas often present with seizures, headache, and lateralizing signs such as hemiparesis, aphasia, or a visual field deficit. On MRI, low-grade gliomas typically appear as diffuse, nonenhancing lesions with a propensity to occur in the frontal lobe and insular cortex. High-grade gliomas, which typically enhance with contrast, occur in the cortical white matter and are accompanied by significant surrounding edema. Glioblastomas frequently have regions of central necrosis (Fig. 199–3), and hemorrhage can occur in 5 to 8% of patients.

Treatment

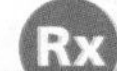

For all gliomas, treatment frequently involves surgery, radiation therapy, and chemotherapy. The surgical goal of complete removal of all visible disease is often impossible. The adequacy of resection is best assessed on a postoperative MRI study, without and with gadolinium, performed within 72 to 96 hours after surgery. Surgical removal usually improves neurologic function and reduces dependency on corticosteroids.

Anaplastic Astrocytomas and Glioblastomas

All anaplastic astrocytomas and glioblastomas should be treated with postoperative radiation therapy to a dose of approximately 60 Gy. In a randomized trial of patients with glioblastoma, the alkylating agent temozolomide (75 mg/m^2 daily), administered concurrently with radiation therapy and followed by adjuvant temozolomide (150 to 200 mg/m^2 for 5 consecutive days every 4 weeks for 6 cycles), significantly improved survival (median 14.6 months) compared with radiation therapy alone (median 12.1 months; $p < .001$), and the 2-year survival rate more than doubled to 26.5%. [3] Patients whose tumors contained a methylated promoter of the 06-methylguanine-DNA methyltransferase (MGMT) DNA repair gene benefited most from the addition of temozolomide. Based on these data, combined treatment is the current standard of care for patients with glioblastoma. Patients with anaplastic astrocytoma should receive radiation therapy followed by temozolomide (150 to 200 mg/m^2 for 5 consecutive days every 4 weeks for at least 6 cycles). Chemotherapy is generally well tolerated and associated with minimal toxicity. Recurrences can be treated with re-resection, additional

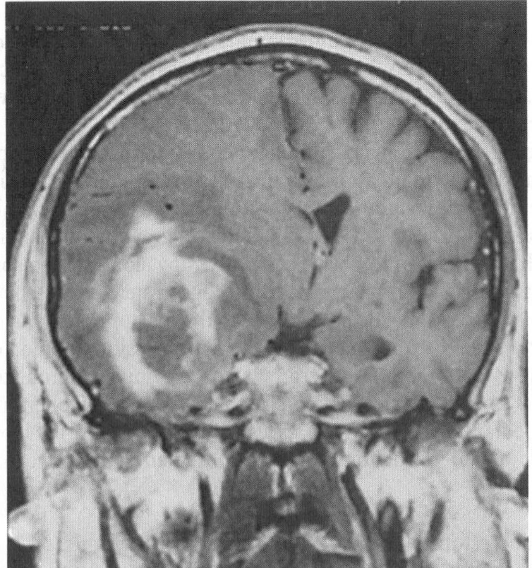

FIGURE 199–3 • Temporal lobe glioblastoma. This T1 gadolinium-enhanced magnetic resonance imaging scan shows a typical ring configuration of contrast with central necrosis and marked mass effect.

chemotherapy, and/or, occasionally, stereotactic radiosurgery. Despite aggressive treatment, disease recurs in almost all patients, and the median survival time is 14 to 15 months for glioblastoma and about 3 years for anaplastic astrocytoma. However, some young patients with anaplastic astrocytoma can survive many years before the tumor recurs.

Optic and Brain Stem Gliomas

Optic gliomas, which can involve the optic nerve or optic chiasm, are usually associated with neurofibromatosis type 1. These gliomas are typically pilocytic tumors that can have an indolent course, including rare spontaneous regression. Often they are not amenable to surgical resection, and they can have a stuttering clinical course, with periods of visual loss punctuated by prolonged periods of visual stability. When necessary, radiation or even chemotherapy may be useful, but often no treatment is required. Brain stem gliomas usually involve the pons, less often the medulla or midbrain. Brain stem gliomas are most commonly seen in children in the first decade of life but can be found even in the elderly; they can have a low-grade or a high-grade histology, but outcome is primarily determined by the location of the tumor. In general, most brain stem gliomas have a dismal outcome with survival of 1 year or less, but relatively benign variants occasionally occur.

Low-Grade Astrocytomas

Low-grade astrocytomas have a variable course. In patients who present with isolated seizures that can be easily controlled with anticonvulsants, treatment with radiation therapy or chemotherapy immediately after surgery does not prolong survival, and patients can be monitored until there is clinical or radiographic evidence of tumor progression. [4] Patients with progressive neurologic symptoms or cognitive impairment require immediate treatment after diagnosis, and focal radiation therapy to a total of about 54 Gy is the optimal choice. An astrocytoma can progress as a low-grade tumor or transform to a higher-grade malignancy, a change that typically is associated with the appearance of contrast enhancement on MRI. Resection or a biopsy may be necessary in these patients, followed by radiation therapy if they have not received it previously; chemotherapy with temozolomide (150 to 200 mg/m^2 for 5 days every 4 weeks for anywhere from 6 to 24 cycles) is also used. Patients with astrocytomas have a median survival of about 5 years.

Oligodendrogliomas

Oligodendrogliomas occur as low-grade tumors and, less commonly, as anaplastic lesions. Treatment of these tumors differs from that of their astrocytic counterparts, because oligodendrogliomas are uniquely chemosensitive, owing to their characteristic loss of chromosomes 1p and 19q. As with the low-grade astrocytomas, treatment should be withheld in patients with low-grade oligodendrogliomas who have no symptoms other than well-controlled seizures. Patients with progressive neurologic symptoms require treatment, and initial therapy is often chemotherapy, usually with single-agent temozolomide (150 to 200 mg/m^2 for 5 days every 4 weeks for 6 to 24 cycles) or the combination of procarbazine, lomustine, and vincristine. Radiation therapy is withheld until chemotherapy fails.

By comparison, all anaplastic oligodendrogliomas require immediate treatment. The standard approach includes focal radiation therapy. Adjuvant chemotherapy significantly prolongs disease-free survival but not overall survival time. 5 However, there is a growing movement toward treating high-grade tumors with chemotherapy alone and, in some cases, using high-dose chemotherapy with autologous stem cell rescue (Chapter 184). Some success has been reported with this approach, but it should still be considered experimental. Tumor progression should be treated with re-resection, radiation therapy if not previously administered, and additional chemotherapy. Patients with low-grade oligodendrogliomas have a median survival time in excess of 15 years, and those who have anaplastic oligodendrogliomas survive a median of 4 to 5 years.

Medulloblastomas

Medulloblastomas usually occur in the vermis of the cerebellum and principally affect children and young adults. Boys outnumber girls by about 2:1, and peak onset is at age 7 years; medulloblastoma in adulthood is rare and usually affects the cerebellar hemisphere.

The most common chromosomal abnormality associated with medulloblastoma is isochromosome 17q, which is found in as many as 60% of tumors. Tumors with an identical histology but different genetics may arise in the cerebral hemispheres and are called *primitive neuroectodermal tumors* (PNETs). PNETs usually have an aggressive course, leading to rapid death despite vigorous treatment.

Medulloblastomas have a characteristic clinical presentation, with ataxia (due to cerebellar and brain stem involvement) and headache, nausea, and vomiting (due to increased ICP from obstructive hydrocephalus). Aggressive surgery with complete excision is strongly associated with improved outcome. Surgery is always followed by neuraxis radiation therapy. Chemotherapy with vincristine, etoposide, carboplatin, and cyclophosphamide significantly improves 5-year event-free survival from 60 to 74% but has not significantly prolonged overall survival, which is about 70 to 80% at 5 years. This vigorous therapy often results in significant delayed complications in survivors, including intellectual deficits, growth impairment, and endocrinologic dysfunction.

Gangliogliomas

Gangliogliomas, as the name implies, possess both a glial component and a neoplastic neural component (ganglion cell). Some low-grade gangliogliomas are indolent and do not require additional treatment after surgical extirpation. Patients with anaplastic tumors may fare better than patients with malignant gliomas, but recurrence is the rule despite surgery and radiation therapy.

Primary Central Nervous System Lymphomas

Primary CNS lymphomas are associated with immunodeficiency states, particularly acquired immunodeficiency syndrome (Chapter 416) and organ transplantation, and are seen with increased frequency among the apparently immunocompetent population as well. Men are more frequently affected than women, and the median age at diagnosis is about 60 years. These tumors are usually large-cell, B-cell non-Hodgkin's lymphomas identical to systemic lymphoma. The tumor can involve the CSF, the eye, and the brain, where it is multifocal in about 40% of patients at presentation. In contrast to all other brain tumors, surgical resection is not associated with improved survival and can cause significant neurologic morbidity; therefore, biopsy, not resection, is the better surgical approach. Chemotherapy is the primary treatment, and high-dose methotrexate (3 to 8 g/m^2 on alternate weeks for 3 to 12 months) is the most important chemotherapeutic agent. In older patients, radiation therapy is avoided because the necessary whole brain irradiation causes significant cognitive impairment when combined with chemotherapy. Furthermore, radiation therapy alone produces a response but is followed by relapse within 1 year. Corticosteroids (e.g., dexamethasone 8 to 16 mg/day), which are frequently used as part of the chemotherapeutic regimen, not only help manage the associated cerebral edema, but also can cause tumor regression. With the use of multiagent chemotherapy, with or without cranial irradiation, median survival times are now in the 3- to 5-year range.

Other Intra-axial Tumors

Rare, intra-axial cerebral tumors include the *ependymoma*, which is optimally treated with surgical excision followed by radiation therapy. *Choroid plexus papillomas* and carcinomas may manifest with hydrocephalus or lateralizing signs. Resection may be sufficient for the benign papilloma, but carcinomas rapidly recur even when postoperative radiation therapy is also used. *Colloid cysts* of the third ventricle are benign tumors that can cause obstructive hydrocephalus; they may be treated with a ventricular peritoneal shunt or with resection using an intraventricular endoscope. *Hemangioblastomas* occur primarily in the cerebellum but can also occur in the spinal cord and the hemispheres. About 15% of patients with a hemangioblastoma have the autosomal dominant disorder, von Hippel–Lindau disease (Chapter 444), which is characterized by hemangioblastomas in the CNS and retina, renal cell carcinoma, pheochromocytoma, endolymphatic sac tumors, and cysts in a variety of visceral organs. Hemangioblastomas are treated by surgical excision and require radiation therapy only for recurrence. Complete removal usually results in cure.

Metastatic Tumors

Brain Metastases

Definition and Epidemiology

Every systemic cancer is capable of metastasizing to the brain. Melanoma (Chapter 214) has the greatest propensity to spread to the CNS, but the most common causes of CNS metastases are cancers of the breast (Chapter 208) and lung (Chapter 201), followed by cancers of the colon (Chapter 203) and kidney (Chapter 207). CNS metastases are being seen with greater frequency as patients with systemic cancers have prolonged survival with better treatments. In most patients with brain metastases, CNS disease develops late in the course of their illness, but a brain metastasis may be the initial presentation of a systemic cancer. In most of the latter patients, lung cancer is the primary site; in some, however, a primary site is never identified (Chapter 215).

Clinical Manifestations and Diagnosis

Patients with brain metastases present with progressive neurologic symptoms and signs that typically include headache, seizures, and lateralizing signs. Metastases are best diagnosed by a cranial MRI with gadolinium enhancement (Fig. 199–4). All lesions can be clearly seen by MRI, which is better than CT scanning for visualizing the posterior fossa. Metastases, which are usually well circumscribed lesions at the gray-white

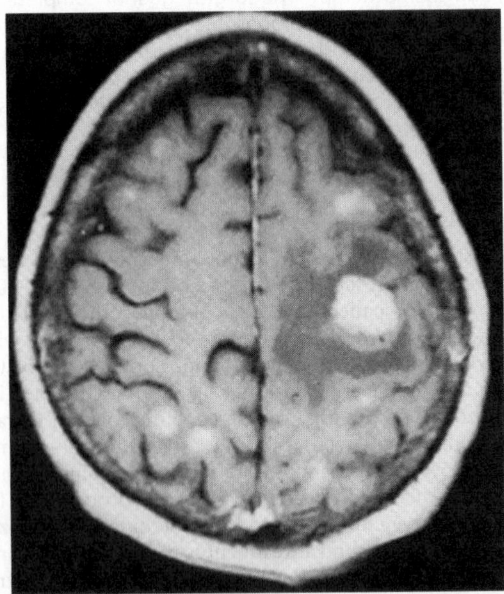

FIGURE 199–4 • Brain metastasis. Multiple metastases from breast carcinoma are seen on this T1 gadolinium-enhanced magnetic resonance imaging scan. The multiple smaller tumors were not visible on computed tomography, even after a contrast agent was given.

matter junction, are often associated with extensive edema. Hemorrhage into a metastasis occurs most frequently with metastases from melanoma, renal cancer, and thyroid cancer; however, because brain metastases from lung cancer are so common, they are the type most commonly associated with hemorrhage. Sometimes, hemorrhage into a brain metastasis is best visualized on a noncontrast head CT.

Treatment

Because brain metastases do not widely infiltrate into brain tissue and tend to have a pseudocapsule around them, they can be completely excised surgically. In randomized controlled studies, complete removal of a single brain metastasis substantially prolonged life and maintained neurologic function for a longer period. [6] Postoperative whole brain radiation therapy significantly improves control of CNS disease after resection of a single brain metastasis, but it does not prolong survival, [7] because patients die of progressive systemic tumor. Consequently, the use of postoperative whole brain radiation therapy is frequently decided on an individual basis. If multiple lesions can be completely resected, these patients do as well as those with a single lesion that has been removed.

Most patients with multiple brain metastases are best treated with a course of whole brain radiation therapy, most commonly 3 Gy in 10 fractions for a total of 30 Gy. Some patients with single brain metastasis are also treated with whole brain irradiation if they are in poor general condition, have uncontrolled systemic disease, or are not good candidates for surgical treatment.

Stereotactic radiosurgery, using either a gamma knife that delivers gamma radiation from multiple cobalt sources or a linear accelerator that delivers x-rays to a highly focused area involving the tumor, has been quite effective for the treatment of one or a few brain metastases. Most patients tolerate radiosurgery without difficulty, but occasionally the procedure is complicated by seizures or acute swelling that causes more neurologic dysfunction. Approximately 20 to 30% of patients develop radionecrosis, which may be indistinguishable clinically and on MRI from recurrent tumor. One advantage of stereotactic radiosurgery is that most of the normal brain is not exposed to the radiation.

Chemotherapy is used to treat brain metastases from only a few chemosensitive primary cancers such as choriocarcinoma, small cell lung cancer, and, to a lesser extent, breast cancer. Because few patients have a significant response to chemotherapy, it is usually used as a last resort. The oral agent, temozolomide (150 to 200 mg/m^2 for 5 days every 4 weeks), has shown some activity against brain metastases from lung cancer and is very well tolerated.

Leptomeningeal Metastases

The brain is the most common intracranial site of metastases, but systemic cancer can spread to the dura and the leptomeninges as well. Dural metastases most commonly arise from breast or prostate cancer, frequently from a metastasis in the overlying calvaria. Metastasis to the leptomeninges often manifests as multifocal neurologic symptoms and signs. These metastases involve the cranial nerves to cause diplopia or bulbar palsy; the cervical and lumbar roots to cause limb pain or weakness; and the intracranial space to cause headache, nausea, vomiting, and elevated ICP. The diagnosis is established by the presence of tumor cells in the CSF or by neuroimaging that definitively outlines tumor in the subarachnoid space (Fig. 199–5). Treatment frequently involves radiation therapy to symptomatic sites; intrathecal chemotherapy, usually through an intraventricular cannula (Ommaya reservoir); or systemic chemotherapy with agents at doses that penetrate into the CSF.

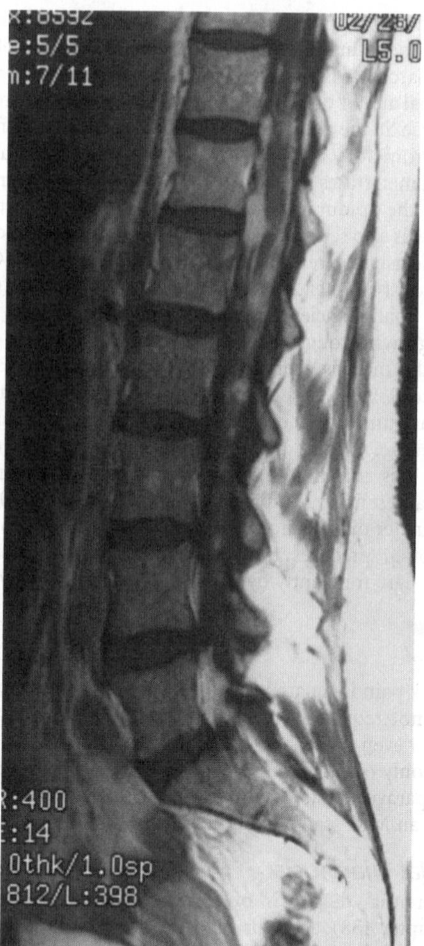

FIGURE 199–5 • Leptomeningeal metastases. Gadolinium-enhanced magnetic resonance imaging scan of the lumbosacral spine in a patient with leptomeningeal metastases from melanoma. Multiple enhancing nodules are seen on the cauda equina, and the conus medullaris and lower spinal cord are encased by tumor.

Spinal Tumors

Tumors involving the spine can be classified according to the anatomic area they involve: extradural, intradural extramedullary, and intramedullary tumors (Table 199–6). Extradural tumors typically arise from the bony elements of the spine and cause neurologic symptoms and signs by spinal cord compression. Intradural but extramedullary tumors arise from the pachymeninges or nerve roots (meningiomas or schwannomas), and they can cause either radicular symptoms or spinal cord compression. Intramedullary spinal cord tumors arise from the spinal cord parenchyma and have a biology similar to brain tumors. Intramedullary tumors are rare.

TABLE 199–6 SPINAL TUMORS

Extradural
Metastasis
Primary bone tumors arising in the spine
Intradural extramedullary
Meningiomas
Neurofibromas
Schwannomas
Lipomas
Arachnoid cysts
Epidermoid cysts
Metastasis
Intramedullary
Ependymoma
Glioma
Hemangioblastoma
Lipoma
Metastasis

Extradural Tumors

Epidemiology and Clinical Manifestations

Most extradural tumors originate from a metastasis to the bony elements of the spine, typically the vertebral body and occasionally the vertebral lamina or spinous process. Less common are primary tumors of the spine, including chordoma, osteogenic sarcoma, plasmacytoma, and chondrosarcoma. Expansile growth of the bone tumor impinges on the spinal canal and, if untreated, compresses the spinal cord or the nerve roots as they exit the intervertebral foramina. Whereas most of these lesions arise from bony metastases, extradural tumors can also arise from paravertebral metastases that can grow through the intervertebral foramina and into the epidural space; very rarely, a direct metastasis to the epidural space is also seen. The most common primary cancers that cause extradural metastases are prostate (Chapter 211), breast (Chapter 208), and lung cancer (Chapter 201), as well as the lymphomas (Chapter 196). Hematologic malignancies may also be associated with paravertebral disease that grows through the intervertebral foramina.

Whether the mass is a primary bone tumor or a metastasis from a distant source, 98% of patients present with pain that is usually local at the site of the tumor. Because there are more thoracic than cervical or lumbar vertebrae, the tumor and pain are likely to be in the middle or high back, a less common site for benign pain (Chapter 423). Motor impairment and sensory symptoms are present in about 50% of patients, whereas sphincter disturbances are found in only about 25% of patients. Back pain often precedes the development of any other neurologic symptom or sign, frequently by weeks and occasionally by months.

Diagnosis

Severe back pain in a patient with cancer should be evaluated by MRI, which does not require intravenous contrast. Plain films of the spine, bone scans, or even CT scans may show bony disease, but epidural tumor can be seen only on MRI. Furthermore, MRI is the only technique that can reveal paravertebral or direct epidural metastasis. Patients who cannot have an MRI scan should be imaged by CT myelography.

Differential Diagnosis

The differential diagnosis of extradural tumors includes epidural abscess (Chapter 438), acute or subacute epidural hematomas (Chapter 423), herniated intervertebral discs (Chapter 423), spondylosis (Chapter 423), epidural lipomatosis, and, rarely, extramedullary hematopoiesis. Occasionally, a percutaneous needle biopsy or decompressive laminectomy is required to make a definitive diagnosis.

Treatment

Rx

Extradural metastases require immediate treatment, because patients can develop acute and unpredictable neurologic deterioration resulting in paraplegia. Patients should be started on high-dose corticosteroids, usually 100 mg IV dexamethasone, which rapidly relieves pain and may contribute to neurologic recovery. Surgery followed by postoperative radiation therapy is superior to radiotherapy alone in preserving the ability to walk [8] and may prolong survival in a wide population of patients with metastatic spinal cord compression. It is much easier to preserve neurologic function than to reverse impairment, so clinically silent areas of extradural tumor that are detected on MRI should be treated before neurologic compromise develops. Patients whose primary tumor arises in the spine, such as an osteogenic sarcoma (Chapter 212), should undergo definitive surgery; the need for postoperative radiation therapy is determined on the basis of the tumor's histology. Patients with extradural metastases can have a good neurologic outcome if treated before the onset of severe neurologic compromise, but their overall survival is usually short due to the presence of widespread metastatic disease.

Intradural Extramedullary Tumors

Meningiomas

Most intradural extramedullary tumors are benign. Meningiomas are benign, slow-growing tumors that occur primarily in middle-aged women and are predominantly located in the thoracic region. Back pain is a common symptom, but about 25% of patients have no pain and present with slowly progressive neurologic dysfunction, typically a gait disorder that has been slowly progressing, frequently for years. Spinal MRI with gadolinium clearly delineates the lesion. Surgical resection is curative, and a complete resection can usually be accomplished easily.

Nerve Sheath Tumors

Nerve sheath tumors include schwannomas and neurofibromas. Both typically arise from the dorsal root, and the first symptom is often radicular pain that precedes symptoms of spinal cord compression by months or even years. Some patients with spinal neurofibroma or schwannoma have neurofibromatosis type 1 (Chapter 444), but the majority do not. The diagnosis is clearly established by gadolinium-enhanced MRI of the spine. The treatment is surgical, and complete removal results in cure.

Metastases

Metastasis to the spinal leptomeninges can manifest as an intradural extramedullary lesion. A single large tumor nodule can cause focal symptoms and signs referable to that spinal level, but in most patients multiple levels of the neuraxis are involved, causing multifocal neurologic symptoms and signs. Cervical and lumbosacral radicular pain, as well as sensory and motor loss, is seen in more than half of patients. The diagnosis is established by gadolinium-enhanced MRI showing multifocal nodules or sometimes a layer of cells coating the spinal cord or nerve roots (see Fig. 199–5). If imaging is negative, the diagnosis can be established by demonstrating tumor cells in the CSF. Treatment is complicated and frequently requires radiation therapy to symptomatic sites of disease, intrathecal chemotherapy best administered through an intraventricular cannula (Ommaya device), and occasionally systemic chemotherapy. Radiation therapy can ameliorate neurologic symptoms, particularly pain, but the disease often has a relentless progressive course, resulting in death in 3 to 6 months despite aggressive therapy. Because of the diffuse nature of the disease, surgery is not an option.

Intramedullary Tumors

Intramedullary spinal cord tumors are similar to neoplasms that arise in brain parenchyma. The most common spinal cord tumors are ependymomas and astrocytomas; hemangioblastomas (particularly in association with von Hippel–Lindau disease; Chapter 444), lipomas, and, rarely, intramedullary metastases are also seen.

Clinical Manifestations and Diagnosis

All intramedullary tumors have a similar clinical presentation, and pain is a common initial symptom. Signs of spinal cord dysfunction subsequently ensue and reflect the location of the lesion. In addition, some intramedullary tumors are accompanied by a syrinx (Chapter 444), which can also contribute to symptoms. The classic signs of intramedullary spinal cord lesions, such as dissociated sensory loss, sacral sparing, and early sphincter problems, are not sufficiently reliable to distinguish intramedullary from extramedullary lesions on the basis of clinical findings. The diagnosis is established by gadolinium-enhanced MRI.

Treatment

Rx

Surgery is the first therapeutic intervention, both to obtain a definitive diagnosis and to resect the lesion. Complete resection of spinal cord tumors is possible, particularly in the case of ependymomas and hemangioblastomas. However, spinal cord tumors are rare, and only neurosurgeons experienced in removal of this type of lesion should perform the procedure. High-grade gliomas and residual ependymomas should be treated with postoperative radiation therapy. Low-grade astrocytomas of the spinal cord can be treated with radiation therapy when the patient develops symptomatic neurologic impairment, but presymptomatic treatment does not prevent the development of impairment nor necessarily delay it. Intramedullary metastases do not require surgery, because the diagnosis is usually straightforward; radiation therapy provides limited benefit, because these patients typically have other CNS metastases.

INTRACRANIAL HYPERTENSION AND HYPOTENSION

CSF is made, in part, by the choroid plexus in the ventricular system; newly formed fluid circulates out the foramina of Luschka and Magendie, at the bottom of the fourth ventricle, to surround the entire spinal cord and cerebrum. It is reabsorbed back into the circulation through the arachnoid granulations over the convexities. Balance between CSF pro-

TABLE 199–7 SYMPTOMS AND SIGNS OF INTRACRANIAL HYPERTENSION

COMMON
Headache
Tinnitus
Vomiting (with or without nausea)
Visual obscurations, visual loss, photopsias
Papilledema
Diplopia
Lethargy and increased sleep
Psychomotor retardation
Pain on eye movement
LESS COMMON
Hearing distortion or loss
Vertigo
Facial weakness
Shoulder or arm pain
Neck pain or rigidity
Ataxia
Paresthesias of extremities
Anosmia
Trigeminal neuralgia

duction and reabsorption keeps the volume relatively constant at about 150 mL in the normal healthy adult. CSF is produced at a rate of roughly 20 mL/hour, implying that the entire volume of CSF is replaced three to four times each day. CSF circulates nutrients to the nervous system and removes waste products from the only organ in the body that lacks a lymphatic system. In addition, CSF performs an important mechanical function by absorbing shock to the brain and spinal cord, cushioning them from the bony surroundings of the skull and spine.

A lumbar puncture provides the opportunity, not only for sampling the CSF composition to detect disease processes, but also for measuring ICP. CSF pressure is normally maintained between 70 and 195 mm H_2O. ICP is maintained within this narrow window because significant fluctuations, either up or down, can cause marked neurologic dysfunction.

Intracranial Hypertension

Elevated ICP causes symptoms by compressing neural tissue, a process that causes ischemia and sometimes hemorrhage due to associated arterial and venous compression. ICP is partially maintained through the autoregulatory mechanisms of the cerebral blood vessels. Low ICP is caused by diminished CSF volume, and symptoms result from the loss of buoyancy of the brain as it floats within the CSF liquid. Pulling or stretching of the dura and cortical veins, which are the pain-sensitive structures in the cranial vault, causes headache; compensatory vasodilation may also contribute to headache.

The principal symptoms and signs associated with increased ICP are headache, nausea, vomiting, and lethargy; other symptoms are less frequent (Table 199–7). Focal mass lesions that cause a herniation syndrome may produce lateralizing signs such as hemiparesis; by comparison, diffuse elevation of ICP, as in communicating hydrocephalus, rarely does. Three main herniation syndromes are (1) herniation of the medial frontal gyrus under the falx; (2) transtentorial herniation of the uncus, pushing the diencephalon and the brain stem downward and laterally; and (3) herniation of the cerebellar tonsils through the foramen magnum. Generalized increased ICP may be due to obstruction of CSF, which may be caused by blockage of the ventricular system (obstructive or noncommunicating hydrocephalus) or by impairment of CSF reabsorption (nonobstructive or communicating hydrocephalus).

Increased ICP of any cause may produce pressure or plateau waves (episodic increases in ICP), leading to transient symptoms such as headache, vertigo, or diminished consciousness. Plateau waves occur normally and are associated with symptoms only when the baseline ICP is elevated. Plateau waves may be precipitated by a change in body position.

TABLE 199–8 CAUSES OF HYDROCEPHALUS

ACUTE
Cerebellar hemorrhage/infarction
Colloid cyst of the third ventricle
Exudative meningitis
Head trauma
Intracranial tumor or hematoma
Spontaneous subarachnoid hemorrhage
Viral encephalitis
CHRONIC
Aqueductal stenosis
Ectasia and elongation of the basilar artery (rare)
Granulomatous meningitis
Head trauma
Hindbrain malformations
Leptomeningeal metastasis
Brain and spinal cord tumors
Spontaneous subarachnoid hemorrhage

Hydrocephalus

Hydrocephalus refers to ventricular dilation caused by accumulated CSF. Hydrocephalus can be acute, resulting from sudden blockage of CSF outflow, or chronic, developing slowly over many months to years (Table 199–8). Patients with chronic hydrocephalus sometimes have normal CSF pressures, whereas those with acute hydrocephalus always have elevated CSF pressure.

Clinical Manifestations

Acute hydrocephalus usually manifests with severe headache, lethargy, nausea, vomiting, papilledema, and diplopia from abducens palsy as well as signs from the causative lesion. Diffuse hyperreflexia and bilateral Babinski's signs are common. Patients with chronic communicating hydrocephalus often have normal CSF pressure, so-called normal pressure hydrocephalus (NPH), and may present with progressive dementia characterized by memory loss and psychomotor retardation, an unsteady gait, and urgency incontinence (Chapter 425). Some patients have features of parkinsonism (Chapter 433) because of the bradykinesia and psychomotor retardation associated with hydrocephalus, but resting tremor is absent.

Diagnosis

Ventriculomegaly is readily diagnosed by MRI or CT scan. In older patients, cerebral atrophy and the associated compensating increase in ventricular volume that accompanies normal aging (hydrocephalus ex vacuo) must be considered. Periventricular hyperintensity on T2-weighted or FLAIR MR images may help separate patients with NPH from those with hydrocephalus ex vacuo. MRI is the best test to identify a cause of hydrocephalus.

Treatment

Rx

If the ICP approaches or exceeds the systolic blood pressure, the cerebral perfusion pressure decreases and ischemia develops. Marked elevation of ICP is a neurologic emergency that requires immediate intervention (Table 199–9) to reduce the volume of the intracranial contents and to prevent permanent brain damage. Hyperventilation to lower the arterial partial pressure of carbon dioxide ($Paco_2$) to 25 to 30 mm Hg causes immediate vasoconstriction, which reduces cerebral blood volume. Intravenous mannitol or hypertonic saline can cause a rapid diuresis, which reduces intravascular plasma volume and helps to withdraw water from the extracellular space in the brain. Glucocorticoids, typically as

TABLE 199–9 EMERGENCY TREATMENT OF ELEVATED INTRACRANIAL PRESSURE IN ACUTELY DECOMPENSATING PATIENTS

Therapy	Treatment	Onset (Duration of Action)	Other
Hyperventilation	Lower Pa_{CO_2} to 25–30 mm Hg	Seconds (minutes)	Usually requires intubation and mechanical ventilation
Osmotherapy	Mannitol 0.5–2 g/kg IV, repeat as necessary	Minutes (hours)	Brisk diuresis Requires Foley catheter Strict attention to electrolytes
Corticosteroids	Dexamethasone 50–100 mg IV, followed by 50–100 mg/day in divided doses	Hours (days)	Most effective on vasogenic edema (tumors, abscesses) Less effective on cytotoxic edema (stroke)

Pa_{CO_2}, arterial partial pressure of carbon dioxide.

Rx

dexamethasone 50 to 100 mg by IV bolus, will require hours to reduce underlying edema; vasogenic edema from brain tumor or brain abscess responds rapidly to corticosteroids, but cytotoxic edema accompanying an acute ischemic stroke or hematoma seldom responds to corticosteroids.

Ultimately, however, definitive treatment of the specific cause is necessary. If such treatment is not immediately feasible, hydrocephalus often responds promptly to ventricular drainage. If temporary drainage is necessary, an external ventricular drain can be placed until the underlying obstruction is relieved. A ventriculoperitoneal shunt is the definitive treatment for chronic hydrocephalus, but it is not reliably effective for "idiopathic" NPH. The clinical response to several days of external lumbar CSF drainage has a high predictive value for determining which patients with NPH are likely to benefit from a shunt. Complications of shunting include subdural hematomas and infection.

Idiopathic Intracranial Hypertension

Definition and Epidemiology

Idiopathic intracranial hypertension, also called benign intracranial hypertension or pseudotumor cerebri, refers to elevated ICP that develops in an otherwise healthy individual without evidence of a structural CNS abnormality. Most patients are obese young women, but the disorder can also occur in men, thin patients, older adults, and children. Idiopathic intracranial hypertension can be associated with a variety of systemic disorders and medications (Table 199–10), but the direct cause of ICP elevation is usually unknown. Chronic elevations of ICP can lead to the "empty sella syndrome" (Chapter 242), which refers to enlargement of the sella turcica due to an incompetent diaphragma sellae, leading to CT or MRI evidence of CSF in the sella; the result is a compressed but functioning pituitary gland.

Clinical Manifestations

Patients usually present with headache that may be accompanied by visual disturbances, including visual loss, nausea, vomiting, diplopia, tinnitus, and vertigo. Examination is notable for bilateral papilledema in an otherwise healthy patient. Loss of vision, which is the most feared complication, is uncommon. Visual fields typically reveal an enlarged blind spot due to the papilledema, but no other visual impairment. Diplopia can occur from an abducens palsy as a false localizing sign.

Diagnosis

The diagnosis is established by excluding any structural cause of elevated ICP by MRI. Magnetic resonance venography (MRV) also should be performed to exclude dural venous sinus thrombosis or stenosis. Lumbar puncture is performed after neuroimaging and is required to confirm the diagnosis by establishing an elevated opening pressure,

TABLE 199–10 SYSTEMIC AND IATROGENIC CONDITIONS ASSOCIATED WITH BENIGN INTRACRANIAL HYPERTENSION

COMMONLY PRESCRIBED DRUGS
Nalidixic acid
Nitrofurantoin
Phenytoin
Sulfonamides
Tetracycline
Vitamin A
Retinoic acid (*cis* or *trans*)
ENDOCRINE AND METABOLIC DISORDERS
Addison's disease
Cushing's syndrome
Hypoparathyroidism
Menarche, pregnancy, oral contraceptives
Obesity (often associated with irregular menses)
Corticosteroid therapy or withdrawal
HEMATOLOGIC DISORDERS
Cryoglobulinemia
Iron deficiency anemia
MISCELLANEOUS DISORDERS
Dural venous sinus obstruction or thrombosis
Head trauma
Internal jugular vein ligation
Systemic lupus erythematosus
Middle ear disease

frequently greater than 300 mm H_2O; however, the composition of the fluid is normal, and the protein concentration is typically in the low-normal range (<20 mg/dL).

Treatment

Rx

The need to treat chronic intractable elevation of ICP is based on the patient's symptoms and serial visual field testing. Headache or new or progressive visual loss on eye examination or perimetry testing should trigger one or more of five treatments: (1) weight reduction (e.g., 20 lb), and/or correction of underlying endocrinologic or hematologic disorders; (2) repeated lumbar punctures; (3) acute pharmacologic treatments, including corticosteroids, loop diuretics, and acetazolamide, although corticosteroids can contribute to weight gain and their tapering may exacerbate the syndrome; (4) ventriculoperitoneal or lumboperitoneal shunt; and (5) fenestration of the optic nerve sheath, especially for patients with persistently elevated ICP and deteriorating vision.

TABLE 199–11 CAUSES OF INTRACRANIAL HYPOTENSION

Postlumbar puncture
CSF leak following CNS surgery or trauma
CSF fistula
Post-thoracotomy leak into pleural space
Spontaneous/idiopathic dural tear

CNS = central nervous system; CSF = cerebrospinal fluid.

Prognosis

Outcome is variable: spontaneous remissions may occur; clinical improvement is not always accompanied by a reduction in CSF pressure; and the CSF pressure may remain persistently elevated despite intervention. Furthermore, patients with chronically elevated ICP from idiopathic intracranial hypertension never develop hydrocephalus, so CSF pressure and ventriculomegaly are not linked.

Intracranial Hypotension

Intracranial hypotension occurs most commonly after lumbar puncture or after an idiopathic tear of the spinal dura. Evidence suggests that new "atraumatic" needles, as well as smaller-bore needles and few passes of the needle to perform the lumbar puncture, are associated with a lower incidence of postspinal headache.

Clinical Manifestations and Diagnosis

Low CSF pressure (Table 199–11) can cause clinical symptoms that are usually mild but occasionally severe and debilitating. Postural headaches occur within 30 seconds after assuming the erect posture and subside completely when the patient lies flat (Chapter 421). The headaches, which are usually bifrontal or occipital, are typically severe, generalized, and throbbing. Headaches may be accompanied by nausea, dizziness, photophobia, neck stiffness, and, rarely, an abducens nerve palsy. All symptoms are relieved when the patient lies down.

Treatment and Prognosis

Rx

In most patients, symptoms resolve spontaneously and can be treated with simple analgesics. Some patients develop persistent, symptomatic intracranial hypotension that does not respond to simple measures.

In patients whose symptoms are persistent or disabling, an epidural blood patch is performed by injecting approximately 10 mL of the patient's own blood into the epidural space to seal the presumed dural leak. Occasionally, CSF radioisotope studies must be performed to identify the site of the leak so that surgical repair of the dura can be performed.

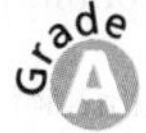

1. Forsyth PA, Weaver S, Fulton D, et al: Prophylactic anticonvulsants in patients with brain tumour. Can J Neurol Sci 2003;30:106–112.
2. Glantz MJ, Cole BF, Forsyth PA, et al: Practice parameter: Anticonvulsant prophylaxis in patients with newly diagnosed brain tumors. Report of The Quality Standards Subcommittee of The American Academy of Neurology. Neurology 2000;54:1886–1893.
3. Stupp R, Mason WP, van den Bent MJ, et al: Radiotherapy plus concomitant and adjuvant temozolomide for glioblastoma. N Engl J Med 2005;352:987–996.
4. Karim AB, Afra D, Cornu P, et al: Randomized trial on the efficacy of radiotherapy for cerebral low grade glioma in the adult. Int J Radiat Oncol Biol Phys 2002;52:316–324.
5. Cairncross G, Berkey B, Shaw E, et al: Phase III trial of chemotherapy plus radiotherapy compared with radiotherapy alone for pure and mixed anaplastic oligodendroglioma: Intergroup Radiation Therapy Oncology Group Trial 9402. J Clin Oncol 2006;24: 2707–2714.
6. Patchell RA, Tibbs PA, Walsh JW, et al: A randomized trial of surgery in the treatment of single metastases to the brain. N Engl J Med 1990;322:494–500.
7. Aoyama H, Shirato H, Tago M, et al: Stereotactic radiosurgery plus whole-brain radiation therapy vs stereotactic radiosurgery alone for treatment of brain metastases: A randomized controlled trial. JAMA 2006;295:2483–2491.
8. Patchell RA, Tibbs, PA, Regine WF, et al: Direct decompressive surgical resection in the treatment of spinal cord compression caused by metastatic cancer: A randomised trial. Lancet 2005;366:643–648.

SUGGESTED READINGS

Behin A, Hoang-Xuan K, Carpentier AF, et al: Primary brain tumours in adults. Lancet 2003;361:323–331. *Overview of genetics, diagnosis, and treatment.*

Khuntia D, Brown P, Li J, et al: Whole-brain radiotherapy in the management of brain metastasis. J Clin Oncol 2006;24:1295–1304. *A comprehensive review.*

Loblaw DA, Perry J, Chambers A, et al: Systematic review of the diagnosis and management of malignant extradural spinal cord compression: The Cancer Care Ontario Practice Guidelines Initiative's Neuro-Oncology Disease Site Group. J Clin Oncol 2005;23:2028–2037. *Literature-based recommendations.*

Schievink WI: Spontaneous spinal cerebrospinal fluid leaks and intracranial hypotension. JAMA 2006;295:2286–2296. *Spontaneous intracranial hypotension remains underdiagnosed.*

Vogelbaum MA, Suh JH: Resectable brain metastases. J Clin Oncol 2006;24:1289–1294. *Review of the surgical literature.*

Whittle IR, Smith C, Navoo P, et al: Meningiomas. Lancet 2004;363:1535–1543. *A comprehensive review.*

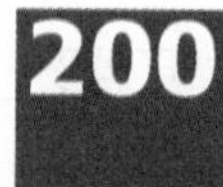

200 HEAD AND NECK CANCER

Marshall Posner

Definition

The principal cancers of the head and neck include squamous cell cancers arising from the mucosal surfaces of the upper aerodigestive tract and a diverse group of salivary gland neoplasms. Unique cancers of the region include nasopharyngeal carcinoma, thyroid malignancies (Chapter 244), esthesioneuroblastoma, and sinonasal undifferentiated carcinoma. A variety of other cancers arise from structures and tissues in the head and neck, including the more common skin cancers (Chapter 214), lymphomas (Chapters 196 and 197), and sarcomas.

Epidemiology

Squamous cell carcinomas account for 95% of all malignancies of the head and neck, whereas salivary gland cancers represent nearly all of the remaining 5%. Approximately 40,000 cases of squamous cell carcinoma of the head and neck occur in the United States each year, or about 4% of all malignancies in the country. The incidence is declining slightly, but the decline has not mirrored the decline in the use of tobacco. Approximately 13,000 deaths are directly attributable each year to squamous cell carcinoma of the head and neck, and the peak incidence occurs between 55 and 65 years of age, although some individuals are in their mid-40s or younger. The disease is about three times more common in men than in women.

The mucosal surfaces of the head and neck are divided into six anatomic regions: the oral cavity, oropharynx, hypopharynx, larynx, nasopharynx, and paranasal sinuses. The site of anatomic origin for a squamous cell carcinoma of the head and neck has important, albeit imperfect implications for diagnosis, spread, prognosis, and treatment because of intrinsic biologic differences in the mucosal cells at the sites of origin, as well as differences in lymphatic drainage patterns and proximity to other structures in this compact region.

Oral Cavity

The oral cavity includes the floor of the mouth, anterior or oral aspect of the tongue, lips, buccal surfaces, hard palate, retromolar trigone, and gums. The oral cavity is easily appreciable by physical examination, and thus tumors in this area can frequently be detected early in their course. Tumors of the oral cavity, which are strongly related to the use of smokeless tobacco and other oral tobacco products (Chapter 30), appear on the buccal and gingival surfaces in the sites where tobacco products are held in contact with the mucosa for long periods. Anterior tongue cancers are more common in smokers. Lip cancers are particularly prevalent in transplant patients and can be caused by DNA damage from solar ultraviolet light.

Oropharynx

The oropharynx consists of the tongue from the midtongue posteriorly to the epiglottis, the tonsils, the associated pharyngeal walls, and the soft palate. The oropharynx has become the most common location for head and neck tumors in the United States and is a common site of origin in Europe. Tumors in this anatomic region are associated with human papillomavirus (HPV), especially in younger, nonsmoking patients.

Hypopharynx

The hypopharynx comprises the piriform sinuses, the lateral and posterior pharyngeal walls, and the posterior surfaces of the larynx. These structures surround the larynx posteriorly and laterally. Tumors in this region can be difficult to detect because of the recesses and spaces surrounding the larynx. As a result, primary hypopharyngeal tumors may be asymptomatic and, like oropharyngeal tumors, may initially be recognized in an advanced state or diagnosed as an "unknown primary" (Chapter 215). These tumors are associated with tobacco (Chapter 30) and alcohol (Chapter 31) use.

Larynx

The larynx includes the vocal cords, the subglottis, and the supraglottic larynx, as well as the thyroid, cricoid, and arytenoid cartilages. The supraglottic larynx is composed of several structures, including the epiglottis, the surrounding aryepiglottic folds, and the false vocal folds. Tumors arising in the true vocal cords are frequently symptomatic early and rarely spread beyond the confines of the larynx, whereas subglottic and supraglottic cancers can be relatively asymptomatic and have a much higher and earlier risk of spread to the lymphatics and regional sites. Laryngeal cancers are strongly associated with smoking (Chapter 30).

Nasopharynx

The nasopharynx includes the mucosal surfaces and structures of the cavity behind the nasal passages. Nasopharyngeal cancers are common in the Pacific Rim, northern Africa, and the Middle East. In some areas of China and Southeast Asia, nasopharyngeal cancers occur with a frequency that rivals lung cancer. In North America, there are about 2000 cases each year, but numbers are increasing as high-risk ethnic populations settle in North America. Nasopharyngeal cancers are frequently associated with the presence of latent infection of the epithelial tumor cells by Epstein-Barr virus (EBV), the etiologic agent of infectious mononucleosis (Chapter 400). Nasopharyngeal cancers are also associated with both environmental and genetic factors in susceptible populations that have migrated to North America and remain at high risk for this disease. Unlike other squamous cell carcinomas of the head and neck, nasopharyngeal cancers can occur at an early age, with a distinct peak in adolescence and young adulthood. Nasopharyngeal cancers are categorized into three histologic subtypes by the World Health Organization (WHO): the undifferentiated (WHO III) and nonkeratinizing forms (WHO II) are latently infected with EBV in 95% of cases and represent the majority of cases in North America and worldwide; the well-differentiated (WHO I) form is rarer and represents about 5% worldwide but about 15 to 25% of all nasopharyngeal cancers in North America, and it is usually associated with traditional risk factors such as smoking. Nasopharyngeal cancers have a high risk for early regional lymph node involvement, a prolonged natural history, and a very high risk of spread to distant sites.

Paranasal Sinuses

The paranasal sinuses comprise the maxillary, ethmoid, sphenoid, and frontal sinuses, as well as the nasal cavity. These are relatively rare locations for tumors of the head and neck in North America, but there is an unexplained higher rate of malignant sinus disease among the Japanese. Squamous maxillary sinus cancers are more common in smokers. Up to 50% of cancers of the sinuses may be of salivary gland origin, often related to exposure to dust from woodworking, tanning, or leather working (Chapter 17). Occasionally, neuroendocrine tumors (including esthesioneuroblastoma, a neuroendocrine sarcoma derived from olfactory neural tissue) and the rare sinonasal undifferentiated carcinoma are found. Sinus cancers are frequently diagnosed late in their course at the time of symptomatic invasion of surrounding structures, including the orbit, nasal cavity, base of the skull, and cranial nerves.

Salivary Glands

Salivary glands occur in all the regions described, as well as in the trachea and esophagus. Tumors can develop in all of the major and minor salivary glands with an incidence that is roughly proportional to the quantity of glandular tissue. The most common single site is the parotid. Although tumors can develop at any age, including childhood, the peak incidence is between 55 and 65 years of age. Salivary gland cancers have diverse histologic findings and manifest different behavior based on their histologic classification. A substantial fraction of parotid salivary tumors can be benign. Among malignant tumors, the three most common histologic types are adenoid cystic carcinoma, mucoepidermoid cancer, and adenocarcinoma. Rare types include acinic cell carcinoma, salivary duct cancer, carcinoma ex pleomorphic adenoma, and squamous cell cancer. Risk factors for salivary gland cancers are poorly understood, but previous radiation therapy in adjacent areas increases the risk (Chapter 18).

Pathobiology

Tobacco products and alcohol are the most important etiologic and risk factors for squamous cell carcinoma of the head and neck, and both show a clear dose response. Any irritating smoked product increases the risk for local cancer, but nicotine in tobacco, as well as in other tobacco leaf components, directly affects the oral mucosa and increases the risk for squamous cancer (Chapter 30). Alcohol is also a carcinogen, and alcohol consumption (Chapter 31), as well as its direct application in mouthwashes, is associated with an increased risk. Moreover, alcohol affects local and systemic detoxification enzymes and may increase the carcinogenic potential of other environmental carcinogens. Other environmental risk factors include radiation exposure and solar radiation; welding, metal refining, diesel exhaust, wood stove, and asbestos exposure; chronic irritants; vitamin A deficiency; and immunosuppression. About 25% of patients have no or only minimal exposure to any risk factors.

Pathogenic HPV subtypes, particularly HPV-16, independently account for approximately 50% of oropharyngeal cancer. Nasopharyngeal cancer is predominantly associated with keratinocyte infection with EBV (Chapter 400). The classic nasopharyngeal cancer, which is also called lymphoepithelioma, is associated with a brisk lymphoid infiltrate that can be confused with a lymphoma. Careful examination reveals the malignant epithelial cells in the tumor. EBV is associated with the early development of dysplasia of the nasopharynx and has been linked to the earliest events in neoplastic transformation in nasopharyngeal cancer. EBV is also rarely associated with epithelial tumors of the oropharynx, tonsil, and salivary gland.

Several inherited diseases and genetic abnormalities are associated with the development of head and neck cancer. Fanconi's anemia (Chapter 171), a rare disorder of a family of related gene products, has been linked to the development of tongue cancer, as has Cowden's syndrome (Chapter 186), which is associated with mutation of the *PTEN* gene. Finally, common inherited allelic variants of the alcohol dehydrogenase and P-450 genes (Chapter 186) may be associated with increased susceptibility to alcohol and other environmental carcinogens.

The development of squamous cell carcinoma of the head and neck is a multistep process in which early genetic changes evolve into frank malignancy. An abnormal premalignant clone of mucosal cells may be localized to a single site within the head and neck, or clones may occur independently in many sites. Clones can also spread from a single site and evolve at other sites within the head and neck to form distinct, but related tumors. Consequently, in about 20% of patients a second primary can develop in the upper aerodigestive tract, most commonly in the head and neck, lung, and esophagus; 5% of patients are initially seen with a synchronous second primary. Tumors frequently show similar genetic alterations as the original primary, thus providing further evidence for the phenomenon of field cancerization. Early changes in mucosal keratinocytes involve genetic damage manifested by aneuploidy and alterations in critical molecular pathways. The cell cycle is dysregulated by the early loss of p16, an inhibitor of cyclin D1, or by upregulation of cyclin

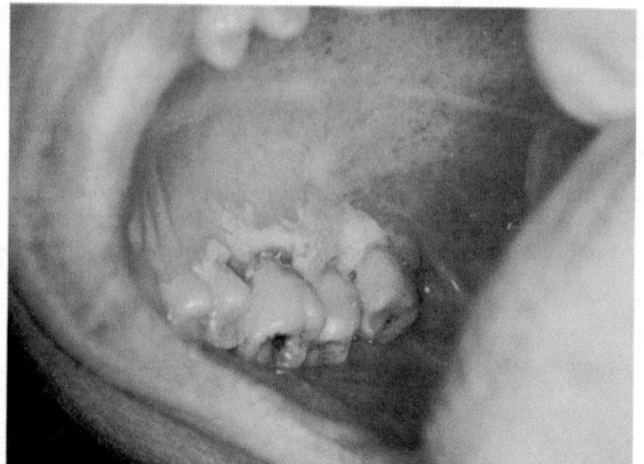

FIGURE 200–1 • Oral leukoplakia.

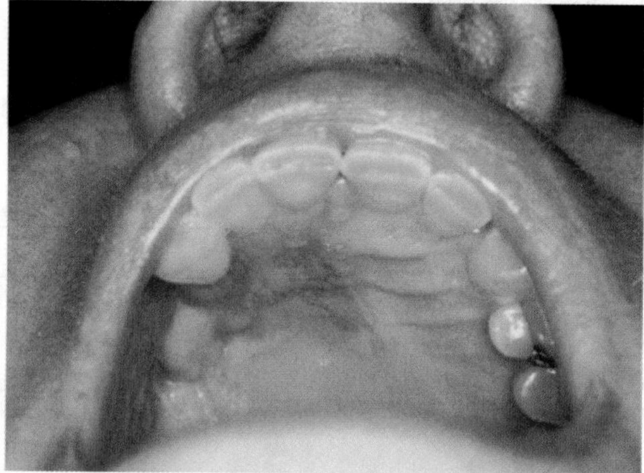

FIGURE 200–2 • Oral erythroplakia.

D1; p53 is disabled through a number of mechanisms preventing programmed cell death; mitogenic signaling is enhanced by upregulation of epidermal growth factor (EGF) receptor function; cyclooxygenase-2 is overexpressed, thereby inhibiting apoptosis and promoting angiogenesis; and chromosomal instability with aneuploidy develops. Many of these early molecular and functional changes occur without obvious alteration in the physical appearance of the oral mucosa, although leukoplakia can occur. Many of these early changes have become targets for novel therapeutics, and molecular changes can be monitored in response to treatment.

Oral premalignancy, which includes leukoplakia and erythroplakia, is a dysplastic state that carries a high risk for the development of squamous cell carcinoma of the head and neck. Leukoplakia (Fig. 200–1), which is diagnosed clinically as a white patch of mucosal tissue in the oral mucosa or larynx, progresses to cancer over a period of several years in approximately 30% of patients; it is most likely to progress when associated with aneuploidy. Erythroplakia (Fig. 200–2), which is a red hyperkeratotic change in the mucosa, is an advanced premalignant lesion with a high rate of aneuploidy and an approximately 60% rate of progression to oral cancer. Unfortunately, surgical resection of leukoplakia or erythroplakia has no effect on the subsequent development of invasive cancer.

There is no proven chemopreventive therapy for persons with oral premalignant lesions. Vitamin A, β-carotene, and vitamin E are all ineffective or harmful. Because continued smoking or alcohol consumption increases the risk for recurrence and second primaries dramatically, patients with prior cancers should stop alcohol and tobacco use.

Patients with a history of squamous cell carcinoma of the head and neck are more at risk for local and regional recurrence and persistent disease than for distant metastases. In addition, although the physical growth rate of tumors may appear to be slow, the cells within the tumor mass double rapidly. If all the cycling tumor cells survived and remained active, the tumors would have the potential to double every 48 hours. Most early tumors have a high rate of cell loss from apoptosis, senescence, differentiation, and inactivation; as a result, tumors may fluctuate in size early in their course. Once therapy is instituted, however, the surviving cells have an increased capacity to grow and repopulate, with less cell loss and more rapid clinical growth. Therefore, curative therapy should be continuous, brisk, and without interruption.

Clinical Manifestations

The symptoms and clinical manifestations of tumors in the head and neck can vary broadly and are related to the structures at the site of the primary tumor, as well as regional lymph node drainage. Small tumors can be easily appreciated because of physical self-discovery or early compromise of the function of a critical structure. As a result of the propensity for squamous cell carcinoma of the head and neck to remain a local and regional disease, it is unusual for this cancer to be associated with abnormalities outside the head and neck. Salivary gland malignancies are less constrained and frequently spread distantly; however, because the primary tumors are also frequently accessible to direct physical examination and discovery, it is still uncommon to identify these tumors as a result of metastatic spread outside the region.

Clinical manifestations of *tumors in the oral cavity* include a painless lump, a painful mass or ulcer, or simple thickening of the mucosa. Small lesions in the lateral aspect of the tongue and the floor of mouth can cause pain referred to the mandible, gums, and ear because of the shared sensory nerves supplying these areas. These symptoms can lead to unnecessary dental procedures or repeated courses of antibiotics if the tumor is not apparent on examination. Antibiotics can relieve symptoms and even reduce the size of a tumor or lymph nodes when superficial infection and inflammation are contributing to the pain; however, recurrent or continued pain in an adult should trigger suspicion about more ominous disease. Speech may be affected late if the tumor causes restricted tongue motion or cranial nerve XII dysfunction. Gingival tumors can loosen teeth and invade the mandible along tooth sockets. Tumors originating in minor salivary glands of the oral cavity are submucosal and less prone to ulceration.

In true vocal cord cancer, hoarseness and other forms of voice change are common and expected early symptoms, but they may be later manifestations of *supraglottic and subglottic laryngeal tumors,* which become relatively large without affecting the voice. Tumors of the piriform sinus can affect voice when they become large, impair the recurrent laryngeal nerve, or are associated with deep local invasion; pain in the ear or pain on swallowing referred to the ear is also a common and important feature of these tumors. Adults with ear pain or persistent hoarseness should be referred to an otolaryngologist for evaluation. Because this posterior area is difficult to assess, primary tumors are frequently missed in routine office examinations. *Tumors of the supraglottic region, subglottic cancers, and cancers of the piriform sinus* can also be manifested as acute, emergency airway obstruction. Frequently, patients have a history of wheezing and mild upper airway distress in the period leading up to the emergency situation. Occasionally, such findings are confused with adult-onset asthma.

A middle ear infection or effusion in an adult should also prompt an ear, nose, and throat (ENT) evaluation. Nasopharyngeal cancer may be manifested as an ear infection in young adults. Hemoptysis or epistaxis may be the only clue to a nasopharyngeal cancer or a *paranasal sinus tumor.* Cranial nerve findings from deep invasion of the base of skull are late events and include lateral gaze abnormalities, diplopia, facial pain, or facial nerve paralysis. *Sinus tumors* can also be associated with these later findings, although nasal stuffiness occurs frequently and can be confused with sinusitis. New and persistent symptoms of sinusitis or facial pain should raise suspicion of sinus disease and prompt an evaluation.

Tumors in the tonsil or base of the tongue can cause local pain and referred ear pain; however, tumors in these areas are frequently asymptomatic and can attain a large size before becoming evident as a result of changes in speech (hot potato voice), a sense of globus, or restriction of tongue movement. Manifestation as a painless lump in the neck is likewise common. Tumors of the tonsil or base of the tongue may also lose their mucosal component, not be seen or felt on direct inspection, and occur as a solid or cystic neck mass, so-called unknown primaries. Isolated neck masses can wax and wane with antibiotics. A mass, especially

TABLE 200–1 AMERICAN JOINT COMMITTEE ON CANCER STAGING FOR HEAD AND NECK SQUAMOUS CELL CARCINOMA

Tumor	Larynx	Lip and Oral Cavity	Oropharynx	Hypopharynx
Tis	Carcinoma in situ	Carcinoma in situ	Carcinoma in situ	Carcinoma in situ
T1	Tumor limited to one subsite of the larynx	Tumor <2 cm	Tumor <2 cm	Tumor <2 cm, limited to one subsite of the hypopharynx
T2	Tumor involving more than one subsite and/or impaired vocal cord mobility	Tumor >2 cm and ≤4 cm	Tumor >2 cm and ≤4 cm	Tumor >2 cm and <4 cm, involving more than one subsite
T3	Vocal cord fixation, cartilage erosion, involvement of pre-epiglottic or postcricoid areas (supraglottic primary)	Tumor >4 cm	Tumor >4 cm	Tumor >4 cm or vocal cord fixation
T4a	Extension outside the larynx, through the thyroid cartilage or into soft tissues	Extension to adjacent structures (soft tissue or bone outside the oral cavity, deep tongue)	Invasion of adjacent structures (larynx, bone, or muscle)	Invasion of adjacent structures (bone, muscle, or cartilage)
T4b	Invasion of the prevertebral space, carotid encasement, or mediastinal invasion	Invasion of the masticator space or pterygoid muscles, carotid encasement, or skull base	Invasion of the pterygoid plates or muscles, carotid encasement, or skull base	Invasion of the prevertebral space, carotid encasement, or mediastinal invasion

Node	Definition
N0	No cervical lymph nodes positive
N1	Single ipsilateral lymph node <3 cm
N2a	Single ipsilateral lymph node >3 cm and <6 cm
N2b	Multiple ipsilateral lymph nodes, each <6 cm
N2c	Bilateral or contralateral lymph nodes, each <6 cm
N3	Single or multiple lymph nodes >6 cm

Metastasis	Definition
M0	No distant metastasis
M1	Distant metastasis present
Mx	Distant metastasis cannot be assessed

Stage	T	N	M
I	T1	N0	M0
II	T2	N0	M0
III	T3	N0	M0
	T1–T3	N1	M0
IVa	T1–T4a	N0–N2	M0
IVb	Any T	N3	M0
IVc	T4b	Any N	M0
	Any T	Any N	M1

a cystic mass, in the neck in an adult is cancer until proved otherwise and should prompt an ENT evaluation, before fine-needle aspiration (FNA) or excisional biopsy.

The staging of squamous cell carcinoma of the head and neck is based on the TNM (tumor, node, metastasis) staging system, and prognosis is related primarily to the N and T stages (Table 200–1). The risk of the cancer spreading to lymph nodes is directly related to the location of the primary and secondarily to the size of the primary. Tumors of the oropharynx have a high risk for nodal metastases, followed in risk by the supraglottic larynx and piriform sinus (hypopharynx), oral portion of the tongue, soft palate, oral cavity/floor of the mouth, and larynx. Nasopharyngeal cancer is highly associated with extensive nodal spread, whereas paranasal sinus cancers rarely spread to the lymph nodes. The location of lymph node spread is determined in part by site. Nasopharyngeal cancer spreads to the posterior cervical lymph nodes, as well as the high cervical nodes. Oropharynx, larynx, and piriform sinus tumors spread to the high cervical nodes. Nodal metastases from these locations can be bilateral. Oral cavity tumors spread to the submental nodes and submandibular nodes. Spread tends to be orderly from the submandibular nodes to the midcervical nodes. Oral cavity cancers can have as high as a 20% risk of clinically unappreciated contralateral spread.

Diagnosis

The relative accessibility of the head and neck to direct inspection makes physical examination critical for diagnosis and staging. Patients with localized symptoms or a sign such as an ulcer or a small mass should have a thorough head and neck office examination performed by their primary physician and by a specialist, including inspection of the visible structures and palpation of the base of the tongue and tonsil areas, as well as the neck. Specialized office examination with fiberoptics should be included in the preliminary assessment by a specialist. Patients with a readily accessible primary can have a diagnostic biopsy performed at the initial examination. Regardless of whether cancer is suspected, excisional biopsies should be discouraged because margins are frequently violated and inadequate, thereby leading to larger re-excisions. A simple punch biopsy is sufficient for diagnosis, particularly in the oral portion of the tongue where tumors can spread readily though lymphatics.

When cancer is highly suspected and before definitive surgical intervention, a computed tomography (CT) scan from the base of the skull to the clavicles, preferably with the spiral technique, and a chest radiograph should be obtained. Magnetic resonance imaging (MRI) provides added information in evaluating soft tissue involvement, especially in the base of the tongue and the parapharyngeal spaces and for sinus tumors. MRI can distinguish between soft tissue masses and retained secretions, whereas CT is more helpful in assessing bone invasion. Positron emission tomography (PET) is a potential adjunct, but its precise role remains to be defined.

When a biopsy indicates cancer or cancer is highly suspected, an examination under anesthesia with endoscopy should be performed to stage the primary tumor before definitive therapy is undertaken. This procedure, which provides information regarding the extent of disease, the appropriateness of the planned definitive procedure, and the presence of second primaries, is an absolute requirement before definitive therapy can be discussed with a patient. Endoscopy and palpation under anesthesia can identify unexpected local spread or a synchronous second primary (found in about 5% of patients), and the procedure should include esophagoscopy or a barium swallow in all patients and bronchoscopy in high-risk patients.

Approach to the Patient with an Unknown Primary Site

Patients frequently seek care from their primary physician because of an enlarged lymph node, a cystic mass, or a collection of lymph nodes in the upper part of the neck (Fig. 200–3). Such masses in an adult should be considered cancer until proved otherwise. Unless there is an obvious symptom or sign that leads the clinician to the identification of a primary site in the head and neck, such patients are considered to have an unknown primary. Masses in the supraclavicular areas represent primary tumors below the clavicles, and masses in the midneck and cervical regions are almost always from the head and neck. Identification of a primary site is critical to focus therapy, reduce morbidity, and determine prognosis.

The most common primary sites for painless lumps are the oropharynx (base of the tongue and tonsil) and piriform sinus. Salivary gland cancers, lymphomas, melanomas, and skin cancers can also be manifested in this manner. Bilateral nodal disease or nodal disease with systemic symptoms may suggest lymphoma. By comparison, pain, warmth, and erythema may suggest an infectious etiology. Intraparotid nodes most likely represent metastases from skin malignancies. Physical examination should include a careful investigation for primary skin cancers. CT and MRI should be part of the initial evaluation. FNA should be performed and repeated if initially negative. CT-guided biopsy may be indicated if the mass is difficult to approach. PET scans may be helpful in this setting. If squamous cells are identified in the FNA or CT-guided biopsy, the tumor is most likely a squamous cell carcinoma of the head and neck. A second FNA is indicated if the first is negative. Next, endoscopy under anesthesia should be performed with bilateral tonsillectomy. The endoscopy should include directed biopsies of any abnormalities, areas of firmness, and the base of the tongue, nasopharynx, and ipsilateral piriform sinus, even if they appear normal. Core or excisional (single node <3 cm in size) biopsy of the lymph node should be performed if the pathology is equivocal and a primary site is not confirmed. Neck dissection can be accomplished if a primary site is not identified and the patient has an N1 or small N2a/b manifestation. Some unknown primaries with squamous histology are never identified. Currently, there are no molecular markers to distinguish head and neck cancer from skin or salivary gland squamous cancer. EBV positivity suggests a nasopharyngeal cancer, and HPV-16 suggests an oropharyngeal primary.

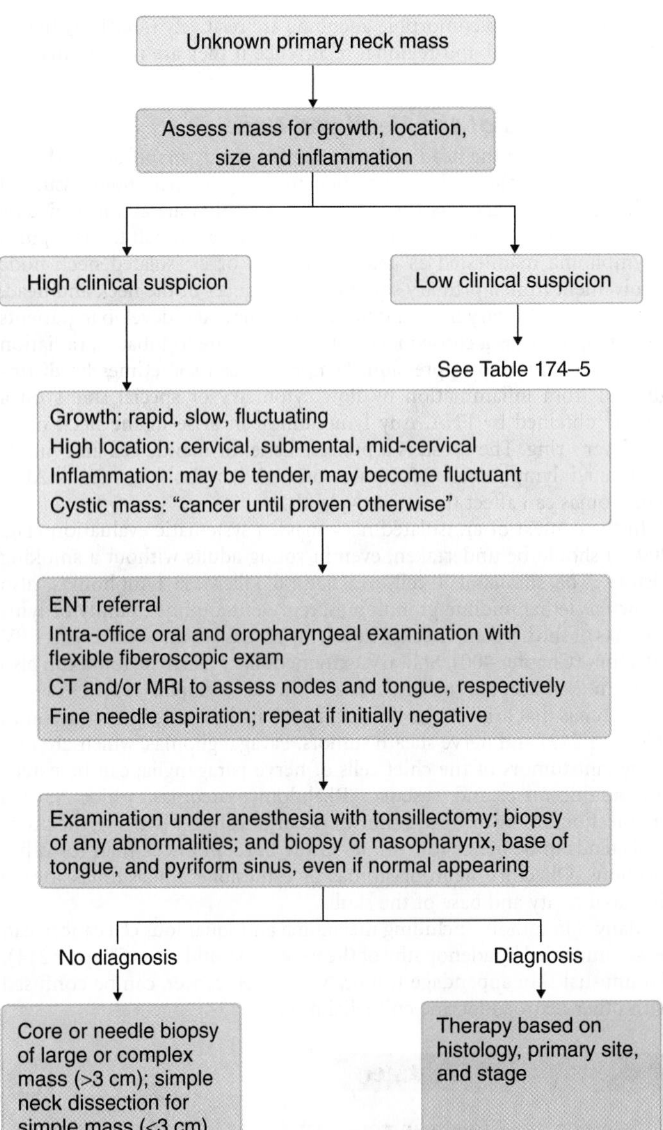

FIGURE 200–3 • Evaluation of an unknown primary neck mass. CT = computed tomography; ENT = ear, nose, and throat; MRI = magnetic resonance imaging.

In contrast to squamous cell carcinoma of the head and neck, salivary gland cancers are heterogeneous in their natural history and treatment. The three most common histologic types are adenoid cystic carcinoma, mucoepidermoid cancer, and adenocarcinoma. Other histologic types include the aggressive salivary duct cancer and squamous cell cancers, whereas less aggressive histologic varieties include adenocarcinoma ex pleomorphic adenoma and acinic cell carcinoma. Because adenoid cystic carcinoma travels along nerves and can spread hematogenously, careful assessment of the cranial nerves and the chest by CT scanning is indicated before major surgery is undertaken. Patients should also be evaluated for bone and liver metastases. Formal lymph node dissection is not indicated. Ethmoid and sphenoid sinus adenoid cystic carcinomas are locally and regionally aggressive and require specialized surgery and radiation therapy techniques for local and regional control. The behavior of mucoepidermoid carcinoma is determined by histology. Low- and intermediate-grade lesions rarely metastasize. Isolated high-grade tumors spread to local lymph nodes and by hematogenous routes and have a high risk for the development of lung metastases. The work-up for high-grade lesions should be similar to that for adenoid cystic carcinoma. Local therapy should be directed at local and regional control with lymph node dissection. Radiation therapy is indicated for close microscopic margins or lymph node involvement. Adenocarcinoma, salivary duct cancers, and squamous cell carcinoma are also poor-prognosis lesions with aggressive local and distant behavior. These tumors should be evaluated in the same fashion as aggressive mucoepidermoid carcinomas. Acinic cell carcinoma and carcinoma ex pleomorphic adenoma are relatively rare. They have a propensity for local and regional recurrence if they are not removed in toto. Metastases are rare and tend to be slow growing.

Other Tumors of the Head and Neck

Lymphomas in the head and neck are frequently manifested either as nodal disease in the neck or as tumor involving the lymphoid tissues of Waldeyer's ring (Chapters 196 and 197). Unless they are accompanied by systemic symptoms or lymphadenopathy, it can be difficult to distinguish a lymphoma manifested as a tonsillar mass or as isolated neck node involvement from a primary squamous cell cancer of the neck and head. In addition, a primary head and neck cancer may later develop in patients with lymphoma as a consequence of past exposure to tobacco, radiation therapy, or immunosuppression. Lymphoma can sometimes be distinguished from inflammation by flow cytometry or special stains on a sample obtained by FNA. Any lymphoma can arise in the neck or in Waldeyer's ring. The tonsil is a preferred site for mantle cell and undifferentiated lymphomas. Mucosa-associated lymphoid tissue (MALT) lymphomas can affect the salivary glands.

In the context of an isolated neck mass, a systematic evaluation (Fig. 200–3) should be undertaken, even in young adults without a smoking history. The sinonasal T-cell and natural killer cell lymphomas, also known as lethal midline granulomas, represent a unique family of lymphomas of the head and neck. These lymphomas are associated with EBV infection (Chapter 400). Solitary, extramedullary plasmacytoma can also occur in the nasopharynx or paranasal sinuses (Chapter 198).

Sarcomas that arise in the head and neck include osteogenic sarcomas (Chapter 212) and nerve sheath tumors. Paragangliomas, which are rare malignant tumors of the chief cells of nerve paraganglia, can be extensive, multicentric, and vascular. Rhabdomyosarcomas, which have a predilection for the orbit and sinuses, occur in younger persons; the prognosis tends to be better for tumors of the head and neck than for other locations. Olfactory neuroblastomas or esthesioneuroblastomas invade the nasal cavity and base of the skull.

Many skin tumors, including melanoma and squamous cell cancer, can be accompanied by adenopathy of the neck or parotid area (Chapter 214). An unusual skin appendage tumor, Merkel cell cancer, can be confused with other neuroendocrine epithelial tumors.

Prevention and Treatment

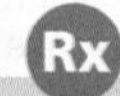

Selection of a treatment program for an individual patient is based on three factors: the primary site and stage of the tumor, the patient's comorbid conditions and preferences, and the biology of the tumor (Table 200–2). Early-stage lesions, T1N0 and T2N0, are defined by their size, and their prognosis is site specific. For example, early *larynx cancer* involving the true vocal cords has an excellent prognosis and can be treated by local excision. Voice-preserving partial laryngectomy is effective for selected patients. Radiation therapy is equally effective for early cancer. When there is a risk of lymph node spread, radiation therapy must be given postoperatively, and the primary value of surgery is diminished. Intensity-modulated radiation therapy (IMRT) allows radiation to be delivered in a more conformal manner to the tumor and areas at risk while sparing critical structures such as the spinal cord and noncritical but important structures such as the salivary glands.

Oral tongue, base of the tongue, and piriform sinus tumors have a worse prognosis and are difficult to stage accurately because of submucosal spread or lymphatic involvement. Stage I and II cancers are cured with local and regional surgery or radiation therapy in 80 to 90% of cases. Surgery may be preferred for limited oral cavity and anterior lesions. In surgically treated patients, those with a positive margin, two or more positive lymph nodes, or extracapsular spread have a poorer survival rate (<30%) at 5 years. Perineural invasion and lymphovascular invasion may also be associated with a poor prognosis. Postoperative cisplatin-based chemoradiation therapy improves local and regional control, as well as survival, and should be given to poor-prognosis patients if their condition permits. [1] At present, no molecular or immunohistochemical finding definitively adds to the information gleaned from pathology, staging, and performance status.

When organ preservation and function are an issue or when radiation therapy is required regardless of surgical outcome, primary chemoradiation therapy should be considered. [2] The curative treatment of intermediate (stage III, T1–3N1, T3N0) and locally advanced (stage IV, T1–3N2–3, T4) disease remains controversial. Long-term (3 years) survival rates in patients with stage III disease are generally between 50 and 75%, whereas only 15 to 50% of stage IV patients survive for 3 years. Intermediate-stage tumors are usually resectable, but organ preservation may be an important consideration. In many of these cases, a combined-modality approach that includes chemotherapy is a standard of care.

Patients with anterior lesions may do better with initial surgical treatment. The oral cavity is easy to assess and is relatively forgiving for surgery and reconstruction; radiation therapy or chemoradiation therapy can be moderated in the absence of bad prognostic features. For intermediate and advanced tumors, radiation therapy or chemoradiation therapy is a necessary adjunct to prevent recurrence. For example, a T3 or N1 lesion of the oropharyngeal tongue or hypopharynx is almost always more extensive than clinically appreciated and may be more suited to a nonsurgical regional and systemic approach. In addition, patients with rapidly growing tumors are more suitable for a combined-modality approach. Patients with extensive N2 or N3 nodal disease (stage IV) should be considered relatively unresectable because of a poor prognosis from regional recurrence and distant metastases. Certain locations such as the nasopharynx and posterior pharynx should also be considered for definitive radiation therapy or chemoradiation therapy.

TABLE 200–2 GENERAL APPROACH TO SQUAMOUS CELL HEAD AND NECK CANCER

Stage	TNM	Disease-Specific Survival	Treatment Approach	Special Conditions
I	T1N0	85–95%	Surgery or radiation therapy	Consider organ function and long-term toxicity
II	T2N0	75–90%	Surgery, radiation therapy, or chemoradiation therapy	Consider organ function Combined modality for high-volume tumor Postoperative chemoradiation therapy for poor prognostic findings on pathologic staging
III	T3N0 T1–3N1	50–75%	Combined-modality treatment	Primary concomitant chemoradiation therapy for organ function Postoperative chemoradiation therapy More aggressive approach (sequential therapy) for high-volume disease or hypopharynx tumors
IV	T1–3N2–3 T4N0–3 Any M1	20–60%	Combined-modality treatment	Combined-modality therapy Limited surgery Postoperative chemoradiation therapy Palliative therapy for M1 (curative therapy for isolated lung metastases)

Rx

Radiation therapy has been proved by randomized trials to yield better local control and disease-free survival if given in twice-daily fractionated treatments rather than as daily therapy. However, the absolute benefit at 5 years is only 3 to 4%. [3]

Induction chemotherapy is the delivery of chemotherapy before definitive local/regional treatment. The most effective induction chemotherapy is cisplatin, 100 mg/m^2 by intravenous bolus, plus 5-fluorouracil, 1000 mg/m^2/day for 5 days by intravenous infusion, repeated every 3 to 4 weeks. Recently, the addition of a taxane to cisplatin and 5-fluorouracil induction chemotherapy has been shown to be better than cisplatin and 5-fluorouracil alone. [3,4] For patients with advanced oropharynx, larynx, and hypopharynx tumors, induction chemotherapy with radiation therapy and nodal surgery improves survival and preserves function when compared with standard radiation therapy. [5]

Chemoradiation therapy integrates chemotherapy and radiation therapy together and has led to significant improvements in overall survival in patients with advanced disease when compared with radiation therapy alone. For example, patients with unresectable disease who received cisplatin (100 mg/m^2 by intravenous bolus) every 3 weeks during radiation therapy have significantly better survival than do those treated with radiation therapy alone. [6] In a trial of patients with oropharyngeal carcinoma, those treated with carboplatin and 5-fluorouracil plus simultaneous radiation therapy had significantly better survival than did those treated by radiation therapy alone. [7]

Patients with locally advanced or unresectable disease (or both) should receive chemotherapy as part of a combined-modality approach. Both induction chemotherapy and chemoradiation therapy prolong survival. A sequential combination of both might be considered as well. Organ preservation should be offered to patients who can tolerate the treatment and participate in the rehabilitation.

Treatment of *tumors of the paranasal sinuses* is a special case. They rarely metastasize, and treatment should focus on chemoradiation therapy or surgical resection with postoperative radiation therapy for resectable stage III and IV disease and on chemoradiation therapy for local and regional control of unresectable disease. Proton beam irradiation may be more suited for tumors in and around the base of the skull and brain.

Follow-up

Patients need lifelong follow-up. A chest radiograph should be performed at least yearly, and surveillance examinations for second primaries and recurrences should be performed monthly to bimonthly in the first year and then less frequently over time. Treatment failure after 3 years is uncommon, but second primaries may continue to be identified. It is important to counsel patients to avoid tobacco products and any exposure to alcohol.

During therapy and immediately after therapy, patients benefit from pain medications, local anesthetics, mucolytics, and saline mouthwash. Patients must avoid alcohol-containing preparations or irritants. Long-acting agents such as fentanyl or time-release narcotics should be added when needed (Chapter 28). A percutaneous endoscopic gastrostomy feeding tube is effective for maintaining weight, improving healing, and managing nutrition during radiation therapy. Because depression is a major problem, psychiatric support and antidepressants may be very helpful (Chapter 420). Salivary function improves over more than 4 years after radiation therapy, but most improvement occurs in the first 2 years. Pilocarpine is an effective stimulant of salivary flow in about 20% of patients.

Long-term sequelae of radiation therapy include dependence on a feeding tube in patients treated with aggressive chemoradiation therapy. Attention should be paid to preserving swallowing function by means of training in speech and swallowing, as well as dilation in selected patients. Hypothyroidism occurs in up to 50% of patients and as early as 3 months after treatment. Patients should be monitored by determining serum thyroid-stimulating hormone levels at regular intervals and then be treated as appropriate (Chapter 244). Patients are at substantial lifelong risk for complications from dental manipulations after radiation therapy. Bone necrosis is painful, can be confused with recurrent tumor, and requires vigorous antibiotic therapy, débridement, and possibly hyperbaric oxygen to promote healing.

Patients with recurrent disease, a second primary, or metastatic disease must be evaluated for potential curability. If patients have a recurrence or second primary, curative treatment options are defined by their current stage, their previous therapy, and the interval from their original therapy. Patients who have previously been treated with surgery but not radiation therapy can undergo surgery, radiation therapy, or chemotherapy as part of a curative treatment plan. Patients with a surgically treatable recurrence in an irradiated field should undergo surgery as appropriate. It is important to recognize that the surgery must encompass the entire recurrence. Symptomatically, persistent pain may be the most important indicator of a recurrence, and repeat biopsy should be considered when a suspicious lesion is observed. Surgical salvage may cure as many as 30% of patients with recurrent oral cavity, larynx, or hypopharyngeal tumors. In some patients a repeat course of radiation therapy is also acceptable.

Patients who are incurable can be managed effectively with palliative therapy to improve quality of life and survival, for example, tracheostomy for airway control, laryngectomy for pain and aspiration, and a percutaneous endoscopic gastrostomy tube for feeding. These maneuvers can improve comfort and care in appropriate patients.

Palliative chemotherapy can provide meaningful benefit to some patients. Response rates with single agents are generally poor, and combination therapy offers higher response rates (30 to 50%), but limited improvement in median and 1-year survival and more toxicity.

Salivary Gland Tumors

In contrast to squamous cell carcinoma of the head and neck, salivary gland cancers are heterogeneous in their natural history and treatment; however, the mainstay of therapy for these tumors is surgery. Early symptoms of local/regional recurrence include cranial nerve dysfunction and progressive pain. A PET scan may be useful in distinguishing recurrence from the neuropathy that may result from radiation therapy.

There are no highly active agents or combinations for treatment of metastatic salivary gland tumors. Local therapy can include surgical removal of isolated metastases, radio frequency ablation, and radiation therapy. Response rates are generally in the 20 to 35% range, but prolonged responses are occasionally seen.

Future Directions

Antibodies that target the EGF receptor and other molecular targets may improve local and regional control, as well as survival, when delivered with radiation therapy. Vaccines against EBV and HPV may prevent malignancy in high-risk populations.

Prognosis

The prognosis for patients with squamous cell carcinoma of the head and neck (see Table 200–2) is directly related to stage and performance status. The risk for recurrence declines dramatically at 2 years after definitive treatment, and survival and possible cure can be defined after 3 years. N (nodal) status is the most important prognostic indicator of recurrence, with T (tumor) stage being next. Stage I patients (T1N0) have a greater than 90% likelihood of tumor control, whereas stage II patients (T2N0) have greater than 85% tumor control. Cancer control in stage III patients (T1–2N1, T3N0–1) is site dependent and varies from 50 to 75%. Patients with stage IVa and IVb disease (T1–3, N2–3, or T4NX) have a 20 to 50% tumor-specific 3-year survival rate. Bad prognostic signs in advanced-stage (IVb) patients are related to N3 nodal disease and invasion of basic structures (carotid artery encasement, base of the skull, pterygoid muscles). Patients with M1 disease are categorized as stage IVc.

Isolated patients with single lung metastases can be cured, whether as a primary or as a recurrence. Patients with recurrent disease and no curative options have a median survival of 6 to 9 months. Death can occur as a result of compromise of local critical structures, including vessels, breathing, and swallowing.

Distant metastases occur in about 15 to 20% of patients, but this rate is increasing as better local and regional control prolongs survival in patients with locally advanced disease. Oropharyngeal, tonsil, and piriform sinus tumors have the highest risk for distant metastases. In approximately 5% of patients a synchronous lung tumor or metastasis develops. A single lung metastasis in a patient at initial evaluation or at follow-up can be cured in about 20% of cases.

Salivary gland cancers vary in behavior, depending on their histology. Adenocarcinoma, salivary duct cancer, salivary squamous cell cancer, and high-grade mucoepidermoid cancer not only spread to lymph nodes but also spread rapidly hematogenously. Except in adenoid cystic carcinoma, the presence of lymph node metastases signals a high risk for distant metastases. Adenoid cystic carcinoma infrequently involves lymph nodes but spreads along nerves. Regional recurrences along cranial nerves are frequent and associated with "skip" lesions. Adenoid cystic carcinoma is also associated with the late development of lung metastases, but these patients can have a prolonged lifespan lasting more than 20 years. Low-grade mucoepidermoid cancer and acinic cell carcinoma have little risk of distant spread and are more notable for local recurrence if not completely removed.

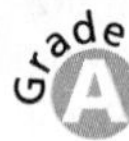

1. Bernier J, Domenge C, Ozsahin M, et al: Postoperative irradiation with or without concomitant chemotherapy for locally advanced head and neck cancer. N Engl J Med 2004;350:1945–1952.
2. Forastiere AA, Goepfert H, Maor M, et al: Concurrent chemotherapy and radiotherapy for organ preservation in advanced larynx cancer. N Engl J Med 2003;349:2091–2098.
3. Bourhis J, Overgaard J, Audry H, et al: Hperfractionated or accelerated radiotherapy in head and neck cancer: A meta-analysis. Lancet 2006;368:843–854.
4. Hitt R, Lopez-Pousa A, Martinez-Trufero J, et al: Phase III study comparing cisplatin (P) & 5-fluorouracil (F) versus P, F and paclitaxel (T) as induction therapy in locally advanced head & neck cancer (LAHNC). J Clin Oncol 2005;23:8636–8645.
5. Zorat PL, Paccagnella A, Cavaniglia G, et al: Randomized phase III trial of neoadjuvant chemotherapy in head and neck cancer: 10-year follow-up. J Natl Cancer Inst 2004;96:1714–1717.
6. Adelstein D, Li Y, Adams G, et al: An Intergroup Phase III comparison of standard radiation therapy and two schedules of concurrent chemoradiotherapy in patients with unresectable squamous cell head and neck cancer. J Clin Oncol 2003;21:92–98.
7. Denis F, Garaud P, Bardet E, et al: Final results of the 94-01 French Head and Neck Oncology and Radiotherapy Group randomized trial comparing radiotherapy alone with concomitant radiochemotherapy in advanced-stage oropharynx carcinoma. J Clin Oncol 2004;22:69–76.

SUGGESTED READINGS

Cooper J, Pajak TF, Forastiere A, et al: Postoperative concurrent radiotherapy and chemotherapy for high-risk squamous-cell carcinoma of the head and neck. N Engl J Med 2004;350:1937–1944. *Postoperative cisplatinum-based chemoradiotherapy improves local-regional control and survival.*

Wei WI, Sham JST: Nasopharyngeal carcinoma. Lancet 2005;365:2041–2054. *A comprehensive overview.*

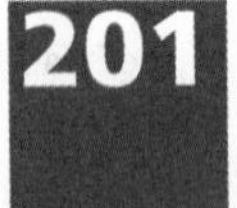

201 LUNG CANCER AND OTHER PULMONARY NEOPLASMS

David S. Ettinger

BRONCHOGENIC LUNG CANCER

Definition

Lung cancer (e.g., bronchogenic carcinoma) arises from the respiratory epithelium. Lung cancer is divided into two major histologic groups: non–small cell lung cancer (NSCLC) and small cell lung cancer (SCLC). NSCLC accounts for approximately 85% of all lung cancer. NSCLC subtypes include adenocarcinoma (40%), squamous cell carcinoma (30%), and large cell carcinoma (15%). SCLC accounts for 15% of all lung cancer. Other less common pulmonary neoplasms include adenosquamous carcinoma, carcinoid tumors, bronchial gland tumors, soft tissue tumors (e.g., sarcomas), pulmonary blastomas, and lymphoma.

Epidemiology

Worldwide, lung cancer accounts for approximately 13% of all cancer; more than 1.1 million cases of lung cancer are diagnosed annually, and over 1 million deaths are caused by the disease. In the United States, about 175,000 new cases are diagnosed annually and about 160,000 deaths, 28% of all annual cancer deaths (31% in men, 25% in women), are due to lung cancer. Lung cancer is the leading cause of cancer death in both men and women, and there are more deaths from lung cancer in the United States than from prostate, breast, and colorectal cancer combined. Although lung cancer is most common in North America and Europe, other regions with a substantial incidence and mortality include Asia, Australia, and South America.

The incidence and mortality of lung cancer in American men and women reflect their smoking habits (Chapter 30). Lung cancer deaths started rising in men in the 1950s and in women 10 to 15 years later. Mortality from lung cancer in men peaked in the late 1980s and is now decreasing. In women, the death rate from lung cancer appears to have stabilized in about the year 2000.

The Surveillance, Epidemiology and End Results (SEER) program estimated that 1 in 13 men and 1 in 17 women will be at risk for the development of lung cancer during their lifetime. Incidence and mortality rates vary by race/ethnicity (Table 201–1), with African American men having a higher incidence and mortality rate than other racial/ethnic groups. Incidence rates of lung cancer for men and women from the period 1996 to 2000 are 80.8 and 49.6 per 100,000 people, respectively. The median age at diagnosis in both sexes is 70 years.

Unfortunately, tobacco use in high-school students increased until the mid-1990s and is slowly declining. However, despite this decline, 38% of high-school seniors smoke. This smoking at an earlier age may in part explain the occurrence of lung cancer in younger patients.

Risk Factors

Tobacco

It is estimated that cigarette smoking is responsible for approximately 85 to 90% of all cases of lung cancer, including 90% of cases in men and 80% in women. More than 40 carcinogens have been identified in cigarette smoke. The risk for development of lung cancer correlates with the number of cigarettes smoked per day, lifetime duration of smoking, age at onset of smoking, degree of inhalation, tar and nicotine content of the cigarettes, and use of unfiltered cigarettes. If a lifelong nonsmoker has a relative risk ratio of 1 for the development of lung cancer, cigarette smokers of less than ½ pack/day, ½ to 1 pack/day, 1 to 2 packs/day and more than 2 packs/day have a risk ratio of 15, 17, 42, and 64, respectively. The risk ratio in ex-smokers is dependent on the duration of abstinence of cigarette smoking; to reach a risk ratio of 1.5 to 2.0 requires abstinence of approximately 30 years.

Pipe and cigar smoking are also risk factors for lung cancer, but the risk is thought to be less than that associated with cigarette smoking, possibly because such tobacco products tend to be inhaled less deeply than cigarette smoke. Marijuana and cocaine smoking probably cause an increased risk for lung cancer, but the carcinogenicity of the two drugs is less well studied than that of cigarette smoking.

Environmental Tobacco Smoke

Exposure to environmental tobacco smoke (i.e., passive smoking) by nonsmokers, especially in the workplace, increases the risk for development of lung cancer. The exposure levels of environmental tobacco smoke depend on the size of the enclosed space and the intensity of smoking.

Other Exposure

The International Agency for Research on Cancer classified the following as group 1 known carcinogens for lung cancer: radon, asbestos, arsenic, beryllium, bis(chloromethyl)ether, cadmium, chromium, nickel, vinyl chloride, and polycyclic aromatic hydrocarbons (PAHs) (Chapters 17 and 93). Group 2A probable carcinogens include acrylonitrile, formaldehyde, and diesel exhaust. Group 2B possible carcinogens include

TABLE 201–1 LUNG CANCER INCIDENCE AND MORTALITY RATES BY RACE/ETHNICITY AND GENDER

	Incidence			Mortality		
	White	African American	Hispanic	White	African American	Hispanic
Male	79.4	120.4	33.2	78.1	107.0	40.7
Female	51.9	54.8	24.4	41.5	40.0	15.1

Incidence and death rates per 100,000 population, 1996 to 2000, from the Surveillance, Epidemiology and End Results (SEER) program.

acetaldehyde, silica, and welding fumes. It is estimated that 9% of lung cancers in men and 2% in women are caused by occupational exposure.

Radon, a gaseous decay product of uranium-238 and radium-226, damages lung tissue by emitting alpha particles. Underground mining of uranium exposes miners to radon and its decay products, thus increasing their risk for lung cancer. Radon may appear in homes, especially basements, because it is present in soil rock and ground water and enters the home through defects in pipes or the foundation. The indoor radon level depends on the soil concentration and ventilation rate. Data are conflicting about the risk for lung cancer with exposure to domestic radon, but the consensus is that the risk is increased.

Exposure to asbestos fibers (Chapter 93) occurs in automobile shops, shipyards, mines, and textile and cement plants and in construction and insulation workers. Workers with asbestosis, not just asbestos exposure, have an increased risk for lung cancer. Cigarette smokers with asbestos exposure have a risk of lung cancer that is multiplicative—a 50-fold relative risk as compared with unexposed nonsmokers. The latency period for the development of lung cancer in workers exposed to asbestos is 25 to 40 years.

Arsenic, a naturally occurring metal, is a byproduct of copper, lead, zinc, and tin ore smelting. The metal is also present in agricultural pesticides and marine organisms. Exposure to arsenic occurs via air, soil, water, and foods. Cigarette smokers exposed to arsenic are at greater risk for the development of lung cancer than those not exposed to arsenic.

Beryllium is a metal used for alloys. Exposure occurs in mining and in the manufacture of ceramics and electronic equipment. The metal is a pulmonary carcinogen.

Bis(chloromethyl)ether is a product of chloromethylation processes used in the manufacture of ion exchange resins, polymers, and plastics. The relative risk for lung cancer in exposed workers is 10, especially for SCLC.

Cadmium is a metal used for electroplating metals, batteries, plastics, and pigments. Studies have shown that exposure to cadmium causes an increased risk for lung cancer.

Chromium is commonly used for metal alloys, paint pigments, electroplating, cement, rubber, photoengraving, and the composition of floor covering. Exposure to chromium increases the risk for lung cancer two- to three-fold.

Nickel is used in electroplating, manufacturing of steel and other alloys, ceramics, storage batteries, electric circuits, and petroleum refining. Nickel exposure increases the risk for lung cancer 1.56-fold.

Vinyl chloride is used to make plastics (e.g., polyvinyl chloride pipe), packaging materials, propellant in cosmetic products, and vinyl floor tiles. Although the risk for development of lung cancer after exposure to vinyl chloride is increased, it is considered small.

PAHs are formed from the incomplete combustion of organic material. Exposure to PAHs occurs with cigarette smoke; smelting of nickel-containing ores; aluminum, iron, steel, and coke production; coal tar; and diesel exhaust. PAHs carry a 1.5 to 2.5 relative risk for lung cancer.

Preexisting Lung Disease

Tobacco smoking causes chronic inflammation and destruction of lung tissue, which results in chronic obstructive pulmonary disease (COPD). Patients with COPD have an approximately four-fold increased risk for lung cancer. In addition, patients in whom idiopathic pulmonary fibrosis or pulmonary fibrosis from asbestosis or silica develops are at increased risk for the development of lung cancer.

Dietary Factors

Increased consumption of fruits and green and yellow vegetables is associated with a reduced risk for lung cancer, whereas low serum concentrations of antioxidant vitamins such as vitamins A and E are associated with the development of lung cancer. However, β-carotene supplementation increases the incidence of lung cancer.

Increased consumption of dietary fat is also associated with an increased incidence of lung cancer. High blood concentrations of selenium, a mineral involved in the protection of cellular membranes, has been associated with a lower risk for lung cancer.

Gender and Racial Differences

Women who smoke have a 1.2- to 1.7-fold higher risk ratio than men do, especially for adenocarcinoma and SCLC. Possible explanations for this difference in lung cancer risk include (1) effects of hormones such as estrogen on the development of lung cancer, (2) gender differences in nicotine metabolism, and (3) gender variations in cytochrome P-450 enzymes involved in the bioactivation of toxic components in cigarette smoke condensate.

The high incidence and mortality of lung cancer in African American males may be due, in part, to (1) increased tobacco use, (2) differences in the metabolism of tobacco smoke, and (3) higher intake of dietary fat.

Human Immunodeficiency Virus Infection

Some studies suggest that the risk for lung cancer is increased in patients infected with human immunodeficiency virus (HIV) (Chapter 416), mostly as a result of cigarette smoking. Most patients are male (10:1) and young, in part reflecting the demographics of HIV infection.

Inheritance

First-degree relatives of patients with lung cancer have a two- to six-fold increase in the risk for lung cancer after adjusting for tobacco use. Second-degree relatives of lung cancer patients have a relative risk of 1.28, and third-degree relatives have a relative risk of 1.14. Nonsmokers with a family history of lung cancer have a two- to four-fold increased risk for lung cancer. The familial risk may be due to shared exposure, such as environmental tobacco smoke, or to shared genetic susceptibility to environmental carcinogens.

Pathobiology

The development of lung cancer is the result of a multistep process from a premalignant lesion to frank cancer (Fig. 201–1) after a number of years. Tobacco smoke or other carcinogens promote sequential genetic and epigenetic changes that result in the loss of normal control mechanisms of cellular growth. These changes affect (1) oncogenes, which are homologues of normal cellular genes and, when mutated, result in activation and gain of function; (2) tumor suppressor genes, which are "cancer" genes in which loss of function by mutation removes inhibitions to control cell growth, and (3) growth factors (Chapter 186).

Oncogenes

The oncogenes that play a role in the pathogenesis of lung cancer include *ras,* the myc family, *HER-2/neu* (c-*erB*), and *Bcl-2*. The *ras* family of oncogenes has three primary members (H-*ras,* K-*ras,* and N-*ras*), one of which, K-*ras,* is activated by point mutations in codon 12 of lung cancer cells. The mutation occurs in 30% of adenocarcinomas of the lung, most often in patients with a history of smoking, but it has not been found in SCLC. Patients who have the K-*ras* mutation have a poorer prognosis, stage for stage.

Amplification and overexpression of the *myc* family oncogenes (a-*myc,* L-*myc,* N-*myc*) are seen in 10 to 40% of SCLC and 10% of NSCLC. The most frequently altered gene, however, is c-*myc,* whose amplification in SCLC tumors that relapse is associated with shorter survival. However,

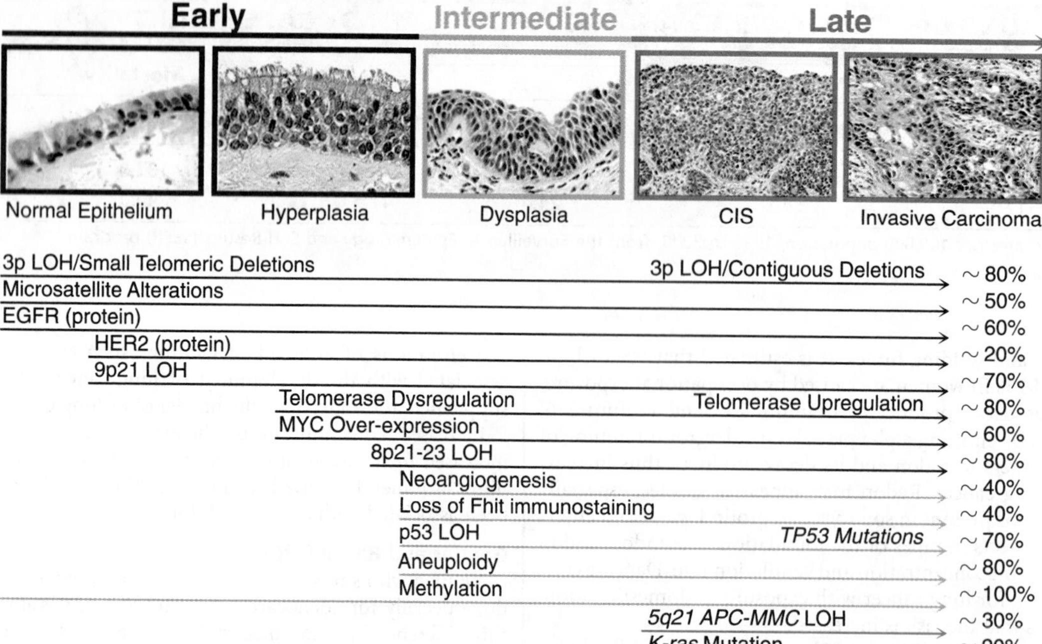

FIGURE 201–1 • Sequential changes during the pathogenesis of lung cancer. (From Hirsch FR, Franklin WA, Gasdar AF, Bunn PA Jr: Early detection of lung cancer: Clinical perspectives of recent advances in biology and radiology. Clin Cancer Res 2001;7:5–22. CIS = carcinoma in situ; LOH = loss of heterozygosity. Updated courtesy of Fred R. Hirsch, MD, PhD, Department of Medical Oncology, University of Colorado Health Sciences Center, and Adi F. Gazdar, MD, Department of Pathology, Southwestern Medical Center.)

overexpression of the *myc* oncogene is not present in the majority of lung cancers, so its overexpression is probably not a primary event.

The *HER-2/neu* (c-*erB*-2) gene, which encodes growth factor receptor or p185 neu (a tyrosine kinase glycoprotein), is activated in NSCLC but not SCLC. Overexpression of *HER-2/neu* in patients with adenocarcinoma of the lung portends a poor survival. *Bcl*-2, an oncogene that encodes a protein that inhibits programmed cell death (apoptosis), is also overexpressed in lung cancer, especially in SCLC.

Tumor Suppressor Genes

Tumor suppressor genes include *p53, Rb, 3p.* The *p53* tumor suppressor gene encodes for a nuclear phosphoprotein that controls cell division in normal as well as malignant cells. If normal cell DNA is damaged, p53 causes cellular arrest in either the G_1/S phase or the G_2/mitosis phase or induces apoptotic death. Normal cells with mutant *p53* lack these normal checkpoints, thereby allowing damaged DNA to be incorporated into the nucleus of daughter cells and causing malignant transformation. The *p53* mutation correlates with cigarette smoking and has been detected in preneoplastic lesions of the lung. Mutations of *p53* are common in both NSCLC (≈50%) and SCLC (≈80%).

The retinoblastoma *(Rb)* gene, located at the chromosome 13q14 region, encodes a nuclear phosphoprotein that regulates G_1/S phase cell cycle checkpoints by binding to cyclin D and various transcription factors. When *Rb* does not function, the G_1/S phase checkpoint is uncontrolled, thereby leading to cell proliferation and malignant transformation. In SCLC, *Rb* is often mutated or deleted, so the Rb protein is not expressed in 90% of SCLC. In NSCLC, Rb is normally expressed, but when Rb is phosphorylated, uncontrolled cell division can occur in NSCLC.

One of the earliest genetic abnormalities in lung cancer occurs with the deletion of genetic material on the short arm of chromosome 3(3p)(p14-p23). The deletion occurs in approximately 50% of NSCLC and 90% of SCLC. The *FHIT* (fragile histidine triad) gene (3p14.2) is abnormal in many lung cancers and may function as a tumor suppressor gene by suppressing tumor growth and causing apoptosis.

Growth Factors

Growth factors secreted by lung cancer cells may reflect adjacent or regional cells (paracrine stimulation) or cause autonomous proliferation of the cells from which they were secreted (autocrine stimulation). Cells that are affected by this autocrine stimulation secrete a biologically active growth factor. Antibodies that bind to this growth factor will inhibit cell growth.

Autocrine (peptide) growth factors that are important in the growth of lung cancer cells, particularly SCLC, include gastrin-releasing peptide (GRP), insulin-like growth factor type I (IGF-I), and hepatocyte growth factor. GRP occurs in approximately 20 to 60% of SCLC and less frequently in NSCLC. Hepatocyte growth factor is expressed mainly in NSCLC.

The oncogene c-*erB*-1 encodes the epidermal growth factor receptor (EGFR), a 170-kD tyrosine kinase glycoprotein. Activation of EGFR initiates autophosphorylation of the receptor and eventually leads to cell cycle proliferation. Overexpression of EGFR occurs more commonly in NSCLC.

Epigenetics

Epigenetics refers to a change in gene expression that is heritable but does not involve a change in DNA sequence. One of these epigenetic modifications involves changes in DNA methylation. These changes, which are very common in lung cancer, can include hypomethylation, dysregulation of DNA methyltransferase I, and hypermethylation. Genes that are methylated in NSCLC include *p16, RAR-β, RASSFIA,* methylguanine-methyltransferase, and death-associated protein kinase (DAP-kinase). This hypermethylation can silence tumor suppressor genes, thereby permitting unregulated cell growth.

Clinical Manifestations

As many as 15% of patients in whom lung cancer is diagnosed are initially asymptomatic. The diagnosis is usually made incidentally on a chest radiograph obtained for other reasons (e.g., a preoperative study). However, the majority of patients have symptoms and signs that are (1) caused by the pulmonary lesion itself—local tumor growth, invasion, or obstruction; (2) intrathoracic—regional tumor spreading to lymph nodes and adjacent structures; (3) extrathoracic—distant spread of disease; and (4) paraneoplastic syndromes. Nonspecific signs and symptoms of lung cancer include anorexia in about 30% of patients, weight loss, fatigue in a third of patients, and anemia and fever in 10 to 20% of patients. More than 80% of patients initially have three or more symptoms or signs as a result of the lung cancer.

Pulmonary Lesion

Symptoms resulting from the primary lung cancer depend on the location and size of the cancer. Such symptoms can be secondary to endobronchial or peripheral growth of the primary tumor. The most common, cough (Chapter 83), occurs in approximately 45% of cases, but it is nonspecific and also common in patients who smoke and have COPD (Chapter 83). Hemoptysis (Chapter 83) occurs in more than 30% of patients, but the most common causes of hemoptysis are bronchitis (Chapter 88) and bronchiectasis (Chapter 90). Dyspnea (Chapter 83) also occurs in 30 to 50% of patients. Wheezing (Chapter 83) is uncommon as an initial symptom in lung cancer and may signify major airway obstruction, which can cause a postobstructive pneumonia that may not initially be evident on chest radiographs and may be diagnosed only when the pneumonia fails to respond to standard therapy (Chapter 97). Lesions may be cavitary and may be associated with an abscess at the time of diagnosis of the lung cancer.

Peripheral lung tumors may be asymptomatic but are more frequently associated with symptoms of cough and pain from involvement of the pleura or chest wall. Chest pain (Chapter 48), which occurs in more than 25% of patients, may be dull in nature, but chest pain that is severe and persists may be due to chest wall involvement.

Intrathoracic Spread

Symptoms associated with intrathoracic spread may be related to direct extension of the tumor or metastasis to regional lymph nodes. Dysphagia may occur secondary to esophageal compression. Although tracheoesophageal or bronchoesophageal fistulas are uncommon, coughing associated with swallowing or the development of aspiration pneumonitis (Chapter 94) should point to this possibility. Hoarseness (Chapter 455), which is associated with recurrent laryngeal nerve paralysis, occurs in less than 20% of cases; it is more common with left-sided lung tumors because the nerve on this side has a longer intrathoracic course than the right-sided nerve does. Phrenic nerve paralysis with hemidiaphragmatic elevation is associated with dyspnea and hiccups. Apical tumors, such as superior sulcus NSCLC (Pancoast's syndrome), may cause Horner's syndrome (Chapter 450), pain secondary to rib destruction, atrophy of hand muscles, and pain in the distribution of the C8, T1, and T2 nerve roots because of tumor invasion of the brachial plexus.

Blockage of the superior vena cava (SVC) (Chapter 100) as a result of compression or direct invasion by the tumor itself or by enlarged mediastinal lymph nodes may cause dyspnea. Signs of SVC syndrome include facial swelling, plethora, upper extremity swelling, dilated neck veins, and a prominent venous pattern on the anterior surface of the chest. Lung cancer accounts for the majority of cases of SVC syndrome, with most cancer being SCLC and located on the right side.

Other manifestations of intrathoracic spread include pleural effusion (Chapter 100) causing dyspnea; pericardial effusion (Chapter 77) and cardiac extension of the tumor (Chapter 59) causing heart failure, arrhythmia, or tamponade; and lymphangitic spread through the lungs causing dyspnea and hypoxemia.

Extrathoracic Spread

At diagnosis, 30 to 40% of patients with NSCLC and approximately 60% of patients with SCLC have extrathoracic hematogenous spread of their tumor. Bone metastasis (Chapter 212) occurs in 30 to 40% of patients with lung cancer and commonly involves the vertebrae, ribs, and pelvic bones. Pain is the primary symptom. Liver metastases can produce right upper quadrant abdominal pain, as well as nonspecific symptoms of fatigue and weight loss. Adrenal metastases can cause pain but most often cause no symptoms. One gland is usually involved, but bilateral metastases may occur. Brain metastasis (Chapter 199), which occurs in 25 to 50% of SCLC and 25% of adenocarcinomas of the lung, may cause no symptoms but is more commonly associated with nausea, vomiting, headaches, seizures, confusion, personality changes, and focal neurologic signs and symptoms, depending on the site of metastatic disease. Epidural, intramedullary spinal cord metastasis and diffuse leptomeningeal involvement are less common than cerebral and cerebellar metastases.

Paraneoplastic Syndromes

Paraneoplastic syndromes (Chapter 189) occur in approximately 10 to 20% of patients with lung cancer. Endocrine syndromes include hypercalcemia (Chapter 266), the syndrome of inappropriate antidiuretic hormone secretion (Chapter 117), and ectopic adrenocorticotropic hormone secretion (Chapter 245). Other endocrine paraneoplastic syndromes of lesser clinical significance produce hormones such as the β-subunit of human chorionic gonadotropin, prolactin, gastrin, growth hormone, thyroid-stimulating factor, insulin-like substance, and calcitonin.

Neurologic syndromes are relatively rare, are most commonly associated with SCLC (Chapter 189), and may have autoimmune mechanisms. Such syndromes include Eaton-Lambert syndrome (Chapter 189), limbic encephalopathy, cerebellar degeneration, subacute sensory neuropathy, autonomic neuropathy (Chapter 445), and optic neuritis (Chapter 450). Skeletal manifestations include digital clubbing (see Fig. 48–10) and hypertrophic pulmonary osteoarthopathy (Chapter 189).

Hematologic/vascular syndromes include hypercoagulable states (Chapter 182), migratory thrombophlebitis (Trosseau's syndrome), and nonbacterial thrombotic endocarditis (Chapter 76). Cutaneous manifestations include dermatomyositis (Chapter 290), acanthosis nigricans, erythema gyratum repens, and hyperkeratosis of the palms and soles of the feet.

Diagnosis

The diagnosis of lung cancer is made by cytologic examination of tissue biopsy specimens, sputum (Fig. 201–2), bronchial washings and brushings of suspicious lesions (Fig. 201–3), bronchoalveolar lavage fluid, and transbronchial and transthoracic needle aspirates (Fig. 201–4). The greater number of viable tumor cells in biopsy specimens from transthoracic, endobronchial, transbronchial, or open biopsy procedures increases the probability of accurate diagnosis. Sputum cytology may be only 20% sensitive for peripheral lung lesions, but it may be 80% sensitive for central lesions. In general, the sensitivity of a single sputum specimen is approximately 50%, whereas examination of three or more specimens increases the sensitivity to nearly 90%. The sensitivity of a single bronchial washing and brushing for detecting lung cancer is approximately 65%. For bronchoalveolar lavage fluid, the sensitivity is 60 to 65%. The sensitivity of fine-needle aspiration biopsy for detecting lung cancer exceeds 85%.

Solitary Pulmonary Nodule

A solitary pulmonary nodule is an asymptomatic lesion less than 3 cm in diameter surrounded by normal lung parenchyma that is incidentally found on a chest radiograph or computed tomography (CT) scan (Fig. 201–5). A solitary pulmonary nodule is found in up to 0.2% of all chest radiographs, and 10 to 70% are malignant. The chance of any solitary pulmonary nodule being cancerous correlates with the size and growth rate of the nodule, the age of the patient, any history of smoking, and a previous history of a malignancy. It is important to compare previous chest radiographs with the one demonstrating the nodule. A nodule that has not changed in size for at least 2 years is probably benign; a high-resolution CT scan with a resolution of 0.3 mm can best assess its size and growth characteristics. Solitary pulmonary nodules smaller than 4 mm have a 1% risk of malignancy, whereas a nodule larger than 8 mm has a 10 to 20% risk. In the latter situation, serial CT scans are indicated;

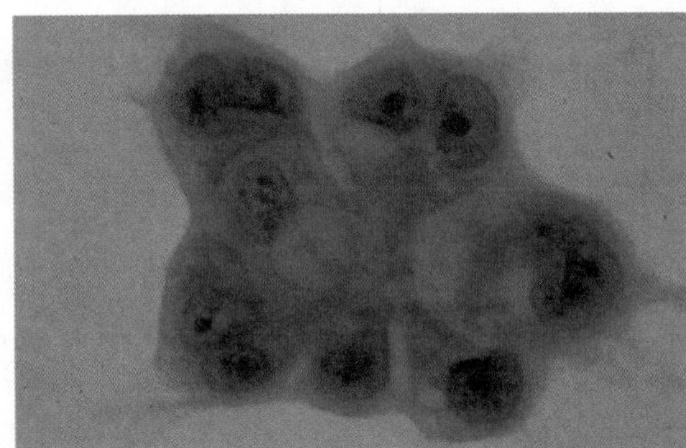

FIGURE 201–2 • Adenocarcinoma cells in a sputum smear. (From Forbes CD, Jackson WF: Color Atlas and Text of Clinical Medicine, 3rd ed. London, Mosby, 2003.)

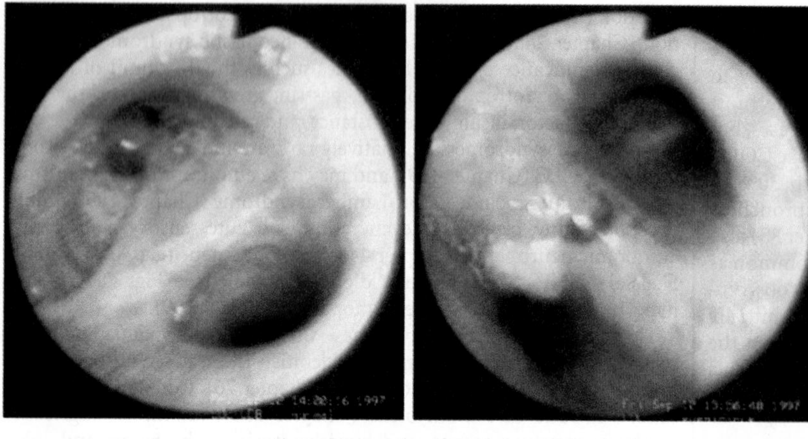

FIGURE 201–3 • Squamous cell carcinoma. Left, Carina between the lingular and upper division bronchus of the left upper lobe. Note the well-defined, sharp features of the carina. **Right,** Carina between the left upper and lower lobes in the same patient. Note the swollen, red, infiltrated appearance of the mucosa and the white exophytic lesion. In addition, there is subepithelial hemorrhage. A biopsy specimen demonstrates squamous cell carcinoma. The patient had increased sputum production, positive sputum cytologic findings, and a nonlocalizing chest radiograph and computed tomography scan.

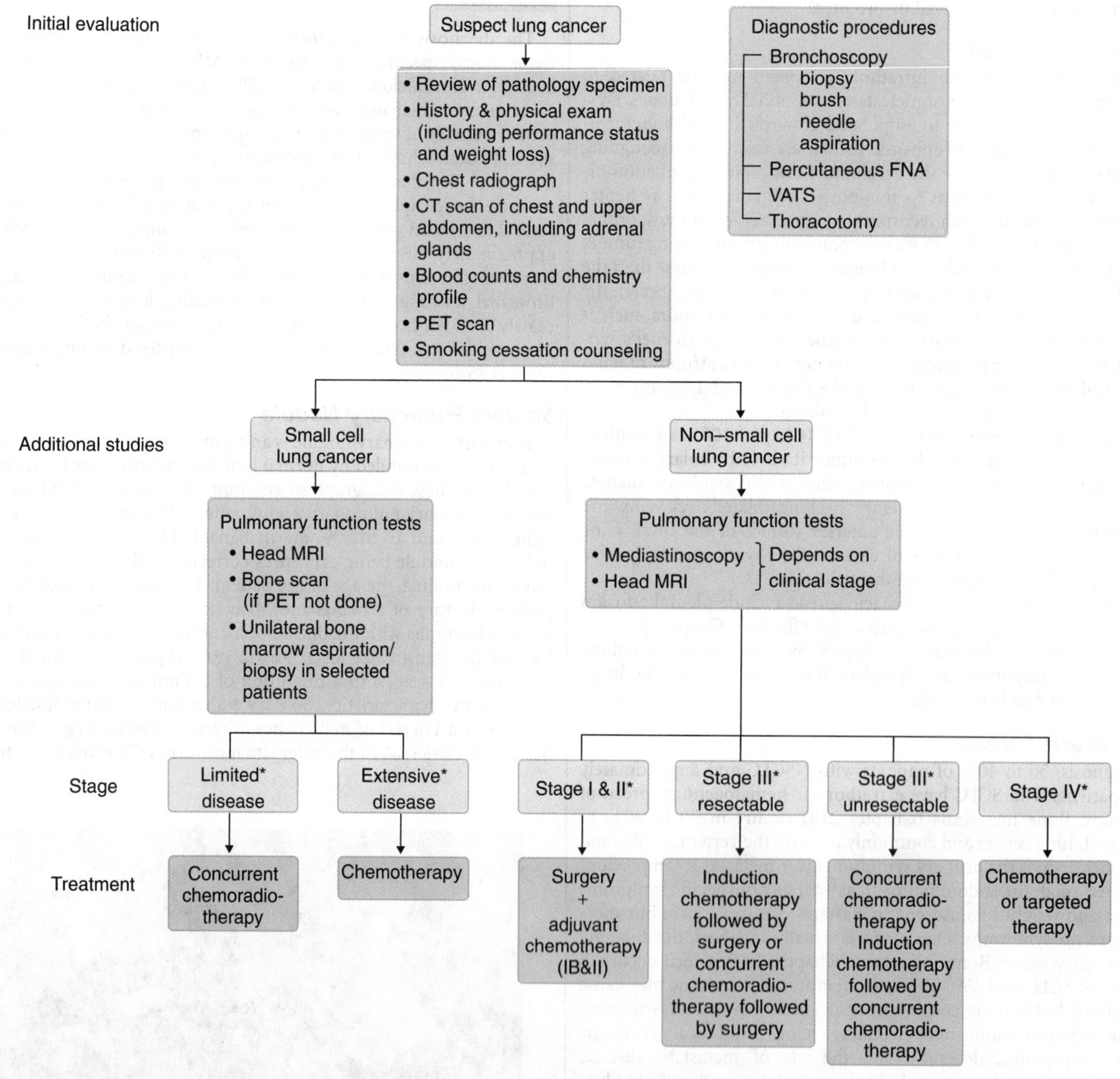

Initial evaluation

Suspect lung cancer

- Review of pathology specimen
- History & physical exam (including performance status and weight loss)
- Chest radiograph
- CT scan of chest and upper abdomen, including adrenal glands
- Blood counts and chemistry profile
- PET scan
- Smoking cessation counseling

Diagnostic procedures
- Bronchoscopy
  - biopsy
  - brush
  - needle aspiration
- Percutaneous FNA
- VATS
- Thoracotomy

Additional studies

Small cell lung cancer

Pulmonary function tests
- Head MRI
- Bone scan (if PET not done)
- Unilateral bone marrow aspiration/biopsy in selected patients

Non–small cell lung cancer

Pulmonary function tests
- Mediastinoscopy
- Head MRI

Depends on clinical stage

	Small cell lung cancer		Non–small cell lung cancer			
Stage	Limited* disease	Extensive* disease	Stage I & II*	Stage III* resectable	Stage III* unresectable	Stage IV*
Treatment	Concurrent chemoradiotherapy	Chemotherapy	Surgery + adjuvant chemotherapy (IB&II)	Induction chemotherapy followed by surgery or concurrent chemoradiotherapy followed by surgery	Concurrent chemoradiotherapy or Induction chemotherapy followed by concurrent chemoradiotherapy	Chemotherapy or targeted therapy

FIGURE 201–4 • Schematic overview for diagnosing, staging, and treating non–small cell and small cell lung cancer. See text for details. (Consult practice guidelines in oncology, non–small cell lung cancer, and small cell lung cancer at www.nccn.org as well for specifics.) *See Tables 201–2 and 201–3. CT = computed tomography; FNA = fine-needle aspiration; MRI = magnetic resonance imaging; PET = positron emission tomography; VATS = video-assisted thoracic surgery.

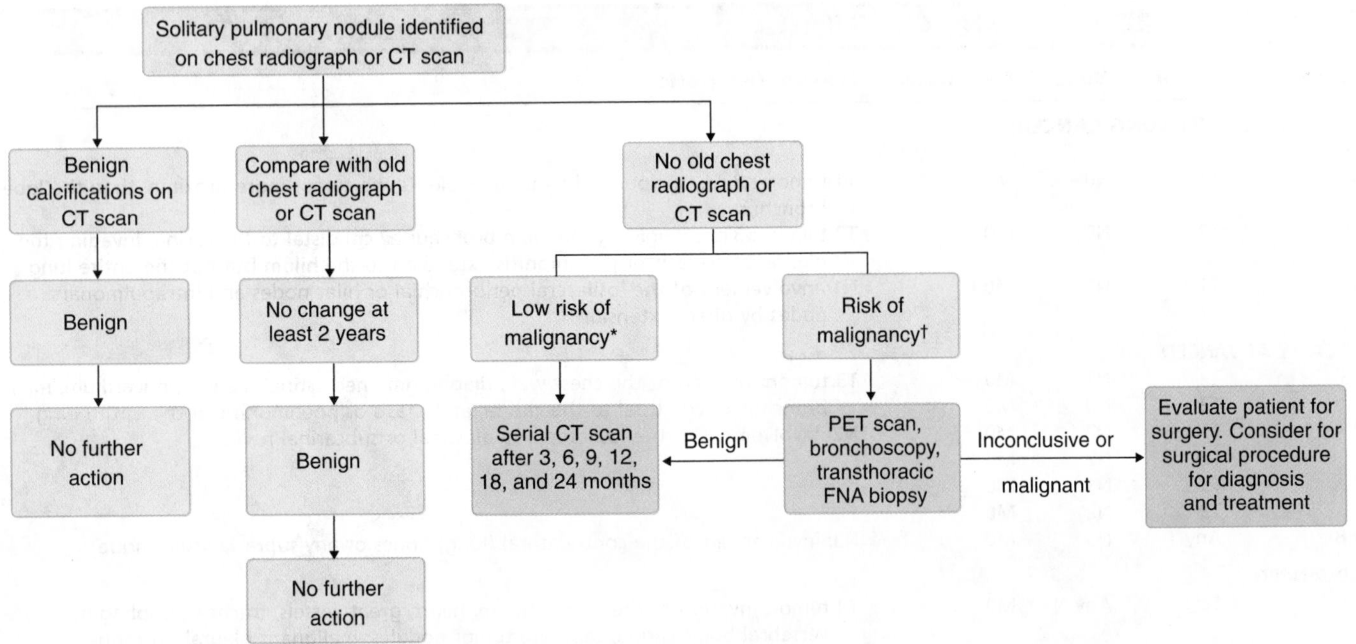

FIGURE 201–5 • Evaluation of a patient with a solitary pulmonary nodule. *Patient with a minimal or absent history of smoking and other known risk factors for the development of lung cancer and a nodule 8 mm or smaller in size. †Patient with a history of smoking and other risk factors for the development of lung cancer and a nodule 8 mm or larger in size. CT = computed tomography; FNA = fine-needle aspiration; PET = positron emission tomography.

position emission tomography (PET) and biopsy should be considered. PET is 96.8% sensitive and 77.8% specific for identifying a malignancy, but because both false-negative and false-positive results can occur, tissue is needed for a definitive diagnosis. Transthoracic fine-needle aspiration biopsy, bronchoscopy, thoracotomy, and video-assisted thoracoscopic surgery (VATS) can establish a diagnosis.

Pathology

The histologic classification of lung cancer includes adenocarcinoma (about 40%), squamous cell (epidermoid) carcinoma (≈30%), large cell carcinoma (≈15%), and small cell carcinoma (≈15%). These four histologic types represent more than 95% of all lung cancer.

Squamous cell carcinoma and adenocarcinoma are further classified by their differentiation: well differentiated, moderately differentiated, and poorly differentiated. The latter types of cells are more aggressive and may have a worse prognosis than well-differentiated tumors. Adenocarcinoma is the most frequent histologic type in women and nonsmokers. Bronchoalveolar carcinoma, a subtype of adenocarcinoma, is well differentiated, grows along intact alveolar septa, and can be localized, multinodular, multifocal, or diffuse.

From a practical perspective based on biologic differences, clinical features, growth properties, and treatment, bronchogenic lung cancer is divided into two main categories: NSCLC and SCLC. In general, all NSCLCs are generally treated the same way based on the stage of the disease. SCLC is usually characterized by more aggressive biology, and treatment is dependent on whether the SCLC is limited stage (i.e., locally advanced) or extensive stage (i.e., metastatic disease).

Staging

Staging of NSCLC involves classification according to T (tumor size), N (regional lymph node involvement), and M (presence or absence of distant metastases) (Table 201–2). For SCLC, TNM staging is not generally used; rather, SCLC is staged as limited disease, defined as disease that can be encompassed by a single radiation portal, or extensive disease, that extending beyond a single radiation portal (usually metastatic).

Staging Procedures

All patients with lung cancer should be clinically staged via a complete history with a focus on performance status and weight loss; physical examination; pathologic review of all biopsied material; completed blood cell and platelet counts; chemistry profile, including renal and liver function tests, electrolytes, glucose, calcium, and phosphorus; and chest radiograph and chest CT (including the upper part of the abdomen and adrenal glands). Magnetic resonance imaging (MRI) of the brain and radionuclide scan of bones should be performed if metastases to these organs are suspected. Radiographs or MRI should be obtained if bone lesions are suggested by radionuclide scanning. PET is used to assess both regional and metastatic spread of tumor. Pulmonary function tests and arterial blood gas determinations should be obtained only if needed for treatment purposes.

For patients with SCLC, the initial pretreatment staging evaluation is similar to that used for NSCLC patients. For patients with peripheral blood count abnormalities, bone marrow aspiration and biopsy are recommended. Twenty to 30% of patients with SCLC will have tumor in bone marrow at the time of diagnosis.

Imaging

Radiography

A standard posteroanterior and lateral chest radiograph, though inexpensive and easy to perform, has limited value in the staging of lung cancer. Although it can detect pulmonary nodules as small as 3 to 4 mm, it is not reliable in detecting hilar or mediastinal lymphadenopathy.

Computed Tomography

A CT scan is commonly used to evaluate whether lung cancer is present in the hilar and mediastinal lymph nodes, liver, and adrenal glands, but its accuracy in identifying mediastinal lymph node involvement is suboptimal (sensitivity of 40 to 65% and specificity of 45 to 90% versus either a PET scan or mediastinoscopy). Most importantly, CT will miss small metastatic foci that do not result in mediastinal lymph node enlargement. Mediastinal lymph nodes that are normal in size (≤1 cm) have an 8 to 15% probability of having metastatic disease, whereas mediastinal lymph nodes that are 1 to 1.5 cm, 1.5 to 2 cm, and greater than 2 cm in size will contain metastases 15 to 30%, approximately 50%, and about 90% of the time, respectively.

Positron Emission Tomography

PET, which uses 2-[^{18}F]fluoro-2-deoxy-D-glucose to identify areas of increased glucose metabolism in lung tumors, is more sensitive than CT in staging lung cancer (see Fig. 201–5); it has a sensitivity of 83%, specificity of 96%, and negative predictive value of 96%. However, increased glucose metabolism also occurs with inflammatory processes. Obtaining both a PET and CT scan can enhance accuracy in the staging of lung cancer. PET also enhances detection of bone, liver, and adrenal metastases. However, if treatment decisions are to be based on PET scan results,

TABLE 201–2 STAGING OF LUNG CANCER

Stage	Tumor	Node	Metastasis	General Description
NON–SMALL CELL LUNG CANCER*				
LOCAL				
IA	T1	N0	M0	T1 tumor: ≤3 cm, surrounded by lung or pleura; no tumor more proximal than the lobe bronchus
IB	T2	N0	M0	T2 tumor: >3 cm, involving the main bronchus ≥2 cm distal to the carina, invading the pleura; atelectasis or pneumonitis extending to the hilum but not the entire lung
IIA	T1	N1	M0	N1: involvement of the ipsilateral peribronchial or hilar nodes and intrapulmonary nodes by direct extension
LOCALLY ADVANCED				
IIB	T2	N1	M0	T3 tumor: invasion of the chest wall, diaphragm, mediastinal pleura, pericardium, main bronchus <2 cm distal to the carina; atelectasis or pneumonitis of the entire lung
	T3	N0	M0	
IIIA	T1	N2	M0	N2: involvement of the ipsilateral mediastinal or subcarinal nodes
	T2	N2	M0	
	T3	N1	M0	
	T3	N2	M0	
IIIB	Any T	N3	M0	N3: involvement of the contralateral (lung) nodes or any supraclavicular node
ADVANCED				
IIIB	T4	Any N	M0	T4 tumor: invasion of the mediastinum, heart, great vessels, trachea, esophagus, vertebral body, carina; separate tumor nodules; malignant pleural effusion
IV	Any T	Any N	M1	Distant metastasis
SMALL CELL LUNG CANCER†				
Limited disease				Evidence of tumor confined to the ipsilateral hemithorax; can be encompassed by a single radiation port
Extensive disease				All other diseases, including metastatic disease

The staging system was developed by the American Joint Commission on Cancer. T = tumor, N = node, M = metastases. SCLC staging was developed by the Veterans Administration Lung Study Group.
*Mountain CF: Revisions in the international system for staging lung cancer. Chest 1997;111:1710–1717.
†Stahel RA, Ginsberg R, Havermann K, et al: Staging and prognostic factors in small cell lung cancer: A consensus. Lung Cancer 1989;5:119–126.

positive PET scan findings require pathologic or other radiologic confirmation.

Evaluation of Mediastinal Tissue

After initial clinical staging, if a patient with NSCLC has potentially surgically resectable disease, the regional lymph nodes (mediastinum) must be sampled for possible metastases. Fiberoptic bronchoscopy to assess the bronchi and transbronchial needle aspirates to evaluate for mediastinal lymphadenopathy are recommended. Transbronchial needle aspirates are positive in 35 to 40% of patients when a CT scan demonstrates hilar or mediastinal lymphadenopathy. The larger the size of the lymph node on CT scan, the greater the chance for the aspirate to be positive.

The gold standard for evaluating the mediastinal lymph nodes for metastatic disease during life is transcervical mediastinoscopy. The subaortic and aortopulmonary window lymph nodes are inaccessible by routine mediastinoscopy, and the subcarinal lymph nodes may be difficult to access. The accuracy of the procedure ranges from 80 to 90%, with a false-negative rate of 10 to 12%. Other procedures used to evaluate the mediastinal lymph nodes include extended cervical mediastinoscopy, anterior mediastinotomy, thoracoscopy, and VATS.

Treatment (Table 201–3 and Fig. 201–4)

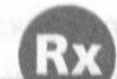

Non–Small Cell Lung Cancer

Stage I and II Disease

For stage I and II NSCLC, surgery is the initial treatment of choice. Before surgical resection, a comprehensive preoperative medical evaluation is mandatory (Chapter 457). This evaluation must be supplemented by pulmonary function tests (forced expiratory volume at 1 second [FEV_1] and diffusing capacity of the lung for carbon monoxide [DLCO]), as well as blood gas analysis (Chapter 85). FEV_1 and DLCO will determine what surgical procedure can be performed safely—pneumonectomy, lobectomy, wedge resection, or segmentectomy. A preoperative FEV_1 less than 40% of predicted and a DLCO less than 40% of normal are associated with an increase in operative mortality. Threshold levels to define resectability include a preoperative FEV_1 greater than 2.0 L and DLCO greater than 60% for pneumonectomy and a preoperative FEV_1 greater than 1.5 L and DLCO greater than 50% for lobectomy. Other factors for determining resectability include exercise tolerance and comorbid disease. The curability of the patient is dependent on the stage of disease and completeness of the resection and not whether lobectomy or pneumonectomy is performed. By comparison, there is a significant risk of local recurrence in patients undergoing wedge resection or segmentectomy rather than more extensive resection of the tumor. Mortality rates for lobectomy and pneumonectomy are 3% and 9%, respectively. For patients older than 70 years, the mortality for pneumonectomy rises to 16 to 25%.

At surgery, a tumor is considered to be unresectable if a metastasis is found in the pleura or contralateral mediastinal lymph nodes or if there is tumor invasion of the mediastinum, heart, great vessels, or other structures. In addition to surgical resection of the tumor, sampling or complete removal of all accessible mediastinal lymph nodes should be performed.

TABLE 201–3 GENERAL APPROACH TO THE TREATMENT OF LUNG CANCER ACCORDING TO STAGE*

Stage	Primary Treatment	Adjuvant Therapy	Outcome
NON–SMALL CELL LUNG CANCER			
I	Surgical resection	Chemotherapy (stage 1B)	5-yr survival rate, >60–70%
II	Surgical resection	Chemotherapy with or without radiation therapy	5-yr survival rate, >40–50%
IIIA (resectable)	Preoperative chemotherapy followed by surgical resection (preferable) or chemotherapy followed by radiation therapy	Chemotherapy with or without radiation therapy	5-yr survival rate, 15–30%
IIIA (unresectable) or IIIB (involvement of the contralateral or supraclavicular lymph nodes)	Chemotherapy plus concurrent radiation therapy (preferable) or chemotherapy followed by radiation therapy	None	5-yr survival rate, 10–20%
IIIB (pleural effusion) or IV	Chemotherapy with 2 agents for 4–6 cycles Chemotherapy + bevacizumab (selected patients) Surgical resection of solitary brain metastasis and surgical resection of primary (T1) lesion	None	Median survival, 8–10 mo 1-yr survival rate, 30–35% 2-yr survival rate, 10–15% 5-yr survival rate, 10–15%
SMALL CELL LUNG CANCER			
Limited disease†	Chemotherapy plus concurrent radiation therapy	None	5-yr survival rate, 15–25%
Extensive disease†	Chemotherapy	None	5-yr survival rate, <5%

*All chemotherapy regimens include either cisplatin or carboplatin. The second drug used as part of the regimen may include etoposide, paclitaxel, docetaxel, vinorelbine, gemcitabine, or irinotecan.
†Prophylactic cranial irradiation is recommended for all patients with a complete response to initial therapy.
Modified from Spira A, Ettinger DS: Multidisciplinary management of lung cancer. N Engl J Med 2004;350:379–392.

Rx

Adjuvant cisplatin-based chemotherapy (e.g., cisplatin, 80 mg/m^2 every 3 weeks for four doses or 100 mg/m^2 every 4 weeks for three or four doses, or cisplatin, 120 mg/m^2 every 4 weeks for three doses, plus etoposide, 100 mg/m^2 for 3 days/cycle, vinorelbine, 30 mg/m^2 weekly, vinblastine, 4 mg/m^2 weekly, or vindesine, 3 mg/m^2 weekly) provides a small absolute increase in overall survival at 5 years for stage I, II, and III disease. 1,2 Treatment with monoclonal antibodies has not yet been consistently beneficial. 3-5

Adjuvant radiation therapy for stage I and II disease is not indicated. However, in patients with stage I NSCLC who for medical reasons are not candidates for surgery, radiation therapy (usually a total dose of 65 to 70 Gy in 2-Gy fractions) can be given with curative intent. Five-year survival rates in patients thus treated range from 10 to 30%.

Stage III—Resectable

For patients with stage III resectable disease (ipsilateral mediastinal spread of disease [N2], tumors [T3] involving the chest wall, diaphragm, or pleura; or superior sulcus tumors [Pancoast's] tumors), surgery alone is suboptimal treatment because of the presence of occult metastatic disease. Neoadjuvant (i.e., induction) chemotherapy given in sequence with or concurrent with radiation therapy before surgery improves survival when compared with surgery alone or surgery plus postoperative radiation therapy. However, concurrent chemoradiation therapy causes significant esophagitis when compared with the use of sequential chemotherapy and radiation therapy.

Stage III—Unresectable

Stage IIIA or IIIB disease may be unresectable. Thoracic radiation therapy (total dose, 60 Gy) relieves symptoms in the chest but has little effect on 5-year survival rates unless combined with induction chemotherapy (e.g., vinblastine plus cisplatin for two cycles), which improves median survival from 9.7 months to 13.8 months and the 5-year survival rate from 7 to 19% when compared with radiation therapy alone. 6

Rx

Concurrent chemotherapy and radiation therapy rather than sequential therapy can improve survival in patients with locally advanced NSCLC but increases side effects, particularly esophagitis, by five-fold. To improve the effectiveness of radiation therapy, different fractionation approaches are under evaluation. Three-dimensional treatment planning permits delivery of higher doses of radiation to the primary tumor and regional lymph nodes without increasing toxicity.

Stage IV—Disseminated Disease

For patients with disseminated NSCLC, treatment generally consists of cisplatin or carboplatin combined with paclitaxel, docetaxel, gemcitabine, vinorelbine, irinotecan, or topotecan. The response rate to such therapy is 20 to 50%, with a median survival of 8 to 10 months, 1-year survival rate of 30 to 35%, and 2-year survival rate of 10 to 15%. Data suggest that two-drug combinations are better than single-agent therapy, but three-drug combinations are not more effective than two-drug combinations. The duration of therapy is four to six cycles, and patients older than 70 years who have good performance status respond to and tolerate chemotherapy as well as younger patients do.

Patients with a solitary metastasis may occasionally benefit from resection of the isolated metastatic lesion. For example, resection of a solitary brain metastasis followed by whole brain irradiation can potentially be curative, with 5-year survival rates as high as 20%. Patients with metastatic NSCLC can benefit from palliative radiation therapy to specific lesions that cause bronchial obstruction, SVC syndrome, bone pain, brain masses, and spinal cord compression.

Small Cell Lung Cancer

The mainstay of treatment of SCLC is chemotherapy because the disease is characterized by its propensity for a rapid growth rate and spread to distant sites. Unfortunately, management of SCLC has changed little in the past decade.

Limited Stage

Thirty to 40% of SCLC patients have limited-stage disease. Management usually consists of chemotherapy and radiation therapy, and surgery is indicated only in the approximately 5% of patients who have a solitary peripheral pulmonary nodule without evidence of mediastinal lymph node involvement with clinical staging. After surgical removal of the SCLC nodule, patients with negative mediastinal lymph nodes at surgery require only postoperative chemotherapy with etoposide and cisplatin. The 5-year survival rate in patients with no mediastinal lymph node involvement is 30 to 60%. If the nodes contain metastases, chest irradiation is recommended in addition to chemotherapy.

For the majority of patients with limited-stage SCLC, concurrent chemotherapy and radiation therapy appears more to be effective than sequential therapy. In the United States, etoposide and cisplatin plus concurrent radiation therapy (i.e., twice-a-day irradiation—total dose of 45 Gy) is the treatment of choice and produces a 5-year survival rate of 26% as compared with 16% when given with the same dose of radiation once a day. 7

In patients who achieve a complete response to therapy, prophylactic cranial irradiation (24 to 36 Gy), recommended because of the high rate of brain metastases with SCLC, reduces the risk for brain metastases and provides about a 5% survival advantage, but its higher risk of precipitating cognitive abnormalities must be taken into consideration, especially in elderly patients.

Extensive Stage

For extensive-stage SCLC, chemotherapy is the treatment of choice. In the United States, etoposide plus cisplatin or carboplatin is commonly used. The latter regimen causes significantly less nausea, vomiting, and neurotoxicity because of the carboplatin. The chemotherapy is administered every 3 weeks for four to six cycles. At this time there is no evidence that maintenance therapy with either chemotherapy or targeted molecular therapy increases survival rates.

Screening and Prevention

Screening

Unfortunately, most patients with lung cancer are initially found to have advanced disease that is not curable. Screening chest radiographs have been unsuccessful in improving outcome.

Spiral CT scanning is four- to five-fold more sensitive than chest radiography for detecting malignant nodules in high-risk patients, but spiral CT also detects seven to eight benign nodules for every malignant nodule found. A large trial is currently ongoing to determine whether current or former smokers benefit from screening with spiral CT.

Prevention

Primary prevention of lung cancer focuses on ways to prevent individuals from smoking and promotion of smoking cessation (Chapter 30). Trials of supplemental doses of β-carotene and vitamin E, stimulated by epidemiologic evidence of lower serum levels of these antioxidants in patients with lung cancer, have not only been unsuccessful but actually produced a higher risk for lung cancer in smokers who received either of these supplements. High concentrations of selenium in blood are associated with a lower risk for lung cancer, and an ongoing trial is comparing selenium with placebo in patients who have survived resection for stage I lung cancer.

Prognosis

Most patients in whom lung cancer is diagnosed have incurable disease, with an overall 5-year survival rate of approximately 15%. What determines the chance for survival is the stage of disease in NSCLC and whether the disease is extensive or limited in the case of SCLC (Table 201–4).

TABLE 201–4 FIVE-YEAR SURVIVAL RATE FOR NON–SMALL CELL LUNG CANCER BY THE CLINICAL AND SURGICAL TNM (TUMOR, NODE, METASTASIS) INTERNATIONAL STAGING SYSTEM FOR LUNG CANCER

		5-Year Survival Rate (%)	
Stage	**TNM Subgroups**	**Clinical Stage**	**Surgical Stage**
IA	T1 N0 M0	61	67
IB	T2 N0 M0	38	57
IIA	T1 N1 M0	34	55
IIB	T2 N1 M0	24	39
IIB	T3 N0 M0	22	38
IIIA	T3 N1 M0	9	25
	T1–3 N2 M0	13	23
IIIB	T4 N0–2 M0	7	—
	Any T N3 M0	3	—
IV	Any T any N M1	1	—

OTHER PULMONARY NEOPLASMS

Neuroendocrine Lung Tumors

Neuroendocrine lung tumors are classified into four types: carcinoid tumors, atypical carcinoids, SCLC, and large cell neuroendocrine carcinomas. Carcinoid tumors are low-grade neuroendocrine tumors with a 10-year survival rate of greater than 90%. Atypical carcinoid tumors are an intermediate-grade tumor, a more aggressive tumor than carcinoid, with survival ranging from 10 months to 3 years. Large cell neuroendocrine carcinoma is an aggressive neuroendocrine tumor that does not meet the criteria for either carcinoid, atypical carcinoid, or SCLC.

Bronchial Carcinoid Tumors

Carcinoid tumors (Chapter 251) of the lung account for 1 to 2% of all lung neoplasms. They are neuroendocrine tumors that trace their origin to the Kulchitsky cell present in bronchial epithelium. Typical and atypical carcinoids differ in the number of mitoses (<2 per 10 high-power fields [HPF] vs. 2 to 10 per 10 HPF, respectively), nuclear pleomorphism (absent vs. present), regional lymph node metastases (5 to 15% vs. 20 to 28%), and distant metastases at initial evaluation (rare vs. 20%). Patients with a typical carcinoid rarely die, whereas patients with atypical carcinoids have a 5-year mortality rate of 27 to 47%. Carcinoid tumors are not associated with cigarette smoking, are twice as common in women as in men, usually occur in patients younger than 40 years, and arise in the perihilar area of the lung. Treatment of bronchial carcinoid tumors is based on the stage of the disease. Usually, mediastinal staging is followed by surgical resection. With mediastinal lymph node involvement, radiation therapy is recommended for typical carcinoid tumors if surgery cannot be performed. For atypical carcinoid or metastatic disease, chemotherapy (etoposide plus cisplatin every 3 weeks for four cycles) plus radiation therapy is commonly used, but there is no evidence for the benefit of one therapy over another.

Malignant Mesothelioma

Pleural mesotheliomas (Chapter 100) are related to asbestos exposure (Chapter 93), with a peak risk 30 to 35 years after the initial exposure to asbestos. Approximately 50% of patients in whom a mesothelioma develops give no history of direct asbestos exposure. Other possible risk factors for mesothelioma include radiation and SV40 virus. Mesothelioma is generally diagnosed in the fifth to seventh decade of life (median age, 60), with the neoplasm developing in men five times more frequently than in women. Common symptoms include shortness of breath (60%) and chest wall pain or discomfort (60%). Chest radiographs usually reveal the presence of a unilateral pleural effusion. When the tumor progresses, it is generally local; symptomatic distant metastases are a late occurrence, if at all. Cytologic evaluation of pleural fluid to establish the diagnosis is difficult and may be inaccurate. The diagnosis is usually made by a biopsy procedure—under CT guidance or thoracoscopically, including VATS if necessary. Several staging systems have been proposed, but none has achieved complete acceptance. Treatment, which depends on the extent of disease, includes surgery (thoracoscopy with sclerosis, pleurectomy, extrapleural pneumonectomy), radiation therapy, and chemotherapy. These three modalities individually have not significantly improved survival rates, so multimodality therapy is being evaluated. Mesothelioma remains a fatal disease with a median survival of 9 to 12 months from the time of diagnosis.

Other Lung Tumors

Carcinomas of the salivary gland type include mucoepidermoid carcinoma and adenoid cystic carcinoma. These tumors are slow-growing neoplasms that arise from the bronchial glands. They represent approximately 0.2% of lung cancers and are usually treated surgically.

Primary sarcomas of the lung are very rare and include malignant fibrous histiocytoma, fibrosarcoma, leiomyosarcoma, rhabdomyosarcoma, epithelioid hemangioendothelioma, angiosarcoma, and liposarcoma. Surgery is the primary treatment, but radiation therapy or chemotherapy, or both, may be necessary, depending on the size and grade of the tumor and whether the margins are clear (Chapter 213).

Primary lymphomas of the lung account for approximately 0.3% of all primary cancers of the lung. The most common type is a low-grade small lymphocytic lymphoma. Surgery and chemotherapy (Chapter 196) are the usual treatments.

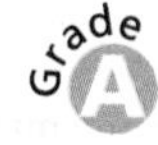

1. The International Adjuvant Lung Cancer Trial Collaborative Group: Cisplatin-based adjuvant chemotherapy in patients with completely resected non–small cell lung cancer. N Engl J Med 2004;350:351–360.
2. Winton T, Livingston R, Johnson D, et al: Vinorelbine plus cisplatin vs. observation in resected non–small-cell lung cancer. N Engl J Med 2005;352:2589–2597.
3. Shepherd FA, Pereira JR, Ciuleanu T, et al: Erlotinib in previously treated non–small cell lung cancer. N Engl J Med 2005;353:123–132.
4. Thatcher N, Chang A, Parikh P, et al: Gefitinib plus best supportive care in previously treated patients with refractory advanced non–small-cell lung cancer: Results from a randomised, placebo-controlled, multicentre study (Iressa Survival Evaluation in Lung Cancer). Lancet 2005;366:1527–1537.
5. Sandler A, Gray R, Perry M, et al: Paclitaxel-Carboplatin alone or with bevacizumab for non–small-cell lung cancer. N Engl J Med 2006;355:2542–2550.
6. Dillman RO, Segren SL, Propert KL, et al: Improved survival of stage III non–small-cell lung cancer: Seven-year follow-up of Cancer and Leukemia Group B (CALGB) 8433 trial. J Natl Cancer Inst 1996;88:1210–1215.
7. Turrisi AT III, Kim K, Blum R, et al: Twice-daily compared with once-daily thoracic radiotherapy in limited small-cell lung cancer treated concurrently with cisplatin and etoposide. N Engl J Med 1999;340:265–271.

SUGGESTED READINGS

Clinical Practice Guidelines in Oncology. Non–Small Cell Lung Cancer and Small Cell Lung Cancer. Version 1. 2006. Available from the National Comprehensive Cancer Network at http://www.nccn.org. *Up-to-date approaches to the treatment of non–small cell and small cell lung cancer.*

Jackman DM, Johnson BE: Small-cell lung cancer. Lancet 2005;366:1385–1396. *A comprehensive review.*

Ost D, Fein AM, Feinsilver SH: The solitary pulmonary nodule. N Engl J Med 2003;348:2535–2542. *An excellent review of approaches to the management of a solitary pulmonary nodule.*

Potti A, Mukherjee S, Petersen RM, et al: A genomic strategy to refine prognosis in early-stage non–small-cell lung cancer. N Engl J Med 2006;355:570–580. *Using lung metagene model to identify and predict recurrence of disease was more effective than clinical prognostic factors.*

Spira A, Ettinger DS: Multidisciplinary management of lung cancer. N Engl J Med 2004;350:379–392. *A review of the treatment of both non–small cell and small cell lung cancer.*

The International Early Lung Cancer Action Program Investigators: Survival of patients with stage I lung cancer detected on CT screening. N Engl J Med 2006;355:1763–1771. *Annual spiral CT screening can detect curable lung cancer.*

202 NEOPLASMS OF THE STOMACH

Anil K. Rustgi

Definition

Gastric neoplasms are predominantly malignant, and nearly 90 to 95% of these tumors are adenocarcinomas. Less frequently observed malignant diseases include lymphomas, especially non-Hodgkin's lymphoma, and sarcomas, such as leiomyosarcoma. Benign gastric neoplasms include leiomyomas, carcinoid tumors, and lipomas.

ADENOCARCINOMA OF THE STOMACH

Epidemiology

The great geographic variation in the incidence of gastric cancer worldwide strongly indicates that environmental factors influence the pathogenesis of gastric carcinogenesis. Further support for this notion comes from observations that groups emigrating from high-risk to low-risk areas, such as Japanese persons moving to Hawaii and Brazil, acquire the low risk of the area into which they emigrate, presumably because of adoption of the endogenous lifestyle and exposure to different environmental factors.

Gastric adenocarcinoma was the most frequently observed malignant disease in the world until the mid-1980s, and it remains extremely common among men in certain regions, such as tropical South America, some parts of the Caribbean, and Eastern Europe. Regardless of gender, it remains the most common malignant disease in Japan and China.

Whereas gastric cancer was the most common cancer in the United States in the 1930s, its annual incidence has steadily decreased; the annual incidence is now fewer than 20,000 new cases per year. However, although the incidence of gastric adenocarcinoma localized to the distal stomach has declined, the incidence of proximal gastric and gastroesophageal adenocarcinomas has been steadily increasing in the United States, a finding that perhaps reflects differences in pathogenic factors. Typically, gastric cancer occurs between the ages of 50 to 70 years and is uncommon before age 30 years. The rates are higher in men than in women by 2 to 1. Five-year survival is less than 20%.

Risk Factors

Risk factors for the development of gastric adenocarcinoma can be divided into environmental and genetic factors, as well as precursor conditions (Table 202–1). For example, *Helicobacter pylori* infection is significantly more common in patients with gastric cancer than in matched control groups. Epidemiologic studies of high-risk populations have also suggested that genotoxic agents such as *N*-nitroso compounds may play a role in gastric tumorigenesis. *N*-Nitroso compounds can be formed in the human stomach by nitrosation of ingested nitrates, which are common constituents of the diet. High nitrate concentrations in soil and drinking water have been observed in areas with high death rates from gastric cancer. Atrophic gastritis (Chapter 141), with or without intestinal metaplasia, is observed in association with gastric cancer, especially in endemic areas. Pernicious anemia (Chapter 141) is associated with a severalfold increase in gastric cancer. Atrophic gastritis and gastric cancer have certain environmental risk factors in common. It is likely that atrophic gastritis and intestinal metaplasia represent intermediary steps to gastric cancer. The achlorhydria associated with gastritis related to *H. pylori* infection, pernicious anemia, or other causes favors the growth of bacteria capable of converting nitrates to nitrites. The nitrosamine *N*-methyl-*N*′-nitro-*N*-nitrosoguanidine causes a high rate of induction of adenocarcinoma in the glandular stomach of rats. At the same time, most patients with atrophic gastritis do not develop gastric cancer, a finding suggesting that neither atrophic gastritis nor achlorhydria alone is responsible.

Benign gastric ulcers do not appear to predispose patients to gastric cancer. However, patients who have a gastric remnant after subtotal gastrectomy for benign disorders have a relative risk of gastric cancer of 1.5 to 3.0 by 15 to 20 years after surgery.

TABLE 202–1 CONDITIONS PREDISPOSING TO OR ASSOCIATED WITH GASTRIC CANCER

ENVIRONMENTAL
Helicobacter pylori infection
Dietary: excess of salt (salted pickled foods), nitrates/nitrites, carbohydrates; deficiency of fresh fruit, vegetables, vitamins A and C, refrigeration
Low socioeconomic status
Cigarette smoking
GENETIC
Familial gastric cancer (rare)
Associated with hereditary nonpolyposis colorectal cancer
Blood group A
PREDISPOSING CONDITIONS
Chronic gastritis, especially atrophic gastritis with or without intestinal metaplasia
Pernicious anemia
Intestinal metaplasia
Gastric adenomatous polyps (>2 cm)
Postgastrectomy stumps
Gastric epithelial dysplasia
Ménétrier's disease (hypertrophic gastropathy)
Chronic peptic ulcer

Pathobiology

Gastric adenocarcinomas can be divided into two types: intestinal and diffuse. The intestinal type is typically in the distal stomach with ulcerations, is often preceded by premalignant lesions, and is declining in incidence in the United States. By contrast, the diffuse type involves widespread thickening of the stomach, especially in the cardia, and it often affects younger patients; this form may present as linitis plastica, a nondistensible stomach with the absence of folds and narrowed lumen caused by infiltration of the stomach wall with tumor. Other conditions may result in linitis plastica, such as lymphoma (Chapters 196 and 197), tuberculosis (Chapter 345), syphilis (Chapter 340), and amyloidosis (Chapter 296). The prognosis is generally worse in the diffuse type.

Key histopathologic features of gastric cancer include degree of differentiation, invasion through the gastric wall, lymph node involvement, and the presence or absence of signet-ring cells within the tumor itself. Other pathologic manifestations include a polypoid mass, which may be difficult to distinguish from a benign polyp. Early gastric cancer, a condition that is not uncommon in Japan and that has a relatively favorable prognosis, consists of superficial lesions with or without lymph node involvement.

The leading hypothesis explaining the way in which *H. pylori* predisposes to gastric cancer risk is the induction of an inflammatory response, in which interleukin-1β may be pivotal. Chronic *H. pylori* infection also leads to chronic atrophic gastritis with resulting achlorhydria, which, in turn, favors bacterial growth that can convert nitrates (dietary components) to nitrites. These nitrites, in combination with genetic factors, promote abnormal cellular proliferation, genetic mutations, and eventually cancer. In a mouse model of gastric cancer, *H. pylori* infection may play a role in the recruitment of bone marrow–derived stem cells that facilitate gastric carcinogenesis.

Genetics

It is clear that genetic factors play a role in gastric cancer. For example, blood group A is associated with a higher incidence rate of gastric cancer, even in nonendemic areas. A threefold increase in gastric cancer has been reported among first-degree relatives of patients with the disease. Furthermore, germline or inherited mutations in the E-cadherin gene have been described in familial diffuse hereditary gastric cancer, which is seen in young patients. In addition, in hereditary nonpolyposis colorectal cancer type II (Chapter 203) patients have associated extracolonic cancers, including gastric cancer.

It now appears that several genetic mechanisms are important in gastric cancer: oncogene activation, tumor suppressor gene inactivation, and DNA microsatellite instability. For example, loss of heterozygosity of the *APC* (adenomatous polyposis coli) gene has been observed in gastric cancers. The p53 tumor suppressor gene product regulates the cell cycle at the G_1/S phase transition and probably also functions in DNA repair and apoptosis (programmed cell death). The *p53* gene is mutated not only in gastric cancer but also in gastric precancerous lesions, a finding suggesting that mutation of the *p53* gene is an early event in gastric carcinogenesis. Microsatellite DNA alterations or instability in dinucleotide repeats that were originally identified in hereditary nonpolyposis colorectal cancer also occur frequently in sporadic gastric carcinoma. Mutations in genes may accumulate as a result of DNA microsatellite instability.

Clinical Manifestations

Symptoms and Signs

In its early stages, gastric cancer may often be asymptomatic or may produce only nonspecific symptoms that make early diagnosis difficult. Later symptoms include bloating, dysphagia, epigastric pain, or early satiety. Early satiety or vomiting may suggest partial gastric outlet obstruction, although gastric dysmotility may contribute to the vomiting in patients with nonobstructive cases. Epigastric pain, reminiscent of that associated with peptic ulcer (Chapter 142), occurs in about one fourth of patients, but in most patients with gastric cancer, the pain is not relieved by food or antacids. Pain that radiates to the back may indicate that the tumor has penetrated the pancreas. When dysphagia is associated with gastric cancer, this symptom suggests a more proximal gastric tumor at the gastroesophageal junction (Chapter 140) or in the fundus.

Signs of gastric cancer include bleeding, which can result in anemia that produces the symptoms of weakness, fatigue, and malaise, as well as more serious cardiovascular and cerebral consequences. Perforation related to gastric cancer is unusual. Gastric cancer metastatic to the liver can lead to right upper quadrant pain, jaundice, and/or fever. Lung metastases can cause cough, hiccups, and hemoptysis. Peritoneal carcinomatosis can lead to malignant ascites unresponsive to diuretics. Gastric cancer can also metastasize to bone.

Physical Examination

In the earliest stages of gastric cancer, the physical examination may be unremarkable. At later stages, patients become cachectic, and an epigastric mass may be palpated. If the tumor has metastasized to the liver, hepatomegaly with jaundice and ascites may be present. Portal or splenic vein invasion can cause splenomegaly. Lymph node involvement in the left supraclavicular area is termed *Virchow's node,* and periumbilical nodal involvement is called *Sister Mary Joseph's node.* The fecal occult blood test may be positive. Metastasis to the ovary is termed *Krukenberg's tumor.*

Paraneoplastic syndromes may precede or occur concurrently with gastric cancer. Examples include the following: Trousseau's syndrome (Chapter 182), which is recurrent migratory superficial thrombophlebitis indicating a possible hypercoagulable state; acanthosis nigricans, which arises in flexor areas with skin lesions that are raised and hyperpigmented; neuromyopathy with involvement of the sensory and motor pathways; and central nervous system involvement with altered mental status and ataxia.

Laboratory Studies

Laboratory studies may reveal iron deficiency anemia. Predisposing pernicious anemia can progress to megaloblastic anemia. Microangiopathic hemolytic anemia has been reported. Abnormalities in liver tests generally indicate metastatic disease. Hypoalbuminemia is a marker of malnourishment. Protein-losing enteropathy is rare but can be seen in Ménétrier's disease, another predisposing condition. Serologic test results, such as those for carcinoembryonic antigen and CA 72.4, may be abnormal. Although these tests are not recommended for original diagnosis, they may be useful for monitoring disease after surgical resection.

Diagnosis

The diagnostic accuracy of upper endoscopy with biopsy and cytologic examination approaches 95 to 99% for both types of gastric cancer. Cancer may arise as a small mucosal ulceration, a polyp, or a mass (Fig. 202–1). In some patients, gastric ulceration may first be noted in an upper gastrointestinal barium contrast study. A benign gastric ulcer is suggested by a smooth, regular base, whereas a malignant ulcer is manifested by a surrounding mass, irregular folds, and an irregular base. Although these and other radiographic characteristics historically helped to predict benign versus malignant disease, upper gastrointestinal endoscopy with biopsy and cytologic examination is mandatory whenever a gastric ulcer is found in the radiologic study, even if the ulcer has benign characteristics.

Staging of gastric cancer and, at times, diagnosis have been greatly enhanced by the advent of endoscopic ultrasonography. The extent of tumor, including wall invasion and local lymph node involvement, can be assessed by endoscopic ultrasonography (Fig. 202–2), which provides information complementary to that from computed tomographic scans. Endoscopic ultrasonography can help guide aspiration biopsies of lymph nodes to determine their malignant features, if any. Computed tomography of the chest and abdomen should be performed to document lymphadenopathy and extragastric organ (especially lung and liver) involvement. In some centers, staging of gastric cancer entails bone scans because of the proclivity of gastric cancer to metastasize to bone.

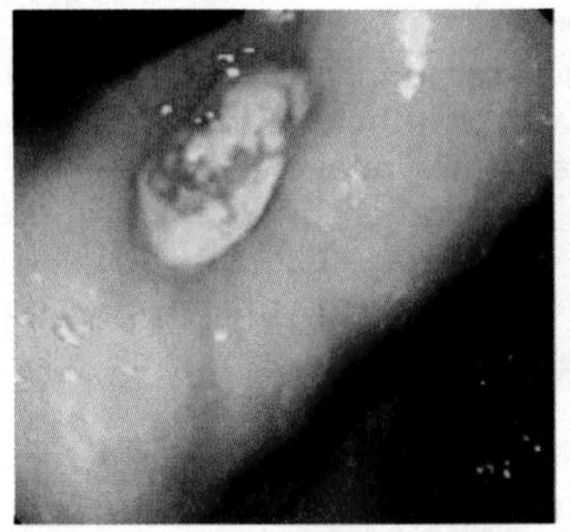
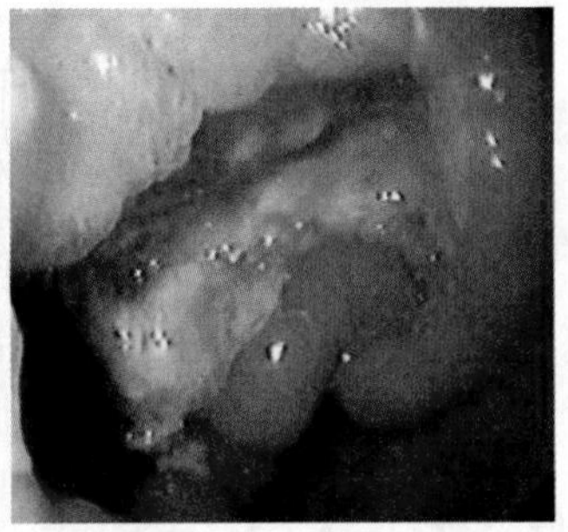

FIGURE 202–1 • Benign (left) and malignant (right) gastric ulcer. Note the shaggy, thickened, and overhanging edges of the cancer. (Courtesy of Pankaj Jay Pasricha, MD.)

Treatment

Surgical Therapy

The only chance for cure of gastric cancer remains surgical resection, which is possible in only 25 to 30% of cases. If the tumor is confined to the distal stomach, subtotal gastrectomy is performed with resection of lymph nodes in the porta hepatis and in the pancreatic head. By contrast, tumors of the proximal stomach merit total gastrectomy to obtain an adequate margin and to remove lymph nodes; distal pancreatectomy and splenectomy are usually also performed as part of this procedure, which carries with it higher mortality and morbidity rates. Limited gastric resection is necessary for patients with excessive bleeding or obstruction. If cancer recurs in the gastric remnant, limited resection may again be necessary for palliation. Most recurrences in both types of gastric cancer are in the local or regional area of the original tumor.

Medical Therapy

Gastric cancer is one of the few gastrointestinal cancers that is somewhat responsive to chemotherapy. Chemotherapy with the combination of epirubicin, cisplatin, and fluorouracil, given both preoperatively and postoperatively, significantly improves 5-year survival from 23% to 36% in patients with resectable gastroesophageal cancer. [1] Similarly, the combination of chemotherapy (fluorouracil and leucovorin) with radiation therapy has been shown to improve median survival from 27 months to 36 months compared with surgery alone in patients with adenocarcinoma of the stomach or gastroesophageal junction. [2]

Single-agent chemotherapy treatment, which provides partial response rates of 20 to 30% and is reserved for patients with a poor performance status, can be given as follows: 5-fluorouracil (a continuous infusion at 200 to 250 mg/m^2/day), mitomycin C (15 to 20 mg/m^2; no more than 40 mg at once), or cisplatin (75 mg/m^2 every 4 weeks). Combination regimens that can yield partial response rates of 35 to 50% include the following: ECF, which is most popular in Europe (epirubicin, 50 mg/m^2 on day 1; cisplatin, 60 mg/m^2 on day 1; 5-fluorouracil, 200 mg/m^2/day as a continuous infusion every 21 days); CF (5-fluorouracil infusion, 1000 mg/m^2/day for 4 days; cisplatin, 75 to 100 mg/m^2 on day 1 every 4 weeks); or TCF (docetaxel [Taxotere], 75 mg/m^2 on day 1; cisplatin, 75 mg/m^2 on day 1; and 5-fluorouracil, 750 mg/m^2/day for 5 days every 3 weeks).

Radiation therapy alone is ineffective and is generally employed only for palliative purposes in the setting of bleeding, obstruction,

Section XV Oncology

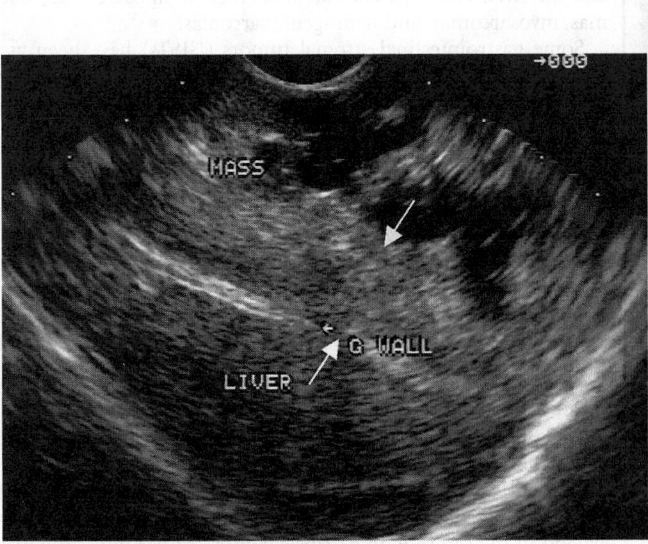

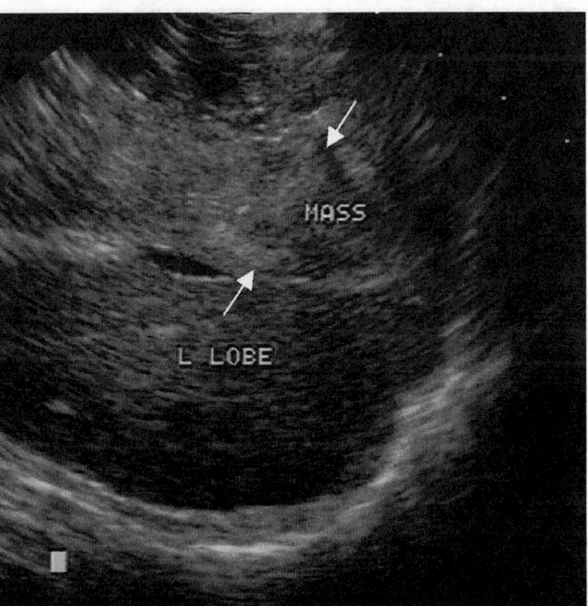

FIGURE 202–2 • Gastric mass. Endoscopic ultrasonography depicting a large gastric mass that is compressing the liver and gallbladder wall **(A)** and, on a different view, the left lobe of the liver **(B)**.

or pain. Gene therapy and immune-based therapy are currently only investigational in animal models.

General Methods

Implicit in the management of the patient with gastric cancer is meticulous attention to nutrition (jejunal enteral feedings or total parenteral nutrition), correction of metabolic abnormalities that arise from vomiting or diarrhea, and treatment of infection from aspiration or spontaneous bacterial peritonitis. To maintain lumen patency, endoscopic laser treatment or prosthesis placement can be utilized in a palliative fashion.

Prognosis

Approximately one third of patients who undergo a curative resection are alive after 5 years. In aggregate, the overall 5-year survival rate in patients with gastric cancer is less than 10%. Prognostic factors include anatomic location and nodal status (Table 202–2); distal gastric cancers without lymph node involvement have a better prognosis than proximal gastric cancers with or without lymph node involvement. Other prognostic factors include depth of penetration and tumor cell DNA aneuploidy. Linitis plastica and infiltrating lesions have a much worse prognosis than polypoid disease or exophytic masses. In the subset of mostly Japanese patients with early gastric cancer that is confined to the mucosa and submucosa, surgical resection may be curative and definitely improves the 5-year survival rate to more than 50%. In fact, when early gastric cancer is confined to the mucosa, endoscopic mucosal resection may be an alternative.

LYMPHOMA OF THE STOMACH

Epidemiology

Gastric lymphoma represents about 5% of all malignant gastric tumors and is increasing in incidence. Most gastric lymphomas are non-Hodgkin's lymphomas (Chapter 196), and the stomach is the most common extranodal site for non-Hodgkin's lymphomas. Patients with gastric lymphoma are generally younger than those with gastric adenocarcinoma, but the male predominance remains.

TABLE 202–2 TUMOR, NODES, AND METASTASIS (TNM) STAGING OF GASTRIC CANCER

TUMOR

T1: Tumor confined to the mucosa or submucosa
T2: Tumor extending into the muscularis propria
T3: Tumor extending through the serosa without involving contiguous structures
T4: Tumor extending through the serosa and involving contiguous structures

NODES

N0: No lymph node metastases
N1: Regional lymph node involvement within 3 cm of the tumor along the greater or lesser curvature
N2: Regional lymph node involvement more than 3 cm from the primary tumor
N3: Involvement of other intra-abdominal lymph nodes not removable at surgery

METASTASES

M0: No distant metastases
M1: Distant metastases

Clinical Manifestations

Patients commonly present with symptoms and signs similar to those of gastric adenocarcinoma. Lymphoma in the stomach can be a primary tumor or it can be secondary to disseminated lymphoma.

B-cell lymphomas (Chapter 196) of the stomach are most commonly large cell with a high-grade type. Low-grade variants are noted in the setting of chronic gastritis and are termed *mucosa-associated lymphoid tissue* (MALT) lymphomas. MALT lesions are strongly associated with *H. pylori* infection.

Diagnosis

Radiographically, gastric lymphomas usually arise as ulcers or exophytic masses; diffusely infiltrating lymphoma is more suggestive of secondary lymphoma. Thus, upper gastrointestinal barium studies usually show multiple nodules and ulcers for a primary gastric lymphoma and typically have the appearance of linitis plastica with secondary lymphoma. As with gastric adenocarcinoma, however, upper endoscopy with biopsy and cytologic examination are required for diagnosis and have an accuracy of nearly 90%. Apart from conventional histopathologic analysis, immunoperoxidase staining for lymphocyte markers is helpful in diagnosis. As with gastric adenocarcinoma, proper staging of gastric lymphoma involves endoscopic ultrasonography, chest and abdominal computed tomographic scans, and bone marrow biopsy as needed.

Treatment

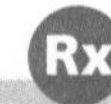

Treatment of gastric diffuse large B-cell lymphoma is best pursued with combination chemotherapy with or without radiation therapy (Chapter 196). In this context, 5-year survival rates of 40 to 60% have been reported. For MALT lesions, eradication of *H. pylori* infection with antibiotics should be attempted (Chapter 142), but patients with refractory lesions require the same treatment as do patients with non-Hodgkin's lymphoma (Chapter 196).

OTHER MALIGNANT TUMORS OF THE STOMACH

Leiomyosarcoma, which constitutes approximately 1% of all gastric cancers, usually occurs as an intramural mass with central ulceration. Symptoms may include bleeding accompanied by a palpable mass. Leiomyosarcomas are often relatively indolent; surgical resection yields a 5-year survival rate of about 50%. Metastasis can occur to lymph nodes and the liver. Other gastric sarcomas include liposarcomas, fibrosarcomas, myosarcomas, and neurogenic sarcomas.

Some gastrointestinal stromal tumors (GISTs) have been associated with activating mutations in the C-*kit* gene. C-*kit* mutations are also found in chronic and acute myelogenous leukemia (Chapters 194 and 195), and approximately 50% of GISTs respond to imatinib mesylate, which is also used in chronic myelogenous leukemia. If imatinib is not successful, sunitinib increases survival. [3] Carcinoid tumors (Chapter 251) may begin in the stomach and are curable by removal if they have not yet spread to the liver.

Primary tumors can also spread to the stomach. In addition to lymphomas, other tumors found in the stomach include primary lung (Chapter 201) and breast (Chapter 208) cancers as well as malignant melanoma (Chapter 214).

LEIOMYOMAS AND BENIGN TUMORS

Leiomyomas, which are smooth muscle tumors of benign origin, occur with equal frequency in men and women and are typically located in the middle and distal stomach. Leiomyomas can grow into the lumen with secondary ulceration and consequent bleeding. Alternatively, they can expand to the serosa with extrinsic compression. Endoscopy may reveal a mass that has overlying mucosa or mucosa replaced by ulceration. On upper gastrointestinal series, leiomyomas are usually smooth with an intramural filling defect, with or without central ulceration. However, benign leiomyomas can be difficult to distinguish from their malignant counterparts radiographically or endoscopically; tissue diagnosis is imperative. Symptomatic leiomyomas should be removed, but those without associated symptoms do not require therapy.

Other benign gastric tumors include lipoma, neurofibroma (Chapter 199), lymphangioma, ganglioneuroma, and hamartoma, the last associated with Peutz-Jeghers syndrome (Chapter 203) or juvenile polyposis (restricted to the stomach).

ADENOMAS

Gastric adenomas and hyperplastic polyps are unusual but may be found in middle-aged and elderly patients. Polyps may be sessile or pedunculated and are also found in nearly 50% of patients with familial adenomatosis polyposis (Chapter 203). Gastric adenocarcinoma arising in the antrum has been described in such patients. Although isolated gastric adenomatous polyps are generally asymptomatic, some patients may have dyspepsia, nausea, or bleeding. Gastric adenomas and hyperplastic polyps are smooth and regular on upper gastrointestinal series, but the diagnosis must be confirmed by upper endoscopy with biopsy. Pedunculated polyps that are larger than 2 cm or that have associated symptoms should be removed by endoscopic snare cautery polypectomy, whereas large sessile gastric adenomatous polyps may merit segmental surgical resection. If polyps progress to an intermediary stage of severe dysplasia or culminate in cancer, treatment is the same as for gastric adenocarcinoma.

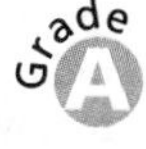

1. Cunningham D, Allum WH, Stenning SP, et al: Perioperative chemotherapy versus surgery alone for resectable gastroesophageal cancer. N Engl J Med 2006;355:11–20.
2. Macdonald JS, Smalley SR, Benedetti J, et al: Chemoradiotherapy after surgery compared with surgery alone for adenocarcinoma of the stomach or gastroesophageal junction. N Engl J Med 2001;345:725–730.
3. Demetri GD, Oosterom AT, Garrett CR, et al: Efficacy and safety of sunitinib in patients with advanced gastrointestinal stromal tumour after failure of imatinib: A randomised controlled trial. Lancet 2006;368:1329–1338.

SUGGESTED READINGS

Carrato A, Gallego-Plazas J, Guillen-Ponce C: Adjuvant therapy of resected gastric cancer is necessary. Semin Oncol 2005;32:S105–108. *Makes the case for adjuvant chemotherapy.*

Demetri GD, von Mehren M, Blanke CD, et al: Efficacy and safety of imatinib mesylate in advanced gastrointestinal stromal tumors. N Engl J Med 2002;347:472–480. *Approximately 50% of these tumors respond to the same therapy used for chronic myelogenous leukemia.*

D'Ugo DM, Pende V, Persiani R, et al: Laparoscopic staging of gastric cancer: An overview. J Am Coll Surg 2003;196:965–974. *A useful approach.*

Kelley JR, Duggan JM: Gastric cancer epidemiology and risk factors. J Clin Epidemiol 2003;56:1–9. *Estimates that* H. pylori *accounts for somewhat less than 50% of cases in western societies.*

Nguyen S, Rebischung C, Van Ongeval J, et al: Epirubicin-docetaxel in advanced gastric cancer: Two phase II studies as second and first-line treatment. Bull Cancer 2006;93:E1–E6. *A promising new regimen.*

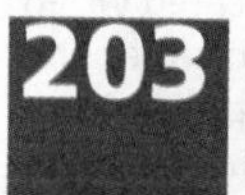

203 NEOPLASMS OF THE LARGE AND SMALL INTESTINE

Raymond N. DuBois

NEOPLASMS OF THE LARGE INTESTINE

A person living in North America faces an average lifetime risk of 6% for developing colorectal cancer. Colorectal cancer is the second leading cause of cancer-related deaths after lung cancer and has a 5-year survival rate of approximately 55%. Cancers of the colon and rectum are the most lethal gastrointestinal malignant diseases in the Western world. Despite these grim statistics, colorectal cancer is preventable and is highly curable if detected early enough, so public health initiatives have emphasized large-scale screening and surveillance.

Major advances in understanding the genetic pathogenesis of colorectal cancer are likely to lead to the development of cell-selective chemotherapeutic agents. By far the two most common and clinically significant neoplastic lesions that appear in the large intestine are adenomatous polyps and adenocarcinomas arising from epithelial cells of the colonic or rectal mucosa. However, the large bowel is also the site of other malignant diseases including anal carcinoma (squamous or transitional cell types; Chapter 148), lymphoma (Chapter 196), leiomyosarcoma (Chapter 213), malignant carcinoid tumor (Chapter 251), and Kaposi's sarcoma (Chapters 213 and 416). Malignant diseases from adjacent sites such as the prostate, ovary, uterus, and stomach may also involve the colon and/or rectum by direct invasion.

Polyps of the Colon

A *polyp* is defined as a grossly visible mass of cells with stroma that protrudes from the mucosal surface into the lumen of the intestine (Fig. 203–1). A polyp may either be sessile or pedunculated when it is attached by a stalk of cells. Polyps are classified as either non-neoplastic or neoplastic, and they are clinically relevant by causing rectal bleeding or partial bowel obstruction (rare) or because of their potential to become malignant.

Nonadenomatous Polyps

Nonadenomatous polyps, which account for approximately 90% of all mucosal polyps detected in the large bowel, can be found in more than 50% of people older than 60 years of age. These polyps, which are also termed *non-neoplastic polyps,* can be further subcategorized into hyperplastic, inflammatory, lymphoid, and juvenile polyps. Most non-neoplastic polyps are hyperplastic polyps, which arise as a result of abnormal maturation of the mucosal epithelial cells; these polyps are usually small in diameter and are found predominantly in the distal sigmoid colon and rectum. Hyperplastic polyps are not malignant and are not thought to be associated with any measurable increase in malignant potential, although the cancer-causing genes in some cells in some subsets of hyperplastic polyps can undergo aberrant methylation. Inflammatory polyps, which arise in the setting of chronic ulcerative colitis and are composed of regions of inflamed mucosa surrounded by areas of ulceration, are associated with an increased risk of cancer. Lymphoid polyps are regions of the mucosa that contain exaggerated intramucosal lymphoid tissue. Juvenile polyps usually develop in the rectum of children younger than 5 years of age and are termed *hamartomatous* because they are focal malformations that resemble tumors but are caused by abnormal development of the lamina propria; these polyps require no

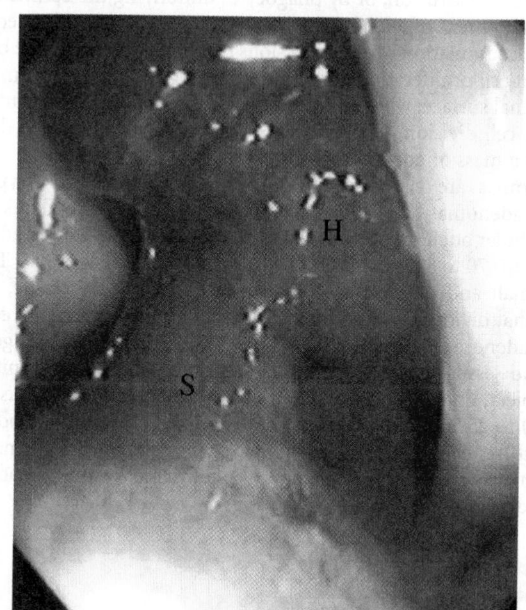

FIGURE 203–1 • Large pedunculated polyp in the rectum. The stalk (S) itself is benign, with the head (H) containing the adenomatous tissue. The polyp was removed safely in a one-step endoscopic procedure. (Courtesy of Pankaj Jay Pasricha.)

therapy unless they cause symptoms such as obstruction or severe bleeding.

Adenomatous Polyps

Definition

Adenomatous polyps (or adenomas), which are neoplastic polyps with malignant potential, are more common in the distal colon and rectum, where their anatomic distribution parallels that of colorectal adenocarcinoma. Adenomatous polyps manifest in a range of sizes; smaller lesions are usually pedunculated, whereas larger polyps can be sessile. Convincing evidence that adenomatous polyps are the precursor lesion to colorectal adenocarcinoma comes from persons with the hereditary polyposis syndromes and from animal studies in which adenomas are induced by either carcinogens or genetic manipulation. Correlative evidence includes the observations that the epidemiology is similar for adenomas and carcinomas, that both lesions are more common in the same anatomic locations, and that adenomatous tissue can often be found in small adenocarcinomas. Intervention studies have shown that removal of adenomatous polyps leads to a significant decrease in risk for colorectal cancer.

Epidemiology

Adenomatous polyps are relatively common, particularly in elderly populations; the prevalence is 20 to 30% in persons in the United States who are less than 40 years old and 40 to 50% in individuals who are more than 60 years old. The prevalence of adenomas tends to be high in regions of the world where colorectal cancer is common, and most autopsy studies indicate a 30% higher prevalence in men. The importance of genetic risk factors is clear in the hereditary polyposis syndromes (see Inherited Colorectal Cancer Syndromes), and sporadic adenomas have a familial component; for example, individuals with a positive first-degree family history are at a four-fold greater risk of developing adenomatous polyps.

Pathobiology

The layer of epithelial cells lining the surface of the normal large bowel undergoes continuous self-renewal with a turnover period of 3 to 8 days. Undifferentiated stem cells located at the base of invaginated crypts give rise to cells that migrate toward the lumen as they differentiate further into specialized enterocytes; these cells are subsequently removed by apoptosis, by extrusion, or by phagocytes underlying the epithelial layer. The development of adenomatous polyps is associated with a sequence-specific accumulation of genetic lesions that cause an imbalance between epithelial cell proliferation and cell death. As a result, cells accumulate at the luminal surface, where they remain undifferentiated and continue to undergo cell division, thus eventually leading to the abnormal development of a mass of adenomatous tissue.

Adenomas are classified into three main histologic subtypes: (1) tubular adenomas, (2) villous adenomas, and (3) tubulovillous adenomas. Tubular adenomas, which are the most common type of adenoma, account for 70 to 85% of all adenomas removed at colonoscopy. They are often small and pedunculated, and they consist of dysplastic, tubular glands that divide and branch out from the mucosal surface. In contrast, villous adenomas are much rarer (<5% of all adenomas), are generally large and sessile, and are composed of strands of dysplastic epithelium that project, finger-like, into the lumen of the gut. Tubulovillous adenomas (10 to 25% of all adenomas) have a mixture of tubular and villous architecture. Small tubular adenomas generally have low malignant potential, whereas approximately 40% of large sessile adenomatous polyps develop into cancer.

Clinical Manifestations

Patients with adenomatous polyps generally remain asymptomatic but may present with an asymptomatic positive stool occult blood test or with evident hematochezia. The lifetime incidence of additional adenomas in a patient with one known adenoma is 30 to 50%. Less than 5% of all adenomas eventually develop into carcinomas. Two critical factors that determine the likelihood that an adenoma will eventually develop into an invasive lesion are the size of the polyp and the grade of dysplasia. For polyps less than 1 cm in size, the risk for carcinoma is 1 to 3%; polyps between 1 and 2 cm have a 10% risk of becoming cancerous; and more than 40% of polyps that are greater than 2 cm progress to an invasive lesion. All adenomatous polyps contain some degree of dysplasia but can be further categorized as low or high grade to indicate the degree of dysplasia and corresponding risk for invasive carcinoma. High-grade dysplasia is associated with a 27% rate for eventual transformation into carcinoma.

Diagnosis

Adenomatous polyps in the colon and rectum can be diagnosed by endoscopy (Chapter 136) or barium radiography (Chapter 135), but multiple studies indicate that colonoscopy is the most accurate tool for diagnosing colorectal polyps. For example, the National Polyp Study reported that barium enema missed 52% of polyps greater than or equal to 1 cm in size. Colonoscopy is thus the preferred method for diagnosing adenomas based on this higher rate of accuracy and because the technique allows for immediate biopsy and resection of most polyps; current evidence supports the use of colonoscopy as a screening tool for the general population older than 50 years of age (Chapter 13). Flexible sigmoidoscopy, which is often used to screen asymptomatic persons at average risk for colorectal adenocarcinoma, detects 50 to 60% of all polyps and cancers. Generally, patients who have polyps detected by barium radiography or flexible sigmoidoscopy should undergo colonoscopy to remove the lesion and to search for additional polyps. However, colonoscopy may not be adequately performed in patients who have advanced diverticulosis or who have had previous pelvic surgery. In these instances, a combination of double-contrast barium radiography and flexible sigmoidoscopy may be an acceptable alternative. Computed tomographic (CT) colonography or virtual colonoscopy was reported to be equivalent in accuracy to conventional colonoscopy for the detection of polyps 6 mm or larger in one large study, but other studies have reported more disappointing sensitivities in the range of 55 to 66%, perhaps owing to different CT techniques (single versus multidetector CT scanners) and interobserver variability in reading the images. Although fiberoptic colonoscopy remains the "gold standard" for polyp detection, CT colonography may emerge as a viable screening tool for certain subsets of patients in the detection of adenomatous polyps and colorectal cancer.

Treatment

Rx

The major goal of treatment for adenomatous polyps is removal or destruction of the lesion during endoscopy by electrocautery. This recommendation is based on the overwhelming evidence that endoscopic polypectomy reduces the subsequent incidence and mortality of colorectal cancer. Pedunculated adenomas are generally removed by snare polypectomy with subsequent submission of the tissue for pathologic analysis. Piecemeal snare resection may be required to remove sessile polyps. Surgical resection of a polyp is indicated when endoscopic resection of an advanced adenoma is not possible. The biopsied polyp must be evaluated histologically so the presence or absence of carcinoma can be determined; if a malignant lesion is found, its histologic grade, vascular and lymphatic involvement, and proximity to the margin of resection should be determined. Polypectomy is the definitive therapy for localized cancers that have not spread beyond the muscularis mucosae layer, are not poorly differentiated, do not involve vascular or lymphatic structures, have margins free of carcinoma cells, and have been completely excised by endoscopic inspection. If invasive carcinoma is present in the stalk of a resected polyp and if it is unclear whether any of the stalk remains after polypectomy, then colonic resection may be indicated. The mortality rate associated with colonic resection is less than 2% in patients between the ages of 50 and 69 years, but it rises to 4%

Rx

in persons older than 70 years of age; it also increases considerably when comorbidities such as chronic liver, renal, or heart disease are present.

Prognosis

Patients who have undergone resection of an adenomatous polyp are at increased risk for subsequent development of adenomas and colorectal adenocarcinoma. In general, a follow-up colonoscopy is recommended in 3 years. Earlier colonoscopies may be warranted in patients who have multiple or large sessile adenomas removed. In contrast, the risk of malignancy is not significantly increased in patients who have had less than three small (<1 cm) tubular adenomas removed; for these individuals, the first follow-up colonoscopy can be delayed to 5 years. If the first follow-up colonoscopy is negative, the second scheduled follow-up can usually be delayed until 5 years.

Inherited Syndromes

Definition

The inherited colorectal cancer syndromes constitute approximately 6% of all cases of colorectal adenocarcinoma. Genetic analyses of these syndromes have led to major advances in understanding how sporadic colorectal cancer develops. Inherited syndromes can be further divided into the following categories: inherited polyposis syndromes, which include familial adenomatous polyposis and its variants Gardner's syndrome and Turcot's syndrome; hereditary nonpolyposis colorectal cancer (HNPCC) or Lynch's syndrome; and hamartomatous polyposis syndromes, which include Peutz-Jeghers syndrome, juvenile polyposis, and the related syndrome of Cowden's disease. Each of these syndromes is characterized by unique genetic lesions, age of onset, and clinical manifestations (Table 203–1). Clinical genetic testing (Chapter 38), which is now part of accepted clinical care of these patients, is indicated (1) in patients in whom the syndrome is clinically apparent or is suspected but not definitively established based on the clinical presentation and (2) in relatives of an individual with an established gene diagnosis. Referral of suspected patients to a genetic counseling service is essential.

Familial Adenomatous Polyposis

Definition and Epidemiology

The hallmark of familial adenomatous polyposis is the development of hundreds to thousands of adenomatous polyps in the large bowel at a relatively young age (Fig. 203–2). Estimates of disease incidence vary from 1 in 6850 to 1 in 31,250.

Pathobiology

The disease, which is autosomal dominant with incomplete penetrance, has been mapped to the adenomatous polyposis coli (*APC*) gene located on the long arm of chromosome 5 (5q21). *APC* is a tumor suppressor gene that is a critical regulator of intestinal epithelial cell growth. Patients with the familial syndrome inherit one mutant copy of *APC;* when a loss-of-function mutation develops in the other *APC* allele, mucosal epithelial cell growth is no longer controlled normally, and polyps develop. Variable phenotypes can be partly attributed to differences in the location of the *APC* mutation.

Clinical Manifestations and Diagnosis

Adenomas begin to appear early in the second decade of life, and gastrointestinal symptoms begin to appear in the third or fourth decade. Polyps are distributed relatively evenly throughout the colon, although a slight predominance has been noted in the distal colon. Almost all patients with familial adenomatous polyposis develop frank colorectal carcinoma by the age of 40 years if the condition is left untreated. Gastric polyps occur in 30 to 100% of patients, and duodenal adenomas are found in 45 to 90% of patients. Periampullary duodenal cancer develops in approximately 10% of cases. Small bowel lesions that are distal to the duodenum rarely progress into malignancy.

TABLE 203–1 GENERAL FEATURES OF THE INHERITED COLORECTAL CANCER SYNDROMES

Syndrome	Polyp Histology	Polyp Distribution	Age of Onset	Risk of Colon Cancer	Genetic Lesion	Clinical Manifestations	Associated Lesions
Familial adenomatous polyposis	Adenoma	Large intestine	16-yr (range 8–34 yr)	100%	5q (*APC* gene)	Rectal bleeding, abdominal pain, bowel obstruction	Desmoids, CHRPE
Gardner's syndrome	Adenoma	Large and small intestine	16-yr (range 8–34 yr)	100%	5q (*APC* gene)	Rectal bleeding, abdominal pain, bowel obstruction	Desmoids, CHRPE
Peutz-Jeghers syndrome	Hamartoma	Large and small intestine	First decade	Slightly above average	19p (*STK11*)	Possible rectal bleeding, abdominal pain, intussusception	Orocutaneous melanin pigment spots
Juvenile polyposis	Hamartoma (rarely adenoma)	Large and small intestine	First decade	Approximately 9%	*PTEN, SMAD4, BMPR1*	Possible rectal bleeding, abdominal pain, intussusception	Congenital abnormalities in 20% of the nonfamilial type
Hereditary nonpolyposis colon cancer	Adenoma	Large intestine	40-yr (range 18–65 yr)	30%	Mismatch repair genes*	Rectal bleeding, abdominal pain, bowel obstruction	Other tumors (e.g., ovary, ureter, pancreas, stomach)

*Including hMSH2, hMSH3, hMSH6, hMLH1, hPMS1, and hPMS2.
CHRPE = congenital hypertrophy of the retinal pigment epithelium.

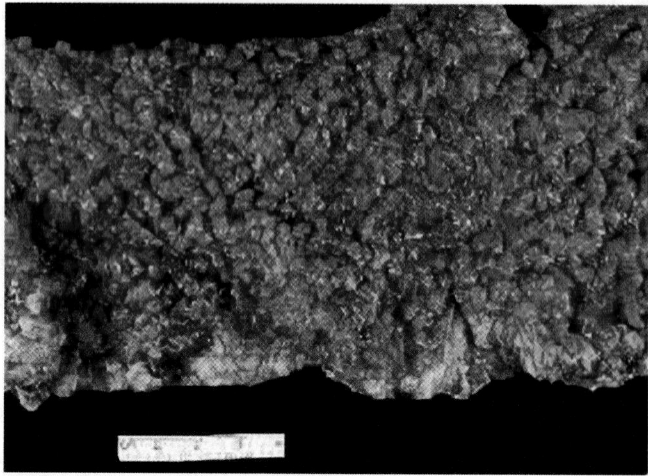

FIGURE 203–2 • A colon lined with hundreds of adenomatous polyps resected from a patient with familial adenomatous polyposis.

Treatment

The primary treatment option is total proctocolectomy with conventional ileostomy or ileoanal (pouch) anastomosis. First-degree relatives of afflicted individuals should be screened. A blood test to detect mutations in the *APC* gene has a sensitivity of 85%, but flexible proctosigmoidoscopy should be performed annually from the ages of 12 to 40 years (and every 3 years after the age of 40 years), even in those who test negative for the *APC* mutation.

Gardner's Syndrome

Gardner's syndrome, which is also caused by mutations in the *APC* gene, differs from familial adenomatous polyposis mainly by the presence of extraintestinal manifestations, including osteomas (particularly mandibular), soft tissue tumors (including lipomas, sebaceous cysts, and fibrosarcomas), supernumerary teeth, desmoid tumors, mesenteric fibromatosis, and congenital hypertrophy of the retinal pigment epithelium. The phenotypic differences between Gardner's syndrome and familial adenomatous polyposis appear to result from variations in the location of the *APC* mutation, the presence of modifying genes, and environmental factors. Adenomatous polyps in Gardner's syndrome have the same malignant potential as those found in familial adenomatous polyposis; hence, colorectal cancer treatment and screening recommendations are similar.

Turcot's Syndrome

A hallmark of Turcot's syndrome is the combination of colorectal polyposis and malignant diseases of the central nervous system. Mutations in the *APC* gene account for two thirds of cases, and the remaining one third of cases result from mutations in the DNA mismatch repair genes that are also mutated in HNPCC. The central nervous system manifestations include medulloblastomas, glioblastomas, and ependymomas.

Hereditary Nonpolyposis Colorectal Cancer

Definition and Epidemiology

HNPCC, also known as Lynch's syndrome, is the most common hereditary colorectal cancer syndrome and accounts for approximately 5% of all cases of colorectal cancer. It is inherited as an autosomal dominant trait and is highly penetrant. Clinically, HNPCC has been defined by the presence of all three of the following: (1) three or more relatives with histologically verified HNPCC-associated cancer (colorectal cancer, or cancer of the endometrium, small bowel, ureter, or renal pelvis), one of whom is a first-degree relative of the other two in the absence of familial adenomatous polyposis; (2) colorectal cancer involving at least two generations; (3) one or more family members with cancer diagnosed before the age of 50 years.

Pathobiology

HNPCC is caused by loss-of-function germline mutations in a set of genes involved in the repair of DNA base pair mismatches that occur during DNA replication (also known as the mutation mismatch repair system). Mutation mismatch repair genes include *hMSH2, hMSH3, hMSH6, hMLH1, hPMS1,* and *hPMS2.* Mutations in these genes lead to the development of DNA microsatellite instability (MSI) that can be detected using genomic techniques. Tumor cells displaying MSI have increased mutation rates in genes that contain small nucleotide repeats; one common gene mutated in HNPCC resulting from the MSI phenotype is the transforming growth factor-β type II receptor, which is an important component of a signaling pathway that regulates normal intestinal epithelial cell growth and differentiation.

Clinical Manifestations and Diagnosis

The median age for diagnosis of HNPCC is in the mid-40s. Although several adenomas may be present, the diffuse polyposis characteristic of familial adenomatous polyposis is not found, hence the name *nonpolyposis.* Adenomatous polyps in HNPCC are located predominantly in the right colon proximal to the splenic flexure. These tumors generally have a better prognosis than similar lesions found in sporadic colorectal cancer. Patients with HNPCC also are at high risk for other malignant diseases, including cancers of the ovary, ureter, pancreas, and stomach, probably partly because of the loss of proper DNA repair. Screening strategies for families with a history suggestive of HNPCC may include the use of genetic testing to identify the MSI phenotype, but approximately 15% of all sporadic colorectal cancers also exhibit increased MSI.

Treatment

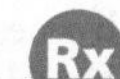

Persons in families with HNPCC should undergo a colonoscopy every 2 years from the ages of 21 to 40 years and every year after the age of 40 years because their risk is quite high and genetic testing is not perfect. Women in HNPCC-affected families should have pelvic examinations every 1 to 3 years beginning at the age of 18 years; annual pelvic examinations, transvaginal ultrasonography, and endometrial biopsy have been recommended beginning at age 25 years.

Peutz-Jeghers Syndrome

Definition and Epidemiology

The defining clinical presentation of Peutz-Jeghers syndrome is intestinal hamartomatous polyposis in association with characteristic mucocutaneous pigmentation. The average age of diagnosis is in the mid-20s.

Pathobiology

The syndrome is inherited in an autosomal dominant fashion with high penetrance. It is rare, with an incidence rate one tenth that of familial adenomatous polyposis. The gene responsible for the syndrome is the serine-threonine kinase *STK11* gene located on chromosome 19p; a mutation in the *STK11* is found in approximately 60% of patients with this syndrome. The hamartomatous polyps in Peutz-Jeghers syndrome are located predominantly in the small intestine (64 to 96%), stomach (24 to 49%), and colon (60%). Histologically, these polyps are benign, and they are unique in that a layer of muscle that extends into the submucosa or muscularis propria may surround the glandular tissue.

Clinical Manifestations and Diagnosis

In rare instances, these polyps may become malignant, particularly in the small bowel. Otherwise, the major gastrointestinal symptoms include recurrent bouts of small bowel intussusception, obstruction, and bleeding that may require surgery. Gastrointestinal bleeding may also occur and lead to iron deficiency anemia. Extraintestinal manifestations include

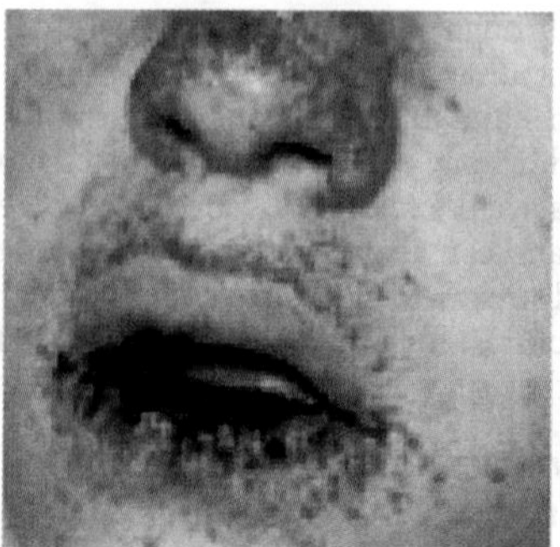

FIGURE 203–3 • Mucosal pigmentation characteristic of a patient with Peutz-Jeghers syndrome.

ovarian sex cord stromal tumors and polyps of the gallbladder, ureter, and nasal passages. More than 95% of patients have a characteristic pattern of melanin spots on the lips, buccal mucosa, and skin (Fig. 203–3); in one large series, 23% of patients were diagnosed on the basis of this typical cutaneous pigmentation.

Treatment

Rx

Standard medical care for patients with Peutz-Jeghers syndrome involves an annual physical examination that includes evaluation of the breasts, abdomen, pelvis, and testes, as well as a complete blood count. Currently, it is suggested that large (>5 cm) or hemorrhagic polyps be removed endoscopically. Surveillance for cancer includes small bowel radiography every 2 years, esophagogastroduodenoscopy and colonoscopy every 2 years, and yearly pancreatic ultrasound scanning. For women, ultrasound scanning of the pelvis is recommended yearly, and mammography should be performed at ages 25, 30, 35, 38 years, then every 2 years until the age of 50 years, after which this should be done annually. Surgical care includes push enteroscopy and intraoperative enteroscopy with polypectomy if needed to defer repeated small bowel resections. Laparotomy and resection, as indicated, are recommended for repeated or persistent small intestinal itussusception, obstruction, or persistent intestinal bleeding.

Juvenile Polyposis

Juvenile (non-neoplastic, hamartomatous) polyposis is a rare syndrome characterized by 10 or more non-neoplastic, hamartomatous polyps throughout the gastrointestinal tract or any number of polyps in a patient with a family history of juvenile polyposis. The syndrome is inherited in an autosomal dominant manner and is caused by mutations in the *SMAD4, PTEN,* or *BMPR1A* gene. The hamartomas are histologically distinct from the polyps seen in Peutz-Jeghers syndrome. Patients generally present with rectal bleeding, anemia, abdominal pain, or intussusception in childhood or early adolescence. Extraintestinal symptoms include pulmonary arteriovenous malformations. The risk of malignancy in juvenile polyposis is reported to be 10%; subtotal colectomy may be necessary in patients with severe dysplasia.

Cowden's Syndrome

Cowden's syndrome (Chapters 186 and 466) is a rare, autosomal dominant syndrome of multiple hamartomatous polyps of the skin and mucous membranes, including gastrointestinal polyps, facial tricholemmomas, oral papillomas, and keratoses of the hands and feet. The rate of associated malignancy is high, particularly in the thyroid and breast. The polyps in Cowden's syndrome are benign. The causative genetic lesion has been mapped to the *PTEN* tumor suppressor gene.

Adenocarcinoma of the Colon and Rectum

Definition and Epidemiology

Adenocarcinomas constitute 98% of the malignant diseases found in the large bowel. Most adenocarcinomas are believed to arise from adenomatous polyps that progress from severe dysplasia to invasive carcinoma. The peak incidence is from 60 to 79 years of age, and fewer than 10% of all cases arise before the age of 50 years. The geographic pattern of colorectal cancer worldwide is highly variable. The highest rates are found in industrialized countries, including the United States, Canada, New Zealand, and the countries of northwestern Europe. Most countries in Asia, Africa, and South America (with the exception of Argentina) have a relatively low rate. This geographic distribution is thought to be primarily the result of environmental factors, because ethnic groups from low-incidence countries in Asia develop rates of disease equivalent to those of white persons in the United States after they migrate to the West. African Americans in the United States also have a much higher risk for disease than do black Africans. Population studies have found positive correlations between the risk for colorectal cancer and the dietary intake of red meat. The rate of colorectal cancer has increased significantly in Japan over the last few decades as the Western diet has become more prominent.

In the United States, about 145,000 new cases of colorectal cancer annually lead to about 55,000 expected deaths, thus making colorectal cancer the second leading cause of cancer-related deaths after lung cancer. The 5-year survival rate for colorectal cancer is approximately 55%, but this varies greatly depending on the stage of disease at the time of diagnosis. Men and women have a similar incidence of adenocarcinoma of the colon, but rectal cancer is more common in men in most parts of the world. The overall rate of deaths related to colorectal cancer has declined since the mid-1980s, perhaps owing to more widespread screening and improved treatment.

TABLE 203–2 LIFESTYLE AND DIETARY RECOMMENDATIONS FOR THE PRIMARY PREVENTION OF COLORECTAL CANCER

Dietary Recommendations	Lifestyle Recommendations
Increase quantity and variety of fruits and vegetables (at least five servings per day)	Maintain normal body weight
Ingest 20–30 g/day of fiber	Exercise daily
Consider supplementation with 3 g/day of calcium carbonate	Avoid smoking
	Avoid excessive alcohol

Environmental Factors

Recommendations for the primary prevention of colorectal cancer are based on risk factors associated with colorectal cancer (Table 203–2); investigators have estimated that adoption of these dietary and lifestyle changes could reduce the incidence of colorectal cancer by 50%. Total energy intake, irrespective of dietary content, is positively associated with the development of colorectal cancer. Colorectal adenomas are associated with tobacco use, and the increased consumption of ethanol, particularly beer, has been associated with a higher risk for colorectal cancer. The higher rates of colorectal cancer in countries that consume "Western-style" diets high in red meat suggests that high dietary fat and low fiber could promote colorectal cancer. However, more recent data show no benefit of low-fat diets on the risk of colorectal cancer despite their other health advantages. The role of dietary fiber is controversial, and major prospective studies have found no correlation between the intake of dietary fiber and the development of colorectal adenomas. Whether diets high in fruits and vegetables can prevent colorectal cancer is under investigation.

Inherited Predisposition

Individuals who have a first-degree relative with colorectal cancer face a two- to three-fold increase in risk for malignancy, and this risk rises to five- or six-fold if two first-degree relatives are affected. Various genetic studies suggest that a large percentage of the population (≤50%) is susceptible to colorectal neoplasia on a familial basis.

Inflammatory Bowel Disease

Adenocarcinoma of the colon is 10 to 20 times more common in persons with ulcerative colitis (Chapter 144) than in the general population. Between 2 and 4% of all patients with long-term ulcerative colitis develop this malignancy, and the cumulative incidence over a 25-year period is approximately 12%. The two most important predictors for eventual development of carcinoma are the duration of the inflammatory disease and the extent of colonic involvement. Identification of dysplasia in the setting of ulcerative colitis is the best indicator of early cancer, but it is difficult to distinguish true dysplastic lesions from areas of intense mucosal regeneration. Dysplasia in a plaque or elevated mass and high-grade dysplasia warrant consideration of colectomy. Most experts agree that colonoscopy every 2 years with multiple biopsies is warranted after 8 years of symptomatic ulcerative colitis with extensive colonic involvement. The recent evolution of surgical procedures, such as ileoanal pull-through, favors the use of prophylactic colectomy in high-risk patients. Individuals with Crohn's colitis have a four to seven times higher risk of colorectal cancer as compared with the general population. Although this risk is less than that seen with ulcerative colitis, routine surveillance is recommended in patients with extensive colonic disease.

Other High-Risk Factors

Persons diagnosed with endocarditis or septicemia caused by *Streptococcus bovis* have a high rate of occult colorectal neoplasias and other upper gastrointestinal malignant diseases; endoscopic or radiographic screening may be warranted in this setting. A 5 to 10% increase in colorectal cancer rates 15 to 30 years after ureterosigmoidostomy to correct congenital exstrophy of the bladder has been reported; the lesions are typically distal to the ureteral implant, where the mucosa is chronically exposed to urine and feces.

Pathobiology

Pathology

The anatomic distribution of carcinoma of the colon (Fig. 203–4) is associated with distinct morphologic patterns. Right-sided tumors commonly grow as polypoid, exophytic masses that bleed, often on an occult basis, and rarely cause obstruction, whereas carcinomas of the distal colon are generally annular, encircling lesions that both bleed and lead to constriction of the bowel ("napkin ring" or "apple core" constriction). Almost all colorectal cancers are adenocarcinomas that exhibit differing degrees of glandular differentiation; most tend to produce mucin that aids in extension of the lesion and worsens prognosis. Lesions spread by direct extension through the wall of the bowel into the pericolonic fat and mesentery, and they can also invade surrounding organs. Alternatively, tumors can enter the lymphatic system and spread to regional lymph nodes, or they may enter the venous system and drain to the liver through the portal vein. Colorectal cancers can spread throughout the peritoneal cavity and can also metastasize to the lung and bone marrow through the blood stream. Rectal cancers can invade the perirectal fat and surrounding structures, including the vagina, prostate, bladder, ureters, and bony pelvis; they may also spread to the lungs and liver.

Molecular Genetics and the Adenoma-to-Carcinoma Sequence

Colorectal cancer is caused by the accumulation of multiple genetic lesions in a specific sequence over time. Both the tissue architecture and the cellular genotype change as the disease progresses (Fig. 203–5). Approximately 80 to 85% of sporadic colorectal cancers are aneuploid tumors that exhibit chromosomal instability. Somatic mutations in the *APC* gene, which is responsible for familial adenomatous polyposis, are

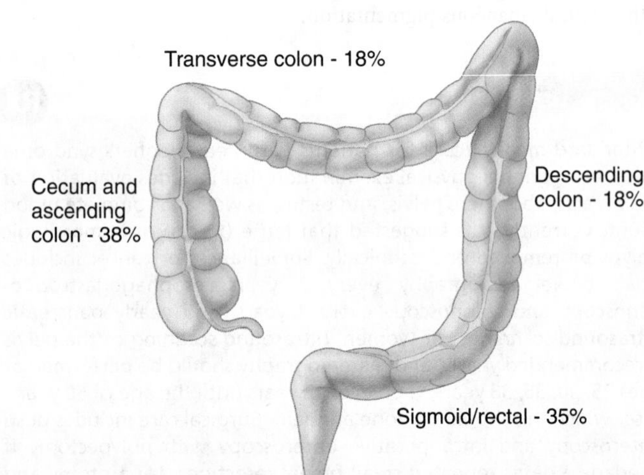

FIGURE 203–4 • Distribution of colorectal cancers in various regions of the large intestine.

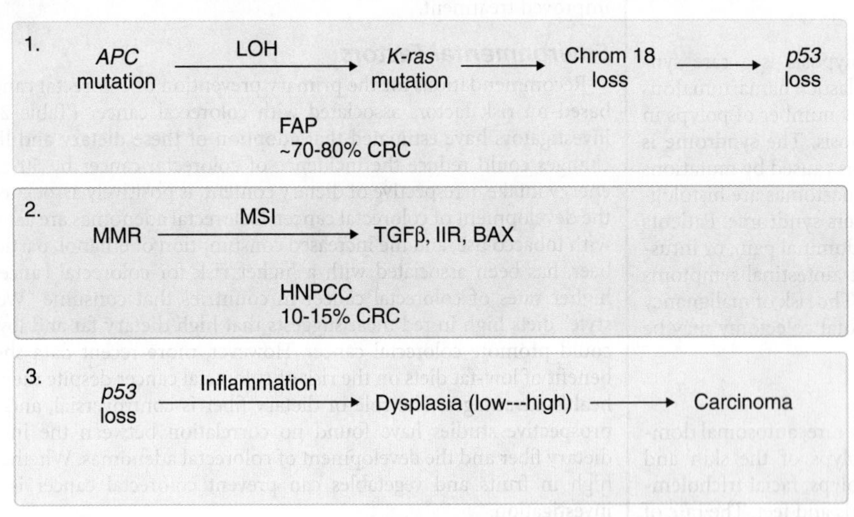

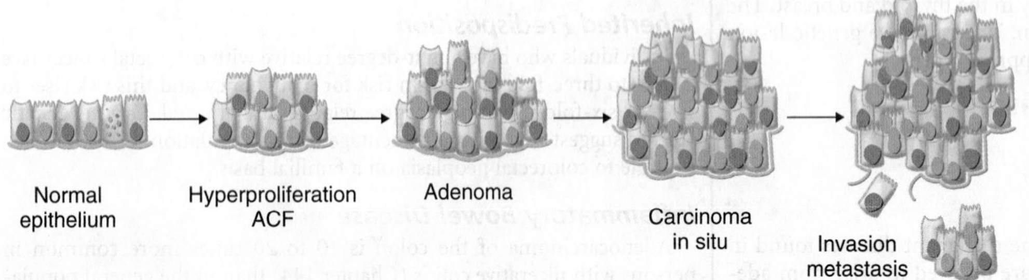

FIGURE 203–5 • The molecular basis of colorectal cancer. Sequence-specific genetic lesions result in the transition from normal large bowel mucosa to invasive carcinoma. BAX = apoptosis-related protein; CRC = colorectal cancer; FAP = familial adenomatous polyposis; HNPCC = hereditary nonpolyposis colorectal cancer; IIR = type II receptor; MMR = mutation mismatch repair; MSI = microsatellite instability; TGFβ = transforming growth factor-β.

common. APC is a multifunctional protein with an essential role in the regulation of the growth of intestinal epithelial cells. One of the important consequences of loss of normal APC is the accumulation of the β-catenin oncogene within the nucleus of cells, where it can participate in the regulation of gene expression that promotes malignancy. Other genomic abnormalities, including gain-of-function mutations in the k-*Ras* proto-oncogene and allelic loss at 18q21 (where several putative tumor suppressor genes reside), herald the progression of the lesion from dysplastic epithelium to early and late adenomas. Loss-of-function mutations in the *p53* tumor suppressor gene are commonly associated with progression to full-blown carcinoma and can occur even after transformation to cancer. Other genetic and epigenetic alterations, including the expression of genes capable of cleaving extracellular matrix and a protein tyrosine phosphatase, lead to metastasis.

The remaining 15 to 20% of colorectal cancers without chromosomal instability exhibit the phenotype of genomic MSI characteristic of the hereditary syndrome HNPCC: mutations in mismatch repair genes and mutations in important growth regulatory genes such as transforming growth factor-β type II receptor. Loss-of-function mutations in *p53* commonly occur in carcinomas that arise in the setting of inflammatory bowel disease.

Clinical Manifestations

Colorectal adenocarcinomas can remain clinically silent for years. When present, symptoms often develop insidiously over a period of months and years. The major symptoms suggesting colorectal cancer are rectal bleeding, pain, and a change in bowel habits. Symptoms typically vary depending on where the lesion resides. Neoplasms in the proximal colon, where intestinal contents are relatively liquid, do not generally cause the abdominal pain or change in bowel habits characteristic of obstructive lesions. These lesions often ulcerate and cause chronic blood loss; patients commonly present with complaints of fatigue, palpitations, or even angina pectoris. Physical examination often reveals Hemoccult-positive stools (Chapter 137), and laboratory testing demonstrates hypochromic, microcytic anemia characteristic of iron deficiency (Chapter 163). Thus, the presence of unexplained iron deficiency anemia in any adult male patient or postmenopausal female patient should prompt a rigorous evaluation for colorectal cancer, that is, endoscopic and/or radiographic visualization of the entire colon. In contrast to right-sided lesions, cancers in the distal colon may bleed, but they often cause constriction of the gut wall and can manifest with abdominal cramping, stool obstruction, or even perforation (Fig. 203–6). Tumors of the rectosigmoid region may manifest with hematochezia, tenesmus, and narrowing of the caliber of the stool. The differential diagnosis for rectal bleeding should include hemorrhoids, angiodysplasia, diverticulosis, and other benign and malignant tumors (Chapter 137).

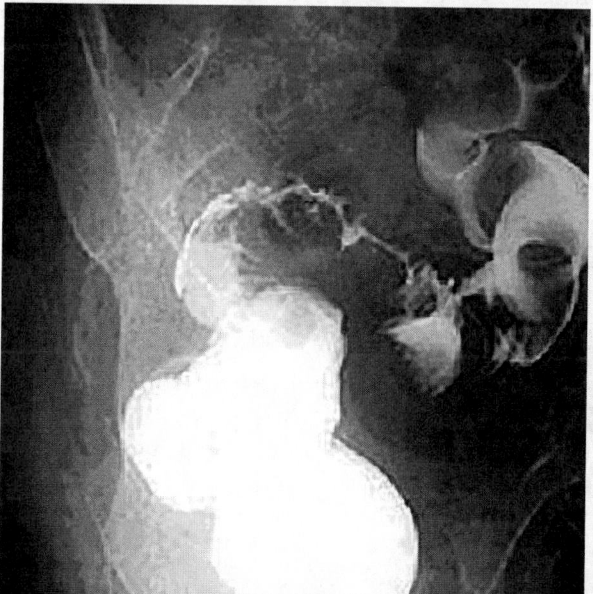

FIGURE 203–6 • A barium enema radiograph in which a colorectal cancer in the distal segment of the large intestine has formed an annular, encircling lesion that leads to constriction of the bowel wall.

Clinically apparent metastatic disease may manifest before or after resection of primary colorectal cancer. Symptoms may include pain related to distention of the liver capsule caused by massive hepatomegaly. If disease has spread to the abdomen, both ascites and bowel obstruction may occur. Metastatic spread to the pelvic region may become evident as bladder dysfunction, sacral or sciatic nerve pain, and vaginal discharge or bleeding. Lesions that have spread to the lung or bone marrow can remain silent until very advanced disease is present.

Diagnosis

The history, physical examination, and judicious use of both laboratory and radiologic tests are important in diagnosing colorectal cancer. Pertinent history should include a prior history of colorectal cancer or adenomatous polyps, inflammatory bowel disease, and any inherited colorectal cancer syndromes, as well as assessing whether the patient has any first-degree relatives with colorectal cancer. On physical examination, extraintestinal lesions characteristic of Peutz-Jeghers or Gardner's syndrome may be noticed. Metastatic disease is suggested by enlargement of the supraclavicular lymph nodes or liver or by the presence of an umbilical mass or ascites. The digital rectal examination may reveal a distal rectal cancer or the spread of tumor to the rectal shelf or pelvis. The stool shows evidence of frank or occult blood in 40 to 80% of advanced cases. Iron deficiency anemia or an elevation in liver enzymes may aid in diagnosis.

Methods for diagnosing colorectal cancer are similar to those used to detect adenomatous polyps. Colonoscopy is the procedure of choice for all patients who have occult blood in their stools or who present with signs and symptoms characteristic of colorectal cancer (Fig. 203–7). Colonoscopy is more accurate than radiographic studies for the detection of colorectal neoplasms of all sizes and has the advantage of enabling the clinician to detect synchronous (simultaneously present, additional) cancers and to obtain tissue for histologic analysis.

The staging of rectal cancers is helped by the use of endoscopic ultrasonography, by which the depth of lesion invasion can be accurately assessed. Patients with colorectal cancers who present with generalized abdominal pain or symptoms characteristic of multiple diseases may be diagnosed initially by CT scanning of the abdomen. A CT scan may also play a role in determining the extent of tumor spread. Both a chest radiograph and a CT scan may detect lung or liver metastases.

Tumor Staging

Accurate anatomic staging of colorectal cancer is essential, because the most important predictive factor for post-surgical outcome and for the need for adjuvant chemotherapy is the stage of disease at the time surgery. Colorectal cancers are staged using both the Dukes method and the universal TNM classification system (Table 203–3). Stage A tumors (T1N0M0) are superficial lesions that do not penetrate the muscularis or involve regional lymph nodes. Neoplasms that are more invasive but have not yet spread to the lymph nodes are categorized as stage B. Stage C cancer involves regional lymph nodes, and stage D indicates distant metastases.

Treatment

Rx

Surgery

Total resection of all malignant tissue is the treatment of choice for most patients with colorectal cancer and is currently the only treatment option that offers a reasonable chance of cure or long-term survival. The primary goal is complete removal of the involved bowel and associated lymphatic drainage. Laparoscopic resection, which is now the most common approach, is equivalent to open colectomy for achieving complete removal of the tumor and leads to a faster recovery. [1,2] A hemicolectomy is performed when lesions are present in the left or right portions of the colon. Tumors located in the sigmoid region and upper rectum are resected anteriorly, with removal of normal colon both proximal and distal to the

Rx

lesion; modern stapling techniques allow a sphincter-saving resection to be performed in a high percentage of cases. Lesions within 5 cm of the anal verge are treated by abdominoperineal resection and permanent colostomy; this approach is also used for large tumors that reside deep in the pelvis, for all neoplasms with high-grade histologic type, and when marked local spread of rectal lesions has occurred.

A palliative colostomy is often helpful in the presence of colonic obstruction caused by a tumor that is unresectable because it is widely metastatic or widely advanced into the peritoneum. Perforated lesions are generally managed by primary resection and colostomy followed by subsequent closure of the colostomy within a few months after the original surgery; in some patients, however, a permanent colostomy may be required. Focal surgical resection of a well-defined single liver metastasis or a wedge resection of a few lesions may be indicated depending on the medical condition of the patient; such procedures are associated with 5-year survival rates of 25 to 30% in patients who do not have advanced liver disease or other significant comorbidities.

Radiation Therapy

For rectal cancer, radiation therapy can be combined with 5-fluorouracil and leucovorin preoperatively to minimize local recurrence and metastasis. Radiation therapy is also useful in reducing tumor size and enabling large, otherwise unresectable lesions to be resected. Postoperative radiation therapy and chemotherapy reduce local recurrence and distant metastasis.

TABLE 203–3 CLASSIFICATION SYSTEMS USED TO STAGE COLON CANCER AND THEIR CORRELATION TO DISEASE OUTCOME

Dukes	TNM*	Stage	Pathology	Prognosis (~5-yr Survival Rate,%)
A	T1N0M0	I	No invasion beyond submucosa	>90
B1	T2N0M0	I	Extension into muscularis	85
B2	T3N0M0	II	Extension into or through the serosa	70–80
C	TxN1M0	III	Involvement of regional lymph nodes	35–65
D	TxNxM1	IV	Distant metastases present	5

*T is the depth of tumor penetration, N is the presence of lymph node involvement, and M indicates the presence of distant metastases.

Chemotherapy

The mainstay of adjuvant chemotherapy for colorectal cancer for decades has been 5-fluorouracil, a compound that targets the enzyme thymidylate synthase. The drug is well tolerated but produces response rates in only 10 to 20% of patients with advanced disease. Leucovorin acts as a biomodulator by enhancing the binding of 5-fluorouracil to its target. Regimens combining 5-fluorouracil with leucovorin can improve disease-free survival in patients with Dukes type C cancers. Direct infusion of the drug into the hepatic artery can improve response rates in patients with hepatic involvement, but the effect on survival is marginal and may not outweigh the cost and toxicity of this approach.

The addition of either irinotecan [3] or oxaliplatin [4] to a 5-fluorouracil/leucovorin protocol improves response rates in advanced colorectal cancer. Irinotecan is a topoisomerase inhibitor, whereas oxaliplatin forms bulky DNA adducts that induce cellular apoptosis. Furthermore, oxaliplatin in combination with bolus 5-fluorouracil and leucovorin is superior to 5-fluorouracil/leuovorin alone as adjuvant therapy in patients with both stage II and stage III disease. [5]

The most recent drugs approved by the U.S. Food and Drug Administration for colorectal cancer, cetuximab and bevacizumab, are both monoclonal antibodies against specific cellular targets. Cetuximab is a monoclonal antibody that targets the extracellular binding domain of the epidermal growth factor receptor. Several phase II clinical trials have shown that cetuximab is synergistic with chemotherapy for advanced colorectal cancers. Bevacizumab is a humanized antibody directed against the vascular endothelial growth factor. The addition of bevacizumab (5 mg/kg given once every 14 days as an intravenous infusion until disease progression is detected) to a regimen of irinotecan, 5-fluorouracil, and leucovorin can provide a statistically significant increase in both response rates and median overall survival. [6]

Follow-up

A primary goal following curative resection for colorectal cancer is to detect curable recurrences or second primary tumors. Patients whose colon cancers have been cured face a 3 to 5% probability of developing an additional cancer of the large intestine during their lifetime and a more than 15% risk of developing an adenomatous polyp. It is also important to detect both synchronous (occurring at the same time) and metachronous (occurring at different times) cancers that may develop later. After curative resection, surveillance colonoscopy should be performed at 3 years and, if negative, at 5-year intervals thereafter. For patients who have had a low anterior

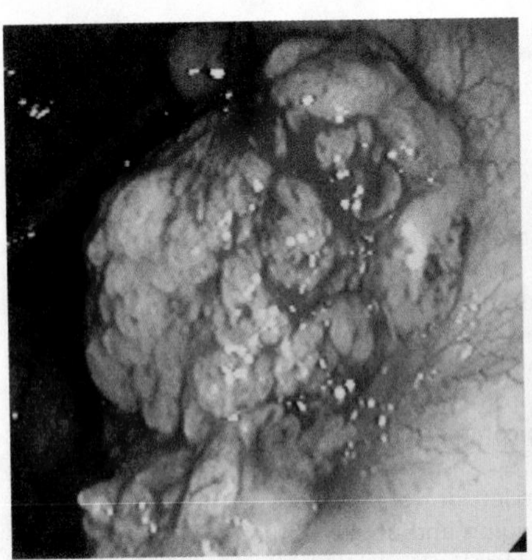
A

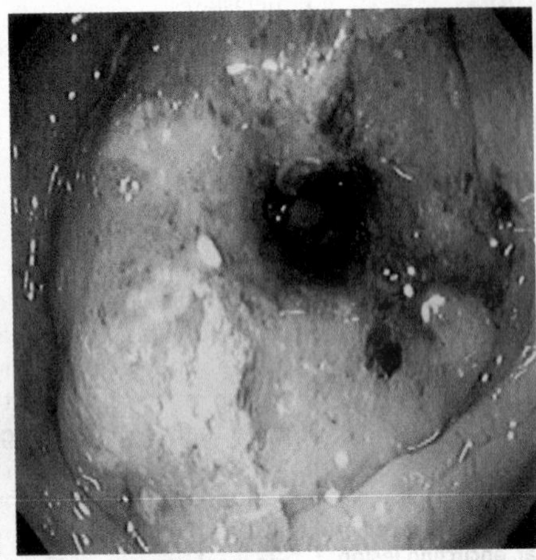
B

FIGURE 203–7 • Two manifestations of colorectal cancer. A, Exophytic growth within the lumen. **B,** "Stricturing" (apple core) lesion.

TABLE 203–4 SCREENING RECOMMENDATIONS FOR COLORECTAL CANCER

Risk	Test	Interval	Age to Begin (yr)
Average	FOBT *or* sigmoidoscopy *or* colonoscopy	Annually Every 5 yr Every 10 yr	50
Familial adenomatous polyposis	Sigmoidoscopy	Every 6–12 mo	10–12
Hereditary nonpolyposis colorectal cancer	Colonoscopy	Every 2 yr until age 40 and annually thereafter	25
Low familial risk for sporadic cancer	FOBT *or* sigmoidoscopy *or* colonoscopy	Annually Every 5 yr Every 10 yr	40
High familial risk for cancer	Colonoscopy	Every 5 yr	40

FOBT = fecal occult blood testing.

Rx

resection of a stage B or C rectosigmoid cancer, flexible sigmoidoscopy should be performed to examine the lower bowel every 3 to 6 months for 2 years, and a colonoscopy will be required to evaluate bowel beyond 60 cm. Additional follow-up measures include semiannual physical examinations and yearly blood chemistry studies. No clear consensus exists on the value of obtaining periodic chest radiographs or CT scans of the abdomen and pelvis in the absence of meaningful symptoms or signs. If the serum carcinoembryonic antigen (CEA) level was normal after the initial resection, a rising CEA suggests recurrent colorectal cancer; some experts advocate periodic assays for blood CEA levels following curative resection.

Prevention

Colorectal cancer is particularly amenable to widespread screening (Table 203–4, Chapter 13). First, it is one of the most common and lethal malignant diseases in many countries, thereby justifying the public health cost associated with a population-wide screening. Second, the natural progression of the lesion from dysplastic mucosa to invasive disease takes on average 10 to 20 years, a range that allows suitable time to detect the disease before it progresses to an incurable state. Finally, clear clinical evidence indicates that early detection of colorectal cancer improves survival. The major approaches to screen for colon cancer are the fecal occult blood test, flexible sigmoidoscopy, and colonoscopy.

Controlled prospective clinical trials performed in Minnesota, New York, Denmark, and the United Kingdom indicate that fecal occult blood test screening is relatively sensitive and reduces the rate of colorectal cancer mortality by 15 to 43%. However, the fecal occult blood test has a low sensitivity for detecting precancerous polyps and cancers of the rectosigmoid or distal rectum. Because many other conditions can cause blood in the stool, the fecal occult blood test is relatively nonspecific. Although no randomized trials have demonstrated the efficacy of flexible sigmoidoscopy for screening of colorectal cancer, case-control and cohort studies have shown a 60 to 85% reduction in the rate of mortality from distal colorectal cancers. Flexible sigmoidoscopy is well tolerated, can be performed relatively quickly, and does not require sedation. It is also highly accurate, with a high positive predictive value. The major drawback of flexible sigmoidoscopy is its inability to detect the 40% or more of large bowel neoplasms that reside beyond its reach; as a result, a full colonoscopy is recommended if flexible sigmoidoscopy reveals a polyp or tumor. Other screening options that may be considered but for which supportive clinical evidence is limited include a barium enema plus flexible sigmoidoscopy every 5 years or a colonoscopy every 10 years. An emerging screening test is to examine recovered DNA from stool for genetic abnormalities. A recent large study found that fecal DNA testing for 21 gene mutations had a sensitivity of 52% and specificity of 94% for the detection of colorectal cancer. The low sensitivity and high cost of this method limit its current use, but ongoing research may allow for more utility of this method in the future.

Because colonoscopy is a required part of any screening strategy, an alternative is to screen only with colonoscopy every 10 years in persons over the age of 50 years. Because screening colonoscopy is now covered by Medicare, it is becoming a standard recommendation that is supported by several professional organizations and by formal quantitative analyses, despite the absence of a randomized trial. Screening recommendations for individuals at high risk because of the presence of inflammatory bowel disease or because of a familial disposition are summarized in Table 203–4.

Chemoprevention

Several chemicals, drugs, and nutraceuticals are being evaluated for either primary or secondary prevention of adenomatous polyps and colorectal cancer. In a randomized trial, calcium provided a moderate 15% reduction for colorectal adenomas as early as 1 year after dietary supplementation. The mechanism may be calcium's blockage of the tumor-promoting effects of bile acids. Long-term intake of aspirin and of other nonsteroidal anti-inflammatory drugs is associated with a reduction in the relative risk for developing colorectal cancer, likely as a result of inhibition of the cyclooxygenase enzyme. Randomized trials of aspirin indicate a reduction in adenoma formation in the aspirin-treated group, 7 but the preferred dose and duration of aspirin therapy remain uncertain. A low-fat diet is not efficacious for preventing colorectal cancer. 8 Several cohort and case-control studies indicate that folic acid may prevent colon cancer by unknown mechanisms. Hormone replacement therapy is associated with lower risk for colorectal cancer, but estrogen and progestin supplementation has thrombogenic side effects that outweigh this benefit.

Epidemiologic data suggest that statins are associated with a 47% relative reduction in the risk of colorectal cancer. Recent observational data indicate that supplementation with vitamin D in people who are deficient may decrease the risk for colorectal cancer.

Prognosis

The 5-year survival rate of colorectal cancer directly correlates with the stage of disease at the time of diagnosis (see Table 203–3). Predictors of poor outcome following surgical resection include poorly differentiated histologic type, perforation, adherence of tumor to adjacent organs, venous invasion, preoperative elevation of CEA to levels greater than 5.0 ng/mL, aneuploidy, and specific chromosomal deletions.

NEOPLASMS OF THE SMALL INTESTINE

Epidemiology

The small intestine represents one of the largest portions of the gastrointestinal tract by tissue mass, but cancer of the small intestine accounts for a very small percentage of gastrointestinal malignant diseases (~2000 cases/year in the United States). The epithelial and stromal elements can give rise to transformed cells directly, or the small intestine can be the site of metastatic disease. Risk factors for cancer of the small intestine include the following: Crohn's disease (Chapter 144), especially after surgical bypass; Gardner's syndrome, specifically periampullary adenocarcinoma; and Peutz-Jeghers syndrome, which carries a 16-fold increased risk for small bowel cancer. Patients who have celiac disease or who are chronically immunocompromised have an increased risk of intestinal lymphoma. Immunoproliferative disease of the small intestine (Mediterranean abdominal lymphoma) occurs primarily in individuals of Middle Eastern origin but can also develop sporadically in others. The lower rate of adenocarcinomas in the small bowel as compared with the large intestine is not understood, but the higher rate of programmed cell death and cell proliferation in the small intestine may result in the shedding of abnormal cells before they become fully transformed.

Pathobiology

Benign lesions of the small intestine include adenomas, leiomyomas, lipomas, and angiomas. Routine upper gastrointestinal endoscopy can detect Brunner's gland adenomas, which are small, benign nodules in the duodenal mucosa that are caused by hyperplasia and hypertrophy of the submucosal duodenal glands. Malignant diseases of the small intestine include adenocarcinomas, carcinoid tumors, lymphomas, and leiomyosarcomas. Adenocarcinomas, which account for almost 50% of all small intestinal malignant diseases, occur most frequently in the duodenum. Carcinoid is the most common tumor of the distal small bowel. Lymphomas typically arise in the ileum.

Clinical Manifestations

Most benign small bowel neoplasms do not result in symptoms and are usually found incidentally at laparotomy or autopsy. Because the small intestinal contents are mostly liquid and the bowel wall is highly distensible, these lesions are unlikely to produce symptoms unless they become quite large. Symptoms can occur when the tumors grow large enough to cause intussusception or volvulus, either of which can lead to partial or complete small bowel obstruction.

The symptoms of cancer of the small intestine include abdominal pain (63%), vomiting (48%), weight loss (44%), and bleeding (23%). Patients with tumors distal to the duodenal bulb often present with symptoms similar to those of peptic ulcer disease, whereas lesions located in the periampullary region can cause obstructive jaundice. Carcinomas in the distal small bowel are usually asymptomatic until intestinal obstruction or gastrointestinal hemorrhage occurs.

Small carcinoid neoplasms (Chapter 251) are often asymptomatic, whereas larger carcinoids can obstruct the lumen or cause bleeding (Fig. 203–8). The carcinoid syndrome can develop after the lesion has metastasized to the liver. Peritoneal involvement is common.

Patients with small intestinal lymphoma can present with symptoms similar to those of adenocarcinomas of similar location. Fever and malabsorption are common (Chapter 196). Large sarcomas of the small bowel can perforate or cause massive hemorrhage.

Diagnosis

Cancer of the small intestine is often associated with an unremarkable or nonspecific physical examination, but patients can also present with obstructive abdominal distention and evidence of augmented peristalsis proximal to the lesion. Patients with advanced cancers may present with cachexia, hepatomegaly, ascites, and jaundice. Advanced lymphomas are commonly accompanied by splenomegaly and/or peripheral lymphadenopathy.

Differential Diagnosis

The same symptoms and signs caused by benign and malignant small bowel tumors are actually more likely to be caused by other conditions. For example, bleeding can result from peptic ulceration, Meckel's diverticulum, or vascular anomalies. Obstructive jaundice is more commonly caused by common duct stones, pancreatitis, or pancreatic cancer. Small bowel obstruction is most often caused by adhesions (especially in patients who have had prior abdominal surgery), internal hernias, volvulus, or intussusception.

Diagnostic Evaluation

Bleeding from neoplasms of the small intestine can lead to hypochromic, microcytic anemia. Hepatic metastases or periampullary tumors that obstruct the ampulla of Vater may lead to elevation of alkaline phosphatase and bilirubin levels. Carcinoid syndrome is associated with increases in the plasma serotonin level and the urinary level of 5-hydroxyindoleacetic acid (Chapter 251). Mediterranean lymphoma is characterized by dysproteinemia in which heavy-chain fragments of immunoglobulin A are present in the serum and urine (Chapter 198).

Upper gastrointestinal endoscopy, barium radiography, selective nasoenteric intubation (enteroclysis), and capsule endoscopy (Chapter 136) can enable the clinician to locate tumors of the small bowel. Colonoscopy can visualize the mucosa of the terminal ileum. Endoscopic ultrasonography can determine the depth of invasion of a particular lesion. Abdominal ultrasonography and CT scanning can allow one to assess intra-abdominal and retroperitoneal spread.

Treatment

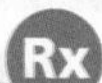

The primary treatment for neoplasms of the small bowel is surgical resection of the lesion. Whipple's procedure (pancreaticoduodenal resection) is used to treat carcinomas or large villous adenomas in the duodenum. Patients with localized lymphoma can be treated with surgical excision, but chemotherapy is necessary for more extensive disease. Adjuvant radiation therapy is recommended for large tumors or localized recurrences. As with any malignant disease, patients with advanced tumors remain at risk for recurrence. Imatinib mesylate has been shown in several early studies to have impressive results in the treatment of patients with unresectable or metastatic stromal tumors of the small bowel.

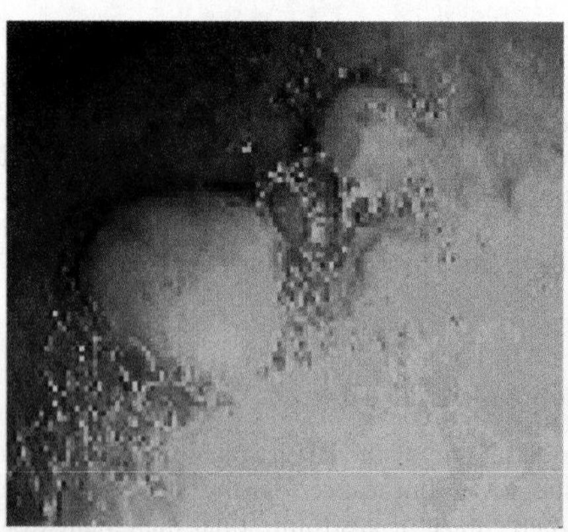

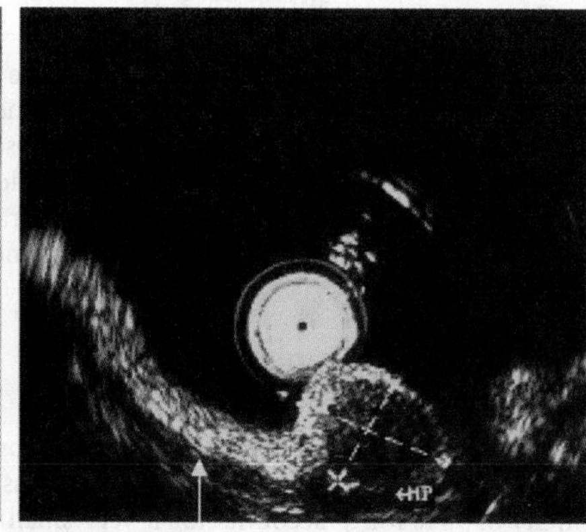

FIGURE 203–8 • Carcinoid nodule. A, Carcinoid nodule in the duodenum. **B,** An endoscopic ultrasonographic image shows that the lesion is confined to the submucosa, because the black stripe (arrow) representing the muscular layer is intact. Based on the endoscopic ultrasonographic findings, the lesion was safely resected endoscopically.

Prognosis

Survival rates and prognosis are good for benign tumors of the intestine if surgical resection is able to treat bleeding and obstruction. The prognosis for adenocarcinomas is poor. Leiomyosarcomas and primary lymphomas have a good prognosis if complete surgical resection is possible, but most such tumors cannot be completely resected. Long-term survival is possible even when hepatic carcinoid tumors involve the liver (Chapter 251).

Mediterranean abdominal lymphoma could be prevented if parasitic infestation could be eliminated. In patients with celiac disease (Chapter 143), early diagnosis and adoption of a gluten-free diet may reduce the incidence of cancer. Rates of periampullary cancers in the hereditary polyposis syndromes may decline with periodic monitoring.

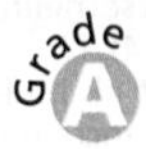

1. Clinical Outcomes of Surgical Therapy Study Group: A comparison of laparoscopically assisted and open colectomy for colon cancer. N Engl J Med 2004;350:2050–2059.
2. Guillou PJ, Quirke P, Thorpe H, et al: Short-term endpoints of conventional versus laparoscopic-assisted surgery in patients with colorectal cancer (MRC CLASICC trial): Multicentre, randomised controlled trial. Lancet 2005;365:1718–1726.
3. Saltz LB, Cox JV, Blanke C, et al: Irinotecan plus fluorouracil and leucovorin for metastatic colorectal cancer: Irinotecan Study Group. N Engl J Med 2000;343:905–914.
4. Giacchetti S, Perpoint B, Zidani R, et al: Phase III multicenter randomized trial of oxaliplatin added to chronomodulated fluorouracil-leucovorin as first-line treatment of metastatic colorectal cancer. J Clin Oncol 2000;18:136–147.
5. André T, Boni C, Mounedji-Boudiaf L, et al: Oxaliplatin, fluorouracil, and leucovorin as adjuvant treatment for colon cancer. N Engl J Med 2004;350:2343–2351.
6. Hurwitz H, Fehrenbacher L, Novotny W, et al: Bevacizumab plus irinotecan, fluorouracil, and leucovorin for metastatic colorectal cancer. N Engl J Med 2004;350:2335–2342.
7. Baron JA, Cole BF, Sandler RS, et al: A randomized trial of aspirin to prevent colorectal adenomas. N Engl J Med 2003;348:891–899.
8. Beresford SA, Johnson KC, Ritenbaugh C, et al: Low-fat dietary pattern and risk of colorectal cancer: The Women's Health Initiative Randomized Controlled Dietary Modification Trial. JAMA 2006;295:643–654.

SUGGESTED READINGS

Bailey AA, Debinski HS, Appleyard MN, et al: Diagnosis and outcome of small bowel tumors found by capsule endoscopy: A three-center Australian experience. Am J Gastroenterol 2006;101:2237–2243. *Detection of small bowel carcinomas on capsule endoscopy frequently alters management and may improve patient outcomes.*

Burt R, Neklason DW: Genetic testing for inherited colon cancer. Gastroenterology 2005;128:1696–1716. *A discussion of the familial colorectal cancer syndromes and the most recent data on genetic testing for these disorders.*

Collins JF, Lieberman DA, Durbin TE, et al: Accuracy of screening for fecal occult blood on a single stool sample obtained by digital rectal examination: A comparison with recommended sampling practice. Ann Intern Med 2005; 142:81–85. *The test detected only 4.9% of patients with advanced colonic neoplasia.*

Levine JS, Ahnen DJ: Adenomatous polyps of the colon. N Engl J Med 2006;355:2551–2557. *A clinical overview.*

Meyerhardt JA, Mayer RJ: Systemic therapy for colorectal cancer. N Engl J Med 2005;352:476–487. *A comprehensive update on systemic therapy for colorectal cancer.*

Ransohoff DF: Colon cancer screening in 2005: Status and challenges. Gastroenterology 2005;128:1685–1695. *A review of the most recent recommendations on colon cancer screening.*

Rockey DC, Paulson E, Niedzwiecki D, et al: Analysis of air contrast barium enema, computed tomographic colonography, and colonoscopy: Prospective comparison. Lancet 2005;365:305–311. *"Virtual colonoscopy" was better than BE, but regular colonoscopy was best by far.*

Weitz J, Koch W, Debus J, et al: Colorectal cancer. Lancet 2005;365:153–165. *A comprehensive review.*

Winawer SJ, Zauber AG, Fletcher RH, et al: Guidelines for colonoscopy surveillance after polypectomy: A consensus update by the US Multi-Society Task Force on Colorectal Cancer and the American Cancer Society. Gastroenterology 2006;130:1872–1885. *Guidelines for colonoscopic surveillance.*

204 PANCREATIC CANCER

Margaret Tempero and Randall Brand

Definition

The term *pancreatic cancer* usually refers to ductal adenocarcinomas, because more than 90% of pancreatic neoplasms are of ductal epithelial origin. Other pancreatic tumors include endocrine tumors (Chapter 188), carcinoid tumors (Chapter 251), lymphomas, and the rare cystic neoplasms, squamous cell carcinomas, giant cell carcinomas, carcinosarcomas, malignant fibrous histiocytomas, solid pseudopapillary neoplasms, sarcomas, and pancreaticoblastomas.

Epidemiology

In the United States, approximately 32,200 pancreatic neoplasms are diagnosed annually, and nearly the same number of persons die each year from cancer-related causes. Carcinoma of the pancreas is the fourth most common cause of cancer death in men and women. Worldwide, pancreatic cancer accounts for 2% of all malignant diseases. Its incidence is higher in developed than in developing countries, but there is less than a two-fold variation in incidence worldwide. The 5-year survival rate for adenocarcinoma of the pancreas is less than 5%, and most patients die within the first 2 years. The risk for developing a pancreatic carcinoma increases with age, with a mean age of onset in the seventh and eighth decades of life. This cancer is slightly more common in women than in men.

Pancreatic cancer is more common in African Americans, Maori New Zealanders, and Polynesians. Cigarette smoking, which is the most significant environmental risk factor, results in a 1.5- to 5.5-fold increased rate of pancreatic cancer. Other risk factors include increased body mass index, chronic pancreatitis (Chapter 147), high intake of animal fat, and prolonged contact with petroleum products and wood pulp. The association between pancreatic cancer and diabetes is complex. Diabetes or impaired glucose tolerance is observed in up to 80% of patients at the time of diagnosis of their pancreatic cancer, and diabetes is often described as a risk factor. However, the diabetes is usually of recent onset and may improve or resolve after resection of the tumor. A population-based study suggests that about 1% of patients who develop diabetes after age 50 years will have a diagnosis of pancreatic cancer within 3 years before or after the onset of diabetes, and most of these individuals will be diagnosed with diabetes within 6 months of detection of the pancreatic cancer. Thus, diabetes may be a sign of underlying pancreatic cancer.

Intraductal papillary mucinous neoplasms occur more frequently in men and are usually located in the head of the pancreas. Other cystic neoplasms most commonly occur in young to middle-aged women and are located in the body or tail of the pancreas.

Pathobiology

Up to 10% of patients with pancreatic cancer have one or more first- or second-degree relatives with the disease. Recognized inherited syndromes include hereditary pancreatitis (Chapter 147), mutation of the *BRCA2* gene (Chapter 208), familial atypical multiple mole-melanoma syndrome and a p16 germline mutation, hereditary nonpolyposis colorectal cancer (Chapter 203), Peutz-Jeghers polyposis (Chapter 203), and ataxia-telangiectasia (Chapter 271).

Tumor suppressor genes that are most frequently mutated in pancreatic adenocarcinoma are *p16* (95%), *p53* (50 to 75%), and *DPC4* (55%). *K-ras*, which is the most commonly activated oncogene, occurs in about 90% of pancreatic cancers. Pancreatic cancers are thought to progress from precursor duct lesions, termed *pancreatic intraepithelial neoplasms*, which have typical histologic features and contain initial genetic alterations, to an invasive adenocarcinoma (Fig. 204–1).

Ductal adenocarcinoma and its variants are characterized by a dense, fibrotic reaction surrounding a compact mass of hard pancreatic tissue that can invade surrounding mesenteric vessels and can involve perineuronal tissue and lymphatic channels or nodes. Because approximately

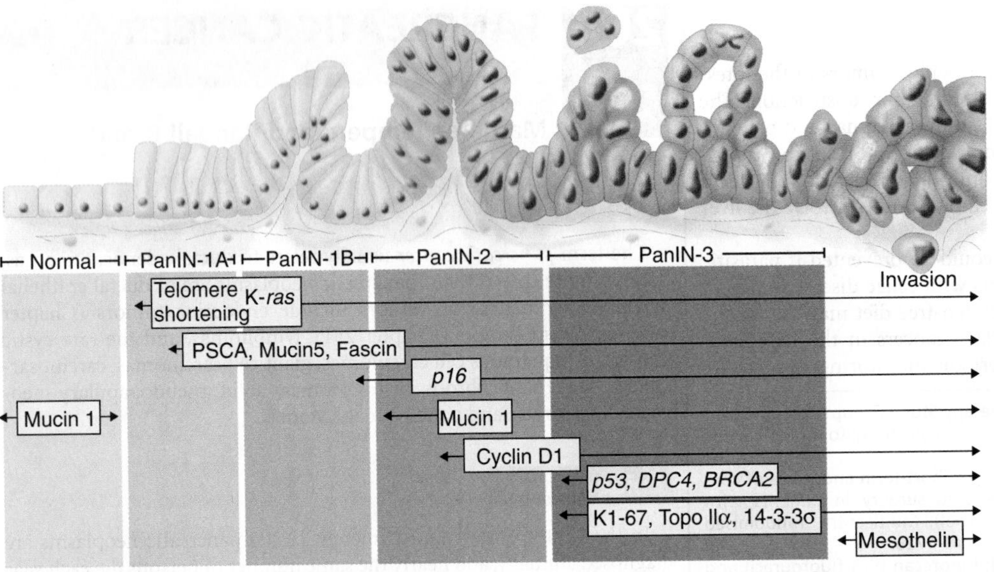

FIGURE 204–1 • Molecular progression model of pancreatic cancer (PanINs). Molecular abnormalities in PanINs can usually be stratified into "early" changes (e.g., expression of MUC5 and prostate stem antigen, or loss of p16), "intermediate" changes (e.g., expression of cyclin D1), and "late" changes (e.g., expression of p53, proliferation antigens, MUC1, mesothelin, and 14-3-3s, or loss of Smad4/Dpc4). (From Maitra A, Adsay NV, Argani P, et al: Multicomponent analysis of the pancreatic adenocarcinoma progression model using a pancreatic intraepithelial neoplasia tissue microarray. Mod Pathol 2003;16: 902–912.)

75% of pancreatic carcinomas are located in the head of the pancreas, the usual clinical presentations are related to invasion or compression of the bile or pancreatic ducts. The duodenum, stomach, and colon may be invaded or compressed. The three common types of cystic neoplasms are serous cystadenomas, mucinous cystic neoplasms, and intraductal papillary mucinous neoplasms. Serous cystadenomas are almost always benign, whereas the other lesions have a high risk of malignancy. Pancreatic cancers other than ductal adenocarcinoma, such as islet cell tumors or lymphomas, tend to be softer and less fibrotic and thus tend to cause distortion rather than encasement or compression of adjacent structures.

Clinical Manifestations

Early symptoms include nonspecific abdominal discomfort, nausea, vomiting, sleeping difficulties, anorexia, and generalized malaise. Despite the historic perception that a mass in the head of the pancreas manifests initially with painless jaundice, the more common presenting symptoms are epigastric pain, obstructive jaundice, and weight loss. Although these symptoms prompt evaluation of the pancreas and biliary tree, they occur late in the disease and are usually associated with advanced tumor at the time of diagnosis. The finding of a palpably distended, nontender gallbladder as a result of obstruction of the distal common bile duct by pancreatic cancer has been called Courvoisier's sign. Patients may manifest superficial or deep venous thrombosis (Trousseau's syndrome; Chapter 189).

The most common laboratory abnormalities include anemia and elevation of serum levels of alkaline phosphatase, bilirubin, and aminotransferases. Approximately 80% of patients have jaundice related to biliary obstruction. Diabetes or hyperglycemia is seen in up to 80% of patients, and pancreatic cancer should be considered in the differential diagnosis of the cause of new-onset diabetes in patients who are more than 50 years old and who do not have a family history of diabetes.

Tumors of other histologic types arising in the pancreas may also cause nonspecific symptoms. Patients with functioning islet cell tumors can present with symptoms related to the overproduction of peptides manufactured in the islets (Chapter 205). Cystic neoplasms generally remain asymptomatic until they become quite large, at which point patients can present with a palpable mass, abdominal pain, nausea, emesis, and weight loss. Obstruction of the common bile duct is less common than with ductal adenocarcinoma. Intraductal papillary mucinous tumors may cause symptoms of acute pancreatitis or pancreatic insufficiency owing to obstruction of the pancreatic duct.

Diagnosis

Differential Diagnosis

The differential diagnosis of pancreatic ductal cancer includes conditions that can manifest as a solid mass in the pancreas, especially acute or, more commonly, chronic pancreatitis (Chapter 147). Ampullary carcinomas and distal cholangiocarcinomas also manifest with biliary obstruction and jaundice (Chapter 159). It may be difficult to differentiate cystic pancreatic neoplasms from non-neoplastic pancreatic pseudocysts based on noninvasive imaging studies; a cystic neoplasm should always be considered in patients who present with isolated cystic lesions and who have no risk factors for pancreatitis, such as alcoholism, abdominal trauma, or a prior history of acute or chronic pancreatitis or biliary tract disease.

Imaging

For all patients with suspected pancreatic tumors, the preferred imaging study is a multidetector computed tomographic (CT) scan with thin cuts through the pancreas (Fig. 204–2). The CT scan provides important information about vascular involvement and metastases, and it is approximately 90% accurate in assessing resectability. Endoscopic ultrasonography may be useful in patients with equivocal findings on the CT scan. When a preoperative biopsy is needed, it is preferable to obtain a fine-needle aspiration under endoscopic guidance to minimize the chance of tumor seeding, but patients with potentially resectable disease can proceed directly to surgery. False-negative biopsy findings can result from the desmoplastic reaction characteristic of pancreatic ductal adenocarcinoma. Patients without a definitive preoperative diagnosis who present with obstructive jaundice and cholangitis should have a temporary plastic stent placed in the bile duct by endoscopic retrograde cholangiopancreatography or by transhepatic cholangiography. Laparoscopy can identify patients who may have occult metastases in the peritoneum or the surface of the liver. Patients whose CT scans indicate an unresectable tumor based on local extension or the presence of metastases should have a definitive diagnosis established by a fine-needle aspiration biopsy of the primary or metastatic site.

Biomarkers

The clinical role for tumor markers (Chapter 190) is limited. CA-19-9, a sialylated Lewis[a] antigen associated with circulating mucins, is the most widely used marker for pancreatic disease. At the most commonly used cutoff level of 37 U/mL, its sensitivity ranges from 81 to 85%, and its specificity ranges from 81 to 90%; CA-19-9 levels higher than 1000 U/mL are associated with unresectable disease. Although this test is not a substitute for a histologic diagnosis, it is useful for monitoring the response to treatment.

The aforementioned radiographic studies also apply to other pancreatic tumors. Endoscopic ultrasonography with fine-needle aspiration can be useful in the evaluation of cystic lesions, and it often provides additional detail not seen by CT and permits sampling of the cystic fluid for tumor marker levels, amylase content, viscosity, and cytologic examination. Carcinoembryonic antigen levels of 192 mg/mL are approximately 80% accurate for identifying mucinous as compared with nonmucinous cystic lesions. For obvious reasons, it is important to clarify whether the lesion is a simple cyst, which would suggest a pseudocyst, or a cystic neoplasm.

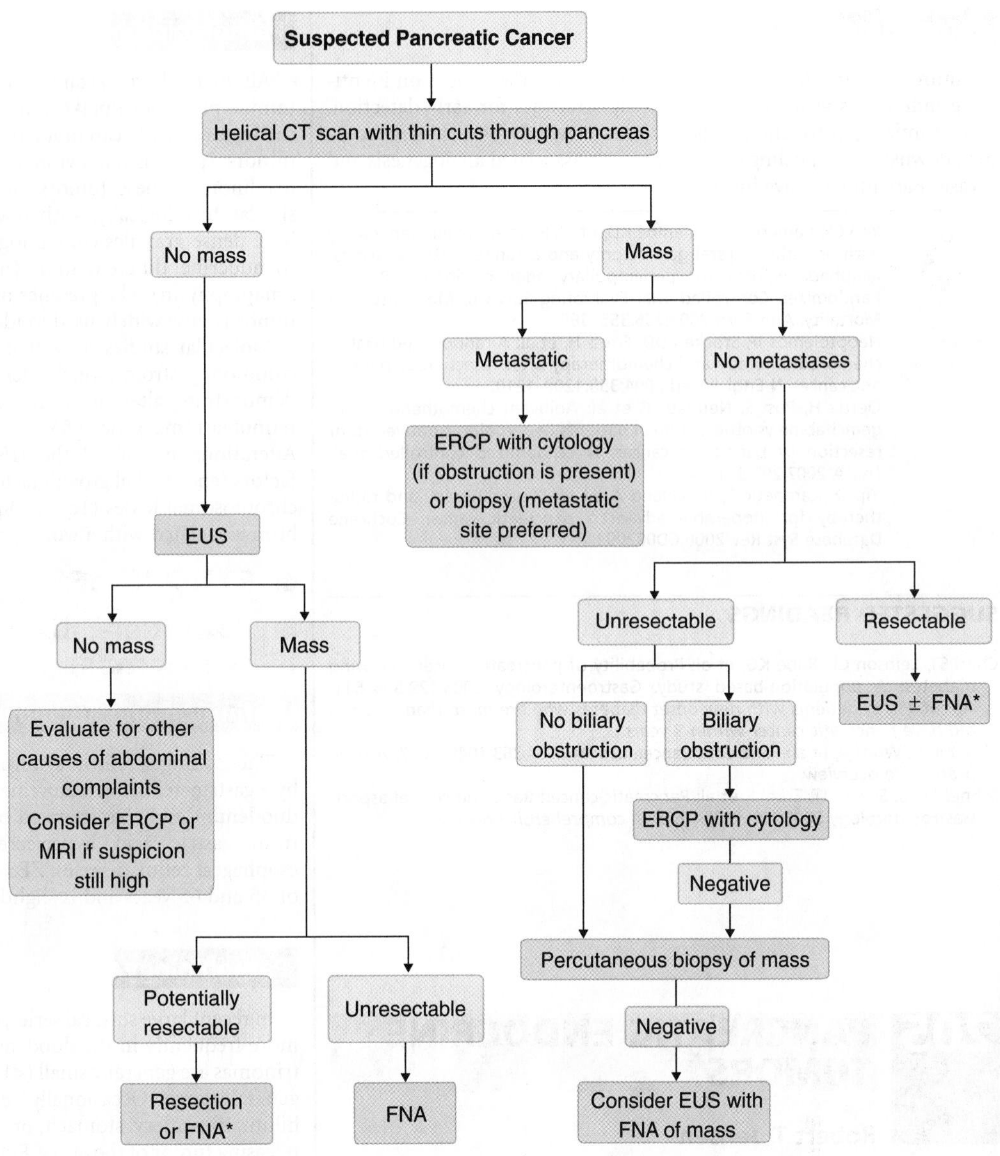

FIGURE 204–2 • Diagnostic algorithm for pancreatic cancer. *Intraoperative fine-needle aspiration (FNA) if the tumor is found to be inoperable during surgery. CT = computed tomographic scan; ERCP = endoscopic retrograde cholangiopancreatography; EUS = endoscopic ultrasonography; MRI = magnetic resonance imaging.

Treatment and Prognosis

Rx

In the absence of metastatic disease, surgical resection is the initial treatment of choice for all patients with pancreatic adenocarcinomas. The procedure should be performed in centers that have a high volume of pancreatectomies, because surgical outcomes are improved with more volume and experience. For periampullary adenocarcinoma, pancreaticoduodenectomy with or without distal gastrectomy and extended lymphadenectomy is now recommended. [1] Preoperative chemotherapy and radiation can be considered, although this approach has not yet become the standard of care.

Tumors are considered resectable if a clear fat plane is present around the celiac and superior mesenteric arteries and if the mesenteric and portal veins are patent. After successful resection, adjuvant therapy using chemoradiation followed by intravenous 5-fluorouracil (425 mg/M²) and folinic acid (20 mg/M²) daily for 5 days and monthly for 6 months has commonly been used, [2] although gemcitabine has recently been shown to increase 3-year disease-free survival from 7.5% to 23.5%. [3] Radiation therapy may not confer any added value beyond 5-fluorouracil alone. In general, successful resection followed by adjuvant therapy results in a 5-year survival rate of approximately 20%.

Surgery can also have an important palliative role. Patients who undergo surgical exploration but who are found not to have a resectable tumor may benefit from a biliary or gastric bypass procedure, depending on the clinical setting. However, there is now substantial experience in the placement of both biliary and luminal (duodenal) stents, so the more invasive operative procedure can be avoided in most instances. In addition, intraoperative, endoscopic ultrasound-guided, or percutaneous chemical splanchnicectomy can provide protracted pain control.

Rx

Patients with locally unresectable disease are usually managed with a combination of chemotherapy and radiation therapy, followed by additional chemotherapy. The most commonly used approach is 5-fluorouracil, given by low-dose continuous infusion, or another fluorinated pyrimidine combined with radiation therapy, but gemcitabine is also being studied. The median survival time for these patients is 10 to 12 months.

For patients with metastatic disease, single-agent gemcitabine (1000 mg/m² intravenously, weekly times 7 for 8 weeks and then weekly times 3 every 4 weeks) remains the standard of care and improves survival, [4] although a small improvement in survival has been observed with the addition of erlotinib (orally, 100 mg/day). For patients with advanced disease, optimal management of pain and of local complications is critical. Biliary obstruction can be managed surgically or with placement of a plastic or expandable metal stent. Narcotic analgesics (Chapter 28) and palliative care (Chapter 3) are cornerstones of therapy.

Most patients with a cystic neoplasm should be considered for surgical resection. The long-term survival rate following resection of malignant pancreatic cystic neoplasms exceeds 70%, and adjuvant therapy is currently not recommended.

Future Directions

Future programs for pancreatic adenocarcinoma will focus on identifying individuals at high risk, developing strategies for early detection, and optimizing treatment. Drugs that interact with tyrosine kinase receptors, downstream signaling events, or tumor-associated angiogenesis and invasion are under active investigation.

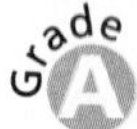

1. Yeo CY, Cameron JL, Lillemoe KD, et al: Pancreaticoduodenectomy with or without distal gastrectomy and extended retroperitoneal lymphadenectomy for periampullary adenocarcinoma: Part 2. Randomized Controlled Trial Evaluating Survival, Morbidity, and Mortality. Ann Surg 2002;236:355–368.
2. Neoptolemos JP, Stocken DD, Friess H, et al: A randomized trial of chemoradiotherapy and chemotherapy after resection of pancreatic cancer. N Engl J Med 2004;350:1200–1210.
3. Oettle H, Post S, Neuhaus P, et al: Adjuvant chemotherapy with gemcitabine vs observation in patients undergoing curative-intent resection of pancreatic cancer: A randomized controlled trial. JAMA 2007;297:311–313.
4. Yip D, Karapetic C, Strickland A, et al: Chemotherapy and radiotherapy for inoperable advanced pancreatic cancer. Cochrane Database Syst Rev 2006;CD002093.

SUGGESTED READINGS

Chari ST, Leibson CL, Rabe KG, et al: Probability of pancreatic cancer following diabetes: A population-based study. Gastroenterology 2005;129:504–511. *About 1% of patients with new-onset diabetes who are more than 50 years old have pancreatic cancer within 3 years.*

Li D, Xie K, Wolff R, et al: Pancreatic cancer. Lancet 2004;363:1049–1057. *A comprehensive overview.*

Schneider G, Siveke JT, Eckel F, et al: Pancreatic cancer: Basic and clinical aspect. Gastroenterology 2005;128:1606–1625. *A comprehensive review.*

205 PANCREATIC ENDOCRINE TUMORS

Robert T. Jensen

Definition

Pancreatic endocrine tumors (PETs) are also called islet tumors or islet cell tumors; however, because the cell of origin of most is unknown, the general term PET is preferred. This term is also a slight misnomer because PETs can also occur outside the pancreas. Eight PETs are well established (Table 205–1). Five additional functional PET syndromes have been rarely reported: PETs causing hypercalcemia (usually secreting parathormone-related peptide), PETs causing the carcinoid syndrome, PETs secreting renin (one case), PETs secreting erythropoietin (one case), and PETs secreting luteinizing hormone that causes virilization (two cases). In addition, PETs synthesizing neurotensin, calcitonin, and ghrelin are reported, but no distinct syndrome has been described.

PETs frequently are classified as functional or nonfunctional depending on whether a clinical syndrome resulting from the autonomously released hormone is present (gastrinoma, insulinoma, glucagonoma, VIPoma, somatostatinoma, GRFoma, ACTHoma). Nonfunctional PETs frequently release hormones and peptides (pancreatic polypeptide, neurotensin, α- and β-subunits of human chorionic gonadotropin, neuron-specific enolase, chromogranin A and breakdown products) that cause no distinct clinical syndromes.

Epidemiology

PETs are uncommon, having a prevalence of less than 10 per million population. Insulinomas, gastrinomas, and nonfunctional PETs are the most common, with an incidence of one to three new cases per million population.

Pathobiology

All PETs share certain features. PETs are classified as APUDomas (amine precursor uptake and decarboxylation), which share cytochemical features with carcinoid tumors, melanomas, and other endocrine tumors (pheochromocytomas, medullary thyroid cancer). Except for insulinomas, these tumors are frequently malignant. All PETs appear similar histologically, with few mitotic figures. Ultrastructurally, they have dense granules containing peptides, amines, and products of neuroendocrine differentiation (neuron-specific enolase, chromogranins, synaptophysin). The presence of chromogranin immunoreactivity in the tumor is now widely used to identify these tumors as endocrine tumors.

Molecular studies show that PETs have a different pathogenesis than common gastrointestinal adenocarcinomas because they infrequently demonstrate alterations in common tumor suppressor genes (e.g., retinoblastoma gene, p53) or common oncogenes (*ras*, *c-Jun*, *c-Fos*). Alterations in $p16^{INK4a}$, the *MEN1* gene, and the expression of growth factors (endothelial growth factor, insulin-like growth factor-I), as well as chromosomal losses (1q, 3p, 3q, 6p, X) and gains (17p, 17q, 20q), have been associated with a worse prognosis in numerous studies.

SYNDROMES

Zollinger-Ellison Syndrome (Gastrinomas)

Definition and Epidemiology

The Zollinger-Ellison syndrome (ZES) is a clinical syndrome caused by a gastrin-releasing endocrine tumor usually located in the pancreas or duodenum and characterized by clinical symptoms and signs resulting from gastric acid hypersecretion (peptic ulcer disease, diarrhea, esophageal reflux disease). ZES occurs most frequently between the ages of 35 and 65 years and is slightly more common in men (60%).

Pathobiology

In recent large surgical series, gastrinomas were found two to five times more frequently in the duodenum than in the pancreas. Duodenal gastrinomas are generally small (<1 cm), whereas pancreatic gastrinomas are generally larger. Occasionally ZES results from a gastrinoma in the splenic hilum, mesentery, stomach, or only in a lymph node or from a gastrin-releasing tumor of the ovary. Extrapancreatic gastrinomas producing ZES have been reported in the heart (two cases) and as a result of small cell lung cancer (one case). As with other PETs, malignancy can be reliably determined only by demonstrating the presence of metastatic disease, and no light microscopic or ultrastructural finding can clearly establish malignant behavior.

Gastrin stimulates parietal cells to secrete acid and also has a growth (trophic) effect on cells of the gastric mucosa. Chronic hypergastrinemia thus leads to increased gastric mucosal thickness, prominent gastric folds, and increased numbers of parietal cells and gastric enterochromaffin-like cells. Patients with gastrinomas have increased basal acid output and an increased maximal acid output, which is a measure of the total number of parietal cells. In contrast to patients with routine peptic ulcers (Chapter 141), *Helicobacter pylori* appears not to be important in the pathogenesis of the ulcer disease in ZES. Diarrhea is common because the large-volume gastric acid output leads to structural damage to the small intestine (inflammation, blunted villi, edema), interference with fat transport, inactivation of pancreatic lipase, and precipitation of bile acids. These same mechanisms, if prolonged, can lead to steatorrhea. If acid hypersecretion is controlled medically, surgically, or with nasogastric suction, the diarrhea will stop at once.

Clinical Manifestations

Abdominal pain resulting from a peptic ulcer is the most common symptom (>80%). Most ulcers occur in the duodenum (>85%), but they occasionally occur in the postbulbar area, jejunum, or stomach, and are occasionally in multiple locations. The pain is usually similar to that of patients with typical peptic ulcers (Chapter 142), especially early in the course of the disease. With time, the symptoms become persistent and,

TABLE 205–1 PANCREATIC ENDOCRINE TUMORS

Name of Tumor	Name of Syndrome	Main Signs or Symptoms	Location	Malignancy	Hormone Causing Syndrome
Gastrinoma	Zollinger-Ellison syndrome	Abdominal pain, diarrhea, esophageal symptoms	Pancreas (30%) Duodenum (60%) Other (10%)	60–90%	Gastrin
Insulinoma	Insulinoma	Hypoglycemic symptoms	Pancreas (100%)	5–15%	Insulin
Glucagonoma	Glucagonoma	Dermatitis, diabetes/glucose intolerance, weight loss	Pancreas (100%)	60%	Glucagon
VIPoma	Verner-Morrison, pancreatic cholera, WDHA	Severe watery diarrhea, hypokalemia	Pancreas (90%) Other: neural, adrenal, periganglionic tissue (10%)	80%	Vasoactive intestinal polypeptide
Somatostatinoma	Somatostatinoma	Diabetes mellitus, cholelithiasis, diarrhea	Pancreas (56%) Duodenum/jejunum (44%)	60%	Somatostatin
GRFoma	GRFoma	Acromegaly	Pancreas (30%) Lung (54%) Jejunum (7%) Other: adrenal, foregut, retroperitoneum (13%)	30%	Growth hormone–releasing factor
ACTHoma	ACTHoma	Cushing's syndrome	Pancreas (4–16% of all ectopic Cushing's)	>95%	Adrenocorticotropic hormone
Nonfunctional	Nonfunctional PPoma	Weight loss, abdominal mass, hepatomegaly	Pancreas (100%)	60–90%	None: pancreatic polypeptide chromogranin released but no known symptoms of hypersecretion

ACTH = adrenocorticotropic hormone; GRF = growth hormone–releasing factor; PP = pancreatic polypeptide; VIP = vasoactive intestinal polypeptide; WDHA = watery diarrhea, hypokalemia, and achlorhydria.

in general, respond poorly to treatments aimed at eliminating *H. pylori* and to conventional doses of histamine (H_2)-receptor antagonists, as well as to the now rarely used surgical treatments for ulcer disease. By comparison, conventional doses of proton pump inhibitors (e.g., omeprazole, lansoprazole, pantoprazole, esomeprazole, rabeprazole) can mask the symptoms of most patients with ZES and can also cause hypergastrinemia as seen in ZES. The widespread use of these drugs has delayed the diagnosis of ZES.

Heartburn resulting from reflux of gastric acid into the esophagus is also common (20%). Diarrhea (60 to 70%) occurs frequently and may precede peptic ulceration in some patients (10 to 20%). Twenty to 25% of patients have ZES as part of the multiple endocrine neoplasia 1 (MEN1) syndrome, an autosomal dominant inherited disease (Chapter 250). These patients have hyperplasia or tumors of multiple endocrine glands and most commonly have parathyroid hyperplasia (>90%), pituitary tumors (60%), and PETs (80%). ZES is the most common functional PET syndrome in these patients (54%), although patients typically first develop renal stones related to hypercalcemia from hyperparathyroidism or have elevated prolactin levels resulting from pituitary tumors and only later develop ZES. However, studies show that 20 to 40% of patients with MEN/ZES initially present with symptoms caused by ZES.

Almost all the symptoms result from the effects of gastric acid hypersecretion, but late in the disease patients can develop cachexia, weight loss, and pain owing to extensive liver metastases. Approximately one third of patients have metastatic liver disease at presentation, but less than 20% of other patients will develop metastatic disease to the liver during a 10-year follow-up period.

Up to 5% of patients with ZES develop Cushing's syndrome as a result of adrenocorticotropic hormone (ACTH) secretion by the gastrinoma. These patients usually have a metastatic gastrinoma in the liver, ZES without MEN1, and a poor prognosis.

Diagnosis

ZES should be suspected in any patient whose peptic ulcer disease is accompanied by diarrhea, is recurrent, does not heal with treatment, is not associated with *H. pylori* infection, is associated with a complication (bleeding, obstruction, esophageal stricture), is multiple or occurs in unusual locations, or is associated with a pancreatic tumor. ZES should also be suspected in patients with chronic secretory diarrhea (Chapter 143), peptic ulcer disease associated with large gastric folds on radiography or endoscopy, a family or personal history of renal stones or endocrinopathies, or the laboratory finding of hypercalcemia, hypergastrinemia, or gastric acid hypersecretion.

If the diagnosis is suspected, the initial test is a fasting serum gastrin level, which is elevated in 99 to 100% of patients with ZES. However, other causes of hypergastrinemia include a physiologic response to achlorhydria or hypochlorhydria because of pernicious anemia, atrophic gastritis, renal failure, *H. pylori* infections, or the use of proton pump inhibitors, which suppress acid for up to 1 week after discontinuation. If the serum gastrin level is elevated, the fasting gastric pH should be determined. If the serum gastrin is greater than 1000 pg/mL (normal <100) and the pH is less than 2.0, then the patient almost certainly has ZES; approximately 40% of patients will have this combination of findings. If the gastrin is elevated less than 10-fold and the pH is less than 2.0, then basal acid output should be measured. Basal acid output is increased in patients with ZES (>10.6 mEq/hour in men and >5.6 mEq/hour in women), and more than 95% will have a value greater than 15 mEq/hour if no previous gastric acid–reducing surgery has been performed. Because of their long duration of action, proton pump inhibitors must be stopped for at least 1 week, if possible, to ensure that the cause of the hypergastrinemia is not the drug itself.

Differential Diagnosis

A secretin test can exclude *H. pylori* infection, retained gastric antrum syndrome, antral G cell hyperfunction or hyperplasia, chronic renal failure, and gastric outlet obstruction that may mimic ZES. Physiologically normal individuals show a less than 120 pg/mL increase in the serum gastrin level after intravenous secretin, whereas 94% of patients who have ZES and a fasting gastrin level that is elevated less than 10-fold above normal have a positive test. No false-positive results have been reported, except in patients with achlorhydria. In all patients with ZES, evaluation must exclude MEN1 syndrome by determining whether the patient has a family history of endocrinopathies and by excluding hyperparathyroidism and pituitary adenomas.

Imaging and Endoscopy

All patients should have imaging studies to localize the tumor. Somatostatin receptor scintigraphy using single photon emission computed tomography after injection of indium-111–[diethylenetriamine pentaacetic acid-D-phenylalanine-1] octreotide is the localization method of choice; it will identify 60% of primary gastrinomas and more than 90% of patients with metastatic disease in the liver with a sensitivity equal to all conventional imaging studies (magnetic resonance imaging, computed tomography, ultrasound, angiography) combined. For pancreatic gastrinomas, endoscopic ultrasound is particularly sensitive. Small duodenal gastrinomas (<1 cm) are frequently not detected by any imaging modality but can be found at surgery if routine duodenotomy is performed.

Treatment

Rx

Medical Therapy

Patients should receive combined medical therapy directed at controlling the gastric acid hypersecretion and if possible, surgical therapy to remove the gastrinoma itself. Proton pump inhibitors (e.g., omeprazole, lansoprazole, pantoprazole, esomeprazole, rabeprazole) are now the drugs of choice. Because of their long duration of action, acid hypersecretion can be controlled in all patients with once- or twice-daily doses. The recommended starting dose for omeprazole is 60 mg once a day. In 30% of patients, higher doses are needed, particularly in patients with MEN1, previous gastric surgery, or a history of severe esophageal reflux. Patients must be treated indefinitely unless they are surgically cured. Long-term therapy is safe, and patients have been treated for up to 20 years with omeprazole without loss of efficacy, although reduced vitamin B_{12} levels, which are common with prolonged treatment, require vitamin B_{12} supplementation (Chapter 170). H_2-receptor antagonists are also effective, but frequent administration (every 4 to 6 hours) and high doses are needed. Total gastrectomy, the historic treatment for this disease, is now performed only for patients who cannot or will not take oral antisecretory medications. Selective vagotomy effectively reduces the acid secretion, but many patients continue to require a low dose of drug. Parathyroidectomy should be performed in patients with hyperparathyroidism, ZES, and MEN1 because it markedly reduces acid secretion and increases the sensitivity to antisecretory drugs.

Surgical Therapy

Surgical exploration for cure is now recommended in all patients without liver metastases, MEN1, or complicating medical conditions that limit life expectancy. Tumors are found by experienced endocrine surgeons in 95% of patients at surgery. Surgical resection decreases the metastatic rate and results in a 5-year cure rate of 30%. Patients with metastatic gastrinoma in the liver have a poor prognosis, with a 5-year survival rate of 30%.

Rx

Metastatic Disease

If the metastatic disease is increasing in size or is symptomatic, treatment with octreotide (100 to 450 μg two to three times daily) alone or in combination with α-interferon (1 to 5 million U 3 to 7 days/week) is effective in inhibiting further tumor growth in 50 to 60% of patients. If this treatment fails, chemotherapeutic agents (streptozotocin, 5-fluorouracil, doxorubicin [Adriamycin]) are recommended. For patients with extensive metastatic disease, somatostatin receptor–directed radiation therapy using analogues labeled with yttrium-90, lutetium-177, or indium-111 is increasingly used. Liver transplantation is occasionally performed in the rare patient with metastases limited to the liver.

Prognosis

Approximately 25% of gastrinomas show aggressive growth. Recent studies show that the most important prognostic predictor is the development of liver metastases. The presence of a large primary tumor, a pancreatic tumor, bone metastasis, or a high fasting gastrin level is associated with more aggressive growth.

Glucagonomas

Definition

Glucagonomas are endocrine tumors of the pancreas that ectopically secrete glucagon.

Pathobiology

Excess glucagon secretion explains the glucose intolerance. The exact origin of the rash is unclear; some studies report that prolonged glucagon infusions can cause the characteristic skin lesions. A role for possible zinc deficiency has been proposed because of the similarity of the rash to that seen with zinc deficiency (acrodermatitis enteropathica) and because the rash improves in some patients who are given zinc. The hypoaminoacidemia is thought to be secondary to the effect of glucagon on amino acid metabolism by altering gluconeogenesis. The wasting and weight loss are intrinsic parts of the glucagonoma syndrome, and recent studies suggest that a novel anorectic substance distinct from glucagon is responsible.

Clinical Manifestations

The clinical syndrome's cardinal features are distinct dermatitis (necrolytic migratory erythema; 70 to 90%), diabetes mellitus or glucose intolerance (40 to 90%), weight loss (70 to 96%), anemia (30 to 85%), hypoaminoacidemia (80 to 90%) with deficiencies of essential fatty acids, thromboembolism (10 to 25%), diarrhea (15 to 30%), and psychiatric disturbances (0 to 20%). The characteristic skin rash is usually found at intertriginous and periorificial sites, especially in the groin and buttocks (Fig. 205–1). It is initially erythematous, becomes raised, and develops central bullae whose tops detach, with the eroded areas becoming crusty. Healing occurs with hyperpigmentation.

Diagnosis

The diagnosis is established by demonstrating elevated plasma glucagon levels. Normal levels are 150 to 200 pg/mL; in patients with glucagonomas, levels usually (>90%) are higher than 1000 pg/mL. However, in some recent studies, up to 40% of patients had plasma glucagon values of 500 to 1000 pg/mL. Increased plasma glucagon levels are also reported in renal insufficiency, acute pancreatitis, hypercorticism, hepatic diseases, celiac disease, severe stress (trauma, exercise, diabetic ketoacidosis), and prolonged fasting, in patients treated with danazol, and in familial hyperglucagonemia. In these conditions, the level does not usually exceed 500 pg/mL except in patients with hepatic diseases, such as cirrhosis, or in those with familial hyperglucagonemia.

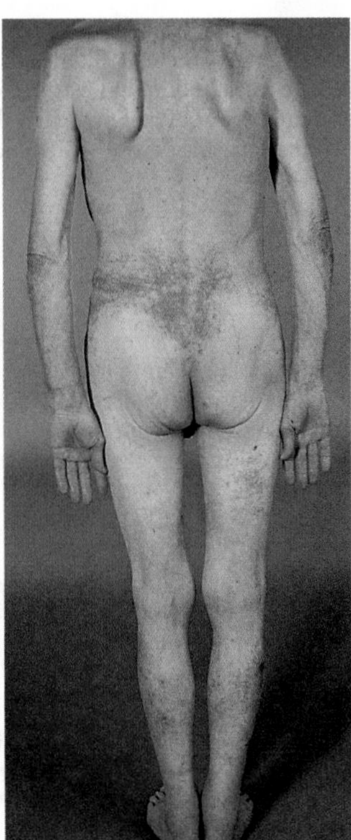

FIGURE 205–1 • A patient with a glucagonoma with the characteristic rash (necrolytic migratory erythema) is shown. The rash is usually at intertriginous areas or periorificial sites and shows various stages of erythema, blistering, and crusting. (From Forbes CD, Jackson WF: Color Atlas and Text of Clinical Medicine, 3rd ed. London, Mosby, 2003, with permission.)

Glucagonomas are generally large when they are discovered (mean size, 5 to 10 cm), and they most frequently occur in the pancreatic tail (>50%). Liver metastases are commonly present at the time of diagnosis (45 to 80%).

Treatment Rx

Subcutaneous administration of the synthetic long-acting somatostatin analogue, octreotide (100 to 400 μg two to three times daily), controls the rash in 80% of patients and improves weight loss, diarrhea, and hypoaminoacidemia, but it usually does not improve the diabetes mellitus. Increasingly, long-acting depot formulations of octreotide [octreotide-LAR] are being given (10 to 30 mg) by monthly injection. Zinc supplementation and infusions of amino acids and/or fatty acids can also diminish the severity of the rash. After tumor localization, surgical resection is preferred; even debulking of metastatic tumor may be of benefit. For advanced disease, chemotherapy (with dacarbazine or streptozotocin and doxorubicin), hepatic embolization, or chemoembolization may control symptoms in refractory cases.

VIPomas

Definition

The VIPoma syndrome, also called the Verner-Morrison syndrome, pancreatic cholera, and the WDHA syndrome (for watery diarrhea, hypokalemia, achlorhydria), results from an endocrine tumor, usually in the pancreas (in adults) that ectopically secretes vasoactive intestinal polypeptide (VIP).

Epidemiology and Pathobiology

VIPomas in adults are found in the pancreas in 80 to 90% of cases; rare cases result from intestinal carcinoids, ganglioneuromas, ganglioneuroblastomas, and pheochromocytomas. Characteristically seen in children younger than 10 years of age and rarely in adults (<5%), the VIPoma syndrome is caused by ganglioneuromas or ganglioneuroblastomas at extrapancreatic sites. VIPomas are usually large and solitary; 50 to 75% of these tumors occur in the pancreatic tail, and 40 to 70% of them have metastasized at diagnosis. VIPomas frequently secrete both VIP and peptide histidine methionine, but VIP is responsible for the symptoms. VIP is a potent stimulant of secretion in both the small and large intestine, and this action is responsible for the cardinal clinical features of the VIPoma syndrome. VIP also causes relaxation of gastrointestinal smooth muscle, and this may contribute to the dilated loops of bowel that are common in this syndrome as well as a dilated, atonic gallbladder that is sometimes seen. Hypochlorhydria is thought to result from the inhibitory effect of VIP on acid secretion, the flushing is related to the vasodilatory effects of VIP, and the hyperglycemia is caused by the glycogenolytic effect of VIP. The mechanism of the hypercalcemia remains unclear.

Clinical Manifestations

The cardinal clinical feature is severe, large-volume, watery diarrhea (>1 L/day) (100%), which is secretory and occurs during fasting (Chapter 143). Hypokalemia (67 to 100%) and dehydration (83%) commonly occur because of the volume of the diarrhea. Achlorhydria is occasionally noted, but hypochlorhydria is usually found (34 to 72% of cases). Flushing occurs in 20% of patients, hyperglycemia in 25 to 50%, and hypercalcemia in 41 to 50%. Steatorrhea is uncommon (16%) despite the volume of diarrhea.

Diagnosis

The diarrhea of VIPomas characteristically persists during fasting and is large in volume (>3 L/day in 70 to 80%); the diagnosis is excluded when fasting stool volume is less than 700 mL/day. To differentiate VIPomas from other causes of large-volume, fasting diarrhea (Chapter 143), fasting plasma VIP levels should be determined. The normal value in most laboratories is less than 190 pg/mL, and elevated levels are present in 90 to 100% of patients in various series. The differential diagnosis of large-volume, fasting diarrhea (>700 mL/day) includes ZES, diffuse islet cell hyperplasia, surreptitious use of laxatives, the pseudopancreatic cholera syndrome, and, rarely, human immunodeficiency virus (HIV) infections (Chapter 143). Serum gastrin levels identify patients with ZES, and plasma VIP levels are normal in most patients who abuse laxatives, in 82% of patients with pancreatic islet cell hyperplasias, and patients with HIV-induced severe secretory diarrhea.

Treatment Rx

The symptoms caused by the VIP can be controlled initially in more than 85% of patients by daily doses of octreotide (50 to 400 μg once to three times daily) or by monthly injections of the depot form, octreotide-LAR (10 to 30 mg), but increased doses may be needed over time. Before the availability of octreotide, small numbers of patients were reported to respond to a variety of agents including high-dose prednisone (60 to 100 mg/day; 40 to 50%), clonidine, lithium carbonate, indomethacin, loperamide, metoclopramide, and phenothiazines. After tumor localization studies, surgical resection should be attempted if it is possible to remove all visible tumor; however, more than 50% of patients have generalized liver metastases at diagnosis, so complete resection may not be possible. For patients with advanced cases and refractory symptoms, chemotherapy with streptozotocin and doxorubicin, hepatic chemoembolization, and hepatic embolization have been beneficial.

Somatostatinomas

Definition and Pathobiology

Somatostatinomas are endocrine tumors that occur in the pancreas or upper small intestine and that ectopically secrete somatostatin. In the gastrointestinal tract, somatostatin inhibits basal and stimulated acid secretion, pancreatic secretion, intestinal absorption of amino acids, gallbladder contractility, and release of numerous hormones including cholecystokinin and gastrin.

Clinical Manifestations

Somatostatinomas cause a distinct clinical syndrome of diabetes mellitus, gallbladder disease, diarrhea, steatorrhea, and weight loss. Sixty percent of somatostatinomas occur in the pancreas, and 40% are found in the duodenum or jejunum. Pancreatic somatostatinomas occur in the pancreatic head in 60 to 80% of cases; 70 to 92% of these tumors have metastasized at diagnosis, and they are usually large (mean, 5 cm) and solitary. In contrast, duodenal somatostatinomas are smaller (mean, 2.4 cm), are more frequently associated with psammoma bodies on histologic examination (11%), and less frequently have metastases at diagnosis (30 to 40%).

Symptoms occur much more commonly (80 to 95% of all cases) in patients with pancreatic than intestinal somatostatinomas. Duodenal somatostatinomas are frequently reported in patients with von Recklinghausen's disease (Chapter 444) and are usually asymptomatic. The diagnosis of *intestinal* somatostatinomas is based on the immunocytochemical finding of somatostatin in the tumor, because the plasma somatostatin is not elevated, and these tumors rarely cause the clinical somatostatinoma syndrome.

Diagnosis

Somatostatinomas are usually found by accident, particularly during exploratory laparotomy for cholecystectomy, during endoscopy, or on imaging studies. The presence of psammoma bodies on histologic examination of a duodenal endocrine tumor or any duodenal lesions in patients with von Recklinghausen's disease should raise the suspicion of a duodenal somatostatinoma. The diagnosis of the somatostatinoma syndrome requires the demonstration of increased concentrations of somatostatin-like immunoreactivity in the plasma and in the resected tumor. However, other tumors outside the pancreas or intestine, such as small cell lung cancer, medullary thyroid carcinoma, pheochromocytomas, and paragangliomas may also have elevated concentrations of somatostatin-like immunoreactivity. Somatostatinomas can be imaged using somatostatin receptor scintigraphy or, if needed, other conventional imaging studies to assess the tumor's location and extent.

Treatment

Treatment with octreotide (50 to 400 μg one to three times daily) can improve symptoms. Surgery, if possible, or chemotherapy, hepatic chemoembolization, or hepatic embolization may be of value.

GRFomas

Definition

GRFomas are endocrine tumors that frequently originate in the pancreas but also occur in other extrapancreatic locations and ectopically release growth hormone–releasing factor (GRF). The GRF causes acromegaly that is clinically indistinguishable from that caused by a pituitary adenoma (Chapters 242 and 243).

Pathobiology

GRFomas most commonly occur in the lung (54%). Most of the remainder occur in the gastrointestinal tract, including 30% in the pancreas. Pancreatic GRFomas are usually large (mean, 6 cm), 39% are metastatic at diagnosis, 40% occur in combination with ZES, and 33% are in patients with MEN1.

Diagnosis

GRFomas are an uncommon cause of acromegaly. These tumors occurred in none of 177 unselected patients with acromegaly in one study. However, any patient with acromegaly and abdominal complaints, with acromegaly but no pituitary tumor, or with acromegaly and hyperprolactinemia (which occurs in 70% of GRFomas) should be suspected of having a GRFoma. The intra-abdominal features of GRFomas result from its metastases and are typical of any malignant PET. The diagnosis is confirmed by performing a plasma assay for GRF and growth hormone.

Treatment

The effects of the GRF can be controlled with octreotide (50 to 450 μg one to three times daily) in more than 90% of patients, using either daily injections or monthly injections (10 to 30 mg) of the depot form, octreotide-LAR. Treatment should be directed at the GRFoma per se, as described for the other more frequent PETs.

Nonfunctional Pancreatic Endocrine Tumors

Definition

Nonfunctional PETs are endocrine tumors that originate in the pancreas and either secrete no peptides or secrete products that do not cause clinical symptoms.

Pathobiology

Frequently secreted, nonfunctional peptides include chromogranin A (100%), chromogranin B (100%), pancreatic polypeptide (60%), and the α-subunit (40%) and β-subunit of human chorionic gonadotrophin. Immunocytochemically, even higher percentages contain these peptides as well as insulin (50%), glucagon (30%), and somatostatin (13%).

Clinical Manifestations

Nonfunctional PETs are frequently diagnosed only late in the course of disease after the patient presents with symptoms or signs of metastatic disease and a liver biopsy reveals metastatic neuroendocrine tumor. Any symptoms or signs result from the tumor per se and include abdominal pain (36 to 56%), abdominal mass or hepatosplenomegaly (8 to 40%), weight loss or cachexia (8 to 46%), and jaundice (27 to 40%). In 20% of asymptomatic patients, tumors are found incidentally at surgery.

Diagnosis

Any patients with a long survival (>5 years) after a diagnosis of metastatic pancreatic adenocarcinoma should be suspected of having a nonfunctional PET. Most primary tumors are large (70% > 5 cm), and 70% occur in the pancreatic head. Liver metastases are frequent (38 to 62%) at presentation. An elevated plasma chromogranin A or pancreatic polypeptide level or a positive somatostatin receptor scintigraphic scan is strong evidence that a pancreatic mass is a PET. Malignancy correlates with vascular or perineural invasion, a proliferative index greater than 2%, a mitotic rate of 2 or greater, a size of at least 4 cm, capsular penetration, nuclear atypia, lack of progesterone receptors, and the presence of calcitonin immunoreactivity in the tumor.

Treatment

Tumor localization, surgical resection, and, for advanced cases, chemotherapy with streptozotocin and doxorubicin, hepatic embolization, or chemoembolization are useful. Survival is better in patients with smaller tumors, patients who are asymptomatic at presentation, in patients with no metastases, and in patients in whom surgical resection can be performed.

ACTHomas and Other Uncommon Tumors

PETs that ectopically secrete ACTH make up 4 to 16% of the causes of ectopic Cushing's syndrome (Chapter 245). Cushing's syndrome occurs in 5% of all cases of ZES, but in patients with sporadic ZES it is invariably a late feature, occurring with metastatic disease to the liver. Its development is associated with a poor prognosis, and the response to chemotherapy is generally poor; however, occasional patients benefit from the use of octreotide.

Paraneoplastic hypercalcemia (Chapter 266) can result from a PET that releases parathormone-related peptide or an unknown hypercalcemic substance. Tumors are generally large and metastatic to the liver at diagnosis. Octreotide may help control the hypercalcemia, but surgery, chemotherapy, hepatic embolization, and chemoembolization are the mainstays of treatment.

PETs causing the carcinoid syndrome (Chapter 251) are usually large, and 68 to 88% are malignant. Octreotide may control the symptoms. Surgery, chemotherapy, or hepatic embolization or chemoembolization may be helpful.

A single case of a PET that secreted renin manifested with severe hypertension; the tumor was localized with somatostatin receptor scintigraphy, and the patient's symptoms improved significantly after tumor resection. A single case of an erythropoietin-secreting PET resulting in polycythemia has been described.

Two symptomatic cases of PETs that secreted luteinizing hormone have been described; virilization occurred in the female patient, whereas the male patient had increased acne and a skin rash. In both cases, the tumors were resectable, and symptoms improved postoperatively.

SUGGESTED READINGS

de Heerder WW, O'Toule D, Rindi G, et al: ENETs consensus guidelines for the management of patients with digestive neuroendocrine tumors. Neuroendocrinol 2006;84:1–66. *Comprehensive guidelines for management.*

House MG, Schulick RD: Endocrine tumors of the pancreas. Curr Opin Oncol 2006;18:23–29. *A review of pathogenesis and molecular markers.*

Warner RR: Enteroendocrine tumors other than carcinoid: A review of clinically significant advances. Gastroenterology 2005;128:1668–1684. *A comprehensive review.*

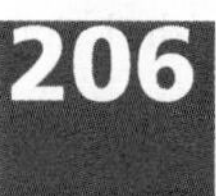

206 LIVER AND BILIARY TRACT TUMORS

Lewis R. Roberts

Liver and biliary tract tumors are a diverse group of benign and malignant tumors that arise from the different epithelial and stromal tissues of the liver. Various malignant diseases of other tissues metastasize to the liver or extend into or metastasize to the vicinity of the biliary tract, but not all mass lesions of the liver and biliary tract are malignant (Table 206–1).

EVALUATION OF MASS LESIONS OF THE LIVER

Diagnostic Approach

Mass lesions of the liver can be classified as benign lesions usually requiring observation only, benign lesions requiring further evaluation and treatment, or malignant lesions requiring appropriate management (see Table 206–1). The clinical approach to liver mass lesions requires careful consideration of the presenting symptoms, physical examination, appropriate laboratory studies, imaging characteristics of the lesion by different imaging modalities, judicious use of liver biopsy for histologic confirmation, and optimal management that considers the patient's age and comorbidities (Fig. 206–1).

History and Physical Examination

Because of the increasing use of imaging techniques for the evaluation of abdominal symptoms, many mass lesions of the liver are discovered incidentally as a result of imaging performed to evaluate nonhepatic diseases, such as abdominal pain or discomfort (Chapter 134). Right upper quadrant discomfort is frequently nonspecific and unhelpful in the evaluation of liver masses. Nevertheless, large liver masses may distend the liver capsule and cause pain, which is occasionally referred to the right shoulder. Patients also may present with episodes of acute, severe pain, which results from bleeding into a hepatic adenoma, a primary hepatocellular carcinoma, or the liver surrounding the lesion. Patients with advanced malignant disease and regional lymph metastases may present with epigastric pain.

Patients with malignant liver disease, whether primary or metastatic, frequently present with constitutional symptoms, which include night sweats, low-grade fever, unintended weight loss (Chapter 134), anorexia, and diarrhea (Chapter 143). In the United States, the most common malignant lesions in the liver are metastases from other primary cancers, including the esophagus (Chapter 140), and stomach (Chapter 202), colon (Chapter 203), pancreas (Chapter 204), breast (Chapter 208), lung (Chapter 201), neuroendocrine tumors (Chapter 205), kidney and bladder (Chapter 207), and melanoma (Chapter 214). Patients with hepatocellular carcinoma often have symptoms related to their underlying liver disease, such as fatigue from chronic hepatitis (Chapter 152) or ascites, spontaneous bacterial peritonitis, variceal bleeding, or hepatic encephalopathy resulting from cirrhosis (Chapter 157) with portal hypertension. Patients with cholangiocarcinoma may present with jaundice from a dominant stricture or with episodes of acute cholangitis in the setting of primary or secondary sclerosing cholangitis (Chapter 159).

When available, previous imaging studies of the liver can be helpful in determining whether a liver lesion is new or enlarging. The patient's characteristics, including age, sex, history of oral contraceptive use (associated with an increased incidence of hepatic adenomas), geographic residence, travel history (relevant in cases of amebic liver abscess and hydatid cysts), and comorbid illnesses (e.g., ulcerative colitis and/or primary sclerosing cholangitis in patients with cholangiocarcinoma) can also provide clues to the diagnosis.

On physical examination, patients with chronic liver disease typically have cutaneous stigmata (spider angiomas and palmar erythema), splenomegaly, and bilobar enlargement of the liver or caudate lobe hypertrophy. They may also have an abdominal bruit over a vascular hepatocellular carcinoma. Patients with metastatic disease may have peripheral or intra-abdominal lymphadenopathy or palpable peritoneal carcinomatosis. Jaundice, peripheral edema, and ascites are nonspecific features that may be related to benign or malignant liver disease.

Laboratory Findings

Laboratory studies are often useful in determining the nature of a liver mass or its underlying cause. Laboratory features of chronic liver disease include the following: thrombocytopenia; elevated levels of serum aminotransferase (elevated in active inflammatory liver disease or infiltrative neoplastic diseases), alkaline phosphatase, and bilirubin (elevated in bile duct obstruction from biliary tumor or mass effect; Chapter 150); low serum albumin levels and an elevated prothrombin time (abnormal in chronic liver disease). Viral markers (e.g., hepatitis B surface antigen and antibody, hepatitis B e antigen and antibody, and hepatitis C antibody), iron studies, and autoimmune markers (e.g., antimitochondrial antibody, antinuclear antibody, and anti–smooth muscle antibody) often help to determine the cause of chronic liver disease (Chapter 149). Finally, tumor markers (Chapter 190) such as α-fetoprotein (AFP; hepatocellular carcinoma), CA 19-9 (cholangiocarcinoma), carcinoembryonic antigen (colorectal metastases or cholangiocarcinoma), and lactate dehydrogenase (lymphoma) have variable sensitivity and utility as screening tests but may be useful in confirming the diagnosis or in predicting prognosis.

TABLE 206–1 LIVER AND BILIARY TRACT TUMORS

Tumor	Characteristics on Imaging
BENIGN TUMORS USUALLY REQUIRING OBSERVATION ONLY	
Cavernous hemangioma	Peripheral enhancement filling into the center on delayed contrast imaging
Focal nodular hyperplasia	Rapid arterial enhancement with return to isointensity in venous phase; possible central scar with feeding vessel
Simple cyst	Hypoechoic on ultrasound
Focal fatty change	Best characterized by in and out of phase sequences on magnetic resonance imaging
Angiolipoma	Arterial enhancement on contrast imaging
BENIGN TUMORS REQUIRING FURTHER EVALUATION AND TREATMENT	
Hepatic adenoma	Heterogeneous lesion with rapid arterial enhancement
Nodular regenerative hyperplasia	Nonspecific and variable
Cystadenoma	Cystic lesion on ultrasonography with solid components, enhancement of cyst wall; possible septations
Hepatic abscess (Chapter 156)	Cystic lesion on ultrasonography
Inflammatory pseudotumor (Chapter 156)	Atypical enhancing mass on contrast imaging
Echinococcal cyst (Chapter 406)	Cystic mass with septations, calcified rims, daughter cysts
MALIGNANT TUMORS REQUIRING APPROPRIATE MANAGEMENT	
Hepatocellular carcinoma	Arterial enhancement with portal venous "washout"
Cholangiocarcinoma	Late arterial enhancement which persists in portal phase
Mixed hepatocellular-cholangiocarcinoma	Early to late arterial enhancement
Liver metastases	Peripheral arterial enhancement, usually bilobar, multifocal disease
Cystadenocarcinoma	Solid enhancing mass in cystic lesion
Sarcoma	Solid mass with arterial enhancement
Mixed hepatic tumor	Solid mass with arterial enhancement; possible areas of calcification
Non-Hodgkin's lymphoma (Chapter 196)	Less intense arterial enhancement than hepatocellular carcinoma; possibly diffuse or mimicking hepatocellular carcinoma with venous invasion

COMMON BENIGN TUMORS OF THE LIVER

Cavernous Hemangioma

Epidemiology

Cavernous hemangioma, which is the most common benign tumor of the liver, is present in up to 7% of individuals in autopsy studies. There is a female predominance of 1.5 to 5:1, and hemangiomas are more common in multiparous women. Hemangiomas are multicentric in up to 30% of cases.

Clinical Manifestations

Cavernous hemangiomas are usually asymptomatic, although large, subcapsular hemangiomas may cause abdominal pain or discomfort. Thrombosis of giant hemangiomas (>10 cm) may cause systemic features of inflammation such as fever, weight loss, and anemia.

Rarely, large hemangiomas are associated with the Kasabach-Merritt syndrome (Chapter 181), which is local or disseminated intravascular coagulation with hypofibrinogenemia and thrombocytopenia, usually in infants. Malignant transformation of cavernous hemangiomas does not occur. Rupture of cavernous hemangiomas is exceedingly rare, considering the high prevalence of hepatic hemangiomas; approximately 30 reported cases of rupture typically involve hemangiomas that are larger than 10 cm in diameter.

Diagnosis

Imaging

Hepatic cavernous hemangiomas have characteristic imaging features. On *ultrasound,* they appear as well-circumscribed, homogeneously hyperechoic lesions with smooth margins. Hemangiomas may also appear hypoechoic in fatty livers. Atypical features include hypoechoic lesions with a thin hyperechoic rim or a thick rind and scalloped borders.

On *dynamic contrast-enhanced multiphasic computed tomography (CT),* hemangiomas are hypoattenuating lesions on nonenhanced scans, with peripheral nodular enhancement during the arterial phase and later filling in toward the center of the lesion. On *contrast magnetic resonance imaging (MRI) with gadolinium,* hemangiomas appear as homogeneous, low-intensity lesions on T1-weighted images and as sharply demarcated, hyperintense lesions on T2-weighted images. In the arterial phase, peripheral enhancement occurs and fills in toward the center of the lesion on delayed images.

Technetium-99m–labeled red blood cell scintigraphy is very specific for hemangiomas. It shows low perfusion on early images and a high concentration of isotope that completely fills the lesion on late images. Larger hemangiomas that are complicated by fibrosis, thrombosis, or bleeding may have incomplete filling in on contrast or technetium-99m studies.

Because the imaging features are often characteristic, biopsy is seldom needed to confirm the diagnosis. Biopsy is occasionally useful for small indeterminate lesions and for large lesions with scarring and atypical imaging features. Histologic examination shows a network of vascular spaces lined by endothelial cells and separated by a thin, fibrous stroma. Large hemangiomas may have areas of thrombosis, scarring, and calcification.

Treatment

Observation is the optimal management for most patients with asymptomatic hemangiomas. Surgical enucleation or anatomic resection is recommended for hemangiomas that cause significant pain, enlarge over time, are of uncertain diagnosis, or are associated with the Kasabach-Merritt syndrome. Rarely, liver transplantation has been used for massive unresectable hepatic hemangiomas, particularly in the presence of Kasabach-Merritt syndrome.

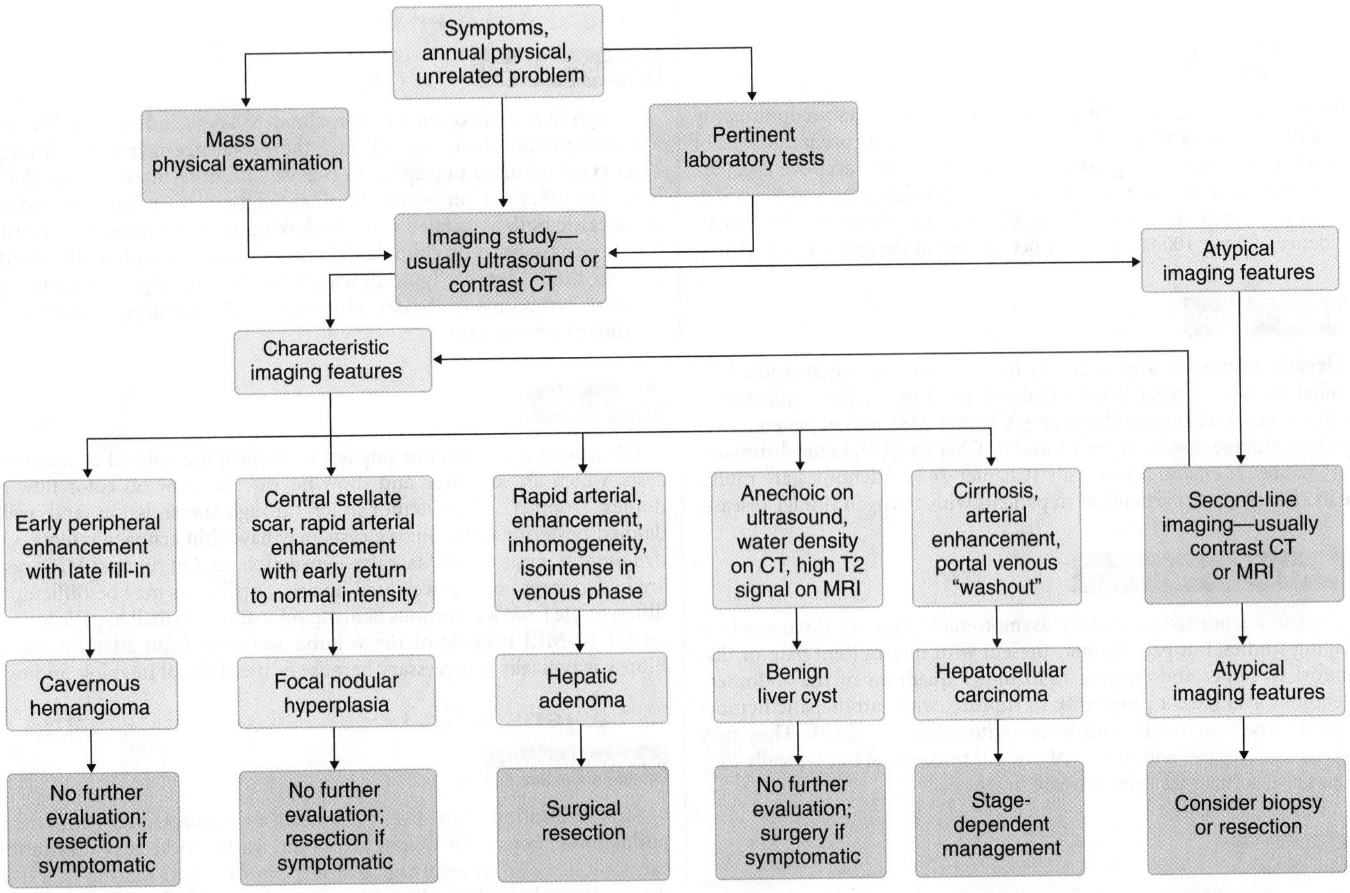

Symptoms, annual physical, unrelated problem

Mass on physical examination

Pertinent laboratory tests

Imaging study—usually ultrasound or contrast CT

Atypical imaging features

Characteristic imaging features

Early peripheral enhancement with late fill-in → Cavernous hemangioma → No further evaluation; resection if symptomatic

Central stellate scar, rapid arterial enhancement with early return to normal intensity → Focal nodular hyperplasia → No further evaluation; resection if symptomatic

Rapid arterial, enhancement, inhomogeneity, isointense in venous phase → Hepatic adenoma → Surgical resection

Anechoic on ultrasound, water density on CT, high T2 signal on MRI → Benign liver cyst → No further evaluation; surgery if symptomatic

Cirrhosis, arterial enhancement, portal venous "washout" → Hepatocellular carcinoma → Stage-dependent management

Second-line imaging—usually contrast CT or MRI → Atypical imaging features → Consider biopsy or resection

FIGURE 206–1 • Approach to evaluating the patient with a mass lesion in the liver. Flow chart showing an algorithm for evaluating and managing common liver mass lesions. CT = computed tomography; MRI = magnetic resonance imaging.

Focal Nodular Hyperplasia

Definition

Focal nodular hyperplasia is a benign reaction to a congenital arterial malformation within the liver. The lesion typically consists of a vascular stellate scar with connective tissue, bile ductules surrounded by proliferated hepatocytes, and Kupffer cells separated by fibrous septa.

Epidemiology

Focal nodular hyperplasia occurs predominantly in women of childbearing age. The relationship with oral contraceptive use is controversial; some studies suggest an association of long-term oral contraceptive use with focal nodular hyperplasia and with complications such as hemorrhage or infarction. However, discontinuation of oral contraceptive use usually does not lead to resolution of focal nodular hyperplasia. There is a female predominance of 2 to 4:1, and the lesions are typically diagnosed in women aged 20 to 50 years. Focal nodular hyperplasias are frequently multiple (10 to 20%) or are associated with cavernous hemangiomas (20%).

Clinical Manifestations

Most focal nodular hyperplasias are asymptomatic. Patients with large or subcapsular lesions may present with abdominal discomfort or an abdominal mass.

Diagnosis

On *ultrasound,* focal nodular hyperplasias are variably hypoechoic, hyperechoic, or isoechoic. The lesions are most commonly hypoechoic except for the central scar. Doppler evaluation frequently shows blood flow within the central stellate scar.

On *dynamic CT,* focal nodular hyperplasias are isoattenuating or slightly hypoattenuating on noncontrast CT. One sees rapid, intense contrast enhancement in the arterial phase and rapid loss of contrast from the lesion, so it becomes isointense in the venous phase. An avascular central scar is often seen, sometimes with a feeding artery coursing into the middle of the lesion.

On *contrast MRI,* the lesions are isointense on T1-weighted images and remain isointense or are slightly hyperintense on T2-weighted images. The central scar is hypointense on T1-weighted images but hyperintense on T2-weighted images. As with contrast CT, rapid, intense contrast enhancement in the arterial phase quickly dissipates. Typically, the central scar has a low signal on T1-weighted images and enhances with contrast.

Technetium-99m–sulfur colloid scintigraphy is occasionally used to characterize focal nodular hyperplasias. Hyperintense or isointense uptake occurs in 50 to 70% of focal nodular hyperplasias because of uptake by Kupffer cells. In contrast, most hepatic adenomas do not have Kupffer cells and so do not take up technetium-99m–sulfur colloid. *Kupffer cell–specific MRI agents* such as ferumoxide are taken up by Kupffer cells and lead to significant signal intensity loss on ferumoxide-enhanced T2-weighted images, which may help to distinguish focal nodular hyperplasia from hepatic adenoma and hepatocellular carcinoma.

When *biopsy* is needed to establish the diagnosis, it is often difficult to distinguish focal nodular hyperplasias from hepatic adenomas, because fine-needle aspirates from both lesions may only show benign-appearing hepatocytes. Histopathologic examination shows a benign hepatic parenchyma with bile ductules in septal fibrosis.

Treatment

The management of asymptomatic focal nodular hyperplasias with characteristic imaging or biopsy features is observation. Patients do not need to discontinue oral contraceptive use, because no convincing evidence indicates that discontinuation leads to reduction in size of the lesions. Surgical resection is recommended for indeterminate or symptomatic lesions.

Hepatic Adenoma

Epidemiology

Hepatic adenoma is a benign liver tumor that occurs predominantly in the third and fourth decade of life. There is a female predominance of 2 to 6:1 as well as a strong association with oral contraceptive use. The relative risk of developing a hepatic adenoma is 2.5 after 3 to 5 years of oral contraceptive use and 25 to 40 after 9 years of use, resulting in an incidence of 4 per 100,000 versus 1 per million in the general population.

Pathobiology

Hepatic adenomas also occur in users of androgenic steroids, in a familial pattern associated with diabetes mellitus, in the syndrome of maturity-onset diabetes of the young (Chapter 248), and in patients with glycogen storage disease types 1A and 3 (Chapter 219), hemochromatosis (Chapter 231), and acromegaly (Chapter 242). Adenomas are multiple in 20% of cases, particularly in patients with glycogen storage disease.

Clinical Manifestations

Hepatic adenomas are usually asymptomatic and are discovered on imaging studies, but patients may present with intermittent pain or discomfort in upper abdomen or right upper quadrant of the abdomen. Adenomas also have a propensity to rupture, with intrahepatic hemorrhage and pain or rarely with hemoperitoneum and shock. They may decrease in size after withdrawal of oral contraceptives, but typically they do not and sometimes even increase in size.

Diagnosis

On *ultrasound,* hepatic adenomas are variably homogeneous or heterogeneous (because of hemorrhage or necrosis within the tumor). On *dynamic CT,* adenomas, like focal nodular hyperplasias, are isoattenuating on nonenhanced scans; with intravenous contrast, they show early enhancement and then become rapidly isoattenuating in the portal venous phase. Adenomas are often hyperattenuating in a fatty liver. Adenomas typically have well-defined borders and are not lobulated. Approximately 40% of adenomas have intralesional hemorrhage with heterogenous regions of high attenuation. Approximately 5% of adenomas show coarse calcifications within the lesion.

On *contrast MRI,* adenomas are hyperintense or isointense on T1-weighted images and are slightly hyperintense on T2-weighted images. They show early enhancement in the arterial phase and become isointense on delayed imaging.

Technetium-99m–sulfur colloid scintigraphy shows no uptake in 70% of adenomas because of the absence of Kupffer cells. Overall, the relatively nonspecific imaging features make adenomas difficult to differentiate from other lesions.

Biopsy is often required for diagnosis, but a significant risk of misdiagnosis exists in differentiating hepatic adenomas from focal nodular hyperplasias, as well as a potential risk of hemorrhage from core biopsies. Histologic examination shows sheets of well-differentiated hepatocytes without bile ductules, fibrous septa, portal tracts, or central veins. Most adenomas do not contain Kupffer cells.

Treatment and Prognosis

Rx

Management of hepatic adenoma is usually by surgical resection because of the risks of hemorrhage (≤30% for large adenomas) and malignant transformation (the exact risk is unknown). Radiofrequency ablation is used in patients who are high surgical risks. Oral contraceptives should be discontinued, and patients should avoid pregnancy until the adenoma is resected, because these lesions often grow during pregnancy. The risk of malignant transformation is small but real.

Benign Liver Cysts

Epidemiology

Benign liver cysts occur in approximately 4% of individuals. There is a female predominance of 4:1, and the prevalence increases with age. Liver cysts are often multiple and coexist with other mass lesions in the liver. The inherited autosomal dominant and recessive polycystic kidney diseases are both associated with the development of multiple liver cysts. Liver cysts are lined by cuboidal bile duct epithelium and are filled with isotonic fluid. Cysts are typically asymptomatic, but large cysts can cause pressure symptoms or biliary obstruction. Hemorrhage, infection, or rupture of cysts is rare.

Diagnosis

Ultrasound is the best imaging test to confirm the fluid-filled nature of cysts, which are anechoic and show no vascular flow on color flow or duplex Doppler. They demonstrate through-transmission and well-defined posterior walls. Simple cysts may have thin echogenic septa. On *dynamic CT,* cysts appear as water-density lesions. On *contrast MRI,* cysts are hyperintense on T2-weighted images. Small cysts may be difficult to differentiate from a cavernous hemangioma or other small hepatic lesions on CT or MRI because of the volume averaging from adjacent tissue. Biopsy is typically unnecessary because of the classical imaging findings.

Lesions with Focal Fat or Fat Sparing

Pathobiology

Fatty infiltration of the liver (Chapter 156) is increasingly common as populations increase in weight across the world. Focal fatty infiltration can look like a mass on imaging studies, as can focal sparing in a liver that is diffusely infiltrated by fat. Associations with fatty change in the liver include obesity (Chapter 239), diabetes mellitus (Chapter 248), high alcohol consumption (Chapter 31), and altered nutritional status as a result of chemotherapy.

Clinical Manifestations

Patients with focal fatty infiltration are typically asymptomatic. The lesions are usually discovered incidentally and are sometimes mistaken for more sinister masses.

Diagnosis

The characteristic imaging feature of focal fat is that it does not distort the contour of the liver, so normal vessels, especially veins, can be seen coursing through the lesion. Focal fat usually occurs in vascular watersheds such as the region around the falciform ligament. Fat sparing usually occurs adjacent to the gallbladder fossa, in subcapsular areas, and in the posterior aspect of segment IV. On ultrasound, fat is usually hyperechoic. On dynamic CT, fatty liver is hypodense compared with the spleen, but not as low in density as adipose tissue. Venous structures can be seen in the lesion on venous phase studies. On contrast MRI, fatty liver is occasionally hyperintense on T1-weighted and T2-weighted images. The decreased signal intensity on out-of-phase gradient imaging is diagnostic of focal fat.

Biopsy is occasionally useful to rule out other lesions. On histologic examination, areas of fatty infiltration show fat-laden cells.

PRIMARY MALIGNANT TUMORS OF THE LIVER AND BILIARY TRACT

Hepatocellular Carcinoma

Epidemiology

Hepatocellular carcinoma, the third most common cause of death from cancer worldwide, accounts for approximately 600,000 deaths annually. There is a male preponderance of 2 to 4:1. The major predisposing factor for the development of hepatocellular carcinoma is cirrhosis of the liver (Chapter 157). The risk factors for the development of hepatocellular carcinoma include chronic hepatitis B or C virus infection (Chapter 152), alcoholic cirrhosis, hereditary hemochromatosis (Chapter 231), α_1-antitrypsin deficiency (Chapter 149), primary biliary cirrhosis (Chapter 159), and autoimmune hepatitis (Chapter 152). The hepatitis B virus almost always integrates into the host genomic DNA and can lead to development of hepatocellular carcinoma in the absence of cirrhosis. The availability of an effective vaccine against hepatitis B has reduced the incidence of hepatitis B–related hepatocellular carcinomas in high-prevalence regions. Long-term exposure to fungal aflatoxins in the diet significantly increases the risk of hepatocellular carcinoma. The aflatoxin-producing fungal species, *Aspergillus flavus* and *Aspergillus parasiticus*, produce at least 13 different types of aflatoxin, with aflatoxin B1 the most potent. The fungi are ubiquitous and invade and grow in grains, legumes, and peanuts when they are stored in conditions of high humidity and temperature. During metabolism of aflatoxin in the liver, an aflatoxin B1-8,9-exo-epoxide intermediate is formed, and it interacts with cellular DNA to mediate formation of specific mutations, most frequently leading to a G-to-T transversion in codon 249 of the p53 tumor suppressor gene. This mutation leads to loss of the p53 tumor suppressor function and an increased tendency to carcinogenesis. Aflatoxin B1 has a synergistic effect with the hepatitis B virus in the development of hepatocellular carcinoma.

In most parts of the world, the most rapidly increasing groups of patients with hepatocellular carcinoma are those with chronic hepatitis C virus infection. More than 90% of individuals with hepatitis C virus infection develop chronic infection, and up to 20% of patients with chronic hepatitis C will develop cirrhosis (Chapter 152). Hepatocellular carcinoma then develops in up to 20% of individuals with cirrhosis from chronic hepatitis C virus, at a rate of 2 to 6% per year. More recently, there has been a progressive increase in obesity-related nonalcoholic fatty liver disease (Chapter 156), which can progress to steatohepatitis, cirrhosis (often previously considered to be of unknown origin or "cryptogenic"), and hepatocellular carcinoma. Diabetes, also obesity-related, has recently been shown to be an independent risk factor for the development of hepatocellular carcinoma.

Pathobiology

Like most other malignant diseases, hepatocellular carcinoma develops as a result of a combination of the activation of cellular oncogenic pathways and abrogation of tumor suppressor pathways. Chronic hepatic injury resulting from viruses, alcohol, and metabolic or autoimmune mechanisms leads to repeated cycles of liver cell death, regeneration, and repair that ultimately lead to premature senescence of the liver.

Cellular senescence is characterized by a progressive decrease in length of the telomeric regions that protect the ends of chromosomes, with resulting development of chromosomal and genetic instabilities that are recognized by cellular stress response pathways and that trigger the apoptosis of senescent cells in a process known as *telomeric crisis*. In some senescent cells, apoptosis is avoided, and the cells become immortal, either through activation of the cellular telomerase enzyme complex, which maintains telomere ends, or through non–telomerase-dependent mechanisms. These genetically unstable, immortal cells are then prone to the development of additional genetic and epigenetic alterations that result in the cancer phenotype of unconstrained cell proliferation, resistance to apoptosis, enhanced cell migration and invasion, and activation of new vessel formation (angiogenesis). Many oncogenic pathways normally have intrinsic tumor suppressor activities that limit their growth-promoting pro-carcinogenic effects; during carcinogenesis, mutations or epigenetic alterations lead to loss of the intrinsic tumor suppressing activity of the oncogenic pathways and result in unconstrained cellular proliferation and the secondary development of the other characteristics of the tumor phenotype. This hypothesis is well illustrated by the phenomenon of aflatoxin-induced mutation of the p53 tumor suppressor, which leads to loss of p53-induced apoptosis. Consequently, oncogenic pathways that normally activate p53 and limit proliferation are left without their natural "brake" on proliferation.

Another important concept in the pathogenesis of malignant liver diseases is that of the development of malignant diseases within the epithelial stem cell compartment. Progenitor oval cells from the canals of Hering in the liver are capable of differentiating into both the hepatic and biliary lineages during liver regeneration. The development of a neoplastic phenotype within this compartment can result in the formation of cells that subsequently mature partially into more differentiated tumor cells and lead to the formation of a cancer with a "parent" clone of more immature progenitor cells and "daughter" clones of more mature cells. The existence of a tumor stem cell compartment has important implications for the development of anticancer therapy, because agents that are active against carcinogenic pathways in the daughter cells but not in the parent clones may be capable of suppressing or arresting tumor growth but will not be curative unless they also target the growth pathways within the tumor stem cell compartment.

Integration of hepatitis B virus into host hepatocyte genomic DNA can lead to the development of hepatocellular carcinoma in the absence of cirrhosis. The pathogenic mechanisms include activation of oncogenic pathways through the activity of hepatitis B virus enhancer sequences and mutational inactivation of tumor suppressor genes by insertional mutagenesis. Certain proteins encoded by the hepatitis viruses have been shown to have oncogenic effects; these include the hepatitis B virus X protein, a truncated carboxy terminal variant of the hepatitis B virus S protein, and the hepatitis C virus core protein.

Specific tumor suppressor and oncogenic molecules and pathways that have been shown to be important in liver carcinogenesis include the p53/p21^{WAF1} pathway, the p16^{INK4a}/CDK4/RB1/E2F pathway, the Wnt/β catenin signaling pathway, transforming growth factor-α, c-myc, the transcription factor NFκB, insulin/insulin-like growth factor-I, and the receptor tyrosine kinases (fibroblast growth factor, hepatocyte growth factor, and vascular endothelial growth factor) and their downstream activators.

Clinical Manifestations

Hepatocellular carcinoma is commonly diagnosed by a surveillance ultrasound, which is recommended every 6 months in patients with cirrhosis of any cause. A serum AFP level greater than 200 ng/mL has a 95 to 100% specificity for hepatocellular carcinoma. However, with recent improvements in imaging technologies and the recognition that the percentage of small hepatocellular carcinomas that are associated with high AFP levels is only 20 to 30%, the AFP level is now generally believed not to be a cost-effective modality for early detection of hepatocellular carcinoma. Most tumors that are discovered by screening are asymptomatic.

Symptoms, when they occur, are typically nonspecific, including anorexia, weight loss, fatigue, low-grade fever, right upper quadrant or epigastric abdominal pain, abdominal fullness, and mild decompensation of cirrhosis. Compression or invasion of the biliary tree can lead to jaundice. The sudden onset of severe abdominal pain may result from hemorrhage within the tumor mass. Rarely, hepatocellular carcinomas can rupture, causing a hemoperitoneum. Signs on physical examination may include a palpable liver mass and a vascular bruit over the tumor. Hepatocellular carcinomas also cause a variety of paraneoplastic syndromes, including hypoglycemia mediated by insulin-like growth factors, erythrocytosis from erythropoietin generation by the tumor, hypercalcemia related to production of a parathyroid-like hormone, and watery diarrhea from tumor production of vasoactive intestinal peptide and other neuroendocrine hormones (Chapters 188 and 189).

Diagnosis

Approximately 80 to 90% of hepatocellular carcinomas occur in a cirrhotic liver, so the early diagnosis of most hepatocellular carcinomas depends on rigorous efforts of intermittent long-term surveillance for cancer in patients with cirrhosis. Surveillance is usually performed using liver ultrasound every 6 months, and any suspicious nodules are then examined with additional contrast imaging studies.

Whether evaluated because of a screening ultrasound scan or as a result of symptoms or signs, small hepatocellular carcinomas are usually hyperechoic, whereas large hepatocellular carcinomas are frequently hypoechoic. Like normal benign liver tissue, cirrhotic nodules and dysplastic nodules receive the major proportion of their blood supply from portal vein radicals. With their transformation into hepatocellular carcinomas, there is a change in the vascularization of malignant hepatocytes, which secrete angiogenic factors, leading to the acquisition of a primarily arterial blood supply.

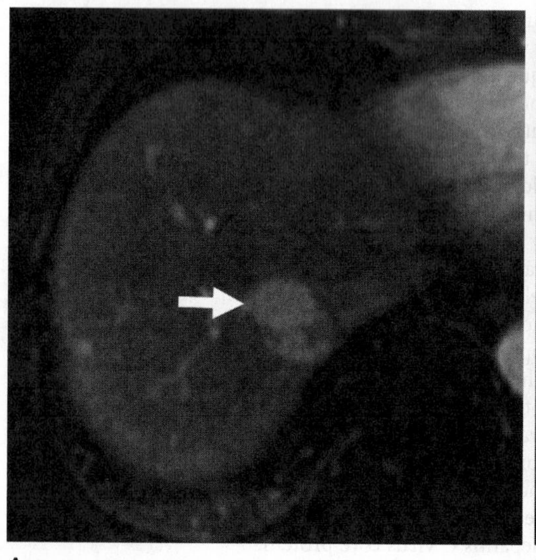

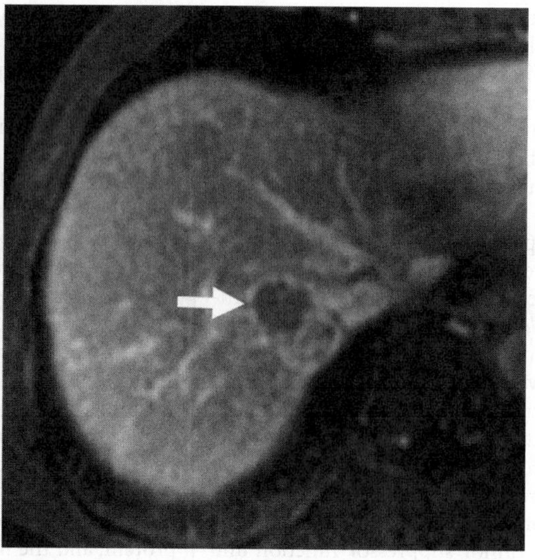

FIGURE 206–2 • Hepatocellular carcinoma. A T1-weighted magnetic resonance imaging scan is shown during the **(A)** arterial and **(B)** portal phases after the administration of intravenous gadolinium contrast. The tumor (white arrow) shows contrast enhancement in the arterial phase and washout in the portal phase.

On contrast imaging studies, including contrast CT, MRI, ultrasound, and angiography, hepatocellular carcinomas are characterized by bright enhancement in the arterial phase, followed by a loss of enhancement as contrast washes out of the arterial circulation, and a characteristic decreased intensity below that of the surrounding liver during the portal phase, when the surrounding liver is perfused by contrast to a higher intensity than that of the tumor nodule. This feature, referred to as *washout,* is highly specific for hepatocellular carcinomas occurring in a cirrhotic liver (Fig. 206–2). In patients with cirrhosis, almost all hepatocellular carcinomas 2 cm or larger can be confidently diagnosed using noninvasive imaging criteria. Hepatocellular carcinomas have a propensity for vascular invasion and frequently invade the hepatic or the portal venous systems.

The diagnosis of small equivocal lesions in a cirrhotic liver can be established by needle biopsy of the lesion. However, because of the small but real risks of tumor seeding (0.5 to 2%), hemorrhage, and false-negative results from biopsy, many centers avoid biopsy in patients who may be candidates for liver transplantation and instead rely on imaging characteristics for the diagnosis of hepatocellular carcinoma.

Prevention

Universal vaccination against hepatitis B has been shown to reduce the incidence of hepatocellular carcinoma. [1] No vaccine is available against the hepatitis C virus. Individuals who have durable responses to treatment for hepatitis C appear to have a reduced risk of developing hepatocellular carcinoma.

Treatment

Rx

Patients who have early-stage hepatocellular carcinoma and who do not have significant underlying liver dysfunction can be treated by surgical resection. Liver transplantation (Chapter 158) of patients who meet the Milan criteria (one tumor mass lesion ≤5 cm or two to three lesions each ≤3 cm, with no evidence of extrahepatic spread) provides long-term survival results no different from those of patients receiving liver transplants for nonmalignant indications. In patients who are not candidates for liver transplantation, local ablation of small tumors up to 3 to 4 cm is performed with percutaneous ethanol injection or radiofrequency ablation, which uses probes with small tines that can be deployed through the tumor and energized with high-frequency electrical current to produce coagulation of the tumor and a surrounding rim of benign tissue. Although surgical resection and the local ablative therapies are effective treatments of small hepatocellular carcinomas, patients with cirrhosis still have a residual molecular defect in the remaining liver that makes them susceptible to recurrent tumor, at a rate of approximately 50% by 3 years after surgical resection or local ablation.

Patients with tumors that do not meet the criteria for surgical resection, liver transplantation, or local ablation, but that are still limited to the liver are considered to have intermediate-stage disease. Intermediate-stage disease is currently treated using transarterial chemoembolization with chemotherapeutic agents, such as doxorubicin, mitomycin C, and/or cisplatin, as well as polyvinyl alcohol (Ivalon) or absorbable gelatin (Gelfoam) particles, sometimes combined with iodized poppyseed oil (Lipiodol or Ethiodol). Randomized trials and meta-analyses have confirmed that transarterial chemoembolization improves survival of patients with intermediate stage hepatocellular carcinoma. [2] Radioembolization with yttrium-90–impregnated glass microspheres, which is an alternative to transarterial chemoembolization, can be used for patients with portal vein thrombosis because, unlike the Ivalon or Gelfoam particles used for chemoembolization, the 20- to 30-μg glass microspheres used for radioembolization do not occlude the hepatic arterial vascular bed. However, radioembolization has not as yet been subjected to rigorous randomized trials.

No reliably effective regimens are available for patients with advanced hepatocellular carcinoma. Treatment using systemic chemotherapy is complicated by the presence of underlying chronic liver disease and a significantly increased risk of drug toxicity. Current efforts are focused on the use of targeted therapies directed against molecular pathways known to be involved in hepatocarcinogenesis, including receptor tyrosine kinases and the Wnt signaling pathway.

Prognosis

Patients with early disease who undergo liver transplantation have an excellent outcome with a 5-year survival of 70 to 80% and 5-year recurrence rate of 10% or less. Patients who are ineligible for liver transplantation who undergo surgical resection or local treatment by radiofrequency ablation or percutaneous ethanol injection also have relatively high 5-year survival rates of 50 to 70%; however, because they still have a cirrhotic liver with a predisposition to cancer, these patients have a 3-year recurrence rate of approximately 50%. Patients with intermediate-stage disease who are treated with transarterial chemoembolization have a 1-year survival of 50 to 80% and a 2-year survival of 25 to 60%. Appropriate selection of individuals with preserved liver function is important for achieving the best outcomes with transarterial chemoembolization, because it can decrease survival by inducing liver decompensation. Patients with advanced-stage disease who are currently candidates for treatment trials or symptomatic treatment have a median survival of only 6 to 8 months and a 1-year survival of 10 to 30%.

Cholangiocarcinoma

Epidemiology

Although the overall incidence of biliary cancers, or cholangiocarcinomas, is relatively low, these tumors are associated with perhaps the most rapidly rising incidence of any cancer in Western industrial nations. The reason for this trend is unknown. Most cholangiocarcinomas occur incidentally, but the known risk factors for cholangiocarcinoma include primary sclerosing cholangitis (Chapter 159), which is often associated with inflammatory bowel disease (Chapter 144), congenital choledochal cysts or other biliary tract abnormalities, Asian cholangiopathies secondary to liver fluke infections, and secondary chronic bacterial cholangitis, which frequently occurs in individuals who have had intrahepatic biliary stones or a prior biliary-enteric anastomosis.

Pathobiology

The pathogenesis of cholangiocarcinoma is not well understood. Current concepts suggest that biliary inflammation results in impairment of DNA repair mechanisms, with the subsequent development of genomic instability and cancer. Genes in pathways shown to be involved in biliary carcinogenesis include *p53, K-ras, c-met, c-erbB2, mcl-1, Bcl-xl,* $p16^{INK4a}$, $p14^{ARF}$, *iNOS,* and *IL-6.*

Clinical Manifestations

Patients with cholangiocarcinomas typically present with painless jaundice resulting from the presence of hilar or distal biliary strictures or with an intrahepatic mass causing abdominal pain, which may be referred to the shoulder. These patients often have associated pruritus, pale stools, and dark urine. Nonspecific symptoms such as weight loss and low-grade fever may also occur.

Diagnosis

Cholangiocarcinomas are classified as intrahepatic or extrahepatic based on the location of the tumor within the biliary tree. The use of MRI with magnetic resonance cholangiography provides a noninvasive means of imaging the obstructed biliary tract before endoscopic retrograde cholangiopancreatography and allows the endoscopist and surgeon to plan an optimal approach for evaluation and therapy. Patients with unilateral biliary obstruction often have atrophy of the involved lobe and compensatory hypertrophy of the other liver lobe, referred to as the *atrophy-hypertrophy complex* (Fig. 206–3). Because of the presence of a dense fibrous stroma around a relatively sparse number of malignant glandular epithelial elements in many cholangiocarcinomas, cytologic examination from brushings of malignant strictures has a relatively low sensitivity, particularly in early cancers most amenable to successful therapy. However, the examination of biliary brush cytology specimens using advanced cytologic techniques such as DNA flow cytometry, digital image analysis, and fluorescence in situ hybridization with DNA probes for the detection of chromosomal polysomy has improved diagnostic accuracy (Fig. 206–4). These techniques can be applied in patients with primary sclerosing cholangitis who present with a new dominant stricture or clinical deterioration to improve the early detection of malignant transformation. Advanced endoscopic methods such as endoscopic ultrasound, intraductal ultrasound, and choledochoenteroscopy also improve visualization and characterization of biliary strictures and associated metastatic lymphadenopathy.

Treatment

Rx

The outcome after development of cholangiocarcinoma is generally poor because the tumor is relatively resistant to chemotherapy and also frequently results in biliary obstruction, which is complicated by episodes of bacterial cholangitis and cholestatic liver dysfunction. The treatment of biliary cancers depends on the extent of involvement of the biliary tree and on the presence of extrahepatic disease.

For disease limited to the liver and biliary tree, with malignant strictures that do not extend beyond the secondary branching of the right or left intrahepatic bile ducts, treatment by surgical resection results in a 5-year survival of approximately 20% after successful resection. Patients with distal biliary cancers without distant spread are usually treated by bile duct resection or by Whipple's pancreaticoduodenectomy.

Patients with unresectable disease are generally treated by palliative biliary stenting using plastic or metal stents. Effective stenting of approximately 25% of the total liver volume using the less affected lobe of the liver is usually sufficient to relieve cholestasis and is significantly less likely to result in repeated episodes of cholangitis.

Adjuvant chemotherapy and radiation, with staging laparotomy followed by liver transplantation for selected patients with early hilar cholangiocarcinomas, have resulted in a remarkable 5-year sur-

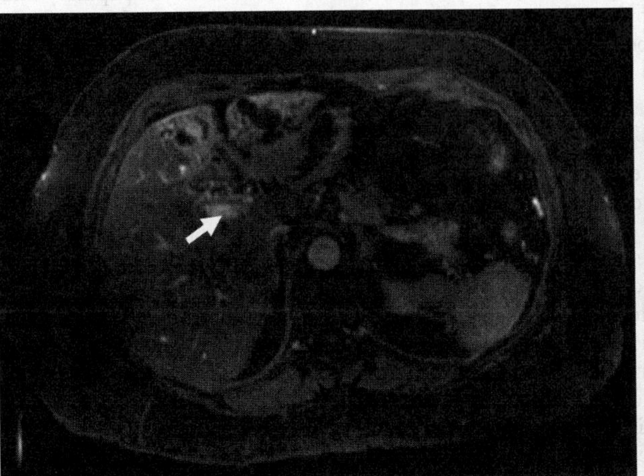
A

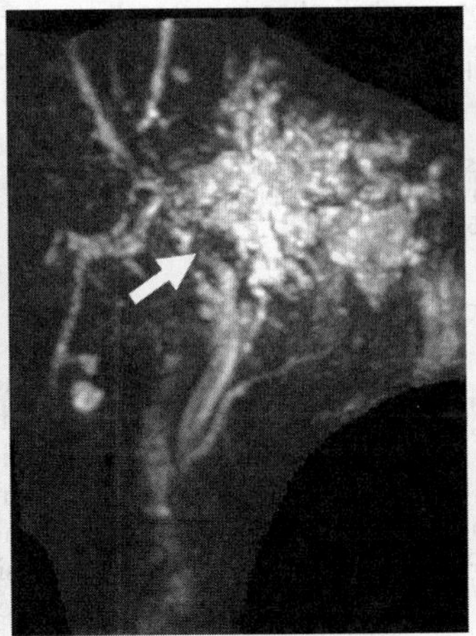
B

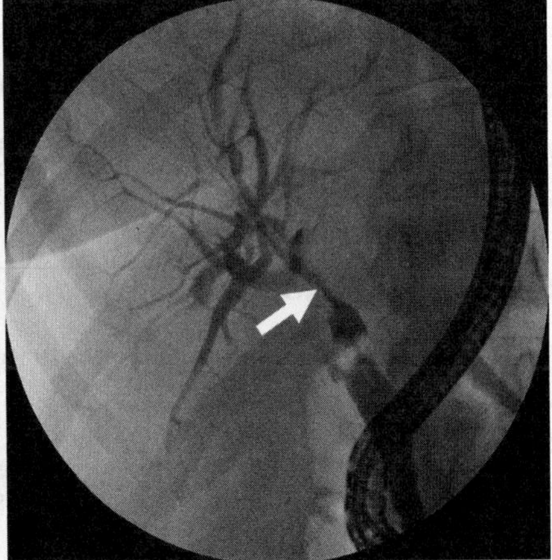
C

FIGURE 206–3 • Cholangiocarcinoma. A, A T1-weighted magnetic resonance imaging scan is shown during the arterial phase after the administration of intravenous gadolinium. The tumor (arrow) occludes the left hepatic duct, thus leading to marked dilation of the left biliary system and atrophy with enhanced contrast enhancement of the left lobe; the right lobe of the liver shows compensatory hypertrophy. This combination of features is called the *atrophy-hypertrophy complex.* **B,** Magnetic resonance cholangiopancreatography from the same patient showing narrowing of the common hepatic duct by the cholangiocarcinoma (arrow) and grossly dilated left biliary system. **C,** Endoscopic retrograde cholangiopancreatography showing filling of the right biliary system through the narrowed common hepatic duct (arrow); the left biliary system is completely isolated and not filled during injection of contrast.

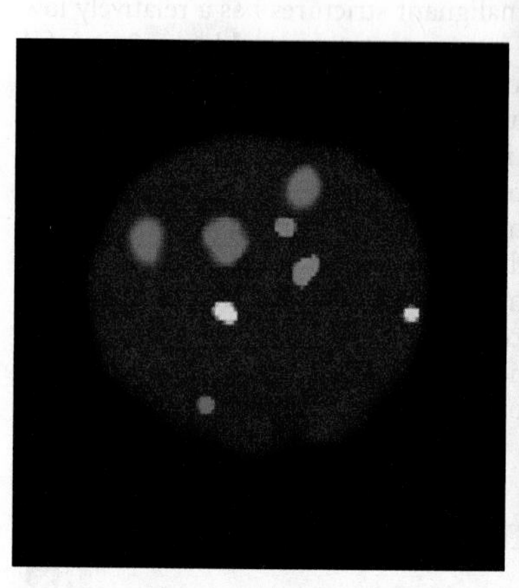

Diploid cell

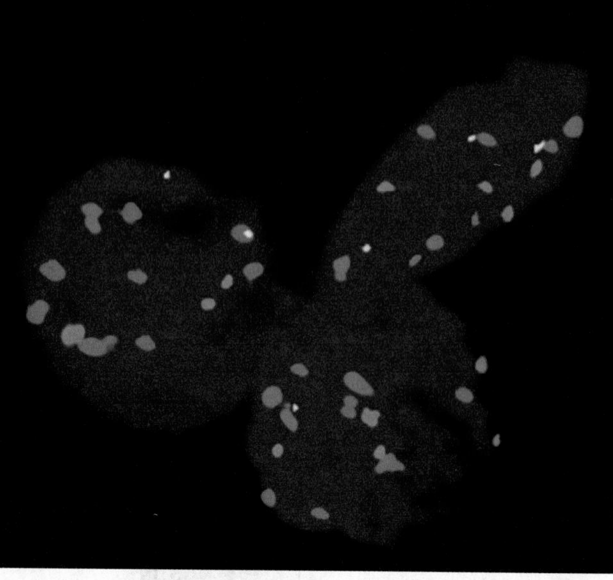

Polysomic cells

FIGURE 206–4 • Fluorescence in situ hybridization for diagnosis of malignancy in biliary strictures. Fluorescent DNA probes for the centromeres of chromosomes 3 (red), 7 (green), 17 (aqua), and the p16 locus at chromosome 9p21 (yellow) are hybridized to brush cytology specimens obtained from biliary strictures at endoscopic retrograde cholangiopancreatography. The normal diploid cell (left) has two copies of each of the probes; the malignant polysomic cells (right) each have multiple copies of chromosomes 3, 7, and 17.

Rx

vival of 80% in patients who can successfully complete the treatment protocol. Photodynamic therapy with 630-nm laser light treatment administered using a fiber inserted across the biliary stricture after intravenous infusion of a photosensitizing porfimer, which is preferentially taken up by malignant cells, can preserve biliary patency and can improve survival in patients with unresectable malignant biliary strictures. [3]

Prognosis

Biliary stenting, photodynamic therapy, and the use of occasionally effective chemotherapy agents such as gemcitabine (used alone or in combination with 5-fluorouracil and leucovorin or capecitabine) generally result in improvements in survival that are measured only in months.

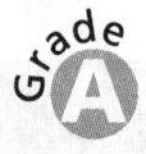

1. Llovet JM, Bruix J: Systematic review of randomized trials for unresectable hepatocellular carcinoma: Chemoembolization improves survival. Hepatology 2003;37:429–442.
2. Chang MH, Shau WY, Chen CJ, et al: Hepatitis B vaccination and hepatocellular carcinoma rates in boys and girls. JAMA 2000;284:3040–3042.
3. Ortner ME, Caca K, Berr F, et al: Successful photodynamic therapy for nonresectable cholangiocarcinoma: A randomized prospective study. Gastroenterology 2003;125:1355–1363.

SUGGESTED READINGS

Choi BY, Nguyen MH: The diagnosis and management of benign hepatic tumors. J Clin Gastroenterol 2005;39:401–412. *A comprehensive review of benign liver masses.*

Colli A, Fraquelli M, Casazza G, et al: Accuracy of ultrasonography, spiral CT, magnetic resonance, and alpha-fetoprotein in diagnosing hepatocellular carcinoma: A systematic review. Am J Gastroenterol 2006;101:513–523. *Meta-analysis of the accuracy of these diagnostic tools in hepatocellular carcinoma screening.*

El-Serag HB, Davila JA, Petersen NJ, et al: The continuing increase in the incidence of hepatocellular carcinoma in the United States: An update. Ann Intern Med 2003;139:817–823. *Documents the increasing incidence of hepatocellular carcinoma in the United States over the past 25 years.*

Khan SA, Thomas HC, Davidson BR, et al: Cholangiocarcinoma. Lancet 2005;366:1303–1314. *A comprehensive review.*

Llovet JM: Updated treatment approach to hepatocellular carcinoma. J Gastroenterol 2005;40:225–235. *A comprehensive review.*

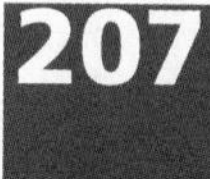

207 TUMORS OF THE KIDNEY, BLADDER, URETERS, AND RENAL PELVIS

Dean F. Bajorin

RENAL CELL CARCINOMA

Definition

Cancers of the kidney are a heterogeneous group of neoplasms, the majority of which are of epithelial origin and malignant. Renal cell carcinoma, classically referred to as clear cell carcinoma or hypernephroma, is not a single entity. Rather, renal cell carcinoma consists of a group of distinguishable malignancies, each with a strong relationship between its morphologic and genetic features (Table 207–1). The metastatic potential, which is dependent on the histologic subtype, ranges from the most virulent conventional clear cell carcinomas (65% of total tumors but accounting for 90% of metastases), to the more indolent papillary and chromophobe carcinomas (25% of the total but only 10% of metastases), to the benign oncocytomas (10% of all tumors).

Epidemiology

It is estimated that more than 35,000 new cases and approximately 13,000 deaths from kidney cancer occur annually in the United States, with a 126% increase in the incidence of renal cancer and a 36.5% increase in annual mortality since 1950. The increase in incidence of renal cell cancers may in part be related to early detection as a consequence of computed tomography (CT) and magnetic resonance imaging (MRI) of the abdomen for other medical conditions. The male-to-female ratio is approximately 2:1 to 3:1, and the incidence is highest in African Americans and lowest in Asian/Pacific Islanders. The mean age at diagnosis is in the sixth to seventh decade of life.

Aside from genetic predisposition, risk factors associated with renal cell carcinoma include cigarette smoking, obesity, hypertension, and the use of diuretics. For cigarette smokers, a dose-response phenomenon has been reported in both men and women; the risk may decrease by about 20 years after smoking cessation. Obese persons have an increased risk for renal cell carcinoma, and the risk rises with increasing body mass index. Although there is an elevated risk associated with diuretic use, this association is difficult to distinguish from the increased risk related to hypertension. Renal cell carcinoma is more prevalent in patients with preexisting renal conditions such as polycystic kidney disease (Chapter 128), horseshoe kidney, and chronic renal failure requiring hemodialysis (Chapter 131).

Pathobiology

A consideration of cytogenetics permits a better understanding of the cell of origin for the various subtypes of renal carcinoma (Fig. 207–1).

Clear Cell Carcinoma

The classic clear cell carcinoma accounts for approximately 65% of tumors and is believed to be derived from the proximal convoluted tubule. It is generally solitary and well circumscribed, with a golden yellow color because of abundant cytoplasmic lipid. Higher-grade tumors contain less lipid and glycogen. About half the tumors exhibit either a solid or an acinar growth pattern consisting of solid sheets of tumor cells and accompanied by a rich capillary vascular network.

TABLE 207–1 CLASSIFICATION OF RENAL CELL NEOPLASMS AND THEIR BENIGN AND MALIGNANT COUNTERPARTS

Benign	Malignant
Oncocytoma	Clear cell (conventional) renal cell carcinoma
Papillary (chromophil) adenoma	Papillary (chromophil) renal cell carcinoma
Metanephric adenoma	Chromophobe renal cell carcinoma
Nephrogenic adenofibroma	Collecting duct carcinoma
	Medullary carcinoma
	Mixed tubular and spindle cell carcinoma
	Renal cell carcinoma, unclassified

Modified from Storkel S, Eble JN, Adlakha K, et al: Classification of renal cell carcinoma: Workgroup No. 1. Union Internationale Contre le Cancer (UICC) and the American Joint Committee on Cancer (AJCC). Cancer 1997;80:987–989.

Clear cell carcinoma is characterized by the loss of genetic material on the short arm of chromosome 3 (3p) and mutations in the von Hippel-Lindau (VHL; Chapter 199) gene. In patients with VHL disease, these losses and mutations occur in virtually all cases. Hereditary clear cell tumors have a mutation in the VHL gene, which is inactivated by a point mutation or by epigenetic gene silencing by promoter methylation. The more common sporadic, unilateral, and unifocal tumors, however, also frequently have somatic mutations or hypermethylation in the same region. The loss of VHL, responsible for ubiquination and degradation of hypoxia-inducible factor (HIF) genes, leads to upregulation of the HIF-responsive genes that are responsible for angiogenesis and cell growth. Two of these upregulated genes are platelet-derived growth factor (PDGF) and vascular endothelial growth factor (VEGF), which are angiogenic factors thought to induce the neovascularity seen in both primary and metastatic clear cell cancer. In contrast to patients with sporadic tumors, patients with VHL syndrome more commonly have tumors at an earlier age and frequently have multiple tumors. Other tumors associated with VHL syndrome include central nervous system hemangioblastomas (Chapter 199), pancreatic neuroendocrine tumors (Chapter 205), pheochromocytomas, retinal angiomas, and epididymal cystadenomas.

Papillary Renal Cell Carcinoma

Papillary renal cell carcinomas represent 7 to 14% of primary epithelial renal neoplasms. The majority of patients have unilateral tumors; multifocality, either bilateral or multifocal lesions in the same kidney, is present in about 45% of cases. Most of these tumors exhibit a broad morphologic spectrum, including papillary, papillary-trabecular, and papillary-solid areas. Associated necrosis is a common finding. The classic papillary pattern is characterized by discrete papillary fronds lined by neoplastic epithelial cells and containing a central fibrovascular core, easily recognized on low magnification. These tumors are divided into type 1 and type 2 lesions based on cytologic features and genetic differences.

The majority of sporadic papillary renal cell carcinomas are characterized by trisomy of chromosomes 7 and 17, as well as loss of chromosome Y. Hereditary papillary renal cancer is a result of germline mutations and activation of the *MET* proto-oncogene, which is located on chromosome 7p. These cells have aberrant hepatocyte growth factor receptors that are unable to deactivate after binding by the growth factor. Somatic *MET* gene amplifications have also been observed in about 10% of sporadic papillary renal cancer. The syndrome of hereditary leiomy-

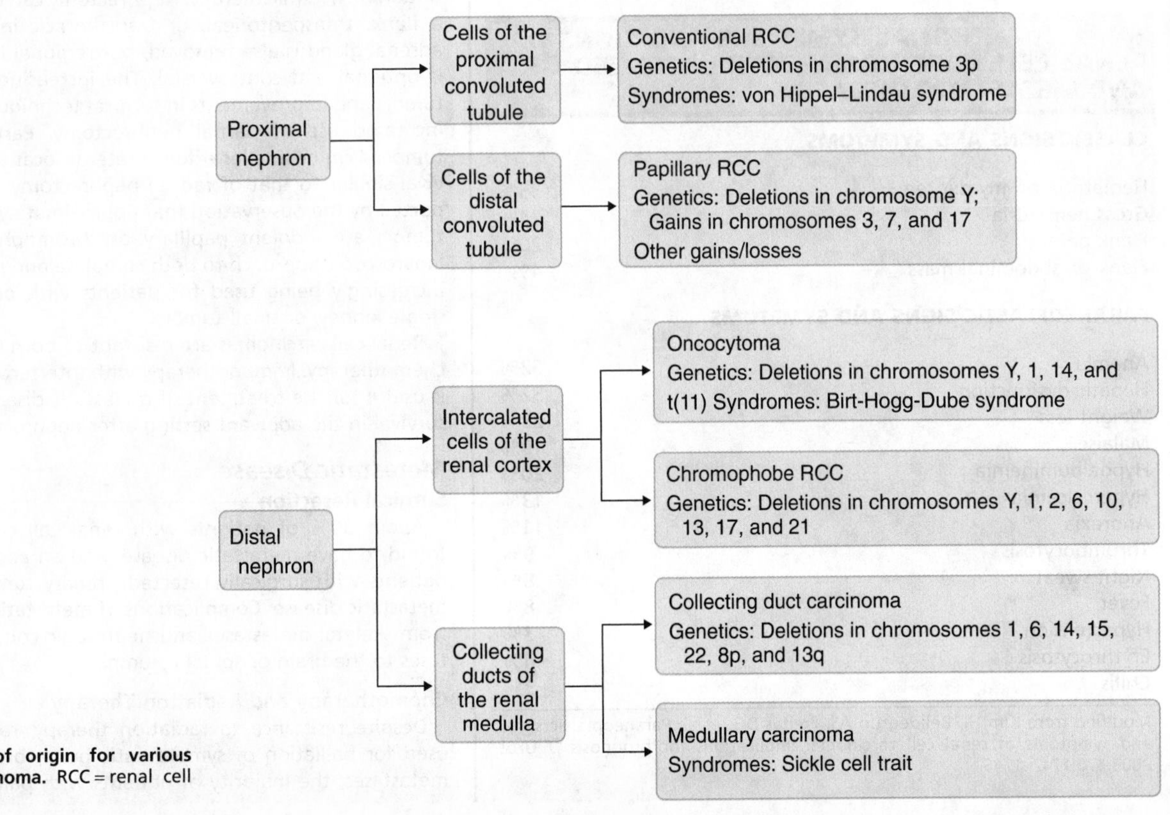

FIGURE 207–1 • Cell of origin for various subtypes of renal carcinoma. RCC = renal cell carcinoma.

omatosis and papillary renal cancer is associated with the gene for fumarate hydratase.

Chromophobe Renal Cancers

Chromophobe renal cancers account for 6 to 11% of renal epithelial tumors. Characteristically, these tumors are solitary and discrete but not encapsulated. The typical histology consists of large round to polygonal cells with well-defined cell borders and pale basophilic cytoplasm admixed with a smaller population of polygonal cells with eosinophilic cytoplasm. These tumors may be quite large at diagnosis, yet still resectable.

Chromophobe renal cell cancers are characterized by genetic loss on chromosomes 1 and Y, as well as combined chromosomal losses affecting chromosomes 1, 6, 10, 13, 17, and 21. Birt-Hogg-Dube syndrome is a rare disorder predominantly associated with chromophobe renal cancers but in which clear cell tumors and chromophobe/oncocytic tumors can develop. The gene associated with Birt-Hogg-Dube syndrome has been mapped to 17p and expresses a novel protein, folliculin, whose function is not yet defined.

Clinical Manifestations

Although renal cell carcinoma has a high propensity for metastases and has associated paraneoplastic syndromes, the majority of patients are asymptomatic at diagnosis. Historically, renal cell carcinoma was characterized by the initial triad of hematuria, a palpable mass, and pain in as many as 10% of patients. Over the last decade, however, there has been a stage migration in which detection of earlier-stage tumors has increased with the use of abdominal imaging for unrelated medical conditions. Up to 48% of tumors may be discovered in this manner, and less than 5% of patients now have a palpable mass at diagnosis. The more common initial symptoms are anemia, weight loss, malaise, and anorexia (Table 207–2), and the presence of these symptoms is associated with decreased disease-free survival.

Patients with renal cell carcinoma frequently have associated paraneoplastic syndromes. Hypercalcemia (Chapter 266) is observed in up to 20% of patients and can be due to the secretion of parathyroid hormone, parathyroid hormone–like peptide, and interleukin-6 (IL-6), which has been shown to stimulate osteoclastic bone resorption. Other associated syndromes include hypertension (Chapter 66), erythrocytosis (Chapter 172) from ectopic production of erythropoietin, and the rare Stauffer syndrome, in which patients without hepatic metastases have abnormal liver enzyme levels (Chapter 150) that resolve after surgical resection of the primary tumor.

TABLE 207–2 INITIAL SYMPTOMS AND SIGNS OF RENAL CELL CARCINOMA (BOTH LOCALIZED AND METASTATIC DISEASE)

CLASSIC SIGNS AND SYMPTOMS	
Hematuria of any degree	35%
Gross hematuria	24%
Flank pain	20%
Flank or abdominal mass	4%
PARANEOPLASTIC SIGNS AND SYMPTOMS	
Anemia	52%
Hepatic dysfunction	32%
Weight loss	23%
Malaise	19%
Hypoalbuminemia	20%
Hypercalcemia	13%
Anorexia	11%
Thrombocytosis	9%
Night sweats	8%
Fever	8%
Hypertension	3%
Erythrocytosis	4%
Chills	3%

Modified from Kim HI, Belldegrun AS, Freitas DG, et al: Paraneoplastic signs and symptoms of renal cell carcinoma: Implications for prognosis. J Urol 2003;170:1742–1746.

Diagnosis

Evaluation of patients with suspected renal cell carcinoma should include a complete blood cell count, a chemistry profile, a bone scan, and a CT scan of the chest, abdomen, and pelvis. CT is the most reliable method for detecting and staging renal cell carcinoma; the most important phases for imaging renal tumors are the precontrast and nephrographic images because renal lesions appear low in density in contrast to the uniformly enhanced renal parenchyma. The arterial phase is helpful in identifying renal arteries and small hypervascular masses. The excretory phase aids in assessing the collecting system and the renal pelvis. CT is also helpful in detecting regional metastases. Three-dimensional CT imaging is now possible in cases in which "nephron-sparing surgery" or partial nephrectomy is planned.

Ultrasonography and MRI can distinguish benign from malignant lesions of the kidney and can help plan treatment. Ultrasound is used to distinguish cysts from solid lesions. MRI has the advantage of imaging tumors in patients with poor renal function, in whom intravenous contrast may be contraindicated. MRI is also helpful for delineating any thrombi that may extend into the renal vein or inferior vena cava. Magnetic resonance angiography can determine the number and location of renal arteries in patients who are candidates for partial nephrectomy.

Once the evaluation is complete, clinical stage is assessed with the TNM (tumor, node, metastasis) system, and staging is the same for all histology subtypes (Table 203–3).

Treatment

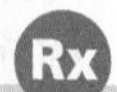

Localized Disease

The historical standard of care for patients with all types of renal cell carcinoma is radical nephrectomy. Tumors routinely selected for radical nephrectomy include large tumors, centrally localized tumors that have effectively replaced the majority of normal renal parenchyma, tumors associated with regional adenopathy (of benign or malignant etiology), tumors with extension into the inferior vena cava or right atrium, and metastatic tumors before the initiation of systemic therapy. Nephrectomy can be performed through a flank, transperitoneal, or transthoracic incision. The ipsilateral adrenal gland is also removed, but regional lymph node dissection is optional and controversial. The increasing percentage of small tumors and improvements in surgical techniques have resulted in an increased use of partial nephrectomy. Partial nephrectomy for tumors 4 cm or smaller offers a rate of local tumor control and survival similar to that of radical nephrectomy. This approach is supported by the observation that approximately 35% of renal cortical tumors are indolent papillary or chromophobe carcinomas. The laparoscopic approach to both complete and partial nephrectomy is increasingly being used for patients with poor renal function, a single kidney, or small tumors.

Renal cell carcinomas are resistant to both radiation therapy and chemotherapy. Immunotherapy with interferon alfa and IL-2, which is useful for the treatment of metastatic disease, does not improve survival in the adjuvant setting after nephrectomy.

Metastatic Disease

Surgical Resection

About 30% of patients with renal cell carcinoma are initially found to have metastatic disease, and an additional 20 to 30% of patients with surgically resected primary tumors will relapse with metastatic disease. Complications of metastatic disease include pain from skeletal metastases and neurologic compromise from metastases to the brain or spinal column.

Chemotherapy and Radiation Therapy

Despite resistance to radiation therapy, radiation is frequently used for palliation of symptomatic bone, brain, or spinal column metastases; the majority of patients with painful bone metastases

TABLE 207–3 TNM STAGING OF RENAL CELL CARCINOMA

TUMOR, NODES, AND METASTASES CLINICAL CLASSIFICATION (2002)

T—PRIMARY TUMOR

TX	Primary tumor cannot be assessed
T0	No evidence of primary tumor
T1a	<4.0 cm; limited to the kidney
T1b	4–7 cm; limited to the kidney
T2	>7.0 cm; limited to the kidney
T3	Tumor extends into the major veins or invades the adrenal gland or perinephric tissues but does not extent beyond Gerota's fascia
T3a	Tumor invades the adrenal gland or perinephric tissues but does not extend beyond Gerota's fascia
T3b	Tumor grossly extends into the renal vein(s) or vena cava below the diaphragm
T3c	Tumor grossly extends into the vena cava above the diaphragm
T4	Tumor invades beyond Gerota's fascia

N—REGIONAL LYMPH NODES

NX	Regional lymph nodes cannot be assessed
N0	No regional lymph node metastasis
N1	Metastasis in a single regional lymph node
N2	Metastasis in more than one regional lymph node

M—DISTANT METASTASIS

MX	Distant metastasis cannot be assessed
M0	No distant metastasis
M1	Distant metastasis

STAGE GROUPING

Stage I	T1	N0	M0
Stage II	T2	N0	M0
Stage III	T1	N1	M0
	T2	N1	M0
	T3a	N0, N1	M0
	T3b	N0, N1	M0
	T3c	N0, N1	M0
Stage IV	T4	N0	M0
	T4	N1	M0
	Any T	N2	M0
	Any T	Any N	M1

Rx

achieve palliation, but benefit for brain metastases is less common. Cytoreductive nephrectomy before starting systemic therapy extends survival in patients with metastatic disease, 1 and palliative nephrectomy is sometimes used to relieve pain from locally extensive disease. Surgical resection of metastatic disease (i.e., metastectomy) may extend survival and even cure a subset of patients. Patients most likely to benefit from surgical resection of metastatic disease are those with a disease-free interval longer than 1 year and those with a solitary site of metastasis. Long-term survival has been observed when the solitary site of resection was the lung (up to 45%) and even the brain (up to 20%). Renal cell carcinoma is resistant to most conventional chemotherapy agents, with responses seen in less than 10% of patients. No single agent or combination of chemotherapy drugs is considered the standard of care.

Immunotherapy

High-dose intravenous IL-2 (600,000 U/kg per dose every 8 hours on days 1 to 5 and 15 to 19) and conventional-dose subcutaneous interferon alfa (most frequently 5 to 9 million IU 3 to 5 days per week) are approved treatments for patients with metastatic disease.

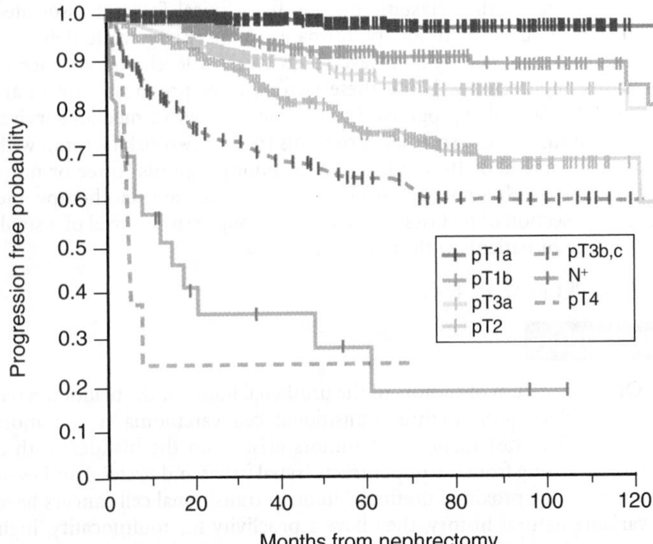

FIGURE 207–2 • Survival distributions for patients undergoing surgery for primary renal cell carcinoma. (From Russo P, Snyder ME, Di Blasio CJ, et al: Changing demographics and the contemporary surgical management of renal cortical tumors. J Urol 2003;169:347A.)

Rx

IL-2 therapy requires a dedicated inpatient setting because of its severe associated toxicities, which include hypotension, pulmonary edema, renal failure, and central nervous system toxicity. However, most toxicities are reversible, complete or partial responses are seen in approximately 15 to 20% of patients, and about 4% of patients achieve long-term, disease-free survival. Lower doses of subcutaneous IL-2 are less toxic, but response rates are also lower. Interferon alfa therapy is more frequently used for metastatic renal cell carcinoma because of less toxicity, ease of administration in the outpatient setting, and an overall response rate of approximately 15%. However, the proportion of patients achieving long-term disease-free remission is less with subcutaneous immunotherapy than with high-dose intravenous IL-2. 2 Reversible toxicities of interferon alfa include fever, chills, myalgias, and mild myelosuppression and hepatic dysfunction. Recently, the Food and Drug Administration has approved two new agents, sorafenib and sunitinib, that function as tyrosine kinase inhibitors and block the actions of the receptors for VEGF and PDGF. Sorafenib is better than placebo, 3 and sunitinib can provide better progession-free survival (11 months vs. 5 months) and quality of life than interferon alfa. 4

Experimental Therapy

Nonmyeloablative allogeneic stem cell transplantation has been successful in approximately 50% of highly selected patients, but this approach has not been widely adopted because of the toxicity and need for a matched donor. Bevacizumab, an antibody that blocks VEGF, has shown activity as a single agent and is currently under study in combination with interferon.

Prognosis

Survival rates for resected nonmetastatic renal cortical tumors range between 60 and 100%, depending on the histology, size, and stage at diagnosis (Fig. 207–2). The prognosis declines considerably for patients who have more advanced disease, with long-term survival seen in only 20% of stage III patients and in 5% or less of stage IV patients. Of the more common histologic subtypes of renal cell carcinoma, the prognosis of clear cell carcinoma is less favorable than that of papillary renal cell carcinoma; chromophobe renal cell carcinoma is the most favorable.

For patients with metastatic disease, five clinical features associated with shorter survival are low performance status, high lactate dehydrogenase level, low hemoglobin level, high calcium level, and absence of previous nephrectomy. Using these factors, three prognostic strata are defined: (1) favorable prognosis (no risk factors), with a median survival of 20 months; (2) intermediate prognosis (one or two risk factors), with a median survival of 10 months; and (3) poor prognosis (three or more risk factors), with a median survival of 4 months. Immunotherapy and surgical resection of metastases can result in long-term survival of a small percentage of patients with metastatic disease.

BLADDER CANCER

Definition

Of the spectrum of tumors of the urothelial lining of the bladder, renal pelvis, ureters, and urethra, transitional cell carcinoma is the most common. The vast majority of tumors arise from the bladder, with a minority arising from the upper tracts (renal pelvis and ureters) and even fewer from the proximal urethra. Although transitional cell cancers have a variable natural history, they have a proclivity for multifocality, high recurrence rates, and progression to higher pathologic stages. These tumors are generally grouped into the three broad categories—superficial, muscle-invasive, and metastatic disease—each of which differs in clinical behavior, prognosis, and primary management. For superficial tumors, the aim is to prevent recurrences and progression to a more advanced stage. In muscle-invasive disease, the medical challenge is to integrate surgery, chemotherapy, or radiation therapy, or any combination of these modalities, to optimize the chance for cure and minimize morbidity. For metastatic disease, chemotherapy is generally used to palliate symptoms, but a subset of patients may be cured. Over the past 30 years, improvements in diagnosis, management, and therapy have increased the 5-year survival rate from 73% in 1974 to 1976 to 82% between 1995 and 2000.

Epidemiology

More than 63,000 estimated new cases of bladder cancer are diagnosed annually in the United States, and 13,000 patients are expected to succumb to their disease. The male-to-female ratio of 3:1 is similar in all racial groups, and it is the fourth most common cancer in men and the ninth in women. The combined bladder cancer incidence for men and women has remained stable from 1986 to 2001 after rising 0.7% per year from 1975 to 1986, whereas the death rate from bladder cancer continues to decline. Bladder cancer is twice as prevalent in whites as in African Americans and is less frequent in Asians. The median age at diagnosis is approximately 70 years, and the disease is rarely diagnosed before the age of 40.

Risk Factors

Carcinogens or their metabolites implicated in the carcinogenesis of bladder cancer are believed to be excreted in urine, where they can act directly on the urothelial lining. Because the latency period from initial exposure to the development of cancer is almost 20 years, it is difficult to establish a definitive cause-and-effect relationship between a putative carcinogen and development of the disease. Cigarette smoking (Chapter 30), which is the leading risk factor for bladder cancer, is believed to contribute to 48% of the cancers in men and 28% of the cancers in women. A longer duration of exposure is associated with higher risk than is more intense exposure (in cigarettes per day) over a shorter period. Overall, smokers have a two- to four-fold higher relative risk for bladder cancer than nonsmokers do.

Polycyclic aromatic hydrocarbons, benzidine, benzene, and exhaust from combustion gases are associated with an increased risk for bladder cancer. Occupations reported to be associated with higher risk include aluminum workers, dry cleaners, manufacturers of preservatives and polychlorinated biphenyls, and pesticide applicators. Arylamines, also implicated in carcinogenesis, are metabolically activated to electrophilic compounds by *N*-hydroxylation in the liver by cytochrome P-450 IA2 and detoxified by *N*-acetylation; studies suggest that individuals with a fast oxidizer and slow acetylator phenotype are at highest risk. Occupations associated with higher exposure to arylamines, such as workers in the dye, rubber, and leather manufacturing industries, are believed to be at higher risk for bladder cancer. *Schistosoma haematobium* (Chapter 376) infection enhances the formation of carcinogenic *N*-nitroso compounds and results in an increased risk for both squamous and transitional cell carcinoma of the bladder. An association has been observed between squamous cell carcinoma (but not transitional cell tumors) and the presence of chronic urinary tract infections in paraplegics and patients with chronic bladder stones and indwelling Foley catheters. The chemotherapy agent cyclophosphamide can increase the risk for bladder cancer nine-fold, and phenacetin-containing compounds have been implicated in the development of tumors of the renal pelvis and ureter.

Pathobiology

More than 90% of urothelial tumors originate in the bladder, 8% in the renal pelvis, and the remaining 2% in the ureter and urethra. Transitional cell carcinomas account for 90 to 95% of urothelial tumors; squamous cell (keratinizing) tumors (3%), adenocarcinomas (2%), and small cell tumors (1%) represent the remainder. Mixed-histology tumors, consisting of predominantly transitional cell carcinoma with areas of squamous, adenocarcinomatous, or neuroendocrine elements, are frequently observed. Squamous cell tumors are more frequent in the distal urethra, and adenocarcinomas occur in the embryonal remnant of the urachus on the dome of the bladder and in periurethral tissues. In endemic areas of *S. haematobium* infection such as Egypt, 40% of tumors are squamous cell carcinomas. Rare tumors of the bladder include lymphoma, sarcoma, and melanoma.

Grading

The majority (70 to 80%) of newly detected bladder cancers are classified as superficial tumors, including exophytic papillary tumors confined to the mucosa (Ta), tumors invading the lamina propria (T1), and carcinoma in situ (CIS, also called Tis). Superficial bladder tumors are typically graded as low (G1), intermediate (G2), or high (G3) grade, with the latter more likely to progress to higher clinical stage. Grading is more important for noninvasive Ta tumors because almost all invasive bladder tumors (T1 or greater) are high grade. Primary Tis, without a concurrent Ta or T1 tumor, constitutes 1 to 2% of new bladder cancer cases but is more frequently found in the presence of multiple papillary tumors, either immediately adjacent to another lesion or involving remote mucosa in the bladder. Tis is regarded as a precursor to more invasive tumors because more invasive disease develops in 60% of untreated tumors within 5 years. T1 tumor is an aggressive, invasive malignancy. Virtually all T1 tumors are grade 3, and 50% have associated Tis. Fifty percent of patients have recurrence by 1 year and 90% within 5 years. A minority of primary tumors are found at diagnosis to invade the muscularis propria (T2), extend to perivesicular fat (T3), or extend into immediately adjacent organs (T4); all primary tumors stage T2 or higher are high grade.

Genetics

The natural history of a urothelial tumor is to recur either at the same location or at a separate site in the urothelial tract, at the same or at a more advanced stage. Several studies support the concept that these recurrences are clonal in origin. Chromosome 9 deletions are the most commonly observed chromosomal changes in bladder cancer. Chromosomal deletions of 17p (the *TP53* locus), 18q (the *DCC* gene locus), and the *RB* gene locus are frequently observed in invasive tumors, whereas deletions of 3p and 11p occur in both superficial and invasive tumors. Associations between specific gene deletions and prognosis have been attempted, but inconsistent findings among studies preclude their routine use in clinical management. The epidermal growth factor receptor is highly expressed (≈80%) on bladder cancer tumors, and the Her2/Neu growth factor receptor is less frequently expressed (≈50%). Studies suggest that higher expression of these receptors in bladder cancer is associated with a more advanced or more aggressive phenotype of disease, or both.

Clinical Manifestations

Hematuria is the initial symptom in 80 to 90% of bladder cancers, but others may have a urinary tract infection. Urinary frequency and nocturia may be present as a consequence of either irritative symptoms or reduced bladder capacity. Pain, when present, typically reflects the location of the bladder tumor. Lower abdominal pain may occur as a result of a bladder mass, whereas rectal discomfort and perineal pain can result from tumors invading the prostate or pelvis. Tumors of the renal pelvis, ureter, or the ureteral orifice of the bladder can cause hydronephrosis, reduced renal function, and flank pain. Patients with more advanced disease may have anorexia, fatigue, weight loss, or pain from a metastatic bone lesion. Physical examination is frequently unremarkable because the vast majority of patients have organ-confined tumors.

Diagnosis

Individuals older than 40 years in whom hematuria develops should undergo evaluation for the presence of urothelial cancer; studies should include urinary cytology and cystoscopy. In selected patients, additional imaging of the urinary tract may be required. Screening asymptomatic subjects for hematuria increases the probability of diagnosing bladder cancer at an earlier stage but does not improve survival; thus, it is not routinely recommended.

Cytology, Cytoscopy, and Biopsy

In all patients with a suspected bladder tumor, urine is obtained to evaluate for the presence of malignant cells (cytology). Cystoscopy is required for a suspected tumor regardless of whether the results of urine cytology are positive or negative. The mainstay of diagnosis and staging of bladder cancer is cystoscopic evaluation, including examination under anesthesia to determine whether there is a palpable mass and, if so, whether it is mobile. A nonmobile tumor mass is indicative of disease extending beyond the wall of the bladder and invading into regional organs such as the prostate, vagina, or the muscles along the pelvic sidewall; these tumors are unlikely to be surgically resectable. The bladder is visually inspected to detail the size, number, location, and growth pattern (papillary or solid) of all lesions. All visible tumors should undergo transurethral resection to determine the histologic subtype and depth of invasion; invasion into muscle requires consideration of surgical cystectomy. Biopsy samples are taken from areas of erythema to assess for CIS. Patients with positive cytologic findings but no apparent tumor within the bladder or negative biopsies should undergo selective retrograde catheterization of the ureters up to the renal pelves to assess for upper tract disease.

Imaging

The decision whether to image the abdomen and pelvis is based on cystoscopy results and the pathology of the tumor. CT or MRI may distinguish whether a tumor extends to the perivesical fat (T3) or the prostate or vagina (T4) and whether regional lymph nodes are involved (N^+). If biopsies are negative, an intravenous pyelogram or CT-urogram can evaluate the upper urinary tracts for the presence of tumors. In the case of larger, invasive tumors, staging to determine the presence or absence of metastases requires CT of the abdomen and pelvis, a chest radiograph, and a radionuclide bone scan.

Staging

Patients with carcinoma of the bladder or related sites are staged with the TNM (tumor, node, metastasis) system advocated by the American Joint Committee on Cancer (Table 207–4).

TABLE 207–4 TNM DEFINITIONS FOR CANCER OF THE BLADDER, URETER, AND RENAL PELVIS

PRIMARY TUMORS OF THE BLADDER (T)

TX	Primary tumor cannot be assessed
T0	No evidence of primary tumor
Ta	Noninvasive papillary carcinoma
Tis	Carcinoma in situ (i.e., flat tumor)
T1	Tumor invades subepithelial connective tissue
T2	Tumor invades muscle
pT2a	Tumor invades superficial muscle (inner half)
pT2b	Tumor invades deep muscle (outer half)
T3	Tumor invades perivesical tissue
pT3a	Microscopically
pT3b	Macroscopically (extravesical mass)
T4	Tumor invades local structures
T4a	Tumor invades the prostate, uterus, vagina
T4b	Tumor invades the pelvic wall, abdominal wall

PRIMARY TUMORS OF THE URETER AND RENAL PELVIS (T)

TX	Primary tumor cannot be assessed
T0	No evidence of primary tumor
Ta	Papillary noninvasive carcinoma
Tis	Carcinoma in situ
T1	Tumor invades subepithelial connective tissue
T2	Tumor invades the muscularis
T3	(For the renal pelvis only) Tumor invades beyond the muscularis into peripelvic fat or the renal parenchyma
T3	(For the ureter only) Tumor invades beyond the muscularis equlige into periureteric fat
T4	Tumor invades adjacent organs or through the kidney into perinephric fat

REGIONAL LYMPH NODES FOR UROTHELIAL TUMORS (N)

NX	Regional lymph nodes cannot be assessed
N0	No regional lymph node metastasis
N1	Metastasis in a single lymph node, ≤2 cm in greatest dimension
N2	Metastasis in a single lymph node, >2 cm but ≤5 cm in greatest dimension, or in multiple lymph nodes, ≤5 cm in greatest dimension
N3	Metastasis in a lymph node, >5 cm in greatest dimension

DISTANT METASTASIS FOR UROTHELIAL TUMORS (M)

MX	Distant metastasis cannot be assessed
M0	No distant metastasis
M1	Distant metastasis

STAGE GROUPINGS FOR BLADDER CANCER

0a	Ta, N0, M0
0is	Tis, N0, M0
I	T1, N0, M0
II	T2a, N0, M0
	T2b, N0, M0
III	T3a, N0, M0
	T3b, N0, M0
	T4a, N0, M0
IV	T4b, N0, M0
	Any T, N1, M0
	Any T, N2, M0
	Any T, N3, M0
	Any T, any N, M1

STAGE GROUPINGS FOR CANCER OF THE RENAL PELVIS AND URETER

0a	Ta, N0, M0
0is	Tis, N0, M0
I	T1, N0, M0
II	T2, N0, M0
III	T3, N0, M0
IV	T4, N0, M0
	Any T, N1, M0
	Any T, N2, M0
	Any T, N3, M0
	Any T, any N, M1

Treatment

Rx

Superficial Disease

Endoscopic Resection and Intravesical Therapy

The standard treatment of superficial tumors is complete endoscopic resection. New tumors develop in the majority of patients, and 30% progress to a higher stage, thus mandating vigilant surveillance at 3-month intervals via cystoscopy and urine cytology and repeat transurethral resection when indicated. Prophylactic or adjuvant intravesical therapy is typically instituted when a patient has shown either a repeated tendency for the development of new lesions in the bladder or is at high risk for recurrence or progression de novo because of multifocal or large lesions, high-grade papillary lesions, T1 tumors, CIS, or any combination of these lesions. Such therapy is never advised for muscle-invasive tumors because agents instilled in the bladder do not penetrate beyond a few layers of cells. Once sufficient time for healing after endoscopic resection has elapsed, intravesical therapy is most frequently initiated with bacille Calmette-Guérin (BCG); typical doses are 81 mg for BCG produced by Connaught Laboratories Limited and 50 mg for BCG manufactured by Tice, weekly for 6 weeks. Maintenance therapy for up to 3 years may be used in responding patients. Occasionally, intravesical chemotherapy with mitomycin, 40 mg weekly for 6 weeks, is used when BCG is contraindicated.

If persistence of disease is shown by repeat cytoscopy at 3 and 6 months, either a repeat course of BCG treatment or even immediate cystectomy may be recommended. Toxicities of BCG include bladder irritability or spasm, hematuria, and pain on urination; a rare complication is the development of systemic tuberculosis requiring treatment (Chapter 345). BCG is highly effective in eradicating Tis, with 70% of patients being disease free at 1 year and 40% at 10 years.

Selected tumors in the ureter or renal pelvis can be managed by ureteroscopic resection, in some cases by instillation of BCG through the renal pelvis, or by nephroureterectomy. Tumors of the prostatic urethra are frequently managed by cystoprostatectomy, particularly if complete resection cannot be accomplished.

Muscle-Invasive Tumors

For tumors infiltrating the muscularis propria, the standard of care in the United States is radical cystectomy and pelvic lymphadenectomy because of the high likelihood of cancer extending into perivesicular fat or into regional lymph nodes; improved survival and decreased local recurrence are associated with an increased number of regional lymph nodes removed. This approach provides 5-year disease-free survival in 75 to 80% of patients with organ-confined disease, in approximately 50% of patients with tumors extending into the perivesical tissues, and in nearly a third of patients with regional lymph node involvement. Prostatectomy is also performed in men; in women, the urethra, uterus, fallopian tubes, ovaries, and anterior vaginal wall are removed. Urinary flow can be directed through either a conduit diversion or a continent reservoir. With a conduit diversion, urine is drained directly from the ureters to a loop of small bowel that is anastomosed to the skin surface with no internal reservoir; urine is collected in an external appliance. Alternatively, a low-pressure continent reservoir can be created from a detubularized segment of bowel attached to the abdominal wall with a continent stoma that can be self-catheterized at regular intervals; low-pressure reservoirs can also be anastomosed to the urethra, thereby creating an internal orthotopic neobladder and permitting the patient to void via the urethra. Complications of cystectomy include recurrent urinary infections, hyperchloremic acidosis, oxalate stones, incontinence, and impotence.

Neoadjuvant chemotherapy for 12 weeks before cystectomy improves 5-year disease-free survival. Neoadjuvant chemotherapy with the four-drug regimen MVAC (methotrexate, 30 mg/m^2 on days 1 and 15; vinblastine, 3 mg/m^2 on days 2 and 15; doxorubicin, 30 mg/m^2 on day 2; and cisplatin, 70 mg/m^2 on day 2, all given for three cycles every 28 days) improves median survival from 46 months to 77 months compared with surgery alone. [5] This therapy requires normal renal function and good performance status.

Rx

Patients with a solitary early-stage lesion and no evidence of hydronephrosis can be treated with simultaneous chemotherapy (usually cisplatin) and 65 Gy of radiation delivered in five daily fractions a week ranging from 2.0 to 2.5 Gy rather than cystectomy after successful, nearly complete transurethral resection of the tumor. Toxicities include inflammation of the skin, impotence, fatigue, and irritative symptoms from the bladder and bowel; persistent proctitis is rare. The 5-year disease-free survival rate with this approach is 50%, with the majority of patients retaining a normally functioning bladder.

Metastatic Disease

For patients with metastatic disease, the two most commonly used regimens are gemcitabine (1000 mg/m^2 on days 1, 8, and 15) plus cisplatin (70 mg/m^2 on day 2) (referred to as GC), recycled every 28 days, and the four-drug regimen of MVAC (doses and schedule as noted earlier); both regimens are given for a total of six cycles of therapy over a 6-month period. The most frequently observed toxicities include anemia, thrombocytopenia, neutropenic fever, mucositis, and fatigue. The two-drug GC regimen is better tolerated and has less severe toxicities; both regimens provide a median survival of approximately 14 months and a 5-year survival rate of about 15%. [6] Patients with good performance status and metastatic disease limited to the lymph nodes have a 20 to 33% 5-year disease-free survival rate.

Prognosis

Superficial Ta grade 1 lesions, easily treated with endoscopic resection alone, almost never progress, whereas aggressive transitional cell CIS can have up to a 60% 5-year disease-free survival rate after intravesical immunotherapy therapy with BCG in addition to endoscopic resection. For muscle-invasive disease, cure rates for T2 tumors can be as high as 80% with cystectomy, pelvic lymphadenectomy, and systemic chemotherapy for micrometastases. Metastatic urinary bladder cancer is a fast-growing and often lethal malignancy; despite aggressive chemotherapy, only a small proportion (≈15%) of patients are disease free at 5 years.

CANCERS OF THE RENAL PELVIS AND URETERS

Approximately 10% of transitional cell carcinomas occur in the ureters and the renal pelvis. These tumors can arise either de novo or in the setting of previous tumors; the risk for development of an upper tract tumor in patients with multifocal CIS of the bladder approaches 25% by 10 years. These tumors are morphologically similar to the tumors in the bladder and behave in a similar manner. Hematuria is the most common initial symptom, although patients with large tumors or ureteral obstruction (or both) can experience flank pain. Intravenous pyelography, CT, or MRI is used to stage the extent of primary disease and to detect regional metastases. Upper tract transitional cell carcinomas are staged according to the TNM system (see Table 207–4).

Low-grade ureteral tumors can be treated endoscopically, and high-grade tumors can be cured with nephroureterectomy. In renal pelvis tumors, nephroureterectomy is performed because of the high risk for multifocal tumors along the entire upper tract and the inability to monitor the ureteral stump with accuracy. Ureteroscopic resection alone without nephrectomy can be considered in patients with low-grade tumors of the renal pelvis. Systemic chemotherapy is used for patients with unresectable primary tumors, regional adenopathy, or recurrent tumors. Treatment of advanced, nonsurgical disease is with chemotherapy as for bladder cancer, with similar response and survival rates, except that carboplatin-based chemotherapy is considered instead of cisplatin if renal insufficiency is present, either from obstruction or from previous nephroureterectomy.

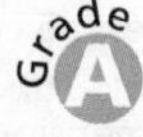

1. Flanigan RC, Salmon SE, Blumenstein BA, et al: Nephrectomy followed by interferon alfa-2b compared with interferon alfa-2b alone for metastatic renal-cell cancer. N Engl J Med 2001; 345:1655–1659.

Section XV Oncology

2. McDermott DF, Regan MM, Clark JI, et al: Randomized phase III trial of high-dose interleukin-2 versus subcutaneous interleukin-2 and interferon in patients with metastatic renal cell carcinoma. J Clin Oncol 2005;23:133–141.
3. Escudier B, Eisen T, Stadler WM, et al: Sorafenib in advanced clear-cell renal-cell carcinoma. N Engl J Med 2007;356:125–134.
4. Motzer RJ, Hutson TE, Tomczak P, et al: Sunitinib versus interferon alfa in metastatic renal-cell carcinoma. N Engl J Med 2007;356:115–124.
5. Grossman HB, Natale RB, Tangen CM, et al: Neoadjuvant chemotherapy plus cystectomy compared with cystectomy alone for locally advanced bladder cancer. N Engl J Med 2003; 349:859–866.
6. von der Maase H, Hansen SW, Roberts JT, et al: Gemcitabine and cisplatin versus methotrexate, vinblastine, doxorubicin, and cisplatin in advanced or metastatic bladder cancer: Results of a large, randomized, multinational, multicenter, phase III study. J Clin Oncol 2000;18:3068–3077.

SUGGESTED READINGS

Cohen HT, McGovern FJ: Medical progress: Renal-cell carcinoma. N Engl J Med 2005;353:2477–2490. *A comprehensive overview of kidney cancer.*

Garcia JA, Dreicer R: Systemic chemotherapy for advanced bladder cancer: Update and controversies. J Clin Oncol 2006;24:5545–5551. *Review of chemotherapy for advanced bladder cancer.*

Parekh DJ, Bochner BH, Dalbagni G: Superficial and muscle-invasive bladder cancer: Principles of management for outcomes assessments. J Clin Oncol 2006;24:5519–5527. *Review of the management of bladder cancer.*

Patel PH, Chaganti RS, Motzer RJ: Targeted therapy for metastatic renal cell carcinoma. Br J Cancer 2006;94:614–619. *A review of newly approved targeted agents for the treatment of metastatic kidney cancer.*

Porter MP, Wei JT, Penson DF: Quality of life issues in bladder cancer patients following cystectomy and urinary diversion. Urol Clin North Am 2005;32:207–216. *A review of quality-of-life studies in patients undergoing cystectomy.*

208 BREAST CANCER AND DIFFERENTIAL DIAGNOSIS OF BENIGN LESIONS

Hyman B. Muss

Epidemiology

Breast cancer is the most common cancer affecting women in the United States. Each year in the United States, approximately 210,000 new cases of invasive breast cancer and approximately 50,000 cases of ductal carcinoma in situ (DCIS) are diagnosed, and approximately 41,000 people die of breast cancer. Although most women treated for breast cancer are cured, late recurrences make the certainty of cure in any individual patient difficult. In patients with low-stage cancer that has an otherwise good prognosis, relapses are occasionally seen as late as 30 or more years after primary therapy. One in every seven women develops breast cancer during her lifetime, and breast cancer accounts for 32% of cases of cancer in women. It accounts for 15% of female cancer deaths and is the second leading cause of female cancer death after lung cancer. Male breast cancer accounts for approximately 1% of all new cases and, stage for stage, has a natural history similar to that of female breast cancer. The incidence of breast cancer continues to increase slowly, but mortality rates have decreased since the early 1990s. This decrease is probably the result of multiple factors, including wider use of mammographic screening, better surgical and radiation therapy, and the use of systemic adjuvant therapy.

It is estimated that, worldwide, more than 1 million new cases of breast cancer are diagnosed yearly. The incidence and mortality rates for breast cancer differ dramatically among nations. In general, more affluent Western nations have the highest incidence rates, whereas developing nations have the lowest. Although racial factors may play a role in its incidence, the differing rates of breast cancer among nations are more likely related to sociodemographic and dietary factors, including per capita income, nutritional status, and dietary composition.

Pathobiology: Pathogenesis

The causes of breast cancer remain elusive. Numerous risk factors have been defined (Table 208–1). The incidence of breast cancer increases dramatically with increasing age; more than 50% of women with breast cancer in the United States are older than 60 years, and more than half of all breast cancer deaths are in women 65 years old and older. Moreover, the number of older women with breast cancer is increasing dramatically as the population ages. Several risk factors, such as younger age at menarche and older age at menopause, are indirect measures of the number of menstrual cycles that a woman has in her lifetime. Increasing the number of cycles could predispose women to greater DNA damage in the proliferating breast ductal tissue and thus could increase the risk of mutations that directly lead to breast cancer. Western cultures are characterized by younger age at menarche, older age at menopause, later age of childbearing or nulliparity, increased obesity, more sedentary lifestyles, increased use of hormone replacement therapy, and a longer life span. A convincing body of data indicates that breast cancer risk directly correlates with serum estradiol concentration. Oral contraceptive use increases breast cancer risk minimally if at all. The use of estrogen-progestin hormone replacement therapy in postmenopausal women increases the risk of breast cancer approximately 1.5 times. It is uncertain whether estrogen replacement alone increases risk. The greatest increase in risk associated with the use of hormone replacement therapy is in leaner postmenopausal women.

The available data suggest that the risk of breast cancer is not affected by dietary saturated fat intake during adulthood or by vitamin A, C, and E consumption. Dietary composition, however, may be important; populations with high intake of soy proteins, which are rich sources of plant estrogen-like compounds (phytoestrogens), have lower rates of hormonally related cancers such as breast, endometrial, and prostate cancer. Alcohol intake is also related to breast cancer, in that women who have several drinks daily have a moderately higher risk than those who abstain. Women whose Hodgkin's disease has been treated with chest irradiation have a risk of breast cancer that is at least two- to three-fold higher than average, with a cumulative lifetime risk of 30 to 40%. Exposure to environmental pollutants (dichlorodiphenyltrichloroethane [DDT], polychlorinated biphenyls [PCBs], and others) may increase the risk of breast cancer, but such a relationship has not been confirmed.

TABLE 208–1 RISK FACTORS FOR BREAST CANCER

Risk Factor	Relative Risk
Any benign breast disease	1.5
Postmenopausal hormone replacement (estrogen with or without progestin)	1.5
Menarche at <12 yr	1.1–1.9
Moderate alcohol intake (two to three drinks/day)	1.1–1.9
Menopause at >55 yr	1.1–1.9
Increased bone density	1.1–1.9
Sedentary lifestyle and lack of exercise	1.1–1.9
Proliferative breast disease without atypia	2
Age at first birth >30 yr or nulliparous	2–4
First-degree relative with breast cancer	2–4
Postmenopausal obesity	2–4
Upper socioeconomic class	2–4
Personal history of endometrial or ovarian cancer	2–4
Significant radiation to chest	2–4
Increased breast density on mammogram	2–4
Older age	>4
Personal history of breast cancer (in situ or invasive)	>4
Proliferative breast disease with atypia	>4
Two first-degree relatives with breast cancer	5
Atypical hyperplasia and first-degree relative with breast cancer	10

Twenty percent of women with breast cancer have a positive family history, and a clear pattern of autosomal dominant inheritance is noted in approximately 5 to 10% of all patients with breast cancer. Most of these patients have mutations of either the *BRCA1* or the *BRCA2* gene (Table 208–2). The *BRCA1* and *BRCA2* genes can be carried and passed to children by men as well as by women. Specific genetic abnormalities appear to be characteristic of specific ethnic groups. For example, only three specific mutations account for 95% of *BRCA1* and *BRCA2* carriers among Ashkenazi Jewish women. The Li-Fraumeni syndrome is a rare disorder of the *p53* gene (Chapter 186); affected patients have a high incidence of breast cancer, brain tumors, sarcomas, and leukemias. Patients with Cowden's syndrome and germline abnormalities of the *PTEN* gene have a 30 to 50% lifetime risk of breast cancer. Patients who carry the ataxia telangiectasia trait (one abnormal *ATM* gene; Chapter 271) may be at increased risk.

Clinical Manifestations

Breast cancer is usually first detected as a palpable mass or as a mammographic abnormality, but it can also be manifested by nipple discharge, changes in the skin over the breast, or breast pain. Palpable masses, including discrete masses and areas of asymmetrical thickening of breast glandular tissue, remain the most common manifestations of breast cancer and are often first detected by the patient. Paget's disease of the nipple is a form of adenocarcinoma involving the skin and lactiferous sinuses of the nipple; it usually appears as an eczematous lesion of the skin of the nipple and is frequently associated with excoriation of the skin and discharge.

Spontaneous bloody or watery discharge from the nipple is commonly associated with underlying breast malignancy. Milky discharge almost always has a benign cause. Patients with a clear or bloody discharge require breast examination and mammography. If the results of mammography and breast examination are normal and the discharge is located within a single or a few well-defined ducts, excisional biopsy of the involved ducts is indicated. A bloody discharge is frequently caused by an intraductal papilloma; a ductogram may help locate such lesions. Breast duct endoscopy has been shown to be an effective way to locate such lesions.

Breast pain is a common symptom in many women and is reported in approximately 10% of patients with breast cancer. In patients with breast cancer, the breast pain typically is associated with a palpable lump or mammographic abnormality. In premenopausal women, breast pain is a common premenstrual symptom. When pain is localized to a specific region of the breast and occurs throughout the menstrual cycle, an underlying lesion should be suspected. All patients with noncyclic breast pain should undergo a breast examination and bilateral mammography. If no abnormalities are found, evaluation of the painful area by ultrasonography or magnetic resonance imaging may help to exclude the small possibility of a malignancy.

TABLE 208–2 CHARACTERISTICS OF THE *BRCA1* AND *BRCA2* GENES

Characteristic	*BRCA1*	*BRCA2*
Chromosome location	17	13
Percentage of all breast cancers	<5%	<5%
Contribution to hereditary breast cancer	20–40%	10–30%
Population frequency (U.S.)		
General	1/345	?
Ashkenazi Jewish	1/40	~1/40
Lifetime cancer risk		
Breast cancer	56–85%	56–85%
Second primary breast cancer	~50%	~50%
Ovarian cancer	15–45%	10–20%
Male breast cancer	Low	6%
Other cancers seen in families		Prostate Pancreas Gastric Melanoma

Diagnosis

Diagnostic evaluation is typically triggered either by symptoms, by the detection of a palpable breast mass by the patient or physician, or by finding a suspicious mass on screening mammography (Fig. 208–1). Breast symptoms in the absence of a mass generally warrant mammography assessment. Most breast masses, especially those found in young premenopausal women, are benign. However, all breast masses require evaluation. In a premenopausal woman, if the mass is small and likely to be a cyst, it can be observed for 2 to 4 weeks until after the next menstrual period. If the mass persists, biopsy is indicated; all masses in postmenopausal women require prompt investigation.

Mammograms, ultrasonographic evaluation, and breast magnetic resonance imaging (Fig. 208–2) may help to characterize a mass as well as

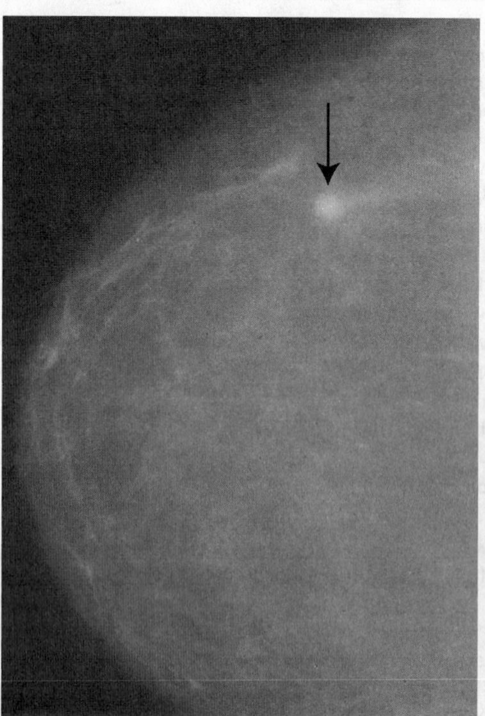

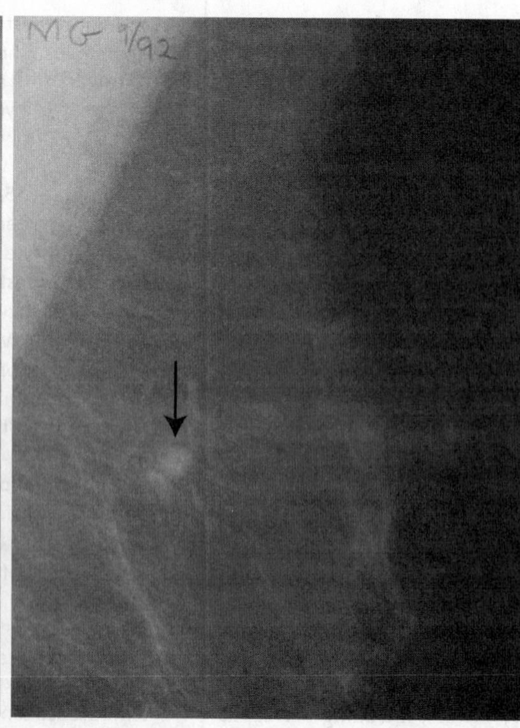

A B

FIGURE 208–1 • A positive mammogram showing a small, nonpalpable breast cancer. A, Cranial caudal view. **B,** Lateral view. The black arrow points to cancer.

to detect abnormalities in noninvolved breast tissues. All persistent masses require biopsy, even when all imaging studies are normal. As many as 15 to 25% of all palpable breast cancers are not detected with mammography.

Aspiration, Biopsy, and Pathology

Fine-needle aspiration should be considered for lesions likely to be cysts; aspiration of the fluid with resolution of the mass is adequate treatment. If the cystic fluid is clear, cytologic evaluation is not usually necessary. Core biopsy is preferable to fine-needle aspiration as a diagnostic tool for solid masses. Core biopsies provide larger tissue samples and, most importantly, are usually able to distinguish in situ from invasive lesions. Because management may be quite different for these lesions (i.e., axillary node evaluation is not indicated for in situ lesions), treatment can be guided by core biopsy. A negative fine-needle or core biopsy of a persistent breast mass should be followed by a repeat biopsy, preferably an excisional biopsy.

Carcinoma in situ accounts for approximately 15 to 25% of malignant breast disease. Carcinoma in situ is characterized by the proliferation of malignant cells within the ducts or lobules of the breast without invasion of stromal tissue. The two major subtypes are DCIS and lobular carcinoma in situ (LCIS) (Table 208–3). The remaining 75 to 85% of breast cancers are invasive. Infiltrating ductal carcinoma accounts for 85% of invasive lesions, infiltrating lobular carcinoma for 5 to 10%, medullary carcinoma for 5 to 7%, mucinous or colloid carcinoma for 3%, and tubular carcinoma for 2%.

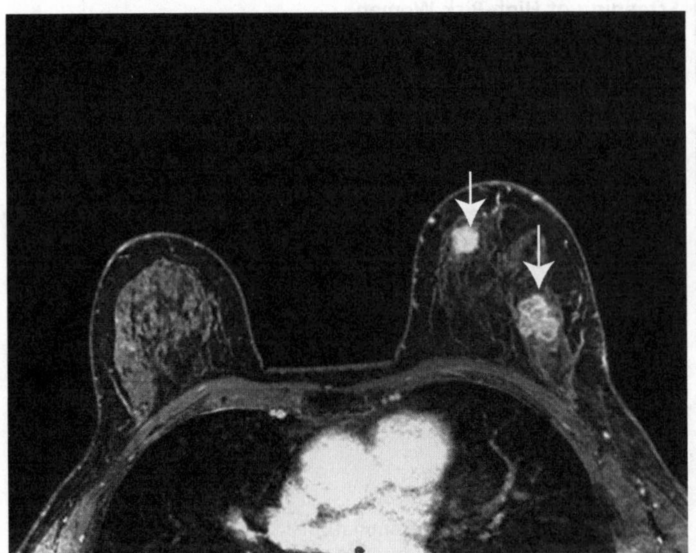

FIGURE 208–2 • A positive breast magnetic resonance image showing two breast cancers (arrows).

When matched for stage, infiltrating ductal carcinoma and infiltrating lobular carcinoma have similar prognoses, and both are more likely to metastasize than is medullary carcinoma. Tubular and colloid carcinomas are usually associated with an excellent prognosis. The histologic grade is important in determining the prognosis for women with infiltrating ductal carcinoma; when matched by stage, patients with high-grade lesions are more likely to develop metastatic disease. A few patients, mainly premenopausal, initially have inflammatory carcinoma. This lesion is associated with an almost 95% risk of distant metastases and is characterized clinically by redness and erythema involving more than half the breast and pathologically by tumor involving the dermal lymphatics of the breast.

Staging

A complete history and physical examination, complete blood cell count and chemistry profile, and chest radiography constitute an appropriate preoperative work-up for asymptomatic women with breast cancer. Women with bone pain, abdominal pain, or other symptoms should have appropriate studies of symptomatic sites. Bilateral mammograms should be performed in all women with biopsy-proven breast cancer to look for other lesions in the involved breast as well as in the opposite breast.

Metastases from invasive breast cancer probably develop early during growth of the primary lesion, proliferate in distant metastatic sites as occult "micrometastases," and become clinically detectable (~1 cm^3) after approximately 30 tumor cell doublings. The axillary lymph nodes are not barriers to metastases; the number of axillary nodes involved by tumor is directly correlated with the risk of both locoregional and distant metastases.

Staging of breast cancer is based on tumor size, the extent of breast involvement, axillary lymph node involvement, and distant metastases (the TNM system). Determination of tumor size is made by the pathologist on review of biopsy, lumpectomy, or mastectomy specimens. The staging system was revised in 2003 (Table 208–4). Survival rates based on the TNM stage are listed in Table 208–5. Currently, approximately 50 to 60% of women with newly diagnosed breast cancer are node negative, and 25 to 40% are node positive; of those who are node positive, approximately 60% have involvement of only one to three nodes. Fewer than 10% of patients are initially seen with distant metastases. Patients who present with involvement of ipsilateral supraclavicular nodes and are treated with chemotherapy, surgery, radiation, and endocrine therapy have a long-term disease-free survival rate of 20 to 30%.

In a small percentage of patients, breast cancer is manifested as an axillary mass without any breast lesion detected on physical examination, mammography, or other breast imaging modality (Chapter 215); these patients characteristically have axillary node involvement by adenocarcinoma. Such patients are best managed by axillary node dissection, ipsilateral breast irradiation (mastectomy is not mandatory and, even when performed, fails to detect a primary lesion in 30% of patients), and appropriate systemic adjuvant therapy. The natural history of disease in such patients may be somewhat better than in node-positive patients with palpable breast lesions.

TABLE 208–3 CARCINOMA IN SITU: DUCTAL VERSUS LOBULAR

Feature	Lobular Carcinoma In Situ	Ductal Carcinoma In Situ
Age	Younger	Older
Palpable mass	No	Uncommon
Mammographic appearance	Not detected on mammography	Microcalcifications, mass
Immunophenotype	E-cadherin negative	E-cadherin positive
Usual manifestation	Incidental finding on breast biopsy	Microcalcifications on mammography or breast mass
Bilateral involvement	Common	Uncertain
Risk and site of subsequent breast cancer	~25% risk for invasive breast cancer in either breast over remaining life span	At site of initial lesion; ~0.5% risk/yr of invasive breast cancer in noninvolved breast
Prevention	Consider tamoxifen	Consider tamoxifen if estrogen receptor positive
Treatment	Yearly mammography and breast examination	Lumpectomy with breast radiation; mastectomy for large or multifocal lesions

Screening

Routine Screening

The routine use of annual screening mammography in women 40 to 74 years of age reduces the likelihood of dying of breast cancer by 10 to 20%. [1] In women 40 to 49 years of age, the use of screening mammography remains controversial, but data from studies of fair quality or better show an approximately 15% reduction in the risk of breast cancer death. More extensive data indicate that a similar reduction is seen in older patients. Approximately 15 to 25% of palpable breast cancers are not imaged by mammography; this phenomenon is most common in premenopausal women and in women with dense breasts. Patients with breast cancer detected by palpation have a poorer prognosis than patients with breast cancer detected by mammographic screening alone. The sensitivity and specificity of screening mammography are also lower in postmenopausal women who are taking hormone replacement therapy and in women with dense breast tissue. The U.S. Preventative Task Force (USPTF) found fair evidence (grade B) that mammography every 12 to 33 months in women 40 to 69 years of age significantly reduced mortality from breast cancer (Chapter 13) and recommends screening mammography every 1 to 2 years in women 40 years of age and older. Screening mammography has not been rigorously tested in clinical trials in women more than 70 years old, but the USPTF recommends mammography for women 70 years of age and older who are in reasonably good health. Newer imaging methods, including digital mammography, magnetic resonance imaging of the breast, radionuclide imaging with sestamibi, and high-resolution ultrasonography are being evaluated in clinical trials but have not yet been shown to be superior to mammography for routine screening.

Physical examination by a health professional should be part of all screening programs. The value of breast self-examination is controversial, and a large randomized trial in Chinese women showed no effect of self-examination for reducing breast cancer mortality. [2] Nevertheless, substantial numbers of cancerous breast masses are first detected by self-examination. Current screening recommendations of the American Cancer Society are listed in Table 208–6; these recommendations, which include annual mammography and breast self-examinations, serve as a reasonable guideline for breast cancer screening.

Screening of High-Risk Women

Genetic tests for *BRCA1* and *BRCA2* are now commercially available (Chapter 186). Consideration of genetic testing is appropriate for women in whom breast cancer develops at a young age, women with a family history of breast or ovarian cancer (Chapter 209) in first-degree relatives, and women who are blood relatives of those with known *BRCA1* or

TABLE 208–4 STAGING OF BREAST CANCER: TNM SYSTEM

TUMOR SIZE: T (LARGEST DIAMETER)

TX	Primary tumor cannot be assessed
T0	No evidence of primary tumor
Tis	Carcinoma in situ: ductal carcinoma in situ, lobular carcinoma in situ, or Paget's disease of the nipple with no tumor
T1	Tumor ≤2 cm in greatest dimension
T2	Tumor >2 cm but not >5 cm in greatest dimension
T3	Tumor >5 cm in greatest dimension
T4	Tumor of any size with direct extension to chest wall* or skin (includes inflammatory carcinoma)

NODAL INVOLVEMENT: N (NODAL STATUS)

NX	Regional lymph nodes cannot be assessed (e.g., previously removed, not removed)
N0	No regional lymph node metastases histologically
N1	Metastasis to one to three ipsilateral axillary nodes
N2	Metastases to four to nine ipsilateral axillary nodes or internal mammary lymph nodes in the absence of axillary lymph node metastases
N3	Metastases to 10 or more ipsilateral internal mammary lymph nodes, or to internal mammary lymph nodes and axillary lymph nodes, to ipsilateral supraclavicular lymph nodes, or to ipsilateral infraclavicular lymph nodes

METASTASES: M

M0	No evidence of distant metastasis
M1	Distant metastases

*The chest wall includes the ribs, intercostal muscles, and serratus anterior but not the pectoral muscle.

From Singletary SE, Allred C, Ashley P, et al: Revision of the American Joint Committee on Cancer staging system for breast cancer. J Clin Oncol 2002;20:3628–3636.

TABLE 208–6 SCREENING RECOMMENDATIONS (AMERICAN CANCER SOCIETY)

Age Group	Examination	Frequency
20–39	Clinical breast examination	Every 3 yr
≥40 yr	Mammography	Every year, for women in good health
	Clinical breast examination	Every year
≥20 yr	Breast self-examination	An option for women but not required

TABLE 208–5 TNM STAGE AND SURVIVAL

Stage	TNM Category*	Recurrence Free at 10 Yr (No Systemic Adjuvant Therapy)
0		TisN0M0 98%
I	T1N0M0	80% (all stage I patients)
	T < 1 cm	90%
	T > 1–2 cm	80–90%
IIA	T0N1M0; T2N0M0	60–80%
IIA	T1N1M0	50–60%
IIB	T2 N1M0	5–10% worse than IIA above and based on node status
IIB	T3N0M0	30–50%
IIIA	T0 or T1 or T2N2M0; or T3N1 or N2M0	10–40%
IIIB	T4N0 or N1 or N2M0	5–30%
IIIC	Any T, N3M0	15–20%
IV	Any T, any NM1	<5%

*See Table 208–5 for TNM definitions.

BRCA2 mutations. All women who are tested for genetic abnormalities should have genetic counseling (Chapter 38). For carriers of mutations in *BRCA1* or *BRCA2,* the use of magnetic resonance mammography has been shown to be superior to standard radiographic mammography or ultrasound in detecting early breast cancers in these high-risk patients.

Most experts have recommended that women with a strong family history of breast cancer have screening performed at an age 5 to 10 years younger than that of the youngest relative in whom breast cancer has developed, but not before age 25 years. At present, no convincing evidence indicates that such screening leads to increased survival. Newer techniques, such as ductal lavage, in which cytologic examination is performed on aspirated specimens from the breast ducts, show promise and are being assessed in large clinical trials.

Prevention

Prevention of breast cancer remains a major goal. Regular exercise may lower estrogen levels and has been associated with a lower risk of breast cancer. Postmenopausal obesity is strongly correlated with an increased risk of breast cancer, probably because it is directly correlated with increased estrogen levels. Maintaining ideal or average body mass decreases risk, and low dietary fat intake may confer a small benefit.

For women who carry the *BRCA1* and *BRCA2* genes, prophylactic mastectomy will eliminate the likelihood of breast cancer in 90% or more of these patients, but it remains a controversial approach. Prophylactic oophorectomy after completion of childbearing lowers the risk of breast cancer and will substantially lower the likelihood of ovarian cancer, although areas of embryonic epithelial tissue in the peritoneal cavity remain a potential source of ovarian cancer even after oophorectomy. Tamoxifen therapy may lower the risk of breast cancer in patients with *BRCA2* mutations but appears ineffective in lowering the risk in patients with *BRCA1* mutations.

For women at high risk, defined as a risk of invasive breast cancer of 1.67% or more over 5 years, tamoxifen, 20 mg daily, reduces the risk of both invasive and noninvasive breast cancer by approximately 50% [3] in all age groups. The benefits of tamoxifen exceed the risk in all premenopausal women whose risk of breast cancer is greater than 1.5% over 5 years. In postmenopausal women who have had a hysterectomy and who therefore are not at risk of endometrial cancer, the benefit of tamoxifen exceeds its risk for women ages 50 to 59 years, 60 to 69 years, and 70 to 79 years who have 5-year risks of invasive breast cancer of 1.5%, 3.5%, and 6.0%, respectively. In postmenopausal women with an intact uterus, tamoxifen's benefit exceeds its risk for those 50 to 59 years of age and those 60 to 79 years of age who have 5-year risks of invasive breast cancer of 4.0% and 7.0%, respectively. A prevention trial comparing tamoxifen, 20 mg daily, with raloxifene, 60 mg daily, for 5 years in nearly 20,000 postmenopausal women showed that each drug reduced the risk of invasive breast cancer by approximately 50%, but raloxifene-treated patients had 36% fewer uterine cancers and 29% less venous thrombosis than tamoxifen-treated patients. [4] However, unlike tamoxifen, raloxifene did not reduce the incidence of noninvasive breast cancer (DCIS and LCIS). Aromatase inhibitors, retinoic acid derivatives, anti-inflammatory agents, phytochemicals, and statins are potential preventive agents, and several are currently being evaluated in clinical trials.

Treatment

Rx

Primary Treatment

Carcinoma In Situ

LCIS is not considered a malignant lesion but rather a marker of increased risk for subsequent breast cancer; it confers an approximately 25% lifetime risk of invasive ductal cancer in either breast. Patients with LCIS alone are currently managed by annual physical examination and mammography without additional surgery or irradiation.

Despite the better prognosis of DCIS than of invasive breast cancer, primary treatment of DCIS remains controversial, and such patients should be managed by surgeons, radiation specialists, and medical oncologists with expertise in breast cancer. Most patients with DCIS are best managed with lumpectomy (excision of the tumor mass with a clear margin around the tumor) and irradiation, but selected patients with very small lesions may be adequately treated with lumpectomy alone. Lumpectomy with or without irradiation allows for breast preservation and is preferred by most patients. At present, the best predictor of in-breast recurrence following lumpectomy alone is the extent of the normal tissue margin around the tumor; patients with DCIS in which the closest margin is 1 cm or larger have a local recurrence rate that is 10% or less. Breast irradiation following lumpectomy lowers the risk of breast recurrence, irrespective of the size of the primary lesion. Patients with lesions larger than 2.5 cm in largest diameter or close margins, or both, and those with multifocal DCIS may be best treated with mastectomy. Metastatic disease occurs in only 1 to 3% of patients with DCIS, but DCIS confers a risk of approximately 0.5% per year for developing contralateral invasive breast cancer. Axillary nodes are rarely involved, so axillary dissection is not indicated. In patients whose DCIS lesions express estrogen or progesterone receptors, tamoxifen decreases the rate of in-breast recurrence as well as the risk of contralateral breast cancer, without any documented survival effect.

In patients who have DCIS or LCIS, tamoxifen decreases the risk of both ipsilateral and contralateral invasive breast cancer by 50%. Patients with atypical ductal hyperplasia, a pathologic abnormality associated with a high-risk of subsequent breast cancer also have their breast cancer risk substantially reduced by tamoxifen.

Invasive Breast Cancer

Estrogen, Progesterone, And Her-2 Expression

Estrogen and progesterone receptor expression is important primarily to define patients who are likely to benefit from endocrine therapy, but it has little effect on long-term survival. HER-2 overexpression, found in 20% of breast cancers, confers a poorer prognosis but is most important in identifying patients who are most likely to benefit from trastuzumab.

Surgery and Radiation Therapy

Most patients with tumors smaller than 5 cm are best managed with lumpectomy followed by radiation therapy to the involved breast. This treatment is as effective as mastectomy, is associated with similar survival, and results in breast preservation. Breast irradiation following lumpectomy reduces the risk of ipsilateral breast tumor recurrence (which usually occurs at the lumpectomy site) from 40% to less than 10%, has a minimal effect on cosmetic results, and improves survival by a few percent, [5] even in patients who also receive tamoxifen. [6] For patients with larger lesions, mastectomy is usually preferred, but preoperative chemotherapy or endocrine therapy (in patients with estrogen receptor-positive tumors) may shrink the tumor and make many of these patients suitable candidates for lumpectomy and irradiation. Patients with large breast cancers or inflammatory breast cancer are best treated with preoperative ("neoadjuvant") chemotherapy followed by mastectomy and by chest wall and nodal irradiation. Patients with DCIS in addition to invasive breast cancer are managed similarly to patients with invasive breast cancer. In patients with lesions that contain both in situ and invasive components, tumor size is defined as the largest diameter of the invasive lesion.

Except in patients with small, well-differentiated primary lesions (≤5 mm) or patients with small tubular carcinomas, axillary node evaluation should be performed on most women who are suitable candidates for preventive (adjuvant) therapy (see later). Options include sentinel node biopsy and axillary node dissection; randomized trials are currently comparing these two techniques for long-term survival, but sentinel lymph node biopsy is associated with fewer complications. In most patients, an injection of isosulfan blue dye, a radioactive isotope, or both around the primary lesion or areolar area will identify the first node (or nodes) draining the primary lesion. In 95% of patients with breast cancer, the sentinel node is in the ipsilateral axilla. Patients whose sentinel node is histologically negative have less than a 5% chance of having histologically positive nodes higher in the axilla. In 60% of patients with a positive sentinel node, only the sentinel node is involved by tumor, and further axillary dissection is recommended to stage the disease in these patients.

TABLE 208–7 INFORMATION RESOURCES

Web Address or Phone Number	Description
1-800-4-CANCER	Access number for the NCI Cancer Information Service
http://www.cancer.gov	Information service of the NCI: Includes PDQ and summaries on treatment, screening, prevention, supportive care, and ongoing clinical trials; also access to CANCERLIT, NCI's bibliographic database
http://www.fda.gov/cder/cancer	U.S. Food and Drug Administration: Variety of information on cancer and approved drug therapies
http://www.ncbi.nlm.nih.gov/entrez/query.fcgi	PubMed: Access to >11,000,000 literature citations from the National Library of Medicine
http://www.asco.org	American Society of Clinical Oncology: Rich source of information for providers and patients; patient follow-up guidelines for breast cancer
http://www.cancer.org/	American Cancer Society: Excellent resources and links for providers and patients
http://www.nccn.org/	National Comprehensive Cancer Network: Treatment guidelines for patients and providers
http://www.adjuvantonline.com	Excellent site for estimating risks for recurrence and benefits of adjuvant therapy
http://www.breastcancerupdate.com/	Excellent resource for new treatment-related information and references
http://www.y-me.org	Y-me National Breast Cancer Organization: Excellent resource for patients with breast cancer
http://www.plwc.org	American Society of Clinical Oncology's website devoted to "People Living with Cancer": An excellent site for patients seeking information on all types of cancer
http://www.komen.org	Susan G. Komen Breast Cancer Foundation: Excellent resource for information about breast cancer

NCI = National Cancer Institute.

Rx

Preoperative chemotherapy, which involves the use of four to eight courses of an active chemotherapy regimen or a single agent before definitive treatment of the primary tumor, can cause tumor regression in as many as 90% of patients, and 5 to 25% of these patients demonstrate complete regression of the tumor pathologically as well as clinically. However, preoperative chemotherapy is not superior to postoperative therapy in preventing metastases. The major use of preoperative chemotherapy is to convert a large primary lesion requiring mastectomy to a smaller lesion that is amenable to lumpectomy and breast conservation. Recent data suggest that preoperative endocrine therapy may be as effective as chemotherapy in shrinking tumors in patients with estrogen or progesterone receptor–positive lesions, even though only a few patients achieve complete pathologic responses to such treatment.

Psychosocial Support

Most patients should be offered psychosocial support shortly after diagnosis because counseling and support groups can help patients, especially those who are most distressed, to cope better with breast cancer, particularly during the first several years after diagnosis. Although some trials suggested that such support may be associated with improved survival, most trials have not shown a survival benefit. Many women may wish to become more involved in advocacy groups (Table 208–7).

Reconstruction

Breast reconstruction, performed at the same time as or after mastectomy, provides an opportunity for women to overcome the psychological damage that frequently follows mastectomy and helps to relieve the patient's sense of deformity. Saline or silicone implants are safe, less costly, and generally easy to perform, whereas flaps from autogenous tissue eliminate the need for the foreign materials and are more suitable for large defects. Excellent evidence now indicates that silicone implants do not increase the risk of breast cancer or connective tissue disorders. The remaining breast frequently requires surgical correction to match the reconstructed side. Although reconstruction frequently achieves excellent results, the cosmetic results of lumpectomy and breast irradiation are usually far superior.

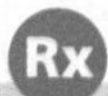

Adjuvant Therapy

Adjuvant therapy is defined as the use of chemotherapy, hormonal therapy, radiation therapy, biologic therapy, or a combination of these before, during, or after definitive treatment of the primary breast cancer. The objective of adjuvant therapy is to destroy small, clinically occult, distant micrometastases. Because micrometastases cannot be detected clinically, patients who have been cured by their primary treatment and patients who truly have micrometastases will both be treated. In addition, adjuvant therapy probably delays disease recurrence for a median of 2 to 3 years in the majority of treated women. [7]

Recommendations for adjuvant therapy are based on menopausal status, tumor size, tumor grade, the presence of lymph node involvement, and the estrogen and progesterone receptor and HER-2 status of the tumor; such recommendations should be made in consultation with a surgical, medical, and/or radiation oncologist (Table 208–8). Adjuvant therapy results in a proportional decrease in risk of recurrence that is similar for all patients irrespective of their risk for metastases, and the reduction varies according to the type of adjuvant therapy. Therefore, the absolute benefit of adjuvant therapy is greater for individuals with greater risk of recurrence.

ADJUVANT ENDOCRINE THERAPY. Tamoxifen (20 mg/day for 5 years) has been the most widely used endocrine agent and, when added to chemotherapy, improves survival in both premenopausal and postmenopausal patients who are estrogen or progesterone receptor positive. Its estrogen-agonist effects on bone and liver help to maintain bone density and to lower cholesterol levels in postmenopausal women, but the drug may cause bone loss in premenopausal women. Over a period of 5 years, use of tamoxifen results in a 1% risk of endometrial cancer and a 1% incidence of deep venous thrombosis; it can cause or exacerbate hot flashes in 10 to 30% of postmenopausal women.

Aromatase inhibitors, including anastrozole (1 mg/day for 5 years), exemestane (25 mg/day for 2 to 3 years after 2 to 3 years of tamoxifen), and letrozole (2.5 mg/day for 5 years initially or after 5 years of tamoxifen), generally show a small but significant 3 to 5% decrease in recurrence rates compared with tamoxifen in postmenopausal women with hormone-positive breast cancer. [8] In addition, letrozole improves survival in women with positive lymph

TABLE 208–8 ADJUVANT TREATMENT GUIDELINES FOR PATIENTS WITH EARLY-STAGE INVASIVE BREAST CANCER*

Patient Group*	Treatment
Favorable Histology (Tubular or Colloid)	
ER- and/or PR-positive breast cancer	
<1 cm	No adjuvant therapy
1–2.9 cm	Consider adjuvant hormonal therapy + adjuvant chemotherapy†
≥3 cm or node-postive	Adjuvant hormonal therapy + adjuvant chemotherapy
ER- and PR-negative	
<1 cm	No adjuvant therapy
1–2.9 cm	Consider adjuvant chemotherapy
≥3 cm or node-positive	Adjuvant chemotherapy
Hormone Receptor Positive Breast Cancer (ER- and/or PR-positive)	
Lymph-nodes negative	
≤0.5 cm	No adjuvant therapy
0.6–1.0 cm well differentiated and no unfavorable features‡	Consider adjuvant hormonal therapy
0.6–1.0 cm moderate or poorly differentiated or unfavorable features	Adjuvant hormonal therapy ± adjuvant chemotherapy
>1 cm	Adjuvant hormonal therapy ± adjuvant chemotherapy
Lymph-nodes positive	Adjuvant hormonal therapy + adjuvant chemotherapy
Hormone Receptor Negative Breast Cancer (ER- and PR-negative)	
≤0.5 cm	No adjuvant therapy
0.6–1.0 cm	Consider chemotherapy
>1 cm or lymph-node positive	Adjuvant chemotherapy
HER-2 positive	Trastuzumab should be added to the suggested treatment above for all node-positive patients; trastuzumab not recommended for tumors ≤1 cm for most node-negative patients; for tumors >1 cm, trastuzumab should be considered for most patients

*Data are insufficient to make chemotherapy recommendations for patients ≥70 yr. Treatment should be individualized for these patients based on life expectancy and comorbidity.
†In ER-positive or PR-positive patients, decisions regarding the added value of chemotherapy in addition to hormonal therapy alone can be aided by accurately assessing the added value of chemotherapy in individual patients using a web-based model: www.adjuvantonline.com.
‡Unfavorable characteristics include high-grade tumor, blood vessel or lymphatic invasion by tumor, and high tumor proliferation rate (high S-phase by flow cytometry or high Ki-67 value by immunohistochemistry) or HER-2–positive status.
ER = estrogen receptor; PR = progesterone receptor.
Modified from National Comprehensive Cancer Network Guidelines. Available at www.nccn.org.

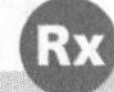

nodes. Unlike tamoxifen, aromatase inhibitors are not associated with an increased risk of thromboembolism or endometrial cancer, but they are associated with a higher risk of arthralgia, myalgia, bone loss, and fractures compared with tamoxifen. Patients treated with aromatase inhibitors should be monitored for osteopenia and osteoporosis and should be managed accordingly (Chapter 264). The optimal use of aromatase inhibitors is uncertain, but it is now recommended that all postmenopausal women with hormone receptor–positive breast cancer receive an aromatase inhibitor at sometime in the course of their adjuvant treatment.

In premenopausal women with estrogen or progesterone-positive tumors, ovarian ablation and older chemotherapy regimens appear equally effective in improving survival. However, there is added value for chemotherapy in most higher-risk premenopausal patients. Current trials are also investigating the addition of ovarian ablation to tamoxifen or aromatase inhibitors in these patients.

Chemotherapy

Combinations of several chemotherapeutic agents given concurrently are superior to single-drug treatment, and short courses of chemotherapy (3 to 6 months) are as effective as longer treatments. The most effective chemotherapy regimens include anthracyclines (epirubicin or doxorubicin), [9] and, for high-risk patients, they integrate new biologic agents or other drugs such as taxanes. More recently, the addition of trastuzumab, a humanized monoclonal antibody targeted against the transmembrane protein encoded by the *HER-2* oncogene, to chemotherapy in patients with HER-2–positive breast cancer resulted in a further 50% reduction in relapse when compared with chemotherapy alone. [10] Trastuzumab can cause myocardial damage and heart failure in a small percentage of patients, so monitoring of left ventricular function is mandatory.

Radiation Therapy

Radiation therapy to the chest wall following mastectomy decreases the rate of local recurrence at the mastectomy site and in the regional nodes in node-positive women with early-stage breast cancer, and it improves these women's survival by a few percentage points. Chest wall irradiation after mastectomy should be offered to all women with large primary lesions (≥5 cm, irrespective of nodal involvement) and to those with extensive nodal involvement (four or more positive lymph nodes). The use of routine chest wall irradiation after mastectomy in patients with one to three positive lymph nodes remains controversial. Although routine post-mastectomy chest wall irradiation is generally well tolerated, it increases the risk of lymphedema in the upper extremity on the side of the mastectomy and is associated with a very small risk of radiation-induced malignancy. Breast radiation after lumpectomy reduces in-breast recurrence by approximately two thirds and also improves survival by a few percentage points.

Follow-up of Early-Stage Patients

Routine follow-up visits provide a forum for patients to discuss their fears and concerns and for physicians to provide reassurance and to obtain annual mammograms (Table 208–9). Intensive follow-up of asymptomatic patients after the diagnosis and treatment of early-stage breast cancer by routine laboratory tests, tumor marker assessment (carcinoembryonic antigen, CA-15.3, and CA-27.29), and imaging studies (e.g., chest radiographs, bone scans, computed tomography, magnetic resonance imaging, or ultrasonography of the liver, or positron emission tomography) may occasionally detect recurrence before signs or symptoms develop, but early detection by these means has not improved survival or quality of life.

Even when frequent imaging and laboratory testing are performed, approximately 75% of recurrences are detected by the physician or the patient from signs and symptoms. Locoregional recurrence on the chest wall or in regional lymph nodes accounts for approximately 20 to 40% of initial recurrences, bone for 15 to 65%, lung for 15 to 25%, liver for 5 to 25%, and the central nervous system for 5 to 15%. Almost one third of initial recurrences occur in soft tissue and nodal areas; physical examination remains the mainstay of such detection.

TABLE 208–9 FOLLOW-UP GUIDELINES FOR PATIENTS WITH EARLY-STAGE BREAST CANCER: AMERICAN SOCIETY OF CLINICAL ONCOLOGY GUIDELINES*

Procedure or Test	Frequency
History and physical examination* (eliciting of symptoms of breast cancer)	Every 3–6 mo for first 3 yr, every 6–12 mo for next yr, then yearly
Mammography	
Mastectomy patients	Yearly
Lumpectomy patients	Yearly
Pelvic examination	Yearly
Breast self-examination	Monthly
Complete blood cell counts and chemistry studies	The literature does not support the use of these tests
Chest radiography, bone scans, PET scans, breast MRI, liver imaging, and tumor marker studies	Not recommended for routine follow-up in asymptomatic patients
Patient education regarding signs and symptoms of recurrence	Each visit

*Limited evaluation: Assess for pain, dyspnea, weight loss, and other major changes in function. The limited examination should include an assessment of nodes, axillae, lumpectomy or mastectomy site, chest, and abdomen. Patients should be instructed regarding symptoms of recurrence.

Modified from Khatcheressian JL, Wolff AC, Smith TJ, et al: American Society of Clinical Oncology 2006 update of the breast cancer follow-up and management guidelines in the adjuvant setting. J Clin Oncol 2006;24:5091–5097.

Treatment of Metastatic Disease

Only 1 to 3% of patients treated with standard endocrine therapy or chemotherapy regimens attain long-term remission. Breast cancer can recur at any site, and the median survival for all patients after recurrence remains 2 to 3 years, with a 5-year survival rate less than 20%. Responses must last for at least 1 month and are defined as complete (disappearance of all metastatic lesions), partial (30% reduction in tumor mass based on the sum of the largest diameters of measurable lesions before and after treatment), stable (<30% reduction or a 25% increase in measurable lesions for 3 to 4 months), and progressing (continued growth or new lesions during therapy).

Endocrine Therapy

Response to endocrine therapy is seen in 30 to 70% of women who are hormone receptor positive and in perhaps 10% who are receptor negative. Women who are older, who have a long disease-free interval (time from diagnosis to metastases), who are progesterone as well as estrogen receptor positive, or who have bone or soft tissue lesions are most likely to respond.

In premenopausal women, tamoxifen (20 mg/day continued until disease progression) and ovarian ablation are the treatments of choice. Aromatase inhibitors are contraindicated in premenopausal women unless ovarian ablation has been performed. Ovarian ablation can be done surgically, with external beam irradiation, or medically, with luteinizing hormone–releasing hormone agonists, such as goserelin, 3.6 mg every 28 days subcutaneously into upper abdominal wall, or leuprolide, 3.75 mg/month intramuscularly. Combining ovarian ablation with tamoxifen or an aromatase inhibitor may provide higher response rates, longer time to tumor progression, and superior survival when compared with treatment with oophorectomy or tamoxifen alone.

In postmenopausal women, aromatase inhibitors are superior to tamoxifen and progestins (megestrol, 160 mg/day orally in four equally divided doses. Fulvestant (250 mg intramuscularly every month) is as effective as an aromatase inhibitor and can also be used. In addition, high-dose estrogens may be helpful in these patients as third- or fourth-line therapy. Ovarian ablation is not effective in postmenopausal women.

Responses to initial hormonal therapy last an average of 6 to 12 months. Patients who respond to one agent have a fair chance of responding to a second hormonal agent after failure of initial therapy.

Chemotherapy

Chemotherapy is best reserved for women who have tumor progression while receiving hormonal therapy or whose cancers lack hormone receptors. Approximately 40 to 80% of patients have a complete or partial response to their initial chemotherapy that generally persists for 6 to 12 months. Responses to second- and third-line chemotherapy are less frequent but usually persist only for several months. Sequential, single-agent therapy, using taxanes (paclitaxel, 175 mg/m^2 intravenously over 3 hours every 3 weeks or 80 to 100 mg/m^2 weekly; docetaxel, 60 to 100 mg/m^2 intravenously over 1 hour every 3 weeks; protein-bound paclitaxel (Abraxane), 260 mg/m^2 intravenously over 30 minutes every 3 weeks), capecitabine (1000 mg/m^2 orally twice daily for 2 weeks then 1 week off in 3-week cycles), gemcitabine (1000 mg/m^2 intravenously over 30 minutes weekly) or vinorelbine (30 mg/m^2 intravenously over 6 to 10 minutes weekly), provides similar survival, better quality of life, and less toxicity compared with combination regimens. High-dose chemotherapy with autologous bone marrow or stem cell transplantation yields results that are generally similar to those of standard chemotherapy and should not be used in women with metastatic disease.

Trastuzumab alone (4 mg/kg intravenously as a 90-minute infusion initially, then 2 mg/kg weekly as a 30-minute infusion) is associated with response rates of approximately 25% when used as first-line therapy in women with HER-2–positive tumors. Single-agent or combination chemotherapy in addition to trastuzumab provides significantly higher response rates, time to tumor progression, and survival times as compared with standard chemotherapy alone in HER-2–positive patients.

Other biologic agents targeted to epidermal growth factor receptor pathways and to blocking tumor angiogenesis are being studied intensely. When added to paclitaxel, the angiogenesis inhibitor bevacizumab (at 5 mg/kg every 14 days intravenously starting 28 days after any major surgery and continuing until disease progression), significantly improves response rates and time to disease progression compared with paclitaxel alone. Numerous new small molecules targeted to key signaling domains related to breast cancer growth and metastases are being developed and tested. Vaccines targeted against transmembrane glycoproteins coded by the *MUC-1* oncogene are also being evaluated in clinical trials.

Centralized Nervous System, Spinal Cord, and Leptomeningeal Metastases

Spinal cord compression is most commonly seen in patients with bone metastases, and almost all patients have back pain and radiographic evidence of spinal metastases. Magnetic resonance imaging is currently the imaging method of choice to establish the diagnosis. For patients with rapid loss of function or major symptoms, emergency surgical decompression is the favored management approach to lower the probability of paraplegia. Patients with leptomeningeal metastases frequently have headaches and lesions of cranial and peripheral nerves; the diagnosis is best made with lumbar puncture and examination of cerebrospinal fluid for malignant cells. Gadolinium-enhanced magnetic resonance imaging of the brain or spinal cord shows enhancement of the meninges in approximately 70% of patients with leptomeningeal spread.

Radiation therapy can be an extremely effective palliative therapy for central nervous system metastases and spinal cord compression. Dexamethasone, in doses of 4 to 10 mg every 6 hours, should be used in conjunction with irradiation. For leptomeningeal metastases, intrathecal chemotherapy (methotrexate and other agents) can lead to brief remission, but the general outlook for such patients remains exceedingly poor.

Rx

Skeletal Metastases

Bisphosphonates (pamidronate, 90 mg over 2 to 4 hours, or zoledronate, 4 mg intravenously every 3 or 4 weeks) significantly reduce complications from skeletal metastases in both premenopausal and postmenopausal patients, but these drugs do not improve survival. Osteonecrosis of the mandible, especially after recent dental procedures, is a potential complication of bisphosphonates in this setting, and patients should be closely monitored for this rare complication.

External beam irradiation results in significant palliation in patients with moderate to severe bone pain at specific metastatic sites. Radioisotopes that localize in bone, such as strontium-89 and samarium-153, also may be effective.

Hypercalcemia is a common complication of metastatic breast cancer (Chapters 188 and 266) and is more likely to occur in patients with skeletal metastases. Initial treatment of symptomatic patients includes hydration, bisphosphonates, and diuresis. Calcitonin (starting at 4 IU/kg every 12 hours, increasing by 8 IU/kg every 12 hours if no response) and glucocorticoids or plicamycin (25 μg/kg/day intravenously for 3 to 4 days) can also be effective in patients who need rapid reduction of their serum calcium level. Ultimate control depends on the response to systemic therapy.

Surgery

Patients with isolated or minimal metastatic disease (one to three lesions) to the central nervous system, lung, or liver and those who have limited or no other metastatic disease may benefit from surgical resection of metastatic lesions. Moreover, patients with locoregional recurrence are best managed by surgical resection of chest wall lesions when feasible, followed by external beam irradiation of the involved area. Chest tube drainage and sclerotherapy are successful in approximately 70% of patients with persistent or recurrent malignant effusions that have not been controlled by systemic therapy. Patients with a recurrent ipsilateral breast tumor after lumpectomy alone may be managed with repeat resection and breast irradiation; tumors recurring after lumpectomy and breast radiation are usually best managed by mastectomy, although further lumpectomy may be appropriate in patients with small recurrences.

Other Issues in Treatment

Breast Cancer in Older Women

Most new breast cancers in the United States occur in women 65 years and older. Older women are less likely to have mammographic screening, to be offered the opportunity for breast preservation, to receive breast radiation after lumpectomy, to be considered for adjuvant therapy, and to be treated aggressively for metastases. However, older women in reasonably good health are able to tolerate and benefit from treatment similar to younger women, so they should be offered the same prevention, diagnostic, and treatment options as their younger peers. Women who are more than 70 years old and who have short estimated life spans and small, node-negative, hormone receptor–positive breast cancers and can be adequately managed with lumpectomy and endocrine therapy, without breast radiation.

Breast Cancer in Men

Men account for approximately 0.8% of cases of breast cancer, and the disease is more common in men with benign breast disease, testicular disease, Klinefelter's syndrome, *BRCA-2* abnormalities, or a positive family history. Treatment recommendations are similar to those for women.

Breast Cancer and Pregnancy

The diagnosis of breast cancer during pregnancy (Chapter 258) is extremely traumatic. Such patients are usually first seen when their disease is at higher stages, probably because of difficulties in diagnosis. After the first trimester, definitive surgical procedures can usually be performed with minimal risk to the mother and fetus. Chemotherapy administered after the first trimester has not been associated with increased fetal loss or birth defects. Limited data suggest that development is normal in children of mothers who have received chemotherapy during pregnancy. Alkylating agents given during pregnancy frequently cause subsequent infertility. Hormonal agents should be avoided during pregnancy. Pregnancy following breast cancer, especially 2 to 3 years after diagnosis, does not appear to increase the risk of metastatic disease. Major considerations relating to childbearing after breast cancer should be based on the risks of recurrence.

Rx

Hormone Replacement Therapy after Breast Cancer

Hormone replacement with estrogen-progestin therapy in women with a diagnosis of breast cancer should be avoided; the safety of estrogens alone after hysterectomy is controversial (Chapter 262). A short course of hormone replacement therapy can be considered in patients with early-stage breast cancer who have truly disabling vasomotor symptoms. The bone benefits of hormone replacement therapy can be accomplished using bisphosphonates.

Lymphedema

Lymphedema develops in the ipsilateral arm in approximately 15% of women with breast cancer following primary therapy. The incidence may be slightly higher in women treated with lumpectomy and radiation and is lower in women managed with sentinel lymph node procedures. Symptoms are usually mild but persistent; slowly progressive edema can lead to functional loss. Early recognition is key, and patients should be asked about this complication at each routine follow-up visit. Affected patients should be referred to physical therapists and other health professionals skilled in the management of lymphedema. Treatment consists of avoidance of trauma, special exercises, elevation of the extremity, and the use of compression pumps and specially fitted compression stockings. Manual lymphatic drainage procedures may be more effective than compression pumping. Diuretics are rarely effective and should be avoided.

Prognosis

The essential prognostic factors for predicting the risk of metastases are (1) invasion (DCIS and other noninvasive tumors have excellent prognoses), (2) tumor size, (3) tumor grade, (4) the number of involved ipsilateral axillary nodes, and (5) histologic grade. Lymphovascular invasion by tumor cells generally also confers a poorer outcome.

Primary tumors with an invasive component 1 cm or smaller in largest diameter generally have a very good prognosis, with an overall survival rate of 90% or more. Poorly differentiated tumors tend to have more aggressive growth patterns and are associated with a poorer prognosis. Evaluation of gene expression with polymerase chain reaction or microarray techniques has shown great promise in helping to define the prognosis of individual patients as well as the likelihood of their response to treatment. Commercial assays to predict outcome for individual patients are now available but are not considered the standard of care.

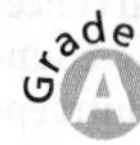

1. Gotzsche PC, Nielsen M: Screening for breast cancer with mammography. Cochrane Database Syst Rev. 2006;4:CD001877.
2. Thomas DB, Gao DL, Ray RM, et al: Randomized trial of breast self-examination in Shanghai: Final results. J Natl Cancer Inst 2002;94:1445–1457.
3. Cuzick J, Powles T, Veronesi U, et al: Overview of the main outcomes in breast-cancer prevention trials. Lancet 2003;361: 296–300.
4. Vogel VG, Constantino JP, Wickerham DL, et al: Effects of tamoxifen vs raloxifene on the risk of developing invasive breast cancer and other disease outcomes: The NSABP study of tamoxifen and raloxifene (STAR) P-2 trial. JAMA 2006;295:2727–2741.
5. Fisher B, Anderson S, Bryant J, et al: Twenty-year follow-up of a randomized trial comparing total mastectomy, lumpectomy, and lumpectomy plus irradiation for the treatment of invasive breast cancer. N Engl J Med 2002;347:1233–1241.
6. Fyles AW, McCready DR, Manchul LA, et al: Tamoxifen with or without breast irradiation in women 50 years of age or older with early breast cancer. N Engl J Med 2004;351:963–970.
7. Early Breast Cancer Trialists' Collaborative Group (EBCTCG): Effects of chemotherapy and hormonal therapy for early breast cancer on recurrence and 15-year survival: An overview of the randomised trials. Lancet 2005;365:1687–1717.

8. Breast International Group (BIG) 1-98 Collaborative Group: A comparison of letrozole and tamoxifen in postmenopausal women with early breast cancer. N Engl J Med 2005;353: 2747–2757.
9. Poole CJ, Earl HM, Hiller L, et al: Epirubicin and cyclophosphamide, methotrexate, and fluorouracil as adjuvant therapy for early breast cancer. N Engl J Med 2006;355:1851–1862.
10. Romond EH, Perez EA, Bryant J, et al: Trastuzumab plus adjuvant chemotherapy for operable HER2-positive breast cancer. N Engl J Med 2005;353:1673–1684.

SUGGESTED READINGS

Adjuvant Online. Available at http://www.adjuvantonline.com. *Estimates of the benefit of adjuvant therapy.*

Arpino G, Laucirica R, Elledge RM: Premalignant and in situ breast disease: Biology and clinical implications. Ann Intern Med 2005;143:446–457. *Overview of premalignant breast lesions, risk for invasive cancer with each type of lesion, predictors of progression, and clinical management.*

Berry DA, Cronin KA, Plevritis SK, et al: Effect of screening and adjuvant therapy on mortality from breast cancer. N Engl J Med 2005;353:1784–1792. *Screening mammography and treatment have helped to reduce the rate of death from breast cancer in the United States.*

Fentiman IS, Fourquet A, Hortobagyi GN: Male breast cancer. Lancet 2006;367:595–604. *A comprehensive review.*

Moss S, Cuckle H, Evans A, et al: Effect of mammographic screening from age 40 years on breast cancer mortality at 10 years' follow-up: a randomised controlled trial. Lancet 2006;368:2053–2060. *Though not statistically significant, the 17% benefit was consistent with the results of other studies.*

Prentice RL, Caan B, Chlebowski RT, et al: Low-fat dietary pattern and risk of invasive breast cancer: The Women's Health Initiative Randomized Controlled Dietary Modification Trial. JAMA 2006;295:629–642. *The rate was 0.03% lower per year in the intervention group (0.42%) than in the control group (0.45%; HR 0.91; 95% CI 0.83–1.01).*

Santen RJ, Mansel R: Benign breast disorders. N Engl J Med 2005;353:275–285. *A comprehensive review.*

Smith RL, Pruthi S, Fitzpatrick LA: Evaluation and management of breast pain. Mayo Clin Proc 2004;79:353–372. *Pain rarely indicates cancer and usually responds to nonpharmacologic therapy.*

U.S. Preventive Services Task Force: Genetic risk assessment and *BRCA* mutation testing for breast and ovarian cancer susceptibility: Recommendation statement. Ann Intern Med 2005;143:355–361. *Recommends genetic risk assessment and BRCA mutation testing for women with a family history associated with an increased risk for deleterious mutations.*

Veronesi U, Boyle P, Goldhirsch A, et al: Breast cancer. Lancet 2005;365: 1727–1741. *A comprehensive review.*

209 GYNECOLOGIC CANCERS

Kelly L. Molpus and Howard W. Jones III

Gynecologic tumors may originate in the vulva, vagina, cervix, uterus, fallopian tubes, ovaries, peritoneum, or placenta. Uterine cancers, which are the most common, frequently arise from the endometrial lining of the uterus and usually are diagnosed when the disease is confined to the uterus. Ovarian carcinoma is the second most frequent; signs and symptoms are nonspecific, and most ovarian cancers are not diagnosed until disease has spread to the abdomen or distant sites. Invasive cervical cancer is one of the most common malignant neoplasms in developing countries but is now uncommon in the United States, where cervical intraepithelial neoplasia is more common. Vulvar carcinoma arises from the external genitalia (vulva) and accounts for only 1 to 2% of all gynecologic cancers. Primary vaginal tumors are rare and manifest like cervical cancers. Primary peritoneal carcinomas can be indistinguishable from ovarian carcinoma. Primary fallopian tube carcinomas are rare and share characteristics of ovarian and primary peritoneal tumors. Gestational trophoblastic tumors range from benign to overtly malignant neoplasms that result from abnormal proliferation of trophoblastic tissue associated with a normal or abnormal pregnancy.

UTERINE CANCER

Epidemiology

Uterine malignant neoplasms usually arise from the glandular component of the endometrial lining. Infrequently, tumors arise from the endometrial stroma or from the smooth muscle and connective tissue within the wall of the uterus. In the United States, an estimated 40,880 new cases of endometrial cancer are diagnosed annually, and about 7300 women die of the disease. The lifetime risk is approximately 2% for the general population. Most women with uterine cancer are postmenopausal, but about 5% of patients are diagnosed before the age of 40 years. For type I endometrial cancers, a risk factor is excessive estrogenic stimuli, and women taking unopposed estrogen replacement therapy have about a 9.5-fold increased risk. Breast cancer patients taking tamoxifen for 5 years have an estimated 1.7- to 4-fold increased relative risk. Women who are 50 pounds above their ideal body weight have an estimated 10-fold increased risk for development of endometrial adenocarcinoma because of prolonged stimulation of the endometrium by estrone, a weak estrogen that is converted from adrenal androstenedione in adipose tissue. Hypertension, diabetes, early menarche, late menopause, and nulliparity are also considered risk factors. In contrast, type II endometrial cancers tend to occur in older, thinner women without exogenous estrogen exposure and tend to be higher grade, clinically aggressive tumors.

Pathobiology

Endometrial hyperplasia with cellular atypia (increased nuclear-to-cytoplasmic ratio, pleomorphism, multinucleated cells) has an approximately 30% chance of malignant transformation, and early adenocarcinomas often arise within a background of atypical endometrial hyperplasia. It is unlikely, however, that all endometrial carcinomas transition through a detectable premalignant phase. Although no genetic cause of uterine cancer has been identified, endometrial carcinomas are the most common extracolonic malignant neoplasms in women with Lynch II/hereditary nonpolyposis colon cancer syndrome (Chapter 203), with an estimated lifetime risk of 22 to 43%.

Clinical Manifestations

Endometrial cancer is often diagnosed at an early stage because more than 90% of patients present with abnormal bleeding. Atrophic changes are the most common cause of postmenopausal bleeding, and only about 10% of women who present with bleeding actually have carcinoma. Nevertheless, any postmenopausal spotting, isolated bleeding episode, or blood-tinged vaginal discharge warrants further evaluation. Younger women commonly present with intermenstrual bleeding (metrorrhagia) or heavy menstrual bleeding (menorrhagia).

Diagnosis

Endometrial tissue sampling is the only definitive way to establish the diagnosis. Endometrial biopsy in the office can obtain adequate tissue samples in 90 to 95% of patients, with an accurate diagnosis rendered in 85% (false-negative rate of 15%). All endometrial surfaces should be sampled. If endometrial biopsy results are inconclusive or inconsistent with the clinical presentation, a dilation and curettage may be necessary. Direct visualization of the uterine cavity and removal of lesions by hysteroscopy may be warranted in selected patients if bleeding persists or the cause of the uterine bleeding remains uncertain. Preoperative hysteroscopy may increase the incidence of positive (malignant) peritoneal cytologic results, the prognostic significance of which remains uncertain.

Transvaginal pelvic ultrasonography and sonohysterography are alternative means to delineate the endometrial anatomy. These diagnostic tests may be useful in identifying women who have uterine bleeding due to atrophy. Endometrial atrophy is the most likely cause of postmenopausal bleeding and can be reliably diagnosed when a symmetrical endometrial stripe is visualized with a thickness of 5.0 mm or less. As the stripe thickness increases above 5.0 mm, the risk of significant disease (atypical hyperplasia, carcinoma) increases proportionately, and an endometrial biopsy is indicated.

The Papanicolaou (Pap) smear has no established role in the screening or diagnosis of uterine carcinoma. Women who have breast cancer and are taking tamoxifen are at increased risk of endometrial cancer. These women should have an annual pelvic examination, but neither ultrasonography nor endometrial biopsy is indicated in the absence of atypical bleeding.

TABLE 209–1 DISTRIBUTION AND PROGNOSIS OF GYNECOLOGIC CANCER

	Stage*	Percentage of Patients	5-Year Survival Rate (%)
ENDOMETRIAL ADENOCARCINOMA			
I	Corpus only	70.2	87.4
II	Cervical involvement	12.4	76.3
III	Pelvic metastases	13.3	56.6
IV	Distant metastases	4.1	17.8
EPITHELIAL OVARIAN CANCER			
IA	Ovary only	12.7	89.9
IIB	Pelvic metastases	3.2	63.7
IIIC	Abdominal metastases >2 cm	40.0	28.7
IV	Extra-abdominal metastases	11.9	16.8
CANCER OF THE CERVIX			
IB-1	Cervix only	33.2	90.5
IIB	Parametrium	23.7	73.3
IIIB	Pelvic sidewall	19.3	46.4
IV	Metastatic	3.9	25.2

*Note: Not all substages are listed in this table.
From Pecorelli S, Benedet JL, Boyle P, et al: FIGO annual report on the results of treatment in gynecological cancer; vol 24. J Epidemiol Biostat 2001;6:7–43.

Prevention and Treatment

Women who have simple or complex hyperplasia without cellular atypia may be treated with progestins to offset the estrogenic stimulation. Because of the risk of associated endometrial cancer, atypical hyperplasia is best treated with hysterectomy. In patients who are medically inoperable or who wish to preserve fertility, however, progestins are an alternative in combination with clinical surveillance. Follow-up biopsy may be indicated to ensure regression of the hyperplasia or nonprogression to carcinoma.

Endometrial carcinoma is treated with hysterectomy and bilateral salpingo-oophorectomy. Additional surgical staging is individualized on the basis of the tumor's grade, size, and depth of myometrial invasion as well as the presence or absence of endocervical extension or extrauterine disease. The most common route of extrauterine spread is to the pelvic lymph nodes; metastases to the para-aortic nodes are uncommon in the absence of positive pelvic nodes. Metastases to the ovary are found in as many as 6 to 10% of women in whom disease appears confined to the uterus, thereby warranting routine salpingo-oophorectomy.

Post-surgical therapy depends on the surgical stage, grade, and extent of disease. Low-grade tumors confined to the uterus have an excellent chance of cure with surgery alone. Lymph node metastases are a poor prognostic finding, and most such patients are treated with postoperative radiation therapy to include the affected lymphatics. Women with advanced-stage, metastatic, or recurrent disease require multimodality therapy and should be included in clinical trials when they are available. Metastatic endometrial adenocarcinoma responds poorly to chemotherapy.

Prognosis

The majority of endometrial cancers can be cured because their presenting symptoms lead to rapid diagnosis and treatment (Table 209–1). Prognosis worsens as the extent of disease is more advanced. Patients who have isolated pelvic or para-aortic lymph node metastases and who are treated with adjunctive radiation therapy have an estimated 40 to 50% 5-year survival.

OVARIAN CARCINOMA

Epidemiology

Ovarian carcinoma is the most deadly of the gynecologic malignant neoplasms. The incidence gradually rises and reaches a peak at about 70 years of age, at which age the incidence is 55 per 100,000 among white women but somewhat lower in African American women. The lifetime risk of ovarian cancer for women in the United States is about 1.4%, but women with one first-degree relative who has had ovarian cancer appear to have an increased risk of 3 to 5%. The cause of ovarian cancer is unknown. *BRCA1* or *BRCA2* (Chapter 208) gene mutations are found in about 10% of women with epithelial ovarian cancer. Rare families with a high incidence of ovarian, breast, endometrial, and colon cancer represent the hereditary nonpolyposis colon cancer syndrome (Lynch syndrome II) (Chapters 186 and 203). Multiple pregnancies and the use of oral contraceptives exert a protective effect, perhaps because of decreased ovulation.

Pathobiology

There are four types of ovarian tumors. Common *epithelial tumors* of the ovary include serous, mucinous, endometrioid, clear cell, and otherwise unspecified adenocarcinomas; these tumors account for almost 90% of ovarian cancers and are most commonly found in postmenopausal women. *Germ cell tumors,* which arise from the totipotent oocytes, are usually benign ("dermoid cysts"); they often occur in young women and are almost always unilateral. When these tumors are malignant (e.g., dysgerminoma, teratoma), they are highly aggressive but respond well to combination chemotherapy. *Stromal tumors* are generally low grade and arise from the granulosa, theca, and Sertoli-Leydig cells of the ovary; they may be hormonally functional. These tumors are usually unilateral and may occur in any age group but most typically occur in the fourth and fifth decades. Surgical excision may be sufficient, but combination chemotherapy is effective for metastatic or recurrent disease. *Metastatic cancer* to the ovary must always be considered in patients with a pelvic mass, which may be the first indication of a primary gastrointestinal, endometrial, or breast carcinoma.

Clinical Manifestations

Early ovarian cancer is usually asymptomatic. On occasion, ovarian enlargement is found on routine examination, and cancer may be discovered incidentally at the time of abdominal or pelvic surgery for other indications. In two thirds of patients, however, widespread intra-abdominal metastases are present by the time the diagnosis is made. Symptoms of abdominal swelling, bloating, and pelvic fullness or pressure are common. Many patients have vague abdominal complaints or nonspecific gastrointestinal symptoms. Ascites or a palpable abdominopelvic mass may be found on examination. The presence of an irregular mass in the pelvis or nodularity in the cul-de-sac accompanied by ascites is often diagnostic. Malignant pleural effusions may be manifested as shortness of breath.

Diagnosis

Screening

Screening tests for ovarian cancer remain controversial. Transvaginal ultrasonography, although effective for diagnosis of ovarian cysts and tumors, is nonspecific, and its use results in surgical exploration of a large number of women with benign ovarian cysts. Serum levels of the tumor-associated antigen CA-125 above 35 U/mL are present in 80% of postmenopausal women with ovarian cancer (Chapter 190). Unfortunately, many low-stage ovarian tumors do not cause elevated levels of CA-125, whereas endometriosis, pelvic inflammatory disease, and some benign ovarian tumors may do so. The relative rarity of ovarian cancer, combined with the nonspecific nature and relative insensitivity of currently available tests, makes ovarian cancer screening unsatisfactory.

Differential Diagnosis

A pelvic mass can be caused by either a benign or a malignant tumor of the ovary as well as by ectopic pregnancy, endometriosis, inflammatory conditions, physiologic cysts, and malignant neoplasms of other pelvic organs and structures. After a complete history has been obtained, a physical examination has been performed, and the size and character of the mass have been confirmed by ultrasonography, several additional studies may be helpful. A chest radiograph is useful to exclude pulmonary metastases and pleural effusions. An abdominal and pelvic computed tomographic scan can identify evidence of upper abdominal metastases or ureteral obstruction, and a barium enema study or colonoscopy is almost always indicated before surgery to exclude a primary lesion or secondary involvement of the colon.

Prevention and Treatment

Rx

Surgery

In almost all cases of suspected ovarian carcinoma, an exploratory laparotomy is the ultimate diagnostic procedure. Laparoscopy may be used by some surgeons to establish a diagnosis, but laparoscopy may disseminate localized cancer, and most experts think that definitive resection cannot be done by laparoscopy. If the diagnosis is confirmed, tumor debulking, including total abdominal hysterectomy and bilateral salpingo-oophorectomy, should be performed if possible to make a definitive diagnosis and to stage the extent of disease. Aggressive tumor debulking, even when all cancer cannot be removed, improves the length and quality of survival. Ideally, this initial surgery should be done by a gynecologic oncologist whose special training and experience provide the optimal management.

Chemotherapy

Except for some patients with stage IA disease, chemotherapy is recommended postoperatively for most women with ovarian cancer. [1] For patients with epithelial ovarian cancer who have been optimally surgically debulked (less than 1 cm greatest diameter residual disease), an intense regimen of combined intraperitoneal and intravenous chemotherapy has been shown to be most effective. [2] This high-dose combination chemotherapy consisting of intravenous and intraperitoneal paclitaxel and intraperitoneal cisplatin should be administered at treatment centers with considerable experience because of the high rate of serious side effects. For patients with more extensive residual disease or who are physically unable to tolerate intraperitoneal therapy, traditional intravenous paclitaxel (175 mg/m^2) and carboplatin (area under the curve = 6) chemotherapy every 3 weeks for 6 cycles is recommended. [3] The mean disease-free interval for women with stage III and stage IV disease is about 18 months, and median survival in women with optimally debulked disease approaches 60 months in recent studies.

Other active drugs include liposomal doxorubicin, gemcitabine, topotecan, and etoposide. A variety of trials involving antiangiogenic agents, growth factor inhibitors, and gene therapy are currently ongoing. Chemotherapy for recurrent, metastatic disease is usually well tolerated, and quality of life is satisfactory until late in the course of the disease. Radiation therapy is associated with significant toxicity and is rarely used because of the volume of disease that needs to be radiated.

Treatment of Recurrent, Metastatic Disease

The overall survival rate of patients treated for ovarian cancer is only about 40%; progressive disease develops in many women despite appropriate primary therapy. Salvage chemotherapy protocols for recurrent disease produce a 20 to 30% response rate. Although almost all women with recurrent disease succumb to cancer, many women live 3 to 5 years with a good quality of life.

Prognosis

The long-term survival rate of patients treated for epithelial ovarian cancer is still disappointing (see Table 209–1). Almost 60% of patients have stage III or stage IV disease at the time of diagnosis. Although the majority of women with advanced disease live several years with a reasonable qualify of life, recurrent cancer usually becomes symptomatic; only about 25% of patients with advanced disease survive for 5 years. By comparison, almost 80% of women with stage I ovarian cancer survive for 5 years.

Future Directions

Early diagnosis of ovarian cancer by accurate screening tests is perhaps the most important area of future investigation.

CERVICAL CANCER

Epidemiology

Cervical cancers originate from the squamous epithelium of the ectocervix or the glandular lining of the endocervix. The prevalence of invasive cervical cancer is much higher in developing countries where health care is not readily available. Cervical cancer is the leading cause of death from gynecologic malignant disease worldwide; about 500,000 cases are diagnosed each year. In the United States, the incidence of cervical cancer has dramatically declined since the introduction of the Pap smear, and there has been a four- to five-fold reduction in death from cervical cancer. Approximately 10,500 new cases of cervical carcinoma are diagnosed annually in the United States, and about 3700 women die each year of this disease. However, despite the availability of effective screening, up to 50% of all women diagnosed with cervical cancer have never had a Pap smear.

Pathobiology

Most if not all cervical cancers are preceded by a phase of cervical intraepithelial neoplasia (CIN) that progresses slowly for years before stromal invasion occurs. Human papillomavirus (HPV) DNA can be identified in at least 95% of dysplastic and malignant cervical lesions (Chapter 396). HPV subtypes 16 and 18 are isolated most frequently in invasive squamous cell carcinoma and adenocarcinoma, respectively. Additional high-risk subtypes have been characterized, such as 31, 33, 35, and others. It is estimated that up to 50% of sexually active women have been exposed to HPV, but only a small fraction of exposed women develop high-grade CIN or invasive cervical cancer. Cofactors for malignant transformation include tobacco use and immunosuppression. For example, cervical cancers are manifested at a more advanced stage and are clinically more aggressive in women infected with human immunodeficiency virus, and cervical carcinoma is an acquired immunodeficiency syndrome–defining illness (Chapter 416).

Clinical Manifestations

Early cervical cancers are asymptomatic. Regular Pap smear screening is vital to detect premalignant and early malignant changes. As the cervical cancer progresses, the patient may complain of intermenstrual spotting, postcoital bleeding, postmenopausal bleeding, or bloody vaginal discharge. Advanced cases may present with severe back or pelvic pain, alteration of bowel and bladder function, enlarged lymph nodes, hemorrhage, or obstructive uremia.

Diagnosis

The Pap smear is a well-established screening test for abnormalities arising from the cervix (Fig. 209–1). Cervical cytology can detect microscopic changes not visible on physical examination. A single Pap test, however, may have a false-negative rate of up to 50% because of problems with sampling, preparation, or interpretation. Despite the low sensitivity of a single Pap test, repeated smears have a high sensitivity, so that a woman with three consecutive negative Pap test results has less than a 1% chance of an undetected cervical lesion. Invasive cancer is usually associated with inflammation, hemorrhage, and necrosis, which may make a Pap test difficult to interpret. Accordingly, biopsy of any suspicious visible lesion should be performed without delay.

HPV testing for high-risk viral types may be the most effective method to evaluate a Pap smear that shows atypical squamous cells. The presence of a high-risk viral type or a Pap smear suggestive of an intraepithelial lesion or carcinoma warrants further investigation by colposcopy and directed biopsy. In patients who have biopsy-confirmed high-grade dysplasia or carcinoma that is not grossly visible, further diagnostic evaluation by cervical conization or a loop electrosurgical excision procedure is recommended. Any woman with evidence of invasive carcinoma should be referred to a gynecologic oncologist.

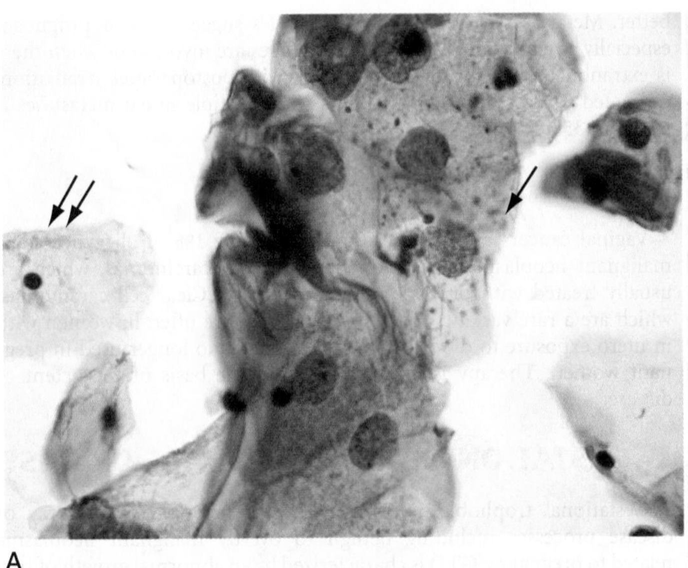
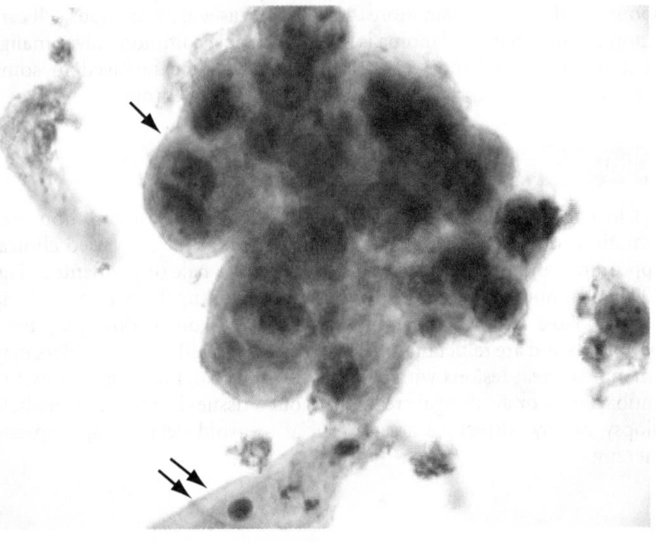

FIGURE 209–1 • Cervical abnormalities on Pap smear. A, Low-grade squamous intraepithelial neoplasia. Note group of mildly dysplastic cells with increased nuclear-to-cytoplasmic ratio (arrow) contrasted by normal squamous epithelial cell (double arrow). Papanicolaou stain, magnification ×400. **B,** Cervical adenocarcinoma. Note three-dimensional cluster of pleomorphic cells with markedly increased nuclear-to-cytoplasmic ratio, dense nuclear chromatin, and macronucleoli (arrow) contrasted by normal squamous epithelial cell (double arrow). Papanicolaou stain, magnification ×400.

Prevention and Treatment

Rx

Screening

The current screening guidelines for cervical cancer recommend that every woman undergo pelvic examination including Pap smear by the age of 21 years or within 3 years of the onset of sexual activity, whichever comes first (Chapter 13). Screening should be continued annually with conventional cervical cytology or every 2 years with liquid-based cytology. After three consecutive normal annual Pap smears, women at low risk may be screened at 3-year intervals at the discretion of the physician. Women at increased risk (i.e., those with previous history of high-risk HPV infection, dysplasia or carcinoma, in utero exposure to diethylstilbestrol, or immunosuppression) may not be good candidates for prolonged screening intervals. Screening should be continued until at least the age of 70 years.

The Food and Drug Administration has recently approved HPV DNA testing for high-risk viral types in women who are at least 30 years old. HPV testing may be combined with cytology, but high-risk viral testing need not be done more frequently than every 3 years.

Early Cervical Intraepithelial Neoplasm

In women who are compliant with follow-up surveillance, CIN-1 and focal CIN-2 lesions do not require immediate treatment because at least half of these lesions will undergo spontaneous regression over time. Extensive CIN-2 and any CIN-3 lesions can be treated by a loop electrosurgical excision procedure or cervical conization. Some squamous dysplastic lesions can alternatively be managed by cryotherapy or laser vaporization. Cold knife conization is the preferred method to evaluate endocervical (glandular) dysplasia.

Vaccines

Well-tolerated monovalent (HPV-16), bivalent (HPV-16/18), and quadrivalent (HPV-6/11/16/18) virus-like particle vaccines (Chapter 16) prevent newly acquired, type-specific HPV infections 3,4 and promote significant resolution of preexisting HPV infections, condylomas, and dysplastic lesions in young women. Duration of follow-up has been relatively short term, but the results are extremely encouraging.

Cervical Cancer

Effective treatment of early-stage cancers with depth of invasion of less than 3 mm (stage IA-1) includes a hysterectomy or the option of cervical conization in women who wish to preserve fertility. Larger tumors that are confined to the cervix or upper vagina (stage IA-2, IB-1, or IIA) can be managed by radical hysterectomy with pelvic lymphadenectomy or by pelvic radiation therapy. Radical trachelectomy (removal of the cervix, parametria, and upper vagina) with uterine preservation may be used in selected patients who have stage I tumors and a strong desire for fertility. Large primary cervical cancers (i.e., bulky stage IB-2 or larger) and invasive tumors in patients who are deemed medically inoperable are best treated with a combination of radiation therapy and cisplatin chemotherapy (cisplatin, 40 mg/m^2 weekly infusion, for 5 to 6 weeks during external irradiation). Patients whose tumors have invaded into the bladder or rectum (stage IVA) or metastasized to distant sites (stage IVB) require multimodality therapy, preferably in a clinical trial if it is available. Cisplatin-based chemotherapy is usually recommended for patients with metastatic or recurrent disease, but the response rates are only 20 to 30% and are of limited duration.

Prognosis

The prognosis is directly related to the clinical stage at the time of diagnosis (see Table 209–1). A large primary tumor, invasion of the lymphovascular space, and lymph node metastases are poor prognostic factors. Overall, patients who are treated when the tumor is confined to the cervix can expect an 85% or better 5-year survival. In contrast, tumors that have spread beyond the cervix to the parametrial tissue and pelvic sidewalls are associated with approximately 70% and 50% 5-year survivals, respectively.

Future Directions

The most exciting development is the HPV vaccine. Future studies will address numerous questions about long-term efficacy, cost, implementation in younger and older women, and ethical issues.

VULVAR CANCER

Epidemiology

Vulvar cancers arise from the external female genitalia (vulva) and account for 1 to 2% of all gynecologic malignant neoplasms. Approximately 4000 new cases are diagnosed annually in the United States, with about 900 deaths per year. More than 90% of cases are squamous cell carcinomas; malignant melanoma is the second most common vulvar malignant neoplasm (Chapter 214). HPV appears to be involved in some squamous cell cancers, especially in the younger age group.

Clinical Manifestations and Diagnosis

Chronic pruritus and a persistent lesion are the most common presentations of vulvar carcinoma. Malignant lesions have a varied clinical appearance and may be eczematoid or ulcerative, pale or pigmented (Fig. 209–2). Tumors may arise from any region, including the perineum, labia minora, labia majora, and mons pubis. Many women downplay their symptoms and are reluctant to seek evaluation. Health care providers may attempt to treat lesions with a variety of steroidal, hormonal, antiviral, antibacterial, or antifungal creams without a tissue diagnosis. Immediate biopsy of any suspicious area is crucial to avoid delay in appropriate therapy.

Prevention and Treatment

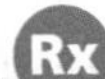

Wide local excision is the preferred management of precancerous vulvar intraepithelial neoplasia. Small lesions that are confined to the vulva and have less than 1.0 mm of invasion are treated by local excision. More deeply invasive lesions and those more than 2 cm in diameter require more radical resection and inguinal-femoral lymphadenectomy. Sentinel lymph node detection is being investigated in the surgical management of vulvar cancers. Postoperative radiation therapy to the pelvis and groin is usually recommended if lymph node metastases are identified. Locally advanced disease (i.e., lesions involving the urethra, vagina, or anus) and metastatic disease should be treated with multimodality therapy, preferably in a clinical trial.

Prognosis

The prognosis of invasive vulvar cancer is directly related to the depth of invasion and size of the lesion, both of which predict the chance of lymphatic spread. Lesions that are confined to the vulva and have minimal invasion can usually be cured with surgical excision. If the primary tumor is less than 2 cm in diameter, 5-year survival is 85% or better. Metastases to regional lymph nodes suggest a poor prognosis, especially when more than two lymph nodes are involved or when there is extranodal extension of disease. Even with postoperative irradiation, estimated 5-year survival of patients with multiple nodal metastases is less than 35%.

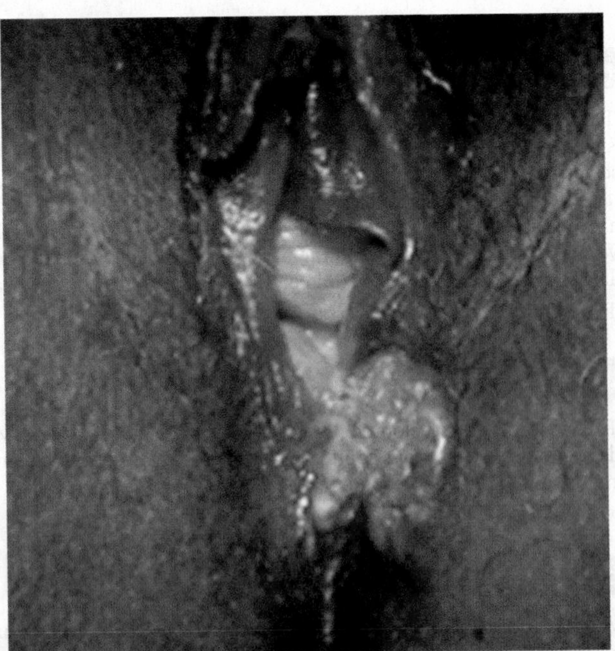

FIGURE 209–2 • Vulvar cancer. Invasive squamous cell carcinoma of the vulva.

VAGINAL CANCER

Vaginal cancers are rare, accounting for only 1% of all gynecologic malignant neoplasms. Most are squamous cell carcinomas, which are usually treated with primary radiation therapy. Clear cell carcinomas, which are a rare variant, occur significantly more often in women with in utero exposure to diethylstilbestrol, which is no longer used in pregnant women. Therapy is individualized on the basis of the extent of disease.

GESTATIONAL TROPHOBLASTIC DISEASE

Gestational trophoblastic disease (GTD) encompasses an array of disease processes including benign to overtly malignant neoplasms related to pregnancy. GTD is characterized by an abnormal growth of trophoblastic (placental) tissue and most commonly manifests in the form of molar pregnancy. Persistent GTD occurs in 20% of molar pregnancies, despite complete uterine evacuation. GTD may also follow any other pregnancy event, including preterm or term birth, miscarriage, abortion, and ectopic pregnancy. GTD includes complete or partial hydatidiform mole, invasive mole, choriocarcinoma, and placental site trophoblastic tumor.

Molar pregnancy commonly presents as second trimester bleeding in a woman whose uterus is larger than expected for the estimated gestational age. A characteristic heterogeneous echogenic pattern ("snowstorm") is evident on ultrasonography. Persistent GTD may manifest as bleeding more than expected subsequent to delivery or uterine evacuation. Pulmonary symptoms may be present because the lungs are involved in 80% of cases with metastatic disease. Distant metastases to other sites are uncommon in the absence of lung metastases. The second most common site of extrauterine disease is the vagina, which occurs in 30% of advanced cases. The characteristic laboratory feature is a persistently elevated β-human chorionic gonadotropin (β-hCG) level. Human placental lactogen level may be elevated with a placental site trophoblastic tumor.

GTD was the first metastatic tumor ever cured with systemic chemotherapy. Nonmetastatic GTD and low-risk metastatic disease usually respond well to single-agent chemotherapy with methotrexate (40 mg/m^2 weekly intramuscular injection) or actinomycin D (1.25 mg/m^2 intravenous infusion every 2 weeks). Alternative effective protocols are available for single-agent therapy. The duration of therapy and treatment intervals are determined by the rate and magnitude of decline in the serum β-hCG level. High-risk metastatic disease and disease unresponsive to single-agent therapy are treated with combination chemotherapy with etoposide, methotrexate, actinomycin D, cyclophosphamide, and vincristine. Hysterectomy is recommended when intrauterine tumor does not respond to chemotherapy and in cases of placental site trophoblastic tumor. The majority of patients with gestational trophoblastic tumors can be placed into complete remission, with cure rates approximating 100% for nonmetastatic and low-risk metastatic disease and 90% for high-risk metastatic disease.

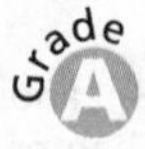

1. Colombo N, Guthrie D, Chiari S, et al: International Collaborative Ovarian Neoplasm trial 1: A randomized trial of adjuvant chemotherapy in women with early-stage ovarian cancer. J Natl Cancer Inst 2003;95:125–132.
2. Armstrong DK, Bundy B, Wenzel L, et al: Intraperitoneal cisplatin and paclitaxel in ovarian cancer. N Engl J Med 2006;354:34–43.
3. Ozols RF, Bookman MA, duBois A, et al: Intraperitoneal cisplatin therapy in ovarian cancer: Comparison with standard intravenous carboplatin and paclitaxel. Gynecol Oncol 2006;103:1–6.
4. Harper DM, Franco EL, Wheeler C, et al: Efficacy of a bivalent L1 virus-like particle vaccine in prevention of infection with human papillomavirus types 16 and 18 in young women: A randomised controlled trial. Lancet 2004;364:1757–1765.
5. Villa LL, Costa RL, Petta CA, et al: Prophylactic quadrivalent human papillomavirus (types 6, 11, 16, and 18) L1 virus-like particle vaccine in young women: A randomised double-blind placebo-controlled multicentre phase II efficacy trial. Lancet Oncol 2005;6:271–278.

SUGGESTED READINGS

Buekers TE, Kao MS, Phillips NJ, et al: The treatment of early stage cervical cancer: An assessment of pre-operative factors. Gynecol Oncol 2007:104:665–669. *Assessment of pre-operative factors that stratify early stage cervical cancers by likelihood for adjuvant radiotherapy.*

Cervical Cancer Screening: Clinical Practice Guidelines in Oncology. J Natl Compr Cancer Network 2005;2:570–587. *Consensus guidelines and evidence to support them.*

Clifford GM, Gallus S, Herrero R, et al: Worldwide distribution of human papillomavirus types in cytologically normal women in the Internal Agency for Research on Cancer HPV prevalence surveys: A pooled analysis. Lancet 2005;366:991–998. *HPV subtypes vary among women from different geographic regions.*

Lukaszuk K, Liss J, Gulczynski J, et al: Predictive value of HPV DNA in lymph nodes in surgically treated cervical carcinoma patients—a prospective study. Gynecol Oncol 2007;104:721–726. *The presence of HPV DNA in lymph nodes is an early sign of metastasis.*

210 TESTICULAR CANCER

Lawrence H. Einhorn

Epidemiology

Testicular tumors are relatively uncommon and account for only 1% of male malignancies in the United States. The highest worldwide incidence occurs in Scandinavian countries; by contrast, testicular cancer is rare in African Americans and Asian Americans. The primary age group is 15 to 35 years for nonseminomatous tumors and a decade older for seminoma.

Male patients with a history of cryptorchidism have a 10- to 40-fold increased risk for development of a testicular cancer. The normally descended testis in these men is also at higher risk, thus suggesting a dysgenetic abnormality.

Pathobiology

More than 95% of tumors of the testis originate from germ cells. Germ cell tumors can be seminomas or nonseminomatous germ cell tumors. Seminomas are more likely to be confined to the testis (stage I) and are exquisitely sensitive to radiation therapy. Pure seminomas never have elevated serum α-fetoprotein (AFP) levels. Nonseminomatous germ cell tumors consist of embryonal cell carcinomas, choriocarcinomas, yolk sac tumors, or teratomas, alone or mixed with other elements. Teratomas do not secrete human chorionic gonadotropin (HCG) or AFP and do not usually metastasize, but they grow by local extension and are completely resistant to radiation therapy and chemotherapy.

Most germ cell testicular cancers in adults are associated with a cytogenetic abnormality, i12p—an isochromosome of the short arm of chromosome 12 that is a highly specific chromosomal finding in germ cell tumors. Sertoli cell tumors, Leydig cell tumors, and lymphomas are the most common non–germ cell tumors. In men older than 60 years, most tumors are non-Hodgkin's lymphoma (Chapter 196), with a predilection for bilateral involvement.

Clinical Manifestations

Most patients with testicular cancer are initially evaluated because of testicular pain or because of a mass or enlargement of one testis. Others are asymptomatic and first detected during a routine physical examination. Less commonly, the diagnosis may initially be made during an evaluation for infertility, in part because testicular cancer can cause oligospermia.

Metastatic spread is either lymphatic or hematogenous. Lymphatic metastases usually go initially to the ipsilateral retroperitoneal lymph nodes, where they may be associated with flank pain. Lymphatic metastases may continue in a superior direction to the posterior mediastinum and eventually to the left supraclavicular lymph nodes. A large retroperitoneal mass or a supraclavicular lymph node may be palpable on physical examination. Hematogenous spread usually occurs first to the pulmonary parenchyma bilaterally. Pulmonary symptoms such as chest pain, shortness of breath, dyspnea on exertion, coughing, or hemoptysis are seen only with extensive pulmonary metastases. Other sites of hematogenous spread include the liver, bone, or brain. Significant elevation of the serum HCG level may produce gynecomastia.

Diagnosis

Patients with a palpable mass in the testis should be suspected of having testicular cancer, especially if there is a history of cryptorchidism. Other causes of testicular and scrotal abnormalities may be included in the differential diagnosis. Acute pain in the testis suggests torsion. Painful enlargement may be due to a hydrocele, which may be caused by an underlying primary testicular malignancy. Pain and tenderness adjacent to the testis may be due to epididymitis or a varicocele. Tenderness of the testis itself on physical examination may reflect orchitis. However, an underlying neoplasm should always be considered.

Any testicular symptoms, including pain or a suspected mass, require evaluation. Testicular ultrasound is the test of choice in all suspicious cases. A hypoechogenic mass within the testis must be presumed to be testicular cancer and requires referral to a urologist (Fig. 210–1).

When orchiectomy reveals the diagnosis of testicular cancer, a staging evaluation is performed to determine the extent of disease and appropriate therapy. Clinical stage I disease is confined to the testis; stage II disease reflects spread to the retroperitoneal lymph nodes; and stage III is supradiaphragmatic disease, with either nodal metastases to the posterior mediastinum or supraclavicular region or hematogenous spread, especially to the lungs.

In addition to a full history and physical examination, serum HCG and AFP levels should be determined. Because the serum half-life is 1 day for HCG and 5 days for AFP, an AFP level of 1000 may take more than a month to normalize after orchiectomy, even if all of the tumor has been completely removed. Imaging studies to define the extent of disease include abdominal and pelvic computed tomography (CT) and a chest radiograph. If the chest radiograph does not show pulmonary metastases, a chest CT scan should be performed. Bone scans and head CT scans can be reserved for patients with symptoms suggestive of osseous or central nervous system metastases, respectively.

Prevention and Treatment

Rx

A careful testicular examination is a mandatory part of the physical examination in men, especially young men (Chapter 13), and serves as the key means for detecting tumors at an early stage. With the patient lying supine or standing up, the testis should be gently palpated with the thumb and second and third fingers; the entire

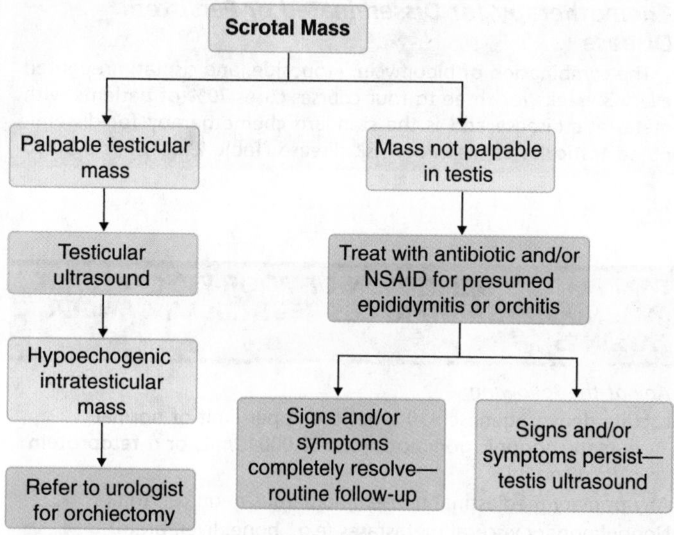

FIGURE 210–1 • Management of a scrotal mass. NSAID = nonsteroidal anti-inflammatory drug.

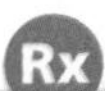

anterior, posterior, and lateral surfaces of the testis should be examined.

Local and Regional Disease

Seminoma

About 70% of seminomas are initially seen in clinical stage I disease. Although the cure rate with orchiectomy alone is 80 to 95%, treatment can also include 2000 cGy para-aortic irradiation [1] or adjuvant carboplatin. [2]

Twenty percent of patients with seminoma are initially found to have stage II disease (positive abdominal CT scan). For these patients, radiation therapy has a 90% cure rate; in patients who are not cured by radiation therapy, subsequent cisplatin combination chemotherapy (cisplatin combined with etoposide with or without bleomycin) is usually curative. If the transverse diameter of the tumor is greater than 3 cm, if there are multiple anatomic levels of nodal metastases, or if stage III disease is present, the preferred initial treatment is cisplatin combination chemotherapy without irradiation, and the cure rate is 70 to 100%, depending on the extent of the disease.

Nonseminomatous Germ Cell Tumors

Management of clinical stage I nonseminomatous germ cell tumors begins with orchiectomy, which has a 70% cure rate, followed by either retroperitoneal lymph node dissection or close surveillance, which can detect metastases early and guide curative chemotherapy. Most relapses occur in the first year, during which meticulous surveillance should include history and physical examination, serum markers, chest radiograph, and abdominal and pelvic CT every 2 months. The same studies are performed every 4 months during the second year, every 6 months during the third to fifth years of surveillance, and annually thereafter. CT scans are discontinued after 5 years. The physical examination should include palpation of the remaining testis because these patients have a 1 to 2% chance of a contralateral primary. The major complication of retroperitoneal lymph node dissection is inadvertent severing of the sympathetic plexus with resultant retrograde ejaculation or failure of ejaculation. Nerve-sparing retroperitoneal lymph node dissection can retain antegrade ejaculation in more than 95% of patients. Some centers advocate primary chemotherapy for high-risk (embryonal predominant or vascular or lymphatic invasion) clinical stage I disease with cisplatin combination chemotherapy.

For clinical stage II disease with persistently elevated serum markers or a transverse diameter greater than 3 cm, chemotherapy is preferred. Other stage II patients are treated with retroperitoneal lymph node dissection, often followed by close surveillance (as noted earlier, but without abdominal CT scans) or adjuvant chemotherapy. Testicular cancer has a higher cure rate with surgery alone despite nodal metastases than any other cancer does.

Chemotherapy for Disseminated or Persistent Disease

The combination of bleomycin, etoposide, and cisplatin repeated every 3 weeks for three to four courses cures 70% of patients with metastatic disease and is the standard chemotherapy for disseminated testicular cancer. Poor-risk disease (Table 210–1) has a 50 to 60% cure rate with standard three-drug therapy, intermediate-risk disease (HCG, 5000 to 50,000 IU/mL, or AFP, 1000 to 10,000 Ng/mL) has a 70% cure rate, and all other forms of metastatic disease (good risk) have a 90 to 100% cure rate.

In the 30% of metastatic germ cell tumors that are not cured by the initial combination chemotherapy, the use of standard-dose salvage therapy (ifosfamide, cisplatin, and either vinblastine or paclitaxel) or high-dose carboplatin and etoposide therapy followed by peripheral blood stem cell transplantation can cure 25 to 70% of refractory cases, depending on the patient's characteristics.

TABLE 210–1 DEFINITION OF POOR-RISK DISEASE (ALL NONSEMINOMATOUS TESTICULAR CANCER PATIENTS)

Any of the following:
Lactate dehydrogenase >10 times the upper limit of normal, human chorionic gonadotropin >50,000 IU/mL, or α-fetoprotein >10,000 ng/mL
Any primary mediastinal nonseminomatous germ cell tumor
Nonpulmonary visceral metastases (e.g., bone, liver, brain)

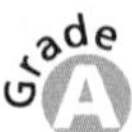

1. Jones WG, Fossa SD, Mead GM, et al: Randomized trial of 30 versus 20 Gy in the adjuvant treatment of stage I testicular seminoma. J Clin Oncol 2005;23:1200–1208.
2. Oliver RTD, Mason MD, Mead GM, et al: Radiotherapy versus single-dose carboplatin in adjuvant treatment of stage I seminoma: A randomised trial. Lancet 2005;366:293–300.

SUGGESTED READINGS

Horwich A, Shipley J, Huddart R: Testicular germ-cell cancer. Lancet 2006;367: 754–765. *A comprehensive review.*

Richie JP: Second cancers among 40,576 testicular cancer patients: Focus on long-term survivors. Urol Oncol 2006;24:171–172. *For patients with seminomas or nonseminomatous tumors at 35 years of age, cumulative risks for solid cancer at 75 years of age were 36% and 31%, respectively, as compared with 23% for the general population.*

Rowland RG: Risk of contralateral testicular cancer: A population-based study of 29,515 U.S. men. Urol Oncol 2006;24:173. *The low risk for contralateral cancer argues against biopsy of the contralateral testis.*

Tyldesley S, Vondue D, McKenzie M, et al: Surveillance of stage I testicular seminoma: British Columbia Cancer Agency Experience 1992 to 2002. Urology 2006;67:594–598. *The annual percentage of patients going onto surveillance increased. The 5-year actuarial relapse-free survival rate was 78%, and relapse was more common in patients with rete invasion or size greater than 4 cm.*

211 PROSTATE CANCER

Eric J. Small

Definition

Prostate cancer is the most common noncutaneous malignant neoplasm in men, with nearly 200,000 new cases per year in the United States. It also causes about 32,000 deaths in the United States each year, thereby making it the second most common cause of cancer death in men. Prostate cancer is a single histologic disease whose marked clinical heterogeneity ranges from indolent, clinically irrelevant disease to a virulent, rapidly lethal phenotype.

Epidemiology

The incidence of clinically diagnosed prostate cancer reflects the effects of screening by the prostate-specific antigen (PSA) assay. Before PSA testing was available, about 19,000 new cases of prostate cancer were reported per year in the United States; this number reached 84,000 by 1993 and peaked at about 300,000 new cases in 1996. Since 1996, the reported annual incidence of prostate cancer in the United States has declined to about 200,000, a number that may more closely estimate the true annual incidence of clinically detectable disease. The death rate due to prostate cancer has declined by about 1% per year since 1990. The age-specific decrease in mortality has been greatest in men younger than 75 years. Men older than 75 years still account for two thirds of all prostate cancer deaths. Whether this decline is due to early detection (screening) or to improved therapy is not proved.

Risk factors for prostate cancer include increasing age, family history, African American race, and dietary factors. Epidemiologic studies have suggested that nutritional factors such as reduced fat intake and increased soy protein, lycopene, vitamin E, and selenium supplementation may have a protective effect against the development of prostate cancer, although prospective data are minimal. The incidence of prostate cancer among African Americans is nearly twice that observed among white Americans. Prostate cancer is diagnosed in African Americans at a more advanced stage, and disease-specific survival is lower in African Americans. The relative contributions of biologic, genetic, and environmental differences as well as differences in health care access are not well established. Prior vasectomy and benign prostatic hypertrophy (Chapter 130) do not increase the risk. Prostatic intraepithelial neoplasia, particularly when it is high grade, is recognized as a premalignant lesion, so its presence on biopsy increases the likelihood of subsequent malignancy.

Pathobiology

Prostate cancer appears to be common among relatives of men with early-onset prostate cancer. At the molecular level, there appears to be a susceptibility locus for the development of prostate cancer at an early age on chromosome 1, band q24, although an abnormality at this locus occurs in less than 10% of patients with prostate cancer. Although many genetic abnormalities with both loss and gain of function have been identified, consistent patterns of changes associated with an increased likelihood for development of prostate cancer have not been identified.

Testosterone is required for maintenance of a normal, healthy prostatic epithelium, but it is also a prerequisite for the development of prostate cancer. Prostate cancers express robust levels of androgen receptor, and signaling through the androgen receptor results in growth, progression, and invasion of prostate cancer. Inhibition of signaling, typically by the surgical or pharmacologic reduction of testosterone levels, results in prostate cancer apoptosis and involution. Ultimately, androgen deprivation therapy loses clinical efficacy. The biologic events surrounding the clinical development of "hormone-resistant prostate cancer" are not well delineated, but amplification of the androgen receptor, which is a common event in these patients, presumably makes the cancer sensitive to minute levels of androgen or other ligands of the androgen receptor.

Clinical Manifestations

Most patients with early-stage, organ-confined disease are asymptomatic. Obstructive voiding symptoms (hesitancy, intermittent urinary stream, decreased force of stream) generally reflect locally advanced disease with growth into the urethra or bladder neck, although these symptoms are indistinguishable from benign prostatic hypertrophy (Chapter 130). Locally advanced tumors can also result in hematuria and hematospermia. Prostate cancer that has spread to the regional pelvic lymph nodes can occasionally cause edema of the lower extremities or discomfort in the pelvic and perineal areas. Metastasis occurs most commonly to bone, where it is frequently asymptomatic, but it can also cause severe and unremitting pain. Bone metastasis can result in pathologic fractures or spinal cord compression. Although visceral metastases are rare as presenting features of prostate cancer, patients can have pulmonary, hepatic, pleural, peritoneal, and central nervous system metastases late in the natural history or after hormonal therapies fail.

Diagnosis

More than 60% of patients with prostate cancer are asymptomatic, and the diagnosis is made solely because of an elevated screening PSA level. A palpable nodule on digital rectal examination, which is the next most common clinical presentation, generally prompts biopsy. Much less commonly, prostate cancer is diagnosed because of advanced disease that causes obstructive voiding symptoms, pelvic or perineal discomfort, lower extremity edema, or symptomatic bone lesions.

Although the digital rectal examination has a low sensitivity and specificity for diagnosis of prostate cancer, biopsy of a nodule or area of induration reveals cancer 50% of the time, suggesting that prostate biopsy should be undertaken in all men with palpable nodules. The PSA level has a far better sensitivity but a low specificity because conditions such as benign prostatic hypertrophy and prostatitis can cause false-positive PSA elevations (Chapter 130). By use of a PSA threshold of 4 ng/mL, 70 to 80% of tumors are detected. However, cancer rates range from 4 to 9% in patients whose PSA level is less than 4 ng/mL. The positive predictive value for a single PSA level above 10 ng/mL is greater than 60% for cancer, but the positive predictive value for a PSA level between 4 and 10 ng/mL is only about 30%. Assays of the PSA fraction that circulates unbound (percentage free PSA) may help distinguish prostate cancer from benign processes; in patients with a PSA level of 4 to 10 ng/mL, the percentage of free PSA appears to be an independent predictor of prostate cancer, and a cutoff value of free PSA less than 25% can detect 95% of cancers while avoiding 20% of unnecessary biopsies.

The search for novel biomarkers of prostate cancer has included characterization of the pattern of proteins produced by cancer cells, although this approach is hampered by an inability to detect low levels of cancer proteins. More recently, a novel method for the detection of prostate cancer based on a patient's antitumor antibody repertoire had 88.2% specificity and 81.6% sensitivity for prostate cancer and added significantly to PSA testing alone. Although it is not yet in widespread clinical use, this approach holds great promise for the future.

Transrectal ultrasonography with biopsies is indicated when the PSA level is elevated, when the percentage of free PSA is less than 25%, or when an abnormality is noted on digital rectal examination. Sextant biopsy specimens (base, midgland, and apex on each side) are generally obtained. Seminal vesicles are sampled in high-risk patients. A bone scan is warranted only in patients with PSA levels above 10 ng/mL, and abdominal and pelvic computed tomographic scanning or magnetic resonance imaging is usually unrevealing in patients with a PSA level below 20 ng/mL.

The prognosis of prostate cancer correlates with histologic grade and extent (stage) of disease. More than 95% of prostate cancers are adenocarcinomas, and multifocality is common. Histologic grade ranges from 1 to 5; the Gleason score, which refers to the sum of the two most common histologic patterns seen on each tissue specimen, ranges from 2 (1 + 1) to 10 (5 + 5). In general, tumors are classified as well differentiated (Gleason scores 2, 3, or 4), of intermediate differentiation (Gleason scores 5, 6, or 7), and poorly differentiated (Gleason scores 8, 9, or 10).

Clinical stage is defined by the extent of disease based on the physical examination, imaging studies, and pathology. Stage T1 is nonpalpable prostate cancer detected only on pathologic examination, either incidentally noted after transurethral resection for benign hypertrophy (T1a and T1b) or on a biopsy specimen obtained because of an elevated PSA level (T1c, the most common clinical stage at diagnosis). Stage T2 is a palpable tumor that appears to be confined to the prostate gland (T2a in one lobe, T2b in two lobes), and stage T3 is tumor with extension through the prostatic capsule (T2a if it is focal, T2b if seminal vesicles are involved). T4 tumors are those with invasion of adjacent structures, such as the bladder neck, the external urinary sphincter, the rectum, the levator muscles, or the pelvic sidewall. Nodal metastases can be microscopic and can be detected only by biopsy or lymphadenectomy, or they can be visible on imaging studies. Distant metastases are predominantly to bone, but occasional visceral metastases occur.

Prevention

Epidemiologic studies suggest that a low-fat diet, high soy protein intake, and supplementation with selenium and vitamin E may reduce the incidence of prostate cancer. Prospective randomized trials are under way. The use of finasteride, a 5α-reductase inhibitor, reduces the risk for development of prostate cancer. ■ However, this approach has not been widely used because of attendant side effects, such as loss of libido and erectile dysfunction. In addition, when prostate cancer develops in patients treated with finasteride, it tends to be higher grade. Whether this is an artifact of the effect of finasteride on the histologic examination of tissue or a real biologic event is not known.

TABLE 211–1 APPROACH TO THE TREATMENT OF PROSTATE CANCER

Extent of Cancer	Therapeutic Options
Organ confined: low risk (usually T1 or T2, GS < 7, PSA < 10 ng/mL)	Surveillance Radical prostatectomy External beam radiotherapy to prostate Brachytherapy
Organ confined: intermediate risk (usually T2, GS = 7, PSA = 10–20 ng/mL)	Radical prostatectomy External beam radiotherapy to prostate, possibly to pelvis, with or without AD Brachytherapy
Organ confined: high risk (usually T3, GS >7, PSA > 20 ng/mL)	Radical prostatectomy (with adjuvant radiotherapy, if needed) External beam radiotherapy to prostate and pelvis (usually with AD) Brachytherapy plus radiotherapy (usually with AD)
Climbing PSA level after local therapy	AD: antiandrogen monotherapy or combined AD Salvage radiation therapy (for patients with prior prostatectomy) Salvage radical prostatectomy (for patients with prior radiation therapy) Surveillance Investigational therapy
Node positive	Surveillance AD Pelvic or prostate radiotherapy + AD Investigational therapy
Metastatic: untreated hormone-refractory prostate cancer	AD Second-line hormones Chemotherapy Investigational therapy

AD = androgen deprivation; GS = Gleason score; PSA = prostate-specific antigen.

Treatment

The approach to the treatment of prostate cancer is detailed in Table 211–1.

Localized Prostate Cancer

Principles of Therapy

The principal therapeutic options for men with localized prostate cancer include the following: watchful waiting; androgen deprivation; retropubic or perineal radical prostatectomy, with or without postoperative radiotherapy to the prostate margins and pelvis; external beam radiotherapy; and brachytherapy (either permanent or temporary radioactive seed implants), with or without external beam radiotherapy to the prostate margins and pelvis.

Treatment options require individualization, taking into account the patient's comorbidity, life expectancy, likelihood of cure, and personal preferences based on an understanding of potential morbidity associated with each treatment. A multidisciplinary approach to integrate surgery, radiation therapy, and androgen deprivation is increasingly recommended. For higher risk patients with a greater likelihood of systemic micrometastases, androgen deprivation is often combined with radiation therapy. In patients at extremely high risk of micrometastatic disease, systemic therapy alone without concurrent local therapy may be appropriate.

PSA screening has led to the early detection of a large number of nonpalpable tumors, for which conventional clinical means of staging are inadequate. Thus, less emphasis is being placed on clinical stage and more emphasis is being placed on PSA value and other predictors of outcome. Careful risk assessment is required to identify patients who are appropriate candidates for definitive local treatment.

Several studies have confirmed that serum PSA level, clinical stage, and biopsy Gleason score can be used to predict final pathologic stage after prostatectomy and that they are independent predictors of survival without PSA elevation after external beam radiation therapy or radical prostatectomy. For example, in a radiation therapy series, clinical stage T3 or higher, PSA level above 10 ng/mL, and biopsy Gleason score of 7 or higher were risk factors for poor outcome (death or PSA elevation); 5-year survival without PSA elevation was 85% for patients with none of these adverse features (good risk), 65% for patients with one adverse feature (intermediate risk), and 35% for patients with two or three adverse features (poor risk). Similar statistics are cited in radical prostatectomy series. The percentage of biopsy specimens that are positive is also an independent predictor of outcome after radical prostatectomy and can be used to counsel patients about therapeutic options (Table 211–2).

Low- to Intermediate-Risk Disease

In a randomized trial of patients younger than 75 years with clinical stage T1b, T1c, or T2 prostate cancer, radical prostatectomy significantly reduced the relative risk of death due to prostate cancer by 50% (a 2% absolute risk reduction) and overall mortality by a similar absolute amount at 8.6 years. 2 Reductions in progressive disease and metastases were also significant. The adverse effects on quality of life differ between the two strategies—more dysfunction and urinary leakage after radical prostatectomy, more urinary obstruction with watchful waiting—but are of similar magnitude. 3 Nerve-sparing radical prostatectomy was not routinely performed in this study, and many patients already had palpable disease, so the implications for less advanced disease with newer surgical techniques are not known. Nonrandomized data suggest that watchful waiting may be judiciously used in patients with Gleason score 2, 3, or 4 tumors who have a life expectancy of 10 years or less. Watchful waiting is probably not appropriate for young, otherwise healthy men with high-risk features as described earlier (PSA >10 ng/mL, Gleason sum of 7, or clinical stage T3 or higher). Whether watchful waiting is appropriate for men with intermediate-risk nonpalpable tumors remains debated. Androgen deprivation has not been carefully studied as primary therapy for localized disease, but it is becoming a more common approach in men who wish to receive some therapy but are not suited for or decline prostatectomy or radiation therapy.

Men with T1 or T2 prostate cancer who otherwise have a life expectancy of more than 10 years and no significant comorbid illnesses usually should have definitive local therapy with either surgery or radiation therapy. Long-term survival is excellent. Men

TABLE 211–2 FOUR-YEAR PROGRESSION-FREE SURVIVAL AFTER RADICAL PROSTATECTOMY AS A FUNCTION OF PERCENTAGE OF POSITIVE BIOPSIES

	≤34% of Biopsies Positive	34–50% of Biopsies Positive	>50% of Biopsies Positive
Good risk (usually T1 or T2, GS < 7, PSA < 10 ng/mL)	95%	88%	74%
Intermediate risk (usually T2, GS = 7, PSA = 10–20 ng/mL)	88%	50%	20%
Poor risk (usually T3, GS >7, PSA > 20 ng/mL)	68%	25%	18%

Modified from D'Amico AV, Whittington R, Malkowicz SB, et al: Clinical utility of the percentage of positive prostate biopsies in defining biochemical outcome after radical prostatectomy for patients with clinically localized prostate cancer. J Clin Oncol 2000;18:1164–1172. See text for definitions of risk.
GS = Gleason score; PSA = prostate-specific antigen.

Rx

with T1 or T2 tumors with Gleason scores of 7 or less have 8-year survival rates of 85 to 95%. Patients with T1 or T2 tumors with Gleason scores of 8 to 10 have 8-year survival rates of about 70%.

Nerve-sparing procedures and careful dissection techniques have decreased the risk of postoperative urinary incontinence and impotence. Postoperative urinary incontinence is reported to occur in less than 10% of cases. Postoperative impotence is dependent on a variety of factors, including the patient's age, preoperative erectile function, extent of cancer, and whether a nerve-sparing procedure was undertaken. In general, impotence rates of 10 to 50% are cited. After a radical prostatectomy, the PSA should become undetectable; a detectable PSA implies the presence of cancer cells, either locally or at a metastatic site. Immediate (adjuvant) postoperative radiotherapy improves biochemical progression-free survival and local control in patients with one or more pathologic risk factors (capsule penetration, positive surgical margins, or invasion of seminal vesicle) after radical prostatectomy. 4

Conventional external beam radiation therapy is being replaced by three-dimensional conformal radiation therapy, which permits higher doses to the target tissue with less toxicity. Randomized trials suggest a benefit to higher doses of radiation. Brachytherapy, which is the placement of permanent or temporary radioactive seeds directly into the prostate, is adequate for intracapsular disease with no more than minimal transcapsular extension; otherwise it can be combined with external beam radiation therapy.

High-Risk Disease

Patients with adverse risk features (Gleason score 8 to 10, PSA >10, stage T3) are at high risk of nodal and micrometastatic disease and are generally treated with aggressive local therapy in combination with androgen deprivation, which is synergistic with radiation therapy. Taken in aggregate, these trials have suggested that 4 months of androgen deprivation with radiation therapy can improve local control and prolong progression-free survival in patients with intermediate-risk features, whereas long-term androgen deprivation (up to 3 years) prolongs local control, progression-free survival, and overall survival in patients with high-risk features compared with radiation therapy. 4,5 Patients assigned to stage T3 with Gleason scores of 7 have intermediate outcomes, with 8-year survival rates of about 70%, whereas patients with stage T3 disease and Gleason scores of 8 to 10 have an 8-year survival after radiation therapy of about 50%. Patients with high-risk disease who are treated surgically and who have capsule penetration, positive margins, or seminal vesicle involvement in general should receive immediate adjuvant radiation therapy.

Recurrent Disease

Nearly 50% of men treated with radiation therapy or prostatectomy have evidence of recurrence, as defined by a climbing PSA level. For selected patients with clear local recurrences, local salvage therapy (surgery for patients previously treated with radiation therapy, radiation therapy for patients previously treated with surgery, 6 and androgen deprivation) can be considered. However, early hormone therapy appears to be better than hormonal salvage therapy in terms of survival.

Rx

Advanced Disease

In patients whose radical prostatectomy surgery reveals microscopic involvement of lymph nodes, immediate androgen deprivation prolongs survival compared with deferment of androgen deprivation until osseous metastases are detected. Similarly, patients who are at high risk of nodal invasion and who undergo external beam radiation benefit from concurrent short-term hormonal therapy. 5

In patients with newly diagnosed metastatic prostate cancer, androgen deprivation is the mainstay of treatment and results in symptomatic improvement and disease regression in approximately 80 to 90% of patients. Androgen deprivation can be achieved by orchiectomy or by medical castration, with a luteinizing hormone–releasing hormone (LHRH) agonist (leuprolide acetate, goserelin acetate), which is safer and as effective as estrogen treatment.

Some LHRH agonists cause a transient worsening of signs and symptoms during the first week of therapy as a result of a surge in luteinizing hormone and testosterone, which peaks within 72 hours; an antiandrogen (flutamide, bicalutamide, or nilutamide) should be given with the first LHRH injection to prevent a tumor flare. Medical castration occurs within 4 weeks. The duration of hormone sensitivity is 5 to 10 years for node-positive or high-risk localized (or recurrent) prostate cancer, but the duration of hormone sensitivity is closer to 18 to 24 months in patients with overt metastatic disease. The most common side effects of androgen ablation are loss of libido, impotence, hot flashes, weight gain, fatigue, anemia, and osteoporosis. Bisphosphonates reduce bone mineral loss associated with androgen deprivation (Chapter 264).

Hormone-Resistant Prostate Cancer

Typically, the first manifestation of resistance to androgen deprivation is a climbing PSA level in the setting of anorchid levels of testosterone. In about 20% of patients, discontinuation of antiandrogen therapy (flutamide, bicalutamide, nilutamide) while continuing with LHRH agonists results in a PSA decline that can be associated with symptomatic improvement and can persist for 4 to 24 months or more. If this approach fails, treatment with secondary hormonal manipulations, such as ketoconazole or estrogens, is appropriate. Thereafter, treatment with chemotherapeutic regimens, such as mitoxantrone plus corticosteroids or estramustine plus a taxane, may be effective. Two randomized phase III trials have demonstrated a survival advantage of approximately 25% in patients receiving docetaxel-based therapy compared with mitoxantrone, 7,8 and docetaxel-prednisone is now considered a standard therapeutic approach in patients with metastatic, hormone-refractory prostate cancer. In general, serial PSA levels are the best although imperfect way to follow up patients, and a decline of 50% or more is probably clinically significant.

Palliative Care

Many patients with advanced prostate cancer have bone pain or functional impairments that adversely affect quality of life, and provision of appropriate palliative care is an integral component of their management. In addition to the usual analgesics, glucocorticoids serve as anti-inflammatory agents and can alleviate bone pain. For patients with widespread bone metastases and pain not easily

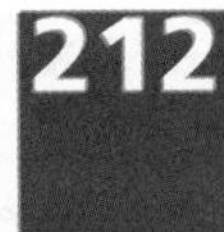

controlled with analgesics or local irradiation (Chapter 28), strontium 89 and samarium 153 are selectively concentrated in bone metastases and alleviate pain in 70% or more of treated patients.

Prognosis

In general, the 10-year PSA progression-free survival is 70 to 80% with Gleason scores of 2 to 4, whether treatment is with radiation therapy or surgery; 50 to 70% for Gleason scores of 5 to 7; and 15 to 30% for Gleason scores of 8 to 10. For patients with a climbing PSA level after radical prostatectomy, time to detectable PSA, Gleason score at the time of prostatectomy, and PSA doubling time are important prognostic variables. The likelihood of bone metastases at 7 years ranges from 20% for good-prognosis patients to 80% for poor-prognosis patients.

For patients with microscopic nodal disease, 10-year survival appears to exceed 80% in men treated with androgen deprivation. Median survival in men treated with androgen deprivation for established metastatic disease ranges from 3 to 5 years. The median survival for men with hormone-resistant disease ranges from 20 months if they are minimally symptomatic to 8 to 12 months if they are severely symptomatic.

Future Directions

Molecular markers help not only in identifying patients at risk for development of progressive disease but also as therapeutic targets. Enhanced understanding of androgen receptor biology may permit the development of specific hormonal therapies and guide the more rational use of existing agents.

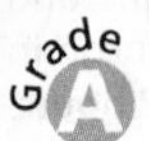

1. Thompson IM, Goodman PJ, Tangen CM, et al: The influence of finasteride on the development of prostate cancer. N Engl J Med 2003;349:215–224.
2. Bill-Axelson A, Holmberg L, Ruutu M, et al: Radical prostatectomy versus watchful waiting in early prostate cancer. N Engl J Med 2005;352:1977–1984.
3. Steineck G, Helgesen F, Adolfsson J, et al: Quality of life after radical prostatectomy or watchful waiting. N Engl J Med 2002;347:790–796.
4. Bolla M, van Poppel H, Collette L, et al: Postoperative radiotherapy after radical prostatectomy: A randomized controlled trial (EORTC trial 22911). Lancet 2005;366:572–578.
5. Roach M 3rd, DeSilvio M, Lawton C, et al: Phase III trial comparing whole-pelvic versus prostate-only radiotherapy and neoadjuvant versus adjuvant combined androgen suppression: Radiation Therapy Oncology Group 9413. J Clin Oncol 2003;21:1904–1911.
6. Stephenson AJ, Shariat SF, Zelefsky MJ, et al: Salvage radiotherapy for recurrent prostate cancer after radical prostatectomy. JAMA 2004;291:1325–1332.
7. Petrylak DP, Tangen CM, Hussain M, et al: Docetaxel and estramustine versus mitoxantrone and prednisone: Results of a Southwest Oncology Group Intergroup Protocol 99-15. N Engl J Med 2004;351:1513–1520.
8. Tannock IF, de Wit R, Berry WR, et al: Docetaxel plus prednisone or mitoxantrone plus prednisone for advanced prostate cancer. N Engl J Med 2004;351:1502–1512.

SUGGESTED READINGS

D'Amico AV, Chen MH, Roehl KA, et al: Preoperative PSA velocity and risk of death from prostate cancer after radical prostatectomy. N Engl J Med 2004;351:125–135. *Men whose PSA level increases more than 2.0 ng/mL during the year before diagnosis may have a relatively high risk of death from prostate cancer despite radical prostatectomy.*

Frankel S, Smith GD, Donovan J, et al: Screening for prostate cancer. Lancet 2003;361:1122–1128. *A concise overview.*

Harris R, Lohr KN: Screening for prostate cancer: An update of the evidence for the U.S. Preventive Services Task Force. Ann Intern Med 2002;137:917–929. *The evidence on which U.S. recommendations are based.*

Pisansky TM: External-beam radiotherapy for localized prostate cancer. N Engl J Med 2006;355:1583–1591. *A clinical overview.*

Sharifi N, Gulley JL, Dahut WL: Androgen deprivation therapy for prostate cancer. JAMA 2005;294:238–244. *A clinical review.*

Thompson IM, Ankerst DP, Chi C, et al: Operating characteristics of prostate-specific antigen in men with an initial PSA level of 3.0 ng/mL or lower. JAMA 2005;294:66–70. *There was a continuum of prostate cancer risk at all values of PSA.*

212 BONE TUMORS: PRIMARY AND METASTATIC BONE LESIONS

Laurence H. Baker

Primary bone tumors are uncommon, whereas metastatic bone cancers are quite common in patients with breast cancer (Chapter 208), prostate cancer (Chapter 211), thyroid cancer (Chapter 244), and other tumors. Primary bone tumors can be benign or malignant.

PRIMARY BONE TUMORS

Definition

A primary bone cancer is any neoplasm that arises from the tissues or cells present within bone and has the capacity to metastasize to distant organs (Table 212–1). Tumors arising from osteoblasts, cartilage cells, fibrous tissue, fat, vascular elements, or hematopoietic and neural tissues of bone are referred to as sarcomas. The three most common primary bone cancers are osteosarcoma, Ewing's family of tumors, and chondrosarcoma. Bone sarcomas are named according to the predominant differentiated tissue type, so bone-forming sarcomas are osteosarcoma and cartilage tumors are chondrosarcomas. The cell of origin of Ewing's sarcoma remains unknown, but a neuroectodermal origin has been assumed on the basis of variable expression of neuronal markers, ultrastructure features, and ability to differentiate in vitro along neural pathways. In the past 30 years, the cure rate for patients with osteosarcoma or Ewing's sarcoma has dramatically improved from 5 to 20% to 50 to 60%, principally owing to integrated care from orthopedic oncologists and pediatric and medical oncologists.

Epidemiology

In the United States, osteosarcoma, Ewing's family of tumors, and chondrosarcoma together affect about 2500 new patients and result in about 1000 deaths annually. The peak age of incidence for osteosarcoma

TABLE 212–1 CLASSIFICATION OF PRIMARY MALIGNANT BONE TUMORS

Osteosarcoma
Intramedullary high grade (conventional)
Intramedullary low grade
Juxtacortical high grade (high-grade surface osteosarcoma)
Juxtacortical intermediate grade, chondroblastic (periosteal osteosarcoma)
Juxtacortical low grade (periosteal osteosarcoma)
Chondrosarcoma
Intramedullary
Juxtacortical
Primitive neuroectodermal tumor, Ewing's sarcoma
Angiosarcoma
Conventional
Epithelioid hemangioendothelioma
Fibrosarcoma, malignant fibrous histiocytoma
Chordoma
Adamantinoma
Conventional
Well-differentiated osteofibrosis, dysplasia-like
Other
Liposarcoma
Leiomyosarcoma
Malignant peripheral nerve sheath tumor
Rhabdomyosarcoma
Malignant mesenchymoma
Malignant hemangiopericytoma
Sarcoma, not otherwise specified

and Ewing's sarcoma is in the second decade of life (typically about the age of 15 years, coincident with adolescent growth spurts), whereas chondrosarcoma has a peak incidence in the sixth or seventh decade. Both osteosarcoma and Ewing's sarcoma have similar incidence rates in both sexes until the age of 13 years, at which point males are more affected. Osteosarcoma occurs with the same prevalence in every country. Ewing's sarcoma is 10 times more common in whites that in individuals of African or Asian descent.

Pathobiology

The increased incidence of bone sarcomas in teenage years supports the assumption that skeletal neoplasms arise in areas of rapid growth. Growing or remodeling bone is susceptible to transformation. The most common location of primary bone sarcomas is adjacent to the growth plate in the metaphyseal region, which is the area of long bones with the most cellular proliferation and remodeling. Nearly two thirds of all bone sarcomas occur in the distal femur or proximal tibia near the knee, areas with the two most active growth plates. Prolonged growth or overstimulation of bone metabolism can result from chronic conditions such as Paget's disease, osteomyelitis, or bone infections and lead to a bone sarcoma. Both external radiation treatment and bone-seeking radioisotopes from occupational or medicinal therapies can lead to osteogenic sarcoma or chondrosarcoma.

Chromosome translocations can allow the creation of fusion proteins that promote tumorigenesis. Almost all Ewing's sarcoma cases are associated with a translocation between chromosomes 11 and 22, which result in a fusion protein between the *EWS* and *FLI1* genes. Loss of tumor suppressor function is also an important mechanism of cancer development. Patients with hereditary retinoblastoma are at great risk for development of a second cancer, which is osteosarcoma in half of the cases, representing a 2000-fold increased risk. Almost one third of patients with osteosarcoma but without retinoblastoma also have mutations in the *RB* gene. Similarly, a significant percentage of patients with osteosarcoma have mutations of *P53*. A minority of patients with osteosarcoma and Ewing's sarcoma have overexpression of *MDM2*, which binds to *P53* and inhibits normal DNA binding.

Primary bone sarcomas are classified according to their cytologic features and cellular products (i.e., osteoid). Osteosarcoma is the most common primary malignant bone sarcoma. Although osteosarcomas can occur as low or high cellular grade lesions, on the basis of their mitotic count, pleomorphism, and cellular atypia, nearly 90% are high grade. The second most common bone sarcoma is chondrosarcoma, which is derived from cartilage cells. Chondrosarcomas, unlike most other primary bone sarcomas, become more frequent with increased age and often involve the axial skeleton. Although chondrosarcomas may be primary, they also can arise from preexisting benign lesions such as enchondromas and osteochondromas. In syndromes with multiple occurrences of these lesions, such as enchondromatosis (Ollier's disease) or hereditary multiple exostosis, the incidence of malignant transformation of one or more of these lesions can be as high as 25%. Although secondary chondrosarcomas are rare in people younger than 50 years, Ollier's disease and multiple hereditary osteochondromatosis frequently occur in young adults. Ewing's sarcoma, which is a primitive neuroectodermal tumor, can also arise in the soft tissues. The morphologic appearance of Ewing's sarcoma is as a primitive undifferentiated neoplasm with monotonous sheets of small round blue cells. There is usually extensive necrosis with viable tumor around blood vessels. Ewing's sarcoma is considered a high-grade neoplasm. Although no routinely used histochemical stain can positively distinguish Ewing's sarcoma from other small round blue cell neoplasms, most express high levels of a cell surface glycoprotein that is encoded by the *MIC2* gene.

Clinical Manifestations

Patients with a bone sarcoma present because of pain, swelling, or a mass. Pain tends not to be associated with activity and is often worse at night. If the lesion is near a joint, an effusion or stiffness of the joint may be the complaint. Systemic or constitutional symptoms, such as weight loss, fever, and malaise, can occur with Ewing's sarcoma but are otherwise rare.

Diagnosis

Important information from the history includes previous radiation treatment or a prior history of cancer. Conventional radiographs of the involved bone are mandatory. Bone lesions may be lytic, destroying bone, or blastic, either inducing reactive bone formation or actively forming bone. Although osteosarcomas are an example of a blastic bone-forming tumor, they can also appear completely lytic radiographically. Important information from the plain film includes whether the lesion is well circumscribed, whether it has a moth-eaten appearance, the degree of permeation, and the presence of a periosteal reaction. To determine the local extent of tumor, magnetic resonance imaging best shows the relationship between normal tissues, neurovascular structures, and the tumor tissue.

Biopsy is critical to diagnosis. Planning for the biopsy is best done jointly by the orthopedic oncologist, the musculoskeletal radiologist, and the bone pathologist. The biopsy should be performed through the compartment in which the tumor has risen to prevent contamination to other structures. Needle biopsies can achieve a diagnostic accuracy of 90% at experienced institutions, but the risk of sampling error makes some centers prefer incisional biopsy.

The most common sites of metastasis of bone sarcomas are to the lung parenchyma and to other bones. Computed tomographic scanning of the chest is recommended to determine if pulmonary metastasis has already occurred. Bone scanning is often performed to evaluate for distant bone metastases and noncontiguous tumors or skip lesions. Important laboratory studies include a white blood cell count, an alkaline phosphatase level, and a lactate dehydrogenase level, which correlates with survival in patients with osteosarcoma and Ewing's sarcoma.

Treatment

Rx

Bone sarcomas are best managed by a combination of surgery, chemotherapy, and radiation therapy. Amputation is performed in only 10% of cases, and limb salvage surgery allows better function and cosmesis without compromise of local control or survival. Chemotherapy has greatly improved the survival of patients with osteosarcoma and Ewing's sarcoma. Most modern treatment plans use initial (neoadjuvant) chemotherapy followed by local treatment and additional chemotherapy. Because most treatment failures are due to distant metastasis, effective systemic therapy is the key to cure. Effective chemotherapies include doxorubicin, cisplatin, high-dose methotrexate, ifosfamide, and etoposide. Even patients presenting with lung metastasis from a Ewing's sarcoma can sometimes be cured. Thus, all patients with Ewing's sarcoma should have the benefit of chemotherapy. Chondrosarcomas are relatively resistant to chemotherapy, so wide surgical excision is the treatment of choice.

Radiation Therapy

Radiation therapy is less often used in osteosarcoma and usually only for those patients unable to undergo definitive surgical resection. However, adjuvant radiation therapy is an essential component of Ewing's sarcoma treatment if the surgical margins are inadequate or very close. Proton beam irradiation for chondrosarcoma at the base of the skull can lead to prolonged progression-free survival and can be an effective treatment strategy.

METASTATIC TUMORS TO BONE

Breast cancer (Chapter 208) is the most common primary tumor to cause bone metastases in women, with lung cancer (Chapter 201) a distant second. Prostate cancer is the most common primary tumor in men, followed by tumors arising in the lung, kidney, gastrointestinal tract, and thyroid.

Clinical Manifestations and Diagnosis

Metastatic tumors to bone typically present with localized or referred pain but can present with a pathologic fracture. These tumors usually produce bone destruction with little or no surrounding soft tissue mass, except when there is direct extension from an adjacent tumor, as is sometimes seen in lung cancer, for example. On plain films, most metastatic tumors cause lytic bone lesions, but breast (Chapter 208) or prostate (Chapter 211) cancers typically produce mixed lytic and blastic changes, and myeloma is usually purely lytic.

A radioisotope bone scan can determine whether more than one lesion is present, as is usual for metastatic disease. For myeloma, a skeletal series with plain films is recommended because its lesions commonly are not seen on radioisotope scans. Otherwise, current clinical practice typically does not recommend radiologic testing to screen for bone metastases in cancer patients with no relevant symptoms or signs.

When bone metastases are suspected but a primary tumor is not evident, needle biopsy of a lesion, if possible, is preferable to a detailed search for an unknown primary (Chapter 215).

Treatment and prognosis

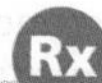

Lesions can be palliated with direct irradiation or with radioisotopes, but treatment otherwise depends on the type of tumor. Bisphosphonates (Chapter 264) can ameliorate symptoms and delay the onset of bone-related clinical events. By comparison, calcitonin appears not to be beneficial. Surgery should be considered to preserve function when there is important structural compromise and the patient's overall condition warrants surgery.

SUGGESTED READINGS

Costelloe CM, Kumar R, Yasko AW, et al: Imaging characteristics of locally recurrent tumors of bone. AJR Am J Roentgenol 2007;188:855–863. *Review of identifying radiologically recurrent tumors of the bone.*

National Comprehensive Cancer Network: The NCCN v.1.2006 Bone Cancer Clinical Practice Guidelines in Oncology. Available at http://www.nccn.org. *Consensus guidelines.*

Roodman GD: Mechanisms of bone metastasis. N Engl J Med 2004; 350:1655–1664. *A comprehensive review.*

Selvaggi G, Scagliotti GV: Management of bone metastases in cancer. A review. Crit Rev Oncol Hematol 2005;56:365–378. *Bisphosphonates significantly increase the time to a first skeleton-related event.*

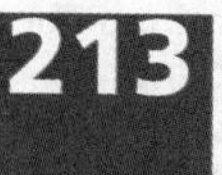

213 SARCOMAS OF SOFT TISSUE

Karen Antman

Definition

Sarcomas include malignant tumors of bone and soft tissue that, like leukemias and lymphomas, arise in tissues of mesodermal origin (Table 213–1). By convention, sarcomas also include a small group of malignant tumors of peripheral nerves, which are of ectodermal origin.

TABLE 213–1 CLASSIFICATION OF SARCOMAS

SARCOMAS OF BONE
Osteosarcomas
Ewing's sarcomas
Chondrosarcomas
SARCOMAS OF SOFT TISSUE
Classic sarcomas of trunk and extremity
Visceral and organ sarcomas (e.g., sarcomas of the gastrointestinal tract, uterus, or breast)
Atypical sarcomas: rhabdomyosarcomas, extraosseous Ewing's sarcoma/peripheral neuroectodermal tumors, Kaposi's sarcoma, gastrointestinal stromal sarcomas, and mesotheliomas

Epidemiology

Soft tissue sarcomas represent 0.7% of adult malignancies and 15% of pediatric malignancies. About 9500 U.S. residents develop soft tissue sarcoma annually, and 3500 die. However, current coding excludes visceral and organ sarcomas (e.g., sarcoma of the stomach or breast); including these tumors would approximately double the numbers of reported sarcomas.

Excluding uterine sarcomas, the ratio of incidence and mortality of classic soft tissue sarcoma in men and women is 1.36:1 and 1.2:1, respectively. Men account for 70% of cases of Kaposi's sarcomas (Chapter 416) and 58% of liposarcomas but only 35% of leiomyosarcomas (Chapter 209).

Known risk factors such as radiation therapy (Chapter 18), chemotherapy, and specific environmental or occupational exposures (Chapters 17 and 20) account for only 5% of sarcomas. Although most radiation-associated sarcomas arise in bone, mixed mesodermal sarcomas of the uterus, mesotheliomas, and other soft tissue sarcomas may develop, usually decades after therapeutic radiation. Angiosarcomas of the breast, however, can develop in radiation ports as early as a few years after breast radiation; lymphedema strongly increases the risk of angiosarcoma. Chemotherapeutic agents (Chapter 192) associated with sarcoma include melphalan, procarbazine, nitrosoureas, and chlorambucil; tamoxifen is a risk factor for endometrial sarcomas.

Angiosarcoma of the liver (Chapter 206) can develop after chronic hemochromatosis (Chapter 231) or after exposure to arsenic or to polyvinyl chloride in the plastics industries (Chapter 20). Chlorophenols, agricultural herbicides, or dioxin (Agent Orange) exposure also may increase the risk of soft tissue sarcomas. Mesotheliomas (Chapter 100) are associated with occupational or household exposure to asbestos (Chapter 93).

Human herpesvirus 8 (Chapter 398) is detected in virtually all patients with Kaposi's sarcoma (Chapter 416). In immunosuppressed patients, leiomyosarcomas are associated with Epstein-Barr virus (Chapter 401). Human herpesvirus 8 and Epstein-Barr virus are closely related gamma herpesviruses. Murine, simian, and avian sarcoma viruses are well documented in other species.

Pathobiology

Familial and Multiprimary Syndromes

Li-Fraumeni syndrome (Chapter 186) is characterized by childhood sarcomas, breast cancer (often bilateral), brain tumors, leukemia, and adrenal cortical carcinomas, many developing before age 45 years. About 70% of these families carry germline *p53* mutations. The *CHK2* gene is mutated in a subset of the remaining families; its protein, a checkpoint serine/threonine kinase, acts upstream of *p53* in response to DNA damage.

Familial gastrointestinal stromal tumors (GISTs; see later) occur in family members who carry a mutation in the *cKit* gene on chromosome 4. Patients with *Gardner's syndrome* (Chapter 203), a variant of familial adenomatous polyposis (Chapter 203), have an increased risk of intra-abdominal desmoid tumors (borderline or low-grade fibrosarcomas), as well as gastrointestinal tract polyps, osteomas, epidermoid cysts, fibromas, and dental abnormalities. A mutated adenomatous polyposis coli *(APC)* gene is inherited as an autosomal dominant.

Werner's syndrome (Chapter 22) is characterized by small stature, genital hypoplasia, and early aging, including juvenile cataracts, gray hair, scleroderma-like skin changes, osteoporosis, and hyperglycemia. Most reported families are Japanese. Patients die of malignant or arteriosclerotic diseases at an average age of 45 years. Up to 25% of patients develop sarcomas and carcinomas. The *WRN* gene is a DNA helicase and exonuclease, but the mechanism for a decline in physiologic functions is unknown.

Neurofibromatosis type 1 (Chapter 444) is associated with a 2 to 16% lifetime risk of malignant sarcoma, most commonly a malignant peripheral nerve sheath tumor, also called malignant or plexiform neurofibroma. About half of patients who develop neurofibrosarcoma have an underlying diagnosis of neurofibromatosis.

Carney's triad includes gastric stromal tumors, pulmonary hamartomas, and functioning extra-adrenal paragangliomas. Pulmonary lesions detected on radiography may be metastases or benign hamar-

TABLE 213–2 TRANSLOCATIONS IN SARCOMA

Sarcoma	Translocation	Fusion Product
Ewing's sarcoma/peripheral neuroectodermal tumor	t(11;22)(q24;q12)	*FLI-1-EWS*
	t(21;22)(q22;q12)	*ERG-EWS*
	t(7;22)(p22;q12)	*ETV1-EWS*
	t(17;22)(q12;q12)	*EIAF-EWS*
	t(2;22)(q33;q12)	*FEV-EWS*
Alveolar rhabdomyosarcoma	t(2;13)(q35;q14)	*PAX3-FKHR*
	t(1;13)(p36;q14)	*PAX7-FKHR*
Myxoid/round cell liposarcoma	t(12:16)(q13;q11)	*CHOP-TLS*
	t(12;22)(q13;q11-12)	*CHOP-EWS*
Desmoplastic small round cell tumor	t(11;22)(p13;q12)	*WT1-EWS*
Synovial sarcoma	t(X;18)(p11.2;q11.2)	*SSX1&2-SYT*
Clear cell sarcoma	t(12;22)(q13;q12)	*ATF-1-EWS*
Extraskeletal myxoid chondrosarcoma	t(9;22)(q22;q12)	*TEC-EWS*
Dermatofibrosarcoma protuberans/giant cell fibroblastoma	t(17;22)(q22;q13)	*PDGFB-COL1A1*
Infantile fibrosarcoma	t(12;15)(p13;q25)	*ETV6-NTRK3*
Alveolar soft part sarcoma	t(X;17)(p11;q25)	*ASPL-TFE3*

TABLE 213–3 STAGING OF SOFT TISSUE SARCOMAS

Stage	Grade	Greatest Diameter	Depth	Involved Lymph Nodes or Metastases
1		Low or intermediate	Any	Any No
2	High	<5 cm	Any	No
	High	>5 cm	Superficial	No
3	High	>5 cm	Deep	No
4	Any	Any	Any	Yes

tomas and must be examined by biopsy before chemotherapy is administered for metastatic disease.

Genetics

Simple reciprocal translocations are virtually diagnostic of about one third of sarcomas, in contrast with 3% of carcinomas but 50 to 60% of lymphomas and leukemias. Such sarcomas tend to develop in younger patients. The remaining two thirds of sarcomas tend to have unbalanced, nonspecific, and complex karyotypes characterized by *Rb* and *p53* inactivation, including sarcomas associated with Li-Fraumeni syndrome and prior radiation exposure (Table 213–2).

Rhabdomyosarcoma has at least three molecular variants. Embryonal rhabdomyosarcoma, most common in the orbit and urinary tract in young children, is characterized by loss of heterozygosity at 11p15. Alveolar rhabdomyosarcoma, however, has two variants: translocations involving the transcription family forkhead *(FKHR)* gene on chromosome 13 with either *Pax 3* on chromosome 2 or Pax 7 on chromosome 1. Patients with the *Pax 3* translocation tend to be older with central lesions and a higher risk of metastases. Synovial sarcoma is characterized by two variant t(X:18) translocations, both of which are aberrant transcriptional regulators and have different histologic patterns and prognoses.

Clinical Manifestations

Most soft tissue sarcomas develop in the lower (30%) or upper (15%) extremity. Approximately 30% arise in the trunk and retroperitoneum, and 15% occur in the head and neck. Soft tissue sarcomas of the extremities or trunk usually develop as a painless mass. Patients may report a lump present for years (particularly with synovial sarcomas), but the median duration of symptoms before diagnosis is approximately 2 months. Sarcomas in the gastrointestinal, genitourinary, and gynecologic tracts manifest with bleeding or pain. Retroperitoneal sarcomas can become very large before they cause sufficient pain, weight loss, or a mass to prompt diagnosis.

Diagnosis

Because sarcomas are relatively uncommon, most physicians are inexperienced in their diagnosis. Whenever possible, patients with possible sarcoma should be referred to an experienced institution.

Biopsy

An incisional biopsy should be planned so the biopsy scar is excised during the definitive resection and included in the radiation port should the biopsy reveal a sarcoma. Once a biopsy-confirmed diagnosis of sarcoma is established, preoperative staging generally requires computed tomography (CT) of the lungs and magnetic resonance imaging (MRI) of the primary lesion. The staging system is based on tumor size, grade, and depth (Table 213–3).

A continuum exists from normal connective tissue to benign lesions, to borderline and very low-grade malignancies, and finally to aggressive, undifferentiated, invasive high-grade sarcomas. Sarcomas do not normally arise within their benign tumor variants, which in most cases have very different molecular genetics (Table 213–4).

Malignant fibrous histiocytoma and leiomyosarcomas were the most common sarcomas until recently. The diagnosis of malignant fibrous histiocytoma became less common with the development of immunocytochemistry, genetic diagnosis, and other techniques that provide specific diagnoses. Similarly, most tumors that were previously called leiomyosarcomas of the gastrointestinal tract are now considered GISTs (see later).

Types of Sarcoma

Leiomyosarcoma, a malignant tumor of smooth muscle, most commonly develops in the uterus, blood vessels, extremities, or trunk. Uterine leiomyosarcomas, which rarely if ever develop in existing uterine fibroids, usually manifest with bleeding or pain. A large mass or a large area of necrosis on CT or MRI suggests a sarcoma. Retroperitoneal and vena cava leiomyosarcomas affect women disproportionately and may grow rapidly during pregnancy.

Liposarcomas, which may be multicentric, develop in the thigh or retroperitoneum, generally in patients older than 50 years. *Synovial*

TABLE 213–4 CONTINUUM OF NORMAL TO MALIGNANT TUMORS OF CONNECTIVE TISSUE

Normal	Benign Tumor	Borderline Malignancy	Low Grade	High Grade (Invasive, Aggressive, Metastasizing)
Smooth muscle	Leiomyoma	Benign metastasizing leiomyoma	Leiomyosarcoma	Leiomyosarcoma
Striated muscle	Rhabdomyoma	—	—	Rhabdomyosarcoma
Fibrous tissue, fascia	Fibroma, Dupuytren's contracture	Desmoid, fibromatosis	Fibrosarcoma	Pleomorphic fibrosarcoma
Blood vessel endothelium	Angioma, hemangioma	Hemangioendothelioma	Angiosarcoma	Angiosarcoma
Vascular pericytes	—	Angioblastic meningioma	Hemangiopericytoma	—
Fat	Lipoma	—	Myxoid liposarcoma	Pleomorphic liposarcoma

sarcoma manifests as a mass, often present for years, adjacent to a joint and involving the joint capsule, bursae, and tendon sheath but not the joint itself, typically in adolescents and young adults. Radiographic calcifications are present in one third of patients.

Neurosarcomas and malignant schwannomas produce a fusiform mass with tumor extending within the nerve sheath. About half of these tumors develop in patients with preexisting neurofibromatosis (Chapter 444).

Angiosarcomas, previously sometimes called hemangioblastomas, hemangiosarcomas, or lymphangiosarcomas, most commonly arise as multicentric scalp lesions in older men or in edematous extremities, typically after mastectomy and axillary dissection for breast cancer. Angiosarcomas of the breast occur in young and middle-aged women, particularly after breast irradiation. Angiosarcomas occur in the liver after exposure to thorium dioxide and polyvinyl chloride. These tumors are also the most common primary malignancy of the myocardium (Chapter 59). Angiosarcomas may produce microangiopathic hemolytic anemia (Kasabach-Merritt syndrome) from traumatic injury of red cells traversing the tumor bed (Chapter 164).

Hemangiopericytomas, derived from vascular pericytes, most commonly develop in the thigh (35%) and retroperitoneum (25%). Intracranial hemangiopericytomas, formerly designated angioblastic meningiomas, grow along the sinuses, locally recur, and may metastasize.

Treatment

Rx

The goals of treatment are to obtain local and systemic control of the sarcoma while preserving function of the involved extremity or organ as well as quality of life. Most soft tissue sarcomas are currently treated similarly grade for grade.

If preoperative evaluation reveals no evidence of metastasis, treatment is surgical, often with preoperative or postoperative radiation therapy. Preoperative chemotherapy is sometimes considered for patients with large primary tumors, particularly if shrinking the tumor would facilitate complete resection.

Wide excision of 3 to 6 cm of normal tissue is required for local control if radiation therapy is not planned. Soft tissue sarcomas are usually pseudoencapsulated (i.e., microscopic projections of tumor extend beyond the apparent tumor capsule). Any excision that merely "shells out" the apparently encapsulated tumor generally leaves behind microscopic residual tumor and results in local regrowth in about 80% of cases. Lymph node dissections are rarely necessary and are considered only if lymph nodes are clinically involved. Low-grade lesions, if adequately resected, are generally curable, as are lesions smaller than 5 cm, even if they are histologically of high grade. However, intra-abdominal and retroperitoneal tumors tend to be large and to invade vital vessels and organs. Even small head and neck sarcomas tend to be difficult to resect with adequate margins. Many primary retroperitoneal and head and neck lesions are unresectable at presentation.

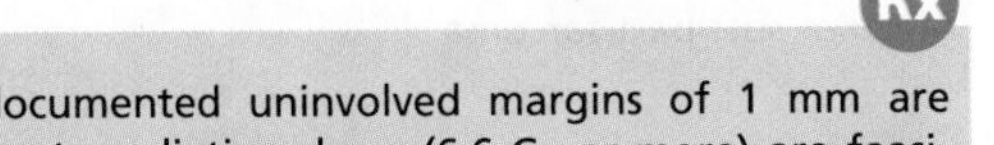
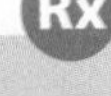

Pathologically documented uninvolved margins of 1 mm are acceptable if adequate radiation doses (6.6 Gy or more) are feasible. Such doses are usually tolerated for lesions on the extremities, but they are less often possible for tumors in the retroperitoneum or abdomen because of damage to neighboring normal structures.

The current standards of limb-sparing surgery combined with radiation therapy, or radical resection or amputation, achieve local control with acceptable function in 90% of patients with extremity lesions at experienced centers. Local control rates remain 50 to 75% for trunk lesions and 30 to 50% for primary retroperitoneal lesions.

Sarcomas tend to spare lymph nodes and to metastasize from trunk and extremities directly to lung or from intra-abdominal sites to liver. The median survival for patients with unresectable or metastatic sarcoma is about 12 months.

Adjuvant Chemotherapy for Resectable Sarcomas

Adjuvant chemotherapy is well established for the treatment of rhabdomyosarcomas, osteosarcomas, and Ewing's sarcomas, but randomized data are equivocal for other soft tissue sarcomas in adults. In a meta-analysis, doxorubicin-based adjuvant chemotherapy for adult soft tissue sarcomas significantly improved recurrence-free survival but not overall survival. [1]

Therapy for Advanced Soft Tissue Sarcomas

Sarcomas that recur locally are generally resected if metastases are not present. Some patients with metastatic sarcoma who are rendered clinically free of disease either surgically or with chemotherapy survive without relapse. Surgical removal of typical subpleural metastases results in disease-free survival in 15 to 20% of carefully selected patients. Patients with fewer than five nodules, a disease-free interval of more than 12 months, and a tumor doubling time of more than 20 days survive longer. Repeated metastasectomy may be necessary.

Single-agent therapy is often used for palliation. With the exception of doxorubicin, drugs are generally discontinued when the tumor progresses or unacceptable toxicity develops. Doxorubicin (25 mg/m^2/day for 3 days with the course repeated every 21 days) is the most active single agent in soft tissue sarcomas, with a response rate of 20%. Because of the risk of doxorubicin-associated cardiomyopathy, use of this drug must be carefully supervised by an experienced physician.

Dacarbazine, 250 mg/m^2/day for 4 days with the course repeated every 21 days, has a response rate of about 16% and is most active in leiomyosarcomas. Giving the drug by continuous infusion somewhat ameliorates the nausea and vomiting. Ifosfamide, 2.5 g/m^2/day for 4 days with the course repeated every 21 days, produces response rates of 15 to 20%; mesna is required to avoid bladder toxicity.

Combination chemotherapy is appropriate if a response would facilitate potentially curative resection or if treatment is needed for palliation, particularly in patients less than 50 years old who have high-grade lesions. Doxorubicin in combination with ifosfamide

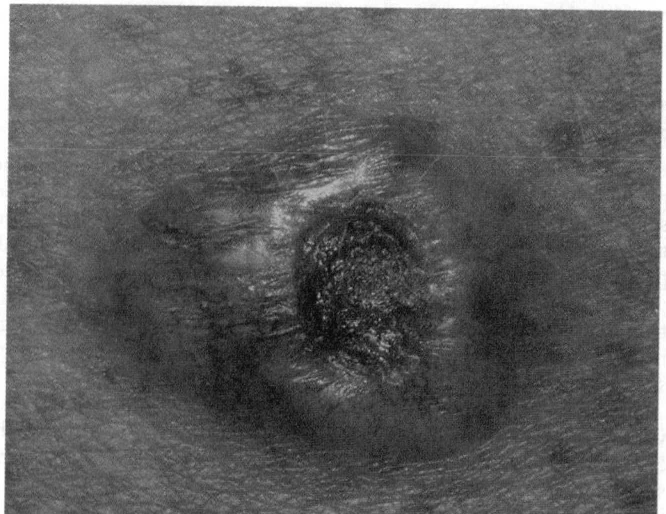

FIGURE 214–6 • Basal cell carcinoma.

(Chapter 18). The timing and pattern of sun exposure are associated with different types of skin cancer. In general, squamous cell carcinoma is associated with cumulative sun exposure and occurs most frequently in areas maximally exposed to the sun (e.g., the face, back of hands, and forearms). Intermittent, intense exposure to the sun, particularly in childhood, is associated with an increased risk of basal cell carcinoma. Individuals who have fair skin, light-colored eyes, red hair, a tendency to burn rather than tan, and a history of severe sunburns are at increased risk for nonmelanoma skin cancers. Other risk factors, primarily for squamous cell carcinoma, include chronic arsenic exposure, therapeutic radiation, chronic inflammatory skin conditions, psoralen plus UVA (PUVA) treatment for psoriasis and other diseases, and immunosuppression. Most cases in African-American patients are associated with scarring or burns rather than UV exposure. Human papillomavirus infection has also been implicated in some squamous cell carcinomas, particularly in the autosomal dominant disorder epidermodysplasia verruciformis.

Basal cell carcinoma can be seen in association with several conditions, including the basal cell nevus syndrome (also called nevoid basal cell carcinoma syndrome or Gorlin's syndrome), albinism, and xeroderma pigmentosum. The basal cell nevus syndrome is a rare autosomal dominant disorder caused by germline mutations in the patched gene *(PTCH)*.

Prevention and Screening

Primary prevention strategies are aimed at reducing long-term sun exposure. Public education and patient education should encourage the regular use of sunscreens with a sun protection factor of 15 or greater, especially in childhood, and sun protective clothing (e.g., a broad-brimmed hat). Avoidance of tanning parlors and minimizing of total sun exposure, especially to the midday sun, is recommended. The thinning of the ozone layer has been linked to increased UV radiation and increases in the incidence of nonmelanoma skin cancers. Currently, no evidence indicates that total body skin examination is effective at reducing mortality or morbidity from nonmelanoma skin cancer.

Clinical Manifestations

Basal Cell Carcinoma

Approximately 90% of basal cell carcinomas occur on sun-exposed areas such as the face, neck, ears, scalp, and arms. The nose is the most common site. Typical basal cell carcinomas appear as slowly growing, shiny, skin-colored to pink translucent papules with telangiectasia and a "pearly" rolled border (Fig. 214–6). As the tumor grows, the center may become ulcerated and bleed, although there is usually no associated pain or tenderness. Basal cell carcinoma rarely metastasizes and is usually curable with a variety of treatments. Although the mortality rate is low, these cancers may result in significant morbidity owing to invasive local growth with potential disfigurement and destruction of skin, bone, and cartilage.

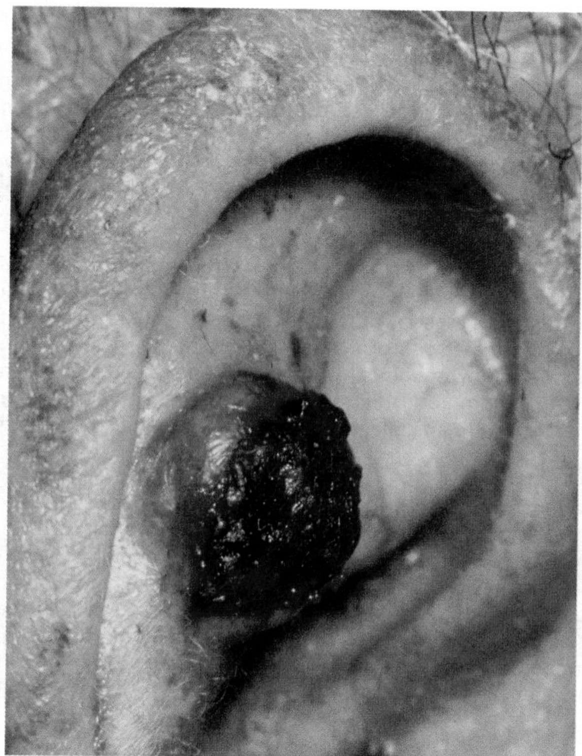

FIGURE 214–7 • Squamous cell carcinoma of the skin.

Squamous Cell Carcinoma

This type of skin cancer usually appears on areas of skin that are heavily damaged by sun exposure. The most common sites include the head or neck, back, forearms, and dorsum of the hand. Clinically, squamous cell carcinoma occurs as a discrete scaly erythematous papule on an indurated base that can develop on normal-appearing skin or on an actinic keratosis (Fig. 214–7). The lesion may grow over time and may become ulcerated, itchy, painful, or bleeding. Keratoacanthoma is a variant that is characterized by rapid growth and a crateriform appear ance with a central plug. Bowen's disease, or squamous cell carcinoma situ, manifests as an erythematous, scaly, sharply defined plaque.

Untreated squamous cell carcinoma may cause significant destruction. However, unlike basal cell carcinoma, squamous ce nomas carry a 0.5 to 5% risk of metastasis. Higher-risk lesions se that are larger than 2 cm, are moderately or poorly different have perineural involvement, are on the ear or the lip, arise in sc s, or occur in immunosuppressed patients. Most metastases develop in regional lymph nodes, although metastases may also occur in lung, liver, brain, skin, or bone. For patients with lymph node metastases, the 5-year survival is less than 50%.

Diagnosis

The diagnosis of basal cell carcinoma and squamous cell carcinoma is frequently suspected by inspection alone, but histologic confirmation is usually indicated. Either a shave or a punch biopsy technique is acceptable (Chapter 462). Care should be taken to include the base of the lesion if a shave biopsy technique is used.

Treatment

Basal Cell Carcinoma

The technique with the lowest recurrence rate and using the least tissue is Mohs' micrographic surgery, which utilizes frozen tissue mapping of the resection margins in stages to locate residual tumor. Mohs' microsurgery should be considered when treating recurrent cases; microscopically aggressive forms, such as the morpheaform subtype; lesions greater than 2 cm in greatest diameter; and tumors of the ears, eyelids, nose, nasolabial folds, and lips. Other options for local lesions include traditional surgical excision, cryosurgery (liquid nitrogen), electrodesiccation and curettage, and radiation therapy. Retinoids, interferon-α, topical 5-fluorouracil, photodynamic therapy, and imiquimod are also used. Cure rates for basal cell carcinoma range between 90 and 99%.

Squamous Cell Carcinoma

As with basal cell carcinoma, Mohs' micrographic surgery provides the lowest recurrence rate, with cure rates greater than 90%. Mohs' microsurgery is especially useful for recurrent tumors or lesions that have an increased risk of metastasis. Squamous cell carcinoma can also be cured by traditional surgical excision and radiation therapy. Topical 5-fluorouracil, photodynamic therapy, or imiquimod may have a role in the management of in situ squamous cell cancers.

Follow-up

Patients with basal cell carcinoma and squamous cell carcinoma require ongoing follow-up to detect local recurrences and to recognize new skin cancers. The likelihood of developing a second basal cell carcinoma or squamous cell carcinoma has been estimated to be 15% over 3 years. In addition, these patients have an increased risk of developing cutaneous melanoma. Patient education regarding modification of risk factors (i.e., sun exposure) is an important component of follow-up.

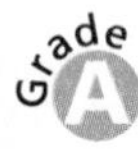

1. Balch CM, Soong S, Ross MI, et al: Long-term results of a multi-institutional randomized trial comparing prognostic factors and surgical results for intermediate thickness melanomas (1.0 to 4.0 mm): Intergroup Melanoma Surgical Trial. Ann Surg Oncol 2000;7:87–97.
2. Thomas JM, Newton-Bishop J, A'Hern R, et al: Excision margins in high-risk malignant melanoma. N Engl J Med 2004;350:757–766.
3. Kirkwood JM, Ibrahim JG, Sosman JA, et al: High dose interferon alfa-2b significantly prolongs relapse free and overall survival compared with the GM2-KLH/QS21 vaccine in patients with resected stage IIB/III melanoma: Results of intergroup Trial E1694/S9512/C509801. J Clin Oncol 2001;19:2370–2380.
4. Morton DL, Thompson JF, Cochran AJ, et al: Sentinel-node biopsy or nodal observation in melanoma. N Engl J Med 2006;355:1307–1317.

Section XV Oncology

SUGGESTED READINGS

Cummins DL, Cummins JM, Pantle H, et al: Cutaneous malignant melanoma. Mayo Clin Proc 2006;81:500–507. *A comprehensive review.*

Curtin JA, Fridyland J, Kageshita T, et al: Distinct sets of genetic alterations in melanoma. N Engl J Med 2005;353:2135–2147. *Identifies genetic alterations in melanomas at different sites and with different levels of sun exposure.*

Ferrone CR, Porat LB, Panageas KS, et al: Clinicopathological features of and risk factors for multiple primary melanomas. JAMA 2005;294:1647–1654. *The incidence was increased in patients with a positive family history and/or dysplastic nevi.*

Tsao H, Atkins MB, Sober AJ: Management of cutaneous melanoma. N Engl J Med 2004;351:998–1012. *An excellent review.*

215 CANCER OF UNKNOWN PRIMARY ORIGIN

John D. Hainsworth and F. Anthony Greco

Definition

The first signs or symptoms of cancer are frequently the result of metastases to visceral or nodal sites. In most such patients, routine clinical evaluation with a comprehensive history, physical examination, complete blood cell count, screening chemistries, and directed radiologic evaluation of specific symptoms or signs identifies the primary tumor. Patients who have no primary tumor located after this routine clinical evaluation are defined as having cancer of unknown primary site. Further clinical and pathologic evaluation will identify the primary site in only a few patients, and approximately 80% will never have a primary site identified during their subsequent clinical course.

Epidemiology

In patients whose primary site of cancer remains undetectable, the primary site presumably has remained small or, less likely, has regressed spontaneously. Large autopsy series before the routine use of computed tomographic scans or magnetic resonance imaging identified small primary sites of cancer in 85% of patients with previously unidentified primary tumors, usually in the pancreas, lung, and various other gastrointestinal sites; with current use of computed tomography and magnetic resonance imaging, however, autopsy series have identified primary sites in only 50 to 70% of patients.

Approximately 3% of all patients with cancer have metastatic disease without a known primary site; the annual incidence is approximately 50,000 to 60,000 cases in the United States. Cancer of unknown primary site occurs with approximately equal frequency in men and women, and it increases in incidence with advancing age.

Diagnosis

The initial clinical and pathologic evaluation should focus on identifying a primary site when possible and on identifying patients for whom specific treatment is indicated. In most patients with cancer of unknown primary site, the diagnosis of advanced cancer is strongly suspected after the initial history and physical examination. A brief additional evaluation, including complete blood cell counts, chemistry profile, and computed tomography of the chest and abdomen should be performed. In addition, specific symptoms or signs should be evaluated with appropriate radiologic and endoscopic studies.

Biopsy

The diagnosis of metastatic cancer should be confirmed by biopsy of the most accessible metastatic lesion. Fine-needle aspiration may or may not provide sufficient material for optimal histologic examination and special pathologic procedures. If tissue is inadequate, a larger biopsy sample should be obtained so all necessary stains and procedures can be performed.

Optimal pathologic evaluation can identify subsets of patient who have chemotherapy-responsive tumors and sometimes can identify a primary site. The initial light microscopic evaluation identifies an adenocarcinoma in approximately 60% of patients with cancer of unknown primary site. Other diagnoses obtained by initial light microscopic examination include poorly differentiated carcinoma (25%), squamous carcinoma (10%), and poorly differentiated neoplasm (inability to distinguish among carcinoma, lymphoma, melanoma, and sarcoma; 5%).

In patients with adenocarcinoma, it is seldom possible for the pathologist to identify a primary site either by light microscopic characteristics or with additional pathologic techniques. Specific exceptions include immunoperoxidase staining for prostate-specific antigen (PSA), which is relatively specific for adenocarcinoma of the prostate (Chapter 211); for estrogen and progesterone receptors, which are suggestive of breast cancer (Chapter 208); and for leukocyte common antigen, which can identify non-Hodgkin's lymphoma (Chapter 196) as the primary tumor in up to 50% of patients with poorly differentiated neoplasms. Other diagnoses suggested by immunoperoxidase staining include neuroendocrine carcinomas, melanomas (Chapter 214), and sarcomas (Chapter 213). Electron microscopy should be considered when light microscopy and immunoperoxidase staining fail to identify the tumor, especially in young patients with anaplastic tumors, specific ultrastructural features of which may suggest neuroendocrine carcinoma (neurosecretory granules), melanoma (premelanosomes), and certain sarcomas.

Occasionally, detection of a tumor-specific chromosomal abnormality can provide a definitive diagnosis. Cancers with recognized specific chromosomal abnormalities include germ cell tumors (i12p; Chapter 210), peripheral neuroepithelioma and Ewing's tumor (t11;22; Chapter 212), and non-Hodgkin's lymphoma (Chapter 196). Chromosomal analysis should therefore be considered, especially in young men who have poorly differentiated mediastinal or retroperitoneal tumors and in whom other pathologic studies have been inconclusive. In the future, gene array profiling will be likely to aid in identifying the primary site and in guiding therapy.

Search for the Primary Site

After completion of the brief and directed initial evaluation outlined previously, further diagnostic studies should be limited (Table 215–1). Positron emission tomography identifies a primary site and guides therapy in about one third of patients, so it should be obtained in all patients with an initially unknown primary tumor. By comparison, other routine radiologic and endoscopic evaluations of asymptomatic areas are not useful in the identification of a primary site and therefore are not recommended. Levels of serum tumor markers, including carcinoembryonic antigen, CA-125, CA-19–9, and CA-15–3, are frequently elevated in patients with carcinoma of unknown primary site; however, these elevations are nonspecific and should not be used to infer a primary site, even though they can be useful in monitoring response to treatment.

All men with metastatic adenocarcinoma should have measurement of serum PSA. Mammograms should be considered in women with metastatic adenocarcinoma, particularly if clinical features are consistent with metastatic breast cancer (e.g., axillary node involvement, pleural effusion, lytic or blastic bone metastases). Patients younger than 50 years of age with poorly differentiated carcinoma should have measurement of serum human chorionic gonadotropin and α-fetoprotein levels. Patients with metastatic squamous carcinoma involving cervical lymph nodes should have thorough endoscopic evaluation of the head and neck, including visualization of the structures from the nasopharynx to the larynx and biopsy of any suspicious areas (Chapter 200). Fiberoptic bronchoscopy should also be considered in patients who have low cervical adenopathy and who do not have a head or neck primary site established by endoscopic examination (Chapter 201). Patients with metastatic squamous carcinoma involving inguinal lymph nodes should have careful inspection of all perineal structures, including anoscopy, a urologic evaluation, and a pelvic examination in women.

Treatment

Rx

Management of Specific Treatable Subsets

Because all patients with cancer of unknown primary site have advanced disease, therapeutic nihilism has been common. However, several subsets of patients who benefit from specific treatment can be identified on the basis of clinical and pathologic features (Table 215–2). These patients are important to recognize and treat appropriately, because some patients in each group have the potential for long-term survival.

Adenocarcinoma

Women with Axillary Lymph Node Metastases

Metastatic breast cancer should be suspected in women who have axillary lymph node involvement with adenocarcinoma, particularly when other metastatic sites are not evident. In these patients, pathologic evaluation of the initial lymph node biopsy should include staining for estrogen and progesterone receptors and for HER-2 expression; elevated levels provide strong evidence for the diagnosis of breast cancer. When no other metastases are identified, these women should be treated as if they had stage II breast cancer, which is potentially curable with appropriate therapy (Chapter 208). Modified radical mastectomy identifies a breast primary site in 44 to 82% of women, even when the breast examination and mammographic findings are normal. Axillary lymph node dissection followed by empirical radiation therapy to the breast appears to give results similar to those of mastectomy, although these two options for primary therapy have not been compared directly. Adjuvant systemic therapy should follow standard guidelines for treatment of patients with stage II breast cancer.

Women with Peritoneal Carcinomatosis

Adenocarcinoma involving the peritoneum in women usually originates from the ovary (Chapter 209), although carcinomas arising in the gastrointestinal tract or breast can occasionally produce this syndrome. However, diffuse peritoneal carcinomatosis occasionally occurs in women who have histologically normal ovaries or who have had previous bilateral oophorectomy. The peritoneum is frequently the only site of tumor involvement, and serum CA-125 levels are usually elevated. When histologic features suggest ovarian cancer, this syndrome has been called *peritoneal papillary serous carcinoma* or *primary extraovarian serous carcinoma*.

Even when the histologic features are not typical, women with adenocarcinoma of unknown primary site involving the peritoneum often have cancers with biologic characteristics similar to those of ovarian cancer (Chapter 209). Treatment of these patients should

TABLE 215–1 RECOMMENDED EVALUATION FOLLOWING INITIAL LIGHT MICROSCOPIC DIAGNOSIS

Diagnosis	Clinical Evaluation*	Special Pathologic Studies
Adenocarcinoma (or poorly differentiated adenocarcinoma)	PET scan CT scans of chest, abdomen Men: serum PSA Women: Mammograms Additional directed radiologic/endoscopic studies to evaluate abnormal symptoms, signs, laboratory values	Men: PSA stain Women: estrogen and progesterone receptor stains (if clinical features suggest metastatic breast cancer)
Poorly differentiated carcinoma	PET scan CT scans of chest, abdomen Serum hCG, AFP Additional directed radiologic/endoscopic studies to evaluate abnormal symptoms, signs, laboratory values	Immunoperoxidase staining Electron microscopy (if immunoperoxidase stains indeterminate) Molecular genetic analysis (consider in young men with features of extragonadal germ cell tumor)
Squamous carcinoma, cervical nodes	PET scan Direct laryngoscopy with visualization/biopsy of nasopharynx, pharynx, hypopharynx, larynx Fiberoptic bronchoscopy (if laryngoscopy is negative)	—
Squamous carcinoma, inguinal nodes	PET scan Complete examination of perineal area (including pelvic examination) Anoscopy Cystoscopy	

*In addition to a history, physical examination, complete blood cell counts, chemistry profile, and chest radiograph.
AFP = α-fetoprotein; CT = computed tomography; hCG = human chorionic gonadotropin; PET = positron emission tomography; PSA = prostate-specific antigen.

TABLE 215–2 SPECIFIC PATIENT SUBSETS AND RECOMMENDED TREATMENT

Specific Subset-Identifying Features		
Histologic	**Clinical**	**Treatment Recommendations**
Adenocarcinoma	Women, isolated axillary adenopathy	Treat as stage II breast cancer
Adenocarcinoma	Women, peritoneal carcinomatosis (?occasionally men)	Treat as stage III ovarian cancer
Adenocarcinoma	Men, elevated PSA and/or blastic bone metastases	Treat as advanced prostate cancer
Adenocarcinoma, poorly differentiated carcinoma	Single metastatic lesion	Definitive local therapy (resection and/or radiation therapy) with or without chemotherapy
Squamous	Cervical adenopathy	Treat as locally advanced head or neck cancer
Squamous	Inguinal adenopathy	Definitive local therapy (node dissection with or without radiation therapy) with or without chemotherapy
Poorly differentiated carcinoma	Young men with midline tumor and/or elevated hCG, AFP	Treat as extragonadal germ cell tumor
Poorly differentiated carcinoma	Diverse clinical features	Empirical chemotherapy with paclitaxel/platinum/etoposide
Neuroendocrine carcinoma, poorly differentiated	Diverse clinical presentations	Treat with platinum/etoposide
Neuroendocrine carcinoma, well differentiated	Usually liver metastases	Treat as metastatic carcinoid tumor

AFP = α-fetoprotein; hCG = human chorionic gonadotropin; PSA = prostate-specific antigen.

Section XV Oncology

Rx

follow guidelines for stage III ovarian cancer. When feasible, a full laparotomy with maximal surgical cytoreduction should be performed, followed by combination chemotherapy with a taxane/platinum-containing regimen. Measurement of serial serum CA-125 levels provides an accurate assessment of the efficacy of treatment. A few of these patients may have complete responses and long-term survival, particularly when initial surgical cytoreduction leaves minimal residual disease. A similar syndrome of peritoneal carcinomatosis that is responsive to chemotherapy for ovarian cancer has occasionally been reported in men.

Men with Skeletal Metastases and/or Elevated Serum Prostate-Specific Antigen Level

Metastatic prostate cancer (Chapter 211) should be suspected in men with adenocarcinoma predominantly involving bone, particularly if the metastases are blastic. An elevated serum level of PSA or tumor immunostaining for PSA provides confirmatory evidence for the diagnosis of prostate cancer. Occasionally, men with adenocarcinoma of unknown primary site and patterns of metastasis unusual for prostate cancer (e.g., lung metastases, mediastinal lymph node metastases) are found to have elevated serum PSA levels. These patients should be treated according to guidelines for advanced prostate cancer. Androgen ablation produces excellent responses and substantial palliation in most patients.

Single Metastatic Lesion

Occasionally, a single metastatic lesion containing adenocarcinoma or poorly differentiated carcinoma is identified, and a complete evaluation reveals no other evidence of disease. Such presentations can include a single lymph node or subcutaneous site or single lesions at various visceral sites, including bone, liver, lung, brain, and adrenal gland. The possibility of an unusual primary site mimicking a metastatic lesion should be considered (e.g., a subcutaneous nodule from a primary apocrine or sebaceous carcinoma rather than a metastasis), but this possibility can usually be excluded on the basis of clinical or pathologic features. Positron emission tomography is useful in excluding other metastatic lesions. For patients with only a single identifiable lesion, definitive local therapy should be used, as guided by the site of tumor involvement. Such therapy may include surgical resection, radiation therapy, or a combination of these modalities. Although most of these patients

Rx

eventually develop other metastatic sites, a significant disease-free interval is often experienced, and local treatment provides substantial palliation. The role of systemic chemotherapy in addition to definitive local therapy is not well defined; younger patients with poorly differentiated carcinoma or poorly differentiated adenocarcinoma are often treated with a short course of a taxane/platinum-based regimen (see Empirical Chemotherapy).

Squamous Carcinoma

Cervical Adenopathy

Squamous carcinoma of unknown primary site is relatively uncommon. Most patients with this syndrome have involvement of cervical lymph nodes, usually in the upper or mid-cervical area. Often, patients with this syndrome are middle-aged or elderly and have a history of substantial tobacco or alcohol use, or both. A primary site in the head and neck region should be suspected (Chapter 200); however, complete endoscopic evaluation fails to identify a primary site in approximately 15% of these patients. Even if other tests are negative, positron emission tomography identifies a primary site in the head and neck region in approximately 25% of such patients and should be part of the initial evaluation.

Even when no primary site is identified, management of these patients should follow standard guidelines for treatment of locally advanced squamous carcinoma arising in head and neck regions. Many reports have documented long-term survival rates of 30 to 60% following definitive local treatment, which should include radiation therapy or combined radiation and cervical lymph node dissection. Outcome of treatment depends on the size and number of involved cervical lymph nodes. Concurrent chemotherapy and radiation therapy are now considered the standard treatment approach for patients with locally advanced head and neck cancers and should be considered in patients with multiple lymph nodes or nodes larger than 2 cm in diameter (Chapter 200).

Inguinal Adenopathy

Occasionally, metastatic squamous cancer is found in inguinal lymph nodes. In most of these patients, a primary site can be located in the perineal or anorectal area. For the occasional patient in whom no primary site is identified, long-term survival can result from local therapy with inguinal lymph node dissection, with or without radiation therapy. Recently, combined modality treatment with concur-

Rx

rent chemotherapy and radiation therapy has improved cure rates in patients with several squamous cancers arising in this region (e.g., cervix, anus, bladder). Although data are incomplete for the uncommon patient without an identified primary site, a reasonable approach is the addition of chemotherapy with a platinum/5-fluorouracil regimen, such as the following: cisplatin, 70 mg/m^2 intravenously on day 1; 5-fluorouracil, 1000 mg/m^2, 24-hour continuous intravenous infusion on days 1 to 4, repeated every 21 days for two cycles (concurrent with radiation therapy) or four cycles (after node dissection).

Poorly Differentiated Carcinoma

Extragonadal Germ Cell Cancer Syndrome

Young men with clinical features of extragonadal germ cell tumors, including tumors that are in the mediastinum or retroperitoneum or are associated with elevated serum levels of human chorionic gonadotropin or α-fetoprotein, should be treated according to guidelines for extragonadal germ cell tumors (Chapter 210). Some of these patients can be proven to have germ cell tumors by molecular genetic analysis, even when the diagnosis is not possible with other standard pathologic techniques. Approximately 30 to 40% of these patients achieve complete responses and long-term survival following chemotherapy with cisplatin, etoposide, and bleomycin, as used for advanced germ cell tumors.

Anaplastic Lymphoma

Appropriate initial pathologic evaluation should identify most histologically atypical lymphomas. Occasionally, immunoperoxidase staining for leukocyte common antigen is negative or cannot be adequately performed in patients with anaplastic lymphoma. The disease in some of these patients can be recognized using other immunoperoxidase stains (e.g., Ki-1 or CD-30) or molecular genetic analysis (detection of immunoglobulin gene rearrangements). All patients with lymphomas identified by special pathologic studies should be treated using standard guidelines for aggressive non-Hodgkin's lymphoma (Chapter 196).

Neuroendocrine Carcinoma

In approximately 10% of poorly differentiated carcinomas, neuroendocrine features are identified either by immunoperoxidase staining or by electron microscopy. Treatment of these patients is discussed later (see Neuroendocrine Carcinoma).

Other Poorly Differentiated Carcinomas

Most patients with poorly differentiated carcinoma do not have clinical or pathologic features that enable them to be assigned to any one of these three subsets. However, this heterogeneous group contains some patients whose carcinomas are highly sensitive to platinum-based chemotherapy. Clinical factors predictive of sensitivity to chemotherapy include site of tumor involvement (lymph nodes as compared with visceral metastases), fewer sites of metastatic disease, and younger age. In selected patients with one or more of these favorable clinical features, treatment with cisplatin-based chemotherapy can produce a greater than 60% response rate, and approximately 15% of patients remain free of disease more than 8 years after completing treatment. Therefore, a brief trial of empirical chemotherapy (see later) is recommended for all patients with poorly differentiated carcinoma, unless they are extremely debilitated at the time of diagnosis. Patients with highly sensitive tumors can be identified within the first 4 to 6 weeks of treatment, and ineffective treatment can be discontinued in the remainder.

Neuroendocrine Carcinoma

Poorly Differentiated Neuroendocrine Carcinoma or Small Cell Anaplastic Carcinoma

These high-grade neuroendocrine tumors are now reliably identified using widely available immunoperoxidase stains. Although the origin of these tumors remains unknown, they are often highly sensitive to combination chemotherapy; with platinum/etoposide chemotherapy, the overall response rate is about 75%, and 25% of patients have complete responses. In patients with locoregional disease, the addition of radiation therapy following chemotherapy is reasonable.

Low-Grade (Carcinoid Type) Neuroendocrine Tumors

Occasionally, low-grade neuroendocrine tumors are found at a metastatic site. In almost all cases, the liver is the site of involvement, and the histologic features suggest a carcinoid (Chapter 251) or islet cell tumor of gastrointestinal origin (Chapter 205). Various clinical syndromes caused by secretion of vasoactive peptides (e.g., serotonin, vasoactive intestinal peptide, gastrin) have been described. Like other carcinoid tumors, these tumors often have indolent biologic characteristics, and patients can frequently survive for several years despite multiple liver metastases. Unlike poorly differentiated neuroendocrine tumors, these tumors are relatively resistant to chemotherapy, and intensive combination regimens should usually be avoided. Management of these patients should follow guidelines for metastatic carcinoid tumors (Chapter 251) and may include the use of somatostatin analogues, local ablative procedures (e.g., surgical resection, radiofrequency ablation, chemoembolization), or fluorouracil-based chemotherapy regimens.

Empirical Chemotherapy

Approximately 60 to 70% of patients with carcinoma of unknown primary site do not fit into any of these defined clinical subsets. In these patients, earlier reports of empirical chemotherapy were discouraging, with overall response rates of only 20 to 25% and short median survival times (5 to 7 months). The combination of paclitaxel (200 mg/m^2 intravenously on day 1) and carboplatin (AUC 6.0 intravenously on day 1), with or without etoposide (50 mg alternating with 100 mg orally on days 1 to 10), all repeated every 21 days for four courses, produces objective responses in 30 to 45% of patients, with median survival in the 9- to 12-month range. In addition, a few patients receive a major benefit from treatment; the 2-year survival rate with taxane-containing regimens is 20 to 25%. A three-drug regimen of cisplatin (35 mg/m^2), gemcitabine (1000 mg/m^2), and vinorelbine (25 mg/m^2) has been reported to increase median survival to 13.6 months.

At present, patients with carcinoma of unknown primary site who have reasonable performance status should be considered for an empirical trial of combination chemotherapy. Patients with responsive tumors can be identified after 4 to 6 weeks of treatment, and they should continue treatment for a standard 4- to 5-month course. Patients who do not respond to initial combination chemotherapy are unlikely to respond to further treatment; palliative care is appropriate in these patients (Chapter 3). For patients who have poor performance status at the time of diagnosis, palliative care alone is an appropriate approach.

SUGGESTED READINGS

Mantaka P, Baum RP, Hertel A, et al: PET with 2-[F-18]-fluoro-2-deoxy-D-glucose (FDG) in patients with cancer of unknown primary (CUP): Influence on patients' diagnostic and therapeutic management. Cancer Biother Radiopharm 2003;18:47–58. *Positron emission tomography was better than computed tomography for detecting unknown primary cancers.*

Palmeri S, Lorusso V, Palmeri L, et al: Cisplatin and gemcitabine with either vinorelbine or paclitaxel in the treatment of carcinomas of unknown primary site: Results of an Italian multicenter, randomized, phase II study. Cancer 2006;107:2898–2905. *The combination with vinorelbine was superior, with a median survival of 13.6 months.*

Pavlidis N, Briasoulis E, Hainsworth J, et al: Diagnostic and therapeutic management of cancer of an unknown primary. Eur J Cancer 2003;39:1990–2005.

Seve P, Billotey C, Broussolke C, et al: The role of 2-deoxy-2-[f-18] fluoro-D-glucose positron emission tomography in disseminated carcinoma of unknown primary site. Cancer 2007;109:292–299. *Summary of evidence supporting its diagnostic value.*

Section XVI

Metabolic Diseases

APPROACH TO INBORN ERRORS OF METABOLISM

Louis J. Elsas II

Definition

Metabolism is a collective term for integrated biochemical processes of the intact organism, differentiated organ, cell, and subcellular organelle. Normal metabolism enables homeostasis for the organism by maintaining anabolic and catabolic flow of substrates to products.

History

In the early 20th century, Garrod recognized heritable blocks in normal human metabolic flow that conformed to mendelian mechanisms of inheritance. He first coined the term *inborn error of metabolism* in his Croonian Lectures of 1908, in which he described four diseases—alkaptonuria, albinism, cystinuria, and pentosuria. Garrod presumed that a patient expressing the full abnormality was homozygous for mutant alleles affecting a specific metabolic flow whereas the parents were heterozygous for this same inherited block but were clinically normal. When he gave patients with alkaptonuria proteins or other precursors of homogentisic acid, excretion of alkaptones increased, as evidenced by darkening of the urine on standing. He theorized that this "block-in-reaction sequence" was controlled genetically because pedigree analyses were consistent with an *autosomal recessive* mode of inheritance. The enzyme defect in alkaptonuria was not discovered until 50 years later, when homogentisic acid oxidase was found impaired in the liver and kidneys of patients with this disease. More recently, the gene for homogentisate 1,2-dioxygenase was cloned, and mutations causing altered function were defined.

First proof that abnormal protein function led to disease came from Gibson's observation in 1948 that erythrocyte methemoglobin reductase was decreased in patients with *methemoglobinemia.* By 1952, Pauling and Ingram had identified an abnormal hemoglobin structure in *sickle cell anemia.* During this same period, Cori and Cori identified a deficiency of hepatic glucose-6-phosphatase in *von Gierke's disease,* or *type I glycogen storage disease,* and confirmed Garrod's theory by defining a block in the flow of hepatic glucose production from its stored glycogen.

Pathobiology

Pathogenesis

Protein Diversity

Variations in human proteins do not usually produce disease. Heritable diversity in hemoglobins, phosphoglucomutase, lactate dehydrogenase, red blood cell acid phosphatase, haptoglobins, and immunoglobins was discovered and defined for normal populations. In some cases, diversity is required for optimal health, for example, the ability of the immune system to produce gamma globulin in response to a wide range of antigenic epitopes. Nucleotide sequence variations may produce different amino acid changes in the primary protein structure without producing a functional change. When no functional change occurs, the alteration is considered a *polymorphism.* The term *single nucleotide polymorphism* is now used to scan diversity of the entire human genome.

Normal Protein Diversity

There are many molecular mechanisms producing normal protein diversity. Normal protein variation can occur through gene rearrangements, as exemplified by the formation of immunoglobins, which give rise to required variations in response to foreign antigens (Chapter 270). Here, gene rearrangements occur in response to antigens to produce protein diversity. Post-transcriptional, alternative splicing of RNA is another mechanism for protein variation. There are many examples of alternative splicing, including the diverse forms of the DNA splicing factors themselves called SFRS. Post-translational modification of proteins produces diversity and is important in directing proteins to subcellular organelles, to the cell surface, or for secretion. Glycosylation of proteins directed to plasma membrane receptors is an example of this post-translational mechanism. As an example of the importance of these mechanisms, consider that humans have more than 250,000 functional proteins but only 35,000 to 37,000 genes predicted from the human genome sequence.

Mutations

The relatively rare circumstance in which a change in a protein impairs function is called a *mutation,* and it may produce an inborn error of metabolism. Naturally occurring mutations that produce pathology also provide insight into the functional role of normal proteins in human metabolism. Inborn errors of metabolism are classified here in accordance with the organ, cell, and subcellular location of normal protein function (Table 216–1) and the abnormal mechanisms that interfere with normal metabolic flow as a result of impaired proteins (Table 216–2).

Therapy for inborn errors of metabolism is aimed at returning homeostasis to the intact organism. In the postgenomic era, new technologies enable microarray analysis of the genome, transcriptome, and proteome. The correlation of genes that are transcribed and translated approaches only 20% of the genome in any cell or organ and helps explain diversity, as well as organ specificity for metabolic pathways in differentiated human organs. A new field known as "metabolomics" studies the effects of changes in the analyte concentration of precursors and substrates of enzyme reactions in a perturbed cell or organism on gene expression and protein translation. Network perturbation models for essential metabolic pathways are being defined, particularly in the context of drug-induced adverse events, where heritable variations may be defined by personalized genomic microarrays before the drug is given and thereby prevent adverse reactions. Microarrays for genomic variation in the cytochrome P-450 genes are now commercially available and will assist in predicting some sensitivities to drugs.

Pathophysiology

One important clinical aspect in defining the genetic component of a metabolic disease is that one can predict, intervene in, and prevent irreversible pathology by a variety of stratagems before the disease is expressed. In general, the severity of an inborn error of metabolism depends on the degree of protein impairment rendered by the genetic mutation and the trauma induced by the environment. A "leaky" mutation may not be expressed until adulthood, whereas a complete block in the same metabolic pathway is lethal in infancy. The age at onset and severity of disease are a result of complex interactions of the gene environment, or other genes that modify the underlying genetic susceptibility. The pathophysiologic mechanisms outlined in Table 216–2 may occur individually or may combine to produce loss in homeostasis and a disease state. The clinical manifestations are usually *pleiotropic,* which means that one blocked reaction produces multiple dysfunctions at the organ level. An example is galactosemia, which causes cataracts, ovarian failure, liver disease, and central nervous system dysfunction. The phenotype (clinical outcome) is also affected not only by the specific genetic block but also by alternative metabolic pathways (*epigenetic* phenomena) that may remove toxic precursors or supply deficient products of a blocked reaction. Outcome may be adversely affected by an alternative pathway that produces a toxic analyte, and a pathophysiologic mechanism may differ among organs. In galactosemia, the accumulation of galactose can produce excess intracellular galactitol through an alternative pathway catalyzed by aldose reductase and, consequently, cell death of optic lens fibers as a result of the osmotic effect of intracellular galactitol. Accumulation of galactitol causes cataracts, whereas accumulation of galactose 1-phosphate produces hepatic cell death.

ERRORS IN METABOLISM THAT CAUSE DISEASES

Plasma Membrane Transporter Protein Mutations

Many disorders are produced by mutant proteins that impair the transport of nutrients into cells (Table 216–3). *Familial glucose-galactose malabsorption syndrome* exemplifies defective transporter protein and results in the accumulation of nontransported glucose in the intestinal lumen and refractory diarrhea secondary to its osmotic effects. Direct evidence for genetic control of intestinal glucose transport in humans was obtained by in vitro studies of jejunal biopsy material from families in

TABLE 216–1 CLASSIFICATION OF PROTEIN FUNCTION BY LOCATION IN ORGANISM

Proteins act as follows:

1. Catalyze plasma membrane functions
   a. Substrate transport
   b. Cellular signaling (receptors)
2. Catalyze integrated metabolic pathways in the cytosol, lysosome, peroxisome, mitochondria, nucleus, and endoplasmic reticulum
3. Circulate in blood and provide and maintain various functions (clotting; metal, lipid, and vitamin transport; immunity; oxygen transport; regulation of proteases, hormones, and adhesion proteins)
4. Maintain structural integrity of organs and organelles (collagen, elastin, actin, dystrophin, fibrillins)

TABLE 216–2 CLASSIC PATHOLOGIC MECHANISMS FOR INBORN ERRORS OF METABOLISM

1. Accumulation of substrates to toxic concentrations in a blocked catabolic reaction. *Examples:* maple syrup urine disease, galactosemia, glucose-galactose malabsorption, Fabry's disease, Gaucher's disease, urea cycle defects
2. Production of toxic byproducts through a normally minor pathway. *Examples:* tyrosinemia type I, adenosine deaminase deficiency
3. Deficiency of an end product in an anabolic pathway. *Examples:* albinism, orotic aciduria, scurvy
4. Loss of regulation resulting in overproduction of intermediates to toxic levels. *Examples:* congenital adrenal hyperplasia, intermittent porphyria, familial hypercholesterolemia

TABLE 216–3 DISEASES CAUSED BY MUTATIONS IN PLASMA MEMBRANE TRANSPORTER PROTEINS

Disease	Tissue Affected	Substrate	Mode of Inheritance	Clinical Expression
B_{12} malabsorption	Ileum	Vitamin B_{12}	Autosomal recessive	Juvenile
Blue diaper syndrome	Gut	Tryptophan	Autosomal recessive	Hypercalcemia
Primary carnitine deficiency	Kidney + gut	Carnitine	Autosomal recessive	Hypoglycemia, hypotonia
Congenital chloridorrhea	Gut	Chloride	Autosomal recessive	Diarrhea, alkalosis
Cystic fibrosis	Apical epithelia	Chloride	Autosomal recessive	Lung, intestinal obstruction
Cystinuria	Kidney + gut	Cystine + lysine, arginine, ornithine	Autosomal recessive	Renal lithiasis (cystine)
Familial hypophosphatemic rickets	Kidney + gut	Phosphate	X-linked dominant	Rickets
Folate deficiency	Lymphocyte, erythrocyte	Methyltetrahydrofolate	Autosomal recessive	Aplastic anemia
Glucose-galactose malabsorption	Gut + kidney	Glucose and galactose	Autosomal recessive	Refractory diarrhea
Hartnup's syndrome	Gut + kidney	Neutral amino acids	Autosomal recessive (pellagra)	Nicotinic acid deficiency
Hereditary hypophosphatemic rickets	Kidney	Phosphate	Autosomal dominant	Growth restriction, rickets, hypercalciuria
Hereditary renal hypouricemia	Kidney	Uric acid	Autosomal recessive	Urolithiasis (uric acid)
Hereditary spherocytosis	Erythrocyte	Sodium	Autosomal recessive	Hemolytic anemia
Hyperdibasic aminoaciduria (type I)	Kidney	Lysine, arginine, ornithine	Autosomal dominant	?Symptoms
Iminoglycinuria	Kidney + gut	Glycine, proline, hydroxyproline	Autosomal recessive	Benign?
Isolated lysinuria	Kidney + gut	Lysine	Autosomal recessive	Growth failure, seizures
Lysinuric protein intolerance (type II)	Kidney, fibroblasts, hepatocytes, gut	Lysine	Autosomal recessive	Growth restriction, hyperammonemia, mental retardation
Methionine malabsorption (oasthouse disease)	Gut	Methionine	Autosomal recessive?	Mental retardation, white hair, failure to thrive
Renal glycosuria	Kidney	Glucose	Autosomal recessive	Benign glycosuria
Renal tubular acidosis (type I)	Distal renal tubule	H^+ secretion, citrate, calcium	Autosomal dominant	Hypokalemia, growth restriction, nephrocalcinosis
Renal tubular acidosis (type II)	Proximal renal tubule	Bicarbonate	"Familial"	Hyperchloremic metabolic acidosis

which the affected members expressed refractory diarrhea on ingesting D-galactose or D-glucose but not fructose. Pedigree analysis conformed to autosomal recessive inheritance. These data predicted a gene that coded for a stereospecific, sodium-dependent, and energy-dependent transporter protein in human jejunal (and proximal renal tubular) microvilli. Expression cloning of active glucose transport has now confirmed the presence of a family of glucose transporter genes, their deduced amino acid sequences, and specific codon changes producing the syndromes of familial glucose-galactose malabsorption and renal glycosuria.

Defects of Glucose Transporters

There are many inherited defects involving the plasma membrane transport of glucose that are caused by mutations of either active or facilitative glucose transport. Glucose transporters are a family of proteins whose definitions of function evolved after their cloning and molecular genetic analysis (Table 216–4). By comparing data from families with renal glycosuria and glucose-galactose malabsorption, it became evident that different Na^+-dependent, active glucose transporters (sodium-glucose transporter [SGLT]) were present in kidney and gut epithelium. SGLT1 is shared by the kidney and gut, whereas SGLT2 functions predominantly in the kidney alone and causes renal glycosuria without glucose-galactose malabsorption (see Table 216–4). An insulin-responsive, facilitative glucose transporter (GLUT4) is not Na^+ dependent and is expressed primarily in insulin-responsive tissues (fat cells, skeletal muscle). More than one glucose transporter is expressed by most cells. The jejunal epithelial cell uses SGLT1 to concentrate glucose from its luminal surface into the cytosol, then effluxes glucose at its basal-lateral surfaces through GLUT2. GLUT2 is also involved in regulating the amount of glucose transported into beta cells of the pancreas, a process that regulates glucose stimulation of insulin release. Indirect evidence suggests that mutations in the *GLUT2* gene are "sensitivity genes" involved in regulating insulin secretion.

Hormone Resistance

Many diseases characterized by "hormone resistance" are caused by a family of proteins that function as receptors in the plasma membrane and as postreceptor transmitters of signals located in the cytosol and nucleus. The concept of failure to respond to hormone stimulation originated in the early 1940s with a description of *pseudohypoparathyroidism* (Chapter 266). Heritability of resistance to parathormone was suggested before the existence of parathormone receptors, hormone-sensitive adenylate cyclases, or guanine nucleotide–binding proteins was known.

Defects in Transmembrane Binding and Signaling

Diseases caused by defective transmembrane binding and signaling include *Laron dwarfism*, which results from growth hormone receptor (GHR) defects. The phenotypic characteristics are *proportionate dwarfism*, hypoglycemia, craniofacial dysmorphology with a doll-like face, balding, frontal bossing, truncal obesity, and wrinkled skin. In this disorder, the growth hormone concentration in blood is elevated, peripheral tissue responses are decreased, and insulin-like growth factor type I concentrations in blood are low. An autosomal recessive mode of inheritance has been defined. Dominant or polygenic symmetrical growth restriction may result from mutations in nuclear transproteins, hypothalamic pituitary trophic proteins, growth hormone, GHR, and postreceptor signaling. The *GHR* gene is found on chromosome 5p13-p12, and many different mutations in this gene account for disorders of stature.

Familial Hypercholesterolemia

Familial hypercholesterolemia defines a phenotype of autosomal dominant hypercholesterolemia and early-onset heart disease (Chapter 79). This disorder affects an estimated 1 in 500 individuals in the general population. An autosomal dominant mode of inheritance for early-onset adult heart disease is caused by many different mutations in the low-density lipoprotein (LDL) cholesterol receptor. Dysfunction of LDL receptors results in a loss of the cell's ability to downregulate endogenous cholesterol synthesis and incorporate LDL cholesterol into cells. Increased intravascular accumulation of LDL cholesterol results in atherosclerosis and heart disease before the sixth decade of life (see Table 216–2). The gene for the LDL cholesterol receptor is found on chromosome 19p13.1-13.2.

Errors of Insulin Resistance

Leprechaunism

Leprechaunism has become a prototypical inborn error of severe insulin resistance and loss of cellular signal transduction through the insulin receptor. Affected infants have low birthweight, acanthosis nigricans, cystic changes in organs, and loss of glucose homeostasis. Affected patients have remarkably elevated plasma insulin concentrations greater than 500 mIU/mL. Specific impairment in iodine 125–labeled insulin binding is evident in cells cultured from patients, and a spectrum of

TABLE 216–4 HUMAN GLUCOSE TRANSPORTERS

Protein	kD (AA)	mRNA Size (kb)	Chromosomal Localization	Expression in Tissue and Cells	Function	Disorder
GLUT1	55 (492)	2.8	lp35 → p31.3	Blood-brain barrier, erythrocyte, fibroblast	Basal glucose transport across most cells, including the blood-brain barrier	Seizures with low cerebrospinal fluid and normal blood glucose
GLUT2	58 (524) 3.4 5.4	2.8	3q26.1 → q26.3	Liver, kidney, intestine, beta cell of the pancreas	Low-affinity glucose transport	Defective insulin secretion in diabetes
GLUT3	54 (496)	2.7 4.1	12p13.3	Neurons, fibroblasts, placenta, testes	Basal glucose transport, high affinity	?
GLUT4	55 (509) 3.5	2.8	17p13	Fat, skeletal muscle, heart	Insulin-stimulated glucose transport	Defective insulin-stimulated transport, ?NIDDM
GLUT5	50 (501)	2.0	1p32 → p22	Small intestine	Fructose transport	?
GLUT7 (rat)	52 (528)	?	?	Liver microsome endoplasmic reticulum	Glucose release from	Type ID glycogen storage disease
CONCENTRATIVE GLUCOSE TRANSPORTERS						
SLGT1	75 (664)	2.2 2.6 4.8	22q11 → qter	Intestine, kidney (medulla)	Intestinal absorption, renal reabsorption, high affinity (2 Na: 1 glucose)	Glucose-galactose malabsorption
SLGT2	76 (672) 3.0 3.5 4.5	2.4	16p11.2	Kidney (cortex)	Low affinity, high capacity (1 Na: 1 glucose)	Renal glycosuria

AA = amino acids; NIDDM = non–insulin-dependent diabetes mellitus.

mutations produces a variety of severe insulin-resistant syndromes (leprechaunism, Rabson-Mendenhall syndrome, and type A diabetes with acanthosis nigricans). Obligate heterozygotes (parents) of patients with leprechaunism have partially impaired insulin binding and glucose tolerance curves suggesting type 2 diabetes mellitus. The insulin receptor transfers its signal by phosphotransfer to the insulin receptor signal protein 1 (IRS-1), and a cascade of anabolic signals occurs.

Pseudohypoparathyroidism

In *Albright's hereditary osteodystrophy,* or *pseudohypoparathyroidism* (Chapter 266), a heterogeneous group of mutations affect the gene for the parathormone receptor's guanine nucleotide–binding protein (G_sa), which links the receptor to adenylate cyclase and stimulates cyclic adenosine monophosphate when the receptor is occupied by parathormone. The gene for G_sa is located on chromosome 20q13, and deletions and missense mutations that produce Albright's hereditary osteodystrophy have been defined. Somatic mutations in arginine 201 of the same gene turn the G_sa protein constitutively "on" and produce another disease, McCune-Albright-Sternberg syndrome. Cells are *mosaic* for the mutation, and the syndrome includes nonossifying bone tumors and premature puberty.

Impaired Cytosolic Enzymes

Inborn errors affecting proteins of the cytosolic compartment within a cell are the more "traditional" inborn errors of metabolism (Table 216–5). They impair the catalytic reactions of anabolic or catabolic pathways and are usually classified by the class of biochemical involved, such as impairment of glucose, lipid, fatty acid, amino acid, purine, organic acid, vitamin, or drug metabolism.

Phenylketonuria

Phenylalanine is essential for growth, and its anabolic products include tyrosine, thyroid hormone, adrenergic neurotransmitters, and melanin. *Phenylketonuria* (PKU) is caused by mutations in the gene encoding phenylalanine hydroxylase, the first enzyme in this anabolic flow that catalyzes tyrosine production. PKU may also occur if coenzymes are deficient in this reaction, such as dihydropteridine reductase or enzymes involved in biopterin biosynthesis.

Albinism

Albinism is an example of an inborn error in an anabolic pathway in which the pathophysiologic mechanism is related directly to the lack of an end product (see mechanism 3, Table 216–2). Tyrosine is converted by the action of a cytosolic tyrosinase first to dopa and then to dopamine. Dopamine can be converted either to the red-yellow pigment pheomelanin or to the black-brown pigment eumelanin. These reactions occur in the melanosomes produced in melanocytes and exported to keratinocytes. Color of skin is an inherited factor that depends on many genes (polygenic) and is a function of the intensity of the pigment in the skin and not the number of melanocytes, which is constant for all humans. Although skin color is a polygenic trait, single genes can have a profound effect on this color, as evidenced by the albino phenotype. In humans, *oculocutaneous albinism* (OCA) is inherited as an autosomal recessive trait. X-linked forms of *ocular albinism* also exist. Individuals with OCA are classified as tyrosinase negative or positive for tyrosine activity in hair bulbs. Tyrosinase-negative individuals form no pigment. The gene for tyrosinase has been localized to chromosome 11q14, and many mutations have been defined. A tyrosine-positive OCA has been associated with an autosomal recessive gene located on chromosome 15q11-13 (the P gene), and X-linked ocular albinism is caused by *OCA-1* gene mutations. Wide variation in the phenotypic expression of albinism ranging from severe neurologic deficiency with ocular and sarcomatous skin cancers to mild cosmetic problems has been reported.

Errors of the Urea Cycle

Inborn errors of the urea cycle (Chapter 226) are represented by defects in the integration of anabolic and catabolic pathways and the distribution of catalytic proteins between mitochondria and cytosol. The role of the urea cycle is to convert ammonia, a byproduct of protein breakdown, to urea and to synthesize arginine and ornithine. Reactions to complete this anabolic cycle require mitochondrial enzymes, cytosolic enzymes, and mitochondrial transporter proteins. Inherited disorders affecting the function of these proteins are known. Individuals with defects in any of the enzymes have varying degrees of hyperammonemia caused by protein ingestion or a nutritional state in which muscle is catabolized. With the exception of the gene for ornithine transcarbamylase found on the short arm of chromosome X, the other proteins are encoded on autosomes, and defects are inherited as autosomal recessive traits. Many principles of diagnosis and therapy for inborn errors of metabolism are exemplified by disorders of the urea cycle.

Errors in Mitochondrial Proteins

A group of inborn errors of metabolism are caused by mutations in nuclear genes that encode mitochondrial proteins. Collectively, they are considered disorders of organic acid metabolism (Table 216–6). Branched-chain α-ketoacid dehydrogenase is a multienzyme complex located on the matrix side of the mitochondrial inner membrane in all tissues. When any of these proteins are impaired, the autosomal recessive disorder *maple syrup urine disease* may result (Chapter 227). In addition to nuclear-encoded genes, 13 proteins of mitochondrial complexes involved in oxidative phosphorylation are encoded in the mitochondrial

TABLE 216–5 SOME DISEASES CAUSED BY IMPAIRED CYTOSOLIC ENZYMES

Disorder	Enzyme Defect	Phenotype	Inheritance
CARBOHYDRATES			
Fructosuria	Fructokinase	Benign	Autosomal recessive
Hereditary fructose intolerance	Fructose 1-phosphate aldolase	Liver dysfunction, early death	Autosomal recessive
Galactosemia	Galactose 1-phosphate uridyltransferase	Liver dysfunction, cataracts, sepsis, mental retardation, death	Autosomal recessive
Hereditary fructose-1,6-bis-phosphate deficiency	Fructose-1,6-bis-phosphatase	Apnea, ketosis, lactic acidosis	Autosomal recessive
AMINO ACIDS			
Phenylketonuria	*p*-Hydroxyphenylalanine hydroxylase	Mental retardation (teratogenic)	Autosomal recessive
Tyrosinemia			
Type II	Tyrosine aminotransferase	Palmar bullae, corneal lesions	Autosomal recessive
Type I	Fumarylacetoacetate hydrolase	Succinyl acetone accumulation	Autosomal recessive
Homocystinuria	Cystathionine β-synthase	Marfanoid habitus, arterial thrombosis, lens dislocation, mental retardation	Autosomal recessive
Hyperornithinemia	Ornithine aminotransferase	Gyrate atrophy of the retina	Autosomal recessive
Lesch-Nyhan syndrome	Hypoxanthine phosphoribosyltransferase	Neurologic dysfunction with self-destructive tendency	X-linked

TABLE 216–6 ORGANIC ACIDEMIAS: DISORDERS OF METABOLISM BY MITOCHONDRIAL PROTEINS

Disorder	Enzyme Defect	Inheritance
Isovaleric acidemia	Isovaleryl-CoA dehydrogenase	Autosomal recessive
Methylcrotonic aciduria	3-Methylcrotonyl-CoA carboxylase	Autosomal recessive
Glutaconic aciduria	3-Methylglutaconyl-CoA hydratase	Autosomal recessive
Glutaric aciduria (1)	3-Hydroxy-3-methylglutaryl-CoA lyase	Autosomal recessive
Mevalonic aciduria	Mevalonate kinase	Autosomal recessive
Thiolase deficiency	2-Methylacetoacetyl-CoA thiolase	Autosomal recessive
Isobutyric aciduria	3-Hydroxyisobutyryl-CoA deacylase	Autosomal recessive
Propionic aciduria	Propionyl-CoA carboxylase	Autosomal recessive
Methylmalonic aciduria	Methylmalonyl-CoA mutase	Autosomal recessive
Lactic acidosis	Pyruvate dehydrogenase	Autosomal recessive
Pyruvate decarboxylase		
Acyl-CoA dehydrogenase deficiencies	Short-, medium-, and long-chain fatty acyl-CoA dehydrogenase	Autosomal recessive
Branched-chain α-ketoacidemia	Branched-chain α-ketoacid dehydrogenase	Autosomal recessive
Glutaric acidemia type II	Electron transfer factor deficiency	Autosomal recessive
Leber's optic atrophy	Mitochondrial oxidative phosphorylation complexes	Maternal
Myoclonic epilepsy and ragged red fibers	Mitochondrial oxidative phosphorylation complexes	Maternal
Leigh's disease	Mitochondrial oxidative phosphorylation complexes	Maternal

DNA genome. Only complex II is encoded entirely by the nuclear genome. A wide range of disorders affecting the eye, brain, and muscle are caused by mutations in mitochondrial DNA that impair oxidative phosphorylation. The inheritance pattern of disorders encoded by the mitochondrial genome is distinguished from disorders caused by mutations in nuclear DNA by being transmitted through an affected mother to all of her offspring. Males do not transmit mitochondrial mutations to their offspring, thus the term *maternal inheritance.* Because there are about 10,000 mitochondrial genomes per cell, variation in disease expression is caused by differences in the ratio of mutant to normal mitochondrial genomes (*heteroplasmy*) and the environment.

Lysosomal Disorders

Another group of inborn errors of metabolism are collectively categorized as *lysosomal disorders* (Chapter 223) to indicate the subcellular localization of these enzymes that function in this acidic environment. Most of these enzymes are involved in the breakdown of endocytosed membrane components, and when defective, their nondegraded substrates accumulate in the lysosomes and macrophages of affected organs.

I-Cell Disease

I-cell disease is an inborn error of post-translational processing of proteins directed to the lysosome. Clarification of this pathophysiology led to an understanding of the mechanisms by which lysosomal enzymes are polarized through phosphorylation to remain in the acidic lysosomes. Patients with I-cell disease have inherited defects in the recognition markers required to direct enzymes to the endocytic receptor of the plasma membrane and to their capture in the acidic milieu of the lysosome. Patients lack all cellular lysosomal enzymes. Instead, empty lysosomes look like inclusion bodies ("I cell"). The misdirected lysosomal enzymes are secreted and are present in excess in plasma but are missing from cells. These extracellular enzymes were found to lack mannose 6-phosphate residues, and this observation led to an understanding of the post-translational mechanisms by which enzymes are directed to the lysosome and recaptured into endosomes by adding phosphorylated mannose to their protein structure. Individuals with I-cell disease lack this phosphotransferase activity.

Disorders of Mucopolysaccharides and Gangliosides

Inborn errors affecting single enzymes in the degradative pathway for mucopolysaccharides and gangliosides helped define the steps required for the breakdown of these complex macromolecules. Disorders of mucopolysaccharide metabolism (Chapter 223) include Hurler's syndrome; Scheie's syndrome; Hunter's syndrome; Sanfilippo's syndrome types A, B, C, and D; Morquio's syndrome types A and B; and Sly's syndrome. Disorders of ganglioside metabolism (Chapter 223) include Fabry's disease, Gaucher's disease, Niemann-Pick disease, Tay-Sachs disease, I-cell disease, fucosidosis, mannosidosis, sialidosis, and aspartylglycosaminuria.

TABLE 216–7 INBORN ERRORS OF PEROXISOMES: DISORDERS OF PEROXISOMAL BIOGENESIS

Zellweger's syndrome (cerebrohepatorenal syndrome)
Neonatal adrenoleukodystrophy
Infantile Refsum's disease
Hyperpipecolic acidemia
Leber's amaurosis
Rhizomelic chondrodysplasia punctata (Conradi's syndrome)
Peroxisomal 3-oxoacyl-CoA thiolase deficiency
Peroxisomal acyl-CoA oxidase deficiency
X-linked adrenoleukodystrophy (impaired lignoceroyl-CoA and hexacosanoyl-CoA ligase)
Adult Refsum's disease (phytanic acid α-hydroxylase deficiency)
Acatalasemia (H_2O_2 oxidoreductase deficiency)

Peroxisomal Diseases

Another group of inborn errors of metabolism defined by altered organelle function are *peroxisomal diseases* (Table 216–7). Peroxisomes are radiodense organelles 0.5 to 1 nm in diameter bounded by a single trilaminar membrane. Anabolic and catabolic reactions occur in this organelle. Primary pathways synthesize plasmalogens (unique fatty acids containing vinyl ethers), cholesterol, and bile acids. Other biosynthetic reactions include gluconeogenesis from amino acids and the formation of oxalic acid by the action of alanine-glyoxylate aminotransferase. Catabolic reactions include breakdown of hydrogen peroxide by peroxisomal catalase, a traditional protein of the peroxisome; polyamine oxidation; purine breakdown; ethanol oxidation; hydroxylation of phytanic acid; and degradation of pipecolic acid. A major function of the peroxisome is β-oxidation of very long chain fatty acids (>24 carbons). Diagnosis of these disorders entails finding an excess of very long chain fatty acids but reduced plasmalogen in blood.

An understanding of the importance of many reactions that occur in the peroxisome has come from identifying patients with either defects in individual biochemical pathways or lack of peroxisomes. The targeting signal for peroxisomal proteins may lie in their carboxyl-terminal end, and mutations in alanine-glyoxylate aminotransferase have resulted in mistargeting of this enzyme to mitochondria with consequent *familial hyperoxaluria* (Chapter 221).

TABLE 216–8 SOME INBORN ERRORS OF PROTEINS THAT CIRCULATE IN BLOOD

Functional Class	Protein	Phenotype
Transport	Ceruloplasmin	Wilson's disease
	Albumin	Analbuminemia
	Hemoglobin	Hemoglobinopathies
	α-Lipoprotein	Analphalipoproteinemia
	β-Lipoprotein	Abetalipoproteinemia
	Transcobalamin II	Megaloblastic anemia
Hormones	Growth hormone	Pituitary dwarfism
	Insulin	Diabetes mellitus (insulin dependent)
	Somatomedin	Pituitary dwarfism
Coagulation	Factors I–XIII	Coagulopathies
	Kininogen	Kininogen deficiency
	Prekallikrein	Prekallikrein deficiency
Immune system	Complement components	Hypocomplementemias
	Immunoglobulins	Hypogammaglobulinemias
Inhibitors	α_1-Antitrypsin	Pulmonary emphysema and/or cirrhosis
	G'1 esterase inhibitor	Angioneurotic edema
Drugs	Pseudocholinesterase	Prolonged paralysis after succinylcholine (Anectine) exposure

TABLE 216–9 APPROACHES TO TREATING INBORN ERRORS OF METABOLISM

Genetic counseling: prospective therapy
Diagnosis, risk assessment, informational transfer, support for resource allocation
Reproductive alternatives: contraception, abstinence, artificial insemination, in vitro fertilization, risk taking with or without prenatal monitoring
Environmental engineering
Avoiding the offending agent
Supplemental physical, speech, occupational therapy
Nutritional management
- Promote anabolism
- Limit toxic precursor
- Detoxify through alternative metabolic route
- Provide feedback inhibitor
- Provide supraphysiologic amounts of vitamin precursor
- Induce protein (enzyme) production
- Chemoprevention

Protein and enzyme replacement
Infuse engineered enzyme
Provide clotting factors and peptide hormones
Transplantation
- Organ transplant
- Bone marrow transplant
- Stem cell transplant (adult, embryonic, nuclear transfer)

Genetic engineering
Somatic gene therapy
- Random insertion
- Homologous recombination (site specific)

Germline therapy

Errors in Nuclear Proteins

Several inborn errors are caused by abnormalities in proteins that function in the nucleus and are involved in DNA repair (see class 2, Table 216–1). Patients expressing these inherited disorders carry a high risk for the development of cancer. Among these inborn errors of DNA repair are rare disorders, such as *xeroderma pigmentosum, Bloom's syndrome, ataxia-telangiectasia,* and *Fanconi's anemia;* diseases associated with early aging, such as *progeria, Cockayne's syndrome,* and *Werner's syndrome;* and more common adult-onset *nonpolyposis colon cancer.* Collectively, the disorders show increased sensitivity and delayed repair of DNA damaged as a result of ultraviolet, x-ray, or alkylating cross-link mechanisms or have "normal" DNA repair requirements.

Errors in Blood-Circulating Proteins

Many inborn errors involve proteins that circulate in blood (see class 3 of Table 216–1). Stable circulating proteins in blood perform a variety of functions, including immunologic, hemostatic, regulatory, hormonal, and interorgan transport of trace metals, lipids, and other nutrients. Some inherited disorders affecting circulating proteins are tabulated in Table 216–8. Proteins involved in oxygen transport, coagulation, and immunity are detailed in other chapters, but the pathophysiologic mechanisms and genetic approaches of screening, diagnosis, and intervention to restore homeostasis and prevent an expected disease state make them appropriate to consider here as inborn errors of metabolism.

Abnormal Matrix Proteins

Abnormal matrix proteins produce inborn errors, such as Marfan syndrome (fibrillin), osteogenesis imperfecta (collagen type I), spondyloepiphyseal dysplasia (collagen type II), and Sachs' disease (collagen type III). These disorders exemplify class 4 of inborn errors of metabolism (see Table 216–1). The enzymes involved in post-translational processing of these proteins can also cause these syndromes. An example is Ehlers-Danlos syndrome type VI, in which collagen lysyl hydroxylase deficiency produces excess poorly hydroxylated lysyl residues in collagen. Inborn errors of matrix proteins are exemplified by disorders of collagen metabolism. More than 20 different genes dispersed on nine chromosomes are currently known to code for more than 13 different types of collagen.

Treatment

Rx

Because the metabolic diseases considered in this chapter have in common the fact that they are caused by genes of large effect that disrupt normal homeostasis, we can consider a general approach to their treatment, as outlined in Table 216–9. The level at which therapy is rendered depends on the level of understanding of the pathophysiologic mechanisms producing disease and the interventional methods available.

Gene Therapy

Somatic Gene Therapy

Somatic cell gene therapy to treat patients with genetic disease has entered the arena of clinical research. Numerous laboratories throughout the world are actively designing strategies by which exogenous DNA can be incorporated into the genomic DNA of specific organs to provide a missing gene function. *Somatic gene therapy* for many inherited metabolic diseases continues to be a goal of the future and awaits a nontoxic, stable vector with which to transfer normally transcribed genes.

Genetic Counseling

Genetic counseling is a unique and fundamental aspect of the management of inherited metabolic diseases and is used for all inherited diseases, even those whose mechanisms are not yet understood and for which no other treatment is available. Patients, their parents, and relatives usually ask questions such as the following: Why did this disease occur? Will this disease happen to me or my children? Can it be cured or prevented? Genetic counseling tries to answer these questions through processes involving several elements. One cannot overemphasize the importance of an accurate family history, clinical diagnosis, and prognosis. A genetic discriminant is necessary for other family members before entering into formal genetic counseling. The genetic discriminant can be at the clinical, histologic, biochemical, or molecular level and must define

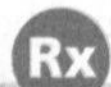

whether an individual family member has or has not inherited the mutant allele or alleles.

Environmental Engineering

Environmental engineering is the most commonly used approach to preventing disease in patients affected by inherited metabolic disease. Environmental factors (nutritional intake, exposure to toxins, sun, stress, climatic variation, and drug therapy) may produce a disease state in individuals who have inherited single genes or polygenic susceptibility to specific environmental stress. Newborn screening for galactose 1-phosphate uridyltransferase deficiency identifies infants susceptible to accumulation of galactose 1-phosphate if they ingest human or cow's milk. Restriction and replacement of lactose with sucrose saves the lives of infants with galactosemia. Pharmacogenetic disorders exemplify the simple treatment of *avoidance* when the genetic susceptibility is identified. Health can be viewed as a continual adaptation between the individual and the environment. Environmental engineering is a form of genetic therapy in which individual genetic susceptibility is identified and the environment is altered to provide optimal health for the individual's unique genetic constitution. The frequency of diseases caused by genetic susceptibility to the environment varies from rare to 100%. *Scurvy* develops in all humans unless ascorbate is provided in the diet because we are all unable to convert glucuronic acid to glucuronolactone and ascorbate. Humans and primates lost this anabolic pathway during evolution. By contrast, humans can usually synthesize tetrahydrobiopterin, a cofactor in many hydroxylase reactions, including phenylalanine hydroxylase. In some rare diseases (about 1 in 500,000) of increased blood phenylalanine and severe neurodegeneration, biopterin is not synthesized.

Surgical Therapy

Surgical intervention may be a useful adjunct for treating heritable disorders. Stabilization of hypoplastic cervical vertebrae may prevent quadriparesis or death in a variety of *chondrodysplasias* and *mucopolysaccharidoses* accompanied by hypoplasia of the odontoid process or atlantoaxial instability. In Marfan syndrome, careful monitoring of aortic root diameter with surgical removal of the aorta and prosthesis may prevent lethal aortic dissection. Evaluation of polyps and early colectomy may prevent disseminated adenocarcinoma in families with the autosomal dominant forms of *familial polyposis coli.* Molecular diagnosis of mutations in the *APC* gene helps identify at-risk family members and reassure members who did not inherit the mutant allele. Preventing heritable cancer by surveillance and early surgical excision is therapeutic for *medullary thyroid carcinoma, Wilms' tumors,* and the neurofibromas of *von Recklinghausen's disease.* Other examples of the benefit of preventive surgery for inborn errors include splenectomy for hemolytic anemias associated with spherocytosis, pyloroplasty for pyloric stenosis, and mastectomy and oophorectomy for patients with *BRCA1* or *BRCA2* mutations.

Transplantation

Organ transplantation for metabolic disorders that are lethal and have no other available therapy may be life-saving. Transplantation with histocompatible organs is clinically available because of advances in immunology that not only allow better tissue typing but also enable long-term immunosuppression with drugs such as cyclosporine, azathioprine, and prednisone to prevent rejection. Adult stem cells from cord blood are being used to treat neurodegenerative disorders in early childhood. Cloned embryonic cells or stem cells that are still naïve to adult antigens are promising therapeutic agents in a research category. Considerable political debate continues regarding the production of stem cells from embryonic blastocysts and from nuclear transfer to enucleated ova.

Several principles are required for successful treatment of an inherited metabolic disorder by organ transplantation: (1) The normal enzyme, protein, or function must be provided by the transplanted organ. (2) The pathogenesis must be understood to decide whether the affected organ should be removed. (3) The host must be immunologically tolerant to the gene product being introduced, in addition to the transplanted organ itself. These principles are particularly relevant when displacement bone marrow transplantation is used. In the latter, normal donor stem cells differentiate and provide their enzymes to the recipient's reticuloendothelial system. Diseases associated with accumulation of products in the central nervous system are not yet ameliorated by bone marrow transplantation, although accumulation in bone, liver, and spleen is reduced. In one group of metabolic diseases, stem cell bone marrow transplantation is performed to prevent leukemia caused by inherited syndromes that are associated with defective DNA repair, such as *Fanconi's anemia, Bloom's syndrome,* and *ataxia-telangiectasia.* Liver or kidney transplantation can reverse growth and developmental delay in type I glycogen storage disease, cystinosis, acute intermittent porphyria, type I tyrosinemia, Fabry's disease, oxalosis, and non-neuronotropic lysosomal storage diseases. Lung transplantation has been successful for cystic fibrosis and α_1-antitrypsin deficiency, and prophylactic aortic transplantation has prevented aortic dissection in patients with Marfan syndrome.

Medical Therapy

Nutritional management and chemoprevention involve correction of the metabolic imbalance and return of the patient to homeostasis through diet manipulation and drug therapy. Many of the diseases mentioned in this chapter are amenable to several concurrent therapeutic approaches listed in Table 216–9. For example, in disorders of the urea cycle, protein intake is limited, and anabolism is encouraged to reduce accumulation of ammonia from either protein intake or catabolism of lean body mass. Arginine is supplemented to provide deficient product of the blocked reaction, and alternative pathways are induced for nitrogen excretion. The latter therapy is made possible by a ubiquitous enzyme, *N*-glycine-acylase, that forms adducts with benzoic acid and glycine to produce hippuric acid, which is excreted, thereby eliminating one nitrogen molecule. Phenylacetylglutamine transferase is also used by giving phenylacetate to produce and excrete two nitrogen molecules as phenylacetylglutamate. Orotic aciduria is caused by mutations in the bifunctional enzyme orotate phosphoribosyltransferase–orotidine-5′-monophosphate decarboxylase. The disease process, which includes severe anemia and immune deficiency, is caused by a deficient end product, uridine, and is treated by replacing 100 to 200 mg/kg/day of uridine up to 1.0 grams three times daily (orally). Feedback inhibition of pituitary adrenocorticotropic hormone production is important in treating congenital adrenal hypertrophy with replacement doses of hydrocortisone to prevent virilization from overproduction of testosterone. Vitamin dependency disorders require supraphysiologic amounts of a specific vitamin as the precursor for an active cofactor required for holoenzyme function. Many vitamin-dependent metabolic disorders are known and include pyridoxine (vitamin B_6)-dependent homocystinuria and vitamin C–dependent Ehlers-Danlos syndrome type VI. In vitamin B_6–dependent homocystinuria, mutant cystathionine β-synthase is stabilized to biologic degradation when saturated with pyridoxal phosphate. Others include vitamin B_{12}–dependent methylmalonic aciduria, thiamine-dependent maple syrup urine disease, biotin-dependent multiple carboxylase deficiency, and biopterin-dependent hyperphenylalaninemia. Some blocked metabolic reactions can be augmented by inducing transcription of their gene. Phenobarbital and several other drugs induce hepatic uridine diphosphate glucuronyl transferase gene expression and reduce the accumulation of unconjugated bilirubin in Gilbert's syndrome. In tyrosinemia type I, the drug NTBC blocks the catabolic pathway by which tyrosine produces the toxin succinylacetone and successfully prevents hepatotoxicity.

If the specific protein or enzyme has been purified and engineered to function in its specified organ or subcellular organelle, it can be used to treat an inherited metabolic disease. One good example is

Rx

glucocerebrosidase, the enzyme that is impaired in Gaucher's disease. This enzyme has been purified in large quantities from the placenta and from recombinant mammalian cells. The secreted enzyme is biochemically engineered to contain the mannose recognition site for cellular uptake into lysosomal compartments. It has been used successfully to prevent and reverse the hypersplenism, pancytopenia, and bone disease of *type I Gaucher's disease* (Chapter 223). Many proteins are now made through recombinant techniques to treat metabolic disease and reduce the risk for viral disease attendant on using human-derived biologic agents. These enzymes now include *glucocerebrosidase*, factor VIII for *hemophilia type A*, growth hormone for *growth hormone deficiency*, α-galactosidase to treat *Fabry's disease*, iduronidase for *Hurler-Scheie syndrome*, and acid maltase for *Pompe's disease*. Several other engineered proteins used to treat inherited metabolic disease include 1-deamino-8-D-arginine vasopressin to treat *X-linked recessive diabetes insipidus* and recombinant α_1-antitrypsin made stable by inactivating methionine 385 for the treatment of *α_1-antitrypsin deficiency*. Some enzymes, such as adenosine deaminase, have been modified with polyethylene glycol to reduce immunogenicity and prolong their biologic half-life in blood. It is used to treat *severe combined immunodeficiency*. Chemoprevention is being developed for heritable cancers. Cyclooxygenase-2 inhibitors may prevent progression of colon polyps to adenocarcinoma, and estrogen receptor inhibitors may prevent some forms of breast cancer.

SUGGESTED READINGS

GeneTests and GeneClinics. Available at http://www.genetests.org/cgi-bin. *This newly merged website offers updated information for physicians and investigators on the availability of diagnostic tests and reviews of diagnosis and intervention for many inherited metabolic disorders.*

Hanley WB: Adult phenylketonuria. Am J Med 2004;117:590–595. *A clinical review.*

Moser HW, Raymond GV, Dubey P: Adrenoleukodystrophy: New approaches to a neurodegenerative disease. JAMA 2005;294:3131–3134. *A clinical review.*

National Center for Biotechnology. Available at http://www3.ncbi.nlm.nih.gov/Omim. *The database can be searched by disease name and contains updated information on the history, biochemistry, and molecular biology of all inherited disorders caused by mutations in single genes.*

Society for Inherited Metabolic Disorders. Available at http://www.simd.org. *This website has linkages to an international collection of websites dealing with diagnosis and treatment guidelines for inherited metabolic disorders. Includes patient support groups.*

217 DISORDERS OF LIPID METABOLISM

Clay F. Semenkovich

In industrialized countries, many adults are aware of the relationship between abnormal lipid metabolism and vascular disease. Terms such as "bad cholesterol" are entrenched in popular culture because of the availability of effective lipid-modifying therapies proved to decrease the risk of cardiovascular disease. Despite considerable progress, morbidity and mortality from vascular diseases are substantial and are likely to increase, given the epidemic of lipid-associated diseases such as obesity and diabetes as well as the export of Western habits to the developing world. Recently discovered mediators of lipid metabolism continue to provide new insight into the mechanisms causing abnormal levels of cholesterol and triglycerides, among the most common problems encountered by practicing physicians. A clear appreciation of the pathways of lipid metabolism is required for appropriate diagnosis and therapy because the optimal treatment for lipid disorders is still undefined.

COMPONENTS OF LIPID TRANSPORT

Cholesterol and Triglycerides

Cholesterol is a critical constituent of eukaryotic cell membranes and the precursor for the synthesis of steroid hormones such as cortisol, estradiol, and testosterone. Triglycerides carry fatty acids, nutrients utilized preferentially by muscle tissue and especially important as an energy source in the fasting state. Both cholesterol and triglycerides are regularly consumed in the diet and are essentially insoluble in water. The lipid transport system evolved because of the simple need to move these fats from one site to another through an aqueous environment.

Lipoproteins

Cholesterol and triglycerides are transported in lipoproteins (Table 217–1), spherical particles that differ in size and composition depending on their site of origin. Each particle is composed of a central core consisting of cholesteryl esters (the product of an esterification reaction between the polar cholesterol molecule and a fatty acid) and triglycerides, both nonpolar compounds. Free cholesterol, phospholipids and apolipoproteins are found on the particle surface.

Chylomicrons and their remnants are the largest lipoproteins. Produced by the intestine, these particles carry fats that are absorbed from the diet. Their residence time in the circulation after a meal is short, on the order of minutes in healthy people. Chylomicrons are large and light; that is, their density is quite low. Other lipoprotein particles have names that more directly reflect their migration in a density gradient following centrifugation. Because fat floats on water, particles with high fat and low protein content have lower density. Very low density lipoprotein (VLDL) is a triglyceride-rich particle produced by the liver. The removal of triglycerides from VLDL converts this particle to intermediate-density lipoprotein (IDL), which is subsequently metabolized to yield low-density lipoprotein (LDL, popularly known as bad cholesterol). A covalent modification of the apolipoprotein (apo) in LDL, apo B100, results in the formation of lipoprotein (a), Lp(a). High-density lipoprotein (HDL, or "good cholesterol") is formed in the blood as a byproduct of the metabolism of triglyceride-rich lipoproteins and the acquisition (followed by its esterification) of cholesterol from peripheral tissues.

Apolipoproteins

Apolipoproteins are amphipathic molecules capable of interacting with both the lipids of the lipoprotein core and the aqueous environment of the plasma. They function as biochemical keys, allowing lipoprotein particles access to specific sites for the delivery, acceptance, or modification of lipids. Major apolipoproteins, their chromosomal locations with sequence accession numbers, and functions are shown in Table 217–2. Serum measurements of apolipoproteins may have clinical utility. For example, increased levels of apo B and decreased levels of apo AI are associated with vascular disease. Apo B48, specific for gut-derived particles, derives its name from the fact that it is about 48% of the size of apo B100. Apo B100 and apo B48 are products of the same gene, with B48 resulting from the post-transcriptional introduction of a premature stop codon in the apo B messenger RNA by apobec1, a cytidine deaminase. Genetic variants in apolipoproteins can be associated with well-defined clinical syndromes.

Receptors and Proteins

Several receptors and proteins required for normal lipid transport are listed in Table 217–3.

Low-Density Lipoprotein Receptor

The LDL receptor mediates the removal of LDL as well as some VLDL and IDL particles by binding to apo B100 and apo E. The most important site of LDL receptor expression is the liver, where its regulation is mediated by sterol regulatory element–binding proteins (SREBPs).

TABLE 217–1 LIPOPROTEIN CHARACTERISTICS

Lipoprotein	Apolipoprotein Content	Major Lipids	Size (nm diameter)	Density (g/mL)
Chylomicrons, chylomicron remnants	Apo B48, apo E, apo AI, apo AII, apo AIV, apo CII, apo CIII	Triglycerides from diet	80–500	<<1.006
VLDL	Apo B100, apo E, apo CII, apo CIII	Triglycerides from liver	30–80	<1.006
IDL	Apo B100, apo E	Cholesteryl esters, triglycerides	25–35	1.006–1.019
LDL	Apo B100	Cholesteryl esters	18–25	1.019–1.063
HDL	Apo AI, apo AII, apo AV	Cholesteryl esters, phospholipids	5–12	1.063–1.210
Lp(a)	Apo B100, apo(a)	Chlolesteryl esters	~30	1.055–1.085

Apo = apolipoprotein; HDL = high-density lipoprotein; IDL = intermediate-density lipoprotein; LDL = low-density lipoprotein; Lp(a) = lipoprotein (a); VLDL = very low density lipoprotein.

TABLE 217–2 MAJOR APOLIPOPROTEINS

Apolipoprotein	Chromosomal Location, GenBank Sequence Identification	Functions
Apo B100	2p24-p23, M14162	Structural component of atherogenic lipoproteins (VLDL, IDL, LDL), VLDL secretion, ligand for LDL receptor, elevated levels associated with vascular disease
Apo B48	Same as apo B100	Chylomicron secretion from intestine
Apo E	19q13.31, K00396	Ligand for binding of triglyceride-rich particles to LDL receptor and LRP, potential roles in Alzheimer's disease and neuronal injury
Apo AI	11q23-q24, X02162	Structural component of HDL, activates LCAT, elevated levels associated with protection from vascular disease
Apo AII	1q21-Q23, NM_001643	Genetically and biochemically associated with familial combined hyperlipidemia
Apo AIV	11q23-qter, NM_000482	Potential role in regulating food intake
Apo AV	11q23, AF202889	Required for normal lipolysis of triglyceride-rich lipoproteins
Apo CII	19q13.2, X00568	Activator of LPL
Apo CIII	11q23-qter, X01388	Inhibitor of LPL
Apo (a)	6q26-q27, X06290	Covalent bond with apo B100 forms Lp(a) and renders particle resistant to uptake by LDL receptor

Apo = apolipoprotein; HDL = high-density lipoprotein; IDL = intermediate-density lipoprotein; LCAT = lecithin-cholesterol acyltransferase; LDL = low-density lipoprotein; Lp(a) = lipoprotein (a); LRP = LDL receptor–related protein; VLDL = very low density lipoprotein.

TABLE 217–3 IMPORTANT RECEPTORS AND PROTEINS IN LIPID TRANSPORT

Protein	Chromosomal Location, GenBank Sequence Identification	Functions
LDL receptor	19p13.3, AY114155	Clearance of apo B100 and apo E–containing lipoproteins, activity increased by statin drugs, deficiency causes familial hypercholesterolemia
LDL receptor-related protein (LRP)	12Q13-Q14, NM_000014	Clearance of apo E–containing lipoproteins
Scavenger receptor B1 (SR-B1)	12q24.32, Z22555	HDL receptor
Lipoprotein lipase (LPL)	8p22, NM_000237	Rate limiting for triglyceride metabolism, deficiency causes chylomicronemia syndrome
Lecithin-cholesterol acyltransferase (LCAT)	16q22.1, NM_000229	Esterifies cholesterol in HDL to increase HDL cholesterol levels, deficiency decreases HDL levels
Cholesteryl ester transfer protein (CETP)	16q13, NM_000078	Exchanges cholesteryl ester in HDL for triglyceride in apo B–containing lipoproteins, deficiency increases HDL levels
ABCA1	9q31, AJ12376	Transfers cholesterol in tissues to nascent HDL particles, deficiency causes Tangier disease

ABCA1 = ATP binding cassette A1; Apo = apolipoprotein; HDL = high-density lipoprotein; LDL = low-density lipoprotein.

SREBPs are found in inactive forms in the endoplasmic re-ticulum (ER). When cellular cholesterol levels rise after the delivery of cholesterol by the LDL receptor, increased ER sterol content causes cholesterol to bind to Scap, a protein that promotes the migration of SREBPs from the ER to the Golgi. SREBPs undergo proteolytic conversion in the Golgi to active forms that move to the nucleus and stimulate the expression of genes involved in cholesterol synthesis. The binding of cholesterol to Scap induces a conformational change that causes it to bind to Insigs, ER anchor proteins. However, when intracellular cholesterol levels are high, the Scap/SREBP complex does not move to the Golgi, SREBPs are not processed, and cholesterol synthesis stops. When cholesterol levels are low, Scap is released from Insigs, the Scap/SREBP complex moves to the Golgi, SREBPs are converted to active forms, and genes important for cholesterol synthesis and acquisition (such as the LDL receptor) are transcribed. Statin drugs effectively lower cholesterol. They inhibit 3-hydroxy-3-methylglutaryl coenzyme A (HMG-CoA) reductase, the rate-limiting enzyme in cholesterol synthesis. Cholesterol levels fall, Scap is free to shepherd SREBPs to the Golgi for activation, an active SREBP stimulates transcription of the LDL receptor gene, and increased levels of the LDL receptor protein on the surface of the hepatocyte bind and remove LDL particles from the circulation.

Low-Density Lipoprotein Receptor–Related Protein

The LDL receptor–related protein (LRP), also called the chylomicron remnant receptor, participates in the removal of intestine-derived lipoproteins by interacting with apo E. Chylomicron remnants carry apo B48, which is missing the LDL receptor binding domain, but these particles are also cleared by the LDL receptor through apo E binding.

Scavenger Receptor B1

Scavenger receptor B1 (SR-B1) is a protein expressed in liver that binds HDL. Unlike the LDL receptor that endocytoses LDL particles, SR-B1 does not appear to internalize HDL particles but instead facilitates the transfer of cholesteryl ester from HDL to the liver. Its genetic manipulation in mice has raised clinically relevant questions regarding the significance of elevated HDL levels. Inactivation of SR-B1 elevates HDL cholesterol levels but promotes atherosclerosis, presumably because of the disruption of the transport of cholesterol from peripheral cells, where it can cause disease, to the liver, where it is excreted. These results suggest that it is not the level of HDL per se but the flux of cholesterol through HDL that affords protection from vascular disease.

Lipoprotein Lipase

Lipoprotein lipase (LPL) is rate limiting for the metabolism of triglyceride-rich lipoproteins and required for the generation of HDL particles because HDL is absent from LPL-deficient mice. Deficient LPL activity thus provides a physiologic explanation for the common association between high triglyceride levels and low HDL cholesterol.

Lecithin-Cholesterol Acyltransferase

Another protein important in HDL metabolism is lecithin-cholesterol acyltransferase (LCAT). LCAT is associated with HDL in the circulation, where it esterifies free cholesterol to form cholesteryl esters that are easily stored in the nonpolar core of the lipoprotein. LCAT deficiency, a rare disorder, is characterized by low HDL as well as anemia and renal failure, clinical features probably related to the disruption of normal membrane function by the accumulation of excessive amounts of unesterified cholesterol.

Cholesteryl Ester Transfer Protein

Cholesteryl ester transfer protein (CETP) exchanges one molecule of cholesteryl ester in HDL for one molecule of triglyceride in apo B–containing particles such as VLDL. The resulting HDL particle is triglyceride enriched, enhancing its clearance (especially by an enzyme related to LPL, hepatic lipase) and lowering HDL. Inhibition of CETP activity increases HDL levels.

ATP Binding Cassette A1

ATP binding cassette A1 (ABCA1) is a cell membrane protein that mediates the transfer of cholesterol and phospholipids from cells to the apolipoproteins of lipid-poor HDL. ABCA1 in liver probably contributes to the genesis of HDL, and ABCA1 in macrophages appears to protect blood vessels from developing atherosclerosis. Heterozygous ABCA1 deficiency is responsible for isolated low HDL cholesterol levels that occur in some kindreds (also known as familial hypoalphalipoproteinemia based on an older term for HDL). Rare homozygotes for ABCA1 mutations have Tangier disease, characterized by the accumulation of cholesteryl esters in macrophages and causing distinctive features including orange-yellow tonsils, neuropathy, and hepatosplenomegaly. HDL is very low to absent. Atherosclerosis is probably increased in these patients, but its extent may be moderated by concomitant low LDL levels.

EXOGENOUS LIPID METABOLISM

Animal products, composed of substantial amounts of cholesterol and triglycerides, are eaten regularly by most people. Dietary fats are broken down in the gut to free cholesterol and fatty acids, which are transported across cell membranes into the enterocyte. Here, they are re-esterified into cholesteryl ester and triglycerides and then packaged onto apo B48. These particles gain access to the plasma through the thoracic duct and acquire other apolipoproteins in part by transfer from HDL, and these mature chylomicrons circulate to peripheral tissues. LPL, bound to the capillary endothelium in tissues such as adipose tissue and muscle, is activated by apo CII on chylomicrons, and fatty acids hydrolyzed from triglycerides by LPL are released and transported into adipose tissue for storage or muscle for energy. This process also requires apo AV, an apolipoprotein transported in HDL that appears to facilitate the interaction between LPL and triglyceride-rich lipoproteins.

Progressive hydrolysis of triglyceride converts chylomicrons into chylomicron remnants, which are relatively enriched in cholesteryl esters. Chylomicron remnants are removed in the liver by species that bind apo E: LRP, the LDL receptor, and cell surface glycosaminoglycans. Chylomicrons are large, and it is unlikely that they contribute to atherosclerosis. Chylomicron remnants are enriched in cholesteryl esters, the major lipid component of the atherosclerotic lesion, and small enough to enter the subendothelial space, where they are taken up by macrophages. Remnants are atherogenic, consistent with the idea that the progression of atherosclerotic lesions can occur in the postprandial state, a potential contributor to morbidity not assessed by current practices that focus on the measurement of fasting lipoproteins.

Chylomicrons are not soluble. Their presence causes the "tomato soup" appearance of blood drawn after a fatty meal. Because they are mostly triglycerides, they float to the top of serum that is refrigerated overnight, leaving a layer of cream on the top of the sample. The detection of chylomicrons in fasting serum has clinical relevance because it indicates a risk for pancreatitis and other elements of the chylomicronemia syndrome.

ENDOGENOUS LIPID METABOLISM

Fats deposited in the liver are further metabolized into component lipid species, re-esterified as cholesteryl ester and triglycerides, and either stored in hepatocytes or exported as lipoproteins (Fig. 217–1). The liver produces the triglyceride-rich lipoprotein VLDL. Its rate of production appears to depend on the availability of triglycerides. Apo B100 is the major apolipoprotein of VLDL, but under normal conditions the regulation of the apo B gene does not appear to play an appreciable role in the control of VLDL synthesis. Apo B transcription appears to be mostly constitutive, and production of the apo B100 protein depends on its cotranslational stabilization. As the message is translated into protein, the presence of triglyceride stabilizes the peptide and allows continued addition of amino acids. In the absence of triglycerides, the apo B molecule is degraded.

The transfer of triglycerides to the growing apo B peptide is mediated by microsomal transfer protein (MTP). Mutations in MTP cause abetalipoproteinemia, a rare disease characterized by the absence of circulating apo B. In the absence of apo B, the metabolism of fat-soluble vitamins (normally carried in lipoproteins) is disrupted and patients suffer from multisystem defects including severe neurologic dysfunction and retinopathy presumably caused by deficiency of vitamins E and A. Drugs that interfere with MTP function lower lipids but, not surprisingly, cause the accumulation of triglyceride in the liver. The apo B gene is normal in patients with abetalipoproteinemia. Mutations in the apo B gene cause another condition known as hypobetalipoproteinemia, caused by shortened forms of the apo B protein. Subjects with hypobetalipoproteinemia have very low, but not absent, levels of circulating lipids and appear to be healthy.

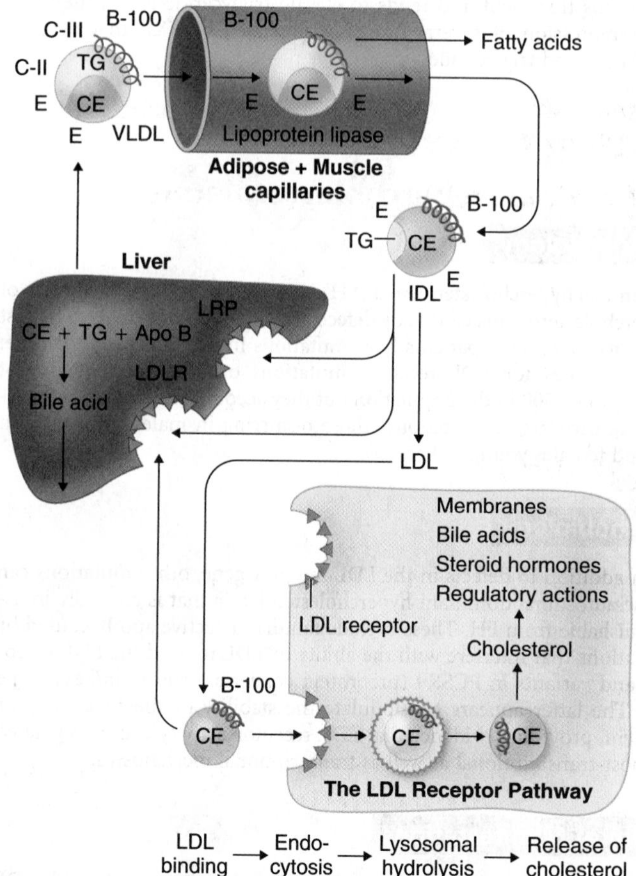

FIGURE 217–1 • Endogenous lipid metabolism. In the liver, triglycerides (TGs), cholesteryl esters (CEs), and apolipoprotein B100 are packaged as very low density lipoprotein (VLDL) particles. TG is hydrolyzed by lipoprotein lipase (LPL) to generate intermediate density lipoprotein (IDL), which is further metabolized to generate low density lipoprotein (LDL). This particle can be removed by the liver or by peripheral cells. Cholesterol derived from LDL regulates several processes and can be used for the synthesis of bile acids, steroid hormones, and cell membranes.

Nascent VLDL containing one apo B100 molecule per particle is secreted into the plasma, where it acquires apo E, apo CII, and apo CIII. In a process analogous to that occurring with chylomicrons, apo CII on VLDL activates LPL, and fatty acids hydrolyzed from triglycerides by LPL are released in capillary beds and transported into tissues. With continued hydrolysis and the loss of both phospholipids and apolipoproteins to HDL, VLDL is converted to IDL, a cholesteryl ester–rich particle with an apolipoprotein complement of only apo B and apo E. These particles, like chylomicron remnants, are thought to have high atherogenic potential. Unlike chylomicron remnants, IDLs are included in current management schemes because reporting of LDL cholesterol levels by most clinical laboratories includes IDL. IDL can be taken up by either the LRP or the LDL receptor in the liver. In the presence of a normal apo E molecule, IDLs are converted to LDL, with one molecule of apo B100 per particle and cholesteryl ester with essentially no triglycerides. About 75% of LDL is removed from the plasma by the LDL receptor pathway, and most of this takes place in the liver. The uptake of LDL results in the migration of LDL particles to lysosomes, where cholesterol is released for (depending on the cell type) plasma membrane localization, bile acid synthesis, steroid hormone synthesis, and interaction with Scap for the control of SREBP activation. A minority of LDL enters the subendothelial space of the vascular wall, where its modification by oxidation or other processes promotes its uptake by macrophages in atherosclerotic lesions.

Most VLDL particles are large and not thought to promote vascular disease. However, some small VLDL particles as well as IDL and LDL are atherogenic. Because the majority of VLDL is triglyceride, most patients with elevated levels of fasting triglyceride have either increased numbers of VLDL particles or increased content of triglycerides in each VLDL. Unlike most other lipoproteins, LDL has a fairly long residence time with

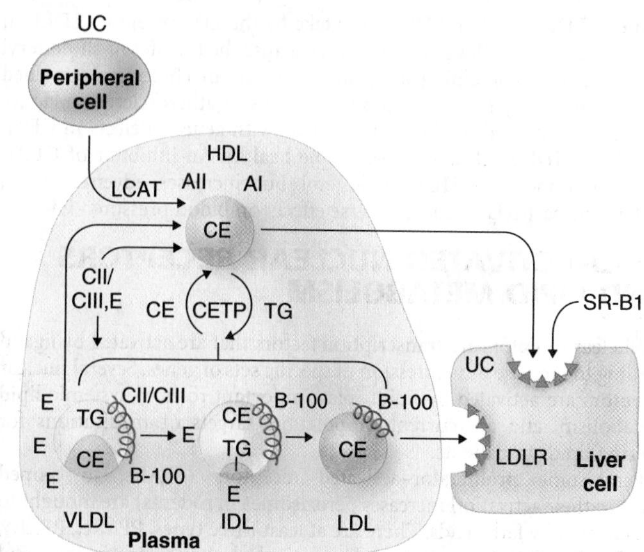

FIGURE 217–2 • Reverse cholesterol transport and high-density lipoprotein (HDL) metabolism. Unesterified cholesterol (UC) in peripheral cells can be transferred to HDL and esterified by lecithin-cholesterol acyltransferase (LCAT). This cholesterol ester (CE) in HDL can be transferred to the liver directly through scavenger receptor B1 (SR-B1). Alternatively, it may be transferred to apolipoprotein B100–containing lipoproteins in exchange for triglycerides (TGs) through the action of cholesteryl ester transfer protein (CETP).

a plasma half-life of 2 to 5 days. Accordingly, the detection of elevated levels of fasting cholesterol usually reflects the presence of either increased numbers of LDL particles or increased cholesteryl ester in each LDL. LDL also exists in a range of sizes. Small dense LDL tends to occur in the setting of concomitant hypertriglyceridemia. This type of lipoprotein is thought to have greater atherogenic potential than larger LDL species, perhaps because of more facile access to the vascular wall and greater susceptibility to oxidative modification. Lipoprotein particle size and number can be quantified by nuclear magnetic resonance techniques, but it is not clear that these data provide diagnostic advantages beyond the determination of total cholesterol, triglycerides, LDL cholesterol, and HDL cholesterol.

REVERSE CHOLESTEROL TRANSPORT AND HIGH-DENSITY LIPOPROTEIN METABOLISM

Lipid metabolism is extremely dynamic. At the same time lipoproteins are processed to modify their nonpolar lipids, particles are interacting with each other, exchanging surface materials, apolipoproteins, and nonpolar lipids. HDL is an important reservoir for components cast off during the metabolism of other lipoproteins as well as lipids discarded by cells. Nascent HDL is generated by the liver and intestine as a phospholipid disc containing apo AI and apo AII. It accepts unesterified (free) cholesterol (UC in Fig. 217–2) and phospholipids shed from cells. This unesterified cholesterol is converted to cholesteryl ester by the action of LCAT and stored in the center of the disc, allowing it to become a spherical particle. The particle is further modified as a consequence of the action of LPL on triglycerides in apo B–containing lipoproteins. As the core triglycerides of VLDL are metabolized, the particle collapses, leaving redundant surface lipids (phospholipid in the form of lecithin and unesterified cholesterol) and excess apolipoproteins such as apo CII, apo CIII, and apo E that are transferred to HDL. LCAT again esterifies the cholesterol to increase the content of cholesteryl ester in the HDL.

Reverse cholesterol transport is the beneficial process by which cholesterol present in peripheral cells such as foam cells in a growing atherosclerotic lesion is transported back to the liver for excretion. There are at least two well-defined pathways mediating this transfer. First, after accepting cholesterol from peripheral cells and esterifying it through the action of LCAT, HDL can interact directly with the liver by binding to SR-B1 and transferring cholesteryl ester to the hepatocyte. Second, HDL can transfer cholesteryl ester to apo B100–containing lipoproteins such as VLDL (bottom of Fig. 217–2) through the action of CETP. This cholesteryl ester can ultimately be transported to the liver after conversion of VLDL to IDL to LDL and uptake by the LDL receptor (LDLR in Fig. 217–2). This pathway is not direct because the transfer of cholesteryl ester to apo B–containing lipoproteins results in cholesterol-enriched particles that may be taken up by foam cells in atherosclerotic plaques before being cleared by the liver. Humans with genetic defects in CETP have high HDL levels and appear to be healthy. An inhibitor of CEPT, torcetrapib increases HDL cholesterol but increases adverse events, perhaps in part related to its adverse effects on blood pressure. 1

LIPID-ACTIVATED NUCLEAR RECEPTORS AND LIPID METABOLISM

Nuclear receptors are transcription factors that are activated by ligand binding to increase the expression of specific sets of genes. Several nuclear receptors are activated by lipids, play important roles in systemic lipid metabolism, and are current or potential targets of medications for altering lipids in patients.

Peroxisome proliferator–activated receptors (PPARs, so named because their activation increases peroxisomes in rodents) are thought to be activated by fatty acids. There are at least three types, PPARα, PPARγ, and PPARδ. PPARα appears to be particularly important in liver and muscle. It stimulates the expression of genes mediating fatty acid oxidation as well as those promoting the formation of HDL. Fibrate drugs such as gemfibrozil and fenofibrate work by activating PPARα. They lower triglycerides, by accelerating the oxidation of fatty acids in the liver so that less lipid is available for stabilizing apo B100 in VLDL secretion, and elevate HDL, by increasing expression of apo AI, LPL, and other genes. PPARγ is expressed mostly in adipose tissue and macrophages but also has measurable effects in other tissues such as muscle. It increases the expression of genes promoting the development of fat tissue and appears to suppress certain mediators of chronic inflammation. Thiazolidinedione drugs such as pioglitazone and rosiglitazone work by activating PPARγ. They lower blood glucose in people with diabetes by decreasing insulin resistance, a complex process that also results in multiple lipid effects including lower triglycerides and higher HDL (expected to be beneficial) and higher LDL (expected to be detrimental). The overall effects appear to be favorable. 2 Combined PPARα-PPARγ agonists are in development. PPARδ is expressed widely, has multiple potential effects that include the regulation of fatty acid oxidation, and is the subject of intense pharmacologic investigation.

Two other nuclear receptors are activated by lipids and modulate lipid physiology. Liver X receptors (LXRα and LXRβ) are activated by oxidized derivatives of cholesterol. In the liver, they promote the synthesis of fatty acids and triglycerides in addition to stimulating both the conversion of cholesterol into bile acids and the excretion of bile acids into the gut. In the intestine, they suppress the absorption of cholesterol. The farnesoid X receptor (FXR) is activated by bile acids. FXR stimulates the secretion of bile acids into bile as well as the reabsorption of bile acids from the intestine.

Together, these receptors help orchestrate two important futile cycles in lipid metabolism. In one, fatty acids exported from the liver (in the form of triglycerides within VLDL) and from the intestine (in chylomicron triglycerides) are released to peripheral tissues by the action of LPL. Some are taken up by muscle, where their activation of PPARα accelerates their oxidation in mitochondria, yielding ATP. Others enter adipose tissue, where they are re-esterified into triglycerides. From here, fatty acids are released in a process stimulated by catecholamines and glucagon. This process is complicated, involving hormone-sensitive lipase, a recently discovered enzyme known as adipose triglyceride lipase, and the remodeling of proteins that coat lipid droplets to alter their accessibility to lipases. Following lipolysis, fatty acids bind to albumin and return to the liver, where they can fuel the production of more VLDL particles. Nicotinic acid improves lipids in part by blocking the release of fatty acids from adipose tissue. A G protein–coupled receptor for nicotinic acid has been identified.

In another futile cycle, bile acids (formed from cholesterol and constituting the major pathway for excretion of cholesterol from the body) are secreted into the intestine through events stimulated by LXR and FXR. Bile acids are reabsorbed in the terminal ileum. Treatment with bile acid sequestrants such as cholestyramine and colesevelam interrupts this enterohepatic circulation, and the increased excretion of cholesterol (in the form of bile acids) depletes cholesterol content in the liver, leading to the induction of LDL receptors resulting in lower circulating levels of LDL. This treatment also tends to elevate triglyceride levels, the result of de-repression of several processes mediated by FXR that decrease fatty acids and triglycerides.

IMPORTANT CLINICAL DISORDERS OF LIPID METABOLISM

Familial Hypercholesterolemia

Epidemiology

Familial hypercholesterolemia (FH) is an autosomal dominant form of hypercholesterolemia caused by defects in LDL receptor activity. The vast majority of affected patients have mutations in the LDL receptor gene. Heterozygotes for LDL receptor mutations occur at a frequency of perhaps 1 in 500 in the population but they account for up to 5% of premature myocardial infarctions (those occurring in males younger than 55 and females younger than 65).

Pathobiology

In addition to defects in the LDL receptor gene, other mutations can cause autosomal dominant hypercholesterolemia that is clinically indistinguishable from FH. These include familial defective apo B, caused by mutations that interfere with the ability of LDL to bind the LDL receptor, and variants in PCSK9 (preprotein convertase subtilisin/kexin type 9a). The latter appears to modulate the stability of the LDL receptor protein, providing evidence that LDL receptor activity can be regulated by post-transcriptional as well as transcriptional mechanisms.

Clinical Manifestations

Total cholesterol levels are usually greater than 300 mg/dL with LDL cholesterol levels greater than 200 mg/dL. Triglycerides are generally normal. Clinical features include thickening of the Achilles tendon as well as xanthomas at the extensor tendons of the knees and hands, reflecting infiltration of lipid-laden macrophages at these sites. There is evidence that clinically apparent tendon xanthomas occur in a minority of patients with FH. Arthralgias are common, perhaps because of the presence of macrophage-mediated inflammation, and tend to improve with cholesterol lowering. Other features include xanthelasmas and corneal arcus, although the latter is also seen in elderly people and certain ethnic populations independent of cholesterol levels. Homozygotes (about 1 in 1,000,000) have total cholesterol levels in the range 800 to 1000 mg/dL and usually do not survive to adulthood without liver transplantation to provide LDL receptors. Children and adolescents with this disease may develop aortic valve disease because of macrophage infiltration at the aortic origin.

The penetrance of cardiovascular events in heterozygous FH is variable, with some subjects presenting with sudden death or accelerated disease in their 20s and others (generally women without other risk factors) surviving beyond menopause without clinically evident disease.

Treatment

Treatment should include aggressive reduction of any associated risk factors for vascular disease such as smoking, hypertension, and diabetes. Patients should be instructed in a diet low in saturated fat and cholesterol, and most require more than one cholesterol-lowering medication to achieve goals. The National Cholesterol Education Program (NCEP) provides periodic updates on the approach to screening and treating hyperlipidemia (Fig. 217–3). It is not uncommon for FH homozygotes to be treated with a statin drug, ezetimibe (which inhibits cholesterol absorption by binding to the enterocyte protein Niemann-Pick C1-like 1), and nicotinic acid. Some with aggressive disease require LDL apheresis, which involves perfusing blood through a column that extracts apo B–containing lipoproteins.

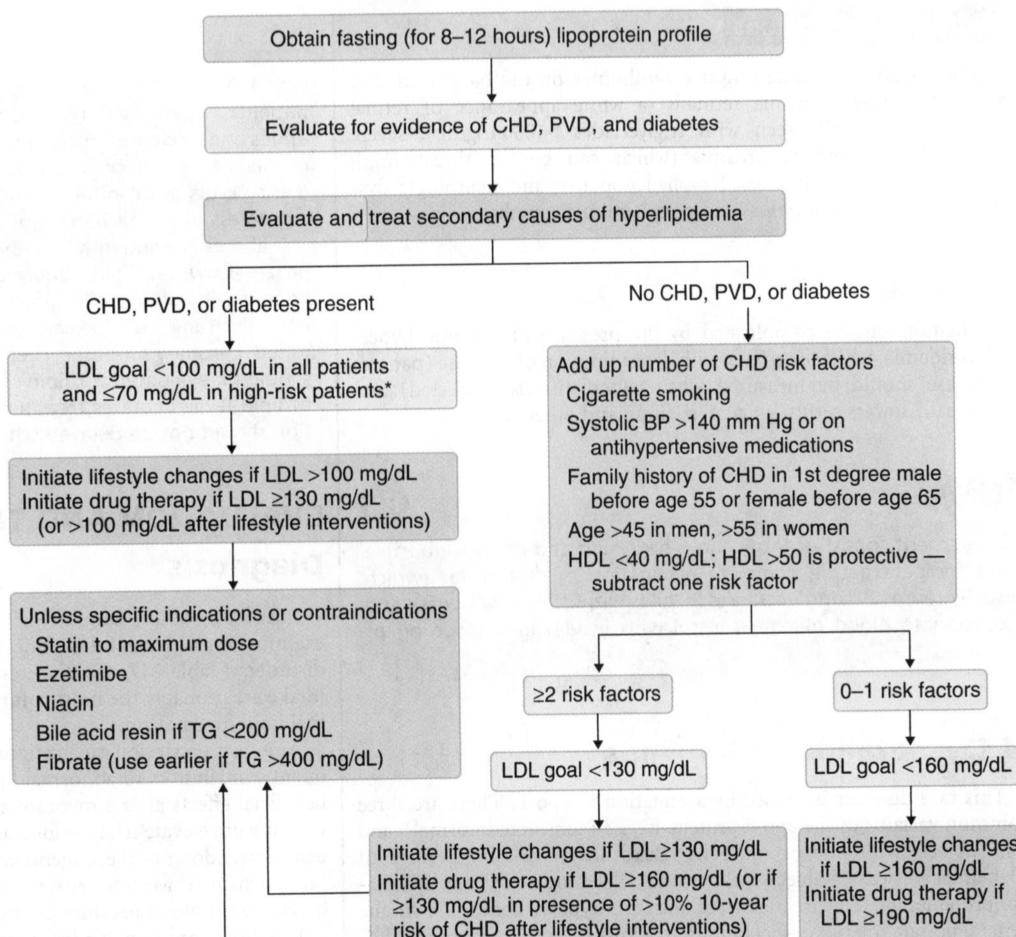

FIGURE 217–3 • Approach to lipid screening and treatment. BP = blood pressure; CHD = coronary heart disease; HDL = high-density lipoprotein; LDL = low-density lipoprotein; PVD = peripheral vascular disease; TG = triglycerides. *See Chapters 70 to 72. (Based on recommendations of the Executive Summary of the Third Report of the National Cholesterol Education Program [NCEP] Expert Panel on detection, evaluation, and treatment of high blood cholesterol in adults [Adult Treatment Panel III]. JAMA 2001;285: 2486–2497.)

Familial Combined Hyperlipidemia

Epidemiology

Familial combined hyperlipidemia (FCH) is an autosomal dominant form of hyperlipidemia that is present in up to 2% of the general population. It accounts for as many as 20% of cases of premature coronary artery disease.

Pathobiology

The specific molecular defect is uncertain, although upstream stimulatory factor 1 (USF1), a member of a family of ubiquitously expressed transcription factors that control lipid and glucose metabolism, may be associated with the disorder. FCH also appears to be associated with the metabolic syndrome (Chapter 248). The disorder is characterized by the primary overproduction of apo B. VLDLs secreted by the liver are small. Small dense LDLs, thought to be particularly atherogenic, accumulate. For a given concentration of LDL cholesterol, FCH patients have greater numbers of LDL particles and an increased apo B concentration.

Diagnosis

The diagnosis is made in the setting of a family history of premature coronary disease with different lipid phenotypes combined in the same family. Affected family members may have elevated triglycerides, elevated LDL cholesterol, both elevated triglycerides and LDL, or hypertriglyceridemia with low HDL cholesterol. Lipid phenotypes commonly change over time.

Familial Hypertriglyceridemia

Familial hypertriglyceridemia is also a common autosomal dominant disorder, occurring in 1 to 2% of the general population. Affected family members have isolated elevated triglycerides. A unifying molecular mechanism is lacking. The phenotype is stable with affected family members consistently showing isolated hypertriglyceridemia on repeated analyses. The disorder is characterized by primary overproduction of triglyceride. Lipoprotein particles tend to be large, consisting of increased amounts of triglyceride relative to apo B. For a given level of cholesterol, these patients have lower numbers of lipoprotein particles and a decreased apo B concentration. The relationship between this disorder and cardiovascular risk is uncertain. Affected kindreds do not appear to have a propensity for premature vascular disease, but these individuals are at risk for the chylomicronemia syndrome when an additional stimulus for hypertriglyceridemia such as uncontrolled diabetes is present.

Chylomicronemia Syndrome

Pathobiology

This syndrome occurs when triglycerides are extremely elevated, usually greater than 2000 mg/dL. Individuals with homozygous defects in the LPL gene can present with the syndrome in infancy, although the penetrance of clinical sequelae is extremely variable. Some individuals suffer repeated episodes of the syndrome throughout life, whereas others with triglycerides consistently above 2000 mg/dL remain completely asymptomatic. The basis for the wide spectrum of symptoms despite similar degrees of severe hypertriglyceridemia is unknown. Other molecular defects responsible for the syndrome include mutations in apo CII and apo AV.

Although defects in LPL, apo CII, and apo AV can cause the syndrome, the disorder is most likely to occur when patients with a common predisposition to hypertriglyceridemia (FCH or familial hypertriglyceridemia) develop another defect associated with elevated triglycerides (such as uncontrolled diabetes, obesity, and treatment with glucocorticoids, estrogens, or other drugs).

Clinical Manifestations

Clinical features include eruptive xanthomas on the back, buttocks, knees, and elbows; lipemia retinalis (a white appearance of retinal blood vessels, usually seen with triglycerides >4000 mg/dL); severe abdominal pain and pancreatitis (which can be life threatening); hepatosplenomegaly; dyspnea; lymphadenopathy; and neurologic dysfunction such as memory loss and peripheral neuropathy.

Diagnosis

Evaluation can be complicated by the presence of extreme hypertriglyceridemia, which interferes with determination of amylase (pancreatic lipase should be measured when pancreatitis is suspected) and artifactually lowers serum glucose, sodium, and other analytes.

Treatment

Rx

Treatment consist of intravenous hydration and other supportive care for pancreatitis, complete elimination of dietary fat (which usually causes striking decreases in lipids within 24 to 48 hours), and appropriate blood glucose control with insulin in the setting of diabetes.

Dysbetalipoproteinemia

This rare disorder is caused by a mutation in apo E. There are three common variants of the apo E protein, E2, E3 (considered normal), and E4. Subjects with one or more E4 alleles are at risk for a form of Alzheimer's disease. Subjects with two E2 alleles are at risk for dysbetalipoproteinemia. The frequency of this genotype is about 1% in the general population but dysbetalipoproteinemia is rare, requiring an additional poorly defined factor. Hypothyroidism is known to precipitate the disorder. Subjects classically present with equal elevations of triglycerides and cholesterol in the range of about 300 to 600 mg/dL and xanthomas, especially in the palmar creases of the hands. They are at substantial risk for coronary artery disease. Unlike patients with FH, patients with dysbetalipoproteinemia are also at risk for severe peripheral vascular disease. Atherosclerosis occurs in part because of the presence of elevated concentrations of chylomicron remnants, which are not removed normally because of the presence of apo E2, and IDL particles, which are not converted normally to LDL in the presence of apo E2. It is unknown why the remnants that accumulate in dysbetalipoproteinemia cause both peripheral vascular disease and coronary disease whereas the LDL particles that accumulate in FH tend to cause only coronary disease.

Diabetic Dyslipidemia

Pathobiology

Insulin is a critical regulator of lipid metabolism, and because diabetes represents impaired insulin signaling, lipid disorders are common in both type 1 and type 2 diabetes. Hypertriglyceridemia is the hallmark of diabetic dyslipidemia. This is driven by two mechanisms. First, LPL is insulin dependent. In the absence of insulin or in the presence of insulin resistance, LPL enzyme activity is deficient and triglyceride-rich lipoproteins cannot be metabolized appropriately. Second, insulin suppresses the release of free fatty acids from adipose tissue stores. Insulin deficiency or resistance results in unabated release of free fatty acids, and these return to the liver, where they stabilize apo B synthesis and increase VLDL production.

Treatment

The lack of insulin in patients with type 1 diabetes causes diabetic ketoacidosis, in which elevated triglycerides can be severe and are corrected by reinstitution of insulin therapy. Intensive insulin therapy in type 1 diabetes decreases triglycerides, LDL, and often Lp(a). Patients gain weight with intensive insulin therapy, and increased adiposity tends to lower HDL levels, which may explain why HDL does not always increase in intensively treated type 1 patients. Patients with type 2 diabetes usually have increased triglycerides and decreased HDL. These abnormalities improve but seldom normalize with improved glycemic control. Most of the improvement occurs with initial pharmacologic glucose-lowering therapy, regardless of its mechanism of action.

Diabetes is frequently classified as a secondary cause of lipid disorders. However, lipid abnormalities are intrinsic to diabetes, and people with diabetes lacking clinical evidence of vascular disease have the same risk for cardiovascular events as those with established coronary disease. Therefore, every person with diabetes should be evaluated for lipid disorders and often adequate control of lipid levels requires treatment with a statin drug. This intervention should not be delayed while glycemic control is optimized.

EVALUATION AND THERAPY

Diagnosis

Initial evaluation should include a complete history and physical examination with careful attention to potential secondary causes of lipid disorders (Table 217–4). Diabetes, hypothyroidism, and excess alcohol intake are probably the most common secondary contributors to abnormal lipid metabolism.

Among prescription medications, β-adrenergic blocking agents are frequent contributors to abnormal lipid profiles. These agents have proven beneficial effects after a myocardial infarction but also tend to promote weight gain, elevate triglycerides, and decrease HDL. Many clinicians are using lower doses of these agents and relying on more lipid-neutral drugs (angiotensin-converting enzyme inhibitors and angiotensin receptor blockers) for blood pressure control.

It is now common for internists to encounter patients with human immunodeficiency virus (HIV) infection with hyperlipidemia. Some series estimate that more than half of HIV patients treated with protease inhibitors for 2 years develop dyslipidemia, frequently with redistribution of fat resembling that in genetic lipodystrophy syndromes. In addition to appropriate management of other risk factors, lipid-lowering therapy should be tailored to the ongoing HIV drug regimen. Some evidence suggests that certain newer agents may be less likely to promote hyperlipidemia. Pravastatin is least likely to interact with protease inhibitors but is less effective at lowering LDL cholesterol. Agents such as simvastatin that are substantially metabolized by the cytochrome P-450 3A4 (CYP3A4) system should not be used in patients treated with protease inhibitors because of delayed clearance of the statin. PPARα agonists such as fenofibrate can be used to lower triglycerides, but effects are limited because their clearance is accelerated by protease inhibitor treatment.

Antipsychotics have complex effects on metabolism. Some of the newer agents used to treat schizophrenia promote hyperlipidemia, obesity, and insulin resistance. Although therapeutic decisions should be based on psychiatric responses, substituting for agents with prominent metabolic side effects such as olanzapine can improve lipid profiles.

Laboratory Evaluation

After an 8- to 12-hour fast (subjects should be told that it is acceptable to drink water and other beverages without calories during this period), total triglycerides, total cholesterol, HDL cholesterol, and LDL cholesterol should be obtained. In most clinical laboratories, LDL cholesterol is still calculated using the formula LDL = total cholesterol − HDL cholesterol − (triglycerides/5). This formula is not valid when triglycerides are over 400 mg/dL. It is also possible to measure LDL directly, which is sometimes useful for monitoring therapeutic effects on LDL alone because this determination does not require patients to fast.

What constitutes "normal" lipid levels is unknown. For triglycerides, Adult Treatment Panel (ATP) III of the National Cholesterol Education Program identified a normal triglyceride level as less than 150 mg/dL. Values from 150 to 199 are borderline high, 200 to 499 is considered high, and above 500 is very high. In patients with fasting triglycerides over 500, triglycerides are a primary target of therapy in order to decrease the risk of pancreatitis and the chylomicronemia syndrome. These individuals are treated with a very low fat diet (usually 15% of calories as fat), an exer-

TABLE 217–4 SECONDARY CAUSES OF LIPID DISORDERS

Condition/Medication	Comments
Diabetes	Common contributor to dyslipidemia. Abnormal lipids are seldom normalized by glycemic control alone.
Hypothyroidism	Thyroid hormone regulates multiple steps in lipid metabolism including LDL receptor expression and LPL activity.
Alcohol	Can cause hypertriglyceridemia in susceptible patients but mild intake linked to decreased risk of vascular disease.
Renal disease	Increased LDL in nephrotic syndrome, hypertriglyceridemia in end-stage renal disease.
Obstructive liver disease	Can be associated with very high cholesterol levels. Some evidence that diseases such as primary biliary cirrhosis not associated with increased vascular events despite dyslipidemia.
Diuretics	Increased LDL with high doses. Current practice of using low doses of thiazides decreases vascular events and has minimal effect on lipids.
β-Adrenergic receptor blockers	Increased triglycerides/decreased HDL probably by inhibiting LPL.
Anabolic steroids	Can result in very low HDL (<10 mg/dL).
Estrogens	Exacerbate hypertriglyceridemia when given orally. This effect is not seen with topical estrogen therapy.
Protease inhibitors	Increased triglycerides/decreased HDL especially in setting of HIV-associated lipodystrophy.
Glucocorticoid excess	Increased triglycerides/decreased HDL probably related to exacerbation of insulin resistance.
Antipsychotics	Increased triglycerides/decreased HDL probably related to increased adiposity and insulin resistance.
Retinoids	Increased triglycerides.
Systemic lupus erythematosus	Chronic inflammation may increase risk of vascular disease independent of effects on lipid metabolism.
Acute intermittent porphyria	Many agents used to treat lipid disorders reported to provoke episodes of abdominal pain.

HDL = high-density lipoprotein; HIV = human immunodeficiency virus; LDL = low-density lipoprotein; LPL = lipoprotein lipase;

cise program, a weight loss regimen in the setting of obesity, glycemic control in the setting of diabetes, and either nicotinic acid or a fibrate drug, alone or in combination with fish oils.

Risk Assessment

ATP III identified therapeutic goals in terms of LDL cholesterol level based on the 10-year risk of coronary heart disease in 2001 and updated these goals in 2004. High risk, with a greater than 20% probability of a vascular event in 10 years, includes those with coronary heart disease (myocardial infarction, angina of any type, previous coronary artery procedure, known myocardial ischemia) or a coronary heart disease equivalent (diabetes, carotid artery disease, abdominal aortic aneurysm, peripheral vascular disease, multiple risk factors indicating a 10-year risk of >20%). For these high-risk patients, the LDL goal is less than 100 mg/dL, and less than 70 mg/dL is an optional goal.

Risk factors for coronary heart disease include smoking, hypertension (or treatment for hypertension), family history of premature coronary heart disease (younger than 55 years in males, 65 in females), low HDL (under 40), age (older than 45 in men, 55 in women). For those with two or more risk factors and a calculated 10-year risk for coronary heart disease under 20%, the LDL goal is less than 130 mg/dL. For those with 0 to 1 risk factor, the LDL goal is less than 160 mg/dL.

These recommendations are likely to be modified as new data are incorporated into practice. The most recent updates, as well as 10-year risk calculators that are useful for customizing recommendations for individuals patients, are available at *http://www.nhlbi.nih.gov/guidelines/cholesterol.*

Treatment

Rx

General Measures

Intensive Lowering of Low-Density Lipoproteins

Randomized clinical trials support the concept that intensive LDL lowering is appropriate for patients with coronary heart disease and its equivalents. In the Heart Protection Study, [3] those who entered the study with LDL less than 100 mg/dL benefited from further lowering of LDL with simvastatin. In the Pravastatin or Atorvastatin Evaluation and Infection Therapy (PROVE IT) trial, [4] patients with acute coronary syndrome derived greater benefit with an LDL of 62 mg/dL achieved with atorvastatin than with an LDL of 95 mg/dL

Rx

achieved with pravastatin. In the Treating to New Targets (TNT) study, [5] patients with stable coronary heart disease had fewer clinical events with an LDL of 77 mg/dL achieved with 80 mg of atorvastatin than with 101 mg/dL achieved with 10 mg of the same drug. In the Incremental Decrease in End Points Through Aggressive Lipid-Lowering (IDEAL) study, [6] there were fewer secondary end points among patients with stable coronary heart disease with an LDL of 81 mg/dL achieved with 80 mg of atorvastatin as compared with 104 mg/dL achieved with 20 mg of simvastatin.

Lifestyle Changes

Therapeutic lifestyle changes should be recommended as part of the treatment regimen. These include smoking cessation, weight reduction, exercise on most days of the week, reduced intake of dietary cholesterol to less than 200 mg/day, reduction of saturated fat to less than 7% of total calories, increased soluble fiber intake (to at least 10 g/day) and consumption of plant stanols or sterols (2 g/day).

Medical Therapy

Medications commonly used to treat lipid disorders are listed in Table 217–5.

Statins

Statins are by far the most effective. An analysis of results from 90,000 participants in statin trials suggested that the 5-year incidence of cardiovascular events decreases by about 1% for each 2 mg/dL decrease in LDL. The benefit appears to be independent of a patient's baseline lipid values. Patients at sufficient risk should be treated so that LDL is lowered by 30 to 40% regardless of initial levels.

Statins are well tolerated. Up to 5% of patients have mildly elevated serum transaminases with therapy, which is usually asymptomatic and resolves spontaneously. Therapy should be discontinued if elevations exceed three times the upper limit of normal or if patients have symptoms of liver dysfunction (especially fatigue and weight loss). Rhabdomyolysis is rare and more likely in the setting of concurrent treatment with azole antifungals, erythromycin, cyclosporine, and several other agents. Common side effects include constipation, abdominal pain, and difficulty sleeping. A substantial

TABLE 217–5 MEDICATIONS USED TO TREAT LIPID DISORDERS

Class	Side Effects	Lipid Effects	Specific Agents
Statins (HMG-CoA reductase inhibitors)	Mildly increased liver enzymes, myalgias without evidence of muscle disease, constipation, insomnia, rhabdomyolysis (rare)	↓↓LDL, 18–55% ↑ HDL, 5–15% ↓ TG, 7–30%	Simvastatin (20–80 mg/d) Atorvastatin (10–80 mg/d) Pravastatin (20–80 mg/d) Fluvastatin (20–80 mg/d) Lovastatin (20–80 mg/d) Rosuvastatin (10–40 mg/d)
Nicotinic acid	Flushing, nausea, diarrhea, hyperglycemia, hyperuricemia, hepatotoxicity (rare)	↑↑HDL, 15–35% ↓↓TG, 20–50% ↓ LDL, 5–25% ↓ Lp(a), variable	Extended release or crystalline niacin (1–2.5 mg/d)
Fibrates	Mildly increased liver enzymes, dyspepsia, gallstones, hepatotoxicity (rare), rhabdomyolysis (rare)	↓↓TG, 20–90% ↑ HDL, 10–20%	Gemfibrozil (1.2 mg/d) Fenofibrate (48–145 mg/d)
Cholesterol absorption inhibitor	Hepatitis, abdominal pain, back pain, arthralgias	↓ LDL, 18%	Ezetimibe (10 mg/d)
Bile acid sequestrants	Constipation, decreased absorption of some drugs	↓ LDL, 15–30% ↑ TG, variable ↑ HDL, 3–5%	Colesevelam (2.6–3.9 mg/d) Cholestyramine (4–16 mg/d) Colestipol (5–20 mg/d)
Fish oils	Eructation, dyspepsia	↓ TG, variable ↑ LDL, variable	ω-3-acid ethyl esters (variable)

HDL = high-density lipoprotein; HMG-CoA = 3-hydroxy-3-methylglutaryl coenzyme A; LDL = low-density lipoprotein; Lp(a) = lipoprotein (a); TG = triglyceride.

Rx

minority of patients treated with statins develop myalgias without physical findings or laboratory evidence of muscle dysfunction. The etiology of this side effect is unknown. Patients with this complaint should be evaluated for hypothyroidism, vitamin D deficiency, rheumatologic disorders, and depression. The problem may be resolved by changing to a different statin or by stopping the medication, allowing symptoms to revolve, and restarting at a much lower dose with gradual increases over weeks.

Given the success of statins, it is not surprising that they are also formulated with other agents. Pravastatin with aspirin, atorvastatin with amlodipine, lovastatin with extended release niacin, and simvastatin with ezetimibe are available as single pills. If both agents are indicated, these combinations can enhance compliance and decrease co-payment costs to patients.

Nicotinic Acid

Nicotinic acid is a B complex vitamin required to prevent pellagra. When administered in high doses, it has potent triglyceride lowering and HDL elevating effects and a modest LDL lowering effect. A once-daily extended release form appears to be safe and effective. The most common side effect is flushing, which frequently diminishes over time. Its intensity can be diminished with aspirin, taking the medication with a small snack, and avoiding hot beverages at that time. Nicotinic acid has been used safely with simvastatin in patients with vascular disease to induce atherosclerotic regression.

Fibrates

Fibrates are effective for lowering triglycerides in patients with very high triglycerides who are at risk for pancreatitis, especially in those who cannot tolerate niacin. These drugs increase HDL (although not as effectively as niacin) but also tend to increase LDL in patients with high triglycerides. The effects of fibrates in clinical trials have been mixed. [7] Many clinicians use fibrates with statins in high-risk patients with mixed hyperlipidemia, which should be done cautiously because of the increased risk of rhabdomyolysis with this combination. The Action to Control Cardiovascular Risk in Diabetes (ACCORD) study is currently testing the efficacy of the statin-fibrate combination in people with diabetes.

Other Agents

Ezetimibe lowers both LDL and triglycerides with minimal effects on HDL. It is effective at providing additional LDL lowering when used in combination with a statin. Coadministration with fibrates was not recommended when this drug was approved.

Bile acid sequestrants have been shown to lower LDL and decrease cardiovascular event rates. They are especially effective when combined with statins. Acceptance by patients is limited because of gastrointestinal side effects. These agents also tend to elevate triglycerides and decrease the absorption of some drugs, an effect that is less of an issue with colesevelam.

Fish oils may be used as an adjunct in the therapy of patients with very high triglycerides. These ω-3 fatty acids, which occur naturally in cold water fish, may work by activating PPARα. They tend to elevate LDL but may also have beneficial anti-inflammatory properties.

Primary Prevention

The results of clinical trials (see Treatment) strongly support lipid lowering for secondary prevention, that is, preventing events in those with known disease. Data are less compelling for primary prevention, that is, preventing events in those without known disease. There is evidence that the use of a statin to lower lipids is effective for primary prevention in at least two groups, patients with multiple risk factors and individuals with type 2 diabetes. In the Anglo-Scandinavian Cardiac Outcomes Trial–Lipid-Lowering Arm (ASCOT-LLA), [8] subjects with hypertension and at least three other risk factors had fewer events with an LDL of 90 mg/dL achieved with atorvastatin than with an LDL of about 130 mg/dL in control subjects. In the Collaborative Atorvastatin Diabetes Study (CARDS), [9] people with type 2 diabetes had fewer events with an LDL of about 75 mg/dL achieved with atorvastatin compared with placebo-treated subjects with an LDL of about 119 mg/dL.

In short, there does not appear to be a threshold effect of LDL on atherogenesis. In people with established coronary heart disease and those with diabetes, reaching very low LDL cholesterol levels is desirable. The absolute value at which maximum benefit is reached is unknown, and higher doses of statins are associated with more side effects (especially increased serum transaminases), but some analyses assume that an LDL of 40 mg/dL represents no increased risk of vascular disease.

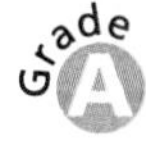

1. Tall AR, Yuan-Charvet L, Wang N: The failure of torcetrapib: Was it the molecule or the mechanism? Arterioscler Thromb Vasc Biol 2007;27:257–260.
2. Dormandy JA, Charbonnel B, Eckland DJ, et al: Secondary prevention of macrovascular events in patients with type 2 diabetes in the PROactive Study (PROspective pioglitAzone Clinical Trial In macroVascular Events): A randomised controlled trial. Lancet 2005;366:1279–1289.
3. Heart Protection Study Collaborative Group: MRC/BHF Heart Protection Study of cholesterol lowering with simvastatin in 20,536 high-risk individuals: A randomised placebo-controlled trial. Lancet 2002;360:7–22.
4. Cannon CP, Braunwald E, McCabe CH, et al: Intensive versus moderate lipid lowering with statins after acute coronary syndromes. N Engl J Med 2004;350:1495–1504.
5. LaRosa JC, Grundy SM, Waters DD, et al: Intensive lipid lowering with atorvastatin in patients with stable coronary disease. N Engl J Med 2005;352:1425–1435.
6. Pedersen TR, Faergeman O, Kastelein JJ, et al: High-dose atorvastatin vs usual-dose simvastatin for secondary prevention after myocardial infarction: The IDEAL study: A randomized controlled trial. JAMA 2005;294:2437–2445.
7. Keech A, Simes RJ, Barter P, et al: Effects of long-term fenofibrate therapy on cardiovascular events in 9795 people with type 2 diabetes mellitus (the FIELD study): Randomised controlled trial. Lancet 2005;366:1849–1861.
8. Sever PS, Dahlof B, Poulter NR, et al: Prevention of coronary and stroke events with atorvastatin in hypertensive patients who have average or lower-than-average cholesterol concentrations, in the Anglo-Scandinavian Cardiac Outcomes Trial–Lipid Lowering Arm (ASCOT-LLA): A multicentre randomised controlled trial. Lancet 2003;361:1149–1158.
9. Colhoun HM, Betteridge DJ, Durrington PN, et al: Primary prevention of cardiovascular disease with atorvastatin in type 2 diabetes in the Collaborative Atorvastatin Diabetes Study (CARDS): Multicentre randomised placebo-controlled trial. Lancet 2004; 364:685–696.

SUGGESTED READINGS

Cholesterol Treatment Trialists' (CTT) Collaborators: Efficacy and safety of cholesterol-lowering treatment: Prospective meta-analysis of data from 90056 participants in 14 randomised trials of statins. Lancet 2005;366:1267–1278. *An extensive analysis of statin use in clinical trials.*

Engelking LJ, Liang G, Hammer RE, et al: Schoenheimer effect explained—Feedback regulation of cholesterol synthesis in mice mediated by Insig proteins. J Clin Invest 2005;115:2489–2498. *The feedback inhibition by dietary cholesterol of hepatic cholesterol synthesis defined in molecular terms by the laboratory that has profoundly affected our understanding of lipid metabolism for 30 years.*

Grundy SM, Cleeman JI, Merz CN, et al: Implications of recent clinical trials for the National Cholesterol Education Program Adult Treatment Panel III guidelines. Circulation 2004;110:227–239. *Updated recommendations for lipid lowering therapy based on recent clinical trials.*

National Heart, Lung, and Blood Institute: National Cholesterol Education Program. Avilable at www.nhlbi.nih.gov/about/ncep/index.htm. *Website with information for health professionals and patients.*

Nicholls SJ, Tuzsu Em, Sipahi I, et al: Statins, high-density lipoprotein cholesterol, and regression of coronary atherosclerosis. JAMA 2007;297:499–508. *Reductions in LDL and increases in HDL are associated with regression of atherosclerosis.*

Shulman AI, Mangelsdorf DJ: Mechanisms of disease—Retinoid X receptor heterodimers in the metabolic syndrome. N Engl J Med 2005;604–615. *A review of nuclear receptors and how their modulation could be useful for the treatment of lipid disorders.*

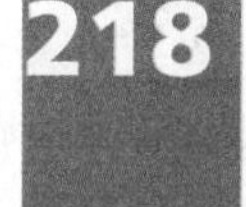

218 GALACTOSEMIA

Louis J. Elsas II

Definition

Classic galactosemia is an autosomal recessive trait characterized by neonatal jaundice, bleeding diathesis, feeding intolerance, lethargy, *Escherichia coli* sepsis, hypotension, and death if untreated. This clinical syndrome is caused by absent function of galactose 1-phosphate uridyltransferase (GALT) (E.C. 2.7.7.12), which results in the accumulation of galactose and galactose 1-phosphate in blood and excretion of excess galactose and galactitol in urine if lactose ingestion continues (Fig. 218–1). Impairment of two other enzymes can cause less severe elevation of blood galactose in this evolutionarily conserved galactose metabolic pathway. Deficiency of uridine diphosphate (UDP)galactose 4-epimerase (GALE) increases erythrocyte galactose 1-phosphate and galactose in the presence of normally functioning GALT. Benign and "generalized" neurologic dysfunctions are described in GALE deficiency. Galactosemia and excess urinary galactitol accumulate in galactokinase (GALK) deficiency. In the absence of galactose 1-phosphate accumulation, patients with GALK deficiency have neonatal and childhood cataracts without hepatocellular dysfunction. For all of these enzyme-deficient, inherited metabolic disorders, lactose (galactose)-restricted diets should be implemented during the first days of life.

Epidemiology

The incidence of GALT deficiency has been defined from many population-based newborn screening programs. Severe mutations in either homozygous or compound heterozygous genotypes have an incidence of about 1 in 35,000 newborns. However, less severe mutations that reduce erythrocyte GALT activity to below 15% of normal and increase erythrocyte galactose 1-phosphate have an incidence of about 1 in 8000 newborns. GALK deficiency has an unknown incidence in the general population, probably less than 1 in 100,000. Within inbred isolates such as the Roma Gypsy, however, the prevalence is 1 in 1600, with the carrier rate being as high as 5% in that population. GALE deficiency has an estimated prevalence of 1 in 23,000 in Japan, but the prevalence is unknown and less frequent in Europe and the United States.

Pathobiology

The galactose metabolic pathway outlined in Figure 218–1 is evolutionarily conserved. In *E. coli* and *Saccharomyces cerevisiae,* the genes for these enzymes are regulated through *operons* and *regulons.* Although humans have maintained structural homology for the proteins, their genes are located on separate chromosomes (Table 218–1). The products of this pathway produce energy and CO_2 from glucose 1-phosphate and maintain the pools of UDPglucose and UDPgalactose that are essential substrates for glycogen synthesis, post-translational production of glycoproteins, and the formation of glycolipids. In brief, this pathway is essential for cellular growth and differentiation. As can be seen in Figure 218–1, several pathways are available to maintain homeostasis of UDPglucose and UDPgalactose concentrations even when GALT is impaired. Recent expression microarray experiments with GALT-deficient yeast and their revertants and cultured human fibroblasts have defined the toxic effects of galactose 1-phosphate when accumulated in millimolar concentrations. Galactose 1-phosphate inhibits glucose-1-phosphate pyrophosphorylase, thus decreasing the amount of UDPglucose and, consequently, UDPgalactose that is available for important neonatal functions such as bilirubin conjugation, brain myelin formation, and the post-translational processing of many secreted proteins, such as follicle-stimulating hormone, and membrane receptors. Other metabolic disturbances are also caused by accumulated galactose 1-phosphate, including initiation of the endoplasmic reticulum (ER) stress reaction through calcium release from the ER. This pleiotropic effect of accumulated intracellular galactose 1-phosphate is severe in GALT deficiency and may occur to a lesser degree in GALE deficiency. Its effects are recognized pathologically in the newborn as rising direct bilirubin (and kernicterus), hepatocellular failure, growth failure, and if untreated, severe neurologic deficits such as mental retardation, tremor, spasticity, and seizures. Approximately 10% of newborns with GALT deficiency have *E. coli* sepsis and die. Public health newborn screening programs have reduced but not eliminated this natural pathologic history because of week-long intervals required for postnatal screening results. Screening newborns with ^{13}C-galactose for their ability to produce $^{13}CO_2$ in expired air is under investigation as a point-of-care solution before nursery discharge. Lethal sepsis may result from reduced glycoprotein cell wall barriers to intestinal bacteria and from decreased cellular resistance secondary to reduced galactosyl and neuraminic acid residues on surface proteins.

Deficiency of GALE has a bias of ascertainment with regard to clinical outcome because most reported families have been identified as a result of evaluation of pervasive mental delays. At a molecular level, some mutations such as V94M are found in more than one family, have been evaluated in vitro, and are presumed to cause disease in humans. Further molecular studies of heterozygous mutations in GALK, GALT, and GALE may reveal

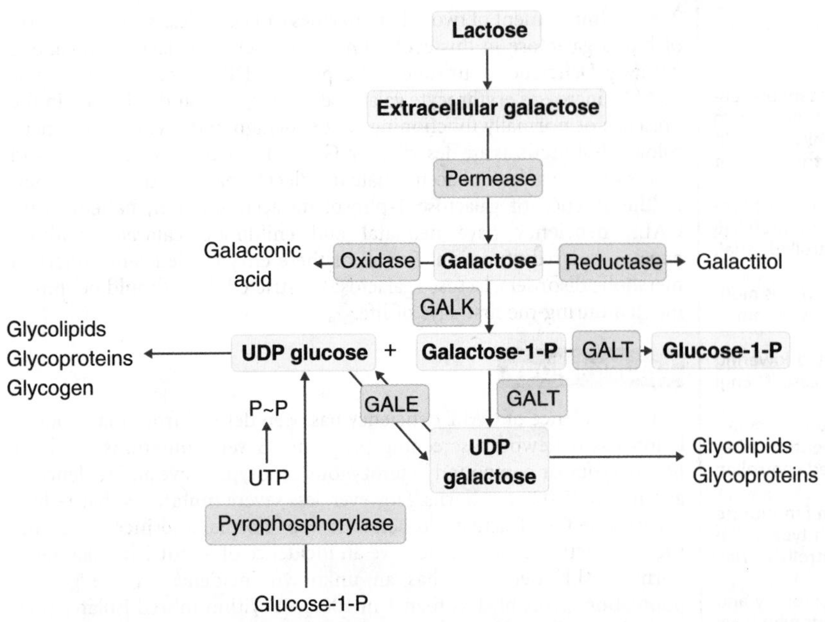

FIGURE 218–1 • Metabolic pathway for conversion of galactose to glucose 1-phosphate (glucose-1-P), uridine diphosphate (UDP)glucose, and UDPgalactose. Trivial names for enzymes are boxed in blue, and substrates and products of galactose metabolism are depicted in yellow. Three enzymes produce galactosemia when impaired in humans: galactose 1-phosphate uridyltransferase (GALT), UDPgalactose 4-epimerase (GALE), and galactokinase (GALK). Normally, end products of galactose metabolism include CO_2 production from glucose-1-P and the synthesis of glycogen, glycolipid, and glycoproteins. Alternative pathways for accumulated galactose are indicated and include the increased production of galactitol and galactonic acid. Galactonic acid is meta-bolized through the pentose pathway, whereas galactitol accumulates in cells as an end product. UTP = uridine triphosphate.

TABLE 218–1 DISORDERS OF GALACTOSE METABOLISM AND ASSOCIATED MUTATIONS

Deficient Enzyme	Chromosomal Location	Some Common Mutations	Geographic or Ethnic Origin	Clinical Symptoms* (Untreated)
GALT (galactose 1-phosphate uridyltransferase)	9p13	Q188R	Northern Europe	Severe
		S135L	Africa	Moderate
		K285N	Southern Germany Croatia	Severe
		L195P	Europe	Severe
		Y209C	Asia	Severe
		F161S	Europe	Severe
		N314D	Panethnic	Benign
		5Kbdel	Ashkenazim	Severe
		IVS2 nt2a → g (167 more)	Hispanic	Moderate
GALK (galactokinase)	17q24	P28T	Roma Gypsies	Cataracts
		R68C	Europe	Cataracts
		T288M	Europe	Cataracts
		R256W	Japan	Cataracts
		A384P	Europe	Cataracts
		T344M	Japan	Cataracts
		G349S	Japan	Cataracts
		410delg	Japan	Cataracts
		509-510delgt (12 more)	Japan	Cataracts
GALE (UDPgalactose 4-epimerase)	1p36	L183P	Pakistani Europe	Late childhood mental retardation
		N34S	Pakistani Europe	Late childhood mental retardation
		G90E	Asia	Mental retardation
		D103G	Asia	Mental retardation
		K257R	Africa	Benign
		V94M	British	Pervasive delays Hepatomegaly
		L313M	Asia	Benign
		D103G	British	Benign

*See text for description in more detail.
UDP = uridine diphosphate.

"sensitivity" genes for more common adult disorders such as ovarian failure, presenile dementia, liver failure, and early cataract formation. Some mutations in GALT and GALE have a "dominant negative" effect on the normal allele, and multiple heterozygous hits on this important glycobiologic pathway could have additive effects and produce organ pathology.

Clinical Manifestations

If an infant with GALT deficiency is detected within a few days of life and galactose removed from the diet, there is rapid remission of hepatocellular damage and normalization of health. However, an enigmatic set of chronic problems occurs later in life, including verbal dyspraxia (56%), reduced IQ (46%), cataracts (10%), ovarian failure (up to 85% in females), ataxia and tremors (18%), and growth delay (before puberty). The pathobiology of these conditions is not known. Some could be embryologic in origin and related to the "toxic" effects of accumulating galactose 1-phosphate on glycoproteins in rapidly dividing embryologic cells. Intracellular accumulation of galactitol is known to cause cataracts and seizures by its osmotic effects on lens epithelium and neurons, respectively.

Cataracts without hepatic, ovarian, or central nervous system pathologic conditions are found in GALK deficiency. When compared with GALT deficiency, galactitol but not galactose 1-phosphate is accumulated through the alternative aldose reductase pathway (see Fig. 218–1). The accumulation of galactitol in lens fibers produces an osmotic gradient, swelling of cells, loss of permeability, cell death, and scarring. This process also occurs in GALT deficiency and is progressive if galactose intake continues.

Diagnosis

Because GALT deficiency can be lethal yet is preventable in the neonatal period, population-based newborn screening is used to identify and urgently treat affected newborns.

Diagnostic Tests

The GALT enzyme is measured in erythrocytes from dried blood on filter paper via enzyme-linked fluorometric methods. In classic galactosemia, there is no GALT activity, but variant galactosemia is also detected with approximately 5 to 25% activity. In hot, humid months, the prevalence of these variant forms is greater because of the instability of mutant GALT dimeric proteins. State-based laboratories also use accumulation of galactose and galactose 1-phosphate as part of the screening process.

A positive screening test should *immediately* be followed by retrieval of the newborn, removal of lactose from the diet, and a more quantitative measurement of GALT activity and its isoforms by isoelectric focusing. Additional studies include quantitation of erythrocyte galactose 1-phosphate, urinary galactitol, and molecular genotyping of GALT. All of these tests are available through commercial laboratories on an emergency status. An additional study, the "breath test," quantitates total body oxidation of ^{13}C-galactose to $^{13}CO_2$ in the infant's breath. GALT enzyme activity below 5% of control, erythrocyte galactose 1-phosphate above 1.5 mg/dL, urinary galactitol above 78 mmol/mol creatinine, and $^{13}CO_2$ in breath below 5% of administered ^{13}C-D-galactose indicate clinically significantly impaired GALT. This full set of diagnostic tests is recommended because they confirm the diagnosis and provide a basis for prognosis. For example, the S135L mutation, common in African Americans with GALT-deficient galactosemia, has no erythrocyte GALT activity, but total body oxidation of ^{13}C-galactose to $^{13}CO_2$ is normal and the prognosis is good if the deficiency is detected and treated in the newborn period. By contrast, the Q188R mutation is common in people of northern European descent and has absent erythrocyte GALT activity, but these patients have less than 5% of ^{13}C-galactose recovered as $^{13}CO_2$ during their breath test. If the Q188R mutation is either homozygous or associated with another "severe" mutant allele listed in Table 218–1, the subsequent development of dyspraxic speech and ovarian failure is increased 10-fold.

Deficiency of GALK will *not* be detected by most public health newborn screening programs and should be suspected in any patient with congenital or early-onset ocular cataracts. The diagnosis is suspected on finding increased urinary galactitol and confirmed by finding reduced GALK in peripheral erythrocytes. Molecular analysis of the GALK gene is available on a research basis. Molecular analysis of GALK is important when considering heterozygosity for GALK deficiency as a diagnosis in patients with later-onset cataracts and a positive family history. Enzyme analysis alone for GALK may not differentiate heterozygosity from homozygous normal, and further molecular analysis is recommended.

Differential Diagnosis

Population newborn screening may not be universal or timely, and thus the diagnosis should be entertained in any infant with jaundice, progressive hepatocellular dysfunction, cataracts, or *E. coli* sepsis. Quantitation of erythrocyte galactose 1-phosphate and urinary galactitol, GALT enzyme assay in erythrocytes, GALT molecular genotype, and galactose oxidation studies are available (*http://www.genetests.org*). The differential diagnosis includes other causes of hepatocellular dysfunction, such as hepatitis, biliary obstruction, and other rare inborn errors such as Niemann-Pick disease, hereditary fructose intolerance, and tyrosinemia type I.

The diagnosis of GALE deficiency is entertained when newborn screening results indicate elevated red blood cell galactose 1-phosphate and galactose but normal erythrocyte GALT activity. Most newborns remain asymptomatic, but cataracts or mental retardation may develop later in life. The diagnosis is made by finding reduced GALE activity in erythrocytes, cultured fibroblasts, or transformed lymphoblasts. Molecular analysis of the GALE gene is available on a research basis.

Treatment

Rx

Treatment of galactosemia is exclusion of galactose from the diet, which involves the elimination of milk and its products. The mainstay of the diet for such an infant is substitution of a soy preparation for all milk products. Because endogenous galactose production continues, strict avoidance of all casein-derived proteins, as well as lactose itself, is necessary in the newborn. Some fruits and vegetables, such as watermelon and tomatoes, contain bioavailable galactosides and are avoided. Education of parents and older children about the galactose content of foods is important. Lists of the galactose content of foods are available and are useful in management. Calcium supplements are necessary, and approximately 500 to 1000 mg of ionized calcium per day should be prescribed as well as 600–1000 IU of cholecalciferol. Lactose must not be used as a filler or as a medication by the pharmacy. For example, lactulose is used in managing the hyperammonemia of liver disease but contains gram quantities of free lactose and thus must be avoided in newborns with liver disease secondary to GALT deficiency. Speech evaluation is indicated at 2 to 3 years of age, and speech therapy can prevent later "learning disabilities" if early intervention is provided. In females, estrogen creams and replacement therapy may be indicated when ovarian failure is present. Ophthalmologic evaluation for cataracts may be required periodically.

Determination of the galactose 1-phosphate content of erythrocytes and urinary galactitol is useful in monitoring adherence to the diet. Erythrocyte galactose 1-phosphate should be kept below 3.5 mg/dL (140 mmol/L). Concentrations above this level increase the odds ratio for the development of dyspraxia and ovarian failure.

Primary Prevention

Primary prevention of galactosemia involves heterozygote detection and prenatal counseling of at-risk family members and parents of galactosemic children. Prenatal monitoring is available in the early second trimester by combined GALT enzyme analysis of cultured amniotic fluid cells or chorionic villous cells. Mutational analysis of DNA from these cells is the most sensitive and specific prenatal diagnostic method. To use mutational analysis, the genotype of the proband must be known. Late trimester analysis of galactitol in amniotic fluid is useful. As measured by gas chromatography/mass spectroscopy or high-pressure liquid chromatography, amniotic fluid from affected fetuses has a range of 5.9 to 10.6 μM galactitol, with normal being 0.23 to 1.6 μM. There is no evidence that restricting maternal lactose intake will influence the intracellular overproduction of either galactose 1-phosphate or galactitol by affected fetal cells.

Prognosis

If a galactose-restricted diet is provided during the first 7 days and continued throughout life, the initial hepatotoxic symptoms resolve quickly and the prognosis is good. If the diagnosis of GALT-deficient galactosemia is not established within days of life, an infant treated only with intravenous antibiotics and partially restricted lactose intake demonstrates relapsing and episodic jaundice and bleeding from altered hemostasis. If treatment is delayed, complications such as mental and growth retardation are likely. Despite early and adequate therapy, the long-term outcome in older children and adults with "severe" galactosemia can include speech defects, poor growth, poor intellectual function, neurologic deficits (predominantly extrapyramidal findings with ataxia), and ovarian failure. Outcome and "disease burden" can be predicted on the basis of the level of GALT activity, GALT genotype, age at which successful therapeutic control was achieved, and compliance with galactose restrictions. The most accurate prognostic test for treated infants is the galactose oxidation breath test. If total body oxidation of ^{13}C-D-galactose to $^{13}CO_2$ during the breath test is greater than 5% at 2 hours, the outcome is good.

SUGGESTED READINGS

Elsas LJ: Prenatal diagnosis of galactose-1-phosphate uridyltransferase (GALT)-deficient galactosemia. Prenat Diagn 2001;21:302–303. *Comprehensive review of ethics, methodology, and outcome of prenatal diagnosis for GALT deficiency.*

Gene Tests/Gene Clinics. www.genetests.org or http:www.geneclinics.org. Updated March 1, 2005. *A review of all syndromes producing galactosemia and their mutations.*

OMIM—Online Mendelian Inheritance in Man. www3.ncbi.nlm.nih.gov/Omim. Accessed May 8, 2003. *Updated history and molecular and clinical manifestations of these autosomal recessive disorders of galactose metabolism.*

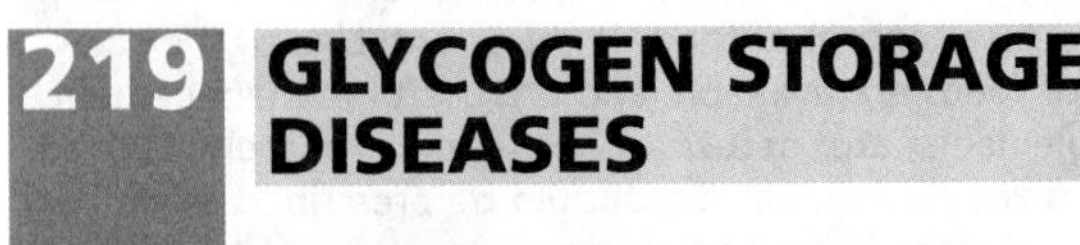

219 GLYCOGEN STORAGE DISEASES

Joseph I. Wolfsdorf

Definition

Glycogen, a highly branched polymer of glucose, is the storage form of glucose in mammals. The major sites of glycogen deposition are skeletal muscle and liver, but many cell types are capable of glycogen synthesis, including cardiac and smooth muscle, the kidney, the brain, and even adipose tissue. Glycogen accounts for approximately 4 to 6% and 1 to 2% of the wet weight of the liver and skeletal muscle, respectively. In the average well-fed man consuming a diet rich in carbohydrate, about 80 g of glycogen is stored in the liver and 400 g in skeletal muscle.

Physiology

Glucose transporter type 2 (GLUT2) predominates in the liver (and pancreatic beta cells) and has a high K_m ($\approx$15 to 20 mmol/L); consequently, the free glucose concentration in hepatocytes increases in direct proportion to the increase in plasma glucose concentration. Glucose is rapidly phosphorylated by glucokinase to form glucose 6-phosphate, which is converted to glucose 1-phosphate, the starting point for glycogen synthesis (Fig. 219–1). Hepatic glycogen synthase catalyzes the formation of α-1,4-linkages, which elongate the chains of glucose molecules. A branching enzyme leads to the formation of α-1,6-linkages at branch points along the chain. The concentration of GLUT4 in the plasma membrane of skeletal muscle markedly increases after exposure to insulin and in response to exercise; as a result, glucose transport into the muscle cell is increased, where it is either oxidized to provide energy for contracting muscle or converted to glycogen.

In the intervals between meals and during the overnight fast, a cascade of enzymatic reactions (including adenylyl cyclase, phosphorylase *b* kinase, and cyclic adenosine monophosphate–dependent protein kinase) activate hepatic glycogen phosphorylase, the rate-limiting enzyme in glycogenolysis, which removes glucose from the outer branches of glycogen and ultimately leads to the formation of glucose 6-phosphate. Glucose-6-phosphatase catalyzes the terminal reaction of both glycogenolysis and gluconeogenesis—hydrolysis of glucose 6-phosphate—thereby allowing glucose to be released from the liver into the systemic circulation. This process is critically important for the maintenance of glucose homeostasis. Because muscle lacks glucose-6-phosphatase, it cannot release glucose for systemic use. Muscle glycogen is used to meet the energy requirement of contracting muscle and is a source of lactate, pyruvate, and alanine for gluconeogenesis early in starvation. The rate of glycogenolysis in muscle is most rapid during the first 5 to 10 minutes of exercise. As exercise continues and blood flow to muscle increases, blood-borne substrates (glucose and free fatty acids) become increasingly important sources of energy.

Epidemiology

The overall frequency of glycogen storage diseases (GSDs) is approximately 1 case per 20,000 to 25,000 births. The GSDs are referred to either by the deficient enzyme or by a number that reflects the historical sequence of their description. Twelve distinct types of GSD have been identified. They are all uncommon and some are extremely rare. Seven types of GSD account for about 97% of cases and will be briefly discussed

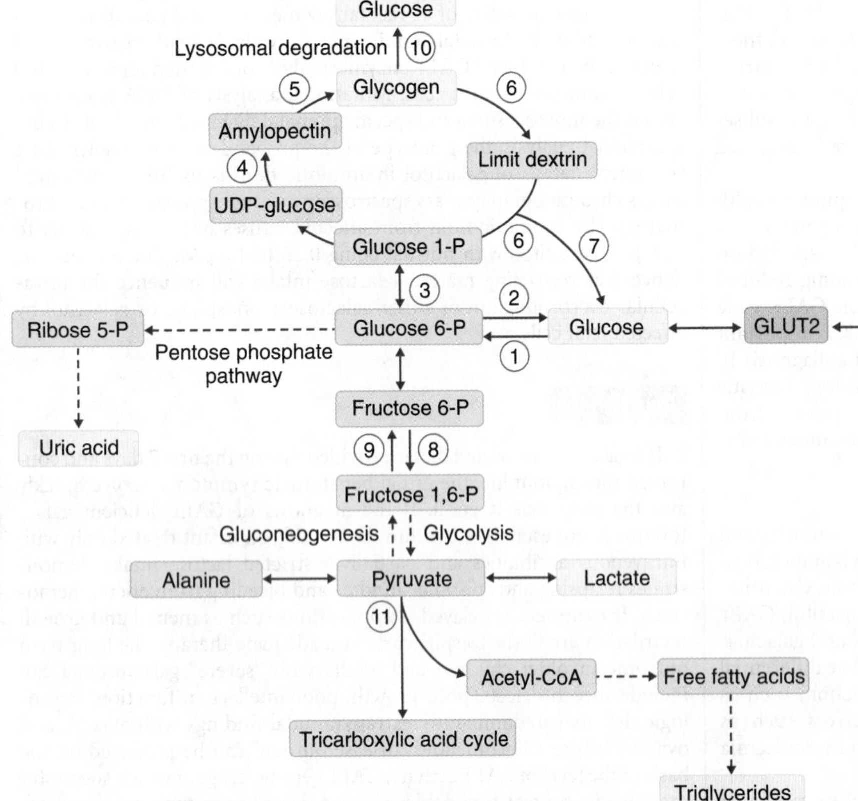

FIGURE 219–1 • Simplified scheme of glycogen synthesis and degradation in the liver. Note that in skeletal muscle, GLUT4 transports glucose across the cell membrane and glucose 6-phosphatase is absent. UDP-glucose = uridine diphosphoglucose. 1, hexokinase/glucokinase; 2, glucose-6-phosphatase; 3, phosphoglucomutase; 4, glycogen synthase; 5, branching enzyme; 6, glycogen phosphorylase; 7, debranching enzyme; 8, phosphofructokinase; 9, fructose-1,6-bisphosphatase; 10, acid maltase; 11, pyruvate dehydrogenase.

in this chapter: GSD 0 (≤1%), GSD I (25%), GSD II (15%), GSD III (24%), GSD IV (3%), and GSD VI and IX (30%).

Pathobiology

GSDs, or glycogenoses, comprise several inherited diseases (all autosomal recessive with the exception of type IX [see later], which is X-linked). GSDs are caused by mutations in the genes that code for enzymes involved in the synthesis or degradation of glycogen in liver or muscle, or both. They are characterized by an abnormal tissue concentration or abnormal structure (or both) of the glycogen molecule. The GSDs may involve skeletal and cardiac muscle and liver.

Clinical Manifestations

Hepatomegaly and hypoglycemia are the principal clinical manifestation of the hepatic glycogenoses, whereas muscle cramps, exercise intolerance, easy fatigability, and progressive weakness are the major manifestations of the muscle glycogenoses. Features of the most common GSDs are listed in Table 219–1.

TABLE 219–1 PRINCIPAL FEATURES OF THE COMMON GLYCOGEN STORAGE DISEASES

Type	Defective Enzyme	Characteristic Clinical Features	Diagnosis	Therapy
0	Hepatic glycogen synthase	Autosomal recessive; liver normal in size, fasting ketotic hypoglycemia, postprandial hyperglycemia and hyperlactatemia	Liver biopsy, enzyme assay, mutation analysis	UCS, especially at bedtime
Ia	Glucose-6-phosphatase	Autosomal recessive; hepatomegaly, failure to thrive, growth retardation, severe hypoglycemia, lactic acidosis, hyperuricemia, hyperlipidemia	Liver biopsy, enzyme assay, mutation analysis	UCS during the day and night or continuous overnight intragastric feeding
Ib	Glucose 6-phosphate transporter	Same as type Ia; also neutropenia, recurrent bacterial infections, and inflammatory bowel disease	Liver biopsy, enzyme assay, mutation analysis	As for type Ia; granulocyte colony-stimulating factor
II	Lysosomal acid maltase (α-glucosidase)	Autosomal recessive; infantile form (Pompe's disease) characterized by severe generalized hypotonia, muscle weakness, and hypertrophic cardiomyopathy leading to cardiorespiratory failure usually by 1 year of age. Skeletal myopathy with slowly progressing muscle weakness is the primary clinical manifestation of the juvenile- and adult-onset forms. Serum creatine kinase is markedly increased	Skin fibroblast or muscle enzyme assay	Supportive care; intravenous enzyme replacement with recombinant human α-glucosidase may be useful
III	Debranching enzyme	Autosomal recessive; hepatomegaly, moderate to severe ketotic hypoglycemia, muscle weakness and wasting, hypertrophic cardiomyopathy (IIIa), increased transaminases without muscle involvement (IIIb)	Skin fibroblast, muscle, or liver enzyme assay; mutation analysis	UCS
IV	Glycogen branching enzyme	Autosomal recessive; a clinically heterogeneous disorder. The typical manifestation is liver disease in early childhood progressing to lethal cirrhosis. The less common neuromuscular manifestation is distinguished by age at onset into 4 groups: perinatal, congenital, childhood, and adult	Liver biopsy shows excessive abnormal glycogen with fewer branching points and longer outer branches, resembling an amylopectin-like structure (polyglucosan); fibrosis and cirrhosis. Skin fibroblast, muscle, or liver biopsy shows absent branching enzyme activity	No specific treatment; liver transplantation has resulted in decreased glycogen storage in heart and skeletal muscle
V	Muscle glycogen phosphorylase	Autosomal recessive; symptoms usually begin in adolescence or early adulthood with exercise intolerance, fatigue, myalgia, muscle cramps, and muscle swelling. Transient	The forearm ischemic lactate test shows a flat venous lactate curve. Muscle enzyme assay shows no phosphorylase activity.	High-protein diet (50% carbohydrate and 25–30% protein); oral sucrose before sustained aerobic exercise appears to be beneficial 1

TABLE 219–1 PRINCIPAL FEATURES OF THE COMMON GLYCOGEN STORAGE DISEASES—cont'd

Type	Defective Enzyme	Characteristic Clinical Features	Diagnosis	Therapy
		myoglobinuria secondary to rhabdomyolysis may occur after exercise. Severe myoglobinuria may lead to acute renal failure. Later in adult life, persistent and progressive muscle weakness and atrophy with fatty replacement. Increased serum creatine kinase	Mutation analysis of DNA from peripheral blood leukocytes	
VI	Hepatic glycogen phosphorylase	Autosomal recessive; hepatomegaly, growth retardation, mild to moderate ketotic hypoglycemia, and increased serum transaminases, cholesterol, and triglycerides	Liver biopsy and enzyme assay	UCS
VII	Muscle phosphofructokinase	Autosomal recessive; manifested in childhood with fatigue, muscle cramps, exercise intolerance; rhabdomyolysis and myoglobinuria with strenuous exertion; increased serum creatine kinase; may have mild hemolytic anemia and mild hyperbilirubinemia; hyperuricemia	Ischemic forearm exercise test shows no increase in lactate; muscle biopsy and enzyme assay; increased subsarcolemmal glycogen with a normal appearance; phosphofructokinase activity is deficient in muscle and reduced in erythrocytes	No specific treatment; avoid strenuous exercise
IX (VIII)*	Phosphorylase *b* kinase	X-linked; hepatomegaly, mild ketotic hypoglycemia, growth retardation, increased serum transaminases, hypercholesterolemia, hypertriglyceridemia	Liver/muscle biopsy and enzyme assay	UCS

*Sometimes classified as type VIII.
UCS = uncooked cornstarch.

Treatment

Rx

The goal of treatment of the hepatic forms of GSD is prevention of hypoglycemia and counter-regulation of glucose. In infants and children with GSD 0, frequent high-protein meals and snacks are given every 3 to 4 hours during the day. Uncooked cornstarch (UCS), 1 to 1.5 g/kg at bedtime, prevents overnight hypoglycemia. Excess glucose cannot be stored as glycogen and is converted to lactic acid. The diet should be rich in protein to provide substrate for gluconeogenesis and contain decreased carbohydrate to minimize postprandial hyperglycemia and hyperlactatemia.

Treatment of GSD I consists of providing a continuous dietary source of glucose to maintain blood glucose levels at 80 to 90 mg/dL before meals and overnight and prevent them from falling below 70 mg/dL, which activates counter-regulation and causes hyperlactacidemia, hyperuricemia, and hypertriglyceridemia. In infants, continuous glucose can be provided by frequent feeding during the day and continuous intragastric feeding at night via a nasogastric or gastrostomy tube. From about 6 to 12 months of age, UCS, which is slowly digested and absorbed into the circulation as glucose, can be used as an alternative method of continuously providing glucose. UCS allows the interval between feeding to be increased eventually to 4 to 6 hours. Galactose and fructose must be restricted because they cannot be converted to glucose and large quantities may exacerbate the biochemical derangements. If optimal dietary management fails to lower serum uric acid and triglycerides to acceptable levels, treatment with allopurinol and gemfibrozil, respectively, is indicated. The neutropenia in type Ib responds well to granulocyte colony-stimulating factor therapy, which is also efficacious for the inflammatory bowel disease that is common in this disorder.

Rx

In GSD III, after infancy, UCS (1.75 g/kg at 6-hour intervals) can be used to maintain normoglycemia, improve growth, and ameliorate the biochemical abnormalities. Amino acids can be used as a substrate for gluconeogenesis, and there is some evidence that a high-protein diet may be beneficial.

GSD VI and GSD IX are both milder than GSD I and GSD III and generally have a good prognosis. Most patients do not require specific treatment. In the unusual patient with nocturnal hypoglycemia and ketosis, UCS (2 g/kg) at bedtime prevents their occurrence. Clinical and biochemical abnormalities gradually disappear with increasing age. Hepatomegaly decreases at puberty, and most adult patients are asymptomatic.

Treatment of the muscle glycogenoses is presented in Table 219–1.

Management of Complications

Long-term complications of GSD I, usually evident in adolescence or early adulthood, may include hepatic adenomas, focal segmental glomerulosclerosis, renal tubular dysfunction, nephrocalcinosis, nephrolithiasis, gout, anemia, and osteoporosis. Poor metabolic control contributes to the pathogenesis of these complications. Hepatic adenomas may gradually enlarge and undergo malignant transformation or hemorrhage into the peritoneal cavity. Ultrasonography is the preferred method to screen for hepatic adenomas. Serum α-fetoprotein is normal in patients with adenomas but may be increased in some cases of hepatocellular carcinoma. Complications of GSD III include short stature, cardiomyopathy, and hepatic adenomas in 25% of patients.

Grade A 1. Vissing J, Haller RG: The effect of oral sucrose on exercise tolerance in patients with McArdle's disease. N Engl J Med 2003; 349:2503–2509.

SUGGESTED READINGS

Association for Glycogen Storage Disease. Available at http://www.agsdus.org. Accessed November 7, 2005. *This website provides basic information about the glycogen storage diseases intended to be of use to people affected by one of the glycogen storage diseases, their families, and other interested parties.*

Chen Y-T: Glycogen storage diseases. *In* Scriver CR, Beaudet AL, Sly WS, et al (eds): The Metabolic and Molecular Bases of Inherited Disease, 8th ed. New York, McGraw-Hill, 2001, pp 1521–1555. *A comprehensive review of the glycogen storage diseases.*

Kishnani PS, Corzo D, Nicolino M, et al: Recombinant human acid α-glucosidase: Major clinical benefits in infantile-onset Pompe disease. Neurology 2007; 68:99–109. *Appears safe and effective in small trial with historical controls.*

Roach PJ: Glycogen and its metabolism. Curr Mol Med 2002;2:101–120. *A detailed review of the biochemistry and molecular biology related to the synthesis and degradation of glycogen in liver and muscle.*

Wolfsdorf JI, Weinstein DA: Glycogen storage diseases. Rev Endocr Metab Disord 2003;4:95–102. *A concise review of the clinical features, diagnosis, and management of the hepatic glycogenoses with special emphasis on nutritional therapy to prevent hypoglycemia.*

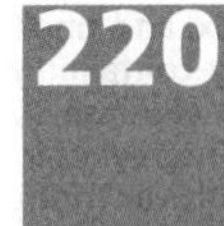

220 DISORDERS OF FRUCTOSE METABOLISM

Beat Steinmann

Fructose is one of the main sweetening agents in the human diet. It is found in free form in honey, fruits, and many vegetables and is associated with glucose in the disaccharide sucrose in numerous foods and beverages. Sorbitol, also widely distributed in fruits and vegetables, is converted to fructose in the liver by sorbitol dehydrogenase. Essential fructosuria, hereditary fructose intolerance (HFI), and fructose-1,6-bisphosphatase (FBPase) deficiency are three known inborn errors in the pathway of fructose metabolism (Fig. 220–1).

ESSENTIAL FRUCTOSURIA—FRUCTOKINASE DEFICIENCY (MIM 229800)

Essential fructosuria is a rare, autosomal recessive inherited disorder. It is detected by routine screening of urine for reducing sugars. Essential fructosuria is caused by a deficiency of fructokinase (see Fig. 220–1) encoded by the *KHK* gene on chromosome 2p23.3-23.2. In cases of deficiency, ingested fructose is partly (10 to 20%) excreted as such in urine, and the rest is slowly metabolized by an alternative pathway, namely, conversion into fructose 6-phosphate by hexokinase in adipose tissue and muscle.

Fructose gives a positive test for reducing sugars and a negative reaction with glucose oxidase. It can be identified and quantitated by various techniques. Fructosuria depends on the time and amount of fructose intake and, thus, is inconstant. Unlike HFI, ingestion of fructose provokes neither an increase in blood glucose, as in normal subjects, nor hypoglycemia or other changes as occur in HFI and FBPase deficiency.

Dietary treatment is not indicated, and the prognosis is excellent.

HEREDITARY FRUCTOSE INTOLERANCE (MIM 229600)

Pathobiology

Metabolic Derangement

HFI is caused by an inability of the isozyme aldolase B (fructose 1,6-bisphosphate aldolase; see Fig. 220–1) to split fructose 1-phosphate (F-1-P) into dihydroxyacetone phosphate and glyceraldehyde and convert the triosephosphates into glucose and lactate. Accumulation of F-1-P has two major effects: it inhibits the production of glucose by blocking gluconeogenesis and glycogenolysis, hence inducing hypoglycemia, and it provokes depletion of adenosine triphosphate.

Residual activity measurable with fructose 1,6-bisphosphate as substrate is mainly due to the isozyme aldolase A. Thus, glycolysis and gluconeogenesis are not impaired in the fasted state in patients with HFI.

Genetics

Aldolase B is the major fructaldolase of the liver, renal cortex, and small intestine and is encoded by the gene *ALDOB* on chromosome 9q22.3. At present, approximately 30 causative mutations are known; among them, three amino acid substitutions, A150P, A175D, and N335K, are relatively common in patients of central European and American descent and have been detected in 65%, 11%, and 8% of mutated alleles, respectively. Molecular genetic neonatal screening studies in England and Germany have calculated the prevalence of HFI to be 1 in 18,000 and 1 in 29,600, respectively.

Clinical Manifestations

Infants, children, and adults with HFI are perfectly healthy and asymptomatic as long as they do not ingest food containing fructose, sucrose, or sorbitol. Thus, during breast-feeding, no metabolic derangement occurs. The younger the child and the higher the dietary fructose load, the more severe the reaction. In the acute form of HFI, an infant who is not breast-fed but receives a cow's milk formula sweetened and enriched with fructose or sucrose is in danger of severe liver and kidney failure and death.

At weaning from breast-feeding or a fructose/sucrose-free infant formula, the first symptoms appear with the intake of fruits and vegetables. They generally consist of gastrointestinal discomfort, nausea, vomiting, restlessness, pallor, sweating, trembling, lethargy, and eventually, apathy, coma, jerks, and convulsions. At this stage, laboratory signs may be those of acute liver failure and generalized dysfunction of the renal proximal tubules. If the condition is not recognized and fructose is not excluded from the diet, the disease takes a chronic, uphill-downhill course with failure to thrive, liver disease manifested by hepatomegaly, jaundice, a bleeding tendency, edema, ascites, and signs of proximal renal tubular dysfunction. Laboratory findings consist of liver failure, proximal renal tubular dysfunction, and derangements of intermediary metabolism. Note that hypoglycemia after fructose ingestion is a short-lived sign and is thus easily missed or masked by concomitant glucose intake.

In young infants, HFI can be suspected if the parents, aware that their baby does not tolerate certain foods, have excluded these foods from the diet so that the infant develops normally. In older children, a distinct aversion toward foods containing fructose may develop. These feeding habits protect them but are sometimes considered neurotic behavior. At school age, HFI is occasionally recognized when hepatomegaly or growth delay is found. The diagnosis may remain undetected in affected subjects, and yet they may have a normal lifespan.

Diagnosis

Whenever HFI is suspected, fructose should be immediately eliminated from the diet. The beneficial clinical and chemical effects of withdrawal, usually seen within days, provide the first diagnostic clue. Laboratory findings in patients with HFI will show a reversal of elevations in serum transaminases and bilirubin, improved levels of blood clotting factors, and amelioration of proximal tubular dysfunction (proteinuria, mellituria, generalized hyperaminoaciduria, metabolic acidosis).

A cornerstone in the diagnosis of HFI is a carefully taken nutritional history, with special emphasis on the time of weaning when fruits and vegetables were introduced. If the nutritional history is suggestive or other aspects are indicative of HFI (e.g., a positive family history), the disorder should be confirmed by molecular diagnosis on DNA from peripheral leukocytes.

Diagnostic Tests

If no mutation can be found despite a strong clinical and nutritional history indicative of HFI, enzymatic determination or a functional test should be undertaken after a few weeks of fructose exclusion. In liver biopsy specimens from HFI patients, the capacity of aldolase to split F-1-P and F-1,6-P is markedly and moderately reduced, respectively. Enzymatic determination of aldolase B in small intestinal mucosa is discouraged.

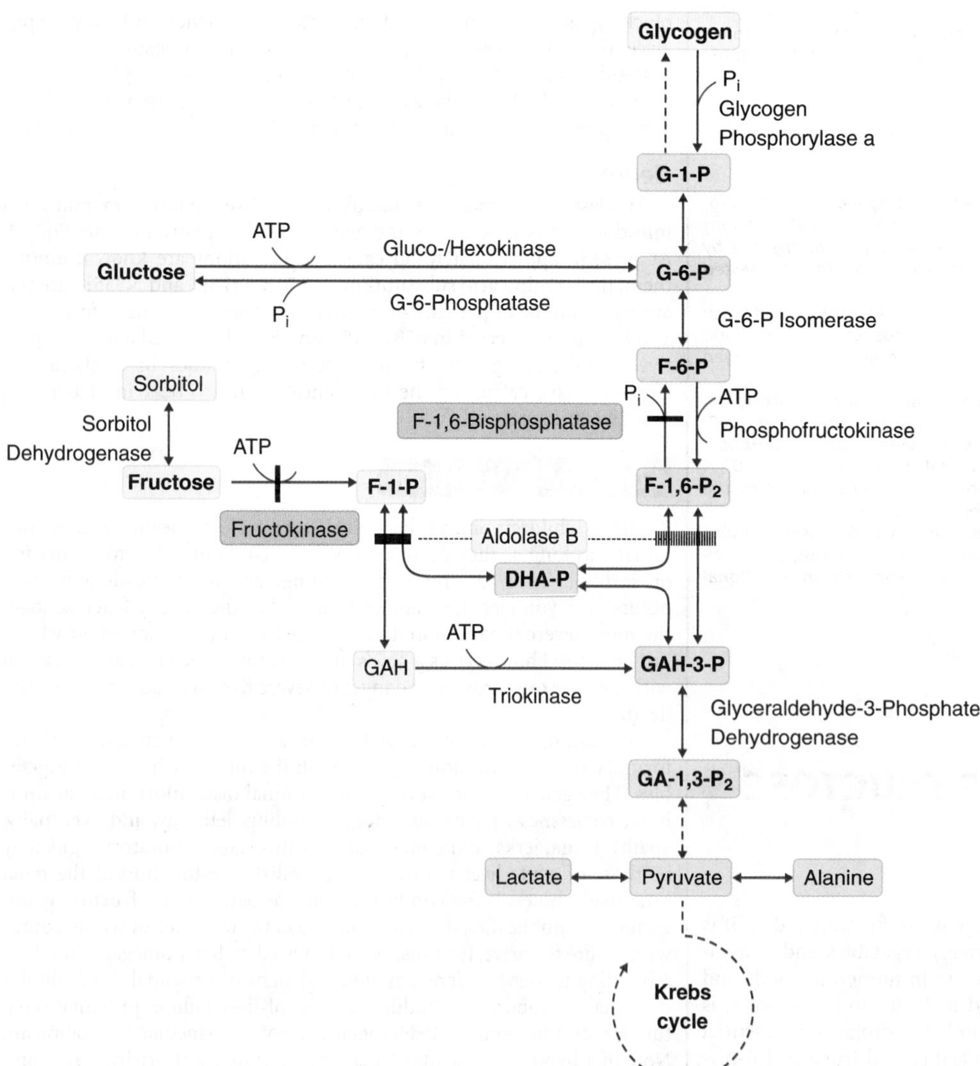

FIGURE 220–1 • Fructose is metabolized mainly in the liver, kidney cortex, and small intestinal mucosa in a pathway containing fructokinase (ketohexokinase), aldolase B, and triokinase. Aldolase B also intervenes in the glycolytic-gluconeogenic pathway (right part of the scheme). The three enzyme defects in fructose metabolism are boxed and depicted by solid bars across the arrows; the diminished activity of aldolase B toward fructose 1,6-bisphosphate in hereditary fructose intolerance is depicted by a broken bar. DHA-P = dihydroxyacetone phosphate; F = fructose; G = glucose; GA = glycerate; GAH = glyceraldehyde; P = phosphate; Pi = inorganic phosphate.

In vivo handling of fructose is best reflected by an intravenous fructose tolerance test. In normal subjects, blood glucose increases by 0 to 40%, with no or minimal changes in phosphate. In patients with HFI, glucose and phosphate levels decrease within 10 to 20 minutes. As a rule, the decrease in phosphate precedes and occurs more rapidly than that of glucose. Oral fructose tolerance tests are not recommended because they provoke more ill effects and are less reliable.

Differential Diagnosis

A high degree of diagnostic awareness is often needed in HFI because the spectrum of symptoms and signs is wide and nonspecific. HFI has been misdiagnosed as pyloric stenosis, gastroesophageal reflux, galactosemia, tyrosinemia, intrauterine infections, glycogen and other storage disorders, and later in life, Wilson's disease, leukemia, and growth retardation. Fructosuria may be secondary to liver damage, as in tyrosinemia. Fructose malabsorption is frequently confused with HFI; its metabolic basis is not well understood, but it is probably due to a defective fructose transporter in the small intestine, and ingestion of fructose leads to abdominal pain and diarrhea. In sucrase-isomaltase deficiency, ingestion of sucrose results in bloating, abdominal cramps, and fermentative osmotic diarrhea; free fructose, however, is well tolerated.

Treatment

Rx

In acute intoxication, intensive care may be required and supportive measures such as fresh-frozen plasma may be needed. The main therapeutic step in HFI, however, is the immediate elimination of all sources of fructose from the diet. This involves the avoidance

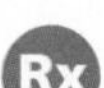

of all types of food in which fructose, sucrose, or sorbitol occur naturally or have been added. It should be borne in mind that fructose and sorbitol may be present in medications (e.g., syrups, immunoglobulin solutions) and infant formulas (without adequate declaration of the carbohydrate composition).

Sucrose should be replaced by glucose, maltose, or starch (or any combination) to prevent the fructose-free diet from containing too much fat. Despite the availability of books and online information on food composition, a dietician should be consulted and practical aspects of the diet should be discussed (e.g., the considerable variability in the fructose content of different food types, the influence of storage temperature or method of preparation, and the manner of cooking on bioavailability). Substitution of the vitamins ascorbic acid and folate should be prescribed to make up for their lack of intake from fruits and vegetables.

Prognosis

After institution of a fructose-free diet, most abnormalities disappear rapidly, except for hepatomegaly, which may persist for months or even years. Fructose intake should be as low as possible, and at least in childhood, its threshold should not be determined by subjective tolerance. For dietary control, regular taking of the nutritional history is still best because of the lack of good sensitive chemical parameters. Needless to say, these patients (and their parents) should report HFI on any hospital admission. The prognosis is excellent, with normal growth, intelligence, and lifespan.

FRUCTOSE-1,6-BISPHOSPHATASE DEFICIENCY (MIM 229700)

Pathobiology

Metabolic Derangement

Deficiency of FBPase, the key enzyme in gluconeogenesis, impairs the formation of glucose from all gluconeogenic precursors, including dietary fructose (see Fig. 220–1). Thus, hypoglycemia is likely to occur when glycogen reserves are limited (as in newborns) or exhausted (as when fasting). The defect also provokes accumulation of the gluconeogenic substrates lactate/pyruvate, glycerol, and alanine.

Children with FBPase deficiency generally tolerate sweet foods, up to 2 g of fructose per kilogram of body weight per day, when given regularly distributed over the day, and in contrast to subjects with HFI, they do thrive on such a diet. Nevertheless, loading tests with fructose do induce hypoglycemia, as in HFI, as a result of the inhibitory effect of the rapidly formed, but slowly metabolized F-1-P on liver glycogen phosphorylase *a*.

Genetics

Deficiency of the liver-type isoform of FBPase is a rare autosomal recessive disorder caused by mutations in the *FBP1* gene on 9q22.2-q22.3; to date, 22 different mutations have been published.

Several FBPase-deficient patients have been reported in whom no mutation could be found in the coding region of *FBP1*. Therefore, it has been supposed that these patients carry mutations within the promoter region of *FBP1*.

Clinical Manifestations

In about half of all cases, FBPase deficiency is manifested in the neonatal period (days 1 to 4) as severe hyperventilation, profound lactic acidosis, and marked hypoglycemia. Later, episodes of irritability, somnolence or coma, apneic spells, dyspnea and tachycardia, muscular hypotonia, and moderate hepatomegaly may occur and are typically triggered by a febrile episode accompanied by refusal to feed and vomiting. In between attacks, patients are usually well. The frequency of the attacks decreases with age, and the majority of survivors display normal somatic and psychomotor development. Once the diagnosis is established and treatment begins, the course is favorable. In contrast to HFI, chronic ingestion of fructose does not lead to gastrointestinal symptoms—hence there is no aversion to sweet foods—or failure to thrive.

Laboratory Findings during an Attack

Analysis of plasma during acute episodes reveals lactic acidosis, an increased lactate-pyruvate ratio, hyperalaninemia, hyperketonemia, and glucagon-resistant hypoglycemia. Urinary analysis reveals increased lactate, alanine, glycerol, and ketones.

Diagnosis

Most affected children experience a number of acute attacks before the diagnosis is made. Whenever FBPase is suspected, adequate amounts of intravenous or oral glucose should be given.

The diagnosis has to be confirmed by molecular diagnosis on DNA from peripheral leukocytes. If no mutation can be found despite the strongly suggestive clinical and laboratory findings, determination of enzymatic activity in a liver biopsy sample should be undertaken. Cultured skin fibroblasts, amniotic fluid cells, and chorionic villi do not exhibit FBPase activity.

Functional studies such as loading with fructose (or with glycerol or alanine) or fasting should not be performed as first-line tests because they provide only a tentative diagnosis. However, they may be useful if mutation analysis and enzyme activity are normal despite a strong clinical and chemical suspicion of FBPase deficiency.

Differential Diagnosis

Other disturbances in gluconeogenesis have to be considered, such as (1) pyruvate dehydrogenase deficiency, characterized by a low lactate-pyruvate ratio and aggravation of lactic acidosis by glucose infusion; (2) pyruvate carboxylase deficiency; (3) phosphoenol pyruvate carboxylase deficiency; (4) respiratory chain disorders; and (5) glycogenosis types Ia and Ib, characterized by hepatonephromegaly, hyperlipidemia, and hyperuricemia.

Treatment

Acute, life-threatening episodes should be treated with an intravenous bolus of 20% glucose followed by a continuous high-rate infusion of glucose (10 to 12 mg/kg/min for newborns) and bicarbonate to control hypoglycemia and acidosis.

Maintenance therapy should be aimed at avoiding fasting periods, particularly during febrile episodes. This involves frequent feeding, the use of slowly absorbed carbohydrates (such as uncooked starch), and a gastric drip, if necessary.

Prognosis

Once FBPase deficiency has been diagnosed and adequate management initiated, its course is usually benign. Growth and psychomotor and intellectual development seem unimpaired, and tolerance to fasting improves with age up to the point that the disorder does not present a problem later in life. Many patients become obese because their concerned parents overfeed them and later they adopt these eating habits.

SUGGESTED READINGS

Cox TM: The genetic consequences of our sweet tooth. Nat Rev Genet 2002;3:481–487. *Discusses fructose intolerance in the context of the rise of sucrose and fructose as preferred sources of energy.*

Steinmann B, Gitzelmann R, van den Berghe G: Disorders of fructose metabolism. *In* Scriver CR, Beaudet AL, Sly WS, Valle D (eds): The Metabolic and Molecular Bases of Inherited Disease, 8th ed. New York, McGraw-Hill, 2001, pp 1489–1520. *Abnormal %CDT values may allow prompt detection of HFI.*

Wong D: Hereditary fructose intolerance. Mol Genet Metab 2005;85:165–167. *A biochemical review.*

221 PRIMARY HYPEROXALURIA

Richard E. Hillman

Definition

Primary hyperoxaluria refers to two different peroxisomal enzyme deficiencies that are characterized by massive synthesis and urinary excretion of oxalic acid.

Epidemiology

Until recently, primary hyperoxaluria was considered a very rare disease. Now, however, more than 350 cases of type I disease have been described, as well as approximately 40 cases of type II disease.

Clinical Manifestations

Primary hyperoxaluria has far more clinical variability than initially thought. Patients with milder cases present as adults, and some unusual presentations are the result of oxalate deposition in tissues other than the kidney. Oxalate is also deposited in the heart, the eye, the skin, and other organs. Of particular interest, oxalate has led to cardiac conduction system abnormalities.

Usually, in type I disease, clinical manifestations appear early in childhood, with nephrolithiasis or nephrocalcinosis, and lead to renal failure within the first decade of life. Type II disease is much more variable.

Diagnosis

Both types of primary hyperoxaluria are inherited as autosomal recessive traits and must be distinguished from secondary hyperoxalurias resulting from increased absorption of oxalate by the gut. These secondary causes include inflammatory bowel disease and fat malabsorption, which alter calcium absorption and convert insoluble calcium oxalate to more absorbable salts. Although most adult patients with calcium oxalate nephrolithiasis excrete normal amounts of oxalate, it is now clear that hyperoxaluria must be considered in the differential diagnosis.

Pathobiology

Type I Disease

Primary hyperoxaluria type I (glycolic aciduria) is caused by a defect in the peroxisomal enzyme alanine glyoxylate amino transferase (gene map locus 2q36-q37). This enzyme normally converts glycolic acid to the amino acid glycine. In its absence, glycolic acid leaves the peroxisome and is converted to oxalic acid by lactic dehydrogenase (Fig. 221–1). Both glycolic and oxalic acids are excreted in large amounts, usually more than 60 mg/1.73 m^2/24 hours. In most cases, this concentration exceeds the solubility of oxalic acid. This enzyme has been cloned, and multiple defects have been demonstrated. Some correlation exists between specific mutations and the severity of the disease.

Type II Disease

Primary hyperoxaluria type II (glyceric aciduria) results from a deficiency of D-glycerate dehydrogenase glyoxylate reductase, a dual functional enzyme whose absence leads to accumulation of both hydroxypyruvate and glyoxylate (gene map 9cen). The hydroxypyruvate is reduced in the cytoplasm to L-glyceric acid, and the glyoxylate, as in type I disease, is converted to oxylate by lactic dehydrogenase. Type II primary hyperoxaluria is a much milder disease than type I and may manifest only after dehydration. A review of 24 cases suggests the variability of the clinical presentation of this defect and indicates that this diagnosis should be considered in any patient with urolithiasis or nephrocalcinosis. Like type I disease, it is inherited as an autosomal recessive trait.

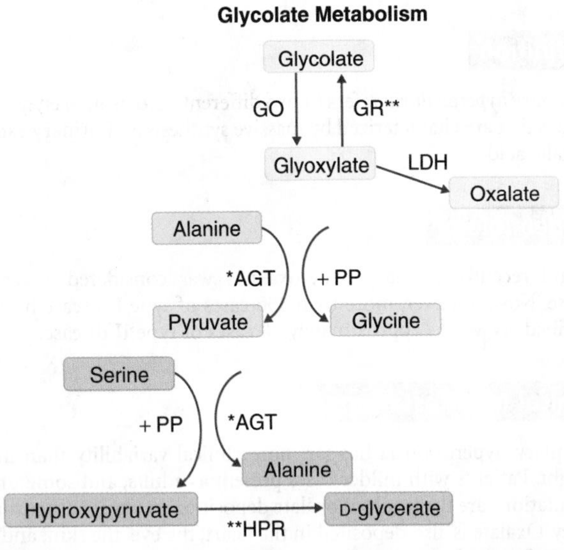

FIGURE 221–1 • Glycolate metabolism. Glyoxylate oxidase (GO) converts glycolate to glyoxylate. Alanine glyoxylate aminotransferase (AGT) catalyzes the conversion of glyoxylate to glycine in the presence of pyridoxal phosphate (PP). The type I enzymatic deficiency of AGT leads to conversion of excess glycolate reductase (GR) to oxalate by lactate dehydrogenase (LDH). The type II deficiency of GR and hydroxyl pyruvate reductase (HPR) also leads to the accumulation of oxalate.

Treatment

Rx

Some patients with mild type I disease respond to large doses of pyridoxine (50 to 200 mg/day), which is effective only in patients with some enzyme. Dilute urine should be maintained by high fluid intake, and some reports suggest that diuretics may help. Attempts to form more soluble salts of oxalate, particularly with magnesium orthophosphate and citrate, have met with some success. *Oxalobacter formigenes* treatment, which may induce secretion of oxalate into the intestinal lumen for degradation there, is a potential new therapy. The only "cure" for this disease has been a combined renal and liver transplant. Renal transplants alone have failed because of the accumulation of oxalate produced in the liver. Therapeutic outcomes in patients with type II disease are variable. Pyridoxine has no effect. Other measures that maintain a dilute urine seem to be sufficient in patients with milder cases.

SUGGESTED READINGS

Bobrowski AE, Langman CB: Hyperoxaluria and systemic oxalosis: Current therapy and future directions. Expert Opin Pharmacother 2006;7:1887–1896. *An overview of options.*

Milliner D: Treatment of primary hyperoxaluria: A new chapter. Kidney Int 2006;70:1198–2000. *Discusses the potential of* Oxalobacter formigenes *treatment.*

Pirulli D, Marangella M, Amoroso A: Primary hyperoxaluria: Genotype-phenotype correlation. J Nephrol 2003;16:297–309. *Homozygous genotypes were more frequent than expected and generally had a less severe form of the disease than compound heterozygotes.*

222 DISORDERS OF PURINE AND PYRIMIDINE METABOLISM

Michael S. Hershfield

PURINE ENZYME DEFICIENCIES AND DISORDERS OF IMMUNE FUNCTION

Adenosine Deaminase Deficiency

Definition

Infants with the usual early-onset form of inherited adenosine deaminase (ADA) deficiency have profound lymphocyte depletion, lack both cellular and humoral immune function, and as a result have severe combined immunodeficiency disease (SCID). Less complete ADA deficiency is associated with T-cell dysfunction and more variable loss of B-cell function, which causes progressive immune dysfunction in children, adolescents, and even adults. Healthy individuals with so-called partial ADA deficiency have been identified by screening for erythrocyte ADA activity in populations and families of immunodeficient patients.

Epidemiology

ADA deficiency accounts for about 15% of all cases of SCID and a third of those with autosomal recessive inheritance. It has been estimated to occur in 1 in 200,000 to 1 in 1 million births.

Pathobiology

Etiology

More than 70 mutations leading to loss of ADA enzymatic activity have been identified in the 12-exon *ADA* gene located on chromosome 20q. About two thirds are single-base changes within the coding region; the remainder are deletions and splicing mutations. Most patients possess two different mutant alleles. The ADA catalytic activity of cloned mutant alleles expressed in *Escherichia coli* correlates well with both clinical severity and the level of specific metabolic abnormalities in the patient's erythrocytes. Some mildly affected patients have shown mosaicism for reversion of a mutant allele in lymphoid cells.

Pathogenesis

ADA catalyzes the irreversible deamination of adenosine to inosine and 2′-deoxyadenosine to 2′-deoxyinosine (Fig. 222–1). In the absence of ADA activity, plasma levels of both ADA substrates are increased to 0.5 to 10 μmol/L; high levels of 2′-deoxyadenosine, but not adenosine, are excreted in urine. Two pathognomonic metabolic abnormalities occur in the erythrocytes of immunodeficient patients with ADA deficiency (but not in healthy individuals with "partial deficiency"): (1) a marked elevation (50- to more than 1000-fold) in the level of 2′-deoxyadenosine triphosphate (dATP) derived from 2′-deoxyadenosine and (2) decreased activity of the enzyme *S*-adenosylhomocysteine hydrolase as a result of its inactivation by 2′-deoxyadenosine.

Lymphocyte depletion and immunodeficiency stem mainly from the preferential phosphorylation of 2′-deoxyadenosine and subsequent accumulation of dATP in immature thymocytes. Expansion of the dATP pool has several cytotoxic effects: (1) it inhibits the enzyme ribonucleotide reductase, thus blocking DNA replication; (2) dATP participates in a cytoplasmic complex with cytochrome *c* released from mitochondria and the protein apoptosis-activating factor I to initiate a caspase proteolytic cascade leading to cell death; and (3) dATP accumulation induces single-strand breaks in DNA. In addition to these effects of dATP, inactivation of *S*-adenosylhomocysteine hydrolase by 2′-deoxyadenosine causes the accumulation of *S*-adenosylhomocysteine, an inhibitor of *S*-adenosylmethionine–dependent transmethylation reactions. Elevated levels of extracellular adenosine, acting through cell membrane adenosine receptors, may interfere with T- and B-lymphocyte differentiation or function by several mechanisms, including blocking of antigen receptor-stimulated activation of the nuclear factor NF-κB.

Clinical Manifestations

ADA-deficient SCID is manifested in infants by failure to thrive and recurrent infections with ordinary pathogens and opportunistic organisms. *Pneumocystis jirovecii* and viral pneumonitis, persistent diarrhea, and candidiasis of the skin and gastrointestinal tract are common, as are cytomegalovirus, varicella virus, and adenovirus infections. Vaccination with live organisms may be fatal, and unirradiated blood products may cause fatal graft-versus-host disease; an increased incidence of B-cell lymphomas has been reported. Serum transaminase elevation or hepatitis and diverse neurologic abnormalities in some cases may be due to the metabolic effects of ADA deficiency, as well as to infection. Lymph nodes and tonsillar tissue are absent, and some infants show prominent costochondral junctions. Chest radiographs reveal the absence of a thymus and cupping and flaring of the rib ends. Peripheral blood shows an absolute lymphopenia, often less than 500/μL, with decreased numbers of T, B, and natural killer cells. Hypogammaglobulinemia and lack of specific antibody response to immunization and infection are found, and in vitro tests reveal absent or decreased lymphocyte function, including proliferative responses to mitogens and antigens. In older children and adults with less complete ADA deficiency, recurring respiratory infections are often the primary manifestation of combined immunodeficiency; chronic pulmonary insufficiency is often present by the time that the diagnosis is made. Elevated serum IgE, asthma, and autoimmune cytopenia also occur as a result of the immune dysregulation.

Diagnosis

The disorder should be considered in individuals of any age with recurrent infections associated with unexplained lymphopenia. The diagnosis is made by measuring ADA activity in the hemolysates of untransfused patients. Finding elevated dATP and decreased *S*-adenosylhomocysteine hydrolase activity in erythrocytes is confirmatory and may help gauge the degree of ADA deficiency. Prenatal diagnosis can be accomplished by assay of ADA activity in cultured amniotic or chorionic villi cells. In kindreds in which *ADA* gene mutations have previously been identified, the diagnosis can be made by DNA sequencing or restriction enzyme digestion. Because of the genetic diversity, however, mutation analysis is not an efficient method of diagnosis in cases in which the genotype is unknown.

Treatment

Rx

Specific antibiotic and antiviral treatment of infections is essential. In addition, patients should receive prophylaxis for *P. jirovecii* and fungal infections and should not receive live virus vaccines or unirradiated blood products. Most patients are also treated with intravenous immunoglobulin. Once the diagnosis is established, the patient is a candidate for either bone marrow transplantation or enzyme replacement therapy with polyethylene glycol (PEG)-conjugated bovine ADA (PEG-ADA, Adagen). Trials of gene therapy have been in progress for 15 years. Within the past 4 to 5 years, correction of immune deficiency has been reported in several patients treated in Italy.

For SCID patients, the long-term survival rate after human leukocyte antigen (HLA)-identical sibling marrow transplantation is 70 to 90%, and this remains the treatment of choice if a donor is available. Transplanting T-cell–depleted marrow from HLA-haploidentical (usually a parent) or matched unrelated donors has been less successful, with long-term survival rates ranging from 28 to 67% at different transplant centers.

Enzyme replacement by intramuscular injection of PEG-ADA once or twice a week is used for patients who lack an HLA-identical donor and are considered poor candidates for transplantation or for whom the risks associated with transplantation are unacceptable. By maintaining high ADA activity in plasma, PEG-ADA eliminates circulating

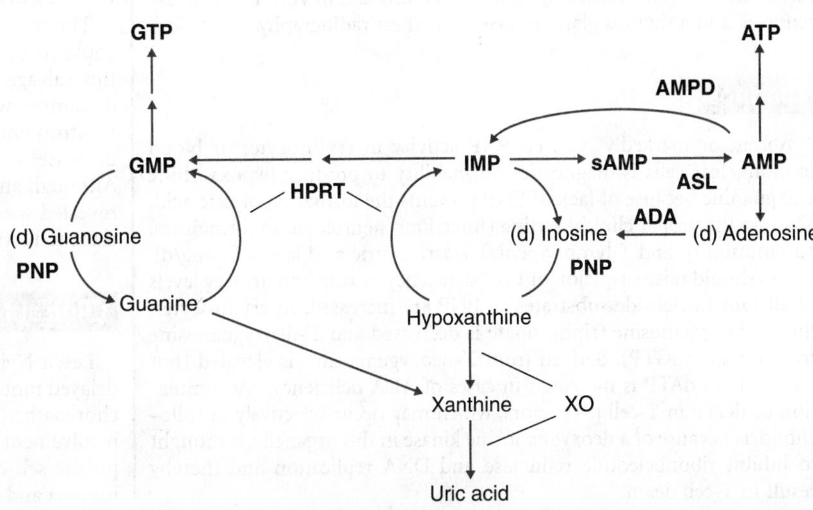

FIGURE 222–1 • Schema of purine metabolism demonstrating metabolic reactions catalyzed by adenosine deaminase (ADA), purine nucleoside phosphorylase (PNP), adenosine monophosphate deaminase (AMPD), adenylosuccinate lyase (ASL), hypoxanthine-guanine phosphoribosyltransferase (HPRT), and xanthine oxidase (XO). AMP = adenosine monophosphate; ATP = adenosine triphosphate; IMP = inosine monophosphate; (d) = 2′-deoxy; GMP = guanosine monophosphate; GTP = guanosine triphosphate; sAMP = succinyl adenosine monophosphate.

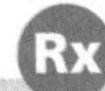

ADA substrates and corrects levels of their toxic metabolites in cells. Improvement in lymphocyte counts and function usually occurs within several weeks to a few months of initiating treatment. Although immune function is often only partly restored, the majority of patients have done well clinically. PEG-ADA is well tolerated, and the overall survival rate among more than 100 patients treated during the first 15 years after its introduction has been comparable to the best results reported with HLA-nonidentical transplantation. PEG-ADA therapy has been limited by the development of neutralizing antibody to PEG-ADA in 8 to 9% of patients. A gradual decline over time in lymphocyte counts and in vitro tests of lymphocyte function may also limit long-term effectiveness.

Experimental gene therapy has been performed in about a dozen patients, who have been treated concomitantly with PEG-ADA. Most of these patients received repeated infusions of autologous T cells that had been transfected ex vivo with a retroviral vector containing human ADA cDNA. Three prenatally diagnosed neonates received transfected $CD34^+$ umbilical cord stem cells shortly after birth. The vector was found to persist for several years in 1 to 10% of the circulating T lymphocytes of some patients, a finding consistent with selection for ADA-expressing lymphocytes. During the past 4 years, stem cell–targeted therapy with retroviral vectors has been effective in restoring lymphocyte counts and immune function in several patients who were not treated with PEG-ADA.

Purine Nucleoside Phosphorylase Deficiency

Definition

Encoded by a six-exon gene on chromosome 14q, purine nucleoside phosphorylase (PNP) catalyzes the reversible phosphorolytic cleavage of inosine and 2′-deoxyinosine (products of the ADA reaction), as well as guanosine and 2′-deoxyguanosine, to their respective purine bases (hypoxanthine or guanine) plus ribose- or deoxyribose-1-PO_4 (see Fig. 222–1).

Epidemiology

PNP deficiency is diagnosed about a tenth as often as ADA deficiency but also causes T-cell depletion and cellular immune dysfunction. B-cell function may be normal but more often is depressed or hyperactive, and autoimmune disorders such as hemolytic anemia or thrombocytopenia develop in about a third of patients. Various neurologic abnormalities (spasticity, ataxia, behavioral abnormalities, hypertonia, hypotonia) occur in more than 50% of patients and may be apparent before immunodeficiency is evident. The most severely affected patients have a SCID-like manifestation as infants, but the disorder may occur at any time in the first decade of life, often with disseminated varicella or other serious recurrent viral infections. T-lymphocyte counts and in vitro function are reduced, and a thymus gland is absent on chest radiography.

Diagnosis

Absent or markedly reduced PNP activity in erythrocytes or blood mononuclear cells is diagnostic. An inability to produce hypoxanthine and guanine because of lack of PNP prevents the formation of uric acid. Thus, in the proper clinical setting (infections, neurologic abnormalities, autoimmunity, and T lymphopenia), a serum uric acid level of 1 mg/dL or less should raise suspicion of PNP deficiency. Serum and urinary levels of all four nucleoside substrates of PNP are increased. In erythrocytes, the level of guanosine triphosphate is decreased and 2′-deoxyguanosine triphosphate (dGTP), derived from 2′-deoxyguanosine, is elevated (but far less than dATP is increased in cases of ADA deficiency). Accumulation of dGTP in T-cell precursors, which may occur selectively in mitochondria because of a deoxyguanosine kinase in this organelle, is thought to inhibit ribonucleotide reductase and DNA replication and thereby result in T-cell death.

Treatment

Treatment with red blood cell transfusions or infusions of deoxycytidine aimed at restoring DNA replication has not resulted in any consistent therapeutic response. Bone marrow transplantation has been curative, but outcomes reported for about a dozen patients suggest a high rate of failure. PEG-conjugated PNP and gene therapy is being investigated in mouse models, but the small number of patients with PNP deficiency makes clinical research on this disorder difficult.

OTHER INHERITED DISORDERS OF PURINE METABOLISM

Lesch-Nyhan Syndrome

Definition

Lesch-Nyhan syndrome is an X-linked disorder caused by absence of the enzyme hypoxanthine phosphoribosyltransferase (HPRT). It is manifested in affected males as uric acid nephrolithiasis or gout and a devastating neurologic disorder consisting of compulsive self-mutilation, choreoathetosis, spasticity, and often mental retardation.

Epidemiology

The syndrome occurs in about 1 in 100,000 male births. Partial deficiency of HPRT also causes hyperuricemia and severe gout, but without severe neurologic deficits; this disorder accounts for less than 1% of patients with gout (Chapter 294).

Pathobiology

Etiology

HPRT deficiency has been attributed to more than 300 different point mutations, splicing defects, and deletions. HPRT catalyzes condensation of the purine bases hypoxanthine and guanine (the PNP reaction products) with ribose-5-PO_4 derived from phosphoribosylpyrophosphate to form the nucleotides inosine monophosphate (IMP) and guanosine monophosphate. In the absence of these "purine salvage" reactions, hypoxanthine and guanine can be catabolized only via xanthine oxidase to uric acid, which causes hyperuricemia and markedly increased uricaciduria. Loss of HPRT also leads to increased intracellular phosphoribosylpyrophosphate and reduced formation of IMP and guanosine monophosphate, which activates the de novo synthesis of purine nucleotides and thus further increases the generation of uric acid. In patients with Lesch-Nyhan syndrome, hyperuricemia and increased uric acid excretion lead to the juvenile onset of uric acid stone formation and gouty arthritis.

Pathogenesis

The pathogenesis of the neurologic defects is not well understood but could involve guanine nucleotide deficiency in neurons that depend on the salvage pathway for purine nucleotide synthesis. Basal ganglia dopamine was decreased by 60 to 90% in three autopsied brains, and positron emission tomography has demonstrated a selective 50 to 70% decrease in dopamine transporters in the caudate and putamen. Although anatomic studies of the brains of affected individuals have not revealed specific structural lesions, imaging studies have shown a significant reduction in caudate volume.

Clinical Manifestations

Lesch-Nyhan syndrome is manifested during the first year of life by delayed motor development, followed by extrapyramidal signs leading to choreoathetosis and, at approximately 1 year of age, by pyramidal tract involvement with hyperreflexia, clonus, and scissoring of the legs. Compulsive self-destructive behavior (such as biting fingers, lips, and buccal mucosa and self-inflicted head trauma) appears some time between early childhood and adolescence. This behavior pattern, which is unique to this disorder, necessitates restraints and in some cases edentulation. Patients are unable to walk, and mental and growth retardation occurs in the majority. Uric acid crystalluria may first be noted as orange crystals in the diaper during the first weeks of life. If untreated, uricaciduria may lead to nephrolithiasis, obstructive uropathy, and azotemia. Hyperuricemia may attain levels of 18 mg/dL. Gout may develop later in the course of the disease, but not generally before puberty. Death generally occurs in the second or third decade from infection or renal failure.

In patients with partial deficiency of HPRT, uric acid crystalluria and renal calculi develop in childhood, and gouty arthritis often begins before the age of 20 years. Neurologic manifestations may occur in 20% of these patients and include mental retardation, mild spastic quadriplegia, dysarthria, cerebellar ataxia, and seizures, but self-mutilation does not develop. Patients with partial HPRT deficiency may seek medical attention after passing a renal calculus or after an attack of gouty arthritis. Life expectancy is normal.

Diagnosis

Lesch-Nyhan syndrome is strongly suggested by the self-mutilation and characteristic choreoathetosis; mental retardation of other origins is rarely accompanied by self-injury, especially in the presence of intact sensation. The finding of hyperuricemia supports the diagnosis. Definitive diagnosis is established by demonstrating a lack of HPRT enzymatic activity in red blood cells or other tissues. Female carriers cannot be definitively identified by assay of HPRT activity in peripheral blood cells but may be detected by analysis of DNA if the mutation has been defined in an affected male relative.

Partial deficiency of HPRT is manifested by the early onset of gouty arthritis or uric acid crystalluria or nephrolithiasis in male patients. In patients with normal renal function, uric acid overexcretion is marked. HPRT activity in red cells is usually in the range of 0.2 to 5% of normal and occasionally as high as 30 to 50%, whereas patients with Lesch-Nyhan syndrome have less than 0.01% of control values.

Treatment

Rx

Uric acid stone formation, tophi, and gouty arthritis can be controlled in patients with both the Lesch-Nyhan syndrome and partial deficiency of HPRT by the administration of allopurinol to inhibit xanthine oxidase activity. Xanthine renal stones may occur with this therapy. No effective pharmacologic treatment of the neurologic disorder has been developed. Neither bone marrow transplantation nor red blood cell transfusions have significantly ameliorated the neurologic disorder, which makes it unlikely that enzyme replacement therapy or hematopoietic stem cell gene transduction will play any role in treatment. Attempts at developing methods for direct delivery of HPRT cDNA to the central nervous system are under way.

Myoadenylate Deaminase Deficiency and Myopathy

Definition

Myoadenylate deaminase is the muscle-specific isoenzyme of adenosine monophosphate deaminase (AMPD). It is the product of one (*AMPD1*) of three distinct genes encoding AMPD isoenzymes. This enzyme, which catalyzes the deamination of adenosine monophosphate (AMP) to IMP plus ammonia (NH_3), is an integral part of the purine nucleotide cycle that appears to play a role in energy production in skeletal muscle (see Fig. 222–1).

Epidemiology

Deficiency of AMPD1 has been found in 2% of all muscle biopsy specimens submitted for histologic examination. Inherited deficiency of myoadenylate deaminase may be associated with exercise-related cramps and myalgias, but these symptoms are often mild and variable. An acquired deficiency of AMPD1 is associated with a number of primary muscle disorders.

Pathobiology

The 16-exon *AMPD1* gene, located on chromosome 1p, is expressed predominantly in skeletal muscle, in which the AMPD1 protein has been shown to bind to myosin heavy chain. *AMPD2* and *AMPD3* are expressed in other tissues. *AMPD1* transcripts normally undergo alternative splicing of the 12–base pair second exon such that 0.6 to 2% of the mRNA in human skeletal muscle lacks exon 2 and encodes a catalytically active protein deficient in four amino acids. A nonsense mutation within this second exon has been found at frequencies of 0.13 to 0.19 in the general population. Homozygosity for this nonsense mutation is responsible for the vast majority of cases of inherited myoadenylate deaminase deficiency. An acquired (secondary) AMPD1 deficiency, associated with decreased *AMPD1* mRNA levels, occurs in a variety of muscle disorders and may be due to a pleiotropic regulatory defect in expression of multiple muscle genes.

During muscle contraction, the AMPD1-catalyzed generation of IMP and NH_3 from AMP increases markedly. After exertion, AMP is regenerated from IMP with the production of fumarate, a citric acid cycle intermediate, by the next two enzymatic steps in the purine nucleotide cycle (see Fig. 222–1). Several mechanisms have been proposed by which these reactions might enhance regeneration of adenosine triphosphate. Patients with complete functional deficiency of AMPD1 do not generate IMP, NH_3, or fumarate in skeletal muscle during exercise. Studies in a few patients have documented greater than normal exertion-dependent depletion of high-energy phosphate in muscle. However, in other studies, complete and partial AMPD1 deficiency did not have such effects and did not affect exercise performance.

Clinical Manifestations

The inherited form of AMPD1 deficiency has been documented in more than 200 individuals. In most, fatigue, cramps, or myalgias develop after vigorous exercise; myoglobinuria has been reported occasionally. The majority of these patients were first evaluated for these symptoms during childhood or as young adults. Given the high frequency of the exon 2 nonsense mutation in the general population, a large number of homozygous mutant individuals must exist whose symptoms are not sufficient to warrant medical evaluation. It has been postulated that the normal alternative splicing of exon 2, which would suppress the effect of the nonsense mutation, could provide sufficient catalytically active AMPD1 protein to prevent or ameliorate the clinical consequences in many homozygous patients. A low level of expression of one of the other AMPD isoforms in skeletal muscle could have the same effect. A secondary deficiency of AMPD1 is found in a number of other muscle diseases, including neurogenic disorders, various myopathies, and collagen vascular disorders. The clinical symptoms of these individuals are dictated by the primary muscle disease. Because of the clinical heterogeneity associated with AMPD1 deficiency, there may be uncertainty, in any given individual, about whether the enzyme deficiency state is responsible for the symptoms.

Diagnosis

Individuals with AMPD1 deficiency do not produce NH_3 on ischemic exercise of the forearm, and an elevated creatine phosphokinase concentration occurs in 50% of cases. Histochemical stains and determination of enzyme activity demonstrate an absence of AMPD1 in muscle biopsy tissue. The genetic abnormality can be detected by finding an altered restriction enzyme digestion site in genomic DNA.

Treatment

No treatment has been demonstrated to be effective. Oral ribose, administered in an attempt to enhance the synthesis of purine nucleotides, has met with variable subjective improvement.

2,8-DIHYDROXYADENINE RENAL STONES

In the absence of the purine salvage enzyme adenine phosphoribosyltransferase (APRT), the substrate adenine accumulates and is oxidized, though inefficiently, by xanthine oxidase to the very insoluble product 2,8-dihydroxyadenine. Patients with autosomal recessive deficiency of APRT are predisposed to radiolucent renal calculi composed of 2,8-dihydroxyadenine, which may develop within the first months of life or as late as the fifth decade, but stones never develop in many APRT-deficient individuals. The composition of the stones is determined by ultraviolet, infrared, or mass spectrometry or by x-ray crystallography. Definitive diagnosis requires demonstrating the absence of APRT activity in erythrocyte lysates. No other biochemical or clinical abnormalities have been reported in individuals with APRT deficiency, and heterozygotes have no clinical abnormalities. Relatively few mutations at the 2.8-kb *APRT* locus on chromosome 16q are responsible for causing enzyme deficiency. The disorder is relatively common in individuals of Japanese ancestry, mainly because of a single base mutation at codon 136 found in 68% of defective alleles, with two other mutations accounting for 28%. APRT mutations in non-Japanese subjects cluster at the intron 4 splice donor site and at codon 87. Therapy for individuals with 2,8-dihydroxyadenine calculi consists of restricting dietary purines, high fluid intake, and treatment with allopurinol to prevent the oxidation of adenine by xanthine oxidase.

Xanthinuria

Classic, or type I, xanthinuria is an often benign disorder that results from deficiency of the enzyme xanthine oxidase (xanthine dehydrogenase), which catalyzes conversion of the "oxypurines" xanthine and hypoxanthine to uric acid, the last step in purine catabolism in humans. Clinical consequences are related to the insolubility of xanthine, the predominant compound excreted by these individuals (hypoxanthine is efficiently reused by cells via the HPRT salvage reaction). About a third of the approximately 100 individuals in whom xanthinuria has been identified have had renal stones composed of xanthine (which in pure form are radiolucent but often also contain calcium). Crystalline deposits of xanthine in muscle have been found in a few xanthinuric individuals with muscle cramps after exercise. Deficiency of xanthine oxidase can be established by direct assay of biopsied liver tissue or small intestinal mucosa, but the diagnosis is strongly suggested by the finding of very low serum and urinary uric acid in conjunction with elevated serum and urinary oxypurines. Xanthine calculi are treated primarily by increasing fluid intake.

A deficiency of xanthine oxidase can also occur in combination with deficiencies of one or both of two other enzymes, aldehyde oxidase and sulfite oxidase, with which it shares a requirement for a molybdenum-containing cofactor for catalytic activity. Xanthine oxidase and aldehyde oxidase have overlapping substrate specificities, and patients deficient in both have so-called type II xanthinuria, which is clinically similar to classic xanthinuria. Patients with type I and type II xanthinuria can be distinguished by a difference in their ability to metabolize allopurinol (type I patients can convert allopurinol to oxypurinol, whereas type II patients cannot) and certain other compounds. Patients with a combined deficiency of xanthine oxidase, aldehyde oxidase, and sulfite oxidase because of defective production of the common molybdenum cofactor have a much more devastating disorder. They are initially seen in infancy with severe neurologic dysfunction characterized by seizures, nystagmus, enophthalmos, ocular lens dislocation, and Brushfield spots. These same clinical findings occur in nonxanthinuric patients with isolated deficiency of sulfite oxidase.

Adenylosuccinate Lyase Deficiency

Variable psychomotor retardation, seizures, autistic features, and in some cases, growth retardation and muscular wasting have been associated in more than 50 patients with a deficiency of adenylosuccinate lyase (ADSL). More than 30 different mutations have been identified in the *ADSL* gene on chromosome 22q. Homotetrameric ADSL catalyzes two late steps in the de novo purine biosynthetic pathway. In each, a nucleotide intermediate formed by the addition of aspartic acid is cleaved to release fumarate with transfer of a nitrogen to the growing purine ring. Levels of the dephosphorylated ADSL substrates succinylamidoimidazolecarboxamide (SAICA) riboside and succinyladenosine (S-Ado) may reach 100 to 500 μM in the cerebrospinal fluid of affected patients, 20- to 100-fold higher than levels in their plasma. More severe clinical phenotypes are associated with higher SAICA riboside levels and with lower ratios of S-Ado/SAICA riboside in cerebrospinal fluid.

DISORDERS OF PYRIMIDINE METABOLISM

Hereditary Oroticaciduria

Hereditary oroticaciduria is a rare disorder of de novo pyrimidine biosynthesis associated with macrocytic, hypochromic anemia, leukopenia, retarded growth and development, and the overexcretion of urinary orotic acid. The last feature is often associated with orotic acid crystalluria or renal stones. The disorder results from mutations in the gene for uridine monophosphate (UMP) synthase on chromosome 3q, which encodes a bifunctional enzyme that in two steps catalyzes the conversion of orotic acid to UMP. Depletion of UMP results in a diminished ability to synthesize both RNA and DNA. Administering the nucleoside uridine is effective treatment because it can be directly converted to UMP via the salvage enzyme uridine kinase.

Pyrimidine 5′-Nucleotidase Deficiency

Pyrimidine 5′-nucleotidase deficiency is a rare autosomal recessive disorder that results in hemolytic anemia and prominent basophilic stippling of red blood cells. Erythrocytes contain high levels of cytidine and uridine monophosphate, the enzyme substrates, as well as pyrimidine nucleotide conjugates, including cytidine diphosphate–choline, cytidine diphosphate–ethanolamine, and uridine diphosphate–glucose. Hemolysis is believed to result in part from increased oxidative stress secondary to inhibition of the pentose phosphate shunt pathway. An acquired pyrimidine 5′-nucleotidase deficiency has been associated with lead toxicity, which is also characterized by anemia and basophilic erythrocyte stippling (as a result of undegraded ribosomal nucleoprotein). Diagnosis of the hereditary disorder is made by measuring erythrocyte pyrimidine 5′-nucleotidase enzymatic activity. A change from normal controls in the ultraviolet absorption spectra of red blood cell lysates, reflecting elevated pyrimidine nucleotides, has been used as a screening test for the disorder.

Dihydropyrimidine Dehydrogenase Deficiency

Dihydropyrimidine dehydrogenase deficiency is a rare autosomal recessive disorder that prevents degradation of the pyrimidine bases uracil and thymidine. High levels of these metabolites are found in urine and may be detected during screening for organic aciduria. Although no consistent clinical symptoms have been associated with this defect, administration of fluoropyrimidines (5-fluorouracil, 5-fluorodeoxyuridine) to enzyme-deficient patients with malignancy can result in severe and prolonged drug-related neurotoxicity.

Mitochondrial Myopathy, Peripheral Neuropathy, Gastrointestinal Disease, and Encephalopathy

The syndrome of *mitochondrial myopathy, peripheral neuropathy, gastrointestinal disease, and encephalopathy (MNGIE)* is an autosomoal recessive disorder of mitochondrial respiratory chain function. Usually seen between the ages of 10 and 40 years, severe diarrhea, cachexia, ptosis, ophthalmoparesis, peripheral neuropathy, and encephalopathy develop in affected patients. Muscle biopsy tissue shows ragged red fibers and focal deficiency of cytochrome *c* oxidase; these findings have been related to multiple point mutations and deletions of mitochondrial DNA. This rare syndrome results from loss-of-function mutations in the chromosome 22q–encoded gene for the cytoplasmic enzyme thymidine phosphorylase, which catalyzes the cleavage of thymidine and deoxyuridine. The disorder may be diagnosed by measuring thymidine phosphorylase activity in buffy coat cells or by demonstrating elevated plasma levels of thymidine and deoxyuridine. It is thought that high levels of these nucleosides cause an elevation in mitochondrial thymidine triphosphate, and this in turn is mutagenic to mitochondrial DNA. No treatment is currently available.

SUGGESTED READINGS

Booth C, Hershfield M, Notarangelo L, et al: Management options for adenosine deaminase deficiency; proceedings of the EBMT satellite workshop (Hamburg, March 2006). Clin Immunol 2007. *A review of the management options for adenosine deaminase (ADA) deficiency.*

Hershfield MS: New insights into adenosine-receptor–mediated immunosuppression and the role of adenosine in causing the immunodeficiency associated with adenosine deaminase deficiency. Eur J Immunol 2005;35:25–30. *Reviews mechanisms by which adenosine-mediated signal transduction may contribute to immune deficiency.*

Nishigaki Y, Marti R, Copeland WC, Hirano M: Site-specific somatic mitochondrial DNA point mutations in patients with thymidine phosphorylase deficiency. J Clin Invest 2003;111:1913–1921. *How imbalances in mitochondrial nucleotide pools may lead to respiratory chain dysfunction.*

Nyhan WL: Disorders of purine and pyrimidine metabolism. Mol Genet Metab 2005;86:25–33. *An overivew of the clinical presentations and mechanisms of the disorders of purine and pyrimidine metabolism.*

Nyhan WL: Lesch-Nyhan disease. Hist Neurosci 2005;14:1–10. *A generalized overview of Lesch-Nyhan disease.*

Pais VM Jr, Lowe G, Lallas CD, et al: Xanthine urolithiasis. Urology 2006;67:1084. *A review of the underlying pathophysiology and approach to treatment in patients with xanthine urolithiasis.*

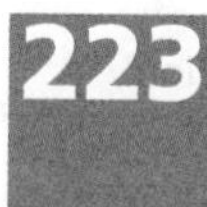

223 LYSOSOMAL STORAGE DISEASES

Margaret M. McGovern and Robert J. Desnick

The lysosomal storage diseases are a family of more than 40 disorders resulting from different defects in lysosomal function. Although most of these disorders are caused by deficiency of a specific hydrolytic enzyme, others are due to impaired receptors or deficiencies of crucial cofactors or protective proteins. Prevalent among these disorders are Fabry's disease, Gaucher's disease, and Niemann-Pick disease (NPD)—lipid storage diseases that result from mutations in specific genes encoding lipid-degrading enzymes. The respective enzymatic defects lead to the storage of specific lipids and their metabolites in lysosomes. All three of these disorders have later-onset forms that can be manifested clinically in adult life. In addition, Gaucher's disease and NPD have severe, fatal infantile forms that are described briefly.

FABRY'S DISEASE

Definition

Fabry's disease is an X-linked recessive inborn error of glycosphingolipid metabolism. The classic phenotype occurs in childhood and is characterized by angiokeratomas (telangiectatic skin lesions), hypohidrosis, corneal and lenticular opacities, acroparesthesias, and vascular disease of the kidney, heart, and brain. The disease has an estimated incidence of about 1 in 40,000 males. Later-onset affected males with residual α-galactosidase A activity may have cardiac or renal disease (or both), including hypertrophic cardiomyopathy and renal failure. Females heterozygous for the classic phenotype can be asymptomatic or as severely affected as males, the variability being due to random inactivation of the X chromosome. There is limited information available on the manifestations in heterozygotes for the later-onset phenotypes.

Pathobiology

The disease results from mutations in the α-galactosidase A gene, which encodes lysosomal hydrolase α-galactosidase A (Table 223–1). The enzyme deficiency in classically affected males leads to the accumulation of globotriaosylceramide and related glycosphingolipids with terminal α-galactosyl moieties in the plasma and lysosomes of endothelial, perithelial, and smooth muscle cells of blood vessels. These glycosphingolipid deposits are also prominent in epithelial cells of the cornea, in the glomeruli and tubules of the kidney, in muscle fibers of the heart, and in ganglion cells of the dorsal roots and autonomic nervous system. The skin lesions are telangiectases. The larger lesions are usually located in the upper dermis, where they may produce elevation, flattening, or hypertrophy of the epithelium along with keratosis, hence the term *angiokeratoma.* Ultrastructurally, the glycosphingolipid inclusions in lysosomes have a concentrically arranged lamellar or myelin-like structure. Later-onset patients lack the vascular endothelial glycosphingolipid deposition that is responsible for the early manifestations in the classic phenotype.

Clinical Manifestations

Affected males with the classic phenotype have the skin lesions, acroparesthesias, hypohidrosis, and ocular changes, whereas males with the later-onset phenotypes lack these findings and have cardiac or renal disease (or both) in adulthood. Angiokeratomas usually occur in childhood, which may lead to early diagnosis. They increase in size and number with age and range from barely visible to several millimeters in diameter. The lesions are punctate, dark red to blue-black, and flat or slightly raised. They do not blanch with pressure, and the larger ones may show slight hyperkeratosis. Characteristically, the lesions are most dense between the umbilicus and the knees, in the "bathing trunk area," but they may occur anywhere, including the oral mucosa. The hips, thighs, buttocks, umbilicus, lower part of the abdomen, scrotum, and glans penis are common sites, and a tendency toward bilateral symmetry is noted. Variants without skin lesions have been described. Sweating is usually decreased or absent. Corneal opacities and characteristic lenticular lesions, observed by slit lamp examination, are present in affected male patients, as well as in about 70 to 80% of heterozygotes for the classic phenotype. Conjunctival and retinal vascular tortuosity is common and results from systemic vascular involvement.

Pain is the most debilitating symptom in childhood and adolescence. Fabry crises, lasting from minutes to several days, consist of agonizing, burning pain in the hands and feet and proximal parts of the extremities and are usually associated with exercise, fatigue, and fever. These painful acroparesthesias usually become less frequent in the third and fourth decades of life, although in some men they may become more frequent and severe. Attacks of abdominal or flank pain may simulate appendicitis or renal colic.

With increasing age, the major morbid symptoms result from progressive involvement of the vascular system. Early in the course of the disease, casts, red blood cells, and lipid inclusions with characteristic birefringent "Maltese crosses" appear in the urinary sediment. Proteinuria, isosthenuria, gradual deterioration in renal function, and the development of azotemia occur in the second to fourth decades. Cardiovascular findings may include hypertension, left ventricular hypertrophy, anginal chest pain, myocardial ischemia or infarction, and congestive heart failure. Mitral insufficiency is the most common valvar lesion. Abnormal electrocardiographic and echocardiographic findings are common. Cerebrovascular manifestations result primarily from multifocal small vessel involvement. Other features may include obstructive airway disease that increases with age, lymphedema of the legs without hypoproteinemia, episodic diarrhea, osteoporosis, retarded growth, and delayed puberty. Death most often results from uremia or vascular disease of the heart or brain. Before the advent of hemodialysis and renal transplantation, the mean age at death in affected men was 40 years.

Patients with later-onset cardiac variants and residual α-galactosidase A activity have cardiac disease and may have mild proteinuria but usually have normal renal function for age. The cardiac manifestations include hypertrophy of the left ventricular wall and interventricular septum and electrocardiographic abnormalities consistent with cardiomyopathy. Others have had hypertrophic cardiomyopathy or myocardial infarction, or both.

Diagnosis

The diagnosis of Fabry's disease in classically affected males should be pursued in individuals who have acroparesthesias, hypohidrosis, characteristic skin lesions, corneal opacities, or lenticular lesions. The diagnosis of classic and variant cases is confirmed biochemically by markedly

TABLE 223–1 BIOCHEMICAL AND PHENOTYPIC CHARACTERISTICS OF LYSOSOMAL STORAGE DISEASES

Disease	Deficiency	Substance Accumulated	Site	Complications
Fabry	α-Galactosidase A	Primarily globotriaosylceramide	Most cells, particularly vascular endothelial and smooth muscle cells	Ischemia, infarction
Gaucher				
Type 1	Acid β-glucosidase	Primarily glucosylceramide	Macrophage-monocyte system hepatosplenomegaly, skeletal complications	Infiltration of bone marrow, progressive
Type 2	Acid β-glucosidase	Primarily glucosylceramide	Macrophage-monocyte system, CNS hepatosplenomegaly, skeletal complications, neurodegeneration	Infiltration of bone marrow, progressive
Type 3	Acid β-glucosidase	Primarily glucosylceramide	Macrophage-monocyte system, CNS	Progressive neurodegeneration
Niemann-Pick				
Type A	Acid sphingomyelinase	Sphingomyelin	Monocyte-macrophage system, CNS	Hepatosplenomegaly, progressive neurodegeneration
Type B	Acid sphingomyelinase	Sphingomyelin	Monocyte-macrophage system	Progressive hepatosplenomegaly, infiltrative lung disease
Type C	Abnormal cholesterol transport	Primarily cholesterol	Most cells, especially liver, CNS	Hepatosplenomegaly, progressive neurodegeneration

CNS = central nervous system.

decreased α-galactosidase A activity in plasma, isolated leukocytes, or cultured fibroblasts or lymphoblasts. Variants lack the early classic manifestations.

Females heterozygous for the classic phenotype may have corneal opacities, isolated skin lesions, and low to normal activities of α-galactosidase A in plasma or cell sources. Rare female heterozygotes may have manifestations as severe as those in affected male subjects. However, in asymptomatic, at-risk female members of families affected by Fabry's disease, optimal diagnosis should be by direct analysis of the family's specific mutation. Prenatal detection of affected male fetuses can be accomplished by demonstrating deficient α-galactosidase A activity or by detecting the family's specific gene mutation in chorionic villi obtained in the first trimester of pregnancy or in cultured amniocytes obtained by amniocentesis in the second trimester.

Differential Diagnosis

Fabry's disease is often misdiagnosed as rheumatic fever, erythromyalgia, or neurosis. The skin lesions must be differentiated from benign angiokeratomas of the scrotum (Fordyce's disease) and from angiokeratoma circumscriptum. Angiokeratomas identical to those of Fabry's disease have been reported in patients with fucosidosis, aspartylglycosaminuria, late-onset GM_1 gangliosidosis, galactosialidosis, α-*N*-acetylgalactosaminidase deficiency, and sialidosis. Diagnosis of later-onset cardiac variants should be considered in individuals with left ventricular hypertrophy or cardiomyopathy. Recently, later-onset variants have been identified in chronic hemodialysis patients.

Treatment

Rx

Clinical trials with recombinant α-galactosidase (Fabrazyme, Genzyme Corporation, Cambridge, MA; Replagal, TKT Corporation, Cambridge, MA) have revealed the safety and effectiveness of enzyme replacement therapy for Fabry's disease at a dose of 1 mg/kg every other week. The enzyme replacement therapy is available in Europe and has been approved by the U.S. Food and Drug

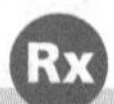

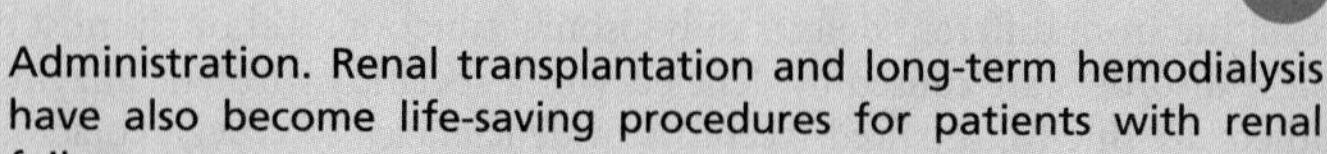
Administration. Renal transplantation and long-term hemodialysis have also become life-saving procedures for patients with renal failure.

GAUCHER'S DISEASE

Definition

Gaucher's disease is a glycolipid storage disease characterized by the deposition of glucocerebroside in cells of the macrophage-monocyte system. Three clinical subtypes are delineated by the absence or presence and progression of neurologic involvement: type 1, the adult non-neuronopathic form; type 2, the infantile or acute neuronopathic form; and type 3, the juvenile or subacute neuronopathic form. All three subtypes are inherited as autosomal recessive traits.

Epidemiology

Type 1 disease is the most common lysosomal storage disease and the most prevalent genetic disorder in Ashkenazi Jewish individuals, with an incidence of about 1 in 1000 and a carrier frequency of about 1 in 16 to 18.

Pathobiology

Etiology

All three subtypes of Gaucher's disease result from deficient activity of lysosomal hydrolase acid β-glucosidase (see Table 223–1). The molecular basis of Gaucher's disease has been identified for more than 95% of Ashkenazi Jewish patients (Table 223–2). Genotype/phenotype correlations have been noted for the different subtypes, particularly type 1 Gaucher's disease. Presumably, the amount of residual enzymatic activity determines the disease subtype and severity. For example, type 1 patients homozygous for the milder *N370S* mutation tend to have a later onset and milder course than do patients with one *N370S* allele and another mutant allele. However, the wide variability in clinical findings among patients with Gaucher's disease cannot be fully explained by the nature of the underlying acid β-glucosidase mutations. The lesions causing the severe type 2 (infantile) disease express little if any enzymatic activity in vitro.

Pathology

The pathologic hallmark is the presence of Gaucher cells in the macrophage-monocyte system, particularly in the bone marrow. These cells, which are 20 to 100 μm in diameter, have a characteristic wrinkled-paper appearance resulting from intracytoplasmic substrate deposition. These cells stain strongly positive with periodic acid–Schiff stain, and their presence in bone marrow or other tissues suggests the diagnosis (Fig. 223–1). The accumulated glycolipid glucosylceramide is derived primarily from the phagocytosis and degradation of senescent leukocytes and to a lesser extent from erythrocyte membranes. Glycolipid storage results in organomegaly and pulmonary infiltration. Neuronal cell loss in patients with type 2 and 3 disease is presumably caused by accumulation of the cytotoxic glycolipid glucosylsphingosine in the brain as a result of the severe deficiency of acid β-glucosidase activity. Accumulation of glucosylceramide in the bone marrow, liver, spleen, lungs, and kidney leads to pancytopenia, massive hepatosplenomegaly, and occasionally, diffuse infiltrative pulmonary disease and nephropathy or glomerulonephritis. The progressive infiltration of Gaucher cells into bone marrow causes thinning of the cortex, pathologic fractures, bone pain, bony infarcts, and osteopenia. Central nervous system involvement occurs only in patients with type 2 and 3 disease.

Clinical Manifestations

A broad spectrum of clinical expression is seen in patients with type 1 disease, in part because of a combination of different mutant alleles and unidentified modifier genes. The onset of clinical manifestations occurs from early childhood to late adulthood. At examination, patients may display easy bruisability because of thrombocytopenia, chronic fatigue secondary to anemia, hepatomegaly with or without elevated liver function test results, splenomegaly, and bone pain or pathologic fractures. Occasional patients have pulmonary involvement. Patients whose disease is diagnosed in the first 5 years of life are frequently non-Jewish and typically have a more malignant disease course. Patients with milder disease are discovered later in life during evaluation for hematologic or skeletal problems or are found to have splenomegaly on routine examination. In symptomatic patients, the splenomegaly is progressive and can become massive. Clinically apparent bone involvement, which occurs in more than 20% of patients, can be manifested as bone pain or pathologic fractures. Most patients have radiologic evidence of skeletal involvement, including an Erlenmeyer flask deformity of the distal end of the femur and osteopenia, which are early skeletal changes. In patients with symptomatic bone disease, lytic lesions can develop in the long bones, ribs, and pelvis, and osteosclerosis may be evident at an early age. Bone crises with severe pain and swelling can occur. Bleeding secondary to thrombocytopenia may be manifested as epistaxis and bruising and is frequently overlooked until other symptoms become apparent. Children with massive splenomegaly are short in stature because of the energy expenditure required by the enlarged organ.

Type 2 disease, which is rare and panethnic in distribution, is characterized by a rapid neurodegenerative course with extensive visceral involvement and death within the first 2 years of life. The disease occurs

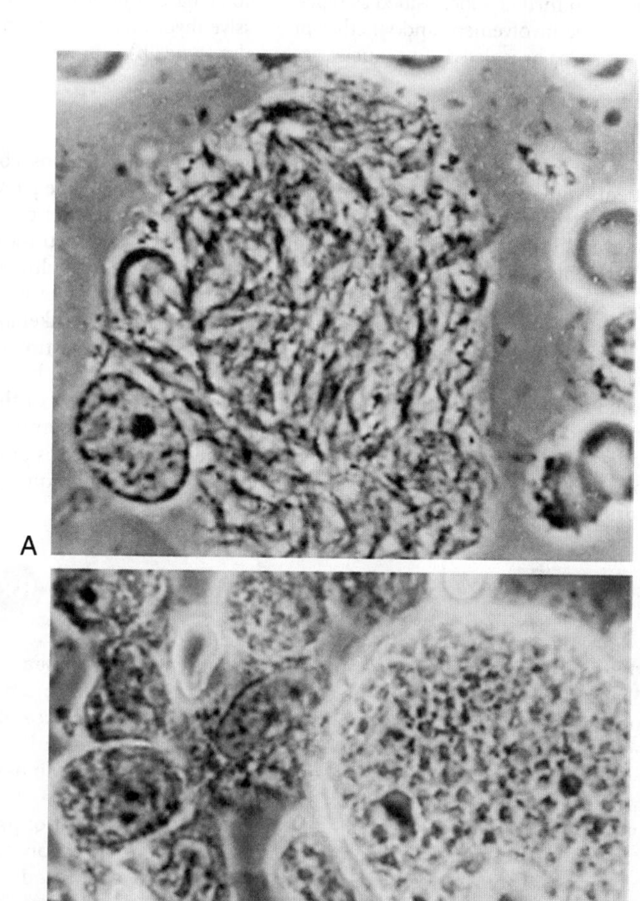

FIGURE 223–1 • Niemann-Pick disease. Gaucher cell (A) and a foam cell (B) seen in a case of Niemann-Pick disease. Both are viewed under phase microscopy with unstained smears of aspirated bone marrow. Magnification can be estimated from adjacent red blood cells.

TABLE 223–2 MOLECULAR GENETICS OF FABRY'S, GAUCHER'S, AND NIEMANN–PICK DISEASES

Disease	Chromosome Assignment	Molecular Characteristics	Comments
Fabry	Xq22.1	cDNA, entire genomic sequences, >450 mutant alleles known	More than 450 private mutations detected in a single or a few families
Gaucher	1q21	cDNA, functional and pseudogenomic sequences, >200 mutant alleles known	Four mutations (N370S, L444P, 84insG, IVS2+1) account for 90 to >95% of mutant alleles in Ashkenazi Jewish patients
Niemann-Pick			
Types A and B	11p15.1 to p15.4	cDNA, entire genomic sequence, >100 mutant alleles known	Four mutations account for >95% of mutant alleles in Ashkenazi Jewish patients with type A disease
Type C	18q11-q12 region	cDNA, entire genomic sequence, >100 mutant alleles known	More than 100 mutations in the *NPC1* gene

cDNA = complementary DNA; mRNA = messenger RNA.

in infancy and is associated with increased tone, strabismus, and organomegaly. Failure to thrive and stridor from laryngospasm are typical. The progressive psychomotor degeneration leads to death, usually secondary to an intercurrent respiratory infection and respiratory compromise.

Type 3 disease is noted in infancy or childhood. In addition to the organomegaly and bone involvement, patients have neurodegenerative manifestations. Type 3 disease is most frequent in Sweden (1 in 50,000), where it has been traced to a common founder in the 17th century. Type 3 has been further subclassified as types 3a and 3b based on the extent of neurologic involvement and whether progressive myotonia and dementia (type 3a) or isolated supranuclear gaze palsy (type 3b) is present.

Diagnosis

Gaucher's disease should be considered in the differential diagnosis of patients with unexplained organomegaly, easy bruisability, or bone pain. Bone marrow examination usually reveals the presence of Gaucher cells; however, all suspected diagnoses should be confirmed by demonstration of deficient acid β-glucosidase activity in isolated leukocytes or cultured cells. For possible genotype/phenotype correlations, the specific acid β-glucosidase mutation may be determined, particularly in Ashkenazi Jewish patients. Carrier identification is best achieved by DNA testing in Jewish families. Testing should be offered to all family members, but it should be kept in mind that heterogeneity, even among members of the same kindred, can be so great that cases may be diagnosed in asymptomatic affected individuals during such testing. Prenatal diagnosis is possible by determining the enzymatic activity or specific mutations in chorionic villi or cultured amniotic fluid cells.

Treatment

Rx

Enzyme replacement with recombinant acid β-glucosidase is available for the treatment of symptomatic patients with type 1 disease. Clinical trials have demonstrated that most extraskeletal symptoms are reversed within 12 to 36 months by an initial debulking dose of enzyme (60 IU/kg) administered by intravenous infusion every other week. Early treatment may be efficacious in normalizing linear growth and bone morphology in affected children. Efforts are also under way to develop gene therapy for type 1 disease. Although enzyme replacement does not alter the neurologic progression of patients with types 2 and 3 Gaucher's disease, it has been used in selected patients as a palliative measure, particularly in type 3 patients with severe visceral involvement. Alternative treatments are also being evaluated, including the use of agents designed to decrease the synthesis of glucosylceramide by chemical inhibition of glucosylceramide synthase.

NIEMANN-PICK DISEASE

Definition

NPD types A and B are lipid storage disorders that result from deficiency of the lysosomal enzyme acid sphingomyelinase and subsequent accumulation of its substrate sphingomyelin. The original description of NPD referred to what is now known as type A NPD, which is a fatal disorder of infancy characterized by failure to thrive, hepatosplenomegaly, and a rapidly progressive neurodegenerative course that leads to death by the age of 2 or 3 years. Type B is a non-neuronopathic form observed in children and adults. Type C NPD results from defective cholesterol transport. Previously, a type D disease was identified in patients from Nova Scotia; however, these patients actually have a form of type C disease. All the subtypes are inherited as autosomal recessive traits and display variable clinical features.

Pathobiology

Etiology

NPD types A and B result from deficient acid sphingomyelinase activity (see Table 223–1). In type C NPD, the genetic defect involves the defective transport of cholesterol from the lysosome to the cytosol. The identification of two different genes causing the altered cholesterol transport in type C disease (*NPC1* and *NPC2*) has permitted more precise diagnosis, carrier detection, and prenatal diagnosis in affected families.

Pathology

The pathologic hallmark in NPD types A and B is the histochemically characteristic lipid-laden foam cell, often referred to as the *Niemann-Pick cell*. These cells, which can be readily distinguished from Gaucher cells by their histologic and histochemical characteristics, are not pathognomonic for NPD because histologically similar cells are found in patients with Wolman's disease, cholesterol ester storage disease, and lipoprotein lipase deficiency, as well as in some patients with GM_1 gangliosidosis type 2. Sphingomyelin is the major lipid that accumulates in the cells and tissues of patients with type A and B NPD. In most normal tissues, sphingomyelin constitutes 5 to 20% of the total cellular phospholipid content; however, in patients with type A and B disease, sphingomyelin levels may be elevated up to 50-fold and thus constitute about 70% of the total phospholipid fraction. Lysosomal sphingomyelin accumulation in the brain, liver, kidneys, and lungs has been documented in organs from patients with NPD types A and B; they contain about the same amount of sphingomyelin, with the notable exception that patients with type B NPD have little or no lipid storage in their central nervous system. In general, patients with type A disease have less than 1% of normal acid sphingomyelinase in cultured fibroblasts and lymphocytes, whereas cells from type B patients typically have some residual activity, which prevents the development of neurologic symptoms.

Clinical Manifestations

The clinical features and course of type A disease are relatively uniform and characterized by normal appearance at birth, with the first signs being hepatosplenomegaly and psychomotor retardation, which are usually evident by 6 months of life and are followed by rapid neurodegeneration. The loss of motor function and deterioration in intellectual capabilities are progressive. In later stages, spasticity and rigidity are evident, with affected infants experiencing complete loss of contact with their environment.

Natural History

In contrast to the predictable natural history of the type A phenotype, the clinical features and course in patients with type B disease are variable. Most cases are diagnosed in infancy or childhood, when enlargement of the liver, spleen, or both is detected during routine physical examination. At diagnosis, type B patients also have evidence of mild pulmonary involvement, usually detected as a diffuse reticular or finely nodular infiltration on chest radiography. In most patients, hepatosplenomegaly is particularly prominent in childhood, but with increasing linear growth the abdominal protuberance decreases and becomes less conspicuous. In mildly affected patients, the splenomegaly may not be noted until adulthood. In most patients with type B disease, decreased pulmonary diffusion secondary to alveolar infiltration becomes evident in childhood and progresses with age. Severely affected individuals may experience significant pulmonary compromise by the age of 15 to 20 years. Such patients have low PO_2 values and dyspnea on exertion. Life-threatening bronchopneumonia may occur, and cor pulmonale has been described. Severely affected patients may also have liver involvement leading to life-threatening cirrhosis, portal hypertension, and ascites. Clinically significant pancytopenia from secondary hypersplenism occurs rarely but may necessitate partial or total splenectomy. However, removal of the spleen can lead to significant worsening of the pulmonary involvement. Cholesterol abnormalities characterized by low high-density lipoprotein cholesterol and increased total cholesterol are found in most patients and can be associated with early atherosclerotic changes. Typically, patients with type B disease do not have neurologic involvement and are intellectually intact.

Patients with NPD type C often have prolonged neonatal jaundice, appear normal for 1 to 2 years, and then experience a slowly progressive and variable neurodegenerative course. Their hepatosplenomegaly is less severe than that in patients with type A or B disease, and they may survive into adulthood.

Diagnosis

Type A disease is diagnosed in the patient's first year of life by failure to thrive, organomegaly, and severe psychomotor retardation. In patients with type B disease, splenomegaly is usually noted early in childhood; however, in very mild cases, the enlargement may be subtle and detection may be delayed until adolescence or adulthood. The presence of the characteristic Niemann-Pick cells in bone marrow supports the diagnosis. However, patients with type C disease also have infiltration of these cells into bone marrow. Thus, all suspected cases should be evaluated enzymatically or molecularly to confirm the clinical diagnosis by measuring the acid sphingomyelinase activity in peripheral leukocytes, cultured fibroblasts, and lymphoblasts or by determining the precise NPD mutations. Patients with type A and B disease have markedly decreased levels of enzymatic activity (1 to 10% of normal), whereas patients with type C disease may have slightly decreased sphingomyelinase activity (50 to 75% of normal). Type C disease can be biochemically documented by demonstrating the cholesterol transport defect in cultured fibroblasts or by determining the specific mutations in the *NPC1* or *NPC2* genes. Enzymatic identification of heterozygotes for types A, B, and C is problematic. However, in families in which the specific molecular lesion has been identified, members can be accurately tested for heterozygote status by DNA analysis. Prenatal diagnosis of type A and B disease can be reliably made by measuring acid sphingomyelinase activity in cultured amniocytes or chorionic villi. In type C disease, the cholesterol defect can be demonstrated by filipin staining, but DNA diagnosis using fetal cells is most accurate.

Treatment

Rx

At present, no specific treatment is available for any of the NPD subtypes. Orthotopic liver transplantation in an infant with type A disease and amniotic cell transplantation in several patients with type B disease have been attempted without success. Bone marrow transplantation in a small number of patients with type B NPD has been shown to be successful in reducing spleen and liver volume, the sphingomyelin content of the liver, the number of Niemann-Pick cells in the marrow, and radiologically detected infiltration of the lungs. However, in one patient, liver biopsy specimens taken up to 33 months after transplantation showed only a moderate reduction in stored sphingomyelin. To date, lung transplantation has not been performed in any severely compromised patient with type B disease, although two patients have been reported who underwent whole lung lavage. The first, an adult, showed initial improvement in resting arterial oxygen tension but was then lost to follow-up, whereas the second, a child, continued to have progressive respiratory failure and succumbed. Future prospects for treatment of type B disease include enzyme replacement and gene therapy. Treatment of type A and C disease is currently precluded by the severe neurologic involvement.

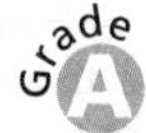

1. Banikazemi M, Bultas J, Waldek S, et al: Agalsidase-beta therapy for advanced Fabry disease: A randomized trial. Ann Intern Med 2007;146:77–886.

SUGGESTED READINGS

Butters TD, Dwek RA, Platt FM: Imino sugar inhibitors for treating the lysosomal glycosphingolipidoses. Glycobiology 2005;15:43R–52R. *Intravenous enzyme supplementation therapy is the treatment of choice for moderate or severe disease, but in mildly affected patients, an oral substrate inhibitor can be considered if intravenous treatment is less attractive.*

Desnick RJ, Brady R, Barranger J, et al: Fabry disease, an under-recognized multisystemic disorder: Expert recommendations for diagnosis, management, and enzyme replacement therapy. Ann Intern Med 2003;138:338–346. *Recommendations for clinicians.*

Eng CM, Fletcher J, Wilcox WR, et al: Fabry disease: Baseline medical characteristics of a cohort of 1765 males and females in the Fabry Registry. J Inherit Metab Dis 2007;30:184–192. *Baseline characteristics of the first 1765 patients in the Fabry Registry.*

Imrie J, Dasgupta S, Besley GT, et al: The natural history of Niemann-Pick disease type C in the UK. J Inherit Metab Dis 2007;30:51–59. *There is a wide range of phenotypic variability and a paucity of treatment options.*

Keating GM, Simpson D: Agalsidase beta: A review of its use iin the management of Fabry disease. Drugs 2007:67:435–455. *An important advance in the treatment of Fabry disease.*

Vellodi A: Lysosomal storage disorders. Br J Haematol 2005;128:413–431. *A detailed review.*

224 DISORDERS OF PHENYLALANINE AND TYROSINE METABOLISM

Stephen D. Cederbaum

Until recently, the inclusion of any disorder of phenylalanine or tyrosine metabolism, except for alkaptonuria, in a textbook of internal medicine would have been considered unnecessary. However, the striking success of treatment for phenylketonuria and, more recently, for hepatorenal tyrosinemia has thrust them both firmly into the realm of adult metabolic disorders. Phenylketonuria (MIM 261600; Online Mendelian Inheritance in Man [catalogues of mendelian traits]; available at *www.ncbi.nlm.nih.gov/OMIM*), the best known of these disorders, may no longer be considered a disease, although it continues to be a risk factor, because its principal manifestations (mental retardation, pigment dilution, mousy odor, neurotransmitter deficiency) occur only in rare cases in patients who escape early diagnosis and/or effective treatment. This satisfactory turn of events came about because the pathogenesis from hyperphenylalaninemia (HPA; the risk factor) is offset by treatment (a low-phenylalanine diet).

Figure 224–1 gives a brief outline of the main catabolic pathway for phenylalanine and tyrosine. The sites of the enzyme deficiency in HPA, alkaptonuria, and hepatorenal tyrosinemia are indicated by number.

HYPERPHENYLALANINEMIAS

Phenylalanine Metabolism

Phenylalanine is an essential amino acid. The normal concentration in plasma is less than 125 μmol/L. Metabolic utilization is largely controlled by a hydroxylation reaction (see Fig. 224-1A), and impaired hydroxylation is the chief explanation for HPA. The reaction requires the apoenzyme phenylalanine hydroxylase (PAH, a monooxygenase), molecular oxygen, and tetrahydrobiopterin (BH4) cofactor; the last-named is consumed in stoichiometric amounts to form tyrosine, the reaction product. The catalytic property of PAH requires both moment-to-moment regeneration of BH4 from 4α-carbinolamine and dihydrobiopterin, consecutive byproducts of the hydroxylation reaction, and long-term renewal of the BH4 pool by synthesis from precursors. The former is achieved by the enzymes 2′-ketotetrahydropterin reductase and dihydropteridine reductase, the latter by a synthesis pathway in which two enzymes act in sequence, guanosine triphosphate cyclohydrolase 1 and 6-pyruvoyl tetrahydropterin synthase. Accordingly, there are several ways to impair phenylalanine hydroxylation. Failure to recognize the biologic heterogeneity of HPA may lead to erroneous counseling and the wrong treatment; all its forms require special management of women during the reproductive years.

Genetic forms of HPA are described here; they are all autosomal recessive disorders. Approximately 0.01% of live births are affected. Physicians of adult patients must be aware of maternal HPA and its consequences for the fetus (see later).

Disorders of Phenylalanine Hydroxylase Integrity

The PAH enzyme is multimeric and homopolymeric. The polypeptide is encoded by a gene on chromosome 12, region q24.1, which is expressed principally in the liver in humans. *PAH* mutations range from "severe"

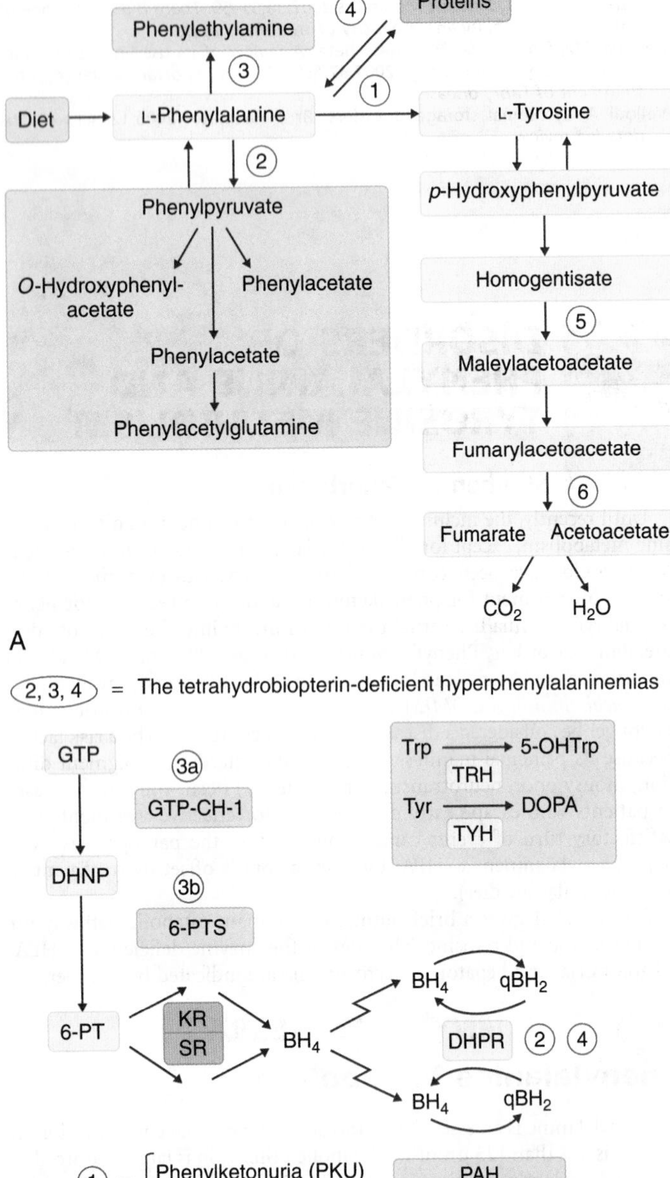

FIGURE 224–1 • Catabolic pathway for phenylalanine and tyrosine. A, Intake of phenylalanine (an essential amino acid supplied only by diet) and its disposal by hydroxylation (1) (representing three fourths of normal runout), transamination (2), decarboxylation (3), and incorporation into proteins (4) (representing a fourth of runout). The subsequent catabolism of tyrosine is depicted on the right side of the panel. The enzymes whose deficiency causes alkaptonuria, homogentisic acid oxidase, and hepatorenal tyrosinemia, fumarylacetoacetate hydrolase, are indicated by numbers 5 and 6. **B,** Interrelations among phenylalanine hydroxylase (PAH), dihydropteridine reductase (DHPR), and the tetrahydrobiopterin (BH4) biosynthesis pathway serving aromatic amino acid hydroxylation reactions. Mutations at the relevant chromosomal loci impair the hydroxylation reactions with effects on PAH activity only (1), DHPR activity (2), guanosine triphosphate (GTP)-cyclohydrolase 1 (GTP-CH-1) activity (3a), 6-pyruvoyl tetrahydropterin synthase activity (6-PTS) (3b), and 4α-carbinolamine dehydratase (4). Disorders 2, 3a, 3b, and 4 can impair function of three hydroxylases: PAH, tyrosine hydroxylase (TYH), and tryptophan hydroxylase (TRH). DHNP = dihydroneopterin triphosphate; KR = 2′-ketotetrahydropterin reductase; 6-PT = 6-pyruvoyl tetrahydropterin; qBH2 = quinonoid dihydrobiopterin; SR = sepiapterin reductase.

and cause phenylketonuria (with plasma phenylalanine values >1 mM on a normal diet) to "mild" and cause nonphenylketonuric HPA (values <1 mM but >0.125 mM). Phenylketonuria is typically associated with mental retardation in the untreated patient. If hydroxylation activity is deficient and dietary intake is not curtailed, free phenylalanine accumulates in the body. Overburden of phenylalanine impairs brain development in ways still not fully understood. The risk of mental retardation without treatment is thought to be quite low in those individuals whose phenylalanine values are consistently lower than 625 μM. The incidence and relative frequencies of the two forms (together ~1 per 10,000 births) vary widely among populations.

Phenylketonuria was first described as a clinical entity in 1934. In the following 3 decades, phenylketonuria was seen as a paradigm for the biochemical basis of mental disease, of disease that could be prevented by deliberately restoring normal metabolism, and of chemical individuality that could be used as the basis for a screening test and early diagnosis. Newborn screening for HPA (and other disorders) is now one of the most widely applied "genetic" tests. The incidence of the risk factor has not changed, but the frequency of the associated disease is now trivial in screened populations.

Tetrahydrobiopterin-Deficient Forms of Hyperphenylalaninemia

Not every case of persistent HPA is explained by a primary hydroxylase deficiency. BH4 insufficiency impairs function of three hydroxylases (for phenylalanine, tryptophan, and tyrosine) and synthesis of their products, notably 5-hydroxytryptophan (the precursor of serotonin) and L-dopa (the precursor of catecholamines) (see Fig. 224–1B). The products function as neurotransmitters in the brain, and a deficiency of them gives rise to central nervous system disease (including retarded psychomotor development, basal ganglion dysfunction, and unstable body temperature), even when the elevated phenylalanine levels are controlled by diet. Deficient activity of guanosine triphosphate cycolohydrolase 1 (GCH1), 6-pyruvoyl tetrahydropterin synthase, 2′-ketotetrahydropterin reductase, or dihydropteridine reductase impairs the synthesis of BH4 and accounts for approximately 1% of cases of HPA ascertained in the newborn period. It is increasingly clear that inherited disorders of neurotransmitter metabolism in the brain may occur in the absence of elevation of plasma phenylalanine and may cause similar neurologic symptoms.

Pathobiology

Mutant alleles (at all relevant loci) are recessive. Their aggregate frequency in the population is approximately 0.01, meaning that 2% of the population is heterozygous. Observed explanations for the high allelic frequency of this "rare" phenotype include founder effect and genetic drift in some populations and possibly a selective advantage for carriers of the mutant trait.

Diagnosis: Screening

Screening newborns for HPA is public policy in all developed and many developing countries. Capillary blood collected on filter paper from heel puncture is analyzed by increasingly modern quantitative methods. Blood phenylalanine values greater than approximately 150 μM or ratios of phenylalanine to tyrosine that are greater than 1.5 on the first day of life or thereafter are considered abnormal and require further investigation. The HPA phenotype test is still the most efficient; DNA-based tests detect more than 498 mutations in the *PAH* gene and dozens in the genes controlling BH4 homeostasis, but none are common to every case of HPA.

Every infant with persistent HPA is investigated in specialized centers to rule out disorders of BH4 homeostasis. Prenatal diagnosis for most of these disorders is possible, particularly if mutations are known.

Mutation databases exist for phenylketonuria (*http://www. pahdb. mcgill.ca*) and for disorders of BH4 homeostasis (*http://www.bh4.org*). Routine mutation analysis in the HPAs is much debated, and the benefits, at the moment, are more abstract than real. Progress in the future may tip the balance more heavily toward DNA testing.

Treatment

Rx

The mainstay of treatment for primary PAH deficiency is dietary restriction of the amino acid. Several semisynthetic dietary products ("orphan foods") are available for this purpose. Phenylketonuric patients can tolerate only 250 to 500 mg of phenylalanine per day (normal intake is >1000 mg) to maintain the blood phenylalanine level at less than the ideal level of 350 μM. Intake, blood levels of phenylalanine, and growth rate are monitored at frequent intervals to avoid undertreatment or overtreatment. Treatment into adult life is now recommended to maintain normal neuropsychologic function. Well-treated patients have normal or near-normal intellectual development.

Patients with the BH4-deficient forms of the disorder require continuous replacement therapy of cofactor alone or in combination with neurotransmitter precursors. Whether postnatal treatment of these disorders is fully effective remains to be seen. Some mutations in the *PAH* gene may be partially or almost completely responsive to BH4 as well. BH4 may soon be more widely available.

Prevention: Maternal Hyperphenylalaninemia

Maternal HPA is a problem relevant to all practitioners who counsel women about pregnancy. Intrauterine HPA places the fetus at risk of microcephaly, mental retardation, and organ malformations (notably cardiac). Accordingly, all female patients with HPA should be identified, followed, counseled about risk when they attain reproductive age, and treated with diet to maintain near-normal blood phenylalanine levels before conception and throughout the pregnancy. When the condition is well treated in the mother, pregnancy outcome for the children of women with HPA is generally good. BH4 treatment may also be applicable in pregnancy, but this form of treatment has not been formally assessed and cannot now be recommended.

ALKAPTONURIA

Definition

Alkaptonuria (MIM 203500) is a rare autosomal recessive disorder in which homogentisic acid oxidase activity is deficient (see Fig. 224-1). Homogentisic acid produced during the metabolism of phenylalanine and tyrosine accumulates and is excreted in the urine. It causes pigmentation of cartilage and other connective tissue (ochronosis) and, in later years, degenerative arthritis of the spine and of the larger peripheral joints. The alkaptonuria gene (symbol *AKU*), encoding homogentisic acid oxidase, has been mapped to human chromosome 3q21-q23, it has been cloned and characterized, and mutations have been identified.

Epidemiology

The trait is rare (<1 per 250,000 births), but cases are still being reported (now >600), including one in a 3500-year-old Egyptian mummy.

Pathobiology

Pathogenesis

The activity of homogentisic acid oxidase in the normal adult human liver is sufficient to metabolize more than 1600 g/day of homogentisic acid. Normally, no homogentisic acid can be detected in plasma or urine. Alkaptonuric patients have little or no detectable activity of this enzyme in liver, kidney, or prostate, where it is normally abundant. Plasma levels of homogentisic acid rise to approximately 175 to 200 μM, and the urinary excretion ranges from 4 to 8 g/day. Mammalian tissue also contains an enzyme called homogentisic acid polyphenyloxidase that catalyzes the oxidation of homogentisic acid to an ochronotic pigment, but pigment can also be produced nonenzymatically in the presence of oxygen and alkali, as, for example, in urine. The homogentisic acid polymer has a high affinity for cartilage and connective tissue macromolecules. The stained tissue is fragile and eventually may break down, thereby leading to degenerative intervertebral disc or joint disease. Homogentisic acid may also have a direct effect on collagen synthesis through inhibition of lysyl hydroxylase.

Pathology

In the adult alkaptonuric patient, costal, laryngeal, and tracheal cartilages are densely pigmented. Pigmentation is also present throughout the body in fibrous tissue, fibrocartilage, tendons, ligaments, epidermis, endocardium, and intima of larger vessels in various organs.

Clinical Manifestations

Homogentisic acid is present in urine from birth. Urine is colorless when passed but darkens when alkaline or after long exposure to air. Generally, the earliest physical sign is a slight pigmentation of the sclerae or the ears, beginning at age 20 to 30 years. The cartilage of the ears may be slate blue or gray and may feel irregular and thickened. Sometimes dusky discolorations of underlying tendons can be seen through the skin over the hands. Pigment in perspiration stains clothing in the axillary and genital regions. The arthritis causes limitation of motion of the hips, knee joints, or shoulders, and there may be periods of acute inflammation. Limitation of motion and ankylosis in the lumbosacral region are late findings. In addition, alkaptonuric patients appear to have a high incidence of cardiovascular disease; at least one degenerated pigmented aortic valve has been replaced with a prosthesis. Other complications include ruptured intervertebral discs, prostatitis, and renal stones.

Radiographic Findings

Almost pathognomonic changes affect vertebral bodies of the lumbar spine, which show degeneration of the intervertebral discs, narrowing of the space, dense calcification of remaining disc material, and variable fusion of vertebral bodies. The degenerative changes of ochronotic arthritis are most severe in the hip, shoulder, and knee, and patients may have calcific deposits in the tendons. Ear cartilage may be calcified.

Diagnosis

The diagnosis is suggested by urine discoloration and by the presence of non–glucose-reducing substance, pigmentation of sclerae or cartilage, arthritic episodes, and typical radiographic changes of the lumbar spine. Homogentisic acid in urine can be identified by chromatographic or enzymatic assays.

Treatment

Rx

A low-protein diet for life would be prudent. Dietary restriction of phenylalanine and tyrosine of the degree necessary to reduce homogentisic aciduria is impractical and is potentially deleterious. Pharmacologic doses of ascorbic acid, early and continuously, may reduce polymerization and pigmentation because ascorbic acid inhibits the polyphenol oxidase. It does not alter the primary metabolic defect. 2-(2-Nitro-4-trifluoromethylbenzoyl)-1,3-cyclohexanedione (NTBC), the potent inhibitor of *p*-hydroxyphenylpyruvic acid oxidase, would prevent excess formation of homogentisic acid by blocking the pathway prior to the mutant step, but it requires reduced protein intake and synthetic amino acid supplementation.

HEPATORENAL TYROSINEMIA (OR TYROSINEMIA TYPE I)

Definition

Hepatorenal tyrosinemia (MIM 276700) is an autosomal recessive disorder in which the final enzyme in tyrosine catabolism, fumarylacetate hydrolase, is deficient. The fumarylacetoacetate that accumulates is converted nonenzymatically to succinylacetone, which is toxic to the liver and kidneys and inhibits the porphyrin synthetic enzyme ALA dehydratase, with resulting sudden neurologic crises in some patients.

Epidemiology

The worldwide incidence is estimated to be less than 1 in 100,000 to 150,000 births. A higher incidence of 1 in 15,000 to 1 in 20,000 occurs in the Canadian Province of Quebec and is as frequent as 1 in 1500 to 1 in 2000 live births in the Saguenay–Lac St. Jean region. This high frequency is the result of the effect of a small, inbred founder population that migrated from France more than 300 years ago.

Pathobiology

The cause of all clinical manifestations is almost certainly the highly toxic succinylacetone that accumulates. Elimination of succinylacetone in humans and in the knockout mouse model substantially eliminates all clinical and biochemical manifestations of the disease.

Clinical Manifestations

The age of onset may vary from infancy to adolescence. Patients present with failure of liver synthetic functions, particularly clotting factors, but they have proportionately less jaundice and hypoglycemia. Cirrhosis and ascites also occur early in the disease course, but transaminase elevations are more modest. α-Fetoprotein levels are quite high, often exceeding 100,000 ng/mL (normal is <10 in children 6 to 9 months of age and thereafter). A more indolent course of gradual onset of cirrhosis occurs as well. Precocious onset of hepatocellular carcinoma is a grave risk; this disease may occur very early, and this situation has led to close scrutiny of surviving patients and, commonly, preemptive liver transplantation.

Neurologic crises resembling those of acute intermittent porphyria occur quite frequently and may be relatively intractable. Renal Fanconi's syndrome occurs in all patients, and rickets follows in most.

Treatment

Rx

Dietary therapy limiting the intake of phenylalanine and tyrosine improved acute symptoms but had little effect on the long-term outlook of the disorder. The first "cure" for this disorder was liver transplantation, in which one disorder was traded for another. The procedure eliminated succinylacetone from blood (but not from urine), eliminated renal Fanconi's syndrome, and eliminated the neurologic crises. An effective acute drug therapy is NTBC (see earlier), which blocks tyrosine catabolism just before formation of homogentisic acid and brings succinylacetone levels to less than the sensitivity of the analytic procedure. Patients with acute disease may improve within hours and are well enough for discharge from the hospital within days. The longer-term effectiveness of this therapy is unknown. It certainly reduces the incidence of hepatocellular carcinoma, but it may not eliminate the risk entirely, especially in patients with a longer pretreatment clinical course. All patients must be followed carefully with α-fetoprotein measurement and sensitive liver imaging techniques. Even with NTBC therapy, liver transplantation specialists particularly are prone to choosing earlier rather than later surgical intervention. Patients with well advanced renal tubular dysfunction may not improve appreciably with treatment.

SUGGESTED READINGS

Farrugia R, Scerri CA, Montalto SA, et al: Molecular genetics of tetrahydrobiopterin (BH[4]) deficiency in the Maltese population. Mol Genet Metab 2007;90:277–283. *A review of a specific population.*

Giovannini M, Verduci E, Salvatici E, et al: Phenylketonuria: Dietary and therapeutic challenges. J Inherit Metab Dis 2007;30:145–152. *Patients with PKU need special attention in the definition of optimal supplementation of nutrients.*

Matalon R, Michals-Matalon K, Bhatia G, et al: Double-blind placebo control trial of large neutral amino acids in treatment of PKU: Effect on blood phenylalanine. J Inherit Metab Dis 2007;30:153–158. *Orally administered LNAA has a role in lowering blood phenylalanine concentrations in patients with PKU, but long-term studies are needed to validate efficacy and safety of such treatment.*

Moller AT, Jensen TS: Neurological manifestations in Fabry's disease. Nat Clin Pract Neurol 2007;3:95–106. *A review that focuses on the importance of recognizing neurological symptoms for the diagnosis of Fabry disease.*

Phornphutkul C, Introne WJ, Perry MB, et al: Natural history of alkaptonuria. N Engl J Med 2002;347:2111–2121. *A review of the natural history of 58 patients with alkaptonuria.*

Pieroni M, Chimenti C, De Cobelli F, et al: Fabry's disease cardiomyopathy: echocardiographic detection of endomyocardial glycosphingolipid compartmentalization. J Am Coll Cardiol 2006;47:1663–1671. *A sensitive and specific diagnostic hallmark of Fabry's disease cardiomyopathy is echocardiographic binary appearance of left ventricular endocardial border, reflecting endomyocardial glycosphingolipids compartmentalization.*

Rutherford P, Poustie VJ: Protein substitute for children and adults with phenylketonuria. Cochrane Database Syst Rev 2005;19:CD004731. *Demonstrates lack of randomized trials examining the benefits and adverse effects of protein substitutes in patients with PKU.*

Watson MS: Current status of newborn screening: Decision-making about the conditions to include in screening programs. Ment Retard Rev Disabil Res Rev 2006;12:230–235. *A comprehensive discussion.*

Yalaz K, Vanli L, Yilmaz E, et al: Phenylketonuria in pediatric neuroology practice: A series of 146 cases. J Child Neurol 2006;21:987–990. *Review of the neurologic manifestations of a cohort of patients with phenylketonuria.*

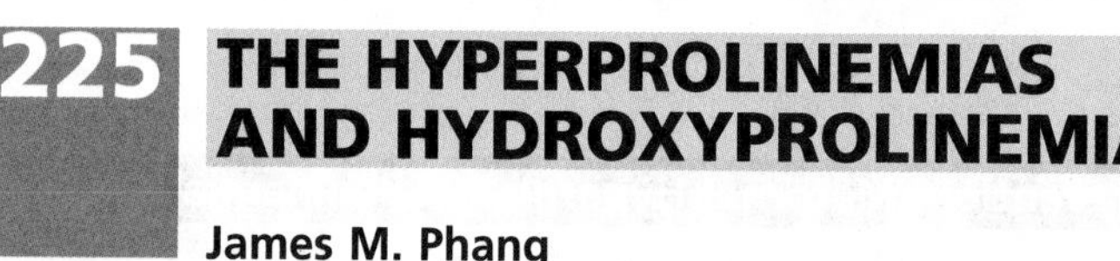

225 THE HYPERPROLINEMIAS AND HYDROXYPROLINEMIA

James M. Phang

Pathobiology

There are three autosomal recessive genetic disorders in the degradative pathways for proline and hydroxyproline. Although these rare disorders are generally benign, the resulting metabolic abnormalities in one of the disorders is associated with neurologic manifestations in childhood.

The α-nitrogen of the imino acids proline and hydroxyproline is incorporated within a pyrrolidine ring. This feature confers structural and functional properties to proteins. Because of the ring structure, the metabolism of proline, including biosynthesis from glutamate and ornithine and degradation back to glutamate, is catalyzed by a specific set of enzymes. Both synthetic and degradative pathways share Δ^1-pyrroline-5-carboxylate as an intermediate. The cycling of proline mediates the transfer of reducing-oxidizing potential, which may be bioenergetically important under certain conditions. Recent studies suggest that with programmed cell death, proline oxidation is increased and generates reactive oxygen species to stimulate both the mitochondrial and "death receptor" pathways for apoptosis. Preformed hydroxyproline is not incorporated into proteins. Instead, hydroxyproline is formed from the peptide-linked proline primarily in collagen. The degradation of hydroxyproline does not yield an amino acid for protein synthesis.

HYPERPROLINEMIAS

The two genetic disorders in proline metabolism, type I and type II hyperprolinemia, are characterized by hyperprolinemia and iminoglycinuria, but they are due to different enzyme deficiencies; only type II hyperprolinemia can be diagnosed directly. This disorder is due to a deficiency of Δ^1-pyrroline-5-carboxylate dehydrogenase, which catalyzes the second step in the degradative pathway for proline (Fig. 225–1); the deficiency in enzyme activity can be determined in extracts of circulating leukocytes or cultured fibroblasts. The hyperprolinemia in type II is more marked than that in type I, but the distinguishing feature of type II is the accumulation of Δ^1-pyrroline-5-carboxylate in plasma and its excretion in urine. The hyperprolinemia in type I is due to a deficiency of the first enzyme in the pathway, proline oxidase (a.k.a. proline dehydrogenase). Although plasma proline is generally lower than in type II, the diagnosis of type I is one of exclusion, that is, hyperprolinemia unaccompanied by Δ^1-pyrroline-5-carboxylate in urine or plasma.

Clinical manifestations have been described with the hyperprolinemias, but the association may be due to chance because in most cases, the hyperprolinemia was identified fortuitously in patients with clinical abnormalities (biased ascertainment). This is especially true for type I hyperprolinemia, where the renal disease and mental retardation found in some pedigrees were shown to segregate independently of hyperprolinemia. Recent reports suggesting a link between susceptibility for schiz-

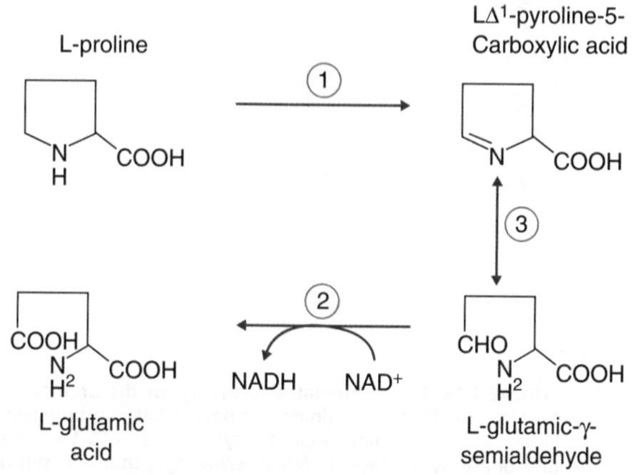

FIGURE 225–1 • Schematic of the degradative pathway for proline. Reaction 1 is catalyzed by proline oxidase (EC number unassigned), reaction 2 is catalyzed by Δ^1-pyrroline-5-carboxylic acid dehydrogenase (EC 1.5.1.12), and reaction 3 is spontaneous. Type I hyperprolinemia is due to blockade at reaction 1 (deficiency of proline oxidase), and type II hyperprolinemia is due to blockade at reaction 2 (deficiency of Δ^1-pyrroline-5-carboxylic acid dehydrogenase).

ophrenia and mutations in the gene for proline oxidase (*PRODH*) have reopened the question. Mutations identified in patients with early onset of mental symptoms yielded translation products with abnormal enzyme function. For type II hyperprolinemia, clinical associations untainted by biased ascertainment have been clearly identified. Screening of a large pedigree in Ireland identified 14 new cases confirmed by elevated plasma Δ^1-pyrroline-5-carboxylate and undetectable enzyme activity in leukocytes. Nine of these 14 new subjects had a history of recurrent childhood febrile seizures requiring hospitalization and treatment with anticonvulsants. Thus, the association of type II hyperprolinemia with a predisposition to seizures appears convincing. Adults in this pedigree were fertile and otherwise normal. Although the mechanism for this association remains unclear, the identification of a high-affinity proline transporter in rat brain suggests that proline or its metabolites may have a neuromodulatory function.

HYDROXYPROLINEMIA

Hydroxyprolinemia with hydroxyprolinuria, but without hyperprolinemia or prolinuria, has been described in members of several families. Although the degradation of hydroxyproline parallels that of proline, the pathway enzymes are distinct except that the second degradation step for both is catalyzed by a common enzyme that dehydrogenates Δ^1-pyrroline-5-carboxylate (see earlier) and 3-OH-Δ^1-pyrroline-5-carboxylate. The first step in their degradation, however, is catalyzed by distinct oxidases. The absence of urinary Δ^1-pyrroline-5-carboxylate or its hydroxylated congener leads to the conclusion that this autosomal recessive disorder is due to a deficiency of hydroxyproline oxidase. In this disorder there are no clinical manifestations related to abnormalities in collagen metabolism or central nervous system function, and therapy is not indicated.

SUGGESTED READINGS

Bender HU, Almashanu S, Steel G, et al: Functional consequences of PRODH missense mutations. Am J Hum Genet 2005;76:409–420. *The severity of hyperprolinemia corresponds with the mutation's effect on proline oxidase activity.*

Delwing D, Chiarani F, Bavaresco CS, et al: Protective effect of antioxidants on brain oxidative damage caused by proline administration. Neurosci Res 2005;52:69–74. *Antioxidant adminstration may help aviod the progression of the neuropsychiatric dysfunction.*

Donald SP, Sun XY, Hu CA, et al: Proline oxidase, encoded by p53-induced gene-6, catalyzes the generation of proline-dependent reactive oxygen species. Cancer Res 2001;61:1810–1815. *Proline-dependent radical oxygen species increase with overexpression of proline oxidase.*

Liu Y, Borchert GL, Donald SP, et al: MnSOD inhibits proline oxidase–induced apoptosis in colorectal cancer cell. Carcinogenesis 2005;26:1335–1342. Superoxide radicals play a crucial role in proline oxidase–induced apoptosis and the process is partially blocked by MnSOD.

Swarna M, Jyothy A, Usha Rani P, et al: Amino acid disorders in mental retardation: A two-decade study from Andhra Pradesh. Biochem Genet 2004;42:85–98. *A study of the prevalence of amino acid disorders in mentally retarded children from a state in India.*

226 DISEASES OF THE UREA CYCLE

Stephen D. Cederbaum

UREA CYCLE DEFECTS

Definition

Ammonia is a highly toxic metabolic product that when present at levels no more than two times the upper limit of normal (20 to 50 μM), may cause symptoms. The urea cycle is an eight-step metabolic pathway in which two molecules of ammonia and one of bicarbonate are converted to urea, which is nontoxic. It is the only major pathway to remove waste nitrogen derived from ingested protein or from normal or augmented endogenous protein turnover. The urea cycle occurs predominantly or possibly exclusively in the liver.

The urea cycle is shown in Figure 226–1. The six primary enzymes generally associated with it are *N*-acetylglutamate synthetase (NAGS), carbamoylphosphate synthetase 1 (CPS-1), and ornithine transcarbamoylase (OTC), all found in the mitochondrion, and argininosuccinate synthetase (ASAS), argininosuccinate lyase (ASAL), and arginase 1, found in the cytoplasm. The ornithine transporter (ORNT1), which recycles ornithine to the mitochondrion, and a mitochondrial aspartate carrier protein (SLC25A13), which presumably transports aspartate out of the mitochondrion when deficient, cause symptomatic hyperammonemia as well. The normal urea cycle can increase its ureagenic capacity greatly in response to an ammonia challenge. The genes for all six enzymes and the two transporters have been cloned and are available for defining mutations, prenatal diagnosis, and population studies.

Epidemiology

Disorders of the urea cycle are estimated to occur in at least 1 in 25,000 births. It is probable that 2 to 4% of the population is heterozygous for a urea cycle defect, although only women who are carriers of OTC deficiency are known to be prone to symptomatic disease. It is unclear whether patients receiving intensive chemotherapy for leukemia, in whom hyperammonemia occurs rarely, or patients receiving valproate anticonvulsant therapy, in whom it occurs more mildly, are heterozygotes for one or another of these enzyme deficiencies (see later discussion). More recently, metabolic centers have been referred adult patients with mild hyperammonemia, usually recipients of polypharmacy for vague symptoms, in whom no urea cycle disorder can be diagnosed.

Pathobiology

In children, the vast majority of cases of hyperammonemia are the result of inborn errors of metabolism (Chapter 216), primarily of the urea cycle. In adults, a larger proportion of cases are due to liver failure and less frequently to toxic ingestion and intensive chemotherapy. Nevertheless, with the wider availability of blood ammonia tests, the increased recognition of urea cycle disorders, and more successful treatment modalities, the inherited disorders of ammonia metabolism are being recognized with greater frequency in adolescents and adults with acute or intermittent organic brain syndrome. Hyperammonemia appears to be better tolerated by infants and young children, in part because the cranium is more compliant. Ammonia levels that leave minimal residual damage in infants may be deadly in adults. Ammonia itself and glutamine, an amino acid in equilibrium with ammonia, appear to be the metabolites that are toxic to the central nervous system. The primary toxic effect appears to be the uptake of fluid into astrocytes, which causes cerebral edema. Death is caused acutely by herniation of the brain through the foramen magnum with consequent cerebral ischemia, but survivors may have various degrees of brain damage.

Clinical Manifestations

Complete deficiency of any of the first five enzymes in the cycle usually leads to severe hyperammonemia in the initial 2 to 4 days of life. Affected

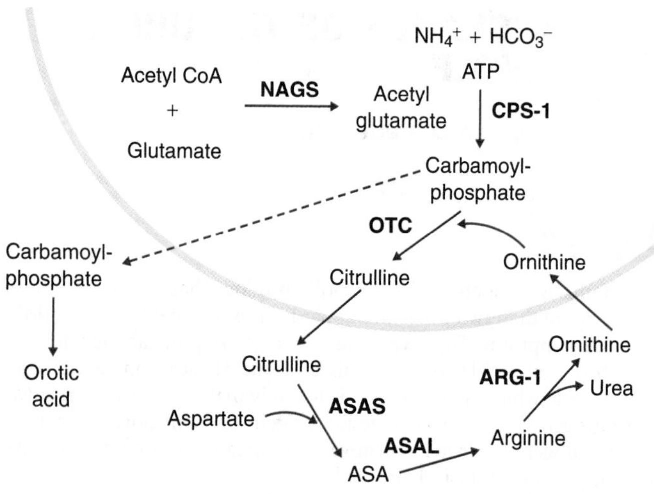

FIGURE 226–1 • Abbreviated pathway for the urea cycle. ARG-1 = arginase 1; ASA = argininosuccinate; ASAL = argininosuccinate lyase; ASAS = argininosuccinate synthetase; CPS-1 = carbamoylphosphate synthetase 1; NAGS = *N*-acetylglutamate synthetase; OTC = ornithine transcarbamoylase. Enzymes within the colored line function within the mitochondrial matrix.

TABLE 226–1 GENETIC CHARACTERISTICS OF DISORDERS OF THE UREA CYCLE

Enzyme Defect	Inheritance Pattern	Heterozygote Detection	Heterozygote Symptoms	Prenatal Diagnosis*
N-Acetylglutamate synthetase	AR	No†	No	Yes
Carbamoylphosphate synthetase	AR	No†	No	Yes
Ornithine transcarbamoylase	X-linked	Yes, in most instances*	Yes	Yes
Argininosuccinate synthetase	AR	No†	No	Yes
Argininosuccinate lyase	AR	Yes	No	Yes
Arginase 1	AR	Yes	No	Yes
Ornithine transporter	AR	No†	No	Yes
Aspartate transporter	AR	No†	No	Yes

*With varying degrees of ease.
†Heterozygotes for all disorders can be detected if the specific base change in the gene has been ascertained. This is not practical at the present time outside the research laboratory.
AR = autosomal recessive.

patients have irritability, lethargy, and poor feeding that progress rapidly to stupor, seizures, coma, and death. The plasma ammonia level often exceeds 1000 μM, and urea levels are extremely low. Episodic hyperammonemia occurs in association with periods of endogenous protein catabolism and severely affects patients, such as those with severe OTC deficiency. They almost certainly die or suffer severe neurologic impairment during one of these episodes. Patients with partial deficiency of urea cycle enzymes or those who avoid hyperammonemia in the neonatal period may initially be identified at any time later in life, from infancy to adulthood. Older patients have irritability, vomiting, and disorientation, which may progress (as in infants) to stupor, seizures, coma, and death. These episodes are often precipitated by severe infection, excessive protein intake, parturition, or rarely, menstruation, or they may have no apparent cause. Some general genetic characteristics of defects in the urea cycle are presented in Table 226–1.

Treatment

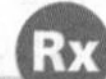

Urea cycle defects, originally considered a pediatric problem, are moving into the realm of internal medicine. Internists must cast aside the lactulose used for the hyperammonemia of liver failure and gastrointestinal bleeding in favor of diversion therapy and hemodialysis. Soon, liver replacement, the artificial liver (perhaps stem cells), and gene therapy will be more widely used.

ENZYME DEFICIENCIES

Deficiency of *N*-Acetylglutamate Synthetase (MIM 237310) and Carbamoylphosphate Synthetase (MIM 2373001*)

NAGS and CPS-1 are considered together because the symptoms and signs of their deficiencies may be indistinguishable. NAGS has, as its only known function, catalysis of the synthesis of acetylglutamate, an obligatory allosteric activator of CPS-1. CPS-1, the second enzyme in the urea cycle, constitutes up to 25% of the mitochondrial matrix protein in liver. Ordinarily, all of the carbamoylphosphate synthesized from ammonium and bicarbonate by CPS-1 is used to produce urea. Orotic acid and pyrimidines are products of carbamoylphosphate as well, which is synthesized by a second, independently regulated cytoplasmic enzyme. Patients with both the neonatal and the later-onset forms of these disorders have been described. The diagnosis may be inferred from hyperammonemia, low to absent levels of citrulline in plasma, and normal or elevated bicarbonate levels. During acute hyperammonemia, there is usually a generalized hyperaminoacidemia with particular prominence of glutamine.

Liver transplantation alone offers definitive treatment. Restriction of dietary protein, supplementation of essential amino acids and citrulline,

* MIM = Mendelian Inheritance in Man; the online catalogs of mendelian traits can be found at www.ncbi.nlm.nih.gov/OMIM.

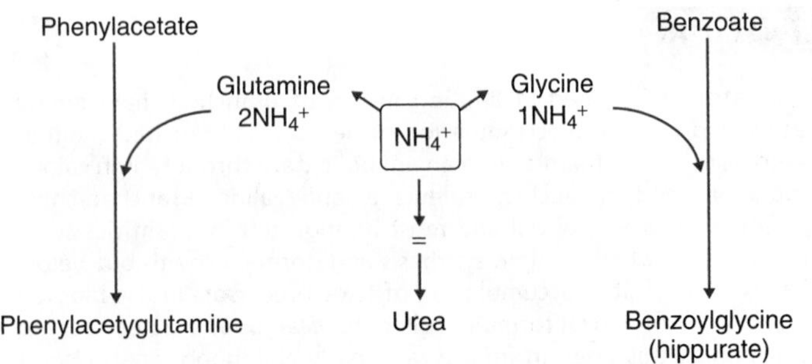

FIGURE 226–2 • Mechanisms of ammonia diversion from the urea cycle with the administration of sodium phenylacetate and sodium benzoate.

hospitalization for "catabolic crises," hemodialysis or peritoneal dialysis, and administration of phenylacetate (or phenylbutyrate) and benzoate to divert ammonia to phenylacetylglutamine and benzoylglycine (hippurate) are used to control symptoms and treat crises (Fig. 226–2). Patients with this and other urea cycle defects are prone to the development of severe hyperammonemia with valproate anticonvulsant therapy. A polymorphism at base 4332 in the mRNA (T1405N) reduces enzyme activity and appears to be associated with the predisposition to hepatic venoocclusive disease, pulmonary hypertension, and hyperammonemia that occurs with intensive chemotherapy. Whether this polymorphism affects metabolism in less stressful conditions is unknown.

Deficiency of Ornithine Transcarbamoylase (MIM 311250)

This mitochondrial enzyme catalyzes the reaction of carbamoylphosphate with ornithine to form citrulline, which is then transported out of the mitochondrion for further metabolism. The acute form of this X-linked enzyme deficiency usually occurs in male subjects. Uncommonly, a newborn female may be severely affected, which is thought to be due to nonrandom, X-chromosome inactivation. Female carriers of this codominant trait generally escape obvious symptoms, but those who have them are usually seen later in life or at parturition with hyperammonemic crises, some of which may be severe enough to be fatal. A number of male patients with partial enzyme deficiency may come to attention later as well, and bariatric surgery is one potential precipitant of symptoms. Patients with this later-onset form of the disease may suffer from severe and otherwise inexplicable protein intolerance. The amino and organic acid profiles resemble those of CPS-1 deficiency. OTC deficiency is distinguished by extraordinarily high levels of orotic acid in urine, formed when the excess carbamoylphosphate accumulating in the mitochondrion leaks into the cytoplasm and is channeled into the pyrimidine biosynthetic pathway (see Fig. 226–1). Orotic acid levels may be normal when ammonia has been controlled. Because of this typical clinical biochemical picture, liver biopsy to confirm enzymes is less frequently undertaken than for NAGS and CPS-1 deficiencies. An allopurinol challenge may help detect carrier females. Treatment is identical to that described for CPS-1 deficiency.

Deficiency of Argininosuccinate Synthetase (Citrullinemia, MIM 215700)

This cytoplasmic enzyme condenses the citrulline synthesized by OTC with aspartate to form argininosuccinate in a reaction that introduces the second ammonia nitrogen for excretion as urea. ASAS deficiency leads to hyperammonemia, greatly increased blood citrulline levels, and excretion of excessive amounts of citrulline and orotic acid in urine. Here, too, neonatal, later-onset, or symptomless deficiency of the enzyme has been reported. A second form of citrullinemia has been described, primarily from Japan and occurring mainly in adulthood. This disorder is due to mutations in the aspartate transporter SLC25A13 (citrin, MIM 603471, 605814).

Treatment is similar to that for CPS-1 and OTC deficiencies, except that arginine is supplemented instead of citrulline. Citrulline excretion is more complete than that of ammonia, and management of this condition is somewhat easier.

Deficiency of Argininosuccinate Lyase (Argininosuccinic Aciduria, MIM 207900)

Argininosuccinate is cleaved into two smaller product molecules, arginine and fumarate, in a reaction catalyzed by ASAL. This enzyme deficiency results in massive accumulation and excretion of argininosuccinate. Variable onset or lack of symptoms characterizes this enzyme deficiency as well. Argininosuccinate is actively secreted by the renal tubules, and its synthesis can be stimulated by stoichiometric amounts of arginine as a source of ornithine to drive the urea cycle. By this means, ammonia levels are rapidly reduced and can be controlled more reliably than in any other urea cycle disorder.

Deficiency of Arginase 1 (Hyperargininemia, MIM 207800)

Arginase, the final enzyme in the urea cycle, catalyzes the hydrolysis of arginine to urea and ornithine, the latter returned to the mitochondrion to participate in another cycle of ammonia detoxification (see Fig. 226–1). Clinical symptoms of hyperargininemia are usually of later onset, are more gradual and relentless in progression, and are less frequently or seriously punctuated by apparent episodes of acute hyperammonemia. Rather typically, gait abnormalities and spasticity begin to develop in normal patients at 2 to 3 years of age, and cortical and pyramidal tract dysfunction progresses slowly. More than 80% of reported patients are still alive, some at 40 years or older. The diagnosis is often suspected when arginine levels are found to be elevated in blood or urine. Hyperammonemia is generally seen only during acute catabolic episodes.

Although most patients have been moderately to severely retarded at detection, treatment by limiting protein and diverting ammonia reverses many of the most severe manifestations of the disease, and presymptomatic treatment has allowed two patients to reach the age of 30 or older without apparent clinical manifestations.

Deficiency of the Ornithine Transporter Protein ORNT1 (Hyperornithinemia, Hyperammonemia, Homocitrullinuria [HHH Syndrome], MIM 238970)

This inherited predisposition to hyperammonemia is due to deficient activity of the mitochondrial ornithine transporter protein coded for by the recently cloned *ORNT1* gene. Patients may be protein intolerant, and many are mildly developmentally delayed, at least. The plasma ornithine level may be no more than two times the upper limit of normal. Treatment of the hyperammonemia is similar to treatment of CPS and OTC deficiencies, but hemodialysis may not be required for lesser degrees of hyperammonemia, and arginine supplementation is not indicated.

SUGGESTED READINGS

Bachmann C: Long-term outcome of patients with urea cycle disorders and the question of neonatal screening. Eur J Pediatr 2003;162(Suppl 1):S29–S33. *A concise overview.*

Hu WT, Kantarci OH, Merritt JL 2nd, et al: Ornithine transcarbamylase deficiency presenting as encephalopathy during adulthood following bariatric surgery. Arch Neurol 2007;64:126–128. *An instructive case report.*

Kleppe S, Mian A, Lee B: Urea cycle disorders. Curr Treat Options Neurol 2003;5:309–319. *Overview of the genetics, pathophysiology, and treatment, including possible cell and gene therapies.*

BRANCHED-CHAIN AMINOACIDURIAS

Louis J. Elsas II

MAPLE SYRUP URINE DISEASE

Definition

Maple syrup urine disease (MSUD), also called *branched-chain α-ketoaciduria*, derives its name from the burnt sugar smell in the urine and earwax of affected patients.

Epidemiology

In surveyed populations, the frequency of MSUD varies from 1 in 760 (in Mennonites) to an average U.S. figure of 1 in 185,000 newborns. The disease is more frequent in Middle Eastern populations, where consanguineous matings are more common than in the United States. Atypical cases with less severe clinical manifestations may be missed in newborn screening and appear with intermittent ataxia in later childhood or early adulthood.

Pathobiology

MSUD is caused by impaired branched-chain α-ketoacid dehydrogenase (BCKD), which catalyzes decarboxylation of the α-ketoacid derivatives of all three of the branched-chain amino acids: leucine, isoleucine, and valine (Fig. 227–1). They are essential amino acids that share branching, aliphatic chains. If BCKD is impaired, branched-chain α-ketoacids and amino acids accumulate throughout the body. Isovaleric acidemia affects the next metabolic step, but only for products of leucine catabolism. Leucine is transaminated to α-ketoisocaproate, which is decarboxylated and transacetylated to isovaleryl coenzyme A (CoA). Isovaleric acidemia is caused by defects in isovaleryl CoA dehydrogenase (see Fig. 227–1). Both disorders conform to autosomal recessive patterns of inheritance. An affected homozygote for MSUD exhibits impaired activity in the BCKD multienzyme complex (Fig. 227–2). MSUD is caused by mutations in one of six genes that code for the six different proteins that make up the BCKD multienzyme complex. A wide range of mutations has been defined, along with the severity of impaired enzyme and consequent clinical manifestations (Table 227–1 and Fig. 227–2).

Although they function in mitochondria, BCKD proteins are encoded in the nuclear genome. Once translated in the cytosol, they are guided to the mitochondria by their intrinsic amino-terminal leader sequences and chaperone proteins. They then transmigrate through the outer and inner mitochondria membranes and assemble as a multienzyme complex in the mitochondrial matrix. The six proteins are (1) E1α and (2) E1β, which produce the dimeric E1α, β; (3) a branched-chain dihydrolipoamide acyltransferase (E2); (4) lipoamide oxidoreductase (E3); (5) E1α-kinase; and (6) E1α-phosphatase (see Fig. 227–2 and Table 227–1).

Several cofactors are involved in the overall reaction, including thiamine pyrophosphate (TP~P), lipoamide covalently bound to E2, CoA, and nicotinamide adenine dinucleotide.

Diagnosis

In typical MSUD, feeding difficulties and apnea develop in a newborn who was normal at birth. Convulsions and decorticate rigidity may develop. The diagnosis should be suspected clinically when a patient has intermittent symptoms related to protein ingestion and sweet-smelling earwax. A positive dinitrophenylhydrazine reaction is seen in affected patients' urine, and the diagnosis is confirmed by abnormal excesses of the branched-chain amino acids and α-keto acids α-ketoisocaproate, α-keto-β-methylisovalerate, and α-ketovalerate in blood and urine. The enzyme defect is demonstrable in leukocytes and cultured, dermal fibroblasts. Prenatal monitoring is accomplished both biochemically and through DNA analysis of specific mutations. Determination of the biochemical phenotype or genotype in an affected sibling's cultured cells is required before attempts at prenatal monitoring.

Treatment

Rx

Treatment is aimed at limiting intake of branched-chain amino acids to prevent the accumulation of neurotoxic branched-chain α-keto acids and at maintaining an anabolic state through high caloric intake limited in leucine, isoleucine, and valine. Branched-chain amino acids are essential and must be ingested in quantities sufficient to allow new protein synthesis and normal growth but below levels that result in accumulation of toxic precursors in the blocked reaction. Commercial formulas called *medical foods* are necessary to accomplish this goal. In infancy and early childhood, anabolism is encouraged by providing excess calories and maintaining branched-chain amino acid–restricted protein intake at the recommended daily allowance. Treatment is monitored clinically in terms of growth and development and biochemically through analysis of plasma amino acid and urine organic acid concentrations. Because leucine residues are more frequent than isoleucine and valine in natural proteins, care must be taken not to over-restrict isoleucine and valine while attempting to lower blood concentrations of leucine.

Many patients respond to pharmacologic excesses of thiamine supplementation (8 mg/kg/day). The presumed mechanism is that by saturating binding sites for thiamine pyrophosphate on E1α, the multienzyme complex is stabilized against biologic degradation. Small increases in enzyme function can provide dramatic improvement in the patient, who will continue to require reduced intake of leucine, isoleucine, and valine.

Thiamine supplements allow increased natural protein intake in thiamine-responsive patients. Chronic acidosis may deplete carnitine, which should also be monitored in blood and supplemented if deficient. Treatment is lifelong.

Prognosis

Before population-based newborn screening, affected infants died or were severely damaged. With newborn screening, retrieval, diagnosis, and diet intervention before 2 weeks of age, these children have reached adulthood with good function.

ISOVALERIC ACIDEMIA

Pathobiology

Isovaleryl CoA is the product formed from the action of BCKD on α-ketoisocaproate (leucine's derivative). Isovaleryl CoA is normally converted to β-methylcrotonyl CoA by isovaleryl CoA dehydrogenase (see Fig. 227–1).

Clinical Manifestations

When isovaleryl dehydrogenase is impaired, isovaleric acid accumulates in blood and urine and produces a foul odor similar to that of rancid cheese or sweaty feet. In the neonatal form, symptoms are severe in the first week of life and consist of vomiting, acidosis, hypoglycemia, tremors, coma, and death. Leukopenia, anemia, thrombocytopenia, and hyperammonemia may occur during acute attacks.

Diagnosis

The diagnosis is suspected as a result of the clinical findings and associated odor and is established by demonstrating excess isovaleric acid and its adducts in urine by mass spectroscopy. Tandem mass spectroscopy of dried blood is used in some states to screen for isovaleric acidemia in normal newborns. The gene has been cloned and sequenced, and some mutations have been defined. The gene is located on chromosome 15q13, and the coding sequence has homology to short- and medium-chain acyldehydrogenase.

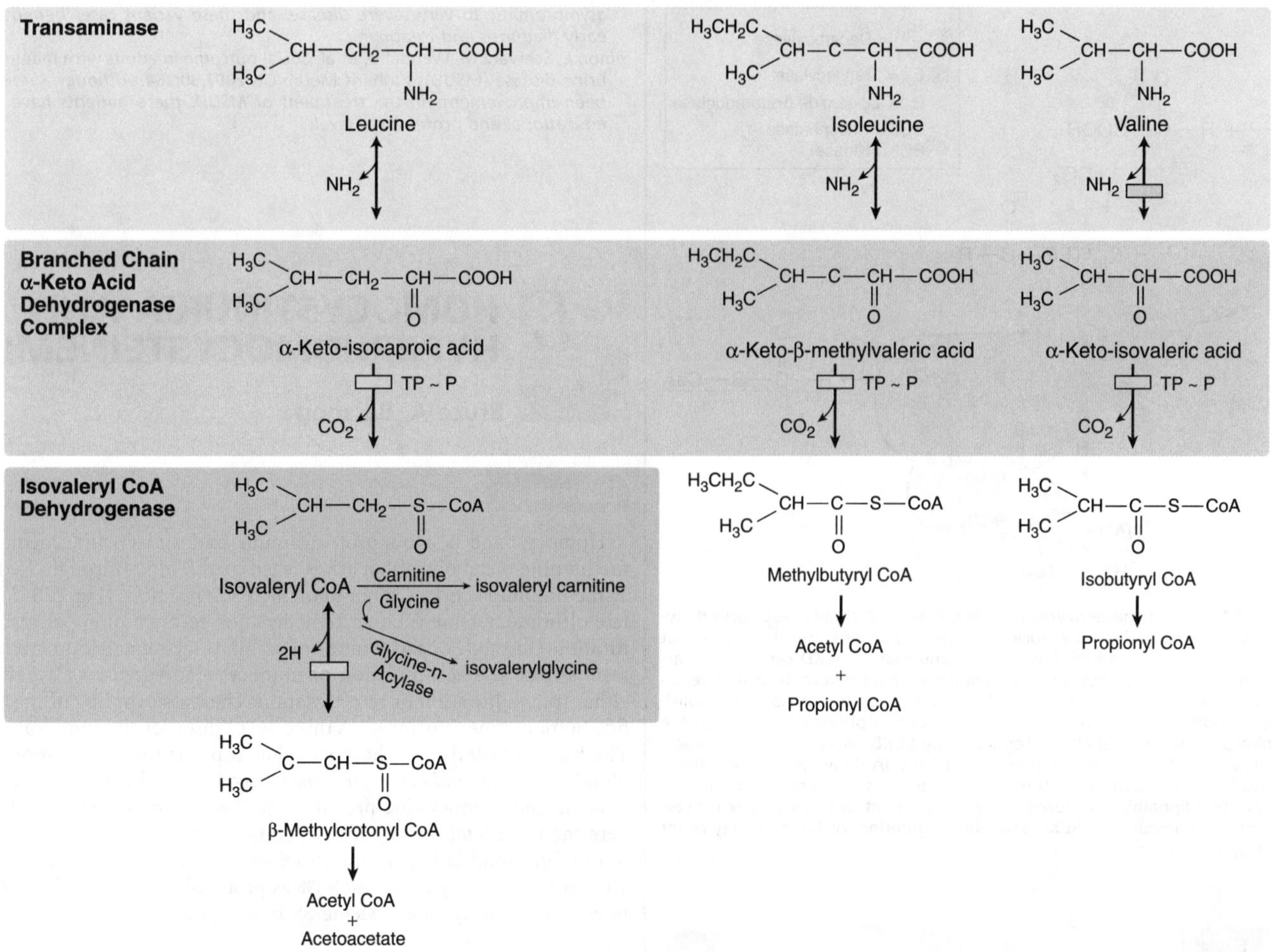

FIGURE 227–1 • Catabolic pathway for the branched chain amino acids. L-Leucine, L-isoleucine, and L-valine are transaminated to their branched chain α-keto acids. Valine transaminase may be impaired in hypervalinemia. The branched chain α-keto acids are decarboxylated and transacylated by a mitochondrial multienzyme complex, the branched chain α-keto acid dehydrogenase (BCKD). Impairment of BCKD results in maple syrup urine disease. This enzyme requires thiamine pyrophosphate (TP≈P) as its active cofactor. When isovaleryl CoA dehydrogenase is impaired, isovaleric acidemia occurs. Accumulated isovaleryl CoA can utilize alternate pathways using carnitine transferase and glycine-n-acylase. These alternate pathways are activated as therapeutic interventions in isovaleric acidemia.

TABLE 227–1 GENES, PROTEINS, AND MUTATIONS IN THE HUMAN BRANCHED-CHAIN α-KETO ACID DEHYDROGENASE COMPLEX

	Chromosome			
Name (Function)	**Locus**	**Gene Size (kb)**	**Mature Protein (kD)**	**Mutation**
E1α (decarboxylase)	19q13.3	55	46	Y438N (Mennonite missense mutation)
E1β (stabilizes decarboxylase)	6q1.4	100	38	11-Base pair deletion (frameshift with premature STOP)
E2 (acyltransferase)	1p31	68	46	E163STOP, R183P (common in Ashkenazim) F215C (exonic and intronic insertions and deletions)
E3 (dehydrogenase)	7q22	20	50	Affects other substrate-specific dehydrogenases (α-ketoglutarate and pyruvate)
E1α kinase (inactivates)	16p13.12	40	43	Inhibited by tumor necrosis factor-α (may cause cachexia in cancer)
E1α phosphatase (activates)	?	?	?	?

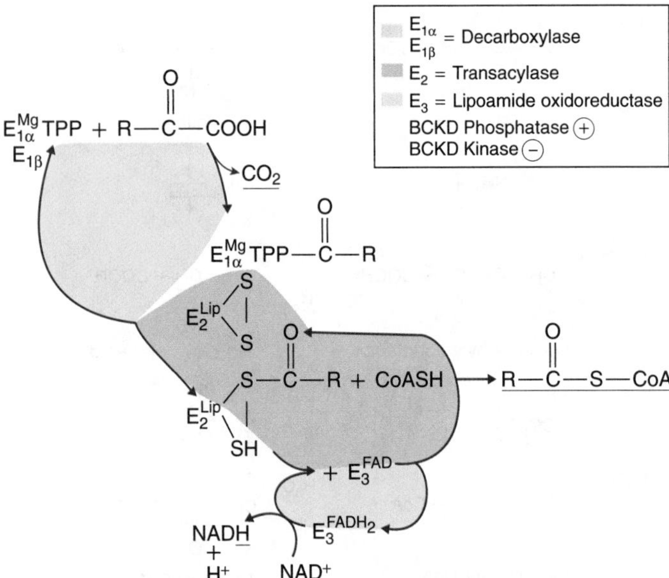

FIGURE 227–2 • The multienzyme complex, branched-chain α-keto acid dehydrogenase (BCKD). At least six nuclear encoded proteins are illustrated that assemble in the mitochondrial, inner-membrane matrix. BCKD catalyzes decarboxylation and transacylation of three branched-chain α-keto acids and reoxidation of lipoic acid. The proteins E1α and E1β decarboxylase accomplish decarboxylation. E1α is positively regulated by dephosphorylation through the BCKD phosphatase and negatively regulated by BCKD kinase. The E2 transacylase transfers CoASH to form the branched-chain CoA derivative. E2 contains a lipoic acid that is reduced in this transacylation process and is reoxidized by the E3 flavoprotein lipoamide oxidoreductase. Impairment of this complex process by mutant genes involved in BCKD assembly, regulation, or function may result in maple syrup urine disease.

Treatment

Emergency Therapy

Emergency therapy consists of eliminating dietary leucine and supplementing with intravenous, oral, and colonic infusion of glycine (300 mg/kg/day) to provide an alternative excretory pathway for the nontoxic adduct isovaleryl glycine. Carnitine (100 mg/kg/day) may provide nontoxic adducts of isovaleryl carnitine (see Fig. 227–1). Both adducts are excreted in urine. Emergency therapy also requires producing anabolism by using excess calories from carbohydrates, fat, and non–leucine-containing protein. As patients mature, they have less frequent attacks and are developmentally normal. "Attacks" are caused by excess leucine ingestion, starvation, infections, or other causes of catabolism. Chronic intermittent forms of this disorder occur in later life and are less severe but have not been differentiated from acute infantile forms at the biochemical or molecular level of enzyme or gene analysis. These differences in clinical expression may result from epigenetic and environmental phenomena.

Long-Term Therapy

Long-term therapy includes reduced intake of leucine. Unlike patients with MSUD, valine and isoleucine are catabolized normally and are required as essential nutrients in normal amounts in the diet. Supplements of glycine (90 to 100 mg/kg/day) and carnitine (30 mg/kg/day) are used as part of chronic dietary management. Outcome is excellent in both the infantile and later-onset forms of isovaleric acidemia disease if the acute, irreversible effects of the neonatal disease are prevented.

SUGGESTED READINGS

Organic acidemias. Available at www.geneclinics.org. *A source for diagnostic testing.*

Simon E, Flaschker N, Schadewaldt P, et al: Variant maple syrup urine disease (MSUD)—the entire spectrum. J Inherit Metab Dis 2006;29:716–724. *In variant maple syrup urine disease, there is a wide spectrum of clinical severity from asymptomatic to very severe disease, and these variant cases benefit from early diagnosis and treatment.*

Simon E, Schwarz M, Wendel U, et al: Social outcome in adults with maple syrup urine disease (MSUD). J Inherit Metab Dis 2007;30:264. *Although there have been improvements in the treatment of MSUD, these patients have lower educational and professional levels.*

228 HOMOCYSTINURIA AND HYPERHOMOCYSTEINEMIA

Bruce A. Barshop

Definition

Homocysteine is a nonprotein amino acid and an intermediate in methionine metabolism that arises when methionine (through *S*-adenosylmethionine) acts as a donor in methylation reactions (Fig. 228–1). The fate of homocysteine is either remethylation to methionine or transsulfuration (through cystathionine) of serine to cysteine. Homocystinuria results from the accumulation of homocysteine because of a defect in either transsulfuration or remethylation. The classic finding of the disulfide homocystine in urine gives this class of disorders its common name. The free sulfhydryl form, homocysteine, is present in lower amounts in blood. The term *total homocyst(e)ine* is used to describe the mix of homocysteine and homocystine present as sulfhydryl and disulfide, although here the term *total homocysteine* is considered equivalent. The defining finding in blood is hyperhomocysteinemia, which is distributed about 10% as free homocysteine and 90% as protein-bound and soluble disulfides (e.g., homocystine, cysteine-SS-homocysteine).

Epidemiology

Etiology

The classic form of homocystinuria is cystathionine β-synthase deficiency, which results in decreased transsulfuration and hypermethioninemic hyperhomocyst(e)inemia. Homocystinuria may also result from defective remethylation, as in a deficiency of methylenetetrahydrofolate reductase, or from a disorder in delivery, generation, or utilization of the methylcobalamin cofactor of methionine synthase. Defects of remethylation give rise to hyperhomocysteinemia with normal or low methionine. All of these disorders are inherited in an autosomal recessive manner (Table 228–1).

Incidence and Prevalence

Minimum estimates of the incidence of cystathionine β-synthase deficiency by newborn screening programs have ranged from 1 in 60,000 to 1 in 300,000 live births, varying with the population and method. Estimates of its incidence in Europe have been in the range of 1 in 40,000, which corresponds to a carrier (heterozygote) frequency of about 1%, but studies screening for known mutations suggest that the prevalence may be more than twice that rate. The incidence of severe homocysteine remethylation defects appears to be less than 1 in 500,000. In contrast, partial remethylation deficiencies seem to have a much greater incidence, which may be clinically relevant in predisposing individuals to thrombotic disorders, because evidence of deficiency has been reported in 15 to 30% in some series of patients with vaso-occlusive disease.

Pathobiology

Homocysteine has effects on vascular endothelium, platelets, and coagulation factors that predispose to thrombosis. Endothelial dysfunction can be elicited in normal patients when hyperhomocysteinemia is induced transiently, and there is evidence of inflammatory mediator activation in experimental systems related to the pro-oxidant effects of homocysteine, but there remains some controversy about the relevance of these factors in humans. Modification of connective tissue proteins

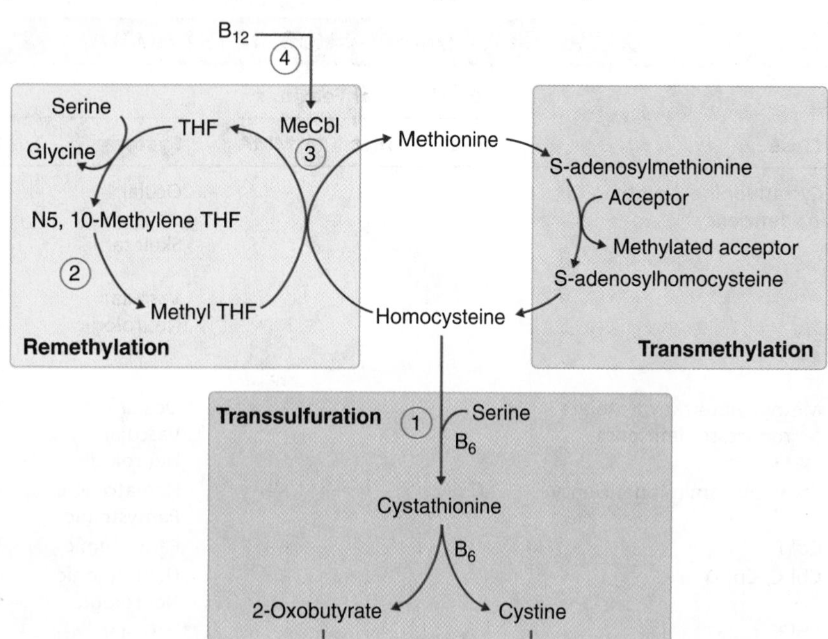

FIGURE 228–1 • **Pathways of homocysteine metabolism.** The systems of transmethylation, remethylation, and transsulfuration are marked. Steps discussed are numbered: (1) cystathionine β-synthase; (2) methylenetetrahydrofolate reductase; (3) methionine synthase and methyltransferase reductase; (4) systems of cobalamin absorption, distribution, and reduction. B_6 = pyridoxine; B_{12} = cyanocobalamin/hydroxocobalamin; MeCbl = methylcobalamin; THF = tetrahydrofolate.

TABLE 228–1 GENETIC DEFECTS ASSOCIATED WITH HOMOCYSTINURIA

Functional Defect	Common Name	Enzyme Defect	Chromosome Locus
Transsulfuration	"Classic" homocystinuria	Cystathionine β-synthase	22q22.3
Remethylation	Folate-dependent homocystinuria	Methylenetetrahydrofolate reductase	1p36.3
	Cbl G	Methionine synthase (methyltransferase)	1q43
	Cbl E	Methyltransferase reductase	5p15.2-p15.3
Cobalamin transport	TC-II	Transcobalamin II	22q11-q13.1
	Cbl F	Lysosomal B_{12} translocase	—
Cobalamin reductase	Cbl C	Unknown	1p34.1
	Cbl D	Unknown	—

may cause the skeletal and ocular manifestations associated with homocystinuria. These effects are probably related to fibrillin, which is a component of the matrix of periosteum and perichondrium, the major component of the zonular fibers of the ocular lens, and a protein singularly rich in cysteine. Fibrillin structure is affected by linking of homocysteine to cysteine; as a result, some features of homocystinuria are also associated with fibrillin mutations (Marfan syndrome). The neurologic effects of homocysteine may be due predominantly to agonism of the *N*-methyl-D-aspartate receptor by homocysteic acid, although cerebral vascular effects may contribute as well.

Clinical Manifestations

Cystathionine β-synthase deficiency is pleiotropic, with effects in the eye, skeleton, and central nervous and vascular systems (Table 228–2). The eye and skeletal system changes resemble those in Marfan syndrome. Nontraumatic dislocation of the ocular lens can be an initial finding. Some abnormality of the skeletal system develops in almost all untreated patients. Between a third and three fourths of untreated patients have mild or moderate mental retardation, and cerebrovascular thrombosis may play a role in the neurologic picture. Affected patients have a lifelong danger of thromboembolic phenomena, which are the major cause of mortality in those with untreated disease. Arterial and venous occlusion, in small or large vessels, may occur at any time in life, including infancy. Treatment with pyridoxine, the cofactor of the enzyme, may be effective in nearly half of these patients, particularly those with relatively high residual activity and spared amounts of immunologically detectable enzyme. Blood total homocysteine concentrations may be intermediately elevated in heterozygotes, especially after a methionine load, and heterozygotes are at some increased risk for vaso-occlusive events. Although increased vascular complications have not been formally demonstrated in outcome studies of obligate heterozygotes, a considerable number of studies show a highly disproportionate fraction of patients with various vaso-occlusive complications who manifest either total blood homocysteine concentrations or fibroblast cystathionine β-synthase activities that fall in the range observed for heterozygotes.

Methylenetetrahydrofolate reductase deficiency has been described in a limited number of patients, and the spectrum of manifestations includes neurologic symptoms, thrombosis, and lens dislocation, but without conspicuous skeletal changes. Partial deficiencies and thermolabile variants have been observed in otherwise normal subjects who have premature vaso-occlusive disorders. Polymorphisms are also found in the methylenetetrahydrofolate reductase gene in association with spinal closure defects, a class of disease that has been known to be influenced by folate. Cobalamin metabolic disorders generally occur in early childhood and are characterized by neurologic symptoms, megaloblastic anemia, and in some cases, methylmalonic acidemia.

Diagnosis

Qualitative detection using sodium nitroprusside led to the recognition of homocystinuria early in the history of biochemical genetics, but it is neither specific nor sensitive. Assay of plasma amino acids by routine methods may not reveal homocysteine as a result of the high degree of protein binding. Because of lower protein concentrations, routine amino acid analysis of urine is more successful, hence the common name *homo-*

TABLE 228–2 CLINICAL FEATURES OF HOMOCYSTINURIA

	Biochemical Features			Clinical Features	
Class	**Hcys**	**met**	**MMA**	**System**	**Signs**
Cystathionine β-synthase deficiency	$\uparrow$	$\uparrow$	–	Ocular	Ectopia lentis, myopia, glaucoma, optic atrophy, retinal detachment
				Skeletal	Elongated and thinned bones, arachnodactyly, genu valgum, pectus malformation, scoliosis
				Vascular	Thromboembolic events (arterial or venous)
				Neurologic	Mental retardation often in untreated cases, cerebrovascular thromboses, seizures Psychiatric disorders, personality disorder
Methylenetetrahydrofolate reductase deficiency	$\uparrow$	$\downarrow$	–	Ocular	Ectopia lentis
				Vascular	Thromboses
				Neurologic	Variable—psychiatric to severe neurologic
Transcobalamin II deficiency	$-/\uparrow$	$-/\downarrow$	+/–	Hematologic	Pancytopenia, macrocytosis
				Pansystemic	MMA, ketoacidosis, stomatitis
Cbl F	$-/\uparrow$	?	+/–	Pansystemic	MMA, macrocytosis, stomatitis
Cbl C, Cbl D	$-/\uparrow$	$-/\downarrow$	+	Hematologic	Pancytopenia
				Neurologic	Mental retardation
Cbl E, Cbl G	$\uparrow$	$-/\downarrow$	–	Vascular	Vaso-occlusive phenomena
				Neurologic	Spasticity, dystonia

Cbl = cobalamin; Hcys = homocyst(e)inemia/homocystinuria; met = plasma methionine; MMA = methylmalonic acidemia.

cystinuria. The preferred diagnostic method is total homocysteine, which is measured in plasma treated with a reducing agent to release bound homocysteine before deproteinization. Plasma amino acids will indicate a transsulfuration or remethylation defect, depending on the presence or absence of hypermethioninemia (see Table 228–2). The clinical diagnosis of remethylation defects is facilitated by detection of urine methylmalonate and blood vitamin B_{12} and folate. The normal range of total homocysteine in blood extends up to around 15 μmol/L and may be more than 50% higher 2 to 4 hours after an oral methionine load. A standard methionine load (100 mg/kg) may identify individuals with partial defects, which could increase the susceptibility to vascular disease.

Treatment

Rx

Cystathionine β-synthase deficiency is responsive to administration of the cofactor pyridoxine in about 50% of cases. Doses of 100 to 500 mg/day have been used successfully. Higher doses of pyridoxine should be given cautiously because of the risk for peripheral neuropathy. Responsiveness is documented by the elimination of free homocysteine in blood and urine as pyridoxine is added, but measurement of total homocysteine demonstrates that the effect is generally far less than complete. Betaine (*N,N,N*-trimethylglycine, Cystadane) is effective in reducing homocysteine through an alternative remethylation step. It is particularly important in pyridoxine-unresponsive cases but may also be used as an adjunct in responsive patients. Betaine is generally given at 6 g/day in divided doses, but considerably higher doses have been used. The dose used in children is generally 100 to 250 mg/kg. There have been two reports of cerebral edema associated with betaine, presumably caused by unusually high levels of methionine or betaine. In the absence of pyridoxine responsiveness, special diets are adopted to restrict methionine and supplement cysteine. Folic acid may be effective in remethylation defects, and it is also generally used as a supplement (10 to 20 mg/day) in all forms of homocystinuria. Vitamin B_{12} preparations may be life-saving in disorders of cobalamin metabolism, although their effectiveness in the most common forms of cobalamin C or D defects is generally far from complete. Initial doses are usually 1000 μg/day, and hydroxocobalamin may be more effective than cyanocobalamin. It is prudent to adopt measures to decrease thrombosis, such as using low-dose aspirin or dipyridamole and avoiding smoking and birth control pills. Nitrous oxide may also be relatively contraindicated inasmuch as it can inhibit methionine synthase. Surgery poses serious risks but can be performed safely as long as attention is paid to hydration and coagulation status.

Prognosis

In cases of cystathionine β-synthase deficiency, pyridoxine responsiveness generally correlates with higher residual activity, and the prognosis is significantly better than that for unresponsive cases, with or without treatment. Skeletal, ocular, vascular, and neurologic risks are all reduced with successful treatment. Without early institution of treatment, the median IQ in a large outcome study was 57 for unresponsive patients and 78 for responsive patients. With early treatment, pyridoxine-unresponsive patients have a nearly normal median IQ. With treatment in responsive patients, the prognosis for intellectual development is very good, but significant increases in total homocysteine still generally persist, and some increased risk for vascular complications probably does remain.

SUGGESTED READINGS

Jacobsen DW: Hyperhomocysteinemia and oxidative stress: Time for a reality check? Arterioscler Thromb Vasc Biol 2000;20:1182–1184. *Balanced discussion of theories of oxidative stress related to homocysteine.*

Miles EW, Kraus JP: Cystathionine β-synthase: Structure, function, regulation, and location of homocystinuria-causing mutations. J Biol Chem 2005; 279:29871–29874. *A minireview of the molecular biology of cystathionine β-synthase.*

Perna AF, Ingrosso D, De Santo NG: Homocysteine and oxidative stress. Amino Acids 2003;25:409–417. *Presents several hypotheses of disease mechanisms associated with hyperhomocysteinemia.*

Vilaseca MA, Cuartero ML, Martinez de Salinas M, et al: Two successful pregnancies in pyridoxine-nonresponsive homocystinuria. J Inherit Metab Dis 2004;27:775–777. *Instructive case reports.*

Yap S, Boers GH, Wilcken B, et al: Vascular outcome in patients with homocystinuria due to cystathionine beta-synthase deficiency treated chronically: A multicenter observational study. Arterioscler Thromb Vasc Biol 2001; 21:2080–2085. *A long-term multicenter observational study that demonstrates the effectiveness of treatment in reducing vascular risk despite imperfect biochemical control.*

229 THE PORPHYRIAS

Karl E. Anderson

Definition

Porphyrias are due to deficiencies of specific enzymes of the heme biosynthetic pathway and, when clinically expressed, are associated with striking accumulations of heme pathway intermediates. Most porphyrias are inherited, but other factors are important in determining their severity. Porphyrias are more prevalent and more often manifested in adults than are most metabolic diseases and are likely to be encountered by physicians in many disciplines. The three most common porphyrias differ considerably from each other and are managed differently.

The Heme Biosynthetic Pathway and the Porphyrias

The genes encoding all eight enzymes of this important pathway (Fig. 229–1) have been sequenced and their chromosome locations identified (Table 229–1). Mutations of the erythroid-specific form of δ-aminolevulinic acid (ALA) synthase, the first enzyme, are found in X-linked sideroblastic anemia. Mutations in genes for the other seven enzymes are found in the porphyrias. (Standard abbreviations for these diseases are shown in Table 229–1.) These diseases are all heterogeneous at the molecular level. Therefore, different mutations are to be expected in unrelated families with any given type of porphyria.

Heme is synthesized in largest amounts in bone marrow and liver, where it is used primarily to make hemoglobin and cytochrome P-450 enzymes, respectively. Hepatic heme biosynthesis is regulated primarily by ALA synthase, which is rate limiting and under sensitive feedback control by a regulatory pool of cellular heme. Hepatic ALA synthase is induced by many of the same drugs and steroids that induce P-450 enzymes. Additional pathway enzymes and cellular uptake of iron are important in regulating heme synthesis in erythroid cells.

Intermediates in the pathway (see Fig. 229–1) are normally conserved during heme synthesis and excreted only in small amounts. The porphyrin precursors ALA and porphobilinogen (PBG) are normally excreted in much larger amounts than porphyrins. Porphyrinogens undergo auto-oxidation outside cells and are excreted primarily as porphyrins. ALA, PBG, and porphyrinogens are colorless and nonfluorescent. Porphyrins are reddish and fluoresce on exposure to long-wave ultraviolet light. ALA, PBG, uroporphyrin, and the heptacarboxyl, hexacarboxyl, and pentacarboxyl porphyrins are excreted mostly in urine; coproporphyrin (a tetracarboxyl porphyrin), in urine and bile; and harderoporphyrin and protoporphyrin, in bile and feces.

Classification

Porphyrias are classified as erythropoietic or hepatic types, depending on whether overproduction of heme pathway intermediates occurs primarily in bone marrow or liver, and also on the basis of clinical features. The acute porphyrias are characterized by neurologic effects. In the cutaneous porphyrias, photosensitivity results from activation of porphyrins by long-wave ultraviolet light (UVA) with generation of oxygen radicals that damage the skin.

THE MOST COMMON PORPHYRIAS

The three most common types of porphyria are likely to be encountered periodically by any physician and differ markedly from each other with regard to major clinical manifestations, exacerbating factors, tests

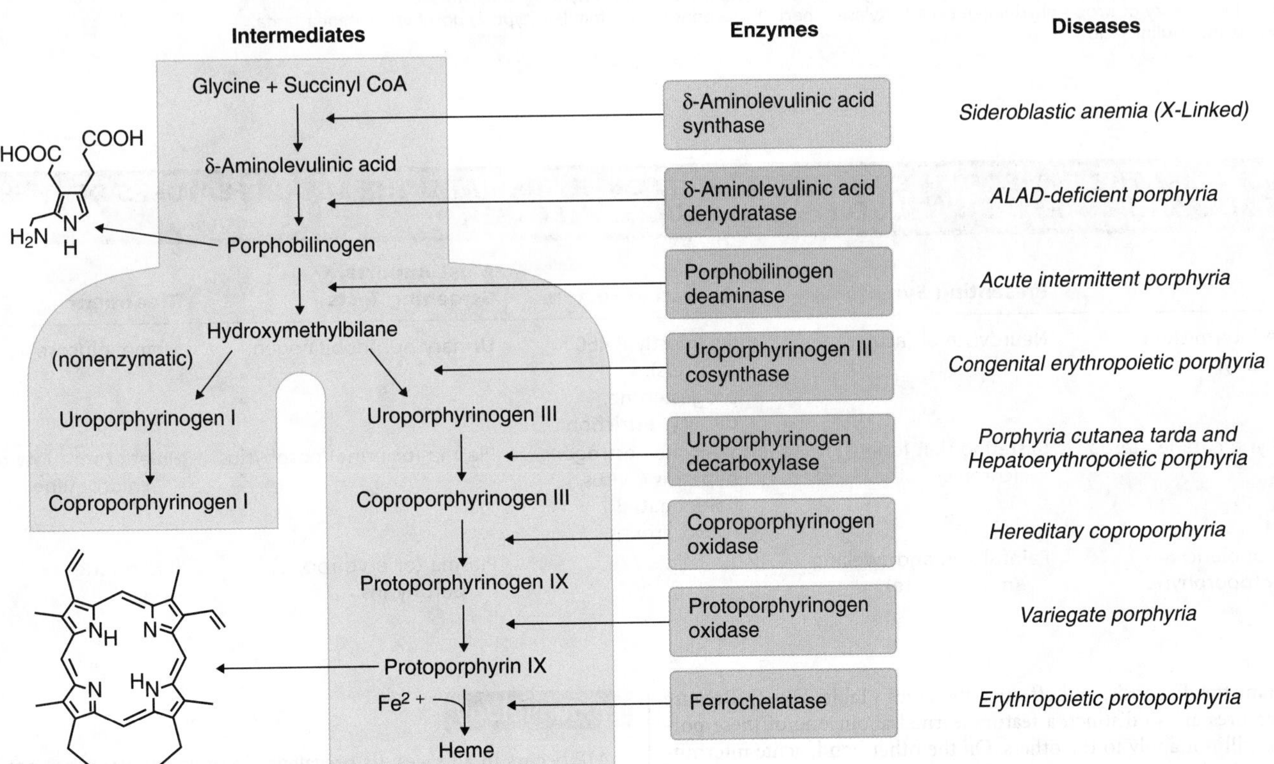

FIGURE 229–1 • Intermediates and enzymes of the heme biosynthetic pathway and the major diseases of porphyrin metabolism that have been associated with deficiencies of specific enzymes. The initial and last three enzymes (in pink) are mitochondrial and the other four (in brown) are cytosolic. Heme is synthesized from glycine and succinyl coenzyme A. Intermediates in the pathway include δ-aminolevulinic acid (an amino acid used exclusively for heme synthesis), porphobilinogen (a pyrrole), and hydroxymethylbilane (a linear tetrapyrrole). Uroporphyrinogen III cosynthase catalyzes closure of hydroxymethylbilane, with inversion of one of the pyrroles, to form a porphyrin macrocycle, uroporphyrinogen III. (Nonenzymatic closure occurs without inversion of this pyrrole, forming uroporphyrinogen I, which is not metabolized beyond coproporphyrinogen I.) The next two enzymes result in decarboxylation of six of the eight side chains of uroporphyrinogen III, with sequential formation of heptacarboxyl porphyrinogen, hexacarboxyl porphyrinogen, pentacarboxyl porphyrinogen, tetracarboxyl porphyrinogen (coproporphyrinogen III), tricarboxyl porphyrinogen (harderoporphyrinogen), and dicarboxyl porphyrinogen (protoporphyrinogen IX). The final two enzymes catalyze oxidation of protoporphyrinogen IX to protoporphyrin IX and insertion of ferrous iron into the porphyrin macrocycle to form heme (iron protoporphyrin IX). With the exception of protoporphyrin IX, all porphyrin intermediates are in their reduced forms (hexahydroporphyrins or porphyrinogens). Chemical structures of two intermediates are shown. ALAD = δ-aminolevulinic acid dehydratase.

TABLE 229–1 ENZYMES OF THE HEME BIOSYNTHETIC PATHWAY AND CLASSIFICATION AND INHERITANCE OF DISEASES ASSOCIATED WITH THEIR DEFICIENCIES*

Enzyme	Chromosome Location	Disease	Inheritance	Classifications of Porphyrias: Hepatic	Erythropoietic	Acute	Cutaneous
ALA synthase							
Erythroid	Xp11.21	Sideroblastic anemia	X-linked recessive				
Nonerythroid	3p21	None known					
ALA dehydratase	9q34	ALA dehydratase–deficient porphyria (ADP)	Autosomal recessive	?X		X	
Porphobilinogen deaminase[1]	11q24.1 → q24.2	Acute intermittent porphyria (AIP)	Autosomal dominant	X		X	
Uroporphyrinogen III cosynthase	10q25.2 → q26.3	Congenital erythropoietic porphyria (CEP)	Autosomal recessive		X		X
Uroporphyrinogen decarboxylase	1p34	Porphyria cutanea tarda (PCT)[2]	Autosomal dominant	X			X
		Hepatoerythropoietic porphyria (HEP)	Autosomal recessive	X	X		X
Coproporphyrinogen oxidase	3q12	Hereditary coproporphyria (HCP)	Autosomal dominant	X		X	X
Protoporphyrinogen oxidase	1q22 or 23	Variegate porphyria (VP)	Autosomal dominant	X		X	X
Ferrochelatase	18q21.3 or 22	Erythropoietic protoporphyria (EPP)	Autosomal dominant		X		X

*The most precise classification is according to the specific enzyme deficiencies. Other classifications based on the major tissue site of overproduction of heme pathway intermediates (hepatic vs. erythropoietic) or the type of major symptoms (acute neurovisceral vs. cutaneous) are useful but not precise or mutually exclusive.

[1]This enzyme is also known as hydroxymethylbilane synthase and formerly as uroporphyrinogen I synthase.

[2]Inherited deficiency of uroporphyrinogen decarboxylase is partially responsible for familial (type 2) porphyria cutanea tarda.

ALA = δ-aminolevulinic acid.

TABLE 229–2 THE THREE MOST COMMON HUMAN PORPHYRIAS AND THE MAJOR FEATURES OF THESE DISORDERS THAT ARE DISTINCTLY DIFFERENT FROM EACH OTHER

	Presenting Symptoms	Exacerbating Factors	Most Important Screening Tests	Treatment
Acute intermittent porphyria	Neurovisceral (acute)	Drugs (mostly P-450 inducers), progesterone, dietary restriction	Urinary porphobilinogen	Heme, glucose
Porphyria cutanea tarda	Blistering skin lesions (chronic)	Iron, alcohol, estrogens, hepatitis C virus, halogenated hydrocarbons	Plasma (or urine) porphyrins	Phlebotomy, low-dose chloroquine
Erythropoietic protoporphyria	Painful skin and swelling (mostly acute)		Plasma (or erythrocyte) porphyrins	β-Carotene

important for diagnosis, and effective therapies (Table 229–2). Because their features are so distinct, a feature learned about one of these porphyrias will not apply to the others. On the other hand, acute intermittent porphyria and porphyria cutanea tarda (see Table 229–2) are prototypical; they share some important features with certain other less common porphyrias. These important differences are evident in the brief descriptions of each of the porphyrias that follow.

Acute Intermittent Porphyria

Acute intermittent porphyria (AIP), an autosomal dominant disorder, results from an approximately 50% deficiency of PBG deaminase. Penetrance is low, that is, the majority of subjects with PBG deaminase deficiency remain asymptomatic.

Epidemiology

AIP occurs in all races. Its prevalence in most countries has not been precisely estimated, but it may be most common (perhaps 5 per 100,000) in northern European populations.

Pathobiology

More than 250 different mutations of the gene encoding PBG deaminase have been identified in unrelated AIP lineages. PBG deaminase is decreased in all tissues of most patients with AIP. However, there are two isoenzymes of PBG deaminase, an erythroid-specific and a nonerythroid or "housekeeping" form, both of which are transcribed by alternative mRNA splicing from the same gene. The erythroid-specific isoenzyme is encoded by exons 2 to 15, and the erythroid promoter, which functions only in erythroid cells, is found immediately upstream from exon 2. The nonerythroid enzyme is encoded by exons 1 and 3 to 15, and the nonerythroid promoter is immediately upstream from exon 1. For some mutations—in or near exons 1 or 3—only the nonerythroid isoenzyme is deficient. Therefore, in individuals with this type of mutation, the enzyme activity is deficient in nonerythroid tissues but normal in erythrocytes.

The fact that most heterozygotes are asymptomatic and have normal levels of ALA and PBG indicates that the partial deficiency of PBG deaminase does not of itself greatly impair hepatic heme synthesis or induce ALA synthase. However, when the demand for hepatic heme is increased by drugs, hormones, or nutritional factors, the deficient enzyme can become limiting for heme synthesis. Induction of hepatic ALA synthase is then accentuated and ALA and PBG accumulate in liver and increase in plasma and urine. Excess porphyrins originate nonenzymatically from PBG or enzymatically from ALA transported to tissues other than the liver.

Most drugs that are harmful in AIP induce hepatic ALA synthase and cytochrome P-450 enzymes. Some, such as sulfonamide antibiotics, are harmful for reasons not understood. Reduced calorie and carbohydrate intakes enhance induction of ALA synthase in animals and can increase ALA and PBG in AIP and precipitate symptoms. The peroxisome proliferator–activated receptor γ coactivator 1α (PGC-1α) mediates induction of ALA synthase by fasting and is an important link between nutritional status and acute porphyrias.

Porphyrias and related disorders associated with increased ALA have similar neurologic manifestations, but the mechanism of neural damage is not established. It seems most likely that ALA or another product of the heme pathway is neurotoxic. ALA is structurally analogous to γ-aminobutyric acid (GABA) and can interact with GABA receptors. Alternatively, heme deficiency in nervous tissue may lead to neurologic dysfunction.

Clinical Manifestations

Symptoms occur intermittently in some heterozygotes as acute attacks lasting for several days or longer, usually followed by complete recovery. Attacks are rare before puberty. Frequently recurring attacks and chronic symptoms sometimes occur. There is often no family history of porphyria. Abdominal pain, the most common symptom, is usually steady and poorly localized, but it may be cramping. Tachycardia, hypertension, restlessness, fine tremors, and excess sweating may be due to sympathetic overactivity. Other manifestations include nausea and vomiting; constipation; pain in the limbs, head, neck, or chest; muscle weakness; and sensory loss. Ileus, with distention and decreased bowel sounds, is common. However, increased bowel sounds and diarrhea may be seen. Because the abdominal symptoms are neurologic rather than inflammatory, tenderness, fever, and leukocytosis are generally absent or mild. Dysuria and bladder dysfunction may occur. Recurrent attacks tend to be similar in a given patient.

Peripheral neuropathy in AIP is primarily motor and results from axonal degeneration. This does not develop in all patients with acute attacks, even when abdominal symptoms are severe. Rarely, neuropathy develops apart from abdominal symptoms. Weakness most commonly begins in proximal muscles (often requiring a careful examination to be detected) and more often in the arms than in the legs. It can be asymmetrical and focal. Tendon reflexes may be little affected or hyperactive in early stages but are usually decreased or absent with advanced neuropathy. Cranial and sensory nerves can be affected. Progression to respiratory and bulbar paralysis and death is unlikely if porphyria is promptly recognized, harmful drugs are discontinued, and appropriate treatment is instituted. Sudden death, presumably from cardiac arrhythmia, sometimes occurs.

The central nervous system can be involved. Anxiety, insomnia, depression, disorientation, hallucinations, and paranoia, which can be especially severe during acute attacks, may suggest a primary mental disorder or hysteria. Seizures may occur as an acute neurologic manifestation of AIP, as a result of hyponatremia, or secondary to causes unrelated to porphyria. Hyponatremia may be due to hypothalamic involvement and inappropriate antidiuretic hormone secretion, vomiting, diarrhea and poor intake, or excess renal sodium loss.

An attack may resolve rapidly after several days. Attacks during the luteal phase of the menstrual cycle usually resolve with onset of menses. Even advanced neuropathy seen with a prolonged attack is potentially reversible. Pain, depression, and other symptoms are sometimes chronic.

Chronic hepatic abnormalities are common in AIP. Risk of hepatocellular carcinoma (not associated with hepatitis B or C) is also increased. AIP may predispose to chronic hypertension and be associated with impaired renal function.

Homozygous AIP is extremely rare. It presents in early childhood primarily with delayed development and neurologic dysfunction, but not with acute attacks.

Precipitating Factors

Recognition of precipitating factors, most importantly drugs, endogenous steroid hormones, and nutritional alterations, is important in management. Features such as onset after puberty and more frequent clinical expression in women suggest that endogenous hormones are important. Recurrent cyclic attacks are troublesome in some women and occur when progesterone levels are highest. Progesterone and its metabolites are potent inducers of ALA synthase, whereas estrogens are not. Exacerbations may be seen after administration of progestin-containing steroid combinations. Although pregnancy is usually well tolerated (despite high progesterone levels), attacks may become more frequent, and hyperemesis gravidarum and reduced calorie intake may contribute.

Drugs remain important as causes of AIP attacks. Barbiturates and sulfonamides are most notorious, whereas benzodiazepines, which have largely replaced barbiturates in clinical practice, are less hazardous. The major drugs known to be harmful or safe in the acute porphyrias are listed in Table 229–3, but many are not easily classified. Advice can be sought from an interactive website maintained by the European Porphyria Initiative (*www.porphyria-europe.com/*) or from the American Porphyria Foundation (*www.porphyriafoundation.com/*). Some drugs may exacerbate porphyria cutanea tarda but not acute porphyrias (see later).

Attacks are also provoked by reduced calorie intake (usually instituted in an effort to lose weight), infections, and major surgery. Cigarette smoke contains chemicals that can induce hepatic heme synthesis and may predispose to attacks. Attacks are almost always due to two or more factors acting in an additive fashion. Probably for this reason, (1) drugs may produce attacks in adults but rarely in children, (2) anticonvulsants do not produce attacks in all PBG deaminase–deficient subjects, and (3) barbiturate anesthetics more frequently exacerbate porphyria if symptoms are present before anesthetic exposure.

Diagnosis

A high index of suspicion is necessary for diagnosis of AIP and other acute porphyrias because they are uncommon, their symptoms are nonspecific, and physical findings are minimal. In some European countries, almost all families with acute porphyrias have been identified and studied, but in the United States, many cases still present without a known family history of porphyria. The diagnosis of acute porphyria is established initially by demonstrating a marked increase in urinary PBG (see the later discussion of laboratory methods). Urinary PBG excretion in excess of approximately 6 mg/day virtually ensures a diagnosis of AIP, variegate porphyria (VP), or hereditary coproporphyria (HCP). Excretion is generally in the range of 50 to 200 mg/day for PBG (reference range, 0 to 4 mg/day) and 20 to 100 mg/day for ALA (reference range, 0 to 7 mg/day) during attacks of AIP, but increases are less in HCP and VP, and these levels generally decrease with clinical improvement. PBG levels become normal after hemin therapy (usually transiently) and sometimes with prolonged clinical latency. Urinary ALA and PBG decrease to normal levels more readily in HCP and VP than in AIP. Fecal porphyrins are usually normal or minimally increased, which distinguishes AIP from HCP and VP. Urinary uroporphyrin and coproporphyrin are often considerably increased and erythrocyte protoporphyrin may be slightly increased in AIP, but these findings are not specific.

TABLE 229–3 DRUGS CONSIDERED UNSAFE AND SAFE IN ACUTE INTERMITTENT PORPHYRIA, HEREDITARY COPROPORPHYRIA, AND VARIEGATE PORPHYRIA

Unsafe	Safe
Angiotensin-converting enzyme inhibitors (especially enalapril)	Acetaminophen
Alcohol	Acetazolamide
Barbiturates[1]	Allopurinol
Calcium-channel blockers (especially nifedipine)	Amiloride
Carbamazepine[1]	Aspirin
Carisoprodol[1]	Atropine
Clonazepam	Bromides
Danazol[1]	Cimetidine
Diclofenac and possibly other nonsteroidal anti-inflammatory drugs[1]	Erythropoietin[1,2]
Ergots	?Estrogens[1,3]
Glutethimide[1]	Gabapentin
Methyprylon	Gentamicin
Ethchlorvynol[1]	Glucocorticoids
Griseofulvin[1]	Insulin
Mephenytoin	Narcotic analgesics
Meprobamate[1] (also mebutamate,[1] tybutamate[1])	Ofloxacin
Metoclopramide[1]	Penicillin and derivatives
Phenytoin[1]	Phenothiazines
Primidone[1]	Ranitidine[1,2]
Progesterone and synthetic progestins[1]	Streptomycin
Pyrazinamide[1]	Tetracycline
Pyrazolones (aminopyrine, antipyrine)	
Rifampin[1]	
Succinimides (ethosuximide, methsuximide)	
Sulfonamide antibiotics[1]	
Valproic acid[1]	

[1]Porphyria is listed as a contraindication, warning, precaution, or adverse effect in U.S. labeling for these drugs. For drugs listed here as unsafe, absence of such cautionary statements in U.S. labeling does not imply lower risk.
[2]Although porphyria is listed as a precaution in U.S. labeling, these drugs are regarded as safe by other sources.
[3]There is little evidence that estrogens alone are harmful in acute porphyrias. They have been implicated as harmful mostly on the basis of experience with estrogen-progestin combinations and because they can exacerbate porphyria cutanea tarda.

Laboratory reports documenting the diagnosis of AIP should remain available for future reference. Because PBG levels often remain variably elevated between attacks of AIP, recurrent attacks are recognized primarily on the basis of recurrent symptoms and signs rather than by a particular level of increased PBG.

Decreased PBG deaminase (most conveniently measured in erythrocytes) confirms a diagnosis of AIP. However, as already noted, some PBG deaminase mutations reduce only the nonerythroid enzyme. Furthermore, erythrocyte PBG deaminase has a wide normal range (up to threefold) that somewhat overlaps the AIP range and is increased by inapparent concurrent conditions that stimulate erythropoiesis. The enzyme is not reduced in HCP and VP, which are also important to consider when acute porphyria is suspected. For these reasons, measurement of erythrocyte PBG deaminase is not useful in acutely ill patients, but it is useful for analysis of pedigrees of known AIP patients if it is established that an index case has a low value. It is now recommended that the specific PBG deaminase mutation be determined in an index case in a family, and then relatives can be tested reliably for latent AIP. Diagnosis in utero is possible but seldom indicated in view of the favorable outlook for most PBG deaminase–deficient subjects.

Laboratory testing for acute porphyrias becomes less sensitive with time after symptoms have subsided. However, in many cases, these disorders may still be recognized and differentiated by more extensive testing to include urinary ALA and PBG, porphyrins in urine and in plasma and feces, and erythrocyte PBG deaminase. An attempt to provoke increases in ALA and PBG for diagnostic purposes by glycine loading or administration of phenobarbital may be dangerous and is not definitive.

Treatment

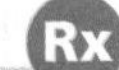

Acute attacks usually require hospitalization for treatment of severe pain, nausea, and vomiting and for the intravenous administration of glucose and hemin. Patients should be observed for neurologic complications, respiratory impairment, electrolyte imbalances, and nutritional status. Precipitating factors—usually multiple—should be identified and removed whenever possible. Symptomatic therapy includes narcotic analgesics, which are usually required for severe abdominal pain, and small to moderate doses of a phenothiazine for nausea, vomiting, anxiety, and restlessness. Chloral hydrate can be used for insomnia. Benzodiazepines in low doses may be safe if a minor tranquilizer is required. Bladder distention may require catheterization. After recovery, continued treatment with a phenothiazine is seldom indicated.

Hemin therapy and carbohydrate loading are specific therapies because they repress hepatic ALA synthase and overproduction of ALA and PBG. Hemin is more effective and should be initiated early, but only after the initial diagnosis of acute porphyria is confirmed by a marked increase in urinary PBG. (Spot samples of urine, plasma, and feces are saved for later differentiation of AIP, HCP, and VP.) Diagnosis is more difficult after hemin is started, which at least transiently is expected to normalize ALA and PBG. In patients with frequent attacks and persistently high levels of PBG, a spot urine sample may be obtained for PBG measurement before hemin is administered and therapy started before the result is available.

The standard regimen for hemin treatment is 3 to 4 mg of hemin per kilogram of body weight infused intravenously once daily for 4 days. A longer course of treatment is seldom necessary if treatment is started early. Efficacy is reduced and recovery less rapid when treatment is delayed and neuronal damage is more advanced. It is not effective for chronic symptoms of AIP. Hemin is available in the United States as a lyophilized hematin (hydroxyheme) preparation. The product is unstable when it is reconstituted with sterile water, and degradation products adhere to endothelial cells, platelets, and coagulation factors, causing a transient anticoagulant effect and frequently a phlebitis at the site of infusion. Reconstitution with human albumin enhances the stability of hematin and prevents these side effects. Heme arginate (available in Europe and South Africa) is more stable and has fewer side effects.

Carbohydrate loading may suffice for mild attacks and can be given orally as sucrose, glucose polymers, or carbohydrate-rich foods. If oral intake is poorly tolerated or contraindicated by distention and ileus, intravenous administration of glucose (at least 300 g daily) is usually indicated, although larger amounts may be more effective. A central venous line facilitates more complete parenteral nutrition support and avoids excess fluid volumes. The effect of glucose is mediated in part by elevation of insulin, which reduces expression of PGC-1α in the liver.

Treatment of seizures is problematic because almost all antiseizure drugs can exacerbate AIP. Bromides, gabapentin, and probably vigabatrin can be given safely. β-Adrenergic blocking agents may control tachycardia and hypertension in acute attacks of porphyria, but they may be hazardous in patients with hypovolemia, in whom increased catecholamine secretion may be an important compensatory mechanism. Cimetidine has been reported to be beneficial, but controlled studies are lacking. Numerous other therapies have been tried in this disease but have not been consistently useful.

Prevention

Some specific measures are helpful in preventing clinical expression of AIP. Family members should be screened, preferably by DNA methods, to detect latent cases. Harmful drugs should be avoided. "Crash diets" for weight reduction and even brief periods of starvation (e.g., during postoperative periods or intercurrent illnesses) should be avoided; diet regimens for obesity should provide for gradual weight loss during periods of clinical remission of porphyria. Gonadotropin-releasing hormone analogues can prevent frequent cyclic attacks in women; oophorectomy is not an acceptable option for preventing cyclic attacks. Single hemin infusions once or twice weekly sometimes prevent frequently recurring attacks. Because suicide is a risk in AIP, a preventive approach is appropriate, especially in patients with chronic symptoms and depression.

Prognosis

If acute attacks are treated promptly, inciting factors removed, and precautions taken to prevent further attacks, the outlook for patients with AIP is usually very good. Recurrent attacks occur in some patients and can be disabling, but they do not occur throughout adult life. Chronic pain, depression, and other symptoms can increase the risk of suicide but may improve in the long term.

The majority of relatives with PBG deaminase deficiency never develop symptoms, especially if they have normal urinary porphyrin precursors. Such individuals with latent AIP may be less sensitive to inducing drugs or other factors that exacerbate AIP than are patients with prior porphyric symptoms, but they should follow the same precautions as those who have had symptoms. Latent AIP should never be construed as a health risk that limits availability of health insurance.

Porphyria Cutanea Tarda

Definition

Porphyria cutanea tarda (PCT), the most common and readily treated form of porphyria, is caused by a deficiency of uroporphyrinogen decarboxylase (UROD) in the liver. It presents with blistering cutaneous lesions on sun-exposed areas.

Pathobiology

PCT is mostly an acquired disorder that is thought to result from generation of a UROD inhibitor in the liver, which reduces the activity of the enzyme to less than 20% of normal. (The hepatic UROD protein remains at its genetically determined level, as measured immunochemically.) A normal or increased amount of hepatic iron is essential for development of PCT, although iron does not directly inhibit UROD. Iron and one or more cytochrome P-450 enzymes are believed to be involved in formation of the UROD inhibitor, and some of the factors that increase susceptibility for development of PCT may increase oxidative stress in hepatocytes. The causative inhibitor has been isolated as a uroporphomethene, derived from uroporphyrinogen. Multiple genetic, viral, and chemical susceptibility factors are known, and at least several are combined in individual patients. Heterozygous carriers of *UROD* mutations are more susceptible, for example, because their genetically determined levels of UROD are half-normal to begin with in all tissues including liver.

Most patients with manifest PCT (~80%) do not have *UROD* mutations and are classified as sporadic (type 1), whereas those with *UROD* mutations are said to have familial (type 2) disease. Most type 2 patients present sporadically (without a family history of PCT) because penetrance of familial PCT is low. Type 2 cases can be distinguished by finding half-normal UROD activity in erythrocytes, but DNA studies are more reliable. Clustering of related individuals with features of type 1 PCT, including absence of *UROD* mutations, has been referred to as type 3, but the genetic basis is not known. Types 1 to 3 are clinically similar, although age at disease onset may on average be earlier in type 2.

Examples of toxic porphyria have resembled PCT. Most notably, an extensive outbreak of porphyria occurred in eastern Turkey in 1955–1958 after seed wheat containing the fungicide hexachlorobenzene was used for food. 2,3,7,8-Tetrachlorodibenzo-*p*-dioxin (TCDD, dioxin) has been implicated in smaller outbreaks. When these chemicals are administered to animals, they decrease UROD activity (only in the liver) and induce a pattern of excess porphyrins resembling PCT. Such exposures are seldom evident in sporadic cases of PCT.

Multiple susceptibility factors contribute to the development of hepatic UROD deficiency, mostly by increasing iron or oxidative stress in the liver. Although the prevalence of most known susceptibility factors is substantially increased in PCT, this disease is found in few individuals with any one of these factors. The following are readily identified clinically in patients with PCT.

- Alcohol in excess has long been recognized as an important contributor and may increase hepatic iron, induce cytochrome P-450 enzymes, and increase activated oxygen species in hepatocytes.
- Smoking has been considered a potential contributor more recently. Constituents of cigarette smoke can induce hepatic cytochrome P-450 enzymes that may be involved in generation of a UROD inhibitor (especially CYP1A2).
- Estrogen use is strongly associated with PCT in women and may also lead to production of reactive oxygen species in hepatocytes.
- The prevalence of hepatitis C, which may cause steatosis and oxidative damage in hepatocytes, may exceed 70% among PCT patients in some geographic areas, including the United States and southern Europe.
- Human immunodeficiency virus infection is less commonly associated but is probably an independent risk factor for PCT.
- Hemochromatosis gene (*HFE*) mutations favor increased iron absorption. Patients with PCT are homozygous or heterozygous for *HFE* gene mutations more commonly than is expected by chance. About 10% of PCT patients of northern European origin may be homozygous for the *C282Y* mutation, which defines them genetically as having hereditary hemochromatosis, and a corresponding number are *C282Y/H63D* compound heterozygotes. *C282Y* heterozygotes and *H63D* homozygotes have some increase in iron absorption, making them somewhat more susceptible for development of PCT.

Other susceptibility factors require more specialized laboratory studies. *UROD* mutations, which identify patients with type 2 disease, are most reliably found by DNA studies; most will have half-normal erythrocyte UROD activity. Reduced levels of antioxidants, such as vitamin C and carotenoids, have been reported. A *CYP1A2* polymorphism that favors induction of this enzyme is more common in PCT and deserves further study.

Almost all patients will have at least several of these susceptibility factors. In addition, drugs may worsen PCT, but this is not commonly observed. Those so indicated in U.S. labeling are several nonsteroidal anti-inflammatory drugs, sulfonylureas, and busulfan. Associations with systemic lupus erythematosus and bone marrow disorders have been described. PCT sometimes occurs in patients with advanced renal disease. Skin lesions may be more severe and plasma porphyrin levels much higher in this setting because urinary excretion of porphyrins is not possible, and they are poorly dialyzed.

As PCT is developing, massive amounts of porphyrins accumulate in the liver, probably during many months, and then excess porphyrins appear in plasma and urine. Thus, this is generally a chronic disease without acute exacerbations. Hepatic ALA synthase may be little increased because the amount of excess porphyrins produced in PCT is small relative to the rate of hepatic heme formation. This contrasts with the acute porphyrias, in which much larger amounts of intermediates are excreted as porphyrin precursors, particularly during attacks, and ALA synthase is substantially induced.

The pattern of porphyrins that accumulate in PCT is complex and characteristic. The enzyme-catalyzed decarboxylation of uroporphyrinogen occurs in four sequential steps. Therefore, when the enzyme is markedly deficient, uroporphyrin and the heptacarboxyl, hexacarboxyl, and pentacarboxyl porphyrins (type I and III isomers derived from the corresponding porphyrinogens) accumulate. In addition, pentacarboxyl porphyrinogen can be metabolized by coproporphyrinogen oxidase (the next enzyme in the pathway) to a series of tetracarboxyl porphyrinogens termed isocoproporphyrinogens. The corresponding isocoproporphyrins are excreted primarily in bile and feces and are diagnostic of UROD deficiency.

Clinical Manifestations

Cutaneous photosensitivity is the major clinical feature. Vesicles and bullae develop on the face, dorsum of the hands and feet, forearms, and legs. Sun-exposed skin becomes friable, and minor trauma may precede the formation of bullae or cause denudation of the skin. Small white plaques (milia) may precede or follow vesicle formation. Involved skin tends to heal slowly. Hypertrichosis and hyperpigmentation sometimes occur even in the absence of vesicles. Thickening, scarring, and calcification of affected skin (pseudoscleroderma) may be striking. Neurologic effects are not observed.

Abnormal liver test results—especially transaminases—are common in PCT and can occur in the absence of hepatitis C. Liver histopathology is nonspecific, other than the finding of fluorescence due to porphyrins, which appear as inclusions in fixed tissue. Liver iron is often increased. Risk of cirrhosis and hepatocellular carcinoma increases with disease duration. Very rarely, hepatic tumors themselves contain and presumably produce excess porphyrins. Some of these cases have resembled PCT.

Diagnosis

Skin lesions in PCT, VP, and HCP are indistinguishable clinically and histologically. It is important to differentiate these conditions by laboratory testing before therapy is started. A predominance of uroporphyrin and heptacarboxyl porphyrin in urine is diagnostic of PCT, and increased isocoproporphyrin in feces provides further confirmation. In PCT, urinary ALA may be slightly increased, whereas PBG is normal. Total fecal porphyrins are usually less increased in PCT than in HCP and VP. Plasma porphyrins are virtually always increased in patients with skin lesions from any type of porphyria with the occasional exception of erythropoietic protoporphyria; the fluorescence spectrum of plasma can distinguish VP and erythropoietic protoporphyria from PCT (see later).

Treatment

Rx

All three types of PCT respond to treatment; with remission, hepatic UROD activity returns to its genetically determined level (which for type 2 is half-normal). A course of phlebotomies is the preferred treatment. Patients are also advised to discontinue alcohol, estrogens, iron supplements, or other contributing factors. Because iron stores in PCT are seldom markedly increased, removal of only 5 to 8 units of blood at 1- to 2-week intervals is usually sufficient. Many more phlebotomies are needed in the minority of patients with very high ferritin levels. Plasma (or serum) ferritin and porphyrin levels should be followed (Fig. 229–2). Deferoxamine, an iron chelator, may be effective but is much less efficient.

A course of low-dose chloroquine (125 mg twice weekly) or hydroxychloroquine (100 mg twice weekly for several months) is usually effective when repeated phlebotomies are contraindicated. The mechanism of their effects in PCT has not been established. One hypothesis is that chloroquine forms complexes with porphyrins and promotes their removal from the liver. If usual doses of these drugs are given to patients with PCT, marked increases in photosensitivity and porphyrin levels in plasma and urine are seen and may be accompanied by nausea, malaise, fever, and hepatocellular damage. Although these adverse effects are generally transient and are followed by complete remission, it is prudent to avoid them by use of a low-dose regimen. These may not be effective in patients with marked iron overload.

Therapy is more difficult when PCT occurs with advanced renal disease because phlebotomy is usually contraindicated by anemia (usually because of erythropoietin deficiency). Treatment with genetic recombinant erythropoietin can mobilize excess iron, support phlebotomy, and lead to remission of PCT in these patients.

Erythropoietic Protoporphyria

Definition

Erythropoietic protoporphyria (EPP) was not clearly described until 1961, perhaps because it seldom causes blistering of the skin and urine porphyrins are not increased. It is now recognized as the third most common porphyria in adults and the most common in children. EPP is due to a deficiency of ferrochelatase (FECH), with increased protoporphyrin in erythrocytes, plasma, bile, and feces.

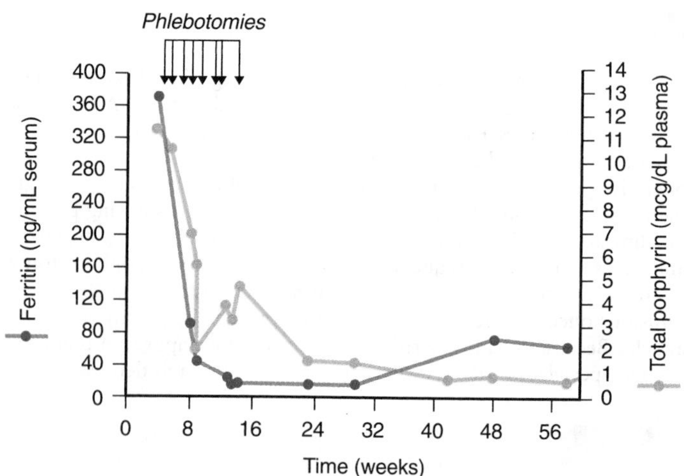

FIGURE 229–2 • Treatment of porphyria cutanea tarda by repeated phlebotomy. The patient was a 37-year-old woman with a history of excess alcohol intake and chronic hepatitis C. Each arrow indicates removal of 450 mL of whole blood. Phlebotomies are stopped when serum ferritin is near the lower limit of normal. Further iron depletion is of no additional benefit and may cause anemia and associated symptoms. Plasma porphyrins become normal and appearance of new skin lesions ceases within several months. After remission, ferritin can return to normal without recurrence, in most cases. In some cases, relapses occur and respond to another course of phlebotomies. (Modified from Anderson KE: The porphyrias. *In* Boyer T, Wright T, Manns M [eds]: Zakim and Boyer's Hepatology. Philadelphia, WB Saunders, 2006, pp 1391–1432.)

Pathobiology

Although EPP is an autosomal dominant disease in most families, it is now established that inheritance of two alleles associated with reduced FECH activity is required for disease expression. This is consistent with FECH activities as low as 15 to 25% of normal in patients with EPP. Many different *FECH* mutations expressing little or no enzyme activity have been identified in various EPP families. In most individuals with manifest EPP, a disabling mutation affecting one *FECH* allele is combined with a common polymorphism affecting the other allele, which produces less than normal amounts of enzyme. This intronic single nucleotide polymorphism, IVS3-48T/C, results in expression of an aberrantly spliced mRNA that is degraded by a nonsense-mediated decay mechanism, which decreases the steady-state level of FECH mRNA. The IVS3-48T/C polymorphism by itself does not cause disease, even when it is homozygous. In a few families, two *FECH* mutations and a pattern of autosomal recessive inheritance have been found, and autosomal recessive inheritance occurs naturally in cattle and in mouse models. In a recently described variant form with clinical features typical of EPP, FECH activity is normal and there are no *FECH* mutations. This form of EPP is probably due to an unidentified genetic defect in iron delivery to the normal FECH enzyme. Late-onset cases of EPP may be associated with a myeloproliferative disorder and a somatic mutation, with expansion of an affected clone of erythroid cells.

Bone marrow reticulocytes are the primary source of the excess protoporphyrin in EPP. Circulating erythrocytes and the liver contribute smaller amounts. Protoporphyrin is increased in plasma and excreted in bile and feces. The large amounts of protoporphyrin in erythrocytes of patients with EPP is free (not complexed with zinc) and diffuses more readily into plasma compared with zinc protoporphyrin (found in lead poisoning, iron deficiency, and some homozygous forms of porphyria). Excretion of protoporphyrin requires hepatic uptake and biliary excretion, and intestinal absorption may result in enterohepatic circulation.

Clinical Manifestations

Photosensitivity typically begins early in childhood and is distinctly different from other cutaneous porphyrias. Burning, itching, erythema, and swelling can occur within minutes of sun exposure. Diffuse edema of sun-exposed areas may resemble angioneurotic edema. Characteristic chronic changes include skin lichenification, leathery pseudovesicles, labial grooving, and nail changes. Scarring is rarely severe or deforming. Vesicles, pigment changes, friability, and hirsutism are unusual. No fluorescence of the teeth and (except with severe hepatic failure) no neuropathic manifestations are present. Drugs that exacerbate hepatic porphyrias are not known to worsen EPP but are generally avoided as a precaution.

Hemolysis is uncommon or mild in uncomplicated cases. Mild anemia with hypochromia and microcytosis is noted in some cases. Gallstones containing protoporphyrin may develop and require cholecystectomy if they are symptomatic. Liver function is usually normal in this condition.

In a minority of patients with EPP (5% or less), liver disease develops in association with hepatic protoporphyrin accumulation, which can progress rapidly to death from liver failure. Excess protoporphyrin itself has cholestatic effects and damages hepatocytes. Intercurrent factors such as viral hepatitis, alcohol, iron deficiency, fasting, and oral contraceptive steroids have played a role in some patients. Marked photosensitivity and skin blistering and even motor neuropathy have developed in some EPP patients with liver failure.

Diagnosis

Protoporphyrin is increased in bone marrow, erythrocytes, plasma, bile, and feces of patients with EPP. An increase in erythrocyte protoporphyrin that is primarily free (not complexed with zinc) is diagnostic of EPP. However, both free and zinc protoporphyrin are increased in the variant form of the disease with normal FECH activity. Urinary porphyrins and porphyrin precursors are normal. Hepatic complications of EPP are often preceded by increasing levels of erythrocyte and plasma protoporphyrin and abnormal liver function test results as marked deposition of protoporphyrin occurs in the liver.

Treatment

Rx

β-Carotene (Lumitene) was originally developed primarily for treatment of EPP and found to be beneficial in large series of patients. Its mechanism of action may involve quenching of singlet oxygen or free radicals. Carotenemia with mild, dose-related skin discoloration is expected. Cholestyramine may reduce protoporphyrin levels by interrupting its enterohepatic circulation. Iron deficiency, calorie restriction, and drugs or hormone preparations that impair hepatic excretory function should be avoided.

Hepatic complications may resolve spontaneously if a reversible cause of liver dysfunction, such as viral hepatitis or alcohol, is contributing. Transfusions or intravenous administration of hemin may suppress erythroid and hepatic protoporphyrin production. Splenectomy, correction of iron deficiency, and cholestyramine or activated charcoal may be beneficial. Liver transplantation is sometimes required. Because liver disease may recur after transplantation, bone marrow transplantation has been recommended if a suitable donor is available. Operating room lights have produced severe skin and peritoneal burns in some patients.

LESS COMMON PORPHYRIAS

ALA Dehydratase–Deficient Porphyria

In this rare autosomal recessive disorder, ALA dehydratase is markedly reduced (usually 1 to 2% of normal). Most of the documented cases have been in adolescent men, with symptoms resembling AIP. More severe cases may have neurologic impairment beginning in childhood. Late-onset cases may be associated with myeloproliferative disorders. Hemolysis is sometimes present. Urinary ALA and coproporphyrin III and erythrocyte zinc protoporphyrin are increased. In this as well as in other disorders in which ALA accumulates, coproporphyrin III may originate from excess ALA by metabolism in tissues other than its tissue of origin.

Lead poisoning and hereditary tyrosinemia type 1 are associated with ALA dehydratase deficiency and can present with symptoms (abdominal pain, ileus, and motor neuropathy) that are strikingly similar to those of the acute porphyrias. Lead concentrates in erythroid cells and deficient erythrocyte ALA dehydratase in lead poisoning can be restored to normal in vitro with dithiothreitol. Erythrocyte protoporphyrin and urinary coproporphyrin are increased, as in ALA dehydratase–deficient porphyria. In hereditary tyrosinemia type 1, a deficiency of fumarylacetoacetase leads to accumulation of succinylacetone (2,3-dioxoheptanoic acid). This structural analogue of ALA is a potent inhibitor of ALA dehydratase. Other heavy metals or styrene exposure can also inhibit ALA dehydratase.

Congenital Erythropoietic Porphyria

Definition

Congenital erythropoietic porphyria (CEP) is an autosomal recessive disorder that is due to a deficiency of uroporphyrinogen III cosynthase (UROS, also known as uroporphyrinogen III synthase). Fewer than 250 cases have been reported. CEP occurs in several animal species (including all fox squirrels).

Pathobiology

Many different mutations of the gene encoding uroporphyrinogen III cosynthase have been identified in CEP. Most patients have unrelated parents and have inherited a different mutation from each parent. The severity of the disease is variable and relates to the degree of enzyme deficiency caused by the particular mutations. There is considerable accumulation of hydroxymethylbilane (the substrate of the deficient enzyme), which is converted nonenzymatically to uroporphyrinogen I. Uroporphyrin I and other porphyrins accumulate in bone marrow erythroid cells that are actively synthesizing hemoglobin and lead to intramedullary and intravascular hemolysis. Even in the most severe cases, some residual UROS activity is present, and heme production is actually increased in response to hemolysis. Splenomegaly can contribute to anemia and cause leukopenia and thrombocytopenia. Sunlight, other sources of ultraviolet light, and minor trauma to friable skin are other determinants of clinical expression. Drugs, steroids, and nutrition have little influence.

Clinical Manifestations

In most cases, reddish urine and severe cutaneous photosensitivity are noted in early infancy. In a few very severe cases, CEP has been manifested as nonimmune hydrops and intrauterine transfusions were administered. Neonatal hyperbilirubinemia may be present at birth, but phototherapy may cause marked photosensitivity and scarring and should be avoided. Late-onset cases are likely to be associated with myeloproliferative disorders and expansion of a clone of cells carrying a UROS somatic mutation.

Lesions on sun-exposed skin resemble those in porphyria cutanea tarda but are usually more severe. Bullae and vesicles are likely to rupture and become infected, which contributes to loss of digits and facial features and corneal scarring. Other features include areas of hypopigmentation or hyperpigmentation and hypertrichosis. Porphyrins are deposited in the teeth (producing a reddish brown color termed erythrodontia) and in bone. Bone demineralization can be substantial and due in part to marrow hyperplasia. Hemolysis and splenomegaly are almost always present, but there are no neurologic manifestations. Life expectancy is often shortened by infections or hematologic complications.

Diagnosis

Porphyrin levels and excretion are generally much greater in CEP than in other forms of porphyria. Porphyrins are primarily uroporphyrin I and coproporphyrin I in urine and mostly coproporphyrin I in feces. ALA and PBG are normal. In most cases, uroporphyrin I predominates in erythrocytes. A predominance of protoporphyrin in red cells has been described in some cases and is characteristic of bovine CEP. CEP is readily distinguished from erythropoietic protoporphyria clinically but may resemble hepatoerythropoietic porphyria and homozygous cases of VP and HCP. These conditions are distinguishable by patterns of porphyrins and porphyrin precursors.

Treatment

Rx

Protection of the skin from sunlight and minor trauma and prompt treatment of secondary bacterial infections help prevent scarring and mutilation. Improvement may occur after splenectomy. Oral charcoal may be helpful by increasing fecal excretion of porphyrins. Blood transfusions, sometimes combined with hydroxyurea, may suppress erythropoiesis sufficiently to reduce porphyrin overproduction. Bone marrow or stem cell transplantation may be the most effective current therapy. Gene therapy may eventually be possible.

Prevention

In affected families, heterozygotes with intermediate deficiencies of UROS can be detected and CEP can be diagnosed in utero. Therefore, options are available to prevent genetic transmission.

Hepatoerythropoietic Porphyria

This rare autosomal recessive disease is clinically similar to CEP but is distinguished by excess isocoproporphyrin in feces and urine and decreased UROD activity in erythrocytes (and other tissues). Mild cases may resemble PCT. Mutations in the gene encoding UROD are found in this disease and are associated with some residual enzyme activity. Increased erythrocyte protoporphyrin probably reflects an earlier accumulation of uroporphyrinogen in erythroblasts, which after completion of hemoglobin synthesis is metabolized to protoporphyrin. A similar explanation can account for increased erythrocyte protoporphyrin in other homozygous forms of porphyria.

Hereditary Coproporphyria and Variegate Porphyria

Epidemiology

These autosomal dominant acute hepatic porphyrias are clinically similar to AIP but are less common in most countries. Unlike AIP, these disorders can cause cutaneous photosensitivity. Variegate porphyria is prevalent in South Africa, where most cases have been traced to a couple who emigrated from Holland in the late 1600s.

Pathobiology

Hereditary coproporphyria (HCP) and variegate porphyria (VP) are due to approximately 50% deficiencies of coproporphyrinogen oxidase (CPO) and protoporphyrinogen oxidase (PPO), respectively. Many different mutations in the genes for these enzymes have been described. A specific mutation of the *PPO* gene (R59W) is common in South Africa. ALA and PBG are increased during acute attacks, although the degree and duration of increases are usually less than in AIP. Increases in ALA and PBG occur when hepatic 5-aminolevulinate synthase (ALAS1) is induced by factors such as endogenous steroids, drugs, and nutritional alterations and because PBG deaminase activity is almost as low as ALAS1 activity even in normal liver. Coproporphyrinogen III may accumulate in VP because of a functional association between CPO and the deficient PPO in mitochondria. Furthermore, coproporphyrinogen is more readily lost from the liver than are other porphyrinogens, and its loss increases further when heme synthesis is stimulated. The excess porphyrinogens are auto-oxidized to the corresponding porphyrins. In one form of HCP, termed harderoporphyria, a structurally altered CPO with reduced substrate affinity results in accumulation of harderoporphyrin as well as coproporphyrin. A few homozygous cases of HCP and VP with severe photosensitivity and developmental abnormalities but few acute attacks have been described.

Clinical Manifestations

Drugs, steroids, and nutritional factors that are detrimental in AIP provoke exacerbations of HCP and VP. Neurologic manifestations are identical to those in AIP. Blistering skin lesions, which are much more common in VP than in HCP, are identical to those in PCT and may occur apart from the neurovisceral symptoms. Impaired biliary excretion by concurrent liver diseases or drugs such as contraceptive steroids can cause porphyrin retention and worsen photosensitivity.

Diagnosis

Urinary ALA and PBG are commonly increased during acute attacks. With resolution of symptoms, ALA and PBG normalize more readily than in AIP. Increases in urinary porphyrins are more persistent. A marked, isolated increase in fecal coproporphyrin (especially isomer III) is distinctive for HCP. Fecal coproporphyrin and protoporphyrin are about equally increased in VP. The fluorescence spectrum of plasma porphyrins (at neutral pH) is characteristic and useful for rapidly distinguishing VP from the other porphyrias. This test is probably the most sensitive porphyrin measurement to detect VP, including latent cases, at least in adults. Identification of specific CPO and PPO mutations is recommended and facilitates screening of relatives.

Treatment

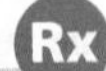

Acute attacks of both HCP and VP are treated as in AIP. The striking decreases in attacks and deaths from VP in South Africa have been attributed to identification of latent cases, avoidance of harmful drugs, and better treatment during acute attacks. Measures that protect the skin from sunlight are helpful for photosensitivity. Cholestyramine may decrease the photosensitivity that occurs with liver dysfunction. Phlebotomies and chloroquine are not effective.

DUAL PORPHYRIA

This term refers to patients with porphyria and deficiencies of more than one enzyme of the heme biosynthetic pathway. Examples include deficiencies of both PBG deaminase and UROD (with symptoms of AIP, PCT, or both), UROS and CPO, and ALA dehydratase and CPO.

LABORATORY DIAGNOSIS OF PORPHYRIAS

Porphyrias are readily detected and misdiagnoses avoided by relying primarily on a few first-line tests that are both specific and sensitive. This avoids overuse of tests and misinterpretation of results. The preferred approach for screening, as outlined in Table 229–4, is to rely on measurement of urinary porphyrin precursors (ALA and PBG) and total porphyrins for patients with neurovisceral symptoms; a fluorometric measurement of plasma total porphyrins is performed when it is suspected that blistering skin lesions might be due to porphyria. Nonblistering photosensitivity in EPP is usually accompanied by increased plasma porphyrins, but measurement of erythrocyte protoporphyrin is more sensitive. More extensive testing is required if an initial screening test provides a positive result or may also be necessary initially if subclinical porphyria is suspected.

In acutely ill patients, it is important to identify or to exclude acute porphyria promptly. Urinary PBG (and ALA) is virtually always substantially increased during acute attacks of AIP. ALA and PBG may be less increased in HCP and VP, but urinary total porphyrins are consistently markedly increased in symptomatic patients. Normal levels of urinary ALA, PBG, and total porphyrins effectively exclude all acute porphyrias as potential causes of current symptoms. Because increases are so striking during an attack, quantitation on a random urine sample is highly informative. Assays for PBG employ Ehrlich's aldehyde (*p*-dimethylaminobenzaldehyde), which forms reddish purple chromogens with PBG, urobilinogen, and other substances in urine. Qualitative methods for increased PBG (e.g., the Watson-Schwartz and Hoesch tests) are considered obsolete. A kit that is reliable for screening for increased PBG in urine includes color standards to aid interpretation (Trace America/Trace Diagnostics, Louisville, Colorado).

TABLE 229–4 FIRST-LINE LABORATORY TESTS FOR SCREENING FOR PORPHYRIAS AND SECOND-LINE TESTS FOR FURTHER EVALUATION WHEN THE INITIAL TEST RESULT IS POSITIVE

	Symptoms Suggesting Porphyria	
Testing	**Acute Neurovisceral Symptoms**	**Cutaneous Photosensitivity**
First line	Urinary ALA, PBG, and total porphyrins (quantitative; random urine)[3]	Total plasma porphyrins[1,2]
Second line	Urinary ALA, PBG, and total porphyrins[3] (quantitative; 24-hour urine) Total fecal porphyrins[3] Erythrocyte PBG deaminase Total plasma porphyrins[1]	Erythrocyte porphyrins Urinary ALA, PBG, and total porphyrins[3] (quantitative, 24-hour urine) Total fecal porphyrins[3]

[1]The preferred method is by direct fluorescent spectrophotometry.
[2]Erythrocyte protoporphyrin should also be measured if erythropoietic protoporphyria is strongly suspected.
[3]Qualitative testing for PBG is often preferred in acutely ill patients (see text). Urinary and fecal porphyrins are fractionated only if the total is increased.
ALA = δ-aminolevulinic acid; PBG = porphobilinogen.

Total plasma porphyrins are virtually always increased in patients with active, blistering skin lesions due to porphyrias. Normal plasma and erythrocyte protoporphyrin levels exclude porphyria as a cause of cutaneous symptoms. Measurement of plasma porphyrins is best carried out by a simple and direct fluorometric method. Plasma porphyrins in VP are mostly covalently bound to plasma porphyrins and may not be detected by other methods. Measurement of erythrocyte protoporphyrin is more sensitive than plasma porphyrins for detecting EPP. Erythrocyte protoporphyrin is increased in many erythrocytic conditions, such as iron deficiency and lead poisoning, but in these conditions it is complexed with zinc rather than metal free, as in EPP.

The interpretation of urine, fecal, or erythrocyte porphyrins results is often problematic. Urine and erythrocyte porphyrins can be increased in many conditions other than porphyria. Fecal porphyrin determinations are semiquantitative and subject to interference by diet and other factors.

Laboratory testing of asymptomatic relatives is usually not appropriate until test results have firmly established a diagnosis of porphyria in an index case. Results of testing of the index case guide the choice of tests for relatives. Consultation with a physician and laboratory with experience in testing for porphyrias is helpful in these situations. Cytosolic heme biosynthetic pathway enzymes (ALA dehydratase, PBG deaminase, UROS, and UROD) can be measured in erythrocytes. These are not recommended for initial screening of patients with symptoms suggestive of porphyria. The other heme pathway enzymes are mitochondrial and can be measured in cells such as lymphocytes. Demonstration of a specific mutation in a family greatly facilitates detection of relatives who carry the same mutation.

Laboratory data that were the basis for an original diagnosis of porphyria should remain available for future reference. Incorrect diagnoses of porphyria are not uncommon when in fact symptoms are due to other diseases. There is little evidence for the suggestion that porphyria is common in disorders such as multiple chemical sensitivity syndrome.

SUGGESTED READINGS

Akagi R, Inoue R, Muranaka S, et al: Dual gene defects involving δ-aminolaevulinate dehydratase and coproporphyrinogen oxidase in a porphyria patient. Br J Haematol 2006;132:237–243. *A patient with acute porphyria and dual enzyme defects documented at the molecular level.*

Akagi R, Kato N, Inoue R, et al: δ-Aminolevulinate dehydratase (ALAD) porphyria: The first case in North America with two novel ALAD mutations. Mol Genet Metab 2006;87:329–336. *A rare and underrecognized form of acute porphyria.*

Anderson KE, Bloomer JR, Bonkovsky HL, et al: Recommendations for the diagnosis and treatment of the acute porphyrias. Ann Intern Med 2005;142:439–450. *Current detailed recommendations on diagnostic methods and treatment for acute porphyrias.*

Goodwin RG, Kell WJ, Laidler P, et al: Photosensitivity and acute liver injury in myeloproliferative disorder secondary to late-onset protoporphyria caused by deletion of a ferrochelatase gene in hematopoietic cells. Blood 2006;107:60–62. *A well-documented example of an erythropoietic porphyria due to a somatic mutation in bone marrow.*

Kauppinen R: Porphyrias. Lancet 2005;365:241–252. *An excellent review of porphyrias.*

Lambrecht RW, Thapar M, Bonkovsky HL: Genetic aspects of porphyria cutanea tarda. Semin Liver Dis 2007;27:99–108. *Recent advances in genetics have allowed DNA testing for porphyria cutanea tarda and are likely to be instrumental in developing improved, gene-based treatments.*

McGuire BM, Bonkovsky HL, Carithers RL Jr, et al: Liver transplantation for erythropoietic protoporphyria liver disease. Liver Transpl 2005;11:1590–1596. *Experience with liver transplantation for protoporphyric hepatic disease.*

Poblete-Gutierrez P, Wiederholt T, Merk HF, et al: The porphyrias: Clinical presentation, diagnosis and treatment. Eur J Dermatol 2006;16:230–240. *An overview of the clinical presentation, diagnosis, and treatment of porphyrias.*

Sassa S: Modern diagnosis and management of the porphyrias. Br J Haematol 2006;135:281–292. *A review of the modern diagnostic techniques for diagnosing porphyrias.*

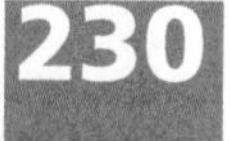

230 WILSON'S DISEASE

Stephen G. Kaler

Definition

Wilson's disease is an autosomal recessive disorder of copper transport. Affected individuals accumulate abnormal levels of copper in the liver and later in the brain as a result of mutations in both alleles of the Wilson disease gene (*ATP7B*). The gene was identified in 1993 and encodes a copper-transporting ATPase expressed primarily in the liver, where its major function is excretion of hepatic copper into the biliary tract.

The clinical condition was first described in 1912 by S. A. K. Wilson, an American-born neurologist working in England. Thirty-six years later, the pathologist J. N. Cummings proposed an etiologic connection with copper overload. Therapy with copper chelation by penicillamine was introduced in 1956 by J. M. Walshe, a British physician working at Boston City Hospital in Massachusetts.

Epidemiology

The incidence of Wilson's disease, defined as the occurrence of new cases, is approximately 1 in 30,000 to 40,000 live births. For special populations in which consanguineous mating is common, the risk of autosomal recessive traits such as Wilson's disease is higher.

In the general population, the prevalence of heterozygous gene carriers (defined as the ratio of all individuals with one mutant *ATP7B* allele to the population at risk of harboring one) is estimated to be 1 in 90. These individuals may represent a susceptible group for liver disease related to copper overload.

Pathobiology

Individuals consume 1 to 3 mg of dietary copper daily, of which approximately 50% is absorbed through the gastrointestinal tract. Most diets contain adequate amounts of copper, and certain foods (e.g., shellfish, liver, mushrooms, chocolate, nuts) contain particularly high quantities. In normal homeostasis, copper is absorbed from the stomach and duodenum, where absorption is mediated by specific copper uptake genes (e.g., *hCTR1*). The Menkes disease gene (*ATP7A*), which encodes a copper-transporting ATPase with high homology to the Wilson gene product, transports copper from within intestinal epithelial cells into the blood stream, where it is bound by albumin and amino acids and carried to the liver through the portal vein.

Within the liver, copper may be

1. incorporated into ceruloplasmin, a multifunctional 132-kD α_2-glycoprotein enzyme containing 0.3% copper—six copper atoms per molecule;
2. used in the synthesis of other copper-requiring enzymes;
3. bound by metallothionein, a low-molecular-weight cysteine-rich protein that provides a storage and detoxification depot for copper and other trace metal elements; or
4. excreted into the bile.

In Wilson's disease, incorporation in ceruloplasmin is usually impaired, resulting in low circulating levels of the ceruloplasmin holoenzyme, whereas excretion into bile is invariably impaired, producing massive hepatic copper overload if the disease is unrecognized. These findings indicate that copper incorporation into ceruloplasmin and biliary excretion of copper are both mediated by the Wilson disease gene product in the normal state.

Circulating levels of functional ceruloplasmin and total serum copper are low in many patients with Wilson's disease. However, these biochemical abnormalities are not necessarily associated with liver disease, as illustrated by the inherited disorders aceruloplasminemia, Menkes' disease, and occipital horn syndrome. A feature that distinguishes Wilson's disease from these conditions is the amount of non–ceruloplasmin-bound serum copper, which is about five-fold normal in Wilson's disease patients.

Thus, the major pathophysiologic component of Wilson's disease is hepatic copper overload resulting from defective biliary excretion of the metal. If this diagnosis goes unrecognized, copper overload subsequently involves other tissues, including brain, which is particularly sensitive to perturbations in trace metal homeostasis.

Clinical Manifestations

Presenting clinical features of Wilson's disease include nonspecific liver disease, neurologic abnormalities, psychiatric illness, hemolytic anemia, renal tubular Fanconi syndrome, and various skeletal abnormalities.

Age influences the specific presentation in Wilson's disease. Nearly all individuals who present with liver disease are younger than 30 years, whereas those presenting with neurologic or psychiatric signs may range in age from the first to the fifth decade. This reflects the sequence of events in the pathogenesis of this disease (see earlier discussion). However, regardless of clinical presentation, some degree of liver disease invariably is present. In one series of 400 adult patients with Wilson's disease, approximately 50% presented with neurologic and psychiatric symptoms, 20% with neurologic and hepatic symptoms, and 20% with purely hepatic symptoms.

In patients with neurologic presentations, abnormalities include speech difficulty (dysarthria), dystonia, rigidity, tremor or choreiform movements, abnormal gait, and uncoordinated handwriting. Wilson's disease may properly be classified as a movement disorder. The neurologic signs and symptoms reflect the predilection for involvement of the basal ganglia (e.g., caudate, putamen) in the brains of these individuals. Parkinson's disease or other movement disorders may be mistakenly diagnosed.

In psychiatric presentations, changes in personality (irritability, anger, poor self-control), depression, and anxiety are common symptoms. Patients presenting in this fashion are typically in their late teens or early 20s, a period during which substance abuse is also a diagnostic consideration. Wilson's disease should be formally excluded in all teenagers and young adults with new-onset psychiatric signs.

In hepatic presentations, signs and symptoms include jaundice, hepatomegaly, edema, and ascites. Secondary endocrine effects of liver disease may include delayed puberty or amenorrhea. Viral hepatitis and cirrhosis are often initial diagnostic considerations in individuals with Wilson's disease.

In addition to the brain and liver, the eye is a primary site of copper deposition in Wilson's disease, producing a pathognomonic sign, the Kayser-Fleischer ring (Fig. 230–1). The Kayser-Fleischer ring is a golden to green-brown annular deposition of copper in the periphery of the cornea. This important diagnostic sign first appears as a superior crescent, then develops inferiorly and ultimately becomes circumferential. Slit lamp examinations are required to detect rings in their early stage of formation. Copper can also accumulate in the lens and produce "sunflower" cataracts.

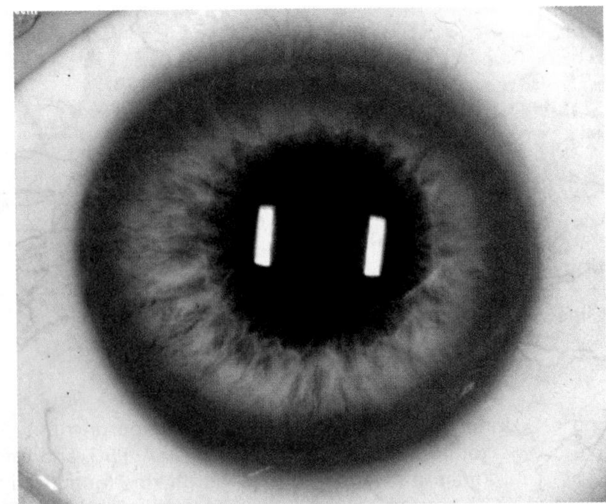

FIGURE 230–1 • Kayser-Fleischer ring in newly diagnosed patient with Wilson's disease.

Approximately 95% of patients with neurologic signs manifest the Kayser-Fleischer ring compared with approximately 65% of those with hepatic presentations. Copper chelation therapy causes fading and even disappearance of corneal copper over time.

Hemolytic anemia resulting from the direct toxic effects of copper on red blood cell membranes has been observed in Wilson's disease. This usually is associated with release of massive quantities of hepatic copper into the circulation, a phenomenon that can be sudden and catastrophic.

Renal dysfunction in Wilson's disease is tubular in nature and leads to abnormal losses of amino acids, electrolytes, calcium, phosphorus, and glucose. This effect is presumably related to copper toxicity. High copper levels have been noted previously in the kidneys of patients with Wilson's disease. Treatment with copper chelation often improves the renal disturbances.

There can be skeletal effects of Wilson's disease, including osteoporosis and rickets; these may be attributable to renal losses of calcium and phosphorus. Osteoarthritis primarily affecting the knees and wrists also occurs in Wilson's disease patients and may involve excess copper deposition in the bone and cartilage.

Diagnosis

The presence of clinical abnormalities described earlier is valuable in the clinical diagnosis of Wilson's disease. Laboratory findings that support the diagnosis include low levels of serum copper and serum ceruloplasmin, elevated hepatic transaminase levels, aminoaciduria, and hemolytic anemia. Incorporation of radiolabeled ^{64}Cu into serum ceruloplasmin, measured as the appearance of copper in the serum after an oral load, is a highly specific diagnostic test; patients with Wilson's disease incorporate very little ^{64}Cu into ceruloplasmin.

Increased urinary excretion of copper (>100 mg/24 hr) is another easily performed and important diagnostic test for this disorder. Acid-washed (copper free) collection containers should be used. A variation involving serial urine copper measurements is the penicillamine "challenge" in which 500 mg of penicillamine is administered orally after collection of a baseline 24-hour urine specimen. The penicillamine dose is repeated after 12 hours, the midpoint of the second 24-hour urine collection. A several-fold increase in copper excretion in the second collection is suggestive of the diagnosis. Some workers think that the challenge does not add enormously to diagnostic discrimination compared with the baseline measurement alone.

Percutaneous needle liver biopsy for measurement of hepatic copper remains a "gold standard" albeit an invasive technique for diagnosis. Hepatic copper values greater than 200 mg per gram of dry weight (normal, 20 to 50 mg/g dry weight) are characteristic of Wilson's disease. Atomic absorption spectrometry is the preferred method; histochemical staining for copper in a liver biopsy specimen is unreliable.

A Wilson's disease mutation database (*http://www.medicalgenetics.med.ualberta.ca/wilson/index.php*) contains nearly 300 different mutations reported at the *ATP7B* locus (January 2007). For families in which the mutant alleles have been determined, molecular diagnosis is highly reliable.

In summary, in the absence of formal molecular evidence, the diagnosis of Wilson's disease can be reliably rendered in the presence of two of the following symptoms: positive family history; Kayser-Fleischer rings; Coombs-negative hemolytic anemia; low serum copper and ceruloplasmin; elevated hepatic copper; increased 24-hour urine copper; and positive result of penicillamine challenge.

Treatment

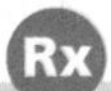

The era of successful treatment of Wilson's disease began in 1956 with Walshe's use of penicillamine, a free thiol that binds (chelates) copper. This drug does not formally correct the basic defect of impaired copper excretion in the bile; however, it greatly enhances urinary excretion of copper and thereby corrects and prevents copper overload and its effects. Faithful compliance with oral penicillamine treatment has enabled the good health of thousands of Wilson's disease patients worldwide during the past 50 years. Pyridoxine (vitamin B_6) is usually prescribed concomitantly to counter the deficiency of this vitamin that tends to develop during long-term penicillamine administration.

Certain individuals are intolerant of penicillamine, however. Significant side effects include nephrotoxicity, hematologic abnormalities, and a distinctive rash, elastosis perforans serpiginosa (which often involves the neck and axillae). Furthermore, in some Wilson's disease patients with neurologic presentations, penicillamine treatment induces paradoxical worsening of the clinical picture.

Even though penicillamine is the Wilson's disease therapy with the longest experience, other pharmaceutical agents are available that may eventually supplant it as a first-line drug. For example, triethylene tetramine dihydrochloride (trien) is a suitable alternative chelating agent with a somewhat less significant side effect profile.

Oral zinc acetate has proved highly effective in Wilson's disease, the mechanism of which involves induction of metallothionein synthesis in intestinal epithelial cells; increased metallothionein synthesis results in greater binding of dietary copper and thus decreased absorption. Zinc therapy has particular value in young, presymptomatic patients; in patients who are pregnant, given the possible fetal teratogenic effects of other compounds; and as maintenance therapy for patients after their initial "decoppering" is accomplished. Zinc acetate has minimal side effects. The only drawback to its use is the relatively long time (4 to 6 months) needed for restoration of proper copper balance when it is used as monotherapy in the initial stages of treatment.

Tetrathiomolybdate is a molecule that forms stable tripartite complexes with protein and copper. This drug both decreases copper absorption and reduces circulating free copper. It is fast acting and can restore normal copper balance within several weeks compared with the several months required with other copper chelators or with zinc. Tetrathiomolybdate is especially appropriate for the initial treatment of patients with neurologic presentations, based on a recently published clincial trial. [1]

Regardless of the specific regimen chosen, treatment of Wilson's disease is lifelong. Noncompliance eventually leads to fulminant liver failure.

Liver transplantation is a rare consideration in Wilson's disease because the condition is typically responsive to medical therapy. This is generally necessary only when delayed diagnosis or poor compliance results in irreversible hepatic damage.

Apart from pharmacologic treatment, there are several other important considerations in Wilson's disease treatment. These include dietary restriction of shellfish and liver, both copper-rich foods. The major sources of patients' drinking water should be tested for copper concentration and avoided if levels approach 1.3 mg/L, which is the current maximum contaminant level goal (MCLG) established by the U.S. Environmental Protection Agency. The MCLG for copper in drinking water is set as a concentration at which no known or expected adverse health effects occur and for which there is an adequate margin of safety.

In newly diagnosed patients, there is also frequent need for speech therapy, physical or occupational therapy, and psychiatric counseling.

Wilson's Disease Heterozygotes

There is some debate about the risk for copper overload faced by individuals who are heterozygous for Wilson's disease. Even though Wilson's disease is a classic autosomal recessive trait, that is, requiring two mutant alleles at the *ATP7B* locus for expression of the disease, a report from the National Academy of Sciences suggested that heterozygous Wilson's disease carriers could represent a relatively sensitive population in terms of copper overload, particularly when dietary or drinking water copper exposures are higher than usual. Abnormally increased urinary copper excretion has been documented among some siblings of Wilson's disease patients, although genetic confirmation of carrier or noncarrier status for these individuals was not available. Further patient and family studies are needed to formally address these questions.

Prognosis

The prognosis in Wilson's disease is generally favorable. Current therapeutic approaches can prevent or reverse most of the significant clinical signs and symptoms, including the Kayser-Fleischer rings. However, if treatment is stopped, irreversible and potentially fatal liver damage inevitably occurs.

Future Directions

Gene therapy for Wilson's disease is a theoretical possibility. Because the Wilson copper transporter is expressed most prominently and functions most critically in the liver, this organ could be specifically targeted by use of adenoviral, adeno-associated viral, or replication-deficient lentiviral vectors. This contrasts with the situation in Menkes' disease, a copper transport disorder in which the normal gene product is highly similar to Wilson's but for which the target organ is the brain.

Hepatocyte transfer is an alternative to adenovirus-, adeno-associated virus-, and lentivirus-mediated gene transfer. It may be applicable to treatment of liver-specific metabolic disorders through a process termed therapeutic liver repopulation.

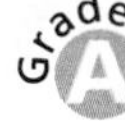

1. Brewer GJ, Askari F, Lorincz MT, et al: Treatment of Wilson disease with ammonium tetrathiomolybdate: IV, comparison of tetrathiomolybdate and trientine in a double-blind study of treatment of the neurologic presentation of Wilson disease. Arch Neurol 2006;63:521–527.

SUGGESTED READINGS

Ala A, Walker AP, Ashkan K, et al: Wilson's disease. Lancet 2007;369:397–408. *An excellent review of Wilson's disease.*

Ferenci P, Caca K, Loudianos G, et al: Diagnosis and phenotypic classification of Wilson disease. Liver 2003;23:139–142. *Consensus report on genetic diagnosis and genotype-phenotype correlations.*

Merle U, Schaefer M, Ferenci P, et al: Clinical presentation, diagnosis and long-term outcome of Wilson's disease: A cohort study. Gut 2007;56:115–120. *A comprehensive review.*

Sutcliffe RP, Maguire DD, Muiesan P, et al: Liver transplantation for Wilson's disease: Long-term results and quality-of-life assessment. Transplantation 2003;75:1003–1006. *Liver transplantation provided excellent results in 21 of 24 patients.*

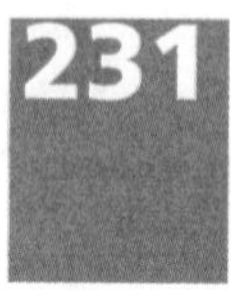

IRON OVERLOAD (HEMOCHROMATOSIS)

Bruce R. Bacon

Definition

Hereditary hemochromatosis (HH) is a common inherited disorder of iron metabolism. It is characterized by an increase in iron absorption from the upper gastrointestinal tract with subsequent tissue iron deposition in parenchymal cells of the liver, heart, pancreas, joints, and endocrine organs.

Classification

The term *hereditary hemochromatosis* should be reserved to describe inherited disorders of iron metabolism that lead to tissue iron loading (Table 231–1). The most common form of this disease, *HFE*-related HH, is caused primarily by homozygosity for the C282Y mutation in the *HFE* gene. Other heritable forms of iron overload (non–*HFE*-related HH) have also been recognized, including (1) autosomal recessive forms of HH characterized by rapid iron accumulation and caused by mutations in the genes for hemojuvelin and hepcidin (also called juvenile hemochromatosis), (2) an autosomal dominant form of HH caused by mutations in the ferroportin gene, (3) an autosomal recessive form of HH resulting from mutations in the gene for transferrin receptor 2 (*TFR2*), and (4) rare forms of HH resulting from mutations in the *DMT1* gene or in the regulatory region of ferritin messenger RNA. Some other types of iron overload may have a familial or inherited component, but the genes involved have not yet been identified. For example, *African iron overload* is a familial disorder of iron loading prevalent in sub-Saharan Africa that is exacerbated by the ingestion of iron-rich home-brewed beer. The degree of iron loading can be similar to that seen in *HFE*-related HH, but the cellular and lobular distribution of iron is different. In addition, a rare disorder termed *neonatal iron overload* is characterized by the presence of increased hepatic iron and severe liver injury at birth.

TABLE 231–1 CLASSIFICATION OF IRON OVERLOAD SYNDROMES

HEREDITARY HEMOCHROMATOSIS
***HFE* related**
C282Y/C282Y
C282Y/H63D
Other mutations
Non–*HFE* related
Hemojuvelin (*HJV*) mutations (autosomal recessive)
Hepcidin (*HAMP*) mutations (autosomal recessive)
Ferroportin (*SLC40A1*) mutations (autosomal dominant)
Transferrin receptor 2 (*TFR2*) mutations (autosomal recessive)
Divalent metal transporter 1 (*SLC11A2*) mutations (rare)
Ferritin regulatory mutations (rare)
Miscellaneous
African iron overload
Neonatal iron overload (rare)
SECONDARY IRON OVERLOAD
Anemia caused by ineffective erythropoiesis
Thalassemia major
Sideroblastic anemias
Congenital dyserythropoietic anemias
Congenital atransferrinemia
Liver disease
Alcoholic liver disease
Chronic viral hepatitis B and C
Porphyria cutanea tarda
Nonalcoholic steatohepatitis
After a portacaval shunt
Miscellaneous
Excessive iron ingestion

Of the more common patients who have *HFE*-linked hemochromatosis, it has been recognized over the last several years that many of them have no evidence of iron overload. With these issues in mind, four stages of HH have been described:

1. Genetic predisposition with no phenotypic abnormality
2. Iron overload (approximately 2 to 5 g) but without symptoms
3. Iron overload with mild or early symptoms
4. Iron overload with organ damage such as cirrhosis

The ability to establish a genetic diagnosis has helped us relate genetic abnormalities to degrees of iron loading.

Epidemiology

The genetic abnormality that is responsible for most patients with typical HH is homozygous in about 1 in 250 persons of northern European descent. The autosomal recessive inheritance pattern of HH was clearly shown in the 1970s, and the gene responsible for most cases of HH was identified in 1996. The gene is called *HFE* and encodes a novel major histocompatibility complex (MHC) class I–like molecule that binds with transferrin receptor (TfR) and affects hepcidin homeostasis. Recent prospective population studies have demonstrated that only about 50% of patients who are homozygous for the major mutation found in *HFE* (C282Y) have evidence of phenotypic expression of iron overload and that in only a small percentage (<10%) does tissue damage from excess iron deposition eventually develop. These studies have changed modern thinking about HH and must be considered when evaluating patients for the disease and when developing national health policy regarding screening for this genetic disorder. The discovery of *HFE* has had a tremendous impact in a number of areas. The ability to accurately diagnose disorders of iron overload has been strengthened, family screening is improved, and the evaluation of patients with other forms of liver disease complicated by moderate to severe iron overload is possible.

Furthermore, with the discovery of *HFE,* a considerable new body of knowledge regarding the mechanisms of iron absorption has been identified, both in normal individuals and in pathologic conditions when *HFE* mutations are present.

Pathobiology

Genetics

Since the classic linkage studies of Simon and colleagues in the mid-1970s, it has been known that the gene for hemochromatosis was located in the human leukocyte antigen (HLA) region on chromosome 6. In 1996, a team of molecular geneticists used positional cloning to identify a candidate gene for HH, which is now called *HFE. HFE* codes for a novel MHC class I–like molecule, which like all MHC proteins, requires interaction with β_2-microglobulin for normal presentation on the cell surface. Two missense mutations were initially identified in *HFE:* one results in a change in cysteine at position 282 to tyrosine (Cys282 → Tyr, C282Y); the second results in a change in histidine at position 63 to aspartate (His63 → Asp, H63D). Several other mutations have been identified in *HFE,* but their frequency is low and their clinical impact appears to be limited. In the original study, 83% of typical phenotypic HH patients were found to be homozygous for the C282Y mutation. Several other studies from around the world in predominantly white populations have demonstrated that of patients with typical hemochromatosis, about 85 to 90% were homozygous for C282Y. Thus, about 10 to 15% of patients with typical HH have some reason other than C282Y homozygosity for their iron overload.

Hepcidin is a 25–amino acid peptide that influences systemic iron status such that it is now considered to be the principal iron regulatory hormone. Dysregulation of hepcidin expression is thought to play a role in the pathogenesis of HH. Patients with *HFE*-related HH have low hepatic expression of hepcidin, as do *HFE* knockout mice, despite excess hepatic iron stores. Conversely, overexpression of hepcidin in *HFE* knockout mice prevents the HH phenotype. The molecular mechanisms by which hepcidin expression is regulated by body iron status have not been determined. It has been hypothesized that TfR-2 in hepatocytes may act as an iron sensor. Mutations in TfR-2 cause a rare form of HH in humans, and TfR-2 mutant mice have an HH phenotype. Similarly, HFE protein and hemojuvelin may participate in the hepcidin-regulated signaling pathway within hepatocytes inasmuch as inactivating mutations of both these proteins result in low hepcidin expression and iron overload.

Pathophysiology

Nearly all absorption of dietary iron occurs in the duodenum, where iron may be taken up either as ionic iron or as heme. Ionic iron requires reduction to the ferrous state, which is accomplished by the ferric reductases (such as Dcytb) expressed on the luminal surface of duodenal enterocytes. This ferrous iron crosses the apical membrane via DMT-1, and iron taken up by the enterocyte is either stored as ferritin or transferred across the basolateral membrane to plasma. This latter process occurs via the iron transporter ferroportin and requires oxidation of iron to the ferric state by the ferroxidase hephaestin.

Regardless of how these mechanisms function, excess iron (both transferrin bound and non–transferrin bound) is avidly taken up by hepatocytes and stored. Iron stores increase to the point where iron-induced oxidative damage occurs and results in cell injury and cell necrosis with phagocytosis by Kupffer cells. Iron-laden Kupffer cells become activated and produce profibrogenic cytokines (transforming growth factor-β, platelet-derived growth factor) that stimulate hepatic stellate cells to synthesize excess collagen and other matrix proteins. Increased fibrosis and then cirrhosis result.

Clinical Manifestations

Several symptoms and clinical findings have been identified in patients with fully established HH, and all physicians should be aware of these symptoms and findings, as summarized in Tables 231–2 and 231–3. Table 231–4 summarizes the typical laboratory findings in symptomatic and asymptomatic patients with HH. Recent series have found that many patients who are C282Y homozygotes are now coming to medical attention without any symptoms or findings because they are being identified by family screening studies, by population surveys, or because of evaluation of abnormal iron studies found on routine blood chemistry testing. It is ideal to identify patients who have some phenotypic expression with abnormal iron studies but who do not have evidence of organ damage. Several large population screening studies have shown evidence of phenotypic expression, although less than 10% of individuals who are C282Y homozygotes actually have signs and symptoms of the disease.

Diagnosis

Because patients with a genetic abnormality can be identified before having evidence of phenotypic expression, the whole discussion of the diagnosis of HH has undergone change. The role of liver biopsy has lessened considerably with the advent of genetic testing. Nonetheless, some general principles should be acknowledged.

Hematologic Testing

If the diagnosis of HH is being considered, blood tests, including fasting transferrin saturation (serum iron ÷ transferrin or total iron-binding capacity × 100%) and ferritin levels, should be obtained. In patients with symptoms (see Table 231–2), both of these values are elevated; however, transferrin saturation is typically the earliest phenotypic marker of HH and may be elevated in young individuals with normal ferritin levels. Serum ferritin can sometimes be elevated in other conditions such as certain cancers and in chronic inflammatory disorders in which there is no evidence of iron overload. Furthermore, in patients with other types of liver disease such as chronic hepatitis C, nonalcoholic steatohepatitis (NASH), and alcoholic liver disease, ferritin levels can be elevated in as many as half of the patients studied. Thus, ferritin is relatively sensitive but not specific for iron overload in the presence of these other disorders. The development of a widely available genetic test has contributed to better characterization of patients with underlying liver disease and abnormal serum iron studies.

TABLE 231–2 SYMPTOMS IN PATIENTS WITH HEREDITARY HEMOCHROMATOSIS

ASYMPTOMATIC
Abnormal serum iron studies on a routine screening chemistry panel
Evaluation of abnormal liver test results
Identified by family screening
Identified by population screening
NONSPECIFIC, SYSTEMIC SYMPTOMS
Weakness
Fatigue
Lethargy
Apathy
Weight loss
SPECIFIC, ORGAN-RELATED SYMPTOMS
Abdominal pain (hepatomegaly)
Arthralgias (arthritis)
Diabetes (pancreas)
Amenorrhea (cirrhosis)
Loss of libido, impotence (pituitary, cirrhosis)
Congestive heart failure (heart)
Arrhythmias (heart)

TABLE 231–3 PHYSICAL FINDINGS IN PATIENTS WITH HEREDITARY HEMOCHROMATOSIS

ASYMPTOMATIC
No physical findings
Hepatomegaly
SYMPTOMATIC
Liver
Hepatomegaly
Cutaneous stigmata of chronic liver disease
Splenomegaly
Liver failure: ascites, encephalopathy
Joints
Arthritis
Joint swelling
Heart
Dilated cardiomyopathy
Congestive heart failure
Skin
Increased pigmentation
Endocrine
Testicular atrophy
Hypogonadism
Hypothyroidism

Liver Biopsy

In the past, if either an elevated transferrin saturation or ferritin level was identified, a liver biopsy would be performed to establish a diagnosis with histochemical iron stains (Perls' Prussian blue stain) and biochemical determination of hepatic iron concentration with calculation of the hepatic iron index (HII). The HII is the ratio of the patient's hepatic iron concentration in μmol/g dry weight divided by the patient's age in years. Previously, when the HII was greater than 1.9, the diagnosis of HH was established. Recent studies with genetic testing have shown that many (>50%) HH patients may have an HII less than 1.9. Thus, the role of the HII is no longer important in the diagnosis of HH.

TABLE 231–4 LABORATORY FINDINGS IN PATIENTS WITH HEREDITARY HEMOCHROMATOSIS

Measurements	Normal Subjects	Patients with Hereditary Hemochromatosis	
		Asymptomatic	Symptomatic
BLOOD (FASTING)			
Serum iron level (μg/dL)	60–180	150–280	180–300
Serum transferrin level (mg/dL)	220–410	200–280	200–300
Transferrin saturation (%)	20–45	45–100	80–100
Serum ferritin level (ng/mL)			
Men	20–200	150–1000	500–6000
Women	15–150	120–1000	500–6000
GENETIC (HFE MUTATION ANALYSIS)			
C282Y/C282Y	wt/wt	C282Y/C282Y	C282Y/C282Y
C282Y/H63D*	wt/wt	C282Y/H63D	C282Y/H63D
LIVER			
Hepatic iron concentration			
μg/g dry weight	300–1500	2000–10,000	8000–30,000
μmol/g dry weight	5–27	36–179	140–550
Hepatic iron index†	<1.0	1.0 to >1.9	>1.9
Liver histology Perls' Prussian blue stain	0, 1+	2+ to 4+	3+, 4+

*Compound heterozygote.
†The hepatic iron index (HII) is calculated by dividing the hepatic iron concentration (in μmol/g dry weight) by the age of the patient (in years). With increased knowledge of genetic testing results in patients with iron overload, the specificity of HII has diminished.

When liver biopsy is performed, iron deposition is found preferentially in a periportal (acinar zone 1) region of the hepatic lobule with a decrease in gradient in acinar zones 2 and 3. With significant iron loading, iron deposition can be identified in sinusoidal lining cells (Kupffer cells), and iron can be found in bile duct cells and in fibrous tissue in the portal tracts or septa. In patients with secondary iron overload related to alcoholic liver disease or chronic viral hepatitis, iron deposition is typically in Kupffer cells, as well as in hepatocytes, and is in a panlobular (as opposed to a periportal) distribution. Histologic evaluation of iron-staining patterns provides complementary information to traditional biochemical testing for iron overload, along with the available genetic information.

Genetic Testing

Currently, when abnormal iron studies are identified, it is reasonable to proceed to genetic testing. If individuals are C282Y homozygotes or compound heterozygotes (C282Y/H63D), liver biopsy is reserved for those with elevated liver enzymes or ferritin levels greater than 1000 ng/mL (Fig. 231–1). Several studies have shown that increased fibrosis or cirrhosis is not seen in HH patients when ferritin levels are less than 1000 ng/mL or when liver enzymes are normal. Accordingly, as genetic testing has become more available, liver biopsy is less necessary.

Treatment

Even though there have been advances in the molecular and cell biologic understanding of HH and the impact of *HFE* mutation analysis on diagnosis has been significant, treatment of HH remains simple, inexpensive, and safe. Patients should undergo therapeutic phlebotomy of 500 mL of whole blood (containing approximately 200 to 250 mg of iron, depending on the hemoglobin concentration) on a weekly basis if tolerated. Therapeutic phlebotomy should be performed until iron-limited erythropoiesis develops, as identified by failure of the hemoglobin level and hematocrit to recover before the next phlebotomy. It is reasonable to monitor transferrin saturation and ferritin levels periodically (every 3 months) to predict the return of iron stores to normal and to provide a means of encouragement to patients who are undergoing phlebotomy. Therapeutic phlebotomy should be continued until the transferrin saturation is less than 50% and the ferritin level is less than 50 ng/mL. It is not necessary for patients to become anemic or iron deficient, just depleted of their excess iron stores. Once the initial therapeutic phlebotomy has been completed, most patients require maintenance phlebotomy to remove 1 U of blood every 2 to 3 months. This requirement is derived empirically with an intent to maintain transferrin saturation at less than 50% and ferritin at less than 50 ng/mL.

With successful iron depletion, patients have an improved sense of well-being, right upper quadrant abdominal pain dissipates, liver test results improve, and diabetes may be easier to manage. Established cirrhosis, arthropathy, and testicular atrophy generally do not improve.

Family Screening

Once an HH proband is recognized, all first-degree relatives should be offered testing. In the past, HLA haplotyping was performed, but now, *HFE* mutation analysis is recommended along with determination of fasting transferrin saturation and ferritin. In probands with children, *HFE* mutation analysis is performed in the spouse to accurately predict the genotype in the child. If the spouse has either mutation, testing of the child is necessary, although the value and availability of genetic testing in children are debated. If an adult relative of a C282Y homozygote is identified and is either a C282Y homozygote or a compound heterozygote and if blood iron studies are abnormal, a presumptive diagnosis can be made and therapeutic phlebotomy can be initiated under the guidelines already discussed.

Population Screening

Because HH is a common disorder with a well-described treatment and a long latent period (i.e., time before disease occurs), it has been suggested that HH would be an ideal disorder to undergo population screening by genetic testing. However, recent studies showing a less than expected phenotypic expression with a decreased number of patients who have clinical manifestations of iron-mediated disease being identified have raised questions about this recommendation. Initial results from a

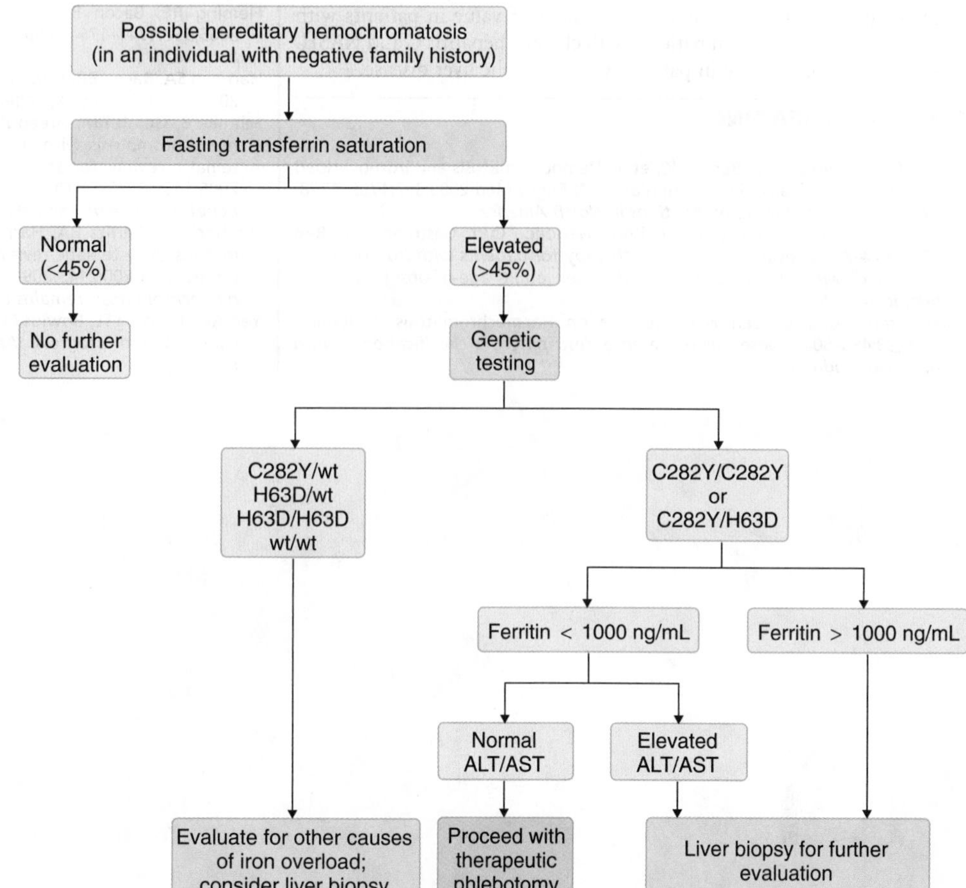

FIGURE 231–1 • Algorithm for evaluation of possible hereditary hemochromatosis in a person with a negative family history. ALT = alanine transaminase; AST = aspartate transaminase.

large National Institutes of Health–sponsored screening study performed in North America have demonstrated a prevalence of C282Y homozygosity of 1 in 227. The C282Y homozygotes had higher ferritin levels than the general population did, but 25% had a normal ferritin level. When screening for iron overload as opposed to screening for *HFE*-linked HH, fasting transferrin saturation should be performed. In this situation, when abnormal iron studies are identified and the patient does not have a mutation in *HFE,* liver biopsy should be considered to clarify the situation relative to iron stores.

Mutation Analysis in Patients with Liver Disease

Many patients with liver disease have abnormalities in serum parameters of iron metabolism. These abnormalities are more commonly seen in patients with hepatocellular liver diseases than in those with cholestatic liver diseases. Several clinical studies have shown that approximately 50% of patients with alcoholic liver disease, chronic viral hepatitis C, and NASH have abnormalities in serum iron studies. Generally, this is an elevation in serum ferritin, but occasionally, elevated transferrin saturation can be seen as well. When liver biopsy is performed, increased iron deposits can be seen, usually in a panlobular distribution with iron in both hepatocytes and sinusoidal lining cells (Kupffer cells). Hepatic iron concentrations may be slightly increased or normal.

Alcoholic Liver Disease

When *HFE* mutations have been evaluated in patients with alcoholic liver disease, there has been no increased incidence of either C282Y or H63D (either heterozygote or homozygote) over that of control populations. Furthermore, there was no increase in *HFE* mutations in patients with alcoholic liver disease who had an increased amount of fibrosis. Thus, the abnormal iron studies frequently seen in patients with alcoholic liver disease are most likely due to mechanisms other than mutations in *HFE.*

Chronic Hepatitis C

In chronic hepatitis C, the relationship of abnormal iron studies and elevated hepatic iron concentrations with treatment response to interferon monotherapy has been known for several years. Numerous studies have shown that patients who failed to respond to interferon monotherapy had a higher hepatic iron concentration than did those who responded. A corollary to this observation involved therapeutic phlebotomy to deplete iron stores in order to enhance a response to therapy. A reduction in iron stores by therapeutic phlebotomy does reduce liver enzymes and has had some marginal beneficial effect on liver histology but does not have any virologic effects. When *HFE* mutation analysis has been investigated in patients with chronic hepatitis C, the frequency of C282Y and H63D has been equivalent to that of control populations. Most studies have shown that when *HFE* mutations are present, they correlate with increased iron stores seen histologically. Some studies have shown a synergistic effect with the development of fibrosis. At present, it is recommended that *HFE* mutation analysis be done when abnormal iron studies are seen in patients with chronic hepatitis C. In addition, iron stains are typically performed on liver biopsy samples when biopsies are done for grading and staging of chronic hepatitis C. If iron stores are increased, it is reasonable to perform therapeutic phlebotomy to deplete excess iron stores before initiating antiviral therapy.

Nonalcoholic Steatohepatitis

In patients with NASH, several studies have provided conflicting results. Some have shown an increase in *HFE* mutations in patients with NASH, whereas others have shown no difference from control populations. When there has been an increased prevalence of *HFE* mutations in NASH, there has been good correlation between abnormal serum parameters of iron and hepatic iron concentrations. Furthermore, some studies have shown an increase in fibrosis in NASH patients with *HFE* mutations. These observations have not been fully confirmed by others, and more investigation in this area is necessary.

Porphyria Cutanea Tarda

Finally, in porphyria cutanea tarda (PCT), the relationship between abnormalities in iron metabolism and the role of therapeutic phlebotomy in treatment has been known for many years. Moreover, it has recently been shown that as many as 70% of patients with PCT are infected with hepatitis C virus and many patients with PCT drink excessive amounts of alcohol. An increased prevalence of *HFE* mutations has been shown in both European and American studies of PCT patients, and the use of phlebotomy to deplete excess iron stores is still recommended.

Thus, the role of *HFE* mutation analysis is of value in patients with PCT and may be of value in patients with chronic hepatitis C and NASH. It is probably not of value in patients with alcoholic liver disease.

SUGGESTED READINGS

Adams PC, Reboussin DM, Barton JC, et al: Hemochromatosis and iron-overload screening in a racially diverse population. N Engl J Med 2005;352:1769–1778. *Definitive study of large populations in North America.*

Barton JC: Chelation therapy for iron overload. Curr Gastroenterol Rep 2007;9:74–82. *A review of chelation therapy for patients with iron overload associated with the HFE gene and other adult age-of-onset types of hemochromatosis.*

EASL International Consensus Conference on Haemochromatosis. J Hepatol 2000;33:485–504. *Consensus conference describing the classification of iron overload syndromes.*

Fleming RE, Bacon BR: Orchestration of iron homeostasis. N Engl J Med 2005;352:1741–1744. *Discussion of current theories of regulation of iron balance.*

Harrison SA, Bacon BR: Hereditary hemochromatosis: Update for 2003. J Hepatol 2003;38:14–23. *A comprehensive review.*

Schmitt B, Golub RM, Green R: Screening primary care patients for hereditary hemochromatosis with transferrin saturation and serum ferritin level: Systematic review for the American College of Physicians. Ann Intern Med 2005;143:522–536. *There is no available evidence to demonstrate that the benefits outweigh the risks and costs of screening for hemochromatosis.*

Whitlock EP, Garlitz BA, Harris EL, et al: Screening for hereditary hemochromatosis: A systematic review for the US Preventive Services Task Force. Ann Intern Med 2006;145:209–223. *The role of genetic screening for hereditary hemochromatosis remains uncertain.*

Yen AW, Fancher TL, Bowlus CL: Revisiting hereditary hemochromatosis: Current concepts and progress. Am J Med 2006;119:391–399. *A comprehensive review.*

Section XVII

Nutritional Diseases

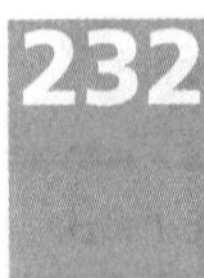

NUTRITION'S INTERFACE WITH HEALTH AND DISEASE

Douglas C. Heimburger

OLD AND NEW PARADIGMS IN THE SCIENCE OF NUTRITION

Nutrition science was characterized by two major phases in the 20th century. During the first phase, nutrition scientists discovered, characterized, and synthesized the various vitamins and described their deficiency syndromes in detail. The dietary requirements for these nutrients were estimated and periodically updated as recommended dietary allowances (RDAs). Beginning in 1997, the RDAs were reformulated in a series of volumes containing dietary reference intakes (DRIs) that in addition to recommended intakes judged to be sufficient to meet the nutrient requirements of nearly all healthy individuals, include estimates of tolerable upper intake levels representing the highest intake level likely not to pose any adverse health risks. 1

More fundamentally, however, the DRIs reflect the second phase of modern nutrition science, which focuses on evidence that is accumulating on the relationships of diet and nutritional status to the diseases that plague Western societies, such as coronary heart disease, cancer, and the other leading causes of death. Whereas the RDAs focused on dietary intakes required to prevent deficiencies, the DRIs recommend levels of intake that not only prevent deficiencies but may also promote long-term health and disease prevention. The expansion in focus from prevention of deficiency to promotion of health and prevention of disease is based on substantial evidence related to nutritional risks for heart disease, cancer, obesity, osteoporosis, congenital neural tube defects, and other conditions.

NUTRITION'S INFLUENCE ON MORTALITY AND MORBIDITY

Evidence for Connection between Diet and Disease

The causal connections between diet and chronic diseases are difficult to tease out of the complex network of other risk factors, including social and behavioral variables, so a wide variety of studies must be relied on to establish these connections with reasonable certainty.

The first links between diet and disease are often derived from epidemiologic studies, but such studies are unable to infer causal relationships and may be confounded by variables that have not been examined. Epidemiologic studies are also challenged by the difficulty of accurately assessing the diets of free-living individuals.

Animal and in vitro studies can overcome some of these drawbacks but may be confounded by experimental conditions that differ from those encountered by humans. A large number of prospective, randomized human intervention trials have been undertaken to test the effects of dietary change on risks for disease. However, even these trials are not always conclusive because of pitfalls associated with selecting study populations and isolating individual dietary factors.

Nevertheless, taken together, epidemiologic, animal, in vitro, and intervention studies are proving that human dietary habits contribute importantly to the pathogenesis of most of the major causes of death in developed countries.

Diseases Influenced by Nutrition

Table 232–1 lists 8 of the top 15 causes of death in the United States that are influenced by nutrition. Five are strongly linked with dietary habits and three are associated with alcohol abuse. The table also outlines dietary contributions to obesity, atherosclerosis, osteoporosis, diverticular disease, and neural tube defects, all of which cause significant morbidity and indirect mortality. Table 232–2 summarizes the 2005 Dietary Guidelines for Americans, and Table 232–3 compares dietary recommendations promulgated by professional societies for risk reduction and/or management of the following major chronic diseases.

Coronary Heart Disease

Nutritional influences on the number one cause of death in the United States, coronary heart disease (CHD), have been the subject of a great deal of research. The overall U.S. mortality rate from CHD peaked in the 1960s and, in a trend that surprised medical science, has declined steadily ever since. Changes in lifestyle, including diet, are responsible for a substantial proportion of this decline. Elevated plasma low-density lipoprotein cholesterol (LDL-C) levels are a major risk factor for CHD and peripheral atherosclerosis and correlate strongly with dietary saturated fat intake and less strongly with cholesterol intake. 2 Intake of both of these substances in the United States is derived largely from foods of animal origin such as meats, dairy products, and eggs. Attempts to produce less atherogenic substitutes for some of these foods have not always proved beneficial. For instance, hydrogenation of vegetable oils to create margarine and shortening results in the formation of *trans* fatty acids, which affect serum cholesterol levels in a manner similar to and perhaps worse than the saturated fatty acids found in butter and lard. LDL-C levels can be lowered modestly by increasing the intake of soluble fiber from legumes, fruits, vegetables, and flax seed, as well as by consuming proteins and isoflavones from soy foods. LDL must be oxidized before it induces injury to the arterial wall. Although adequate dietary levels of the antioxidant vitamins C and E and β-carotene have been shown to inhibit LDL oxidation, pharmacologic doses of these vitamins have not reduced CHD events when tested in randomized trials. In fact, pharmacologic doses of vitamin E (>400 IU/day) and other antioxidants have no benefit and may often increase all-cause mortality. 3

Epidemiologic evidence suggests that fish consumption may reduce CHD risk, perhaps through the action of ω-3 fatty acids. Evidence also indicates that moderate consumption of alcohol, especially wine, is associated with decreased risk for CHD, possibly through increasing high-density lipoprotein (HDL) cholesterol levels or preventing oxidation of LDL, or both. The polyphenols in red wine are also apparently beneficial. Circulating levels of the amino acid homocysteine, which are asymptomatically elevated in 20 to 25% of Americans, have been strongly correlated with risk for CHD. Homocysteine levels can be reduced by increasing the intake of folic acid (mainly from legumes, vegetables, and fortified grain) and decreasing the intake of methionine (principally from animal protein). Folic acid supplements, however, have not reduced CHD rates. A conservative estimate suggests that moderate dietary modification by the U.S. population, consisting mainly of replacing saturated fats with complex carbohydrates, fiber, monounsaturated fats, and fish, could easily lead to another 10% reduction in serum cholesterol levels and a 20% or greater reduction in CHD. The actual risk reduction could be much greater.

Cancer

Nutrients, non-nutritive dietary constituents, and nutritional status can influence the risk for cancer in a variety of ways. Nutrition interacts with each step of carcinogenesis (carcinogen activation and tumor initiation, promotion, and progression). Humans are exposed to countless potential carcinogens, but to many anticarcinogens as well, each day through dietary and other means. Excess energy intake may favor the generation of free radicals and reduce the body's ability to detoxify carcinogens. By contrast, antioxidant nutrients scavenge free radicals and other (pre)carcinogens and may thereby inhibit their activation or their ability to initiate mutations, or both. Folic acid may improve a cell's ability to preserve, repair, and methylate its DNA, either preventing or reversing the tendency to mutation. Obesity has emerged as a major risk factor for many cancers, perhaps by inducing insulin resistance and elevating serum levels of insulin and related hormones. Excessive alcohol intake promotes tumor growth.

Lung Cancer

Evidence indicates that the number one cancer killer, lung cancer, is influenced by diet. Although the most important causal factor is cigarette smoking, consumption of fruits and vegetables is inversely associated with lung cancer risk in both smokers and nonsmokers. It is probable that both nutrients and the non-nutritive phytochemicals in fruits and vegetables are responsible for the protective effects. However, in view of the disappointing results of randomized trials of supplementation with β-carotene, which increased mortality from lung cancer and other causes, antioxidant supplements should not be relied on to reduce disease risk.

TABLE 232–1 DIETARY INFLUENCES ON MAJOR CAUSES OF DEATH AND MORBIDITY IN THE UNITED STATES

Cause of Death or Morbidity	Factors Associated with Decreased Risk	Factors Associated with Increased Risk
DEATH		
Heart diseases	Intake of complex carbohydrates, particular fatty acids (e.g., monounsaturated, polyunsaturated, and ω-3 fatty acids from fish), soluble fiber, polyphenols, soy proteins, antioxidants (vitamins E, C; β-carotene; selenium), folic acid, moderate alcohol	Intake of saturated fat, cholesterol; excess calories, sodium; abdominal distribution of body fat
Cancer	Intake of fruits and vegetables (for β-carotene; vitamins A, C, D, and E; folic acid; calcium; selenium; phytochemicals), fiber	Intake of excess calories, fat, alcohol, red meat, salt- and nitrite-preserved meats, possibly grilled meats; abdominal distribution of body fat
Cerebrovascular diseases	Intake of potassium, calcium, ω-3 fatty acids	Sodium, alcohol consumption (as with hypertension)
Accidents		Excess alcohol consumption
Diabetes mellitus	Fiber intake	Intake of excess calories, fat, alcohol; abdominal distribution of body fat
Suicide		Excess alcohol consumption
Chronic liver disease and cirrhosis		Excess alcohol consumption
Hypertension and hypertensive renal disease	Intake of fruits and vegetables, potassium, calcium, magnesium, ω-3 fatty acids	Intake of sodium, alcohol, excess calories, total and saturated fat; abdominal distribution of body fat
MORBIDITY		
Obesity		Intake of excess calories and fat
Osteoporosis	Intake of calcium, vitamin D, vitamin K	Intake of excess vitamin A, sodium, protein
Diverticular disease, constipation	Fiber intake	
Neural tube defects	Folic acid intake	

TABLE 232–2 DIETARY GUIDELINES FOR AMERICANS 2005: KEY RECOMMENDATIONS FOR THE GENERAL POPULATION

ADEQUATE NUTRIENTS WITHIN CALORIE NEEDS

- Consume a variety of nutrient-dense foods and beverages within and among the basic food groups while choosing foods that limit the intake of saturated and *trans* fats, cholesterol, added sugar, salt, and alcohol.
- Meet recommended intakes within energy needs by adopting a balanced eating pattern, such as the U.S. Department of Agriculture (USDA) Food Guide or the Dietary Approaches to Stop Hypertension (DASH) Eating Plan.

WEIGHT MANAGEMENT

- To maintain body weight in a healthy range, balance calories from foods and beverages with calories expended.
- To prevent gradual weight gain over time, make small decreases in food and beverage calories and increase physical activity.

PHYSICAL ACTIVITY

- Engage in regular physical activity and reduce sedentary activities to promote health, psychological well-being, and a healthy body weight.
- To reduce the risk for chronic disease in adulthood, engage in at least 30 minutes of moderate-intensity physical activity, above usual activity, at work or home on most days of the week.
- For most people, greater health benefits can be obtained by engaging in physical activity of more vigorous intensity or longer duration.
- To help manage body weight and prevent gradual, unhealthy body weight gain in adulthood, engage in approximately 60 minutes of moderate- to vigorous-intensity activity on most days of the week while not exceeding caloric intake requirements.
- To sustain weight loss in adulthood, participate in at least 60 to 90 minutes of daily moderate-intensity physical activity while not exceeding caloric intake requirements. Some people may need to consult with a health care provider before participating at this level of activity.
- Achieve physical fitness by including cardiovascular conditioning, stretching exercises for flexibility, and resistance exercises or calisthenics for muscle strength and endurance.

TABLE 232-2 DIETARY GUIDELINES FOR AMERICANS 2005: KEY RECOMMENDATIONS FOR THE GENERAL POPULATION—cont'd

FOOD GROUPS TO ENCOURAGE

- Consume a sufficient amount of fruits and vegetables while staying within energy needs. Two cups of fruit and 2½ cups of vegetables per day are recommended for a reference 2000-calorie intake, with higher or lower amounts depending on the calorie level.
- Choose a variety of fruits and vegetables each day. In particular, select from all five vegetable subgroups (dark green, orange, legumes, starchy vegetables, and other vegetables) several times a week.
- Consume 3 or more ounce-equivalents of whole grain products per day, with the rest of the recommended grains coming from enriched or whole grain products. In general, at least half the grains should come from whole grains.
- Consume 3 cups per day of fat-free or low-fat milk or equivalent milk products.

FATS

- Consume less than 10% of calories from saturated fatty acids and less than 300 mg/day of cholesterol, and keep *trans* fatty acid consumption as low as possible.
- Keep total fat intake between 20 and 35% of calories, with most fats coming from sources of polyunsaturated and monounsaturated fatty acids, such as fish, nuts, and vegetable oils.
- When selecting and preparing meat, poultry, dry beans, and milk or milk products, make choices that are lean, low fat, or fat free.
- Limit intake of fats and oils high in saturated and/or *trans* fatty acids, and choose products low in such fats and oils.

CARBOHYDRATES

- Choose fiber-rich fruits, vegetables, and whole grains often.
- Choose and prepare foods and beverages with little added sugar or caloric sweeteners, such as amounts suggested by the USDA Food Guide and the DASH Eating Plan.
- Reduce the incidence of dental caries by practicing good oral hygiene and consuming sugar- and starch-containing foods and beverages less frequently.

SODIUM AND POTASSIUM

- Consume less than 2300 mg of sodium (approximately 1 teaspoon of salt) per day.
- Choose and prepare foods with little salt. At the same time, consume potassium-rich foods, such as fruits and vegetables.

ALCOHOLIC BEVERAGES

- Those who choose to drink alcoholic beverages should do so sensibly and in moderation—defined as the consumption of up to one drink per day for women and up to two drinks per day for men.
- Alcoholic beverages should not be consumed by some individuals, including those who cannot restrict their alcohol intake, women of childbearing age who may become pregnant, pregnant and lactating women, children and adolescents, individuals taking medications that can interact with alcohol, and those with specific medical conditions.
- Alcoholic beverages should be avoided by individuals engaging in activities that require attention, skill, or coordination, such as driving or operating machinery.

FOOD SAFETY

- To avoid microbial food-borne illness:
  - Clean hands, food contact surfaces, and fruits and vegetables. Meat and poultry should not be washed or rinsed.
  - Separate raw, cooked, and ready-to-eat foods while shopping, preparing, or storing foods.
  - Cook foods to a safe temperature to kill microorganisms.
  - Chill (refrigerate) perishable food promptly and defrost foods properly.
  - Avoid raw (unpasteurized) milk or any products made from unpasteurized milk, raw or partially cooked eggs or foods containing raw eggs, raw or undercooked meat and poultry, unpasteurized juices, and raw sprouts.

Breast Cancer

The second largest cause of cancer deaths in women, breast cancer, is positively associated with obesity, especially when it predominantly affects the abdomen, and with physical inactivity. Epidemiologic evidence suggests that alcohol intake may also be a risk factor for this disease, particularly in women with lower intake of folic acid.

Colorectal Cancer

Colorectal cancer is the third leading cause of cancer mortality in men and women. Its risk correlates positively with intake of red meat (especially when it is overcooked) and dietary fat and with obesity and inversely with intake of calcium and folic acid. Evidence regarding the effect of dietary fiber is somewhat equivocal, but the preponderance of evidence points to a protective effect. Higher physical activity is associated with a 30 to 50% lower risk for colon cancer and may also reduce breast cancer risk.

The interaction of all these influences is powerful enough to suggest that diet and physical inactivity contribute to well over 35% of cancer deaths in Western countries. Even though the independent influences of potentially protective nutrients such as carotenoids, vitamins C and E, folic acid, and fiber are not known with certainty because they are all present in vegetables and fruits, the evidence that liberal intake of fruits and vegetables reduces cancer risk is compelling. A very large randomized trial indicated that lowering dietary fat intake did not reduce rates of breast [4] or colon cancers. [5]

Hypertension

Elevated blood pressure is a major risk factor for stroke, CHD, heart failure, peripheral vascular disease, and renal disease. It is often associated with obesity, especially abdominal obesity, and weight reduction in obese hypertensives generally leads to improvement in blood pressure. Sodium restriction also usually reduces blood pressure levels. The DASH

TABLE 232–3 DIETARY GUIDELINES PROMULGATED BY NATIONAL ORGANIZATIONS*

	Organization				
	U.S. Department of Agriculture and Department of Health and Human Services Dietary Guidelines for Americans 2005	**National Cholesterol Education Program ATP III Therapeutic Lifestyle Change (Tlc) Diet (2002)**	**National High Blood Pressure Education Program/Joint National Committee 7 Dietary Approaches to Stop Hypertension (DASH, 2003)**	**American Diabetes Association (2004)**	**American Cancer Society (2002)**
Indication or objective	General health promotion and disease prevention	Elevated cholesterol/heart disease prevention	Prehypertension and hypertension	Diabetes	Cancer prevention
NUTRIENT/FOOD GROUP					
Total energy	Adequate energy intake to maintain a healthy weight		Reduce energy intake to lose weight if overweight	Reduced energy intake and modest weight loss can improve glycemia and insulin resistance	Choose foods that help you maintain a healthful weight
Fruits/vegetables	2 cups of fruit and 2.5 cups of vegetables per 2000 calories per day		8–10 servings per day		≥5 servings per day
Meat			2 servings or less per day; limit red meat intake		Limit consumption of red meats, especially those high in fat and processed
Dairy	2–3 servings per day of low-fat dairy		2–3 servings per day of low-fat dairy		
Grains	3 or more ounce-equivalents of whole grain products		7–8 servings of whole grains and whole grain products		Choose whole grains in preference to refined grains
Fat	20–35% of daily energy intake	25–35% of daily energy intake	Less than 27% of daily energy intake		
Saturated fats	Less than 10% of daily energy intake	Less than 7% of daily energy intake	Less than 7% of daily energy intake	Less than 10% of daily energy intake; those with LDL cholesterol ≥100 may benefit from lowering saturated fat to <7%	

Polyunsaturated fats	Up to 10% of daily energy intake	Up to 10% of daily energy intake	Up to 10% of daily energy intake	Up to 10% of daily energy intake	
Monounsaturated fats	10–20% of daily energy intake	Up to 20% of daily energy intake	Up to 20% of daily energy intake	15–20% of daily energy intake; combination of MUFA and carbohydrates should equal 60–70% of total energy intake	
Trans fats	Less than 1% of daily energy intake	Intake should be kept low		Intake should be minimized	
Cholesterol	Less than 300 mg/day	Less than 200 mg/day	150 mg/day	Less than 300 mg/day; those with LDL cholesterol ≥100 may benefit from lowering cholesterol intake to 200 mg/day	
Carbohydrates	45–65% of daily energy intake	50–60% of daily energy intake	55% of daily energy intake	Total amount of carbohydrate is more important than the source or type	
Sugar	Limit added sugars			Sucrose and sucrose-containing foods do not need to be restricted	
Protein		Approximately 15% of daily energy intake	18% of daily energy intake	10–20% if renal function is normal	
Alcohol	Up to 2 drinks per day for men and up to 1 drink per day for women; persons in special circumstances (e.g., pregnancy, history of alcoholism) should abstain		Less than 2 drinks per day for men and less than 1 drink per day for women	If individuals choose to drink, limit to 2 drinks per day for men or 1 drink per day for women	For people who drink, limit to 2 drinks per day for men or 1 drink per day for women
Sodium	Up to 2300 mg/day		Less than 2400 mg/day	Less than 2400 mg/day	
Potassium			4700 mg/day		
Calcium			1200 mg/day	1000–1500 mg/day	
Magnesium			500 mg/day		

*For further detail, see the websites listed in this chapter.
LDL = low-density lipoprotein; MUFA, monounsaturated fatty acid.
From Heimburger DC, Ard JD (eds): Handbook of Clinical Nutrition, 4th ed. Philadelphia, Elsevier, 2006.

(Dietary Approaches to Stop Hypertension) diet, rich in fruits, vegetables, and low-fat dairy products and with reduced saturated and total fat content, can also decrease blood pressure levels; reduced sodium intake provides additional benefit when included as part of the DASH diet. Because alcohol intake elevates blood pressure, its use should be limited in hypertensive patients.

Diabetes Mellitus

Type 2 diabetes mellitus is strongly associated with obesity, especially abdominal obesity. Sugar consumption does not lead to diabetes except to the extent that it may promote weight gain. Previous recommendations to restrict total carbohydrate intake in diabetics have been abandoned for lack of evidence; 55 to 60% of a diabetic's energy intake should come from carbohydrates, preferably unrefined carbohydrates that include fiber. Because higher-fat diets tend to promote both obesity and CHD, for which diabetics are at high risk, dietary fat intake should be kept low. Alcohol can cause hypoglycemia, hyperglycemia, and increased triglyceride levels in diabetics, and its use should be limited. In both diabetics and nondiabetics, excess alcohol intake is responsible for many deaths, particularly from accidents and liver disease, and is a factor in some suicidal deaths.

Osteoporosis

Osteoporosis is influenced by several dietary factors. Inadequate calcium intake during adolescence can result in suboptimal peak bone mass in early adulthood, and during later life it can lead to accelerated bone loss, thereby increasing the risk for osteoporosis. Sodium and protein, which are consumed by Americans in greater quantities than required, may promote excess bone loss. Excessive supplementation with vitamin A reduces bone mass and increases fracture risk. Vitamin D, vitamin K, and magnesium assist in maintaining optimal bone mass.

Other Conditions

Obesity

The causes and health effects of obesity, the most prevalent nutritional disorder in the United States, are reviewed in Chapter 239. The metabolic syndrome, a constellation that includes obesity with an enlarged waist circumference, increased serum glucose, triglycerides, and blood pressure, and reduced HDL cholesterol—variously referred to as the "metabolic syndrome" or "syndrome X," among other terms—is strikingly prevalent in the United States and is a major risk factor for CHD, cancer, type 2 diabetes, and hypertension (Chapter 248).

Intestinal Diverticular Disease

Low dietary fiber intake causes constipation, and it is thought to be a cause of intestinal diverticular disease.

Congenital Neural Tube Defects

Inadequate maternal folic acid intake has been definitively proved to be a major risk factor for congenital neural tube defects such as spina bifida and myelomeningocele. For this reason, cereal and grain products have been fortified in the United States with folic acid since 1998.

TRANSLATING EVIDENCE INTO DIETARY CHANGE

Thus, the evidence is strong that dietary habits can influence the incidence and severity of many incapacitating or lethal diseases in the United States. No justification exists for the belief that modification of the "usual" American diet is unnecessary or futile. The only questions are whether change is feasible and what is required to effect it. Various health agencies and the U.S. government have used public education, particularly the publication of dietary goals, as their primary means (see Table 232–3). The U.S. Department of Agriculture and the Department of Health and Human Services have developed and periodically revised the Dietary Guidelines for Americans (see Table 232–2) and a food guidance system, now called MyPyramid (Fig. 232–1). Although some have commented that MyPyramid, released in 2005, is complex and overly ambitious, both it and the Dietary Guidelines for Americans are more evidence based than previous versions, and MyPyramid provides detailed recommendations tailored to individual characteristics entered online by the user.

Physicians can influence their patients' health by encouraging them to optimize their dietary habits and providing them with instructional materials and assistance from dietitians to help them make needed changes. A significant barrier to practical nutritional interventions could be removed if health insurers would reimburse dietitians' services.

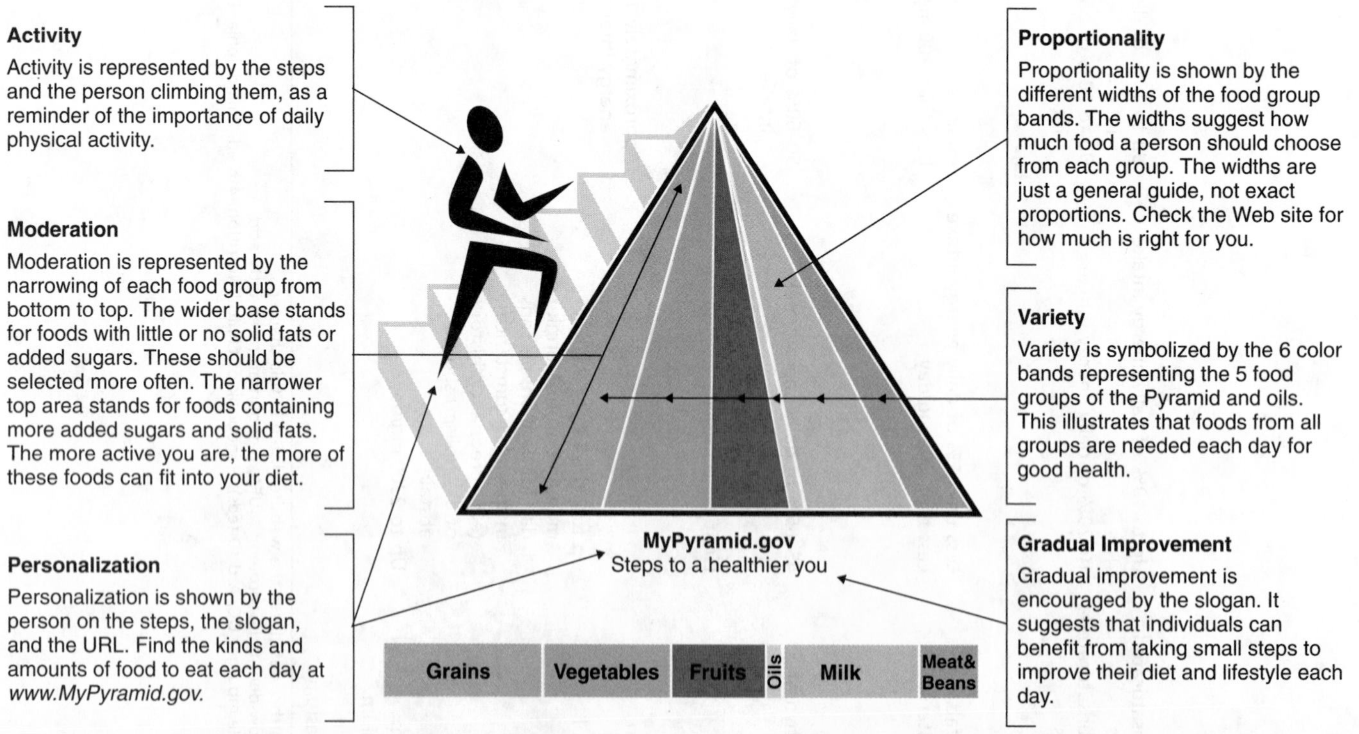

Activity
Activity is represented by the steps and the person climbing them, as a reminder of the importance of daily physical activity.

Moderation
Moderation is represented by the narrowing of each food group from bottom to top. The wider base stands for foods with little or no solid fats or added sugars. These should be selected more often. The narrower top area stands for foods containing more added sugars and solid fats. The more active you are, the more of these foods can fit into your diet.

Personalization
Personalization is shown by the person on the steps, the slogan, and the URL. Find the kinds and amounts of food to eat each day at *www.MyPyramid.gov.*

Proportionality
Proportionality is shown by the different widths of the food group bands. The widths suggest how much food a person should choose from each group. The widths are just a general guide, not exact proportions. Check the Web site for how much is right for you.

Variety
Variety is symbolized by the 6 color bands representing the 5 food groups of the Pyramid and oils. This illustrates that foods from all groups are needed each day for good health.

Gradual Improvement
Gradual improvement is encouraged by the slogan. It suggests that individuals can benefit from taking small steps to improve their diet and lifestyle each day.

MyPyramid.gov
Steps to a healthier you

Grains | Vegetables | Fruits | Oils | Milk | Meat& Beans

FIGURE 232–1 • USDA MyPyramid. One size doesn't fit all. USDA's new MyPyramid symbolizes a personalized approach to healthy eating and physical activity. The symbol has been designed to be simple. It has been developed to remind consumers to make healthy food choices and to be active every day. An interactive version of MyPyramid, with individually tailored nutrition information, is available at *www.MyPyramid.gov.*

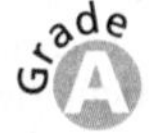

1. Food and Nutrition Board, Institute of Medicine: Dietary Reference Intakes. Available at http://www.nal.usda.gov/fnic/etext/000105.html.
2. Executive Summary of the Third Report of the National Cholesterol Education Program (NCEP) Expert Panel on Detection, Evaluation, and Treatment of High Blood Cholesterol in Adults (Adult Treatment Panel III). JAMA 2001;285:2486–2497.
3. Bjelakovic G, Nikolova D, Gluud LL, et al: Mortality in randomized trials of antioxidant supplements for primary and secondary prevention: Systematic review and meta-analysis. JAMA 2007;297:842–857.
4. Prentice RL, Caan B, Chlebowski RT, et al: Low-fat dietary pattern and risk of invasive breast cancer. JAMA 2006;295:629–642.
5. Beresford SA, Johnson KC, Ritenbaugh C, et al: Low-fat dietary pattern and risk of colorectal cancer. JAMA 2006;295:643–654.
6. Sacks FM, Svetkey LP, Vollmer WM, et al: Effects on blood pressure of reduced dietary sodium and the Dietary Approaches to Stop Hypertension (DASH) diet. N Engl J Med 2001;344:3–10.

SUGGESTED READINGS

Heimburger DC, Ard JD (eds): Handbook of Clinical Nutrition, 4th ed. Philadelphia, Elsevier, 2006. *A source for clinically useful information on nutritional risks for and nutritional management of disease.*

U.S. DHSS, USDA: Dietary Guidelines for Americans, 2005. Washington, DC, Government Printing Office, 2005. Available at http://www.healthierus.gov/dietaryguidelines/. *A detailed expansion of the recommended dietary habits covered in this chapter to promote health and prevent disease.*

Zarraga IG, Schwarz ER: Impact of dietary patterns and interventions on cardiovascular health. Circulation 2006;114:691–673. *Comprehensive review.*

SUGGESTED WEBSITES

American Cancer Society, *www.cancer.org*
American Diabetes Association, *www.diabetes.org*
American Heart Association, *www.americanheart.org*
National Cholesterol Education Program, *www.nhlbi.nih.gov/about/ncep/index.htm*
National High Blood Pressure Education Program, *www.nhlbi.nih.gov/guidelines/hypertension/*
Nutrition Data.com, *www.nutritiondata.com*
USDA MyPyramid, *www.MyPyramid.gov*
US DHHS/USDA Dietary Guidelines for Americans 2005, *www.healthierus.gov/dietaryguidelines/*

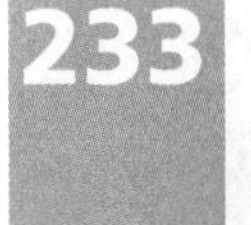

233 NUTRITIONAL ASSESSMENT

Bruce R. Bistrian

GOALS AND IMPORTANCE OF NUTRITIONAL ASSESSMENT

Nutritional assessment in clinical medicine has three primary goals: to identify the presence and type of malnutrition, to define health-threatening obesity, and to devise suitable diets as prophylaxis against disease later in life. The focus of this chapter is on the diagnosis of protein-energy malnutrition because of its wide prevalence and major impact on disease outcome. Other deficiency diseases are of much less relevance in that most occur in conjunction with protein-energy malnutrition or in specific disease states, such as thiamine deficiency in alcoholic liver disease and fat-soluble vitamin deficiency in malabsorptive states. The classic deficiency diseases, whether primary or secondary, are considered elsewhere in those chapters specifically dealing with the diseases mentioned here. The widespread availability of parenteral and enteral therapeutic measures since the mid-1980s that can provide adequate feeding regimens for virtually any disease condition makes a rudimentary knowledge of the pathophysiology of protein-energy malnutrition and its nutritional assessment essential for all primary care practitioners (Chapter 234).

CLINICAL NUTRITIONAL ASSESSMENT

Clinical assessment of protein nutritional status is based principally on the clinical history, physical examination including simple anthropometry, and measurement of the levels of several secretory proteins.

Clinical History

Although detailed dietary assessment can at times be helpful, in most circumstances physicians can safely limit their diet questions to whether patients have been following a prescribed diet, how much alcohol they drink, and whether they habitually take dietary supplements, including vitamins, minerals, and herbs. In ambulatory patients, the ability to maintain usual and adequate weight generally indicates that serious micronutrient deficiency is probably not the result of dietary inadequacy. Isolated vitamin deficiencies in the absence of weight loss or symptoms are rare, except perhaps for folate and vitamin B_{12}. Although nutritional anemias do exist, the role of dietary deficiency in folic acid–related or vitamin B_{12}–related anemias is minimal in the absence of underlying disease or weight loss. Only iron deficiency is a reasonable cause of dietary anemia. By contrast, full dietary assessment and diet prescriptions are likely to help patients with conditions such as fat malabsorption accompanied by weight loss, cramps, or diarrhea. Such evaluations are most effectively carried out by dietitians. Thus, detailed nutritional assessment of protein-energy malnutrition with secondary assessment of vitamin and mineral deficiencies is usually needed only when protein-energy malnutrition or a specific disorder known to interfere with nutrient metabolism coexists, such as celiac disease, pernicious anemia, or nutrient-drug interactions. Even then, the assessment should emphasize the likely deficiencies. For fat malabsorption, one should check levels of the fat-soluble vitamins A, D, E, and K, important divalent and trivalent cations (calcium [Ca^{2+}] zinc [Zn^{2+}], magnesium [Mg^{2+}], and iron [Fe^{3+}]), and phosphorus and alkaline phosphatase. When ileal resection has occurred, serum vitamin B_{12} levels should be measured, and the potential for bile salt depletion should be considered. Weight loss resulting from short-gut syndrome should prompt assessment of the fat-soluble vitamins, folic acid, vitamin B_{12}, calcium, magnesium, phosphorus, zinc, and iron. At least initially, levels of the water-soluble vitamins likely to have clinical impact such as thiamine and ascorbic acid should be checked, but provision of the full complement of vitamins should be routine in the management of this condition. Measurements of body water status (blood urea nitrogen, serum creatinine, serum sodium) and acid-base balance (serum carbon dioxide combining power, chloride and potassium, and urine and arterial pH) should be obtained if the diarrhea is profuse.

Clinically obvious marasmus and hypoalbuminemic malnutrition affect 25 to 50% of patients hospitalized for acute care and are secondary to the underlying disease in most instances. Many of these patients can benefit from nutritional support and require a thorough clinical nutritional assessment, including a dietary history, physical examination, and laboratory tests that serve to confirm clinical impressions. The history should list information about the timing and amount of weight loss, medical illnesses, medications, gastrointestinal symptoms (abdominal pain, diarrhea, dysphagia), diet habits (eating fewer than two meals per day, alcohol consumption, dietary supplement intake, dental status), social habits (eating alone, needing assistance in self-care), economic status (having enough money for food), and mental status, particularly the presence of depressive symptoms. A special focus should be reserved for the elderly, in whom protein-energy malnutrition secondary to these last factors is more common.

Nutritional Support

Four factors principally determine the timing, need, and appropriateness of nutritional support: (1) the presence and severity of protein-energy malnutrition, defined primarily by degree of weight loss and weight-to-height ratio as a percentage of standard or body mass index (BMI); (2) the presence and severity of the systemic inflammatory response, defined principally by the serum albumin level but also by the presence of fever, leukocytosis, and increased band forms; (3) the actual or expected duration of inadequate nutritional intake; and (4) the prognosis of the underlying condition. Well-nourished individuals have a 7- to 10-day reserve of energy and protein to withstand a moderate systemic inflammatory response without adverse nutritional consequences. Greater degrees of systemic inflammatory response and preexisting protein-energy malnutrition dramatically shorten the period that semistarvation, defined as consuming less than 50% of the energy and protein needs, can be tolerated.

Weight Loss

A recent unintended weight loss of 10 lb, or more than 5% of usual weight, should prompt efforts to diagnose the underlying disorder or social circumstance. Weight loss alone does not distinguish the composition of tissue loss, which can range from 25 to 30% lean tissue in semistarvation alone to 50% lean tissue loss following semistarvation plus injury and as much as 75% of the weight loss with the severest forms of injury, severe sepsis, major body burns, severe closed head injury, and multiple trauma. Therefore, unintentional weight loss of more than 10 lb indicates a need for thorough nutritional assessment. Weight loss in excess of 10% of usual weight should be considered to represent protein-energy malnutrition that will impair physiologic function, particularly muscle strength and endurance. Weight loss in excess of 20% should be considered severe protein-energy malnutrition that will substantially impair most organ systems. If major elective surgery is planned, such individuals would benefit from adequate feeding preoperatively or at least early nutritional intervention postoperatively. If palliative or curative radiation therapy or systemic chemotherapy is planned, adequate feeding during therapy with the use of supplemental formulas, tube feeding, or parenteral nutrition (in that order) is indicated. However, if the weight loss represents end-stage systemic illness (e.g., cancer, end-stage liver, renal, or lung disease, acquired immunodeficiency syndrome) for which no primary therapy is planned or is effective, then invasive nutritional support is rarely indicated.

TABLE 233–1 CLINICAL SIGNS AND SYMPTOMS OF NUTRITIONAL INADEQUACY IN ADULT PATIENTS

	Clinical Sign or Symptom	Nutrient
General	Wasted, skinny appearance	Calorie
	Loss of appetite	Protein-energy, zinc
Skin	Psoriasiform rash, eczematous scaling	Zinc, vitamin A, essential fatty acids
	Pallor	Folate, iron, vitamin B_{12}, copper
	Follicular hyperkeratosis	Vitamin A, vitamin C
	Perifollicular petechiae	Vitamin C
	Flaking dermatitis	Protein-energy, niacin, riboflavin, zinc
	Bruising	Vitamin C, vitamin K
	Pigmentation changes	Niacin, protein-energy
	Scrotal dermatosis	Riboflavin
	Thickening and dryness of skin	Linoleic acid
Head	Temporal muscle wasting	Protein-energy
Hair	Sparse and thin, dyspigmented	Protein
	Easy to pull out	Protein
	Corkscrew hairs	Vitamin C
Eyes	History of night blindness (also impaired visual recovery after glare)	Vitamin A, zinc
	Photophobia, blurring, conjunctival inflammation	Riboflavin, vitamin A
	Corneal vascularization	Riboflavin
	Xerosis, Bitot's spots, keratomalacia	Vitamin A
Mouth	Glossitis	Riboflavin, niacin, folic acid, vitamin B_{12}, pyridoxine
	Bleeding gums	Vitamin C, riboflavin
	Cheilosis	Riboflavin, pyridoxine, niacin
	Angular stomatitis	Riboflavin, pyridoxine, niacin
	Hypogeusia	Zinc
	Tongue fissuring	Niacin
	Tongue atrophy	Riboflavin, niacin, iron
	Nasolabial seborrhea	Pyridoxine
Neck	Goiter	Iodine
	Parotid enlargement	Protein
Thorax	Thoracic rosary	Vitamin D
Abdomen	Diarrhea	Niacin, folate, vitamin B_{12}
	Distention	Protein-energy
	Hepatomegaly	Protein-energy
Extremities	Edema	Protein, thiamine
	Softening of bone	Vitamin D, calcium, phosphorus
	Bone tenderness	Vitamin D
	Bone ache, joint pain	Vitamin C
	Muscle wasting and weakness	Protein, calorie, vitamin D, selenium, sodium chloride
	Muscle tenderness, muscle pain	Thiamine
Nails	Spooning	Iron
	Transverse lines	Protein
Neurologic	Tetany	Calcium, magnesium
	Paresthesias	Thiamine, vitamin B_{12}
	Loss of reflexes, wristdrop, footdrop	Thiamine
	Loss of vibratory and position sense	Vitamin B_{12}
	Ataxia	Vitamin B_{12}
	Dementia, disorientation	Niacin
Blood	Anemia	Vitamin B_{12}, folate, iron, pyridoxine
	Hemolysis	Phosphorus, vitamin E

Physical Examination

Although the patient's external appearance and a check of the skin, eyes, mouth, hair, and nails often provide clues to the presence of nutritional abnormalities (Table 233–1), the physical findings of deficiency syndromes of vitamins, essential fatty acids, and trace metals are relatively insensitive and nonspecific. With respect to protein-energy malnutrition, only the marasmic form of semistarvation is evident at examination. Loss of subcutaneous fat and skeletal muscle is manifested by sunken temples, thin extremities, wasting of the muscles of the hand, and, rarely, edema. Although kwashiorkor in children is characterized by severe edema and a potbelly appearance from hepatomegaly and ascites, one rarely encounters these clinical signs in cases of hypoalbuminemic malnutrition that develops in the setting of systemic inflammation resulting from disease in industrialized societies.

Body Weight

The most useful element in the physical examination is body weight, which is expressed as a relative value to evaluate the patient in relation to the healthy population. Weight and height are easily obtained, and standards for comparison have been established (Table 233–2). Although newer standards are available, they reflect the increasing prevalence of obesity in the U.S. population. Use of the 1959 standards allows the same tables to be used to diagnose significant protein-energy malnutrition (<85% of desirable weight, which approximates the fifth percentile) and significant obesity, defined as obesity predisposing to excessive mortality risk (>130% of desirable weight or BMI of ≥30). Although severe protein-energy malnutrition often occurs at levels greater than 85% of desirable weight because of the greater likelihood of preexisting obesity, this condition is generally detected by percentage of weight loss or by upper arm anthropometry. Height can be measured in a reclining patient with a tape measure, and in certain situations the clinician may rely on the patient's history. The major confounding variable that limits the value of weight and height as an index of protein-energy malnutrition is the tendency for water retention with disease, and thus weight gain may not reflect an increase in lean body mass or protein content. Fluid retention is particularly a problem in patients with hypoalbuminemic malnutrition because of the effects of aldosterone, antidiuretic hormone, and insulin stimulated by the stress response, which causes sodium and fluid retention. Fluid retention, however, does not usually confound weight assessment in patients who are first seen at the physician's office except in those patients with diseases such as cardiac failure, end-stage liver disease, and severe renal disease in whom the disturbance in water metabolism results from the underlying disease and not principally from the hormonal response to systemic inflammation.

Body Mass Index

The BMI, which is the weight in kilograms divided by the height in meters squared, has gained favor as a nutritional measure because of two valuable attributes. The measure is relatively independent of height, and the same standards apply to male and female patients. The following BMI values are used: normal nutrition, BMI of 20 to less than 25; significant protein-energy malnutrition, less than 18.5; overweight, from 25 to less than 30; and obesity, 30 or greater, with morbid obesity defined as a BMI of 40 and greater. Evidence from developing countries suggests that the BMI is better correlated with outcome than are weight and height.

Upper Arm Anthropometry

Approximately 50% of body fat is subcutaneous. The use of skinfold calipers to define the triceps skinfold (TSF) is the most practical technique to estimate body fat. Standards for skinfold measurement are available from the National Health and Nutrition Examination Surveys I and II and were derived from a probability sample of the U.S. population. Generally, a value lower than the fifth percentile is used to define abnormality (Table 233–3). The principal value of the TSF measurement is to determine the arm muscle circumference (AMC) or arm muscle area.

$$\text{AMC (cm)} = \text{arm circumference} - (\pi)(\text{TSF [mm]})/10$$

The AMC is a specific measure of protein-energy malnutrition if the fifth or tenth percentile is chosen as the cutoff point, and it is particularly valuable in patients in edematous states or in amputees, in whom

TABLE 233–2 DESIRABLE WEIGHT IN POUNDS IN RELATION TO HEIGHT FOR MEN AND WOMEN 25 YEARS OR OLDER*

Men, Medium Frame				Women, Medium Frame			
Height		Weight (lb)		Height		Weight (lb)	
ft	in	Range	Midpoint	ft	in	Range	Midpoint
				4	8	93–104	98.5
				4	9	95–107	101
				4	10	98–110	104
				4	11	101–113	107
				5	0	104–116	110
5	1	113–124	118.5	5	1	107–119	113
5	2	116–128	122	5	2	110–123	116.5
5	3	119–131	125	5	3	113–127	120
5	4	122–134	128	5	4	117–132	124.5
5	5	125–138	131.5	5	5	121–136	128.5
5	6	129–142	135.5	5	6	125–140	132.5
5	7	133–147	140	5	7	129–144	136.5
5	8	137–151	144	5	8	133–148	140.5
5	9	141–155	148	5	9	137–152	144.5
5	10	145–160	153	5	10	141–156	148.5
5	11	149–165	157				
6	0	153–170	161.5				
6	1	157–175	166				
6	2	162–180	171				
6	3	167–185	176				

*Corrected to nude weights and heights by assuming 1-inch heel for men, 2-inch heel for women, and indoor clothing weight of 5 and 3 lb for men and women, respectively.
Adapted from the Metropolitan Life Insurance Company Statistical Bulletin 1959;4:1.

TABLE 233–3 FIFTH, TENTH, AND 50TH PERCENTILE FOR TRICEPS SKINFOLD AND MID-UPPER ARM MUSCLE CIRCUMFERENCE OF U.S. MEN AND WOMEN FROM THE FIRST NATIONAL HEALTH AND NUTRITION EXAMINATION SURVEY

	MUAMC (cm) Percentile			TSF (mm) Percentile		
Age Group	**5th**	**10th**	**50th**	**5th**	**10th**	**50th**
MEN						
18–24	23.8	24.8	27.9	4.5	6	11
18–24	23.5	24.4	27.2	4	5	9.5
25–34	24.2	25.3	28	4.5	5.5	12
35–44	25	25.6	28.7	5	6	12
45–54	26	26.9	28.1	5	6	11
55–64	22.8	26.4	27.9	5	6	11
65–74	22.5	23.7	26.9	4.5	5.5	11
WOMEN						
18–24	13.4	19	21.8	11	13	22
18–24	17.7	18.5	20.6	9.4	11	18
25–34	18.3	18.9	21.4	10.5	12	21
35–44	18.5	19.2	22	12	14	23
45–54	18.8	19.5	22.2	13	15	25
55–64	18.6	19.5	22.6	11	14	25
65–74	18.6	19.5	22.5	11.5	14	23

MUAMC = mid-upper arm muscle circumference; TSF = triceps skinfold.
From Bishop CW, Bowen PE, Ritchey SJ: Norms for nutritional assessment of American adults by upper arm anthropometry. Am J Clin Nutr 1981;34:2530–2539.

weights are inaccurate or insensitive. The TSF and AMC measurements are most useful in initially defining marasmic-type malnutrition or the mixed disorder. Many dietitians are skilled in upper arm anthropometry.

Serum Proteins

Despite many concerns, the serum albumin level remains the traditional standard for nutritional assessment by virtue of its extensive history and its continued use to separate the two principal forms of protein-energy malnutrition. Hypoalbuminemia is a strong predictor of risk for morbidity and mortality in both hospitalized and ambulatory patients. In almost all cases, except perhaps for hereditary analbuminemia, excessive loss secondary to nephrosis, and, occasionally, protein-losing enteropathy, hypoalbuminemia identifies the recent or ongoing presence of a systemic inflammatory response. A value for serum albumin less than 3.5 g/dL is considered to indicate a mild systemic inflammatory response, whereas a value less than 2.4 g/dL represents a severe systemic inflammatory response, reflecting systemic inflammation that produces anorexia (limiting food intake) and increases protein catabolism and thus accelerates the development of protein-calorie malnutrition. With a half-life for albumin of 18 to 20 days and the fractional replacement rate of about 10% per day, the return of serum albumin to normal takes about 2 weeks of feeding when the stress response remits. Adequate feeding in the presence of systemic inflammation will not increase the serum albumin concentration, even though substantial nutritional benefit will occur in terms of wound healing and immune function. Levels of other proteins such as transferrin, prealbumin, and retinol-binding protein with respective half-lives of 7 days, 2 days, and half a day, also fall acutely with injury and respond more quickly when systemic inflammation remits. Serum transferrin also varies with iron status, however, and prealbumin and retinol-binding protein vary with dietary carbohydrate and renal function. As a result, these proteins do not reliably identify the presence and severity of the systemic inflammatory response any better than does albumin, but they reflect the nutritional response more quickly when inflammation lessens.

Composite Screening Tools

Investigators have made numerous attempts to combine the various components of nutritional assessment including clinical history, physical examination, anthropometry, and serum proteins into a single score. Some of the more widely used tools include the following: the Subjective Global Assessment, which classifies patients as A, B, or C or as having normal, mild, or moderate malnutrition; the Nutritional Risk Index, which is based on weight loss and serum albumin only; and the more extensive evaluations with Mini-Nutritional Assessment and Malnutrition Universal Screening Tool. A clear advantage of one technique over another has not been established.

NUTRITIONAL THERAPY AND ITS ASSESSMENT

The same indices that are used in the baseline nutritional assessment can be used to assess response to therapy, provided certain points are kept in mind.

Assessing Lean Body Mass and Total Body Water

In a stressed, hospitalized patient receiving nutritional support, day-to-day weight changes generally reflect changes in fluid balance rather than energy balance. In an ambulatory setting, weight increases or decreases are most likely to reflect changes in protein nutritional status and body fat because the underlying illness is usually less severe. Even the most sensitive research methods for assessing changes in lean body mass, however, do not offer major improvements in diagnosis in the more seriously ill patients. Techniques that measure total body water such as isotope dilution and underwater weighing, from which lean tissue is extrapolated, fail to account for the distortion in hydration of lean tissue with illness. Surrogate measures of total body protein to estimate lean tissues such as total body potassium measurement do not adjust for differing potassium-to-nitrogen ratios with disease. A newer method, single-frequency or multifrequency body impedance analysis, does show promise as a simple, accurate, noninvasive method that may allow distinction between intracellular and extracellular water, with the former used to estimate lean tissue for an initial assessment, However, the inherent difficulties resulting from the greater disturbance of total body water in critically ill patients have not been overcome with this technique.

Restoration of Lean Tissue

In an unstressed patient with marasmus, appropriate protein and calorie intake should cause a positive nitrogen balance of 2 to 6 g/day (60 to 180 g lean tissue) and slow weight gain, depending on the positive energy balance. For instance, a 300-kcal excess of intake over expenditure would provide approximately 120 g of lean tissue (100-kcal equivalent) in addition to 200 kcal (22 g) as fat, for a total of approximately 140 g, or approximately one third of a pound of weight per day. Weight gains in excess of this number usually reflect sodium and thus water retention from the insulin stimulated by dietary carbohydrate. Such overhydration can be improved by reducing salt and limiting fluid intake. In patients with hypoalbuminemic malnutrition who are no longer stressed, a similar nutritional regimen will lead to a comparable gain of tissue, but weight change is often less as edema becomes mobilized, with normalization of serum albumin in 2 to 4 weeks and of retinol-binding protein, prealbumin, and transferrin more quickly. In stressed patients with hypoalbuminemic malnutrition, appropriate nutritional support often does not restore lean tissue but does improve other important functions, such as wound healing and immunocompetence. These are important treatment goals, and they improve the ultimate clinical outcome. Both the systemic inflammatory response and the limited activity level reduce the efficiency of skeletal muscle repletion, which represents 30% of body weight and 75% of actively metabolizing lean tissue. Functional testing of muscle strength and endurance such as hand dynamometry can be useful as a means of assessing this response but has not found wide clinical acceptance. Similarly, any reduction in other physiologic functions or impairment in the patient's ability to perform the usual activities of daily living will accentuate the consequences of protein-energy malnutrition.

Measures of Energy Expenditure and Caloric Need

Although caloric expenditure can now be reliably and easily measured with portable indirect calorimeters, estimated energy expenditure is sufficient in most clinical situations. The three components of total energy expenditure are basal energy expenditure (~55 to 65% of total energy expenditure), thermal effect of feeding (~10% of total energy expenditure), and activity energy expenditure (25 to 33%). An energy intake of 30 to 35 kcal/kg of body weight will maintain weight in most sedentary ambulatory patients, with adjustments upward or downward in 200- to 300-kcal increments as prompted by biweekly changes in weight. Although young, severely burned, or traumatized patients may require 35 to 40 kcal/kg in the acute phase to meet total energy expenditure, providing energy intakes principally as carbohydrates that exceed 35 kcal/kg substantially increases the likelihood of hyperglycemia. Evidence strongly implicates hyperglycemia in excess of 180 mg/dL as a major risk factor for nosocomial infection, thus emphasizing the importance of better glycemic control by the use of insulin infusions or by reducing the level of energy intake, or both. Most postoperative patients who require invasive nutritional support for mechanical or infectious complications usually require approximately 25 kcal/kg to meet energy needs and not more than 30 kcal/kg because of their older age and reduced activity and energy expenditure. Overfeeding should be avoided in such patients.

SUGGESTED READINGS

Alberda C, Graf A, McCargar L: Malnutrition: Etiology, consequences, and assessment of a patient at risk. Best Pract Res Clin Gastroenterol 2006;20:419–439. *Review of nutritional assessment and monitoring in patients with gastrointestinal diseases.*

Pablo AM, Izaga MA, Alday LA, et al: Assessment of nutritional status on hospital admission: Nutritional scores. Eur J Clin Nutr 2003;57:824–831. *Malnutrition is common and can be assessed by several different readily available methods.*

Stratton RJ, Hackston A, Longmore D, et al: Malnutrition in hospital outpatients and inpatients: Prevalence, concurrent validity and ease of use of the "malnutrition universal screening tool" ("MUST") for adults. Br J Nutr 2004;92:799–808. *A comparison of various composite models for nutritional assessment.*

Wansink B, Chandon P: Meal size, not body size, explains errors in estimating calorie content of meals. Ann Intern Med 2006;145:326–332. *Obese individuals generally underestimate the size of their meals.*

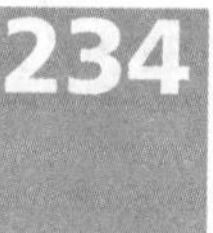

PROTEIN-ENERGY MALNUTRITION

Samuel Klein

Definition

Normal nutritional status represents a healthy relationship between nutrient intake and nutrient requirements. An imbalance between intake and requirements over time can lead to malnutrition, manifested by alterations in intermediary metabolism, organ function, and body composition. The term *protein-energy malnutrition* has been used to describe macronutrient deficiency syndromes, which include kwashiorkor, marasmus, and nutritional dwarfism in children and wasting associated with illness or injury in children and adults.

Pathobiology

Primary protein-energy malnutrition is caused by lack of access to adequate nutrient intake and usually affects children and elderly persons. The functional and structural abnormalities associated with primary protein-energy malnutrition are often reversible with nutritional therapy. However, prolonged primary protein-energy malnutrition can cause irreversible changes in organ function and growth.

Secondary protein-energy malnutrition is caused by illnesses that alter appetite, digestion, absorption, or nutrient metabolism and can be divided into three general, but often overlapping, categories: (1) diseases that affect gastrointestinal tract function, (2) wasting disorders, and (3) critical illness. Gastrointestinal disease can cause protein-energy malnutrition by premucosal (maldigestion), mucosal (malabsorption), or postmucosal (lymphatic obstruction) defects (Table 234–1). The nutritional status of patients with protein-energy malnutrition caused by gastrointestinal tract dysfunction can often be restored to normal if adequate nutritional support can be provided by dietary manipulations, enteral tube feeding, or parenteral nutrition. Wasting disorders, such as cancer, acquired immunodeficiency syndrome, and rheumatologic diseases, are characterized by involuntary loss of body weight and muscle mass in the setting of a chronic illness. These patients often experience wasting because of (1) inadequate nutrient intake related to anorexia and possibly gastrointestinal tract dysfunction and (2) metabolic abnormalities caused by alterations in regulatory hormones and cytokines. The alterations in metabolism are responsible for the greater loss of muscle tissue observed in these patients than in those with pure starvation or semistarvation. Restoration of muscle mass is unlikely with nutritional support unless the underlying inflammatory disease is corrected. Weight gain that occurs after nutritional support is initiated is usually caused by increases in fat mass and body water, without significant increases in lean tissue. Patients with critical illness exhibit marked metabolic alterations, manifested by increased energy expenditure, altered endogenous glucose production and lipolytic rates, and protein breakdown. Therefore, protein and energy requirements are increased in critically ill patients. However, providing aggressive nutritional support may ameliorate but does not prevent net lean tissue losses without correction of the underlying illness or injury.

METABOLIC RESPONSE TO STARVATION

The adaptive response to starvation involves specific metabolic alterations that enhance the chance for survival by increasing the use of body fat as a fuel, sparing the use of glucose, minimizing body nitrogen losses, and decreasing energy expenditure. A marked shift in fuel use occurs during the first day of starvation. By 24 hours of fasting, the use of glucose as a fuel has decreased; only 15% of liver glycogen stores remain, and the rates of hepatic glucose production and whole body glucose oxidation have decreased. Conversely, endogenous fat stores become the body's major fuel, and the rates of adipose tissue lipolysis, hepatic ketone body production, and fat oxidation are increased. After 3 days of fasting, the rate of glucose production is reduced by one half, and the rate of lipolysis is more than double the value found at 12 hours of fasting. The increase in fatty acid delivery to the liver, in conjunction with an increase in the ratio of plasma glucagon to insulin concentration, enhances

TABLE 234–1 CLASSIFICATION OF MALDIGESTIVE AND MALABSORPTIVE DISORDERS

Primary Abnormality	Pathophysiology	Representative Disorders
Premucosal defect	Pancreatic insufficiency	Chronic pancreatitis
		Cystic fibrosis
		Pancreatic duct obstruction
	Bacterial overgrowth	Motility diseases
		Blind loop syndromes
		Small intestine diverticula
	Rapid gastric emptying and intestinal transit	Post–gastric surgery syndrome
Mucosal defect	Inadequate bowel syndrome	Intestinal resection
		Gluten-sensitive enteropathy
		Immunoproliferative small bowel disease
		Radiation enteritis
		Intestinal ischemia
		AIDS enteropathy
Postmucosal defect	Lymphatic obstruction	Congenital intestinal lymphangiectasia
		Milroy's disease
		Secondary intestinal lymphangiectasia
		Retroperitoneal carcinoma
		Lymphoma
		Retroperitoneal fibrosis
		Chronic pancreatitis
		Tuberculosis
		Sarcoidosis
		Crohn's disease
		Whipple's disease
		Constrictive pericarditis
		Chronic congestive heart failure

AIDS = acquired immunodeficiency syndrome.

hepatic ketone body production. By 7 days of fasting, plasma ketone body concentrations have increased 75-fold, and ketone bodies provide 70% of the brain's energy needs.

In contrast to fatty acids, ketone bodies can cross the blood-brain barrier and provide a water-soluble fuel derived from water-insoluble adipose tissue triglycerides. The use of ketone bodies by the brain greatly diminishes glucose requirements and thus reduces the need for muscle protein degradation to provide glucose precursors. Furthermore, thyroid hormone inactivation and plasma ketones inhibit muscle protein breakdown and prevent rapid protein losses. If postabsorptive protein breakdown rates were to continue throughout starvation, a potentially lethal amount of muscle protein would be catabolized in less than 3 weeks. As fasting continues, the kidney becomes an important site for glucose production; glutamine, released from muscle, is converted to glucose in the kidney and accounts for almost half of total glucose production. Resting metabolic rate decreases by approximately 15% at 7 days.

Adaptation is maximal during more prolonged starvation (>14 days of fasting). At this time, adipose tissue provides more than 90% of daily energy requirements. Total glucose production has decreased to about 75 g/day, providing fuel for glycolytic tissues (40 g/day) and the brain (35 g/day). Muscle protein breakdown has decreased to less than 30 g/day, which causes a marked decrease in urea nitrogen production and excretion. The diminished urea load to the kidneys decreases urine volume to 200 mL/day, thereby minimizing fluid requirements. Resting energy expenditures decrease by approximately 25%.

UNDERNUTRITION-INDUCED ALTERATIONS IN TISSUE MASS AND FUNCTION

BODY COMPOSITION. All body tissue masses are affected by undernutrition, but fat mass and muscle mass are the most severely affected. In lean adults, these two tissues account for almost two thirds of body weight. Therefore, the loss of weight that occurs in malnourished patients is principally the result of a loss in muscle and fat mass. Body adipose tissue can be almost completely depleted and up to half of muscle mass can be consumed before death from starvation occurs.

BODY WATER. Many patients who are malnourished have intravascular volume depletion because of inadequate water and sodium intake. However, the percentage of body weight that is composed of water may be increased. Decreased plasma proteins, leaky capillaries, leaky cells, and increased interstitial ion content may cause intravascular volume depletion and expansion of the interstitial space. Therefore, malnourished patients may have diminished intravascular volume in the presence of whole body fluid overload.

SKIN. The skin is a large organ that regenerates rapidly: a basal cell of the dermis reaches the cornified layer and dies in 10 to 14 days. Frequently, undernutrition causes the skin to be dry, thin, and wrinkled, with atrophy of the basal layers of the epidermis and hyperkeratosis. Severe malnutrition may cause considerable depletion of skin protein and collagen. Patients with kwashiorkor experience sequential skin changes in different locations. Hyperpigmentation occurs first, followed by cracking and stripping of superficial layers and leaving behind hypopigmented, thin, and atrophic epidermis that is friable and easily macerated.

HAIR. Scalp hair becomes thin and sparse and is pulled out easily. In contrast, the eyelashes become long and luxuriant, and there may be excessive lanugo hair in children. Children with kwashiorkor experience hypopigmentation with reddish brown, gray, or blond discoloration. Adults may lose axillary and pubic hair.

GASTROINTESTINAL TRACT. Starvation and malnutrition cause structural and functional deterioration of the intestinal tract, pancreas, and liver. The total mass and protein content of the intestinal mucosa and pancreas are markedly reduced. Mucosal epithelial cell proliferation rates decrease, and intestinal mucosa becomes atrophic with flattened villi. The synthesis of mucosal and pancreatic digestive enzymes is reduced. Intestinal transport and absorption of free amino acids are impaired, whereas hydrolysis and absorption of peptides are maintained. Gastric and biliary secretions are diminished. The abdomen may become protuberant because of hypomotility and gas distention. Hepatomegaly is common in severe malnutrition because of excessive fat accumulation caused by decreased very low density lipoprotein synthesis and triglyceride export. Synthesis of most hepatic proteins is decreased.

HEART. Chronic undernutrition affects cardiac mass and function. Cardiac muscle mass decreases, and the decrease is accompanied by fragmentation of myofibrils. Bradycardia (heart rate can decrease to less than 40 beats/min) and decreased stroke volume can cause a marked decrease in cardiac output and low blood pressure. For example, a hypocaloric diet in physiologically normal volunteers that caused a 24% decrease in body weight was associated with a 38% decrease in cardiac index.

LUNGS. Respiratory muscle function is altered by malnutrition, as evidenced by a decrease in vital capacity, tidal volume, and minute ventilation.

KIDNEYS. Renal mass and function are relatively well preserved during undernutrition, provided adequate water is consumed to prevent a severe decrease in renal perfusion and acute renal failure. However, when malnutrition is severe, decreases are noted in kidney weight, glomerular filtration rate, the ability to excrete acid, the ability to excrete sodium, and the ability to concentrate urine. Mild proteinuria may also occur.

BONE MARROW. Severe undernutrition suppresses bone marrow red blood cell and white blood cell production and leads to anemia, leukopenia, and lymphocytopenia.

MUSCLE. Muscle function is impaired by malnutrition because of both a loss of muscle mass and impaired metabolism. Decreased sodium pump activity causes an increase in intracellular sodium and a decrease in intracellular potassium, which affects myocyte electrical potential, contributing to fatigue.

BRAIN. The weight and protein content of the brain remain relatively stable during long-term starvation. Therefore, the integrity of the brain is preserved at the expense of other organs and tissues. However, data from one study found that cerebral atrophy was associated with protein-energy malnutrition in children, a finding suggesting that the brain is not completely protected from malnutrition during childhood.

IMMUNE SYSTEM. Severe undernutrition causes atrophy of all lymphoid tissues, including thymus, tonsils, and lymph nodes. Cell-mediated immunity is diminished more than antibody production. Alterations in cell-mediated immunity cause impaired delayed cutaneous hypersensitivity and anergy. The ability to kill bacteria is diminished because of decreased complement and impaired neutrophil function. Gastrointestinal immunoglobulin A secretion is also decreased. Malnourished patients are at increased risk for opportunistic infections and should be considered immunocompromised.

ENDOCRINE SYSTEM. Decreased plasma insulin concentrations and glucose intolerance are common in severe malnutrition. Growth hormone is usually increased and is much greater in the kwashiorkor type than the marasmic type of protein-energy malnutrition. Serum thyroxine levels are low, and the conversion of thyroxine to triiodothyronine is decreased, with increased conversion to reverse triiodothyronine. Plasma cortisol concentration is usually greater than normal. The decrease in plasma leptin concentration that occurs early during energy restriction may be an important initiator of the neuroendocrine response to fasting.

ENERGY METABOLISM. Starvation and undernutrition decrease basal energy expenditure because of diminished organ size and function, increased conversion of active thyroid hormone to its inactive form, decreased sodium pump activity, decreased protein turnover, decreased body core temperature, absence of shivering and nonshivering thermogenesis, and suppression of sympathetic nervous system activity. Energy is also conserved by the onset of fatigue, which causes physical activity to diminish.

DEATH FROM STARVATION

At the terminal phase of starvation, body fat mass, skeletal muscle mass, and the size of most organs are markedly decreased. During this final phase of starvation, body fat stores are nearly depleted, energy derived from body fat decreases, and muscle protein catabolism is accelerated. The mechanism responsible for death from starvation in humans is not well understood, but many patients ultimately succumb to infection. It has been suggested that there are lethal levels of body weight loss (loss of 40% of body weight), of protein depletion (loss of 30 to 50% of body protein), of fat depletion (loss of 70 to 95% of body fat stores), or of body size (body mass index of 13 kg/m^2 for men and 11 kg/m^2 for women) in humans. The duration of survival depends on the amount of available endogenous fuels and the amount of lean tissue. Data from Irish Republican Army hunger strikers demonstrate that death occurs in lean men after approximately 2 months of starvation when more than 35% (~25 kg) of body weight is lost. Obese persons can survive much longer periods of starvation because of their increased fat stores and lean tissue mass. The longest reported fast is that of a severely obese (207-kg) man who safely lost 61% (126 kg) of his initial weight after completing a 382-day fast in which he ingested only acaloric fluids, vitamins, and minerals.

Clinical Manifestations

Protein-Energy Malnutrition in Children

Undernutrition in children differs from that in adults because it affects growth and development. Much of our understanding of undernutrition in children comes from observations and studies in developing nations where poverty, inadequate food supply, and unsanitary conditions lead to a high prevalence of protein-energy malnutrition. The Waterlow classification of malnutrition takes into account that undernutrition affects childhood growth. Therefore, nutritional status can be assessed by comparing a child's weight for height (wasting) and height for age (stunting) with normal standards (Table 234–2). The characteristics of the three major clinical syndromes of protein-energy malnutrition in children are outlined in Table 234–3. Although these three syndromes are classified separately, they may coexist in the same patient. The use of mid-upper arm circumference has been proposed as a useful screening tool in underserved areas, because height is difficult to measure accurately in ill children and accurate assessment of weight depends on access to functioning scales. Mid-upper arm circumference of up to 11.5 cm in children 1 to 5 years old can predict subsequent inpatient mortality as reliably as the Waterlow classification.

MARASMUS. Weight loss and marked depletion of subcutaneous fat and muscle mass are the characteristic features in children with marasmus. Loss of fat and muscle makes ribs, joints, and facial bones prominent. The skin is thin, loose, and lying in folds.

KWASHIORKOR. The word *kwashiorkor* comes from the Ga language of West Africa and can be translated as "disease of the displaced child" because it was commonly seen after weaning. The presence of peripheral edema distinguishes children with kwashiorkor from those with marasmus and nutritional dwarfism (Fig. 234–1). Children with kwashiorkor also have typical skin and hair changes (see earlier sections on hair and skin changes). The abdomen is protuberant because of weakened abdominal muscles, intestinal distention, and hepatomegaly, but these children

TABLE 234–2 WATERLOW CLASSIFICATION OF PROTEIN-ENERGY MALNUTRITION IN CHILDREN

Measure	Normal	Mild	Moderate	Severe
WEIGHT FOR HEIGHT (WASTING)				
Percent of median NCHS standard	90–110	80–89	70–79	<70
Standard deviation from the NCHS median	+Z–-Z	−1.1Z–-2Z	−2.1Z–-3Z	<−3Z
HEIGHT FOR AGE (STUNTING)				
Percent of median NCHS standard	95–105	90–94	85–89	<85
Standard deviation from the NCHS median	+Z–-Z	−1.1Z–-2Z	−2.1Z–-3Z	<−3Z

NCHS = National Center for Health Statistics; Z = 1 standard deviation.

TABLE 234–3 FEATURES OF PROTEIN-ENERGY MALNUTRITION SYNDROMES IN CHILDREN

Characteristic	Kwashiorkor	Marasmus	Nutritional Dwarfism
Weight for age (% expected)	60–80	<60	<60
Weight for height	Normal or decreased	Markedly decreased	Normal
Edema	Present	Absent	Absent
Mood	Irritable when picked up Apathetic when alone	Alert	Alert
Appetite	Poor	Good	Good

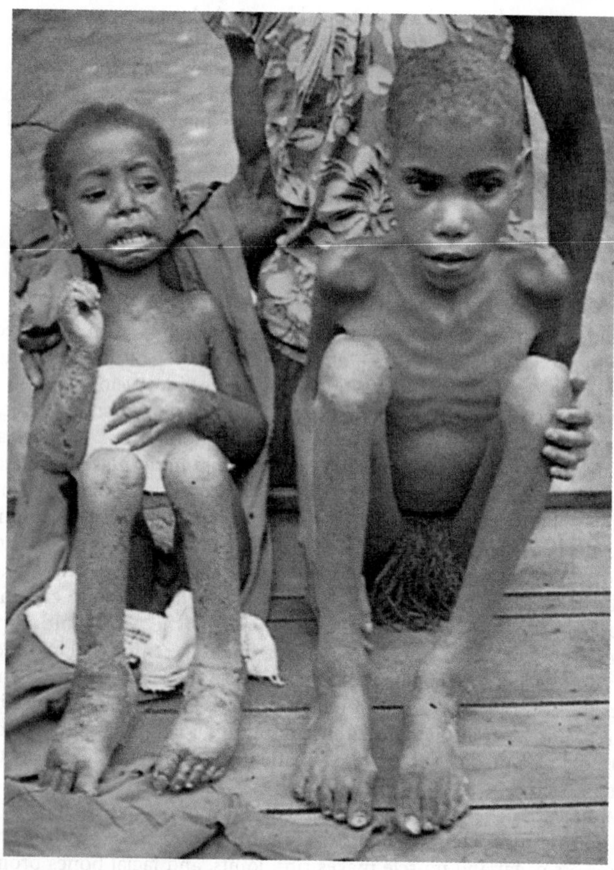

FIGURE 234–1 • Kwashiorkor and marasmus in brothers. The younger brother, on the left, has kwashiorkor with generalized edema, skin changes, pale reddish yellow hair, and an unhappy expression. The older child, on the right, has marasmus, with generalized wasting, spindly arms and legs, and an apathetic expression. (From Peters W, Pasvol G [eds]: Tropical Medicine and Parasitology, 5th ed. London, Mosby, 2002, Fig. 986.)

do not have ascites. In fact, the presence of ascites should prompt the clinician to search for liver disease or peritonitis. Children with kwashiorkor are typically lethargic and apathetic when left alone but become quite irritable when they are picked up or held. Kwashiorkor is not caused by a relative deficiency in protein intake, as was previously believed; in fact, protein and energy intakes are similar in children with kwashiorkor and marasmus. The pathogenesis of kwashiorkor is not clear, but it is likely related to the physiologic stress of an infection that induces a deleterious metabolic cascade in an already malnourished child. This explains why kwashiorkor is an acute illness compared with the chronicity of undernutrition alone and why marasmus and kwashiorkor overlap. Kwashiorkor is characterized by leaky cell membranes that permit the movement of potassium and other intracellular ions to the extracellular space. The increased osmotic load in the interstitium causes water movement and edema.

NUTRITIONAL DWARFISM. The child with failure to thrive may be of normal weight for height but has short stature and delayed sexual development. Providing appropriate feeding can stimulate catch-up growth and sexual maturation.

TABLE 234–4 CLASSIFICATION OF PROTEIN-ENERGY MALNUTRITION IN ADULTS BY BODY MASS INDEX

Body Mass Index (kg/m^2)	Nutritional Status
18.5–24.9	Normal
17.0–18.4	Mildly malnourished
15.0–16.9	Moderately malnourished
<15.0	Severely malnourished

Protein-Energy Malnutrition in Adults

The diagnosis of protein-energy malnutrition in adults is different from that in children because adults are no longer growing in height. Therefore, undernutrition in adults causes wasting rather than stunting and can be assessed by determining body mass index, defined as the patient's weight (in kilograms) divided by the patient's height (in meters squared) (Table 234–4). In addition, although kwashiorkor and marasmus can occur in adults, most studies of adult protein-energy malnutrition have evaluated hospitalized patients with secondary protein-energy malnutrition and coexisting illness or injury. The current methods that are used clinically to evaluate protein-energy malnutrition in hospitalized adult patients shift nutritional assessment from a diagnostic to a prognostic instrument in an attempt to identify patients who can benefit from nutritional therapy. Therefore, common nutritional assessment parameters are affected by non-nutritional factors that make it difficult to separate the influence of the disease itself from the contribution of inadequate nutrient intake. At present, no "gold standard" exists for determining protein-energy malnutrition in ill patients. The most commonly used methods include a careful history, physical examination, and selected laboratory tests.

Treatment

INITIAL EVALUATION. A careful clinical examination is needed to identify life-threatening complications of protein-energy malnutrition that require immediate treatment. The presence of fluid, plasma glucose, electrolyte, and acid-base abnormalities should be determined. A search for infections (e.g., obtaining a white blood cell count, urine analysis and culture, blood cultures, and chest radiograph) should be considered even in the absence of physical findings because many patients are not able to mount a normal inflammatory response. The evaluation must also include a careful analysis of the possible route for nutritional support and whether the gastrointestinal tract can be used or parenteral nutrition is needed for refeeding.

INITIAL SUPPORTIVE CARE. Judicious resuscitation with fluids and electrolytes may be necessary before beginning feedings, with frequent evaluations to prevent congestive heart failure from excessive fluid. Vitamin supplementation should be given routinely. Severely malnourished patients are poikilothermic, and a warm ambient temperature and warming blankets may be necessary to raise their core temperature slowly. However, if warming blankets are used, patients must be carefully monitored to avoid hyperthermia.

REFEEDING. The goal of feeding the severely malnourished patient can be divided into three phases: (1) to prevent further deteriora-

Rx

tion and correct life-threatening abnormalities, (2) to restore normal organ function and metabolism, and finally (3) to replete deficient nutrient stores. Oral or enteral tube feedings are preferred to parenteral feeding because of fewer serious complications and enhanced gastrointestinal tract recovery. Feedings should be given in small amounts at frequent intervals to avoid overwhelming the body's limited capacity for nutrient processing and to prevent hypoglycemia, which can occur during brief nonfeeding intervals. Therefore, small amounts of oral feeding should be given frequently (every 1 to 4 hours), enteral tube feeding by continuous drip, or parenteral nutrition by continuous infusion. Sodium intake should be limited during early refeeding, but liberal amounts of phosphorus, potassium, and magnesium should be given to patients who have normal renal function. Daily monitoring of body weight, fluid intake, urine output, and plasma glucose and electrolyte values is critical during the first few days of refeeding so that nutritional therapy can be appropriately adjusted when necessary. Appetite has usually improved during the second phase. Protein and energy intake should be marginally higher than estimated requirements to provide for adequate maintenance and repair. Additional protein and energy should be provided during phase 3 for repletion and synthesis of new tissue.

REFEEDING COMPLICATIONS. Refeeding can be harmful and may even cause death because of impaired organ function and depleted nutrient stores resulting from previous starvation. The adverse consequences caused by initiating feeding too aggressively are known as the refeeding syndrome and usually occur within the first 5 days. Refeeding syndrome complications include fluid overload, electrolyte imbalances, glucose intolerance, cardiac arrhythmias, and diarrhea.

Fluid Overload. Severely malnourished patients are at increased risk for fluid retention and congestive heart failure after nutritional therapy because of compromised cardiac and renal function. Because the ability to excrete sodium is impaired, even normal amounts of dietary sodium intake can be excessive. In addition, carbohydrates increase the concentration of circulating insulin, which stimulates sodium and water reabsorption by the renal tubule. The presence of heart failure requires discontinuation of feeding until cardiac status is stabilized.

Mineral Depletion. Carbohydrate refeeding stimulates insulin release and intracellular uptake of phosphate, which is used for protein synthesis and glucose metabolism. Therefore, plasma phosphorus concentrations can sometimes fall precipitously to less than 1 mg/dL after initiating nutritional therapy if adequate phosphate is not given. Severe hypophosphatemia, associated with muscle weakness, paresthesias, seizures, coma, cardiopulmonary decompensation, and death, has occurred in severely malnourished patients after they received enteral or parenteral nutritional therapy.

Decreased body cell mass and decreased sodium, potassium–adenosine triphosphatase activity or leaky cell membranes in the malnourished patient lead to depletion of the major intracellular cations, potassium and magnesium. Nonetheless, serum potassium and magnesium concentrations may remain normal or near normal during starvation because of their release from tissue and bone stores. During refeeding, increases in protein synthesis, body cell mass, and glycogen stores require generous intakes of potassium and magnesium. In addition, hyperinsulinemia during refeeding increases cellular uptake of potassium and can cause a rapid decline in extracellular concentrations.

Glucose Intolerance. Malnourished patients are predisposed to hypoglycemia because of decreased hepatic glucose production. However, starvation and malnutrition impair insulin's ability to suppress endogenous glucose production and stimulate glucose uptake and oxidation. Therefore, providing enteral or parenteral carbohydrates can cause hyperglycemia, glucosuria, dehydration, and hyperosmolar coma. Furthermore, because of the importance of thiamine in glucose metabolism, carbohydrate refeeding in patients who are thiamine deficient can precipitate Wernicke's encephalopathy.

Cardiac Arrhythmias. Sudden death from ventricular arrhythmias can occur during the first week of refeeding in severely malnourished patients and has been reported in conjunction with severe hypophosphatemia. A prolonged QT interval may be a contributing cause of the rhythm disturbances.

Gastrointestinal Dysfunction. Alterations in gastrointestinal tract function limit the ability of the gastrointestinal tract to digest and absorb food. Mild diarrhea after initiating oral-enteral feeding usually resolves and is not clinically important if fluid and electrolyte homeostasis can be maintained. However, in some severely malnourished patients, oral feeding is associated with severe diarrhea and death. Therefore, aggressive fluid and electrolyte replacement and a search for enteric pathogens should be considered in patients with prolonged or severe diarrhea.

SUGGESTED READINGS

Berkely J, Mwangi I, Griffiths K, et al: Assessment of severe malnutrition among hospitalized children in rural Kenya. JAMA 2005;294:591–597. *This study demonstrates the usefulness of using mid-upper arm circumference as a practical tool for identifying severe malnutrition in children in sub-Saharan Africa.*

Collins S, Dent N, Binns P, et al: Management of severe acute malnutrition in children. Lancet 2006;368:1992–2000. *Comprehensive review of acute malnutrition.*

Keusch GT: The history of nutrition: Malnutrition, infection and immunity. J Nutr 2003;133:336S–340S. *This article reviews the relationship between malnutrition and susceptibility to infection.*

Muller O, Krawinkel M: Malnutrition and health in developing countries. CMAJ 2005;173:279–286. *Review of epidemiology, pathophysiology, and management of malnutrition in children.*

Pauly L, Stehle P, Volkert D: Nutritional situation of elderly nursing home residents. Z Gerontol Geriatr 2007;40:3–12. *Though studies vary, this is a remarkably common problem.*

Persson M, Hytter-Landahl A, Brismar K, Cederholm T: Nutritional supplementation and dietary advice in geriatric patients at risk of malnutrition. Clin Nutr 2007;26:216–224. *A standardized approach to counseling and supplementation can improve outcomes.*

235 ENTERAL NUTRITION

John L. Rombeau

Enteral nutrition is the provision of liquid formula diets into the gastrointestinal tract. When compared with total parenteral nutrition, enteral nutrition measurably increases intestinal mucosal growth and function and is less costly. Because of these acknowledged benefits, enteral nutrition is used with increasing frequency in medical patients. It is therefore incumbent on physicians to be familiar with the rationale, indications, administration, and complications of enteral nutrition.

PROVISION OF ENTERAL NUTRIENTS

Rationale

The most important stimulus for gut growth and function is the presence of nutrients within the gastrointestinal tract. Enteral nutrients mediate such effects both directly and indirectly. The presence of nutrients within the intestinal lumen directly increases epithelial proliferation and enhances mucosal cell renewal. In the absence of luminal stimuli or intestinal nutrients, the small and large bowels atrophy not only in the absorptive cells and brush border enzymes but also in the mucus-secreting cells and the gut-associated lymphoid tissue. These entities are important protective components of the intestinal barrier against bacteria, endotoxins, and other antigenic macromolecules and may provide a rationale for using small volumes (e.g., 10 mL/hour) of continuous enteral feeding in critically ill patients even if these patients cannot tolerate larger volumes and must be fed parenterally as well.

Enteral nutrients mediate many of their indirect enterotropic effects by stimulating gut hormones such as gastrin, neurotensin, bombesin, and enteroglucagon. Gastrin exerts trophic effects on the stomach, duodenum, and possibly the colon. Enteral nutrients given to animal models increase the production of additional enterotropic hormones such as glucagon-like peptide 2. Furthermore, because of reduced manufacturing costs of its nutrient components, enteral feeding is less costly than total parenteral nutrition and may be more cost-effective than hand feeding disabled or debilitated patients.

Indications

General indications for enteral nutrition include the following: (1) the presence of protein-energy malnutrition (Chapter 234), (2) a gastrointestinal tract that can safely tolerate enteral formulas, and (3) anticipated inadequate oral intake for at least 7 days. Safe use of the gastrointestinal tract is possible in the absence of obstruction, severe intractable diarrhea, or massive bleeding. The anticipated duration of inadequate oral intake is based solely on the clinical judgment of the primary physician. Table 235–1 lists examples of specific medical indications for enteral nutrition. In patients with functioning gastrointestinal tracts, enteral nutrition is as effective as parenteral nutrition with fewer complications and lower costs 1 (Fig. 235–1).

TABLE 235–1 INDICATIONS FOR THE USE OF ENTERAL NUTRITION IN ADULT MEDICAL PATIENTS

Protein-energy malnutrition with anticipated significantly decreased oral intake for at least 7 days
Anticipated significantly decreased oral intake for 10 days
Severe dysphagia
Massive small bowel resection (used in combination with total parenteral nutrition)
Low-output (<500 mL/day) enterocutaneous fistula

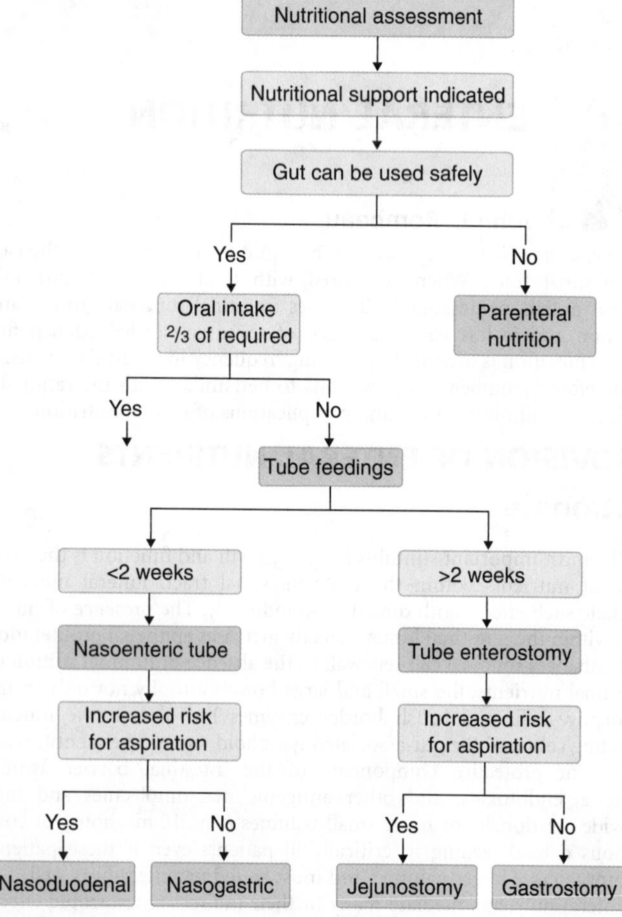

FIGURE 235–1 • Decision approach for the type and route of nutritional support.

Dietary Formulas

Commercial enteral formulas have proliferated rapidly. Table 235–2 outlines the nutrient composition of some of these agents, including polymeric balanced diets, modified formulas, and modular supplements.

POLYMERIC BALANCED FORMULAS. Polymeric formulas are "complete," balanced, isotonic diets containing 100% of the Recommended Dietary Allowance for substrates, vitamins, and minerals when these formulas are prescribed in the recommended amounts. These formulas are palatable and are the first choice for oral supplementation or tube feeding when digestion and absorption are reasonably normal. The nitrogen source consists of an intact or partially hydrolyzed natural protein (e.g., soy, egg, lactalbumin) that requires the patient's ability to digest protein in addition to carbohydrate and fat. The caloric density of these formulas is usually 1 kcal/mL, but it can be as high as 1.5 or 2 kcal/mL. Calorie-dense formulas are reasonable choices for patients who have unusually high caloric requirements, can tolerate only limited feeding volumes, or require fluid restriction. Most importantly, polymeric balanced formulas are less expensive than the other formulas. Their major disadvantage is a fixed nutrient composition.

MODIFIED FORMULAS. Conventional modified diets are also "complete" diets. Composed primarily of predigested or elemental nutrients, they require minimal digestion and are almost completely absorbed. Although the protein source can be crystalline amino acids, some pancreatic function is required to digest carbohydrates (oligosaccharides and disaccharides) and fats (≤30% of which are provided as medium-chain triglycerides). In addition, absorption of glucose, sodium, amino acids, fat, vitamins, and trace elements requires intact mucosal transport systems.

Unlike the polymeric balanced diets, modified diets are hyperosmolar, unpalatable, and relatively expensive. They cost between three and 10 times as much per calorie as polymeric balanced formulas. Modified diets may produce osmotic diarrhea if they are administered too rapidly, and they require flavoring supplements for oral use. Modified diets may be indicated in patients with conditions of digestive or absorptive insufficiency, in whom polymeric diets are not well tolerated. Examples of such limiting conditions include chronic pancreatitis, short-bowel syndrome, and prolonged ileus.

DISEASE-SPECIFIC FORMULAS. Certain modified formulas are designed for patients with specific nutritional needs. Formulas that contain only essential amino acids as the protein source are designed for patients with renal failure. Formulas that are high in fat content (~55% of calories) and low in carbohydrate content (~28% of calories) have been recommended for patients with respiratory insufficiency because their oxidation produces less carbon dioxide. The high fat content of these formulas may produce diarrhea in critically ill patients. Diets supplemented with fish oils, arginine, and nucleotides have been developed, allegedly to enhance the immune response of critically ill and postoperative patients. These diets are very expensive. Well-controlled and properly designed clinical trials are needed before the use of these diets can be recommended. Little objective evidence justifies the use of any of these expensive, disease-specific formulas. Their use should be restricted to patients with specific nutrient needs who cannot tolerate polymeric and conventional modified diets.

MODULAR SUPPLEMENTS. Modular supplements, which consist of single or multiple nutrients, can be added to existing "fixed-ratio" diets without affecting the quality or quantity of other nutrients. These supplements are designed for patients for whom standard fixed-ratio formulas are suboptimal. Commercially available modules include carbohydrate, fat, protein, mineral, electrolyte, and vitamin formulations.

Administration

ACCESS. Selection of the access site for delivery of enteral nutrients is based on the anticipated duration of forced feeding and the potential risk of aspiration.

Oral Route. Ideally, enteral nutrition is given by the oral route to conscious patients with intact gag reflexes who require nutritional supplementation only with meals. For patients who cannot tolerate oral nutrition, other access techniques include nasogastric tube, nasoenteric tube, and tube enterostomy.

Nasogastric/Nasoenteric Route. Nasogastric or nasoenteric tubes are ideal for patients who require short-term (<2 weeks) enteral nutrition.

TABLE 235–2 COMMONLY USED ADULT COMMERCIAL ENTERAL FEEDING FORMULAS*

Category	Formulation			
	1.0 kcal/mL	1.2 kcal/mL	1.5 kcal/mL	2.0 kcal/mL
Polymeric balanced ≤16% protein	Ensure, Resource, Isocal, Osmolite, Nutren 1.0		Nutren 1.5, Ensure Plus, Resource Plus, Boost Plus, Comply	Nutren 2.0, Deliver, Magnacal
17–20% protein	Osmolite HN, Isocal HN, Ensure HN, Ultracal, Jevity		Ensure Plus HN	TwoCal HN
≥20% protein	Sustacal, Replete, Promote, Protain XL (22%), Isosource VHN (25%)		TraumaCal	
Modified conventional ≤16% protein	Peptamen, Reabilan, Vivonex Plus, Criticare HN			
17–20% protein	Vital HN, Reabilan HN, Alitra Q			
Peptide based	Peptamen (16%), Reabilan (12.5%), Criticare HN (14%), Peptamen VMP (25%), Reabilan HN (17.5%), Alitra Q (21%), Vital HN (16%), SandaSource Peptical (20%)		Crucial (25%)	
Elemental	Tolerex (8%), Vivonex T.E.N. (15%), Vivonex Plus (18%)			
Modified disease specific (% protein)[†]				
Critical care	Immun-Aid (32%), Impact (22%), Impact/Fiber (22%)	Perative (20%)		
Glucose intolerance	Glytrol (18%), Choice dM (17%), Glucerna (16.7%), Diabeta Source (20%)			
Hepatic	Travasorb Hepatic (11%), Hepatic-Aid (15%)	Hepatic-Aid II (15%)	Nutrihep (11%)	
Malabsorption			Lipisorb (17%), Travasorb	Renal Cal (6–9%)
Renal			Renal (7%)	Amin-Aid (4%)
Pulmonary			NutriVent (18%), Respalor (20%), Pulmocare (16.7%)	
Modular supplements				
Protein	Casec, ProMod			
Carbohydrate	Moducal, Polycose Microlipid, MCT oil fat			

*This table includes only a partial listing of commercial products.
[†]Manufacturers market these products as disease specific. My use of this designation is intended neither to endorse the manufacturer's claims of special efficacy in the diseases specified nor to deny that the polymeric-balanced or modified-conventional formulas may be appropriate or even superior in these conditions.
MCT = medium-chain triglyceride.

To use these access routes safely, patients must have intact gag reflexes and competent lower esophageal sphincters. Ideal candidates are those with poor oral intake such as occurs with cancer of the head and neck and the lung. The stomach is the preferred site of delivery, but the nasoenteric tube should be advanced into the jejunum in patients with gastroparesis and a high risk of aspiration.

Tube Enterostomies. Permanent access through tube enterostomies is the preferred route of delivery for long-term enteral nutrition (>2 weeks). Tube enterostomies are inserted endoscopically, laparoscopically, or operatively into the stomach and jejunum.

The percutaneous endoscopic approach is the preferred method for gastrostomy placement. It has the advantage of decreased procedure time, use of local anesthesia, absence of an incision, and avoidance of ileus. The speed, simplicity, low cost, and low complication rate of percutaneous endoscopic gastrostomy have resulted in its replacing surgical gastrostomy in most hospitals. Surgical gastrostomy for feeding is indicated for patients unable to tolerate percutaneous endoscopic gastrostomy or for individuals undergoing concomitant gastrointestinal surgery.

Jejunostomy. Jejunostomy is indicated for patients who need long-term enteral nutrition and who have chronic aspiration, gastric outlet obstruction, or stomach or duodenal cancer and for patients who have had a gastrectomy.

DELIVERY. Feeding formulas are delivered intermittently or continuously.

Intermittent Feeding. Intermittent feeding is preferred for delivery into the stomach because it is more physiologic and "frees" the patient from the feeding equipment. Feedings of polymeric diets in a volume of 240 to 400 mL every 4 hours are well tolerated. The disadvantages of intermittent feedings consist of an initial requirement for nursing supervision, such as monitoring for gastric residuals, and a higher risk of aspiration if gastric emptying is delayed. Slow administration of small volumes into the stomach (25 to 40 mL/hour) is well tolerated and avoids the abdominal discomfort often caused by the increased rate and volume of intermittent feedings.

Continuous Feeding. Continuous feeding, administered by infusion pump over 18 to 24 hours, requires less nursing supervision and results in smaller residual volumes and a lower risk of aspiration than does intermittent feeding. When patients are fed into the duodenum or jejunum, continuous feeding is required to avoid distention of the bowel, fluid and electrolyte shifts, and diarrhea, all of which can occur with intermittent feeding. Feedings into the small bowel usually consist of isotonic polymeric solutions, initially at a rate of 30 mL/hour. The rate is increased approximately 25 mL/hour/day until the desired volume is achieved to meet the patient's nutrient requirements. Infusions should be initiated at very low rates (10 mL/hour) in critically ill patients. Disadvantages of continuous feeding include the expense of the volumetric infusion pump and the limitation it places on ambulatory patients.

MONITORING. Patients receiving enteral feedings require the same careful monitoring as do those who receive parenteral nutrition. This need for monitoring is especially true in critically ill patients. Routine monitoring is best accomplished by following a protocol that ensures

TABLE 235–3 STANDARD ORDER FORM FOR PATIENTS RECEIVING ENTERAL NUTRITION

Obtain an abdominal radiograph to confirm tube location before feeding.
Elevate the head of the patient's bed 30 degrees when feeding into the stomach.
Record the name, volume, and strength of the formula and the duration and rate (mL/hr) of feeding.
Check the gastric residual every 4 hr in patients receiving gastric feedings. Withhold feedings for 4 hr if the residual is greater than 150 mL. Notify the physician if two consecutive measurements detect excessive residual.
Weigh the patient on Monday, Wednesday, and Friday.
Record input and output daily. Every 8 hr, chart the volume of formula administered separately from water or other oral intake.
Change administration tubing daily.
Irrigate the feeding tube with 20 mL of water at the completion of each intermittent feeding, when the tube is disconnected, after delivery of crushed medications, or if feeding is stopped for any reason.
When the patient is ingesting oral nutrients, request calorie counts daily.
Obtain a complete blood cell count with red blood cell indices, SMA-12, serum iron, serum magnesium, albumin, transferrin, and prealbumin every Monday.
Obtain an SMA-6 every Thursday.
Hold feedings for nausea, vomiting, or distention. Call a house officer.

SMA-6, sequential multiple analyzer, 6 tests; SMA-12 = sequential multiple analyzer, 12 tests.

complete and detailed surveillance to reduce the possibility of error in the choice of formula and nutrient administration and to assess progress toward nutritional goals (Table 235–3).

Tolerance. Special attention must be paid to gastrointestinal tolerance to the formula. The patient's condition should be evaluated daily for diarrhea, constipation, nausea, cramping, vomiting, and abdominal distention. Clinical evidence of abdominal distention is a contraindication to enteral feeding. One must give close attention to the patient's metabolic status and fluid and electrolyte balance. In many instances, potential complications can be avoided by simple maneuvers such as changing the infusion rate, caloric density, or formulation.

Nutritional Adequacy. Periodic nutritional assessment is required to evaluate the adequacy of the nutritional support. Nitrogen balance, body weight change, and serum protein status should be monitored and the nutrient prescription amended when indicated. Because of frequent disruptions in feeding attempts, it is not uncommon for hospitalized patients to receive as little as 70% of the enteral calories ordered on a daily basis. These considerations may make it necessary to increase the infusion rate or to supplement infusions with parenteral feeding until satisfactory enteral intake is achieved.

COMPLICATIONS

Clinically significant complications of enteral feeding, although few, should be promptly recognized and treated aggressively. As noted, a standardized monitoring protocol helps prevent and detect possible problems. Complications of enteral feeding are grouped into four major categories: gastrointestinal, metabolic, infectious, and mechanical.

Gastrointestinal Complications

Definition

Diarrhea, defined as stool weight (or volume) of more than 500 mL/24 hours, is the most common complication of enteral nutrition and occurs in 10 to 20% of patients.

TABLE 235–4 CAUSES OF DIARRHEA IN TUBE-FED PATIENTS

COMMON CAUSES UNRELATED TO TUBE FEEDING
Elixir medications containing sorbitol Magnesium-containing antacids Antibiotic-induced sterile gut Pseudomembranous colitis
POSSIBLE CAUSES RELATED TO TUBE FEEDING
Administration of concentrated medications through feeding tube Inadequate fiber to form stool bulk High fat content of formula (in the presence of fat malabsorption syndrome) Bacterial contamination of enteral products and delivery systems (causal association with diarrhea not documented) Rapid advancement in rate (after the gastrointestinal tract is unused for prolonged periods)
UNLIKELY CAUSES RELATED TO TUBE FEEDING
Formula hyperosmolality (proven not to be a cause of diarrhea) Lactose (absent from nearly all enteral feeding formulas)

Pathobiology

The possible causes of diarrhea are listed in Table 235–4. Factors related to tube feeding that have been suggested to predispose patients to diarrhea but are not documented by controlled studies include formula hyperosmolality, lactose in the presence of relative lactase deficiency, and bacterial contamination of the enteral products and delivery systems. Although contamination is not a frequent cause of diarrhea, formula containers and administration tubing should be changed daily to avoid this complication. High-fat formulas may cause diarrhea when patients suffer from fat malabsorption (as in pancreatic exocrine insufficiency, biliary obstruction, ileectomy, or ileitis). Enterally administered medications, including antibiotics, hyperosmolar drug solutions such as sorbitol-containing elixirs, and magnesium-containing antacids, can cause diarrhea. Many elixir medications contain substantial amounts (up to 65%) of sorbitol, although the agent is listed in the drug information insert only as an "inactive" ingredient. For this reason, all elixir medications must be considered potential causes of diarrhea in tube-fed patients, and it is often prudent to discontinue these medications or to change them to tablet or intravenous forms to determine whether they are the etiologic agent.

Treatment

Treatment of diarrhea is directed at the underlying cause; however, several therapeutic options are available when no cause is clearly identifiable. Decreasing the feeding flow rate may alleviate diarrhea by allowing time for intestinal mucosal adaptation to occur when the gastrointestinal tract has not been used for extended periods (in cases of starvation and intestinal atrophy induced by total parenteral nutrition). The flow rate is then slowly increased over several days. Parenteral feeding may be necessary to meet full nutrient requirements during this interval. Nonspecific treatment with antidiarrheal agents can also be tried cautiously. Supplementation of formulas with fiber may help to solidify the stool and slow transit time in patients not receiving broad-spectrum antibiotics. The fiber contained in some commercial formulas (usually soy polysaccharide) has not been shown to reduce the incidence of diarrhea.

Metabolic Complications

Definition

Metabolic complications include abnormalities in fluid and electrolyte balance, hyperglycemia, trace element deficiencies, vitamin K deficiency, and abnormalities in protein tolerance.

Diagnosis

Abnormalities of most electrolytes and trace elements have been reported. Routine screening of many of these substances permits early detection before clinical manifestations are apparent. Such screening is especially important in patients with renal, cardiac, or hepatic insufficiency.

Treatment

Overhydration occurs in 20 to 25% of patients receiving enteral nutrition. Cardiac failure and renal insufficiency aggravate the problem and complicate its management. Slowing of the infusion rate or substitution of a 1.5 to 2 kcal/mL formula usually provides adequate treatment, and diuretics are rarely necessary for acute control. Although uncommon, hypertonic dehydration also can occur in patients fed calorie-dense formulas, especially when these patients cannot communicate their thirst.

Hyperglycemia occurs in 10 to 30% of tube-fed patients. High-calorie enteral diets may unmask type 2 diabetes mellitus. Hyperglycemia is corrected by decreasing the formula flow rate, administering insulin, or implementing both these measures. Because hyperglycemia can cause osmotic diuresis, the patient's fluid status must be carefully monitored.

Infectious Complications

Aspiration Pneumonia

The most common infectious complication of enteral nutrition is aspiration pneumonia, which is potentially fatal. Its incidence varies from 1 to 44%, depending on how it is defined.

Diagnosis

Aspiration can occur subtly, without witnessed episodes of vomiting, and it should be suspected with new onset of tachycardia, tachypnea, fever, hypoxemia, or chest radiographic changes. Patients fed nasogastrically appear to have a higher likelihood of aspiration than do patients fed by gastrostomy or jejunostomy. Those with an endotracheal tube or a tracheostomy have an especially high risk. Feeding beyond the duodenum probably lowers the incidence of aspiration, although no conclusive evidence supports this premise. A chest radiograph should be obtained before feeding is initiated in every patient with a newly inserted nasogastric or nasoenteric tube if gastric contents cannot be withdrawn through the tube. Methods for detecting "silent" aspiration of enteral formulas in intubated patients include checking tracheal aspirations for the presence of glucose with the use of oxidant reagent strips or placing methylene blue dye in the formula as a potential marker in tracheal aspirates.

Prevention

Preventive measures include elevating the head of the bed to 30 degrees, periodic measuring of gastric residuals, and inflating the endotracheal tube cuff. Correct techniques to insert the soft feeding tubes and careful observation of the tube's position may prevent potentially lethal bronchopleural complications.

Mechanical Complications

Mechanical complications associated with enteral nutrition generally relate to the tube itself or to its anatomic position. Nasoenteric tubes can cause nasopharyngeal erosions and discomfort, sinusitis, otitis media, gagging, esophagitis, esophageal reflux, tracheoesophageal fistulas, and rupture of esophageal varices. Feeding tubes can become knotted or clogged. Gastrostomy or jejunostomy tubes can cause mechanical obstruction of the pylorus or small bowel. Additional complications of percutaneous tubes include leakage around the tube, dislodgment to an intraperitoneal position, and occlusion, especially of small-bore needle-catheter jejunostomies.

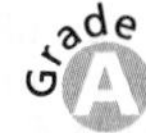

1. Zaloga GP: Parenteral nutrition in adult inpatients with functioning gastrointestinal tracts: Assessment of outcomes. Lancet 2006;367:1101–1111.
2. Dan A, Jacques TC, O'Leary MJ: Enteral nutrition versus glucose-based or lipid-based parenteral nutrition and tight glycaemic control in critically ill patients. Crit Care Resusc 2006;8:283–288.

SUGGESTED READINGS

Heyland DK, Dhaliwal R, Drover JW, et al: Canadian clinical practice guidelines for nutrition support in mechanically ventilated, critically ill adult patients. JPEN J Parenter Enteral Nutr 2003;27:355–373. *A review of established guidelines for nutritional support in critically ill, ventilated patients.*

Kieft H, Roos AN, van Drunen JDE, et al: Clinical outcome of immunonutrition in a heterogeneous intensive care population. Intensive Care Med 2005;31:524–532. *There was no significant benefit of immunonutrition when compared with isocaloric, less expensive conventional formulas.*

Koretz RL, Avenell A, Lipman TO, et al: Does enteral nutrition affect clinical outcome? A systematic review of the randomized trials. Am J Gastroenterol 2007;102:412–429. *Review of randomized trials of enteral nutrition in the patient with difficult medical problems.*

Mackenzie SL, Zygun DA, Whitemore BL, et al: Implementation of a nutrition support protocol increases the proportion of mechanically ventilated patients reaching enteral nutrition targets in the adult intensive care unit. JPEN J Parenter Enteral Nutr 2005;29:74–80. *A structured protocol significantly improved the delivery of enteral nutrients.*

236 PARENTERAL NUTRITION

Alexander Wilmer and
Greet Van den Berghe

Malnutrition is a pathologic state resulting from unmet metabolic needs. It is associated with reduced body mass, reduced organ function, abnormalities in blood chemistries, and increased morbidity and mortality. Malnutrition is common in clinical practice, among both chronically and acutely ill patients. On admission to the hospital, 30 to 60% of patients have some degree of malnutrition, and it may be severe in 10 to 25%. Many patients, especially the elderly, those with prolonged hospitalization, and those with severe disease, are at increased risk for development of malnutrition in the hospital. Frequent reasons for malnutrition include increased catabolism or losses and decreased calorie intake or impaired anabolism.

Since the 1960s, parenteral provision of nutritional support has been widely accepted as a means to modulate the catabolic response and to correct or to prevent nutritional deficits associated with disease. A state of malnutrition induced by starvation can usually be reversed by parenteral nutrition. However, in disease states associated with hypercatabolism, such as in the critically ill, the provision of parenteral nutrients can at best be supportive. The use of parenteral nutrition is costly and associated with risks. It is also a practice that has grown into a standard of care in spite of a lack of objective evidence for a beneficial effect on outcome.

INDICATIONS AND NUTRITIONAL SCREENING

All patients who are malnourished or at risk for malnutrition should receive specialized nutritional care on the basis of the premise that this will improve outcome. A nutritional screening process should always precede the provision of artificial nutrition. The initial screening should be a rapid and simple process aimed at identifying those patients who might benefit from a more in-depth assessment. This assessment should determine whether parenteral nutrition is truly necessary and whether nutritional treatment is likely to influence outcome. In the practice guidelines of 2002, the American Society for Parenteral and Enteral Nutrition suggests that nutritional screening should incorporate data such as height, weight, weight change, primary diagnosis, and comorbidities for all patients in an ambulatory, hospital, home, or alternative site care setting. If nutritional screening identifies a patient to be at risk, a formal assessment should be performed, including a combination of clinical (history and physical examination) and biochemical parameters. However, there is no single method with sufficient sensitivity and specificity to screen for nutritional risk or to assess malnutrition, and none of the existing screening systems has been validated with respect to outcome. The Nutritional Risk Screening 2002 is a scoring system developed to detect the presence of malnutrition and the risk for development of malnutrition in the hospital (Tables 236–1 and 236–2). This system has good reliability, high practicability, and reasonably good predictive validity to identify patients who will benefit from nutritional support (likelihood ratio, 1.4 [1.9–1.0]).

TABLE 236–1 NUTRITIONAL RISK SCREENING (NRS 2002): INITIAL SCREENING

	Yes	No
1. Is BMI < 20.5?		
2. Has the patient lost weight within the last 3 months?		
3. Has the patient had a reduced dietary intake in the last week?		
4. Is the patient severely ill? (e.g., in intensive therapy)		

Yes: If the answer is yes to any question, the screening in Table 236–2 is performed.
No: If the answer is no to all questions, the patient is rescreened at weekly intervals. If the patient is scheduled for a major operation, a preventive nutritional care plan is considered to avoid the associated risk status.
From Kondrup J, Allison SP, Elia M, et al: ESPEN guidelines for nutritional screening 2002. Clin Nutr 2003;22:415–421.

Parenteral nutrition should be initiated only when the gastrointestinal tract is nonfunctional or when it is impossible to obtain enteral access. However, enteral nutrition frequently results in hypocalorie feeding. Even though there is no evidence for or against it, it seems reasonable to supplement enteral with parenteral nutrition as a safe and effective means to achieve earlier optimal calorie intake when the enteral approach does not deliver the estimated calories. There is also no evidence that patients without risk factors will benefit from enteral or parenteral feeding if the expected duration of inability to tolerate enteral feeding is less than 7 to 10 days.

ORDERING PARENTERAL NUTRITION

Estimation of Fluid and Calorie Needs

Before parenteral nutrition is ordered, the fluid requirements of the patient should be evaluated. These will vary according to the age of the patient, the disease itself, and the impact of the disease on organ function. Fluid requirements will generally be met with 30 to 40 mL/kg per day or at 1 to 1.5 mL/kcal expended. A more accurate formula for patients with a body weight of 20 kg or more is 1500 mL + 20 mL/kg for each kilogram above 20 kg.

A second step in ordering parenteral nutrition is to estimate the calorie needs of a patient, which remains a difficult task. The total calorie intake should be determined in relation to the energy expenditure. Age, gender, body size, physical activity, fever, and severity of the disease are factors that modulate energy expenditure. Total energy expenditure is the amount of calories burned during 24 hours and can be measured directly by heat loss (direct calorimetry) or indirectly by the relation between oxygen consumption and carbon dioxide production (indirect calorimetry). Calorimetry is viewed as the "gold standard" in measuring energy expenditure. Unfortunately, time limitations and financial constraints preclude this method for everyday clinical practice. Total energy

TABLE 236–2 NUTRITIONAL RISK SCREENING (NRS 2002): FINAL SCREENING

Impaired Nutritional Status		Severity of Disease (= increase in requirements)	
Absent Score 0	Normal nutritional status	Absent Score 0	Normal nutritional requirements
Mild Score 1	Weight loss > 5% in 3 months *or* Food intake below 50–75% of normal requirement in preceding week	Mild Score 1	Hip fracture* Chronic patients, in particular with acute complications: cirrhosis,* COPD* *Chronic hemodialysis, diabetes, oncology*
Moderate Score 2	Weight loss > 5% in 2 months or BMI 18.5–20.5 + impaired general condition *or* Food intake 25–60% of normal requirement in preceding week	Moderate Score 2	Major abdominal surgery* Stroke* *Severe pneumonia, hematologic malignancy*
Severe Score 3	Weight loss > 5% in 1 month (>15% in 3 months) or BMI < 18.5 + impaired general condition *or* Food intake 0–25% of normal requirement in preceding week	Severe Score 3	Head injury* Bone marrow transplantation* *Intensive care patients (APACHE > 10)*
Score:	+	Score:	= Total score
Age	If ≥70 years: add 1 to total score above		= age adjusted total score

Score ≥ 3: the patient is nutritionally at risk and a nutritional care plan is initiated.
Score < 3: weekly rescreening of the patient. If the patient is scheduled for a major operation, a preventive nutritional care plan is considered to avoid the associated risk status.
NRS 2002 is based on an interpretation of available randomized clinical trials.
*Indicates that a trial directly supports the categorization of patients with that diagnosis.
Nutritional risk is defined by the present **nutritional status** and risk of impairment of present status due to **increased requirements** caused by stress metabolism of the clinical condition.
A nutritional care plan is indicated in all patients who are (1) severely undernourished (score = 3), or (2) severely ill (score = 3), or (3) moderately undernourished + mildly ill (score 2 + 1), or (4) mildly undernourished + moderately ill (score 1 + 2).
Diagnoses shown in *italics* are based on the following prototypes:
Prototypes for severity of disease
Score = 1: a patient with chronic disease admitted to the hospital because of complications. The patient is weak but out of bed regularly. Protein requirement is increased but can be covered by oral diet or supplement in most cases.
Score = 2: a patient confined to bed because of illness (e.g., after major abdominal surgery). Protein requirement is substantially increased but can be covered, although artificial feeding is required in many cases.
Score = 3: a patient in intensive care with assisted ventilation, for example. Protein requirement is increased and cannot be covered even by artificial feeding. Protein breakdown and nitrogen loss can be significantly attenuated.
Modified from Kondrup J, Allison SP, Elia M, et al: ESPEN guidelines for nutritional screening 2002. Clin Nutr 2003;22:415–421.

expenditure is the sum of cold- and diet-induced thermogenesis, energy consumed by physical activity, and resting energy expenditure. In hospitalized patients, resting energy expenditure is the most variable component and is highly influenced by body composition and degree of inflammation. The variability for the same disease can be as much as 100%, depending very much on the severity of the disease and the time course. This is why all of the frequently cited equations to predict energy expenditure are often inaccurate in patients with more acute and severe disease and can be associated with a substantial risk for overfeeding or underfeeding.

The Harris-Benedict equation, which was developed in normal individuals and calculates resting energy expenditure, is the most popular of these equations:

Females: $655 + (9.6 \times \text{weight in kg}) + (1.8 \times \text{height in cm}) - (4.7 \times \text{age in yr})$

Males: $66.5 + (13.8 \times \text{weight in kg}) + (5.0 \times \text{height in cm}) - (6.8 \times \text{age in yr})$

Stress and activity factors are added to this calculation. The predicted amount usually falls between 20 and 35 kcal/kg per day. A more practical method, for unstressed subjects, is to calculate calorie needs on the basis of an average value of 1 kcal/kg per hour for men; in women, subtract 5 to 10%. Yet another simple method is given by the following formulas (calculated for ideal body weight):

$$\text{Women} > 60 \text{ yr} = 20 \text{ kcal/kg/day}$$
$$\text{Women} < 60 \text{ yr} = 25 \text{ kcal/kg/day}$$
$$\text{Men} > 60 \text{ yr} = 25 \text{ kcal/kg/day}$$
$$\text{Men} < 60 \text{ yr} = 30 \text{ kcal/kg/day}$$

Forty percent to 50% of Americans are obese, and obesity makes accurate prediction of calorie needs even more difficult. Based on empirical data, a possible approach is to calculate the ideal body weight and to add a percentage (25 to 45%) of the excess body weight to the ideal weight. A formula to calculate ideal body weight is

$$\text{Women} = 45.5 + 0.91 \times (\text{length in cm} - 152.4)$$
$$\text{Men} = 50 + 0.91 \times (\text{length in cm} - 152.4)$$

Formulations

Total parenteral nutrition is the term used to describe a means of feeding whereby all or almost all of the estimated calorie needs are met solely by intravenous administration of nutrients. Supplementary parenteral nutrition refers to a patient who is receiving part of his or her nutritional needs through the gastrointestinal tract and the rest by parenteral infusion. Parenteral nutrition administered through a central vein is referred to as central parenteral nutrition (often also called total parenteral nutrition); when it is given through a peripheral vein, it is referred to as peripheral parenteral nutrition. The main difference is that formulations for peripheral parenteral nutrition need to be isotonic with blood to avoid phlebitis. Hypertonic parenteral formulas are given through a central vein, in which the high flow rapidly dilutes the contents. The main limitation of peripheral parenteral nutrition is that larger volumes are necessary for the nutritional needs of the patient to be met.

The products found in parenteral nutrition formulations typically include macronutrients (protein, carbohydrates, fat emulsions) and micronutrients (vitamins, minerals, and trace elements) (Table 236–3).

Carbohydrates

Carbohydrates are the main source of calories in almost all parenteral nutrition formulations. In the body, glucose is the main metabolic fuel. In the food industry, the natural form of glucose (D-glucose) is also frequently referred to as dextrose. The brain, renal medulla, leukocytes, erythrocytes, bone marrow, and peripheral nerves use glucose as their main source of oxidative energy. Provision of parenteral glucose has a protein-sparing effect because it decreases the need for skeletal muscle breakdown to provide amino acid precursors for gluconeogenesis. Glucose also stimulates insulin release, thus decreasing lipolysis. Glucose oxidation results in a respiratory quotient of 1 (respiratory quotient = moles of produced carbon dioxide/moles of consumed oxygen), which is higher than the respiratory quotient of 0.7 associated with oxidation of long-chain fatty acids. In patients with limited pulmonary function, the elimination of this extra load of carbon dioxide might be an important additional burden.

The oxidation of 1 g of glucose yields 4 kcal. To meet the needs of the brain, the minimum daily amount of glucose is estimated to be 100 to 150 g. Parenteral nutrition formulations classically contain glucose concentrations ranging from 5 to 70%; the selection depends on the estimated calorie needs and the total volume requirement. In the stressed patient, maximum oxidation rate of glucose is 4 to 7 mg/kg/min (for a 70-kg patient, 400 to 700 g/day). To decrease the risk for metabolic alterations, the maximum rate of glucose infusion should not exceed 5 mg/kg/min.

Protein

In parenteral nutrition, nitrogen is administered as amino acids containing all essential and almost all nonessential amino acids. Amino acids are a source of calories and precursors for the biosynthesis of proteins involved in almost every body function. Protein can be oxidized and yields 4 kcal/g. In steady-state conditions, protein oxidation equals protein intake, and under such conditions, exogenous protein serves as an energy supply. However, in Europe, it is generally assumed that in critically ill patients, the structural or biosynthetic function of amino acids outweighs their function as a metabolic fuel. Therefore, parenteral protein in that part of the world is usually not included in the calculation of calorie needs. The dietary reference intake for healthy adults is 0.8 g per kilogram of body weight per day, assuming that total calorie intake is adequate. In patients with more severe disease, such as the critically ill, 1.2 to 1.5 g/kg may seem more appropriate. Burn patients or patients with important gastrointestinal losses presumably fare better with high-protein regimens (>1.5 g/kg).

The standard formulations for amino acids include solutions containing amino acids only or combinations of amino acids with glucose. Standard amino acid solutions are also available with or without electrolytes. Within the amino acid solutions, different formulations have been tailored to specific disease states. For example, patients with hepatic encephalopathy may benefit from solutions with increased amounts of branched-chain amino acids (valine, leucine, and isoleucine) and reduced amounts of aromatic amino acids. Branched-chain amino acids are oxidized in muscle tissue and therefore may decrease the metabolic burden on the liver. A few clinical studies have shown improved outcome with parenteral glutamine, and current evidence tends to favor its use in subgroups of critically ill patients. There is no convincing evidence for specific amino acid compositions in patients with acute renal failure, who may need as much as 1.5 g/kg/day of protein when undergoing renal replacement therapies. This is in contrast with stable patients and chronic renal failure, for which a moderate protein restriction (0.7 to 1.0 g/kg/day) is recommended.

Lipids

Lipids are fat emulsions used for provision of energy and to supply linoleic acid and linolenic acid, which are essential, polyunsaturated fatty acids. Linoleic acid is the basic substance of the long-chain ω-6 fatty

TABLE 236–3 MACRONUTRIENTS IN PARENTERAL NUTRITION

Macronutrient	Minimum Need	Maximum Not to Be Exceeded	Total Calories
Carbohydrate	100–150 g/day	4–5 g/kg/day	40–70%
Protein	0.8 g/kg body weight	2 g/kg/day	15–20%
Lipids	2–4% of total calories	2.5 g/kg/day	15–40%

acids, and linolenic acid is the equivalent of the ω-3 fatty acid family. Lipid emulsions are iso-osmolar and contain a core made essentially of triglycerides stabilized by a layer of phospholipids. Phospholipids serve as an emulsifying agent; glycerol is used to make the emulsion isotonic. Fat emulsions are available in concentrations of 10%, 20%, and 30%. Conventional lipid emulsions use soybean oil or safflower oil or a mixture of both containing only long-chain triglycerides. More recent emulsions contain a mixture of both medium- and long-chain triglycerides. Medium-chain triglycerides are derived from coconut oil and contain mainly saturated fatty acids. They have a number of advantages, such as faster clearance from the blood stream, faster oxidation for energy production, no accumulation in liver tissue, and no storage in adipose tissue. However, hepatic metabolism results in ketogenesis and may lead to acidosis. Olive oil has recently been introduced into fat emulsions. Olive oil is rich in monounsaturated oleic acid and, compared with safflower or soybean oil, may have beneficial influences on inflammatory and immunologic mechanisms. Research on the importance of ω-6 and ω-3 fatty acids in the standard Western diet has led to the development of lipid emulsions based on fish oil. Deep-sea fish oil is an important source of the very long chain, polyunsaturated ω-3 fatty acids eicosapentaenoic acid and docosahexaenoic acid. An increased incorporation of ω-3 fatty acids into plasma membranes derived from fish oil, compared with ω-6 fatty acids derived from vegetable oils and animal fats, increases the release of eicosapentaenoic acid rather than arachidonic acid. The lipid mediators derived from these substances differ markedly. Those derived from eicosapentaenoic acid are mainly anti-inflammatory; those derived from arachidonic acid are more pro-inflammatory. The ratio of ω-6 to ω-3 fatty acids in soybean emulsions and in mixtures of long- and medium-chain triglycerides is 7 to 1; in olive oil emulsions, it is 9 to 1. Outside the United States, manufacturers are marketing lipid emulsions with a ratio of ω-6 to ω-3 fatty acids of less than 4 to 1 with the hope of improved nutritional immunomodulation.

Use of lipids as an energy source can have important benefits. Oxidation of 1 g of intravenous fat supplies 9 kcal. It allows a reduced prescription of parenteral glucose and can thereby reduce the risk or severity of hyperglycemia, especially in stressed patients with insulin resistance. Because of a lower respiratory quotient of 0.7, less carbon dioxide is produced during oxidation of 1 g of lipids compared with 1 g of glucose, although substrate oxidation of glucose is probably not decreased. Only 10% of parenteral nutrition is needed as fat to meet essential fatty acid needs. However, most parenteral nutrition formulations now contain 15 to 40% as lipids. Adults usually receive 0.5 to 1.5 g/kg/day. In patients with hypertriglyceridemia (more than 4 to 5 mmol/L or 350 to 400 mg/dL), lipid emulsions should not be started or should be temporarily interrupted.

Micronutrients

Vitamins are essential organic micronutrients, and most of them are used as necessary precursors of coenzymes. Thirteen different vitamins are required in the diet of human beings; nine of these are water soluble and four are fat soluble. The essential trace elements include iron, iodine, copper, manganese, zinc, cobalt, molybdenum, selenium, vanadium, and nickel. These trace elements are needed as enzyme cofactors or prosthetic groups.

Vitamins and trace elements are usually administered as combination products; some are also commercially available as single-item injection. The ideal amount of micronutrients remains poorly defined. The American Medical Association has issued guidelines for the composition of intravenous administration of vitamins and trace elements. These were amended by the Food and Drug Administration in recognition of increased demands in disease states. It is commonly recommended and accepted that all patients should receive daily micronutrient supplementation in standard doses routinely with parenteral nutrition. In critically ill patients, it may be advantageous to increase the dose of vitamins C and E and of selenium because of their role as nonenzymatic reactive oxygen species scavengers. Unless there is clear clinical suggestion of potential deficiency, routine monitoring of serum levels of vitamins or trace elements is not recommended.

PARENTERAL NUTRITION DELIVERY

Total parenteral nutrition can be given in different ways: as separate solutions for carbohydrates, amino acids, and lipids; as a primary amino acid and glucose solution (two-in-one) with the lipid component as piggyback; or as a three-in-one admixture (all-in-one infusion). Several manufacturers now make all-in-one infusions of varying volumes and varying but predefined contents of lipids, glucose, and protein. These have become popular in many institutions because pharmacy and handling costs are decreased and potential breaks in sterility are avoided. However, compared with prescriptions tailored specifically to an individual patient, these all-in-one infusions are less precise in meeting individual nutritional needs.

Because faster infusion rates are associated with a higher incidence of acute adverse effects, during the first days, lipid emulsions should not be infused at a rate faster than 0.1 g/kg/hr with long-chain triglycerides and 1.5 g/kg/hr with mixed medium- and long-chain triglycerides.

Vascular Access

Solutions for peripheral parenteral nutrition are hypertonic to blood, and their osmolality should not exceed 900 mOsm/L. When solution osmolality exceeds 900 mOsm/L, the incidence of phlebitis, inflammation, and pain is clearly increased. Adding 5000 units of heparin to a peripheral parenteral nutrition solution may prolong the duration of the peripheral line.

In most cases, parenteral nutrition is delivered through a central venous access. The selection of the site for catheter insertion and the type of catheter needs to be individualized. If the aim of the intervention is to provide an access for parenteral nutrition only, a single-lumen catheter is preferred. In general, the favored site for insertion is the subclavian vein. Placement in the internal jugular vein, compared with the subclavian vein, appears to be associated with a slightly higher risk of infection and a clearly higher risk of thrombosis. It is also less comfortable for mobile patients. Placement in the subclavian vein is associated with a small risk for pneumothorax and a slightly higher risk of stenosis. The femoral vein should be used only when placement in the jugular or subclavian vein is contraindicated or not possible. A femoral vein access is associated with the highest risk of infection or thrombosis. Most catheters are introduced by skin puncture; catheters intended for long-term use are placed surgically. Peripherally inserted catheters are inserted through a peripheral, usually antecubital vein and then advanced into a central vein. They can be placed if the intended duration of parenteral nutrition is more than 2 weeks, and they can be used for up to 6 months in stable patients. The main advantage of these catheters is the avoidance of the risks associated with the puncture of a central vein, but it may lead to a higher rate of phlebitis.

Before placement of a vascular access, patients should be well hydrated and the coagulation status checked. Strict aseptic technique is necessary, and correct positioning of the catheter should be controlled by a chest radiograph before central parenteral nutrition is initiated. Proper catheter care includes regular inspection of the insertion site and dressing with gauze or transparent, semipermeable dressings.

Mechanical complications during placement include arterial puncture, pneumothorax, and hematoma. Infectious complications related to a central venous access occur in 4 to 20% of hospitalized patients, especially in immunocompromised patients or in the critically ill. In patients with central parenteral nutrition, any sign of fever or sepsis should prompt the thought of catheter-related septicemia or catheter infection. Thrombosis detected by ultrasound examination is frequent, but its clinical relevance remains unclear.

METABOLIC COMPLICATIONS AND MONITORING OF PARENTERAL NUTRITION

The metabolic complications related to parenteral nutrition can be serious, but they can be minimized with adequate monitoring. Acute metabolic complications include electrolyte deficiencies, particularly potassium, magnesium, phosphorus, and calcium. These deficiencies are common but can be prevented by adequate monitoring of plasma levels. The same is true for trace elements and vitamin deficiencies, particularly thiamine. Excess glucose can aggravate hyperglycemia, which has been associated with poor outcome after cardiac surgery, myocardial infarction, and stroke and an impaired leukocyte function contributing to an increased nosocomial infection rate. Randomized trials in critically ill patients have shown that tighter blood glucose control significantly reduces morbidity 1 and may reduce mortality. In these patients, blood glucose concentration should be monitored frequently, every 2 to 4 hours, with the aim of maintaining blood glucose concentration below 110 mg/dL (6.1 mmol/L). Insulin will often be required to achieve the desired glycemic levels and is a second reason for frequent monitoring to detect possible hypoglycemia. If central parenteral nutrition needs to be interrupted, it should be replaced with glucose 10% until it can be restarted. A guideline for insulin titration in critically ill patients is described in Table 236–4. Hypertriglyceridemia can increase the risk for liver steatosis. Infusion of lipids during a period of 4 to 8 hours can result in pulmonary hypertension. Serum triglyceride levels should be determined before parenteral nutrition is started and once a week thereafter. When parenteral nutrition is instituted, patients with renal failure are more susceptible to uremia and those with volume depletion to metabolic acidosis.

Liver steatosis is usually caused by overfeeding and may give rise to elevated aminotransferases and parenchymal abnormalities on ultrasonography. Cholestatic liver disease may be serious and should be suspected in the setting of elevated γ-glutamyltransferase and alkaline phosphatase, often also in combination with hyperbilirubinemia. The etiology is

TABLE 236–4 INSULIN PROTOCOL FOR GLYCEMIC CONTROL IN CRITICALLY ILL PATIENTS

INSULIN INFUSION

Concentration and mode of administration:

Insulin is given only by continuous IV infusion through a central venous line by use of a 50-mL syringe-driven pump.

The standard concentration is 50 IU of insulin in 50 mL of 0.9% NaCl.

Prepared solutions are not stable after 24 hours.

MEASUREMENT OF BLOOD GLUCOSE LEVELS

Whole blood glucose levels are measured in undiluted arterial blood.

Undiluted samples are obtained by removal of at least four times the flush-volume in the line between the sampling point and the arterial puncture site before the actual sample is taken.

After admission to the intensive care unit and until normoglycemia (80–110 mg/dL or 4.4–6.1 mmol/L) is reached (usually within the first 12–24 hours), hourly or 2-hourly measurement of blood glucose concentration is advised. Thereafter, measurement of blood glucose concentration every 4 to 6 hours suffices.

In case of hypoglycemia or steep falls or rises in glycemia, more frequent control than every 4 hours is advised.

TITRATION SCHEDULE

Starting up insulin infusion and initial stabilization of blood glucose level

- When blood glucose level exceeds 110 mg/dL (6.1 mmol/L), insulin infusion is initiated at a starting dose of 2 IU/hr. If the blood glucose level on which insulin is started is >220 mg/dL, the starting dose of insulin can be set at 4 IU/hr.
- If a next blood glucose level is >140 mg/dL, increase the insulin infusion rate with 2 IU/hr.
- If a next blood glucose level is between 110 and 140 mg/dL, increase the insulin infusion rate with 0.5–1 IU/hr.
- If blood glucose approaches the normal range, adjust with increments or decrements of 0.1–0.5 IU/hr.
- When blood glucose level is within the normal range, leave insulin dose unaltered.

Dose adjustments after initial stabilization

- If blood glucose level falls steeply (>50% change) after a dose adjustment, reduce the insulin dose to half and check blood glucose level more frequently.
- If blood glucose is 60–80 mg/dL, reduce the dose adequately (rate depending on the previous blood glucose level) and check the blood glucose level within the next hour.
- If blood glucose is 40–60 mg/dL, stop the insulin infusion, ensure adequate baseline glucose intake, and check the blood glucose level within the next hour.
- If blood glucose is <40 mg/dL, stop the insulin infusion, ensure adequate baseline glucose intake, administer glucose per 10-g IV boluses, and check the blood glucose level within the next hour.
- Insulin sensitivity usually improves with time in the intensive care unit. Hence, in a patient in whom stable normoglycemia was reached, the need for insulin may decrease again at a later stage. If in such a case glycemia starts to fall, even though it is still within the normal range, beware of improved insulin sensitivity, reduce the insulin dose by 20%, and check blood glucose level.
- Increase in body temperature is always accompanied by an increased insulin requirement, particularly if this is caused by infection. Conversely, the need for insulin decreases again when an infection is under control.
- Maximal insulin dose is arbitrarily set at 50 IU/hr.
- Blood glucose levels are usually controllable below 110 mg/dL within 24 hours. On average, the insulin requirement is 6 IU/hr during the first 6 hours (about 10% of patients need more than 20 IU/hr) and 3 IU/hr from the second day of intensive care onward (10% of patients need more than 6 to 8 IU/hr).
- At discharge from the intensive care unit, a less strict approach is best adopted (glycemia ≤200 mg/dL) to avoid hypoglycemia in the less well controlled setting of a regular ward (see What to Do When a Patient Is Ready for Discharge to a Regular Ward).

SPECIAL CONCERNS REGARDING ALTERATIONS IN CALORIE INTAKE

Adequate calorie and glucose intake is essential. To avoid fluctuating blood glucose levels and too frequent need for readjustment of the insulin dose, administer IV glucose-containing solutions always by an infusion pump.

At the time of interruptions of tube feeding, the insulin dose should be reduced proportionately to avoid hypoglycemia. In a patient receiving full enteral tube feeding, this means that during the standard once-a-day, 2-hourly interruptions of tube feeding in our unit, insulin is virtually stopped, although in some patients (including those who had insulin-requiring diabetes before admission to the intensive care unit), a low (0.5 IU/h) maintenance dose is needed during that time.

At the time of transportation of a patient to an investigation or to the operating room for surgery, all IV and enteral administration of feeding is usually stopped, and insulin infusion should also be stopped. Check blood glucose level after having done so and ensure an adequate level before transport.

Whenever a patient is extubated and assumed to restart normal oral food intake, the IV or tube feeding is usually reduced to allow appetite to recur. In those patients, it is crucial to reduce the insulin dose proportionately (or often to stop it temporarily).

Continued

TABLE 236–4 INSULIN PROTOCOL FOR GLYCEMIC CONTROL IN CRITICALLY ILL PATIENTS—cont'd

SPECIAL CONCERNS ABOUT CONCOMITANT DRUGS

Glucocorticoids, particularly in high doses (>90 mg/day hydrocortisone or its equivalent), aggravate insulin resistance in patients in the intensive care unit. The dose of insulin to maintain normoglycemia will always need to be increased whenever such treatments are initiated.

To avoid annoying, recurrent fluctuations in insulin need, the total daily dose of glucocorticoids is best administered as a continuous infusion.

WHAT TO DO WHEN A PATIENT IS READY FOR DISCHARGE TO A REGULAR WARD

If a previously non–insulin-requiring patient is normoglycemic while receiving <2 IU/hr of insulin, the insulin infusion can be stopped. Control blood glucose level before discharge should be <200 mg/dL.

If insulin is required to maintain blood glucose level <200 mg/dL, it is most likely that the patient has preexisting diabetes. Follow-up by an endocrinologist should be planned, and the regimen of insulin should be arranged with the consulting physician to guarantee adequate follow-up on the regular ward.

unclear; the best solution is to decrease parenteral nutrition and to reinstitute enteral feeding as soon as possible. Other complications of the hepatobiliary tract associated with parenteral nutrition are gallbladder stasis that leads to increased risk for gallbladder sludge, gallstones, and acalculous cholecystitis. The best way to prevent these complications is to give small amounts of oral or enteral nutrition to stimulate gallbladder contraction.

The refeeding syndrome is a potentially life-threatening complication of parenteral nutrition. This syndrome comprises a series of metabolic and physiologic derangements resulting from reinstitution of nutrition, possibly because the provision of full specialized nutritional support is initiated too rapidly. Patients who have lost a large amount of weight or who are chronically malnourished are at greatest risk for this syndrome. This syndrome usually manifests itself within the first 2 weeks after the start of parenteral nutrition with malaise, edema, weakness, and cardiac arrhythmias. Typical metabolic complications are hypophosphatemia, hypokalemia, hypomagnesemia, thiamine deficiency, and fluid overload. Refeeding syndrome seems to be the result of a metabolic shift from use of stored energy as fat to exogenous energy in the form of carbohydrates. Infused glucose is associated with a rise in plasma insulin levels, which in turn causes intracellular shifts of electrolytes.

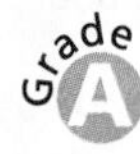

1. Van den Berghe G, Wilmer A, Hermans G, et al: Intensive insulin therapy in the medical ICU. N Engl J Med 2006;54:449–461.

SUGGESTED READINGS

Newton AF, DeLegge MH: Home initiation of parenteral nutrition. Nutr Clin Pract 2007;22:57–64. *Review of the indications and complications of home parenteral nutrition.*

Zaloga GP: Parenteral nutrition in adult inpatients with functioning gastrointestinal tracts: Assessment of outcomes. Lancet 2006;367:1101–1111. *Enteral nutrition generally results in reduced rates of infection and sepsis, as well as length of stay and costs.*

VITAMINS, TRACE MINERALS, AND OTHER MICRONUTRIENTS

Joel B. Mason

MICRONUTRIENTS IN NUTRITIONAL SCIENCE

Dietary Requirements

Micronutrients are a diverse array of dietary components necessary to sustain health. The physiologic roles of micronutrients are as varied as their composition; some micronutrients are used in enzymes as either coenzymes or as prosthetic groups, others as biochemical substrates or hormones, and, in some instances, the functions are not well defined. Under normal circumstances, the average daily dietary intake for each micronutrient that is required to sustain normal physiologic operations is measured in milligrams or smaller quantities. In this manner, micronutrients are distinguished from macronutrients, which encompass carbohydrates, fats, and proteins, as well as the macrominerals calcium, magnesium, and phosphorus.

Optimal Intake

For orderly homeostasis to proceed, most dietary nutrients must be ingested in quantities that are neither too small nor too great. Disorders may arise, therefore, when this physiologic window is either not met or exceeded. The size of this physiologic window varies for each micronutrient and should be kept in mind, particularly in this era when the administration of large quantities of certain micronutrients is increasingly explored for possible therapeutic implications. The dietary requirement for a particular micronutrient is determined by many factors, only one of which is the amount needed to sustain those physiologic functions for which it is used (Table 237–1). The U.S. Institute of Medicine Food and Nutrition Board regularly updates dietary guidelines that define the quantity of each micronutrient that is "adequate to meet the known nutrient needs of practically all healthy persons." These *recommended dietary allowances* (RDAs) were revised between 1998 and 2001, and the values for adults appear in Tables 237–2 and 237–3. Also established for the first time for each micronutrient were *tolerable upper limits* (TULs), which are the maximal daily levels of oral intake likely to pose no adverse health risks (see Tables 237–2 and 237–3). *Adequate intake,* the amount necessary to prevent a deficiency state, is not necessarily synonymous with *optimal intake.*

TYPES AND FUNCTION OF MICRONUTRIENTS

Vitamins

Vitamins have long been categorized as either fat soluble (A, D, E, K) or water soluble (all the others), as shown in Table 237–2. This manner of categorization remains physiologically meaningful. None of the fat-soluble vitamins appear to serve as coenzymes. Absorption of the fat-soluble vitamins is primarily through a micellar route, and pathophysiologic conditions associated with fat malabsorption frequently are associated with selective deficiencies of the fat-soluble vitamins. In contrast, most of the functions of the water-soluble vitamins are as coenzymes. Furthermore, the water-soluble vitamins are not absorbed through the lipophilic phase in the intestine.

Trace Elements

Fifteen trace elements have been identified as essential for health in animal studies: iron, zinc, copper, chromium, selenium, iodine, fluorine, manganese, molybdenum, cobalt, nickel, tin, silicon, vanadium, and arsenic (see Table 237–3). Nevertheless, only for the first 10 of these has compelling evidence indicated that they are essential nutrients in

Text continued on p. 1633.

TABLE 237–1 FACTORS THAT DETERMINE DIETARY REQUIREMENT OF A MICRONUTRIENT

PHYSIOLOGIC FACTORS

Bioavailability: Proportion of a micronutrient that is ingested and is capable of being assimilated and used for physiologic purposes
Quantity required to fulfill physiologic roles
Extent to which the body can reuse the micronutrient
Distribution of nutrient in the body: storage compartments
Gender
Stage of life cycle: Intrauterine development, childhood, adulthood, elder adulthood, pregnancy, lactation

PATHOPHYSIOLOGIC AND PHARMACOLOGIC FACTORS

Inborn errors of metabolism that variously affect assimilation, utilization, or excretion of micronutrients
Acquired disease states that alter the amounts required to sustain homeostasis (e.g., malabsorption, maldigestion, states that increase use)
Lifestyle habits such as smoking, ethanol consumption
Drugs that may alter bioavailability or utilization

TABLE 237–2 VITAMINS AND THEIR FUNCTIONS

	Biochemistry and Physiology	Deficiency [RDA*]	Toxicity [TUL†]	Assessment of Status
FAT-SOLUBLE VITAMINS				
Vitamin A	A subset of the retinoid compounds, each member having biologic activity qualitatively similar to retinol, a member of the family. Carotenoids are structurally related to retinoids. Some carotenoids, most notably β-carotene, are metabolized into compounds with vitamin A activity and are therefore considered to be provitamin A compounds. Vitamin A is an integral component of rhodopsin and iodopsins, light-sensitive proteins in rod and cone cells in the retina. It is needed for the induction and maintenance of cellular differentiation in certain tissues. It serves as a signal for appropriate morphogenesis in the developing embryo and is needed for maintenance of cell-mediated immunity. One microgram of retinol is equivalent to 3.33 IU of vitamin A.	Follicular hyperkeratosis and night blindness are early indicators. Conjunctival xerosis, degeneration of the cornea (keratomalacia), and de-differentiation of rapidly proliferating epithelia are later indications of deficiency. *Bitot's spots* (focal areas of the conjunctiva or cornea with foamy appearance) are an indication of xerosis. Blindness from corneal destruction and retinal dysfunction ensues if the deficiency is left uncorrected. Increased susceptibility to infection is also a consequence. [F: 700 μg; M: 900 μg]	In adults, >150,000 μg may cause *acute* toxicity: fatal intracranial hypertension, skin exfoliation, and hepatocellular necrosis. *Chronic* toxicity may occur with habitual daily intake of >10,000 μg: alopecia, ataxia, bone and muscle pain, dermatitis, cheilitis, conjunctivitis, pseudotumor cerebri, hepatocellular necrosis, hyperlipidemia, and hyperostosis are common. Single, large doses of vitamin A (30,000 μg) or habitual intake of >4500 μg/day in early pregnancy can be teratogenic. Chronic excessive intake of β-carotene can cause yellowish skin discoloration and is implicated in enhancing lung carcinogenesis in smokers. Habitually large doses of canthaxanthin may induce a retinopathy. [3000 μg]	Retinol concentration in the plasma and vitamin A concentrations in the milk and tears are reasonably accurate measures of adequate status. Toxicity is best assessed by elevated levels of retinyl esters in plasma. A quantitative measure of dark adaptation for night vision and an electroretinogram are useful functional tests.
Vitamin D	A group of sterol compounds whose parent structure is cholecalciferol (vitamin D_3). Cholecalciferol is formed in the skin from 7-dehydrocholesterol (provitamin D_3) by	Deficiency results in disordered bone modeling called *rickets* in childhood and *osteomalacia* in adults. Expansion of the epiphyseal growth	Excess amounts result in abnormally high concentrations of calcium and phosphate in the serum: metastatic calcifications, renal damage, and altered	The serum concentration of the major circulating metabolite, 25-hydroxy vitamin D, is an excellent indicator of systemic status except in chronic renal failure, in

Continued

TABLE 237–2 VITAMINS AND THEIR FUNCTIONS—cont'd

	Biochemistry and Physiology	Deficiency [RDA*]	Toxicity [TUL†]	Assessment of Status
	exposure to ultraviolet B radiation. A plant sterol, ergocalciferol (provitamin D_2) can be similarly converted into vitamin D_2 and has similar vitamin D activity. The vitamin undergoes sequential hydroxylations in the liver and kidney at the 25 and 1 positions, respectively, producing the most bioactive form of the vitamin, 1,25-dihydroxy vitamin D. It maintains intracellular and extracellular concentrations of calcium and phosphate by enhancing intestinal absorption of the two ions and, in conjunction with parathyroid hormone, promoting their mobilization from bone mineral. Vitamin D retards proliferation and promotes differentiation in certain epithelia. One microgram is equivalent to 40 IU.	plates and replacement of normal bone with unmineralized bone matrix are the cardinal features of rickets; the latter feature also characterizes osteomalacia. Deformity of bone and pathologic fractures occur. Decreased serum concentrations of calcium and phosphate may occur. [5 μg, ages 19–50 yr; 10 μg, ages 51–70 yr; 15 μg, age >70 yr]	mentation may occur. [50 μg]	which the impairment of renal 1-hydroxylation results in disassociation of in the mono- and dihydroxyvitamin concentrations. Measuring the serum concentration of 1,25-dihydroxy vitamin D is then necessary.
Vitamin E	A group of at least 8 naturally occurring compounds, some of which are tocopherols and some of which are tocotrienols. At present, the only dietary form thought to be biologically active in humans is α-tocopherol. It acts as an antioxidant and free radical scavenger in lipophilic environments, most notably in cell membranes. It acts in conjunction with other antioxidants such as selenium.	Deficiency from dietary inadequacy is rare in developed countries. It is usually seen in (1) premature infants, (2) individuals with fat malabsorption, and (3) individuals with abetalipoproteinemia. RBC fragility occurs and can produce hemolytic anemia. Neuronal degeneration produces peripheral neuropathies, ophthalmoplegia, and destruction of posterior columns of the spinal cord. Neurologic disease is frequently irreversible if deficiency is not corrected early enough. It may contribute to hemolytic anemia and retrolental fibroplasia in premature infants. It has been reported to suppress cell-mediated immunity. [15 mg]	Depressed levels of vitamin K–dependent procoagulants and potentiation of oral anticoagulants has been reported, as has impaired WBC function. Doses of 800 mg/day have been reported to increase the incidence of hemorrhagic stroke slightly. [1000 mg]	Plasma or serum concentration of α-tocopherol is most commonly used. Additional accuracy is obtained by expressing this value per milligrams of total plasma lipid. The RBC cell peroxide hemolysis test is not entirely specific but is a useful functional measure of the antioxidant potential of cell membranes.

TABLE 237–2 VITAMINS AND THEIR FUNCTIONS—cont'd

	Biochemistry and Physiology	Deficiency [RDA*]	Toxicity [TUL†]	Assessment of Status
Vitamin K	A family of naphthoquinone compounds with similar biologic activity. Phylloquinone (vitamin K_1) is derived from plants; a variety of menaquinones (vitamin K_2) is derived from bacterial sources. It serves as an essential cofactor in the post-translational γ-carboxylation of glutamic acid residues in many proteins. These proteins include several circulating procoagulants and anticoagulants as well as proteins in the bone matrix.	Deficiency syndrome is uncommon, except in (1) breast-fed newborns, in whom it may cause "hemorrhagic disease of the newborn," (2) adults with fat malabsorption or who are taking drugs that interfere with vitamin K metabolism (e.g., coumarin, phenytoin, broad-spectrum antibiotics), and (3) individuals taking large doses of vitamin E and anticoagulant drugs. Excessive hemorrhage is the usual manifestation. [F: 90 μg; M: 120 μg]	Rapid intravenous infusion of vitamin K_1 has been associated with dyspnea, flushing, and cardiovascular collapse, likely related to the dispersing agents in the solution. Supplementation may interfere with coumarin-based anticoagulation. Pregnant women taking large amounts of the provitamin menadione may deliver infants with hemolytic anemia, hyperbilirubinemia, and kernicterus. [no TUL established]	Prothrombin time is typically used as a measure of functional K status; it is neither sensitive nor specific for vitamin K deficiency. Determination of undercarboxylated prothrombin in the plasma is more accurate for detecting deficiency but less widely available.
WATER-SOLUBLE VITAMINS				
Thiamine (vitamin B_1)	A water-soluble compound containing substituted pyrimidine and thiazole rings and a hydroxyethyl side chain. The coenzyme form is thiamine pyrophosphate. It serves as a coenzyme in many α-ketoacid decarboxylation and transketolation reactions. Inadequate thiamine availability leads to impairments of the foregoing reactions, resulting in inadequate adenosine triphosphate synthesis and abnormal carbohydrate metabolism, respectively. It may have an additional role in neuronal conduction independent of aforementioned actions.	The classic deficiency syndrome ("beriberi") is described in Asian populations consuming a polished rice diet. Alcoholism and chronic renal dialysis are common precipitants; can also occur after bariatric surgery complicated by persistent vomiting. Mild deficiency commonly produces irritability, fatigue, and headaches. More pronounced deficiency produces various combinations of peripheral neuropathy, cardiovascular dysfunction, and cerebral dysfunction. Cardiovascular involvement ("wet beriberi") includes congestive heart failure and low peripheral vascular resistance. Cerebral disease includes nystagmus, ophthalmoplegia, and ataxia (Wernicke's encephalopathy) as well as hallucinations, impaired short-term memory, and confabulation ("Korsakoff's psychosis"). The deficiency syndrome responds within 24 hr to parenteral thiamine but is partially or wholly irreversible after a certain stage. [F: 1.1 mg; M: 1.2 mg]	Excess intake is largely excreted in the urine, although parenteral doses of >400 mg/day are reported to cause lethargy, ataxia, and reduced tone of the gastrointestinal tract. [TUL not established]	The most effective measure of vitamin B_1 status is the RBC transketolase activity coefficient, which measures enzyme activity before and after addition of exogenous thiamine pyrophosphate: RBCs from a deficient individual express a substantial increase in enzyme activity with addition of thiamine pyrophosphate. Thiamine concentrations in blood or urine are also used.

Continued

TABLE 237–2 VITAMINS AND THEIR FUNCTIONS—cont'd

	Biochemistry and Physiology	Deficiency [RDA*]	Toxicity [TUL†]	Assessment of Status
Riboflavin (vitamin B_2)	A compound consisting of a substituted isoalloxazine ring with a ribitol side chain. The vitamin serves as a coenzyme for a diverse array of biochemical reactions. The primary coenzymatic forms are flavin mononucleotide and flavin adenine dinucleotide. Riboflavin holoenzymes participate in oxidation-reduction reactions in a myriad of metabolic pathways.	Deficiency is usually seen in conjunction with deficiencies of other B vitamins. Isolated deficiency of riboflavin produces hyperemia and edema of nasopharyngeal mucosa, cheilosis, angular stomatitis, glossitis, seborrheic dermatitis, and normochromic, normocytic anemia. [F: 1.1; M: 1.3]	Toxicity is not reported in humans. [TUL not established]	The most common method of assessment is determining the activity coefficient of glutathione reductase in RBCs (the test is invalid for individuals with glucose-6-phosphate dehydrogenase deficiency). Measurements of blood and urine concentrations are less desirable methods.
Niacin (vitamin B_3)	Refers to nicotinic acid and the corresponding amide, nicotinamide. The active coenzymatic forms are composed of nicotinamide affixed to adenine dinucleotide, forming NAD or NADP. More than 200 apoenzymes use these compounds as electron acceptors or hydrogen donors, either as a coenzyme or a cosubstrate. The essential amino acid tryptophan is used as a precursor of niacin; 60 mg dietary tryptophan yields approximately 1 mg niacin. Dietary requirements thus depend partly on the tryptophan content of the diet. The requirement is often determined on the basis of caloric intake (i.e., niacin equivalents/1000 kcal). Large doses of nicotinic acid (1.5–3 g/day) effectively lower low-density lipoprotein cholesterol and elevate high-density lipoprotein cholesterol.	*Pellagra* is the classic deficiency syndrome and is often seen in populations where corn is the major source of energy. It is still endemic in parts of China, Africa, and India. Diarrhea, dementia (or associated symptoms of anxiety or insomnia), and pigmented dermatitis that develops in sun-exposed areas are typical features. Glossitis, stomatitis, vaginitis, vertigo, and burning dysesthesias are early signs. It is reported to occur occasionally in carcinoid syndrome, because tryptophan is diverted to other synthetic pathways. [F: 14 mg; M: 16 mg]	Human toxicity is known largely through studies examining hypolipidemic effects. It includes vasomotor phenomenon (flushing), hyperglycemia, parenchymal liver damage, and hyperuricemia. [35 mg]	Assessment of status is problematic: blood levels of the vitamin are not reliable. Measurement of urinary excretion of the niacin metabolites, *N*-methylnicotinamide and 2-pyridone, are thought to be the most effective means of assessment at present.
Vitamin B_6	Refers to several derivatives of pyridine, including pyridoxine, pyridoxal, and pyridoxamine, which are interconvertible in the body. The coenzymatic forms are PLP and pyridoxamine-5-phosphate. As a coenzyme, vitamin B_6 is involved in many transamination reactions (and thereby in gluconeogenesis), in the synthesis of niacin from	Deficiency is usually seen in conjunction with other water-soluble vitamin deficiencies. Stomatitis, angular cheilosis, glossitis, irritability, depression, and confusion occur in moderate to severe depletion; normochromic, normocytic anemia has been reported in severe deficiency.	Long-term use with doses exceeding 200 mg/day (in adults) may cause peripheral neuropathies and photosensitivity. [100 mg]	Many useful laboratory methods of assessment exist. The plasma or RBC PLP levels are most common. Urinary excretion of xanthurenic acid after an oral tryptophan load and activity indices of RBC alanine or aspartic acid transaminases are functional measures of vitamin B_6–dependent enzyme activity.

TABLE 237–2 VITAMINS AND THEIR FUNCTIONS—cont'd

	Biochemistry and Physiology	Deficiency [RDA*]	Toxicity [TUL†]	Assessment of Status
	tryptophan, in the synthesis of several neurotransmitters, and in the synthesis of δ-aminolevulinic acid (and therefore in heme synthesis). It also has functions unrelated to coenzymatic activity: pyridoxal and PLP bind to hemoglobin and alter oxygen affinity; PLP also binds to steroid receptors, inhibiting receptor affinity to DNA, and thereby modulates steroid activity.	Abnormal electroencephalograms and, in infants, convulsions have been observed. Some sideroblastic anemias respond to vitamin B_6 administration. Isoniazid, cycloserine, penicillamine, ethanol, and theophylline can inhibit vitamin B_6 metabolism. [Ages 19–50 yr: 1.3 mg; >50: 1.5 mg for women, 1.7 mg for men]		
Folate	A group of related pterin compounds. More than 35 forms of the vitamin are found naturally. The fully oxidized form, folic acid, is not found in nature but is the pharmacologic form of the vitamin. All folate functions relate to its ability to transfer one-carbon groups. It is essential in the de novo synthesis of nucleotides, in the metabolism of several amino acids, and is an integral component for the regeneration of the "universal" methyl donor, S-adenosylmethionine. Inhibition of bacterial and cancer cell folate metabolism is the basis for the sulfonamide antibiotics and chemotherapeutic agents such as methotrexate and 5-fluorouracil, respectively.	Women of childbearing age are most likely to be deficient. The classic deficiency syndrome is megaloblastic anemia. The hematopoietic cells in bone marrow become enlarged and have immature nuclei, reflecting ineffective DNA synthesis. The peripheral blood smear demonstrates macro-ovalocytes and polymorphonuclear leukocytes with an average of more than 3.5 nuclear lobes. Megaloblastic changes also occur in other epithelia that proliferate rapidly (e.g., oral mucosa, gastrointestinal tract, producing glossitis and diarrhea, respectively). Sulfasalazine and diphenytoin inhibit absorption and predispose to deficiency. [400 μg of dietary folate equivalents (DFE); 1 μg folic acid = 1 μg DFE; 1 μg food folate = 0.6 μg DFE]	Doses >1000 μg/day may partially correct the anemia of vitamin B_{12} deficiency and may therefore mask (and perhaps exacerbate) the associated neuropathy. Large doses are also reported to lower seizure threshold in individuals prone to seizures. Parenteral administration is rarely reported to cause allergic phenomena, which is probably the result of dispersion agents. [1000 μg]	Serum folate measures short-term folate balance, whereas RBC folate is a better reflection of tissue status. Serum homocyst(e)ine rises early in deficiency but is nonspecific because vitamin B_{12} or B_6 deficiency, renal insufficiency, and older age may also cause elevations.
Vitamin C (ascorbic and dehydroascorbic acid)	Ascorbic acid readily oxidizes to dehydroascorbic acid in aqueous solution. Because the latter can be reduced in vivo, it possesses vitamin C activity. Total vitamin C is therefore measured as the sum of ascorbic and dehydroascorbic acid concentrations. Because of its reductant properties,	Overt deficiency is uncommon in developed countries. The classic deficiency syndrome is *scurvy*: characterized by fatigue, depression, and widespread abnormalities in connective tissues, such as inflamed gingivae, petechiae,	Quantities 500 mg/day (in adults) sometimes cause nausea and diarrhea. Acidification of the urine with supplementation and the potential for enhanced oxalate synthesis have raised concerns about nephrolithiasis, but this has yet to be demonstrated.	Plasma ascorbic acid concentration reflects recent dietary intake, whereas WBC levels more closely reflect tissue stores. Women's plasma levels are approximately 20% higher than men's for any given dietary intake.

Continued

TABLE 237–2 VITAMINS AND THEIR FUNCTIONS—cont'd

	Biochemistry and Physiology	Deficiency [RDA*]	Toxicity [TUL†]	Assessment of Status
	it serves primarily as a biologic antioxidant in aqueous environments. Biosyntheses of collagen, carnitine, bile acids, and norepinephrine, as well as proper functioning of the hepatic mixed-function oxygenase system, depend on this property. Vitamin C in foodstuffs increases the intestinal absorption of nonheme iron.	perifollicular hemorrhages, impaired wound healing, coiled hairs, hyperkeratosis, and bleeding into body cavities. In infants, defects in ossification and bone growth may occur. Tobacco smoking lowers plasma and leukocyte vitamin C levels. [F: 75 mg; M: 90 mg; increase requirement for cigarette smokers by 35 mg/day]	Supplementation may interfere with laboratory tests based on redox potential (e.g., fecal occult blood testing, serum cholesterol, and glucose). Withdrawal from long-term ingestion of high doses of vitamin C supplements should occur gradually over a month because accommodation seems to occur, raising a concern of "rebound scurvy." [2 g]	
Vitamin B_{12}	A group of closely related cobalamin compounds composed of a corrin ring (with a cobalt atom in its center) connected to a ribonucleotide via an aminopropanol bridge. Microorganisms are the ultimate source of all naturally occurring vitamin B_{12}. The two active coenzyme forms are desoxyadenosyl-cobalamin and methylcobalamin. These coenzymes are needed for the synthesis of succinyl CoA, which is essential in lipid and carbohydrate metabolism, and for the synthesis of methionine. The latter reaction is essential for amino acid metabolism, for purine and pyrimidine synthesis, for many methylation reactions, and for the intracellular retention of folates.	Dietary inadequacy is a rare cause of deficiency except in strict vegetarians. Most deficiencies arise from loss of intestinal absorption: this may be a result of pernicious anemia, pancreatic insufficiency, atrophic gastritis, small bowel bacterial overgrowth, or ileal disease. Megaloblastic anemia and megaloblastic changes in other epithelia (see Folate) are the result of sustained depletion. Demyelination of peripheral nerves, posterior and lateral columns of spinal cord, and nerves within the brain may occur. Altered mentation, depression, and psychoses occur. Hematologic and neurologic complications may occur independently. Folate supplementation, in doses of 1000 μg/day, may partly correct the anemia, thereby masking (or perhaps exacerbating) the neuropathic complication. [2.4 μg]	A few allergic reactions have been reported to crystalline vitamin B_{12} preparations and are probably caused by impurities, not by the vitamin. [TUL not established]	Serum, or plasma, concentrations are generally accurate. Subtle deficiency with neurologic complications, as described in the Deficiency column, can best be established by concurrently measuring the concentration of plasma vitamin B_{12} and serum methylmalonic acid, because the latter is a sensitive indicator of cellular deficiency.
Biotin	A bicyclic compound consisting of a ureido ring fused to a substituted tetrahydrothiophene ring. Endogenous synthesis by intestinal flora may contribute significantly to	Isolated deficiency is rare. Deficiency in humans has been produced experimentally (by dietary inadequacy), by prolonged total parenteral nutrition	Toxicity has not been reported in humans with doses as high as 60 mg/day in children. [TUL not established]	Plasma and urine concentrations of biotin are diminished in the deficient state. Elevated urine concentrations of methyl citrate,

TABLE 237–2 VITAMINS AND THEIR FUNCTIONS—cont'd

	Biochemistry and Physiology	Deficiency [RDA*]	Toxicity [TUL†]	Assessment of Status
	biotin nutriture. Most dietary biotin is linked to lysine, a compound called biotinyl lysine, or biocytin. The lysine must be hydrolyzed by an intestinal enzyme called biotinidase before intestinal absorption occurs. It acts primarily as a coenzyme for several carboxylases; each holoenzyme catalyzes an adenosine triphosphate–dependent carbon dioxide transfer. The carboxylases are critical enzymes in carbohydrate and lipid metabolism.	lacking the vitamin, and by ingestion of large quantities of raw egg white, which contains avidin, a protein that binds biotin with such high affinity that it renders it biounavailable. Alterations in mental status, myalgias, hyperesthesias, and anorexia occur. Later, seborrheic dermatitis and alopecia develop. Biotin deficiency is usually accompanied by lactic acidosis and organic aciduria. [30 μg]		3-methylcrotonylglycine, and 3-hydroxyisovalerate are also observed in deficiency.
Pantothenic acid	Pantoic acid linked to β-alanine through an amide bond. It serves as an essential component of CoA and phosphopantetheine, which are needed for synthesis and β-oxidation of fatty acids, as well as for synthesis of cholesterol, steroid hormones, vitamins A and D, and other isoprenoid derivatives. CoA is also involved in the synthesis of several amino acids and δ-minolevulinic acid, a precursor for the corrin ring of vitamin B_{12}, the porphyrin ring of heme, and of cytochromes. CoA is also necessary for the acetylation and fatty acid acylation of a variety of proteins.	Deficiency is rare, reported only as a result of feeding semisynthetic diets or an antagonist to the vitamin. Experimental, isolated deficiency in humans produces fatigue, abdominal pain, vomiting, insomnia, and paresthesias of the extremities. [5 mg]	In doses of 10 g/day, diarrhea is reported to occur. [TUL not established]	Whole blood and urine concentrations of pantothenate are indicators of status; serum levels are not thought to be accurate.

*Recommended dietary allowance (RDA) established for female (F) and male (M) adults by the U.S. Food and Nutrition Board, 1999 to 2001. In some instances, insufficient data exist to establish an RDA, in which case the adequate intake (AI) established by the board is listed.
†Tolerable upper intake (TUL) established for adults by the U.S. Food and Nutrition Board, 1999 to 2001.
CoA, coenzyme A; PLP = pyridoxal-5-phosphate; RBC = red blood cell; WBC = white blood cell.

humans. Cobalt seems to be essential solely as a component of vitamin B_{12}, but an isolated deficiency state has never been described. Deficiency syndromes for several of the other essential trace elements were not recognized until recently because of their exceedingly small requirements and because of the ubiquitous nature of these elements in foodstuffs. Only under exceptional circumstances, such as long-term reliance on total parenteral nutrition lacking these elements, have some of the deficiency syndromes been observed.

The biochemical functions of trace elements have not been as well characterized as those for the vitamins, but most of their functions appear to be as components of prosthetic groups or as cofactors for enzymes. Determination of essential trace element status is problematic with the exception of iron. The vanishingly low concentrations of these elements in bodily fluids and tissues, the finding that blood levels frequently do not correlate well with levels in the target tissues, and the fact that functional tests cannot be devised until their biochemical functions are better understood preclude an accurate and convenient laboratory method of assessing most of the trace elements.

Additional Compounds with Nutritional Relevance

Evidence indicates that humans also have an absolute requirement for the dietary component choline, which is a necessary precursor for acetylcholine and phospholipids and is needed to sustain normal levels of biologic methylation. To date, the most significant adverse effect of dietary inadequacy has been hepatic inflammation. Deficiency is nevertheless thought to be extremely rare, although pregnancy, and particularly lactation, increase the apparent requirement. Individuals whose long-term nutritional requirements are solely derived from total parenteral nutrition

Text continued on p. 1637.

TABLE 237–3 NUTRITIONAL TRACE ELEMENTS AND THEIR CLINICAL IMPLICATIONS

	Biochemistry and Physiology	Deficiency [RDA*]	Toxicity [TUL†]	Assessment of Status
Chromium	Dietary chromium consists of both inorganic and organic forms. Its primary function in humans is to potentiate insulin action. It accomplishes this function as a circulating complex called "glucose tolerance factor," thereby affecting carbohydrate, fat, and protein metabolism.	Deficiency in humans is described only in patients receiving long-term TPN with insufficient chromium. Hyperglycemia or impaired glucose tolerance is uniformly observed. Elevated plasma free fatty acid concentrations, neuropathy, encephalopathy, and abnormalities in nitrogen metabolism are also reported. Whether supplemental chromium may improve glucose tolerance in mildly glucose-intolerant but otherwise healthy individuals remains controversial. [F: 25 μg; M: 35 μg]	Toxicity after oral ingestion is uncommon and seems confined to gastric irritation. Airborne exposure may cause contact dermatitis, eczema, skin ulcers, and bronchogenic carcinoma. [no TUL established]	Plasma or serum concentration of chromium is a crude indicator of chromium status; it appears to be meaningful when the value is markedly higher or lower than the normal range.
Copper	Copper is absorbed by a specific intestinal transport mechanism. It is carried to the liver where it is bound to ceruloplasmin, which circulates systemically and delivers copper to target tissues in the body. Excretion of copper is largely through bile, and then into the feces. Absorptive and excretory processes vary with the levels of dietary copper, providing a means of copper homeostasis. Copper serves as a component of many enzymes, including amine oxidases, ferroxidases, cytochrome *c* oxidase, dopamine β-hydroxylase, superoxide dismutase, and tyrosinase.	Dietary deficiency is rare; it has been observed in premature and low-birthweight infants fed exclusively a cow's milk diet and in individuals receiving long-term TPN without copper. Clinical manifestations include depigmentation of skin and hair, neurologic disturbances, leukopenia, hypochromic microcytic anemia, and skeletal abnormalities. Anemia arises from impaired utilization of iron and is therefore a conditioned form of iron deficiency anemia. The deficiency syndrome, except the anemia and leukopenia, is also observed in Menkes' disease, a rare inherited condition associated with impaired copper utilization. [900 μg]	Acute copper toxicity has been described after excessive oral intake and with absorption of copper salts applied to burned skin. Milder manifestations include nausea, vomiting, epigastric pain, and diarrhea; coma and hepatic necrosis may ensue in severe cases. Toxicity may be seen with doses as low as 70 μg/kg/day. Chronic toxicity is also described. Wilson's disease is a rare, inherited disease associated with abnormally low ceruloplasmin levels and accumulation of copper in the liver and brain that eventually leads to damage to these two organs. [10 mg]	Practical methods for detecting marginal deficiency are not available. Marked deficiency is reliably detected by diminished serum copper and ceruloplasmin concentrations as well as low RBC superoxide dismutase activity.
Fluorine	Known more commonly by its ionic form, fluoride. It is incorporated into the crystalline structure of bone, thereby altering its physical characteristics.	Intake of <0.1 mg/day in infants and <0.5 mg/day in children is associated with an increased incidence of dental caries. Optimal intake in adults is between 1.5 and 4 mg/day. [F: 3 mg; M: 4 mg]	Acute ingestion of >30 mg/kg body weight is likely to cause death. Excessive long-term intake (0.1 mg/kg/day) leads to mottling of teeth (dental fluorosis), calcification of tendons and ligaments, and exostoses and may increase the brittleness of bones. [10 mg]	Estimates of intake or clinical assessment are used because no good laboratory test exists.

Iodine	Readily absorbed from the diet, concentrated in the thyroid, and integrated into the thyroid hormones, thyroxine and triiodothyronine. These hormones circulate largely bound to thyroxine-binding globulin. They modulate resting energy expenditure and, in the developing human, growth and development.	In the absence of supplementation, populations relying primarily on food from soils with low iodine content have endemic iodine deficiency. Maternal iodine deficiency leads to fetal deficiency, which produces spontaneous abortions, stillbirths, hypothyroidism, cretinism, and dwarfism. Rapid brain development continues through the second year, and permanent cognitive deficits may be induced by iodine deficiency over that period. In the adult, compensatory hypertrophy of the thyroid goiter occurs along with varying degrees of hypothyroidism. [150 μg]	Large doses (>2 mg/day in adults) may induce hypothyroidism by blocking thyroid hormone synthesis. Supplementation with >100 mg/day to an individual who was formerly deficient occasionally induces hyperthyroidism. [1.1 mg]	Iodine status of a population can be estimated by the prevalence of goiter. Urinary excretion of iodine is an effective laboratory means of assessment. Thyroid-stimulating hormone blood level is an indirect, and therefore not entirely specific, means of assessment.
Iron	Conveys the capacity to participate in redox reactions to a number of metalloproteins such as hemoglobin, myoglobin, cytochrome enzymes, and many oxidases and oxygenases. Primary storage form is ferritin and, to a lesser degree, hemosiderin. Intestinal absorption is 15–20% for "heme" iron and 1–8% for iron contained in vegetables. Absorption of the latter form is enhanced by the ascorbic acid in foodstuffs; by poultry, fish, or beef; and by an iron-deficient state. It is decreased by phytate and tannins.	This is the most common micronutrient deficiency in the world. Women of childbearing age are the highest-risk group because of menstrual blood losses, pregnancy, and lactation. The classic deficiency syndrome is hypochromic, microcytic anemia. Glossitis and koilonychia ("spoon" nails) are also observed. Easy fatigability often is an early symptom, before anemia appears. In children, mild deficiency of insufficient severity to cause anemia is associated with behavioral disturbances and poor school performance. [M and postmenopausal F: 8 mg; premenopausal F: 18 mg]	Iron overload typically occurs when habitual dietary intake is extremely high, intestinal absorption is excessive, repeated parenteral administration occurs, or a combination of these factors exists. Excessive iron stores usually accumulate in the reticuloendothelial tissues and cause little damage (hemosiderosis). If overload continues, iron eventually begins to accumulate in tissues such as the hepatic parenchyma, pancreas, heart, and synovium, thus causing hemochromatosis (Chapter 231). Hereditary hemochromatosis results from homozygosity of a common recessive trait. Excessive intestinal absorption of iron is seen in homozygotes. [45 mg]	Negative iron balance initially leads to depletion of iron stores in the bone marrow: a bone marrow biopsy and the concentration of serum ferritin are accurate and early indicators of such depletion. As the severity of deficiency proceeds, serum iron (SI) decreases and total iron-binding capacity (TIBC) increases: an iron saturation (SI/TIBC) of <16% suggests iron deficiency. Microcytosis, hypochromia, and anemia ensue as latter stages of the deficient state. Elevated levels of serum ferritin or an iron saturation >60% suggest iron overload, although systemic inflammation elevates serum ferritin regardless of iron status.
Manganese	A component of several metalloenzymes. Most manganese is in mitochondria, where it is a component of manganese superoxide dismutase.	Manganese deficiency in the human has not been conclusively demonstrated. It is said to cause hypocholesterolemia, weight loss, hair and nail changes, dermatitis, and impaired synthesis of vitamin K–dependent proteins. [F: 1.8 mg; M: 2.3 m g]	Toxicity by oral ingestion is unknown in humans. Toxic inhalation causes hallucinations, other alterations in mentation, and extrapyramidal movement disorders. [11 mg]	Until the deficiency syndrome is better defined, an appropriate measure of status will be difficult to develop.
Molybdenum	A cofactor in several enzymes, most prominently xanthine oxidase and sulfite oxidase.	A probable case of human deficiency is described as being secondary to parenteral administration of sulfite and resulted in hyperoxypurinemia, hypouricemia, and low sulfate excretion. [45 μg]	Toxicity is not well described in humans, although it may interfere with copper metabolism at high doses. [2 mg]	Laboratory means of assessment will not be meaningful until the deficiency syndrome is better described.

Continued

TABLE 237–3 NUTRITIONAL TRACE ELEMENTS AND THEIR CLINICAL IMPLICATIONS—cont'd

	Biochemistry and Physiology	Deficiency [RDA*]	Toxicity [TUL†]	Assessment of Status
Selenium	Most dietary selenium is in the form of an amino acid complex. Nearly complete absorption of such forms occurs. Homeostasis is largely performed by the kidney, which regulates urinary excretion as a function of selenium status. Selenium is a component of several enzymes, most notably glutathione peroxidase and superoxide dismutase. These enzymes appear to prevent oxidative and free radical damage of various cell structures. Evidence suggests that the antioxidant protection conveyed by selenium operates in conjunction with vitamin E because deficiency of one seems to enhance damage induced by a deficiency of the other. Selenium also participates in the enzymatic conversion of thyroxine to its more active metabolite, triiodothyronine.	Deficiency is rare in North America but has been observed in individuals receiving long-term TPN lacking selenium. Such individuals have myalgias or cardiomyopathies. Populations in some regions of the world, most notably some parts of China, have marginal intake of selenium. In these regions, *Keshan's disease*, a condition characterized by cardiomyopathy, is endemic; it can be prevented (but not treated) by selenium supplementation. [55 μg]	Toxicity is associated with nausea, diarrhea, alterations in mental status, peripheral neuropathy, loss of hair and nails: such symptoms were observed in adults who inadvertently consumed 27–2400 mg. [400 μg]	RBC glutathione peroxidase activity and plasma, or whole blood, selenium concentrations are the most commonly used methods of assessment. They are moderately accurate indicators of status.
Zinc	Intestinal absorption occurs by a specific process that is enhanced by pregnancy and corticosteroids and is diminished by co-ingestion of phytates, phosphates, iron, copper, lead, or calcium. Diminished intake of zinc leads to an increased efficiency of absorption and decreased fecal excretion, thus providing a means of zinc homeostasis. Zinc is a component of more than 100 enzymes, among which are DNA polymerase, RNA polymerase, and transfer RNA synthetase.	Zinc deficiency has its most profound effect on rapidly proliferating tissues. Mild deficiency causes growth retardation in children. More severe deficiency is associated with growth arrest, teratogenicity, hypogonadism and infertility, dysgeusia, poor wound healing, diarrhea, dermatitis on the extremities and around orifices, glossitis, alopecia, corneal clouding, loss of dark adaptation, and behavioral changes. Impaired cellular immunity is observed. Excessive loss of gastrointestinal secretions through chronic diarrhea and fistulas may precipitate deficiency. *Acrodermatitis enteropathica* is a rare, recessively inherited disease in which intestinal absorption of zinc is impaired. [F: 8 mg; M: 11 mg]	Acute zinc toxicity can usually be induced by ingestion of >200 mg of zinc in a single day (in adults). It is manifested by epigastric pain, nausea, vomiting, and diarrhea. Hyperpnea, diaphoresis, and weakness may follow inhalation of zinc fumes. Copper and zinc compete for intestinal absorption: long-term ingestion of >25 mg zinc/day may lead to copper deficiency. Long-term ingestion of >150 mg/day has been reported to cause gastric erosions, low high-density lipoprotein cholesterol levels, and impaired cellular immunity. [40 mg]	No accurate indicators of zinc status exist for routine clinical use. Plasma, RBC, and hair zinc concentrations are often misleading. Acute illness, in particular, is known to diminish plasma zinc levels, in part by inducing a shift of zinc out of the plasma compartment and into the liver. Functional tests that determine dark adaptation, taste acuity, and rate of wound healing lack specificity.

*Recommended dietary allowance (RDA) established for female (F) and male (M) adults by the U.S. Food and Nutrition Board, 1999 to 2001. In some instances, insufficient data exist to establish an RDA, in which case the adequate intake (AI) established by the board is listed.
†Tolerable upper limit (TUL) established for adults by the U.S. Food and Nutrition Board, 1999 to 2001.
RBC = red blood cell; TPN = total parenteral nutrition.

appear to be susceptible to choline deficiency. Both an RDA (425 mg, women; 550 mg, men) and a TUL (3.5 g) have now been established.

L-Carnitine is a dietary component that participates in fatty acid metabolism in mitochondria. Although no evidence exists for a dietary requirement in children or adults, infants receiving formulas lacking this compound have low serum levels of carnitine and biochemical evidence of altered fatty acid metabolism. It is unclear whether this finding has any clinical relevance.

CONDITIONS THAT INCREASE REQUIRED DIETARY INTAKE

Many physiologic, pathophysiologic, and pharmacologic factors increase the dietary requirements for micronutrients (see Table 237–1), thereby enhancing the risk of developing a deficiency state.

Physiologic Factors

Stages of the life cycle frequently have a significant impact on the requirements of nutrients. Phases of rapid growth and development, such as in utero development, infancy, adolescence, and pregnancy are associated with remarkable increases in the utilization of certain micronutrients on a per kilogram basis.

Pregnancy

Requirements for most micronutrients are increased in pregnancy, but, proportionately, the observed increases in the maternal requirements for iron and folate are particularly great and are related to the rapid proliferation of the placental and fetal tissues. Periods of lactation are similarly associated with remarkable increases in requirements; a lactating woman experiences disproportionately large increases in her requirements for zinc and vitamins A, E, and C to meet the metabolic demands incurred by milk production in addition to the aforementioned needs observed in pregnancy.

Infancy

Infancy carries particular vulnerabilities to specific micronutrient inadequacies. Healthy infants in the United States are typically supplemented with vitamin K at birth and with iron and vitamin D during the course of the first year because of their particular susceptibility to deficiencies of these nutrients.

Women of Childbearing Age

The ability to maintain adequate iron status from menarche through menopause is compromised in women by the additional losses incurred by menstruation, pregnancy, and lactation. Therefore, it is not surprising that the population subset that almost invariably displays the highest rate of iron deficiency is women of childbearing age.

Elderly Persons

Specific dietary recommendations for the elderly have been formally incorporated into the RDAs because the continuous evolution of physiology that occurs during the life cycle has a concrete impact on the requirements for certain micronutrients. Vitamin B_{12} status, for instance, declines significantly with aging because of the high prevalence of atrophic gastritis and its associated impairment in protein-bound vitamin B_{12} absorption. Estimates suggest that 10 to 20% of the elderly population is at risk of clinically significant vitamin B_{12} deficiency because of this phenomenon. Consequently, elderly persons should consume some of their vitamin B_{12} requirement in the crystalline form rather than solely from the naturally occurring protein-bound forms found in food because absorption of the former is not impaired by atrophic gastritis. The elderly also require greater quantities of vitamins B_6 and D to maintain health compared with younger adults, as reflected in the new RDAs (see Table 237–3). For instance, adequate intake for vitamin D in persons aged 51 to 70 years is 10 μg/day (400 international units), double the value for younger adults; this value increases to 15 μg in persons older than 70 years. This increase appears largely to result from diminished cutaneous synthesis of vitamin D by senile skin and from decreased sun exposure, the latter of which is particularly important in elderly patients in long-term institutional facilities. The need for crystalline vitamin B_{12} and for a quantity of vitamin D that is difficult to achieve without resorting to a supplement suggests that universal use of a daily multivitamin pill would benefit the elder population. This approach remains a matter of controversy but is supported by existing evidence. However, elders with chronic renal failure appear to have a vulnerability to vitamin A toxicity, a finding suggesting that use of supplements containing this vitamin is contraindicated among this segment of the geriatric population.

PATHOPHYSIOLOGIC AND PHARMACOLOGIC FACTORS

Diseases of the Gastrointestinal Tract

Intestinal malabsorptive and maldigestive states predispose to multiple micronutrient deficiencies. Both fat-soluble and water-soluble micronutrients (except vitamin B_{12}) are absorbed predominantly in the proximal small intestine. Therefore, diffuse mucosal diseases affecting the proximal portion of the gastrointestinal tract are likely to result in deficiencies. However, even in the absence of mucosal disease of the proximal small intestine, extensive ileal disease, small bowel bacterial overgrowth, and chronic cholestasis can each interfere with the maintenance of adequate intraluminal conjugated bile acid concentrations and can thereby impair absorption of fat-soluble vitamins. Maldigestion is usually the result of chronic pancreatitis. Untreated, it frequently causes malabsorption and deficiencies of fat-soluble vitamins. Vitamin B_{12} malabsorption can often be demonstrated in this setting, a result of inadequate R-protein digestion, but clinical vitamin B_{12} deficiency is rarely reported.

Inborn Errors of Metabolism

Myriad rare inborn errors of metabolism have been described for vitamins and minerals that impair an individual's ability to assimilate, utilize, or retain a particular micronutrient (Chapter 216). Such defects are usually partial and can often be overcome, to a certain extent, by administering doses of the nutrient that are several degrees of magnitude greater than usually required. Suspicion for such defects should be entertained if (1) a known defect exists in the family, (2) a deficiency syndrome arises at birth or during infancy, or (3) the deficiency syndrome is present despite adequate dietary intake and the absence of any disease that would impair the ability to assimilate the nutrient.

Medications

Long-term administration of many drugs may adversely affect micronutrient status and may either induce an overt deficiency syndrome or predispose patients to one. The manner in which drug-nutrient interactions occur varies; some of the more common mechanisms are outlined in Table 237–4. Some drugs exert their therapeutic effects by specifically inhibiting the actions of a micronutrient. Examples include coumarin, which inhibits γ-carboxylation reactions mediated by vitamin K, and methotrexate, which binds tightly to dihydrofolate reductase, thereby inhibiting folate metabolism.

Toxins

Tobacco smoking alters the metabolism of several vitamins, including folate and vitamins C and E. In large surveys, diminished plasma levels of folate and ascorbic acid have been observed in chronic smokers. Smoking is also associated with diminished levels of folate in cells of the oral mucosa, diminished ascorbic acid levels in leukocytes, and decreased concentrations of vitamin E in the alveolar fluid, findings providing evidence that many tissues can be affected by smoking and that the effect does not simply represent a shift of these micronutrients out of the plasma compartment.

ADVANCES IN NUTRITIONAL SCIENCE

New Frontiers in Marginal Deficiency States of Micronutrients

New Definitions of Deficiency

An interesting and important evolution in the understanding of micronutrient requirements has occurred over the past century. As nutritional science has expanded its appreciation for additional physiologic functions of micronutrients, an ever-increasing need to redefine the concept of deficiency has ensued. The original means by which the

TABLE 237–4 DRUG-MEDIATED EFFECTS ON MICRONUTRIENT STATUS: EXAMPLES

Drug	Nutrient	Mechanism of Interaction
Dextroamphetamine, fenfluramine, levodopa	Potentially all micronutrients	Induces anorexia
Cholestyramine	Vitamin D, folate	Adsorbs nutrient, decreases absorption
Omeprazole	Vitamin B_{12}	Causes modest bacterial overgrowth, decreases gastric acid, impairs absorption
Sulfasalazine	Folate	Impairs absorption and inhibits folate-dependent enzymes
Isoniazid	Pyridoxine	Impairs utilization of vitamin B_6
Nonsteroidal anti-inflammatory agents	Iron	Causes gastrointestinal blood loss
Penicillamine	Zinc	Increases renal excretion

necessary intake of these nutrients was defined was typically based on a disease entity that occurred as a result of a flagrant deficiency of that nutrient, the so-called classic deficiency syndrome. In retrospect, this approach was naive because it is now evident that most micronutrients serve important functions in a wide variety of distinct biochemical systems. As the science of nutrition has come to appreciate such diversity in function, so has the appreciation grown for definitions of new deficiency syndromes based on disordered physiology other than those described by the classic definitions.

Do Optimal Micronutrients Optimize Health?

Nevertheless, the redefinition of micronutrient deficiencies and the closely related reexamination of recommended daily intakes have proved difficult for several reasons. In some instances, the evidence for the role of a particular micronutrient in a newly proposed function continues to be less than definitive. However, even if a novel biochemical or physiologic role is well demonstrated for a nutrient, an appropriate question is whether optimization of such function translates into optimization of health. For example, providing supplemental vitamin E to elderly individuals who are vitamin E replete enhances T-lymphocyte responsiveness to mitogens; nevertheless, it is unclear whether this effect diminishes infection rates among the elderly. Another difficult problem pertains to the use of micronutrients in supraphysiologic quantities, that is, intakes that greatly exceed all conventional concepts of what is necessary for health. Some micronutrients, when taken in such large quantities, have effects on physiologic functions that impart apparent health benefits. The ingestion of gram quantities of niacin to reduce low-density lipoprotein (LDL) cholesterol is an example. Such physiologic effects are not observed at more conventional levels of intake and are therefore usually considered pharmacologic effects of the nutrient. Nevertheless, if the dietary requirement of a nutrient is strictly defined as the dose necessary for the maintenance of optimal health, then supraphysiologic doses would have to be considered the dietary requirement in such instances. Thus, the determination of optimal nutrient intake is highly dependent on which physiologic effect is sought. Furthermore, if only a segment of the population will benefit from supraphysiologic quantities of a nutrient, should dietary guidelines for the remainder of the population be established according to this effect?

Determining an adequate level of intake implies the existence of a means of measuring nutrient status. In seeking an appropriate measure of nutrient status, the diversity of function often makes it difficult to decide which measurement is the most germane. Tobacco smoking, for example, appears to diminish vitamin E levels significantly in alveolar fluid but not in the serum. Thus, the concepts of localized nutrient deficiencies and tissue-specific requirements add an additional level of complexity to the determination of nutrient status.

Redefinition of Nutritional Requirements

Folate

A cogent example of the redefinition of vitamin deficiency is the water-soluble vitamin folate. In the past, guidelines regarding the necessary intake of the vitamin were based on the prevention of megaloblastic anemia. Measuring serum and erythrocyte folate concentrations has been the most common means of assessing status; maintaining such levels within accepted normative ranges provides good assurance that folate status is adequate to prevent anemia.

However, degrees of deficiency that are insufficient to cause anemia may still disturb normal biochemical and physiologic homeostasis and, in some instances, cause clinical disease. Clinical trials have demonstrated that women taking folate supplements at the time of conception have a markedly lower chance of delivering a baby with a neural tube defect compared with women who are not folate supplemented but whose folate status falls within a conventionally accepted range. This observation compelled the U.S. government to mandate the fortification of flour, beginning in 1998. Present recommendations are that women of childbearing age consume 400 μg/day of folic acid in the form of supplements or fortified foods, although the dose-response curve of this effect is ill defined. Less than optimal intake of folate is also evidenced by an increase in serum homocysteine, an amino acid that is normally metabolized by a folate-dependent pathway. Before the federally mandated fortification of flour, the median intake of folate among adults was one half of the present RDA, and a substantial minority of Americans had significantly elevated serum homocysteine levels. An elevation in homocysteine reflects a less than optimal disposal of this amino acid, an alteration that has been consistently associated with the development of occlusive vascular disease. Vitamins B_6 and B_{12} are also important components of the biochemical pathways by which the body disposes of homocysteine. In randomized clinical trials, however, dietary supplementation of folate, vitamin B_{12}, and vitamin B_6 has shown no benefit against cardiovascular disease despite their ability to lower homocysteine levels. [1] Such supplementation also has no clear benefit for cognitive function, except perhaps in patients with low baseline folate levels. [2]

A more controversial observation is the inverse relationship between the ingestion of folate and the incidence of epithelial neoplasia of the uterine cervix, the breast, and the colorectum. This inverse relationship is observed even when folate status (or dietary intake) falls within the range of conventionally accepted normative values.

The aforementioned considerations prompted the U.S. RDA for folate to be raised from 200 to 400 μg/day, and some indications suggest that further increases are warranted. Substantial increases in the suggested intake of any micronutrient must be tempered, however, by the consideration of toxicity. With folate, this is primarily related to its ability to mask vitamin B_{12} deficiency when folate is taken in doses exceeding 1000 μg/day (see Table 237–2).

Antioxidant and Free-Radical Scavenging Vitamins and Provitamins

Vitamins A, C, and E, as well as many of the carotenoids, are effective antioxidants. In addition, it is clear that vitamins C and E and some of the carotenoids can scavenge free radicals when these nutrients are taken in adequate quantities. Such properties have long been appreciated, but it is only recently that oxidation and free radical damage have been implicated as important contributors to common degenerative illnesses such as atherosclerosis, cancer, cataract of the lens, and retinal degeneration. Clinical trials to test the efficacy of antioxidant supplements have shown no benefit and oftentimes harm, [3] although growing evidence indicates that the adverse effects of the large doses used in many trials may have obscured the health benefits of these nutrients and that populations with marginal antioxidant status may benefit from such supplements.

TABLE 237–5 NEWLY IDENTIFIED ROLES FOR VITAMINS

Vitamin or Provitamin	Classical Role	New Role
β-Carotene	Provitamin A	Antioxidant, free radical
Niacin	NAD/NADP coenzyme	Reduction of low-density lipoprotein, elevation of high-density lipoprotein and cholesterol
Folate	Hemopoietic factor	Diminishes homocyst(e)inemia
Vitamin A	Transduction of visual input in retina	Induction and maintenance of epithelial differentiation, signal in embryogenesis
Vitamin D	Regulator of calcium	Retards epithelial proliferation; promotes differentiation
Vitamin B_6	Coenzyme for transamination	Modulation of steroid activity

NAD = nicotinamide adenine dinucleotide; NADP = nicotinamide-adenine dinucleotide phosphate.

The point is well exemplified by two large-scale clinical intervention trials with β-carotene supplements that were conducted in the 1990s, each of which observed increased rates of lung cancer among the recipients of the carotenoid. Subsequent mechanistic studies indicated that the large doses administered (~30 mg/day) result in asymmetrical cleavage of the carotenoid into unnatural products that antagonize normal signaling pathways in the lung epithelium, whereas lower supplemental doses do not undergo asymmetrical cleavage and protect against neoplastic transformation.

LDL can undergo oxidation in vivo, and the LDL thus transformed appears to be particularly atherogenic. Prevention of LDL oxidation, at least in animal models, retards the process of atherogenesis. Supplementation of human subjects with several times the RDA of α-tocopherol, and perhaps some of the other antioxidant micronutrients, is an effective means of preventing LDL oxidation. However, human intervention trials with vitamin E as well as other antioxidant nutrients have been unable to demonstrate clinical benefits in the reduction of cardiovascular events.

An enormous body of epidemiologic studies indicates that occurrence of cancers of the oral cavity, lung, esophagus, and stomach (and perhaps the colorectum) is inversely related to dietary intake of fresh vegetables and fruits. Careful dissection of dietary data suggests that β-carotene and vitamin E content are strongly predictive components of these foodstuffs. High doses of vitamin A and some of its synthetic analogues (e.g., 13-*cis*-retinoic acid) can effectively reduce the recurrence of head and neck cancers, although hepatic toxicity is sometimes a limiting factor in such cancer preventive therapy. Similarly, these agents, as well as β-carotene or vitamin E, when taken in large doses have been shown significantly to promote the regression of oral leukoplakia, a premalignant lesion. Daily supplementation with one to three times the U.S. RDA of β-carotene, selenium, and vitamin E has been shown to reduce the incidence of adenocarcinoma of the stomach in a region of China where the disease, as well as marginal vitamin status, is particularly prevalent. However, as mentioned earlier, trials conducted in developed Western countries have observed no diminution of lung cancer among smokers with daily supplementation of β-carotene and vitamin E.

Epidemiologic associations also suggest an inverse relationship between lens cataract or macular degeneration and the intake of vitamins C, E, and β-carotene. Considerable experimental evidence indicates that these common degenerative conditions of the eye are caused, at least in part, by photo-oxidation. Some evidence in animal models indicates that these degenerative processes can be retarded by supraphysiologic supplementation with vitamins C or E. Individuals who ingest quantities of vitamin C that exceed the U.S. RDA have a lower incidence of cataract than those ingesting the RDA, a finding suggesting a potential preventive role for doses of these nutrients that are larger than conventionally recommended. Nevertheless, insufficient interventional data exist to assume a preventive role for antioxidants in cataract and macular degeneration conclusively.

Further investigation is necessary to define the circumstances more clearly under which antioxidant nutrients can be used to prevent or treat chronic degenerative diseases.

Vitamin B_{12} and Neuropsychiatric Disease

Plasma vitamin B_{12} concentrations are considered to be an accurate indication of vitamin B_{12} status. The normative range for a healthy population has typically been reported to be 150 to 900 pg/mL; values greater than 150 pg/mL (or 200 pg/mL in some laboratories) were thought, until recently, to exclude vitamin B_{12} deficiency as a cause of neurologic or psychiatric syndromes. Recent observations now indicate that 7 to 10% of individuals who have plasma vitamin B_{12} values between 150 and 400 pg/mL may develop neuropsychiatric complications of vitamin B_{12} deficiency in the absence of any indications of megaloblastic anemia. Such individuals can be identified by the demonstration of an elevated level of methylmalonic acid in the blood that decreases to normal levels with parenteral vitamin B_{12} administration. An elevation in serum methylmalonic acid is both a sensitive and a specific indication of cellular vitamin B_{12} deficiency. An alternative approach, although one that is less scientifically objective, is to administer several parenteral injections of vitamin B_{12} to an individual who has an otherwise unexplained neuropsychiatric syndrome and whose plasma vitamin B_{12} level falls in the range of 150 to 400 pg/mL. Awareness of this phenomenon is particularly important because it is has become clear that atrophic gastritis, an asymptomatic condition that affects approximately 30% of the elderly population, frequently produces a modest decrease in vitamin B_{12} status.

Table 237–5 lists several examples of biochemical functions of vitamins that have only recently been identified. As the clinical significance of each of these new roles is defined and as quantities of each vitamin needed to optimize such functions are determined, redefinition of the desirable range of vitamin status is likely to occur.

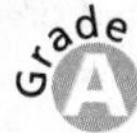

1. Lonn E, Yusuf S, Arnold MJ, et al: Homocysteine lowering with folic acid and B vitamins in vascular disease. N Engl J Med 2006;354:1567–1577.
2. Balk EM, Raman G, Tatsioni A, et al: Vitamin B_6, B_{12}, and folic acid supplementation and cognitive function: A systematic review of randomized trials. Arch Intern Med 2007;167:21–30.
3. Bjelakovic G, Nikolova D, Gluud LL, et al: Mortality in randomized trials of antioxidant supplements for primary and secondary prevention: Systematic review and meta-analysis. JAMA 2007;297:842–857.

SUGGESTED READINGS

Bartali B, Semba RD, Frongillo EA, et al: Low micronutrient levels as a predictor of incident disability in older women. Arch Intern Med 2006;166:2335–2340. *Elderly women with low serum concentrations of vitamins B_6, B_{12}, and selenium are at risk for subsequent disability in their ADLs.*

Huang HY, Caballero B, Chang S, et al: The efficacy and safety of multivitamin and mineral supplement use to prevent cancer and chronic disease in adults: A systematic review for a National Institutes of Health state-of-the-science conference. Ann Intern Med 2006;145:372–385. *A review of the efficacy and safety of multivitamin and mineral supplement use to prevent cancer and chronic disease in adults.*

238 EATING DISORDERS

Marsha D. Marcus

Definition

The eating disorders are psychiatric syndromes characterized by abnormal eating behavior and maladaptive attitudes or beliefs about eating, shape, or weight. The *Diagnostic and Statistical Manual of Mental Disorders,* 4th edition (DSM-IV), of the American Psychiatric Association includes two eating disorders, anorexia nervosa and bulimia nervosa. A third diagnostic category, eating disorders not otherwise specified, includes all other presentations of clinically significant eating problems that do not meet criteria for anorexia nervosa or bulimia nervosa. Diagnostic criteria for anorexia nervosa and bulimia nervosa are presented in Tables 238–1 and 238–2.

Anorexia Nervosa

The hallmark of anorexia nervosa is persistent unwillingness or inability to maintain a minimally adequate body weight, which is defined in DSM-IV as less than 85% of that expected, coupled with an intense fear of gaining weight. Anorexia nervosa has two subtypes, binge eating/purging and restricting. In the binge eating/purging subtype, individuals regularly engage in binge eating or purging, whereas in the restricting type, they do not.

Bulimia Nervosa

Bulimia nervosa is characterized by persistent and recurrent episodes of binge eating (defined as the intake of an exceptionally large amount of food given the context and paired with a sense of loss of control over eating) that are coupled with compensatory behaviors (e.g., self-induced vomiting, fasting) intended to undo the effects of the binge episodes. Bulimia nervosa also has two subtypes. In the purging type, the individual induces vomiting or misuses laxatives, diuretics, or enemas; in the nonpurging type, individuals use inappropriate behaviors, such as fasting or excessive exercise, to offset the effects of binge eating.

TABLE 238–1 DSM-IV DIAGNOSTIC CRITERIA FOR ANOREXIA NERVOSA

A. Refusal to maintain body weight at or above a minimally normal weight for age and height (e.g., weight loss leading to maintenance of body weight less than 85% of that expected or failure to make expected weight gain during period of growth resulting in body weight less than 85% of that expected).
B. Intense fear of gaining weight or becoming fat even though underweight.
C. Disturbance in the way in which one's body weight or shape is experienced, undue influence of body weight or shape on self-evaluation, or denial of the seriousness of the current low body weight.
D. In post-menarchal females, amenorrhea, i.e., the absence of at least three consecutive menstrual cycles. (A woman is considered to have amenorrhea if her periods occur following only hormone, e.g., estrogen, administration.)

Specify type:

Restricting type: During the current episode of anorexia nervosa, the person has not regularly engaged in binge eating or purging behavior (i.e., self-induced vomiting or the misuse of laxatives, diuretics, or enemas).

Binge eating/purging type: During the current episode of anorexia nervosa, the person has regularly engaged in binge eating or purging behavior (i.e., self-induced vomiting or the misuse of laxatives, diuretics, or enemas).

TABLE 238–2 DSM-IV DIAGNOSTIC CRITERIA FOR BULIMIA NERVOSA

A. Recurrent episodes of binge eating. An episode of binge eating is characterized by both of the following:
   1. Eating, in a discrete period (e.g., within any 2-hour period), an amount of food that is definitely larger than most people would eat during a similar period and under similar circumstances.
   2. A sense of lack of control over eating during the episodes (e.g., a feeling that one cannot stop eating or control what or how much one is eating).
B. Recurrent inappropriate compensatory behavior to prevent weight gain such as self-induced vomiting; misuse of laxatives, diuretics, enemas, or other medication; fasting; or excessive exercise.
C. The binge eating and inappropriate compensatory behaviors both occur, on average, at least twice a week for 3 months.
D. Self-evaluation is unduly influenced by body shape and weight.
E. The disturbance does not occur exclusively during episodes of anorexia nervosa.

Specify type:

Purging type: During the current episode of bulimia nervosa, the person has regularly engaged in self-induced vomiting or the misuse of laxatives, diuretics, or enemas.

Nonpurging type: During the current episode of bulimia nervosa, the person has used other inappropriate compensatory behaviors, such as fasting or excessive exercise, but has not regularly engaged in self-induced vomiting or the misuse of laxatives, diuretics, or enemas.

Eating Disorders Not Otherwise Specified

A complete discussion of the residual category of eating disorders, eating disorders not otherwise specified (ED NOS), is beyond the scope of this chapter; however, it is important to note that ED NOS is the most common diagnosis at many university-based eating disorders clinics, reflecting the considerable fluidity of the clinical picture of disordered eating over time in a given individual and the limitations of the current diagnostic criteria. For example, there is little evidence to support the binge or purge frequencies required for the diagnosis of bulimia nervosa. Similarly, the utility of the amenorrhea criterion for diagnosis of anorexia nervosa has been questioned. Consequently, most cases of ED NOS probably are subsyndromal variants of anorexia nervosa or bulimia nervosa, but there also are other patterns of disordered eating. Binge eating disorder, which is included in the DSM-IV as a proposed diagnosis requiring further study and as one example of ED NOS, has received a considerable amount of research attention. The disorder is characterized by persistent and frequent binge eating in the absence of purging or regular inappropriate compensatory behavior. Recently, purging disorder, or recurrent purge behavior in the absence of binge eating, has been described. It is not clear how or whether the next version of the *Diagnostic and Statistical Manual* will incorporate additional eating disorder syndromes, and additional research is needed to explicate the spectrum of disordered eating.

Epidemiology

Epidemiologic data on the incidence and prevalence of eating disorders are limited. Anorexia nervosa is not common, and depending on case definition, lifetime prevalence estimates range from 0.3% (for narrowly defined anorexia nervosa) to 3.7% (for broadly defined anorexia nervosa) in women. Lifetime prevalence estimates for bulimia nervosa range from 1 to 4.2%. Evidence suggests that the prevalence of anorexia nervosa may be increasing, whereas the prevalence of bulimia nervosa appears to have decreased slightly in recent years. Eating disorders are significantly more common among women than among men, with ratios of approximately

10:1. In contrast, differences between sexes in rates of binge eating disorder appear to be less pronounced, with the ratio estimated at 3:1 for women and men, respectively. Available evidence suggests that anorexia nervosa and bulimia nervosa are equally common in white, Hispanic, and Native American women and less common in African American and Asian women. However, binge eating disorder appears to occur with equal frequency in white, African American, and Hispanic women. Large-scale community-based studies are needed to document the prevalence of symptoms and syndromes of disordered eating in multiethnic samples of men and women.

Age at onset of anorexia nervosa typically is during adolescence, but prepubertal onset does occur. New-onset anorexia nervosa is not common in adult women, but there are reports of anorexia nervosa onset after the age of 40 years; these cases often appear to be triggered by life crisis. The onset of bulimia nervosa typically is during later adolescence or early adulthood. Bulimia nervosa is rare in younger children, and although new cases are not common in later adulthood, the symptoms of disordered eating—such as restrictive dieting, binge eating, and preoccupation with eating, shape, and weight—occur with reasonable frequency in older women.

Pathobiology

The etiology of eating disorders is unknown, but there is consensus that the causality is complex and may include genetic, constitutional, psychological, family, and sociocultural factors. Research focusing on the genetics of eating disorders has proliferated, and family history and twin studies have implicated genetic factors in the pathogenesis of disordered eating. The results are particularly compelling in the case of restricting anorexia nervosa. However, evidence also suggests that bulimia nervosa and binge eating run in families and that much of the variance in observed cases is explained by genetic factors. Although the exact mechanisms of transmission are not known, genetic linkage and association studies have implicated several susceptibility loci for anorexia nervosa and bulimia nervosa, and association studies have led to the identification of numerous polymorphisms that appear to affect activation, mood, or reward systems.

Multiple psychological traits, including neuroticism and perfectionism, have been identified as putative risk factors for disordered eating. Family factors including a tendency to overweight and parental concerns about eating, shape, and weight also have been implicated as potential contributors to the vulnerability for disordered eating. A history of victimization (sexual, physical, or emotional abuse) is a potent risk factor for the development of psychiatric disorder in women, in general, and for disordered eating, in particular. Finally, in the United States and other industrialized nations, the sociocultural emphasis on shape and weight and a marked preference for a thin, lithe body type have been implicated in the complex pathogenesis of eating disorders. Thus, a given case of eating disorder is likely to reflect some combination of risk or vulnerability factors whose expression may be promoted by a cultural milieu in which thinness is overvalued.

Clinical Manifestations

Symptoms and Signs

Patients with eating disorders often present with other common psychiatric symptoms, including depression, anxiety, and social withdrawal, as well as with the specific symptoms of disordered eating. In anorexia nervosa, the hallmark symptoms are low body weight and denial of the seriousness of the problem. Many of the associated signs and symptoms are secondary to malnutrition and semistarvation. Psychiatric symptoms such as irritability, obsessionality, and preoccupation with food may be secondary to semistarvation and may remit with refeeding. Physical symptoms of semistarvation or malnutrition affect virtually all systems and may include osteopenia or osteoporosis, dehydration, hypothermia, cardiovascular or renal irregularities, gastrointestinal and endocrine disturbances, and changes in neuropsychological functioning. Laboratory results may be normal, especially in restricting anorexia nervosa, but patients may still be at risk for cardiac events resulting from malnutrition.

Signs and symptoms of bulimia nervosa are most commonly associated with purging behavior and include dental enamel erosion secondary to vomiting, gastrointestinal symptoms, salivary gland hypertrophy, and electrolyte disturbances. Misuse of stimulant laxatives can cause hypomagnesia or hypophosphatemia and ultimately disruption of normal bowel functioning. Binge eating is associated with gastric distention and, in rare cases, gastric rupture.

Natural History

Information about the natural history of eating disorders is limited because there is a dearth of prospective community-based research. One Scandinavian study has provided some information about the outcome of anorexia nervosa among individuals in the community. It showed that about half of the individuals with anorexia nervosa recovered completely during a period of 10 years, but the remainder had significant psychiatric morbidity including depression, obsessive-compulsive disorder, autism spectrum symptoms, and personality disorders. Evidence also suggests that there is some spontaneous improvement in symptoms of bulimia nervosa in untreated community individuals during a 5-year period. However, although about half will no longer meet criteria for a diagnosis of bulimia nervosa, most individuals continue to report significant eating disorder symptoms.

Diagnosis

As is the case in all psychiatric disorders, the clinical interview is the primary diagnostic tool in the assessment of eating disorders. Diagnoses are documented by careful review of the patient's history, symptoms, and behaviors in the course of a collaborative interview. Evaluation of comorbid psychiatric problems, particularly mood, anxiety, and substance use disorders, is critical. Assessment for the presence of suicidal ideation or behavior also is warranted. Involvement of the family is viewed as critical for all children and adolescents who present for assessment of disordered eating. A complete physical examination is recommended for all patients with particular attention to body mass index (weight in kilograms divided by height in meters squared), vital signs, cardiovascular function, hematologic assessment, and blood chemistries.

Patients with eating disorders frequently are examined for gastrointestinal problems or amenorrhea; however, these symptoms often remit with successful treatment of the eating disorder. Marked weight loss in young women in the absence of substance dependence, severe depression, or other documented illness suggests the need for an eating disorder evaluation.

Treatment

Anorexia Nervosa

Research evidence to guide the treatment of anorexia nervosa is limited. For emaciated patients, the cornerstone of treatment is medical monitoring and supervised nutritional rehabilitation to restore body weight and to normalize eating behavior. Markedly underweight individuals may require a hospital-based program to achieve weight restoration, which usually is accomplished with supervised meals and snacks provided in a supportive and reassuring environment. When patients refuse to eat, nasogastric feeding may be used; continuous feeding is better tolerated than bolus feeding.

With regard to psychotherapy, which remains the mainstay for treatment of anorexia nervosa when adequate nutrition is restored, several small clinical trials have documented the benefit of family therapy in the treatment of adolescent anorexia nervosa of short duration, but research suggests that younger patients, in general, fare better than older patients do. The Maudsley model of family therapy, in which families are helped to play a central role in the management of anorexia nervosa, has shown promise, but replication of the positive results in larger samples is required. [1] The evidence base for psychotherapeutic interventions for adults with anorexia nervosa is meager. One trial has documented the potential utility of cognitive-behavioral therapy for weight-restored adults with anorexia nervosa [2]; a second trial [3] yielded additional evidence that cognitive-behavioral therapy might be helpful for adults with acute anorexia nervosa and also provided initial evidence that specialist supportive care warrants further study. However, there is

Rx

no compelling evidence for the efficacy of any form of psychotherapy for adults with anorexia nervosa.

Similarly, there is no strong positive evidence favoring the use of any particular medication in treating anorexia nervosa. Numerous trials have examined the potential utility of numerous classes of drugs including antidepressants, anxiolytic agents, antipsychotic agents, and hormones with disappointing results. Although some evidence has suggested the potential utility of selective serotonin reuptake inhibitors in preventing relapse, a recent well-controlled clinical trial failed to show any benefit of fluoxetine treatment. Several small studies have suggested that second-generation antipsychotic agents (e.g., olanzapine, risperidone, and quetiapine) may be helpful in reducing resistance to weight regain and ameliorating obsessional thinking among patients with anorexia nervosa, but again, the findings require corroboration in controlled clinical trials. Hormone treatment and vitamin supplements are not considered useful, although supplemental calcium and vitamin D often are recommended.

Bulimia Nervosa

The evidence base for treatment of bulimia nervosa is stronger than that for anorexia nervosa, but the quality of extant studies is variable. Several forms of psychotherapy have been studied, and available evidence indicates that cognitive-behavioral therapy aimed at restoring a healthy pattern of eating and modifying the maladaptive attitudes about eating, shape, and weight is effective in reducing aberrant eating and psychological symptoms. [4] Almost all studied antidepressant agents have a moderate impact on the symptoms of bulimia nervosa, but as is the case with psychotherapy, there is a significant nonresponse rate. Fluoxetine at 60 mg/day is the best studied agent, and there is a Food and Drug Administration–approved indication for its use at that dose in the treatment of bulimia nervosa. There is no strong evidence that provides support for use of medications other than antidepressants, but small trials have suggested the potential utility of the anticonvulsant agent topiramate for the treatment of normal-weight patients with bulimia nervosa, and one trial has indicated the possible benefit of ondansetron. In clinical practice, antidepressant medication is often provided in addition to some form of psychotherapy, but there is no compelling support for the benefits of combined treatment.

Eating Disorders Not Otherwise Specified

Cases of ED NOS that reflect subsyndromal variants of anorexia nervosa and bulimia nervosa usually are treated with methods appropriate for management of anorexia nervosa or bulimia nervosa. However, numerous trials have examined the use of cognitive-behavioral therapy, interpersonal therapy, behavioral weight management, antidepressants, and anorectic agents in the treatment of binge eating disorder. Available research indicates that most overweight patients can be helped with either a behavioral weight control program or an eating disorders treatment. Pharmacotherapy may also reduce binge eating but generally does not add to the effectiveness of psychosocial treatment.

Prognosis

Anorexia Nervosa

There are numerous studies that have observed cohorts of treated patients with anorexia nervosa, although included treatments have varied and many studies have significant methodologic limitations. Extant data suggest that about half of the individuals in patient cohorts did not meet criteria for anorexia nervosa at follow-up, but most had eating disorder symptoms, with a poor outcome in 10 to 20% of individuals. Up to 50% of patients with anorexia nervosa develop bulimic symptoms over time, but information relating to the temporal onset of binge eating or purging is limited. Studies consistently indicate better outcomes for adolescent patients, but time to recovery nevertheless may be protracted (5 to 6 years). Mortality rates of anorexia nervosa are elevated and as high as those for any psychiatric disorder; individuals with co-occurring substance problems appear to be at highest risk for premature death. The primary causes of death are suicide and problems related to chronic starvation.

Bulimia Nervosa

The outcome of bulimia nervosa appears to be better than that for anorexia nervosa, but on average, eating behavior also persists for several years in treated patients. Cognitive-behavioral therapy is regarded as the treatment of choice and is associated with 80% reductions in binge eating and purging; approximately 50% of patients are abstinent from binge eating at 1 year after treatment. However, there is a significant nonresponse rate, with up to one third of patients failing to benefit. Antidepressant treatment studies also have documented significant improvements in eating disorder symptoms, but improvements from cognitive-behavioral therapy generally are superior to those shown in medication trials. Several studies have examined combining medication and psychotherapeutic interventions. Findings have been mixed, but overall, there is not strong evidence that combination treatment enhances treatment outcome. The only consistent predictor of poorer treatment outcome in bulimia nervosa has been depression. In contrast to anorexia nervosa, bulimia nervosa does not appear to be associated with an increased risk of premature death.

Future Directions

Given the morbidity and mortality associated with anorexia nervosa, there is a compelling need for research focusing on the development and evaluation of treatments for this illness. However, additional study of treatments for bulimia nervosa aimed at documenting optimal treatment combinations and duration and evaluating the efficacy of interventions that target nonresponders to current treatments also is needed. Finally, research studies that include cases of eating disorders not otherwise specified are necessary to provide information about this understudied but significantly large group of patients.

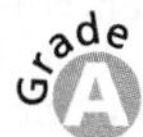

1. Eisler I, Dare C, Hodes M, et al: Family therapy for adolescent anorexia nervosa: The results of a controlled comparison of two family interventions. J Child Psychol Psychiatry 2000;41:727–736.
2. Pike KM, Walsh BT, Vitousek K, et al: Cognitive behavior therapy in the posthospitalization treatment of anorexia nervosa. Am J Psychiatry 2003;16:2046–2049.
3. McIntosh VV, Jordan J, Carter FA, et al: Three psychotherapies for anorexia nervosa: A randomized controlled trial. Am J Psychiatry 2005;162:741–747.
4. Agras WS, Walsh BT, Fairburn CG, et al: A multicenter comparison of cognitive-behavioral therapy and interpersonal psychotherapy for bulimia nervosa. Arch Gen Psychiatry 2000;57:459–466.

SUGGESTED READINGS

American Psychiatric Association: Practice Guidelines for the Treatment of Patients with Eating Disorders, 3rd ed. Washington, DC, American Psychiatric Association, 2006. *Comprehensive summary of treatment for the eating disorders reflecting clinical consensus and available evidence.*

Berkman ND, Bulik CM, Brownley KA, et al: Management of Eating Disorders. Evidence Report/Technology Assessment No. 135 (prepared by RTI International–University of North Carolina Evidence-Based Practice Center under contract no. 290-02-0016). Rockville, MD, Agency for Healthcare Research and Quality, April 2006. AHRQ publication 06-E010. Available at http://www.ahrq.gov/downloads/pub/evidence/pdf/eatingdisorders/eatdis.pdf. *Provides a systematic review of evidence relating to the treatment of eating disorders.*

National Institute for Clinical Excellence: Eating Disorders: Core Interventions in the Treatment and Management of Anorexia Nervosa, Bulimia Nervosa and Related Eating Disorders: Clinical Guideline 9. London, National Institute for Clinical Excellence, 2004. Available at http://www.nice.org.uk/pdf/cg009niceguidance.pdf. *Provides guidance on the treatment and management of eating disorders.*

239 OBESITY

Michael D. Jensen

Obesity is the most common nutritional disorder in the United States, costing more that $100 billion per year in health-related expenses. Unfortunately, training for physicians in the evaluation and management of obesity is not at a level commensurate with the fact that more than half the patients they encounter are likely to be overweight or obese. Although progress has been made in understanding the pathophysiology and treatment of obesity, it nonetheless remains a difficult disease to treat. The safest and most effective treatment approaches (lifestyle changes and behavior modification) are not those commonly employed by physicians.

Definition

The National Institutes of Health/National Heart, Lung, and Blood Institute report entitled "Clinical Guidelines on the Identification, Evaluation, and Treatment of Overweight and Obesity" (*http://www.nhlbi.nih.gov/guidelines/*) provides clear, scientifically based definitions of overweight and obesity. Body mass index (BMI) is now the recommended means to categorize weight relative to height for adults. BMI is calculated as weight (in kilograms)/height squared (in meters). To calculate BMI by pounds and inches, the formula is modified as follows: weight (pounds)/height (inches^2) × 703. The weight classifications according to BMI are summarized in Table 239–1. Individuals who are overweight (BMI of 25.0 to 29.9) may or may not have excessive fat. Some men may be overweight because of increased muscle mass, which is a straightforward clinical judgment. Although in general the risk of developing weight-related health problems increases with a BMI above 25, the guidelines point out that intervention or discussion of weight issues with the patient may not be necessary for overweight adults who are entirely healthy or who are not overfat. On the other hand, some individuals in the BMI range of 27 to 29.9 develop serious metabolic complications of obesity that could be expected to improve with weight loss. These individuals are candidates for more aggressive treatment, including pharmacotherapy if it is needed.

The risk of comorbidities increases considerably at BMIs above 30, the level at which an individual is defined as obese. Obesity is divided into three classes, also depending on BMI. Treatment approaches may differ for those who are overweight and for different classes of obesity. For example, current Food and Drug Administration guidelines indicate that pharmacotherapy can be adjunct treatment for any class of obesity, even if medical complications are not present. Although some would argue that treating obese patients without medical complications is a lower priority than treating those with medical complications, familiarity with the guidelines is important; supervisory agencies and third-party payers use them to determine who is eligible for treatment benefits. Extreme obesity (BMI > 40) is one of the key features that prompts consideration of a patient for bariatric surgery when medical treatments have failed. Patients with class II obesity (BMI of 35.0 to 39.9) may be considered for bariatric surgery if medical treatments have failed and if severe, life-threatening complications are present.

In addition to BMI, the National Heart, Lung, and Blood Institute guidelines recommend the waist circumferences as another office assessment tool that can help with the treatment decision-making process. A waist circumference of more than 102 cm or 40 inches for men and of more than 88 cm or 35 inches for women is an additional indication of risk for overweight and obesity. This measure is primarily relevant to disease risk in overweight and class I obesity categories, however. In overweight individuals, a large waist circumference changes the relative risk from increased (relative to someone with a normal BMI) to high. In class I obesity, a large waist circumference increases the risk of disease from high to very high. A large waist circumference does not affect disease risk in those with class II or class III obesity. These definitions of overweight, obesity, and high-risk waist circumference are generally applicable to those of European and African descent, but different (lower) values are recommended for those of Asian and Southeast Asian descent because the onset of metabolic abnormalities occurs at lower BMIs and waist circumferences in these populations.

TABLE 239–1 CLASSIFICATION OF OVERWEIGHT AND OBESITY BY BMI

	Obesity Class	BMI (kg/m^2)
Underweight		<18.5
Normal		18.5–24.9
Overweight		25.0–29.9
Obesity	I	30.0–34.9
Obesity	II	35.0–39.9
Extreme obesity	III	≥40

Epidemiology

Prevalence

The number of overweight and obese adults in the United States has increased dramatically during the past 20 years. It is estimated that approximately 60% of adult Americans are either overweight or obese. Approximately 60% of U.S. men and 51% of U.S. women are overweight or obese, although a greater percentage of women than of men are obese, whereas a larger percentage of men than of women are overweight. There are substantial differences in the prevalence of obesity by age, race, and socioeconomic status. The prevalence of obesity in adults tends to rise steadily from the ages of 20 to 60 years but does not increase and, in fact, begins to decrease in later years. It has been estimated that almost 75% of men aged 60 to 69 years in the United States have a BMI above 25. The increase in mean BMI with age may not be as much of a threat to population health as might first be anticipated. Whereas it is true that young adults with BMIs in the lower part of the normal range have the lowest mortality rates, this changes with age. The BMI associated with the lowest mortality rates is actually at or somewhat above 25 kg/m^2 for those in their 60s and 70s. Clearly, weight recommendations for a given individual will depend on whether adverse health consequences associated with obesity have developed.

The differences in overweight and obesity between African Americans, Mexican Americans, and European Americans are not subtle. African American women and Mexican Americans of both sexes have the highest rates of overweight and obesity in the United States. In interpreting these data, however, it is important to keep in mind that there is an inverse relationship between socioeconomic status and obesity, especially among women. Women in lower socioeconomic classes are much more likely to be obese than those in higher socioeconomic classes, particularly in the United States. This association reduces but does not eliminate the racial differences in the prevalence of obesity. Whether the remaining racial differences in the prevalence of obesity are due to genetic, constitutional, or social factors not related to income is not yet clear.

Constitutional Influences on Obesity

A number of environmental influences can result in long-term, gene-like effects on body weight regulation and the tendency to be susceptible to obesity-related health problems. The effect of the intrauterine environment and the perinatal period on subsequent weight and health is best studied. For example, undernutrition in the last trimester of pregnancy and in the early postnatal period results in a decreased risk of adult obesity. Unfortunately, the low birthweight that is associated with undernutrition (or smoking) in late pregnancy also increases the risk of hypertension, abnormal glucose tolerance, and cardiovascular disease in adulthood. In contrast, undernutrition limited to the first two trimesters of pregnancy is associated with an increased probability of adult obesity. Other early "environmental" effects are that infants of diabetic mothers tend to be fatter than those of nondiabetic mothers, and children of diabetic mothers have a greater prevalence of obesity when they are 5 to 19 years old, independent of their mother's obesity status. Finally, intrauterine exposure to the diabetic environment results in an increased risk of diabetes mellitus and obesity in the offspring. Thus, the issue of genes versus environment with respect to obesity and metabolic complications of obesity is blurred in the intrauterine and perinatal time intervals. One of the striking and worrisome aspects of these metabolic effects is not only the long-term effects on weight regulation and health but the suggestion that these traits can be passed on to future generations.

TABLE 239–2 ENVIRONMENTAL FACTORS PROMOTING OBESITY

Dietary	Activity
↑ Energy density of foods	↑ Sedentary behavior
↑ Portion size	↓ Activities of daily living
↑ Variety*	↓ Employment physical activity
↑ Palatability	
↑ Availability	
↓ Cost	
↑ Caloric beverages (soft drinks, juices)	

*Variety of sweets, snacks, and entrees.

Environmental Contributors to Human Obesity

Few would argue that there have been dramatic changes in the environment during the last 50 years. These changes allowed reduced physical activity for most Americans. In addition, alterations in the food supply have either increased energy intake or failed to allow the expected decrease in energy intake that would be needed to match the reduced energy expenditure.

Food

A number of environmental factors can influence food intake (Table 239–2). Consuming energy-dense foods results in greater energy intake because many adults respond to the volume of food taken in rather than to the energy content of food. This factor probably accounts for the association between high-fat diets and excess body weight; many high-fat foods are also energy dense. When humans consume diets that are high in fat but low in energy density, energy intake is not greater than would be expected on the basis of the energy density of the foods. Larger food portion size has also been shown to increase food intake. Given the trend in the United States to serve larger portions of food and beverage, this could be a contributing variable toward obesity. Food variety can also affect energy intake. An increased variety of entrees, sweets, snacks, and carbohydrates in the diet is associated with an increase in body fatness and food intake. In contrast, an increase in the variety of vegetables available does not result in an increased energy intake and is not associated with increased body fatness. Another factor that may have broad population effects in the United States is the reduced cost of food relative to increased availability and palatability of foods. Finally, there is evidence that consumption of beverages such as soft drinks and fruit juices is not accompanied by a decrease in food intake to offset the extra energy intake. The implication is that these types of beverages will add to the energy intake during the day and promote weight gain. Evidence suggests that dairy products do not share this property and that consumption of low-fat dairy products in the context of a weight loss program may be beneficial under some circumstances.

Several individual factors may also influence how properties of food affect energy intake. Individuals vary with respect to their dietary restraint (the tendency to consciously limit food intake to control weight), their feelings of hunger, or their disinhibition (the tendency to overeat opportunistically). It has been proposed that interindividual differences in these factors may modify how food variety and portion size affect the eating profile. In addition to these environmental influences on food consumption, there are also effects of the social context under which food is consumed and the emotional state of the individual. These effects are not yet well quantified.

Physical Activity

Physical activity can be broadly divided into exercise (fitness and sports-related activities) and nonexercise activities, both employment and nonemployment. Tables are widely available that allow one to calculate energy expenditure on the basis of an individual's weight as well as the type and duration of exercise in which the individual engages. Only a fraction of Americans engage in exercise at the recommended frequency, intensity, or duration that could be expected to have a protective effect on the development of obesity and other health problems. The portion of Americans who exercise regularly is approximately 30%. This does not appear to be changing; therefore it seems unlikely that a change in exercise habits during the past several decades is causing the increase in obesity. To the extent that reduced physical activity is contributing to the epidemic of obesity, it is likely the nonexercise component that is changing.

It is difficult to measure the energy expended in nonexercise activity. Although it seems obvious that employment physical activity has decreased with the advent of more automated systems in the workplace, there are few data in this regard. One estimate suggests that between 1982 and 1992, energy expenditure at work decreased by approximately 50 kcal/day. The additional changes in the workplace since that time have likely further reduced employment physical activity.

The other component of nonexercise physical activity, the activities of daily living, is equally difficult to measure. A plethora of labor-saving conveniences (drive-through food and banking, escalators, remote controls, e-mail, and online shopping) have been introduced into the modern environment. Each of these further reduces the energy humans must expend to get through the day. Again, there are few hard data to assess how much of a change has actually occurred, although a reduction in daily walking trips and an increase in daily automobile trips have been documented.

Perhaps because it is easier to assess, information as to how differences in sedentary activity (television watching, video games, and computer use) relate to obesity is more readily available. There is compelling evidence that more time spent in sedentary pursuits is associated with an increased risk of overweight and obesity. The striking aspect to these studies is that the adverse effect of sedentary activities is independent of participation in traditional exercise activities.

Understanding the contributions of decreases in work-related physical activity, decreases in activity of daily living, and increases in sedentary behavior can help the physician working with the patient to uncover patterns that may relate to weight gain.

In summary, there are clearly dramatic changes in the Western environments that are conspiring to bring out tendencies toward obesity in those with constitutional or genetic susceptibility. Physicians who are aware of these environmental factors are in a better position to help their obese patients identify which of these environmental factors are contributing to the problem and develop plans for intervention.

Pathobiology

Etiology

In one sense, the etiology of obesity can be considered simplistically; if energy intake exceeds energy expenditure, and if lean body mass remains stable, body fat must increase. Unfortunately, obesity is a much more complex issue. There are significant genetic and constitutional susceptibility aspects to obesity that are heavily affected by environmental factors. Evidence from family studies and studies of twins strongly supports the concept that within a given environment, a significant portion of the variation in weight is genetic. That said, however, the tremendous increase in the prevalence of obesity in the United States during the last several decades can hardly be ascribed to mass changes in the genetic makeup of Americans.

Genetics

There is strong evidence for a hereditary tendency toward the regulation of body weight. The multiple gene defects resulting in obesity include a number of classic genetic syndromes, such as Prader-Willi and Laurence-Moon-Biedl. More recently, rare monogenic forms of human obesity due to mutations in the leptin gene and leptin receptor gene have been described. The result is an actual or functional leptin deficiency, much like that seen in *ob/ob* or *db/db* mice, the animal models that stimulated the discovery of leptin. There have also been reports of inherited forms of human obesity due to mutations of genes that regulate appetite neuropeptide synthesis. Doubtless, reports of single-gene mutations associated with human obesity will continue to appear. However, the overwhelming majority of human obesity is related to the combination of polygenic susceptibility traits and environmental conditions.

Regulation of Body Weight and Energy Balance

Not all of the factors that contribute to the regulation of adult body weight are fully understood; however, this must be a well-balanced process. For example, the typical U.S. adult will take in and expend approximately 2000 to 3000 kcal/day. If there were a consistent error of even 1% in overconsumption of food, this would result in the gain of approximately 25 to 30 pounds of fat every 10 years if there were no change in energy expenditure. It follows that most adults regulate the average energy balance with greater than 1% precision. There appears to be regulation of both energy intake and energy expenditure by conscious and unconscious processes.

The excess energy consumed by adults is generally stored as triglyceride in adipocytes. The primary means by which adipose tissue mass expands is to increase the amount of fat stored in each cell (adipocyte hypertrophy). This process can store only a limited amount of fat, however, because there is an upper limit to the size of fat cells. If sufficient fat is deposited, eventually new fat cells are recruited from preadipocytes present in the stromovascular component of adipose tissue. Some adults recruit new adipocytes more readily than others do and thus gain weight more so from adipocyte hyperplasia than from hypertrophy. Those who gain fat with large adipocytes are more likely to display inflammatory responses, both in adipose tissue (greater numbers of macrophages and increased expression of cytokines) and systemically (increased C-reactive protein). Adipose tissue, rather than being static, is slowly but continuously being turned over. It is possible that genetic or constitutional variations in this process contribute to the metabolic complications of obesity.

The discovery of leptin, a protein from the cytokine family that is secreted almost exclusively by adipocytes, was the first confirmation that adipose tissue can secrete hormones that have central nervous system effects on food intake. Leptin also has other hypothalamic and pituitary functions and is proposed to have diverse peripheral physiologic actions. The leptin-deficient animal model of obesity, the *ob/ob* mouse, is severely obese, hyperphagic, hypometabolic, and sexually immature and has low levels of spontaneous activity. Administration of leptin to this animal corrects all of these defects. A few humans have been found also to have leptin deficiency due to mutations in the leptin gene. These children had low plasma leptin concentrations and were hyperphagic and severely obese. They responded to exogenous leptin administration with dramatic weight loss, reduced food intake, and accelerated maturation of the pituitary-gonadal axis. With the exception of these rare mutations, however, obese humans are not leptin deficient. In fact, because plasma leptin concentrations increase logarithmically with the percentage of body fat, obesity results in high plasma leptin concentrations. Likewise, because women normally have more body fat than men do, they also have higher plasma leptin concentrations. From what is currently known, screening for leptin deficiency is not warranted except in severe, hyperphagic obesity beginning in early childhood that is accompanied by sexual immaturity (in adolescents or older age groups) and in the absence of other known causes (e.g., Prader-Willi syndrome).

Some animal models of genetic obesity (the *db/db* mouse and *fa/fa* rat) have defective leptin receptors, making them unresponsive to leptin. These observations raised the possibility that human obesity, rather than being a condition of leptin deficiency, is a state of leptin resistance. Although rare cases of obese humans with defective leptin receptor genes have been reported, again it appears that leptin resistance due to leptin receptor defects (or genetic postreceptor signaling abnormalities) is extremely uncommon. Clinical screening for leptin receptor mutations is not warranted given that no treatment exists.

In humans, leptin is secreted in a diurnal fashion that is regulated by the effects of insulin and glucose on adipocytes. Leptin secretion can be increased by 30 to 40% with brief periods of overfeeding (before changes in body composition) and is reduced by 50% in response to periods of underfeeding that do not result in significant changes in body composition. Clinical studies indicate that low or absent leptin results in extreme hunger; treatment of congenital leptin deficiency with physiologic doses of recombinant leptin markedly reduces hunger and allows significant fat loss. In contrast, treatment of overweight patients with recombinant leptin does not show promising weight loss results despite achieving peak serum leptin concentrations more than 30 times basal. In animals, falling leptin secretion plays an important role in modulating the hypothalamic-pituitary response to undernutrition, such as mediating the endocrine adaptation to starvation with reduced thyroid-stimulating hormone and gonadotrophin secretion. Clinical studies suggest that leptin may play a similar role with regard to the hypothalamic-pituitary-gonadal axis in humans.

In summary, the discovery of leptin has been an important advance in understanding the biology of obesity. However, defects in leptin secretion or inherited defects in leptin action appear to be the cause of only a tiny fraction of human obesity. The subsequent discovery of a plethora of adipose-derived hormones (see later) emphasizes the complexity of regulation of fat mass.

Energy Intake

Much has been learned about the biologic regulation of food intake, mostly from the study of animal models. There are a series of peripheral "satiety" signals that act to inhibit further food intake at some point during meal consumption (Fig. 239–1). Some of the signals reach the brain through the vagus nerve and some through the systemic circulation. Examples of the proposed factors modulating appetite are listed in Table 239–3. The compounds range from gut (ghrelin, cholecystokinin, glucagon-like peptide 1) and pancreas-derived (insulin) hormones to peptides such as apolipoprotein A-IV, which is secreted with chylomicrons. The signals are thought to be triggered by mechanical stimuli (e.g., the fullness of the stomach) as well as by the presence of nutrients in the jejunum and ileum.

The central nervous system regulation of food intake is also better understood. A number of neuropeptides, lipid derivatives, and monoamines have been identified that have either anabolic (increased food intake with or without decreased energy expenditure) or catabolic (decreased food intake with or without increased energy expenditure) properties. A list of these molecules is provided in Table 239–4. Many of these compounds serve more than one function, such as regulation of hormone secretion (thyrotropin-releasing hormone and corticotropin-releasing hormone), wakefulness (norepinephrine), or behavior reinforcing systems (endocannabinoids). Understanding the process of appetite regulation has allowed the discovery of therapeutic agents that inhibit or stimulate central appetite regulation pathways.

TABLE 239–3 SUGGESTED BIOLOGIC MODULATORS OF FOOD INTAKE

Peripheral Signal	Proposed Effect on Food Intake
Vagal	–
Cholecystokinin	–
Apolipoprotein A-IV	–
Insulin	–
Glucagon-like peptide 1	–
Other glucagon-related peptides	–
Leptin	+ when leptin ↓↓
Ghrelin	+
Tumor necrosis factor-α	–
Obestatin	–

TABLE 239–4 CENTRAL NERVOUS SYSTEM MODULATORS OF ENERGY BALANCE

Central Anabolic (↑ intake)	Central Catabolic (↓ intake)
Neuropeptide Y	α-Melanocyte–stimulating hormone
Agouti-related protein	Corticotropin-releasing hormone
Melanin-concentrating hormone	Thyrotropin-releasing hormone
Hypocretins/orexins	Cocaine- and amphetamine-regulated transcript
Galanin	Interleukin-1β
Norepinephrine	Urocortin
Endogenous endocannabinoids (anandamide and 2-arachidonoylglycerol)	Oxytocin
	Neurotensin
	Serotonin

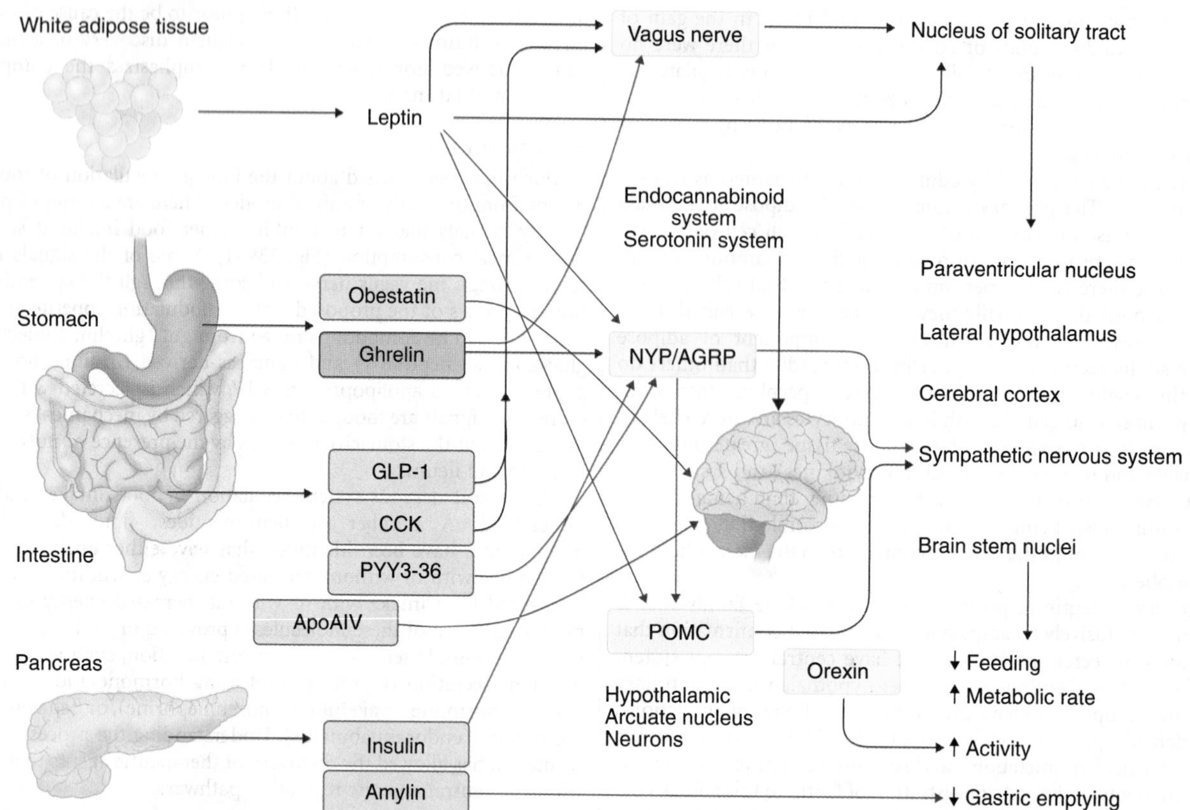

FIGURE 239–1 • Energy balance regulation. AGRP = agouti-related protein; ApoAIV = apolipoprotein A-IV; CCK = cholecystokinin; GLP-1 = glucagon-like peptide 1; NPY = neuropeptide Y; POMC = proopiomelanocortin. (Modified from Neary NM, Goldstone AP, Bloom SR: Appetite regulation: From the gut to the hypothalamus. Clin Endocrinol [Oxf] 2004;60:153–160.)

Energy Expenditure

There is a wide range of daily energy expenditure in adults, from less than 1400 kcal/day to more than 5000 kcal/day; larger, more physically active individuals have the greatest energy needs. Typically, daily energy expenditure is divided into resting (or basal) metabolic rate, the thermic effect of food, and physical activity energy expenditure.

Basal Metabolic Rate

The basal metabolic rate (BMR) is the energy expenditure of laying still at rest, awake, in the overnight postabsorptive state. A true BMR is measured after awakening but before arising from bed. The resting metabolic rate (RMR) is similarly defined but is not necessarily measured before arising from bed. For most sedentary adult Americans, the RMR represents the major portion of energy expended during the day and may range from less than 1200 to more than 3000 kcal/day. Most (~80%) of the BMR is directly proportional to the amount of lean tissue mass.

Not all components of lean tissue consume oxygen at the same relative rates. Visceral or splanchnic bed tissues account for approximately 25% of RMR but a much smaller proportion of body weight. The brain, which is only a small percentage of body weight, accounts for almost 15% of RMR. Likewise, the heart (~7%) and kidneys (~5 to 10%) account for greater portions of resting energy needs than their relative contribution to body mass. In contrast, resting muscle makes up 40 to 50% of lean tissue mass but accounts for only 25% of RMR. This contribution changes dramatically with exercise, at which time muscle can account for 80 to 90% of energy expenditure, especially during high-intensity exercise. Adipose tissue is a minor contributor to daily energy expenditure, consuming only approximately 3 kcal/kg/day.

Although most of the RMR can be accounted for by the mass of lean tissue, there are also other, more subtle influences. Age, sex (women have slightly lower BMRs even corrected for fat-free mass), and fat mass affect RMR. Small changes in BMR occur during the menstrual cycle (luteal phase > follicular phase). There is also evidence that heritable or family factors do influence BMR, accounting for as much as 10% of the interindividual differences.

There are both obligatory and facultative components to RMR. With an energy-restricted diet, significant reductions in BMR relative to the amount of fat-free mass occur. Reductions in the production of triiodothyronine from thyroxine are thought to contribute to this phenomenon. Likewise, during brief periods of overfeeding, it has been shown that RMR increases above that which would be expected for the amount of lean tissue present.

It has been proposed that individuals with BMRs lower than predicted are at increased risk of future weight gain. Published data suggest that the relative risk is small, and clinical effort to identify such patients is not warranted at this time. Measurement of BMR is sometimes helpful in the evaluation of patients who insist they are unable to lose weight while following diets of less than 1000 kcal/day. Almost without fail, their BMR is substantially greater than their reported food intake. This underscores the fact that most adults are notoriously unreliable in assessing their own food intake.

The Thermic Effect of Food

Approximately 10% of the energy content of food is expended in the process of digestion, absorption, and metabolism of nutrients. There is a significant interindividual variability in this value, however, ranging from a low of approximately 5% to a high of approximately 15% of meal calories that are "wasted" in the postprandial interval. The thermic effect of a meal is related to the carbohydrate and protein calorie content of the meal (the fat content has little stimulatory effect). Both obligatory and facultative components of the thermic effect of food have been identified. The obligatory components no doubt reflect the energy costs of digestion, absorption, and storage of nutrients. Approximately 60 to 70% of the thermic effect of meals is obligatory, and the remaining 30 to 40% is facultative thermogenesis. The two factors thought to play a role in the facultative component of the thermic effect of food are the postprandial insulin response and activation of the sympathetic nervous system. The thermic effect of food is somewhat lower in insulin-resistant obese humans, but there have been no reported links between reduced postprandial thermogenesis and future obesity.

Physical Activity Energy Expenditure

The energy expenditure of physical activity is a product of the amount of work done and the work efficiency of the individual. Because there is not much variability in work efficiency, the published values for estimating the energy costs of work performed are generally accurate. The common means to express work units is as metabolic equivalents (METs), a multiple of the RMR. If an individual's RMR is 1 kcal/min, a workload of 5 METs is 5 kcal/min. Highly trained athletes can work at extremely high METs (>16) for extended periods, but most sedentary individuals can work only for a limited time at much lower workloads. The peak work capacity refers to the maximum number of calories that can be expended (or the maximum amount of oxygen that can be consumed, $\dot{V}O_2max$). There is tremendous variability in peak work capacity that is largely but not solely related to how much and what type of physical activity is performed.

Another important concept in understanding the capacity for physical activity (and thus exercise prescriptions) is the lactate threshold. The lactate threshold can be thought of as the level at which exercise begins to become so uncomfortable that it cannot be maintained much longer. The biochemical definition relates to the progressive rise in blood lactate concentrations. The lactate threshold may range from 50 to 90% of an individual's peak work capacity. Training raises the lactate threshold closer to the maximum workload and thus allows individuals to work at higher rates for longer periods. Obese, sedentary individuals typically have low lactate thresholds (sometimes on the order of 4 or 5 METs), and the threshold can be even less in obese patients with type 2 diabetes.

Exercise (fitness and sports-related activities) is commonly considered the main component of physical activity thermogenesis. Although a large amount of energy can be expended in relatively brief periods in fit individuals, most adults do not exercise at high levels or for a sufficient duration to expend a large amount of energy. Thus, rather than focusing solely on "exercise" as the main component of physical activity energy expenditure, it is important to consider the energy costs of nonexercise activity.

Nonexercise activity thermogenesis (NEAT) is the calorie expense of performing all activities other than exercise. The range of observed NEAT under controlled (metabolic chamber) conditions has been from less than 100 to up to approximately 800 kcal/day. There is probably a much wider range in free-living individuals. NEAT is not a static component of daily energy expenditure. It has been shown that NEAT can increase in response to increased food intake in an unconscious manner. In fact, modulation of NEAT can be a significant factor that acts to stabilize weight despite variations in food intake. Low levels of NEAT have been reported to predict future weight gain in some populations, and there may be differences between lean and obese persons in the daily amount of NEAT, which could relate to differential tendencies to regulate weight. There is virtually no information as to what the regulatory systems are that stimulate or inhibit NEAT.

Pathogenesis

Secondary Causes of Obesity

Medications

A growing number of medications cause weight gain in some or most of those patients for whom they are prescribed. Awareness of the medications that have this potential can facilitate weight loss treatment in some patients. Table 239–5 lists a number of medications that are associated with weight gain as well as alternative treatment approaches, if any, for the underlying condition.

Diseases

Less than 1% of obese patients have an underlying disease that can explain the development of their obesity. Endocrinopathies are the most common secondary cause of obesity. These include Cushing's syndrome, hypothalamic damage resulting in overeating (most commonly after pituitary surgery), insulinoma, and hypothyroidism. A Cushing's syndrome–like fat distribution is common; therefore, other aspects of the patient are the best clues to test for this condition. These include the classic purple striae, thinning skin, easy bruising, and proximal muscle weakness. Correction of Cushing's syndrome commonly results in substantial loss of excess body fat. Insulinoma is a rare tumor, and only a

TABLE 239–5 PHARMACOLOGIC INFLUENCES IN WEIGHT GAIN AND ALTERNATIVE THERAPIES

Drugs That May Promote Weight Gain	Alternative Treatments—Weight Neutral or Weight Loss
Psychiatric-neurologic medications	Alternative psychiatric-neurologic medications
Antipsychotics: olanzapine, clozapine, risperidone, quetiapine, aripiprazole	Ziprasidone
Antidepressants	
Tricyclics: imipramine, amitriptyline	Nortriptyline, bupropion, nefazodone, fluvoxamine, sertraline, duloxetine
Triazolopyridines: trazodone	
Serotonin reuptake inhibitors: paroxetine, fluoxetine, citalopram	
Tetracyclics: mirtazapine	
Monoamine oxidase inhibitors	
Antiepileptic drugs: gabapentin (higher doses), valproic acid, carbamazepine, divalproex	Topiramate, zonisamide (weight loss), lamotrigine (less weight gain)
Mood stabilizers: lithium, carbamazepine, lamotrigine, gabapentin (higher doses)	
Steroid hormones	Alternatives to steroid hormones
Progestational steroids	Barrier methods, intrauterine device
Corticosteroids	Nonsteroidal anti-inflammatory drugs
Hormonal contraceptives	
Anti-diabetes agents	Alternative anti-diabetes agents
Insulin (most forms)	Metformin
Sulfonylureas	Acarbose, miglitol
Thiazolidinediones	Pramlintide
Antihistamines—commonly reported with older agents; also oxatomide, loratadine, and azelastine	Decongestants, mast cell stabilizers, antagonists of endogenous mediators of inflammation
Antihypertensive agents	Alternative antihypertensive agents
α- and β-Adrenergic receptor blockers	Angiotensin-converting enzyme inhibitors
Calcium-channel blockers: nisoldipine	Calcium-channel blockers—most other agents
	Angiotensin receptor blockers
	Diuretics
Highly active antiretroviral therapy	

small portion of patients with insulinoma present with obesity; only some patients consciously prevent spells by eating more often and thus become obese. The weight gain associated with hypothyroidism is virtually always due to fluid retention and resolves dramatically with thyroid hormone replacement. Unfortunately, successful treatment is not available for hyperphagia due to hypothalamic damage. On occasion, adult patients with growth hormone deficiency, most commonly after hypophysectomy, will lose excess body fat with growth hormone replacement therapy.

Psychosocial Aspects of Obesity

Sexual, physical, and emotional abuse, especially in women, can result in long-term adverse consequences that include obesity. The effects of the abuse tend to be most profound if it occurs in childhood and adolescence. These women may be severely obese, suffer from chronic depression, and experience a number of psychosomatic symptoms, particularly chronic gastrointestinal distress. Identification of these issues before initiation of weight loss programs is important because successful weight loss may actually aggravate the distress experienced by these women. In addition, appropriate referral for psychiatric help may be needed before initiation of treatment for obesity.

Pathophysiology

Metabolic Complications of Obesity

The properties of excess adipose tissue that contribute to the metabolic complications of obesity are now better understood. A key observation has been that a central or upper body fat distribution, more so than total fat mass, is predictive of the metabolic complications of obesity. It also has been noted that obese individuals with enlarged fat cells (adipocyte hypertrophy) are more likely to suffer the metabolic complications than are obese persons with normal-sized fat cells (adipocyte hyperplasia). In vitro studies have shown that lipolysis, which results in the release of fatty acids and glycerol, is less well regulated in large adipocytes than in normal-sized adipocytes. The finding that upper body obesity is associated with adipocyte hypertrophy and lower body obesity with adipocyte hyperplasia has provided a potential link between fat distribution differences and adipose tissue function in regard to its fuel export function.

Adipose tissue release of free fatty acids and glycerol into the circulation by lipolysis provides the majority (in a kinetic sense) of the energy derived from fat stores. Lipolysis is capable of providing 50 to 100% of daily energy needs. Adipose tissue lipolysis is regulated primarily by insulin (inhibition) and catecholamines (stimulation), although growth hormone and cortisol also can stimulate lipolysis to a lesser extent. Upper body obesity is associated with several abnormalities of adipose tissue lipolysis, most remarkably with higher free fatty acid concentrations due to excess release in the postabsorptive and postprandial periods. Abnormally high free fatty acid concentrations can contribute to or account for a number of the metabolic complications of obesity.

Insulin Resistance

The term *insulin resistance* is typically used in reference to the ability of insulin to promote glucose uptake, oxidation, and storage as well as to inhibit the release of glucose into the circulation. The primary site of insulin-stimulated glucose uptake, oxidation, and storage is skeletal muscle. The principal site of glucose production is the liver. Insulin resistance initially leads to hyperinsulinemia and may eventually lead to the development of type 2 diabetes mellitus if there is subsequent pancreatic β-cell loss.

The ability of insulin to promote glucose uptake, oxidation, and storage in muscle and to suppress plasma concentrations of free fatty acids is reduced in upper body obesity. High plasma concentrations of free fatty acids can induce a state of insulin resistance both in the muscle (glucose uptake) and in the liver (glucose release), independent of obesity. Thus, abnormal regulation of adipose tissue export of free fatty acids can potentially explain much of the insulin resistance with respect to glucose metabolism.

Dysregulated production of a number of adipose-derived hormones has also been hypothesized to contribute to insulin resistance and the metabolic complications of obesity (Table 239–6). For example, reduced secretion of adiponectin, an adipocyte-derived hormone that improves insulin action in animals, is seen in obesity and diabetes. Increased production of resistin, interleukin-6, tumor necrosis factor-α, and retinol binding protein 4 by adipose tissue has been linked to insulin resistance in animal models. Visfatin, another adipocyte hormone secreted preferentially by omental and mesenteric adipocytes, appears to function to increase insulin action, albeit by a mechanism different from that of adiponectin. To date, there is insufficient experimental evidence from human studies to know what role these so-called adipokines play in the metabolic complications of obesity.

TABLE 239–6 NOVEL HORMONE REGULATORS OF INSULIN ACTION

Promotes Insulin Sensitivity	Promotes Insulin Resistance
Adiponectin	Resistin
Visfatin	Retinol binding protein 4
	Tumor necrosis factor-α
	Interleukin-6

Islet Cell Failure and Type 2 Diabetes Mellitus

Type 2 diabetes is generally the result of defects in both insulin secretion and insulin action. Many obese individuals are insulin resistant, yet only a subset will develop diabetes mellitus. It follows that those who develop type 2 diabetes have pancreatic β-cell decompensation with subsequent hyperglycemia. Rodent studies have suggested that a process referred to as lipotoxicity is involved in pancreatic β-cell failure. In this model, increased free fatty acids are proposed to contribute to the insulin secretory abnormalities seen in obesity and ultimately lead to β-cell failure. Free fatty acids have clearly been shown to modulate insulin secretion in humans, and a small number of studies have suggested that free fatty acids have adverse effects on islet β-cell function in humans. There are a number of important differences between rodent models of diabetes and human diabetes that require consideration of other possibilities. Another explanation for the development of β-cell failure in obesity is the overproduction of islet amyloid polypeptide. This protein is co-secreted with insulin, and because of its tertiary structure (which is different in humans and rodents), it can form toxic amyloid deposits in β cells. Amyloid deposits have been found in the pancreatic islets obtained at autopsy from patients with type 2 diabetes mellitus.

Hypertension

Blood pressure can be increased by a number of mechanisms. Increased circulating blood volume, abnormal vasoconstriction, decreased vascular relaxation, and increased cardiac output may all contribute to hypertension in obesity. The effect of hyperinsulinemia to increase renal sodium absorption may contribute to hypertension through increased circulating blood volume. Abnormalities of vascular resistance also contribute to the pathophysiologic process of obesity-related hypertension. Under some experimental conditions, elevated free fatty acids have been found to cause increased vasoconstriction and reduced nitric oxide–mediated vasorelaxation, similar to that seen in the metabolic syndrome. Some obese adults have increased sympathetic nervous system activity, which could contribute to obesity-associated hypertension. Finally, angiotensinogen (also produced by adipocytes) is a precursor of the vasoconstrictor angiotensin II, and its increased secretion has been proposed to contribute to elevated blood pressure.

Dyslipidemia

Upper body obesity and type 2 diabetes mellitus are associated with increased triglycerides, decreased high-density lipoprotein cholesterol, and a high proportion of small, dense low-density lipoprotein particles. This dyslipidemia contributes to the increased cardiovascular risk observed in the metabolic syndrome. Fasting hypertriglyceridemia is caused by increased hepatic very low density lipoprotein secretion, which may be driven by increased delivery of free fatty acids to the liver coming from both visceral fat and upper body subcutaneous fat. The reduced high-density lipoprotein cholesterol concentrations and the increased small, dense low-density lipoprotein particle concentrations associated with upper body obesity are likely to be an indirect consequence of elevated triglyceride-rich very low density lipoprotein. Increased cholesterol ester transfer protein activity and hepatic lipase activity can theoretically account for the atherogenic shifts in triglycerides and cholesterol between lipoproteins. Genetic influences play a significant role in the expression of these lipid abnormalities. Polymorphisms in the genes for apolipoprotein E, lipoprotein lipase, apolipoprotein B-100, and apolipoprotein A-II are reported to affect the expression of increased triglycerides and decreased high-density lipoprotein of upper body obesity.

Endocrine Manifestations of Obesity

Obesity can cause abnormalities of the endocrine system. One of the most common abnormalities is polycystic ovarian syndrome. This syndrome is characterized by mild hirsutism and irregular menses or amenorrhea with anovulatory cycles. It is most commonly linked with obesity and often improves with weight loss or other treatments that improve insulin resistance. Thus, it is thought that the insulin resistance associated with obesity may trigger the development of polycystic ovarian syndrome in susceptible individuals.

Whereas mild to moderate androgen overproduction is a feature of upper body obesity in women, obese men may suffer from mild hypothalamic hypogonadism. This androgen deficiency improves with weight loss and does not seem to benefit substantially from testosterone replacement. There has been some concern that testosterone treatment of obese men may increase the risk of obstructive sleep apnea.

Estrogens are not elevated in obese premenopausal women, but they remain somewhat above postmenopausal levels in obese postmenopausal women. This may contribute to some of the increased prevalence of malignant neoplasms (see later).

Serum growth hormone concentrations are commonly low in obese adults, but insulin-like growth factor 1 concentrations are often normal, and growth hormone concentrations increase with weight loss. Treatment of these patients with growth hormone has been reported to worsen insulin resistance and glucose intolerance and cannot be justified at this time, considering the costs and poor risk-to-benefit ratio.

Mechanical Complications of Obesity

The excess body weight associated with obesity is thought to be responsible for the increased prevalence of lower extremity degenerative joint disease seen in obesity. Extreme obesity can result in premature degenerative joint disease, and this may be especially difficult to treat surgically given the greater stress on joint replacements. Severely obese individuals may also have severe problems with venous stasis, which is occasionally aggravated by right-sided heart failure (see later).

Obstructive Sleep Apnea

Sleep apnea is common in severely obese patients, tending to be more common in men and more common in women with an upper body obese phenotype. Sleep apnea is most likely explained by enlargement of upper airways soft tissue, resulting in collapse of the upper airways with inspiration during sleep. The obstruction leads to apneas, with hypoxemia, hypercapnia, and a stress response (high catecholamine and endothelin levels). The frequent arousals to restore breathing result in poor sleep quality. Sleep apnea is associated with an increased risk of hypertension, and if sleep apnea is severe, it can lead to right-sided heart failure and sudden death. A history of daytime hypersomnolence, loud snoring, restless sleep, or morning headaches is suggestive of obstructive sleep apnea. Treatment of sleep apnea is important to improve cardiovascular risk, and the failure to recognize and to treat this complication may make weight loss intervention strategies much less successful.

Cancer

The risk of breast cancer and endometrial cancer is increased in obese women. It is thought that this may be due to the increased estrogen levels associated with obesity in the postmenopausal woman. Obese men also have a higher mortality of cancers of the prostate and colon. The reasons for these associations are unknown.

Gastrointestinal Disorders

Gastroesophageal reflux disease and gallstones are more prevalent in obese patients. Likewise, fatty liver and nonalcoholic steatohepatitis are more common in obesity. Nonalcoholic steatohepatitis can eventually progress to cirrhosis and can be fatal. Weight loss and interventions that improve insulin sensitivity appear to improve fatty liver and nonalcoholic steatohepatitis.

Diagnosis

Evaluation

In the office practice, obtaining an accurate height and weight allows calculation of BMI; under some circumstances, measurement of the patient's waist circumference can be useful in assessing risk (see earlier). Accurate measurement of blood pressure, which may require a large blood pressure cuff, is important. Identification of the adverse health consequences of obesity should be a routine part of office evaluation of a patient who is overweight or obese. The presence or absence of dyslipidemia (high-density lipoprotein cholesterol level below 45 mg/dL for women or below 35 mg/dL for men and triglycerides above 150 mg/dL), hypertension, glucose intolerance or diabetes, and hyperuricemia should be documented. Three or more of these health problems (or two with evidence of insulin resistance) are considered criteria for diagnosis of the metabolic syndrome. A history suggestive of sleep apnea should prompt a referral for overnight oximetry or a sleep disorder evaluation.

History

After the level of health risk facing the patient with obesity is determined, a review of the patient's lifestyle, including an assessment of physical activity level and eating habits, may help provide information about why the patient is obese. A family history of obesity, or longstanding obesity, provides evidence against a secondary cause of obesity. A careful medication history and social history may help the clinician identify precipitating factors that can be modified to enhance the success of treatment.

Treatment

Rx

Obesity represents an individual's response to the environment based on genetics and learned behavior. It is seldom a temporary condition and is best viewed as a chronic disease. Therefore, treatment must be considered a long-term issue, much like diabetes, hypertension, or dyslipidemia. Substantial weight loss can be induced by severe calorie restriction; but without approaches to ensure behavioral changes, body fat is invariably regained. To the extent that environmental factors contribute to a patient's overweight status and to the extent that the macroenvironment is unlikely to change, patients must learn how to make permanent lifestyle changes (eating and activity behavior) to hope for permanent weight loss. Behavior modification approaches often seek to help patients recognize and circumvent environmental cues for sedentary behavior and overeating as a means to accomplish these lifestyle changes.

Evaluation of Potential Success of Treatment

Before a weight management program is instituted, it is important to ensure that the patient is interested and ready to make lifestyle changes and has realistic goals and expectations. Patients often expect to lose large amounts of weight in a short time. Medical treatment programs, even if they include pharmacotherapy, do not often result in greater than 10% weight loss. This degree of weight loss is sufficient to markedly reduce the medical complications of obesity; however, disappointment with "only" 10% weight loss may cause patients to quit a medically successful program. Helping the patient to realize and to accept that 10% weight loss is a reasonable, initial goal can be one of the more challenging aspects for a physician but can prevent unnecessary disappointment later on.

It is sometimes necessary to delay entry into treatment programs if a patient is not ready to make changes in lifestyle. In this case, a reasonable strategy is periodically to remind the patient of the potential health benefits of improved activity and eating habits. Once a willingness to make changes is apparent, treatment is more likely to succeed.

General Measures

Reducing energy intake is the most efficient and effective means to lose weight. For example, creating a 500 kcal/day deficit by reduced food intake can allow the loss of 1 pound of fat per week.

Rx

Although possible, it is much more difficult to increase energy expenditure by 500 kcal/day through exercise. Higher levels of physical activity can prevent weight gain (or weight regain after weight loss). Some patients, given the proper information, are able to change eating and activity habits on their own; others require formal or informal behavior modification interventions (see earlier) to help make these changes. In some instances, pharmacotherapy or surgery may be needed for treatment of obesity. A flow diagram of how to evaluate and to manage patients with overweight and obesity is presented in Figure 239–2.

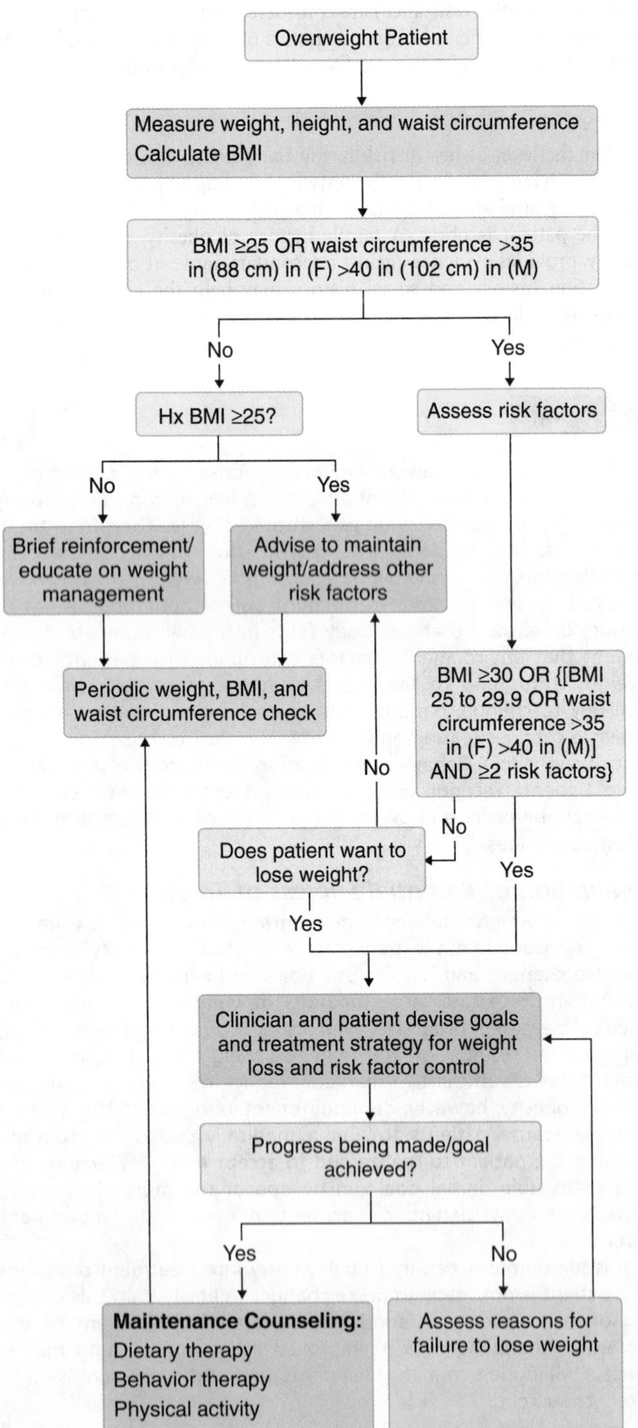

FIGURE 239–2 • Evaluation and management of patients with overweight and obesity. BMI = body mass index. (Modified from the National Institutes of Health/National Heart, Lung, and Blood Institute: Clinical Guidelines on the Identification, Evaluation, and Treatment of Obesity in Adults: The Evidence Report. Obes Res 1998;6:51S–209S.)

Rx

Diet

Changes in eating habits must be permanent if weight loss is to be maintained. An experienced registered dietitian can be helpful in the evaluation of a patient's eating habits and will be able to provide the needed education. The diet history may identify a few eating behaviors that are resulting in excess energy intake. Specific recommendations can then focus on the most blatant poor eating habits. Although it is important to address specific adverse eating behaviors, the patients need to understand some general principles regarding diet. Reducing the energy density of food (most commonly accomplished by reducing dietary fat) can allow patients to feel satiated while consuming fewer calories. A common mistake, however, is for patients to consume large quantities of easy to eat "nonfat" foods, thereby offsetting the expected benefits of the diet. In addition to reducing the intake of high-fat foods, patients should understand that increasing the consumption of foods high in water and fiber (fruits, vegetables, legumes, and soups) can provide satiety without excess calories. It is also important to avoid the excess intake of beverages containing substantial calories with little or no satiety. Finally, a regular pattern of eating should be encouraged.

New, fad diets are continually being promoted with the promise of easy weight loss. A common feature of these diets is the claim that special properties of certain foods help people lose weight or are the cause of obesity. If followed, most of these diets result in weight loss because of a reduced energy intake. The reduced intake can be related to the monotony of the diet, and there have been no diets identified that cause persons to lose weight not in accordance with physiologic principles and the laws of physics. No published data exist to support the use of fad diets in the long-term treatment of obesity.

Very low calorie diets (less than 800 calories per day) have been used for years to achieve accelerated weight loss. The rationale for this approach is now in question, given that the long-term results of these diets are no better and sometimes worse than the results from the standard low-calorie diet combined with behavior modification. The expensive laboratory monitoring required for very low calorie diets without an improved long-term outcome raises questions as to the cost/benefit of this approach.

Physical Activity

Long-term increase in physical activity, either through the activities of daily living or through regular exercise, is key to prevent weight regain after successful weight loss. Unfortunately, many overweight and obese patients are unfit, being unable to walk even 1 mile continuously. It is not possible for most adults to burn large numbers of calories. For example, only about 100 kcal is expended by a 70-kg adult walking 1 mile. Losing weight solely by increasing exercise is impractical for most patients; however, increasing physical activity as a means of maintaining weight loss is an attainable goal for most patients.

Successful maintenance of weight loss requires that daily energy expenditure be an average of 80 to 90% above RMR. This is a considerable increase for most patients. For example, someone with an RMR of 1500 kcal/day would need to expend approximately 1000 kcal/day in physical activity to meet this target. Activities other than "exercise" are important means to achieve this goal. The most commonly applicable approach is by increasing the amount of walking done throughout the day.

There are important health benefits from regular physical activity over and above the effects on weight. These include lower cardiovascular and all-cause mortality, independent of weight. The options for increasing physical activity include exercise (sports or fitness pursuits) and lifestyle approaches. Both methods can improve fitness and allow weight stability; however, persuading obese patients to become more active is not easy. Physicians can begin by asking patients about their current and past activity habits as well as what barriers they see to increasing physical activity. This accomplishes the goal of stimulating patients to think about the issue in a tactful manner. It can help to ask the patient what personal benefits are envisioned as a result of increasing the level of activity. If patients

Rx

agree to begin an exercise or physical activity program, they will need to monitor their activity and set realistic goals for the amount of exercise they are going to achieve. The ready availability of step counters offers a practical means for patients to track physical activity throughout the day and to assess the effects of changes in lifestyle on their activity level. Self-monitoring of how many steps are taken each day for 1 to 2 weeks can give the patient a good sense of the level of activity. Many Americans get as few as 4000 to 5000 steps per day, whereas it may take as many as 15,000 to 17,000 steps per day to help those who have lost significant amounts of weight to maintain that lower weight. Gradually increasing the number of steps regularly taken during the day through a series of changes in habits (parking farther away and walking during work breaks) is more likely to result in long-term success for most persons than is setting aside 2 hours or more for continuous walking.

Behavior Modification

Patients who are unable to make changes in eating activity habits on their own or with informal office counseling may benefit from referral to a behavior therapist. The goals of behavior modification are to help patients modify their eating, activity, and thinking habits that predispose to obesity. The goals of behavioral therapy focus on achieving selected results in regard to eating and activity habits and focusing on specific pathways of how to achieve the goals. These pathways may include identification and removal of barriers to the development of better eating or activity habits. Small, incremental and consistent changes in behavior are encouraged as opposed to large, inconsistent changes in behavior. Self-monitoring of food and activity is considered a key feature to success because most obese patients underestimate food intake and overestimate exercise in the absence of objective measures. Cognitive restructuring has been introduced as a way to help overcome the thought processes that can lead to failure of a weight management program. Patients are taught to identify, to challenge, and to correct self-defeating thoughts.

Medical Therapy

Pharmacotherapy

A limited number of drugs are currently available to help patients with weight loss. The disastrous experience with fenfluramine and dexfenfluramine (pulmonary hypertension and cardiac valvar disease) seems to have dampened the enthusiasm of many physicians to prescribe weight loss drugs, even under circumstances that justify their use. That said, not all overweight or obese patients are candidates for pharmacologic treatment of obesity. Table 239–7 provides criteria that should help select patients for pharmacologic treatment. Because pharmacologic treatment of obesity exposes patients to some risks and expense, it is reasonable to require an objective benefit. A rational argument can be made that prioritization should be given to those with one or more medical complications or conditions that are likely to improve with weight loss. Numerous studies have shown that medications used alone are much less effective than when they are used as a part of a comprehensive program that includes diet, exercise, and behavior modification. In prescribing antiobesity medications, it is important to set clear goals with respect to both weight loss and health benefits. Just as with other classes of medications, continued use of ineffective or suboptimally effective drugs does not serve the patient.

Medications

The medications currently available for long-term use act either through appetite reduction (sibutramine) or by inhibition of pancreatic lipase (orlistat), which results in fat malabsorption. Phentermine, an appetite suppressant, is currently approved for short-term (3 months) use. Because weight that is lost with pharmacotherapy (especially when it is used without a comprehensive program) is quickly regained once the medication is discontinued, agents that are approved for long-term use (sibutramine and orlistat) are more rational therapeutic choices.

The effect of sibutramine on appetite is typically described as earlier satiety, resulting in less food intake, but not less hunger. The usual starting dose for sibutramine is 10 mg in the morning, with a

TABLE 239–7 INDICATIONS FOR PHARMACOLOGIC TREATMENT OF OBESITY

BMI > 27 kg/m^2
One or more complications or conditions that are likely to improve with weight loss
Previous failure of conservative treatment with diet and exercise
Agree to 2- to 4-week trial of making initial changes in diet and exercise before starting pharmacotherapy
Agree to continued treatment with diet, exercise, and behavioral modification while receiving pharmacologic treatment
Agree to periodic follow-up
Premenopausal women (able to have children) must use some form of contraception
Consider a pregnancy test when treatment is initiated if there is any possibility of pregnancy
No contraindications to the specific drug used for pharmacologic treatment

Rx

maximum dose of 15 mg if the response is suboptimal. Monthly monitoring for the first 3 months is needed to ensure a good response and to detect adverse effects. A minority of patients will have cardiovascular responses (hypertension and tachycardia) that contraindicate continued use of the medication. Failure to lose weight during the first 1 to 2 months is a strong indicator of drug treatment failure and should also prompt the physician to discontinue sibutramine.

Orlistat facilitates weight loss through a different mechanism. At the typical dose of 120 mg three times daily with meals, approximately 30% of dietary fat is malabsorbed. As expected, adverse gastrointestinal side effects such as oily spotting, abdominal pain, excess flatus, fecal urgency, and fatty or oily stools are not uncommon. These side effects decrease over time, and the concomitant use of bulk-forming laxatives (psyllium or methylcellulose) can reduce these symptoms. A daily multivitamin is recommended for those receiving long-term orlistat therapy. It is not necessary to take orlistat if a nonfat meal is being consumed.

Both sibutramine and orlistat improve the results of medical treatment programs that include diet, exercise, and behavior modification. The addition of either agent results in almost twice as many patients achieving goal weight loss (10% of body weight). There appears to be no additive effect of sibutramine and orlistat. Rimonabant, a cannabinoid-1 receptor blocker, also can produce modest but sustained weight loss. [1]

Success of Medical Therapy

It has been estimated that more than 95% of those embarking on self-diets or fad diets fail to maintain a significant weight loss for a time that would have meaningful health benefits. The published results of commercial programs are not impressively better, mostly because of high dropout rates. In contrast, organized, scientifically based weight management programs that employ behavior modification in addition to dietary instruction, physical activity, and medications (when indicated) can achieve impressive results, and the combination of lifestyle modification and pharmacotherapy is better than either alone. [2] Although these programs tend to be more selective (accepting only motivated patients), the dropout rates can be acceptable (<30%); and of those remaining in the program, a weight loss of more than 10% can be achieved and maintained for more than 1 to 2 years in 40 to 60% of patients. These results are more impressive than those reported with older, less comprehensive programs, wherein almost all patients regained all weight in less than 6 months.

Surgical Therapy

Bariatric Surgery

Surgical treatment may be indicated for severely obese patients with severe medical complications that could be expected to improve with successful weight loss. Patients with a BMI of 35 to 40 with life-threatening complications can be considered, but more typically patients with a BMI above 40 and several complications are candidates for surgery, assuming past attempts at medical treatment have failed. Because the risks and costs of surgical treatment are greater than for medical treatment, it is reasonable practice to select patients who stand to obtain more potential benefit from surgery. Contraindications to surgery include active substance abuse, defined noncompliance or inability to comply with medical care, and certain psychiatric disorders (schizophrenia, borderline personality disorder, uncontrolled depression).

A multidisciplinary team, including a physician, a dietitian, a psychologist or psychiatrist with expertise in this area, and a surgeon experienced in bariatric procedures, is important for optimal outcome. Defining realistic expectations is an important part of the evaluation process. Patients undergoing bariatric surgery are not likely to be reduced to their ideal body weight. Successful weight loss is typically defined as an average of 50 to 60% of excess body weight. For example, if someone is 100 kg *overweight,* a reasonable definition of success is to lose 50 kg.

A variety of bariatric surgical procedures have been used. The jejunoileal bypass has been abandoned for decades because of delayed, severe complications, including liver failure, renal failure, and arthropathy. If these complications are identified before end-stage organ failure, reversal of the procedure can improve or stabilize organ function. Several procedures that modify the capacity of the stomach (gastroplasty, vertical stapling, vertical banded gastroplasty, and gastric banding) but that do not cause malabsorption of nutrients are employed but are generally less effective than the Roux-en-Y gastric bypass in terms of long-term weight loss and outright surgical failure. Nevertheless, laparascopic gastric banding is better than nonsurgical therapy for sustaining weight loss in mildly to moderately obese patients. [3] The partial pancreaticobiliary bypass and the duodenal switch procedures have become popular because they do not severely restrict the volume of food consumed, but they are more frequently associated with severe, even fatal vitamin and mineral deficiencies. These procedures can be performed either as the standard, open procedure or laparoscopically. Each approach has its advantages and disadvantages in the perioperative interval, but the open procedures are more likely than the laparoscopic approach to result in later incisional hernias.

After surgery, almost all of the weight loss that occurs will happen during the first 1 to 2 years. Long-term (>5 years) success rates are outstanding in good programs. Virtually all patients with successful weight loss will have a dramatic improvement in the medical complications of obesity. For these reasons, bariatric surgery has become an important tool in the treatment of severe, medically complicated obesity.

The results of the Roux-en-Y gastric bypass for treatment of morbid obesity have been favorable. Approximately 70% of patients achieve success, as defined before, with this procedure. The mortality and morbidity (i.e., infection, anastomotic leak, wound dehiscence) of this procedure are low in centers with expertise, despite the high-risk population. A variety of approaches to this basic procedure are used. In addition to the standard Roux-en-Y gastric bypass, surgeons may increase the length of intestine that is bypassed before the anastomosis that allows pancreatic and biliary juices to combine with the alimentary contents for digestion and absorption. These variations are commonly referred to as long-limb and very long-limb gastric bypass procedures. Although greater amounts of weight loss are obtained with these procedures, the degree of maldigestion or malabsorption increases with potentially serious consequences to the patient's long-term nutritional status. Follow-up to support the necessary changes in long-term behavior is recommended to optimize weight loss outcomes. After any of the malabsorptive procedures, the patients must have permanent follow-up to ensure adequate protein, calorie, vitamin, and mineral nutrition. After the gastric bypass procedures, supplemental vitamin B_{12}, iron, and calcium are routinely added to standard multivitamins. The most common nutritional consequences of malabsorptive procedures are disorders of calcium and vitamin D metabolism. An increase in bone alkaline phosphatase may signal calcium or vitamin D deficiency. Low plasma vitamin D levels and low urinary calcium excretion should prompt aggressive replacement therapy. Iron deficiency, other fat-soluble vitamin deficiencies, and cases of copper deficiency occurring more than 5 to 10 years postoperatively have been described. There have also been cases of pancreatogenous hypoglycemia that develop after bariatric surgical procedures. The symptoms are primarily postprandial and may be severe enough to warrant partial pancreatectomy. Findings at the time of surgery in these cases have ranged from islet hyperplasia and hypertrophy to multiple, small insulinomas. Thus, it is important not to dismiss symptoms of postprandial cognitive dysfunction in patients having undergone gastric bypass surgery.

Future Directions

The dramatic increase in the prevalence of obesity during the past few decades strongly suggests that preventive strategies will become more important in the future. Public health approaches that emphasize education have been almost uniformly unsuccessful at preventing weight gain or producing weight loss. Public health strategies that virtually impose behavior change are more successful in this regard. Unless widespread efforts are made to address the problem of obesity, it is likely that its prevalence and the complications of obesity will become an ever-increasing health burden in the United States.

1. Pi-Sunyer FX, Aronne LJ, Heshmati HM, et al: Effect of rimonabant, a cannabinoid-1 receptor blocker, on weight and cardiometabolic risk factors in overweight or obese patients: RIO-North America: A randomized controlled trial. JAMA 2006;295:761–775.
2. Wadden TA, Berkowitz RI, Womble LG, et al: Randomized trial of lifestyle modification and pharmacotherapy for obesity. N Engl J Med 2005;352:2111–2120.
3. O'Brien PE, Dixon JB, Laurie C, et al: Treatment of mild to moderate obesity with laparoscopic adjustable gastric banding or an intensive medical program: A randomized trial. Ann Intern Med 2006;144:625–633.

SUGGESTED READINGS

Adams KF, Schatzkin A, Harris TB, et al: Overweight, obesity, and mortality in a large prospective cohort of persons 50 to 71 years old. N Engl J Med 2006;355:763–778. *Excess body weight during midlife, including overweight, is associated with an increased risk of death.*

Thompson WG, Cook DA, Clark MM, et al: Treatment of obesity. Mayo Clin Proc 2007;82:93–101. *Review of the multimodal approach to managing obesity in the primary care setting.*

Wu JC, Mui LM, Cheung CM, et al: Obesity is associated with increased transient lower esophageal sphincter relaxation. Gastroenterology 2007;132:883–889. *Obesity is associated with increased transient lower esophageal sphincter relaxation and acid reflux during the postprandial period in subjects without GERD.*

Section XVIII

Endocrine Diseases

240 PRINCIPLES OF ENDOCRINOLOGY

Gordon N. Gill and David R. Clemmons

OVERVIEW OF HORMONES AND RECEPTORS

Communication between cells is necessary for development from a single fertilized egg to a mature adult, for an orderly reproductive cycle, and for homeostatic adjustments to a constantly changing environment. Hormones are the distinct chemical messengers that communicate information from one cell to another to coordinate homeostatic adaptations, growth, development, and reproduction; the word *hormone* is derived from Greek, meaning "excite" or "set in motion." Hormones bind with high affinity and specificity to receptors, which are allosteric proteins. Receptor proteins have two essential functional characteristics: (1) a recognition site, which binds hormones with high specificity and affinity; and (2) an activity site, which transduces the information received into a biochemical message. Allosteric receptor proteins adopt various conformational states; binding of the hormone ligand results in the transition to the active conformational state. The initial event in hormone action is thus a bimolecular reaction dependent on the concentration of hormone, the concentration of receptor, and the affinity of receptor for hormone. Therefore, factors that control the concentration of both hormone and receptor determine biologic responses of cells, of organs, and of the whole organism.

Many hormones are produced in specialized glands and are transported to distant target cells and tissues. Hormone synthesis and secretion as well as factors regulating transport and metabolic inactivation determine the effective hormone concentration that reaches target cells. Diseases of endocrine glands that impair hormone production result in deficiency states, whereas diseases that cause excessive production result in states of hormone excess. Expression of hormone receptors is equally important in regulating the formation of the active hormone-receptor complex. Genetic and acquired diseases that impair receptors cause deficiency states, even though hormone concentrations are increased in a compensatory manner. Increased receptor expression or constitutive activation results in an excess state.

Hormones are produced not only by the specialized glands of internal secretion but also by a variety of cells throughout the body. Neurohormones, produced in the hypothalamus, are produced in cells throughout the nervous system and modulate neuronal function. Gastrointestinal hormones are produced within the nervous system. Hormones that regulate production and maturation of cells of the hematopoietic and immune systems are made in cells of these lineages and in endothelial and mesenchymal cells. Growth-promoting and growth-inhibiting hormones (growth factors and growth inhibitors) are produced by macrophages and mesenchymal cells. Many of these signaling molecules do not travel long distances through the blood to reach target cells as do classic hormones (endocrine) but act on target cells in the vicinity of the producer cell (paracrine) or even on the producer cell itself (autocrine). During development, cell surface hormones may act on the cell surface receptor of a neighboring cell, thereby functioning as a cell-cell communication system. Regardless of signaling distance, the same principles of hormone-receptor interactions apply.

HOW HORMONES WORK

Two classes of hormones operate via two distinct types of receptors (Fig. 240–1). *Peptide hormones* are synthesized as parts of larger protein molecules and are processed to smaller proteins that are secreted. They act through receptors located in the cell membrane with the recognition and binding site exposed on the cell surface and the activity domain facing the inside of the cell. Activated cell surface receptors use a variety of strategies to transduce signal information, and they often activate second messengers that amplify and distribute the molecular information. Many peptide hormones ultimately signal by regulation of protein phosphorylation, a process through which proteins are covalently modified when a phosphate group is donated to the protein by adenosine triphosphate (ATP). This allows peptide hormones to change the conformation and thus the function of existing intracellular signaling intermediates rapidly. It also induces somewhat slower changes in gene transcription, which regulate the concentration of regulatory cellular proteins (e.g., enzymes). Biogenic amines function like peptide hormones and bind to cell surface receptors.

Steroid hormones are synthesized from precursor cholesterol. Thyroid hormone, retinoic acid (vitamin A), and vitamin D are synthesized through separate pathways but act through the same family of receptors and mechanisms as do steroid hormones. This group of hormones acts through structurally related receptors that bind to DNA recognition sites to regulate transcription of target genes. This results in changes in the concentration of cellular proteins, primarily enzymes, and thus in the metabolic activity underlying the physiologic response.

Peptide Hormone Binding and Signal Transduction

Peptide hormone receptors have one of three general structures (Fig. 240–2): (1) a seven-membrane-spanning structure in which the recognition site is formed by exterior sequences between membrane-spanning helices and the activity site is formed by interhelical regions inside the cell; (2) a single membrane-spanning helical structure separating the extracellular recognition domain from the cytoplasmic domain, which contains an intrinsic enzyme activity; and (3) a single membrane-spanning helix that separates the recognition domain from an intracellular domain that couples to second messenger systems, as do the seven-membrane-spanning receptors. The protein coupled may be an intracellular tyrosine kinase or another enzyme.

Hormone ligands and receptors bind with high affinities (equilibrium dissociation constants of nanomolar to picomolar), thus providing the specificity necessary for cells to decode the information provided by the low concentration of hormone present among the many other circulating and extracellular proteins. The conformational change resulting from peptide hormone binding activates receptors to signal from the cell surface. Removal of receptors from the cell surface results in downregulation and attenuation of the response. Binding affinities and dose-response curves for the initial event in cell signaling are the same. Biologic responses consequent to these initial events occur through a series of amplifications. The result is a dose-response curve for a biologic response that is more sensitive than that for binding and initial activation of the receptor. Full biologic responses may thus occur at a low concentration of hormone, with a resulting occupancy of only 10% of receptors or less. This provides high sensitivity to small changes in hormone concentration. It also provides significant reserve. Hormone-induced downregulation may remove 90% of receptors from the cell surface. This process renders the cell refractory to the initial hormone concentration, but if the need is great enough, hormone concentrations can increase and can activate the residual 10% of receptors, thereby increasing the biologic response. Such a response system provides high initial sensitivity, buffering through downregulation against excessive hormone responses, but it also leaves a reserve that can operate when the signal strength is strong enough.

Receptors are mobile in the plane of the membrane. Following ligand binding, the mobility is reduced, and they become relatively fixed while transducing signals. Ligand binding may induce sequestration of receptors and may result in their retention inside the cell through interactions with cell proteins, as occurs with rhodopsin and adrenergic receptors. Ligand binding may induce endocytosis through clathrin-coated pits with ultimate degradation of receptors by lysosomal enzymes, as occurs with the insulin and epidermal growth factor receptors. The concentration of cell surface receptors is regulated by interaction with hormone ligand and by other signals that regulate their synthesis and affinity. The concentration of receptors is an important determinant of the responsiveness of cells. Antagonists compete with hormones for binding to receptors, but in general they do not induce desensitization. When antagonists are removed, receptor concentrations are high, and cells are very responsive to hormone exposure. The changes can result in clinically significant changes, such as excessive adrenergic responses when β-blockers are rapidly withdrawn, or downregulation of insulin receptors resulting in insulin resistance in type 2 diabetes. Regulation of receptor synthesis is an important mechanism by which one hormone regulates responsiveness to another to coordinate their biologic effects.

A class of cell surface receptors serves to modulate nutrient delivery rather than perform an informational function. These molecules include the low-density lipoprotein (LDL) receptor and the transferrin receptor. LDL and transferrin receptors, which are clustered in coated pits, internalize, deliver LDL (cholesterol) and iron to the cell interior, and then recycle to the cell surface. Such receptors are not downregulated by ligand but undergo repeated rounds of recycling to provide the cell with essential nutrients. The concentration of these receptors is regulated in response to changes in the metabolic state.

Intracellular Second Messengers

Cyclic Adenosine Monophosphate and Cyclic Guanosine Monophosphate

The concept of second messengers was established by Earl Sutherland, who discovered cyclic adenosine monophosphate (AMP), an intracellular allosteric effector that mediates the action of many peptide hormones. Hormone receptors are coupled to catalytic adenylate cyclase through guanosine nucleotide binding (G) proteins, the β-adrenergic receptor being a paradigm for this signaling pathway (Fig. 240–3). More than 600 human genes encode receptors of this class and mediate responses to a variety of ligands and physical stimuli (hormones, biogenic amines, light, sound, touch, pain, taste, smell). These receptors belong to the seven-membrane-spanning class. On ligand binding, the receptor interacts with a G protein trimer consisting of α, β, and γ subunits. Because G proteins bind guanosine diphosphate (GDP) with higher affinity than guanosine triphosphate (GTP), guanine nucleotide exchange is triggered by proteins that facilitate exchange of GTP for GDP; activity is reversed by hydrolysis of GTP to GDP. Binding of hormones to receptors that operate through the cyclic AMP second messenger system results in a conformational change and causes receptors to bind to G proteins. Ligand-activated receptors facilitate exchange of GTP for GDP, so the activated Gαs (the stimulating GTP-binding subunit) dissociates from the β and γ subunits. The [ligand·hormone receptor]·[Gαs·GTP] complex activates adenylate cyclase to catalyze formation of cyclic AMP from ATP. Each hormone ligand induces formation of multiple cyclic AMP molecules through this mechanism. Inhibitory G proteins operate in a similar manner to decrease cyclic AMP formation. In both cases, ligand-activated receptors act to exchange GTP for GDP, analogous to proteins that catalyze this process to regulate protein synthesis.

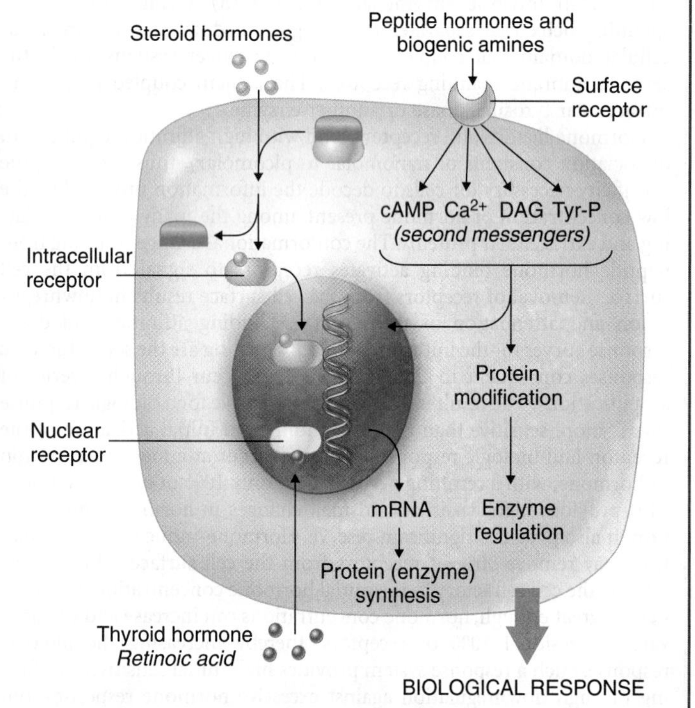

FIGURE 240–1 • Mechanisms by which peptide and steroid hormones signal.

Adenylate cyclase is a large complex molecule with a 12-membrane-spanning structure. The two large cytoplasmic domains have internal sequence similarities and are related to sequences in guanylate cyclase. Activation of adenylate cyclase is buffered and terminated by several mechanisms. First, hormone dissociates from receptor. Binding of Gα·GTP to the receptor decreases affinity for hormone approximately one order of magnitude to facilitate this dissociation. Second, receptors desensitize and are removed from the cell surface by a process involving phosphorylation and interaction with cell proteins termed *arrestins.* If hormone exposure is short, receptors are dephosphorylated and reappear on the cell surface; if exposure is prolonged, receptors are degraded, and resensitization requires synthesis of receptors. Third and most importantly, Gα proteins possess intrinsic GTPase activity so GTP is hydrolyzed to GDP, and, on GDP binding, Gα is inactivated and reassociates with the β/γ subunits. A family of proteins, the regulators of G protein signaling (RGS), enhances this GTPase activity to facilitate the "off" switch. Some RGS proteins are specific for the various G proteins (Gαs, Gαi, Gαq, Gα12).

There are many consequences when this mechanism of signal transduction is perturbed. Mutations in seven-membrane-spanning receptors may inactivate so signaling is defective; some mutations, such as those observed in thyroid-stimulating hormone (TSH) receptors in hyperfunctioning thyroid nodules, may activate so that receptors signal in the absence of hormone. Continuous exposure to hormone results in desensitization or tachyphylaxis. Deficiency of a G protein, which occurs in certain forms of pseudohypoparathyroidism, results in insensitivity to hormone. Cholera toxin, which activates adenosine diphosphate (ADP) ribosylation of Gαs, inhibits GTPase activity and interferes with reversibility so profound and prolonged elevations in cyclic AMP occur. Mutations in Gα proteins that are predicted to impair GTPase activity have been described in tumors that occur in endocrine glands.

Cyclic AMP, an intracellular allosteric effector, binds to the regulatory subunit of cyclic AMP–dependent protein kinase A. This kinase is a

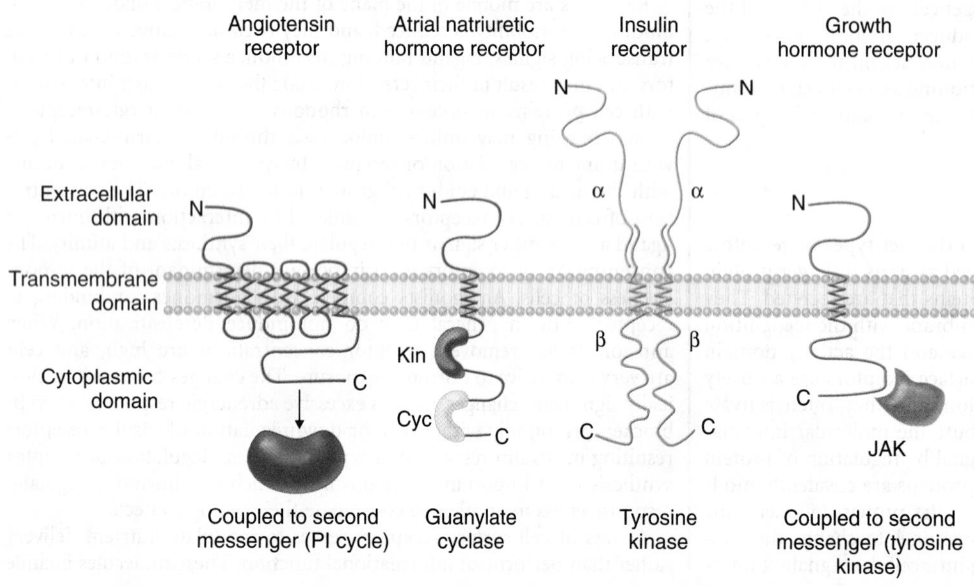

FIGURE 240–2 • Structures of peptide hormone receptors.

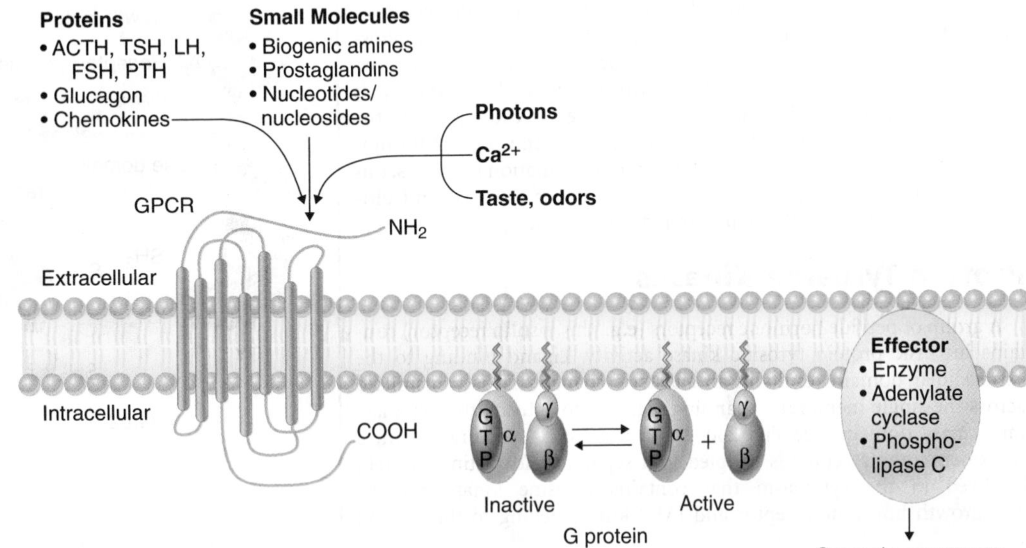

FIGURE 240–3 • G protein–coupled signal transduction. Various hormones and other stimuli bind to seven-membrane-spanning receptors that activate G protein switches by exchanging guanosine diphosphate for guanosine triphosphate (GTP). GTP-bound G proteins then couple to a variety of signaling machines that transmit information. GTP hydrolysis turns off the switch. (Adapted from Bockaert J, Pin JP: Molecular tinkering of G protein–coupled receptors: An evolutionary process. EMBO J 1999;18:1723–1729, by permission of Oxford University Press.)

tetrameric protein consisting of two regulatory and two catalytic subunits. Binding of cyclic AMP dissociates the inhibitory regulatory subunits as a dimer from the two catalytic subunits. The latter then catalyzes the transfer of the γ phosphate of ATP to serine and threonine residues in proteins. This covalent modification by phosphorylation causes an allosteric conformational change in the substrate protein that results in a change in its activity. The hormonal signal is transduced into an alteration in enzyme activity and thus in cellular function. Phosphorylation of cytoplasmic proteins results in alterations such as glycolysis; the activated catalytic kinase subunit also migrates to the nucleus to phosphorylate and activate transcription factors such as the cyclic AMP response element–binding protein (CREB).

Cyclic AMP actions are reversed by hydrolysis of cyclic AMP by phosphodiesterase to 5′ AMP, and protein phosphorylation is reversed by the action of phosphatases. Phosphodiesterases are regulated and are a frequent target of inhibitor drugs such as methylxanthines, which prolong cyclic AMP action by blocking its degradation. Phosphatases are regulated by phosphatase-inhibitor proteins, which are refined by phosphorylation of these molecules.

A conceptually similar but structurally distinct system provides signal transduction through the second messenger cyclic guanosine monophosphate (GMP). Two forms of guanylate cyclase catalyze formation of cyclic GMP from GTP. The best characterized mammalian enzyme is the receptor for atrial natriuretic hormone. The binding site for atrial natriuretic hormone is located on the extracellular portion of its receptor and is separated by a single membrane-spanning domain from the cytoplasmic guanylate cyclase (see Fig. 240–2). In contrast to adenylate cyclase, receptor and catalytic activities reside in the same molecule. Activity is regulated primarily by ligand binding but also depends on phosphorylation of the enzyme, with dephosphorylation causing desensitization. Cyclic GMP acts by binding to the regulatory domain of cyclic GMP–dependent protein kinase. G-kinase, a dimeric enzyme that is evolutionarily related to A-kinase, is allosterically activated on cyclic GMP binding. Like A-kinase, it catalyzes protein phosphorylation to alter enzyme function and physiologic responses. Reactions are terminated by cyclic GMP phosphodiesterase and protein phosphatases. Cyclic GMP phosphodiesterase is activated by binding of calcium and calmodulin. This is an example of a mechanism that provides biochemical communication between two signaling systems.

Calcium and Diacylglycerol

Hormone receptors that activate the phosphatidylinositol (PI) cycle transmit information to the interior of the cell by two second messengers: calcium (Ca^{2+}) and diacylglycerol (DAG). The cycle of PI metabolism consists of synthesis of this phospholipid, its breakdown, and its resynthesis. PI is composed of a three-carbon glycerol backbone with long-chain fatty acids esterified at carbons 1 and 2 and an inositol ring esterified by a phosphoester bond at carbon 3. Distinct kinase enzymes catalyze phosphorylation of the inositol ring at positions 3, 4, and 5. Quantitatively, the principal phosphorylations occur sequentially at positions 4 and then 5. The principal function of activated hormone receptors is to stimulate phosphoinositidase (phospholipase C), which releases the phosphorylated inositol to generate inositol trisphosphate (IP_3, inositol 1,4,5 P_3) and DAG (the glycerol backbone with fatty acids attached at carbons 1 and 2). IP_3 increases the concentration of cytoplasmic Ca^{2+}. It mobilizes stored intracellular Ca^{2+} by binding to specific receptors on intracellular membranes and by facilitating opening of calcium channels. The concentration of basal cytoplasmic Ca^{2+} is at least 1000-fold less than that in storage sites and outside the cell. The release from intracellular stores or entry of Ca^{2+} into the cell rapidly increases cytoplasmic Ca^{2+}.

Ca^{2+} plays a regulatory role in muscle contraction, in neuromuscular transmission, and in hormone signaling. Ca^{2+} binds to calmodulin and alters its conformation, causing the Ca^{2+}·calmodulin complex to bind to a variety of enzymes to regulate their activities. Ca^{2+}·calmodulin regulates protein kinases, including myosin light chain kinase involved in smooth muscle contraction, phosphorylase kinase involved in breakdown of glycogen, and calmodulin-dependent protein kinase important in synaptic transmission. Ca^{2+}·calmodulin regulates cyclic nucleotide phosphodiesterase and adenylate and guanylate cyclases to influence cyclic AMP and cyclic GMP concentrations, and it is involved in microtubule assembly and disassembly. Ca^{2+}·calmodulin is thus able to bind to a variety of other proteins and to alter their activity in response to information provided by the cytoplasmic Ca^{2+} concentration.

DAG acts as a second messenger by binding to protein kinase C to activate this important regulatory enzyme. Protein kinase C also requires Ca^{2+} for activation, so both second messengers of this pathway cooperate to increase the activity of this enzyme. Tumor promoters, such as active phorbol esters, are DAG analogues and act through protein kinase C.

The components of this second messenger system are diverse and complex. There are several isoenzyme forms of protein kinase C and of phosphoinositidase. Although one isoenzyme form of phosphoinositidase is activated by receptor-coupled G proteins, another is activated by binding to receptor tyrosine kinases and undergoing tyrosine phosphorylation. Additional kinases phosphorylate alternate positions on the inositol ring; PI_3-kinase is activated by certain tyrosine kinases to yield unique PI metabolites with functions distinct from Ca^{2+} mobilization. Phosphatidylinositol (PtdIns), which is phosphorylated at the 4,5 position, functions in recognizing PH domains to localize and activate kinases and other proteins, and phosphatidylinositol (3) phosphate (PtdIns [3] P) binds to FYVE in proteins. PX domains also bind to phosphorylated PtdIns. PtdIns kinases thus create membrane docking sites for signal transduction complexes that assemble through proteins that contain PH, FYVE, and PX domains. This process also assembles protein complexes that direct trafficking through the membrane compartments of the cell. Sphingosine, a component of glycosphingolipid metabolism, inhibits protein kinase C, which provides dual regulation of this protein. A major mechanism to regulate inositol phosphate function is provided by specific phosphatases that remove the phosphate groups from the inositol ring to terminate its activity. PtdIns 3 phosphatase is one such phosphatase, and deletion of the gene, which occurs frequently in cancer, removes an essential "off" switch, thus leaving growth and survival signals in the "on" position. Lithium has the opposite effect because it blocks the activity of one of these phosphatases to enhance accumulation of the biologically active inositol phosphates. Like other information pathways, this one generates coordinated cellular responses and is buffered and ultimately turned off when the signal strength decreases.

Protein Tyrosine Kinases

A group of peptide hormone receptors (e.g., this insulin receptor) contains intrinsic protein tyrosine kinase activity. Ligand binding to the extracellular domain results in an allosteric change that is transmitted across the single membrane-spanning segment to activate the cytoplasmic kinase domain (see Fig. 240–2). In a second structural motif, a transmembrane receptor is coupled to a separate and distinct protein localized in the cytoplasm that contains tyrosine kinase activity. The growth hormone receptor and JAK2 kinase belong to this second class.

Within the cell, the majority of protein-bound phosphate is attached to serine and threonine residues, with only a small fraction attached to tyrosine. Numerous kinases, however, covalently modify tyrosine residues in proteins as a central regulatory function in cell proliferation, developmental processes, and differentiated function. The extracellular ligand binding domains of receptors of this class contain cysteine-rich regions that create the binding sites either as monomers (epidermal growth factor receptor) or as dimers (insulin receptor) or contain immunoglobulin-like structures (platelet-derived growth factor and fibroblast growth factor receptors). The cytoplasmic protein tyrosine kinase domains are highly homologous and contain ATP and substrate binding sites, but different receptors recognize distinct substrates to give specific biologic responses. For example, insulin stimulates glucose uptake, whereas epidermal growth factor stimulates cell proliferation. The tyrosine kinases contain variable domains on both sides of the tyrosine kinase core as well as inserts within the kinase domain, which provide regulatory sites that modulate ligand-activated tyrosine kinase activity.

Information received by a cell surface tyrosine kinase receptor is transmitted through a signal transduction pathway that begins with direct physical coupling of the receptor ligand and proceeds through the GTP-binding protein ras (Fig. 240–4). In response to ligand binding, receptor tyrosine kinases either self-phosphorylate or phosphorylate a linker substrate. Proteins that contain a 100-amino acid domain homologous to a region in src, SH2, bind tightly to these sites of tyrosine phosphorylation. The growth factor receptor binding protein 2 (Grb2) is a molecular coupler containing an SH2 domain that plugs into a tyrosine phosphorylation site. Shc is another molecular coupler that is frequently used. Grb2 also contains two SH3 domains that act as a receptacle for proline-rich domains of the guanine nucleotide exchange protein SOS. These high-affinity protein-to-protein interactions bring SOS to the cell membrane where ras is present in its inactive GDP-bound form. Activated GTP-bound ras then couples to a serine/threonine protein kinase cascade involving first raf-1, then MEK and MAP (mitogen-activated protein) kinases. Information is thus relayed, expanded, and is fused ultimately to control gene expression and cell division. Operative mechanisms for this, as for other hormone-signaling pathways, include ligand or protein-protein interactions, activated GTP-bound G proteins, and protein phosphorylation. Receptor tyrosine kinases also couple to additional signaling pathways through SH2 domains in other proteins and through tyrosine phosphorylation of these proteins including phospholipase C-γ, transcription control proteins termed signal transducers and activators of transcription (STAT), and PI_3-kinase. Different hormone receptors utilize different combinations of the signaling elements to activate their target cell responses. For example, the growth hormone receptor uses the JAK-STAT pathway, whereas the insulin receptor uses insulin receptor substrate 1 (IRS-1)/Grb-2 RAS and MAP kinase.

Increased tyrosine kinase activity is reversed by four principal mechanisms: (1) ligand-induced endocytosis and downregulation of surface receptors; (2) tyrosine phosphatases, which specifically remove phosphate from tyrosine residues; (3) reversal of the kinase reaction to transfer the phosphate from tyrosine residues in protein to ADP; and (4) hydrolysis of ras-bound GTP to GDP.

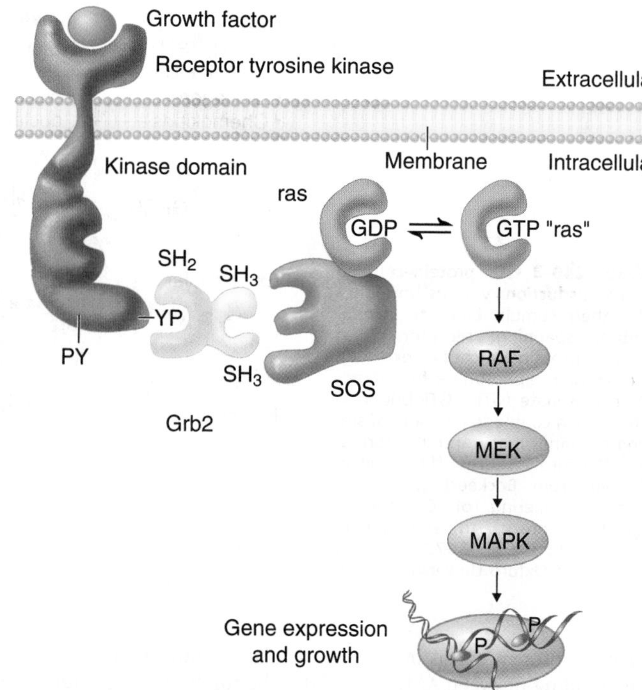

FIGURE 240–4 • Information transfer through a receptor tyrosine kinase pathway. Sites of receptor tyrosine self-phosphorylation, Y-P, are recognized by the SH2 domain of the linker Grb2, which brings the guanine nucleotide exchange factor SOS to the membrane where ras is located. Activated guanosine triphosphate (GTP)–bound ras initiates signaling by contacting raf, a serine threonine kinase, to initiate a cascade of kinase activations.

Regulation and reversibility of ligand-activated tyrosine kinases are important. Mutations involving these proteins occur frequently in cells transformed from normal to cancerous patterns of growth. These mutations can bypass the normal regulatory mechanisms and result in constitutive kinase activation. The kinases may be overexpressed, most frequently owing to gene amplification but also to enhanced transcription, or the ligand may be constitutively expressed, resulting in continuous receptor activation. Mutant ras proteins may be constitutively active owing to decreased GTPase activity or to a defect in a protein that stimulates the GTPase activity of ras. Any of these changes converts a normal regulatory protein into an oncoprotein, one capable of causing neoplastic transformation.

Steroid Hormones Act through Nuclear Receptors

Superfamily of Steroid Hormone Receptors

All steroid hormone receptors share structural similarities indicative of a common ancestral molecule. Some bind their steroid ligand in the cell cytoplasm and move into the nucleus, whereas others encounter their ligand in the nucleus (see Fig. 240–1). The most conserved structural feature is the DNA-binding domain that contains zinc "fingers." The spatial location of cysteine residues within this domain creates a structure coordinately linked to a zinc atom that forms a helix that binds to the major groove of DNA. Because the energy of protein-DNA interaction depends on the area of contact, most proteins bind DNA as complexes. Steroid hormone receptors of the glucocorticoid receptor subfamily bind to DNA as homodimers; receptors of the thyroid hormone receptor subfamily may bind as homodimers, but they more commonly bind as heterodimers with a common partner, the retinoid X receptor (RXR) (Fig. 240–5).

The DNA recognition element consists of two half-sites of six base pairs, each half binding one monomer surface of the dimeric receptor protein. The half-sites are arranged as direct, inverted, or everted repeats. Receptors of the glucocorticoid receptor subfamily most often bind to palindromic sites, whereas receptors of the thyroid hormone receptor subfamily most often bind to sites made up of directly repeated DNA sequences. Small variations in the DNA-binding domain and in the DNA recognition element provide specificity for hormone action. One impor-

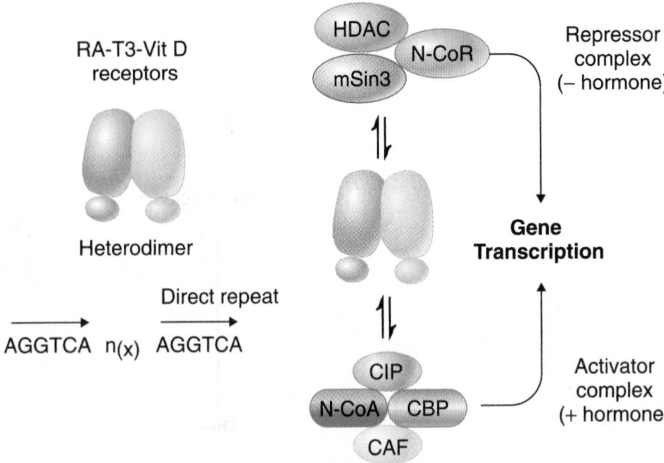

FIGURE 240–5 • How steroid hormone receptors work. Left, Glucocorticoid receptor family members bind as homodimers to palindromic DNA sites. Thyroid hormone receptor family members bind primarily as heterodimers with retinoid X receptor to direct repeat DNA sites separated by varying numbers of base pairs. Right, As a result of hormone binding, repressor complexes dissociate and activator complexes bind to nuclear receptors. Repressor complexes contain histone deacetylase (HDAC) and activator complexes contain histone acetylase (CAF). The coactivator and corepressor complexes contain multiple proteins; only a few are shown.

tant determinant for receptor binding and activity is the spacing between the two half-sites for dimeric receptor binding. The spacing rules for DNA recognition elements that are arranged as direct repeats (DR) indicate that a spacing of 1 (DR+ 1) directs RXR homodimer binding and 9-*cis*-retinoic acid responses, DR + 3 directs vitamin D receptor·RXR binding and vitamin D responses, DR + 4 directs thyroid hormone receptor·RXR binding and thyroid hormone responses, and DR + 5 directs retinoic acid receptor·RXR binding and all-*trans*-retinoic acid responses. RXR binds to the upstream half, and the hormone-specific receptor binds to the downstream half of these DNA response elements to mediate hormone-dependent changes in transcription. Spacing between these sites is crucial for binding homodimeric receptors of the glucocorticoid receptor class, but the sequence of the half-site also provides an essential discriminant. Specificity is quantitative, not absolute. For example, progesterone receptors bind to glucocorticoid response elements, and retinoic acid receptors bind to thyroid hormone receptor DNA response elements. Specificity is sufficient for generating hormone-specific responses but may permit overlapping functions as in ligand-activated progesterone receptor induction of glucocorticoid-regulated genes.

Hormone binding activates the biologic function of the receptor. Cortisol receptors exist in inactive complexes with other proteins; cortisol binding induces an allosteric change that facilitates dissociation, thus allowing the ligand-bound receptor to bind to DNA. Thyroid hormone and retinoic acid receptors exist bound to DNA rather than complexed to protein; hormone binding results in an allosteric change that activates the receptor, so it interacts with other components of the transcription machinery. Binding of triiodothyronine (T_3) to the thyroid hormone receptor results in dissociation of a repressor complex that binds to the empty receptor and binding of an activator complex to the liganded receptor. The thyroid hormone receptor and activator interact with proteins such as the CREB-binding protein (CBP) that integrate information from multiple transcription factors, including CREB, STAT, and the thyroid hormone receptor family.

The steroid hormone receptor family is large and includes subfamilies of receptors: at least six for retinoic acid, two for thyroid hormone, several for 1,25$(OH)_2$ vitamin D and for fatty acids or metabolites causing peroxisome proliferation, and a group of "orphans" whose ligands remain to be identified. As ligands are identified, many orphan receptors are being adopted. Among these are the receptors that heterodimerize with RXR and regulate cholesterol, bile acid, and xenobiotic metabolism. Metabolism of cholesterol to bile acids in the liver, the major route for cholesterol catabolism, is stimulated by oxysteroids acting through oxysterol (lipid) receptors (LXR) (Fig. 240–6). LXRα stimulates transcription of the cytochrome P-450 CYP7A gene that catalyzes formation of bile acids. The bile acid receptor farnesoid X receptor (FXR), in turn, blocks this activation to provide a feedback loop between cholesterol catabolism and bile acid formation. This receptor also regulates the transport proteins that facilitate bile acid uptake and egress in gut and liver.

Two receptors that regulate detoxification and elimination of toxic endogenous substances and xenobiotics are the constitutive androstane receptor (CAR), which mediates responses to phenobarbital-like inducers by enhancing transcription of the *CYP2B* gene, and steroid and xenobiotic receptor (SXR)/pregnane X receptor (PXR), which senses xenobiotics and induces *CYP3A* gene expression, thus metabolizing more than 50% of prescribed drugs and toxic lithocholic bile salts (see Fig. 240–6). SXR/PXR also induces expression of ABC transporters to export toxic compounds from cells. The steroid receptor family of proteins thus regulates many aspects of metabolism beyond those regulated by products of classic endocrine organs.

Regulation of Gene Transcription

Hormone-activated receptor proteins bound to their DNA response element targets act as *cis*-active enhancers. They act from various positions relative to the start of transcription and in various combinations with other regulatory proteins to control the rate of initiation of gene transcription. Gene promoters lie upstream of the site where eukaryotic RNA polymerase II initiates transcription of messenger RNA. The best characterized promoter contains a TATA box that binds a protein, transcription factor II-D (TF II-D), which directs accurate transcription by RNA polymerase II approximately 30 base pairs downstream. Seven proteins (TATA-associated factors [TAFs]) associate with TF II-D in a specific complex that provides a molecular surface for interaction with the transcription regulatory proteins, which are bound elsewhere to DNA. Other promoter motifs include a basal initiator and GC-rich regions in which multiple transcription start sites exist. Gene expression is induced by increasing the rate of transcription. Mechanisms involved in enhancing rates of initiation of transcription include summing of multiple weak protein-protein interactions and acetylating histones to change their interaction with DNA at the transcription start site.

Hormone-activated receptors can also repress transcription. Negative feedback loops operate through this process. Activated cortisol receptors repress transcription of the gene encoding the adrenocorticotropic hormone (ACTH) precursor; activated thyroid hormone receptors inhibit transcription of both α and β-TSH subunit genes. The principle of ligand-activated receptors binding to specific DNA target sequences in the regulated gene is the same as that required for inductive responses. The hormone receptor may inhibit transcription by multiple mechanisms, including deacetylating histones, to increase their interaction with DNA.

Many other proteins regulate initiation of transcription, both as inducers and as inhibitors. These bind to DNA through specific sequences, as do steroid receptors, or they may interact with proteins that do. These proteins may be modified in response to hormonal signals initiated at the cell surface. Such alterations account for the changes in gene transcription resulting from hormones acting through surface receptors. Two general and cooperative mechanisms exist: phosphorylation and translocation of transcription factors from cytoplasm to nucleus. Genes regulated by cyclic AMP contain DNA sequences that specify binding of a specific nuclear transcription regulator (CREB). CREB, which undergoes changes in activity on phosphorylation, is a required final mediator of gene induction by peptide hormones that act at the cell surface to activate adenylate cyclase and cyclic AMP–dependent protein kinase. STAT and related proteins are phosphorylated on tyrosine residues and, when phosphorylated, enter the nucleus to activate transcription of specific genes. This chain of effects alters transcription of messenger RNAs and cell protein concentrations to dictate changes in cell function and organ physiology.

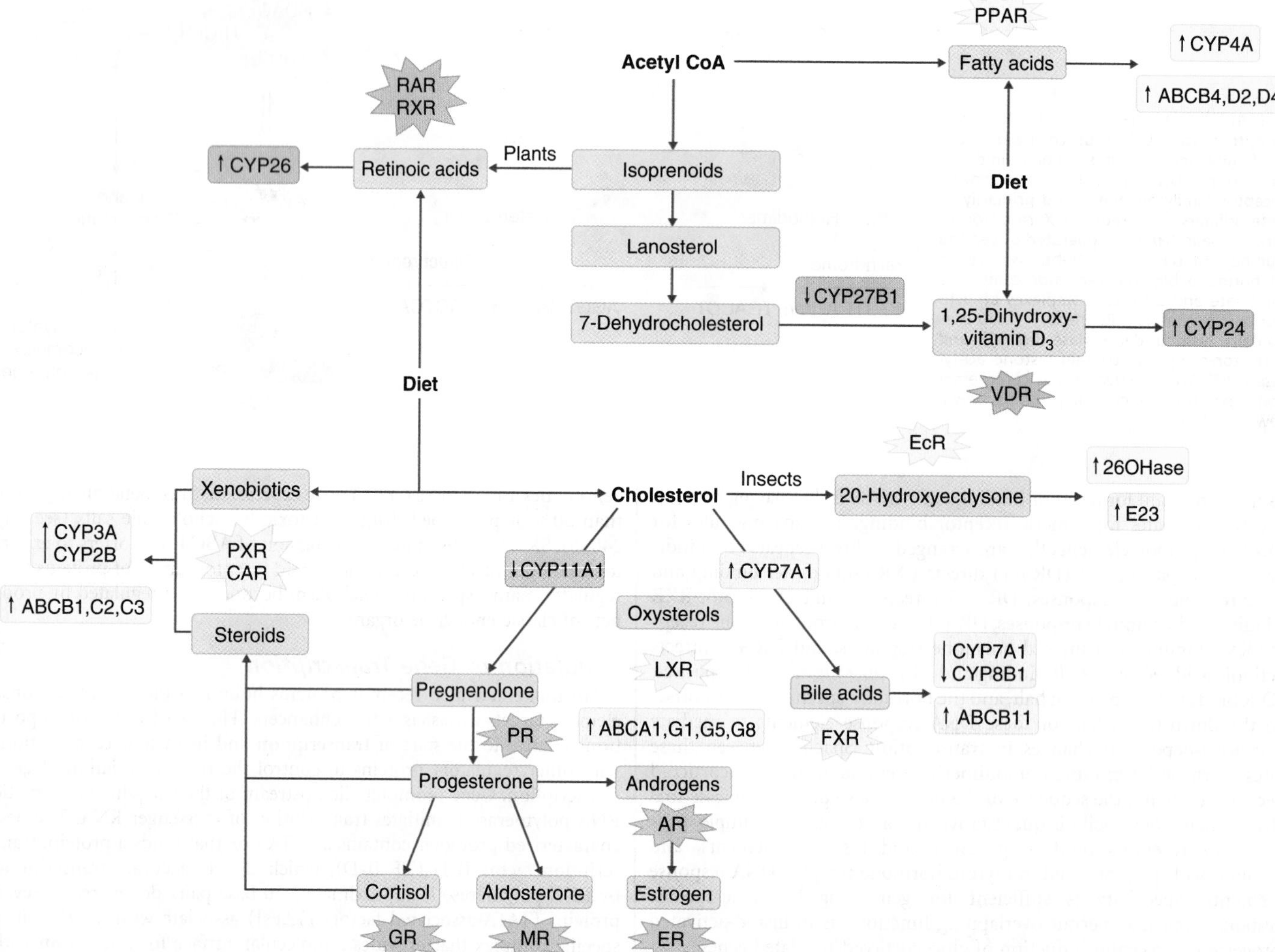

FIGURE 240–6 • Steroid receptor family proteins regulate multiple metabolic processes. CYP genes are cytochrome P-450 proteins involved in hepatic metabolism and steroid endocrine gland hormone biosynthesis. Peroxisome proliferator–activated receptors (PPARs) are activated by polyunsaturated fatty acids, prostaglandins, eicosanoids, and thiazolidinediones. Oxysterol (lipid) receptors (LXRs) are activated by oxidized derivatives of cholesterol. Farnesoid X receptor (FXR) is activated by bile acids. Pregnane X receptor (PXR) is the rodent orthologue of human SXR, the steroid xenobiotic receptor that binds a variety of xenobiologic ligands. Constitutive androstane receptor (CAR) responds to phenobarbital-like inducers. Classic steroid receptors for androgens (AR), estrogens (ER), glucocorticoids (GR), mineralocorticoids (MR), progesterone (PR), vitamin D (VDR), and retinoic acid (RAR, RXR) are indicated. (Adapted from Chawla AJ, Repa J, Evans RM, Mangelsdorf D: Nuclear receptors and lipid physiology: Opening the X-files. Science 2001;294:1866–1870, with permission.)

BIOSYNTHESIS OF HORMONES AND RECEPTORS

Synthesis and Delivery of Peptide Hormones

Peptide hormone biosynthesis and secretion occur through the same processes as other nonhormonal secretory proteins. In general, peptide hormones are synthesized as part of larger precursor proteins that contain additional information. The precursor protein is cleaved, covalently modified, and folded into the form for ultimate secretion.

The precursor structure may have a variety of functions. Precursors for antidiuretic hormone (ADH) and oxytocin contain specific neurophysins that serve as carriers of the peptides from the site of synthesis in the hypothalamus to storage granules in axon terminals in the posterior pituitary. The ACTH precursor, pro-opiomelanocortin, contains information for several peptides that may be coordinately involved in stress responses. Structures in the precursor protein may serve to fold the peptide correctly. The precursor of the hormone ghrelin encodes a peptide termed obestatin that functions to antagonize the actions of ghrelin and this presumably functions to maintain homeostasis. The connecting peptide in the insulin precursor between the β and the α subunits facilitates folding for formation of mature insulin with correctly formed disulfide bonds between and within the two chains. The connecting peptide is then excised and removed from mature α-β insulin.

Following their synthesis, certain peptide hormones such as TSH, luteinizing hormone (LH), follicle-stimulating hormone (FSH), and human chorionic gonadotropin are glycosylated, and this occurs within the endoplasmic reticulum and Golgi apparatus. Secretory granules containing highly concentrated hormone accumulate in the unstimulated cell. During secretion, the membrane of the secretory granule fuses with the plasma membrane and stored hormone is discharged into the circulation, a process termed *exocytosis.* Rapid release of hormone in response to specific stimuli reflects discharge of secretory granules, whereas prolonged secretion reflects release of newly synthesized hormone.

Peptide hormones may also be derived from precursors with receptor-like structures or from circulating forms. Epidermal growth factor and transforming growth factor-α are made as a part of the surface domain of a transmembrane protein with a receptor-like structure. They are released by proteolysis, although they may act on adjacent cells without processing to provide cell-to-cell communication. Renin, an enzyme released from juxtaglomerular cells, acts on angiotensinogen secreted from liver. Angiotensin II is synthesized by a series of proteolytic cleavage reactions of precursor forms that occur outside of cells: for example, renin cleaves angiotensin to yield angiotensin I and angiotensin-converting enzyme cleaves it to yield angiotensin II, the active peptide.

Secreted peptide hormones often have a short half-life of 3 to 7 minutes in the circulation. Glycoprotein hormones may have longer half-lives of 1 to 4 hours. The short circulating half-life and peptide degradation by gastric acid and intestinal enzymes have precluded oral use of this class of hormones. Several attempts to prolong half-lives have met with partial success. Complexing with zinc and protamine creates a slowly absorbed and longer-acting form of injectable insulin; and removing the amino group from the N terminal amino acid and substituting a D-arginine creates a longer-acting ADH, which can be absorbed from nasal mucous membranes. At present, direct use of most peptide hormones is limited to injectable forms. Prolonged action results in receptor desensitization, so recreation of the normal cyclic secretory pattern typical of endogenous production presents a second difficulty. For example, use of gonadotropin-releasing hormone must be both by the parenteral route and pulsatile to induce ovulation and successful pregnancy. Peptide hormones may achieve a prolonged half-life by binding to binding proteins in plasma. The class of insulin-like growth factors binds to a group of high affinity binding proteins that prolongs their half-lives from less than 10 minutes to 16 hours.

Synthesis and Transport of Steroid Hormones

Steroid hormones are derived from cholesterol provided by de novo cellular synthesis from acetate or by uptake of circulating cholesterol made in the liver and delivered to cells by means of LDL particles. Synthesized steroid hormones are not stored, so secretory rates directly reflect production rates. In adrenal and gonadal tissues, the rate-limiting step for increased steroid hormone biosynthesis is transfer of substrate cholesterol to the side-chain cleavage enzyme located in the inner mitochondrial membrane. Cleavage of the side chain of cholesterol is catalyzed by a cytochrome P-450 enzyme that resembles other steroid hydroxylases. These enzymes progressively modify the cholesterol nucleus by the sequential addition of hydroxyl groups to specific sites. The rate-limiting step is stimulated in target cells by ACTH, LH, and FSH to result in rapid increases in steroid hormone biosynthesis. These trophic stimulatory hormones also maintain the structure of the target glands and induce each of the enzymes involved in hormone biosynthesis. With hypophysectomy or appropriate feedback, inhibition of pituitary hormone production and all the components of the steroid biosynthetic pathway decrease. If trophic hormone suppression is prolonged, atrophy of the adrenal, ovary, or testis will occur. Repeat addition of trophic hormones induces enzymes and regrowth of target glands. Induction of biosynthetic enzymes appears directly mediated through second messenger pathways, primarily cyclic AMP, but target organ growth requires coordinate provision of growth factors.

The pattern of biosynthetic enzymes expressed during cell differentiation determines which steroid hormone is produced and is the basis of the differentiated functions of the adrenal and gonads. The fascicularis zone of the adrenal cortex expresses cytochrome P-450 enzymes that catalyze hydroxylations at carbons 21, 17, and 11. They also express 3β-hydroxysteroid dehydrogenase, Δ4, 5 isomerase, which forms cortisol. The zona glomerulosa of the adrenal cortex makes aldosterone through a similar series of reactions, but the pathway lacks 17α-hydroxylase and contains a hydroxylase that acts at carbon 18. The testis lacks 21- and 11β-hydroxylases, so reactants flow to testosterone. Ovarian synthesis of estradiol requires cooperation between adjacent theca interna and granulosa cells. Granulosa cells express aromatase, the enzyme that catalyzes placement of three double bonds in the A ring of estrogens but cannot provide precursor androstenedione, which is synthesized in the theca interna cell located adjacent to the granulosa cell. Granulosa cells efficiently convert precursor androstenedione provided by the theca interna to estrone and estradiol.

The active form of vitamin D, $1,25(OH)_2$ vitamin D, is also made from cholesterol, but the biosynthetic enzymes are located in three separate organs: skin, liver, and kidney. Vitamin D_3 is formed from 7-dehydrocholesterol by ultraviolet irradiation of skin. Vitamin D_3 is then hydroxylated at carbon 25 in the liver to yield 25(OH) vitamin D. This is converted by 1α-hydroxylase to $1,25(OH)_2$ vitamin D in proximal tubule cells of the kidney. In this unique endocrine system, the major site for regulation is the final 1α-hydroxylation in renal proximal tubule cells, a step controlled by parathyroid hormone (PTH) and phosphate.

In contrast to most peptide hormones, steroid hormones have longer circulating half-lives and may be active when they are administered orally. After secretion into the circulation, steroid hormones are bound to transport glycoproteins made in the liver. The transport proteins, which have a binding but not an activity site, provide a reservoir of hormone that is protected from metabolism and renal clearance and therefore can be released to cells. Four transport proteins have been characterized: CBG, which binds cortisol and progesterone, sex steroid hormone–binding globulin (SHBG), which binds testosterone with greater affinity than estradiol, and vitamin D–binding protein, which binds precursor 25(OH) vitamin D with greater affinity than $1,25(OH)_2$ vitamin D. Thyroid-binding globulin (TBG) binds L-thyroxine (T_4) to provide its uniquely long half-life of 7 days. Estrogens induce and androgens inhibit synthesis of these transport proteins. Albumin provides a large carrier system that weakly binds hormones.

Free steroid hormone, which is in equilibrium with that bound to transport protein, enters cells to bind intracellular receptors and generate biologic responses. The free fraction is also the active one in feedback regulation, so the concentration of free hormone is altered in homeostatic responses. The free fraction is very small compared with the bound fraction, but total hormone concentrations from both fractions are measured in most clinical assays. In general, the concentration of the free hormone is proportional to bound hormone, and conditions that increase or decrease the total measured hormone also change the free fraction. The exceptions are conditions such as pregnancy, which alter binding protein concentrations, and thus alter total measured hormone but not the biologically relevant free hormone concentration. In these special clinical situations, measurement of binding protein concentration and the free hormone may be required for accurate assessment.

Steroid hormones are metabolized principally in the liver to inactive water-soluble metabolites. Cortisol is inactivated by reduction of the double bond in the A ring and conjugation to glucuronide or sulfate at carbon 3 to make it water soluble for renal excretion. However, not all peripheral metabolic alterations are inactivating. 5α-Reductase converts testosterone to 5α-dihydrotestosterone, which is the biologically active species in male reproductive tract and skin. Androstenedione produced in the ovary and the adrenal gland can be converted to testosterone in peripheral tissues. Significant quantities of estradiol are produced by conversion of less active circulating precursors.

As with their hormonal ligands, receptor synthesis is highly regulated to control cellular responses and sensitivity to hormones. Receptor synthesis is increased in response to environmental or developmental need or is repressed in negative feedback loops and during stages of development. Receptor concentration is as important as hormone concentration in determining cell responses. Regulation of receptor synthesis is therefore central to providing coordinated and appropriate endocrine responses.

ENDOCRINE RESPONSES AND FUNCTION

Integration of Endocrine Responses

Feedback Loops

Multiple hormones cooperate to coordinate growth, development, reproduction, and homeostasis. When a hormone has elicited an appropriate response, the signal must be terminated. In addition to the buffering that occurs in target cells, feedback control is the principal mechanism through which this occurs (Fig. 240–7). Feedback loops are especially important for communication between organs that are spatially separated. The hormonal products of peripheral endocrine glands such as thyroid, adrenal cortex, ovary, and testis exert negative feedback control over the synthesis and secretion of the stimulatory pituitary hormone. Feedback, which occurs at the level of the pituitary cell and in the hypothalamus, operates by control of several essential steps. The neurohormone thyrotropin-releasing hormone (TRH) stimulates thyrotropes of the anterior pituitary to synthesize and secrete TSH, which, in turn, increases synthesis and secretion of thyroid hormone. Increased production of thyroid hormone induces appropriate metabolic responses in target organs; it also inhibits production of TSH to return the system to baseline. The prohormone T_4 is converted in the pituitary thyrotrope to active T_3, and T_3 binds to nuclear T_3 receptors to inhibit transcription of both α- and β-TSH subunit genes. T_3-bound receptors also decrease synthesis of TRH receptors and render cells less responsive to stimulatory TRH. In addition, T_3 inhibits hypothalamic production of TRH. Conversely, when thyroid hormone concentrations are low, feedback inhibition is relieved, and TRH stimulates increased production of TSH, which increases production of T_4 and thus reestablishes homeostasis. Feedback principles provide an exquisitely sensitive system for

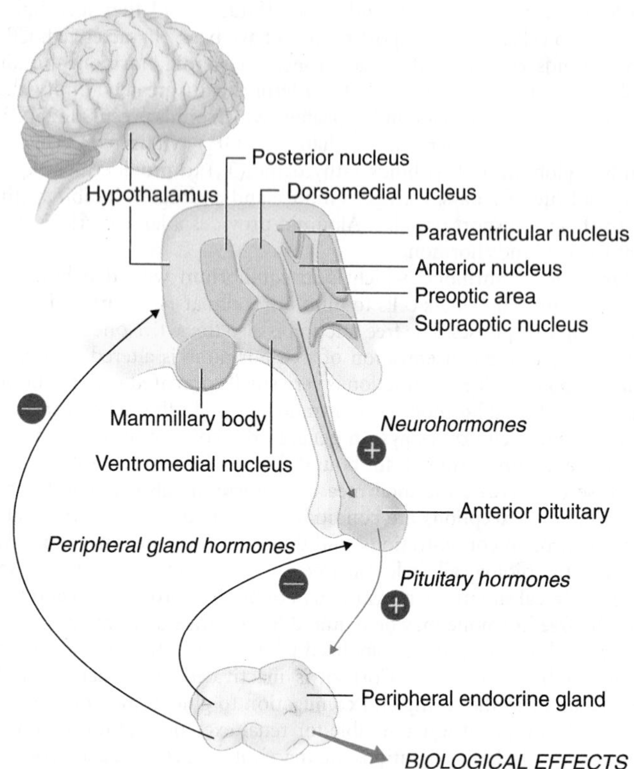

FIGURE 240–7 • Forward regulation and negative feedback.

making appropriate changes and then returning to the homeostatic set point.

Feedback operates not only through steroid and thyroid hormones but also through peptides and ions. Pituitary FSH production is feedback regulated by the ovarian steroid hormone estrogen and by the ovarian peptide hormone inhibin. PTH regulates serum Ca^{2+} concentrations; with hypocalcemia, PTH increases and reestablishes normocalcemia. The increase in serum $[Ca^{2+}]$ acts through a calcium sensing receptor to inhibit PTH synthesis and secretion to reestablish serum PTH concentrations appropriate to normocalcemia. With mutations in the $[Ca^{2+}]$ sensing receptor, feedback sensing is impaired, and excessive PTH is secreted.

Recruitment of Coordinate Responses

Physiologic responses result from many different cell types and organs acting in concert. The necessary coordination is provided both by a hormone acting at multiple sites and by each hormone eliciting multiple responses, which sum to give the overall effect. Integrated responses require that one hormone regulate the synthesis or action of another; the nervous system is integrated into the overall response. Paradigms of such coordinated responses include stress, fasting, and reproduction.

A major stress, such as trauma with pain and hypovolemia, initiates a central nervous system response that includes synthesis and secretion of corticotropin-releasing hormone (CRH) and ADH. CRH is the major stimulus to increase pituitary secretion of ACTH, which increases adrenal cortisol production. Cortisol maintains not only blood glucose but also vascular responsiveness to epinephrine and norepinephrine. It limits excessive inflammatory responses to prevent further volume loss and tissue damage. In the central nervous system, CRH acts to stimulate the peripheral sympathetic nervous system. Increased sympathetic nervous system activity mediates adaptive cardiovascular responses, including increased blood pressure and pulse rate. It also induces appropriate behavioral responses. ADH increases permeability of the collecting duct of the distal nephron to conserve water and intravascular volume. It facilitates CRH-stimulated ACTH secretion. In hypovolemia, the renin-angiotensin-aldosterone system is also activated to enhance vasoconstriction and to conserve sodium and intravascular volume. These responses of the hypothalamus, pituitary, and adrenal cortex work together to facilitate survival from stresses.

During fasting, blood glucose concentrations are maintained for 12 to 24 hours by glucagon- and epinephrine-mediated release of glucose from glycogen stores. During more prolonged fasting, cortisol-stimulated gluconeogenesis is the major mechanism that sustains blood glucose. Insulin secretion is suppressed. Metabolic demands are decreased by inhibition of 5′-deiodinase to decrease conversion of T_4 to active T_3 in peripheral tissues. Growth-promoting hormones, such as insulin-like growth factor-I, are also suppressed under conditions of nutrient insufficiency. In starvation, gonadotropin secretion decreases, and reproductive capacity is diminished.

Female reproductive cycles result from coordinated signaling by hypothalamic, pituitary, and ovarian hormones. Pulsatile secretion of gonadotropin-releasing hormone stimulates pituitary production of LH and FSH. During the follicular phase of the menstrual cycle, these peptide hormones regulate ovarian secretion of estrogen and direct maturation of follicles, one of which increases 1000-fold in diameter and becomes dominant for ovulation. FSH induces LH receptors in ovarian granulosa cells, and both LH and FSH induce aromatase as part of the mechanism that enhances estrogen production. LH and FSH increase during the follicular phase, and, with follicle development, estrogen secretion increases. Positive feedback effects of estrogen result in the midcycle surge of LH and FSH, which induces ovulation. The remaining granulosa and theca cells reorganize to form the corpus luteum, which produces progesterone as well as estrogen. Concentrations of these hormones negatively inhibit FSH and LH production and induce additional uterine changes necessary for implantation. Ovarian inhibin also inhibits FSH production. If fertilization and implantation occur, the corpus luteum is regulated by human chorionic gonadotropin until placental steroidogenesis is established. If fertilization does not occur, negative feedback of estrogen and progesterone inhibits LH and FSH, and the luteal phase of the menstrual cycle ends after approximately 10 days when the corpus luteum, now deprived of trophic stimulation, decreases estrogen and progesterone production. Menstruation occurs, and, in the absence of negative feedback, FSH and LH again increase to initiate a subsequent reproductive cycle.

Cycles and Rhythms

Nervous system rhythms are evident within feedback loops and coordinate hormonal responses. Several pituitary hormones are secreted with a frequency of 15 to 60 minutes, owing to pulsatile secretion of hypothalamic hormones. Longer rhythms are superimposed on these pulses. Pulsatile secretion of peptide hormones maximizes target cell responses by preventing excessive receptor downregulation. ACTH and, consequently, cortisol exhibit a diurnal rhythm, with early morning secretion exceeding evening secretion by at least twofold. Growth hormone is entrained to deep sleep; maximal daily production is coincident with electroencephalographically defined slow-wave sleep. Cycles also occur at different stages of development. At puberty, nocturnal increases in gonadotropins occur, a rhythm much less pronounced in adult life. Measured hormone levels must be interpreted relative to these rhythms and cycles, as well as to stages of the menstrual cycle when one assays reproductive hormones.

Assessment of Endocrine Function

Quantification of Circulating Hormones and Metabolic Products

Endocrine function is assessed by accurately measuring the concentration of hormones present in blood. Even though circulating concentrations are low (nanomolar to micromolar for steroid hormones and thyroxine and picomolar to nanomolar for peptide hormones), precise assays based on competitive protein binding are widely available. Improved sensitivity and accuracy of hormone measurements reduce the need to perform more complex stimulation and suppression tests. Even with sensitive and precise assays of hormone concentration, clinical assessment is essential. Measured values must be interpreted in relation to clinical signs and symptoms. It is also extremely helpful to measure both arms of a feedback loop. Most hormone concentrations exhibit a gaussian distribution of normal values, so an individual measurement at either end of the normal range may be normal or abnormal for that individual. Coincident measurement of TSH and T_4, LH and testosterone, ACTH and cortisol, and PTH and Ca^{2+} gives greater information than either measurement alone. A T_4 value at the lower end of the normal range with an elevated TSH concentration indicates thyroid gland failure, whereas the same T_4 value with a normal TSH value likely indicates a euthyroid state. An elevated cortisol value with suppressed ACTH indicates autonomous production of cortisol by an adrenal tumor. Cycles and rhythms of hormone secretion must also be considered. Evening cortisol concentrations are half or less of peak morning values. Coincident measurement of ACTH clarifies whether a low cortisol level represents diurnal rhythm or adrenal insufficiency; an elevated ACTH level when the cortisol level is low suggests adrenal insufficiency. Measurement of gonadotropins, estradiol, and progesterone must be related to normal values for follicular and luteal phases of the menstrual cycle.

Steroid and thyroid hormones are bound to carrier proteins. In pregnancy, in which estrogen increases hepatic production of carrier proteins, total cortisol and T_4 values are elevated, but ACTH and TSH values are normal. On occasion, it is necessary to measure the free, active hormone concentration. Because the free fraction is very small relative to the total amount, careful separation of bound from free fractions is necessary, and very sensitive detection systems are required. Assays for free T_4 and for ionized Ca^{2+} are available for specialized clinical circumstances. One can assess the amount of binding globulin directly or can indirectly measure unoccupied binding sites (T_3 resin uptake test).

Measurement of urinary excretion of some hormones provides an integrated value for daily production rates. Measurement of urinary free cortisol is particularly useful because cortisol-binding globulin, which binds one cortisol molecule per molecule of protein, is approximately saturated at the peak morning cortisol concentration. Free unbound cortisol that exceeds binding capacity is filtered at the glomerulus, so an elevated 24-hour urine free cortisol determination provides an accurate assessment in cortisol excess syndromes. Measurement of metabolic effects is an essential component of endocrine evaluation. Insulin function is assessed by measuring plasma and urine glucose concentrations, PTH by measuring serum Ca^{2+}, aldosterone by measuring serum potassium, and ADH by measuring serum and urine osmolalities.

Stimulation and Suppression Tests

Measurement of both arms of a feedback loop provides sufficient laboratory information to confirm the diagnosis in most endocrine deficiency or excess states. Additional diagnostic information can be gained, however, by perturbing the feedback system through administration of hormones. For stimulation tests, a hormone is administered, and the ability of the target gland to respond is assessed by measuring its product. This approach provides an estimate of the ability of the target gland to synthesize hormone, of its trophic maintenance, and of its exposure to feedback inhibition. Baseline measurements are made before hormone administration and at the established normal time of peak target gland response. Ranges of normal responses have been established for comparison. Examples include TRH stimulation tests, in which levels of pituitary-produced TSH are measured. In hypopituitarism, serum TSH fails to increase in response to a standard intravenous injection of TRH. In primary hypothyroidism, in which feedback inhibition by thyroid hormone is small, TSH increases excessively, whereas in hyperthyroidism, excessive feedback inhibition results in minimal or no increases in TSH. For ACTH stimulation tests, $ACTH_{1-24}$ is administered as an intravenous injection to assess the ability of the adrenal cortex to produce cortisol. A low baseline cortisol level that fails to increase indicates adrenal insufficiency. Interpretation requires integration of clinical information because failure to respond to ACTH may also occur when the adrenal cortex has been suppressed, owing to prolonged treatment with synthetic glucocorticoids. A variation of stimulation tests involves interruption of the feedback loop by metabolic inhibitors of hormone biosynthesis. Metyrapone, an inhibitor of 11β-hydroxylase, decreases serum cortisol, thus relieving feedback suppression of ACTH production. The resulting increase in ACTH can be measured directly; or ACTH-stimulated 11-deoxycortisol, the precursor of cortisol, can be measured as an indicator of increased ACTH. The metyrapone test provides an assessment of pituitary corticotrope function and reserve. Stimulation tests are most useful in suspected endocrine deficiency states.

Suppression tests, which measure the ability of administered hormone to provide feedback inhibition, are most useful in evaluating hormone excesses. Dexamethasone, a potent synthetic glucocorticoid, is administered to inhibit ACTH production. Because dexamethasone is not detected in cortisol assays, more easily measured cortisol rather than ACTH can be used as an end point. In Cushing's syndrome, the source of cortisol excess can be deduced using dexamethasone suppression. Pituitary tumors that produce excess ACTH frequently retain a susceptibility to feedback inhibition. These tumors are resistant to doses of dexamethasone that suppress normal corticotrope ACTH production but are inhibited by higher doses of dexamethasone. In contrast, adrenal gland tumors and tumors that ectopically produce ACTH are resistant to even high doses of dexamethasone.

Anatomic Assessment

Imaging of endocrine glands is important, especially when surgical therapy is considered. The high sensitivity and precision of computed tomography and nuclear magnetic resonance imaging allow detection of even small endocrine tumors such as pituitary, parathyroid, and adrenal adenomas. Ultrasonographic techniques are also useful for imaging the thyroid gland, ovaries, testes, and pancreas. Radionuclide imaging may also be useful. Radioactive isotopes of iodine (^{123}I, ^{131}I) or compounds that are concentrated by the thyroid gland similar to iodine, such as technetium-99m, are used to determine anatomy and to assess thyroid gland function.

Measurement of hormone concentrations in venous effluent of glands may be useful in specialized circumstances to localize the source of abnormal production. Measurement of ACTH in petrosal sinus blood may be helpful in localizing pituitary tumors, of PTH in neck and chest veins in localizing unusually located parathyroid adenomas, and of insulin in mesenteric venous drainage in localizing pancreatic insulinomas.

Cytologic and immunocytochemical techniques are important. Fine-needle aspiration of thyroid nodules with cytologic examinations analogous to those used in Papanicolaou smears has become the procedure of choice to distinguish benign and malignant thyroid nodules. Staining of surgical tissues with antihormone antibodies provides proof of hormone production by a tumor, and it can be an important guide to future therapy.

Receptors are not routinely measured but can be quantitated using immunologic techniques. Recombinant DNA technologies can be used to define inherited defects in receptors. When oncogenes are identified in specific endocrine neoplasms, these can be measured and mutations identified using DNA hybridization techniques. Autoimmune endocrine diseases can be documented by quantitating antibodies directed against specific organs (thyroid-stimulating immunoglobulin, anti–islet cell antibodies, antiadrenal antibodies).

ENDOCRINE ABERRATIONS IN DISEASE

Deficiency States

The most prevalent endocrine disorders result from hormone deficiencies. Various disease states impair or destroy endocrine glands: defects in organ development, genetic defects in biosynthetic enzymes, immune-mediated destruction, neoplasia, infections, hemorrhage, nutritional deficits, and vascular insufficiency. Endocrine gland failure may be acute, with rapid development of symptoms, or chronic, with slower development of symptoms but more pronounced physical changes. Defects in a gland such as the thyroid may result in a multisystem disorder resulting from failure to produce a single hormone, whereas defects in the hypothalamus or pituitary may result in a multisystem disorder, including thyroid deficiency, resulting from failure to produce many hormones. Multiple endocrine gland deficiencies may also be caused by autoimmune-mediated mechanisms in the polyglandular autoimmune deficiency syndromes. Because hormones participate in coordinated responses, secondary changes in other endocrine responses often result from deficiency of a single hormone.

Deficiency states also result from defects in hormone receptors and in signaling mechanisms. Defects may be inherited or acquired. Genetic abnormalities in androgen receptors result in unresponsiveness to androgens and an XY male with a female phenotype; defects in vitamin D receptors result in vitamin D–resistant rickets; defects in thyroid hormone receptors result in the resistance to thyroid hormone of Refetoff's syndrome; and defects in growth hormone receptors result in ateliotic dwarfism of Laron's syndrome. Acquired receptor defects most often result from immunologic mechanisms wherein antibodies bind to receptors and block ligand access. Postreceptor defects may occur. A defect in $G\alpha s$ results in pseudohypoparathyroidism, characterized by unresponsiveness to PTH. Such patients fail to respond normally to other hormones whose receptors couple to adenylate cyclase (TSH, glucagon,

LH). Type 2 diabetes mellitus, which is inherited, is characterized by insulin resistance. The molecular defect has not yet been characterized, but understanding this pathophysiology underlies therapeutic approaches directed at reducing resistance to and augmenting secretion of insulin. Because receptor and postreceptor defects are characterized by hormone resistance, feedback does not occur; and producer glands enlarge and circulating hormone concentrations are high despite clinical evidence for deficiency.

Excess States

Excessive production of hormone and clinical evidence of such excess imply failure of normal feedback mechanisms. This situation occurs most commonly with neoplasia and with autoimmunity, in which antireceptor antibodies act as hormone agonists. Tumors of endocrine glands characteristically produce excessive amounts of the hormone made by the cell of origin but are no longer subject to normal feedback controls. Some tumors, such as pituitary adenomas that produce ACTH, retain feedback but require higher concentrations of cortisol to suppress ACTH. Prolactinomas retain dopamine suppression, and both their function and growth can be inhibited by dopamine agonists. Tumors arising in peripheral endocrine glands that are under pituitary trophic hormone regulation are autonomous because they are not normally subject to negative feedback. Tumors that contain highly undifferentiated cells may also be insensitive to feedback regulation.

Hormones may be produced in excess by tumors arising from cells that do not normally produce the hormone. Ectopic production of peptide hormones is common in a variety of neoplasms, and symptoms of hormone excess may contribute significantly to morbidity. Because steroid hormones are made through a multienzyme pathway, excesses of these hormones occur only with tumors arising in the producer gland or with excessive production of the trophic peptide hormone. Cortisol excess may result from adrenocortical tumors or from excessive stimulation by ACTH produced by pituitary or ectopic neoplasms.

The most prevalent disease resulting from agonistic antibodies is Graves' disease, in which antibodies are produced that activate the TSH receptor and thus lead to hyperthyroidism. Because many hormones are available as therapeutic agents, some patients take excessive amounts and present with an endocrine excess syndrome.

Genetic Determinants of Disease

Many endocrine diseases result from genetic mutations. Genetic defects in biosynthetic enzymes may result in deficiency states: Hypothyroidism may result from thyroid peroxidase or deiodinase enzyme defects; adrenal insufficiency may result from 21-hydroxylase deficiency or a defect in other steroid biosynthetic enzymes; a form of male hypogonadism may result from 5α-reductase deficiency. Receptor defects are less common, but they have been demonstrated to occur in all major classes of hormone receptors. They may lead to mild or severe phenotypes, depending on their location. Type 2 diabetes, the most common endocrine abnormality, is inherited, but its molecular basis is not yet known. Autoimmune endocrine diseases also have a genetic basis involving an inherited defect in immune surveillance. Multiple endocrine neoplasia syndromes are caused by activating mutations in the ret tyrosine kinase receptor, so cell growth and function are constitutively stimulated without ligand.

Methods using nucleic acid probes can be implemented to make precise diagnoses in disease states and to provide predictive information before overt disease develops. Because genetic defects are present in all DNA, peripheral blood cells and skin fibroblasts provide ready sources of material for assay. Acquired mutations can be assessed by assay of material obtained by biopsy.

SUGGESTED READINGS

Chawla AJ, Repa J, Evans RM, Mangelsdorf D: Nuclear receptors and lipid physiology: Opening the X-files. Science 2001;294:1866–1870. *An overview of the role of many of the steroid receptors in metabolic regulation.*

Marx S, Simonds WF: Hereditary hormone excess: Genes, molecular pathways and syndromes. Endocr Rev 2005;26:615–661. *A review of how constitutive activation of hormone signaling pathways occurs and the clinical consequences of abnormal activation.*

Pascussi JM, Gerbal-Chaloin S, Drocourt L, et al: The expression of CYP2B6, CYP2C9 and CYP3A4 genes: A tangle of networks of nuclear and steroid receptors. Biochim Biophys Acta 2003;3:243–253. *A review of steroid hormone receptors and how they function cooperatively to control steroid hormone actions.*

Smith CL, O'Malley BW: Coregulator function: A key to understanding tissue specificity of selective receptor modulators. Endocr Rev 2004;25:45–71. *A clear presentation of how steroid hormone action is modified by coregulators.*

Turgeon JL, McDonnell DP, Martin KA, et al: Hormone therapy: Physiological complexity belies therapeutic simplicity. Science 2004;304:1269–1273. *Review of the lessons to learn from the emerging data on the safety of hormone replacement therapy.*

Wettschureck N, Offermanns S: Mammalial G proteins and their cell type specific functions. Physiol Rev 2005;85:1159–1204. *A comprehensive review of G protein function as it relates to hormone action.*

241 NEUROENDOCRINOLOGY AND THE NEUROENDOCRINE SYSTEM

Mark E. Molitch

NEUROENDOCRINE REGULATION

Neuroendocrinology refers to the general area of endocrinology in which the nervous system interacts with the endocrine system to link aspects of cognitive and noncognitive neural activity with metabolic and hormonal homeostatic activity. Neural cells that can secrete hormones, that is, *neurosecretory* cells, serve as the final common pathway linking the brain with the endocrine system. The *neurohypophysial* neurons originate from the paraventricular and supraoptic nuclei, traverse the hypothalamic-pituitary stalk, and release vasopressin and oxytocin from nerve endings in the posterior pituitary. The *hypophysiotropic* neurons, localized in specific hypothalamic nuclei, project their axons to the median eminence to secrete their peptide and bioamine releasing and inhibiting hormones into the proximal end of the hypothalamic-pituitary portal vessels (Fig. 241–1). Neurons from other nuclei within the hypothalamus and other parts of the brain influence pituitary hormone secretion by interacting with these specific neurons. The median eminence receives its blood supply from the superior hypophysial artery, which arborizes into a rich capillary bed. The capillary loops extend into the median eminence and coalesce to form the long portal veins that traverse the pituitary stalk and end in the pituitary. The capillary walls are "fenestrated" and allow entry of the peptides secreted by the axon terminals. At the pituitary end of the stalk, the portal vessels again branch to form an extensive capillary plexus.

The neuroendocrine system operates through a series of feedback loops that control pituitary and target organ hormone levels precisely. Target organ hormones can feed back at both the hypothalamic and the pituitary levels to complete the loop, and efferent controller factors from the hypothalamus may include both stimulatory and inhibitory substances. The feedback loops can be perturbed and result in temporary or prolonged alterations of set points by such factors as length of day (circadian periodicity), stress, nutritional status, and systemic illness. The suprachiasmatic nuclei, located just above the optic chiasm, are important in regulating circadian rhythms of the body.

Hypophysiotropic Hormones

Regulation of pituitary hormones by the hypophysiotropic hormones is quite complex, in part because of the multiplicity of substances present in the hypothalamus that can affect pituitary hormone secretion and in part because of the redundancy and overlapping nature of the feedback loops alluded to earlier. In addition, some hypophysiotropic hormones exert effects on more than one pituitary hormone (Fig. 241–2). Some of the hypophysiotropic hormones are also found elsewhere in the body, particularly the gastrointestinal tract and placenta, where they may have significant physiologic functions. All the hypophysiotropic hormones are also present in extrahypothalamic brain tissue and function as neurotransmitters. Several hormones can occur in the same hypothalamic nucleus. In each instance, the action of the hypophysiotropic hormone is mediated first by binding to specific receptors and then by alteration of intracellular transduction mechanisms.

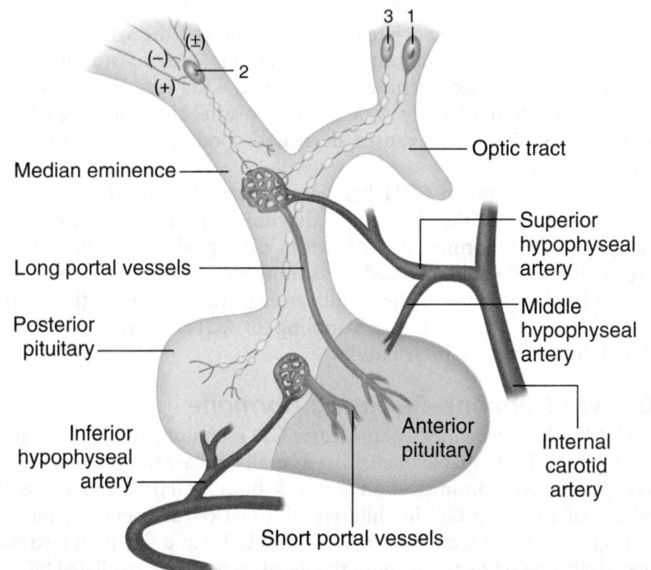

FIGURE 241–1 • Neuroendocrine organization of the hypothalamus and pituitary gland. The posterior pituitary is fed by the inferior hypophyseal artery and the hypothalamus by the superior hypophyseal artery, both branches of the internal carotid artery. A small portion of the anterior pituitary also receives arterial blood from the middle hypophyseal artery. Most of the blood supply to the anterior pituitary is venous by way of the long portal vessels, which connect the portal capillary beds in the median eminence to the venous sinusoids in the anterior pituitary. Hypophysiotropic neuron 3 in the parvocellular division of the paraventricular nucleus and neuron 2 in the arcuate nucleus are shown to terminate in the median eminence on portal capillaries. These neurons of the tuberoinfundibular system secrete hypothalamic releasing and inhibiting hormones into the portal veins for conveyance to the anterior pituitary gland. Neuron 2 is innervated by monoaminergic neurons. The multiple inputs to such neurons, using neuron 2 as an example, can be stimulatory, inhibitory, or neuromodulatory, in which another neuron may affect neurotransmitter release. Neuron 1 represents a peptidergic neuron originating in the magnocellular division of the paraventricular nucleus or supraoptic nucleus and projecting directly to the posterior pituitary by way of the hypothalamic-neurohypophyseal tract, where it releases vasopressin or oxytocin. (Adapted from Gay VL: The hypothalamus: Physiology and clinical use of releasing factors. The American Society for Reproductive Medicine [Fertility and Sterility, 1972, Vol 23, pp 50–63].)

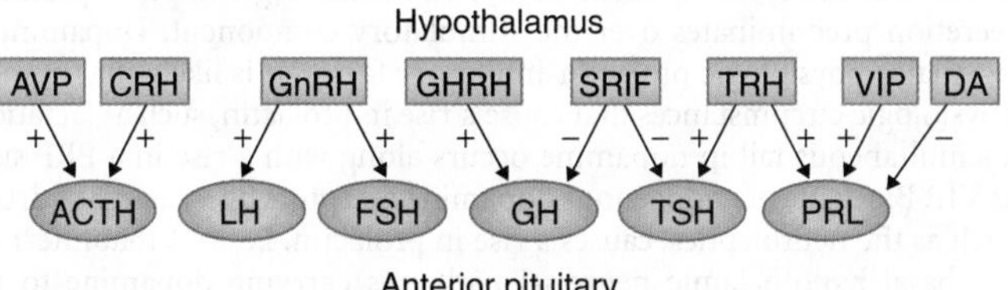

FIGURE 241–2 • Interrelationships between hypothalamic and pituitary hormones. Plus signs indicate stimulatory effects, and minus signs indicate inhibitory effects. ACTH = adrenocorticotropic hormone; AVP = arginine vasopressin; CRH = corticotropin-releasing hormone; DA = dopamine; FSH = follicle-stimulating hormone; GH = growth hormone; GHRH = growth hormone-releasing hormone; GnRH = gonadotropin-releasing hormone; LH = luteinizing hormone; PRL = prolactin; SRIF = somatotropin release–inhibiting factor (somatostatin); TRH = thyrotropin-releasing hormone; TSH = thyroid-stimulating hormone; VIP = vasoactive intestinal polypeptide.

Thyrotropin-Releasing Hormone

Thyrotropin-releasing hormone (TRH) is a tripeptide whose secretion is stimulated by norepinephrine and dopamine but is inhibited by serotonin. The primary neuroendocrine function of TRH is to stimulate the synthesis and release of thyroid-stimulating hormone (TSH) and prolactin. It has been estimated that a single molecule of TRH, through its TSH-releasing effect, induces the release of more than 100,000 molecules of thyroxine from the thyroid. In cases of hypothyroidism, the increased TRH synthesis and binding to the pituitary result in elevated basal and TRH-stimulated TSH and prolactin levels. Correction of the hypothyroidism with thyroid hormones decreases the elevated TSH and prolactin levels. Conversely, in cases of hyperthyroidism, basal and TRH-stimulated TSH levels are markedly suppressed; basal prolactin levels are not low, but the prolactin response to TRH is significantly blunted and returns to normal with correction of the hyperthyroidism. Therefore, although the feedback effects of thyroid hormones occur primarily at the pituitary, they also occur at the hypothalamus.

Although TRH is the major regulator of TSH synthesis and secretion, the role of TRH as a physiologic prolactin-releasing factor (PRF) remains questionable. TRH can also stimulate growth hormone (GH) secretion in patients with acromegaly, as well as in several states associated with decreased insulin-like growth factor-I (IGF-I) feedback on GH secretion, such as cirrhosis, renal insufficiency, anorexia nervosa, poorly controlled type 1 diabetes mellitus, and malnutrition. Such responses are also seen in patients with depression and schizophrenia, which may be associated with disordered central bioaminergic regulation. Moreover, TRH can stimulate follicle-stimulating hormone (FSH) secretion in some patients with gonadotroph adenomas, but not in physiologically normal individuals. Obviously, somatotroph and gonadotroph cells must have TRH receptors, but "activation" of such receptors, which may involve alteration of intracellular transduction mechanisms, occurs only in special circumstances.

Gonadotropin-Releasing Hormone

Gonadotropin-releasing hormone (GnRH) is a 10–amino acid peptide. Embryologic studies suggest that GnRH neurons originally develop in the epithelium of the medial part of the olfactory placode. During fetal development, these cells migrate across the cribriform plate, enter the forebrain with the nervus terminalis and vomeronasal nerves, travel medial to the olfactory bulbs, and eventually enter the septal-preoptic region of the hypothalamus. This demonstration of the origin of GnRH-producing neurons from olfactory epithelium is of clinical interest with respect to the entity of Kallmann's syndrome, in which GnRH deficiency is associated with anosmia secondary to agenesis of the olfactory bulbs. At least one form of Kallmann's syndrome has now been found to be caused by a gene defect resulting in loss of function of a protein that facilitates the embryologic migration of these GnRH-producing neurons. GnRH secretion is stimulated by dopamine and norepinephrine and is inhibited by serotonin.

The primary function of GnRH is to stimulate the secretion of luteinizing hormone (LH) and FSH. Although early studies suggested the presence of separate LH and FSH releasing factors, only one GnRH has been identified, and the differential secretion of LH and FSH results from variations in sensitivity of the feedback effects of steroid and peptide hormones and variations in sensitivity to GnRH. GnRH pulsatile secretion also directly upregulates its own receptors; that is, it causes an increase in GnRH receptor number. In contrast, continuous administration of GnRH is associated with a downregulation of gonadotropin synthesis and secretion as a result of decreased receptor numbers, as well as postreceptor mechanisms.

In women, positive and negative steroid hormone feedback regulation of the hypothalamic-pituitary-gonadal axis occurs at both the pituitary and the hypothalamic levels. The hypothalamic effect is alteration of GnRH pulse amplitude and frequency, and the pituitary effect is modulation of the gonadotropin response to GnRH. In the follicular phase of the menstrual cycle, estrogen feeds back negatively on gonadotropin secretion. At midcycle, estrogen feedback becomes positive, and rising estrogen levels from the developing follicle stimulate the ovulatory surge of LH and FSH. Following ovulation, the feedback again becomes negative, and the estrogen and progesterone produced by the corpus luteum result in decreasing levels of LH and FSH. In men, testosterone decreases GnRH pulsatile secretion, with a resultant decline in gonadotropin pulse amplitude and frequency, as well as a diminished gonadotropin response to exogenous GnRH.

The negative-feedback effects of inhibin, a peptide produced by testicular Sertoli cells and ovarian granulosa cells, are predominantly on FSH at the pituitary. Inhibin causes a dose-related decrease in the sensitivity of gonadotrophs to GnRH, but a hypothalamic site of action may also be present. The related ovarian protein activin stimulates basal and GnRH-stimulated FSH synthesis and release from the pituitary, but its primary action is to facilitate the response of ovarian granulosa cells to FSH. Another gonadal peptide, follistatin, also inhibits the oophorectomy- and GnRH-induced rise in FSH selectively, primarily by binding to activin. These ovarian peptides are also found in the pituitary and may therefore have additional local effects on gonadotropin secretion.

The hormone levels and feedback loops mentioned are primarily those of mature adults. In children, gonadotropin and gonadal steroid levels are very low. At puberty, negative feedback of steroid hormones decreases, and gonadotropin and steroid levels gradually rise. During this pubertal development, variation in negative and positive estrogen feedback develops in girls and eventually precipitates the changes that result in the ovulatory menstrual cycle. At menopause, ovarian estrogen and inhibin production cease, gonadotropin levels rise markedly, and the symptoms associated with estrogen deficiency develop. In men, aging sometimes produces a decrease in testosterone production with a modest rise in gonadotropins, but no clinical syndrome similar to menopause affects men.

GnRH itself has been administered in pulsatile fashion to individuals with hypogonadotropic hypogonadism secondary to GnRH deficiency. This approach has had great success, that is, restoration of normal sexual function and fertility. Long-acting GnRH agonists have been used to downregulate GnRH receptors and gonadotropin secretion in a variety of conditions, including precocious puberty, prostate cancer, breast cancer, uterine fibroids, and endometriosis. Direct GnRH antagonists that compete for the GnRH receptor are being explored for similar conditions.

Somatostatin

Somatostatin (also known as *somatotropin release–inhibiting factor*) is a tetradecapeptide: a 28–amino acid precursor also has GH inhibitory properties. Somatostatin blocks the rise in GH that occurs with all stimuli in a dose-dependent fashion. The interaction of somatostatin and GH-releasing hormone (GHRH) on GH secretion is complex. GH secretory episodes are associated with increased GHRH secretion, often accompanied by low somatostatin levels; the basal or trough GH levels are associated with low GHRH concentrations and more elevated somatostatin levels. Somatostatin also inhibits basal and stimulated TSH secretion. However, dose-response studies using somatostatin infusions in humans have shown that GH is about 10-fold more sensitive to inhibition by somatostatin than is TSH, a finding thus suggesting that the physiologic role of somatostatin in inhibiting TSH secretion is limited.

Somatostatin is also present in the D cells of the pancreatic islets and the gut mucosa, as well as the myenteric neural plexus. Through paracrine and endocrine actions, somatostatin suppresses the secretion of insulin, glucagon, cholecystokinin, gastrin, secretin, vasoactive intestinal polypeptide (VIP), and other gastrointestinal hormones, as well as such functions as gastric acid secretion, gastric emptying, gallbladder contraction, and splanchnic blood flow. Analogues of somatostatin have been developed for the treatment of acromegaly, carcinoid tumors, VIP-secreting tumors, TSH-secreting pituitary tumors, islet cell tumors, and diarrhea of numerous causes.

Corticotropin-Releasing Hormone

Corticotropin-releasing hormone (CRH) releases adrenocorticotropic hormone (ACTH), β-endorphin, β-lipotropin, melanocyte-stimulating hormone (MSH), and other peptides generated from proopiomelanocortin (POMC) in equimolar amounts. CRH mediates 75% of the ACTH response to stress, and the remaining 25% is mediated by vasopressin. CRH and vasopressin have synergistic effects on ACTH release. In fact, CRH and vasopressin coexist in about half of the CRH-containing paraventricular neurons and even in the same neurosecretory granules. CRH and vasopressin are not always released coordinately, however, and stress has been shown to activate the vasopressin-containing subset of CRH neurons selectively.

Cortisol feeds back to decrease ACTH secretion at both the hypothalamic and the pituitary levels. ACTH and β-endorphin also feed back negatively to decrease CRH release by the hypothalamus. Morphine suppresses the ACTH response to CRH in humans, presumably acting through opioid μ-receptors. Central bioamines and peptides also influence CRH secretion. Acetylcholine, dopamine, norepinephrine, and epinephrine stimulate and γ-aminobutyric acid inhibits hypothalamic CRH secretion. Norepinephrine and epinephrine also stimulate pituitary ACTH secretion directly and are additive to the stimulatory effect of CRH.

Monokines released by inflammatory tissue, such as interleukin-1, interleukin-6, and tumor necrosis factor-α, stimulate the synthesis and release of CRH and vasopressin from the hypothalamus and the release of ACTH by the pituitary. The consequent increase in cortisol then reduces the intensity of the inflammatory response and release of these monokines, thus completing the feedback loop. Therefore, this neuroendocrine-immune loop serves to modulate the inflammatory response.

CRH and CRH receptors are widely distributed in the brain, and increases in CRH are associated with activation of the sympathetic and suppression of the parasympathetic nervous system, stimulation of arousal, and increased learning performance. CRH may also be involved in the regulation of body weight; with overfeeding, increased leptin stimulates CRH, which causes decreased food intake and increased energy expenditure.

Biosynthetic human CRH has become available for clinical use. Its major utility is in the differential diagnosis of Cushing's disease and ectopic ACTH syndrome. Patients with Cushing's disease respond with a greater than 35% increment, whereas those with ectopic ACTH secretion have a lesser response. If the results are equivocal, CRH testing during bilateral inferior petrosal sinus sampling for ACTH often provides additional discriminatory information.

Growth Hormone–Releasing Hormone

GHRH dose dependently stimulates GH secretion, and in some individuals GHRH is capable of eliciting a small increase in prolactin as well. With repetitive administration every 3 hours, GHRH can cause the release of sufficient GH in children with GHRH deficiency to increase IGF-I levels and to accelerate growth. Both IGF-I and GH itself feed back negatively on GH secretion, with the negative feedback mediated by both a decrease in GHRH and an increase in somatostatin. This feedback effect of IGF-I is clinically relevant, as documented by the high circulating GH levels that occur in IGF-I–deficient states, such as renal insufficiency and cirrhosis. In children with mutations of the GH receptor that result in a lack of response to GH (GH insensitivity syndrome, also known as Laron-type dwarfism), IGF-I levels are very low and GH levels are correspondingly elevated. α_2-Adrenergic receptors and serotonin activate GHRH and GH secretion, but γ-aminobutyric acid inhibits GHRH secretion.

A separate GH-stimulating system for GH secretion involves a distinct receptor, termed the *GH secretagogue* (GHS) receptor that interacts with a 28–amino acid peptide called ghrelin that was initially isolated from the stomach. GHS receptor and ghrelin mRNA are both present in the pituitary and hypothalamus of humans. The interaction of ghrelin physiologically with GHRH and somatostatin is complex but appears to be of minor importance. However, ghrelin may play a more important role in the regulation of appetite and food intake.

Prolactin-Inhibitory Factor

The inhibitory component of hypothalamic regulation of prolactin secretion predominates over the stimulatory component. Dopamine is the major physiologic prolactin-inhibitory factor. It is likely that in most physiologic circumstances that cause a rise in prolactin, such as lactation, a simultaneous fall in dopamine occurs along with a rise in a PRF such as VIP. Blockade of endogenous dopamine receptors by a variety of drugs, such as the neuroleptics, causes a rise in prolactin. Lesions that interrupt the basal hypothalamic neuronal pathways carrying dopamine to the median eminence or that interrupt portal blood flow, such as craniopharyngiomas or other large mass lesions, cause less dopamine to reach the pituitary and lead to hyperprolactinemia.

Prolactin-Releasing Factor

Hypothalamic peptides other than TRH have also been shown to have PRF activity. VIP stimulates prolactin synthesis and release at concentrations found in hypothalamic-pituitary portal blood. Within the VIP precursor is another similarly sized peptide known as *peptide histidine methionine,* which also has PRF activity. Complicating the role of VIP as a PRF is the finding that VIP is actually synthesized by anterior pituitary tissue. The precise roles of VIP versus peptide histidine methionine and hypothalamic VIP versus pituitary VIP are still not clear. A 31–amino acid peptide termed prolactin (PRL)-releasing peptide that releases PRL from the pituitary has also been found to be present in the hypothalamus and pituitary. Its G protein–coupled receptor has also been demonstrated in human pituitaries. However, studies to date have shown that this PRL-releasing peptide is of negligible physiologic importance in humans.

Endogenous Opioid Peptides

In the mid-1970s, discovery of the opiate receptors and the finding that some of the endogenous opioid peptide ligands for these receptors were present within POMC, the precursor to ACTH, prompted widespread speculation about the importance of this system in neuroendocrine

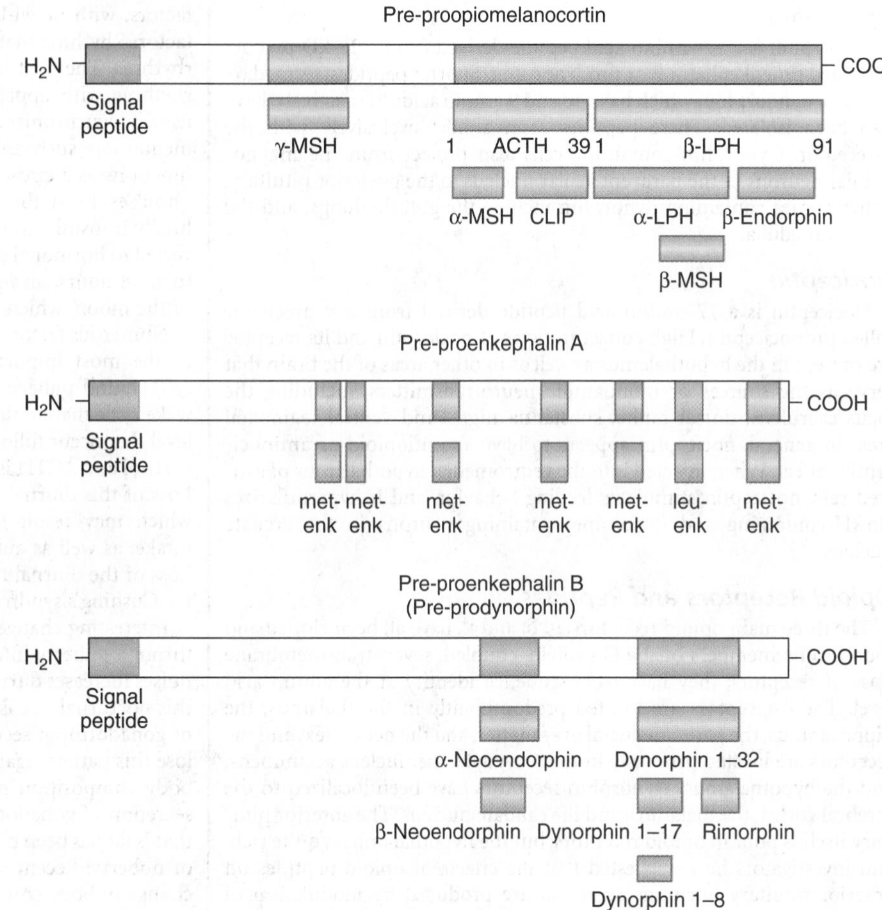

FIGURE 241–3 • Structures of the precursors of the endogenous opioid peptides. Pre-proopiomelanocortin generates several peptides, including β-lipotropin (β-LPH), β-endorphin, adrenocorticotropic hormone (ACTH), α-melanocyte-stimulating hormone (α-MSH), β-MSH, γ-MSH, and corticotropin-like intermediate lobe peptide (CLIP). Pre-proenkephalin A generates six copies of methionine enkephalin (met-enk) and one copy of leucine-enkephalin (leu-enk). Pre-proenkephalin B (pre-prodynorphin) generates α- and β-neoendorphins; dynorphins 1–8, 1–17, and 1–32; and rimorphin.

regulation, as well as the interaction of neuroendocrinology, mental illness, and opiate addiction. Most data now suggest at most a modest role for endogenous opioid peptides in neuroendocrine regulation, however.

The endogenous opioid peptides have a common five–amino acid sequence at their amino termini (Tyr-Gly-Gly-Phe-Met [or Leu]) that is important for their binding to endogenous opioid receptors and bioactivity. Three major opioid peptide receptors and three major groups of opioid peptides (Fig. 241–3) are recognized, but the correspondence is not 1:1. The μ-receptor mediates most of the endocrine effects and analgesia; morphine is its prototypical agonist, and naloxone is its prototypical antagonist. The primary peptide ligand for the μ-receptor is β-endorphin, which is derived from POMC, although β-endorphin also binds to the δ-receptor and the enkephalins can also bind to the μ-receptor. The δ-receptor mediates behavioral, analgesic, and some endocrine effects and has as its primary peptide ligands met- and leu-enkephalins, which are derived from proenkephalin A. It is much less well blocked by naloxone than is the μ-receptor. The κ-receptor mediates sedation and ataxia and binds primarily dynorphin and the neoendorphins, which are derived from proenkephalin B (prodynorphin). A fourth receptor has recently been described that has considerable sequence homology with the δ-receptor and binds to an endogenous 17–amino acid peptide called nociceptin (also known as orphanin FQ). This system also appears to be important in analgesia.

Proopiomelanocortin

POMC is a 31-kD precursor peptide that harbors within it ACTH, β-lipotropin, and β-endorphin; the last substance corresponds to the C-terminal 31 amino acids of β-lipotropin. POMC undergoes tissue-specific post-translational processing. In other words, in the anterior pituitary the major cleavage products are β-lipotropin and ACTH, with a significant proportion of β-lipotropin further processed to β-endorphin, but in the intermediate lobe of the pituitary, the major products are α-MSH, corticotropin-like intermediate peptide, β-endorphin, and γ-lipotropin. Brain POMC, however, is processed primarily to β-endorphin, γ-lipotropin, and ACTH, with most of the ACTH further processed to corticotropin-like intermediate peptide and α-MSH. All neuronal perikarya containing POMC-derived peptides are located in the arcuate nucleus, from which β-endorphin– and α-MSH–containing fibers project to the following: the median eminence; the ventromedial, dorsomedial, paraventricular, and periventricular nuclei of the hypothalamus; the amygdala; the preoptic area; the periaqueductal gray matter; the reticular formation; the stria terminalis; the locus caeruleus; the striatum; and the hippocampus. The projection to the median eminence results in the presence of significant quantities of β-endorphin in portal blood. POMC-derived peptides are also found in the placenta, thyroid C cells, pancreas, testes, ovaries, adrenal medulla, gastric antrum, and macrophages. Anterior pituitary β-endorphin is secreted with ACTH after CRH and vasopressin stimulation (see earlier discussion), but the only factors known to decrease hypothalamic β-endorphin are dopamine and estradiol.

Pentapeptide Enkephalins

The pentapeptide enkephalins are derived from the 28-kD precursor proenkephalin A, which contains six copies of the met-enkephalin sequence and one copy of the leu-enkephalin sequence. Other extended cleavage products with biologic activity may also exist, and the ratio of met- to leu-enkephalin ranges between 5:1 and 10:1 in various places in the brain, possibly representing evidence of differences in tissue-specific cleavage or degradation. Neuronal perikarya containing the enkephalins are widely distributed throughout the brain, as are fiber networks. Most enkephalinergic neurons are short and have the characteristics of interneurons. Rich enkephalinergic neural fiber networks can be found in the globus pallidus, the amygdala, and the midbrain, with specific areas of innervation including the origin of the central noradrenergic system, the locus caeruleus, the origin of the central serotoninergic system, the raphe nuclei, and the origin of the striatal dopaminergic system, the substantia nigra. Enkephalinergic neurons in the magnocellular portion of the paraventricular and supraoptic nuclei project to the posterior pituitary. Within the pituitary, enkephalins have been detected primarily in the posterior pituitary. Enkephalins have also been found in the adrenal medulla, gut, heart, lung, sympathetic ganglia, vagus, and retina.

Dynorphin

Dynorphin is a 17–amino acid peptide derived from a 28-kD precursor called proenkephalin B or prodynorphin. Shorter peptides, termed α- and β-neoendorphin, which have 10 and 9 amino acids, respectively, have also been isolated. These peptides react almost exclusively with the κ-receptor. Dynorphin-containing cells also project from the magnocellular neurons of the paraventricular nucleus to the posterior pituitary. Other tissues containing dynorphin include the gut, the lungs, and the adrenal medulla.

Nociceptin

Nociceptin is a 17–amino acid peptide derived from a κ precursor called pronociceptin. High concentrations of nociceptin and its receptor are present in the hypothalamus as well as in other areas of the brain that serve as the sources of monoamine neurotransmitters, including the locus caeruleus, dorsal raphe, substantia nigra, and ventral tegmental area. In general, nociceptin appears to have an antiopioid or antinociceptive effect. When injected into the ventromedial hypothalamus of satiated rats, nociceptin stimulates feeding behavior, and it hyperpolarizes GnRH-containing and dopamine-containing neurons in the arcuate nucleus.

Opioid Receptors and Peptides

The three main opioid receptors, μ, δ, and κ, have all been cloned and found to be members of the G protein–coupled, seven-transmembrane class of receptors; they have 61% sequence identity at the amino acid level. The δ-receptors are located predominantly in the thalamus, the hippocampus, the periaqueductal gray matter, and the neocortex, and the receptors are located primarily in the amygdala, the nucleus accumbens, and the hypothalamus. Dynorphin receptors have been localized to the cerebral cortex, the thalamus, and the caudate nucleus. The anterior pituitary itself is poor in opioid receptors, but the hypothalamus is quite rich, and investigators have suggested that the effects of opioid peptides on anterior pituitary hormone secretion are produced by modulation of hypothalamic bioamines and hypophysiotropic factors.

The specific functions of the various opioid peptides and the opioid receptors are still not completely understood, although evidence links them to certain body functions, including stress, mental illness, narcotic tolerance and dependence, eating, drinking, gastrointestinal function, learning, memory, reward, cardiovascular responses, respiration, thermoregulation, seizures, brain electrical activity, locomotor activity, pregnancy, and neuroimmune activity. More specific functions regarding neuroendocrine regulation have been documented, however. In general, endogenous opioids have an inhibitory influence on gonadotropin secretion through action on GnRH secretion, probably by inhibition of noradrenergic neuronal input. Exogenous β-endorphin and enkephalin analogues increase serum GH and prolactin levels, but blockade of endogenous opioid pathways with naloxone does not alter basal or stimulated GH or prolactin levels. Opioids feed back negatively on ACTH and β-endorphin secretion, and naloxone can increase basal and stimulated ACTH levels. Opioids have virtually no effect on TSH secretion. Overall, the effects of the endogenous opioids on normal physiologic regulation of the various pituitary hormones appear quite minimal. In some states of pathologic gonadotropin dysfunction, it is possible that increased opioid peptidergic tone is present, but this increased tone appears to be somewhat inconsistent.

Central Nervous System Rhythms and Neuroendocrine Function

Pituitary hormones are secreted in a pulsatile fashion with numerous rhythms superimposed. The pulse amplitude of a pituitary hormone reflects the amount of releasing hormone, as well as factors that may alter sensitivity to that releasing hormone. Thus, the amplitude can be altered by the presence of inhibitory factors (e.g., GHRH versus somatostatin), nutritional factors, feedback effects of target organ hormones, and prior stimulation that depletes a readily releasable pool of hormone. The frequency is generally governed by the frequency of release of the hypophysiotropic factor, which is regulated by the hypothalamic pulse generator system.

The pituitary has an intrinsic rhythm of small amplitude with a frequency of every 2 to 10 minutes. Superimposed on this intrinsic rhythm is a rhythm caused by the pulsatile release of hypophysiotropic releasing factors, with or without the withdrawal of a corresponding inhibitory factor. Rhythms that are shorter than a day are referred to as *ultradian* rhythms. The next layer of rhythmicity is the *circadian* rhythm, that is, rhythms with approximately 24-hour periodicity. These rhythms are usually synchronized with the 24-hour period by a periodic environmental cue such as the dark-light cycle. The suprachiasmatic nucleus functions as a circadian pacemaker and receives light-induced electrical impulses from the retina through the retinohypothalamic tract and finally transmits those impulses to the pineal gland, where they are converted to hormonal signals. Signals for a rhythm with a periodicity longer than 24 hours, an *infradian* rhythm, include the gravitational influence of the moon, which gives rise to the menstrual cycle.

Numerous factors may influence circadian and infradian rhythms. One of the most important is the sleep-wake cycle. GH, TSH, prolactin, ACTH, and pubertal LH secretion are all entrained more to the sleep-wake cycle than to the dark-light cycle. Each has an increase and maximal level that occur following sleep onset. The profound diurnal variation in cortisol and ACTH is often used as an index of "normality" of the system. Loss of this diurnal rhythm occurs with disordered regulation by CRH, which may result from endogenous depression or excessive alcohol intake, as well as autonomous secretion of ACTH in Cushing's disease. Loss of the diurnal rhythm of cortisol has been used as a diagnostic test for Cushing's syndrome.

Interesting changes occur in gonadotropin secretion as a child passes through puberty into adulthood. Early in puberty, the amplitude of the pulses increases during sleep at night, especially for LH, but in adulthood this nocturnal rise is lost. In patients with anorexia nervosa, the pattern of gonadotropin secretion often reverts to this pubertal pattern, only to lose this pattern again with weight gain. This phenomenon suggests that body composition may in some way affect regulation of the pulsatile secretion of gonadotropins. In fact, the percentage of body composition that is fat has been proposed as being important in the timing of the onset of puberty. Recent studies implicate leptin as the signal indicating this change in body composition.

Endocrine rhythms appear to reflect a rather primitive organizing influence that helps an animal adapt to the environment. Circadian synchronization with the light-dark cycle and sleep and infradian synchronization with seasonal changes are present very early phylogenetically. However, because humans are able to alter the light-dark cycles, they are less tied to environmental changes. This adaptation has led to modern problems with these rhythms, such as jet lag, which involves rapid resynchronization of the rhythms with several-hour time zone displacements. Because not all rhythms resynchronize at the same rates, some of the disorientation and other symptoms associated with jet lag may result from abnormal phase relations of various body rhythms to each other and to the dark-light cycle.

NEUROENDOCRINE DISEASE

Diseases of the Hypothalamus

Pathobiology

Diseases may affect the hypothalamus by being localized to the hypothalamus, by being part of more generalized central nervous system (CNS) disease such as neurosarcoidosis, or by indirect means such as by causing hydrocephalus (Table 241–1). Furthermore, hormonal changes mediated by functional alterations in hypothalamic regulation may occur in a variety of psychiatric disorders or systemic illnesses.

The axons projecting to the median eminence that contain the various hypophysiotropic factors are concentrated in the basal portion of the hypothalamus. Thus, lesions located within this final common pathway may be expected to cause significant decreases in secretion of some or all of the pituitary hormones except prolactin, which may increase because of the elimination of tonic inhibition by dopamine. Diabetes insipidus may also occur. Other functions of the hypothalamus are more diffusely located, such as the regulation of temperature, food intake, and blood pressure.

Symptoms resulting from hypothalamic dysfunction are related to the size of the lesion and consequently to the area of the hypothalamus involved, as well as to the rapidity of the increase in lesion size. Slowly growing lesions tend to cause problems of hormone dysregulation rather than dramatic symptoms. Large, slowly growing lesions can cause more

TABLE 241–1 ETIOLOGY OF HYPOTHALAMIC DISEASE

NEONATES
Congenital embryopathic disorders: agenesis of the corpus callosum, cleft palate (*Hesx1*)
Congenital disorders: isolated hormone and receptor mutations, combined pituitary hormone deficiency (*Pit-1, Prop-1*), Laurence-Moon-Bardet-Biedl syndrome, Prader-Labhart-Willi syndrome
Tumors: glioma, hemangioma
Trauma
Hydrocephalus, hydranencephaly, kernicterus
1 MONTH–2 YEARS
Tumors: glioma, especially optic glioma, hemangiomas
Infiltrative disease: Langerhans cell histiocytosis, meningitis
Hydrocephalus
2–10 YEARS
Tumors: craniopharyngioma, glioma, dysgerminoma, hamartoma, leukemia, ganglioneuroma, ependymoma, medulloblastoma
Infiltrative disease: Langerhans cell histiocytosis, meningitis, tuberculosis, encephalitis
Irradiation: for nasopharyngeal tumors, intracranial tumors, leukemia
Functional conditions: psychosocial deprivation
10–25 YEARS
Congenital disorders: Kallmann's syndrome, gonadotropin-releasing hormone receptor defects
Tumors: craniopharyngioma, pituitary tumors, glioma, hamartoma, dysgerminoma, dermoid, lipoma, neuroblastoma
Trauma: subarachnoid hemorrhage, vascular aneurysm, arteriovenous malformation
Infiltrative diseases: Langerhans cell histiocytosis, sarcoidosis, tuberculosis, meningitis, encephalitis, leukemia
Chronic hydrocephalus or increased intracranial pressure
Functional conditions: hypogonadotropic hypogonadism associated with weight loss, exercise
25–50 YEARS
Tumors: pituitary tumors, meningioma, craniopharyngioma, Rathke's cleft cyst, glioma, lymphoma, angioma, colloid cyst, ependymoma
Infiltrative diseases: sarcoidosis, Langerhans cell histiocytosis, tuberculosis, viral encephalitis
Subarachnoid hemorrhage, vascular aneurysms, arteriovenous malformation
Irradiation: for pituitary adenoma, nasopharyngeal tumors, intracranial tumors
Nutritional disorders: Wernicke's disease
Functional conditions: hypogonadotropic hypogonadism associated with weight loss, exercise
50 YEARS AND OLDER
Tumors: pituitary tumors, meningioma, craniopharyngioma, sarcoma, glioblastoma, lymphoma, colloid cysts, ependymoma
Vascular disorders: infarct, subarachnoid hemorrhage, pituitary apoplexy, aneurysm
Irradiation: for pituitary adenoma, nasopharyngeal tumors, intracranial tumors
Infiltrative diseases: encephalitis, sarcoidosis, meningitis
Nutritional disorders: Wernicke's disease

Adapted from Plum F, Van Uitert R: Non-endocrine diseases of the hypothalamus. *In* Reichlin S, Baldessarini RJ, Martin JB (eds): The Hypothalamus. New York, Raven Press, 1978, p 415.

acute problems, however, when a slight increment in growth eliminates the remaining vestiges of vasopressin or ACTH secretion or completely occludes the aqueduct of Sylvius and precipitates hydrocephalus.

Diagnosis

The best way of discerning lesions affecting the hypothalamus is by magnetic resonance imaging (MRI) with gadolinium enhancement, although computed tomographic scanning with intravenous contrast is also quite good. Formal visual field testing may discern impingement of the optic nerves and chiasm by hypothalamic lesions, including the suprasellar extension of pituitary tumors. Detailed testing of hypothalamic-pituitary function may reveal evidence of functional hypothalamic disruption with great sensitivity.

Congenital Embryopathic Disorders

Midline Cleft Syndromes

The most common embryopathic disorders to affect the hypothalamus are the midline cleft syndromes, which cause varying degrees of defects of midline structures, especially the optic and olfactory tracts, the septum pellucidum, the corpus callosum, the anterior commissure, the hypothalamus, and the pituitary.

Pathobiology

Genetics

Mutations responsible for the developmental defects of the embryopathic disorders are the subject of active investigation. One possible mutation that has been found is in the *Hesx1* gene (also called *Rpx*, for Rathke's pouch homeobox), which is a member of the paired-like class of homeobox genes expressed in the thickened layer of oral ectoderm that gives rise to Rathke's pouch. A C→T substitution in one position in the human *Hesx1* gene was found to cause agenesis of the corpus callosum and panhypopituitarism in one kindred. Many other transcription factors have been described that are expressed sequentially during embryogenesis in Rathke's pouch that are important in the ultimate development of the normal pituitary cell lineages. Mutations have been found in many of these transcription factor genes, including the following: *Pit-1,* which causes hypoplasia of somatotrophs, lactotrophs, and thyrotrophs; *Prop-1,* which causes hypoplasia of these same cell populations and, in addition, gonadotrophs; *Lhx3* and *Lhx4,* which give similar clinical findings to *Prop-1* mutations but have additional cervical spine and skull base abnormalities; and *Sox3,* which gives rise to isolated GH deficiency and variable mental retardation and facial abnormalities (Chapter 242). Case reports of mutations in other transcription factors, such as *Pitx2* (Rieger's syndrome) and *Gli2,* describe patients with brain and skull developmental abnormalities along with varying degrees of hypopituitarism. Combined pituitary hormone deficiency has an incidence of about 1 in 8000 births, and about 10% of patients have an affected relative; more than half of these cases appear to result from *Pit-1* or *Prop-1* deficiencies.

Clinical Manifestations

The clinical features of patients with midline cleft defects vary in severity from cyclopia to cleft lip and from isolated hypothalamic hormone defects to panhypopituitarism. The combination of absent septum pellucidum associated with optic nerve hypoplasia is referred to as *septo-optic dysplasia* and is associated with abnormalities of hypothalamic and other diencephalic structures. Some patients with septo-optic dysplasia and hypothalamic hypopituitarism have sexual precocity, presumably caused by a lack of inhibitory influences from other parts of the hypothalamus and intact GnRH-producing structures. Children with very mild midline cleft defects consisting of just cleft lip, cleft palate, or both have been found to have a markedly increased risk of having GH and other pituitary hormone deficiencies. Recent MRI studies of patients with "idiopathic" GH deficiency show an absence of the infundibulum in nearly 50%.

Kallmann's Syndrome

Kallmann's syndrome is a condition characterized by anosmia or hyposmia and hypogonadotropic hypogonadism. The diagnosis is made by finding anosmia and low gonadotropin levels, and MRI shows absence or hypoplasia of the olfactory bulbs. The X-linked form of Kallmann's syndrome, comprising about 85% of cases, is caused by a gene defect (*KAL-1*) resulting in loss of function of a protein called anosmin that facilitates the embryologic migration of GnRH-producing neurons from the olfactory placode to the hypothalamus and the olfactory nerves to the olfactory bulbs. The pituitary is usually intact in this condition, and treatment with pulsatile GnRH therapy or gonadotropins results in spermatogenesis and normal gonadal function. In some patients, other neurologic abnormalities may be present, including cerebellar ataxia, nerve deafness, color blindness, cleft lip and palate, mental retardation, and disordered thirst.

Tumors

Pituitary Adenomas

The most common tumors affecting the hypothalamus are *pituitary adenomas* that have significant suprasellar extension. These tumors can cause varying degrees of hypopituitarism, diabetes insipidus, and hyperprolactinemia, either by compressing the normal pituitary or, more commonly, by affecting the pituitary stalk and mediobasal hypothalamus. Evidence that hypopituitarism is caused by pituitary compression includes a low serum prolactin level and a lack of TSH response to TRH; pituitary function in such cases usually does not improve after treatment. In patients with normal or elevated prolactin levels, pituitary function often returns following therapy.

Craniopharyngiomas and Rathke Cleft Cyst

Craniopharyngiomas are the next most common tumors affecting the hypothalamus. Microscopically, craniopharyngiomas consist of cysts alternating with stratified squamous epithelium. The cyst fluid is usually thick and dark, and the material is often calcified. These tumors arise from remnants of Rathke's pouch. A closely related lesion is a *Rathke cleft cyst,* which develops from the space between the anterior and rudimentary intermediate lobes. Rathke's cleft cysts are lined with cuboidal as opposed to squamous epithelium, and the cyst fluid is usually a white, mucoid fluid. Craniopharyngiomas may be difficult to remove in their entirety, and postoperative radiation reduces recurrences. Rathke's cleft cysts less commonly recur. Craniopharyngiomas most commonly arise during childhood, but they may also occur in adults and even in elderly persons. These tumors come to attention because of mass effects, including headache, vomiting, visual disturbance, seizures, hypopituitarism, and polyuria. Some patients have galactorrhea, amenorrhea, and hyperprolactinemia, features suggestive of a prolactinoma. Careful endocrine testing reveals varying degrees of hypopituitarism in 50 to 75% and modest hyperprolactinemia in 25 to 50%. Surgical extirpation of craniopharyngiomas commonly causes a worsening of pituitary function, often resulting in complete panhypopituitarism and diabetes insipidus because of stalk section, and it may damage hypothalamic centers regulating thirst, body temperature, and food intake. Irradiation may also be helpful, especially in children.

Suprasellar Dysgerminomas

Suprasellar dysgerminomas arise from primitive germ cells that have migrated to the CNS during fetal life and are structurally identical to germ cell tumors of the gonads. These tumors most commonly occur in children, in whom they cause decreased growth because of hypopituitarism, as well as diabetes insipidus and visual problems. Hyperprolactinemia occurs in more than 50% of affected children, and 10% have precocious puberty from the production of human chorionic gonadotropin by the tumor. The finding of an elevated human chorionic gonadotropin level in the spinal fluid may be diagnostic. As opposed to craniopharyngiomas, these tumors are very radiosensitive, and radiation therapy is the preferred treatment.

Hamartoma

A hypothalamic *hamartoma* is a nodule of growth of hypothalamic neurons attached by a pedicle to the hypothalamus between the tuber cinereum and the mammillary bodies and extending into the basal cistern. Asymptomatic hamartomas may be present in up to 20% of random autopsies; rarely, these lesions may enlarge and disrupt hypothalamic function because of compression of adjacent tissue. A variant of hamartoma consisting of similar tissue present within the anterior pituitary but without a neural attachment to the hypothalamus is called a *choristoma* or *gangliocytoma*. These neuronal tumors are of particular endocrine interest because they can produce hypophysiotropic hormones. Several cases associated with precocious puberty have been reported in which the hamartomas produced GnRH. Successful treatment has been reported with surgery and with the administration of a long-acting GnRH analogue, which suppresses gonadotropin secretion but does not affect the tumor itself. If the hamartoma does not cause other problems from mass effects, medical therapy with the GnRH analogue may be the best choice, because surgery can be noncurative or even fatal. Some gangliocytomas have been reported that produced GHRH and acromegaly or CRH and Cushing's syndrome.

Other Tumors

Other tumors and space-occupying lesions occurring in the suprasellar area include arachnoid cysts, meningiomas, gliomas, astrocytomas, chordomas, infundibulomas, cholesteatomas, neurofibromas, lipomas, and metastatic cancer (particularly from the breast and lung). Any such lesion may be manifested by varying degrees of hypopituitarism, diabetes insipidus, and hyperprolactinemia, and surgical therapy often worsens the hormonal deficit and may cause other hypothalamic damage.

Inflammatory Disorders

Sarcoidosis

CNS involvement in cases of *sarcoidosis* occurs in 1 to 5% of patients, as determined on clinical grounds, and in up to 16% of cases at autopsy. Isolated CNS sarcoidosis is quite uncommon, however. When sarcoidosis does involve the CNS, the hypothalamus is affected in 10 to 20% of cases. Sarcoid granulomas can involve the hypothalamus, stalk, or pituitary and may be infiltrative or occur as a mass lesion. Rarely, sarcoid granulomas can be manifested as an expanding intrasellar mass mimicking a pituitary tumor. The most common endocrine findings are varying degrees of hypopituitarism, diabetes insipidus, and hyperprolactinemia. Obesity secondary to hypothalamic involvement by sarcoidosis has also been reported. In patients with isolated CNS sarcoidosis, the diagnosis may be extremely difficult. Examination of cerebrospinal fluid usually shows elevated protein levels, low glucose levels, pleocytosis, and variable elevations of angiotensin-converting enzyme. However, biopsy is often necessary. Although corticosteroid therapy has been reported to reverse the thirst disorders at least partially, anterior pituitary hormone deficits usually do not respond to treatment.

Langerhans Cell Histiocytosis

Langerhans cell histiocytosis or eosinophilic granulomatous infiltration of the hypothalamus may cause diabetes insipidus, varying degrees of hypopituitarism, and hyperprolactinemia. It is the most common cause of diabetes insipidus in children. Usually, this infiltration appears as a thickening of the pituitary stalk, but it may also appear as a mass lesion of the hypothalamus or the pituitary. Osteolytic lesions may be present in the jaw or mastoid, so radiographs of the jaw are a worthwhile part of the diagnostic evaluation of an unknown suprasellar mass or diabetes insipidus for this reason. Therapy consists of local surgery, focal irradiation, or chemotherapy with alkylating agents and high-dose corticosteroids.

Vascular Disease

An enlarging aneurysm may be manifested as a mass lesion of the hypothalamic-pituitary area and may cause hypopituitarism and visual field defects. Obviously, the distinction must be made before surgery. Tumors and aneurysms may also coexist, and careful radiologic evaluation with MRI is necessary to discern such association. Hypothalamic disease caused by vascular infarction is extremely rare.

Trauma

Head trauma can cause defects ranging from isolated ACTH deficiency to panhypopituitarism with diabetes insipidus. Within the first 72 hours of trauma, GH, LH, ACTH, TSH, and prolactin levels may actually be elevated in blood, perhaps because of acute release. These levels subsequently fall, and either pituitary function returns to normal or hypopituitarism develops. In patients dying of head injury, anterior pituitary infarction has been found in 16% of cases, posterior pituitary hemorrhage in 34%, and hypothalamic hemorrhage or infarction in 42% of cases. The paraventricular and supraoptic nuclei and median eminence are particularly involved with microhemorrhages, hence the high frequency of panhypopituitarism with diabetes insipidus. With frontal injuries, the brain travels backward but the pituitary cannot move; consequently, the pituitary stalk becomes avulsed, with interruption of the portal vessels. Most patients with head injury are hyperprolactinemic, a finding that clinically confirms that the hypothalamus or stalk is the primary site of injury.

Irradiation

Whole brain irradiation for intracranial neoplasms frequently results in hypothalamic dysfunction, as evidenced by endocrine abnormalities and behavioral changes. The most common endocrine abnormality is hyperprolactinemia, but hypopituitarism can also occur. When the radiation therapy is targeted to the hypothalamic area, as in patients with tumors in that area or nasopharyngeal carcinomas, hypopituitarism occurs even more frequently. The frequencies of loss of pituitary function are so high that all patients who have had their pituitary and hypothalamic areas irradiated must be monitored periodically for the purpose of detecting these deficits when they occur. However, the development of such deficiencies may take many years, so yearly testing is warranted for up to 20 years. It appears that stereotactic irradiation using the gamma knife apparatus or a linear accelerator for pituitary and other parasellar tumors causes a risk of hypopituitarism similar to that of conventional irradiation.

Effects of Hypothalamic Disease on Pituitary Function

Hypothalamic disease can cause both pituitary hyperfunction and hypofunction in varying degrees of severity. Although severe disease can cause absolute deficiencies of the various hormones, milder disease may produce a subtle alteration in feedback loops and timing such that, for example, the integration of signals necessary for menstrual cycling is lost, with subsequent hypothalamic amenorrhea. Furthermore, the hypothalamic defects may be interrelated. The common finding of hyperprolactinemia occurring with hypothalamic dysfunction causes hypogonadotropic hypogonadism that is reversible when the elevated prolactin levels are brought down to normal. In many cases, no structural lesion can be found on MRI, and a functional defect caused by altered neurotransmitter regulation is invoked.

Growth Hormone

Loss of normal GH secretion is the most common hormonal defect occurring with structural hypothalamic disease. Congenital idiopathic GH deficiency is a heterogeneous disorder consisting of hypothalamic and pituitary defects, and it has a reported incidence between 1 in 3500 and 1 in 10,000 live births. The diagnosis is usually made between 1 and 3 years of age because of impaired growth. Between 5 and 30% of subjects with idiopathic GH deficiency have an affected relative, and thus their defect is thought to have a genetic basis. One autosomal dominant form of complete GH deficiency has been found to be associated with deletion of the gene for GH. About three fourths of patients with GH deficiency have a normal GH response to exogenous GHRH, a finding implying that the defect is probably disordered hypothalamic regulation. Defects in the gene for GHRH have not been found, but a rare form of GH deficiency has been determined to be caused by a mutation in the GHRH receptor. As noted earlier, nearly half of children with "idiopathic" GH deficiency have midline cleft defects, and MRI scans should be performed routinely as part of the evaluation.

Emotional Deprivation Syndrome

A reversible form of idiopathic GH deficiency caused by inadequate parental care and affection is referred to as the *emotional deprivation syndrome* or *psychosocial dwarfism*. Restoration of a proper social environment for such a child results in prompt normalization of GH secretion and growth. Investigators have hypothesized that the disordered GH regulation results from psychogenic alteration of the neurotransmitter balance necessary for normal GHRH and somatostatin secretion. Other systemic illnesses such as inflammatory bowel disease, often occult, may also decrease GH secretion and growth; treatment of the systemic illness corrects the growth abnormality. Treatment of children and adults with GH deficiency is discussed in Chapter 242.

Gonadotropins

Both hypogonadism and hypergonadism can occur as a result of hypothalamic dysfunction.

Hypothalamic Hypogonadism

Pathobiology

The primary defect in this group of disorders is thought to involve the secretion of GnRH, with resultant impairment in pituitary gonadotropin secretion and gonadal function. The disorders causing these conditions may be primary, that is, congenital defects, or acquired. Depending on the time of onset, they are manifested as delayed puberty, interruption of pubertal progression, or loss of adult gonadal function. The lesions responsible for these disorders may cause loss of other hormones or may be isolated to GnRH. Loss of gonadotropin secretion as the result of hypothalamic structural damage is the second most common defect after GH deficiency. However, many of these defects are the result of hyperprolactinemia and are reversible with correction of the hyperprolactinemia. In some cases, the defect is idiopathic.

Lesions occurring prepubertally result in the failure of onset of puberty or, if the defect is partial, in incomplete progression of puberty. If the disorder is limited to GnRH and the gonadotropins, prior growth and development are normal, but the growth spurt occurring at puberty is lost. Undescended testes are present in 50% of patients with GnRH deficiency, probably secondary to the absence of gonadotropins during fetal development. The most common congenital lesion causing prepubertal GnRH deficiency is Kallmann's syndrome, which affects 50% of boys and 37% of girls seen with isolated gonadotropin deficiency (see earlier). In other patients with idiopathic GnRH deficiency, the gene for GnRH appears to be normal, but the gene for the GnRH receptor may be abnormal. Indirect measures of functional GnRH secretion show, however, that disorders of pulse amplitude or frequency, or both, may be present. When hyperprolactinemia occurs before puberty, it can prevent the onset of puberty and must always be looked for in this setting.

Treatment Rx

The ideal therapy for patients with GnRH deficiency is replacement of GnRH by subcutaneous administration every 2 hours with a portable pump. This treatment causes a rapid rise in LH and FSH responses to GnRH, a rise in testosterone to normal, and the development of normal spermatogenesis in men. Similar approaches in women result in ovulatory cycles in 80%. The success of such therapy confirms the original hypothesis of a primary defect of GnRH secretion. In men, comparable results can be obtained with exogenous gonadotropins given three times per week. GnRH therapy is not successful in patients with GnRH receptor mutations. Replacement with testosterone alone causes adequate androgenization but does not increase testicular size or enhance spermatogenesis.

Loss of formerly normal GnRH secretion in adults may result from structural hypothalamic damage such as a tumor, a functional change unassociated with a detectable lesion, or hyperprolactinemia. Structural disease must be excluded in such patients by computed tomography or MRI. Most but not all cases of functional hypogonadotropic hypogonadism occur in women, and the most common causes are weight loss, excessive exercise, psychogenic stress, and systemic illness. In some women, the exercise results in a loss of body fat not detected with total body weight measures, and it is unclear whether the hypogonadism is directly caused by the loss of body fat or by the exercise per se. Studies of pulsatile gonadotropin secretion in such patients reveal absent pulses. Usually, the gonadotropin response to injected GnRH is normal. Regain of weight and cessation of the exercise result in resumption of normal gonadal function. Furthermore, the administration of leptin to such women results in resumption of normal gonadotropin pulsatile secretion and ovulation, a finding confirming leptin's key role in mediating the influence of body energy stores on reproductive function. Hyperprolactinemia occurring postpubertally can also decrease GnRH and the pulsatile secretion of LH and FSH and can thereby result in anovulation with oligomenorrhea or amenorrhea in women and impotence and infertility in men.

Therapy should be directed at the underlying process, if possible. Efforts at weight gain and exercise restriction should be made when appropriate. Two goals in the treatment of idiopathic, functional

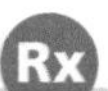

hypogonadotropic amenorrhea are (1) restoration of a normal estrogen status to promote well-being and to prevent osteoporosis and (2) facilitation of ovulation for fertility. The former can generally be achieved with cyclic estrogen and progesterone, whereas the latter may require clomiphene or GnRH or gonadotropin therapy. In men, similar goals may be achieved with testosterone or GnRH or gonadotropins.

Hypothalamic Hypergonadism (Precocious Puberty)

Precocious puberty is defined as the onset of puberty before the age of 8 years in girls or 9 years in boys. "Pseudo"-precocious puberty is that resulting from peripheral (gonadal or adrenal) causes. Central, "true," or GnRH-dependent precocious puberty is characterized by hormonal changes similar to those that occur at the time of normal puberty, that is, an increase in the pulsatile release of LH, an increase in the gonadotropin response to GnRH, and an increase in gonadal steroid secretion. GnRH-dependent precocious puberty therefore represents premature activation of this GnRH pulse generator by a variety of lesions, or it may also be idiopathic.

Pathobiology

Fewer than one fourth of cases of central precocious puberty occur in boys, but boys tend to have more serious underlying disease. In boys with central, GnRH-dependent precocious puberty, hypothalamic hamartomas account for 38% of cases, other CNS lesions represent 31%, familial disease accounts for 23%, and idiopathic disease accounts for only 8%. The picture is quite different in girls, however: hypothalamic hamartomas account for only 15% of cases, other CNS lesions represent 14%, the McCune-Albright syndrome (polyostotic fibrous dysplasia) accounts for 6%, and fully 65% of cases are idiopathic. Dysgerminomas in the suprasellar or pineal region can produce chorionic gonadotropin, which acts like LH in its stimulation of gonadal function. Usually, such tumors cause increased sex steroid formation but fail to cause ovulation.

Treatment

Rx

Therapy for central GnRH-dependent precocious puberty consists of surgical removal of the tumor or medical therapy with a long-acting GnRH analogue. The latter can suppress gonadotropin and sex steroid hormone levels and cause stabilization or even regression of secondary sex characteristics and a slowing of growth and bone maturation in most cases. When therapy is discontinued at the normal time of puberty, sex steroid levels increase, secondary sexual characteristics again develop, growth increases, and regular menses occur spontaneously. For patients who do not respond to GnRH analogues, treatment with medroxyprogesterone acetate or testolactone, an aromatase inhibitor, is indicated.

Hypothalamic Hyperprolactinemia

Diagnosis

Structural or infiltrative lesions of the hypothalamus, such as those discussed earlier, can decrease the amount of dopamine reaching the lactotrophs and thus cause modest hyperprolactinemia. Prolactin elevations resulting from such lesions rarely exceed 150 ng/mL and are usually less than 100 ng/mL. Similar elevations are also seen in patients with the empty sella syndrome.

Because their therapy is quite different, it is very important to differentiate nonsecreting pituitary adenomas with extensive suprasellar extension causing prolactin elevations in this range from prolactin-secreting adenomas, which, when of such a large size, usually cause prolactin elevations 5 to 50 times higher. A peculiarity of two-site immunoassays, referred to as the *hook effect,* can sometimes cause a very high prolactin level to read falsely normal or just mildly elevated; a 1:100 dilution of the serum sample with saline will show the true level when the specimen is reevaluated. In all patients with very large tumors, prolactin should be measured undiluted and at 1:100 dilution to avoid this important spurious finding. Numerous medications, antipsychotic agents in particular, can cause hyperprolactinemia, primarily by interfering with central catecholamines (Table 241–2).

Treatment

prolactinemia itself may impair gonadal function, so efforts may also be made to lower prolactin levels with dopamine agonists. Prolactin levels usually fall quite readily in such patients. Restoration of gonadal function is not automatic, however, because the primary

TABLE 241–2 ETIOLOGY OF HYPERPROLACTINEMIA

PITUITARY DISEASE
Prolactinomas
Acromegaly
Empty sella syndrome
Lymphocytic hypophysitis
Cushing's disease
Pituitary stalk section
HYPOTHALAMIC DISEASE
Craniopharyngiomas
Meningiomas
Dysgerminomas
Nonsecreting pituitary adenomas
Other tumors
Sarcoidosis
Eosinophilic granuloma
Neuraxis irradiation
Vascular disorders
NEUROGENIC FACTORS
Chest wall lesions
Spinal cord lesions
Breast stimulation
OTHER CONDITIONS
Pregnancy
Hypothyroidism
Chronic renal failure
Cirrhosis
Pseudocyesis
Adrenal insufficiency
Idiopathic conditions
MEDICATIONS
Antipsychotic agents
Atypical antipsychotic agents
Monoamine oxidase inhibitors
Tricyclic antidepressants
Reserpine
Methyldopa
Metoclopramide
Domperidone
Cocaine
Verapamil
Serotonin reuptake inhibitors

Adapted from Molitch ME: Medication-induced hyperprolactinemia. Mayo Clin Proc 2005;80:1050–1057.

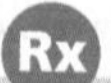

hypothalamic lesion may also directly impair release of GnRH. In that circumstance, both dopamine agonists and sex steroid replacement may be necessary. When administration of psychotropic medications that cause the hyperprolactinemia cannot be stopped, dopamine agonists may be used, but they may exacerbate the patient's psychosis. In such cases and in other patients in whom fertility is not an issue, treatment with cyclic estrogen and progestin replacement can be carried out safely.

Idiopathic Hyperprolactinemia

Idiopathic hyperprolactinemia is a diagnosis of exclusion. Prolactin levels in this condition are usually lower than 100 ng/mL. In such cases, small pituitary or hypothalamic tumors could exist that are beyond the resolution of current imaging techniques, but when such patients are monitored for many years, it is very uncommon for tumors to be visualized later. Idiopathic hyperprolactinemia can cause amenorrhea, galactorrhea, impotence, infertility, and loss of libido, just as occurs with hyperprolactinemia of other causes, so the condition may need to be treated. Premature osteoporosis related to the estrogen deficiency may also occur. The only possible treatment is with dopamine agonists, and these agents are successful in more than 90% of cases. Alternatively, cyclic estrogen and progesterone replacement may be given, but fertility will not be restored.

Thyroid-Stimulating Hormone

Hypothalamic hypothyroidism, also referred to as *tertiary hypothyroidism,* is the result of a central lesion that impairs the secretion of TRH, usually along with the loss of other hormones. It occurs considerably less commonly than hypothalamic GH and gonadotropin deficiency. Defects in the gene for TRH have not been detected, but a case has been reported of a TRH receptor mutation causing hypothyroidism. TSH levels in this syndrome are generally normal or even slightly elevated, and the response to TRH is delayed, peaking at 60 to 120 minutes rather than at 20 to 30 minutes. TSH in these patients is biologically less active than normal and binds to the TSH receptor less well because of altered glycosylation as a result of the TRH deficiency. Treatment is with L-thyroxine and therapy is monitored solely by measurement of free thyroxine levels and not TSH levels.

Adrenocorticotropic Hormone

Hypothalamic ACTH deficiency caused by hypothalamic lesions is uncommon. It may occur with the loss of other hormones, but it may also appear as an isolated deficiency. In the absence of CNS lesions or a history of trauma, most cases of isolated ACTH deficiency appear to be a pituitary autoimmune disorder. However, in patients with hypothalamic disease as the cause, basal ACTH levels are low, and the ACTH response to injected CRH may be prolonged and exaggerated, much as is the TSH response to TRH. The best test remains a comparison of ACTH responses to hypoglycemia, which is clearly mediated by the hypothalamus, and to CRH. The ACTH response is low in response to hypoglycemia but is increased and delayed in response to CRH in most patients with hypothalamic CRH deficiency. Treatment is with glucocorticoids, and mineralocorticoids are not needed.

A transient form of ACTH deficiency may be seen in 10 to 20% of patients with sepsis and possibly other severe illness. Although controlled studies are lacking, treatment with glucocorticoids appears to improve the rate of mortality in those with very low cortisol levels. On resolution of the sepsis, the hypothalamic-pituitary-adrenal axis recovers in most patients.

Vasopressin

Diabetes insipidus can develop as a result of destructive lesions in the supraoptic and paraventricular nuclei or in the mediobasal hypothalamus in the path of the neural fibers containing vasopressin (Chapter 243) that are passing on to the posterior pituitary. Irritative lesions can trigger the release of vasopressin in an unregulated fashion and thereby can result in the syndrome of inappropriate antidiuretic hormone (vasopressin) secretion.

Effects of Hypothalamic Disease on Other Neurometabolic Functions

Numerous functions that affect the internal milieu, in addition to anterior and posterior pituitary function, are regulated, at least in part, by the hypothalamus and include temperature control, behavior, consciousness, memory, sleep, food intake, and carbohydrate metabolism.

Alterations in Food Intake

Body weight is kept relatively constant in nonobese individuals through the integration of certain factors relating to the intake of nutrients and the output of energy; these functions are also affected by hormonal, environmental, and genetic factors. As with the regulation of hormone secretion, regulation of food intake can be conceptually regarded as an adjustment of food intake and energy expenditure around set points that may be different for body weight, total body fat, and lean body mass. The primary regulatory system involves production of the hormone leptin by adipocytes; leptin binds to hypothalamic leptin receptors and feeds back negatively on food intake and energy expenditure, but other peptides are involved as well (Chapter 239). Several areas of the hypothalamus are involved in the regulation of energy balance.

Hypothalamic Obesity

Destruction of the mediobasal hypothalamus sometimes inhibits satiety and may result in hyperphagia and hypothalamic obesity. The hyperphagia is the result of destruction of noradrenergic fibers originating in the paraventricular nucleus and passing through the mediobasal hypothalamus. Because of their location, such lesions also usually produce hypopituitarism and diabetes insipidus. In certain rare syndromes with obesity as a major characteristic, a hypothalamic cause has been postulated. Prader-Willi syndrome is the most common and occurs in 1 in 25,000 births. It is characterized by hypotonia, obesity, short stature, mental deficiency, hypogonadism, and small hands and feet. Approximately 70% of patients with Prader-Willi syndrome have a chromosome 15 deletion (15q11-q13) on the paternally derived chromosome. In the few cases studied at autopsy, no discernible hypothalamic lesions were detected. In the other syndromes (Laurence-Moon-Biedl-Bardet, Alström-Hallgren), no specific hypothalamic lesions have been found.

Hypothalamic Anorexia

Lesions of the lateral hypothalamus, which destroy nigrostriatal dopaminergic fibers that pass through this area, produce hypophagia along with an increase in peripheral norepinephrine turnover and metabolic rate. This syndrome is very rare, probably owing to the requirement of bilateral lesions. All the hormonal changes that occur in anorexia nervosa appear to be secondary to the weight loss, and no evidence for a primary hypothalamic disorder in this syndrome has been found.

Hyperglycemia

Hypothalamic activation as part of the generalized response to stress can cause release of GH, prolactin, and ACTH, which serve as counterregulatory hormones with respect to insulin. These hormones promote lipolysis, gluconeogenesis, and insulin resistance, with resulting glucose elevation. Of more importance in the acute response to stress, this hypothalamic response results in sympathetic activation with release of catecholamines that inhibit insulin secretion and stimulate glycogenolysis. In rare circumstances of acute hypothalamic injury from trauma, stroke, or infection, severe hyperglycemia can occur that is similar to the hyperglycemia seen in animals when the floor of the fourth ventricle is pricked with a needle, a phenomenon referred to as "piqûre" diabetes by Claude Bernard.

Temperature Regulation

The anterior hypothalamus and preoptic area contain temperature-sensitive neurons that respond to internal temperature changes by initiating certain thermoregulatory responses necessary to restore a constant temperature. Measures that dissipate heat include cutaneous vasodilation, sweating, panting, and behavioral changes that result in attempts to alter the environment. Measures that increase body heat include increasing metabolic heat production, shivering, cutaneous vasoconstriction, and similar behavioral changes. In humans, much of the increase in metabolic heat production occurs through sympathetic activation. The thermosensitive neurons are affected by endogenous pyrogens and drugs that alter thermoregulation, as well as by input from thermoreceptors in the skin and spinal cord.

Tumors

Rare patients have been reported with anterior hypothalamic lesions that caused sustained hypothermia from failure of heat generation by shivering and vasoconstriction but who had intact heat dissipation or resetting of the temperature set point lower. Paroxysmal hypothermia lasting for minutes to days from the sudden onset of sweating, vasodilation, and a fall in core temperature has been reported in numerous patients in association with demonstrated lesions such as tumors and agenesis of the corpus callosum. Some of these patients had evidence of other hypothalamic dysfunction, including diabetes insipidus, hypogonadism, and precocious puberty.

Fever

Fever as a manifestation of hypothalamic disease is uncommon but has been reported in association with trauma or bleeding into the region of the anterior hypothalamus. Such fevers rarely persist more than 2 weeks. Paroxysmal hyperthermia secondary to hypothalamic dysfunction also occurs. Some patients with paroxysmal hypothermia and hyperthermia respond to anticonvulsant medications, a finding suggesting that the neuronal discharges effecting the temperature changes resemble seizures.

Poikilothermy

Poikilothermy results from an inability to dissipate or generate heat to keep the body temperature constant in the presence of varying ambient temperatures. This condition results from bilateral lesions in the posterior hypothalamus and rostral mesencephalon, which are the areas responsible for the final integration of thermoregulatory neural efferents. Patients with this condition do not feel discomfort with temperature changes and are unaware of having a problem. Depending on the ambient temperature, they may experience life-threatening hypothermia or hyperthermia. Mild poikilothermy is normally present in infants and frequently occurs in elderly individuals.

SUGGESTED READINGS

Bonadanelli M, Ambrosio MR, Zatelli MC, et al: Hypopituitarism after traumatic brain injury. Eur J Endocrinol 2005;152:679–691. *This article reviews the changes in pituitary hormone secretion that occur following brain injury.*

Crowell MD, Decker GA, Levy R, et al: Gut-brain neuropeptides in the regulation of ingestive behaviors and obesity. Am J Gastroenterol 2006;101:2848–2856. *Review of the peptides involved in weight regulation.*

Engel JB, Schally AV: Drug insight: Clinical use of agonists and antagonists of luteinizing hormone-releasing hormone. Nat Clin Pract Endocrinol Metab 2007;3:157–167. *Review of the indications for and efficacy of these medications.*

Gregory SJ, Kaiser UB: Regulation of gonadotropins by inhibin and activin. Semin Reprod Med 2004;22:253–267. *A review of inhibin, activin, and follistatin and their interactions in the hypothalamic-pituitary-gonadal axis.*

Huhtaniemi I: Mutations affecting gonadotropin secretion and action. Horm Res 2003;60(Suppl 3):21–30. *This article reviews the various genetic abnormalities that can result in central hypogonadism.*

Karavitaki N, Brufani C, Warner JT, et al: Craniopharyngiomas in children and adults: Systematic analysis of 121 cases with long-term follow-up. Clin Endocrinol 2005;62:397–409. *This is a report of a large series of patients with this hypothalamic tumor with emphasis on its clinical features and treatment.*

Molitch ME: Medication-induced hyperprolactinemia. Mayo Clin Proc 2005;80: 1050–1057. *The various medications that can cause hyperprolactinemia are reviewed here.*

242 ANTERIOR PITUITARY

Mark E. Molitch

ANATOMY AND EMBRYOLOGY

The pituitary is divided into anterior (adenohypophysis) and posterior (neurohypophysis) lobes, with the anterior lobe accounting for approximately 80% of the gland. Superiorly, the pituitary is covered by the diaphragma sellae, a reflection of the dura mater that forms the roof of the sella and has a central opening that is penetrated by the pituitary stalk and its blood vessels. The optic chiasm, formed by the decussation of the optic nerves, is positioned directly above the pituitary gland and below the third ventricle. The lateral boundaries of the sella are formed by the cavernous sinuses, which contain the internal carotid artery and cranial nerves III, IV, V_1, V_2, and VI.

The blood supply to the pituitary gland is derived from the superior and inferior hypophyseal arteries, branches of the internal carotid arteries. Specialized vascular structures located in the median eminence of the hypothalamus drain into portal veins that course down the pituitary stalk to join the sinusoidal capillaries of the anterior lobe. Hypothalamic hormones enter fenestrations in these capillaries to flow from the hypothalamus to the anterior pituitary. Venous drainage from the anterior lobe is into the cavernous sinuses. The cavernous sinuses are interconnected by means of channels that encircle the pituitary, and drain into the petrosal sinuses which can be catheterized for hormone sampling.

The six major pituitary cell types include somatotrophs (growth hormone [GH] producing), lactotrophs (prolactin [PRL] producing), corticotrophs (adrenocorticotropic hormone [ACTH] producing), thyrotrophs (thyroid-stimulating hormone [TSH] producing), gonadotrophs (follicle-stimulating hormone [FSH] and luteinizing hormone [LH] producing), and folliculostellate cells that do not produce the classic pituitary hormones. The biochemical characteristics of the major anterior pituitary hormones are summarized in Table 242–1.

The pituitary is formed early in embryonic life from the fusion of Rathke's pouch (which gives rise to the anterior pituitary) and a portion of the ventral diencephalon (which gives rise to the posterior pituitary). Rathke's pouch is an ectodermal evagination in the roof of the primitive oropharynx. The ontogeny of hormone production during anterior pituitary development has been characterized in detail. The pituitary anlage expresses the glycoprotein hormone α gene even as the progenitor cells are arising from Rathke's pouch. Subsequently, pro-opiomelanocortin (POMC)-producing cells can be seen in the hypothalamus and in the pituitary. An evanescent group of TSH-producing cells appears, but then fades away, to be followed later by a distinct population of TSH cells in a different location in the pituitary. After gonadotrophs develop, GH- and PRL-producing cells appear and later form distinct populations of somatotrophs and lactotrophs. Several transcription factors are important in the development of the various types of pituitary cells. Lhx3 is present in somatotrophs, lactotrophs, and thyrotrophs, and mutations in this gene result in complete deficits of GH, PRL, TSH, and the gonadotropins along with a rigid cervical spine. Mutations in *HESX1* are associated with dysplasia of the septum pellucidum and optic tracts in addition to multiple pituitary hormone deficits. The transcription factor Pit-1, a member of the Pou-Homeodomain family, is produced in somatotrophs, lactotrophs, and thyrotrophs. Mutations in the *Pit-1* gene prevent the development of these cells and cause deficiencies of GH, PRL, and TSH. This lineage relationship probably accounts for the observation that some GH-producing tumors also secrete PRL and approximately one third of TSH-producing tumors co-secrete GH. Prop-1 is another transcription factor critical for the development of somatotrophs, lactotrophs, and thyrotrophs that may in addition be important for gonadotrophs. Mutations in *PROP-1* result in deficiencies of GH, PRL, and TSH, and some affected individuals have delayed puberty. Combined pituitary hormone deficiency (GH, PRL, TSH) has an incidence of approximately 1 in 8000 births, and 10% of patients have an affected relative. More than half of these cases result from *Pit-1* or *Prop-1* mutations.

Somatotrophs, which constitute 40 to 50% of anterior pituitary cells, and lactotrophs, which make up 15 to 25%, are located predominantly in the lateral aspects of the anterior pituitary. Corticotrophs constitute 10 to 20% of anterior pituitary cells and are located mainly in the central region of the anterior pituitary. Gonadotrophs, which account for approximately 10% of pituitary cells, produce both FSH and LH, although a few gonadotrophs appear selectively to secrete only one of the hormones. Only 5% of pituitary cells are thyrotrophs. The folliculostellate cells have been shown to produce growth factors such as basic fibroblast growth factor, vascular endothelial growth factor, and follistatin, among others.

RADIOLOGIC IMAGING

Radiologic imaging of the pituitary gland primarily involves computed tomography (CT) and magnetic resonance imaging (MRI). CT scans are performed using high-resolution (1.5-mm), contrast-enhanced procedures with direct coronal sections. Although CT provides excellent resolution, problems include artifacts from metallic objects and dental fillings, and some patients have difficulty assuming the position required

TABLE 242–1 FEATURES OF THE MAJOR ANTERIOR PITUITARY HORMONES*

Hormone	Amino Acids	Molecular Weight (kD)	Serum Half-Life (min)	Cell Type	Target Gland
Growth hormone (GH)	191	22	20	Somatotroph	Multiple
Prolactin (PRL)	198	23	20	Lactotroph	Breast
Adrenocorticotropic hormone (ACTH)	39	4.5	8	Corticotroph	Adrenal
Thyroid-stimulating hormone (TSH)	α subunit, 92 β subunit, 118	14 17	50	Thyrotroph	Thyroid
Luteinizing hormone (LH)	α-subunit, 92 β subunit, 121	14 18	50	Gonadotroph	Gonad
Follicle-stimulating hormone (FSH)	α subunit, 92 β subunit, 111	14 18	220	Gonadotroph	Gonad

*The amino acid lengths are based on the cloned complementary DNAs and differ in some cases from the lengths of the sequenced proteins, perhaps because of proteolysis. The indicated molecular weights include the contributions of the carbohydrates in the case of the glycoprotein hormones (TSH, LH, FSH). The serum half-lives assume single-compartment monoexponential decay.

TABLE 242–2 FACTORS THAT REGULATE PITUITARY HORMONE SECRETION

Hormone	Releasing Factors	Inhibiting Factors
Growth hormone	GHRH	Somatostatin, IGF-I
Prolactin	TRH, VIP, E_2	Dopamine
Adrenocorticotropic hormone	CRH, vasopressin	Cortisol
Thyroid-stimulating hormone	TRH	T_4, T_3, somatostatin, dopamine
Luteinizing hormone	GnRH	E_2, testosterone
Follicle-stimulating hormone	GnRH, activin	Inhibin, E_2, testosterone

CRH = corticotropin-releasing hormone; E_2 = estradiol; GHRH = growth hormone–releasing hormone; GnRH = gonadotropin-releasing hormone; IGF-I = insulin-like growth factor-I (formerly called somatomedin C); T_4 = thyroxine; T_3 = triiodothyronine; TRH = thyrotropin-releasing hormone; VIP = vasoactive intestinal polypeptide. The gonadal steroids E_2 and testosterone exert much of their inhibitory effects on gonadotropin secretion at the hypothalamic level.

for coronal sections. Pituitary adenomas are hypodense on both unenhanced and contrast-enhanced CT scans. Overall, MRI is the technique of choice for evaluating the sellar region. MRI provides multiplanar imaging and excellent resolution of the pituitary and surrounding cerebrospinal fluid and vascular and central nervous system structures. Radiation exposure with MRI is less, thus allowing repeated imaging as required for follow-up. Bone structures are not well defined by MRI. The normal anterior pituitary appears isointense with brain white matter, whereas the posterior pituitary exhibits high signal intensity ("bright spot"). The optic chiasm can be readily identified superior to the pituitary gland because it is surrounded by hypodense areas. MRI detects pituitary microadenomas (tumors <1 cm) in most patients with surgically proven tumors. Pituitary adenomas typically appear hypointense on T1-weighted images and show less enhancement with gadolinium than surrounding normal tissue. Focal hypodense areas are also seen in approximately one fourth of physiologically normal individuals. These areas may correspond to cysts or small adenomas that have been described in autopsy series, thus emphasizing the importance of endocrine evaluation in making the diagnosis of pituitary tumors.

REGULATION OF THE PITUITARY AXIS

The pituitary gland integrates the influences of an array of positive and negative signals to modulate hormone secretion within a narrow range (Table 242–2). The major hypothalamic-pituitary-target gland axes include the thyrotropin-releasing hormone (TRH)-TSH–thyroid hormone axis, the corticotropin-releasing hormone (CRH)-ACTH-cortisol axis, the gonadotropin-releasing hormone (GnRH)-LH/FSH-gonadal axis, and the GH-releasing hormone (GHRH)-GH–insulin-like growth factor-I (IGF-I) axis. PRL is the only major pituitary hormone that is not subject to feedback inhibition by hormones produced in target tissues. However, it is controlled by positive and negative input from the hypothalamus, the latter being dominant.

The principles of feedback regulation are well illustrated by the hypothalamic-pituitary-thyroid axis. Hypothalamic TRH stimulates TSH secretion from the pituitary. TSH increases thyroid hormone secretion, which, in turn, suppresses hypothalamic TRH as well as pituitary TSH. A typical regulatory loop therefore has both positive (TRH, TSH) and negative (thyroxine [T_4], triiodothyronine [T_3]) components, thereby allowing a high degree of control of hormone levels. The pituitary gland integrates positive TRH signals and the negative effects of thyroid hormone. The concept of feedback regulation is important not only for understanding pituitary physiology but also because it provides the basis for analyzing pituitary gland function using stimulation and suppression tests.

The feedback regulatory systems just described are superimposed on hormonal rhythms used for adaptation to the environment. Seasonal changes, the daily light-dark cycles, and stress are but a few of many environmental events that have major impacts on the secretion of pituitary hormones. Some hormonal pathways, such as ACTH, GH, and PRL secretion, are entrained to the sleep-wake cycle and cause characteristic peaks of ACTH and cortisol production in the early morning with a nadir in the late afternoon and evening. The menstrual cycle provides an example of a pituitary rhythm that occurs on a much longer time scale (e.g., 28 days). The pattern of the menstrual cycle is coupled to cycles of follicular development in the ovary. As follicular development progresses, levels of gonadal steroids and inhibin feed back on the hypothalamus and pituitary to modulate LH and FSH secretion.

Because many hormones are released in a pulsatile manner and in a rhythmic fashion, it is important to be aware of these characteristics of secretion when attempting to relate serum measurements to normal values. Although it is possible to characterize pulsatile patterns of hormone secretion using frequent blood sampling, this is not practical in a clinical setting. Alternative approaches include stimulation and suppression tests or the use of "integrated" measurements of hormone production such as 24-hour urine free cortisol as an index of ACTH secretion or IGF-I as a biologic marker of GH action.

HYPOPITUITARISM

Hypopituitarism implies diminished production of one or more anterior pituitary hormones. Although the recognition of panhypopituitarism is usually straightforward, the detection of partial or selective hormone deficiencies is more challenging. Pituitary hormone deficiencies can be caused by loss of hypothalamic stimulation (tertiary hormone deficiency) or by direct loss of pituitary function (secondary hormone deficiency). When hypopituitarism is accompanied by diabetes insipidus or hyperprolactinemia, hypothalamic causes of pituitary dysfunction should be considered.

Pathogenesis

Numerous congenital and acquired causes of hypopituitarism have been described (Table 242–3). Sporadic and familial forms of panhypopituitarism occur, but the underlying genetic or developmental defects have not been elucidated. *Congenital deficiencies* of multiple pituitary hormones are often caused by mutations in the genes for the transcription factors mentioned earlier. Gene mutations have been found at several steps leading to pituitary hormone secretion, including the following: those for the hypophysiotropic releasing factor receptors for GnRH, GHRH, and TRH; those for the pituitary hormone structures for GH, ACTH, and the β subunits of FSH, TSH, and LH; and those for the target organ receptors for GH, ACTH, TSH, and LH. Best studied are mutations of the GH gene, which are heterogeneous. Some include large deletions of the GH gene that are inherited in an autosomal recessive manner. Point mutations have also been described in the GH gene, and some of these can be inherited in an autosomal dominant manner, apparently because the mutant hormone impairs normal GH biosynthesis. The congenital embryopathic disorders causing hypopituitarism are discussed in Chapter 241.

TABLE 242–3 CAUSES OF HYPOPITUITARISM

GENETIC DEFECTS

Hypophysiotropic hormone gene defects
Hypophysiotropic hormone receptor gene defects
- GHRH receptor defect
- GnRH receptor defect
- TRH receptor defect

Pituitary hormone gene defects
- Gonadotropins: LH and FSH β-subunit gene defects
- Growth hormone: defects in GH gene
- Thyrotropin: defects in TSH β subunit
- Multiple hormone (GH, PRL, TSH) defects: mutation in *Pit-1* gene and *Propl* gene

Pituitary hormone receptor genetic defects
- Growth hormone receptor defects: GH insensitivity syndrome (Laron-type dwarfism)
- ACTH receptor defects: congenital insensitivity to ACTH
- LH receptor defects
- FSH receptor defects
- TSH receptor defects

CONGENITAL EMBRYOPATHIC DEFECTS

Anencephaly
Midline cleft defects: septo-optic dysplasia, basal encephalocele, cleft lip and palate
Pituitary aplasia
Kallmann's syndrome (GnRH defect with anosmia)

ACQUIRED DEFECTS

Tumors: pituitary adenomas, craniopharyngiomas, dysgerminomas, meningiomas, gliomas, metastatic tumors, hamartomas, Rathke's cleft cysts
Irradiation
Trauma: surgery, external blunt trauma
Empty sella syndrome
Vascular disorders
- Pituitary apoplexy
- Sheehan's syndrome
- Internal carotid aneurysm
- Vasculitis

Inflammatory/infiltrative diseases
- Sarcoidosis
- Langerhans cell histiocytosis (histiocytosis X, eosinophilic granuloma)
- Tuberculosis, syphilis
- Meningitis
- Lymphocytic hypophysitis, infundibulohypophysitis

Metabolic disorders
- Hemochromatosis
- Amyloidosis
- Critical illness
- Malnutrition
- Anorexia nervosa
- Psychosocial deprivation

Idiopathic conditions

ACTH = adrenocorticotropic hormone; FSH = follicle-stimulating hormone; GH = growth hormone; GHRH = growth hormone–releasing hormone; GnRH = gonadotropin-releasing hormone; LH = luteinizing hormone; PRL = prolactin; TRH = thyrotropin-releasing hormone; TSH = thyroid-stimulating hormone.

Neoplastic lesions, particularly pituitary macroadenomas, are the most common causes of acquired hypopituitarism. Pituitary adenomas cause hypopituitarism in several different ways. In some cases, the normal pituitary is directly destroyed or compressed. Compression of the pituitary stalk can impair blood supply to the pituitary as well as decrease input from hypothalamic hormones. Hemorrhage into tumors can lead to pituitary infarction. A mild degree of hyperprolactinemia is characteristic of disorders that cause stalk compression, and hyperprolactinemia further impairs gonadotropin secretion. Various other neoplasms that occur near the sella, such as craniopharyngiomas, can also cause hypopituitarism (see Table 242–3).

Radiation causes hypopituitarism primarily because of its effects on hypothalamic function, although high-dose radiation (e.g., proton beam) can also cause direct pituitary damage. The sellar region is subjected to radiation in the treatment of pituitary adenomas, craniopharyngiomas, clivus chordomas, optic gliomas, meningiomas, dysgerminomas, and neoplasms of the oropharynx. Importantly, the effects of radiation can be delayed for several years, and patients at high risk should be evaluated yearly for hypopituitarism. Although GH and gonadotropin deficiencies usually develop first, ACTH or TSH deficiencies can occur, a finding emphasizing the need to evaluate each of the major axes.

Empty sella syndrome can occur as a primary or as an acquired condition. It is caused by defects in the diaphragma sellae that allow herniation of the arachnoid membrane into the hypophyseal fossa. In long-standing cases, sellar enlargement occurs, probably because of persistent transmission of intracranial pressure. With appropriate imaging studies, the pituitary gland is seen as a flattened rim of tissue along the floor of the sella. Primary empty sella occurs most commonly in women and may be associated with features of benign intracranial hypertension. Pituitary function in patients with primary empty sella syndrome is usually but not always normal; 10% of patients may have mild hyperprolactinemia resulting from stretching of the pituitary stalk. Acquired forms may occur as a result of surgery, radiation, or pituitary infarction (usually of an adenoma).

Pituitary apoplexy is usually caused by hemorrhage into a tumor with associated infarction. In the absence of a tumor, predispositions to apoplexy include trauma, pregnancy, anticoagulation, sickle cell anemia, and diabetes mellitus. Pituitary infarction in the peripartum period is referred to as *Sheehan's syndrome* and is usually associated with significant obstetric hemorrhage and hypovolemia. Although Sheehan's syndrome may manifest acutely with vascular collapse, it more commonly has a subacute manifestation consisting of postpartum inability to lactate, amenorrhea, and symptoms of adrenal insufficiency. Sheehan's syndrome is now infrequent, owing to improvements in obstetric care.

Infiltrative diseases such as sarcoidosis, histiocytosis, and tuberculosis usually cause hypopituitarism by infiltrating the hypothalamus and stalk rather than the pituitary (discussed in Chapter 241). In *lymphocytic hypophysitis,* the pituitary is infiltrated by lymphocytes and plasma cells, with destruction of the parenchyma; this disorder is believed to have an autoimmune basis. The lesion that develops is usually large, and patients present with symptoms or signs of hypopituitarism or those of a mass lesion (i.e., visual field defects and/or headaches). Some patients may have mild hyperprolactinemia and diabetes insipidus. Patients have a predilection for damage to corticotroph cells, resulting in ACTH/adrenal insufficiency. Most cases occur in women, usually first seen during or after pregnancy. In pregnancy, such lesions may be confused with prolactinomas, but the mild PRL elevation points to a nonsecretory lesion. MRI cannot reliably differentiate pituitary adenoma from hypophysitis, although hypophysitis usually manifests with a diffuse enlargement of the pituitary, rather than as a focal lesion. Diagnosis is usually made by biopsy, but the lesion may be suspected clinically if it manifests during or just after pregnancy. Careful pituitary function testing is mandatory, because undiagnosed cases have died of adrenocortical insufficiency. Although the prognosis is not clear, a number of cases have resolved spontaneously. An entity with similar histologic findings involving the stalk and posterior pituitary, referred to as *infundibuloneurohypophysitis*, can cause diabetes insipidus.

The pituitary may undergo damage because of iron deposition in patients with *hemochromatosis* and amyloid fibrils in patients with *systemic amyloidosis*. Functional, reversible hypopituitarism of varying degrees occurs in patients with severe systemic illness, severe psychosocial and emotional deprivation, and severe weight loss, particularly in those with anorexia nervosa.

Diagnosis

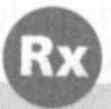

The diagnosis of hypopituitarism rests on the stimulation tests that are summarized in Table 242–4.

Treatment

Therapy for hypopituitarism depends on the nature and severity of the hormone deficiencies as well as on the desired clinical end points. The goal is to replace hormones in a physiologic manner, with efforts to avoid the consequences of overreplacement. Examples of hormonal replacement paradigms are provided in Table 242–5. Adjustment of hormone doses is done primarily based on clinical findings, and the TSH level is not helpful for adjusting thyroxine doses in patients with central hypothyroidism. Even when conventional hormone replacement (adrenal, thyroid, gonadal) is carried out appropriately, an approximately twofold excess risk of death is reported in patients with hypopituitarism. Although untreated GH deficiency has been hypothesized to be the cause of this excess risk, this has not been proved. The benefits of GH therapy are less clear than those for the other pituitary hormones and include improvements in body composition, bone, and quality of life; although adverse effects are few, treatment involves daily injections.

TABLE 242–4 TESTS OF PITUITARY INSUFFICIENCY

Hormone	Test	Interpretation
Growth hormone (GH)	Insulin tolerance test: Regular insulin (0.05–0.15 U/kg) given IV and blood drawn at −30, 0, 30, 45, 60, and 90 min for measurement of glucose and GH	If hypoglycemia occurs (glucose <40 mg/dL), GH should increase to >5 µg/L*
	L-Arginine test: 0.5 g/kg (maximum, 30 g) IV over 30 min with GH measurements at 0, 30, 60, and 120 min	Normal response: GH > 5 µg/L
	Arginine-GHRH test: GHRH 1 µg/kg IV bolus followed by 30 min infusion of L-arginine (30 g)	Normal response: GH > 4.1 µg/L
Adrenocorticotropic hormone (ACTH)	Insulin tolerance test: Regular insulin (0.05–0.15 U/kg) given IV and blood drawn at −30, 0, 30, 45, 60, and 90 min for measurement of glucose and cortisol	If hypoglycemia occurs (glucose <40 mg/dL), cortisol should increase by >7 µg/dL or to >20 µg/dL
	CRH test: 1 µg/kg ovine CRH IV at 8 AM with blood samples drawn at 0, 15, 30, 60, 90, and 120 min for measurement of ACTH and cortisol	Normally, basal ACTH usually increases twofold to fourfold and reaches a peak (20–100 pg/mL); ACTH responses may be delayed in cases of hypothalamic dysfunction; cortisol levels usually reach 20–25 µg/dL
	Metyrapone test: Metyrapone (30 mg/kg; maximum, 2 g) at midnight with measurements of plasma 11-deoxycortisol and cortisol at 8 AM; ACTH can also be measured; a 3-day test is also available. Basal cortisol should be >5–6 µg/dL before test	Normal response: 11–deoxycortisol >7.5 µg/dL or ACTH >75 pg/mL; plasma cortisol should fall to <4 µg/dL to ensure adequate response
	ACTH stimulation test: $ACTH_{1-24}$ (cosyntropin), 0.25 mg IM or IV; cortisol measured at 0, 30, and 60 min	Normal response: cortisol >18 µg/dL; in suspected hypothalamic-pituitary deficiency, low-dose (1 µg) test may be more sensitive
Thyroid-stimulating hormone (TSH)	Basal thyroid function tests: free T_4, free T_3, TSH	Low free thyroid hormone levels in the setting of TSH levels that are not appropriately increased
Luteinizing hormone (LH), follicle-stimulating hormone (FSH)	Basal levels of LH, FSH, testosterone, estrogen	Basal LH and FSH should be increased in postmenopausal women; low testosterone levels in conjunction with low or low-normal LH and FSH are consistent with gonadotropin deficiency
	GnRH test: GnRH (100 µg) IV with measurements of serum LH and FSH at 0, 30, and 60 min	Normally, LH usually increases by 10 IU/L and FSH by 2 IU/L; normal responses are variable, and repeated stimulation may be required 50% increase should occur in LH and FSH, usually by day 5
	Clomiphene test: Clomiphene citrate (100 mg) given orally for 5 days; serum LH and FSH measured on days 0, 5, 7, 10, and 13	
Multiple hormones	Combined anterior pituitary test: GHRH (1 µg/kg), CRH (1 µg/kg), GnRH (100 µg), given sequentially IV; blood samples drawn at 0, 15, 30, 60, 90, and 120 min for measurements of GH, ACTH, LH, and FSH	Combined or individual releasing hormone responses must be evaluated in the context of basal hormone values and may not be diagnostic (see text)

*Values are with polyclonal assays.
CRH = corticotropin-releasing hormone; GHRH = growth hormone–releasing hormone; GnRH = gonadotropin-releasing hormone; IM = intramuscularly; IV = intravenously; T_3 = triiodothyronine; T_4 = thyroxine; TRH = thyrotropin-releasing hormone.

TABLE 242–5 HORMONAL REPLACEMENT THERAPY IN HYPOPITUITARISM*

Pituitary Axis	Hormonal Replacements
Growth hormone (GH)	In children, GH (0.025 mg/kg) SC daily; in adults, GH (0.3–1.2 mg) SC daily; titrate dose to achieve IGF-I levels in upper part of normal range; women receiving oral estrogens require higher doses
Prolactin	None
Adrenocorticotropic hormone–cortisol	Prednisone (2.5 mg PO QAM; 2.5 mg PO QPM) or hydrocortisone (10–20 mg PO QAM; 5–10 mg PO QPM); dose adjusted on clinical basis; stress dosing: 50–75 mg hydrocortisone IV q8h
Thyroid-stimulating hormone–thyroid	L-Thyroxine (0.075–0.15 mg) PO qd
Gonadotropins–gonads	Pulsatile GnRH (via pump) can be used for GnRH-deficient subjects, or FSH and LH (or hCG) can be used to induce ovulation in women; hCG alone, or FSH and LH, can be used to induce spermatogenesis in men In men, testosterone enanthate (100–300 mg) IM q1–3 wk or testosterone cyclopentylpropionate (100–300 mg) IM q1–3 wk; testosterone transdermal patches can also be used (5 mg qd); testosterone gel (1%) 1–2 packets (5–10 g)/day In women, conjugated estrogens (0.625–1.25 mg) or mestranol (35 mg) PO days 1–25 each month cycled with medroxyprogesterone acetate (5–10 mg) PO days 15–25 each month; low-dose contraceptive pills may also be used Estrogen-containing transdermal patches also available
Posterior pituitary	Desmopressin, 0.5–0.2 mL (5–20 μg) intranasally once or twice daily, or tablets (0.1–0.4 mg every 8–12 hr) or 0.5 mL (2 μg) SC

*Replacement therapy is dictated by the types of hormone deficiencies and by the clinical circumstances. In each case, the recommended preparations and doses are representative but need to be adjusted for individual patients. Other hormonal preparations are also available.
FSH = follicle-stimulating hormone; GnRH = gonadotropin-releasing hormone; hCG = human chorionic gonadotropin; IGF-I = insulin-like growth factor-I; IM = intramuscularly; IV = intravenously; LH = luteinizing hormone; PO = orally; SC = subcutaneously.

TABLE 242–6 PREVALENCE OF DIFFERENT TYPES OF PITUITARY ADENOMAS

Type of Pituitary Adenoma	Disorder	Hormone Produced	Prevalence*
Somatotroph	Acromegaly/gigantism	Growth hormone	10–15%
Lactotroph (prolactinoma)	Hypogonadism, galactorrhea	Prolactin	25–40%
Corticotroph	Cushing's disease	Adrenocorticotropic hormone	10–15%
Gonadotroph	Mass effects, hypopituitarism	Follicle-stimulating hormone and luteinizing hormone	15–20%
Thyrotroph	Hyperthyroidism	Thyroid-stimulating hormone	<3%
Nonfunctioning/null cell	Mass effects, hypopituitarism	None	10–25%

*The prevalence rates represent ranges described in several different large series. Mixed tumors (e.g., growth hormone and prolactin) and plurihormonal adenomas are not shown. Rates vary depending on methods used to establish the diagnosis. Prolactinomas were underestimated in most recent pathologic series because they are largely managed medically. Most glycoprotein hormone–producing pituitary tumors were classified as nonfunctioning adenomas until the application of immunohistochemical studies.

PITUITARY TUMORS

Classification

Pituitary tumors are classified according to the hormones that they produce and their size: microadenomas, less than 10 mm in diameter; macroadenomas, more than 10 mm in diameter; and macroadenomas with extrasellar extension. In general, the levels of hormones produced by the tumors parallel the size of the tumors. The prevalence of the different types of pituitary adenomas, based on surgical data, is summarized in Table 242–6. Immunohistochemical studies have been used to define tumor phenotype. Pituitary adenomas are very rarely malignant but can be locally invasive.

Most pituitary tumors are monoclonal. This finding does not exclude a role for hormonal stimulation as a predisposing factor for somatic mutations, and the hormonal environment may also affect the rate of tumor growth (e.g., Nelson's syndrome). Supporting the concept that somatic mutations lead to pituitary tumorigenesis, a subset (35 to 40%) of somatotroph adenomas has activating mutations in the gene for the Gsα subunit, resulting from two different amino acid (Arg201 and Glu227) substitutions. Either mutation causes the Gsα subunit to stimulate adenylyl cyclase in a constitutive manner, and the elevated intracellular cyclic adenosine monophosphate levels lead to increased cell growth as well as GH production. Mutations in other oncogenes, such as *ras*, *Rb*, and *p53*, are uncommon in pituitary tumors. The nature of the somatic defects in most pituitary tumors remains unknown.

Two types of inherited predispositions to pituitary tumors are recognized. Patients with *McCune-Albright syndrome* occasionally develop pituitary adenomas as well as characteristic abnormalities in other tissues, particularly the ovary, bone, and thyroid. The McCune-Albright syndrome is also caused by mutations in the gene for the Gsα subunit. However, the somatic mutations in McCune-Albright occur early during development, rather than only in the pituitary gland, so multiple tissues are affected. In *multiple endocrine neoplasia type 1* (MEN1) (Chapter 250), the predisposition to pituitary tumors is inherited in an autosomal dominant manner and occurs in conjunction with tumors of the parathyroid and pancreas. The *MEN1* gene codes for the protein menin, which is thought to act as a constitutive tumor suppressor. Individuals with *MEN1* are thought to inherit one mutant allele, with tumorigenesis occurring after a "second hit" mutates or deletes the normal *MEN-1* gene. It is thought that several different tumor suppressor genes may play a role in the development of pituitary tumors.

Clinical Manifestations

The mass effects of the enlarging tumor can also lead to specific signs and symptoms. Particularly in the case of nonfunctioning tumors or those that produce gonadotropins, the primary clinical manifestations are related to effects of the tumor on surrounding structures.

Headaches are common in patients with macroadenomas and appear to be caused by expansion of the diaphragma sellae or by invasion of bone. The sudden onset of severe headache associated with nausea, vomiting, and altered consciousness can also be caused by hemorrhagic infarction with sudden enlargement of a pituitary adenoma. In severe cases, pituitary apoplexy can occur, requiring glucocorticoid treatment and possible surgical decompression.

The effects of pituitary tumors on the visual fields are well explained by the relationship of the optic chiasm with the sella turcica. Expansion of macroadenomas into the suprasellar region exerts pressure on the optic chiasm, usually in the central region where nerves emanating from the inferior and medial part of the retina (superior and temporal visual fields) cross. Consequently, bitemporal hemianopia is the most common visual field abnormality associated with pituitary adenomas. However, the exact pattern of visual field loss is variable and is affected by the location and flexibility of the chiasm as well as by the direction and extent of tumor growth. Large tumors may grow asymmetrically and may invade the cavernous sinus or surround an optic nerve, thus leading to other patterns of visual field changes or loss of visual acuity. The size and direction and degree of extrasellar extension are best evaluated with MRI with gadolinium infusion. If the tumor abuts the chiasm on MRI, then formal visual field testing should be performed by an ophthalmologist. Even long-standing visual field changes may be reversible by surgical or medical decompression.

The normal pituitary is often compressed into a thin rim of tissue by large adenomas. Hypopituitarism probably results more from compression of the hypothalamic-pituitary stalk than from direct pressure on the normal pituitary. GH deficiency and gonadotropin deficiency are common. Slightly elevated PRL levels (e.g., <100 ng/mL) occur in cases of stalk compression because of diminished inhibition by dopamine. It is important not to mistake such tumors for prolactinomas, because they will not decrease in size in response to medical therapy with dopamine agonists. Preoperative hypopituitarism caused by a large pituitary mass is reversible in half of patients after surgical decompression. Diabetes insipidus (vasopressin deficiency) is rarely caused by pituitary tumors and should raise the suspicion of a craniopharyngioma or other disorders likely to cause hypothalamic dysfunction.

Treatment Rx

Surgery

Except for prolactinomas, surgical removal is the primary mode of therapy for most pituitary tumors that warrant intervention. Indications for surgery include reduction in hormone levels and decompression to relieve mass effects or to prevent further tumor expansion. The transsphenoidal route is used almost exclusively. Because of substantially greater morbidity, subfrontal craniotomy is reserved for patients with tumors that require extensive exploration of the suprasellar region and surrounding structures. The transsphenoidal approach usually involves a sublabial incision allowing ready access to the sphenoidal sinus that leads to the floor of the sella, but an endoscopic, endonasal approach is becoming used more widely. In experienced hands, transsphenoidal surgery is effective, and complications are uncommon (<5%). These complications include cerebrospinal fluid leak, hemorrhage, optic nerve injury, hypopituitarism, and sinusitis. Transient diabetes insipidus occurs in 5% of patients after surgery but rarely persists in the long term. Mortality rates are less than 1%. Complication rates increase with increasing size of the tumor and when a craniotomy is performed.

Surgical cure rates are a function of the size and location of the pituitary mass. When stringent hormonal criteria are used to assess surgical success rates, fewer than 30% of macroadenomas are cured by surgery, although considerable improvements in hormone levels or mass effects can be achieved. Conversely, hormone hypersecretion by microadenomas can be corrected completely in 80 to 90% of patients.

Radiation Therapy

Irradiation is usually used as adjunctive therapy after surgery or in combination with medical therapy. Radiation is typically adminis-

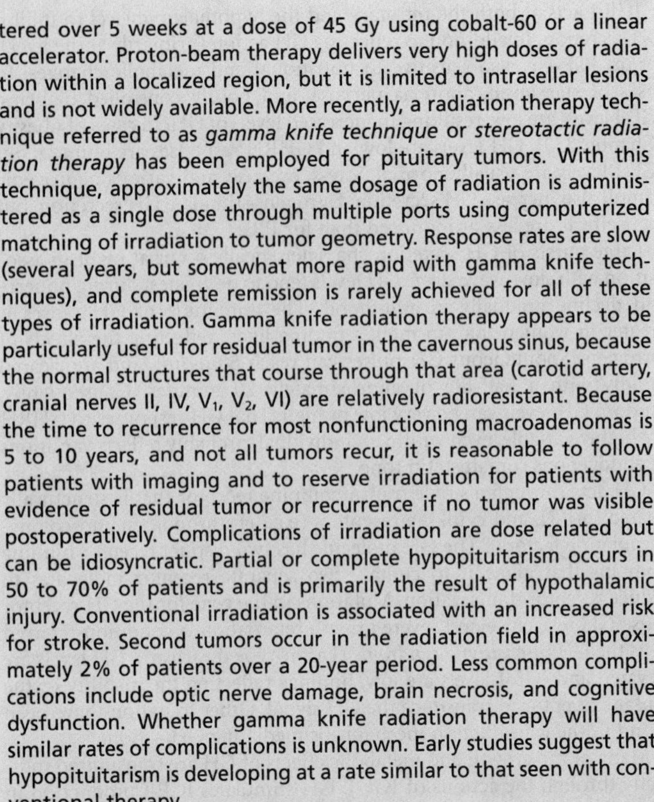

Rx

tered over 5 weeks at a dose of 45 Gy using cobalt-60 or a linear accelerator. Proton-beam therapy delivers very high doses of radiation within a localized region, but it is limited to intrasellar lesions and is not widely available. More recently, a radiation therapy technique referred to as *gamma knife technique* or *stereotactic radiation therapy* has been employed for pituitary tumors. With this technique, approximately the same dosage of radiation is administered as a single dose through multiple ports using computerized matching of irradiation to tumor geometry. Response rates are slow (several years, but somewhat more rapid with gamma knife techniques), and complete remission is rarely achieved for all of these types of irradiation. Gamma knife radiation therapy appears to be particularly useful for residual tumor in the cavernous sinus, because the normal structures that course through that area (carotid artery, cranial nerves II, IV, V_1, V_2, VI) are relatively radioresistant. Because the time to recurrence for most nonfunctioning macroadenomas is 5 to 10 years, and not all tumors recur, it is reasonable to follow patients with imaging and to reserve irradiation for patients with evidence of residual tumor or recurrence if no tumor was visible postoperatively. Complications of irradiation are dose related but can be idiosyncratic. Partial or complete hypopituitarism occurs in 50 to 70% of patients and is primarily the result of hypothalamic injury. Conventional irradiation is associated with an increased risk for stroke. Second tumors occur in the radiation field in approximately 2% of patients over a 20-year period. Less common complications include optic nerve damage, brain necrosis, and cognitive dysfunction. Whether gamma knife radiation therapy will have similar rates of complications is unknown. Early studies suggest that hypopituitarism is developing at a rate similar to that seen with conventional therapy.

Medical Therapy

The emergence of medical therapies for pituitary tumors has dramatically affected the management of these patients. Dopamine agonists, which include bromocriptine, pergolide, and cabergoline, have a primary role in the management of prolactinomas. These drugs induce a rapid fall in PRL levels and decrease tumor size. Dopamine agonists are also used in the management of acromegaly, although the GH responses and effects on tumor size are generally much less pronounced than in prolactinomas. Somatostatin analogues, such as octreotide and lanreotide, act to suppress the secretion of certain hormones, including GH and TSH, and have been used to treat patients with acromegaly and TSH-producing tumors. Medical therapy for Cushing's disease is primarily directed toward inhibition of steroid biosynthesis. These drugs include ketoconazole, metyrapone, aminoglutethimide, mifepristone, etomidate, and mitotane. Because of substantial side effects and because patients with Cushing's disease tend to escape from the cortisol-suppressing effects of these drugs by producing more ACTH, medical therapy is used primarily as an adjunctive treatment.

GROWTH HORMONE

The pituitary gland contains large amounts of stored GH (5 to 10 mg), a 191–amino acid, single-chain protein that contains two intramolecular disulfide bonds (see Table 237–1). GH is complexed in the circulation to two different binding proteins. The high-affinity binding protein has been identified as a circulating form of the extracellular domain of the GH receptor. In addition to reducing the clearance of GH greatly, this binding protein may also modulate GH action.

Production of GH is controlled by a complex interplay of hypothalamic stimulatory and inhibitory peptides, neurotransmitters, growth factors, sex steroids, and nutritional conditions. The most important regulators of GH are the hypothalamic hormones: GHRH, which is stimulatory; and somatostatin, which is inhibitory. A hypothalamic peptide, ghrelin, releases GH in humans but is of uncertain physiologic significance. GH increases the production of IGF-I, which, in turn, inhibits GH production. GHRH causes somatotroph proliferation as well as increasing GH biosynthesis and secretion. The Gsα subunit, which is coupled to the GHRH receptor, is one of the targets for activating mutations that lead to somatotroph adenomas.

IGF-I acts at both the pituitary and the hypothalamic level to inhibit GH secretion. In addition to reflecting GH action (primarily at the liver), serum IGF-I is also sensitive to nutritional and metabolic changes. In cases of starvation, anorexia nervosa, and poorly controlled diabetes, IGF-I levels are low, resulting in increased levels of GH. In cases of obesity (Chapter 239), GH levels are low and GHRH responses are blunted, but IGF-I levels are usually normal. Stress, exercise, and various neurogenic stimuli also increase GH secretion. Estrogens stimulate GH secretion, but their effects are less pronounced than for PRL.

Large bursts of GH secretion characteristically occur at night in association with slow-wave sleep. GH levels tend to be greatest during puberty and decline gradually in adulthood. The amplitude of GH pulses is greater in women than in men, a finding likely reflecting the effects of estrogens. Spontaneous GH pulses can reach 50 ng/mL and are cleared rapidly with a half-life of approximately 20 minutes. Consequently, random GH levels can be very low or high. That GH responses to GHRH are highly variable, even within an individual, probably reflects variations in endogenous somatostatin tone.

GH acts through a single transmembrane receptor that is structurally related to PRL and cytokine receptors (e.g., erythropoietin and colony-stimulating factors). The GH molecule has two distinct receptor binding domains that allow it to contact two separate receptor molecules to induce receptor dimerization. Mutations in the gene for the GH receptor cause GH resistance and severe growth retardation, a condition referred to as the *GH insensitivity syndrome* (Laron-type dwarfism). GH levels are elevated and IGF-I levels are low, findings reflecting the inability of the mutant receptor to transduce the GH signal. Other mutations have been found in the transduction mechanisms mediating GH action.

Many of the growth and metabolic effects of GH are transmitted indirectly through the actions of IGF-I. GH stimulates IGF-I production in most tissues, where it then exerts autocrine or paracrine effects. Circulating IGF-I is derived predominantly from the liver and is a useful marker of GH action because it has a longer half-life and integrates the effects of GH pulses. Although IGF-I levels are used in the diagnosis of acromegaly and to assess the integrity of the GH axis, factors other than GH (e.g., malnutrition) can alter IGF-I levels. IGF-I acts through widely distributed receptors that are structurally related to insulin receptors. In addition to its growth-promoting and anabolic effects, IGF-I also stimulates mitogenesis in many tissues. The bioactivity of IGF-I is itself modulated by six IGF binding proteins (IGFBPs). These IGFBPs can inhibit or enhance IGF-I actions. IGFBP-3 is the major IGFBP in plasma; it is regulated by GH, and its levels generally parallel those of IGF-I, both reflecting GH bioactivity.

GH has major effects on linear growth but also influences a variety of metabolic pathways. Some of these effects are mediated by GH directly, whereas others are conferred by IGF-I. Although the relative roles of GH and IGF-I are debated, their actions are cooperative in many cases. The effects of GH on linear growth appear to be mediated largely by IGF-I, which has been used to stimulate growth in patients with the GH insensitivity syndrome. Linear growth in the fetus and neonate is not GH dependent, as illustrated by the finding that GH-deficient infants have normal birth lengths, although intrauterine IGF-I and IGF-II may be important for fetal growth. In contrast, normal postnatal linear growth requires GH, as illustrated by the clinical manifestations of GH deficiency. GH and IGF-I act together to accelerate linear growth markedly, particularly at the time of puberty when sex steroids enhance GH and IGF-I levels.

GH also induces lipolysis and stimulates anabolic activity, including amino acid uptake and protein synthesis. As a result, it reduces body fat, increases lean body mass, and leads to positive nitrogen balance. These properties of GH are most strikingly seen in GH-deficient children who have undergone GH replacement. GH opposes many of the actions of insulin and can be considered diabetogenic. In patients with diabetes, nocturnal GH secretion accounts in large part for the *dawn phenomenon,* in which a decrease in glucose utilization causes a tendency toward hyperglycemia.

GROWTH HORMONE DEFICIENCY

Causes of GH deficiency include hypothalamic and pituitary disorders, GHRH receptor mutations, GH gene mutations, combined pituitary hormone deficiencies, GH receptor mutations, IGF-I receptor mutations, radiation, and psychosocial deprivation (Chapter 241). The clinical manifestations of GH deficiency depend on the time of onset and the severity of hormone deficiency. Children with complete GH deficiency have slow linear growth rates (e.g., 3 cm/year), and they rapidly fall to less than normal values on standardized growth charts. GH-deficient children have normal skeletal proportions, and many have a pudgy, youthful appearance because of decreased lipolysis. These patients have a predisposition to hypoglycemia, particularly in the setting of cortisol deficiency.

Basal GH does not provide a reliable measure of GH reserve, whereas low IGF-I and low IGFBP-3 levels are consistent with GH deficiency. Conversely, not all patients documented to have GH deficiency by stimulation testing have IGF-I levels that are lower than the normal range. GH deficiency is most frequently assessed using insulin-induced hypoglycemia, which activates central nervous system pathways and leads to stimulation of both GH and ACTH secretion (see Table 242–4). The insulin tolerance test requires careful monitoring for symptoms of severe hypoglycemia, such as confusion or depressed consciousness. This test should be avoided in patients with seizure disorders or coronary artery disease. Insulin doses (0.1 to 0.15 U/kg) may need to be decreased if glucocorticoid deficiency is suspected or increased in conditions of insulin resistance (e.g., obesity). Alternatives to the insulin tolerance test for evaluation of GH include stimulation by L-dopa or arginine. Stimulation tests using a combination of arginine and GHRH have become standardized as well, especially in adults.

Treatment

Rx

In children with well-documented GH deficiency, GH replacement is effective and is essential to increase final adult height. In a typical regimen, recombinant GH (0.025 mg/kg) is given daily as subcutaneous injections. The efficacy of GH treatment depends on when it is initiated as well as on replacement of other hormone deficiencies, if they coexist. In the setting of multiple hormone deficiencies, replacement of thyroid hormone and cortisol is necessary for effective GH action. In contrast, sex steroids (estrogen in particular) lead to epiphyseal closure and limit linear growth. Consequently, GH is more effective before puberty; if exogenous sex steroids are given, low doses should be used. GH has also been shown to increase the final height of girls with Turner's syndrome (chromosomal XO state) and children with end-stage renal disease. These are U.S. Food and Drug Administration (FDA)–approved indications.

Although the potential role of GH replacement in adults is debated, this therapy has been approved by the FDA for the treatment of adults with GH deficiency. Only approximately one third of children with isolated, idiopathic GH deficiency are found to be GH deficient on retesting as adults. Thus, all such patients should be retested before GH therapy is continued or restarted unless proven molecular defects were the cause of their GH deficiency. Studies show that GH treatment can increase lean body mass, decrease fat mass, and improve the sense of well-being in adults with documented GH deficiency. Safety data for long-term GH administration show negligible adverse effects. Whether GH treatment in adults will affect the increased mortality rate associated with hypopituitarism is unknown. Adverse effects occur at lower doses in adults compared with children; a starting dose of 0.2 to 0.3 mg/day has been recommended, with gradual titration guided by clinical benefits, adverse effects, and IGF-I levels.

GROWTH HORMONE EXCESS: ACROMEGALY AND GIGANTISM

Etiology and Pathogenesis

GH-producing pituitary tumors, which account for 10% of pituitary tumors (see Table 242–6), can secrete more than one hormone. PRL is produced in approximately 40% of somatotroph adenomas, and some patients may present because of symptoms of hyperprolactinemia (i.e., amenorrhea and/or galactorrhea). A subset of these tumors is categorized morphologically as mammosomatotroph adenomas. GH-producing

TABLE 242–7 CLINICAL FEATURES OF ACROMEGALY

Clinical Features	No. of Subjects	Years or Frequency
Age at diagnosis	885	42 yr
Delay to diagnosis	680	8.7 yr
Gender (% male)	1,331	48%
Acral/facial changes	595	98%
Oligo/amenorrhea (females)	366	72%
Hyperhidrosis	751	64%
Headaches	825	55%
Paresthesias/carpal tunnel	725	40%
Impotence (males)	355	36%
Hypertension	630	28%
Goiter	705	21%
Visual field defects	993	19%

From Molitch ME: Clinical manifestations of acromegaly. Endocrinol Metab Clin North Am 1992;21:597–614.

tumors can also co-secrete glycoprotein hormones, most frequently the common α subunit (10 to 30%) or, rarely, TSH.

Ectopic production of GHRH (usually carcinoid or pancreatic islets) is a well-documented but rare (<1%) cause of acromegaly that can result in somatotroph hyperplasia. Activating Gsα subunit mutations occur in 35 to 40% of somatotroph adenomas. Molecular defects in the remaining 60 to 65% of somatotroph adenomas remain unidentified.

Clinical Manifestations

Tumors that secrete GH cause acromegaly in adults and gigantism in children in whom GH excess occurs before epiphyseal closure. The annual incidence of acromegaly has been estimated at three per million. Acromegaly affects men and women with equal frequency and is most often recognized when patients are in their 30s or 40s, usually after a decade of GH excess. The clinical features of acromegaly are summarized in Table 242–7. The most striking features usually involve the face, hands, and feet. The diagnosis is often suspected because of changes in facial appearance that include enlargement of the lower jaw (prognathism), the nose and lips, and the sinuses (causing frontal bossing) (Fig. 242–1). Oral cavity changes including malocclusion and increased spacing between the teeth, and enlargement of the tongue may lead to recognition of the disorder by dentists. A hollow, resonant voice is caused by changes in the vocal cords and the soft tissues of the hypopharynx. Sleep apnea may occur in patients with soft tissue obstruction of the pharynx but also because of a central disorder. Few acromegalic patients wear rings because they have long since outgrown them, and they usually have a history of progressive increase in shoe size and width. In addition to bony enlargement, the soft tissues of the hands and feet increase markedly. A moist, doughy, enveloping handshake is characteristic of acromegaly. Heel pad thickness (which can be assessed radiographically) correlates well with IGF-I levels and other clinical features of the disease. Arthritis (hands, feet, hips, knees) is common (75%) and is caused by cartilage and synovial overgrowth. Some degree of carpal tunnel syndrome is seen in 50%. Skin changes include increased skinfolds, particularly over the brow and forehead. The skin is usually oily, owing to increased sebaceous activity and sweating. Skin tags are common, and their presence correlates with the presence of colonic polyps. Galactorrhea may be seen in women, and reproductive dysfunction occurs in both women and men when PRL levels are elevated. Headaches, visual field defects, and other neurologic symptoms depend on the location and extent of tumor growth.

Acromegaly causes as much as a two- to threefold increase in the rate of mortality. Most of the increased mortality can be attributed to cardiovascular and cerebrovascular diseases and may be related in part to the increased prevalence of hypertension (25 to 35%) and diabetes mellitus (10 to 25%). Evidence indicates cardiac hypertrophy in the majority of patients, and symptomatic heart disease, consisting of cardiomyopathy or congestive heart failure or both, occurs in 15 to 20% of patients. Sleep apnea may predispose patients to cardiac dysrhythmias. Some analyses have found an increased risk of premalignant polyps and colon cancer in patients with acromegaly, and screening with colonoscopy is recommended. The disfigurement, metabolic complications, and increased mortality associated with acromegaly emphasize the importance of early diagnosis and implementation of appropriate therapy to lower the GH levels into the normal range.

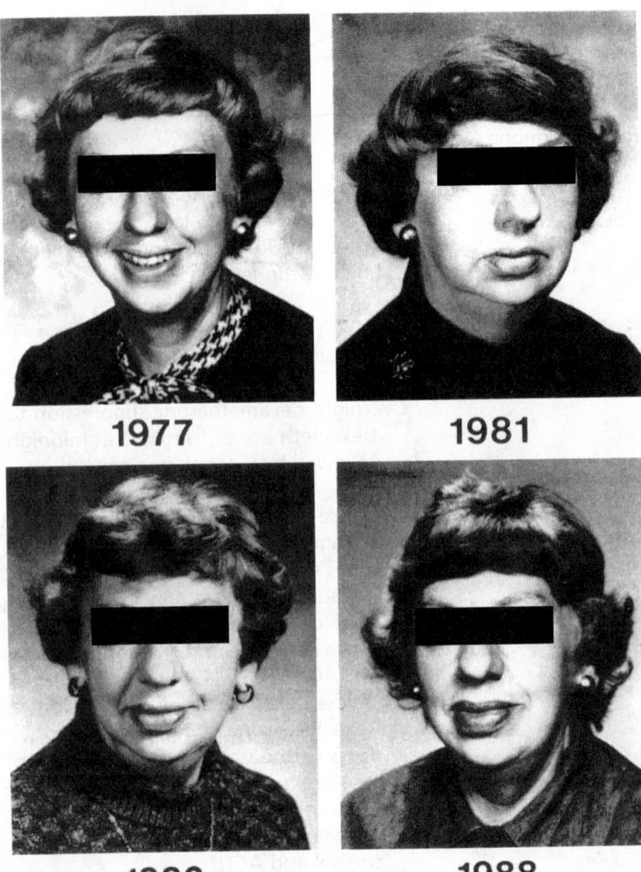

FIGURE 242–1 • Clinical features of acromegaly. Serial photographs of a 64-year-old woman with acromegaly. Over an 11-year period, the patient had a progressive coarsening of facial features, including enlargement of the nose and lips and development of prognathism. She also experienced hypertension, arthropathy, and enlargement of the hands (not shown). (From Molitch ME: Clinical manifestations of acromegaly. Endocrinol Metab Clin North Am 1992;21:597–614.)

Diagnosis

Because GH is secreted in a pulsatile manner, and because the amplitude of normal GH pulses can be large (>50 ng/mL), random GH level measurements are not useful in making the diagnosis of acromegaly. IGF-I levels provide an integrated index of GH production and provide a better screening test for acromegaly. IGF-I levels are normally elevated during puberty and pregnancy and decrease with age, so normal ranges must be age adjusted. IGF-I levels correlate well with 24-hour GH production and with disease activity. The most reliable test for acromegaly is the glucose tolerance test (Table 242–8). In acromegaly, increased glucose levels fail to suppress GH levels to less than 1 ng/mL with polyclonal antibody immunoassays and to levels lower than 0.4 ng/mL using newer monoclonal antibody two-site assays. Co-secretion of PRL should be evaluated. After diagnosis, radiologic studies, preferably using MRI, should be used to evaluate the extent of tumor growth. Unlike in Cushing's disease and prolactinomas, most patients with acromegaly have macroadenomas. In the absence of an apparent pituitary tumor, the possibility of ectopic GHRH secretion causing somatotroph cell hyperplasia should be considered.

TABLE 242–8 SELECTED TESTS OF EXCESS PITUITARY FUNCTION

Hormone	Test	Interpretation
Growth hormone (GH)	Basal IGF-I	Elevated IGF-I levels are consistent with acromegaly when interpreted in the context of age and nutritional status
	Oral glucose suppression test: After 75-g glucose load, GH measured at –30, 0, 30, 60, 90, and 120 min	GH should be suppressed to <1 μg/L normally, with polyclonal radioimmunoassays; <0.4 μg/L with two-site monoclonal assays; GH may paradoxically increase in acromegaly
Prolactin	Basal prolactin levels	Elevated prolactin (>200 μg/L) is consistent with prolactinoma; with prolactin levels 20–200 μg/L, other causes of hyperprolactinemia should also be considered
Adrenocorticotropic hormone (ACTH)	Measurement of 24-hr urine free cortisol	Elevated urine free cortisol level is suggestive of Cushing's syndrome, but it has several other causes as well
	Overnight dexamethasone suppression test: Dexamethasone (1 mg) PO at midnight followed by 8 AM plasma cortisol	Normally, AM cortisol should be suppressed to <5 μg/dL; normal dexamethasone suppression excludes Cushing's syndrome; several other disorders can cause failure to suppress normally
	Low-dose dexamethasone suppression test: Dexamethasone (0.5 mg) q6h for eight doses with basal and end of treatment measurements that may include 24-hr urine collections for free cortisol or 17-hydroxysteroids and AM plasma cortisol and ACTH	17-Hydroxysteroids should be suppressed to <4 mg/24 hr; urine free cortisol should be <20 μg/24 hr; serum cortisol should be suppressed to <6 μg/dL; failure to suppress cortisol production is consistent with the diagnosis of Cushing's syndrome
	High-dose dexamethasone suppression test: Dexamethasone (2 mg) q6h for eight doses with basal and end of treatment measurements that may include 24-hr urine collections for free cortisol or 17-hydroxysteroids and AM plasma cortisol and ACTH	High-dose test is intended to distinguish Cushing's disease (pituitary adenoma), ectopic ACTH production, and adrenal adenoma; 50% suppression of 17-hydroxysteroids or 90% suppression of urine free cortisol production is suggestive of Cushing's disease; <50% suppression suggests ectopic ACTH or adrenal adenoma; low ACTH levels are consistent with adrenal adenoma
	CRH test: Ovine CRH (1 μg/kg) administered IV and ACTH and cortisol drawn at –15, 0, 15, 30, 60, 90, and 120 min	In Cushing's disease, there is usually a 50% increase in ACTH and a 20% increase in cortisol; adrenal adenoma is associated with suppressed ACTH; ectopic ACTH is associated with high basal ACTH and cortisol levels that are not affected by CRH
	Petrosal sinus ACTH sampling: inferior petrosal sinus is catheterized, ideally bilaterally, and plasma ACTH is compared with simultaneous peripheral samples; sampling can be done in conjunction with CRH stimulation	In Cushing's disease, ratio of ACTH in the petrosal sinus/periphery is at least 2 basally and at least 3 after CRH; in ectopic ACTH, ratio of petrosal sinus/peripheral level is <1.5
Thyroid-stimulating hormone (TSH)	Basal thyroid function tests	Inappropriate normal or elevated TSH in the setting of increased free thyroid hormone levels is consistent with a TSH-producing tumor or other causes of inappropriate TSH secretion
	Free α-subunit level	Elevated free α-subunit levels associated with inappropriately elevated TSH are suggestive of a TSH-producing tumor
Follicle-stimulating hormone (FSH), luteinizing hormone (LH)	Basal FSH, LH, testosterone	Increased LH and testosterone levels in male patients are consistent with LH-secreting tumors; elevated FSH and low-normal testosterone are suggestive of an FSH-producing tumor if primary gonadal failure is not present; in female patients, assessment of excess hormone secretion is difficult because of changes during the menstrual cycle and at menopause
	TRH test: TRH (200 μg) given IV with measurements of serum FSH, LH, FSH β, and LH β subunits at 0, 20, and 60 min	Stimulation of LH, FSH, or their free β subunits is suggestive of a gonadotropin-producing adenoma

CRH = corticotropin-releasing hormone; IGF-I = insulin-like growth factor-I; IV = intravenously; PO = orally; TRH = thyrotropin-releasing hormone.

Treatment

The goals of therapy in acromegaly are to reverse or prevent tumor mass effects and to reduce the long-term morbidity and mortality that result from excess GH production. Correction of the disorder prevents further physical disfigurement and can result in substantial resolution of soft tissue changes and improvements in metabolic derangements. Although reductions in GH levels are associated with improvements in symptoms, the ultimate goal is to achieve normal GH and IGF-I levels and to prevent tumor recurrence without incurring hypopituitarism.

Transsphenoidal surgery results in GH levels lower than 2.5 ng/mL in approximately 80% of patients with microadenomas. This level, along with GH suppression to less than 1 ng/mL during an oral glucose tolerance test, and a normal IGF-I level have been associated with a normalization of the increased mortality of acromegaly.

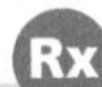

Patients with macroadenomas are less often cured by surgery (<30%), but they usually have reductions in GH levels.

Medical therapies for acromegaly include dopamine agonists, such as cabergoline, somatostatin analogues, such as octreotide and lanreotide, and a GH receptor antagonist, pegvisomant. Although cabergoline reduces GH and IGF-I levels, normal levels are achieved in only 10 to 20% of patients. Long-acting preparations of octreotide and other somatostatin analogues that can be given by intramuscular injection every 2 to 4 weeks reduce GH and IGF-I levels in almost all patients, with normal levels of IGF-I achieved in approximately 60% of cases. Tumor size is reduced in approximately one half of cases. Somatostatin analogues are useful as adjunctive therapy in patients who are not cured by surgery or radiation. Side effects of somatostatin analogues include diarrhea and an increased risk of cholelithiasis, although cholecystitis and the need for cholecystectomy are less common. Some patients experience additive beneficial effects from combining these two classes of medications while keeping the dose of each drug low enough to avoid adverse effects. Pegvisomant is a biosynthetic GH analogue that prevents binding of GH to its receptor. It is capable of normalizing IGF-I levels in 97% of patients with corresponding clinical benefits, but it has no effects on the tumor itself. Pegvisomant is given by daily subcutaneous injection, and long-term experience is limited, so the drug generally used in patients who do not respond optimally to other treatment modalities.

Radiation is not recommended as primary therapy for acromegaly because of the long time (5 to 10 years) required for reductions in GH levels and the high incidence of hypopituitarism and other complications. Adjunctive radiation therapy may be required for patients with macroadenomas when GH levels or mass effects persist after transsphenoidal surgery and medical therapy. Recent data suggest that gamma knife radiation therapy may be the most efficacious form of radiation therapy for acromegaly.

PROLACTIN

PRL and GH appear to be derived from a common ancestral gene, and this accounts for the similarities in their present-day structures and some overlap in their functional properties. Estrogen stimulates lactotroph proliferation, and the number of lactotrophs is consequently greater in women than in men and during pregnancy (e.g., 70% of pituitary cells).

Secretion of PRL is controlled by tonic inhibition by dopamine, which acts through D_2-type receptors on lactotrophs. PRL biosynthesis and secretion are stimulated by the hypothalamic peptides TRH and vasoactive intestinal polypeptide. Hypothyroidism causes increased TRH output and increased sensitivity of the lactotrophs to TRH and can result in hyperprolactinemia. Vasoactive intestinal polypeptide, which acts through receptors that increase cyclic adenosine monophosphate, may be responsible, along with a decrease in dopamine, for PRL increases associated with suckling. Vasoactive intestinal polypeptide is also found in the pituitary, where it may act as an autocrine or paracrine regulator of PRL secretion. On balance, dopamine inhibition is the dominant influence for PRL secretion, so PRL is the one pituitary hormone that increases after pituitary stalk section. Numerous pharmacologic agents can stimulate PRL secretion, often by impairing dopamine secretion or action (see Table 242–2).

Secretion of PRL is pulsatile and increases with sleep, stress, chest wall stimulation, and pregnancy. PRL levels are usually less than 15 to 20 ng/mL in women and 10 to 15 ng/mL in men. The primary function of PRL is to induce and sustain lactation. However, PRL binds to specific receptors that are located in several tissues, including breast, gonads, lymphoid cells, and liver. During pregnancy, PRL levels increase, and, in conjunction with other hormones (estrogens, progesterone, thyroid hormone, cortisol, and insulin), breast epithelium is stimulated to proliferate and milk synthesis is induced. High levels of estrogen and progesterone inhibit lactation during pregnancy. The rapid decline in these steroids in the postpartum period permits lactation to occur. Neural pathways leading to the secretion of oxytocin provide the "let-down" reflex that induces lactation in response to suckling. Early in the postpartum period, PRL secretion is stimulated by suckling, but this response becomes damped with time. PRL also suppresses gonadotropins, by a direct action on GnRH-secreting neurons. Consequently, breast-feeding can suppress ovulation. High levels of PRL are present in amniotic fluid, and PRL is produced in the decidual layer of the placenta.

PROLACTIN DEFICIENCY

PRL deficiency is rare and occurs primarily in the setting of combined hormone deficiencies. The only recognized consequence of PRL deficiency is the absence of postpartum lactation. This situation may be found in patients with pituitary infarction occurring as a result of obstetric hemorrhage (Sheehan's syndrome). No effects on breast development or other tissues have been described in PRL deficiency.

HYPERPROLACTINEMIA

Etiology and Pathogenesis

Hyperprolactinemia can occur as a consequence of pharmacologic alterations in the pathways that control PRL secretion, of physiologic or metabolic effects on PRL production and clearance, or of neoplastic conditions (see Table 241–2 in Chapter 241). PRL-producing adenoma is the most common type of pituitary tumor (25 to 40%). Estrogen is a potent stimulus for lactotroph proliferation and may cause prolactinomas in rats; however, in humans, no clear association exists between estrogens (e.g., oral contraceptive use) and the incidence of prolactinomas. Estrogen can stimulate the growth of preexisting prolactinomas, and the very high estrogen levels present during pregnancy may cause approximately 25% of large prolactinomas to enlarge during pregnancy. Diminished dopamine tone results in increased PRL but has not been shown to cause prolactinomas.

Microprolactinomas constitute the great majority of tumors in premenopausal women. In contrast, macroadenomas are more commonly seen in men and in postmenopausal women. The predominance of smaller tumors in premenopausal women may be accounted for by a bias of ascertainment, because elevated PRL levels in this group lead to clinical manifestations (amenorrhea, galactorrhea, or infertility). Subclinical prolactinomas exist in men and in many older women, and approximately 10% of apparently healthy individuals have PRL-positive microadenomas in autopsy series.

Clinical Manifestations

Hyperprolactinemia causes galactorrhea and oligomenorrhea or amenorrhea in premenopausal women. Estrogen facilitates PRL-induced galactorrhea, and this feature explains why the condition is less common in postmenopausal women and in women with prolonged hypogonadism. Amenorrhea is primarily a consequence of PRL suppression of GnRH, although PRL may also have inhibitory effects at the level of the pituitary and the gonad. Amenorrhea is associated with infertility, and PRL levels should be a routine part of the hormonal evaluation of infertility. Estrogen deficiency can cause decreased libido, vaginal dryness, and dyspareunia. Long-standing estrogen deficiency also leads to osteopenia in some women. A subset of patients has hirsutism and can exhibit elevations of adrenal androgens. Oral contraceptives may mask PRL-induced oligomenorrhea or amenorrhea, which becomes apparent when these drugs are discontinued. In postmenopausal women, prolactinomas are often identified because of mass effects rather than because of their hormonal effects.

In men, hyperprolactinemia causes hypogonadism with suppressed LH and FSH levels and low testosterone levels. Hypogonadism causes diminished libido, impotence, infertility, and, rarely, gynecomastia or galactorrhea. Diminished libido may also reflect suppression of GnRH because testosterone replacement is not as effective as suppression of hyperprolactinemia. Hyperprolactinemia is found in 1 to 2% of men evaluated for sexual dysfunction.

Diagnosis

Four primary categories of causes of hyperprolactinemia must be distinguished if the correct therapy is to be instituted: (1) physiologic or metabolic hyperprolactinemia, (2) pharmacologic hyperprolactinemia, (3) hypothalamic or pituitary stalk compression, and (4) prolactinoma (see Table 241–2). With the exception of pregnancy and renal failure, physiologic causes of increased PRL result in minor elevations in PRL (usually <50 ng/mL). Primary hypothyroidism should be excluded as a cause of mild hyperprolactinemia. A careful drug history should be obtained in all patients with hyperprolactinemia because of the large number of agents that can stimulate PRL secretion. Psychotropic medications, in particular, can increase PRL either by reducing dopamine production or by blocking its action. In most cases, the degree of hyperprolactinemia caused by drugs is less than 150 ng/mL. Various suprasellar and parasellar mass lesions cause mild hyperprolactinemia (e.g., 20 and 100 ng/mL) because of compression of the hypothalamus or pituitary stalk. Unless very good evidence for physiologic or drug-induced hyperprolactinemia exists, even patients with mild hyperprolactinemia should be evaluated with CT or MRI to distinguish among idiopathic hyperprolactinemia, microprolactinomas, and other large mass lesions that cause stalk compression and decrease the amount of dopamine that reaches the lactotrophs. However, a specific caution is needed when two-site assays are used, because patients with very high PRL levels may appear to have PRL levels that are normal or only modestly elevated, owing to the "hook effect." To avoid this problem, PRL levels should always be measured again at 1:100 dilution in patients with macroadenomas and normal to modestly elevated PRL levels. When no pituitary lesions are seen by radiographic studies and physiologic and pharmacologic causes of hyperprolactinemia cannot be identified, the diagnosis of idiopathic hyperprolactinemia is made. Idiopathic hyperprolactinemia may represent microprolactinomas too small to be detected accurately by current imaging techniques or altered hypothalamic regulation of PRL secretion. Whether such patients should be treated depends on the clinical effects of hyperprolactinemia. Over several years, few of these patients develop large tumors, only 10 to 15% show MRI evidence of microadenomas, and in one third of cases the hyperprolactinemia resolves.

Treatment

Rx

The natural history of prolactinomas has been evaluated in several series. Although large prolactinomas clearly must evolve from smaller lesions, it is uncommon (7%) for microprolactinomas to progress to macroadenomas. When patients with microadenomas are observed over 3 to 5 years but are not treated, PRL levels decrease in 20 to 30% and increase in less than 10% of patients. PRL levels may decrease because of spontaneous tumor infarction. Because of the slow rate of growth, it is reasonable to monitor patients with microprolactinomas without treatment by periodic measurement of PRL levels unless the hyperprolactinemia is causing symptoms that warrant therapy.

When hyperprolactinemia causes hypogonadism, osteopenia, or infertility, a dopamine agonist such as cabergoline or bromocriptine is the therapy of choice. Dopamine agonists normalize PRL levels and correct amenorrhea and galactorrhea in 80 to 90% of patients. Cabergoline is more effective and has fewer adverse side effects than bromocriptine and has the additional advantage of once- or twice-weekly administration. Bromocriptine must be started in low doses with gradual increases to avoid side effects (nausea, dizziness, somnolence, and nasal stuffiness).

Cabergoline may cause a considerable reduction in tumor size in patients with macroprolactinomas. Approximately 80 to 90% of patients have a greater than 50% reduction in tumor size but such size reduction is seen in only approximately two thirds of patients treated with bromocriptine. Visual field defects are a very sensitive index of tumor size, and improvements can be seen in approximately 90% of patients. Thus, cabergoline is used as first-line therapy even in patients with visual field defects as long as visual acuity is not threatened by rapid progression or recent tumor hemorrhage. In patients treated with cabergoline whose tumors shrink to the point of nonvisualization on MRI and whose PRL levels are normal for at least 2 years, approximately three fourths can maintain normal PRL levels and not experience tumor re-expansion with cessation of therapy. In some cases, prolactinomas appear to be resistant to a dopamine agonist, but it is important to ensure compliance with therapy and to be certain that the underlying lesion is a prolactinoma and not some other cause of hyperprolactinemia. In these patients, an alternative dopamine agonist may be successful. Pergolide is another dopamine agonist with proven efficacy in decreasing PRL levels and prolactinoma size, but it has not been approved by the FDA for treatment of this condition. Recently, some patients treated with high doses of pergolide and cabergoline for Parkinson's disease have been reported to have developed cardiac valvular lesions. No such cases have been reported with doses usually used in patients with prolactinomas. However, if higher than normal doses are used, monitoring with echocardiography may be warranted. Alternatively, transsphenoidal surgery may be used. Although initial remission rates (70 to 80%) for transsphenoidal surgery of microprolactinomas are good, approximately 20% of patients have long-term recurrence of their tumors. For macroprolactinomas, the initial remission rates are 30%, with a similar recurrence rate. Radiation therapy, usually gamma knife, is reserved for those patients with macroadenomas not responding to either medical or surgical treatment.

Bromocriptine therapy for infertility, or when a possibility of pregnancy exists, deserves special consideration. Bromocriptine can induce ovulation in 80 to 90% of patients with hyperprolactinemia. Although bromocriptine has not been associated with congenital malformations or complications during pregnancy, most physicians and patients prefer to avoid its use during pregnancy if possible. A form of barrier contraception is usually recommended until two to three regular menstrual cycles have occurred. Subsequently, pregnancy can be confirmed if a menstrual period is missed, thus allowing discontinuation of bromocriptine with exposure of the fetus to the drug for only 3 to 5 weeks. At present, the safety data for pregnancy outcome are much more limited for cabergoline; therefore, some clinicians prefer bromocriptine when fertility is desired. Fewer than 2% of patients with microadenomas, but 31% of patients with macroadenomas, develop symptoms of tumor enlargement (headaches, visual field defects) during pregnancy. If symptoms develop, MRI and formal visual field testing should be performed. If evidence of visual field compromise or tumor growth is noted, then bromocriptine therapy should be restarted to shrink the tumor. PRL levels are not very useful because they are normally increased in pregnancy, and an enlarging tumor may not cause PRL production to increase substantially. Because problems of tumor growth occur most often in patients with macroadenomas, consideration can also be given to the option of transsphenoidal decompression before pregnancy in women with large tumors, as long as fertility can be preserved.

ADRENOCORTICOTROPIC HORMONE

Structure

ACTH is a 39–amino acid peptide that is derived from a precursor polypeptide POMC (241 amino acids), which encodes several peptides, including an amino-terminal peptide, joining peptide, ACTH, and β-lipotropin (β-LPH) (Chapter 241). The functional roles of some of the POMC-encoded peptides other than ACTH have been defined. β-LPH may stimulate melanocytes and may contribute to hyperpigmentation in conditions of POMC stimulation. β-LPH can be processed further to yield γ-lipotropin and β-endorphin. The biologically active portion of ACTH resides within the first 18 of its 39 amino acids. However, because a synthetic peptide (cosyntropin) that includes the first 24 amino acids has a longer half-life, it is used clinically to assess adrenocortical function. The half-life of ACTH is relatively short (<10 minutes), and pulses of ACTH secretion are discrete. Levels of precursor peptides, such as β-LPH, do not always parallel those of ACTH because of their slower clearance rates. In cases with neoplastic ectopic production of ACTH, the levels of precursor peptides may be elevated. The POMC gene can also be expressed from alternate transcription start sites, thus giving rise to aberrant POMC transcripts in ectopic tumors.

The primary effect of ACTH is to stimulate the adrenal gland to produce cortisol. It also stimulates secretion of adrenal androgens and mineralocorticoids, but mineralocorticoid production is controlled primarily through the renin-angiotensin system (Chapter 245). Consequently, mineralocorticoid function is preserved in ACTH deficiency, in contrast to primary adrenal insufficiency, which is characterized by loss of glucocorticoid and mineralocorticoid function. Long-term stimulation by ACTH causes adrenal hyperplasia and enlargement. Conversely, ACTH deficiency leads to adrenal atrophy, and several days of ACTH stimulation are required before steroid synthesis returns to normal.

The secretion of ACTH is regulated by the hypothalamic-pituitary-adrenal axis. Hypothalamic CRH is the most important stimulator of ACTH secretion. CRH is a 41–amino acid peptide that is produced in the paraventricular nucleus of the hypothalamus and in other sites in the nervous system (Chapter 241). Chronic stimulation by CRH causes corticotroph cell hyperplasia, which is seen in cases of ectopic CRH production.

Arginine vasopressin weakly stimulates ACTH, but when administered with CRH, it acts synergistically and functions as a physiologic stimulus to ACTH secretion along with CRH. Some CRH-containing paraventricular neurons also contain arginine vasopressin. CRH and vasopressin are not always released coordinately, however, and stress has been shown selectively to activate the vasopressin-containing subset of CRH neurons. Cortisol inhibits ACTH secretion, blunts the ACTH response to CRH, and inhibits CRH production. After prolonged glucocorticoid suppression of the hypothalamic-pituitary-adrenal axis, the amount of endogenous CRH secretion appears to be rate limiting and can require several months to recover.

Plasma ACTH is secreted in discrete pulses that occur approximately once an hour. Because of the marked variation in ACTH levels, random measurements are of little value, and most clinical tests are therefore based on levels of cortisol or its metabolites, which tend to integrate the effects of ACTH. ACTH secretion exhibits a marked diurnal rhythm, greatest at night several hours after the initiation of sleep. ACTH, in turn, induces a diurnal pattern of cortisol secretion. Cortisol levels are greatest in the early morning and reach a nadir in the late afternoon and evening. Patients with Cushing's disease lose or exhibit a blunted diurnal rhythm of ACTH secretion. ACTH secretion can be stimulated by a variety of different forms of stress, including psychological stimuli, such as fright, and surgery. Depression is associated with activation of the hypothalamic-pituitary-adrenal axis and impaired dexamethasone suppressibility. Hypoglycemia induces ACTH secretion through a central mechanism. The resulting increase in cortisol secretion represents one of several counter-regulatory mechanisms that increase glucose production. Insulin-induced hypoglycemia provides a mechanism for testing the integrity of the hypothalamic-pituitary-adrenal axis (see Table 242–4). Serious trauma and infection activate an array of cytokines that stimulate CRH and ACTH secretion. Because cortisol levels can be increased up to 10-fold in these circumstances, adjustments in cortisol replacement doses are required in seriously ill patients with adrenal insufficiency.

ADRENOCORTICOTROPIC HORMONE DEFICIENCY: SECONDARY HYPOCORTISOLISM

Secondary hypocortisolism causes symptoms of glucocorticoid deficiency, including nausea, vomiting, weakness, fatigue, fever, and hypotension. In addition to reduced levels of cortisol, abnormal laboratory test findings can include hyponatremia, hypoglycemia, and eosinophilia. Depending on its cause, the severity of cortisol deficiency in cases of secondary adrenal insufficiency is often not as marked as in primary adrenal insufficiency. In addition, mineralocorticoid function is preserved in secondary adrenal deficiency. Consequently, the clinical manifestations of volume depletion are less pronounced, and hyperkalemia is not a feature of ACTH deficiency. Because ACTH levels are low in cases of secondary adrenal insufficiency, hyperpigmentation is not seen, as in primary adrenal insufficiency. In women, reduced adrenal androgens can decrease libido and can cause loss of axillary and pubic hair.

The most common cause of ACTH deficiency is treatment with exogenous glucocorticoids, which suppress the hypothalamic-pituitary-adrenal axis. Sudden withdrawal of glucocorticoids or an increased requirement induced by the superimposition of severe illness can elicit symptoms of glucocorticoid deficiency. Congenital forms of ACTH deficiency are rare and usually occur in combination with the loss of other pituitary hormones. Acquired, isolated ACTH deficiency does occur, particularly in women with lymphocytic hypophysitis.

ACTH reserve is most often evaluated using CRH or the *insulin tolerance test.* Caution should be exercised before inducing hypoglycemia in patients with suspected adrenal insufficiency. Insulin-induced hypoglycemia stimulates central responses to neuroglycopenia and mimics some, but not all, stresses that activate ACTH secretion. *CRH testing* (ovine CRH, 1 μg/kg intravenously) may be useful for distinguishing hypothalamic and pituitary causes of ACTH deficiency, because it will still induce an ACTH response in most patients with hypothalamic dysfunction and blunted responses to hypoglycemia. The *metyrapone test* provides an alternative to the insulin tolerance test. By blocking the 11-hydroxylation step, metyrapone inhibits cortisol production, resulting in stimulation of ACTH secretion and an increase in precursor adrenal steroids (e.g., 11-deoxycortisol). Patients should be monitored closely for evidence of adrenal insufficiency, and metyrapone should be used only in patients with at least some evidence of adrenocortical function. *ACTH stimulation tests* using $ACTH_{1-24}$ (cosyntropin) can accurately evaluate primary adrenocortical insufficiency but do not accurately assess secondary adrenal insufficiency. A variation of the ACTH simulation test using the low dose of 1 μg has been found to be useful for diagnosing secondary adrenal insufficiency in some studies.

Deficiency of ACTH is treated by replacement with glucocorticoids. Doses need to be individualized and are based largely on clinical criteria in which symptoms of glucocorticoid deficiency are balanced against features of glucocorticoid excess. Patients should wear MedicAlert tags and should be instructed about the warning signs of cortisol deficiency, including nausea, vomiting, abdominal pain, low-grade fever, fatigue, and postural dizziness. Stress doses of steroids should be used during times of illness. Recent studies suggest that doses of 50 to 75 mg every 8 hours for severe stress are required. Mineralocorticoid replacement is not required in patients with ACTH deficiency.

CUSHING'S DISEASE

Etiology and Pathogenesis

Cushing's disease results from a pituitary adenoma that causes excess production of ACTH. It should be distinguished from other causes of Cushing's syndrome (glucocorticoid excess), which include adrenal causes of cortisol excess, ectopic production of ACTH and CRH, and physiologic states that result in overproduction of cortisol (Chapter 245). Cushing's disease accounts for 60 to 70% of cases of Cushing's syndrome. Ten to 15% of pituitary tumors secrete ACTH. For unknown reasons, Cushing's disease occurs approximately eight times more often in women than in men.

Most ACTH-producing pituitary neoplasms, like other pituitary tumors, are monoclonal, implying a primary defect in corticotroph cells. This concept is supported by the observation that most patients who undergo successful removal of a corticotroph adenoma exhibit suppression of the hypothalamic-pituitary-adrenal axis after surgery. In addition, rare cases of corticotroph hyperplasia causing Cushing's syndrome are secondary to CRH production by either adjacent CRH-producing intrasellar gangliocytomas or ectopic CRH-producing cancers.

In contrast to other pituitary tumors, 80 to 90% of ACTH-secreting tumors are microadenomas. The clinical features of cortisol excess may allow detection of these tumors before they enlarge. High levels of cortisol may also restrain tumor growth. ACTH-secreting macroadenomas tend to be locally invasive.

Clinical Manifestations

The clinical features of Cushing's disease are caused by the effects of excess glucocorticoids and by the hypersecretion of ACTH and other POMC peptide products. The severity of the features of Cushing's disease varies greatly and appears to reflect not only the level of free cortisol but also the duration of the disease and perhaps the sensitivity to glucocorticoid action. In florid cases of Cushing's disease (Fig. 242–2), the constellation of symptoms and physical features is readily recognized. Early in the disease or in mild cases, however, it can be difficult to distinguish the clinical features of Cushing's disease from similar traits that are seen in the normal population. Clinical suspicion is of paramount importance and leads to appropriate screening before laboratory studies are performed. Conversely, one must be discriminating and not formally evaluate everyone with obesity, hypertension, and glucose intolerance. Of the many features listed in Table 242–9, some are relatively specific for Cushing's disease. For example, the centripetal distribution of fat, with the characteristic "buffalo hump," "moon facies," and deposition of fat in the supraclavicular area but not in the extremities, is more specific than

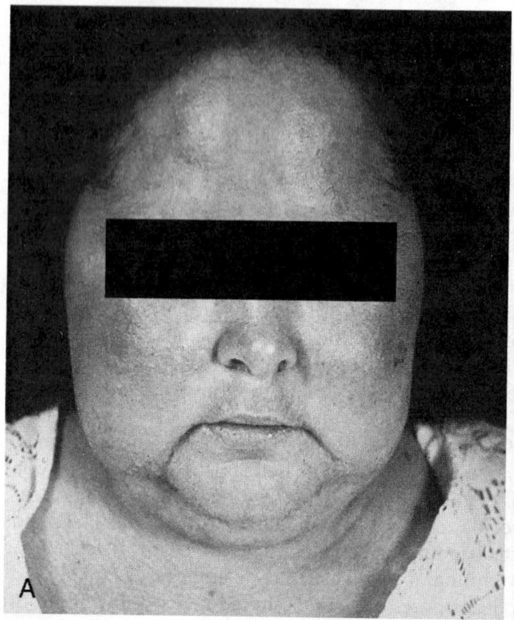

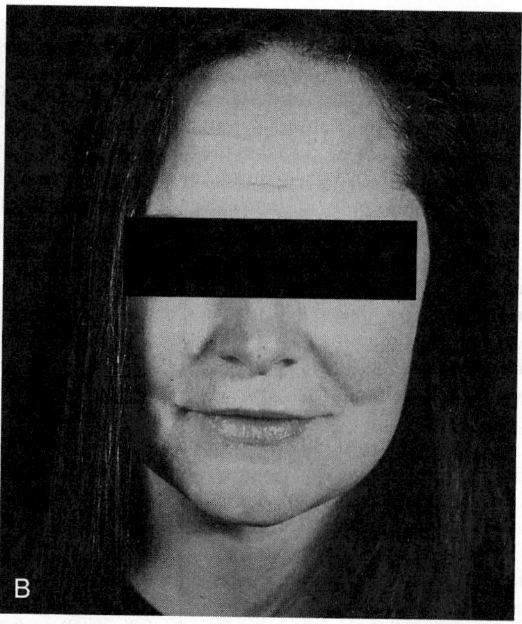

FIGURE 242–2 • Clinical features of Cushing's disease. A 25-year-old woman presented with severe Cushing's disease. **A,** Facial features of Cushing's syndrome including plethora, moon facies, and hirsutism are evident. **B,** Dramatic resolution of the manifestations of cortisol excess after successful transsphenoidal surgery. (Photographs courtesy of Dr. Beverly M. K. Biller.)

TABLE 242–9 CLINICAL FEATURES OF CUSHING'S DISEASE

GENERAL FEATURES
Obesity (centripetal distribution)
"Moon facies" and mild proptosis
Increased supraclavicular fat and "buffalo hump"
Hypertension
SKIN
Hyperpigmentation
Facial plethora
Hirsutism
Violaceous striae and thin skin
Capillary fragility and easy bruising
Acne
Edema
MUSCULOSKELETAL CHANGES
Muscle weakness (proximal)
Osteoporosis and back pain
REPRODUCTIVE FEATURES
Decreased libido
Oligomenorrhea/amenorrhea
NEUROPSYCHIATRIC FEATURES
Depression
Irritability and emotional lability
Psychosis
METABOLIC CHANGES
Hypokalemia and alkalosis
Hypercalciuria and renal stones
Glucose intolerance or diabetes mellitus
Impaired wound healing
Impaired resistance to infection
Granulocytosis and lymphopenia
TUMOR MASS EFFECTS
Headache
Visual field loss
Hypopituitarism

generalized obesity. Striae that are wide (>1 cm) and purple reflect steroid-induced thinning of the dermis and can be distinguished from the more common "stretch marks." Numerous spontaneous ecchymoses also occur because of thinning of the skin and capillary fragility. Proximal muscle weakness represents another manifestation of glucocorticoid excess. Osteopenia and hypokalemia, when present, provide objective evidence consistent with ACTH excess. Hypokalemia results from the effects of ACTH on mineralocorticoid production but also from the ability of high levels of cortisol to saturate 11β-dehydrogenase, an enzyme in the kidney that inactivates cortisol. As a result, cortisol can "spill over" and act on mineralocorticoid receptors in the distal tubule. Hirsutism and acne are caused by the increased production of adrenal androgens and are more prominent in patients with Cushing's disease than in those with adrenal adenomas, in whom glucocorticoids tend to be the predominant product. Oligomenorrhea and amenorrhea probably have several causes, including androgen effects on the reproductive axis and glucocorticoid inhibition of GnRH, which may also account for diminished libido. Hypertension and glucose intolerance are caused by glucocorticoid excess. Immunosuppression, opportunistic infections, and impaired wound healing can lead to considerable morbidity. Neuropsychiatric symptoms, including depression, can be prominent effects of Cushing's disease. Suicide occurs with increased frequency in persons who receive no treatment for the disease.

Diagnosis

The screening tests and differential diagnosis of Cushing's syndrome represent some of the greatest diagnostic challenges in endocrinology (Chapter 245). The first step is to determine whether a patient truly has cortisol excess. After confirmation of Cushing's syndrome, one must distinguish among (1) adrenal causes of cortisol excess, (2) pituitary causes of ACTH excess (Cushing's disease), (3) ectopic sources of ACTH, and (4) ectopic CRH (Table 242–10).

In screening for hypercortisolism, random cortisol levels are not useful because of diurnal variation of the hormone. The overnight dexamethasone test is the most widely used screening test (see Table 242–8). A normal result of the dexamethasone test essentially excludes Cushing's syndrome. However, abnormal overnight dexamethasone suppression can be seen in up to 30% of hospitalized patients and in many patients with depression or during alcohol withdrawal. An elevated 24-hour urine free cortisol value provides an alternative, or additional, screening test for hypercortisolism. Often, two sequential specimens are collected because of day-to-day variations in hormone production. The sensitivity and specificity of urinary free cortisol measurements are greater than those of the overnight dexamethasone suppression test, particularly in hospitalized patients. A third test takes advantage of the observation that the diurnal variation of cortisol levels is lost in all forms of Cushing's syndrome. This test consists of finding elevation of a midnight cortisol level

TABLE 242–10 TESTS USED IN THE DIFFERENTIAL DIAGNOSIS OF CUSHING'S SYNDROME*

Etiology	Overnight Dexamethasone Suppression Test	Plasma ACTH	Low-Dose Dexamethasone	High-Dose Dexamethasone	Corticotropin-Releasing Hormone Stimulation of ACTH	Petrosal/ Peripheral ACTH Ratio
Normal	Suppression	Normal	Suppression		Normal	
Pituitary	No suppression	Normal or high	No suppression	Suppression	Normal or increased	>2
Ectopic	No suppression	High or normal	No suppression	No suppression	No response	<1.5
Adrenal	No suppression	Low	No suppression	No suppression	No response	

*Classic responses are indicated. Certain cases of ectopic adrenocorticotropic hormone (ACTH) production are suppressed by high-dose dexamethasone or are stimulated by corticotropin-releasing hormone. In these cases, petrosal sinus sampling is the most reliable method for distinguishing pituitary and ectopic sources of ACTH.

in the serum or saliva. Kits are available for patients to obtain a late-night salivary cortisol sample.

After demonstrating cortisol excess, the next step is to determine the source of excess ACTH or cortisol. The classic approach is to perform a low-dose, followed by a high-dose, dexamethasone suppression test (see Tables 242–8 and 242–10). The low-dose dexamethasone test excludes or confirms the presence of Cushing's syndrome. On the second day of the test, normal individuals suppress plasma cortisol to less than 5 μg/dL and reduce the urinary 17-hydroxysteroids to less than 2.5 mg/24 hours or urinary free cortisol to less than 20 μg/24 hours. Patients with all forms of Cushing's syndrome fail to show suppression according to these criteria.

The high-dose dexamethasone test is one of several means to distinguish between ACTH-independent and ACTH-dependent causes of Cushing's syndrome and to discriminate between pituitary and ectopic causes of ACTH-dependent Cushing's syndrome (see Table 242–10). Because adrenal sources of cortisol excess are autonomous and ACTH independent, plasma and urinary cortisol levels are not affected by dexamethasone suppression, even at high doses. In addition, plasma ACTH levels are low in adrenal causes of Cushing's syndrome because the hypothalamic-pituitary axis is suppressed. Pituitary and ectopic causes of Cushing's disease are both ACTH dependent but respond differently to high-dose dexamethasone. Pituitary adenomas have an altered set point for glucocorticoid inhibition but retain a partial ability to respond to high-dose dexamethasone. The exact criteria for dexamethasone suppression in the high-dose test are debated. In most patients with ACTH-producing pituitary adenomas, urinary 17-hydroxysteroids are suppressed to less than 50% of baseline, and urinary free cortisol is suppressed to less than 90% of baseline during the high-dose dexamethasone test.

The *ectopic ACTH syndrome* should be suspected in patients with known malignant disease, particularly the following: small cell carcinoma of the lung; bronchial, thymic, or gastrointestinal carcinoids; islet cell tumors; and medullary carcinoma of the thyroid. Plasma ACTH levels are often very high (>200 pg/mL) and can be associated with hyperpigmentation. Clinical features of Cushing's syndrome may be altered by the rapid onset of extreme hypercortisolemia coincident with elements of tumor cachexia. Pronounced weakness, fluid retention, glucose intolerance, hypokalemia, and poor skin integrity are often seen.

Ectopic ACTH syndrome is readily recognized in its classic form. However, some patients with tumors, particularly carcinoids, exhibit dexamethasone suppression that is similar to that seen in patients with pituitary adenomas. When suspected, carcinoids can sometimes be detected by CT or MRI, but many are too small to be seen even with these techniques. Because of these exceptions to the high-dose dexamethasone test, various procedures have been devised in an attempt to distinguish ectopic and pituitary-dependent sources of ACTH further. The metyrapone test takes advantage of the finding that inhibition of 11β-hydroxylase blocks cortisol production. As a result, negative feedback is reduced, and pituitary-dependent sources of ACTH typically exhibit an increase in ACTH that stimulates the production of precursor adrenal steroids (e.g., 11-deoxycortisol) (see Table 242–4). Although most ectopic causes of ACTH exhibit a blunted response to the decreased cortisol levels, patients with the subset of ectopic tumors that respond atypically to dexamethasone are most likely to give a positive response in the metyrapone test. CRH testing may also prove useful; patients with pituitary tumors exhibit an increase in ACTH, and those with tumors that make ACTH ectopically have little or no response.

In recent years, inferior petrosal sinus sampling has been used to distinguish pituitary from ectopic sources of ACTH when the source of ACTH is not obvious based on the clinical circumstances, biochemical evaluation, and imaging studies. This test requires an experienced radiologist for safe and effective catheterization of the petrosal sinuses (which drain the pituitary venous effluent). Blood samples are taken simultaneously from the left and right petrosal sinuses and from the periphery. In the case of ACTH-producing pituitary adenomas, there is a gradient in ACTH levels between the central and peripheral blood specimens. Administration of CRH stimulates ACTH and tends to enhance the gradient. A gradient of 2:1 (central to peripheral) basally or 3:1 after CRH administration on either the left or the right is consistent with a pituitary source of ACTH. When clinical and biochemical studies suggest the presence of a pituitary adenoma, pituitary imaging should be performed using CT or MRI. Most ACTH-secreting pituitary adenomas are small, and results of scans are normal in more than half of patients.

Treatment

Rx

The efficacy of transsphenoidal surgery for Cushing's disease is greatly aided by making the correct diagnosis preoperatively. In experienced hands, surgical cures of ACTH-producing microadenomas occur in 75 to 90% of patients undergoing a first operation. As in other pituitary tumors, complete remissions with macroadenomas are much less common. In the event of surgical remission or cure, postoperative hypocortisolism is to be expected because of suppression of the hypothalamic-pituitary axis. After coverage for steroid withdrawal in the postoperative period, cortisol replacement should gradually be decreased to allow recovery of the hypothalamic-pituitary-adrenal axis.

If transsphenoidal surgery is unsuccessful, reoperation may be indicated and can result in remission in up to 50% of patients; in this circumstance, consideration should be given to performing a total hypophysectomy at reoperation. If transsphenoidal surgery cannot be performed or has failed, alternative forms of therapy should be used to prevent the long-term consequences of hypercortisolism. Pituitary irradiation is usually the second line of treatment for patients with Cushing's disease. It is more efficacious in children and in younger patients, but even in older adults remissions can be achieved in 50 to 60% within 2 years. To prevent the continued ravages of hypercortisolism during this period, however, concomitant medical therapy is usually given. Bilateral adrenalectomy represents another alternative for patients with severe hypercortisolism after transsphenoidal surgery. It rapidly and effectively lowers cortisol levels but is associated with relatively high morbidity and mortality rates (≤5%) because of the associated metabolic and immune system alterations caused by hypercortisolism. The morbidity has been reduced in recent years by introduction of the laparoscopic approach. After adrenalectomy, patients must take maintenance glucocorticoids and mineralocorticoids, and they risk developing Nelson's syndrome.

Medical therapy for Cushing's disease has its primary role in preparation for surgery or for control of hypercortisolism during the interval when radiation therapy is taking effect. Because most pituitary adenomas are responsive to changes in cortisol levels, they have a tendency to "escape" from adrenal blockade caused by some therapies by producing higher levels of ACTH. The antifungal agent ketoconazole is highly effective in decreasing glucocorticoid biosynthesis, and it also inhibits ACTH secretion, so it has become the medical therapy of choice. Alternative medications include metyrapone, aminoglutethimide, mifepristone, etomidate, and mitotane.

NELSON'S SYNDROME

Nelson's syndrome was initially described as the appearance of a pituitary adenoma after bilateral adrenalectomy. In addition to an enlarging pituitary mass, the syndrome is characterized by very high ACTH levels and hyperpigmentation. It is caused by a preexisting ACTH-producing tumor that grows in the absence of feedback inhibition by high levels of glucocorticoids. The incidence of clinically significant Nelson's syndrome after adrenalectomy for Cushing's disease varies from 10 to 50% in different series. Patients with Cushing's disease who have undergone adrenalectomy should be followed with imaging studies and plasma ACTH levels because tumors that cause Nelson's syndrome can be very aggressive. When evidence shows mass effects or rapid growth, transsphenoidal surgery should be performed. Postoperative irradiation may provide additional benefit, although it appears to be less efficacious than in other ACTH-producing adenomas.

GONADOTROPINS (FOLLICLE-STIMULATING HORMONE AND LUTEINIZING HORMONE)

The pituitary glycoprotein hormones include FSH, LH, and TSH. Each of the glycoprotein hormones has a specific β subunit that forms a non-covalent dimer with the common α subunit. The α and individual β subunits are encoded by separate genes. The β-subunit genes are evolutionarily related and share a common gene structure as well as having nucleotide and amino acid sequence homology. Similarities in the structures of the β subunits account for their ability to form non-covalent dimers with the common α subunit. The α and β subunits each undergo glycosylation, which is important for correct hormone folding, intracellular transport, and secretion. Glycosylation is also required for biologic activity, presumably because it affects tertiary structure. The half-life of LH (50 minutes) is shorter than that of FSH (220 minutes), thus accounting for the more rapid secretory dynamics of LH, even though both hormones are secreted together.

The gonadotropins are involved in sexual differentiation, sex steroid production, and gametogenesis. The regulation and physiologic roles of gonadotropins are quite different in males and females. In boys and men, receptors for FSH are located on Sertoli cells and seminiferous tubules, where FSH acts to stimulate sperm maturation. LH receptors are located on Leydig cells in the testis, where they stimulate androgen production. Thus, FSH and LH act together to induce spermatogenesis (Chapter 253).

In girls and women, ovarian FSH receptors are located on granulosa cells, where they induce enzymes involved in estrogen biosynthesis. LH receptors are located predominantly on thecal cells in the ovary and stimulate the production of ovarian androgens and steroid precursors that are transported to granulosa cells for aromatization to estrogens. The pattern of FSH and LH secretion during the menstrual cycle results in follicular recruitment and maturation (largely FSH mediated), followed by ovulation (largely LH mediated) and steroid production by the corpus luteum.

Gonadotropin secretion is regulated primarily by the hypothalamic decapeptide GnRH. The gonadotroph cell is very sensitive to the pattern of GnRH stimulation. Continuous, rather than pulsatile, exposure to GnRH causes gonadotroph desensitization and suppression of LH and FSH. Gonadotroph sensitivity to GnRH is modulated by sex steroids and other hypothalamic peptides, such as neuropeptide Y. Increased GnRH secretion, in combination with a higher density of GnRH receptors and rising estradiol concentrations, accounts for the dramatic release of gonadotropins that induces ovulation.

The hypothalamic-pituitary-gonadal axis is activated during fetal development. After birth, LH and FSH levels fall and remain suppressed until puberty. This suppression involves tonic inhibition of the GnRH pulse generator by the central nervous system because the pituitary gland is still responsive to GnRH. Most theories hold that the onset of puberty reflects disinhibition of the pulse generator. Puberty occurs between the ages of 8 and 13 years in girls and between the ages of 9 and 14 years in boys. In the peripubertal period, bursts of LH secretion are first detected during sleep. Subsequently, LH pulse frequency and amplitude increase, and LH pulses are detected during the day and at night.

In women, the pattern of GnRH pulse frequency varies across the menstrual cycle (Chapter 256). The combination of GnRH stimulation and ovarian feedback regulation results in a complex orchestration of positive and negative hormonal signals that converge at the gonadotroph to regulate LH and FSH secretion. The typical 28-day menstrual cycle is divided into follicular and luteal phases that are separated by ovulation on day 14. Unlike chronic exposure to low concentrations of estrogens, which exert negative feedback regulation and inhibit GnRH, the increasing concentration of estrogen before the LH surge exerts positive feedback that results in increased GnRH pulse frequency. Increased GnRH, in combination with increased gonadotroph sensitivity to GnRH, results in the surge of LH and FSH. During the luteal phase, the gonadotropin pulse frequency is reduced. In addition to feedback regulation by steroids, ovarian peptides such as inhibin also play a role in control of the reproductive axis. Inhibin causes selective suppression of FSH, without affecting LH secretion. A homodimer of inhibin β-subunits, referred to as *activin,* has opposite actions and selectively stimulates FSH, but its predominant physiologic action is to increase ovarian granulosa cell responsivity to FSH. Circulating inhibin provides one of the negative feedback inputs that leads to FSH suppression as the follicle develops.

The perimenopause is characterized by a gradual cessation of ovarian function. After several years of menstrual cycles that are sometimes anovulatory or irregular, menses cease, thereby defining the menopause (Chapter 262). Although there is considerable variation, menopause usually occurs at approximately age 50 years. At this point, ovarian follicles have been depleted, and the production of sex steroids changes such that production of estrogen and progesterone is minimal, but ovarian androgens continue to be made at lesser levels, primarily by stromal cells. The chronic decline in estrogen and progesterone causes loss of feedback inhibition and a marked increase in LH and FSH levels.

In males, the regulation of the pituitary-gonadal axis is relatively constant. After early puberty, LH and FSH pulses occur approximately once an hour during the night and day. Testosterone inhibits the hypothalamic-pituitary axis, although its actions are mediated, in part, by aromatization to estrogens, as shown in rare patients who are unable to convert testosterone to estrogen because of a deficiency of aromatase. Much of the inhibition by gonadal steroids occurs at the hypothalamic level, but evidence also suggests weak inhibition of the gonadotroph at the level of the pituitary gland. In contrast to menopause in women, no analogous abrupt change in hormone levels occurs in men. However, a gradual decline in testosterone levels is associated with an increase in LH and FSH with aging.

HYPOGONADOTROPIC HYPOGONADISM

Clinical features of hypogonadotropic hypogonadism in women are primarily the result of estrogen deficiency and include breast atrophy, vaginal dryness, and diminished libido. Hot flashes are uncommon, in contrast to postmenopausal estrogen deficiency. In premenopausal women, normal menstrual cycles provide evidence for an intact hypothalamic-pituitary-gonadal axis. LH and FSH levels should be increased in postmenopausal women and normal levels may indicate deficiency. Hypogonadism in men causes decreased libido and sexual function. In men, low testosterone without elevation of LH and FSH is consistent with impaired hypothalamic-pituitary reserve. GnRH stimulation can distinguish hypothalamic and pituitary deficiency but may require multiple injections to prime the pituitary, if GnRH deficiency is of long standing.

Treatment

Rx

In premenopausal women, preparations of estrogen and progestins should be used for hormonal replacement and to allow cyclical growth of the endometrium. Pulsatile GnRH (for GnRH-deficient subjects) or gonadotropins can be given to induce ovulation if fertility is desired. Testosterone can be replaced in men using intramuscular injections that are given at 2- to 4-week intervals. Doses and the intervals between injections should be adjusted on an individual basis using libido and testosterone levels as a guide. Oral preparations of androgens should be avoided because of hepatotoxicity. Transdermal patch and gel preparations are available and give more even testosterone levels but are more expensive than depot injections. Induction of spermatogenesis requires pulsatile GnRH (for GnRH-deficient subjects) or injections of gonadotropins.

A congenital form of hypogonadotropic hypogonadism is caused by deficiency of GnRH, which, in turn, causes deficiencies of LH and FSH. When associated with anosmia (absent sense of smell), the condition is referred to as Kallmann's syndrome (Chapter 241). Pulsatile GnRH has been used to induce puberty and fertility in both male and female patients with Kallmann's syndrome and other forms of GnRH deficiency.

Secondary hypogonadotropic hypogonadism is relatively common. In most cases, it is reversible and is caused by weight loss, anorexia nervosa, stress, heavy exercise, or severe illness. Reversible forms of secondary hypogonadotropic hypogonadism are caused by GnRH deficiency and are more common in women. The condition is ideally treated by correcting the underlying cause. Many women have a discrete threshold for weight or exercise level that will cause loss of menstrual periods. When it is not possible to correct the underlying abnormality, hormonal replacement can be used in women for protection against osteopenia and to cycle the endometrium.

Various pathologic conditions can cause secondary hypogonadotropic hypogonadism, often in association with deficiencies of other pituitary hormones (see Table 242–3). These include hypothalamic lesions or central nervous system irradiation. Pituitary tumors can suppress gonadotropins because of stalk compression and disruption of pulsatile GnRH input as well as by direct destruction of normal pituitary tissue. Hyperprolactinemia can suppress GnRH and can lead to reduced gonadotropin levels.

In contrast to the aforementioned causes of hypogonadotropic hypogonadism, which result from GnRH deficiency, primary deficiencies of LH and FSH are uncommon. An acquired form of isolated gonadotroph deficiency is rarely encountered and may have an autoimmune basis. Mutations in the *LHβ* or *FSHβ* genes have been described and cause selective hormonal loss. Inactivating mutations in the GnRH receptor and the LH and FSH receptors causing hypogonadotropic hypogonadism have also been reported.

TUMORS PRODUCING FOLLICLE-STIMULATING HORMONE AND LUTEINIZING HORMONE

Etiology and Pathogenesis

Although most early series suggested that gonadotropin-producing adenomas were uncommon, more recent studies using sensitive techniques to characterize tumor phenotype show a prevalence (15 to 20%) that is greater than that of corticotroph or somatotroph adenomas (see Table 242–6). Most (70 to 80%) of pituitary tumors classified previously as nonfunctioning adenomas can be shown to produce low levels of intact glycoprotein hormones or their uncombined α or β subunits. Biosynthetic defects in the tumor cells account for relatively inefficient hormone secretion as well as the propensity to produce uncombined subunits. FSH is produced more commonly than LH. Elevated levels of free α subunits are noted more often than increased free β subunits.

Clinical Manifestations

Gonadotropin-producing tumors are somewhat more common in men than women and increase in prevalence with age. FSH- and LH-producing tumors do not usually cause a characteristic hormone excess syndrome. The tumors are typically large macroadenomas and manifest as clinically nonfunctioning tumors with symptoms and signs related to local mass effects. Visual field loss resulting from suprasellar extension and compression of the optic chiasm is found in more than 70% of patients. Many of these tumors are detected incidentally by CT and MRI performed for unrelated indications. Symptoms of hypopituitarism, including hypogonadism with loss of libido, are also common. Men with predominantly FSH-secreting tumors may present with testicular enlargement from hypertrophy of the seminiferous tubules, but they also can paradoxically present with hypogonadal features that are related to low levels of testosterone. These patients must be distinguished from those with primary hypogonadism who have testicular dysfunction. Tumors that primarily secrete LH are rare but can cause increased testosterone levels. Premenopausal women with gonadotropin-producing tumors may experience menstrual irregularity or secondary hypogonadism. Postmenopausal women often show reduced gonadotropin levels because the mass effects of the gonadotropin-producing tumors cause stalk compression, thus impairing GnRH stimulation of gonadotropins from normal pituitary cells.

Diagnosis

Because of the absence of a clinical syndrome in most patients, the preoperative diagnosis of gonadotropin-producing pituitary tumors has relied on imaging studies and laboratory tests. Unfortunately, the laboratory diagnosis of gonadotropin-producing tumors is less than satisfactory. First, the tumors synthesize gonadotropins inefficiently, and hormone levels are usually not markedly elevated. Second, because the secretion of gonadotropins is pulsatile, random LH and FSH values are difficult to interpret. Furthermore, gonadotropin levels vary widely and are normally elevated in postmenopausal women. GnRH stimulation tests also do not clearly distinguish subjects with gonadotropin-producing tumors from physiologically normal subjects, and suppression tests have not proved useful. Paradoxical responses to TRH have helped to identify gonadotropin-secreting tumors. In contrast to its effect in physiologically normal persons, TRH stimulates secretion of intact gonadotropins or the uncombined FSH β and LH β subunits in most patients with gonadotropin tumors. Once identified, the uncombined α or β subunits can serve as tumor markers and can be useful for monitoring responses to therapy.

Men with proven gonadotropin-producing tumors typically have high-normal or elevated FSH levels but low levels of testosterone. Moderately elevated PRL levels are common and are caused by tumor mass effects. It is important to distinguish this group from patients with true prolactinomas. Women, including those in the postmenopausal group, may have paradoxically low gonadotropin levels. Thus, the absence of elevated gonadotropins does not exclude the diagnosis of a gonadotropin-producing tumor.

The postoperative diagnosis of gonadotropin-producing tumors can be made based on immunohistochemical analyses or using more sophisticated studies of gonadotropin gene expression. These types of analyses confirm that most clinically nonfunctioning tumors are composed of gonadotropin-producing cell types.

Treatment

Because the major symptoms of the gonadotropin-producing tumors result from extrasellar extension and local mass effects, the main aim of treatment is reduction in the size of the tumor. Complete or partial reversal of visual field defects and hypopituitarism can be accomplished surgically, unless these conditions are chronic. Transsphenoidal surgery is rarely curative of this group of macroadenomas. Patients with significant residual tumor may benefit from radiation therapy. Because most tumors are slow growing, when no tumor is visible postoperatively by MRI, the patient may be followed with yearly monitoring for tumor recurrence using CT or MRI. If tumor markers such as free α- or β-subunit levels are available, they can also be used to monitor tumor function. When follow-up studies show tumor regrowth, repeat surgery or radiation therapy, or both, is indicated.

Great interest has been shown in medical therapies that could be useful as adjuncts to surgery or even as primary therapies in patients who do not require immediate decompression. The success of dopamine agonists and somatostatin analogues in treating hormone oversecretion and tumor mass in prolactinomas and acromegaly has not been seen in patients with gonadotropin-producing tumors, although exceptions have been described in selected patients. GnRH antagonists have been shown to suppress FSH levels in small series of patients, but these agents have not been found to reduce tumor size.

THYROID-STIMULATING HORMONE

Like the other glycoprotein hormones, TSH is a heterodimer composed of the common α subunit and the unique TSH β subunit. TSH is produced in thyrotroph cells. TSH is measured by highly sensitive immunoradiometric assays that use antisera directed toward the TSH β subunit. Normal levels of TSH range from 0.4 to 4.0 μU/mL. The detection limit for current TSH assays is less than 0.01 μU/mL, thus allowing measurement of suppressed TSH levels in patients with hyperthyroidism.

TSH controls thyroid hormone (T_4 and T_3) synthesis and secretion from the thyroid gland. TSH stimulates cyclic adenosine monophosphate production and acts as a trophic hormone as well as stimulating hormone synthesis. TSH secretion from the pituitary gland is regulated by the hypothalamic-pituitary-thyroid axis. Hypothalamic TRH is a tripeptide that stimulates TSH synthesis and secretion. Various other hypothalamic hormones including somatostatin and dopamine can inhibit TSH secretion, but their roles in normal physiology have not been clearly elucidated.

Thyroid hormones have an inhibitory effect on the production of TRH and TSH and constitute a powerful negative feedback loop in the hypothalamic-pituitary-thyroid axis. The direct effects of thyroid hormone at the level of the pituitary gland are well illustrated by TSH responses to TRH stimulation tests. In hypothyroidism, TSH responses to exogenous TRH are exaggerated. In hyperthyroidism, TSH responses to TRH are blunted or flat, a finding indicating that the inhibitory effects of thyroid hormone override the stimulatory effects of TRH. Thyroid hormones act through nuclear receptors that function at the transcriptional level to suppress expression of the TRH gene as well as the α- and β-subunit genes of TSH. In hypothyroidism, expression of the *TSHα* and *TSHβ* genes is stimulated, and hormone production is markedly enhanced.

Secretion of TSH is pulsatile, but the amplitude of the pulses is relatively small and does not create the difficulties in measurement of TSH that are encountered with measurements of other pituitary hormones. TSH levels are elevated in infants in the immediate postpartum period. Thereafter, thyroid function tests remain remarkably constant throughout life. TSH secretion has a diurnal rhythm with a small increase at night. Because of the integrated nature of the hypothalamic-pituitary-thyroid axis, thyroid function tests are best interpreted when concentrations of TSH, free T_4, and free T_3 levels are known. Except in conditions of secondary hypothyroidism or TSH-secreting pituitary tumors, TSH levels provide an excellent screening test for thyroid dysfunction. In cases of primary hypothyroidism, TSH levels are elevated as TSH increases logarithmically in response to falling thyroid hormone levels. In hyperthyroidism, TSH is suppressed to levels lower than or near the detection limits of most sensitive assays.

CENTRAL HYPOTHYROIDISM

Central forms of hypothyroidism include secondary hypothyroidism, which is caused by TSH deficiency, and tertiary hypothyroidism, which is caused by TRH deficiency. Three different types of congenital TSH deficiency are caused by genetic mutations. One type involves mutations in the *TSHβ* gene, in which several different types of mutations have been described. A second involves mutations in *Pit-1*, which causes combined deficiencies of GH, PRL, and TSH (see earlier). A third involves a mutation in the gene for TRH. Acquired, central forms of hypothyroidism are often associated with other pituitary hormone deficiencies, and usually goiter is absent because of low TSH levels.

Tests for TSH deficiency are best interpreted by analyzing free T_4 levels in combination with TSH. Low free T_4 without elevated TSH is consistent with central hypothyroidism. Free T_4 measurements should be used, rather than total T_4, to avoid confusion caused by thyroxine-binding globulin deficiency. In some patients with hypothalamic disease, the TSH level is partially elevated in the presence of low levels of free T_4, but the bioactivity of the TSH is reduced. Central forms of hypothyroidism must be distinguished from the sick-euthyroid condition (Chapter 244). Laboratory tests in patients with the sick-euthyroid syndrome progress through several phases but can include prolonged periods when both TSH and free thyroid hormone levels are low. It can be very difficult in these patients to exclude central hypothyroidism unequivocally. In addition to the clinical setting in which thyroid function tests are measured, the presence of normal thyroid function tests before the illness and the absence of known hypothalamic or pituitary disease make true central hypothyroidism unlikely. Increased levels of reverse T_3 are suggestive of sick-euthyroidism, and free T_4 and T_3 may be in the normal or low normal range in sick-euthyroid patients. When TSH deficiency is documented, thyroid hormone is replaced using daily doses of L-thyroxine (0.05 to 0.15 mg/day). Because TSH cannot be used as an end point, one monitors serum levels of free T_4 and T_3.

TUMORS SECRETING THYROID-STIMULATING HORMONE

Etiology and Pathogenesis

TSH-secreting tumors are rare and account for 1 to 3% of pituitary tumors. TSH-producing tumors may be plurihormonal. GH and PRL are co-secreted most often, a finding perhaps reflecting the common cellular lineage for thyrotrophs, somatotrophs, and lactotrophs. Long-standing severe hypothyroidism can cause thyrotroph hyperplasia and pituitary enlargement. These hyperplastic masses regress with thyroid hormone replacement therapy. Most true TSH-producing tumors are relatively autonomous and respond weakly to TRH stimulation or to thyroid hormone suppression.

Clinical Manifestations

TSH-secreting tumors are usually macroadenomas by the time a diagnosis has been made. Consequently, many patients exhibit mass effects of the tumor and hyperthyroidism. Now that measurement of TSH is used as the initial assessment for hyperthyroidism, however, smaller tumors are seen more commonly than previously. The clinical features of TSH-secreting tumors resemble those of Graves' disease, except features of autoimmunity such as ophthalmopathy are absent. Circulating levels of T_4 and T_3 range widely but can be elevated as much as two- to threefold. Diffuse goiter is present in the majority of patients with TSH-producing tumors, and the 24-hour uptake of radioiodine is elevated.

Diagnosis

Because feedback inhibition of TSH is impaired in TSH-producing tumors, TSH levels are inappropriately elevated in the presence of high levels of T_4 and T_3. TSH levels produced by tumors range from the low normal to as high as 500 μU/mL, but most levels are minimally elevated. Free α-subunit measurements can be very helpful in confirming the diagnosis of a TSH-secreting tumor. Most TSH-producing tumors (>80%) secrete excess free α subunit. Thus, the diagnosis of a TSH-secreting tumor can usually be made by demonstrating that a hyperthyroid patient has a detectable serum TSH level associated with excess secretion of the free α subunit. The finding of a mass lesion on CT or MRI confirms the diagnosis. Several other causes of inappropriate TSH secretion should be considered, including resistance to thyroid hormone and familial dysalbuminemic hyperthyroxinemia and other disorders that alter serum thyroid hormone–binding proteins.

Treatment Rx

The goals of therapy are to treat the underlying TSH-secreting tumor and to correct the hyperthyroidism. Transsphenoidal surgery alone is rarely curative because of the large size of most tumors, but it can alleviate mass effects and lower TSH levels. As in other large pituitary tumors, adjunctive irradiation may be required to control tumor growth. Somatostatin analogues have been used as adjunctive medical therapy, and they decrease TSH and α-subunit levels in approximately 80% of patients with TSH-secreting tumors. However, consistent effects on tumor growth have not been demonstrated. Hyperthyroidism caused by TSH-secreting tumors can be treated using antithyroid drugs or radioiodine.

NULL CELL PITUITARY TUMORS

Null cell adenomas, or clinically nonfunctioning tumors, are variably defined depending on the criteria used to analyze tumor cell phenotype. The majority of clinically nonfunctioning adenomas can be shown to produce low levels of the free α subunit, free β subunits of FSH and LH, and intact FSH and LH when analyzed by immunocytochemistry or for messenger RNA expression. A smaller fraction can be shown to produce low levels of other pituitary hormones, particularly ACTH or GH. Even with detailed analyses of hormone production, a subset (10 to 20%) of nonfunctioning adenomas does not appear to produce one of the major pituitary hormones.

The clinical features and management of null cell tumors are similar to those for gonadotropin-producing tumors. The major signs and symptoms result from tumor mass effects that cause visual field defects, headache and other neurologic symptoms, and hypopituitarism. Transsphenoidal surgery is the primary mode of treatment, with a goal of debulking the tumor to relieve mass effects. Because no serum tumor markers are known, patients must be followed by CT or MRI in conjunction with visual field tests.

SUGGESTED READINGS

Arafah BM: Medical management of hypopituitarism in patients with pituitary adenomas. Pituitary 2002;5:109–117. *Review of the treatment of hypopituitarism.*

Beck-Peccoz P, Persani L: Medical management of thyrotropin-secreting pituitary adenomas. Pituitary 2002;5:83–88. *Emphasizes role of somatostatin analogues.*

Caturegli P, Newschaffer C, Olivi A, et al: Autoimmune hypophysitis. Endocr Rev 2005;26:599–614. *A detailed review of this unusual entity.*

Findling JW, Raff H: Cushing's syndrome: Important issues in diagnosis and management. J Clin Endocrinol Metab 2006;91:3746–3753. *Comprehensive review of the diagnosis and treatment of Cushing's syndrome.*

Melmed S: Medical progress: Acromegaly. N Engl J Med 2006;14:2558–2573. *Comprehensive review of acromegaly.*

Molitch ME: Medical management of prolactinomas. Pituitary 2002;5:55–65. *Most prolactinomas are treated medically, and these aspects are reviewed here.*

Sheehan JP, Niranjan A, Sheehan JM, et al: Stereotactic radiosurgery for pituitary adenomas: An intermediate review of its safety, efficacy, and role in the neurosurgical treatment armamentarium. J Neurosurg 2005;102:678–691. *This article reviews the outcomes of 1621 patients who had been treated by stereotactic radiation therapy from 35 studies.*

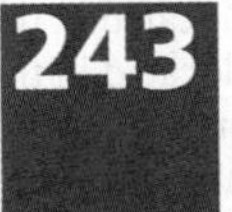

243 POSTERIOR PITUITARY

Joseph G. Verbalis

ANATOMY AND HORMONE SYNTHESIS

The hormones of the posterior pituitary, vasopressin and oxytocin, are synthesized in specialized neurons in the hypothalamus, the neurohypophysial neurons. These neurons are specialized for synthesis and secretion of each hormone and are notable for their large size, hence their designation as magnocellular neurons. In the hypothalamus, the neurohypophysial magnocellular neurons are clustered in the paired paraventricular and supraoptic nuclei (Fig. 243–1). Vasopressin and oxytocin are also synthesized in parvicellular (i.e., small cell) neurons of the paraventricular nuclei, and vasopressin (but not oxytocin) is also synthesized in the suprachiasmatic nucleus.

Transcription of vasopressin and oxytocin mRNA and translation of the vasopressin and oxytocin prohormones occur entirely in the cell bodies of the neurohypophysial neurons. The pre-prohormones are cleaved from the signal peptide in the endoplasmic reticulum, and the prohormones provasopressin and pro-oxytocin are packaged along with processing enzymes into neurosecretory granules. The neurosecretory granules are transported out of the perikaryon of the neurohypophysial neurons through microtubules down the long axons that form the supraopticohypophysial tract to terminate in axon terminals in the posterior pituitary. The entire unit including the magnocellular neurons in the supraoptic and paraventricular nuclei, the supraopticohypophysial tract, and the axon terminals in the posterior pituitary is called the neurohypophysis. During transport, the processing enzymes cleave provasopressin into vasopressin (9 amino acids), vasopressin-neurophysin (95 amino acids), and vasopressin glycopeptide (39 amino acids). Pro-oxytocin is similarly cleaved to oxytocin (which differs from vasopressin by only two of nine amino acids) and oxytocin-neurophysin, but there is

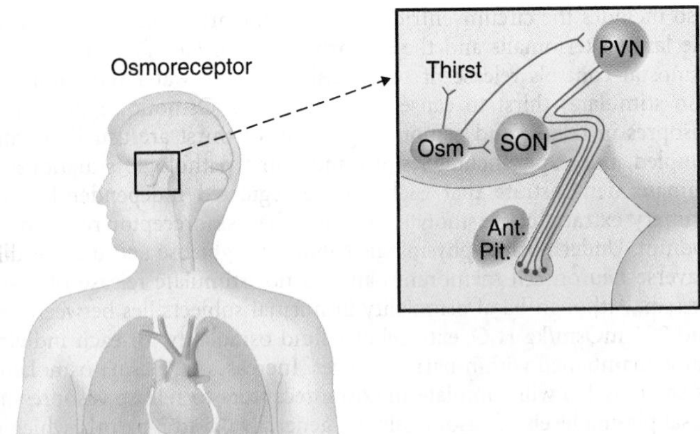

FIGURE 243–1 • Sagittal view of the head demonstrating the position of the neurohypophysis. The magnocellular neurons are clustered in two paraventricular nuclei (PVN) and two supraoptic nuclei (SON). Only one nucleus of each pair is illustrated. The supraoptic nuclei are lateral to the edge of the optic chiasm, whereas the paraventricular nuclei are central along the wall of the third ventricle. The axons of the four nuclei combine to form the supraopticohypophysial tract as they course through the pituitary stalk to their storage terminals in the posterior pituitary. The osmostat (Osm) is in the hypothalamus anterior to the third ventricle; the thirst center (Thirst) is distributed across different brain areas. Ant. Pit. = anterior pituitary. (From Buonocore CM, Robinson AG: Diagnosis and management of diabetes insipidus during medical emergencies. Endocrinol Metab Clin North Am 1993;22:411–423.)

no glycopeptide contained in pro-oxytocin. Within the neurosecretory granules, neurophysins form neurophysin-hormone complexes that stabilize the hormones. Crystallography has demonstrated that tetramers of neurophysin form specific binding sites for five molecules of hormone, so the hormone within the granules is always bound. Stimulatory (e.g., glutamatergic, cholinergic, and angiotensin) neurotransmitter terminals and inhibitory (e.g., γ-aminobutyric acid and noradrenergic) neurotransmitter terminals control the release of vasopressin by the activity of synaptic contacts on the cell bodies. Physiologic release of vasopressin or oxytocin into the general circulation occurs at the level of the posterior pituitary, where, in response to an action potential, intracellular calcium is increased and causes the neurosecretory granules to fuse with the axon membrane, thereby releasing the entire contents of the granule through exocytosis into the pericapillary space. Once it is released, each hormone has no further association with its respective neurophysin, and each of the peptide products can be independently detected in the general circulation. Although vasopressin and oxytocin compose only small parts of their respective prohormones, they are the only known biologically active components of the prohormones. Factors that stimulate the release of neurohypophysial hormones also stimulate their synthesis; however, whereas release is instantaneous, synthesis requires a longer time. Because synthesis is delayed, maintenance of a large store of hormone in the posterior pituitary is essential for the instantaneous and massive release of each hormone that is necessary with acute hemorrhage (vasopressin) or during parturition (oxytocin). In most species, sufficient vasopressin is stored in the posterior pituitary to support maximum antidiuresis for several days and to maintain baseline levels of antidiuresis for weeks without ongoing synthesis of new hormone.

The axons of the parvicellular neurons of the paraventricular nuclei project to different areas within the brain rather than to the posterior pituitary. Some terminate in the median eminence of the basal hypothalamus, where, similar to other hypothalamic releasing factors, the hormones are secreted into the portal capillary system and where vasopressin serves as one of the regulators of secretion of adrenocorticotropic hormone. Other neurons project to the limbic system, the brain stem, and the spinal cord, where vasopressin and oxytocin serve neurotransmitter and neuromodulatory roles. Still other axons secrete hormones into the cerebrospinal fluid of the third ventricle, the function of which is unknown.

Vasopressin

Vasopressin and Regulation of Osmolality

The primary physiologic action of vasopressin is its function as a water-retaining hormone. The central sensing system (osmostat) for control of release of vasopressin is anatomically discrete, located in a small area of the hypothalamus just anterior to the third ventricle that also includes the circumventricular organs the organum vasculosum of the lamina terminalis and the subfornical organ (see Fig. 243–1). The osmostat controls release of vasopressin to cause water retention and also stimulates thirst to cause water repletion. Osmotic regulation of vasopressin release and osmotic regulation of thirst are usually tightly coupled, but experimental lesions and some pathologic situations in humans demonstrate that each can be regulated independently. The primary extracellular osmolyte to which the osmoreceptor responds is sodium. Under normal physiologic conditions, glucose and urea readily traverse neuron cell membranes and do not stimulate release of vasopressin. Although basal osmolality in normal subjects lies between 280 and 295 mOsm/kg H_2O, extracellular fluid osmolality for each individual is maintained within narrow ranges. Increases in plasma osmolality as small as 1% will stimulate the osmoreceptors to release vasopressin. Basal plasma levels of vasopressin are generally 0.5 to 2 pg/mL, which is sufficient to maintain urine osmolality above plasma osmolality and urine volume in the range of 2 to 3 L/day. When vasopressin levels are suppressed below 0.5 pg/mL, maximum urine osmolality decreases to less than 100 mOsm/kg H_2O and a free water diuresis ensues to levels approaching 800 to 1000 mL/hr (18 to 24 L/day). Increases in plasma osmolality cause a linear increase in plasma vasopressin and a corresponding linear increase in urine osmolality. At a plasma osmolality of approximately 295 mOsm/kg H_2O, urine osmolality is maximally concentrated to 1000 to 1200 mOsm/kg H_2O. Thus, the entire physiologic range of urine osmolality is accomplished by relatively small changes in plasma vasopressin of 0 to 5 pg/mL, as illustrated in Figure 243–2.

To maintain fluid balance, water must be not just conserved but consumed as well to replace insensible water losses and obligate urine output.

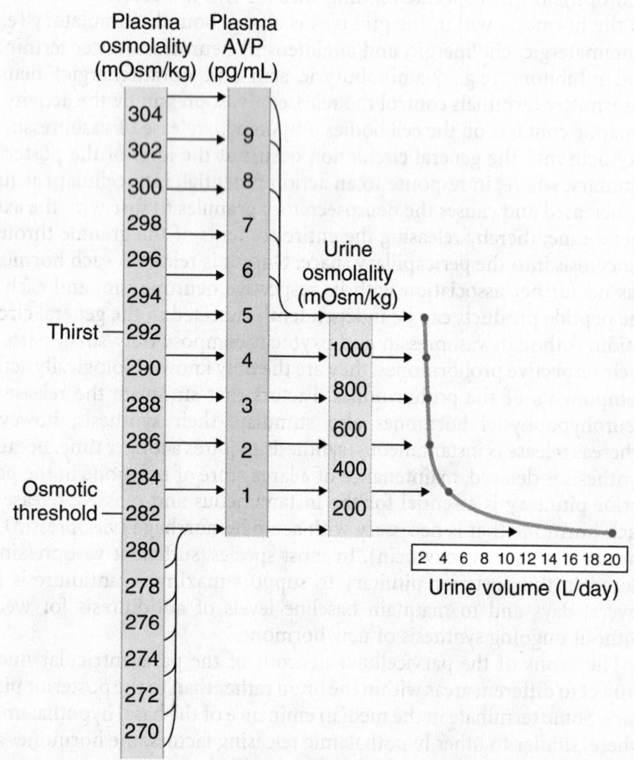

FIGURE 243–2 • Idealized schematic of the normal physiologic relationships among plasma osmolality, plasma vasopressin (AVP), urine osmolality, and urine volume. The entire physiologic range of urine osmolality occurs with plasma vasopressin levels from 0 to 5 pg/mL. Increases in plasma osmolality above approximately 290 to 295 mOsm/kg H_2O result in increases in plasma vasopressin but no further concentration of the urine, which is limited by the maximal osmolality in the inner medulla. The relation of volume (calculated on the basis of a constant osmolar load) is inversely exponential to the other parameters. Because of this relationship, urine volume does not change substantially until there is nearly absent vasopressin secretion, after which urine volume increases dramatically. The shaded area represents the normal range and the interrelationships among the various parameters. (Calculated from formulae presented in Robertson GL, Shelton RL, Athar S: The osmoregulation of vasopressin. Kidney Int 1976;10:25–37. Figure drawn by J. G. Verbalis, Georgetown University, Washington, DC.)

Most studies have indicated that thirst is not stimulated until a somewhat higher plasma osmolality (5 to 10 mOsm/kg H_2O) than the threshold for release of vasopressin. During the course of a normal day, most humans derive sufficient water from habitual fluid intake and catabolism of food to maintain plasma osmolality below the threshold required to activate thirst. Therefore, under normal physiologic conditions, water balance (and hence plasma osmolality) is regulated more by secretion of vasopressin than by true thirst. However, with more severe degrees of dehydration, thirst is essential to restore body water deficits.

Vasopressin acts on V_2 or antidiuretic receptors in the collecting duct cells of the kidney to cause water retention, or antidiuresis. Vasopressin V_2 receptors are G protein–coupled receptors that activate adenylate cyclase with subsequent increased intracellular cyclic adenosine monophosphate (cAMP) levels upon ligand activation of the receptor. The increased cAMP initiates the movement of aquaporin-2 water channels from the cytoplasm to the apical (luminal) membrane of the collecting duct cells. Once they are inserted into the apical membrane, these channels allow facilitated rapid transport of water from the collecting duct lumen into the cell along osmotic gradients. The water then exits the cell through the basolateral membrane, into the kidney medullary circulation through aquaporin-3 and aquaporin-4 water channels, which are constitutively present in the basolateral membrane. This entire process is termed antidiuresis. In the absence of vasopressin, the aquaporin-2 channels are reinternalized from the apical membrane into subapical vesicles. This prevents active reabsorption of water from the collecting duct lumen, resulting in diuresis. In addition to this rapid "shuttling" of the aquaporin-2 channels to regulate water reabsorption on a minute-to-minute basis, vasopressin also acts through V_2 receptors to regulate long-term stores of aquaporin-2; that is, increased vasopressin stimulates aquaporin-2 synthesis, and the absence of vasopressin results in decreased aquaporin-2 synthesis. The hypertonic medullary interstitium determines the maximum concentration of the urine, which is isotonic with the inner medulla of the kidney under conditions of maximal antidiuresis (Chapter 116).

Vasopressin and Pressure and Volume Regulation

In contrast to the osmoregulatory system, volume regulation is anatomically more diffuse. High-pressure baroreceptors are located in the aorta and carotid sinus, and low-pressure baroreceptors are located in the right and left atria. Stimuli for pressure and volume receptors are carried through the glossopharyngeal (ninth) and vagal (tenth) cranial nerves to the nucleus tractus solitarius in the brain stem. Subsequent secondary and tertiary projections converge on the magnocellular neurons, where they provide inhibitory as well as excitatory inputs. Decreases in blood pressure or vascular volume stimulate vasopressin release, whereas situations that increase blood volume or left atrial pressure (e.g., negative-pressure breathing) decrease secretion of vasopressin. The release of vasopressin in response to changes in volume or pressure is less sensitive than the release in response to osmoreceptors, and generally a 10 to 15% reduction in blood volume or pressure is needed to stimulate release of vasopressin. However, once arterial pressure falls below this threshold, the stimulated response is exponential, and plasma levels of vasopressin achieved are markedly greater than those achieved by osmotic stimulation. Other nonosmotic stimuli, such as nausea and intestinal traction, probably act through similar nonosmotic neural pathways to release vasopressin.

The pressor effects of vasopressin are mediated through V_{1a} receptors on vascular smooth muscle. For V_{1a} and V_{1b} receptors, the mechanism of action of vasopressin is to increase intracellular calcium rather than to stimulate adenylate cyclase. In intact animals, the pressor activity of vasopressin is weak because of compensatory vasodilatory systems that act to modulate vasopressor actions. The relatively insensitive regulation of vasopressin secretion by changes in volume and pressure and the modest role of vasopressin to regulate blood pressure are consistent with the notion that regulation of body sodium homeostasis by the renin-angiotensin-aldosterone system is more important for control of extracellular and blood volume than is regulation of water homeostasis. However, the action of vasopressin to regulate blood pressure can become prominent when other blood pressure regulatory systems are deficient (e.g., autonomic neuropathy or renin-angiotensin-aldosterone system blockade) or in states of pathologic vasodilation (e.g., liver cirrhosis, septic shock).

Vasopressin and Adrenocorticotropic Hormone

Vasopressin in the parvicellular neurons whose axons terminate in the median eminence is released into the pituitary portal capillaries and carried to the anterior pituitary. Anterior pituitary corticotrophs are stimulated through V_{1b} receptors to release adrenocorticotropic hormone. Although the major regulator of adrenocorticotropic hormone secretion is corticotropin-releasing hormone, because vasopressin and corticotropin-releasing hormone activate different signal transduction systems in the corticotrophs, each hormone has synergistic effects on the actions of the other to release adrenocorticotropic hormone.

Interaction of Osmotic and Volume Regulation

The vasopressin system has been adapted to optimize mammalian drinking behavior. Water is consumed as available in the absence of stimulated thirst, then vasopressin regulates water excretion to maintain plasma osmolality; this allows extensive geographic movement without thirst that would produce time-consuming and potentially dangerous water-seeking behavior. Yet, thirst serves as a back-up if dehydration becomes excessive. Similarly, because pressure-volume regulation of vasopressin is less sensitive, modest changes in pressure or volume, which are exacerbated by upright posture, do not interfere with regulation of osmolality. Yet, the pressor effect of high vasopressin serves as a back-up if volume depletion or hypotension becomes excessive. Usually, the physiologic regulation of osmolality and pressure-volume are synergistic. Dehydration causes an increase in osmolality and a decrease in volume, both of which stimulate release of vasopressin. Excess administration of fluid causes both a decrease in osmolality and an expansion of volume, both of which inhibit vasopressin secretion. However, other pathologic situations can result in opposing signals to vasopressin secretion (e.g., hyponatremia resulting from diuretic use with a decreased extracellular fluid volume or from cardiac failure or cirrhosis due to a decreased effective arterial blood volume). In these situations, vasopressin secretion represents a balance between the excitatory and inhibitory inputs provided by the osmotic and volume-pressure stimuli.

In addition, other factors can modulate the osmotic release and action of vasopressin. With volume expansion, natriuretic factors such as atrial natriuretic peptide and brain natriuretic peptide are released from atrial myocytes and act at the kidney to induce natriuresis. Atrial natriuretic peptide is also synthesized in the hypothalamus, where it may act to decrease vasopressin secretion. During pregnancy, there is a decrease of plasma osmolality by approximately 10 mOsm/kg H_2O as a result of a resetting of the osmostat, whereby vasopressin increases and decreases appropriately around the lower plasma osmolality; the osmostat for thirst is reset in parallel. Data suggest that this effect may be mediated by the placental hormone relaxin.

Abnormalities in water and electrolyte balance are common in elderly humans. This is in part due to age-related changes in body volume (as much as a 50% decrease in total body water above the age of 75 years) and renal function. However, elderly humans also have a decreased appreciation for thirst; and although there is a normal or even increased ability to secrete vasopressin with age, there is a decreased ability to achieve either maximum urine concentration to retain water or maximum dilution of urine to excrete water. Consequently, the elderly are particularly prone to hypernatremia or hyponatremia with diseases that affect water balance or from the drugs used as therapy for these diseases.

Oxytocin

Oxytocin is also synthesized in the magnocellular neurons of the neurohypophysis and differs in structure from vasopressin by only two of nine amino acids. Oxytocin has similar concentrations in the posterior pituitary of both men and women, but to date a physiologic function for oxytocin has been described only in women.

Prolactin is the main hormone necessary for milk production, but oxytocin is essential for milk secretion. Suckling stimulates tactile receptors in the nipple, producing an afferent signal to the hypothalamus that causes release of oxytocin from the posterior pituitary. Oxytocin binds to oxytocin receptors in the breast and induces contraction of myoepithelial cells around the alveoli and ductules to eject milk. Oxytocin also participates in parturition, although this action is more complex and is variable among species. In all species, there is interaction of oxytocin with gonadal steroid hormones, prostaglandins, and relaxin. In addition, upregulation of the uterine receptors for oxytocin dramatically increases the response to oxytocin at the end of pregnancy. The interaction of these various hormones in a cross-stimulation feed-forward cascade to support parturition is important to ensure survival of the species, so it is understandable that during parturition, lack of any single hormone (including oxytocin) is generally not sufficient to inhibit delivery. The greatest release of oxytocin occurs with, not before, delivery of the infant, probably secondary to stretching of the vaginal wall. This Fergusson reflex may aid delivery of subsequent fetuses in animals with multiple births; in humans, oxytocin release may be more important to induce uterine contraction to inhibit blood loss after delivery than to initiate parturition.

No pathologic syndromes of either increased or decreased secretion of oxytocin have yet been defined. Women with diabetes insipidus secondary to traumatic damage of the magnocellular neurons often have normal pregnancy and delivery and can breast-feed their infants; but it may be that in these cases, oxytocin neurons survive better than vasopressin neurons. In animal studies, administration of oxytocin to males increases sperm transport, but this function has not been documented in humans. Although only a single receptor for oxytocin has been identified, similar to the receptors for vasopressin, the receptors for oxytocin in the breast and in the myometrium are independently regulated. Because of the structural similarity between vasopressin and oxytocin, at high plasma levels, oxytocin can activate vasopressin receptors and vasopressin can activate oxytocin receptors. One example of this is that administration of oxytocin to induce labor can stimulate V_2 receptors of the kidney and cause water retention and hyponatremia if excess fluids are administered simultaneously.

Although peripheral effects of oxytocin have been described only in females, parvicellular oxytocin neurons in the paraventricular nuclei, like those of vasopressin, project to multiple different areas within the brain where oxytocin serves as a neurotransmitter and neuromodulator. Evidence in animals has strongly implicated brain oxytocin in the production of maternal behaviors in females and in affiliative (i.e., affection and bonding) behaviors in both sexes. These may prove to be of equal or greater importance than the peripheral actions of this hormone.

SYNDROME OF INAPPROPRIATE ANTIDIURETIC HORMONE SECRETION

Excess secretion of vasopressin can be caused by abnormal secretion from the posterior pituitary or by ectopic synthesis and secretion of vasopressin by a tumor. The inappropriate secretion of vasopressin causes renal water retention and volume expansion of body fluids, with a secondary natriuresis and consequent hyponatremia. This disorder is called the syndrome of inappropriate antidiuretic hormone secretion and is discussed in Chapter 117.

DIABETES INSIPIDUS

Definition

Diabetes insipidus is the excretion of a large volume of hypotonic, insipid (tasteless) urine, usually manifested by polyuria (increased urination) and polydipsia (increased thirst). The large volume, usually in excess of 50 to 60 mL/kg/day, must be distinguished from increased frequency of small volumes and from large volumes of isotonic or hypertonic urine, both of which have other clinical significance.

Pathobiology

Four pathophysiologic mechanisms must be considered in the differential diagnosis of diabetes insipidus.

1. Central diabetes insipidus is caused by the inability to secrete (and usually to synthesize) vasopressin in response to increased osmolality. No concentration of the dilute glomerular filtrate takes place in the renal collecting duct, and consequently a large volume of urine is excreted. This produces an increase in serum osmolality with stimulation of thirst and secondary polydipsia. Levels of vasopressin in plasma are unmeasurable or inappropriately low for plasma osmolality.
2. Nephrogenic diabetes insipidus is caused by the inability of an otherwise normal kidney to respond to vasopressin. As in hypothalamic diabetes insipidus, the dilute glomerular filtrate entering the collecting duct is excreted as a large volume of hypotonic urine. The

rise in plasma osmolality that occurs stimulates thirst and produces polydipsia. Unlike central diabetes insipidus, however, measured levels of vasopressin in plasma are high or appropriate for plasma osmolality.

3. Gestational diabetes insipidus is a rare condition produced by elevated levels or activity of placental cystine aminopeptidase (oxytocinase or vasopressinase) during pregnancy. The rapid destruction of vasopressin produces diabetes insipidus with polyuria and secondary stimulation of thirst with polydipsia. Because of the circulating vasopressinase, plasma vasopressin levels usually cannot be measured.
4. Primary polydipsia is a disorder of thirst stimulation rather than of vasopressin secretion or activity. Excessive ingested water produces a mild decrease in plasma osmolality that shuts off secretion of vasopressin. In the absence of vasopressin action on the kidney, urine does not become concentrated, and a large volume of dilute urine is excreted. The amount of vasopressin in plasma is unmeasurable or low but is appropriate for the low plasma osmolality.

Although the pathophysiologic mechanisms for each of these four disorders are distinct, patients in each category usually manifest polyuria and polydipsia. The serum sodium level is normal because the normal thirst mechanism is sufficiently sensitive to maintain water homeostasis in the first three disorders, and the normal kidney has sufficient capacity to excrete the excess water load in the fourth.

Clinical Manifestations

Central Diabetes Insipidus

The sudden appearance of hypotonic polyuria after transcranial surgery in the area of the hypothalamus or after head trauma with basal skull fracture and hypothalamic damage obviously suggests the diagnosis of central diabetes insipidus. In these situations, if the patient is unconscious and unable to recognize thirst, hypernatremia is a common accompaniment. However, even in patients with more insidious progression of a specific disease or in patients with idiopathic central diabetes insipidus, the onset of polyuria is often relatively abrupt and occurs during several days or weeks. The initial problem is the volume of urine and polydipsia, not the decrease in urine osmolality. Most patients do not report polyuria until urine volume exceeds 4 L/day, and as illustrated in Figure 243–2, urine volume does not exceed 4 L/day until the ability to concentrate the urine is severely limited and plasma vasopressin is nearly absent. As few as 10% of the normal number of vasopressinergic neurons in the hypothalamus can maintain asymptomatic urine volume, but the further loss of these few neurons produces a rapid increase in urine volume and symptomatic polyuria. Urine volume seldom exceeds the amount of dilute fluid delivered to the collecting duct (about 18 to 24 L in humans), and in many cases urine volume is less because patients voluntarily restrict fluid intake, which causes some mild volume contraction and increased proximal tubular reabsorption of fluid. Patients often express a preference for cold liquids, which are more effective in assuaging thirst. Both thirst and increased urine output persist through the night. Patients with partial central diabetes insipidus have some ability to secrete vasopressin, but this secretion is markedly attenuated at normal levels of plasma osmolality. Therefore, these patients have symptoms and urine volume similar to those of patients with complete central diabetes insipidus. Because most patients with central diabetes insipidus have sufficient thirst to drink fluid to match urine output, few laboratory abnormalities are present at the time of initial evaluation. Serum sodium level may be in the high-normal range, whereas blood urea nitrogen level may be low secondary to large urine volume. Uric acid is relatively high due to the modest volume contraction and the lack of action of vasopressin on V_{1a} receptors in the kidney, which stimulate clearance of uric acid. Uric acid levels greater than 5 mg/dL have been reported to distinguish diabetes insipidus from primary polydipsia.

A variant of central diabetes insipidus is the syndrome of osmoreceptor dysfunction. This syndrome has been referred to as essential hypernatremia and adipsic hypernatremia because such patients have a chronically increased serum sodium concentration and an absence of thirst. Physiologic maneuvers demonstrate that when the patients are euvolemic, an increase in plasma osmolality produces neither secretion of vasopressin nor a sensation of thirst. However, vasopressin is still synthesized by the hypothalamus and stored in the posterior pituitary because stimulation of baroreceptors by hypovolemia or hypotension results in prompt secretion of vasopressin; the kidney is responsive because vasopressin release by volume receptor stimulation causes urinary concentration. Because patients lack thirst, they are chronically dehydrated, with increased serum sodium levels. However, it is the dehydration-induced volume depletion, not the increased osmolality, that eventually stimulates secretion of vasopressin. The volume of urine output depends on the degree of dehydration-induced secretion of vasopressin. If sufficient fluid replacement is given to return extracellular fluid volume to normal, these patients are unable to regulate vasopressin by osmolality and then become markedly polyuric, thereby manifesting their underlying diabetes insipidus.

Central diabetes insipidus can be inherited as an autosomal dominant disease that is typically characterized by an asymptomatic infancy but onset later in childhood. Most genetic defects are either in the signal peptide of the pre-prohormone or in the neurophysin portion of the prohormone. Mutations involving the vasopressin sequence itself are few. Abnormal packaging of vasopressin and neurophysin might also produce increased degradation of both the mutant and the normal wild-type prohormone and hence inadequate secretion of vasopressin. However, most cases are believed to result from disruption of cleavage from the signal peptide or abnormal folding of the neurophysin, which slows trafficking of the mutant prohormone through the endoplasmic reticulum, thereby leading to neuronal cell dysfunction and death by virtue of accumulation of the unprocessed mutant protein within the magnocellular neurons. Because this is a cumulative process, this accounts for the later onset of central diabetes insipidus with these types of mutations.

Myxedema and adrenal insufficiency both impair the ability to excrete free water by renal mechanisms. The simultaneous occurrence of either of these diseases with central diabetes insipidus (as can occur with a tumor of the hypothalamus or pituitary) may decrease an otherwise large urine output, thereby masking the symptoms of the diabetes insipidus. Replacement treatment for the anterior pituitary deficiency, especially glucocorticoids, can then cause a sudden and massive excretion of dilute urine. Similarly, the onset of either hypothyroidism or adrenal insufficiency during the course of diabetes insipidus can decrease the need for vasopressin replacement and in some cases even cause hyponatremia. Central diabetes insipidus is extremely common in patients with severe brain ischemia and is usually indicative of brain death. Treatment of the diabetes insipidus along with any coexistent anterior pituitary hormone deficiencies has been advocated to preserve donor organs in such cases.

Nephrogenic Diabetes Insipidus

Nephrogenic diabetes insipidus is caused by mutations of the vasopressin V_2 receptor or the vasopressin-induced water channel, aquaporin-2, or impairments in the signal transduction system linking the V_2 receptor and aquaporin-2. Familial nephrogenic diabetes insipidus is a rare disease, most cases of which (>90%) are due to mutations of the V_2 receptor. More than 100 different V_2 receptor mutations have been described, which can be classified into four general categories on the basis of differences in transport to the cell surface and vasopressin binding or stimulation of adenylate cyclase: (1) the mutant receptor is not inserted in the membrane; (2) the mutant receptor is inserted in the membrane but does not bind or respond to vasopressin; (3) the mutant receptor is inserted in the membrane and binds vasopressin but does not activate adenylate cyclase; or (4) the mutant protein is inserted into the membrane and binds vasopressin but responds subnormally in terms of adenylate cyclase activation. Because the gene for the V_2 receptor is located on the Xq28 region of the X chromosome, this is an X-linked recessive disease. Symptoms are noted only in affected males, who present with vomiting, constipation, failure to thrive, fever, and polyuria during the first week of life. Hypernatremia is found with a hypo-osmolar urine. The phenotype is similar in the less than 10% of patients with mutations of the aquaporin-2 water channel, but because the aquaporin-2 gene is located on chromosome 12, mutations cause autosomal recessive disease; consequently, consanguinity and a family history of the disease in men and women is common, and this disorder should be suspected when the proband is a girl.

Nephrogenic diabetes insipidus can also be acquired during treatment with certain drugs, such as demeclocycline (which is used to treat inappropriate secretion of vasopressin), lithium carbonate (used to treat bipolar disorders), and fluoride (previously used in fluorocarbon anesthetics), and from electrolyte abnormalities such as hypokalemia and hypercalcemia. All causes of acquired nephrogenic diabetes insipidus have in common decreased synthesis and function of aquaporin-2 due to impaired vasopressin signaling from V_2 receptor binding and activation. Other diseases of the kidney produce polyuria and inability to concentrate the urine secondary to altered renal medullary blood flow or to other disorders that inhibit maintenance of the hyperosmolar concentrating gradient in the inner medulla. Renal manifestations of such disorders (e.g., sickle cell disease, sarcoidosis, pyelonephritis, multiple melanoma, analgesic nephropathy) are discussed in Chapter 123.

Gestational Diabetes Insipidus

In pregnancy, there is an increased metabolism of vasopressin due to cystine aminopeptidase (oxytocinase or vasopressinase), an enzyme that is normally produced by the placenta to degrade circulating oxytocin and prevent premature uterine contractions. Because of the close structural similarity between vasopressin and oxytocin, this enzyme degrades both peptides. Normally, this can be overcome by increased synthesis of vasopressin. Rarely during pregnancy, women with normal regulation of vasopressin develop diabetes insipidus because of nonphysiologic, markedly elevated levels of vasopressinase. Some of these patients have been noted to have accompanying preeclampsia, acute fatty liver, and coagulopathies, but causal relations between the diabetes insipidus and these abnormalities have not been identified. In general, diabetes insipidus is not found after the pregnancy ends or in subsequent normal pregnancies.

Polyuria can also become manifest in patients who have limited vasopressin reserve because of a decreased ability either to secrete vasopressin (partial central diabetes insipidus) or to respond to vasopressin action (compensated nephrogenic diabetes insipidus). In these cases, vasopressin synthesis cannot keep up with even physiologic circulating levels of vasopressinase during pregnancy. Treatment may be required only during the pregnancy, and the patient often returns to previous baseline function without need for therapy when the pregnancy ends. Less commonly, central diabetes insipidus of another cause first becomes symptomatic during pregnancy and then persists with the usual course of the diabetes insipidus.

Primary Polydipsia

Excessive fluid intake also causes hypotonic polyuria and, by definition, polydipsia. Consequently, this disorder must be differentiated from the various causes of diabetes insipidus. It is apparent that despite normal pituitary and kidney function, nonetheless patients with this disorder share many characteristics of both central diabetes insipidus (i.e., vasopressin secretion is suppressed as a result of the decreased plasma osmolality) and nephrogenic diabetes insipidus (kidney aquaporin-2 expression is decreased as a result of the suppressed plasma vasopressin levels). Many different names have been used to describe patients with excessive fluid intake, but primary polydipsia remains the best descriptor because it does not presume any single etiology for the increased fluid intake.

Primary polydipsia is sometimes due to a severe mental illness such as schizophrenia, mania, or an obsessive-compulsive disorder, in which case it is called psychogenic polydipsia. These patients usually deny true thirst and attribute their polydipsia to bizarre motives, such as a need to cleanse their body of poisons. Series of patients in psychiatric hospitals have shown an incidence as high as 42% of patients with some form of polydipsia, and there is no obvious explanation for the polydipsia in most reported cases. However, primary polydipsia can also be caused by an abnormality in the osmoregulatory control of thirst, in which case it has been termed dipsogenic diabetes insipidus. These patients have no overt psychiatric illness and invariably attribute their polydipsia to a nearly constant thirst. Dipsogenic diabetes insipidus is usually idiopathic, but it can also be secondary to organic structural lesions in the hypothalamus identical to any of the disorders described as causes of central diabetes insipidus, such as neurosarcoidosis of the hypothalamus, tuberculous meningitis, multiple sclerosis, or trauma. Consequently, all polydipsic patients should be evaluated with a magnetic resonance imaging (MRI) scan of the brain before it is concluded that excessive water intake is due to an idiopathic or psychiatric cause. Primary polydipsia can also be produced by drugs that cause a dry mouth or by any peripheral disorder causing marked elevations of renin or angiotensin.

Finally, primary polydipsia is sometimes caused by physicians, nurses, lay practitioners, or health writers who recommend a high fluid intake for valid (e.g., recurrent nephrolithiasis) or unsubstantiated health reasons. These patients lack overt signs of mental illness but also deny thirst and usually attribute their polydipsia to habits acquired from years of adherence to their drinking regimen. Patients with primary polydipsia may drink even greater amounts of fluid (e.g., >20 L/day) during the day than patients with central diabetes insipidus do yet characteristically do not manifest nocturia and often sleep through the night with minimal disruption. The disorder may be exacerbated during times of stress, yet not be bothersome during normal intervals. Laboratory studies in these patients are generally normal, although serum sodium concentration can sometimes be at the low end of the normal range and the level of uric acid is lower than in patients with other forms of diabetes insipidus.

Diagnosis

Physiologic Diagnosis

Diabetes insipidus should be considered in all patients presenting with significant polyuria (i.e., urine output of more than 50 mL/kg/day). Although osmotic diuresis secondary to hyperglycemia, intravenous contrast agents, or renal injury is a more common clinical cause of polyuria, the medical history, an isotonic urine osmolality, and routine clinical laboratory tests generally distinguish these disorders from diabetes insipidus. A diagnosis of diabetes insipidus can be made when urine osmolality is inappropriately low in the presence of an elevated plasma osmolality as a result of increased serum sodium concentration. These criteria are sometimes met at the initial examination, especially in cases of acute diabetes insipidus occurring after trauma or after surgery in which fluid replacement has not been adequate. In such patients with hypernatremia and hypotonic urine osmolality with normal renal function, one need only administer a vasopressin agonist to differentiate central diabetes insipidus, in which a renal response with decreased urine volume and increased urine osmolality occurs, from nephrogenic diabetes insipidus, in which a subnormal renal response is seen. Sometimes in the postoperative state, a water diuresis occurs as a result of water retention during the surgical procedure. Vasopressin is normally secreted in response to surgical stress, causing fluid administered intravenously during the procedure to be retained. During recovery, vasopressin levels fall, and a diuresis of the retained fluid occurs. In this case, however, the serum sodium level is almost always normal; but if further fluid is administered to match the urine output, persistent polyuria might be mistaken for diabetes insipidus. In this situation, the physician should decrease the rate of fluid administered and follow the urine output and serum sodium level. If urine output decreases and the serum sodium level remains normal, no treatment is necessary; if serum sodium rises above the normal range and the urine remains hypotonic, diabetes insipidus is likely, and the response to a vasopressin agonist will ascertain the type.

Most outpatients with diabetes insipidus will not be hypernatremic because the polydipsia produced by a normal thirst response is generally sufficient to maintain water homeostasis. Instead, they will present with polyuria, polydipsia, and a normal sodium level. In these patients, it is necessary to perform further testing to increase serum osmolality and then measure the plasma vasopressin level or the urinary response to an administered vasopressin agonist. The best described test is the water deprivation test (Fig. 243–3). The test should be carried out under controlled observation in the hospital or an appropriately equipped outpatient area. The timing of the test depends on the symptoms of the patient. If the patient has marked polyuria during the night, it is best to begin the test during the day because the patient may become dehydrated overnight. However, if the patient has only two or three episodes of nocturia per night, it is best to begin the test in the evening so that the major part of the dehydration takes place when the patient is asleep. In either case, the patient is weighed at the beginning of the test, and all subsequent fluids are withheld. The volume and osmolality (measured directly by freezing point depression) of all excreted urine are measured and the

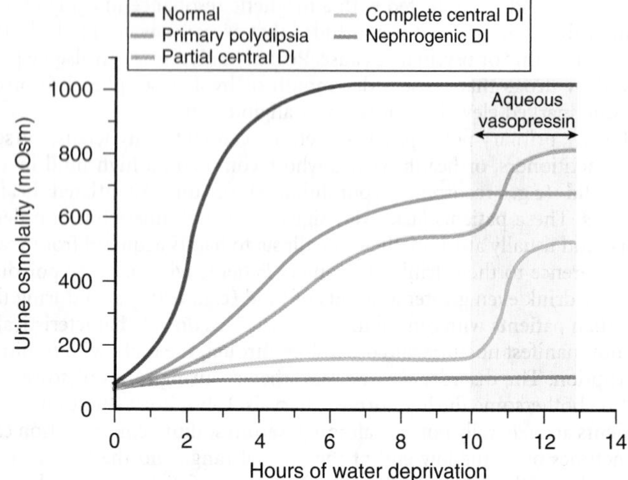

FIGURE 243–3 • Responses to the water deprivation test to differentiate various types of diabetes insipidus and primary polydipsia (as described by Miller and associates, Ann Intern Med 1970;73:721). The response to dehydration shows a plateau, and the subsequent change in urine osmolality in response to administered vasopressin is illustrated. See discussion in the text. DI = diabetes insipidus.

patient is re-weighed after each liter of urine output. When three consecutive urine samples have an osmolality differing by no more than 10% and the patient has lost at least 2% of body weight, a blood sample is obtained for measurement of serum osmolality, sodium, and plasma vasopressin. The patient is then given 2 mg of desmopressin intravenously or intramuscularly and observed for an additional 2 hours.

Adults with normal vasopressin secretion will be able to concentrate their urine to above 800 mOsm/kg H_2O and will have less than a 10% increase in urine osmolality in response to administered desmopressin. Patients with complete central diabetes insipidus have minimal concentration of the urine with dehydration and a marked increase in urine osmolality (usually >50%) in response to administered desmopressin. Patients with nephrogenic diabetes insipidus usually have no increase in urine concentration in response to administered desmopressin, although in some cases of acquired nephrogenic diabetes insipidus, some increased urinary concentration (generally <10%) can occur. Nephrogenic diabetes insipidus is best distinguished from central diabetes insipidus by measurement of vasopressin in the plasma; plasma vasopressin levels are elevated normally in cases of nephrogenic diabetes insipidus, especially after dehydration.

In patients with partial central diabetes insipidus and patients with primary polydipsia, the urine is often somewhat concentrated in response to dehydration, but not to the maximum of a normal person because the chronically reduced level of vasopressin downregulates the synthesis of aquaporin-2 water channels, and the large urine volume, regardless of cause, washes out the medullary osmotic gradient that determines the maximum urine concentration. When desmopressin is administered, patients with partial central diabetes insipidus have a further increase (usually >10% but <50%) in urine osmolality, whereas most patients with primary polydipsia have no further increase (i.e., <10%). However, the reliability of distinguishing between these last two disorders by the water deprivation test is suboptimal. Some patients with primary polydipsia may not become sufficiently dehydrated with the test to secrete maximum vasopressin and hence have an increase in urine osmolality in response to administered desmopressin. Alternatively, some patients with partial central diabetes insipidus can become sufficiently dehydrated that their maximal concentration of urine is reached during the test and no further concentration is seen with administered desmopressin. Plasma vasopressin levels at the end of dehydration offer a better means to discriminate between these two disorders, but only at high serum sodium concentrations (i.e., >145 mmol/L). Consequently, some investigators advise a limited infusion of hypertonic (3%) NaCl solution to achieve these levels if they are not achieved by the water deprivation itself. It is important to maintain adequate follow-up of patients with suspected partial central diabetes insipidus to ensure that during treatment with vasopressin, a good therapeutic response is obtained. In some difficult cases, the response to treatment with a vasopressin agonist can be an adjunct to the diagnosis. If a decrease in polyuria and thirst with maintenance of normal serum sodium concentration occurs, a diagnosis of partial central diabetes insipidus is confirmed; however, if polydipsia persists and hyponatremia develops, a diagnosis of primary polydipsia is confirmed.

Etiologic Diagnosis

If the water deprivation test confirms that inadequate vasopressin secretion or function is responsible for the polyuria, the underlying cause must be determined. MRI of the hypothalamic-pituitary area is the most important diagnostic tool in these cases. The three areas of interest are the immediate suprasellar region of the hypothalamus, the pituitary stalk, and the posterior pituitary within the sella turcica. As noted in the discussion of anatomy, vasopressin is synthesized in the paired paraventricular nuclei high on the walls of the third ventricle and the paired supraoptic nuclei lateral to and above the optic chiasm and then transported to the posterior pituitary for storage and release. Transection or damage of these axons at the level of the posterior pituitary causes an accumulation of neurosecretory material in the axon proximal to the site of the injury as well as outgrowth of axons in the median eminence, where vasopressin can be secreted into the pituitary portal capillaries. Therefore, most slow-growing tumors that are confined to the sella do not cause diabetes insipidus. To cause central diabetes insipidus, tumors in the hypothalamic area immediately above the sella must be either sufficiently large to destroy 80 to 90% of the vasopressin cells or located where the paths of the four nuclear groups converge at the origin of the pituitary stalk just above the diaphragma sellae. Primary tumors, especially craniopharyngioma, suprasellar germinoma, metastatic tumors, and infiltrative diseases, can also cause diabetes insipidus by infiltration of the pituitary stalk, which is then thickened on MRI scanning. In addition, on T1-weighted MRI images, the vasopressin and oxytocin stored in neurosecretory granules in the posterior pituitary are visualized as a "bright spot" in the sella turcica. Most but not all normal subjects have this bright spot; and in most but not all patients with central diabetes insipidus, the bright spot is lost. Thickening of the stalk and absence of the bright spot are therefore especially suggestive of a hypothalamic disease process.

Tumors that cause central diabetes insipidus are most often benign primary intracranial tumors, such as craniopharyngioma, ependymoma (suprasellar germinoma), and pinealoma, that arise in the third ventricle. Primary tumors of the anterior pituitary cause diabetes insipidus only when substantial suprasellar extension is present. However, rapidly growing intrasellar lesions, such as metastases from carcinomas of the lung, breast, and melanoma or hemorrhage into pituitary adenomas, can cause diabetes insipidus because of insufficient time to allow vasopressin axons to adapt by releasing hormone into the vasculature of the median eminence. Metastasis to the hypothalamus can also lodge in the portal capillaries of the median eminence, thereby destroying the supraopticohypophysial tract and producing diabetes insipidus. Granulomatous diseases, such as Langerhans cell histiocytosis, sarcoidosis, and tuberculosis, and leukemic infiltrates and lymphomas of the hypothalamus can cause diabetes insipidus by destroying vasopressin cells in the hypothalamus. In such patients with diseases having peripheral manifestations, the diagnosis is usually suspected on the basis of general medical findings.

Lymphocytic infundibuloneurohypophysitis is an autoimmune disease similar to lymphocytic hypophysitis of the anterior pituitary in which lymphocytes infiltrate the neurohypophysis to produce diabetes insipidus. The hallmarks of this process are a thickened pituitary stalk and an absence of the pituitary bright spot in a patient with abrupt onset of polyuria and polydipsia, particularly in a postpartum female. The diagnosis was originally demonstrated by pituitary biopsy but now is generally made by regression of the thickened stalk with continued follow-up. When no cause is found, the diagnosis of exclusion is idiopathic diabetes insipidus, but most such cases probably also are caused by an autoimmune disease, and other autoimmune diseases are often recognized in affected patients. When central nervous system disease is suspected but not diagnosed by MRI or general physical examination, cerebrospinal fluid obtained by lumbar puncture may be helpful in identifying tumor cells or markers of tumors or inflammatory processes (e.g., elevated angiotensin-converting enzyme levels in neurosarcoidosis).

Treatment

Because excess diuresis of water is the primary manifestation of diabetes insipidus, water replacement in adequate quantities avoids the metabolic complications of this disease. However, oral or intravenous administration of the volume of fluid required to replace urinary losses in diabetes insipidus is difficult and inconvenient. The goal of therapy is to reduce the amount of polyuria and polydipsia to a tolerable level while avoiding overtreatment, which can produce water retention and hyponatremia. The best therapeutic agent for treatment of hypothalamic diabetes insipidus is the vasopressin agonist desmopressin. Desmopressin is different from vasopressin in that the amino group of the N-terminal cystine residue has been removed to prolong the duration of action, and D-arginine has been substituted for L-arginine in position 8 to decrease vasopressor effects. At therapeutic dosages, this agent acts on V_2 or antidiuretic receptors with minimal activity at V_{1a} or pressor receptors. Desmopressin is available in tablets of 0.1 mg or 0.2 mg for oral administration and in either a spray bottle that delivers a fixed dose of 10 μg in 100 μL or in a bottle with a rhinal catheter that can deliver 50 to 200 μL (5 to 20 μg for intranasal administration). When therapy is initiated, it is generally best to begin with a low dose (e.g., half of a 0.1-mg tablet, 5 μg by the rhinal tube, or a single 100 μL spray of 10 μg) at bedtime to allow the patient to sleep through the night, then to determine the duration of action by quantifying the polyuria the next day. The duration of action of a single dose varies between patients from 6 to 24 hours; but in most patients, a dosage can be determined that provides a good therapeutic response on an every-12-hour schedule for the nasal spray and an 8- or 12-hour schedule for the tablets. If patients are never polyuric on a fixed schedule, it may be advisable to delay administration of a dose once a week to allow diuresis of any accumulated water. Desmopressin is also available for parenteral use in 1-mL vials of 4 μg/mL. Parenteral administration is especially useful postoperatively or when a patient is unable to take the nasal preparation. In hospitalized patients, some physicians add vasopressin directly to a crystalloid solution to infuse doses in the range of 0.25 to 2.7 mIU/kg/hr to cause modest but persistent urinary concentration as a treatment of diabetes insipidus. With any parenteral administration, serum sodium levels should be monitored frequently to prevent the development of hyponatremia.

Some orally administered pharmacologic agents are also useful in treating diabetes insipidus. Chlorpropamide in doses of 100 to 500 mg daily enhances the effect of vasopressin at the renal tubule and is especially useful in patients with partial central diabetes insipidus. An antidiuretic effect is noted in 1 to 2 days, but maximum antidiuresis may not be achieved until after several days of administration. Thiazide diuretics cause sodium depletion and volume contraction and decrease urine volume by increasing proximal tubular reabsorption of glomerular filtrate. Prostaglandin synthase inhibitors (e.g., indomethacin) block the action of prostaglandin E to inhibit the action of vasopressin on the kidney. Although use of a prostaglandin synthase inhibitor is not a primary treatment of central diabetes insipidus, it can alter the antidiuretic response of other agents. Chlorothiazide, amiloride, and prostaglandin synthase inhibitors are useful to reduce polyuria in nephrogenic diabetes insipidus. However, none of these agents has approval of the Food and Drug Administration for treatment of diabetes insipidus; therefore, the prescribing physician should be aware of potential toxicities and side effects. In cases of drug-induced nephrogenic diabetes insipidus, the most direct therapy is discontinuation of the offending agent, if possible. Symptomatic nephrogenic diabetes insipidus is usually treated with a thiazide diuretic, which is enhanced by the coadministration of the potassium-sparing diuretic amiloride. Amiloride can be especially beneficial in cases of nephrogenic diabetes insipidus induced by lithium because the drug decreases the entrance of lithium into cells in the distal tubule. When diuretics are used to treat nephrogenic diabetes insipidus, special attention should be paid to the possibility that the induced dehydration may increase the concentration of other drugs.

Some situations require special attention during therapy. Rarely, if patients with diabetes insipidus are unable to drink or are given a hypertonic solution, severe hypernatremia can develop acutely. Osmotic equilibrium with the intracellular water of neurons and glia produces shrinking of the brain. The brain is in a closed vault (i.e., the skull), and when the brain shrinks, traction on the vasculature of the central nervous system can cause rupture of blood vessels and subarachnoid or intracerebral hemorrhage. If the hypernatremia persists for a longer time, the neurons accommodate by production of organic osmolytes, previously called idiogenic osmoles, which limit the amount of brain shrinkage. Once this adaptation has occurred, too rapid lowering of osmolality in the extracellular fluid will produce a shift of water into the brain and cause cerebral edema. In this situation, desmopressin can be administered to produce constant antidiuresis, and the amount of water given can be regulated to decrease osmolality by no more than approximately 1 mEq every 2 hours. Postoperatively or after head trauma, diabetes insipidus can be transient (see prognosis in the next section), and the need for long-term maintenance therapy cannot be immediately established. During pregnancy, vasopressinase increases the metabolism of vasopressin but not of desmopressin, so desmopressin is the drug of choice. The vasopressinase activity subsides by a few weeks after delivery, and patients with the onset of partial diabetes insipidus during pregnancy may become asymptomatic after delivery. An additional advantage of desmopressin is that it has little action on the oxytocin receptors of the uterus. During pregnancy, normal plasma osmolality decreases by approximately 10 mOsm/kg H_2O because of changes in serum sodium, so pregnant patients with diabetes insipidus require sufficient desmopressin only to maintain their serum sodium at this lower level.

Prognosis

The prognosis of properly treated diabetes insipidus is excellent. Historical complications of bladder hypertrophy and hydroureter secondary to voluntarily decreasing urine frequency are largely unseen with modern therapy. If nephrogenic diabetes insipidus is diagnosed and treated early, intracranial calcification and mental retardation do not occur. When the diabetes insipidus is secondary to a recognized disease process, it is that disease which generally determines the ultimate prognosis. In some specific clinical situations, the course is different and characteristic. The development of diabetes insipidus after surgical or traumatic injury to the neurohypophysis can follow any of several different well-defined patterns (Fig. 243–4). In some patients, polyuria develops 1 to 4 days after injury and resolves spontaneously. Less often, the diabetes insipidus is permanent and continues indefinitely. Most interestingly, one can see a "triphasic" response that has been well described after pituitary stalk transection. The initial diabetes insipidus (first phase) is due to axon shock and lack of function of the damaged neurons. This phase lasts several hours to several days and then is followed by an antidiuretic phase (second phase) that is due to the uncontrolled release of vasopressin from the disconnected and degenerating posterior pituitary or from the remaining severed neurons. Overly aggressive administration of fluids during this second phase does not suppress the uncontrolled vasopressin release from the damaged neurohypophysis and can lead to hyponatremia. The antidiuresis can last 2 to 14 days, after which diabetes insipidus recurs after depletion of the vasopressin from the degenerating posterior pituitary gland (third phase). Transient hyponatremia without preceding or subsequent diabetes insipidus has been reported recently after transsphenoidal surgery for pituitary microadenomas. This generally occurs 5 to 10 days postoperatively, and the incidence may be as high as 30% when such patients are carefully observed, although the majority of cases are mild and self-limited. This is due to inappropriate vasopressin secretion by the same mechanism as the triphasic response, except that in these cases, only the second phase occurs ("isolated second phase") because the neural lobe or pituitary stalk damage does not impair vasopressin secretion sufficiently to produce clinical manifestations of diabetes insipidus.

Once a deficiency of vasopressin secretion has been present for more than a few days or weeks, it rarely improves even if the underlying cause of the neurohypophysial destruction is eliminated. The major exception to this is in patients with postoperative diabetes insipidus, when sponta-

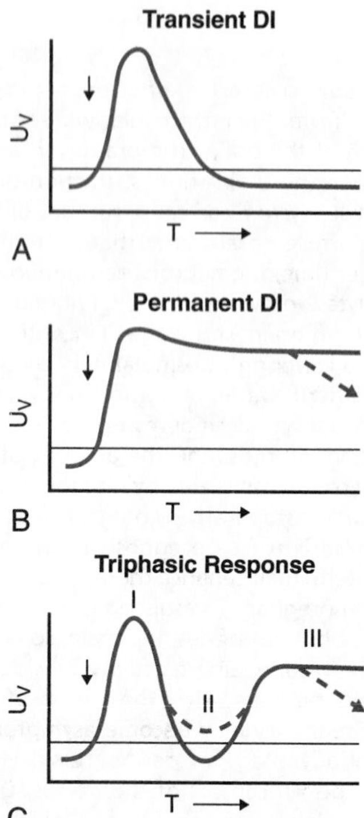

FIGURE 243-4 • Diagrammatic summary of the major patterns of postoperative and post-traumatic diabetes insipidus. The abscissa represents time after the initial injury (arrow); the ordinate represents urinary volume relative to a hypothetical "normal" urine output of 2 to 3 L/24 hr (solid line). See discussion in text. During the triphasic response, uncontrolled release of vasopressin from the disconnected or damaged posterior pituitary gland causes an antidiuresis that can lead to water retention and a dilutional hyponatremia. Diabetes insipidus returns as the third phase after the stored hormone in the posterior pituitary has been depleted. DI = diabetes insipidus. (From Verbalis JG, Robinson AG, Moses AM: Postoperative and post-traumatic diabetes insipidus. In Czernichow AP, Robinson A [eds]: Diabetes Insipidus in Man: Frontiers of Hormone Research. Basel, S Karger, 1985, p 247.)

neous resolution is the rule. Although recovery from diabetes insipidus that persists more than several weeks postoperatively is less common and is distinctly uncommon after 1 year of continued diabetes insipidus, well-documented cases of long-term recovery have been reported as long as 10 years after the initiating event. The reason for amelioration and resolution is apparent from pathologic and histologic examination of neurohypophysial tissue after pituitary stalk section in both animals and humans. Neurohypophysial neurons that have intact perikarya are able to regenerate axons and form new nerve terminal endings capable of releasing vasopressin into nearby capillaries. Potential return of function is another reason for occasionally withholding therapy during long-term treatment. Diabetes insipidus should not be considered idiopathic until at least 4 years of follow-up. During this interval, annual computed tomography or MRI scans are indicated to test for the appearance of a tumor or infiltrative process that may not have been detected at the initial examination.

SUGGESTED READINGS

Fujiwara TM, Bichet DG: Molecular biology of hereditary diabetes insipidus. J Am Soc Nephrol 2005;16:2836–2846. *Comprehensive review of hereditary nephrogenic diabetes insipidus caused by mutations of the V_2 receptor or the aquaporin-2 water channels.*

Ghirardello S, Malattia C, Scagnelli P, Maghnie M: Current perspective on the pathogenesis of central diabetes insipidus. J Pediatr Endocrinol Metab 2005;18:631–645. *Review of etiologies of central diabetes insipidus in pediatric patients, emphasizing that 35 to 50% of spontaneous cases are idiopathic.*

Makaryus AN, McFarlane SI: Diabetes insipidus: Diagnosis and treatment of a complex disease. Cleve Clin J Med 2006;73:65–71. *Review of central and nephrogenic diabetes insipidus.*

Pivonello R, De Bellis A, Faggiano A, et al: Central diabetes insipidus and autoimmunity: Relationship between the occurrence of antibodies to arginine vasopressin–secreting cells and clinical, immunological, and radiological features in a large cohort of patients with central diabetes insipidus of known and unknown etiology. J Clin Endocrinol Metab 2003;88:1629–1636. *In one third of cases, an autoimmune cause is likely.*

244 THYROID

Paul Ladenson and Matthew Kim

EMBRYOLOGY

The embryonic thyroid gland develops from endoderm at the foramen cecum that migrates downward and elongates to form two clusters of spherical follicles. The follicles proliferate to form the lobes of the thyroid gland.

Ectopic thyroid tissue can remain at the base of the tongue to form a lingual thyroid or may remain along the thyroglossal duct. It can migrate as far inferiorly as the diaphragm. A thyroglossal duct cyst can present as a fluctuant midline cervical mass that elevates with extension of the tongue.

ANATOMY

The adult thyroid gland contains two lobes that wrap along the right and left anterolateral aspects of the trachea midway between the thyroid cartilage and the suprasternal notch. Each lobe is demarcated into upper, middle, and lower poles. The right and left lobes are connected by an isthmus on the anterior aspect of the trachea just below the cricoid cartilage. The normal terminus of the thyroglossal duct can persist as a pyramidal lobe. A pyramidal lobe is often palpably enlarged in diffuse thyroid disorders, such as autoimmune thyroiditis and Graves' disease. The adult thyroid gland weighs 15 to 20 g. Each lobe measures approximately 4 cm in length, 2 cm in width, and 1.5 cm in depth.

After thyroid enlargement, the attachment of the sternothyroid muscle to the trachea limits upward expansion of the superior aspect of each lobe. Lateral and posterior growth may cause inferior expansion that may extend into the superior mediastinum, compressing the trachea and veins at the thoracic outlet. The parathyroid glands usually lie beneath the posterior aspects of each thyroid lobe. The recurrent laryngeal nerves course upward along the tracheoesophageal groove, from which branches pass behind each thyroid lobe to innervate the larynx.

HISTOLOGY

Thyroid tissue is composed of clustered spherical follicles, each containing a single layer of follicular epithelial cells known as thyrocytes that surround a lumen containing colloid. The principal component of colloid is thyroglobulin, a thyrocyte-specific protein. Microvilli on the luminal surface of thyrocytes play active roles in thyroid hormone synthesis and secretion. Aggregated clusters of follicles are surrounded by dense networks of capillaries innervated by sympathetic and parasympathetic nerve fibers. Parafollicular C cells, which are derived from neural crest tissue and produce calcitonin, are widely dispersed between follicles.

PHYSIOLOGY

Thyroid Hormone Synthesis and Secretion

Dietary iodine in the form of iodide (I^-) or iodate (IO_3^-) is absorbed from the gastrointestinal tract and distributed in the extracellular fluid. The median urinary iodide level in an iodine-sufficient population is 10 μg/dL. The current average daily intake of iodine in the United States equals the recommended daily intake of 150 μg because of widespread use of iodized salt, iodate as a preservative in baked goods, and dairy products that contain iodine. Circulating iodide is actively transported into the thyrocyte by the sodium-iodide symporter. Within the thyrocyte, iodide is rapidly oxidized by H_2O_2 in a reaction catalyzed by thyroid peroxidase. The reactive intermediate formed is covalently bound to tyrosyl residues present in thyroglobulin to generate monoiodotyrosine and diiodotyrosine residues through a process known as organification. Thyroid peroxidase also catalyzes the coupling of the monoiodotyrosine and diiodotyrosine residues to generate thyroxine (T_4) and triiodothyronine (T_3). Exposure to excessive amounts of circulating iodide may transiently inhibit thyroid hormone synthesis by disrupting organification. T_4 and T_3 are secreted after proteolysis of thyroglobulin. This hydrolytic process may be inhibited by exposure to excessive amounts of iodide or lithium. In the normal state, 100 μg of T_4 and 5 μg of T_3 are directly released into the circulation each day.

Thyroid Hormone Transport and Metabolism

Circulating thyroid hormones are more than 99% bound to one of three classes of plasma proteins. Thyroxine-binding globulin (TBG) synthesized by the liver functions as the principal transport protein. Pregnancy and exposure to pharmacologic doses of estrogens can increase TBG levels, as can hepatitis, familial TBG excess, and certain medications including 5-fluorouracil, tamoxifen, and methadone. Conversely, decreased TBG levels may occur with systemic illness, severe hepatic disease, nephrotic syndrome, and treatment with androgens, glucocorticoids, and slow-release nicotinic acid. Whereas total T_4 and T_3 levels rise and fall with changes in the TBG level, free T_4 and T_3 levels remain relatively constant. Familial dysalbuminemic hyperthyroxinemia is an autosomal dominant disorder characterized by the production of albumin that binds T_4 with a high affinity. Affected individuals may present with high total T_4 levels and normal free T_4 levels. Thyroxine-binding prealbumin and albumin make lesser contributions to T_4 and T_3 transport in blood.

The receptor binding and biologic activity of T_3 is eightfold greater than that of T_4. More than 80% of the T_3 present in target tissues is derived from T_4 through the action of deiodinase enzymes. Type 1 deiodinase, present in the liver and kidneys, converts T_4 to T_3, which contributes to the pool of T_3 in the circulation. The activity of type 1 deiodinase may be inhibited by systemic illness, iodide-containing compounds including amiodarone and radiocontrast agents, glucocorticoid therapy, and selenium deficiency. Type 2 deiodinase is present in the pituitary gland and brain. Type 3 deiodinase is present in the glial cells of the central nervous system. It deactivates thyroid hormone by inner ring monodeiodination, a process that converts T_4 to inactive reverse triiodothyronine (rT_3) and T_3 to inactive diiodothyronine (T_2).

Control of Thyroid Function

The growth of thyroid tissue and the synthesis and secretion of thyroid hormones are controlled by the hypothalamus and the pituitary gland. Thyrotropin-releasing hormone (TRH) synthesized in the supraoptic and paraventricular nuclei of the hypothalamus is transported to the anterior pituitary gland through the hypophysial portal system. TRH binds to receptors on thyrotrophic cells in the anterior pituitary, stimulating the synthesis and secretion of thyroid-stimulating hormone (TSH). TSH is a heterodimeric glycoprotein composed of a unique β subunit coupled to an α subunit identical to that present in follicle-stimulating hormone, luteinizing hormone, and human chorionic gonadotropin. It is transported in the circulation to the thyroid gland, where it binds to the extracellular domain of TSH receptors on thyrocytes. The binding of TSH to the TSH receptor stimulates growth of individual thyrocytes, iodide transport and organification, hydrolysis of thyroglobulin, and secretion of thyroid hormone. Circulating T_4 and T_3 exert negative feedback at the levels of both the hypothalamus and the pituitary gland, inhibiting the synthesis and secretion of TRH and TSH, respectively.

Thyroid Hormone Action

Thyroid hormone binds receptors that are members of the nuclear receptor superfamily, regulating expression of thyroid hormone–responsive genes. Isoforms of the thyroid hormone receptors (α_1, β_1, and β_2) bind to a specific hexameric oligonucleotide sequence in the transcriptional regulatory region of thyroid hormone–responsive genes. Thyroid hormone increases oxygen consumption, thermogenesis, and expression of the low-density lipoprotein (LDL) receptor, resulting in accelerated LDL cholesterol degradation. In myocardium, T_3 increases myocyte contractility and relaxation by altering myosin heavy chain and sarcoplasmic reticulum adenosine triphosphatase (ATPase). In the cardiac conducting system, T_3 increases the heart rate by altering sinoatrial node depolarization and repolarization. Other physiologic effects of thyroid hormone include increased mental alertness, ventilatory drive, gastrointestinal motility, and bone turnover. During fetal development, thyroid hormone plays a critical role in brain development and skeletal maturation.

Diagnosis

Physical Examination

Examination of the thyroid begins with inspection of the lower anterior portion of the neck to check for diffuse or asymmetrical gland enlargement, tracheal deviation, lymphadenopathy, and jugular venous distention. Palpation can be performed by an anterior or posterior approach. Anterior palpation can be performed by using the thumb of one hand to locate the isthmus of the gland beneath the cricoid cartilage. The right lobe of the thyroid gland can be palpated by placing the left thumb along the left side of the trachea to brace the contralateral lobe, using the tips of the fingers of the right hand to laterally retract the right sternocleidomastoid muscle at the level of the isthmus, and using the pads of the fingers of the right hand to explore and define the tissue composing the lobe. The mass of tissue that moves beneath the fingertips when the patient swallows represents the lobe. This maneuver can be reversed to examine the left lobe.

Laboratory Findings

TSH and Thyroid Hormone Levels

The log-linear negative relationship between levels of $T_4 + T_3$ and TSH makes it a sensitive indicator of primary thyroid gland dysfunction. Current TSH immunoassays with a functional sensitivity of less than 0.02 mIU/L permit accurate detection of all common causes of thyroid hormone deficiency and excess. Indeed, TSH levels become abnormal when patients' thyroid hormone levels remain within broad reference ranges, conditions termed subclinical hypothyroidism and subclinical thyrotoxicosis. In most patients with primary thyroid gland dysfunction, measurement of a single TSH level permits accurate classification of thyroid status. Limitations of TSH testing occur when there is TSH-mediated secondary thyroid dysfunction, reduced biologic activity of T_3 or TSH itself, temporary disequilibrium of the hypothalamic-pituitary-thyroid axis, or analytical derangements affecting the TSH immunoassay.

Measurements of T_4 and T_3 levels confirm the significance of an abnormal TSH level, define the severity of thyroid dysfunction, and provide a clue to the underlying etiology. Thyroid hormone measurements are also essential to define patients' thyroid status when TSH levels cannot be trusted. Immunoassays are available to measure total and free levels of T_4 and T_3. Whereas assays that measure total T_4 and T_3 levels are accurate, their results do not distinguish between large plasma protein–bound and free fractions of each hormone. Consequently, congenital and acquired derangements of TBG (and less commonly transthyretin and albumin) can alter total but not free T_4 and T_3 levels. These conditions can be misdiagnosed as abnormal thyroid function unless a discordance in TSH is noted or one of these underlying conditions is suspected (Tables 244–1 and 244–2).

There are several methods of estimating unbound T_4 and T_3 levels. Free T_4 and free T_3 immunoassays are widely employed for this purpose and yield reliable results in common conditions that alter plasma protein

TABLE 244–1 CAUSES OF EUTHYROID HYPERTHYROXINEMIA (INCREASED TOTAL T_4, NORMAL TSH, NORMAL FREE T_4)

Increased synthesis of thyroxine-binding globulin
Pregnancy
Hepatitis
Acute intermittent porphyria
Drugs
Estrogens
Tamoxifen
Raloxifene
Methadone
5-Fluorouracil
Increased binding of thyroid hormone to albumin
Familial dysalbuminemic hyperthyroxinemia
Increased binding of thyroid hormone to transthyretin
Hereditary variants
Pancreatic neuroendocrine tumors

TABLE 244–2 CAUSES OF EUTHYROID HYPOTHYROXINEMIA (DECREASED TOTAL T_4, NORMAL TSH, NORMAL FREE T_4)

- Increased metabolism of thyroid hormone
  - Drugs
    - Phenytoin
    - Phenobarbital
    - Carbamazepine
    - Rifampin
- Decreased synthesis of thyroxine-binding globulin
  - Severe liver disease
  - Malnutrition
  - Drugs
    - Androgens
    - Danazol
    - L-Asparaginase
- Increased clearance of thyroxine-binding globulin
  - Nephrotic syndrome
  - Protein-losing enteropathy
- Decreased binding of thyroid hormone to thyroxine-binding globulin
  - Drugs
    - Salicylates (high dose)
    - Phenytoin (high dose)
    - Furosemide (intravenous)

levels, such as estrogen-induced TBG excess. Free T_4 measurement after equilibrium dialysis of serum is the most accurate approach but is technically demanding and not readily available in most settings.

Other Laboratory Tests

Measurement of thyroid autoantibody titers can be useful in the evaluation of thyroid dysfunction. Antithyroid peroxidase and antithyroglobulin antibody titers can confirm a diagnosis of autoimmune thyroiditis. Thyroid-stimulating immunoglobulin activity levels can be measured to evaluate Graves' disease. The erythrocyte sedimentation rate can be helpful in the diagnosis of subacute thyroiditis. Serum thyroglobulin and calcitonin levels are used as tumor markers in observing patients with treated differentiated and medullary thyroid cancers, respectively.

Imaging

Anatomic Imaging

Ultrasonography provides detailed views that help measure the size of the thyroid gland, characterize its texture, and identify structural abnormalities including solid nodules and simple or partially cystic nodules. Diffuse heterogeneity may suggest autoimmune thyroiditis. Certain characteristics of nodules—including the appearance of capsules, vascularity, and patterns of calcification—can alter the probability of malignancy but do not confirm or exclude thyroid cancer with certainty. Imaging of surrounding structures may identify cervical lymphadenopathy not detectable on physical examination.

Computed tomographic (CT) and magnetic resonance imaging (MRI) scans can also define the size and anatomic relationships of thyroid tissue but are less sensitive than ultrasonography in characterizing thyroid lesions. The value of these modalities is their ability to delineate tracheal deviation, narrowing, and substernal extension of the thyroid into the mediastinum. Cervical CT scanning can also help define and localize regional lymphadenopathy. Positron emission tomography (PET) plays a role in the localization of residual thyroid cancer.

Functional Imaging

Radionuclide scanning takes advantage of the fact that gamma ray–emitting tracers transported into thyrocytes by the sodium-iodide symporter can generate images that reflect the regional activity of thyroid tissue. Technetium Tc 99m and iodine 123 are commonly used. ^{99m}Tc-pertechnetate is rapidly trapped by thyrocytes, and ^{99m}Tc scans can be acquired 20 to 30 minutes after injection. ^{123}I and ^{131}I thyroid scans generate images providing a more accurate representation of regional thyroid tissue function that can indicate whether a nodule is hypofunctioning (cold), hyperfunctioning (hot), or equivalent in function to extranodular tissue (warm). Radionuclide imaging no longer plays a central role in the differential diagnosis of most thyroid nodules. When it is necessary, ^{123}I is the preferred tracer for use because of its lower thyroidal and whole body radiation dose.

TABLE 244–3 ETIOLOGIES OF HYPOTHYROIDISM

- Primary hypothyroidism
  - Insufficient functioning thyroid tissue
    - Congenital absence of thyroid tissue
    - Autoimmune destruction of thyroid tissue
      - Autoimmune thyroiditis (Hashimoto's thyroiditis)
    - Surgical removal of thyroid tissue
    - Radioablation of thyroid tissue by radioactive iodine or external beam radiation
    - Infiltrative destruction of thyroid tissue
      - Hemochromatosis
      - Scleroderma
      - Amyloidosis
  - Impaired thyroid hormone synthesis
    - Iodine deficiency
    - Congenital enzymatic defects that disrupt thyroid hormone synthesis
    - Drug-mediated inhibition of thyroid hormone production and release
      - Thionamides
      - Amiodarone
      - Lithium
      - Aminoglutethimide
- Secondary hypothyroidism
  - Insufficient secretion of TRH or TSH
    - Hypothalamic disorders
      - Tumor (lymphoma, germinoma, glioma)
      - Irradiation
      - Inflammation (sarcoidosis, vasculitis)
    - Hypopituitarism
      - Mass lesions
      - Pituitary surgery
      - Pituitary radiation
      - Hemorrhagic apoplexy (Sheehan's syndrome)
      - Infiltration (hemochromatosis, tuberculosis, fungal infection)
      - Lymphocytic hypophysitis
- Thyroid hormone resistance syndrome

Thyroid Uptake

The fraction of an administered radioactive iodine or technetium dose taken up and retained by the thyroid gland during a defined period represents an index of the gland's activity. Typically, technetium pertechnetate uptakes are determined at 20 minutes and range from 0.5 to 3%; radioiodine uptakes are usually determined at 6 or 24 hours and range from 8 to 28%. These fractional thyroid uptakes can be useful in the differential diagnosis of thyrotoxicosis. Radioiodine uptake values are also used to calculate effective ^{131}I doses for treatment of hyperthyroidism and thyroid cancer.

HYPOTHYROIDISM

Definition

Primary hypothyroidism (termed myxedema when it is severe) refers to hormone deficiency caused by intrinsic dysfunction of the thyroid gland that disrupts the synthesis and secretion of T_4 and T_3 (Table 244–3). Overt hypothyroidism is characterized by an elevated TSH level, usually greater than 10 mIU/L, in conjunction with a free T_4 level below the lower limit of the reference range. In mild or subclinical hypothyroidism, the TSH level is only modestly elevated; the free T_4 level remains in the low-normal to normal range.

Secondary or central hypothyroidism refers to deficient thyroid gland function that is the result of inadequate stimulation by TSH. This is due, in turn, to production of either insufficient or ineffective TSH from a number of congenital or acquired pituitary and hypothalamic disorders.

Epidemiology

Primary hypothyroidism is common. Population-based surveys reveal that it is present in almost 5% of individuals. It is more commonly diagnosed in women and with advancing age, although it occurs in men and younger individuals. It is more prevalent among whites and Latinos. Secondary hypothyroidism is rare, representing less than 1% of all cases.

Pathobiology

Dietary iodine deficiency is the chief cause of primary hypothyroidism in certain underdeveloped regions of the world. The most common cause of primary hypothyroidism in the United States and most other countries is autoimmune (or Hashimoto's) thyroiditis, a condition in which altered T cell–mediated immunity causes destruction of thyroid tissue and impaired gland function. On histologic examination, the condition is characterized by a lymphocytic infiltrate and fibrosis. Circulating antithyroid antibodies directed against thyroid peroxidase and thyroglobulin are clinically useful markers of the disease, but glandular inflammation is principally the result of altered T cell–mediated function. There is a genetic predisposition to the condition. Linkage studies suggest a polygenic basis. Patients with autoimmune thyroiditis may have other endocrine and nonendocrine autoimmune disorders. It may be a component of the type 2 polyglandular autoimmune syndrome associated with autoimmune adrenal insufficiency and type 1 diabetes mellitus. It is less commonly a component of the type 1 syndrome that includes adrenal insufficiency, hypoparathyroidism, and chronic mucocutaneous candidiasis. Other nonendocrine autoimmune conditions associated with autoimmune thyroiditis include atrophic gastritis, pernicious anemia, systemic sclerosis, Sjögren's syndrome, and vitiligo. Individuals treated with interferon alfa may develop autoimmune thyroiditis with transient or permanent hypothyroidism.

Surgical resection of thyroid tissue to treat thyroid disorders or other head and neck cancers predictably leads to hypothyroidism. Radioactive iodine therapy for treatment of hyperthyroidism commonly destroys sufficient thyroid tissue to cause postablative hypothyroidism. External beam radiation therapy for head and neck cancer also commonly causes thyroid gland failure. Exposure to certain pharmacologic and radiocontrast agents that contain large amounts of iodine, such as the antiarrhythmic agent amiodarone, radiocontrast dyes, and some expectorants and topical disinfectants, can disrupt key steps in thyroid hormone production. Lithium used to treat affective disorders inhibits secretion of T_4 and T_3, leading to hypothyroidism in 10% of treated patients. Other pharmacologic agents reported to cause hypothyroidism include stavudine, thalidomide, and aminoglutethimide.

There are a number of other rare causes of primary hypothyroidism. Agenesis or dysgenesis of the thyroid gland and defects in thyroid hormone synthesis cause congenital hypothyroidism. Infiltrative disorders can disrupt thyroid function, including hemochromatosis, amyloidosis, systemic sclerosis, and invasive fibrous thyroiditis (also known as Riedel's thyroiditis). The thyroid gland inflammation that occurs with subacute thyroiditis and painless (postpartum) thyroiditis causes transient hypothyroidism, from which most patients recover.

Secondary or central hypothyroidism may be caused by a number of disorders that impair normal hypothalamic or pituitary control of the thyroid gland. Infiltrative disorders affecting the hypothalamus that can interfere with TRH secretion include sarcoidosis, hemochromatosis, and histiocytosis. Masses that impinge on the pituitary stalk can impede TRH delivery through the hypophysial portal system. Compression of thyrotrophic cells by pituitary adenomas and other masses in the sella turcica can inhibit synthesis and secretion of TSH. Surgery and radiotherapy to treat pituitary adenomas can destroy thyrotrophic cells, leading to secondary hypothyroidism that develops as a component of panhypopituitarism. Other disorders that may be associated with secondary hypothyroidism include lymphocytic hypophysitis, pituitary metastases from primary malignant neoplasms, apoplexy, infarction caused by hemorrhage at the time of delivery in women (also known as Sheehan's syndrome), and head trauma.

Clinical Manifestations

Symptoms and Signs

Symptoms of hypothyroidism include fatigue, lethargy, weight gain despite poor appetite, cold intolerance, hoarseness, constipation, weakness, myalgias, arthralgias, paresthesias, dry skin, and hair loss. Females may develop precocious puberty, menorrhagia, amenorrhea, and galactorrhea. Affected individuals may experience depressed mood with limited initiative and sociability. Cognitive deficits can range from mild lapses in memory to delirium, dementia, seizures, and coma. The nonspecific nature of most of these symptoms makes it difficult to determine which patients presenting with them have hypothyroidism compared with other causes. In most cases, hypothyroidism is insidious in onset, making its recognition difficult. Symptoms that are new, progressive, or present in combination are more likely to be due to hypothyroidism.

The physical findings associated with hypothyroidism vary according to the age at onset and disease severity. Children may present with delayed linear growth despite weight gain, precocious or delayed puberty, and pseudohypertrophy of muscle. Adults can present with bradycardia, diastolic hypertension, and mild hypothermia. The skin may be coarse, dry, yellow, and cool to the touch as a result of peripheral vasoconstriction. Diffuse thinning of scalp hair accompanied by thinning of the lateral eyebrows may occur. The nails may be brittle. Examination of the chest may reveal distant heart sounds. Examination of the extremities may reveal diffuse nonpitting edema caused by the deposition of glycosaminoglycans. Neurologic examination may reveal slow dysarthric speech and diffuse slowing of deep tendon reflexes with a marked delay in the terminal relaxation phase.

Examination of the neck may reveal a range of findings. Healed transverse or lateral incisional scars in this region indicate a history of surgical resection of thyroid tissue. The thyroid gland may be normal in size, diffusely enlarged, or atrophic to the point at which it may be difficult to palpate with any degree of certainty. It may be soft and smooth with a lobular texture or firm and irregular with a variegated nodular texture.

Other Routine Test Abnormalities

Blood tests may reveal anemia, hyponatremia, hypoglycemia, and elevated creatine phosphokinase, prolactin, homocysteine, triglyceride, and total and LDL cholesterol levels. Electrocardiography may show sinus bradycardia with low voltage in the limb leads. Chest radiography and echocardiography may demonstrate a pericardial effusion.

Diagnosis

Suspected primary hypothyroidism is confirmed by an elevated TSH level (Fig. 244–1). Established reference ranges for TSH levels typically extend from 0.5 to 4.5 mIU/L. However, the distribution of values within this range is skewed toward the lower half, such that the mean TSH level is estimated to be 1.5 mIU/L. Measurement of the free T_4 level confirms the diagnosis of primary hypothyroidism and characterizes its severity. A low free T_4 level in conjunction with a persistently elevated TSH level establishes the diagnosis of overt primary hypothyroidism, whereas a low-normal free T_4 level with an elevated TSH level is termed mild primary hypothyroidism. Other uncommon causes of isolated TSH elevation should be considered in appropriate settings, including recovery from severe systemic illness, renal failure, and adrenal insufficiency.

Testing to determine the underlying cause of primary hypothyroidism is usually unnecessary. The condition can almost always be ascertained from the patient's history, and if not, autoimmune thyroiditis is usually the etiology. When confirmation is required (e.g., to convince a patient that the condition is permanent), serum antithyroid antibodies may be assessed. Measurement of antithyroid peroxidase antibody is a more sensitive test than antithyroglobulin antibody for this purpose. Ten percent of patients with histologic autoimmune thyroiditis will not have any circulating antithyroid antibodies.

When clinical findings suggest the possibility of secondary hypothyroidism, the TSH level cannot be relied on to provide an accurate index of thyroid function. These circumstances include presence of a sellar mass, previous pituitary surgery or irradiation, other pituitary axis hormone deficiencies, and conditions known to cause hypothalamic or pituitary dysfunction. In these settings, the serum free T_4 level must be assessed, and a low or even low-normal free T_4 level can confirm the diag-

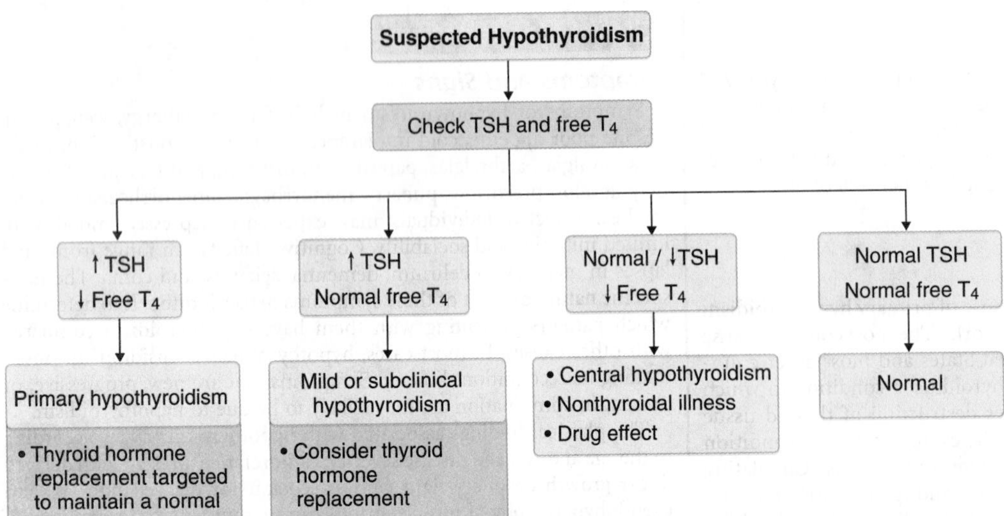

FIGURE 244–1 • Laboratory assessment of suspected hypothyroidism.

nosis. The TSH level in patients with secondary hypothyroidism can be low, normal, or even modestly elevated.

Treatment

Rx

The goals of thyroid hormone replacement therapy are straightforward: to replace endogenous thyroid hormone production, to avoid iatrogenic thyrotoxicosis, and rarely to treat systemic complications of severe hypothyroidism. Levothyroxine sodium (hereafter thyroxine) is the hormonal preparation of choice for both primary and secondary hypothyroidism. Thyroxine has a number of favorable pharmacokinetic characteristics. It is well absorbed, and its plasma protein binding gives it a 7-day half-life, permitting daily dosing. Thyroxine is physiologically deiodinated to the more biologically active T_3 in peripheral tissues. However, thyroxine is a narrow therapeutic index drug, and doses differing by as little as 12% can have clinical consequences. Tablets of multiple dose strengths ranging from 25 to 300 µg are available in the United States. Whereas regulatory standards ensure pharmaceutical equivalence in terms of mass of thyroxine, bioavailability may differ by as much as 12% among different preparations. Consequently, adherence to a single thyroxine formulation is advisable.

The optimal dose of thyroxine for replacement therapy is related to lean body weight, with most adults requiring a daily dose of 1.8 µg/kg. The dose requirement for elderly adults is typically lower (e.g., 1.0 µg/kg/day) because of reduced metabolic clearance. Patients with postsurgical or postablative hypothyroidism usually require a higher daily dose than patients with autoimmune thyroiditis who may have some residual gland function. Patients with coexisting malabsorptive disorders may require higher and variable doses. Certain medications, mineral supplements, and foods can interfere with thyroxine absorption, including ferrous sulfate, calcium carbonate, aluminum hydroxide, sucralfate, cholestyramine, and soy-containing foods (Table 244–4). Thyroxine doses should be separated from these substances by 4 or more hours.

Thyroxine dose requirements may increase as a result of accelerated metabolic clearance in several circumstances. Patients with nephrotic syndrome and other systemic illnesses that lead to rapid clearance of thyroid hormone require higher daily doses. Dose requirements increase by an average of 75% in most pregnant women, probably as a result of placental metabolism of thyroxine. Simultaneous treatment with phenytoin, phenobarbital, carbamazepine, or rifampin also typically accelerates thyroxine metabolism. One third of postmenopausal women beginning estrogen replacement therapy have increased dose requirements.

Most adults without known or suspected coronary artery disease can be started on a full replacement dose of thyroxine. The initial dose can be calculated on the basis of the patient's weight and age, rounding down to the nearest available dose strength. For patients with primary hypothyroidism, adequacy of thyroxine therapy can be assessed by TSH measurement 4 to 6 weeks after the dose is started or adjusted. The target TSH level for most individuals should be the lower half of the reference range (i.e., 1.0 to 2.0 mIU/L). Once an adequate dose has been established, a TSH level should be checked annually. In patients with secondary hypothyroidism, the serum free T_4 level should be monitored 2 to 4 weeks after the thyroxine dose is started or adjusted, with a target free T_4 level in the upper half of the reference range.

TABLE 244–4 INTERFERENCE WITH THYROXINE REPLACEMENT THERAPY

- Factors contributing to underreplacement
  - Inadequate prescribed dose
  - Limited compliance
  - Decreased absorption due to ingestion of agents that bind thyroxine
    - Ferrous sulfate
    - Calcium carbonate
    - Aluminum hydroxide
    - Sucralfate
    - Cholestyramine
    - Soy protein
  - Increased metabolism of thyroxine
    - Pregnancy
    - Drugs
      - Phenytoin
      - Phenobarbital
      - Carbamazepine
      - Rifampin
  - Diminishing residual thyroid function
  - Changing formulations
- Factors contributing to overreplacement
  - Excessive prescribed dose
  - Factitious ingestion of additional doses
  - Decreased metabolism of thyroxine due to aging
  - Increasing residual thyroid function
  - Changing formulations

Rx

Management of Complications

Complications of thyroxine therapy are limited to iatrogenic thyrotoxicosis and rarely adverse effects of restoring euthyroidism. Typical symptoms and signs of thyrotoxicosis accompany overtreatment. Even a modestly excessive thyroxine dose can induce bone mineral loss, especially in postmenopausal women, and can increase the risk of atrial fibrillation in older individuals. In patients with underlying coronary artery disease, the positive chronotropic and inotropic effects of thyroxine may exacerbate myocardial ischemia. Adults with known or suspected ischemic heart disease should be started on a low dose that is titrated upward in small increments once tolerance is ensured (e.g., starting with 25 μg daily, then increasing the dose by 12.5 to 25 μg every 4 to 6 weeks). In some cases, β-blocker therapy may need to be intensified to counter the induction of myocardial ischemia. Deliberate suboptimal dosing of thyroxine should be avoided. If necessary, coronary revascularization may be required before euthyroidism can be fully restored. Coexisting adrenal insufficiency associated with hypopituitarism or the type 2 polyglandular autoimmune syndrome may be unmasked when cortisol clearance is accelerated by a return to a euthyroid state. Other adverse effects that infrequently occur with thyroxine therapy include transient hair loss, acute sympathomimetic symptoms that resolve with dose reduction and slow advancement, and pseudotumor cerebri in children.

A minority of patients with thyroxine-treated hypothyroidism report bothersome symptoms ascribed to hypothyroidism, despite biochemical evidence of adequate thyroid hormone replacement. Some of these patients improve with prescription of a higher thyroxine dose that restores the serum free T_4 level to the upper limit of normal. It was anecdotally suggested that combination thyroxine and T_3 therapy could aid such patients. Several studies have shown that provision of a physiologic T_3 supplement is not superior to placebo when iatrogenic thyrotoxicosis is avoided and depressed patients are excluded. Consequently, combination T_4 and T_3 therapy, including the use of desiccated thyroid, appears to offer no advantage.

Mild Hypothyroidism

Whether individuals diagnosed with mild hypothyroidism (i.e., an elevated or high-normal TSH level with a free T_4 level within the reference range) benefit from thyroxine therapy is controversial. Proponents argue that treatment with thyroxine relieves symptoms, lowers cholesterol, avoids the emergence of overt hypothyroidism, and is relatively safe. Detractors counter that these purported benefits have not been confirmed in adequately powered, randomized controlled trials. In practice, many providers opt for a trial of therapy in mildly hypothyroid patients who are symptomatic, have underlying hypercholesterolemia, or demonstrate a high likelihood of progressing to overt hypothyroidism. Predictors of progressive thyroid failure include age older than 65 years, TSH level higher than 10 mIU/L, and the presence of circulating antithyroid antibodies indicating underlying autoimmune thyroiditis.

Myxedema Coma

Severe hypothyroidism can culminate in myxedema coma, a life-threatening condition characterized by hypothermia, bradycardia, hypotension, altered mental status, and multisystem organ failure. Risk factors include advanced age, poor access to health care, and other underlying major organ system diseases. Most patients have long-standing thyroid hormone deficiency. Treatment should include thyroxine (1.8 μg/kg daily with or without a 500-μg loading dose). Some experts advocate coadministration of triiodothyronine in divided doses to compensate for impaired conversion of T_4 to T_3. No controlled trials have been performed to evaluate the relative benefits and risks of these different approaches. Glucocorticoids should be administered in stress doses after a cosyntropin stimulation test has been performed to check for evidence of concomitant adrenal insufficiency. Care should be taken to avoid exposure to potent sedative or analgesic agents that may exacerbate altered mental status. Hypothermia should be treated with external warming to reduce the risk of circulatory collapse.

Nonthyroidal Illness

In patients with severe nonthyroidal illness, a characteristic constellation of thyroid function test changes occur that often appear to be consistent with hypothyroidism (Fig. 244–2). The T_3 level usually declines as a result of decreased extrathyroidal T_4 to T_3 conversion. With increasingly severe disease, total T_4 and free T_4 levels also decline. TSH levels are usually low to low-normal. During the course of recovery, the TSH level can rise above the upper limit of the normal range, producing a profile that can be mistaken for primary hypothyroidism. Clinical correlation is essential to assess thyroid function in severely ill patients (e.g., a history of preexisting thyroid or pituitary disease, the presence of a goiter, or features suggesting other elements of hypopituitarism). Because no benefit of thyroid hormone treatment has been shown for these patients, observation with retesting 6 to 8 weeks after recovery is the preferred approach.

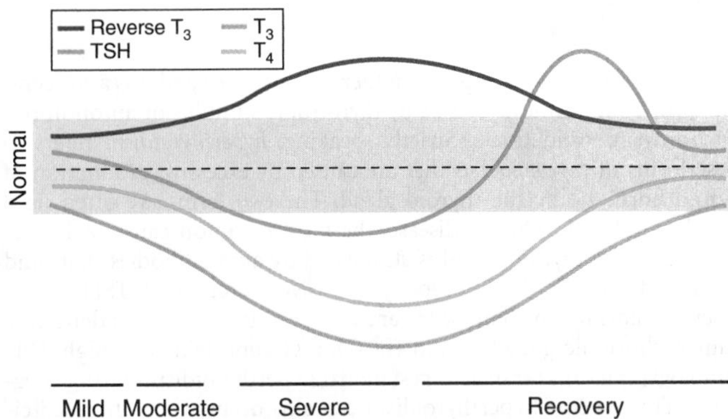

FIGURE 244–2 • Changes in thyroid hormone levels during nonthyroidal illness.

TABLE 244–5 ETIOLOGIES OF THYROTOXICOSIS

- Hyperthyroidism
  - Antibody-mediated stimulation of thyroid tissue
    - Graves' disease
  - Autonomously functioning thyroid tissue
    - Toxic multinodular goiter
    - Toxic adenoma
    - Iodine exposure
  - Autonomously functioning heterotopic thyroid tissue
    - Struma ovarii
    - Metastatic differentiated thyroid cancer
  - Excessive secretion of TSH
    - TSH-secreting pituitary adenoma
- Nonhyperthyroid thyrotoxicosis
  - Ingestion of exogenous thyroid hormone
    - Pharmacologic
      - Levothyroxine
      - Liothyronine
      - Combination preparations
    - Nonpharmacologic
      - Dietary supplements
    - Improperly processed meat products
  - Inflammation causing release of endogenous thyroid hormone
    - Subacute thyroiditis
    - Autoimmune thyroiditis

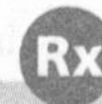

THYROTOXICOSIS

Definition

Thyrotoxicosis is defined as a systemic syndrome caused by exposure to excessive amounts of thyroid hormone (Table 244–5).

Epidemiology

It presents in 1 of every 2000 adults, affecting 1% of all individuals during the course of a lifetime.

Pathobiology

Hyperthyroidism develops when there is excessive synthesis and secretion of thyroid hormone caused by thyrotropic stimulus or autonomous function of thyroid tissue. Strictly speaking, *hyperthyroidism* refers to those forms of *thyrotoxicosis* that are caused by excessive production of thyroid hormone by the thyroid gland. The two terms are often used interchangeably. In Graves' disease, the most common cause of hyperthyroidism, the thyroid gland is stimulated by autoantibodies that bind to and activate the TSH receptor. Excessive secretion of TSH causes hyperthyroidism in patients with rare TSH-secreting pituitary adenomas. Human chorionic gonadotropin (hCG), a glycoprotein with high TSH homology, can cause transient gestational hyperthyroidism during pregnancy. This type of hyperthyroidism can also occur when choriocarcinoma, molar pregnancy, or a germ cell tumor produces variant forms of hCG that are more active, or when mutant TSH receptors bind hCG more avidly, as occurs in familial gestational thyrotoxicosis.

Autonomous production of thyroid hormone occurs when thyrocytes function independently of TSH receptor activation. This can occur as a result of growth of a benign functioning thyroid adenoma, as a result of growth of multiple autonomously functioning nodules forming a toxic multinodular goiter, or in rare cases when patients with well-differentiated thyroid cancer present with functioning metastases. In some toxic adenomas, somatic mutations in the TSH receptor gene lead to constitutive activation. In patients whose thyroid glands have the potential for autonomous function, exposure to excessive amounts of iodine in the form of amiodarone or iodinated contrast agents can sometimes provoke hyperthyroidism.

Transient thyrotoxicosis also can be caused by inflammatory conditions that release excessive amounts of thyroid hormone stored in the gland. These include subacute thyroiditis that is believed to be caused by a viral infection, acute or suppurative thyroiditis caused by bacterial infection, radiation-induced thyroiditis, and pharmacologic thyroiditis precipitated by exposure to amiodarone. Autoimmunity can also provoke an inflammatory thyroiditis that causes transient thyrotoxicosis. This commonly occurs in the setting of lymphocytic thyroiditis (also known as silent, painless, or postpartum thyroiditis). It rarely occurs in the setting of autoimmune thyroiditis (also known as Hashimoto's thyroiditis).

In rare cases, excess thyroid hormone can be secreted by ectopic thyroid tissue located anywhere from the base of the tongue to the mediastinum, or by heterotopic thyroid tissue that develops as part of an ovarian teratoma (a condition known as struma ovarii).

Thyrotoxicosis can also be caused by ingestion of excessive amounts of thyroid hormone. This is most often the result of prescription of excessive doses of pharmacologic preparations of thyroid hormone, but it can rarely be due to surreptitious or accidental ingestion.

Clinical Manifestations

Symptoms and Signs

When classic symptoms of thyrotoxicosis are present, including weight loss despite a hearty appetite, heat intolerance, palpitations, tremor, and hyperdefecation (increased frequency of formed bowel movements), clinical diagnosis should be straightforward. Thyrotoxicosis can escape early detection because of presentation with common nonspecific symptoms such as fatigue, insomnia, anxiety, irritability, weakness, atypical chest pain, or dyspnea on exertion. Delayed recognition may also occur when atypical symptoms such as headache, weight loss, periodic paralysis, or nausea and vomiting dominate the clinical picture. Elderly patients may present with apathetic thyrotoxicosis typified by weight loss and the absence of sympathomimetic symptoms and signs.

Signs of thyrotoxicosis include resting tachycardia, systolic hypertension with a widened pulse pressure, warm moist skin with a velvety texture, onycholysis, and staring gaze with lid lag (noted to be present when a rim of sclera is visible between the upper eyelid and superior margin of the iris on downward gaze). Cardiac examination may reveal a prominent apical impulse and a systolic flow murmur. Neurologic findings may include a restless impatient demeanor, pressured speech, proximal muscle weakness, distal hand tremor, and brisk deep tendon reflexes.

Clinical findings often provide a strong indication of the underlying cause of thyrotoxicosis. In Graves' disease, the gland is diffusely enlarged with a smooth or slightly lobulated contour and may manifest an audible bruit. Ophthalmopathy and dermopathy are also unique to Graves' disease. In patients with toxic nodular goiter, one or more discrete nodules may be appreciated. In subacute thyroiditis, the gland is modestly enlarged, extremely tender, and firm. A history of recent pregnancy suggests possible painless thyroiditis. Recent exposure to amiodarone, other iodine-containing compounds, interferon alfa, or pharmacologic preparations of thyroid hormone may suggest the characteristic forms of thyrotoxicosis associated with these agents.

Graves' Disease

Definition

Graves' disease is an autoimmune disorder characterized by a variable combination of hyperthyroidism, ophthalmopathy (also known as thyroid eye disease), and dermopathy.

Epidemiology

Graves' disease is more common among women but also affects men. It can develop at any time, but onset most often occurs between 30 and 60 years of age.

Pathobiology

The proximate cause of hyperthyroidism is production of thyroid-stimulating immunoglobulins that bind to and activate the TSH receptor, promoting thyroid hormone secretion and growth of the thyroid gland. Other thyroid autoantibodies also commonly identified in the setting of Graves' disease include antithyroid peroxidase antibodies, antithyroglobulin antibodies, and anti–TSH receptor antibodies that block TSH binding. The fundamental pathogenesis of Graves' disease remains unknown. A genetic predisposition is implicated by a higher incidence in monozygotic twins and first-degree relatives of affected individuals. Environmental factors implicated in triggering the onset of Graves' disease include exposure to cigarette smoke, high dietary iodine intake, stressful life events, and certain antecedent infections.

Clinical Manifestations

Affected individuals usually present with thyrotoxicosis and a thyroid gland that is diffusely enlarged with a rubbery consistency, smooth contour, definable pyramidal lobe, and audible bruit or palpable thrill due to increased blood flow. When it is clinically evident, thyroid eye disease usually presents within a few months of the onset of hyperthyroidism. In rare cases, it may develop long before, long after, or without any biochemical confirmation of hyperthyroidism.

Prognosis

The hyperthyroidism associated with this condition often follows a persistent and progressive course, but approximately one fourth of patients with Graves' disease demonstrate spontaneous disease remission.

Ophthalmopathy

Definition

Thyroid eye disease is a distinctive disorder characterized by inflammation and swelling of the extraocular muscles and orbital fat, eyelid retraction, periorbital edema, episcleral vascular injection, conjunctival swelling (chemosis), and proptosis (also called exophthalmos). Swelling of soft tissues within the confines of the orbits precipitated by fibroblast growth and inflammatory cell infiltrate can cause proptosis, entrapment of extraocular muscles, and compression of the optic nerve.

Clinical Manifestations

Affected individuals typically complain of a change in eye appearance, ocular irritation, foreign body sensation, dryness, and, ironically, excessive tearing. More severe involvement may cause exposure keratitis with corneal ulceration, diplopia, and blurred vision. On examination, patients may have staring gaze; a rim of sclera visible between the upper eyelid and superior margin of the iris during downward gaze (lid lag); signs of conjunctival inflammation; periorbital edema; and abnormalities of conjugate gaze, color vision, and visual acuity. The precise degree of proptosis can be measured by an exophthalmometer. Orbital imaging with CT scanning or ultrasonography can confirm the diagnosis, which must sometimes be distinguished from other causes of bilateral and unilateral proptosis.

Treatment

Rx

Treatment of mild thyroid-related eye disease focuses on protecting the corneas from exposure and desiccation with moisturizing drops and ointment, glasses, and sometimes taping the eyelids closed at bedtime to prevent exposure during sleep. High-dose systemic glucocorticoid therapy can attenuate orbital inflammation but does not represent an attractive long-term solution. Orbital irradiation may be helpful in controlling inflammatory symptoms in some patients. Persistent corneal exposure, diplopia, altered vision due to optic nerve compression, and cosmetic issues may require surgery to decompress the orbits and readjust the extraocular muscles. Immunosuppressive agents and plasmapheresis have been used in severely affected patients with anecdotal success.

Dermopathy

Infiltrative dermopathy, the least commonly seen complication of Graves' disease, is precipitated by the deposition of glycosaminoglycans in the dermis of the skin. Affected individuals usually present with mildly pruritic, orange peel–like thickening of the skin along the anterior aspects of the shins, commonly known as pretibial myxedema. The dorsal aspects of the feet and fingers, the extensor surface of the elbows, and the face are more rarely affected.

When the diagnosis is not clinically obvious, it can be confirmed by skin biopsy. Treatment of early infiltrative dermopathy with topical glucocorticoids under an occlusive wrap may limit its progression. Treatments involving the use of intradermal or systemic glucocorticoids, long-acting somatostatin analogues, and even surgical resection of soft tissue have shown limited success.

Toxic Adenoma

A toxic adenoma is a solitary, autonomously functioning thyroid neoplasm that synthesizes and secretes excessive amounts of thyroid hormone independent of TSH stimulation. These neoplasms are almost always benign, although rare cases of malignant conversion have been reported. Most grow large enough to be palpated by the time they present with thyrotoxicosis. Somatic gene mutations causing constitutive activation of the TSH receptor and the stimulatory subunit of the guanine nucleotide ($G_{s\alpha}$) have been identified in a subset of toxic adenomas. The hyperthyroidism caused by a toxic adenoma does not remit, except in unusual cases complicated by hemorrhagic infarction of the neoplasm.

Toxic Multinodular Goiter

A toxic multinodular goiter is composed of multiple autonomously functioning thyroid nodules that collectively synthesize and secrete excessive amounts of thyroid hormone. In some patients with nontoxic multinodular goiters, hyperthyroidism can be precipitated by exposure to excessive amounts of iodine. Most affected individuals have a goiter with multiple palpable thyroid nodules. Progressive enlargement may go undetected when there is substernal extension of nodular tissue. Toxic multinodular goiters are more common among older individuals.

TSH-Secreting Pituitary Adenomas

TSH-secreting pituitary adenomas (also known as thyrotropinomas) represent less than 1% of all functioning pituitary tumors. By the time of diagnosis, most patients have developed macroadenomas that are larger than 1 cm in diameter. Smaller microadenomas may also be identified. Patients may present with typical clinical manifestations of thyrotoxicosis, a diffuse goiter, symptoms and signs precipitated by an expanding sellar mass, syndromes associated with co-secretion of other anterior pituitary hormones (growth hormone, prolactin, or adrenocorticotropic hormone), or symptoms and signs of hypopituitarism. The key to suspecting the condition is usually recognition of an inappropriately nonsuppressed TSH level in a patient with thyrotoxicosis. The diagnosis is confirmed in most cases when laboratory testing reveals an elevated circulating level of the pituitary glycoprotein α subunit in conjunction with a radiographically definable sellar mass.

Diagnosis

Laboratory Findings

Abnormalities detected in routinely ordered laboratory tests are often the first clues that suggest thyrotoxicosis. Thyrotoxic patients may have hypercalcemia or hypercalciuria, increased alkaline phosphatase levels, modestly elevated transaminase levels, and low or declining total and LDL cholesterol levels. When they are measured, ferritin and angiotensin-converting enzyme levels are often increased. Electrocardiography typically reveals resting sinus tachycardia or other atrial tachyarrhythmias, particularly atrial fibrillation with a rapid ventricular response. In severe cases, chest radiography may reveal cardiomegaly.

In most patients with suspected thyrotoxicosis, the diagnosis can be determined by measurement of TSH (Fig. 244–3). Sensitive TSH immunoassays with a detection limit less than 0.02 mIU/L can accurately discriminate between clearly suppressed TSH levels characteristic of all common forms of thyrotoxicosis and mildly suppressed levels that fall just beneath the reference range, as may occur in otherwise sick and elderly euthyroid individuals. Only the rare conditions associated with TSH-mediated hyperthyroidism (TSH-secreting pituitary tumors and isolated pituitary resistance to thyroid hormone) will yield false-negative TSH results in screening for thyrotoxicosis. Conversely, there are other conditions that present with suppressed TSH levels. In these conditions, serum free T_4 and T_3 levels will not be elevated on subsequent testing.

Measurement of serum free T_4 and total or free T_3 levels will confirm a diagnosis of thyrotoxicosis, define its severity, and occasionally provide a clue to its underlying etiology. *Overt thyrotoxicosis* is characterized by free T_4 or T_3 levels above the upper limit of the reference range, whereas *mild* or *subclinical thyrotoxicosis* is characterized by a suppressed TSH level with free T_4 and T_3 levels within the normal reference range. When only the free T_4 or T_3 concentrations are elevated, the terms *T_4 toxicosis* and *T_3 toxicosis* are applied, respectively.

Differential Diagnosis

Once a diagnosis of thyrotoxicosis has been confirmed, it is important to define its underlying cause to determine the most appropriate treatment. The relative degrees of T_4 and T_3 elevation sometimes can be helpful. Predominantly T_3 toxicosis is typical of Graves' disease and can also occur with toxic nodular goiter. In contrast, predominantly T_4 toxicosis is more typical of subacute or painless thyroiditis. T_4 toxicosis also is more common in patients with iodine-induced hyperthyroidism.

Other laboratory tests sometimes can be helpful in differential diagnosis. Thyroid-stimulating immunoglobulins are pathognomonic of Graves' disease. An elevated erythrocyte sedimentation rate typically is seen in subacute thyroiditis.

Imaging studies can also help establish a differential diagnosis. The fractional thyroidal uptake of radiotracer within the thyroid gland on scintigraphic scanning often helps establish a definitive diagnosis (Table 244–6). Thyroid ultrasonography can confirm the presence of solitary or multiple thyroid nodules. Chest radiography and CT scanning may help delineate a substernal goiter.

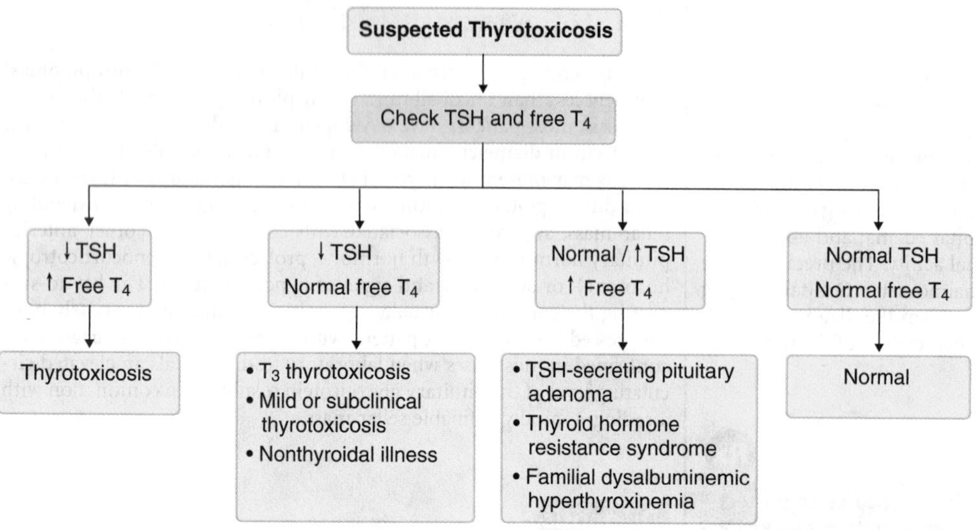

FIGURE 244–3 • Laboratory assessment of suspected thyrotoxicosis.

TABLE 244–6 RADIOGRAPHIC EVALUATION OF SUSPECTED THYROTOXICOSIS

Etiology	Fractional 24-Hour Radioiodine Uptake	Thyroid Scan Appearance
Graves' disease	35–95%	Diffuse increased homogeneous uptake; visible pyramidal lobe extending from the isthmus
Toxic adenoma	20–60%	Solitary focus of intense uptake; suppression of uptake in the remainder of the thyroid
Toxic multinodular goiter	20–60%	Patchy heterogeneous foci of increased uptake interspersed with regions of diminished uptake
Subacute thyroiditis	0–2%	Minimal to absent uptake
Autoimmune thyroiditis	0–2%	Minimal to absent uptake; patchy heterogeneous uptake during recovery
Iodine-induced hyperthyroidism	0–2%	Minimal to absent uptake
Exogenous thyroid hormone intoxication	0–2%	Minimal to absent uptake
Metastatic differentiated thyroid cancer	0–5%	Focal uptake in metastases
TSH-secreting pituitary adenoma	30–80%	Diffuse increased homogeneous uptake

Treatment

Selection of the most effective treatment for a specific condition causing thyrotoxicosis requires an understanding of the underlying pathophysiologic process and natural history. For example, a toxic multinodular goiter will not remit and requires radioiodine treatment or surgery; subacute thyroiditis will subside spontaneously and requires only temporizing symptomatic therapy.

β-Blockers

β-Blockers help alleviate the sympathomimetic manifestations of thyrotoxicosis, regardless of the underlying cause. Palpitations, tremor, and anxiety can often be promptly controlled. However, certain other clinical features of thyrotoxicosis, including weight loss, heat intolerance, and fatigue, are not ameliorated by these agents. In thyrotoxic patients with marked sinus tachycardia or atrial fibrillation with a rapid ventricular response rate, β-blockers can be used as rate-controlling agents. Propranolol also partially inhibits extrathyroidal conversion of T_4 to T_3, which may be of added benefit in patients with severe thyrotoxicosis.

Propranolol can be started at a dose of 20 to 40 mg every 8 hours and titrated upward to a maximal daily dose of 240 mg on the basis of symptom control. Sustained-release propranolol or longer-acting β-blockers, such as metoprolol and atenolol, can also be used. Esmolol can be used when a short-acting parenteral agent is required. β-Blockers should be used with caution in thyrotoxic patients with a history of heart failure, obstructive pulmonary disease, or Raynaud's phenomenon.

For patients with transient forms of thyrotoxicosis (subacute thyroiditis, autoimmune thyroiditis, or exogenous thyroid hormone intoxication), a β-blocker may be the only treatment required. In patients with more sustained conditions, such as Graves' disease or toxic nodular goiter, β-blockers provide prompt initial relief of symptoms while definitive treatment with antithyroid drugs, radioiodine, or surgery is planned and implemented.

Antithyroid Drugs

The thionamides inhibit thyroid hormone biosynthesis by competitively inhibiting iodine organification and iodotyrosine coupling in thyrocytes. These agents are used for the treatment of thyrotoxicosis caused by glandular overproduction of thyroid hormones. Because the thionamides block only new thyroid hormone synthesis, glandular stores of preexisting thyroid hormone must be exhausted before they are fully effective. Secretion of preexisting thyroid hormone may continue for up to 3 to 8 weeks in patients with Graves' disease or toxic multinodular goiters. Although antithyroid drugs can provide long-term control of hyperthyroidism, they are most appropriately used when there is a possibility that the underlying condition will remit, as in Graves' disease, or when thyrotoxicosis must be attenuated before radioiodine treatment or surgery.

Rx

Two thionamide agents are currently available, methimazole and propylthiouracil. Methimazole may be taken as a single daily dose because of its longer half-life and higher effective intrathyroidal concentration. This can bolster adherence of patients and drug effectiveness. Propylthiouracil acts to partially inhibit extrathyroidal conversion of T_4 to T_3, an effect that may be beneficial in patients with severe complicated thyrotoxicosis. Propylthiouracil is also preferred for treatment of pregnant women with thyrotoxicosis because it crosses the placental barrier less readily than methimazole does. However, the shorter half-life of propylthiouracil necessitates administration of three or four daily doses.

For patients with mild to moderate hyperthyroidism, methimazole is usually started at a dose of 10 to 30 mg once daily that can be increased to as much as 90 mg once daily. For patients with more severe hyperthyroidism, thyrotoxicosis complicated by cardiac disease, or concomitant pregnancy, propylthiouracil should be started at doses of 50 to 200 mg every 6 to 8 hours. Methimazole may be given rectally if necessary. The anticipated duration of treatment depends on the underlying cause. In patients with toxic multinodular goiters, antithyroid drugs are generally used only to restore euthyroidism in anticipation of definitive therapy. An effective dose can be continued for a period of 6 to 24 months in a patient with Graves' disease before it is tapered off to determine whether there has been a remission of the patient's autoimmune thyroid disease. Patients most likely to respond are those presenting with mild clinical and biochemical hyperthyroidism, a small thyroid gland, and no active ophthalmopathy.

Patients treated with antithyroid drugs should have thyroid function tests checked every 3 to 12 weeks during dose titration to monitor for iatrogenic hypothyroidism. Common side effects include rash, pruritus, fever, and arthralgias, which affect 5% of thionamide-treated patients. Agranulocytosis and hepatitis are rare but potentially fatal adverse reactions to thionamide medications. Their presentations are relatively sudden in onset and unpredictable. Monitoring of leukocyte counts and liver function test results is not useful as a preventive measure. Patients who are prescribed antithyroid drugs should be cautioned about manifestations of these adverse reactions and should be instructed to discontinue treatment and to seek medical attention if they develop a high fever, pharyngitis, jaundice, or abdominal pain.

Radioactive Iodine

The selective uptake and concentration of iodide in thyrocytes permits the use of radioactive iodine to treat hyperthyroidism. Once it is concentrated in the gland after oral administration, ^{131}I emits β particles that cause localized destruction of thyroid tissue, effectively controlling hyperthyroidism. A dose of ^{131}I can be calculated on the basis of the fractional uptake of radioiodine, but the outcome of dosimetry has not been shown to be superior to administration of 10 mCi. Patients can be treated on an outpatient basis with precautions to prevent exposure of others. Approximately three quarters of patients will be cured with a single dose of radioiodine.

The principal side effect of radioactive iodine therapy is postablative hypothyroidism, which develops in most individuals receiving treatment for Graves' disease and a lesser proportion of patients treated for toxic nodular goiter. Lifelong monitoring of thyroid function is important, as patients who initially remain euthyroid after treatment continue to develop postablative hypothyroidism at a rate of 3% per year. Another less common complication is a transient exacerbation of thyrotoxicosis that occurs in one quarter of patients during the first month after treatment as a result of radiation thyroiditis. Long-term follow-up studies have shown that radioiodine-treated patients with Graves' disease do not have any greater risk of thyroid cancer or other malignant neoplasms. However, hyperthyroid children and adolescents treated with radioactive iodine are more likely to develop benign nodules. Among hyperthyroid women treated with radioiodine, incidences of infertility, spontaneous abortion, and children with birth defects are not increased. Diagnostic or therapeutic radioactive iodine is contraindicated in women during pregnancy, and treated women should avoid pregnancy until euthyroidism has been confirmed 3 to 6 months after administration of a dose.

Other Drugs

A saturated solution of potassium iodide (SSKI) or Lugol's solution transiently inhibits the synthesis and release of thyroid hormone from the gland. It may be used to accelerate recovery after radioactive iodine treatment, to prepare patients for thyroidectomy, and to augment other treatments used to control severe thyrotoxicosis (see later). Iodinated radiocontrast agents inhibit release of thyroid hormone while blocking peripheral conversion of T_4 to T_3. Lithium carbonate also inhibits glandular release of thyroid hormone. These agents are rarely used in combination with thionamides to treat patients with severe thyrotoxicosis. They may also help provide temporary control of hyperthyroidism when severe allergies preclude continued use of thionamides. Cholestyramine can be used to bind thyroid hormone in the gut to interrupt enterohepatic circulation in cases of suspected exogenous thyroid hormone intoxication.

Surgical Therapy

Surgery has a limited role in treatment of hyperthyroid patients because of its potential for injury to the adjacent recurrent laryngeal nerves and parathyroid glands. Resection of a toxic adenoma by lobectomy is curative and often preserves sufficient normal thyroid tissue for euthyroidism to be maintained. Consequently, it is often recommended for treatment of younger individuals. Toxic multinodular goiters causing compressive symptoms or cosmetic disfigurement may be appropriately managed with surgical resection. Although surgery is seldom recommended for the treatment of hyperthyroid Graves' disease, it may be appropriate when other modalities are contraindicated, or when a thyroid nodule thought to be malignant or hyperparathyroidism also requires surgical intervention.

Specific Treatment Scenarios

Pregnancy

Pregnant patients with hyperthyroidism present special challenges. Diagnosis requires careful assessment of symptoms, especially heat intolerance, palpitation, and vomiting, which also occur during normal pregnancy. The serum total T_4 level is elevated because of increased TBG, and the TSH level can be suppressed in the first trimester as a result of hCG-mediated thyroid stimulation. Diagnostic radioiodine studies are contraindicated. After diagnostic confirmation, hyperthyroidism must be treated because it is associated with an increased risk of spontaneous abortion, premature labor, low birthweight, and toxemia. β-Blockers should be used only transiently to treat severe symptoms. Propylthiouracil is the preferred thionamide for treatment of Graves' disease during pregnancy because it is less likely to cross the placenta. Treatment with methimazole during pregnancy may be associated with aplasia cutis. Because Graves' disease often remits later in pregnancy, antithyroid drug dose requirements decline as gestation progresses. Measurement of maternal thyroid-stimulating immunoglobulin levels can help predict the risk of an infant's developing neonatal Graves' disease.

Mild Hyperthroidism

Patients with mild hyperthyroidism may have symptoms that justify treatment. In patients with TSH levels suppressed to less than 0.1 mIU/L, there may be skeletal and cardiac consequences of even mild thyroid hormone excess. Atrial fibrillation occurs more commonly in mildly hyperthyroid patients aged 60 years and older. Osteoporosis can be associated with chronic mild hyperthyroidism, particularly in postmenopausal women. It is less clear, however, that asymptomatic patients with modestly suppressed TSH levels (e.g., 0.1 to 0.5 mIU/L) require anything more than periodic monitoring.

Thyrotoxic Crisis

Thyrotoxic crisis, also known as thyroid storm, is a potentially life-threatening syndrome that is usually the end result of severe and

Rx

sustained thyrotoxicosis. It can affect patients with other medical conditions that render them vulnerable to the cardiovascular, neuropsychiatric, and gastrointestinal effects of exposure to excessive amounts of thyroid hormone. Thyrotoxic crisis typically develops in the setting of inadequately treated Graves' disease and may be precipitated by intercurrent illness, surgery, or treatment with radioactive iodine. Affected individuals present with fever, atrial tachyarrhythmias, congestive heart failure, nausea and vomiting, diarrhea, and seizures. Mental status changes can include agitation, delirium, psychosis, and coma. Prompt recognition and treatment in a monitored setting is crucial. A multifaceted treatment regimen should incorporate antipyretics, β-blockers, thionamides, iodinated contrast agents, and glucocorticoids as well as aggressive evaluation and management of underlying medical problems.

THYROIDITIS

Subacute (de Quervain's) Thyroiditis

Pathobiology

Transient thyrotoxicosis results from uncontrolled leakage of thyroid hormone from the inflamed gland. After 2 to 8 weeks, when the supply of stored hormone is exhausted, thyrotoxicosis resolves spontaneously. Hypothyroidism ensues as the gland's biosynthetic capabilities remain impaired. This is also transient, lasting approximately 1 month, with subsequent restoration of normal thyroid function in most patients.

Clinical Manifestations

Subacute thyroiditis is characterized by painful enlargement of the thyroid, systemic inflammatory symptoms, and transient thyrotoxicosis that is often followed by transient hypothyroidism. The histologic pattern shows inflammatory cell infiltrates that are believed to be the result of a viral infection. Many patients with subacute thyroiditis report antecedent upper respiratory infections.

Patients usually present with pain localized to the thyroid or radiating to the throat, ears, or jaw. Constitutional symptoms, including fever, chills, sweats, and malaise, are generally present. On occasion, these features may dominate the presentation. Examination of the thyroid typically reveals an exquisitely tender, modestly enlarged, and woody hard gland.

Diagnosis

Differential Diagnosis

The differential diagnosis of thyroid pain must be considered in the evaluation of patients presenting with pain and tenderness localized to the lower anterior neck. In addition to subacute thyroiditis, potential causes of thyroid pain include acute (suppurative) thyroiditis; hemorrhage into an existing thyroid nodule; and rapid growth of anaplastic thyroid cancer, diffusely infiltrating thyroid cancer, or thyroid lymphoma.

Laboratory Findings

Laboratory testing in patients with subacute thyroiditis reveals a profile of overt thyrotoxicosis. Elevated T_4 levels are usually proportionately higher than T_3 levels. Patients typically have an elevated erythrocyte sedimentation rate during the acute phase. The fractional uptake of radioiodine is typically less than 2% at 24 hours.

Treatment

Rx

High-dose aspirin or naproxen sodium can be used to treat thyroid pain and systemic inflammatory symptoms. Patients who fail to respond may require glucocorticoid therapy, but it must be tapered over several weeks or patients will relapse, prolonging the overall course of their illness. Symptoms ascribed to transient thyrotoxicosis may respond to treatment with a β-blocker continued for a limited course of 1 to 3 weeks. Patients who progress to symptomatic hypothyroidism may then need short-term thyroxine replacement therapy, but most will not require long-term thyroid hormone replacement.

Lymphocytic (Postpartum, Painless, Silent) Thyroiditis

Epidemiology

Lymphocytic thyroiditis occurs most commonly in postpartum women, affecting as many as 6% of women 2 to 12 months after delivery or termination. Rarely, this condition occurs in non-postpartum women or in men. Predisposing factors include a history of previous episodes of postpartum thyroiditis, type 1 diabetes mellitus, and circulating antithyroid autoantibodies.

Pathobiology

This painless inflammation of the thyroid gland can cause transient thyrotoxicosis followed by transient or persistent hypothyroidism. These phases of thyroid dysfunction typically last 2 to 8 weeks. This condition is believed to reflect transient autoimmunity.

Diagnosis

The diagnosis of lymphocytic thyroiditis is often overlooked when nonspecific symptoms of thyrotoxicosis (e.g., weight loss, insomnia, and anxiety) or hypothyroidism (e.g., fatigue and depression) are misinterpreted as common postpartum complaints. The thyroid gland is nontender and either normal in size or modestly enlarged. Once it is considered, a diagnosis of lymphocytic thyroiditis can be readily confirmed or excluded by laboratory testing, which will reveal a suppressed TSH level during phases of thyrotoxicosis and an elevated TSH level during phases of hypothyroidism. This condition must be distinguished from Graves' disease, which can also present in the same timeframe after delivery. Relative degrees of T_4 and T_3 elevation can sometimes provide a clue as to which condition is present; lymphocytic thyroiditis is typically characterized by predominant increases in T_4 levels. Fractional uptake of radioiodine is either absent or very low in the setting of lymphocytic thyroiditis but increased in active Graves' disease, thus providing a useful diagnostic test.

Treatment

Rx

Lymphocytic thyroiditis can sometimes be managed with reassurance and observation alone. Symptomatic thyrotoxicosis can be treated with a limited course of β-blocker therapy. Overt hypothyroidism may require transient thyroxine replacement.

Prognosis

Whereas most affected patients eventually return to a euthyroid state, 25% develop persistent hypothyroidism due to classic autoimmune thyroiditis.

Acute (Suppurative) Thyroiditis

Infection of the thyroid gland is a rare condition that typically presents with severe thyroid pain, fever, and other systemic manifestations of infection. Bacterial infection of thyroid tissue can be the result of direct spread of gram-positive or gram-negative pathogens through fistulas communicating with the piriform sinus or the skin. Hematogenous spread of bacterial, mycobacterial, fungal, or parasitic organisms, especially *Pneumocystis carinii,* can occur in immunocompromised individuals. On examination, affected patients are typically febrile with asymmetrical swelling of a thyroid that is tender, warm, and fluctuant to firm in consistency beneath erythematous skin. Ultrasonography may reveal an abscess that can be aspirated to identify a pathogen. Patients with suppurative thyroiditis require prompt treatment with appropriate antibiotics. Surgical drainage of abscesses may be required.

Other Forms of Thyroiditis

Certain drugs can cause thyroid gland inflammation. Amiodarone can produce a painless thyroiditis associated with thyrotoxicosis. Whenever possible, this should be distinguished from the iodine-induced form of thyrotoxicosis that can also be associated with amiodarone therapy. The former is optimally treated with glucocorticoid therapy, whereas the latter is managed with antithyroid drugs. Interferon alfa can provoke a painless thyroiditis associated with transient thyrotoxicosis similar to lymphocytic thyroiditis. This must be differentiated from interferon alfa–induced Graves' disease, as the former is managed with β-blockers and the latter with antithyroid drugs.

Riedel's thyroiditis or struma is characterized by fibrotic replacement of the thyroid with adherence and infiltration of adjacent structures that causes local compressive symptoms. In this idiopathic condition, the thyroid is substantially enlarged, hardened, and fixed. Affected patients may also develop mediastinal and retroperitoneal fibrosis, sclerosing cholangitis, or orbital pseudotumor. Diagnosis requires open biopsy. Surgical excision is difficult or impossible. Glucocorticoid therapy and tamoxifen therapy have been anecdotally reported to be effective.

GOITER

Definition

Goiters can be classified as diffuse or nodular, nontoxic or toxic (i.e., associated with thyroid hormone overproduction), and benign or malignant. Thyroid enlargement can be the result of thyrocyte proliferation stimulated by circulating factors (e.g., TSH and thyroid-stimulating immunoglobulins), infiltration of the gland by inflammatory or malignant cells, or benign or malignant neoplastic changes arising within the gland itself. In a patient with a goiter, three potential clinical issues must be considered: local compressive or cosmetic problems, gland hyperfunction or hypofunction, and potential malignancy.

Epidemiology

Dietary iodine deficiency represents the most common cause of endemic goiter worldwide. It is encountered in the United States only among immigrants from iodine-deficient regions. Younger patients present with diffuse or simple goiters that shrink in response to adequate iodine supplementation. In older individuals, iodine-deficient goiters typically become multinodular and do not decrease in size with iodine repletion. Excessive iodine exposure can provoke thyrotoxicosis in these patients.

Pathobiology

Benign multinodular goiter and its histologic correlate, benign adenomatous hyperplasia, can be the result of genetic defects that lead to dyshormonogenesis including mutations in the thyroglobulin, thyroid peroxidase, and pendrin genes. Similarly, exposure to goitrogenic substances in foodstuffs, water, or drugs (e.g., lithium carbonate) that inhibit normal steps in thyroid hormone synthesis can lead to goiter. In most patients with benign nodular goiter, the underlying cause is unknown.

Autoimmune thyroiditis typically produces a modest goiter as a result of glandular infiltration with lymphocytes, inflammatory changes in thyrocytes, and fibrosis. The hypothyroid state caused by autoimmune thyroiditis results in increased TSH that further stimulates thyroid enlargement. Graves' disease is also characterized by diffuse thyroid enlargement due to the action of thyroid-stimulating immunoglobulins. Other forms of thyroiditis can also present with goitrous enlargement of the thyroid gland, including subacute, lymphocytic, and acute (suppurative) thyroiditis.

Malignant neoplasms that involve the gland diffusely, including thyroid lymphoma and infiltrative papillary, medullary, and anaplastic thyroid cancer, may present as rapidly enlarging goiters. Affected patients often experience local pain and symptoms related to tumor expansion and invasion.

Diagnosis

Clinical Examination

The first step in evaluating a suspected goiter is to confirm whether the observed swelling represents enlargement of the thyroid. Redundant skin and subcutaneous fat in the lower anterior neck can be mistaken for an enlarged thyroid. These findings can usually be distinguished from true thyroid enlargement by palpating a normal thyroid beneath the misleading soft tissue and by observing that the fullness does not rise and fall with deglutition. Ultrasonography may help resolve uncertainty.

A patient's history can provide important clues to the underlying cause. A childhood medical and social history may confirm previous iodine deficiency. Symptoms of hypothyroidism may suggest autoimmune thyroiditis, whereas clinical evidence of thyrotoxicosis may suggest Graves' disease or toxic multinodular goiter. Clinical findings may lead to recognition of one of the various forms of thyroiditis (e.g., pain in subacute thyroiditis or postpartum status in lymphocytic thyroiditis). Symptoms suggesting invasion of adjacent structures may raise concern for malignant disease or Riedel's thyroiditis.

Careful examination of the thyroid is informative. Diffuse enlargement favors one of the forms of thyroiditis, Graves' disease, or a diffusely infiltrating malignant neoplasm. Nodular enlargement is more likely to reflect a benign multinodular goiter or malignant neoplasm. The precise size of the gland should be documented. Dysphonia, tracheal deviation, cervical lymphadenopathy, and venous engorgement in the neck should be noted. Dynamic obstruction of the thoracic outlet may be revealed by having the patient touch the hands together above the head (Pemberton's maneuver) while checking for signs of facial plethora and cervical venous distention.

Laboratory Findings

A TSH level will determine whether there is primary hypothyroidism or thyrotoxicosis. Elevated antithyroid peroxidase antibody titers can confirm suspected autoimmune thyroiditis. In asymptomatic patients with a modest diffuse goiter, no further evaluation may be indicated. Other blood tests (e.g., erythrocyte sedimentation rate for subacute thyroiditis or calcitonin for medullary thyroid cancer) can be useful when clinical clues suggest specific diagnoses.

Imaging

Cervical ultrasonography is usually the best imaging technique to define the character and extent of a goiter limited to the neck. It can help determine if a goiter is diffuse or nodular, if the thyroid is impinging on other cervical structures, and if lymphadenopathy is present. When a goiter extends posteriorly or beneath the sternal notch into the thorax, CT or MRI scanning may be required. Administration of iodine-containing radiocontrast dye should be avoided in the evaluation of patients with goiters because the stable iodide load may interfere with subsequent radioiodine imaging or therapy. Thyroid uptake studies may help define whether quantitative tracer uptake is subnormal or supranormal. Radioiodine scanning can help determine if a superior mediastinal mass is thyroid tissue. Barium swallow radiographs with fixed-diameter markers and pulmonary function testing with flow-volume loops can help determine if symptoms are directly related to compression of the esophagus or trachea. Laryngoscopy is useful to evaluate vocal cord function in patients with potential recurrent laryngeal nerve involvement.

Treatment

Rx

Once thyroid dysfunction and malignant disease have been excluded, asymptomatic patients with goiters can be observed conservatively with periodic clinical assessment. Ultrasonography can be relied on as a reproducible technique for monitoring the size of an enlarged thyroid gland. Thyroxine therapy to suppress TSH levels is effective in shrinking goiters only in a minority of patients. Furthermore, chronic thyroid hormone treatment carries with it risks of symptomatic thyrotoxicosis, atrial fibrillation, and bone mineral loss.

Patients with benign multinodular goiters causing local compressive symptoms or cosmetic concerns may be treated with surgery or radioactive iodine therapy. Surgery is often preferred when a patient has substantial gland enlargement causing compressive complications, especially when there is substernal extension of the goiter

Rx

or acute obstructive symptoms. When surgery may be contraindicated by a patient's health status, radioactive iodine therapy has been shown to reduce goiter size by an average of 50% over a period of 12 to 24 months.

THYROID NODULES

Epidemiology

Thyroid nodules are common, being detected by palpation in 6% of women and 2% of men. Furthermore, contemporary high-resolution ultrasonography identifies thyroid nodules in as many as 50% of all adults. Although the majority of these represent small benign adenomatoid nodules or cysts, 5 to 10% of thyroid nodules are malignant. Less commonly, thyroid nodules are clinical problems by virtue of being hyperfunctioning or by causing local compressive symptoms or cosmetic dissatisfaction.

Diagnosis

Thyroid nodules are usually noted by the patient or physician in the absence of any other complaints. It is also common for thyroid nodules to be incidentally detected on imaging procedures, such as carotid ultrasonography and cervical spine CT or MRI scans. Symptoms suggesting compression or invasion of adjacent tissues suggest that a nodule may be malignant. These include pain in the lower anterior neck, cough or dyspnea due to tracheal compression, hemoptysis due to tracheal invasion, dysphonia due to recurrent laryngeal nerve encasement, and dysphagia or odynophagia due to esophageal compression. Certain other symptoms and signs lead to consideration of specific underlying conditions. A toxic adenoma should be suspected in a patient with a thyroid nodule who has classic clinical manifestations of thyrotoxicosis. Hypothyroid symptoms and signs suggest the possibility of autoimmune thyroiditis with asymmetrical thyroid enlargement. Hypercalcitonemia associated with the metastatic spread of medullary thyroid cancer can cause pruritus, flushing, and diarrhea. Clinical assessment should also check for symptoms and signs related to common sites of thyroid cancer metastasis, such as chest pain, dyspnea, bone pain, and neurologic findings. Thyroid nodules rarely can be due to metastasis from other primary malignant neoplasms, including kidney, colon, and breast cancer.

History

Special predisposition to thyroid cancer is suggested by a personal history of therapeutic neck irradiation in childhood. Family history can be informative if relatives have had medullary or papillary thyroid cancers, which are familial in 50% and 10% of cases, respectively. The possibility of medullary thyroid cancer should also be considered when there is a personal or family history of clinical problems associated with the multiple endocrine neoplasia type 2 (MEN 2) syndrome, including hyperparathyroidism and pheochromocytoma.

Physical Examination

Physical examination of the thyroid nodule should seek to define its size, consistency, surface texture, mobility, and tenderness. The presence of malignant disease is suggested by fixation and ipsilateral regional adenopathy or vocal cord paresis. Multinodularity of the gland may reflect benign nodular goiter, but it is not sufficiently reassuring to avoid further diagnostic testing. This is particularly true for a so-called dominant nodule, which is larger, enlarging faster, or more symptomatic than others present in the thyroid.

Laboratory Findings

Routine laboratory testing includes measurement of TSH levels to identify patients with hyperthyroidism or hypothyroidism. When the TSH level is low or undetectable, the possibility of a benign autonomously functioning toxic adenoma can be pursued with radionuclide thyroid scanning. If an elevated TSH level indicates primary hypothyroidism, antithyroid peroxidase antibody titers should be measured to confirm whether the patient has autoimmune thyroiditis. Ultrasonography can often distinguish asymmetrical enlargement caused by autoimmune thyroiditis from a discrete encapsulated nodule. Calcitonin levels should be measured in patients with a known or suspected family history of MEN 2 or familial medullary thyroid cancer. Serum thyroglobulin measurement is not helpful in distinguishing benign from malignant thyroid abnormalities as it can be elevated in both settings.

Imaging

Cervical ultrasonography is not required before biopsy, but it can help confirm that a mass is within the thyroid, accurately define its size, classify it as cystic or solid, and determine whether additional nodules are present. Ultrasonography occasionally reveals other suspicious findings, such as fine calcifications, irregular nodule borders, and cervical adenopathy.

Radionuclide scanning with radioiodine or technetium pertechnetate is helpful only in certain cases. In patients with a thyroid nodule and a suppressed TSH level, scanning can confirm that the nodule is hyperfunctioning or "hot," in which case biopsy is usually not required. CT, MRI, and PET imaging are generally unnecessary in the evaluation of patients with thyroid nodules. Furthermore, administration of iodinated radiocontrast dye can interfere with the subsequent management of patients who prove to have thyroid cancer.

Invasive Evaluation

Fine-Needle Aspiration Biopsy

Fine-needle aspiration biopsy is the most accurate test to exclude or confirm malignant disease in patients who have a nodule and a normal TSH level (Fig. 244–4). Most solid nodules and complex cysts larger than 1.0 to 1.5 cm in diameter should be sampled. Although aspiration can be directed by palpation alone when a nodule is readily definable, ultrasonography provides more certain guidance for sampling of poorly localized lesions, often revealing additional nodules that should be assessed.

The cytologic assessment of aspirated material must first confirm that there is adequate material for assessment (e.g., six clumps of 10 cells on two slides). Biopsies with inadequate specimens, which are more common in cystic lesions, must be repeated. Ultrasonographic guidance and on-site preliminary cytologic assessment can improve the yield of biopsy. When adequate cytologic material is obtained, a sampled nodule can be categorized as benign, malignant, or indeterminate (suspicious).

Benign adenomatoid nodules typically yield samples containing clusters of normal-appearing follicular epithelial cells with colloid. Pure colloid cysts may have scant epithelium. These benign cytologic categories are highly accurate, with a false-negative rate of less than 3%, and surgical resection is not required. In most cases, conservative observation based on yearly clinical or sonographic reassessment can be recommended. Further enlargement during observation should prompt repeated biopsy. If a nodule is determined to be benign, a trial of thyroxine therapy to suppress the TSH level to the low but detectable range (e.g., 0.1 to 0.5 mIU/L) can be considered, although this approach is likely to shrink nodules in less than 50% of cases. Surgical resection should be considered if a cytologically benign nodule continues to grow, causing compressive symptoms or cosmetic disfigurement.

Cytologic material categorized as malignant typically contains abundant epithelial cells with atypical nuclear features and scant or absent colloid. This is also a highly reliable finding, with 95% of such lesions found to be thyroid cancers on subsequent resection. Consequently, bilateral thyroidectomy is indicated in patients without contraindication to operation.

One in five biopsies yields adequate but diagnostically indeterminate cytologic material. Such uncertain findings include abundant follicular or Hürthle cells in microfollicles with little or no colloid and minor degrees of nuclear atypia potentially indicative of papillary cancer. Although the majority of such indeterminate nodules are benign follicular adenomas, up to 20% represent thyroid carcinomas. Consequently, surgery is advisable in most otherwise healthy patients with nodules that fall within this diagnostic category. Unilateral thyroid lobectomy has the advantage of a lower incidence of surgical complications and postoperative hypothyroidism when the lesion is benign but necessitates a subsequent completion thyroidectomy for most patients who prove to have cancer. For patients with no clinical features of malignancy, particularly women in or beyond middle life with multinodular glands in whom the

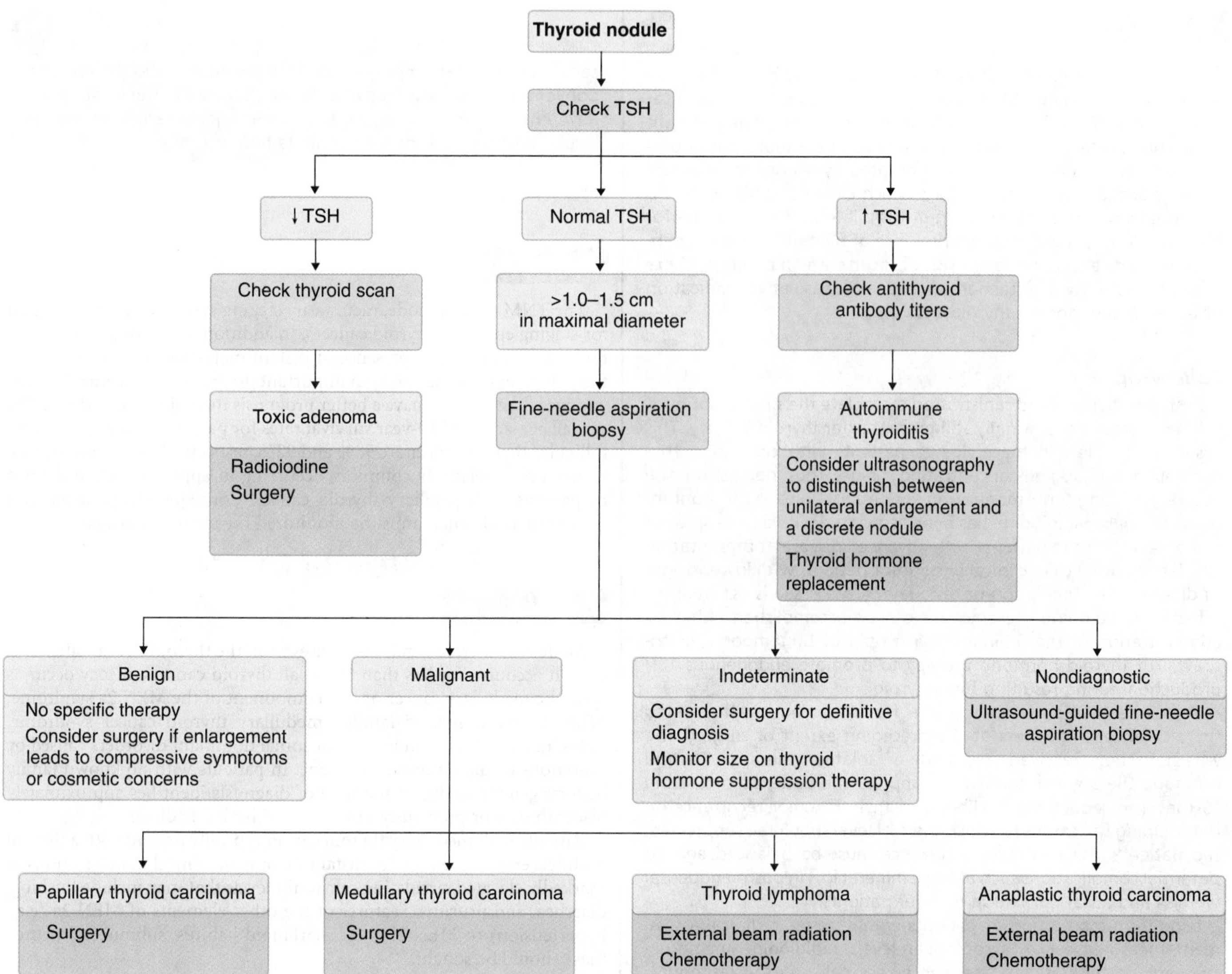

FIGURE 244–4 • Evaluation of a thyroid nodule.

prevalence of malignancy is 5% or less, vigilant observation with serial sonography is an alternative.

THYROID CANCER

Cancers of the thyroid gland have a spectrum of behavior that ranges from incidentally detected and clinically inconsequential microcarcinomas to aggressive and virtually untreatable anaplastic malignant neoplasms. Approximately 25,000 new cases are diagnosed annually in the United States. Thyroid cancer is three times more common in women. When it is diagnosed early, treatment of most thyroid cancer types is effective. There are an estimated 350,000 U.S. thyroid cancer survivors, who require lifelong follow-up for recurrence. Most thyroid cancers present as thyroid nodules that are either asymptomatic or associated with local cervical symptoms or adenopathy. Less often, thyroid cancers first present with manifestations of metastatic disease, such as a pulmonary mass or bone pain.

Epithelial (Papillary and Follicular) Thyroid Carcinomas

Papillary and follicular thyroid cancers arise from follicular epithelium and often retain responsiveness to TSH, produce thyroglobulin, and concentrate iodide. They are distinguished by their histopathologic appearances and characteristic patterns of progression. Hürthle cell carcinoma of the thyroid is composed of thyrocytes with abundant cytoplasm and behaves like a follicular thyroid cancer, although it typically does not retain iodine-concentrating ability.

Epidemiology

Papillary thyroid carcinoma is the most common form of thyroid cancer, representing more than 80% of cases. Whereas the mean age at diagnosis is 45 years, papillary thyroid carcinoma does occur in children and increases in incidence with age.

Pathobiology

Irradiation of the thyroid gland in childhood is a risk factor, as evidenced by the epidemics of thyroid cancer that followed both external beam radiotherapy for benign childhood conditions and radioiodine exposure after nuclear incidents. A substantial body of evidence now implicates RET/PTC and B-Raf kinase gene mutations that activate the MAP kinase signaling pathway in the pathogenesis of papillary thyroid cancer. Most papillary thyroid carcinomas are slow growing and either remain confined to the gland or metastasize to a few cervical lymph nodes. Papillary microcarcinomas are a common incidental pathologic finding in 5% of thyroid glands excised for other reasons. Some papillary thyroid carcinomas are more aggressive, with extension into adjacent tissues, extensive nodal involvement, and distant metastatic spread, most commonly to the lungs. This is more common in older patients.

Follicular and Hürthle cell thyroid carcinomas account for 10% of all thyroid cancers. When these tumors show histologic evidence of only invading the tumor capsule, they are termed minimally invasive and behave like papillary thyroid carcinomas. However, follicular and Hürthle cell carcinomas with vascular invasion are more likely to be associated with distant metastatic disease, which most commonly involves the lungs and skeleton.

Treatment

Rx

Treatment of epithelial thyroid cancer entails surgery, often followed by radioiodine ablation of remnant thyroid tissue. Total or nearly total thyroidectomy with selective central compartment lymph node resection is usually the appropriate initial surgical procedure. Thyroid surgery can be complicated by hypoparathyroidism or recurrent laryngeal nerve injury, which causes hoarseness if it is unilateral and airway obstruction if it is bilateral. The rationale for bilateral surgery is the frequent presence of bilateral disease in papillary thyroid cancer and lower risk of recurrence. In addition, there is greater accuracy in detection of residual disease after eradication of all remaining normal thyroid tissue.

Follow-up

Postoperatively, ^{131}I administration can ablate the small amount of normal thyroid tissue usually still present after thyroid surgery. This tissue, if it is left in place, leaves patients with circulating thyroglobulin and iodine-concentrating tissue, thus decreasing the accuracy of long-term monitoring for residual disease. In nonrandomized trials, radioiodine has been associated with a lower rate of tumor recurrence in patients with advanced disease at presentation (see later) but no clear clinical benefit for patients with lower stages of disease. TSH stimulation of residual thyroid tissue is essential for effective radioiodine therapy. This can be accomplished either by administration of recombinant thyrotropin or by temporary withdrawal of thyroid hormone therapy to promote endogenous TSH production during resulting hypothyroidism.

Thyroxine therapy is appropriate for all patients with treated thyroid cancer, regardless of the preceding extent of surgery and whether they received radioiodine ablative therapy. Thyroid hormone therapy is intended to suppress the patient's circulating TSH level to reduce the likelihood of thyroid tumor recurrence. In determining the extent to which the TSH level should be suppressed, the patient's risk of cancer recurrence must be balanced against potential complications such as bone mineral loss in postmenopausal women and atrial fibrillation in older patients.

Long-term monitoring of patients entails periodic clinical assessment, measurement of thyroglobulin levels, radioiodine imaging in the early postoperative phase, and occasional use of ultrasonography. Clinically, patients should be assessed for local neck symptoms or recurrent cervical masses as well as for optimization of thyroid hormone therapy. For patients with treated epithelial thyroid cancers, thyroglobulin is a tumor marker that is more specific if all remaining normal thyroid tissue has been ablated. For patients with undetectable thyroglobulin levels on TSH-suppressive thyroid hormone therapy, thyroglobulin measurement after recombinant TSH stimulation can sometimes reveal residual disease. Radioiodine scanning after TSH stimulation can be helpful in patients who have previously undergone radioiodine ablation, but once iodine imaging is normal, it offers little or no advantage over measurement of stimulated thyroglobulin levels. This is particularly true in recurrent papillary thyroid cancers, which often lose the ability to concentrate iodine. Unfortunately, thyroglobulin testing is impossible in the 20% of patients who have circulating thyroglobulin autoantibodies that interfere with thyroglobulin immunoassays. Because most epithelial thyroid cancer recurrences are in cervical nodes or soft tissues, ultrasonography is useful in postoperative monitoring, particularly for patients who presented with extensive cervical disease or who have persistent detectable serum thyroglobulin. CT scanning of the chest should be employed to detect intrathoracic disease in patients whose findings suggest recurrence outside the neck. In patients with substantial detectable thyroglobulin levels (e.g., >10 ng/dL) and normal findings on standard imaging studies, PET scanning can identify sites of residual disease in more than 50% of patients.

Localization of recurrent cervical disease is usually an indication for modified lateral neck dissection. Distant and nonresectable metastases that are iodine avid, as occur more commonly in patients with invasive follicular thyroid cancer, can be treated with repeated doses of ^{131}I. Symptomatic hilar node and bone metastases can be treated palliatively with external beam radiation therapy. Surgery can sometimes be employed for isolated metastatic disease sites. Conventional chemotherapy has limited efficacy in the treatment of differentiated thyroid cancer, but newer agents targeting the molecular pathogenesis of these tumors hold promise.

Prognosis

The TNM (tumor, node, metastasis) staging system is commonly used for staging epithelial thyroid cancers. In addition to tumor size, extent of node involvement, and presence of distant metastatic disease, the age of the patient at presentation is an important predictor of outcome. Patients younger than 45 years have a better prognosis than older individuals. The overall age-adjusted 10-year survival rates for patients with papillary and follicular thyroid cancer are 98% and 92%, respectively. However, disease recurrence is relatively common, occurring in approximately one third of patients with papillary thyroid cancer. Consequently, patients with treated thyroid cancer must be monitored for recurrent disease.

Medullary Thyroid Carcinoma

Pathobiology

Medullary thyroid carcinoma arises from the thyroid's parafollicular C cells. It accounts for less than 5% of all thyroid cancers. It may occur as sporadic medullary cancer or as a component of the MEN 2a syndrome, MEN 2b syndrome, or familial medullary thyroid cancer syndrome. These inherited syndromes are autosomal dominant disorders caused by mutations of the *ret* proto-oncogene. In patients with no known family history, genetic testing at the time of diagnosis identifies approximately 6% with new or previously unrecognized heritable disease.

Patients with medullary thyroid cancer typically present with a thyroid nodule, cervical adenopathy, distant disease, or clinical manifestations of markedly elevated circulating calcitonin levels that may include flushing, diarrhea, and pruritus. Features of the other elements of MEN 2a (e.g., hypertension) or MEN 2b (e.g., marfanoid habitus, submucosal neuromas) should be sought.

Treatment

Rx

Initial treatment is surgical resection of the thyroid and regional lymph nodes, which are involved in 50% of affected patients at the time of diagnosis. The high risk of extrathyroidal disease and limited availability of secondary treatment options mandate aggressive initial surgery, including central neck compartment dissection, unilateral or bilateral modified neck dissection, and even superior mediastinal exploration to extirpate suspicious lymphadenopathy. The risk for development of medullary thyroid carcinoma has been determined to be so high in children with inherited *ret* proto-oncogene mutations that prophylactic thyroidectomy is advisable during childhood. Distant metastases involving the liver are present in a small minority of patients and can often be established by laparoscopically guided liver biopsy.

Follow-up

Because medullary thyroid carcinoma cells produce calcitonin and carcinoembryonic antigen, these tumor markers can be measured serially to monitor patients for recurrence and progression of disease. Surgery can be repeated to treat significant cervical and mediastinal node disease. External beam radiation therapy has been used for nonresectable cervical disease, but its value has not been established in controlled trials. Radioiodine therapy is ineffective, and thyroid hormone therapy is intended only to maintain euthyroidism as TSH suppression is not required. Somatostatin analogues can be used to control the diarrhea and flushing associated with hypercalcitonemia.

Anaplastic Thyroid Carcinoma

Anaplastic thyroid carcinoma is a rare histologically undifferentiated and clinically aggressive malignant neoplasm that typically arises in older patients, one fourth of whom present with evidence of a preceding or concurrent differentiated type of thyroid cancer. Affected patients present with a rapidly enlarging mass in the anterior or lateral neck associated with pain, tenderness, and compressive symptoms including dysphagia, dysphonia, and stridorous dyspnea. Fine-needle aspiration biopsy of the mass usually yields large pleomorphic undifferentiated cells, but open surgical biopsy is sometimes required to confirm the diagnosis.

Most cases are unresectable at presentation because of invasion of cervical structures. Surgery is not curative and should aim to secure the patient's airway. A percutaneous gastrostomy tube is often placed to ensure adequate nutrition in the face of esophageal impingement. Conventional therapy consisting of combined external beam radiation therapy and chemotherapy with doxorubicin with or without cisplatin produces an initial response in 25% of patients. Those with disease limited to the neck may have extended survival, but almost all patients relapse within a few months and succumb to their disease, with median survival rates ranging from 3 to 7 months. Current research initiatives are focused on the use of targeted antiangiogenic agents to treat unresponsive disease.

Thyroid Lymphoma

Lymphoma rarely arises in the thyroid gland, typically presenting in older persons as a rapidly enlarging and painful diffuse goiter. Patients often have a preceding history of autoimmune thyroiditis. The diagnosis is further suspected when fine-needle aspiration biopsy yields abundant lymphocytes without other cellular features of autoimmune thyroiditis. Immunohistochemical staining and flow cytometry of sampled material can serve to characterize a monoclonal lymphocyte population. Surgical biopsy is sometimes required to establish the diagnosis. In 50% of cases, lymphoma is primary to the thyroid gland, usually an intermediate-grade non-Hodgkin's type lymphoma.

Surgical resection of the thyroid is not indicated, but elective tracheostomy should be considered as a prophylactic measure when tracheal compression is imminent. Most patients respond to treatment with combined external beam radiation therapy and chemotherapy. Disease-free survival rates vary with the disease stage at diagnosis and the initial response to combination therapy.

SUGGESTED READINGS

AACE/AME Task Force on Thyroid Nodules: American Association of Clinical Endocrinologists and Associazione Medici Endocrinologi medical guidelines for clinical practice for the diagnosis and management of thyroid nodules. Endocr Pract 2006;12:63–102. *Guidelines for the treatment and management of thyroid nodules.*

Alexander EK, Hurwitz S, Heering JP, et al: Natural history of benign solid and cystic thyroid nodules. Ann Intern Med 2003;138:315–318. *Retrospective series demonstrating that changes in the size of identified thyroid nodules do not reliably predict malignancy.*

Caturegli P, Kimura H, Rocchi R, et al: Autoimmune thyroid diseases. Curr Opin Rheumatol 2007;19:44–48. *Review of recent advances in the pathophysiology of autoimmune thyroid disease.*

Escobar-Morreale HF, Botella-Carretero JI, Escobar del Rey F, et al: Treatment of hypothyroidism with combinations of levothyroxine plus liothyronine. J Clin Endocrinol Metab 2005;90:4946–4954. *Systematic review of randomized controlled trials evaluating impact of combination treatments incorporating variable fractions of thyroxine and liothyronine.*

Imaizumi M, Akahoshi M, Ichimaru S, et al: Risk for ischemic heart disease and all-cause mortality in subclinical hypothyroidism. J Clin Endocrinol Metab 2004;89:3365–3370. *Cross-sectional analysis identifying an association between mild hypothyroidism and coronary artery disease.*

Kinder BK: Well differentiated thyroid cancer. Curr Opin Oncol 2003;15:71–77. *Overview of standard and experimental therapies.*

O'Neill JP, O'Neill B, Condron C, et al: Anaplastic (undifferentiated) thyroid cancer: Improved insight and therapeutic strategy into a highly aggressive disease. J Laryngol Otol 2005;119:585–591. *Review detailing the limitations of available treatment options.*

Pearce EN: Diagnosis and management of thyrotoxicosis. BMJ 2006;332:1369–1373. *Clinical review.*

Peeters RP, Wouters PJ, Kaptein E, et al: Reduced activation and increased inactivation of thyroid hormone in tissues of critically ill patients. J Clin Endocrinol Metab 2003;88:3202–3211. *Study documenting changes in thyroid hormone levels and deiodinase expression in severe nonthyroidal illness.*

Wartofsky L: Myxedema coma. Endodrinol Metab Clin North Am 2006;35:687–698. *Comprehensive review.*

245 ADRENAL CORTEX

Lynnette K. Nieman

The adrenal glands are two small structures adjacent to the upper kidneys that weigh 6 to 8 g in adults (Fig. 245–1). Each contains a cortex, which makes steroid hormones, and a medulla, which produces catecholamines. Diseases of the adrenal medulla are discussed in Chapter 246. In the adrenal cortex, production of the three major classes of steroids occurs in specific zones: the outermost layer, the glomerulosa, produces mineralocorticoids, primarily aldosterone; the middle layer, the fasciculata, produces glucocorticoids, primarily cortisol; the innermost layer, the reticularis, produces adrenal "androgens," primarily dehydroepiandrosterone (DHEA) and its sulfated conjugate (DHEA-S) (Fig. 245–2). This zonation reflects the fact that although most of the steroidogenic synthetic machinery is present in all three zones, certain critical enzymes are restricted to specific zones, resulting in the ability or inability to synthesize end products.

FUNCTION

The actions and regulation of these steroid classes differ. Aldosterone and other steroids with mineralocorticoid activity act through the renal mineralocorticoid receptor to promote the reabsorption of sodium and the secretion of potassium. Its secretion is primarily stimulated by hyperkalemia and by angiotensin II (which itself is stimulated by hypovolemia and excess renin). These agents increase the production of aldosterone synthase and its activity in the glomerulosa to restore homeostasis through this feedback loop. Aldosterone is stimulated to a much smaller degree by adrenocorticotropic hormone (ACTH).

Cortisol and other glucocorticoids act through the glucocorticoid receptor type 2 and its isoforms to support physiologic integrity. The actions of this class of steroids are much broader, including effects on carbohydrate handling, lipid and calcium metabolism, and the immune and nervous systems. Cortisol production is regulated primarily by ACTH, which is secreted in a circadian rhythm so that cortisol levels are highest in the morning and fall to a nadir around midnight. Cortisol itself helps coordinate ACTH production through negative feedback and corticotropin-releasing hormone (CRH). Vasopressin secretion also plays a role in stimulating ACTH release.

Although DHEA and DHEA-S are the most abundant products of the adrenal gland, no specific receptor has been identified. They appear to exert their estrogenic and androgenic effects as prohormones, being converted to estrogens and testosterone in the peripheral tissues and activating the androgen and estrogen receptors. There is no clear physiologic regulator of DHEA synthesis, but its production declines with age.

DISORDERS OF ADRENAL FUNCTION

Most disorders of the adrenal cortex reflect overproduction or underproduction of the products of a single synthetic zone—cortisol, aldosterone, or testosterone or estrogen (Fig. 245–3). The congenital adrenal hyperplasias are an exception and present with both overproduction and underproduction. Abnormal secretion is suggested by clinical features of each disorder and reflected in plasma or urine levels of the relevant hormones or by the consequent increases or decreases in feedback systems, which form the basis of the biochemical diagnostic tests.

Glucocorticoid Excess: Cushing's Syndrome

Clinical Manifestations

Cushing's syndrome is a symptom complex that reflects excessive tissue exposure to cortisol. Classic features of Cushing's syndrome include weight gain, plethora, hypertension, and striae (Table 245–1). Not all patients have all features; the number and severity of features correlate roughly with the duration and severity of hypercortisolism. Because many of the signs and symptoms are nonspecific or common in the general population, the diagnosis may be confused with psychiatric disorders, polycystic ovary syndrome, the metabolic syndrome, simple obesity, fibromyalgia, or acute illness. However, because worsening hyper-

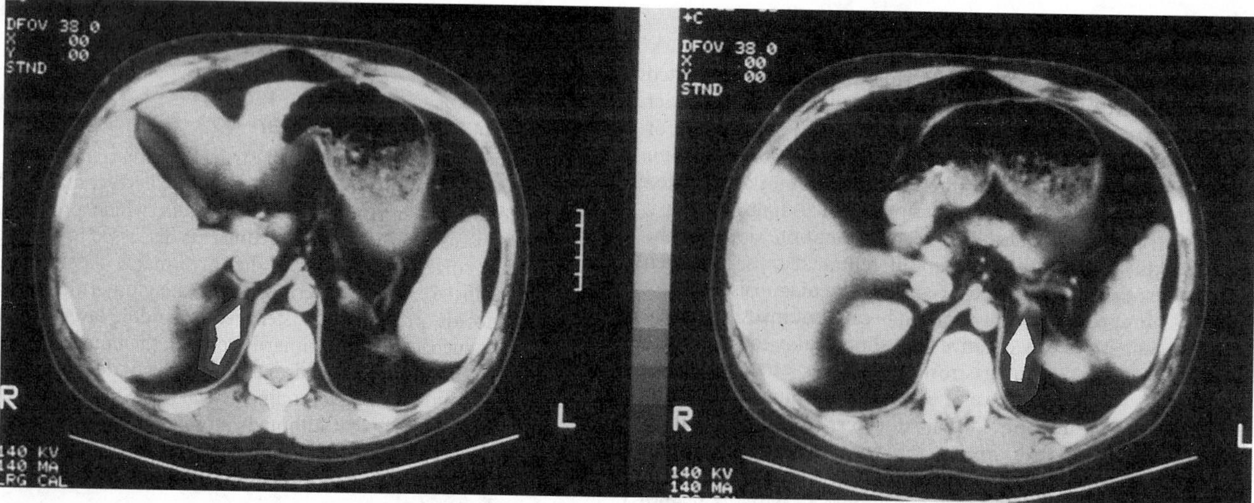

FIGURE 245–1 • Magnetic resonance images of the abdomen showing the position and relative size of the normal adrenal glands.

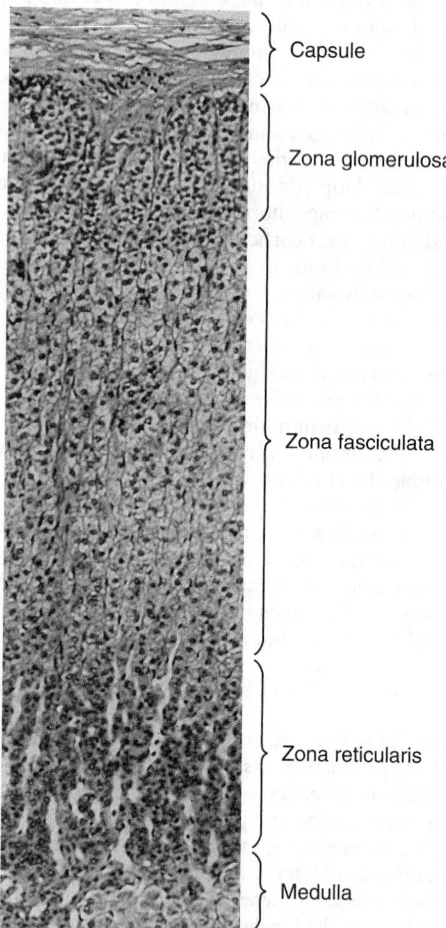

FIGURE 245–2 • Histologic section through a normal adult adrenal gland showing the progression, outside-in, of the zona glomerulosa, zona fasciculata, zona reticularis, and medulla.

cortisolism may precipitate hypertension, glucose intolerance, infections, psychiatric disturbances, impaired cognition, and hypercoagulability, it is important to identify this treatable disorder to prevent its associated morbidity and mortality.

Changes in mood and cognition are useful markers of hypercortisolism. These include irritability, crying, and restlessness; depressed mood; decreased libido; insomnia; anxiety; and decreased concentration and impaired memory (especially for recent events). Serial 7 subtractions and recall of three cities (or three objects) are useful bedside strategies to identify some of these changes.

Diagnosis

Clinical Examination

In the absence of a florid clinical presentation, biochemical tests are needed to establish the diagnosis. Cushing's syndrome screening is most likely to be positive in the presence of signs that are most typical of glucocorticoid excess, such as abnormal fat distribution in the supraclavicular and temporal fossae, proximal muscle weakness, wide (>1 cm) purple striae, and new irritability, decreased cognition, and decreased short-term memory. Testing is indicated when clinical features have progressed over time. For example, oligomenorrhea is more suggestive of Cushing's syndrome if a woman had previously regular menses.

Laboratory Findings

Urine free cortisol excretion during 24 hours is a good screening test. Specific, structurally based assay techniques such as high-performance liquid chromatography and tandem mass spectrometry are becoming the "gold standard." Their upper normal limit is much lower and more specific than that of antibody-based assays, in which steroids other than cortisol may cross-react.

However, urine free cortisol excretion also may be increased in the so-called pseudo-Cushing states, including psychiatric disorders (depression, anxiety disorder, obsessive-compulsive disorder), chronic pain, severe exercise, alcoholism, uncontrolled diabetes, and morbid obesity. Here, it is hypothesized that higher brain pathways stimulate CRH release and activation of the entire hypothalamic-pituitary-adrenal axis. Cortisol negative feedback inhibition on CRH and pituitary ACTH release restrains the resulting hypercortisoluria to less than four-fold greater than normal. Thus, Cushing's syndrome cannot be diagnosed with certainly unless values reach this threshold. Conversely, patients with Cushing's syndrome may have normal urine free cortisol excretion because of intermittent hypercortisolism or altered renal metabolism of cortisol. If urine free cortisol is only mildly elevated and clinical features are minimal, it is best to treat any pseudo-Cushing state and to remeasure urine free cortisol excretion with the expectation that it will normalize. Alternatively, if urine free cortisol excretion is normal but clinical suspicion is high, repeated measurement might disclose intermittent hypercortisolism.

Dexamethasone Suppression Tests

The 1-mg dexamethasone suppression test is a simple screening test that takes advantage of the negative feedback effect of glucocorticoids to reduce ACTH (and hence serum cortisol). It involves giving dexamethasone, 1 mg, orally between 2300 and midnight and measurement of plasma cortisol concentration between 0800 and 0900 the following morning. The test has an 8% false-negative rate in patients with Cushing's disease and a 30% false-positive rate in chronic illness, obesity, psychiatric disorders, and normal individuals. As a result, Cushing's syndrome cannot be diagnosed by this test alone unless the result is extremely abnormal.

The two-day 2-mg dexamethasone suppression test discriminates patients with a pseudo-Cushing state if plasma cortisol end points of less

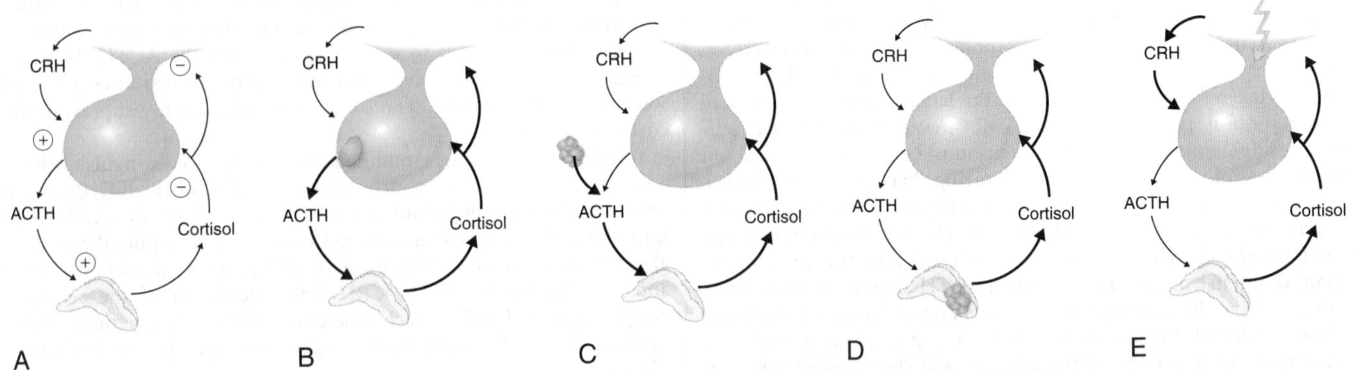

FIGURE 245–3 • The physiology of the adrenal axis in health, Cushing's syndrome, and pseudo-Cushing states. A, In healthy individuals, cortisol production is stimulated by increased hypothalamic release of CRH, which then travels down the pituitary stalk to stimulate corticotrope ACTH secretion and release. Circulating ACTH stimulates adrenal gland production and secretion of cortisol. Cortisol then functions in a negative feedback mechanism to inhibit both CRH and ACTH. **B,** In Cushing's disease, a pituitary tumor releases excessive amounts of ACTH, which results in increased cortisol secretion by the adrenal glands. **C,** In ectopic ACTH secretion, a nonpituitary ACTH-secreting tumor releases excessive amounts of ACTH, which results in increased cortisol secretion by the adrenal glands. **D,** In ACTH-independent adrenal forms of Cushing's syndrome, the adrenal tumor autonomously releases excess amounts of cortisol. In all forms of Cushing's syndrome, the negative feedback effects of excessive cortisol inhibit endogenous CRH and ACTH secretion, so that circulating ACTH levels reflect the underlying tumor (levels normal or increased) or independent cortisol production (levels suppressed). **E,** In pseudo-Cushing states, a central stimulation increases CRH secretion, which in turn increases ACTH and hence cortisol production. In this setting, the negative feedback effects of excessive cortisol inhibit endogenous CRH and ACTH secretion so that cortisol levels are ultimately constrained, albeit at an increased level.

TABLE 245–1 THE FREQUENCY OF CLINICAL SIGNS AND SYMPTOMS OF CUSHING'S SYNDROME

Sign or Symptom	%
Decreased libido in men and women	100
Obesity or weight gain	97
Plethora	94
Round face	88
Menstrual changes	84
Hirsutism	81
Hypertension	74
Ecchymoses	62
Lethargy, depression	62
Striae	56
Weakness	56
Electrocardiographic changes or atherosclerosis	55
Dorsal fat pad	54
Edema	50
Abnormal glucose tolerance	50
Osteopenia or fracture	50
Headache	47
Backache	43
Recurrent infections	25
Abdominal pain	21
Acne	21
Female balding	13

TABLE 245–2 ETIOLOGY OF CUSHING'S SYNDROME

Exogenous	Endogenous
Most common cause of Cushing's syndrome	ACTH independent—autonomous adrenal activation (20% of all cases)
Glucocorticoid or ACTH driven	Adrenal adenoma (40–50%)
May be factitious or iatrogenic	Adrenal carcinoma (40–50%)
	Primary pigmented nodular adrenal disease
	McCune-Albright syndrome
	Massive macronodular adrenal disease
	Gastric inhibitory polypeptide or food induced
	ACTH dependent—adrenal activation by excessive ACTH (80% of all cases)
	Corticotrope adenoma (80%)
	Ectopic ACTH secretion (20%)
	Ectopic CRH secretion (rare)

than 1.4 or 2.2 μg/dL are used. The test involves the administration of dexamethasone, 500 μg, orally every 6 hours for eight doses and measurement of plasma cortisol 2 or 6 hours after the last dose. The test has excellent sensitivity (90 to 100%) and specificity (97 to 100%) for discriminating Cushing's syndrome but has the disadvantage of high cost and the requirement for excellent compliance of the patient. The immediate subsequent administration of CRH (1 μg/kg body weight intravenously) and measurement of cortisol 15 minutes later increased the sensitivity and specificity to 100% in a small study of 58 patients, with use of values above 1.4 μg/dL to indicate Cushing's syndrome. Whereas this combined dexamethasone-CRH test has a high diagnostic accuracy, it has the disadvantages of the 2-day dexamethasone suppression test and the added cost of CRH testing. Because of these drawbacks, in the United States, these tests usually are reserved for patients with ambiguous or confusing results of urine free cortisol measurement or the 1-mg dexamethasone suppression test. CRH is available commercially (Acthrel) with Food and Drug Administration–approved labeling for the differential diagnosis of Cushing's syndrome. Its use in the dexamethasone-CRH test is an off-label use.

Any dexamethasone test may give false results in patients with abnormal metabolic clearance of the drug. Agents that induce the cytochrome P-450 CYP3A4 enzymes (alcohol, rifampin, phenytoin, and phenobarbital) increase dexamethasone clearance, whereas renal or hepatic failure decreases it. Measurement of a dexamethasone level can determine whether its clearance has been altered.

Measurement of plasma cortisol at midnight distinguishes pseudo-Cushing states from Cushing's syndrome, with 95% diagnostic accuracy by a criterion of more than 7.5 μg/dL for the diagnosis of Cushing's syndrome. Measurement of salivary cortisol at bedtime or midnight works as well as the plasma cortisol. However, the criteria for interpretation differ in various studies, so each assay must be validated before it is used for this purpose.

Differential Diagnosis

The causes of endogenous Cushing's syndrome may be divided broadly into ACTH-dependent (80%) and ACTH-independent (20%) forms (Table 245–2). Hypercortisolism from autonomously functioning adrenal tumors suppresses ACTH, whereas in primary ACTH excess disorders, the adrenal glands respond passively to ACTH. Plasma ACTH concentration measured by a sensitive two-site sandwich assay distinguishes between these causes. ACTH is usually less than 10 pg/mL in primary adrenal disorders but is also suppressed by exogenous steroids, whether they are prescribed intentionally (iatrogenic Cushing's syndrome) or taken factitiously. Patients in the latter group often have had multiple surgical procedures and do not reveal that they are self-administering steroids. As a result, patients must be queried closely about exogenous steroid administration, recognizing that parenteral, inhaled, and topical steroids may all cause glucocorticoid excess. Patients with endogenous Cushing's syndrome and low ACTH concentrations undergo adrenal imaging to identify the site of adrenal abnormality. Nonautonomous adrenal tissue atrophies when ACTH support is subnormal. Because of this, the common ACTH-independent forms of Cushing's syndrome, adrenal adenoma and carcinoma, present as a unilateral adrenal mass, with atrophy of the adjacent and contralateral tissue on magnetic resonance or computed tomographic scan. If there is a question about bilateral function, an iodocholesterol scan may exclude non-functioning masses.

Bilateral forms of primary adrenal disease are rare and may present with small or large adrenal nodules. Primary pigmented nodular adrenal disease occurs primarily in children and young adults and is characterized by small to normal-sized adrenal glands containing small (<5 mm) black-brown cortical nodules. About half of these patients have additional features, termed Carney's complex, that are often inherited in an autosomal dominant fashion. The clinical features of Carney's complex include myxomas of the skin, breast, and heart; spotty pigmentation, such as lentigenes and blue nevi; and other endocrine overactivity, such as acromegaly and testicular tumors. Some of these patients have mutations leading to a truncated form of protein kinase A regulatory 1α subunit. The resultant increase in protein kinase A activation by cyclic adenosine monophosphate presumably allows tumor formation. Bilateral nodular hyperplasia with Cushing's syndrome can occur in the setting of McCune-Albright syndrome, mostly in infants. Massive macronodular adrenal disease generally presents after the age of 40 years with huge adrenal glands with aberrant expression of "illicit" receptors for various ligands (gastric inhibitory polypeptide, β-adrenergic, vasopressin), which presumably mediates autonomous cortisol production.

A normal or elevated plasma ACTH level (>15 pg/mL; 3.3 pmol/L) is consistent with an ACTH-producing tumor. Intermediate ACTH concentrations between 5 and 15 pg/mL (1.1 to 3.3 pmol/L) are not diagnostic. In these patients, suboptimal cortisol responses to CRH stimulation may identify the minority of cases of ACTH-independent Cushing's syndrome with borderline basal ACTH value. In addition, a suppressed plasma DHEA-S value supports the diagnosis of an ACTH-independent disorder.

Cushing's disease, an ACTH-secreting pituitary adenoma, is the most common cause of Cushing's syndrome. It is more common in women than in men (6:1), with a mean age at onset in the fourth decade. ACTH also may be secreted ectopically by a variety of neuroendocrine tumors as shown in Table 245–3.

Pituitary magnetic resonance imaging shows a tumor in only about 40 to 50% of patients with Cushing's disease, but it is obtained routinely in patients with ACTH-dependent disease to exclude a macroadenoma or abnormal anatomy before petrosal sinus sampling or surgery. Biochemical tests must be used to distinguish between the ACTH-dependent causes of Cushing's syndrome and must be performed after a 4- to 6-week period of sustained hypercortisolism sufficient to suppress normal corticotrope function.

Inferior petrosal sinus sampling is the best test to distinguish between a pituitary and an ectopic source of excess ACTH; worldwide, the overall sensitivity and specificity are about 94%. The test involves catheterization of a peripheral vein and the petrosal sinuses draining the pituitary gland, simultaneous measurement of ACTH levels at each site before and after administration of CRH, and calculation of the central to peripheral ACTH ratio at each time point. Ratios of more than 2 before or more than 3 after CRH administration are consistent with Cushing's disease.

Although it is accurate in experienced hands, inferior petrosal sinus sampling carries a small risk of stroke and is expensive and not widely available. Other tests, such as the CRH test and the 8-mg dexamethasone suppression test, may be useful if both responses indicate Cushing's disease. In this setting, the likelihood of ectopic ACTH secretion is low. However, the diagnosis is not clear if the responses are mixed or both negative.

If endocrine tests suggest ectopic ACTH secretion, imaging is obtained to localize the tumor. Computed tomographic and magnetic resonance scans of the chest are the best initial screen because these tumors are most often in the thoracic cavity. Octreotide scintigraphy is a useful adjunctive test. Measurement of serum calcitonin and gastrin and of plasma or urine catecholamines may identify medullary carcinoma of the thyroid, gastrinoma, and pheochromocytoma. The process may be repeated every 6 to 12 months; tumors that make ACTH ectopically have a spectrum of malignant potential, and annual screening should continue, regardless of treatment for hypercortisolism.

TABLE 245–3 THE INCIDENCE AND TYPES OF TUMORS CAUSING THE SYNDROME OF ECTOPIC ACTH SECRETION

Tumor Type	Percentage
Carcinoma of lung (small cell or oat cell)	19–50
Carcinoid of bronchus	2–37
Carcinoid of thymus	8–12
Pancreatic tumors, carcinoid and islet cell	4–12
Pheochromocytoma, neuroblastoma, ganglioma, paraganglioma	5–12
Medullary carcinoma of the thyroid	0–5
Miscellaneous*	<1

*Miscellaneous tumors reported to secrete ACTH in 1 to 10 cases include carcinoma of ovary, prostate, breast, thyroid, kidney, salivary glands, testes, gallbladder, esophagus, and appendix; gastric carcinoid and renal carcinoid; acute myeloblastic leukemia; melanoma; and cloacogenic carcinoma of anal canal.

Treatment

Rx

Surgical Therapy

The optimal treatment of Cushing's syndrome is surgical resection of the lesion that is producing excessive ACTH or cortisol. In ACTH-dependent Cushing's syndrome, if this is unsuccessful or cannot be done, bilateral adrenalectomy is an option. Medical therapy also may be used for patients with occult ectopic ACTH-secreting tumors and in combination with pituitary irradiation to treat Cushing's disease.

Transsphenoidal resection of a microadenoma is the optimal therapy for the patient with Cushing's disease, with up to a 90% chance of cure in the hands of an experienced neurosurgeon. A successful outcome is less likely if the initial surgery was not curative, in recurrence, and in macroadenomas. Controversy exists about criteria for remission; although a low postoperative cortisol level is encouraging, it does not preclude later recurrence. If recurrence develops, additional resection and alternative therapy should be considered.

Radiation Therapy

Radiation therapy to the pituitary gland with adjunctive medical therapy to normalize cortisol levels is a good option for patients who cannot undergo surgery, for those in whom the risk of Nelson's syndrome is deemed great, and for recurrent disease. This is usually delivered in 200-rad daily increments to a total dose of 4500 cGy. The disadvantage of radiotherapy is the length of time needed for full response, up to 10 years, and the possibility of hypopituitarism. There is less experience with high-energy radiotherapy, such as the gamma knife. Adrenalectomy is preferable if rapid normalization of hypercortisolism is needed and may be chosen by patients who have concerns about radiation-induced hypopituitarism and loss of reproductive function.

Medical Therapy

Combination Surgical and Medical Therapy

Medical therapy alone is rarely appropriate for Cushing's disease because it requires close monitoring and adjustment of dose and has low long-term efficacy.

Rx

Patients with ectopic ACTH secretion can be cured if the tumor can be removed and is not metastatic. Otherwise, adrenalectomy or medical therapy is chosen. Adrenalectomy is appropriate when the patient cannot tolerate the cost, medical toxicity, or adverse psychological effects of long-term medical therapy and monitoring or if the patient requires rapid correction of hypercortisolism. Adrenalectomy is appropriate when maximal daily doses of ketoconazole (1600 mg), aminoglutethimide (2 g), and metyrapone (2 g) given in combination do not render the patient eucortisolemic.

Nonmalignant primary adrenal causes of Cushing's syndrome are cured by resection of the abnormal tissue, whether unilateral or bilateral. Laparoscopy is the preferred approach for adults and children. Surgery is the mainstay in the treatment of adrenal cancer; multiple operations may be needed to resect primary lesions, local recurrences, and hepatic, thoracic, and intracranial metastases. Adjuvant adrenolytic therapy with mitotane may provide chemotherapeutic benefit.

Mineralocorticoid Excess

Diagnosis

Patients with mineralocorticoid excess often have few clinical symptoms apart from fatigue or muscle weakness or cramps related to hypokalemia. Most often the condition is suspected because of hypertension, especially if it occurs at an early age in association with spontaneous hypokalemia or is difficult to control. Mineralocorticoid excess can result from primary adrenal disease, in which aldosterone (or another mineralocorticoid) is produced autonomously (and renin levels are appropriately low), or it may be due to nonadrenal causes as a result of elevated renin values, which stimulate aldosterone secretion. The latter situations include states of contracted arterial volume such as congestive heart failure or cirrhosis with ascites, decreased renal arterial blood flow, and tumoral production of renin; they are not considered further here (Table 245–4).

Renin-Independent Mineralocorticoid Excess

Diagnosis

Although most of these conditions result from excessive aldosterone production by one or both adrenal glands, excessive production of other mineralocorticoids or constitutive activation of the renal sodium channel must be excluded. In these conditions, both aldosterone and renin values are low, resulting in the so-called syndrome of apparent mineralocorticoid excess. In this setting, diagnostic information is obtained by history (licorice ingestion) or measurement of other mineralocorticoids (see Table 245–4).

The diagnosis of primary hyperaldosteronism rests on demonstration of an increased plasma aldosterone value of more than 15 pg/mL with an increased ratio of aldosterone to plasma renin activity (>20). If both renin and plasma or urinary aldosterone concentrations are low, excessive production of other mineralocorticoids should be sought. Salt loading can be used to confirm primary hyperaldosteronism by demonstrating lack of aldosterone response to this physiologic suppression. Two liters of saline, 0.9%, is infused during 4 hours; plasma aldosterone concentration at the end of the infusion should be less than 5 ng/dL in normal individuals.

Differential Diagnosis

Having made the diagnosis of aldosterone-dependent mineralocorticoid excess, one must differentiate between the two most common adrenal causes, hyperplasia and adenoma, after excluding potential rare causes of hyperaldosteronism. Glucocorticoid-suppressible hyperaldosteronism is a rare cause of aldosterone excess caused by a genetic swap of the promoter for *CYP11B1* (11β-hydroxylase) with that of *CYP11B2* (aldosterone synthase), forming a chimeric gene in which ACTH stimulates aldosterone synthase. Glucocorticoid-suppressible hyperaldosteronism should be suspected in the setting of familial hyperaldosteronism, particularly in the setting of a history of cardiovascular accidents at an early age. Serum 18-hydroxycortisol and 18-oxocortisol concentrations are elevated in glucocorticoid-suppressible hyperaldosteronism, and gene testing confirms the diagnosis (*http://www.brighamandwomens.org/gra*).

For the more common conditions, adrenal computed tomographic scans may show nonfunctioning nodules and falsely suggest an adenoma. The responses to physiologic maneuvers such as upright posture and salt loading with oral or intravenous sodium tend to be preserved in patients with hyperplasia, but there is significant overlap between groups of patients. The best diagnostic test involves measurement of cortisol and aldosterone in bilateral adrenal venous effluent and a peripheral vein before and during an ACTH infusion. Cortisol is used to evaluate catheter placement in the adrenal veins as levels from the two sides should be similar. When an adenoma is present, the aldosterone-to-cortisol ratio on one side is usually at least five-fold greater than the other, which may be similar to the periphery, indicating suppression. Bilateral hyperplasia tends to produce similar values on each side.

TABLE 245–4 CAUSES OF MINERALOCORTICOID EXCESS

PRIMARY HYPERALDOSTERONISM: HIGH ALDOSTERONE, LOW RENIN

Aldosterone-producing adenomas (30–50%)
Bilateral zona glomerulosa hyperplasia
Familial hyperaldosteronism
- Type 1: glucocorticoid-remediable hyperaldosteronism. This results from formation of a chimeric gene containing the regulator portion of 11β-hydroxylase (normally regulated by ACTH) and the synthetic region of aldosterone synthase; as a result, ACTH stimulates aldosterone synthase and hence aldosterone production.
- Type 2: adrenal adenomas or hyperplasia expressed in a familial pattern

Aldosterone-producing adrenal carcinoma
Ectopic aldosterone secretion (rare): kidney, ovary

SECONDARY HYPERALDOSTERONISM: HIGH ALDOSTERONE, HIGH RENIN

Renovascular hypertension and aortic stenosis
Diuretic use
Renin-secreting tumors
Severe cardiac failure

APPARENT MINERALOCORTICOID EXCESS: LOW ALDOSTERONE, LOW RENIN

Licorice ingestion: Licorice (candy or flavored tobacco) containing glycyrrhetinic acid (or similar compounds such as carbenoxolone) inhibits renal 11β-hydroxysteroid dehydrogenase type 2, reducing cortisol conversion to cortisone and enabling cortisol to act as an endogenous mineralocorticoid.
Severe hypercortisolism: This is similar in mechanism to licorice ingestion. Very high cortisol levels are thought to overwhelm the ability of 11β-hydroxysteroid dehydrogenase type 2 to convert cortisol to cortisone in the kidney; cortisol itself then acts as a potent mineralocorticoid.
Liddle's syndrome (mutation of β or γ subunit of collecting tubule sodium channel leading to constitutive increase in sodium reabsorption and potassium excretion)
11β-Hydroxylase deficiency form of congenital adrenal hyperplasia; 11-deoxycortisol accumulates because of an inability to convert it to cortisol.
17-Hydroxylase deficiency form of congenital adrenal hyperplasia; deoxycorticosterone and corticosterone are increased.

Treatment

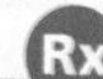

Treatment of primary hyperaldosteronism includes laparoscopic resection for adenomas. Afterwards, hypokalemia generally resolves, but hypertension persists in up to 65% of patients. The mineralocorticoid antagonist spironolactone or amiloride is used to treat patients unable to undergo surgery or those with hyperplasia. Antihypertensive agents are continued. Eplerenone is a newer, more selective mineralocorticoid antagonist (hence fewer side effects of sexual dysfunction and gynecomastia compared with spironolactone). It is currently approved by the Food and Drug Administration for the treatment of hypertension and congestive heart failure; trials are ongoing for the treatment of primary hyperaldosteronism.

Androgen Excess

Definition

Women with excess circulating androgens or increased sensitivity to androgens present with complaints of hirsutism, acne, and anovulation or infertility. When testosterone is secreted in great excess, women may virilize and show deepened voice, clitorimegaly, masculinized body habitus, and alopecia. These issues are considered more fully in Chapter 261.

Diagnosis

The adrenal causes of hyperandrogenism—congenital adrenal hyperplasia, Cushing's disease, adrenal cancer, and androgen-producing adrenal adenoma—are uncommon. Most women have no clear-cut etiology (idiopathic hirsutism) or polycystic ovary syndrome. Rarely, androgen-secreting ovarian tumors, hyperprolactinemia, glucocorticoid resistance, or exogenous drugs cause hyperandrogenism. Patients with an adrenal source of hyperandrogenism usually have increased serum levels of DHEA-S or androstenedione, in contrast to the testosterone excess that is more typical of an ovarian source. DHEA and DHEA-S are weak androgens that can be converted locally to testosterone in the hair follicles. As DHEA and DHEA-S levels decline through adult life, these values must be interpreted with age-specific normal ranges. Although a tumor is more likely if DHEA-S is greater than 500 μg/dL or testosterone is greater than 200 ng/mL, it is not excluded at lower levels.

Imaging identifies nearly all adrenal tumors but may miss a small intraovarian one. Urine free cortisol may be elevated in patients with virilizing adrenal carcinoma or Cushing's disease (see earlier) and in those with glucocorticoid resistance.

By contrast, androgen-secreting adrenal adenomas do not have glucocorticoid excess. Women suspected of having nonclassic forms of congenital adrenal hyperplasia should undergo measurement of precursor and product hormones before and after ACTH to confirm the diagnosis.

Treatment

Treatment of adrenal causes of hyperandrogenism varies according to the disorder. Tumors are resected. Late-onset congenital adrenal hyperplasia is treated by glucocorticoids to normalize ACTH and hence androgen levels (typically dexamethasone, 0.125 to 0.375 mg at bedtime). Additional medical and local or topical therapy is reviewed in Chapter 261.

Mixed Mineralocorticoid and Glucocorticoid Deficiency: Adrenal Insufficiency

Clinical Manifestations

The clinical presentation of adrenal insufficiency reflects the etiology and the duration of this uncommon condition. Primary adrenal insufficiency eventually destroys the entire adrenal cortex, with loss of both glucocorticoid and mineralocorticoid activity. By contrast, secondary adrenal insufficiency reflects an inability of the hypothalamic-pituitary unit to deliver CRH or corticotropin (ACTH), thus reducing trophic support to otherwise normal glands. As a result, only cortisol production decreases as mineralocorticoid production is not very ACTH dependent.

The characteristic clinical presentation of acute primary adrenal insufficiency includes orthostatic hypotension, agitation, confusion, circulatory collapse, abdominal pain, and fever. These features are most likely to be caused by hemorrhage, metastasis, or acute infection and can lead to death if not treated. In contrast, the typical history and clinical findings of chronic primary adrenal insufficiency include a longer history of malaise, fatigue, anorexia, weight loss, joint and back pain, and darkening of the skin (especially in the creases of the hands, extensor surfaces, recent scars, buccal and vaginal mucosa, and nipples). Patients may crave salt and develop unusual food preferences, such as drinking the brine surrounding pickles. Associated biochemical features for both presentations include hyponatremia, hypoglycemia, hyperkalemia, unexplained eosinophilia, and mild prerenal azotemia.

Chronic secondary adrenal insufficiency presents in a similar way without hyperpigmentation or mineralocorticoid abnormalities.

Diagnosis

Biochemical testing confirms the diagnosis of adrenal insufficiency. A morning serum cortisol measurement is an inexpensive but relatively insensitive screening test for adrenal insufficiency in patients who are not acutely ill. Adrenal insufficiency is virtually excluded by values more than 19 μg/dL (524 nmol/L) and is likely if the value is less than 3 μg/dL (83 nmol/L). However, because of the pulsatile nature of cortisol secretion, both healthy individuals and patients with adrenal insufficiency may have results in the intermediate range of 3 to 19 μg/dL, requiring additional evaluation.

Patients with acute adrenal insufficiency should be evaluated for sepsis or hemorrhage or metastasis in the adrenal glands. Imaging of the glands and other testing may reveal an infectious etiology. Individuals thought to have congenital adrenal hyperplasia should undergo additional measurement of ACTH-stimulated precursor and product hormones to delineate the site of enzymatic deficiency. In acute adrenal insufficiency, a serum cortisol value generally is inappropriately normal or subnormal in the setting of hypotension (in which cortisol values are usually well above 18 μg/dL). There is controversy about the best test for the diagnosis of chronic adrenal insufficiency. Many use the cortisol response to exogenous ACTH as a "gold standard" test of adrenal steroidogenic ability. In the classic test, 250 μg of ACTH (1–24, cosyntropin) is given intravenously or intramuscularly, at any time of day. This supraphysiologic dose of ACTH is a maximal stimulus to the adrenal gland, so that the peak serum cortisol level measured 30 to 60 minutes later is greater than 18 μg/dL. Lower values indicate adrenal insufficiency. Insulin-induced hypoglycemia and lower doses of the ACTH stimulation test have been proposed as better tests for patients with mild or recent secondary adrenal insufficiency who may respond to pharmacologic doses of ACTH. Insulin testing has significant risks in patients without normal counter-regulatory processes and in those with coronary artery disease or epilepsy. Also, because there is no commercial formulation of ACTH for the lower dose tests, the product must be diluted and delivered on site, leading to concerns about accuracy of the administered dose and the validity of the results.

Cerebral adrenoleukodystrophy, presenting in childhood, is characterized by cognitive and gait disturbances; the adult form, adrenomyeloneuropathy, is characterized by spinal cord and peripheral nerve demyelination. In both forms, accumulation of very long chain fatty acids in the adrenal cortex alters membrane function and inhibits signal transduction by ACTH. Because a substantial minority of patients in both groups present first with adrenal insufficiency, boys and young men with adrenal insufficiency should be screened for adrenoleukodystrophy.

Differential Diagnosis

Primary and secondary adrenal insufficiency may be distinguished by measurement of plasma ACTH. In primary adrenal insufficiency, ACTH levels generally are above the normal range and may exceed the normal range before the cortisol response to exogenous ACTH stimulation is subnormal. In addition, hyperkalemia and elevated renin values are characteristic of primary but not of secondary adrenal insufficiency.

Pathobiology

Primary Adrenal Insufficiency

Autoimmune Destruction

Autoimmune destruction is the most common cause of primary adrenal insufficiency in industrialized countries and may occur alone or, rarely, in association with autoimmune polyglandular syndromes. These syndromes tend to present either in childhood (type 1), in association with hypoparathyroidism and mucocutaneous candidiasis, or in adulthood (type 2), in association with insulin-dependent diabetes mellitus, autoimmune thyroid disease, alopecia areata, and vitiligo.

Adrenoleukodystrophy

Adrenoleukodystrophy, a rare (1/25,000) X-linked condition, is characterized by deficiency of peroxisomal membrane adrenoleukodystrophy protein, which transports activated acyl coenzyme A derivates into the peroxisomes, where they are shortened by β oxidation. This deficiency results in accumulation of very long chain fatty acids in the central nervous system and other tissues and increased plasma $C_{26:0}$ fatty acids. Incomplete penetrance of the genetic defect and variable accumulation of very long chain fatty acids in adrenal gland, brain, testis, and liver account for the clinical phenotypes, which differ by age and presentation.

Infection

Infections cause about 15% of primary adrenal insufficiency and typically include tuberculosis and systemic fungal diseases (histoplasmosis, coccidioidomycosis, blastomycosis), in which the adrenal tissue is replaced by caseating granulomas. End-stage AIDS-associated opportunistic infections, such as cytomegalovirus or *Mycobacterium avium-intracellulare,* may reduce adrenal function. Adrenal tissue may be replaced by bilateral metastases (most commonly primary carcinoma of the lung, breast, kidney, or gut or primary lymphoma), although adrenal insufficiency is uncommon. Intra-adrenal hemorrhage may also lead to insufficient steroidogenesis. Hemorrhage usually occurs in the setting of a stressed hospitalized patient receiving long-term prophylactic anticoagulation and is often accompanied by back pain. The adrenal glands tend to be large on computed tomographic scan; those affected by autoimmune destruction are small.

Congenital Adrenal Hyperplasias

The congenital adrenal hyperplasias are a disparate group of diseases caused by a genetic deficiency of one of the enzymes needed for adrenal steroidogenesis. Patients with nearly complete deficiency of an enzyme required for cortisol synthesis present in childhood with adrenal insufficiency and salt-wasting crisis. This is most problematic in patients with mutation of the 21-hydroxylase (*CYP21*) or 11β-hydroxylase (*CYP11B1*) gene. The increase in ACTH levels caused by cortisol deficiency drives the intact steroidogenic pathways so that there is excessive production of the steroids just proximal to the enzymatic block, 17-hydroxyprogesterone and 11-deoxycortisol, respectively, in 21-hydroxylase and 11β-hydroxylase deficiency. Because of the increased levels of precursor steroids, adrenal androgen levels increase. As a result, severely affected girls may be virilized in utero. Girls and women with nonclassic congenital adrenal hyperplasia have greater enzyme activity so that cortisol production is adequate but increased ACTH values cause hyperandrogenism after puberty.

Rare Causes

Other rare causes of primary adrenal insufficiency include ACTH resistance, congenital adrenal hypoplasia, Smith-Lemli-Opitz syndrome, and amyloidosis. Patients with primary adrenal insufficiency should undergo further evaluation to determine its etiology (Table 245–5). Detection of antibodies to 21-hydroxylase identifies nearly all patients with idiopathic

TABLE 245–5 CAUSES OF ADRENAL INSUFFICIENCY AND ANCILLARY TESTS

Specific Causes	Suggestive Clinical Features	Useful Ancillary Tests
Primary adrenal insufficiency	Hyperpigmentation, orthostatic hypotension	Hypokalemia, elevated ACTH
Idiopathic autoimmune destruction	The most common cause (80%) in developed countries; with or without other endocrinopathy as below	Antibodies to 21-hydroxylase are present. On imaging, these adrenal glands are small.
Polyglandular failure type 1	Hypoparathyroidism, mucocutaneous candidiasis, vitiligo; age < 20 years	
Polyglandular failure type 2	Insulin-dependent diabetes, autoimmune thyroid disease, alopecia areata, vitiligo; age > 40 years	On imaging, these adrenal glands are small.
Infections: tuberculosis, systemic fungal diseases, and AIDS-associated opportunistic infections such as cytomegalovirus	15% of patients in U.S. series	These adrenal glands tend to be large on CT scan and may be calcified.
Space-occupying adrenal lesions	Metastases from carcinoma of lung, breast, kidney, gut; lymphoma or hemorrhage (heparin use)	Abnormal shape of adrenal glands on CT scan; evidence of hemorrhage.
Bilateral adrenalectomy or treatment with steroidogenesis inhibitors	Ketoconazole, mitotane, aminoglutethimide, trilostane, and metyrapone reduce cortisol levels	
Adrenoleukodystrophy	X-linked—screen males; in childhood, cognitive and gait disturbances; in adults, spastic paraparesis	Deficiency of peroxisomal very long chain acyl coenzyme A synthetase leads to elevated plasma $C_{26:0}$ fatty acid levels.
Secondary adrenal insufficiency		
Suppression of the adrenal axis by exogenous or endogenous glucocorticoids	Medication history; history of Cushing's syndrome	Adrenal glands are small on imaging.
Structural lesions of the hypothalamus or pituitary gland (tumors, destruction by infiltrating disorders, x-irradiation, and lymphocytic hypophysitis)	Other pituitary deficiencies	Adrenal glands are normal or small on imaging; MR/CT scan may show pituitary or hypothalamic lesion.
Isolated ACTH deficiency		

CT = computed tomography; MR = magnetic resonance.

disease. If this test result is negative in a male, a measurement of very long chain fatty acids will detect all cases of adrenoleukodystrophy. Taken together, these measurements can identify the etiology in nearly all adult patients with idiopathic adrenal insufficiency. Patients with autoimmune disease should be tested for other endocrine deficiencies, and those with adrenoleukodystrophy require neurologic evaluation.

Secondary Adrenal Insufficiency

Suppression of the Pituitary Axis

Suppression of the hypothalamic-pituitary-adrenal axis by exogenous or endogenous glucocorticoids is the most common cause of secondary adrenal insufficiency. This phenomenon depends on the dose, duration, and schedule of glucocorticoid administration. Thus, adrenal suppression is unusual with "replacement" doses of glucocorticoid that are roughly equivalent to daily production (e.g., total daily doses of 20 mg of hydrocortisone, 5 mg of prednisone, or 0.3 to 0.5 mg of dexamethasone). At higher doses, adrenal suppression is not usually seen before 3 weeks of administration, and a single morning administration is less suppressive than are divided doses given during the entire day. When potentially suppressive doses of glucocorticoids are stopped, symptoms of adrenal insufficiency may occur within 48 hours, and the entire axis may not recover for up to 18 months after discontinuation of medication. During this time, the patient should receive replacement glucocorticoid treatment or supplemental steroids at times of physiologic stress, depending on the degree of impairment (see later).

Lesions of the Hypothalamus or Pituitary

Secondary adrenal insufficiency also may result from structural lesions of the hypothalamus or pituitary gland that interfere with CRH production or transport or with corticotrope function. This includes tumors, destruction by infiltrating disorders, x-irradiation, and lymphocytic hypophysitis. In general, these are not reversible conditions. Patients with secondary adrenal insufficiency not ascribed to glucocorticoid use should undergo imaging of the pituitary and hypothalamus to exclude a structural or infiltrating lesion and tests of other pituitary function to exclude additional deficiencies.

Treatment

Acute Adrenal Insufficiency

In suspected acute adrenal insufficiency, hydrocortisone is the treatment of choice because it has both glucocorticoid and mineralocorticoid activity. Treatment with intravenous saline for volume expansion, glucose for hypoglycemia, and intravenous hydrocortisone, 100 mg, is started immediately after placement of an intravenous line and withdrawal of blood for documentation of the cortisol value.

Chronic Adrenal Insufficiency

Therapy for chronic adrenal insufficiency should provide physiologic replacement of steroids. Glucocorticoid replacement is achieved by administering 12 to 15 mg/m^2 of hydrocortisone daily in one or two oral doses that attempt to mimic the physiologic diurnal variation of cortisol concentrations. Hydrocortisone offers the advantage of multiple-dose tablets, which allows fine adjustment and splitting of the daily dose. Ideally, the morning dose is given as soon after waking as possible; for individuals who feel extremely fatigued in the morning before the agent is absorbed, a strategy of taking the medication 30 minutes before arising may be helpful. Although many patients do well with a single dose, others complain of pronounced fatigue in the afternoon and evening. For them, a split-dose regimen, in which about one third of the daily dose is given around 4:00 PM, may be useful.

Other glucocorticoids may be used for daily replacement therapy. Prednisone, 5 to 7.5 mg daily, has the advantage of a long half-life and may be particularly helpful in patients with afternoon or evening fatigue. Dexamethasone may be used but has a disadvantage of variable interindividual metabolism so that it is difficult to recommend a specific replacement dose; in addition, few options for fixed doses are available so that it is difficult to adjust the dose.

Patients with primary adrenal insufficiency should be encouraged to salt their food and not to limit salt intake. Most also require mineralocorticoid as fludrocortisone, 50 to 300 μg/day. The dose is adjusted until plasma renin activity is normal. If mineralocorticoid is not given, the dose of hydrocortisone or other steroid with mineralocorticoid activity is often mistakenly increased to reduce hyperkalemia or salt craving. The problem with this approach is that the amount of glucocorticoid increases beyond physiologic replacement, and the patient becomes cushingoid.

Patients with primary adrenal insufficiency also have decreased serum DHEA levels. Replacement of DHEA at a 50-mg daily dose may improve overall well-being as well as self-reported scores for fatigue, depression, and anxiety. In women but not in men, there is improvement in sexual interest and satisfaction.

Ensuring Proper Dosing

Education of the Patient

All patients receiving chronic glucocorticoid replacement therapy should be instructed that they must take glucocorticoids as prescribed and that failure to take or to absorb the medication will lead to adrenal crisis and possibly death. They should obtain a medical information bracelet or necklace that identifies this requirement.* It is important to educate patients and their families about glucocorticoid adjustment during physiologic stress conditions, including emergency administration of intramuscular glucocorticoid by a kit containing prefilled syringes with injectable steroid.

Dosing for Stress

The daily oral glucocorticoid dose is usually doubled for "stressful" physiologic conditions such as fever, nausea, and diarrhea, although there are few data to support this strategy. In addition, this practice may lead to chronic overmedication by the patient because of a liberal interpretation of what constitutes physical stress. Thus, education of when and how to change the dose of steroid should be reinforced periodically, preferably with written material, and the dangers of excessive steroid use should be emphasized. If the patient is vomiting, has severe diarrhea, or has collapsed, intramuscular glucocorticoids should be given before transport to a medical facility.

The glucocorticoid dose is increased further in proportion to the amount of stress. Thus, during maximally stressful situations (adrenal crisis, major surgery, trauma, or labor and delivery), the daily hydrocortisone dose will be 100 to 300 mg. (Few data support the need for this pharmacologic rather than physiologic replacement dose, but the safety of not following this practice has not been established.) The dose is usually tapered by 50% per day as long as the patient is clinically stable. For more moderate stress, such as that of cholecystectomy, the dose is reduced to 75 to 100 mg hydrocortisone on the day of surgery, and the dose is tapered more rapidly. Patients undergoing minimal stress, such as tooth extraction or short operative orthopedic procedures, may not require any additional supplementation.

Clinical Assessment to Ensure Proper Dosing

Clinical assessment is the best way to judge whether the glucocorticoid dose is correct. Symptoms of adrenal insufficiency improve with adequate therapy. The development of cushingoid features or osteopenia suggests frank or subtle overreplacement, respectively, and the presence of adrenal insufficiency symptoms (fatigue, anorexia, weight loss) suggests underreplacement. In women, DHEA replacement increases testosterone levels, so that hirsutism, acne, or other signs of androgen excess may suggest overreplacement. In primary adrenal insufficiency, with adequate hormone replacement, plasma ACTH levels decrease but remain elevated in the range of 100 to 200 pg/mL. Renin values, however, normalize completely and may be used to judge the adequacy of mineralocorticoid replacement. Although hydrocortisone is metabolized to cortisol, plasma

*MedicAlert Foundation, 2323 Colorado Ave, Turlock, CA 95382; telephone 1-800-432-5378.

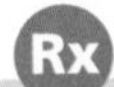

cortisol values should not be used to monitor therapy because clearance from the blood stream is rapid and circulating values are low for most of the day. Urine free cortisol does not reflect adequate replacement; the increase in plasma cortisol levels after a single daily dose may exceed corticosteroid-binding globulin capacity, resulting in excessive urine levels and overestimation of integrated cortisol levels.

Mineralocorticoid Deficiency

Definition

Hypoaldosteronism may be classified as a low-normal renin or high renin state on the basis of plasma renin activity after 4 hours of upright posture. Renin deficiency is the most common cause of hypoaldosteronism, occurring most often in older patients with mild, nonoliguric renal disease, who often have insulin-dependent diabetes and potentially diabetic nephropathy. Indomethacin and other prostaglandin synthesis inhibitors as well as autonomic dysfunction associated with prolonged bedrest can also result in hyporeninemic hypoaldosteronism.

Clinical Manifestations

There are few clinical features associated with mineralocorticoid deficiency; as a result, it is usually suspected when laboratory results reveal hyperkalemia, hyponatremia, and a mild metabolic alkalosis. If glucocorticoid deficiency is excluded, isolated hypoaldosteronism is established if the circulating level of aldosterone is inappropriately low.

High renin states of hypoaldosteronism include congenital adrenal hyperplasias with mineralocorticoid deficiency and primary adrenal insufficiency, when it is treated with pure glucocorticoid replacement.

Treatment

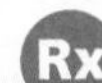

Treatment of these conditions involves sodium replacement with at least 10 mEq/kg/day, roughly equivalent to the 4 g of sodium chloride found in a typical diet in the United States. For individuals who do not maintain such a diet, often the elderly or the young, fludrocortisone can be given at doses used in primary adrenal insufficiency.

SUGGESTED READINGS

Arlt W, Allolio B: Adrenal insufficiency. Lancet 2003;361:1881–1893. *An overview including presentation, diagnosis, and therapy.*

Arnaldi G, Angeli A, Atkinson AB, et al: Diagnosis and complications of Cushing's syndrome: A consensus statement. J Clin Endocrinol Metab 2003;88:5593–5602. *A consensus statement on diagnosis and differential diagnosis.*

Berger J, Moser HW, Forss-Petter S: Leukodystrophies: Recent developments in genetics, molecular biology, pathogenesis and treatment. Curr Opin Neurol 2001;14:305–312. *A review of pathophysiology, presentation, and treatments.*

Bouillon R: Acute adrenal insufficiency. Endocrinol Metab Clin North Am 2006;35:767–775. *Comprehensive review.*

Fulmer BR: Diagnosis and management of adrenal cortical carcinoma. Curr Urol Rep 2007;8:77–82. *Overview of the medical and surgical treatments for these tumors.*

Jacobi J: Corticosteroid replacement in critically ill patients. Crit Care Clin 2006;22:245–253. *Up-to-date review of the literature regarding the use of corticosteroids in critical illness.*

Malchoff CD: Carney complex—clarity and complexity. J Clin Endocrinol Metab 2000;85:4010–4012. *A balanced update on this syndrome.*

Mattsson C, Young WF Jr: Primary aldosteronism: Diagnostic and treatment strategies. Nat Clin Pract Nephrol 2006;2:198–208. *Comprehensive review.*

Shen WT, Sturgeon C, Duh QY: From incidentaloma to adrenocortical carcinoma: The surgical management of adrenal tumors. J Surg Oncol 2005;89:186–192. *Laparoscopic adrenalectomy has become the gold standard for nearly all procedures.*

Speiser PW, White PC: Congenital adrenal hyperplasia. N Engl J Med 2003;349:776–788. *An overview of this condition, including presentation in adolescence and adulthood.*

Young WF Jr: Clinical practice: The incidentally discovered adrenal mass. N Engl J Med 2007;356:601–610. *Comprehensive review of the work-up for adrenal masses.*

246 ADRENAL MEDULLA, CATECHOLAMINES, AND PHEOCHROMOCYTOMA

William F. Young, Jr.

ADRENAL MEDULLA AND CATECHOLAMINES

The adrenal medulla occupies the central portion of the adrenal gland and accounts for 10% of total adrenal gland volume. Adrenomedullary cells are called chromaffin cells (stain brown with chromium salts). Chromaffin cells differentiate in the center of the adrenal gland in response to cortisol; some chromaffin cells also migrate to form paraganglia, collections of chromaffin cells on both sides of the aorta. The largest cluster of chromaffin cells outside the adrenal medulla is near the level of the inferior mesenteric artery and is referred to as the organ of Zuckerkandl.

The term *catecholamine* refers to substances that contain catechol (*o*-dihydroxybenzene) and a side chain with an amino group—the catechol nucleus (Fig. 246–1). Epinephrine is synthesized and stored in the adrenal medulla and released into the systemic circulation. Norepinephrine is synthesized and stored not only in the adrenal medulla but also in the peripheral sympathetic nerves. Dopamine, the precursor of norepinephrine found in the adrenal medulla and peripheral sympathetic nerves, acts primarily as a neurotransmitter in the central nervous system.

Catecholamines affect many cardiovascular and metabolic processes, including increasing the heart rate, blood pressure, myocardial contractility, and cardiac conduction velocity. Specific receptors mediate the biologic actions. The three types of adrenergic receptors are α, β, and DA; their receptor subtypes are α_1, α_2, β_1, β_2, β_3, DA_1, and DA_2. The α_1 subtype is a postsynaptic receptor that mediates vascular and smooth muscle contraction; stimulation causes vasoconstriction and increased blood pressure. The α_2 receptors are located on presynaptic sympathetic nerve endings and, when activated, inhibit release of norepinephrine; stimulation causes suppression in central sympathetic outflow and decreased blood pressure. Stimulation of the β_1 receptor causes positive inotropic and chronotropic effects on the heart, increased renin secretion in the kidney, and lipolysis in adipocytes as well as bronchodilation, vasodilation in skeletal muscle, glycogenolysis, and increased release of norepinephrine from sympathetic nerve terminals. The β_3 receptor regulates energy expenditure and lipolysis. DA_1 receptors are localized to the cerebral, renal, mesenteric, and coronary vasculatures; stimulation causes vasodilation in these vascular beds. DA_2 receptors are presynaptic and localized to sympathetic nerve endings, sympathetic ganglia, and brain; stimulation inhibits the release of norepinephrine, inhibits ganglionic transmission, and inhibits prolactin release, respectively.

Catecholamines are synthesized from tyrosine by a process of hydroxylation and decarboxylation (see Fig. 246–1). Tyrosine is derived from ingested food or synthesized from phenylalanine in the liver, and it enters neurons and chromaffin cells by active transport. Tyrosine is converted to 3,4-dihydroxyphenylalanine (dopa) by tyrosine hydroxylase, the rate-limiting step in catecholamine synthesis. α-Methyl-*p*-tyrosine (metyrosine) is a tyrosine hydroxylase inhibitor that may be used therapeutically in patients with catecholamine-secreting tumors. Aromatic L–amino acid decarboxylase catalyzes the decarboxylation of dopa to dopamine. Dopamine is actively transported into granulated vesicles to be hydroxylated to norepinephrine by the copper-containing enzyme dopamine β-hydroxylase. These reactions occur in the synaptic vesicle of adrenergic neurons in the central nervous system, the peripheral nervous system, and the chromaffin cells of the adrenal medulla. In the adrenal medulla, norepinephrine is released from the granule into the cytoplasm, where the cytosolic enzyme phenylethanolamine *N*-methyltransferase converts it to epinephrine. Expression of phenylethanolamine *N*-methyltransferase is regulated by the presence of glucocorticoids, which are in high concentration in the adrenal medulla. Thus, catecholamine-secreting tumors that secrete primarily epinephrine are localized to the adrenal medulla. In normal adrenal medullary tissue, approximately 80% of the catecholamine released is epinephrine.

Catecholamines are among the shortest lived signaling molecules in plasma; the initial biologic half-life of circulating catecholamines is between 10 and 100 seconds. Approximately half of the catecholamines

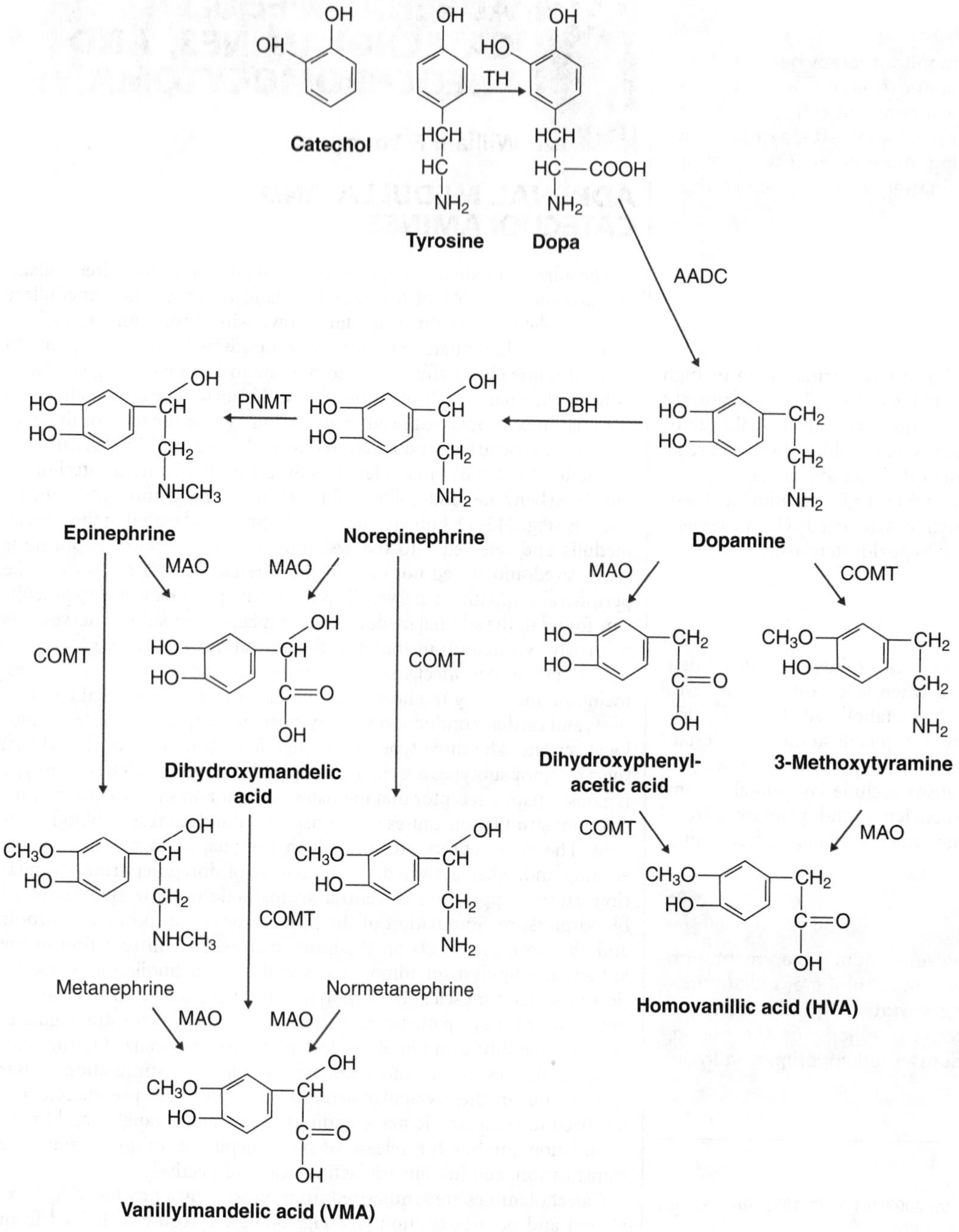

FIGURE 246–1 • Biosynthetic and metabolic pathways for catecholamines. The term *catecholamine* comes from the catechol (o-dihydroxybenzene) structure and a side chain with an amino group—the catechol nucleus (top left). Tyrosine is converted to 3,4-dihydroxyphenylalanine (dopa) in the rate-limiting step by tyrosine hydroxylase (TH). Aromatic L-amino acid decarboxylase (AADC) converts dopa to dopamine. Dopamine is hydroxylated to norepinephrine by dopamine β-hydroxylase (DBH). Norepinephrine is converted to epinephrine by phenylethanolamine *N*-methyltransferase (PNMT); cortisol serves as a cofactor for phenylethanolamine *N*-methyltransferase, and this is why epinephrine-secreting pheochromocytomas are almost exclusively localized to the adrenal medulla. Metabolism of catecholamines occurs through two enzymatic pathways. Catechol-*O*-methyltransferase (COMT) converts epinephrine to metanephrine and norepinephrine to normetanephrine by *meta-O*-methylation. Metanephrine and normetanephrine are oxidized by monoamine oxidase (MAO) to vanillylmandelic acid by oxidative deamination. Monoamine oxidase also may oxidize epinephrine and norepinephrine to dihydroxymandelic acid, which is then converted by catechol-*O*-methyltransferase to vanillylmandelic acid. Dopamine is also metabolized by monoamine oxidase and catechol-*O*-methyltransferase, with the final metabolite homovanillic acid.

circulate in plasma in loose association with albumin. Thus, plasma concentrations of catecholamines fluctuate widely. Catecholamines are removed from the circulation either by reuptake by sympathetic nerve terminals or by metabolism through two enzyme pathways (see Fig. 246–1), followed by sulfate conjugation and renal excretion. Almost 90% of catecholamines released at sympathetic synapses are taken up locally by the nerve endings (uptake 1). Uptake 1 can be blocked by cocaine, tricyclic antidepressants, and phenothiazines. Extraneuronal tissues also take up catecholamines, and this is termed uptake 2. Most of these catecholamines are metabolized by catechol-*O*-methyltransferase. Metanephrine and normetanephrine are oxidized by monoamine oxidase to vanillylmandelic acid by oxidative deamination. Monoamine oxidase may also oxidize epinephrine and norepinephrine to 3,4-dihydroxymandelic acid, which is then converted by catechol-*O*-methyltransferase to vanillylmandelic acid. Monoamine oxidase is located on the outer membrane of mitochondria. In the storage vesicle, norepinephrine is protected from metabolism by monoamine oxidase. Monoamine oxidase and catechol-*O*-methyltransferase metabolize dopamine to homovanillic acid (see Fig. 246–1).

PHEOCHROMOCYTOMA AND PARAGANGLIOMA

Definition

Catecholamine-secreting tumors that arise from chromaffin cells of the adrenal medulla and the sympathetic ganglia are referred to as pheochromocytomas and extra-adrenal catecholamine-secreting paragangliomas (extra-adrenal pheochromocytomas), respectively. Because the tumors have similar clinical presentations and are treated with similar approaches, many clinicians use the term *pheochromocytoma* to refer to both adrenal pheochromocytomas and extra-adrenal catecholamine-secreting paragangliomas. However, the distinction between pheochromocytoma and paraganglioma is an important one because of implications for associated neoplasms, risk for malignant transformation, and genetic testing.

Epidemiology

Catecholamine-secreting tumors are rare; the annual incidence is 2 to 8 cases per million people. Nevertheless, it is important to suspect, confirm, localize, and resect these tumors. The associated hypertension is curable with surgical removal of the tumor; a risk of lethal paroxysm exists; at least 10% of the tumors are malignant; and 15 to 20% are familial, and detection of this tumor in the proband may result in early diagnosis in other family members.

Pathobiology

Genetics

Approximately 15 to 20% of patients with catecholamine-secreting tumors have germline mutations (inherited mutations present in all cells of the body) in genes associated with genetic disease. Hereditary catecholamine-secreting tumors typically present at a younger age than sporadic neoplasms do. Sporadic pheochromocytoma typically is diagnosed on the basis of symptoms or an incidental discovery on computed imaging, whereas syndromic pheochromocytoma is frequently diagnosed earlier in the course of disease because of biochemical surveillance or genetic testing.

Multiple Endocrine Neoplasia

Multiple endocrine neoplasia (MEN) type 2a is an autosomal dominant disorder; the phenotype includes adrenal pheochromocytoma (usually bilateral and may be asynchronous), medullary carcinoma of the thyroid, and hyperparathyroidism. Medullary carcinoma of the thyroid is usually detected before pheochromocytoma. Numerous activating mutations throughout the *RET* proto-oncogene have been documented in persons with MEN type 2a. MEN type 2b is also an autosomal dominant disorder, and it represents approximately 5% of all MEN type 2 cases; the phenotype includes pheochromocytoma (usually bilateral), medullary carcinoma of the thyroid, mucosal neuromas, thickened corneal nerves, intestinal ganglioneuromatosis, and marfanoid body habitus. MEN type 2b is associated with mutations in codon 918 (in exon 16) of the *RET* proto-oncogene. Overall, pheochromocytoma occurs in approximately 50% of patients with MEN type 2.

Von Hippel–Lindau Disease

Von Hippel–Lindau disease (VHL) is an autosomal dominant disorder characterized by pheochromocytoma (frequently bilateral), paraganglioma (rarely), retinal angiomas, cerebellar hemangioblastoma, epididymal cystadenoma, renal and pancreatic cysts, and renal cell carcinoma. Pheochromocytoma is reported to occur in about 10 to 20% of patients with VHL. Nearly 100% of patients with VHL have an identifiable gene mutation (VHL tumor suppressor gene). Certain missense mutations appear to be associated with a "pheochromocytoma only" presentation of VHL.

Neurofibromatosis

Neurofibromatosis type 1 (NF1) is an autosomal dominant disorder characterized by neurofibromas, café au lait spots, axillary and inguinal freckling, and iris hamartomas (Lish nodules). Approximately 2% of patients with NF1 develop catecholamine-secreting tumors. In these patients, the catecholamine-secreting tumor is usually a solitary benign adrenal pheochromocytoma, occasionally bilateral adrenal pheochromocytoma, and rarely an abdominal paraganglioma. Inactivating *NF1* mutations cause the disorder (NF1 tumor suppressor gene).

Familial Paraganglioma

Familial paraganglioma is an autosomal dominant disorder characterized by paragangliomas that are located in the head and neck, thorax, abdomen, and pelvis. Most cases of familial paraganglioma are caused by mutations in the succinate dehydrogenase (SDH; succinate : ubiquinone oxidoreductase) subunit genes (*SDHB, SDHC, SDHD*), which compose portions of mitochondrial complex II. Inactivating germline mutations in *SDHD* have been identified in multigenerational families with head and neck parasympathetic paragangliomas that are usually nonfunctional and occasionally with adrenal pheochromocytoma. In patients with *SDHD* mutations, penetrance depends on the mutation's parent of origin. Hence, the disease is not manifested when the mutation is inherited from the mother but is highly penetrant when it is inherited from the father. This phenomenon is known as maternal imprinting. Missense mutations in *SDHC*, located on chromosome 1q21, have been reported in families with head and neck parasympathetic paragangliomas that are usually nonfunctional. The gene associated with paraganglioma syndrome type 2 has not been identified, although it has been mapped to chromosome 11q13.1. Like families with mutations in *SDHD*, families with paraganglioma syndrome type 2 also exhibit maternal imprinting. Inactivating mutations in the tumor suppressor gene *SDHB*, located on chromosome 1p35-36, are associated with paragangliomas in the abdomen, pelvis, and mediastinum. Adrenal pheochromocytomas may also be found in patients with *SDHB* mutations. Patients with *SDHB* mutations are at an increased risk for malignant paraganglioma.

Genetic Testing

Genetic testing should be considered if a patient has one or more of the following: paraganglioma; bilateral adrenal pheochromocytoma; unilateral adrenal pheochromocytoma and a family history of pheochromocytoma or paraganglioma; unilateral adrenal pheochromocytoma onset at a young age (<20 years); or other clinical findings suggestive of one of the previously discussed syndromic disorders. Genetic testing can be complex; testing of one family member has implications for related individuals. Genetic counseling is recommended to help families understand the implications of genetic test results; to coordinate testing of at-risk individuals; and to help families work through the psychosocial issues that may arise before, during, or after the testing process. The clinician may obtain a list of clinically approved molecular genetic diagnostic laboratories at *www.genetests.org.*

Clinical Manifestations

Catecholamine-secreting tumors occur with equal frequency in men and women, primarily in the third, fourth, and fifth decades. These tumors are rare in children; when discovered, they may be multifocal and associated with a hereditary syndrome. When symptoms are present, they are due to the pharmacologic effects of excess concentrations of circulating catecholamines (Table 246–1). The resulting hypertension may be sustained (in approximately half of the patients) or paroxysmal (in approximately a third of the patients). The remaining patients have normal blood pressure. Episodic symptoms may occur in spells, or paroxysms, that can be extremely variable in presentation but typically include forceful heartbeat, pallor, tremor, headache, and diaphoresis. The spell may start with a sensation of a "rush" in the chest and a sense of shortness of breath, followed by a "pounding" heartbeat in the chest that typically progresses to a throbbing headache. Peripheral vasoconstriction with a spell results in cool or cold hands and feet and facial pallor. Increased sense of body heat and sweating are common symptoms that occur toward the end of the spell. Spells may be either spontaneous or precipitated by postural change, anxiety, medications (e.g., metoclopramide, anesthetic agents), exercise, or maneuvers that increase intra-abdominal pressure (e.g., change in position, lifting, defecation, exercise, colonoscopy, pregnancy, trauma). Although the types of spells experienced across the population of patients are highly variable, spells tend to be stereotypical for each patient. Spells may occur multiple times daily or as infrequently as once monthly. The typical duration of a pheochromocytoma spell is 15 to 20 minutes, but it may be much shorter or last several hours. However, the clinician must recognize that most patients with spells do not have a pheochromocytoma.

Additional clinical signs of catecholamine-secreting tumors include hypertensive retinopathy, orthostatic hypotension, angina, nausea, constipation (megacolon may be the presenting symptom), hyperglycemia, diabetes mellitus, hypercalcemia, Raynaud's phenomenon, livedo reticularis, erythrocytosis, and mass effects from the tumor. The fasting hyperglycemia and diabetes mellitus are caused in part by the α-adrenergic inhibition of insulin release. Painless hematuria and paroxysmal attacks induced by micturition and defecation are associated with urinary bladder paragangliomas. Some of the co-secreted hormones that may dominate the clinical presentation include adrenocorticotropic hormone (Cushing's syndrome), parathyroid hormone–related peptide (hypercalcemia), vasopressin (syndrome of inappropriate antidiuretic hormone secretion), vasoactive intestinal peptide (watery diarrhea), and growth hormone–releasing hormone (acromegaly) (see Table 246–1). Cardiomyopathy and congestive heart failure are the symptomatic presenta-

TABLE 246–1 SIGNS AND SYMPTOMS ASSOCIATED WITH CATECHOLAMINE-SECRETING TUMORS

SPELL RELATED
Anxiety and fear of impending death
Diaphoresis
Dyspnea
Epigastric and chest pain
Headache
Hypertension
Nausea and vomiting
Pallor
Palpitation (forceful heartbeat)
Tremor
CHRONIC
Anxiety and fear of impending death
Cold hands and feet
Congestive heart failure—dilated or hypertrophic cardiomyopathy
Constipation
Diaphoresis
Dyspnea
Ectopic hormone secretion–dependent symptoms (e.g., CRH/ACTH, GHRH, PTH-RP, VIP)
Epigastric and chest pain
Fatigue
Fever
General increase in sweating
Grade II to IV retinopathy
Headache
Hyperglycemia
Hypertension
Nausea and vomiting
Orthostatic hypotension
Painless hematuria (associated with urinary bladder paraganglioma)
Pallor
Palpitation (forceful heartbeat)
Tremor
Weight loss
NOT TYPICAL OF PHEOCHROMOCYTOMA
Flushing

ACTH = adrenocorticotropic hormone; CRH = corticotropin-releasing hormone; GHRH = growth hormone–releasing hormone; PTH-RP = parathyroid hormone–related peptide; VIP = vasoactive intestinal polypeptide.
Modified from Young WF Jr: Pheochromocytoma: 1926–1993. Trends Endocrinol Metab 1993;4:122–127.

tions caused by pheochromocytoma that perhaps are most frequently unrecognized by clinicians. The cardiomyopathy, whether it is dilated or hypertrophic, may be totally reversible with tumor resection. Some patients with pheochromocytoma may be asymptomatic despite high circulating levels of catecholamines, probably reflecting adrenergic receptor desensitization related to chronic stimulation.

Pheochromocytomas are localized to the adrenal glands, with an average diameter of 4.5 cm (Fig. 246–2). Paragangliomas are found where there is chromaffin tissue: along the para-aortic sympathetic chain, within the organs of Zuckerkandl (at the origin of the inferior mesenteric artery), in the wall of the urinary bladder, and along the sympathetic chain in the neck or mediastinum. Paragangliomas in the head and neck region (e.g., carotid body tumors, glomus tumors, chemodectomas) usually arise from parasympathetic tissue and typically do not hypersecrete catecholamines and metanephrines, whereas paragangliomas in the mediastinum, abdomen, and pelvis usually arise from sympathetic chromaffin tissue and usually do hypersecrete catecholamines and metanephrines.

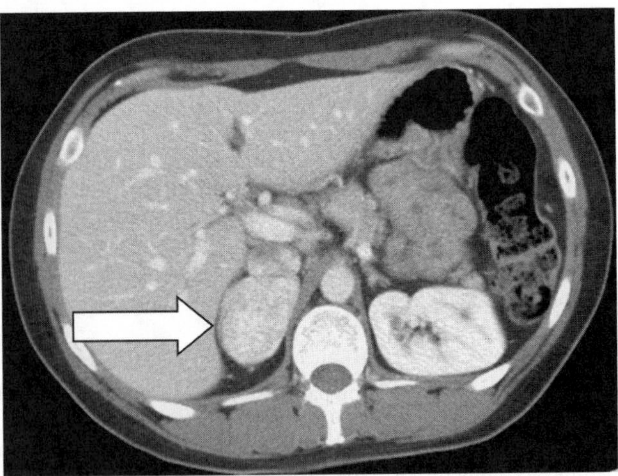

FIGURE 246–2 • A computed tomographic scan of the abdomen with intravenous administration of a contrast agent in a 32-year-old second-year medical student with a peripartum discovery of pheochromocytoma. The fractionated plasma free metanephrines were abnormal: metanephrine, 0.19 nmol/L (normal, <0.5 nmol/L); and normetanephrine, 28.6 nmol/L (normal, <0.9 nmol/L). The 24-hour urine studies were abnormal: norepinephrine, 781 μg (normal, <170 μg); epinephrine, 2.4 μg (normal, <35 μg); dopamine, 197 μg (normal, <700 μg); metanephrine, 117 μg (normal, <400 μg); and normetanephrine, 8760 μg (normal, <900 μg). The axial image shows a typical 5-cm heterogeneously enhancing right adrenal mass consistent with pheochromocytoma (arrow). After α- and β-adrenergic blockade, a 5.3 × 5.0 × 2.0-cm 40-g pheochromocytoma was removed laparoscopically.

TABLE 246–2 MEDICATIONS THAT MAY INCREASE MEASURED LEVELS OF CATECHOLAMINES AND METANEPHRINES

Tricyclic antidepressants
Levodopa
Drugs containing adrenergic receptor agonists (e.g., decongestants)
Amphetamines
Buspirone and most psychoactive agents
Prochlorperazine
Reserpine
Withdrawal from clonidine and other drugs
Ethanol
Acetaminophen (may increase measured levels of fractionated plasma metanephrines in some assays)

Diagnosis

Differential Diagnosis

Numerous disorders can cause signs and symptoms that may trigger the clinician to test for pheochromocytoma. The disorders span much of medicine and include endocrine disorders (e.g., primary hypogonadism), cardiovascular disorders (e.g., idiopathic orthostatic hypotension), psychological disorders (e.g., panic disorder), pharmacologic causes (e.g., withdrawal from an adrenergic inhibitor), neurologic disorders (e.g., postural orthostatic tachycardia syndrome), and miscellaneous disorders (e.g., mast cell disease). Indeed, most patients tested for pheochromocytoma do not have it. In addition, fractionated catecholamines and metanephrines may be elevated in several clinical scenarios: withdrawal from medications or drugs (e.g., clonidine, alcohol), any acute illness (e.g., subarachnoid hemorrhage, migraine headache, preeclampsia), and many drugs and medications (e.g., tricyclic antidepressants, cocaine, phencyclidine, lysergic acid diethylamide, amphetamines, ephedrine, pseudoephedrine, phenylpropanolamine, isoproterenol) (Table 246–2).

Pheochromocytoma should be suspected in patients who have one or more of the following: hyperadrenergic spells (e.g., self-limited episodes of nonexertional palpitations, diaphoresis, headache, tremor, or pallor);

resistant hypertension; a familial syndrome that predisposes to catecholamine-secreting tumors (e.g., MEN 2, NF1, VHL); a family history of pheochromocytoma or a history of a previously resected pheochromocytoma and a present history of recurrent hypertension or spells; an incidentally discovered adrenal mass; hypertension and diabetes; pressor response during anesthesia, surgery, or angiography; onset of hypertension at a young age (e.g., before 20 years); and idiopathic dilated cardiomyopathy.

Laboratory Findings

The diagnosis must be confirmed biochemically by increased concentrations of fractionated catecholamines and fractionated metanephrines in the urine or plasma (Fig. 246–3). Most laboratories now measure fractionated catecholamines (dopamine, norepinephrine, and epinephrine) and metanephrines (metanephrine and normetanephrine) by high-performance liquid chromatography with electrochemical detection or tandem mass spectroscopy. These techniques have overcome the problems with fluorometric analysis (e.g., false-positive results caused by α-methyldopa, labetalol, sotalol, and imaging contrast agents). One of the most reliable case-finding methods for identifying catecholamine-secreting tumors is measurement of metanephrines and catecholamines in a 24-hour urine collection (sensitivity, 98%; specificity, 98%). If clinical suspicion is high, fractionated plasma free metanephrines should also be measured. Some groups have advocated that fractionated plasma free metanephrines should be measured as a first-line test for pheochromocytoma; the predictive value of a negative test result is extremely high, and the finding of normal fractionated plasma metanephrine levels excludes pheochromocytoma except in patients with early preclinical disease and those with strictly dopamine-secreting neoplasms. A plasma test is also attractive because of simplicity. Although measurement of fractionated plasma metanephrines has a sensitivity of 96 to 100%, the specificity is poor at 85 to 89%; the specificity falls to 77% in patients older than 60 years. It has been estimated that 97% of patients with hypertension seen in a tertiary care clinic who have an abnormal fractionated plasma metanephrine measurement will not have a pheochromocytoma. This high rate of false-positive tests results in excessive health care expenditures because of subsequent imaging and potentially inappropriate surgery. Thus, fractionated plasma free metanephrines lack the necessary specificity to be recommended as a first-line test; therefore, this measurement is reserved for cases for which the index of suspicion is high.

The index of suspicion for pheochromocytoma should be high (see Fig. 246–3) in patients with the clinical scenarios described before and in those patients with an incidentally discovered adrenal mass that has imaging characteristics consistent with pheochromocytoma. These include marked enhancement with intravenous contrast medium on computed tomography (CT), high signal intensity on T2-weighted magnetic resonance imaging (MRI), cystic and hemorrhagic changes, bilaterality, and larger size (e.g., >4 cm) (see later). In addition, measurement of fractionated plasma free metanephrines is a good first-line test for children because it is difficult to obtain a complete 24-hour urine collection.

Although it is preferred that patients not receive any medication during the diagnostic evaluation, treatment with most medications may be continued. Tricyclic antidepressants interfere most frequently with the interpretation of 24-hour urinary catecholamines and metabolites. For effective screening of catecholamine-secreting tumors, treatment with tricyclic antidepressants and other psychoactive agents listed in Table 246–2 should be tapered and discontinued at least 2 weeks before any hormonal assessments. Furthermore, catecholamine secretion may be appropriately increased in situations of physical stress or illness (e.g.,

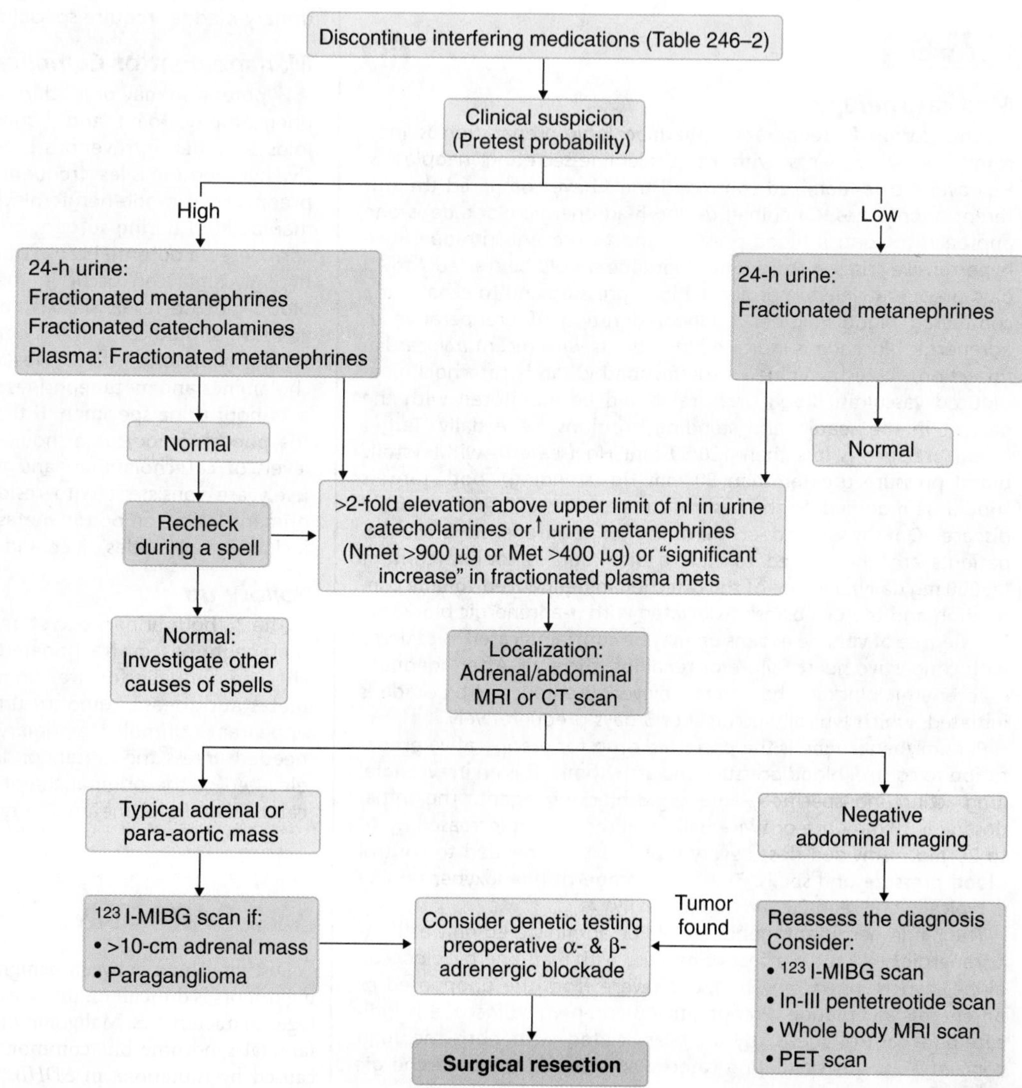

FIGURE 246–3 • Evaluation and treatment of catecholamine-secreting tumors. Clinical suspicion is triggered by the following: paroxysmal symptoms (especially hypertension); hypertension that is intermittent, unusually labile, or resistant to treatment; family history of pheochromocytoma or associated conditions; or incidentally discovered adrenal mass. The details are discussed in the text. CT = computed tomography; ^{123}I-MIBG = ^{123}I-metaiodobenzylguanidine; mets = metanephrines; MRI = magnetic resonance imaging; nl, normal; Nmet = normetanephrine; PET = positron emission tomography. (Modified from Young WF Jr: Pheochromocytoma: 1926–1993. Trends Endocrinol Metab 1993;4:122, with permission.)

stroke, myocardial infarction, congestive heart failure, obstructive sleep apnea). Therefore, the clinical circumstances under which catecholamines and metanephrines are measured must be assessed in each case.

Imaging

Localization studies should not be initiated until biochemical studies have confirmed the diagnosis of a catecholamine-secreting tumor (see Fig. 246–3). Computer-assisted imaging of the adrenal glands and abdomen with MRI or CT should be the first localization test (sensitivity, >95%; specificity, >65%) (see Fig. 246–3). Approximately 85% of these tumors are found in the adrenal glands, and 95% are found in the abdomen. Although CT is still the primary adrenal imaging modality, MRI has advantages in certain clinical situations. Early in the history of abdominal MRI, it became clear that with low- or mid-field strength magnets, T1- and T2-weighted imaging could be used to differentiate pheochromocytoma and malignant neoplasms from benign adenomas. If the results of abdominal imaging are normal, scintigraphic localization with ^{123}I-labeled metaiodobenzylguanidine (^{123}I-MIBG) is indicated (see Fig. 246–3). This radiopharmaceutical agent accumulates preferentially in catecholamine-producing tumors (sensitivity, 80%; specificity, 99%). If a typical (<10 cm) unilateral adrenal pheochromocytoma is found on CT or MRI, ^{123}I-MIBG scintigraphy is superfluous and the results may even confuse the clinician. If the adrenal pheochromocytoma is larger than 10 cm in diameter or if a paraganglioma is identified on CT or MRI, ^{123}I-MIBG scintigraphy is indicated because the patient has increased risk of malignant disease and additional paragangliomas.

Localizing procedures that also can be used but are rarely required include computer-assisted imaging of the chest, neck, and head; somatostatin receptor imaging with [^{111}In] pentetreotide; and positron emission tomography scanning with [^{18}F]fluorodeoxyglucose, [^{11}C] hydroxyephedrine, or 6-[^{18}F]fluorodopamine (see Fig. 246–3).

Treatment

Rx

Medical Therapy

Some form of preoperative pharmacologic preparation is indicated for all patients with catecholamine-secreting neoplasms. However, no randomized controlled trials have compared the different approaches. Combined α- and β-adrenergic blockade is one approach to control blood pressure and to prevent intraoperative hypertensive crises. α-Adrenergic blockade should be started 7 to 10 days preoperatively to normalize blood pressure and to expand the contracted blood volume. A longer duration of preoperative α-adrenergic blockade is indicated in patients with recent myocardial infarction, catecholamine cardiomyopathy, and catecholamine-induced vasculitis. Blood pressure should be monitored with the patient in the seated and standing positions twice daily. Target blood pressure is less than 120/80 mm Hg (seated), with systolic blood pressure greater than 90 mm Hg (standing); both targets should be modified on the basis of the patient's age and comorbid disease. On the second or third day of α-adrenergic blockade, patients are encouraged to start a diet high in sodium content (≥5000 mg daily) because of the catecholamine-induced volume contraction and the orthostasis associated with α-adrenergic blockade. This degree of volume expansion may be contraindicated in patients with congestive heart failure or renal insufficiency. After adequate α-adrenergic blockade has been achieved, β-adrenergic blockade is initiated, which typically occurs 2 or 3 days preoperatively.

Phenoxybenzamine is the preferred drug for preoperative preparation to control blood pressure and arrhythmia. It is an irreversible, long-acting, nonspecific α-adrenergic blocking agent. The initial dosage is 10 mg once or twice daily, and the dose is increased by 10 to 20 mg in divided doses every 2 or 3 days as needed to control blood pressure and spells. The final dosage of phenoxybenzamine is typically between 20 and 100 mg daily.

The β-adrenergic antagonist should be administered only after α-adrenergic blockade is effective because with β-adrenergic blockade alone, hypertension may be more severe from the unopposed α-adrenergic stimulation. Preoperative β-adrenergic blockade is indicated to control the tachycardia associated with both the high concentrations of circulating catecholamines and the α-adrenergic

Rx

blockade. The clinician should exercise caution if the patient is asthmatic or has congestive heart failure. Chronic catecholamine excess can produce a cardiomyopathy that may become evident with the initiation of β-adrenergic blockade, resulting in acute pulmonary edema. Therefore, when the β-adrenergic blocker is administered, it should be used cautiously and at a low dose. Other agents that may be used to prepare the patient with pheochromocytoma for surgery include α-methyl-*p*-tyrosine (metyrosine) and calcium-channel blockers. Acute hypertensive crises may occur before or during an operation, and they should be treated intravenously with sodium nitroprusside, phentolamine, or nicardipine.

Surgical Therapy

The treatment of choice for pheochromocytoma is complete surgical resection. Surgical survival rates are 98 to 100% and are highly dependent on the skill of the endocrinologist–endocrine surgeon–anesthesiologist team. Careful preoperative pharmacologic preparation is crucial for successful treatment. Most catecholamine-secreting tumors are benign and can be totally excised. Tumor excision usually cures hypertension.

In the past, an anterior midline abdominal surgical approach was generally used to resect adrenal pheochromocytoma. However, the laparoscopic approach to the adrenal gland is currently the procedure of choice for patients with solitary intra-adrenal pheochromocytomas smaller than 8 cm in diameter. Laparoscopic adrenalectomy for pheochromocytoma should be converted to open adrenalectomy for difficult dissection, invasion, adhesions, or inexperience of the surgeon. An anterior midline abdominal surgical approach is indicated for abdominal paragangliomas. The midline abdomen should be inspected carefully. Paragangliomas of the neck, chest, and urinary bladder require specialized approaches.

Management of Complications

Hypotension may occur during and after surgical resection of the pheochromocytoma, and it should be treated with fluids and colloids and then intravenous pressor agents if necessary. Postoperative hypotension is less frequent in patients who have had adequate preoperative α-adrenergic blockade. If both adrenal glands were manipulated during surgery, adrenocortical insufficiency should be considered a potential cause of postoperative hypotension. Because hypoglycemia can occur in the immediate postoperative period, blood glucose levels should be monitored, and fluid given intravenously should contain 5% dextrose.

Approximately 1 to 2 weeks after surgery, fractionated catecholamines and metanephrines should be measured by collection of a 24-hour urine specimen. If the levels are normal, the resection of the pheochromocytoma should be considered complete. Increased levels of catecholamines and metanephrines detected postoperatively are consistent with residual tumor due to either a second primary lesion or occult metastases. Common sites of metastasis include lymph nodes, liver, and bone.

Follow-up

The 24-hour urinary excretion of fractionated catecholamines and metanephrines or fractionated plasma metanephrines should be checked annually for life. Annual biochemical testing assesses for metastatic disease, tumor recurrence in the adrenal bed, or delayed appearance of multiple primary tumors. Follow-up CT or MRI is not needed unless the metanephrine or catecholamine levels become elevated or the original tumor was associated with minimal or no catecholamine or metanephrine excess.

MALIGNANT PHEOCHROMOCYTOMA AND PARAGANGLIOMA

Distinguishing between benign and malignant catecholamine-secreting tumors is difficult on the basis of clinical, biochemical, or histopathologic characteristics. Malignant disease is rare in patients with an adrenal familial syndrome but common in those with familial paraganglioma caused by mutations in *SDHB*. Although the 5-year survival rate for patients with malignant pheochromocytoma is less than 50%, the prognosis is variable; approximately 50% of patients have an indolent form of the disease, with a life expectancy of more than 20 years, and the other 50% of patients have rapidly progressive disease, with death occurring within 1 to 3 years after diagnosis. The clinician should first assess the pace of the malignant disease and target the level of therapy to the aggressiveness of the tumor behavior. A multimodality multidisciplinary individualized approach is indicated to control catecholamine-dependent symptoms, local mass effects, and overall tumor burden.

PHEOCHROMOCYTOMA IN PREGNANCY

Pheochromocytoma in pregnancy can cause the death of both the fetus and the mother. The approach to the biochemical diagnosis is the same as for the nonpregnant patient. MRI is the preferred imaging modality, and ^{123}I-MIBG is contraindicated. The treatment of hypertensive crises is the same as for nonpregnant patients except that use of nitroprusside should be avoided. Although the most appropriate management is debated, adrenal pheochromocytomas should be removed promptly if diagnosis is made during the first two trimesters of pregnancy. The preoperative preparation is the same as for a nonpregnant patient. If the pregnancy is in the third trimester, one operation is recommended for a cesarean delivery and removal of the adrenal pheochromocytoma at the same time. Spontaneous labor and delivery should be avoided. The management of catecholamine-secreting paragangliomas in pregnancy may require modification of these guidelines, depending on tumor location.

SUGGESTED READINGS

Erickson D, Kudva YC, Ebersold MJ, et al: Benign paragangliomas: Clinical presentation and treatment outcomes in 236 patients. J Clin Endocrinol Metab 2001;86:5210–5216. *Comprehensive report from the Mayo Clinic on patients with benign paragangliomas.*

Gumbs AA, Gagner M: Laparoscopic adrenalectomy. Best Pract Res Clin Endocrinol Metab 2006;20:483–499. *The role for laparoscopic surgery in adrenal diseases.*

Kudva YC, Sawka AM, Young WF Jr: Clinical review 164: The laboratory diagnosis of adrenal pheochromocytoma: The Mayo Clinic experience. J Clin Endocrinol Metab 2003;88:4533–4539. *Extensive review and update of the laboratory diagnosis of pheochromocytoma.*

Pawlu C, Bausch B, Reisch N, Neumann HP: Genetic testing for pheochromocytoma-associated syndromes. Ann Endocrinol (Paris) 2005;66:178–185. *Summary of the role for genetic testing in patients with pheochromocytoma or paraganglioma.*

Pecak K, Eisenhofer G, Ahlman H: Pheochromocytoma: Recommendations for clinical practice from the First International Symposium. Nat Clin Pract Endocrinol Metab 2007;3:92–102. *Comprehensive review.*

Young WF Jr: The incidentally discovered adrenal mass. N Engl J Med 2007; 356:601–610. *How to work-up adrenal masses.*

247 TYPE 1 DIABETES MELLITUS

Silvio E. Inzucchi and Robert S. Sherwin

TYPE 1 DIABETES MELLITUS

Definition

Diabetes mellitus is a chronic disorder characterized by the impaired metabolism of glucose and other energy-yielding fuels as well as by the late development of vascular and neuropathic complications. Diabetes comprises a group of disorders involving distinct pathogenic mechanisms, for which hyperglycemia is the common denominator. Regardless of its cause, the disease is associated with a common hormonal defect, namely, insulin deficiency, which may be absolute or relative in the context of coexisting insulin resistance. Insufficient insulin effect plays a primary role in the metabolic derangements linked to diabetes; hyperglycemia in turn plays an important role in disease-related complications.

Classification

The American Diabetes Association classification scheme for diabetes mellitus is summarized in Table 247–1. Clinical diabetes is divided into four general subclasses: type 1, primarily caused by autoimmune pancreatic β-cell destruction and characterized by absolute insulin deficiency; type 2, characterized by insulin resistance and relative insulin deficiency; "other" specific types of diabetes (associated with identifiable clinical conditions or syndromes); and gestational diabetes mellitus. In addition to these clinical categories, two forms of pre-diabetes—impaired glucose tolerance and impaired fasting glucose—have been defined to describe intermediate metabolic states between normal glucose homeostasis and overt diabetes. Both impaired glucose tolerance and impaired fasting glucose significantly increase the future risk for development of diabetes mellitus and in many cases are part of the disease's natural history. Patients with any form of diabetes may require insulin therapy; for this reason, the previously used terms *insulin-dependent diabetes* (for type 1) and *non–insulin-dependent diabetes* (for type 2) have been eliminated.

TABLE 247–1 CLASSIFICATION OF DIABETES MELLITUS

ESTABLISHED DIABETES MELLITUS
Type 1 diabetes, formerly known as insulin-dependent diabetes mellitus or juvenile-onset diabetes (primarily due to β-cell destruction, usually leading to absolute insulin deficiency)
Immune mediated
Idiopathic
Type 2 diabetes, formerly known as non–insulin-dependent diabetes or adult-onset diabetes (may range from predominantly insulin resistance with relative insulin deficiency to predominantly secretory defect with insulin resistance)
Other specific types
Genetic defects of β-cell function (e.g., maturity-onset diabetes of the young, types 1 to 6; point mutations in mitochondrial DNA)
Genetic defects in insulin action (e.g., type A insulin resistance, leprechaunism, Rabson-Mendenhall syndrome, lipoatrophic diabetes)
Disease of the exocrine pancreas (e.g., pancreatitis, trauma, pancreatectomy, neoplasia, cystic fibrosis, hemochromatosis, fibrocalculous pancreatopathy)
Endocrinopathies (e.g., acromegaly, Cushing's syndrome, hyperthyroidism, pheochromocytoma, glucagonoma, somatostatinoma, aldosteronoma)
Drug or chemical induced (e.g., vacor, pentamidine, nicotinic acid, glucocorticoids, thyroid hormone, diazoxide, β-adrenergic agonists, thiazides, phenytoin, interferon alfa)
Infections (e.g., congenital rubella, cytomegalovirus)
Uncommon forms of immune-mediated diabetes (e.g., "stiff-man" syndrome, anti–insulin receptor antibodies)
Other genetic syndromes (e.g., Down syndrome, Klinefelter's syndrome, Turner's syndrome, Wolfram's syndrome, Friedreich's ataxia, Huntington's disease, Laurence-Moon-Biedl syndrome, myotonic dystrophy, porphyria, Prader-Willi syndrome)
Gestational diabetes mellitus
RISK CATEGORIES FOR DIABETES MELLITUS
Impaired fasting glucose
Impaired glucose tolerance

Epidemiology

In 2005, the Centers for Disease Control and Prevention estimated that nearly 21 million Americans (or nearly 7% of the U.S. population) fulfilled the diagnostic criteria for diabetes mellitus. Of these, most (90 to 95%) have type 2 diabetes (Chapter 248). In those older than 60 years, the prevalence is now estimated at 21%. Approximately 6 million of those currently affected (nearly 30%) do not know they have diabetes. An additional 41 million Americans have pre-diabetes. Since 1980, the prevalence of diabetes in the United States has more than doubled. The number of affected patients continues to rise, with current estimates exceeding 1.4 million new cases per year. It is estimated that one of every three Americans born in 2000 will develop diabetes in their lifetime. Diabetes is the fourth most common reason for contact of a patient with an American physician, accounting for approximately 14% of U.S. health care dollars and total annual costs exceeding $132 billion in 2002—$92 billion in direct medical costs and another $40 billion in indirect costs due to losses in productivity. Worldwide, diabetes affects more than 194 million people; this figure is projected to reach 366 million cases by the year 2030. Unfortunately, the rate of growth of diabetes is largest in developing nations because of increased urbanization and westernization of lifestyle habits but where barriers still exist to proper diagnosis and treatment.

Diabetes is a leading cause of both mortality and early disability; in the United States, it is the leading cause of blindness among working-age adults, end-stage renal disease, and nontraumatic limb amputations. Diabetes increases the risk of cardiac, cerebral, and peripheral vascular disease two- to seven-fold and is a major contributor to neonatal morbidity and mortality and in the obstetric setting. A growing body of evidence, however, suggests that most if not all of the debilitating complications of diabetes can be prevented or delayed by the prospective treatment of hyperglycemia and other cardiovascular risk factors. In treating diabetes, the timing of therapy is crucial; clinical outcomes depend on early recognition and treatment of the disease.

Incidence and Prevalence

Prevalence rates for type 1 diabetes are relatively accurate because these patients invariably become symptomatic; current estimates for the United States hover between 0.3 and 0.4%. Type 1 diabetes is more prevalent in Finland, Scandinavia, and Scotland; less prevalent in most of Southern Europe and the Middle East; and uncommon in Asian nations. The annual incidence appears to have risen in the last half-century, which could imply the introduction of an unidentified environmental factor. Prevalence rates are strikingly different among ethnic groups living in the same geographic region, probably because of genetic differences in susceptibility to the disease.

Recent recognition that type 1 diabetes has a protracted preclinical phase has shed new light on some epidemiologic characteristics of the disease. Type 1 diabetes has an increased incidence in the winter months and may be associated with specific viral epidemics. These observations may in part be explained by the superimposition of illness-provoked insulin resistance in patients with marginal β-cell function. Similarly, the common appearance of type 1 diabetes during puberty may also be attributed to insulin resistance; even under normal circumstances, puberty is accompanied by impaired insulin-stimulated glucose metabolism. New methods for tracking islet-directed autoimmunity have led to a reappraisal of the age at which type 1 diabetes first appears. Although the age-specific incidence rises progressively from infancy to puberty and then declines, incidence rates persist at low levels for many decades; in fact, nearly 30% of patients are diagnosed after the age of 20 years. In the patients with later onset, the clinical syndrome tends to evolve more slowly; in addition, islet-directed antibody titers may be lower, and HLA types may be different from those of younger patients. As a result, type 1 diabetes is initially misdiagnosed as type 2 in many of these patients.

Pathobiology

Insulin Secretion and Action

The gene coding for human insulin is located on the short arm of chromosome 11. Insulin is initially synthesized in pancreatic β cells as proinsulin, a single-chain, 86–amino acid polypeptide. Subsequent cleavage of proinsulin removes a connecting strand (C-peptide) to form the smaller, double-chain insulin molecule, which contains 51 amino acid residues. Both insulin and the C-peptide remnant are packaged in membrane-bound storage granules; stimulation of insulin secretion results in the discharge of equimolar amounts of insulin and C-peptide (and a small amount of proinsulin) into the portal circulation. Whereas insulin is heavily metabolized during its first pass through the liver, the C-peptide fragment largely escapes hepatic metabolism; as a result, peripheral C-peptide levels provide a more precise marker of endogenous insulin secretion.

Glucose Concentration

Glucose concentration is the key regulator of insulin secretion. For activation of secretion, a glucose molecule must first be transported by a protein (GLUT 2) into the β cell, phosphorylated by the enzyme glucokinase, and metabolized. The precise triggering process is poorly understood but probably involves activation of signal transduction pathways and mitochondrial signals, closure of adenosine triphosphate–sensitive potassium channels, and calcium entry into the cytoplasm of the β cell. Normally, when blood glucose concentration rises even slightly above fasting levels, β cells secrete insulin, initially from preformed (stored) insulin and later from de novo insulin synthesis as well. The magnitude of the insulin response is determined by the level of glucose as well as by the mode of glucose entry; compared with intravenous administration, higher insulin levels are produced when glucose is given orally because of the simultaneous release of gut peptides known as incretins (e.g., glucagon-like peptide 1, gastric inhibitory polypeptide) that amplify the insulin response (see later).

Other Secretagogues

Other insulin secretagogues include amino acids (e.g., leucine), vagal stimulation, sulfonylurea drugs, repaglinide, nateglinide, and agents that modulate the incretin system, such as GLP-1 agonists and DPP-IV inhibitors (Chapter 248). Once it is secreted into the portal vein, 50% or more of insulin is removed by first pass through the liver. The consequence of this hepatic metabolism is that portal vein insulin levels are at least two- to four-fold higher than levels in the peripheral circulation. This point has clinical relevance with regard to insulin therapy; whereas insulin secreted by pancreatic β cells directly enters the portal circulation, peripherally administered insulin cannot adequately raise portal insulin levels and therefore may be less efficient in inducing hepatic effects.

Insulin Action

Insulin acts on its target tissues (liver, muscle, and fat, primarily) through a specific insulin receptor, which is a heterodimer containing two α and two β chains linked by disulfide bridges. The α subunits of the receptor reside on the extracellular surface and are the sites of insulin binding. The β subunits span the membrane and can be phosphorylated on serine, threonine, and tyrosine residues on the cytoplasmic face. The intrinsic protein tyrosine kinase activity of the β subunit is essential for the function of the insulin receptor. Rapid receptor autophosphorylation and tyrosine phosphorylation of insulin receptor substrates (IRS-1 and IRS-2) are important early steps in insulin action. Thereafter, a series of phosphorylation and dephosphorylation reactions are triggered, leading to insulin's ultimate effects. A variety of postreceptor signal transduction pathways are activated by insulin, including phosphatidylinositol 3-kinase, an enzyme whose product appears to be critical for the eventual translocation of glucose transport proteins (GLUT 4) from inside the cell to the cell surface to facilitate glucose uptake.

A number of so-called counter-regulatory hormones oppose the metabolic actions of insulin, including glucagon, growth hormone, cortisol, and catecholamines. Among these, glucagon and, to a lesser extent, growth hormone play a role in the expression of the diabetic state. Glucagon is normally secreted by pancreatic α cells in response to hypoglycemia, amino acids, and activation of the autonomic nervous system. Its chief effects are on the liver, where it stimulates glycogenolysis, gluconeogenesis, and ketogenesis through cyclic adenosine monophosphate–dependent mechanisms. Glucagon release is normally inhibited by hyperglycemia; however, in both types of diabetes, glucagon levels are absolutely or, more commonly, relatively *elevated* despite the presence of hyperglycemia. Growth hormone secretion by the anterior pituitary gland is also inappropriately increased in type 1 diabetes, a result (at least in part) of the body's attempt to overcome a defect in insulin-like growth factor type 1 generation caused by insulin deficiency. The major metabolic actions of growth hormone are on peripheral tissues, where it acts to promote lipolysis and to inhibit glucose use. In type 1 diabetic patients with reduced portal insulin levels, growth hormone is also capable of stimulating hepatic glucose production.

Metabolic Effects of Insulin

Insulin deficiency—whether it is relative or absolute—plays a pivotal role in the pathophysiologic process of diabetes mellitus. The effects of insulin lack are best appreciated by first examining the normal role of insulin in fuel homeostasis.

Fasted State

After an overnight fast, low basal insulin levels result in diminished glucose uptake in peripheral insulin-sensitive tissues (e.g., muscle and fat). In the fasted state, most glucose uptake occurs in insulin-insensitive tissues, primarily the brain, which because of its inability to use long-chain free fatty acids is critically dependent on a constant supply of glucose for oxidative metabolism. Maintenance of stable blood glucose levels is achieved through the release of glucose by the liver (and, to a small extent, by the kidney); production rates of 7 to 10 g/hr (~2 mg/kg/min) match those of the consuming tissues. The hepatic processes involved are glycogenolysis and gluconeogenesis; both play a significant role, and both depend critically on the balance between insulin and glucagon in the portal circulation. Reduced portal insulin levels decrease glycogen synthesis, which allows glucagon's stimulatory effect on glycogenolysis to prevail. Glucagon predominance also stimulates gluconeogenesis, whereas concurrent low insulin levels promote the peripheral mobilization of gluconeogenic precursors (amino acids, lactate, pyruvate, glycerol) and alternative energy sources (free fatty acids).

Fed State

Ingestion of a large glucose load triggers multiple homeostatic mechanisms to minimize glucose excursions, including suppression of endogenous glucose production, stimulation of hepatic glucose uptake, and acceleration of glucose uptake by peripheral tissues, predominantly muscle. Each of these mechanisms depends principally on insulin. In the liver, meal-stimulated insulin levels rapidly suppress glucose production. At least 30% of ingested glucose is deposited directly in the liver by glycogen synthesis and storage; concurrently, hepatic triglyceride synthesis increases. Peripherally, insulin-stimulated glucose transport across the cell membrane of both adipose and muscle tissue is attributable to the recruitment of glucose transport proteins (i.e., GLUT 4) from the cytosolic compartment to the plasma membrane. In muscle, glucose may then be metabolized or converted to glycogen for storage. In adipose tissue, glucose is used primarily for the formation of α-glycerophosphate, which is necessary for the esterification of free fatty acids to form triglycerides for storage in adipose tissue.

The scenario described—the ingestion of large quantities of pure glucose—is not representative of conditions during ordinary meals. If the quantity of carbohydrate consumed and resulting insulin response are small, glucose homeostasis is maintained largely by reduced hepatic glucose production rather than by increased glucose uptake because glucose production is much more sensitive than glucose uptake to the effects of small changes in insulin secretion. The rise in insulin that accompanies the consumption of mixed meals also facilitates protein and fat storage. Because muscle is in negative nitrogen balance in the fasting state, repletion of muscle nitrogen depends on the net uptake of amino acids in response to protein feeding. In muscle, insulin acts to promote positive nitrogen balance by facilitating amino acid uptake, by inhibiting the breakdown of protein, and (to a lesser extent) by stimulating new protein synthesis. In adipose tissue, the action of insulin accelerates triglyceride incorporation by stimulating lipoprotein lipase while simultaneously inhibiting the hormone-sensitive lipase, which catalyzes the hydrolysis of stored triglycerides. In adipose tissue, the net effect of insulin is to inhibit lipolysis and to promote the synthesis and storage of triglycerides.

The Role of the Incretins

It has long been recognized that an equivalent amount of carbohydrate administered by mouth generates a more robust pancreatic insulin response than when it is administered by vein. This "incretin" effect is the result of the secretion of insulinotropic peptides by the gut, in response to meals that augment insulin output. The best studied of these hormones, glucagon-like peptide 1, has additional beneficial effects on glucose homeostasis, including the attenuation of glucagon secretion, a slowing of gastric emptying, and, most likely, a central effect to promote satiety.

Metabolic Defects in Diabetes

Fasting Hyperglycemia

In both type 1 and type 2 diabetes, fasting hyperglycemia results mainly from an inappropriate increase in hepatic glucose production; this effect is magnified in type 1 diabetes due to absolute portal insulin deficiency. Increased hepatic glucose production in both types of diabetes is due mostly to accelerated gluconeogenesis; the loss of insulin's restraining effect on the α cell leads to a relative increase in portal glucagon levels, resulting in increased uptake and conversion of glycogenic substrates to glucose within the liver. Insulin deficiency in type 1 diabetes leads to the hypersecretion of growth hormone as well, which further accentuates glucose overproduction. In the extreme situation of total insulin lack, marked increases in counter-regulatory hormone release further stimulate gluconeogenesis while blocking compensatory increases in glucose disposal. The clinical correlate is profound hyperglycemia and glycosuria (Fig. 247–1).

Postprandial Hyperglycemia

Diabetes is also characterized by marked postprandial hyperglycemia. In type 2 diabetes, delayed insulin secretion and hepatic insulin resistance join forces to impair both suppression of hepatic glucose production and the liver's ability to store glucose as glycogen. Hyperglycemia ensues, even though insulin levels may eventually rise to levels above those seen in nondiabetic individuals (insulin secretion remains deficient relative to the prevailing glucose level), because insulin resistance also reduces the capacity of myocytes to extract and to store the ingested carbohydrate calories and the excess glucose released from the liver.

Under normal circumstances, insulin increases the levels of glucose 6-phosphate in muscle; this rise is markedly attenuated in diabetes, which implies that the block in glycogen synthesis and glucose metabolism precedes glucose 6-phosphate formation and thus is mediated at the level of glucose transport (by GLUT 4). The conversion of glucose to glucose 6-phosphate (by hexokinase) may contribute as well. These defects are more pronounced in patients with severe hyperglycemia, in whom insulin secretion is further reduced.

Type 1 patients show the most marked and prolonged elevations in blood glucose after ingestion of carbohydrates. These individuals have low portal vein insulin levels, which cannot be reversed by subcutaneous insulin therapy. Consequently, during hyperglycemia, the liver fails to arrest glucose production and fails to appropriately take up glucose for storage as glycogen. In addition, glucose uptake by peripheral tissues is impaired by the lack of insulin and by the development of insulin resistance secondary to chronic insulin deprivation and the toxic effects of chronic hyperglycemia. The net result is a gross defect in glucose disposal that can be compensated only partially by renal glycosuria.

Free Fatty Acids

In addition to hyperglycemia, fasting free fatty acid levels are also elevated in diabetes because of accelerated mobilization of fat stores. In type 2 diabetes, elevated free fatty acid levels occur in the presence of normal

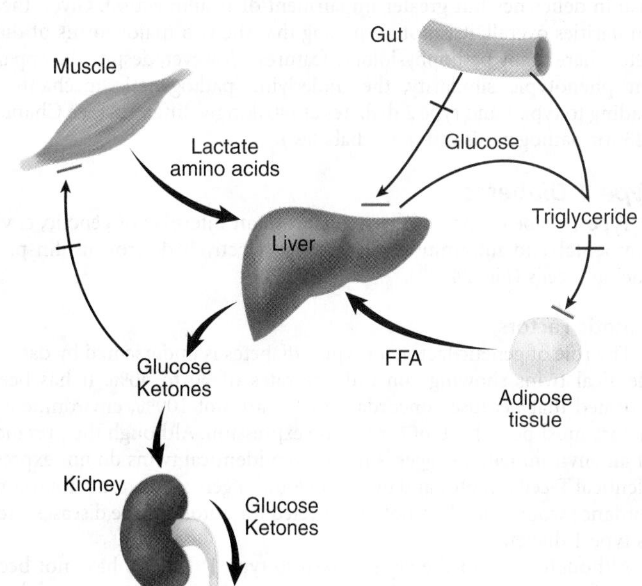

FIGURE 247–1 • The effects of severe insulin deficiency on body fuel metabolism. Lack of insulin leads to mobilization of substrates for gluconeogenesis and ketogenesis from muscle and adipose tissue, accelerated production of glucose and ketones by the liver, and impaired removal of endogenous and exogenous fuels by insulin-responsive tissues. The net results are severe hyperglycemia and hyperketonemia that overwhelm renal removal mechanisms. FFA = free fatty acids.

or even increased insulin levels, suggesting that adipocytes become resistant to insulin's inhibitory effect on lipolysis. This adipocyte resistance ultimately leads to the mobilization and inappropriate deposition of triglyceride into liver and muscle, especially under conditions of a hypercaloric diet, which in turn is linked to insulin resistance in these organs.

Although free fatty acids are not directly converted to glucose, they do promote hyperglycemia by providing the liver with energy to support gluconeogenesis as well as by impairing insulin signaling in muscle and thus interfering with muscle glucose uptake (predominantly by inhibiting glucose transport) and insulin production at the level of the pancreatic β cell. Endogenous insulin secretion in type 2 diabetes provides sufficient portal levels of insulin to suppress the conversion of free fatty acids to ketones in the liver. In type 1 diabetes, however, mobilized free fatty acids are more readily converted to ketone bodies. The combined effects of insulin deficiency and the presence of glucagon suppress fat synthesis in the liver. This suppression of fat synthesis reduces intrahepatic malonyl coenzyme A, which together with carnitine stimulates the activity of hepatic carnitine acyltransferase I and thereby facilitates the transfer of long-chain fatty acids into mitochondria, where they are broken down by β-oxidation and converted to ketone bodies. In addition, hypoinsulinemia, by decreasing ketone turnover, enhances the magnitude of the ketosis for any given level of ketone production. During diabetic ketoacidosis, ketone levels are further increased because of the concurrent release of counter-regulatory hormones. Glucagon levels rise, accelerating hepatic ketogenesis, whereas elevations of catecholamines, growth hormone, and cortisol act in concert to increase lipolysis and subsequent delivery of free fatty acids to the liver (see Fig. 247–1). The increase in substrate delivery may become so pronounced that it saturates the oxidative pathway, thus leading to hepatic steatosis and severe hypertriglyceridemia.

Hyperaminoacidemia

In addition to disordered glucose disposal, type 1 diabetic patients may exhibit defects in the disposal of ingested proteins and fats as well. In the absence of the normal rise in insulin, meal ingestion may produce hyperaminoacidemia, because of a failure to stimulate the net uptake of amino acids in muscle, and hypertriglyceridemia, through the reduced activity of lipoprotein lipase. Thus, diabetes should be viewed not only as a disorder of glucose tolerance but as a disorder of protein and fat tolerance as well.

Pathogenesis

Type 1 diabetes produces profound β-cell failure with secondary insulin resistance, whereas type 2 diabetes is associated with less severe insulin deficiency but greater impairment of insulin action. Given their similarities overall, it is not surprising that the two major forms of diabetes share many pathophysiologic features. However, despite the apparent phenotypic similarity, the underlying pathogenetic mechanisms leading to type 1 and type 2 diabetes are strikingly different. (See Chapter 248 for pathogenesis of type 2 diabetes.)

Type 1 Diabetes

Type 1 diabetes most likely results from an interplay of genetic, environmental, and autoimmune factors that selectively destroy insulin-producing β cells (Fig. 247–2).

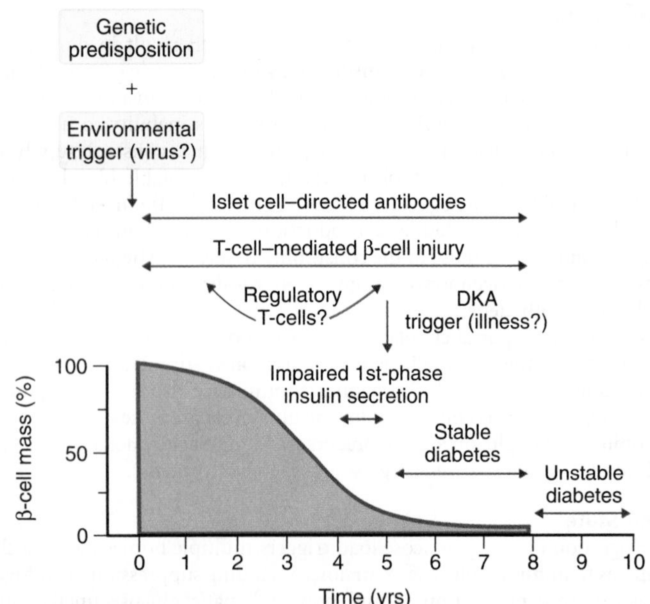

FIGURE 247–2 • A summary of the sequence of events that lead to pancreatic β-cell loss and ultimately to the clinical evolution of type 1 diabetes. DKA = diabetic ketoacidosis.

Genetic Factors

The role of genetic factors in type 1 diabetes is underscored by data in identical twins showing concordance rates of 30 to 40%. It has been assumed that because concordance rates are not 100%, environmental factors must be important for disease expression. Although the presence of an environmental trigger is likely, even identical twins do not express identical T-cell receptor and immunoglobulin genes; as a result, total concordance would therefore not be expected for autoimmune diseases such as type 1 diabetes.

Although many of the genes linked to type 1 diabetes have not been identified, some are known. HLA genes, located on the short arm of chromosome 6, clearly play a dominant role; in nonaffected siblings, the risk for development of diabetes is 15 to 20% if they are HLA identical, approximately 5% if they share one HLA gene, and less than 1% if no HLA genes are shared. Specific HLA haplotypes have been linked to type 1 diabetes; 90 to 95% of type 1 patients express DR3 or DR4 class II HLA molecules (compared with 50 to 60% of the general population), whereas 60% express both alleles, a rate more than 10-fold that of the general population. Another class II allele, DQB1*0602, has a negative association with the disease. Specific class II DQ haplotypes (e.g., DQ8 and DQ2) even more strongly correlate with disease susceptibility in white individuals; this susceptibility is associated with polymorphisms of the allele encoding the β chain of the DQ class II HLA molecule. The presence of aspartic acid at position 57 protects against disease, whereas substitution of a neutral amino acid at this position is associated with higher disease frequency. Other polymorphisms, such as the substitution of arginine at position 52 of the DQ α chain, may confer additional risk. Overall, it seems clear that significant genetic heterogeneity exists and that no single class II HLA gene accounts for all HLA-associated susceptibility to disease. Association of the disease with specific class II HLA genes implies the involvement of $CD4^+$ T cells in the autoimmune process because these molecules are critical for both the presentation of antigenic peptides to $CD4^+$ T cells and the selection of the $CD4^+$ T-cell repertoire in the thymus.

Other genes are likely to contribute to genetic susceptibility to type 1 diabetes. *IDDM2* (chromosome 11p), a noncoding promoter region of the insulin gene, may influence insulin gene expression in the thymus and may therefore affect thymic selection of insulin-reactive T cells. *CTLA4* (chromosome 2q) plays a role in T-cell action and regulation. Protein tyrosine phosphatase N22 (*PTPN22*) on chromosome 1 is also a regulator of T-cell activation. Many other genes have also been implicated, underscoring the polygenic nature of this disease.

Environmental Factors

Although environmental factors such as diet and toxins have been proposed as triggers of diabetes, most of the scientific attention has focused on putative viruses. Epidemics of mumps, congenital rubella, and coxsackievirus infection have been associated with an increased frequency of type 1 diabetes. In one instance, coxsackievirus B4 was isolated from the pancreas of a child who died of diabetic ketoacidosis, and inoculation of the virus into mice caused diabetes, fulfilling Koch's postulates. However, it is likely that acute, lytic viral infections are responsible for only an occasional case of diabetes. Instead, if viruses are involved, it is far more likely that they trigger an autoimmune response. If a virus contains an epitope resembling a β-cell protein, viral infection could theoretically abrogate self-tolerance and trigger autoimmunity.

Autoimmune Factors

About 80% of patients with new-onset type 1 diabetes have islet cell antibodies. Antibodies to a variety of β-cell constituents have been identified, including insulin, isoforms of glutamic acid decarboxylase (GAD 65 and GAD 67), and the secretory granule protein islet cell antigen (ICA) 512 or IA-2, which contains a tyrosine phosphatase–like domain. The idea that type 1 diabetes is a chronic autoimmune disease with acute clinical manifestations is supported by the fact that islet antigen–directed antibodies may be present in asymptomatic first-degree relatives of patients. Such antibody-positive individuals are at risk for the development of type 1 diabetes, although clinical onset may be delayed by many years. The likelihood of type 1 diabetes is greater than 50% if autoantibodies are present to more than one β-cell antigen (i.e., insulin, GAD 65, ICA 512); diabetes rarely develops in antibody-negative relatives. If antibodies appear at a young age, the risk for clinical diabetes is particularly high.

The listed antibodies appear to be markers for rather than the cause of β-cell injury. β-Cell destruction (by apoptotic and cytotoxic mechanisms) is mediated by a variety of cytokines or by direct T-lymphocyte activity. Supporting this notion, type 1 diabetes has been transferred through bone marrow cells from a diabetic patient to a nondiabetic recipient. In addition, autopsies performed on patients dying soon after disease onset have shown islet-restricted monocytic cellular infiltrates (termed insulitis) that are composed of $CD8^+$ and $CD4^+$ T cells, macrophages, and B cells. Usually, as the disease progresses, the islets become completely devoid of β cells and inflammatory infiltrates; α, δ, and pancreatic polypeptide cells are left intact, thus illustrating the exquisite specificity of the autoimmune attack. At the time of clinical diagnosis, about 10 to 20% of the original β-cell mass typically remains (see Fig. 247–2). In most patients, there is gradual loss of these remaining β cells; some patients continue to exhibit residual insulin production for many years.

A critical role for T cells is supported by studies involving pancreatic transplantation in identical twins. Monozygotic twins with diabetes who received kidney and pancreas grafts from their nondiabetic, genetically identical sibling required little or no immunosuppression for graft acceptance. Nevertheless, the islets were soon selectively invaded with mononuclear cells, predominantly $CD8^+$ T cells, with the subsequent recurrence of diabetes. Thus, decades after the original onset of disease, the immune system retained the ability to selectively destroy β cells. Evidence implicating T cells also derives from clinical trials using immunosuppressive drugs. Drugs such as cyclosporine or antibodies directed against a component of the T-cell receptor slow or prevent the progression of recent-onset diabetes, but this effect is not sustained if immunosuppression is withdrawn. Further supporting data for a primary role for T cells derive from NOD mice, in which insulitis and islet autoantibodies develop at about 4 weeks of age and diabetes ultimately develops after 12 to 24 weeks; in these mice, a variety of treatments designed to deplete T cells can prevent diabetes. Most important, adoptive transfer of T cells isolated from diabetic mice donors into immune-incompetent NOD mice rapidly produces diabetes. Both $CD4^+$ and $CD8^+$ T cells are generally required for transfer of disease, which suggests that both are necessary for disease expression. These diabetogenic T cells target specific β-cell antigens, including insulin and glutamic acid decarboxylase. A likely role for glutamic acid decarboxylase or insulin is also suggested by data showing that if NOD mice are made tolerant to glutamic acid decarboxylase or to insulin (or to peptides derived from these molecules) early in life, insulitis and diabetes fail to develop. Finally, the chronic, smoldering nature of type 1 diabetes suggests the presence of regulatory or protective influences. In keeping with this observation, T cells that release immunoregulatory cytokines and, in turn, protect the islet from immune attack have been isolated from the islets of NOD mice. Such findings suggest that the rate of appearance and clinical expression of disease may be modulated by the balance between diabetogenic and protective populations of T cells. "Tipping the scales" in favor of protective T-cell proliferation is the goal of protective immunization.

Clinical Manifestations

Patients with type 1 diabetes mellitus have little or no insulin secretory capacity and depend on exogenous insulin to prevent metabolic decompensation and death. Classically, symptoms appear abruptly (i.e., during days or weeks) in previously healthy, nonobese children or young adults who may have close relatives with the disease but more commonly do not. Older patients, however, often present more gradually. At the time of initial evaluation, most type 1 diabetic patients are ill and symptomatic, most commonly presenting with polyuria, polydipsia, polyphagia, and weight loss; such patients may also present with ketoacidosis. Type 1 diabetes is believed to have a prolonged asymptomatic preclinical phase (often lasting years), during which pancreatic β cells are gradually destroyed by an autoimmune attack influenced by HLA and other genetic factors as well as by the environment (see Fig. 247–2). In some patients, an acute illness may speed the transition from the preclinical phase to clinical disease.

Initially, most type 1 patients will require high-dose insulin therapy to restore a disordered metabolism. However, a so-called honeymoon period may follow (lasting weeks or months), during which smaller doses of insulin are needed because of partial recovery of β cell function and reversal of the insulin resistance caused by acute illness. Thereafter, insulin secretory capacity is gradually lost; in some patients, particularly older individuals, this process commonly takes several years. The rate of decline is slowed by intensive insulin therapy targeting near-normoglycemia.

That type 1 diabetes is an autoimmune disease is supported by its association with specific immune response (HLA) genes and by the presence of autoantibodies to islet cells and their constituents (e.g., insulin, glutamic acid decarboxylase, ICA 512). Type 1 diabetes accounts for less than 10% of diabetes in the United States. See Chapter 248 for more detailed discussion of the non–type 1 forms of diabetes.

Diagnosis

Because diagnosis and screening are topics more germane to the evaluation of the patient with type 2 diabetes or other forms of diabetes, this area is reviewed in Chapter 248. Briefly, current criteria of the American Diabetes Association and the World Health Organization for the diagnosis of diabetes include a fasting plasma glucose concentration in excess of 125 mg/dL and a "casual" (i.e., random, without specific relationship to meals) or, during an oral glucose tolerance test, a 2-hour plasma glucose concentration in excess of 199 mg/dL. In most patients with type 1 diabetes, the hyperglycemia at presentation is severe, sometimes in conjunction with frank metabolic decompensation. As a result, the diagnosis is usually straightforward.

Treatment

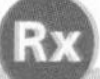

Treatment of diabetes mellitus involves changes in lifestyle and may require pharmacologic intervention with insulin or oral glucose-lowering drugs. In type 1 diabetes, the primary focus is to replace the insulin secretion that has been lost. A healthy lifestyle is also required to facilitate insulin therapy and to optimize health. In the short term, the goals of diabetes treatment are to optimize metabolic control and to improve the patient's sense of clinical well-being. Long-term therapeutic goals focus on the prevention of complications, including cardiovascular disease, nephropathy, retinopathy, and neurologic disease.

Management of Complications

Relation between Diabetes Control and Its Complications

Whether the vascular and neuropathic complications of diabetes mellitus can be prevented or delayed by improved glycemic control was debated for more than half a century. To answer the question, the National Institutes of Health initiated the Diabetes Control and Complications Trial (DCCT), a 9-year multicenter study involving 1441 type 1 patients aged 13 to 39 years who were randomly assigned to either intensive insulin therapy or conventional care. Intensive therapy consisted of three or more insulin injections per day (or an insulin pump), self-monitoring of blood glucose concentration at least four times per day, and frequent contact with a diabetes health care team. Conventional care consisted of one or more (commonly two) injections of insulin per day, less frequent monitoring of glucose concentration, standard education, and less frequent health care visits. The target goals of therapy were different as well. The intensive therapy group sought pre-meal blood glucose levels of 70 to 120 mg/dL, postprandial blood levels of less than 180 mg/dL, and glycohemoglobin values as close as possible to normal. In the conventional care group, the primary goal was simply to maintain clinical well-being. Patients were divided into two groups: a primary prevention group, with diabetes for 1 to 5 years and no detectable

Rx

complications; and a secondary intervention group, with diabetes for 1 to 15 years and mild retinopathy.

The DCCT achieved a clear separation of glucose levels between the groups during the entire study period. Glycohemoglobin (HbA_{1c}) and mean glucose levels in the intensive therapy group were 1.5 to 2.0% and 60 to 80 mg/dL lower, respectively, than in those receiving conventional care. Although considerable variability was noted among individual patients, most of the intensive care group failed to achieve normal glucose levels (glycohemoglobin averaged 1.1% above normal, or a glucose level of about 155 mg/dL). Nevertheless, intensive therapy reduced the development of retinopathy by 76% in the primary prevention group and the progression of retinopathy by 54% in the secondary intervention group (Fig. 247–3); 1 the latter effect became apparent after only 4 years. In addition, intensive therapy reduced the risk of microalbuminuria by 39%, frank proteinuria by 54%, and clinical neuropathy by 60%. The incidence of major cardiovascular events also tended to be lower, but the number of events was insufficient for statistical proof; at the very least, intensive therapy did not pose a risk for macrovascular complications. An exponential relationship over time between the average blood glucose level (as reflected by HbA_{1c}) and the progression of retinopathy in the intensive care group suggests that there may be no threshold level at which complications occur. These findings imply that any degree of improvement in glycemic control has benefit and that normalization of glucose levels is not required to slow the progression of diabetic complications.

The benefits achieved by intensive control in the DCCT were not without risk, however. Weight gain was more common in the intensive care group. In addition, the frequency of severe hypoglycemia (including multiple episodes in some patients) was three-fold higher in the intensive care group; in many cases, such episodes occurred without classic warning symptoms, often while the patient was asleep. It is reasonable to conclude that in some patients, the risks of intensive therapy may outweigh the benefits; possibly included are patients with recurrent severe hypoglycemia and decreased perception of hypoglycemia, patients with advanced complications, young children, and patients who are unable or unwilling to participate in their management (e.g., self-monitoring of blood glucose level). Such individuals are likely to benefit from less aggressive therapy designed to lower glucose levels moderately without the risk of hypoglycemia. Despite the higher rate of hypoglycemia, intensive therapy in the DCCT had no detectable long-term effects on cognitive function.

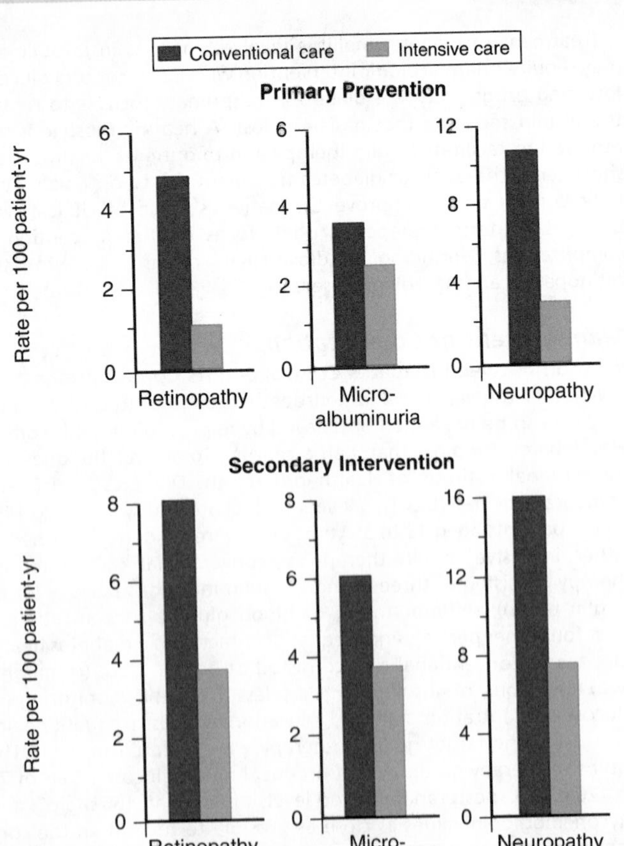

FIGURE 247–3 • A summary of the results of the Diabetes Control and Complications Trial (DCCT).

Translating these results into clinical practice remains a challenge because significant motivation is needed on the part of the patient to comply with the intensive monitoring and insulin administration regimens required. Significant expertise is also required on the part of the practitioner to manage these individuals properly on an ongoing basis. An important lesson from these studies was that successful treatment of diabetes is largely accomplished through the efforts of the patients themselves as well as by nurse educators, dietitians, and diabetes counselors. It makes sense, then, to encourage the use of physician-directed health care teams to translate the findings of the DCCT into clinical practice.

In an update involving the original DCCT cohort, the Epidemiology of Diabetes Interventions and Complications (EDIC) study, the benefit from intensive glycemic control on microvascular complications persisted. 2 Even more important, the group that had been intensively treated had long-lived cardiovascular benefits. Among the 1375 volunteers who agreed to continue in this observational extension of the DCCT, the intensively treated patients had less than half of the cardiovascular events (myocardial infarction, coronary revascularization, and stroke) than those previously assigned to the conventionally treated group had (46 compared with 98 events) during a total of 17 years of follow-up. These results were all the more impressive because the mean HbA_{1c} in the intensive group had actually risen to about 8% from about 7% during the EDIC study, whereas the conventional therapy group in the DCCT improved their mean HbA_{1c} from about 9% to about 8%. Therefore, despite nearly equal glycemic control during most of the EDIC study, a persistent benefit on these macrovascular end points was observed after intensive treatment.

Medical Therapy

Insulin Preparations and Pharmacokinetics

A variety of highly purified insulin preparations are commercially available (Table 247–2). Premixed insulin preparations are also available and may offer added convenience for selected patients. Nearly all insulin preparations contain 100 U/mL (U-100), although a more concentrated preparation of regular insulin of 500 U/mL (U-500) can be obtained for severely resistant patients. Human insulin is now the only form of insulin sold in North America and other industrialized countries, largely because of immunologic concerns and the higher production costs of animal insulins. The same insulin preparation can produce variable responses in a single patient because the peak and duration of most insulin preparations are influenced by the site of administration and the magnitude of the insulin dose.

Short- and Rapid-Acting Insulin Preparations

After subcutaneous injection, regular (R) insulin begins to act in about 30 minutes and should therefore be administered 20 to 30 minutes before a meal. Because it acts quickly and has a relatively short duration of action (5 to 8 hours), it is effective for blunting postprandial glucose excursions and for facilitating rapid dose adjustments based on measured blood glucose values. The properties of regular insulin are especially helpful in managing glucose elevations that occur during illness or after the consumption of large meals. Given intravenously, regular insulin is also effective in the perioperative period and in the management of severely ill hospitalized patients and acute hyperglycemic complications.

In regular insulin preparations, insulin molecules exist predominantly in hexameric form. Before being absorbed, insulin hexamers must first be diluted in subcutaneous interstitial fluid, then dissociate into single molecules; this property accounts for the slightly delayed absorption of regular insulin from subcutaneous injection

TABLE 247-2 INSULIN PREPARATIONS: EFFECT ONSET, PEAK, AND DURATION AFTER SUBCUTANEOUS ADMINISTRATION

Class	Preparation	Onset of Effect	Peak Effect (hr)	Duration of Action (hr)
Rapid acting	Lispro, aspart, or glulisine	10–15 min	1–2	3–4
Short acting	Regular (R)	30 min	2–4	5–8
Intermediate acting	NPH (N) or Lente	2–4 hours	6–12	16–24
Long acting	Ultralente (U)	4–6 hours	8–16	~24
	Glargine	2–4 hours	No peak	>30
	Detemir	1 hour	No peak	Up to 24

Rx

sites. Advances in recombinant DNA technology led to the development of insulin analogues intended to bypass this property, allowing more rapid absorption in an effort to more closely mimic the normal brisk increase in endogenously secreted insulin in response to meals. Insulin lispro was the first analogue approved by the Food and Drug Administration (FDA), with amino acids in positions B28 [lysine] and B29 [proline] reversed. Lispro thereby has a reduced capacity for hexameric self-association and is therefore more rapidly absorbed. Its effects begin within 10 to 15 minutes of administration and generally wane within 3 to 4 hours. In insulin aspart, a neutral proline residue at position B28 is replaced by negatively charged aspartic acid, resulting in a reduced capacity for self-association and faster absorption. The pharmacokinetic properties of insulin aspart are similar to those of insulin lispro; insulin aspart may have a slightly longer duration of effect. In insulin glulisine, the asparagine at position B3 is replaced by lysine and the lysine in position B29 is replaced by glutamic acid. Because of their rapid onset, these rapid-acting insulin analogues can be given just before eating (as opposed to 30 minutes prior), a feature that greatly simplifies the planning and consumption of meals; also, because the effects wane more rapidly, there is a reduced risk of "late" hypoglycemia if the next meal is delayed. With their use, postprandial glucose and HbA_{1c} reductions are equal to or better than those achieved with regular insulin, and there is a reduced incidence of delayed hypoglycemia. For these reasons and because of greater convenience and flexibility, rapid-acting analogues are being used with increasing frequency in intensive treatment regimens. However, these differences in responses are small, and long-term safety and efficacy data are not yet available. 3

Intermediate- and Long-Acting Insulin Preparations

The longer acting insulin preparations have been modified to delay their absorption from injection sites, resulting in a longer duration of insulin activity. The addition of protamine and zinc yields intermediate-acting neutral protamine Hagedorn (NPH) insulin; enlargement of the size of the zinc-insulin crystal yields Lente (intermediate acting) and Ultralente (long acting) insulins, both of which are no longer widely available. NPH and Lente, the intermediate-acting insulins, have a similar time course of action; given twice per day, they offer a compromise between some degree of meal coverage (coinciding with peak activity) and the provision of basal insulin levels. Ultralente insulin, because of its longer duration and less evident peaks, offers some advantages for basal insulin replacement and can be given once daily in many patients. However, the pharmacokinetics of Ultralente can be unpredictable in clinical practice (even within a single patient), and its effects may wane before 24 hours, necessitating twice-daily dosing and limiting its utility. Lente and Ultralente are no longer widely available.

Insulin glargine, the first long-acting, basal insulin analogue, differs from human insulin both at position A21, where asparagine is replaced by glycine, and at the carboxyl terminus of the B chain, where two arginine residues have been added. Insulin glargine is soluble at acidic pH and less so in physiologic conditions; injected at a pH of 4, it is neutralized in subcutaneous tissue and forms microprecipitates, delaying its absorption and prolonging its duration of activity. The primary advantages of glargine insulin are more than 24-hour activity (allowing once-daily dosing) and the lack of peak concentrations; both characteristics are desirable for the provision of consistent basal insulin levels. Disadvantages include the higher cost, a higher incidence of mild injection site discomfort (compared with NPH, 6.0% vs. 0.3%), and the inability to mix glargine with other insulins. Clinical trials in type 1 diabetic patients suggest that insulin glargine may produce larger reductions in HbA_{1c} compared with NPH; comparative trials have also shown a reduced incidence in both symptomatic and nocturnal hypoglycemia when insulin glargine is used.

Insulin detemir is a more recent basal insulin analogue. It has been engineered with a unique fatty acid side chain that facilitates self-association at the injection site and, once absorbed, binding to circulating serum albumin. Both of these features allow a smooth basal profile, taken once or twice daily.

Insulin Regimens

Although it is a simple concept, the clinical use of insulin to treat diabetes mellitus, especially in the absolutely insulin-deficient type 1 diabetes, can be extraordinarily complex. There are many important interpatient (and intrapatient) variables, so a predictable algorithm cannot be uniformly applied to all patients or to a single patient at all times. In general, subcutaneous insulin regimens for type 1 diabetes may be classified as conservative or intensive. Continuous subcutaneous insulin infusion with insulin pumps is becoming increasingly popular, mainly in patients with type 1 diabetes, and this mode of therapy provides the most refined insulin replacement regimen to date.

Conservative Insulin Therapy

Through the early stages of type 1 diabetes, some degree of β-cell function is usually preserved, allowing many patients to achieve glycemic control with less intensive effort. During this initial phase, when many patients have residual β-cell function, CD3-antibody therapy may reduce insulin requirements. 4 Because intermediate-acting insulins are not generally sustained during a 24-hour period, and because insulin requirements tend to increase early in the morning, most of these patients should start with two daily injections, consisting of a mixture of intermediate-acting and short- or rapid-acting human insulins administered before breakfast and before dinner. Regardless of the initiation method used, insulin dose adjustments will inevitably be required. Initially, doses of the intermediate-acting insulin should be adjusted to optimize pre-dinner and fasting (morning) glucose levels. Once these goals are accomplished, short- or rapid-acting insulin doses should then be adjusted to optimize postprandial, pre-lunch, and bedtime glucose values. Patients should generally inject in the same anatomic region at the same time each day (e.g., in the abdomen in the morning, in the thigh at night) to ensure consistent insulin delivery; an effort should also be made to avoid exact duplication of injection sites within a 1-week period. Some patients may experience a brief "honeymoon" period, during which β-cell function partially recovers and insulin needs are temporarily reduced. Such an improvement should not be used as a signal to reduce efforts aimed at glycemic control because continuation of optimal insulin therapy will help preserve residual β-cell function.

Premixed combinations of intermediate insulins and short- or rapid-acting insulins are also available (NPH/regular 70/30, neutral protamine lispro/lispro 75/25, and neutral protamine aspart/aspart 70/30).

Multiple Subcutaneous Injections

Several years after the onset of type 1 diabetes, residual insulin secretion typically ceases. When this occurs, twice-daily insulin injections are no longer acceptable, even if they continue successfully to control marked hyperglycemia and diabetic symptoms. For optimal glycemic control, insulin delivery should more closely simulate the "normal" pattern of insulin secretion; continuous or "basal" insulin levels are required throughout the day, whereas brief increases in insulin levels ("boluses") should coincide with the ingestion of meals. The primary problem with twice-daily insulin regimens is that the glucose-lowering effect of the pre-dinner intermediate-acting insulin is greatest when insulin requirements are at their lowest (i.e., around 3:00 AM). In addition, when requirements are increasing in the predawn hours, insulin levels are declining. The net results of this poorly matched insulin supply and demand are the production of nocturnal hypoglycemia and fasting (morning) hyperglycemia.

Successful management of diabetes begins with fasting glucose control. Failure to control the morning glucose level often results in the stubborn perpetuation of hyperglycemia throughout the day. Once hepatic gluconeogenesis has been activated in the morning, it is not readily suppressed by insulin injections. The key factors responsible for fasting hyperglycemia are inadequate overnight delivery of insulin and sleep-associated growth hormone release. The "dawn phenomenon" is most pronounced in patients with type 1 diabetes because of their inability to compensate by raising endogenous insulin secretion. The magnitude of the dawn phenomenon can be attenuated by designing insulin regimens to ensure that the effects of exogenous insulin do not peak in the middle of the night and dissipate by morning. Several approaches to insulin therapy can deal with this problem; some of the more common regimens are displayed in Figure 247–4. One common approach is to use three injections (i.e., a mixture of intermediate NPH and short- or rapid-acting insulin before breakfast, short- or rapid-acting insulin before dinner, and NPH at bedtime). The primary disadvantage of this approach is that meal sizes and schedules must be fixed rigidly. Alternative multidose regimens incorporate short- or rapid-acting insulin injections before each meal, with one or two daily doses of intermediate- or long-acting insulin. Pen-style insulin injectors are also available; these may help make multidose regimens more convenient and tolerable for patients.

Pramlintide

Amylin is a natural peptide that is normally secreted by the pancreatic β cell with insulin in response to meals. It has several beneficial effects on glucose homeostasis, including the suppression of glucagon secretion, the retardation of gastric emptying, and the promotion of satiety. Pramlintide, a synthetic amylin analogue, is currently approved for use in patients with type 1 diabetes (as well as insulin-requiring type 2 diabetes) who are inadequately controlled with their current regimens. It is given before meals, usually in conjunction with prandial insulin, but in a separate subcutaneous injection. Its major role is to decrease postprandial glucose excursions, stabilizing glycemic control. In clinical trials, the absolute reduction in HbA_{1c} is modest (–0.3 to 0.5%), although it is associated with mild weight loss, which distinguishes it from insulin therapy. Side effects include nausea and vomiting, especially at higher doses. A frequent dosing schedule (three times daily) also makes it inconvenient for many patients. At this time, its niche appears to be in poorly controlled type 1 (and type 2) diabetes for patients already on intensive insulin regimens but whose glucose profile shows postprandial hyperglycemia not adequately addressed by increasing the dose of pre-meal rapid-acting insulin. Because of its effect on body weight, it seems to be most attractive for patients who are overweight.

Continuous Subcutaneous Insulin Infusion

In continuous subcutaneous insulin infusion, rapid-acting insulin is administered around-the-clock by an externally worn, battery-powered, computer-controlled infusion pump (see Fig. 247–4). The pump delivers a continuous basal rate and can be programmed to vary the flow rate automatically for set periods, such as reducing the flow rate after bedtime and increasing flow to compensate for increased insulin requirements in the predawn hours. Boluses, determined by self-monitoring of blood glucose concentration and expected meals, are given by manual pump activation. Most insulin pumps contain an insulin reservoir attached to a subcutaneous catheter (the catheter is inserted subcutaneously by an introducing needle, which is then removed). Catheters are generally best placed in the abdomen to standardize absorption and to maximize visibility. Overall, the continuous subcutaneous insulin infusion method provides diabetic patients with the highest degrees of lifestyle flexibility and glucose control. Newer units communicate by radio frequency to separate capillary blood glucose–monitoring meters, even offering supplemental insulin dosing suggestions. Ultimately, subcutaneous interstitial sensors may one day communicate continuously with pumps, allowing a nearly "artificial pancreas." Several hurdles in terms of precision, accuracy, and safe, reliable interfaces will need to be passed before such closed-loop devices will be ready for commercial use.

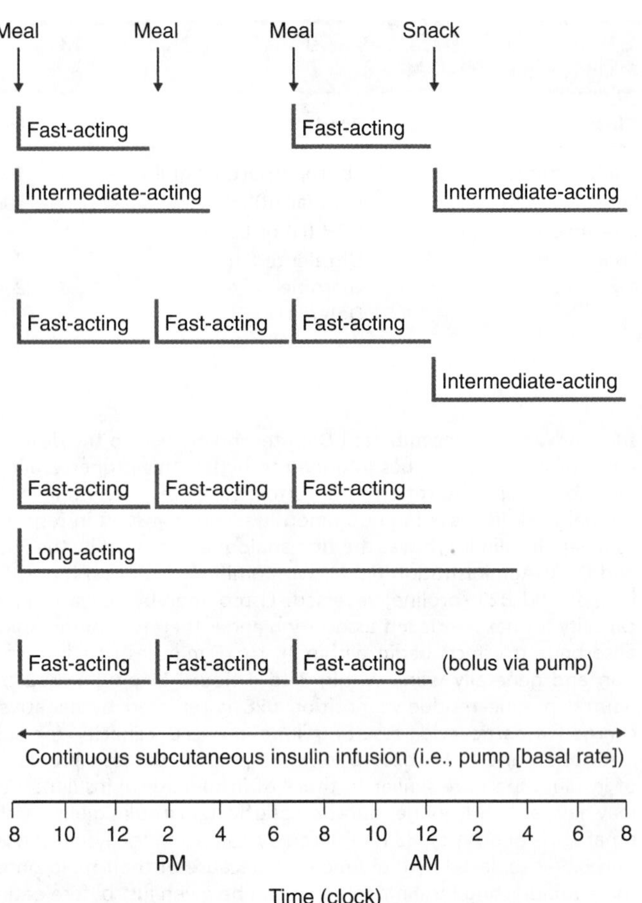

FIGURE 247–4 • Several intensive insulin regimens commonly used in the treatment of diabetes. Each is designed to provide a continuous supply of insulin around-the-clock and to make extra insulin available at the time of meals, thereby simulating more closely the normal physiologic pattern of insulin secretion.

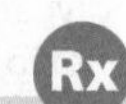

The continuous subcutaneous insulin infusion approach has several limitations. One obvious disadvantage of pump therapy is the wearing of the pump itself; the device may be undesirable for patients during intense exercise, contact sports, submersion in water, or personal intimacy. Furthermore, because continuous subcutaneous insulin infusion uses rapid-acting insulin, any interruption in flow (most commonly because of occlusions within or at the terminus of the catheter) can lead to rapid deterioration of metabolic control. Local infections at the catheter site occasionally occur, necessitating a site change every 2 or 3 days. Furthermore, maintenance of the pump and appropriate insulin infusion rates requires significant effort by the patient and sophistication.

The intensive treatment regimens described are not for everyone. In appropriate patients, however, intensive insulin therapy should be strongly encouraged to reduce the risk of late diabetic complications. Pregnancy is an absolute indication for intensive therapy, and reduction of the excess neonatal morbidity and mortality associated with diabetic pregnancies requires tight glycemic control. Ideally, intensive insulin therapy should be instituted in type 1 patients before conception to minimize the risk of fetal anomalies. After conception, blood glucose targets are more stringently applied than at other times, with the specific aim of maintaining glucose levels in the normal range.

Inhaled insulin is an alternative to subcutaneous insulin. However, it is generally not quite as effective as subcutaneous insulin and is generally not recommended for type 1 diabetics who can tolerate subcutaneous insulin. 5

General Measures

Lifestyle Changes

Diet and exercise contribute importantly to the care of patients with type 1 diabetes. Patients should be educated about balancing calorie intake (diet) with energy expenditure (exercise) and should understand the basic concepts of insulin therapy as it relates to stress and physical activity. If they are properly managed and sufficiently motivated, diabetic patients should be able to consume the foods they enjoy and should be able to participate fully in exercise and sports.

Diet

The introduction of intensive insulin regimens has increased meal flexibility by allowing more latitude in varying the size, content, and timing of meals. New approaches offer the opportunity for a more normal lifestyle, thus reducing compliance problems and optimizing acceptance and satisfaction of patients. Meals should be nutritionally sound, designed to reduce cardiovascular risk, and should provide sufficient calories to meet the energy needs of growing children, active young adults, and pregnant women; the 1800-kcal diet classically prescribed for overweight type 2 diabetic patients is grossly insufficient in these and other individuals. Furthermore, diabetic diets should specifically aim to minimize long-term cardiovascular risk by minimizing the ingestion of sodium, cholesterol, and saturated fats (Table 247–3).

Because type 1 patients depend on exogenous insulin, proper management is facilitated by a meal plan designed to match the time course of the selected insulin regimen. Patients should learn to compensate for departures from the meal plan by adjusting their insulin doses and for periods of altered activity by adjusting their consumption of food. Even in patients on basal-bolus regimens or receiving continuous subcutaneous insulin infusion, an effort should be made to avoid long delays between meals, and small snacks may still be helpful at times of peak insulin action to avoid hypoglycemia. Most patients, regardless of their regimen, should incorporate a bedtime snack to reduce the risk of nocturnal hypoglycemia. Finally, the potential for insulin-induced weight gain requires special emphasis on portion control; to control hypoglycemia, patients should master the use of appropriate carbohydrate intake and avoid overcompensation.

Exercise

Regular exercise is important to promote overall health and to reduce cardiovascular complications. Surprisingly, there is little evidence to suggest that exercise itself substantially improves glycemic control in type 1 diabetes, although it is known to reduce overall insulin requirements by further enhancing insulin sensitivity. Through accelerated insulin absorption (due to increased local blood flow at the injection site) and increased muscle glucose consumption, exercise can rapidly reduce blood glucose levels, particularly when it coincides with the peak action of an insulin injection. In nondiabetic individuals, blood glucose levels remain stable during exercise, as decreased endogenous insulin secretion promotes increased hepatic glucose production to match the increased rate of

TABLE 247–3 LIFESTYLE MODIFICATIONS FOR PATIENTS WITH DIABETES

DIETARY PRESCRIPTION

Weight reduction, gain, or maintenance to achieve and to maintain ideal body weight

Restriction of saturated fat to less than 10% of total calories, to be replaced in the diet by carbohydrates and monounsaturated fats; if low-density lipoprotein reduction is also desired, saturated fats should be further restricted to less than 7% of daily calorie intake

Decreased cholesterol intake to less than 300 mg/day; if low-density lipoprotein reduction is also desired, cholesterol intake should be further restricted to less than 200 mg/day

Sodium restriction (<2.4 g/day) in patients with hypertension; with overt nephropathy, sodium intake should be further restricted to less than 2.0 g/day

Protein restriction to less than 20% of total calories; with nephropathy, protein intake should be further restricted to less than 0.8 mg/kg/day or to about 10% of daily calorie intake

EXERCISE PRESCRIPTION*

A combination of aerobic exercise and resistance training is preferred. Avoid heavy lifting, straining, and Valsalva maneuvers, which can raise blood pressure and may aggravate proliferative diabetic retinopathy.

Intensity: Increase heart rate "moderately" to at least 55% of "maximal" heart rate (220 minus age in years), with adjustments based on the patient's cardiovascular fitness. Patients with improved cardiovascular fitness can proceed to "harder" activities, achieving heart rates exceeding 70% of maximum.

Duration: 30 minutes, preceded and followed by stretching and flexibility exercises for a minimum of 5 to 10 minutes.

Frequency: at least 3 days per week. Results are best if exercise occurs nearly every day.

Avoid strenuous exercise if fasting glucose levels are 250 mg/dL or higher. Avoid all forms of exercise if glucose levels are 300 mg/dL or higher or ketosis is present.

Monitor blood glucose level before, during, and after exercise to learn responses to different exercise conditions and to identify when changes in insulin or food intake are necessary.

Consume added foods as needed to avoid hypoglycemia. A rapidly absorbed carbohydrate source should be readily available during exercise and for up to 8 hours after exercise is completed.

*Exercise limitations are imposed by preexisting coronary or peripheral vascular disease, proliferative retinopathy, peripheral or autonomic neuropathy, and poor glycemic control.

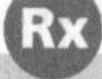

glucose consumption. In diabetic patients receiving exogenous insulin, however, this finely tuned homeostatic mechanism is perturbed. The continued presence of exogenous insulin during exercise further accelerates glucose uptake and, more important, blocks the compensatory increase in glucose production; as a result, circulating glucose levels can fall precipitously during exercise. Because the magnitude of this fall is not easily titrated, hypoglycemia may occur if the patient is unable to adjust diet and insulin appropriately before, during, and after physical activity. Some general guidelines useful in regulating the glycemic response to exercise are summarized in Table 247–3.

Monitoring

Self-monitoring of Blood Glucose Concentration

Self-monitoring of blood glucose concentration has revolutionized the management of diabetes. It actively involves patients in the treatment process, allows more rapid treatment adjustments, and reinforces dietary changes. Self-monitoring provides the patient with the tools necessary to assist in management of the disease; it is especially useful during periods of stress and for patients who are susceptible to hypoglycemia. Urine glucose testing provides only a gross approximation of recent glucose status and should be used only in patients who cannot or refuse to test their blood.

Newer glucose meters are small, portable, and reliable; they give a digital readout and have computerized memory to facilitate recordkeeping. Blood sampling is facilitated (and made less painful) by automated, spring-operated lancet devices. "Alternate-site" testing is available with many meters so that blood sampling can be obtained on nonfinger skin sites, such as the arm, which is less painful. Self-monitoring of blood glucose concentration is of maximal value if the patient performs tests on a regular basis, can accurately measure glucose levels, and can make use of the results. The patient must become familiar with what a normal glucose value is, what the glucose targets are, and how levels can vary with changes in diet or activity and insulin absorption. For most insulin-dependent patients, day-to-day adjustments in short-acting insulin based on pre-meal values and an adjusted scale (applying a "correction factor") can be readily accomplished. These patients also need to examine the effects of their longer acting insulin injections and to make adjustments if glucose levels (e.g., pre-breakfast and pre-dinner values) are not within the target range. At a minimum, patients should be able to adjust to repetitive patterns of hypoglycemia or hyperglycemia as well as to periods of stress and illness ("sick days"). For patients in the latter circumstance, urine testing for ketones should also be routinely performed.

The success of insulin therapy depends on the frequency with which the patient performs self-monitoring. Patients with type 1 diabetes should be encouraged to monitor before each meal and at bedtime and whenever symptoms occur. Periodic checks 120 minutes after meals help control postprandial hyperglycemia, and patients should occasionally monitor predawn (e.g., 3 AM) glucose levels to assess for asymptomatic nocturnal dips. Testing should be more frequent during the initiation of treatment, after changes in therapy, and during any time that altered metabolic control is suspected.

Continuous Glucose Monitoring

Traditional self-monitoring of blood glucose concentration is often inadequate to optimize metabolic control. Continuous glucose monitoring of interstitial fluid has revealed that tight glycemic control is often being achieved at the expense of unacceptably high rates of nocturnal hypoglycemia, and postprandial glucose excursions are often larger than expected. To minimize these highs and lows, despite some limitations in accuracy, continuous glucose monitoring systems have been approved for clinical use. The first generation of "real-time" glucose sensors were worn during a 72-hour period. Their data were evaluated post hoc, similar to a cardiac Holter monitor, to alert clinicians to previously undetected nocturnal hypoglycemia and postprandial glucose elevations. Armed with this additional information, patients and clinicians could then adjust the therapeutic regimen to minimize glucose excursions and to maximize the patient's safety. Live-read glucose sensors have recently been approved. These units provide frequent digital readouts of the patient's current interstitial glucose concentrations along with trend information. The precise role of these devices will certainly evolve as they become more accurate, available, and widely accepted by insurers.

Glycohemoglobin

Glycohemoglobin (glycosylated hemoglobin) assays have emerged as the "gold standard" for long-term glycemic control. The test does not rely on a patient's ability to self-monitor blood glucose levels and is not influenced by acute glycemic changes or by recent meals. Glycohemoglobin is formed when glucose reacts nonenzymatically with the hemoglobin A molecule; it is composed of several fractions, the largest being hemoglobin A_{1c} (HbA_{1c}). HbA_{1c} (expressed as the percentage of total hemoglobin) varies in proportion to the average level of glucose during the lifespan of the red blood cell, thereby providing an index of glycemic control during the preceding 6 to 12 weeks. Several assay methods have been developed and yield different ranges for nondiabetic control subjects. Clinicians should therefore become familiar with the specific assays used for testing their patients.

Although ambient glucose levels are the dominant influence on glycohemoglobin levels, other factors can confound the interpretation of the test result. For example, any condition that increases red blood cell turnover (e.g., pregnancy, hemolytic anemia) spuriously lowers glycohemoglobin levels, regardless of the assay used. Some assays yield spuriously low values in patients with hemoglobinopathies (e.g., sickle cell disease or trait, hemoglobin C or D) or high values when either hemoglobin F is increased (e.g., thalassemia, myeloproliferative disorders) or large doses of aspirin are consumed. Thus, for unexpectedly high or low values encountered in clinical practice, factors that alter the specific assay should be excluded. In most cases, discrepancies between self-monitoring of blood glucose concentration and glycohemoglobin results reflect problems with the former rather than the latter. In clinical practice, frequent blood glucose measurements in conjunction with glycohemoglobin are essential for proper adjustment of the therapeutic regimen.

Treatment Planning

A management plan should take into consideration the life patterns, age, work and school schedules, psychosocial needs, educational level, and motivation of each individual patient. The plan should include lifestyle changes, a meal plan, medications, monitoring instructions (including sick-day management), and education about the prevention and treatment of hypoglycemia. Importantly, all components of the plan must be both understood and accepted by the patient. Active participation of the patient in problem solving as well as ongoing support from a health care team is critical for the successful management of diabetes. In this regard, active and ongoing support from diabetes centers, certified diabetes educators, nutritionists, and exercise physiologists can be invaluable.

At each visit, the management plan should be reviewed and an assessment should be made of the patient's progress in achieving glucose targets. If goals are not being met, causes need to be identified, and the plan should then be modified accordingly. At each visit, the history and physical examination should focus on early signs and symptoms of retinal, cardiovascular, neurologic, and podiatric complications and on reinforcement of the diet and exercise prescription. A complete ophthalmologic examination, assessment of cardiovascular risk factors, and measurement of urinary albumin excretion (through either a timed collection or the more convenient spot urine albumin-to-creatinine ratio) should be performed annually. Specialized podiatric care is also recommended for all patients with evidence of peripheral neuropathy, foot deformities, history of ulcerations, or evidence of peripheral vascular disease. Table 247–4 presents target glycemic guidelines for nonpregnant diabetic patients as well as targets for other clinical factors (e.g., blood pressure, lipids) that are related to the development of diabetic complications.

Surgical Therapy

Pancreas or Islet Transplantation

Intensive insulin therapy rarely if ever restores glucose homeostasis to levels achieved in nondiabetic individuals. As a result, a more effective method of treatment remains a crucial long-term goal of diabetes research. Pancreas transplantation is promising in this regard; with growing experience in recent years, there have been substantial improvements in the outcome of pancreas transplantation surgery. In major centers, 80 to 90% of patients emerge from the perioperative period with a functioning graft; once insulin independence is established, the majority of patients remain stable for several years. Successful pancreas transplantation improves the quality of life of patients with diabetes, primarily by eliminating the need for dietary restrictions, insulin injections, and frequent

TABLE 247–4 THERAPEUTIC TARGETS FOR NONPREGNANT DIABETIC PATIENTS

Parameters	Normal	Target*
Preprandial plasma glucose (mg/dL)	<100	90–130
2-hour postprandial glucose (mg/dL)	<140	<160–180
Bedtime plasma glucose (mg/dL)	<120	110–150
Hemoglobin A_{1c} (%)†	<6	<7
LDL cholesterol (mg/dL)	<130	<100
HDL cholesterol (mg/dL)	>40 (m), >50 (w)	>45 (m), >55 (w)
Fasting triglycerides (mg/dL)	<150	<150
Blood pressure (mm Hg)	<140/90	<130/85

*Clinical targets vary for individual patients, depending on assessment of overall health and the risk-benefit ratio.

†Whereas the hemoglobin A_{1c} goal for patients in general is less than 7%, a goal as close as possible to normal (<6%) without significant hypoglycemia is advisable for an individual patient. Also, less stringent goals may be appropriate for some patients (history of severe hypoglycemia, limited life expectancy, very young children or older adults, and those with significant comorbidities).

HDL = high-density lipoprotein; LDL = low-density lipoprotein; m = men; w = women.

Rx

self-monitoring of glucose concentration. Although pancreas transplantation is only partially able to reverse long-term diabetic complications, it effectively eliminates acute complications such as hypoglycemia and diabetic ketoacidosis.

Unfortunately, because of the need for long-term immunosuppression, pancreas transplantation is at present an option for only a select group of patients, mainly type 1 diabetics who will already require immunosuppression for a renal allograft. In such individuals, successful pancreas transplantation may also be effective in preventing nephropathy in the grafted kidney. In the absence of indications for kidney transplantation, pancreas transplantation alone should generally be considered only in rare diabetic patients with a history of frequent, severe metabolic complications (e.g., life-threatening hypoglycemia with or without recurrent ketoacidosis), in whom insulin therapy consistently fails to achieve metabolic control. It should be considered, however, that in many patients with so-called brittle diabetes, educational, social, and emotional (rather than biologic) factors may provide the greatest obstacles to the patient's achieving control of his or her diabetes. This would obviously need to be considered carefully before committing the patient to lifelong immunosuppression.

Pancreatic islet cell transplantation holds many potential advantages over whole-gland transplantation because it is simpler to perform and less costly. Initially, this experimental procedure involving the intraportal injection of isolated islets from cadaveric sources had disappointing results with regard to long-term insulin independence. In 2000, a series from Edmonton, Alberta, Canada, reported that insulin independence could be achieved in the majority of type 1 diabetic patients. In subsequent follow-up, however, it has become apparent that beyond 1 to 2 years, most patients resume some insulin therapy and many have little or no β-cell function. Of note, compared with patients with type 1 diabetes, islet cell transplantation has been more successful in patients with chronic pancreatitis, many of whom have successfully undergone total pancreatectomy followed by intraportal injection of their pancreatic islets. The implication here is that with diabetes, the use of immunosuppressive drugs, chronic low-grade rejection of the foreign islet grafts, or the activation of an autoimmune response may account for the high incidence of transplant failure. If these inferences are correct, the future of islet transplantation therapy for diabetes depends mainly on manipulating the islet or the immune response rather than on technical surgical advances. These will indeed be difficult tasks.

TABLE 247–5 PRECIPITANTS OF DIABETIC KETOACIDOSIS AND THE HYPEROSMOLAR HYPERGLYCEMIC STATE

THE MOST COMMON PRECIPITANTS

Infections (30–50%): pneumonia, urinary tract infections, sepsis, gastroenteritis
Inadequate insulin treatment (20–40%): includes noncompliance, insulin pump failure
Myocardial ischemia or infarction (3–6%): often clinically "silent" in diabetic patients

OTHER PRECIPITANTS

Cerebrovascular accident
Intracranial bleeding (e.g., subdural hematoma)
Acute pulmonary embolism
Intestinal or mesenteric thrombosis
Intestinal obstruction
Acute pancreatitis
Alcohol intoxication or abuse
Severe burns, hyperthermia or hypothermia
Endocrine disorders: Cushing's syndrome, thyrotoxicosis, acromegaly
Total parenteral nutrition
Drugs
  Cardiovascular: β-blockers, calcium-channel blockers, diuretics, diazoxide, encainide
  Immunosuppressant drugs, including corticosteroids
  Miscellaneous: antipsychotics, phenytoin, cimetidine, pentamidine, L-asparaginase

ACUTE METABOLIC COMPLICATIONS

Hyperglycemic States

Metabolic decompensation in diabetes is generally classified into one of two broad clinical syndromes, diabetic ketoacidosis (DKA) or the hyperosmolar hyperglycemic syndrome (HHS). Although DKA is generally seen in type 1 patients, whereas the HHS affects patients with type 2 diabetes (Chapter 248), lines of classification are commonly blurred. For example, the HHS can present with variable degrees of ketosis and acidosis, and DKA is being seen with increasing frequency in obese type 2 patients. Criteria for both conditions can be met by some patients who experience an overlap syndrome. Despite aggressive treatment, mortality rates remain high for both conditions, approaching 5% for DKA and 15% for the HHS. Mortality is associated with advanced age and comorbidity and is usually due to an associated catastrophic illness (e.g., myocardial infarction, cerebrovascular accident, sepsis) or acute complications including aspiration, cardiac arrhythmias, and cerebral edema. Treatment of hyperglycemic states therefore involves far more than the administration of insulin to reverse hyperglycemia; it also depends critically on prompt attention to the accompanying fluid and electrolyte disturbances as well as the detection and treatment of any precipitating illness.

Diabetic Ketoacidosis

Pathobiology

DKA may herald the onset of type 1 diabetes but most often occurs in established diabetic patients as a result of intercurrent illness (e.g., infection), inappropriate reduction in insulin dosage, or missed insulin injections (especially in adolescents). A common scenario is a patient who fails to adjust insulin therapy or to maintain adequate volume status during an illness, typically a viral gastroenteritis or an influenza-like syndrome. Other common precipitants of DKA (and the HHS) include myocardial infarction, cerebrovascular accident, and alcohol intoxication or abuse; a more extensive list of common precipitants appears in Table 247–5.

The three cardinal biochemical features of DKA—hyperglycemia, ketosis, and acidosis—result from the combined effects of deficient circulating insulin activity and the excessive secretion of counter-regulatory hormones. These hormonal imbalances mobilize the delivery of substrates from muscle (amino acids, lactate, pyruvate) and adipose tissue (free fatty acids, glycerol) to the liver, where they are actively converted to glucose or to ketone bodies (β-hydroxybutyrate, acetoacetate, acetone). Both are ultimately released into the circulation at rates that greatly exceed the capacity of tissues to use them. The end results are hyperglycemia (>250 mg/dL), ketoacidosis (pH < 7.30), and an osmotic diuresis that promotes dehydration and electrolyte loss.

Clinical Manifestations

The clinical history of DKA typically involves deterioration during several days, with advancing polyuria, polydipsia, and other symptoms of progressive hyperglycemia. Other common clinical features are weakness, lethargy, nausea, and anorexia. Abdominal pain in the setting of DKA is classically periumbilical and can mimic an acute abdomen. Reduced motility of the gastrointestinal tract or, in severe cases, paralytic ileus may further contribute to diagnostic confusion. Vomiting is an ominous symptom because it precludes oral replacement of fluid losses; severe volume depletion may follow quickly. Physical findings in DKA are mainly secondary to dehydration and acidosis; these include dry skin and mucous membranes, reduced jugular venous pressure, tachycardia, orthostatic hypotension, depressed mental function, and Kussmaul (deep, rapid) respirations. Ketosis may be recognizable by a sweet, sickly smell on the patient's breath.

Diagnosis

The diagnosis of DKA is usually straightforward and needs to be made promptly. The clinical picture and the presence of hyperglycemia should alert the clinician to test for ketones, to assess the acid-base status, and to measure arterial pH. Initial laboratory tests to be performed include routine serum chemistries (including divalent cations), complete blood count with differential, and urinalysis. Cardiac enzymes and liver and pancreatic function tests should also be considered. An electrocardiogram and a chest x-ray are also routinely obtained, and culture specimens should be taken from blood, urine, and other potential sources as clinically indicated. In DKA, glucose levels vary from 250 to more than 1000 mg/dL, serum bicarbonate concentration drops below 18 mEq/L, and there is an excess anion gap that is generally proportional to the decrease in serum bicarbonate. Hyperchloremia may be superimposed if the patient maintains an adequate glomerular filtration rate and is able to exchange keto acid anions for chloride in the kidney. The degree of depression of arterial pH depends largely on respiratory compensation. In mild cases, the pH may range from 7.20 to 7.30; in severe cases, it can fall below 7.00. In general, clinical severity of DKA depends more on the magnitude of acidosis than on hyperglycemia; as a result, arterial pH is widely used as a reference indicator of DKA severity (Table 247–6). On occasion, a degree of superimposed metabolic alkalosis (e.g., caused by vomiting or diuretic use) may obscure the true severity of the ketoacidosis. An increased anion gap out of proportion to the fall of bicarbonate should suggest this possibility. Other laboratory abnormalities commonly seen in DKA include a reduced measured serum sodium concentration (due to hyperosmolarity and the resulting osmotic shift of intracellular water into the intravascular space), prerenal azotemia, and hyperamylasemia. The last is usually of nonpancreatic origin and can lead to an erroneous diagnosis of pancreatitis. Normal, elevated, or reduced concentrations of potassium, phosphate, and magnesium may exist when DKA is diagnosed; however, large deficits of these electrolytes invariably accompany the osmotic diuresis and become readily apparent during the course of treatment. The serum triglyceride concentration is frequently elevated, a reflection of deranged lipid metabolism in the setting of insulin deficiency. The white blood cell count is typically elevated, sometimes with a predominance of neutrophils. The hemoglobin and hematocrit may be elevated, reflecting volume contraction.

Special care should be taken in interpreting serum or urine ketone results. Because quantitative measurements of β-hydroxybutyrate and acetoacetate are not readily available, rapid diagnosis usually requires *qualitative* assessment of serum ketones by use of serum dilutions and reagent strips (Ketostix) or tablets (Acetest), which depend on a nitroprusside reaction with acetoacetate. However, acetone reacts weakly with nitroprusside, and β-hydroxybutyrate reacts not at all; as a result, qualitative testing for ketones can be misleadingly low. Furthermore, because of the presence of intracellular acidosis, β-hydroxybutyrate levels are often much higher than levels of acetoacetate, which may further conceal the true degree of ketoacidosis. Conversely, after insulin therapy begins, the nitroprusside reaction may give the "false" impression of sustained ketoacidosis for hours or even days. This results because nonacidic acetone is slowly cleared from the circulation and also because, as acidosis improves, β-hydroxybutyrate is converted to acetoacetate, giving the illusion of worsening ketonemia.

HHS is discussed in Chapter 248.

Treatment

The initial goals of therapy for both hyperglycemic states are to replace fluid and electrolyte deficits and to slowly correct hyperglycemia. Unless it is severe, ketoacidosis will generally be corrected with these measures and requires no specific therapy. Current management guidelines of the American Diabetes Association are presented in Figure 247–5 and summarized here. In the treatment of hyperglycemic states, special attention must be paid both to treatment of precipitating illness and to potential complications that may arise during (or as a result of) medical therapy.

Conventional Medical Therapy

In the early hours of treatment, the primary considerations are to restore intravascular volume, to correct tissue hypoperfusion, and to restore insulin sensitivity. With DKA, massive total body deficits of water (5 to 10 L), sodium (5 to 10 mEq/kg), and other electrolytes (see later) may exist. (These losses are even more profound in the HHS, which typically develops during a longer time.) Although water

TABLE 247–6 DIAGNOSTIC CRITERIA FOR DIABETIC KETOACIDOSIS AND THE HYPEROSMOLAR HYPERGLYCEMIC STATE

	Mild DKA	Moderate DKA	Severe DKA	HHS
Plasma glucose (mg/dL)	>250	>250	>250	>600
Effective serum osmolality (mOsm/kg)*	Variable	Variable	Variable	>320
Urine or serum ketones (NP reaction)	Positive	Positive	Positive	Negative to trace
Arterial pH	7.25–7.30	7.00–7.24	<7.00	>7.30
Serum bicarbonate (mEq/L)	15–18	10–15	<10	>15
Anion gap (mEq/L)	>10	>12	>12	<12
Typical mental status	Alert	Drowsy	Stupor or coma	Stupor or coma

*Effective serum osmolality (mOsm/kg) = 2 [measured serum sodium (mEq/L)] + [serum glucose (mg/dL)/18]. Normal range = 285 ± 5 mOsm/kg. Urea nitrogen is an "ineffective osmole" (i.e., it diffuses freely across compartments) and is therefore purposely excluded from this equation.
DKA = diabetic ketoacidosis; HHS = hyperosmolar hyperglycemic state; NP = nitroprusside.
Modified from Kitabchi AE, Umpierrez G, Murphy MB, et al: Management of hyperglycemic crises in patients with diabetes. Diabetes Care 2001;24:131–153.

Rx

loss usually exceeds the loss of sodium, it is almost always preferable to begin fluid replacement with isotonic normal saline (0.9% NaCl solution) for efficient intravascular volume restoration. Fluid replacement regimens vary, but it is common to administer 1 liter of normal saline within the first hour, followed by continuous infusion with either 0.45% NaCl or 0.9% NaCl, depending on the corrected serum sodium concentration and the patient's hemodynamic status and the clinical assessment of tissue perfusion. Likewise, the rate of infusion (commonly 250 to 500 mL/hr) should be adjusted according to both biochemical responses and the age and clinical status of the

Adult patient with DKA or HHS

Complete initial evaluation, including (but not limited to):
- Medical history and physical examination
- Complete blood count with differential
- Fingerstick blood glucose
- Serum chemistries ("Chem-10" plus serum ketones)
- Urine for urinalysis and ketones
- Cultures as indicated (wound, blood, urine, etc.)
- Chest ± abdominal x-ray
- 12-lead ECG

→

- Concurrently, begin empirical fluid resuscitation with 0.9% NaCl at 1000 mL/hr
- Consider volume expanders if hypovolemic shock is present
- Continue fluid resuscitation until volume status and cardiovascular parameters (pulse, BP) have been restored

IV Fluids
- Based on corrected serum sodium*
- If high/normal, use 0.45% NaCl
- If low/normal, use 0.9% NaCl
- Continue IV fluids at 250–1000 mL/hr, depending on volume status, cardiovascular history, and cardiovascular status (pulse, BP)

Insulin Therapy
- Regular insulin bolus, 0.15 U/kg
- IV infusion, 0.10 U/kg hr
- Check serum glucose hourly—should fall by 50–80 mg/dL/hr
- If serum glucose falling too rapidly, back off on insulin infusion
- If serum glucose rising or falling too slowly, increase insulin infusion rate by 50–100%

When Serum Glucose Reaches 250–300 mg/dL:
- Add dextrose to IV fluids. Continue IV fluids at 150–250 mL/hr, and adjust insulin infusion to maintain serum glucose ~200 mg/dL until metabolic control is achieved:
- For DKA, continue until anion gap has closed and acidosis has resolved
- For HHS, continue until plasma osmolality drops below 310 mOsm/kg
- Begin more exhaustive search for precipitant of metabolic decompensation

←

Continuing Management:
- Follow and replete serum electrolytes (including divalent cations) q2–4h until stable
- After resolution of hyperglycemic state, follow blood glucose q4h and initiate sliding scale regular insulin coverage
- Convert IV insulin to subcutaneous injections (or resumption of prior therapy), ensuring adequate overlap
- Begin clear liquid diet and advance as tolerated. Encourage resumption of ambulation and activity
- Review and update diabetes education, with special attention to prevention of further hyperglycemic crises

Potassium (K^+) Repletion
- Obtain baseline serum potassium
- Obtain 12-lead ECG

$[K^+] \geq 5.5$ mEq/L → Hold K^+ therapy → Treat hyperkalemia if ECG changes present → Recheck $[K^+]$ in 2 hr

$[K^+] < 5.5$ mEq/L and adequate urine output → Add K^+ to IV fluids (Use KCl and/or KPhos)
- $[K^+] = 4.5$–5.4: add 20 mEq/L IV fluids
- $[K^+] = 3.5$–4.4: add 30 mEq/L IV fluids
- $[K^+] < 3.5$: add 40 mEq/L IV fluids

- Follow serum $[K^+]$ every 2–4 hours until stable: anticipate rapid drop of serum $[K^+]$ during therapy, due to dilution and intracellular shifting
- Ensure adequate urine output to avoid over-repletion and hyperkalemia
- Continue K^+ repletion until serum $[K^+]$ is stable at between 4–5 mEq/L
- If refractory hypokalemia, ensure concurrent magnesium repletion
- Repletion may need to be continued for several days, as total body losses may reach up to 500 mEq

Bicarbonate Therapy
- Obtain ABG
- Obtain baseline serum bicarbonate

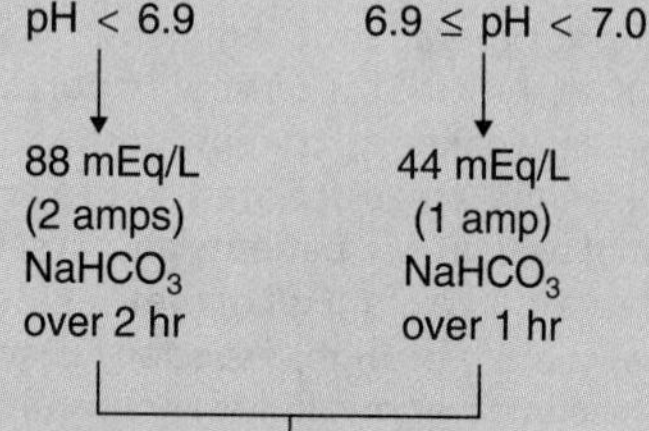

- pH < 6.9 → 88 mEq/L (2 amps) $NaHCO_3$ over 2 hr
- 6.9 ≤ pH < 7.0 → 44 mEq/L (1 amp) $NaHCO_3$ over 1 hr
- pH ≥ 7.0 → Assess need for bicarbonate

- Repeat ABG after bicarbonate administration
- Repeat $NaHCO_3$ therapy until pH ≥ 7.0, then discontinue therapy
- Follow serum bicarbonate q4h until stable

*Sodium correction: Serum sodium should be corrected for hyperglycemia. For every 100 mg/dL of glucose elevation above 100 mg/dL, add 1.6 mEq/L to the measured sodium value; this will yield the corrected serum sodium concentration.

FIGURE 247–5 • Management of diabetic ketoacidosis (DKA) and the hyperosmolar hyperglycemic syndrome (HHS). ABG = arterial blood gases; BP = blood pressure; ECG = electrocardiogram; IV = intravenous.

patient (e.g., oliguria or underlying cardiovascular disease). In pediatric patients with DKA, isotonic solutions are generally preferred because they are less likely than hypotonic solutions to accelerate water shifts into the intracellular space and contribute to cerebral edema. During the course of treatment, once blood glucose concentration falls to below 250 mg/dL, glucose should be added to intravenous fluids to avoid eventual hypoglycemia because continued insulin delivery will still be required to correct often persistent acidosis.

Although insulin resistance is present in both DKA and HHS, supraphysiologic doses of insulin are unnecessary and are more likely to provoke hypokalemia, hypophosphatemia, and delayed hypoglycemia. A typical insulin replacement regimen uses an intravenous bolus of 0.15 U/kg of rapid-acting (e.g., regular) insulin, followed by 0.1 U/kg/hr thereafter. Intravenous administration is the most predictable way of delivering insulin to target tissues, particularly in severely hypovolemic patients with reduced peripheral blood flow. If intravenous administration is not possible, intramuscular or subcutaneous routes of administration can be used. It is ideal if blood glucose levels fall at a steady and predictable rate (50 to 80 mg/dL/hr), so it is important to monitor blood glucose levels hourly during insulin therapy to ensure an appropriate rate of decline. Blood glucose levels should not fall too rapidly, especially in young children, in whom accelerated glucose correction has been associated with cerebral edema.

Treatment Planning

In reviewing the progress of treatment, it is important to consider a failure in insulin delivery if blood glucose concentration fails to drop appropriately. In some patients, persistent hyperglycemia may be due to severe insulin resistance and necessitates an increase in the insulin dose. However, because the primary mechanism for lowering plasma glucose concentration in the early stages of treatment is urinary glucose disposal (rather than insulin-stimulated glucose consumption), the problem may simply reflect inadequate replacement of intravascular volume, in which case insulin rates may not need to be increased. After a stable blood glucose level below 250 mg/dL is achieved, with resolution of the anion gap acidosis, subcutaneous administration of insulin can be started and the intravenous insulin infusion may be discontinued. With DKA, it is important to overlap the intravenous and subcutaneous routes by 1 to 2 hours to avoid the return of ketoacidosis. After the return of normoglycemia, long-term medical management should be initiated (or resumed), with both long-acting and short-acting insulins, to approximate what the discharge regimen will be. A temporary "regular insulin sliding scale" is no longer advised as such therapy will likely allow the glucose levels to rise into the hyperglycemic range before insulin is administered. More proactive insulin replacement regimens are preferred. The eventual dosage and frequency of insulin will depend on multiple factors, including body habitus, comorbidity, insulin sensitivity, and effectiveness of prior therapeutic regimens.

Potassium replacement in DKA (and HHS) is of vital importance. Hypokalemia can result in muscle weakness, cramps, and nausea; both hyperkalemia and hypokalemia are associated with cardiac arrhythmias. At the time of initial evaluation, patients have a severe total body potassium deficit (about 3 to 7 mEq/kg), yet measured serum potassium levels may be normal, or high, especially if acidosis or renal failure is present. Once intravenous fluids and insulin are started, serum potassium levels fall quickly because of an insulin-mediated shift of potassium into the intracellular space. In addition, fluid replacement causes extracellular dilution of potassium, leading to improved renal perfusion and increased urinary potassium excretion. This rapid decline can be countered by potassium replacement based on measured serum levels. A low potassium level (<3.5 mEq/kg) requires prompt treatment with up to 40 mEq/hr, whereas "normal" serum levels (3.5 to 5.0 mEq/kg) call for less aggressive repletion (10 to 30 mEq/hr), assuming adequate urine output. In patients who may have lost potassium for additional reasons, such as diuretic use or gastrointestinal loss, one should anticipate the need for greater potassium supplementation. Serial electrocardiograms are valuable because they provide a more direct assessment of *intracellular* potassium concentration; flat to inverted T waves and U waves suggest a low potassium level, and peaked T waves and QRS prolongation may indicate hyperkalemia. The intracellular potassium deficit in renal tubular cells further promotes potassium loss through the kidneys; this abnormality may take several days to be corrected. As a result, excess urinary potassium losses may continue for days to weeks and may call for prolonged oral supplementation for normokalemia to be maintained.

In the majority of patients with mild to moderate DKA, keto acids clear spontaneously with standard therapeutic measures, and artificial correction with alkali (bicarbonate) is unnecessary. Suppression of lipolysis by insulin reduces free fatty acid flux to the liver and blocks ketogenesis. The remaining keto acids are then cleared or oxidized, with subsequent regeneration of bicarbonate and restoration of pH. In cases of severe acidosis (pH < 7.0), however, bicarbonate administration may be indicated; the hyperventilatory drive of severe acidosis is uncomfortable, and severe acidosis also impairs cardiac functions and peripheral vasodilation. Bicarbonate therapy should be used with caution because it can further provoke hypokalemia, which in turn can precipitate cardiac arrhythmias. In addition, by causing a sudden left shift of the dissociation curve for oxyhemoglobin, bicarbonate may impair oxygen delivery to the tissues. If alkaline therapy is given, small amounts should be administered, and slowly: 44 mEq (one ampule) of $NaHCO_3$ during 1 hour for pH 6.9 to 7.0 and 88 mEq during 2 hours for pH below 6.9. After bicarbonate administration, arterial pH (and serum potassium levels) should be rechecked every 2 hours, and alkaline therapy should be discontinued when the pH rises above 7.0.

In the setting of DKA, phosphate losses average 3 to 7 mmol/kg; magnesium losses reach 1 to 2 mEq/kg. (Magnitudes of depletion for both ions may be greater for the HHS because of a more prolonged osmotic diuresis.) Phosphate is shifted extracellularly during hyperosmolar states, so initial serum levels may be falsely elevated and may drop rapidly during therapy. Complications of hypophosphatemia generally occur at serum levels below 1.0 mg/dL and include respiratory and skeletal muscle weakness, impaired cardiac systolic performance, and hemolytic anemia. Phosphate depletion may also contribute to depressed concentrations of 2,3-diphosphoglycerate, thus shifting the oxygen dissociation curve to the left and further limiting tissue oxygen delivery. Although *prophylactic* phosphate replacement has shown no clinical benefit in trials, phosphate repletion should be given to patients with serum phosphate levels below 1.0 mg/dL and to patients with evidence of cardiac or respiratory compromise, hypoxia, or hemolytic anemia. An effective means of replacing phosphate is to replace one third of potassium losses (discussed before) as potassium phosphate; in general, 20 to 30 mEq/L of potassium phosphate can be added to intravenous fluids and given during several hours. Because of calcium binding, hypocalcemic tetany may complicate phosphate therapy unless magnesium supplements are also provided; for this reason, serum calcium, phosphate, and magnesium levels should be monitored periodically during any phosphate infusion.

Management of Complications

The most common complications of therapy for hyperglycemic states are hypoglycemia, hypokalemia, hypophosphatemia, and fluid overload; precautions to avoid these complications have been described earlier. Two other rare but potentially fatal complications deserve special mention.

Cerebral edema, which occurs primarily in pediatric patients, is associated with overaggressive correction of hyperglycemia and with hypotonic fluid replacement. It is likely to be the result of osmotically driven movement of water into the central nervous system when plasma osmolarity declines too rapidly. Clinically, cerebral edema is characterized by lethargy and headache, with progressive decline in mental status and neurologic deterioration.

The acute respiratory distress syndrome is also attributed to rapid reductions in colloid osmotic pressure, causing increased lung water content, decreased lung compliance, and noncardiogenic pulmonary

Rx

edema. These patients present clinically with respiratory distress, hypoxemia with an elevated alveolar-arterial oxygen gradient, and bilateral pulmonary congestion on the chest film.

In practice, a suspicion for either cerebral edema or acute respiratory distress syndrome requires prompt diagnosis. All such patients should be transferred to an intensive care unit for immediate and aggressive management.

Prevention

Prevention of DKA requires extensive education in sick-day insulin and fluid management as well as home-based assessment of urine ketones whenever severe hyperglycemia or physical illness is noted.

Hypoglycemia

Definition

Hypoglycemia is the most frequent complication resulting from insulin therapy for type 1 diabetes. Nearly all patients are symptomatically affected at least once per year, and a significant percentage have severe hypoglycemia requiring medical assistance. Studies using continuous glucose monitoring of type 1 diabetics have shown alarmingly high rates of hypoglycemia, especially at night, when sleeping patients are unaware of its existence.

Pathobiology

Symptoms of low blood glucose concentration result from changes in autonomic activity and brain function. Autonomic symptoms, including sweating, tremor, and palpitations, are often the earliest subjective warning signs of hypoglycemia. Central nervous system symptoms and signs of glucose deficiency, termed neuroglycopenia, may be nonspecific (e.g., fatigue or weakness) or more clearly neurologic (e.g., double vision, oral paresthesias, slurring of speech, apraxia, personality change, or behavioral disturbances). Hypoglycemia affects type 2 patients as well; most cases occur during treatment with insulin or insulin secretagogues, especially the longer acting sulfonylureas. Because of the long-acting nature of the oral agents, low blood glucose concentration can recur up to 48 hours after drug withdrawal, and a more extended course of therapy is often required.

It is well known that prolonged, severe hypoglycemia can cause irreversible brain damage. What is less clear, however, is whether significant neurologic damage results from shorter, milder episodes of low blood glucose concentration. Studies have suggested that electroencephalographic abnormalities and reduced cognitive function are more prevalent in young children with a history of recurrent hypoglycemia. The DCCT, however, reported no evidence of neuropsychological impairment in patients with recurrent severe hypoglycemic episodes, after an average of 7 years of intensified treatment. Nevertheless, hypoglycemia may provoke seizures, accidental injury, and a catecholamine response that can induce cardiac ischemia or arrhythmias in patients with underlying cardiac disease. Overall, hypoglycemia is thought to account for 3 to 4% of deaths in insulin-treated diabetic patients. Hypoglycemia also has far-reaching social implications. On a personal level, it can induce great fear, preclude comfortable engagement in routine activities (e.g., driving), and lead both patient and clinician to aim deliberately for less than optimal glycemic control. From a practical standpoint, the growing body of evidence that tight glucose control prevents long-term complications of diabetes has led to more aggressive treatment regimens, inevitably resulting in a greater incidence of clinical hypoglycemia. This, in turn, has necessitated further study of the physiology, consequences, and prevention of hypoglycemia in diabetic patients.

In *non*diabetic persons, hypoglycemia provokes a rapid, multi-tiered metabolic response intended to restore normal blood glucose levels. The brain cannot store more than a few minutes' supply of energy; in the short term, its function is exclusively dependent on a constant supply of glucose for fuel. To preserve central nervous system function, spontaneous recovery from hypoglycemia involves both the activation of endogenous glucose production and reduced peripheral glucose use. Three fundamental mechanisms are responsible for this process: dissipation of endogenous insulin; counter-regulatory hormone activity; and subjective awareness of hypoglycemia, resulting in hunger and subsequent carbohydrate ingestion. Early hormonal changes are triggered when plasma glucose concentration approaches the hypoglycemic range (65 to 70 mg/dL). A rise in glucose production, attributable mainly to stimulation of hepatic glycogenolysis, is initiated by the release of glucagon from pancreatic α cells in conjunction with falling levels of endogenous insulin. Catecholamines are also released, which produce "alarm" symptoms for hypoglycemia (e.g., hunger, tremor, palpitations) and further promote the synthesis of glucose through stimulation of hepatic glycogenolysis, mobilization of substrates for gluconeogenesis, and further suppression of insulin production. When hypoglycemia is sustained, additional counter-regulatory hormones such as growth hormone and corticosteroids are released; through a variety of complementary mechanisms, these hormones also help promote continued glucose availability. Reduced peripheral glucose uptake results from an interplay of factors, including low circulating insulin levels, epinephrine's inhibitory effect on insulin-stimulated glucose uptake, elevated free fatty acid levels, and hypoglycemia per se. For a more in-depth discussion of metabolic responses to hypoglycemia, refer to Chapter 249.

Patients with type 1 diabetes are more likely to have hypoglycemia for several reasons. First, injected insulin enters the circulation from a nonphysiologic source (e.g., a subcutaneous depot), which is therefore unaffected by any counter-regulatory response to falling glucose levels, as may occur in type 2 patients with endogenous insulin secretion. In addition, patients with type 1 diabetes, as a rule, are insulin sensitive, as opposed to their type 2 counterparts. Type 1 patients also lose their glucagon response to hypoglycemia, for unclear reasons; this appears to be a stimulus-specific phenomenon because their glucagon response to other stimuli may be unaffected. Defective glucagon responses develop in most type 1 patients 2 to 5 years after diagnosis (usually at about the same time that they become completely insulin deficient), after which time counter-regulation relies heavily on epinephrine release. Unfortunately, half of type 1 patients also undergo a stimulus-specific diminution in their epinephrine response to hypoglycemia, further predisposing them to severe episodes. Finally, the ability of type 1 diabetic patients to recognize hypoglycemia and to take corrective action may also be impaired. In some cases, the irritability and confusion that occur during hypoglycemia may prevent the patient's awareness of its cause. In other cases, patients may lose the autonomic warning symptoms of hypoglycemia and may recognize (or even fail to recognize) the condition only when somatic neurologic function becomes impaired. This so-called hypoglycemic unawareness syndrome has been associated with a number of factors, including duration of diabetes and autonomic neuropathy.

Hypoglycemia unawareness may also occur when patients are switched to intensive insulin regimens. The introduction of intensified treatment regimens can lower the glucose level that triggers epinephrine release and adrenergic symptoms, which at least partly explains the increased frequency of severe hypoglycemia reported in the DCCT. The mechanism underlying the changes is an increased incidence of iatrogenic hypoglycemia during intensified insulin therapy. It has been shown that even brief periods of antecedent hypoglycemia can suppress counter-regulatory responses during subsequent hypoglycemic episodes. Defective glucose counter-regulation induced by intensive insulin regimens, however, appears to be reversible by scrupulous avoidance of hypoglycemia and readjustment of treatment goals for several weeks. This underscores the need to prevent iatrogenic hypoglycemia by improving patients' self-management skills. Continuous glucose monitoring, by allowing more precise adjustments in the insulin regimen, can be expected to improve hypoglycemia unawareness and the diminished counter-regulatory response.

CHRONIC DIABETIC COMPLICATIONS

The pathogenesis of the microvascular and neuropathic complications of diabetes is complex and poorly understood. However, these complications are undoubtedly mediated in large part by the metabolic derangements associated with diabetes, especially hyperglycemia. It has been suggested that glucose-induced cell injury is particularly pronounced in those cell types that are unable to regulate their intracellular glucose concentration (e.g., endothelial cells and neurons) and that this leads to increased production of reactive oxygen species (superoxide) as well as advanced glycation end products (AGEs) and an accelerated polyol pathway with consequent protein kinase C activation.

Studies suggest that hyperglycemia-mediated intracellular overproduction of reactive oxygen species may be the common mechanism triggering a variety of pathways thought to contribute to cell injury in diabetes. In addition, a variety of proteins are nonenzymatically glycosylated in vivo (including hemoglobin, collagen, laminin, low-density lipoprotein particles, and peripheral nerve proteins) in direct proportion to prevailing levels of glucose. AGE cross-linking capabilities render them resistant to natural degradation. The consequent AGEs accumulate in a variety of tissues (including the kidneys and blood vessels), where they bind to a receptor for AGE (RAGE). Of particular interest, the binding of AGEs to RAGE is thought to contribute to cell injury through a variety of mechanisms, including stimulation of oxidative reactions as well as proinflammatory cytokines, complement, and growth factors. In the polyol pathway, increased activity of intracellular aldose reductase leads to accumulation of sorbitol and fructose, resulting in decreased glutathione antioxidant activity (through decreased NAD^+), and enhanced formation of diacylglycerol. Diacylglycerol formation can in turn activate specific isoforms of protein kinase C, which stimulate transforming growth factor-β release and play an important role in cell proliferation and vascular permeability. In experimental diabetic animals, prevention of superoxide accumulation, inhibition of AGE formation, and specific protein kinase C inhibitors reduce diabetic complications.

Other potential mechanisms through which glucose could impair cell function include (but are not limited to) activation of cytokines (angiotensin II, endothelin), growth factor stimulation (transforming growth factor-β, vascular endothelial growth factor), and depletion of basement membrane glycosaminoglycans. It is likely that each of these factors plays a variable and interrelated role in the development and progression of microvascular complications in diabetes.

Hemodynamic changes in the microcirculation may also contribute to microangiopathy. In the diabetic kidney, glomerular filtration rate is increased out of proportion to renal plasma flow owing to an elevation in the transglomerular pressure gradient. It is assumed that raised glomerular pressures promote the passage of proteins and AGEs; with time, their accumulation in the mesangium is likely to trigger the proliferation of mesangial cells and matrix production, eventually leading to glomerulosclerosis. Compensatory hyperfiltration and a decreasing number of functional glomeruli would exacerbate matters, increasing intraglomerular pressure, further resulting in progressive glomerular damage. Clinical studies support this view. Unilateral renal artery stenosis diminishes diabetic pathologic lesions in the affected kidney, and angiotensin-converting enzyme (ACE) inhibitors and angiotensin II receptor antagonists (which reduce intraglomerular pressures) are known to slow the progression of diabetic nephropathy. The diabetes-associated increase in microcirculatory hydrostatic pressure may also contribute to generalized capillary leakage of macromolecules in diabetic patients.

These theories would predict the benefits of optimal glycemic control reported by the DCCT in patients with few or no complications. Whether similar benefits can be expected once severe damage has occurred is less clear. Extensive glycosylation of proteins with slow turnover rates would not be readily affected by correction of hyperglycemia. Moreover, the hemodynamic theory for nephropathy predicts that once glomerular injury causes compensatory hyperfiltration, progressive injury may continue in the remaining glomeruli, regardless of the prevailing metabolic state.

Although the microvascular complications of diabetes may affect patients with type 1 or type 2 diabetes, they are discussed in this chapter. The macrovascular complications, which are particularly common in type 2 diabetes, are discussed in Chapter 248.

Diabetic Retinopathy

Definition

Diabetic retinopathy refers to progressive pathologic alterations in the retinal microvasculature, leading to areas of retinal nonperfusion, increased vascular permeability, and the pathologic proliferation of retinal vessels.

Epidemiology

In the United States, diabetes is the leading cause of blindness in persons aged 20 to 74 years. Retinopathy in poorly controlled type 1 diabetics occurs in about 25% of patients 5 years after diagnosis, 60% at 10 years, and more than 95% at 15 years. Blindness occurs 25 times more frequently in diabetic patients than in control subjects and is seen most often after the disease has been present for at least 15 years, in the setting of advanced retinopathy. Approximately 10 to 15% of type 1 diabetic patients will become legally blind (visual acuity of 20/200 or worse in the better eye). In type 2 diabetes, although the incidence of blindness is lower, higher disease prevalence results in an even larger number of patients affected with severe visual loss.

Clinical Manifestations

Nonproliferative Diabetic Retinopathy

The earliest pathologic changes associated with retinopathy are termed mild nonproliferative diabetic retinopathy. In type 1 patients, these changes generally begin no sooner than 5 years after diagnosis. The first signs of mild nonproliferative diabetic retinopathy are microaneurysms, which arise most often in areas of capillary occlusion. Subsequently, increasing vascular permeability leads to retinal blot hemorrhages (round, with blurred edges) and "hard" exudates (sharply defined and yellow). Infarctions of the nerve fiber layer, known as soft exudates or cotton-wool spots, appear as white or gray, rounded swellings. At this early stage of retinopathy, visual acuity is generally unaffected, and the risk of progression to high-risk proliferative diabetic retinopathy (see following) is about 15% at 5 years.

Moderate nonproliferative diabetic retinopathy is characterized by intraretinal microvascular abnormalities, including venous caliber changes, beading, and increased capillary dilation and permeability. Later changes, termed severe or very severe nonproliferative diabetic retinopathy, include progressive retinal capillary loss and ischemia, with further development of extensive hemorrhages, exudates, and microaneurysms. At 5 years, moderate and severe nonproliferative diabetic retinopathy are associated with a 30% and 60% risk of progression to high-risk proliferative diabetic retinopathy, respectively.

Proliferative Diabetic Retinopathy

Proliferative diabetic retinopathy involves neovascularization, the growth of fine tufts of new blood vessels and fibrous tissue from the inner retinal surface or the optic head. Early proliferative changes are confined to the retina, but later invasion of the vitreous body constitutes high-risk proliferative diabetic retinopathy; during this end stage, fibrosis and contracture of the neovasculature result in retinal detachment and hemorrhage, the most important determinants of blindness. On occasion, new vessels can invade the iris and anterior chamber, leading to sight-threatening closed-angle glaucoma.

Clinically Significant Macular Edema

Clinically significant macular edema results from vascular leakage at the macula and can occur either with or without the stages of retinopathy described before. Clinically significant macular edema is suggested by hard macular exudates on funduscopic examination and can be confirmed with slit-lamp biomicroscopy. In general, maculopathy is more common in type 2 patients, in whom it is an important contributor to the loss of visual acuity. As will be discussed, the treatment of clinically significant macular edema runs parallel to the treatment of other forms of diabetic retinopathy.

Treatment

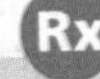

Medical Therapy

At present, medical management of diabetic retinopathy is aimed at controlling risk factors for progression. The value of tight glycemic control was proved by the DCCT, whose primary prevention arm demonstrated an impressive 76% risk reduction for the onset of retinopathy with intensive therapy. In the secondary

Rx

prevention arm, patients with early nonproliferative diabetic retinopathy undergoing intensive therapy demonstrated a 47% risk reduction in the development of severe nonproliferative diabetic retinopathy or proliferative diabetic retinopathy, a 51% risk reduction in the need for laser treatment, and a 26% risk reduction in the development of clinically significant macular edema. Other targets for medical management, all associated with accelerated retinal damage, include hypertension, hyperlipidemia, treatment of nephropathy, and careful follow-up during pregnancy, when accelerated retinal disease has been linked to preexisting diabetes (but not gestational disease). Recently, inhibitors of protein kinase C-β (e.g., ruboxistaurin) have shown some promise in delaying progression in advanced forms of retinopathy.

Surgical Therapy

Surgical management of retinopathy is aimed at slowing disease progression as baseline visual acuity is difficult to recover. In the 1980s, large-scale prospective clinical trials such as the Diabetic Retinopathy Study and the Early Treatment Diabetic Retinopathy Study established photocoagulation as the treatment of choice when retinopathy threatens vision. Most patients with proliferative diabetic retinopathy, and selected patients with severe nonproliferative diabetic retinopathy, are now treated primarily with scatter (panretinal) photocoagulation; cryotherapy or vitrectomy may be required if laser treatment is unfeasible for technical reasons or because of extensive disease. Clinically significant macular edema is nearly universally treated with focal photocoagulation, with the possible exception of patients exhibiting, concurrently, no or minimal nonproliferative diabetic retinopathy. In such patients, close follow-up in a 2- to 4-month interval is an acceptable option. A treatment chart, adapted from a thorough technical review by Aiello and colleagues, is shown in Table 247–7. Note that the decision to treat depends not only on stage of retinopathy and extent of clinically significant macular edema but also on the type of diabetes, general medical status, compliance with follow-up, and status of the contralateral eye.

These considerations make it imperative for physicians *prospectively* to identify diabetic patients at risk for retinopathy and visual loss. Nonspecialists, including house officers, internists, and diabetologists, are known to have difficulty diagnosing the stages of retinopathy; studies show that such physicians arrive at the correct diagnosis in less than half of cases. Accordingly, patients should be referred to an experienced eye specialist for a complete examination to include a dilated funduscopic examination, tonometry, and slit-lamp biomicroscopy. The most recent guidelines of the American Diabetes Association recommend initial eye examination within 3 to 5 years of diagnosis of type 1 diabetes and at the time of diagnosis in type 2 patients.

Follow-up

Follow-up of all patients should occur *at least* on a yearly basis, with the possible exception of those with retinopathy-free type 2 diabetes. Even in the latter cases, the American Diabetes Association does recommend yearly examinations to avoid lost follow-up and to identify patients with more aggressive ocular disease. Of special note, because retinopathy rarely develops in children before puberty, patients with early-onset type 1 diabetes generally do not require screening before 10 years of age. Also, the acceleration of retinopathy during pregnancy demands that all patients with preexisting diabetes be examined during the first trimester.

Diabetic Nephropathy

Epidemiology

End-stage renal disease (ESRD) from diabetic nephropathy is a major cause of morbidity and mortality, particularly in patients with type 1 diabetes, of whom 30 to 35% are susceptible to this complication. Although the risk of nephropathy is somewhat less frequent in type 2 diabetics (~20%, partially due to a shortened life expectancy), patients with type 2 diabetes still make up the majority of diabetic patients seeking therapy for ESRD. Reports suggest a decline in the incidence of ESRD, at least in whites with type 1 diabetes, from strategies (see later) to reduce its progression. Nevertheless, diabetes is the leading cause of ESRD in the United States, accounting for more than one third of cases.

Risk Factors

There are several known risk factors for the development of diabetic nephropathy: duration of disease; elevated glycohemoglobin levels; and concurrent hypertension, hyperlipidemia, and tobacco use. Race is known to play a major role as well, as demonstrated by a higher prevalence of nephropathy in African American, Hispanic, and Native American patients. There is also a high concordance rate in families; studies in both type 1 and type 2 diabetic families revealed a three- to four-fold increase in the prevalence of nephropathy with affected siblings. Strong associations have been noted with several other factors as well, including a deletion polymorphism of the ACE gene, increased sodium-lithium countertransport, and degree of insulin resistance.

Clinical Manifestations

Natural History

Details are less clear in type 2 diabetes, but the natural history of diabetic nephropathy in type 1 diabetes is well described (Fig. 247–6). The period immediately after diagnosis is best characterized by glomerular hyperfiltration. During this time, there is renal hypertrophy, increased renal blood flow, increased glomerular volume, and increased transglomerular pressure gradient, all contributing to a rise in glomerular filtration rate. Importantly, these changes depend at least in part on

TABLE 247–7 GUIDELINES FOR TREATMENT AND FOLLOW-UP OF DIABETIC RETINOPATHY

Stage of Retinopathy	Panretinal PC	If CSME, Focal PC*	Follow-up
No or minimal NPDR	Not recommended	Possible	12 mo†
Mild to moderate NPDR	Not recommended	Probable	6–12 mo†
Severe to very severe NPDR	Possible	Recommended	2–4 mo
Early PDR	Probable	Recommended	2–4 mo
High-risk PDR	Recommended	Recommended	2–4 mo

*If retinopathy and CSME coexist, focal PC for CSME should always precede panretinal PC.
†In these patients, follow-up is recommended in just 2 to 4 months if CSME is also present.
CSME = clinically significant macular edema; NPDR = nonproliferative diabetic retinopathy; PC = photocoagulation; PDR = proliferative diabetic retinopathy.
Modified from Aiello LP, Gardner TW, King GL, et al: Diabetic retinopathy [technical review]. Diabetes Care 1998;21:143.

Diagnosis →	3 Years →	5 Years →	15 Years →	25 Years → ESRD
Renal hypertrophy (gross) Normal microarchitecture Normal microvasculature	Thickened GBM Mesangial matrix expansion Early arteriolosclerosis	Early GS K-W nodules Advanced arteriolosclerosis	Progressive GS (End-stage fibrosis) Vessel obliteration	
Increased GFR Normal serum CR Normoalbuminuria Normotensive	Increased GFR Normal serum CR Reversible albuminuria Mostly normotensive	"Pseudonormalization" of GFR Normal serum CR Microalbuminuria ~50% hypertensive	Declining GFR Rising serum CR Albuminuria ~100% hypertensive	

FIGURE 247–6 • Pathogenesis of diabetic nephropathy. CR = creatinine; ESRD = end-stage renal disease; GBM = glomerular basement membrane; GFR = glomerular filtration rate; GS = glomerulosclerosis; K-W = Kimmelstiel-Wilson.

hyperglycemia, as they are diminished by intensive diabetes treatment. Three to 5 years after diagnosis, early glomerular lesions appear, characterized by thickening of glomerular basement membranes, mesangial matrix expansion, and arteriolosclerosis. Albumin excretion remains low during early glomerular changes; however, as pathologic changes mount, the glomeruli lose their functional integrity, resulting in glomerular filtration defects and increased glomerular permeability. Although the results of routine tests of renal function (creatinine concentration and urinalysis) still remain normal, microalbuminuria (30 to 300 mg/day) appears. Systemic hypertension is also present at this time in more than 50% of cases.

After several years, most diabetic patients exhibit diffuse glomerulosclerosis, although a minority will have pathognomonic Kimmelstiel-Wilson nodular lesions. Although pathologic changes continue to mount throughout the disease, glomerulosclerosis extensive enough to cause ESRD develops in a minority of patients; in these cases, overt albuminuria (>300 mg/day) begins approximately 15 years after diagnosis. Soon after, following a variable period on the order of 3 to 5 years, glomerular filtration rate begins a relentless decline (10 mL/min per year or more), which is eventually reflected by an increase in serum creatinine concentration. The appearance of massive proteinuria and the nephrotic syndrome is common in this context and often heralds progression to ESRD. Once the serum creatinine concentration rises (reflecting an approximately 50% decline in glomerular filtration rate), ESRD develops in most patients within 10 years. This course is highly variable, however, particularly in type 2 diabetics, who may exhibit moderate proteinuria for several years without a substantial deterioration of renal function. A simple but useful method of monitoring progression to renal failure is to plot the reciprocal of the serum creatinine concentration as a function of time. This technique allows better assessment of both therapeutic interventions and the time when renal replacement therapy will become necessary.

Treatment

Early Stage Treatment

Treatment of nephropathy has become an important focus of recent research and depends heavily on stage of disease. Early in the course of diabetes (before the onset of microalbuminuria), strict glycemic control is of the utmost importance. The DCCT demonstrated that intensive therapy reduced microalbuminuria by 39% and overt albuminuria by 54% in type 1 diabetics, with a mean follow-up of 6.5 years. A similar result was demonstrated in the United Kingdom Prospective Diabetes Study (UKPDS) of patients with type 2 diabetes (Chapter 248), in which a less dramatic improvement in glycemic control reduced microalbuminuria and overt albuminuria by 24% and 33%, respectively, with a mean follow-up of 9 years. In normotensive, normoalbuminuric type 2 diabetics, treatment with ACE inhibitors retards microalbumin production, but

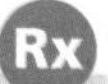

studies achieving similar results with β-blockers and calcium-channel blockers suggest that blood pressure lowering may be responsible for this effect. Studies using ACE inhibitors and angiotensin II receptor blockers have consistently shown that both drug classes can delay the progression of both proteinuria and declining glomerular filtration rate. These drugs are therefore widely favored in diabetic patients, in whom systolic blood pressure should be maintained at 120 mm Hg or less if possible. 6

Later Stage Treatment

Once clinical nephropathy becomes evident, aggressive efforts at strict glycemic control have marginal value in slowing the progression of nephropathy. As described before, efforts aimed at reducing hypertension and glomerular pressure become the mainstay of therapy. Dietary protein restriction (i.e., 0.8 g per kilogram of body weight) may add limited benefit, and adherence is difficult. Aggressive lipid management is useful in preventing both renal and extrarenal vascular complications. As ESRD approaches, long-term treatment plans should proceed much as they would in nondiabetic uremic patients, but therapy should usually be initiated sooner. It is well known that diabetic patients have a poorer tolerance for uremia than their nondiabetic counterparts do. Protein wasting is accelerated, hypertension becomes more difficult to control, and there is acceleration of generalized atherosclerosis with extensive cardiovascular morbidity. Current options for ESRD patients include hemodialysis, peritoneal dialysis, kidney transplantation, and combined kidney-pancreas transplantation (Chapter 133). Decisions among these options are complex and must be made on an individual basis. Finally, mortality associated with both dialysis and organ transplantation is higher in diabetic than in nondiabetic patients, usually because of cardiovascular comorbidity and the more rapid development of complications such as vascular insufficiency.

Management of Complications

Glomerular nephropathy is not the only entity that commonly affects the genitourinary system in diabetic patients. Asymptomatic bacteriuria and pyelonephritis are twice as common in diabetic women because of several factors, including autonomic bladder dysfunction, impaired organ perfusion, and glycosuria. Papillary necrosis is also associated with diabetes, and renal artery stenosis is more common as well. Hyperkalemia, another frequent complication of diabetes, is due to a variety of factors including insulin deficiency, metabolic acidosis, reduced glomerular filtration rate, use of pharmacologic modulators of the renin-angiotensin axis, and the syndrome of hyporeninemic hypoaldosteronism commonly seen in elderly patients with impaired renal function. Finally, diabetic patients are at notable risk for azotemic complications after the injection of contrast dye for radiologic studies. For this reason, aggressive hydration before and after the study with intravenous fluids, especially those containing sodium bicarbonate, or the prophylactic use of *N*-acetylcysteine is critical in these cases.

Diabetic Neuropathy

Epidemiology

Symptomatic, potentially disabling neuropathy affects about 50% of diabetic patients. It is usually symmetrical but can be focal and frequently involves the autonomic nervous system as well. The prevalence of symmetrical neuropathy is similar in type 1 and type 2 diabetes; focal syndromes are more common in older, type 2 patients. Diabetes is the most common cause of neuropathy in developed nations and the leading cause of nonhealing skin ulcers and limb amputation.

Pathobiology

The term *diabetic neuropathy* describes a wide variety of clinical syndromes representing a complex interplay of pathogenic factors. Chronic, more insidious neuropathies may be mediated by metabolic factors, whereas the more acute, self-limiting neuropathies most likely have a vascular cause. Also, nerve growth factor is diminished in neurons of patients with neuropathy, perhaps limiting regenerative capacity. Autoimmune mechanisms may also be involved; in affected type 1 diabetics, autonomic nerve bundles may show monocytic infiltration, and the sera may contain complement-fixing antibodies to sympathetic ganglia. Because of the multifactorial nature of diabetic neuropathy, current classification schemes are based largely on clinical presentation. Current taxonomy includes focal, diffuse, and autonomic neuropathies. Our suboptimal understanding of the causes of diabetic neuropathy has disadvantaged the development of appropriate medical therapies.

Clinical Manifestations

Focal Diabetic Neuropathies

Focal diabetic neuropathies (mononeuropathies) typically present with pain, but motor losses and abnormal deep tendon reflexes can be present. They usually begin suddenly, suggesting a vascular cause. Although any cranial or peripheral nerve can be involved, the most common sites include the oculomotor, median, radial, and lateral popliteal nerves. Painful radiculopathy may also occur in the distribution of one or more spinal roots and can easily be confused clinically with internal organ disease or postherpetic neuralgia. Because of the self-limited nature of focal neuropathy, treatment is generally aimed at pain control, with physical therapy as needed to maintain function of affected muscle groups. Focal neuropathies are generally self-limited, with an average duration of 6 to 8 weeks; chronicity can occur but is less common.

Entrapment syndromes are also common in diabetics and may be distinguished by their more gradual onset, slow progression, and persistence with time. Frequent entrapment sites include the median (carpal tunnel syndrome), ulnar, and radial nerves; lower extremity nerves, such as the lateral popliteal, peroneal, and plantar nerves, can also be involved. Conservative treatment of entrapment syndromes involves splinting and the use of anti-inflammatory medication. Surgical correction is often curative.

Distal Symmetrical Polyneuropathy

Distal symmetrical (sensorimotor) polyneuropathy (Chapter 446) is the most common neurologic syndrome seen in diabetes. This process involves all somatic nerves but has a strong predilection for distal sensorimotor nerves of the feet and hands. Sensory fibers are generally preferentially affected; disease affects both small, unmyelinated C fibers (transmitting pain and temperature) and larger, myelinated Aδ/Aβ fibers, which carry touch, vibration, and proprioception. Early on, most patients with distal neuropathy are asymptomatic, with subtle examination abnormalities including the loss of vibration sense, light touch, two-point discrimination, and thermal sensitivity. Once symptomatic, patients typically report numbness and tingling of the distal extremities, often in the classic "stocking-glove" distribution. Pain is also common, involving either C fibers (burning, dysesthesia, and allodynia) or the large fibers, usually described as gnawing or like a toothache. Severe, spontaneous, short-lived lancinating pains may also occur. Left unchecked, all types of pain may gradually gain in intensity, with a tendency to worsen at night, and there may be progressive loss of sensorimotor function as well. Later stages of disease can involve severe sensory loss, small muscle wasting of the hands and feet, sensory ataxia, and neuropathic arthropathy (Charcot joints).

Acute sensory neuropathy, a rapid-onset variant of symmetrical polyneuropathy, usually occurs in the setting of altered metabolic control (e.g., DKA) or during initiation of insulin therapy (insulin neuritis). In this condition, C-fiber symptoms predominate, although large-fiber pains can occur. Acute sensory neuropathy carries a better prognosis than its chronic counterpart, with many patients achieving complete resolution.

Proximal Motor Neuropathy

Proximal motor neuropathy (diabetic amyotrophy), although classified as a polyneuropathy, is a unique condition that deserves special mention. This syndrome primarily affects elderly type 2 patients and is more common in men. It classically begins with pain in bilateral thighs, hips, and buttocks, followed by weakness and atrophy of the proximal pelvic muscle groups. Iliopsoas, obturator, and adductor muscles of the pelvis are preferentially affected, with relative preservation of the hamstrings and gluteal muscles. Weight loss may also occur.

Proximal motor neuropathy can be secondary to a number of other diseases, all more common in diabetics but not directly related to hyperglycemia. These include chronic inflammatory demyelinating polyneuropathy, monoclonal gammopathy, and vasculitis, all of which should be ruled out before the diagnosis of diabetic amyotrophy is made. This form of neuropathy has a good prognosis, with most cases resolving spontaneously in 12 to 24 months. Therapy is primarily supportive.

Autonomic Neuropathy

Symptomatic autonomic diabetic neuropathy (Chapter 445) carries a poor prognosis. Autonomic neuropathy typically accompanies other chronic complications of diabetes and may play a pathogenetic role through disturbed regulation of local blood flow. The manifestations of autonomic neuropathy are protean. Common syndromes are discussed here, grouped by organ system.

Cardiac

Common cardiovascular abnormalities seen with autonomic neuropathy include resting tachycardia (due to preferential dysfunction of parasympathetic fibers), diminished heart rate variability, prolonged QTc, and silent myocardial ischemia. Diabetic patients will often have defective heart rate and blood pressure responses to exercise, and their lack of autonomic regulation places them at high risk for myocardial infarction, congestive heart failure, and sudden cardiac death. Unfortunately, there are currently no specific treatments available for these conditions. Recent efforts to identify patients at risk for cardiac complications will allow only coronary artery disease screening, closer clinical follow-up, and appropriate treatment of coexisting cardiovascular risk factors.

Vascular

Postural hypotension is probably caused by an impaired sympathetic vasoconstrictor response and impaired cardiac reflexes. Non-neurogenic causes of orthostasis, such as volume depletion, impaired cardiac function, and infectious causes, should be ruled out before the diagnosis is made. Tilt-table testing can be useful to confirm the diagnosis (Chapter 61). Nonpharmacologic measures, such as a raised-head position at night, reduction of rapid positional changes, and supportive elastic stockings, can be useful in mild cases. Disabling disease may require pharmacologic intervention; first-line agents include mineralocorticoids (9-α-fluorohydrocortisone), α-agonists (midodrine), and β-blockers with intrinsic sympathomimetic activity (pindolol). Clonidine, ergotamine-caffeine combinations, yohimbine, octreotide, and desmopressin can be tried in selected cases. Often, the side effects of these agents limit their use; caution must be exercised before any of these agents is prescribed to patients with diabetes.

Gastrointestinal

Altered gastrointestinal function is commonly seen in diabetes. Constipation is the most common clinical syndrome. Diarrhea is another frequent complaint and can be caused by a variety of conditions, including hypermotility (impaired sympathetic inhibition), hypomotility with bacterial overgrowth, pancreatic insufficiency, and bile salt irritation. Treatment is generally aimed at the underlying condition and may include antidiarrheals, intermittent use of broad-spectrum antibiotics, pancreatic enzymes, and bile acid sequestrants (cholestyramine).

Gastroparesis is a particularly disabling condition, often presenting with bloating, early satiety, nausea, and vomiting. Labile glycemic control can result from delayed delivery of nutrients to the small bowel. Treatment of gastroparesis begins with small, frequent meals and the use of metoclopramide, a central dopaminergic agonist with gastric cholinergic activity. Early treatment is useful, but the drug's effect may diminish over time. Cisapride, another promotility agent, can be useful in severe cases, but concerns about cardiotoxicity and drug interactions have led the FDA to restrict this agent to compassionate use only. In selected cases, erythromycin, which acts on the motilin receptor to promote gastric motility, may also be considered.

Genitourinary

Impaired parasympathetic innervation leads to bladder hypotonia, incomplete bladder emptying, dribbling, and overflow incontinence. Bethanechol, a parasympathomimetic agent, can be helpful to reverse these symptoms, but its use is often limited by side effects including salivation, lacrimation, diarrhea, and bronchoconstriction. α-Blockers help by relaxing the urinary sphincter, but these agents will potentiate postural hypotension, already prevalent in diabetic patients. Advanced cases of bladder dysfunction often require intermittent straight catheterization or, if absolutely necessary, the placement of an indwelling catheter.

Erectile dysfunction is commonly seen in male diabetic patients. Selective oral inhibitors of phosphodiesterase type 5 (sildenafil, tadalafil, vardenafil) inhibit local breakdown of cyclic guanosine monophosphate, which in the presence of nitric oxide leads to selective engorgement of the corpus callosum. These agents have demonstrated efficacy in the context of diabetes, but caution should be used in patients with suspected coronary disease, and such drugs are contraindicated in combination with nitrate therapy. In men who do not respond to these drugs, intrapenile injections of locally acting vasomotor agents, such as alprostadil and papaverine, have been used with moderate success but carry the risk of priapism, infection, and local fibrosis with repeated use. In refractory cases, referral to a urologist for a penile prosthetic implant should be considered.

Sudomotor Dysfunction

Abnormal sweat production in diabetic patients can result in xerosis and cracking of the skin, further predisposing these patients to cutaneous infections. Distal anhidrosis with compensatory truncal-facial sweating may occur, whereas generalized anhidrosis can produce heat intolerance and increase the risk of hyperthermia and heat stroke. An impaired sweat response can also further impair the diabetic patient's ability to recognize hypoglycemia. Current therapy for sudomotor dysfunction is limited to behavioral modification (i.e., heat avoidance), topical moisturizers, and intensive skin care. Local sympathectomy for hyperhidrosis should be considered only in severe, refractory cases.

Diagnosis

Diagnosis of diabetic neuropathy can be a difficult task. It begins with a careful history and detailed neurologic examination, including detailed sensory testing (10-g Semmes-Weinstein monofilament, two-point discrimination, 128-cps tuning fork, thermal discrimination), motor and gait examination, and documentation of deep tendon reflexes. Electrophysiologic studies, such as nerve conduction velocity studies and electromyography, are of use in confirming the diagnosis, but unmyelinated C-fiber neuropathy is undetectable with these methods. Nerve biopsy can occasionally be helpful to rule out other causes of neuropathy but is generally not recommended for diagnosis. If diffuse neuropathic symptoms are predominantly sensory in nature, serologic work-up for additional causes of neuropathy should include testing for human immunodeficiency virus infection, VDRL, vitamin B_{12} levels, and serum protein electrophoresis; additional testing is performed when it is indicated in suspected cases of porphyria, heavy metal intoxication, and paraneoplastic syndromes. Of note, and in contrast to other forms of diabetic microvascular disease, is the recent finding that distal somatosensory neuropathy can be seen in patients with milder degrees of hyperglycemia, such as pre-diabetes.

Treatment

Early treatment of diabetic neuropathy should include tight glycemic control. In the DCCT, intensive therapy slowed the onset of neuropathy by 70% and the progression of early neuropathy by 57%; in the UKPDS, glucose control was associated with improved vibratory sensation. Experimental therapies (e.g., aldose reductase inhibitors) have shown limited efficacy in slowing the progression of neuropathy; however, none of these agents is currently approved for clinical use. Other potential treatments still mainly in investigational stages include ACE inhibitors, the antioxidant α-lipoic acid, and γ-linoleic acid, an important constituent of neuronal membrane phospholipids.

The use of several therapies for neuropathic pain (Chapters 28 and 446) has been supported by randomized controlled trials. Tricyclic antidepressants, including amitriptyline, desipramine, and nortriptyline, are moderately effective and well tolerated at low doses, but dose escalation can result in drowsiness, anticholinergic effects, potentiation of cardiac arrhythmias, and worsening of glaucoma. Anticonvulsants, such as carbamazepine and gabapentin, are also effective, but carbamazepine can cause hematologic abnormalities, and patients taking gabapentin may report dizziness, fatigue, headaches, or diarrhea. Recently, two drugs have been approved by the FDA for use in diabetic neuropathy. The first, duloxetine, is a selective serotonin and norepinephrine reuptake inhibitor (related to venlafaxine) that is also approved as an antidepressant. The second, pregabalin, an analogue of γ-aminobutyric acid (GABA; related to gabapentin), modulates calcium channels and GABAergic neurotransmission. Both are modestly effective in decreasing neuropathic pain. Topical therapies, such as capsaicin cream (which depletes stores of axonal substance P) and clonidine and lidocaine gels, can be moderately effective. Additional oral agents to be considered include mexiletine, an oral lidocaine analogue, and tramadol, a centrally acting reuptake inhibitor with opiate activity. In refractory cases, long-term opiate use and consultation with a specifically trained pain specialist may be required.

The Diabetic Foot

Definition

The diabetic foot is characterized by slowly healing plantar ulcers that result from apparently insignificant trauma. Left untreated, superficial ulcers may penetrate to underlying tissues, leading to complications including cellulitis, abscess formation, joint sepsis, and osteomyelitis. Gangrene may occur, and amputation may be required in severe cases.

Epidemiology

Overall, about 15% of diabetic patients experience clinically significant foot ulceration. Risk factors for ulcer development include long-standing diabetes, poor glycemic control, and concurrent diabetic complications. Visual loss and severe obesity may also contribute to difficulties with self-care. Many affected diabetic patients will eventually require amputation, with diabetes accounting for more than half of nontraumatic lower extremity amputations in the United States. In the United States, the total costs of caring for diabetic foot ulcers are estimated at more than $6 billion annually.

Clinical Manifestations

To varying degrees, the diabetic foot is characterized by the combination of chronic sensorimotor neuropathy, vascular disease, autonomic neuropathy, and impaired immune function. Sensory neuropathy prevents the detection of minor traumatic events, so that ill-fitting shoes (or sharp objects in the shoe) may erode the skin surface without signaling pain. Pedal neuropathy also produces abnormalities in both proprioception and intrinsic muscle motor function, pathologically altering weight distribution on the metatarsal heads and leading to "clawing" of the metatarsophalangeal joints. In advanced cases, abnormal loading of the

TABLE 247–8 FOOT CARE PRESCRIPTION FOR DIABETIC PATIENTS WITH LOWER EXTREMITY SENSORY NEUROPATHY

Never walk barefoot.
Do not apply hot water or heating pads to the feet.
Inspect the feet daily, using a mirror for plantar surfaces.
Wash the feet daily, drying thoroughly between the toes.
Lubricate dry skin to avoid cracking.
Wear clean, soft, cotton socks.
Wear properly fitting, well-cushioned shoes (insoles).
Break in new shoes slowly.
Consider a second pair of shoes at night (larger size for dependent edema).
Cut toenails straight across, to conservative lengths.
Schedule regular visits to a diabetic foot care specialist.

foot can result in repeated painless fractures and the displacement of normal joint surfaces, producing the so-called Charcot foot or Charcot joint. Aortic and peripheral vascular disease often coexist. Diminished cardiac output or disturbed autoregulatory mechanisms of the microcirculation may further contribute to impaired blood flow and delay ulcer healing. Finally, abnormal immune function (secondary to hyperglycemia) can predispose to prolonged inflammation and infection, further slowing wound closure and increasing the likelihood of ulcer complications.

Prevention

Prevention of the diabetic foot parallels general diabetes care, with emphasis on proper nutrition, tight glycemic control, and medical risk factor modification, including smoking cessation. A general foot care prescription (Table 247–8) is valuable, and office visits should routinely include careful examination of the feet. In affected patients, examination by a specialist is recommended at least once per year. In cases of deformed feet, pressure relief (offloading) is essential and may include the use of orthotics, specialty shoes, assistive devices, or a total contact cast to direct pressure away from a high-risk area.

Treatment

Rx

Once an ulcer has formed, it should be treated aggressively with antibiotics, appropriate local wound care, and débridement of necrotic tissue. In selected cases, newer FDA-approved treatments should also be considered. Local application of recombinant human platelet–derived growth factor can moderately accelerate wound healing. Bioengineered tissue therapies, containing human dermal-epidermal components, are also effective in refractory cases. These products act as biologic dressings and contain live human fibroblasts that deliver growth factors and extracellular matrix components directly to damaged skin. For extensive cases of gangrene or deep tissue infections, surgical amputation may be required. A compromised peripheral circulation makes such an outcome more likely. If poor circulation is a dominant clinical feature, a vascular surgeon should be consulted for consideration of revascularization.

In caring for patients with type 1 diabetes mellitus, the primary long-term goals are to minimize complications and to preserve the patient's sense of clinical well-being. These goals are attained by early initiation of metabolic control as close as possible to the euglycemic range while minimizing the risk of hypoglycemia. In concert with the management of blood glucose concentrations should be a rigorous program of cardiovascular risk factor reduction (Chapter 248). Because most microvascular complications of diabetes develop slowly and are not easily reversible, it is crucial for clinicians to take a prospective, preventive approach to diabetes care. Key elements of a comprehensive management plan for the care of diabetic patients are summarized in Table 247–9.

TABLE 247–9 KEY ELEMENTS OF A COMPREHENSIVE MANAGEMENT PLAN FOR PATIENTS WITH DIABETES MELLITUS

LIFESTYLE CHANGES

Healthy diet
Aerobic exercise
Weight control
Smoking cessation
Stress reduction

CONTROL OF MODIFIABLE METABOLIC FACTORS

Glucose control
Lipid management
Blood pressure control
Aspirin prophylaxis

PREVENTIVE CARE

Regular medical screening examinations
Regular screening for albuminuria
Regular ophthalmologic examinations
Regular podiatric examinations (and self-examinations)
Regular dental check-ups
Yearly influenza vaccinations
Pneumococcus vaccination

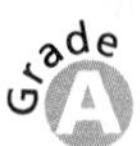

1. Diabetes Control Complications Trial Research Group: The effect of intensive treatment of diabetes on the development and progression of long-term complications of insulin-dependent diabetes mellitus. N Engl J Med 1993;329:927.
2. Diabetes Control and Complications Trial/Epidemiology of Diabetes Intervention and Complications (DCCT/EDIC) Study Research Group: Intensive diabetes treatment and cardiovascular disease in patients with type 1 diabetes. N Engl J Med 2005;353:2643.
3. Siebenhofer A, Plank J, Berghold A, et al: Short-acting insulin analogues versus regular insulin in patients with diabetes mellitus. Cochrane Database System Rev 2006;(2):CD003287.
4. Keymeulen B, Vandemeulebroucke E, Ziegler AG, et al: Insulin needs after CD3-antibody therapy in new-onset type 1 diabetes. N Engl J Med 2005;352:2598–2608.
5. Ceglia L, Lau J, Pittas AG: Meta-analysis: Efficacy and safety of inhaled therapy in adults with diabetes mellitus. Ann Intern Med 2006;145:665–675.
6. Strippoli GF, Bonifati C, Croig M, et al: Angiotensin converting enzyme inhibitors and angiotensin receptor antagonists for preventing the progression of diabetic kidney disease. Cochrane Database Syst Rev 2006;(4):CD006259.

SUGGESTED READINGS

American Diabetes Association: Standards of medical care in diabetes—2007. Diabetes Care 2007;30:S4–S41. *An up-to-date summary of the current classification of diabetes and clinical practice recommendations for the management of diabetic patients, including goals of treatment.*

Camilleri M: Clinical practice. Diabetic gastroparesis. N Engl J Med 2007;356:820–829. *Review of management strategies.*

Jawa A, Kcomt J, Fonseca VA: Diabetic nephropathy and retinopathy. Med Clin North Am 2004;88:1001. *A comprehensive overview of the two major microvascular complications of diabetes.*

Kitabchi AE, Umpierrez G, Murphy MB, et al: Management of hyperglycemic crises in patients with diabetes. Diabetes Care 2001;24:131–153. *A thorough technical review of the pathophysiology, diagnosis, and treatment of acute hyperglycemic crises in patients with diabetes.*

McMahon GT, Arky RA: Inhaled insulin for diabetes mellitus. N Engl J Med 2007;356:497–502. *A clinical review.*

Mooradian AD, Bernbaum M, Albert SG: Narrative review: A rational approach to starting insulin therapy. Ann Intern Med 2006;145:125–134. *A practical review.*

Vinik AI, Mehrabyan A: Diabetic neuropathies. Med Clin North Am 2004;88:947. *Outstanding review of the diagnosis and management of a major diabetic complication.*

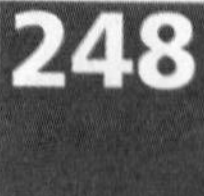

248 TYPE 2 DIABETES MELLITUS

Silvio E. Inzucchi and Robert S. Sherwin

Definition

In this chapter, we discuss the pathogenesis and treatment of type 2 diabetes and other forms of the disease. See Chapter 247 for a general overview of normal carbohydrate metabolism and the complex physiology of insulin secretion and action. Although type 2 diabetes has many similarities to type 1 diabetes, there are many important differences from the vantage point of both biology and therapeutics.

Type 2 diabetes accounts for the majority of diabetes encountered in clinical practice. Patients retain some endogenous insulin secretory capacity; however, their insulin levels are low relative to their ambient glucose concentrations and magnitude of insulin resistance. Type 2 patients are not dependent on insulin for immediate survival, and ketosis rarely develops, except under conditions of great physical stress. Nevertheless, many of these patients will require insulin therapy for proper glycemic control. Although type 2 diabetes has recently been found with increasing frequency in children, adolescents, and young adults, it is usually associated with advancing age; most cases are diagnosed after the age of 45 years. Type 2 diabetes has a high rate of genetic penetrance unrelated to HLA genes and is associated with obesity and a lack of physical activity. The clinical features of type 2 diabetes can be insidious; classic symptoms may be mild. Fatigue, weakness, dizziness, blurred vision, and other nonspecific complaints may dominate the clinical picture and may be tolerated for many years before the patient seeks medical attention. Moreover, if the degree of hyperglycemia is insufficient to produce any symptoms at all, the diagnosis can be made only after the development of vascular or neuropathic complications.

The general classification scheme for diabetes mellitus is summarized in Table 247–1.

Other Specific Types of Diabetes

This category encompasses a wide variety of diabetic syndromes attributed to a specific disease, drug, or condition. Categories include genetic defects of β-cell function or insulin action, diseases of the exocrine pancreas (e.g., chronic pancreatitis), other endocrinopathies (e.g., Cushing's syndrome, acromegaly), drug- or chemical-induced diabetes (e.g., due to glucocorticoids), infections, and other immune-mediated and genetic syndromes associated with diabetes mellitus.

Maturity-onset diabetes of the young (MODY), formerly classified as a subtype of type 2 diabetes, has now been more accurately described as a consequence of genetic research. Clinically, patients with MODY generally present in adolescence or young adulthood; unlike patients with classic type 2 diabetes, they are usually nonobese, normotensive, and normolipidemic at the time of diagnosis. MODY is a heterogeneous disorder encompassing several monogenic defects of β-cell function; autosomal dominant inheritance and penetrance exceed 80%. Mutations at several genetic loci have been identified. The most common form, MODY type 3, is associated with a mutation of hepatocyte nuclear factor 1α, a gene transcription factor encoded on chromosome 12. A subgroup of MODY type 2 patients has a mutation in the gene encoding glucokinase, the key enzyme responsible for the phosphorylation of glucose within the β cell and the liver. A variety of glucokinase mutations, each capable of interfering with the transduction of the glucose signal in the β cell, have been identified in different families. Other described forms of MODY are shown in Table 248–1; the existence of additional forms of MODY is suggested by clusters of patients with similar clinical findings whose genetic basis for disease remains unknown.

Severe illness (e.g., burns, trauma, sepsis) can provoke stress hyperglycemia as a result of the hypersecretion of insulin antagonistic hormones (e.g., catecholamines, cortisol). Although this may represent the unmasking of underlying diabetes, the metabolic disturbance may be self-limited and should therefore not be formally classified as diabetes until the precipitating illness has resolved. Whereas most patients can be readily classified on clinical grounds, a small subgroup of patients are difficult to categorize because they display features common to both type 1 and type 2 diabetes. Such patients are classically nonobese, with reduced insulin secretory capacity but little tendency for ketosis. Many of these patients initially respond to oral agents; however, nearly all of them will eventually require insulin therapy. Many of these patients appear to have a slowly evolving form of type 1 diabetes, with measurable titers of autoimmune markers.

Gestational Diabetes Mellitus

The term *gestational diabetes mellitus* (Chapter 259) describes women with abnormal glucose tolerance that appears or is first detected during pregnancy. Women with known diabetes before conception are not classified as having gestational diabetes. Gestational diabetes mellitus usually appears in the second or third trimester, when pregnancy-associated insulin antagonistic factors (many placentally derived) reach their peak. After delivery, glucose tolerance generally (but not always) reverts to normal. However, within 10 years, type 2 diabetes develops in most women with prior gestational diabetes; on occasion, pregnancy can precipitate type 1 diabetes as well. As a whole, gestational diabetes occurs in approximately 7% of U.S. pregnancies, accounting for approximately 200,000 cases per year; local prevalence rates may rise as high as 14% in high-risk populations. Although patients with gestational diabetes generally present with mild, asymptomatic hyperglycemia, rigorous treatment is indicated to protect against hyperglycemia-associated fetal morbidity. Insulin is often required.

Epidemiology

Systematic screening for asymptomatic type 2 diabetes mellitus is generally limited to high-risk populations, rendering broader prevalence estimates imprecise. Total U.S. prevalence is now estimated at 7% but probably exceeds 15% in persons older than 50 years. Type 2 diabetes is more common in Native Americans, Hispanic Americans, and African Americans than in whites; these patients also typically present at an earlier age. Prevalence rates vary worldwide; type 2 diabetes has a propensity for Asiatic Indians, Polynesians-Micronesians, and Latin Americans. Interestingly, African blacks, Australian Aborigines, Asians, and Pacific Islanders all have an increased risk of diabetes after emigration to the

TABLE 248–1 CLASSIFICATION OF CURRENTLY RECOGNIZED GENETIC DEFECTS OF β-CELL FUNCTION: MATURITY-ONSET DIABETES OF THE YOUNG (MODY)

MODY Type	Chromosome	Defective Gene Product	Molecular Defect	Most Common Therapy
1	20q	HNF-4α	β-cell mass, insulin secretion	Oral hypoglycemic agent, insulin
2	7p	Glucokinase	Glucose phosphorylation	Diet and exercise
3	12q	HNF-1α	β-cell mass, insulin secretion	Oral hypoglycemic agent, insulin
4	13q	IPF-1 (PDX-1)	β-cell development and function	Oral hypoglycemic agent, insulin
5	17cen-q	HNF-1β	β-cell mass, insulin secretion	Insulin
6	2q	NeuroD1/BETA2	β-cell development and function	Insulin

HNF = hepatocyte nuclear factor; IPF = insulin promoter factor; NeuroD1 = neurogenic differentiation factor 1; PDX = pancreatic-duodenal homeobox factor.
Modified from Fajans SS, Bell GI, Polonsky KS: Molecular mechanisms and clinical pathophysiology of maturity-onset diabetes of the young. N Engl J Med 2001;345:971–980.

United States; this may be attributable to a genetically determined inability to adapt metabolically to "Western" behavior patterns (i.e., reduced physical activity and a high-fat, high-calorie diet).

Although relatively little is known about the specific genetic abnormalities associated with type 2 diabetes, the personal factors promoting disease expression are well established. Increased age, reduced physical activity, and especially obesity promote the expression of disease in genetically susceptible persons. The severity and duration of obesity contribute significantly to diabetes risk; patients with high waist-to-hip ratios (i.e., central or upper body obesity) are also more prone to the disease. Family history is also important because type 2 diabetes occurs more frequently in persons with diabetic parents or siblings. Identical twin concordance rates approach 100%; in these cases, affected twins will even develop diabetes at a similar age.

Impaired Fasting Glucose and Impaired Glucose Tolerance

In 2000, the Centers for Disease Control and Prevention estimated that a total of 41 million adults had pre-diabetes in the United States. There is overlap between the impaired fasting glucose (IFG) and impaired glucose tolerance (IGT) groups, as demonstrated by the fact that approximately 37% of patients with IFG also have IGT, whereas approximately 24% of patients with IGT also have IFG. Because of the insidious nature of both conditions, precise rates of progression to overt diabetes are difficult to establish; current estimates approach 5 to 10% per year for each condition, with even higher rates if both conditions are present. In general, IGT seems to have a greater sensitivity for the future development of diabetes; IFG has a higher positive predictive value. IGT is also an independent risk factor for cardiovascular complications.

Pathobiology

Whereas the pathogenesis of hyperglycemia in patients with type 1 diabetes is reasonably straightforward (lack of insulin due to islet destruction), the metabolic underpinnings of type 2 diabetes are comparatively more enigmatic, involving defects in both insulin action and secretion. Hyperglycemia in type 2 diabetes probably results from complex genetic interactions, the expression of which is modified by environmental factors such as body weight and exercise. With type 2 diabetes, identical twin concordance rates approach 100%, although disease onset and course can vary greatly on the basis of environmental factors. Hyperglycemia itself is known to impair insulin secretion and action; elevated free fatty acid levels also play an important pathogenic role. By the time that hyperglycemia is detected, nearly all type 2 patients exhibit both defective insulin secretion and insulin resistance; this makes it difficult to determine which of the two factors is primarily responsible for the vicious circle leading to disease (Fig. 248–1).

Genetics

Although monogenic forms of diabetes have been identified (e.g., MODY types 1 to 6), most cases are likely to be polygenic in nature. Type 2 diabetes shows clear familial aggregation but does not segregate in classic mendelian fashion; this implies that the disease results either from a combination of genetic defects or from the simultaneous presence of multiple susceptibility genes and predisposing environmental factors. Candidate gene mutations for polygenic forms of type 2 diabetes include mutations of the coding region of the insulin gene, peroxisome proliferator–activated receptor (PPAR)–γ, β-cell adenosine triphosphate–sensitive potassium channel, intestinal fatty acid–binding protein 2, calpain 10, and β_3-adrenergic receptor. These and other mutations have been associated with isolated clusters of patients with type 2 diabetes.

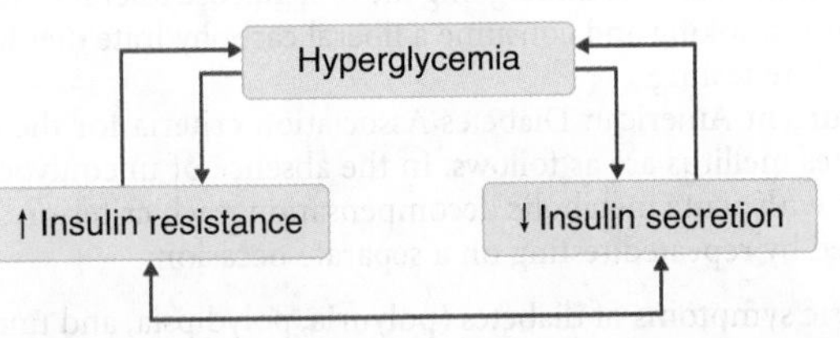

FIGURE 248–1 • Elevations of circulating glucose initiate a vicious circle in which hyperglycemia begets more severe hyperglycemia.

Pathogenesis

Insulin Secretion

It is now apparent that the driving force in the progression from normal glucose tolerance to IGT to frank type 2 diabetes is the progressive loss of insulin secretory capacity. Once type 2 diabetes becomes manifested, fasting insulin levels in type 2 diabetes generally appear normal or elevated, yet they are *relatively* low given the degree of coexisting hyperglycemia. As the disease progresses and hyperglycemia becomes more severe, basal insulin levels eventually fail to keep up and may even decline. Indeed, autopsy studies demonstrate that β-cell mass is reduced by 50% in such patients. The insulin secretory defect usually correlates with the severity of fasting hyperglycemia and is more evident after carbohydrate ingestion. In its mildest form, the β-cell defect is subtle, involving the loss of the "first-phase" insulin response and the normal oscillatory pattern of insulin secretion. Although the overall insulin response may appear to be fairly intact, this "normal" response is actually totally inadequate to maintain glucose tolerance when it is viewed in the context of simultaneous insulin resistance. During this early stage, the β-cell defect is usually specific for glucose; other secretagogues (e.g., amino acids) maintain their potency, and insulin deficiency is thus less pronounced during the ingestion of mixed meals. Patients with more severe fasting hyperglycemia lose this capacity to respond to the other insulin secretagogues; thus, their secretory defect worsens as their disease progresses. Unfortunately, the underlying cause of the secretory defect remains uncertain and is probably multifactorial, involving both functional and anatomic defects.

Studies in rodents suggest that the loss of glucose-stimulated insulin secretion is associated with a decreased expression of GLUT 2, the primary glucose transport protein of the pancreatic β cell. Pathologic studies of islets from patients with long-standing type 2 diabetes have demonstrated amyloid-like deposits composed of islet amyloid polypeptide, or amylin, a peptide synthesized in the β cell and co-secreted with insulin. Chronic hypersecretion of amylin may lead to intraislet precipitation of the peptide, which over time might also contribute to impaired β-cell function. Experiments in gene knockout mice suggest a potential role for impaired insulin receptor signaling in the development of impaired β-cell function. A link between insulin resistance and secretion is also suggested by the accumulation of fat within the β cell, which appears to interfere with normal insulin secretion. Finally, studies in patients with type 2 diabetes demonstrate reduced circulating glucagon-like peptide 1 (GLP-1) concentrations, particularly in response to meals. Whether this phenomenon contributes to abnormal insulin secretion and glucagon physiology is not known.

Insulin Resistance

With few exceptions (e.g., a subgroup of African American patients), type 2 diabetes is characterized by impaired insulin action. The insulin dose-response curve for augmenting glucose uptake in peripheral tissues is shifted to the right, representing decreased insulin sensitivity, and maximal response is reduced, particularly in the setting of severe hyperglycemia. Other insulin-dependent processes, such as inhibition of hepatic glucose production and lipolysis, also show reduced sensitivity to insulin. The mechanisms responsible for insulin resistance remain poorly understood. Studies suggest that an important contributory factor is impaired mitochondrial function and the resulting accumulation of free fatty acids in insulin-responsive tissues.

Early studies of insulin resistance focused on defects of the insulin receptor. Mutation of the insulin receptor gene can produce leprechaunism, characterized by severe growth retardation, extreme insulin resistance, and early infant death. Other syndromes related to mutated insulin receptors include the Rabson-Mendenhall syndrome, also associated with tooth and nail abnormalities and pineal gland hyperplasia, and "type A insulin resistance," most often affecting young females with acanthosis nigricans, polycystic ovaries, and hirsutism. Another example of extreme insulin resistance involves the presence of anti–insulin receptor antibodies; it is associated clinically with acanthosis nigricans and a number of other autoimmune phenomena.

Although insulin receptors are abnormal in a few type 2 patients, defects in more distal "postreceptor" pathways play a far greater role in insulin resistance. One important aspect of insulin resistance is a reduced capacity for translocation of GLUT 4 to the cell surface in muscle cells. A separate defect in glycogen synthesis also is likely to be present. Whether the defects uncovered are primary or secondary to the disturbance in glucose metabolism is uncertain; possibly, a variety of genetic abnormalities in cellular transduction of the insulin signal may individually or in concert produce an identical clinical phenotype. It is uncertain whether mechanisms of insulin resistance in nonobese patients are identical to those of their obese counterparts; however, the coexistence of obesity clearly accentuates the severity of the resistant state. In particular, upper body or abdominal (compared with lower body or peripheral) obesity is associated with insulin resistance and diabetes. Intra-abdominal visceral fat deposits, detected by computed tomography or magnetic resonance imaging, have a higher lipolytic rate than peripheral fat and are more resistant to insulin. The resulting increase in circulating free fatty acid levels promotes fat deposits within the liver and muscle, worsening insulin resistance. Intracellular free fatty acid metabolites appear to promote insulin resistance through complex mechanisms involving serine (rather than tyrosine) phosphorylation of insulin signaling molecules. Cortisol hypersecretion or hereditary factors may also influence the distribution of body fat, the latter contributing an additional genetic influence on the expression of disease.

Adipocyte-Derived Hormones and Cytokines

Adipocytes, once thought of as inert fat storage cells, are now known to produce a number of metabolically active hormones that may affect insulin sensitivity. Leptin, for example, acts on the hypothalamus to promote satiety and energy expenditure and may accelerate glucose metabolism. Adiponectin, another fat-derived hormone, circulates at levels that correlate inversely with both adiposity and degree of insulin resistance. The administration of adiponectin to obese mice causes a transient, dose-dependent, insulin-independent decrease in circulating glucose levels; adiponectin also improves insulin sensitivity by decreasing triglycerides in the liver and muscle, probably by increasing the expression of molecules (e.g., adenosine monophosphate kinase) involved in fatty acid combustion and energy dissipation. Weight loss paradoxically increases adiponectin, as does pharmacologic therapy that improves insulin sensitivity. Interestingly, adiponectin may have some beneficial effects on atherosclerosis, which may explain at least to some degree the increased prevalence of cardiovascular disease in obesity and type 2 diabetes. Finally, adipose tissue is an abundant source of the cytokine tumor necrosis factor-α, which is known to inhibit muscle glucose metabolism by inducing serine phosphorylation of insulin-signaling molecules. The precise impact that these and other adipocyte-derived factors (resistin, angiotensinogen, interleukin-6, transforming growth factor-β, plasminogen activator inhibitor 1) exert on insulin resistance and on diabetes and its vascular complications is an active area of scientific research but has yet to be firmly established.

Glucotoxicity and Lipotoxicity

Hyperglycemia per se impairs the β-cell response to glucose and promotes insulin resistance. Reversal of glucotoxicity can disrupt the vicious circle that perpetuates hyperglycemia (see Fig. 248–1). Circulating lipids can also adversely affect glucose metabolism; increased free fatty acid levels accelerate hepatic gluconeogenesis, inhibit muscle glucose metabolism, and impair pancreatic β-cell function. As is the case with glucotoxicity, the reversal of lipotoxicity can rapidly improve metabolic control and facilitate favorable therapeutic outcomes.

What Is the Primary Defect?

It remains uncertain whether insulin resistance or defective insulin secretion is the primary defect in type 2 diabetes (Fig. 248–2). This issue is difficult to resolve once diabetes has developed; therefore, research attention has focused primarily on high-risk nondiabetic subjects. Studies in high-risk populations (e.g., Pima Indians, Mexican Americans) have suggested that insulin resistance is the initial defect; similar findings have been reported in first-degree relatives of type 2 diabetic patients and in healthy pre-diabetic offspring of two diabetic parents. Interestingly, hyperinsulinemia has been detected in pre-diabetic subjects as early as one to two decades before clinical onset, suggesting that the development of diabetes can be exceedingly slow. Although these studies support the view that insulin resistance generally antedates insulin deficiency, the presence of insulin resistance alone is generally insufficient to generate disease; this implies that for diabetes to occur, impaired insulin secretion is required (see Fig. 248–2). It is possible that the appearance of a secretory defect is a secondary phenomenon resulting from "β-cell exhaustion," excess fatty acid delivery, or amylin accumulation. Perhaps more likely, diminished insulin secretion may result from an independent defect that becomes evident only on chronic β-cell stimulation, such as a subtle genetic defect in insulin signaling or β-cell replication.

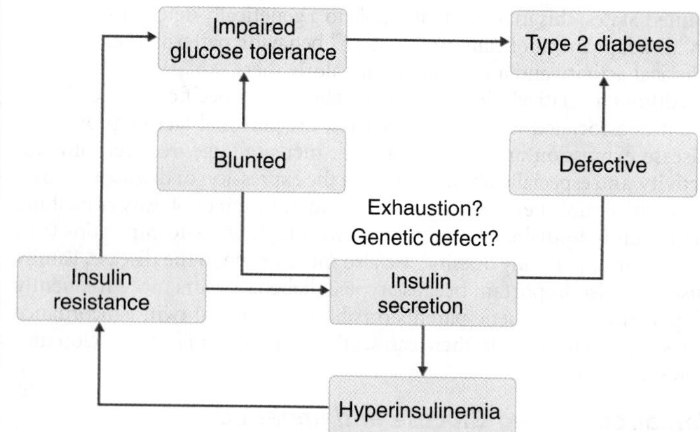

FIGURE 248–2 • A proposed sequence of events leading to the development of type 2 diabetes. Insulin resistance resulting from genetic influences, central obesity, inactivity, or a combination of these factors leads over time to a progressive loss of the β cell's capacity to compensate for this defect.

The sequence of events described—underlying insulin resistance followed by a secretory defect—is common but clearly does not describe all type 2 diabetic patients. For example, a subgroup of African American patients exhibits little or no insulin resistance. (An insulin deficiency–predominant phenotype is also encountered not infrequently in clinical practice in other racial groups, although, admittedly, many of these individuals may have a slowly progressive form of type 1 diabetes.) In addition, diminished glucose-stimulated insulin secretion is seen in women with gestational diabetes in whom type 2 diabetes later develops. Finally, the demonstration of functional β cell–associated gene mutations in patients with MODY indicates that primary β-cell defects are capable of producing a similar phenotype. Taken together, these lines of evidence strongly suggest that type 2 diabetes cannot be explained by insulin resistance alone or by any single pathogenic mechanism.

Diagnosis

The diagnosis of diabetes mellitus is straightforward when classic symptoms of polyuria, polydipsia, and unexplained weight loss are present. In these cases, a random (or "casual") plasma glucose measurement of 200 mg/dL or more is sufficient to confirm the diagnosis. Although glycosuria is strongly suggestive of diabetes, urine test results should never be used exclusively to diagnose diabetes because an altered renal threshold for glucose can produce similar findings. If suspected diabetes is not confirmed through random glucose determination, additional diagnostic testing should be performed.

An 8-hour (overnight) fasting plasma glucose measurement is most convenient; diabetes is established if fasting glucose levels are 126 mg/dL or higher on two separate occasions. Alternatively, a 75-g oral glucose tolerance test may be employed. The oral glucose tolerance test should be performed after an overnight fast, with use of a glucose load containing 75 g of anhydrous glucose dissolved in water; 2-hour postload glucose levels of 200 mg/dL or higher confirm the presence of diabetes. An important note about the oral glucose tolerance test: although it is able to detect diabetes in its earliest stage, this test should be performed under controlled conditions to ensure its accuracy. Common factors that nonspecifically deteriorate the oral glucose tolerance test result include antecedent dietary carbohydrate restriction, bedrest or severe inactivity, medical or surgical stress, drugs (e.g., thiazides, β-blockers, glucocorticoids, phenytoin), smoking, and anxiety from repeated phlebotomies. As a result, the oral glucose tolerance test should not be performed in acutely ill patients, and patients undergoing the oral glucose tolerance test should ideally stop smoking and consume a liberal carbohydrate diet for at least 3 days before testing.

The current American Diabetes Association criteria for the diagnosis of diabetes mellitus are as follows. In the absence of unequivocal hyperglycemia with acute metabolic decompensation, each criterion should be confirmed by repeated testing on a separate occasion:

1. classic symptoms of diabetes (polyuria, polydipsia, and unexplained weight loss) *plus* random plasma glucose concentration ≥ 200 mg/dL (≥11.1 mmol/L);

TABLE 248–2 DIAGNOSTIC CATEGORIES: IMPAIRED FASTING GLUCOSE, IMPAIRED GLUCOSE TOLERANCE, AND DIABETES MELLITUS

Fasting Plasma Glucose Level	2-Hour (75-g) OGTT Result		
	<140 mg/dL	140–199 mg/dL	≥200 mg/dL
<100 mg/dL	Normal	IGT	DM
100–125 mg/dL	IFG	IGT *and* IFG	DM
≥126 mg/dL	DM	DM	DM

These diagnostic categories are based on the combined fasting plasma glucose level and a 2-hour, 75-g oral glucose tolerance test result. Note that a confirmed random plasma glucose level of 200 mg/dL or higher in the appropriate clinical setting is diagnostic of diabetes and precludes the need for further testing.
DM = diabetes mellitus; IFG = impaired fasting glucose; IGT = impaired glucose tolerance; OGTT = oral glucose tolerance test.

or

2. fasting (≥8-hour) plasma glucose concentration ≥ 126 mg/dL (≥7.0 mmol/L);

or

3. a 2-hour postload plasma glucose concentration ≥ 200 mg/dL (≥11.1 mmol/L) during a 75-g oral glucose tolerance test.

In recent years, increasing emphasis has been placed on two "risk categories" for diabetes, IFG and IGT. Because both conditions are associated with an increased risk for development of diabetes as well as subsequent vascular disease, all patients with IFG or IGT should be treated with diet and exercise and screened annually for progression to diabetes. As detailed, diabetes mellitus is established if fasting glucose levels are 126 mg/dL or higher; however, a fasting glucose concentration of 99 mg/dL, not 125 mg/dL, is now designated the upper limit of normal. Although somewhat arbitrary, this level was chosen because fasting glucose levels above 99 mg/dL are associated with an increased risk for development of diabetes. Patients with fasting glucose levels between 100 and 125 mg/dL are classified as having IFG (Table 248–2). Because individuals with IFG may exhibit severe postprandial hyperglycemia, a 75-g oral glucose tolerance test may be considered to rule out diabetes. During the 75-g oral glucose tolerance test, 2-hour postload glucose concentrations of 200 mg/dL or higher are diagnostic of diabetes; patients with levels between 140 and 199 mg/dL are defined as having IGT. Patients displaying IFG and IGT simultaneously have a greater risk for development of diabetes. Table 248–2 summarizes the diagnosis of IFG, IGT, and overt diabetes mellitus.

With regard to screening, the clinical utility and cost-effectiveness of screening for diabetes mellitus have never been directly demonstrated. However, because patients with diabetes may harbor the disease for many years before symptoms are appreciated, the American Diabetes Association has endorsed the screening at 3-year intervals beginning at 45 years of age (Table 248–3). More frequent screening is advised for "high-risk" individuals, such as those with a personal history of IFG, IGT, gestational diabetes mellitus, obesity, hypertension, or dyslipidemia, or those in high-risk ethnic groups and patients with first-degree relatives with diabetes. In most cases, a fasting plasma glucose level is the screening test of choice; however, the oral glucose tolerance test has the advantage of detecting patients with IGT and early diabetes.

Gestational Diabetes Mellitus

Because even mild glucose elevations can have serious adverse effects on a developing fetus, an aggressive screening approach is recommended during pregnancy (Chapter 259). Women with a high clinical risk of gestational diabetes (personal history of gestational diabetes mellitus, obesity, glycosuria, or a strong family history of diabetes) should undergo screening as soon as possible after conception; in these patients, screening *before* pregnancy is preferred if possible. At 24 to 28 weeks of gestation, screening is recommended for *all* pregnant women, except those in the lowest risk category who meet *all* of the following clinical characteristics:

- age younger than 25 years
- weight normal before pregnancy
- member of an ethnic group with a low risk of gestational diabetes (e.g., whites)
- no known diabetes in first-degree relatives
- no history of abnormal glucose tolerance and
- no history of poor obstetric outcome

TABLE 248–3 CRITERIA FOR DIABETES SCREENING IN ASYMPTOMATIC INDIVIDUALS

Testing for diabetes should be considered in all individuals at the age of 45 years and older. If results are normal, testing should be repeated at 3-year intervals.

Testing should be considered at a younger age or be carried out more frequently in individuals who

- are obese (>120% desirable body weight or a body mass index > 27 kg/m²)
- have a first-degree relative with diabetes
- are members of a high-risk ethnic population (e.g., African American, Hispanic American, Native American, Asian American, Pacific Islander)
- have delivered a baby weighing more than 9 pounds or have been diagnosed with gestational diabetes mellitus
- have systemic hypertension (BP > 140/90)
- have an HDL cholesterol level below 35 mg/dL or a triglyceride level above 250 mg/dL
- on previous testing, had impaired glucose tolerance or impaired fasting glucose

A fasting plasma glucose level or an oral glucose tolerance test may be used for diagnosis. In most clinical settings, the fasting plasma glucose level is preferred because of ease of administration, convenience, acceptability to patients, and lower cost.
Modified from Report of the expert committee on the diagnosis and classification of diabetes mellitus. Diabetes Care 2000;23 (Suppl. 1):S4–S19.

In pregnant women, a casual plasma glucose level of 200 mg/dL or higher or a confirmed fasting plasma glucose level of 126 mg/dL or higher establishes the diagnosis of gestational diabetes mellitus and precludes the need for a glucose challenge. In the absence of overt hyperglycemia, a screening 1-hour 50-g glucose challenge test should be performed between 24 and 28 weeks of gestation. If the fasting glucose level is 105 mg/dL or higher or the 1-hour postload value is 140 mg/dL or higher, a diagnostic 3-hour 100-g oral glucose tolerance test is indicated. Gestational diabetes is then diagnosed if two or more values equal or exceed the upper limits of normal: fasting, 95 mg/dL; 1 hour, 180 mg/dL; 2 hour, 155 mg/dL; and 3 hour, 140 mg/dL. To save time and effort, proceeding directly to the 100-g diagnostic oral glucose tolerance test is an acceptable alternative, particularly in those deemed at higher risk.

Treatment

Rx

Complications

As discussed in Chapter 247, the Diabetes Control and Complications Trial (DCCT), involving solely patients with type 1 diabetes, conclusively determined that improved glucose control reduces the risk of microvascular complications. It was assumed but not concluded that the same relationship would apply to patients with type 2 diabetes. Ultimate evidence for such a benefit came from the United Kingdom Prospective Diabetes Study (UKPDS).  The UKPDS recruited 5102 patients with newly diagnosed type 2 diabetes between 1977 and 1991. After 3 months of diet therapy, the 3867 patients with fasting glucose levels between 6.1 and 15.0 mmol/L (110 and 270 mg/dL) were randomized to a more intensive regimen, consisting of sulfonylurea and metformin (for obese patients only) or insulin, or a conventional treatment regimen focused primarily on symptom reduction. Subjects were monitored for an average of 10 years. Although glycemic control gradually deteriorated in both groups, the intensified treatment group had lower mean hemoglobin A_{1c} (HbA_{1c}) than their conventionally treated counterparts did (7.0% vs. 7.9%). This modest improvement significantly reduced microvascular complications by 25% and reduced all diabetes-related events by 12%. The intensified treatment group also had a 16% reduction in a combined end point—nonfatal or fatal myocardial

Rx

infarction or sudden death—that did not quite reach statistical significance (P = .052). A continuous relationship was again noted between glycemic control and diabetic complications. Also similar to the DCCT, no glycemic threshold for microvascular complications was observed. Importantly, serious adverse events were rare for all of the treatment arms in the UKPDS, and only a single death from hypoglycemia occurred in more than 27,000 patient years of intensive therapy.

What conclusions can be drawn from the UKPDS as well as from the DCCT and the Epidemiology of Diabetes Interventions and Complications (EDIC) study? The primary message is that "glucose matters." In both type 1 and type 2 diabetic patients who are willing and able to participate actively in their management, the goal should be to achieve the best possible level of glycemic control as rapidly as possible without undue risk. These studies also demonstrate that most patients benefit from lower glucose levels, even if normalization is not achieved; for most type 2 patients, effective glucose reductions can be achieved by diet, oral agents, or less complicated insulin regimens than are required in type 1 patients. Although a statistically significant benefit on macrovascular outcomes could not be detected in the tight control arm of the UKPDS, it is noteworthy that epidemiologic data showed a linear relationship between glycemia and cardiovascular events (even into the "normal" range for glucose). Finally, a central conclusion from the UKPDS was that β-cell function continues to decline after the diagnosis of diabetes is made, mandating more aggressive treatment regimens.

General Measures

As in individuals with type 1 diabetes, the primary long-term goals in type 2 patients are to minimize complications and to preserve the patient's sense of clinical well-being. Glucose control should not be addressed in a vacuum. Lifestyle modification should be the primary focus of the patient's care. Also, aggressive lowering of lipids and blood pressure should be routinely incorporated into the treatment program.

In many type 2 diabetic patients, diet and exercise are the only therapeutic interventions required to restore metabolic control. As a result, the temptation to use pharmacologic agents should be restrained at the outset if the patient is asymptomatic and the hyperglycemia is mild. On the other hand, the clinician must also resist the temptation to avoid pharmacologic therapy if glucose levels are not approaching the nondiabetic range after several months.

Diet

Irrespective of initial weight, modest weight reduction (on the order of 5 kg) in obese diabetic patients leads to improved glycemic control. The dramatic impact of weight loss is mediated by changes in insulin-responsive tissues as well as by enhanced β-cell activity; insulin resistance diminishes, glucose production declines, and lower glucose levels improve glucose-stimulated insulin secretion. The beneficial effects of weight loss are not restricted to glucose; dietary therapy also yields improved lipoprotein profiles and reductions in systemic blood pressure. In general, it matters little how weight loss is achieved, provided good health is preserved and adequate nutrition is maintained. Successful weight loss (Chapter 239) is best achieved by the combination of a supportive environment that emphasizes long-term goals, regular exercise to increase energy expenditure, and long-term behavior modification.

In sedentary diabetic patients, maintenance calorie requirements can be as low as 20 to 25 kcal per kilogram of body weight per day. In these individuals, depending on baseline weight, the classically prescribed 1800-kcal diet is often ineffective in producing weight loss. It is sensible to begin with a nutritionally sound, individually tailored diet that is aimed at producing a calorie deficit of about 500 kcal/day. Because a calorie deficit of about 3500 kcal is required to lose 1 pound of body fat, weight loss by this method can be expected at 1 pound per week. For obese patients with a history of multiple failed weight loss attempts, very low calorie diets (<1000 kcal/day) can be useful when they are carried out under medical supervision. Orlistat, a gastrointestinal lipase inhibitor that reduces dietary fat absorption, can be an effective adjunct for achieving weight loss in some patients; it may also improve glycemic control and lipoprotein profiles. Most patients are unable to maintain low-calorie diets for an extended period; if they are successful, the majority of patients will resume higher calorie diets and regain lost weight. In patients with type 2 diabetes, metabolic factors may also contribute to difficulty maintaining weight loss. Dieting reduces glycosuria and therefore lessens urinary calorie loss. Also, the expected decrease in basal metabolic rate during weight loss is accentuated in diabetic patients because weight loss reverses both accelerated gluconeogenesis and the futile cycling of substrates; these conditions, commonly seen in poorly controlled diabetes, decrease use of excess energy that has been ingested in the hyperglycemic state.

Even when diabetic patients cannot lose weight, a careful meal plan is a valuable tool for reducing their risk of cardiovascular disease. This benefit is best achieved by restricting saturated fats and cholesterol and by raising the dietary content of carbohydrates and monounsaturated fats. It is now appreciated that a diet high in carbohydrate (>50%) may improve insulin action and glycemic control, particularly in patients with mild hyperglycemia. In patients with more severe fasting hyperglycemia or with triglyceride elevations aggravated by high-carbohydrate diets, reduced carbohydrate intake (<45% of total calories) and greater reliance on monounsaturated fats may be preferable. It has also been assumed that carbohydrate intake should be focused on complex carbohydrates (starches) and that sucrose should be avoided; however, evidence supporting these assumptions is scarce. Simple sugars raise glucose levels to an extent similar to that with complex carbohydrates; thus, total carbohydrate intake, rather than type of carbohydrate, should be the primary consideration. Fiber-containing carbohydrates such as oats, gums, legumes, and fruit pectin may also be beneficial because fiber blunts meal-induced glucose excursions by delaying gastric emptying and carbohydrate absorption. Fiber helps prevent constipation and may also contribute to lowering of triglyceride and low-density lipoprotein (LDL) cholesterol levels.

Diabetic patients with normal lipid profiles are encouraged to follow the recommendations of the National Cholesterol Education Program (NCEP) by limiting total fat intake to less than 30% of total calories, with less than 10% of calories as saturated fat and less than 300 mg/day of dietary cholesterol (see Table 247–3). If LDL levels are elevated, stricter recommendations apply (NCEP Step II diet), with less than 7% of calories as saturated fat and less than 200 mg/day of dietary cholesterol. Despite a lack of supporting scientific evidence, moderation of dietary protein is also currently recommended for patients with diabetes; this issue assumes greater importance in patients with proteinuria and overt diabetic nephropathy.

Exercise

Regular exercise is a powerful adjunct in the treatment of type 2 diabetes. Long-term studies demonstrate consistent beneficial effects of regular exercise on carbohydrate metabolism and insulin sensitivity that can be maintained for several years. Exercise also facilitates weight loss and its maintenance, which further improves glycemic control and also has beneficial effects on cardiovascular risk. Regular exercise lowers triglyceride-rich very low density lipoprotein (VLDL) levels, raises high-density lipoprotein (HDL) levels, and improves fibrinolytic activity. In general, "moderate" levels of exercise should be prescribed most days of the week (see Table 247–3 in Chapter 247). Limitations may be imposed by preexisting coronary or peripheral vascular disease, proliferative retinopathy, peripheral or autonomic neuropathy, and poor glycemic control.

Medical Therapy

Oral Glucose-Lowering Agents

Sulfonylureas were the only oral agents available in the United States for more than four decades. Since the 1995 approval of metformin by the Food and Drug Administration (FDA), several new

classes of oral agents have become available for the treatment of type 2 diabetes (Table 248–4 and Fig. 248–3). Oral agents are indicated in patients in whom diet and exercise fail to achieve treatment goals and may be favored over insulin in older patients with relatively mild degrees of hyperglycemia. Patients with more severe hyperglycemia may require insulin during the initial phases of treatment; once glucose levels have stabilized and the "toxic" effects of severe hyperglycemia on β-cell function and insulin action have been minimized, many of these patients may then be converted to oral agents.

Sulfonylureas

Sulfonylureas are insulin "secretagogues" that act through specific sulfonylurea receptors on the β-cell surface. Drug-receptor

TABLE 248–4 CHARACTERISTICS OF ORAL ANTIHYPERGLYCEMIC AGENTS

Class and Agent	Total Daily Dose (mg/day)	Doses per Day	Metabolism and Excretion	Duration of Action (hr)
SULFONYLUREAS				
Insulin secretagogues. Administer 30 minutes before meals.				
Principal side effects: hypoglycemia, weight gain, hyperinsulinemia (?)				
First generation				
Chlorpropamide	100–500	1	K > L	~60
Tolazamide	100–1000	1–2	L > K	12–24
Tolbutamide	500–3000	2–3	L > K	6–12
Second generation				
Glimepiride	1–8	1	L > K	24
Glyburide	1.25–20	1–2	L > K	12–24
Glyburide micronized	1.5–12	1–2	L > K	12–24
Glipizide	5–40	1–2	L > K	12–24
Glipizide GITS	5–20	1	L > K	24
NON-SULFONYLUREA SECRETAGOGUES				
Insulin secretagogues. Administer 15 minutes before meals.				
Principal side effects: hypoglycemia, weight gain, hyperinsulinemia (?)				
Repaglinide	1.5–16	3	L > K	4–6
Nateglinide	180–360	3	K > L	4
BIGUANIDE				
Inhibits hepatic gluconeogenesis. Administer with meals.				
Principal side effects: gastrointestinal disturbances (abdominal pain, nausea, diarrhea), lactic acidosis				
Metformin	500–2550	2–3	K	12–18
Metformin XR	500–2000	1	K	24
Metformin-glyburide	250–2000/1.25–20	2	K/L > K	12–24
Metformin-glipizide	250–2000/2.5–20	2	K/L > K	12–24
Metformin-rosiglitazone	500–2000/2–8	2	K/L	12–24
Metformin-pioglitazone	500–2550/15–45	2–3	K/L	12–24
THIAZOLIDINEDIONES				
Insulin sensitizers (PPAR-γ agonists). Administer with meals.				
Principal side effects: fluid retention, weight gain, congestive heart failure, edema, anemia				
Due to the troglitazone experience, periodic monitoring of LFTs is recommended				
Pioglitazone	15–45	1	L	24
Pioglitazone-glimepiride	30/2, 30/4	1	L/L>K	24
Rosiglitazone	4–8	1–2	L	Up to 24
Rosiglitazone-glimepiride	4/1, 4/2, 4/4	1–2	L/L>K	Up to 24
α-GLUCOSIDASE INHIBITORS				
Delay carbohydrate absorption. Administer just before meals.				
Principal side effects: gastrointestinal disturbances (abdominal pain, nausea, diarrhea), LFT elevation				
Acarbose	75–300	3	Gut/K*	2–3
Miglitol	75–300	3	K	2–3
DIPEPTIDYL PEPTIDASE (DPP) IV INHIBITORS				
Increases insulin secretion; decreases glucagon secretion				
Principal side effects: none				
Sitagliptin	100	1	K	24

*The small fraction (<2%) of acarbose that is absorbed is eliminated by the kidneys.
K = kidney; L = liver; LFT = liver function test.

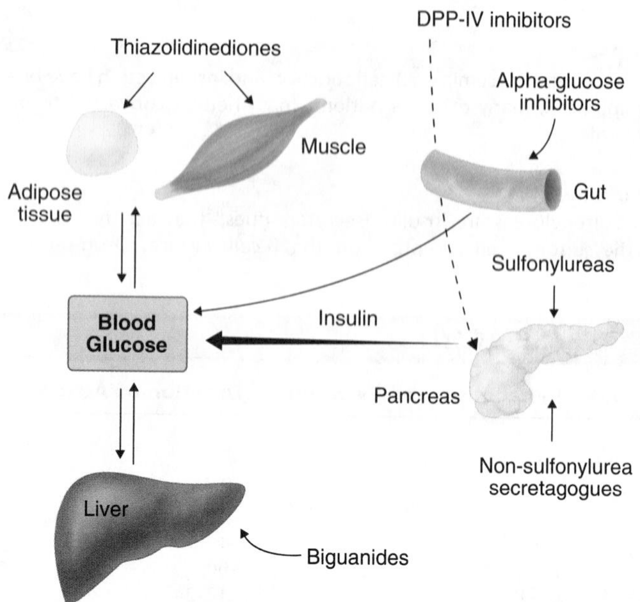

FIGURE 248–3 • Mechanism of action of oral glucose-lowering agents.

Rx

binding acts to close adenosine triphosphate–dependent potassium channels, resulting in cellular depolarization, calcium influx, and translocation of insulin secretory granules to the β-cell surface. The resulting release of insulin into the portal vein rapidly suppresses hepatic glucose production and later facilitates peripheral glucose use. Insulin resistance commonly diminishes as a secondary result of the reversal of glucotoxicity. Because sulfonylureas rely on a preserved β-cell response, they are ineffective in the treatment of type 1 diabetes. They are also ineffective in type 2 diabetic patients with markedly impaired β-cell function.

Although the sulfonylureas differ in relative potency, effective dosage, metabolism, and duration of action, these differences have marginal significance from a clinical standpoint (see Table 248–4). Each drug has similar hypoglycemic effects; at maximally effective doses, an average drop in HbA_{1c} of 1 to 2% is expected, correlating to average fasting plasma glucose reductions of 40 to 80 mg/dL. Drugs that are hepatically metabolized and have a shorter duration of action have advantages in elderly patients with impaired renal function (who are more vulnerable to hypoglycemia) but may be less effective in practice because of noncompliance with multiple dosing schedules. Conversely, longer acting agents can be dosed once daily, enhancing compliance but increasing the risk of prolonged hypoglycemia. After the appropriate drug is chosen, treatment is initiated at low doses, with dose increases every 1 to 2 weeks until either treatment goals are met or "maximally effective" doses are reached. Note that for all sulfonylureas, efficacy plateaus at about 50% of the listed maximum dose; above these maximally effective doses, little clinical benefit is derived from dose escalation, and additional therapies should be considered.

The majority of type 2 patients initially respond to sulfonylureas with improved glycemic control. However, 10 to 20% of patients show little or no response and are referred to as primary drug failures. Many other patients will experience the loss of drug effect after years of successful therapy; these secondary drug failures occur at rates of 5 to 10% per year because of progressive β-cell failure, drug tolerance, lack of enthusiasm for diet and exercise, or the superimposition of comorbid illness. Glucotoxicity itself can also contribute to worsening glucose control. In clinical practice, early signs of secondary drug failure should provoke renewed attempts to reinforce diet and exercise as well as a reassessment of drug dosage. The reappearance of hyperglycemia despite maximally effective drug doses signals the need to add another class of oral agent or to transition to insulin therapy. Overall, only about 25% of patients reach glucose targets with a sulfonylurea alone; stated another way, three of four patients will require additional modes of therapy. As shown in Table 248–4, advantages of sulfonylureas include low cost (especially with generics), convenience (once-daily dosing), and proven reduction of microvascular end points (retinopathy, nephropathy, and probably neuropathy). Disadvantages include hypoglycemia and weight gain.

Rx

Nonsulfonylurea Secretagogues

Repaglinide and nateglinide are non-sulfonylureas that interact with a different portion of the sulfonylurea receptor to stimulate insulin secretion. The major advantage of the non-sulfonylureas over sulfonylureas is their rapid and relatively short duration of action, which may attenuate postprandial glucose excursions and reduce the risk of fasting hypoglycemia. Both drugs require frequent daily dosing and should be taken 0 to 15 minutes before meals. Repaglinide is a somewhat stronger secretagogue than nateglinide and similar to the sulfonylureas in glucose-lowering power, with an expected average HbA_{1c} improvement of 1 to 2%. Both agents have a favorable side effect profile and typically produce less clinical hypoglycemia than traditional sulfonylureas do. The primary disadvantages of the non-sulfonylureas are their high cost and multiple dosing schedules and the lack of long-term outcomes data with these agents.

Biguanides

Metformin is the only biguanide available for use in the United States. Unlike sulfonylureas, this agent is considered an insulin sensitizer that acts mainly to reduce hepatic glucose production by suppressing gluconeogenesis. Metformin may also augment peripheral glucose use, although this effect may be secondary to reversal of glucotoxicity. Metformin exhibits a glucose-lowering effect similar to that of the sulfonylureas, with expected HbA_{1c} reductions of 1 to 2%. As with sulfonylureas, however, only about 25% of patients will be adequately controlled with monotherapy. Metformin has a relatively short half-life (it is eliminated exclusively by the kidney) and is therefore given in two or three divided doses with meals. An extended-release metformin product allows more convenient once-daily dosing.

Because the effects of metformin are extrapancreatic, insulin levels generally fall, a potential advantage if the theory implicating hyperinsulinemia in the development of atherosclerosis proves correct. Other advantages of metformin include mild weight loss, mild (<10%) LDL and triglyceride reductions, and no hypoglycemia when it is used as monotherapy. Small studies have also demonstrated a benefit on fibrinolytic activity and endothelial dysfunction, which may provide a cardiovascular benefit. Side effects are primarily gastrointestinal, including abdominal pain, bloating, nausea, diarrhea, and anorexia; these may be partially responsible for the weight loss effect. Metformin can also very rarely produce lactic acidosis (approximately 0.03 case per 1000 patient years) and should therefore not be given to patients with renal insufficiency (serum creatinine ≥ 1.5 in males or ≥ 1.4 in females), liver disease, severe congestive heart failure, metabolic acidosis, or history of alcohol abuse. The drug should also be held in dehydrated patients and for 48 to 72 hours before either surgery or the administration of intravenous radiocontrast agents. Recent observational data sets suggest that the current prescribing guidelines in patients with mild renal insufficiency and heart failure may be overly conservative.

With regard to evidence-based medicine, metformin has the most proven track record among the oral agents. Like sulfonylureas, metformin reduced microvascular end points in the UKPDS; unlike sulfonylureas, it may also have produced statistically significant reductions in myocardial infarction, diabetes-related death, and overall mortality. Furthermore, in the Diabetes Prevention Program (see later), metformin showed an ability to delay the progression to diabetes in patients with IGT.

Thiazolidinediones

Thiazolidinediones (TZDs) reduce insulin resistance, most likely through activation of PPAR-γ, a nuclear receptor that regulates the transcription of several insulin-responsive genes that regulate carbohydrate and lipid metabolism. The biologic effect of TZDs is prin-

Rx

cipally mediated by stimulation of peripheral glucose metabolism. PPAR-γ activation also reduces lipolysis and enhances peripheral adipocyte differentiation, thereby redistributing fat stores from the liver and muscle to subcutaneous depots; this effect may be largely responsible for the "insulin-sensitizing" effects of the TZDs. There is a concomitant modulation in the circulating levels of adipocytokines, particularly in adiponectin, which is increased two- to threefold in TZD-treated patients. In 1997, troglitazone was the first TZD approved for use in the United States; although effective, the drug was withdrawn from the market in 1999 because of concerns about idiosyncratic hepatotoxicity. Rosiglitazone and pioglitazone were later approved; these agents have no significant hepatotoxicity and are currently in widespread use.

Compared with sulfonylureas and metformin, TZDs, when used as monotherapy, have more delayed glucose-lowering effects that are ultimately similar in degree. Clinical advantages of TZDs include convenience (once-daily dosing), little hypoglycemia, and reduced levels of circulating insulin. TZDs have many other potentially beneficial effects: lower triglyceride levels (particularly with pioglitazone); higher HDL levels; reductions in small, dense LDL cholesterol; small reductions in blood pressure; improved endothelial function; reduced vascular inflammation; and enhanced fibrinolytic activity. At a more fundamental level, TZDs have also been demonstrated, mainly in in vitro models, to attenuate the expression of a variety of locally derived factors that promote the atherosclerotic process. In the first outcomes study to assess the effect of TZDs on cardiovascular events (PROactive), the addition of pioglitazone to baseline antihyperglycemic therapy modestly reduced the time to all-cause mortality, myocardial infarction, and stroke in high-risk patients with type 2 diabetes. 2 In this study involving more than 5000 patients, the primary end point, however, consisted of more outcomes including procedure-based end points such as coronary and peripheral artery revascularizations was not significantly altered. HbA_{1c} was 0.5% lower in the pioglitazone group, making the impact of the insulin-sensitizing properties of the TZD difficult to know fully. Moreover, an increase in heart failure diagnosis was observed in active therapy patients, attenuating widespread enthusiasm for the routine use of TZDs in all high-risk patients. Certainly, these early data concerning the effects of the TZDs on atherosclerosis need to be confirmed in subsequent studies.

Finally, there is some evidence that TZDs may also slow the decline of β-cell function, thus delaying the clinical progression from IGT to overt diabetes mellitus. This has been suggested in a small diabetes prevention trial using the TZD troglitazone, which is no longer available.

Compared with other oral hypoglycemic agents, TZDs are more costly. Side effects of the TZDs are largely related to fluid retention and fat redistribution and include weight gain, edema, mild anemia, and worsening of heart failure. These side effects develop most commonly in patients receiving concomitant insulin therapy. These drugs are therefore not recommended for use in patients with New York Heart Association class III-IV heart failure or with severe anemia. As mentioned, the two newer agents appear to be free of hepatic toxicity; however, because of the troglitazone experience, they should not be used in patients with active liver disease or with elevated serum transaminases (alanine transaminase ≥ 2.5 times the upper limit of normal). The manufacturers of both rosiglitazone and pioglitazone currently recommend periodic monitoring liver function tests according to clinical judgment. TZDs should be discontinued if transaminases are three times or more the upper limit of normal. Somewhat paradoxically, these agents reduce hepatic fat content and might actually improve the histologic and biochemical abnormalities in the liver condition encountered most frequently in obese, type 2 diabetic patients, nonalcoholic steatohepatitis. This, however, remains to be proved.

α-Glucosidase Inhibitors

Acarbose and miglitol are competitive inhibitors of α-glucosidases, brush border enzymes in the proximal small intestine that serve to break down complex carbohydrates into monosaccharides to facilitate transmucosal absorption. These agents delay the absorption of carbohydrates such as starch, sucrose, and maltose but do not affect the absorption of glucose and other monosaccharides. To be effective, acarbose and miglitol must be taken at the beginning of each carbohydrate-containing meal, usually three or four times per day. Acarbose is minimally absorbed systemically, whereas miglitol is absorbed and rapidly excreted (unchanged) in the urine. Perhaps as a result of improved glycemic control, both of these agents are associated with modest (<10%) reductions in circulating triglyceride levels and have no appreciable effects on LDL or HDL cholesterol.

In controlled trials performed in patients with type 2 diabetes, α-glucosidase inhibitors reduced postprandial glucose excursions and produced small (0.5 to 1.0%) but meaningful reductions in HbA_{1c}. Their most prominent effect is on postprandial blood glucose levels. It has been suggested that the postprandial glucose level may be more closely aligned with cardiovascular risk than fasting glucose concentration is. It is of interest that in a post hoc analysis from the Study to Prevent Non–Insulin-Dependent Diabetes Mellitus (STOP-NIDDM diabetes prevention trial), acarbose therapy was associated with a marked reduction (~50%) in the incidence of cardiovascular events in these pre-diabetic subjects. There have been no long-term studies employing an α-glucosidase inhibitor in diabetic patients, however, to assess if such a seeming vasculoprotective effect might be confirmed.

The most common side effects associated with both acarbose and miglitol are abdominal pain, bloating, flatulence, and diarrhea; these adverse events can be minimized by initiating therapy at low doses and by using a slowly escalating dose titration schedule. Still, the manufacturers of both drugs discourage their use in patients with inflammatory bowel disease, colonic ulceration, or any other significant chronic gastrointestinal disorder. They are also to be avoided in patients with advanced liver disease.

DPP-IV Inhibitors

The most recently available oral agents for the management of type 2 diabetes are the DPP-IV inhibitors (e.g., sitagliptin). This class of drug inhibits the activity of dipeptidyl peptidase 4, the enzyme responsible for the breakdown of the naturally occurring incretins, GLP-1 and GIP. As monotherapy and in combination with other oral agents, gliptins reduce HbA1c by 0.7 to 0.8% versus placebo therapy. However, since the baseline HbA1c in these trials (8 to 8.5%) was lower than in most studies previously conducted with more traditional agents, it is difficult to compare the results. In head-to-head comparisons, the gliptins appear to fare favorably to most other available oral antihyperglycemic medications. The advantage of this therapeutic class is the relative absence of major side effects, including lack of hypoglycemia. They may be of greatest use in patients with mild elevations of blood glucose. The DPP-IV inhibitors are currently approved for use as monotherapy and in combination with metformin and thiazolidinediones. There are no data on micro- or macrovascular outcomes, and the long-term safety of DPP-IV inhibition is not known.

Exenatide

Exenatide is a member of the class of drugs known as incretin mimetics. Specifically, exenatide is a GLP-1 mimetic and, as a result, stimulates insulin secretion in a glucose-dependent fashion, inhibits glucagon secretion, slows gastric emptying, and may have a central satiety effect. It is available only in an injectable form, administered twice daily. Exenatide is approved for use in combination with oral agents in type 2 diabetes. It reduces HbA_{1c} by nearly 1% compared with placebo and also promotes weight loss, a feature distinguishing it from most other antihyperglycemic agents. Side effects include nausea and vomiting. Exenatide does not by itself lead to hypoglycemia, but it may increase the risk when it is used with oral insulin secretagogues. In preliminary studies in animals, incretin mimetics appear to preserve β-cell function and therefore might be useful earlier in the disease course than is currently recommended. At present, however, exenatide has a niche as an alternative to the initiation of insulin for those patients whose treatment with oral

Rx

agents is failing. Other incretin mimetics under active development include several injectable GLP-1 analogues and the oral dipeptidyl peptidase IV inhibitors; the latter inhibit the enzyme that rapidly inactivates endogenous GLP-1.

Insulin Therapy In Type 2 Diabetes

Insulin is commonly used as first-line therapy for nonobese, younger, or severely hyperglycemic type 2 diabetic patients and is often temporarily required during times of severe stress (e.g., injury, infection, surgery) or during pregnancy. Insulin should not be used as first-line therapy for patients who are poorly compliant, unwilling to self-monitor glucose levels, or at high risk for hypoglycemia (e.g., the very elderly). In obese patients, profound insulin resistance often necessitates the use of large doses of insulin, which can interfere with efforts to restrict calorie intake and achieve weight loss. In leaner patients and in patients with relatively mild fasting hyperglycemia (who continue to maintain endogenous insulin secretory capacity), relatively small doses of basal insulin (e.g., 0.3 to 0.4 U per kilogram of body weight per day) given once or twice per day may be sufficient to achieve glucose targets. Many of these patients retain some degree of meal-stimulated endogenous insulin secretion and may therefore require none or less rapid-acting insulin as well.

Although it is common practice to administer a single dose of intermediate-acting insulin (e.g., NPH) in the morning, the glucose-lowering effect of this regimen does not usually extend during a full 24-hour period. Because a key element of successful insulin treatment is to counteract accelerated rates of endogenous glucose production in the morning, it is generally more effective to split the dose and to administer sufficient amounts of intermediate-acting insulin in the evening (preferably at bedtime) to optimize control. Alternatively, a single dose of intermediate-acting insulin given at bedtime may be effective throughout the following day in patients who have retained the capacity to secrete insulin with meals. This approach has the advantage of greater simplicity and compliance and may be combined with oral glucose-lowering agents during the day to facilitate endogenous insulin release and action. More recently, with the availability of long-acting, basal insulins, such as glargine and detemir, one injection per day is an increasingly favored approach in many patients. This is typically also provided at bedtime but can actually be administered at any time of day.

With regard to the initiation of more advanced insulin replacement regimens, which are required in certain insulin-deficient type 2 patients, there are many acceptable approaches. As a first step, the total daily dose of insulin should be estimated from body weight; total insulin requirements range between 0.5 and 1.0 U/kg/day, typically higher than those used in type 1 diabetes. One classic method for starting insulin is to divide the total daily dose unevenly, with two thirds given before breakfast and the remaining third before dinner. Each of the two doses is then further subdivided: at breakfast, two thirds of the dose is given as intermediate-acting insulin and the other third as a short- or rapid-acting preparation; at dinner, the dose is divided into two equal parts. As an example, for a 90-kg man with estimated requirements of 0.67 U/kg/day, 60 U of insulin may be required. By use of this method, the patient might receive 27 units of NPH with 13 units of a rapid-acting insulin analogue (e.g., lispro, aspart, or glulisine) before breakfast, then 10 units of NPH with 10 units of analogue before dinner. Note that this is only one of many "rule-of-thumb" methods for the initiation of insulin. Most insulin-treated patients have more severe hyperglycemia, and oral agent therapy has already failed. As a result, they may require more refined "basal-bolus" regimens that offer more physiologic insulin replacement. The regimen in the most motivated and capable patients is ideally adjusted on the basis of the anticipated carbohydrate intake ("carbohydrate counting") as well as the pre-meal blood glucose level. These regimens are certainly more complex and inconvenient and do require frequent dosage adjustments. Thus, in the absence of hyperglycemic complications, clinicians should generally begin with more conservative doses of insulin to minimize hypoglycemia and to smooth the patient's transition to multiple-dose subcutaneous insulin therapy.

Rx

In short, the complexity of the regimen should be individualized according to the clinical context, the patient's abilities and capacities to perform self-care, and most important, the patient's level of education and motivation. Experience with the use of intensified insulin treatment, including continuous subcutaneous insulin infusion pumps and multiple subcutaneous injection regimens, is growing in patients with type 2 diabetes. Preliminary results suggest that intensified treatment may be successfully applied to selected patients. Inhaled insulin may become a reasonable alternative for type 2 diabetic patients who are unable or unwilling to inject insulin but who will benefit from its addition. [3]

In many cases, the combination of intensive insulin therapy with oral hypoglycemic agents (e.g., TZDs or metformin) may reduce insulin dose requirements and improve glycemic control. Although this is growing in acceptance, the potential benefit of reducing circulating insulin levels (by combination therapy) on the development of atherogenesis remains to be established. As in patients with type 1 diabetes, weight gain and hypoglycemia are potential side effects of insulin therapy. It is noteworthy, however, that the incidence of severe hypoglycemia is markedly lower (<5%) compared with that seen in patients with type 1 diabetes.

Pramlintide

See Chapter 247 for a brief description of this newer agent, which is also approved for insulin-requiring patients with type 2 diabetes.

Treatment Strategies for Type 2 Diabetes

In contrast to type 1 diabetes, in which insulin therapy is required, several pharmacologic options exist for the management of type 2 diabetes. The pros and cons of the various oral hypoglycemic agents were discussed earlier; often, it is difficult to justify the use of one oral agent over another, although the consensus of most diabetologists is to favor metformin as first-line therapy, given the lack of hypoglycemia associated with its use as monotherapy, its low cost, and a slight degree of weight loss that often accompanies its use. In the literature, few studies have compared the glucose-lowering power of one oral agent with another, and even fewer studies have compared the drugs in terms of relevant clinical outcomes such as mortality, cardiovascular disease, or microvascular complications. To date, the largest study to address such outcomes in type 2 diabetes was the UKPDS.

In the UKPDS, improved outcomes produced by intensified therapy were similar for patients given insulin, sulfonylureas, or metformin therapy. The ability of the study to detect differences among the various treatments was limited because of drug crossovers and the frequent need for drug combinations as the study progressed. The use of metformin in the UKPDS deserves specific mention here because of conflicting results. In the study, patients initially assigned to metformin therapy showed decreased rates of microvascular complications, combined diabetes-related end points, diabetes-related deaths, all-cause deaths, and myocardial infarction compared with conventionally treated patients. In contrast, patients treated with insulin or sulfonylureas demonstrated reductions in only two of the five categories, microvascular complications and combined diabetes-related end points. Thus, metformin therapy appeared advantageous. Late in the study, however, 537 patients failing sulfonylurea therapy were randomly assigned to continuation of the sulfonylurea alone or the addition of metformin. Compared with the sulfonylurea subgroup, this combined-therapy subgroup had an unexpected 60% *increase* in all-cause mortality. The results of this "substudy" have been called into question because it was unblinded and lacked a placebo control. In addition, 25% of the patients assigned to continue monotherapy eventually required metformin to achieve glucose targets. In summary, on the basis of the UKPDS, it is difficult to offer an unequivocal recommendation for metformin compared with sulfonylureas or insulin therapy.

The choice of initial pharmacologic therapy for type 2 diabetes should be influenced mainly by the severity of fasting hyperglycemia, the degree of obesity, and the presence and magnitude

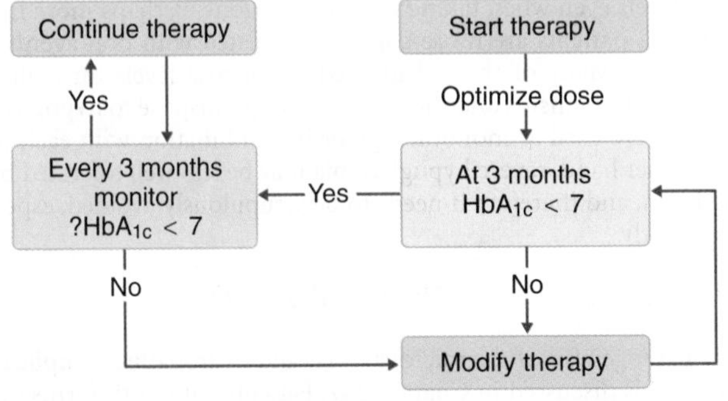

FIGURE 248-4 • Strategy for the treatment of type 2 diabetes.

of hyperglycemic symptoms. Other factors such as age, education, motivation, comorbid conditions, and drug cost and convenience should also be considered. To determine the effectiveness of the therapy selected, drug regimens should be adjusted during a 2- to 3-month period on the basis of self-monitoring of glucose concentration; failure to meet glucose targets within 3 months suggests the need for combination therapy (Fig. 248–4). Published clinical trials comparing drug combinations with monotherapy have generally shown additive reductions in HbA_{1c}; with few exceptions, the magnitude of A_{1c} reduction approximates that achieved when the added agent is used as monotherapy. As is the case with monotherapy, there is no convincing evidence favoring one combination regimen over another, and most combinations have been approved by the FDA. "Triple-therapy," or combining three agents to achieve glucose targets, is also used in clinical practice (although not formally with FDA approval) and appears to be effective. Ultimately, if glucose targets cannot be met by combining oral agents, insulin remains an effective treatment option.

Monitoring

See Chapter 247. Patients with type 2 diabetes generally require less frequent self-monitoring of blood glucose concentration, particularly those managed with oral agents or less intensive insulin regimens. Glucose and HbA_{1c} targets should be the same as in type 1 diabetes (see Table 247–4), although there are few data on the effectiveness and safety of strict glycemic targets in the elderly. Accordingly, each patient's desirable glucose range must be an individual decision between the practitioner and the patient. Elements of this decision must take into account the motivation and capacities of the patient, propensity for hypoglycemia and its unawareness, presence or absence of complications, and other established comorbidities.

Inpatient Management of Diabetes

Much attention has been paid recently to the inpatient management of hyperglycemia, both in patients with an established diagnosis of diabetes and in those whose glucose elevations are a response to illness. Observational studies previously have correlated the degree of hyperglycemia and outcomes in a variety of settings, including after cardiac surgery, in the critically ill, and in patients with acute myocardial infarction and stroke. Acutely, hyperglycemia has a notable detrimental effect on the immune system, wound healing, endothelial function, and cardiac metabolism. When glucose elevations are severe, dangerous fluid shifts and electrolyte fluxes may occur. Randomized clinical trials suggest improved short-term outcomes in critically ill patients managed with intensive insulin infusions to reduce the blood glucose concentration to or near the euglycemic range. [4] Whether this target should be applied to all hospitalized patients is a controversial point. Although it is clearly achievable in the intensive care unit, such rigorous therapy may not be practical on general medical-surgical wards. Until more information is available, at the very least, all reasonable attempts should be made to avoid moderate to marked hyperglycemia (>200 mg/dL) in all hospitalized patients. Those in the intensive care unit would benefit from stringent control, which can be achieved most reliably with intravenous insulin. Multidisciplinary inpatient diabetes management teams have been shown to be useful in assisting hospitals to improve the quality of their diabetes care and in reducing the length of stay of diabetic patients.

Prevention

With our increasing understanding of the pathogenesis of type 2 diabetes and our appreciation of the often lengthy period between impaired glucose metabolism and overt diabetes, there has been significant attention on the possibility of preventing this disease in at-risk individuals.

In the Diabetes Prevention Program, more than 3000 overweight subjects with IGT were randomized into four treatment arms: (1) intensive lifestyle changes aimed at reducing body weight by 7% through a low-fat diet and 150 minutes of weekly exercise; (2) treatment with metformin, 850 mg twice per day; (3) treatment with placebo pills, twice per day; and (4) treatment with troglitazone, 400 mg once per day (this arm was discontinued because of concerns about liver toxicity). [5] The last three groups also received standard information about diet and exercise. On the advice of the Diabetes Prevention Program's external data monitoring board, the trial was stopped a year early because of definitive results. In the placebo group, 29% of patients developed diabetes during the average follow-up period of 3 years, compared with 22% of patients taking metformin and only 14% of patients undergoing intensive diet and exercise. The relative risk reduction for patients taking metformin was 31% versus standard care, whereas patients undergoing intensive lifestyle interventions reduced their risk by an impressive 58%. This risk reduction was identical to that measured by Finnish investigators in the Diabetes Prevention Study, involving a similar study design but focusing on lifestyle change alone. [6] This suggests that patients with IGT can sharply lower their immediate risk of diabetes with intensive lifestyle changes (or in some cases with metformin).

Whether screening, identifying, and then treating patients with IGT in routine clinical practice is cost-effective or even doable remains somewhat controversial. Certainly, if recommendations regarding healthy lifestyle changes were followed by high-risk patients, the incidence of type 2 diabetes will decrease. If such therapy is durable, this would necessarily translate to fewer microvascular complications over time. Whether such interventions will mitigate the risk of macrovascular disease is less clear, although Diabetes Prevention Program participants on diet and exercise did experience some amelioration in cardiovascular risk factors.

How drug therapy fits into this equation is similarly a point of controversy. Notably, after metformin therapy was washed out in Diabetes Prevention Program participants for 2 weeks, 25% of those whose diabetes was apparently prevented developed the disease. Similarly, in the STOP-NIDDM diabetes prevention trial involving the α-glucosidase inhibitor acarbose, a 25% decrease in the appearance of type 2 diabetes during a 3-year period was demonstrated. In the Troglitazone in Prevention of Diabetes (TRIPOD) study, troglitazone therapy for high-risk women with a prior history of gestational diabetes reduced the risk of type 2 diabetes by 55%, and this more substantial effect appeared to persist many months after the discontinuation of the drug. The results of ongoing studies involving currently available TZDs should be available soon.

ACUTE METABOLIC COMPLICATIONS

Diabetic Ketoacidosis

See Chapter 247 for a discussion of diabetic ketoacidosis.

Hyperosmolar Hyperglycemic Syndrome

Clinical Manifestations

The metabolic state formerly known as the hyperglycemic hyperosmolar nonketotic state or coma has been renamed the hyperosmolar hyperglycemic syndrome (HHS) to highlight two important points: (1) ketosis (and acidosis) may be present to varying degrees in HHS and (2) alterations in sensorium most commonly occur in the absence of coma. In fact, only 10% of HHS patients present with frank coma, and an equal percentage show no signs whatsoever of mental status change.

As shown in Table 247–6, the hallmarks of the HHS are severe hyperosmolarity (>320 mOsm/L) and hyperglycemia (>600 mg/dL) (see also Chapter 247). Severe hyperglycemia occurs because patients cannot drink enough liquid to keep pace with a vigorous osmotic diuresis. The resulting impairment in renal function eventually further reduces glucose excretion through the kidney, leading to remarkable blood glucose elevations, sometimes exceeding 1000 mg/dL. In contrast to diabetic ketoacidosis, even though glucose concentrations are generally higher, severe acidosis and ketosis are generally absent in the HHS. This is probably explained by the residual insulin secretory capacity retained by patients with even decades of type 2 diabetes. Their insulin levels remain sufficient to suppress lipolysis and to avoid significant keto acid production. However, some type 2 patients with depressed endogenous insulin secretion may be unable to suppress ketone production fully in the face of elevated counter-regulatory hormones produced by physical illness. Because HHS patients have higher portal vein insulin concentrations than patients with diabetic ketoacidosis do, keto acid production by the liver is relatively mild, yielding only mild acidosis. In the HHS, in the absence of concurrent acid-base disturbances, arterial pH rarely drops below 7.30, and serum bicarbonate levels rarely fall below 18 mEq/L.

In the hyperosmolar hyperglycemic state, clinical severity and levels of consciousness generally correlate with the severity and duration of hyperosmolarity. Clinical signs indicate profound dehydration; gastrointestinal symptoms are less frequently seen than in diabetic ketoacidosis. A variety of often reversible neurologic abnormalities may exist, including grand mal or focal seizures, extensor plantar reflexes, aphasia, hemisensory or motor deficits, and worsening of a preexisting organic mental syndrome. The laboratory picture is dominated by the effects of uncontrolled diabetes and dehydration; renal function is impaired, hemoglobin is elevated, and liver function test results may be abnormal because of baseline hepatic steatosis. Although severe hyperglycemia would be expected to lower measured serum sodium concentration, it is not uncommon to see "normal" or even "elevated" sodium levels because of the severity of dehydration. The serum osmolarity itself can be measured directly or estimated by the following formula, which excludes urea because it is freely diffusible throughout the body and therefore has little influence on the osmotic pressure gradient:

$$\text{Effective osmolarity (mOsm/L)} = 2\ [\text{measured serum Na}^{+}\ (\text{mEq/L})] + [\text{glucose (mg/dL)}/18]$$

Treatment Rx

Patients with HHS should be treated as aggressively as those with diabetic ketoacidosis are, although they tend to have more dramatic volume contraction (Chapter 247). By definition, acidosis is not present or is minimal in degree. Accordingly, patients may not require clamping. Also, it is important to volume resuscitate the patient adequately before insulin is administered for fear that intracellular fluid shifts that occur as glucose levels are reduced may worsen systemic tissue perfusion. Because, by definition, there is no significant acidosis to clear in HHS, patients may be transitioned directly from insulin infusion to subcutaneous injections, without need for any coadministration of dextrose as is necessary in diabetic ketoacidosis to allow further clearance of ketone bodies. Some patients with HHS may ultimately be able to be managed with oral agents alone. However, the development of HHS signifies a significant degree of insulin deficiency. As a result, it is always best to prescribe insulin injections before the patient is discharged and to reserve judgment about the appropriateness of oral agents until the patient's progress can be monitored in the outpatient setting.

HYPOGLYCEMIA

See Chapter 247 for a full discussion of this complication of diabetes therapy. As previously mentioned, hypoglycemia is encountered less frequently in patients with type 2 diabetes because of biologic as well as practical reasons. Because the typical type 2 patient retains some residual endogenous insulin secretion, the development of mild hypoglycemia will lead to its abrupt reduction. Accordingly, type 2 diabetic patients can autoregulate to a degree not possible in the absolutely insulin deficient type 1. Also, patients with type 2 diabetes are, almost by definition, insulin resistant and therefore less likely to develop abnormally low blood glucose levels even when taking insulin injections. Perhaps more important, type 2 patients are more commonly treated with oral agents than with insulin. Many of these drugs reduce glucose levels through nonpancreatic mechanisms and therefore do not predispose to hypoglycemia when they are used as monotherapy or in combination with each other. On the other hand, severe hypoglycemia may be less well tolerated by the aging brain, and therefore it needs to be scrupulously avoided, especially in the elderly.

CHRONIC DIABETIC COMPLICATIONS

The pathogenesis of the microvascular and neuropathic complications of diabetes is discussed in Chapter 247. Patients with both forms of diabetes are at risk for retinopathy, nephropathy, and nerve dysfunction.

Atherosclerosis

Atherosclerosis (Chapter 69) involving the coronary, cerebral, and peripheral (lower extremity) arteries is the predominant cause of diabetes-related mortality, responsible for up to 70% of all deaths in patients with this disease. The atherosclerotic process in diabetes is indistinguishable from that of the nondiabetic population, but it begins earlier and is often more extensive and more severe. A predilection to cardiovascular disease is observed over the entire spectrum of diabetes, from poorly controlled insulin-dependent patients to those with mild, diet-controlled hyperglycemia. For unclear reasons, the disparity between diabetic and normal subjects is more pronounced in women. When it is accompanied by other major cardiovascular risk factors such as hypertension, dyslipidemia, and smoking, diabetes markedly increases the incidence of macrovascular complications. For example, the observed 2- to 3-fold greater risk of myocardial infarction with diabetes rises to 8-fold in the presence of hypertension and to nearly 20-fold if both hypertension and dyslipidemia are present; smoking increases these risks even further. As a result, the diagnosis of diabetes mellitus should quickly prompt both an exhaustive search for coexisting cardiovascular risk factors and the initiation of aggressive preventive measures.

Diabetes is an *independent* risk factor for accelerated atherosclerosis. Its association with vascular disease is not solely attributable to an increased prevalence of other recognized vascular risk factors such as hypertension, smoking, and dyslipidemia. Many abnormalities induced by the diabetic state may contribute to atherosclerosis, including lipid abnormalities (e.g., increased total VLDL and LDL, increased small dense [atherogenic] LDL, decreased HDL, increased lipoprotein oxidation, increased lipoprotein glycosylation, decreased lipoprotein lipase activity), accentuated platelet aggregation and adhesion, endothelial cell dysfunction, and induced procoagulant state (e.g., increased clotting factors and fibrinogen; decreased levels of antithrombin III, protein C, and protein S; and decreased fibrinolytic activity). It has been suggested that hyperinsulinemia per se may contribute to macrovascular disease; proposed pathogenetic mechanisms include insulin-induced stimulation of vascular endothelial and smooth muscle cells, enhanced insulin-like growth factor 1 expression, and augmented synthesis of atherogenic factors such as endothelin and plasminogen activator inhibitor. Moreover, in type 2 diabetes, insulin resistance is an independent risk factor for vascular events and may exert its effect through many of these disease intermediaries.

ASSOCIATED CONDITIONS

Hypertension

In patients with diabetes, systemic hypertension (Chapter 66) is an important cofactor in the development of cardiovascular disease, nephropathy, and retinopathy. The prevalence of hypertension in type 2 patients is more than twice that of the nondiabetic population, largely due to the clustering of both disorders in patients with obesity and insulin resistance. Type 1 patients, in contrast, are usually normotensive in the absence of renal disease; if nephropathy develops, the majority of affected patients will then develop secondary hypertension. The importance of aggressive blood pressure management in diabetes has been established by the UKPDS (see earlier); in the study, blood pressure reduction (with angiotensin-converting enzyme [ACE] inhibitors or β-blockers) in type 2 diabetic patients with hypertension produced striking decreases in both cardiovascular and microvascular outcomes. Subsequent prospective trials, including the Systolic Hypertension in the Elderly Program (SHEP), the Systolic Hypertension in Europe (Sys-Eur) trial, and the

Hypertension Optimal Treatment (HOT) trial, have confirmed the value of aggressive blood pressure goals in reducing major cardiovascular events in diabetic patients. On the basis of these and other studies, the Seventh Report of the Joint National Committee on Prevention, Detection, Evaluation, and Treatment of High Blood Pressure (JNC 7) has established blood pressure targets of less than 130/85 for patients with diabetes mellitus; even stricter reductions (<125/75) are recommended in the presence of established nephropathy (Chapter 66).

The choice of antihypertensive agent for diabetic patients has for years been the subject of considerable research and debate. Among the various therapeutic options, ACE inhibitors and angiotensin II receptor blockers (ARBs) may offer special advantages; they have consistently demonstrated the ability to lower intraglomerular pressures and to slow the progression of albuminuria and diabetic nephropathy. These agents are advocated by the American Diabetes Association as first-line agents, including their use in normotensive diabetic patients with albuminuria. In addition to ACE inhibitors and ARBs, JNC 7 has additionally endorsed low-dose diuretics, β-blockers, and calcium-channel blockers as preferred agents in diabetic patients with hypertension. β-Blockers should also be strongly considered in the setting of concurrent cardiovascular disease, including prior myocardial infarction, mild to moderate congestive heart failure, and cardiac arrhythmias. Prospective trials comparing antihypertensive agents in diabetic patients have yielded mixed results. In the UKPDS, β-blockers were as effective as ACE inhibitors in reducing adverse cardiac and microvascular outcomes. Conversely, several large trials, including the Appropriate Blood Pressure Control in Diabetes (ABCD) trial, the Captopril Prevention Project (CPP), the Heart Outcomes Prevention Evaluation (HOPE) study (MICRO-HOPE substudy), [7] and the Fosinopril versus Amlodipine Cardiovascular Events Trial (FACET), suggest improved cardiovascular outcomes with the specific use of ACE inhibitors as first-line therapy. On the basis of currently available evidence, ACE inhibitors are recommended as first-line antihypertensive therapy in patients with diabetes, especially in the presence of microalbuminuria or overt nephropathy. ARBs are an excellent alternative, especially in patients who are unable to tolerate ACE inhibitors.

Dyslipidemia

Dyslipidemia (Chapter 217) is another crucial therapeutic target in the management of diabetes. The most common lipid disorder associated with diabetes is an increased level of triglyceride-rich lipoproteins (e.g., VLDL), low levels of HDL, and the presence of small dense and, as a result, more atherogenic LDL particles. The third report of the NCEP Expert Panel continues to identify LDL cholesterol as the primary target for therapy on the basis of overwhelming evidence from clinical trials. [8] This panel has established diabetes as a coronary heart disease "equivalent," meaning that all diabetic patients should strive for LDL levels below 100 mg/dL. In addition, HDL levels should generally exceed 40 mg/dL (50 mg/dL in women); triglyceride levels should fall below 150 mg/dL. Recommendations from the American Diabetes Association are similar. Both organizations endorse more aggressive LDL reduction (to below 70 mg/dL) in high-risk patients with overt cardiovascular disease. Such a target is based on the findings of randomized clinical trials in patients with known coronary artery disease. Achieving this goal may require combination therapy with a statin plus a cholesterol absorption inhibitor, such as ezetimibe.

Hydroxymethylglutaryl–coenzyme A reductase inhibitors (i.e., statins) are generally used as first-line therapy for lowering LDL cholesterol in patients with diabetes; of note, many of the statins at high doses have a modest triglyceride-lowering effect as well. Randomized clinical trials involving diabetic patients alone (Collaborative Atorvastatin Diabetes Study [CARDS], diabetic subset of the Heart Protection Study) have confirmed equal if not greater benefit of statin therapy in this important subgroup of patients. [9] If statins are contraindicated or poorly tolerated, a cholesterol absorption inhibitor can be used to lower LDL. Nicotinic acid, although it is also effective at lowering LDL (and triglycerides), is less useful in diabetic patients because it can worsen insulin resistance and adversely affect glycemic control.

Although most published trials involving diabetic patients involve statins to lower LDL, the characteristic lipid profile in the diabetic patient is an elevated triglyceride concentration and suppressed HDL cholesterol, both risk factors for coronary artery disease. Initial steps in treating diabetic dyslipidemia should include optimization of glycemic control, dietary reinforcement, and a prescription of aerobic exercise. Strict dietary parameters for diabetic patients with dyslipidemia call for less than 35% of daily calories as fat, with less than 7% of total calories as saturated fat and less than 200 mg/day of dietary cholesterol (the NCEP Step II diet). Regular aerobic exercise will help by raising HDL levels, and weight loss achieved through exercise can further attenuate lipid abnormalities. Prospective trials using the fibric acid derivative gemfibrozil to lower triglyceride levels and to raise HDL levels have produced improved cardiovascular outcomes (Veterans Affairs HDL Intervention Trial), although a study involving the fibrate fenofibrate in diabetic patients with normal to modestly elevated triglycerides yielded mixed results. On the basis of these data, although few would argue that marked hypertriglyceridemia (>400 mg/dL) should not be treated pharmacologically, it remains unclear which diabetic patient with mild to moderate hypertriglyceridemia (150 to 400 mg/dL) would benefit from aggressive intervention. Unless triglyceride levels are severely elevated, the management of hypertriglyceridemia should always begin with lifestyle change, including the incorporation of a low saturated fat diet, weight reduction, minimization of ethanol use, and, when it is present, the treatment of any underlying hypothyroidism.

Clearly, the prevention of cardiovascular disease in type 2 diabetes requires a comprehensive and multifactorial approach. Such an approach has been shown to reduce cardiovascular events by almost 50% (Steno-2 study). [10]

The measures described are largely aimed at *preventing* coronary artery disease in diabetic patients; once coronary artery disease has been *established,* it should also be aggressively treated. Compared with the general population, a higher proportion of diabetic patients die within a year of an acute myocardial infarction. Furthermore, while there has recently been a considerable decline in overall coronary artery disease–related mortality, a similar decline in patients with diabetes has not been observed. Low-dose aspirin therapy (81 to 325 mg/day) should be routinely recommended for the majority of adult patients with diabetes (especially with concurrent coronary artery disease) because of proven reductions in cardiovascular morbidity and mortality. After myocardial infarction, particularly in the setting of left ventricular systolic dysfunction, β-blockers and ACE inhibitors (or ARBs) may offer additional benefits. Finally, although angioplasty is often a viable option in diabetic patients with coronary disease, there is evidence to suggest that diabetic patients may derive greater than expected comparative benefit from coronary bypass procedures. However, with the recent development of advanced stenting procedures and the use of drug-eluting stents, which markedly attenuate stent restenosis rates, and adjunctive antiplatelet therapy, this distinction is becoming less important. Whether asymptomatic patients with diabetes should be routinely screened for coronary artery disease remains controversial. A study showed that more than one in five type 2 diabetic patients with no symptoms of angina and with normal findings on electrocardiography had an abnormality on screening myocardial perfusion imaging, indicative of underlying coronary artery disease. Whether their identification will improve ultimate clinical outcomes is unknown.

Unfortunately, the known association between diabetes mellitus and premature atherosclerosis may be only the "tip of the iceberg" with regard to linking glucose metabolism and vascular risk. Insulin resistance (i.e., impaired insulin-stimulated glucose metabolism) is common in "healthy" people living in Western nations; in such individuals, insulin resistance is often counterbalanced by increased insulin secretion, preventing the emergence of overt diabetes mellitus. Although this state of insulin resistance and chronic hyperinsulinemia may successfully defend against diabetes, a heavy price may be paid, including adverse effects on other insulin-related systems, such as sympathetic nervous system activity, renal sodium reabsorption, hepatic triglyceride synthesis, vascular endothelial function, and cellular events that mediate the atherosclerotic process, including arterial smooth muscle proliferation, expression of vascular adhesion molecules, matrix metalloproteinases, and a variety of cytokines and chemokines that appear to accelerate atherogenesis. This much is known: nonobese, nondiabetic individuals with insulin resistance have higher blood pressure, glucose concentration, and triglyceride levels (and lower HDL cholesterol concentrations) than those of matched subjects with normal insulin levels. The term *metabolic syndrome* is used by some to describe this phenomenon, namely, the clustering within one person of hyperinsulinemia, mild glucose intolerance, dyslipidemia, and hypertension, each of which is probably an independent risk factor for atherosclerosis (Fig. 248–5). Whether identifying such individuals as having metabolic syndrome as opposed to treating the composite risk

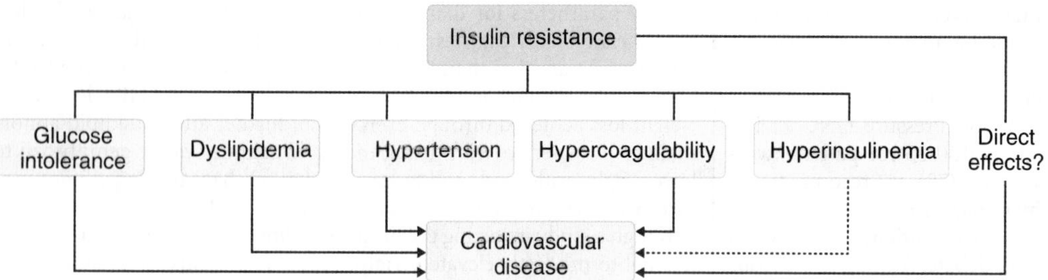

FIGURE 248-5 • Metabolic syndrome and the theoretical construct of the link between insulin resistance and cardiovascular disease.

factors individually is of any benefit remains controversial. Prospective population studies have confirmed that chronic hyperinsulinemia predicts the development of cardiovascular disease. Although such statistical associations do not prove causality, they suggest that insulin resistance itself may play a role in promoting atherosclerosis. If true, this hypothesis further underscores the importance of lifestyle changes in the treatment of type 2 diabetes and suggests that proper diet and exercise could also benefit insulin-resistant patients with more subtle metabolic abnormalities (i.e., metabolic syndrome, IGT, and IFG). The answer to the obvious question of whether insulin-sensitizing drugs decrease atherosclerosis risk in this setting remains unknown.

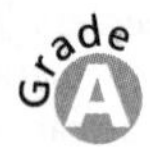

1. UK Prospective Diabetes Study (UKPDS) Group: Intensive blood-glucose control with sulphonylureas or insulin compared with conventional treatment and risk of complications in patients with type 2 diabetes (UKPDS 33). Lancet 1998;352:837–853.
2. Dormandy JA, Charbonnel B, Eckland DJ, et al, for the PROactive investigators: Secondary prevention of macrovascular events in patients with type 2 diabetes in the PROactive study (PROspective pioglitAzone Clinical Trial In macroVascular Events): A randomised controlled trial. Lancet 2005;366:1279.
3. Ceglia L, Lau J, Pittas AG: Meta-analysis: Efficacy and safety of inhaled insulin: Therapy in adults with diabetes mellitus. Am Intern Med 2006;145:665–675.
4. Van den Berghe G, Wilmer A, Hermans G, et al: Intensive insulin therapy in the medical ICU. N Engl J Med 2006;354:449–461.
5. Knowler WC, Barrett-Connor E, Fowler SE, et al; Diabetes Prevention Program Research Group: Reduction in the incidence of type 2 diabetes with lifestyle intervention or metformin. N Engl J Med 2002;346:393–403.
6. Lindstrom J, Ilanne-Parikka P, Peltonen M, et al: Sustained reduction in the incidence of type 2 diabetes by lifestyle intervention: Follow-up of the Finnish Diabetes Prevention Study. Lancet 2006;368:1673–1679.
7. Heart Outcomes Prevention Evaluation Study Investigators: Effects of ramipril on cardiovascular and microvascular outcomes in people with diabetes mellitus: Results of the HOPE study and MICRO-HOPE substudy. Lancet 2000;355:253.
8. Collins R, Armitage J, Parish S, et al; Heart Protection Study Collaborative Group: MRC/BHF Heart Protection Study of cholesterol lowering with simvastatin in 5963 people with diabetes: A randomised placebo controlled trial. Lancet 2003;361:2005–2016.
9. Colhoun HM, Betteridge DJ, Durrington PN, et al: Primary prevention of cardiovascular disease with atorvastatin in type 2 diabetes in the Collaborative Atorvastatin Diabetes Study (CARDS): Multicentre randomised placebo-controlled trial. Lancet 2004;364:685.
10. Gaede P, Vedel P, Larsen N, et al: Multifactorial interventions and cardiovascular disease in patients with type 2 diabetes. N Engl J Med 2003;348:383.

SUGGESTED READINGS

American Diabetes Association: Medical Management of Type 2 Diabetes, 5th ed. Alexandria, VA, American Diabetes Association, 2005. *A monograph that reviews the diagnosis, pathogenesis, and treatment of type 2 diabetes.*

Clement S, Braithwaite SS, Magee MF, et al; American Diabetes Association Diabetes in Hospitals Writing Committee: Management of diabetes and hyperglycemia in hospitals. Diabetes Care 2004;27:553–597. *An excellent overview of an increasingly popular topic.*

Gami AS, Witt BJ, Howard DE, et al: Metabolic syndrome and risk of incident cardiovascular events and death: A systematic review and meta-analysis of longitudinal studies. J Am Coll Cardiol 2007;49:403–414. *RR of cardiovascular death for patients with the metabolic syndrome was 1.78.*

Kitabachi AE, Nyenwe EA: Hyperglycemic crises in diabetes mellitus: Diabetic ketoacidosis and hyperglycemic hyperosmolar state. Endocrinol Metab Clin North Am 2006;35:725–751. *A practical review.*

Sowers JR: Treatment of hypertension in patients with diabetes. Arch Intern Med 2004;164:1850. *A comprehensive and evidence-based review of blood pressure management in the diabetic patient.*

Wackers FJ, Young LH, Inzucchi SE, et al; Detection of Ischemia in Asymptomatic Diabetics Investigators: Detection of silent myocardial ischemia in asymptomatic diabetic subjects: The DIAD study. Diabetes Care 2004;27:1954–1961. *A multicenter investigation that conclusively showed the high rate (22%) of silent heart disease in patients with type 2 diabetes.*

249 HYPOGLYCEMIA/ PANCREATIC ISLET CELL DISORDERS

Robert A. Rizza and F. John Service

HYPOGLYCEMIA

Definition

Hypoglycemia is a clinical syndrome of diverse causes in which low levels of serum glucose can eventually lead to neuroglycopenia.

Pathobiology

Regulation of Carbohydrate Metabolism

Interactions between Insulin and Counter-Insulin Hormones

Under normal circumstances, serum glucose concentration averages 70 to 100 mg/dL before meals and rarely exceeds 140 to 150 mg/dL after meals. The brain is almost totally dependent on glucose for energy, although over the long term it can adapt to substrates other than glucose (e.g., ketone bodies). Because severe hypoglycemia can impair mental function and, if prolonged, can cause permanent brain damage, a series of well-developed, and at times redundant, homeostatic processes defends against hypoglycemia. Insulin suppresses glucose production by inhibiting both glycogenolysis and gluconeogenesis. Insulin also stimulates glucose uptake in muscle, liver, and fat. Glucagon, epinephrine, cortisol, and growth hormone, collectively referred to as the counter-regulatory or counter-insulin hormones, oppose the effects of insulin.

In healthy nondiabetic subjects, insulin concentration increases as glucose concentration increases and falls as glucose concentration falls. In contrast, counter-regulatory hormone concentrations change (in general) in the opposite direction of insulin, by falling as glucose rises and rising as glucose falls. By doing so, insulin and the counter-insulin hormones act in concert to ensure that the amount of glucose entering and leaving the blood stream is closely matched in both the fed and the fasted state. Excess amounts of insulin or insulin-like material (e.g., insulin-like growth factor [IGF]-1 or IGF-2), inadequate secretion of counter-insulin hormones, insufficient substrate, or defects in the gluconeogenic or glycogenolytic pathways alone or in combination can disrupt this balance and can cause hypoglycemia.

Regulation of Glucose Concentration in the Fed State

After an overnight fast (e.g., 8 to 10 hours), rates of glucose production and utilization average about 2 mg/kg/minute. At this time, the majority of the glucose is released from the liver, and a small amount is produced by the kidney. Carbohydrate ingestion increases glucose concentration, which stimulates secretion of insulin from the pancreatic β cells and suppresses secretion of glucagon from the pancreatic α cells. The resultant rise in the insulin-to-glucagon ratio increases hepatic glycogen synthesis and inhibits both glycogenolysis and gluconeogenesis, thereby increasing hepatic glycogen content. Glucose concentrations continue to rise until the rate of glucose uptake by peripheral tissues exceeds the net amount of glucose (meal-derived and endogenously produced) released from the splanchnic bed. Glucose concentration then begins to fall toward preprandial levels. This results in a progressive fall in insulin and a progressive rise in glucagon concentration, which, in turn permit a gradual increase in endogenous glucose production and a gradual fall in glucose utilization to basal rates. Depending on the amount and type of food ingested, both glucose concentration and turnover are generally back to basal levels between 4 and 6 hours after the start of a meal.

Thus, the rate of carbohydrate absorption, the timing as well as the amount of insulin and glucagon secreted, the ability of the liver to store and subsequently release glucose, and the response of the liver, muscle, and fat to insulin and counter-insulin hormones all interact to minimize the rise in glucose concentration after a meal as well as to ensure a smooth return of glucose concentrations to preprandial levels during the transition from the fed to the postabsorptive state.

Regulation of Glucose Concentrations in the Fasted State

The contribution of gluconeogenesis becomes progressively more important as the duration of fast is extended and hepatic glycogen stores are depleted. The rate of glycogen depletion depends on a variety of factors, including antecedent diet and exercise, but the process is nearly complete after 24 to 48 hours of fasting. Anything that lowers the demand for glucose lessens the need to break down protein stores. This is accomplished by changing from a primarily carbohydrate-based metabolism in the fed state to a primarily fat-based metabolism in the fasted state.

As hepatic glycogen is depleted, the glucose concentration falls and insulin decreases. Concentrations of glucagon, growth hormone, and cortisol all increase. This change in the hormonal milieu stimulates lipolysis and ketogenesis, which result in an increase in plasma glycerol, free fatty acid, and ketone body concentrations. Glycerol serves as a gluconeogenic substrate, thereby sparing amino acids. Free fatty acids are metabolized by muscle, liver, and other tissues in place of glucose. Free fatty acids also are converted by means of ketogenesis to acetoacetate and β-hydroxybutyrate, which can substitute for glucose as a fuel for the brain. These metabolic adaptations normally permit glucose to decrease gradually to 40 to 50 mg/dL during a fast without provoking symptoms of hypoglycemia. Inadequate glycogen stores or breakdown, insufficient gluconeogenesis resulting from defects in enzyme activity, lack of substrate availability, and persistent elevations of insulin or of insulin-like activity, alone or in combination, can cause or exacerbate hypoglycemia.

Recovery from Hypoglycemia

If counter-regulation is intact, hypoglycemia (regardless of the cause) will result in a decrease in insulin secretion and an increase in glucagon, epinephrine, cortisol, and growth hormone secretion. Glucagon provides the major defense against acute hypoglycemia. Epinephrine appears to become progressively more important when hypoglycemia is prolonged or severe. Permissive amounts of cortisol and growth hormone are required for a normal hepatic response to glucagon and epinephrine. Drugs or diseases that inhibit counter-regulatory secretion or action predispose patients to hypoglycemia.

Clinical Manifestations

Symptoms of hypoglycemia have been classified into two major groups: those arising from activation of the autonomic nervous system (autonomic) and those related to insufficient glucose supply to the brain (neuroglycopenic). During acute insulin-induced hypoglycemia in healthy persons, autonomic symptoms are recognized at a threshold of approximately 60 mg/dL (3 mM), and impairment of brain function manifested by neuroglycopenic symptoms occurs at a threshold of approximately 50 mg/dL (2.8 mM) in arterialized venous blood (Fig. 249–1). Comparable venous levels would be about 3 mg/dL (0.16 mM) less. The rate of glucose descent has little if any influence on the occurrence of symptoms and signs of hypoglycemia in nondiabetic persons.

Variations among reports regarding allocation of symptoms to the autonomic and neuroglycopenic types may be ascribed to the specific groups of patients examined. These include patients with diabetes versus those without it, patients with type 1 versus type 2 diabetes, clinical versus experimental conditions, and, most importantly, differences among persons regarding their perception of symptoms. During experimentally induced hypoglycemia in 20 persons with and 25 persons without diabetes, a principal component analysis allocated sweating, trembling, feeling of warmth, anxiety, and nausea to the autonomic group and dizziness, confusion, tiredness, difficulty with speaking, headache, and inability to concentrate to the neuroglycopenic group. Hunger, blurred vision, drowsiness, and weakness could not be allocated to either group with any confidence. [1] In another study of 10 nondiabetic persons, partitioning of symptoms during insulin-induced hypoglycemia allocated the categories of shaky/tremulous, heart pounding, nervous/anxious, sweaty, hungry, and tingling to the autonomic group and warm, weak, difficulty thinking/confused, and tired/drowsy to the neuroglycopenic group. [2]

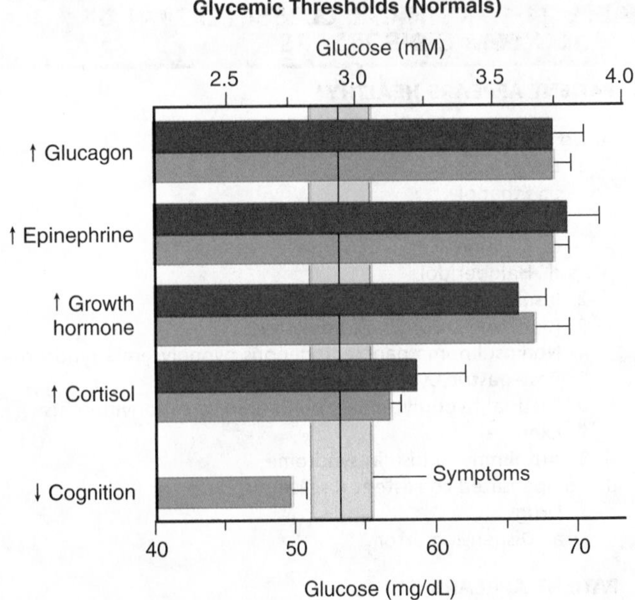

FIGURE 249–1 • Arterialized (blue) and venous (green) glycemic (mean ± standard error) thresholds for increments in plasma glucagon, epinephrine, growth hormone, and cortisol for symptoms of hypoglycemia and for impairment of cognitive function during decrements in serum glucose in normal humans from two independent studies. (From Cryer PE: Glucose counterregulation: The physiological mechanisms that prevent or correct hypoglycemia. *In* Frier B, Fisher BM [eds]: Hypoglycaemia and Diabetes: Clinical and Physiological Aspects. London, Edward Arnold, 1993, pp 34-55, with permission.)

In a retrospective analysis of 60 patients with insulinoma, 85% had various combinations of diplopia, blurred vision, sweating, palpitations, and weakness; 80% had confusion or abnormal behavior; 50% were amnesic for the episode or had coma; and 12% had generalized seizures. [3] None of the symptoms noted earlier, regardless of type, is specific for hypoglycemia. It is unlikely that autonomic symptoms alone, in the absence of at least one event of neuroglycopenia, are indicative of a hypoglycemic disorder.

Diagnosis

Classification

A useful approach for the clinician is a classification based on clinical characteristics (Table 249–1). Persons who appear healthy are likely to have hypoglycemic disorders that are different from those of persons who are ill. Hospitalized patients are at additional risk for hypoglycemia, often from iatrogenic factors.

Evaluation

The direction and extent of evaluation depend on the clinical presentation. The healthy-appearing patient with no coexistent disease who has a history of episodic symptoms suggestive of hypoglycemia requires an approach quite different from the hospitalized patient with acute hypoglycemia.

The Healthy-Appearing Patient

Serum Glucose

Because symptoms of hypoglycemia are not specific, it is essential to document a low serum glucose concentration at the time of the occurrence of spontaneous symptoms and relief of symptoms through correc-

TABLE 249–1 CLINICAL CLASSIFICATION OF HYPOGLYCEMIC DISORDERS

I. PATIENT APPEARS HEALTHY*

A. No coexistent disease
1. Drugs
a. Ethanol
b. Salicylates
c. Quinine
d. Haloperidol
2. Insulinoma
3. Islet hypertrophy/nesidioblastosis
4. Noninsulinoma pancreatogenous hypoglycemia syndrome
5. Post–gastric bypass hypoglycemia
6. Factitial hypoglycemia from insulin or sulfonylurea use
7. Exercise
8. Autoimmune insulin syndrome

B. Compensated coexistent disease
1. Drugs
a. Dispensing error

II. PATIENT APPEARS ILL

A. Drugs
1. Pentamidine and *Pneumocystis* pneumonia
2. Sulfamethoxazole/trimethoprim and renal failure
3. Propoxyphene and renal failure
4. Quinine and cerebral malaria
5. Quinine and malaria
6. Topical salicylates and renal failure
7. Unripe ackee fruit and undernutrition

B. Predisposing illness
1. Infant small for gestational age
2. Beckwith-Wiedemann syndrome
3. Erythroblastosis fetalis
4. Infant of diabetic mother
5. Glycogen storage disease
6. Defects in amino acid and fatty acid metabolism
7. Reye's syndrome
8. Cyanotic congenital heart disease
9. Hypopituitarism
10. Isolated growth hormone deficiency
11. Isolated adrenocorticotropic hormone deficiency
12. Addison's disease
13. Hereditary fructose intolerance
14. Carnitine deficiency
15. Defective type 1 glucose transporter in the brain
16. Acquired severe liver disease
17. Non–islet cell tumor hypoglycemia
18. Sepsis
19. Renal failure
20. Congestive heart failure
21. Lactic acidosis
22. Starvation
23. Anorexia nervosa
24. Postoperative removal of pheochromocytoma
25. Insulin receptor antibody hypoglycemia
26. Spinal muscular atrophy

C. Hospitalized patient
1. Diseases predisposing to hypoglycemia
2. Total parenteral nutrition and insulin therapy
3. Questran interference with glucocorticoid absorption
4. Shock

*Mutations in the β-cell sulfonylurea receptor gene, glutamate dehydrogenase gene, and glucokinase gene are rare causes of hyperinsulinemic hypoglycemia, usually manifested in infancy or childhood.

TABLE 249–2 PROTOCOL FOR 72-HOUR FAST

1. Date the onset of the fast as of the last ingestion of calories; discontinue all nonessential medications.
2. The patient may drink calorie-free and caffeine-free beverages.
3. The patient must be active during waking hours.
4. Measure plasma glucose, insulin, C-peptide, and β-hydroxybutyrate (on the same venipuncture specimen) every 6 hours until plasma glucose reaches ≤60 mg/dL (3.3 mM), when frequency should be every 1 to 2 hours.
5. End the fast when the plasma glucose is ≤45 mg/dL (2.5 mM) and the patient has symptoms or signs of hypoglycemia, or plasma glucose is ≤55 mg/dL if Whipple's triad had been demonstrated previously.
6. At the end of the fast, measure plasma glucose, insulin, C-peptide, β-hydroxybutyrate, and sulfonylurea (on the same venipuncture specimen); then inject glucagon, 1 mg intravenously, and measure plasma glucose every 10 minutes three times. After this, feed the patient.

tion of the low serum glucose concentration (Whipple's triad) before concluding that a patient has a hypoglycemic disorder. Furthermore, reliance solely on a low blood glucose value to diagnose a hypoglycemic disorder fails to take into consideration the possibility of laboratory error, artifactual hypoglycemia, and, indeed, the finding that physiologically normal persons may have serum glucose levels much lower than 50 mg/dL (2.8 mM) during prolonged fasting. A normal serum glucose concentration (when measured reliably) obtained during the occurrence of spontaneous symptoms absolutely eliminates the possibility of a hypoglycemic disorder; no further evaluation is required. Although hypoglycemic disorders are uncommon, symptoms suggestive of hypoglycemia are quite common.

Often, measurement of serum glucose is not feasible while spontaneous symptoms are occurring during ordinary life activities. Under such circumstances, judging whether to proceed with further evaluation depends on a detailed history. Elicitation of a history of neuroglycopenic symptoms or evidence of a confirmed low serum glucose concentration warrants further testing.

Seventy-two-Hour Fast

The prolonged supervised (72-hour) fast is an important diagnostic test. It should be conducted in a standardized fashion. A suggested protocol is shown in Table 249–2. For patients who experience signs or symptoms of hypoglycemia and who have simultaneously measured serum glucose in the hypoglycemic range, the fast should be terminated at that point. Studies in patients who have neither should not be extended beyond 72 hours.

The decision to end the fast may not be easy. Some patients have slightly depressed glycemic levels without symptoms or signs of hypoglycemia. Other patients may experience the symptoms they have had in ordinary life but have serum glucose levels higher than the hypoglycemic range. Young, lean, healthy women and, to a lesser degree, men may have serum glucose levels in the range of 40 mg/dL during prolonged fasting. Careful examination and testing for subtle signs of symptoms of neuroglycopenia should be conducted repeatedly when the patient's serum glucose level is near or in the hypoglycemic range. The 72-hour fast may be ended when the serum glucose concentration is 55 mg/dL or less if Whipple's triad had previously been demonstrated. β-cell polypeptides are suppressed in healthy persons when serum glucose is 55 mg/dL or less. Although most patients with insulinoma become hypoglycemic before 72 hours (33% in 12 hours, 65% in 24 hours, 84% in 36 hours, 93% in 48 hours, and 99% in 72 hours in a group of 170 patients with insulinoma), continuation of the fast to 72 hours is necessary to rule out the likelihood of organic hypoglycemia. Although the 72-hour fast has usually been considered to be an inpatient procedure, it may be initiated in an endocrine testing center after an overnight fast. Forty percent of patients have had positive results of the fast in the outpatient setting. Those patients whose fast result is not positive by the end of the outpatient evaluation period are admitted to the hospital to complete the 72-hour fast.

The interpretation of concentrations of β-cell polypeptides (insulin, C-peptide, and proinsulin) during the 72-hour fast is predicated on the concomitant serum glucose concentration. The normal overnight fasting ranges for these polypeptides do not apply when the serum glucose level is low (e.g., ≤55 mg/dL).

Insulin-mediated hypoglycemic disorders are characterized by plasma insulin concentrations greater than or equal to 3 μU/mL (immunochemiluminometric assay) (Fig. 249–2). Persons with insulinomas have insulin concentrations that rarely exceed 100 μU/mL. Values of 1000 μU/mL or greater suggest recent insulin administration or the presence of insulin antibodies. Ratios of glucose to insulin, and vice versa, including the "amended ratio," have been used in an effort to identify relative hyperinsulinemia when the insulin concentration is in the normal overnight fasting range. Unfortunately, these ratios have very poor diagnostic utility (see Fig. 249–2).

Criteria for hyperinsulinemia using C-peptide and proinsulin (each measured by immunochemiluminometric assays) are 200 pmol/L or more and 5 pmol/L or more, respectively (see Fig. 249–2). The molar ratio of insulin to C-peptide is the same for patients with insulinomas as it is for healthy individuals (~0.2). Although the molar ratio of proinsulin to insulin is increased in patients with insulinoma, it appears to have no diagnostic utility.

Because of the antiketogenic effect of insulin, plasma β-hydroxybutyrate measurement at the end of the fast (72 hours in healthy individuals and at Whipple's triad in patients with a hypoglycemic disorder) is useful. This parameter is considered to be an insulin surrogate. Patients with insulin-mediated hypoglycemia have concentrations of less than 2.7 mmol/L, whereas others (healthy individuals or those with non–insulin-mediated hypoglycemia) have higher levels (see Fig. 249–2). The progressive rise of β-hydroxybutyrate concentration early in the 72-hour fast in persons destined to have a negative test, in contrast to the sustained suppressed level in patients with insulinoma (Fig. 249–3), provides the opportunity to end the fast before the 72-hour point either by attaining a level of 2.7 mmol/L or higher or by having two successive concentrations measured at 6-hour intervals that exceed the concentration at the 18-hour time point. Another insulin surrogate is the response of serum glucose to 1 mg of glucagon injected intravenously at the end of the fast. The rationale for this procedure is that insulin is glycogenic and antiglycogenolytic. Patients with insulin-mediated hypoglycemia have a maximum increment of at least 25 mg/dL greater than the terminal fasting serum glucose, whereas others (healthy individuals or those with non–insulin-mediated hypoglycemia) have lower increments (see Fig. 249–2). When the serum glucose concentration exceeds 60 mg/dL at the end of the fast, measurement of the β-cell polypeptides and insulin surrogates is uninformative and unnecessary.

Measurement of sulfonylureas in the plasma at the end of the fast is an essential component of the prolonged supervised fast. The pattern of serum glucose and β-cell polypeptides in sulfonylurea-induced hypoglycemia is identical to that observed in persons with insulinoma. A liquid chromatographic tandem mass spectrography method provides a sensitive measurement of first and second-generation sulfonylureas and meglitinides. See Table 249–3 for diagnostic interpretation.

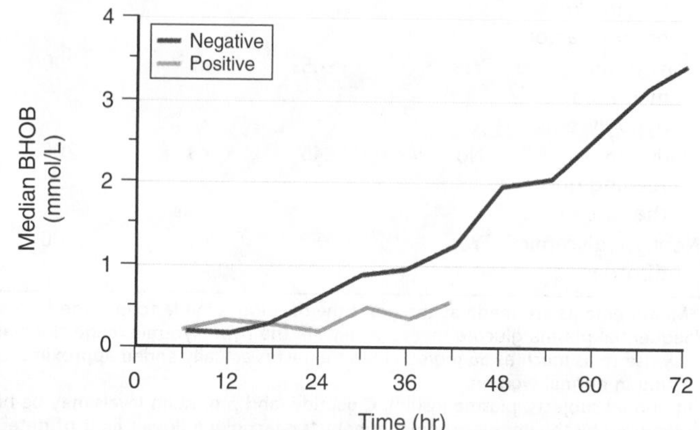

FIGURE 249–3 • Median concentrations of β-hydroxybutyrate (BHOB) during 72-hour fasts are shown for patients with insulinoma, all of whom had positive fasts, and for persons with negative fasts. (From Service F: Increasing serum B-hydroxybutyrate. J Clin Endocrinol Metab 2005;90:4555–4558. Copyright 2005, The Endocrine Society.)

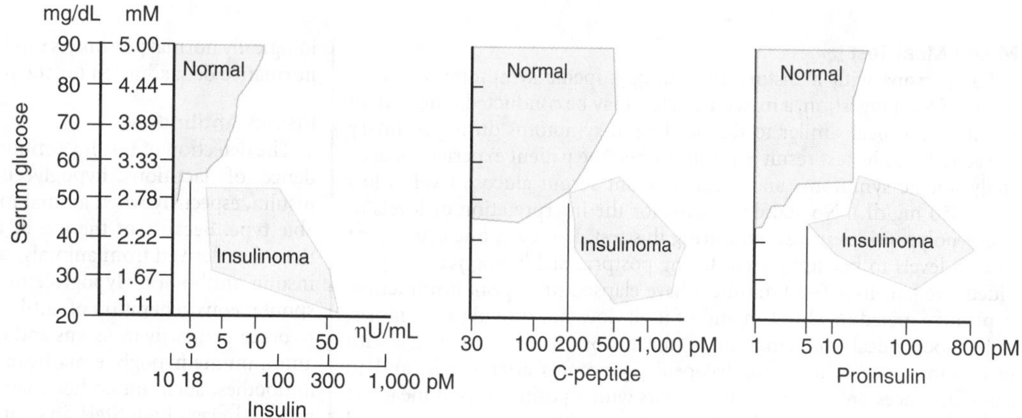

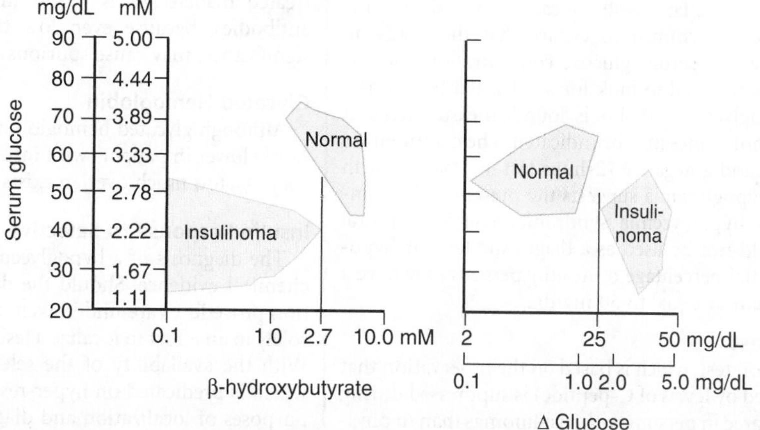

FIGURE 249–2 • Distributions of plasma insulin, C-peptide proinsulin, β-hydroxybutyrate, and serum glucose (Δ glucose) response to intravenous glucagon versus serum glucose at the end of the prolonged fast (72 hours in normal persons [n = 25] or at Whipple's triad for patients with histologically confirmed insulinoma [n = 40]) are shown. The shaded area represents serum glucose level less than or equal to 50 mg/dL (2.8 mM). The vertical line represents the diagnostic level for insulinoma. Criteria for insulinoma are insulin level greater than or equal to 3 μU/mL (18 pM), C-peptide level greater than or equal to 200 pM, proinsulin level greater than or equal to 5 pM, β-hydroxybutyrate level less than or equal to 2.7 mM, and Δ glucose level greater than or equal to 25 mg/dL (1.4 mM).

TABLE 249–3 DIAGNOSTIC INTERPRETATION OF THE RESULTS OF A 72-HOUR FAST*

	Signs and Symptoms	Glucose[†] (mg/dL)	Insulin[‡‡] (μU/mL)	C-Peptide[‡§] (pmol/L)	Proinsulin[‡‖] (pmol/L)	β-Hydroxybutyrate (mmol/L)	Glucose[¶] (mg/dL)	Sulfonylurea in Plasma
Normal	No	≥40	<3	<200	<5	>2.7	<25	No
Insulinoma	Yes	≤45	≥3[r]	≥200	≥5	≤2.7	≥25	No
Factitious hypoglycemia from insulin	Yes	≤45	≥3**	<200	<5	≤2.7	≥25	No
Sulfonylurea-induced hypoglycemia	Yes	≤45	≥3	≥200	≥5	≤2.7	≥25	Yes[††]
Hypoglycemia mediated by insulin-like growth factor	Yes	≤45	≤3	<200	<5	≤2.7	≥25	No
Non–insulin-mediated hypoglycemia	Yes	≤45	<3	<200	<5	>2.7	<25	No
Inadvertent feeding during the fast	No	≤45	<3	<200	<5	≤2.7	≥25	No
Nonhypoglycemic disorder	Yes	≥40	<3	<200	<5	>2.7	<25	No

*Measurements are made at the point the decision is made to end the fast.
[†]Sequential plasma glucose measurements in the hypoglycemic range fluctuate. Plasma glucose levels ≤45 mg/dL at the time a decision is made to end the fast may rise to as much as 56 mg/dL when the fast is actually ended approximately 1 hour later. Plasma glucose levels may be as low as 40 mg/dL during prolonged fasting in normal women.
[‡]In normal subjects, plasma insulin, C-peptide, and proinsulin levels may be higher if the plasma glucose level is >60 mg/dL.
[§]Measured by the immunochemiluminometric technique (lower limit of detection, 33 pmol/L).
[‖]Measured by the immunochemiluminometric technique (lower limit of detection, 0.2 pmol/L).
[¶]In response to intravenous glucagon (peak value minus value at end of fast).
[r]Ratios of insulin to glucose are of no diagnostic value in patients with insulinomas.
**Plasma insulin levels may be very high (>100 μU/mL or even = 1000 μU/mL) in factitious hypoglycemia produced by insulin.
[††]Unlike the first generation of sulfonylurea drugs, which were easily measured, second-generation drugs are difficult to measure.
[‡‡]Measured by immunochemiluminometric assay, lower limit of detection is 0.1 μU/mL.
Reprinted with permission from Service FJ: Hypoglycemia disorder. N Engl J Med 1995;332:1144–1152.

Mixed Meal Test

For persons with a history of neuroglycopenic symptoms within 5 hours of food ingestion, a mixed meal test may be conducted. The patient should eat a meal similar to that leading to symptoms during ordinary life activities. The test result is positive when the patient experiences neuroglycopenic symptoms and a concomitant serum glucose level is low (e.g., ≤50 mg/dL). No standards exist for the interpretation of levels of β-cell polypeptides measured during this test. However, one can expect insulin levels to be suppressed during postprandial hypoglycemia, provided five half-lives (~30 minutes) have elapsed from peak insulinemia. A positive mixed meal test in and of itself does not provide a diagnosis, only biochemical confirmation of the history. Because patients with insulinoma may have neuroglycopenic symptoms after meals, and in some instances only after meals, patients with a positive mixed meal test may require a 72-hour fast. For those patients with a positive mixed meal test result and a negative 72-hour fast result, glucagon levels during the mixed meal test should be determined to ensure that there was an increase in response to the low serum glucose concentration. Gastric emptying studies may be performed to look for accelerated transit as a cause of postprandial hypoglycemia. If this is found, measurement of prokinetic gastrointestinal hormones may be indicated. The combination of positive mixed meal test and a negative 72-hour fast in a patient with a history of postprandial hypoglycemia suggests the presence of noninsulinoma pancreatogenous hypoglycemia syndrome. The 5-hour oral glucose tolerance test should not be used as a diagnostic test for hypoglycemia because a substantial percentage of healthy persons may have a serum glucose nadir less than or equal to 50 mg/dL.

C-Peptide Suppression Test

The C-peptide suppression test, which is based on the observation that β-cell secretion (as measured by levels of C-peptide) is suppressed during hypoglycemia to a lesser degree in persons with insulinomas than in physiologically normal persons, is rarely used anymore. Interpretation requires normative data adjusted for the patient's body mass index and age.

Insulin Antibodies

The detection of insulin antibodies was once considered to be firm evidence of factitious hypoglycemia resulting from self-administered insulin, especially when animal insulin was the only commercially available type. Because of the use of human insulin, which is less antigenic than that derived from animals, such patients usually have no detectable insulin antibodies. Hypoglycemia that can be directly attributed to the spontaneous generation of antibodies to native insulin has been reported to occur primarily in Asians and rarely in whites. In patients with insulin autoimmune hypoglycemia from the spontaneous generation of insulin antibodies, such antibodies may be monoclonal or polyclonal and are present in very high titers, in contrast to the much lower titers in insulin-treated diabetes. It is important to test for the presence of insulin antibodies, because even low titers, which may have no diagnostic significance, may cause spurious results of the assay for insulin.

Glycated Hemoglobin

Although glycated hemoglobin concentrations are statistically significantly lower in patients with insulinomas than in physiologically normal subjects, too much overlap exists to provide a diagnostic criterion.

Insulin Response to Selective Arterial Calcium Injection

The diagnosis of a hypoglycemic disorder is made entirely from biochemical evidence. Should the data point to insulinoma, then localization procedures are undertaken. Standard radiologic tests are conducted solely in an effort to localize a lesion, rather than for diagnostic purposes. With the availability of the selective arterial calcium stimulation test, which is predicated on hyper-responsive β cells for a positive result, the purposes of localization and diagnosis of β-cell hyperfunction are both served. This test requires access to various intra-abdominal vessels including the right hepatic vein, splenic artery, gastroduodenal artery, and superior mesenteric artery. A two- to threefold increase in insulin concentration in the right hepatic vein in response to calcium injection into one or more of the arteries suggests that the region of the pancreas served by that artery harbors abnormally functioning β cells, whether from insulinoma or islet hypertrophy or nesidioblastosis.

The Ill-Appearing Patient

Hypoglycemia in persons with coexistent disease sometimes occurs as a discrete episode, which may be asymptomatic if the patient has preexisting blunting of consciousness. Recognition of the underlying disease and its propensity for hypoglycemia and action taken to minimize recurrence may be sufficient. Confirmation of the suspected mechanism for the hypoglycemia may be pursued, such as low insulin and C-peptide levels in cases of non–insulin-mediated hypoglycemia as in ethanol hypoglycemia, elevated IGF-II in cases of non–β-cell tumor–related hypoglycemia, low levels of cortisol in cases of adrenal insufficiency, and blunted serum glucose responses to intravenous glucagon in cases of hypoglycemia resulting from abnormal liver function, glycogen storage disease, sepsis, or congestive heart failure.

With the progressively restrictive limitations for admissions to hospital, those patients who are in hospitals generally are severely ill and have multisystem disease. These patients are at risk for iatrogenic hypoglycemia in addition to the potential risk generated from the underlying disease. In one tertiary medical center, 1.2% of all patients admitted over a 6-month period experienced hypoglycemia (serum glucose ≤49 mg/dL). The primary causes among persons without diabetes were renal insufficiency, malnutrition, liver disease, infection, and shock. Several patients had more than one risk factor. Not infrequently, nondiabetic patients become hyperglycemic because of treatment with enteral or parenteral nutrition or glucocorticoids. Use of insulin to control hyperglycemia puts patients at risk of hypoglycemia, especially if feedings are interrupted, the dose of glucocorticoid is abruptly reduced or stopped, or glucocorticoid availability is diminished through simultaneous administration of a bile acid sequestrant. In ferreting out the cause of hypoglycemia in the seriously ill hospitalized patient, diligent examination of the record is profitable.

Treatment

Rx

The treatment of hypoglycemic disorders encompasses two distinct components: (1) relief of neuroglycopenic systems by restoration of the low serum glucose level to the normal range and (2) correction of the underlying cause of the hypoglycemia. Unlike diabetes, in which restoration of euglycemia is the ideal goal, overtreatment of hypoglycemia in a nondiabetic person has no sequelae. For the patient with an as-yet undiagnosed disorder, blood by venipuncture should be obtained for measurement of glucose, β-cell polypeptides, and β-hydroxybutyrate before treatment. Both diagnosis and treatment can be achieved by intravenous injection of glucagon with monitoring of the serum glucose response. Depending on the response, the patient may require intravenous glucose administration as a bolus of 50% or a continuous infusion of 5 or 10% or may recover sufficiently to take oral nutrition.

Treatment of the underlying cause of the hypoglycemia depends on the specific cause. Once a biochemical diagnosis of insulinoma has been made, preoperative localization should be attempted. Because of the rarity of insulinoma, only a few referral centers have generated sufficient experience to assess the effectiveness of various localization procedures: computed tomography, magnetic resonance imaging, endoscopic and transabdominal ultrasonography, octreotide scan, celiac axis angiography, and selective arterial calcium stimulation and transhepatic portal venous sampling. Experts differ in their preferred approaches because of differences in experience and skill level. Ultrasonography has the advantage of precise localization, especially in relation to the pancreatic duct. Magnetic resonance imaging and octreotide scanning are not useful. Transhepatic portal venous sampling has been abandoned in centers that once used this technique. There is general agreement that intraoperative ultrasonography combined with careful palpation of the pancreas by an experienced surgeon provides the highest success rate in localization.

Specific Causes

Insulinoma is a rare tumor. The incidence is estimated to be 4 cases per 1 million person-years, similar to that of pheochromocytoma. Insulinoma occurs at any age, is slightly more common in women (59%), and is associated with low rates of malignancy (6%), multiplicity (9%), multiple endocrine neoplasia syndrome (8%), and recurrence (8%). After successful removal of an insulinoma, the patient can look forward to a normal life expectancy. Medical therapy for the patient whose insulinoma is missed at pancreatic exploration, for the patient unsuitable for surgery, or for the patient with metastatic insulinoma may include diazoxide, verapamil, phenytoin, propranolol, or octreotide. Insulinoma is occasionally suspected in patients with labile diabetes, especially when insulin therapy has apparently been suspended. One case of documented insulinoma in a person with type 1 diabetes and a few cases in persons with type 2 diabetes have been reported. Optimal treatment is surgical resection.

Adults with episodes of hyperinsulinemic hypoglycemia resulting in neuroglycopenia may harbor islet hypertrophy/nesidioblastosis but no insulinoma (noninsulinoma pancreatogenous hypoglycemia syndrome). The clinical features are uniquely different from those of insulinoma: predominance of male patients, postprandial neuroglycopenia, negative 72-hour fast result, negative radiologic localization studies, positive selective arterial calcium stimulation test, and relief of symptoms with gradient guided partial pancreatectomy. A subgroup of these patients has been identified who have the unique characteristic of a history of Roux-en-Y gastric bypass surgery.

Insulin factitial hypoglycemia usually is manifested by neuroglycopenic symptoms that occur erratically. This disorder is observed more often in women, usually those in a health-related occupation. Once confronted with the diagnosis, about half of the patients admit to self-abuse, and most cease this activity. Insulin autoimmune hypoglycemia may be very difficult to distinguish from insulin factitial hypoglycemia because of similar biochemical features. However, some patients with the former have evidence of another autoimmune disease, and the insulin antibody titers are very high.

Mutations in the β-cell sulfonylurea receptor gene, glutamate dehydrogenase gene, and glucokinase gene have been reported to cause hyperinsulinemic hypoglycemia (i.e., inappropriately elevated insulin and C-peptide concentrations). Patients usually present at an early age, and often a familial pattern is detected. Physical exercise–induced hypoglycemia also has been described in some families. Insulin-like material can be secreted by some malignant tumors (e.g., hemangiopericytomas, fibromas, fibrosarcomas, hepatomas). In such instances, plasma insulin and C-peptide concentrations are low at the time of hypoglycemia, whereas pro–IGF-II concentrations are elevated.

ISLET CELL TUMORS

Definition

Tumors of the endocrine pancreas generally are malignant. Insulin-producing tumors are the exception because they are usually benign. Islet cell tumors are commonly referred to as either functioning or nonfunctioning. Functioning tumors release one or more hormones in amounts sufficient to raise plasma concentrations. Nonfunctioning tumors may contain one or more hormones but, by definition, do not release substantial amounts into the systemic circulation.

Functioning tumors generally manifest with symptoms relating to the hormones secreted, whereas nonfunctioning tumors generally manifest as a pancreatic mass or as a metastasis. Nonfunctioning tumors tend to be larger and more advanced at the time of diagnosis because their presence is not heralded by symptoms generated by hormone excess.

Pathobiology

Functioning islet cell tumors are commonly associated with one of five widely recognized syndromes (Table 249–4). The insulinoma, Zollinger-Ellison, glucagonoma, VIPoma, and somatostatinoma syndromes are believed to result (at least in part) from excess secretion of insulin, gastrin, glucagon, vasoactive intestinal polypeptide (VIP), and somatostatin, respectively. However, additional symptoms also can occur because these tumors frequently secrete more than one hormone (e.g., pancreatic polypeptide, adrenocorticotropin, calcitonin, neurotensin, human chori-

TABLE 249–4 CHARACTERISTICS OF FUNCTIONING ISLET CELL CARCINOMAS

Syndrome	Clinical Presentation	Biochemical Diagnosis	Rate of Malignancy (%)	Metastases at Diagnosis (%)	Localization (Radiographic)	Ectopic Sites (Nonpancreatic)
Insulinoma	Neuroglycopenia Adrenergic response	Blood glucose ≤45 mg/dL Insulin >3 μU/mL Absence of insulin antibodies elevated C-peptide	<10	<10	Ultrasonography, spiral CT, selective calcium stimulation test	Rare
Zollinger-Ellison syndrome	Dyspepsia/ulcer Diarrhea	Elevated basal gastrin Elevated basal acid output Positive secretin test	50–60	50–80	Ultrasonography, CT, angiography, PVS	Duodenum, rarely other
WDHA (VIPoma)	Profuse, secretory diarrhea Hypokalemia Hypochlorhydria/achlorhydria, hypercalcemia, hyperglycemia	Elevated VIP	50	50	CT, occasionally, PVS angiography	Retroperitoneum, lung
Glucagonoma	Dermatitis Diabetes Weight loss Anemia	Elevated glucagon	75	60–70	CT	Rare
Somatostatinoma	Diabetes Cholelithiasis Diarrhea Steatorrhea	Elevated somatostatin	90–100	50–75	CT	Duodenum

CT = computed tomography; PVS = portal venous sampling; VIP = vasoactive intestinal peptide; WDHA = watery diarrhea, hypokalemia, achlorhydria.
Adapted from Grant CS: Surgical management of malignant islet cell tumors. World J Surg 1993;17:498–503.

onic gonadotropin, growth hormone–releasing factor, prostaglandins, and parathyroid hormone), and the amount and type of the hormone secreted can change over time. Islet cell tumors are either sporadic or can occur in association with other known genetic syndromes, such as multiple endocrine neoplasia type 1. Sporadic tumors occur at any age but most commonly are detected between 40 and 60 years of age. The diagnosis can be confirmed by obtaining tissue during surgical resection or by needle biopsy.

Treatment

Rx

With the exception perhaps of insulinomas, the optimal treatment of islet cell tumors is currently not known because their rarity has made the conduct of randomized therapeutic trials extremely difficult. Furthermore, in the absence of metastases, no reliable histologic criteria distinguish benign from malignant lesions. Islet cell tumors most commonly metastasize to the liver and adjacent lymph nodes. Metastases to lung, bone, adrenal gland, kidney, and ovary may also occur. Fortunately, the rate of growth of malignant islet cell tumors is generally slow. Therefore, many clinicians recommend surgery if the pancreatic tumor is resectable and if the extent of metastatic disease (if present) is limited. "Debulking" of metastases, whether by surgery or by hepatic embolization, may improve symptoms by lowering circulating hormone concentrations. Treatment with chemotherapeutic agents such streptozotocin (alone or in combination with 5-fluorouracil), doxorubicin, dacarbazine, or interferon-β also may improve symptoms and, in some instances, perhaps improve survival. Somatostatin is a potent inhibitor of hormone secretion. Treatment with long-acting analogues of somatostatin can result in a dramatic, albeit at times temporary, decrease in symptoms, particularly those associated with glucagonomas and VIPomas.

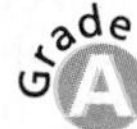

1. Hepburn DA, Deary IJ, Frier BM, et al: Symptoms of acute insulin-induced hypoglycemia in humans with and without IDDM: Factor-analysis approach. Diabetes Care 1991;14:949–957.
2. Towler DA, Havlin CE, Craft S, et al: Mechanism of awareness of hypoglycemia: Perception of neurogenic (predominantly cholinergic) rather than neuroglycopenic symptoms. Diabetes 1993;42:1791–1798.
3. Service FJ, Dale AJ, Elveback LR, et al: Insulinoma: Clinical and diagnostic features of 60 consecutive cases. Mayo Clin Proc 1976;51:417–429.

SUGGESTED READINGS

Guettier JM, Gorden P: Hypoglycemia. Endocrinol Metab Clin North Am 2006;35:753–766. *Comprehensive review.*

House MG, Schulick RD: Endocrine tumors of the pancreas. Current Opin Oncol 2006;18:23–29. *Comprehensive review.*

Otonkoski T, Kaminen N, Ustinov J, et al: Physical exercise-induced hyperinsulinemic hypoglycemia is an autosomal-dominant trait characterized by abnormal pyruvate-induced insulin release. Diabetes 2003;52:199–204. *A newly described syndrome.*

Service FJ, O'Brien PC: Increasing serum beta-hydroxybutyrate concentrations during the 72 hour fast: evidence against hyperinsulinemic hypoglycemia. J Clin Endocrinol Metab 2005;4555–4558. *Means to truncate a negative 72-hour fast.*

Service GJ, Thompson GB, Service FJ, et al: Hyperinsulinemic hypoglycemia with nesidioblastosis after gastric-bypass surgery. N Engl J Med 2005;353:249–254. *Newly discovered sequela of gastric bypass surgery.*

Vella A, Service FJ, O'Brien PC: Glucose counterregulatory hormones in the 72-hour fast. Endocr Pract 2003;9:115–118. *Approach to the diagnosis of glucagon deficiency.*

250 POLYGLANDULAR DISORDERS

Henry M. Kronenberg

Internists need to recognize diseases that involve independent abnormalities of more than one endocrine gland for several reasons. First, the known patterns of multiglandular disease can alert the clinician to look for a second disorder when one is diagnosed. Second, the treatment of many of the individual diseases in polyglandular disorders may differ from the treatment appropriate for the same diseases when they manifest in isolation. Third, because many of these diseases appear in characteristic familial patterns, the recognition of the syndromes can lead to useful family screening. Fourth, an understanding of the pathogenesis of these unusual disorders is likely to clarify the pathogenesis of more common single-gland disorders as well. This chapter discusses the best-characterized polyglandular disorders with these four considerations as the primary focus. Other chapters should be consulted for more detailed discussion of the diseases of individual glands.

NEOPLASTIC SYNDROMES

Three mechanistically distinct neoplastic syndromes involve more than one endocrine gland. Although given a variety of different names in the past, they are now most frequently called *multiple endocrine neoplasia type 1, multiple endocrine neoplasia types 2a and 2b,* and *McCune-Albright syndrome.*

Multiple Endocrine Neoplasia Type 1

Definition

Multiple endocrine neoplasia type 1 (MEN 1) is an autosomal dominant disorder characteristically involving the parathyroid glands, the pancreatic islets, and the anterior pituitary. Less commonly, adrenal cortical neoplasia and foregut carcinoids (primarily of thymus and lung) occur. Nonendocrine manifestations include lipomas, facial angiofibromas, and collagenomas.

Pathogenesis

The gene for MEN 1 is located at chromosome 11, band 11q13, and it encodes a 610–amino acid protein called menin. Menin is a widely expressed nuclear protein that forms complexes with proteins that methylate histones in chromatin and also binds many transcription factors. Menin increases gene transcription by poorly understood mechanisms. Although the normal physiologic role of menin is unknown, the abnormalities in MEN 1 suggest that the menin gene is a tumor suppressor gene. The inherited mutations in the menin gene vary widely, are located throughout the gene, and often generate truncated, presumably nonfunctional, menin peptides. In addition to this genetic abnormality that is present in all cells in the body, MEN 1 tumors usually harbor deletions of the normal allele of the menin gene. Presumably, loss of both copies of the tumor suppressor gene, one by inherited mutation and one by mutation of one particular cell, confers a selective advantage to the cell that proliferates to become a clonal tumor. Such clonal deletions have been found in 100% of parathyroid tumors removed at surgery from patients with MEN 1. Other acquired genetic abnormalities accumulate in these tumors; thus, the tumors in MEN 1 follow the pattern of multistep tumorigenesis found in malignant tumors. The two-hit tumor suppressor model has been confirmed by the generation of mice missing one or both copies of the menin gene in specific target cell types.

The two-hit tumor suppressor model can explain many of the clinical features of MEN 1. Clinical presentation of an inherited disorder in adulthood can be explained by the requirement for second mutations before clonal expansion. The asymmetrical but relentless nature of the parathyroid disease may be explained by asynchronous but inevitable somatic mutations in each of the parathyroid glands. Multiple islet tumors may result from the same process. What remains completely unexplained is the particular vulnerability of parathyroid, pancreatic islet, and pituitary cells, given the widespread expression of the menin gene.

The menin gene is mutated in about 20% of sporadic parathyroid adenomas, a fraction of sporadic malignant endocrine tumors of the pancreas, and some sporadic carcinoid tumors of the lung as well. Because these mutations occur only in the tumor and not in the patients' normal cells, no familial clustering occurs.

Diagnosis

Screening

Genetic screening for menin gene mutations is now available in reference laboratories. Because inactivating mutations can occur anywhere within the gene, standard surveys of the borders of exons and introns detect only 70% of the genetic abnormalities in families affected by MEN 1. Thus, the specific mutation in an index case should be ascertained before family members are screened. Because no safe and effective therapies are available for asymptomatic MEN 1 tumors, the precise role for genetic screening has not been established.

Detection

To detect active disease, the most useful single test to complement a thorough history and physical examination is measurement of blood calcium, particularly ionized calcium, at intervals after the age of 15 years. Prolactin, gastrin, and fasting blood glucose measurements can also be useful.

PARATHYROID DISEASE. Hyperparathyroidism, the most common abnormality in MEN 1, is found in more than 90% of patients. Elevation of blood calcium levels generally first appears between the ages of 20 and 40 years, considerably earlier than in sporadic primary hyperparathyroidism; however, the disease does not usually present during childhood. At first, the disease is asymptomatic but then can lead to all the expected consequences of primary hyperparathyroidism. Unlike sporadic hyperparathyroidism, the disease is relentlessly progressive and, with prolonged follow-up, always involves all four parathyroid glands. The involvement is characteristically asymmetrical and asynchronous. This pattern can lead to inappropriately limited parathyroid surgery. If fewer than three parathyroid glands are removed, hypercalcemia always recurs, although not necessarily immediately. Surgical results in patients with MEN 1 are generally less satisfactory than in patients with sporadic four-gland parathyroid disease. At some centers, all four glands are removed, and a portion of one gland is reimplanted in the easily accessible forearm in an attempt to avoid the hazards of too much or too little surgery. The difficulty in attaining long-term normocalcemia has led many clinicians to postpone surgery when the disease is asymptomatic. This strategy may need to be modified if the patient develops Zollinger-Ellison syndrome (see later), because hypercalcemia can dramatically increase the gastrin levels in such patients.

PANCREATIC ISLET DISEASE. As many as 80% of patients have pancreatic abnormalities at autopsy; many correspondingly have increased blood levels of gastrin, insulin, pancreatic polypeptide, somatostatin, vasoactive intestinal polypeptide, or glucagon during stimulation or suppression tests. The pancreas is often diffusely involved with microadenomas and macroadenomas and apparently hyperplastic lesions. Characteristically, more than one islet hormone is secreted from these multiple tumors. Despite this underlying pattern of multiple cellular involvement, patients characteristically present with symptoms of only one hormonal disorder. The most common disease is Zollinger-Ellison syndrome, a peptic ulcer disease associated with gastrin-producing tumors. Identification of disease-causing tumors has proved difficult. The gastrinomas in MEN 1 are often multiple, very small, and found in the duodenal wall. Macroadenomas observed in the pancreas by computed tomography or intraoperative ultrasonography in patients with MEN 1 who have Zollinger-Ellison syndrome may well synthesize hormones other than gastrin.

Although some centers continue to experiment with aggressive attempts at surgical cure, the high recurrence rate after surgery has limited the role for surgery in this disease. Medical therapy with histamine (H_2)–receptor antagonists and hydrogen, potassium–adenosine triphosphatase inhibitors can usually adequately control the secretion of stomach acid. The tumors are slow growing but frequently metastasize locally and to the liver. Chemotherapy is only partially effective and does not cure the disease.

Insulinomas are the second most common clinically important islet tumor in patients with MEN 1. These tumors are often small and multiple and are much less frequently malignant than the gastrinomas. Despite the frequently diffuse nature of the disease, dominant insulin-producing tumors can often be identified by selective portal venous sampling. Removal of the dominant tissue or, if necessary, subtotal (80%) pancreatectomy is the primary therapeutic strategy.

PITUITARY DISEASE. As in sporadic disease, pituitary disease can manifest with a hypersecretion syndrome or with symptoms resulting from a sellar mass or from hypopituitarism. Pituitary tumors occur in about one third of patients with MEN 1. Prolactinomas are the most common tumors. Adrenocortical hyperfunction can result from a pituitary adenoma or from production of adrenocorticotropic hormone or corticotropin-releasing hormone by a foregut carcinoid. Although nonfunctioning adrenal neoplasms are common in patients with MEN 1, primary adrenal neoplasms causing glucocorticoid excess are rare. Acromegaly can result from a pituitary neoplasm or as a consequence of production of growth hormone–releasing hormone by pancreatic islet tumors. After consideration of ectopic hormone and releasing hormone production by nonpituitary tumors, the course and treatment of pituitary disease in MEN 1 resemble those of sporadic pituitary disease.

Prognosis

The most life-limiting disorders in MEN 1 are the malignant tumors of the pancreatic islets. Whereas sporadic gastrinomas causing the Zollinger-Ellison syndrome can sometimes be cured surgically, the gastrinomas in MEN 1 have not been cured by any surgical approach reported thus far. Although vigorous acid control is possible and has dramatically increased life expectancy, these tumors metastasize to the liver and have been poorly responsive to chemotherapy. Other functioning and nonfunctioning pancreatic islet tumors can metastasize and cause death as well. Thus, periodic computed tomography scans of the abdomen to detect, monitor, and remove growing islet tumors is common practice. The parathyroid tumors are almost always benign but recur with a relentlessness much greater than in sporadic multiple gland parathyroid disease. Thus, even after resection of three and one half glands, recurrence of hyperparathyroidism is common. The course of pituitary tumors, in contrast, resembles the course of sporadic pituitary tumors of analogous hormonal type.

Multiple Endocrine Neoplasia Types 2a and 2b

Definition

Multiple endocrine neoplasia type 2a is an autosomal dominant disease that manifests with medullary carcinoma of the thyroid (MCT), pheochromocytoma, and, less commonly, hyperparathyroidism. MEN 2b is closely related to MEN 2a because it also manifests with MCT and pheochromocytoma and because both diseases involve mutations in the *RET* proto-oncogene (see later). Patients with MEN 2b present with certain abnormalities not found in patients with MEN 2a, however. These include mucosal neuromas of the tongue, lips, eyelids, and gastrointestinal tract and a marfanoid habitus. Hyperparathyroidism rarely occurs in patients with MEN 2b. MEN 2b is less common than MEN 2a.

Pathogenesis

In MEN 2a and 2b, the MCTs and the pheochromocytomas often appear bilaterally. Careful prospective analysis of families with MEN 2a has demonstrated that diffuse C-cell hyperplasia precedes a clinically obvious appearance of MCT. C-cell hyperplasia can be detected during the first decade of life by measurement of calcitonin after administration of gastrin, although this test has been supplanted clinically by genetic screening (see later). Virtually all patients with MEN 2a eventually develop C-cell disease. Complete thyroidectomy of patients with C-cell hyperplasia has dramatically decreased the incidence of MCT, which has been the major cause of death in patients with MEN 2a.

Almost all patients with MEN 2a have been found to harbor point mutations in the *RET* proto-oncogene, found in the pericentromeric region of chromosome 10. *RET* encodes a member of the tyrosine protein kinase family of cell surface receptors. The gene is expressed in spinal cord, in certain cultured blood cell lines, and in all tested medullary thyroid cancer and pheochromocytoma cell lines (both from patients with MEN 2 and from those with sporadic tumors). *RET* interacts with other transmembrane receptors, which, in turn, bind ligands of the glial cell line–derived neurotrophic factor (GCNF) family. This complicated system of ligands and receptors controls the migration, proliferation, and survival of neural crest cells that populate the thyroid gland, the adrenal gland, and the intrinsic nervous system of the gut. Mutations in *RET* have been found in five different cysteines located in the portion of the receptor that forms the extracellular, ligand-binding domain. The mutant *RET* gene signals in a ligand-independent manner, thereby acting as an oncogene. The mutant *RET* genes can transform cultured cells and cause MCT in transgenic mice.

The transition from diffuse hyperplasia of C cells or adrenal medullary cells to clonal neoplasms of the thyroid or adrenal gland probably requires subsequent somatic mutations. Such mutations include the loss of genetic markers on chromosomes 1p, 3p, 3q, and 22q that frequently occur in these tumors.

Patients with MEN 2b harbor point mutations in the substrate binding pocket of the *RET* kinase, most commonly a change of methionine-918 to threonine. These mutations activate the kinase and change its substrate specificity.

Familial MCT, without tumors of the adrenal or parathyroid gland, is also caused by mutations of the *RET* gene. These mutations include the same mutations that cause MEN 2a, as well as unique mutations in the *RET* gene's kinase domain. Systematic analysis of the *RET* gene has demonstrated that inheritable *RET* gene abnormalities can occur in patients with apparently sporadic MCT as well. Inherited *RET* gene abnormalities are sometimes found in patients with apparently isolated pheochromocytomas but not in those with sporadic parathyroid adenomas. Remarkably, some patients with familial Hirschsprung's disease, associated with absence of neurons in the enteric sympathetic nervous system, have inactive *RET* genes.

Diagnosis

Screening

Direct genetic testing has now replaced calcitonin testing as a screening tool in families with MEN 2. These genetic studies have shown that calcitonin testing and even histologic analysis of thyroid tissue can lead to false-positive and false-negative assignment of disease within families. The limited numbers of sites in the *RET* gene that cause inherited disease make genetic testing routinely feasible.

Half the patients with MEN 2a develop pheochromocytomas. Family screening allows the detection of pheochromocytoma before the development of hypertension. Plasma metanephrine levels are elevated consistently in patients with MEN 2a pheochromocytomas, as they are in patients with sporadic pheochromocytomas. The tumors are usually found in the adrenal glands and can be documented preoperatively by computed tomography, magnetic resonance imaging, and [iodine-131]–metaiodobenzylguanidine scanning.

Treatment

Surgery to prevent MCT is now performed before the age of 5 years in patients with MEN 2a, with some variation depending on the specific *RET* mutation, and before 6 months of age in patients with the more severe MEN 2b disease.

Prognosis

Because of early detection and curative surgery, MCT can be prevented or cured in virtually all children with MEN 2a or 2b after appropriate genetic testing at young ages. When tumors are seen clinically, however, because such testing was not performed or the patient represents an index case in a family, then the prognosis resembles that of sporadic tumors, except for the high frequency of multiple primary tumors. Similarly, the pheochromocytomas and parathyroid tumors are multiple but otherwise resemble their sporadic counterparts in prognosis.

McCune-Albright Syndrome

Definition

The McCune-Albright syndrome is a noninherited disorder consisting of the triad of polyostotic fibrous dysplasia, light brown pigmented skin lesions (café-au-lait spots), and an endocrinopathy, usually precocious puberty. Multiple endocrine abnormalities can occur.

Pathogenesis

Precocious puberty, more often seen in girls than boys, is gonadotropin independent. Hyperthyroidism is caused by autonomous thyroid nodules. Acromegaly is caused by pituitary adenomas that produce growth hormone and, usually, prolactin. Adrenocortical hyperfunction is caused by adrenocorticotropic hormone–independent adrenal adenomas. Hypophosphatemic rickets, with normal blood calcium level, phosphate wasting, and low or inappropriately normal levels of 1,25-dihydroxyvitamin D, may result from release of fibroblast growth factor 23 from the dysplastic fibrous tissue.

This somewhat bewildering array of endocrine abnormalities has been rationalized by the observation that cells in the involved tissues harbor mutations in the α subunit of the G_S protein. The G_S protein links cell surface receptors to the activation of adenylate cyclase. The mutations in McCune-Albright syndrome are point mutations at arginine-201 in the G_S subunit; these mutations lead to prolonged activity of G_S and inappropriate activation of adenylate cyclase. Increased levels of cyclic adenosine monophosphate lead to cellular proliferation and hormone secretion. Patients with McCune-Albright are genetic mosaics. Presumably, at an early stage in embryonic development, a point mutation occurs in the G_S gene of a cell that then proliferates, differentiates, and variably populates normal bone, skin, and endocrine tissues. In cell types in which elevations in cyclic adenosine monophosphate lead to proliferation, abnormal cells become predominant and lead to disease. Because the disease is not inherited, the mutation is presumably lethal when it is present in all cells of the embryo. In contrast, the very same mutations at arginine-201 have been found in cases of isolated acromegaly and autonomous thyroid nodules. One can therefore speculate that McCune-Albright syndrome is the most dramatic example of a spectrum of disorders that vary in severity and presentation, depending on the stage of development of the original mutant cell.

Treatment Rx

The treatment of the individual hormonal disorders is identical to that of the corresponding sporadic tumor. The polyostotic bone lesions require orthopedic correction when functional disability occurs, and bisphosphonate therapy may slow their growth.

Prognosis

The prognosis of each hormonal component of the syndrome is similar to that of the corresponding sporadically occurring disorder.

AUTOIMMUNE SYNDROMES

Organ-specific autoimmune disease, characterized by lymphocytic infiltration and organ-specific autoantibodies, commonly results in endocrine hypofunction or hyperfunction. Clinical manifestations of disease are usually limited to one gland. Not uncommonly, however, disorders of more than one endocrine gland appear in families or in individual patients. Characteristic patterns of disease presentation and genetic inheritance allow the definition of two syndromes with overlapping manifestations (Table 250–1).

Autoimmune Polyglandular Syndrome Type 1

Definition

Autoimmune polyglandular syndrome type 1 is a rare disease that is also known as autoimmune polyendocrinopathy, candidiasis, and ectodermal dystrophy syndrome. It typically manifests in early childhood.

TABLE 250–1 CLINICAL FEATURES OF AUTOIMMUNE POLYGLANDULAR SYNDROMES

Feature	Type 1	Type 2
Mucocutaneous candidiasis	Very common	Not seen
Hypoparathyroidism	Common	Rare
Addison's disease	Common	Common
Primary hypogonadism	Common	Occurs
Autoimmune thyroid disease	Rare	Common
Autoimmune diabetes	Occurs	Common
Hypophysitis	Occurs	Occurs
Autoimmune hepatitis	Occurs	Not seen
Pernicious anemia	Occurs	Occurs
Vitiligo	Occurs	Occurs
Malabsorption syndrome	Occurs	Occurs in celiac disease
Alopecia	Common	Occurs
Myasthenia gravis	Not seen	Occurs
Keratopathy	Common	Not seen
Tympanic membrane calcification	Common	Not seen
Inheritance	Autosomal recessive	HLA association
Age at onset	Usually childhood	Usually adulthood

HLA = human leukocyte antigen.

Pathogenesis

Autoimmune polyglandular syndrome type 1 is an autosomal recessive disorder, caused by a variety of inactivating mutations in the gene encoding autoimmune regulator-1 (AIRE-1), a nuclear protein that influences gene transcription, perhaps by acting as an enzyme, an E3 ubiquitin ligase, that ligates the protein, ubiquitin, to other nuclear proteins. AIRE-1 is expressed in epithelial cells of the thymus, cells that normally express a wide variety of genes usually expressed only in peripheral tissues. The synthesis of these "peripheral" proteins by thymic epithelial cells may be important for the normal ablation of lymphocytes reactive to these "self" proteins. In an animal model of AIRE-1 gene ablation, the thymic epithelial cells fail to express many of these "peripheral" proteins, perhaps leading to the persistence of lymphocytes responsible for autoimmune attack. The appearance of organ-specific autoantibodies precedes disease presentation and predicts the development of specific end-organ damage. The role of these antibodies is unknown, however.

Clinical Manifestations

Mucocutaneous candidiasis occurs in virtually all patients and is usually the first manifestation of disease. Hypoparathyroidism and Addison's disease are the most common endocrine manifestations; each of these diseases occurs in 70 to 80% of patients. Hypoparathyroidism usually precedes Addison's disease; both diseases typically manifest before the age of 15 years. Premature ovarian failure (in 60% of affected women) usually appears as secondary amenorrhea; testicular failure occurs less frequently. Insulin-dependent diabetes mellitus occurs in 12% of patients, usually in adulthood; hypothyroidism is uncommon.

Nonendocrine components of this syndrome, in addition to the mucocutaneous candidiasis, include alopecia, vitiligo, corneal opacities, autoimmune hepatitis, enamel hypoplasia of teeth, tympanic membrane calcification, nail dystrophy that correlates only loosely with obvious candidiasis, parietal cell atrophy and vitamin B_{12} malabsorption, and more general intestinal malabsorption with steatorrhea. Asplenism, with Howell-Jolly bodies on peripheral blood smears, has been noted in several patients. Each of the disease components should be sought when any patient presents with hypoparathyroidism, primary adrenal insufficiency, or mucocutaneous candidiasis.

Treatment

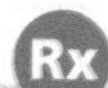

The hypoparathyroidism is treated like the sporadic disease with oral calcium and 1,25-dihydroxyvitamin D, although variable intestinal malabsorption can present a particular therapeutic challenge. The candidiasis can be satisfactorily controlled with ketoconazole.

Prognosis

The prognosis of the variably expressed hormonal disorders is similar to that of the sporadic counterparts. When the diagnosis of autoimmune polyglandular syndrome type 1 is made, of course, then surveys for other components of the syndrome can allow treatment earlier than would otherwise occur.

Autoimmune Polyglandular Syndrome Type 2

Pathogenesis

Autoimmune polyglandular syndrome type 2 is usually inherited in families with characteristic human leukocyte antigen (HLA) associations. The HLA associations do not predict disease absolutely, even in identical twins, so environmental factors must contribute to disease presentation. Abnormal expression of the gene encoding cytotoxic T-lymphocyte antigen-4 (CTLA-4) can also predispose to autoimmune polyglandular syndrome type 2. Typically, several different autoimmune diseases occur in each family. Autoimmune vulnerability rather than specific organ disease is inherited.

Clinical Manifestations

Autoimmune polyglandular syndrome type 2 is considerably more common than the type 1 syndrome and typically manifests in adulthood. Insulin-dependent diabetes mellitus and thyroid dysfunction, either autoimmune hypothyroidism or Graves' disease, are the most frequent manifestations. Addison's disease is the third major endocrine component of this disorder. Although most patients who present with autoimmune diabetes or thyroid disease have clinical involvement of only one gland, many patients with autoimmune Addison's disease develop clinically evident disease in other endocrine glands. Less common components of the type 2 polyglandular syndrome include primary hypogonadism and hypophysitis. Pernicious anemia, vitiligo, celiac disease, alopecia, and myasthenia gravis are also associated with this syndrome.

Treatment

The treatment of each component of this syndrome is identical to the treatment of each disorder in isolation, although possible clustering of diseases must be kept in mind during the evaluation and follow-up of all patients with each individual component disorder. Thyroid hormone therapy can precipitate symptoms of adrenal insufficiency in patients with both disorders. Consequently, careful history, including family history, physical examination, and a low threshold for specific laboratory testing for adrenal insufficiency should be part of the evaluation of every patient with autoimmune hypothyroidism. Further, combinations of hypothyroidism, adrenal insufficiency, and hypogonadism can mimic hypopituitarism, although specific hormonal testing can easily distinguish these disorders. Because multiple components of the syndrome can appear asynchronously, periodic evaluation for the early appearance of further disease components is indicated.

Organ-specific antibodies appear before clinical disease and predict subsequent disease. The role of these antibodies in organ hypofunction has not been established, however.

Prognosis

The prognosis of the individual components of autoimmune polyglandular syndrome type 2 is the same as for the sporadic versions of each component.

SUGGESTED READINGS

Eisenbarth GS, Gottlieb PA: Autoimmune polyendocrine syndromes. N Engl J Med 2004;350:2068–2079. *Excellent overview.*

Marx SJ: Molecular genetics of multiple endocrine neoplasia types 1 and 2. Nat Rev Cancer 2005;5:367–375. *Concise summary of molecular understanding of these disorders.*

Villasenor J, Benoist C, Mathis D: AIRE and APECED: Molecular insights into an autoimmune disease. Immunol Rev 2005;204:156–164. *Overview of molecular underpinning of autoimmune polyendocrine syndrome type 1.*

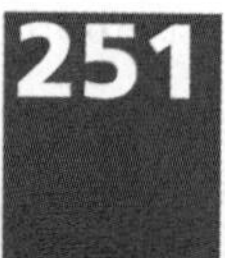

251 MULTIPLE-ORGAN SYNDROMES: CARCINOID SYNDROME

Kenneth R. Hande

Carcinoid syndrome is the term used for the systemic signs and symptoms resulting from the release of neuroendocrine mediators by some carcinoid tumors. Cutaneous flushing, diarrhea, and cardiac valvular lesions are the most common endocrine consequences of these tumors.

THE NEOPLASMS

Carcinoids are neuroendocrine tumors that arise from enterochromaffin cells. Enterochromaffin cells are located throughout the body; however, carcinoid tumors occur primarily in the lung (15% of all carcinoid tumors), stomach (3%), small intestine (22%), appendix (35%), and rectum (10%). Carcinoid tumors demonstrate a histologic pattern of dense nests of cells with uniform size and nuclear appearance. Ultrastructural examination of carcinoid tumors reveals electron-dense secretion granules. Only 8 to 10% of all carcinoid tumors are associated with the carcinoid syndrome. The neurosecretory granules in carcinoid tumors associated with the carcinoid syndrome typically contain 5-hydroxytryptamine (serotonin) and tachykinins such as substance P. Histochemically, these granules typically exhibit an argentaffin reaction in which the cells convert a silver salt to metallic silver. Tumors associated with carcinoid syndrome usually arise from the ileum and have metastasized to the liver. The carcinoid syndrome also can be produced by neoplasms arising from the remainder of the small intestine, from organs derived from the embryonic foregut (e.g., bronchus, stomach, pancreas, and thyroid), and from ovarian or testicular teratomas. Carcinoid tumors arising from organs of the embryonic foregut may contain few if any argentaffin cells. Carcinoids from the distal large intestine may metastasize but rarely exhibit endocrine effects and are argentaffin negative.

Pathogenesis

Endocrine Function of Carcinoid Tumors

SEROTONIN. The most constant biochemical feature of carcinoid tumors is the presence of tryptophan hydroxylase, which catalyzes the formation of 5-hydroxytryptophan (5-HTP) from tryptophan (Fig. 251–1). The typical ileal carcinoid tumor also contains aromatic L-amino acid decarboxylase, which catalyzes the conversion of 5-HTP to 5-hydroxytryptamine (serotonin). Gastric carcinoids, however, are frequently deficient in this decarboxylase and release 5-HTP from the tumor. Following its release from the tumor, serotonin is inactivated primarily by monoamine oxidase; uptake in the platelets also contributes to removal of free serotonin from blood. Monoamine oxidase oxidizes serotonin to 5-hydroxyindoleacetaldehyde, which is rapidly converted to 5-hydroxyindoleacetic acid (5-HIAA) by aldehyde dehydrogenase (see Fig. 251–1). This acid is rapidly excreted into the urine, and almost all circulating serotonin can be accounted for as urinary 5-HIAA.

TACHYKININS. Peptides of the tachykinin family are stored in carcinoid tumors and are released during flushing. Several tachykinins are derived

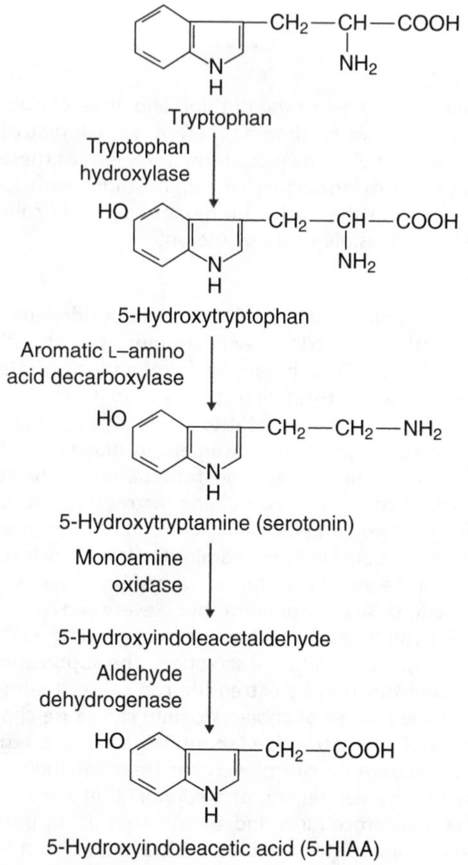

Tryptophan

Tryptophan hydroxylase

5-Hydroxytryptophan

Aromatic L-amino acid decarboxylase

5-Hydroxytryptamine (serotonin)

Monoamine oxidase

5-Hydroxyindoleacetaldehyde

Aldehyde dehydrogenase

5-Hydroxyindoleacetic acid (5-HIAA)

FIGURE 251–1 • Synthesis and degradation of serotonin.

from a common precursor β-preprotachykinin; of these, neuropeptide K, neurokinins A and B, and substance P have been identified in tumors and blood from patients with the carcinoid syndrome.

OTHER BIOLOGICALLY ACTIVE SUBSTANCES. Some carcinoid tumors, particularly those of gastric origin, release excessive amounts of histamine. This can be detected by an increased urinary excretion of histamine or its metabolite, *N*-methylhistamine. Carcinoid tumors have been associated with a number of ectopic endocrine syndromes, including hyperadrenocorticism, which results from ectopic production of adrenocorticotropic hormone and acromegaly in response to secretion of growth hormone–releasing hormone by the tumor.

MECHANISM OF THE FLUSH. Flushing can be triggered by catecholamines, and this probably accounts for the association of flushing with exercise and emotional stimuli. Injection of isoproterenol, in amounts as little as 0.5 μg, or pentagastrin, in doses as small as 0.25 μg, also can trigger flushing, an action that may explain the provocation of flushes by eating in some patients. Because the hemodynamic changes associated with such pharmacologically induced attacks can be severe, epinephrine and other β-adrenergic amines as well as pentagastrin should be administered with great caution. Flushing episodes can be blocked by somatostatin.

Most evidence points to the tachykinins as mediators of the carcinoid flush. Tachykinins, particularly neuropeptide K, can be identified in plasma during flushing. Tachykinin levels have been shown to be increased during pentagastrin-induced flushing, and when pentagastrin-induced flushing is inhibited by somatostatin, the rise in tachykinin levels also is blocked. Tachykinins are known vasodilators.

Serotonin does not cause flushing. In patients with gastric carcinoids that secrete histamine, the flushing attacks can be attributed to histamine.

PATHOPHYSIOLOGY OF SEROTONIN OVERPRODUCTION. Serotonin contributes to the intestinal hypermotility and diarrhea. A secondary effect of serotonin overproduction occurs when a large fraction of dietary tryptophan is shunted into the hydroxylation pathway, thus leaving less tryptophan available for the formation of nicotinic acid and protein. When urinary excretion of 5-HIAA exceeds 100 mg/day, low levels of plasma tryptophan and evidence of nicotinic acid deficiency (pellagra) can be seen.

The interaction of serotonin with platelets and the cardiac endothelium is considered the cause of carcinoid heart disease. This hypothesis is supported by the finding of valvular heart disease in patients taking appetite suppressants, such as fenfluramine, that release serotonin. The risk of valvular heart disease in patients with the carcinoid syndrome is correlated with the amount of 5-HIAA excreted in the urine.

Clinical Manifestations

Carcinoid tumors typically have a slow rate of growth, and many patients with carcinoid syndrome survive for years after the disease is recognized. The carcinoid syndrome occurs when mediators produced by the tumor and normally metabolized by the liver escape into the systemic circulation. For much of the duration of the illness, morbidity results largely from the endocrine functions of the tumor. Death usually is caused by cardiac or hepatic failure and by complications associated with tumor growth.

VASODILATOR PAROXYSMS. Cutaneous flushing, occurring in 80% of patients with the carcinoid syndrome, is the most common clinical feature. The typical flush is dark red to violaceous and involves the head, neck, and upper trunk (blush area). The flush usually lasts for 30 seconds to 3 minutes. Carcinoid tumors of the foregut produce a slightly different flush, characteristically bright salmon pink to red. Prolonged flushing attacks may be associated with lacrimation and periorbital edema. The flush may be accompanied by tachycardia. The blood pressure usually falls or does not change. A rise in blood pressure during flushing is rare, and carcinoid syndrome is not a cause of sustained hypertension. Flushing may be provoked by excitement, exertion, eating, and ethanol ingestion. In patients with the bronchial carcinoid variant, flushing may last for hours.

TELANGIECTASIA. In addition to paroxysms of cutaneous vasodilatation, some patients also develop telangiectasia, primarily on the face and neck, which is most marked in the malar area. These patients may have the characteristic features of rosacea.

GASTROINTESTINAL SYMPTOMS. Intestinal hypermotility with borborygmi and cramping occurs in 50 to 70% of patients with carcinoid syndrome. Explosive secretory diarrhea may occur, although chronic diarrhea with a secretory component is more common. When diarrhea is severe, malabsorption may occur. Gastrointestinal transit times through the small and large bowel are two- to sixfold faster than in physiologically normal patients.

CARDIAC MANIFESTATIONS. Symptomatic valvular heart disease is present in 15 to 20% of patients with the carcinoid syndrome. Up to 50% of patients with carcinoid syndrome have echocardiographic evidence of heart disease. Plaquelike thickening of the endocardium of the valvular cusps and cardiac chambers occurs primarily on the right side of the heart but may involve the left side to a minimal degree. The endocardial thickening is composed of smooth muscle cells embedded in a stroma rich in mucopolysaccharides. The thickening and deformation of the valve cusps, chordae tendineae, and papillary muscles interfere with valvular function and may lead to regurgitation, stenosis, or combined functional lesions. Lesions of the tricuspid valve (usually regurgitation) are present in 65% of patients with carcinoid heart disease, and pulmonic valvular disease (again, usually regurgitation) is seen in 20% of those with heart disease. Cardiac function may be further compromised by impaired atrial and ventricular compliance and by the occasional occurrence of a high cardiac output that probably results from continuing release of a vasodilator.

PULMONARY SYMPTOMS. Bronchoconstriction, usually most pronounced during flushing attacks, is a less common feature of the syndrome, but it may be severe.

GENERAL FEATURES. Intestinal obstruction may result from the primary tumor or from the desmoplastic reaction in the surrounding mesentery; infrequently, the primary tumors cause gastrointestinal bleeding. Necrosis of hepatic tumor masses may produce an acute syndrome of abdominal pain, tenderness, fever, and leukocytosis. Hepatomegaly from the metastatic disease is usually present, but extensive metastatic involvement of the liver by the slowly growing tumors may occur before liver function tests become abnormal. Generalized fatigue and debilitation are underappreciated features of carcinoid syndrome. Attacks of severe and sustained flushing with life-threatening hemodynamic compromise and bronchoconstriction may occur and are referred to as *carcinoid crisis.*

Precipitating factors include anesthesia or surgery, tumor necrosis, and catecholamine infusion.

Diagnosis

When all its clinical features are present, carcinoid syndrome is easily recognized. The diagnosis also must be considered when any one of its clinical manifestations is present.

The diagnostic hallmark consists of overproduction of 5-hydroxyindoles accompanied by increased excretion of urinary 5-HIAA in a patient with a carcinoid tumor. Normally, excretion of 5-HIAA does not exceed 9 mg/day. Ingestion of foods containing serotonin may complicate the biochemical diagnosis of carcinoid syndrome; bananas, walnuts, and certain other foods contain enough serotonin to produce abnormally elevated urinary excretion of 5-HIAA after their ingestion. Selected drugs may also falsely elevate urinary 5-HIAA measurements. Instructions to avoid these foods during collection of urine for analysis of 5-HIAA will prevent the concern and costs engendered by falsely elevated levels of urinary 5-HIAA. When dietary 5-hydroxyindoles are excluded, urinary excretion of 25 mg/day of 5-HIAA is diagnostic of carcinoid syndrome. Elevation in the range of 9 to 25 mg may be seen with carcinoid syndrome, nontropical sprue, vomiting, or acute intestinal obstruction. Measurement of serotonin in blood or platelets is of interest but has less diagnostic value than assay of the major metabolite of serotonin in the urine.

Plasma chromogranin A levels may be elevated by neuroendocrine tumors, including carcinoids, and may serve as a marker of tumor mass. The diagnostic value of plasma chromogranin A is relatively low, however, because this substance may be elevated in a variety of neuroendocrine tumors. Assessment of the extent and localization of both primary and metastatic tumor is aided by computed tomographic scans of the abdomen and chest and by imaging with radionuclide-labeled somatostatin receptor ligands.

DIFFERENTIAL DIAGNOSIS. Attacks of flushing in a patient with normal urinary excretion of 5-HIAA raise other diagnostic possibilities. Systemic mastocyte activation disorders, including systemic mastocytosis and idiopathic anaphylaxis, produce flushing and diarrhea and should be considered when 5-HIAA excretion is not elevated. Flushing also occurs in genetically predisposed individuals following ethanol ingestion, in the postmenopausal state, and in conjunction with other neuroendocrine tumors such as VIPomas (vasoactive intestinal peptide [VIP]) and medullary carcinoma of the thyroid.

VARIANTS OF THE CARCINOID SYNDROME. The origin of the tumor influences the biologically active substances produced and their storage and release. The typical carcinoid syndrome usually results from tumors of midgut origin, which almost invariably secrete serotonin. Tumor serotonin content is likely to be high, and the tumor usually contains dense nests of argentaffin-positive cells. In contrast, tumors arising from the embryonic foregut contain fewer argentaffin cells, have a lower serotonin content, and may secrete 5-HTP. Ectopic hormone production (e.g., Cushing's syndrome and acromegaly) and multiple endocrine adenomas are more likely to be associated with tumors of embryonic foregut.

Patients with gastric carcinoids frequently exhibit unique flushing, which begins as bright, patchy erythema with sharply delineated serpentine borders; these patches tend to coalesce as the blush heightens. Food ingestion is especially likely to produce flushes. The tumors are usually deficient in decarboxylase enzyme and secrete 5-HTP; histamine secretion is also common, as is a high incidence of peptic ulceration. In these patients, histamine is the principal factor causing flushing.

With carcinoid tumors arising from the bronchus, attacks of flushing tend to be prolonged and severe and may be associated with periorbital edema, excessive lacrimation and salivation, hypotension, tachycardia and tachyarrhythmias, anxiety, and tremulousness. Nausea, vomiting, explosive diarrhea, and bronchoconstriction may progress to a severe degree. This group is therapeutically unique in that severe flushes often can be prevented by corticosteroids.

Treatment

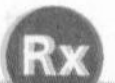

Treatment of the carcinoid syndrome is directed toward (1) pharmacologic therapy for humorally mediated symptoms and (2) the reduction of tumor mass.

Somatostatin

Somatostatin can prevent the flushing and other endocrine symptoms of the carcinoid syndrome. Therapy with somatostatin analogues has been a major advance in the treatment of these patients. The development of analogues of somatostatin, with longer biologic half-lives than the native hormone, has made subcutaneous administration a feasible route of therapy.

Octreotide

One of the somatostatin analogues, octreotide, improves the flushing and other endocrine manifestations in most patients with carcinoid syndrome. This therapy is frequently associated with a reduction in urinary 5-HIAA excretion and in tachykinin levels in blood. With the improvement of these endocrine symptoms, including fatigue, a considerable improvement in quality of life may be achieved. A long-acting octreotide formulation (octreotide LAR), consisting of microspheres containing octreotide, permits once-monthly dosing. Two to 4 weeks may be required to achieve steady-state levels of octreotide from administration of octreotide LAR, during which time supplementation with subcutaneous octreotide may be needed. An uncommon but severe adverse effect of octreotide is hypoglycemia, probably as a result of the inhibition of glucagon and growth hormone secretion. The suppression of pancreatic exocrine function by octreotide can cause steatorrhea, and inhibition of the release of cholecystokinin can cause cholelithiasis. In patients receiving octreotide, about 5% achieve a regression in tumor mass. Octreotide can prevent or treat carcinoid crises that accompany the massive release of mediators that sometimes occurs during operative procedures and tumor necrosis. In patients with histamine-secreting gastric carcinoids, blockade of both H_1- and H_2-histamine receptors markedly ameliorates flushing.

Surgery

Early diagnosis of the carcinoid syndrome has led to complete surgical cure in a few patients with tumors arising in ovarian or testicular teratomas or in the bronchus. By releasing their humoral mediators directly into the systemic circulation, these tumors can produce the syndrome before metastatic disease occurs. In contrast, tumors that release humoral substances into the portal circulation, to be largely metabolized by the liver, usually produce the syndrome only after liver metastases occur. Given the slow progression of this neoplasm, effective reduction in tumor mass can ameliorate morbidity and improve the quality of life even after metastases have occurred. In selected patients, this goal can be achieved by surgical debulking of tumor, including hemihepatectomy for unilobar metastases, excision of large superficial hepatic metastases, and removal of the primary tumor together with regional lymph nodes containing metastases. Elective cholecystectomy during the surgical intervention will prevent the complications of cholelithiasis that may result from octreotide treatment. Because the blood supply of hepatic metastases is largely arterial, percutaneous embolization of the hepatic arterial supply to the most involved hepatic lobe sometimes can reduce inoperable hepatic metastases; the procedure carries a high risk of complications.

Chemotherapy

Chemotherapy with single or combination cytotoxic agents given on a short-term basis has produced little benefit. For patients who exhibit tumor progression or whose clinical syndrome has failed to improve following cytoreduction and octreotide, interferon-α may be considered as adjunctive therapy.

Prognosis

A concerted strategy consisting of removal of the primary tumor, reduction in tumor bulk, and the administration of octreotide (with or without interferon-α) can lead to considerable amelioration of symptoms and improvement in the quality of life, reduction of the release of the humoral substances that engender the cardiac lesions, and prolongation of survival.

SUGGESTED REFERENCES

Crocetti E, Paci E: Malignant carcinoids in the USA, SEER 1992–1999: An epidemiological study with 6830 cases. Eur J Cancer Prev 2003;12:191–194. *Thirteen percent of patients had metastases at diagnosis, 24% had multiple tumors, and 5-year survival was 82%.*

Delaunoit T, Rubin J, Necporenko F, et al: Somatostatin analogs in the treatment of gastroenteropancreatic neuroendocrine tumors. Mayo Clin Proc 2005; 80:502–506. *Reviews the use of somatostatin analogues in the treatment of neuroendocrine tumors, including carcinoid syndrome.*

Moller JE, Connolly HM, Rubin J, et al: Factors associated with progression of carcinoid heart disease. N Engl J Med 2003;348:1005–1015. *Higher serotonin levels carry a worse prognosis in patients with carcinoid heart disease.*

Ramage JK, Davies AHG, Ardill J, et al: Guidelines for the management of gastroenteropancreatic neuroendocrine (including carcinoid) tumours. Gut 2005;54 (Suppl. 4):1–16. *Recommendations of a panel of experts on the diagnosis, staging, and management of carcinoid tumors.*

Turner GB, Johnston BT, McCance DR: Circulating markers of prognosis and response to treatment in patients with midgut carcinoid tumors. Gut 2006;55:1586–1591. *Neurokinin A, urinary 5-hydroxyindolacetic acid output, age, and number of liver metastases are predictors of outcome.*

252 DISORDERS OF SEXUAL DIFFERENTIATION

Perrin C. White

Definition

This chapter reviews the concepts underlying the initial evaluation and management of the intersex patient. By definition, such an individual has lack of concordance of various aspects of gender. These include chromosomal sex (46XX, 46XY, or other), gonadal/reproductive sex (ovaries, Fallopian tubes, and uterus versus testes, seminal vesicles, prostate gland, and ejaculatory ducts), genital sex (vagina and clitoris versus scrotum and penis), and gender-specific behavior. Depending on chromosomal sex, most patients may be classified either as incompletely masculinized males (46XY, male pseudohermaphrodites, or males with micropenis), excessively virilized females (46XX, female pseudohermaphrodites), and patients with abnormalities of sex chromosomes such as those with mixed gonadal dysgenesis. Many conditions may be associated with intersex states (Table 252–1).

Normal Sexual Differentiation

Gonadal Differentiation

At 5 to 6 weeks' gestation, the gonadal primordia (gonadal ridges) develop from the coelomic epithelium overlying the medial surface of the mesonephros (primitive kidneys; Fig. 252–1). These primitive gonads are apparently identical in both sexes. Germ cells form at 3 to 4 weeks' gestation and migrate through the gut mesentery into the gonads at this early bipotential stage. Whether germ cells are directed toward male or female gametogenesis depends largely on the environment generated by surrounding somatic cells rather than on factors intrinsic to the germ cells.

During the seventh week, XY male gonads begin to differentiate under the influence of a series of testis-determining genes. The first to be expressed is *SRY*, the key gene on the Y chromosome controlling male differentiation. *SRY* expression depends on the WT1 transcription factor. SRY initiates the development of Sertoli cells by indirectly (perhaps by altering chromatin structure) or directly increasing expression of SOX9, a related transcription factor encoded not on the Y chromosome but on chromosome 17. SOX9 expression also requires an intermediate level of expression of the transcription factor DAX1 but is inhibited by high DAX1 levels.

Sertoli cells surround germ cells to form testis cords, which nourish primordial germ cells and direct them into the pathway for male gametogenesis. In testes, germ cells (before spermatogonia) undergo mitotic arrest and are blocked from entering meiosis until after birth. Sertoli cells secrete several possibly redundant factors that induce migration of additional cells from the mesonephros into the testis, and they also stimulate proliferation of cells in the coelomic epithelium. These may include nerve growth factors, hepatocyte growth factor, platelet-derived growth factors (PDGF), and fibroblast growth factors (FGF), particularly FGF9.

TABLE 252–1 CAUSES OF INTERSEX STATES*

I. VIRILIZATION OR SEX REVERSAL IN XX FEMALES

- A. Virilizing forms of congenital adrenal hyperplasia
  1. 21-Hydroxylase deficiency (1:15,000 births) [*CYP21*]: salt-wasting or simple virilizing forms
  2. 11β-Hydroxylase deficiency [*CYP11B1*]
  3. 3β-Hydroxysteroid dehydrogenase deficiency [*HSD3B2*]
  4. Cytochrome P-450 oxidoreductase deficiency (also maternal effect) [*POR*]
- B. Maternal or exogenous androgens:
  1. Drugs (danazol, progestins)
  2. Luteoma
  3. Aromatase deficiency [*CYP19*]
  4. Transcription factor mutations
- C. Mutations in genes affecting gonadal differentiation
  1. *SRY* (translocation to X)
  2. *SOX9* (duplication)
  3. *WT1* (Denys-Drash syndrome)
- D. Structural/idiopathic

II. UNDERVIRILIZATION OR SEX REVERSAL IN XY MALES

- A. Biosynthetic defects
  1. Lipoid adrenal hyperplasia [*STAR*]
  2. 17α-Hydroxylase/17,20 lyase [*CYP17*]
  3. 3β-Hydroxysteroid dehydrogenase [*HSD3B2*]
  4. 17-Ketosteroid reductase [*HSD17B3*]
  5. 5α-Reductase [*SRD5A2*]
  6. Cytochrome P-450 oxidoreductase deficiency [*POR*]
  7. Smith-Lemli-Opitz syndrome (1:20,000) [*DHCR7*]
- B. Androgen insensitivity (1:20,000) [*AR*]: complete or partial
- C. LH insensitivity [*LHR*]
- D. Mutations in genes affecting gonadal differentiation
  1. *SRY*
  2. *SOX9* (camptomelic dysplasia)
  3. *SF1* (associated with adrenal hypoplasia)
  4. *WT1* (WAGR and Denys-Drash syndromes)
  5. *DAX1* or *WNT4* duplications
  6. *DHH* (associated with peripheral neuropathy)
- E. Exposure to 5α-reductase inhibitors, other endocrine disruptors

III. MICROPENIS

- A. Panhypopituitarism [including *PROP1* mutations]
- B. Septo-optic dysplasia [including *HESX* mutations]
- C. Hypogonadotropic hypogonadism
  1. Kallmann's syndrome [*KAL1*]
  2. Prader-Willi syndrome [paternal chromosome 15q11 deletion]
  3. Congenital adrenal hypoplasia [*DAX1*]
- D. Vanishing testes (may also cause ambiguous genitalia)

IV. OTHER SYNDROMES AFFECTING REPRODUCTIVE SYSTEMS

- A. Chromosomal aneuploidy
  1. Turner's syndrome (1:2,500): 45 X, 45X/46XX mosaics, 46XXr, 46XXq–
  2. Klinefelter's syndrome (1:1,000): 47 XXY
  3. Mixed gonadal dysgenesis: 45X/46XY, 45X/47XXY
  4. Other: trisomy 13, trisomy 18, triploidy, 4p–, 13q–
- B. Persistent müllerian duct syndrome in XY males
  1. Type 1 [*AMH*]
  2. Type 2 [*AMHR2*]
- C. Mayer-Rokitansky-Kuster-Hauser syndrome (vaginal atresia) [*WNT4*]

*Frequencies of relatively common (at least 1 : 20,000) diseases are noted in parentheses. Where causative genetic mutations have been identified, the affected locus is noted in square brackets.

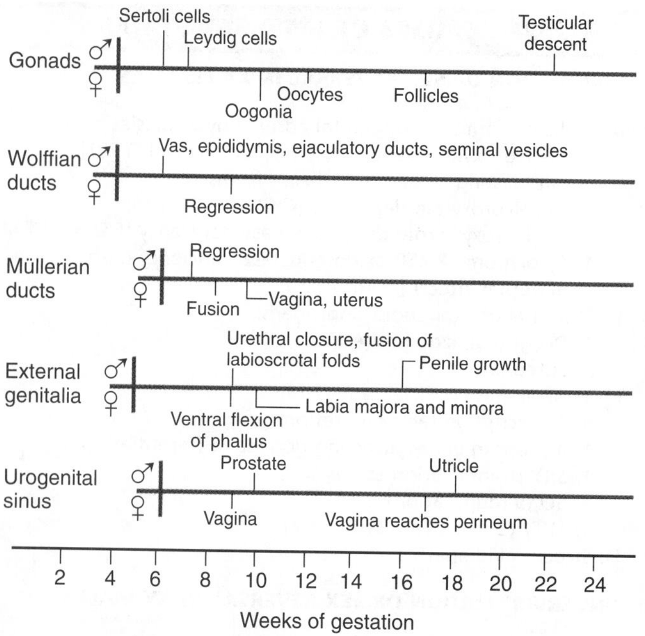

FIGURE 252–1 • Time course of prenatal sexual differentiation in male and female fetuses. (Adapted from Barthold JS, Gonzalez R: Intersex states. *In* Gonzales ET, Bauer SB [eds]: Pediatric Urology Practice. Philadelphia, Lippincott Williams & Wilkins, 1999.)

Recruitment of additional endothelial cells leads to development of a testis-specific vasculature that is required for development of the normal organization of the testis.

Steroidogenic cells develop from the mesonephros, a process requiring the SF1 transcription factor, and these cells migrate into the developing adrenal cortex and testis at about 8 weeks' gestation. In the testis, they become Leydig cells, which secrete the testosterone required for the subsequent development of the male reproductive system. Other factors required for Leydig cell differentiation and growth include DHH (desert hedgehog) and PDGFA ("A" being the first of four ligands termed A to D) secreted by Sertoli cells, as well as the ARX transcription factor expressed in interstitial cells surrounding the testis cords. In the first trimester, testosterone secretion is mainly under the control of human chorionic gonadotropin (hCG), whereas it subsequently requires luteinizing hormone (LH) secreted by the fetal anterior pituitary.

Ovaries are recognizable at about 10 weeks. The signaling molecule WNT4 plays an active role in ovarian development. It represses expression of testis-specific genes such as *SOX9* and *DHH,* as well as testis-specific vascular development. It also represses migration of Leydig cell precursors into the developing ovary. Some of these may be direct effects of WNT4 but others a consequence of increased expression of DAX1. Germ cells in the ovary continue into the first meiotic prophase beginning at 12 weeks' gestation and continuing until 7 months' gestation.

Development of Male and Female Internal Reproductive Tracts

The reproductive tracts are derived from intermediate mesoderm. The male reproductive tract develops from the mesonephric (wolffian) ducts, whereas the female reproductive tract develops from the paramesonephric (müllerian) ducts (Fig. 252–2). Both sets of ducts are originally present in normal embryos.

Further development of wolffian or müllerian structures depends on the presence or absence of normally functioning testes. The Sertoli cells secrete antimüllerian hormone (AMH, also termed müllerian inhibiting substance) starting when the testes differentiate. As with other members of the transforming growth factor-ß superfamily, this glycoprotein interacts with a heterodimeric receptor. The type II subunit, AMHR2, is specific for AMH. It is a serine/threonine kinase that recruits and phosphorylates a type I receptor, which then phosphorylates downstream targets. The type I receptors have not been identified with certainty but may be identical with the activin A type I receptor (ACVR1) or bone morphogenetic protein receptors. Expression of AMH is controlled by several transcription factors: SF1 and WT1 (Wilms' tumor locus) synergize to promote transcription, whereas DAX1 antagonizes it.

The molecular events engendered by AMH signaling are not well understood, although this signaling does increase expression of matrix

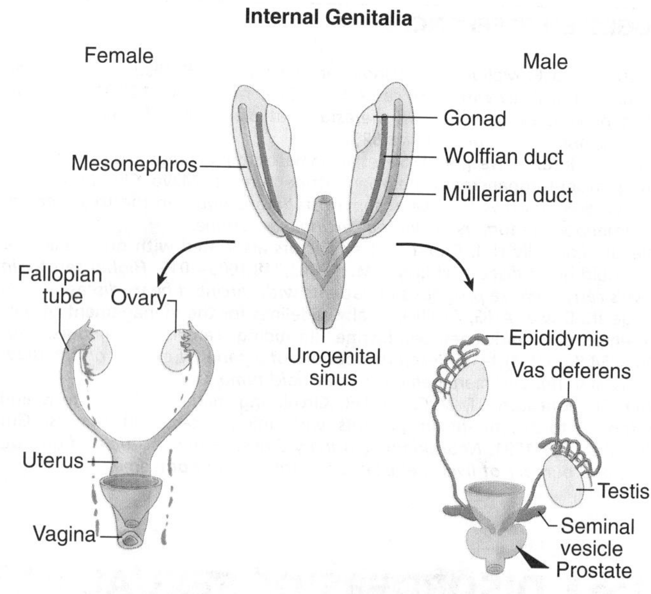

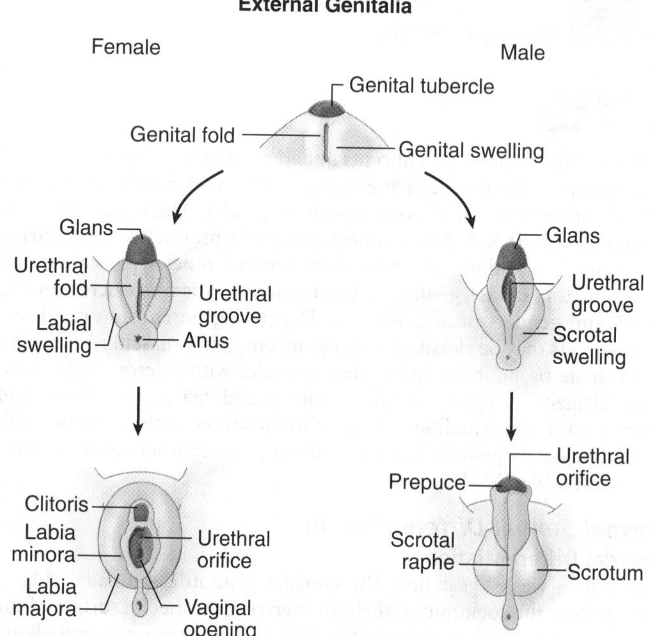

FIGURE 252–2 • Differentiation of the internal and external genitalia of the human fetus. (Adapted from Griffen JE, Ojeda SR [eds]: Textbook of Endocrine Physiology. New York, Oxford University Press, 1996.)

metalloproteinase 2 (MMP2). The overall effect is to induce regression of müllerian structures between 8 and 12 weeks' gestation. Otherwise, development of the müllerian ducts proceeds, and the female internal structures (fallopian tubes, uterus, cervix, and upper vagina) are formed. Müllerian development requires several transcription factors including LIM1, PAX2, EMX2, and WNT4.

In contrast, development of male genital structures derived from the wolffian ducts, including the epididymis, ductus deferens, ejaculatory ducts, and seminiferous tubules, requires high local concentrations of testosterone secreted from Leydig cells of the testis beginning at about 7 weeks' gestation. In the absence of testosterone, wolffian ducts regress. Levels of testosterone in the circulation are insufficient to develop wolffian structures. Thus, in conditions in which the gonads develop asymmetrically (e.g., true hermaphroditism or mixed gonadal dysgenesis; see later), wolffian structures develop asymmetrically as well.

Development of wolffian structures requires an intact androgen receptor. As with other steroid hormone receptors, the androgen receptor is a "nuclear" hormone receptor that, when occupied by its ligand, is translocated to the nucleus, where it interacts with DNA and other transcription factors to influence expression of target genes.

Development of the External Genitalia

External genital structures are also bipotential in early gestation, and consist of the genital tubercle, genital folds (later, urethral-labial folds), and genital swelling (later, the labioscrotal folds) (see Fig. 252–2). Differentiation to male genitalia occurs from 8–9 to 13–14 weeks of gestation under the influence of dihydrotestosterone, which must interact with an intact androgen receptor. The genital tubercle becomes the glans penis; the genital folds fuse to become the shaft of the penis and penile urethra, and the labioscrotal folds (derived from the genital swelling) fuse to become the scrotum. Without androgens, these structures become the clitoris, labia minora, and labia majora, respectively.

Normal Gonadal and Adrenal Steroidogenesis

Many forms of genital ambiguity result from defects in steroid biosynthesis in the testes or adrenal cortex or from defective steroid metabolism in the placenta or in target tissues (Fig. 252–3). The human ovary does not synthesize appreciable levels of steroid hormones until puberty.

Steroid biosynthesis in the testes and adrenals begins with importation of cholesterol into mitochondria, a highly regulated process controlled largely by the steroidogenic acute regulatory (StAR) protein; levels of StAR are controlled within the adrenal by adrenocorticotropic hormone (ACTH) and within the testis by hCG during the first trimester and by LH later in pregnancy.

Within mitochondria, the side chain of cholesterol is cleaved between carbons 20 and 22 by the cholesterol side-chain cleavage enzyme (cholesterol desmolase, CYP11A), a cytochrome P-450 enzyme that utilizes electrons donated from reduced nicotinamide-adenine dinucleotide phosphate (NADPH) via two accessory proteins, adrenodoxin reductase and adrenodoxin. The product of this reaction is pregnenolone, which is transported to the endoplasmic reticulum. Some pregnenolone is converted by 17α-hydroxylase (CYP17) to 17-hydroxypregnenolone. As with other microsomal P-450 enzymes, but unlike mitochondrial P-450s, CYP17 receives electrons from an NADPH-dependent cytochrome P-450 oxidoreductase (POR). Both 17-hydroxypregnenolone and the remaining pregnenolone are converted by 3ß-hydroxysteroid dehydrogenase (HSD3B2) to 17-hydroxyprogesterone and progesterone, respectively.

The side chains of 17-hydroxypregnenolone are cleaved by the 17,20-lyase activity of CYP17 to dehydroepiandrosterone (DHEA). DHEA may also be converted to androstenedione by HSD3B2.

All the preceding steps can occur in the adrenal cortex, in Leydig cells of the testis, and (after puberty) in theca cells of ovarian follicles. Subsequent biosynthetic steps are specific to different glands. In the adrenal cortex, 17-hydroxyprogesterone is converted by 21-hydroxylase (CYP21, a microsomal P-450) to 11-deoxycortisol, which is then converted in mitochondria to cortisol by 11ß-hydroxylase (CYP11B1). Additionally,

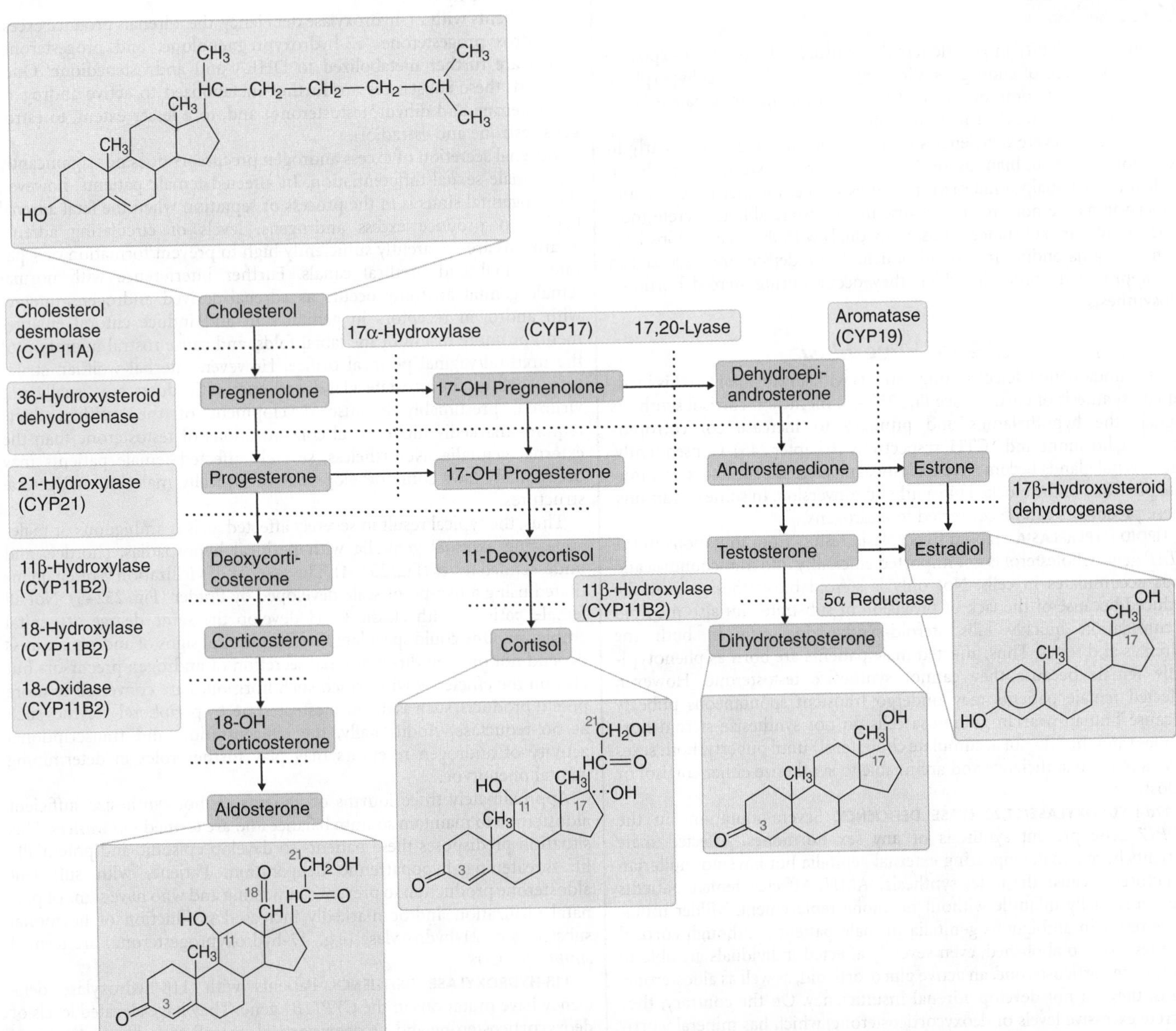

FIGURE 252–3 • Steroidogenesis. The pathways for synthesis of progesterone and mineralocorticoids (aldosterone), glucocorticoids (cortisol), androgens (testosterone and dihydrotestosterone), and estrogens (estradiol) are arranged from left to right. Planar structures are shown for cholesterol and the end products of each pathway. The enzymatic activities catalyzing each bioconversion are written in boxes. For those activities mediated by specific cytochrome P-450 subsets, the systematic name of the enzyme (CYP followed by a number) is listed in parentheses. CYP11B2 and CYP17 have multiple activities.

progesterone is converted to deoxycorticosterone by CYP21, which is then converted to aldosterone by aldosterone synthase (CYP11B2). DHEA may be converted to DHEA sulfate by steroid sulfotransferase. This reaction is particularly prominent in the fetal adrenal gland.

In Leydig cells of the testis, androstenedione is converted to testosterone by 17-ketosteroid reductase (17ß-hydroxysteroid dehydrogenase type 3 [HSD17B3]); the same reaction occurs in theca cells of the ovary, catalyzed by 17ß-hydroxysteroid dehydrogenase type 1 (HSD17B1). In granulosa cells of the ovary (after puberty), androstenedione and testosterone are converted by aromatase (CYP19) to estrone and estradiol, respectively. In skin of the developing male external genitalia, steroid 5α-reductase (SRD5A2) converts testosterone to a more powerful androgen, dihydrotestosterone.

The placenta is a steroid-synthesizing and metabolizing tissue as well; it has high steroid sulfatase activity that converts DHEA sulfate from the fetal adrenal gland back to DHEA. This is then successively converted by 3ß-hydroxysteroid dehydrogenase type 1 (HSD3B1) and aromatase (CYP19) to androstenedione and estrone, respectively, which are then converted to estradiol by HSD17B1.

DEFECTS OF SEX DIFFERENTIATION

Defects of Steroidogenesis

Pathobiology

Genital ambiguity in genetic females is usually the result of exposure to excessive levels of androgens. Virilizing congenital adrenal hyperplasia (CAH), the most common cause of genital ambiguity in female infants, occurs in approximately 1 in 15,000 births.

Conversely, severe deficiencies of androgens, if present since early in gestation, cause ambiguous or female-appearing external genitalia in male infants. Usually, müllerian structures such as the uterus, cervix, and upper vagina are not present because the testes are able to secrete müllerian inhibitory substance. Thus, individuals with these conditions have a short vagina ending in a blind pouch. These defects are discussed in the approximate order in which they occur during steroid hormone biosynthesis.

Congenital Adrenal Hyperplasia

The fundamental defect among patients with any form of CAH is inadequate synthesis of cortisol (see Fig. 252–3). Inefficient cortisol synthesis signals the hypothalamus and pituitary to increase corticotropin-releasing hormone and ACTH, respectively (Chapter 245). Consequently, the adrenal glands become hyperplastic, and steroid precursors accumulate proximal to the blocked biosynthetic conversion. In some conditions, these precursors can be converted to androgens.

LIPOID HYPERPLASIA. Lipoid hyperplasia results from mutations in the *STAR* gene. Cholesterol is not imported efficiently into mitochondria and thus accumulates in cells. Not only is steroid biosynthesis drastically reduced because of the lack of provision of substrate, but also the lipid accumulation quickly kills steroid-synthesizing cells in both the adrenals and testes. Thus, affected male patients are born as phenotypically female because they cannot synthesize testosterone. However, affected female patients may undergo transient spontaneous puberty because human ovarian granulosa cells do not synthesize steroid hormones (and thus do not accumulate cholesterol) until puberty. Both sexes have adrenal insufficiency and are unable to synthesize either cortisol or aldosterone

17α-HYDROXYLASE/17,20 LYASE DEFICIENCY. Severe mutations in the *CYP17* gene prevent synthesis of any sex hormones. Affected male patients have female-appearing external genitalia but have no müllerian structures because the testes synthesize AMH. Affected female patients remain sexually infantile without hormone replacement. Milder mutations result in ambiguous genitalia in male patients. Although cortisol synthesis is also abolished, even severely affected individuals are able to synthesize corticosterone, an active glucocorticoid, as well as aldosterone. Thus, they do not develop adrenal insufficiency. On the contrary, they secrete excessive levels of deoxycorticosterone, which has mineralocorticoid activity, and are therefore prone to develop hypertension.

3β-HYDROXYSTEROID DEHYDROGENASE DEFICIENCY. Severe mutations in the *HSD3B2* gene prevent synthesis of aldosterone, cortisol, testosterone, and estrogens. Because DHEA, a weak androgen, is synthesized and secreted at high levels, some degree of phallic growth is permitted. Thus, affected male patients have severely ambiguous genitalia, but affected female patients may have clitoromegaly. Both sexes develop adrenal insufficiency if they are untreated.

Because many children with premature adrenarche (early development of axillary and pubic hair), as well as many women with polycystic ovarian syndrome, have elevated levels of DHEA, it was thought at one time that such individuals could have a mild form of HSD3B2 deficiency. However, mutations in *HSD3B2* are rarely if ever found in such individuals, who instead seem to have an imbalance in the relative levels of HSD3B2 and CYP17 activity within the adrenal cortex.

21-HYDROXYLASE DEFICIENCY. More than 90% of cases of CAH are caused by 21-hydroxylase deficiency resulting from mutations in the *CYP21* gene. The relatively high incidence of this condition is a consequence of the proximity of a highly homologous pseudogene, CYP21P, which contains approximately 10 mutations that are deleterious to expression, mRNA processing, or enzymatic activity. CYP21 and CYP21P are located within the major histocompatibility complex on chromosome 6p21.3, a genomic region noteworthy for a high rate of recombination. More than 90% of all mutations are the result of intergenic recombination between *CYP21* and *CYP21P*. Most are transfers of deleterious mutations from *CYP21P* to *CYP21*, a process termed *gene conversion*, whereas approximately 20% are net deletions of *CYP21* resulting from unequal meiotic crossing over.

In patients with 21-hydroxylase deficiency, the adrenals produce excess 17-hydroxyprogesterone, 17-hydroxypregnenolone, and progesterone, which are further metabolized to DHEA and androstenedione. Once secreted, these substances are further metabolized to active androgens (testosterone and dihydrotestosterone) and, to a lesser extent, to estrogens (estrone and estradiol).

Adrenal secretion of excess androgen precursors does not significantly affect male sexual differentiation. In affected female patients, however, the urogenital sinus is in the process of septation when the fetal adrenal begins to produce excess androgens; levels of circulating adrenal androgens are apparently sufficiently high to prevent formation of separate vaginal and urethral canals. Further interference with normal female genital anatomy occurs as adrenal-derived androgens interact with androgen receptors in genital skin and induce clitoral enlargement, promote fusion of the labial folds, and cause rostral migration of the urethral/vaginal perineal orifice. However, internal wolffian structures such as the prostate gland and spermatic ducts are usually not virilized, presumably because development of the wolffian ducts requires markedly higher local concentrations of testosterone than the external genitalia. Nevertheless, severely affected female patients may occasionally have some development of typically male internal genital structures.

Thus, the typical result in severely affected girls is ambiguous or male-appearing external genitalia with perineal hypospadias, chordee, and undescended testes (Fig. 252–4). The severity of virilization is often quantitated using a five-point scale developed by Prader (Fig. 252–5). Not all female patients with classic CAH develop the same degree of genital ambiguity. One could speculate that the physical signs of androgen excess depend not only on direct adrenal secretion of androgen precursors but also on the efficiency with which such hormones are converted to more potent products, such as dihydrotestosterone, by peripheral enzymes such as 5α-reductase. Additionally, the concentration and transcriptional activity of androgen receptors may play further roles in determining genital phenotype.

Approximately three fourths of patients cannot synthesize sufficient aldosterone to maintain sodium balance and are termed *salt wasters.* This situation predisposes these patients to develop episodic and potentially life-threatening hyponatremic dehydration. Patients with sufficient aldosterone production to prevent salt wasting and who have signs of prenatal virilization and/or markedly increased production of hormonal substrates of 21-hydroxylase (e.g., 17-hydroxyprogesterone) are termed *simple virilizers.*

11β-HYDROXYLASE DEFICIENCY. Patients with 11β-hydroxylase deficiency have mutations in the *CYP11B1* gene. They have elevated levels of deoxycorticosterone and 11-deoxycortisol, as well as earlier cortisol precursors such as 17-hydroxyprogesterone. Thus, these patients secrete excess adrenal androgens, with consequences similar to those seen in 21-hydroxylase deficiency. However, patients with 11β-hydroxylase deficiency synthesize aldosterone normally and do not have problems with salt wasting. Instead, they are likely to become hypertensive as a result of elevated levels of deoxycorticosterone and its metabolites.

Defects of Androgen Biosynthesis

Lipoid hyperplasia, 17-hydroxylase/17,20 lyase deficiency, and HSD3B2 deficiency affect biosynthesis of both corticosteroids and sex hormones. In contrast, two enzymatic defects affect only androgen biosynthesis. They have similar phenotypes. Affected male patients are born with ambiguous genitalia, but they virilize at puberty and often reassign themselves to a male gender if they were raised as females. They have absent müllerian structures as a result of secretion of AMH by the testes.

17-KETOSTEROID REDUCTASE (17-HYDROXYSTEROID DEHYDROGENASE 3) DEFICIENCY. This disorder is caused by mutations in the *HSD17B3* gene. Although testosterone is not synthesized well, androstenedione, an active androgen (affinity for the androgen receptor ~1.5% that of dihydrotestosterone), is synthesized. Because several other isozymes have 17-ketosteroid reductase activity in other tissues, some testosterone is invariably synthesized, especially at puberty, when circulating levels of androstenedione increase.

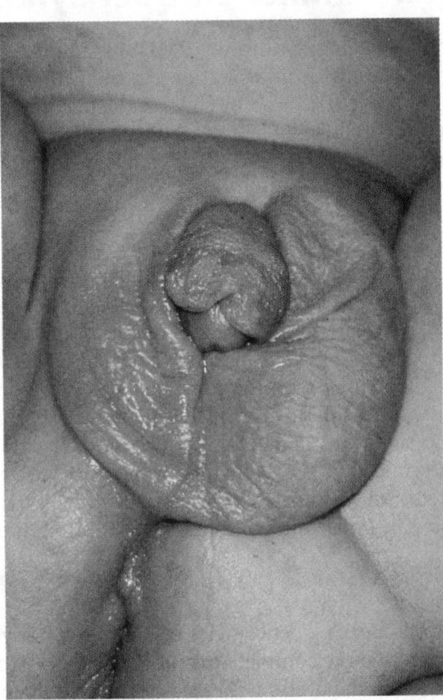

FIGURE 252–4 • Virilized external genitalia in a female infant with congenital adrenal hyperplasia caused by 21-hydroxylase deficiency. No gonads are present in the scrotum.

5α-REDUCTASE DEFICIENCY. Patients with 5α-reductase deficiency resulting from mutations in the *SRD5A2* gene synthesize entirely normal amounts of testosterone, but they cannot synthesize adequate amounts of dihydrotestosterone, the most potent naturally occurring androgen. This enzyme is not expressed at high levels in the testes (circulating levels of dihydrotestosterone are relatively low), but instead in genital skin. Internal wolffian structures do not require this enzyme and are intact; high testosterone levels at puberty induce significant phallic growth without 5α-reductase activity.

Other Defects of Steroidogenesis

AROMATASE DEFICIENCY. Mutations in *CYP19* cause aromatase deficiency in both the fetus and the placenta. The placenta can convert DHEA sulfate to androstenedione and testosterone normally, but it cannot convert these androgens to estrone and estradiol, respectively. These androgens accumulate in both the fetal and maternal circulations and virilize both the mother and the affected fetus if it is female. Affected male infants are phenotypically normal. Affected female patients virilize further at puberty if they are untreated. The lack of aromatase activity within bone leads to tall stature in both sexes, because estrogens are required to close the growth plates, and later to osteoporosis.

CYTOCHROME P-450 OXIDOREDUCTASE DEFICIENCY. POR deficiency is a recently recognized subset of Antley-Bixler syndrome. This syndrome is characterized by skeletal anomalies and craniosynostosis, and most patients have ambiguous genitalia associated with mutations in the *POR* gene. Antley-Bixler syndrome without genital abnormalities is caused by mutations in the FGF receptor *(FGFR2)* gene.

Because this disorder affects the activity of all microsomal cytochrome P-450 subsets, complete deficiency of POR is lethal, and identified mutations in humans yield POR with partial activity. The mechanism by which this causes skeletal anomalies is not understood. Genital ambiguity is caused by several mechanisms. Decreased activity of 17α-hydroxylase/17,20 lyase (CYP17) affects androgen synthesis and leads to undervirilization in male patients. Conversely, decreased activity of 21-hydroxylase (CYP21) can virilize affected female patients. These two deficiencies can also cause adrenal insufficiency. Finally, decreased activity of aromatase (CYP19) virilizes both the mother and the affected fetus (if female).

SMITH-LEMLI-OPITZ SYNDROME. This relatively frequent (1 in 20,000 Northern Europeans) disorder of the final step of cholesterol biosynthesis (conversion from 7-dehydrocholesterol) is caused by mutations in the *DHCR7* gene encoding 7-dehydrocholesterol reductase. The syndrome is characterized by multiple congenital anomalies including short stature, microcephaly, mental retardation, aggressive behavior, seizures, hypotonia, polydactyly, cleft palate, cardiac defects, lung hypoplasia, and renal anomalies. Male patients have ambiguous genitalia. The range of clinical severity is wide and depends on the nature of the mutations.

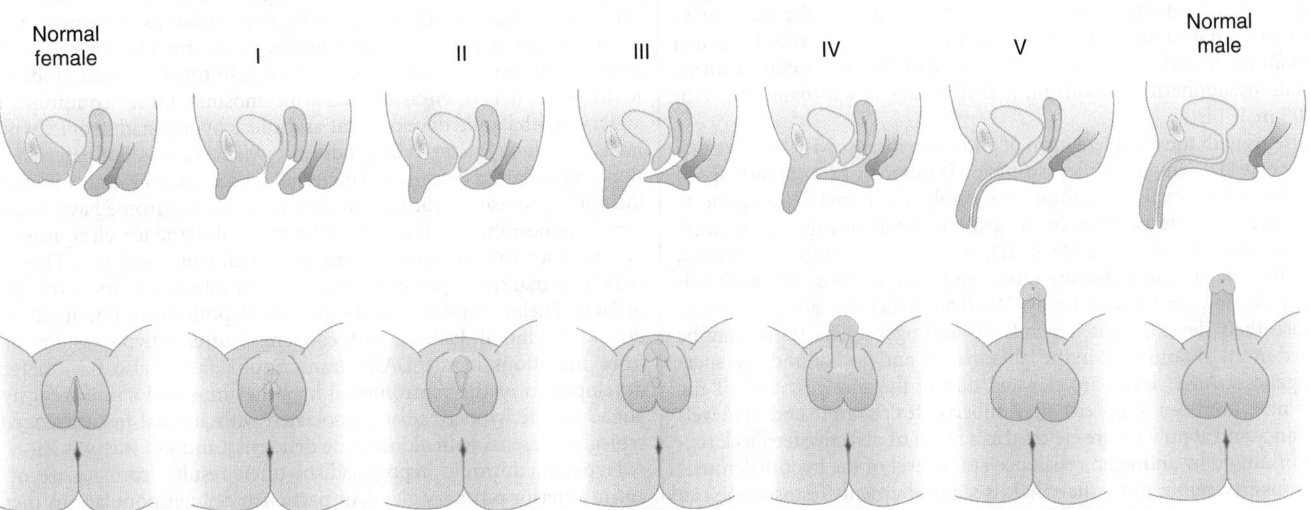

FIGURE 252–5 • Abnormal differentiation of the urogenital sinus and external genitalia. Schematic representations of normal female and male anatomy flank a series of schematics illustrating different degrees of virilization of females, graded using the scale developed by Prader. The uterus (shaded) persists in virilized female patients even when the external genitalia have a completely masculine appearance (Prader grade 5). (From Prader A: Der Genitalbefund beim Pseudohermaphroditismus femininus der kengenitalen adrenogenitalen Syndroms. Helv Paediatr Acta 1954;9:231–248).

Pathogenetic mechanisms for the ambiguous genitalia may include insufficient provision of cholesterol for steroid hormone biosynthesis or toxic effects of the precursor, 7-dehydrocholesterol, on steroidogenic cells. Moreover, cholesterol is a required cofactor for the hedgehog family of morphogens including DHH, which is required for Leydig cell differentiation.

MATERNAL CONDITIONS AFFECTING THE FETUS

Aromatase deficiency and POR deficiency both virilize the mother and directly affect the fetus (see previous section).

Luteoma of Pregnancy

Luteomas are probably the most common causes of maternal virilization during pregnancy. They are not true tumors; their cellular origin is uncertain. They often occur bilaterally. Although many luteomas are discovered incidentally during cesarean sections or postpartum tubal ligations, one fourth of mothers virilize during the latter half of pregnancy, and half of female infants born to these mothers also exhibit signs of virilization, most typically clitoromegaly and labial fusion. Spontaneous regression of the luteoma generally begins within days after delivery.

Drug Exposure

Depending on the agent, maternal drug exposure may affect either male or female fetuses. Females may be virilized by androgens such as 19-nor-testosterone or progestins administered to prevent spontaneous abortion. Undervirilized males can be born to women exposed to 5α-reductase inhibitors such as finasteride. The antifungal agent, fluconazole, can inhibit many cytochrome P-450 enzymes and can lead to a condition closely resembling Antley-Bixler syndrome.

The synthetic estrogen, diethylstilbestrol, was used several decades ago to attempt to prevent spontaneous abortion (it was actually ineffective for this purpose). Males exposed to this agent in utero were born with testicular hypoplasia, cryptorchidism, hypospadias, and/or microphallus. Females had uterine, cervical, and vaginal abnormalities and an increased risk of clear cell adenocarcinoma of the vagina. These defects may have resulted in part from disrupted expression of important transcription factors including WNT7A and several homeobox factors including HOXA10 and HOXA11. Considering that many cases of genital ambiguity are idiopathic, it is likely that additional endocrine disruptors in the environment have not yet been identified.

HORMONE INSENSITIVITY SYNDROMES AND OTHER HORMONE DEFICIENCIES

Androgen Insensitivity

Males normally carry a single copy of the X-linked androgen receptor gene. Thus, a single mutation can completely inactivate the receptor in males and can lead to complete androgen insensitivity (formerly termed *testicular feminization syndrome*). This is one of the most frequent forms of male pseudohermaphroditism, and it occurs in approximately 1 in 20,000 male births.

Patients with the complete form of androgen insensitivity have normal female external genitalia. Unless suspicion is raised by prior knowledge of the infant's karyotype, the condition is rarely discovered before puberty unless the testes are palpated in the groin or labia on routine examination. Because the testes secrete AMH, müllerian structures are absent, including the uterus, fallopian tubes, and cervix. Thus, the vagina is usually shallow and ends blindly. Wolffian structures are also absent because their development depends on androgens. The testes may be located in the abdomen or in the labia majora and do not undergo spermatogenesis. AMH levels are elevated during the first year and (if the testes have not been removed) after puberty. Testosterone and LH levels in infancy and at puberty are elevated as a result of defective feedback regulation caused by androgen resistance at the level of the hypothalamus.

At puberty, pubic and axillary hair is scant or absent. Testosterone can be aromatized to estradiol by CYP19 in breast fat, and estrogen receptors are unaffected in this condition. Thus, breast development is that of a normal female.

Partial androgen insensitivity (Reifenstein's syndrome) is characterized by a variable degree of genital ambiguity, and both virilization and breast development occur at puberty. Mild androgen insensitivity can also occur with a male phenotype, with gynecomastia and infertility as the sole manifestations. Mutations in the androgen receptor are not detected in many mild cases, which may result from defects in other factors affecting actions of the receptor.

Leydig Cell Agenesis

Leydig cell agenesis or hypoplasia is a rare autosomal recessive syndrome caused by mutations in the *LHGCR* gene encoding the LH receptor. Without stimulation by LH (or by hCG early in gestation), Leydig cells do not differentiate normally and do not secrete testosterone. Thus, affected male infants are born with female-appearing or ambiguous external genitalia. Müllerian structures are absent because of unaffected secretion of AMH by Sertoli cells. LH levels are high in infancy and at puberty, and they respond normally to gonadotropin-releasing hormone, whereas testosterone levels are low and do not respond to stimulation by hCG. Affected female patients are phenotypically normal but may have oligomenorrhea resulting from primary ovarian dysfunction.

Persistent Müllerian Duct Syndrome

Persistent müllerian duct syndrome (PMDS) is a rare autosomal recessive condition that results from mutations in the genes for either AMH (PMDS type I) or the AMH receptor (*AMHR2* gene, PMDS type II). The two are distinguished clinically by low or absent AMH levels in patients with AMH mutations and by AMH levels high in the normal range in patients with AMH receptor mutations.

Affected male patients have unimpaired testosterone secretion and thus have normal external genitalia and wolffian structures. However, the lack of AMH action prevents regression of müllerian structures, and thus these patients retain a uterus and fallopian tubes. These structures are often closely approximated to the vasa deferentia. The müllerian structures are usually dragged into the inguinal canal by the descending testes. However, these structures typically prevent the testes from descending into the scrotum and thus cause bilateral inguinal hernias (with the uterus on one side) and bilateral or occasionally unilateral cryptorchidism. The condition is usually discovered only at surgery. Fertility in affected patients may be normal or impaired, with an increased risk of malignant disease in undescended testes left in the abdomen.

Hypogonadotropic Hypogonadism

Milder or later-appearing deficiencies of androgen biosynthesis (after 13 to 14 weeks) may allow complete fusion of the labioscrotal folds and normal positioning of the urethral meatus, but subsequent growth of the phallus is suboptimal. Such individuals have a micropenis. The most common cause is lack of gonadotropin (specifically, LH) secretion; even when LH is lacking, early male development is normal because testosterone secretion is controlled mostly by hCG during the first trimester.

Defective LH and follicle-stimulating hormone (FSH) secretion can result from failure of migration into the hypothalamus of the neurons that normally secrete gonadotropin-releasing hormone. This condition, Kallmann's syndrome, is most often X-linked, resulting from mutations in the *KAL1* gene. It is often associated with anosmia. Other conditions that affect hypothalamic development and cause hypogonadotropic hypogonadism include Prader-Willi syndrome, which is a result of paternal deletions, methylation defects, and maternal uniparental disomy of imprinted loci on chromosome 15q12. Children with this syndrome have a characteristic appearance with a narrow bitemporal diameter, almond-shaped eyes with an anti-mongoloid slant, and small hands and feet. They typically have marked hypotonia as infants with subsequent moderate developmental delay and slow somatic growth. Hypothalamic obesity develops during childhood. Patients with congenital adrenal hypoplasia resulting from mutations in the DAX1 transcription factor also have defective development of the ventromedial hypothalamus and consequent hypogonadotropic hypogonadism, associated with adrenal insufficiency that typically presents with aldosterone deficiency and salt wasting.

Hypogonadotropic hypogonadism often results from failure of the entire anterior pituitary gland, or particular cellular populations therein, to develop. Pituitary gland abnormalities can be associated with other midline defects including hypoplasia of the optic nerves and the septum pellucidum, a condition termed *septo-optic dysplasia* or *de Morsier's syndrome*. Associated pituitary hormone deficiencies may include growth hormone, ACTH (and therefore cortisol), and thyroid-stimulating hormone (TSH) (and therefore thyroxine). These deficiencies may present in the neonatal period as hypoglycemia; hypothyroidism is usually detected by newborn screening programs that measure thyroxine levels. Optic nerve dysfunction is difficult to detect by routine examination in the neonatal period, but it causes a characteristic wandering nystagmus after a few months of age.

Although panhypopituitarism is most often sporadic, mutations in transcription factors controlling pituitary development have been documented (Chapter 242) particularly PROP1, and septo-optic dysplasia has been associated with mutations in the *HESX* gene. Rarely, mutations in the gene encoding the β subunit of LH may yield a phenotype similar to hypogonadotropic hypogonadism.

OTHER GENETIC CONDITIONS

Aneuploidy of Sex Chromosomes

TURNER'S SYNDROME. Patients with Turner's syndrome have normal female external genitalia and a normal uterus and fallopian tubes, but they have dysgenetic streak ovaries. Most fetuses with Turner's syndrome spontaneously abort, but the incidence in live births is approximately 1 in 2500. Classically, the karyotype is 45,X, but many patients retain an abnormal second X chromosome or even a fragment of a Y chromosome lacking SRY. Other patients are mosaic for 46,XX and 45,X cells and may have relatively mild phenotypes.

Untreated patients are short. Many have typical dysmorphic features including lymphedema of the neck at birth, webbed neck, low posterior hairline, increased carrying angle of the arms, shield chest with widely spaced nipples, low-set ears, and micrognathia. Patients typically have primary amenorrhea and are infertile, but occasionally they can have menarche followed by premature ovarian failure.

KLINEFELTER'S SYNDROME. In this condition, male patients have normal development of the penis and scrotum, but the testes are small and firm. Patients tend to be tall. At adolescence, gynecomastia is frequent. Signs of testosterone deficiency occur in most affected adults, and most have azoospermia. The usual karyotype is 47,XXY. Hormonal findings include elevated gonadotropin levels and decreased serum testosterone concentration. Klinefelter's syndrome is a common disorder that occurs in 1 in 500 to 1000 men.

Mixed Gonadal Dysgenesis

Mixed gonadal dysgenesis, a frequent cause of sexual ambiguity, occurs in approximately 1 in 20,000 births. The karyotype is usually mosaic 45,X/46,XY. Gonadal pathologic features can vary from fibrous streaks indistinguishable from those in Turner's syndrome to normally developed testes and a normal male phenotype. Typically, patients have a testis on one side and a fibrous streak on the other. Some patients may have a Turner-like phenotype. A fallopian tube is usually present on the side of the streak gonad. Leydig cell function, evaluated by testosterone response to hCG, and Sertoli cell function, evaluated by serum AMH levels, vary from poor to normal.

XX Male Syndrome

Males with a 46,XX karyotype have normal external and internal male genitalia; however, they resemble patients with Klinefelter's syndrome in that they have small testes, azoospermia, and infertility. Translocation of the *SRY* gene to the X chromosome is detected in 75 to 90% of sporadic cases; this can occur because the gene is located very near the pseudoautosomal region in which the short arms of the X and Y chromosomes are homologous and meiotic recombination is possible. Duplication of the SOX9 transcription factor may be responsible for some familial cases of XX sex reversal.

XY Female Syndromes

Patients with pure XY gonadal dysgenesis (Swyer's syndrome) have a normal female phenotype, including uterus and fallopian tubes, but they have streak gonads. These patients are free of Turner-like malformations and attain normal height. Mutations of the *SRY* gene have been identified in 15% of cases. Unlike 45,X patients with Turner's syndrome, these patients have an increased risk of gonadoblastoma.

Similar phenotypes result from duplication of the region of the X chromosome containing the *DAX1* gene, from duplication of the *WNT4* gene, or from haploinsufficiency of the SF1 transcription factor (associated in some cases with adrenal hypoplasia). XY sex reversal can also result from mutations in the SOX9 transcription factor, associated with a form of dwarfism, camptomelic dysplasia. Mutations of *DHH* cause XY gonadal dysgenesis, associated with peripheral neuropathy.

Other 46,XY patients with absent gonads have various degrees of sexual ambiguity and no müllerian derivatives. The implication that some testicular tissue was functional at least up to 10 weeks and subsequently regressed led to the name *fetal testicular regression syndrome.* Testicular regression may occur in late pregnancy or even postnatally; these fully virilized male patients have isolated anorchia.

Vaginal Atresia

Mutation of *WNT4* affects development of müllerian structures but permits normal ovarian development, thus causing vaginal atresia and uterine abnormalities. This disorder is termed *Mayer-Rokitansky-Kuster-Hauser syndrome.*

True Hermaphroditism

True hermaphroditism, a rare and usually sporadic disorder, is defined as the coexistence of seminiferous tubules and ovarian follicles in the same subject. Most patients have an ovotestis with either an ovary or a testis on the opposite side; a gonad in the scrotum is usually a testis but may be an ovotestis.

The genitalia are usually ambiguous, but they may appear completely masculine or feminine. The anatomy of the internal reproductive tract depends on the nature of the gonads, particularly whether they secrete AMH. A uterus or uterine horn is present in approximately 90% of cases. Testosterone response to hCG is variable, and AMH levels are usually low. Most patients experience breast development, ovulation, and even menstruation at puberty; pregnancy and successful childbirth are possible if selective removal of testicular tissue is feasible. Unless gender has already been assigned, male orientation should be restricted to patients with no uterus and descended testicular tissue because testicular tissue is usually dysgenetic and prone to malignant degeneration. Most true hermaphrodites have a 46,XX karyotype. Despite the presence of testicular tissue, true hermaphrodites usually lack SRY, a finding suggesting that the condition, at least in familial cases, is the result of constitutive activation of a gene normally triggered by SRY.

MANAGEMENT OF INTERSEX INDIVIDUALS: GENDER ROLE AND IDENTITY

The influence of prenatal sex steroid exposure on personality is controversial. In considering this question, it is important to distinguish among gender role, sexual orientation, and gender identity.

Gender Role

Gender role refers to gender-stereotyped behaviors such as choice of play toys by young children. For example, parents of young girls with CAH often report that their daughters prefer to play with trucks as compared with dolls and tend to be tomboyish later in childhood. Decreased interest in maternal behavior, beginning with infrequent doll play in early childhood and extending in older girls and women to lack of interest in childrearing, occurs frequently.

Sexual Orientation

Sexual orientation refers to homosexual versus heterosexual preferences. In many studies, small but significant percentages of women with CAH have been actively homosexual or bisexual or have an increased tendency to homoerotic fantasies. These characteristics occur more frequently in women with the salt-wasting form of 21-hydroxylase deficiency.

Gender Identity

Gender identity refers to self-identification as male or female. Spontaneous gender reassignment back to male has been reported in cases of male patients with penile trauma or exstrophy of the bladder who were raised as girls. Gender reassignment may also occur in male pseudohermaphrodites raised as girls, especially in cases of 5α-reductase or 17-

ketosteroid reductase deficiencies, in which the brain may be exposed to high circulating levels of androgens. Conversely, female-to-male transsexuals may have relatively high levels of androgens and a high incidence of polycystic ovary syndrome. However, self-reassignment to the male gender is unusual in women with CAH. When it occurs, it may be related to delays in gender assignment or genital surgery or to inadequate suppression of adrenal androgens with glucocorticoid therapy. Severely virilized girls are more likely to be raised as boys in cultures that value boys more highly and/or in developing countries in which the diagnosis is likely to be delayed. Few studies have directly compared psychosexual functioning in severely virilized genetic female patients with CAH who were raised as girls or boys, but it does not appear that those raised as boys are psychologically better adjusted than those raised as girls. The role of external genital anatomy before and after genital surgery in causing problems relating to gender identity is unclear compared with the roles of prenatal hormone exposure, rearing by the family, and community attitudes.

Diagnosis

Management of the child born with ambiguous genitalia presents a difficult challenge to medical personnel. It is important to refrain from assigning the sex until diagnostic information can be gathered. Usually, test results can be obtained within 24 to 48 hours, and parents can be advised about the child's chromosomal and gonadal sex and about the anatomy of internal sexual structures.

In addition, the physician must keep in mind that intersex conditions may be associated with life-threatening biochemical or anatomic abnormalities. In particular, the most common cause of severely masculinized external genitalia in female patients, the salt-wasting form of CAH resulting from steroid 21-hydroxylase deficiency, may cause hyponatremia, hyperkalemia, hypovolemia, and shock. In contrast, male patients with ambiguous genitalia may have lipoid adrenal hyperplasia or a salt-wasting form of HSD3B2 deficiency. Males with micropenis may have panhypopituitarism, in which case they are at risk of significant hypoglycemia resulting from low cortisol (because of low ACTH) and low growth hormone levels, or they may have congenital adrenal *hypo*plasia, in which case they could have adrenal insufficiency. Finally, patients with ambiguous genitalia are at increased risk of renal anomalies, or they may have chromosomal syndromes with other associated anomalies.

History

The gestational history should concentrate on potential exposure to agents that could interfere with normal sexual differentiation. For a female infant with virilized genitalia, these include progestational agents, whereas the mother of a male with incompletely masculinized genitalia may have been exposed to a 5α-reductase inhibitor through her husband's use of such an agent for alopecia or prostate enlargement. It should be determined whether amniocentesis and karyotype have been performed. A family history should elicit similar cases of genital ambiguity or cases of sudden death, which could raise suspicion of undiagnosed salt-wasting CAH.

PHYSICAL EXAMINATION. The physical examination should document the size of the phallus (clitoris or penis), the degree of chordee (ventral bowing of the phallus), and the extent of fusion of the labioscrotal folds. The urethral meatus should be identified, and there must be careful palpation for gonads in the inguinal canals and labia or scrotum. Bilateral cryptorchidism, even if an isolated finding in a phenotypic male patient, should always engender evaluation for a possible intersex condition. Vital signs and other anatomic anomalies (if present) should be documented.

Rapid Diagnostic Tests

In many centers, fluorescence in situ hybridization of interphase nuclei using sex chromosome–specific probes can be obtained within 24 hours. This technique accurately counts sex chromosomes, although it cannot detect translocations or some chromosomal fragments; these require a full karyotype on metaphase chromosomes. If a reliable operator is available, a pelvic and abdominal sonogram can be performed in the first 1 to 2 days of life. This will detect the kidneys and a uterus, if present; it may also locate the gonads and determine the size of the adrenal glands. A magnetic resonance imaging scan of the abdomen is a more expensive alternative that requires sedation of the patient. A radiologic dye study is often performed subsequently to define the internal genitourinary anatomy further.

At this point, the chromosomal sex and gonadal sex of the child are usually clear even before the fluorescence in situ hybridization results are available. If gonads are palpable, it is very likely that the child is genetically male, whereas demonstrating a uterus by sonography means that the child is probably female. However, these tests usually do not identify the cause of the intersex condition, and this requires further biochemical evaluation.

Biochemical Evaluation of the Virilized Female

At the least, diagnostic tests should include measurement of basal serum 17-hydroxyprogesterone, androstenedione, and testosterone. Preferably, a complete profile of adrenocortical hormones is obtained before and 1 hour after stimulation of the adrenal cortex with 125 to 250 μg of cosyntropin ($ACTH_{1-24}$). These assays should be deferred past the first 24 hours of life. They will identify potential defects in adrenal steroidogenesis (i.e., CAH); 21-hydroxylase deficiency is identified by elevations in 17-hydroxyprogesterone, whereas 11-deoxycortisol and 11-deoxycorticosterone are high in 11β-hydroxylase deficiency.

After testing is completed, the child's vital signs should be monitored for any indication of adrenal crisis. It is rare for salt-wasting crisis to occur before 7 days of life, but many clinicians obtain electrolyte measurements to assess hyponatremia and hyperkalemia in CAH-affected newborns during the first week. Plasma renin activity and aldosterone are elevated in many normal infants and do not usually add much useful information within the first days of life.

Biochemical Evaluation of the Undervirilized Male

In intersex males, it is necessary to test adrenal and gonadal function as well as extragonadal androgen metabolism. With regard to adrenal defects, 11-deoxycorticosterone and the ratio of pregnenolone to 17-hydroxypregnenolone are high in 17α-hydroxylase deficiency; 17-hydroxypregnenolone and DHEA are high in HSD3B2 deficiency, and all steroids are low in lipoid hyperplasia.

Defects in gonadal steroidogenesis are best evaluated after stimulation with hCG (1500 IU intramuscularly on days 1, 3, and 5, with blood drawn on day 6). However, 17-hydroxylase and HSD3B2 deficiencies affect both the gonads and the adrenal cortex and thus are often diagnosed by cosyntropin stimulation testing. Low levels of all androgen precursors suggests 17α-hydroxylase/17,20 lyase deficiency or a generalized defect in testicular function such as the vanishing testis syndrome or gonadotropin insensitivity. A high ratio of androstenedione to testosterone is indicative of 17-ketosteroid reductase (also called HSD17B) deficiency, and a high ratio of testosterone to dihydrotestosterone is diagnostic of 5α-reductase deficiency. The diagnosis of androgen insensitivity syndrome is suspected when a 46,XY patient has ambiguous or female-appearing external genitalia despite normal or high circulating levels of testosterone and dihydrotestosterone.

Patients with micropenis rarely have defects in steroid biosynthesis, but instead they often have low levels of gonadotropins (i.e., hypogonadotropic hypogonadism). Because gonadotropins are usually higher in neonates than in older children, these levels can be measured directly. If they are low, or if there is any history of hypoglycemia, pituitary function should be completely evaluated by measuring thyroid-stimulating hormone and thyroxine, as well as cortisol, in a random blood sample (ACTH may also be measured, but it often takes longer for results to be returned). If the cortisol level is equivocal, a low-dose (1 μg/1.73 M^2) cosyntropin stimulation test may be performed. This test differs from the cosyntropin stimulation test used to diagnose adrenal steroidogenic defects by using a more physiologic dose of cosyntropin that can detect mild atrophy of the adrenal cortex resulting from chronic deficiency of ACTH. Growth hormone cannot be measured accurately in random blood samples unless the patient is hypoglycemic, but levels of insulin-like growth factor-I (IGF-I) and IGF-binding protein 3 are readily measured surrogates; growth hormone can be measured after appropriate stimulation if suspicion of growth hormone deficiency is high. Any patient with suspected hypopituitarism should have magnetic resonance imaging of the head and an ophthalmologic examination to look for associated abnormal development of the optic nerves (septo-optic dysplasia). Patients with hypogonadotropic hypogonadism should have normal testicular function documented with an hCG stimulation test.

Gonadal Biopsies

Patients with mixed gonadal dysgenesis, true hermaphroditism, or unclear diagnoses should undergo bilateral gonadal biopsies (the two gonads often are not identical in their histology). Dysgenetic gonads have a high potential for malignant transformation and will usually need to be removed in childhood.

Treatment

Initial Medical Management

Patients with CAH resulting from 21-hydroxylase or HSD3B2 deficiencies, or lipoid hyperplasia, require replacement of both glucocorticoids and mineralocorticoids, usually with hydrocortisone (15 to 20 mg/M^2/day in divided doses) and fludrocortisone (usually 0.1 mg/day, but as much as 0.4 mg/day in neonates with salt-wasting crises), respectively. Neonates with severe salt losing may require sodium chloride supplementation (≤8 mEq/kg/day). Patients with 11β-hydroxylase or 17α-hydroxylase deficiencies have normal aldosterone biosynthesis and require only glucocorticoids. Patients with panhypopituitarism usually require treatment with hydrocortisone, thyroxine, and growth hormone.

All male infants with ambiguous genitalia or micropenis in whom rearing as a boy is contemplated should have a 3-month therapeutic trial of monthly depot testosterone injections (25 mg) to attempt to increase the size of the phallus during infancy. This treatment may improve social acceptability of the genitalia later in childhood and adolescence and/or may make reconstructive surgery easier. In cases of suspected partial androgen insensitivity, this treatment will also document the degree to which the patient is androgen responsive and thus may provide useful information on whether rearing as a boy is feasible. Higher doses of testosterone (75 mg every 4 weeks) may be used under these circumstances.

Considerations for Sex Assignment

In large medical centers, a team consisting of a neonatologist, a pediatric endocrinologist, a urologist, and preferably an experienced social worker and/or child psychiatrist should promptly review the early diagnostic data and should make a recommendation to the family as to the sex of rearing and any medical and/or surgical treatments. These recommendations should be based on both current knowledge of psychosexual development in intersex individuals and the feasibility of surgical correction (see later).

Adequate time in a private room must be allotted for this discussion; the relevant biologic concepts are complex for most laypersons, and the topic is emotionally fraught. With the ready availability of fetal sonography and/or chorionic villus sampling, many parents may have had expectations of several months' duration regarding the sex of their child, and they may have bought sex-specific clothing or nursery decorations, may have settled on a name, and may have imparted this information to grandparents and other relatives and friends. These matters should be ascertained by the physician early in the discussion and sympathetically addressed. In cases not diagnosed neonatally, changing the sex of rearing becomes progressively more difficult with age. It should be attempted only with extreme caution in children who are more than a few months old.

In general, the recommended sex assignment should be that of the genetic/gonadal sex, if for no other reason than to retain the possibility of reproductive function. This is especially true for female infants with CAH who have normal internal genital structures and a potential for childbearing. An exception to this may be considered in the genetically female infant with completely male-appearing genitalia, especially if the child has been raised as a boy for more than a few months. Such children will need to be castrated at puberty to avoid feminization.

Conversely, genetic male infants with completely female-appearing external genitalia (usually resulting from complete androgen insensitivity syndrome but also seen with severe testosterone biosynthetic defects) should be raised as female because the potential for reconstruction of male genitalia is poor. They, too, need to be castrated by early adulthood to avoid malignant transformation of the testes. However, male infants with 17-ketosteroid reductase or 5α-reductase deficiency should usually be reared as boys because they have normal levels of androstenedione or testosterone, respectively, and often virilize significantly at puberty. Indeed, many of these patients reassign themselves to the male gender when they are made aware of the diagnosis. The same considerations pertain to male patients with normal testosterone biosynthesis who have penile trauma or anatomic abnormalities such as bladder exstrophy.

Moreover, recommendations for sex assignment are to some extent culture specific. In cultures that value infant boys over girls, parents may strongly resist rearing a female infant with ambiguous genitalia as a girl, and many girls with severely virilized external genitalia will be raised as boys.

Corrective Surgery

Surgery for Ambiguous Genitalia

Whether, how, and when to intervene surgically in the correction of genital anomalies is the subject of continuing debate. Some adult patients with intersex conditions have been unhappy with their gender assignment or surgical outcome. They, as well as some physicians, have advocated postponing genital surgery until the affected individual is able to provide informed consent for cosmetic genital surgery, thus keeping all options open if the adult patient wishes to function sexually with abnormal genitalia that have sensation undiminished by surgery or to reassign his or her gender. Declining or postponing surgery should not be confused with raising the child with an indeterminate gender, a concept currently well outside the mainstream. The option of deferring surgery should always be presented as part of the informed consent process. Nevertheless, most parents want their child to look as "normal" as possible, and they often resist suggestions to postpone corrective surgery.

In addressing this question, it is best to consider the various general types of genital surgery separately. The greatest change in practice over the past few decades has probably been with male infants with ambiguous (but not completely female) external genitalia. Physicians are now far less likely to assign such patients to a female sex of rearing because it is now recognized that many of these patients will reassign themselves as male at puberty. Thus, the ambiguous genitalia in such patients should rarely be "corrected" to female. On the contrary, surgical techniques for hypospadias repair have advanced significantly, and reconstruction of male genitalia is attempted more often, particularly if the infant responds to a course of testosterone with significant phallic growth.

Surgery for female infants with ambiguous genitalia may need to address both an enlarged clitoris and the lack of a vaginal introitus, as well as the presence of a urogenital sinus. The clitoris is normally prominent in many infant girls. Even when enlarged in a girl with virilizing CAH, the clitoris can be prevented from growing larger with adequate suppression of adrenal androgens by glucocorticoids, and it will become less prominent as the patient grows. Thus, mild to moderate clitorimegaly is often best managed without surgery. When attempted, clitoroplasty must be approached keeping in mind the important role of clitoral sensation in the female sexual response. Such surgery must be performed only by experienced operators with scrupulous attention to preservation of clitoral innervation.

Consensus is still lacking regarding the best age for vaginoplasty. Although many surgeons advocate a first procedure in infancy, it is difficult to maintain a functionally adequate introitus in the absence of estrogen exposure and mechanical dilation (with dilators or through sexual intercourse), and many patients require reoperation as young adults.

There is a dearth of large longitudinal studies comparing outcomes in patients who have had early genital surgery versus those who have had no surgery or surgery in adolescence. According to self-assessment surveys among sexually active women with CAH who have had genital surgery, most are able to have satisfactory sexual intercourse. As surgical and medical treatment regimens have improved in recent years, more women with CAH have successfully conceived spontaneously, completed pregnancies, and given birth. Most often, delivery is by cesarean section because of an inadequate introitus, but vaginal delivery is possible in some cases.

Rx

Hypospadias repair is usually begun in the first year of life, after testosterone treatment (if necessary to increase phallic size). Depending on the degree of hypospadias, more than one surgical procedure may be required.

Removal of Intra-abdominal Testes in Male Pseudohermaphrodites

Intra-abdominal testes are at increasing risk of malignant transformation with time. In a boy with cryptorchidism who is being reared as male, orchidopexy should be performed as quickly as possible; this will also maximize the possibility of fertility when the underlying condition does not preclude it. Dysgenetic gonads that cannot be brought into the scrotum should be removed soon after diagnosis because the risk of malignant transformation in childhood is relatively high.

There is a lack of consensus regarding non-dysgenetic testes in severely undervirilized genetic male infants in whom a female sex of rearing is planned. In patients with complete androgen insensitivity or complete defects in testosterone biosynthesis, no possibility of fertility exists, and so there would seem to be no reason to retain the testes. Conversely, the risk of malignant transformation in such gonads is low before puberty, and patients with complete androgen insensitivity can undergo spontaneous breast development at puberty. Then, patients themselves can assent or consent to gonadectomy, which may usually be accomplished laparoscopically. This is of particular importance in genetic male patients with partial androgen insensitivity or incomplete defects of testosterone biosynthesis, because such patients may eventually desire a male gender role.

Patients with PMDS have a reduced but still appreciable potential for fertility, and virilization is unaffected. Thus, the testes should be removed only if they cannot be brought into the scrotum. Because the müllerian and wolffian structures are closely approximated in these patients, surgical excision of the uterus and fallopian tubes may result in ischemic and/or traumatic damage to the vasa deferentia and testes, and thus salpingectomy and hysterectomy are indicated only in patients whose müllerian structures limit intrascrotal placement of the testes.

Prenatal Diagnosis and Treatment

Many conditions causing ambiguous genitalia can be detected by karyotyping of chorionic villus samples (for chromosomal abnormalities) or by direct molecular genetic testing. In most cases, this information is useful only for counseling purposes. In the case of virilizing forms of CAH (particularly 21-hydroxylase deficiency), the mother of an affected female fetus can take dexamethasone (20 μg/kg/day), which can cross the placenta and suppress the fetal adrenal gland, thus reducing secretion of androgens and ameliorating virilization of the external genitalia. To be most effective, this treatment should be started by the sixth week of gestation, before the sex or genotype of the fetus is known. Thus, seven of eight pregnancies known to be at risk will be unnecessarily treated until chorionic villus sampling can be performed. Although effective in reducing prenatal virilization, this dose of dexamethasone can cause Cushing's syndrome in the mother, and the long-term sequelae of this treatment in the fetus are not known. Therefore, many endocrinologists believe that this treatment should be used only under approved research protocols that allow for case registries and long-term follow-up.

Psychosocial Support

Families of intersex patients should be assessed for emotional health, initially by the pediatrician and/or pediatric endocrinologist. Parents should be offered psychological counseling soon after the diagnosis is made. Intermittent assessment of family functioning may be a useful tool in predicting future problems. Children should, as they mature, be repeatedly informed about their condition by parents and physicians in a sensitive and age-appropriate manner. When psychotherapy is undertaken, medical and psychiatric caregivers should maintain communication so both are aware of the patient's and family's status. Unfortunately, many locales lack mental health professionals with experience in counseling patients and families with intersex conditions.

To minimize feelings of self-consciousness or embarrassment associated with genital abnormalities, follow-up examinations of genitalia in patients past infancy should be limited to those that are medically indicated. Demonstrations of physical findings to large audiences on hospital rounds should be avoided.

Although psychosexual development of intersex individuals cannot be predicted with confidence, patients' families should receive anticipatory counseling. For example, counseling of parents of girls affected with CAH should initially address the high likelihood that such girls will exhibit tomboyish behavior, masculine play preferences, and perhaps, when older, a preference for a career over domestic activities. In the contemporary United States, these preferences usually have a high degree of social acceptance. Parents should also be told that most (but not all) girls with CAH function heterosexually, although they may require repeated genital surgical procedures to have satisfactory sexual intercourse. The endocrinologist and/or mental health professional (depending on inclination and experience) caring for the adolescent girl with CAH should address sexual orientation, both fantasized and actual. Health care professionals should accept that a few women with CAH may be most comfortable as homosexuals and that such individuals should be helped to come to terms with their situation. Adult patients should also be made aware of relevant patient advocacy groups.

SUGGESTED READINGS

Bondy CA, Turner syndrome study group: Care of girls and women with Turner syndrome: A guideline of the Turner syndrome study group. J Clin Endocrinol Metab 2007;92:10–25. *Clinical review.*

Hughes IA, Deeb A: Androgen resistance. Best Pract Res Clin Endocrinol Metab 2006;20:577–598. *Comprehensive review.*

Merke DP, Bornstein SR: Congenital adrenal hyperplasia. Lancet 2005;365: 2125–2136. *Comprehensive review.*

Wilhelm D, Palmer S, Koopman P: Sex determination and gonadal development in mammals. Physiol Rev 2007;87:1–28. *The developmental biology of the reproductive organs.*

253 THE TESTIS AND MALE SEXUAL FUNCTION

Ronald S. Swerdloff and Christina Wang

The testis is a bifunctional organ serving as the site of sex steroid (i.e., testosterone) synthesis and sperm production in the male. Thus, the testis controls both sexuality and the perpetuity of the species (fertility). In addition, androgens and their metabolites (including estrogens) serve essential metabolic roles and may be important inducers and effectors of brain function in men. The discussion in this chapter focuses on male reproductive physiology and its disorders: androgen deficiency, sexual dysfunction, infertility, and androgen excess states.

PHYSIOLOGY

The male reproductive axis consists of six main components: (1) extrahypothalamic central nervous system (CNS), (2) hypothalamus, (3) pituitary, (4) testes, (5) sex steroid–sensitive end organs, and (6) sites of androgen transport and metabolism (Fig. 253–1). The components of this system function in an integrative fashion to control the concentrations of circulating gonadal steroids required for normal male sexual development and function; for androgen- and estrogen-mediated metabolic effects on critical end organs such as brain, bone, muscle, liver, skin, and bone marrow; and for immune systems. The reproductive axis is also responsible for normal germ cell maturation and sperm transport necessary for male fertility.

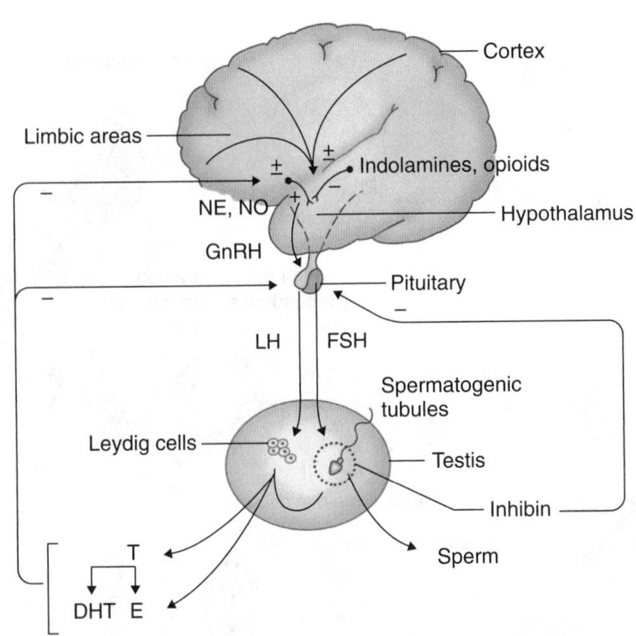

FIGURE 253–1 • The hypothalamic-pituitary-gonadal axis in the male. DHT = dihydrotestosterone; E = estrogen; FSH = follicle-stimulating hormone; GnRH = gonadotropin-releasing hormone; LH = luteinizing hormone; NE = norepinephrine; NO = nitric oxide; T = testosterone.

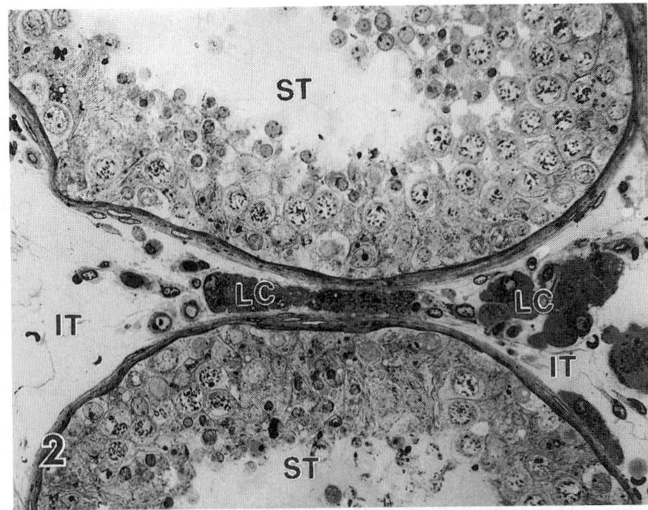

FIGURE 253–2 • Testis. Light micrograph of the glutaraldehyde-fixed, epoxy-embedded testicular section from a normal man showing seminiferous tubules (ST) and interstitium (IT). The seminiferous tubules contain Sertoli cells and germ cells at various phases of maturation. The interstitium consists of Leydig cells (LC), blood vessels, and lymphatic space.

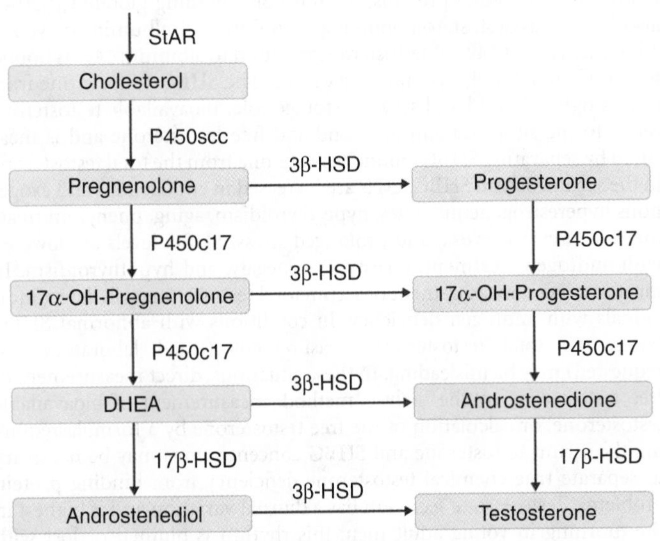

FIGURE 253–3 • The steroid acute regulatory (StAR) protein mobilizes cholesterol from cellular stores to the mitochondria. Intratesticular steroidogenic pathways for synthesis of testosterone. Although both the Δ^5 (left) and Δ^4 (right) pathways exist, the Δ^5 pathway predominates in the testis. DHEA = dehydroepiandrosterone; HSD = hydroxysteroid dehydrogenase.

Hypothalamic Pituitary Function

The hypothalamus is the principal integrative unit responsible for the normal pulsatile secretion of gonadotropin-releasing hormone (GnRH), which is delivered through the hypothalamic-hypophyseal portal blood system to the pituitary gland (Chapter 241). Although GnRH has been identified in many areas of the CNS, it is most concentrated in the medial basal, arcuate, and suprachiasmatic nuclei in the hypothalamus and travels by axonomic flow to the axon terminals of the median eminence. The pulsatile release of GnRH provides the signals for the timing of the release of luteinizing hormone (LH) and follicle-stimulating hormone (FSH), which in normal circumstances occurs approximately every 60 to 90 minutes. The secretion of GnRH is regulated in a complex fashion by neuronal input from higher cognitive and sensory centers and by circulating levels of sex steroids and peptide hormones such as prolactin and leptin. The local effectors of GnRH synthesis and release include a number of neuropeptides (galanin-like peptide, kisspeptins, neuropeptide Y, vasoactive intestinal peptide, corticotropin-releasing peptide), catecholamines, indolamines, nitric oxide and excitatory amino acids, γ-aminobutyric acid, and dopamine. Testosterone either directly or through its metabolic products (i.e., estradiol and dihydrotestosterone) has inhibitory effects on the secretion and release of GnRH as well as direct inhibitory effects on secretion and release of LH and FSH. Prolactin is a potent inhibitor of GnRH secretion, thus explaining its role in inhibiting LH and testosterone secretion in conditions of hyperprolactinemia.

LH and FSH are glycopeptides consisting of two subunits (α and β). They share the same α subunit, with specificity endowed by the β subunit. The heterodimer is required for biologic activity; the subunits can be detected in serum and may be increased in certain pathologic conditions (e.g., α subunit elevations in gonadotropin-secreting pituitary adenomas). LH and FSH are synthesized in the same pituitary cell (gonadotrophs) and secreted in a pulsatile pattern. The clearance of these two gonadotrophic hormones differs, with LH having a shorter half-life than FSH. LH and FSH are secreted in a pulsatile pattern regulated by GnRH pulse generator in the hypothalamus. Puberty is heralded by nighttime pulsatile serum patterns before obvious increases are noted in the daytime. Feedback regulation of LH and FSH secretion also occurs at the pituitary, with testosterone, dihydrotestosterone (DHT), and estrogens inhibiting the synthesis or release of both gonadotropins. Circulating testicular peptide products of the Sertoli cell (i.e., inhibin) also produce selective inhibition of FSH. LH and FSH circulate unbound to carrier proteins and act predominantly through specific cell surface receptors on the Leydig and Sertoli cells of the testes, respectively.

Testis Function

The testis is a complex organ consisting of (1) seminiferous tubules containing Sertoli cells and germ cells in various stages of maturation and (2) the interstitium, where the steroid-secreting cells (Leydig), macrophages, myoid cells, and blood vessels reside (Fig. 253–2). The Leydig cells synthesize steroid hormones under the regulation of LH. The LH receptors on the cell surface of the Leydig cells lead to G protein/cyclic adenosine monophosphate–mediated events. This process involves a steroid acute regulatory (StAR) protein essential for steroidogenesis in the gonads and adrenal glands (Fig. 253–3).

TESTOSTERONE SYNTHESIS. Testosterone is the principal male hormone secreted by the testes; about 7 mg is produced per day in adult men. Testosterone synthesis occurs in the human testes through either the Δ^4 or the Δ^5 pathway (see Fig. 253–3); the Δ^5 pathway is predominant. The enzymatic rate-limiting step in the process is the LH-inducible StAR

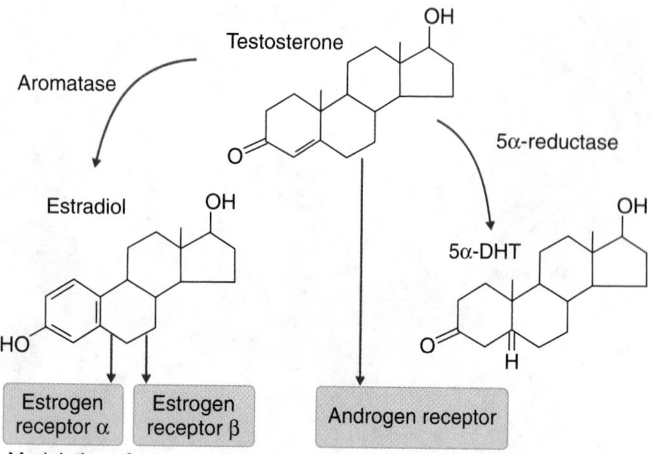

FIGURE 253–4 • Testosterone action is mediated directly (androgen receptor), after conversion to estradiol (estrogen receptor α or β), or after conversion to DHT (androgen receptor). (From Kuiper GCJM, Carlquist M, Gustafsson JA: Estrogen is a male and female hormone. Sci Med 1998;5:36–45; with permission.)

protein and the conversion of cholesterol to pregnenolone by the cholesterol side-chain cleavage enzyme P450SCC.

TESTOSTERONE TRANSPORT IN BLOOD. Testosterone circulates mainly bound to two plasma proteins, sex hormone–binding globulin (SHBG; also known as testosterone-binding globulin) and albumin. In young adult men, about 54% of testosterone is bound to albumin, 44% is bound to SHBG, and 2 to 3% is unbound or free. The SHBG-testosterone fraction is tightly bound and serves a storage role. Bioavailable testosterone refers to the sum of albumin-bound and free testosterone and is measured by separating SHBG-bound testosterone from the total testosterone in the serum. Serum SHBG levels are increased in endogenous and exogenous hyperestrogenemic states, hyperthyroidism, aging, phenytoin treatment, anorexia nervosa, and prolonged stress. SHBG levels are lowered with androgen treatment, obesity, acromegaly, and hypothyroidism. In most instances, measurement of serum total testosterone will detect individuals with androgen deficiency. In conditions with abnormal SHBG levels, the total testosterone measurement (usual laboratory test requested) may be misleading. In these situations, direct measurement of free testosterone by the dialysis method, measurement of bioavailable testosterone, or calculation of the free testosterone by a formula requiring the serum testosterone and SHBG concentrations may be necessary to separate true chemical testosterone deficiency from binding protein problems. Testosterone secretion has a diurnal variation and is highest in the morning in young adult men; this rhythm is blunted or lost with aging.

TESTOSTERONE ACTION. Testosterone exerts its effects at different end organs either through direct action or after conversion to an active metabolite such as DHT by 5α-reductase or estradiol by the aromatase enzyme (Fig. 253–4). Thus, testosterone can act as an androgenic hormone or as a precursor for DHT with effects mediated by the intracellular androgen receptor. Different tissues may also have coactivators or coinhibitors that modify the action of the androgen-receptor complex, providing tissue selectivity. Testosterone can also serve as a precursor for estradiol in some tissues, and subsequently, after conversion, estrogen binds the estrogen receptors (α or β) to induce its effects. Various end organs differ in their 5α-reductase and aromatase activity and in their requirements for conversion of testosterone to DHT for androgenic activity. Congenital and acquired defects in these two enzymes as well as in the estrogen and androgen receptors result in distinct syndromes with characteristic phenotypes (Chapter 252).

SPERMATOGENESIS. The spermatogenic compartment consists of the Sertoli and germ cells and is intimately interactive with the interstitial compartment (Fig. 253–5). The Sertoli cells bridge the entire space between the basement membrane and the lumen of the tubules (see Fig. 253–2). They are the target of androgenic and FSH stimulation of spermatogenesis and also the source of a multitude of paracrine regulators of spermatogenesis (e.g., inhibin, activin, growth factors, cytokines).

Germ cell maturation is dependent on the proper hormonal (FSH) and paracrine (testosterone) milieu for proliferation to occur. Not all germ

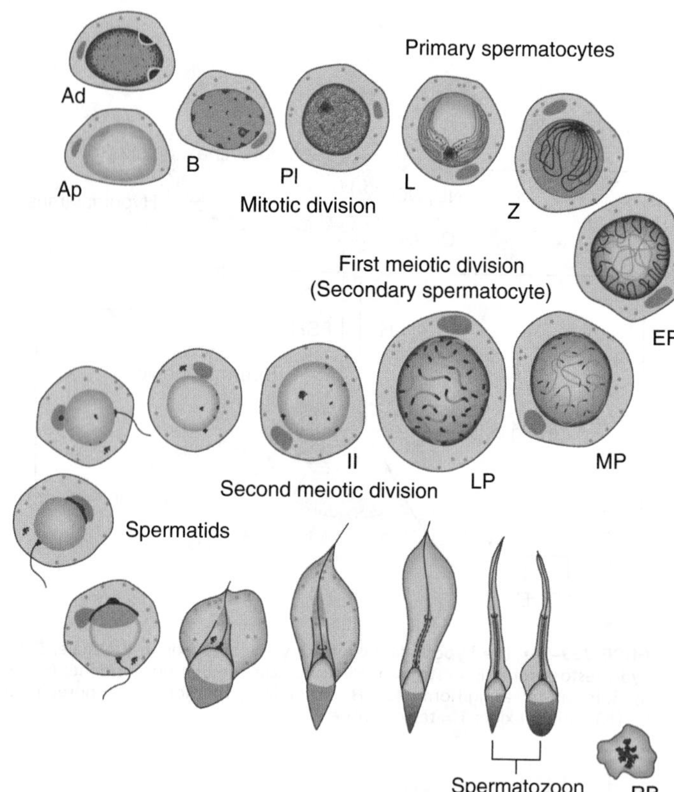

FIGURE 253–5 • Stages of human spermatogenesis. (From Hermo L, Clemont Y: How are germ cells produced and what factors control their production? *In* Robaine B, Pryor J, Trasler J [eds]: Handbook of Andrology. New York, American Society of Andrology, 1995, pp 13–15.)

cells reach maturity. Spontaneous death of certain germ cells is a constant feature of germ cell homeostasis. In fact, considerable data indicate that major effects of both testosterone and FSH are to limit the amount of germ cell death (apoptosis).

SPERM TRANSPORT. After spermatogenesis is completed, mature spermatozoa are released into the excretory system and travel through the rete testes and epididymis, where they functionally mature before traversing the vas deferens. The semen gains constituents from the seminal vesicles, prostate, and bulbourethral glands before ejaculation.

Normal Sexual Function and Erectile Physiology

Normal sexual function in men requires normal sexual desire (libido) and erectile, ejaculatory, and orgasmic capacity. The process is complex, involving cognitive, sensory, hormonal, autonomic neuronal, and penile vascular integrative actions for normal function. Defects occur at multiple levels. Although considerable progress has occurred in the past few years in therapeutic options, an understanding of the normal physiology is essential for proper assessment and treatment of men with sexual dysfunction.

The brain is the integrative center of the sexual response system. It processes sensory input, stored fantasy information, purposeful thoughts, spontaneous nocturnal reflex activity, and hormonal signals (e.g., testosterone) to create the hypothalamic neuronal message that traverses the spinal cord to the thoracic 9–12 sympathetic and sacral parasympathetic outflow tracts. The nonadrenergic, noncholinergic autonomic plexus nerves initiate vasodilation of the cavernosal arterial and corpora cavernosal sinusoids of the penis through release of local vasodilators such as nitric oxide and vasoactive intestinal peptide from the vascular endothelium and the smooth muscle cells of the sinusoids (Fig. 253–6). A family of enzymes (nitric oxide synthetases) regulates nitric oxide synthesis, which produces smooth muscle dilation through activation of cyclic guanosine monophosphate (cGMP) and modification of calcium flux. The cGMP levels are rapidly reversible through inactivation by phosphodiesterase. The neurogenic mechanisms leading to vasodilation of the cavernosal arterioles and sinusoids lead to a rapid increase in penile blood flow and expansion of the vascular channels; this, in turn, inhibits venous return through compression of the venous channels against the tunica albuginea and limits drainage of the obliquely penetrating veins. After orgasm, detumescence occurs owing to less vasodilatory (nitric oxide) and greater vasoconstrictive (α_2-adrenergic, endothelins) signals.

Testosterone seems to have its primary effect on erectile function by enhancing libido with secondary effects on penile nitric oxide synthase activity. Sexual desire and fantasy are highly sensitive to testosterone, thus explaining the preservation of erectile capacity in many men with partial androgen deficiency. In contrast, erectile dysfunction is common in older men despite normal serum testosterone levels; this effect appears to be the result of impaired penile vasodilatory capacity. This is often reversible through local (intracavernosal or transurethral) administration of potent vasodilators (prostaglandins, papaverine, and phentolamine) or by oral administration of penile-selective phosphodiesterase-5 inhibitors (i.e., sildenafil, vardenafil, and tadalafil). Combined androgen deficiency with decreased libido and decreased penile responsiveness due to impaired nitric oxide synthase activity may be common in elderly men. With the availability of effective penile vasodilatory medications to ensure erectile capacity, complaints of diminished libido may be effectively treated with androgen supplementation.

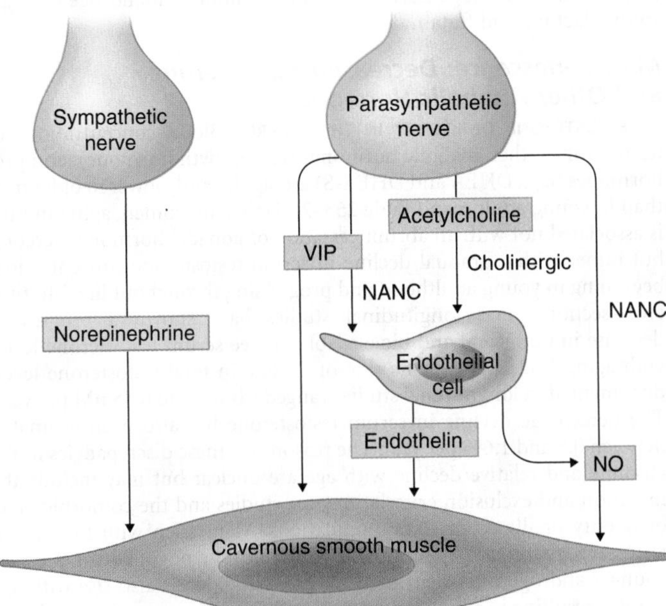

FIGURE 253–6 • The interaction among cholinergic, adrenergic, and nonadrenergic, noncholinergic (NANC) neuronal pathways and their contribution to penile smooth muscle contraction (patterned arrows) and dilation (open arrows). NO = nitric oxide; VIP = vasoactive intestinal polypeptide. (From Lue TF: Physiology of penile erection and pathophysiology of erectile dysfunction and priapism. *In* Walsh P, Retick A, Vaughn E, Wein A [eds]: Campbell's Urology, 7th ed. Philadelphia, WB Saunders, 1998, p 1164.)

Physiology in Development and Aging

Reproductive Axis during Fetal Development, Childhood, and Puberty

SEXUAL DIFFERENTIATION IN THE FETUS. Normal male sexual differentiation is complex and includes the establishment of genetic and phenotypic sex (Chapter 252).

ADRENARCHE AND PUBERTY. Adrenarche occurs at about 7 or 8 years of age when the zona reticularis of the adrenal gland undergoes maturation, leading to increased secretion of androgen precursors, such as androstenedione, dehydroepiandrosterone (DHEA), and DHEA sulfate (DHEA-S). Although the physiologic events initiating adrenarche are incompletely understood, the process is probably under the control of adrenocorticotropic hormone and independent of the control of LH and FSH. Adrenarche usually heralds subsequent activity in the hypothalamic-pituitary-gonadal axis. Androstenedione and DHEA are technically androgenic prehormones and do not bind to the androgen receptor. In part, the prepubertal growth spurt and the early development of pubic and axillary hair are mediated by conversion of these precursors to testosterone and DHT at the peripheral tissue sites.

Puberty occurs when a hypothalamic clock is activated, resulting in increased GnRH and gonadotropin secretion. In the interval before the onset of puberty, LH and FSH are secreted in low amounts and are subject to feedback control by the small amounts of circulating testosterone from the testes. Initiation of puberty is determined by increase in the pulsatile pattern of hypothalamic GnRH secretion. This is marked by nocturnal bursts of LH secretion when puberty begins. As puberty progresses, feedback sensitivity of the hypothalamus and pituitary to circulating steroids lessens, and increasing concentrations of both gonadotropins and gonadal steroids ensue. The increasing concentrations of intratesticular testosterone and circulating FSH stimulate the Sertoli cell to produce factors leading to the maturation of spermatogenesis and inhibition of germ cell apoptosis. The phenotypic equivalents of the hormonal changes in puberty have been well documented. Pediatricians and endocrinologists routinely perform staging of the genital and pubic hair development (Table 253–1). The majority of the extratesticular end-organ events of puberty are secondary to the increased circulating levels of testosterone and its metabolic products (DHT and estradiol). The penis and scrotum grow and become pigmented. As spermatogenesis advances, the testes increase in size from 1 to 2 mL at the outset of puberty to 15 to 35 mL in adulthood. There is a progressive increase in facial, axillary, chest, abdominal, thigh, and pubic hair; frontal scalp hair regresses, and the voice deepens (Fig. 253–7). Genital and sexual hair development as well as temporal scalp hair regression requires conversion of testosterone to DHT for its full effects.

ABERRATIONS OF TIMING OF PUBERTY. Delayed puberty in boys is usually defined as a temporary (physiologic) form of hypothalamic hypogonadotropic hypogonadism in which sexual development has not begun by the age of 13.5 years. These children usually have a height age (the age that is representative for 50% of normal children at the patient's height) that is delayed with respect to their chronologic age and is concordant with their bone age. Once it is initiated, puberty should be completed within 4.5 years. Although delayed sexual maturation is an inevitable component of prepubertal onset of hypogonadism or androgen resis-

TABLE 253–1 PUBERTAL STAGES IN BOYS

	Pubic Hair	Genital
Stage 1	Absence of pubic hair	Childlike penis, testes, and scrotum (testes 2 mL)
Stage 2	Sparse, lightly pigmented hair mainly at the base of the penis	Scrotum enlarged with early rugation and pigmentation; testes begin to enlarge (3–5 mL)
Stage 3	Hair becomes coarse, darker, and more curled and more extensive	Penis has grown in length and diameter; testes now 8–10 mL; scrotum more rugated
Stage 4	Hair adult in quality, but distribution does not include medial aspect of thighs	Penis further enlarged with development of the glans; scrotum and testes (10–13 mL) further enlarged
Stage 5	Hair is adult and extends to thighs	Penis and scrotum fully adult; testes 15 mL and greater

Modified from Marshall WA, Tanner JM: Variation in pattern of pubertal changes in boys. Arch Dis Child 1970;45:13–23.

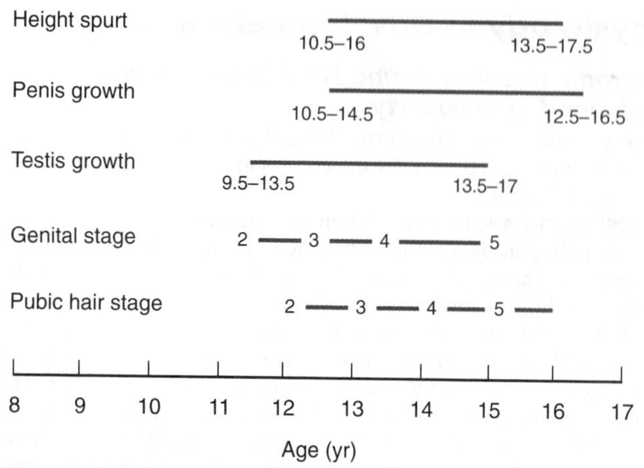

FIGURE 253–7 • Diagram of the timing of the various components of puberty. The range of ages in which each parameter begins and is completed is shown for each bar. These data are from European children obtained 30 years ago. There may be a slight trend for earlier onset of puberty during the past 30 years. (From Marshall WA, Tanner JM: Variations in the pattern of pubertal changes in boys. Arch Dis Child 1970;45:13–23.)

tance, the majority of boys with delayed development have a constitutional delayed physiologic clock and eventually attain full sexual adulthood. There is often a family history of a parent or sibling being a "late bloomer." The physiologic stimuli responsible for the initiation of puberty are not fully understood, but increases in leptin precede the maturation of the GnRH pulse generator, possibly as a signal of the availability of metabolic fuel. The *GPR54* gene encodes a kisspeptin-responsive G protein–coupled receptor whose absence results in hypogonadotropic hypogonadism due to impaired secretion of GnRH. The kisspeptin-GPR system has been proposed as a stimulus for pubertal awakening of the reproductive axis. Careful documentation of changing physical findings and measurement of serum LH, FSH, and testosterone concentrations may provide valuable clues of the beginning of puberty. An increase in testicular size to more than 3 mL usually heralds other signs of pubertal onset. Inquiring and testing for hyposmia or anosmia and other midline defects may indicate a common variant of congenital hypogonadotropic hypogonadism (Kallmann's syndrome). A family history of delay in puberty may encourage patience and observation. The decision of how early to treat depends on the perceived degree of psychological stress associated with the maturational delay. The major concern about treatment is early fusion of the epiphyses, which compromises optimal height. With proper dosing and monitoring of bone age, this is unusual because bone age is usually retarded in delayed puberty. In adolescent boys with delayed puberty and low levels of gonadotropins, periodic withdrawal of treatment is used to determine whether spontaneous puberty has occurred. Many adult men diagnosed with and treated for hypogonadotropic hypogonadism at the age of 15 to 19 years have proved to have normal reproductive function when they discontinue testosterone therapy many years later.

Precocious puberty in boys is defined as the onset of pubertal (genital and secondary sexual) development before 9 years of age (2.5 SD above the mean age of progression to stage 2). Sexual precocity can be subcategorized to true (complete and incomplete) isosexual precocious puberty and pseudoprecocious puberty. The distinction is that true precocious puberty is associated with increases in GnRH-stimulated LH and FSH secretion (hypothalamic-pituitary origin), whereas pseudoprecocious puberty is independent of GnRH stimulation of LH and FSH secretion. True precocious puberty is often associated with CNS disease (two thirds of boys and less than 10% of girls), including hypothalamic tumors, cysts, inflammatory conditions, and seizure disorders. The diagnosis is based on the finding of sexual precocity, inappropriately elevated serum LH levels, and associated elevations of serum testosterone. CNS visualizations by magnetic resonance imaging can localize most lesions. Pseudoprecocious puberty is characterized by increased testosterone with suppressed β-LH levels. Causes of precocious puberty include human chorionic gonadotropin secretory tumors (i.e., testicular, hepatic, hypothalamic, and pineal tumors), congenital virilizing adrenal hyperplasia, testicular testosterone-secreting neoplasms, and constitutively active LH receptor mutations, resulting in uncontrolled testosterone secretion

TABLE 253–2 HORMONAL CHANGES ASSOCIATED WITH AGING

GnRH–LH/FSH/T	CRH–ACTH–DHEA-S	GHRH-GH-IGF Axis
↑LH,* ↑FSH	No change in ACTH	↓GHRH message and receptor
↓T (↓Leydig cells)	↓DHEA and DHEA-S	↓GH secretory pulses
↓Free T	↓DHEA and DHEA-S	↓Circulating GH
↑SHBG	Response to ACTH	↓Serum IGF-I

*Decreased LH pulse amplitude and decreased responsiveness to GnRH. ACTH = adrenocorticotropic hormone; CRH = corticotropin-releasing hormone; DHEA = dehydroepiandrosterone; DHEA-S = DHEA sulfate; FSH = follicle-stimulating hormone; GH = growth hormone; GHRH = growth hormone–releasing hormone; GnRH = gonadotropin-releasing hormone; IGF-I = insulin-like growth factor I; LH = luteinizing hormone; SHBG = sex hormone–binding globulin; T = testosterone.

(testotoxicosis). Treatment of true precocious puberty is removal of the CNS lesion if possible and treatment with GnRH analogues. Treatment of pseudoprecocious puberty depends on the cause but includes glucocorticoids for congenital virilizing adrenal hyperplasia and ketoconazole (suppresses steroidogenesis) with or without antiandrogens (e.g., spironolactone and flutamide).

Male Senescence: Decreased Testosterone and Other Anabolic Hormones

TESTOSTERONE DEFICIENCY IN THE ELDERLY. Blood concentrations of testosterone, other anabolic hormones (e.g., growth hormone), and prehormones (e.g., DHEA and DHEA-S) are significantly lower in older men than in young adult men (Table 253–2). Unlike in women, aging in men is associated not with an abrupt cessation of gonadal hormone secretion but rather with a gradual decline in serum testosterone concentration, beginning in young adulthood and progressing throughout life. Multiple cross-sectional and longitudinal studies have shown a progressive decrease in both total and bioavailable or free serum testosterone levels with aging (Fig. 253–8). The rate of decline in total testosterone levels documented in longitudinal studies ranged from 0.1 to 0.38 nM per year. The percentage decline in serum testosterone has also been estimated between 0.8 and 1.6% per year. The reasons for these discrepancies in the absolute and relative decline with age are unclear but may include the inclusion and exclusion criteria in some studies and the comorbid state of obesity or illness in some populations. Many men with low serum testosterone are not symptomatic of typical hypogonadism seen in younger androgen-deficient men. Serum SHBG levels also rise with age in men, resulting in a higher percentage of circulating testosterone tightly bound and less bioavailable. Recent data indicate that between 40 and 80% of men older than 70 years have blood levels of bioavailable or free testosterone below the normal range for young adults (Fig. 253–9).

The effects of low testosterone levels in aging men are similar to those observed in younger hypogonadal men. These include decreases in muscle mass, muscle strength, bone mass, libido, and erectile function and impaired mood and sense of well-being. Older men have increased body fat, particularly visceral fat. The effect of reduced androgen levels on cognition and memory is unknown. The benefits of testosterone treatment of symptomatic older men with low serum testosterone levels remain controversial because randomized, controlled large-scale international trials have not been performed. In recent years, a number of studies have demonstrated the beneficial effects of testosterone replacement in elderly men with relatively low serum testosterone levels. Testosterone replacement therapy (up to 3 years) decreases fat mass, increases lean body mass, improves strength, and increases bone mineral density in some studies. Data on fracture rates with androgen replacement therapy for older men with low serum biologically active testosterone levels are not yet available. Because erectile dysfunction in the older man is multifactorial, with impaired vasodilatory function in the penis predominating in many cases (see section on sexual dysfunction), testosterone replacement therapy in older men may enhance libido but often does not improve erectile dysfunction. Improved sense of well-being and increased energy levels have been reported but are not consistently observed after treatment with testosterone. More data are clearly needed to prove

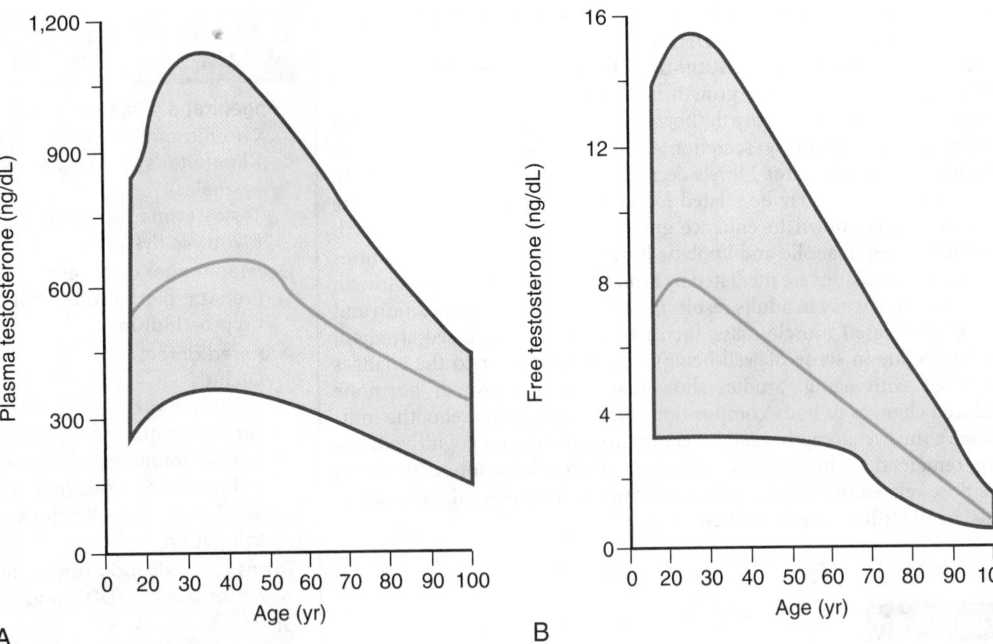

FIGURE 253–8 • Relationship between plasma testosterone (A) and free testosterone (B) levels and age in normal males. (From Baker HWG, Berger HG, DeKretser DM, et al: Changes in the pituitary-testicular system with age. Clin Endocrinol 1996; 5:349–372.)

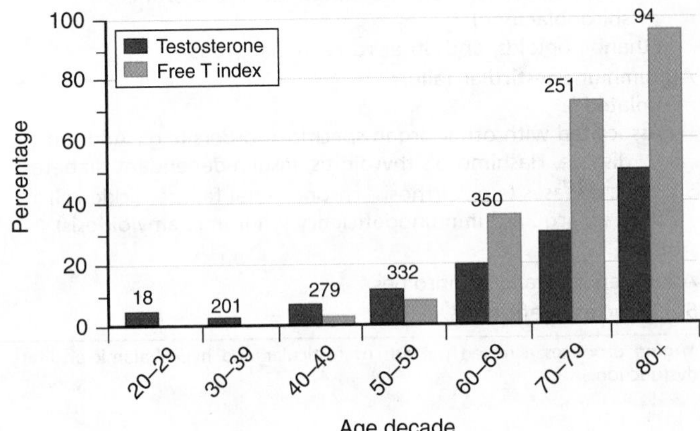

FIGURE 253–9 • Hypogonadism in aging men. Bar height indicates the percentage of men in each 10-year interval, from the third to the ninth decades, with at least one testosterone value in the hypogonadal range. The criteria used for these determinations are total testosterone less than 11.3 nmol/L (325 ng/dL) and testosterone and SHBG (free T index) less than 0.153 nmol/nmol. The numbers above each pair of bars indicate the number of men studied in the corresponding decade. The fraction of men who are hypogonadal increases progressively after the age of 50 years by either criterion. More men are hypogonadal by free T index than by total testosterone after 50 years, and there seems to be a progressively greater difference, with increasing age, between the two criteria.

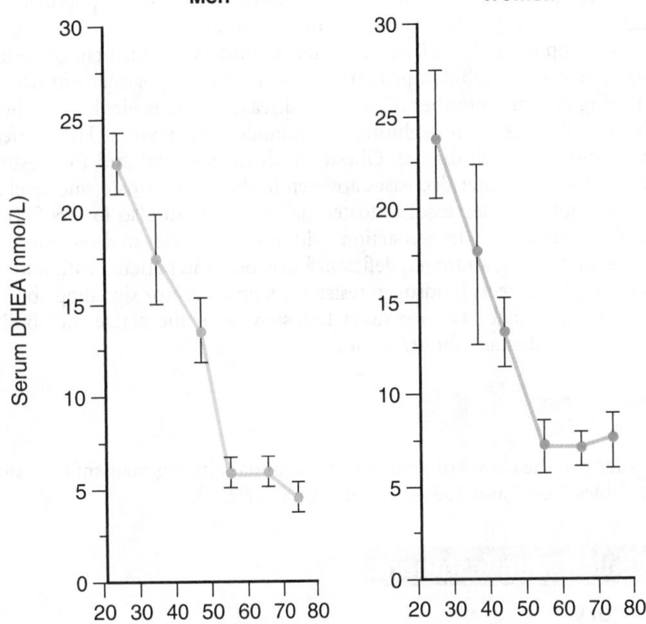

FIGURE 253–10 • Declining serum DHEA concentration with aging. Serum DHEA-S levels (not shown) parallel the decrease in DHEA. (Modified from Labrie F, et al: Marked decline in serum concentrations of adrenal C19 sex steroid precursors and conjugated androgen metabolites during aging. J Clin Endocrinol Metab 1997;82:2396–2402. © The Endocrine Society.)

efficacy as well as to properly evaluate risks of treatment with testosterone. At present, testosterone treatment is not recommended for men known to have or suspected of having prostate cancer, severe and uncorrected sleep apnea, and high red blood cell mass.

Digital rectal examination should be performed, prostate-specific antigen level determined, and symptoms of severe urinary tract obstruction evaluated to ensure that there are no findings suggestive of severe benign prostatic hypertrophy or prostate cancer (nodules, irregularities).

DEFICIENCY OF ADRENAL ANDROGEN IN OLDER MEN. In recent years, a marked decline in the circulating levels of adrenal androgens, especially DHEA and DHEA-S, has been recognized in elderly men and women (Fig. 253–10) (Chapter 252). Serum levels of DHEA and DHEA-S peak at about the third decade of life and then decline at about 2% per year, resulting in levels 10 to 20% of baseline by 80 years of age. This decline in DHEA and DHEA-S is not accompanied by a decrease in adrenocorticotropic hormone. DHEA is a precursor to true androgens such as testosterone and DHT but does not bind to the androgen receptor itself. It is unclear whether DHEA binds to a unique nuclear receptor to initiate its action. Studies have reported that DHEA administered to aging experimental animals and humans may improve the sense of well-being, reduce anxiety and depression, enhance memory, prevent development of cancer, decrease body fat, decrease risk of cardiovascular disease, and provide other beneficial effects on immune function. Most studies in humans used oral doses of 1 to 5 mg/kg/day. An oral dose of 50 mg/day will increase testosterone and DHT to or above the normal physiologic range for women but not for men. Much higher doses of DHEA can increase testosterone to male ranges but at the expense of very high serum DHEA concentrations. Studies showed that oral administration of 50 mg of DHEA to older men raised serum DHEA and DHEA-S concentrations to the levels found in young men but had no beneficial effects on quality of life, sexual function, mood, body composition, or exercise capacity. In the United States, DHEA is available without prescription as a health supplement and is widely used, creating a situation in which large-scale multicenter, prospective, placebo-controlled trials are difficult to perform.

There is no documented benefit to the administration of DHEA to older men who may have low serum DHEA levels.

GROWTH HORMONE AND INSULIN-LIKE GROWTH FACTOR I DEFICIENCY IN OLDER MEN. Hypothalamic growth hormone–releasing hormone messenger RNA, pituitary growth hormone–releasing hormone receptor concentrations, pituitary secretion of growth hormone, and serum insulin-like growth factor I levels decrease with aging (see Table 253–2). Part of the decline may be related to falling testosterone levels because testosterone is known to enhance growth hormone secretion. Growth hormone is an anabolic and lipolytic hormone, and many of its actions on peripheral tissues are mediated by insulin-like growth factor I. Growth hormone deficiency in adults results in changes in body composition and mood (decreased muscle mass, increased body fat, decreased strength, and a decline in sense of well-being), which are similar to the changes observed with aging. Studies show that although growth hormone induced changes in body composition compared with placebo, the individual's muscle strength, exercise endurance, mood, and cognitive function remained unchanged. The side effects of growth hormone treatment are dose related but include edema of lower extremities, diffuse arthralgias, hand stiffness, and tiredness.

MALE HYPOGONADISM

Definition

Hypogonadism refers to low circulating levels of testosterone. Most androgen-deficient men are infertile. Primary hypogonadism indicates that the abnormality originates in the testis; secondary hypogonadism indicates a defect at the hypothalamus or pituitary, resulting in decreased gonadotropins (LH, FSH, or both) and secondary impairment of testicular function. Combined primary and secondary hypogonadism occurs in aging and in a number of systemic diseases, such as alcoholism, liver disease, diabetes mellitus, human immunodeficiency virus (HIV) infection, and sickle cell disease. Obesity leads to low total and free testosterone levels. Greater decreases are seen in the total testosterone level as obesity not only decreases testosterone secretion but also lowers SHBG levels. Decreased androgen action, with normal or elevated testosterone levels, mimicking androgen deficiency may occur in patients with androgen receptor defects (androgen resistance), postreceptor signaling abnormalities, and inability to convert testosterone to the active metabolite DHT (5α-reductase abnormalities).

TABLE 253–3 CAUSES OF PRIMARY TESTICULAR FAILURE AND END-ORGAN RESISTANCE

- Congenital disorders
  - Chromosome disorders
  - Klinefelter's and related syndromes (e.g., XXY, XXY/XY, XYY, XX males)
  - Testosterone biosynthetic enzyme defects
  - Myotonic dystrophy
- Developmental disorders
  - Prenatal diethylstilbestrol syndrome
  - Cryptorchidism
- Acquired defects
  - Orchitis
  - Mumps and other viruses
  - Granulomatous (e.g., tuberculosis, leprosy)
  - Human immunodeficiency virus infection
  - Infiltrative diseases (e.g., hemochromatosis, amyloidosis)
  - Surgical, traumatic injuries, and torsion of testis
  - Irradiation
- Toxins (e.g., alcohol, fungicides, insecticides, heavy metals, cottonseed oil, DDT, and other environmental estrogens)
- Drugs
  - Cytotoxic agents
  - Inhibitors of testosterone synthesis and antiandrogens (e.g., ketoconazole, cimetidine, flutamide, cyproterone, spironolactone)
  - Ethanol, opioids, and other recreational drugs
- Autoimmune testicular failure
  - Isolated
  - Associated with other organ-specific disorders (e.g., Addison's disease, Hashimoto's thyroiditis, insulin-dependent diabetes)
- Systemic diseases (e.g., cirrhosis, chronic renal failure, sickle cell disease, acquired immunodeficiency syndrome, amyloidosis)
- Aging*
- Androgen resistance syndromes
- 5α-Reductase deficiency

*Aging produces a mixed pattern of testicular and hypothalamic-pituitary dysfunction.

Etiology

Many of the causes of primary and secondary hypogonadism are listed in Tables 253–3 and 253–4 (see also Chapter 252).

Clinical Manifestations

History

The medical history should focus on testicular descent, pubertal development, shaving frequency, changes in body hair, and present and past systemic illnesses. A complete sexual history includes changes in libido, erectile and ejaculatory functions, and frequency of masturbation, coital activity, and fertility (including that of present and previous partners). Information should be obtained on previous orchitis, sinopulmonary complaints, sexually transmitted diseases, HIV status, genitourinary infections, and previous surgical procedures that might affect the reproductive tract (e.g., vasectomy, hernia repair, prostatectomy, varicocele ligation). Social history should include tobacco and alcohol intake. Medication and drug history should include any agent that could affect hormonal, spermatogenic, and erectile function. These include recreational drugs; anabolic steroids; psychiatric, antihypertensive, antiandrogenic, cytotoxic, alternative medicine therapies; environmental toxins; and exposure to heat (including saunas and Jacuzzis) and irradiation.

Physical Examination

The general physical examination is supplemented by height and span measurements; assessment of muscle mass and adiposity; characterization of facial, pubic, and body hair distribution; presence of acne and facial wrinkling; breast examination for gynecomastia; examination of the scrotal contents; measurement of penile length and urethral integrity; digital rectal prostate examination; and visual field assessment. The scrotal examination should include assessment of midline fusion (e.g., bifid scrotum, hypospadias); measurement of testicular size (a ruler will suffice, but Prader or Takihara orchidometers are preferred) and consistency; presence of intratesticular masses; abnormalities of the epididymis; bilateral presence of vas deferens; and presence of varicoceles, hydroceles, or hernias. Normal testicular size ranges from 3.6 to 5.5 cm in length, 2.1 to 3.2 cm in width, and 15 to 35 mL in volume in white and black men. Asian men have slightly smaller mean testicular size. A decrease in testicular volume usually implies decreased spermatogenic cells because the seminiferous tubules account for more than 80% of testicular volume.

Laboratory Studies

Because a strong diurnal rhythm in testosterone secretion results in the highest serum levels in the morning hours and the lowest levels in the evening, the measurement of testosterone, LH, and FSH is routinely determined from morning blood samples. The value of free testosterone measurements when symptoms suggest hypogonadism but serum total testosterone concentrations are borderline was discussed in an earlier section of this chapter. Some of the variability in the normal ranges for testosterone as determined by immunometric assays may disappear when measurements of testosterone based on gas-liquid chromatography–tandem mass spectroscopy become more readily available. Elevated LH and FSH levels distinguish primary from secondary hypogonadism (both have low serum testosterone levels), but many older men with low serum testosterone levels have normal LH concentrations. Serum prolactin levels should be measured in all cases of hypogonadotropic hypogonadism, pituitary mass lesions, and galactorrhea. DHT is measured in cases of abnormal differentiation of the genitalia and when DHT defi-

TABLE 253–4 CAUSES OF HYPOGONADOTROPIC HYPOGONADISM

IDIOPATHIC OR CONGENITAL

Isolated deficiency of gonadotropin-releasing hormone
- With anosmia (Kallmann's syndrome)
- With other abnormalities (Prader-Willi syndrome, Laurence-Moon-Biedl syndrome, basal encephalocele)

Partial deficiency of gonadotropin-releasing hormone (fertile eunuch syndrome)
Multiple hypothalamic and pituitary hormone deficiency
Pituitary hypoplasia or aplasia

ACQUIRED

Trauma, postsurgery, postirradiation
Neoplastic
Pituitary adenomas (prolactinomas, other functional and nonfunctional tumors)
Craniopharyngiomas, germinomas, gliomas, leukemia, lymphomas
Pituitary infarction, carotid aneurysm
Infiltrative and infectious diseases of hypothalamus and pituitary (sarcoidosis, tuberculosis, coccidioidomycosis, histoplasmosis, syphilis, abscess, histiocytosis X, hemochromatosis)
Autoimmune hypophysitis
Aging*
Obesity
Malnutrition and systemic disease
Anorexia nervosa, starvation, renal failure, liver failure
Exogenous hormones and drugs
Antiandrogens, estrogens and antiestrogens, progestogens, glucocorticoids, cimetidine, spironolactone, digoxin, drug-induced hyperprolactinemia (metoclopramide, tranquilizers, antihypertensives)

*Aging produces a mixed pattern of central and testicular dysfunction.

ciency is suspected. Serum estradiol should be measured in cases of gynecomastia. Assessment of other testosterone precursors and products may be required in special circumstances, including suspected congenital enzyme defects. The semen analysis is the "cornerstone" of the laboratory examination for infertility.

Hypogonadism and Androgen Resistance

Primary Testicular Hypogonadism

Definition

Primary hypogonadism refers to a condition of androgen deficiency with or without infertility in which the pathologic process lies at the testis level. A list of common causes is given in Table 253–3.

Pathogenesis

Congenital Disorders

See Chapter 252.

Acquired Defects

MUMPS, ORCHITIS, LEPROSY, HIV INFECTION, AND HEMOCHROMATOSIS. After puberty, mumps is associated with clinical orchitis in 25% of cases, and 60% of those affected become infertile. During acute orchitis, the testes are inflamed, painful, and swollen. After the acute inflammatory phase, the testes gradually decrease in size, although swelling can persist for months. The testes may return to normal size and function or undergo atrophy. Spermatogenic changes occur more often and earlier than Leydig cell dysfunction. Thus, patients with postorchitic infertility may have normal testosterone and LH levels with increased serum FSH levels. With time, elevations in LH and lowered serum testosterone levels may appear. Leprosy may also cause orchitis, and gonadal insufficiency. HIV infection is often associated with hypogonadism, which can be either hypogonadotropic or hypergonadotropic (Chapter 416). Hemochromatosis and amyloidosis are examples of infiltrative diseases of the testis that can result in hypogonadism.

TRAUMA. The exposed position of the testes in the scrotum makes them particularly susceptible to injury. Surgical injury during scrotal surgery for hernias, varicocele, and vasectomy can result in permanent testicular damage.

IRRADIATION. Irradiation to the testes from accidental exposure in the treatment of an associated malignant disease will produce testicular damage.

Drugs

Chemotherapy, in particular with alkylating agents such as busulfan, for malignant disorders frequently leads to irreversible germ cell damage. Toxins may also directly damage the testes. Many agents, such as fungicides and insecticides (e.g., DBCP, metabolites of DDT), heavy metals (lead, cadmium), and cottonseed oil (gossypol), produce damage to the germ cells. Leydig cells are relatively less susceptible to most chemotherapeutic drugs than are Sertoli and germ cells. Serum testosterone levels are usually normal despite infertility in the exposed men.

Some medications may interfere with testosterone biosynthesis (e.g., ketoconazole, spironolactone) or action (cyproterone, flutamide). Ethanol, independent of its effect in causing liver disease, will inhibit testosterone biosynthesis. Marijuana, heroin, methadone, medroxyprogesterone acetate, other progestins, and estrogens lower testosterone, but mainly by decreasing the pituitary secretion of LH. Medical treatment with androgens such as testosterone, DHT, and synthetic anabolic steroids or their illicit use (e.g., in athletes, body builders) will lower serum LH and FSH levels and lower sperm counts in the absence of clinical signs and symptoms of androgen deficiency. Serum testosterone levels will be normal to elevated after testosterone treatment but will be low after use of DHT and synthetic anabolic agents.

Autoimmune Testicular Failure

Antibodies against the microsomal fraction of the Leydig cells may occur either as an isolated disorder or as part of a multiglandular disorder involving, to variable degrees, the thyroid, pituitary, adrenals, pancreas, and other organs.

Testicular Defects Associated with Systemic Diseases

Abnormalities of the hypothalamic-pituitary-testicular axis occur in a number of systemic diseases. These include liver failure, renal failure, severe malnutrition, sickle cell anemia, advanced malignant disease, severe obesity, diabetes, cystic fibrosis, and amyloidosis. About half of men undergoing chronic hemodialysis for renal failure experience decreased libido, infertility, and impotence. The effects of cirrhosis of the liver on testicular function are complex and may be either independent or associated with direct toxic effects of continued use of alcohol. Gynecomastia, testicular atrophy, and impotence are concomitant signs of cirrhosis. Decreased spermatogenesis with peritubular fibrosis occurs in at least 50% of patients. In contrast to the decrease in serum testosterone levels, estradiol levels are usually elevated. This results in an increased ratio of serum estradiol to testosterone with an increased proclivity for gynecomastia. Patients with sickle cell anemia often have impaired testicular function. Boys with sickle cell anemia may have impaired sexual maturation, and men are often infertile. The defect in sickle cell anemia seems to be ischemic in origin, probably with accelerated apoptosis; it may occur either at the testicular or at the hypothalamic-pituitary level. Diabetes and obesity are two major factors in hypogonadism. Emerging data show that diabetes is associated with low blood testosterone levels and that the decrease in serum testosterone correlates with the degree of hyperglycemia.

Secondary Gonadal Insufficiency (Hypogonadotropic Hypogonadism)

Definition

Hypogonadotropic hypogonadism represents a deficiency in the secretion of gonadotropins (LH and FSH) due to an intrinsic or functional abnormality in the hypothalamus or pituitary glands (see earlier and Chapter 252). Such disorders result in the secondary Leydig cell dysfunction (see Table 253–4). The clinical manifestations depend on the age of the patient at the onset of the disorder.

Acquired Hypogonadotropic Disorders and Functional Disorders

ANOREXIA NERVOSA AND WEIGHT LOSS. Anorexia nervosa and weight loss are examples of functional defects resulting in low serum testosterone levels. Anorexia nervosa, predominantly a disorder of adolescent girls, is characterized by excessive weight loss as a result of dietary restriction or bulimia. On occasion, anorexia nervosa is seen in men, but in such an instance, it usually implies a variant of a more severe psychiatric disorder. Men and women present with manifestations of hypogonadotropic hypogonadism. Starvation from other than a psychological basis may also reduce gonadotropic secretion, although women seem more susceptible to this disorder. Although strenuous exercise commonly produces reproductive dysfunction in female athletes (e.g., long-distance runners and dancers), it has minimal effects on testicular function in men.

STRESS AND ILLNESS. Severe stress and systemic illness also lower gonadotropin and testosterone levels. Organic hypothalamic-pituitary disorders include neoplastic, granulomatous, infiltrative, and post-traumatic lesions in the region of the hypothalamus and pituitary.

MALIGNANT DISEASE. Prolactinomas present differently in men and women (Chapter 242). Unlike in women, in whom small tumors can be detected early because of symptoms of amenorrhea and galactorrhea, in men the tumors are usually large (>1 cm in diameter [macroadenomas]) by the time they are detected. It is unclear whether the large size of the adenoma at the time of presentation in men is due to the late diagnosis, caused by failure of patients and physicians to appreciate early signs, or the more rapid growth of these tumors in men. Male patients with prolactin-secreting macroadenomas usually present with hypogonadism, erectile dysfunction, and visual manifestations from suprasellar extension. Hypogonadism in microprolactinomas is usually the result of prolactin suppression of GnRH secretion. In macroadenomas, the suppression of gonadotropins and hypogonadotropic hypogonadism may be due to the GnRH suppressive effects described earlier or a mass effect damaging the non-neoplastic gonadotrophs.

Large non–prolactin-secreting pituitary tumors (growth hormone, adrenocorticotropic hormone, glycopeptide, and null cell) may also produce gonadotropin insufficiency from damage to the adjacent normal pituitary gland (Chapter 242), resulting in decreased serum LH and testosterone levels.

Androgen Resistance (Androgen-Sensitive End-Organ Deficiency)

Certain conditions have clinical phenotypes mimicking testosterone deficiency in the absence of lowered testosterone levels. These are either drug induced (antiandrogens) or congenital defects in the androgen receptor, postreceptor defects, or 5α-reductase deficiency (Chapter 252).

Diagnosis

The diagnosis is based on clinical symptoms and signs and a reduced serum testosterone level. The most available and commonly used blood measurement of testosterone is serum total testosterone. The normal range of a young adult male population varies for different laboratories but should be in the general range of 300 to 1000 ng/dL (10 to 38 nmol/L). Accurate measurements of testosterone in the female or severely hypogonadal range are best done by tandem mass spectroscopy. Total testosterone measurements may be misleading indicators of Leydig cell status in conditions in which SHBG levels are abnormal (see earlier section). In these circumstances, a measurement of free testosterone (by dialysis method), bioavailable testosterone (free and albumin bound), or calculated free testosterone (by total testosterone and SHBG measurements) is useful to characterize circulating bioactive testosterone levels.

The following rules apply to most young and middle-aged men thought to have hypogonadism. If a morning serum total testosterone level is repeatedly below 250 ng/dL (8.5 nmol/L), the patient is most probably hypogonadal, and testosterone replacement is indicated. If the serum testosterone level is between 250 and 300 ng/dL with normal serum LH levels, the patient may not be hypogonadal, and androgen replacement may not improve the symptoms (e.g., sexual dysfunction). Thus, when serum total testosterone is borderline and LH is not increased, measurement of one of the bioactive testosterone levels is indicated. The guidelines for men older than 60 years are less certain; because SHBG levels are increased in this age group, total testosterone levels may overestimate the biologically active forms of circulating testosterone. In men older than 60 years with signs or symptoms of androgen deficiency, a serum total testosterone level above 400 ng/dL argues strongly against hypogonadism; a serum level below 200 ng/dL is almost always a clinically significant level, and total testosterone concentrations between 200 and 400 ng/dL deserve further testing with one of the tests of bioactive testosterone.

Treatment

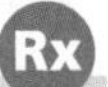

The main medical indication for androgen replacement therapy is male hypogonadism (Table 253–5).

Contraindications to Testosterone Therapy

Absolute contraindications to androgen replacement therapy include carcinoma of the prostate and the male breast. These cancers are androgen dependent for growth and proliferation. Androgens should be used with caution in older men with enlarged prostates and urinary symptoms, elevated hematocrit, and sleep-related breathing disorders.

Androgen Preparations

Testosterone esters such as testosterone enanthate (or cypionate) are widely used preparations in the United States and throughout the world (Table 253–6). The recommended dose is 150 to 200 mg administered intramuscularly once every 2 to 3 weeks.

Modified 17α-alkylated androgens (methyltestosterone and many anabolic steroids), which are available in oral preparations, are not recommended as androgen replacement. These agents may lead to abnormalities in liver function and marked decreases in high-density lipoprotein cholesterol and increases in total cholesterol levels compared with the testosterone esters. Orally active testosterone undecenoate is not available in the United States but is used in Canada, Europe, and other places in the world. This ester is absorbed into the lymphatics and has variable bioavailability; it must be taken with fatty food or liquid at least twice daily for optimal blood testosterone levels. Transbuccal delivery of testosterone by mucoadhesive tablets (30 mg applied twice daily) gives physiologic-range testosterone levels through absorption directly into the systemic circulation, thus avoiding first-pass effects on the liver.

Testosterone Implants

Implants are pellets of crystalline testosterone. The serum testosterone levels are maintained in the physiologic range for 4 to 6 months. Implants are not popular in the United States but are widely used in Australia and the United Kingdom.

Transdermal testosterone delivery through skin patches and hydroalcoholic gels is available and widely used throughout the

TABLE 253–5 INDICATIONS FOR ANDROGEN THERAPY

Androgen deficiency (hypogonadism)
Microphallus (neonatal)
Delayed puberty in boys
Elderly men with low total or bioavailable or free testosterone levels
Angioneurotic edema
Other possible uses or under investigation
Hormonal male contraception
Wasting disease associated with cancer, human immunodeficiency virus infection, chronic infection
Postmenopausal women

TABLE 253–6 ANDROGEN PREPARATIONS

Route	Preparation	Dose and Frequency of Administration
Oral*	Testosterone undecenoate (not available in United States; available in Canada, Mexico, Europe, Asia)	40–80 mg orally two or three times per day
Injectable	Transbuccal testosterone, mucoadhesive tablets (Striant)	30 mg two times daily
	Testosterone enanthate and cypionate	100 mg intramuscularly per week or 150–200 mg intramuscularly per 2–3 weeks
Implants	Testosterone implants	200-mg pellets, four inserted once every 4 to 6 months
Transdermal	Scrotal patch	One patch delivering 4 or 6 mg of testosterone per day
	Nonscrotal patch, Androderm	Two patches delivering 2.5 mg of testosterone each per day or one patch delivering 5 mg of testosterone per day
	Testoderm TTS	One patch delivering 5 mg of testosterone per day
Transdermal hydroalcoholic gels	AndroGel or Testogel; Testim	5–10 g containing 5-10 mg of testosterone is applied once daily

*Oral modified 17α-alkylated androgens such as methyltestosterone, fluoxymesterone, oxymetholone, stanozolol, and oxandrolone are not recommended for use in treatment of androgen deficiency states because of potential hepatotoxicity and adverse effects on serum lipids.

Rx

world. The nonscrotal patches deliver 5 mg of testosterone per day, which is the physiologic production rate. Some patches use alcohol-based absorption enhancement systems that decrease the patch size. These patches deliver levels of testosterone within the normal range but have a high incidence of skin irritability (redness, swelling, and blisters). Other patches are large and less likely to cause skin irritation but have a tendency to fall off with activity. Hydroalcoholic testosterone gels have been developed for transdermal application. They have become the most widely used testosterone formulations in the United States. The usual dosage is 5 to 10 g of 1% testosterone gel applied daily. Transfer from user to others through direct contact is possible. They give reasonably constant serum concentrations and cause little skin irritation.

Benefits versus Risks of Androgen Therapy

Table 253–7 shows the benefits and potential side effects of androgen treatment. In hypogonadal men, androgen replacement leads to the development and maintenance of secondary sexual characteristics. Testosterone has important anabolic effects on muscle and bone and improves libido and sexual dysfunction. It has less effect on erectile dysfunction (see later section on sexual dysfunction).

TABLE 253–7 ANDROGEN THERAPY: RISKS VERSUS BENEFITS

Benefits	Risks
Development or maintenance of secondary sex characteristics	Fluid retention Gynecomastia
Improves libido and sexual function	Acne, oily skin
Increases muscle mass and strength	Increases hematocrit
Increases bone mineral density	Decreases high-density lipoprotein cholesterol (oral 17-alkylated agents produce the greatest effect)
Decreases body and visceral fat	
Improves mood	
Effect on cognition (?)	
Effect on quality of life (?)	
	Sleep apnea
	Prostate diseases Benign prostate hyperplasia (?) Carcinoma of prostate (aggravate existing cancer) Aggressive behavior (?)

MALE INFERTILITY

Definition

Infertility is defined as the failure of a couple to achieve a pregnancy after at least 1 year of frequent unprotected intercourse. If a pregnancy has not occurred after 3 years, infertility most likely will persist without medical treatment.

Incidence and Prevalence

Studies in the United States and Europe showed a 1-year prevalence of infertility in 15% of couples. The prevalence in developing countries is likely to be higher because of the higher prevalence of genital tract infection. As shown in multicenter studies, 30 to 35% of subfertility can be attributed to predominantly female factors, 25 to 30% to male factors, and 25 to 30% to problems in both partners; in the remaining cases, no cause can be identified.

Etiology

Hypothalamic-pituitary disorders are infrequent causes of male infertility and are discussed in the section on hypogonadism and androgen deficiency. Primarily, testicular disorders are the most frequent identifiable cause of infertility (see Table 253–3).

Diagnosis

The approach to the diagnosis of an infertile couple includes management of the male and the female partner (Figs. 253–11 and 253–12).

Examination of the ejaculate is the cornerstone for the investigation of an infertile man (Table 253–8). Semen samples are collected when possible at the physician's office or at home, preferably after 2 to 7 days of abstinence from sexual intercourse.

The generally accepted reference values for a semen analysis are given in Table 253–9. A normal sperm concentration is greater than 20 million/mL; however, men with lower sperm counts can be fertile. More than 50% of the spermatozoa should be motile, and more than 25% should demonstrate a rapidly progressive motility pattern.

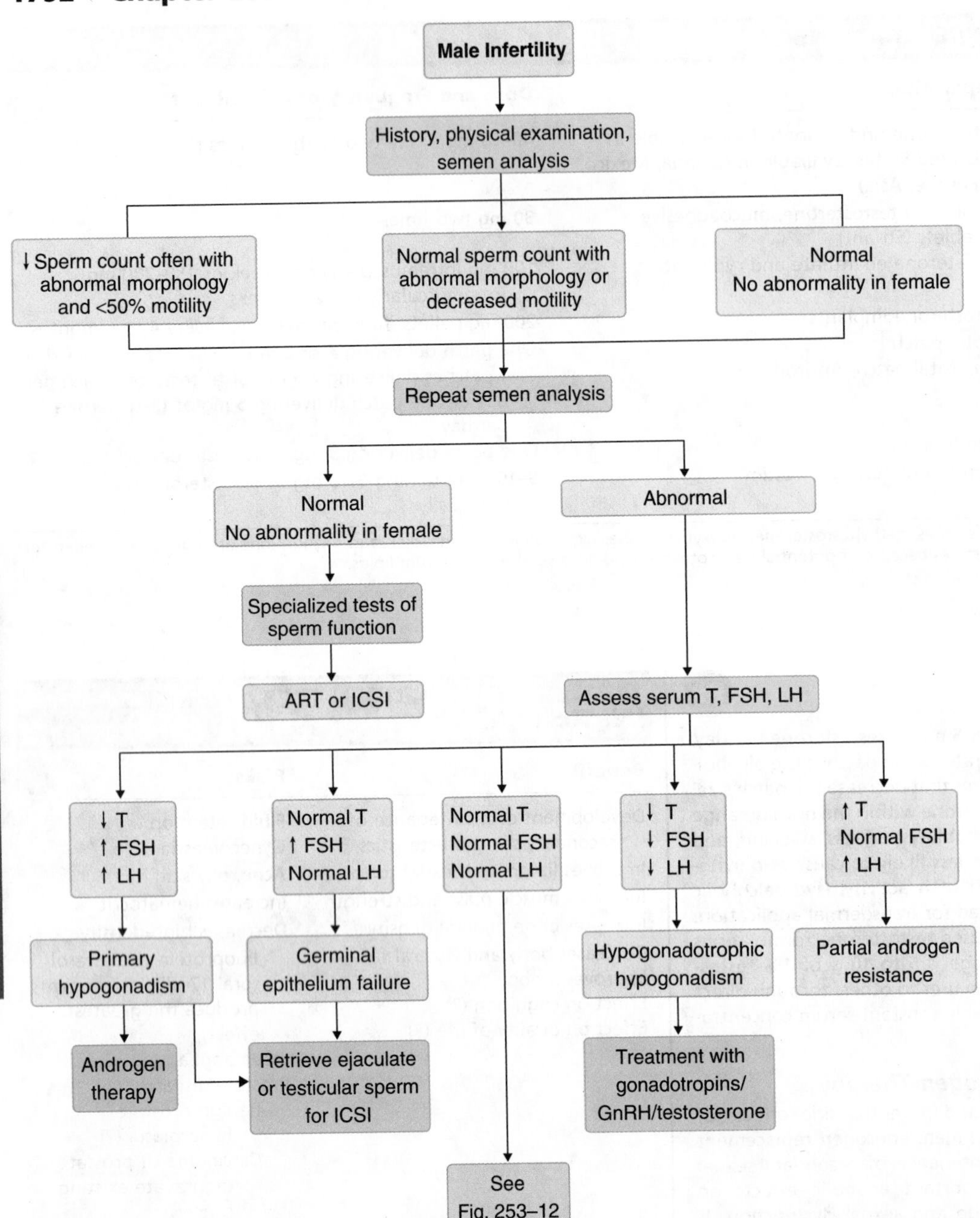

FIGURE 253–11 • Algorithmic approach to the diagnosis and treatment of male infertility. ART = assisted reproductive technology; FSH = follicle-stimulating hormone; GnRH = gonadotropin-releasing hormone; ICSI = intracytoplasmic sperm injection; LH = serum luteinizing hormone; T = serum testosterone.

TABLE 253–8 MALE INFERTILITY: BASIC LABORATORY TESTS

Semen Analyses	Hormone Analyses (in patients with abnormal semen analyses)
Volume, pH	Serum luteinizing hormone and follicle-stimulating hormone
Microscopy: agglutination, debris	Serum testosterone
Sperm: concentration, motility, morphology, vitality	If luteinizing hormone and testosterone levels are low, serum prolactin
Leukocytes	
Immature germ cells	
Sperm autoantibodies (sperm and semen biochemistry, sperm function tests)	

Numerous studies have demonstrated that considerable overlap is observed in the semen quality of fertile and subfertile men. No definite threshold is defined below which a man would be infertile except when azoospermia is present.

In patients with abnormal semen analyses, measurements of serum FSH, LH, and testosterone are indicated (see Fig. 253–10). Elevated FSH levels usually indicate severe germinal epithelium damage and may be associated with a guarded prognosis. A decreased serum inhibin β level also reflects poor Sertoli cell function and may be a marker of spermatogenic dysfunction. Elevated serum LH and FSH concentrations together with a low serum testosterone level indicate pantesticular failure. Low serum FSH, LH, and testosterone concentrations suggest hypothalamic pituitary dysfunction; serum prolactin should be measured, and additional appropriate investigations (as discussed in the section on sec-

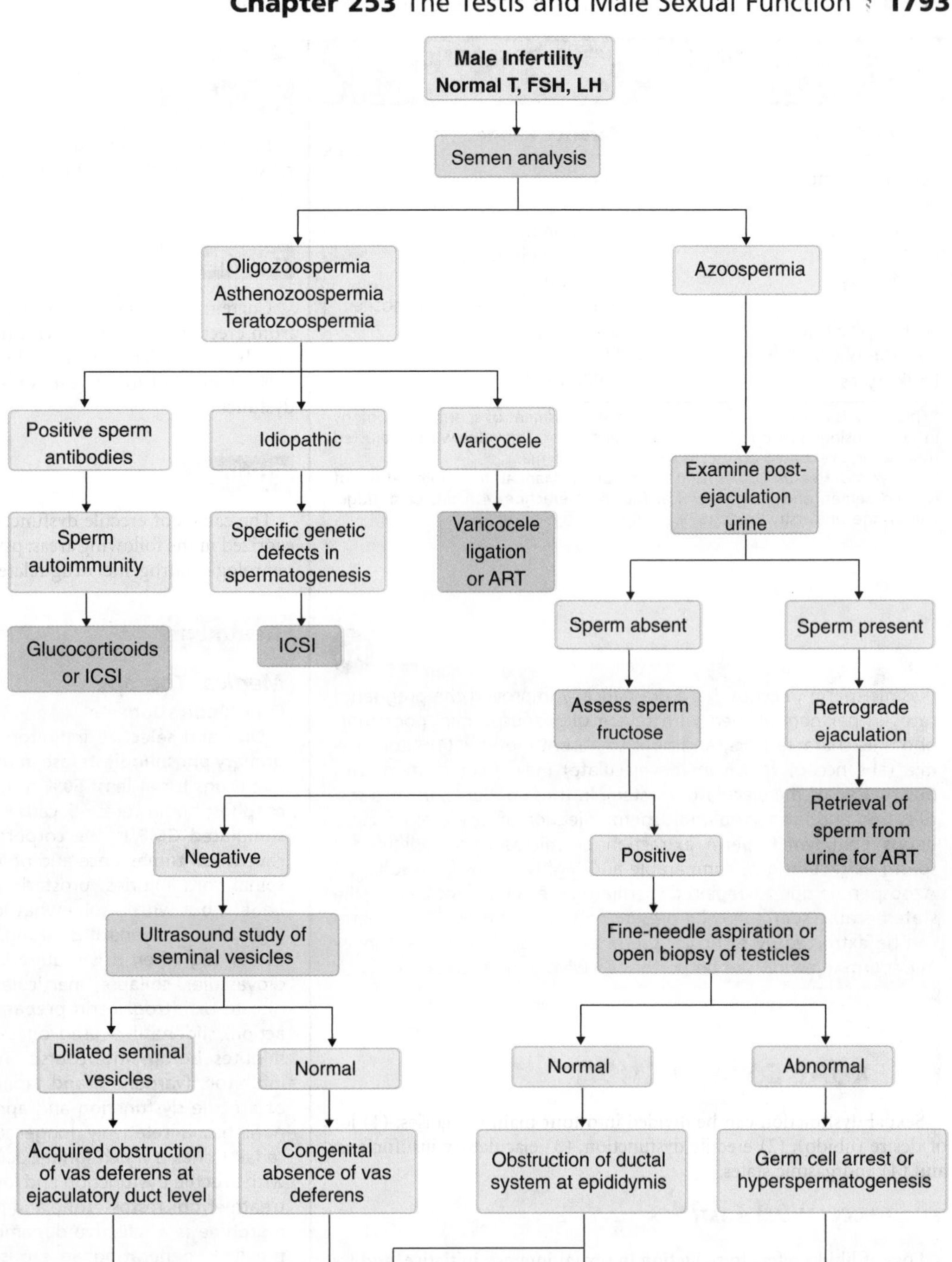

FIGURE 253–12 • Algorithmic approach to the diagnosis and treatment of male infertility in patients with normal serum hormone concentrations. ART = assisted reproductive technology; FSH = follicle-stimulating hormone; ICSI = intracytoplasmic sperm injection; LH = serum luteinizing hormone; T = serum testosterone.

ondary hypogonadism) may be required. The low sperm concentration and suppressed LH level with increased, normal, or low serum testosterone level (without clinical manifestations of androgen deficiency) may suggest exogenous androgen therapy. The hormonal pattern in androgen insensitivity (an uncommon cause of male infertility) is elevated LH, normal FSH, and high-normal to increased serum testosterone levels. Normal hormonal parameters in azoospermic (no sperm in the ejaculate) men with normal-sized testes may suggest congenital or acquired obstruction in the epididymis or vas deferens. Studies have shown that up to 20% of men with azoospermia or severe oligospermia (<1 to 3 million germ cells per milliliter of ejaculate) have microdeletions in the long arm of the Y chromosome (often in the AZF regions).

Treatment

Rx

An algorithmic approach to the treatment of male infertility is illustrated in Figures 253–11 and 253–12. The principles of management of male factor infertility can be summarized as follows. (1) Men with mild to moderate oligozoospermia with or without decreased sperm motility and some impairment of motility are subfertile rather than infertile. Spontaneous pregnancies occur in this group. (2) Reliable medical treatment is limited to the 1 to 2% of infertile men with gonadotropin insufficiency. (3) Assisted reproductive technologies including in vitro fertilization and intracyto-

TABLE 253–9 SEMEN ANALYSIS: REFERENCE RANGE

Parameter	Reference Range
Semen volume	>2 mL
Sperm	
Concentration	>20 million/mL
Total count	>40 million/ejaculate
Motility	>50% motile
	>25% rapid progressively motile
Morphology	>15% normal*
Vitality (live)	>75%
Leukocytes	<1 million/mL

*This value is based on the strict criteria for assessment of sperm morphology in studies using in vitro fertilization as an end point. This value will be adjusted to a lower level based on recent studies in fertile men.

From World Health Organization Laboratory Manual for Examination of Human Semen and Sperm–Cervical Mucus Interaction, 4th ed. Cambridge, Cambridge University Press, 1999.

Rx

plasmic sperm injection have dramatically improved the pregnancy rates in partners of men with severe oligozoospermia, poor morphologic characteristics, and poor to absent motility. (4) Azoospermia (absence of sperm in the ejaculate) may occur in men with obstruction of the ejaculatory system. In these patients, in vitro fertilization and intracytoplasmic sperm injection after either percutaneous epididymal sperm extraction or microsurgical epididymal sperm extraction give comparable and highly successful results. (5) Azoospermia due to impaired spermatogenesis may not be a sterile state because sperm may be present within the testes. These sperm can be extracted by testicular sperm extraction, and intracytoplasmic sperm injection can be performed with good success.

SEXUAL DYSFUNCTION

Sexual dysfunction can be divided into four main categories: (1) loss of desire (libido), (2) erectile dysfunction, (3) ejaculatory insufficiency, and (4) anorgasmic states.

Decreased Libido

Loss of libido refers to reduction in sexual interest, initiative, and frequency and intensity of responses to internal or external erotic stimuli. Causal factors include psychogenic factors, CNS disease, androgen deficiency and resistance, and side effects from medications (e.g., antihypertensives, psychotropics, alcohol, narcotics, dopamine blockers, antiandrogens). Treatment is directed toward the causal mechanism.

Ejaculatory Failure and Impaired Orgasm

Ejaculatory insufficiency refers to absent or reduced seminal emission or impaired ejaculatory contraction. It is usually associated with neurologic conditions and medication therapy. Anorgasmic state is a distressing but relatively uncommon condition in men when the normal process of erection and ejaculation occurs in the absence of the subjective sensation of pleasure initiated at the time of emission and ejaculation. Premature ejaculation is the most common form of male sexual dysfunction. Estimates of prevalence vary, but 25 to 30% seems a reasonable estimate. The *Diagnostic and Statistical Manual of Mental Disorders,* fourth edition, defines the diagnostic criteria for premature ejaculation as follows: persistent or recurrent ejaculation with minimal sexual stimulation that (1) occurs before, upon, or shortly after penetration and before the person wishes, (2) is associated with marked distress or interpersonal difficulty, and (3) is not a direct effect of substance abuse such as opiate withdrawal.

Erectile Dysfunction

Definition

Erectile dysfunction can be defined as the inability of a man to obtain rigidity sufficient to permit coitus of adequate duration to satisfy himself and his partner.

Prevalence

Current estimates suggest that 10 to 15% of all American men suffer from erectile dysfunction, with the incidence progressively increased as men become older. Data from the Massachusetts Aging Study report that 52% of men 40 to 70 years of age experience some degree of erectile dysfunction.

Etiology

The causes of erectile dysfunction are many but can be generally categorized in the following areas: psychological, endocrine, systemic illness, neurologic, iatrogenic, drug related, and aging.

Treatment

Rx

Medical Therapy

Oral Medications

Oral and selective inhibitors of cGMP phosphodiesterase-5 (the primary phosphodiesterase in the penile cavernosal tissue) are effective drugs for at least 50% of the men with this disorder. Inhibition of phosphodiesterase-5 causes persistence of normally (sexually) stimulated GMP in the corpora cavernosa, resulting in protracted cavernosal tumescence and rigidity. Patients with diabetes mellitus, spinal cord injuries, prostatic surgery, and pelvic irradiation also benefit but with a somewhat lower response rate. The usual starting dose of sildenafil is 50 mg, increasing in 25-mg increments up to 100 mg when it is required. The most serious side effect is cardiovascular collapse, particularly in patients taking long-acting nitrate or nitroglycerin preparations. Because of its mechanism of action, sildenafil is used on demand; it is administered 20 to 60 minutes before intercourse. Two additional phosphodiesterase-5 inhibitors (vardenafil and tadalafil) are widely used for treatment of erectile dysfunction and appear to be equally effective. Vardenafil has a relatively longer duration of action (4 to 6 hours); tadalafil has a much longer action (17.5 hours). Hypogonadal men with erectile dysfunction and low libido may benefit from combined treatment of testosterone and phosphodiesterase-5 inhibitors. Apomorphine is a selective dopamine receptor agonist that stimulates the CNS, generating an arousal response that includes a penile erection. Apomorphine has not been approved by the Food and Drug Administration and appears inferior to phosphodiesterase-5 inhibitors. Yohimbine is an indolalquinolonic alkaloid with central-acting effects, including α_2-adrenergic blockade and cholinergic and dopaminergic stimulation. Despite its widespread use, placebo-controlled studies have shown variable degrees of success, and yohimbine seems most useful in conditions in which there is a mechanism of organic disease. Trazodone, an antidepressant, possesses both serotonin and α_2-adrenergic antagonistic properties. It appears to be moderately effective in approximately one third of patients; the main side effect is sedation.

The intraurethral prostaglandin E_1 suppository alprostadil is believed to work locally on the corpora cavernosa as a vasodilatory agent. The suppository is apparently successful in improving erectile function in one third to two thirds of cases.

Intracavernosal Injections of Vasodilating Drugs

Until the recent availability of oral phosphodiesterase-5 inhibitors, intracavernosal injection with prostaglandin E_1 and other vasodilators (papaverine, phentolamine) was the mainstay of pharmacologic therapy for erectile dysfunction. The medications are injected with a 27- to 30-gauge needle and may be useful in men who are refractory to oral agents.

SUGGESTED READINGS

Beckman TJ, Abu-Lebdeh HS, Mynderse LA: Evaluation and medical management of erectile dysfunction. Mayo Clin Proc 2006;81:385–390. *A clinical review.*

Frajese GV, Pozzi F: New achievement and novel therapeutic applications of PDE5 inhibitors in older males. J Endocrinol Invest 2005;28:45–50. *Description of uses of PDE5 inhibitors for erectile dysfunction in older men.*

Haddad RM, Kennedy CC, Caples SM, et al: Testosterone and cardiovascular risk in men: A systematic review and meta-analysis of randomized placebo-controlled trials. Mayo Clin Proc 2007;82:29–39. *Limited number of studies and follow-up suggesting no adverse CV effects of therapeutic testosterone use.*

Harman SM, Metter EJ, Tobin JD, et al: Longitudinal effects of aging on serum total and free testosterone levels in healthy men. J Clin Endocrinol Metab 2001;86:724–731. *Largest longitudinal evaluation of the effects of normal aging on circulating gonadal hormone levels.*

Liu PY, Swerdloff RS, Veldhuis JD: The rationale, efficacy and safety of androgen therapy in older men: Future research and current practice recommendations. J Clin Endocrinol Metab 2004;89:4789–4796. *Review of the status of testosterone intervention for hypogonadism in the older man.*

Liverman CT, Blazer DG: Testosterone and Aging: Clinical Research Directions. Washington, DC, National Academies Press, 2004. *The Institute of Medicine report on the topic of testosterone deficiency and replacement therapy in the older male population.*

Qoubaitary A, Swerdloff RS, Wang C: Advances in male hormone substitution therapy. Expert Opin Pharmacother 2005;6:1493–1506. *A review of this topic.*

Selvin E, Burnett AL, Platz EA: Prevalence and risk factors for erectile dysfunction in the US. Am J Med 2007;120:151–157. *Overall prevalence of 18.4%, higher in those with CV risk factors.*

Setter SM, Iltz JL, Fincham JE, et al: Phosphodiesterase 5 inhibitors for erectile dysfunction. Ann Pharmacother 2005;39:1286–1295. *A review of the role of this class of drugs for erectile dysfunction.*

Section XIX

Women's Health

APPROACH TO WOMEN'S HEALTH

Janet B. Henrich

Women's health has emerged as a rapidly expanding field of scientific inquiry and knowledge with important implications for clinical practice and for the education and training of physicians. Women's health can be viewed broadly as the study of the effect of sex and gender on health and disease that occurs across the spectrum of the biologic, behavioral, and social sciences. Increasing scientific information about the influence of sex and gender differences on health and disease has expanded our concept of women's health beyond the traditional focus on reproductive organs and their function. This broader interdisciplinary perspective has created a new area of knowledge and scholarship that is distinct from or more detailed than the knowledge base of existing disciplines. It has provided a new model to study the interactions between biologic mechanisms and psychosocial and environmental factors and their influence on human growth and development and response to health challenges. The clinical application of this information to women across all age groups highlights the interdisciplinary nature of this field.

BASIC PRINCIPLES UNDERLYING WOMEN'S HEALTH

The importance of the effect of sex and gender differences on health and disease is outlined in the Institute of Medicine Report *Exploring the Biological Contributions to Human Health: Does Sex Matter?* Complex interactions exist among sex hormones, normal and abnormal physiologic processes, and the physical and emotional well-being of women. As early as the embryonic period, there are structural differences between female and male brains. Many of these differences are programmed during fetal life by hormones. During the reproductive years, the influence of sex hormones on sexual development and reproductive function differentiates a category of health issues that are unique to women. As women age and sex hormones decrease during the menopause, women's risk factors for disease change dramatically and become more similar to men's. Although women develop the diseases that affect men, biologic mechanisms and psychosocial factors influence the course of disease differently in women.

Until recently, most of the information used to make clinical decisions in women was based on studies conducted primarily in men. Women were excluded from research on diseases that are important to both sexes because of misconceptions about women's health, legal and ethical issues, and cultural biases. Because women, on average, live longer than men and are affected by major diseases at a later age, it was often perceived incorrectly that women were healthier than men. In fact, throughout life, women experience poorer health than men do, especially in the advanced years. The lack of information concerning women had important implications. Information based primarily on studies done in men was often applied inappropriately to women or resulted in different standards of care. To rectify this gap in knowledge, the National Institutes of Health implemented a policy in 1994 that requires the inclusion of women and minorities in all human research studies funded by the National Institutes of Health. Substantial progress has been made in this area. Recent efforts have focused on ensuring that adequate numbers of women are included and that findings related to sex and gender differences are reported.

Efforts to increase our knowledge about women's health issues require an integrated approach that acknowledges the diversity among women and considers the social factors that influence their lives. One of the important social trends during the past 50 years is the increasing participation of women in the work force. Currently, it is estimated that 59% of women aged 16 years or older are in the work force, including 71% of women with children younger than 18 years, and 60% of working women are employed full-time throughout the year. The full effects of multiple roles, work stress, and new environmental exposures on women's health and reproductive status are largely unknown but are certain to have important health and social ramifications. Paralleling the growing numbers of women in the work force is the increasing number of single-parent families headed by women, especially minority women. Many of these families live in poverty. Increasing evidence indicates that socioeconomic factors are major indicators of health and that for some health outcomes, poverty and lack of education are more important determinants of health than ethnicity is. However, important ethnic and racial differences remain in women's susceptibility and response to certain diseases that cannot be explained wholly by socioeconomic status. For example, mortality rates for coronary heart disease, stroke, and breast cancer are higher in black than in white women, whereas death rates from lung cancer are higher in white women.

The increasing diversity of the population will affect health trends in the United States and the health status of women specifically. Regardless of their racial or ethnic designation, minority group women have a lower life expectancy than white women do and experience greater health problems. These differences are most pronounced in areas related to reproductive issues and childbearing, the occurrence and course of chronic disease, the incidence and outcome of cancer, and acts of interpersonal violence. Along with changes in our society, human immunodeficiency virus (HIV) infection is an additional special health concern of minority group women.

One of the most important factors underlying the current interest in women's health is the increasing number of women entering the health professions, especially the discipline of medicine. During the last century, the proportion of women represented in the population of physicians increased four-fold, from 6% in the early 1900s to 24% in 2000. Contributing to this growing population, the proportion of women graduates from medical schools increased from 6% in 1960 to 43% in 2001. Currently, women constitute 49% of entering medical school students. Although significant barriers remain to their attaining equal professional and academic status, the potential for women to influence the structure of their profession, the delivery of health care, and the direction of medical research is considerable.

MORBIDITY AND MORTALITY IN WOMEN

Mortality

At the turn of the 20th century, the average lifespan of women in the United States was 48 years, compared with 46 years in men. Since then, the life expectancy in women has increased more than 30 years and is now close to 80 years, compared with 74 years in men. The reasons for the dramatic increase in overall life expectancy are thought to be related to the control of infectious diseases and progress in the treatment of chronic diseases such as diabetes and cardiovascular disease.

Table 254–1 shows the leading causes of death in U.S. women of all ages and races.

Heart Disease

Despite a dramatic decline in mortality rates for heart disease that has occurred in both sexes during the past two decades, heart disease remains the leading cause of death for women and accounts for 30% of all deaths in women. Heart disease occurs 10 to 15 years later in women than in men. This delayed onset is thought to be due primarily to the protective effect of estrogens in premenopausal women and accounts for the fact that 90% of heart disease mortality in women occurs after the menopause. There are significant racial and ethnic differences in mortality among women. Black women are more likely than white women to die of heart disease up to the age of 85 years; thereafter, death rates are higher in white women. In contrast, Hispanic, Native American, and Asian–Pacific Islander women have significantly lower rates of death from heart disease. Evidence suggests that heart disease, once it develops, is more serious in women than in men, resulting in higher mortality rates. In addition to biologic factors, the poorer survival of women may be due to the older age of women at the time of diagnosis and increased prevalence of comorbid conditions as well as less well defined social factors that influence the diagnosis and treatment of heart disease in women.

Cancer

Cancer is the second leading cause of death in women and is the most common cause of premature death. The mortality rate for all cancers combined in women changed little during the last half of the 20th century. Major advances in the diagnosis and treatment of cervical and uterine cancers in women were offset by an increase in mortality rates for lung and breast cancer. Although breast cancer is the most common cancer diagnosed in women, lung cancer is the overall leading cause of

TABLE 254–1 LEADING CAUSES OF DEATH AND NUMBER OF DEATHS IN U.S. WOMEN: UNITED STATES, 2002

Cause of Death	Deaths	Percentage of Total Deaths
All causes	1,244,123	100.0
Cardiovascular diseases	356,014	28.6
Malignant neoplasms	268,503	21.6
Cerebrovascular diseases	100,050	8.0
Chronic lung diseases	64,103	5.2
Alzheimer's disease	41,877	3.4
Diabetes mellitus	38,948	3.1
Accidents (unintentional injuries)	37,485	3.0
Pneumonia, influenza	36,763	3.0
Nephritis, nephrotic syndrome, nephrosis	21,279	1.7

From National Center for Health Statistics: Health, United States, 2004, with Chartbook on Trends in the Health of Americans. Hyattsville, MD, U.S. Department of Health and Human Services, Centers for Disease Control and Prevention, 2004.

cancer deaths. It is estimated that 90% of lung cancer deaths can be attributed to cigarette smoking and are therefore potentially preventable. Whereas deaths from lung cancer in men have begun to decline as the result of a decrease in male cigarette use, death rates for women continue to rise.

Breast Cancer

Breast cancer is the second overall leading cause of cancer deaths in women and the most common cause in women younger than 55 years. Although the incidence of breast cancer continues to rise, mortality rates have begun to decline for the first time since cancer registries began tracking this disease in the 1940s. This disparity is thought to be related partly to the widespread use of screening mammography and the detection of cancers in earlier stages that have a more favorable prognosis. There are significant racial differences in breast cancer incidence. White women continue to have the highest rates of breast cancer, followed closely by black women. Hispanic and Asian–Pacific Islander women are at intermediate risk, and Native American women are at lowest risk. There are also significant racial differences in breast cancer mortality. Although breast cancer incidence rates are 22% higher in white women than in black women, mortality rates are 36% higher in black women. Reasons for racial differences in breast cancer incidence and mortality are unclear but may be related to socioeconomic and biologic factors as well as certain health behaviors, such as participation in screening mammography. Although it has been shown that breast cancer screening with mammography and clinical breast examination decreases mortality from breast cancer and that 70% of American women 40 years and older report having had a recent mammogram, screening rates are lower in women who are poor or less well educated.

Stroke

Although stroke-related deaths have declined by more than 60% in the United States during the past 25 years, deaths from stroke still account for 8% of all deaths in women and rank third as a cause of mortality. Striking racial differences exist in stroke mortality; death rates in black women are almost twice those for white women up to the age of 75 years. Most of the stroke deaths in women result from thromboembolic disease and occur in older women. However, aneurysmal subarachnoid hemorrhage, a less frequent form of stroke that is more common in women than in men, contributes to stroke mortality, particularly in younger or pregnant women.

Respiratory Disease

Death rates from chronic lower respiratory diseases have increased steadily for both women and men during the past 25 years; however, the increase has been greater in women. Because this increase has been linked to patterns in cigarette smoking, death rates in women for pulmonary disease as well as for lung cancer are expected to continue to rise. Death rates from pneumonia and influenza closely parallel pulmonary-related deaths and vary over time on the basis of the epidemiology of these acute illnesses.

Diabetes

Diabetes has consistently ranked as a leading cause of death in women. Moreover, the reported death rate from diabetes most likely underestimates the impact of this disease on mortality because of its strong association with other life-threatening medical conditions, such as cardiovascular disease, stroke, and kidney failure. Close to 9% of all women 20 years or older have diabetes; however, prevalence rates are higher in black, Hispanic, and Native American women. Separate from disease-related death rates, diabetes is a significant cause of morbidity and, in women of childbearing age, has important adverse effects on pregnancy and pregnancy outcome, resulting in an increased risk of toxemia, macrosomia, hydramnios, congenital malformations, cesarean section, and fetal and perinatal mortality.

Human Immunodeficiency Virus Infection

Although mortality rates from HIV infection and acquired immunodeficiency syndrome (AIDS) began to decline in the mid-1990s as a result of highly effective combination treatment of HIV infection and better prevention of opportunistic infections, HIV infection remains a leading cause of death in younger women. Women overall account for an increasing proportion of AIDS cases, and ethnic minority women are disproportionately affected. As the features of this epidemic change, with heterosexual transmission accounting for the majority of new cases of HIV infection in women, these rates are expected to continue to rise.

Morbidity

Mortality rates alone do not provide a complete picture of women's health status. Although women live longer than men do, overall measures of health status are worse in women. On the basis of estimates from the 2002 National Health Interview Survey, more women than men report symptoms or seek care for acute medical conditions and are more disabled by these self-limited illnesses as measured by number of bed days or days lost from work. In addition, several chronic conditions occur more frequently in women and cause significant disability, such as arthritis, pain syndromes (including migraine and neck, back, and face pain), and chronic respiratory disorders (including chronic bronchitis, sinusitis, and asthma). Women are also more likely than men to experience severe psychological stress. Data from the National Institute of Mental Health show that affective disorders, especially major depressive episodes, and the anxiety disorders are significantly more prevalent in women. Most important, women's perception of their health status is lower than men's. According to estimates from the National Health Interview Survey, women are less likely than men to rate their health excellent and more likely to rate it poor to good.

LIFESPAN GROUPS

Many of the important health issues in women have their onset or greatest impact at certain ages and are intricately linked with women's psychosocial and sexual development. To develop a more integrated concept of women's health, it is instructive to look at the important health issues in women within the major lifespan groups. Several governmental and institutional sources were used to compile this information. Of these, the themes developed by the *Report of the National Institutes of Health: Opportunities for Research on Women's Health,* known as the Hunt Valley Report, form the basis of this section.

Birth to Young Adulthood

As young women reach puberty, the health issues that emerge are related primarily to developmental changes involving physical and sexual growth and changing relationships within and outside the family. Central to the psychosocial development of young women is the process of gender identification and orientation and the development of self-esteem. Intentional and unintentional injuries, including an increasing frequency of acts of physical and sexual violence, are the primary cause of death and disability in young women. A small proportion of girls develop a chronic disease or disability. Most of these conditions are related to autoimmune disorders, such as lupus erythematosus, juvenile rheumatoid arthritis, and thyroid disease. Because of hormonal influences, many of these conditions first occur or are exacerbated during puberty.

Ages 15 to 44 Years

During young adulthood, mortality rates in women are relatively low and deaths due to injury predominate.

Cancer

As women progress through this age group, cancers of the breast and reproductive tract emerge as the leading causes of death, followed by unintentional injury and heart disease.

Injury

Among the unintentional and intentional injuries in this age group, motor vehicle accidents, homicide, and suicide account for three fourths of all injury deaths. The death rate from motor vehicle accidents is highest in women 15 to 24 years of age; more than half of these deaths are alcohol related. Although there is a downward trend in death rates from homicide and suicide in young women, black women are most likely to be homicide victims, and firearms are used in more than half of these deaths. Because 30% of murders in women are perpetrated by a family member or acquaintance, the contribution of ongoing family violence to these fatal events is thought to be substantial.

Human Immunodeficiency Virus Infection

The most dramatic trend in this age group, beginning in the 1980s and peaking in the mid-1990s, was the emergence and rapid rise of HIV infection as a major cause of death. Although overall AIDS incidence and mortality rates have decreased yearly since 1996, the rate of decline has been smaller in women. The biologic and social aspects of HIV infection are difficult to separate; however, current evidence suggests that gender differences in the presentation and clinical course of HIV infection are related to women's limited access to care and lower acceptance of or adherence to treatment more than to true biologic differences. The consequences of this disease for gynecologic care and reproductive counseling in women are unique. Because of the interrelationships between the degree of immunosuppression related to HIV infection, the presence of coinfection with human papillomavirus (HPV), and an increased risk of cervical neoplasia, the Centers for Disease Control and Prevention and the Agency for Health Care Policy and Research recommend that newly diagnosed HIV-infected women have an initial pelvic examination and Papanicolaou (Pap) smear that are repeated in 6 months. If the findings of these examinations and prior Pap smears are normal and the woman has no AIDS-defining condition or evidence of HPV infection, subsequent annual screening is adequate. Women who are at higher risk because they do not meet these criteria require more frequent surveillance or additional studies, depending on the Pap smear findings.

Primary physicians play a unique role in counseling HIV-infected women of childbearing age. Because HIV can be transmitted during pregnancy and more than 40% of pregnancies are unintended, routine medical care should include discussions about effective contraceptive methods, the effects of pregnancy on HIV infection and treatment, and the potential for perinatal transmission of HIV. Treatment strategies in women who may become or are pregnant should take into consideration regimens that maximally suppress maternal viral load and reduce transmission to the fetus while minimizing toxicity. In 1994, the Pediatric AIDS Clinical Trials Group demonstrated that a three-part regimen of zidovudine reduces the risk of perinatal transmission by 70% and is effective even in women with advanced disease. Current U.S. Public Health Service recommendations for antiretroviral chemoprophylaxis to reduce perinatal transmission of HIV are evolving rapidly and take into consideration the now standard use of more aggressive combination drug therapies to treat HIV infection as well as the clinical status and antiviral drug history of the woman. Zidovudine should be part of the antepartum drug regimen in all pregnant HIV-infected women if feasible. (Treatment guidelines are updated periodically and are available at *http://AIDsinfo.nih.gov.*) Despite these advances, the social consequences of this disease are enormous and result in loss of productive life, disruption of family structure, and premature death. The challenge to primary physicians to help control the transmission of HIV is an essential part of national prevention efforts.

Risk-taking and Unhealthy Behaviors

An important role of physicians in the care of young women is to recognize and to reduce risk-taking and other unhealthy behaviors. Health habits become established during early adulthood. Unhealthy behaviors not only place women at risk for life-threatening events but also have important implications for the development of illness later in life. For example, early or unprotected sexual activity increases women's risk for sexually transmitted diseases. Not only are these diseases transmitted more easily from men to women, but women are disproportionately affected because of infectious complications that can lead to disorders of reproductive function, such as pelvic inflammatory disease, ectopic pregnancy, and infertility. Unfortunately, efforts at risk reduction, particularly in the use of harmful substances, are hampered by industry and market forces and other social factors that influence women's lives. For example, the adverse effects of cigarette smoking on lung cancer and other respiratory diseases, heart disease, osteoporosis, and reproductive function are well documented, yet 20% of women continue to smoke, and 18% of teenage mothers smoke during pregnancy.

Eating Disorders

Social and cultural factors have also contributed to the increasing prevalence of dieting and eating disorders. The American Psychiatric Association Work Group on Eating Disorders estimates that up to 4% of young women suffer from anorexia nervosa or bulimia, and an additional 5% have less specific eating disorders characterized by aberrant eating patterns and weight management habits. These disorders are often refractory to treatment and can be life-threatening. The statistics most likely underestimate the prevalence of eating disorders in young women. According to findings from the 2003 Youth Risk Behavior Surveillance System developed by the Centers for Disease Control and Prevention, 56% of adolescent women reported that they had attempted dieting in the previous month, 18% had gone more than 24 hours without eating, 11% had taken diet aids without professional advice, and 8% had induced vomiting or taken laxatives for weight control.

Reproductive Health

This lifespan group delineates women's reproductive years. In addition to traditional childbearing and family responsibilities, women are increasingly assuming new roles. The effect of multiple and often conflicting roles on women's mental and physical health remains to be determined but is closely linked to reproductive freedom and health. Thus, physicians need to understand the safety, effectiveness, and acceptability of current methods of contraception in culturally diverse women, including emergency contraception. 1 Because of an increased understanding of many other common disorders of reproductive function, it is also clear that general physicians can no longer view these disorders as exclusively gynecologic problems. The association of the polycystic ovary syndrome with insulin resistance and an increased risk of diabetes and cardiovascular disease and the contribution of nonreproductive causes to chronic pelvic pain highlight the general medical nature of these disorders.

Autoimmunity

One of the themes linking many of the medical disorders that have the highest prevalence in women in this age group is the role of autoimmunity. Most of the autoimmune diseases are more common in women than in men and cause greater morbidity. Many are influenced by changes in estrogen levels, particularly during pregnancy. Among the collagen vascular diseases, rheumatoid arthritis, systemic lupus erythematosus, and scleroderma have prevalence rates that are three to nine times higher in women. Many autoimmune-related endocrinopathies, such as Hashimoto's thyroiditis and Graves' disease, have a female-to-male ratio as high as 10:1. Less well recognized is the role of autoimmunity in recurrent pregnancy loss and infertility in women.

Mental Disorders

Among the mental disorders, depressive illnesses are twice as common in women as in men. An estimated 6.5% of women experience a major depressive episode each year, and twice that many have chronic low-grade symptoms of depression. The excess risk of depression in women begins at puberty and declines after the menopause. In addition, many women experience mood, cognitive, or behavioral changes associated with cyclic changes in hormone levels during the menstrual cycle or with marked changes in levels during the postpartum period and the menopausal transition. The genetic, biologic, and environmental contributions to women's susceptibility to depression are not fully understood; however, hormonal factors are thought to play a major role. Women are also twice as likely as men to be diagnosed with an anxiety disorder, including panic disorder, post-traumatic stress disorder, generalized anxiety, agoraphobia, and simple phobia.

Physical and Sexual Abuse

A major cause of psychosocial morbidity in women is physical and sexual abuse. On the basis of the National Violence Against Women Survey conducted by the National Institute of Justice and the Centers for Disease Control and Prevention in 1998, 52% of women have been physically assaulted at some time during their life, and 18% have experienced a rape. Young women are at particular risk for rape; of those women who have been raped, more than half were younger than 18 years when rape first occurred. Physical and sexual assault in women is primarily a problem of partner violence. Three fourths of women who experience physical or sexual abuse after the age of 18 years are assaulted by a current or former spouse or male intimate. On the basis of this finding, states are developing legal and other preventive strategies to protect women. Unfortunately, owing to lack of knowledge and training and misconceptions about physical and sexual violence, physicians often fail to recognize or to address symptoms of abuse. Adequate screening tools are especially crucial in the emergency department, where up to one third of women who have been assaulted seek care. To ensure widespread detection of abuse, screening should become a regular part of the medical history in any setting.

Ages 45 to 64 Years

Death rates for women in this age group have declined by 30% in the past 25 years. Previously, the leading cause of death was heart disease; however, cancer is now ranked number one. This shift in mortality rates reflects primarily a decline in death rates for heart disease that has been observed in both sexes and is attributed to changes in lifestyle, such as better control of hypertension and lower blood cholesterol levels.

Many of the important chronic conditions in women first appear in this age group, and the prevalence of some increases markedly during this period. There are significant racial and ethnic differences in the prevalence of many of these conditions.

Obesity

Associated with the dramatic increase in obesity in the U.S. population during the past 20 years, 62% of women are now overweight or obese, and 34% are obese. The prevalence of obesity in particular is disproportionately high in minority women; close to 50% of black and 39% of Mexican American women are obese, compared with 31% of white women. Because obesity is a major risk factor for diabetes, heart disease, stroke, gallbladder disease, sleep apnea, and some cancers (endometrial, breast, and colon cancer) and may be a factor in osteoarthritis, weight control in women is an important public health issue.

Menopause

The emergence of many of these conditions, such as heart disease, osteoporosis, and cancer, is inextricably linked to the menopause and the marked decline in estrogen levels that occur during this age period. Hormone replacement is the most effective therapy for vasomotor and vaginal symptoms associated with the menopause and decreases bone loss and the risk of osteoporotic fractures. [2] On the basis of data from a large number of observational studies, expectations were that hormone therapy would also protect women from heart disease and stroke and may protect women from the development of colon cancer. Data from a smaller number of studies also suggested that hormone therapy may protect the brain from cognitive decline and dementia, increase quality of life, and protect the urinary tract from aging problems such as urinary incontinence.

These hopes were not borne out by findings from the National Institutes of Health–sponsored Women's Health Initiative Trial, the first large randomized trial designed to look at the role of hormone therapy in altering the risk for development of these disorders. The combined estrogen-progesterone arm of this multicenter study was halted early in 2002 because of an increased incidence of breast cancer in women receiving active therapy, a potentially adverse outcome of hormone therapy that was confirmed in the study. [3] Rates of heart disease, stroke, dementia, and urinary problems were also increased in women receiving hormone therapy compared with women taking placebo, whereas rates of hip fracture and colon cancer were reduced. [4-8] Because the risks of hormone therapy outweigh its benefits, combined estrogen and progesterone should not be used as preventive therapy in postmenopausal women. The estrogen-only arm of the trial was halted 1 year later, when investigators found that even though the harmful effects of hormone therapy were less pronounced in women who used estrogen without progesterone, the risks still outweighed the benefits. [9]

Transitions in Social Roles and Life Circumstances

Whereas the menopause encompasses many of the physiologic changes that define this period, women also experience major transitions in social roles and life circumstances that profoundly affect their physical and mental health. Children leave home, many women become widowed or divorced, parenting roles change as women are called on to care for aging parents, and disabilities increase, making it difficult for some women to function within and outside the home. An understanding of these life events is essential to the comprehensive care of mature women.

Ages 65 Years and Older

Heart disease is the leading cause of death in older women, followed by cancer and stroke. Mortality rates for all three disorders rise steeply after the age of 65 years and begin to approach the rates for men. Chronic pulmonary disease and pneumonia continue to cause high death rates because of the increase and severity of infections associated with an age-related decline in immune function. Injury is the sixth leading cause of death in older women; most of these deaths are related to falls.

Illnesses of the Very Old

As women's longevity increases, they bear the burden of illnesses that are seen primarily in the very old. Of these, the neurologic degenerative diseases, such as dementia, sleep disorders, and neurosensory and movement disorders, are particularly common in women. Unfortunately, the added years of life in women are often spent in a frail or dependent state and often result in institutionalization. Currently, women residing in nursing homes outnumber men by three to one. In particular, urinary incontinence and osteoporosis put women at high risk for institutionalization. Prevalence rates of urinary incontinence are twice as high in women as in men and affect up to half of community-dwelling women. Osteoporosis is associated with deformity and pain secondary to vertebral fractures; however, hip fracture, usually the result of a fall, is the most serious consequence of osteoporosis in older women. According to the National Osteoporosis Foundation, 85% of women older than 50 years with a hip fracture cannot walk unassisted 6 months after a fracture, and one fourth never live independently again.

Social and Psychological Changes

The social and psychological changes that women experience as they age add to the burden of illness. Social isolation increases because of death of loved ones, loss of financial stability, and increasing physical disabilities. In addition to an increasing incidence of dementia with age, mental health problems become more prevalent or serious. The role of the primary physician is to recognize and help reduce the impact of these accumulated conditions on women's ability to function and on their quality of life.

PRIMARY PREVENTION GUIDELINES IN NONPREGNANT WOMEN

Many of the conditions that cause the greatest morbidity and mortality in women can be prevented or delayed by the early recognition and treatment of risk factors and the identification of individuals who might benefit the most from early intervention. The U.S. Preventive Services Task Force (USPSTF) publishes primary preventive guidelines that can assist clinicians in providing care to women. The recommendations are conservative and represent the minimum level of preventive services that should be offered.

On the basis of recommendation from the USPSTF, all women should have periodic blood pressure evaluation, height and weight measurements, and screening for obesity and depression. Cervical cancer screening with Pap smears is recommended in sexually active women. Although guidelines about when to start or to stop Pap smear screening and the optimal screening interval in low-risk women differ among policymaking organizations, the USPSTF recommends initiation of screening 3 years after sexual activity begins or at the age of 21 years, whichever occurs first, and screening of low-risk women at least every 3 years after two or three annual normal Pap smears. Routine screening is not recommended in low-risk women after the age of 65 years if they have had adequate recent screening or in women who have had a total hysterectomy for benign reasons. Newer screening methods using liquid-based cytology offer advantages over conventional Pap smears, such as the option of reflex HPV testing, but are more expensive. Until more information is available from trials assessing the role of HPV testing in cervical cancer screening, the USPSTF's position is that the evidence is insufficient at this time to recommend the use of this new technology over the routine Pap smear. Prophylactic vaccines shown in clinical trials to be highly effective against HPV infection are now available for widespread immunization; guidelines for their use are being developed. [10, 11] Sexually active women younger than 25 years should be screened routinely for chlamydia; screening for chlamydia, gonorrhea, syphilis, and HIV infection should be done in any woman with risk factors for these diseases.

Breast cancer screening with mammography, with or without clinical breast examination, is recommended every 1 to 2 years starting at the age of 40 years, although women aged 50 to 65 years and those at increased risk for breast cancer benefit the most. Clinicians should discuss the risks and benefits of breast cancer chemoprophylaxis in high-risk women. Routine screening for ovarian cancer is not recommended.

Cholesterol screening is recommended every 5 years in women starting at the age of 45 years; those with hypertension or hyperlipidemia should be screened further for diabetes. As in men, colorectal screening is recommended beginning at the age of 50 years. Routine screening for osteoporosis in women is recommended starting at the age of 65 years; however, many younger women have conditions that put them at increased risk for osteoporotic fractures. In these women, screening is recommended starting at the age of 60 years. Periodic vision and hearing screening is recommended in both women and men after the age of 65 years.

On the basis of findings from studies that were conducted primarily in men, the USPSTF currently recommends that clinicians discuss the use of aspirin for the primary prevention of coronary heart disease with postmenopausal women and younger women with risk factors for coronary heart disease. However, results from the first randomized trial that assessed the risks and benefits of aspirin as chemoprevention for coronary heart disease in women found a beneficial effect only in women aged 65 years or older. [12] In younger women, aspirin reduced the risk of thromboembolic stroke but had little effect on coronary heart disease, findings opposite to those described in men. Similar to its use in men, the use of aspirin in older women was associated with an increased risk of hemorrhagic stroke and major gastrointestinal hemorrhage. Until more information is available about aspirin's effects in women, discussions about its use should be individualized for each patient.

The USPSTF recommends counseling women of childbearing age about folic acid supplementation to reduce the risk of neural tube defects and women of all ages about adequate calcium and vitamin D intake. All women should be counseled about tobacco and other substance use, strategies to decrease the transmission of sexually transmitted diseases, effective methods of contraception, healthy diet and increased physical activity, and injury prevention, with a focus in older individuals on falls and the potential dangers of multiple medication use.

EDUCATION AND TRAINING IN WOMEN'S HEALTH FOR PHYSICIANS

Among academic medical institutions, there is increasing awareness of the importance of women's health. However, there is often uncertainty about what actually constitutes women's health and the best way to train physicians to provide more comprehensive care to women. As a foundation for addressing women's health conditions, it is essential that physicians understand basic female physiology and reproductive biology. In addition, they need to appreciate the complex interaction between the environment and the biology and psychosocial development of women. Among the conditions that are not specific to women, physicians need to be aware of those aspects of disease that are different in women or have important gender implications. The ability to apply this information requires that physicians adopt attitudes and behavior that are culture and gender sensitive. Women's relationship to the medical system is also changing and requires physicians to understand women's patterns of health seeking and forms of communication and interaction as well as to appreciate gender differences in clinical decision making.

To provide models that may assist academic institutions in implementing these recommendations, the U.S. Department of Health and Human Services has funded the establishment of 21 National Centers of Excellence in Women's Health within academic health centers. These centers are designed to facilitate the development of innovative clinical models, integrated curricula, and interdisciplinary research in women's health and to foster the development of women faculty. The impact of the centers on curriculum reform, clinical care, and research initiatives is currently being evaluated.

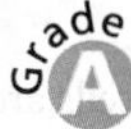

1. Raine TR, Harper CC, Rocca CH, et al: Direct access to emergency contraception through pharmacies and effect on unintended pregnancy and STIs: A randomized controlled trial. JAMA 2005; 293:54–62.
2. Cauley JA, Robbins J, Chen Z, et al: Effects of estrogen plus progestin on risk of fracture and bone mineral density: The Women's Health Initiative randomized trial. JAMA 2003;290: 1729–1738.
3. Rossouw JE, Anderson GL, Prentice RL, et al: Risks and benefits of estrogen plus progestin in healthy postmenopausal women: Principal results from the Women's Health Initiative randomized controlled trial. JAMA 2002;288:321–333.
4. Manson JE, Hsia J, Johnson KC, et al: Estrogen plus progestin and the risk of coronary heart disease. N Engl J Med 2003;349: 523–534.
5. Hendrix SL, Wassertheil-Smoller S, Johnson KC, et al: Effects of conjugated equine estrogen on stroke in the Women's Health Initiative. Circulation 2006;113:2425–2434.
6. Shumaker SA, Legault C, Rapp SR, et al: Estrogen plus progestin and the incidence of dementia and mild cognitive impairment in postmenopausal women: The Women's Health Initiative Memory Study: A randomized controlled trial. JAMA 2003;289:2651–2662.
7. Rapp SR, Espeland MA, Shumaker SA, et al: Effect of estrogen plus progestin on global cognitive function in postmenopausal women: The Women's Health Initiative Memory Study: A randomized controlled trial. JAMA 2003;289:2663–2672.
8. Hendrix SL, Cochrane BB, Nygaard IE, et al: Effects of estrogen with and without progestin on urinary incontinence. JAMA 2005; 293:935–948.
9. Anderson GL, Limacher M, Assaf AR, et al: Effects of conjugated equine estrogen in postmenopausal women with hysterectomy: The Women's Health Initiative randomized controlled trial. JAMA 2004;291:1701–1712.
10. Koutsky LA, Ault KA, Wheeler CM, et al: A controlled trial of a human papillomavirus type 16 vaccine. N Engl J Med 2002;347: 1645–1651.
11. Harper DM, Franco EL, Wheeler C, et al: Efficacy of a bivalent L1 virus-like particle vaccine in prevention of infection with human papillomavirus types 16 and 18 in young women: A randomised controlled trial. Lancet 2004;364:1757–1765.
12. Ridker PM, Cook NR, Lee IM, et al: A randomized trial of low-dose aspirin in the primary prevention of cardiovascular disease in women. N Engl J Med 2005;352:1293–1304.

SUGGESTED READINGS

Grady D: Clinical practice. Management of menopausal symptoms. N Engl J Med 2006;355:2338–2347. *A clinical review.*

National Center for Health Statistics: Health, United States, 2004, with Chartbook on Trends in the Health of Americans. Hyattsville, MD, U.S. Department of Health and Human Services, Centers for Disease Control and Prevention, 2004. *A report on the health status and trends of the nation.*

U.S. Preventive Services Task Force website. Available at http://www.ahrq.gov/clinic/uspstfix.htm. *Provides the latest recommendations for evidence-based preventive services and links to major resources, including the Guide to Clinical Preventive Services.*

255 OVARIES AND DEVELOPMENT

Robert W. Rebar and Gregory F. Erickson

Definition

The ovaries episodically release female gametes (oocytes or eggs) and secrete sex steroid hormones, principally androstenedione, estradiol, and progesterone. Oocytes are released only during the adult reproductive years, when sex steroid secretion is also greatest, but the ovaries are physiologically active throughout life.

Sex steroids affect the growth, differentiation, and function of a variety of tissues and organs throughout the body; therefore, abnormalities of the ovaries and of sex steroid secretion should be recognized by all physicians. A rational approach to the diagnosis and treatment of reproductive disorders in women requires an understanding of the functions of the ovaries and of their most important unit, the follicle, throughout life.

Physiology

Embryology

Embryogenesis and Differentiation

Organogenesis of the ovaries occurs during fetal life. Ovarian cells are derived from two different sources: (1) primordial germ cells (PGCs) originate at a site outside the prospective gonads, and (2) somatic cells differentiate from the coelomic epithelium and gonadal mesenchyme. In females, PGCs become oocytes, whereas somatic cells differentiate into a variety of cell types, including granulosa, theca, and vascular cells.

PGCs in the human embryo can be distinguished at the gastrula stage (Fig. 255–1). Shortly after formation, PGCs migrate through the dorsal mesentery to the genital ridges. Chemotaxis plays a role in directing PGCs to the gonads. During migration, PGCs proliferate in response to growth factors, most notably kit ligand. The importance of kit is demonstrated by the finding that loss-of-function mutations result in a paucity of PGCs, which in turn results in premature ovarian failure.

The genital ridges are characterized by a thickening of the coelomic epithelium and underlying primary mesenchyme. Initially, the gonads are sexually indifferent. Male gonadal differentiation is triggered by the Y chromosome–encoded testis-determining factor, SRY. SRY expression results in the differentiation of Sertoli cells and the secretion of müllerian-inhibiting substance, which induces regression of the müllerian ducts. Testicular interstitial cells differentiate into Leydig cells, which secrete testosterone, which in turn stimulates wolffian duct development. In the female, absence of müllerian-inhibiting substance and testosterone leads to the degeneration of the wolffian ducts and to the development of the müllerian ducts. Thus, the development of the ovaries and female reproductive system is considered a "default" pathway.

When PGCs enter the genital ridges, they begin gametogenesis (see Fig. 255–1). In females, this process is termed oogenesis and involves the differentiation of PGCs into oogonia and oocytes. When sex-specific differentiation of the ovary commences, the inactive X chromosome in the PGCs becomes active. This denotes the formation of mitotically active oogonia. The importance of two functional X chromosomes during oogenesis is emphasized by the fact that 45,X females lack oocytes and undergo premature menopause.

After repeated mitosis, oogonia initiate meiosis and become oocytes (see Fig. 255–1). At approximately the same time, granulosa cells differentiate within the gonadal mesenchyme and establish intimate associations with oocytes. Oocytes that become surrounded by granulosa cells stop meiosis after diplotene, and the bivalents enter an interphase state known as dictyotene. If an oocyte is not surrounded by granulosa cells, meiosis continues to diakinesis and the oocyte dies by apoptosis. Granulosa cells, therefore, are critical for oocyte survival. The majority of oocytes die during fetal ovary development (Fig. 255–2), apparently from a lack of contact with granulosa cells.

With further development, the oocyte–granulosa cell complex becomes a primordial follicle. This occurs between the sixth and ninth months of gestation (Fig. 255–3). A primordial follicle consists of a single layer of squamous granulosa cells, a small (about 15 μm in diameter) dictyotene oocyte, and a thin basal lamina (see Fig. 255–3). In the human female, all potential future eggs have entered diplotene of meiosis at the time of birth, and no reserve oogonia remain.

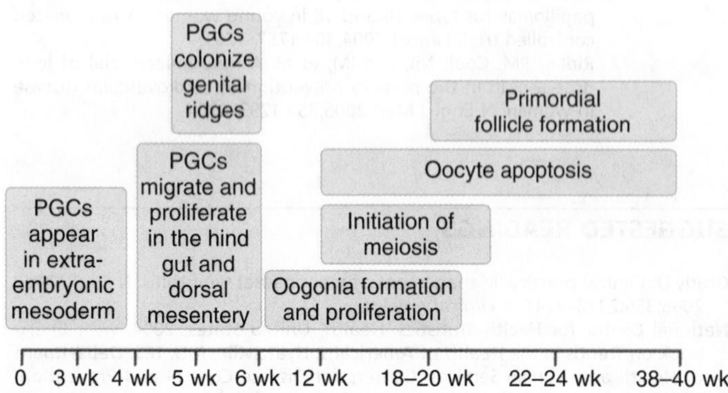

FIGURE 255–1 • Diagram illustrating the developmental timetable of the major events that ultimately lead to the formation of primordial follicles during the process of human ovary organogenesis. PGC = primordial germ cell.

Anatomy

The Adult Ovary

The ovaries of normal cycling women are oval bodies that each measure 2.5 to 5.0 cm in length, 1.5 to 3 cm in width, and 0.6 to 1.5 cm in thickness. The medial edge is attached by the mesovarium to the broad ligament, which in turn extends from the uterus laterally to the wall of the pelvic cavity. The ovary is covered by cuboidal epithelium. Beneath the epithelium is a layer of dense connective tissue, the tunica albuginea, which contains the primordial follicles.

The ovaries are organized into two principal parts. A central zone, the medulla, is surrounded by a prominent peripheral zone, the cortex (Fig. 255–4). Growing follicles at different stages of development are present in the cortex. Typically, one follicle per cycle reaches maturity and ovulates its ovum. After ovulation, the follicle transforms into a corpus luteum. The corpus luteum of the cycle lasts for about 14 days, after which

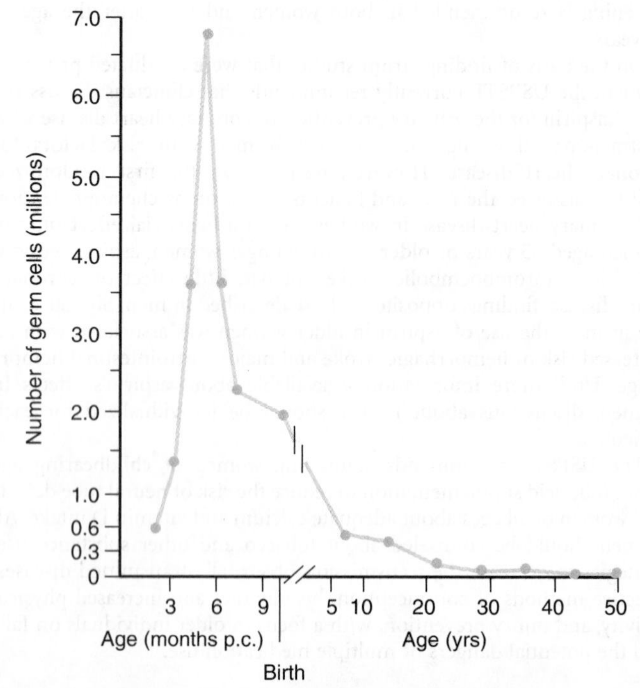

FIGURE 255–2 • Changes in the total number of germ cells in the human ovaries during aging. At early to mid gestation, the number of germ cells increases to almost 7 million; shortly thereafter, the number declines rapidly to about 2 million at birth. The number continues to decline until no oocytes are detected at 50 years of age. (From Baker TG: Radiosensitivity of mammalian oocytes with particular reference to the human female. Am J Obstet Gynecol 1971;110:746–761, with permission.)

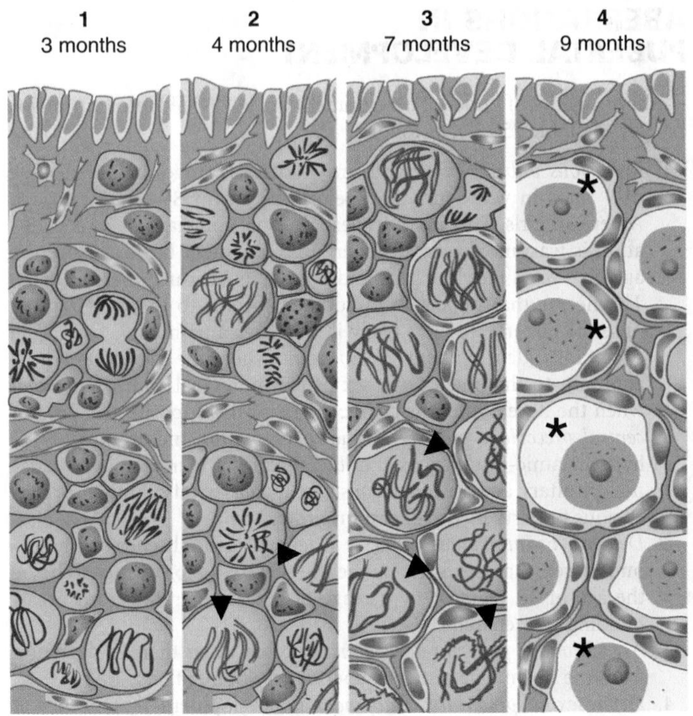

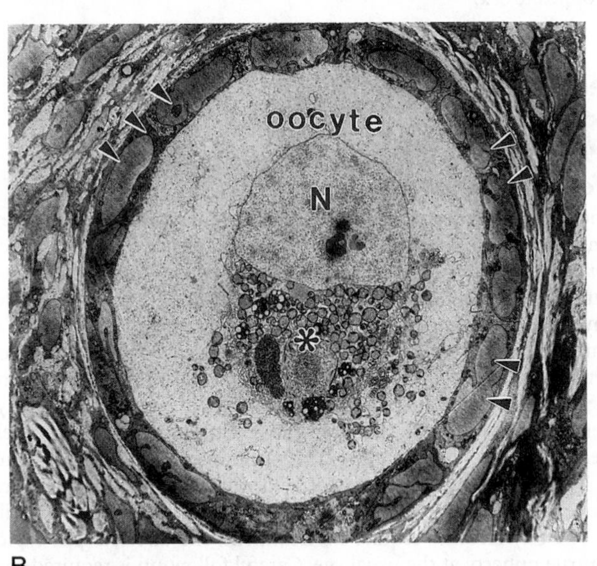

FIGURE 255–3 • A, Drawing showing gametogenesis in the human fetal ovary leading to the formation of primordial follicles. At 3 months (1), oogonia divide mitotically. At 4 months (2), some oogonia deep within the cortical cords enter meiosis (arrowheads). At 7 months (3), the cords are no longer distinct and all germ cells are in meiotic prophase I. At 9 months (4), some oocytes become associated with granulosa cells and appear as primordial follicles (asterisks). **B,** Electron micrograph of human primordial follicle. Granulosa cells (arrowheads), oocyte nucleus (N), and Balbiani body (asterisk) are shown. (From Erickson GF: The ovary: Basic principles and concepts. *In* Felig P, Baxter JD, Broadus AE, et al [eds]: Endocrinology and Metabolism, 3rd ed. New York, McGraw-Hill, 1995, with permission.)

it dies and becomes a nodule of dense connective tissue, the corpus albicans (see Fig. 255–4).

The medulla is composed of loose connective tissue with numerous blood vessels and associated nerves. The arterial supply to the ovary originates from two principal sources, the ovarian artery and the uterine artery. These two vessels, which enter the medulla from opposite directions, form an anastomotic trunk and become a common vessel called the ramus ovaricus artery. This artery gives rise to a series of primary branches (spiral arteries) that enter the hilum. In the hilum, numerous secondary and tertiary branches are given off to supply the medulla and the follicles and luteal tissue in the cortex (see Fig. 255–4). The hilum also

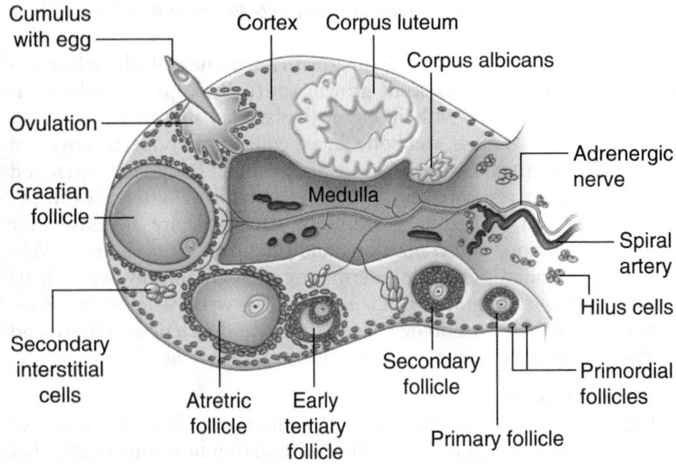

FIGURE 255–4 • Diagram showing the anatomy of the human ovary during the reproductive years. Developing follicles and corpora lutea are located in the cortex; the hilus cells, autonomic nerves, and spiral arteries are present in the medulla. (From Erickson GF: The ovary: Basic principles and concepts. *In* Felig P, Baxter JD, Broadus AE, et al [eds]: Endocrinology and Metabolism, 3rd ed. New York, McGraw-Hill, 1995, with permission.)

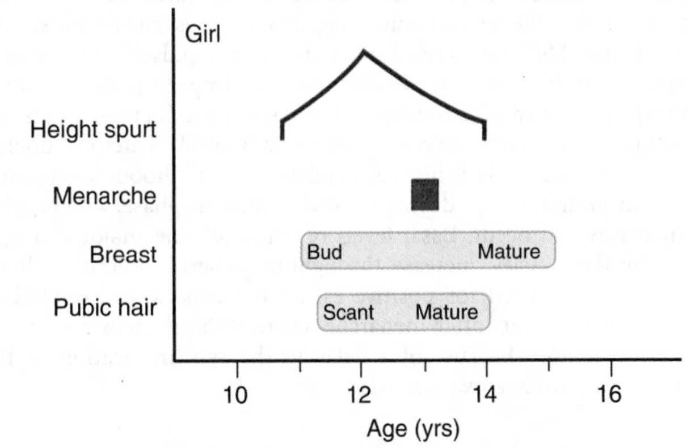

FIGURE 255–5 • Temporal sequence of events for the "average" girl during puberty. (From Rebar RW: Practical evaluation of hormonal status. *In* Yen SSC, Jaffe RB, Barbieri RL [eds]: Reproductive Endocrinology: Physiology, Pathophysiology, and Clinical Management, 4th ed. Philadelphia, WB Saunders, 1999, p 710.)

contains the hilus cells (see Fig. 255–4), which, like the testicular Leydig cells, contain Reinke crystals and secrete testosterone. The physiologic role of the hilus cells is still unknown.

Ovarian Function in Childhood and Puberty

Physical Changes at Puberty

Puberty extends from the earliest signs of sexual maturation until the attainment of physical, mental, and emotional maturity. Pubertal changes in girls result directly or indirectly from maturation of the hypothalamic-pituitary-ovarian unit. Human puberty is characterized hormonally by a resetting of the negative gonadal steroid feedback loop, the establishment of new circadian and ultradian (frequent) gonadotropin rhythms, and the acquisition in the female of a positive estrogen feedback loop controlling the menstrual cycle as interdependent expressions of the gonadotropins and ovarian steroids. In girls, pubertal development generally occurs between 8 and 14 years of age. The age at onset and the rate of progress through puberty are variable and depend on genetic, socioeconomic, nutritional, physical, and psychological factors.

Physical changes occur in an orderly sequence during a definite time frame in puberty (Fig. 255–5). Breast budding in girls is usually the first pubertal change, followed shortly by the appearance of pubic hair, with menarche occurring late in pubertal development. The time from breast budding (median age at onset, 9.8 years) to menarche approximates 2 years. Breast development results from increasing ovarian estrogen production, and pubic and axillary hair from increasing ovarian androgen production. Estrogens are required for growth of pubic hair as well.

The ovarian sex steroids join with growth hormone and adrenal androgens to produce the adolescent growth spurt. Peak growth velocity is achieved relatively early with little growth observed after menarche. Lean body mass, skeletal mass, and body fat are equal in prepubertal boys and girls, but by maturity, women have twice as much body fat as men and less lean body mass and skeletal mass as a result of differences in sex steroid secretion beginning at puberty. Estrogens are necessary for normal formation, mineralization, and maturation of bones. Well-established standards exist for determining radiographically, typically by examination of radiographs of the bones of the wrist, whether bone age is appropriate for chronologic age. Estrogen deficiencies retard and excesses advance bone age in relation to chronologic age.

Hormonal Changes

The ovaries function even in early childhood. The low levels of luteinizing hormone (LH) and follicle-stimulating hormone (FSH) that are normally present increase if the ovaries are removed before puberty, just as they do later in life, indicating exquisite sensitivity of the hypothalamic-pituitary unit to extremely low circulating sex steroid levels. As puberty nears, there is a progressive decrease in sensitivity of the hypothalamic-pituitary unit to sex steroids, leading to increased secretion of pituitary gonadotropins, stimulation of sex steroid output, and development of secondary sex characteristics. Increased secretion of both LH and FSH initially occurs at night with sleep and is associated with increased estradiol secretion the next morning (Fig. 255–6). As is true for most hormones, LH and FSH are secreted in an episodic or pulsatile rather than in a continuous fashion. It is possible that the sleep-entrained pulsatile secretion of gonadotropins commences in response to increased pulsatile secretion of gonadotropin-releasing hormone (GnRH). Later in puberty, secretion of LH and FSH is increased, relative to childhood, throughout the 24-hour period, except during the early follicular phase, when nighttime increases still occur. Basal levels of estradiol, the major estrogen secreted by the ovaries, increase throughout puberty. A "critical body mass" may be required for positive estrogen feedback and ovulation. During the first 2 years after menarche, up to 90% of menstrual cycles may be anovulatory because of a delay in the synchronization of the hypothalamic-pituitary-ovarian axis.

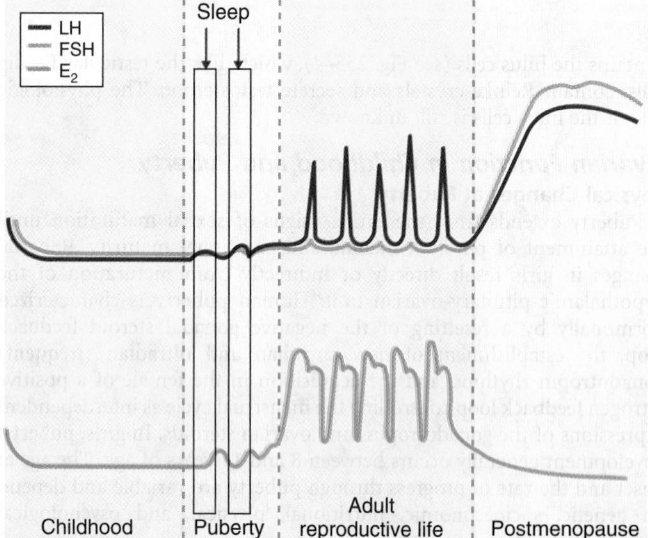

FIGURE 255–6 • The changing patterns of LH, FSH, and estradiol (E_2) concentrations in peripheral blood throughout the life of a woman. Not shown is the fact that both LH and FSH are secreted in a pulsatile fashion. The pubertal period has been expanded to illustrate the sleep-associated increases in LH and FSH followed by morning increases in E_2 that are observed during puberty. (Reprinted with permission from Endocrine and Metabolism Continuing Education Quality Control Program, 1982. Copyright American Association for Clinical Chemistry, Inc.)

ABERRATIONS IN PUBERTAL DEVELOPMENT

Abnormalities of pubertal development can be divided into four major categories (Table 255–1), as follows.

1. *Precocious puberty* represents any pubertal changes before the age of 9 years in white girls and before the age of 8 years in African American girls. This is controversial. Some clinicians believe evaluation is warranted only if pubertal development begins before the age of 7 years in white girls and 6 years in African American girls. The nearer that pubertal development begins to the mean age at onset of puberty, the less likely it is to have a pathologic basis. The precocious development is *isosexual* when the development is common to the phenotypic sex of the individual and *heterosexual* when the development is characteristic of the opposite sex. *True* or *central precocious puberty* is due to premature maturation of the hypothalamic-pituitary axis. In the absence of increased hypothalamic-pituitary activity, *precocious pseudopuberty* (also known as precocious puberty of peripheral origin) exists.
2. *Delayed* (or *interrupted*) *puberty* is defined as the absence of any secondary sex characteristics by the age of 13 years or of menarche by the age of 16 years or by passage of 5 years or more from breast budding to menarche.
3. *Asynchronous pubertal development* occurs when there is deviation from the normal pattern of pubertal development.
4. *Heterosexual pubertal development* is development that occurs at the appropriate time but with some features characteristic of the opposite sex.

Precocious Puberty

Diagnosis

Differential Diagnosis

The temporal sequence in which the signs and symptoms of sex steroid hormone excess appear is most important. *Incomplete isosexual precocious puberty* indicates premature development of only a single pubertal feature. If breast budding occurs before the age of 8 years in the absence of any other development, the diagnosis may be *premature thelarche.* Premature thelarche is believed to be due to transient increases in estrogen secretion or increased breast sensitivity to the small quantities of circulating estrogens present before puberty. Simple ovarian cysts may be present in some girls with this disorder. If pubic or axillary hair develops alone and persists, *premature pubarche* and *adrenarche* must be considered. These abnormalities are associated with slight increases in adrenal androgen secretion but not with clitorimegaly or other signs of virilization. These syndromes require no treatment, and affected girls typically begin true puberty at the usual age. Careful follow-up is required to distinguish these disorders from true precocious puberty.

When precocious development is isosexual, the purpose of evaluation is to determine if the cause is central (true precocious puberty). Careful questioning of the patient and her parents may indicate inadvertent ingestion or absorption of sex steroids (iatrogenic or factitious). About 10% of individuals with true precocious puberty have one of several organic brain diseases, including neoplasms, tuberous sclerosis, neurofibromatosis, encephalitis, meningitis, and hydrocephalus. The seriousness of intracranial lesions mandates that girls with precocious puberty have radiographic evaluation of the central nervous system, most effectively by magnetic resonance imaging. In almost 90% of girls with true precocious puberty, however, no cause is identified (idiopathic or constitutional).

The physical examination may also provide critical information about the cause of the precocious development. Cutaneous café au lait spots, facial asymmetry, polyostotic fibrous dysplasia and other skeletal abnormalities, cranial nerve deficits, and multiple ovarian follicular cysts suggest *McCune-Albright syndrome* in a girl with precocious puberty. It is now known that various clones of cells in the endocrine glands of girls with this disorder function autonomously with respect to cyclic adenosine monophosphate production as a consequence of a mutation within exon 8 of the G protein α subunit. This same mutation probably accounts for the bone lesions and café au lait hyperpigmentation. Precocious

TABLE 255–1 ABERRATIONS OF PUBERTAL DEVELOPMENT

PRECOCIOUS DEVELOPMENT

- Isosexual precocity
  - Incomplete sexual precocity
    - Premature thelarche
    - Premature pubarche
    - Premature adrenarche
  - True (central) precocious puberty
    - Idiopathic (constitutional)
    - Due to central nervous system lesions
    - Primary hypothyroidism
    - Silver-Russell syndrome
  - Precocious pseudopuberty (of peripheral origin)
    - Ovarian neoplasms
    - Adrenal neoplasms
    - Iatrogenic (estrogen-containing preparations)
    - Human chorionic gonadotropin–secreting neoplasms distinct from central nervous system and ovarian tumors
    - McCune-Albright syndrome
- Heterosexual precocity
  - Ovarian neoplasms
  - Adrenal neoplasms
  - Congenital adrenal hyperplasia
  - Other rare disorders of sexual differentiation

DELAYED PUBERTAL DEVELOPMENT (no development by age 13 yr; absence of menarche by age 16 yr; passage of 5 yr or more from breast budding without menarche)

- Anatomic abnormalities
  - Müllerian agenesis or dysgenesis (Rokitansky-Küster-Hauser syndrome)
  - Distal genital tract obstruction
    - Transverse vaginal septum
    - Imperforate hymen
    - Vaginal agenesis
- Hypergonadotropic hypogonadism (follicle-stimulating hormone >30–40 mIU/mL)
  - Gonadal dysgenesis
    - With stigmata of Turner's syndrome
    - Pure (46,XX or 46,XY)
    - Mixed
  - Ovarian failure with normal ovarian development
    - Autoimmune disorders
    - Gonadotropin receptor or postreceptor defects (? resistant ovary or Savage's syndrome)
    - Enzymatic defects (17α-hydroxylase deficiency, galactosemia)
    - Physical causes
      - Irradiation
      - Chemotherapeutic agents
      - Viral agents
    - Idiopathic
- Hypogonadotropic or normogonadotropic hypogonadism (luteinizing hormone and follicle-stimulating hormone <10 mIU/mL or luteinizing hormone and follicle-stimulating hormone 6–25 mIU/mL with at least one being >10 mIU/mL)
  - Isolated gonadotropin deficiency
    - In association with midline defects (Kallmann's syndrome)
    - Independent of associated disorders
  - Neoplasms of the hypothalamic-pituitary axis
    - Craniopharyngiomas
    - Pituitary tumors
    - Others
  - Infiltrative processes (Langerhans-type histiocytosis)
  - Idiopathic hypopituitarism
  - "Hypothalamic" forms of amenorrhea
    - Psychogenic
    - Exercise associated
    - Associated with malnutrition
    - Anorexia nervosa
  - Miscellaneous disorders
    - Prader-Labhart-Willi syndrome
    - Lawrence-Moon-Bardet-Biedl syndrome
    - Primary hypothyroidism
  - Constitutional delayed puberty

ASYNCHRONOUS PUBERTAL DEVELOPMENT

- Incomplete forms of androgen insensitivity
- Complete forms of androgen insensitivity

HETEROSEXUAL PUBERTAL DEVELOPMENT

- Polycystic ovary syndrome
- Congenital adrenal hyperplasia (female pseudohermaphroditism)
  - 21-Hydroxylase deficiency
  - 11β-Hydroxylase deficiency
  - 3β-ol-Hydroxysteroid dehydrogenase deficiency
- Male pseudohermaphroditism due to 5α-reductase deficiency
- Male pseudohermaphroditism due to partial androgen insensitivity
- Mixed gonadal dysgenesis
- Androgen-producing neoplasms
  - Ovarian
  - Adrenal
- Cushing's syndrome

development associated with short stature, congenital body asymmetry, triangular facies, and clinodactyly suggests the *Silver-Russell syndrome.* Characteristic signs and symptoms may suggest the coexistence of primary hypothyroidism and precocious puberty, especially if galactorrhea is also present. In these patients, thyroid hormone replacement therapy halts progression of pubertal development until the expected age of puberty. (Enigmatically, primary hyperthyroidism may also lead to delayed pubertal development.)

Abdominal and rectal examination may reveal a mass, suggesting an adrenal or ovarian tumor. Because palpable ovarian cysts may develop rarely before ovulation in true precocious puberty, the presence of a mass need not confirm the diagnosis of precocious pseudopuberty.

When vaginal bleeding is the only sign of development, the diagnosis of sexual precocity should be suspect. Common causes of bleeding in this age group include irritation from a vaginal infection or foreign body, sexual assault, prolapse of the urethral meatus, and ingestion of estrogen-containing medications (most commonly, oral contraceptive preparations). A vaginal or cervical neoplasm is also a rare possibility. Thus, vaginal bleeding dictates the need for vaginal examination, often best performed under anesthesia, before further evaluation is undertaken.

Heterosexual precocity in an apparent prepubertal female is almost always due to congenital adrenal hyperplasia or to an androgen-secreting adrenal or ovarian neoplasm. Only very rarely must another disorder of sexual differentiation be considered (Chapter 252). It is important to examine the external genitalia carefully because congenital adrenal hyperplasia is usually associated with some degree of sexual ambiguity.

Excessive androgens produced endogenously by abnormal fetal adrenal glands in utero or diffusing across the placenta to the fetus from the mother can virilize the external genitalia and result in female pseudohermaphroditism. The extent of virilization varies from an enlarged clitoris only to sexual ambiguity sufficient to make gender assignment difficult.

Excessive maternal androgen secretion, typically from an ovarian or adrenal neoplasm, can lead to virilization of a female fetus. This occurs very rarely because of the great capacity of the placenta to aromatize naturally occurring androgens to estrogens. Virilization of a female fetus is much more likely to occur if a pregnant woman has ingested a synthetic steroid preparation with androgenic properties because available synthetic compounds generally cannot be aromatized.

Excessive androgen secretion beginning in utero is usually associated with defective cortisol synthesis. As a consequence, pituitary corticotropin secretion is increased, resulting in congenital adrenal hyperplasia and excessive androgen secretion. The three different enzyme defects in the steroidogenic pathway that can lead to virilization of the female fetus are described in Chapter 252. 21-Hydroxylase deficiency is the most common form of congenital adrenal hyperplasia, accounting for the disorder in more than 90% of affected individuals. The defect may vary from partial to complete deficiency of the enzyme.

Diagnostic Tests

Measurement of Peptide and Steroid Hormones

Increased levels of immunoreactive human chorionic gonadotropin (hCG) may suggest an hCG-secreting neoplasm, most commonly an ovarian teratoma or dysgerminoma. In such cases, the hCG, which is antigenically and biologically similar to LH, stimulates ovarian steroid secretion and pseudopubertal development. Because even specific LH immunoassays show some cross-reactivity with hCG, values for serum LH may be elevated in individuals with hCG-secreting tumors. Immunoreactive hCG is always elevated in the presence of such tumors. Levels and ratios of FSH and LH typical of pubertal as opposed to prepubertal girls help in diagnosis of true precocious puberty. Timed urine collections rather than blood samples can be used to measure gonadotropin secretion if necessary. The use of exogenous GnRH to stimulate endogenous LH and FSH secretion can help differentiate gonadotropin-dependent from gonadotropin-independent precocious puberty. Excessively high circulating levels of estrogen suggest an estrogen-producing neoplasm. High levels of serum testosterone suggest an ovarian source of excess androgen in girls with heterosexual development, whereas increased levels of dehydroepiandrosterone or its sulfate (the principal precursors of 17-ketosteroids) suggest an adrenal source. High levels of serum 17-hydroxyprogesterone imply congenital adrenal hyperplasia secondary to 21-hydroxylase deficiency, whereas high levels of serum 11-deoxycortisol imply an 11β-hydroxylase deficiency. In congenital adrenal hyperplasia, these hormone levels should decrease promptly after oral administration of suppressive doses of dexamethasone. Suppression in response to exogenous corticoids occurs much less consistently in individuals with adrenal cortical adenomas and carcinomas and rarely in those with ovarian androgen-secreting neoplasms (Chapters 252 and 258).

Additional Studies

Ultrasonic scanning of the adrenals and ovaries and computed tomography of the adrenals may be indicated to confirm clinical suspicions. In girls with ovarian or adrenal neoplasms, the tumor can almost always be localized radiographically. Catheterization of the ovarian and adrenal veins and measurements of the effluent steroids from each gland should be pursued only when computed tomography, ultrasonography, or magnetic resonance imaging fails to identify what is suspected to be a neoplasm. Although plain skull films may be of use in screening for pituitary and parapituitary tumors, computed tomography or magnetic resonance imaging of the skull is indicated in the presence of definite neurologic deficits or if true precocious puberty is suspected. Radiographic estimation of bone age is indicated in all cases and serves as a useful tool to follow the results of treatment.

Treatment

Treatment of precocious puberty should be initiated promptly so that (1) the patient's ultimate height is not compromised as a result of sex steroid–induced premature epiphyseal closure and (2) emotional disturbances in the patient and her parents are prevented or attenuated.

GnRH analogues are now the preferred therapy for suppressing gonadotropin secretion and also may prevent early bone maturation. The analogues are not effective in children with McCune-Albright syndrome, and ketoconazole and testolactone have been only marginally successful. Aqueous depot medroxyprogesterone acetate (100 to 200 mg intramuscularly every 2 to 4 weeks) also may be used to suppress gonadotropin secretion. Medroxyprogesterone acetate, however, does not always prevent premature epiphyseal closure and the resultant short stature.

Individuals with central nervous system or steroid-secreting neoplasms must undergo therapy appropriate for the particular lesion. Girls with congenital adrenal hyperplasia are appropriately managed with glucocorticoids (plus mineralocorticoids when indicated) as outlined in Chapter 252.

Delayed Puberty

Girls with delayed puberty typically present at age 16 years or later because of primary amenorrhea, but younger girls may present because of failure to initiate pubertal development. Because of the anxiety generated by delayed puberty, some evaluation is always indicated regardless of the age of the patient.

When pubertal development progresses normally but menstruation does not begin, an abnormality in the genital tract should be considered. Congenital malformations of the müllerian ducts are uncommon, occurring in 0.02% of all women. Most do not cause amenorrhea, and many do not impair reproduction. The anomalies associated with amenorrhea vary in severity from an imperforate hymen to complete aplasia of all müllerian duct derivatives with vaginal atresia. Although aplasia generally involves all of the müllerian duct derivatives, defects may involve only a single part of the distal genital tract. Family aggregates of the most common disorders of müllerian differentiation in females—müllerian aplasia and incomplete müllerian fusion—do occur and are best explained by polygenic or multifactorial inheritance. It is clear that the *HOX* genes, a family of regulatory genes that encode transcription factors, are essential for proper development of the müllerian tract.

A müllerian duct anomaly is suggested by (1) normal levels of serum gonadotropins and steroids, (2) an abnormal outflow tract, (3) a history of cyclic abdominal pain with or without a palpable mass, and (4) normal development of secondary sex characteristics. Normal ovarian function still induces endometrial growth and shedding after menarche if the uterus is normal. In the absence of a normal outflow tract, however, the menstrual effluent is retained and may or may not be able to escape into the abdominal cavity. Free in the abdominal cavity, the effluent may cause endometriosis. Constrained to the uterine cavity, the effluent causes hematometra and a large abdominal mass. In the absence of a mass or cyclic pain, a karyotype is indicated in girls with evidence of an abnormal genital tract to rule out any of several disorders of sexual differentiation (Chapter 252). Such disorders, however, almost never occur together with completely normal pubertal development. In girls with a normal karyotype and a genital tract anomaly, examination under anesthesia and diagnostic laparoscopy should be undertaken to delineate the extent of the defect. When the abnormality consists of an imperforate hymen or transverse vaginal septum only, surgical restoration can be accomplished relatively simply. Attempts to provide an outflow tract for the uterus should not be undertaken if there is no cervix because of the high risk of recurrent pelvic infection. Even with a functional cervix, the construction of an outflow tract that permits successful pregnancy is unlikely. A functional vagina can be constructed surgically or by the daily use of ever-larger dilators. To prevent shrinkage and scarring, surgery should be deferred until the patient is willing to use dilators postoperatively on a daily basis or she is about to become sexually active.

Other causes of delayed puberty and primary amenorrhea are the same as those that may cause amenorrhea in older women (Chapter 256).

When no apparent cause of delayed development is found, constitutional delayed puberty must be entertained as a diagnosis of exclusion. A strong family history of delayed maturation adds support to this presumption. Small doses of estrogen may be administered to induce some pubertal development but may obscure a pathologic cause of the delay and may compromise linear growth and ultimate height.

Asynchronous Pubertal Development

Asynchronous pubertal development is characteristic of male pseudohermaphroditism due to androgen insensitivity, especially complete testicular feminization. This syndrome of androgen insensitivity is inherited either as an X-linked recessive or as a sex-limited autosomal dominant trait. Despite the presence of intra-abdominal or inguinal testes, there is complete failure of virilization. Affected individuals develop breasts (but only to Tanner stage 3) and a typical female habitus with unambiguous female external genitalia but with absence of internal female structures, generally having only a foreshortened blind-ending vagina. Little or no pubic and axillary hair develops. The karyotype is 46,XY in these individuals. Circulating testosterone levels are equivalent to or higher than those found in normal men, and LH levels are elevated while FSH levels are normal compared with those in menstruating women.

For a more detailed description, see Chapter 252.

Heterosexual Pubertal Development

Polycystic Ovary Syndrome

Polycystic ovary syndrome, by far the most common cause of heterosexual pubertal development, is associated with the development of some secondary sex features characteristic of males at the normal age of puberty. Feminization occurs in affected girls, and they develop normal breasts and a typical female habitus, but masculinization also occurs. (In contrast, girls with congenital adrenal hyperplasia generally show little if any female development at puberty.) A heterogeneous syndrome, polycystic ovary syndrome most typically begins at or near puberty with hirsutism and irregular menses from the time of menarche. Many girls who develop polycystic ovary syndrome are overweight in childhood, and obesity is clearly a risk factor. Menarche may be delayed as well, so that young women may present with primary amenorrhea. Basal LH levels tend to be somewhat elevated in perhaps 80% of cases, and circulating levels of all androgens are elevated moderately. Some degree of insulin resistance is almost invariably present as well, and hypercholesterolemia may predispose to cardiovascular disease later in life. This is discussed more completely in Chapter 261.

Congenital Adrenal Hyperplasia

Congenital adrenal hyperplasia is generally diagnosed before puberty, and heterosexual precocious pseudopuberty is typical. However, if the defect is mild and changes to the external genitalia are minimal, masculinization may occur at the expected age of puberty. This attenuated or nonclassic form of 21-hydroxylase deficiency seems to occur in families with a strong family history of hirsutism. Affected girls generally have some defeminization with flattening of the breasts, severe hirsutism, relatively short stature, and obesity.

For a more detailed description, see Chapter 252.

Mixed Gonadal Dysgenesis

Mixed gonadal dysgenesis designates asymmetrical gonadal development, with a germ cell tumor or a testis on one side and an undifferentiated streak, rudimentary gonad, or no gonad on the other. The extent of genital virilization before puberty is variable in this rare disorder. Most individuals are reared as girls, in whom virilization occurs at puberty; some may note breast development as well. Affected individuals generally have a mosaic karyotype, with 45,X/46,XY being most common. Short stature and other stigmata associated with a 45,X karyotype in Turner's syndrome are less common in patients with tumors than in patients with testes. Gonadectomy is indicated in all individuals with a Y chromosome to eliminate the increased neoplastic potential of such dysgenetic gonads and in all patients in whom virilization occurs at puberty to remove the source of androgen. Estrogen replacement therapy is warranted after gonadectomy. Other causes of male pseudohermaphroditism associated with heterosexual pubertal development are described in Chapter 252.

Other Causes

An androgen-producing adrenal neoplasm or Cushing's syndrome may occur rarely during the pubertal years and lead to heterosexual development.

SUGGESTED READINGS

Chumlea WC, Schubert CM, Roche AF, et al: Age at menarche and racial comparisons in U.S. girls. Pediatrics 2003;111:110–113. *Analysis of the most recent developmental data in U.S. girls.*

Elmlinger MW, Kuhnel W, Ranke MB: Reference ranges for serum concentrations of lutropin (LH), follitropin (FSH), estradiol (E_2), prolactin, progesterone, sex hormone–binding globulin (SHBG), dehydroepiandrosterone sulfate (DHEAS), cortisol and ferritin in neonates, children and young adults. Clin Chem Lab Med 2002;40:1151–1160. *A useful guide to normal values of reproductive hormones in children and adolescents.*

Erickson GF: The role of growth factors in ovary organogenesis. J Soc Gynecol Investig 2001;8:S13–S16. *Overview that emphasizes the role of the primordial follicles, which vary in number among women, and how this number influences fertility and menopause.*

Merke DP, Bornstein SR: Congenital adrenal hyperplasia. Lancet 2005;365:2125–2136. *A clinical review.*

Selevan SG, Rice DC, Hogan KA, et al: Blood lead concentration and delayed puberty in girls. N Engl J Med 2003;348:1527–1536. *Increased lead levels correlated with delays in multiple pubertal measures.*

Speroff L, Fritz MA: Abnormal puberty and growth problems. *In* Speroff L, Fritz MA: Clinical Gynecologic Endocrinology and Infertility, 7th ed. Philadelphia, Lippincott Williams & Wilkins, 2005, pp 361–399. *A detailed discussion of normal and abnormal pubertal development.*

Wang Y: Is obesity associated with early sexual maturation? A comparison of the association in American boys versus girls. Pediatrics 2002;110:903–910. *The importance of obesity in the timing of pubertal development is documented in this analysis of data from a national U.S. survey.*

256 MENSTRUAL CYCLE AND FERTILITY

Robert W. Rebar and Gregory F. Erickson

THE NORMAL MENSTRUAL CYCLE

Between menarche at the age of approximately 12 years and the menopause at about 51 years, the reproductive organs of normal women undergo a series of closely coordinated changes at approximately monthly intervals that together constitute the normal menstrual cycle. The menstrual cycle is the expression of the coordinated interactions of the hypothalamic-pituitary-ovarian axis, with associated changes in the target tissues (endometrium, cervix, vagina) of the reproductive tract.

A menstrual cycle begins with the first day of genital bleeding (day 1; menses) and ends just before the next menstrual period. The median menstrual cycle length is 28 days, but normal ovulatory menstrual cycles may range from about 21 to 40 days in length. Menstrual cycles vary most greatly in length in the years immediately after menarche and in the years immediately preceding menopause, largely because of an increased incidence of anovulatory cycles. Irregularities in menstrual cycle length may also be caused by abrupt changes in diet, exercise, or environment; serious emotional disturbances; and parturition or abortion. The menstrual cycle can be divided into three distinct phases: follicular, ovulatory, and luteal.

Follicular (Preovulatory) Phase

Variable in length, the follicular phase begins with the first day of menstrual bleeding and extends to the day before the preovulatory luteinizing hormone (LH) surge. A rise in serum follicle-stimulating hormone (FSH) begins in the late luteal phase of the previous menstrual cycle, continues into the early follicular phase, and initiates growth and development of a group of follicles (Fig. 256–1). The preovulatory follicle destined for ovulation is selected from this cohort. Circulating LH levels rise slowly throughout the follicular phase, but FSH levels fall after the early follicular phase. Approximately 7 to 8 days before the preovulatory LH surge, estradiol and estrone increase, generally reaching a maximum on the day before or the day of the LH surge. The divergence in LH and

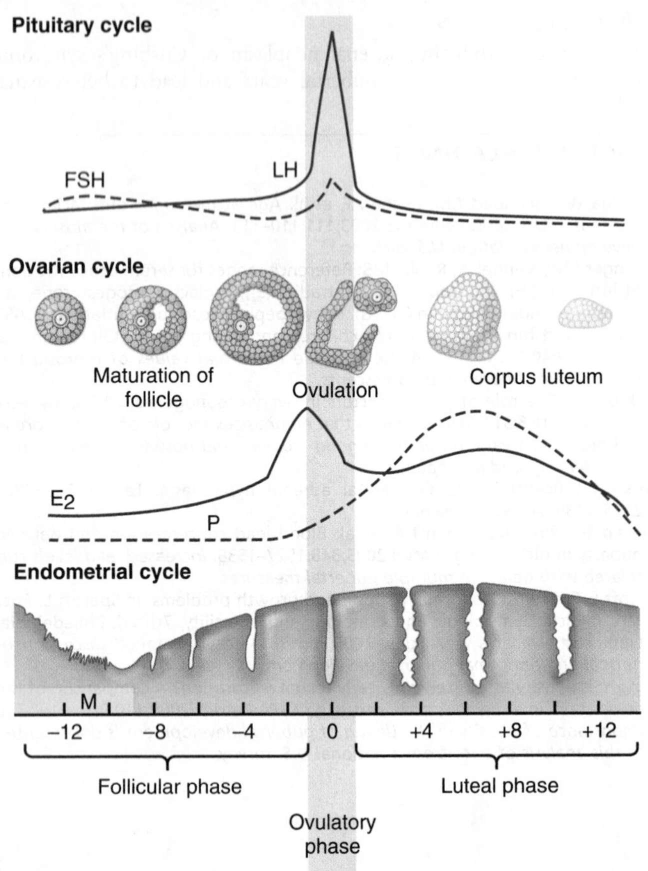

FIGURE 256–1 • The idealized cyclic changes observed in gonadotropins, estradiol (E_2), progesterone (P), and uterine endometrium during the normal menstrual cycle. The data are centered on the day of the luteinizing hormone (LH) surge (day 0). Days of menstrual bleeding are indicated by M. FSH = follicle-stimulating hormone. (Reprinted with permission from Endocrine and Metabolism Continuing Education Quality Control Program, 1982. Copyright American Association for Clinical Chemistry, Inc.)

FSH levels may be related to the follicular secretion of inhibin B, a hormone that specifically inhibits the release of FSH. Several days before the LH surge, plasma androgens (androstenedione and testosterone) and some progestins (17α-hydroxyprogesterone and 20α-dihydroprogesterone) begin to increase. They peak on the day of the LH surge. Progesterone itself does not increase until just before the onset of the LH surge.

Ovulatory Phase

During this phase, the ovum is released from the mature graafian follicle about 32 to 34 hours after the onset of the preovulatory surge of LH. The ovulatory phase extends from 1 day before the LH surge to 1 day after the LH surge (see Fig. 256–1). Some women experience brief (a few minutes to a few hours in length), dull, unilateral pelvic pain near the time of ovulation, termed *mittelschmerz.* The association of this pain with ovulation is unknown, but it may be due to leakage of follicular fluid into the abdominal cavity at ovulation. Mittelschmerz may occur before or after actual ovulation or not at all. During the ovulatory phase, a rapid rise in plasma LH in response to positive estrogen feedback leads to final maturation of the follicle and to ovulation. As peak LH levels are reached, estradiol levels drop but progesterone levels continue to increase.

Luteal (Postovulatory) Phase

The more constant half of the menstrual cycle, the luteal phase, is approximately 14 days in length and ends with the onset of menses (see Fig. 256–1). This phase represents the functional lifespan of the corpus luteum of the ovary, which supports the released ovum by secreting progesterone. In the luteal phase, progesterone secretion increases to a peak 6 to 8 days after the LH surge. Parallel but smaller increases in 17α-hydroxyprogesterone, estradiol, and estrone levels also occur. Progesterone levels decrease before menses unless the ovum is fertilized and pregnancy results. The finding of serum progesterone levels greater than 10 ng/mL 1 week before menses is probably diagnostic of normal ovulation. Progestins increase basal morning body temperature so that a "thermogenic shift" of more than 0.3° C occurring after a nadir is a presumptive sign of ovulation and progesterone secretion. Unfortunately, taking basal temperatures on a daily basis is tedious, subject to error, and not very reliable.

CYCLIC CHANGES IN TARGET ORGANS

Endometrium

During the menstrual cycle, the endometrium undergoes remarkable histologic and cytologic changes that culminate with menstrual bleeding when the corpus luteum ceases to secrete progesterone (see Fig. 256–1). The basal layer of the endometrium, which is not lost during menses, then regenerates the superficial layer of compact epithelial cells lining the uterine cavity and an intermediate layer of spongiosa, both of which are shed at each menstruation. Endometrial glands in these layers proliferate under the influence of estrogen in the follicular phase so that the mucosa thickens. In the luteal phase, under the influence of progesterone, the glands become coiled and secretory, with increased vascularity and edema of the stroma. As both estradiol and progesterone decline in the late luteal phase, the stroma becomes increasingly edematous, endometrial and blood vessel necrosis occurs, and endometrial bleeding ensues. Local release of prostaglandins may initiate vasospasm and ischemic necrosis in the endometrium as well as the uterine contractions accompanying menstrual flow. Thus, prostaglandin synthetase inhibitors can relieve dysmenorrhea (menstrual cramping). Fibrinolytic activity in the endometrium also peaks at the time of menstruation, accounting for the noncoagulability of menstrual blood. Because the histologic changes during the menstrual cycle are so characteristic, endometrial biopsies are used to characterize the stage of the cycle and to assess the tissue response to gonadal steroids.

Cervix and Cervical Mucus

During the follicular phase, cervical vascularity, congestion, and edema increase progressively under the influence of estrogen. The external cervical os opens to a diameter of 3 mm at ovulation and then decreases to 1 mm. Cervical mucus increases in quantity (10- to 30-fold) and in elasticity. Arborization (ferning) becomes prominent just before ovulation (if cervical mucus is allowed to dry on a glass slide and examined microscopically). Under the influence of progesterone during the luteal phase, cervical mucus thickens, becomes less watery, and loses its elasticity and ability to fern. The characteristics of cervical mucus are useful in evaluating the stage of the cycle and the amount of estrogen present.

Vagina

When ovarian estrogen secretion is low, as in the early follicular phase, vaginal epithelium is pale and thin. In the follicular phase under the influence of estrogens, the epithelium thickens, and the number of mature cornified epithelial cells increases. During the luteal phase, progesterone causes a decrease in the percentage of cornified cells and an increase in the number of precornified intermediate cells and polymorphonuclear leukocytes. There is also increased cellular debris and clumping of shed desquamated cells. Histologic changes in the vaginal epithelium and in the cervical mucus are the most sensitive indicators of estrogen status in the body. However, the reliability of vaginal smears depends on the absence of infection or exogenously administered steroid hormones that have antiestrogenic effects. Steroid hormones also facilitate progression of spermatozoa toward the ovaries and of ova toward the uterine cavity through effects on the fallopian tubes.

Ovary

During the reproductive years, the human ovaries regularly produce a single dominant graafian follicle that grows and develops to the preovulatory stage during the follicular phase of the menstrual cycle. This process is brought about by combined action of FSH and LH on the follicle wall to cause the biosynthesis of increasing quantities of estradiol. At about midpoint in the menstrual cycle, the surge of LH acts on the preovulatory follicle to cause the secretion of a mature fertilizable oocyte by a process termed ovulation. After ovulation, the follicle wall transforms into the corpus luteum, which produces considerable quantities of progesterone and estradiol during the luteal phase of the cycle. If implantation does not occur, the corpus luteum undergoes luteolysis and stops hormone production. In the late luteal phase, another dominant follicle develops and a new menstrual cycle begins. The potential to produce a dominant follicle stops at the menopause, when few or no reserve oocytes remain.

Chronology of Folliculogenesis

The preovulatory follicle arises by folliculogenesis. It begins its development when a primordial follicle is recruited into the pool of growing follicles. As a consequence of successive primordial follicle recruitments, the ovaries contain a pool of small graafian follicles with the potential to develop into the preovulatory follicle. In the human female, folliculogenesis is a long process. In each menstrual cycle, the preovulatory follicle arises from a primordial follicle that was recruited to grow about 1 year earlier (Fig. 256–2). The mechanism responsible for recruitment is poorly understood, but studies in rodents indicate that specific molecules from the granulosa cells, namely, kit ligand and müllerian inhibiting substance, play stimulatory and inhibitory roles, respectively.

There are two major phases of folliculogenesis, the preantral (gonadotropin-independent) and the antral or graafian (gonadotropin-dependent) period. The first phase is characterized by growth of the oocyte within the follicle and the onset of granulosa proliferation. The early stages of preantral folliculogenesis (class 1, primary and secondary follicle states; class 2, tertiary or cavitation state) proceed slowly. It requires 300 days or more for a recruited primordial follicle to complete the preantral or gonadotropin-independent period of folliculogenesis (see Fig. 256–2). During the second phase of folliculogenesis, the granulosa and theca cells proliferate extensively and the antrum enlarges greatly. The size of the graafian follicle increases relatively rapidly as it grows and develops through the small (classes 3, 4, and 5), medium (class 6), and large (classes 7 and 8) stages. The mature graafian follicle that will ovulate requires 40 to 50 days to complete the antral phase of follicular growth. The follicles that do not participate in ovulation undergo atresia and die by apoptosis. Atresia can occur at any stage of antral follicle development but appears most prominent in the small graafian follicles at the class 5 stage.

Selection

The dominant follicle is selected from a cohort of class 5 follicles (4.7 ± 0.7 mm in diameter) at the end of the luteal phase of the menstrual cycle. A typical class 5 follicle consists of a fully grown oocyte surrounded by a zona pellucida, about 1 million granulosa cells, a theca interna containing several layers of differentiated theca interstitial cells, and a band of smooth muscle cells termed the theca externa (Fig. 256–3). Once it is selected, a dominant follicle requires about 20 days to develop to the ovulatory stage.

The mechanism responsible for selection involves a high sustained rate of granulosa and theca cell proliferation. Shortly after the midluteal phase of the cycle, the granulosa cells in all of the cohort class 5 follicles show a sharp increase (approximately two-fold) in the rate of granulosa mitosis. The first indication of a selection is that the granulosa cells within the chosen follicle continue dividing at a high rate while proliferation slows in the other cohort follicles. Because this event occurs in the late luteal phase, it is believed that the selection occurs at this point in the menstrual cycle. As a consequence of the high sustained mitotic rate and the progressive accumulation of follicular fluid, the dominant follicle undergoes remarkable growth, reaching 6.9 ± 0.5 mm in diameter at days 1 to 5, 13.7 ± 1.2 mm at days 6 to 10, and 18.8 ± 0.5 mm at days 11 to 14 of the menstrual cycle. In nondominant follicles, growth and expansion proceed more slowly, and atresia becomes increasingly more evident with time. Rarely does an atretic human follicle reach 9 mm or more in diameter.

FSH is required for selection of the next dominant follicle. It is the increase in plasma FSH levels that begins at the end of luteal phase and continues through the early follicular phase that evokes follicle selection (Fig. 256–4). This rise in plasma FSH results in an increase in the concentration of FSH in the follicular fluid of the healthy (dominant) follicle as it moves through the cycle. By contrast, the levels of FSH remain low or undetectable in the follicular fluid of the nondominant atretic follicles. Such evidence has led to the concept that selection is controlled by a selective increase in the concentration of FSH in the follicular fluid of one cohort follicle. The manner in which this selective increase in FSH is controlled is unknown.

Mechanism of Follicle-Stimulating Hormone Action

FSH exerts its influence on follicle growth and development by stimulating granulosa cell mitosis and cytodifferentiation. FSH regulates biologic responses through activation of specific high-affinity FSH receptors on the surface of the granulosa cell. The binding event is transduced into an intracellular signal through the cyclic adenosine monophosphate–dependent protein kinase A signal transduction pathway (Fig. 256–5). This process leads to the activation of a large body of genes that results in increases in cell number and regulatory molecules leading to cytodifferentiation.

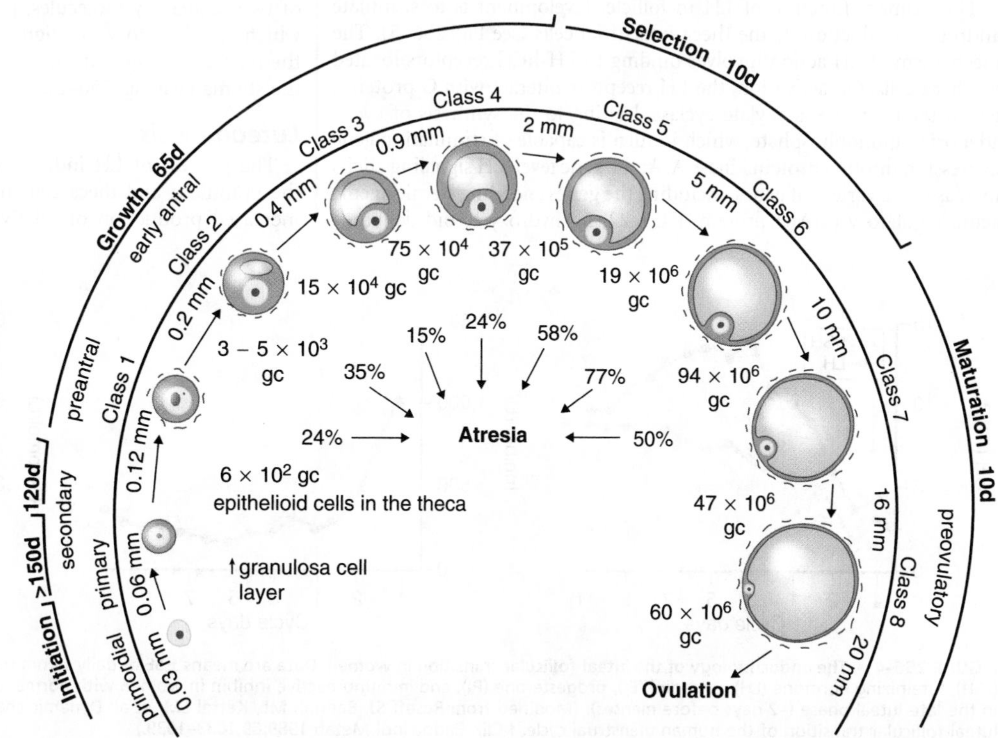

FIGURE 256–2 • The chronology of folliculogenesis in the human ovary. Folliculogenesis is divided into two major periods, preantral (gonadotropin independent) and antral (gonadotropin dependent). In the preantral period, a recruited primordial follicle develops to the primary-secondary (class 1) and early tertiary (class 2) stage, at which time cavitation or antrum formation begins. The antral period includes the small graafian (0.9 to 5 mm, classes 3, 4 and 5), medium graafian (6 to 10 mm, class 6), large graafian (10 to 15 mm, class 7), and preovulatory (16 to 20 mm, class 8) follicles. Time required for completion of preantral and antral periods is approximately 300 and approximately 40 days, respectively. gc = number of granulosa cells; millimeters indicate follicle diameter; percentage of atresia is indicated. (Modified from Gougeon A: Dynamics of follicular growth in the human: A model from preliminary results. Hum Reprod 1986;1:81–87.)

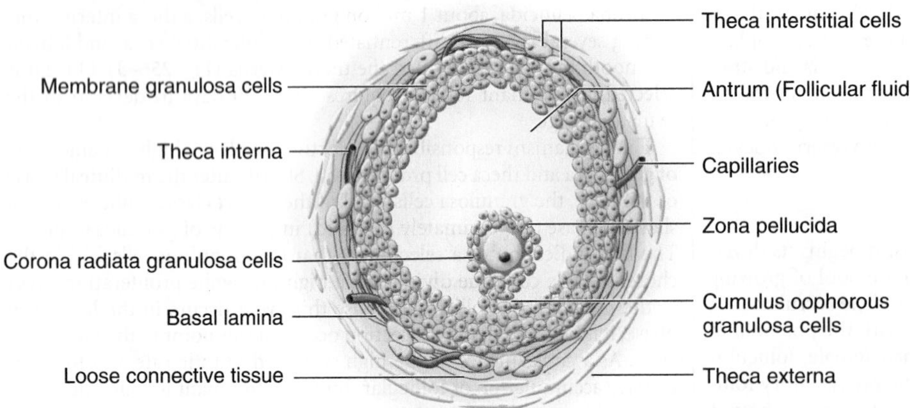

FIGURE 256–3 • Schematic cross section of a healthy graafian follicle. (From Erickson GF: Primary cultures of ovarian cells in serum-free medium as models of hormone-dependent differentiation. Mol Cell Endocrinol 1983;29:21–49.)

The granulosa cells in the chosen follicle continue to divide at a relatively rapid rate throughout the follicular phase of the cycle, increasing from about 1×10^6 cells at selection to more than 50×10^6 cells at ovulation. The high mitotic rate in the granulosa cells during dominant follicle growth can be accounted for by the relatively high concentrations of FSH in follicular fluid.

FSH is also the major inducer of granulosa cytodifferentiation in the dominant follicle. The gene encoding cytochrome P-450 aromatase (P450arom) is one of the physiologically important genes whose expression is induced by FSH (see Fig. 256–5). The temporal pattern of expression of P450arom is a critical determinant of when and how much estradiol is produced by the developing dominant follicle during the follicular phase of the menstrual cycle. Another major FSH-dependent transcriptional event is the expression of LH receptors. Typically, this expression is delayed until the dominant follicle is fully differentiated at around day 12 of the cycle. The presence of a large number of LH receptors in the granulosa cells is essential for the LH–human chorionic gonadotropin (hCG) surge to trigger ovulation. The terminal differentiation of the granulosa cells is also characterized by the increasing synthesis and accumulation of a wide variety of FSH-regulated gene products in addition to P450arom and LH receptors. Examples include inhibin B, activin, and follistatin.

Mechanism of Luteinizing Hormone Action

The primary function of LH in follicle development is to stimulate androgen production by the theca interstitial cells (see Fig. 256–5). The mechanism of LH action involves binding to LH-hCG receptors located on theca cells. On activation, the LH receptors interact with G proteins, which then activate adenylate cyclase, leading to the synthesis of cyclic adenosine monophosphate, which in turn is capable of stimulating gene expression through protein kinase A. At the gene level, LH signaling elicits increases in a variety of genes, including the genes encoding steroidogenic acute regulatory (StAR) protein, P450c22, 3β-hydroxysteroid dehydrogenase, and P450c17. The biologic outcome of this LH response is increased conversion of cholesterol to androstenedione. Theca cells express insulin receptors with protein tyrosine kinase activity. Activation of the insulin receptor signaling pathway leads to increased theca androgen production. The crosstalk between the insulin and LH receptor signaling is clinically relevant because of the relationship between hyperinsulinemia and hyperandrogenism in women.

One of the most important consequences of FSH and LH action on the dominant follicle is the production of estradiol. This physiologically important process is called the two gonadotropin–two cell concept of follicular estrogen production (see Fig. 256–5).

Ovulation

At about midpoint in the menstrual cycle, the preovulatory surges of LH and FSH act on the preovulatory follicle to initiate the events leading to ovulation (Fig. 256–6). During this process, the LH surge induces meiotic maturation, a process that converts the oocyte into a fertilizable egg arrested at the second meiotic metaphase. As the egg undergoes meiotic maturation, the granulosa cells juxtaposed to the oocyte are stimulated by high levels of FSH to produce hyaluronic acid and undergo cumulus expansion. Cumulus expansion is a prerequisite for the egg's pickup and transport by the oviduct. Another important effect of the LH surge is to stimulate the production of proteolytic enzymes in the vicinity of the presumptive stigma. This process requires the LH stimulation of two regulatory molecules, progesterone and prostaglandins, both of which are obligatory for stigma formation. After a 36-hour time course, the fertilizable egg and surrounding cumulus cells are secreted through the stigma (see Fig. 256–6).

Luteogenesis

The process of LH-induced ovulation leads to dramatic changes in the granulosa and theca cells of the ovulated follicle that result in the increased production of relatively large amounts of progesterone and

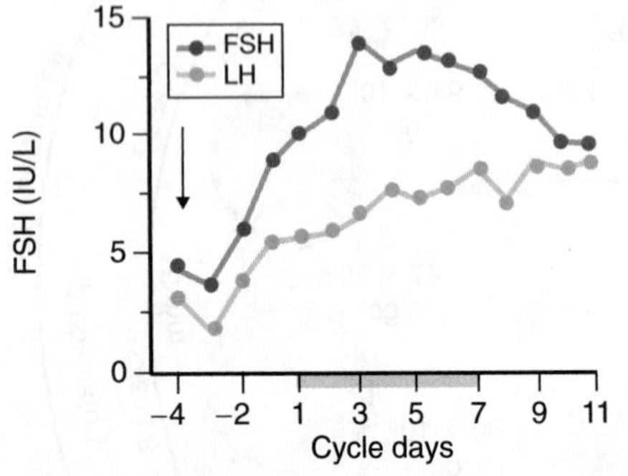

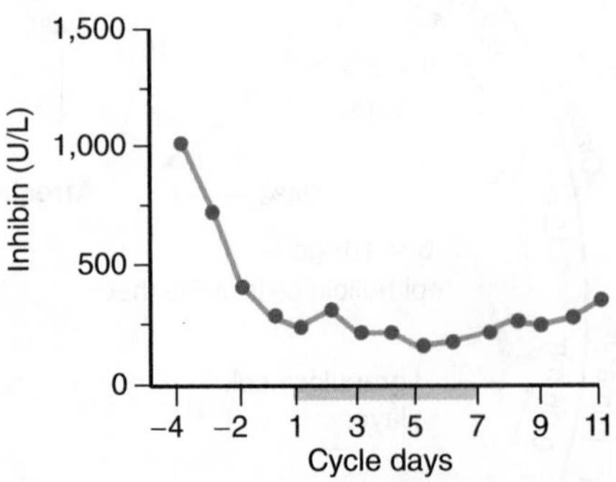

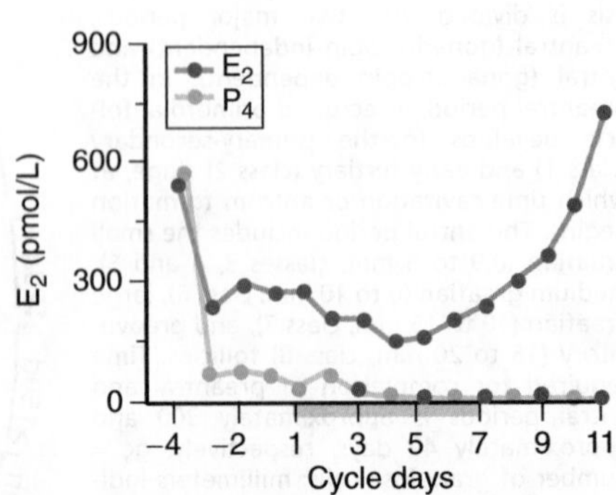

FIGURE 256–4 • The endocrinology of the luteal-follicular transition in women. Data are means ± SE of daily serum concentrations of follicle-stimulating hormone (FSH), luteinizing hormone (LH), estradiol (E_2), progesterone (P_4), and immunoreactive inhibin in women with normal cycles. Note the secondary rise in plasma FSH in the late luteal phase (–2 days before menses). (Modified from Roseff SJ, Bangah ML, Kettel LM, et al: Dynamic changes in circulating inhibin levels during the luteal-follicular transition of the human menstrual cycle. J Clin Endocrinol Metab 1989;69:1033–1039.)

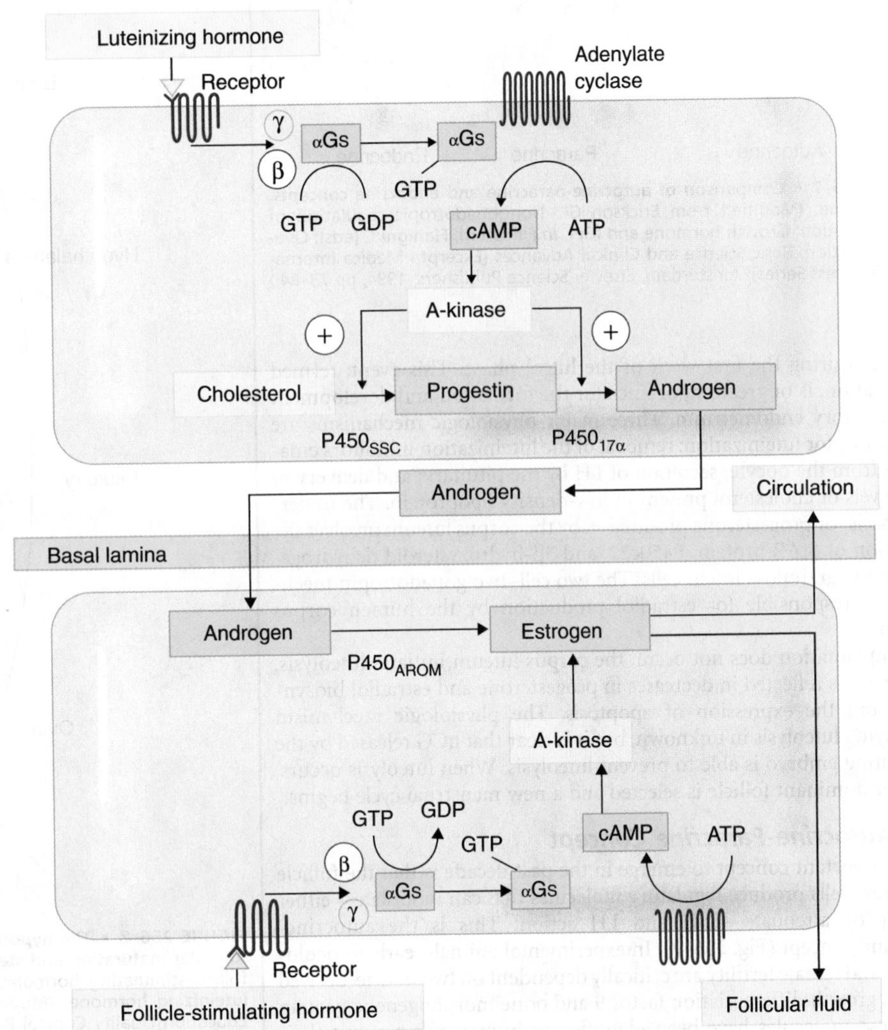

FIGURE 256-5 • The two gonadotropin–two cell concept of follicle estrogen production. ATP = adenosine triphosphate; cAMP = cyclic adenosine monophosphate; GDP = guanosine diphosphate; GTP = guanosine triphosphate. (Modified from Erickson GF: Normal ovarian function. Clin Obstet Gynecol 1978;21:31–52.)

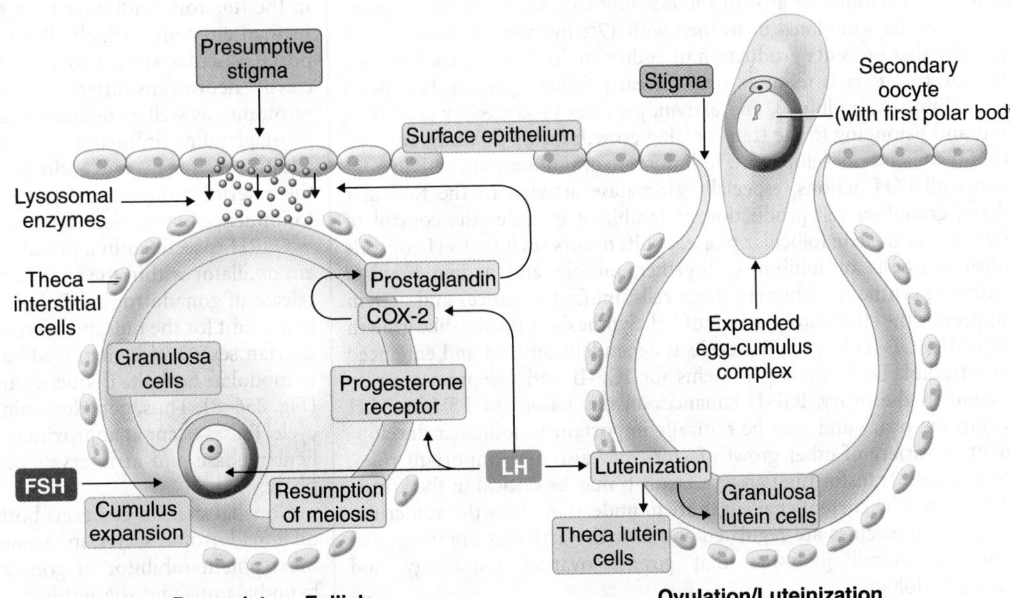

FIGURE 256-6 • The mechanism of ovulation. COX-2 = cyclooxygenase 2; FSH = follicle-stimulating hormone; LH = luteinizing hormone. (Modified from Erickson GF: The ovary: Basic principles and concepts. *In* Felig P, Baxter JD, Broadus AE, Frohman LA [eds]: Endocrinology and Metabolism, 3rd ed. New York, McGraw-Hill, 1995, pp 973–1015.)

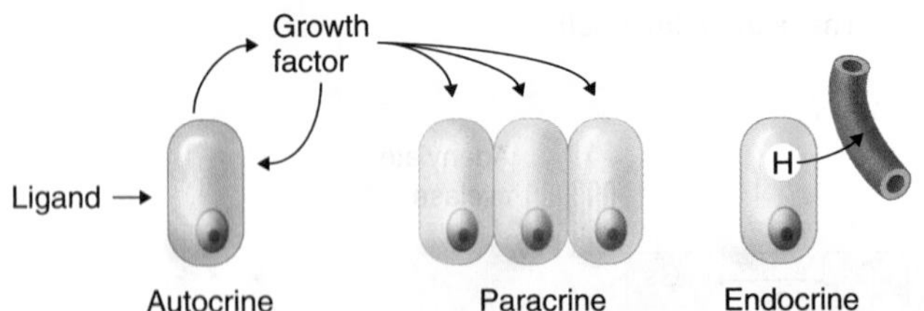

FIGURE 256–7 • Comparison of autocrine-paracrine and endocrine concepts. H = hormone. (Modified from Erickson GF: Nongonadotropic regulation of ovarian function: Growth hormone and IGFs. *In* Filicori M, Flanigni C [eds]: Ovulation Induction: Basic Science and Clinical Advances [Excerpta Medica International Congress Series]. Amsterdam, Elsevier Science Publishers, 1994, pp 73–84.)

estradiol during the first week of the luteal phase. This event, termed luteinization, is of great importance for the formation and development of a secretory endometrium. Three major physiologic mechanisms are responsible for luteinization: removal of the luteinization inhibitors emanating from the oocyte; secretion of LH by the pituitary; and delivery of high levels of cholesterol present in low-density lipoprotein. The underlying basis for progesterone production by the corpus luteum involves the induction of StAR protein, P450c22, and 3β-hydroxysteroid dehydrogenase in the granulosa lutein cells. The two cell–two gonadotropin mechanism is responsible for estradiol production by the human corpus luteum.

If implantation does not occur, the corpus luteum initiates luteolysis. This event is reflected in decreases in progesterone and estradiol biosynthesis and the expression of apoptosis. The physiologic mechanism underlying luteolysis in unknown, but it is clear that hCG released by the implanting embryo is able to prevent luteolysis. When luteolysis occurs, another dominant follicle is selected and a new menstrual cycle begins.

The Autocrine-Paracrine Concept

An important concept to emerge in the past decade is that the follicle and luteal cells produce regulatory molecules that can modulate—either amplify or attenuate—FSH and LH action. This is the autocrine-paracrine concept (Fig. 256–7). In experimental animals, early folliculogenesis and female fertility are critically dependent on two oocyte-derived factors, growth differentiation factor 9 and bone morphogenetic protein 15. These molecules have been identified in human oocytes, but their importance for ovarian function is unknown.

In contrast, evidence has accumulated to indicate that other autocrine-paracrine peptides play major roles in regulating ovarian follicle growth and development. Estradiol may not be important for follicular development. Normal follicular growth and development, with subsequent pregnancy, can be stimulated in women with 17α-hydroxylase deficiency, a disorder that prevents production of androgens and estrogens. The data indicate that FSH is required only for early folliculogenesis. It appears that inhibin-A, inhibin-B, and activin, peptides produced by granulosa cells and belonging to the transforming growth factor-β family, are critical for follicular development. In immature granulosa cells, activin augments all FSH actions, especially aromatase activity. In the follicular phase, granulosa cell production of inhibin-B is under the control of FSH; but in the late follicular phase, a shift occurs such that LH controls luteal synthesis of inhibin-A. Together, inhibin and activin regulate androgen synthesis in human theca cells; inhibin enhances and activin suppresses the stimulatory action of LH. Synthesis of insulin-like growth factor II (IGF-II) by granulosa cells is dependent on FSH and enhanced by estradiol. Both binding proteins for IGF-II and receptors are also present in the ovary. IGF-II enhances all the actions of FSH and LH within the ovary and may be critically important to follicular development. A variety of other growth factors may also play important roles; for example, transforming growth factor-β may be critical in the atresia of follicles. The current challenges are to understand how the autocrine-paracrine molecules are regulated and how the activities are integrated into the overall pathways that govern ovarian physiology and pathophysiology.

Neuroendocrine Regulation of the Ovaries

Neurons containing various peptide hormones that can release or inhibit secretion of the gonadotropins are found in the hypothalamus (Chapter 241). Specifically, cells containing gonadotropin-releasing hormone (GnRH) occur in the area including the arcuate nucleus and median eminence and the preoptic area. Axons from these neurons run in the tuberoinfundibular tract and terminate on capillaries within the median eminence, which allows delivery of their products through the portal vascular system to the anterior pituitary gland. It appears that classic neurotransmitters, including norepinephrine, dopamine, and serotonin, as well as neuromodulators, such as endogenous opiates and prostaglandins, influence secretion of GnRH by the hypothalamus. In addition, estrogens and androgens bind to cells in the hypothalamus and the anterior pituitary and progestins bind to cells in the hypothalamus to influence hypothalamic-pituitary regulation of ovarian function.

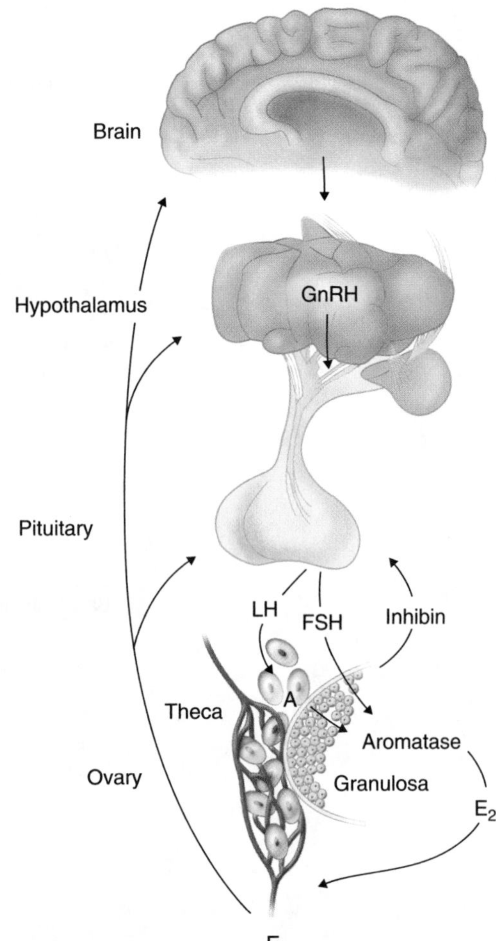

FIGURE 256–8 • The hypothalamic-pituitary-ovarian axis in the regulation of follicular maturation and steroidogenesis. A = androgens; E_2 = estradiol; FSH = follicle-stimulating hormone; GnRH = gonadotropin-releasing hormone; LH = luteinizing hormone. (Modified from Endocrine and Metabolism Continuing Education Quality Control Program, 1982. Copyright American Association for Clinical Chemistry, Inc.)

GnRH is secreted in a pulsatile fashion (perhaps because of an inherent oscillator within the arcuate nucleus) and is responsible for pulsatile release of gonadotropins. Pulsatile gonadotropin release in turn appears to account for the pulsatile secretion of sex steroids from the ovaries. The ovarian sex steroids then feed back on the hypothalamic-pituitary unit to modulate both the frequency and amplitude of the gonadotropin pulse (Fig. 256–8). Thus, gonadotropin pulses vary throughout the menstrual cycle. Pulses occur at approximately 60- to 90-minute intervals in the follicular phase and at intervals of more than 180 minutes in the luteal phase.

Gonadal steroids can exert both negative and positive feedback effects on gonadotropin secretion. Among ovarian steroids, 17β-estradiol is the most potent inhibitor of gonadotropin secretion, acting on both the hypothalamus and the pituitary. For women to ovulate, estradiol must also elicit a positive feedback effect on gonadotropin release. The feedback effects are both time and dose dependent. In the normal menstrual cycle, the positive feedback action of estradiol leading to the LH surge is preceded by a period when lower estradiol levels are present with their negative feedback effects.

It appears that the ovary is the "clock" for the timing of ovulation, with the hypothalamus stimulating pulsatile release of the gonadotropins. The follicle complex and corpus luteum develop in response to gonadotropin stimulation. For appropriate ovarian regulation of reproductive function in women, three biologic characteristics are necessary: an appropriate balance and sequence of negative and positive feedback actions; differential feedback effects on the release of LH and FSH; and local intraovarian controls on follicular growth and maturation, separate from but interrelated with the effects of gonadotropins on the ovaries.

ABNORMALITIES OF THE REPRODUCTIVE YEARS

Dysmenorrhea and Endometriosis

Definition

Dysmenorrhea, perhaps the most common of all gynecologic disorders, affects about 50% of postpubertal women. Dysmenorrhea can be classified as primary or secondary.

Endometriosis, which may result in dysmenorrhea, infertility, and/or dyspareunia (i.e., painful intercourse), is the ectopic occurrence of endometrial tissue, most commonly within the abdominal cavity but sometimes in surgical scars, on the vulva, in the umbilicus, and elsewhere.

Pathobiology

Primary dysmenorrhea occurs only in ovulatory cycles. Prostaglandins that are released from the endometrium just before and during menstruation cause contraction of uterine smooth muscle and produce dysmenorrhea by initiating painful, exaggerated uterine contractions and myometrial ischemia. Associated systemic symptoms include nausea, diarrhea, headache, and emotional changes. Primary dysmenorrhea is much more common than secondary dysmenorrhea.

In secondary dysmenorrhea, there is a pathologic cause of the dysmenorrhea. Endometriosis is the most common cause. Other possible causes include pelvic inflammatory disease; congenital abnormalities, such as atresia of a portion of the distal genital tract and cystic duplication of the paramesonephric ducts; and cervical stenosis.

Treatment

Rx

Prostaglandin synthetase inhibitors such as naproxen, ibuprofen, mefenamic acid, and indomethacin are the mainstays of treatment of primary dysmenorrhea. If the dysmenorrhea is still severe, addition of an oral contraceptive preparation to inhibit ovulation and limit prostaglandin release is generally effective. In cases in which the pelvic pain still remains intractable, additional evaluation is warranted. If thorough evaluation of the gastrointestinal and urinary tracts fails to reveal a definitive cause, examination under anesthesia and diagnostic laparoscopy may be indicated.

If endometriosis is diagnosed at laparoscopy, treatment varies according to the severity of the disease and the goals of the patient regarding fertility. It may be possible to fulgurate implants or to lyse adhesions through the laparoscope. In general, endometriosis should be treated medically, with additional surgery deferred until infertility (if present) becomes manifested. Medical therapy can consist of continuous suppression with GnRH analogues, progestins, oral contraceptive agents, or danazol for 3 to 6 months. Selective estrogen and progesterone receptor modulators are now in various stages of testing for the treatment of endometriosis. GnRH analogues have become the most frequent form of medical suppressive therapy. After a course of therapy, use of oral contraceptive agents should probably be continued until fertility is desired. Conservative surgical resection of endometriotic tissue should almost always be deferred until it is established as the cause of infertility. Surgery may be required, however, for continuing severe pain, severe endometriosis, or large ovarian cysts containing endometriosis (endometriomas). If symptoms continue despite adequate treatment or if psychological overlay is suspected, psychiatric evaluation may be indicated. Medical causes of dysmenorrhea, however, should be eliminated first.

TABLE 256–1 COMMON SYMPTOMS OF CYCLIC PREMENSTRUAL SYNDROME

SOMATIC SYMPTOMS	
Abdominal bloating	Constipation or diarrhea
Acne	Headache
Alcohol intolerance	Peripheral edema
Breast engorgement and tenderness	Weight gain
Clumsiness	
EMOTIONAL AND MENTAL SYMPTOMS	
Anxiety	Insomnia
Change in libido	Irritability
Depression	Lethargy
Fatigue	Mood swings
Food cravings (especially salt and sugar)	Panic attacks
	Paranoia
Hostility	Violence toward self and others
Inability to concentrate	Withdrawal from others
Increased appetite	

Premenstrual Syndrome

Definition

Premenstrual syndrome (PMS), also known as premenstrual tension, is a complex of physical and emotional symptoms that occur repetitively in a cyclic fashion before menstruation and that diminish or disappear with menstruation.

Diagnosis

The cyclic symptoms typically are sufficiently severe to interfere with some aspects of life. Women with established psychiatric disturbances probably should not be included among those with PMS. More than 150 different symptoms are now thought to vary with the menstrual cycle (Table 256–1). Estimates of the prevalence of PMS range from 25 to 100%. The American Psychiatric Association has defined a disorder that should be regarded as similar to but more severe than PMS and termed it premenstrual dysphoric disorder (PMDD). Certain specific symptoms must be present for diagnosis of PMDD. For most women, PMS is merely annoying; severe PMS (or PMDD) causes serious difficulties for no more than 5 to 10% of women of reproductive age. The diagnosis of PMDD is best established by requiring patients to keep prospective daily records of symptoms during a 2- to 3-month period. Less than 50% of women complaining of PMS are found to have the syndrome when such records are examined.

Most women seek help for PMS in their 30s after 10 or more years of symptoms. Many report that their symptoms began at menarche; approximately half state that symptoms followed childbirth. Severity and duration of symptoms are often reported to increase after each successive pregnancy and to become more severe with advancing age. Women with severe long-standing PMS almost always describe associated psychological reactions, including social difficulties, such as marital discord, difficulty relating to their children, difficulty maintaining friendships, and withdrawal from social activities.

Treatment

General Measures

The cause of PMS is unknown, and patients should be informed that no one therapy has been effective in all women. Women with mild premenstrual symptoms often benefit from simple changes in lifestyle, including daily mild aerobic exercise; reduction in intake of xanthine-containing beverages, salt, and refined sugar, particularly in the luteal phase; stress reduction; and adequate rest.

Medical Therapy

Women with more severe PMS may benefit from symptomatic treatment of predominant complaints. Thus, bromocriptine* (generally 2.5 mg twice a day) or danazol (100 to 400 mg/day in two divided doses) may be given continuously for relief of mastalgia, with the understanding that both may have unpleasant side effects. Prostaglandin synthetase inhibitors may help reduce dysmenorrhea and may alleviate headaches. Mild sedatives and tranquilizers may help reduce insomnia and anxiety. Low doses of fluoxetine (20 mg) and other selective serotonin reuptake inhibitors, administered either daily or for the last 2 weeks of each menstrual cycle, often reduce the emotional symptoms associated with PMS. Mild diuretics (especially spironolactone at doses up to 100 mg each morning) may benefit cyclic edema if that can be confirmed.

Natural progesterone, particularly in the form of vaginal suppositories given at doses of up to 800 mg/day, has been used, but results of double-blind placebo-controlled trials have provided no evidence of efficacy. Likewise, the value of large quantities of multiple vitamins or of oil of evening primrose, containing the essential fatty acid γ-linolenic acid, a precursor of prostaglandins, is unsubstantiated.

Surgical Therapy

Because PMS requires the occurrence of cyclic ovulation, oophorectomy is occasionally considered for patients with particularly intractable symptoms. However, oophorectomy may create new problems related to estrogen deficiency for women with PMS treated in this permanent fashion. Several trials employing a GnRH agonist together with exogenous steroids (so-called add-back therapy) have been described as reducing PMS. Whether such therapy can be used in the long term remains to be determined.

*This use is not listed in the manufacturer's directive or approved by the FDA.

Abnormal Uterine Bleeding

Diagnosis

Differential Diagnosis

The causes of abnormal uterine bleeding in the reproductive years include complications from the use of oral contraceptives; complications of pregnancy, especially threatened, incomplete, or missed abortion and ectopic pregnancy; coagulation disorders, most commonly idiopathic thrombocytopenic purpura and von Willebrand's disease; and pelvic disease, such as intrauterine polyps, leiomyomas, and tumors of the vagina and cervix. Clear cell adenocarcinoma of the vagina or cervix may occur in women exposed to diethylstilbestrol during fetal life as a result of maternal ingestion. Affected women may also have congenital abnormalities of the upper vagina, cervix, and uterus. Because a history of diethylstilbestrol exposure is not always obtained and because this malignant tumor may be fatal, clinical suspicion should remain high. Women with a history of diethylstilbestrol exposure should be reassured, however, that the incidence of malignant change is extremely low. Trauma (coital or otherwise), foreign bodies, systemic illnesses including various endocrinopathies (such as diabetes mellitus, hypothyroidism and hyperthyroidism, Cushing's syndrome, and Addison's disease), leukemia, and renal disease may also be associated with abnormal bleeding as the presenting manifestation.

So-called dysfunctional uterine bleeding, abnormal uterine bleeding with no demonstrable organic genital or extragenital cause (75% of cases), is most frequently associated with anovulation and might more appropriately be termed anovulatory bleeding. Postmenarchal bleeding in adolescents secondary to immaturity of the hypothalamic-pituitary-ovarian axis accounts for about 20% of all cases, and perimenopausal bleeding consequent to incipient ovarian failure constitutes more than half of the cases. Most anovulatory bleeding is due to either estrogen withdrawal or estrogen breakthrough bleeding. In anovulatory women, estrogen stimulates the endometrium unopposed by progesterone. As a consequence, the endometrium proliferates, becomes thicker, and may shed irregularly, especially if estrogen levels drop. Anovulatory bleeding tends to occur at less frequent intervals, and organic lesions tend to cause bleeding more frequently than cyclic menses.

Clinical Evaluation

All cases of abnormal bleeding should be evaluated, including obtaining a thorough history with special emphasis on the amount and duration of blood loss. Prospective charting of the days on which bleeding occurs may be required to evaluate the bleeding pattern. Complications of pregnancy or a bleeding diathesis must always be ruled out.

The findings on physical examination (including the Papanicolaou smear) are normal in dysfunctional bleeding except for signs of anemia in the more severe cases. Laboratory tests should include a complete blood count, platelet count, coagulation studies, thyroid function tests, and fasting blood glucose concentration. Dysfunctional uterine bleeding must be a diagnosis of exclusion. Management of dysfunctional uterine bleeding depends on the age of the patient and the extent of the bleeding. A sample of the endometrium should be obtained by biopsy or by dilation and curettage from all women older than 35 years and from those at increased risk for endometrial carcinoma because of prolonged anovulatory bleeding.

Treatment

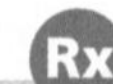

Even profuse bleeding in anovulatory women can almost always be successfully treated by the administration of one combination oral contraceptive pill every 6 hours for 5 to 7 days.* Bleeding should cease within 24 hours, but patients should be warned to expect heavy bleeding 2 to 4 days after therapy is stopped. If anemia and signs of acute blood loss are profound, blood transfusion may be necessary. If the bleeding continues despite therapy, curettage can be carried out. Recurrence can be prevented by giving the patient combination oral contraceptive agents cyclically for 3 months or more. If spontaneous cyclic menses do not resume and pregnancy is not desired, the patient can be treated with cyclic progestin (medroxyprogesterone acetate, 5 to 10 mg for 10 to 14 days each month) or oral contraceptive agents. If pregnancy is desired, ovulation can be induced, as discussed subsequently.

Acute episodes of anovulatory bleeding can also be treated with conjugated estrogens administered intravenously (25 mg every 4 hours for up to three doses) until bleeding ceases.* Progestin therapy (medroxyprogesterone acetate, 5 to 10 mg orally for 10 days) should be started simultaneously. Withdrawal bleeding occurs after cessation of therapy, and the patient can then be treated with oral contraceptive agents for at least three cycles.

For individuals with anovulatory bleeding without an episode of profuse bleeding, treatment with cyclic oral contraceptive agents or progestin can be provided unless pregnancy is desired, in which case ovulation must be induced.

Endometrial ablation by any of several methods is being used increasingly to treat persistent bleeding, especially because it is not a major operation. However, ablation is not 100% effective, and medical management remains the first line of therapy for most women. Hysterectomy may be an appropriate choice for a small number of women.

*These uses are not listed in the manufacturer's directive or approved by the FDA.

Amenorrhea

Definition

Amenorrhea is the absence of menstruation for 3 months or more in women with past menses (secondary amenorrhea) or the absence of menarche by the age of 16 years regardless of the absence or presence of secondary sex characteristics (primary amenorrhea).

Pathobiology

If an intact genital outflow tract exists and there is no primary disease of the uterus, amenorrhea is a sign of failure of the hypothalamic-pituitary-ovarian axis to produce cyclically the hormones necessary for menses. Amenorrhea is a sign of any of several disorders involving different organ systems. Amenorrhea is physiologic in the prepubertal girl, during pregnancy and early in lactation, and after the menopause. At any other time, it is pathologic and demands evaluation. Use of the term *post-pill amenorrhea* to refer to failure to resume menses within 3 months of discontinuation of oral contraceptives is inappropriate. Women so affected should be evaluated in the same manner as any woman with amenorrhea. Similarly, individuals with menses occurring at infrequent intervals of more than 40 days or having fewer than nine menses per year, termed oligomenorrhea, should be evaluated identically to women with amenorrhea.

Diagnosis

Clinical Evaluation

In patients with amenorrhea, even subtle hormonal abnormalities may be manifested by obvious signs and symptoms. Breast development indicates exposure to estrogens, and the presence of pubic and axillary hair indicates androgenic stimulation.

Patients should be questioned especially closely for evidence of psychological disturbances, dietary and exercise habits, lifestyle, environmental stresses, family history of genetic anomalies, and abnormal growth and development. Patients should also be asked about and examined for any signs of hyperandrogenism, including hirsutism, temporal balding, deepening of the voice, increased muscle mass, clitorimegaly, and increased libido, as well as for signs of defeminization, including decreasing breast size and vaginal atrophy. Any history of galactorrhea, the nonpuerperal secretion of milk from the breasts, should be determined. A history of symptoms related to thyroid and adrenal dysfunction should also be sought (Chapters 242, 244, 245).

The physical examination should focus on the evaluation of body dimensions and habitus, extent and distribution of body hair, breast development and secretions, and genitalia. In normal adult women, the arm span is similar to the height; in hypogonadal women, the span is generally more than 5 cm greater than the height. The general appearance of the patient should be evaluated to determine whether the habitus is that of an adult female. The distribution and quantity of body hair should be considered in view of the family history. The extent of any hirsutism should be recorded, preferably by photographs. Other signs of virilization should be sought carefully. Breast development should be graded according to the method of Tanner (Table 256–2). Breast secretion should be sought by applying pressure to the breasts while the patient is seated. Any secretion should be examined microscopically for the presence of perfectly round fat globules of varying size, which are always present in milk and indicate galactorrhea. Finally, the female genitalia should be examined carefully because they are such sensitive indicators of hormonal milieu. The Tanner stage of pubic hair development should be noted (see Table 256–2).

Because the sensitivity of the genitalia to androgens decreases onward from early in fetal development, the extent of any virilization is important. Fusion of the labia and enlargement of the clitoris with or without formation of a penile urethra are observed in women exposed to androgens during the first 3 months of fetal development (Chapter 252). Significant clitorimegaly in the absence of other signs of sexual ambiguity and in the presence of other signs of virilization requires marked androgenic stimulation and strongly implicates an androgen-secreting neoplasm in the absence of a history of ingestion of exogenous steroids. The development of the labia minora in postpubertal women indicates the influence of estrogens. Overt anomalies of the distal genital tract and especially any evidence of obstruction to the escape of menstrual blood should be sought in the remainder of the pelvic examination. The vaginal mucosa and the cervical mucus are exquisitely sensitive to estrogen. Under the influence of estrogen, the vaginal mucosa changes during sexual maturation from a tissue with a shiny, bright red appearance with sparse, thin secretions to a dull, gray-pink rugated surface with copious, thick secretions.

The history and physical examination quickly differentiate among several causes of amenorrhea, regardless of the age of the patient (Table 256–3). The various disorders of sexual differentiation and the other anatomic causes are often apparent on inspection. Distal genital tract obstruction should be identified at the time of pelvic examination even if the specific abnormality is not obvious. The physical stigmata of Turner's syndrome, discussed subsequently, generally make the diagnosis simple. Any sexual ambiguity indicates the need for chromosomal analysis and the measurement of 17α-hydroxyprogesterone to rule out congenital adrenal hyperplasia. Pregnancy and gestational trophoblastic disease may be suspected and confirmed by measurement of circulating concentrations of hCG. The possibility of intrauterine synechiae or adhesions (Asherman's syndrome) must be considered in individuals in whom amenorrhea develops after curettage or endometritis. Tuberculous endometritis, especially in younger women, may also lead to this disorder. Without hormonal measurements, it may be impossible to distinguish between individuals with chronic anovulation, in whom hypothalamic-pituitary-ovarian function is insufficiently coordinated to produce cyclic ovulation, and those with ovarian failure, in whom in most cases the ovaries are devoid of oocytes. Still, it is generally possible to form some strong clinical impressions about the cause of the amenor-

TABLE 256–2 CRITERIA FOR DISTINGUISHING TANNER STAGES 1 TO 5 DURING PUBERTAL MATURATION

Tanner Stage	Breast	Pubic Hair
1 (prepubertal)	No palpable glandular tissue or pigmentation of areola; elevation of areola only	No pubic hair; short, fine vellus hair only
2	Glandular tissue palpable with elevation of breast and areola together as a small mound; areolar diameter increased	Sparse, long, pigmented terminal hair chiefly along the labia majora
3	Further enlargement without separation of breast and areola; although more darkly pigmented, areola still pale and immature; nipple generally at or above midplane of breast tissue when individual is seated upright	Dark, coarse, curly hair, extending sparsely over mons
4	Secondary mound of areola and papilla above breast	Adult-type hair, abundant but limited to mons and labia
5 (adult)	Recession of areola to contour of breast; development of Montgomery's glands and ducts on areola; further pigmentation of areola; nipple generally below midplane of breast tissue when individual is seated upright; maturation independent of breast size	Adult-type hair in quantity and distribution; spread to inner aspects of the thighs in most racial groups

Data from Ross GT: Disorders of the ovary and female reproductive tract. *In* Wilson JD, Foster DW (eds): Textbook of Endocrinology, 7th ed. Philadelphia, WB Saunders, 1985, p 206; Speroff L, Glass RH, Kase N: Clinical Gynecologic Endocrinology and Infertility, 3rd ed. Baltimore, Williams & Wilkins, 1983, p 377; and Kustin J, Rebar RW: Menstrual disorders in the adolescent age group. Primary Care 1987;14:139–166.

rhea. It can be noted whether the patient has absence of, incomplete, or complete development of secondary sex characteristics. The presence of excess body hair or galactorrhea may provide clinical evidence of the pathogenesis of the amenorrhea. Signs and symptoms of adrenal or thyroid dysfunction may be important as well.

Administration of a progestin (typically medroxyprogesterone acetate, 5 to 10 mg given orally for 5 to 10 days, or progesterone in oil, 100 mg given intramuscularly) has been advocated to assess the level of endogenous estrogen. This test is of limited value, however, because almost half the young women with premature ovarian failure experience withdrawal bleeding in response to progestin.

To ascertain whether the outflow tract is intact, an orally active estrogen, such as 2.5 mg of conjugated estrogen daily for 21 days, with 5 to 10 mg of oral medroxyprogesterone acetate for the last 5 to 10 days, may be administered. Withdrawal bleeding should occur if the endometrium is normal. Still, hysterosalpingography and hysteroscopy may be required for the diagnosis of Asherman's syndrome because some patients continue to have some withdrawal bleeding.

TABLE 256–3 CAUSES OF AMENORRHEA

ANATOMIC CAUSES
Pregnancy
Various disorders of sexual differentiation
Distal genital tract obstruction (müllerian agenesis or dysgenesis)
Gonadal dysgenesis*
Ambiguity of external genitalia (male and female pseudohermaphroditism)
Intrauterine adhesions (Asherman's syndrome)
Gestational trophoblastic disease
CHRONIC ANOVULATION
Due to CNS-hypothalamic-pituitary dysfunction
With inappropriate steroid feedback (e.g., polycystic ovary syndrome)
Due to thyroid or adrenal disorders
OVARIAN "FAILURE"
Menopause
Genetic abnormalities
Physical and environmental causes (e.g., chemotherapeutic agents, irradiation)
Idiopathic

*Gonadal dysgenesis may be viewed as both a disorder of sexual differentiation and a form of gonadal "failure."
CNS = central nervous system.

Laboratory Findings

Basal levels of FSH, prolactin, and thyroid-stimulating hormone (TSH) should be measured in all amenorrheic and oligomenorrheic women to confirm the clinical impression (Fig. 256–9).

Increased TSH levels with or without increased levels of prolactin imply primary hypothyroidism, and further evaluation for this disorder is indicated (Chapter 244). Although hypothyroidism commonly results in anovulation, amenorrhea occurs in only some hypothyroid women. Menorrhagia and oligomenorrhea may occur as well. The sensitive immunoassays for TSH permit identification of women with hyperthyroidism as well because TSH levels are suppressed in those individuals.

If the prolactin concentration is increased (typically more than 20 to 30 ng/mL) and the TSH level is normal (generally less than 5 μU/mL), measurement of the prolactin concentration in the basal state should be repeated before more extensive evaluation is undertaken. This is the case because prolactin levels are increased by nonspecific stressful stimuli, sleep, and food ingestion. Prolactin levels may be elevated in as many as one third of women with amenorrhea.

Increased FSH levels (generally above 30 to 40 mIU/mL) imply ovarian failure and require further evaluation. Chromosomal evaluation is indicated in all individuals with elevated FSH levels who are younger than 30 years at the time the amenorrhea begins.

If prolactin and TSH concentrations are within normal ranges and FSH levels are low or normal, the measurement of total testosterone levels may be helpful whether or not there is any evidence of hirsutism or virilization. Hyperandrogenic women need not be hirsute because some have relative insensitivity of the hair follicles to androgens. Mildly increased levels of testosterone (and perhaps dehydroepiandrosterone sulfate as well) suggest polycystic ovary syndrome. However, total circulating androgen levels are rarely not elevated because of the alterations in metabolic clearance rate and sex hormone–binding globulin that are present in polycystic ovary syndrome. Consequently, some clinicians prefer to measure circulating free testosterone levels.

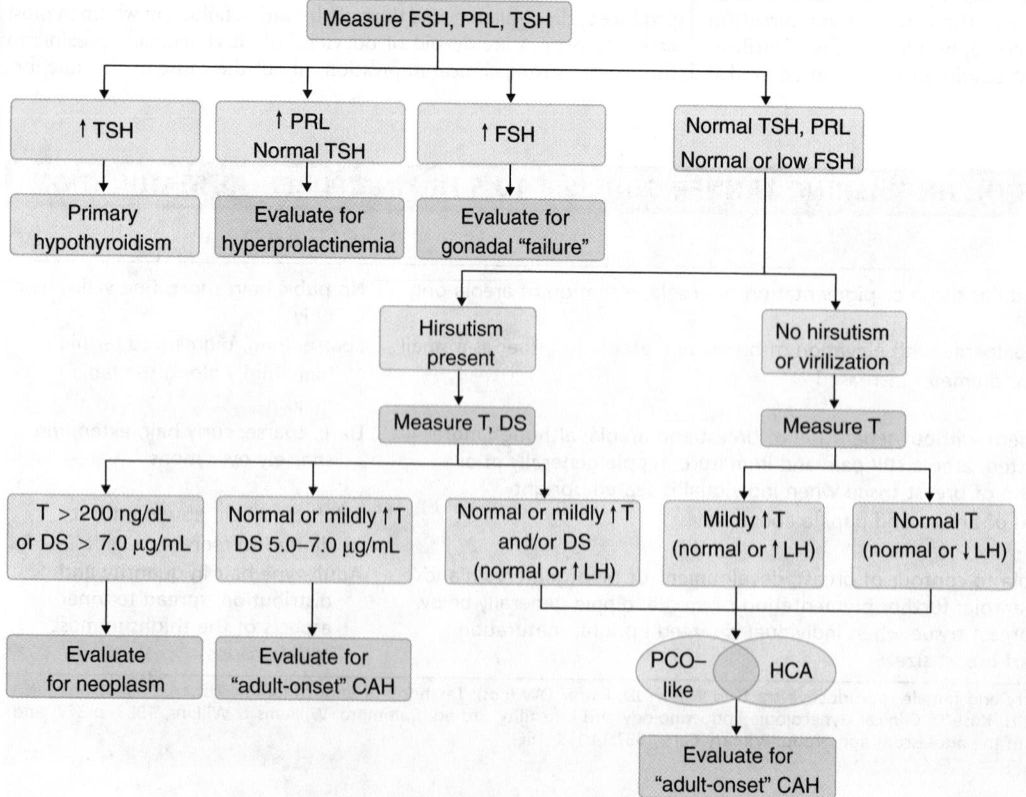

FIGURE 256–9 • Biochemical evaluation of amenorrhea. This schema must be considered an adjunct to the clinical evaluation of the patient. See text for details. CAH = congenital adrenal hyperplasia; DS = dehydroepiandrosterone sulfate; FSH = follicle-stimulating hormone; HCA = hypothalamic chronic anovulation; LH = luteinizing hormone; PCO-like = polycystic ovarian–like; PRL = prolactin; T = testosterone; TSH = thyroid-stimulating hormone.

Circulating levels of LH and FSH may aid in differentiation of polycystic ovary syndrome from hypothalamic-pituitary dysfunction. LH levels are frequently elevated in polycystic ovary syndrome so that the ratio of LH to FSH is increased; however, LH levels may be identical to those observed in normal women in the follicular phase. In contrast, levels of LH and FSH are normal or slightly reduced in hypothalamic-pituitary dysfunction. There is some overlap between women with "polycystic ovarian–like" disorders and those with hypothalamic-pituitary dysfunction. Radiographic assessment of the sella turcica is indicated in all amenorrheic women in whom both LH and FSH levels are very low (both below 10 mIU/mL) to exclude a pituitary or parapituitary neoplasm. Other pituitary functions should be evaluated in any individual with significantly impaired LH and FSH secretion, as detailed subsequently. Both total testosterone and dehydroepiandrosterone sulfate levels should be measured in hirsute or virilized women. Testosterone levels greater than 200 ng/dL should lead to investigation for an androgen-producing neoplasm, most likely of ovarian origin. Dehydroepiandrosterone sulfate levels greater than 7.0 μg/mL should lead to evaluation for an adrenal neoplasm, and levels between 5.0 and 7.0 μg/mL should lead to evaluation for adult-onset congenital adrenal hyperplasia (Chapter 252).

Hypergonadotropic Amenorrhea (Presumptive Ovarian Failure, Primary Hypogonadism, Primary Ovarian Insufficiency)

Diagnosis

Differential Diagnosis

Gonadal failure may begin at any time during embryonic or postnatal development and may result from many causes (Table 256–4). Normally, the ovaries fail at menopause, when virtually no functioning follicles remain. However, premature loss of oocytes before the age of 40 years may occur and lead to premature ovarian failure, possibly from abnormalities in the recruitment and selection of oocytes. Because FSH is the principal regulator of folliculogenesis, most causes of premature ovarian failure may somehow involve FSH secretion or action. Circulating gonadotropin levels increase whenever ovarian failure occurs because of decreased negative estrogen feedback to the hypothalamic-pituitary unit.

TABLE 256–4 CLASSIFICATION OF HYPERGONADOTROPIC AMENORRHEA (FSH >30 MIU/ML)*

- Menopause
- Genetic abnormalities
  - Genetically reduced germ cell endowment
  - Accelerated atresia
  - Gonadal dysgenesis
    - With stigmata of Turner's syndrome (45,X)
    - Pure (46,XX or 46,XY)
    - Mixed
  - Trisomy X with or without chromosomal mosaicism
  - Premutations of the *FMR1* (fragile X) gene
  - In association with myotonia dystrophica or other abnormalities
  - Enzymatic defects
    - 17α-Hydroxylase deficiency
    - Galactosemia
    - 20,22-lyase and aromatase deficiency
  - Known genetic alterations of other specific genes
- Physical and environmental causes
  - Gonadal irradiation
  - Chemotherapeutic (especially alkylating) agents
  - Viral agents
  - Surgical extirpation
- Autoimmune disorders
  - Polyglandular, involving ovarian failure and any combination of thyroiditis, hypoadrenalism, hypoparathyroidism, diabetes mellitus, myasthenia gravis, vitiligo, mucocutaneous candidiasis, and pernicious anemia
  - Isolated ovarian failure
  - In association with congenital thymic dysplasia
  - Circulating gonadotropin antibodies
- Defective gonadotropin secretion or action
  - Resistant ovary or Savage's syndrome
  - Secretion of biologically inactive forms
  - α or β subunit defects
  - FSH receptor mutations
- Idiopathic premature ovarian failure

FSH = follicle-stimulating hormone.
*Some disorders may fit in more than one place in this schema.

Pathobiology

Genetics

Several pathologic conditions with dysgenetic gonads involve elevated gonadotropin levels and amenorrhea. The term *gonadal dysgenesis* refers to individuals with undifferentiated streak gonads without any association with either extragonadal stigmata or sex chromosome aberrations. Because individuals with gonadal dysgenesis have the normal complement of oocytes at 20 weeks of fetal age but virtually none by birth, this disorder is a form of premature ovarian failure.

Turner's Syndrome

Turner's syndrome describes patients with streak gonads composed of fibrous stroma and four cardinal features: a female phenotype; sexual infantilism; short stature; and several physical abnormalities, sometimes including webbed neck, low-set ears, multiple pigmented nevi, double eyelashes, micrognathia, epicanthal folds, shield-like chest with microthelia, short fourth metacarpals, increased carrying angle of the arms, and certain renal and cardiovascular defects (most commonly coarctation of the aorta and aortic stenosis). The diagnosis can sometimes be made at birth because of unexplained lymphedema of the hands and feet. The syndrome is associated with an abnormality of sex chromosome number, morphology, or both. Most commonly, the second sex chromosome is absent (45,X). This is the single most common chromosome disorder in humans, but more than 95% of such fetuses are aborted, so that the incidence in newborns is approximately 1 in 3000 to 5000. Chromosome breakage and mosaicism occur frequently as well. In mosaic individuals with a normal 46,XX cell line, sufficient follicles may persist postnatally to initiate pubertal changes and to cause ovulation so that pregnancy is possible.

Pure Gonadal Dysgenesis

Pure gonadal dysgenesis is the term given to phenotypically female individuals with streak gonads who are of normal stature and have none of the physical stigmata associated with Turner's syndrome. Such individuals have either a 46,XX or 46,XY karyotype. The 46,XX defect may be inherited as an autosomal recessive, with 10% having associated nerve deafness. The 46,XY defect may be inherited as an X-linked recessive, with clitorimegaly occurring in 10 to 15% and gonadal tumors developing in 25% if the gonads are not removed.

Trisomy X

Trisomy X (46,XXX karyotype) is also associated with premature menopause, although many such individuals have normal reproductive lives. Premature menopause can also occur in mosaic individuals with cell lines with excess X chromosomes. When gonadal abnormalities occur in women with excess X chromosomes, they seem to occur after ovarian differentiation so that some ovarian function is possible. Only later in life do such women develop secondary amenorrhea and premature ovarian failure.

In girls with the rare syndrome of 17α-hydroxylase deficiency involving *p450c17* who survive until the expected age of puberty, sexual infantilism and primary amenorrhea occur together with elevated levels of gonadotropins. Increased synthesis of desoxycorticosterone leads to hypertension with hypokalemic alkalosis; serum progesterone levels are elevated as well. As with other causes of congenital adrenal hyperplasia, the hypertension is controlled by replacement therapy with glucocorticoids (Chapter 252). Defects in the 20,22-lyase (*p450scc*) or aromatase (*p450arom*) enzymes may also lead to ovarian failure. Women with galactosemia also experience ovarian failure early in life, even when a galactose-restricted diet is introduced early in infancy (Chapter 218).

It now appears that more than 5% of women with 46,XX spontaneous premature ovarian failure will have mutations of the *FMR1* gene, the gene responsible for the fragile X syndrome. This risk is increased if there is a family history of premature ovarian failure. Moreover, a family history of fragile X syndrome, unexplained mental retardation, dementia, developmental delay of a child, or tremor-ataxia syndrome is reason for genetic counseling. Mutations in the *FMR1* gene are known to be associated with a neurodegenerative disorder. Women with mutations in the *FMR1* gene are at risk of having a child with mental retardation, should they be one of the 6 to 8% of women with premature ovarian failure who conceive spontaneously.

Known Genetic Alterations of Specific Genes

Mutations to several other specific genes in addition to those already discussed are now known to result in premature ovarian failure. These include mutations involving *FSHR* (the FSH receptor gene), *FOXL2* (a forkhead transcription factor associated with the blepharophimosis/ptosis/epicanthus inversus syndrome), *INHA* (the inhibin alpha gene), *E1F2B* (a family of genes associated with central nervous system leukodystrophy and ovarian failue), *BMP15* (the gene for bone morphogenetic protein 15 known to be associated with follicular development), *PMM2* (the gene for phosphomannomutase), and *AIRE* (leading to the autoimmune polyendocrinopathy-candidiasis-ectodermal dystrophy syndrome). No doubt other mutations causing ovarian failure will be discovered in the future.

Other Causes

Physical and Environmental

Irradiation and chemotherapeutic agents, especially alkylating agents, used to treat various malignant diseases may also cause premature ovarian failure. Ovulation and cyclic menses return in some of these patients even after prolonged intervals of hypergonadotropic amenorrhea associated with signs and symptoms of profound hypoestrogenism. Rarely, mumps affects the ovaries and causes ovarian failure.

Autoimmune Disorders

Premature ovarian failure may occur in conjunction with a variety of autoimmune disorders. The most well known syndrome involves hypoadrenalism, hypoparathyroidism, and mucocutaneous candidiasis together with ovarian failure (Chapter 250). Testing for adrenal antibodies by indirect immunofluorescence will identify the approximately 4% of women with spontaneous premature ovarian failure who have steroidogenic cell autoimmunity and are at risk of adrenal insufficiency. Thyroiditis is the most commonly associated abnormality. Antibodies to the FSH receptor have been identified in a few cases. These associations make it mandatory to rule out other potentially life-threatening endocrinopathies in young women with hypergonadotropic amenorrhea.

Defective Gonadotropin Secretion or Action

The resistant ovary (Savage's) syndrome occurs in young amenorrheic women who have elevated peripheral gonadotropin concentrations, normal (although immature) follicles present on ovarian biopsy, 46,XX karyotype with no evidence of mosaicism, fully developed secondary sex characteristics, and ovarian resistance to stimulation with human menopausal or pituitary gonadotropins. There seems to be some block to gonadotropin action within the ovary in this syndrome.

At least one form of premature ovarian failure is caused by mutations in the FSH receptor. Affected individuals present with primary or secondary amenorrhea and elevated levels of FSH and may still have ovarian follicles detectable on transvaginal ultrasonography. One specific mutation on chromosome 2p (C566T:alanine to valine) in exon 7 of the FSH receptor has been identified in several Finnish families, but the mutation has not been detected in any other populations.

Treatment

Rx

Women with hypergonadotropic amenorrhea and ovarian failure should be treated identically whether or not they have signs of hypoestrogenism or desire pregnancy. Ovarian biopsy is not indicated to document the existence of follicles because only a small portion of each ovary can be sampled and because pregnancies have resulted in patients who had biopsy samples devoid of follicles. Estrogen replacement is warranted to prevent the accelerated bone loss known to occur in affected women (Chapter 264). The estrogen should be given sequentially with a progestin to prevent endometrial hyperplasia. Young women with ovarian failure may require twice as much estrogen as postmenopausal women for relief of signs and symptoms of hypoestrogenism.

Women with hypergonadotropic amenorrhea are rarely able to become pregnant. It is not clear why pregnancy may rarely occur in

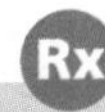

such women, but the pregnancy rate is less than 10%. The most successful treatment of young women with hypergonadotropic amenorrhea involves hormone replacement to mimic the normal menstrual cycle and embryo transfer by use of donor oocytes. Pregnancy rates are higher than in other women undergoing in vitro fertilization and typically exceed 30% per cycle. Whether women with gonadal dysgenesis should be offered pregnancy by use of donor oocytes is now the subject of debate because a markedly increased incidence of aortic rupture during pregnancy secondary to medial necrosis has been detected. Clearly women with Turner's syndrome contemplating pregnancy should be counseled about the risks appropriately.

CHRONIC ANOVULATION

Chronic anovulation, the most frequent form of amenorrhea encountered in women of reproductive age, implies that functional ovarian follicles remain and that cyclic ovulation can be induced or reinitiated with appropriate therapy (Table 256–5). Appropriate management requires that the cause of the anovulation be determined. The pathophysiologic bases for several forms of anovulation are unknown, but the anovulation

TABLE 256–5 CAUSES OF CHRONIC ANOVULATION

Chronic anovulation of hypothalamic-pituitary origin
Hypothalamic chronic anovulation
Psychogenic
Exercise associated
Associated with diet, weight loss, or malnutrition
Anorexia nervosa and bulimia
Pseudocyesis
Forms of isolated gonadotropin deficiency (including Kallmann's syndrome)
Due to hypothalamic-pituitary damage
Pituitary and parapituitary tumors
Empty sella syndrome
Following surgery
Following irradiation
Following trauma
Following infection
Following infarction
Idiopathic hypopituitarism
Hypothalamic-pituitary dysfunction or failure with hyperprolactinemia (multiple causes)
Due to systemic diseases
Chronic anovulation due to inappropriate feedback (i.e., polycystic ovary syndrome)
Excessive extraglandular estrogen production (i.e., obesity)
Abnormal buffering involving sex hormone–binding globulin (including liver disease)
Functional androgen excess (adrenal or ovarian)
Neoplasms producing androgens or estrogens
Neoplasms producing chorionic gonadotropin
Chronic anovulation due to other endocrine and metabolic disorders
Adrenal hyperfunction
Cushing's syndrome
Congenital adrenal hyperplasia (female pseudohermaphroditism)
Thyroid dysfunction
Hyperthyroidism
Hypothyroidism
Prolactin or growth hormone excess
Hypothalamic dysfunction
Pituitary dysfunction (microadenomas and macroadenomas)
Drug induced
Malnutrition

can be interrupted transiently by nonspecific induction of ovulation in the majority of affected women. Anovulation can result in either amenorrhea or irregular (generally less frequent) menses.

Hypothalamic Chronic Anovulation

Definition

Hypothalamic chronic anovulation (HCA) represents a heterogeneous group of disorders with similar manifestations. Emotional and physical stress, exercise, diet, weight loss, body composition, malnutrition, environment, and other unrecognized factors may contribute in varying proportions to the anovulation.

Anorexia Nervosa

Individuals with amenorrhea and significant weight loss should be examined for the possibility of anorexia nervosa (Chapter 238). This disorder may be the most severe form of functional HCA, or it may be a distinct entity.

Kallmann's Syndrome

Kallmann's syndrome (isolated gonadotropin deficiency or familial hypogonadotropic hypogonadism) is a familial disorder consisting of gonadotropin deficiency, anosmia or hyposmia, and color blindness in men or, more rarely, in women. Other midline defects, such as cleft lip and palate, can occur in the affected individual or in family members. The trait is transmitted as an X-linked recessive or a male-limited autosomal dominant trait, but genetic heterogeneity may occur. Partial or complete agenesis of the olfactory bulb is present on autopsy, accounting for use of the term *olfactogenital dysplasia*. The disorder affects only gonadotropin secretion, and all other pituitary hormones are secreted normally. Isolated gonadotropin deficiency in the absence of anosmia occurs as well. Sexual infantilism with a eunuchoid habitus is the clinical hallmark of this disorder, but moderate breast development may occur. Circulating LH and FSH levels are low but almost always detectable. Ovulation induction requires use of exogenous gonadotropins and hCG or pulsatile GnRH. Estrogen replacement therapy is indicated in these women until pregnancy is desired. It may not be possible to distinguish between partial isolated gonadotropin deficiency and functional HCA in all cases.

Hypopituitarism

Hypopituitarism may be obvious on cursory inspection or sufficiently subtle to require endocrine testing (Chapter 242). The clinical presentation depends on the age at onset, the cause, and the nutritional status of the individual. Failure of development of secondary sex characteristics or failure of development to progress once puberty is initiated must always raise the question of hypopituitarism. Ovulation can be induced successfully with exogenous gonadotropins when pregnancy is desired and after the hypopituitarism is treated appropriately. Replacement therapy with estrogen is indicated to prevent signs and symptoms of estrogen deficiency.

Galactorrhea

Galactorrhea associated with hyperprolactinemia, whatever the cause, almost always occurs together with amenorrhea caused by hypothalamic-pituitary dysfunction or failure. Many conditions can cause excess prolactin secretion (Chapter 242). Hirsutism may be observed occasionally in association with amenorrhea-galactorrhea and hyperprolactinemia. Elevated levels of the adrenal androgens dehydroepiandrosterone and dehydroepiandrosterone sulfate may be observed and may account for the polycystic-type ovaries present in some hyperprolactinemic women.

Failure of the Hypothalamic-Pituitary Unit

The hypothalamic-pituitary unit may also fail to function normally in a number of stressful, debilitating, systemic illnesses that interfere with somatic growth and development. Chronic renal failure, liver disease, and diabetes mellitus are the most prominent examples.

Diagnosis

Abrupt cessation of menses in women younger than 30 years who have no anatomic abnormalities of the hypothalamic-pituitary-ovarian axis and no other endocrine disturbances suggests a diagnosis of HCA. Affected individuals tend to be bright, educated, and engaged in intellectual occupations and may well give a history of psychosexual problems and socioenvironmental trauma. HCA is characterized by low to normal levels of gonadotropins and relative hypoestrogenism. Rarely, however, do affected women present with signs and symptoms of estrogen deficiency.

Treatment

Rx

Psychological counseling or a change in lifestyle, especially for women engaged in strenuous exercise programs, may be effective in inducing cyclic ovulation and menses. For women desiring pregnancy, ovulation can also be induced with clomiphene citrate (50 to 100 mg/day for 5 days beginning on the third to fifth day of withdrawal bleeding). Treatment with exogenous purified or synthetic gonadotropins to induce follicular maturation followed by hCG to induce follicular rupture or GnRH administered in a pulsatile fashion may be effective in women who do not ovulate in response to clomiphene. Because women with HCA have low circulating levels of leptin, investigators have given recombinant leptin and documented that ovulation may resume in some affected women. Given the heterogeneous nature of the disorder, it is not surprising that exogenous leptin is not effective in all affected women.

Most physicians advocate the use of exogenous steroids to prevent osteoporosis. A regimen can consist of daily oral conjugated or esterified estrogens (0.625 to 1.25 mg), ethinyl estradiol (20 μg), or micronized estradiol-17β (1 to 2 mg) or transdermal estradiol-17β (0.05 to 0.10 mg) daily, with oral medroxyprogesterone acetate (5 to 10 mg) added for the first 12 to 14 days of each month. Sexually active women can be given oral contraceptive agents as an alternative. If steroid therapy is administered, patients must be informed that the amenorrhea will probably be present when therapy is discontinued. Other physicians believe that only periodic observation is indicated, with barrier methods of contraception recommended for fertility control. Adequate ingestion of calcium should be ensured regardless of therapy. Contraception is needed for sexually active women with HCA because the functional defect is mild in these disorders and may resolve spontaneously at any time, with ovulation occurring before any episode of menstruation.

Chronic Anovulation Related to Inappropriate Feedback

Definition

Polycystic ovary syndrome, which causes anovulation because of inappropriate feedback signals to the hypothalamic-pituitary unit, is a heterogeneous disorder in which there is considerable clinical and biochemical variability among affected individuals. Polycystic ovary syndrome is now considered to exist in women with any two of the following: (1) oligo- or anovulation, (2) hyperandrogenism, or (3) polycystic ovaries on ultrasound, and in whom other etiologies have been eliminated.

Pathobiology

The cause of polycystic ovary syndrome is unknown, but current evidence suggests that the hypothalamic-pituitary unit is intact and that a functional derangement, perhaps involving insulin-like growth factors such as IGF-I within the ovary, results in abnormal gonadotropin secretion. Polycystic ovary syndrome is characterized by insulin resistance and compensatory hyperinsulinemia. The insulin resistance has been found in affected women of many racial and ethnic groups, implying that it is a universal characteristic and that a common defect may be present. There is increasing evidence of specific genetic abnormalities in some women with polycystic ovary syndrome.

Clinical Manifestations

Although patients usually present with amenorrhea, hirsutism, and obesity, affected women may instead complain of irregular and profuse uterine bleeding, may not have hirsutism, and may be of normal weight.

Excess androgen from any source or increased extraglandular conversion of androgens to estrogens can lead to the typical findings of polycystic ovary syndrome. Included are such diverse disorders as Cushing's syndrome, mild congenital adrenal hyperplasia, virilizing tumors of adrenal or ovarian origin, hyperthyroidism and hypothyroidism, obesity, and primary polycystic ovary syndrome with no other recognizable cause.

In the primary syndrome, the irregular menses, mild obesity, and hirsutism begin during puberty and typically become more severe with time. Obesity alone can lead to a polycystic ovarian–like syndrome, with the degree of obesity required to cause anovulation varying widely from individual to individual. All such patients are well estrogenized regardless of whether they present with primary or secondary amenorrhea or dysfunctional bleeding. As noted, LH concentrations tend to be elevated, with relatively low and constant FSH levels, but both may be in the normal range compared with levels in women in the follicular phase of the menstrual cycle. Levels of most circulating androgens, especially testosterone, tend to be mildly elevated.

Diagnosis

A consensus conference in Rotterdam in 2003 concluded that after exclusion of other etiologies, two of the following three are required for diagnosis of polycystic ovary syndrome:

1. hyperandrogenism (clinical or biochemical)
2. oligo-ovulation or anovulation
3. polycystic ovaries on ultrasound examination or at surgery

This definition is confusing to clinicians because it implies that hirsute women with polycystic ovaries on ultrasound examination who ovulate regularly should be considered to have polycystic ovary syndrome. Moreover, it is clear that polycystic ovaries may be identified on ultrasound examination in some otherwise apparently normal women.

In any case, the aim of the diagnostic evaluation is to rule out any causes (such as neoplasms) that require definitive therapy. Hirsutism should be evaluated as detailed in Chapter 261.

A particularly severely affected subset of women present with marked obesity, anovulation, mild glucose intolerance, and high levels of circulating insulin with insulin resistance, acanthosis nigricans, hyperuricemia, and severe hirsutism with markedly elevated circulating androgen levels. These women have hyperthecosis of the ovaries, in which the androgen-producing cells in the stromal, hilar, and thecal components of the ovaries are increased greatly in number. Although it is considered a separate entity by some clinicians, hyperthecosis should probably be viewed as a part of the spectrum of disorders constituting polycystic ovary syndrome.

Treatment

Rx

Patients generally require therapy for hirsutism, for induction of ovulation if pregnancy is desired, and for prevention of estrogen-induced endometrial hyperplasia and cancer. No ideal therapy exists; the therapeutic approach must be individualized to the needs of each patient. In addition, the risks of cardiovascular disease and of diabetes mellitus are increased in women with polycystic ovary syndrome, presumably at least in part because of the increased androgens and insulin resistance invariably present. Moreover, many affected women have elevated cholesterol levels, related at least in part to the other metabolic alterations present.

Medical Therapy

In the anovulatory woman not desiring pregnancy who is not hirsute, therapy with intermittent progestin administration (such as medroxyprogesterone acetate, 5 to 10 mg orally for 10 to 14 days each month) or oral contraceptives can be provided to reduce the increased risk of endometrial carcinoma that is present in such a woman with unopposed estrogen. All women using intermittent progestin administration should be cautioned about the need for effective contraception if they are sexually active because these agents do not inhibit ovulation when they are administered intermittently.

Rx

It is now apparent that improvements in insulin sensitivity in women with polycystic ovaries, either through lifestyle changes (i.e., exercise and diet) or through pharmacologic intervention, consistently result in improvements in the reproductive and metabolic abnormalities associated with polycystic ovaries. Resumption of ovulation may occur in up to 60 to 70% of affected women.

Metformin

The longest and largest published experiences with any agent that improves insulin sensitivity in polycystic ovary syndrome is with metformin, a biguanide that works primarily by suppressing hepatic gluconeogenesis and also improves insulin sensitivity in the periphery (primarily skeletal muscle). Its use in women with polycystic ovaries leads to reductions in circulatory insulin and androgen levels and resumption of menses in some women. Divided doses of 1500 to 2000 mg/day have proved effective.

Some clinicians advocate giving metformin (or another insulin-sensitizing agent) to all women with polycystic ovaries, whereas others would administer such an agent only to those with documented insulin resistance. Some clinicians also advocate giving metformin first to women who desire pregnancy and then adding an agent to induce ovulation if the metformin proves ineffective. This is an evolving field; these agents are not approved for use in pregnant women or for the induction of ovulation.

Treatment Considering Pregnancy

The approach to the hirsute anovulatory woman not desiring pregnancy is detailed in Chapter 261. Oral contraceptive agents are the first line of therapy for such women with mild hirsutism and offer protection from endometrial hyperplasia. In women with polycystic ovary syndrome desiring pregnancy, clomiphene citrate can be used to induce ovulation. Approximately 75 to 80% conceive with such therapy. In addition to insulin-sensitizing agents, other possible methods of inducing ovulation include use of exogenous gonadotropins and hCG, pulsatile GnRH, wedge resection of the ovaries at laparotomy, and laser or cautery destruction of follicles at laparoscopy. A large clinical trial documented that clomiphene citrate is more effective than metformin in inducing ovulation and resulting in pregnancy; there was no further improvement statistically when the two agents were used concurrently. [1]

Surgical Treatment

Surgical treatment is warranted rarely and only in women in whom all other methods fail, in whom there is a question of an ovarian tumor because of ovarian size or circulating androgen levels, and in whom fertility is not an issue (because of the risk of infertility due to pelvic adhesions from the surgery).

Chronic Anovulation Related to Other Endocrine and Metabolic Disorders

Adrenal hyperfunction appears to cause chronic anovulation by inducing a polycystic ovarian–like syndrome secondary to increased adrenal androgen secretion, but other possible mechanisms also exist.

Both hyperthyroidism and hypothyroidism are associated with a variety of menstrual disturbances, including dysfunctional uterine bleeding and amenorrhea as a result of alterations in the metabolism of androgens and estrogens. These metabolic changes in turn result in inappropriate steroid feedback and chronic anovulation.

Disorders of Folliculogenesis

Recognized disorders of folliculogenesis cannot be identified before ovulation begins. They are believed to reflect abnormalities in follicular development.

Luteinized Unruptured Follicle Syndrome

The luteinized unruptured follicle syndrome refers to the development of a dominant follicle without its subsequent disruption and release of the ovum. The abnormality can be diagnosed by ultrasonography or by the absence of evidence of ovulation when the ovary is viewed at laparoscopy. The disorder is believed to occur infrequently and sporadically and is probably not a significant cause of infertility. Menstrual cycles in which no ovum is released are characterized by presumptive evidence of ovulation, including biphasic basal body temperatures, secretory endometrium, normal LH surge, and normal progesterone production in the luteal phase. In fact, although the syndrome is believed to occur, data to substantiate its existence are only circumstantial (although strongly suggestive) at present.

Luteal Phase Dysfunction

Pathobiology

Progesterone secretion in the luteal phase may be reduced in duration (termed luteal phase insufficiency) or in amount (termed luteal phase inadequacy). More rarely, the endometrium may be unable to respond to secreted progesterone because of the absence of progesterone receptors. These disorders are believed to represent causes of infertility (because of inability of fertilized ova to implant) in much less than 5% of infertile couples. Abnormalities of the follicular phase, especially in the frequency of gonadotropin pulses, may account for most luteal phase defects. Luteal phase defects may also occur sporadically in normally ovulating women approximately once each year.

Diagnosis

Luteal phase dysfunction may be associated with several clinical entities, including mild or intermittent hyperprolactinemia (of any cause), strenuous physical exercise, inadequately treated 21-hydroxylase deficiency, and habitual abortion. Luteal dysfunction occurs more commonly at the extremes of reproductive life and in the first menstrual cycles after full-term delivery, abortion, or discontinuation of oral contraceptives. It may also occur during ovulatory cycles induced with clomiphene citrate or exogenous gonadotropins and hCG.

Although it is clear that this disorder exists in rare circumstances, just how and if the diagnosis of luteal phase dysfunction can be made with accuracy has been challenged by studies documenting that histologic evaluation of endometrial biopsy specimens is inaccurate. Endometrial biopsy had been regarded as the "gold standard" in making the diagnosis. The absolute concentration that progesterone must achieve and the length of time progesterone must be increased in the luteal phase to exclude luteal dysfunction are unclear. Luteal dysfunction is extremely rare in women with menstrual cycles longer than 25 days in whom a single random progesterone determination is greater than 15 ng/mL.

Treatment

Rx

Treatment of luteal dysfunction is controversial. Any underlying defect should be treated. If subsequent luteal function depends on prior follicular development, modification of follicular development with either clomiphene citrate (25 to 100 mg daily by mouth for 5 days beginning on cycle day 3 to 5) or FSH (75 to 300 IU intramuscularly for 3 to 5 days beginning on cycle day 3 to 5) is reasonable; hCG (2500 to 5000 IU intramuscularly at 2- to 3-day intervals beginning with the shift in basal body temperature) or progesterone (12.5 mg intramuscularly in oil daily or 25 mg twice a day as rectal or vaginal suppositories) can be used as well. Bromocriptine may correct the abnormality in individuals with hyperprolactinemia. Synthetic progestational agents should not be used to treat luteal phase defects because of their possible (although unproven) association with congenital anomalies. Furthermore, the synthetic progestins produce an abnormal endometrium. None of these agents has been shown to increase the pregnancy rate.

Infertility

Definition

Infertility may be defined as involuntary inability to conceive. Sterility is total inability to reproduce. In either case, the situation may or may not be correctable, especially for each particular couple. Failure to reproduce thwarts a basic human instinct and causes anger, guilt, and depression. More than 10% of couples in the United States seek medical assistance for infertility.

The requirements for pregnancy to occur are several:

- The male must produce adequate numbers of normal, motile spermatozoa.
- The male must be capable of ejaculating the sperm through a patent ductal system.
- The sperm must be able to traverse an unobstructed female reproductive tract.
- The female must ovulate and release an ovum.
- The sperm must be able to fertilize the ovum.
- The fertilized ovum must be capable of developing and implanting in appropriately prepared endometrium.

Infertility is too frequently viewed primarily as a problem of the female. In fact, in approximately 40% of cases, infertility is caused by the male (Table 256–6). In perhaps one third of couples, more than one cause contributes to the infertility.

Peak age for fertility in the female is 25 years. For nulliparous women of this age, the average time during which unprotected intercourse occurs until conception is 5.3 months. For parous women, the average duration of intercourse until conception is 2.7 months. The reproductive performance of couples is influenced by the ages of the female and male partners, the frequency of intercourse, and the length of time the couple has been attempting to conceive. There is a decline in both female and male reproductive performance after the age of 25 years.

Diagnosis

Couples who complain of infertility merit evaluation regardless of the length of infertility. If the couple believes there is a problem, it is the physician's responsibility to reassure them by appropriate evaluation and subsequent explanation of all findings and the prognosis.

The evaluation begins with a detailed history obtained from both partners and physical examinations of both individuals. The couple should be seen together for the first visit. Each couple should be questioned together and separately because separate interviews may uncover information that would not be imparted in the presence of the partner.

Initial evaluation for infertility generally includes assessment of semen; documentation of ovulation by basal body temperature, serum progesterone determination approximately 6 to 8 days before menses, or endometrial biopsy less than 3 days before onset of menses; and evaluation of the female genital tract by hysterosalpingography or sonohysterography, also known as saline infusion sonography. Basal serum levels of thyroid hormones should be measured. Diagnostic laparoscopy with tubal dye instillation may be performed if results of all previous tests are normal because 30 to 50% of women are found to have endometriosis or tubal disease on surgical evaluation.

Treatment

Treatment must be predicated on the findings of the infertility evaluation. Abnormalities of sperm are among the more difficult disorders to treat. Low sperm count or poor motility are best treated either by donor insemination or in vitro fertilzation with intracytoplasmic injection of a single viable sperm into each oocyte. Obstruction of the fallopian tubes may be amenable to surgical intervention, but success rates are often greater with in vitro fertilization. Endometriosis causing infertility may be treated by surgery and/or various suppressive drugs as indicated; however here, too, in vitro fertilization may prove indicated.

Induction of ovulation is one of the most successful therapies when used appropriately in anovulatory women.

Induction of Ovulation

Induction of ovulation should never be attempted until serious disorders precluding pregnancy are ruled out or treated. Further-

TABLE 256-6 CAUSES OF INFERTILITY AND THEIR APPROXIMATE INCIDENCE

Male factors (40%)
- Decreased production of spermatozoa
  - Varicocele
  - Testicular failure
  - Endocrine disorders
  - Cryptorchidism
  - Stress, smoking, caffeine, nicotine, recreational drugs
- Ductal obstruction
  - Epididymal (after infection)
  - Congenital absence of vas deferens
  - Ejaculatory duct (after infection)
  - After vasectomy
- Inability to deliver sperm into vagina
  - Ejaculatory disturbances
  - Hypospadias
  - Sexual problems (i.e., impotence), medical or psychological
- Abnormal semen
  - Infection
  - Abnormal volume
  - Abnormal viscosity
- Immunologic factors
  - Sperm-immobilizing antibodies
  - Sperm-agglutinating antibodies

Female factors
- Fallopian tube disease (20–30%)
  - Pelvic inflammatory disease or puerperal infection
  - Congenital anomalies
  - Endometriosis
  - Secondary to past peritonitis of nongenital origin
- Amenorrhea and anovulation (15%)
- Minor ovulatory disturbances (<5%?)
- Cervical and uterine factors (10%)
  - Leiomyomas and polyps
  - Uterine anomalies
  - Intrauterine synechiae (Asherman's syndrome)
  - Destroyed endocervical glands (after surgery or after infection)
- Vaginal factors (<5%)
  - Congenital absence of vagina
  - Imperforate hymen
  - Vaginismus
  - Vaginitis
- Immunologic factors (<5%)
  - Sperm-immobilizing antibodies
  - Sperm-agglutinating antibodies
- Nutritional and metabolic factors (5%)
  - Thyroid disorders
  - Diabetes mellitus
  - Severe nutritional disturbances

Idiopathic or unexplained (<10%)

Rx

more, ovulation induction should be used only in women with chronic anovulation because women with ovarian failure are unresponsive to any form of ovulation induction. In general, the use of pharmaceutical agents does not improve the quality of an ovum, and thus the chance of pregnancy is not improved in women who ovulate regularly.

Clomiphene citrate is the agent that usually induces ovulation most easily. Clomiphene should be used in individuals without hyperprolactinemia who have the ability to release LH and FSH. A typical course of clomiphene therapy is begun on the fifth day after either spontaneous or induced uterine bleeding. The initial dosage is 50 mg daily for 5 days. Clomiphene appears to act as an antiestrogen and stimulates gonadotropin secretion by the pituitary gland to initiate follicular development. If ovulation is not achieved in the first cycle of treatment, the daily dosage is increased to 100 mg. If ovulation is still not achieved, dosage is increased in a stepwise fashion in 50-mg increments to a maximum of 200 to 250 mg daily for 5 days. The highest dose should be continued for 3 to 6 months before the patient is regarded as unresponsive to clomiphene. The quantity of drug and the length of time that it can be used, as suggested here, are greater than those recommended by the manufacturers and the FDA but conform to published series.

The ovulatory surge of LH may occur 5 to 12 days (average, 7 days) after the completion of the last day of clomiphene treatment in each course. Couples are advised to have intercourse every other day during this interval. Ovulation can be documented by monitoring changes in basal body temperature or preferably by measuring serum progesterone concentration approximately 14 days after the last clomiphene tablet is taken. In addition, menses should occur about 3 weeks after the last day of therapy. Withdrawal bleeding with progestin can be induced if the patient fails to bleed within 4 weeks of therapy and if a serum hCG level documents that the patient is not pregnant. Testing the urine for an LH surge with any of several commercially available tests may also be useful in timing ovulation.

Some clinicians give 5000 to 10,000 IU of hCG intramuscularly 7 days after the last day of clomiphene therapy to trigger ovulation, but this approach has not been established to increase effectiveness. The administration of hCG, however, does serve to time ovulation and may be helpful in selected couples. Ovulation can be expected to occur approximately 36 hours after hCG administration.

Of appropriately selected patients, 75 to 80% ovulate and 40 to 50% can be expected to become pregnant. About 15% of pregnancies can be expected with each ovulatory cycle. The multiple pregnancy rate is about 8%, with almost all being twins. The incidence of congenital anomalies is not increased.

Side effects of clomiphene are uncommon and rarely serious. The most serious ones include vasomotor flushes (10%), abdominal discomfort (5%), breast tenderness (2%), nausea and vomiting (2%), visual symptoms (1.5%), and headache (1%). Ovarian enlargement may occur but is rare (5%). Concern has been raised about the potential for clomiphene to increase the risk of epithelial ovarian cancer. The bulk of the evidence now indicates that clomiphene does not increase this risk, but research in this area continues.

The addition of dexamethasone, 0.5 mg orally at bedtime to blunt the nighttime secretion of adrenocorticotropic hormone, may be useful in hyperandrogenic women with an adrenal component who fail to ovulate in response to clomiphene. Other individuals who do not respond to clomiphene typically require exogenous gonadotropins and hCG or perhaps pulsatile GnRH to induce ovulation.

Both bromocriptine and cabergoline, two dopamine agonists, are effective in inducing ovulation in hyperprolactinemic women. The drug should be stopped when pregnancy is confirmed. Ovulatory menses and pregnancy are achieved in about 80% of patients with galactorrhea and hyperprolactinemia. The majority of women with prolactin-secreting pituitary tumors remain asymptomatic during pregnancy. It is rare for a patient with either a microadenoma or a macroadenoma to develop a problem related to the tumor that affects either the mother or the fetus during pregnancy. Monitoring during pregnancy need consist only of questioning the patient about the development of visual symptoms and headaches. Formal assessment of visual fields and computed tomography or magnetic resonance imaging should be carried out in any patient experiencing suggestive symptoms. Symptoms generally abate with institution of therapy with a dopamine agonist. No adverse effects of dopamine agonists on fetuses or pregnancies have been reported. Concerns have been raised that ergot-derived dopamine agonists, in the large doses used in the treatment of Parkinson's disease may increase the risk of cardiac valve regurgitation. Although there is no evidence of risk in women treated with much lower doses for hyperprolactinemia, they should be counseled about this potential side effect.

Several preparations of purified and synthetic biochemically engineered gonadotropins for use for induction of ovulation now exist.

Rx

Synthetic preparations consist entirely of FSH, whereas most purified preparations contain some LH as well. Each vial typically contains 75 IU of the appropriate gonadotropin. Individuals with gonadotropin deficiency require a preparation containing some LH. Exogenous gonadotropins are typically administered at doses of two to four vials (intramuscularly or subcutaneously, depending on the preparation) for 5 to 12 days to achieve follicular development as monitored by ultrasonography and serum or urinary estradiol concentrations; hCG, 5000 to 10,000 IU, is administered as a single intramuscular dose when follicular maturation is apparent. The hCG should be withheld if more than three follicles mature together. GnRH analogues are now being used to suppress endogenous follicular activity before initiation of therapy with exogenous gonadotropins and continued until hCG is given in older women and those with poor responses to exogenous gonadotropins. Use of the analogues necessitates administration of larger quantities of exogenous gonadotropins. Success rates, however, seem to be somewhat improved with this combined therapy. GnRH analogues are also being used experimentally to induce an endogenous LH surge.

Because of the expense and the complication rate, thorough evaluation should be carried out to exclude other causes of infertility before exogenous gonadotropins and hCG are used. Ovulation can be induced in almost 100% of patients, but pregnancy occurs in only 50 to 70%. There is no increased risk of congenital anomalies with exogenous gonadotropins and hCG. Concerns have been raised that exogenous gonadotropins may increase the risk of ovarian epithelial cancer, but more recent data do not support this possibility.

The rate of multiple pregnancies with exogenous gonadotropins and hCG may approach 30%, with 5% being triplets or more. Ovarian hyperstimulation is the major side effect and may be life-threatening. The ovaries enlarge remarkably in this treatment-induced syndrome, and multiple follicle cysts, stromal edema, and multiple corpora lutea are present. There is a shift of fluid from the intravascular space into the abdominal cavity with resultant hypovolemia and hemoconcentration. The cause of the ascites is unknown. Treatment is conservative, with monitoring of fluid and electrolyte status. Pelvic examinations should not be performed for fear of rupturing the ovaries. The hyperstimulation generally resolves slowly during about 7 days but lasts longer if the cycle results in pregnancy.

GnRH, administered intravenously or less effectively subcutaneously at doses of 5 to 20 μg every 60 to 120 minutes, can also be used to induce ovulation in women with an intact pituitary gland. It is most effective in individuals with HCA; hCG can be administered to support the corpus luteum after ovulation at a dose of 1500 IU intramuscularly every 3 days for three or four doses. The advantage of GnRH rests in the fact that hyperstimulation is extremely unlikely. However, reported pregnancy rates have been no greater than those achieved with exogenous gonadotropins and hCG. Furthermore, some patients do not tolerate wearing the infusion pump that must be used. GnRH is not now marketed for this use in the United States.

Use of clomiphene citrate or exogenous gonadotropins together with intrauterine insemination of spermatozoa is increasing in women with unexplained infertility. The intent is to stimulate several oocytes to be ovulated, but multiple (sometimes high order) gestations are a significant risk. At this time, there is no evidence that this approach helps more couples to conceive than would spontaneously, but the time to pregnancy seems reduced.

Assisted Reproductive Technologies

The assisted reproductive technologies, in which by definition both eggs and sperm are handled outside of the body, are being used with increasing frequency to treat infertile couples with tubal disease, endometriosis, oligospermia and azoospermia, sperm antibodies, and unexplained infertility. The procedure generally consists of in vitro fertilization and several variants. In vitro fertilization involves ovarian hyperstimulation, oocyte retrieval, fertilization, embryo culture, and embryo transfer. Ovarian hyperstimulation with clomiphene citrate and exogenous gonadotropins, gonadotropins alone, or a GnRH agonist or antagonist plus gonadotropins typically causes 1 to 20 oocytes to mature, depending on the patient's age and ovarian "reserve." After follicular growth is judged sufficient by ultrasound examination, hCG is given to induce final follicular maturation. About 34 hours after hCG administration, the oocytes are retrieved by direct needle puncture of each follicle, usually transvaginally with ultrasound guidance. The oocytes are then inseminated in vitro with washed sperm, or a single sperm is injected directly into a single egg (so-called intracytoplasmic sperm injection). Next the embryos are cultured for about 40 hours, after which one or more embryos are transferred to the uterine cavity. Sometimes embryos are cultured to the blastocyst stage before transfer, and controversy exists as to the optimal time to culture embryos for optimal pregnancy rates. Additional embryos can be frozen in liquid nitrogen for transfer in a subsequent natural cycle. Despite the transfer of multiple embryos, the average term-pregnancy rate is about 20 to 25% per attempt. The greatest current problem with in vitro fertilization involves the number of high-order (three or more) multiples resulting. Efforts to limit the number of embryos transferred are occurring throughout the world, either voluntarily or as the result of regulation.

It is now possible to test the early embryo for genetic abnormalities by removal of either a single cell (i.e., blastomere) or a polar body from the embryo in vitro and testing it with probes by fluorescent in situ hybridization or with the assistance of polymerase chain reaction. Identification of normal and abnormal embryos allows only normal embryos to be transferred in families with recognized and testable genetic abnormalities.

SEXUAL FUNCTION AND DYSFUNCTION

Sexual Function

Definition

Although sexual responses begin after puberty, they can continue for the duration of a woman's life. Sexual responses historically have been divided into four phases: excitement, plateau, orgasm, and resolution. With sexual arousal and excitement, vasocongestion and muscle tension increase progressively, primarily in the genitals, manifested by vaginal lubrication in the female. The lubrication is due to formation of a transudate in the vagina. Sexual excitement is initiated by any of a variety of psychogenic or somatogenic sexual stimuli and must be reinforced to result in orgasm. With continued stimulation, the excitement phase increases in intensity into a plateau phase during which a high state of sexual interest is maintained. The plateau phase may be short or long, and it is from this phase that an individual can shift to orgasm. The orgasmic phase tends to be brief and is characterized by rapid release from the developed vasocongestion and muscle tension. The orgasmic release is also known as the climax because peak psychological and physical intensity is achieved and there is an attendant feeling of satisfaction. Copious secretions and transudate may flow during orgasm in women. Although women may resolve toward sleep after orgasm, many remain responsive to sexual stimulation and may return to plateau and subsequent orgasm.

Characteristic genital and extragenital responses occur during these phases. Estrogens magnify the sexual responses, but responses may occur in estrogen-deficient women. For women, these changes occur in the breasts and in the pudendal region and are variable from one response cycle to another. For some women, excitement proceeds quickly through plateau to orgasm, and orgasm is explosive and accompanied by vocalization and involuntary contractions of the pelvic skeletal muscles. For other women, the responses are slow in building, controlled in amplitude, and long lasting. For a few women, orgasm never occurs; for many, it is intermittently absent.

The somatic sensate focus enabling orgasmic release is variable and may include stimulation of the breasts, vagina, or clitoris. The psychological aspect of coitus may involve concentration on the current partner or act or fantasies about other times and persons. Although orgasms may vary in physiologic intensity, what is important is psychological satisfaction. Satisfaction for both men and women may be had without orgasm.

Many clinicians have noted several limitations of this traditional human sex response cycle. In general, the genital focus and the linear sequence do not accurately reflect women's sexual experiences. Moreover, this model fails to reflect the various relationships between the mind and the body when men and women are sexual. Sexual motivation is complex, influenced by many cognitive, societal, and emotional factors. More and more clinicians and researchers see the cycle as circular with stimuli of different types leading to arousal. Clinicians in this field now have extended this theory to include desire and arousal. Women seek sexual experiences for intimacy as well as for sexual gratification. Women may be receptive to or seek out sexual stimuli to enhance intimacy. Biologic and psychological factors contribute to the processing of these stimuli and can enhance arousal and desire simultaneously.

Sexual Dysfunction

Women may seek consultation because of disturbances in normal sexual arousal or orgasm. Such sexual dysfunction may be due to either organic or functional disturbances.

A variety of diseases affecting neurologic function, including diabetes mellitus and multiple sclerosis, may prevent sexual arousal. So, too, may local pelvic disorders, such as endometriosis and vaginitis, which cause dyspareunia and lead to sexual avoidance. Estrogen deficiency causing vaginal atrophy and dyspareunia is a relatively common cause of sexual dysfunction. Debilitating systemic diseases such as malignant disease may also affect sexual function indirectly.

In most cases, the cause of sexual dysfunction is psychological. For instance, vaginismus involves involuntary contractions of the muscles surrounding the introitus and leads to dyspareunia. It is a conditioned response engendered by a previous imagined or real traumatic sexual experience. Feelings of guilt (caused by incest or rape, as examples), of inadequacy (caused by hysterectomy or mastectomy), or of depression or anxiety may lead to failure to be aroused. Failure to achieve orgasm may be viewed as a dysfunction if the woman is frustrated or dissatisfied.

Treatment 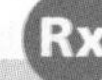

Treatment of sexual dysfunction is best accomplished by eliminating functional causes and providing the patient, often together with her partner, with appropriate psychological counseling. Behavioral modification is effective in treating many women with psychological sexual dysfunction.

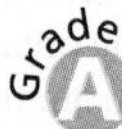

1. Legro RS, Barnhart HX, Schlaff WD, et al: Clomiphene, metformin, or both for infertility in the polycystic ovary syndrome. N Engl J Med 2007;356:551–566.

SUGGESTED READINGS

Aboulghar MA, Mansour RT, Serour GI, et al: Diagnosis and management of unexplained infertility: An update. Arch Gynecol Obstet 2003;267:177–188. *A practical overview.*

Basson R, Berman J, Burnett A, et al: Report of the international consensus developmental conference on female sexual dysfunction: Definitions and classifications. J Urol 2000;163:888–893. *A summary of the classification of disorders of female sexual function.*

Dawood MY: Primary dysmenorrhea: Advances in pathogenesis and management. Obstet Gynecol 2006;108:428–441. *A practical review of the pathophysiology, diagnosis, and treatment of this common disorder.*

Ehrmann DA: Medical progress: Polycystic ovary syndrome. N Engl J Med 2005;352:1223–1236. *Addresses the current knowledge regarding the diagnosis, cause, and treatment of polycystic ovary syndrome.*

Johnson SR: Premenstrual syndrome, premenstrual dysphoric disorder, and beyond: A clinical primer for practitioners. Obstet Gynecol 2004;104:845–859. *Describes the diagnostic approach and treatment strategies for this spectrum of disorders.*

Van Voorhis BJ: In vitro fertilization. N Engl J Med 2007;356:379–386. *A comprehensive review of the strategies and evidence for in vitro fertilization.*

Zapantis G, Santoro N: The menopausal transition: Characteristics and management. Best Pract Res Clin Endocrinol Metab 2003;17:33–52. *A summary of characteristic features and bleeding disorders occurring during the later reproductive years just before menopause.*

257 CONTRACEPTION

Daniel R. Mishell, Jr.

CONTRACEPTIVE USE AND EFFECTIVENESS

Contraceptive Use

Reversible contraception, the temporary prevention of fertility, includes all contraceptive methods except sterilization. Sterilization should be considered permanent despite the possibility of surgical reversal. There are advantages and disadvantages of each contraceptive method. During contraceptive counseling, these advantages and disadvantages should be thoroughly explained so that the individual will choose the most acceptable method and not discontinue use prematurely and have an unwanted pregnancy.

In the United States in 2002 (the latest year for which data are available), there were about 61.5 million women in the reproductive age group (15 to 44 years), and 38 million (62%) were using a method of contraception. Of the remainder, about 3% were sterile (prior hysterectomy), 9% were pregnant or trying to conceive, and 18% were never sexually active or had no recent sexual activity. About 7.4% of women who were sexually active were not using a method of contraception, an increase from the 5.2% incidence of this group in 1995.

In the United States in 2002, the most common methods of fertility prevention were oral contraceptives (OCs) and female sterilization, used by 18.9% and 16.7% of women aged 15 to 44 years. Next in frequency of use was the male condom, followed by male sterilization (Table 257–1). The injectable progestin was used by about 2 million women, but the intrauterine device (IUD), the most effective method of reversible contraception, was used by only 800,000 women. Between 1982 and 2002, there was a marked decrease in diaphragm and IUD use and an increase in condom use. Between 1995 and 2002, diaphragm use virtually disappeared, IUD use doubled, and condom use stabilized. About 80% of reproductive-age women who have had intercourse have used OCs at some time.

Contraceptive Effectiveness

Despite an increased use of contraceptive methods by U.S. women since 1982, more than half the pregnancies that occur are unwanted. Of the 6.4 million pregnancies that occurred in the United States in 2002 (the most recent data available), about half were unintended and 42% of these pregnancies were terminated by elective abortion. Of the women with an unintended pregnancy, 50% stated they were using a method of contraception in the month they conceived.

Typical Use versus Perfect Use

The terms *method effectiveness* and *use effectiveness* (or *method failure* and *patient failure*) were previously used to describe the frequency of conceptions that occurred while the method was being used correctly or incorrectly. These terms have been replaced by the terms *typical use* and *perfect use*. Methods used at the time of coitus have higher failure rates in the first year of use than OCs, implants, injections, the IUD, and sterilization. First-year typical use failure rates with the latter methods are 8% or less (Table 257–2). Cumulative failure rates for use of long-acting methods are low. The pregnancy rate for 10 years' use of the copper T380 IUD is 1.7%. The cumulative failure rate of all types of tubal sterilization is 1.31% during the first 5 years after the procedure and 1.85% after 10 years, being highest for tubal fulguration and lowest for segmental resection. When women conceive while using these long-acting methods, the ectopic pregnancy rates are high: about 30% with tubal sterilization failure and 5% with copper IUD failure.

TYPES OF CONTRACEPTIVES

Spermicides and Barriers

All spermicidal agents contain a surfactant, usually nonoxynol 9, that immobilizes or kills sperm on contact. They also provide a mechanical barrier and need to be placed into the vagina before each coital act. There

TABLE 257–1 NUMBER OF WOMEN 15 TO 44 YEARS OF AGE AND PERCENTAGE DISTRIBUTION (WITH STANDARD ERROR) BY CURRENT CONTRACEPTIVE STATUS AND METHOD: UNITED STATES, 1982, 1995, AND 2002

Contraceptive Status and Method	Year of Survey		
	1982	1995	2002
	Number in Thousands		
All women	54,099	60,201	61,561
	Percentage Distribution (with standard error)		
Total	100.00	100.00	100.0
Using contraception (contraceptors)	55.7 (1.0)	64.2 (0.6)	61.9 (0.8)
Female sterilization	12.9 (0.6)	17.8 (0.4)	16.7 (0.6)
Male sterilization	6.1 (0.4)	7.0 (0.3)	5.7 (0.4)
Pill	15.6 (0.8)	17.3 (0.4)	18.9 (0.7)
Implant, Lunelle, or patch[1]	NA	0.9 (0.1)	0.8 (0.1)
3-month injectable (Depo-Provera)	NA	1.9 (0.1)	3.3 (0.3)
Intrauterine device	4.0 (0.4)	0.5 (0.1)	1.3 (0.2)
Diaphragm	4.5 (0.4)	1.2 (0.1)	0.2 (0.1)
Condom	6.7 (0.8)	13.1 (0.4)	11.1 (0.5
Periodic abstinence—calendar rhythm	1.8 (0.3)	1.3 (0.1)	0.7 (0.1)
Periodic abstinence—natural family planning	0.3 (0.3)	0.2 (0.1)	0.2 (0.1)
Withdrawal	1.1 (0.3)	2.0 (0.2)	2.5 (0.3)
Other methods[2]	2.7 (0.3)	1.1 (0.1)	0.6 (0.1)
Not using contraception	44.3 (1.0)	35.8 (0.6)	38.1 (0.8)
Surgically sterile—female (noncontraceptive)	6.3 (0.4)	3.0 (0.2)	1.5 (0.2)
Nonsurgically sterile—female or male	1.2 (0.3)	1.7 (0.2)	1.6 (0.2)
Pregnant or post partum	5.0 (0.3)	4.6 (0.2)	5.3 (0.4)
Seeking pregnancy	4.2 (0.4)	4.0 (0.2)	4.2 (0.3)
Other nonuse			
Never had intercourse or no intercourse in 3 months before interview	19.5 (0.8)	17.1 (0.5)	18.1(0.7)
Had intercourse in 3 months before interview	7.4 (0.4)	5.2 (0.2)	7.4 (0.4)
All other nonuse[3]	0.7 (0.3)	0.2 (0.0)	0.0 (0.0)

Note: Percentages may not add up to 100 because of rounding. 0.0 = quantity greater than zero but less than 0.05. NA = data not available (method not available in the United States in that year).
[1]1995 percentage includes only Norplant Implant.
[2]Includes Today sponge, cervical cap, female condom, and other small groups, not shown separately.
[3]Includes male sterility of unknown origin and other small groups, not shown separately.
From Mosher WD, Martinez GM, Chandra A, et al: Use of contraception and use of family planning services in the United States: 1982–2002. Adv Data 2004;350:1–36. U.S. Department of Health and Human Services, Centers for Disease Control and Prevention, National Center for Health Statistics.

is no increased risk of birth defects in the offspring of women who conceive while using spermicides.

Diaphragm

A diaphragm must be carefully fitted by the health care provider. The largest size that does not cause discomfort or undue pressure on the vagina should be used. The diaphragm should not be left in place for more than 24 hours because it may cause ulceration of the vaginal epithelium. Diaphragm users have an increased risk of urinary tract infection.

Male Condom

Use of the latex male condom by individuals with multiple sex partners should be encouraged because it is the most effective way to prevent sexually transmitted infections. The natural membrane condoms do not prevent sexually transmitted infections, but polyurethane condoms do.

Female Condom

The female condom consists of a soft, loose-fitting prelubricated sheath and two flexible polyurethane rings. The female condom can be inserted before beginning sexual activity and left in place for a longer time than the male condom after ejaculation occurs. Because the female condom covers the external genitalia, it may prevent transmission of genital herpes. Because polyurethane is stronger than the latex used in most male condoms, the female condom is less likely to rupture. Both polyurethane and latex do not allow virus transmission and should reduce the risk of acquiring human immunodeficiency virus infection.

Oral Steroid Contraceptives

There are three major types of OC formulations: fixed-dose combination, combination phasic, and daily progestin. The combination formulations are the most widely used and most effective. They consist of tablets containing both an estrogen and a progestin usually given continuously for 3 weeks. No steroids are given for the next 7 days (except for one formulation in which estrogen alone is given for an additional 5 days), after which time the active combination is given for an additional 3 weeks. Two recently introduced formulations provide active tablets for 24 days with 4 days inactive tablets. Another formulation provides active tablets for 84 days followed by 7 days without active tablets to allow withdrawal bleeding. The endometrium usually begins to slough 1 to 3 days after steroid ingestion is stopped, causing withdrawal bleeding, which usually lasts 3 to 4 days. The uterine blood loss with OC use averages about 25 mL per cycle, less than the 35 mL average for ovulatory cycles.

Constituents and Action

All formulations are made from synthetic steroids. There are two major types of synthetic progestins: derivatives of 19-nortestosterone (which are used in OCs) and derivatives of 17α-acetoxyprogesterone (pregnanes). Pregnanes are structurally related to progesterone and are used in injectable contraceptives but are not used in OCs.

The 19-nortestosterone progestins used in OCs are of two major types, estranes and gonanes, and both have androgenic activity. The estranes

TABLE 257–2 PERCENTAGE OF WOMEN EXPERIENCING AN UNINTENDED PREGNANCY DURING THE FIRST YEAR OF TYPICAL USE AND THE FIRST YEAR OF PERFECT USE OF CONTRACEPTION AND PERCENTAGE CONTINUING USE AT THE END OF THE FIRST YEAR, IN THE UNITED STATES

Method	Women Experiencing an Unintended Pregnancy in the First Year of Use (%)		Women Continuing Use at 1 Year (%)[c]
	TYPICAL USE[a]	PERFECT USE[b]	
No method[d]	85	85	
Spermicides[e]	29	18	42
Withdrawal	27	4	43
Periodic abstinence	25		51
Calendar		9	
Ovulation method		3	
Symptothermal[f]		2	
Post ovulation		1	
Cap[g]			
Parous women	32	26	46
Nulliparous women	16	9	57
Sponge			
Parous women	32	20	46
Nulliparous women	16	9	57
Diaphragm[g]	16	6	57
Condom[h]			
Female (Reality)	21	5	49
Male	15	2	53
Combined pill and minipill	8	0.3	68
Ortho-Evra patch	8	0.3	68
NuvaRing	8	0.3	68
Depo-Provera	3	0.3	56
Lunelle	3	0.05	56
Intrauterine device			
ParaGard (copper T)	0.8	0.6	78
Mirena (levonorgestrel-containing intrauterine system)	0.1	0.1	81
Norplant or Norplant-2	0.05	0.05	84
Female sterilization	0.5	0.5	100
Male sterilization	0.15	0.10	100
Emergency contraceptive pills: Treatment initiated within 72 hours after unprotected intercourse reduces risk of pregnancy by at least 75%[i]			

Lactational amenorrhea method: A highly effective, *temporary* method of contraception[j].

[a]Among *typical* couples who initiate use of a method (not necessarily for the first time), the percentage who experience an accidental pregnancy in the first year if they do not stop use for any other reason. Estimates of the probability of pregnancy during the first year of typical use for spermicides, withdrawal, periodic abstinence, the diaphragm, the male condom, the pill, and Depo-Provera are taken from the 1995 National Survey of Family Growth corrected for underrated abortion.

[b]Among couples who initiate the use of a method (not necessarily for the first time) and who use it *perfectly* (both consistently and correctly), the percentage who experience an accidental pregnancy during the first year if they do not stop for any other reason.

[c]Among couples attempting to avoid pregnancy, the percentage who continue to use a method for 1 year.

[d]The percentages becoming pregnant in columns two and three are based on data from populations in which contraception is not used and from women who cease use of contraception to become pregnant. Among such populations, about 89% become pregnant within 1 year. This estimate was lowered slightly (to 85%) to represent the percentage who would become pregnant within 1 year among women now relying on reversible methods of contraception or if they abandon contraception altogether.

[e]Foams, creams, gels, vaginal suppositories, and vaginal film.

[f]Cervical mucus (ovulation) method supplemented by calendar in the preovulatory phase and basal body temperatures in the postovulatory phase.

[g]With spermicidal cream or jelly.

[h]Without spermicides.

[i]The treatment schedule is one dose within 120 hours after unprotected intercourse and a second dose 12 hours after the first dose. Both doses of Plan B are taken at the same time. Plan B (one dose is one white pill) is the only dedicated product specifically marketed for emergency contraception. The U.S. Food and Drug Administration has in addition declared the following 18 brands of oral contraceptives to be safe and effective for emergency contraception: *** or Ovral (one dose is two white pills); Alesse, Lessina, or Levlite (one dose is five pink pills); Levlen or Nordette (one dose is four light-orange pills); Crystells, ***, Low-Ogestrel, or Lo/Ovral (one dose is four white pills); Tri-Levlen or Triphasil (one dose is four yellow pills); Portia, Seasonale, or Trivora (one dose is four pink pills); Avaine (one dose is five orange pills); and Empresse (one dose is four orange pills).

[j]However, to maintain effective protection against pregnancy, another method of contraception must be used as soon as menstruation resumes, frequency or duration of breast-feeding is reduced, bottle feedings are introduced, or the baby reaches 6 months of age.

From Trussell J: Contraceptive efficiency. *In* Hatcher RA, Trussell J, Stewart F, et al (eds): Contraceptive Technology, 18th revised ed. New York, Ardent Media, 2004.

currently used in several OCs are norethindrone and its acetates, norethindrone acetate and ethynodiol diacetate. Gonanes have greater progestational activity per unit weight than estranes, and thus a smaller amount of these progestins is used in OC formulations. The parent compound of the gonanes is DL-norgestrel, but only the levo isomer is biologically active. Gonanes used in OCs include both norgestrel and levonorgestrel and three less androgenic derivatives of levonorgestrel: desogestrel, norgestimate, and gestodene. One other progestin that is structurally related to spironolactone has been formulated in an OC. This progestin is called drospirenone and has antimineralocorticoid and antiandrogenic activity as well as progestational activity without androgenic activity.

With the exception of two daily progestin-only formulations, the progestins are combined with varying dosages of two estrogens, ethinyl estradiol and its 3-methyl ether, called mestranol. All the older higher dosage OC formulations contained mestranol, and this steroid is still present in some 50-μg formulations. All formulations with less than 50 μg of estrogen (20 to 35 μg) contain ethinyl estradiol.

The estrogen-progestin combination is the most effective type of OC formulation because these preparations consistently inhibit the midcycle gonadotropin surge and thus prevent ovulation. The progestin-only formulations have a lower dose of progestin than the combined agents and do not consistently inhibit ovulation, even though they are ingested every day. Both types of formulations also act on the cervical mucus and tubal motility to interfere with sperm transport. Progestins also alter the endometrium so if fertilization occurs, implantation may be prevented. For contraceptive effectiveness to be maintained with the combination formulations, it is important that the pill-free interval be limited to no more than 7 days. This is best accomplished by ingestion of either a placebo or an iron tablet daily during the steroid-free interval.

Metabolic Effects

The synthetic steroids in OC formulations have many metabolic effects in addition to their contraceptive actions. These effects can cause the more common, less serious side effects as well as the rare, serious complications. The magnitude of these effects is directly related to the dosage and potency of the steroids in the formulations.

Symptoms Due to Estrogen and Progestin

The most frequent symptoms produced by the estrogen component include nausea, breast tenderness, and fluid retention (bloating). The progestins can produce certain androgenic effects, such as weight gain, acne, and nervousness. Because estrogens decrease sebum production, women who have acne should be given a formulation with a low progestin-estrogen ratio. Unscheduled (breakthrough) bleeding is usually produced by insufficient estrogen, too much progestin, or a combination of both. This problem is more common with formulations containing 20 μg of estrogen than with those containing 30 to 35 μg and is increased in women who also smoke cigarettes. Shortening the pill-free interval to 3 or 4 days should prevent ovarian follicular development and may decrease the incidence of unscheduled bleeding with low-estrogen formulations.

The synthetic estrogens used in OCs cause an increase in the hepatic production of several proteins. The progestins do not affect protein synthesis except to reduce levels of sex hormone–binding globulin. Some of the proteins that are increased by ethinyl estradiol, such as factors V, VIII, and X and fibrinogen, have the potential to enhance thrombosis, whereas an increase in angiotensinogen levels may elevate blood pressure in some users. Blood pressure should be monitored in all users of OCs and the agent discontinued if there is a clinically significant increase. The incidence of both venous and arterial thrombosis in OC users is higher with 50-μg estrogen formulations than with those with 20 to 35 μg of estrogen. Changes in the coagulation parameters with most low-dose OCs are small or nonexistent.

Glucose Metabolism

The effect of OCs on glucose metabolism is directly related to the dose, potency, and type of progestin. Although high-progestin formulations caused peripheral insulin resistance, the low-progestin formulations in current use do not significantly alter levels of glucose, insulin, or glucagon after a glucose load. The risk for development of diabetes mellitus is not increased in women with a history of gestational diabetes who take OCs compared with control subjects. The risk for development of type 2 diabetes is not increased among current or former OC users compared with age-matched control subjects.

The estrogen component of OCs causes an increase in high-density lipoprotein cholesterol levels, a decrease in low-density lipoprotein cholesterol levels, and an increase in total cholesterol and triglyceride levels. The progestin component causes a decrease in high-density lipoprotein levels, an increase in low-density lipoprotein levels, and a decrease in total cholesterol and triglyceride levels. High-progestin formulations have an adverse effect on the lipid profile; because of the direct beneficial effect of estrogen on the arterial wall, however, users of these agents do not have an increased risk of cardiovascular disease. The newer combination formulations with less androgenic progestins have a more favorable effect on the lipid profile.

Complications and Risk Factors

Thrombosis

The cause of the increased incidence of both venous and arterial cardiovascular disease in users of OCs is thrombosis, not atherosclerosis. The background rate of venous thrombosis and embolism in women of reproductive age is about 0.8 per 10,000 woman years. Among users of OCs with 30 or 35 μg of ethinyl estradiol, it is 3 per 10,000 woman years, about four times the background rate but half the rate of 6 per 10,000 woman years that occurs in association with pregnancy. Although the risk of venous thrombosis and embolism is higher among women ingesting OCs with 50 μg of ethinyl estradiol than those with 30 to 35 μg, studies to date indicate that the risk of venous thrombosis and embolism with OCs containing 20 μg of ethinyl estradiol is similar to that of OCs with 30 to 35 μg of ethinyl estradiol. In the presence of an inherited coagulopathy disorder, the risk of venous thrombosis is increased several-fold. Because only 1 in 300 women with activated protein C resistance will develop venous thrombosis with OC use, it is not recommended that screening for coagulation deficiencies be undertaken before patients are started on OC use unless the individual patient has a personal or strong family history of thrombotic events. Women with known inherited or acquired thrombophilic conditions should not use estrogen-containing steroid contraceptives in pills, rings, or patches as each of these agents has thrombophilic effects.

Myocardial Infarction

The use of high-dose OCs by women who smoke cigarettes significantly increases the risk of myocardial infarction. Therefore, combination OCs should not be prescribed to women older than 35 years who smoke cigarettes or use alternate forms of nicotine. Epidemiologic studies indicate that use of low-dose OCs by nonsmoking women without hypertension is not associated with a significantly increased incidence of either myocardial infarction or hemorrhagic or thrombotic stroke.

Delayed Fertility

For about 2 years after the discontinuation of contraceptives, the rate of return of fertility is slightly lower for users of OCs than for users of barrier methods. OCs do not cause permanent infertility or adversely affect pregnancies that occur after their discontinuation. OCs are not teratogenic if they are accidentally ingested during pregnancy.

Breast Cancer

An analysis of worldwide epidemiologic data in 1988 showed that the risk of breast cancer diagnosis was increased by about 25% in young women who were currently using OCs, but this increased risk was no longer present 10 years or more after they stopped using OCs. A large case-control study reported that if OC use was started before 1974, the year when formulations with less than 50 μg of estrogen were first introduced, the relative risk of breast cancer was 3.1 in OC users. However, if OC use was initiated in 1974 or later, the relative risk for development of breast cancer in OC users was 0.74. Furthermore, there was no significant increase in risk of breast cancer with initiation of OC use at a very young age, use before a first birth, or use by women with a family history of breast cancer (Chapter 208). A large study of women aged 35 to 64 years in the United States reported that there was no significantly increased risk of breast cancer among current and former OC users compared with women who had not used OCs.

Cervical Cancer

The epidemiologic data regarding the risk of invasive cervical cancer as well as cervical intraepithelial neoplasia and OC use are conflicting. Nonetheless, the majority of well-controlled studies indicate that there is no change in risk of cervical intraepithelial neoplasia and OC use. However, it is likely that a causal relationship exists between OC use and a reported increased risk of cervical adenocarcinoma. OC users need annual cervical cytologic screening (Chapter 209).

Endometrial Cancer

Several studies have shown that the use of OCs has a protective effect against endometrial cancer. Moreover, the decrease in risk persists for many years after OCs are stopped. Women who use OCs for at least 1 year have a 50% reduced risk of endometrial cancer development between the ages of 40 and 65 years compared with nonusers. This protective effect is related to duration of use, increasing from a 20% reduction with 1 year of use to a 60% reduction with 4 years of use.

Epithelial Ovarian Cancer

In addition, OCs reduce the risk for development of epithelial ovarian cancer as well as cancers with low malignant potential. The magnitude of the decrease in risk is directly related to the duration of OC use, increasing from about a 40% reduction with 4 years of use to a 60% reduction with 12 years of use. The protective effect continues for at least 20 years after the use of OCs ends. As with endometrial cancer, the protective effect occurs only in women of low parity (fewer than four), who are at greatest risk for this type of cancer. Studies have reported that OCs significantly reduce the risk for development of colorectal cancer by about 20%.

Benign Hepatocellular Adenoma

The development of a benign hepatocellular adenoma was a rare occurrence in long-term users of high-dose OCs containing mestranol, but it is not increased by use of ethinyl estradiol OCs. There is no increased risk of liver cancer associated with OC use. OC use also does not increase the risk for development of malignant melanoma or prolactin-secreting pituitary adenomas.

Contraindications

The OCs can be prescribed for the majority of women of reproductive age. An absolute contraindication is a history of vascular disease, including systemic diseases that affect the vascular system, such as lupus erythematosus and diabetes with retinopathy or nephropathy. Cigarette smoking by OC users older than 35 years and uncontrolled hypertension are also contraindications, as are a personal history of cancer of the breast or endometrium and cholestatic jaundice of pregnancy. Pregnancy and any undiagnosed cause of uterine bleeding are also contraindications. Women with functional heart diseases should not use OCs because the fluid retention could result in congestive heart failure. There is no evidence, however, that individuals with asymptomatic mitral valve prolapse should not use OCs. Women with active liver disease should not take OCs. However, women who have recovered from liver disease, such as viral hepatitis, and whose liver function test results have returned to normal, can safely take OCs. The presence of migraine headaches without aura is not a contraindication to OC use, but if auras are present, combination OCs should not be prescribed because of a possible increased risk of stroke. Relative contraindications to OC use include undiagnosed causes of amenorrhea and depression. Use of OCs does not cause enlargement of prolactin-secreting pituitary microadenomas or worsen functional hyperprolactinemia (Chapter 242) as was previously believed.

Initiation of Therapy and Surveillance

If a healthy woman has no contraindications to OC use, it is unnecessary to perform any laboratory tests, including cervical cytology, before use unless these are necessary for routine health maintenance. Routine use of laboratory tests is not indicated unless the woman has a family history of diabetes or arterial vascular disease at a young age, in which case a fasting glucose or lipid panel should be obtained. After the first three cycles of OC use, a nondirected history should be obtained and blood pressure measured. After this visit, the woman should be seen annually; at each visit, a nondirected history should again be taken, blood pressure and body weight measured, and a physical examination (including breast, abdominal, and pelvic examination with cervical cytology) performed. It is not necessary to measure lipids, other than the routine cholesterol screening every 5 years, in women with no cardiovascular risk factors, even if they are older than 35 years. There is no reason to discontinue OC use unless pregnancy is desired. Intermittent discontinuation is unnecessary and may result in an unwanted pregnancy.

Although synthetic sex steroids can retard the biotransformation of certain drugs (e.g., phenazone and meperidine) as a result of substrate competition, such interference is usually not important clinically. However, some drugs can interfere clinically with the action of OCs by inducing liver enzymes that convert the steroids to more polar and less biologically active metabolites. These drugs include barbiturates, sulfonamides, cyclophosphamide, griseofulvin, and rifampin. There is a high incidence of OC failure in women ingesting rifampin, and these two agents as well as systemic griseofulvin should not be given concurrently. There is no reliable evidence that other antibiotics (including ampicillin and tetracycline), analgesics, or barbiturates inhibit OC effectiveness. Products containing St. John's wort reduce contraceptive effectiveness and cause breakthrough bleeding. Women taking medication for epilepsy should be treated with 50-μg estrogen formulations because many antiepileptic medications lower ethinyl estradiol levels and cause breakthrough bleeding, which may cause premature discontinuation of use. Because of their many health benefits, including reduction in risk of endometrial and ovarian cancer and induction of regular cyclic uterine bleeding, the continued use of OCs until menopause should be encouraged in women without contraindications.

Transdermal and Intravaginal Steroid Contraceptives

Transdermal Patch

Two novel long-acting methods of delivering contraceptive steroids other than the oral route have recently been marketed in the United States. One of these is a transdermal patch with an area of 20 cm^2, which delivers 150 μg of the progestin norelgestromin, the active metabolite of norgestimate, and 20 μg of ethinyl estradiol daily into the systemic circulation for 7 days. After this time span, the patch is removed and another is attached to a different area of the skin. The steroids are absorbed into the circulation at a constant rate, yielding fairly constant circulatory levels of each steroid while the patch is attached. This pharmacodynamic pattern differs from the peaks and valleys of steroid levels that occur after ingestion of an OC. After three patches are applied, no patch is used for the fourth week to allow withdrawal bleeding. Contraceptive efficacy, bleeding patterns, and side effects are similar to those associated with OCs, but in one comparative study, compliance was better with the patch than with the OC.

Intravaginal Ring

Another method of administering contraceptive steroids at a constant rate is by use of a flexible vaginal ring, which is 58 mm in outside diameter and 4 mm thick. The ring is composed of ethinyl vinyl acetate and contains the progestin etonogestrel and ethinyl estradiol. The rings are all the same size and do not have to be fitted. The ring is inserted and removed by the woman herself and is left in place for 3 weeks, after which time it is removed for 1 week to allow withdrawal bleeding. Each day, 120 μg of etonogestrel and 15 μg of ethinyl estradiol is released from the ring, and bleeding with the ring in place is uncommon. Contraceptive efficacy and side effects are similar to those of OCs.

Injectable Steroid Contraceptives

Constituents and Use

Several types of injectable steroid formulations are in use for contraception throughout the world. The one most widely used in the United States is depot medroxyprogesterone acetate (DMPA). The initial formulation of this contraceptive was administered as an intramuscular injection of 1 mL of an aqueous suspension containing 150 mg of crystalline medroxyprogesterone acetate once every 3 months. A recently developed formulation that is administered subcutaneously (DMPA-SC) contains 105 mg of DMPA in 0.15 mL of solution. This lower dose formulation has a lower peak medroxyprogesterone acetate concentration than DMPA and a long duration of action that suppresses ovulation for at least 13 weeks and is not affected by body mass. Other injectable contraceptives include norethindrone enanthate, given in a dose of 200 mg every 2 months, and several once-a-month injections of combinations of different progestins and estrogens. DMPA has a low failure rate, 0.1% at 1 year and 0.4% at 2 years. There were no pregnancies during 1 year in two large trials of DMPA-SC (16,073 woman cycles of exposure). The major contraceptive action of both formulations is inhibition of ovulation. These agents also impede sperm transport by keeping the cervical mucus thick and inhibit endometrial growth and glycogen production. With DMPA and DMPA-SC, serum medroxyprogesterone levels rapidly increase to contraceptively effective blood levels (>0.5 ng/mL) within 24 hours after the injection. With DMPA, medroxyprogesterone levels plateau for about 3 months, after which there is a gradual decline until levels become undetectable 7 to 9 months after the injection. With DMPA-SC, medroxyprogesterone levels steadily decline after the initial peak and reach 0.2 ng/mL 3 to 4 months after the injection.

Side Effects

With both formulations, mean endogenous estradiol levels remain above the postmenopausal range (40 to 60 pg/mL), and symptoms of estrogen deficiency do not occur. Although many women using DMPA have a decreased amount of bone mineral density during use, bone mineral density increases to normal levels after DMPA is stopped, and there are no reports of an increased risk of fracture with DMPA use. It is unnecessary to measure bone mineral density or to administer bone antiresorptive agents in DMPA users because the bone loss is temporary.

Because of the lag time it takes to clear DMPA from the circulation, resumption of ovulation is delayed for a variable time after the last injection. It may take as long as 1 year for ovulatory cycles to return. After this initial delay, fecundity resumes at a rate similar to that found after discontinuation of a barrier contraceptive.

Disruption of the Menstrual Cycle

The major side effect of DMPA is complete disruption of the menstrual cycle. Since this formulation contains only a progestin, without an estrogen, endometrial integrity is not maintained and uterine bleeding occurs at irregular and unpredictable intervals. The bleeding is usually light in amount and does not cause anemia. As duration of therapy increases, the incidence of frequent bleeding steadily declines and the incidence of amenorrhea steadily increases, so that at the end of 2 years, about 70% of users are amenorrheic. Women who use this method of contraception should be counseled that with time, the irregular bleeding episodes will cease and amenorrhea will most likely occur. Most DMPA users gain between 1.5 and 4 kg in their first year of use and continue to gain weight thereafter. If weight gain occurs, calorie intake should be decreased. Because there is no estrogen in DMPA, its use does not cause hypertension or thromboembolism.

In cycling women, the initial injection should be given no later than day 5 of the cycle to be certain to inhibit ovulation in the initial treatment cycle. The first injection should be given within 5 days after delivery in nonlactating women but not until after 6 weeks in lactating women.

Because the major reason for discontinuance of all progestin-injectable contraceptives is menstrual irregularity, several combined progestin-estrogen injectables that are given once monthly and produce regular withdrawal bleeding have been developed. A combination of medroxyprogesterone acetate, 25 mg, and an estradiol ester, estradiol cypionate 5 mg, was marketed for use in the United States after extensive clinical trials but is currently unavailable. A 0.5-mL aqueous suspension of this formulation is injected intramuscularly into the deltoid, thigh, or gluteal muscle once every 28 days ± 5 days. Pregnancy rates are reported to be about 0.1% after 1 year of use. The estradiol is cleared about 2 weeks after the injection, and withdrawal bleeding usually occurs between 2 and 3 weeks after each injection. Because the amount of medroxyprogesterone is markedly less than that used in DMPA, the progestin is cleared more rapidly, and ovulation and resumption of fertility occur within a few months of discontinuation.

Subdermal Implants

Constituents and Use

Several types of subdermal implants containing only progestins are effective long-acting methods of contraception. The initial formulation that was marketed consisted of six 3.4-cm polydimethylsiloxane (Silastic) capsules, each containing 36 mg of levonorgestrel, and was very effective. Subcutaneous insertion in the upper arm is performed in an outpatient setting by a small skin incision with local anesthesia. The capsules are removed when desired by the user or at the end of 5 years, which is the duration of maximal contraceptive effectiveness. Return to ovulation is prompt after implant removal. These capsules are no longer marketed in the United States.

Side Effects

The major side effect is the totally irregular pattern of uterine bleeding. Bleeding episodes are more prolonged and irregular during the first year of use, after which they become more regular as ovulatory cycles occur.

Pregnancy Rates

Annual pregnancy rates for the first 5 years of use are about 0.2 per 100 women. The cumulative 5-year pregnancy rate is 1.1%.

Silastic Rods

A formulation containing levonorgestrel in two 4-cm Silastic rods has a pharmacologic pattern similar to that of the six capsules with similar effectiveness and side effects. The two rods are easier to insert and to remove than the six capsules. A single 4-cm by 2-mm ethylene vinyl acetate rod containing 68 μg of etonogestrel, the active metabolite of desogestrel, provides effective contraception for 3 years. This rod is packaged in a disposable metal trocar inserter and does not require a skin incision for insertion, only for removal. Ovulation is inhibited by the circulating etonogestrel levels, and no pregnancies were reported in three large clinical trials. As with other progestin-only implants, irregular bleeding is the most common clinical complaint. This implant has recently become available in the United States and is the only implant marketed in the United States.

Emergency Contraception

For a woman not using contraception, if emergency contraception is given within 72 hours after a single coitus in midcycle, about 75 to 85% of pregnancies will be prevented. If more than one episode of coitus has occurred, or if treatment was initiated later than 72 hours after coitus, the method is less effective. Until recently, the most commonly used regimen was ingestion of four tablets of the OC containing 50 μg of ethinyl estradiol and 0.5 mg DL-norgestrel, in doses of two tablets 12 hours apart. The pregnancy rate with this regimen is 2%, about one fourth that of the 8% expected rate. Another formulation consisting of a 750-μg single tablet of levonorgestrel given once every 12 hours is more effective than the two tablets of the combination steroid formulation without the estrogenic side effects. This formulation is marketed for use as an emergency contraceptive in the United States and elsewhere and prevents about 85% of the expected pregnancies, for a pregnancy rate of 1%.

Intrauterine Devices

Constituents and Use

The main benefits of IUDs are a high level of effectiveness, a lack of systemic metabolic effects for copper IUDs, and the need for only a single act of motivation for long-term use. Despite these advantages, only about 1% of reproductive-age women use the IUD in the United States, compared with 15 to 30% in most European countries and Canada. The copper T380A IUD is the only copper-bearing IUD currently marketed in the United States, but the Multiload CU 375 is widely used in Europe. The copper T380A is approved for use in the United States for 10 years and maintains its high levels of effectiveness for at least 12 years. A levonorgestrel-releasing IUD is also marketed in the United States and elsewhere. A dose of 20 μg of levonorgestrel diffuses from the device into the endometrial cavity each day. Because of the progestational effect on the endometrium, the amount of uterine bleeding is markedly reduced with use of this device, and it has been used therapeutically to treat menorrhagia. This device has a high level of effectiveness for 5 years, which is the approved duration of use.

The main mechanism of contraceptive action of copper-bearing IUDs is spermicidal. This effect is caused by a local sterile leukocytic response produced by the copper as well as the plastic IUD itself. Because of the spermicidal action of IUDs, few if any spermatozoa reach the oviducts, and the ovum usually does not become fertilized. The levonorgestrel-releasing IUD acts mainly by preventing transport of spermatozoa through the cervical mucus and thus preventing fertilization of the ovum. After removal of each type of IUD, the inflammatory reaction rapidly disappears and resumption of fertility is prompt.

Pregnancy Rate

In the first year of use, IUDs have less than a 1% pregnancy rate, a 10% expulsion rate, and a 15% rate of removal for medical reasons, mainly bleeding and pain. The incidence of each of these events, especially expulsion, diminishes steadily in subsequent years. Mefenamic acid ingested in a dosage of 500 mg three times a day during the days of menstruation has been shown to significantly reduce the amount of uterine bleeding in IUD users.

Side Effects

Development of acute salpingitis more than a month after insertion of the IUD is due to infection with a sexually transmitted pathogen and is unrelated to the presence of the device. All IUD-related upper genital tract infections occur only during the insertion process. If there is clinical suspicion that cervicitis is present, the endocervix should be cultured and the insertion delayed until the results reveal that no pathogenic organisms are present. It is not cost-effective to routinely administer antibiotics with IUD insertion.

The IUD is not associated with an increased incidence of either endometrial or cervical carcinoma. The IUD is a particularly useful method of contraception for women who have completed their families, and its effectiveness is similar to that of tubal sterilization. It was calculated that after 5 years of use, the IUD is the most cost-effective of all methods of contraception, including sterilization.

SUGGESTED READINGS

Peterson HB, Curtis KM: Long-acting methods of contraception. N Engl J Med 2005;353:2169–2175. *Discusses the role of IUDs, progestin implants, tubal sterilization, and vasectomy in contraception.*

Petitti DB: Combination estrogen-progestin oral contraceptives. N Engl J Med 2003;349:1443–1450. *A review of the appropriate use and risks associated with oral contraceptives.*

Westhoff C: Emergency contraception. N Engl J Med 2003;349:1830–1835. *Reviews the different medical regimens available for emergency contraception, as well as their timing of use, safety, and outcomes.*

258 MANAGEMENT OF NEOPLASTIC DISEASES DURING PREGNANCY

Edward C. Grendys, Jr.

Epidemiology

Although cancer is uncommon in a relative sense, it remains a leading cause of death in women of reproductive age (Table 258–1). Overall cancer-related deaths account for 13% of mortality in women between the ages of 15 and 34 years and 38% in women aged 35 to 54 years. It is estimated that 1 in 1000 to 1 in 1500 live births is complicated by maternal malignant disease. However, it has been suggested that as women continue to delay childbearing, this incidence may rise in concordance with the direct relationship of age and cancer incidence (Fig. 258–1).

Given these statistics, it is imperative that physicians involved in the care of pregnant women be knowledgeable about and attentive to current screening recommendations, especially regarding the cervix, colon, and breast malignant neoplasms. Subtle signs of malignancy can occasionally be mistaken for side effects of pregnancy, thus possibly leading to diagnostic and treatment delay.

TABLE 258–1 REPORTED DEATHS IN U.S. WOMEN AGED 15 TO 54 YEARS

Cause	No. of Cases/Year
Cancer	34,361
Cardiac disease	13,900
Trauma	12,154

Data from Landis SH, Murray T, Bolden S, Wingo PA: Cancer statistics, 1998. CA Cancer J Clin 1998;48:6–29.

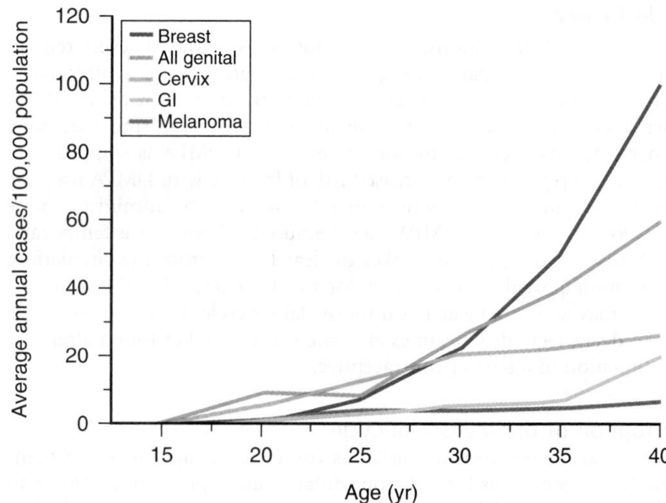

FIGURE 258–1 • Incidence of common malignant neoplasms in pregnancy. (Data from Landis SH, Murray T, Bolden S, Wingo PA: Cancer statistics, 1998. CA Cancer J Clin 1998;48:6–29.)

Treatment Planning

The diagnosis of cancer in pregnancy presents a unique management dilemma that ultimately affects two patients. The decision process is complicated by the significant risks to the fetus in terms of developmental abnormalities and preterm delivery and to the mother in terms of the malignant process itself. Multiple social, ethical, moral, and religious issues also play an important part in the decision tree.

The treatment of these patients should remain unbiased, well researched, and above all multidisciplinary. Basic aspects of cancer screening must be maintained even during pregnancy, and signs and symptoms of serious neoplastic processes must not be overlooked.

When a cancer occurs in a gravid woman, it obviously carries with it enormous pressures on both the patient and her family as well as on the treating team of physicians. Treatment decisions are complicated by multiple issues including medical (risk versus benefit to mother and fetus), ethical, cultural, and religious.

The approach to a pregnant patient diagnosed with a concomitant malignant process requires a concerted multidisciplinary approach. This team should include, at a minimum, obstetricians with experience in high-risk pregnancies and oncologists with a keen understanding of the potential teratogenic risk in fetal development and maturation. Also, significant input from psychosocial, religious, and even legal personnel can be invaluable to maximize the outcome of mother, fetus, and family. An integrated care plan should be formulated, and communication between all team members must be encouraged. The medical and psychological sequelae of this process are complex and not to be taken lightly. Decisions regarding pregnancy preservation, type and timing of diagnostic and therapeutic interventions, use of antepartum lung-maturing corticosteroids, and timing and mode of delivery must be carefully planned and executed.

When pregnancy is complicated by a diagnosis of malignancy, timing in terms of treatment becomes critical. Risks versus benefits of potential life-saving therapeutic intervention and early delivery with subsequent fetal immaturity must be weighed carefully. It must also be understood that certain interventions, including radiographic imaging, surgery, and cytotoxic chemotherapy, are safe during pregnancy if they are performed in an appropriate manner. Impetuous and biased decisions in terms of pregnancy termination or delivery must be avoided. Recent data suggest that a delay in delivery for even a few weeks may have a dramatic impact on fetal well-being (see later).

Two fundamental issues must be contemplated when one approaches the care of a gravid patient diagnosed with a malignant process. The impact of the disease on the patient is obviously of paramount importance, and therefore an understanding of the natural history of the disease is critical. Treatment options, success rates, and risk of treatment modifications or delays must be considered. Equally important are the mater-

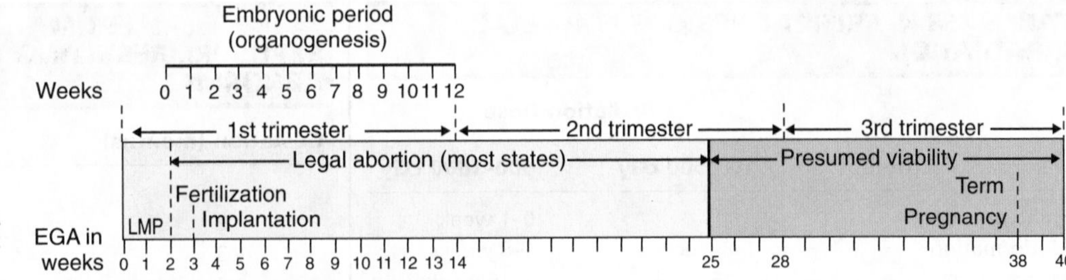

FIGURE 258–2 • Fetal development. EGA = estimated gestational age; LMP = last menstrual period.

nal and paternal desires of pregnancy preservation and the risk of the chosen treatment regimens on fetal health, including sequelae resulting from elective early delivery or potential for in utero fetal harm from toxic side effects of therapy. Patients need to be presented with unbiased information about risks to both mother and fetus and with all potential options of intervention, including pregnancy termination if it is required and desired. Most likely, these management issues are best left to a tertiary care center with a high-risk neonatal nursery (level III) that can adequately manage a preterm yet viable infant if it is necessary.

Fetal Development

Physicians involved with the treatment of cancer in the pregnant patient must possess an in-depth understanding of embryonic development as well as of the disease process and the available therapeutic options. The terminology adopted by embryologists and clinical obstetricians also must be understood.

Fetal age is the most critical concept in terms of prediction of fetal survival and subsequent morbidity. In clinical obstetrics, estimated gestational age (EGA) is defined as the time from the last day of the last menstrual period (Fig. 258–2). Embryonic age from a developmental biologist's viewpoint begins at fertilization and is thus 2 weeks shorter in duration. This 2-week differential is critical and potentially legally important in considering fetal viability and age at which termination (abortion) can be performed. Ovulation and subsequent fertilization do not occur until approximately 2 weeks after the last menstrual period. Thus, the normal gestation is 40 weeks; clinical viability generally has been defined as an EGA of more than 25 weeks. For accurate clinical communication, fetal age should be documented in terms of EGA (in weeks). Gestation is further subdivided into 14-week trimesters, as shown in Figure 258–2. In most states, abortion can legally be performed in the first trimester, whereas some states allow termination until 24 weeks (late abortion).

The most vulnerable portion of development, in terms of teratogenicity, is believed to be during the embryonic period (see Fig. 258–2). During this time, major organ systems are forming (organogenesis), and it appears that the conceptus is susceptible to outside teratogenic influences. For this reason, most clinicians believe that therapeutic intervention is best delayed until after this period to lessen fetal risk in a patient desirous of preserving her pregnancy.

After the embryonic period, fetal development is focused on organ growth and maturation. Certain basic physical and metabolic capabilities appear to be required to maintain extrauterine life. Most commonly, viability is defined as 25 weeks of EGA, although fetal survival before this age has been reported. Subsequent fetal morbidity and mortality are linearly correlated with gestational age and weight (Tables 258–2 and 258–3). Obviously, preterm infants require care in a specific neonatal unit prepared for such complicated management (level III nurseries). Significant literature supports the concept of maximizing in utero fetal life to decrease fetal morbidity, mortality, and long-term developmental delay.

Although the short-term major risk to the fetus appears to be secondary to poor lung development, subsequent development of hyaline membrane disease, and bronchopulmonary dysplasia, reports are confirming increased risk of intraventricular hemorrhage and significant long-term motor and neurologic sequelae associated with survival of a preterm delivery. Infants weighing less than 1500 g at birth appear to suffer from significant long-term deficiencies in intelligence quotient, visual-motor integration, and reading performance. Similar data reveal significant neurologic impairment in infants documented with intraventricular hemorrhage. In one study, only 26% of low-birthweight children with subsequent intraventricular hemorrhage had normal developmental abilities at the time of preschool testing. Predelivery use of corticosteroids (at an EGA of 24 to 34 weeks) decreases the risk of pulmonary complications as well as intraventricular hemorrhage. It is important for parents to understand the potential ramifications of early delivery for their child and to realize that survival can be associated with significant long-term morbidity.

Diagnostic and Therapeutic Procedures in the Pregnant Patient with Cancer

Commonly accepted practices of diagnostic imaging, surgery, therapeutic radiation therapy, and chemotherapy have profoundly different implications in the pregnant versus nonpregnant patient. The risk-benefit profiles of each modality must be carefully considered before implementation.

Radiation Therapy

It appears that ionizing radiation poses significantly more risk to fetal development than do the environmental sources of both ionizing and nonionizing radiation to which one is constantly exposed. Ionizing radiation can cause both direct and indirect intracellular damage and is typically expressed in terms of radiation absorbed dose or relative biologic equivalent. Direct radiation damage is believed to be a relatively minor component of these detrimental effects. Rather, the large amount of intracellular water that undergoes radiation-induced ionization leads to free radical formation with subsequent chemical intracellular reaction and damage. In vitro studies indicate that dividing cells, specifically near the mitotic phase, appear to be most vulnerable.

TABLE 258–2 SURVIVAL STATISTICS IN RELATION TO FETAL WEIGHT

Weight (g)	% Survival
401–500	11
501–600	29
601–700	62
701–800	75
801–900	88

TABLE 258–3 SURVIVAL STATISTICS IN RELATION TO ESTIMATED GESTATIONAL AGE (EGA)

EGA (weeks)	% Survival
25	75
26	80
27	90
28	92
29	95
30	97

TABLE 258–4 CRITICAL PERIODS FOR FETAL IRRADIATION

	Radiation Dose	
Disorder or Problem	**100–500 cGy**	**500–1000 cGy**
Embryonic death		0–1 week
Malformation	1–8 weeks	1–8 weeks
Microcephaly	1–15 weeks	1–15 weeks
Mental retardation	8–15 weeks	8–25 weeks
Growth retardation	1–15 weeks	1–25 weeks
Late-onset cancer	?	1–39 weeks
Genetic aberrations	?	?

TABLE 258–5 ESTIMATED TOTAL RADIATION EXPOSURE RESULTING IN MAJOR ABNORMALITIES

Gestation (months)	Radiation Dose (cGy)
1	40
2	90
3	140
4	200
5	250
6	350
7	No published data
8	500
9	600

At therapeutic doses, radiation does not significantly directly damage cellular microstructures, membranes, or metabolic processes. The primary toxic effects appear to result primarily from free radical–induced damage at the DNA level. The damage is most likely secondary to double-stranded breaks in DNA leading to replication errors, which are presumably lethal and potentially teratogenic.

At doses of radiation less than 100 cGy, cell death results from direct inhibition of cell division and is most prevalent in cells undergoing active division. Radiation-induced mutations increase as a linear function of single doses of 400 to 600 cGy. Because of the acute toxicity to cells, radiation is considered a weak teratogen. Clinical retrospective studies suggest some association of spontaneous abortion with early fetal irradiation.

The fetal effects of radiation appear to be related to the gestational age at the time of exposure as well as to total dose received. An analysis of children exposed in utero to atomic bomb–produced radiation revealed that most long-term neurologic sequelae occurred in children exposed between an EGA of 8 and 15 weeks, with no cases reported in children exposed before 8 weeks. Exposure at an earlier gestational age most likely resulted in miscarriage.

Fetal exposure to radiation between 11 and 16 weeks of gestation appears to result in an increased risk of microcephaly and mental retardation. Exposure in the third trimester may be associated with longer term developmental abnormalities (Tables 258–4 and 258–5). In general, third-trimester fetal doses should not exceed 100 cGy.

Typical sources of medically indicated ionizing radiation are both diagnostic and therapeutic. The fetal exposure during most diagnostic radiographic imaging modalities is relatively small and generally exaggerated by both clinicians and patients, leading to unwarranted fear. In the appropriate setting, the procedures are thought to be safe if they are clinically indicated. Estimated fetal radiation exposures for standard radiographic procedures are listed in Table 258–6. A risk-benefit assessment must be performed before any radiographic evaluation is undertaken in a pregnant patient.

Because of the relatively high fetal exposure associated with pelvic-abdominal computed tomography, it is not recommended in early pregnancy. However, pulmonary imaging with contrast enhancement to evaluate for possibly life-threatening pulmonary emboli is associated with minimal fetal exposure, as are ventilation-perfusion scans.

Mammography (see Table 258–6) presents essentially no risk to the developing fetus. Therefore, its use as a diagnostic modality in the patient with a clinically suspicious breast lesion is recommended.

Perhaps the most commonly employed imaging procedure in the pregnant patient is real-time ultrasonography. Its use in fetal anatomic observation and age determination has been well studied and is considered safe throughout the gestational period.

Ultrasonography can also be an important instrument for maternal evaluation of suspected renal, abdominal, pelvic, hepatic, cardiac, vascular, and breast tissues. Hepatic ultrasonographic evaluation can detect occult liver metastasis with a sensitivity of 76% without fetal risk. Breast ultrasonography is a useful adjunct in characterizing breast lesion architecture noted on physical examination or mammography (see section on breast cancer).

Magnetic resonance imaging, because of its lack of ionizing radiation, is believed to be acceptable in pregnancy. No adverse fetal or maternal sequelae have been described to date.

The maternal effects of radiation are well documented. Direct ovarian exposures of 1000 cGy are associated with permanent sterilization in more than 90% of women. Lower doses also result in sterility but appear to be dependent on the patient's age and menstrual and reproductive history. Ovarian suppression with oral contraceptives or gonadotropin hormone antagonists may help preserve ovarian function and subsequent reproductive potential, especially in the adolescent woman, although randomized trials are lacking. This effect appears to be less pronounced as age increases. Therapeutic megavoltage radiation therapy has a pivotal role in the management of many malignant neoplasms, such as breast and cervical cancer and lymphoma. Its use in pregnancy must be regarded as a completely separate entity from diagnostic radiographic procedures. Depending on the specific anatomic area to be treated, the fetal exposure can range from minimal to substantial (Table 258–7).

Surgical Therapy

Most common solid tumor cancers affecting the pregnant patient are treatable; many are curable by a surgical approach. Fetal risk appears to be most dependent on the anatomic location of the neoplasm and the risk of subsequent stimulation of preterm labor, which is most affected by timing of the procedure. Pelvic and abdominal radical procedures can be safely undertaken with appropriate planning.

TABLE 258–6 ESTIMATED FETAL DOSE FROM COMMON DIAGNOSTIC RADIOGRAPHIC PROCEDURES

Examination	Fetal Dose (cGy)
Chest (posteroanterior, lateral)	0.006
Abdomen	0.15–0.26
Lumbar spine	0.65
Pelvis	0.2–0.35
Hip	0.13–0.2
Intravenous pyelography	0.47–0.82
Upper gastrointestinal tract	0.17–0.48
Barium enema	0.82–1.14
Mammography	Undetectable
Ventilation-perfusion scan	0.35
CT of abdomen (early pregnancy)	0.4
CT of pelvis	2.5
^{99m}Tc-MDP bone scan	0.15
Spiral CT pulmonary angiography	0.2

CT = computed tomography.

TABLE 258–7 ESTIMATED FETAL DOSES FROM EXTRAPELVIC AND EXTRA-ABDOMINAL MATERNAL IRRADIATION

Radiation Site/Prescribed Dose	Estimated Gestational Age	Fetal Dose (cGy)
Tibia sarcoma/50 Gy	25 weeks	1.5
Brain glioblastoma/60 Gy	13 weeks	3.9
Hodgkin's disease (mantle fields)/38 Gy	34 weeks	42
Hodgkin's disease with mediastinum/neck/40 Gy	18–31 weeks	20
Breast cancer/50 Gy	Ovarian dose	9

Data from Greer BE, Goof BA, Kuh W, et al: Cancer in the pregnant patient. *In* Hoskins WJ, Perez CA, Young RC (eds): Principles and Practice of Gynecologic Oncology, 2nd ed. Philadelphia, Lippincott-Raven, 1997, pp 463–485.

Surgical approaches to breast, ovarian, gastrointestinal, thyroid, melanoma, neurologic, and vulvar cancer have been well described, along with a multitude of benign surgical conditions. The current anesthetic agents in common use are believed to be without risk of fetal teratogenicity, and certainly minor procedures with local or regional analgesia (epidural, spinal, nerve block) are essentially without risk. Exclusive of cesarean section, it has been estimated that approximately 35,000 pregnant women undergo some surgical procedure each year.

An issue that should be considered by the surgeon and anesthesiologist is the critical nature of the uteroplacental unit, which is susceptible to blood pressure changes and intravascular volume depletion. Major changes in blood flow to the placenta can lead to subsequent fetal hypoxia and potentially precipitate neurologic sequelae. Therefore, the supine position is best avoided in the gravid patient (especially after an EGA of 20 weeks) owing to decreased cardiac return associated with uterine compression on the inferior vena cava. Patients are best maintained in the left lateral decubitus position (30 degrees) to decrease this compressive effect. Diagnostic procedures including fine-needle aspiration, core biopsy, and surgical removal of suspicious lesions should rarely if ever be deferred because of pregnancy.

Equally critical is the increased thrombogenic state associated with pregnancy as brought about by decreases in plasma fibrinolytic activity, increases in coagulation factors, and increased pelvic and lower extremity stasis. These factors combine for a five- to six-fold increased risk of thromboembolic phenomena in the pregnant patient, and thus appropriate thromboprophylaxis should be undertaken. Current acceptable techniques include subcutaneous heparin (5000 units three times a day), low-molecular-weight heparin (enoxaparin, 40 mg/day), and inflatable compression stockings. Non–custom fit elastic stockings (e.g., TED hose) have no role in thromboprophylaxis.

Medical Therapy

Chemotherapy

Chemotherapy, by definition, is the use of chemical agents to treat or to control disease. Therefore, any medication from acetaminophen to zinc has the potential to cause fetal effects, both beneficial and harmful. The U.S. Food and Drug Administration has established labeling of prescription drugs to provide information about potential fetal risks. These five categories (A, B, C, D, and X) indicate risk of fetal teratogenicity (Table 258–8). A similar classification system has been adopted by the Australian Drug Evaluation Committee as well as by the German Health Care Administration. From a practical standpoint, drugs in Food and Drug Administration categories A, B, and C are prescribed with impunity.

Chemotherapy specifically as an antineoplastic agent has an integral role in the management of many of the cancers encountered during pregnancy. Some agents are used as adjuvant therapy after primary surgery (e.g., breast cancer), whereas others are the primary treatment modality (e.g., Hodgkin's disease). The potential toxicity to the developing fetus must be considered in discussing potential treatment regimens in the pregnant patient.

All chemotherapeutic agents, by virtue of their mechanism of action, have the ability to be both mutagenic and teratogenic to the actively dividing cells of the embryo and fetus. Most of these agents are considered category D or X. Unfortunately, controlled data on their effects on the developing fetus are limited. Most information has come from retrospective reviews, clinical observation, and laboratory experiments on gravid animals.

It appears that the first trimester is the most susceptible to deleterious chemotherapy influences. Overall, it appears that approximately 20% of fetuses exposed to cytotoxic agents in the first trimester will manifest major anomalies, compared with 3% in an unexposed population.

Chemotherapeutic agents primarily act by interrupting various portions of vital cell processes. This reproductive cell cycle is divided into five phases, each with specific actions leading to cell duplication (Table 258–9). Cancer cells are thought to replicate at a higher rate and therefore should be more susceptible to the cytotoxic or cytostatic effects of chemotherapy. Specific chemotherapeutic agents are often categorized by their interaction within the cell cycle and are traditionally classified into alkylating agents, antitumor antibiotics, antimetabolites, vinca alkaloids, biologic response modifiers, hormones, and taxanes. Specific agents and their actions are listed in Table 258–10.

The timing of chemotherapy administration in relationship to anticipated delivery must be carefully planned to avoid delivery around the time of the maternal hematopoietic nadir. Hematopoietic suppression (anemia, leukopenia, and thrombocytopenia) may occur in the fetus as a result of transplacental passage of cytotoxic agents from the mother to the fetus, and the neonatology team should be advised accordingly.

TABLE 258–8 U.S. FOOD AND DRUG ADMINISTRATION PREGNANCY CATEGORY DEFINITIONS

Category	Definition
A	Controlled studies in women fail to demonstrate a risk to the fetus in the first trimester, and the possibility of fetal harm appears remote.
B	Animal studies do not indicate a risk to the fetus, and there are no controlled human studies. Animal studies do show an adverse effect on the fetus, but well-controlled studies in pregnant women have failed to demonstrate a risk to the fetus.
C	Studies have shown that the drug exerts animal teratogenic or embryocidal effects, but there are no controlled studies in women, or no studies are available in either animals or women.
D	Positive evidence of human fetal risk exists, but benefits in certain situations may make use of the drug acceptable.
X	Studies in animals or humans have demonstrated fetal abnormalities or there is evidence of fetal risk based on human experience, and the risk of drug administration clearly outweighs any possible benefit.

Taxanes (paclitaxel and docetaxel) have significant activity in many solid tumor malignant neoplasms. Case reports describing safe administration of paclitaxel (Taxol) have been published, but great caution must still be exercised. Appropriate consent must be obtained before administration, and careful risk-versus-benefit analysis must be undertaken. Given its activity of microtubular assembly, concern for its effect on fetal development is significant.

Breast-feeding is contraindicated during chemotherapeutic administration. These systemically administered antineoplastic agents may reach significant levels in breast milk.

SPECIFIC MALIGNANT NEOPLASMS IN PREGNANCY

The most common malignant neoplasms encountered during pregnancy are uterine and cervical cancer, breast cancer, melanoma, ovarian cancer, thyroid cancer, leukemia, lymphoma, and colorectal cancer (Table 258–11). Specific reviews of these common malignant neoplasms encountered in this population are presented here, along with various strategies employed in their management.

Cervical Cancer

Epidemiology

Cervical cancer remains the most common malignant neoplasm encountered during pregnancy. It occurs with an incidence of approximately 1.2 cases per 10,000 pregnancies. With the expanded knowledge of the natural history of this disease, the majority of patients with early cervical carcinoma can be managed with fetal preservation (if desired) without undue maternal morbidity or mortality.

Diagnosis

Initial prenatal evaluation should routinely include a Papanicolaou (Pap) smear. This simple, inexpensive, and extremely effective screening procedure has significantly decreased the incidence of invasive squamous cell carcinoma of the cervix in the United States. In countries where this procedure is not widely practiced, cervical cancer remains one of the leading causes of death. After intense investigation and numerous clinical observations, the natural progression from a preinvasive dysplastic lesion to overt invasive cervical carcinoma is well understood. The success of Pap smear screening has been in its ability to diagnose dysplastic lesions, thus allowing simple ablative and curative measures.

All clinicians who practice Pap smear screening should have an understanding of the Bethesda system of Pap smear interpretation as well as diagnostic and treatment algorithms. The in utero presence of a fetus should not dramatically change the initial diagnostic approaches to an abnormal Pap smear.

Cytologic evidence of squamous intraepithelial lesions is most commonly evaluated with cervical colposcopy. Colposcopy during pregnancy is safe and effective and in the majority of cases (>90%) provides adequate diagnostic information. As in the nonpregnant patient, any area of gross abnormality, even in the presence of a normal Pap smear, requires biopsy, which again is safe in pregnancy if it is performed by experienced personnel.

Treatment

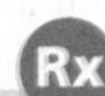

Given the knowledge of the natural history of cervical dysplasia, observational strategies have been developed to allow the pregnancy to continue without need for intervention. Even in the patient with biopsy-proven carcinoma in situ, excision or cervical ablation can most commonly be deferred until after delivery. Importantly, a diagnosis of cervical dysplasia is not an indication for cesarean delivery because there has been no demonstrable increased risk to mother or fetus with vaginal delivery.

TABLE 258–9 CELL CYCLE

Cell Phase	Approximate Time	Activity
G_1 (gap 1)	Variable	RNA manufacture, preparation for DNA synthesis
S (synthesis)	8 hours	DNA duplication
G_2 (gap 2)	3 hours	Spindle apparatus formation
M (mitosis)	1 hour	Mitosis
G_0 (gap 0)		Resting (quiescent)

TABLE 258–11 INCIDENCE OF CANCER IN PREGNANCY

Site and Type	Estimated Incidence per 1000 Pregnancies
Cervix uteri	
Noninvasive	1.3
Invasive	1.0
Breast	0.33
Colorectal	0.2
Melanoma	0.14
Ovary	0.10
Leukemia	0.1
Lymphoma	0.1

From Allen HH, Nisker JA (eds): Cancer in Pregnancy: Therapeutic Guidelines. Mt. Kisco, NY, Futura, 1986.

TABLE 258–10 SPECIFIC CHEMOTHERAPEUTIC AGENTS AND THEIR ACTIONS

Agent	Cell Cycle Action	Potential Fetal Toxicity
Alkylating agent: cyclophosphamide, ifosfamide, chlorambucil, nitrogen mustard, cisplatin	Nonspecific	14% fetal malformations in first trimester; chlorambucil syndrome of renal aplasia, cleft palate, skeletal anomalies
Antitumor antibiotics: dactinomycin, mitomycin C, bleomycin, doxorubicin	Variable	None reported
Antimetabolites: 5-fluorouracil, methotrexate, cytarabine	Cell cycle specific	Multiple defects: cranial dysostosis, hypertelorism, micrognathia, cleft palate; contraindicated in pregnancy
Taxanes: paclitaxel	Cell cycle specific	No data in pregnancy
Biologic response modifiers: interleukins, interferons	Nonspecific	Contraindicated in pregnancy
Hormones: tamoxifen, megestrol	Nonspecific	Contraindicated in pregnancy

Rx

Locally advanced cervical carcinoma not amenable to surgical resection requires treatment with radical radiation therapy. The standard external high-energy teletherapy radiation often exceeds 4500 cGy and is not compatible with fetal life. Again, decisions regarding fetal age, risk of early delivery versus waiting, and parental desires must be weighed, given the curability of this disease. With most lesions confined to the cervix, careful observation with expedited delivery after fetal maturation followed by radical treatment appears reasonable.

Ovarian Neoplasms

Epidemiology

The incidence of adnexal masses associated with pregnancy has been reported to range from 1 in 81 to 1 in 2500. With the use of ultrasonography for routine fetal surveillance, the detection of previously unrecognized adnexal masses in both early and late gestation is likely to increase.

The lifetime risk of ovarian carcinoma for an American woman is approximately 1 in 70, with an age-adjusted annual incidence of approximately 13.7 cases per 100,000 women. This results in approximately 24,000 new cases of ovarian cancer and 14,500 deaths per annum.

These malignant neoplasms can occur at any age, including infancy and childhood; however, the overall age-specific incidence increases dramatically with age. In women 40 years of age, there are approximately 10 cases per 100,000, increasing to a peak incidence of approximately 45 cases per 100,000 women between the ages of 60 and 65 years. Given this age distribution, the discovery of ovarian carcinoma in pregnancy is still distinctly uncommon.

Pathobiology

Of the adnexal masses noticed in pregnancy, approximately 50% are smaller than 5 cm in diameter, whereas 25% are between 5 and 10 cm and 25% are larger than 10 cm at the time of discovery. Ninety-five percent of these also are unilateral.

Unilateral, mobile, noncomplex masses smaller than 5 cm, noticed in the first trimester, will resolve in more than 90% of cases. It therefore is reasonable to observe nonsuspicious masses conservatively with repeated ultrasonography into the second trimester (when elective surgical intervention is safest) to document spontaneous resolution.

A subgroup of patients undergoing assisted reproductive therapy with various ovulation-inducing medications presents a unique situation. Because of the induced ovarian hyperstimulation and increased ultrasonographic surveillance, these patients commonly have ovarian cysts noted in the first trimester. Spontaneous resolution of benign-appearing ovarian cysts can be expected in more than 90% of patients who have undergone ovulation induction. Reports of possible associations between ovulation induction and an increased incidence of ovarian neoplasms should be kept in mind, however, although this is considered most likely to occur after the pregnancy.

Diagnosis

Adnexal masses can originate from multiple sources, and the differential diagnosis is complex, including multiple gynecologic and nongynecologic entities. Fortunately, modern pelvic imaging, especially ultrasonography, aids greatly in differentiating the primary origins of these masses. The common types of neoplastic and non-neoplastic ovarian masses noticed during pregnancy are described in Tables 258–12 and 258–13. Most ovarian tumors occurring during early pregnancy are benign; the most common neoplastic ovarian mass is a benign cystic teratoma.

Imaging

The key to evaluation of the pelvic or adnexal mass in pregnancy is to attempt to differentiate benign from malignant processes to avoid unnecessary intervention. Other than the acute presentation of abdominal pain associated with ovarian torsion, most commonly between weeks 6 and 14 of gestation, these masses often are clinically inapparent and may be accompanied only with the vague nonspecific abdominal discomfort common to pregnancy. Discovery of a mass in the first trimester in most situations should prompt repeated ultrasonography in the early second trimester to confirm resolution or stability.

Two to 5% of adnexal masses persisting after the first trimester are pathologically confirmed as being malignant, resulting in an overall malignancy rate of 1 in 5000 to 1 in 18,000 women who have live births.

Laboratory Findings

Tumor Markers

The use of CA-125 to differentiate malignant from benign adnexal masses has been well described (Chapter 190). Unfortunately, in the premenopausal woman, the high rate of false-positive serum elevations in CA-125 makes this a relatively poor screening test. It is also commonly

TABLE 258–12 DIFFERENTIAL DIAGNOSIS OF THE PELVIC MASS

GYNECOLOGIC

- Ovary
  - Benign (functional)
  - Neoplastic (benign, malignant)
- Fallopian tube
  - Hydrosalpinx
  - Tubo-ovarian abscess
  - Ectopic pregnancy
- Uterine
  - Benign (leiomyomas)
  - Malignant (sarcoma)

NONGYNECOLOGIC

- Gastrointestinal
  - Colon (including stool, diverticular disease)
  - Small bowel
  - Appendix
- Mesothelial tumors
- Lymphoma
- Retroperitoneal neoplasm
- Pelvic kidney
- Urachal cyst
- Mesenteric cyst
- Metastatic disease
- Sacral meningocele
- Distended bladder

TABLE 258–13 HISTOLOGIC TYPE OF NON-NEOPLASTIC OVARIAN TUMORS IN PREGNANCY

Histologic Type	Frequency (%)
Endometriotic	14
Paraovarian	11
Simple cyst	12
Corpus luteal	50
Unknown	6
Miscellaneous	
Luteoma	1
Ovarian edema	1
Thecal lutein	5

Data from Stedman C, Kline R: Intraoperative complications and unexpected pathology at the time of cesarean section. Obstet Gynecol Clin North Am 1988;15:745–769.

elevated because of the pregnancy itself, and therefore its use in the pregnant patient to aid in the differentiation of benign from malignant ovarian neoplasm is not recommended. This same principle applies to assessment of α-fetoprotein and human chorionic gonadotropin, both of which are routinely elevated in pregnancy and are therefore of limited value in attempting to identify a germ cell ovarian neoplasm.

Treatment

Rx

Surgical Therapy

The timing of surgical intervention cannot always be controlled, and emergency situations occasionally arise. If laparotomy is required during the first trimester, spontaneous abortion is more likely, possibly because of disruption of the delicate corpus luteum. After 7 to 10 weeks of gestation, the trophoblast is capable of supplying sufficient quantities of specific steroid hormones for the maintenance of the gestation.

Should surgical extirpation of the corpus luteum be required in the first trimester, progestin support is recommended. A daily intramuscular injection of 100 mg of progesterone in oil or a 100-mg transvaginal suppository every 12 hours provides adequate progestin replacement. A mass that is first noted in the third trimester is best managed by awaiting fetal maturity if the clinical suspicion of malignant disease is low.

The optimal timing of elective surgical intervention is during the second trimester. Apparent risk of preterm labor with subsequent fetal morbidity seems to be lessened. Uterine size at this gestational age does not preclude appropriate aortic and upper abdominal surgical exposure. Severe third-trimester complications are associated with failure to remove significant ovarian masses during mid-pregnancy.

Ovarian Carcinoma

Treatment

Rx

Surgery

Although uncommon, there are unfortunate instances in which both epithelial and germ cell carcinomas are diagnosed during pregnancy. The mainstay of management is still surgery, with removal of the neoplasm as well as appropriate surgical staging and debulking as indicated. It is strongly recommended that this procedure be undertaken as a team approach, including both an experienced gynecologic oncologist and a maternal-fetal medicine specialist.

Medical Therapy

After completion of the initial surgical effort, consideration of chemotherapy is warranted, depending on stage of disease, estimated fetal age, and desires of the mother. Chemotherapeutic intervention, most commonly with a platinum-based regimen (cisplatin), has been well described and appears to be safe for both mother and fetus. Taxanes (paclitaxel and docetaxel) have significant activity in many solid tumor malignant neoplasms, including epithelial ovarian cancer. Case reports describing safe administration of paclitaxel (Taxol) have been published, but great caution must still be exercised. Appropriate consent must be obtained before administration, and careful risk-versus-benefit analysis must be undertaken.

Breast Cancer

Epidemiology

Cancer of the breast during pregnancy or within the first year after delivery is considered pregnancy-associated breast carcinoma. Breast carcinoma remains the second most common malignant neoplasm occurring in the pregnant patient and affects approximately 1 in 3000 pregnancies in the United States (Chapter 208).

Traditionally, pregnancy-associated breast carcinoma has been thought to carry a poorer prognosis, although recent matched controlled data do not support this claim. Women with pregnancy-associated breast carcinoma are, however, more commonly diagnosed with locally advanced node-positive disease at the time of diagnosis (61% vs. 38%). The obvious adverse effect of advanced disease is reflected by a decrease in the 5-year survival rate from 82% in the node-negative group to 47% in the node-positive group. Pregnant patients are also 2.5 times more likely to present with distant metastatic disease at the time of diagnosis, compared with their nonpregnant counterparts.

Diagnosis

Both the patient and the clinician must be continually vigilant to subtle breast changes. Most pregnancy-associated breast carcinomas initially manifest as a painless mass, and more than 90% are detected during the patient's self-examination of the breast. Similar diagnostic algorithms should be applied in both the pregnant and the nonpregnant patient with a suspicious breast lesion. Fine-needle aspiration, diagnostic mammography, ultrasonography, and open-breast biopsy pose no documented fetal risk. The historical reluctance to aggressively pursue histologic diagnosis of breast masses in pregnancy is unwarranted and perhaps detrimental.

A recent series of 134 breast biopsies performed during pregnancy revealed a 21% incidence of malignancy, thereby confirming the need for aggressive measures. As in nonpregnant women, infiltrating ductal carcinoma continues to be the most common histologic subtype encountered.

Breast ultrasonography is an important adjunct in the evaluation of the palpable or mammographically demonstrated breast lesion. Its ability to differentiate cystic from solid lesions can provide useful information and can guide subsequent diagnostic decisions. On characterization of a breast mass, the most common initial diagnostic modality of choice is the fine-needle aspiration.

Treatment

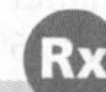

The initial approach to breast carcinoma is most commonly surgical. Depending on the clinical stage, either breast-conserving lumpectomy or mastectomy, both with axillary lymph node dissection, is classically undertaken.

After surgical resection and lymph node evaluation, a decision about adjuvant therapy must be made. In surgically documented, early-stage disease, a complete metastatic work-up is not warranted, given the low yield. Therefore, decisions regarding the need for adjuvant therapy are usually based on the initial choice of surgical procedure. Again, given the potential harm of radiation therapy to the developing fetus, a radical mastectomy with lymph node dissection is usually the procedure of choice, thereby eliminating the need for postoperative radiation therapy.

Chemotherapeutic intervention has been advocated in cases of locally advanced and advanced carcinoma of the breast. As described previously, it is prudent to avoid chemotherapeutic intervention during the critical period of organogenesis in a desired pregnancy (see section on chemotherapy).

Melanoma

Epidemiology

The overall incidence of cutaneous melanoma appears to be increasing, and it has been estimated that 1 in 90 persons were diagnosed with this neoplasm in 2000 (Chapter 214). Some literature suggests that the incidence of melanoma complicating pregnancy will exceed that of cervical carcinoma.

TABLE 258–14 RISK FACTORS ASSOCIATED WITH DEVELOPMENT OF CUTANEOUS MELANOMA

Fair complexion
Tendency toward easy sunburning
Early age at first sunburn
Inability to tan
Familial history of malignant melanoma
Personal history of melanoma
Environmental exposure to ultraviolet B irradiation

Diagnosis

Risk factors documented to increase the risk of melanoma development are outlined in Table 258–14. Increased awareness among physicians and patients as well as improved screening appears to have led to a tendency toward earlier diagnosis. These lesions tend to occur in sun-exposed areas; however, 17% of melanomas diagnosed in the female population are found on the vulva and perineum. This high incidence provides the basis for aggressive biopsy of suspicious pigmented vulvar lesions.

Treatment

Rx

Initial treatment of a melanotic lesion is the same in a pregnant or a nonpregnant patient. Wide local excision with adequate surgical margins remains the procedure of choice. Adjuvant therapy remains controversial in this setting.

The fetal risk of maternal melanoma is not well defined. It remains the most common malignant neoplasm to metastasize to the placenta and fetus. Although overall the incidence appears to be extremely low (approximately 60 cases reported), careful pathologic examination of the placenta is warranted. In documented cases of placental spread, the fetal risk appears to be as high as 40 or 50%. An altered clinical course in the pregnant patient with melanoma has also been suggested. Observational data imply a potential hormonal influence on the melanotic process. Given the well-documented cutaneous manifestations of pregnancy, including increased pigmentation of the vulva, areola, and linea nigra, some investigators have postulated that the increased levels of estrogen, progesterone, adrenocorticotropic hormone, and melanin-stimulating hormone may somehow influence melanoma growth.

Thyroid Cancer

Epidemiology

Thyroid cancer is the most commonly diagnosed endocrinologic malignant neoplasm, with approximately 16,100 cases noted in 1997, of which about 11,000 were in women (Chapter 244). Of these cases, almost half were documented in reproductive-age women (15 to 44 years); thus, thyroid carcinoma complicating pregnancy is not uncommon. Thyroid nodules are common and are often encountered during initial prenatal evaluation (they represent benign entities in approximately 90% of cases).

Diagnosis

Diagnostic evaluation of a thyroid nodule in a pregnant patient is usually limited to physical examination, laboratory studies, and thyroid ultrasonography followed by fine-needle or excisional biopsy. Specifically, nuclear medicine scintigraphy scans are omitted because of concerns about the effects of radioactive ^{123}I or ^{131}I on the fetal thyroid. Transplacental passage of iodine is well documented.

Treatment

After an appropriate diagnosis, surgical resection remains the primary mode of treatment. The timing of this intervention remains an important decision. A retrospective review suggests equivalent outcomes in patients who undergo thyroidectomy during pregnancy and those who wait until the postpartum state. Radionuclide thyroid ablation is contraindicated during pregnancy.

Colorectal Cancer

Epidemiology

The lifetime risk of colorectal carcinoma in women is 1 in 17 (6%), with most of these being diagnosed after the age of 50 years (Chapter 203). Only 8% of cases are noted in the reproductive-age group (<40 years). A similar increase in incidence may be noted as childbearing is delayed.

Diagnosis

More than 80% of colorectal carcinomas associated with pregnancy occur in the rectum (commonly below the peritoneal reflection and thus palpable on digital rectal examination). Diagnostic delays are usually attributed to the increased frequency of rectal bleeding episodes common to pregnancy (usually hemorrhoid related) and thus decreased clinical suspicion. Symptoms associated with advanced disease, such as abdominal pain, distention, and constipation, are rarely encountered.

The diagnosis of colorectal carcinoma depends on a detailed history of risk factors, such as history of polyps or family history of carcinoma (including gastrointestinal and breast); complete lymph node survey; digital rectal examination with Hemoccult testing; and sigmoidoscopy or colonoscopy. Determination of a serum marker such as carcinoembryonic antigen is of no value in pregnancy because it is elevated in the normal gestation.

Treatment

Management of colorectal carcinoma is most commonly surgical. Surgical practices similar to those outlined previously are followed.

The prognosis for a woman diagnosed with colorectal carcinoma in pregnancy is similar to that of matched nonpregnant control subjects. Postoperative local adjuvant pelvic radiation therapy is obviously contraindicated in a desired pregnancy.

Hematologic Malignant Neoplasms

Epidemiology

Hematologic malignant neoplasms complicating pregnancy are rare (Chapters 196 and 197). Hodgkin's disease, considered a primary lymph node malignant neoplasm, commonly affects young adults and is the most common hematologic malignant neoplasm associated with pregnancy. An incidence of 1 in 5000 live births has been reported.

Diagnosis

More than 70% of patients diagnosed with Hodgkin's disease initially present with painless lymphadenopathy, commonly noted in the cervical, submaxillary, or axillary chains. Systemic signs often associated with advanced disease include night sweats, fever, weight loss, and fatigue. Diagnosis depends on appropriate lymph node biopsy and documentation of the pathognomonic Reed-Sternberg cell.

Staging modalities include physical examination; computed tomography of chest, abdomen, and pelvis; lymphangiography; and occasional staging laparotomy with splenectomy. Abdominal-pelvic computed tomography is not recommended in pregnant patients, although magnetic resonance imaging can be performed safely. Both the surgeon and the oncologist must carefully consider the risk versus benefit for both fetus and mother in making decisions about staging laparotomy.

Treatment

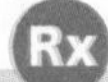

Chemotherapy can be toxic to ovarian function, and its risk seems to be related to the age of the patient. Commonly used protocols consisting of mechlorethamine, vincristine, procarbazine, and prednisone (MOPP) result in amenorrhea in one third of patients; permanent ovarian failure occurs in 75% of patients older than 30 years at the time of treatment. It appears that the doxorubicin, bleomycin, vinblastine, dacarbazine (ABVD) regimen is potentially less toxic, with an approximate risk of amenorrhea of 5%. The role of ovarian suppression and subsequent functional preservation has already been described.

Pheochromocytoma

Although it is only rarely encountered in pregnancy, pheochromocytoma represents a unique neoplastic event with significant morbidity and mortality to both mother and fetus. It most commonly represents a nonmalignant entity, although malignant transformation can occur. Pheochromocytomas are most commonly found within the adrenal medulla, although they can also arise from the chromaffin cell within sympathetic ganglia (Chapter 246).

In pregnancy, the syndrome is manifested by severe episodes of hypertension usually not associated with significant proteinuria. It can be easily confused with an atypical presentation of preeclampsia. Associated signs and symptoms include tachycardia, palpitations, headache, diaphoresis, and anxiety. Given its rarity, the diagnosis is often unsuspected. If the pheochromocytoma is undiagnosed and therefore not treated, maternal and fetal mortality rates exceed 16 and 26%, respectively.

SUGGESTED READINGS

Germann N, Haie-Meder C, Morice P, et al: Management and clinical outcomes of pregnant patients with invasive cervical cancer. Ann Oncol 2005;16: 397–402. *Pregnancy does not seem to influence the prognosis, and treatment delays may be considered in specific situations.*

Lishner M: Cancer in pregnancy. Ann Oncol 2003;14 (Suppl. 3):iii31–36. *A practical overview of management strategies.*

Oduncu FS, Kimmig R, Hepp H, et al: Cancer in pregnancy: Maternal-fetal conflict. J Cancer Res Clin Oncol 2003;129:133–146. *Reviews the effects of cancer on the mother and fetus, with emphasis on an interdisciplinary approach.*

Ring AE, Smith IE, Ellis PA: Breast cancer and pregnancy. Ann Oncol 2005;16:1855–1860. *Available data suggest that diagnosis and surgery may be carried out as for the nonpregnant patient, with some limitations on staging investigations.*

259 PREGNANCY: HYPERTENSION AND OTHER COMMON MEDICAL PROBLEMS

Diane L. Elliot

Caring for women of reproductive age requires knowing how to diagnose pregnancy and how to provide the appropriate initial care during a pregnancy. Managing pregnant women's medical problems necessitates understanding gestation's influence on illnesses, a condition's effects on pregnancy, and the appropriate management to optimize the well-being of both the mother and fetus.

DIAGNOSIS AND MANAGEMENT OF PREGNANCY

History

Historical information (e.g., last menses, sexual activity, contraceptive practices) will not reliably exclude pregnancy. For example, when seen in an acute care setting, approximately 10% of pregnant adolescents reported no sexual activity.

Laboratory Findings

Laboratory testing for pregnancy is suggested for women with suspected pregnancy, amenorrhea, pelvic pain, and scheduled radiographic studies.

Serum and urine pregnancy tests use monoclonal antibodies for the intact human chorionic gonadotropin (hCG) molecule or its β subunit. At implantation, the syncytiotrophoblast begins producing hCG. Two weeks after conception, the hCG level is approximately 80 mIU/mL, with comparable serum and urine values. During a normal early intrauterine pregnancy, the level doubles every 2 days. The lower limit of detection for most assays is approximately 30 mIU/mL, which yields a sensitivity of more than 90% for pregnancy when performed a week after the first missed menses. Home pregnancy tests have similar sensitivity and these tests may claim 99% accuracy, but for inexperienced users, pregnancy was diagnosed with a sensitivity of 80% and a specificity of 70%. Clinical assessment and home pregnancy test results should be confirmed by measurement of hCG.

Imaging

Transvaginal ultrasonography can detect a gestational sac 5 weeks after conception or when the hCG level is greater than 2000 mIU/mL. Before that time, sequential hCG levels may be needed to distinguish an ectopic from an intrauterine pregnancy. A fetal heartbeat is detectable with ultrasonography by 7 to 8 weeks and is audible with Doppler ultrasonography at 10 to 12 weeks. Quickening and fetal heart tones by fetoscope both occur between 16 and 20 weeks of gestation.

Management

When pregnancy is diagnosed, issues to address include the woman's feelings about the pregnancy and the importance of early and continuous prenatal care. The clinician should assess the patient's nutrition, review her medications for contraindicated drugs, and emphasize discontinuing smoking and alcohol. Supplemental folic acid before conception and early in gestation reduces the risk for neural tube defects such as spina bifida and anencephaly by half. All women of childbearing age should receive additional folate, either as a daily multivitamin or in fortified breakfast cereal. Laboratory tests, such as a complete blood cell count, Rh determination, screening for rubella, hepatitis, cytomegalovirus, and toxoplasmosis antibodies, and a Papanicolaou smear and vaginal cultures, are usually deferred and obtained by the health care provider who will care for the woman during pregnancy and delivery.

HYPERTENSION

Epidemiology

Hypertension (Chapter 66) is a common medical problem during pregnancy, with a prevalence of 6 to 8%. It is diagnosed when blood pressure is greater than 140/90 mm Hg measured with the patient in the sitting position on two occasions. Previously, an increase of more than 30/15 mm Hg during pregnancy was also considered a criterion for hypertension, and although patients with such an increase need close follow-up, that finding alone has poor predictive value.

Diagnosis

Hypertension during pregnancy can be classified as (1) preeclampsia, (2) chronic hypertension, (3) chronic hypertension plus preeclampsia, and (4) gestational hypertension or nonproteinuric hypertension of pregnancy. During a normal pregnancy, blood pressure declines during the first and second trimesters and rises to prepregnancy levels near term. Because of the initial blood pressure decrement, when readings before pregnancy are not available, an elevation during the third trimester could represent any of these four categories. Laboratory tests, including serum uric acid levels, do not reliably predict the development of preeclampsia, nor do they differentiate among the different hypertensive disorders of pregnancy.

Preeclampsia and Gestational Hypertension

Definition

Preeclampsia is hypertension that develops during pregnancy accompanied by proteinuria greater than 0.3 g/24 hr or 1+ on a random specimen. Edema was removed as a criterion for preeclampsia because of its high prevalence during pregnancy and lack of specificity for preeclampsia. Hypertension without other manifestations of preeclampsia is termed gestational hypertension or nonproteinuric hypertension of pregnancy.

Epidemiology

The incidence of preeclampsia varies in different groups of women, with rates of 6 to 10% in Western countries. Risks include previous preeclampsia, chronic hypertension, multifetal gestation, and diabetes. Severe preeclampsia is defined by a blood pressure higher than 160/110 mm Hg, proteinuria greater than 5 g/24 hr, oliguria, thrombocytopenia, abdominal pain, or pulmonary edema. Women with nonproteinuric hypertension are at increased risk for preeclampsia and require close monitoring for its other manifestations because the disorder develops in approximately a fourth during the pregnancy. By definition, gestational hypertension resolves by 3 months postpartum, and blood pressure often normalizes within 2 weeks of delivery.

Pathobiology

During a normal pregnancy, the implanted placenta alters the endothelium, internal elastic lamina, and tunica media of the maternal uterine spiral arteries to allow them to become unresponsive to circulating vasoconstrictors and to dilate to five times their prepregnant state. This trophoblastic invasion and arterial change do not occur with preeclampsia. Accordingly, the placenta is chronically underperfused. In addition, the normal increased blood volume and reduced systemic vascular resistance of pregnancy fail to develop in women with preeclampsia. Alterations in circulating levels of proangiogenic and antiangiogenic proteins have been found to precede the clinical development of preeclampsia. The effect of these circulating factors on the kidney may result in hypertension, and their effects on vascular endothelium may relate to the multiorgan manifestations of preeclampsia and activation of platelets and the coagulation cascade.

Clinical Manifestations

Preeclampsia usually develops during the third trimester, often after 32 weeks. Typically, diastolic pressure increases more than systolic, and systolic levels are often less than 160 mm Hg. Blood pressure readings that although elevated would not be alarming for nonpregnant individuals should not be considered reassuring. Severe organ system dysfunction can occur with what would be only moderate hypertension in nonpregnant women. Intravascular coagulation and hepatic ischemia can cause a constellation of findings called the HELLP syndrome (hemolysis, elevated liver enzymes, and low platelets). The occurrence of seizures defines eclampsia. Although delivery is the treatment of preeclampsia, a small percentage of manifestations are seen immediately postpartum.

Treatment

Rx

Transient gestational hypertension is treated with bedrest, close monitoring of the mother and fetus, and medications when necessary. When to initiate antihypertensive drug treatment is controversial. Many authorities recommend drug therapy when the blood pressure persistently exceeds 140/90 mm Hg. The experience with antihypertensive medication in pregnancy is presented in Table 259–1. The definitive treatment of preeclampsia and transient gestational hypertension is delivery. Before 34 weeks of gestation, that benefit is weighed against the advantages of prolonging intrauterine development.

Prevention

Both supplemental calcium (2 g elemental calcium per day) and low-dose acetylsalicylic acid have been shown to decrease the risk for preeclampsia and can be considered for women with low calcium intake and those at increased risk for preeclampsia. Intravenous magnesium is used to prevent eclamptic seizures and is more effective than both phenytoin and diazepam.

Chronic Hypertension

Epidemiology

Chronic hypertension is present in 1 to 5% of pregnant women. Most cases are due to essential hypertension. For the unusual individual with secondary hypertension, causes include intrinsic renal disease, renal artery stenosis, aortic coarctation, connective tissue diseases, and Cushing's disease.

Although fewer than 250 cases have been reported, pheochromocytoma during pregnancy produces significant morbidity and mortality. Its features (headache, excessive perspiration, and palpitations) overlap those of pregnancy, and measurement of urinary catecholamines is indicated for all women with newly diagnosed hypertension before 34 weeks of pregnancy.

Treatment

Women with chronic hypertension who are considering pregnancy should not receive angiotensin-converting enzyme inhibitors or receptor blockers. Among women with preexisting hypertension, the usual blood pressure decrease during the first trimester often allows discontinuation of antihypertensive medications. Pharmacologic treatment has not been shown to prevent preeclampsia or improve pregnancy outcome. Accordingly, blood pressure can be monitored and medications reinstituted if needed at a threshold of 150 to 160/100 mm Hg. Chronic hypertension newly diagnosed during pregnancy can be differentiated from transient gestational hypertension in that the former persists more than 3 months postpartum.

Prognosis

Although the majority of hypertensive women have uncomplicated pregnancies, the risk for abruptio placentae, intrauterine growth restriction, preterm delivery, perinatal death, and superimposed preeclampsia is increased. The preeclampsia rate varies with the severity of hypertension, with some series reporting an incidence of more than 50%. For women with mild hypertension, however, the incidence is approximately 15%. Women with chronic hypertension, especially those with long-standing disease and coincident additional medical problems, are evaluated at least twice weekly during gestation, often with additional home blood pressure monitoring. Superimposed preeclampsia is suggested by a sudden increase in blood pressure, elevations to greater than 160/110 mm Hg, new or worsening proteinuria, and new laboratory abnormalities, including a platelet count less than 100,000/mm^3, abnormal liver enzymes, and creatinine level increasing to more than 1.2 mg/dL.

TABLE 259–1 ANTIHYPERTENSIVE DRUG USE DURING PREGNANCY

Medication	Safety of Use during Pregnancy	Comments
CENTRAL SYMPATHOLYTIC		
Methyldopa	++++	Extensive use, most studied, and best safety record of any antihypertensive used during pregnancy. It reduces vascular resistance while preserving maternal cardiac output and uteroplacental perfusion. Considered safe to use when breast-feeding
Clonidine	+++	Not assessed for chronic hypertension during pregnancy. No adverse effects when used for hypertension during the third trimester. Potential for rebound when discontinued abruptly
α- AND β-BLOCKERS		
Labetalol	++++	Used in several trials without adverse effects. α-Blocking results in vasodilation (including uteroplacental blood vessels), and β-blockade prevents reflex tachycardia. Cardiac output is unchanged. Low concentration in breast milk
β-BLOCKERS		
Atenolol, metoprolol, pindolol, propranolol	+++	Probably safe for third-trimester use, but neonatal bradycardia, respiratory distress, and hypoglycemia have been reported. Use earlier in gestation may result in intrauterine growth retardation. Atenolol and metoprolol are concentrated in breast milk; propranolol has low concentrations in breast milk
DIRECT ARTERIAL VASODILATOR		
Hydralazine	++++	Extensively used during pregnancy. It causes vascular dilation and reflex tachycardia. Primarily used parenterally for acute management of hypertension or with methyldopa or a β-blocking agent
CALCIUM-CHANNEL BLOCKERS		
Nifedipine (most commonly used because of its primarily peripheral effects), diltiazem, verapamil	+++	Probably safely used in the third trimester. Their use maintains uteroplacental perfusion; may also have tocolytic effects. Sublingual nifedipine has been associated with hypotension and fetal distress. Avoid use with magnesium sulfate because combination risks profound hypotension
DIURETICS		
Hydrochlorothiazide, chlorthalidone, furosemide	++	Use during pregnancy is controversial and often discontinued as blood pressure decreases early in pregnancy. If used before pregnancy, it can be continued, but its use should not be initiated during pregnancy. Concentrations in breast milk are low. May reduce milk production
ANGIOTENSIN-CONVERTING ENZYME INHIBITORS AND ANGIOTENSIN II RECEPTOR BLOCKERS		
Captopril, lisinopril, benazepril, enalapril, losartan, valsartan, candesartan	0	Use is contraindicated during pregnancy because it affects renal development in the second and third trimesters. Miscarriage, fetal death, malformations, and neonatal renal failure can result. No reports of adverse effects from brief use, limited to the first trimester. Few data on the effects of angiotensin II receptor antagonists, but presumed similar and also contraindicated

Drugs listed have established effects during pregnancy. Antihypertensive agents not listed may be safe during pregnancy; however, until safety is known, those drugs should be switched to one of the safely used listed agents.

CARDIAC DISEASE

Epidemiology

The prevalence of heart disease during pregnancy is approximately 1%. In Western countries, congenital problems have surpassed rheumatic heart disease as its most common cause. (The chapters in Section VIII discuss cardiovascular disease in detail, and in particular, adult congenital heart disease is discussed in Chapter 68.)

Pathobiology

Understanding the hemodynamic changes during normal pregnancy permits interpretation of the history and physical examination findings and anticipation of pregnancy's effect on preexisting cardiac abnormalities. During gestation, cardiac output increases 30 to 50%, with a peak near week 27. This increased output is due to increases in heart rate and stroke volume, plus a decrease in systemic vascular resistance. Blood volume also expands, and the greater increase in plasma volume than red blood cell mass results in the physiologic anemia of pregnancy.

A woman's previous cardiac functional status is a guide to the effects of pregnancy. Women with New York Heart Association Functional Class I or II disease (no symptoms with normal daily activities) can usually withstand pregnancy. Because of the decreased systemic vascular resistance, regurgitant lesions are tolerated better than stenotic abnormalities. At greatest risk are women with pulmonary hypertension (either primary or Eisenmenger's syndrome) with limitations in right-sided output. The mortality rate during pregnancy in this last group approaches 50%.

Clinical Manifestations

Normal pregnancy results in effects that can mimic heart disease. More than half of normal pregnant women report dyspnea. Physical findings of heart disease are also common during pregnancy. The increased stroke volume results in a systolic flow murmur in the majority of pregnant women, and an S_3 is also audible in a significant percentage. The electrocardiogram can show anterior T wave changes as a result of the heart's leftward rotation late in gestation. However, clinical findings should not be dismissed because the additional cardiac demands of pregnancy may also worsen previously unrecognized problems. Echocardiography, including transesophageal studies, is well tolerated, retains its utility, and may be needed to characterize abnormal findings during pregnancy.

Treatment

Rx

Pregnancy is proarrhythmic, and both atrial and ventricular ectopy increases. Among women with structurally normal hearts, premature contractions are benign and managed expectantly. Drug therapy is needed only for intolerable symptoms or threats to maternal or fetal well-being. The therapy for most arrhythmias is not altered during pregnancy. Most antiarrhythmic drugs are not contraindicated during pregnancy, and cardioversion does not present an increased risk for the mother or fetus. Adenosine can be used safely for terminating atrioventricular node–dependent tachyarrhythmias. Most class I agents are also safe. The digoxin dosage usually requires an increase because of the reduced protein binding and increased renal excretion during pregnancy. Amiodarone should be avoided during gestation. As with most antiarrhythmic drugs, it crosses the placenta and can cause fetal goiter, growth retardation, and neonatal hypothyroidism. β-Blocker and calcium-channel blocker use is discussed in the preceding section on hypertension.

Certain cardiac abnormalities pose unique considerations. For women with Marfan syndrome, pregnancy's connective tissue changes and hyperdynamic state can increase their risk for aortic dissection. However, with β-blockers and follow-up echocardiograms during pregnancy, the risk is acceptably low when the prepregnancy aortic diameter is less than 4.0 cm. Women with repaired aortic coarctation usually have successful pregnancies and an incidence of preeclampsia similar to that of the general population when the difference in arm and leg blood pressure is less than 20 mm Hg. Ischemic cardiac disease is rare during gestation, with a prevalence of 1 in 10,000 pregnancies. When present, it is usually associated with cocaine use or accelerated atherosclerotic vascular disease (e.g., long-standing type 1 diabetes or untreated hyperlipidemia).

Peripartum cardiomyopathy is defined as the onset of global dilated cardiomyopathy during the third trimester to 6 months postpartum. Its prevalence is 1 in 4000 pregnancies. Risk factors for peripartum cardiomyopathy include obesity, African American heritage, and multiple previous pregnancies. Its cause is not understood, and the prognosis is variable. Overall, approximately a third of patients stabilize, a third progress, and a third improve. Both recurrence and normal outcomes have been described with subsequent pregnancies.

Prognosis

A retrospective review of 276 pregnancies in 221 women with heart disease (excluding isolated mitral valve prolapse) showed that 96% of individuals had functional class I or II disease. Overall, approximately 25% of pregnancies resulted in an adverse cardiac event in the mother or neonate (or both). Based on clinical and echocardiographic assessment, independent predictors of cardiac problems during pregnancy were prior cardiac events, previous arrhythmias, functional class greater than II, left-sided heart obstruction, and myocardial dysfunction. With none, one, or more than one of these five factors, the rate of maternal events was 3, 30, and 66%, respectively. These predictors have not been prospectively validated, and few women with certain cardiac problems were included in the cohort. However, the results are consistent with pregnancy's hemodynamic changes and can be combined with lesion-specific considerations when one advises women with heart disease about the risk of pregnancy.

An additional prognostic consideration for women with congenital heart disease is the risk of similar problems arising in their children because congenital heart disease is six times more likely in their offspring, or a risk of approximately 10%. However, because this rate varies with different abnormalities, referral for genetic counseling is appropriate.

THROMBOEMBOLIC DISEASE

Epidemiology

Thrombotic disorders are discussed in Chapter 182, and pulmonary embolism is the topic of Chapter 99. Thromboembolism (deep venous thrombosis [DVT] and pulmonary embolism) is uncommon during pregnancy, with a prevalence of approximately 1 per 1500 pregnancies and the greatest risk during the days postpartum. Death from pulmonary embolism is one of the leading causes of maternal mortality and occurs in 2 or 3 women per 100,000 births.

Pathobiology

Pregnancy results in physical and biochemical changes that increase clot formation. During gestation, the venous system dilates, and stasis is increased by venous obstruction from the gravid uterus. Plasma concentrations of coagulation factors, fibrinolysis inhibitors, and procoagulants shift to promote coagulation. Women with a hereditary thrombophilic disorder (such as activated protein C resistance, protein C and S deficiency, factor V mutations, and antithrombin III deficiency) have high rates of thrombosis during pregnancy.

Antiphospholipid antibodies result in platelet activation and, despite these patients' prolonged partial thromboplastin time, lead to thrombosis. During pregnancy, these patients are prone to placental thrombosis and infarction, which causes recurrent pregnancy loss, intrauterine growth retardation, fetal death, severe preeclampsia, and maternal arterial and venous thromboembolism.

Clinical Manifestations

The symptoms and signs of DVT and pulmonary embolism retain their low sensitivity and specificity during pregnancy, and findings are limited further by the fact that lower extremity edema is a feature of many normal pregnancies. In addition, for unexplained reasons the pulmonary alveolar-arterial oxygen gradient may be normal in more than 50% of pregnant women with documented pulmonary emboli. This percentage is much greater than the rate of 2 to 20% observed in nonpregnant patients. Patient position should be noted when arterial blood gases are measured because during the third trimester, arterial P_{O_2} is approximately 15 mm Hg higher when the subject is sitting than when the subject is supine.

Diagnosis

Pregnancy does not alter the range of diagnostic options for DVT and pulmonary embolism, which include noninvasive lower extremity studies (e.g., compression ultrasonography, Doppler studies, and impedance plethysmography), lung ventilation-perfusion scanning, computed tomography, magnetic resonance imaging, and pulmonary angiography. The operating characteristics of noninvasive studies of the lower extremities appear to be similar to the results in nonpregnant women, provided that the women are evaluated in the lateral decubitus position to minimize the effects of the gravid uterus. Magnetic resonance imaging has been used successfully to detect iliac and ovarian vein thrombosis during pregnancy.

D-dimer levels may be elevated during pregnancy, particularly with concomitant problems such as preeclampsia. However, a low level suggests the absence of venous thrombosis.

Fetal radiation exposure is a consideration when selecting diagnostic tests, and most procedures can be performed with minimal risk. Ventilation-perfusion scanning is a sensitive, but not specific test for pulmonary emboli. A normal scan effectively excludes the diagnosis. However, low- and indeterminate-probability scans are frequent and necessitate additional testing. Ventilation-perfusion lung scans result in fetal radiation exposure of approximately 40 mrad. Fetal exposure during helical computed tomography depends on the height of the uterus and how low on the lung images are obtained. The radiation exposure to the fetus can be up to 200 mrad but is often less than 20 mrad and comparable to ventilation-perfusion scanning. Pulmonary angiography is the "gold standard" means of diagnosing pulmonary emboli. Its use (by the brachial route with appropriate shielding) exposes the fetus to approximately 100 mrad. This is a low amount of radiation; for comparison, fetal exposure during plain abdominal radiography is 240 mrad.

Treatment

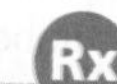

Traditional therapy for thromboemboli has been initial anticoagulation with intravenous unfractionated heparin, followed by oral anticoagulation with warfarin (Coumadin). Warfarin causes an embryopathy, especially if used between the 6th and 12th weeks, and as a result, its use is avoided at that time. Heparin contains large charged molecules that do not cross the placenta. A more uniform dose response, reduced need for monitoring, and lower complication rates, including risk for thrombocytopenia and osteoporosis, have resulted in low-molecular-weight (LMW) heparin replacing unfractionated heparin. LMW heparin is usually administered at a dose of 1 mg/kg twice daily, and anti–factor Xa levels should be obtained 4 hours after the third dose to monitor therapy. The dose should be reassessed every 2 to 4 weeks until delivery.

During labor and delivery, subcutaneous dosing can be withheld for 24 hours or changed to low-dose intravenous heparin (500 U/hr). Eight hours after delivery, subcutaneous LMW heparin therapy can be resumed and continued for an additional 12 weeks. Alternatively, warfarin can be started the evening of delivery, overlapped with heparin therapy, and monitored as usual. Women may breast-feed safely while taking warfarin because only an inactive metabolite is excreted into breast milk.

Risks associated with heparin therapy include thrombocytopenia, a finding that also raises concern about preeclampsia and osteopenia. Heparin-associated osteoporosis can occur when individuals receive more than 3 months of heparin therapy, and that risk may be less with LMW heparin than with unfractionated heparin.

Prevention

Women with DVT during pregnancy should be evaluated for a hypercoagulable state, and because pregnancy also affects these results, interpretation of test results may require expert consultation. When a woman has experienced a previous DVT during pregnancy, has a hereditary thrombophilic disorder, or has antiphospholipid antibodies, her risk for DVT during pregnancy is increased significantly. The indications for and preferred method of prophylaxis have not been established. Subcutaneous unfractionated heparin has been used at a dose of 5000 to 7500 U twice a day. For prophylaxis, the heparin level (measured as anti-factor X_a activity) should be 0.08 to 0.20 U/mL, measured 3 hours after an injection. Often, the dose must be increased by 2500 U each trimester to achieve that level. More recently, LMW heparin has been replacing this therapy. For example, enoxaparin and dalteparin in doses comparable to surgical prophylaxis or dose-adjusted LMW heparin to achieve anti-X_a levels of 0.2 to 0.6 U/mL have been used. Management of pregnant women with antiphospholipid antibodies is dependent on the presence of previous problems and associated conditions. At a minimum, low-dose acetylsalicylic acid is administered. Aspirin and prophylactic heparin may be given if the woman has experienced thromboembolic problems during a previous pregnancy, and for some women intravenous immunoglobulin G also may be a therapeutic consideration. Individualized management is needed for these high-risk patients.

ASTHMA

Epidemiology

Asthma (Chapter 87) is the most common chronic respiratory illness during pregnancy, with a prevalence of 3 to 8%.

Clinical Manifestations

In general, pulmonary function does not change during gestation, including forced expiratory volume in 1 second and peak expiratory flow rate. The course of asthma during pregnancy is variable and cannot be predicted from patient characteristics. Overall, a third of women with asthma remain stable, a third improve, and a third worsen. Those with more severe disease and a history of previous exacerbation during pregnancy are at greater risk for deterioration during gestation. This unpredictable course necessitates that all women with asthma be monitored more closely when pregnant.

Treatment

Management is similar to the usual stepwise approach to caring for individuals with asthma. Table 259–2 lists therapies commonly prescribed for asthma, with comments about their use during pregnancy. Up to 50% of women with asthma do not require drug treatment during pregnancy. When indicated, medication use is similar to that in nonpregnant individuals. Inhaled and oral β_2-agonists can be used during pregnancy. These agents are tocolytic in higher doses and rarely have been reported to inhibit labor. Inhaled cromolyn sodium can be continued. Theophylline crosses the placenta, but other than rare reports of newborn jitteriness, it is used safely during pregnancy. Because its clearance is reduced as pregnancy progresses, serum levels should be monitored. Values of 5 to 12 μg/mL are optimal during pregnancy. Branded products are preferred to reduce variability in absorption. The use of leukotriene modifiers is limited to a few cases; animal studies also raise concern about the use of zileuton.

Exacerbations of asthma should be treated early and aggressively, with a lower threshold for hospitalization. Maternal hypoxia, hypocapnia, and alkalemia are detrimental to the fetus. Oxygen is needed if maternal pulse oximetry is less than 95% or if Pao_2 is less than 75 mm Hg. Fetal well-being should be assessed continuously with an external electronic monitor. The typical triggers for worsening of asthma are respiratory infection and gastroesophageal reflux. Hormonal changes during pregnancy relax the lower esophageal sphincter, and more than a third of pregnant women experience reflux symptoms. Histamine H_2-receptor antagonists, other than nizatidine, are used safely during pregnancy, and ranitidine is the preferred drug. Experience with proton pump inhibitor use during gestation is limited. Although they appear to be safe, their use is reserved for those whose symptoms fail to be relieved with H_2-blockers. Allergic rhinitis can be managed with intranasal corticosteroids and second-generation antihistamines. The rate of sinusitis is six times greater during pregnancy, and because it may not be manifested with its usual findings, a higher index of suspicion is needed. During pregnancy, bronchopulmonary infections can be treated with erythromycin (avoiding the estolate esters), penicillins, and first- and second-generation cephalosporins. Azithromycin is an alternative for patients who cannot use penicillins and cephalosporins. Tetracycline, trimethoprim-sulfamethoxazole, and fluoroquinolones are contraindicated.

TABLE 259–2 DRUG TREATMENT OF ASTHMA DURING PREGNANCY

Therapy	Comments
Desensitization or immunotherapy ("allergy shots")	Ongoing therapy can be continued. However, skin testing, initiating treatment, and increasing therapy should be avoided. Reducing exposure to environmental irritants and allergens remains important.
Antihistamines (chlorpheniramine and tripelennamine preferred and nonsedating agents used when sedation must be minimized)	More information is available for older antihistamines. Recommendations for newer agents, with less sedation, are based on limited animal and human data.
Disodium cromoglycate and nedocromil	Less than 10% of the drug is absorbed. No reported adverse effects from use during pregnancy.
Theophylline	Distribution and clearance are altered during pregnancy, and levels should be checked monthly. It crosses the placenta; rarely, neonatal toxicity has been reported despite therapeutic maternal levels.
β-Agonists (albuterol, metaproterenol, terbutaline; no data on salmeterol)	Use is safe during pregnancy. Rare reports of tocolytic effects.
Inhaled ipratropium	Little data on use during pregnancy, although it is probably safe.
Antileukotriene (zafirlukast, montelukast, zileuton)	No human information; zileuton had adverse effects in animal studies and is not recommended for use during pregnancy.
Inhaled corticosteroids (beclomethasone and budesonide best studied)	Regular use reduces asthma exacerbations during pregnancy.
Oral corticosteroids	May be used safely when indicated. Ninety percent of prednisone is inactivated by the placenta, thus reducing fetal exposure. Betamethasone does not undergo placental 11-oxidation and is the preferred corticosteroid when promoting fetal lung maturation.

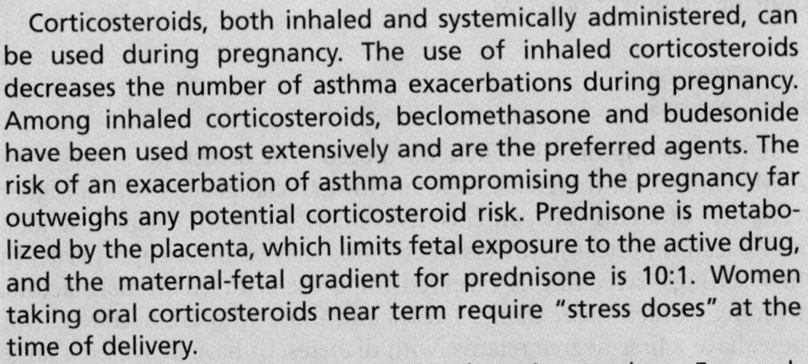

Rx

Corticosteroids, both inhaled and systemically administered, can be used during pregnancy. The use of inhaled corticosteroids decreases the number of asthma exacerbations during pregnancy. Among inhaled corticosteroids, beclomethasone and budesonide have been used most extensively and are the preferred agents. The risk of an exacerbation of asthma compromising the pregnancy far outweighs any potential corticosteroid risk. Prednisone is metabolized by the placenta, which limits fetal exposure to the active drug, and the maternal-fetal gradient for prednisone is 10:1. Women taking oral corticosteroids near term require "stress doses" at the time of delivery.

Asthma treatment is not altered in lactating mothers. For medications used to treat reactive airway disease, the amount reaching an infant through breast milk is less than exposure before birth through the placenta. Corticosteroids are largely protein bound, and their use does not contraindicate breast-feeding.

Prognosis

With current therapy and avoidance of hypoxia, the maternal and fetal morbidity associated with asthma is usually low. The risk for antepartum and postpartum hemorrhage is increased slightly, and gestational hypertension is more likely to develop in women requiring corticosteroids. The offspring of asthmatic women are more susceptible to hyperbilirubinemia.

THYROID DISORDERS (See Chapter 244)

The placenta is impermeable to thyroid hormones and thyroid-stimulating hormone (TSH), and the fetus independently produces and regulates its thyroid hormone levels. The critical period for thyroid hormone's effects on fetal brain maturation is 1 month before birth through the first year of life. Pregnancy alters certain indices of maternal thyroid function. Thyroid-binding globulin increases during gestation, thereby leading to an elevation in total thyroxine and decreased triiodothyronine resin uptake. However, free thyroxine and the calculated thyroid index accurately reflect thyroid function during pregnancy. TSH levels are altered only slightly and remain a useful means of screening for hypothyroidism and for assessing the adequacy of thyroid hormone replacement therapy.

Hypothyroidism

Epidemiology

Hypothyroidism is frequently associated with anovulation and thus results in reduced fertility. Hence, the coexistence of untreated hypothyroidism and pregnancy is rare.

Treatment

Rx

Women undergoing thyroid replacement therapy should have their TSH levels monitored each trimester. Approximately 20% will require a dose increase during pregnancy. Absorption of levothyroxine is inhibited by iron, and women should be reminded to let at least 2 hours pass between taking thyroid replacement medicine and prenatal vitamins, which contain additional iron.

Hyperthyroidism

Epidemiology

Hyperthyroidism develops during 0.02 to 0.3% of pregnancies, and it follows diabetes as the most common endocrine disorder during pregnancy.

Etiology

Women who are hyperthyroid during pregnancy are presumed to have Graves' disease. hCG and TSH share the same β subunit, and hCG weakly cross-reacts with TSH. This resemblance is of clinical importance with a molar pregnancy, during which extremely high hCG levels can be a rare cause of hyperthyroidism.

Clinical Manifestations

Certain findings of hyperthyroidism (e.g., tachycardia, sensation of warmth, fatigue) are features of a normal pregnancy. Rather than the traditional symptom of weight loss, hyperthyroidism during pregnancy can cause inappropriately low weight gain. Treating gestational hyperthyroidism significantly improves maternal and fetal outcomes. Thus, a low threshold for performing thyroid function tests is appropriate.

Treatment

Rx

Thyroid scanning is contraindicated during pregnancy. A hyperthyroid pregnant woman is treated medically with propylthiouracil (PTU) or methimazole. Radioactive iodine is absolutely contraindicated during pregnancy because it will also affect the fetus. Surgical treatment of hyperthyroidism is reserved for the unusual individual who has complications from medical therapy.

In the United States, medical therapy is generally initiated with a PTU dose of 100 mg three times a day. PTU is preferred because of the rare report of aplasia cutis with methimazole and the lower placental permeability of PTU. β-Blockers may be necessary transiently to control the initial symptoms. PTU treatment usually reduces the thyroid hormone level within 3 to 4 weeks, at which time the dose can generally be reduced. Thyroid function is monitored monthly, and the therapeutic goal is the lowest PTU dose needed to maintain maternal thyroid hormone levels in the high-normal range.

PTU crosses the placenta, whereas thyroid hormones and TSH do not. Infants are at risk for a neonatal goiter when the prenatal PTU dosage is more than 100 mg/day. Because of the "immunosuppression" of pregnancy, tapering the PTU dose is usually possible later in pregnancy, and approximately a third of women can discontinue PTU therapy in the last trimester. PTU (at a dose less than 450 mg/day) and methimazole (up to 20 mg/day) appear to be safe with breast-feeding. To minimize potential effects, the mother should take antithyroid drugs just after breast-feeding.

Prognosis

Graves' disease may become worse postpartum. Because fetal exposure is no longer a consideration, many clinicians empirically increase the PTU dose after delivery. Neonatal Graves' disease is uncommon and occurs in approximately 2% of offspring. Because of residual effects of maternal PTU, the disorder may not be apparent at birth and may be manifested 2 weeks after delivery. Assessment of thyroid-stimulating immunoglobulin in mothers with existing or previous Graves' disease is appropriate because levels greater than three times control values are predictive of fetal hyperthyroidism.

Postpartum Thyroid Dysfunction

Epidemiology

Postpartum thyroid dysfunction occurs in 5 to 10% of pregnancies. Risk is increased with a family or personal history of postpartum thyroid dysfunction, a goiter (which is not normally present during pregnancy), and the presence of antimicrosomal antibodies. The recurrence rate in subsequent pregnancies is approximately 50%.

Pathobiology

Postpartum thyroid dysfunction is associated with a "flare" of the woman's preexisting autoimmune thyroid disease. Transient hyperthyroidism associated with low iodine uptake (avoid thyroid scanning if breast-feeding) typically develops in affected individuals 6 to 12 weeks after delivery.

Treatment

Because the hyperthyroidism is self-limited, the usual treatment is symptomatic and consists of β-blockers. Hyperthyroidism is generally followed by hypothyroidism, and that condition is also often temporary. Despite the hypothyroidism not being permanent, thyroid hormone replacement should not be withheld. Six months after initiating replacement, it is appropriate to taper and attempt to discontinue therapy.

Prognosis

For some individuals, the hypothyroidism will be permanent.

DIABETES MELLITUS

Epidemiology

Diabetes (Chapters 247 and 248) is present in 5% of pregnant women, more than 90% of whom have gestational diabetes mellitus (GDM). GDM is defined as glucose intolerance detected during pregnancy, and it is the most common medical complication of pregnancy.

Pathobiology

Pregnancy is characterized by insulin resistance, which begins in the second trimester and increases to term. Decreased maternal responsiveness to insulin may have a role in providing carbohydrates to the fetus because maternal metabolism is shifted toward greater use of lipids. Both greater resistance to insulin and inadequate beta cell function contribute to the development of GDM.

Diagnosis

GDM is asymptomatic when diagnosed. The screening strategy for GDM remains controversial. Among ethnic/racial groups with a higher prevalence of GDM (Hispanic, Native American, Asian, Pacific Islander, and African American), universal screening may be most appropriate. In other settings, screening is reserved for those with GDM risk factors, including women older than 25 years and those who are overweight or obese, have a first-degree relative with diabetes, or have delivered a large infant (more than 9 lb at birth). The screening usually occurs at 24 to 28 weeks' gestation with a glucose measurement obtained 1 hour after the ingestion of 50 g of oral glucose. A serum glucose level greater than 140 mg/dL or whole blood glucose level greater than 170 mg/dL is considered positive. This cutoff value is 90% sensitive and 80% specific, and a 100-g 3-hour glucose tolerance test is used to confirm the presence of GDM.

With the rising prevalence of type 2 diabetes, its prevalence is equal to that of type 1 diabetes in pregnant women with preexisting diabetes. White's classification stratified diabetic women's pregnancy risks according to the duration of diabetes and the presence of retinopathy, nephropathy, or heart disease. This classification has been simplified to uncomplicated type 1 and type 2 diabetes and those with hypertension or any diabetes-associated complication.

Risk Assessment

Risk factors for maternal morbidity and relative contraindications to pregnancy include established renal disease (creatinine greater than 2.0 mg/dL or proteinuria of more than 2 g/day), uncontrolled hypertension, severe gastroparesis, and atherosclerotic vascular disease. If creatinine clearance is less than 80 mL/min or proteinuria is greater than 2 g/day, up to 50% of women will experience permanent further renal impairment during pregnancy. Because diabetic retinopathy progresses in 10 to 50% of pregnant women, an ophthalmologist should examine patients before pregnancy and each trimester.

Treatment

Rx

"Tight" blood glucose control begins before conception because organogenesis occurs early in the first trimester and tighter blood sugar control may decrease the incidence of congenital malformations and miscarriages. Hemoglobin A_{1c} should be normal for at least 2 months before conception. Both angiotensin-converting enzyme inhibitors and receptor blockers should be discontinued because of their potential teratogenic effects. Measurement of urinary protein and creatinine, along with an ophthalmologic examination, is appropriate.

When pregnancy is diagnosed during a period of overt hyperglycemia associated with existing or newly diagnosed diabetes, hospitalization for rapid metabolic correction may be appropriate. Therapeutic goals are fasting blood glucose values of less than 90 mg/dL and 1-hour postprandial values of less than 120 to 140 mg/dL. Women must be able to participate in intensified monitoring, including measuring their blood glucose several times per day (fasting, after meals, evening, and middle of the night when morning values are elevated).

General Measures

Dietary therapy is the initial management of those with GDM. The recommended diet during gestation is 30 to 35 kcal/kg/day based on ideal body weight, with a composition of 40 to 50% carbohydrate, 20% protein, and 30 to 40% fat. Calories are divided into three meals and three snacks a day, with calories partitioned as 10% at breakfast, 30% at lunch, 30% at dinner, and 10% during each snack. Reducing breakfast calories, when insulin resistance is greatest, decreasing the percentage of calories from carbohydrates, and avoiding foods with a high glycemic index can lower maternal glucose levels. With GDM, low-intensity aerobic exercise may reduce maternal glucose levels and is advised, as long as it is not contraindicated for medical or obstetric reasons. Mild caloric restriction to an intake of 25 kcal/kg actual weight per day is appropriate for obese women with GDM. Excessive caloric restriction should be avoided. Ketonemia adversely affects the fetus, and care must be taken to prevent starvation ketosis.

Medical Therapy

Approximately 15% of women with GDM will have fasting glucose levels higher than 105 mg/dL on two occasions and require additional therapy. When nutritional therapy is inadequate, human insulin is the standard treatment, and the usual initial dose is 0.7 U/kg (based on prepregnancy weight), administered as a combination of short- and intermediate-acting insulin given in two to four injections per day to reach the fasting and postprandial target levels.

Older sulfonylureas, such as chlorpropamide and tolbutamide, cross the placenta and were contraindicated during pregnancy. However, second-generation oral hypoglycemic agents, such as glyburide, do not cross the placenta and have been used in pregnancy. In general, the control achieved may be comparable to that with insulin therapy. Their use seems to be safe and as effective as insulin therapy. However, before groups such as the American Diabetes Association and American College of Obstetricians and Gynecologists recommend such therapy, more experience is needed to exclude rare, but clinically important adverse effects.

For women already taking insulin, their requirements usually decrease slightly during the first trimester and then increase until term. During the ninth month, insulin needs are approximately 50% greater than at preconception, and the increase is greater in patients with type 2 diabetes, for whom the additional insulin resistance of pregnancy may increase requirements up to 2 U/kg/day.

Insulin requirements decrease after delivery, and a week postpartum, insulin needs are reduced by approximately 50%. To avoid hypoglycemia, intravenous glucose should be constantly infused, with hourly glucose monitoring. Women with GDM usually normalize their blood glucose immediately postpartum, and follow-up fasting glucose values should be obtained after approximately 2 months to reassess glucose status. Breast-feeding generally improves glycemic control and should be encouraged.

Prognosis

Most women with uncomplicated type 2 diabetes do well during pregnancy. However, maternal risks (including accelerated retinopathy, preeclampsia, and pyelonephritis), sudden fetal death, and perinatal mortality are slightly increased. Despite careful management, congenital malformations complicate 6 to 10% of pregnancies in diabetic women.

Two thirds of women with GDM will have a recurrence in subsequent pregnancies, and diabetes will develop in up to 50% over the next 15 years. Maintaining optimal weight and regular physical activity should be encouraged to reduce this risk.

HEPATIC DISEASE

Most liver function test results are unchanged by pregnancy. Mean levels of alanine aminotransferase, aspartate aminotransferase, γ-glutamyl transpeptidase, and bilirubin are slightly lower during pregnancy. Alkaline phosphatase, coming primarily from the placenta, increases slowly during the first and second trimesters and rises to four times prepregnant values at term. Because of the expanded plasma volume, the serum albumin value decreases 10 to 50%.

New-Onset Jaundice during Pregnancy

Epidemiology

Jaundice is seen in approximately 1 in 2000 pregnancies. Conditions unique to pregnancy, including gestation-associated life-threatening hepatic disorders, are additional diagnostic considerations. Features of the usual causes of newly occurring jaundice during pregnancy are listed in Table 259–3.

Diagnosis

Approximately half of cases of jaundice during pregnancy are due to viral hepatitis, and episodes are distributed evenly among trimesters. The natural history of most viral hepatitides (types A, B, C, and D) is not altered by pregnancy, nor are their serologic diagnoses changed. Hepatitis B can be transmitted to the newborn at the time of delivery. Treating newborns with hepatitis B immunoglobulin and hepatitis B vaccine can prevent vertical transmission of hepatitis B. Rates of hepatitis C vertical transmission vary, with some figures as high as 36%. Quantitative viral RNA assay may allow stratification of that risk. Women with undetectable levels are unlikely to transmit the infection, whereas those whose titers are greater than 1 million copies per milliliter have the greatest risk. Preventive therapy, as used for hepatitis B, is not available for hepatitis C. Hepatitis E is a water-borne infection that can occur in developing areas after flooding. For reasons that are not understood, the fatality rate in pregnant women with hepatitis E is markedly higher than with other types of hepatitis and reaches 20%.

Other causes of pregnancy-associated jaundice are intrahepatic cholestasis of pregnancy, the HELLP syndrome, hepatic rupture, and acute fatty liver of pregnancy. Each typically occurs in the third trimester. During the first trimester, hyperemesis gravidarum may cause jaundice. However, its clinical manifestations usually suggest the diagnosis, and abnormalities resolve within days of improved nutrition.

Ultrasonography is an important noninvasive assessment tool during pregnancy. It can detect biliary tract disease, duct dilation, and hepatic subcapsular hematomas. In addition, the liver's appearance can suggest fatty infiltration, mass lesions, and cirrhosis. However, although findings of acute fatty liver are helpful, ultrasonography and computed tomography each have low sensitivity in detecting acute fatty liver of pregnancy, and liver biopsy may be needed to confirm that diagnosis.

Cholelithiasis occurs during approximately 5% of pregnancies, and choledocholithiasis accounts for approximately 7% of jaundice during pregnancy. Symptoms of cholelithiasis are not changed by gestation. During the first and second trimesters, laparoscopic cholecystectomy can be performed safely. Uterine enlargement makes surgery more difficult in the third trimester, and endoscopic retrograde cholangiopancreatography and sphincterotomy, performed while minimizing fluoroscopy and with appropriate shielding, has been used successfully in this setting.

TABLE 259–3 CAUSES OF NEW-ONSET JAUNDICE DURING PREGNANCY*

Diagnosis	Prevalence	Symptoms and Signs	Laboratory Findings	Management	Maternal and Fetal Outcome
Viral hepatitis (A, B, C, and D)	Leading cause of jaundice during pregnancy, accounting for half of pregnant women with jaundice. Acute hepatitis B in 2 per 1000 pregnancies and acute A or C in 1 per 1000	Natural history of viral hepatitis is unchanged by pregnancy. The typical symptoms and signs occur. Chronic HBV carriers usually have normal pregnancies, unless they also have chronic hepatitis. Unless cirrhosis is present, chronic hepatitis C does not affect pregnancy, nor does pregnancy influence the natural history of hepatitis C	Serologic diagnosis is not changed with pregnancy. Liver function abnormalities are comparable to those in nonpregnant individuals	Supportive and similar to guidelines for viral hepatitis in nonpregnant patients. Any potential for transmission of HBV at delivery is an indication for passive (hepatitis B immunoglobulin) and active (hepatitis B vaccine) immunization of the newborn. No analogous treatment is available for hepatitis C, but vertical transmission uncommon unless coinfected with HIV virus. Discontinue interferon use	Maternal outcomes with hepatitis A, B, C, and D comparable to outcomes in nonpregnant individuals Newborn concern is potential vertical transmission at the time of delivery
Intrahepatic cholestasis of pregnancy (IHCP)	Second leading cause of jaundice during gestation Occurrence rate varies with ethnicity (e.g., 0.1% of pregnancies in the United States, 20% in pregnant Chilean women, and rare in black women)	Usually in the third trimester, pruritus of the entire body develops, typically beginning with the palms and soles. Twenty percent become jaundiced approximately 2 weeks after the onset of pruritus	Bilirubin not elevated greater than 5 mg/dL, transaminase levels increased 2- to 10-fold, alkaline phosphatase increased 4-fold	Parenteral vitamin K plus ursodeoxycholic acid, which reduces pruritus and liver function abnormalities but has not been proved to alter outcome. Small trials demonstrate no benefits for *S*-adenosylmethionine, dexamethasone, and guar gum	No increase in maternal morbidity but associated with increased prematurity, fetal distress, and perinatal infant death. Resolves 2 days to 2 weeks after delivery. Disorder recurs in 60% of subsequent pregnancies
Preeclampsia with HELLP syndrome (*h*emolysis, *e*levated *l*iver enzymes, and *l*ow *p*latelets) plus the rare occurrence of associated hepatic rupture	Preeclampsia occurs during the late second or third trimesters (usually earlier in gestation than AFLP). HELLP seen in 4–12% of women with preeclampsia. Hepatic rupture seen in 5 per 10,000 pregnancies	Nausea, vomiting, right upper quadrant pain, and other findings of preeclampsia (hypertension [absent in 15%], proteinuria [absent in 10%], hyperreflexia) occur. Acute abdominal pain and shock signal hepatic rupture. Imaging of rupture has been reported with ultrasonography, computed tomography, and magnetic resonance imaging	Transaminases increased 2- to 10-fold, and alkaline phosphatase increased 1 to 10 times normal. Platelets are less than 100,000/mm^3, with microangiopathic hemolytic anemia and disseminated intravascular coagulation. Hemolysis results in elevated bilirubin and lactate dehydrogenase levels	Delivery and other therapeutic measures for preeclampsia. Condition may transiently worsen after delivery, then improve over a period of several days	Maternal mortality is 2%, and prematurity and perinatal mortality occur in 5–30%. Recurrence rate is approximately 5%. Maternal mortality with hepatic rupture is more than 50%, and therapy is supportive, with surgery when needed

Acute fatty liver of pregnancy (AFLP)	Occurs in 1 per 13,000 pregnancies, with onset late in the third trimester	Average age is 30 years, and first pregnancy in 40%. Malaise, nausea, vomiting, epigastric pain; may be findings of hepatic encephalopathy. Right upper quadrant is tender	Transaminase levels increased 1- to 5-fold, and alkaline phosphatase increased 2–8 times normal. Increased international normalized ratio. White blood cell count greater than 15,000; platelets often less than 100,000. Hypoglycemia and disseminated intravascular coagulation may be present. Ultrasonography and computed tomography can suggest AFLP, but sensitivity is less than 50% for that diagnosis	Delivery and supportive care	Maternal mortality and fetal mortality approximately 20%. If mother survives, normal liver function is restored soon after delivery. Based on limited information, usually does not recur during next pregnancy. May be associated with long-chain 3-hydroxyacyl-CoA dehydrogenase deficiency (an error of mitochondrial fatty acid metabolism), and offspring should be screened for its presence
Choledocholithiasis	Accounts for approximately 7% of jaundice during pregnancy	Manifestations are not altered by pregnancy	Laboratory findings similar to those when not pregnant. Ultrasonography can reveal abnormality, with same limitations in visualizing the problem as when not pregnant	Uterine enlargement makes surgery more difficult in the third trimester, and endoscopic retrograde cholangiopancreatography and sphincterotomy, performed while minimizing fluoroscopy and with appropriate shielding, has been used successfully in that setting	If obstruction relieved, maternal and fetal outcomes are not adversely affected by the disorder

*Additional considerations are drug-induced hepatitis, Budd-Chiari syndrome, and preexisting chronic liver disease.

SUGGESTED READINGS

Duley L, Henderson-Smart DJ, Meher S: Drugs for the treatment of very high blood pressure during pregnancy. Cochrane Database Syst Rev 2006;3:CD001449. *Patients given calcium channel blockers rather than hydralazine were less likely to have persistent high blood pressure.*

Kaaja RJ, Greer IA: Manifestations of chronic disease during pregnancy. JAMA 2005;294:2751–2757. *Given the physiologic changes that occur during pregnancy, it is an important screening opportunity for cardiovascular and metabolic disease risk factors.*

Langer O, Yogev Y, Xenakis EMJ, Rosenn B: Insulin and glyburide therapy: Dosage, severity level of gestational diabetes, and pregnancy outcome. Am J Obstet Gynecol 2005;192:134–139. *Outcomes are related to glucose control.*

NAEPP Expert Panel Report: Managing asthma during pregnancy: Recommendations for pharmacologic treatment—2004 update. J Allergy Clin Immunol 2005;115:34–46. *Stepwise therapy and evidence on the safety of medication use.*

Sibai B, Dekker G, Kupferminc M: Pre-eclampsia. Lancet 2005;365:785–799. *Discusses the diagnosis, risk factors, pathogenesis, and management of pre-eclampsia.*

Van Mook WNKA, Peeters L: Severe cardiac disease in pregnancy, part II: Impact of congenital and acquired cardiac diseases during pregnancy. Curr Opin Crit Care 2005;11:435–448. *Recent review of conditions and their management.*

260 HUMAN IMMUNODEFICIENCY VIRUS IN PREGNANCY

Stephen A. Spector

Epidemiology

The World Health Organization and the Joint United Nations Programme on HIV/AIDS (UNAIDS) estimated that by the end of 2004 approximately 40 million people were living with human immunodeficiency virus (HIV) infection, including 1 in every 100 adults in the sexually active ages of 15 to 49 years. Overall, approximately 14,000 new HIV infections occur daily, more than 95% of them in developing countries. In sub-Saharan Africa, 57% of infected persons are women. In the United States, the Centers for Disease Control and Prevention (CDC) reports that approximately 22% of persons living with the acquired immunodeficiency syndrome (AIDS) are women. Women also comprise 27% of those with new infections, and AIDS is the fifth most common cause of death in women between 24 and 44 years of age (Chapter 410).

Pregnant women are at risk of transmitting HIV to their newborns; approximately 25% of exposed infants will become infected unless intervention occurs. The exact timing of HIV transmission from mother to infant is unknown. The best estimate is that in developed countries, approximately one third of infections occur in utero, usually late in pregnancy, and two thirds occur intrapartum. Risk factors for increased mother-to-child transmission include women with low $CD4^+$ lymphocyte counts, high HIV RNA loads, the presence of active sexually transmitted diseases, rupture of amniotic membranes beyond 4 hours, and prematurity of birth. Of all risk factors, plasma HIV RNA load is most important in determining the risk for mother-to-child transmission.

Women can also transmit HIV through their breast milk, and such transmission accounts for one third of all infections in infants in developing countries, where most HIV-infected women breast-feed their infants. In developing countries, the benefits of exclusive breast-feeding are believed by some experts to outweigh the risk of transmission of HIV through milk. Although exclusive breast-feeding may decrease the risk of transmission from an infected mother to her infant, few women are able to maintain a regimen of exclusive breast-feeding. Therefore, most experts believe that substitute feeding should be used whenever possible to prevent mother-to-child transmission of HIV. HIV-infected women in developed countries should be strongly discouraged from breast-feeding their newborns.

Antepartum
ZDV 100 mg 5 × daily PO initiated after 14 wks gestation (preferable alternatives: 200 mg 3 × daily PO or 300 mg 2 × daily PO)

↓

Intrapartum
IV ZDV 1 hr loading of 2 mg/kg followed by continuous infusion of 1 mg/kg/hr until delivery

↓

Postpartum to Infant
ZDV syrup 2 mg/kg every 6 hr for first 6 wks of life beginning 8–12 hr after birth

FIGURE 260–1 • Pediatric AIDS Clinical Trials Group (PACTG 076) zidovudine (ZDV) regimen for prevention of mother-to-infant transmission of human immunodeficiency virus.

Treatment

Rx

Use of Antiretroviral Agents during Pregnancy

Treatment recommendations for HIV-infected pregnant women are based on the premise that therapies known to be of benefit should not be withheld during pregnancy unless they are known to be harmful to the mother or fetus (Chapter 412). Thus, unless specific reasons exist for withholding antiretroviral therapy, pregnant women should be given optimal combination therapy, usually including two reverse transcriptase inhibitors and a protease inhibitor. When possible, one of the reverse transcriptase inhibitors should include zidovudine because it has clearly been demonstrated to decrease vertical transmission and to be safe for mother and infant. In a controlled trial conducted by the Pediatric AIDS Clinical Trials Group (PACTG 076), HIV infection occurred in 25% of infants when the mother and infant received placebo compared with 8% of infants when mother and infant received zidovudine. [1] The treatment regimen used for the PACTG 076 study and the currently used preferable zidovudine regimens are summarized in Figure 260–1. The intervention involves three parts: (1) treatment of the mother with oral zidovudine during pregnancy, (2) administration of intravenous zidovudine during labor, and (3) 6 weeks of oral zidovudine administered to the infant after birth. Each of these three parts is thought to contribute to decreasing transmission, and all three parts of the intervention should be administered whenever possible.

In another study (PACTG 185), blocking mother-to-infant transmission with zidovudine intervention was shown to be even more effective, and the regimen decreased transmission to approximately 5%. [2] The use of HIV-specific immunoglobulin provides no additional benefit over the use of zidovudine alone. A study in Thailand found that mother-to-child transmission can be reduced when women receive zidovudine only in their last month of pregnancy. [3] These data indicate that HIV-infected women identified at any stage of pregnancy should receive zidovudine to decrease the risk of perinatal transmission. However, this approach is suboptimal, and women and infants should minimally receive the full PACTG 076 regimen whenever possible.

The treatment regimen of zidovudine, 100 mg, administered five times daily in the PACTG 076 study was based on the standard dose of zidovudine for adults in 1989. The current recommended dosing for zidovudine of 200 mg three times daily or 300 mg twice daily has been associated with a comparable clinical response and is the recommended dosing schedule for use by pregnant women.

In non–breast-feeding women in Thailand, a short-course regimen of zidovudine consisting of 300 mg twice daily from 36 weeks' gestation and 300 mg administered every 3 hours during labor decreased transmission to 9%. Another study using a four-arm factorial design compared administration of zidovudine antenatally

Rx

starting at 28 or 36 weeks' gestation, orally intrapartum, and to the neonate for 3 days or 6 weeks. The long-long arm (beginning at 28 weeks antenatally and 6 weeks of treatment to the infant) was found to be significantly superior to the other arms of the trial, with a resulting transmission rate of 4%. A third study (performed in Africa) in HIV-infected women of whom 73% breast-fed their infants demonstrated that the combination of zidovudine and lamivudine (3-TC) beginning at 36 weeks gestation, orally intrapartum, and for 1 week postpartum to the mother and infant reduced transmission to 6% for infants at 6 weeks of age. However, with the high rate of breast-feeding, by 18 months of age, 15% of infants were identified as infected, and 19% were infected or had died.

Additional trials have demonstrated that intrapartum and postpartum regimens with either zidovudine and lamivudine or nevirapine are also useful in decreasing transmission when these drugs are administered to an HIV-infected pregnant woman late in pregnancy or while in labor. In an African cohort of women and infants, the intrapartum administration of zidovudine to the mother and postpartum to the breast-feeding mother and infant for 1 week decreased transmission at 6 weeks of age from 17% in the placebo group to 6% in the treated group. In this trial, the administration of zidovudine and lamivudine to the mother alone failed to decrease transmission to the infant. In another study performed in Uganda, the administration of a single 200-mg dose of nevirapine to the mother at onset of labor combined with a single 2 mg/kg dose of nevirapine to her infant at 24 to 72 hours of age reduced transmission at 6 weeks to 12%. 4 The ease of administration and the low cost of single-dose nevirapine given to pregnant women and infants have made this equally good medication 5 the intervention of choice in the developing world for programs targeted at reducing mother-to-child transmission. Recently, concern has been expressed about the risk for the development of HIV strains resistant to nevirapine (and other currently available non-nucleoside reverse transcriptase inhibitors) that may occur in virtually all women who receive single-dose nevirapine. However, most experts currently believe that the risk of resistance is outweighed by the clear benefit of protecting a large proportion of infants from HIV infection. Additionally, preliminary studies suggest that when women or babies are treated with zidovudine in combination with lamivudine for 4 or 7 days, the risk for development of nevirapine-resistant virus can be significantly decreased.

In the United States and other developed countries, combination therapy, usually comprising two nucleoside reverse transcriptase inhibitors and a protease inhibitor, when administered to a woman beginning in the second trimester of pregnancy and combined with intrapartum intravenous zidovudine and 6 weeks of zidovudine administered to the infant, has decreased mother-to-child transmission to less than 2%. The addition of nevirapine was of no further benefit in circumstances in which women receive perinatal care and antenatal antiretroviral therapy and in which cesarean section can be safely performed (PACTG 316).

Optimal medical management of the HIV-infected pregnant woman should include treatment with antiretroviral agents, usually including two nucleoside reverse transcriptase inhibitors and a protease inhibitor, to achieve an HIV plasma RNA load of less than 400 copies/mL. Studies done before the availability of combination antiretroviral therapy generally demonstrated a reduction in HIV mother-to-child transmission when the infant was delivered by cesarean section before rupture of amniotic membranes. More recent data indicate that for women with a plasma HIV RNA load of less than 1000 copies/mL, cesarean section confers no additional benefit. Additionally, nonelective cesarean section performed after the onset of labor or rupture of amniotic membranes has not been associated with a significant reduction in infection in infants when compared with vaginal delivery.

Although the use of antiretroviral agents has been shown to be highly effective in decreasing mother-to-child transmission and in the short term to be safe for both mother and infant, the long-term impact on infants, most of whom are uninfected with HIV, is unknown. Additionally, treatment of women who are likely to become pregnant should take into account the possible consequences to a fetus exposed to these antiretrovirals in utero. For example, efavirenz (Sustiva) was shown in primate studies to be associated with neural tube defects, and several reports have noted babies born with predictable neural tube abnormalities. Because the neural tube closes in the first month of gestation, many women do not know that they are pregnant before the time that damage could occur to the fetus. Another non-nucleoside reverse transcriptase inhibitor, nevirapine, has not been associated with human teratogenicity; however, nevirapine is associated with a rash, as well as an increased risk of symptomatic and potentially fatal liver toxicity. The serious liver toxicity occurs in women with $CD4^+$ lymphocyte counts greater than 250/μL when treatment is first initiated. Thus, nevirapine should be initiated in pregnancy for women with more than 250 cells/μL only if the potential benefits outweigh the risk to the mother. Women who become pregnant while they are receiving nevirapine-containing regimens and who are tolerating the regimen need not discontinue this treatment. Additionally, no toxicity has been observed with the use of single-dose nevirapine to prevent mother-to-child transmission. Thus, a decision to use any antiretroviral therapy during pregnancy should be made by the woman after a thorough discussion of risks and benefits with her health care provider. Infants born to HIV-infected women should be followed by or seen in consultation with health care providers experienced in the care of HIV-infected children. Infants identified as infected should be treated as outlined in the CDC's "Guidelines for the Use of Antiretroviral Agents in Pediatric HIV Infection."

Possible Adjustments to the Standard Care of Women Infected with Human Immunodeficiency Virus

Pregnant Women Infected with Human Immunodeficiency Virus Who Have Not Had Prior Antiretroviral Therapy

The recommendation for antiretroviral therapy should be made after standard clinical, immunologic, and virologic evaluation (see first suggested reading). The three-part zidovudine chemoprophylaxis regimen should be recommended for all pregnant women. If the woman's HIV plasma RNA load is greater than 1000 copies/mL, combination therapy with an additional nucleoside reverse transcriptase inhibitor and a protease inhibitor is recommended. Decisions regarding combination antiretroviral treatment should be made after a full review of risks and benefits of treatment. At present, most HIV experts recommend combination antiretroviral therapy, including zidovudine, although recent studies indicate that other nucleoside reverse transcriptase inhibitors, including didanosine and stavudine, may also provide benefit. Some HIV experts recommend beginning antiretroviral therapy after the first trimester (the period of organogenesis) in an attempt to minimize risk to the fetus. If a woman's HIV disease status has not progressed to meet the current guidelines for initiation of antiretroviral therapy (i.e., her $CD4^+$ lymphocyte count is >350 cells/mL and plasma HIV RNA is <100,000 copies/mL), some experts recommend the discontinuation of therapy after delivery. If HIV treatment is to be discontinued, all antiretroviral agents should be stopped at the same time, to minimize the risk for development of antiretroviral resistance.

Women in Late Pregnancy Who Are Infected with Human Immunodeficiency Virus and Who Are Not Receiving Antiretroviral Therapy

A woman who presents late in pregnancy (>~36 weeks' gestation) should have her plasma HIV RNA level and $CD4^+$ lymphocyte count evaluated. The woman should be started on antiretroviral therapy including at least zidovudine. However, most experts recommend instituting three antiretroviral agents, including two nucleoside reverse transcriptase inhibitors and a protease inhibitor. If the RNA load around the expected delivery date is not less than 1000 copies/mL, an elective cesarean section should be considered. During delivery and postpartum to the infant, the PACTG 076 regimen is recommended.

Women Infected with Human Immunodeficiency Virus Who Have Viral Loads Greater Than 1000 Copies/Ml Despite Receiving Antiretroviral Therapy at 36 Weeks' Gestation

If the plasma HIV RNA load is declining at the time of assay, the current antiretroviral therapy should be continued. However, if the viral load is considerably greater than 1000 copies/mL at 36 weeks' gestation, it is unlikely that it will decline to less than 1000 copies/mL at the time of delivery. The woman should be counseled that elective cesarean section may be of benefit in decreasing the risk of intrapartum transmission. During delivery and postpartum to the infant, the PACTG 076 regimen is recommended.

Pregnant Women Infected with Human Immunodeficiency Virus Who Are Receiving Antiretroviral Therapy

Women receiving antiretroviral therapy and who are identified as being pregnant should continue their current antiretroviral therapy, provided plasma HIV RNA levels are lower than 400 copies/mL. Women who are identified as pregnant during the first trimester should be counseled regarding the potential risks of taking an antiretroviral agent during this period. If therapy is discontinued, all drugs should be stopped and reintroduced at the same time to avoid the development of resistance. If the current antiretroviral regimen does not include zidovudine, substituting zidovudine or adding it to the regimen should be considered after 14 weeks' gestation. If the previous antiretroviral therapy had not resulted in plasma HIV RNA levels lower than 400 copies/mL, a regimen usually consisting of three drugs of at least two different classes including at least two new drugs should be instituted during pregnancy. If resistance testing is available, pregnant women should be prescribed antiretroviral agents to which their virus is known to be susceptible.

Women Infected with Human Immunodeficiency Virus Who Are in Labor and Who Have Had No Prior Therapy

Several treatment options are available for women who present with HIV infection in labor; however, transplacental infection of the fetus may have already occurred. Treatment regimens include administration of intrapartum intravenous zidovudine, followed by the 6-week zidovudine regimen for the newborn. Some experts also add nevirapine in a single dose before delivery to the pregnant woman and following delivery to the infant. Some experts recommend cesarean section before rupture of amniotic membranes in this situation, to prevent intrapartum transmission. The benefit to the infant must be weighed against the potential risk to the mother of a cesarean section. After delivery, the woman should have a full evaluation of her HIV status and, when appropriate, antiretroviral therapy recommended for her own health.

Infants Born to Mothers Who Received No Antiretroviral Therapy during Pregnancy or Intrapartum

The 6-week neonatal course of zidovudine is recommended as soon after birth as possible for infants born to HIV-infected women. Most HIV experts recommend three-drug combination regimens, including two reverse transcriptase inhibitors and an antiprotease compound for 6 weeks. Following delivery, the woman should have a full evaluation of her HIV status and, when appropriate, antiretroviral therapy recommended for her own health. All pregnant women, regardless of plasma HIV RNA load, should be advised that the use of antiretroviral prophylaxis has been found to provide benefit in preventing perinatal transmission.

Follow-Up

Testing and Supportive Care

After delivery, HIV-infected women should receive comprehensive care and support services required for management of their HIV infection and for care of their family. This care should begin before pregnancy, with continuity of care ensured throughout pregnancy and postpartum.

Testing for HIV and counseling are essential to any successful plan for identification and treatment of pregnant women. All pregnant women, regardless of their sexual or social history, should be offered HIV antibody testing (Chapter 408). Patients whose test results are negative should be informed that false-negative results may occur because of the latent phase between HIV exposure and development of antibody. The false-negative rate depends on the prevalence of risk-related behavior in the tested population. Patients whose test result is negative should be encouraged to practice low-risk behavior to minimize their risk of infection. A pregnant woman whose test result is positive should have a confirmatory test performed. After confirmation, the patient should have counseling regarding whether to continue the pregnancy, potential risks to the fetus, and benefits of antiretroviral intervention and treatment for herself and her newborn. After identification of HIV infection, care for the infected woman should be the same as for any other person newly identified as HIV positive. Prophylaxis for opportunistic pathogens and treatment of infections should be recommended as for other persons infected with HIV.

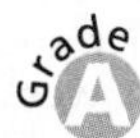

1. Shapiro DE, Sperling RS, Mandelbrot L, et al: Risk factors for perinatal human immunodeficiency virus transmission in patients receiving zidovudine prophylaxis: Pediatric AIDS Clinical Trials Group protocol 076 Study Group. Obstet Gynecol 1999;94: 897–908.
2. Connor EM, Sperling RS, Gelber R, et al: Reduction of maternal-infant transmission of human immunodeficiency virus type 1 with zidovudine treatment. N Engl J Med 1994;331:1173–1180.
3. Lallemant M, Jourdain G, Le Coeur S, et al: A trial of shortened zidovudine regimens to prevent mother-to-child transmission of human immunodeficiency virus type 1. N Engl J Med 2000; 343:982–991.
4. Guay LA, Musoke P, Fleming T, et al: Intrapartum and neonatal single-dose nevirapine compared with zidovudine for prevention of mother-to-child transmission of HIV-1 in Kampala, Uganda: HIVNET 012 randomised trial. Lancet 1999;354:795–802.
5. Volmink J, Siegfried N, van der Merwe L, et al: Antiretrovirals for reducing the risk of mother-to-child transmission of HIV infection. Cochrane Database Syst Rev 2007;1:CD003510.

SUGGESTED READINGS

Centers for Disease Control and Prevention: U.S. Public Health Service Recommendations for the Use of Antiretroviral Drugs in Pregnant Women for Maternal Health and Interventions to Reduce Perinatal HIV-1 Transmission in the United States. Available at www.aidsinfo.nih.gov. *Reviews current guidelines for the use of antiretroviral agents during pregnancy for the health of the mother and for reduction of mother-to-infant transmission of HIV. This is a living document that is continuously being updated.*

Centers for Disease Control and Prevention: U.S. Public Health Service Guidelines for the Use of Antiretroviral Agents in Pediatric HIV Infection. March 2005. Available at www.aidsinfo.nih.gov. *Reviews guidelines for treatment of HIV-infected infants and children. This is a living document that is continuously being updated.*

Centers for Disease Control and Prevention: U.S. Public Health Service Report of the NIH Panel to Define Principles of Therapy of HIV Infection and Guidelines for the Use of Antiretroviral Agents in HIV-Infected Adults and Adolescents. April 2005. Available at www.aidsinfo.nih.gov. *Reviews principles and guidelines for treatment of HIV-infected adults and adolescents. This is a living document that is continuously being updated.*

Chou R, Smits AK, Huffman LH, et al: Prenatal screening for HIV: A review of the evidence for the U.S. Preventive Services Task Force. Ann Intern Med 2005;143:38–54. *Review of evidence supporting routine screening for HIV in pregnancy.*

Lockman S, Shapiro RL, Smeaton LM, et al: Response to antiretroviral therapy after a single, peripartum dose of nevirapine. N Engl J Med 2007;356:135–147. *Increased resistance to nevirapine-based regimens occurs only when antiretroviral therapy is begun within 6 months of peripartum treatment.*

Richardson BA, John-Stewart GC, Hughes JP, et al: Breast-milk infectivity in human immunodeficiency virus type 1-infected mothers. J Infect Dis 2003;187:736–740. *This study demonstrated that the risk of transmission of HIV depends on the viral load within breast milk and not on infant age.*

UNAIDS/World Health Organization (WHO): AIDS Epidemic Update 2001. Available at www.unaids.org. *Reviews worldwide AIDS epidemic to December 2002.*

261 HIRSUTISM

Ricardo Azziz

Definition

Hirsutism is defined as the presence of terminal (coarse) hairs in women in a male-like pattern, and it affects between 5 and 22% of women. Hirsutism is often a sign of an androgen excess disorder, including the polycystic ovary syndrome (PCOS), nonclassic adrenal hyperplasia (NCAH), the hyperandrogenic insulin-resistant acanthosis nigricans syndrome, and androgenic-secreting tumors (ASNs), or more rarely the use or abuse of androgenic drugs. Nonetheless, in some patients the presence of hirsutism may not reflect central dysfunction in androgen production or metabolism, and rather it may result from increased skin sensitivity to normal circulating androgens, such as in idiopathic hirsutism (IH).

Physiology

Normal Hair Physiology

Hair is composed of a column of keratinized melanocytes (keratinocytes) forming the hair shaft, which grows within the outer hair root sheath (Fig. 261–1). Structurally, the three types of hair are *lanugo, vellus,* and *terminal* hairs. Terminal hairs make up the eyebrows, the eyelashes, and the scalp, pubic and axillary hair, and when present in an excessive or male-like pattern in women, they represent hirsutism

Hormonal Control of Hair Growth and Differentiation

Androgens are the most important determinants of the type and distribution of hairs throughout the body. Circulating androgens, particularly testosterone and androstenedione are converted in the hair follicle to dihydrotestosterone through the action of 5α-reductase.

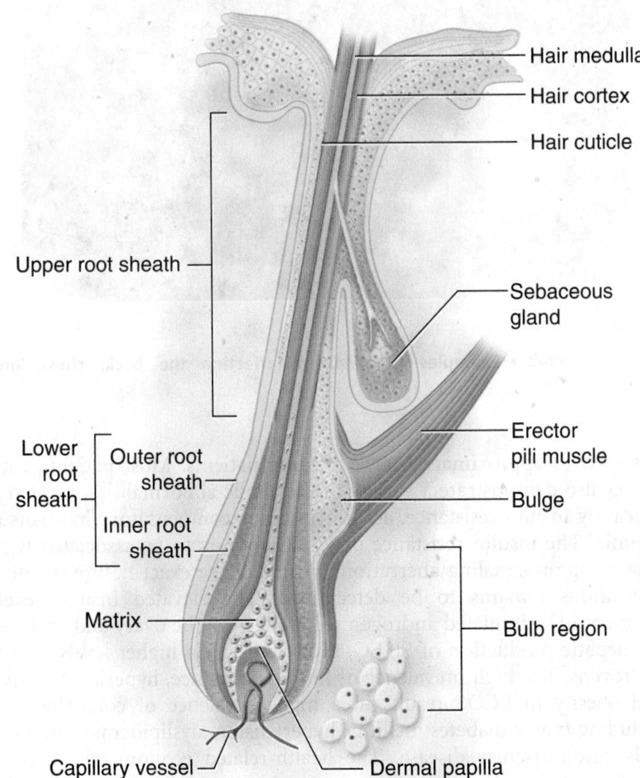

FIGURE 261–1 • Anatomy of a pilosebaceous unit containing a terminal hair follicle. (Adapted from Sanchez LA, Perez M, Azziz R: Laser hair reduction in the hirsute patient: A critical assessment. Hum Reprod Update 2002;8:169–181).

Dihydrotestosterone and, to a limited extent, testosterone, androstenedione, and dehydroepiandrosterone (DHEA) then act on the dermal papilla of androgen-sensitive hair follicles and sebaceous glands to increase the growth rate and thickness of terminal hairs and sebum production, respectively. Androgens also transform vellus-producing follicles to terminal hair–producing follicles, although the process of terminalization may take numerous hair growth cycles before it is complete (and becomes generally irreversible).

Pathobiology and Pathogenesis

Most women with hirsutism demonstrate androgen excess (i.e., hyperandrogenism), although not all hyperandrogenic women demonstrate hirsutism, most notably Asian women and adolescent girls. The causes of hirsutism can be divided into the following categories: those that have nonandrogenic causes (e.g., acromegaly, chronic skin irritation, and use of certain nonandrogenic drugs that stimulate generalized growth in hair, such as phenytoin, cyclosporine, minoxidil, calcium-channel blockers, diazoxide, and erythropoietin); those related to excessive production or ingestion of androgens (i.e., androgenic causes); and IH (Table 261–1).

Rare Androgenic Causes

Rare androgenic causes include male pseudohermaphroditism (e.g., XY gonadal dysgenesis and incomplete androgen insensitivity syndrome), adrenocorticotropic hormone (ACTH)-dependent Cushing's syndrome (i.e., Cushing's disease or ectopic ACTH-producing tumors), and the use or abuse of androgenic drugs (e.g., danazol, stanozolol, oxandrolone, androstenedione, DHEA, and testosterone and its derivatives).

Androgen-producing neoplasms (ASNs), either ovarian or adrenal, are also relatively rare. They should be suspected when the onset of androgenic symptoms is rapid and sudden, when virilization and masculinization ensue, or when significant symptoms develop later in life. Ovarian ASNs are usually palpable on pelvic examination and/or are associated with unilateral ovarian enlargement as seen on an ultrasound scan, and they are generally not malignant (e.g., Sertoli-Leydig cell and lipoid cell tumors). Adrenal ASNs are less common than ovarian neoplasms and include adenomas and carcinomas. Adrenal adenomas secreting solely androgens are exceedingly rare. More common are adrenal carcinomas, which usually cause cushingoid features; these tumors can be diagnosed as large (generally >6 cm), irregular adrenal masses on adrenal computed tomography scanning or magnetic resonance imaging (Chapter 245).

Circulating androgen levels, including testosterone and DHEA sulfate, have limited predictive value for ASNs, and basal androgen levels in these patients often overlap with those of women without a tumor. Likewise, suppression and stimulation tests (including corticosteroid, oral contraceptive, human chorionic gonadotropin, and ACTH administration) can be misleading and are not encouraged for the screening or diagnosis of these neoplasms. Overall, the clinical presentation is the single most important predictive marker. Transvaginal ultrasound and computed tomography scanning, for ovarian and adrenal ASNs, respectively, usually detect these tumors.

Another cause of hyperandrogenism and hirsutism is type C insulin resistance or the hyperandrogenic insulin-resistant acanthosis nigricans (HAIRAN) syndrome, which affects approximately 3% of hyperandrogenic women. These patients demonstrate extreme insulin resistance, with

TABLE 261–1 FREQUENCY OF THE MOST COMMON CAUSES OF HIRSUTISM

Cause	Proportion of Total Patients
Polycystic ovary syndrome	70–85%
Idiopathic hirsutism	5–15%
Hyperandrogenic insulin-resistant acanthosis nigricans syndrome	2–4%
Nonclassic adrenal hyperplasia (21-hydroxylase deficient)	1–10%
Ovarian tumors	1/300–1/1000
Others	Very rare

secondary hyperinsulinemia and hyperandrogenism. Although exact diagnostic guidelines for the HAIRAN syndrome have yet to established, it appears that the disorder can be diagnosed by the presence of extremely high circulating levels of insulin, generally higher than 80 to 100 μU/mL in the fasting state and higher than 300 to 500 μU/mL following a 2- or 3-hour oral glucose tolerance challenge. Overall, both morbidity and mortality are significant, and these patients require intensive counseling, treatment, and long-term follow-up.

NCAHs are autosomal recessive disorders that result in defects in adrenal enzymatic action and cause symptomatic hyperandrogenism (e.g., hirsutism, acne, oligomenorrhea) beginning peripubertally or postpubertally, in the presence of normal female external genitalia. Defects in HSD3B2, encoding for 3β-hydroxysteroid dehydrogenase activity, and CYP11B1, encoding for cytochrome P450c11, which determines 11β-hydroxylase activity, have also been reported to cause the NCAH, although they are extremely rare. The most common type results from a defect in CYP21 encoding P450c21, the enzyme responsible for 21-hydroxylase (21-OH). NCAH resulting from 21-OH deficiency affects between 1 and 10% of hyperandrogenic women, depending on ethnicity; the prevalence is highest among Ashkenazi Jews and patients from the Middle East.

In 21-OH deficient NCAH the production of the appropriate amount of the enzymatic product (e.g., 11-deoxycortisol and cortisol) requires greater concentrations of precursor (i.e., 17α-hydroxyprogesterone [17-HP] and progesterone) as a result of changes in enzymatic activity. The measurement of a morning 17-HP level in the follicular phase of the menstrual cycle can be used to screen for 21-OH deficient NCAH; most untreated patients have basal 17-HP levels greater than 2 ng/mL. If used to screen for 21-OH deficient NCAH, the basal 17-HP should be obtained in the follicular phase of the menstrual cycle, because this progestogen increases in the luteal phase. Patients who demonstrate a basal follicular phase 17-HP level higher than 2 ng/mL merit an ACTH stimulation test to rule out NCAH. If the 17-HP level 30 or 60 minutes following the intravenous administration of one vial (0.25 ng) of $ACTH_{1-24}$ is greater than 10 to 12 ng/mL, then the diagnosis of 21-OH–deficient NCAH is established.

Clinical Manifestations

Hirsutism is characterized by the presence of terminal hairs in women in a male-like pattern (Fig. 261–2). The areas most often affected include the following: the chin, cheek, sideburn, and neck areas; the upper and lower back; the chest; the upper and lower abdomen (i.e., male escutcheon); the upper thighs and buttocks; and the upper arms. Excessive growth of coarse hairs of the lower forearms and lower legs alone does not constitute hirsutism, although women suffering from hirsutism may note increased growth and pigmentation of hairs in these body areas. Other hyperandrogenic features observed alone or in combination with hirsutism include acne, androgenic alopecia, and ovulatory and menstrual dysfunction, and rarely virilization and/or masculinization.

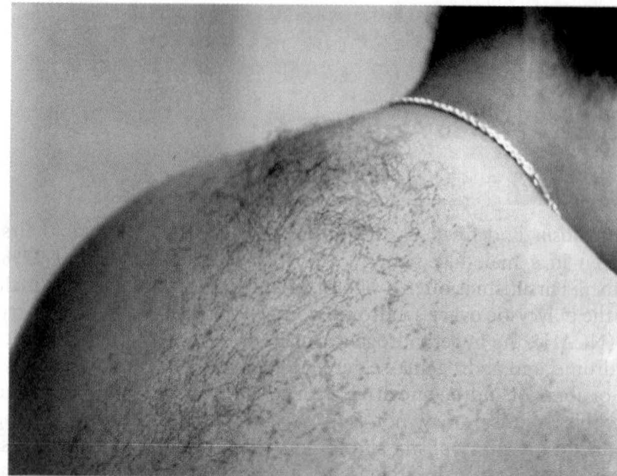
A

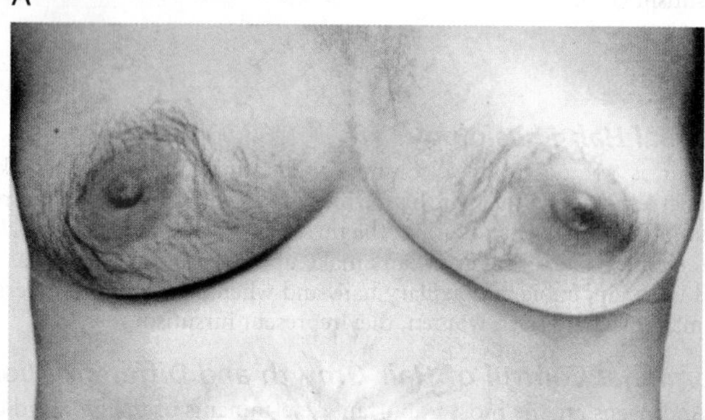
B

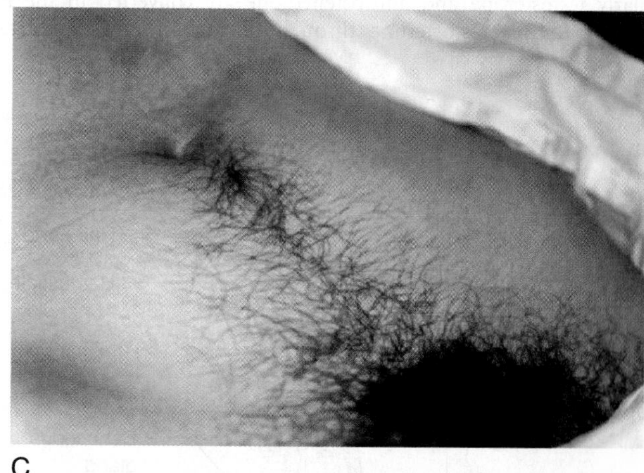
C

FIGURE 261–2 • Examples of hirsutism affecting the back, chest, and abdomen.

Diagnosis

Polycystic Ovary Syndrome

PCOS affects at least 6 to 7% of reproductive-aged women in the United States and is one of the most common causes of oligo-ovulatory infertility and hirsutism (Chapter 255). Patients with PCOS comprise between 60 and 80% of all hyperandrogenic or hirsute women seen clinically. In general, the diagnosis of PCOS is established by the presence of hyperandrogenic oligo-ovulation, after other causes of androgen excess or oligo-ovulation, such as NCAH, hyperprolactinemia, and thyroid dysfunction, have been excluded.

Pathologically, the ovarian cortex contains multiple intermediate and atretic follicles, measuring 2 to 5 mm in diameter, that give the ovary its "polycystic" appearance. Using transvaginal ultrasonography, between 70 and 90% of patients with endocrinologically defined PCOS demonstrate polycystic ovaries.

Biochemically, patients with PCOS frequently, but not always, have elevated circulating levels of free testosterone and a reduction in sex hormone–binding globulin (SHBG), accompanied by variable increases in total testosterone and DHEA sulfate. An elevated ratio of luteinizing hormone (LH) to follicle-stimulating hormone (FSH) that exceeds 2:1 is observed in approximately 60% of these patients. Most patients with PCOS also demonstrate a variety of metabolic abnormalities, most significantly insulin resistance, accompanied by compensatory hyperinsulinemia. The insulin resistance of PCOS appears to be associated with post-receptor signaling aberrations, although the exact nature of these aberrations remains to be determined. The elevated insulin levels augment LH stimulated androgen secretion from the ovary and decrease the hepatic production of SHBG, thus resulting in higher levels of free androgens. The high prevalence of insulin resistance, hyperinsulinemia, and obesity in PCOS results in a high prevalence of comorbidities, including type 2 diabetes mellitus, hypertension, dyslipidemia, and possibly cardiovascular disease. The health-related economic burden of PCOS has been estimated to be at least 4.3 billion dollars annually in the United States alone.

PCOS has a strong familial component, and it appears to be inherited as a complex genetic trait. For example, if a patient has PCOS, her sister will have an approximately 40% risk of also having the disorder. Hence, patients should be counseled appropriately. Efforts to determine the molecular genetic abnormality, or likely abnormalities, underlying PCOS are ongoing, and although some promising associations have been reported, no single mutation has yet been found to account for the disorder in even a subgroup of patients.

Idiopathic Hirsutism

By definition, IH is hirsutism not caused by systemic hyperandrogenism, and it is thought to result from excessive sensitivity of the skin to normal levels of circulating androgens. The diagnosis of IH is reached when an obviously hirsute patient demonstrates normal ovulatory function, normal ovarian morphology, and normal circulating androgen levels. Using this strict definition, approximately 5% of hirsute women will be diagnosed as suffering from IH. It is critical to confirm the presence of normal ovulatory function (e.g., by using a basal body temperature chart and luteal progesterone measurements) in those hirsute patients who claim to have regular menstrual cycles because up to 40% of these individuals actually are oligo-ovulatory if they are studied more carefully.

History

The history is probably the single most important part of the evaluation of the hirsute woman, and the cause of hirsutism can often be suspected from the history alone. In addition to the usual components of the medical history, evaluation of the hirsute patient should include determination of the onset and pace of pubertal development, and its relation to the onset of hirsutism, acne, and/or obesity. A history of drug or medication use and exposure, or use of skin irritants, should be elicited. The onset and progression of hirsutism, acne, balding, and hair loss, and past and present use of treatments for the unwanted hair should be established. Any change in extremity or head size and changes in face contour should be noted. A detailed family history including assessment of endocrine, reproductive, or metabolic disorders should be obtained.

Menstrual and ovulatory function should be determined by assessing whether the episodes of vaginal bleeding are regular and predictable and whether they are preceded by premenstrual molimina (e.g., feeling of swelling or puffiness, breast tenderness, and/or mood changes) reflecting the production of progesterone in the luteal phase of the cycle. The examiner should keep in mind that episodes of vaginal bleeding do not necessarily constitute "menstrual periods or cycles," and episodes of vaginal bleeding can occur that are more or less regular in women who are not necessarily normo-ovulatory. Thus, it is imperative that normal ovulation be confirmed by serial progesterone serum levels in the hirsute eumenorrheic woman, obtained in the luteal phase of the cycle.

Physical Examination

Overall, during the physical examination, it is most important to determine whether hirsutism and other hyperandrogenic features are truly present, and whether the patient has signs or symptoms of other related disorders. The excessive growth of vellus hairs that produces a "fuzzy" appearance is termed *vellus hypertrichosis* and should not be considered hirsutism. Although certain medical problems or medications can lead to vellus hypertrichosis, it is more commonly an ethnic variant noted particularly in individuals of Scandinavian or Mediterranean extraction. Furthermore, excessive hair growth affecting only the lower legs or forearms does not constitute hirsutism, because these areas are normally covered by a mixture of terminal and vellus hairs. Terminal hairs can be identified because they are coarse, pigmented, and generally greater than 1 cm in length (if not cut or trimmed). The type and pattern of excessive terminal hair growth should be scored (Fig. 261–3). The presence of alopecia, acne, acanthosis nigricans, lipodystrophy, clitoromegaly, virilization and/or masculinization, pelvic and/or abdominal masses, abdominal and generalized obesity, cushingoid features, coarseness or bluntness of facial features, galactorrhea, thyroid enlargement, and signs of systemic illness should also be noted.

Laboratory Findings

The laboratory evaluation of the hirsute woman should not be excessive or unfocused. For diagnostic purposes, at a minimum the levels of thyroid-stimulating hormone and 17-HP should be measured, to exclude thyroid dysfunction and 21-OH–deficient NCAH, respectively. In addition, a prolactin level should be assessed in hirsute patients who are oligo-ovulatory (established either because of frank oligomenorrhea or after confirmation of occult oligo-ovulation) to exclude hyperprolactinemia. As noted earlier, patients who are hirsute and who claim to have regular menstrual cycles should also have their ovulatory function assessed, because approximately 40% of these women actually have occult oligo-ovulation. Confirmation of ovulation can be easily achieved by measuring a serum progesterone level once sometime between days 20 and 24 after the first day of vaginal bleeding (i.e., the start of the "menstrual cycle"); a level greater than 4 ng/mL confirms ovulation. For maximum diagnostic accuracy, it is preferable to confirm ovulation in at least two consecutive cycles.

Total and free testosterone and DHEA sulfate levels are often measured, although the added diagnostic value of these tests in the hirsute patient is limited, because hirsute women are already deemed hyperandrogenic. As noted earlier, androgen measures by themselves, in the absence of clinical indicators, are poor predictors of an ASN.

Patients with features suggestive of acromegaly, Cushing's syndrome, thyroid dysfunction, or hyperprolactinemia should be evaluated further, as indicated. In patients suspected of suffering from male pseudohermaphroditism or XY gonadal dysgenesis, owing to the presence of a blind vaginal pouch and/or abnormality of the external genitalia, a karyotype should be obtained.

Finally, if the diagnosis of PCOS is confirmed, assessment of the patient's metabolic status should be made. At a minimum, this may include measuring the fasting glucose level. However, because basal glucose levels are relatively insensitive for the diagnosis of glucose intolerance in patients with PCOS, preferably a 2-hour oral glucose tolerance test should be performed, to measure both insulin and glucose. In addition to diagnosing impaired glucose tolerance and type 2 diabetes mellitus, the oral glucose tolerance test also provides a measure of hyperinsulinemia and, indirectly, insulin resistance. Insulin levels higher than 100 μIU/mL are generally abnormal, and levels higher than 300 μIU/mL indicate severe hyperinsulinemia. Although specific guidelines do not exist, it is appropriate also to obtain a lipid profile every 2 to 3 years in women with PCOS, at least in those who are more than 35 years old, are obese, or have a strong family history of type 2 diabetes mellitus or cardiovascular disease.

Treatment

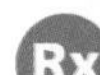

Therapy for hirsutism consists of combinations of hormonal and cosmetic means. The treatment of hirsutism should be undertaken as soon as the diagnosis is established. Although in young children or teenagers the degree of hair growth may not necessarily qualify as hirsutism, one must remember that these disorders are usually progressive, and the development of terminal hairs is not reversible. Furthermore, the presence of hirsutism can be cosmetically disfiguring, with a significant negative impact on a young woman's social and emotional development.

Evidence-Based Treatments

Hormonal Treatments

Current hormonal therapy consists of drugs that primarily suppress androgen secretion from the ovary, and drugs that primarily inhibit the action of androgens at the periphery (i.e., the skin). Often, these drugs are combined simultaneously to suppress androgen production while peripherally blocking their effect.

Suppression of Androgen Production

Suppression of androgen production in the hirsute patient can be accomplished using oral contraceptive pills, insulin sensitizers, and rarely, long-acting gonadotropin-releasing hormone analogues. Oral contraceptive pills remain the mainstay of androgen excess treatment. By suppressing the secretion of LH, the use of oral contraceptive pills leads to a decrease in ovarian androgen production and, through the action of the estrogen contained in the pill, increases SHBG production and blood levels. The result is a decrease in circulating free testosterone levels. [1]

Because up to 70% of patients with PCOS demonstrate overt insulin resistance, hyperinsulinism, and dyslipidemia, the administration of insulin-sensitizing agents, principally metformin and thiazolidinediones, has been proposed for the treatment of this disorder. Insulin sensitizers in patients with PCOS may also have a positive therapeutic effect on hirsutism, albeit generally modest. [2,3]

Hyperandrogenic Features Evaluation Record

Modified Ferriman-Gallwey Hirsutism Score

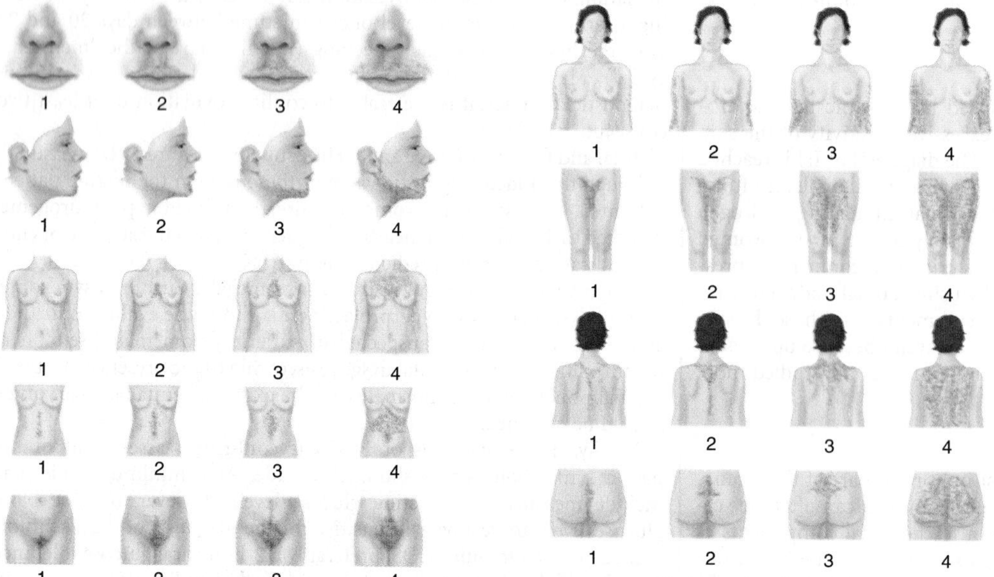

Total modified F-G score:

Acne: Back: ______ Face: ______ Chest: ______

Other (describe): ______

Score: 1-3 of 3

Acanthosis: Neck: ______ Axilla: ______ Abdomen: ______

Other (describe): ______

Check all areas where present

Patient Name: ______

MRN: ______

Date: ______ Examiner initials: ______

© R. Azziz, 2005

FIGURE 261-3 • Evaluation score sheet used to evaluate women suspected of hirsutism. The degree of terminal hair growth is scored in each of nine body areas from 0 to 4, and the scores in each area are summed (if no excess terminal hairs are noted in an area the score is zero and left blank). The presence of acne (using a scale from 1 to 4) and acanthosis is also recorded. (Courtesy of Ricardo Azziz, copyright 2005.)

Rx

Blockade of Androgen Action

Drugs in this category include antiandrogens and 5α-reductase inhibitors. Antiandrogens include spironolactone, flutamide, and cyproterone acetate; these drugs competitively inhibit the binding of androgens to the androgen receptor. Alternatively, finasteride reduces hirsutism by inhibiting 5α-reductase and the conversion of testosterone to dihydrotestosterone. Although side effects vary, teratogenicity (i.e., feminization of a male infant) is a major concern with these drugs when they are used in women of reproductive age, and all at-risk patients should be counseled to use a barrier or hormonal form of contraception during therapy. Overall, androgen receptor blockers have similar success in treating hirsutism, [4, 5] although finasteride appears to be somewhat less effective. [6, 7] Principally, the most important differences center on the type and prevalence of side effects. Combination therapy, including oral contraceptive pills, antiandrogens, and/or metformin, may be more effective than single-agent therapy. [8]

Rx

Mechanical Therapy

Cosmetic treatments, in combination with hormonal therapy, are important to maximize the effectiveness of therapy. Shaving and bleaching may be useful, as is treatment with eflornithine hydrochloride 13.9% cream (Vaniqa, SkinMedica, Inc., Carlsbad, CA). Alternatively, plucking or waxing should be discouraged because these practices may stimulate the growth of surrounding follicles, at least in animal models, and may lead to folliculitis with the subsequent development of ingrown hairs. Excessive use of depilating agents, particularly on the face, can result in chronic irritation and worsening of the skin condition. Electrolysis and laser epilation can be used to achieve a more permanent destruction of unwanted hairs, although data concerning the long-term efficacy of these therapies are scant.

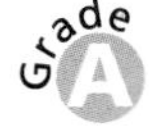

1. Breitkopf DM, Rosen MP, Young SL, et al: Efficacy of second versus third generation oral contraceptives in the treatment of hirsutism. Contraception 2003;67:349–353.
2. Azziz R, Ehrmann D, Legro RS, et al: Troglitazone improves ovulation and hirsutism in the polycystic ovary syndrome: A multicenter, double blind, placebo-controlled trial. J Clin Endocrinol Metab 2001;86:1626–1632.
3. Moghetti P, Castello R, Negri C, et al: Metformin effects on clinical features, endocrine and metabolic profiles, and insulin sensitivity in polycystic ovary syndrome: A randomized, double-blind, placebo-controlled 6-month trial, followed by open, long-term clinical evaluation. J Clin Endocrinol Metab 2000;85:139–146.
4. Venturoli S, Marescalchi O, Colombo FM: A prospective randomized trial comparing low dose flutamide, finasteride, ketoconazole, and cyproterone acetate-estrogen regimens in the treatment of hirsutism. J Clin Endocrinol Metab 1999;84:1304–1310.
5. Moghetti P, Tosi F, Tosti A, et al: Comparison of spironolactone, flutamide, and finasteride efficacy in the treatment of hirsutism: A randomized, double blind, placebo-controlled trial. J Clin Endocrinol Metab 2000;85:89–94.
6. Muderris II, Bayram F, Guven M: A prospective, randomized trial comparing flutamide (250 mg/d) and finasteride (5 mg/d) in the treatment of hirsutism. Fertil Steril 2000;73:984–987.
7. Falsetti L, Gambera A, Legrenzi L, et al: Comparison of finasteride versus flutamide in the treatment of hirsutism. Eur J Endocrinol 1999;141:361–367.
8. Gambineri A, Pelusi C, Genghini S, et al: Effect of flutamide and metformin administered alone or in combination in dieting obese women with polycystic ovary syndrome. Clin Endocrinol (Oxf) 2004;60:241–249.

SUGGESTED READINGS

Azziz R: The evaluation and management of hirsutism. Obstet Gynecol 2003;101:995–1007. *Comprehensive review of the evaluation and management of the hirsute patient.*

Rosenfield RL: Clinical practice. Hirsutism. N Engl J Med 2005;353:2578–2588. *A clinical review.*

Setji TL, Brown AJ: Polycystic ovary syndrome: Diagnosis and treatment. Am J Med 2007;120:128–132. *A clinical review.*

262 MENOPAUSE

Deborah Grady and Elizabeth Barrett-Connor

Definition

All healthy women transition from a reproductive or premenopausal period marked by regular ovulation and cyclic menstrual bleeding to a postmenopausal period marked by infertility and amenorrhea (Fig. 262–1). The onset of the menopausal transition is generally marked by subtle changes in the length of the menstrual cycle and in the duration or amount of menstrual flow. As the menopausal transition progresses, menstrual cycles are missed until complete amenorrhea occurs, but the pattern of missed cycles is not predictable. Amenorrhea for a few months is not a good indicator of menopause, because half to three fourths of middle-aged women who are amenorrheic for 6 months resume cycles. Thus, menopause is typically defined retrospectively after 12 months of amenorrhea.

Epidemiology

The menopausal transition usually begins in the middle to late 40s and lasts approximately 4 years, with menopause occurring at a median age of 51 years and ranging in age from approximately 45 to 57 years. Age at menopause has not changed significantly over the past century. However, a century ago, most women in the United States did not live beyond menopause. A gradual increase in life expectancy to the low 80s now means that the average woman is postmenopausal for more than a third of her life. Age at menopause does not vary significantly by race or ethnicity, but on average, cigarette smokers experience menopause approximately 2 years earlier than nonsmokers.

Biology

During the early menopausal transition, estrogen levels are generally normal (50 to 200 pg/mL, depending on the stage of the menstrual cycle) or even slightly elevated, whereas the levels of follicle stimulating hormone (FSH) and luteinizing hormone (LH) begin to increase (see Fig. 262–1). As the menopause transition progresses, estrogen levels fall markedly, and FSH continues to increase. After menopause, women do not ovulate, and their ovaries do not produce estradiol or progesterone. However, a small amount of estrogen may be produced by

Final menstrual period (between Menopause Transition and Postmenopause)

	Reproductive			Menopause Transition		Postmenopause	
Reproductive stage	Early	Peak	Late	Early	Late	Early	Late
				Perimenopause			
Menstrual cycle	Variable or regular	Regular		Cycle length variable, 1 or 2 missed cycles per year	3 or more missed cycles	None	
Age (duration)	Puberty to mid 40s			Mid 40s to mid 50s (4 yrs)		Mean of 51 years to death	
Steroid hormones	Estradiol 50 to 200 pg/mL Testosterone 400 pg/mL			Same or slightly higher Same		40 pg/mL same	0–15 pg/mL same
Pituitary hormones	FSH 10 mIU/mL day 2–4 LH 10 mIU/mL day 2–4			Same or higher Same or higher		>100 mIU/mL >100 mIU/mL	

FIGURE 262–1 • Stages of the menopause transition. FSH = follicle-stimulating hormone; LH = luteinizing hormone.

metabolism of adrenal steroids to estradiol in peripheral fat tissue. In the early postmenopausal period, mean estradiol levels average approximately 40 pg/mL, and they fall to less than 15 pg/mL in the late postmenopausal period. Depending on the measurement method, approximately 15 to 30% of older postmenopausal women have unmeasurable estradiol levels. Testosterone levels after menopause are similar to premenopausal levels.

It is not clear what causes menopause, but two leading theories have been proposed. Age-related depletion of ovarian follicles may lead to decreased production of estrogen and inhibin and may thus cause altered hypothalamic-pituitary feedback that results in menopause. Alternatively, age-related changes in hypothalamic production of gonadotropin-releasing hormone and subsequent effects on FSH and LH may be responsible for the increased rate of loss of ovarian follicles, declining ovarian function, and menopause.

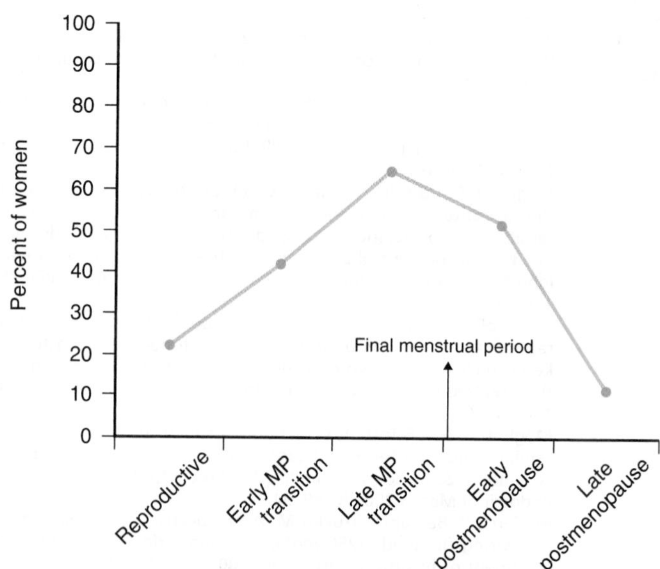

FIGURE 262–2 • Prevalence of hot flushes during the menopause (MP) transition.

MENOPAUSAL SYMPTOMS

Menopause is a very positive occurrence in the life of many women. It marks the end of cyclic bleeding and the need for birth control. It occurs at an age when children generally have become independent adults, thereby reducing family and child-care responsibilities. Conversely, menopause is a notable sign of aging in a culture that values youth. In addition, it often occurs with other stresses such as caring for elderly or ill parents. Women in the menopausal transition commonly report a wide variety of symptoms, including hot flushes, night sweats, vaginal dryness, trouble sleeping, sexual dysfunction, depression, anxiety, labile mood, memory loss, fatigue, headache, joint pains, weight gain, and urinary incontinence. However, in longitudinal studies, the prevalence of most of these symptoms does not differ across the menopausal transition after adjusting for age and other confounding variables. Only vasomotor symptoms, vaginal dryness, and sleep disturbance are consistently associated with the menopausal transition. [1] Other reported symptoms may result from aging or stress associated with menopause. Some symptoms, such as depression, anxiety, memory loss, and fatigue, may be the consequence of frequent hot flushes or poor sleep.

VASOMOTOR SYMPTOMS

Definition

Vasomotor symptoms include hot flushes, chills, and sweats. A *hot flush* is a sudden feeling of warmth, generally most intense over the face, neck, and chest. The duration is variable, but it averages approximately 4 minutes. It is often accompanied by sweating that can be profuse and followed by a chill.

Epidemiology

The prevalence of hot flushes is maximal in the late menopausal transition, occurring in approximately 50% of women (Fig. 262–2). However, prevalence varies markedly, depending on the definition of flushing (any flushing, daily flushing, troublesome flushing) and the population studied. Lower prevalence is reported among women in China, Japan, and other Asian countries. The reason for this variation is not clear, but investigators have suggested that it may result from differences in biology, cultural influences on experiencing or reporting flushes, or diet and lifestyle. In the United States, flushes are more common in African American and Latina women and less common in Chinese and Japanese women compared with white women. Approximately 15% of women with menopausal symptoms consult a physician.

Cigarette smoking increases the likelihood of flushing, but other potential risk factors, including surgical menopause, physical activity, body mass index, alcohol consumption, and socioeconomic status, have been inconsistently associated with hot flushes. [1] Currently, there is no way to predict whether an individual woman will suffer from hot flushes.

Natural History

In most women, hot flushes are transient. Approximately 30 to 50% of women note an improvement within a few months, and symptoms resolve in 85 to 90% within 4 to 5 years. However, some women continue to have frequent and severe flushes many years after menopause. Approximately 10 to 15% of women in their middle to late 60s report significant flushing. It is not clear why flushes persist for many years in some women and resolve in others.

Pathobiology

In humans, body temperature is regulated by inducing vasodilation and sweating to release heat and vasoconstriction and shivering to conserve heat (Fig. 262–3). Thermoregulation is complex and depends on central stimuli from the anterior hypothalamus and local changes in cutaneous vasoconstriction or dilation. A hot flush is very similar to a heat dissipation response, because both result in vasodilation, sweating, and reduction in core body temperature. The core body temperature at which postmenopausal women with hot flushes vasodilate and sweat is lower than in premenopausal women or in postmenopausal women without hot flushes. Variability in core body temperature does not appear to be greater in postmenopausal women with hot flushes than in premenopausal women or in postmenopausal women without hot flushes, but normal small fluctuations in core body temperature may exceed the lowered threshold for vasodilation and result in hot flushes.

The cause of altered thermoregulation in postmenopausal women with hot flushes is not clear. One theory suggests that changes in estrogen levels associated with menopause alter central nervous system adrenergic neurotransmission. This theory is supported by studies showing that metabolites of norepinephrine increase during spontaneous and experimentally induced hot flushes, and that systemic administration of yohimbine, an α_2-adrenergic antagonist that increases norepinephrine release, provokes hot flushes, whereas administration of clonidine, an α_2-adrenergic agonist that decreases norepinephrine release, reduces the frequency of hot flushes. Alternatively, some evidence indicates that declining estrogen levels during the menopause transition result in changes in serotonergic neurotransmission that could cause hot flushes. Lower estrogen levels are associated with lower levels of serotonin (5-hydroxytryptamine) in blood, resulting in increased sensitivity of 5-hydroxytryptamine-$_{2A}$ receptors in the hypothalamus. Stimulation of these receptors can alter the thermoregulatory set point in animals. Mild stressors, such as heat or anxiety, cause a brief release of 5-hydroxytryptamine that may stimulate central 5-hydroxytryptamine-$_{2A}$ receptors, lower the thermoregulatory set point, and cause flushing. This hypothesis is supported by the finding that several drugs that

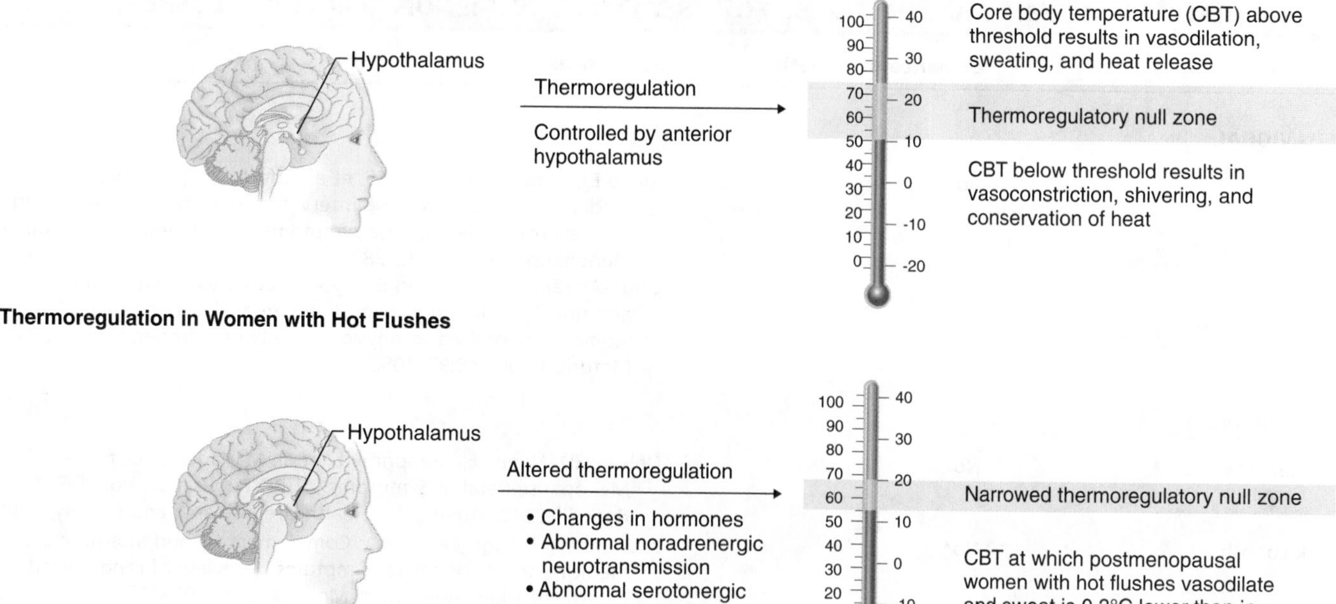

FIGURE 262–3 • Menopausal hot flushes resemble normal heat dissipating responses with a narrowed thermoregulatory null zone.

increase central serotonin levels may be effective in the treatment of hot flushes.

Estrogen treatment effectively relieves hot flushes, but the exact role of estrogen in flushing is not clear. Fluctuations in estrogen levels in an individual woman do not correlate with the onset of flushes. Prepubertal girls with very low levels of endogenous estrogen, premenopausal women with marked fluctuations in estrogen during the menstrual cycle, and most postmenopausal women with low, constant levels of estradiol do not experience flushing. However, women with gonadal dysgenesis who are treated with estrogen for several months experience flushing when treatment is discontinued. Thus, withdrawal of estrogen, rather than the absolute estrogen level, seems to play a key role in the etiology of hot flushes.

In addition to changes in estradiol, menopause is associated with multiple other hormonal changes. In the Study of Women's Health Across the Nation (SWAN), a large cohort study in the United States, lower estradiol was associated with flushing in middle-aged women in univariate models. However, higher FSH was the only measure independently associated with flushing after adjustment for other hormone levels. Hot flushes correlate with pulsatile increases in LH, but suppression of LH with gonadotropin-releasing hormone agonists does not eliminate flushing. Androgens may also play a role, because men who are treated with androgen deprivation therapy for prostate cancer frequently report severe flushing.

Diagnosis

Vasomotor symptoms are classic manifestations of the menopause transition, and the diagnosis is generally obvious from a woman's age and description of the symptoms. No abnormal physical findings are associated with hot flushes. Estradiol, FSH, and LH levels may be in the normal premenopausal range during the menopausal transition (see Fig. 262–1). A woman in her middle 40s to middle 50s who complains of classic hot flushes does not require any specific physical or laboratory evaluation unless there is good reason to suspect another cause of flushing (Table 262–1). However, an FSH determination may be helpful in assessing the risk of pregnancy. A woman in her middle 40s to middle 50s with an FSH level obtained on the third day after menses that is higher than 20 IU/L is not at risk of becoming pregnant.

TABLE 262–1 DIFFERENTIAL DIAGNOSIS OF HOT FLUSHES

Alcohol consumption
Carcinoid syndrome
Dumping syndrome
Hyperthyroidism
Narcotic withdrawal
Pheochromocytoma
Medications
Aromatase inhibitors
Gonadotropin-releasing hormone agonists or antagonists
Nicotinic acid
Nitrates
Selective estrogen receptor modulators (tamoxifen and raloxifene)

Treatment

Rx

Because self-reported frequency and severity of hot flushes improve markedly with placebo, conclusive evidence of efficacy of treatments requires randomized, blinded trials. Clinical trials of treatments for hot flushes have typically been small and of short duration, limiting information about potential adverse effects.

General Measures

Behavioral and Alternative Therapies

Many women have mild flushes and obtain adequate relief with simple measures such as lowering ambient temperature and wearing lighter clothing. Moderate exercise does not improve flushing (Table 262–2).

There is no convincing evidence that acupuncture, Chinese herbs, dong quai, evening primrose oil, ginseng, kava, or red clover extract improve hot flushes (see Table 262–2).  Evidence regarding black cohosh is mixed but primarily negative. 1 Multiple trials have been performed using different phytoestrogen preparations. Although

Section XIX Women's Health

TABLE 262–2 EVIDENCE FROM RANDOMIZED, CONTROLLED CLINICAL TRIALS OF THE EFFICACY OF BEHAVIORAL AND ALTERNATIVE THERAPIES FOR TREATMENT OF MENOPAUSAL HOT FLUSHES

Therapy	Evidence of Benefit	References
BEHAVIORAL		
Exercise	No	Aiello EJ, Yasui Y, Tworoger SS, et al: Effect of a yearlong, moderate-intensity exercise intervention on the occurrence and and severity of menopause symptoms in postmenopausal women. Menopause 2004;11:382–388. Lindh-Astrand L, Nedstrand E, Wyon Y, et al: Vasomotor symptoms and quality of life in previously sedentary postmenopausal women randomised to physical activity or estrogen therapy. Maturitas 2004;48:97–105.
ALTERNATIVE		
Acupuncture	No	Nelson HD, Haney E, Humphrey L, et al: Management of Menopause-Related Symptoms. AHRQ Publication No. 05-E016-2. Rockville, MD, Agency for Healthcare Research and Quality, 2005.
Black cohosh	No*	Kronenberg F, Fugh-Berman A: Complementary and alternative medicine for menopausal symptoms: A review of randomized, controlled trials. Ann Intern Med 2002;137:805–813. Nelson HD, Haney E, Humphrey L, et al: Management of Menopause-Related Symptoms. AHRQ Publication No. 05-E016-2. Rockville, MD, Agency for Healthcare Research and Quality, 2005.
Chinese herbal compounds	No	Kronenberg F, Fugh-Berman A: Complementary and alternative medicine for menopausal symptoms: A review of randomized, controlled trials. Ann Intern Med 2002;137:805–813. Nelson HD, Haney E, Humphrey L, et al: Management of Menopause-Related Symptoms. AHRQ Publication No. 05-E016-2. Rockville, MD, Agency for Healthcare Research and Quality, 2005.
Dong quai	No	Kronenberg F, Fugh-Berman A: Complementary and alternative medicine for menopausal symptoms: A review of randomized, controlled trials. Ann Intern Med 2002;137:805–813. Nelson HD, Haney E, Humphrey L, et al: Management of Menopause-Related Symptoms. AHRQ Publication No. 05-E016-2. Rockville, MD, Agency for Healthcare Research and Quality, 2005.
Evening primrose oil	No	Kronenberg F, Fugh-Berman A: Complementary and alternative medicine for menopausal symptoms: A review of randomized, controlled trials. Ann Intern Med 2002;137:805–813. Nelson HD, Haney E, Humphrey L, et al: Management of Menopause-Related Symptoms. AHRQ Publication No. 05-E016-2. Rockville, MD, Agency for Healthcare Research and Quality, 2005.
Ginseng	No	Kronenberg F, Fugh-Berman A: Complementary and alternative medicine for menopausal symptoms: A review of randomized, controlled trials. Ann Intern Med 2002;137:805–813. Nelson HD, Haney E, Humphrey L, et al: Management of Menopause-Related Symptoms. AHRQ Publication No. 05-E016-2. Rockville, MD, Agency for Healthcare Research and Quality, 2005.
Kava	No	Nelson HD, Haney E, Humphrey L, et al: Management of Menopause-Related Symptoms. AHRQ Publication No. 05-E016-2. Rockville, MD, Agency for Healthcare Research and Quality, 2005.

TABLE 262–2 EVIDENCE FROM RANDOMIZED, CONTROLLED CLINICAL TRIALS OF THE EFFICACY OF BEHAVIORAL AND ALTERNATIVE THERAPIES FOR TREATMENT OF MENOPAUSAL HOT FLUSHES—cont'd

Therapy	Evidence of Benefit	References
Phytoestrogens	No*	Kronenberg F, Fugh-Berman A: Complementary and alternative medicine for menopausal symptoms: A review of randomized, controlled trials. Ann Intern Med 2002;137:805–813. Nelson HD, Haney E, Humphrey L, et al: Management of Menopause-Related Symptoms. AHRQ Publication No. 05-E016-2. Rockville, MD, Agency for Healthcare Research and Quality, 2005. Krebs EE, Ensrud KE, MacDonald R, et al: Phytoestrogens for treatment of menopausal symptoms: A systematic review. Obstet Gynecol 2004;104:824–836.
Red clover	No	Nelson HD, Haney E, Humphrey L, et al: Management of Menopause-Related Symptoms. AHRQ Publication No. 05-E016-2. Rockville, MD, Agency for Healthcare Research and Quality, 2005. Krebs EE, Ensrud KE, MacDonald R, et al: Phytoestrogens for treatment of menopausal symptoms: A systematic review. Obstet Gynecol 2004;104:824–836.
Vitamin E	Yes†	Barton DL, Loprinzi CL, Quella SK, et al: Prospective evaluation of vitamin E for hot flashes in breast cancer survivors. J Clin Oncol 1998;16:495–500.

*Some studies had positive findings, but the weight of evidence is not convincing.
†One trial in survivors of breast cancer found a 17% greater reduction in frequency of hot flushes with vitamin E 800 IU compared with placebo.

TABLE 262–3 EFFICACY OF TREATMENT WITH VARIOUS DOSES OF ESTROGEN FOR HOT FLUSHES

Estrogen	Daily Dose (mg)	Percentage of Reduction in Frequency of Hot Flushes with Treatment*	Percentage of Reduction in Frequency of Hot Flushes with Placebo*
Oral conjugated equine estrogens[5]	0.625	94%	44%
	0.45	78%	
	0.3	78%	
Oral 17β-estradiol[3]	2.0	96%	55%
	1.0	89%	
	0.5	79%	
	0.25	59%	
Transdermal 17β-estradiol[4]	0.1	96%	45%
	0.05	96%	
	0.025	86%	

*Estimated from figures provided in each reference.

Rx

some of these studies have reported benefit, the weight of evidence, especially from good quality trials with blinded comparisons, suggests little benefit. 1 One trial of vitamin E supplementation found an improvement in flushes, but the decrease was only one hot flush per day. Many women prefer alternative medications because they believe that these treatments are harmless, but phytoestrogens and, possibly, black cohosh bind estrogen receptors and theoretically could cause adverse outcomes similar to those observed with estrogen. No studies of these preparations have been of adequate size or duration to document safety.

Rx

Medical Therapy

Estrogens

Multiple randomized trials have demonstrated that estrogen markedly improves the frequency and severity of hot flushes. 2 All types, preparations, and routes of administration of estrogen are effective. The benefit is dose related, but even low doses are often effective (Table 262–3). Higher doses of estrogen may control symptoms more rapidly, but they are also associated with a higher rate of side effects including uterine bleeding, breast tenderness, and headache. 3-5

TABLE 262–4 ESTROGEN AND PROGESTIN PREPARATIONS FOR TREATMENT OF MENOPAUSAL VASOMOTOR SYMPTOMS

Hormones	Generic Name	Brand Name	Dose (mg/day)
Estrogens*			
Oral	Conjugated estrogens	Premarin	0.3, 0.45, **0.625**, 0.9, 1.25
	17β-Estradiol	Estrace/generics	0.5, **1.0**, 2.0
Transdermal	17β-Estradiol	Alora†	0.025, **0.05**, 0.075, 0.1
		Climara‡	0.025, 0.0375, **0.05**, 0.075, 0.1
Vaginal	Estradiol acetate	Femring Vaginal Ring§	**0.05**, 0.1
Progestins			
Oral	Medroxyprogesterone acetate	Provera/generics	2.5, 5.0, 10.0
	Micronized progesterone	Prometrium	100, 200 (in peanut oil)
Vaginal	Progesterone	Prochieve 4%	45 every other day
Combination Preparations			
Oral sequential‖	Conjugated estrogens and medroxyprogesterone acetate	Premphase	0.625 + 5.0
Oral continuous¶	Conjugated estrogens and medroxyprogesterone acetate	Prempro	0.625 + 5.0 0.45 + 2.5 or 1.5
	17β-Estradiol and norethindrone acetate	Activella	0.3 + 1.5 1.0 + 0.5
Transdermal continuous¶	17β-Estradiol and levonorgestrel	ClimaraPro‡	0.045 + 0.015
	17β-Estradiol and norethindrone acetate	CombiPatch†	0.05 + 0.14 or 0.25

*Approximately equivalent doses of estrogens are shown in **bold**.
†Patch applied twice per week.
‡Patch applied once per week.
§Vaginal ring inserted every 90 days: note that Femring, as opposed to the vaginal preparations listed in Table 262–5, delivers systemic levels of estrogen and should be opposed by a progestin in women with a uterus.
‖Each pill contains estrogen days 1 to 14 and estrogen with progestin days 15 to 28.
¶Each pill or patch contains estrogen and progestin.

At similar biologically active doses, oral and transdermal estrogens are approximately equally effective for treatment of vasomotor symptoms. Oral estrogens undergo "first pass" metabolism in the liver that results in changes in hepatic proteins and enzymes. Hepatic effects are responsible for the beneficial effects of estrogen on lipoproteins (reduced low-density lipoprotein cholesterol and increased high-density lipoprotein cholesterol) but also for potentially adverse effects such as increases in clotting factors. The transdermal route may be safer because it minimizes these changes.

Many estrogen preparations are approved for treatment of vasomotor symptoms (Table 262–4). To individualize treatment, physicians should become familiar with several of these preparations, including at least one oral and one transdermal preparation.

Treatment with estrogen alone generally increases the risk of uterine hyperplasia and cancer. The risk of endometrial abnormalities appears not to be increased with the use of vaginal estrogens that deliver low systemic doses, especially if they are used only a few times per week, as is generally suggested for long-term use (Table 262–5).

Adding a progestin to the estrogen regimen prevents the increased risk of uterine cancer. For this reason, a woman with a uterus who takes estrogen should also be given a progestin. There is no reason to add progestins to the hormone regimen in women who have had a hysterectomy. Several progestins are approved by the U.S. Food and Drug Administration for this purpose and are available either to add to estrogen or in preparations combined with estrogen (see Table 262–4). Two general approaches are used to prescribing progestins to protect the endometrium. Sequential therapy (estrogen given daily with a progestin added on the last 14 days of a 28-day cycle) results in endometrial shedding and cyclic bleeding resembling a menstrual period in approximately 80% of women. Alternatively, the progestin can be added to the estrogen every day. This continuous regimen results in endometrial atrophy and unpredictable uterine spotting or bleeding that can be difficult for the woman to anticipate and manage. Bleeding occurs in approximately 80% of women in the first 6 months of continuous treatment. Amenorrhea becomes more common with prolonged use, but some women continue to bleed or spot for many years.

The most commonly used progestins in sequential regimens in women using standard doses of estrogens (0.625 mg oral conjugated estrogens, 1 mg oral estradiol, or 0.05 mg transdermal estradiol) are medroxyprogesterone acetate, 5 mg, norethindrone, 0.5 mg, and micronized progesterone, 200 mg, for 10 to 14 days per month. Continuous regimens generally include half these progestin doses given daily. In some situations, it may be slightly less costly to prescribe estrogen and progestins separately, but the convenience of taking a single pill and the assurance that the estrogen is adequately opposed by progestin indicate that combination preparations are preferred.

SIDE EFFECTS AND RISKS OF POSTMENOPAUSAL HORMONE THERAPY. Estrogen is generally well tolerated, but it may cause headache (especially in women with a history of migraine) and breast tenderness. Added progestins tend to make these side effects more severe and also cause uterine bleeding.

Based on the results of multiple observational studies, postmenopausal hormone therapy was formerly thought to reduce the risk of coronary events, fracture, and dementia and to increase risk of breast cancer (see Table 262–6). Effects on disease outcomes

TABLE 262–5 ESTROGEN VAGINAL PREPARATIONS FOR TREATMENT OF VAGINAL DRYNESS*

Preparation	Generic Name	Brand Name	Dose
Vaginal cream	Conjugated estrogens	Premarin	0.625 mg/2 g cream: 2 g/day for 2 weeks, then 1–2 g 2 to 3 times/wk
	17β-Estradiol	Estrace	0.1 mg/2 g cream: 2 g/day for 2 wk, then 1–2 g 2 to 3 times/wk
Vaginal tablet	Estradiol hemihydrate	Vagifem	0.025 mg tablet: 1 tablet/day for 2 wk, then 1 tablet twice/wk
Vaginal ring	17β-Estradiol	Estring†	0.0075 mg/day

*Most oral, transdermal, and vaginal products listed in Table 262–4 for treatment of vasomotor symptoms are also approved for treatment of vaginal dryness.
†Vaginal ring is inserted every 90 days.

TABLE 262–6 RESULTS OF OBSERVATIONAL STUDIES AND THE WOMEN'S HEALTH INITIATIVE RANDOMIZED TRIALS OF THE EFFECTS OF POSTMENOPAUSAL HORMONE THERAPY ON DISEASE OUTCOMES

Outcomes	Relative Risk (95% Confidence Interval) Observational Studies*	Women's Health Initiative†[6,7] Estrogen and Progestin	Women's Health Initiative‡[8,9] Estrogen
Coronary heart disease events	0.66 (0.53–0.84)[a]	1.29 (1.02–1.63)	0.91 (0.75–1.12)
Stroke	1.12 (1.01–1.23)[b]	1.41 (1.07–1.85)	1.39 (1.10–1.77)
Pulmonary embolism	2.14§ (0.89–8.75)[b]	2.13 (1.39–3.25)	1.34 (0.87–2.06)
Breast cancer	1.35¶ (1.21–1.45)[c]	1.26 (1.00–1.59)	0.77 (0.59–1.01)
Colon cancer	0.80 (0.74–0.86)[d]	0.63 (0.43–0.92)	1.08 (0.75–1.55)
Hip fracture	0.75 (0.68–0.84)[e]	0.66 (0.45–0.98)	0.61 (0.41–0.91)
Dementia	0.71 (0.53–0.96)[f]	2.05 (1.21–3.48)	1.49 (0.83–2.66)
Death	0.81 (0.71–0.92)[b]	0.98 (0.82–1.18)	1.04 (0.88–1.22)

*Results of multiple observational studies among postmenopausal hormone users and non-users summarized in systematic reviews as listed in the sources below.
†Results of the Women's Health Initiative estrogen plus progestin randomized trial: 16,608 postmenopausal women without hysterectomy randomized to 0.625 mg conjugated estrogen plus 2.5 mg medroxyprogesterone acetate per day or identical placebo and followed for 5.2 years.
‡Results of the Women's Health Initiative estrogen only randomized trial: 10,739 postmenopausal women with hysterectomy randomized to 0.625 mg conjugated estrogen per day or identical placebo and followed for 6.8 years.
§Relative risk is for all venous thromboembolic events.
¶Relative risk for 5 or more years of estrogen use.
Sources:
a. Barrett-Connor E, Grady D: Hormone replacement therapy, heart disease, and other considerations. Ann Rev Public Health 1998;19:55–72.
b. Nelson HD, Humphrey LL, Nygren P, et al: Postmenopausal hormone replacement therapy: Scientific review. JAMA 2002;288:872–881.
c. Collaborative Group on Hormonal Factors in Breast Cancer: Breast cancer and hormone replacement therapy: Collaborative reanalysis of data from 51 epidemiological studies of 52,705 women with breast cancer and 108,411 women without breast cancer. Lancet 1997;350:1047–1059.
d. Grodstein F, Newcomb PA, Stampfer MJ: Postmenopausal hormone therapy and the risk of colorectal cancer: A review and meta-analysis. Am J Med 1999;106:574–582.
e. Torgerson DJ, Bell-Syer SEM: Hormone replacement therapy and prevention of nonvertebral fractures: A meta-analysis of randomized trials. JAMA 2001;285:2891–2897.
f. Yaffe K, Sawaya G, Lieberburg I, et al: Estrogen therapy in postmenopausal women: Effects on cognitive function and dementia. JAMA 1998;279:688–695.

Rx

have now been evaluated among generally healthy postmenopausal women in the Women's Health Initiative (WHI) randomized trials (Table 262–6). 6-9 The results of these trials support observational findings with regard to fracture risk: both estrogen and estrogen in combination with progestin reduced the risk of hip fracture 35 to 40%. In contrast to the findings of observational studies, neither estrogen alone nor estrogen with a progestin reduced the risk for coronary events, and both increased the risk for stroke approximately 40%.

Compared with estrogen alone, added progestin appears to increase the risk for coronary events, pulmonary embolism, breast cancer, and dementia (see Table 262–6). This finding suggests that adding a progestin should be avoided, but treatment with unopposed estrogen in women with a uterus markedly increases the risk of uterine hyperplasia and cancer, as well as the rate of gynecologic procedures and hysterectomy.

The excess risk of any one of the adverse events listed in Table 262–6 in the WHI trials was 2 per 1000 women treated for 1 year with estrogen in combination with progestin (4.3 per 1000/year in women more than 65 years old if dementia is included), and 0.6 strokes per 1000 women treated with unopposed estrogen. These risks are relatively small, but they cumulate such that treatment for 5 years is associated with an excess risk of 1 event per 100 women treated with estrogen in combination with progestin and 3 strokes per 1000 women treated with unopposed estrogen. Based on the findings of the WHI trials and the availability of other effective and safe drugs (e.g., bisphosphonates) for prevention of osteoporotic fractures, postmenopausal hormone therapy currently has a very limited role for prevention of disease (i.e., bisphosphonate failures).

The mean age of the women included in the WHI trials was 63 years, whereas the average age of women treated for menopausal vasomotor symptoms is approximately a decade younger. Because the risk for most diseases approximately doubles with each decade of age, the absolute risk for the outcomes listed in Table 262–6 is less for younger than for older women, and the absolute risk increase is proportionately smaller. However, hormone therapy is relatively contraindicated in women with a history of stroke, breast cancer, and venous thromboembolic events and should be avoided in women at high risk of these conditions.

STOPPING HORMONE THERAPY. Given the possible adverse effects of hormone therapy, current guidelines recommend that women use the lowest effective dose for the shortest time necessary. Vasomotor symptoms improve or resolve spontaneously within a few months to a few years of onset in the majority of women, a finding suggesting that most women should be able to discontinue hormone therapy within a few years of starting. Women using hormone therapy for treatment of symptoms should stop every 6 to 12 months to determine whether symptoms have improved to the point that treatment is no longer needed. Most women are able to stop hormone therapy after a few years of treatment, but some women are unable to stop, mainly because vasomotor symptoms recur.

Women experiencing intolerable symptoms after stopping hormone treatment can be told to resume therapy and either to begin a slow taper or to wait 6 months before trying again to stop. Tapering can be accomplished by decreasing the dose of hormone therapy, but it may be easier to slowly decrease the number of days per week that hormone therapy is used. The *dose taper* involves progressively reducing the dose of hormone therapy, for example by reducing the dose of conjugated estrogens from 0.625 mg/day to 0.45 to 0.3 mg/day and then discontinuing therapy. If changing to a lower dose is associated with symptoms, the next reduction in dose should not occur until symptoms improve and are easily tolerable, which may require 3 to 6 months in some women. The *day taper* involves decreasing the number of days per week of hormone therapy use and effectively decreasing the weekly dose. For example, therapy with the same dose of hormone therapy may be continued, but only Monday through Friday. If this reduced weekly dose is tolerated, therapy may be discontinued on Thursday, and so on. As with the dose taper, if symptoms develop, the weekly dose should be maintained until symptoms improve. Both these approaches to tapering can require many months or even years until therapy is discontinued. The day taper has the advantages of allowing smaller reductions in weekly dose, ensuring that the estrogen dose is appropriately opposed by a progestin in women using combined continuous therapy and does not require multiple new prescriptions for different doses of hormone therapy. For women who cannot tolerate even a slow taper, the value of symptom relief likely outweighs the risks of hormone therapy.

OTHER PRESCRIPTION DRUGS. A drug that appears to be as effective as estrogens for treatment of hot flushes is tibolone, a steroid hormone that is not marketed in the United States but is widely available elsewhere (Table 262–7). Tibolone also preserves bone density, but its effects on fracture, cardiovascular disease, and uterine and breast cancer risk have not been adequately investigated. The progestins megestrol and medroxyprogesterone acetate are effective for the treatment of hot flushes, but they have frequent side effects, and progestin use was associated with increased risk of adverse effects in the WHI trials. Several selective serotonin/norepinephrine reuptake inhibitors and gabapentin have been studied. [10] Paroxetine and gabapentin seem to have modest efficacy in relieving hot flushes (see Table 262–7). Although these therapies are thought to be safe, clinical trials have not been adequately large or prolonged to detect uncommon adverse effects.

Summary of Approach to Treatment of Vasomotor Symptoms

Women with mild vasomotor symptoms may find adequate relief by wearing layered clothing and keeping the home and bedroom cool. Women with moderate symptoms may choose a low dose of estrogen or a nonestrogen therapy. Paroxetine is modestly effective and probably has the best side effect profile of the nonhormonal drugs. For women with severe symptoms, hormone therapy is the most effective treatment.

Vaginal Dryness

Epidemiology

The prevalence of vaginal dryness, discomfort, itching, and dyspareunia increases as women transition through the menopause. Up to 30% of perimenopausal and early postmenopausal women and a higher proportion of older menopausal women express these complaints. Urologic symptoms, including urgency, frequency, dysuria, incontinence, and increased risk of urinary tract infections, are not clearly correlated with the menopause transition.

Pathobiology

Vaginal symptoms generally correlate with findings (often called vaginal atrophy) including pallor, dryness, friability, and decreased rugosity of the vaginal mucosa. Vaginal fluid in premenopausal women is acidic, ranging from a pH of approximately 4.5 to 5.5 with mild alkalinization to approximately 6.0 before ovulation. Acidity is produced by proton excretion from the vaginal epithelial cells and by metabolism of glycogen stored in vaginal epithelial cells by *Lactobacillus* species, the normal vaginal flora. The acid environment of the vagina inhibits growth of *Escherichia coli* and other enteric gram-negative bacteria that are a potential cause of urinary tract infections. Vaginal pH can easily be measured from lateral vaginal wall fluid.

In postmenopausal women, vaginal pH is generally neutral, and the predominant flora is often *E. coli* and other gram-negative bacteria. This appears to occur because estrogen deficiency associated with menopause causes vaginal epithelial cell dysfunction, including decreased storage of glycogen, less ability to acidify the vaginal fluid, and lowered production of vaginal lubrication. Vaginal epithelial cells, which are primarily superficial and intermediate cells in premenopausal women, shift to predominately immature parabasal cells in postmenopausal women. Treatment with estrogen improves or relieves vaginal dryness, lowers vaginal pH, and increases the proportion of superficial cells in the vaginal epithelium.

Diagnosis

Diagnosis is primarily based on typical complaints of vaginal dryness, discomfort, itching, or dyspareunia in women undergoing the menopause transition or older postmenopausal women. Pelvic examination should exclude other causes of discomfort, including infections, lesions, and trauma. Physical findings of vaginal dryness, pallor, friability, and vaginal pH greater than 5.5 support the diagnosis. Cytologic examination of the proportion of superficial, intermediate, and parabasal cells from a scraping of the lateral vaginal wall (vaginal maturation index) showing primarily parabasal cells also supports the diagnosis, but the accuracy of this test is not clear.

Treatment

Many women with vaginal symptoms obtain adequate relief with use of over-the-counter vaginal moisturizers, such as Repleus. Estrogen therapy is highly effective. Topical therapy is efficacious [11] and is preferred because it generally results in smaller increases in systemic estrogen levels than oral or transdermal therapy. Estrogen vaginal creams, tablets, and rings approved for treatment of vaginal dryness are listed in Table 262–5.

Most clinicians do not add a progestin to protect the uterus in women treated with vaginal estrogen, but evidence to support the uterine safety of vaginal estrogen is limited to very short-term studies. Low-dose, intermittent treatment (e.g., 1 to 2 g conjugated estrogen cream or 0.025 mg estradiol tablet twice/week) results in very small increases in systemic estrogen levels that appear not to cause endometrial stimulation. However, full-dose daily treatment has been shown to increase estradiol levels to 50 pg/mL or higher in approximately half of treated women and has been associated with uterine bleeding and hyperplasia.

Sleep Disturbance

The prevalence of self-reported sleep disturbance increases from about 40% of premenopausal women to approximately 60% of postmenopausal women. [1] Sleep disturbances including trouble falling asleep and early awakening are reported by menopausal women, but awakening during the night appears to be most bothersome.

TABLE 262–7 EVIDENCE FROM RANDOMIZED, CONTROLLED CLINICAL TRIALS OF THE EFFICACY OF NON-ESTROGEN DRUGS FOR TREATMENT OF MENOPAUSAL HOT FLUSHES

Treatment	Evidence of Benefit	Comments	References	Side Effects*
ANTIDEPRESSANTS				
Citalopram	No	No benefit of 30 mg citalopram compared with placebo	Suvanto-Luukkonen E, Koivunen R, Sundstrom H, et al: Citalopram and fluoxetine in the treatment of postmenopausal symptoms: A prospective, randomized, 9-month, placebo-controlled, double-blind study. Menopause 2005;12:18–26.	Selective serotonin reuptake inhibitors fluoxetine, paroxetine, and citalopram: nausea, vomiting, diarrhea, insomnia or somnolence, anxiety, decreased libido, dry mouth, worsening depression, mania, suicidality, serotonin syndrome, withdrawal syndrome, and possible decreased tamoxifen effectiveness
Fluoxetine	Mixed	One trial among breast cancer survivors found the frequency of hot flushes was reduced 50% with fluoxetine 20 mg/day compared to 36% with placebo, whereas another found no benefit among women without breast cancer who were treated with 30 mg fluoxetine compared with placebo	Loprinzi CL, Sloan JA, Perez EA, et al: Phase III evaluation of fluoxetine for treatment of hot flashes. J Clin Oncol 2002;20:1578–1583. Suvanto-Luukkonen E, Koivunen R, Sundstrom H, et al: Citalopram and fluoxetine in the treatment of postmenopausal symptoms: A prospective, randomized, 9-month, placebo-controlled, double-blind study. Menopause 2005;12:18–26.	
Paroxetine	Yes	One trial found the frequency of hot flushes was reduced 62% with 12.5 mg and 65% with 25 mg paroxetine CR compared with 38% in placebo; a crossover trial in which 81% of participants had a history of breast cancer found that paroxetine 10 mg reduced hot flush frequency by 41% compared to 14% with placebo and paroxetine 20 mg reduced hot flush frequency by 52% compared with 27% with placebo	Stearns V, Beebe KL, Iyengar M, et al: Paroxetine controlled release in the treatment of menopausal hot flashes: A randomized controlled trial. JAMA 2003;289:2827–2834. Stearns V, Slack R, Greep N, et al: Paroxetine is an effective treatment for hot flashes: Results from a prospective clinical trial. J Clin Oncol 2005;23:6919–6930.	
Sertraline	No	One trial among women with a history of breast cancer found no benefit of treatment with 50 mg of sertraline compared with placebo; another trial among generally healthy women found no benefit of 100 mg of sertraline compared with placebo.	Kimmick GG, Lovato J, McQuellon R, et al: Randomized, double-blind, placebo-controlled crossover study of sertraline (Zoloft) for the treatment of hot flashes in women with early stage cancer taking tamoxifen. Breast J 2006;12:114–122. Grady D, Cohen B, Tice J, et al: Ineffectiveness of sertraline for treament of hot flushes. Obstet Gynecol 2007;109:823–830.	

Continued

TABLE 262–7 EVIDENCE FROM RANDOMIZED, CONTROLLED CLINICAL TRIALS OF THE EFFICACY OF NON-ESTROGEN DRUGS FOR TREATMENT OF MENOPAUSAL HOT FLUSHES—cont'd

Treatment	Evidence of Benefit	Comments	References	Side Effects*
Venlafaxine	Mixed	One trial among survivors of breast cancer found the frequency of hot flushes to be reduced 61% with 75 or 150 mg venlafaxine compared with 27% with placebo; another trial among women without breast cancer found no effect on frequency of flushes with 75 mg venlafaxine, but women treated with venlafaxine were more likely to report that flushes improved compared with placebo	Loprinzi CL, Kugler JW, Sloan JA, et al: Venlafaxine in management of hot flashes in survivors of breast cancer: A randomised controlled trial. Lancet 2000;356:2059–2063. Evans ML, Pritts E, Vittinghoff E, et al: Management of postmenopausal hot flushes with venlafaxine hydrochloride: A randomized, controlled trial. Obstet Gynecol 2005; 105:161–166.	In addition to the side effects noted above, the selective serotonin/norepinephrine reuptake inhibitor venlafaxine can also cause hypertension
ANTIHYPERTENSIVES				
Clonidine	Mixed	Several small trials suggest little or no benefit	Nelson HD, Haney E, Humphrey L, et al: Management of Menopause-Related Symptoms. AHRQ Publication No. 05-E016-2. Rockville, MD, Agency for Healthcare Research and Quality, 2005. Goldberg RM, Loprinzi CL, O'Fallon JR, et al: Transdermal clonidine for ameliorating tamoxifen-induced hot flashes. J Clin Oncol 1994;12:155–158. Pandya KJ, Raubertas RF, Flynn PJ, et al: Oral clonidine in postmenopausal patients with breast cancer experiencing tamoxifen-induced hot flashes: A University of Rochester Cancer Center Community Clinical Oncology Program Study. Ann Intern Med 2000;132:78–93.	α–Adrenergic antagonist: dry mouth, drowsiness, dizziness, hypotension, rebound hypertension
Methyldopa	No		Nelson HD, Haney E, Humphrey L, et al: Management of Menopause-Related Symptoms. AHRQ Publication No. 05-E016-2. Rockville, MD, Agency for Healthcare Research and Quality, 2005.	
HORMONES				
Medroxyprogesterone acetate	Yes	One trial found the frequency of hot flushes was reduced 74% with 20 mg medroxyprogesterone acetate compared with 26% with placebo	Schiff I, Tulchinsky D, Cramer D, et al: Oral medroxyprogesterone in the treatment of postmenopausal symptoms. JAMA 1980;244: 1443–1445.	Progestins megestrol and medroxyprogesterone: nausea, vomiting, constipation, somnolence, depression, breast tenderness, uterine bleeding; possible increased risk of venous thromboembolism, cardiovascular events, and breast cancer

TABLE 262–7 EVIDENCE FROM RANDOMIZED, CONTROLLED CLINICAL TRIALS OF THE EFFICACY OF NON-ESTROGEN DRUGS FOR TREATMENT OF MENOPAUSAL HOT FLUSHES—cont'd

Treatment	Evidence of Benefit	Comments	References	Side Effects*
Megestrol	Yes	One trial in breast cancer survivors found the frequency of hot flushes was reduced 74% with 20 mg megestrol twice/day compared to 27% with placebo	Loprinzi CL, Michalak JC, Quella SK, et al: Megestrol acetate for the prevention of hot flashes. N Engl J Med 1994;331:347–352.	
Tibolone†	Yes	Several trials reported improved hot flushes compared with placebo and efficacy equivalent to standard doses of estrogens with 1.25–5.0 mg tibolone	Modelska K, Cummings S: Tibolone for postmenopausal women: Systematic review of randomized trials. J Clin Endocrinol Metab 2002;87:16–23. Nelson HD, Haney E, Humphrey L, et al: Management of Menopause-Related Symptoms. AHRQ Publication No.05-E016-2. Rockville, MD, Agency for Healthcare Research and Quality, 2005.	Steroid hormone: headache, weight gain, uterine bleeding; effects on venous thromboembolism, cardiovascular disease, and breast and uterine cancer unclear
OTHER DRUGS				
Gabapentin	Yes	One trial found the frequency of hot flushes was reduced 45% with gabapentin 300 mg three times/day compared with 29% with placebo; another found the frequency of hot flushes was reduced 31% more than placebo among breast cancer survivors	Guttuso TJ, Kurlan R, McDermott MP, et al: Gabapentin's effects on hot flashes in postmenopausal women: A randomized controlled trial. Obstet Gynecol 2003;101:337–345. Pandya JK, Morrow GR, Rosco JA, et al: Gabapentin for hot flashes in 420 women with breast cancer: A randomized double-blind, placebo-controlled trial. Lancet 2005;366:818–824.	Nausea, vomiting, somnolence, dizziness, rash, ataxia, fatigue, leukopenia

*Side effects were reported in clinical trials of the therapy or from Epocrates Rx drug reference (available at *www.epocrates.com*).
†This drug had not been approved by the U.S. Food and Drug Administration at the time of publication

The etiology of sleep disturbance associated with menopause is unclear. Postmenopausal women with hot flushes are more likely to report sleep disturbance than are those without flushes, and women commonly report that they are awakened by hot flushes. However, studies using actigraphy and polysomnography find that nocturnal hot flushes do not consistently occur at the same time as sleep disturbance. Thus, disturbed sleep appears to be part of a menopausal syndrome, but it may not be caused by flushing.

Menopause-related sleep disturbance can be treated using standard approaches to sleep hygiene and prescription medications. Both oral and transdermal estrogen preparations improve sleep in perimenopausal and postmenopausal women with hot flushes.

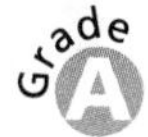

1. Nelson HD, Haney E, Humphrey L, et al: Management of Menopause-Related Symptoms. AHRQ Publication No. 05-E016-2. Rockville, MD, Agency for Healthcare Research and Quality, 2005.
2. MacLennan A, Lester S, Moore V: Oral estrogen replacement therapy versus placebo for hot flushes: A systematic review. Climacteric 2001;4:58–74.
3. Notelovitz M, Lenihan JP, McDermott M, et al: Initial 17-beta estradiol dose for treating vasomotor symptoms. Obstet Gynecol 2000;95:726–731.
4. Utian WH, Burry KA, Archer DF, et al: Efficacy and safety of low, standard, and high dosages of an estradiol transdermal system (Esclim) compared with placebo on vasomotor symptoms in highly symptomatic menopausal patients: The Esclim Study Group. Am J Obstet Gynecol 1999;181:71–79.
5. Utian WH, Shoupe D, Bachmann G, et al: Relief of vasomotor symptoms and vaginal atrophy with lower doses of conjugated equine estrogens and medroxyprogesterone acetate. Fertil Steril 2001;75:1065–1079.
6. Rossouw JE, Anderson GL, Prentice RL, et al: Risks and benefits of estrogen plus progestin in healthy postmenopausal women: Principal results from the Women's Health Initiative randomized controlled trial. JAMA 2002;288:321–333.
7. Shumaker SA, Legault C, Thal L, et al: Estrogen plus progestin and the incidence of dementia and mild cognitive impairment in postmenopausal women: The Women's Health Initiative Memory Study. A randomized controlled trial. JAMA 2003;289:2651–2662.
8. Shumaker SA, Legault C, Kuller L, et al: Conjugated equine estrogens and incidence of probable dementia and mild cognitive impairment in postmenopausal women. JAMA 2004;291: 2947–2958.
9. Women's Health Initiative Steering Committee: Effects of conjugated equine estrogen in postmenopausal women with hysterectomy: The Women's Health Initiative Randomized Controlled Trial. JAMA 2004;291:1701–1712.
10. Nelson HD, Vesco KK, Haney E, et al: Nonhormonal therapies for menopausal hot flashes: Systematic review and meta-analysis. JAMA 2006;295:2057–2071.
11. Suckling J, Lethaby A, Kennedy R: Local oestrogen for vaginal atrophy in postmenopausal women. Cochrane Database Syst Rev 2006;4:CD001500.

SUGGESTED READINGS

Grady D: Management of menopausal symptoms. N Engl J Med 2006;355: 2338–2347. *Reviews the epidemiology, pathophysiology, and treatment of hot flushes.*

North American Menopause Society: Treatment of menopause-associated vasomotor symptoms: Position statement of The North American Menopause Society. Menopause 2004;11:11–33. *Reviews evidence on behavioral, prescription, and nonprescription treatments and provides practice guidelines.*

Proceedings from the NIH State-of-the-Science Conference on Management of Menopause-Related Symptoms, March 21–23, 2005, Bethesda, Maryland, USA. Am J Med 2005;118(Suppl 2):1–171. *This supplement includes articles on a variety of topics on menopause presented at this 2005 NIH conference.*

Society of Obstetricians and Gynaecologists of Canada: The detection and management of vaginal atrophy. J Obstet Gynaecol Can 2004;26:503. *Consensus guidelines.*

Stearns V, Ullmer L, Lopez JF, et al: Hot flushes. Lancet 2002;360:1851–1861. *Review of the knowledge of the epidemiology, pathophysiology, and treatment of hot flushes.*

U.S. Preventive Services Task Force: Hormone therapy for the prevention of chronic conditions in postmenopausal women: Recommendations from the U.S. Preventive Services Task Force. Ann Intern Med 2005;142:855–860. *Summary of recommendations and the supporting scientific evidence.*

Section XX

Diseases of Bone and Mineral Metabolism

263 MINERAL AND BONE HOMEOSTASIS

Murray J. Favus

HOMEOSTATIC SYSTEMS FOR CALCIUM, MAGNESIUM, AND PHOSPHATE

Metabolic bone diseases and mineral disorders my arise from the following: excesses or deficiencies of the calciotropic hormones, which are vitamin D and its metabolites and parathyroid hormone (PTH), or of the steroid or peptide hormones that have direct actions on bone; or altered intake of the key minerals of the bone matrix, that is, calcium (Ca), magnesium (Mg), and phosphorus (P). Genetic or acquired defects in osteoblast or osteoclast function, bone matrix synthesis, mineralization, turnover, or repair may also cause metabolic bone diseases. Under physiologic conditions, maintenance of Ca, Mg, and P (because most biologic forms of P are in the form of inorganic phosphate, P is expressed as PO_4) homeostasis is achieved through a coordinated trafficking of the ions across intestine and kidney to ensure delivery of sufficient amounts to support mineralization of the bone matrix. Disorders that impair any one of the organs involved (intestine, kidney, parathyroid, bone) may disturb homeostasis and may cause bone or mineral disorders. Measurements of blood levels of PTH, vitamin D metabolites, 25-hydroxyvitamin D [25(OH)-D], and 1,25-dihydroxyvitamin D_3 [$1,25(OH)_2D_3$], other key steroid and peptide hormones, biomarkers of bone turnover, and the blood and urine levels of Ca, Mg, and PO_4 are critical for accurate diagnosis. From the measurements of the mineral ions in blood and urine, we are able to make inferences about mineral balance, intestinal absorption, renal handling, and bone mineralization and resorption. This knowledge of homeostasis allows us to understand how it is perturbed by a specific disorder. This chapter reviews the homeostatic systems for Ca, Mg, and PO_4 and the mechanisms whereby each system adapts to changing body requirements. Bone cellular functions and turnover and matrix composition are discussed in the chapter on osteoporosis (Chapter 264). Details of parathyroid gland function and regulation of PTH secretion are discussed in Chapter 266.

DISTRIBUTION OF ELEMENTS

Total Body

Calcium

In a physiologically normal 70-kg man, the total body Ca content is approximately 25 mmol (mg/40 = mmol), of which 99% exists in the mineral phase of bone as a variation of the hydroxyapatite [$Ca_{10}(PO_4)_6(OH)_2$] crystal (Table 263–1). The mineralized skeleton confers the structural and mechanical weight-bearing properties of bone. A portion of bone, estimated to be approximately 1%, composes a labile reservoir that serves as a rapidly available source of Ca, Mg, and PO_4 that can be mobilized to support the ions' many functions in a variety of biologic systems. The molar ratio of Ca to P in $Ca_{10}(PO_4)_6(OH)_2$ is approximately 2 : 1, so as bone is resorbed and $Ca_{10}(PO_4)_6(OH)_2$ is dissolved, Ca and P ions are released into the extracellular fluid (ECF) at a ratio of approximately 2 : 1. Soft tissue and the ECF space including blood contain the remaining 1% of Ca.

In the blood, the serum total Ca concentration is 10^{-3} mol/L Ca is present in the freely ionized state (48%) and is protein bound (46%) largely to albumin, a feature that accounts for 70% of the Ca bound to protein. The remainder of the total Ca (6%) is complexed to citrate and PO_4 ions (Table 263–2). Clinical laboratories measure total serum Ca by automated techniques that are quite reproducible. The ionized fraction of Ca would be the most informative measurement, because the biologic actions of Ca are attributed to ionized Ca, which is readily exchangeable with pools of Ca in bone, blood, and intracellular sites. Because pitfalls in drawing and processing of blood samples call into question the accuracy of ionized Ca, automated methods for measurement of total Ca may be more reliable if the albumin level is not reduced and pH is normal.

Magnesium

The average adult body contains approximately 1.0 mol of Mg, of which 54% is located within the skeleton, 45% is intracellular in other tissues, and 1% is within the extracellular compartment (see Table 263–1). Mg is a major constituent of what has been called the *labile ion pool of bone.* This functional portion of bone is thought to be located at the crystal surface in equilibrium with ECF, but it is not consistently incorporated into the $Ca_{10}(PO_4)_6(OH)_2$ crystal structure. Mg is the most abundant intracellular divalent cation; it functions as a cofactor that regulates enzymes and neuromuscular networks. The cellular cytosolic Mg concentration is approximately 5×10^{-4} M, which approaches the concentration in the ECF. Mg concentration in both the intracellular fluid and the ECF is regulated but has not been well characterized. Serum Mg is partitioned into ionic, protein-bound, and complexed fractions that vary more than similar fractions of blood Ca (see Table 263–2). Ionic Mg is the fraction that most closely correlates with Mg-dependent biologic actions. However, serum total or ionic Mg levels do not accurately estimate the Mg concentrations in the intracellular, soft tissue, or total body spaces.

Phosphate

P exists in tissues and blood primarily as PO_4. Approximately 17,500 mmol of PO_4 are found in adult humans. In bone, PO_4 is a major constituent of the $Ca_{10}(PO_4)_6(OH)_2$ crystal structure and accounts for approximately 85% of total body PO_4. The soft tissue contains 15% of total body PO_4, and only 0.3% is present in the ECF (see Table 263–1). In soft tissues, PO_4 is in the form of PO_4 esters. In contrast to the steep transmembrane gradients for Ca, PO_4 gradients across the plasma membrane are modest, with concentrations in the ECF of 10^{-4} M and cytosol of approximately 2×10^{-4} M.

Serum PO_4 levels are not tightly controlled within a narrow range as are those of Ca, but rather they fluctuate widely depending on age, sex, dietary intake, and growth rate. Serum levels of PTH, $1,25(OH)_2D_3$, growth hormone, insulin-like growth factor-I, and a group of newly discovered regulators called *phosphotonins,* which includes fibroblast growth factor-23 (FGF-23), control serum PO_4 levels primarily by regulating the efficiency of renal proximal tubule reabsorption of filtered PO_4. In addition, $1,25(OH)_2D_3$ increases serum PO_4 through stimulation of intestinal PO_4 absorption, and PTH and $1,25(OH)_2D_3$ release bone PO_4 through stimulation of bone resorption. Serum PO_4 decreases in the postprandial state and during intravenous glucose administration through insulin-mediated cellular PO_4 entry. P in serum is mainly in the inorganic form of PO_4 as ionic, protein bound, and complexed to sodium (Na), Ca, or Mg (see Table 263–2).

Normal serum PO_4 contributes to the maintenance of the Ca × PO_4 ion product at levels sufficient to create the physicochemical forces that drive bone mineralization. Low serum PO_4 may lower the Ca × PO_4 ion product and may thus impair mineralization. A high serum and ECF Ca × PO_4 product may result in ectopic or extraskeletal soft tissue calcification.

Cellular Distribution

Calcium

Fluctuations in cytosolic ionic Ca (Ca^{2+}) are buffered to maintain levels at approximately 10^{-6} M. Blood and ECF Ca concentration is maintained within a narrow range of approximately 10^{-3} M, which creates a 1000-fold chemical gradient favoring Ca entry into the cell. The electrical gradient across the plasma membrane of 50 mV (cell interior negative) generates an electrical gradient that also favors Ca entry. The electrochemical gradients drive Ca influx from the ECF and can, if excessive, present a major threat to cell viability. Excess cellular Ca influx is extruded from the cell through energy-dependent Ca channels, Ca-dependent adenosine triphosphate (ATP)–driven Ca pumps, Na-Ca exchangers, and through active uptake into cell organelles including the endoplasmic reticulum and mitochondria. In addition, intracellular Ca-binding proteins buffer excess cytosolic Ca and thereby prevent Ca toxicity and cell death. Ca reservoirs in mitochondria and endoplasmic reticulum mobilize Ca stores and maintain cytosolic Ca^{2+} when a tendency exists for Ca^{2+} levels to fall. In addition, intracellular Ca may function as a signal through pulsatile release from binding sites on the plasma membrane and within intracellular organelles in response to plasma membrane receptor activation.

Cell Ca homeostasis may also be linked to specialized cellular function. In skeletal and cardiac muscle, Ca facilitates the linking of excitation and contraction by mobilizing large Ca intracellular stores located in the sarcoplasmic reticulum. In other nonskeletal cells, Ca may signal activated

TABLE 263–1 TOTAL BODY DISTRIBUTION OF CALCIUM, MAGNESIUM, AND PHOSPHATE*

Compartment	Calcium (%)	Magnesium (%)	Phosphate (%)
Bone	99	54	85
Extracellular fluid space	0.1	1.0	0.3
Intracellular	1.0	45	15

*Values are the percentage of total body content for a healthy 70-kg man. Phosphorus is mostly in the form of phosphate; the extracellular fluid space includes the blood.

TABLE 263–2 DISTRIBUTION OF CALCIUM, MAGNESIUM, AND PHOSPHATE IN HUMAN PLASMA*

State in Blood	Calcium (%)	Magnesium (%)	Phosphate (%)
Total	2.1–2.55	0.65–1.05	0.87–1.45†
Ionized or free	1.18 (48)	0.52 (62)	1.89 (54)‡
Protein-bound	1.14 (46)	0.26 (31)	0.14 (12)
Complexed	0.08 (3)	0.6 (7)	0.40 (34)§
Unknown	0.08 (3)	0	0

*Values are in mmol/L (mM) and represent normal ranges.
†Values are higher in cord blood and during childhood.
‡Free ionic phosphate (PO_4) is composed of HPO_4^{2-} and $H_2PO_4^-$ at a ratio of 4.4 : 1.0 at pH 7.4.
§Complexed PO_4 is composed of $NaHPO_4^-$, $CaHPO_4$, and $MgHPO_4$ at a ratio of 11.0 : 1.33 : 1.0.

plasma membrane receptors to carry out diverse functions such as hormone and enzyme secretion, neurotransmitter release and uptake, and phosphorylation of a variety of enzymes, transporters, and molecules that store energy.

Magnesium

Cytosolic Mg is a small portion (5 to 10%) of total cellular Mg and is regulated through uptake and binding to intracellular organelles. Mitochondria contain the majority (60%) of intracellular Mg, and there Mg serves as a cofactor in a number of enzymes involved in PO_4 transport, transcription, translation, and energy utilization. The intracellular localizations and concentrations of Mg are maintained by a network of transporters and channels that are poorly understood.

Phosphate

Cytosolic free PO_4 ion concentration is a small fraction of total cellular PO_4. The majority of cell PO_4 resides in mitochondria, mainly in the form of Ca PO_4 salts. Intracellular PO_4 ion may also exist as PO_4 esters, as plasma membrane phospholipids, or as phosphorylated molecules involved in energy generation, storage, and transfer.

BONE MATRIX COMPOSITION AND CELLULAR ELEMENTS

Matrix and the Mineral Phases

One of the main functions of the mineral homeostatic system is to deliver sufficient Ca, Mg, and PO_4 to bone mineralization sites to support growth, maturation, remodeling, and repair of the skeleton at all stages of the life cycle. The connective tissue and mineral compositions of bone are responsible for its mechanical, protective, and mineral homeostatic functions. The bone organic matrix, the largest collection of connective tissue in the body, is unique for its highly organized mineralization phase and the lifelong process of regeneration and replacement or turnover. Bone composition varies with age, state of maturation and turnover, skeletal location, diet, and health, but it is generally 50 to 70% mineral, 20 to 40% organic matrix, 5 to 10% water, and less than 3% lipids. The mineral phase of apatite is similar to the geologic variety of $Ca_{10}(PO_4)_6(OH)_2$, but with a lower Ca and OH^- content. Bone apatite crystals are extremely small (i.e., 200 angstroms), and they contain other divalent cations and anions such as carbonate, Mg, and acid phosphate that occupy sites in the apatite matrix and thereby create an irregular crystal lattice. As a result, the apatite is more readily solubilized, and this property permits the mineral phase to participate in the homeostatic process as a virtually unlimited source of Ca, Mg, and PO_4. Ninety-five percent of the organic matrix is composed of type I collagen, which provides the bone its elasticity and flexibility. Both collagen and the noncollagen proteins play crucial roles in bone mineralization and remodeling. The initial process of mineralization involves deposition of ions followed by crystal formation at specific sites between the collagen fibrils. Because the driving force for mineral deposition in bone is the creation of a supersaturated state with respect to the key ions of apatite including Ca and PO_4, and because blood and ECF are undersaturated with respect to apatite, the bone matrix must contain molecules that facilitate mineral accumulation and apatite deposition. Osteocalcin, the most abundant noncollagen protein in bone, contains a high content of γ-carboxyglutamic acid. This amino acid has a high affinity for Ca and may confer on osteocalcin the important function of ion localization during the early phases of mineralization. Other classes of matrix molecules with high affinity for Ca including the highly anionic glycoproteins and proteoglycans may play roles in calcification and the attachment of the apatite crystals to the collagen fibrils.

The mechanical properties of bone are influenced by the distribution, size, and density of the apatite crystals. Optimal size and content of the apatite are required to maintain the mechanical weight-bearing strength. Disease states associated with too many crystals or with very large crystals favor a brittle bone, whereas disorders leading to sparse crystal distribution or to very small crystals compromise bone mechanical strength.

Cellular Elements

Bone remodeling or the process of replacement of bone is conducted along the surfaces of bone, primarily on the endosteal surface. The internal (endosteal) and external (periosteal) surfaces of bone are each lined with cellular layers called the *endosteum* and *periosteum,* respectively. Cortical and trabecular bone are the two types of bone composing the adult skeleton. Both are composed of the same cells and bone matrix, but they differ structurally and functionally. In cortical bone, 80 to 90% of the volume is mineralized, in contrast to trabecular bone, of which only 15 to 25% is mineralized. These structural differences create a large interface with soft tissue, with approximately 70 to 85% located at the endosteal surface. As a result, trabecular bone and its greater surface area conduct more metabolic functions in mineral homeostasis, whereas the more dense cortical bone contributes more to the mechanical and protective functions.

Three major cell types are responsible for the formation, resorption, and remodeling of bone. *Osteoblasts* line the bone surfaces and synthesize and secrete type I collagen, the accompanying proteins, and small molecules that compose the matrix. Osteoblasts differentiate from multipotential mesenchymal stem cells residing in the marrow in response to local growth factors, such as bone morphogenic proteins and FGFs. The precursor cells then proliferate and differentiate into preosteoblasts and eventually mature osteoblasts. Clusters of osteoblasts are found along the surface of bone setting on newly synthesized unmineralized matrix. There is a delay of 7 to 10 days from the time of matrix secretion until mineralization begins. Full mineralization of an area of newly secreted matrix may take 3 to 4 months to complete.

Osteocytes are mature osteoblasts that have completed matrix protein secretion and subsequent mineralization and are now surrounded by cortical bone. Although mature and no longer capable of bone formation, osteocytes can be stimulated to resorb bone from the surrounding canalicular walls that encase them.

Osteoclasts are large, multinucleated cells on trabecular surfaces that are responsible for bone resorption. The mononuclear and phagocytic cell lineages proliferate and differentiate into preosteoclasts and then become terminally differentiated osteoclasts under the stimulation of monocyte colony-stimulating factor, expression of the RANK surface receptor to bind the osteoblast-generated RANKL, and downstream mediators of RANKL. Specific integrin receptors ($\alpha_v\beta_3$) are expressed on the cell surfaces and serve to bind the mature osteoclasts to the underlying mineralized bone. PTH and $1,25(OH)_2D_3$ are known stimulators of osteoclast-mediated bone resorption.

HOMEOSTASIS

The homeostatic systems for Ca, Mg, and PO_4 maintain total body and intracellular ion distributions and sufficient ion delivery to bone to support matrix mineralization during growth, development, and remodeling. Each ion is regulated by components of a homeostatic system that include the parathyroid glands, bone, intestine, and kidney, as well as PTH and vitamin D and its metabolites. Blood levels of Ca are tightly controlled by the homeostatic system. Blood levels of Mg are less tightly controlled than are those of Ca. Serum PO_4 is important in maintaining the blood Ca × PO_4 ion product that generates the critical driving force for matrix mineralization.

Maintenance of Blood Levels

Calcium

Ca homeostasis has two goals: sufficient delivery of Ca to support skeletal mineralization and maintenance of blood ionized Ca (Ca^{2+}) within a narrow normal range to avoid fluctuations in many different Ca-dependent biologic systems. Because diet Ca intake and skeletal Ca requirements vary widely from day to day and across the various stages of the life cycle, the Ca homeostatic system is constantly adjusting delivery of sufficient Ca, Mg, and PO_4 from intestine and kidney into the ECF and then to bone to meet changing skeletal requirements while at the same time maintaining a constant ECF Ca concentration. This ECF fraction controls cellular biologic functions and therefore has the highest priority. Indeed, the homeostatic system maintains ECF Ca^{2+} even at the expense of the integrity of the bone mineral content.

Because the environment is relatively Ca deficient, and Ca-rich foods are largely confined to dairy products, a decline in Ca^{2+} is defended against by all the actions of PTH (Table 238–3). PTH secretion is regulated by the parathyroid cell plasma membrane Ca-sensing receptor (CaR), which detects ambient serum Ca^{2+} and thus regulates minute-to-minute PTH secretion (Chapter 266). The calcemic actions of PTH increase Ca influx into the ECF through several mechanisms, each with its own time course of appearance. PTH stimulation of renal tubule reabsorption of filtered Ca occurs within minutes. If PTH secretion is sustained, then increased osteoclastically and osteocytically mediated bone resorption will appear within minutes to hours. Finally, PTH stimulates intestinal Ca absorption indirectly through increased renal proximal tubule $1,25(OH)_2D_3$ synthesis that appears with a lag time of approximately 12 to 24 hours. $1,25(OH)_2D_3$ may increase serum PO_4 levels by stimulating both intestinal PO_4 absorption and bone resorption with mineral dissolution that releases bone Ca and PO_4. A large PO_4 load could increase blood PO_4 and lower Ca^{2+}, but PTH mediates a decrease in renal proximal tubule PO_4 reabsorption and so dissipates the PO_4 load by increasing urinary excretion.

On the parathyroid cells, hypercalcemia stimulates cell surface CaR signaling and thereby suppresses PTH secretion. Elevated Ca^{2+} also stimulates distal nephron CaR, which reduces net tubule Ca reabsorption, increases urine Ca excretion, and thus provides a mechanism to lower Ca^{2+} to normal. Elevated Ca^{2+} normally reduces PTH secretion, which, in turn, decreases tubular Ca reabsorption, decreases intestinal Ca absorption through reduction in $1,25(OH)_2D_3$ production, and decreases osteoclast-mediated bone resorption.

Magnesium

Mg blood levels are regulated largely by the quantitative influx and efflux of Mg across intestine, bone, and kidney, rather than by the elaborate PTH and $1,25(OH)_2D_3$ system that has evolved to control Ca^{2+}. Like Ca^{2+}, Mg can also downregulate PTH secretion, but it is less potent than Ca^{2+}. Serum Mg levels are regulated primarily by renal proximal tubular reabsorption.

Phosphate

Serum PO_4 levels decline rapidly during periods of low dietary PO_4 intake, but proximal tubule reabsorption becomes more efficient and thereby lowers urine PO_4 losses to 1 to 2% of the filtered load within 2 to 4 days of ingesting a diet low in PO_4. Whether the parathyroid glands are directly sensitive to ambient PO_4 levels remains controversial.

Mineral Intake and Intestinal Absorption

Calcium

The major source of dietary Ca intake is milk and other dairy products. Some vegetables, including spinach, kale, broccoli, and seaweed, contain Ca, but these foods also contain large amounts of oxalate that bind Ca and prevent a large portion of its absorption. Therefore, Ca intake largely depends on the amount of dairy products in the diet. In humans, the efficiency of absorption (fractional Ca absorption) has been measured experimentally using numerous techniques, including external 6-day balance studies, segmental small intestinal perfusion through a multiple-lumen tube, and single- or double-Ca isotope kinetics. Although these techniques have been widely used in clinical studies, none is available for use in patient care. All these techniques confirm that dietary Ca is incompletely absorbed, with an efficiency of absorption between 30 and 60%. The range reflects the influence of age, habitual Ca intake, skeletal requirements, vitamin D status, the state of the homeostatic system, and the bioavailability of Ca contained in foods. Fractional Ca absorption is directly correlated with ambient $1,25(OH)_2D_3$ circulating levels. The high efficiency of Ca absorption in children and adolescents during periods of rapid skeletal growth and in young women during pregnancy and lactation is mediated by increased circulating $1,25(OH)_2D_3$. Low dietary Ca intake or an increase in Ca requirements stimulates the adaptive increase in fractional Ca absorption. The intestinal adaptation is lost with age in adults, and thus the practice of increasing dietary Ca or using Ca supplements in postmenopausal women and in older men is an attempt to compensate for the age-related decline in fractional intestinal Ca absorption and $1,25(OH)_2D_3$ production. Negative Ca balance (urine Ca + fecal Ca > net intestinal Ca absorption) develops as Ca net absorption falls to less than 5.0 mmol/day. Fecal Ca is the sum of unabsorbed dietary Ca, Ca in secreted pancreatic and biliary juices, and mucosal secretions. Fecal Ca losses are between 2.5 and 5.0 mmol/day and are not regulated by Ca^{2+}, PTH, or $1,25(OH)_2D_3$.

Sites and Mechanisms of Absorption

The rapid transit time across the duodenum and jejunum may limit Ca absorption; however, the large surface areas of these regions are responsible for approximately 90% of Ca absorbed during adequate Ca intake. The physiologic adaptation to certain stimuli increases fractional Ca absorption from 25 to 45% to 55 to 70%. The increases are largely in the duodenum and ileum and, to a lesser extent, in the jejunum and colon.

Intestinal perfusion studies show that net Ca absorption increases with luminal Ca concentration, with a tendency to plateau at higher concentrations. The curvilinear relationship between net Ca absorption and Ca intake reflects the sum of two absorptive mechanisms: a cell-mediated, saturable active transport that dominates absorption at low luminal Ca concentrations; and a passive, diffusional, paracellular absorption that is driven by transepithelial electrochemical gradients and dominates at normal and high luminal Ca concentrations greater than 1.0 mM. Variations in the Ca active transport component may account for the wide range in net Ca absorption in healthy adults at any level of Ca intake. $1,25(OH)_2D_3$ stimulation of the Ca active transport in subjects with increased Ca requirements can be appreciated from the greater net Ca absorption at the same level of luminal Ca concentration as those subjects fed a diet adequate in Ca. Very high Ca intakes are primarily absorbed by passive diffusion, because serum $1,25(OH)_2D_3$ levels are low. Diffusional Ca flow along the paracellular pathway is in part dictated by the permeability of each intestinal segment, which is highest across the duodenum, jejunum, and ileum, is lowest in the cecum, and is intermediate across the colon.

Intestinal epithelial transcellular Ca transport is stimulated by high ambient $1,25(OH)_2D_3$ and by upregulation of the vitamin D receptor. The vitamin D receptor mediates expression of vitamin D–dependent genes encoded for proteins that are required for Ca active transport. Epithelial brush border membrane Ca influx is facilitated by the Ca transport protein TRPV6. The potential importance of this Ca channel is suggested by its dual independent regulation by $1,25(OH)_2D_3$ and estradiol through their intestinal receptors. Once within the cell, Ca is bound to the high-affinity Ca binding protein calbindin 9 kD, which is located within vesicles that move from the base of the brush border across the cell interior to the basolateral plasma membrane, where they fuse with the plasma membrane. Extrusion of Ca from the cell interior may require the low-affinity, high-capacity Na-Ca exchanger and the high-affinity Ca-, Mg-dependent ATPase.

Phosphate

PO_4 is found in most food groups, and PO_4 absorption increases linearly with dietary PO_4 intake. At normal to high dietary PO_4 intake, absorption is largely by a passive diffusional mechanism that depends on the luminal PO_4 concentration. During low PO_4 intake when the luminal concentration is less than 2.0 mM (mg/31 = mmol PO_4), PO_4 absorption largely occurs through an active, cell-mediated transport process that is stimulated by $1,25(OH)_2D_3$. PO_4 is a major constituent of cellular tissues; therefore, dietary PO_4 intake is usually greater than 20 mmol/day. During adequate intake (25 to 60 mmol/day), PO_4 absorption is highly efficient, with 60 to 80% of dietary PO_4 absorbed, and net secretion occurs only when diet PO_4 is quite low (<10 mmol/day). $1,25(OH)_2D_3$ stimulates jejunal PO_4 absorption when luminal concentrations are low. For example, in patients with vitamin D deficiency or during chronic renal failure with low $1,25(OH)_2D_3$ serum levels, $1,25(OH)_2D_3$ administration increases net PO_4 absorption. Net PO_4 absorption is readily detectable when luminal concentrations are normal or increased, even when serum $1,25(OH)_2D_3$ levels are low to undetectable, as in patients with chronic renal failure.

Transcellular PO_4 transport begins with influx across the brush border by overcoming the electrochemical gradients through either an energy-dependent transport process or a secondary active transport process coupled to the influx of a cation such as Na. $1,25(OH)_2D_3$ stimulates net PO_4 absorption by increasing brush border PO_4 uptake that is saturable with an affinity coefficient of 1.0 mM. Therefore, at luminal PO_4 concentrations greater than 1.0 mM, diffusional PO_4 absorption predominates, but when the luminal PO_4 concentration is low, then the transcellular mechanism is active. The saturable active transport mechanism is present primarily in the proximal duodenum and jejunum and, to a lesser extent, in the distal ileum. No net PO_4 absorption occurs in the colon.

Magnesium

Mg is abundant in highly cellular foods, and intake is linearly related to total caloric intake. During usual Mg intake of 7 to 30 mmol (mg/24 = mmol)/day, fractional Mg absorption averages 35 to 40%, and net intestinal Mg absorption increases in direct relation to dietary Mg. Net Mg absorption occurs when secretion is exceeded at Mg intakes greater than 2 mmol/day. $1,25(OH)_2D_3$ does not stimulate Mg absorption, and serum $1,25(OH)_2D_3$ and net Mg absorption do not co-vary. Dietary PO_4 and some other dietary anionic constituents form nonabsorbable complexes with Mg and reduce Mg absorption.

Absorptive and secretory Mg fluxes across small intestine and colon are composed of voltage-dependent and voltage-independent constituents, which are thought to represent paracellular and cellular pathways, respectively. Passive diffusional absorption along the paracellular pathway is driven by intestinal luminal Mg concentrations, and saturable cellular Mg transport is small compared with the total Mg absorptive flux.

Renal Handling and Urinary Excretion

The fine adjustments of Ca, Mg, and PO_4 balances occur at the level of the kidney, where filtered loads and tubular reabsorptions are highly regulated under changing body mineral requirements and wide variations in intakes and net absorptions.

Calcium

Approximately 98% of the Ca glomerular filtrate undergoes tubular reabsorption that results in precise regulation of serum Ca^{2+} and urine excretion. Ultrafiltrable Ca is composed of the serum complexed and ionized Ca fractions and undergoes complete filtration at the glomerulus when Ca concentration is approximately 1.5 mM. The high level of Ca filtered each day, more than 270 mmol, is far in excess of the Ca content contained in the ECF, and it also exceeds net intestinal Ca absorption. Therefore, approximately 98% of the filtered Ca must be reabsorbed to maintain neutral Ca balance. Approximately 70% of filtered Ca is reabsorbed in the proximal tubule through predominantly passive mechanisms. Another 20% of filtered Ca is reabsorbed in the thick ascending limb of the loop of Henle (TALH). The CaR is located on the basolateral membranes of the TALH and is stimulated by increases in ECF and peritubular Ca. CaR reduces lumen-positive voltage and thereby reduces Ca reabsorption. In the distal tubules, the Ca-selective renal epithelial TRPV5 channel is more permeable to Ca than Na and is increased by $1,25(OH)_2D_3$ and estradiol. In the distal tubule segments, calbindin 28 kD and calbindin 9 kD facilitate Ca diffusion, and the Na-Ca exchanger and a Ca-ATPase extrude Ca across the plasma membrane. Whereas Ca generally follows Na in this segment, reabsorption and excretion of Ca and Na can be dissociated. The collecting duct is the final site of Ca reabsorption in which less than 5% of the filtered load is absorbed. The several tubular segments that reabsorb Ca result in a final urine that contains only approximately 2% of the filtered Ca load.

Factors that increase or decrease urine Ca excretion are listed in Table 263–3. Volume expansion increases and volume contraction decreases urine Ca and Na excretions. Hypercalcemia increases ultrafiltrable Ca but decreases glomerular filtration rate (GFR). Hypercalcemia also decreases proximal tubule, TALH, and distal convoluted tubule Ca reabsorption, and the result is greater urinary excretion of Ca than Na. In the TALH, CaR activation by hypercalcemia decreases Ca reabsorption; Ca may also alter paracellin-1–regulated Ca and Mg permeability with decreased reabsorption of both ions. PTH is also the principal regulator of Ca reabsorption by reducing GFR and stimulating tubule reabsorption. Moreover, PTH increases TALH active Ca transport and opens TRPV5 in the distal convoluted tubule for reabsorption. Although PTH increases net Ca reabsorption, patients with primary hyperparathyroidism are often hypercalciuric, because increased tubule Ca reabsorption worsens the hypercalcemia and increases the filtered load of Ca, with resulting hypercalciuria (Table 263–3). PTH-related peptide (PTHrP), which is secreted by certain malignant tumors, mimics the actions of PTH along the nephron. $1,25(OH)_2D_3$ actions on the kidney are incompletely understood but include stimulation of CaR expression, which decreases Ca reabsorption, and increase of calbindin 28 kD, which increases Ca reabsorption. Vitamin D deficiency reduces Ca reabsorption independent of PTH levels. PO_4 administration reduces urine Ca excretion by increasing distal Ca reabsorption and stimulating PTH. Restricted dietary PO_4 causes hypercalciuria by actions in the distal nephron. Acute and chronic metabolic acidosis increase urine Ca excretion and alkalosis decreases urine Ca excretion.

TABLE 263–3 FACTORS THAT INCREASE OR DECREASE RENAL CALCIUM EXCRETION

Increased	Decreased
Glomerular Filtration	
Increased	**Decreased**
Hypercalcemia	Hypocalcemia Renal insufficiency
Tubular Reabsorption	
Increased	**Decreased**
Extracellular fluid volume depletion	Extracellular fluid volume expansion
Hypocalcemia	Hypercalcemia
Thiazide diuretics	Loop diuretics
Phosphate administration	Dietary phosphate deprivation
Metabolic alkalosis	Metabolic acidosis
Parathyroid hormone	Autosomal dominant hypocalcemia
Parathyroid hormone–related peptide	Dent's disease
Familial hypocalciuric hypercalcemia	Bartter's syndrome

TABLE 263–4 FACTORS THAT INCREASE OR DECREASE RENAL MAGNESIUM REABSORPTION

Glomerular Filtration	
Increased	**Decreased**
Hypermagnesemia	Hypomagnesemia Renal insufficiency
Tubular Reabsorption	
Increased	**Decreased**
Extracellular fluid volume expansion	Extracellular fluid volume depletion
Hypomagnesemia	Hypermagnesemia
Hypocalcemia	Hypercalcemia
Metabolic alkalosis	Phosphate depletion
Parathyroid hormone	Loop diuretics Aminoglycoside antibiotics Cisplatin Cyclosporine Ethanol Gitelman's syndrome

TABLE 263–5 FACTORS THAT INCREASE OR DECREASE RENAL PHOSPHATE REABSORPTION

Glomerular Filtration	
Increased	**Decreased**
Hyperphosphatemia Mild hypercalcemia	Hypophosphatemia Moderate hypercalcemia Renal insufficiency
Tubular Reabsorption	
Increased	**Decreased**
Diet phosphate reabsorption	Phosphate excess
Hypercalcemia	Hypocalcemia
Extracellular fluid depletion	Chronic metabolic acidosis
Chronic metabolic alkalosis	Acute metabolic alkalosis Parathyroid hormone Parathyroid hormone–related peptide Fibroblast growth factor-23 1,25-Dihydroxyvitamin D_3 Thiazide diuretics Hypophosphatemic states

Thiazide and related diuretics (hydrochlorothiazide, chlorthalidone), indapamide, and amiloride increase urine Na excretion and decrease urine Ca through an increase in renal distal tubule Ca reabsorption. Loop diuretics (furosemide, torsemide, ethacrynic acid) increase urine Ca and Na excretion by inhibiting the Na-potassium-2Chloride transporter in the TALH. Hypercalciuria continues as long as urinary Na losses are replaced.

Magnesium

Ultrafiltrable Mg, composed of ionized and complexed Mg, makes up approximately 70% of total serum Mg. Urine Mg averages approximately 24 mmol/day, a finding indicating that approximately 95% of the GFR is reabsorbed. The proximal tubule reabsorbs only approximately 15% of the Mg ultrafiltrate. Approximately 70% of Mg is reabsorbed in the cortical TALH, and no reabsorption occurs in the medullary TALH. High serum Mg may decrease Mg reabsorption through stimulation of CaR. Approximately 10% of filtered Mg is reabsorbed in the distal convoluted tubule.

Urine Mg reabsorption is highly regulated by numerous conditions (Table 263–4). ECF volume expansion decreases Mg reabsorption and increases urine Mg. High serum Mg increases urine Mg excretion in part through activation of CaR. Hypomagnesemia increases TALH Mg reabsorption and thereby decreases urine Mg. Hypercalcemia decreases Mg reabsorption in the proximal tubule and the TALH. PTH increases Mg reabsorption, but the hypercalcemia in primary hyperparathyroidism reduces Mg reabsorption. Vitamin D and metabolites have no known actions on Mg reabsorption. Thiazide diuretics have a minimal effect on Mg excretion, and loop diuretics markedly increase urine Mg excretion.

Phosphate

Ultrafiltrable PO_4 makes up approximately 85% of total serum PO_4, and approximately 12.5% of the filtrate appears in the final urine (25 to 33 mmol/day; mg/31 = mmol). Eighty-five percent of PO_4 reabsorption occurs in the proximal tubule through an Na-PO_4 cotransporter, which reabsorbs PO_4 against the brush border electrochemical PO_4 gradients. Three genes encode for related Na gradient-dependent PO_4 transporters *(Npt1-Npt3)*, and the apical brush border membrane Npt2 accounts for approximately 85% of proximal tubule PO_4 reabsorption. The *Npt2* gene is regulated by FGF-23. A full discussion of phosphotonins, including FGF-23 and disorders of hypophosphatemia and renal PO_4 wasting, is found in Chapter 265. Only a small fraction of PO_4 reabsorption occurs in the distal convoluted tubule. The tubular maximum for the reabsorption of PO_4 (expressed as TMP/GFR) is approximately equal to the concentration of filtered PO_4. Therefore, any increase in filtered PO_4 increases urinary PO_4 excretion.

The major factors that regulate Na-dependent PO_4 reabsorption are PTH, FGF-23, and dietary PO_4 (Table 263–5). Each sets the maximal capacity of the kidney to reabsorb filtered PO_4. Low PO_4 intake stimulates reabsorption, whereas high PO_4 intake inhibits reabsorption and increases urine PO_4. Within hours of a change in PO_4 intake, PO_4 reabsorption adapts through brush border Npt2 cotransporter expression. Hypercalcemia and hypocalcemia decrease and increase renal PO_4 reabsorption, respectively. The renal response to hypercalcemia includes a decrease in GFR, and therefore filtered PO_4. The phosphaturic actions of PTH are mediated through suppression of the brush border Npt2 cotransporter, which decreases proximal tubule PO_4 reabsorption. $1,25(OH)_2D_3$ increases intestinal PO_4 absorption and decreases renal PO_4 reabsorption. Serum FGF-23 levels are positively correlated with serum PO_4 and suggest a role in normal physiologic control of renal PO_4 reabsorption.

Mineral Balance and Adaptation to Changing Requirements

Mineral homeostasis is the dynamic state of mineral ion balance (retention or loss) maintained by the calciotropic hormones PTH and $1,25(OH)_2D_3$ through adjustments to changing mineral requirements (see Table 238–3). Dietary supply of one or more of the mineral ions may be insufficient and thus may require adjustment or adaptation of the homeostatic systems through hormonal changes to maintain external balance (balance = net absorption − [fecal excretion + urine excretion]). Mineral balance becomes positive (intake and retention exceed urinary and intestinal losses) during rapid skeletal growth in childhood and adolescence, as well as during pregnancy and lactation. Negative balance (gastrointestinal and/or urinary losses exceed intake and retention) may occur during high rates of bone remodeling, as seen during estrogen deficiency, with aging, and accompanying diseases such as hyperthyroidism and primary hyperparathyroidism. PTH and $1,25(OH)_2D_3$ mediate adaptation of the homeostatic system through increased intestinal Ca, Mg, and PO_4 absorption and by regulation of renal tubule Ca, PO_4, and Mg reabsorption. With respect to Ca, the homeostatic system is sufficiently flexible to maintain blood ionized Ca within the normal range without being disturbed by wide variations in dietary Ca intake and changing rates of bone mineralization.

External mineral balance is measured by feeding patients diets of known Ca, Mg, and PO_4 content. Patients are fed the diets for 7 to 10 days to permit adaptation to any new levels of intake that differ from their habitual intake. External balance is then calculated from data collected during at least 6 days while the diet remains fixed, and all feces and urine passed are collected and analyzed for Ca, Mg, and PO_4 content. The completeness of fecal collection is determined by measuring a nonabsorbable marker that is administered with each meal during the balance period. Net intestinal absorption of Ca, Mg, and PO_4 is calculated as dietary intake minus average daily fecal excretion. Physiologic adaptations and alterations by diseases in Ca, Mg, and PO_4 balance provide insight into the pathophysiologic changes of urine excretions, blood levels, and changes in bone mass.

Neutral Balance

Neutral mineral balance is defined as the state in which fractional mineral ion absorptions match the sum of urinary and fecal mineral losses. Neutral balance is expected in men who are less than 65 years old and in premenopausal, nonpregnant women after they have reached peak bone mass. An example of maintenance of neutral Ca balance is the physiologic adaptation of the homeostatic system to low dietary Ca (Fig. 263–1). The major signal for change is Ca balance, and such hormonal changes also alter the balance and handling of Mg and PO_4.

Positive Balance

In *positive mineral ion balance,* mineral absorption and retention exceed fecal and urine mineral losses. Positive balance of Ca, Mg, and PO_4

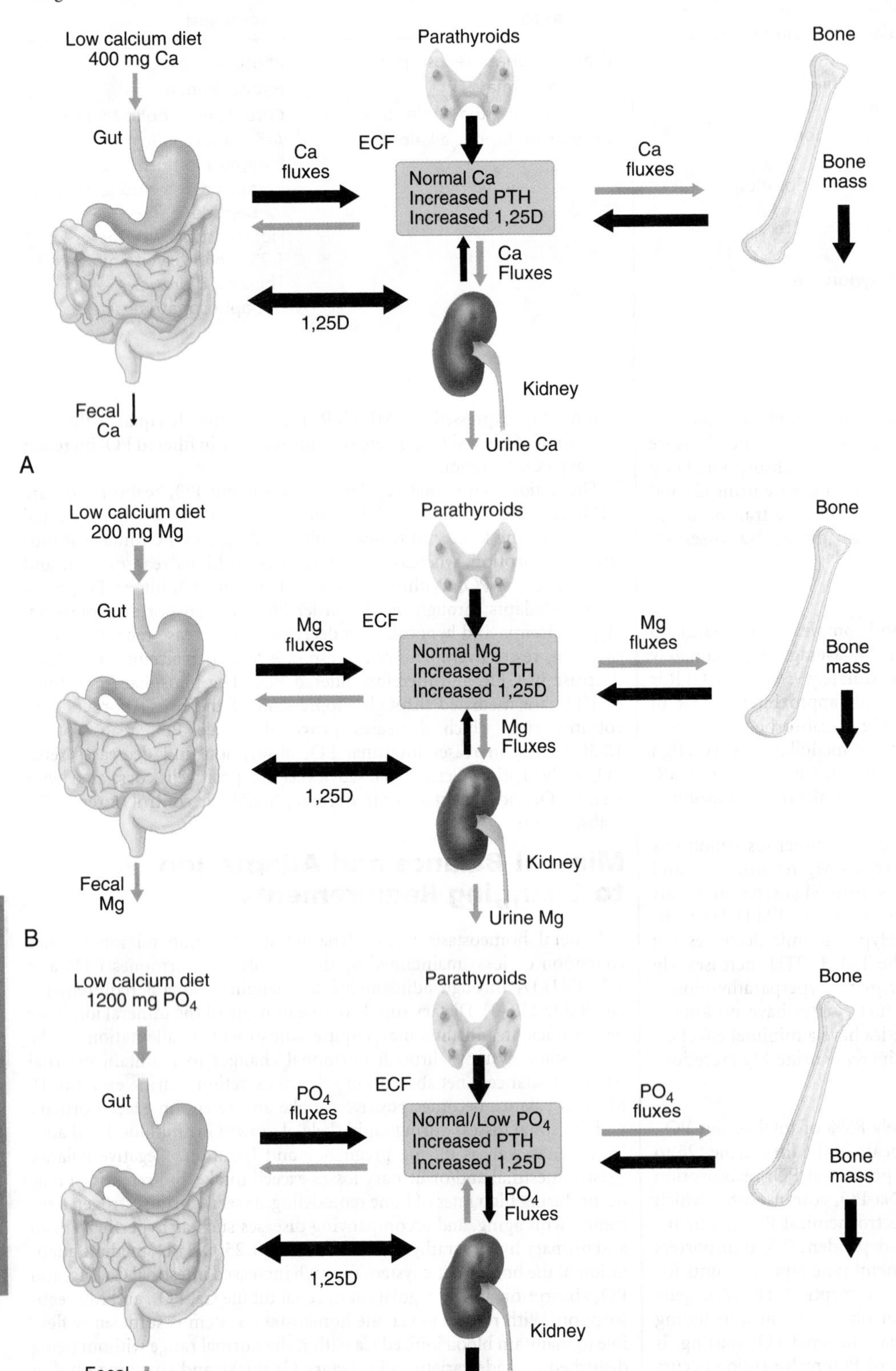

FIGURE 263–1 • Effects of a low-calcium (Ca) diet. Representative changes in Ca **(A)**, magnesium (Mg; **B**), and phosphate (PO_4; **C**) fluxes, distributions, and serum hormone levels during a low-Ca diet and the maintenance of a neutral mineral balance in young adults. When the arrows are paired, the green arrows are unidirectional net fluxes; the black arrows show the direction of the net flux; and the size of the arrow is the relative magnitude of the flux. The solid unidirectional arrows indicate increases from normal, and the small green arrows indicate decreases from normal. For bone, the upward and downward arrows are increased and decreased bone mass, respectively. For the parathyroids, the arrows indicate that parathyroid hormone (PTH) secretion is increased (black arrows) or normal (green arrows). For 1,25-dihydroxyvitamin D_3, serum levels are increased (black arrows) or decreased (small green arrows). ECF = extracellular fluid.

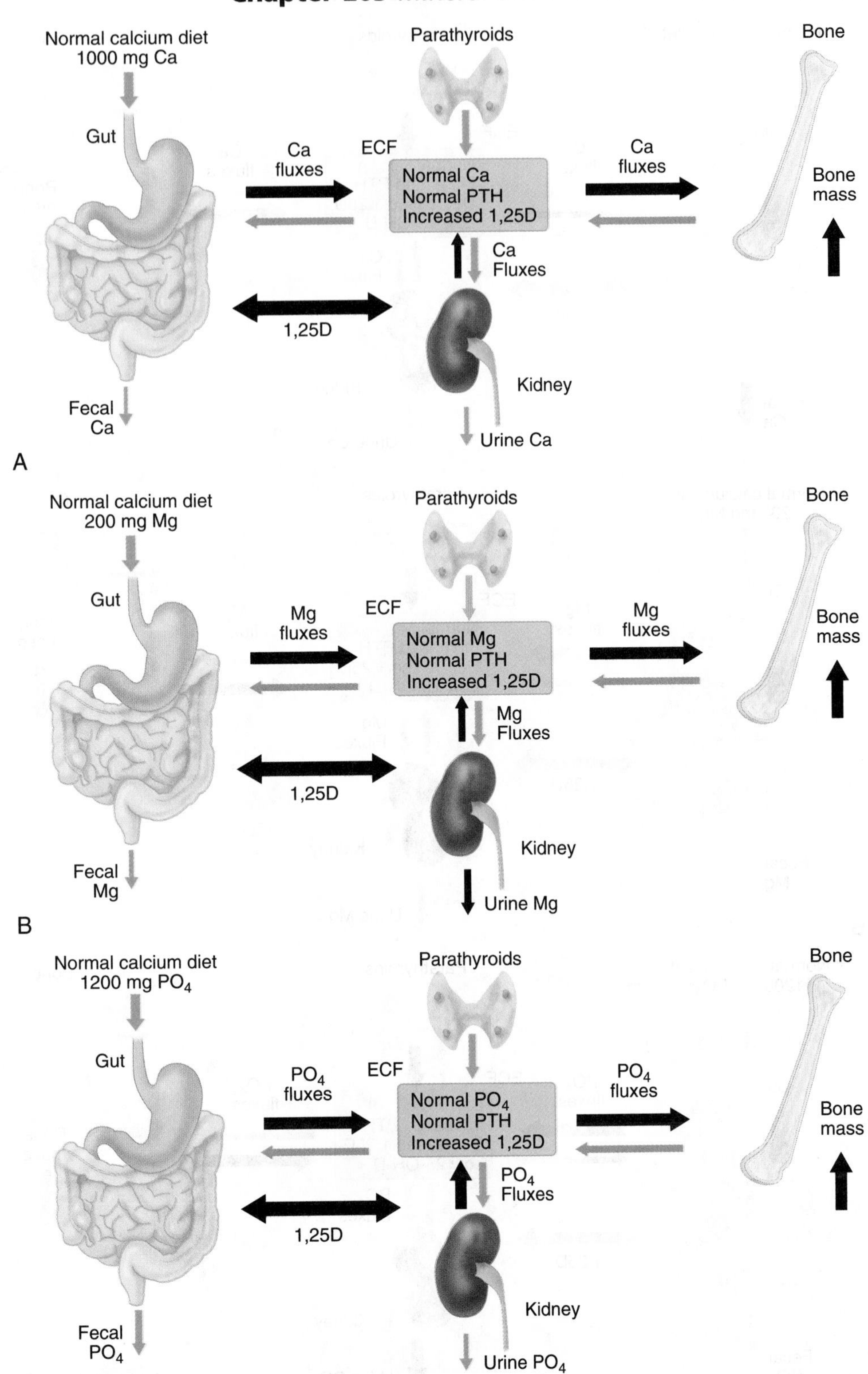

FIGURE 263–2 • Effects of skeletal growth in adolescence. Development of positive calcium (Ca; **A**), magnesium (Mg; **B**), and phosphate (PO_4; **C**) balance and increased bone mass during accelerated skeletal growth in adolescents. Fluxes and hormone levels are as described in Figure 263–1A. ECF = extracellular fluid; PTH = parathyroid hormone.

occurs under conditions of rapid skeletal growth as during childhood and adolescence and during pregnancy and lactation. Intestinal and renal adaptations refer to the following: increased efficiency of intestinal mineral absorption with greater influx of ions into the ECF; reduction of urine mineral ion losses through increased renal tubule reabsorption; and increased serum ion levels to enhance delivery to bone sites of active skeletal mineralization (Fig. 263–2). In these examples, all the homeostatic changes provide sufficient minerals to meet the increased mineral requirements of the growing skeleton, the fetal skeleton, or the breast-feeding newborn. PTH and $1,25(OH)_2D_3$ stimulate insertion of ion channels and transporters into intestinal and renal epithelial membranes to enhance transepithelial fluxes and thereby increase ion fluxes into the ECF.

Negative Balance

Negative Ca, Mg, and PO_4 balance is defined as loss of mineral ions (fecal plus urine) that exceeds retention. Bone loss may accompany the changes in bone ion fluxes. Pregnancy is an example of negative mineral

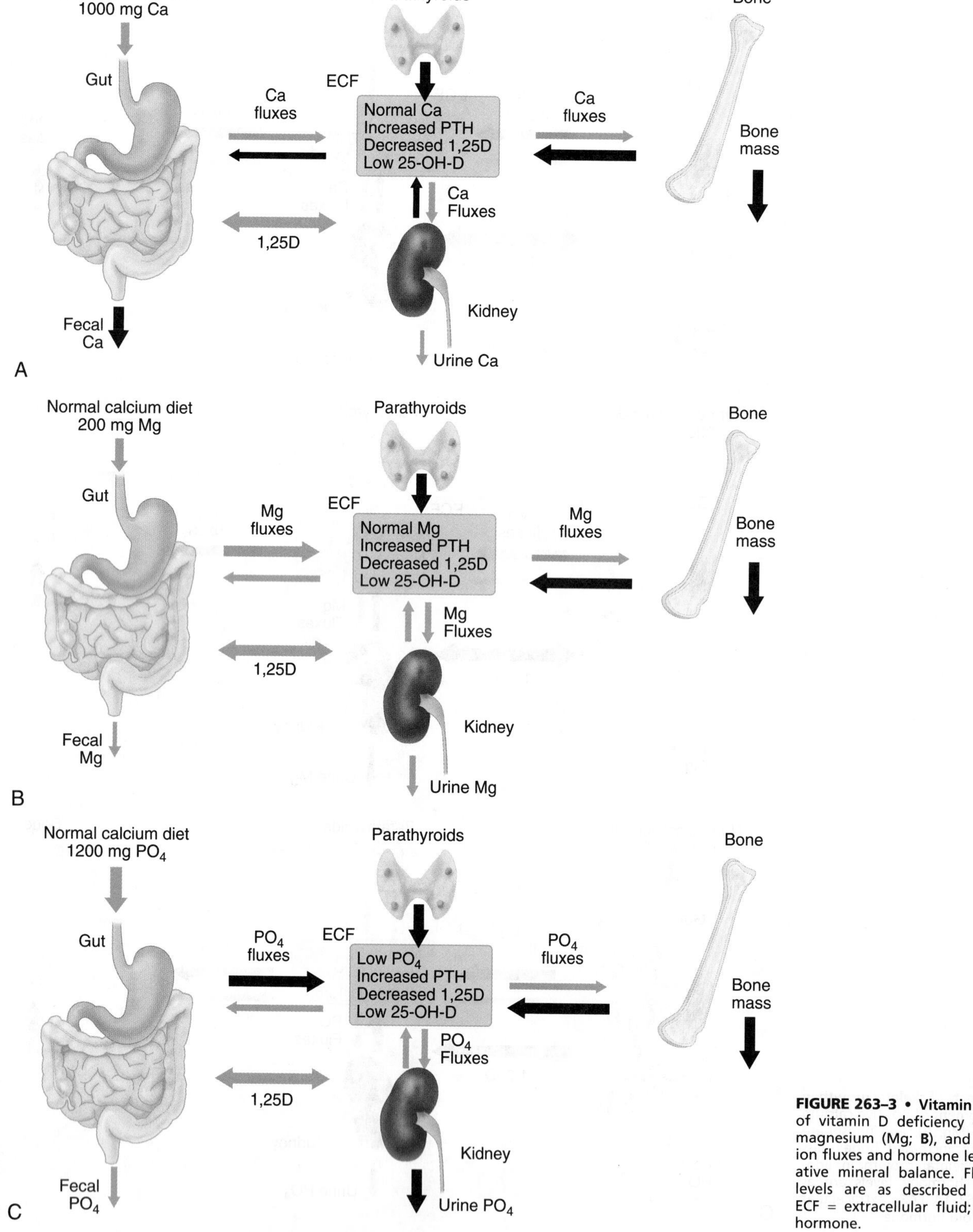

FIGURE 263–3 • Vitamin D deficiency. Effects of vitamin D deficiency on calcium (Ca; **A**), magnesium (Mg; **B**), and phosphate (PO_4; **C**) ion fluxes and hormone levels that cause negative mineral balance. Fluxes and hormone levels are as described in Figure 263–1A. ECF = extracellular fluid; PTH = parathyroid hormone.

ion balance as a result of the transfer of these ions from the mother's skeleton across the placenta to the rapidly growing fetal skeleton. External balance studies conducted on pregnant women reveal that the maternal-fetal unit is in strong positive mineral balance. Estrogen deficiency at the time of menopause results in accelerated bone loss and negative balance as a result of increased bone resorption and defective renal mineral tubule reabsorption. Other causes of negative mineral ion balance include chronic glucocorticoid excess, hyperthyroidism, and vitamin D deficiency (Fig. 263–3). In glucocorticoid excess and hyperthyroidism, reduced intestinal mineral ion absorption and excessive urinary ion excretion contribute to and may cause the bone loss. Vitamin D deficiency is associated with low intestinal absorption and low urine Ca losses. In all three conditions, mineral fluxes into bone are exceeded by bone mineral ion efflux.

SUGGESTED READINGS

Eghbali-Fatourechi GZ, Lamsam J, Fraser D, et al: Circulating osteoblast-lineage cells in humans. N Engl J Med 2005;352:1959–1966. *Characterization of a previously unrecognized circulatory component of bone formation.*

Hadjidakis DJ, Androulakis II: Bone remodeling. Ann NY Acad Sci 2006 Dec;1092:385–396. *A scientific overview.*

Heller HJ, Zerwekh JE, Gottschalk FA, et al: Reduced bone formation and relatively increased bone resorption in absorptive hypercalciuria. Kidney Int

2007;71:808–815. *In addition to increased intestinal absorption, bone resorption is a contributing factor.*
Joost GJ, Muller D, Suzuki M, et al: Epithelial calcium channel: Gate-keeper of active calcium reabsorption. Curr Opin Nephrol Hypertens 2000;9:335–340. *Describes the molecular basis for renal epithelial Ca transport including Ca channels and transporters that were initially described by the authors.*
Shimada T, Kakitani M, Yamazaki Y, et al: Targeted ablation of FGF23 demonstrates an essential physiological role of FGF23 in phosphate and vitamin D metabolism. J Clin Invest 2004;113:561–568. *Some initial descriptions of the functions and regulation of FGF-23, the newly discovered regulator of phosphate homeostasis.*
Steingrimsdottir L, Gunnarsson O, Indridason OS, et al: Relationship between serum parathyroid hormone levels, vitamin D sufficiency, and calcium intake. JAMA 2005;294:2336–2341. *Serum PTH is inversely related to calcium stores as reflected by serum 25-hydroxyvitamin D levels.*

264 OSTEOPOROSIS

Clifford Rosen

Definition

Osteoporosis is a disorder characterized by enhanced skeletal fragility as a result of reduced bone quantity and quality. The clinical symptoms of this disease may include back pain, height loss, and/or a history of fractures. Bone mineral density (BMD), which can be determined by several techniques, is often markedly reduced in osteoporotic patients with fractures. The World Health Organization (WHO) defines osteoporosis as a condition in which a BMD is less than −2.5 standard deviations (SD) below peak bone mass (i.e., a T-score measured as the units of SD below the normative mean of a 35-year-old woman). However, several large observational studies have shown that osteoporotic fractures can occur across a wide spectrum of BMD. These events are likely related to altered bone quality, as a result of microarchitectural changes in the trabecular and cortical skeleton. Qualitative determinants of osteoporotic fractures include trabecular perforations, microcracks, mineralization defects, bone size, and/or rapid bone turnover (Fig. 264–1). Unfortunately, qualitative changes in the skeleton cannot be captured by clinical measurements, even though they strongly influence overall fracture risk. Hence although low BMD defines osteoporosis, this diagnosis should not be excluded in susceptible individuals, particularly those with a history of a low-impact fracture. Finally, although the WHO defined *osteopenia* as a condition with a T-score between −1.0 and −2.5, and therefore places a given individual at a greater risk of fracture, the clinical significance of this term is nebulous. In summary, low BMD is a strong risk factor for subsequent fractures, but there is no threshold BMD above or below which fractures occur. Other risk factors such as a previous fracture history, age greater than 65 years, a strong family history, and recent significant weight loss must be considered.

Epidemiology

By the age of 50 years, the lifetime risk of a fracture resulting from osteoporosis in a white woman is nearly 40%, similar to that for coronary heart disease; in men, the corresponding figure is 13%. In the United States, approximately 350,000 hip fractures, close to 1 million vertebral fractures, and 200,000 wrist fractures occur every year. In addition, other fragility-related fractures, particularly those of the pelvis and humerus, are a significant cause of morbidity in elderly persons. The incidence of osteoporotic fractures increases markedly with age. In women, this increase is seen after the age of 45 years and is mainly the result of forearm fractures. After the age of 65 years, the incidence of hip fractures rises exponentially. In men, the incidence of fragility-related fractures increases after the age of 75 years, and in both sexes the hip is the most common fracture site after the age of 85 years. The incidence of vertebral fractures is less well documented, because many such patients are asymptomatic, but for clinical fractures, an exponential increase occurs with age in men, whereas a more linear age-related increase is noted in women. The increase in fracture prevalence with age is independent of the change in BMD; age alone is an independent risk factor for fracture.

Marked geographic variations in the incidence of osteoporotic fractures are reported. This characteristic may partly be explained by racial differences in skeletal size; osteoporosis is most common in Asian and white populations and is less frequent in African and American blacks. In many parts of the world, evidence indicates that osteoporotic fractures have increased considerably, even after allowing for aging of the population. Although this age-specific increase may now be stabilizing in some countries, greater life expectancy alone is expected to at least double the number of hip fractures over the next 50 years.

Ethnic and gender differences play a major role in the epidemiology of fractures. Men have higher bone density than women, and African Americans have significantly greater BMD during their adult life than whites, both in the cortical and trabecular compartments. These differences are related in part to the effects of body composition including muscle strength, body fat distribution, and bone size. Hence, significantly fewer fractures occur in African Americans than in Asians or whites, particularly whites of European descent.

Pathobiology

As previously mentioned, low BMD is one of the most important predisposing factors for osteoporotic fractures. Adult BMD is determined both by the acquisition of peak bone mass during adolescence and by the

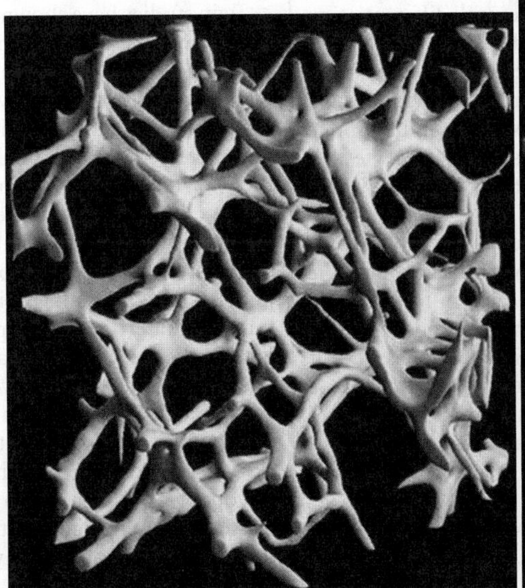
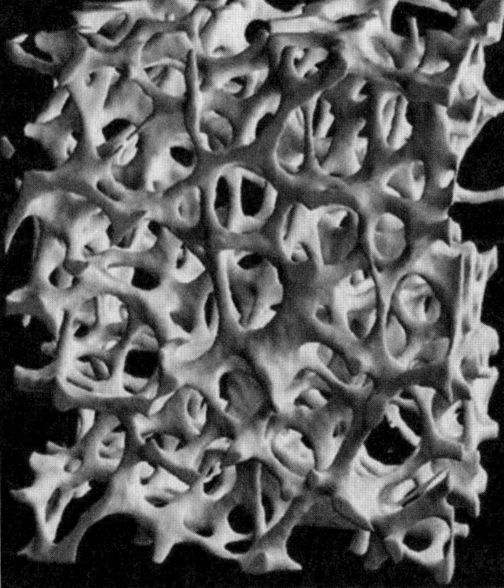

FIGURE 264–1 • Microcomputed tomography images of trabecular bone from the vertebrae of an osteoporotic individual (left) and a healthy age-matched normal woman (right).

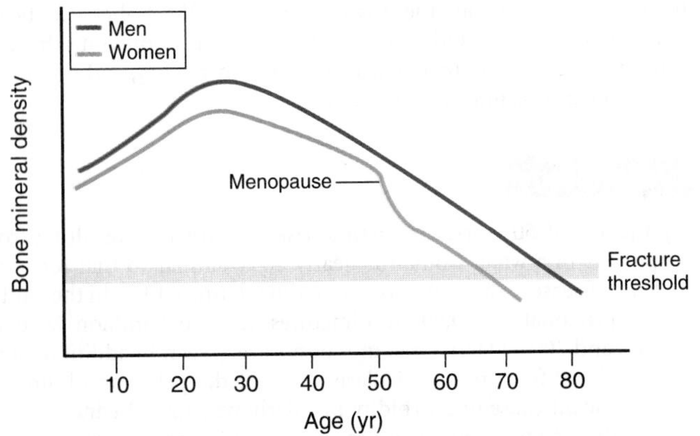

FIGURE 264–2 • Cortical bone mineral density versus age in men and women. Women have lower peak cortical bone density than men and experience a period of rapid bone loss at menopause, thus reaching the fracture threshold (the level of bone density at which the risk of developing osteoporotic fractures begins to increase) earlier than men.

degree of subsequent bone loss over a lifetime (Fig. 264–2). These two processes are regulated at the level of the bone remodeling unit, which is composed of bone-forming osteoblasts, bone-resorbing osteoclasts, and deeply imbedded osteocytes capable of sensing gravitational forces. The remodeling sequence is tightly orchestrated at several levels by the interaction of genetic and environmental and hormonal factors. Even small changes in bone formation or bone resorption can result in bone loss or impairment in the capacity to acquire peak bone mass during adolescence.

Although an osteoporotic fracture inevitably occurs as a result of trauma—major or minor—to a bone with reduced bone quantity and/or quality, a strong inverse relationship exists between BMD and fractures. Hence, changes in remodeling that lead to lower bone mass are major factors in determining the risk of osteoporosis.

Bone Remodeling

Even though trauma is the principal cause of fracture, factors that alter the quality or quantity of bone predispose an individual to osteoporotic fractures. Thus, an understanding of bone remodeling is essential for determining how bone mass can be altered by heritable and environmental influences. Skeletal remodeling preserves serum calcium and bone strength after longitudinal growth ceases. This cyclic process occurs in microscopic elements called remodeling or *basic multicellular units.* Bone remodeling begins with bone dissolution or resorption and ends with new bone formation. Bone resorption is carried out by osteoclasts, which originate from the monocyte-macrophage lineage. New bone is formed by osteoblasts, cells of the fibroblast-stromal lineage that produce several bone matrix proteins and synthesize a lattice for subsequent mineralization. Stromal cells are found in the marrow and are destined to become either fat or bone cells under the influence of several differentiation factors with the marrow milieu. Osteocytes are "old" osteoblasts that are entombed within the bone matrix. Although these cells were originally considered inert, it is now clear that they communicate with resting surface osteoblasts and, under the proper circumstances, initiate bone remodeling. Microcanaliculi connect the osteoblast and osteocyte and likely serve as the conduit for signals that originate from osteocytes in response to gravitational forces.

In adulthood, each remodeling unit is balanced—resorption equals formation—and lasts between 90 and 130 days. Maintenance of bone mass during remodeling ensures a ready source of calcium for the body and a persistent reservoir of stored calcium. However, remodeling units can become imbalanced, and over several cycles, this situation can result in significant bone loss. These imbalances are a result of greater bone resorption relative to bone formation, and they can be traced to changes in systemic hormones, dietary intake, or mechanical loading.

Peak Bone Mass

Acquisition of peak bone mass occurs between 12 and 15 years of age. During this time, there is a tremendous increase in bone mass as a result of growth and modeling of the skeleton. In addition, remodeling favors the formation of bone, thereby permitting a further significant and critical increase in bone mass. Pubertal surges of gonadal steroids and growth hormone are considered critical for such a dramatic increase in bone mass with adolescence. Longitudinal studies suggest that several factors regulate peak bone density, including dietary intake of specific nutrients, physical activity, and, most importantly, genetic determinants (Table 264–1). This view was established in several ways in both humans and animal models. Daughters of mothers with severe osteoporosis have low BMD. Monozygotic twins have much greater concordance in bone mass than dizygotic pairs, and inbred strains of mice differ significantly in peak BMD. However, despite intense efforts over the past decade to identify the heritable determinants of bone mass, little progress has been made. Polymorphic differences in the most promising candidate genes, including the vitamin D and estrogen receptors, insulin-like growth factor-I (IGF-I), parathyroid hormone (PTH), collagen A1a, and others, have not been shown to have major effects on bone acquisition.

TABLE 264–1 FACTORS THAT MAY AFFECT PEAK BONE MASS

Gender
Race
Genetic factors
Gonadal steroids
Growth hormone
Timing of puberty
Calcium intake
Exercise

Rate of Bone Formation

Investigators have uncovered two new pathways in the osteoblast that are genetically regulated and affect the rate of bone formation. These are (1) the Wnt/Lrp5/β-catenin signaling system and (2) the lipoxygenase pathways. In the former, activating mutations of the lipoprotein receptor protein 5 (LRP5) cause high bone mass, whereas inactivating mutations lead to the osteoporosis pseudoganglioma syndrome, a condition related to low bone mass in children. The canonic LRP5 signaling pathway is stimulated by Wnt ligands and leads directly to greater osteoblast proliferation and differentiation. In the latter system, two critical enzymes determine when and how stromal cells enter into either the fat or bone lineage: *12,15-lipoxygenase* (*12 LO* or *Alox 12,15*) produces prostaglandins and other endogenous ligands that bind to the nuclear receptor, Pparg, that stimulates adipocyte differentiation; and *5′LO*, or *Alox 5*, produces leukotrienes that can also activate Pparg and can influence stromal cell differentiation. Polymorphisms in these two genes in mice and humans have been associated with differences in peak bone mass. Studies are currently under way to understand more fully the signaling networks necessary for optimal bone acquisition.

Twin studies have shown that the genetic regulation of peak bone mass can be modified by both hormonal and environmental factors. In particular, adequate and timely secretion of sex steroids, balanced nutrient intake, and physical activity can optimize peak BMD even in people with a genetic predisposition to low bone mass. In fact, small trials have shown that increased calcium intake during peak bone acquisition can enhance BMD in the spine and hip. Similarly, jumping exercises in prepubertal girls are associated with greater peak bone acquisition.

It is likely that perturbations in peak bone acquisition contribute to osteoporosis later in life. For example, men with constitutionally delayed puberty have lower BMD in their 30s and 40s than do men who went through puberty at the appropriate age. Women with anorexia nervosa during their teen years have significantly lower BMD at the time of menopause than do healthy adolescents who do not develop amenorrhea. Women with delayed menarche also have lower BMD in adulthood than do women with a normal timing of menses onset. One area of controversy relates to whether childhood fractures are a sign of subsequent osteoporosis. At least two studies have shown that adolescent radial fractures are associated with lower area bone density and reduced cortical bone size compared with findings in children who do not have fractures. These determinants could predispose children to fractures with relatively low impact and may provide some indication of future risk, although more studies are needed.

Pathophysiology

Bone loss occurs when the bone remodeling unit is uncoupled such that bone resorption exceeds formation. The timing of bone loss is a critical determinant of future fracture risk. For example, rapid bone loss in elderly persons puts them at very high risk for fracture independent of BMD. Conversely, accelerated bone turnover over a short period (such as that related to transient glucocorticoid excess in young adulthood) may lead to reversible changes in bone mass. Once the inciting event has passed or the treatments have stopped, fracture risk returns to baseline, and BMD can be restored. However, bone loss can also be incessant, particularly in postmenopausal women, in whom estrogen deprivation results in markedly increased osteoclastic activity and high-turnover remodeling. Although the basic multicellular unit is tightly coupled, rapid bone resorption over a prolonged period results in an imbalance, because formation cannot be maintained at the same accelerated rate as resorption. During the first few years of menopause, as estrogen levels decline precipitously, trabecular bone loss occurs first. This is followed by cortical thinning. Both conditions are a result of a mismatch between resorption and formation. During menopause, bone loss averages about 1% per year, but in a few women, loss of spine BMD can be as great as 5% per year. At present, it is impossible to identify those women prospectively. Moreover, premature menopause, chemotherapeutically induced ovarian dysfunction, and/or amenorrhea related to heavy exercise result in even higher rates of bone resorption that cannot be matched by bone formation. However, tremendous heterogeneity exists in the response to estrogen deprivation among postmenopausal women. A few women during their first few years of menopause may lose bone at a rate of 2 to 4% per year. Even among "fast losers," this decline slows over time. Estrogen replacement prevents postmenopausal bone loss even among "fast users," although the popularity of this type of prevention waned in the years following publication of the Women's Health Initiative (WHI).

Bone Loss in Elderly Persons

Later in life, particularly in the eighth and ninth decades, bone loss can accelerate dramatically. Several potential mechanisms are responsible for this change. First and foremost, elderly individuals generally have reduced vitamin D and calcium intake, as well as less sun exposure. This finding, combined with a reduced capacity to generate previtamin D in the skin, results in secondary hyperparathyroidism and enhanced bone resorption. Remarkably, more than 50% of women who are more than 70 years old and who live in northern latitudes have insufficient or deficient levels of vitamin D (i.e., serum 25[OH] vitamin D). Other factors also play a role in the accelerated bone turnover of senescence. Increasing levels of homocyst(e)ine may enhance bone resorption or may alter the nature of reactive oxygen species within the skeletal milieu. Inflammatory cytokines such as interleukin-6 (IL-6) and tumor necrosis factor (TNF) also increase with age and can stimulate bone turnover.

The uncoupling of the bone remodeling unit in an older person may be associated with a defect in bone formation, because both osteoblast number and function decline with age. These changes may be related to low levels of circulating and/or skeletal IGF-I or to other trophic factors that either enhance osteoblast survival or stimulate stromal cell recruitment. As a result of impaired osteoblast function, the remodeling deficit becomes more pronounced particularly in the setting of greater bone resorption. Irrespective of the cause of bone loss with aging, estrogen and other antiresorptive therapies are effective in inhibiting bone resorption and in resetting the bone remodeling unit toward a new balance.

Type I and Type II Osteoporosis

Earlier work proposed two types of osteoporosis, based on age of onset: type I or postmenopausal osteoporosis, caused by estrogen deprivation around the time of menopause; and type II osteoporosis, related to high turnover from calcium and vitamin D insufficiency. However, it has become apparent that this type of classification is outdated and has little clinical purpose. Many younger postmenopausal women can have vitamin D deficiency, and elderly individuals may suffer just as much from bone loss as a result of progressive estrogen insufficiency as younger women. Similarly, even though wrist fractures are more common, as are vertebral fractures, in younger, healthy postmenopausal women, these fractures are very characteristic of any type of osteoporosis, and they represent skeletal failure related to impaired bone quantity and/or quality, irrespective of age.

Molecular and Cellular Mechanisms of Normal Remodeling

To understand the pathophysiologic mechanisms of bone loss more fully, it is necessary to define the key molecular and cellular events that occur during normal adult remodeling. Mesenchymal stromal cells or osteoblast precursor cells undergo a series of differentiation stages that culminate in a mature osteoblast capable of laying down matrix and secreting growth factors. During those stages of differentiation, the stromal cells release a series of cytokines that target osteoclast progenitors, resulting in the differentiation of multinucleated cells from the macrophage lineage. Once these cells become osteoclasts, they have the capacity to cause bone resorption by secreting protons and enzymes that dissolve the bone matrix. Within the matrix are several key trophic factors, activated by bone dissolution; as these enter the skeletal milieu, cells of the osteoblast lineage are pushed into differentiation. In this manner, bone resorption is coupled to bone formation.

Several cytokines, including IL-1, IL-6, TNF, receptor activator of nuclear factor-κB (RANKL), and the soluble receptor of RANKL, osteoprotogerin, are secreted by preosteoblasts during their process of differentiation. RANKL is expressed on the surface of the osteoblast precursors,

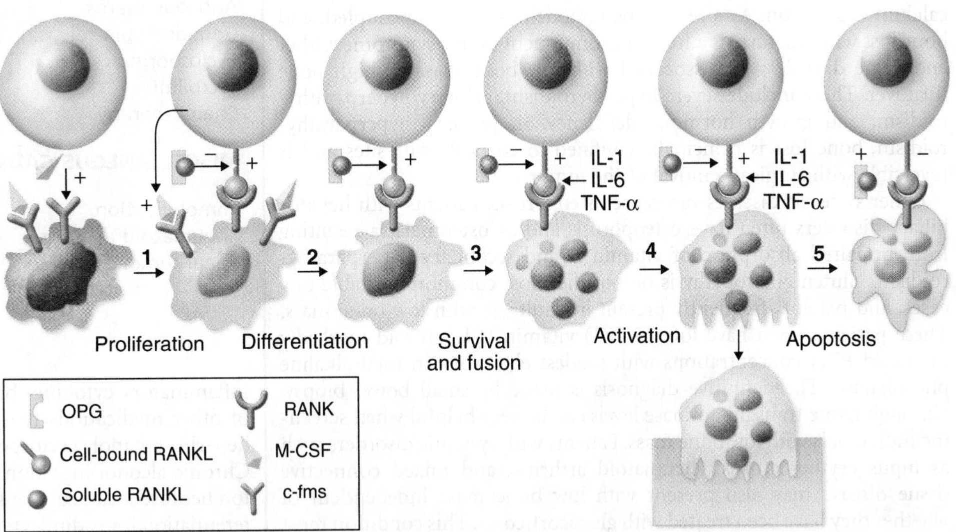

FIGURE 264–3 • Regulation of osteoclast development by receptor activator of nuclear factor-κB ligand (RANKL), receptor activator of nuclear factor-κB (RANK), and osteoprotegerin (OPG). c-fms = receptor for M-CSF; IL = interleukin; M-CSF = macrophage colony-stimulating factor; TNF-α = tumor necrosis factor-α. (From Hofbauer LC, Heufelder AE: The role of receptor activator of nuclear factor-κ ligand and osteoprotegerin in the pathogenesis and treatment of metabolic bone diseases. J Clin Endocrinol Metab 2000;85:2355–2363.)

and its receptor RANK is on the surface of the osteoclast, a convenient match that actually permits cell-cell interaction (Fig. 264–3). Binding of RANKL to RANK in the presence of permissive levels of another cytokine, macrophage colony-stimulating factor stimulates the differentiation of osteoclasts into mature bone resorbing cells. In contrast, OPG, a circulating protein also produced by stromal cells, can bind to RANKL and can prevent its occupation of RANK, thereby reducing osteoclastogenesis.

Cellular and Molecular Mechanisms of Bone Loss

Declining estrogen levels during menopause or after oophorectomy result in an upregulation of all the stromal cytokines, particularly RANKL. Conversely, OPG secretion is suppressed. This situation results in greater osteoclastogenesis and accelerated bone resorption. Because bone formation is coupled to resorption, the entire remodeling unit is activated. Bone resorption is a rapid process, taking about 2 weeks for the osteoclasts to attach and resorb matrix. Formation is much more deliberate, meaning that with the release of soluble cytokines, an imbalance in remodeling occurs that favors resorption. Eventually, this imbalance leads to increased breakdown of collagen and matrix and an inability to match this loss with increased formation. Estrogen administration can prevent bone loss by enhancing OPG production as well as by suppressing RANKL expression. Other systemic and local factors can contribute to imbalanced remodeling. For example, glucocorticoid excess stimulates RANKL production, but it also suppresses stromal cell differentiation into the osteoblast lineage. Aging causes a reduction in several osteoblastic trophic factors such as IGF-I and thus impairs the rate of new bone formation.

Pathogenesis

Secondary Causes of Bone Loss in the Adult

Although most cases of osteoporosis can be labeled "idiopathic" and result from the cellular and molecular processes that are related to estrogen deprivation and/or aging, it is important to exclude secondary causes, primarily because these disorders are sometimes reversible with resolution of the underlying disease (Table 264–2). Hypogonadism of any cause, in either men or women, is probably the most frequent secondary cause of osteoporosis, particularly in younger patients. Anorexia nervosa, hypothalamic amenorrhea, hyperprolactinemia, and exercise-induced amenorrhea lead to early and rapid bone loss that can result in subsequent osteoporotic fractures if these conditions are sustained over a prolonged period. In male patients, primary or secondary hypogonadism results in low peak bone mass and can cause significant bone loss during middle life. Hormonal disorders that interfere with the normal hypothalamic gonadal axis, such as hypercortisolemia, also lead to reduced bone mass. Cushing's syndrome, which results in excess cortisol, dampens gonadotropin-releasing hormone signaling, thereby lowering estrogen or androgen levels and enhancing bone resorption; these changes are accompanied by alterations in osteoblast recruitment and function, increased marrow adiposity, reduced IGF-I signaling, and impaired calcium absorption. As a result, the remodeling unit is uncoupled, and bone loss with fractures is a frequent component of this syndrome. Other endocrine disorders are associated with low bone mass or high bone turnover. These include severe hyperthyroidism, primary hyperparathyroidism, and growth hormone deficiency. In primary hyperparathyroidism, bone loss is principally confined to cortical bone sites and is reversible with surgical removal of the tumor.

Other systemic diseases can cause osteoporosis. Patients with hepatobiliary disorders often have osteoporosis and/or osteomalacia resulting from impaired absorption of vitamin D and secondary hyperparathyroidism. Gluten enteropathy is one of the most common heritable diseases, and patients frequently present in adult life with low bone mass. These patients often have low 25(OH) vitamin D levels and markedly increased PTH concentrations with modest elevations in total alkaline phosphatase. The definitive diagnosis is made by small bowel biopsy, although tissue transglutaminase levels can be very helpful when screening individuals with low bone mass. Patients with systemic disorders such as lupus erythematosus, rheumatoid arthritis, and mixed connective tissue disease may also present with low bone mass independent of whether they have been treated with glucocorticoids. This condition most likely results from the combination of immobility and the release of inflammatory cytokines both locally and systemically, as well as the use of other medications that may be detrimental to the skeleton, such as heparin, ethanol, cyclosporine, tacrolimus, and anticonvulsant agents. Chronic alcohol ingestion may be particularly detrimental to the skeleton because it can suppress osteoblast function, increase stromal cell differentiation into adipocytes, and enhance bone resorption. Many patients who suffer from chronic alcoholism are hypogonadal and frequently have

TABLE 264–2 SECONDARY CAUSES OF OSTEOPOROSIS

ENDOCRINE DISEASES

Female hypogonadism
- Hyperprolactinemia
- Hypothalamic amenorrhea
- Anorexia nervosa
- Premature and primary ovarian failure

Male hypogonadism
- Primary gonadal failure (e.g., Klinefelter's syndrome)
- Secondary gonadal failure (e.g., idiopathic hypogonadotropic hypogonadism)
- Delayed puberty

Hyperthyroidism
Hyperparathyroidism
Hypercortisolism
Growth hormone deficiency
Vitamin D deficiency
Idiopathic hypercalciuria
Diabetes mellitus

GASTROINTESTINAL DISEASES

Subtotal gastrectomy
Malabsorption syndromes
Chronic obstructive jaundice
Primary biliary cirrhosis and other cirrhoses
Alactasia

BONE MARROW DISORDERS

Multiple myeloma
Lymphoma
Leukemia
Hemolytic anemias
Systemic mastocytosis
Disseminated carcinoma

CONNECTIVE TISSUE DISEASES

Osteogenesis imperfecta
Ehlers-Danlos syndrome
Marfan's syndrome
Homocystinuria

DRUGS

Alcohol
Heparin
Glucocorticoids
Thyroxine
Anticonvulsants
Gonadotropin-releasing hormone agonists
Cyclosporine
Tacrolimus
Chemotherapy

MISCELLANEOUS CAUSES

Immobilization
Rheumatoid arthritis
Renal tumor acidosis

low vitamin D levels. Male patients with hypercalcuria and/or kidney stones are also at risk for low bone mass and osteoporotic fractures. The pathogenesis of this relationship is not entirely clear, but secondary hyperparathyroidism in patients with hypercalcuria leads to enhanced bone resorption and gradual bone loss.

Malignancy

Metastatic neoplasms to the skeleton can sometimes manifest as an osteoporotic fracture or as a lytic lesion of uncertain significance. Usually, these lesions are atypical in location (e.g., midshaft of long bones, or pelvis), and the underlying disease frequently is obvious. Less commonly confused with osteoporosis are osteoblastic lesions of vertebrae or long bones. However, primary hematopoietic and lymphoproliferative disorders are often insidious and can be associated with low bone mass and fractures. Multiple myeloma is the most common hematologic malignant disease related to osteoporosis because patients with this disease often have diffuse osteopenia, occasionally with classic osteoporotic fractures of the spine or long bones. The pathogenesis of the skeletal manifestations of multiple myeloma has been clarified. Unlike other metastatic processes to bone, multiple myeloma is associated with very high rates of bone resorption but no change or suppression in bone formation. This situation can lead to rapid bone loss. Plasma cells release cytokines, particularly TNF-α, IL-1, and IL-6, that stimulate osteoclastogenesis. Simultaneously, these cells produce Dickopf I and III, soluble factors that block that critical Wnt/LRP5/β-catenin canonic network. Hence patients have dramatic uncoupling of bone remodeling, rapid bone loss, and fractures. Debate is still ongoing about the relationship of osteoporosis with monoclonal gammopathies of uncertain significance. Other secondary causes of osteoporosis are noted in Table 264–2.

Clinical Manifestations

Although osteoporosis is often considered a silent disease, its presentation has changed dramatically in the last 2 decades. Previously, fractures of the vertebrae, with or without height loss, were the most frequent presenting complaints. Until recently, hip fractures in elderly patients, which can be a late manifestation of osteoporosis, often were considered traumatic but not metabolic. Similarly, wrist fractures in early postmenopausal women that are a sentinel indication of underlying osteoporosis were treated by orthopedic surgeons without regard for any underlying skeletal pathologic processes. However, these patterns began to change in the early part of the 21st century, particularly with the availability of dual energy x-ray absorptiometry (DXA), the method of choice for measuring BMD. Now, the most frequent presenting complaint to a provider regarding osteoporosis is a low BMD measurement, done either routinely or for screening purposes. Because bone mass is only one of several risk factors for osteoporosis, other clinical manifestations of this disease must be considered. Loss of more than 2 inches in height is a reasonable surrogate of previous vertebral fractures. A clinical history of wrist or ankle fractures is another indication of underlying osteoporosis and may be the first manifestation of the disease in younger postmenopausal women. Compression fracture of the spine with minimal stress is another presenting complaint of osteoporosis. Such fractures cause significant midlumbar and lower thoracic back pain that may radiate to the flanks or anteriorly. Sharp, knifelike back pain after an acute injury is disabling, frequently requires narcotics, and often subsides over a period of weeks to months unless a new fracture intervenes. Patients have an approximately 20% likelihood of a new vertebral fracture in the first year after a spinal fracture. In addition, some patients have chronic back pain as a result of one or more vertebral fractures. Low bone mass in and of itself does not result in back pain, and other diagnoses should be considered in that situation. Cervical lordosis and dorsal kyphosis are the classic manifestations of "dowager's hump" but are less frequently seen in young women. Hip fractures resulting in femoral neck, trochanteric, or cervical injuries generally occur following a fall. The direction and height of the fall are critical elements in determining the type of hip fracture, the ensuing surgery, and disability. Hip fractures can be extremely catabolic, both because of the trauma and because of the resultant major surgery. These factors, combined with underlying illnesses, enhance the mortality of hip fractures in older individuals to approximately 20% in the first year alone.

Osteoporosis can also be diagnosed by a radiologist or a primary care provider from plain radiographs, as shown in Figure 264–4. Most often, patients have an obvious loss of bone mass, resulting in the radiographic term *osteopenia,* although at that stage BMD by DXA is usually well below −2.5 SD. Radiographs of the spine can demonstrate kyphosis, osteopenia, and compression fractures in the thoracic or lumbar vertebrae. For the upper lumbar or lower thoracic areas that are the most vulnerable to injury, compression fractures can frequently be visualized. Collapse of either the anterior or posterior elements is often visible on lateral radiographs of the spine; anterior wedging or the so-called "codfish" deformity results from weakening of the subchondral plates and expansion of the intervertebral discs (see Fig. 264–4). Computed tomography (CT) scan of the spine for other reasons will sometimes be able to detect fractures, and can be used clinically to measure density. Magnetic resonance imaging (MRI) is now more frequently utilized as a diagnostic tool; it may demonstrate a compression fracture with or without marrow edema resulting in a bright signal on T1-weighted images. Technetium-99m bone scans are very sensitive to fracture and can be used to detect stress fractures in the pelvis, femur, or tibia. However, because of its high sensitivity, this test is not a useful tool for diagnosis of osteoporosis. In fact, it is rare for the bone scan to be the initial clue to osteoporosis, and in the setting of a positive bone scan, alternative diagnoses including malignant disease should be considered.

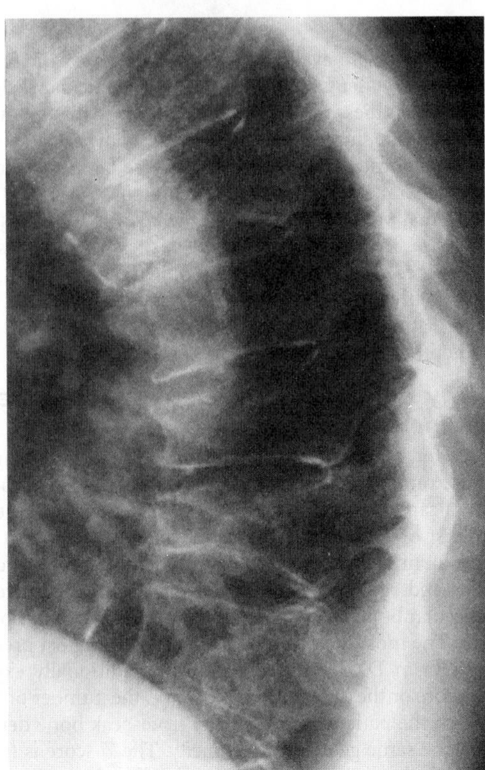

FIGURE 264–4 • Radiograph showing radiolucency, compression fractures, and kyphosis in the spine of a patient with osteoporosis.

Diagnosis

A recent fragility-related fracture of the spine, hip, wrist, ankle, shoulder, or other appendicular sites in postmenopausal women or men would lead to a diagnosis of osteoporosis. However, secondary causes of this condition (as discussed earlier and listed in Table 264–2) should be excluded before therapy is initiated. Similarly, because the WHO has established that a BMD at any site lower than −2.5 SDs from the young normal value meets the definition of osteoporosis, a diagnosis can be made from a densitometry report or measurement. However, this finding must be interpreted in relation to the patient's age, ethnicity, fracture history, family background, previous medications, timing of menopause, and other concomitant disorders. Currently, based on the WHO criteria, most providers make the diagnosis of osteoporosis by measuring bone density with or without biochemical markers of bone turnover.

Bone Densitometry

Several techniques are available for measuring area BMD (i.e., two-dimensional measurements) in the axial and appendicular skeleton. Multiple prospective studies have convincingly shown that a low BMD at virtually any site (i.e., hip, spine, radius, total body, calcaneus) predicts subsequent osteoporotic fractures whether these be in the same area or elsewhere. In general, regardless of the technology, for every 1 SD below the young normal value (i.e., T-score), the risk of future osteoporotic fractures increases by nearly 50%. However, site-specific measurements, for example, spine BMD, usually predict spine fractures better than a hip BMD. Because of the inverse relationship between fracture risk and BMD, a very strong rationale exists for measuring bone mass at least once during the lifetime of every postmenopausal woman.

Dual-Energy X-Ray Absorptiometry Measurements of Bone Mineral Density

Techniques for measuring bone mass include the following: DXA of the spine, hip, radius, or total body; CT of the spine; ultrasound scanning of the calcaneus or wrist; finger DXA; and peripheral quantitative CT of the wrist or tibia. Other experimental techniques that are being tested for evaluating trabecular bone and bone quality include MRI of the calcaneus and radius, virtual MRI using computerized reconstructions of trabecular bone, and "extreme CT" with high-resolution imaging of the radius. The most popular, least expensive, and most precise tool is DXA. Results from DXA measurements are traditionally expressed as either the T-score or the Z-score. The T-score is the number of SDs below or above which the patient's BMD differs from peak bone density of an individual of the same gender and ethnicity. The Z-score is the number of SDs by which the patient's bone density differs from that of an individual matched for age, gender, and ethnicity. Not surprisingly, there can be disparity in absolute BMD by skeletal site within the same individual. This disparity can be attributed to the relative proportion of trabecular and cortical bone at a particular site. Therefore, for example, the vertebra is 85% trabecular bone, whereas the femoral shaft or neck is principally cortical bone. Several studies have shown that nearly one in three subjects has disparate hip and spine T-scores. This finding can be attributed to the differences in skeletal composition; in other words, cortical or outer shell bone is thicker and remodels less frequently, whereas trabecular bone, which is the inner spongiform bone bathed by marrow elements, is metabolically very active. DXA integrates both skeletal compartments as an area measurement. However, because skeletal sites often differ in composition and function, this disparity is frequently noted. Furthermore, age-related changes in the two skeletal compartments differ, and their genetic determinants may be completely distinct. In general, it is recommended that the lowest BMD measurement at any site be used for fracture risk assessment.

The two most common skeletal sites recommended for measuring BMD by DXA are spine and hip. For the spine, both anteroposterior and lateral spine DXAs can be obtained, although most providers use the anteroposterior spine, which is both a sensitive indicator of early bone loss and a precise measure. However, anteroposterior spine DXA can often show high bone mass resulting from increases in degenerative arthritis, disc collapse, vertebral fracture, and/or calcification of the aorta. Hence, in patients who are more than 65 years old, femoral neck and total hip BMD measurements are preferable. Both have good precision, are accurate, and are not complicated by the foregoing processes. Either site has strong predictive value for subsequent fractures.

Other Tools for Measuring Bone Mass

Other means of measuring BMD are available, and each provides T-score equivalents, although these cannot easily be translated across technologies. Quantitative CT scanning of the vertebrae provides a true volumetric measure of bone mass, can detect early bone loss, is accurate, and is available at many centers. However, its reproducibility is not as good as that of DXA, and T-scores can be quite disparate from DXA measurements. Moreover, significantly greater radiation exposure occurs with CT than DXA, and CT requires more time. Ultrasound scanning of peripheral sites has the advantages of portability and ease of operation, and the technique enables the clinician to predict fractures; however, the parameters used to measure sound transmission do not change much with age, or with treatment, thereby making this tool difficult to use for follow-up examination. Peripheral quantitative CT is expensive but accurate; it has greater radiation exposure but provides information about both cortical and trabecular elements. Fewer data on fracture risk are available with this technique, which is primarily a research tool.

In summary, DXA provides the most accurate and precise tool to assess fracture risk. The DXA measurement, combined with age, history of previous fracture, and family history, gives the clinician the most accurate assessment of osteoporotic risk. For follow-up, BMD measurements by DXA are preferable to other technologies because of the low precision error and greater reproducibility.

Biomarkers: Biochemical Markers of Bone Turnover

Newer methods of measuring bone breakdown and synthesis products have been developed since the mid-1980s. Previously, urinary calcium and hydroxyproline were the two urinary markers used to assess bone resorption; both were nonspecific, and their precision was poor. Subsequently, serum and urine markers have emerged with potential clinical utility. Markers of bone resorption mediated by osteoclasts include urinary pyridinoline and deoxypyridinoline, as well as urine cross-links of the C- and N-terminal peptides of type I collagen (C-TX and N-Tx). The latter can be measured either in urine or in serum. Markers of osteoblast-mediated bone formation include bone-specific alkaline phosphatase, osteocalcin, type I procollagen amino-terminal propeptide, and type I procollagen carboxy-terminal propeptide. Immediately after estrogen production ceases from whatever mechanism, markers of bone formation and bone resorption increase significantly. Similarly, later in life, and during states of secondary hyperparathyroidism, these markers can be extremely elevated. In addition, antiresorptive drugs such as estrogen or the bisphosphonates significantly lower urinary and circulating concentrations of these markers. Both longitudinal and cross-sectional studies have demonstrated that high turnover markers predict fracture in elderly women. These markers are independent of BMD risk, a finding suggesting that accelerated bone turnover itself is a risk for fracture. Moreover, several groups have shown that suppression in turnover markers with bisphosphonates can predict fracture risk reduction in older postmenopausal women. However, the use of these markers in clinical practice has been disappointing for several reasons. First, the variability in individual measurements, particularly for the urine studies, is quite high. Therefore, even a single measurement has significant measurement error; follow-up to assess change from baseline is often even more confusing because of the variability issue. Second, most women have turnover marker values within the normal range, thus making interpretation very difficult. Third, the number of older women with high bone turnover has probably been overestimated, particularly in the early postmenopausal period. These issues have limited enthusiasm for a single blood or urine test to help determine risk and assist in management once therapy has commenced. Occasionally, these tests can be helpful: in the young woman who undergoes premature menopause resulting from chemotherapy, for example, knowledge not just of the BMD, but also of the rate of bone turnover, could help in managing her condition with either aggressive antiresorptive therapy or a more measured approach using calcium and vitamin D. It is not recommended that these markers be used routinely to assess compliance with antiresorptive therapies.

Diagnostic Evaluation

The diagnosis of osteoporosis is usually made by bone mass measurements and/or a history of previous osteoporotic fractures. Secondary causes of osteoporosis must be excluded, and follow-up is required to ensure that the disease is not rapidly progressive. Routine profiles for renal and thyroid function are indicated. A serum 25-hydroxyvitamin D measurement in an older individual, particularly in northern latitudes, is recommended because deficiencies can be corrected with vitamin D supplementation. At present, DXA represents the best tool for assessing overall fracture risk and determining the course of therapy. Biochemical markers may be helpful in rare cases.

Treatment

Treatment Plan

A comprehensive management plan for osteoporosis includes diagnosing those at highest risk, excluding secondary causes of low BMD, and selecting appropriate treatment. Decision making should also take into account several caveats. First, osteoporosis therapy can reduce fracture risk by as much as 50%, but some women will con-

Rx

tinue to have fractures despite treatment. Identifying those women at greatest risk of progressive disease is mandatory. Second, lifestyle and pharmacologic interventions are lifetime commitments such that cost, compliance, and safety must be factored into therapeutic decisions. Studies suggest that even with weekly bisphosphonate therapy, more than 40% of individuals treated will not continue therapy beyond 1 year. Third, it is not uncommon for women with T-scores higher than −2.5 to have fractures. In fact, in the National Osteoporosis Risk Assessment cohort of more than 140,000 postmenopausal women in the United States, almost one third of the women who had fractures also had BMD scores in the "osteopenic" range. Thus, treatment decisions should not be based solely on BMD.

Therapy for postmenopausal osteoporosis is framed in terms of *primary prevention* when it is prescribed for those at risk who do not have low bone mass (T-score < −2.5) or fractures and in terms of *treatment* for those with established disease including previous osteoporotic fractures and/or markedly reduced BMD. Thus, selection of an appropriate treatment regimen depends on whether the therapy is designed principally to prevent bone loss or to reduce the likelihood of a new spine or nonvertebral fracture in high-risk individuals.

General Measures

Diet

Calcium

Calcium supplementation should be an adjunct to drug treatments for women with established osteoporosis and must be part of any prevention strategy to ameliorate bone loss. Increased calcium intake reduces the secondary hyperparathyroidism often seen with advancing age and can enhance mineralization of newly formed bone. Evidence that calcium and vitamin D together or individually reduce fracture risk in the osteoporotic individual remains controversial. A meta-analysis of 15 calcium intervention trials demonstrated a nearly 2% increase in spine BMD but a nonsignificant reduction in vertebral fracture risk after 2 years. Calcium supplementation alone has not been shown in small studies to reduce the incidence of nonvertebral fractures in high-risk women. Recently, a very large calcium intervention trial from WHI did not demonstrate hip fracture reduction with daily calcium supplements. [1] Currently, an average total calcium intake of 1200 to 1500/day is still recommended by the National Institute of Medicine for all postmenopausal women.

Vitamin D

Vitamin D is essential for skeletal maintenance and for enhancement of calcium absorption. Insufficiency of this vitamin is a growing problem; as many as two thirds of all patients who have hip fractures are classified as vitamin D deficient. Elderly people in chronic care living situations are particularly vulnerable. One large randomized placebo-controlled trial (RPCT) demonstrated a 33% reduction in hip fractures for nursing home residents who received calcium and vitamin D compared with those receiving placebo. [2] In another trial, high-dose intermittent vitamin D reduced nonvertebral fractures by nearly one third among ambulatory elderly persons. [3] In older New England men and women, the combination of calcium citrate and vitamin D was shown to lessen the risk of nonvertebral fractures. [4] However, in a large, recent population-based study with calcium and vitamin D, supplementation had no effect on nonvertebral fractures, [5] although compliance and assessment of vitamin D levels were not sufficiently well documented to exclude an effect conclusively. Besides the potentially positive effects of vitamin D supplementation on the skeleton, particularly in older women, vitamin D can also enhance muscle strength and has been shown to reduce the risk of falling. For most individuals with osteoporosis, 800 IU/day of vitamin D is sufficient to maintain adequate levels of 25(OH) vitamin D. However, in those patients with low bone mass and insufficient or deficient 25-hydroxyvitamin D levels (i.e., <20 ng/mL), administration of 50,000 IU of ergocalciferol (vitamin D_2) or cholecalciferol (vitamin D_3) given once weekly is a safe and effective way to restore vitamin D levels to the normal range.

Vitamin D analogues have been used in the treatment of osteoporosis since the early 1980s. However, this remains a controversial area. High doses of 1,25-dihydroxyvitamin D increase bone mass, but many patients develop hypercalciuria and/or hypercalcemia. At doses of 0.5 μg/day, rocaltriol reduced the rate of both vertebral and nonvertebral fractures, and it increased bone density in a very small trial. Other studies have found little benefit with a narrow therapeutic window, particularly in relation to renal function and hypercalcemia.

Physical Activity

Bedrest or immobility, particularly in elderly persons, can result in rapid bone loss. Moreover, the number of falls increases with age, and the number of falls that result in fractures also rises. A meta-analysis by the Cochrane Review Group demonstrated that muscle strengthening, balance retraining, home hazard assessment, withdrawal of psychotropic medications, and use of a multidisciplinary risk factor assessment program are beneficial in protecting against falls. An alternative approach is to reduce loads applied to the hip during a fall by padding. Hip protectors have been shown to reduce the risk of hip fractures in at least one population, although compliance is generally poor. A more recent study failed to demonstrate the efficacy of these devices in older women in an assisted living facility. Regular physical activity, including aerobic, weight-bearing, and resistant exercises, is effective in increasing spine BMD and in strengthening muscle mass in postmenopausal women, but no large-scale studies have established whether these interventions reduce fracture risk.

Lifestyle

Other interventions including smoking cessation and reduction of alcohol intake should be considered within the framework of an individual's preventive health strategy. However, studies to date have been inconclusive in respect to understanding how changes in these lifestyles affect overall fracture risk.

Medical Therapy

Abundant evidence indicates that an aggressive intervention program can be successful in reducing fracture risk and in improving quality of life among postmenopausal women with preexisting osteoporosis. Several pharmacologic options are available, and these can be classified by their mechanism of action. The two major classes of osteoporosis drugs are (1) *antiresorptives* (i.e., agents that block bone resorption by inhibiting osteoclasts) and (2) *anabolics* (i.e., drugs that stimulate bone formation by primarily acting on osteoblasts).

Antiresorptive Agents

Antiresorptives inhibit bone resorption by suppressing osteoclast activity. Slowing the remodeling cycle allows bone formation to catch up to resorption, thereby enhancing matrix mineralization and stabilizing trabecular microarchitecture. The antiresorptives increase BMD and reduce fracture risk, but their efficacy varies.

Estrogen

Estrogen replacement therapy was long considered the cornerstone of therapy for postmenopausal women with osteoporosis. It works by slowing bone resorption through inhibition of cytokine signaling from the osteoblast to the osteoclast, thereby increasing BMD. Estrogen replacement inhibits both cortical and trabecular bone loss, and BMD generally increases by 3 to 5% after 3 years. [6] There does not appear to be an additive effect from progesterone on bone mass in women also receiving estrogen. Conversely, progesterone is a necessary part of hormone replacement therapy in women with a uterus because it prevents the development of endometrial hyperplasia and carcinoma. In the WHI, estrogen and progesterone lowered hip fracture risk by one third. [7] Low-dose conjugated estrogens (0.3 or 0.45 mg/day) and ultralow-dose estradiol increase BMD and have been approved for the prevention of bone loss, but antifracture efficacy for these preparations has not been established. Discontinuation of estrogen results in measurable bone loss, although it is not certain whether that translates into a greater fracture risk.

Significant concern has been expressed about the nonskeletal risks associated with long-term estrogen and estrogen in combination with progesterone. Particularly troublesome is the increased risk of breast cancer with the long-term use of estrogen and progesterone. In the WHI, there was a 26% increase in risk of invasive breast cancer over a 5.2-year period of follow-up. [7] Hence estrogen replacement is contraindicated in any woman with a history of breast cancer; yearly mammograms are indicated in all women receiving hormone replacement therapy. Previous case-control and retrospective studies suggested that estrogen could reduce the risk of coronary artery disease; however, in the WHI, the risk of myocardial infarction or death from coronary artery disease was 29% higher in women receiving combination therapy. [7] Thromboembolic disease is also increased more than threefold by hormone replacement therapy. [7] Hence, the use of estrogen and/or estrogen in combination with progestins for the prevention and/or treatment of osteoporosis has fallen dramatically. Moreover, the availability of newer and effective antiresorptive drugs for the treatment of osteoporosis has lessened enthusiasm for primary hormonal therapy in osteoporotic women.

Selective Estrogen Receptor Modulators

Selective estrogen receptor modulators such as tamoxifen and raloxifene also inhibit bone resorption by blocking cytokine release from the osteoblast. Both have been shown to reduce bone loss in postmenopausal women with breast cancer, but only raloxifene is approved by the U.S. Food and Drug Administration (FDA) for the prevention and treatment of osteoporosis.

Both these agents block the actions of estrogen on the breast but act like an estrogen agonist in bone; tamoxifen, but not raloxifene, has estrogen agonistic properties on the uterus and is associated with a greater risk of endometrial carcinoma with long-term use. Both agents have been associated with a reduction in new cases of breast cancer when they are administered as prophylaxis for high-risk patients. [8] Low-density lipoprotein cholesterol levels are also reduced in patients receiving these selective estrogen receptor modulators. Raloxifene increases spine BMD slightly (as does tamoxifen) and lowers the risk of vertebral fracture by 40%, although it has no effect on nonvertebral fracture risk. [9] Hot flashes, leg cramps, and a greater risk of deep venous thrombosis can occur with raloxifene therapy. The recommended dose of raloxifene is 60 mg once daily.

Tissue selectivity with these selective estrogen receptor modulators and others being investigated is a subject of great scientific interest. Raloxifene and estrogen both bind to the same region of the estrogen receptor, but they induce different conformational changes in that receptor. Co-activating and co-repressing proteins are recruited to the receptor ligand complex, and it is thought that these transcription factors ultimately determine the activity of the nuclear complex. Because recruitment also depends on location, it is highly likely that significant tissue selectivity exists for these partners. Newer agents have been designed to facilitate particular complexes and re-arrangements within the nucleus; these are being studied at both the preclinical and the clinical levels.

Bisphosphonates

The bisphosphonates are the most widely prescribed antiresorptives and are often considered first-line therapy for the treatment of severe postmenopausal osteoporosis. These drugs are carbon-substituted analogues of pyrophosphate that bind tightly to hydroxyapatite crystals. It is thought these agents directly suppress resorption by inhibiting osteoclast attachment and enhancing programmed cell death. The first-generation bisphosphonates include etidronate and clodronate. Neither is approved for the treatment of osteoporosis, although etidronate is widely used "off label" and in Europe. The dose of etidronate is 400 mg/day for 2 weeks every 3 months. The drug has few gastrointestinal side effects, and vertebral fracture risk reduction is significant with this agent. Alendronate and risedronate, two second-generation nitrogen-containing bisphosphonates, are effective in suppressing bone resorption and increasing BMD. In RPCTs of postmenopausal women with established osteoporosis, alendronate and risedronate reduced vertebral, hip, and nonvertebral fractures by nearly 50%, particularly during the first year of treatment. [10, 11] Like other antiresorptive drugs, increases in BMD with alendronate or residronate account for a small fraction of their antifracture efficacy. Hence, follow-up DXA measurements may significantly underestimate fracture risk reduction. Recent clinical trials have shown these drugs can be safely administered for at least 7 years without adversely affecting bone strength. Moreover, discontinuation of alendronate after 5 years results in minimal bone loss over the ensuing 5 years. Both drugs have excellent safety profiles, although erosive esophagitis is a serious complication of all nitrogen-containing bisphosphonates. Once-weekly administration of alendronate has been shown to reduce the prevalence of drug-induced esophagitis, and currently both bisphosphonates are marketed as once-weekly treatments.

Other bisphosphonates are available for off-label use or are being studied for the treatment of osteoporosis. Intravenous pamidronate has been available since the mid-1990s for the treatment of Paget's disease and malignant hypercalcemia. It is currently also used to treat osteoporotic women who cannot tolerate oral bisphosphonates, although it has not been formally approved by the FDA, and its antifracture efficacy has not been established. The dose ranges from 30 to 90 mg given every 3 to 9 months. Acute and delayed-type hypersensitivity reactions can occur with this drug, and its use is contraindicated in patients who are vitamin D deficient because it can precipitously drop serum calcium. Ibandronate, administered daily as a 2.5-mg tablet, was approved in 2004 for both the prevention and treatment of postmenopausal osteoporosis. It has been shown to reduce the incidence of vertebral fractures by nearly 50%. [12] Ibandronate, given once monthly at a dose of 150 mg per tablet, is now widely available. First-dose hypersensitivity can occur with ibandronate, and because it is a nitrogen-containing bisphosphonate, it is also associated with esophageal reflux. Intravenous zoledronate has been approved for the treatment of malignant hypercalcemia, multiple myeloma, and skeletal metastases. A once-yearly dose of zoledronate has been shown to suppress bone resorption and increase BMD in postmenopausal women. Phase III trials to test its safety and antifracture efficacy in osteoporosis have been conducted and are currently being analyzed for fracture efficacy.

Calcitonin

Calcitonin is a 32–amino acid peptide normally produced by the thyroid C cells. Osteoclasts have calcitonin receptors, and calcitonin can rapidly inhibit bone resorption. Salmon calcitonin is more potent than human and is the preferred treatment choice. Nasal and subcutaneous calcitonin are both approved for the treatment of postmenopausal osteoporosis. However, the evidence favoring a strong effect from this hormone on either bone loss or fracture efficacy is lacking. In an RPCT of women with postmenopausal osteoporosis, 200 IU/day of nasal calcitonin reduced vertebral fracture incidence by one third. [13] However, methodologic flaws in that trial have limited enthusiasm for this agent as a primary treatment for osteoporosis. In at least one placebo-controlled study, nasal calcitonin reduced the pain associated with new spine fractures. The recommended dose of nasal calcitonin is 200 IU/day, and that of subcutaneous calcitonin is 100 IU/day. Side effects are uncommon with intranasal calcitonin and include nasal stuffiness and flushing. With subcutaneous administration, nausea is not infrequent.

Strontium Ranelate

Strontium ranelate is orally administered and stimulates calcium uptake in bone while it inhibits bone resorption. It is thought to have some anabolic activity, although the precise mechanism of action in the skeleton, where it is incorporated, is not known. In an RPCT of postmenopausal women with established disease, daily strontium reduced the risk of vertebral fractures by 40%. [14] However, a statistically significant effect on nonvertebral fractures was limited to a small subset of women in a post hoc analysis. This

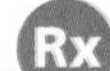

drug is approved by European regulatory agencies but not by the U.S. FDA.

Anabolic Agents

A new class of antiosteoporosis drugs was introduced in 2002. These are the so-called anabolics, agents that stimulate bone formation more than bone resorption. As such, these agents enhance bone remodeling and contrast sharply with the antiresorptives, which slow bone turnover. PTH 1-34 (teriparatide) was the first of this class of drugs to be approved by the FDA.

The prototypical anabolic drug was sodium fluoride, which saw widespread use in the 1970s and 1980s because of its ability to stimulate new bone formation. However, an RPCT in 1990 established that although there were dramatic increases in BMD, nonvertebral fracture risk actually increased. Unlike sodium fluoride, synthetic PTH (PTH_{1-34}) was approved by the U.S. FDA for the treatment of postmenopausal osteoporosis because it not only increases bone mass but also reduces fractures. In the largest RPCT using teriparatide in postmenopausal women with severe osteoporosis, 20 μg/day of PTH, administered subcutaneously, reduced spinal and nonvertebral fractures by more than 50% while it substantially increased (i.e., 8%/year) lumbar BMD. [15] Similar findings were noted in men with osteoporosis who were treated for 11 months. Unfortunately, the PTH trial in postmenopausal women was stopped after 20 months because of concerns related to the development of osteosarcoma in rats treated with high doses of PTH_{1-34}. However, retrospective studies have found no association between osteosarcoma and primary or secondary hyperparathyroidism, and no cases of osteosarcoma in PTH-treated patients have been reported. More recently recombinant human PTH (PTH_{1-84}) has shown similar benefits. [16] Currently, it is recommended that PTH therapy should be limited to those individuals with moderate to severe osteoporosis, and then only for 2 years.

Despite the appeal of using an anabolic with an antiresorptive, no evidence indicates that combinations of classes of drugs are additive or synergistic. Unlike the bisphosphonates, discontinuation of PTH can result in bone loss of 3 to 4% in the first year after PTH cessation. This post-treatment effect is prevented by adding an antiresorptive drug after PTH is stopped. In general, PTH is well tolerated, although nausea, flushing, hypotension, and mild but asymptomatic hypercalcemia (i.e., serum calcium <11.0 mg/dL) can occur. Cost and compliance have been major limiting factors.

GLUCOCORTICOID-INDUCED OSTEOPOROSIS

The most common secondary cause of osteoporosis is glucocorticoid induced. This is often a result of pharmacologic doses of steroids used to treat inflammatory or autoimmune disorders. Generally, it is considered that glucocorticoids have a dose-dependent effect on the skeleton, such that longer duration and higher doses of steroids are most likely to cause bone loss and fractures. However, there clearly are subsets of individuals who are more or less sensitive to the skeletal effects of high doses of glucocorticoids. As a general clinical rule, those individuals with a cushingoid appearance and fat redistribution almost always have low bone mass and/or fractures.

The effects of glucocorticoids on the skeleton are multifaceted and are particularly devastating because these agents cause uncoupling in the remodeling unit. Besides the indirect suppressive effects of glucocorticoids on the hypothalamic-gonadal axis, and inhibition of calcium absorption in the gut, high doses of steroids can stimulate osteoclastogenesis, increase RANKL production, and decrease OPG. This situation results in higher rates of bone resorption. Additionally, glucocorticoids also have a strong negative effect on bone formation by suppressing expression of IGF-I in bone cells and by shifting marrow stromal cells into the fat lineage, rather than down the osteoblast differentiation pathway. It is presumed that just as fat redistribution is a clinical hallmark of Cushing's syndrome in the supraclavicular and mediastinal area, enhanced adiposity in the bone marrow is a characteristic feature, almost certainly as a function of increased stromal cell differentiation into adipocytes. Bone strength is markedly compromised by the uncoupling in remodeling, and bone loss can be rapid over a short time period, particularly with high doses of glucocorticoids. Although there is no true dose-dependent effect on bone resorption, it is thought that prednisone doses as low as 5 mg/day may increase fracture risk. Indeed, in this syndrome, baseline BMD is not predictive of fractures and can often be normal even in the presence of ongoing resorption and recurrent fractures. Trabecular bone suffers the most in this syndrome, and spine DXA is the most sensitive indicator of bone loss. Markers of bone turnover are not helpful in the management of these patients.

Therapy for steroid-induced bone loss centers on treating the underlying disease and/or reducing the dose of glucocorticoids to the lowest possible regimen. Barring that, several interventions have been shown to retard bone loss and prevent fractures. Adequate calcium and vitamin D intake is critical for every patient receiving glucocorticoids. However, these measures alone are not sufficient. Three bisphosphonates have been shown to have efficacy in glucocorticoid-induced osteoporosis: etidronate, alendronate [17], and risedronate, and they are now considered the standard of care for this disease. These drugs are administered either weekly or cyclically to prevent bone loss and to reduce the risk of fractures. Some anecdotal data support the use of gonadal steroids in this condition, but clearly the bisphosphonates are superior. PTH_{1-34} in one trial was shown to reduce the rate of bone loss in combination with hormone replacement therapy. More studies are needed to establish its efficacy in this disease, particularly because secondary hyperparathyroidism is a frequent accompaniment of steroid-induced osteoporosis.

Future Directions

Several new agents in development offer hope for patients with osteoporosis. AMG 162, a synthetic RANKL antibody that works like OPG and is administered twice yearly subcutaneously, has great potential. It prevents bone loss in women with severe disease, and fracture studies are ongoing. PTH-related protein (PTHrp), a peptide that is structurally similar to PTH, binds to the same receptor, and is responsible in some cases for hypercalcemia of malignancy, has been shown to have significant anabolic properties when administered intermittently. Both these agents are being studied in large phase III clinical trials.

OSTEOPOROSIS IN MEN

Epidemiology

Osteoporosis in men is now more frequently recognized. This may stem from greater awareness in respect to the clinical presentation, the role of bone density screening, and a better understanding of the pathogenesis of osteoporosis, particularly in older men. Thirty percent of all hip and vertebral fractures occur in men, and one in six men in later life will suffer a hip fracture.

Clinical Manifestations

The clinical presentation is often different from that in women, especially in relation to the time to diagnosis after symptoms begin. Back pain with vertebral compression is the most common presenting complaint. Bone density measurements are less frequently obtained in men, but they are performed after symptoms occur, a far different situation than in postmenopausal women.

Pathobiology

Secondary causes of osteoporosis dominate this disease in men. Hypogonadism and hypercortisolemia are the major etiologic factors in male osteoporosis and must be considered regardless of the phenotypic presentation. However, certain other conditions, including gluten enteropathy, gastric resection or bypass, and ethanol abuse, are more common in men than women with osteoporosis. Hypercalciuria (with or without kidney stones) that is associated with secondary hyperparathyroidism almost always occurs in men and is a frequent cause of low bone mass in young men. In contrast, anorexia in male patients is extremely rare, and the athlete's triad so characteristic of women runners (i.e., exercise, hypogonadism, and low bone mass) is infrequent, although not unheard of, in men.

The role of androgens in the male and female skeleton has been examined carefully but remains an area of some controversy, even though it is clear that lack of androgens results in a skeletal deficit. Peak bone mass is clearly reduced in androgen-insufficient young male patients whether the condition results from idiopathic hypogonadotropic hypogonadism, Klinefelter's syndrome, or constitutional delayed puberty. The use of long-acting gonadotropin-releasing hormone analogues that block androgen production and are administered in the treatment of prostate cancer is also associated with significant bone loss in later life. Men with primary gonadal failure, hemochromatosis, hyperprolactinemic hypogonadism, and other disorders of the hypothalamus or pituitary often have very low bone mass. Androgens act by directly stimulating bone formation because osteoblasts have androgen receptors. However, testosterone probably also blocks bone resorption and can dampen the release of TNF, IL-6, and IL-1. Not surprisingly, estrogen also plays an important role in the male skeleton. Inhibition of aromatization of testosterone (i.e., aromatase P-450) to estrogen, whether caused by a genetic mutation, or drugs, leads to significant bone loss. Investigators have also shown that men with low estradiol levels are at greater risk for osteoporosis. Thus, it appears that both estrogen and androgen are necessary for the development and maintenance of the male skeleton.

Treatment

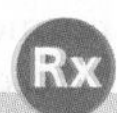

Therapies for osteoporosis in male patients center on identifying any underlying cause and then treating with drugs that are also used in women. Hypogonadism can be effectively treated with androgen replacement, although caution must be used in elderly men because of the risk of prostate cancer. Hypercalciuria can be diminished by use of hydrochlorthiazide, which may also enhance bone density in men. Alendronate has been shown to prevent bone loss and to reduce fractures in men with idiopathic osteoporosis or osteoporosis resulting from androgen deficiency states. [18] PTH_{1-34} has also been approved for the treatment of male osteoporosis, because it too can enhance bone density and reduce bone loss. Selective androgen receptor modulators are currently under development and may offer a new approach for male osteoporosis.

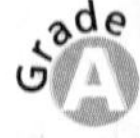

1. Jackson, RD, LaCroix, AZ, et al: Calcium plus vitamin D supplementation and the risk of fractures. N Engl J Med 2006;354:669–683.
2. Chapuy MC, Arlot ME, Duboeuf F, et al: Vitamin D_3 and calcium to prevent hip fractures in the elderly woman. N Engl J Med 1992;327:1637–1642.
3. Trivedi DP, Doll R, Khaw KT: Effect of four monthly oral vitamin D_3 (cholecalciferol) supplementation on fractures and mortality in men and women living in the community: Randomised double blind controlled trial. BMJ 2003;326:469.
4. Dawson-Hughes B, Harris SS, Krall EA, Dallal GE: Effect of calcium and vitamin D supplementation on bone density in men and women 65 years of age or older. N Engl J Med 1997;337:670–676.
5. Grant AM, Avenell A, Campbell MK, et al, and RECORD Trial Group: Oral vitamin D_3 and calcium for secondary prevention of low-trauma fractures in elderly people (Randomised Evaluation of Calcium Or vitamin D, RECORD): A randomised placebo-controlled trial. Lancet 2005;365:1621–1628.
6. Writing Group for the PEPI: Effects of hormone therapy on bone mineral density: Results from the Postmenopausal Estrogen/Progestin Interventions (PEPI) Trial. JAMA 1996;276:1389–1396.
7. Rossouw JE, Anderson GL, Prentice RL, et al: Risks and benefits of estrogen plus progestin in healthy postmenopausal women: Principal results from the Women's Health Initiative randomized controlled trial. JAMA 2002;288:321–333.
8. Cummings S, Eckert S, Krueger K, et al: The effect of raloxifene on risk of breast cancer in postmenopausal women: Results from the MORE randomized trial. JAMA 1999;281:2189–2197.
9. Ettinger B, Black D, Mitlak B, et al: Reduction of vertebral fracture risk in postmenopausal women with osteoporosis treated with raloxifene. JAMA 1999;282:637–645.
10. McClung MR, Geusens P, Miller PD, et al: Effect of risedronate on the risk of hip fracture in elderly women: Hip Intervention Program Study Group. N Engl J Med 2001;344:333–340.
11. Black D, Cummings S, Karpf D, et al: Randomised trial of effect of alendronate on risk of fracture in women with existing vertebral fractures: Fracture Intervention Trial Research Group. Lancet 1996;348:1535–1541.
12. Chesnut IC, Skag A, Christiansen C, et al: Effects of oral ibandronate administered daily or intermittently on fracture risk in postmenopausal osteoporosis. J Bone Miner Res 2004;19:1241–1249.
13. Chesnut CH 3rd, Silverman S, Andriano K, et al: A randomized trial of nasal spray salmon calcitonin in postmenopausal women with established osteoporosis: The prevent recurrence of osteoporotic fractures study. PROOF Study Group. Am J Med 2000;109:267–276.
14. Meunier PJ, Roux C, Seeman E, et al: The effects of strontium ranelate on the risk of vertebral fracture in women with postmenopausal osteoporosis. N Engl J Med 2004;350:459–468.
15. Neer RM, Arnaud CD, Zanchetta JR, et al: Effect of parathyroid hormone (1-34) on fractures and bone mineral density in postmenopausal women with osteoporosis. N Engl J Med 2001;344:1434–1441.
16. Greenspan SL, Bone HG, Ettinger MP, et al: Effect of recombinant human parathyroid hormone (1-84) on vertebral fracture and bone mineral density in postmenopausal women with osteoporosis: A randomized trial. Ann Intern Med 2007;146:326–339.
17. de Nijs RNJ, Jacobs JWG, Lems WF, et al: Alendronate or alfacalcidol in glucocorticoid-induced osteoporosis. N Engl J Med 2006;355:675–684.
18. Orwoll ES, Ettinger M, Weiss S, et al: Alendronate for the treatment of osteoporosis in men. N Engl J Med 2000;343:604–610.

SUGGESTED READINGS

Black D, Greenspan S, Ensrud K, et al: The effects of PTH and alendronate alone or in combination in post-menopausal osteoporosis. N Engl J Med 2003;349:1207–1215. *The combination of PTH and alendronate is not better than PTH alone.*

Bischoff-Ferrari HA, Dawson-Hughes B, Willett WC, et al: Effect of vitamin D on falls: A meta-analysis. JAMA 2004;291:1999–2006. *The best summary of evidence to date on the nonskeletal effects of vitamin D.*

Bone HG, Hosking D, Devogelaer JP, et al: Ten years' experiences with alendronate for osteoporosis in postmenopausal women. N Engl J Med 2004;350:1189–1199. *The longest study to date examining the effects of alendronate on the skeleton.*

Center JR, Bliuc D, Nguyen TV, et al: Risk of subsequent fracture after low-trauma fracture in men and women. JAMA 2007;297:387–394. *Increase in risk of subsequent fracture persisted for 10 years.*

Finkelstein JS, Hayes A, Hunzelman JL, et al: The effects of parathyroid hormone, alendronate, or both in men with osteoporosis. N Engl J Med 2003;349:1216–1226.

Odvina CV, Zerwekh JE, Rao DS, et al: Severely suppressed bone turnover: A potential complication of alendronate therapy. J Clin Endocrinol Metab 2005;90:1294–1301. *One of the most controversial articles in the bone literature; an anecdotal review of nine cases suggesting impaired fracture healing and very low bone turnover in patients receiving long-term alendronate therapy. The difficulty is the small numbers of subjects and the huge implications, which have not been borne out from clinical trials.*

Riggs BL, Hartmann LC: Selective estrogen-receptor modulators: Mechanisms of action and application to clinical practice. N Engl J Med 2003;348:618–629. *An outstanding and up-to-date review of the molecular, cellular, and skeletal actions of the selective estrogen receptor modulators.*

Sambrook P, Cooper C: Osteoporosis. Lancet 2006;367:2010–2018. *A comprehensive overview.*

Siris ES, Harris ST, Rosen CJ, et al: Adherence to bisphosphonate therapy and fracture rates in osteoporotic women: Relationship to vertebral and nonvertebral fractures from 2 US claims databeses. Mayo Clin Proc 2006;81:1013–1022. *Increasing refill compliance was associated with a reduced risk of fracture.*

Surgeon General Bone Health and Osteoporosis: A Report of the Surgeon General. Rockville, MD: U.S. Department of Health and Human Services, 2004, p 436. *A comprehensive evaluation of the implications of osteoporosis on society and includes diagnosis, treatment, and prevention recommendations as well as newer public health initiatives.*

Uitterlinden AG, Ralston SH, Brandi ML, et al: The association between common vitamin D receptor gene variations and osteoporosis: A participant-level meta-analysis. Ann Intern Med 2006;145:255–264. *The cdx2 polymorphism was associated with a reduced fracture risk.*

OSTEOMALACIA AND RICKETS

Marc K. Drezner

Definition

Rickets and osteomalacia are diseases characterized by defective bone and cartilage mineralization in children and bone mineralization in adults. The abnormal calcification of cartilage occurs at epiphyseal growth plates. Delayed maturation of the cartilage cellular sequence and disorganization of cell arrangement are also present. The resultant profusion of disorganized, nonmineralized, degenerating cartilage causes widening of the epiphyseal plates with flaring or cupping and irregularity of the epiphyseal-metaphyseal junctions. The abnormal calcification of bone is restricted to the organic matrix at the bone-osteoid interfaces of remodeling tissue. The insufficient mineralization of newly formed matrix paradoxically results in enhanced bone volume and increased susceptibility to fractures or bone deformities. The various disorders associated with rickets and osteomalacia identified and characterized to date are numerous (Table 265–1). Although the phenotypic expression of the defective bone and cartilage mineralization is similar in each of these disorders, the associated biochemical abnormalities and the therapeutic approaches differ according to the pathogenetic defect. Therefore, when diagnosing rickets and/or osteomalacia, further systematic analysis is needed to determine the cause and appropriate therapy for the disorder.

Pathobiology

Mineralization of cartilage and bone is a complex process in which the calcium-phosphorus inorganic mineral phase is deposited in an organic matrix in a highly ordered fashion. Such mineralization depends on the following: (1) the availability of sufficient calcium and phosphorus from the extracellular fluid; (2) adequate metabolic and transport function of chondrocytes and osteoblasts to regulate the concentration of calcium, phosphorus, and other ions at the mineralization sites; (3) the presence of collagen with unique type, number, and distribution of cross-links, remarkable patterns of hydroxylation and glycosylation, and abundant phosphate content, which collectively permit and facilitate deposition of mineral at gaps, in hole zones, and between the distal ends of two collagen molecules; (4) maintenance of an optimal pH (~7.6) for deposition of calcium-phosphorus complexes; and (5) low concentration of calcification inhibitors (e.g., pyrophosphates, proteoglycans) in bone matrix.

Many of the disorders of mineralization occur secondary to known defects in these control steps. In this regard, most diseases resulting in rickets and/or osteomalacia stem from abnormalities in the vitamin D endocrine system. Traditionally, a direct role has been assumed for vitamin D or, more properly, its active metabolite, 1,25-dihydroxyvitamin D, for production of normal collagen matrix and regulation of bone mineralization. However, it is more likely that the abnormal mineralization in these disorders results from an associated calcium and phosphorus deficiency that diminishes the driving force for calcification. Primary disorders of phosphate homeostasis also underlie many of the rachitic/osteomalacic disorders. Diminished gastrointestinal absorption or renal wasting of phosphorus limits this essential mineral in such disorders. The isolated deficiency of phosphorus alone or in conjunction with a frequently occurring aberration in vitamin D metabolism is the basis for defective mineralization. In accord with the complex regulation of bone mineralization, however, decreases in calcium or phosphorus do not account for rickets and osteomalacia in all forms of the disease. Indeed, certain forms of rickets and osteomalacia occur in spite of a normal or even elevated calcium-phosphate product. In such diseases, altered pH, abnormal collagen matrix, or excessive concentration of calcification inhibitors underlie the abnormal mineralization. In other forms of the disease, the precise mechanism causing the defective mineralization remains unknown.

Inadequate mineralization in rickets occurs in the matrix of cartilage in the growing epiphyseal plate. These characteristic changes are confined to the maturation zone of the cartilage, whereas the resting and proliferative zones of the epiphyses exhibit normal histologic features. In the maturation zone, the height of the cell columns is increased, and the cells are closely packed and irregularly aligned. Moreover, calcification in the interstitial regions of this hypertrophic zone is defective.

In bone, the abnormal mineralization results in accumulation of excess osteoid, a sine qua non for the diagnosis of osteomalacia in most instances (Fig. 265–1). A supranormal amount of osteoid may also occur in disease states associated with accelerated bone turnover, such as hyperparathyroidism, however. In addition, reduced mineralization activity may be observed without hyperosteoidosis in patients with osteoporosis. Establishing the histopathologic diagnosis of osteomalacia, therefore, requires documentation of abnormal mineralization with excess osteoid. These defects are manifest in bone by an increase in the bone-forming surface covered by incompletely mineralized osteoid, an increase in osteoid volume and thickness, and a decrease in the mineralization front (the percentage of osteoid-covered bone-forming surface undergoing calcification) or the mineral apposition rate. The amount of osteoid in bone and the mineralization dynamics are determined in 3- to 5-μm thick sections of decalcified bone by special stains and the fluorescence of previously ingested tetracycline that is deposited at calcification fronts.

Clinical Manifestations

The clinical features of rickets, although variable to some degree according to the underlying disorder, are primarily related to skeletal pain and deformity, bone fractures, slipped epiphyses, and abnormalities of growth. In addition, hypocalcemia, when present, may be severe enough to produce tetany, laryngeal spasm, and seizures.

In infants and young children, symptoms include listlessness, irritability, and, in some forms of metabolic rickets, profound hypotonia and proximal muscle weakness. Indeed, as the disease progresses and muscle weakness is present, delayed motor milestones are evident, children often are unable to walk without support, and lower respiratory infections become frequent. Throughout early life, classic skeletal deformities appear. By 6 months of age, frontal bossing with flattening at the back is evident. Later, a lateral collapse of both chest walls (Harrison's sulcus) and a rachitic rosary may appear. When the condition is left untreated, progressive bony deformities result in bowing (see Fig. 265–1), particularly in the tibia, femur, radius, and ulna, and fractures. In addition, dental eruption may be delayed, and, in those forms of the disease with hypocalcemia or hereditary hypophosphatemia, enamel defects and inadequate dentin calcification occur, respectively.

In contrast, clinical signs of osteomalacia are nondescript. Indeed, the disease-specific abnormalities may be overlooked, and features of an underlying disorder (e.g., malabsorption) may predominate. Symptoms, when present, may include diffuse skeletal pain and muscular weakness. The pain, often described as dull and aching, is generally worsened by activity and prominent around the hips, with a resulting antalgic gait. The muscle weakness is primarily proximal and is frequently associated with wasting, hypotonia, and a waddling gait. This myopathy is seen in almost all forms of rickets and osteomalacia, with X-linked hypophosphatemic rickets (XLH) and osteomalacia the notable exceptions. Clinical improvement in the myopathy usually results from specific therapy, such as vitamin D repletion in patients with nutritional osteomalacia, phosphate supplementation in disorders marked by renal phosphate wasting, or correction of acidosis. Fractures of the ribs, vertebral bodies, and long bones may occur and may lead to progressive deformities as well as point tenderness on palpation.

The radiographic abnormalities in both rickets and osteomalacia reflect the histopathologic changes. In rickets, alterations are most evident at the growth plate, which is wide and flared and displays an irregular, hazy appearance at the diaphyseal line secondary to uneven invasion of the recently calcified cartilage by adjacent bone tissue (see Fig. 265–1). The trabecular pattern of the metaphyses is also abnormal, the cortices of the diaphyses are thinned, and the shafts frequently are bowed (see Fig. 265–1).

In osteomalacia, a moderate decrease in bone density is usually associated with coarsening of the trabeculae and blurring of their margins. When secondary hyperparathyroidism is present, subperiosteal resorption in the phalanges and metacarpals, erosion of the distal ends of the clavicles, and bone cysts may be observed. A more specific radiographic abnormality is the presence of Looser's zones, also called *pseudofractures* or *Milkman's fractures*, in the shafts of long bones. These are ribbon-like

TABLE 265–1 RICKETS AND OSTEOMALACIA SYNDROMES

I. Disorders of the vitamin D endocrine system
  A. Decreased bioavailability of vitamin D
    1. Deficient endogenous production
      a. Inadequate sunlight exposure
      b. Aging
    2. Nutritional deficiency
    3. Loss of vitamin D metabolites
      a. Nephrotic syndrome
      b. Peritoneal dialysis
  B. Vitamin D malabsorption
    1. Gastrointestinal disorders
      a. Partial/total gastrectomy
      b. Small bowel disease (e.g., celiac disease)
      c. Intestinal bypass
    2. Pancreatic insufficiency
    3. Hepatobiliary disease
      a. Biliary atresia
      b. Biliary obstruction
      c. Biliary fistula
      d. Cirrhosis
  C. Abnormal vitamin D metabolism
    1. Impaired hepatic 25-hydroxylation of vitamin D
      a. Liver disease
      b. Anticonvulsant therapy
    2. Impaired renal 1α-hydroxylation of 25-hydroxyvitamin D
      a. Hereditary vitamin D–dependent rickets type 1 (pseudo–vitamin D deficiency)
      b. Chronic renal failure
      c. Pseudohypoparathyroidism
  D. Target organ resistance to vitamin D and metabolites
    1. Hereditary vitamin D–dependent rickets type 2
      a. Hormone binding negative
      b. Defect in hormone binding capacity
      c. Defect in hormone binding affinity
      d. Deficient hormone receptor nuclear localization
      e. Decreased affinity of the hormone receptor complex
II. Disorders of phosphate homeostasis
  A. Dietary
    1. Low phosphate intake
    2. Ingestion of phosphate-binding antacids
  B. Impaired renal tubular phosphate reabsorption
    1. Hereditary
      a. X-linked hypophosphatemic rickets/osteomalacia
      b. Hereditary hypophosphatemic rickets/osteomalacia with hypercalciuria
      c. Autosomal dominant hypophosphatemic rickets
      d. Hypophosphatemic bone disease (nonrachitic hypophosphatemic osteomalacia)
      e. Adult-onset hypophosphatemic rickets
      f. Autosomal recessive hypophosphatemic rickets (X-linked hypercalciuric nephrolithiasis)
      g. X-linked recessive hypophosphatemic rickets (X-linked hypercalciuric nephrolithiasis)
    2. Acquired
      a. Tumor-induced osteomalacia (oncogenous osteomalacia)
        i. Mesenchymal, epidermal, and endodermal tumors
        ii. Fibrous dysplasia of bone
        iii. Neurofibromatosis
        iv. Linear nevus sebaceous syndrome
        v. Light-chain nephropathy
      b. Sporadic hypophosphatemic osteomalacia
  C. General renal tubular disorders
    1. Fanconi's syndrome type 1
      a. Hereditary
        i. Familial idiopathic
        ii. Cystinosis (Lignac-Fanconi syndrome)
        iii. Hereditary fructose intolerance
        iv. Tyrosinemia
        v. Galactosemia
        vi. Glycogen storage disease
        vii. Wilson's disease
        viii. Oculocerebral renal syndrome (Lowe's syndrome)
      b. Acquired
        i. Renal transplantation
        ii. Multiple myeloma
      c. Intoxication
        i. Cadmium
        ii. Lead
        iii. Tetracycline (outdated)
        iv. Antiretroviral drugs
    2. Fanconi's syndrome type 2
III. Metabolic acidosis
  A. Distal renal tubular acidosis
    1. Primary
      a. Sporadic
      b. Familial
    2. Secondary
      a. Galactosemia (after galactose ingestion)
      b. Hereditary fructose intolerance with nephrocalcinosis (after chronic fructose ingestion)
      c. Hypergammaglobulinemic states
      d. Medullary sponge kidney
    3. Acquired
      a. Drug induced
        i. Acetazolamide
        ii. Ammonium chloride
IV. Disorders of calcium homeostasis
  A. Dietary calcium deficiency
V. Abnormal bone matrix
  A. Fibrogenesis imperfecta ossium
  B. Axial osteomalacia
VI. Primary mineralization defects
  A. Hereditary
    1. Hypophosphatasia
      a. Perinatal disease
      b. Infantile disease
      c. Childhood disease
      d. Adult-onset disease
      e. Pseudohypophosphatasia
VII. Mineralization inhibitors
  A. Etidronate
  B. Fluoride
  C. Aluminum

zones of rarefaction, ranging from a few millimeters to several centimeters in length and usually oriented perpendicular to the bone surface. Often, they occur symmetrically and most commonly are present at the medial aspect of the femora near the femoral heads, in the metatarsals, or in the pelvis. Long-standing osteomalacia may also result in additional characteristic radiographic abnormalities, including biconcave collapsed vertebrae and a trefoil (or triangular) pelvis.

In patients with renal tubular disorders (Chapter 129), increased rather than decreased bone density may be present. Despite the increased bone mass, histopathologic evaluation of biopsies reveals an abundance of unmineralized osteoid, and bones remain subject to fracture. Thus, the increased density likely reflects replacement of marrow air space with osteoid.

Biochemical abnormalities in patients with rickets and osteomalacia vary with the cause of the disorder. However, the rachitic and osteomalacic syndromes may be divided into calcipenic and phosphopenic forms, as well as those in which mineral availability is apparently normal. In general, patients with the calcipenic diseases exhibit a low or marginally

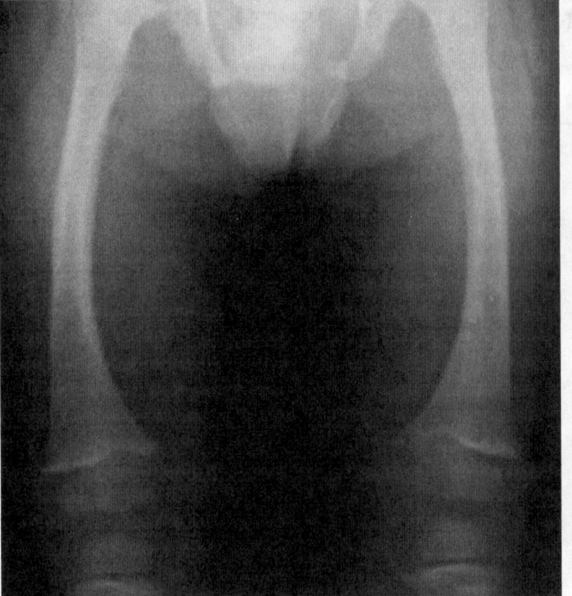

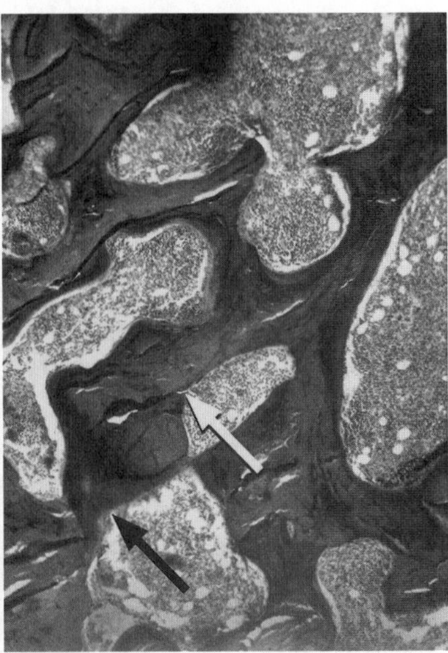

FIGURE 265–1 • A, Radiographic appearance of the lower extremities in a youth with rickets. The bowed femora are evident bilaterally. In addition, at the distal ends of the femora, the growth plates are wide and flared and display an irregular hazy appearance at the diaphyseal line secondary to uneven invasion of the recently calcified cartilage by adjacent bone tissue. **B,** Microscopic appearance of bone biopsy sections from a patient with osteomalacia. Stained sections exhibit mineralized bone (white arrow) covered by unmineralized osteoid seams (black arrow). Such observations are representative of the abnormal mineralization that characterizes the osteomalacic bone disorder.

normal serum calcium level, a decreased serum phosphorus concentration, and (secondary) hyperparathyroidism. When vitamin D deficiency prevails, the serum 25-hydroxyvitamin D levels are characteristically low, generally less than 10 ng/mL but occasionally 10 to 20 ng/mL. In contrast, the serum 1,25-dihydroxyvitamin D concentration may not be overtly decreased secondary to the prevailing hyperparathyroidism. Alternatively, a defect in vitamin D metabolism often results in an isolated deficiency of 1,25-dihydroxyvitamin D, whereas end-organ resistance to this active vitamin D metabolite increases the circulating level of calcitriol.

A primary abnormality of transepithelial phosphate transport in the nephron, resulting in renal phosphate wasting, underlies most of the phosphopenic disorders. As a rule, patients with these disorders maintain a normal serum calcium concentration, whereas the serum phosphorus level is characteristically low. In contrast to the calcipenic forms of disease, the serum 25-hydroxyvitamin D and parathyroid hormone (PTH) levels are normal in patients with hypophosphatemic disease. Moreover, affected subjects commonly maintain a normal (or mildly decreased) serum 1,25-dihydroxyvitamin D level despite the prevailing hypophosphatemia, which should increase production of this active vitamin D metabolite. However, an elevated serum 1,25-dihydroxyvitamin D concentration has been reported in several rare genetic phosphopenic disorders, hereditary hypophosphatemic rickets with hypercalciuria (HHRH), Fanconi's syndrome type 2, and X-linked recessive hypophosphatemic rickets. Whereas the elevated calcitriol level underlies increased gastrointestinal absorption of calcium and hypercalciuria in these diseases, the impact of abnormal vitamin D metabolism on the phenotypic expression of the phosphopenic disorders is less certain. In patients with those diseases with normal serum calcium and phosphorus concentrations, laboratory abnormalities are unique to each form of the disease. Nevertheless, alkaline phosphatase activity in plasma is generally elevated in all forms of rickets and osteomalacia. Even severe forms of disease, however, particularly those caused by renal tubular disorders, may be associated with normal or only marginally elevated enzyme activity.

DISORDERS OF THE VITAMIN D ENDOCRINE SYSTEM

Rickets and osteomalacia resulting from disorders of the vitamin D endocrine system are caused by a wide variety of calcipenic diseases. The variable biochemical abnormalities associated with these disparate disorders are summarized in Table 265–2. Although many of these diseases are no longer common causes of rickets and osteomalacia, others are often hidden causes of bone disease in a varying population of patients.

Decreased Bioavailability of Vitamin D: Inadequate Sunlight and Nutritional Vitamin D Deficiency

Adequate exposure to sunlight and fortification of dairy products with vitamin D have eliminated vitamin D deficiency secondary to inadequate endogenous production or nutrition in the majority of countries. However, in several populations, such as Asian immigrants in Britain, rickets and osteomalacia secondary to vitamin D deficiency occur in neonates and infants, in adolescents during pubertal growth, and, less frequently, among adults. In addition, over the past 20 years, a resurgence of vitamin D deficiency rickets has been observed in North America and Europe. Insufficient vitamin D intake secondary to using unfortified foods, naturally dark pigmentation (which interferes with ultraviolet transmission through the skin), genetic factors, and social customs (such as avoiding sun exposure) contribute to the development of disease in these subjects. Moreover, occurrence of disease in neonates is virtually always the result of vitamin D deficiency in mothers with ethnocultural risk factors for such deficiency. In the United States and other developed countries, a surprisingly frequent occurrence of vitamin D deficiency osteomalacia has also been recognized recently in alcoholic patients, institutionalized patients, and elderly persons. Poor diet, in some cases including avoiding milk and milk products because of lactose intolerance, lack of sunlight exposure, and an age-related decline in the dermal synthesis of 7-dehydrocholesterol are among the factors predisposing to the vitamin D deficiency and consequent bone disease.

The clinical sequelae of decreased vitamin D bioavailability are generally preceded by a fall in circulating 25-hydroxyvitamin D levels and begin to occur in the first 18 months of life. Whereas such a deficiency is caused in most patients by inadequate circulating vitamin D, Asian Indians in the United States also manifest increased 25-hydroxyvitamin D-24-hydroxylase activity, which may limit circulating 25-hydroxyvitamin D levels. In any case, measurement of 25-hydroxyvitamin D serves to identify populations at risk for, and facilitates early detection of, vitamin D deficiency rickets and osteomalacia. However, it has become increasingly clear that nutritional rickets exists along a spectrum ranging from isolated vitamin D deficiency to isolated calcium deficiency. Moreover, along the spectrum, it is likely that relative deficiencies of calcium and vitamin D interact with genetic and/or environmental factors to stimulate the development of rickets. Thus, vitamin D supplementation alone may not prevent or treat rickets in populations with limited calcium intake.

Treating clinically evident vitamin D–deficient rickets and osteomalacia invariably results in healing of the bone disease. The disorder is best treated with vitamin D and restoration of normal dietary calcium and

TABLE 265–2 BIOCHEMICAL ABNORMALITIES OF THE CALCIOPENIC RACHITIC/OSTEOMALACIC DISORDERS

	VDDR	CRF	HVDDR 1	HVDDR 2	HP	PSH
BIOCHEMICAL FINDINGS						
Calcium	⇓	⇓	⇓	⇓	⇓	⇓
Phosphorus	N/⇓	⇑	N/⇓	N/⇓	⇑	⇑
Alkaline phosphatase	⇑	⇑	⇑	⇑	N/⇑	N/⇑
Parathyroid hormone	⇑	⇑	⇑	⇑	⇓	⇑
25(OH)D	⇓	N/⇓	N	N	N	N
$1,25(OH)_2D$	N/⇑	⇓	⇓	⇑	⇓	⇓
RENAL FUNCTION						
Urinary phosphorus	⇑	⇓	⇑	⇑	⇓	⇓
Urinary calcium	⇓	⇓	⇓	⇓	⇓	⇓
GASTROINTESTINAL FUNCTION						
Calcium absorption	⇓	⇓	⇓	⇓	⇓	⇓
Phosphorus absorption	⇓	⇓	⇓	⇓	⇓	⇓

$1,25(OH)_2D$ = 1,25-dihydroxyvitamin D; 25(OH)D = 25-hydroxyvitamin D; ⇓ = decreased; ⇑ = increased; CRF = chronic renal failure; HP = hypoparathyroidism; HVDDR 1 = hereditary vitamin D–dependent rickets type 1; HVDDR 2 = hereditary vitamin D–dependent rickets type 2; N = normal; N/⇓= normal or decreased; N/⇑= normal or increased; PSH = pseudohypoparathyroidism; VDDR = vitamin D–deficiency rickets (including sunlight or nutritional deficiency, vitamin D malabsorption, inhibition of 25-hydroxylation).

phosphorus intake. Ergocalciferol (vitamin D_2) is preferred to calcitrol because it provides the missing substrate that submits to physiologic regulation of vitamin D metabolite production.

Vitamin D Malabsorption

Gastrointestinal malabsorption associated with diseases of the small intestine, hepatobiliary tree, and pancreas may result in decreased absorption of vitamin D and/or depletion of endogenous 25-hydroxyvitamin D stores owing to abnormal enterohepatic circulation. In general, malabsorption of vitamin D occurs as a consequence of steatorrhea, which disturbs fat emulsification and chylomicron-facilitated absorption (Chapter 143). Such abnormalities often are associated with rickets and/or osteomalacia. However, most affected patients are asymptomatic, and many exhibit only reduced bone volume rather than evidence of defective bone mineralization. Intestinal bypass surgery and adult celiac disease are common instances in which vitamin D malabsorption occurs and in which the suspicion for osteomalacia should remain high. In contrast, patients with cholestatic liver disease, extrahepatic biliary obstruction, and diseases of the distal portions of the small intestine, such as regional enteritis, may develop bone disease secondary not only to poor vitamin D absorption but also to disruption of enterohepatic circulation.

Osteomalacia may also develop in patients who have had partial or total gastrectomy for peptic ulcer disease or other indications. Loss of gastrointestinal acidity or malfunction of the proximal small bowel underlies the vitamin D malabsorption in such circumstances. The absence of sufficient absorbing surface or the failure of intestinal mucosal cells to respond to vitamin D or its metabolites may also cause vitamin D malabsorption and consequent bone disease. In addition, after bariatric surgery, malabsorption may result in vitamin D deficiency and abnormal calcium metabolism occur in up to 60% of untreated patients, whereas osteomalacia develops in a substantial subset of the affected subjects.

Treatment of established disease generally requires pharmacologic amounts of vitamin D or its metabolites to overcome the defective absorption and/or the aberrant enterohepatic circulation or to offset end-organ resistance at the intestinal mucosa. Most patients respond well to calcium supplements, 1 to 1.5 g/day, and ergocalciferol, 1250 to 5000 μg/day. If the severity of malabsorption makes oral vitamin D ineffective, parenteral ergocalciferol, 12,500 to 25,000 μg, given intramuscularly once a month, is a practical alternative. Because magnesium deficiency often coexists in patients with malabsorptive diseases and may slow healing of the osteomalacia, adjunctive therapy with magnesium oxide may facilitate bone mineralization.

Abnormal Vitamin D Metabolism

Liver Disease

Because vitamin D is hydroxylated in the liver to form 25-hydroxyvitamin D, patients with severe parenchymal or obstructive hepatic disease (Chapter 154) may have reduced production of this metabolite. These patients, however, rarely manifest biochemical or histologic evidence of osteomalacia. Indeed, an overt decrease of 25-hydroxyvitamin D generally requires concomitant nutritional deficiency or interruption of the enterohepatic circulation. Consequently, therapy for biopsy-proven osteomalacia, when present, is similar to therapy for osteomalacia that is secondary to malabsorption of vitamin D.

Drug-Induced Disease

Decreased circulating levels of 25-hydroxyvitamin D may also occur in patients treated with drugs such as phenytoin, phenobarbital, carbamazepine, and rifampin. This defect in vitamin D metabolism results from induction of hepatic microsomal enzymes that metabolize 25-hydroxyvitamin D to inactive metabolites. Evidence suggests that such drugs activate the orphan nuclear receptor, pregnane X receptor, with consequent transactivation of the CYP24 promoter, enhanced CYP24 expression, and increased 25-hydroxyvitamin D-24-hydroxylase activity. Such increased enzyme activity would be expected to decrease the serum 25-hydroxyvitamin D levels. Secondary to this abnormality and/or to the direct inhibitory effects of these drugs on intestinal calcium absorption and PTH-mediated calcium mobilization from bone, treated patients often exhibit a decreased level of ionized calcium. These multiple influences commonly result in a bone disorder that may be mild osteomalacia or hyperparathyroid bone disease. Treatment of the bone disease and of hypocalcemia generally requires modest vitamin D supplementation (150 to 400 μg/week).

Vitamin D–Dependent Rickets Type 1 (Pseudovitamin D Deficiency)

Limited production of 1,25-dihydroxyvitamin D consequent to hereditary or acquired diseases represents another abnormality of vitamin D metabolism that invariably results in rickets or osteomalacia. Vitamin D–dependent rickets type 1 is such a genetic disorder, transmitted as an autosomal recessive trait and characterized by hypocalcemia, hypophosphatemia, and elevated alkaline phosphatase activity. As a result of the hypocalcemia, PTH levels are elevated, and, consequently, urinary excretion of amino acids and phosphate is enhanced. In addition to these biochemical abnormalities, within the first year of life patients exhibit muscle weakness and hypotonia, motor retardation, and stunted growth. As the condition progresses, patients develop the classic radiographic signs of vitamin D–deficiency rickets and bone biopsy evidence of osteomalacia. Further, affected subjects generally have a decreased serum 1,25-dihydroxyvitamin D concentration, resulting from inactivating missense and null mutations in the 1α-hydroxylase gene, as well as deletions, duplications, and splice site mutations, which abolish enzyme activity and limit production of this active vitamin D metabolite. This abnormality has been substantiated by (1) experiments in humans that demonstrate that serum calcitriol levels do not increase in response to classic stimuli of enzyme activity, (2) the absence of enzyme activity in renal cortical homogenates from the porcine homologue of this disease, and (3) the development of classic disease in mice following targeted ablation of 25-hydroxyvitamin D–1α-hydroxylase activity. More recently, however, two mutations have been identified, which result in only partial inactivation of enzyme activity and produce a mild form of the disease with normal serum levels of calcium and calcitriol but elevated circulating concentrations of PTH.

A physiologic dose of calcitriol (1 μg/day) generally promotes complete healing of the bone disease and resolution of the biochemical abnormalities, whereas a pharmacologic dose of vitamin D (20,000 to 100,000 U/day) or 25-hydroxyvitamin D (0.1 to 1.0 mg/day) is required to achieve similar effects. Regardless of the therapy used, in the majority of affected patients, therapy with vitamin D or its metabolites must be continued for life to prevent relapse.

Chronic Renal Failure

Osteomalacia is common in patients with chronic renal failure and often tends to be the predominant type of renal osteodystrophy in younger patients (Chapter 132). The abnormal mineralization may be part of mixed uremic osteodystrophy, or it may exist in isolation as a low-turnover osteomalacia. In the latter, the defect in mineralization almost certainly results in part from a decreased conversion of 25-hydroxyvitamin D to 1,25-dihydroxyvitamin D. Such abnormal vitamin D metabolism occurs secondary to either insufficient viable renal cortical tissue or the inhibitory effects of hyperphosphatemia on renal 25-hydroxyvitamin D–1α-hydroxylase activity. In addition, in some patients aluminum accumulated in bone underlies the abnormal mineralization. Indeed, the presence of aluminum may render the bone abnormality resistant to vitamin D. Under such circumstances, treatment with deferoxamine may be necessary to mobilize the aluminum from bone and other tissues and to improve mineralization.

Hypoparathyroidism

Osteomalacia only rarely occurs in patients with hypoparathyroidism (Chapter 266). Hypocalcemia and low or low-normal serum 1,25-dihydroxyvitamin D are usually present and appear important in the pathogenesis of the bone disease. However, the underlying reason for the variable occurrence of bone disease remains uncertain. The low serum 1,25-dihydroxyvitamin D concentration results from the PTH deficiency. Bone pain suggests the diagnosis, and generally the diagnosis depends on histomorphometric analysis of a bone biopsy. Most patients respond well to treatment with vitamin D and calcium supplements, but for reasons that are not clear, some require therapy with 1,25-dihydroxyvitamin D.

Pseudohypoparathyroidism

In pseudohypoparathyroidism, apparent bone and kidney resistance to PTH results in hypocalcemia, retention of phosphate, and low serum 1,25-dihydroxyvitamin D levels (Chapter 266). Surprisingly, however, affected patients often manifest bone disease marked by increased resorptive activity and osteomalacia. Indeed, severe demineralization, including frank osteitis fibrosa cystica and occasionally rickets or osteomalacia, has been observed in 24 patients with pseudohypoparathyroidism. More commonly, the bone disease is silent, and diagnosis often depends on histomorphometric analysis of a bone biopsy sample. Undoubtedly, hypocalcemia, secondary hyperparathyroidism, and low serum 1,25-dihydroxyvitamin D levels are important cofactors in the pathogenesis of the disease. Patients respond well to pharmacologic amounts of vitamin D or to replacement doses of 1,25-dihydroxyvitamin D.

Target Organ Resistance to Calcitriol

Vitamin D–Dependent Rickets Type 2

Patients with clinical and biochemical abnormalities similar to those of patients with vitamin D–dependent rickets type 1, but with elevated 1,25-dihydroxyvitamin D levels, have been described. They have not only calcipenic rickets and osteomalacia but also variably associated abnormalities, including alopecia (in 60% of patients) and, in a minority of subjects, additional ectodermal anomalies, such as multiple milia, epidermal cysts, and oligodontia. The disease is a rare autosomal recessive disorder caused by mutations in the DNA and ligand-binding domains of the vitamin D receptor, which results in a decreased target organ responsiveness to 1,25-dihydroxyvitamin D through heterogeneous mechanisms. The genetic defects identified to date consist largely of point mutations in the conserved zinc finger region that reduce or abolish the affinity of the receptor for the DNA response element and, less often, point mutations that introduce a premature stop codon in the hormone binding domain of the receptor, which limits binding of 1,25-dihydroxyvitamin D to the receptor. As a consequence, affected patients manifest (1) failure of 1,25-dihydroxyvitamin D binding to available receptors, (2) a reduction in 1,25-dihydroxyvitamin D receptor binding sites, (3) abnormal binding affinity of 1,25-dihydroxyvitamin D to receptor, (4) inadequate translocation of the 1,25-dihydroxyvitamin D receptor complex to the nucleus, and (5) diminished affinity of the 1,25-dihydroxyvitamin D receptor complex for the DNA binding domain secondary to changes in the structure of receptor zinc binding fingers. It appears that complete loss of vitamin D receptor function by DNA binding domain mutations generally causes the alopecia or hair loss, whereas patients with mild impairment of the vitamin D receptor function from ligand binding domain mutations do not develop alopecia.

The role of the vitamin D receptor in the pathogenesis of this disorder has been confirmed in mice by targeted ablation of the DNA binding domain of the receptor; this procedure caused hypocalcemia, hyperparathyroidism, and alopecia within the first month of life. Effective treatment of this disease likely depends on the nature of the underlying abnormality. Thus, patients with deficient affinity of 1,25-dihydroxyvitamin D to receptor and inadequate nuclear translocation respond to high-dose vitamin D or 1,25-dihydroxyvitamin D with complete clinical and biochemical remission. In contrast, patients with other forms of the disease generally remain refractory to treatment with vitamin D or its analogues. However, every patient should receive a 6-month trial of therapy with supplemental calcium (1 to 3 g/day) and vitamin D (400,000 to 1,200,000 U/day), 25-hydroxyvitamin D (0.05 to 1.5 mg/day), or, in more severe cases, 1,25-dihydroxyvitamin D (5 to 60 μg/day). If the abnormalities of the syndrome do not normalize in response to this treatment, clinical remission may be achieved by administering high-dose oral calcium or long-term intracaval infusion of calcium. In addition, studies indicate that phosphate restriction in vitamin D–resistant null mice, the murine homologue of the human disease, effects normal bone mineralization.

DISORDERS OF PHOSPHATE HOMEOSTASIS

Rickets and osteomalacia occur in association with a variety of disorders in which phosphate depletion predominates (Chapter 120). Most typically, these diseases have in common abnormal proximal renal tubular function, which results in an increased renal clearance of inorganic phosphorus and hypophosphatemia. However, the biochemical abnormalities characteristic of these disorders are quite variable (Table 265–3).

Impaired Renal Tubular Phosphate Reabsorption

X-Linked Hypophosphatemic Rickets/Osteomalacia

XLH represents the prototypic phosphate-wasting disorder, characterized in general by progressively severe skeletal abnormalities, growth retardation, and X-linked dominant inheritance. However, the clinical expression of the disease varies widely. The mildest abnormality is hypophosphatemia without clinically evident bone disease, and the most common clinically evident manifestation is short stature. Nevertheless, most children with the disease exhibit enlargement of the wrists and/or knees secondary to rickets, as well as bowing of the lower extremities. Additional early signs of the disease may include late dentition, tooth abscesses secondary to poor mineralization of the interglobular dentine, and premature cranial synostosis. Despite marked variability in the

TABLE 265–3 BIOCHEMICAL ABNORMALITIES OF THE PHOSPHOPENIC RACHITIC/OSTEOMALACIC DISORDERS

	XLH	HHRH	ADHR	XRHR	FS 1	FS 2	TIO
BIOCHEMICAL FINDINGS							
Calcium	N	N	N	N	N	N	N
Phosphorus	⇓	⇓	⇓	⇓	⇓	⇓	⇓
Alkaline phosphatase	N/⇑	N/⇑	N/⇑	N/⇑	N/⇑	N/⇑	N/⇑
Parathyroid hormone	N	⇓	N	⇓	N	⇓	N
25(OH)D	N	N	N	N	N	N	N
$1,25(OH)_2D$	(⇓)	⇑	(⇓)	⇑	(⇓)	⇑	⇓
RENAL FUNCTION							
Urinary phosphorus	⇑	⇑	⇑	⇑	⇑	⇑	⇑
Urinary calcium	⇓	⇑	⇓	⇑	⇓	⇑	⇓
GASTROINTESTINAL FUNCTION							
Calcium absorption	⇓	⇑	⇓	⇑	⇓	⇑	⇓
Phosphorus absorption	⇓	⇑	⇓	⇑	⇓	⇑	⇓

$1,25(OH)_2D$ = 1,25-dihydroxyvitamin D; 25(OH)D = 25-hydroxyvitamin D; ⇓= decreased; ⇑= increased; (⇓) = decreased relative to the serum phosphorus concentration; ADHR = autosomal dominant hypophosphatemic rickets; FS 1 = Fanconi's syndrome type 1; FS 2 = Fanconi's syndrome type 2; HHRH = hereditary hypophosphatemic rickets with hypercalciuria; N = normal; N/⇑= normal or increased; TIO = tumor-induced osteomalacia; XLH = X-linked hypophosphatemic rickets; XRHR = X-linked recessive hypophosphatemic rickets.
Adapted from Econs MJ, Drezner MK: Bone disease resulting from inherited disorders of renal tubule transport and vitamin D metabolism. *In* Coe FL, Favus MJ (eds): Disorders of Bone and Mineral Metabolism. New York, Raven Press, 1992, p 937.

clinical presentation, bone biopsies in affected children and adults invariably reveal osteomalacia, the severity of which has no relation to gender, the extent of the biochemical abnormalities, or the severity of the clinical disability. In untreated youths and adults, the serum 25-hydroxyvitamin D level is normal, and the concentration of 1,25-dihydroxyvitamin D is in the low-normal range. The paradoxical occurrence of hypophosphatemia and normal serum calcitriol levels results from aberrant regulation of renal 25-hydroxyvitamin D–1α-hydroxylase activity, caused by abnormal phosphate transport or a circulating factor central to the genesis of the disease (see later).

A primary inborn error that results in an expressed abnormality in the renal proximal tubule (and perhaps the intestine), which impairs phosphate reabsorption (and absorption), underlies the pathogenesis of XLH. Although controversy exists regarding the character of the inborn error, studies in *Hyp* mice suggest that elaboration of a humoral factor is the basis for the observed inhibition of phosphate transport in affected patients. In this regard, investigations resulted in the cloning and identification of the disease gene as *PHEX*, a *ph*osphate-regulating gene with homologies to *e*ndopeptidases located on the *X* chromosome. Deactivating mutations of this gene, which alters a membrane localized protein, clearly underlie the phenotypic expression of XLH by a mechanism that is incompletely understood. However, recognition of a humoral factor as essential to the pathogenesis of the disease suggests that the PHEX gene product may function normally to inactivate phosphatonin, a presumed phosphaturic hormone. An excess of this hormone would occur secondary to PHEX protein dysfunction and would result in renal phosphate wasting and perhaps abnormal bone mineralization. Despite these apparent advances, further progress has been limited by the inability to identify physiologically relevant PHEX substrates, which may function as phosphatonins. The search for candidate substrates has been guided, in part, by the knowledge that related endopeptidases have substrates that are coexpressed in an organ/cell type–specific fashion. In this context, physiologically relevant PHEX substrate is likely produced in osteoblasts, the site of predominant *PHEX* expression. Indeed, genes regulating extracellular matrix production, bone mineralization, and renal P transport (i.e., stanniocalcin I) are co-localized to the osteoblast. However, efforts to date have not identified a PHEX/Phex substrate in osteoblasts that influences renal P transport or bone mineralization. Nevertheless, various studies have identified circulating proteins, including fibroblast growth factor-23 (FGF-23), matrix, extracellular phosphoglycoprotein (MEPE), and secreted frizzled-related protein 4 (sFRP-4), which have actions consistent with those of presumptive phosphatonins. Moreover, circulating levels of FGF-23 are elevated in affected subjects with XLH and the *Hyp*-mouse.

Current treatment strategies for children with the disease directly address the combined calcitriol and phosphorus deficiency. Generally, the regimen includes a period of titration to achieve a maximum dose of calcitriol, 40 to 60 ng/kg/day in two divided doses, and phosphorus, 1 to 2 g/day in four or five divided doses. Although youths occasionally prove refractory to such therapeutic intervention, combined therapy often improves growth velocity, normalizes lower extremity deformities, and induces healing of the attendant bone disease. Of course, treatment involves a significant risk of toxicity that is generally expressed as abnormalities of calcium homeostasis and/or detrimental effects on renal function. Therapy in adults is reserved for episodes of intractable bone pain and refractory nonunion bone fractures. The observations that long-term growth hormone administration in affected youths may benefit growth, phosphate retention, and bone density suggest that a subgroup of patients may benefit from adjunctive treatment with this hormone.

Hereditary Hypophosphatemic Rickets with Hypercalciuria

This rare autosomal recessive genetic disease is marked by hypophosphatemic rickets with hypercalciuria. In contrast to other diseases in which renal phosphate transport is limited, patients with HHRH exhibit increased 1,25-dihydroxyvitamin D production. The resultant elevated serum calcitriol levels enhance the gastrointestinal calcium absorption, which, in turn, increases the filtered renal calcium load and inhibits PTH secretion. The clinical expression of the disease is heterogeneous, although initial symptoms generally consist of bone pain and/or deformities of the lower extremities. Additional features of the disease include short stature, muscle weakness, and radiographic signs of rickets/osteomalacia and/or osteopenia. The various symptoms and signs may exist separately or in combination and may be present in a mild or severe form. In general, the severity of the bone mineralization defect correlates inversely with the prevailing serum phosphorus concentration. Relatives of patients with evident HHRH may exhibit an additional mode of disease expression. These persons manifest hypercalciuria and hypophosphatemia, but the abnormalities are less marked and occur in the absence of discernible bone disease.

Studies have mapped the disease genetic locus to the end of the long arm of chromosome 9, which contains *SLC34A3*, the gene encoding the renal sodium-phosphate cotransporter NaPi-IIc, located in renal proximal tubule cells. Nucleotide sequence analysis in multiple families has revealed disease-associated mutations. In individuals homozygous for the mutation, loss of *SLC34A3* function presumably ensues, resulting in a primary renal tubular defect, which is compatible with the HHRH phenotype. Individuals heterozygous for the *SLC34A3* mutation manifest the hypercalciuria and mild hypophosphatemia observed in relatives of patients with evident HHRH.

Patients with HHRH have been treated successfully with high-dose phosphorus (1 to 2.5 g/day in five divided doses) alone. In response to therapy, bone pain disappears, and muscle strength improves substantially. Moreover, most treated patients exhibit accelerated linear growth, and radiologic signs of rickets are completely absent within 4 to 9 months. Despite this favorable response, limited studies indicate that such treatment does not completely heal the associated osteomalacia. Therefore, further studies are necessary to determine whether phosphorus treatment alone is truly sufficient for this disorder.

Autosomal Dominant Hypophosphatemic Rickets

Not all familial renal phosphate wasting disorders are X-linked; several studies have documented an autosomal dominant inheritance of a hypophosphatemic disorder similar to XLH. The phenotypic manifestations of this disorder include the expected hypophosphatemia resulting from renal phosphate wasting, lower extremity deformities, and rickets/osteomalacia. Affected patients also demonstrate normal serum levels of PTH and 25-hydroxyvitamin D, while maintaining an inappropriate normal concentration of 1,25-dihydroxyvitamin D, in the presence of hypophosphatemia. Long-term studies indicate that a few of the affected female patients demonstrate delayed penetrance of clinically apparent disease and an increased tendency for bone fracture, which are uncommon occurrences in XLH. In addition, among patients who manifest disease in childhood, rare individuals lose the renal phosphate-wasting defect after puberty. Limited information is available regarding other aspects of the disease. However, recent studies have identified the gene locus for this disease on chromosome 12p13.3 in an 1.5-Mb region between the markers D12S1685 and D12S1594. Mutation screening of the genes in this region ensued and direct sequencing of *FGF-23* exons from families affected by autosomal dominant hypophosphatemic rickets (ADHR) revealed three unique missense mutations, which were not found in 214 sequenced control alleles and more than 1400 control alleles evaluated by RFLP analysis. Moreover, mutations in FGF-23 have been discovered in patients with ADHR. These mutations protect the protein from proteolysis, thereby potentially elevating circulating levels of the FGF-23, which likely leads to P wasting. This discovery suggests that FGF-23 may function not only as a phosphaturic factor in ADHR but also as phosphatonin in XLH.

X-Linked Recessive Hypophosphatemic Rickets (X-Linked Hypercalciuric Nephrolithiasis)

The initial description of X-linked recessive hypophosphatemic rickets involved a family in which male family members presented with rickets or osteomalacia, hypophosphatemia, and a reduced renal threshold for phosphate reabsorption. In contrast to patients with XLH, affected patients exhibited hypercalciuria, elevated serum 1,25-dihydroxyvitamin D levels, and proteinuria of up to 3 g/day. Patients also developed nephrolithiasis and nephrocalcinosis with progressive renal failure in early adulthood. Female carriers in the family were not hypophosphatemic and lacked any biochemical abnormalities other than hypercalciuria. Three related syndromes have been reported independently: X-linked recessive nephrolithiasis with renal failure, Dent's disease, and low-molecular-weight proteinuria with hypercalciuria and nephrocalcinosis. These syndromes differ in degree from each other, but common themes include proximal tubular reabsorptive failure, nephrolithiasis, nephrocalcinosis, progressive renal insufficiency, and, in some cases, rickets or osteomalacia. Identification of mutations in a gene in all four syndromes, *CLCN5*, whose product is involved in chloride transport, has established that they are phenotypic variants of a single disease and are not separate entities. However, the varied manifestations that may be associated with mutations in this gene, particularly the presence of hypophosphatemia and rickets/osteomalacia, underscore that environmental differences, diet, and/or modifying genetic backgrounds may influence phenotypic expression of the disease.

Tumor-Induced Osteomalacia (Oncogenous Osteomalacia)

Since the initial recognition of this disease, reports have been published of more than 125 patients in whom rickets and/or osteomalacia were associated with a coexisting tumor. The coexistent tumors were of mesenchymal origin in the majority of patients. The cardinal feature of this disease is remission of the unexplained bone disease after tumor resection. In general, affected patients present with bone and muscle pain, muscle weakness, and, occasionally, recurrent fractures of long bones. Biochemical abnormalities include renal phosphate wasting marked by an abnormally low renal tubular maximum for the reabsorption of phosphate, decreased gastrointestinal absorption of phosphate, and consequent hypophosphatemia. In general, serum 25-hydroxyvitamin D levels are normal, and serum calcitriol is profoundly decreased or is inappropriately normal relative to the hypophosphatemia. Generalized osteopenia, pseudofractures, and coarsened trabeculae, as well as widened epiphyseal plates in children, are the common radiographic abnormalities of the syndrome.

Most investigators agree that tumor production of a humoral factor or factors that may affect multiple functions of the proximal renal tubule, particularly phosphate reabsorption (resulting in hypophosphatemia), underlies the pathogenesis of this syndrome. This possibility is supported by (1) the presence of phosphaturic activity in tumor extracts in patients with tumor-induced osteomalacia, (2) the occurrence of hypophosphatemia and increased urinary phosphate excretion in heterotransplanted tumor-bearing athymic nude mice, and (3) the demonstration that extracts of the heterotransplanted tumor inhibit renal 25-hydroxyvitamin D–1α-hydroxylase activity in cultured kidney cells. Indeed, extensive analysis of tumors from patients with tumor-induced osteomalacia have revealed constitutively high expression of several genes that potentially are involved in the systemic regulation of inorganic phosphate and calcitriol levels, including FGF-23, MEPE, and sFRP-4 and excessive production of proteins with known functions related to regulation of renal phosphate excretion (FGF-23, sFRP-4). Although such evidence supports the existence of several circulating factors, or phosphatonins, that play a pathogenetic role in the regulation of inorganic phosphate and vitamin D homeostasis in tumor-induced osteomalacia, the interaction of these factors and the predominant or coincident roles that they play in generating the phenotype of this disease remain under active investigation.

Regardless, studies indicate that in many affected patients, the secretion of the phosphatonins may be modulated by somatostatin receptors. Hence, tumor identification is possible on octreotide scanning, and octreotide therapy (50 to 100 μg subcutaneously three times a day) may ameliorate the biochemical and perhaps bone abnormalities of the syndrome if tumor resection is not possible.

Adding to the complexity of the syndrome, patients with tumor-associated osteomalacia secondary to hematogenous malignancy exhibit abnormalities of the syndrome secondary to a distinctly different mechanism. In these subjects, the nephropathy associated with light-chain proteinuria results in decreased renal phosphate reabsorption and consequent hypophosphatemia. At least 15 patients with this form of the disorder have been reported.

The primary treatment of this disorder is complete resection of the associated tumor. However, recurrence or metastasis of tumors often precludes such definitive therapy. In such cases, calcitriol (1.5 to 3.0 μg/day) alone or combined with phosphorus supplementation (2 to 4 g/day) completely heals the attendant bone disease or significantly improves the biochemical and histologic abnormalities. Careful serial assessment of parathyroid function, serum and urinary calcium, and renal function are essential to ensure safe therapy in affected subjects.

Fanconi's Syndrome

Rickets and osteomalacia are frequently associated with Fanconi's syndrome, a disorder characterized by phosphaturia and consequent hypophosphatemia, aminoaciduria, renal glycosuria, albuminuria, and proximal renal tubular acidosis (Chapter 129). Although many diverse congenital and acquired diseases are associated with this syndrome (see Table 265–1), damage to the proximal renal tubule represents the common underlying mechanism of disease. Resultant dysfunction produces renal wasting of those substances primarily reabsorbed at the proximal tubule. The associated bone disease in this disorder is likely secondary to hypophosphatemia and/or acidosis, abnormalities that occur in association with aberrantly regulated (Fanconi's syndrome type

1) or normally regulated (Fanconi's syndrome type 2) vitamin D metabolism. Most recently, several investigators have recognized that antiretroviral therapeutic regimens in human immunodeficiency virus–positive patients cause Fanconi's syndrome in a subset of the treated patients. Regardless of the underlying cause, patients with osteomalacia associated with adult-acquired Fanconi's syndrome appear to respond well to treatment with phosphate alone or in combination with vitamin D replacement. In fact, these patients do not appear to require 1,25-dihydroxyvitamin D.

PRIMARY DISORDERS OF BONE MATRIX

Intrinsic disorders of bone in which apparently abnormal matrix is produced but is not normally mineralized are extremely rare and are poorly understood. These diseases may result from presumed abnormalities of collagen or other proteins in the matrix or aberrant enzyme activity essential for normal mineralization.

Abnormal Bone Matrix

Fibrogenesis Imperfecta Ossium

Fibrogenesis imperfecta ossium is a rare, sporadically occurring disorder characterized by the gradual onset of intractable skeletal pain in middle-aged men and women. Pathologic fractures are a prominent clinical feature, and patients typically become bedridden. Although the serum calcium and phosphorus levels are normal, the alkaline phosphatase level is invariably elevated. The bones have a dense, amorphous, mottled appearance radiologically and a disorganized arrangement of collagen with decreased birefringence histologically. Most likely, the disorganized collagen matrix limits normal bone mineralization.

Axial Osteomalacia

Axial osteomalacia is another unusual, sporadically occurring disorder that generally affects only middle-aged men. Most patients present with only vague, dull, chronic axial discomfort that typically affects the cervical region most severely. Abnormal radiographic findings are limited to the pelvis and spine, where the coarsened trabecular pattern is characteristic of osteomalacia. Although the alkaline phosphatase level may be increased, histopathologic studies reveal a normal lamellar pattern of collagen. However, the osteoblasts appear flat and inactive, a finding suggesting that an osteoblastic defect and perhaps an attendant abnormal matrix inhibit normal mineralization.

Abnormal Enzyme Activity

Hypophosphatasia

Hypophosphatasia is a heritable disorder characterized by a deficiency of the tissue-nonspecific (liver, bone, kidney) isoenzyme of alkaline phosphatase, increased urinary excretion of phosphorylethanolamine, and skeletal disease that includes osteomalacia and rickets. The severity of clinical expression is remarkably variable and spans intrauterine death from profound skeletal hypomineralization at one extreme to lifelong absence of symptoms at the other. As a consequence, six clinical disease types are distinguished (see Table 265–1). The age at which skeletal disease is initially noted delineates, in large part, the perinatal (lethal), infantile, childhood, and adult variants of the disorder. However, affected children and adults may manifest only the unique dental abnormalities of the syndrome and, accordingly, are classified as having odontohypophosphatasia. Finally, patients with the rare variant, pseudohypophosphatasia, have the clinical, radiologic, and biochemical features of the classic disease without a decrease in the circulating levels of alkaline phosphatase. These individuals have defects in cellular localization and substrate specificity of the enzyme.

Affected infants exhibit hypercalcemia, hypercalciuria, enlarged sutures of the skull, craniosynostosis, delayed dentition, enlarged epiphyses, and prominent costochondral junctions. Genu valgum or genu varum may develop subsequently. In older children, disease may be limited to rickets. Surprisingly, the disorder in adults is mild despite the presence of osteopenia. Indeed, the disease may be limited to slowly healing metatarsal fractures or loss or fracture of teeth. Nevertheless, 50% of patients have a history of early exfoliation of deciduous teeth and/or rickets, and disease may reflect re-expression of the childhood disorder.

The perinatal and infantile forms of disease are inherited as autosomal recessive traits. The modes of inheritance for odontophosphatasia, adult hypophosphatasia, and childhood hypophosphatasia remain unclear, although an autosomal dominant disease transmission has been described in some kindreds with mild or severe disease. In many of these families, studies indicate that the existent mutations exhibit a negative dominant effect, thereby inhibiting the enzymatic activity of the heterodimer. The variability in disease apparently depends on the degree of heterodimeric inhibition with highly negative dominant effects associated with severe hypophosphatasia. The physiologic basis for the bone disease likely relates to the role of alkaline phosphatase in cleaving pyrophosphate, an inhibitor of bone mineralization. Failure to hydrolyze this physiologic substrate results in inorganic pyrophosphate elevated to levels sufficiently high to inhibit the mineralization process. The consequence of this pathophysiologic process is a block of the vectorial spread of mineral from initial nuclei within matrix vesicles outward into the matrix of growth cartilage and bone. Confirmation of this pathophysiologic mechanism has been obtained in mice with deletion of the tissue-nonspecific alkaline phosphatase gene. These animals have hypophosphatasia, elevated levels of pyrophosphate, and poorly mineralized bone, rescued by deletion of nucleotide pyrophosphatase phosphodiesterase 1, which generates pyrophosphate.

Therapy of this disease has been generally unrewarding. Thus, supportive treatment is important and may include craniotomy in children (to manage craniosynostosis) and, in adults, insertion of load-sharing intramedullary rods to treat fractures. Expert dental care is also crucial to minimize tooth loss and to prevent consequent malnutrition in youth.

MINERALIZATION INHIBITORS

ETIDRONATE. Disturbances in mineralization may be seen in patients who consume etidronate daily at doses greater than 5 mg/kg of body weight. The etidronate is deposited at the bone surface and inhibits osteoblast function; it also directly inhibits calcium-phosphate crystallization.

FLUORIDE. Although multiple studies document that fluoride stimulates new bone formation, administering the drug in high doses without adequate calcium supplementation results in poorly mineralized bone, consistent with osteomalacia. The mechanisms by which fluoride alters osteoblast function and/or directly inhibits mineralization remains unknown.

ALUMINUM. Excess aluminum accumulation in bone inhibits mineralization and is a potential mechanism for the osteomalacia observed in patients with chronic renal failure, as discussed earlier. In addition, accumulation of aluminum in bone likely underlies the osteomalacia observed in patients treated with total parenteral nutrition. In such cases, aluminum contamination of casein hydrolysate, as well as albumin, phosphate, and calcium solutions, provides the major source of the mineral. Changing total parenteral nutrition solutions from those with casein hydrolysate to those with purified amino acids has markedly reduced the incidence of clinically evident bone disease.

SUGGESTED READINGS

Baroncelli GI, Bertelloni S, Ceccarelli C, Saggese G: Effect of growth hormone treatment on final height, phosphate metabolism, and bone mineral density in children with X-linked hypophosphatemic rickets. J Pediatr 2001;138:236–243. *Review of the underlying concepts and the specific details of treatment for hypophosphatemic rickets, including use of growth hormone.*

Gartner LM, Greer FR, for the Section on Breastfeeding and Committee on Nutrition. American Academy of Pediatrics: Prevention of rickets and vitamin D deficiency: New guidelines for vitamin D intake. Pediatrics 2003;111:908–910. *Recommends 200 IU/day of vitamin D be continued throughout childhood and adolescence.*

Holick MF: Resurrection of vitamin D deficiency and rickets. J Clin Invest 2006;116:2062–2072. *Summarizes the role of vitamin D in the prevention of rickets.*

Jonsson KB, Zahradnik R, Larsson T, et al: Fibroblast growth factor 23 in oncogenic osteomalacia and x-linked hypophosphatemia. N Engl J Med 2003;348:1656–1663. *FGF-23 is markedly elevated in these patients.*

Wharton B, Bishop N: Rickets. Lancet 2003;362:1389–1400. *Details the effects of genes, stage of development, and environment on clinical expression of this disease.*

White KE, Larrson TM, Econs MJ: The roles of specific genes implicated as circulating factors involved in normal and disordered phosphate homeostasis: Frp-4, MEPE, and FGF23. Endocr Rev 2006;27:221–241. *FGF-23, Frp-4, and MEPE can be markedly elevated in oncogenic osteomalacia or X-linked hypophosphatemia and may have a role in phosphate homeostasis.*

266 THE PARATHYROID GLANDS, HYPERCALCEMIA, AND HYPOCALCEMIA

John J. Wysolmerski and Karl L. Insogna

CALCIUM AND CALCIUM METABOLISM

Calcium serves two principal physiologic functions. First, insoluble calcium salts (primarily hydroxyapatite) provide the structural characteristics that allow bones to protect internal organs, to bear weight, and to function as the levers on which muscles act during locomotion. Second, soluble calcium ions in the extracellular fluid (ECF) and cytosol are critical for a myriad of biochemical reactions, signaling cascades, and electrical systems that are necessary for life. An adult human contains about 1000 g of calcium, the majority of which (~99%) is found in bone. Only approximately 1% of total body calcium is contained within the ECF and soft tissues. Therefore, the skeleton is called on as a source of calcium when the ECF concentration falls and as a storehouse for excess calcium. Of the total circulating calcium, the ionized fraction is generally estimated to be approximately 50%, with the remainder of the total serum calcium bound to serum proteins, primarily albumin, and to a lesser extent complexed with anions, such as citrate or sulfate. Only the ionized fraction of total serum calcium is physiologically important, and this component is regulated on a minute-to-minute basis. Although it is possible to measure ionized calcium routinely in large clinical laboratories, the specimen must usually be obtained anaerobically and analyzed promptly. Therefore, total serum calcium is often used as an indirect assessment of the ionized calcium fraction.

Roughly 1% of skeletal calcium is in active equilibrium with the ECF under normal physiologic conditions. A complicated homeostatic system involving multiple organs and several hormones regulates both the calcium concentration of the ECF and the calcium content of the skeleton (Chapter 263). The organs involved in the regulation of calcium metabolism are the parathyroid glands, the kidneys, the skeleton, and the gut. The hormones include parathyroid hormone (PTH), vitamin D, and PTH-related protein (PTHrP). Abnormalities in these organs, the hormones, or their receptors can all cause disturbances in calcium metabolism and can lead to hypercalcemia or hypocalcemia. In this chapter, we review calcium homeostasis in humans and then discuss the most common causes of hypercalcemia and hypocalcemia.

Calcium Homeostasis

Parathyroid Glands and Parathyroid Hormone

The four parathyroid glands are located in the neck, closely apposed to the posterior capsule of the four poles of the thyroid gland. Embryologically, they are derivatives of the third and fourth branchial pouches. The pair of glands located at the upper poles of the thyroid is derived from the fourth pouch, whereas those located at the lower poles migrate downward from the third pouch, along with the thymus gland. Extra parathyroids or parathyroid glands in aberrant locations are not uncommon, especially along the path of embryologic migration.

The parathyroid glands make PTH, an 84-amino acid protein encoded by a single gene. PTH is initially synthesized as a single chain, pre-proparathyroid peptide. The 25-residue presequence is cleaved on entry of pre-pro-PTH into the endoplasmic reticulum. The shorter, 6-residue prosequence is subsequently cleaved to generate the mature, 84-amino acid, full-length protein (PTH 1-84). PTH (1-84) is packaged into cytoplasmic granules that also contain several proteases to await secretion. Full-length PTH is the biologically active form of the hormone. It has a very short half-life (minutes) in the circulation and is degraded by the liver and kidney. This degradative process releases carboxy-terminal (C-terminal) fragments of PTH into the circulation. In addition, in response to hypercalcemia, the proteases found within parathyroid secretory granules digest the amino-terminal portion of PTH and secrete inactive C-terminal fragments. Therefore, the concentration of circulating inactive C-terminal species is a product of both parathyroid cell secretion and peripheral metabolism of full-length PTH. These fragments are cleared by the kidney and accumulate in the circulation in renal failure.

The secretion of PTH is regulated by the extracellular ionized calcium concentration. A steep inverse sigmoidal relationship exists between PTH secretion and calcium concentration that can be defined by four parameters (Fig. 266–1). The first is the maximum secretory rate of the parathyroid glands. The second is the slope of the curve at the midpoint. The third is the set point, or the calcium concentration at which PTH secretion is half maximal. The final parameter is the minimal, nonsuppressible rate of PTH secretion. The steep part of this curve encompasses the physiologic range for extracellular calcium, over which small changes in the concentration of ionized calcium elicit large changes in the rate of PTH secretion.

For parathyroid cells to regulate PTH secretion, they must have the ability to sense changes in extracellular calcium concentration. This is accomplished through a G protein–coupled receptor (GPCR) known as

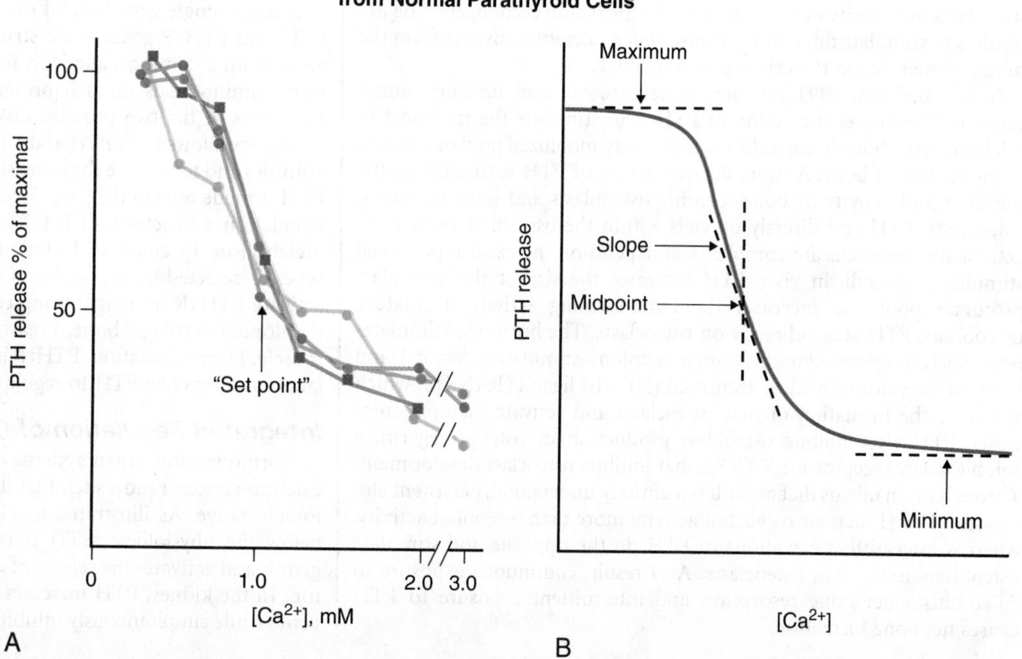

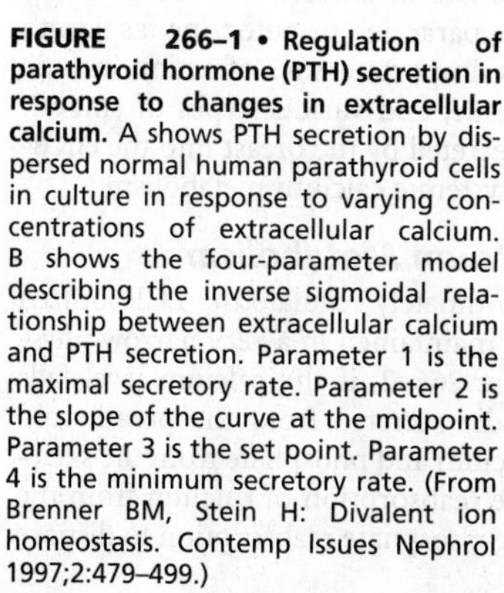
FIGURE 266–1 • Regulation of parathyroid hormone (PTH) secretion in response to changes in extracellular calcium. A shows PTH secretion by dispersed normal human parathyroid cells in culture in response to varying concentrations of extracellular calcium. B shows the four-parameter model describing the inverse sigmoidal relationship between extracellular calcium and PTH secretion. Parameter 1 is the maximal secretory rate. Parameter 2 is the slope of the curve at the midpoint. Parameter 3 is the set point. Parameter 4 is the minimum secretory rate. (From Brenner BM, Stein H: Divalent ion homeostasis. Contemp Issues Nephrol 1997;2:479–499.)

the *calcium-sensing receptor* (CaR). The calcium ion is a ligand for this receptor. Ligand binding to the CaR activates downstream signaling pathways (primarily induction of phospholipases and intracellular calcium transients) in response to increases in extracellular calcium concentration. This process, in turn, suppresses PTH secretion. If calcium levels are persistently elevated, activation of this receptor also reduces PTH mRNA levels and inhibits parathyroid cell proliferation. In addition to parathyroid cells, the CaR is also prominently expressed in the kidney, where it regulates calcium handling by the renal tubules. In this way, hypercalcemia directly promotes the excretion of calcium in the urine, and hypocalcemia directly enhances its reabsorption.

The actions of PTH are mediated by the type 1 PTH/PTHrP receptor (PTH1R). The calcium-regulating effects of the receptor appear to be primarily the result of activation of adenylate cyclase downstream from the PTH1R. It is activated equally well by the amino-terminal portions of PTH and PTHrP (see below). It is most abundant in bone and kidney, where it mediates the systemic functions of PTH. However, PTH1R is also expressed at lower levels in many other cells in the body, where it serves as a PTHrP receptor. In this capacity, PTH1R has important functions during bone and mammary development and mediates many of PTHrP's effects on cellular proliferation, apoptosis, and differentiation (see later).

PTH exerts direct effects on kidney and bone cells and indirect effects on enterocytes. The integrated action of PTH on these organs results in an increase in the circulating concentration of ionized calcium. In the kidney, PTH has three principal effects. First, it acts on proximal tubular cells to inhibit the reabsorption of phosphate. Phosphate transport depends on the actions of sodium-phosphate cotransporters 2a and 2c (NPT2a, NPT2c), which are located in the luminal membranes of proximal tubular cells. PTH acts to inhibit phosphate reabsorption by causing NPT2a to be removed from the luminal membrane and be degraded. PTH also stimulates the activity of the renal 1α-hydroxylase in proximal tubular cells. This is a microsomal cytochrome P-450 enzyme that leads to the formation of biologically active $1,25(OH)_2$ vitamin D from its circulating precursor 25(OH) vitamin D. PTH also inhibits 24-hydroxylase, thus preventing the formation of the inactive metabolite, $24,25(OH)_2$ vitamin D. Both these actions increase the circulating concentrations of $1,25(OH)_2$ vitamin D, an increase that, in turn, stimulates intestinal calcium absorption. Finally, PTH acts to increase the reabsorption of calcium by the kidney. The majority of calcium is reclaimed from the glomerular filtrate in the proximal tubule through a PTH-independent paracellular process linked to the reabsorption of sodium. PTH helps to promote some calcium reabsorption in the cortical thick ascending loop of Henle by increasing the net positive charge on the luminal side of the tubule, which enhances paracellular calcium and magnesium reabsorption. However, the distal tubule is the primary target of PTH's actions to promote calcium transport. In these cells, PTH leads to insertion of calcium channels into the apical membrane of the cell and stimulates the activity of basolateral sodium/calcium exchangers. The net result is to stimulate directional, transcellular calcium transport from the tubule lumen, across the cell and into the ECF.

In the skeleton, PTH activates bone turnover and liberates stored calcium. The immediate action of PTH is to stimulate the transport of calcium across bone lining cells from an easily mobilized pool of calcium at the surface of bone. A more delayed action of PTH is to increase the numbers and activity of bone-forming osteoblasts and bone-resorbing osteoclasts. PTH acts directly on cells within the osteoblast lineage. Its actions on these cells are complex and depend on the exact type of cell stimulated. Overall, in vivo, PTH increases the size of the osteoblast precursor pool and increases the bone-forming activity of mature osteoblasts. PTH acts indirectly on osteoclasts. The hormone stimulates osteoblasts to release cytokines, such as colony-stimulating factor 1 and receptor activator of nuclear factor-κB (NF-κB) ligand (RANKL), which stimulate the formation of new osteoclasts and activate mature osteoclasts. PTH also inhibits osteoblast production of osteoprotegerin, a soluble decoy receptor for RANKL that inhibits osteoclast development. Through mechanisms that are still not entirely understood, persistent elevations of PTH increase osteoclast activity more than osteoblast activity, whereas intermittent elevations in PTH do the opposite and stimulate osteoblasts more than osteoclasts. As a result, continuous exposure to PTH causes net bone resorption and intermittent exposure to PTH causes net bone formation.

Vitamin D

In response to ultraviolet light, keratinocytes in the epidermis convert 7-dehydrocholesterol, the immediate precursor of cholesterol, into vitamin D_3. Cutaneous production of vitamin D_3 is affected by a variety of factors such as latitude, season, use of sunscreen, concentration of melanin, and type of clothing, all of which vary the amount of ultraviolet light that penetrates the skin. Aging also reduces the ability of the skin to synthesize vitamin D. Most foods contain little vitamin D, although some is found in oily fish and in fish liver oils. In the United States, vitamin D is also found in fortified foods, including certain cereals, milk, and bread. Given these restrictions on its production and availability, vitamin D deficiency is very common in the winter months in elderly populations living at higher latitudes.

Vitamin D_3 produced in the skin is biologically inert and must be hydroxylated in two successive steps to become active. The first hydroxylation is performed in the liver by the cytochrome P-450 vitamin D 25-hydroxylase and generates 25-hydroxyvitamin D_3. This has little biologic activity but is metabolized by cells in the proximal renal tubule to form the active hormone, $1,25(OH)_2$ vitamin D_3. The cytochrome P-450 mono-oxygenase, 25(OH)D-1α-hydroxylase (1α-hydroxylase) enzyme catalyzes this final hydroxylation step. The hepatic 25-hydroxylation step occurs through mass action, whereas the renal 1α-hydroxylation step is tightly regulated. As noted earlier, PTH stimulates the activity of the renal 1α-hydroxylase. This enzyme is also stimulated by phosphate and is inhibited by hypercalcemia.

Vitamin D is a steroid hormone and interacts with specific nuclear receptors to regulate gene expression. The vitamin D receptor is a member of the steroid hormone receptor family of ligand-binding transcription factors. It heterodimerizes with the retinoic acid X receptor, and, in the presence of $1,25(OH)_2$ vitamin D, the vitamin D receptor–retinoic acid X receptor complex binds to specific DNA recognition sequences within target genes. The main function of $1,25(OH)_2$ vitamin D is to support the circulating calcium concentration through two actions. The first is to stimulate calcium absorption from the gut lumen by enterocytes. The active vitamin D metabolite stimulates the expression of calcium channels within intestinal cells that allow calcium to enter the apical surface of the cell. It also enhances the production of proteins that shuttle calcium through the cytoplasm and stimulates the activity of calcium pumps that extrude calcium across the basolateral membrane of the cells. Vitamin D also enhances the absorption of phosphorus from the diet. The second important action of $1,25(OH)_2$ vitamin D is to increase bone resorption by stimulating osteoblastic production of RANKL. This latter effect is clinically important only when production of $1,25(OH)_2$ vitamin D is elevated to pathologic levels.

Parathyroid Hormone–Related Protein

PTHrP was discovered in the course of studies exploring the pathogenesis of humoral hypercalcemia of malignancy (HHM) (see later). In humans, a single gene located on chromosome 12 encodes PTHrP. The PTH and PTHrP genes share structural features that suggest that they arose from a common ancestor. In particular, of the first 13 amino-terminal amino acids in each protein, eight are identical; after this, the sequences of the two proteins diverge completely. The amino-terminal homology allows both PTH and PTHrP to bind to the PTH1R with equal affinities and to activate the same signaling pathways. As discussed earlier, PTH is made only in the parathyroid glands, is secreted into the systemic circulation, and activates PTH1R in bone and kidney to regulate calcium metabolism. In contrast, PTHrP is made in a variety of different cell types, is secreted locally, and acts in a paracrine or autocrine fashion to activate PTH1R on neighboring cells. Important sites of action include developing cartilage, bone, breast tissue, and various types of smooth muscle. During lactation, PTHrP is secreted by the breast into the circulation and acts like PTH to regulate systemic calcium metabolism.

Integrated Regulation of Calcium Metabolism

Hormones and organ systems coordinately regulate the ECF ionized calcium concentration such that it is maintained in a very narrow physiologic range. As illustrated in Figure 266–2, if the calcium level falls below the physiologic, PTH is rapidly secreted from the parathyroid glands and activates the release of calcium and phosphate from the skeleton. In the kidney, PTH increases the reabsorption of calcium from the urine while simultaneously inhibiting phosphate reabsorption to dispose

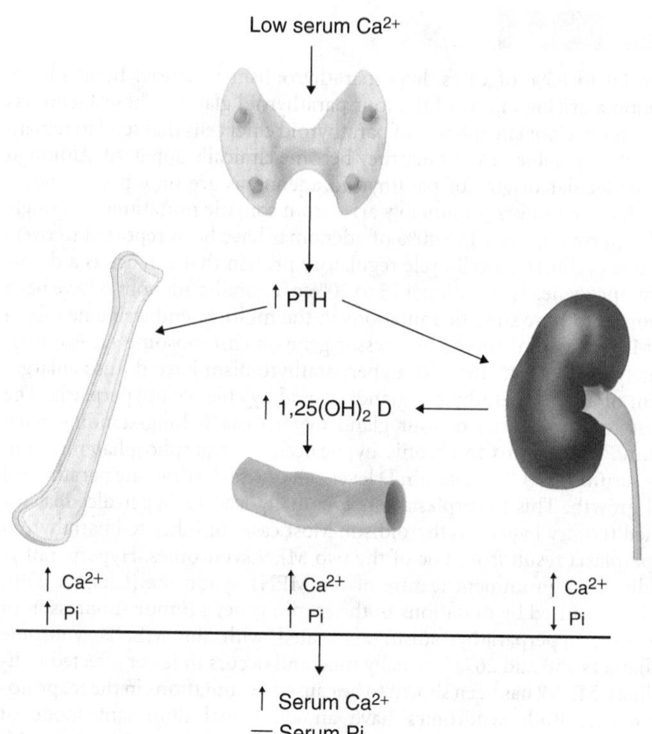

FIGURE 266–2 • Homeostatic response to a fall in serum calcium (Ca^{2+}). PTH = parathyroid hormone; Pi = inorganic phosphate.

of the phosphate released from the skeleton. This process prevents serum phosphate from rising, an action that would otherwise inhibit a rise in serum calcium by inducing the precipitation of calcium phosphate salts in soft tissues. In addition, alterations in CaR signaling within the kidney activate calcium reabsorption independent of changes in PTH. Combined, these actions return the calcium concentration back toward normal and thus inhibit further PTH release. When hypocalcemia persists, PTH also stimulates the renal production of $1,25(OH)_2$ vitamin D, which increases intestinal calcium absorption. In the presence of hypercalcemia, PTH secretion is suppressed, and the various organs alter their calcium handling in an opposite fashion so circulating calcium levels fall.

HYPERCALCEMIA

Pathobiology

The long list of potential causes of hypercalcemia is provided in Table 266–1. However, most cases of hypercalcemia (>90%) are caused either by primary hyperparathyroidism or by malignancy-associated hypercalcemia (MAHC). These two diseases, as well as a few other selected causes, are discussed in detail. The interested reader should consult a subspecialty text for a more detailed discussion of other disorders.

Several of the less common causes of hypercalcemia are worth noting briefly. First, abnormalities in serum proteins and severe thrombocytosis (platelet counts >700,000) can cause *pseudohypercalcemia,* defined as elevations in total calcium without elevations in ionized calcium. Several *endocrine disorders* including thyrotoxicosis, pheochromocytoma, adrenal insufficiency, and islet cell tumors of the pancreas can manifest with mild to moderate hypercalcemia. An increasingly common cause of hypercalcemia is the *milk-alkali syndrome.* Patients with this disorder present with a triad of hypercalcemia, systemic alkalosis, and renal insufficiency associated with the ingestion of large amounts of calcium and absorbable alkali. The disorder was originally described in the 1930s as a complication of the treatment of peptic ulcer disease, but, in its modern form, it is associated with the ingestion of calcium carbonate for the treatment or prevention of osteoporosis. In some patients, this syndrome can be precipitated by the daily intake of as little as 2 g of calcium. Immobilization uncouples bone turnover by inhibiting bone formation. Thus, in patients with elevated rates of bone resorption, immobilization can worsen or precipitate hypercalcemia. Patients most at risk appear to be

TABLE 266–1 CAUSES OF HYPERCALCEMIA IN ADULTS

HYPERPARATHYROIDISM
Adenoma
Hyperplasia
Carcinoma
Familial hypocalciuric hypercalcemia
Tertiary hyperparathyroidism of renal failure
MALIGNANCY-ASSOCIATED HYPERCALCEMIA
Humoral hypercalcemia of malignancy
Local osteolytic hypercalcemia
GRANULOMATOUS DISORDERS
Tuberculosis
Leprosy
Cryptococcosis
Histoplasmosis
Cytomegalovirus infection
Sarcoidosis
Wegener's granulomatosis
ENDOCRINE DISORDERS
Hyperthyroidism
Adrenal insufficiency
Pheochromocytoma
Vasoactive intestinal polypeptide tumor (VIPoma)
MEDICATIONS
Vitamin D preparations
Thiazides
Lithium
Aminophylline
Vitamin A
Tamoxifen
Total parenteral nutrition
MISCELLANEOUS CAUSES
Milk-alkali syndrome
Immobilization
Aluminum toxicity
Acute renal failure
Rhabdomyolysis (recovery phase)
Systemic lupus erythematosus
Breast hyperplasia

adolescents with physiologic elevations in bone turnover and patients with preexisting Paget's disease or subtle primary hyperparathyroidism. Finally, several *medications* other than calcium carbonate can cause hypercalcemia. The most commonly implicated drugs include thiazide diuretics, lithium carbonate, and vitamin D preparations. Several well-documented episodes of vitamin D intoxication have been caused by errors in the fortification of dairy products or the preparation of dietary supplements.

Clinical Manifestations

Patients with mild hypercalcemia (<1 mg/dL above normal) are usually asymptomatic unless they have concomitant cerebral dysfunction. The likelihood of developing symptoms from the hypercalcemia is related to both the degree of elevation in serum calcium and the rapidity with which the calcium level rises. When present, symptoms are caused by dehydration secondary to urinary losses of calcium, water, and other electrolytes and to an increase in membrane potential caused by the elevation in ECF ionized calcium concentration. Dehydration develops because an increase in the filtered load of calcium leads to variable degrees of hypercalciuria. Loss of calcium in the urine obligates the loss of anions and water. In addition, hypercalcemia causes nephrogenic diabetes insipidus because stimulation of the CaR in the collecting ducts of the kidney interferes with the trafficking of aquaporin water channels in response to vasopressin. Consequently, patients with hypercalcemia frequently report symptoms of polyuria and polydipsia. If significant dehydration ensues, hypercalcemia can worsen quickly because any impairment of glomerular filtration reduces the ability of the kidneys to excrete excess calcium. Patients with moderate to severe hypercalcemia often complain of nausea and vomiting, symptoms likely related to dehydration as well as to the effects of the hypercalcemia on central nervous system function. Because hypercalcemia tends to hyperpolarize membranes, a range of neurologic and neuromuscular signs and symptoms can occur. Patients with mild hypercalcemia often complain of fatigue, depressed affect, and asthenia. With further increases in serum calcium, these complaints progress to impaired concentration and memory, difficulty with cognitive function, stupor, and coma. Muscle weakness can be seen, which can occasionally progress to flaccid paralysis if hypercalcemia becomes severe. Gastrointestinal motility is impaired, and this commonly results in constipation and likely contributes to nausea and vomiting. Occasionally, pancreatitis can be the cause of abdominal pain in patients with hypercalcemia. Finally, cardiovascular function can be impaired, as manifested by bradycardia and sensitivity to the effects of digitalis. Electrocardiographic changes include shortening of the QT interval, varying degrees of atrioventricular block, and bradyarrhythmias and tachyarrhythmias.

Diagnosis

As noted previously, most patients with hypercalcemia have either hyperparathyroidism or MAHC. If the patient has hyperproteinemia or hypoproteinemia, or if the platelet count is markedly elevated, hypercalcemia should be confirmed by measuring the serum ionized calcium concentration. Otherwise, the first test that should be ordered is a serum intact PTH level. An elevated PTH in the presence of hypercalcemia establishes the diagnosis of hyperparathyroidism. If PTH levels are suppressed and the patient has a known malignant disease, then the diagnosis of MAHC is entertained. If skeletal metastases are not widespread, this diagnosis may be confirmed by measuring PTHrP levels. If the patient has a suppressed PTH level in the absence of a known malignant disease, then a serum PTHrP level should be measured, and a careful screen for occult malignant disease should be performed. If the PTHrP level is normal in this setting, a careful history of prescription and over-the-counter medications should be taken, and laboratory tests to investigate other causes of hypercalcemia should be performed as dictated by the clinical situation.

Primary Hyperparathyroidism

Definition

Primary hyperparathyroidism is a disorder of calcium metabolism caused by the overproduction of PTH by the parathyroid glands and is therefore characterized by simultaneous elevations in both circulating PTH and calcium levels.

Epidemiology

Historically, hyperparathyroidism was thought to be a rare disorder associated with severe complications. However, with the introduction of routine measurements of serum calcium concentrations in the 1970s, investigators recognized that many more patients had milder forms of the disease. Hyperparathyroidism is currently estimated to have an incidence between 1 in 500 and 1 in 1000 persons. After the age of 50 years, women are more frequently affected then men; the female-to-male ratio in that age group is 3 : 1. Although hyperparathyroidism can manifest at any age, it is more common in older individuals, and the peak incidence is in the sixth decade. As these statistics demonstrate, it is primarily a disease of postmenopausal women. Typically, hyperparathyroidism occurs sporadically, but in a few patients it is part of a familial syndrome. Apart from these genetic disorders, the only other known risk factor is exposure to external neck irradiation during childhood.

Pathobiology

In 80 to 85% of cases, hyperparathyroidism is caused by a solitary adenoma arising in one of the four parathyroid glands. These adenomas are benign, clonal neoplasms of parathyroid chief cells that tend to remain remarkably stable in size once they become clinically apparent. Although the molecular origins of parathyroid adenomas are only partly understood, these tumors presumably arise from somatic mutations in a single cell. Approximately 20 to 40% of adenomas have been reported to overexpress cyclin D1, a cell-cycle regulatory protein that can act as a dominant oncogene. An additional 25 to 30% of sporadic adenomas have been reported to have somatic mutations in the multiple endocrine neoplasia 1 (MEN1; menin) tumor suppressor gene on chromosome 11. Approximately 15% of patients with hyperparathyroidism have diffuse enlargement of all four parathyroid glands caused by chief cell hyperplasia. The most common cause of four gland hyperplasia is long-standing renal failure, which leads to chronic hypocalcemia, hyperphosphatemia, and low serum $1,25(OH)_2$ vitamin D levels, all of which stimulate parathyroid cell growth. This hyperplasia can eventually lead to hypercalcemia, so-called tertiary hyperparathyroidism. Most cases of inherited parathyroid hyperplasia result from one of the two MEN syndromes. Hyperparathyroidism is a prominent feature of the MEN1 syndrome (Chapter 250), which is caused by mutations in the menin gene, a tumor suppressor. In contrast, hyperparathyroidism associated with the MEN2 syndrome (Chapters 250 and 267) is usually mild and occurs in fewer affected individuals. MEN2 has been shown to be caused by mutations in the *ret* proto-oncogene. Both syndromes have an autosomal dominant mode of inheritance. Hyperplasia in these syndromes can be asynchronous, with unequal enlargement of the individual glands over time that gives the misimpression of single-gland disease. Approximately 0.5% of all patients with hyperparathyroidism have parathyroid carcinoma. Typically, these patients have severe hypercalcemia and hyperparathyroidism that recurs following initial therapy. It can be very difficult to distinguish a parathyroid carcinoma from an adenoma by pathologic evaluation alone, but local tissue invasion, local lymph node involvement, and the presence of mitotic figures are clues to the diagnosis. Parathyroid carcinoma occurs with increased frequency in a rare genetic syndrome known as *hyperparathyroid jaw-tumor syndrome,* which is characterized by primary hyperparathyroidism in association with mesenchymal tumors of the mandible. This syndrome was found to be caused by mutations in the gene encoding the tumor suppressor, parafibromin, and emerging data suggest that mutations in this gene may also cause a significant proportion of sporadic cases of parathyroid carcinoma.

Clinical Manifestations

The presentation of hyperparathyroidism includes the characteristic symptoms of hypercalcemia combined with the variable occurrence of skeletal and renal complications. Hypercalcemia is caused by the chronic overproduction of PTH by the abnormal parathyroid cells. An important component of this abnormal secretion is a shift of the set point and slope of the calcium-PTH response curve; that is, adenoma cells become less sensitive to calcium's ability to suppress PTH production. Parathyroid adenomas still do respond to calcium, but only at higher ambient levels of the ion, thereby resulting in the establishment of a new equilibrium at abnormally high levels of calcium and PTH.

The most common complication of hyperparathyroidism besides hypercalcemia is nephrolithiasis. Approximately 20% of patients present with kidney stones. Nephrocalcinosis, which is the diffuse deposition of calcium phosphate complexes in the renal parenchyma, is seen less commonly. The most common stone type seen in hyperparathyroidism is calcium oxalate. However, stones of mixed chemical composition (calcium oxalate and calcium phosphate) are often observed. The risk factors for stone disease in patients with hyperparathyroidism are hypercalciuria (>4 mg/kg calcium excretion over 24 hours) and a tendency to waste bicarbonate, which leads to a relatively alkaline urine. Precipitation of calcium phosphate is favored in an alkaline urine. Whether mild hyperparathyroidism directly impairs renal function is unclear. In the majority of patients followed conservatively with this disease, renal function remains stable.

The classic skeletal presentation of hyperparathyroidism is *osteitis fibrosa cystica,* which is defined as the combination of subperiosteal bone resorption, especially in the distal phalanges and skull, bone cysts, brown tumors of the long bones, osteoporosis, and fractures. This form of bone disease is now uncommon, occurring in less than 5% of patients. However, up to 25% of otherwise asymptomatic patients with hyperparathyroidism develop progressive bone loss and are at risk for osteoporosis. Thus, bone mineral density should be measured in all patients with hyperparathyroidism. Cortical bone is more sensitive to the effects of hyperparathyroidism, so bone mineral density in the distal forearm is typically more severely affected than is bone mineral density in the spine or total hip.

Patients with severe hyperparathyroidism can develop muscle weakness and myopathy. Patients with mild disease often complain of weakness, fatigue, listlessness, and trouble concentrating, and they have abnormal neuropsychiatric test results. However, the specificity and origin of these symptoms are debated. Occasionally, patients with hyperparathyroidism develop acute or subacute monoarticular inflammatory arthritis resulting from calcium pyrophosphate dihydrate crystal arthropathy. Finally, some reports have suggested that patients with hyperparathyroidism have excess body fat, are insulin resistant, and suffer from an increased incidence of cardiovascular events. Investigators have demonstrated that serum levels of the inflammatory cytokine interleukin-6 (IL-6) are elevated in patients with hyperparathyroidism. Elevations in serum IL-6 have been linked to insulin resistance and adverse cardiac outcomes. Thus, is it possible that IL-6 provides a pathogenic link between hyperparathyroidism and these complications, although this connection remains to be demonstrated.

Diagnosis

The diagnosis of hyperparathyroidism is made by documenting simultaneous elevations in the circulating levels of calcium and PTH in a patient with normal renal function. If abnormalities of serum proteins are noted, then it may be necessary to measure ionized calcium to be certain that hypercalcemia is present. Again, C-terminal fragments of PTH are excreted by the kidney and may accumulate in renal failure. This was historically a problem in assays that used antisera directed at the midregion or C-terminal portions of PTH and therefore gave falsely elevated results in patients with renal insufficiency. In addition, investigators have discovered that the first-generation immunoradiometric assays for intact PTH detected large, biologically inactive fragments of PTH that were missing only the first several amino-terminal residues. This finding has led to the introduction of newer, "biointact" PTH assays, which avoid this problem and should be used to measure PTH in any patient with abnormal renal function. Patients with hyperparathyroidism also may have slightly low or low-normal serum phosphorus concentrations, and mild hyperchloremic metabolic acidosis. Alkaline phosphatase levels may be elevated in patients with overt bone disease.

Once a diagnosis of hyperparathyroidism is made, patients should be screened for end-organ complications. Renal ultrasonography or spiral computed tomography scans can be used to determine whether the patient has kidney stones. Bone mineral density measurements should be done to detect skeletal disease, preferably using dual energy x-ray absorptiometry, at the spine, hip, and wrist. A 24-hour urine collection should be performed to determine whether hypercalciuria is present. Hyperparathyroid myopathy can be diagnosed by electromyography.

Treatment

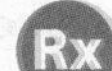

Traditionally, this involved bilateral neck exploration, during which the surgeon identified all four parathyroid glands before resecting the abnormal gland. In the past several years, however, minimally invasive parathyroidectomy has begun to supplant traditional neck exploration in referral centers. This requires preoperative localization of the offending adenoma. Technetium-99m–sestamibi scans, ultrasonography, and magnetic resonance imaging can all be used as preoperative localization studies; we prefer the first two. If parathyroid hyperplasia is suspected, a minimally invasive approach is not appropriate because the surgeon must remove either three and one half parathyroid glands or all four glands with autotransplantation of some parathyroid tissue to the forearm. Complications of parathyroid surgery include damage to the recurrent laryngeal nerve and permanent hypoparathyroidism. Activity of the unaffected parathyroid glands is suppressed by the hypercalcemia associated with hyperparathyroidism, and the remaining glands take several days to recover normal secretory activity after removal of the adenoma. This can result in postoperative hypocalcemia in the first 24 to 48 hours. If significant bone disease is present, the influx of calcium into the skeleton as it heals following parathyroid adenomectomy can lengthen the duration and increase the severity of hypocalcemia. This phenomenon is known as the *hungry bones syndrome*. Operative and postoperative complications are much less frequent when parathyroidectomy is performed by an experienced surgeon. Therefore, patients should be referred to centers that perform this operation frequently.

Many patients with mild hyperparathyroidism are asymptomatic and have no evidence of end-organ damage. In addition, studies suggest that most patients with mild forms of the disease do not develop more severe disease over time. Therefore, it is not clear that all patients necessarily benefit from surgery. However, concern lingers over the possibility of excess vascular disease in these patients as well as over the subtle neurocognitive effects ascribed to hyperparathyroidism in some studies. Given the ongoing uncertainty about this topic, a group of experts met at the National Institutes of Health in 2002 to review and update guidelines for parathyroidectomy first formulated by a consensus conference in 1990. Table 266–2 lists the criteria for surgery in otherwise asymptomatic patients, and Table 266–3 provides the guidelines for managing nonsurgical patients as suggested by the 2002 consensus conference. These guidelines are not rigid, and each patient must be approached with his or her unique circumstances in mind. Studies have demonstrated that most patients who do not meet criteria for surgery remain stable from the standpoint of both biochemical parameters and bone density over 10 years of follow-up. However, approximately 25% of asymptomatic patients have biochemical progression of their disease and/or demonstrate progressive bone loss. Therefore, patients who do not undergo surgical treatment should have biannual measurements of serum calcium and yearly measurements of serum creatinine and bone density. If patients demonstrate worsening of hypercalcemia, deterioration of renal function, or progressive bone loss, they should be referred for surgery.

Several adjunct medical therapies exist for patients who meet the criteria for surgery but who either decline parathyroidectomy or are poor operative candidates. Maintenance of hydration and physical activity are important in all patients. Bisphosphonates have been shown to prevent and even reverse, to a limited extent, low bone mass in patients with

TABLE 266–2 GUIDELINES FOR PARATHYROID SURGERY IN ASYMPTOMATIC PRIMARY HYPERPARATHYROIDISM: 2002 NATIONAL INSTITUTES OF HEALTH CONSENSUS CONFERENCE

Serum calcium >1.0 mg/dL above upper limit of normal
24-hour urine calcium excretion >400 mg
Reduction of creatinine clearance by ≥30%
Bone mineral density T-score of <–2.5 at any site
Age <50 yr

TABLE 266–3 MONITORING GUIDELINES FOR PATIENTS WITH ASYMPTOMATIC HYPERPARATHYROIDISM NOT MEETING CRITERIA FOR SURGERY—2002 NIH CONSENSUS CONFERENCE

Measurement of serum calcium biannually
Measurement of serum creatinine annually
Measurement of bone density at spine, hip, and forearm annually

hyperparathyroidism. Finally, cinacalcet has been shown to lower serum calcium levels in patients with primary hyperparathyroidism. This drug is an allosteric activator of the CaR and directly inhibits PTH release by parathyroid adenomas. It is not yet clear whether calcimimetic agents will be appropriate for the long-term medical treatment of hyperparathyroidism, but cinacalcet showed good efficacy in controlling serum calcium in a 1-year clinical trial in patients with this disease.

Hypercalcemia of Malignancy

Definition

The most common cause of elevated calcium levels in hospitalized patients is MAHC. MAHC has two pathophysiologic subgroups: humoral hypercalcemia of malignancy (HHM), which is caused by tumor-cell secretion of a bone-resorbing factor (usually PTHrP) into the systemic circulation; and local osteolytic hypercalcemia (LOH), which is caused by localized bone resorption surrounding tumor cells within the skeleton.

Epidemiology

Hypercalcemia, a frequent complication of cancer, occurs in up to 20 to 30% of patients sometime during the course of their malignant disease. MAHC is usually a manifestation of advanced disease, and investigators have estimated that patients with MAHC have a 50% 30-day mortality. HHM is classically associated with squamous cell tumors of the lung, head and neck, esophagus and cervix, urothelial malignant diseases (both renal cell and transitional cell), and breast cancers. However, almost every tumor type has been reported to secrete PTHrP and to cause HHM. LOH is most frequently diagnosed in patients with multiple myeloma or breast cancer.

Pathobiology

The principal cause of hypercalcemia in MAHC is increased bone resorption. In HHM, patients have a generalized increase in osteoclast numbers and activity, whereas in LOH, osteoclast numbers and activity are increased only in the vicinity of skeletal metastases. In both instances, hypercalcemia develops when the efflux of calcium from the skeleton exceeds the kidneys' ability to excrete the excess calcium that enters the ECF. Patients with MAHC often suffer from nausea and anorexia and have hypercalcemia-induced polyuria. Therefore, dehydration is an important component of the presentation of all patients with MAHC.

In most cases, HHM is caused by the secretion of PTHrP into the systemic circulation by tumor cells. As noted earlier, PTH and PTHrP bind and activate the PTH/PTHrP receptor with equal affinity. Thus, when PTHrP gains access to the systemic circulation, it activates PTH/PTHrP receptors in the bone and stimulates bone resorption throughout the skeleton, as occurs in hyperparathyroidism. However, in contradistinction to patients with hyperparathyroidism, patients with HHM have suppressed bone formation. Because no compensatory increase in bone formation occurs, patients with HHM tend to be more severely hypercalcemic than do patients with hyperparathyroidism. Another important biochemical difference between these two diseases is that, in HHM, $1,25(OH)_2$ vitamin D levels are either low normal or low, so intestinal calcium absorption is not increased. Therefore, bone is the main and often sole source of the excess calcium in this disease.

In LOH, tumor cells within the skeleton secrete various cytokines into the local microenvironment that recruit new osteoclasts into the area surrounding the tumor cells. This process leads to osteolysis, which releases growth factors from the bone matrix that stimulate the growth of the adjacent tumor cells. This pernicious, positive feedback loop both sustains the pathologic bone resorption and leads to expansion of the bone metastasis and can ultimately result in local pain and pathologic fracture. Once the size and number of metastases reach a point at which the release of calcium from the skeleton exceeds the ability of the kidney to excrete it, systemic hypercalcemia ensues. Much research has been directed at elucidating the nature of the osteoclast-activating factors secreted by bone metastases. In the case of multiple myeloma, several cytokines, including MIP-1α, transforming growth factor-α, IL-1, IL-3, and IL-6 have been implicated. More recent work has suggested that myeloma cells also secrete Dickkopf 1 (DKK-1), an inhibitor of the Wnt signaling pathway that suppresses osteoblast activity and bone formation. In the case of breast cancer, local production of PTHrP, IL-8, and IL-11 has been suggested to be important in mediating local osteolysis.

Diagnosis

Patients with HHM typically present with moderate to severe elevations in serum calcium levels, low to low-normal levels of serum phosphorus, low levels of $1,25(OH)_2$ vitamin D, suppressed levels of PTH, and elevated circulating levels of PTHrP. These patients, by definition, have no (or only a few) skeletal metastases. In contrast, patients with LOH have many skeletal metastases. They also have moderate to severe hypercalcemia, but they do not have elevations in PTHrP, and they also have normal serum phosphorus concentrations. Because MAHC is a late manifestation of malignant disease, the offending tumor is usually clinically obvious, and detailed laboratory investigations are not needed. However, because hyperparathyroidism is common in the general population, it should be ruled out by measuring PTH levels in all hypercalcemic patients, even those with cancer. In patients with suspected HHM, documentation of elevated PTHrP levels confirms the diagnosis. This approach is not needed in all cases, but it can be helpful in patients with unusual tumor types and the rare occurrence of HHM in association with benign tumors.

Treatment

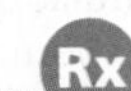

Rehydration is the first step in the acute treatment of MAHC. This often requires the infusion of isotonic saline at rates of 200 to 300 mL/hour, and it should be accompanied by close monitoring of electrolytes and cardiovascular status. Once volume depletion is corrected, treatment with loop diuretics can be initiated to induce natriuresis, which increases the renal calcium excretion. Rehydration and forced saline diuresis can result in lowering of the serum calcium on the order of 1 to 1.5 mg/dL. The only cure for MAHC is successful treatment of the underlying malignant disease; hypercalcemia will resolve with successful surgery or chemotherapy. If the tumor cannot be successfully treated, pharmacologic therapy can be used to lower calcium levels transiently. Because the principal cause of MAHC is increased bone resorption, antiresorptive drugs have shown the greatest efficacy for this condition. Calcitonin is the most rapidly acting antiresorptive agent. It can be given in doses of 4 to 8 IU/kg subcutaneously or intramuscularly every 6 to 12 hours. This treatment can lower serum calcium by 1 to 2 mg/dL within several hours, but tachyphylaxis to calcitonin occurs within 24 to 48 hours. Bisphosphonates are now the standard treatment for MAHC. Pamidronate has been the most commonly used medication for the past decade. Intravenous infusion of 60 or 90 mg of pamidronate begins to lower serum calcium after 24 to 72 hours, and nadir calcium levels are reached within 5 to 6 days. Up to 70% of patients experience a normalization of calcium levels that can last up to 18 days. More recently, zoledronate has become the treatment of choice. Intravenous infusions of 4 to 8 mg of zoledronate result in the normalization of calcium within 3 to 5 days in approximately 90% of patients, with a duration of response lasting for up to 32 days. In a head-to-head trial, zoledronate resulted in more rapid and more durable remission of hypercalcemia in patients with MAHC than did pamidronate. Dialysis against a calcium-free bath can be useful in patients with MAHC and renal failure or in patients who cannot tolerate bisphosphonates.

HYPOCALCEMIA

Definition

Hypocalcemia is defined as an abnormally low serum concentration of ionized calcium.

Pathobiology

Hypocalcemia can (1) be caused by abnormalities of PTH availability, (2) result from PTH resistance due to PTH receptor or postreceptor defects, or (3) occur in the setting of normal or increased PTH activity

TABLE 266–4 CAUSES OF HYPOCALCEMIA

HYPOCALCEMIA RESULTING FROM REDUCED OR ABSENT PTH SECRETION
Surgical damage or destruction of the parathyroid glands
Infiltrative diseases and deposition of heavy metals
High-dose radiation
Failure of organogenesis: DiGeorge sequence
Idiopathic hypoparathyroidism
Molecular abnormalities in the PTH gene (loss of function mutations)
Molecular abnormalities in the calcium-sensing receptor gene (gain of function mutations)
Autoimmune polyglandular syndrome type 1
Functional defects in PTH secretion
HYPOCALCEMIA RESULTING FROM RESISTANCE TO THE ACTIONS OF PTH
Pseudohypoparathyroidism
Hypomagnesemia
HYPOCALCEMIA IN THE SETTING OF NORMAL OR INCREASED SERUM PTH LEVELS AND NORMAL PTH RECEPTOR FUNCTION
Hypocalcemia induced by hyperphosphatemia
Nutritional vitamin D deficiency
Vitamin D malabsorption
Loss of function mutations in the 1α-hydroxylase enzyme
Hereditary resistance to $1,25(OH)_2$ vitamin D
Hypocalcemia resulting from accelerated skeletal mineralization (hungry bones syndrome)
Medical illness (sepsis)
Medications

PTH = parathyroid hormone.

and normal PTH receptor function. A full listing of specific causes of hypocalcemia is given in Table 266–4. Selected disorders are discussed in the following subsections.

Hypocalcemia Resulting from Abnormalities of Parathyroid Hormone Availability

Various congenital or acquired disorders can lead to developmental failure of the parathyroid glands, failure of functional hormone production, or destruction of the glands. These disorders all manifest as hypocalcemia, usually with attendant hyperphosphatemia and undetectable or inappropriately low levels of circulating PTH.

Destruction of the Parathyroid Glands

Surgical destruction of the parathyroid glands is the most common cause of hypoparathyroidism. Given the close anatomic relationship of the parathyroid glands with the thyroid, complete or near-complete extirpation of the thyroid gland as part of the management of either Graves' disease or thyroid cancer can be complicated by destruction or vascular compromise of parathyroid tissue and varying degrees of hypoparathyroidism. Aggressive surgical treatment of head and neck cancer can also cause parathyroid damage. Permanent destruction of the parathyroid glands should be a rare complication of neck surgery, and for experienced surgeons it occurs with a frequency of less than 10%. More common is transient parathyroid dysfunction, so-called stunned parathyroids, which can cause a decline of approximately 1 mg/dL in total serum calcium in the first 24 to 48 postoperative hours. The presumed cause is temporary vascular compromise or mechanical damage to the glands.

Infiltrative diseases, granulomatous diseases, metastases to the parathyroids, and deposition of heavy metals are all uncommon but recognized causes of parathyroid destruction and hypoparathyroidism. Although the parathyroid glands are quite resistant to radiation, hypoparathyroidism following radioactive iodine treatment for hyperthyroidism has been described.

Hypomagnesemia

Magnesium is an important cofactor for PTH secretion, apparently required for release of the stored hormone from secretory granules. In severe cases of hypomagnesemia (i.e., serum levels <1 mg/dL), suppressed parathyroid secretion can occur. This is most often seen in chronic gastrointestinal disease, nutritional deficiency, especially alcoholism, or with *cis*-platinum therapy. Resistance to the actions of PTH at the level of bone and kidney may also contribute to the hypocalcemia seen with magnesium deficiency. Replenishment of magnesium stores promptly restores parathyroid function to normal.

Idiopathic Hypoparathyroidism

Isolated failure of parathyroid gland development is a rare genetic cause of hypoparathyroidism. Molecular abnormalities in PTH biosynthesis can cause genetic absence of the hormone in the presence of apparently normal parathyroid glands. In addition, activating mutations in the CaR can lead to inappropriate suppression of PTH secretion, a condition referred to as *autosomal dominant familial hypocalcemia.* In affected individuals, the mutant receptor constitutively signals and leads to continuous suppression of PTH secretion despite hypocalcemia.

Autoimmune Polyglandular Syndrome Type 1

This autoimmune disorder is characterized by early development of hypoparathyroidism in association with Addison's disease and mucocutaneous candidiasis. Most affected individuals manifest hypocalcemia by the age of 10 years. In addition to Addison's disease, one third of these patients develop other endocrine disorders such as diabetes mellitus, pernicious anemia, or premature ovarian failure. This disorder is now known to be caused by mutations in the gene encoding an autoimmune regulatory protein (AIRE).

Hypocalcemia Resulting from Resistance to the Actions of Parathyroid Hormone

Pseudohypoparathyroidism

Peripheral tissue resistance to PTH was classically termed *pseudohypoparathyroidism* (PHP). The characteristic biochemical manifestations of PHP are hypocalcemia and hyperphosphatemia, just as in parathyroprivic hypoparathyroidism; however, circulating levels of PTH are elevated, rather than low or undetectable. The renal tubule is the primary site of PTH resistance, although variable degrees of skeletal resistance have also been reported. When the skeleton retains sensitivity to PTH, lesions characteristic of hyperparathyroidism, including osteitis fibrosa cystica, can develop. PTH stimulates renal cyclic adenosine monophosphate (cAMP) production, and levels of cAMP increase in the urine following administration of the hormone. A direct correlation has been demonstrated between the degree of PTH resistance (as assessed by the magnitude of the change in cAMP excretion or renal phosphate threshold) and the ambient circulating PTH level.

The renal cAMP response is the basis of a diagnostic test that allows partial classification of this heterogeneous group of disorders. Individuals with PHP who demonstrate a blunted urinary cAMP response have type I PHP. Those who generate a normal cAMP response have type II PHP.

PHP type I has been further characterized into types Ia, Ib, and Ic. Type 1a describes those individuals with the *Albright's hereditary osteodystrophy* phenotype, defined by short stature and large frame, broad facies, and shortened fourth metacarpals (Fig. 266–3). Soft tissue calcifications and multiple endocrine abnormalities are often present. These individuals frequently have a mutation in the α subunit of the stimulatory guanine nucleotide binding regulatory protein, G_s. This regulatory protein couples membrane receptors to adenylate cyclase, thereby regulating receptor-dependent cAMP production. The presence of G_s in various cell types accounts for the generalized hormone resistance that may occur. For example, affected patients often have elevated thyrotropin levels with a compensated euthyroid state. Variable degrees of gonadotropin, antidiuretic hormone, adrenocorticotropic hormone, and glucagon resistance have been described. Patients with type Ib PHP only have PTH resistance, without the Albright's hereditary osteodystrophy

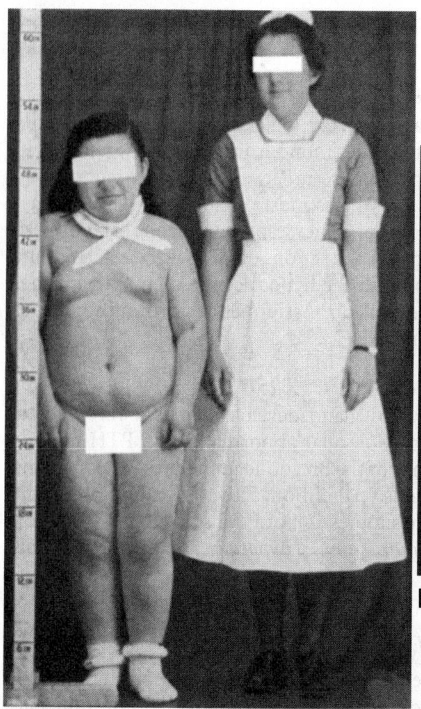

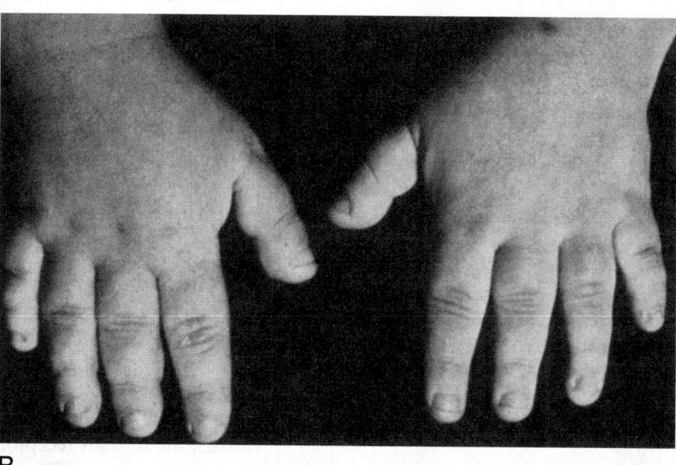

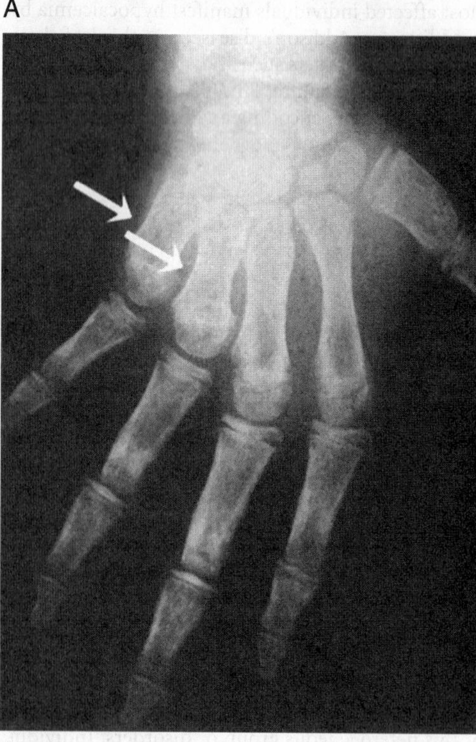

FIGURE 266–3 • Patients with Albright's hereditary osteodystrophy. A, Note short stature and round facies in this patient. **B,** Hands of the patient shown in **A.** Note that the third and fourth fingers are shorter than the second. This is because of short metatarsals. **C,** Hand radiograph of another patient; note the short fourth and fifth metatarsals (arrows). **(A and B,** From Albright F, Burnett CH, Smith PH, Parson W: Pseudoparathyroidism—an example of Seabright-Bantam syndrome. Endocrinology 1942;30:922; **C,** from Kolb FO, Steinbach HL: Pseudohypoparathyroidism with secondary hyperparathyroidism and osteitis fibrosa. J Clin Endrinol Metab 1962;22:59–70.)

phenotype. It has been suggested that this phenotype may result from abnormalities in the tissue-specific imprinting of the G_s α gene, such that $G_{s\alpha}$ function is specifically lost in the kidney but is retained in other tissues. Patients without a mutation in $G_{s\alpha}$ but with associated hormonal abnormalities and/or Albright's hereditary osteodystrophy have been classified as having type Ic PHP. The catalytic subunit of adenylate cyclase is a possible site for the defect in this latter condition.

Type II PHP appears to result from a variety of defects distal to cAMP generation in the intracellular PTH signaling cascade. No distinct phenotype exists, although various autoimmune findings have been described in some patients. Finally, other investigators have suggested that a circulating PTH inhibitor may play a role in the pathogenesis of PHP and have indicated that this inhibitor may be generated by parathyroid tissue itself. Resistance to PTH has also been described in hypomagnesemia, as noted previously.

Hypocalcemia in the Setting of Normal or Increased Parathyroid Hormone Activity and Normal Receptor Function

Despite normal PTH function and downstream signaling from its receptor, hypocalcemia can still result from disturbances in skeletal homeostasis, vitamin D metabolism, and a variety of medical illnesses.

Hypoproteinemia

The most common cause of a low serum calcium level in hospitalized patients is a reduction in the concentration of serum proteins (particularly albumin). In these patients, the ionized calcium is unaffected, and signs and symptoms of hypocalcemia are absent. Low serum albumin concentrations are often seen in patients with nephrotic syndrome, chronic illness, malnutrition, cirrhosis, and volume overexpansion. One commonly cited rule of thumb used to correct for the effects of decreased serum albumin on total serum calcium concentration is to add 0.8 mg/dL to the total serum calcium for every 1 g/dL decline in serum albumin to less than 4.0 g/dL. However, this estimate has been shown to be somewhat inaccurate, and it is preferable to determine the ionized calcium concentration directly in this setting.

Vitamin D Deficiency

Vitamin D synthesis in the skin requires adequate exposure to ultraviolet light. Thus, vitamin D deficiency is uncommon in settings where sunlight exposure is abundant. In extremes of latitude (e.g., northern climates in North America), and where industrial pollution can interfere with transmission of ultraviolet light, normal vitamin D status depends on adequate dietary vitamin D intake. Supplementation of milk products with vitamin D has significantly reduced the incidence of vitamin D deficiency in North America. Although this condition is much more common in children, adults occasionally present with nutritional vitamin D deficiency. Elderly persons in particular are at risk for this complication, because of general nutritional compromise and limited sunlight exposure.

Overt hypocalcemia is seen only in severe vitamin D deficiency. PTH levels are high in this setting. Serum levels of alkaline phosphatase (of bone origin) can be elevated as a result of associated osteomalacia, which is manifested by painful pseudofractures, particularly in weight-bearing long bones. The best way to assess vitamin D status is by measuring circulating levels of 25(OH) vitamin D. Levels of this metabolite are low in vitamin D deficiency. Levels lower than 20 ng/mL indicate vitamin D deficiency, although hypocalcemia is not usually seen until serum levels are lower, often less than 10 ng/mL. Circulating $1,25(OH)_2$ vitamin D levels may be low, normal, or elevated in the setting of vitamin D deficiency. This finding may appear paradoxical, but $1,25(OH)_2$ vitamin D circulates in 1000-fold lower concentrations than 25(OH) vitamin D.

Because vitamin D is a fat-soluble vitamin, generalized fat malabsorption can also lead to vitamin D deficiency. Gastrointestinal diseases such as Crohn's disease, celiac sprue, and pancreatic insufficiency can be accompanied by hypocalcemia resulting from vitamin D malabsorption. Interruption of the enterohepatic circulation of both 25(OH) vitamin D and $1,25(OH)_2$vitamin D may lower body vitamin D stores in these diseases. Mild hypocalcemia and secondary hyperparathyroidism are also seen in cholestatic liver diseases such as primary biliary cirrhosis. Circulating levels of 25(OH) vitamin D are reduced in this setting because of impaired hydroxylation of vitamin D in the liver and because of intestinal malabsorption of vitamin D.

Hyperphosphatemia

Since the 1930s, clinicians have appreciated that oral or parenteral phosphate can induce a decline in serum calcium concentrations, and hyperphosphatemia can lead to frank hypocalcemia. Clinical settings in which this can occur include (1) excessive enteral or parental phosphate administration, (2) the tumor lysis syndrome, and (3) rhabdomyolysis-induced acute renal failure. Hypocalcemia induced by either oral or parental phosphate administration is often associated with soft tissue calcification. Such ectopic calcification has been observed during the treatment of hypophosphatemia resulting either from diabetic ketoacidosis or from acute alcoholism. Adults receiving phosphate-containing enemas may also become hypocalcemic. Under most circumstances, discontinuation of exogenous phosphate intake leads to a prompt return of the serum calcium level to normal. Hypocalcemia in the setting of massive tumor lysis results from the release of intracellular phosphate as a consequence of chemotherapy-induced cell death, usually during the treatment of rapidly proliferating neoplasms. The hypocalcemia may continue beyond the period of hyperphosphatemia and appears to be aggravated by suppressed $1,25(OH)_2$ vitamin D levels. Rhabdomyolysis-induced acute renal failure occurs with trauma and drug or alcohol abuse. Marked hypocalcemia can occur in the early oliguric phase, and moderate to severe hypercalcemia is noted in the subsequent polyuric phase. The appearance of hypercalcemia and high serum $1,25(OH)_2$ vitamin D levels during the diuretic phase may result from rapid development of secondary hyperparathyroidism during the initial hypocalcemic period.

Pancreatitis

Hypocalcemia and tetany were first reported in patients with pancreatitis in the early 1940s. Pancreatic lipase released from the damaged gland is believed to liberate free fatty acids that chelate calcium, thereby removing it from the ECF. Hypomagnesemia resulting from poor oral intake, alcohol use, or vomiting may contribute to the hypocalcemia. Hypocalcemia in the setting of pancreatitis often suggests a poor clinical course. Treatment consists of parental calcium and magnesium when indicated.

Chronic Kidney Disease

Progressive renal disease is associated with a decline in serum calcium resulting from several factors. Important among these are a rise in serum phosphate as the ability of the kidney to clear absorbed phosphate declines and a fall in serum levels of $1,25(OH)_2$ vitamin D because of diminishing renal production of this metabolite. The consequent stimulation of parathyroid function can lead to severe secondary and even tertiary hyperparathyroidism, and therefore early intervention with phosphate binders and calcitriol or calcitriol analogues is now the standard of care for patients with significantly impaired renal function. The challenges of managing hypocalcemia in the patient treated with dialysis are beyond the scope of this chapter, and the reader is referred to specialty texts on this clinical problem.

Sepsis

Up to 20% of septic patients have reductions in ionized serum calcium. Hypocalcemia is associated with a worse prognosis. This phenomenon is most often reported with gram-negative sepsis, but it has occurred in toxic shock syndrome caused by staphylococcal infection. The pathophysiology of hypocalcemia in this setting is unknown.

Clinical Manifestations

Manifestations of hypocalcemia are primarily related to increased neuromuscular irritability. Tetany is the classic sign of hypocalcemia, but it is not always present. Paresthesias are more common and often first occur around the mouth or in the fingertips. They may progress to overt muscle spasm in the face and extremities, the latter typified by carpopedal spasm. The term *latent tetany* refers to signs elicited by provocative stimuli such as ischemia (Trousseau's test: induction of carpal spasm within 3 minutes of inflating a sphygmomanometer above systolic blood pressure) or percussion of the facial nerve to induce involuntary contraction of the facial muscles including the corner of the mouth, nose, and eye (Chvostek's sign). Neither the degree of hypocalcemia nor the rapidity with which it develops necessarily correlates with clinical manifestations, although the frequency of overt signs increases when serum calcium falls to less than 7.5 mg/dL.

Patients with hypomagnesemia or hyperkalemia may present with similar findings, which can be exacerbated by hypocalcemia. In contrast, hypermagnesemia or hypokalemia can mask symptoms in a hypocalcemic individual. Abnormalities of cardiac repolarization are seen in hypocalcemic individuals reflected by a prolonged QT interval on the electrocardiogram.

Basal ganglia calcifications are typical findings in long-standing hypoparathyroidism. Osteoporosis and dental abnormalities have also been reported in chronic untreated hypoparathyroidism. Dry skin, coarse hair, and a form of psoriasis that responds to correction of hypocalcemia have all been described in this clinical setting.

Diagnosis

The initial step in evaluating hypocalcemia is to confirm that the ionized calcium level is low. If the serum albumin concentration is within the normal range, then the total serum calcium can be considered an accurate reflection of the ionized fraction. Otherwise, ionized serum calcium must be measured. Once it has been established that the patient is hypocalcemic, a serum PTH level should be measured. A low or undetectable PTH level in the presence of hypocalcemia confirms the diagnosis of hypoparathyroidism. The diagnostic focus in this setting should be on destructive, infiltrative, and autoimmune diseases of the parathyroid glands, as well as on genetic disorders leading to the absence of the parathyroid glands or (as in the case of activating mutations of the CaR) their functional absence. If the serum PTH level is elevated, then the differential diagnosis should focus on factors inducing resistance to the actions of PTH. The presence of hyperphosphatemia suggests concomitant renal failure or excessive ingestion or administration of phosphate salts. A low serum phosphorus level in the setting of hypocalcemia and an elevated PTH suggests the possibility of vitamin D deficiency, and a serum 25(OH) vitamin D level should be checked early in the evaluation. The presence of vitamin D deficiency indicates nutritional deficiency or intestinal malabsorption. The diagnosis of hypomagnesemia should be excluded. In the absence of any of these accompanying changes, phenotypic abnormalities such as those seen in Albright's hereditary osteodystrophy should be looked for because PHP is a likely diagnostic possibility.

Treatment

Rx

Acute Management

Hypocalcemia-induced seizures, laryngospasm, and tetany are examples of clinical settings in which immediate correction of hypocalcemia is required. In these emergencies, 10 to 20 mL of 10% calcium gluconate should be infused over a 10- to 15-minute period. This treatment can be followed, if necessary, by an infusion of calcium. For this purpose, 10 ampules of calcium gluconate can be diluted in 1 L of 5% dextrose, and, beginning at a rate of 50 mL/hour, the infusion rate can be titrated to maintain the serum calcium in the low-normal range.

In patients with hypomagnesemia, magnesium therapy may be required to restore PTH secretion and peripheral activity. Before administration of magnesium salts, adequate renal function and urinary output should be ensured. In the acute setting, magnesium may be infused slowly with up to 2.4 mg of elemental magnesium/kg body weight given over a 20-minute period (to a maximum of 180 mg). The length of parenteral therapy must be individualized, and maintenance with oral magnesium salts should be implemented when ongoing hypomagnesemia is anticipated.

The administration of intravenous calcium or magnesium should be carefully monitored. The patient's cardiac status should be followed and the infusions stopped if electrocardiographic changes occur. Deep tendon reflexes can be used to monitor for magnesium toxicity, and therapy should be halted if reflexes diminish. Intravenous calcium gluconate is a useful antidote for magnesium intoxication and should be available at the bedside.

Long-Term Treatment

Many of the causes of hypocalcemia discussed earlier are corrected by treating the underlying disorder (e.g., vitamin D deficiency, tumor lysis syndrome). However, some patients require maintenance therapy for hypocalcemia, including hypoparathyroidism, PHP, and vitamin D–resistant states.

Hypoparathyroidism, whether primary or secondary to trauma or surgery, is the most frequently encountered condition that requires long-term therapy to support circulating calcium concentrations. In these individuals, the goal is to maintain serum calcium in the low-normal range (8.5 to 9.2 mg/dL). This approach will reduce the likelihood of symptoms such as circumoral tingling, signs such as carpopedal spasm, and more long-term complications such as cataracts. Increasing the serum calcium level into the middle to high-normal range can result in significant hypercalciuria, nephrocalcinosis, and nephrolithiasis.

There is no single best way to achieve target calcium levels, although the combination of a vitamin D metabolite with calcium supplements is generally preferred. Many different preparations of both are available. Because of the prolonged toxicity that occurs with excessive ingestion of either ergocalciferol or 25(OH) vitamin D, the use of rapid-acting preparations of vitamin D is generally preferred for the treatment of hypoparathyroidism. Calcitriol [1,25$(OH)_2D_3$] and dihydrotachysterol are two preparations suited to this purpose. Both are fully active in vivo. In general, it is best to establish a stable dose for one of these agents and to refine the serum calcium level by adjusting the intake of supplemental calcium, rather than by making repeated changes in vitamin D metabolite therapy. Calcitriol can be used in most patients. The dose of calcitriol

Rx

can range from as little as 0.25 up to 2.0 µg/day. The biologic half-life of the drug is 12 to 14 hours. When hypercalcemia develops during therapy with calcitriol, it usually resolves within 3 to 4 days after discontinuing the drug, although it can persist for more than 1 week. In addition to a high-calcium diet, calcium supplements are important for the treatment of hypoparathyroidism. Doses of 1000 to 2000 mg/day of calcium may be necessary. Preparations including the carbonate, citrate, lactate, gluconate, and glucobionate salts are suitable for this purpose. In some patients with hypoparathyroidism, a thiazide diuretic may be useful in augmenting serum calcium levels and in reducing the hypercalciuria that can occur with the institution of treatment. Long-term treatment of hypoparathyroidism with synthetic human PTH is not yet practical, although short-term therapy has been successful. Various stresses such as trauma, infection, and pregnancy can increase the therapeutic requirements of patients with chronic hypocalcemia, and the clinician should be alert to this possibility.

SUGGESTED READINGS

Bilezikian JP, Silverberg SJ: Asymptomatic primary hyperparathyroidism. N Engl J Med 2004;350:1746–1751. *A case-based discussion.*

Goldmuntz E: DiGeorge syndrome: New insights. Clin Perinatol 2005;32:963–978. *A comprehensive review.*

Jacobs TP, Bilezikian JP: Rare causes of hypercalcemia. J Clin Endocrinol Metab 2005;90:6316–6322. *A source for the less common causes of hypercalcemia.*

Marx SJ: Hyperparathyroid and hypoparathyroid disorders. N Engl J Med 2000;343:1863–1875. *A comprehensive review.*

Potts JT: Parathyroid hormone: Past and present. J Endocrinol 2006;188:135–153. *Discusses the history, physiology, and function of this hormone.*

Stewart AF: Hypercalcemia associated with cancer. N Engl J Med 2005; 352:373–379. *A clinical update.*

Strippoli GF, Tong A, Palmer SC, et al: Calcimimetics for secondary hyperparathyroidism in chronic kidney disease patients. Cochrane Database Syst Rev 2006:(4):CD006254. *Treatment improves biochemical parameters, but patient-based benefits have not yet been demonstrated.*

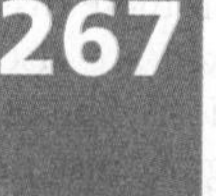

267 MEDULLARY THYROID CARCINOMA AND CALCITONIN

Leonard J. Deftos and Robert F. Gagel

Definition

Medullary thyroid carcinoma (MTC) is a rare tumor of the calcitonin-producing cells of the thyroid gland that often occurs in association with other endocrine tumors. Calcitonin is a 32-amino acid peptide secreted primarily by these thyroidal C cells in mammals and thus serves as a serum marker for this tumor. In submammals, calcitonin is secreted by the embryologically related ultimobranchial gland. The main biologic effect of calcitonin is to decrease bone resorption by inhibiting the osteoclast. This effect, along with a lesser calciuric action, decreases the concentration of blood calcium, with a nadir directly related to bone turnover; thus, the hypocalcemia may be slight in physiologically normal adults but considerable when bone resorption is increased pathologically in disease states or physiologically during bone growth. This property of calcitonin makes it an effective drug for hyperresorptive diseases, such as Paget's disease, osteoporosis, and hypercalcemia. The physiologic significance of other reported effects of calcitonin is not well established. The calciuric effect of calcitonin is seen primarily with pharmacologic doses of the hormone. An analgesic effect of calcitonin continues to receive considerable attention and may be related to neuroendocrine actions of the hormone. In addition to its role in skeletal physiology and treatment, calcitonin is a serum marker and tumor marker for MTC, and its serum concentrations are increased whether MTC occurs sporadically or as a component of multiple endocrine neoplasia (MEN) 2 and its variants (Table 267–1).

TABLE 267–1 COMPONENTS OF MULTIPLE ENDOCRINE NEOPLASIA 2 AND THEIR FREQUENCY BASED ON AVERAGE FIGURES FROM THE LITERATURE

Component	Type 2a	Type 2b
Medullary thyroid carcinoma	95%	90%
Pheochromocytoma	50%	45%
Hyperparathyroidism	25%	Rare
Mucosal neuroma syndrome	—	90%

CALCITONIN

Biochemistry

The 32-amino acid structure of calcitonin, determined for several species, reveals a common 1,7-amino-terminal disulfide bridge and carboxy-terminal proline. Seven of the nine amino-terminal residues are identical in all calcitonin molecules. The interspecies structural differences in the rest of the molecule cause the submammalian (ultimobranchial) calcitonin molecules to be more potent in mammals than the mammalian calcitonin molecules. Thus, the potent salmon form of the hormone is the one used for treatment of osteoporosis, hypercalcemia, and Paget's disease of bone. The greater chemical basicity of these submammalian calcitonin species probably accounts for their increased potency. In contrast to the other major bone-active peptides, parathyroid hormone and parathyroid hormone–related protein that have bioactive moieties processed from their precursors, a biologically active fragment of calcitonin has not been identified, and the entire molecule seems to be necessary for biologic activity.

Secretion and Production

The most important secretory regulation of calcitonin is mediated by ambient calcium. An acute elevation in blood calcium concentration increases the secretion of calcitonin, and an acute decrease in blood calcium level reduces the secretion of calcitonin. This action is mediated through the calcium-sensing receptor expressed by the thyroidal C cells. The effects of chronic changes in blood calcium concentration on secretion have not been as well defined. Chronic hypercalcemia may stimulate calcitonin production, but this compensatory response may be limited. Chronic hypocalcemia seems to increase calcitonin storage in C cells. Although various other factors have been reported to stimulate calcitonin secretion, only pentagastrin and its related peptides are consistent additional secretagogues. The high concentration of pentagastrin necessary to stimulate secretion does not support the presence of a normal entero–C cell secretory pathway, although mildly elevated calcitonin levels have been observed in chronic hypergastrinemia (e.g., ulcer drugs). Pentagastrin and calcium are clinically important agents for evaluating calcitonin secretion by both normal and malignant C cells. Although both are used for provocative testing of calcitonin secretion, the former is not widely available.

The effect of gonadal steroids and age on calcitonin production remains controversial. It is well established that blood concentrations of calcitonin are higher in males than in females and in children than in adults. Some studies report a decline in calcitonin secretion during adulthood and a stimulation of calcitonin production by estrogens and testosterone. These observations have led to the hypothesis that age- and menopause-related declines in calcitonin production contribute to the corresponding declines in bone mass seen in elderly persons, especially postmenopausal women. These observations provide a rationale for use of calcitonin in treating osteoporosis, but more complex hormonal abnormalities underlie this skeletal disorder.

MEDULLARY THYROID CARCINOMA

Definition

MTC, a rare tumor of the calcitonin-producing C cells of the thyroid gland, accounts for approximately 5 to 10% of thyroid cancers. These cells migrate from the neural crest to the thyroid gland and to other sites of the diffuse neuroendocrine system during embryogenesis in mammals. In submammals, these cells form their own distinct organ, the ultimobranchial gland. The neural crest origin of C cells accounts for their production of a variety of biologically active substances. This embryologic origin may also explain the common association of MTC with other neuroendocrine tumors. Thus, MTC can occur as part of MEN type 2 or sporadically, the latter being more common. Whereas early reports emphasized sporadic tumors, the growing appreciation of the inherited nature of the tumor has resulted in an increased diagnosis of familial cases. Even in apparently sporadic cases in patients with no family history of the tumor, approximately 6% are found to have a genetic basis.

Pathobiology

A palpable tumor is the most common physical finding in the patient with MTC. The tumor is usually firm and is located in the middle or upper lobes of the gland. Bilateral and multicentric tumors are common in patients with MEN, whereas a unilateral and single site is more common in sporadic cases. In hereditary MTC, multifocal C-cell hyperplasia is a precursor to frank malignancy. Calcification can be present in the tumor, and this may result in a radiographic pattern that is characteristic enough to help in its clinical diagnosis. Similarly, the presence of amyloid in the tumor can assist in histologic diagnosis. However, cytologic diagnosis is made difficult by the finding that the cells of MTC can be arranged in a variety of patterns. Therefore, the diagnosis of MTC is conclusively made by demonstrating calcitonin in the tumor by immunohistologic testing with a calcitonin antibody. The presence of abnormal calcitonin-producing cells may be revealed by diagnostic fine-needle aspiration of the thyroid. Hyperplasia of the C cells can antedate the frank malignancy of MTC, especially in the familial forms of the tumor. C-cell hyperplasia is often too subtle to be appreciated by light microscopy, and immunohistology for calcitonin is necessary to make this diagnosis. The advent of genetic testing for MEN 2 has provided additional strategies for distinguishing MTC from other thyroid tumors.

Clinical Manifestations and Natural History

The natural history of the tumor is variable. The clinical behavior of MTC is usually intermediate between that of aggressive anaplastic thyroid cancer and that of indolent papillary and follicular thyroid cancer. Local lymph node spread is common, and metastases to lung, liver, and bone occur with some frequency. MTC in which all or most of the cells produce calcitonin generally has a better prognosis than more heterogeneous tumors in which calcitonin production is not uniform. Even in the most aggressive tumors, calcitonin production is usually sufficient to serve as a specific marker for this thyroid cancer. However, there may be rare instances in which calcitonin production has ceased. The 5-year survival rate of patients with metastatic MTC approximates 50%. Survival can vary from several months to 3 decades after diagnosis.

In hereditary MTC, a germline mutation of the *RET* proto-oncogene leads to development of microscopic carcinoma as early as 2 to 3 years of age. Palpable hereditary MTC is most commonly identified in the 15- to 30-year range. Approximately 25% of sporadic MTCs appear to be initiated by a somatic *RET* mutation; although such a mutation could occur at any age, sporadic MTC most commonly presents in the third or fourth decade, with a range from less than 2 years to more than 80 years.

One of the interesting features of MTC is its variable aggressiveness. In general, hereditary MTC associated with MEN 2a is less aggressive than either sporadic MTC or that associated with MEN 2b (discussed later). Sporadic MTCs with somatic codon 918 *RET* proto-oncogene mutations or MTCs associated with MEN 2b (codon 918 germline mutation of the *RET* proto-oncogene) are the most aggressive and are associated with a shorter survival time. Serum calcitonin or carcinoembryonic antigen doubling times can be useful for prognosticating survival. A calcitonin or carcinoembryonic antigen doubling time of less than 1 year, measured over a period of several years because of the variability of calcitonin measurements, is generally an indication of an aggressive tumor.

TABLE 267–2 MULTIPLE ENDOCRINE NEOPLASIA 2

MEN 2a (Sipple's syndrome)
Medullary thyroid carcinoma
Pheochromocytoma
Parathyroid neoplasia
Variants of MEN 2a
MEN 2a with cutaneous lichen amyloidosis
MEN 2a with Hirschsprung's disease
Familial medullary thyroid carcinoma
MEN 2b
Medullary thyroid carcinoma
Pheochromocytoma
Parathyroid disease (rare)
Marfanoid habitus
Intestinal ganglioneuromatosis and mucosal neuromas

MEN = multiple endocrine neoplasia.

Multiple Endocrine Neoplasia

Definition

In addition to sporadic tumors, MTC can occur in association with other endocrine tumors as part of a MEN syndrome, designated MEN 2, to distinguish it from MEN 1, which consists of parathyroid, pancreatic, and pituitary tumors (Chapter 250). MEN 2 (Sipple's syndrome) is an autosomal dominant syndrome that can be clinically classified into two subtypes, 2a and 2b (Table 267–2).

Clinical Manifestations

Pheochromocytoma

Pheochromocytoma is a component of MEN 2a and 2b, in which the tumor can be bilateral or unilateral (Chapter 246). Bilateral and multifocal pheochromocytomas are very common in this clinical setting, with an incidence of more than 50%. This figure contrasts with a usual bilateral incidence of less than 10% for sporadic pheochromocytomas and only 20 to 50% for other familial pheochromocytomas. Other hereditary forms of bilateral pheochromocytoma include von Hippel–Lindau disease, hereditary paraganglioma syndromes, and, rarely, MEN 1 and neurofibromatosis type 1. Adrenal medullary hyperplasia is a predecessor of the pheochromocytomas seen with MTC. The increase in adrenal medullary mass results from diffuse or multifocal proliferation of adrenal medullary cells, primarily those found within the head and body of the glands. The biochemical and clinical manifestations of this tumor may be elusive, so diagnostic tests for pheochromocytoma should be pursued vigorously in patients with MEN 2, with appropriate testing and retroperitoneal imaging. Decades of routine screening for pheochromocytomas in patients with MEN 2 have led to a change in the clinical presentation. Large pheochromocytomas that put patients at high risk for sudden death are seen only in rare patients with previously undiscovered MEN 2 or in patients with known MEN 2 who decline screening. More commonly, patients are identified by subtle clinical features or modest abnormalities of catecholamine or metanephrine production. Measurement of plasma metanephrine is the most convenient diagnostic procedure for identifying these tumors, and the measurement of serum chromogranin A may have diagnostic value. Early diagnosis and appropriate treatment combined with the routine use of adrenergic blockade have rendered death or serious morbidity from pheochromocytoma uncommon in this disorder. For a more detailed description and evaluation of pheochromocytoma, see Chapter 246.

Hyperparathyroidism

Hyperparathyroidism occurs in 10 to 20% of patients with MEN 2; it is more common in MEN 2a and rarely occurs in MEN 2b. It also occurs in patients with MEN 1. The presence of hyperparathyroidism thus should always make one consider the possibility of MEN. The differential diagnosis of hereditary hypercalcemia includes familial hypercalcemic hypocalciuria, familial parathyroid adenoma–jaw tumor syndromes, familial parathyroid hyperplasia, MEN 1, and MEN 2a. Parathyroid hyperplasia is more common than adenoma, an important consideration for surgical exploration of all parathyroid glands. The *RET* proto-oncogene is expressed in parathyroid tissue and is likely to account for the neoplastic changes.

Multiple Mucosal Neuromas

The presence of neuromas with a centrofacial distribution is the most consistent nonendocrine component of MEN 2b (Chapter 246). The most common location of neuromas is the oral cavity. The oral lesions are almost invariably present by the first decade and in some cases even at birth. Mucosal neuromas can also be present in the eyelid, conjunctiva, cornea, and other mucosal surfaces. The most prominent microscopic feature of neuromas is an increase in the size and number of nerves. These hypertrophied nerve fibers are readily seen with a slit lamp and occasionally by direct ophthalmologic examination. Hypertrophied corneal nerves have also been identified in MEN 2a, although no mucosal neuromas have been reported in this syndrome.

Gastrointestinal tract abnormalities are part of the multiple mucosal neuroma syndrome. The most common of these is gastrointestinal ganglioneuromatosis, which usually occurs in the small and large intestines but has also been noted in the esophagus and stomach. Neurologic dysfunction is frequently associated with swallowing abnormalities, megacolon, diarrhea, and constipation, and it is the most common presenting manifestation in childhood. The diarrhea may also result from excess production of bioactive substances by the MTC. In any case, diarrhea is the most common symptom of MTC. The association of MTC with Hirschsprung's disease is also recognized.

Marfanoid Habitus

Some patients with MEN 2b have a tall, slender body with long arms and legs, an abnormal ratio of upper to lower body segments, and poor muscle development. Other features associated with the marfanoid habitus may include dorsal kyphosis, pectus excavatum or pectus carinatum, pes cavus, and a high-arched palate. In contrast to patients with true Marfan's syndrome, these patients do not have aortic arch abnormalities, ectopia lentis, homocyst(e)inuria, or mucopolysaccharide abnormalities.

Pathobiology and Pathogenesis

Hereditary Medullary Thyroid Carcinoma (Familial Medullary Thyroid Carcinoma and Multiple Endocrine Neoplasia 2)

Genetic linkage studies mapped the gene for MEN 2 to a centromeric chromosome 10 locus, and *RET* proto-oncogene mutations were subsequently identified for the associated clinical syndromes (see Tables 267–1 and 267–2). The gene encodes a receptor tyrosine kinase. Two broad classes of mutations have been identified (Fig. 267–1). Six specific codons (609, 611, 618, 620, 630, and 634) in the extracellular domain of the tyrosine kinase receptor encoded by *RET* change a conserved cysteine to another amino acid. Codon 634 mutations, and by inference other extracellular domain mutations, cause receptor dimerization and activation and initiate the transformation of C cells. A second class of less common mutations involves the intracellular domain, with the most common located at codon 918 (see Fig. 267–1). This coding change results in receptor activation in the absence of dimerization. Other intracellular domain mutations occur at codons 768, 790, 791, 804, 883, and 891. Identification of the mutation in a family member can be a guide to the appropriate genetic diagnosis. The clinical syndromes associated with each of these mutations are described in Figure 267–1. Mutations of other components of the *RET* signaling system (glial cell–derived neurotrophic factor and the glial cell–derived neurotrophic factor-α_1 receptor) have not been identified in MTC (see Fig. 267–1).

In familial MTC, the earliest identified histologic abnormality associated with the *RET* proto-oncogene mutations is C-cell hyperplasia. It appears that a second genetic event at the *RET* locus may hasten or facilitate transformation. These events include loss of the normal *RET* allele or amplification of the mutant *RET* allele. The specific somatic mechanisms for amplification include trisomy 10 (two mutant chromosome 10 copies) or tandem duplication of the mutant *RET* gene. Evidence for loss of normal copies of genes on chromosomes 1p, 3q, 13q, and 22q suggests that other as yet unidentified genes are likely involved in the progression observed in hereditary MTC.

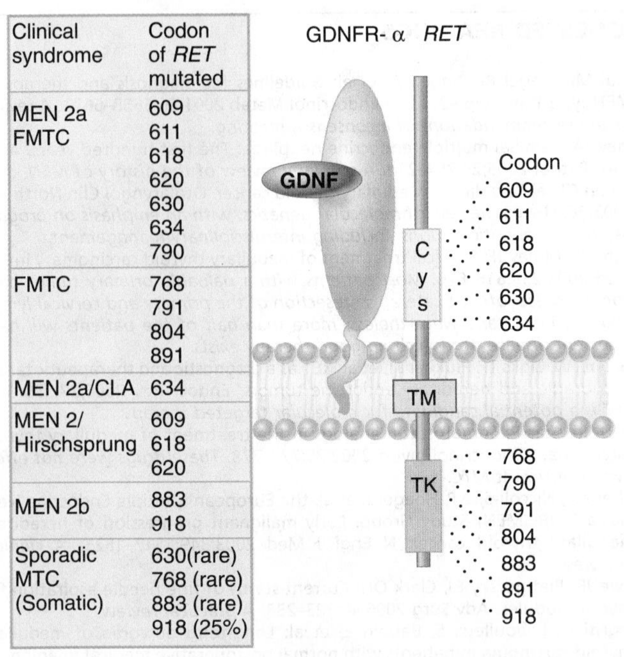

FIGURE 267–1 • The RET proto-oncogene/glial cell–derived neurotrophic factor receptor (GDNFR)-α_1 complex. Mutations of the RET proto-oncogene receptor are causative for multiple endocrine neoplasia type 2a (MEN 2a), familial medullary thyroid carcinoma (FMTC), MEN 2a/cutaneous lichen amyloidosis (MEN 2a/CLA), MEN 2 associated with Hirschsprung's disease, or MEN 2b. Mutations of the extracellular cysteine-rich region of the receptor (Cys) and intracellular tyrosine kinase domain (TK) have been identified as germline mutations in the indicated syndromes. Somatic mutations of the RET proto-oncogene have also been identified in sporadic MTC. GDNF is a small peptide ligand for the RET/GDNF receptor complex.

Because most familial cases have an identifiable *RET* mutation, as can occur in even apparently sporadic cases, screening should be vigorously pursued by routine testing of *RET* exons 10, 11, 13, 14, 15, and 16, with sequencing of the remaining 15 exons if indicated. The clinician should be aware that technical errors can occur in testing and should be prepared to use more than one laboratory for confirmation studies.

Germline RET *Mutations in Apparently Sporadic Medullary Thyroid Carcinoma*

The discovery of *RET* proto-oncogene mutations in MTC has uncovered unidentified kindreds with hereditary MTC in which the proband masqueraded as sporadic MTC. Approximately 6% of patients with apparently sporadic MTC have germline *RET* mutations indicative of familial MTC. Although most are members of previously unidentified kindreds, some are examples of de novo mutations, most commonly of codon 634. This finding has led to the identification of additional family members at risk for development of MTC. A consensus has evolved that all patients with apparently sporadic MTC should have a germline *RET* analysis.

Somatic Mutations in Sporadic Medullary Thyroid Carcinoma

Somatic mutations (non-germline mutations acquired during cell growth) of *RET* codon 918 are found in approximately 25% of sporadic tumors (see Fig. 267–1), and evidence suggests that sporadic MTCs with this mutation are more aggressive and are associated with shorter survival. In the aggressive tumors with a codon 918 mutation, it is not clear whether the mutation is the initiating abnormality or one that is acquired in the progression from a less to a more malignant phenotype.

Diagnosis

Genetic Testing

Genetic testing is used to identify individuals, especially children, at risk for development of familial MTC and MEN 2. These tests are available from a variety of commercial sources (http://www.genetests.org). Testing is best performed on peripheral blood leukocytes. The presence of a specific mutation and the propensity to develop the clinical syndrome of MEN 2 or familial MTC essentially indicate full concordance. Genetic testing can be complicated by numerous laboratory or sampling errors. Because genetic testing has become the "gold standard" for diagnosis of hereditary MTC and decisions regarding thyroidectomy are based on these results, it is prudent to repeat the genetic test on a separate peripheral blood sample, preferably in more than one laboratory. It is reasonable to exclude an individual with two or more negative genetic test results in the context of a family with hereditary MTC from further screening efforts. Although genetic testing has a great impact on the diagnosis and treatment of MTC, it has little impact on the management of adrenal medullary and parathyroid disease, in which manifestations generally develop later.

Calcitonin

Expression of the calcitonin gene is the molecular hallmark of MTC. This expression results in the production of calcitonin by the tumor and secretion of the hormone into blood. Most patients with MTC have an increased circulating concentration of calcitonin that can be detected by immunoassay and that reflects the increase in tumor mass. Usually, the basal blood concentration of calcitonin is sufficiently elevated to be diagnostic of the presence of the tumor. In the early stages of the disease, however, the basal concentrations of calcitonin may not be readily distinguished from normal values. In these circumstances, provocative testing of calcitonin secretion can reveal the presence of the abnormal C cells. Such testing is also clinically indicated for the relative of a patient with familial MTC when early diagnosis is sought, although, as discussed, genetic testing has largely replaced calcitonin testing in MEN 2 kindreds with an identifiable *RET* mutation. Family screening is no longer recommended for patients with apparently sporadic tumors and a negative *RET* proto-oncogene analysis. The predicted probability that a patient with sporadic MTC with a negative *RET* test will have hereditary MTC is very low, probably in the 0.1% range, thus making calcitonin testing largely unnecessary in this situation. The two most commonly used provocative agents for calcitonin secretion are calcium and the synthetic gastrin analogue pentagastrin (not generally available for clinical use in United States at present), alone or in combination. Most tumors respond to either agent with a diagnostic increase in calcitonin secretion. Calcitonin blood measurements can also be used to evaluate therapy and monitor tumor recurrence. Interpretation must be made according to the specific performance of the assay procedure used.

Treatment Rx

Surgical Therapy

Surgery is the treatment of choice for the three types of neoplasia in MEN 2. Because all these conditions are potentially lethal, especially MTC and pheochromocytoma, but can be cured in their early stages, aggressive therapy is warranted. Early surgery is effective treatment and can be curative. Management of the individual components of MEN 2 generally follows the accepted procedures for each neoplasm. The sequence of treatment, however, is guided by several important principles. In adults with the fully formed MEN 2a syndrome, pheochromocytomas, commonly bilateral, should be treated first because they can be life-threatening. Management of thyroid and parathyroid disorders follows. Accepted surgical procedures include unilateral or bilateral adrenalectomy for diseased glands by anterior, posterior, or laparoscopic approaches or unilateral cortical sparing adrenalectomy in an attempt to preserve adrenal cortical function. Bilateral adrenalectomy at an early age is recommended in the rare kindred with a history of malignant pheochromocytoma. In adults with palpable MTC (>1 cm), metastasis to local lymph nodes is common, and total thyroidectomy and compartment-oriented lymph node dissection should be performed to enhance the likelihood of complete removal of all tumor. Hyperparathyroidism may be managed by either subtotal parathyroidectomy or total parathyroidectomy with transplantation of parathyroid tissue to the nondominant forearm.

Medical Therapy

Various agents have been tried for the treatment of MTC, but the results have been generally disappointing. Chemotherapy, radiopharmaceuticals, immunotherapy, and chemoembolization can be

Rx

palliative or stabilizing, but the disease usually progresses. Phase I and II studies of small organic molecules that inhibit phosphorylation of the *RET* receptor showed preliminary evidence of efficacy for those tumors with germline or somatic mutations of *RET*. Multiple pharmaceutical corporations have produced competing molecules. Clinical trials over the next several years should provide clarity on the efficacy of these compounds.

Gene Therapy

Hereditary MTC is currently unique among genetic malignant diseases in that identification of a genetic abnormality leads to a specific therapeutic intervention. In other genetic malignant diseases such as colon or breast carcinoma, the identification of a germline mutation leads to increased surveillance, but this information is only rarely used to direct a specific therapy.

The identification of a mutation of the *RET* proto-oncogene indicates that the affected individual has a greater than 90% probability of developing MTC at some point during life. A 25-year history of prospective screening for MEN 2 has provided reasonable evidence that more than 85% of children who have had total thyroidectomy in the teenage years currently have no evidence of disease. This experience has been sufficiently positive that the consensus in the endocrine community is that total thyroidectomy and central node dissection should be performed in most children with MEN 2a and a germline *RET* mutation (codons 611, 618, 620, 634, or 891) by the age of 6 years. Other rarer mutations (609, 768, 790, 791, and 804) that cause MEN 2a or familial MTC appear to be associated with less aggressive MTC, and in some kindreds with these mutations, death or serious morbidity from MTC is rare. Deferral of thyroidectomy until the teenage years or until calcitonin abnormalities appear in these unique kindreds may be appropriate.

Death from MTC in MEN 2a or hereditary MTC before prospective screening with calcitonin testing occurred in the fourth or fifth decade, with rare deaths caused by MTC in the third or fourth decade. Thus, the results of prospective studies that were initiated 25 years ago are only now providing meaningful evidence that early intervention is beneficial. Even though a still longer period of observation will be required before definitive conclusions can be drawn, there is growing confidence that early thyroidectomy combined with appropriate care of pheochromocytomas can restore lifespan close to normal for most patients with hereditary MTC and can render death from metastatic MTC a rare event.

Management of Complications: Persistent Postoperative Calcitonin Measurements in Patients with Medullary Thyroid Carcinoma

A vexing problem for clinicians is the persistence of calcitonin elevations following primary surgical management. The major question is whether reoperation to remove all identifiable lymph nodes in the neck (compartment-oriented dissection) has value. Some experience supports reoperative strategy in patients with persistent disease who have not previously had a lymph node dissection. In the selection of these patients, it is important to perform a careful search for distant metastatic disease and to exclude hepatic, bone, and pulmonary metastasis by appropriate imaging studies. Imaging procedure, both general (e.g., computed tomography, magnetic resonance imaging, positron emission tomography) and specific (e.g., labeled calcitonin and carcinoembryonic antigen antibodies and octreotide scanning), can be useful in identifying local spread and distant metastases. Some physicians perform laparoscopy with direct hepatic visualization to identify hepatic metastasis. In patients with no evidence of distant metastatic disease, reoperative compartment-oriented lymphadenectomy may be appropriate. Approximately one of five carefully selected patients will have normalized serum calcitonin levels following microsurgical dissection (calcitonin values nondetectable following pentagastrin). No long-term follow-up studies in this group of patients have been performed to determine whether this type of surgical intervention affects morbidity or mortality related to MTC, yet the lack of other effective therapy for this disease makes it a reasonable consideration.

SUGGESTED READINGS

Brandi ML, Gagel RF, Angeli A, et al: Guidelines for diagnosis and therapy of MEN type 1 and type 2. J Clin Endocrinol Metab 2001;86:5658–5671. *A review of the recommendations of a consensus meeting.*

Carney JA: Familial multiple endocrine neoplasia: The first hundred years. Am J Surg Pathol 2005;29:254–274. *A scholarly review of the history of MEN.*

Clayman GL, el-Baradie TS: Medullary thyroid cancer. Otolaryngol Clin North Am 2003;36:91–105. *Review of molecular genetics, with an emphasis on prognosis and therapeutic options, including interdisciplinary management.*

Cohen MS, Moley JF: Surgical treatment of medullary thyroid carcinoma. J Intern Med 2003;253:616–626. *Most patients with a palpable primary tumor have nodal disease, often bilateral, so resection of the primary and cervical lymph nodes is important. Nevertheless, more than half of the patients will have recurrent disease, for which no good therapy exists.*

de Groot JW, Links TP, Plukker JT, et al: RET as a diagnostic and therapeutic target in sporadic and hereditary endocrine tumors. Endocr Rev 2006;27:535–560. *RET is a potential candidate for molecular targeted therapy.*

Diez JJ, Iglesias P: Somatostatin analogs in the treatment of medullary thyroid carcinoma. J Endocrinol Invest 2002;25:773–778. *These drugs were not effective in recurrent MTC.*

Machens A, Niccoli-Sire P, Hoegel J, et al, the European Multiple Endocrine Neoplasia (EUROMEN) Study Group. Early malignant progression of hereditary medullary thyroid cancer. N Engl J Med 2003;349:1517–1525. *A cliinical overview.*

Ogilvie JB, Piatigorsky EJ, Clark OH: Current status of fine needle aspiration for thyroid nodules. Adv Surg 2006;40:223–238. *A practical review.*

Pellegriti G, Leboulleux S, Baudin E, et al: Long-term outcome of medullary thyroid carcinoma in patients with normal postoperative medical imaging. Br J Cancer 2003;88:1537–1542. *Elevated postoperative calcitonin levels and evidence of tumor extension were critical prognostic factors for a high risk of imaging-detected relapse.*

Quayle FJ, Moley JF: Medullary thyroid carcinoma: including MEN 2A and MEN 2B syndromes. J Surg Oncol 2005;89:122–129. *A general review emphasizing approaches to treatment.*

Sanso GE, Domene HM, Garcia R, et al: Very early detection of RET proto-oncogene mutation is crucial for preventive thyroidectomy in multiple endocrine neoplasia type 2 children. Cancer 2002;94:323–330. *Potential use of this diagnostic approach to select patients for prophylactic thyroidectomy.*

Skinner MA, Moley JA, Dilley WG, et al: Prophylactic thyroidectomy in multiple endocrine neoplasia type 2A. N Engl J Med 2005;353:1105–1113. *Lower incidence of persistent or recurrent medullary thyroid cancer in those that had the surgery.*

268 PAGET'S DISEASE OF BONE

G. David Roodman

Definition

Paget's disease is a focal disorder of the skeleton that is the second most common bone disease, exceeded only by osteoporosis. It affects approximately 1 to 2% of adults older than 55 years in the United States and up to 4 to 6% of adults 55 years old or older in certain areas of the United Kingdom. Paget's disease is the most exaggerated form of bone remodeling, with increases in all phases of the bone remodeling process. The initial phase is characterized by markedly increased bone resorption, followed by exuberant new bone formation. The bone that is formed is abnormal and woven, with disorganized collagen. This increased bone formation results in bone enlargement and deformity because of the poor quality of the bone.

Epidemiology and Etiology

The cause of Paget's disease is unknown. However, a genetic predisposition to Paget's disease has been clearly established. Approximately 40% of patients with Paget's disease have an affected first-degree relative, and large numbers of families with vertical transmission of Paget's disease and an autosomal dominant pattern of inheritance have been described. At least six genetic loci have been linked to Paget's disease, and mutations in the sequestosome-1 gene *(SQSTM1)*, also known as p62, are the most frequent. *SQSTM1* mutations have been detected in 30% of patients with familial Paget's disease and in 10% of patients with sporadic Paget's disease. Although the penetrance for Paget's disease is high, it can vary in families with a genetic predisposition. Elderly patients with *SQSTM1* mutations may have no evidence of Paget's disease even though they are homozygous for the mutation.

The primary cellular abnormality in Paget's disease resides in the osteoclast. These cells contain nuclear inclusions that resemble paramyxoviral nucleocapsids. Both measles virus and respiratory syncytial virus nucleocapsid proteins and transcripts have been detected in osteoclasts from patients with Paget's disease, but some studies have not detected paramyxoviral transcripts or proteins in pagetic osteoclasts. Furthermore, a cause-and-effect relationship between Paget's disease and paramyxovirus infection has not been definitively established. Nevertheless, in vitro studies in which normal osteoclast precursors were transfected with measles virus transcripts or infected with measles virus have demonstrated that osteoclast precursors containing the measles virus nucleocapsid gene can form pagetic-like osteoclasts.

As noted earlier, Paget's disease is the second most common bone disease. However, the prevalence of Paget's disease varies among different populations. In the United Kingdom, for instance, Paget's disease affects up to 6% of the population older than 55 years. Further, the frequency of symptomatic Paget's disease increases with age. Similarly, Paget's disease occurs in Western Europe and in the white populations in New Zealand and Australia. However, Paget's disease is extremely rare in Scandinavia and in the Far East, and it does not affect indigenous populations in either Australia or New Zealand. The prevalence of Paget's disease appears to have decreased since the early 1980s. In England and New Zealand, the prevalence of Paget's disease was reported to have decreased from approximately 8 to 4% and from 5 to approximately 3%, respectively. The basis for this decrease in prevalence in England and New Zealand is unknown. In addition, the severity of Paget's disease in these populations has decreased.

Pathobiology

Bone remodeling is increased five- to tenfold in patients with Paget's disease. Paget's disease is highly localized, with focal areas of involvement. In pagetic lesions, osteoclast numbers are increased, and the osteoclasts are hyper-multinucleated with up to 100 nuclei/cell. This finding is in contrast to normal osteoclasts, which contain 3 to 20 nuclei/osteoclasts. The bone resorbing capacity of pagetic osteoclasts is decreased compared with normal osteoclasts. However, because of the large numbers of osteoclasts in the pagetic lesion, bone resorption is markedly increased (Fig. 268–1). The increased bone resorption phase is followed by new bone formation. As the disease progresses, the bone formation begins to predominate, and the bones become enlarged (Fig. 268–2). Large numbers of osteoblasts are often found near areas of resorbed bone and may even be prominent in a lesion that appears purely osteolytic by roentgenogram. The osteoblasts contain abundant rough endoplasmic reticulum, mitochondria, and a well-developed Golgi zone. These features of heightened cellular activity are consistent with the increased bone formation in active lesions. In addition to the increased numbers of osteoclasts and osteoblasts, the marrow in pagetic lesions is often grossly abnormal. The normal hematopoietic elements are usually absent and are replaced by mononuclear cells of indeterminate origin intermixed with highly vascular connective tissue. The bone matrix structure in Paget's disease is extremely abnormal and arises as a consequence of disordered bone resorption and formation. The matrix consists of a "mosaic" of irregularly shaped pieces of lamellar bone with an erratic pattern of cement lines. The matrix is interspersed with numerous foci of woven bone, which, in adults, is ordinarily found associated with fracture healing. After a long time, the lesions become sclerotic. This rapid and abnormal deposition of bone results in the characteristic irregular cement lines that give rise to the mosaic appearance on radiographs and on tissue sections. Marrow vascularity is markedly increased in pagetic

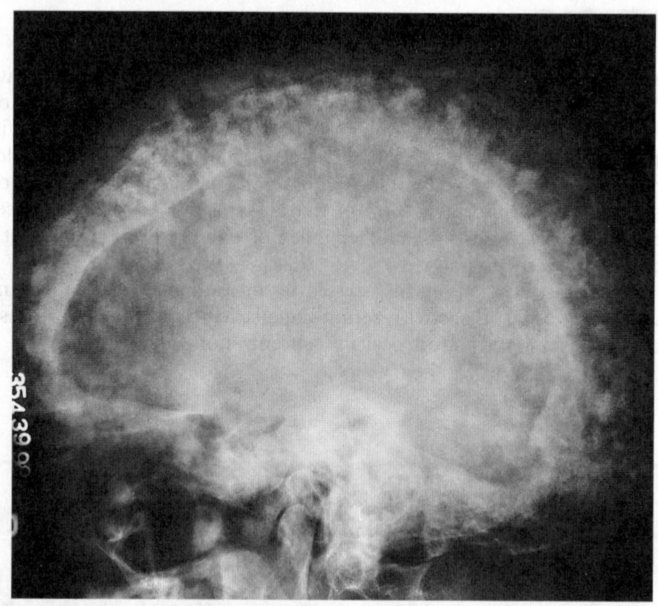

FIGURE 268–2 • Advanced involvement of the skull with marked thickening of the entire vault, areas of osteolysis, and patchy new bone formation resulting in a "cotton-wool" appearance.

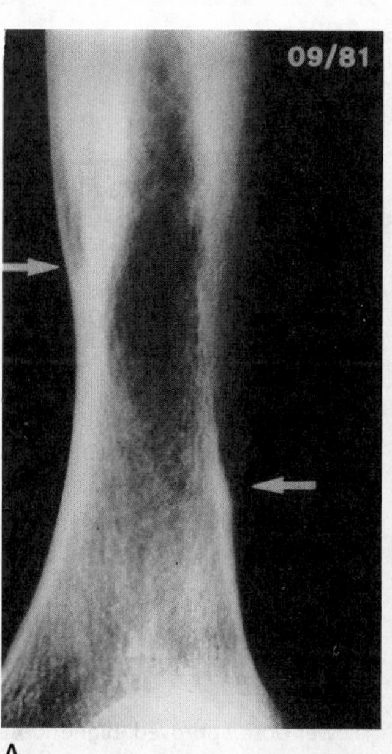

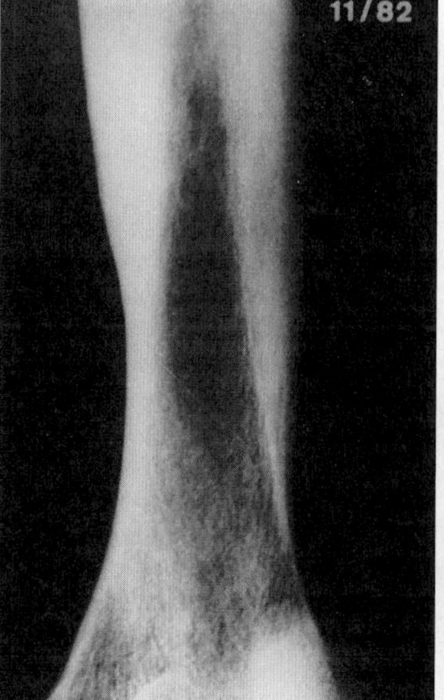

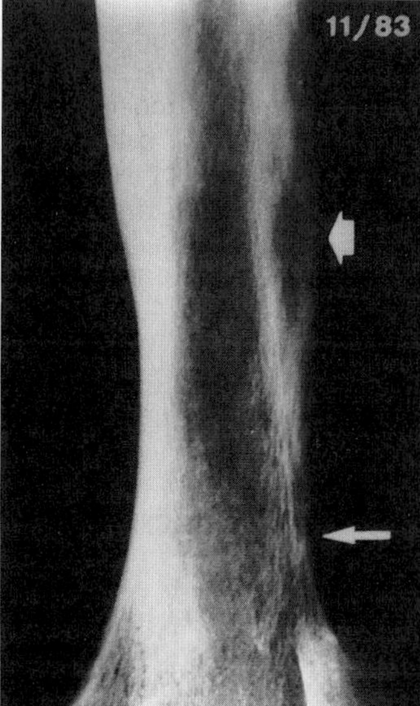

FIGURE 268–1 • Sequential radiographs of the distal end of the femur at the dates shown. A, Distinction between Paget's and normal bone (arrows), the osteolytic front, and expansion of bone diameter at the affected site. **B,** Treatment with a bisphosphonate induced in-filling of the resorption font. **C,** Relapse after treatment was associated with a new area of osteolysis (thick arrow) and progression of the resorption front. (From Kanis JA: Pathophysiology and Treatment of Paget's Disease of Bone, 2nd ed. London, Martin Dunitz, 1998.)

lesions such that the involved bones often feel warm to the touch. Electron microscopy studies of pagetic osteoclasts show nuclear inclusions that resemble paramyxovirus nucleocapsids. However, these nuclear inclusions are not unique to Paget's disease and have been reported in rare cases of osteopetrosis and other bone diseases such as giant cell tumors of bone.

Clinical Manifestations

Most patients with Paget's disease are elderly, and the age at diagnosis is usually greater than 50 years. Paget's disease affects both men and women, with a slight male predominance. Although Paget's disease is often asymptomatic, 10 to 30% of patients experience pain, skeletal deformity, neurologic symptoms, pathologic fractures, or deafness. Patients may have only one affected bone or pagetic lesions in multiple bones. Patients with familial Paget's disease tend to have more bones affected and more deformity than patients with sporadic Paget's disease. Paget's disease remains highly localized, and patients rarely develop new lesions in previously unaffected bones after diagnosis. Table 268–1 lists the common clinical features and complications of Paget's disease.

Diagnosis

The biochemical findings in Paget's disease reflect the cellular events occurring throughout the skeleton of affected patients. Measurement of collagen cross-link degradation products in urine provides a specific measurement of skeletal matrix degradation. Urinary N-telopeptide, pyridinoline, and deoxypyridinoline have all been used as measures of skeletal matrix resorption. Serum tartrate–sensitive acid phosphatase, released by osteoclasts, is another index of bone resorption in Paget's disease research laboratories.

Osteoblast activity can be assessed by measurement of total serum alkaline phosphatase activity, serum bone-specific alkaline phosphatase concentration, serum osteocalcin concentration, and serum type 1 carboxy-terminal procollagen peptide concentration. The most useful of these are the total serum alkaline phosphatase and bone-specific alkaline phosphatase determinations. Total serum alkaline phosphatase measurements are routinely used to monitor disease activity in the clinic.

TABLE 268–1 CLINICAL FEATURES AND COMPLICATIONS OF PAGET'S DISEASE

COMMON
Pagetic or articular bone pain
Fracture of long bones and vertebral bodies
Neurologic deafness
Deformity and enlargement of bones
UNCOMMON
Spinal neurologic syndromes
Hypercalciuria of immobilization or fracture
Vascular bleeding from bone during surgery
Extraskeletal (aortic) calcification
Osteosarcoma and other bone tumors
RARE
Cardiovascular disease
Cranial nerve lesions (except VIII)
Brain stem and cerebellar lesions
Hypercalcemia of immobilization
Extramedullary hematopoiesis
Epidural hematoma
SIGNIFICANCE UNCERTAIN
Gout
Pseudogout
Angioid streaks
Hyperparathyroidism
Urolithiasis

Treatment

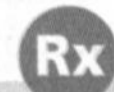

Medical Therapy

Patients with Paget's disease who are symptomatic require treatment. No data support treatment of asymptomatic patients except in the presence of rapidly advancing osteolytic lesions in long bones that are weight bearing, in which the risk of pathologic fractures is increased. Because the osteoclast is the primary cell involved in Paget's disease, medical treatment focused on inhibiting osteoclast activity, in particular the use of bisphosphonates, calcitonin, and mitomycin, has been successful in treating Paget's disease. Salmon calcitonin by injection, which has been used since the early 1980s, is an effective treatment for Paget's disease. This treatment suppresses the biochemical parameters of the disease by 50%. Bisphosphonates, which can inhibit osteoclast formation but predominantly induce osteoclast apoptosis, are the most frequently used treatments for Paget's disease. Bisphosphonates are pyrophosphate derivatives with a high affinity for bone. They are incorporated into sites of bone resorption, released during the resorption process, and taken up by osteoclasts. This process results in the death of osteoclasts. In addition, bisphosphonates have been shown to affect angiogenesis as well as cytokine production by osteoclasts. Because biochemical markers strongly correlate with disease activity, following serum alkaline phosphatase activity is a simple method for monitoring the activity of the disease. Some treatments may result in normalization of both some skeletal abnormalities and the bone scan in these patients. With the availability of more potent bisphosphonates to treat patients with Paget's disease, the prognosis has greatly improved (Table 268–2). A single intravenous dose of 5 mg of zoledronic acid can provide a 96% response rate for the next 6 months and is more effective than 2 months of oral risedronate. 1

Patients treated with bisphosphonates can usually attain remission of the disease. However, after variable periods of time, patients suffer a relapse and require treatment.

Surgical Therapy

Surgery is used to treat fractures and to correct deformity of bowed bones as well as to treat bone disease in the hip. In addition, surgical treatment may relieve the neurologic complications of overgrowth of pagetic bone with resultant nerve root compression. Before elective surgery, patients with Paget's disease are usually treated with bisphosphonates to decrease the vascularity and activity of the bone and to prevent increased bleeding.

TABLE 268–2 BISPHOSPHONATES USED IN TREATMENT OF PAGET'S DISEASE

Agent	Route	Dose (mg/day)	Duration of Effect
Alendronate	Oral	40	6 mo
Clodronate*	Oral	1600	3–6 mo
	Intravenous	300	5 days
Etidronate	Oral	400	6 mo
Pamidronate	Intravenous	30–60†	3 days
Risedronate	Oral	30	2 mo
Tiludronate	Oral	400	3 mo
Zoledronic arid	Intravenous	5 one-time dose	6 mo

*Has not been approved by the Food and Drug Administration at the time of publication.
†Lower dose approved; higher dose used by investigators.

Prognosis

Pagetic bone pain responds to medical treatment. Much of the bone pain associated with Paget's disease results from arthritis or joint pain arising from the bone deformity, rather than pain from the pagetic bone per se. Unless treated, pagetic lesions continue to increase in size, but rarely if ever do patients develop new lesions in a previously unaffected bone. In patients for whom analgesic or other specific treatments are unsuccessful, joint replacement can be performed. The most dreaded complication in Paget's disease is the development of osteosarcoma in the pagetic lesion. Although osteosarcoma is an extremely rare complication, affecting less than 1% of patients with Paget's disease, it is the most common cause of osteosarcoma in adults. Once patients develop osteosarcoma, their prognosis is extremely poor, and the outcome is usually fatal. Active treatment of Paget's disease decreases the biochemical abnormalities, with near normalization of alkaline phosphatase activity, and improves the neurologic syndromes associated with this disease.

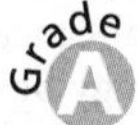

1. Reid IR, Miller P, Lyles K, et al: Comparison of a single infusion of zoledronic acid with risedronate for Paget's disease. N Engl J Med 2005;353:898–908.

SUGGESTED READINGS

Doyle T, Gunn J, Anderson G, et al: Paget's disease in New Zealand: Evidence for declining prevalence. Bone 2002;31:616–619. *The declining prevalence over the past 2 decades suggests important environmental determinants in its development.*

Roodman GD, Windle JJ: Paget disease of bone. J Clin Invest 2005;115:200–208. *Overview of the pathophysiology of Paget's disease.*

Whyte MP: Paget's disease of bone. N Engl J Med 2006;355:593–600. *There is no cure, but antiresorptive treatment reduces pain.*

269 OSTEONECROSIS, OSTEOSCLEROSIS/HYPEROSTOSIS, AND OTHER DISORDERS OF BONE

Michael P. Whyte

OSTEONECROSIS

Definition

Osteonecrosis (aseptic, avascular, or ischemic necrosis of bone) refers to skeletal infarction. Bone infarcts may be asymptomatic, cause self-limited discomfort, or engender painful collapse of subarticular bone that leads to joint destruction.

Pathobiology and Pathogenesis

Many conditions are associated with osteonecrosis (Table 269–1). In adults, the most common causes are ethanol abuse and long-term glucocorticoid therapy, both of which have dose-dependent effects.

Skeletal infarction may result from blood vessel destruction (e.g., joint dislocation, fracture), obstruction (e.g., thromboemboli, sickle cell disease, fat emboli, caisson disease), or, hypothetically, compression from local expansion of fatty tissue (e.g., ethanol abuse, glucocorticoid treatment, diabetes mellitus). However, symptoms may not occur unless, weeks later, resorption of dead bone during skeletal repair leads to pathologic fracture. Certain skeletal sites (often subarticular) are predisposed to osteonecrosis but differ for traumatic and nontraumatic processes and for children and adults. *Osteochondrosis* refers to necrosis of ossification centers; more than 50 eponymic types are recorded. The susceptibility of children to osteochondrosis and its pathogenesis are poorly understood. At all ages, however, the femoral head is especially prone to infarction. Nontraumatic osteonecrosis also commonly affects the femoral condyles, distal end of the tibia, humeral head, and talus.

TABLE 269–1 CAUSES OF ISCHEMIC NECROSIS OF CARTILAGE AND BONE

Endocrine/metabolic
Ethanol abuse
Glucocorticoid therapy
Cushing's disease
Diabetes mellitus
Hyperuricemia
Osteomalacia
Hyperlipidemia
Bisphosphonate therapy
Storage diseases (e.g., Gaucher's disease)
Hemoglobinopathies (e.g., sickle cell disease)
Trauma (e.g., dislocation, fracture)
Human immunodeficiency virus infection
Dysbaric conditions (e.g., caisson disease)
Collagen-vascular disorders
Irradiation
Pancreatitis
Organ transplantation
Hemodialysis
Burns
Intravascular coagulation
Idiopathic, familial

Clinical Manifestations

Pain occurs acutely on skeletal collapse. Chronic arthralgia results from desquamated necrotic tissue and articular destruction.

Diagnosis

Magnetic resonance imaging demonstrating bone marrow edema is especially sensitive for detecting early osteonecrosis. Bone scintigraphy discloses skeletal reconstitution with or without fracture. Relatively late in the pathologic process, radiographs first show patchy areas of osteopenia and osteosclerosis that reflect skeletal repair. A linear subchondral radiolucency (crescent sign) indicates bony collapse.

Treatment

Non-weight-bearing is advisable for an affected limb. Decompression by trephine insertion is used for some sites. Arthrotomy to remove debris, transpositional osteotomy, arthroplasty, or joint replacement may be necessary.

OSTEOSCLEROSIS/HYPEROSTOSIS

Many conditions are associated with radiographic evidence of increased bone density. Skeletal dysplasias, metabolic disturbances, and various other disorders can cause generalized or focal increases in bone mass (Table 269–2). Aberrations in skeletal growth, modeling (shaping), and/or remodeling (turnover) may be at fault. *Osteosclerosis* refers to thickening of trabecular (spongy, cancellous) bone. *Hyperostosis* describes widening of cortical (compact) bone. Increases in trabecular or cortical bone or both may augment skeletal density.

Osteosclerosis

Neoplastic, hematologic, and metabolic disorders may preferentially cause sclerosis in trabecular bone because it houses marrow and remodels more rapidly than cortical bone.

TABLE 269–2 DISORDERS THAT CAUSE DENSE BONES

DYSPLASIAS
Central osteosclerosis with ectodermal dysplasia
Craniodiaphyseal dysplasia
Craniometaphyseal dysplasia
Dysosteosclerosis
Endosteal hyperostosis
van Buchem's disease
Sclerosteosis
Worth-type (LRP5 activation)
Frontometaphyseal dysplasia
Infantile cortical hyperostosis (Caffey's disease)
Juvenile Paget's disease
Lenz-Majewski syndrome
Melorheostosis
Metaphyseal dysplasia (Pyle's disease)
Mixed-sclerosing-bone dystrophy
Oculodento-osseous dysplasia
Osteodysplasia of Melnick and Needles
Osteopathia striata
Osteopetrosis
Osteopoikilosis
Progressive diaphyseal dysplasia (Engelmann's disease)
Pycnodysostosis
METABOLIC CONDITIONS
Carbonic anhydrase II deficiency
Fluorosis
Heavy metal poisoning
Hepatitis C–associated osteosclerosis
Hypervitaminosis A, D
Hyperparathyroidism, hypoparathyroidism, and pseudohypoparathyroidism
Hypophosphatemic rickets or osteomalacia
Milk-alkali syndrome
Renal osteodystrophy
OTHER DISORDERS
Axial osteomalacia
Fibrogenesis imperfecta ossium
High bone mass (with or without torus palatinus): LRP5 activation
Ionizing radiation
Lymphoma
Mastocytosis
Multiple myeloma
Myelofibrosis
Osteomyelitis
Osteonecrosis
Paget's bone disease
Sarcoidosis
Skeletal metastases
Tuberous sclerosis

From Whyte MP: Skeletal disorders characterized by osteosclerosis or hyperostosis. *In* Avioli LV, Krane SM (eds): Metabolic Bone Disease, 3rd ed. San Diego, Academic Press, 1998.

Fibrogenesis Imperfecta Ossium

Definition

This rare, sporadic condition features generalized osteopenia, but coarsening of remaining trabeculae places it among disorders of increased bone mass.

Pathobiology

The cause is unknown. Subperiosteal bone formation and collagen synthesis in nonosseous tissues seem to be normal.

Clinical Manifestations

Typically, intractable skeletal pain begins gradually during middle age or later and then rapidly increases with a debilitating course and immobility. Spontaneous fractures are a prominent complication. Physical examination reveals marked bony tenderness.

Diagnosis

On radiographic study, only the skull is spared. Initially, osteopenia and a slightly abnormal appearance of trabecular bone are noted. Subsequently, the changes suggest osteomalacia. Corticomedullary junctions become indistinct as compact bone is replaced by an abnormal cancellous pattern. Generalized osteopenia causes the remaining spongy bone to appear coarse and dense in a fishnet pattern of mixed lytic and sclerotic areas. Alkaline phosphatase activity in serum is increased.

The skeletal lesion is a localized form of osteomalacia that varies considerably in severity from area to area. In diseased regions, polarized light microscopy shows collagen fibrils that lack birefringence, and electron microscopy reveals that they are thin and randomly organized.

Hyperostosis

Progressive Diaphyseal Dysplasia (Camurati-Engelmann Disease)

Pathobiology

Progressive diaphyseal dysplasia (Camurati-Engelmann disease) affects all races and is inherited as an autosomal dominant trait with variable penetrance. New bone formation gradually envelops both the periosteal and endosteal surfaces of long bone diaphyses. In patients with severe disease, osteosclerosis also occurs in the axial skeleton.

Mutations compromise the gene that encodes transforming growth factor-β. Osteoblast differentiation may also be deranged.

Clinical Manifestations

During childhood, limping or a broad-based and waddling gait is noted. Muscular dystrophy can be diagnosed erroneously. Severely affected individuals may have a characteristic body habitus featuring an enlarged head with prominent forehead, proptosis, and thin limbs with little subcutaneous fat or muscle mass and tender thickened bones. Cranial nerve palsies and raised intracranial pressure can occur. Some patients have hepatosplenomegaly, Raynaud's phenomenon, and additional findings suggestive of vasculitis. Symptoms may remit after puberty.

Diagnosis

Irregular hyperostosis of the diaphyses of the major long bones slowly develops as a result of periosteal and endosteal new bone formation. Femora and tibiae are most commonly affected. Metaphyses may eventually become involved. The age of onset, rate of progression, and severity are variable. Clinical, radiographic, and bone scan findings are generally concordant. Routine biochemical parameters of bone and mineral metabolism are typically normal, although serum alkaline phosphatase activity, urinary hydroxyproline levels, and the erythrocyte sedimentation rate can be elevated. Histopathologic study reveals newly formed woven bone that matures and becomes incorporated into cortical bone. Electron microscopy of muscle may show myopathic changes and vascular abnormalities.

Treatment 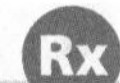

Glucocorticoid therapy (typically a low dose of prednisone on alternate days) can relieve bone pain and may normalize skeletal histology. Bisphosphonates have sometimes been useful.

Endosteal Hyperostosis

Pathobiology

Sclerosteosis and van Buchem's disease, autosomal recessive disorders, are the principal types of endosteal hyperostosis. Sclerosteosis and van Buchem's disease both map to chromosome 17q12-q21. Sclerosteosis is caused by mutations in a gene called *SOST.* Van Buchem's disease involves a downstream deletion. Enhanced osteoblast activity with failure of osteoclasts to compensate for the increased bone formation seems to explain the skeletal changes.

Clinical Manifestations

Sclerosteosis (cortical hyperostosis with syndactyly) occurs primarily in Afrikaners of South Africa. Elsewhere, Dutch ancestry is also common. Gender distribution appears equal. Patients are tall and heavy beginning in childhood, have a prominent and square mandible, and have deafness and facial nerve palsy from cranial nerve entrapment. Raised intracranial pressure and headache may reflect a small cranial cavity that can shorten life expectancy. Van Buchem's disease causes progressive asymmetrical enlargement of the jaw during puberty, but prognathism is not a feature. Patients may be symptom free, or, beginning as early as infancy, they may have recurrent facial nerve palsy, deafness, and optic atrophy from narrowing of cranial foramina. Long bones may hurt with applied pressure but are not fragile.

Diagnosis

In sclerosteosis, the skeleton is radiographically normal in early childhood, except when bony syndactyly is present. Syndactyly is common, most often involving the index and third fingers. Progressive bony thickening widens the skull and causes prognathism. Long bones have thickened cortices. The pelvis, vertebral pedicles, ribs, and other tubular bones may become dense. Computed tomography has shown fusion of ossicles and narrowing of the internal auditory canals and cochlear aqueducts. In van Buchem's disease, endosteal thickening homogeneously widens diaphyseal cortices and narrows medullary canals. Bones are properly modeled. Osteosclerosis involves the skull base, facial bones, vertebrae, pelvis, and ribs. Serum alkaline phosphatase activity can be increased from enhanced skeletal formation.

Treatment 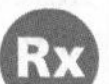

Surgical decompression of narrowed foramina may alleviate cranial nerve palsies.

Pachydermoperiostosis

Pathobiology

Pachydermoperiostosis (hypertrophic osteoarthropathy, primary or idiopathic) is an autosomal dominant disorder that features clubbing of the digits, hyperhidrosis with thickening of the skin (especially of the face), and periosteal new bone formation prominently in the distal ends of the limbs. Autosomal recessive inheritance also seems to occur. Not all patients manifest all three principal features.

The genetic defect is unknown. A controversial hypothesis suggests that initially some circulating factor acts on the vasculature to cause hyperemia and thereby alters soft tissues, but later blood flow is reduced.

Clinical Manifestations

Men seem to be more severely affected than women and blacks more commonly than whites. Symptoms typically begin during adolescence, intensify during the next decade, but then become quiescent. Arthralgia and fatigue are common. Stiffness and limited mobility occur in both the appendicular and the axial skeleton. Clubbing, with slowly progressive enlargement of the hands and feet, results in a pawlike appearance. Cutaneous changes include thickening, furrowing, pitting, and oiliness, especially of the scalp and face.

Diagnosis

Periostitis thickens the distal portions of the tibia, fibula, radius, and ulna. Clubbing is obvious, and acro-osteolysis can occur. Periosteal proliferation is exuberant, with irregular texture, and it often involves the epiphyses, whereas secondary hypertrophic osteoarthropathy (pulmonary or otherwise) typically causes a smooth and undulating periosteal reaction. Ankylosis of joints, especially in the hands and feet, may trouble older patients. Bone scanning in either condition reveals symmetrical, diffuse, regular uptake along the cortical margins of long bones, especially in the legs—the "double-stripe" sign.

Treatment 

Patients with painful synovial effusions may respond to nonsteroidal anti-inflammatory drugs. Contractures or neurovascular compression by osteosclerotic lesions may require surgical intervention.

OSTEOSCLEROSIS WITH HYPEROSTOSIS

Osteopetrosis

Pathobiology

Osteopetrosis (marble bone disease) occurs in two major clinical forms: the autosomal recessive or "malignant" type, which kills during infancy or early childhood if it is untreated; and the autosomal dominant or "benign" type, which causes fewer problems. Other autosomal recessive types feature intermediate severity, neuronal storage disease, stillbirth, or renal tubular acidosis with cerebral calcification secondary to carbonic anhydrase II isoenzyme deficiency. Bisphosphonate-induced osteopetrosis has been reported.

Pathogenesis

The defective gene causing autosomal dominant osteopetrosis encodes a chloride channel important for osteoclast activity. Abnormalities in this gene or one that encodes a subunit of a vacuolar proton pump can also result in malignant disease. Carbonic anhydrase II deficiency is caused by deactivating mutations in the gene that encodes this isoenzyme.

Histopathologic studies show that all true forms of osteopetrosis feature profound deficiency of osteoclast action. Primary spongiosa (calcified cartilage deposited during endochondral bone formation) persists away from growth plates and constitutes the pathognomonic finding. Defective endosteal bone resorption impairs the formation of marrow space. Quiescent skeletal remodeling leads to bone fragility from diminished interconnection of osteons and from delayed conversion of immature (woven) bone to mature (compact) bone. Studies of animal models of osteopetrosis suggest that, rarely, some patients have abnormalities as distal as the marrow microenvironment that compromise osteoclast precursor cell growth and differentiation or abnormalities as proximal as bone tissue itself, with resistance to degradation. Neuronal storage disease (ceroid lipofuscin) could reflect a lysosomal defect. Deficient superoxide production (necessary for bone resorption) may also be a pathogenetic factor. Viral-like inclusions in osteoclasts are of uncertain significance.

Clinical Manifestations

Malignant osteopetrosis can first manifest during infancy as nasal "stuffiness" from underdeveloped mastoid and paranasal sinuses. Small cranial foramina may cause optic, oculomotor, or facial nerve palsy. Failure to thrive, delayed dentition, and fracture are common. Hypersplenism and recurrent infection, bruising, and bleeding reflect myelophthisis. Short stature, large head, frontal bossing, nystagmus, hepatosplenomegaly, and genu valgum are characteristic physical features. Untreated children usually die during the first decade of life of hemorrhage, pneumonia, severe anemia, or sepsis. Benign osteopetrosis occasionally causes fracture, facial palsy, deafness, mandibular osteomyelitis, bone marrow failure, impaired vision, psychomotor delay, carpal tunnel syndrome, or osteoarthritis. Carbonic anhydrase II deficiency can result in failure to thrive, fracture, developmental delay, mental subnormality, and short stature. Cerebral calcification develops during childhood, but defective skeletal modeling and osteosclerosis may correct spontaneously. Both proximal renal tubular acidosis and distal renal tubular acidosis have been described.

Diagnosis

A generalized increase in bone density is the radiographic hallmark. In severe disease, modeling defects in long bones produce an "Erlenmeyer flask" deformity (Fig. 269–1). Alternating dense and lucent bands commonly occur in the metaphyses and pelvis. The cranium is usually thickened and dense, especially at the base, and the paranasal and mastoid sinuses are underpneumatized. Vertebrae may show, on lateral view, a "bone-in-bone" (endobone) configuration or end-plate sclerosis causing a "rugger jersey" appearance. Skeletal scintigraphy can disclose fractures and osteomyelitis. Magnetic resonance imaging helps the clinician to monitor the response to bone marrow transplantation because successful engraftment normalizes bone marrow signals.

Serum levels of acid phosphatase and creatine kinase (brain isoenzyme), apparently from osteoclasts, are abnormal. In malignant osteopetrosis, hypocalcemia with secondary hyperparathyroidism and elevated serum concentrations of calcitriol can accompany radiographic changes that resemble rickets. In benign osteopetrosis, biochemical indices of mineral homeostasis are typically unremarkable, although serum parathyroid hormone levels may be increased.

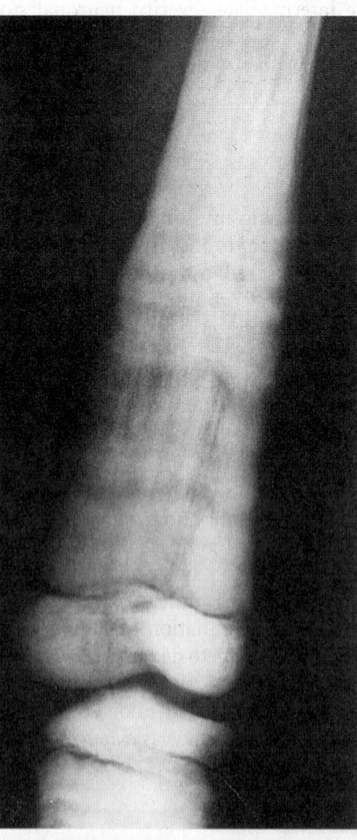

FIGURE 269–1 • Osteopetrosis. An anteroposterior radiograph of the distal end of the femur shows a widened metadiaphyseal region with characteristic alternating dense and lucent bands. (From Whyte MP, Murphy WA: Osteopetrosis and other sclerosing bone disorders. *In* Avioli LV, Krane SM [eds]: Metabolic Bone Disease, 2nd ed. Philadelphia, WB Saunders, 1990.)

Treatment

Rx

Because the origin, pathogenesis, and prognosis of the osteopetroses differ, correct classification is crucial. It may be necessary to evaluate disease progression and to study the family. For the malignant form, human leukocyte antigen (HLA)–identical bone marrow transplantation to supply functional osteoclasts has remarkably benefited some children. Calcium-deficient diets have been used but may be limited by hypocalcemia and rickets. Massive oral doses of calcitriol (1,25-dihydroxyvitamin D_3), together with dietary calcium restriction (to prevent hypercalciuria/hypercalcemia) or human interferon-γ, which enhances superoxide production, have successfully stimulated osteoclast activity. Prednisone, alone or with a low-calcium, high-phosphate diet, may also be effective. Glucocorticoid therapy stabilizes pancytopenia and hepatosplenomegaly. Hyperbaric oxygenation helps in the treatment of osteomyelitis. Surgical decompression of optic and facial nerves can be beneficial. Early prenatal diagnosis, radiographically or by ultrasound, has not been successful. Mutation analysis is now useful in many affected families.

Pycnodysostosis

Epidemiology

Pycnodysostosis is believed to have troubled the French impressionist painter Henri de Toulouse-Lautrec (1864–1901). Most descriptions have come from Europe and the United States, but the disorder seems to be especially common in Japan.

Pathobiology

This autosomal recessive condition is caused by defects in the gene that encodes cathepsin K. Diminished rates of collagen degradation and skeletal turnover are reported. In chondrocytes and osteoblasts, abnormal inclusions have been described.

Clinical Manifestations

Characteristic features seen during infancy or early childhood are disproportionate short stature, a relatively large cranium, fronto-occipital prominence, proptosis, bluish sclerae, a beaked and pointed nose, small facies and chin, an obtuse mandibular angle, a high-arched palate, and dental malocclusion with retention of primary teeth. Cranial sutures remain open. Fingers are short and clubbed from acro-osteolysis or aplasia of the terminal phalanges, and the hands are small and square. Repeated fractures cause knock-knee deformity. Mental retardation is noted in approximately 10% of patients. Adult height ranges from 4 ft 3 in to 4 ft 11 in. Life expectancy can be shortened by recurrent respiratory infections and right-sided heart failure from chronic upper airway obstruction secondary to micrognathia.

Diagnosis

Osteosclerosis is uniform, first becoming apparent in childhood and increasing with age. Skeletal modeling defects do not occur, although long bones appear to have thick cortices because of narrow medullary canals. Clavicles are gracile and hypoplastic at their lateral segments. The calvarium and base of the skull are sclerotic, orbital ridges are dense, and wormian bones are present. Serum calcium and inorganic phosphate levels and alkaline phosphatase activity are typically normal. Anemia is not a problem.

Treatment

No effective medical therapy is documented. Fractures of the long bones usually mend satisfactorily. Internal fixation of long bones is formidable because of their hardness. Tooth extraction is difficult. Osteomyelitis of the mandible may require antibiotic, surgical, and/or hyperbaric therapy.

Hepatitis C–Associated Osteosclerosis

Rarely, achy and tender limbs develop in individuals who are infected with hepatitis C virus. Radiographic studies reveal a marked generalized increase in bone mass from osteosclerosis and hyperostosis. Disturbances in the insulin-like growth factor system may explain the enhanced bone formation. Calcitonin or bisphosphonate therapy has benefited some patients.

FOCAL OSTEOSCLEROSIS/HYPEROSTOSIS

Osteopoikilosis

Osteopoikilosis ("spotted bones") is a radiologic curiosity inherited as a highly penetrant autosomal dominant trait resulting from a deactivating mutation of the *LEMD3* gene. The bony lesions are asymptomatic. However, incorrect diagnosis may lead to confusion with serious conditions, including metastatic disease. Some patients have connective tissue nevi called *dermatofibrosis lenticularis disseminata* (i.e., Buschke-Ollendorff syndrome). Radiologically, numerous small round or oval foci of bony sclerosis appear in cancellous bone in the tarsal, carpal, pelvic, and metaepiphyseal regions of tubular bones.

Osteopathia Striata

This autosomal dominant curiosity features linear striations in the metaphyseal regions of long bones and in the ilium. Clinically important syndromes include osteopathia striata with cranial sclerosis or with focal dermal hypoplasia (Goltz's syndrome). Goltz's syndrome is an X-linked recessive condition featuring widespread linear areas of dermal hypoplasia and various bony defects in the limbs of affected male patients.

Melorheostosis

Definition

Melorheostosis causes bony changes likened to wax that has dripped down a candle. No mendelian basis for this disorder has been established. The anatomic distribution suggests a segmentary embryogenic defect.

Clinical Manifestations

Usually, monomelic involvement is noted; bilateral disease is generally asymmetrical. Cutaneous changes over affected bones are common (e.g., linear scleroderma-like areas and hypertrichosis). Soft tissue abnormalities often appear before the hyperostosis. Symptoms typically begin during childhood, with pain and stiffness the major complaints. Joints may become contracted and deformed. Leg length inequality results from soft tissue contractures and premature fusion of epiphyses. Skeletal changes seem to progress most rapidly throughout childhood. During adult life, melorheostosis may or may not gradually spread, although pain is especially common.

Diagnosis

As seen radiographically, irregular, very dense, eccentric periosteal and endosteal hyperostosis affects a single bone or several adjacent bones. The lower limbs are most commonly involved. Endosteal thickening predominates during infancy and childhood, and periosteal new bone formation is prominent during adulthood. Ectopic bone formation may occur, particularly near joints.

Treatment

Rx

Surgical correction of contractures is difficult. Recurrent deformity is common.

Mixed-Sclerosing-Bone Dystrophy

This typically sporadic disorder features combinations of osteopoikilosis, osteopathia striata, melorheostosis, cranial sclerosis, or other skeletal defects in one individual. Patients may experience problems associated with the individual patterns of osteosclerosis or hyperostosis, such as nerve palsy with cranial sclerosis and bone pain with melorheostosis.

OTHER DISORDERS OF BONE

Fibrous Dysplasia

This sporadic, developmental disorder features an expansile fibrous lesion within bone. Polyostotic disease is typically seen before the age of 10 years; monostotic disease begins in adolescence or early adult life. *McCune-Albright syndrome* refers to a condition characterized by polyostotic fibrous dysplasia, café au lait spots (Fig. 269–2), and endocrine hyperfunction.

Pathobiology

Postzygotic mosaicism for an activating mutation in the gene that encodes the α subunit of the receptor subunit/adenylate cyclase–coupling G protein causes fibrous dysplasia and the McCune-Albright syndrome. Imperfect bone forms because mesenchymal cells do not fully differentiate to osteoblasts. Endocrinopathy generally results from end-organ hyperactivity.

Clinical Manifestations

Monostotic fibrous dysplasia is more common than polyostotic disease. The skull and long bones are affected most often. The skeletal lesions can deform bones, cause fractures, and occasionally entrap nerves. Sarcomatous degeneration is rare (incidence, <1%), but it typically occurs within the facial bones or femur and is more frequent when polyostotic disease is present. Pregnancy may reactivate previously quiescent lesions. McCune-Albright syndrome usually causes pseudoprecocious puberty in girls. Less commonly, one sees pseudoprecocious puberty in boys or thyrotoxicosis, Cushing's disease, acromegaly, hyperprolactinemia, or hyperparathyroidism. In some patients, acquired renal phosphate wasting causes hypophosphatemic rickets or osteomalacia.

Diagnosis

As seen radiographically, in the long bones, lesions are found in either the metaphysis or the diaphysis. They are typically well defined with thin cortices and have a ground-glass appearance (Fig. 269–3).

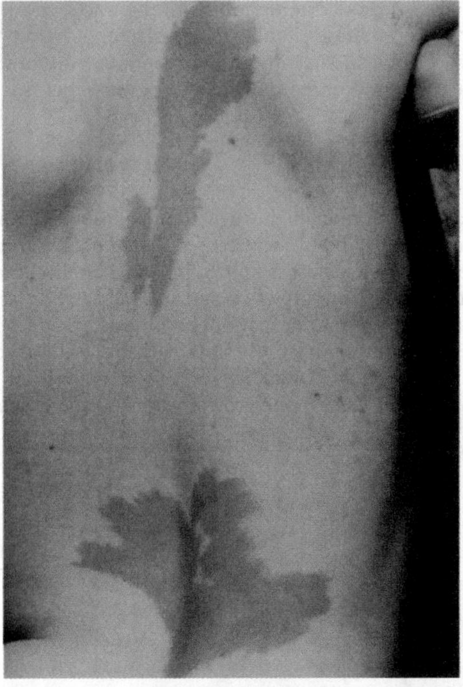

FIGURE 269–2 • McCune-Albright syndrome. Typical rough-border ("coast-of-Maine") pigmented café au lait spots. (From Whyte MP: Metabolic and dysplastic disorders. *In* Coe FL, Favus MJ [eds]: Disorders of Bone and Mineral Metabolism. New York, Raven Press, 1992.)

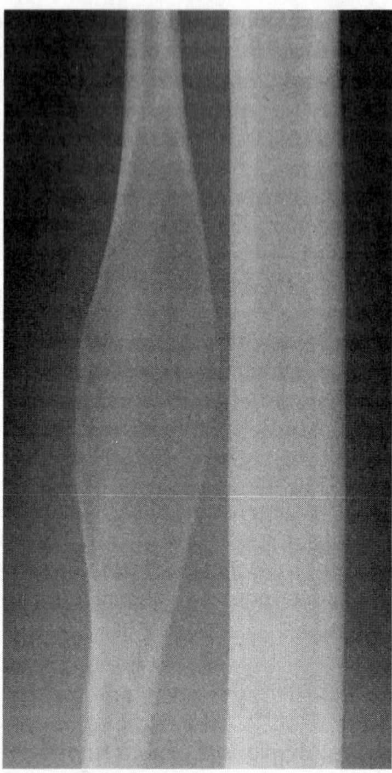

FIGURE 269–3 • Fibrous dysplasia. A characteristic expansile lesion with a ground-glass appearance has caused thinning of the cortex in the mid-diaphysis of the fibula. (From Whyte MP: Fibrous dysplasia. *In* Favus MJ [ed]: Primer on the Metabolic Bone Diseases and Disorders of Mineral Metabolism, 3rd ed. Philadelphia, Lippincott-Raven, 1996.)

Occasionally, the defects are lobulated, with trabeculated areas of radiolucency.

Treatment

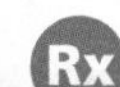

In patients with mild disease, bone lesions may not expand. In severe cases, individual defects can progress and new ones may appear. Spontaneous healing does not occur, but pathologic fractures generally mend well. Stress fractures, however, can be difficult to detect and treat. When the skull is involved, nerve compression may require surgical intervention. In the McCune-Albright syndrome, the aromatase inhibitor testolactone helps to control pseudoprecocious puberty in girls. Intravenous infusions of the bisphosphonate pamidronate have helped some patients.

Hereditary Multiple Exostoses

This relatively common, highly penetrant, autosomal dominant disorder features irregular bony excrescences that protrude from expanded metaphyses. The gene defect is known in some families. Osteocartilaginous exostoses arise from growth plates and increase in size until linear growth ceases. Lesions may or may not become detached from the parent bone. Their structure is relatively unremarkable, with an outer cortex and an inner spongiosa. Disability results primarily from limb length discrepancies when linear bone growth suffers at the expense of transverse expansion. Compression of nerves, the spinal cord, or the vascular system occurs occasionally. Sarcomatous degeneration (0.5 to 2% of patients) should be suspected when an exostosis enlarges rapidly, especially during adult life.

Enchondromatosis (Dyschondroplasia, Ollier's Disease)

This sporadic disorder features cartilaginous masses within the trabecular bone that arise from growth plates. The condition begins in childhood with localized swelling and interferes with linear bone growth. At puberty, expansion of cartilage masses ceases, and these masses can be replaced by mature bone. Enchondromas appear radiographically as lucent defects in flat bones or in metaphyses of tubular bones, often with central calcific stippling. When enchondromatosis occurs with multiple hemangiomas (Maffucci's syndrome), the enchondromas or hemangiomas undergo malignant transformation in approximately 15% of cases.

Achondroplasia

Chondrodystrophies are disorders of cartilage growth that result in disproportionate short stature. Achondroplasia is the most common. A defect occurs in the gene that encodes fibroblast growth factor receptor type 3. Approximately 80% of cases are new mutations for this autosomal dominant defect, which increases in frequency with increasing paternal age. Short, tubular bones form because of abnormal endochondral ossification in the limbs. In the chondrocranium, membranous ossification is undisturbed, hence the skull vault is normal. However, the cranial base and foramen magnum are small. Lumbar lordosis is greatly exaggerated, and the spinal canal narrows from the upper to lower segments of the vertebral column. This disturbance is revealed radiographically by decreasing interpediculate distance. The head is large with frontal bossing and midface hypoplasia. The trunk is of relatively normal length, but the limbs show rhizomelic shortening, and the hands have a trident configuration. The long bones appear massive owing to their disproportionately normal width. Surprisingly, growth plates are not grossly disorganized in achondroplasia, and chondrocytes appear normal. Complications can include hydrocephalus or compression of the brain stem, spinal cord, or nerve roots. Minimal impingement by a disk or osteophyte on the small spinal canal can cause neurologic disturbances. Despite its problems, achondroplasia is compatible with good health and a normal life span.

SUGGESTED READINGS

Bilezikian JP: Osteonecrosis of the jaw—do bisphosphonates pose a risk? N Engl J Med 2006;355:2278–2281. *An observed side effect of nitrogen-containing bisphosphonates.*

Hernigou P, Bachir D, Galacteros F: The natural history of symptomatic osteonecrosis in adults with sickle-cell disease. J Bone Joint Surg Am 2003;85:500–504. *When osteonecrosis develops, the deterioration is rapid, and, in most patients, operative intervention is necessary because of intractable pain.*

Lieberman JR, Berry DJ, Mont MA, et al: Osteonecrosis of the hip: Management in the 21st century. Instr Course Lect 2003;52:337–355. *Recommended procedures include core decompression, vascularized and nonvascularized bone grafting procedures, and arthroplasty.*

Mader R: Clinical manifestations of diffuse idiopathic skeletal hyperostosis of the cervical spine. Semin Arthritis Rheum 2002;32:130–135. *Patients often present with abnormalities of the pharynx, larynx, and esophagus.*

Tolar J, Teitelbaum SL, Orchard PJ: Osteopetrosis. N Engl J Med 2004;351: 2839–2849. *A scholarly review.*

Section XXI

Diseases of Allergy and Clinical Immunology

270 APPROACH TO THE PATIENT WITH ALLERGIC OR IMMUNOLOGIC DISEASE

Stephen I. Wasserman

Allergic diseases and disorders of the immune system affect multiple organ systems and may arise in a variety of manners. The reader is directed to Chapters 42 to 47 for detailed discussion of the immune system and for specific autoimmune and acquired immune disorders. This chapter addresses allergic disorders, the most common manifestation of immune system dysfunction, and primary immune deficiencies, which are uncommon manifestations of immune dysfunction. For clarity, these two issues are treated separately.

ALLERGIC DISEASE

Definition

Allergic disorders are common, and their prevalence is increasing, particularly in urbanized, Western societies. It is said that allergic diseases are the most common disorders seen by a primary care physician. Moreover, even in nonallergic patients, consideration of allergy frequently enters the differential diagnosis of a problem under consideration. Therefore, an appreciation of how to approach the diagnosis and treatment of allergic patients is of major importance to the practice of internal medicine. Allergic disorders are those caused by the interaction of a sensitized host (one who has made immunoglobulin E [IgE] antibody recognizing a specific antigen) with a specific allergen. Not all patients possessing specific IgE antibody react adversely on interaction with the allergen, and such individuals are termed *sensitized* but not *allergic.* The primary allergic conditions are seasonal allergic rhinoconjunctivitis (hay fever), perennial allergic rhinitis or sinusitis, asthma, anaphylaxis (especially secondary to foods, medications, and hymenopteran stings), urticaria or angioedema, atopic dermatitis (eczema), and food allergy.

Epidemiology

It is currently estimated that more than 50% of the population is atopic (i.e., able to mount an IgE immune response and to exhibit a positive prick puncture immediate hypersensitivity response to common aeroallergens). Clinically, 10 to 20% of the general population will develop allergic rhinoconjunctivitis, 5 to 7% will have active asthma, and 20% will experience urticaria at some time.

The increase in allergic diseases noted in the past 2 decades is thought to result from advancing hygienic conditions, decreases in infant and childhood infections, and an increasingly sedentary and indoor lifestyle. These changes appear to be associated with a less effective activation of the innate immune system, thereby altering the protective maturation of the acquired immune system. The immune bias in utero and in infancy is toward a type 2 helper T-lymphocyte (T_H2)-directed immune response, which is the immune pathway required for the expression of allergic disease. Ineffective generation of regulatory T lymphocytes underlies the genesis and persistence of allergy. It is therefore postulated that without sufficient early childhood infection to induce a switch to an effective and protective T_H1 immune response, allergic disease is more likely to emerge during childhood. Substantial epidemiologic evidence has been gathered to support this concept, now termed the *hygiene hypothesis.* Thus, allergy is more prevalent in individuals of higher socioeconomic status, in those living in urban areas, in less polluted communities (e.g., Western Germany), in first-born children compared with later siblings, in those multiply immunized, and in those free of mycobacterial disease. Conversely, children living on farms, in rural communities, and in more highly polluted areas (e.g., Eastern Germany), as well as those children with mycobacterial infection and those who have experienced multiple early childhood infections, are less likely to develop allergic disorders. A concentration-effect relationship appears to exist between exposure to endotoxin (as a marker for hygiene) and the incidence of allergic sensitization. Low and very high levels of exposure to endotoxin are associated with abnormal immune maturation and allergic expression, whereas moderate levels of exposure predispose to a nonallergic phenotype.

Pathobiology

The persistence or aberrant activation of T_H2 lymphocytes leads to the generation of cytokines (e.g., interleukins-4, 5, 13) that stimulate B-lymphocyte synthesis of IgE antibody and the production of eosinophilic polymorphonuclear leukocytes. The expression of allergic disorders results from the interaction of specific allergen with allergen-reactive IgE bound to high-affinity receptors on mast cells and basophils. This interaction leads to activation of these target cells and to their release of preformed, granule-associated mediators (exemplified by histamine), synthesis of lipid mediators from membrane lipids (sulfidopeptide leukotrienes), and the transcription and secretion of cytokines including tumor necrosis factor-α and interleukins-4, 5, and 13. These mediators directly induce smooth muscle contraction, vascular dilation, and endothelial leakage; they also cause vascular adhesion molecule expression, and they attract and activate inflammatory leukocytes, particularly $CD4^+$ T lymphocytes, basophils, and eosinophils. These and other IgE-dependent mediators are thought to be responsible for stimulating smooth muscle proliferation and tissue remodeling.

Diagnosis

Allergy is a systemic immune disorder, and thus its expression can be multifocal. It is essential to remember this fact during the approach to the patient with suspected allergic problems because a focus only on the major presenting symptom may be insufficient to identify all the pertinent medical issues present in a given patient.

History

Allergic disease has a high degree of heritability, with a great degree of concordance in identical twins. The risk of expressing allergic disease is highest if both parents are atopic. The inheritance of specific manifestations of allergy and of the specific allergen to which a patient is sensitized is less simple. Quite often, the diagnosis of allergic disorders is straightforward and may be made by asking about the nature of the patient's complaints, when and where reactions occur, and what exposures the patient believes are relevant to symptom induction or exacerbation (Table 270–1).

Seasonal and Perennial Rhinitis

Patients with seasonal and perennial rhinitis commonly present with complaints of itchy nose and palate, sneezing, watery rhinorrhea, itching, watery and burning eyes, and nasal obstruction, which, when severe, may cause anosmia. In the evaluation of possible causes of seasonal rhinoconjunctivitis or sinusitis, the time of the year when symptoms occur is pertinent to the association of symptoms with pollination of trees (early spring), grasses (late spring and summer), and weeds (fall). In some patients with perennial symptoms, the multiple overlapping pollen seasons are responsible for their symptoms. Indoor exposures at home, school, workplace, or recreational site to furred animals, house dust mites or insects, and mold should be addressed in the search for additional causes of perennial symptoms. Molds and mites are to be expected in humid environments, and mites are nearly ubiquitous in bedding and in homes with pets, carpeting, and overstuffed furnishings. Additional occupational or recreational exposures may be pertinent in selected situations (i.e., bakers, health care workers, food handlers, horse fanciers, laboratory animal handlers, and others) in which specific, inciting allergens may be identified. Because many patients with rhinitis have concomitant asthma, it is important to obtain historical information regarding the presence of this disease in patients with rhinitis.

Asthma

Patients with asthma (Chapter 87) may present with cough or wheeze with dyspnea, which is reversible spontaneously or with treatment. In addition to the historical associations noted for rhinitis, the influence of exercise, exposure to tobacco smoke, the effect of respiratory infection (particularly viral), occupational exposures (e.g., ≤30% of atopic animal handlers develop asthma), and medication use (e.g., β-adrenergic blocking drugs) are of particular pertinence. Because most patients with asthma have concurrent rhinitis, it is essential that the physician evaluate this issue in all asthmatic patients. Wheezing may accompany other disorders besides asthma, including pulmonary edema in congestive heart failure.

TABLE 270–1 SYMPTOMS, SIGNS, AND TREATMENT OF ALLERGIC DISEASE

Symptoms	Approach to Treatment
Cutaneous: itch, rash	H_1-antihistaminic agent
Ocular: gritty sensation, itch	Topical H_1-antihistaminic or mast cell stabilizing agent
Upper respiratory: palatal pruritus, clear rhinorrhea, sneeze, nasal obstruction	Topical corticosteroid, oral H_1-antihistaminic agent, leukotriene receptor antagonist, topical nasal H_1-antihistaminic agent
Lower respiratory: wheeze, cough, dyspnea	B_2-agonist, inhaled corticosteroid, inhaled B_2-agonist, leukotriene receptor antagonist, oral methylxanthine, parenteral corticosteroid, parenteral anti–immunoglobulin E
Gastrointestinal: nausea, vomiting, cramping pain	Epinephrine (if caused by anaphylaxis), oral corticosteroid, oral cromolyn
SIGNS	
Cutaneous: flushing, urticaria, angioedema, eczema	
Ocular: conjunctival erythema, chemosis	
Upper respiratory: pallor, edema, clear rhinorrhea, polyps	
Lower respiratory: wheeze	

Urticaria and Angioedema

Patients with urticaria (Chapter 273) describe pruritic, erythematous cutaneous lesions with regular or irregular borders occurring anywhere on the body that may vary in size from small (1 × 1 mm) to extremely large. Skin lesions are often preceded by intense intertriginous pruritus. Individual urticarial lesions generally persist for a few hours and rarely last for more than 24 hours. However, many disorders can cause a sensation of itching; skin and systemic diseases associated with pruritus are listed in Table 461–3. Angioedema (Chapter 273) is most frequently appreciated in the face, hands, and other soft tissues and is generally accompanied by symptoms of stretching, tingling, and tightness of the skin rather than pruritus. Lesions, especially in the face, typically last 24 to 36 hours. Although most cases of urticaria or angioedema are not IgE mediated, it is nonetheless important to identify foods and medications used by patients with acute urticaria or angioedema, particularly those substances ingested within 2 to 4 hours of the development of lesions, and to inquire about insect stings. Chronic urticaria is less often IgE mediated; questions about medications, especially nonsteroidal anti-inflammatory drugs, recent infection (especially with Epstein-Barr virus), and the presence of autoantibodies to the IgE receptor must be addressed. Approximately one half to two thirds of patients with such autoantibodies also have antibodies to thyroid antigens. In angioedema, the use of angiotensin-converting enzyme inhibitors must be sought. Atopic dermatitis is another allergic cutaneous disorder in which patients complain of intense pruritus, especially in flexural surfaces. In adults, foods (IgE mediated) and cutaneous infection with *Staphylococcus aureus* (superantigen mediated) are the most commonly identified precipitating events for atopic dermatitis.

Anaphylaxis

Anaphylaxis (Chapter 274) is the most important allergic emergency and is potentially fatal. It is an acute allergic response associated with cutaneous (urticaria, angioedema, flushing), respiratory (laryngeal edema, asthma), cardiovascular (arrhythmia, hypotension, extravascular fluid loss), gastrointestinal (nausea, vomiting, abdominal pain, diarrhea), and nonspecific symptoms (metallic taste, sense of impending doom) that may occur singly or together. Historical information of note includes all medications, foods, and other encounters occurring within 2 hours of the reaction. Epidemiologic data suggest that foods (especially peanuts, tree nuts, shellfish, milk, and egg), hymenoptera stings, and medications (antibiotics, muscle relaxants, radiocontrast media) are the most frequently identified causes of this important problem.

Food Allergy

Patients presenting with food allergy often complain of oral pruritus and the specific gastrointestinal manifestations of nausea, vomiting, diarrhea, and abdominal pain. Eczema, urticaria, and anaphylaxis, as noted previously, may also be consequences of food allergy. In general, allergic symptoms consequent to foods occur within minutes to 2 hours of ingestion of the causative food; delayed symptoms are unlikely to be mediated by IgE-allergen interaction. Other symptoms attributable to foods are less easily explained by allergic mechanisms and are termed food intolerance.

Physical Examination

The physical examination of the patient with suspected allergic disease should emphasize the organ systems pertinent to the complaints of the patient. The skin should be examined for the presence of urticarial or angioedematous lesions and for signs of atopic dermatitis including flexural papules, excoriations, and lichenification. Keratosis pilaris, particularly on the outer aspect of the upper arm, commonly accompanies atopic dermatitis. Urticaria typically consists of small, pink, irregular lesions that blanch on pressure and clear, leaving normal skin. In a patient with urticaria, a simple test for dermatographism should be undertaken. Angioedematous lesions are larger, more diffuse, and pale, and they are most often found affecting the face and acral areas.

The eyes, ears, nose, and throat should be examined in all patients suspected of having allergic disease, particularly in those whose symptoms suggest seasonal or perennial allergic rhinoconjunctivitis-sinusitis or asthma. In allergic disease, the conjunctivae are often injected and may be edematous. "Cobblestoning" of the epithelium may be present. The periorbital tissues may be swollen and darkened. Examination of the nares may show pale and edematous nasal mucous membranes and swollen turbinates, and polyps may be seen. Secretions, generally clear, may be seen in the nasal passages or in the posterior pharynx. Such secretions generally contain copious numbers of eosinophils (see later), and their absence is a point against allergic causation. Fever and discolored secretions, particularly thick and yellow or green, in the presence of neutrophilic polymorphonuclear leukocytes suggest infection. Percussion over the maxillary or frontal sinuses may elicit tenderness in acute sinusitis, and in such a case transillumination of the sinus, albeit a test of low sensitivity, may be impaired. In chronic sinusitis, the physical examination may be unrevealing. In acute otitis media, patients may have erythema and bulging or perforation of the tympanic membrane with fluid in the canal, and in chronic cases the drum may be scarred and retracted. Alteration in air-bone conduction may be noted as well.

Patients with acute asthma may display tachypnea and auditory wheezes, and they may be unable to speak in full sentences because of shortness of breath. Use of accessory muscles of respiration and evidence of cyanosis should be sought. Examination of the chest includes inspection for evidence of chronic hyperinflation and auscultation for wheezing (which, if unilateral, may suggest a foreign body or tumor). In mild asthma, the examination may be normal, or the only physical finding may be wheezing on forced expiration and a slight prolongation of the expiratory phase.

Patients experiencing acute anaphylaxis usually demonstrate flushing, and concomitant urticaria and angioedema are often present. Assessment of vital signs may disclose hypotension and tachycardia. In some situations, hoarseness or stridor related to laryngeal edema or wheezing secondary to asthma can be identified. Hyperactive bowel sounds may be noted. Progressive hypoxia and cyanosis may ensue. In severe anaphylaxis, cardiovascular collapse secondary to hypoxia and hypotension may result in death.

Laboratory Evaluation

In the evaluation of patients with allergic disorders, the laboratory may be of assistance in both the identification and the quantification of the degree of specific organ dysfunction, as well as in the assessment of the presence and specificity of IgE antibody.

Assessment of Total and Allergen-Specific Immunoglobulin E

Essentially all (>95%) IgE antibody is bound to specific high-affinity receptors on tissue mast cells and circulating peripheral blood basophils. The small amount of free serum IgE antibody circulates in nanogram quantities and can be identified only with techniques of sufficient sensitivity. Generally, such tests employ a solid phase to which an antibody to human IgE is coupled. The patient's serum is then added, the contained IgE is bound, and nonbound materials are removed by washing. The amount of IgE bound is then determined by addition of a second antibody to IgE to which a quantifying reagent, such as a radioactive isotope or an enzyme capable of creating a colorimetric end point, is bound. A large proportion of IgE in a given individual may be directed toward a single antigen, and thus total IgE levels may be normal in the presence of allergic disease. Therefore, the measurement of total serum IgE is rarely of help in diagnosis. In a few situations, such as adult atopic dermatitis or allergic bronchopulmonary aspergillosis, measurement of total serum IgE levels may give insight into disease severity or into the risk of disease exacerbation.

Of more importance is the identification of allergen-specific IgE in a patient in whom allergic disease is suspected (Table 270–2). Such specific IgE may be identified in vitro or in vivo. A search for allergen-specific IgE is particularly useful in the evaluation of patients with suspected allergic rhinitis, asthma, eczema, food reactions, and anaphylaxis. In vitro assessment is performed much as for the quantification of total IgE, except the initial capture reagent bound to a solid phase is a specific pollen, mold, insect, venom, food, or other allergen. Development of the assay is identical to that used to quantify total IgE, and results are generally reported in a semiquantitative manner. The magnitude of the reaction is weakly correlated with the degree of sensitization and expression of allergy, although for certain foods more precise correlative data exist on the risk of allergy and the amount of the allergen-specific IgE detected. The in vivo assessment of allergen-specific IgE is undertaken by introducing into the skin a minute quantity of the allergen in question by a prick puncture technique and assessing the cutaneous response 15 to 30 minutes thereafter. A positive response is one in which a wheal and flare at least 2 mm larger than those caused by a saline control occur at the injection site. In vivo tests are rapid and inexpensive; they require the absence of dermatographism, that patients not be using antihistaminic medications, and that patients display a positive response to a control employing histamine. In some situations (e.g., penicillin or hymenopteran sting), a more diluted allergen is directly injected intradermally, and wheal-and-flare responses are assessed similarly. The presence of allergen-specific IgE antibody and a clear temporal correlation of exposure to allergen and genesis of symptoms are required to conclude that a patient is allergic to a specific allergen. In the absence of symptoms, the patient with allergen-specific IgE is termed sensitized but not allergic.

Specific in vivo challenge tests may also be used to identify allergen responsiveness. Such tests in the presence of specific IgE antibody may be useful in research settings, or they may be used clinically to clarify the exact relationship between exposure and symptoms. Such tests may be dangerous because they introduce the allergen to which the patient is presumed allergic. In food allergy, such challenges, best done in a double-blind and placebo-controlled manner, may be useful in separating allergy from sensitization or in eliminating a suspect food from consideration. However, food challenge tests are unnecessary in the situation of anaphylaxis and a positive test for IgE antibody to the putative allergen. Because many patients falsely believe that foods are responsible for their symptoms, such double-blind challenges may be useful in directing patients' concerns to more productive areas. Inhalation tests employing specific allergens or chemicals have been helpful in elucidation of some cases of occupational allergy or asthma.

Other Laboratory Aids in Allergic Disease

In a patient with acute asthma, chest radiographs generally demonstrate hyperinflation. In some instances, evidence of bronchiectasis may be present, a finding that raises the specter of allergic bronchopulmonary aspergillosis. The presence of a tumor or radiopaque foreign body may be noted on a chest radiograph and should be sought in a patient with unilateral localized wheezing. In the examination of the patient with asthma, assessment of both airflow and volumes can provide a clear picture of the severity of asthma and its response to treatment. Flow-volume loops can also identify the presence of vocal cord dysfunction. When patients with airway obstruction are evaluated, their response to inhaled β_2-adrenergic agonist medication can be helpful in elucidating the reversible nature of their disorder. Essentially all asthmatic patients exhibiting bronchoconstriction display a bronchodilatory response to inhalation of such agents. In suspected cases of asthma, when pulmonary function is normal, challenge with histamine or methacholine can be performed. These agents take advantage of the nonspecific bronchial hyperresponsiveness characteristic of patients with asthma. Failure of a patient to develop bronchoconstriction on inhalation of either of these agents strongly argues against the diagnosis of this disorder.

Other laboratory tools may be of benefit to the clinician in the identification and classification of allergic disorders. Audiometry may clarify the degree of hearing loss caused by otitis media in a patient with allergic rhinitis. When sinusitis is suspected, computed tomography of the sinuses gives the most complete imaging and has the highest degree of sensitivity for the identification of mucosal thickening, opacification of air spaces, and the presence of polyps and bone erosions. Computed tomography is particularly useful in the examination of the ethmoid and sphenoid sinuses, which are often affected in chronic allergic disease and are difficult to assess on physical examination or with plain radiographs.

The hematology and biochemistry laboratory may also be helpful in the evaluation of a patient with allergic disease. The quantification of

TABLE 270–2 ADVANTAGES AND DISADVANTAGES OF DIFFERENT ALLERGY TESTING METHODS

Method	Patient Selection	Clinical Advantages	Clinical Disadvantages
Skin testing	Clinical indication suggesting allergic disease	Rapid (15–30 min) turnaround Sensitive and specific; prick puncture for aeroallergens, prick puncture followed by intradermal testing for drugs, sera, and venoms	Patient must not be taking H_1-antihistaminic agents for 5–7 days Not interpretable in the presence of dermatographism Requires sufficient normal skin to enable testing
In vitro testing	Clinical indication suggesting allergic disease	Antihistaminic therapy not contraindicated Dermatographism not a problem Sensitive and specific; equal to prick puncture skin testing	Requires blood drawn Slow turnaround (7–14 days)

blood, sputum, nasal mucus, or tissue eosinophilia and the response to corticosteroid therapy are useful correlates in the identification and management of allergic disease. The quantification of tryptase, a mast cell–specific protease with a serum half-life of 2 hours, if performed on serum or plasma obtained within hours of a systemic response with associated hypotension, can assist in the diagnosis of anaphylaxis.

IMMUNOLOGIC DISEASE

Epidemiology

Diseases related to disordered immune function (immunodeficiency) are far less common than allergic disorders. The most frequent is IgA deficiency, which occurs in approximately 1 in 1000 individuals and is often asymptomatic. Next most frequently encountered are disorders of B and T lymphocytes such as common variable hypogammaglobulinemia, and other disorders including DiGeorge's syndrome and severe combined immunodeficiency (Chapter 271). Much less common are defects in neutrophil function or complement.

Diagnosis

In essence, the clinical expression of immune deficiency disorders is primarily infection related to impaired host defense. Thus, the evaluation of suspected immune deficiency is the evaluation of recurrent, persistent, severe, and otherwise unexplained infections. Although many immune disorders arise in early childhood, not all do so, and with improved management many patients presenting in childhood live into adulthood. It is important for the general internist and internal medicine subspecialist to be cognizant of the presentation of these disorders.

History

The most important historical information includes the following: the age of onset of the problem in question; a family history of frequent infection or death at an early age from infection; the number, sites, and type of infection; and the presence of other physical abnormalities (Table 270–3). The earlier the onset of infections, the more severe the immune defect is likely to be. T-lymphocytic defects, with or without B-cell deficiencies, usually arise in the first 3 to 5 months of life, whereas B-cell function is supported by maternal antibody until after the first 6 months of life. Many of the immune disorders are X-linked, and a careful family history is critical in such situations. Death related to infection of a male sibling of the patient or of the patient's mother should lead to the question of such an X-linked disorder.

In a patient with a T-cell disorder, viral, fungal, mycobacterial, and other opportunistic infections (*Pneumocystis jirovecii, Toxoplasma gondii*) are most commonly noted, and live virus vaccination may be associated with disseminated and progressive viral disease. Persistent thrush, diarrhea, malabsorption, and failure to thrive occurring in early childhood may suggest the presence of T-cell abnormalities.

In B-cell or antibody deficiency, pyogenic bacterial infections predominate, particularly infections involving encapsulated microorganisms. Usually, such infections affect the upper and lower respiratory tract and skin and are severe and persistent. Infections with unusual organisms, with unexpected complications, or involving multiple sites (lung, sinus, joint, bone, meninges, abscess formation, or sepsis) should raise the index of suspicion. In adults, the most common disorder in this class is termed *common variable immunodeficiency.*

As in any patient with infection, information should be sought about exposure to ill individuals or to irritants such as tobacco smoke, the hygiene of the environment to which the patient is exposed, and the presence of an anatomic abnormality or allergy that could predispose to infection.

Physical Examination

Physical examination beyond that necessary to assess the extent and severity of a particular infection should be focused on immune organs. Assessment of tonsillar tissue and determination of the presence and size of lymph nodes, spleen, and liver is important. Patients with common variable immunodeficiency often present with hepatosplenomegaly and lymph node hyperplasia, whereas in X-linked hypogammaglobulinemia lymph tissue is absent. Telangiectasia (ataxia-telangiectasia), cardiac defects (DiGeorge's syndrome), chronic eczema (Wiskott-Aldrich syndrome), and chronic periodontitis (neutrophil defects) all suggest immune deficiency syndromes.

Laboratory Evaluation

The proper use of the laboratory is essential in the elucidation of a suspected immune deficiency disorder. Screening tests appropriate to the generalist's initial approach include complete blood count, total neutrophil and lymphocyte enumeration, quantitative immunoglobulin levels, and assessment of isohemagglutinins (especially when common variable immunodeficiency is suspected). In some situations, quantification of IgG subclasses may be warranted to identify specific subclass deficiency. In consideration of T-lymphocyte defects, it is important to enumerate total T cells and specific T-cell subsets. Delayed hypersensitivity skin testing to recall antigens is also helpful in assessing cellular immunity. When neutrophil defects are suspected, a nitroblue tetrazolium test or measurement of phagocytic potency can be performed. Complement defects are best addressed by obtaining a CH_{50} level. CH_{50} is the amount of patient serum required to cause lysis of 50% of test erythrocytes. It is compared with the amount of pooled normal serum required to cause the same degree of lysis. Tests for specific individual components of complement, or of complement regulatory proteins, can also be obtained under special circumstances.

Additional tests of antibody production to defined stimuli, including vaccinations, may be helpful when selective antibody deficiency is suspected or when borderline immunoglobulin levels are encountered in the presence of frequent infection. In some situations, assessment of T-cell proliferation to mitogens or antigen may be of benefit. Further testing could include assessment of natural killer cell function and the production of cytokines by activated lymphocytes. In general, such additional laboratory tests should be performed in conjunction with consultation with an expert in immune disorders.

TABLE 270–3 KEY POINTS REGARDING IMMUNOLOGIC DISORDERS

ANTIBODY DEFICIENCY DISORDERS
Onset after 6 mo of age
Recurrent respiratory infection
Infection with bacteria, especially encapsulated organisms
Absence of isohemagglutinins
Evaluation of B-cell function, not numbers
CELLULAR IMMUNE DEFECTS
Onset before 6 mo of age
Recurrent viral, fungal, or parasitic (opportunistic) infection
Defective delayed hypersensitivity skin responses
Malabsorption or diarrhea
COMPLEMENT DEFICIENCIES
Recurrent bacterial infection
Recurrent neisserial infection (deficiency of late components)
Associated rheumatic disorder (especially systemic lupus erythematosus)
FACTORS SUGGESTING NEUTROPHIL DYSFUNCTION
Late separation of umbilical cord
Persistent neutrophilic leukocytosis
Recurrent or persistent gingivitis or periodontitis
Recurrent bacterial infection with granuloma formation

SUGGESTED READINGS

DiRenzo M, Pasqua AL, Anteri A: Common variable immunodeficiency disease: A review. Clin Exp Med 2004;3:211–217. *A review of the most common adult immunodeficiency.*

Jiang H, Chess L: Regulation of immune responses by T cells. N Engl J Med 2006;354:1166–1176. *A comprehensive review of these processes.*

Riminton DL, Limaye S: Primary immunodeficiency disease in adulthood. Intern Med J 2004;34:348–354. *A review of adult immunodeficiency disorders and protocols for evaluation.*

Shearer WT, Li JT: Preface to the fifth primer on allergic and immunologic diseases. J Allergy Clin Immunol 2003;111:441–778. *An overview of and approach to allergy and immunologic disease.*

Wen L, Atkinson JP, Gicles PR: Clinical and laboratory evaluation of complement deficiency. J. Allergy Clin Immunol 2004;113:585–593. *Protocols for evaluation of complement disorders.*

271 PRIMARY IMMUNODEFICIENCY DISEASES

Mark Ballow

Definition

A diverse group of abnormalities of the immune system leads to increased susceptibility to infection. More than 100 primary immunodeficiency diseases have been described, and in many of these disorders, the genetic defect has been delineated. Immunodeficiency diseases are relatively uncommon; it is important to rule out other underlying conditions, such as secondary immunodeficiencies that could lead to recurrent infections. Immunodeficiencies are generally divided into the following categories: B-cell or antibody immunodeficiencies, T-cell or cellular immunodeficiencies, immunodeficiencies associated with the phagocytic system, and immune abnormalities associated with the complement system. Many immune abnormalities, such as those associated with the T-cell immune system, have associated B-cell immune abnormalities as well. Although many primary immunodeficiencies are first noticed in infants and young children, the most frequent B-cell (humoral) immunodeficiencies become evident later in life, especially in young adults whose characteristic presentations should be recognized by the physician so diagnosis and treatment can be initiated.

It is not the purpose of this chapter to present an encyclopedic list of all the known immunodeficiencies, but rather to identify the most common presenting clinical characteristics, to define the initial laboratory evaluation, and to discuss the approach to treatment briefly. Antibody deficiencies make up approximately 65% of all primary immunodeficiency diseases, combined T-cell and B-cell immunodeficiencies constitute approximately 15%, cellular immunodeficiencies approximately 5%, phagocytic cell abnormalities 10%, and complement deficiencies only 5% (Fig. 271–1).

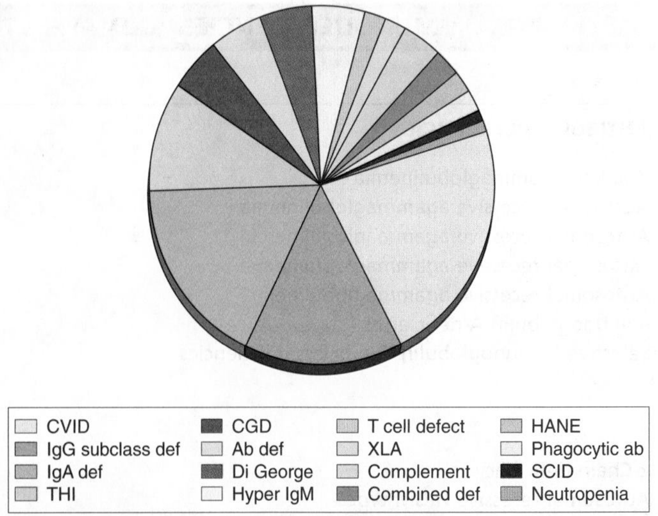

FIGURE 271–1 • The relative number of subjects who present with primary immunodeficiency diseases are shown. Subjects who have common variable immunodeficiency (CVID), immunoglobulin G (IgG) subclass deficiency, or IgA deficiency (IgA def) represent about half of the total group. Other deficiencies include transient hypogammaglobulinemia of infancy (THI), chronic granulomatous disease (CGD), antibody deficiency (Ab def), DiGeorge syndrome, hyper-IgM syndrome, other T-cell defects, X-linked agammaglobulinemia (XLA), complement deficiencies, combined defects (def), hereditary angioedema (HANE), phagocytic abnormality (ab), severe combined immunodeficiency (SCID), and the neutropenias.

Pathobiology

Genetics

The defective gene has been identified in more than 100 primary immunodeficiency disorders (Table 271–1). The mode of inheritance has often been identified in many of the immunodeficiencies as X-linked recessive, autosomal recessive, or autosomal dominant. Many of the immunodeficiencies are caused by mutations of genes required for the development of T cells or B cells or genes needed for the development of precursor cell lineages that differentiate into different types of immune cells. Other genetic abnormalities are widely expressed in many tissues that result in complex multisystem disorders along with the immunodeficiency. Some gene mutations that occur in the same immunologic pathway result in similar clinical manifestations and laboratory findings, such as common γ-chain defect of the interleukin-2 (IL-2) receptor and Janus kinase 3 (JAK3). Conversely, other genetic defects, depending on the nature and the location of the mutation, may result in different clinical phenotypes. An example of the latter is mutations in recombination activating gene (RAG)-1 and RAG-2, which result in severe combined immunodeficiency disease and Omenn's syndrome. The Wiskott-Aldrich syndrome is another example in which variations in the location of the mutation along the gene sequence, such as a missense mutation that allows expression of a mutated protein, result in different clinical phenotypes and a spectrum of the disease.

Clinical Manifestations

This chapter concentrates on presenting to the practicing physician the common clinical signs and the important details of the history and physical examination for the evaluation of a patient with recurrent infections. The association of particular bacterial and viral pathogens with certain immunodeficiencies is also helpful in directing the physician toward a differential diagnosis and an appropriate choice of screening laboratory tests.

History

Clues from the Infecting Pathogen and the Organ System Involved

The organ systems affected by the infection and identification of the isolated pathogens can give clues to the nature of the possible defect. A patient presenting with lymphadenitis or recurrent abscesses caused by low-virulence gram-negative organisms such as *Escherichia coli, Serratia,* or *Klebsiella,* may have an abnormality in phagocyte function. Infections with unusual pathogens such as *Staphylococcus epidermidis* or *Pseudomonas,* especially *Burkholderia cepacia,* can suggest a leukocyte phagocytic disorder. Another characteristic presentation of patients with a phagocyte defect is a history of recurrent skin infections with catalase-positive *Staphylococcus aureus,* a finding underscoring the importance of effective phagocytosis and intracellular superoxide-mediated killing in controlling these infections. A history of delayed separation of the umbilical cord of more than 6 to 8 weeks or poor wound healing suggests the diagnosis of a leukocyte adhesion defect. Suppurative adenitis is common in patients with chronic granulomatous disease, and it can be an important clue in the diagnosis when gram-negative bacteria are recovered from the tissues. The mucous membranes can also be involved in patients with an immunodeficiency of a phagocytic cell. Gingivostomatitis and dental erosions are characteristic of patients with a phagocytic cell defect such as in leukocyte adhesion deficiency. Recurrent oral ulcers are characteristic of patients with cyclic neutropenia. Defects in the late complement components, C5 to C9, are classically associated with infections with neisserial species such as meningitis caused by *Neisseria meningitidis* or septic arthritis caused by *Neisseria gonorrhoeae.* Patients with C3 deficiency can present with overwhelming septicemia, especially with gram-negative organisms, a finding consistent with the important role of complement, particularly C3b, in opsonization and the facilitation of phagocytosis.

B-cell abnormalities most commonly lead to recurrent sinopulmonary infections that are frequently caused by encapsulated bacteria, such as

TABLE 271–1 IMMUNODEFICIENCIES AND AFFECTED GENES

Disease	Gene/Proteins	Chromosome Locus
ANTIBODY DEFICIENCIES		
X-linked agammaglobulinemia	BTK	Xq21.3-q22
Autosomal recessive agammaglobulinemia	Constant region of μ heavy chain	14q32.33
Autosomal recessive agammaglobulinemia	IGLL1/λ5 or 14.1(CD179b)	22q11.21
Autosomal recessive agammaglobulinemia	Igα/ B29 (CD79A)	1q13.2
Autosomal recessive agammaglobulinemia	BLNK	10q23.22
Immunoglobulin A deficiency	IGAD1	6p21.3
Selective Immunoglobulin G subclass deficiencies	IGHG1	14q32.33
	IGHG2	14q32.33
	IGHG3	14q32.33
	IGHG4	14q32.33
κ-Chain deficiency	IGKC	2P12
Autosomal recessive HIGM type3	TNFRSF5/CD40	20q12-q13.2
Autosomal recessive HIGM type 2	AICDA	12p13
Autosomal recessive HIGM	UNG	
COMBINED IMMUNODEFICIENCIES		
T-B⁻ SCID		
RAG-1	RAG1	11p13
RAG-2	RAG2	11p13
Adenosine deaminase deficiency	ADA	20q13.11
Athabaskan SCID	Artemis	10p13
T-B⁺ SCID		
X-linked SCID	IL2Rγ/common γ chain receptor	Xq13
JAK3 deficiency	JAK3	19p13.1
IL-7 receptor α-chain deficiency	IL-7RA/α chain	5p13
OTHER COMBINED IMMUNODEFICIENCIES		
Purine nucleoside phosphorylase deficiency	PNP	14q13.1
ZAP-70 deficiency	ZAP70	2q12
CD3γ deficiency	CD3G	11q23
CD3ε deficiency	CD3E	11q23
CD25 deficiency	Il-2Rα	
CD45 deficiency	CD45	1q31-32
TAP2 peptide transported deficiency	TAP2	6p21.3
MHCII deficiency (defect in CIITA)	MHC2TA	16p13
MHCII deficiency (defect in RFX5)	RFX5	1q21.1-q21.3
MHCII deficiency (defect in RFXAP)	RFXAP	13q14
MHCII deficiency (defect in RFXANK)	RFXANK	19p12
X-linked immunodeficiency with increased immunoglobulin M	TNFSF5/CD40Ligand	Xq26.3q27.1
OTHER WELL-DEFINED IMMUNODEFICIENCIES		
Wiskott-Aldrich syndrome	WASP	Xp11.23-p11.22
DiGeorge syndrome	DGCR	22q11.2
Ataxia-telangiectasia	ATM	11q22.3
X-linked lymphoproliferative syndrome	SH2DIA/SAP	Xq25
Familial hemophagocytic lymphohistiocytosis	PRF1	10q21-22
ICF syndrome	DNMT3B	20q11.2
X-linked immune dysregulation with polyendocrinopathy syndrome	FOXP3	Xp11.23-q13.3
Hyper-immunoglobulin M with hypohidrotic ectodermal dysplasia	NEMO/IKK γ chain	Xq28
APECED	AIRE	21q22.3
WHIM	CXCR4	2q21
Nijmegan breakage syndrome	NBS1/nibrin	8q21
Cartilage-hair hypoplasia	RMRP	9p21-p12
Griscelli's syndrome	MYO5A/RAB27A	15q21

TABLE 271–1 IMMUNODEFICIENCIES AND AFFECTED GENES—cont'd

Disease	Gene/Proteins	Chromosome Locus
AUTOIMMUNE LYMPHOPROLIFERATIVE SYNDROME (ALPS)		
Fas defect	TNFRSF6/CD95	10q24.1
Fas ligand defect	TNFSF6/FasL/CD95L	
Caspase 10 defect	CASP10	
Caspase 8 defect	CASP8	
PHAGOCYTIC IMMUNODEFICIENCIES		
LAD type I	ITGB2 (CD18)	21q22.3
LAD type II	GDP-fucose transporter	11
LAD Rac2 deficiency	Rac2	22q12.3
Chédiak-Higashi syndrome	CHS1	1q42.1-q42.2
CD16 deficiency	CD16 (FcγRIII)	1q23
Cyclic neutropenia	Neutrophil elastase/ELA2	19p13.3
Neutrophil-specific granule deficiency	C/EBPε	14q11.2
Mannose-binding protein deficiency	MBP	10q11.2-q21
X-linked CGD gp91 phox	CYBB/ CD18	Xp21.1
Autosomal recessive CGD p22^{phox}	CYBA	16q24
Autosomal recessive CGD p47 ^{phox}	NCF1	7q11.23
Autosomal recessive CGD p67 ^{phox}	NCF2	1q25
Myeloperoxidase deficiency	MPO	17q23.1
IFN-γ RECEPTOR/IL-12 PATHWAY DEFICIENCY		
IFN-γ1 receptor deficiency	IFNGR1	6q23-q24
IFN-γ2 receptor deficiency	IFNGR2	21q22.1-q22.2
IL-12p40 deficiency	IL12RB1	19p13.1-33.1
IL-12 receptor β1 deficiency	IL12B	5q31.1-q33.1
STAT 1 deficiency	STAT1	2q32.2-q32.3

APECED = autoimmune polyendocrinopathy with candidiasis and ectodermal dystrophy; CGD = chronic granulomatous disease; HIGM = hyper-immunoglobulin M; ICF = immunodeficiency, centromeric region instability, and facial anomalies; IFN = interferon; IL = interleukin; JAK = Janus kinase; LAD = leukocyte adhesion deficiency; MHC = major histocompatibility complex; RAG = recombinase activating gene; SCID = severe combined immunodeficiency; STAT = signal transducers and activators of transcription 1; WHIM = warts, hypogammaglobulinemia, infections, myelokathexis syndrome.

Streptococcus pneumoniae or *Haemophilus influenzae.* Examination of the pharynx and nasal cavities for signs of sinusitis including posterior pharyngeal cobblestoning, postnasal drainage, or purulent nasal discharge is important. Tympanic membranes can appear scarred and disfigured as a sign of recurrent and chronic infection of the middle ear. Rales on auscultation of the chest may suggest bronchiectasis occurring as a complication of recurrent lung infections. Digital clubbing points to significant lung disease. Pulmonary hypertension can occur in patients with chronic lung disease. These types of infection underscore the importance of immunoglobulins in opsonization for effective phagocytosis and killing of the microorganism. A characteristic feature of patients with X-linked agammaglobulinemia (XLA) is an unusual susceptibility to a viral meningoencephalitis caused by enteroviruses (e.g., coxsackievirus, echovirus). Chronic gastrointestinal symptoms caused by *Giardia lamblia* are likely related to impaired mucosal immunity and lack of secretory IgA, and they commonly occur in patients with common variable immunodeficiency (CVID) and IgA deficiency. Small bowel bacterial overgrowth and infections with *Yersinia* and *Campylobacter* can lead to chronic gastrointestinal symptoms; diarrhea and occasionally malabsorption are frequent presenting symptoms in patients with CVID.

T cells are essential not only in controlling viral, fungal, mycobacterial, and protozoal infections but also in providing crucial signals to help B cells produce immunoglobulins. Extensive mucous membrane candidiasis would suggest a T-cell defect. Patients with cellular immune defects often present with opportunistic infections such as *Mycobacterium avium intracellulare* and *Pneumocystis jirovecii.*

Lymphatic System in Patients with Immunodeficiency

The examination of the lymphatic system for hepatosplenomegaly and for the presence or absence of lymphoid tissue is an important aspect of the physical examination in a patient suspected of immunodeficiency. Patients with severe combined immunodeficiency disease or infantile XLA do not have palpable lymphoid tissue or visible tonsils. However, the presence of lymphoid tissue can be misleading: adult patients with common variable hypogammaglobulinemia may actually have enlarged lymphoid tissue and even hepatosplenomegaly. This occurs because the reticuloendothelial system undergoes hyperplasia in the absence of opsonic antibody. Draining abscesses of the lymph nodes suggest a phagocyte defect.

Immunodeficiency and Autoimmunity

Deficiencies of the early complement components, such as C4 and C2, are associated with autoimmune disease often first manifesting with arthritis, frequently in conjunction with dermal vasculitis. A lupus-like rash with negative or low-titer antinuclear antibodies may occur in deficiencies of the early components of the classical complement pathway. Patients with some primary immunodeficiencies can present with features of autoimmunity involving hematopoietic or other organ systems. For example, the diagnosis of CVID can be preceded by autoimmune hemolytic anemia.

Immunodeficiency and Gastrointestinal Disease

Many patients with primary immunodeficiency disease have symptoms and clinical findings referable to the gastrointestinal tract. In a survey of 248 patients with CVID, 21% had significant gastrointestinal disease. Liver disease occurred in an additional 12%. Bacterial overgrowth of the small bowel, including infections with *Yersinia* and *Campylobacter,* parasitic infestations with such organisms as *G. lamblia,* and chronic viral enteritis caused by enteroviruses and cytomegalovirus are relatively common in patients with B- or T-cell immune defects. The incidence of lactose intolerance is higher in patients with immunodeficiency than in the immunologically normal population. Patients with the X-linked syndrome of immune dysregulation, polyendocrinopathy, and enteropathy (IPEX) have protracted diarrhea.

Immunodeficiency and Family History

A detailed family history in patients suspected of immunodeficiency can add valuable information. Numerous immunodeficiencies are X-linked; therefore, a family history of maternal male relatives affected with unusually frequent infections or who died in early infancy should alert the physician to the possibility of an X-linked form of immunodeficiency. The mother in these cases would be expected to be a carrier, although the rate of new mutations for X-linked disorders is significant, so a negative family history may not exclude this inheritance pattern. CVID and IgA deficiency are familial disorders and are often seen in a setting of other family members with autoimmune disorders, such as pernicious anemia, rheumatoid arthritis, systemic lupus erythematosus, or autoimmune hematologic diseases.

DEFECTS IN THE INNATE IMMUNE SYSTEM: COMPLEMENT AND PHAGOCYTE DEFICIENCIES

Deficiencies of Complement Proteins

Definition

The complement (C) system is important in host defense and is composed of a complex system of plasma proteins and cell surface receptors (Chapter 47). Important functions of the complement system include opsonization to enhance phagocytosis, clearance of immune complexes, the induction of the humoral immune response, and the clearance of apoptotic cells. Complement deficiencies present as severe or recurrent invasive infection with encapsulated bacteria (resulting from loss of the opsonic function of C3 fragments), immune complex disease (because complement is important in the clearance and solubilization of immune complexes and in their removal from the circulation), angioedema, or the loss of bactericidal and bacteriolytic functions leading to recurrent or invasive infection with *Neisseria* species.

Epidemiology

The proportion of patients with primary immunodeficiency who have complement deficiencies is approximately 5%. Although rare, C2 deficiency is the most common of the classical early complement component diseases; it occurs in 1:10,000 whites. C6 deficiency is the most common of the late complement component disorders. The frequency of complement deficiency in sporadic cases of systemic meningococcal infection has been estimated to be 15%. In patients with recurrent meningococcal disease, the prevalence is as high as 40%.

Clinical Manifestations

These disorders are usually inherited as autosomal codominant traits, in which the parents of the patients have half-normal levels of the involved complement component, whereas the patient has a complete absence of the component in question. The complement deficiencies can be broadly divided into those of the early classical complement pathway (C1, C2, and C4), the components of the alternative complement pathway (factors B, D, and P), the mannose binding proteins and their associated proteases (MASP-1 and MASP-2), the late complement components (C5, C6, C7, C8, and C9), and the complement regulatory proteins (C1 inhibitor and others). Persons deficient in C3 share characteristics of both early and late component complement deficiencies. Patients lacking one of the early complement components often present with a rheumatic disease. Patients often have the typical features of systemic lupus erythematosus, except they often may be seronegative, that is, anti-DNA antibodies are absent, and antinuclear antibodies are present in low titer. Individuals with C2 deficiency may have systemic lupus erythematosus or discoid lupus. Other rheumatic disorders associated with complement deficiencies of the early complement components include dermatomyositis, scleroderma, vasculitis, and membranoproliferative glomerulonephritis. Homozygous factor H deficiency, a complement regulatory protein, may manifest as hemolytic-uremic syndrome. Likewise, deficiencies of late complement components may occasionally be associated with vasculitis or other lupus-like illnesses. Less frequently, patients with late component deficiencies have developed Raynaud's syndrome, scleroderma, or dermatomyositis.

Patients with deficiencies in the late complement components usually present with recurrent infections caused by *Neisseria* species, with invasive meningococcal or gonococcal infection, such as recurrent meningococcal meningitis, gonococcal arthritis, or gonococcal septicemia. However, patients with deficiencies of early or alternative pathway complement components, such as properdin deficiency, may also present with recurrent or invasive neisserial infections.

Diagnosis

Individuals with recurrent blood-borne infection with encapsulated bacteria (e.g., *S. pneumoniae, H. influenzae,* invasive meningococcal or gonococcal disease) or immune complex disease should be screened for complement deficiency by determining the total hemolytic complement activity (CH_{50}) in the serum, a test of classical pathway activity. The CH_{50} should be undetectable. If the CH_{50} is normal, alternative pathway function should be tested with the AH_{50}. Hemolytic activity is very sensitive to heat degradation, so blood samples must be handled appropriately, and the serum should be separated and frozen at −70° C as soon as possible. Abnormalities in CH_{50} or AH_{50} could be pursued by analysis of specific component concentrations in serum.

Treatment

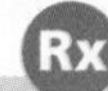

Patients should be immunized with the meningococcal vaccine. Some debate exists on whether to use prophylactic antibiotics because of the emergence of resistant strains.

C1 Esterase Inhibitor Deficiency

Definition

C1 esterase inhibitor (C1 INH) deficiency is associated with life-threatening edema and is inherited as an autosomal dominant disorder (Chapter 273). This complement regulatory plasma protein inhibits the enzymatic activity of C1r and C1s and thus regulates the activation of the early complement cascade. Type I C1 INH deficiency in 85% of patients is associated with diminished serum levels of C1 INH protein and therefore with deficient functional activity. In type II C1 INH deficiency (15%), the protein level is normal, but it possesses little or no functional activity. In acquired C1 INH deficiency, the clinical presentation is similar to the hereditary type but patients have developed an antibody to C1 INH. Many of these patients have an underlying lymphoproliferative disease.

Phagocytic Cell Defects

Patients with defects in phagocyte function experience repeated infections at locations where the body surface interfaces with the environment. The evaluation of the patient with suspected phagocyte dysfunction requires an understanding of the steps involved in normal antimicrobial activity of these cells. Normal function of the phagocyte compartment of host defense requires adequate numbers of neutrophils and monocytes, as well as the normal performance of a number of closely integrated functions to result in the effective killing of a pathogen by the leukocyte. Defects in neutrophil number (neutropenia, cyclic neutropenia, Kostmann's syndrome, Shwachman-Diamond syndrome), adherence, deformability, locomotion, chemotaxis, recognition of foreign particles and attachment, phagocytosis, oxidative respiratory metabolism, and intracellular microbial killing have all been reported. Data from the history and physical examination will help the clinician to focus attention on which phagocyte function is most likely to be defective. Absence of pus at the sites of infection, for example, suggests that the patient either has a decreased number of granulocytes or that these cells have an impaired ability to concentrate at the site of bacterial invasion, that is, defective chemotaxis or adhesion. A critical aspect of host defense is the accumulation of neutrophils at the site of infection. This process requires both the elaboration of chemotactic substances and a normal response

TABLE 271–2 CLINICAL CHARACTERISTICS OF DISEASES OF PHAGOCYTIC CELL DYSFUNCTION

Range from mild skin infections to severe systemic infections
Skin infections, furunculosis, visceral or perirectal abscess with granuloma formation, lymphadenitis, gingivitis
Poor wound healing, lack of pus
Mainly susceptible to low-grade virulent bacterial infections
Staphylococcus species
Gram-negative organisms

by leukocytes to chemoattractants. Chemotactic substances important in vivo include complement activation fragments and the chemotactic peptides and lipids released by a variety of inflammatory cells including mast cells in the allergic response. A history of persistent abscesses with exudates, conversely, suggests that the phagocytes can migrate to the appropriate site but are defective in intracellular bacterial killing. A history of recurrent gingivitis, skin infections with furunculosis, abscesses of the viscera or perirectal tissues, and lymphadenitis should prompt evaluation of the phagocyte host immune defenses. Because of defective phagocyte function, the manifestations of infections may be blunted; erythema, swelling, and pus formation may be limited or absent. Phagocyte defects frequently manifest as infections caused by bacteria of relatively low virulence, such as *S. aureus,* fungi, and gram-negative enteric bacteria, including *Klebsiella, E. coli, B. cepacia,* and *Serratia* species. Infections often fail to respond optimally to the usual courses of antimicrobial agents. Many patients also have a history of poor wound healing, a finding reflecting the critical role of phagocytes in tissue repair. The clinical features of phagocytic cell defects are shown in Table 271–2. The spectrum of phagocyte defects is discussed in more detail in Chapter 175.

Interferon-γ/Interleukin-12 Pathway Deficiencies

These patients have increased susceptibility to infections with nontuberculous mycobacteria, *Salmonella,* and certain viruses, as well as disseminated infection following bacille Calmette-Guérin vaccination. Several genetic defects of the monocyte-macrophage-T_H1 T-cell pathway have been identified (see Table 271–1). Patients with receptor defects have severe impairment in interferon-γ signaling and fail to form tuberculoid granulomas. Patients with a partial defect have a better prognosis. Other patients with a similar clinical phenotype have an IL-12p40 deficiency or a mutation in the IL-12 receptor.

DEFICIENCIES OF T-CELL IMMUNITY

Profound defects in T-lymphocyte function, or defects arresting development of T cells early in ontogeny, not only affect cell-mediated immunity but also impair the development of B-lymphocyte function (humoral immunity) resulting from the absence of T-cell help and T-cell–derived cytokines. The clinical syndromes resulting from these more profound immune defects are referred to as *severe combined immunodeficiency disease.* Recurrent infections with organisms of relatively low virulence in an immunologically normal host (opportunistic infections) occur. Patients with T-cell immunodeficiency also have infection with *Candida albicans* involving the mucous membranes and skin, but this infection is not invasive. Other fungal infections, severe viral diseases, and infection with opportunistic pathogens such as *P. carinii* or *M. avium intracellulare* should prompt an evaluation for disorders in T-cell function. Graft-versus-host disease can be a significant problem in patients with severe T-cell immunodeficiency either after transfusion of lymphocyte-containing blood products or as a result of intrapartum or prenatal maternal-fetal transfusion. The clinical characteristics of patients with T-cell deficiency are shown in Table 271–3.

Patients should be evaluated for T-cell deficiency by enumerating peripheral blood T cell subsets and natural killer cells (NK cells) by flow cytometry, as well as functionally by lymphocyte proliferative responses to mitogens and specific antigens in vitro. Delayed hypersensitivity skin testing can serve as an initial screening test for T-cell immunity. Intracutaneous injection of 0.1 mL of recall antigens including *Candida* at 1:100 dilution wt/vol, tetanus toxoid at 1:100 dilution wt/vol, or

TABLE 271–3 CLINICAL CHARACTERISTICS OF T-CELL DEFICIENCIES

Onset of symptoms frequently in early infancy (4–5 mo)
Recurrent infections with fungi *(Candida),* viruses, and mycobacterial pathogens
Infections with opportunistic organisms: *Pneumocystis jirovecii*
Failure to thrive, often fatal in childhood
Fatal infections from live virus vaccines or bacille Calmette-Guérin vaccination
Graft-versus-host disease from transfusion of blood products containing viable T lymphocytes

Trichophyton at 1:30 dilution to a patient who was previously sensitized to these antigens should produce a reaction of redness and induration greater than 5 mm with a maximum response at 48 to 72 hours. Negative results are seen in patients with impaired T-cell responses, but they can also be seen because of lack of prior antigen exposure. Severe illness or systemic steroid use can also diminish delayed hypersensitivity responses (anergy).

Once the diagnosis of T-cell immunodeficiency has been established in cooperation with a clinical immunologist, the physician needs to be aware of several important issues in providing care to these patients. First, prompt recognition of infections and aggressive treatment is essential to avoid life-threatening complications and to improve prognosis and quality of life. This approach may include initiation of early empirical antibiotic coverage for suspected pathogens, obtaining appropriate cultures, and continued communication with the consulting immunologist. Prophylactic antibiotics are recommended for patients with significant T-cell defects because of the risk of *P. jirovecii* pneumonia; trimethoprim-sulfamethoxazole is the most commonly used antibiotic for *P. carinii* pneumonia prophylaxis. Live vaccines such as oral polio, varicella, and bacille Calmette-Guérin should not be given to patients with suspected or diagnosed antibody or T-cell immunodeficiency because vaccine-induced infection is a risk in these patients. Inactivated polio vaccine instead of oral polio vaccine should be given to household members, to prevent transmission of the virus that can occur via shedding of the attenuated virus in the stool. If patients with T-cell defects need blood transfusions, only irradiated, leukocyte-poor, and virus-free (cytomegalovirus) products should be used, to avoid graft-versus-host disease and cytomegalovirus infection. In patients with T-cell deficiency, varicella-zoster immunoglobulin may be indicated following varicella exposure.

With regard to T-cell immunodeficiency disorders, great strides have been made in the delineation of defects in the immune pathways because of advances in molecular biology (see Table 271–1). Although these patients usually present with these disorders early in life, advances in immune reconstitution by bone marrow transplantation enable patients to live into adulthood. The impact of the corrected T-cell defect on the occurrence of adult-type disorders, such as cardiovascular disease and others, is currently unknown. These profound T-cell immunodeficiencies manifest in early childhood and are not discussed in this chapter except for ataxia-telangiectasia.

Ataxia-telangiectasia is a form of SCID that manifests in childhood. The disease is due to a mutated gene that encodes for a DNA-dependent protein kinase involved in multiple intracellular functions. The clinical characteristics of this disorder are progressive cerebellar ataxia, ocular and cutaneous telangiectasias, and chronic sinus and lung infections. Patients may also develop a malignancy, either a B-cell lymphoma or T-cell leukemia. Immunoglobulin levels may be variably decreased or absent, and specific antibody levels may be normal or decreased. Patients also exhibit degrees of lymphopenia, decreased cellular immunity, a hypoplastic thymus, and elevated serum levels of α-fetoprotein. Treatment is supportive to include intravenous gamma globulin in those patients with immunoglobulin deficiencies.

B-CELL IMMUNODEFICIENCIES

Unlike patients with severe combined immunodeficiency disease, in whom the onset of symptoms is at 4 or 5 months of age, patients with severe B-cell deficiencies usually do not have problems with infections

TABLE 271–4 CLINICAL CHARACTERISTICS OF B-CELL DEFICIENCIES

Recurrent infections with encapsulated organisms
Sinopulmonary infections, otitis media, meningitis, sepsis, abscess, osteomyelitis, cellulitis
No problems with fungal or viral infections (except enteroviral infection in XLA)
Lymphoid tissues: absent in patients with XLA, hypertrophied in CVID
Increased incidence of atopy and autoimmune disease
Granulomatous lung disease in CVID
Gastrointestinal disease
Celiac disease
Lactose intolerance
Bacterial overgrowth of small bowel
Nodular lymphoid hyperplasia in CVID
Higher incidence of malignancy in CVID

CVID = common variable immunodeficiency; XLA = X-linked agammaglobulinemia.

until 7 to 9 months of age. The later onset of problems with infections in this group of patients occurs because they are protected initially by the maternal antibodies that passed through the placenta during the third trimester of pregnancy. These patients usually have infections with encapsulated bacterial organisms such as pneumococci and *H. influenzae* type b. The types of infection, as discussed previously, include otitis media, meningitis, septicemia, sinusitis, pneumonia, abscess, and osteomyelitis. Occasionally, these patients may have problems with fungal or viral pathogens. Male patients with infantile XLA have an unusual susceptibility to enteroviruses and may develop chronic enteroviral encephalomyelitis. Generally, one does not see severe growth failure in patients with B-cell deficiency, as in T-cell–deficient patients. Patients with antibody deficiency can survive into adulthood and can lead normal lives with the use of replacement intravenous immunoglobulin (IVIG) therapy.

Patients with severe B-cell deficiency, such as infantile XLA, typically have a paucity of lymphoid tissue (tonsils, adenoids, and peripheral lymph nodes). In contrast, patients with CVID often have lymphoid hypertrophy or hepatosplenomegaly. The incidence of allergy and autoimmune disease is increased, particularly in patients with IgA deficiency and CVID. The primary antibody deficiency disorders are shown in Table 271–1, and the clinical characteristics of patients with B-cell deficiency are shown in Table 271–4.

X-Linked Agammaglobulinemia

Definition

XLA is an X-linked recessive B-cell immunodeficiency with agammaglobulinemia and absent circulating B cells.

Epidemiology

Worldwide, the incidence appears to be approximately 1 in 100,000 to 200,000 or 5 to 10 cases per 1 million population. The prevalence is 1 in 10,000.

Pathobiology

The gene responsible for XLA is located on the X-chromosome, and it has been identified as a cytoplasmic tyrosine kinase (i.e., Bruton's tyrosine kinase [Btk]), which is expressed mainly in lymphocytes of the B-cell lineage. Btk is critical in B-lymphocyte signal transduction pathways and B-cell differentiation. Numerous distinct mutations of the *BTK* gene have been described in patients with XLA, most involving the kinase domain. Mutations in the *BTK* gene lead to a block in B-cell maturation from pro-B cells to pre-B cells.

Some patients with Btk mutations may not present until later in life. This variation may reflect different types of Btk mutations. In fact, the block in B-cell differentiation may be "leaky," and the result may be some immunoglobulin synthesis. Study of one family showed marked phenotypic variation among the male members who had the same gene mutation; serum immunoglobulins also showed variability. A subgroup of patients with CVID may also present with profound hypogammaglobulinemia and markedly reduced numbers of B cells. In a study of male patients with recurrent infections and low numbers of B cells (<1%) by flow cytometry using a monoclonal antibody to the Btk protein, 10 patients were older than 15 years of age (~9%). Investigators have estimated that approximately 10% of adult patients with CVID may be misdiagnosed and may have XLA with deficient Btk.

Clinical Manifestations

Infections occur predominantly in the sinopulmonary tract (60% of patients), including otitis media, chronic sinusitis, and pneumonia. Other types of infections include pyoderma (25%), chronic conjunctivitis (8%), gastroenteritis (35%), arthritis (20%), meningitis or encephalitis (16%), and, less commonly, osteomyelitis (3%) and septicemia (10%). The most common pathogens are *H. influenzae* and *S. pneumoniae.* Young male patients who are untreated experience repeated pulmonary tract infections, leading eventually to bronchiectasis. Infections may also occur with *G. lamblia.* Because cellular immunity is intact, most viral infections, fungal infections, and tuberculosis do not seem to be a problem in patients with XLA. Exceptions to this include viral hepatitis, disseminated polio, and chronic enteroviral encephalitis.

Physical findings relate to the occurrence of repeated bacterial infections of susceptible target organs, such as the middle ear, sinuses, and lungs. Patients have a paucity of lymphoid tissues, for example, adenoids, lymph nodes, and spleen, unlike patients with CVID, who often have lymphoid hyperplasia. Unusual complications in XLA include arthritis, a dermatomyositis-like syndrome, and meningoencephalitis, which are usually manifestations of chronic enterovirus infections, including the echoviruses and occasionally coxsackievirus.

Arthritis occurs in fewer than half of the patients with XLA, and it is usually an acute bacterial infection affecting the large joints. Sedimentation rates may be normal, and serologic tests are negative. In some patients, the joint inflammation results from infections with enteroviruses or with *Ureaplasma urealyticum.* Joint symptoms usually improve or resolve with IVIG therapy. Patients with XLA are highly susceptible to poliovirus infection; vaccine-associated poliomyelitis has been reported in XLA.

Unlike patients with CVID, autoimmune disorders do not seem to be a frequent problem in patients with XLA. Although a predisposition to various cancers seems to be common with many types of immunodeficiencies, it is less clear whether patients with XLA have the same predisposition. The primary immunodeficiency registry reported that only 4.2% of registry patients with malignancy had XLA; lymphoreticular and gastrointestinal malignant diseases were more common.

Patients with XLA have a total absence or marked deficiency in serum immunoglobulins, and they fail to make antibodies to even potent protein antigens. Circulating B cells or surface membrane immunoglobulin-positive lymphocytes are extremely low (<2%) or absent. However, pro-B cells in the bone marrow are normal or even increased in number. T lymphocytes and other lymphoid subpopulations and delayed skin reactivity to recall antigens are normal. The response of peripheral blood mononuclear cells to mitogens and allogeneic cells is normal. Lymphoid tissues show an absence of plasma cells, lymphoid follicles, and germinal centers.

Diagnosis

Serum immunoglobulins should be quantified; patients with XLA usually have a profound hypogammaglobulinemia or agammaglobulinemia. Flow cytometry for B-cell numbers shows absent or very low numbers of B cells (e.g., <2%). Molecular analysis for Btk genetic abnormalities, especially those that involve the early stages of B-cell maturation in patients who present with absent B cells, can be very helpful in diagnostic evaluations. T-cell function is normal.

Treatment

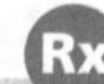

Early diagnosis, broad-spectrum antibiotics, and replacement therapy with IVIG have changed the outcome of this disease. Infections, especially chronic enteroviral infections and chronic pulmonary disease, are still the two major complications of XLA. However, with the availability of IVIG in the early 1980s, the management of this disease became much easier. Early IVIG replacement therapy with nadir serum IgG levels higher than 500 mg/dL is important in preventing severe acute bacterial infections and bronchiectasis. Trough serum IgG levels higher than 800 mg/dL may be necessary to prevent chronic sinusitis and enteroviral infections adequately.

Agammaglobulinemia with Absent B Cells

Approximately 10% of patients with agammaglobulinemia and absent B cells are female, and they present clinically similarly to patients with XLA. Any mutation of a gene involved in the early stages of B-cell differentiation could result in an XLA-like phenotype. Mutations that block the early stages of B-cell differentiation are listed in Table 271–1. Female patients who present with absent B cells and agammaglobulinemia appear to have more severe disease than do boys with Btk mutations. More details can be found in the review by Conley.

Immunodeficiency with Hyper-Immunoglobulin M

Definition

Immunodeficiency with hyper-IgM is characterized by severe recurrent bacterial infections with decreased serum levels of IgG, IgA, and IgE but with normal or elevated levels of serum IgM. The X-linked form of this syndrome is more common (type 1), but a similar phenotype with an autosomal recessive inheritance occurs in female patients (type 3).

Pathobiology

Mutations in the CD40 ligand (CD154) gene are responsible for the X-linked form of hyper-IgM (type 1), whereas mutations in the CD40 ligand receptor (e.g., CD40) are responsible for hyper-IgM type 3.

Clinical Manifestations

Recurrent bacterial infections of the sinopulmonary tract usually begin in the first or second year of life. The clinical history of infection often resembles patients with XLA. Stomatitis and mouth ulcers may occur in association with the neutropenia. *P. jirovecii* has been reported in patients with this disease. Other opportunistic pathogens include cytomegalovirus, *Cryptococcus,* and mycobacteria. Patients are susceptible to opportunistic organisms and have a high incidence of autoimmune diseases such as thrombocytopenia, hemolytic anemia, neutropenia, nephritis, and arthritis. Diarrhea is a frequent finding, occurring in more than 50% of patients, often as a result of cryptosporidiosis. Hepatitis B and hepatitis C viral infections produce chronic hepatitis in these patients. Unlike in patients with XLA, these patients have marked hypertrophy of the lymphoid tissues, including the tonsils, lymph nodes, and spleen. However, the lymph nodes are poorly organized, with absence of the germinal centers. Proliferation of IgM-producing plasma cells with extensive invasion of the gastrointestinal tract and liver may occur by the second decade of life. Patients also have an increased risk of malignant diseases, especially lymphomas. An increased incidence of liver and biliary tumors is a unique feature of X-linked hyper-IgM.

Diagnosis

Serum levels of IgM are markedly increased and may exceed 1000 mg/dL; however, early in life, the level of serum IgM may be normal. Patients can produce IgM antibody, but the secondary IgG response is usually markedly diminished or absent. Surface immunoglobulin-positive lymphocytes in the peripheral blood are primarily positive for IgM; IgA- and IgG-bearing lymphocytes are decreased or absent. T-lymphocyte numbers and mitogen responses are normal. Patients with X-linked hyper-IgM, such as those with as type 1, lack CD40 ligand on activated T cells as a result of mutations in the gene for CD40 ligand. Patients with hyper-IgM type 3 lack the receptor for CD40 ligand (CD40) on B cells and antigen-presenting cells.

Treatment

Supportive care, use of prophylactic antibiotics for *P. carinii*, and recognition and treatment of other opportunistic infections are all important. Parenteral nutrition may be necessary for patients with severe gastrointestinal disturbances. Treatment consists of IVIG replacement therapy. The autoimmune neutropenia responds well to treatment with IVIG and granulocyte colony-stimulating factor. Bone marrow transplantation has been used in the treatment of patients with this disease.

Other Forms of Hyper-Immunoglobulin M Phenotypes

Several female patients have been described, a finding suggesting an autosomal form of the disease. These patients normally express CD40L on T cells and CD40 on B cells. Molecular studies have shown that the defects in the autosomal variant of the hyper-IgM syndrome are mutations in the activation-induced cytidine deaminase gene *(AICDA)* and the uracil DNA glycosylase gene *(UNG)* (see Table 271–1). These patients differ from those with the X-linked form by lymphoid hyperplasia with marked follicular hyperplasia, enlarged germinal centers with highly proliferating B cells, defective immunoglobulin variable region gene somatic mutation generation, and defective immunoglobulin class switch recombination.

Another rare form of X-linked hyper-IgM syndrome is associated with ectodermal dysplasia characterized by the absence or hypoplasia of hair, teeth, and sweat glands and by the presence of immunodeficiency. Patients have increased susceptibility to bacterial infections, including atypical mycobacteria, and herpes viral infections. Most patients have low serum levels of IgG with variable levels of IgM and IgA and poor antibody production; NK cell function is also defective. This disorder is related to mutations in the gene that encodes the nuclear factor-κB (NF-κB) essential modulator (NEMO or IKKγ) that is required for activation of the transcription factor NF-κB. Genetic diagnosis and genetic counseling are important, including carrier testing of the patient's mother, sisters, and aunts. Treatment consists of IGIV and mycobacterial prophylaxis.

Common Variable Immunodeficiency

Definition

CVID comprises a heterogeneous group of disorders involving both B-cell and T-cell immune function whose predominant manifestation is hypogammaglobulinemia. CVID is characterized by recurrent bacterial infections, decreased serum immunoglobulin levels (at least two immunoglobulin isotypes more than 2 SD lower than normal for age), and abnormal antibody responses. These patients may present in early childhood, during adolescence, or as young adults. In most patients, the onset of symptoms is in the second and third decade of life. In a large study, the average age of onset of symptoms was 25 years, and the average age at diagnosis was 28 years.

Pathobiology

Several mechanisms have been proposed to explain the immune abnormalities in patients with CVID, including an intrinsic B-cell defect, excessive T-suppressor cell activity, deficient helper T-lymphocyte function, cytokine deficiencies, and suboptimal T-cell–B-cell interactions through deficient expression of the CD40 ligand. T cells in CVID have diminished production of IL-2, IL-4, IL-5, and interferon-γ, and they express lower levels of the IL-2 receptor. A signaling defect may be intrinsic to the B cells, or it may occur between a poorly expressed CD40 ligand on T cells and the CD40 receptor on B cells. Whether these abnormalities are a cause or a consequence of CVID remains to be determined. The number of immune deviations described in patients with CVID underscores the heterogeneous nature of the immune defect or defects in this syndrome. A homozygous deletion in the gene encoding ICOS, a T-cell costimulatory molecule of the CD28 family that enhances the activation of T cells and is important in T-cell–B-cell interactions, was found in a small number of patients with CVID. The clinical phenotype of ICOS deficiency is similar to that of other patients with CVID. Other recent findings are the lack of memory B cells, such as $CD27^+$, and the absence of class-switched B cells in 75% of patients with CVID. These findings have led to the hypothesis that patients with CVID have a defect in the germinal centers of their secondary lymphatics.

Family members of patients with CVID have an unusually high incidence of IgA deficiency, autoimmune diseases, autoantibodies, and malignant disease. Some patients with IgA deficiency and CVID have one or both of two extended major histocompatibility complex (MHC) haplotypes: haplotype 1, HLA-DQB1*0201, HLA-DR3, C4B-Sf, C4A-0, G11-15, Bf-0,4, C2-a, HSP-7.5, TNF-α-a2b3, HLA-B8 and HLA-A1; or the second haplotype, HLA-DQB1*0201, HLA-DR7, C4B-S, C4A-L, G11-4.5, Bf-0.6, C2-b, HSP-9, TNF-α-a7b4 or a11b4, HLA-B44 and HLA-A29. One or more genes within the MHC region on chromosome 6 (e.g., one near or within the class II region and one in the class III region near the class I locus) may be involved in the pathogenesis of CVID and IgA deficiency. An inheritance pattern of autosomal dominance with variable penetrance has been suggested.

Clinical Manifestations

The most frequent presenting infections in adults with CVID involve the respiratory tract, including recurrent otitis media, chronic sinusitis, and recurrent pneumonia, often with resulting bronchiectasis. The bacterial pathogens are similar to those described in XLA. The gastrointestinal tract is affected in approximately half the patients with CVID; patients present with malabsorption or chronic diarrhea. These symptoms can be related to numerous underlying abnormalities, including lactose intolerance, protein-losing enteropathy, and superimposed infection of the small bowel with bacteria such as *Campylobacter* or *Yersinia,* with the parasite *G. lamblia,* or with flora of the large bowel (small bowel bacterial overgrowth syndrome). Atrophic gastritis with achlorhydria may lead to pernicious anemia.

Approximately 5 to 10% of patients with CVID present with noncaseating granulomatous lesions that infiltrate the liver, lymph nodes, lung, and skin. These lesions are often confused with sarcoidosis. Chronic gastrointestinal disease is often associated with nodular lymphoid hyperplasia, characterized by hypertrophy of the Peyer's patches in the small bowel, and diffuse lymphoid infiltration. Hypertrophy of other lymphoid tissues, including the peripheral lymph nodes, the spleen, and occasionally the liver, are also seen. Rarely, hepatosplenomegaly may be severe enough to result in secondary neutropenia or thrombocytopenia. The pathogenesis of this process is not known, but it may be related to increased production of TNF-α. Patients with granulomatous-lymphocytic interstitial lung disease have a worse prognosis, a restrictive pulmonary pattern with a low-normal diffusing lung capacity for carbon monoxide, and diminished T-cell function. High-resolution computed tomography of the chest is helpful in identifying these patients, who require higher replacement doses of IVIG.

Autoimmune disorders occur frequently in CVID (20 to 25% of patients), and they include rheumatic diseases, autoimmune hematologic disorders, autoimmune neurologic diseases, chronic active hepatitis, and autoimmune endocrinopathies. The incidence of malignant disease is increased (11% to 13%) in CVID during the fifth and sixth decades of life. Most of these malignant diseases involve the gastrointestinal tract and the lymphoid tissues (e.g., non-Hodgkin's lymphoma).

Diagnosis

The serum immunoglobulin levels are markedly diminished in patients with CVID. However, one can see tremendous variability in the degree of hypogammaglobulinemia. Specific antibodies are usually lacking, and isohemagglutinin titers are generally diminished. The proportions of circulating B cells in the peripheral blood are usually normal, but a subset of patients may lack circulating B lymphocytes. T-cell function can be quite variable: it is normal in half of the patients and depressed in the other half, with absent delayed hypersensitivity skin reactivity to recall antigens, low numbers of circulating peripheral blood $CD4^+$ T cells, often with a decrease in the CD4 : CD8 ratio, and depressed in vitro responses to mitogens and specific antigens.

Treatment

Rx

Patients with CVID are treated with doses of IVIG of 400 to 600 mg/kg every 4 weeks. Generally, this regimen should achieve a trough serum IgG level higher than 500 mg/dL. Patients who continue to have recurrent infections or who have bronchiectasis should be treated with higher doses of IVIG.

Prognosis

The prognosis is generally very good for patients whose illness is diagnosed early and who undergo replacement IVIG therapy. The reported mortality rate over a 25-year period was 24%, mostly because of lymphoma (18%) and chronic pulmonary disease (11%). The mean age at the time of death was 45.5 years in women and 40 years in men. The patients who died were more likely to have lower levels of IgG at the time of diagnosis and poorer T-cell proliferative responses to phytohemagglutinin (PHA). Twenty-year survival after diagnosis of CVID was 64% for men and 67% for women compared with 92 to 94% for the general population.

Immunodeficiency with Thymoma

Immunodeficiency with thymoma was first described in 1954 (Good's syndrome). It is a disorder of adults, typically between the ages of 40 and 70 years. This immunodeficiency presents with recurrent sinopulmonary infections. Affected individuals have hypogammaglobulinemia, which may affect all major immunoglobulin isotypes. A thymoma may be discovered during the initial investigation of hypogammaglobulinemia by the detection of a mediastinal mass on a routine chest radiograph. Occasionally, the thymoma predates the hypogammaglobulinemia. The thymic tumors are predominantly of the spindle cell type and are usually benign. The clinical symptoms are similar to those found in patients with CVID. In contrast to CVID, however, frequently associated disorders include aregenerative (pure red cell) anemia, agranulocytosis, and myasthenia gravis. These conditions may improve after thymectomy; however, the immunodeficiency persists. Infections commonly associated with T-cell abnormalities can be seen in this disease, including mucocutaneous candidiasis, cytomegalovirus infection, herpes zoster, and *P. carinii* pneumonia.

Immunoglobulin A Deficiency

Definition

Deficiency in serum IgA is one of the most common B-cell immunodeficiencies, with an approximate incidence of 1 in 400 to 2000 individuals in the general population. IgA deficiency is defined as a serum IgA concentration lower than 7 mg/dL, with normal serum levels of IgM and IgG.

Pathobiology

The genetic defect responsible for IgA deficiency is not known. IgA deficiency shares with CVID the inheritance of a restricted MHC extended haplotype. Although the pathogenesis of IgA deficiency is still unknown, it may share a common origin with CVID because these two disorders have many immune aspects in common. IgA deficiency may occur in association with the administration of drugs such as phenytoin, sulfasalazine, hydroxychloroquine, and D-penicillamine. IgA deficiency has also been described in association with partial deletion of the long arm of chromosome 18 (18q syndrome) or with a ring chromosome 18.

Clinical Manifestations

Many individuals with selective IgA deficiency do not have symptoms. The variability in clinical expression may be related to two factors. First, the IgA-deficient patients who tend to be relatively asymptomatic appear to have a compensatory increase in secretory monomeric IgM in their saliva, upper respiratory tract secretions, and gastrointestinal fluids. Second, the association of IgG2/IgG4 or IgG4 subclass deficiencies with IgA deficiency may predispose IgA-deficient patients to more severe and recurrent sinopulmonary infection than is seen in those patients with isolated selective IgA deficiency.

Symptoms of IgA deficiency include sinopulmonary infections and involvement of the gastrointestinal tract with giardiasis, nodular lymphoid hyperplasia, ulcerative colitis, Crohn's disease, or a spruelike disease. An increased frequency of autoimmune disorders has also been associated with IgA deficiency, including arthritis, a lupus-like illness, autoimmune endocrinopathies, chronic active hepatitis, and autoimmune hematologic disorders. IgA-deficient patients are at risk for the development of anti-IgA antibodies on receipt of blood products. Caution must be exercised in the administration of IVIG for replacement of IgG subclass deficiency in IgA-deficient patients because most of these preparations contain small amounts of IgA. However, this risk does not appear to be a problem in those patients with partial IgA deficiency.

Diagnosis

IgA deficiency is defined as serum IgA levels lower than 7 mg/dL. The peripheral blood B cells of IgA-deficient patients coexpress IgA, IgM, and IgD, an immature phenotype. However, the lymphoid tissues are deficient in IgA-producing plasma cells. Studies of T-cell function have been normal in most patients with selective IgA deficiency.

Treatment

Rx

No specific treatment for IgA deficiency exists. Prophylactic antibiotics may be helpful in patients with recurrent sinopulmonary tract infections. Patients with chronic lung disease should receive conventional therapy, to prevent the development of bronchiectasis. IVIG is not indicated in patients with isolated IgA deficiency. Other supportive treatments are aimed at associated diseases. Patients should be transfused only with washed red cells, to avoid sensitization to the IgA in plasma products.

Prognosis

The prognosis is good in most cases. Respiratory infections and autoimmune disease are more common in IgA-deficient patients. A few patients with IgA deficiency presenting in childhood may recover spontaneously; other patients may develop CVID.

Immunoglobulin G Subclass Deficiencies and Selective Antibody Deficiency

Definition

Considerable controversy exists over the biologic significance of IgG subclasses and the clinical significance of an isolated IgG subclass outside the normal range. Because healthy individuals without recurrent infections may have an abnormally low serum IgG subclass concentration, investigators question whether IgG subclass deficiency represents a true immunodeficiency disease. Deficiency in an IgG subclass is defined as a serum IgG subclass concentration that is more than 2 SD lower than the normal mean for age. The age at which each of the IgG subclasses reaches adult levels varies. Gm allotype also influences serum concentrations of certain IgG subclasses, particularly IgG2 and IgG3. In adults, deficiencies in IgG3 subclass are most common, whereas in children, IgG2 is the most prevalent IgG subclass deficiency. IgG subclass deficiency may be seen in conjunction with other primary immunodeficiency disorders, such as ataxia-telangiectasia and IgA deficiency. IgG subclass deficiency occurs in approximately 18% of IgA-deficient patients. An IgG subclass deficiency may occur as an isolated immune defect, or two or more IgG subclass deficiencies may coexist (e.g., IgG2 and IgG4 deficiency).

Patients with selective antibody deficiency have abnormal responses to immunization with polysaccharides such as *H. influenzae* type b (Hib) capsular antigen or to the pneumococcal polysaccharide antigens, but they have normal serum immunoglobulin and IgG subclass concentrations. However, patients immunized to Hib-conjugate vaccine responded normally in that the antibody response to the conjugate vaccine falls principally within the IgG1 subclass instead of the IgG2 subclass. Similar observations have been made for selective antibody deficiency after immunization with a pneumococcal polysaccharide vaccine in patients presenting with recurrent sinusitis or chronic sinusitis.

Clinical Manifestations

The most frequent clinical problems associated with IgG subclass deficiency are recurrent infections of the upper and lower respiratory tracts. Pathogens are generally limited to bacteria and respiratory viruses. Because IgG2 is important in the response to polysaccharide antigens, patients with IgG2 deficiency typically have infections with *H. influenzae* or *S. pneumoniae.* Patients may be unable to produce specific antibodies after immunization with purified polysaccharide antigens (e.g., Pneumovax). Some patients with IgG2 subclass deficiency may be asymptomatic. In part, this may result from a shifting of the antibody response to another IgG subclass or immunoglobulin isotype, which compensates for the selective IgG2 subclass deficiency. IgG3 deficiency has been associated with recurrent upper and lower respiratory tract infections and may occur in combination with IgG1 deficiency. Several studies have suggested that IgG3 is especially important in the primary response to viral respiratory agents. IgG3 is also the predominant antibody response in *Moraxella catarrhalis,* an organism frequently isolated from patients with chronic sinusitis. IgG4 deficiency occurs in the general population at a rate of approximately 10 to 15%. The clinical significance of IgG4 deficiency is not known.

Diagnosis

Serum immunoglobulin concentrations should be measured by quantitative techniques (nephelometry). Values in children must be compared with laboratory normals for age. Immunoelectrophoresis is semiquantitative and should not be used to evaluate the patient with suspected antibody deficiency. Immunoelectrophoresis should be used only to examine serum for paraproteins such as those found in Waldenström's macroglobulinemia or multiple myeloma. IgG subclass quantitation may be helpful, although debate continues over the utility of these measurements. A careful history and physical examination are important in determining the clinical significance of an IgG subclass deficiency. In addition, the measurement of functional or specific antibodies is important in indicating the clinical relevance of an IgG subclass deficiency.

Patients may have normal levels of total serum immunoglobulins and normal IgG subclasses yet may fail to make specific antibodies to bacterial or common viral pathogens. Therefore, the assessment of specific antibody formation following vaccine administration is an important part of the laboratory evaluation in patients with suspected B-cell deficiency. Usually, repeat titers are obtained 4 weeks after immunization, to assess the specific antibody response. Isohemagglutinins are naturally occurring IgM antibodies to the ABO blood group substances. Responses to protein antigens generally fall in the IgG1 subclass, whereas the immune response to the polysaccharide antigens resides within the IgG2 subclass. With the conjugated vaccines for Hib and pneumococcal polysaccharides, antibody responses occur primarily in the IgG1 rather than IgG2 subclass. Therefore, these conjugate vaccines may not be helpful in the functional evaluation of an IgG2 subclass deficiency or a selective polysaccharide antibody deficiency. Because a common complaint of many of these patients is recurrent upper respiratory tract infections, one can test the serum for the presence of antibodies to common respiratory viral agents such as influenza A and B, mycoplasma, respiratory syncytial virus, adenovirus, and the parainfluenza viruses.

Treatment

Replacement IVIG should be considered only if patients demonstrate poor antibody responses to vaccine immunization such as Pneumovax. Often, prophylactic antibiotics are useful in this group of patients, at least for the winter months.

SUGGESTED READINGS

Ballow M: Primary immunodeficiency disorders: Antibody deficiency. J Allergy Clin Immunol 2002;109:581–591. *A comprehensive review of antibody immunodeficiencies.*

Bonilla FA, Bernstein IL, Khan DA, et al: Practice parameter for the diagnosis and management of primary immunodeficiency. Ann Allergy Asthma Immunol 2005;94:S1–S63. *A helpful reference for practitioners to evaluate patients with recurrent infection and to assist in the diagnosis and management of these patients.*

Buckley RH: Primary cellular immunodeficiencies. J Allergy Clin Immunol 2002;109:747–757. *A comprehensive review of T-cell immunodeficiencies.*

Castigli E, Geha RS: Molecular basis of common variable immunodeficiency. J Allergy Clin Immunol 2006;117:40–46. *Discusses the known genetic defects.*

Castigli E, Wilson SA, Garibyan L, et al: TACI is mutant in common variable immunodeficiency and IgA deficiency. Nat Genet 2005;37:829–834. *An important paper that identifies a new gene defect related to IgA deficiency and common variable immunodeficiency, and may help understand the immunobiology of these immunodeficiencies.*

272 ALLERGIC RHINITIS AND SINUSITIS

Larry Borish

Definition

Allergic rhinitis (AR) refers to the nasal and ocular symptoms that occur as a result of the development of an inflammatory hypersensitivity reaction to aeroallergens deposited on the nasal mucosa and conjunctiva.

Epidemiology

AR, the most common chronic disease in the United States, affects between 9 and 24% of adults and up to 42% of children. Each year, nearly 80 million people in the United States experience 7 or more days of nasal or ocular symptoms as a result of AR. Although it is not a severe disorder, the socioeconomic costs of AR are substantial. AR is one of the chief reasons for visiting a primary care physician, it adversely affects work productivity and school performance, and it limits socialization. Its impact also reflects the involvement of AR with a variety of comorbid conditions, including asthma (Chapter 87), chronic sinusitis, nasal polyposis, secretory otitis media, and sleep disorders. Adequately addressing AR requires a thorough understanding of its pathophysiology, its relation to these comorbid conditions, and the effects of various therapeutic options on the pathophysiology of AR and its associated comorbidities.

Pathobiology

Airborne Allergens

Allergic respiratory diseases result from a hypersensitivity immune reaction to airborne allergens. These include the seasonal pollens and molds that are responsible for seasonal AR (SAR) and the indoor allergens, such as house dust mites and animal proteins, that are responsible for perennial AR (PAR) (Table 272–1).

In any area, the specific pollens that are likely to cause symptoms can be predicted from the number of days that a particular pollen is airborne in large numbers. All these pollens utilize a windborne mechanism to produce fertilization. Insect-borne pollens, specifically those produced by flowers, are not significantly airborne and therefore are not inhaled in sufficient concentrations to generate immune responses. In the United States, grass pollens (May to June) and ragweed (mid-August to October) are the most important causes of SAR. Tree pollens vary locally but typically start in late February and continue through April. The major trees implicated in allergy include birch in the North, oak in the mid-Atlantic region, live oak in the South, and mountain cedar in the Southwest. In addition to pollens, outdoor molds, particularly *Alternaria* and *Cladosporium* can produce symptoms. These molds have variable sporing seasons, depending on the weather, and high levels of airborne fungi are common at any time between March and October.

TABLE 272–1 ALLERGENS CAUSING ALLERGIC RHINITIS

Seasonal Allergens	
Common Name	**Season**
TREES	
Birch	March–May
Cottonwood	April–May
Elm	February–May
Cedars	March–May
Oak	May–June
Maple	March–May
GRASSES	
Kentucky blue	mid-May–June
Timothy	mid-May–June
Orchard	mid-May–June
Sweet vernal	mid-May–June
Fescue	mid-May–June
WEEDS	
Ragweed	August–September
Kochia	July–September
Russian thistle	July–September
Sage	July–September
Marsh elder	July–September
English plantain	July–September
OUTDOOR MOLDS	
Alternaria	Spring–fall
Cladosporium	Spring–fall
Perennial Allergens	
HOUSEHOLD ALLERGENS	
Cockroaches (German and American)	
Dust mites: *Dermatophagoides farinae, Dermatophagoides pteronyssinus, Blomia tropicalis*	
Other insects (spiders, ladybugs)	
ANIMALS	
Cats	
Other pets (guinea pigs, ferrets, hamsters, horses)	
Rodents	
Dogs	
? Chicken feathers	
INDOOR MOLDS	
Aspergillus	
Cladosporium	
Penicillium	

PAR may continue year round, but the term is applied to any rhinitis that does not have a clearly defined seasonal association. The most common causes include the following: (1) indoor fungi, which are related to periods of high indoor humidity and the availability of sites to grow; (2) animal danders, the most important being cats, but rodents (mice, rats, guinea pigs, ferrets, hamsters), rabbits, dogs, and birds may also be significant; (3) dust mites of the genus *Dermatophagoides* that grow in carpets, bedding, pillows, sofas, and so forth and that are semiseasonal, with maximum levels from August to December; and (4) other insects (the best studied is the cockroach, but gypsy moths, crickets, ladybugs, spiders, and beetles may also be locally important). Dust mites and cats produce the most important indoor allergens. Dust mites grow well only with a relative humidity higher than 55%. Dust mite allergy is therefore of major importance in the southeastern United States and also on the West Coast, Hawaii, and the Gulf Coast. It is probably relevant in all areas with more than 6 humid months in the year.

Immunoglobulin E/Mast Cell/Basophil Activation

Traditionally, AR is viewed as caused by triggering mast cell degranulation resulting from cross-linking of surface-bound immunoglobulin E (IgE) molecules by the aeroallergen. As with all antibody-mediated immune responses, the initial exposure to the antigen results in B-lymphocyte secretion of low-affinity IgM antibodies. Subsequent exposure to the allergen, in genetically predisposed subjects, leads to a secondary immune response characterized by the isotype switch to IgE. The resulting release of IgE antibodies into the circulation, however, does not cause allergic symptoms. It is only after the binding of these IgE antibodies to their high-affinity receptors on basophils and mast cells that symptoms can develop with subsequent allergen exposures. It takes cross-linking of approximately 300 IgE receptors/cell to stimulate degranulation. As such, it often requires several allergy seasons before sufficient numbers of allergen-specific IgE molecules are present on the mast cell surface to drive degranulation. The development of symptomatic AR is therefore a protracted process, generally requiring at least three or four exposures. As a result, SAR generally is not observed in infants until they are approximately 4 years of age. Similarly, in adults, symptomatic responses to local allergens may not develop until approximately 4 years after moving to the relevant region. PAR, however, can develop much faster.

Within minutes of allergen exposure, IgE-sensitized mast cells degranulate and release preformed and newly synthesized mediators, including histamine, proteases (tryptase and chymase), cysteinyl leukotrienes, prostaglandins, and cytokines. Some of these mediators produce the characteristic early-phase symptoms of AR, namely, sneezing, pruritus, rhinorrhea, and, to some extent, congestion, whereas other mediators stimulate infiltration of the nasal mucosa with inflammatory cells, including basophils, eosinophils, neutrophils, additional mast cells, and mononuclear cells. This infiltration of inflammatory cells and their subsequent release of a secondary wave of mediators sustain the inflammatory reaction with the continued recruitment of inflammatory cells and produce the late-phase response of AR. This slowly developing inflammatory response is primarily characterized by nasal congestion. The inflammation that develops over the course of an allergy season is associated with an approximately 10-fold increase in the numbers of mast cells present in nasal epithelial and submucosal tissue (Fig. 272–1C). This reflects the migration of preexisting mast cells into the epithelium and the differentiation and influx of newly synthesized mast cells into the nasal mucosa under the influence of cytokine growth factors. In the course of chronic allergen stimulation, these mast cells also display increased *priming* that reflects increases in numbers of IgE receptors and surface-bound IgE, as well as enhancement of signal transduction pathways. As the allergen season progresses, less and less allergen is required to trigger mast cell degranulation. In addition, as a result of priming, perennial allergens that are not sufficient by themselves to trigger an allergic reaction may exacerbate symptoms present during an allergy season.

Although mast cells play an important role during the initial AR response, they do not play as substantive a role in sustaining this response. Histamine secretion occurs during both early and late phases after allergen exposure, whereas prostaglandin D_2 increases only during the early phase. Because mast cells synthesize prostaglandin D_2, the absence of this mediator during the late phase indicates that mast cells are not responsible for the late-phase increase in histamine. Basophils

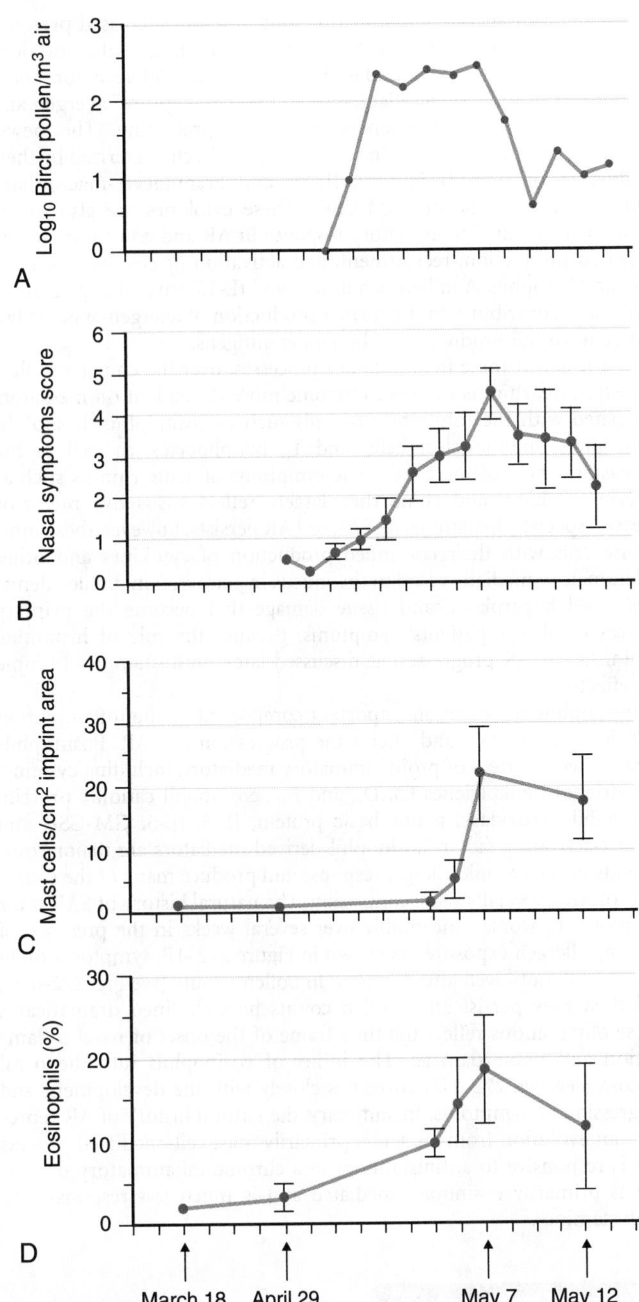

FIGURE 272–1 • Findings in allergy. During an allergy season when birch pollen was elevated **(A)**, associated nasal symptom scores gradually increased **(B)** and correlated significantly with the logarithm of the pollen count ($r = 0.68$; $P < .01$). A significant increase of the number of mast cells in the imprint area **(C)** and percentage of eosinophils in nasal lavage **(D)** also occurred during the allergy season compared with preseason values. (From Pipkorn U, Karlsson G, Enerback L: The cellular response of the human allergic mucosa to natural allergen exposure. J Allergy Clin Immunol 1988;82:1046–1054.)

release histamine, but, in contrast to mast cells, they do not produce prostaglandin D_2 and presumably are the source of this later histamine release.

Antigen-Presenting Cell/Helper T-Lymphocyte Activation

In addition to their interaction with mast cells, allergens also behave like any other foreign antigen and are processed and presented by antigen-presenting cells to helper T (T_H) lymphocytes. Activation of these antigen-presenting cells, including mononuclear phagocytic cells, B lymphocytes, and especially dendritic cells, is an important source of cytokines, especially those associated with innate immunity such as interleukin (IL)-1, IL-6, and tumor necrosis factor-α (TNF-α). With the development of allergic inflammation, one notes an increased presence of B cells expressing allergen-specific surface immunoglobulin and dendritic cells expressing IgE bound to their high-affinity IgE receptor. These antibodies can function as allergen receptors that "capture" allergen and increase these cells' effectiveness in antigen processing. The newly activated T lymphocytes tend to resemble $T_H{}^2$ cells, characterized by their production of IL-4, IL-5, IL-9, IL-13, and granulocyte-macrophage colony-stimulating factor (GM-CSF). These cytokines are also major components of the inflammatory response in AR and contribute to the increased production, recruitment, and activation of eosinophils, mast cells, and basophils. A milieu rich in IL-4 and IL-13 drives the IgE isotype switch and contributes to the further production of allergen-specific IgE and de novo IgE production to bystander antigens.

As a result of these inflammatory processes, over the course of allergen exposure, rhinitis evolves to become more dependent on mediators associated with the infiltration of cells such as eosinophils, basophils, neutrophils, mononuclear cells, and T_H lymphocytes, as well as the increasingly primed mast cells. The symptoms of acute rhinitis such as sneezing, itching, and rhinorrhea largely reflect vasoactive mediator release, especially histamine. As SAR or PAR persists, however, these infiltrating cells with their continued production of cytokines and other inflammatory mediators lead to the mucus hypersecretion, tissue edema, goblet cell hyperplasia, and tissue damage that become the primary sources of allergy patients' symptoms. Because the role of histamine diminishes as AR progresses, as discussed later, antihistamines become less effective.

Eosinophils represent an important component of the inflammation that develops in PAR and affects the progression of SAR. Eosinophils release a wide variety of proinflammatory mediators, including cysteinyl leukotrienes (leukotrienes C_4, D_4, and E_4), eosinophil cationic protein, eosinophil peroxidase, major basic protein, IL-3, IL-5, GM-CSF, and platelet-activating factor. Eosinophil-derived mediators are major components of the chronic allergic response and produce many of the symptoms of AR, especially nasal congestion. The natural history of SAR is for symptoms to worsen inexorably over several weeks in the presence of ongoing allergen exposure. As shown in Figure 272–1B, symptoms often do not peak until well after the peak in pollen counts (see Fig. 272–1A), and then they persist after pollen counts have declined dramatically. These observations reflect the time frame of the onset of nasal inflammation and tissue damage. The influx of eosinophils into the nasal mucosa (see Fig. 272–1D) correlates closely with the development and progression of symptoms. In summary, the natural history of AR represents an evolution from an acute, primarily mast cell–mediated process that is responsive to antihistamines to a chronic inflammatory process that is primarily eosinophil mediated and is much less responsive to antihistamines.

Clinical Manifestations

The diagnosis of AR is based on a history of sneezing, which is often paroxysmal, rhinorrhea with clear watery secretions, nasal congestion, and itching in the nares and palate. These symptoms are generally associated with allergic conjunctivitis manifested by ocular itching, lacrimation, and conjunctival injection. Severe conjunctivitis is less common in PAR, in contrast to SAR. The best explanation for this difference is that pollen grains affect the eyes when they are *blown* into them. Indoor allergens are less likely to be blown into the eyes because the air is relatively still. Indoor aeroallergens are drawn into the nose by breathing.

What historically has been less well appreciated is that AR is a systemic disease associated with circulating activated T lymphocytes and mononuclear phagocytic cells. The activation of these cells is demonstrated by their production of cytokines associated with innate immunity such as IL-1, TNF-α, and IL-6. These cytokines are responsible for the lethargy, fatigue, arthralgias, and myalgias that frequently accompany AR. AR is also associated with cognitive impairment in schoolchildren and adults. These systemic symptoms, which are often the chief complaints of allergy sufferers, contribute to the complaints of diminished quality of life and are often severe enough to make normal activities difficult, including work or school. Although fever is not regarded as a feature of AR, it is intriguing that the lay terminology for this condition is hay fever, a designation reflecting the pronounced flulike nature of this disease.

Diagnosis

AR is primarily a clinical diagnosis based on symptoms and exposure history. It is a complex genetic disorder, and affected patients generally give a positive family history. Physical examination reveals the nasal mucosa to be pale, cyanotic, and swollen with clear secretions. In children, a transverse nasal crease, a high arched palate, mouth breathing, and dental malocclusion are often observed. Periorbital venous dilation produces "allergic shiners." Nasal smears (Hansel stains) of nasal secretions are seldom required, but when performed they typically reveal eosinophils.

The diagnosis of AR is confirmed by demonstration of specific IgE antibodies reactive to the relevant pollen through either positive allergy skin tests or IgE immunoassays. In addition to confirming the diagnosis of AR, identification of specific triggering allergens is essential for recommending appropriate environmental controls specific to the causative allergen. Prick skin testing is safe, specific, rapid, and the diagnostic test of choice for identifying relevant allergens. Intradermal testing is rarely associated with potentially life-threatening systemic reactions. A positive intradermal test in the presence of a negative prick skin test is often a false-positive result and requires careful interpretation. If a referral for prick skin testing is not available or if the test cannot be performed (e.g., patients with eczema or dermatographism, patients using antihistamines, antiemetics, antipsychotic agents, or young children), in vitro testing (IgE immunoassays) can provide useful data. These tests are less sensitive than skin testing; however, positive IgE immunoassays correlate with symptoms on natural exposure, they establish the diagnosis of AR, and they can form the basis for environmental therapy and therefore should be extensively used by primary care physicians who manage patients with AR. However, a negative IgE immunoassay with a strong clinical suspicion should suggest the need for referral.

Differential Diagnosis

Other causes of rhinitis are shown in Table 272–2, and the approach to the patient with sneezing and rhinorrhea is displayed in Figure 272–2. *Viral rhinitis* may be difficult to distinguish from SAR. Viral rhinitis is not associated with release of mast cell mediators. The main mediators present in nasal secretions from patients with the common cold are kinins, whereas leukotrienes and prostaglandins are generally less prevalent. The presence of these different mediators is in keeping with the observation that most allergic patients can distinguish the symptoms of the common cold from those caused by allergen exposure. Pruritus, paroxysmal sneezing, and clear secretions help to distinguish SAR from viral rhinitis, along with the distinct recurrent seasonal nature of SAR. Viral rhinitis produces thicker, purulent secretions, with neutrophils present on the nasal smear. Conjunctival symptoms are less pronounced, and on physical examination the nasal mucosa is erythematous and swollen. *Hormonal influences* that may produce chronic nasal congestion and rhinorrhea include hypothyroidism, birth control pill use, pregnancy, and menopause. Abuse of topical nasal decongestants (e.g., oxymetazoline) with chronic reflex vasodilatation has historically been the most common cause of *rhinitis medicamentosa;* however, cocaine abuse may have surpassed decongestants as the most common cause of this condition. Chronic *unilateral* nasal blockage suggests an anatomic defect, typically a deviated or fractured septum, but such blockage can also result from *polyps, tumors,* and *foreign bodies.* This history necessitates evaluation with computed tomographic scanning of the nose and sinuses and possibly rhinoscopy. *Nasal septum deviation* hardly ever causes *bilateral* nasal congestion, and surgical therapy has little role in the treatment of rhinitis that is producing symptomatic congestion.

An abnormal neurogenic response to irritants (e.g., cold air, pollutants, cigarette smoke, strong odors, alcohol, and foods) is the predominant feature of *vasomotor rhinitis.* This disorder is characterized by nasal autonomic nerve dysfunction. Patients with this vasomotor rhinitis typically have chronic nasal congestion and posterior pharyngeal drainage, but they lack the sneezing, rhinorrhea, pruritus, conjunctivitis, and systemic complaints typical of patients with AR. Patients with vasomotor rhinitis have negative allergen skin tests and an absence of eosinophils in their nasal mucus. Topical antihistamines (nasal azelastine) are often effective in vasomotor rhinitis. Patients with this condition occasionally respond to therapy with topical corticosteroids or atropine (nasal ipratropium).

TABLE 272–2 DIFFERENTIAL DIAGNOSIS OF RHINITIS

ALLERGIC
Seasonal allergic rhinitis (SAR)
Perennial allergic rhinitis (PAR)
INFLAMMATORY
Infectious rhinitis (viral)
Nonallergic rhinitis with eosinophilia syndrome (NARES)
Chronic sinusitis with or without nasal polyposis
HORMONAL
Pregnancy, oral contraceptive use, perimenopause
Hypothyroidism
Hyperthyroidism
RHINITIS MEDICAMENTOSA
Topical decongestants
Antihypertensives
Antidepressants
Cocaine
VASOMOTOR
Irritant induced (pollution, cigarette smoke)
Cold air induced
Gustatory (food induced)
ANATOMIC
Nasal septal deviation
Tumor, neoplasm
Foreign body
Cerebrospinal fluid leak
Atrophic (postsurgical or trauma)

Chronic sinusitis with or without *nasal polyposis* produces a spectrum of symptoms that includes rhinorrhea, mucopurulent posterior pharyngeal drainage, and nasal congestion that can be confounded with PAR. A computed tomographic scan is often required to establish the diagnosis of sinusitis. *Atrophic rhinitis* is characterized by atrophy of the nasal epithelium and is associated with complaints of nasal congestion and a perceived bad odor. It is observed in elderly patients, but the most common cause is devascularization secondary to nasal surgery or trauma. Finally, a nonallergic nasal disease characterized by prominent eosinophilic inflammation has been described and termed *non-AR with eosinophilia syndrome* (or NARES). On further analysis, many of these patients prove to have chronic sinusitis and nasal polyps. Patients with NARES present with symptoms similar to those of vasomotor rhinitis. NARES is diagnosed by performing a nasal smear (Hansel stain) for eosinophils. In contrast to vasomotor rhinitis, NARES is more often responsive to intranasal cromolyn and corticosteroids.

Systemic Manifestations of Allergic Rhinitis

Allergic inflammation associated with AR can lead to obstruction of the sinus ostia and is an important cause of acute (bacterial) sinusitis. More important is the association of AR with chronic sinusitis. Chronic sinusitis represents many disease processes including those caused by chronic bacterial infections, cystic fibrosis, immotile cilia syndrome, immune deficiencies, nonspecific inflammation, hypersensitivity to colonized fungi, and a manifestation termed *chronic hyperplastic eosinophilic sinusitis* (CHES). Approximately half of all patients with chronic sinusitis have CHES, and this discussion focuses on the underlying allergic mechanisms.

CHES, which generally occurs in association with nasal polyposis, is an inflammatory disorder characterized by the accumulation of eosinophils, fibroblasts, mast cells, goblet cells, and T_H2-like lymphocytes. The prominent accumulation of eosinophils, however, is the diagnostic feature of this condition (Fig. 272–3). The sinus tissue is infiltrated with a marked increase in cells, including lymphocytes, fibroblasts, and eosinophils, which are expressing cytokines responsible for eosinophilopoiesis (IL-5), survival (IL-3, IL-5, and GM-CSF), recruitment (CCL11 [eotaxin]), and activation (CCL11, CCL5 [RANTES], IL-3, IL-4, IL-5, GM-CSF, and TNF-α). Both sensitivity to multiple allergens and, more specifically, sensitivity to perennial allergens, such as dust mites, increase the risk of developing CHES. More than 50% of individuals with PAR have abnormal sinus radiographs. Allergens are unlikely to gain access to the sinus cavities in healthy subjects (they are not inhaled into the sinuses with breathing, and diffusion is not efficient), and they are even less likely to do so in the presence of the occlusions of the sinus openings that are characteristic of sinusitis. Studies performed with insufflation of radiolabeled ragweed particles confirm the inability of these pollens to enter the sinuses. The link between AR and sinusitis is thought to involve a systemic inflammatory process (Fig. 272–4).

AR is not just a localized inflammatory disorder of the nasal mucosa, but rather it is associated with systemic inflammation; consequently, it is often seen with other inflammatory conditions, such as asthma (Chapter 87), secretory otitis media, and CHES. For example, in patients with SAR who also have asthma, nasal allergen provocation, done such that the allergen does not gain access to the lungs, leads to increased adhesion molecule expression, eosinophil infiltration, and increased bronchial hyperreactivity. As illustrated in Figure 272–4, in sensitized subjects, allergen exposure activates immune cells, including T_H lymphocytes, dendritic cells, mononuclear cells, mast cells, and others both within the nares and in nasal-associated lymphatic tissues. These cells also include locally produced eosinophil precursors. Some of these T_H cells migrate to the bone marrow, where they stimulate the bone marrow to produce inflammatory cells, including basophils, eosinophils, and mast cell precursors. Thus, allergen challenges increase the bone marrow concentrations of both cytokines and eosinophil/basophil progenitor cells. Ultimately, these newly generated inflammatory cells enter the circulatory system, from which they are selectively recruited to the sinuses in CHES (and lungs in asthma). This selective recruitment of inflammatory cells into the sinuses occurs only in individuals with preexisting CHES in whom specific adhesion molecules, such as vascular cell adhesion molecule-1 (VCAM-1), and chemoattractants, such as CCL11 (eotaxin), are already present. Persons without CHES do not have these addressins in their sinuses and thus do not have the machinery in place to recruit inflammatory cells in response to their AR. This model explains the absence of CHES in approximately half of AR sufferers, but it does not explain the precipitating event that initiates CHES and allows AR to perpetuate the sinus inflammation once it is established.

In support of these concepts, nasal allergen challenges in sensitive individuals produce radiographic changes within the maxillary sinuses, including edema and opacification. Similarly, during seasonal exacerbations of AR, worsening of CHES can be demonstrated. Nasal allergen challenges in allergic individuals produce significant increases in eosinophils, eosinophil cationic protein, histamine, and albumin not only in the nose but also in the maxillary sinus. In one study, sinus lavage fluid from both maxillary sinuses was collected and analyzed after a nasal allergen challenge was performed in only one side of the nose. Both albumin levels and eosinophil counts were significantly increased in these specimens, with no significant differences detected in specimens obtained from the ipsilateral *and contralateral* maxillary sinuses. Similar systemic mechanisms could produce an interaction between AR and secretory otitis media or asthma. It is not known whether treating AR can lessen severity of CHES, but the observation that nasal-directed therapies can attenuate bronchial inflammation and symptoms of asthma suggest that such a linkage is plausible.

Prevention

Avoidance and Environmental Control

When feasible, avoidance or elimination of the source of allergen is the treatment of choice for patients with AR. Avoidance studies in AR are limited (as opposed to asthma), and the amount of allergen reduction needed to reduce symptoms effectively is unknown. Avoidance studies in asthma (Chapter 87) provide compelling evidence for beneficial effects

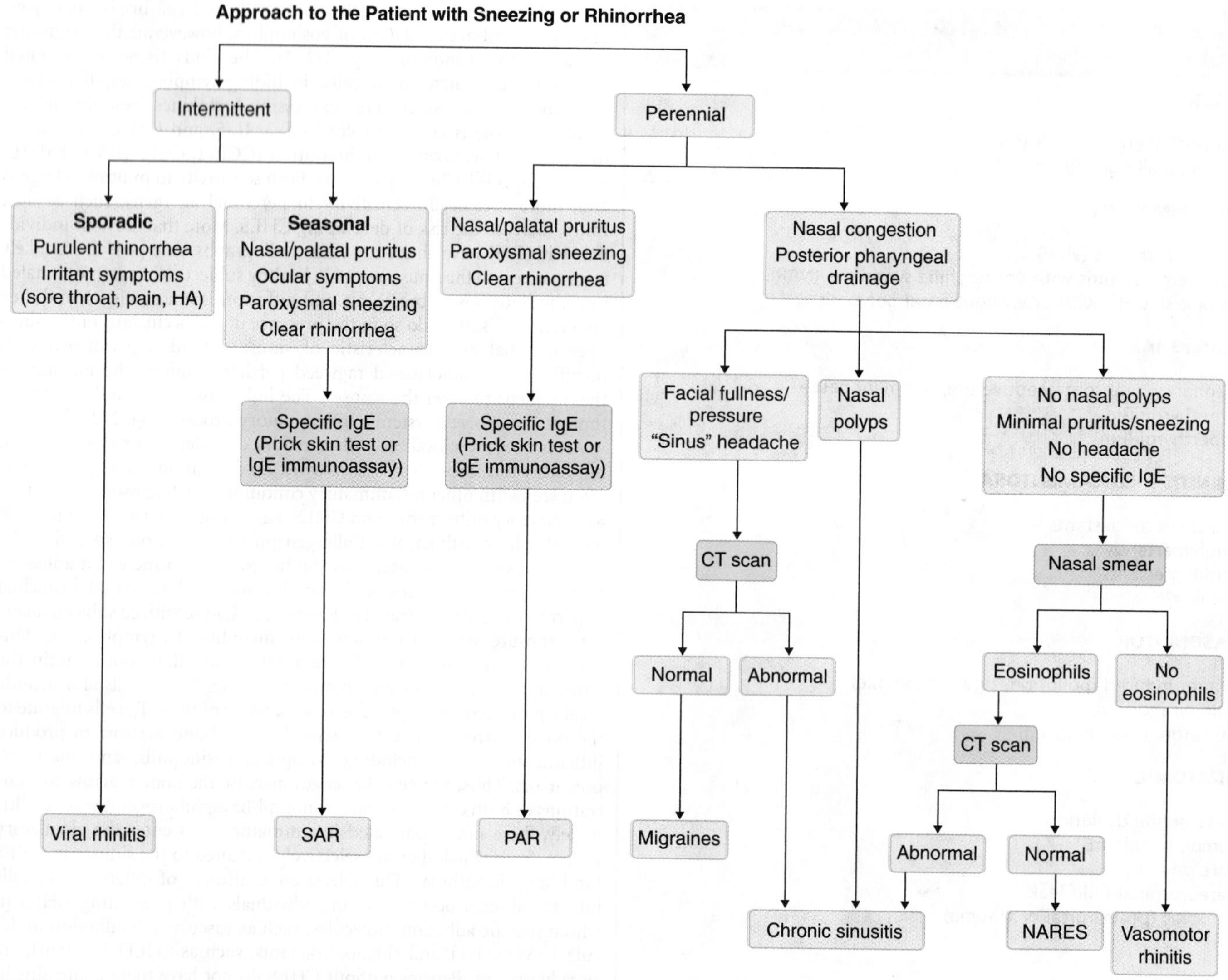

Approach to the Patient with Sneezing or Rhinorrhea

- Intermittent
  - **Sporadic** — Purulent rhinorrhea; Irritant symptoms (sore throat, pain, HA) → Viral rhinitis
  - **Seasonal** — Nasal/palatal pruritus; Ocular symptoms; Paroxysmal sneezing; Clear rhinorrhea → Specific IgE (Prick skin test or IgE immunoassay) → SAR
- Perennial
  - Nasal/palatal pruritus; Paroxysmal sneezing; Clear rhinorrhea → Specific IgE (Prick skin test or IgE immunoassay) → PAR
  - Nasal congestion; Posterior pharyngeal drainage
    - Facial fullness/pressure; "Sinus" headache → CT scan
      - Normal → Migraines
      - Abnormal → Chronic sinusitis
    - Nasal polyps → Chronic sinusitis
    - No nasal polyps; Minimal pruritus/sneezing; No headache; No specific IgE → Nasal smear
      - Eosinophils → CT scan
        - Abnormal → Chronic sinusitis
        - Normal → NARES
      - No eosinophils → Vasomotor rhinitis

FIGURE 272–2 • Approach to the patient with rhinitis symptoms. CT = computed tomography; HA = headache; IgE = immunoglobulin E; NARES = nonallergic rhinitis with eosinophilia syndrome; PAR = perennial allergic rhinitis; SAR = seasonal allergic rhinitis.

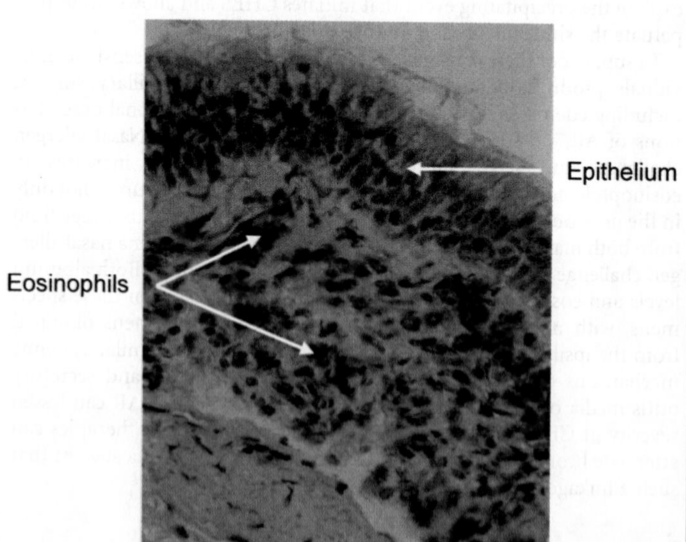

FIGURE 272–3 • Immunohistochemical analysis of a sinus biopsy from a patient with sinusitis and chronic allergic rhinitis. Eosinophils were labeled with an antibody to eosinophil cationic protein and were localized as aggregates within and beneath the epithelium. (Original magnification ×400.) (From Demoly P, Crampette L, Mondain M, et al: Assessment of inflammation in noninfectious chronic maxillary sinusitis. J Allergy Clin Immunol 1994;94:95–108.)

on bronchial hyperreactivity, symptom severity, and need for β-agonist rescue therapy. Dust mite avoidance involves four principles: (1) remove reservoirs for mite growth (i.e., cover mattresses and pillows with allergen-impermeable covers and remove fitted carpets and upholstered furniture from the bedroom); (2) keep the relative humidity lower than 50%; (3) wash bedding in a hot cycle (130° F) because cool cycle washing of bedding does not kill mites, nor does the dryer; (4) wear a simple mask at times when dust is being disturbed and for 10 minutes afterward, to allow large particles to settle. Many of the measures suggested for mites are also helpful for fungi, especially dehumidification. Windows, shower curtains, and indoor plants are important sites for fungal growth and can be treated with mild fungicides (dilute household bleach).

In some houses, and particularly urban apartment blocks, large numbers of cockroaches are present, and IgE sensitivity to cockroach allergen extracts is common. Although it may be difficult to kill cockroaches in an apartment, it is usually possible to keep a house clear of cockroaches by using chemical sprays and traps, for example. Care must be taken when using chemical sprays because they may prove to be an irritant to asthmatic patients. Air conditioning with closed windows is useful for reducing seasonal allergens, and the dehumidification provided by air conditioning also mitigates mite and indoor mold load.

Pets, especially cats, are the most preventable source of allergic diseases and should be eliminated from the home of the patient with AR. Animal dander accumulates in houses over a prolonged period and takes many months to eliminate after the cat, dog, or pet rodent is removed. Although it is difficult to persuade patients to get rid of animals, it may be possible to move the pet out into the garage or restrict the range of pets in the house. Dogs kept outside, washed regularly, and allowed into the house

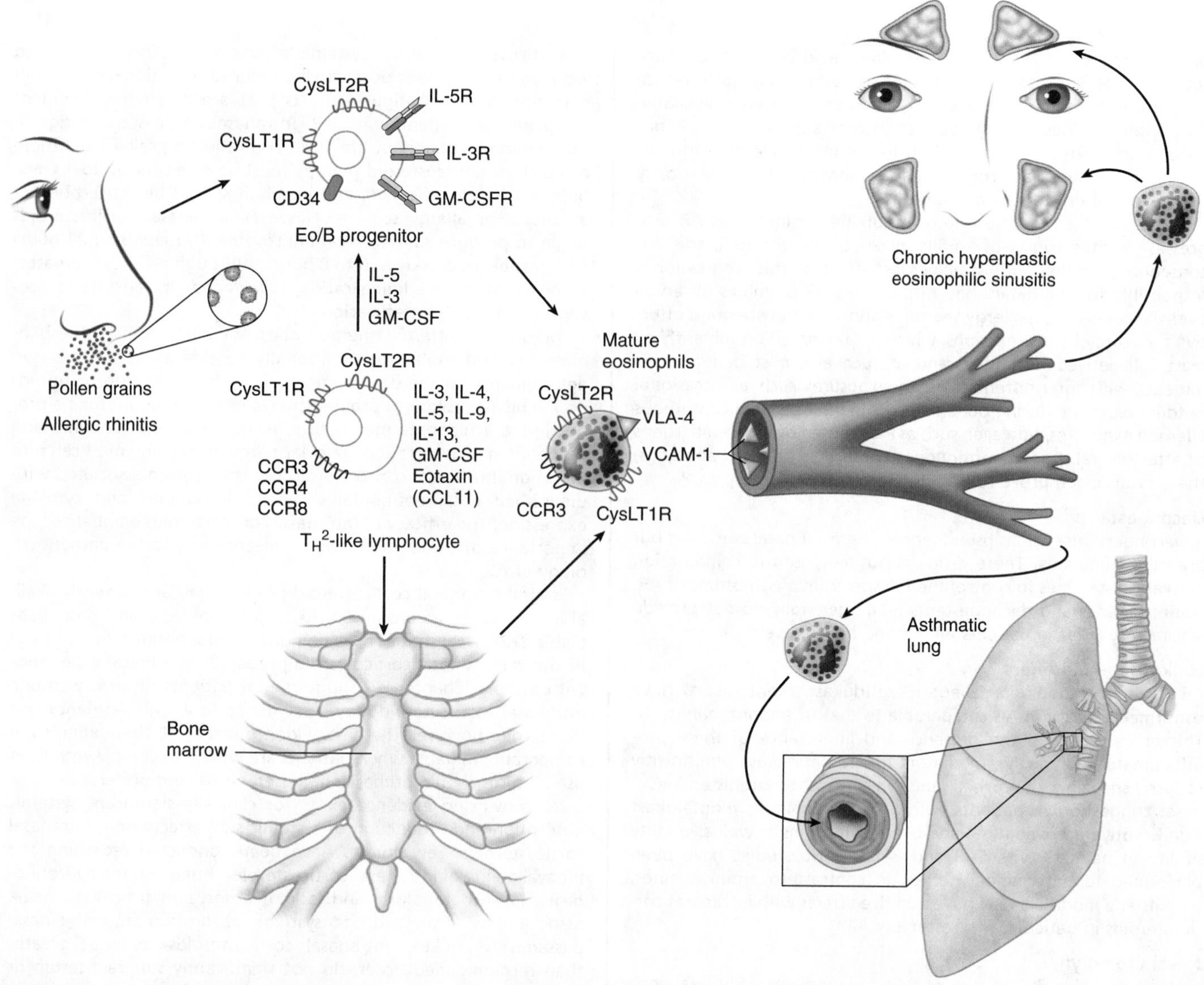

FIGURE 272-4 • In sensitized subjects, allergen exposure activates immune cells including helper T (T_H) lymphocytes, dendritic cells, mononuclear phagocytic cells, mast cells, and others both within the nares and in nasal-associated lymphatic tissues. These cells may also include locally produced $CD34^+$ interleukin-5 receptor-positive ($IL\text{-}5R^+$) eosinophil/basophil (Eo/B) progenitors. These newly activated T_H lymphocytes will have the phenotype of $T_H{}^2$-like cells characterized by their production of IL-3, IL-4, IL-5, IL-9, IL-13, CCL11 (eotaxin), and granulocyte-monocyte colony-stimulating factor (GM-CSF). Some of these T_H cells migrate to the bone marrow, where they stimulate the bone marrow to produce inflammatory cells including basophils, mast cells, and—most importantly—eosinophils. Ultimately, these newly generated inflammatory cells enter the circulatory system from which they are selectively recruited back to the nose, but also to the sinuses (and lungs), thus exacerbating inflammation. This selective recruitment of inflammatory cells into the sinuses and lungs occurs only in individuals with preexisting chronic hyperplastic eosinophilic sinusitis and asthma in whom specific adhesion molecules, such as vascular cell adhesion molecule-1 (VCAM-1), and chemoattractants, such as CCL11, already exist. VLA-4 = $\alpha_4 B_1$ integrin; very late antigen-4. (From Borish L: Allergic rhinitis: Systemic inflammation and implications for management. J Allergy Clin Immunol 2003;112:1021–1032.)

only occasionally do not appear to be an important cause of sensitization or symptoms. Cat allergy is a much more serious problem because a single cat deposits a huge concentration of allergens. Cat owners themselves can, in turn, deposit sufficient concentrations of allergen in schoolrooms and other environments to induce symptoms in their allergic colleagues. The dominant rodent allergen is a urinary protein, and, like cats, rodents can deposit large quantities of allergen in patients' houses.

Treatment

Rx

Although avoidance interventions significantly reduce allergen levels, as single interventions they often fail to produce clinically significant improvements. 1,2 As a result, pharmacotherapy is frequently required.

Evidence-Based Treatments

Antihistamines

Antihistamines are the oldest drugs used in the treatment of AR and are considered first-line therapy. Antihistamines compete with histamine for the H_1-receptor sites that contribute to sneezing, itching, rhinorrhea, and conjunctivitis. Oral antihistamines therefore ameliorate these symptoms of AR but in general do not improve nasal congestion. They also inhibit mast cell activation as manifested by diminished histamine, cysteinyl leukotrienes, and mast cell tryptase secretion. First-generation antihistamines cross the blood-brain barrier and have significant sedative and anticholinergic effects. In addition to causing sleepiness, they interfere with school, work, driving, or use of machinery. Whereas only 10 to 15% of treated patients complain of sedation, virtually all subjects demonstrate decreased motor skills, diminished driving ability, and slower electroencephalographic response times when they are given first-generation antihistamines (e.g., chlorpheniramine, diphenhydramine, and clemastine). Therefore, the use of these drugs is no longer recommended. Second-generation antihistamines have a longer duration of action, do not cross the blood-brain barrier, and are nonsedating. These agents include fexofenadine, descarboxyloratadine, and loratadine. Although it is less sedating than its

Rx

parent compound hydroxyzine, cetirizine may occasionally produce sedation. The intranasal antihistamine azelastine may not produce a significantly more rapid onset of action than currently available oral antihistamines, but in contrast to oral antihistamines, it has decongestant efficacy and is often useful in nonallergic forms of rhinitis. No studies have convincingly demonstrated the superiority of one oral antihistamine over another.

As discussed earlier, the role of histamine diminishes as AR progresses over the course of an allergy season or with PAR, and this consequently makes antihistamines less effective. This progression is responsible for the diminished efficacy of antihistamines observed over the course of an allergy season. Antihistamines are quite effective for acute allergic reactions, which are mediated prominently by mast cell–derived histamine, and as such are most beneficial in patients with intermittent allergen exposures such as occasional outdoor exposure during pollen season. In patients with continuous allergen exposures, however, such as PAR caused by indoor allergens or after several days of continuous exposure to seasonal allergens, these drugs often prove to be little better than placebo. [3, 4]

Decongestants

Decongestants such as pseudoephedrine treat nasal stuffiness but are mild stimulants. These drugs are usually used in combination with antihistamines to control the full spectrum of symptoms of AR. Antihistamines and decongestants alone generally do not provide satisfactory relief in patients with moderate to severe AR.

Leukotriene Modifiers

Leukotriene modifiers (zileuton, zafirlukast, montelukast) have confirmed efficacy in AR comparable to that of antihistamines. [4] This efficacy reflects the presence and importance of these proinflammatory vasoactive mediators to AR. Zafirlukast significantly reduced sneezing, rhinorrhea, and—in contrast to antihistamines—nasal congestion in patients with SAR. [5] Similarly, montelukast significantly improved nasal and ocular symptoms as well as quality of life in patients with SAR and PAR. [4] No studies have been performed to determine whether, in contrast to antihistamines, leukotriene modifiers may have additive effects with intranasal corticosteroids in patients with refractory AR.

Nasal Cromolyn

Nasal cromolyn stabilizes mast cells and mediates additional anti-inflammatory activities toward macrophages and T lymphocytes. Although not as effective as intranasal corticosteroids, cromolyn provides relief in patients with mild to moderate symptoms, [6] and it may be effective in combination with corticosteroids in the treatment of refractory symptoms. The value of cromolyn is mitigated by the need for frequent doses (four times/day), a lack of efficacy in approximately 30 to 40% of recipients, and the superior efficacy of intranasal corticosteroids in controlled studies. Cromolyn (one to two sprays in each nostril every 3 to 4 hours) may be especially useful preventively (e.g., immediately before cat exposure or 1 to 2 weeks before the start of the allergen season). Unlike antihistamines, cromolyn controls nasal congestion. Ocular cromolyn has been especially useful in the treatment of allergic conjunctivitis. No significant side effects are associated with its use.

Intranasal Corticosteroids

Intranasal corticosteroids (fluticasone [Flonase], triamcinolone [Nasacort], flunisolide [Nasarel], budesonide [Rhinocort], and mometasone [Nasonex]) are the most effective treatments of AR and are considered the treatments of choice for patients with moderate to severe SAR or PAR. [6, 7] Comparative studies of antihistamines and intranasal corticosteroids consistently favor the corticosteroids and show insignificant additive effects when antihistamines are combined with optimal topical corticosteroids. [8] In well-performed placebo-controlled studies, intranasal corticosteroids provided a 50 to 90% reduction in symptoms (compared with 15 to 20% for antihistamines). In contrast to antihistamines, topical corticosteroids reduce nasal congestion, in addition to their relieving itching, rhinorrhea, sneezing, and, in some studies, allergic conjunctivitis. Unfortunately, few studies have addressed the influences of corticosteroids on the systemic effects of AR—including missed work and school, poor productivity, reduced cognition, poor school performance, and fatigue—effects that are often the dominant complaints of patients with AR. Intranasal corticosteroids significantly improve quality of life, a finding reflecting relief from these complaints. Corticosteroid therapy must be given for up to 1 week before it is fully effective, and ideally it should be started before exposures or allergy seasons. However, intranasal corticosteroids begin to produce some clinical improvement in less than 24 hours and possibly as quickly as 6 to 8 hours. Although efficacy is greatest with continuous administration, as-needed intranasal corticosteroids have proven efficacious.

Topical corticosteroid therapy does not inhibit IgE synthesis or mast cell degranulation, traditionally considered to be the two determinants for the development of AR. However, corticosteroids do inhibit T-lymphocyte proliferation, chemokine and cytokine production, arachidonate metabolism, recruitment of eosinophils and basophils, mucus secretion, vascular permeability, and mast cell proliferation. Intranasal corticosteroid use is therefore associated with diminished nasal eosinophilia, mast cell number, and cytokine expression. The efficacy of intranasal corticosteroids emphasizes the importance of these nonhistamine mechanisms to the pathophysiology of AR.

Several intranasal corticosteroid preparations are currently available and differ according to dose, approval age, and propellant (Table 272–3). No studies have demonstrated superior efficacy of any of the various nasal corticosteroid preparations. Clinical experience with asthma (Chapter 87) suggests that patients refractory to one intranasal corticosteroid may be switched to a higher-potency corticosteroid; however, the best evidence is that all these agents are comparably valuable when patients are willing to comply with their use. Choices should primarily be based on patient preference.

No convincing evidence exists for clinically significant systemic absorption and production of systemic side effects from intranasal corticosteroids. Few studies have been conducted regarding the bioavailability of intranasal corticosteroids, but given the hydrophobicity, local metabolism, and lack of absorption from lung tissue associated with these drugs, systemic absorption from the nasal passages is unlikely. Intranasal corticosteroids, even at greater than recommended doses, do not significantly suppress serum or urinary cortisol levels or adrenocorticotropic hormone stimulation tests. Studies have reported a small but statistically significant effect of intranasal corticosteroids on short-term growth velocity in children with PAR. The impact of this finding on ultimate adult height will await further clinical experience, but based on the asthma experience, this is not likely to be shown. Nasal corticosteroids cause minimal topical side effects, including local irritation, dryness, an unpleasant aftertaste, and epistaxis. Adverse side effects may differ based on formulation; aqueous formulations usually produce fewer adverse reactions than aerosols. Nasal biopsy studies do not demonstrate nasal atrophy or decreased ciliary function. Nasal perforation has been reported primarily in the setting of underlying devascularization (previous trauma, surgery, or cocaine abuse).

TABLE 272–3 INTRANASAL CORTICOSTEROIDS

Generic Name	Dose (per Actuation)	Minimum Approved Age	Usual Dosing
Flunisolide	25 μg	6 yr	Twice daily
Triamcinolone	55 μg	6 yr	Once daily
Budesonide	32 μg	6 yr	Twice daily
Fluticasone	50 μg	4 yr	Once daily
Mometasone	50 μg	12 yr	Once daily

*Intranasal corticosteroids are generally administered at two sprays per nostril.

Rx

Immunotherapy

The clinical efficacy of immunotherapy for AR caused by grass, ragweed, many other pollens, cat dander, and dust mites has been categorically established in innumerable well-designed controlled studies. Immunotherapy decreases the severity of AR, reduces the need for pharmacotherapy, and significantly improves quality of life. In patients with severe AR and conjunctivitis poorly controlled by antihistamines and intranasal corticosteroids, immunotherapy reduced allergen sensitivity by more than 10-fold, as well as significantly decreasing total symptoms and reducing total antiallergic drug usage. Immunotherapy has also been convincingly established to have efficacy in allergen-exacerbated (extrinsic) asthma (Chapter 87) in studies showing decreased symptoms and the need for β-agonist rescue therapy. Efficacy depends on delivery of the correct antigen, regular injections for 3 to 5 years, and administration of an adequate dose of the allergen (~10 to 15 μg), a dose significantly higher than those historically utilized.

Immunotherapy is primarily indicated in patients with refractory rhinitis or in patients with unacceptable side effects from standard medications. Because intranasal corticosteroids are not universally effective and do not provide complete relief in all patients, consideration of immunotherapy is necessary. In addition, despite the excellent safety profile of intranasal corticosteroids, many patients remain reluctant to use them. Patients should normally go through at least one full pollen season before the decision is made to consider immunotherapy. An additional indication for immunotherapy is derived from recognition that it is the only treatment that produces long-term immune modulation. Both avoidance and pharmacotherapy are effective only as long as they are sustained. The effects of immunotherapy, in contrast, persist for many years after a 3- to 5-year course of treatment has been discontinued and could be lifelong. [9,10] A 5-year course of immunotherapy will have cost advantages over lifelong pharmacotherapy. Many patients are attracted to immunotherapy by this potential for long-term immune modulation, remission of symptoms, and the ability to discontinue daily pharmacotherapy.

Immunotherapy is associated with a small risk for fatal anaphylaxis (~3 fatalities/year in the United States out of ~2 million people receiving this form of treatment). Because of this risk of anaphylaxis, immunotherapy must be administered only in a facility where resuscitation equipment and trained personnel are available. Asthmatic patients are uniquely at risk for fatal anaphylaxis, and as such immunotherapy should be recommended cautiously to these patients.

Future Directions

Many patients have multiple antigen sensitivities, and specific immunotherapy at effective doses may not be practical. Furthermore, immunotherapy has poor efficacy for many antigens, such as molds. These issues have led to a search for new immune-based therapies capable of attenuating allergic inflammation. In addition to the future treatments discussed in the following paragraphs, many experimental approaches being developed for asthma, including various anticytokine therapies, hold the potential to provide efficacy for AR.

Anti–immunoglobulin E Antibodies (Omalizumab)

Omalizumab has been evaluated in the treatment of SAR. In patients with pollen-induced AR, anti-IgE significantly improved nasal symptom scores, use of rescue antihistamines, and quality of life. Clinical trials with omalizumab support its safety, including the absence of immune complex formation, serum sickness, or other significant untoward side effects. Omalizumab reduces the risk of anaphylaxis in patients who are receiving immunotherapy, a possibility that could lead to additional uses of this treatment. Reducing the risk of anaphylaxis could make immunotherapy available to high-risk patients with asthma and could plausibly increase the efficacy of immunotherapy by permitting utilization of even higher doses. At present, omalizumab is approved only for adults with moderate to severe asthma. The limiting feature of this therapy for AR will be its cost.

Novel Forms of Immunotherapy

Future strategies for immunotherapy are aimed at delivering increased efficacy with less risk for IgE-mediated systemic side effects. The challenge is to deliver a sufficiently high dose of protein to the T cell, to induce T-cell tolerance, without concomitantly delivering the allergen to mast cells in a form that can cross-link IgE and thereby induce anaphylaxis. Recognition of the importance of T-cell–dependent mechanisms in immune modulation after immunotherapy is leading to the development of reagents that interact with the T lymphocyte without engaging mast cell/basophil–bound IgE. Short *peptide fragments* derived from genetically engineered allergens have been successfully utilized in immunotherapy studies. These peptides retain the ability to be recognized and processed by antigen-presenting cells, to be presented to T_H lymphocytes, and to drive the T cells into a tolerant state. Because these short peptides lack the complex structure of their parent compound, they cannot be recognized by mast cell/basophil–bound IgE and are generally not associated with risk for immediate-phase, anaphylactic responses. Studies with peptides in patients with cat and bee venom sensitivity have demonstrated induction of T-cell tolerance and therapeutic efficacy. However, these compounds have been frustrated by their tendency initially to activate allergen-specific T_H2-like cells and thereby produce delayed allergic reactions including asthma exacerbations. More recent studies have utilized allergenic peptides coupled to synthetic bacterial DNA sequences. These are based on the concept that engagement of these *immunostimulatory DNA sequences* to their specific receptors (toll-like 9 [TLR9] receptors) provides a potent signal to drive the ensuing immune responses away from T_H2 immunity. Initial studies have been extremely promising regarding efficacy, safety, and long-term immune modulation with these agents.

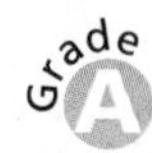

1. Woodcock A, Forster L, Matthews E, et al: Control of exposure to mite allergen and allergen-impermeable bed covers for adults with asthma. N Engl J Med 2003;349:225–236.
2. Terreehorst I, Hak E, Oosting AJ, et al: Evaluation of impermeable covers for bedding in patients with allergic rhinitis. N Engl J Med 2003;349:237–246.
3. Bernstein DI, Schoenwetter WF, Nathan RA, et al: Efficacy and safety of fexofenadine hydrochloride for treatment of seasonal allergic rhinitis. Ann Allergy Asthma Immunol 1997;79:443–448.
4. Meltzer EO, Malmstrom K, Lu S, et al: Concomitant montelukast and loratadine as treatment for seasonal allergic rhinitis: A randomized, placebo-controlled clinical trial. J Allergy Clin Immunol 2000;105:917–922.
5. Donnelly AL, Glass M, Minkwitz MC, Casale TB: The leukotriene D_4-receptor antagonist, ICI 204,219, relieves symptoms of acute seasonal allergic rhinitis. Am J Respir Crit Care Med 1995;151:1734–1739.
6. Welsh PW, Stricker WE, Chu CP, et al: Efficacy of beclomethasone nasal solution, flunisolide, and cromolyn in relieving symptoms of ragweed allergy. Mayo Clin Proc 1987;62:125–134.
7. Weiner JM, Abramson MJ, Puy RM: Intranasal corticosteroids versus oral H_1 receptor antagonists in allergic rhinitis: Systematic review of randomised controlled trials. BMJ 1998;317:1624–1629.
8. Ratner PH, van Bavel JH, Marti BG, et al. A comparison of the efficacy of fluticasone propionate aqueous nasal spray and loratadine, alone and in combination, for the treatment of seasonal allergic rhinitis. J Fam Pract 1998;47:118–125.
9. Durham SR, Walker SM, Varga EM, et al: Long-term clinical efficacy of grass-pollen immunotherapy. N Engl J Med 1999;341:468–475.
10. Creticos PS, Schroeder JT, Hamilton RG, et al: Immunotherapy with a ragweed–toll-like receptor 9 agonist vaccine for allergic rhinitis. N Engl J Med 2006;355:1445–1455.

SUGGESTED READINGS

Borish L: Allergic rhinitis: Systemic inflammation and implications for management. J Allergy Clin Immunol 2003;112:1021–1031. *A discussion of pathogenesis and its influence on treatment options.*

Plaut M, Valentine MD: Allergic rhinitis. N Engl J Med 2005;353:1934–1944. *Reviews the evaluation of and pharmacotherapies available for this condition.*

Prenner BM, Schenkel E: Allergic rhinitis: Treatment based on patient profiles. Am J Med 2006;119:230–237. *A comprehensive review.*

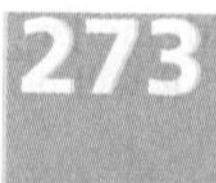

273 URTICARIA AND ANGIOEDEMA

Stephen C. Dreskin

URTICARIA

Urticaria (hives) are pruritic, edematous, erythematous, blanching papules that are round or oval in shape, have pale raised centers (wheals), are of several millimeters to a few centimeters in size, and are transient, lasting minutes to days (Fig. 273–1). Angioedema appears as a brawny, nonpitting edema, typically without well-defined margins and without erythema. Angioedema can be accompanied by a sense of burning, pressure, or aching but not pruritus, and it is distinguished from other edematous states by often involving the lips, tongue, eyelids, hands, feet, or genitalia and rarely occurring in dependent areas of the body. Episodes (daily or almost daily symptoms) of recurrent hives and/or angioedema lasting less than 6 weeks are considered acute, and those lasting longer are said to be chronic. The terms urticaria and urticaria/angioedema are used interchangeably here to refer to illnesses in which mast cells are activated.

Epidemiology

Urticaria/angioedema occurs in 15 to 25% of individuals at some times during their life and can affect both genders and all races. Acute urticaria is more common in young adults and children. Chronic urticaria is more common in adults, affecting women (75% of cases) more often than men.

Pathobiology

Mast cells, the primary effector cells in urticaria/angioedema, are found in high numbers throughout the body and particularly within the subcutaneous tissue. After activation of mast cells there is a rapid release (<10 minutes) of histamine, leukotriene C_4 (LTC_4), and prostaglandin D_2 (PGD_2) leading to vasodilation, subcutaneous and intradermal leakage of plasma from postcapillary venules, and pruritus. In addition, there is a more delayed (4 to 8 hours) production and secretion of inflammatory cytokines such as tumor necrosis factor α (TNF-α), interleukin-4 (IL-4), and IL-5, leading to an inflammatory infiltrate and perpetuation of longer-lived lesions. Angioedema is formed by a similar extravasation of fluid, not superficially in the skin but in the deeper dermal and subdermal sites.

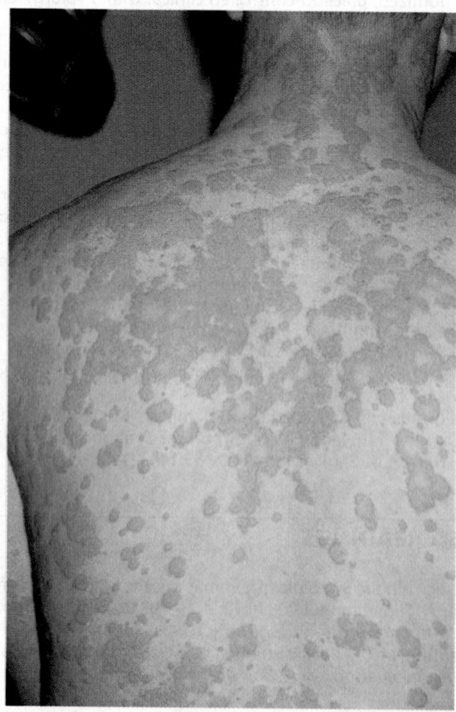

FIGURE 273–1 • Extensive urticaria. Many presentations are more subtle. (From Roitt I, Brostoff J, Male D [eds]: Immunology, 6th ed. London, Mosby, 2001, Figure 21–2.)

Lesions of acute urticaria typically show subcutaneous edema with widened dermal papillae, swollen collagen fibers, and rare inflammatory cells. Most episodes of acute urticaria/angioedema are caused by immediate hypersensitivity reactions to drugs or foods or are a result of inflammatory processes initiated by viral illnesses. The most common drugs that cause acute urticaria/angioedema are penicillins, sulfonamides, muscle relaxants, diuretics, and nonsteroidal anti-inflammatory drugs (NSAIDs), although any drug acting as a hapten can generate an allergic response. The predominant allergenic foods are milk, egg, and peanut for children and peanut, tree nuts, fish, and shellfish for adults, although sensitization can occur to many other foods as well. These allergens cross-link immunoglobulin E (IgE) bound to the high-affinity receptor for IgE (FcεRI), leading to activation of mast cells. Some drugs (e.g., opioids, vancomycin, NSAIDs) and radiocontrast dye can activate mast cells by an IgE-independent (pseudoallergic) mechanism. Ingestion of fish contaminated with bacteria that produce histamine leads to hives as part of a toxic reaction to the histamine (scombroid food poisoning).

Lesions of chronic urticaria are characterized by similar edematous findings, with the addition of a dense perivascular inflammatory infiltrate consisting of CD4- and CD8-positive T lymphocytes, eosinophils, basophils, and neutrophils. A minority of patients have urticarial vasculitis with lesions characterized by vascular destruction with leukocytoclasis (e.g., neutrophils with ingested cellular debris).

The two largest subgroups of chronic urticaria/angioedema are autoimmune urticaria and idiopathic urticaria, each accounting for approximately 40% of cases. Patients in the autoimmune group have symptoms in the absence of a specific physical trigger, allergen exposure, or coexistent disease; autoimmune urticaria is characterized by the presence of IgG antibodies that can cross-link FcεRI. Patients with idiopathic urticaria have symptoms in the absence of specific physical triggers, allergens, coexistent disease, or evidence of autoimmunity.

Physical stimuli activate mast cells by unknown mechanisms and account for about 20% of cases of chronic urticaria. The most common of the physical urticarias is dermographism (also called dermatographism), in which wheals can be "written on the skin" by simple stroking or scratching. Cholinergic urticaria is often included as a physical urticaria, although the trigger leading to mast cell activation is related to cholinergic stimuli occurring after exposure to heat or after exercise. Other physical stimuli can cause urticaria, including cold, solar radiation, pressure, vibration, and water. Cold-induced urticaria is rarely caused by cryoglobulinemia.

In approximately 5% of patients with chronic urticaria/angioedema, symptoms appear to be caused by ingestants (e.g., foods, medications, dietary supplements), contactants (e.g., soaps, detergents, cosmetics, hair or nail products, latex), concomitant infections, hormonal changes, or systemic illnesses. A food must be consumed regularly to cause chronic urticaria. Wheat is occasionally found to be a trigger. Multicellular parasites (e.g., strongyloidiasis, filariasis) elicit strong IgE responses and are important causes of chronic urticaria in endemic areas. Rare patients report that their urticaria occurs only during their menses or is worsened by menses. Some of these patients have immediate hypersensitivity to progesterone (positive skin tests), and others may be reacting to NSAIDs taken for uterine cramping. Chronic urticaria/angioedema can be associated with flares of rheumatic conditions, other autoimmune conditions (including Hashimoto's thyroditis), or neoplastic conditions. Occult neoplasia is exceedingly unlikely to be the cause of chronic urticaria.

Clinical Manifestations

Patients often report that the first sensation of urticaria is poorly localized pruritus that quickly develops into the typical lesions of urticaria. The intensity of the pruritus varies from a minimal inconvenience to an unbearable intensity that can lead to self-inflicted abrasion of the skin. Groups of hives often appear together over a short period, and episodes of hives can come in waves starting several times a day. Patients with cholinergic urticaria usually have a distinctive clinical presentation of diffuse erythema with elevated and pale monomorphic urticarial lesions of a few millimeters in diameter on exertion sufficient to cause sweating. The pruritus is particularly intense, and all of the symptoms are generally limited to the skin. A self-rated quality-of-life survey of patients with chronic urticaria revealed dramatic impairment in the areas of loss of sleep, fatigue, and emotional discomfort. Angioedema, when it occurs, can originate near a wheal or independently in other parts of the body. Symptoms vary from minor discomfort to an intense sense of pressure and may lead to other symptoms, such as severe shortness of breath if there is compromise of the airway.

Diagnosis

The first episode of acute urticaria/angioedema may occur in the absence of an identifiable stimulus. If hives occur within 5 to 30 minutes after ingestion of a drug or a food, the patient often can identify the association. If a physician is consulted, the best approach is to take a careful history with attention to ingestants and intercurrent illnesses. Unnecessary drugs and food supplements should be discontinued, and any recently added medication should be changed to a structurally different agent. Most often, no etiologic agent is identified, and the hives are treated symptomatically (see later discussion) for days or weeks before a spontaneous resolution occurs.

Differential Diagnosis

The differential diagnosis of chronic urticaria/angioedema includes the subgroups of urticaria discussed earlier: idiopathic, autoimmune, physical, ingestant-mediated, and associated with a variety of systemic illnesses. Other conditions that can be confused with chronic urticaria/angioedema include diffuse pruritus complicated by dermographism, flushing disorders, urticarial vasculitis, urticaria pigmentosa, systemic mastocytosis, exercise-induced anaphylaxis, exercise-induced food-associated anaphylaxis, idiopathic anaphylaxis, hereditary angioedema, acquired angioedema, and angioedema associated with angiotensin-converting enzyme (ACE) inhibitors (Table 273–1).

TABLE 273–1 CLASSIFICATION OF URTICARIA AND ANGIOEDEMA

- I. Acute urticaria/angioedema
  - A. Hypersensitivity reactions
    - 1. Drug allergy
    - 2. Food allergy
    - 3. Insect allergy
  - B. Idiopathic
  - C. Pseudoallergic reactions
    - 1. Drugs
    - 2. Radiocontrast dye
  - D. Toxic reactions
  - E. Immune complex
    - 1. Serum sickness
    - 2. Transfusion-related
    - 3. Postviral
- II. Chronic urticaria/angioedema
  - A. Autoimmune
    - 1. Anti-IgE receptor (FcεRI)
    - 2. Anti-IgE
  - B. Idiopathic
  - C. Physical
    - 1. Dermographism
    - 2. Cholinergic
    - 3. Exercise-induced anaphylaxis
    - 4. Delayed pressure
    - 5. Solar
    - 6. Cold
    - 7. Vibratory
    - 8. Aquagenic
  - D. Immune complex
    - 1. Thyroid disease
    - 2. Urticarial vasculitis
    - 3. Malignancy-associated
    - 4. Collagen vascular disease–associated
- III. Urticaria pigmentosa and systemic mastocytosis
- IV. Complement-related and kinin-mediated angioedema
  - A. Hereditary angioedema
  - B. Acquired angioedema
  - C. Angiotensin-converting enzyme inhibitor–induced angioedema

Approximately 95% of patients with urticaria/angioedema are not reacting to an ingestant and do not have another illness causing their hives. However, it is sometimes difficult for patients (and some physicians) to accept this fact, prompting an extensive, invasive, expensive, and unnecessary investigation. The best “test” to identify most of those with a specific underlying cause (i.e., physical trigger, autoimmune condition, allergen, or systemic disease) is a careful and detailed history and physical examination by a specialist knowledgeable in urticarial disease.

A good place to begin is by excluding possible physical triggers. Specific tests are available to establish the diagnosis of most physical urticarias, including scratching the skin and exposing the skin to heat, ice, vibration, pressure, ultraviolet radiation, or water. Acquired cold urticaria must be distinguished from the familial cold autoinflammatory syndrome, which is characterized by a cold-induced papular rash (not urticaria) and is now classified in the family of hereditary periodic fever syndromes. Solar urticaria must be distinguished from other types of light sensitivity, including metabolic abnormalities (e.g., erythrogenic porphyria) and photosensitivity due to drugs.

Even though foods and drugs are infrequent causes of chronic urticaria, many patients focus on ingestants and are not satisfied until these causes are ruled out. As in the evaluation of acute urticaria, the patient must discontinue all food supplements and medications that are not absolutely necessary and, if possible, change essential medications to structurally unrelated compounds. The patient then keeps a food diary to identify suspect foods that can be eliminated. Some allergists use skin tests with foods to identify “suspects.” For highly motivated patients, 2 weeks of a severely restrictive diet, often based on lamb and rice, is recommended. Antihistamines and other medications used to control the urticaria must be discontinued. If the urticaria resolves, it is critical to reintroduce foods in a controlled fashion, to identify the specific food causing the urticaria and to reinstate a healthy diet.

Chronic infections have also been considered as possible associations, including sinus infection, dental abscess, *Helicobacter pylori* gastric infection, cholecystitis, onychomycosis, and tinea pedis. Case reports relate resolution of urticaria after treatment of these infections, although rigorous proof of these associations is lacking. The natural history of chronic urticaria probably accounts for coincidental spontaneous improvement after treatment of these conditions, at least in some cases.

Laboratory evaluation for a patient with typical urticaria should always include a complete blood count with differential, a basic metabolic panel, liver enzymes, and a urinalysis. Specialists are not in full agreement regarding the necessity for further laboratory testing. Levels of thyroid-stimulating hormone and antithyroid antibodies may be measured in otherwise euthyroid-appearing patients to screen for occult hypothyroidism and for antithyroid autoantibodies. Skin tests for immediate hypersensitivity to foods may be ordered for patients with a suggestive history. Some specialists order no “screening” tests at all. As in vitro tests for anti-FcεRI autoantibodies become more available, it is likely that many specialists will obtain this test. The presence of a positive test for anti-FcεRI autoantibodies is useful, because this reassures the patient that the urticaria is being driven by an internal process and is not caused by an ingestant or occult illness. Also, this finding helps direct the physician toward immunomodulatory therapies. Beyond this, other tests should be ordered only as a result of positive findings in the history and physical examination.

Although not routinely indicated in every case of chronic urticaria, a skin biopsy can provide useful information. The most common indication for this procedure is to rule out urticarial vasculitis when the hives are more painful than pruritic, last longer than 24 hours, or leave discolored skin. The presence of vascular destruction, fibrinoid necrosis, and immune complex deposition on microscopic examination (including immunofluorescence) should lead to consideration of specific causes of the urticarial vasculitis (e.g., systemic lupus erythematosus) and to rapid initiation of more aggressive treatment.

Primary mast cell disorders rarely manifest as chronic urticaria (see Chapter 276). Systemic mastocytosis is a very rare condition resulting in increased numbers of atypical mast cells in the bone marrow, skin, and other organs. Levels of tryptase (an enzyme specific for mast cells) are usually elevated in the serum. This condition is frequently accompanied by episodic flushing, urticaria pigmentosa, prominent gastrointestinal symptoms, neuropsychiatric symptoms, and/or recurrent anaphylaxis. Urticaria pigmentosa is characterized by distinctive pigmented cutaneous lesions containing nests of mast cells and is not easily confused with urticaria/angioedema.

Hereditary angioedema, acquired angioedema, and angioedema associated with ACE inhibitors are discussed later in this chapter. Briefly, these syndromes are characterized by episodic swelling without urticaria and are best identified by a careful history, physical examination, and focused laboratory evaluation.

Treatment

Rx

Acute urticaria is usually self-limited and responds well to histamine 1 (H_1)-type antihistamines. Antihistamines work better if they are taken prophylactically rather than after histamine has been released and is bound to the receptor. Patients often self-medicate with or are prescribed diphenhydramine (25 to 50 mg every 6 hours) and hydroxyzine (25 to 50 mg every 6 hours) but may experience significant sedation. Second-generation antihistamines such as cetirizine (10 mg nightly at bedtime), fexofenadine (180 mg every day), and loratadine (10 mg every day) are much better tolerated and can be effective, although doses two to three times larger than the standard doses are sometimes necessary. Occasionally, a brief course of corticosteroids is warranted to control severe symptoms. Epinephrine (0.3 mL of 1:1000, IM) will quickly (but transiently) reverse the signs and symptoms of urticaria and angioedema. Patients who have experienced potentially life-threatening angioedema or anaphylaxis should maintain ready access to epinephrine and be knowledgeable of its indications, administration, and brief duration of action. β-Blockers not only can aggravate urticaria but can interfere with the action of epinephrine. NSAIDs and codeine can lead to IgE-independent mast cell activation. These medications should all be discontinued if it is clinically safe to do so.

H_1 antihistamines are the cornerstone of therapy for chronic urticaria/angioedema but are frequently inadequate to control symptoms. Certain H_1 antihistamines have been proposed as "preferred" for particular subtypes of chronic urticaria, such as hydroxyzine for cholinergic urticaria or cyproheptadine (2 to 4 mg every 6 hours) for cold-induced urticaria. Some have advocated using multiple H_1 antihistamines, changing or "rotating" agents, or using them in dosages well above those approved by U.S. Food and Drug Administration (FDA) labeling procedures.

Approximately 15% of histamine receptors in the skin are of the H_2 subtype, and therefore the addition of an H_2 antihistamine, such as ranitidine (150 mg twice daily) or famotidine (20 mg twice daily), is a logical adjunct to H_1 antihistamine therapy, providing additional clinical benefit. The tricyclic antidepressant doxepin (10 to 100 mg nightly at bedtime) has highly potent H_1 and H_2 antihistamine activity, with an H_1 receptor affinity almost 800 times that of diphenhydramine and an H_2 receptor affinity six times that of cimetidine, but its use can be limited by significant sedation.

Symptoms often persist despite the use of maximal or supramaximal doses of antihistamines. This is not surprising, considering the number of vasoactive and pruritogenic mediators released by mast cells, of which histamine is only one. Antileukotriene medications, such as montelukast (10 mg every day) or zafirlukast (20 mg twice daily) may be added to antihistamines with some success. Especially severe symptoms may require systemic corticosteroids (prednisone, 10 to 60 mg every day) to achieve symptomatic control, but concerns about side effects from chronic administration limit their usefulness.

Rx

Refractory symptoms have been treated with a wide variety of other medications. Some of these medications (adrenergic agents, calcium-channel blockers) are thought to decrease the ability of mast cells to release mediators. Others drugs are anti-inflammatory (hydroxychloroquine, sulfasalazine, dapsone, colchicine), immunomodulatory (cyclosporine, tacrolimus, mycophenolate), or antimetabolic (azathioprine, cyclophosphamide, methotrexate). Other treatments of refractory autoimmune chronic urticaria include intravenous immunoglobulin, plasmapheresis, or both.

Evidence-Based Treatments

Multiple randomized placebo-controlled studies of chronic urticaria/angioedema have shown efficacy of both sedating and nonsedating antihistamines. If sedating antihistamines must be used, doxepin has been demonstrated to be more effective than diphenhydramine, but it must be titrated carefully to avoid significant sedation. Prednisone is generally accepted as a mainstay of therapy in difficult cases but has not been formally studied. Cyclosporine (4 mg/kg/day) was shown to be effective in a randomized, placebo-controlled, parallel study of 30 patients with autoimmune urticaria. [1] LTC_4 receptor antagonists (montelukast and zafirlukast) do not provide any incremental benefit when added to an antihistamine, [2] sulfasalazine, hydroxychloroquine, dapsone, colchicine, methotrexate, azathioprine, and intravenous gamma globulin.

Prevention

As an adjunct to pharmacologic therapy, it is essential to encourage patients with chronic urticaria to accept the long-term nature of their illness and focus on achieving reasonable symptomatic control with effective treatments and the fewest possible side effects. Many patients with physical urticarias can learn to avoid or minimize triggers. The few patients with systemic illness may find relief from their urticaria if the underlying condition is appropriately treated. An excellent example is that chronic urticaria in patients with clinically apparent thyroid disease often resolves once the thyroid disease is treated. For many patients, there are other factors that can be identified as exacerbating their specific symptoms. These factors include stress or anxiety, hormonal fluctuations, aspirin and other NSAIDs, and cutaneous vasodilation (e.g., alcohol, hot baths or showers, exercise, heated waterbeds). Psychosocial stress, in particular, is a commonly reported trigger of worsening symptoms. A plausible biochemical mechanism may include increased release of cutaneous neuropeptides known to lower the threshold for mast cell degranulation.

Prognosis

The prognosis for most patients with chronic urticaria/angioedema is excellent. Spontaneous resolution occurs within 12 months in 50% of patients and within 5 years in an additional 20%. However, 10 to 20% of patients, particularly those with physical urticarias or autoimmune urticaria, continue to have symptoms for as long as 20 years. Patients who have had one episode of chronic urticaria that lasted for months or years and resolved may experience one or more similar recurrences later in life.

Future Directions

For urticaria/angioedema, the current trend is to use multiple antihistamines and other agents that block the actions of the mediators produced by mast cells. In the near future, it is likely that patients will be treated earlier with anti-inflammatory and immunomodulatory drugs. Some agents under development for asthma and rhinitis may be useful for the treatment of urticaria/angioedema, including 5-lipoxygenase inhibitors, PGD receptor antagonists, and more potent nonsedating antihistamines. Agents that decrease the sensitivity of mast cells to degranulation, such as phosphodiesterase 4 inhibitors and syk kinase inhibitors, may also find a role in the treatment of this condition.

HEREDITARY ANGIOEDEMA AND RELATED DISEASES

Definition

Hereditary angioedema (HAE) and related illnesses are characterized by recurrent attacks of angioedema mediated by vasoactive peptides such as bradykinin.

Epidemiology

HAE affects approximately 1 in 50,000 people. It is an autosomal dominant disease and therefore affects 50% of offspring of both genders. Frequently, a history of several generations with this disease is obtained, but new mutations occur, and a negative family history is not uncommon. Acquired angioedema (AAE) is more rare and is not inherited; it affects older persons who often have paraproteinemia or malignancies such as lymphoma. Angioedema associated with ACE inhibitors occurs in 0.1 to 0.2% of treated patients.

Pathobiology

HAE and AAE are caused by either low levels or abnormal function of a regulatory protein in the plasma, C1 inhibitor (C1 INH), which exerts control of the complement, fibrinolytic, and kinin-generating pathways. Because there is one normal gene, levels of C1 INH are detectable but are not sufficient to control generation of kinins. The C1 esterase enzyme, when activated, cleaves two complement products, C4 and C2; without proper inhibition, this leads to low levels of circulating C4 and C2. C1 INH is also a critical modulator of the bradykinin pathway, and decreased C1 INH function leads to increased levels of bradykinin. Increased generation of bradykinin, and not mediators from mast cells or activation of complement, leads to capillary leakage and angioedema.

In HAE type I (85% of patients), the abnormal gene does not produce C1 INH. In HAE type II (15%), an antigenically detectable C1 INH protein is produced, but it is not functional. In HAE type III (very rare), C1 INH is present and functional, but there is a yet-to-be-defined abnormality in the generation of vasoactive compounds. In AAE, unknown factors activate C1 and deplete the C1 INH activity in plasma, or there is an autoantibody to C1 INH that interferes with its function. In ACE inhibitor–associated angioedema, the underlying problem is lack of catabolism of bradykinin; the complement pathway is unaffected.

Clinical Manifestations

Children with HAE can have attacks shortly after birth, but these tend to be mild. For most patients, the severity of the attacks worsens at puberty, with episodic attacks of swelling that can affect any external body surface, including the genitalia. Mucosal surfaces are also affected, and patients can have life-threatening swelling of the uvula and posterior pharynx leading to asphyxiation. Swelling of the submucosa of the gastrointestinal tract can cause symptoms of an "acute abdomen," leading to unnecessary exploratory laparotomy. About half of patients report that trauma, particularly that associated with local pressure, precipitates an attack, and about half of patients note an increased frequency of attacks during times of emotional stress. Attacks in patients with AAE are clinically similar to those in patients with HAE. Patients taking ACE inhibitors may have angioedema that manifests as severe swelling or simply as a chronic cough beginning days to months after ACE inhibitor therapy is initiated.

Diagnosis

The best tests to support the diagnosis of HAE or AAE are measurements of C1 INH level, C1 INH function, and C4 level, particularly during an attack. The distinguishing features of AAE are lack of a family history, late onset, and the presence of a malignancy or paraproteinemia, as mentioned earlier. However, patients with AAE, in addition to having low C2 and C4, can have profound depressions in C1, a protein that is commonly normal in HAE. Patients with ACE inhibitor–associated angioedema can present within hours after initiation of therapy or after many months. The angioedema seen in urticaria/angioedema is distinctive in that it is usually associated with urticaria and is pruritic, responding to antihistamines, steroids, and epinephrine.

Treatment

Rx

C1 INH concentrate (500 U) is available in Europe to treat acute attacks of HAE and is the treatment of choice, but this drug has not yet been approved by the FDA. In the United States, treatment of acute attacks of angioedema is currently suboptimal. Epinephrine is only modestly effective but is the safest agent available. Treatment should include nebulized racemic epinephrine delivered in the airway (1:1000 given by nebulization) and by intramuscular injections (0.2 to 0.3 mL of 1:1000 at intervals of 20 to 30 minutes). The addition of antihistamine for sedation may be helpful. Treating physicians must be prepared to perform nasotracheal intubation, preferably in the operating room under conditions in which tracheostomy can be performed if needed. Acute attacks can be terminated by administering 2 units of fresh-frozen plasma (FFP) to supply the missing C1 INH, but in rare instances patients become more edematous, presumably reflecting increased availability of the substrates for generation of kinins. Therefore, although FFP can be useful for treating non–life-threatening acute attacks, it is not recommended for treatment of life-threatening laryngeal edema.

Patients treated prophylactically with attenuated androgens, antifibrinolytic agents, FFP, or C1-INH concentrate have fewer attacks. Attenuated androgens, such as danazol (100 to 200 mg twice daily), increase the production of C1 INH and lead to marked amelioration of symptoms. Masculinizing side effects are usually mild but can be problematic. FFP (USA) or C1 INH concentrate (Europe) should be used before surgical or dental procedures to minimize edema attack due to trauma. Symptomatic treatment of AAE is similar to that for HAE, but definitive treatment requires amelioration of the underlying disease. Treatment of angioedema associated with the use of an ACE inhibitor includes antihistamines, epinephrine, or both, as appropriate, and discontinuation of the ACE inhibitor. Rare patients also will have angioedema when taking angiotension receptor blockers. An approach to the evaluation and treatment of patients with urticaria and angioedema is summarized in Figure 273–2.

Evidence-Based Treatments

Current therapy for HAE in the United States is directed toward prophylactic treatments, including attenuated androgens, antifibrinolytics, and FFP. Danazol was shown in a double-blind, placebo-controlled trial to significantly reduce the number of acute attacks. C1 INH has been used widely and successfully in Europe. In a study of 193 episodes of laryngeal edema treated with C1 INH concentrate, 192 responded within 60 minutes, and the remaining 1 case responded at 4 hours. 2

Prognosis

The long-term outlook for patients with HAE depends greatly on the phenotype of the illness (more or fewer laryngeal attacks), the patient's willingness to take attenuated androgens, and how well the patient tolerates attenuated androgens. For most patients, life expectancy should be normal. AAE usually resolves with treatment of the underlying condition, but the ultimate prognosis for the patient depends on the nature of that illness. Angioedema associated with the use of an ACE inhibitor resolves after the medication is removed.

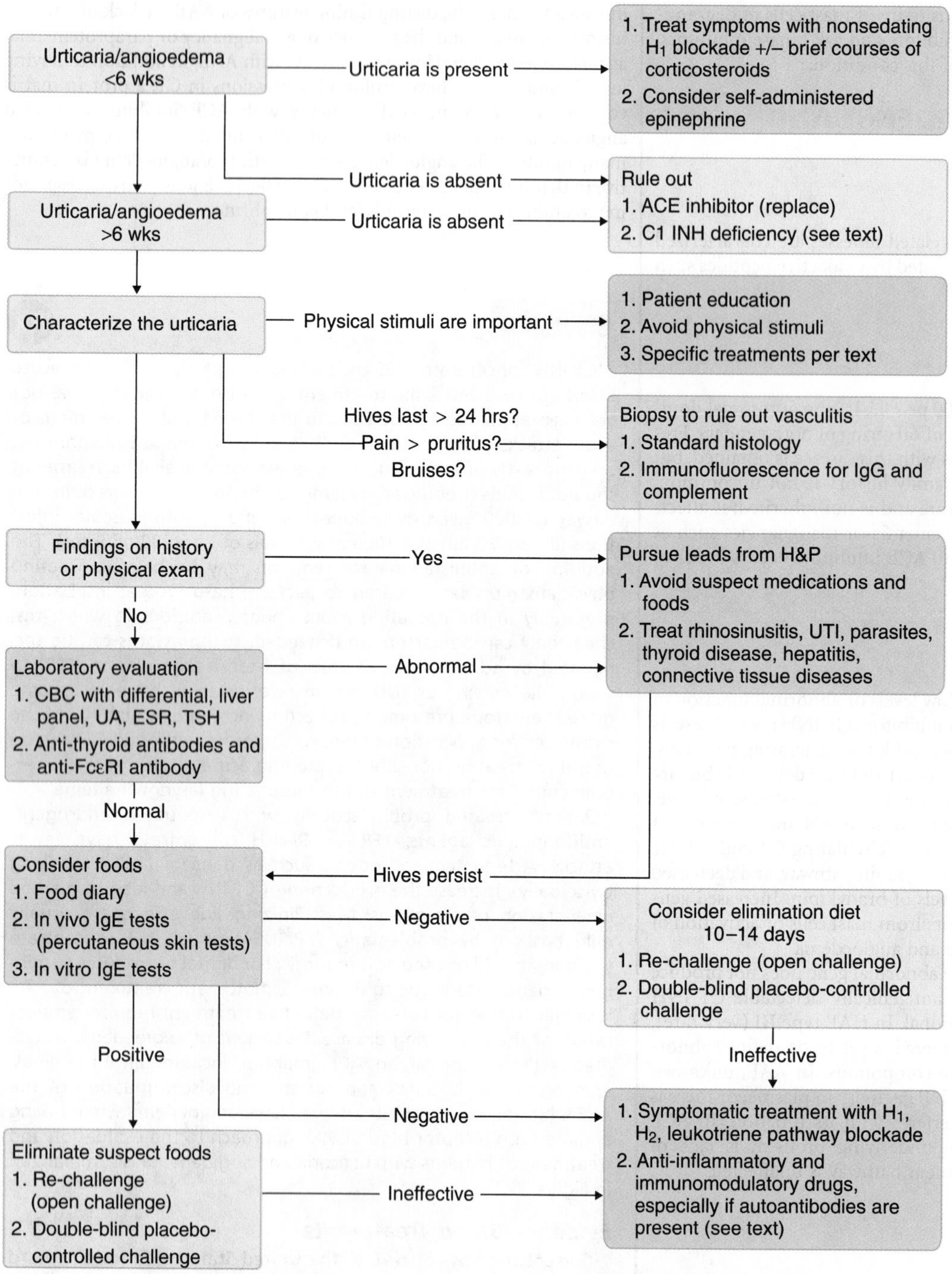

Urticaria/angioedema <6 wks — Urticaria is present → 1. Treat symptoms with nonsedating H_1 blockade +/– brief courses of corticosteroids 2. Consider self-administered epinephrine

Urticaria/angioedema <6 wks — Urticaria is absent → Rule out 1. ACE inhibitor (replace) 2. C1 INH deficiency (see text)

Urticaria/angioedema >6 wks — Urticaria is absent → Rule out 1. ACE inhibitor (replace) 2. C1 INH deficiency (see text)

Urticaria/angioedema >6 wks ↓ Characterize the urticaria

Characterize the urticaria — Physical stimuli are important → 1. Patient education 2. Avoid physical stimuli 3. Specific treatments per text

Characterize the urticaria — Hives last > 24 hrs? Pain > pruritus? Bruises? → Biopsy to rule out vasculitis 1. Standard histology 2. Immunofluorescence for IgG and complement

Characterize the urticaria ↓ Findings on history or physical exam

Findings on history or physical exam — Yes → Pursue leads from H&P 1. Avoid suspect medications and foods 2. Treat rhinosinusitis, UTI, parasites, thyroid disease, hepatitis, connective tissue diseases

Findings on history or physical exam — No ↓ Laboratory evaluation 1. CBC with differential, liver panel, UA, ESR, TSH 2. Anti-thyroid antibodies and anti-FcεRI antibody

Laboratory evaluation — Abnormal → Pursue leads from H&P

Pursue leads from H&P — Hives persist → Consider foods

Laboratory evaluation — Normal ↓ Consider foods 1. Food diary 2. In vivo IgE tests (percutaneous skin tests) 3. In vitro IgE tests

Consider foods — Negative → Consider elimination diet 10–14 days 1. Re-challenge (open challenge) 2. Double-blind placebo-controlled challenge

Consider elimination diet — Ineffective ↓ 1. Symptomatic treatment with H_1, H_2, leukotriene pathway blockade 2. Anti-inflammatory and immunomodulatory drugs, especially if autoantibodies are present (see text)

Consider foods — Negative → 1. Symptomatic treatment with H_1, H_2, leukotriene pathway blockade 2. Anti-inflammatory and immunomodulatory drugs, especially if autoantibodies are present (see text)

Consider foods — Positive ↓ Eliminate suspect foods 1. Re-challenge (open challenge) 2. Double-blind placebo-controlled challenge

Eliminate suspect foods — Ineffective → 1. Symptomatic treatment with H_1, H_2, leukotriene pathway blockade 2. Anti-inflammatory and immunomodulatory drugs, especially if autoantibodies are present (see text)

FIGURE 273–2 • Evaluation and treatment of urticaria/angioedema. Treatment of urticaria with or without angioedema (AE) is similar. Treatment of AE without urticaria depends on the cause. If the AE is caused by an angiotensin-converting enzyme (ACE) inhibitor, discontinuation of the medication is required. Treatment of AE that is caused by a deficiency or dysfunction of C1 inhibitor (C1 INH) is discussed in the text. Idiopathic AE often responds to treatments described for urticaria/angioedema. ESR = erythrocyte sedimentation rate; FcεRI = high-affinity receptor for IgE; H_1 = histamine 1; H_2 = histamine 2; IgE = immunoglobulin E; TSH = thyroid-stimulating hormone; UA = urinalysis; UTI = urinary tract infection.

Future Directions

For treatment of HAE and related disorders, there is a strong effort to have the C1 INH concentrate approved for use in the United States. Finally, new therapies are being developed, including kallikrein inhibitors, bradykinin receptor antagonists, and recombinant C1 INH.

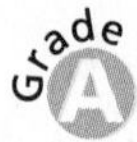

1. Grattan CE, O'Donnell BF, Francis DM, et al: Randomized double-blind study of cyclosporin in chronic "idiopathic" urticaria. Br J Dermatol 2000;143:365–372.
2. Kunschak M, Engl W, Maritsch F, et al: A randomized, controlled trial to study the efficacy and safety of C1 inhibitor concentrate in treating hereditary angioedema. Transfusion 1998;38:540–549.

SUGGESTED READINGS

Bork K, Meng G, Staubach P, Hardt J: Hereditary angioedema: New findings concerning symptoms, affected organs, and course. Am J Med 2006;119:267–274. *A comprehensive review.*

Dibbern DA Jr, Dreskin SC: Urticaria and angioedema: An overview. Immunol Allergy Clin North Am 2004;24:141–162. *An overview of acute and chronic urticaria offering guidance to the evaluation of difficult patients.*

Joint Task Force on Practice Parameters: The diagnosis and management of urticaria: A practice parameter. I. Acute urticaria/angioedema. II. Chronic urticaria/angioedema. Ann Allergy Asthma Immunol 2000;85:S521–S544. *These guidelines are being updated in 2007 and will be available at* www.aaaai.org.

Kaplan AP: Chronic urticaria, pathogenesis and treatment. J Allergy Clin Immunol 2004;114:465. *A concise guide to the evaluation and treatment of chronic urticaria.*

Kozel MM, Sabroe RA: Chronic urticaria: Aetiology, management and current and future treatment options. Drugs 2004;64:2515–2536. *Contains references to many earlier double-blind, placebo-controlled studies of antihistamines as treatment for urticaria.*

Zuberbier T, Bindsley-Jensen C, Canonica W, et al: Management of urticaria. Allergy 2006;61:321–331. *A consensus guideline.*

274 SYSTEMIC ANAPHYLAXIS, FOOD ALLERGY, AND INSECT STING ALLERGY

Lawrence B. Schwartz

Definition

Systemic anaphylaxis, a form of immediate hypersensitivity, arises when mast cells and possibly basophils are provoked to secrete mediators with potent vasoactive and smooth muscle contractile activities that evoke a systemic response. Although mast cells in any organ system may be involved, depending on the distribution of the instigating stimulus, the principal targets are the cardiovascular, cutaneous, respiratory, and gastrointestinal systems, sites where mast cells are most abundant. The terms *anaphylactic* and *anaphylactoid* refer, respectively, to mast cell activation initiated by allergen and immunoglobulin E (IgE), or classical immediate hypersensitivity, and mast cell activation initiated by alternative pathways.

Epidemiology

Assessments of the annual incidence of systemic anaphylaxis and the prevalence of those at risk for systemic anaphylaxis are compromised by imprecise diagnostic measures. Approximately 1500 to 2000 deaths occur per year from systemic anaphylaxis in the United States. Nonfatal cases are much more common, estimated to occur at an incidence of between 10 and 100 cases per 100,000 person-years. Further analyses suggest that between 3 and 43 million people (1 to 15% of the U.S. population) may be at risk for such reactions. Drug reactions account for many of these cases. β-Lactam antibiotics and radiocontrast media provoke most such events, but the list of offending agents is lengthy and ever-increasing. During general anesthesia, systemic anaphylactic reactions occur with a frequency of about 1 in 3500, and muscle relaxants, latex, and induction drugs are the three classes of agents most commonly implicated.

Anaphylaxis to foods and insect stings each account for about 100 deaths per year. Most fatal anaphylactic reactions to injected venom proteins begin within 30 minutes after the sting. In those with suspected anaphylactic reactions, insect venom allergies can be tested by venom skin tests and by in vitro measurements of venom-specific IgE. Sting challenges have been performed experimentally but are not recommended for routine evaluations.

Food allergy is found in about 6% of children younger than 3 years of age and in half that percentage of adults, and these individuals are at risk for food-induced anaphylaxis. Most children lose their allergic sensitivities to cow's milk, egg, wheat, or soy by 5 years of age, whereas sensitivities to peanut, tree nuts, or seafood are typically long-lasting. About 20% of children lose peanut sensitivity by school age, but a small portion of these regain peanut sensitivity later in life, particularly if they continued to avoid this food. Food allergies are evaluated by testing for food allergen-specific IgE using prick skin testing and in vitro measurements; larger wheal-and-flare responses and higher IgE titers to specific allergens are associated with more severe reactions. Oral food challenges are performed under certain circumstances, taking care to minimize the risk of systemic anaphylaxis. These food-allergic reactions involve IgE sensitization and IgE-dependent mechanisms and should be distinguished from a variety of other types of adverse food reactions, including lactose intolerance due to a deficiency in lactase, food-induced enterocolitis in infants (in reaction to cow's milk, soy, or grains), and celiac disease associated with ingestion of gluten in wheat and other grains.

Latex provokes anaphylaxis in a small but significant group of individuals, particularly patients who have undergone multiple surgical procedures early in life such as those with spina bifida or congenital urinary tract disorders, and those with frequent exposure later in life, such as medical personnel. Estimates of the prevalence of latex hypersensitivity range from 1% to 6% in the general population and about 10% among regularly exposed health care workers. Over a 5-year period, the Food and Drug Administration (FDA) collected approximately 1100 reports of latex-induced anaphylaxis, including 15 deaths. Contact hypersensitivity is diagnosed by patch testing, and immediate hypersensitivity by latex-specific IgE tests performed in vitro. Latex allergen skin test reagents have not yet received FDA approval.

Pathobiology

Etiology

Although the mediators elicited from mast cells overlap extensively in anaphylaxis and anaphylactoid reactions, and thereby invoke similar acute therapies, understanding of differences in causation is likely to affect therapeutic interventions aimed at preventing future attacks. Cells other than mast cells also undoubtedly participate in systemic anaphylaxis, particularly those armed with antigen-specific IgE. Basophils, like mast cells, constitutively express substantial amounts of the high-affinity receptor for IgE, FcεRI; when activated through this pathway, also release mediators within minutes. Eosinophils, monocytes, antigen-presenting cells, and epithelial cells may be induced to express this receptor and thereby affect the intensity, duration, or character of anaphylactic reactions. It is theoretically possible that some cases of systemic anaphylaxis occur through one or more of these cell types without involving mast cells, but this remains controversial.

Most IgE-dependent mast cell activation events occur at local sites and result in local disease. For example, allergic conjunctivitis, allergic rhinitis, or allergic asthma typically occurs when allergen lands on the corresponding mucosal surface of a sensitive individual. Systemic anaphylaxis presumably requires the allergen (or nonallergen agonist) to distribute systemically to activate mast cells at remote sites. This is most likely to occur when allergen is administered parenterally; it is less likely after oral ingestion, inhalation, or topical cutaneous or ocular contact. Activation of mast cells in perivascular locations should have the greatest effect on systemic vascular responses, even though large amounts of mediators released locally could, in theory, spill into the circulation and affect remote sites. Accordingly, intravenous penicillin is more likely than oral penicillin to elicit a severe anaphylactic reaction. However, the precise distributions of mast cells that are activated during anaphylactic reactions are undetermined.

Allergens

The most common allergens causing systemic anaphylactic reactions include drugs, insect venoms, foods, radiocontrast media, allergen immunotherapy injections, and latex (Table 274–1). Most allergens are typically proteins or glycoproteins that serve as complete antigens, capable of eliciting immediate hypersensitivity reactions in a sensitized subject without further processing. The protease activity of some allergens may facilitate their penetration at mucosal sites. In contrast to complete antigens, most drugs act as haptens. They become covalently linked to self-proteins in the circulation, in tissues or on cells, emerging as multivalent allergens. Multivalency is important for immediate hypersensitivity, because cross-linking of two IgE molecules on the surface of cells brings together at least two FcεRI molecules, which then transmit an activating signal into the cell. Monovalent antigens fail to elicit mediator release because they bind IgE molecules without cross-linking them.

An allergen exposure must lead to sensitization before an immediate hypersensitivity reaction can occur. This process, which takes 1 to 2 weeks, involves antigen processing by antigen-presenting cells, which then present peptide antigens to T_H2 cells (helper T lymphocytes), which

TABLE 274–1 CAUSES OF SYSTEMIC ANAPHYLAXIS

IgE-Mediated (Anaphylaxis)	Non–IgE-Mediated (Anaphylactoid)
Insect stings	Aspirin
Foods	Radiocontrast media
Drugs	Exercise
Latex	Narcotics/vancomycin
Allergen extracts	Idiopathic (?autoimmune)

in turn select, nurture, and instruct allergen-specific B cells to switch from production of IgM or IgG to IgE. Consequently, anaphylaxis does not occur on first exposure to an allergen (sensitization phase) but may occur after subsequent exposures.

Most cases of food-induced anaphylaxis in children occur in response to egg, peanut, cow's milk, wheat, or soy, whereas peanuts, tree nuts, and seafood account for most reactions in adults. Reactions to seeds such as sesame seem to be growing in importance, and a variety of different foods have proved to be important allergens in specific individuals. Some have the oral allergy syndrome, which results from allergic reactions with food contact that rarely progress to systemic reactions. Many of these reactions are associated with cross-reactivities between food and pollen allergens, such as melon with ragweed pollen and peach or apple with birch pollen. Also, the food epitopes associated with this syndrome are typically conformational (rather than linear) and therefore are more easily destroyed by heating, protease degradation, and acid denaturation.

Hymenoptera families primarily responsible for anaphylactic reactions include the Apidae (honey bees and bumble bees), Vespidae (hornets, yellow jackets, and paper wasps), and Formicidae (fire ants). Major allergens of honey bees include phospholipase A_2 (Api m 1), hyaluronidase (Api m 2), and melitin (Api m 4). Bumble bee venom proteins exhibit immunologic cross-reactivity with those of the honey bee, even though melitin is lacking. Vespid venoms cross-react among themselves and include a protein named antigen 5, phospholipase, and hyaluronidase, the latter allergen cross-reacting with bee hyaluronidase. Fire ant venom toxicity is caused principally by various alkaloids, which are not allergenic. Immediate hypersensitivity reactions to fire ant venom target a phospholipase that cross-reacts with the comparable vespid enzyme and various other proteins that do not cross-react with vespid or bee venom proteins. Allergens in fire ant venom cross-react with those in scorpion venom. A person may exhibit an anaphylactic reaction on first exposure to an insect's sting if previously sensitized to cross-reactive venom from a different insect. In contrast to stinging insects, allergens from biting insects of the Diptera order (mosquitoes, gnats, midges, true flies) are salivary in origin and do not cross-react with Hymenoptera venom allergens. Anaphylaxis to these salivary proteins appears to be uncommon, but precise epidemiologic data are problematic because people are often unaware of an ongoing mosquito bite, and commercial diagnostic reagents of high quality are not yet available.

Latex allergens are derived from the rubber tree, *Hevea brasiliensis*. Irritant dermatitis is the most frequent contact reaction and does not involve acquired immunity. Contact hypersensitivity, which results from cell-mediated immunity to haptenic chemicals added to latex during processing, produces a poison ivy–like local reaction. In contrast, immediate hypersensitivity occurs when IgE is made against proteins naturally found in this plant-derived product. Cutaneous (elastic materials), mucosal or intravascular (catheters), oral (balloon), and inhaled (powdered latex gloves) routes of exposure have been well-documented. IgE-mediated cross-reactivities between latex proteins and allergens in certain fresh foods such as banana, chestnut, avocado, kiwi, peach, bell pepper, and tomato have been reported and may necessitate avoidance of these foods.

Non–IgE-Dependent Agonists

Most non–IgE-dependent foreign agents do not require antigen processing and can elicit a mast cell activation response on first exposure. These include radiocontrast dyes, narcotics such as codeine and morphine, and vancomycin (see Table 274–1). The dose and rate of administration and individual variations in sensitivity are determinants of severity. For radiocontrast dyes, media of low ionic strength are less likely than those of high ionic strength to elicit a systemic reaction. Vancomycin produces a mast cell activation event known as "red man syndrome," typically involving urticaria without cardiovascular compromise, which usually can be avoided by reducing the rate of administration of the antibiotic.

Endogenous mast cell activators include neuropeptides such as substance P, neurokinin A, calcitonin gene-related peptide, and the complement anaphylatoxins C3a and C5a. Whether a magnitude of mast cell activation sufficient to cause systemic anaphylaxis can result from endogenous secretion or generation of these peptides by themselves is unproven. For example, an anaphylactic shock–like syndrome occurred in hemodialysis patients exposed to a contaminated hemodialysis membrane that was associated with complement activation, but mast cell activation was not detected.

Aspirin hypersensitivity typically manifests as either a respiratory or a cardiovascular reaction, although sometimes overlap is observed. Respiratory reactions include bronchospasm, nasal congestion, and rhinorrhea and may extend beyond the respiratory tract to include abdominal cramping, watery diarrhea, and urticaria. Cardiovascular reactions that are identical clinically to allergen-induced systemic anaphylaxis and shock also can occur. In most cases, such reactions appear to be pharmacologically (not IgE) mediated, and in sensitive subjects they can occur in response to any of the cyclooxygenase 1 (COX1) inhibitors. Although cyclooxygenase inhibitors may shunt arachidonic acid metabolism to the lipoxygenase pathway, a mechanism to explain mast cell activation has not yet emerged. COX2-selective inhibitors appear to be relatively safe in aspirin-sensitive asthmatics and also are less likely to cause cardiovascular collapse. Less commonly, sensitivity occurs to only one of the drugs within this class and is caused by IgE against an associated unique chemical moiety.

Autoimmunity

Spontaneous episodes of anaphylaxis, those without an apparent external trigger, also occur. In some cases, such episodes may be an extension of a physical urticaria, occurring in response to stimuli such as exercise, heat, solar radiation, vibration, pressure, or cold. Exercise-dependent anaphylaxis is sometimes associated with food ingestion, occurring within several hours after eating, particularly if sensitivity to the food is present, and might be avoided by delaying exercise until several hours after eating. Progesterone-induced anaphylaxis, which tends to occur just before menses, is uncommon but has been well documented. In other cases, occurrences are not associated with an obvious stimulus. Some cases of chronic urticaria are known to be associated with IgG and IgM antibodies against FcεRI or IgE. In such cases, complement activation leading to the generation of complement anaphylatoxins at the surface of mast cells has been postulated to synergize with FcεRI-mediated activation. These reactions may occur preferentially in the skin because of the expression of anaphylatoxin receptors on the type of mast cell that is predominant in the skin but not on the type predominant in lung. An analogous, albeit speculative, autoimmune process might activate mast cells localized in blood vessel walls, the result being anaphylaxis.

Pathophysiology

Mast cells participate in both acquired and innate forms of immunity. They develop in peripheral tissues from bone marrow progenitors, primarily under the influence of stem cell factor, the ligand for the tyrosine kinase receptor called Kit. Armed with allergen-specific IgE, mast cells are activated by multivalent allergens that cross-link IgE and associated FcεRI molecules on the cell surface. This may be important in the defense against certain parasites that elicit a strong IgE response. Experiments performed in rodents suggest that mast cells also can be directly activated by certain bacterial products, leading to the secretion of mediators that recruit neutrophils. This innate immune response may restrain bacterial dissemination until a more potent acquired immune response develops. Activation of mast cells by endogenous peptides such as substance P or calcitonin gene-related peptide may influence basic biologic processes such as wound healing and angiogenesis. Whether mast cells have a critical, nonredundant role in these biologic and immunologic processes remains controversial. However, their central role in immediate hypersensitivity is clear.

Mediators released by mast cells include preformed mediators stored in secretory granules, newly generated products of arachidonic acid, and an array of cytokines and chemokines. Histamine, formed from histidine by histidine decarboxylase, is the sole biogenic amine stored in all granules of human mast cells and basophils. Histamine released by mast cells or basophils diffuses freely and interacts with H_1, H_2, H_3, and H_4 receptors. H_1 receptors are found on endothelial cells, smooth muscle cells, and sensory nerves; when stimulated, they lead to bronchial and gastrointestinal smooth muscle contraction, vascular smooth muscle relaxation, increased permeability of postcapillary venules, coronary artery vasoconstriction, and pruritus—signs and symptoms often associated with systemic anaphylaxis. In the central nervous system (CNS), blockade of H_1 receptors appears to cause drowsiness. H_2 receptors reside on gastric parietal cells and at lower levels on inflammatory cells, bronchial epithelium, and endothelium and in the CNS. H_2-receptor–mediated increased acid production in the stomach, albeit transient, may occur during systemic anaphylaxis, but it is more likely to become clinically significant if histamine levels are chronically elevated, as observed in patients with systemic mastocytosis. H_3 receptors are found primarily on cells in the CNS. H_4 receptors are found on hematopoietic cells such as mast cells, basophils, and eosinophils and may modulate certain aspects of inflammation, such as eosinophil recruitment. Histamine, after its secretion from mast cells and basophils, is rapidly metabolized to inactive methyl histamine and indole acetic acid.

Prostaglandin D_2 (PGD_2) is the principal COX-catalyzed product of arachidonic acid secreted by activated mast cells, but it is not made by basophils. It binds to the G protein–coupled receptors, CRTH2 and DP. Both COX1 and COX2 are involved in PGD_2 production by mast cells. Consequently, a COX inhibitor that is bipotent might be better than one that is selective at blocking PGD_2-mediated responses during anaphylaxis, which may include hypotension, bronchospasm, and inhibition of platelet aggregation.

Leukotriene C_4 (LTC_4), is released by both mast cells and basophils after its formation from arachidonic acid and glutathione; its formation is sequentially catalyzed first by 5-lipoxygenase and 5-lipoxygenase–activating protein and then by LTC synthase. Conversion to LTD_4 and LTE_4, which also are bioactive, occurs in the extracellular space. These sulfidopeptide leukotrienes bind to the G protein–coupled receptors cysteinyl leukotriene 1 ($CysLT_1$), on bronchial smooth muscle, epithelial and endothelial cells, and leukocytes, and $CysLT_2$, on vascular smooth muscle, endothelial and epithelial cells, leukocytes, and heart muscle. Sulfidopeptide leukotrienes cause bronchoconstriction, mucus secretion, eosinophil recruitment, vasopermeability, diminished cardiac contractility, vasoconstriction of coronary and peripheral arteries, and vasodilation of venules. Antagonists of $CysLT_1$ (montelukast, zafirlukast) but not of $CysLT_2$, as well as a 5-lipoxygenase inhibitor (zileuton), are currently available to patients.

Mast cells also are the sole or principal source of heparin proteoglycan and certain proteases. All express β-tryptase, and a subset also expresses chymase, mast cell carboxypeptidase, and cathepsin G (like neutrophils and monocytes). Mast cells that express only tryptase are called MC_T cells; those that also express the other proteases are called MC_{TC} cells. Mature tryptase is stored in the secretory granules of all mast cells and is released during degranulation of activated cells; levels in serum serve as a clinical marker for mast cell activation. In contrast, precursor forms of tryptase (protryptase) are spontaneously secreted by mast cells at rest; levels in serum serve as a clinical marker of the total body burden of mast cells. MC_{TC} cells express CD88 and therefore are activated by C5a generated during complement activation. Basophils are relatively deficient in these proteases but also express CD88.

Cytokines (tumor necrosis factor-α [TNF-α]; interleukin [IL]-4, -5, -6, -8, -13, and 16; granulocyte-macrophage colony-stimulating factor [GM-CSF]; basic fibroblast growth factor [bFGF]; vascular endothelial growth factor [VEGF]) and chemokines (IL-8, monocyte chemotactic protein-1, monocyte inflammatory protein-1α) represent another dimension of the mediators released by mast cells and basophils. Although these mediators are not selectively produced by these cell types, their vasoactive and inflammatory potential could affect the severity and duration of anaphylaxis. As selective antagonists of the relevant cytokines and chemokines become available and are tested for therapeutic benefits, the roles of these mediators in the pathogenesis of anaphylaxis will be better understood.

Diagnosis

Systemic anaphylaxis, with various combinations of hypotension, tachycardia, urticaria, flushing, bronchoconstriction, laryngeal edema, colics, diarrhea, and vomiting—often associated with a sense of doom and beginning within minutes after the provoking stimulus—can be precisely confirmed in the laboratory by demonstration of antigen-specific IgE (sensitization) and an increased level of mature tryptase (mast cell activation) in serum. Skin testing or in vitro measurements of antigen-specific IgE should be delayed for at least 2 weeks after the precipitating event to prevent false-negative results. An increased level of mature tryptase in serum, which peaks 15 to 60 minutes after the onset of anaphylaxis and then declines with a half-life of about 2 hours (normal levels being undetectable), indicates that mast cell activation has occurred. During a study of experimental insect sting–induced anaphylaxis, the increased level of mature tryptase correlated closely with the drop in mean arterial pressure, indicating that the magnitude of mast cell activation is a primary determinant of clinical severity. Although an increased serum mature tryptase level may be useful for distinguishing anaphylaxis from other conditions in the differential diagnosis, it does not occur in some cases of putative anaphylaxis, particularly after food ingestion. This observation raises questions of whether there are anaphylactic pathways that bypass mast cells, perhaps involving basophil activation. Plasma histamine, because it is rapidly metabolized, is not as practical as serum or plasma mature tryptase for detecting anaphylaxis. Urinary histamine or methylhistamine levels also may reflect overall levels of released histamine, but they are affected by ingested histamine-containing foods, histamine-producing mucosal bacteria, and variability in histamine metabolism.

Differential Diagnosis

Anaphylaxis should be distinguished from a variety of disorders with overlapping presentations. Vasovagal syncope causes diaphoresis, nausea, hypotension, and bradycardia, but without urticaria. Flushing disorders may be benign and unrelated to anaphylaxis, or they could be a manifestation of pathologic conditions such as the carcinoid syndrome, with which urticaria and profound hypotension are not typically associated, or pheochromocytoma, which causes episodic hypertension. Precise detection of these latter conditions involves determination of serum levels of serotonin and urinary levels of 5-hydroxyindole acetic acid, catecholamines, and vanillylmandelic acid. Panic attacks and vocal cord dysfunction can be a challenge to distinguish from anaphylaxis, especially by history alone, but nevertheless must be considered. Acute attacks of hereditary and acquired angioedema caused by C1 esterase inhibitor deficiency are not associated with pruritic urticaria and persist longer than attacks of anaphylaxis. Shock due to complement activation by contaminated hemodialysis tubing, without involving mast cell activation, also has been reported. Scombroidosis occurs 5 to 90 minutes after ingestion of histamine in poorly stored fish and manifests with flushing, palpitations, headache, and gastrointestinal symptoms. The condition lasts several hours, both duration and severity depending on the amount of histamine ingested, and usually responds to H_1-receptor and H_2-receptor antihistamines but occasionally requires epinephrine and intravenous fluids. Acute serum sickness, various cell activation syndromes, endotoxin-mediated septic shock, and superantigen-mediated toxic shock syndromes manifest with fever, which is not characteristic of anaphylaxis by itself. Also, hypoglycemia, seizure, and primary pulmonary or cardiac events should be considered.

In some cases, systemic anaphylaxis occurs together with another disorder. For example, a 65-year-old man, after being stung by a wasp, complained of dizziness and shortness of breath, was hypotensive with urticaria, and responded to treatment with subcutaneous epinephrine, but then complained of chest pressure; electrocardiography indicated an inferior wall infarction. Serum levels of both mature tryptase and cardiac enzymes were elevated, indicating that both anaphylaxis and myocardial infarction had occurred.

Systemic mastocytosis is an important condition to consider in the differential diagnosis of anaphylaxis. In adults, a somatic activating mutation in the gene for Kit in mast cell progenitors results in an excessive body burden of mast cells. In children with this disorder, the disease may regress spontaneously. Patients with too many mast cells are at increased risk for anaphylaxis, and anaphylaxis may be a presenting manifestation of systemic mastocytosis. For example, anaphylaxis in response to an insect sting, particularly in the absence of venom-specific IgE (due to direct mast cell agonists), should raise the possibility of systemic mastocytosis. Diagnostic tests for systemic mastocytosis might include a biopsy of a skin lesion suspected to be urticaria pigmentosa, a bone marrow biopsy stained for mast cells (antitryptase immunohistochemistry being most sensitive), detection by flow cytometry of mast cells in the bone marrow aspirate that express surface CD2 and CD25, and measurement of an elevated serum level (≥20 ng/mL) of total tryptase (mature plus precursor forms of tryptase) during a nonacute interval.

Treatment

Rx

Fatal outcomes in anaphylaxis are principally the result of either airway constriction or hypotension. Accordingly, the acute treatment of systemic anaphylaxis requires that airway patency, blood pressure, and cardiac status be addressed (Table 274–2). Intubation, tracheostomy, volume expanders, and vasopressors may be needed. Patients exhibiting signs and symptoms of hypotension should immediately assume the Trendelenburg position, which may prevent progression to anaphylactic shock or what has been called the empty ventricle syndrome—because almost all hypotensive anaphylactic deaths are preceded by syncope occurring in a sitting or upright posture. Epinephrine injected intramuscularly into the thigh (0.2 to 0.5 mg for adults, 0.01 mg/kg up to 0.3 mg for children, repeated every 5 to 30 minutes as indicated) is the most critical drug to administer, the earlier during the course of an anaphylactic event the better. Alternatively, intravenous administration of a solution of epinephrine (1 mg/100 mL solution starting at 30 to 100 mL/hour), titrated to the lowest effective rate of infusion, can be considered. Epinephrine relaxes bronchial smooth muscle and improves vasomotor tone and vasopermeability, thereby counteracting bronchospasm, hypotension, and tissue edema. However, the benefits of epinephrine need to be weighed against its disadvantages in elderly subjects and in those with cerebrovascular or coronary artery disease, hypertension, diabetes, hyperthyroidism, cardiomyopathy, or narrow-angle glaucoma, in whom it can precipitate myocardial infarction, stroke, or pulmonary edema. Also, patients taking a β-blocker may be resistant to epinephrine; in such a case, glucagon (1 mg IV, or 1 to 5 mg/hour IV) or vasopressin (5 to 40 IU IV) may be used. Oxygen should be administered by nasal cannula. Inhaled bronchodilators can relieve bronchospasm. Parenteral administration of H_1-receptor (diphenhydramine, 1 to 2 mg/kg up to 50 mg) and H_2-receptor (ranitidine, 300 mg IV over 5 minutes) antihistamines may prevent progression of some of the signs and symptoms, particularly urticaria and pruritus, but is not likely to reverse hypotension or tissue edema. Prednisone (20 mg PO) or Solu-Medrol (40 mg IV) may reduce the risk of a protracted reaction or the late phase of biphasic anaphylaxis but is unlikely to be of benefit acutely.

Prevention

Patients who have experienced an anaphylactic reaction are at greatest risk for another episode. Such individuals should wear a Medic-Alert bracelet and be instructed in the use of epinephrine (e.g., EpiPen), which they should carry. Avoidance of β-blockers and ACE inhibitors is recommended, because either may worsen the severity of an anaphylactic episode, and β-blockers clearly interfere with β-agonist treatment. In subjects with recurrent anaphylaxis, prophylactic use of H_1- and H_2-receptor antihistamines is beneficial. A leukotriene antagonist and cyclooxygenase inhibitor theoretically would provide additional benefit, but this has not been systematically studied. Finally, cyclosporin A (3 to 5 mg/kg/day) might be considered in difficult cases of recurrent anaphylaxis because of its ability to inhibit mast cell activation in vitro. Whether glucocorticosteroids, which do not inhibit mast cell activation in vitro or immediate skin test responses to allergens in vivo, provide a major benefit in most patients with recurrent anaphylaxis is debatable.

Specific anaphylactic syndromes have unique considerations. Anti-IgE therapy can increase the threshold of sensitivity from the equivalent of half a peanut to almost nine peanuts. 1 Insect venom sensitivity can be selectively treated by immunotherapy that dramatically decreases the risk of anaphylaxis in response to future stings. Reactions to radiocontrast media can be prevented or attenuated by prior administration of prednisone and H_1- and H_2-receptor antihistamines. Patients who are hypersensitive to penicillin should avoid β-lactam antibiotics in general but can be desensitized if an antibiotic in this class is critically needed (e.g., penicillin for neurosyphilis). However, desensitization is temporary; once the drug has cleared, sensitivity is likely to return. Progesterone-induced anaphylaxis may respond to the luteinizing hormone–releasing hormone analog, Lupron, or to oophorectomy. Patients with systemic mastocytosis, in addition to prophylactic pharmacologic measures, should avoid using direct mast cell agonists such as codeine, morphine, and vancomycin. Aspirin-sensitive subjects can be desensitized but then must continue to ingest a daily dose of aspirin to maintain their desensitization status. Food- and latex-sensitive subjects must practice avoidance of the provocative agent, though preliminary data with anti-IgE neutralization therapy indicates that modest protection for peanut-sensitive subjects against small inadvertent exposures might be achieved. It is hoped that future research will yield more effective and long-lasting desensitization therapies than are currently available for most patients at risk for IgE- and non–IgE-mediated anaphylaxis.

TABLE 274–2 TREATMENT OF ACUTE SEVERE SYSTEMIC ANAPHYLAXIS

HYPOTENSION	AIRWAY CONSTRICTION
Trendelenburg position Epinephrine (IM/IV) Volume expanders Oxygen	**Laryngeal Edema (LE)/Bronchospasm (B)** Epinephrine (IM) (LE/B) or nebulized bronchodilator (B) Oxygen (LE/B)
	Progressive Blockage of Airflow Intubation (B,LE) Tracheostomy (LE)
Urticaria H1R/H2R antihistamines	**Possible Prevention of Late Reactions** Glucocorticosteroids (B,LE)
Possible Prevention of Late Reactions Glucocorticosteroids	
Epinephrine-Resistant β-Blocker Glucagon Vasopressin	

B = bronchospasm; H1R = histamine 1 receptor; H2R = histamine 2 receptor; LE = laryngeal edema.

Future Directions

Ongoing research will provide more precise diagnostic tools that also delineate different pathways of anaphylaxis, indicating which cell types and biochemical pathways are involved. The factors that increase risk for an anaphylactic response will be better understood. Consequently, interventions that reduce anaphylactic risk (including better desensitization regimens) and that more effectively reverse the signs and symptoms of this potentially fatal disorder will be developed.

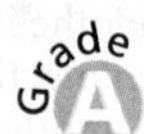

1. Leung DYM, Sampson HA, Yunginger JW, et al: Effect of anti-IgE therapy in patients with peanut allergy. N Engl J Med 2003;348:986–993.

SUGGESTED READINGS

Bilo BM, Rueff F, Mosbech H, et al: Diagnosis of hymenoptera venom allergy. Allergy 2005;60:1339–1349. *Discusses the diagnostic approach to patients with a history of a systemic sting reaction.*

Brown SK, Blackman KE, Stenlake V, Heddle RJ: Insect sting anaphylaxis: Prospective evaluation of treatment with intravenous adrenaline and volume resuscitation. Emerg Med J 2004;21:149–154. *Prospective study to assess the utility of intravenous epinephrine and volume expansion in anaphylaxis from experimental ant stings.*

Galli SJ, Nakae S, Tsai M: Mast cells in the development of adaptive immune responses. Nat Immunol 2005;6:135–142. *Reviews new insights from both animal and human studies on mast cell involvement in immunity.*

Joint Task Force on Practice Parameters; American Academy of Allergy, Asthma and Immunology; American College of Allergy, Asthma and Immunology; Joint Council of Allergy, Asthma and Immunology: The diagnosis and management of anaphylaxis: An updated practice parameter. J Allergy Clin Immunol 2005;115:S483–S523. *A recent comprehensive and practical review of anaphylaxis.*

Sicherer SH, Leung DY: Advances in allergic skin disease, anaphylaxis, and hypersensitivity reactions to foods, drugs, and insects. J Allergy Clin Immunol 2005;116:153–163. *Reviews recent advances in immediate hypersensitivity disorders pertinent to anaphylaxis.*

275 DRUG ALLERGY

Leslie C. Grammer

Definition

Adverse drug reactions (ADRs) are recognized as an important public health problem in that they may be life-threatening. An ADR is defined by the World Health Organization (WHO) as an unintended, noxious response to a drug that occurs at a dose usually prescribed for human patients. The classic pharmacologic definition of ADRs by Rawlins and Thompson separates these into two major subtypes: type A reactions, which are predictable and dose dependent, and type B reactions, which are unpredictable and not dose dependent.

Most ADRs are type A reactions. Type B reactions account for 10 to 15% of all ADRs and include drug allergy (i.e., hypersensitivity reactions to drugs). According to the WHO Nomenclature Review Committee, *drug allergy* refers to a hypersensitivity reaction for which a definite immunologic mechanism, either a B-cell–mediated (antibody) or a T-cell–mediated process, is documented. Most published epidemiologic studies refer to ADRs in general and not to drug allergy specifically because the demonstration of drug-specific B-cell– or T-cell–mediated mechanisms is often quite difficult, and the immunologic culprit may be a drug metabolite.

Epidemiology

Drug allergy is responsible for significant mortality, morbidity, and socioeconomic costs that are probably underestimated. Current data must be evaluated carefully, because they involve different populations, different definitions of ADRs/drug allergy, and different methodologies, especially in terms of data analyses. The Boston Collaborative Drug Surveillance Program collected information on all ADRs in 4031 hospitalized patients during a period of 6 months. An incidence of 6.1%, 247 ADRs, was reported, of which 42% were severe; 1% of the severe reactions resulted in the death of a patient. Using an automatic detection system in a Salt Lake City hospital, Claussen and coinvestigators identified 731 ADRs among 36,653 hospitalized patients. Of note, only 12.3% of these were reported by physicians in the hospital. In a meta-analysis of 33 U.S. prospective studies from 1966 to 1996, Lazarou reported that 15% of hospitalized patients incurred an ADR and that the frequency of drug-related hospital admissions varied from 3 to 6%. Most other studies that followed reported similar data. Epidemiologic information on drug allergy in nonhospitalized people and in the general population is even more limited and is mainly confined to studies of antibiotics.

Risk Factors

Some risk factors have been identified for the development of drug allergy. Certain drugs more commonly cause adverse reactions, and some drugs lead to more severe reactions (Table 275–1). The dosage and route of administration of a drug can also be risk factors; intermittent, repeated administrations of a drug can be more sensitizing than uninterrupted therapy. Some ethnic groups appear to be more prone to certain ADRs. White Americans are at a higher risk for hypersensitivity reactions to abacavir than other ethnic groups. In a study of drug allergy caused by angiotensin-converting enzyme (ACE) inhibitors, the vulnerable population was African American.

In the United States, approximately 10% of individuals who seek health care have a history of penicillin allergy. However, if tested with an appropriate panel of skin tests, fewer than 10% of those individuals would be deemed positive for penicillin allergy. Individuals with a positive history and negative skin tests tolerate penicillin-type antibiotics at the same rate as the general population with a negative history; in addition, there is a very low rate of resensitization.

Pathobiology

Hypersensitivity reactions to drugs can be classified according to the type of immunologic reaction. An immunologic response to any antigen may be diverse, and the resulting reaction complex. Drugs are no exception, and they have been associated with each of the mechanisms of immune disorders discussed in Chapter 44. Drugs that are more frequent perpetrators of significant allergy are listed in Table 275–1.

TABLE 275–1 DRUGS FREQUENTLY IMPLICATED IN ALLERGIC DRUG REACTIONS

Allopurinol	β-Lactam antibiotics
Amiodarone	Cisplatin
Anesthetic agents (muscle relaxants, thiopental)	Enzymes (L-asparaginase, streptokinase, chymopapain)
Antiarrhythmic drugs (procainamide, quinidine)	Heavy metals (gold salts)
Anticonvulsants (hydantoin, phenobarbital, carbamazepine)	Nitrofurans
Antihypertensive agents (angiotensin-converting enzyme inhibitors)	Radiocontrast media
Antipsychotic tranquilizers	Recombinant proteins (insulin, other hormones)
Antisera (antitoxins, monoclonal antibodies)	Sulfonamides
Anti-tuberculous drugs (isoniazid, rifampicin)	Vaccines (egg-based, gelatin)
Aspirin and nonsteroidal anti-inflammatory drugs (NSAIDs)	

Most pharmacologic agents are simple structures with molecular weights of less than 1000 D. Alone, they are unable to induce hypersensitivity-type immunologic responses. However, most of these agents have the ability to covalently bind to proteins, forming hapten–carrier complexes, with the low-molecular-weight agent acting as the hapten and the protein being the carrier. The hapten–carrier complexes are able to induce immunologic responses, with most responses being directed at the hapten.

A well-known example of such an agent is penicillin. Benzylpenicillin has a molecular weight of approximately 300 D and is metabolized into a penicilloyl hapten moiety. The penicilloyl moiety, which constitutes about 95% of all penicillin metabolites, is referred to as the major determinant because it is the major metabolite in terms of quantity. It has been conjugated to poly-D-lysine to form penicilloyl-polylysine, which has been commercially available as Pre-Pen (Hollister Stier, Spokane, WA) for skin testing. However, since 2000 the availability of Pre-Pen has been unpredictable. In the absence of reliable skin test reagents, patients who carry a diagnosis of penicillin allergy are often prescribed antibiotics that are more expensive and have a broader spectrum, contributing to increased health care expenses and to antibiotic resistance.

The other 5% of penicillin metabolites are referred to as the minor determinants. Although they are minor in quantity, these determinants actually are the cause of most of the immediate-type anaphylactic reactions, whereas the major determinant is associated with reactions that are less severe and later in onset. Minor determinant reagents have never been commercially available in the United States. Penicillin skin testing has not been widely used by U.S. physicians; annually, only 40,000 doses of the major determinant have been sold. The potential market for a complete set of penicillin skin test reagents is estimated to be approximately 30 million tests in the United States alone.

In contrast to simple low-molecular-weight drugs, therapeutic agents that are proteins of greater than 5000 D in molecular weight can be recognized by the human immune system and can result in sensitization and hypersensitivity reactions on subsequent exposure. Because these proteins are complete antigens, they can be used as skin testing reagents or as antigens/allergens in in vitro assays. Included among therapeutic protein reagents that have been reported to cause hypersensitivity are porcine insulin, antithymocyte globulin (rabbit or equine), chymopapain, streptokinase, latex, and vaccines such as tetanus toxoid, influenza, yellow fever, pertussis, rubella, and MMR (measles, mumps, rubella). Unexpectedly, a variety of human recombinant proteins, including insulin and monoclonal antibodies, have been reported to cause hypersensitivity reactions. The most plausible explanation is that B cells recognize and mount an immunologic response to an alteration of tertiary or quaternary structure of the recombinant human proteins. These immunologic responses are unlikely to be T-cell driven, because the primary amino acid sequence, which is what T cells recognize, is an exact copy of the endogenously produced protein.

Clinical Manifestations

The clinical manifestations of drug allergy often include a dermatologic component. It is estimated that 80 to 90% of drug allergy results in one of the following cutaneous manifestations: exanthematous or morbilliform eruption; urticaria or angioedema or both; contact dermatitis; fixed drug eruption; erythema multiforme–like eruption; or photosensitivity. There are, however, organ-specific drug hypersensitivity reactions that do not include cutaneous manifestations (Table 275–2).

Diagnosis

The diagnosis of drug allergy requires a complete and exhaustive history, along with a physical examination. It also requires compatible clinical manifestations and temporal eligibility. In vitro tests are rarely clinically useful. In vivo testing such as cutaneous tests and provocative test dosing may be clinically indicated in some situations.

Differential Diagnosis

To distinguish drug allergy from other ADRs, several criteria are helpful. Allergic reactions occur in a tiny fraction of individuals who receive the drug and cannot be predicted. The observed clinical effects do not resemble known pharmacologic actions of the drug. In the absence of prior exposure to the drug, allergic or hypersensitivity symptoms rarely appear before 1 week of continuous therapy. In general, drugs used with no reactions for several months or longer are rarely responsible.

The reaction often resembles other allergic/hypersensitivity reactions such as anaphylaxis, urticaria, and serum sickness–like reactions. Although most drug reactions include cutaneous manifestations, some involve only other organ systems, examples being pulmonary infiltrates with eosinophilia, hepatitis, and acute interstitial nephritis. A list of drugs that cause organ-specific reactions can be found in Table 275–2. Drug-specific antibodies or T-cell receptors or T lymphocytes have been identified that react with the suspected drugs or relevant drug metabolites. As with ADRs in general, the reaction often subsides after the drug is discontinued. However, a hypersensitivity reaction may persist because of the formation of drug metabolites, which act as haptens and bind to carrier proteins such as human serum albumin.

Treatment

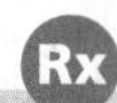

Evidence-Based Treatments

There is a paucity of evidence-based information regarding drug allergy. One study, evaluating the evidence for premedication before administration of antivenom snake bite toxins, concluded that routine prophylactic adrenaline for polyvalent antivenom, known to have high adverse event rates, seems sensible, based on one clinical trial. [1] Antihistamines appear to be of no obvious

TABLE 275–2 ORGAN-SPECIFIC REACTIONS AND IMPLICATED DRUGS

Reactions	Implicated Drugs
PULMONARY MANIFESTATIONS	
Pulmonary infiltrates with eosinophilia	Nitrofurantoin
Pneumonitis and fibrosis	Bleomycin, amiodarone
Noncardiogenic pulmonary edema	Hydrochlorothiazide, cocaine, heroin, methadone
HEMATOLOGIC MANIFESTATIONS	
Eosinophilia	Gold salts, allopurinol, digitalis
DRUG-INDUCED IMMUNE CYTOPENIAS	
Thrombocytopenia	Quinidine, gold salts, sulfonamides, heparin
Hemolytic anemia	Penicillin, methyldopa
Agranulocytosis	Sulfonamides, propylthiouracil, quinidine, procainamide, phenytoin
HEPATIC MANIFESTATIONS	Aminosalicylic acid, dapsone
Cholestasis	Phenothiazines, erythromycin
Hepatocellular damage	Halothane, isoniazid, phenytoin
Mixed pattern	Phenytoin, sulfonamides
RENAL MANIFESTATIONS	
Nephrotic syndrome	Gold salts, captopril, NSAIDs, penicillamine
Acute interstitial nephritis	β-Lactam antibiotics, NSAIDS, sulfonamides
LYMPHOID SYSTEM MANIFESTATIONS	
Pseudolymphoma	Phenytoin
Infectious mononucleosis-like syndrome	Aminosalicylic acid, dapsone
CARDIAC MANIFESTATIONS	Sulfonamides, β-lactam antibiotics
NEUROLOGIC MANIFESTATIONS	Colchicine, nitrofurantoin, sulfonamides
Peripheral neuritis	

NSAIDs = nonsteroidal anti-inflammatory drugs.

Rx

benefit in preventing acute reactions from antivenoms. A second study, evaluating treatment for toxic epidermal necrolysis (TEN), concluded that there are no randomized controlled trials of the most commonly used therapies (i.e., systemic steroids, cyclosporin A, and intravenous immunoglobulins). Furthermore, treatment with thalidomide was not shown to be effective and was associated with higher mortality in a randomized controlled trial.

Although not entirely evidence-based, there are published clinical guidelines for management of infusion-related hypersensitivity reactions caused by the administration of chemotherapeutic or biologic therapy. These guidelines were developed as part of a performance improvement initiative and resulted in a standardized approach to management of reactions and reporting of ADRs.

Prevention

Although the outcome of allergic drug reactions is generally favorable, prevention is the obvious goal. The physician should prescribe medications only if they are clinically appropriate and should, if possible, avoid drugs that are known to produce significant hypersensitivity reactions (see Table 275–1). Before prescription or administration of a medication, the patient should be asked about prior ADRs to the medication or to other pharmacologically related medications. If appropriate, oral administration is probably preferable to parenteral administration; anaphylaxis is less likely, as is sensitization. Protocols for skin testing to foreign antisera and for management of medication hypersensitivity reactions (e.g., premedication, test dosing, desensitization) are available in the Suggested Readings. Therapeutic guidelines regarding treatment of the most important and common allergic drug reactions are also reviewed in those references. A general algorithm is provided in Figure 275–1.

The risk of an anaphylactic reaction to a drug such as penicillin is a function of the history of onset, severity, and proximity (Table 275–3). If an individual experienced an immediate-type reaction that was rapid in onset, involved life-threatening symptoms or signs, and occurred relatively recently, that individual is at high risk for a severe anaphylactic reaction on subsequent exposure.

Because there are no commercially available reagents for penicillin skin testing, the approach to a patient who needs a β-lactam antibiotic, such as a patient with neutropenic fever requiring *Pseudomonas* coverage, usually depends on the risk. Risks and benefits should be thoughtfully discussed and documented. In a low-risk individual, cautious test dosing could be performed. In a high-risk individual, desensitization could be considered if the clinical risks and benefits so warrant.

Prognosis

Most drug allergies involve cutaneous eruptions that are self-limited and resolve shortly after the offending agent has been discontinued. However, severe, life-threatening reactions occur in approximately 1 in every 1000 hospitalized patients. In the United States in 1994, 0.32% of hospitalized patients (106,000 people) died from ADRs. The proportion of ADRs that were allergic reactions was not determined in this study but could be estimated to be about one fourth. The incidence of adverse cutaneous reactions to drugs is higher in women than in men. There also is an increased incidence of ADRs in the elderly.

One of the most severe reactions associated with drug allergy fatalities is anaphylactic shock. It is usually immunoglobulin E (IgE) mediated, but it may occur with non–IgE-mediated reactions to drugs such as nonsteroidal anti-inflammatory drugs (NSAIDs) or radiocontrast media. It is estimated that approximately 1500 deaths occur annually in the United States due to anaphylaxis from medications. In the United Kingdom, drugs are the leading cause of anaphylactic fatalities (88 of 202 fatalities in 2001).

TABLE 275–3 RISK OF ANAPHYLACTIC REACTION TO PENICILLIN OR OTHER PHARMACOTHERAPEUTIC AGENT

Risk	Low	High
Onset of previous reaction	>24 hr	<30 min
Signs and symptoms of previous reaction	Morbilliform eruption Urticaria alone	Life-threatening symptom: hypotension, upper airway angioedema, bronchospasm
Time elapsed since reaction	>20 yr	<1 yr

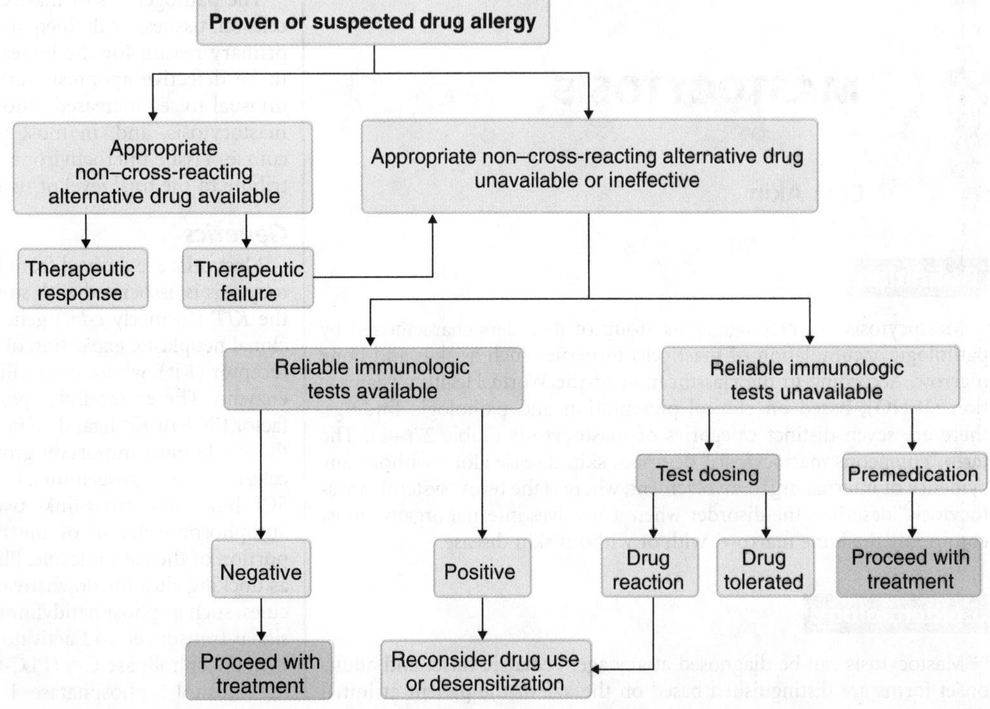

FIGURE 275–1 • Guidelines for the treatment of patients with a history of a drug allergy. In patients with a history of a suspected or known drug allergy, the first choice would be to use an appropriate non–cross-reacting drug. If such a drug is not available, or if the patient does not respond to it, a schema is presented for further evaluation, based on the availability of a reliable immunologic test to detect drug hypersensitivity.

Anaphylaxis is not the major cause of mortality due to allergic drug reactions. Erythema multiforme major, also known as Stevens-Johnson syndrome, has a mortality rate of about 5%, and TEN has a mortality rate of about 30%, mostly due to sepsis. There is an estimated incidence of 0.4 to 1.2 cases per million people per year for Stevens-Johnson syndrome, and 1.2 to 6 cases per million annually for TEN.

Future Directions

Pharmacogenomics is an important future direction to identify those individuals who are at risk for a significant allergic reaction to a given drug. Human leukocyte antigen (HLA) genotyping has been reported to identify individuals who are at increased risk for drug hypersensitivity. As an example, individuals with HLA-B*5701, are at a greater risk (odds ratio, 117; confidence interval, 29 to 481) for a drug hypersensitivity reaction to abacavir, a human immunodeficiency virus (HIV) transcriptase inhibitor. In another example, severe cutaneous adverse reactions to allopurinol are highly associated with the genetic marker HLA-B*5801. Other avenues by which individuals with specific susceptibility to developing allergy to a given medication may be identified include polymorphisms in immune recognition molecules, drug-metabolizing enzymes (DME), and macromolecular adduct repair systems.

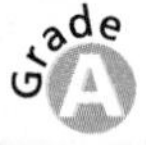
1. Premawardhena AP, de Silva CE, Fonseka MM, et al: Low dose subcutaneous epinephrine to prevent acute adverse reactions to antivenom serum in people bitten by snakes: Randomised, placebo-controlled trial. BMJ 1999;318:1041–1043.

SUGGESTED READINGS

Aberer W, Bircher A, Romano A, et al: Drug provocation testing in the diagnosis of drug hypersensitivity reactions: General considerations. Allergy 2003;58:854–863. *An overview of this approach.*

Brockow K, Christiansen C, Kanny G, et al: Management of hypersensitivity reactions to iodinated contrast media. Allergy 2005;60:150–158. *A comprehensive review.*

Gruchalla RS: Drug allergy. J Allergy Clin Immunol 2003;111:S548–S549. *A comprehensive review.*

Gruchalla RS, Pirmohamed M: Antibiotic allergy. N Engl J Med 2006;354:601–609. *Discusses the strategies and evidence for antibiotic allergy diagnosis and treatment.*

Messaad D, Sahla H, Benahmed S, et al: Drug provocation tests in patients with a history suggesting an immediate drug hypersensitivity reaction. Ann Intern Med 2004;140:1001–1006. *Reporting results of drug provocation tests in 898 patients; more than three-quarters could not be confirmed.*

Pirmohamed M, James S, Meakin S, et al: Adverse drug reactions as a cause of admission to hospital: Prospective analysis of 18,820 patients. Br Med J 2004;329:15–19. *In a large population, several epidemiologic aspects of ADRs are reviewed and classified.*

276 MASTOCYTOSIS

Cem Akin

Definition

Mastocytosis is a heterogeneous group of disorders characterized by pathologic accumulation of mast cells in tissues such as skin and bone marrow. According to the classification of the World Health Organization (WHO), based on clinical presentation and pathologic findings, there are seven distinct categories of mastocytosis (Table 276–1). The term "cutaneous mastocytosis" describes skin disease alone without any evidence of internal organ involvement, whereas the term "systemic mastocytosis" describes the disorder when it involves internal organs (most commonly the bone marrow) with or without skin disease.

Epidemiology

Mastocytosis can be diagnosed at any age. Pediatric-onset and adult-onset forms are distinguished based on the age of the patient at initial diagnosis. These forms display differences in their clinical course, molecular pathology, and prognosis. The most common clinical scenario leading to diagnosis in the pediatric population is a child presenting with skin lesions of cutaneous mastocytosis within the first year of life. Patients with a later onset of skin lesions are more likely to have systemic mastocytosis, as are most patients with adult-onset mastocytosis. The disease has been diagnosed in all ethnic populations. Pediatric-onset mastocytosis appears to be diagnosed more commonly in males (approximately 60%). Estimates of the prevalence of patients with cutaneous mastocytosis range from 1 in 500 to 1 in 8000 patients presenting in dermatology clinics. The prevalence of systemic mastocytosis is more difficult to estimate, because the diagnosis requires biopsy of an involved tissue and a high degree of clinical suspicion. Systemic mastocytosis is likely to be underdiagnosed, considering the fact that there are neither physical examination findings nor routine hematologic or chemistry laboratory abnormalities specifically associated with the disease. Consequently, it is not unusual to encounter several years' delay after the onset of symptoms in many patients before a diagnosis of mastocytosis is reached. The disease is sporadic, although rare cases of familial occurrence have been described.

TABLE 276–1 WORLD HEALTH ORGANIZATION CLASSIFICATION OF MASTOCYTOSIS

Cutaneous mastocytosis
Indolent systemic mastocytosis
Systemic mastocytosis with associated clonal hematologic non–mast cell lineage disease
Aggressive systemic mastocytosis
Mast cell leukemia
Mast cell sarcoma
Extracutaneous mastocytoma

From Valent P, Horny H-P, Li CY, et al: Mastocytosis (mast cell disease). *In* Jaffe ES, Harris NL, Stein H, Vardiman JW (eds): World Health Organization (WHO) Classification of Tumours: Pathology and Genetics. Tumours of Haematopoietic and Lymphoid Tissues. France, Lyon, International Agency for Research on Cancer, 2001, pp 291–302.

Pathobiology

Pathogenesis

The pathogenesis of mastocytosis involves the accumulation of mast cells in tissues, with mediators released by activated mast cells. The primary reason for the increased mast cell numbers in tissues appears to be defective apoptosis rather than uncontrolled proliferation. It is unusual to see increased mitotic activity in biopsies from patients with mastocytosis, and, in most patients, the disease follows an indolent course. Tissue microenvironment and altered chemotaxis may also contribute to the final level of tissue mast cell burden.

Genetics

Mast cells are derived from hematopoietic progenitors. Systemic mastocytosis is associated with somatic gain-of-function point mutations in the *KIT* (formerly *c-kit*) gene of the mast cell progenitor, leading to a clonal neoplastic expansion of mast cells. *KIT* encodes a transmembrane receptor (Kit), whose intracellular portion functions as a tyrosine kinase enzyme. The extracellular portion of Kit binds the cytokine stem cell factor (SCF or Kit ligand). The interaction between SCF and Kit provides the single most important growth and differentiation stimulus for mast cells from their progenitors. Under physiologic conditions, homodimeric SCF binds and cross-links two Kit receptor molecules, which leads to autophosphorylation of the tyrosine amino acids of the intracellular portion of the Kit molecule. Phosphorylated tyrosine residues in turn act as docking sites for downstream adaptor and signal transduction molecules, such as phosphatidylinositol 3 (PI3) kinase, Janus kinase 2 (JAK2), signal transducer and activator of transcription 1 (STAT1) and STAT5, Lyn, phospholipase C-γ (PLC-γ), and Src homology 2 domain–containing inositol-5-phosphatase 1 (SHIP1). These molecules regulate the differentiation, proliferation, chemotaxis, and functional activation of mast cells.

The majority of the mutations reported in systemic mastocytosis involve codon 816 in *KIT*, resulting in the replacement of an aspartic acid by a valine residue (D816V) in the Kit protein. D816 is a critical residue involved in the kinase activity of Kit. Substitution of the wild-type aspartic acid residue in this location by another amino acid results in constitutive activation and autophosphorylation of the receptor molecule without the need for cross-linking by its ligand, SCF. The D816V mutation has been shown in lesional mast cells from the skin and bone marrow tissue of patients with mastocytosis, as well as from other hematopoietic lineages in patients with extensive disease. This aspect of the pathobiology of systemic mastocytosis is similar to the multilineage involvement observed in myeloproliferative disorders.

Codon 816 *KIT* mutations have been reported in various categories of mastocytosis, including those with benign and poor prognoses. Most patients with adult-onset mastocytosis were found to carry this mutation when an appropriate tissue sample from an involved site such as skin or bone marrow was analyzed. In contrast, it has been reported in fewer patients with pediatric-onset cutaneous disease (up to 42%, depending on the study and detection method). Other pathogenetic factors, some yet to be determined, appear to be responsible for the final disease phenotype, because the presence of the D816V *KIT* mutation alone does not explain the remarkable heterogeneity in the clinical presentation and prognosis of the disease. For example, a common polymorphism in the interleukin-4 (IL-4) receptor α-chain (Q576R) has been described as being associated with a milder form of the disease that is limited to the skin.

Symptomatology

The symptomatology of mastocytosis is primarily manifested by the release of mast cell mediators and rarely by a destructive infiltration of mast cells into tissues. Mast cell activation results in the release of various preformed mediators stored in mast cell granules, de novo synthesis of sulfidopeptide leukotrienes such as LTC_4 and prostaglandins (mostly PGD_2) from membrane lipids, and cytokine synthesis. Preformed mediators stored in mast cell granules include histamine; proteases such as tryptase, chymase, and carboxypeptidase A; and proteoglycans such as heparin and chondroitin sulfate. Vasoactive mediators such as histamine, LTC_4, and PGD_2 at local or distant tissues cause vasodilation, which may lead to flushing, tachycardia, hypotension, presyncope, and syncope. Histamine also causes pruritus and stimulates gastric acid hypersecretion from parietal cells. Mast cells are rich sources of cytokines. Elevated serum levels of tumor necrosis factor-α (TNF-α) and IL-6 have been found in patients with mastocytosis and may contribute to the pathophysiology of fatigue and accelerated osteoporosis observed in some patients. Rare aggressive categories of mastocytosis may be associated with an extensive destructive infiltration of mast cells into tissues such as the gastrointestinal tract, which may result in malabsorption, and the liver, which may cause portal fibrosis with associated portal hypertension.

Mast cell activation and mediator release may occur after triggers such as temperature changes (e.g., hot showers); exercise; ingestion of alcohol or spicy foods; emotional stress; insect stings; exposure to certain drugs such as opioid analgesics, nonsteroidal anti-inflammatory drugs (NSAIDs), or muscle relaxants; and sometimes spontaneously without an obvious trigger. The prevalence of atopic disease in patients with mastocytosis is similar to that of the general population, and the serum immunoglobulin E (IgE) level is often found to be low.

Clinical Manifestations

Mastocytosis is a disease with protean clinical manifestations. Although in some patients the only complaint is the cosmetic appearance of urticaria pigmentosa lesions, others suffer from frequent episodes of vascular instability or have life-threatening hematologic disease. In general, patients with mastocytosis belong to one of two broad categories, according to the site of tissue involvement: those with cutaneous disease alone, and those with systemic disease with or without skin involvement. Cutaneous mastocytosis (i.e., disease limited to the skin in the absence of internal organ involvement) is commonly diagnosed in children within the first year of life, whereas systemic mastocytosis is mostly diagnosed in adults by a bone marrow biopsy and aspirate.

Cutaneous Manifestations

Skin lesions of urticaria pigmentosa are the most common presentation of cutaneous mastocytosis (Fig. 276–1). They are also present in 50 to 90% of patients with systemic mastocytosis, depending on the disease category. Remarkably different in appearance from urticaria or hives, lesions of urticaria pigmentosa are fixed, tan- to salmon-colored, maculopapular lesions varying in size from a few millimeters to a few centimeters. They are most prominently observed on the trunk and extremities and tend to spare the face and the sun-exposed areas of the skin, although facial involvement may be seen in children. Blistering of the lesions may occur in children in the first 3 years of life. The lesions are generally not pruritic at rest but may urticate after exposure to a number of triggers (see Pathobiology). Many patients note that the skin lesions become more prominent after exposure to heat or after physical irritation such as rubbing. The lesions may be found concentrated in skin areas that are prone to irritation, such as the axillae and groin.

Uncommon presentations of cutaneous mastocytosis include mastocytomas, diffuse cutaneous mastocytosis, and telangiectasia macularis eruptiva perstans (TMEP). Mastocytomas are benign and generally solitary mast cell tumors, although they have been known to precede urticaria pigmentosa lesions in some cases. They occur almost exclusively in children, and physical irritation of the lesion may result in generalized flushing and other symptoms of mast cell mediator release. Diffuse cutaneous mastocytosis (DCM) is another form of skin involvement seen exclusively in children. It is characterized by diffuse thickening of the skin and appendages with a peau d'orange appearance without individual urticaria pigmentosa lesions. TMEP is a rare form of cutaneous mastocytosis characterized by the presence of diffuse telangiectatic macules. Because TMEP lesions are generally seen in the presence of urticaria pigmentosa, there is debate about whether TMEP represents a distinct form of cutaneous mastocytosis.

Patients with cutaneous mastocytosis may manifest systemic symptoms such as abdominal pain or diarrhea. They also may experience hypotensive episodes resulting from triggered or spontaneous mast cell mediator release, even in the absence of histopathologic mast cell infiltration in the internal organs.

Systemic Manifestations

Symptoms caused by mast cell degranulation may be experienced as brief, recurrent, and self-limited episodes with multiorgan manifestations or as chronic complaints over a prolonged time course. A typical mast cell degranulation episode may variably involve flushing, conjunctival hyperemia, nausea, vomiting, abdominal cramping, diarrhea, tachycardia, and lightheadedness. Hypotension may develop, and the episode may progress to full loss of consciousness in some patients. Therefore, mastocytosis should be ruled out in all patients with recurrent anaphylaxis before a diagnosis of idiopathic anaphylaxis can be made. Tryptase, a protease stored in mast cell granules, may be elevated above the patient's baseline level in the serum or plasma if measured within 3 hours after the onset of the episode in patients with suspected mast cell degranulation or anaphylaxis, regardless of the cause. Angioedema, hives, and wheezing are uncommon in mastocytosis, in contrast to idiopathic anaphylaxis. Flushing usually involves the face and upper chest area. A consistent trigger can be identified in only a small number of patients (see

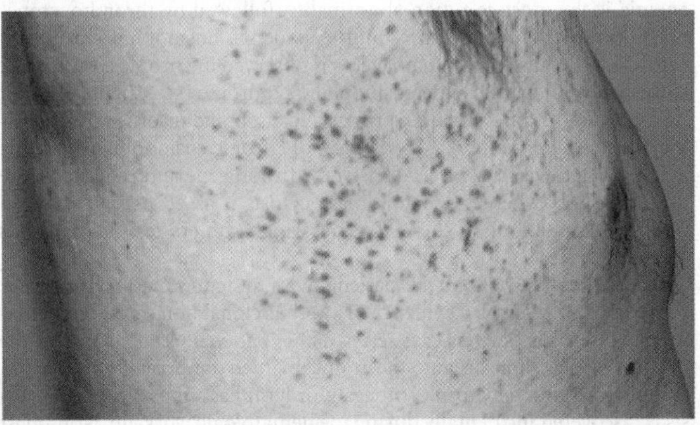

FIGURE 276–1 • Urticaria pigmentosa.

Pathobiology). The episodes usually last for 30 minutes to a few hours. Patients with systemic mastocytosis frequently complain of fatigue, which may last several hours to days after an episode; impaired memory; irritability; and depressed mood. The pathogenesis of these problems is poorly understood, but it may be related to mediators or cytokines released from mast cells, or it may represent the psychological manifestations of having a chronic illness. Hypotensive episodes can be life-threatening, particularly in the presence of comorbidities such as cardiac or pulmonary disease.

Gastrointestinal Symptoms

Gastrointestinal symptoms are observed in more than 50% of patients with mastocytosis. Epigastric pain, lower abdominal cramping, nausea, vomiting, or diarrhea can occur episodically in the context of an acute mast cell degranulation episode or on a chronic basis. Gastric acid hypersecretion induced by mast cell–derived histamine may lead to esophagitis, gastritis, and peptic ulcer disease, although measurements of basal acid output have shown great variability in different studies, ranging from hypersecretion in the range of Zollinger-Ellison syndrome to achlorhydria. Mucosal edema, thickened gastric or duodenal mucosal folds, or nodular lesions may be observed in radiographic or endoscopic evaluations. Diarrhea alternating with constipation may be seen. Severe persistent diarrhea may be complicated by clinically significant malabsorption in patients with aggressive systemic mastocytosis. Hematochezia, hematemesis, and melena are uncommon symptoms and should prompt endoscopic evaluation to rule out coexisting pathology. Mast cells are constituents of the normal lamina propria in gastrointestinal mucosa, and their numbers may be increased in inflammatory states affecting the gastrointestinal tract. However, quantitation of mast cell numbers in gastrointestinal biopsies is generally not helpful, and diagnosis of mast cell disease via a gastrointestinal biopsy, in the absence of typical bone marrow findings, should be avoided. Mild to moderate hepatomegaly with or without abnormalities in serum transaminases may be observed, although portal hypertension and ascites are rare and indicate the presence of advanced categories of mastocytosis. Jaundice and findings on cholangiography resembling those of primary sclerosing cholangitis have been reported in some patients.

Musculoskeletal Symptoms

Musculoskeletal pain is common in patients with mastocytosis and is mostly caused by soft tissue pain resembling fibromyalgia. Accelerated osteoporosis may be seen in a subgroup of patients, particularly in those with other risk factors, such as postmenopausal women, and in those receiving glucocorticoid therapy. Mastocytosis should be considered in the differential diagnosis of patients with premature osteoporosis or pathologic fractures, because the initial clinical finding in some patients is compression fractures of the vertebrae. A bone densitometry measurement should be recommended as part of the standard evaluation of women with mastocytosis and of any patient with a history of pathologic fractures. Radiographic abnormalities have been reported in up to 75% of patients with mastocytosis. In addition to generalized osteoporosis, bone surveys may show a mixture of sclerotic or lytic lesions, and skeletal scintigraphy may reveal focal or diffuse radiotracer uptake.

Hematologic Manifestations

Peripheral blood abnormalities have been noted in up to 50% of patients with systemic mastocytosis. Mild normochromic normocytic anemia is the most common abnormality, followed by thrombocytopenia, eosinophilia, monocytosis, and leukopenia. Eosinophilia in mastocytosis rarely causes organ damage, as is observed in chronic eosinophilic leukemia or idiopathic hypereosinophilic syndrome (see Chapter 176). It is important to differentiate a primary eosinophilic disorder from mastocytosis with eosinophilia. Some cases of chronic eosinophilic leukemia are associated with the *FIP1L1-PDGFRA* fusion gene and respond to the drug imatinib, whereas systemic mastocytosis is associated with codon 816 point mutations of the *KIT* gene, which confers resistance to this drug.

Approximately 20% of the patients with systemic mastocytosis have been reported to display evidence of another clonal non–mast cell hematologic disease in various case series. These patients usually come to the physician's attention because of an unexplained abnormality in peripheral blood count, hepatosplenomegaly, or lymphadenopathy; mastocytosis is discovered incidentally during the hematologic work-up. Non–mast cell clonal hematologic neoplasms associated with mastocytosis are commonly myeloid in nature (myeloproliferative disorders, myelodysplastic syndromes, or myeloid leukemias) but may also involve lymphoproliferative disorders such as lymphomas, myelomas, and lymphocytic leukemias.

Diagnosis

The diagnosis and classification of mastocytosis is carried out according to the guidelines published by the WHO. A suggested algorithm for the diagnosis of mastocytosis is shown in Figure 276–2.

Cutaneous Mastocytosis

Diagnosis of cutaneous mastocytosis is made by observing the typical hyperpigmented maculopapular lesions of urticaria pigmentosa and is confirmed by skin biopsy, which shows infiltration of mast cells in the upper dermis, particularly in perivascular locations. It should be noted that mild increases in mast cell numbers can be observed in inflammatory and neoplastic skin diseases, and establishing a diagnosis of cutaneous mastocytosis by a blind skin biopsy or biopsy of a lesion that does not have the typical appearance of urticaria pigmentosa should be avoided. A localized wheal-and-flare reaction limited to the lesional skin within a few minutes after rubbing or scratching the skin is known as "Darier's sign." Diagnosis of urticaria pigmentosa in adults should always prompt investigation of possible systemic mastocytosis.

Systemic Mastocytosis

Biopsy

A bone marrow biopsy and aspiration is the recommended diagnostic procedure to evaluate the presence of WHO diagnostic criteria for systemic disease (discussed later). This procedure is recommended for all patients with adult-onset urticaria pigmentosa, patients with recurrent symptoms suggestive of mast cell degranulation (such as flushing and hypotension accompanied by abdominal complaints), patients with unexplained osteoporosis, and patients with suspected hematologic disease (see Clinical Manifestations). Children with an onset of lesions within the first year of life usually do not require a bone marrow biopsy unless they have an abnormal complete blood count, lymphadenopathy, hepatomegaly, or splenomegaly. Children with late-onset skin lesions and those who experience persistence of urticaria pigmentosa into adulthood should be considered for diagnostic evaluation for systemic disease.

World Health Organization Diagnostic Criteria

WHO guidelines for diagnosis of systemic mastocytosis consist of one major and four minor criteria (Table 276–2). Presence of the major cri-

TABLE 276–2 WORLD HEALTH ORGANIZATION DIAGNOSTIC CRITERIA FOR SYSTEMIC MASTOCYTOSIS

MAJOR
Multifocal, dense infiltrates of mast cells consisting of 15 or more mast cells in aggregates detected in sections of bone marrow and/or other extracutaneous organs, confirmed by tryptase immunohistochemistry or other special stains
MINOR
More than 25% of mast cells in biopsy sections or bone marrow aspirate smears showing spindle shape or atypical morphology
Detection of a *KIT* codon 816 point mutation in bone marrow, blood, or other extracutaneous organs
Expression of CD2 and/or CD25 by mast cells in bone marrow, blood, or extracutaneous organs
Persistent elevation of serum total tryptase >20 ng/mL*

*Criterion not valid if there is an associated clonal myeloid disorder.
From Valent P, Horny H-P, Li CY, et al: Mastocytosis (mast cell disease). *In* Jaffe ES, Harris NL, Stein H, Vardiman JW (eds): World Health Organization (WHO) Classification of Tumours: Pathology and Genetics. Tumours of Haematopoietic and Lymphoid Tissues. Lyon, France, International Agency for Research on Cancer, 2001, pp 291–302.

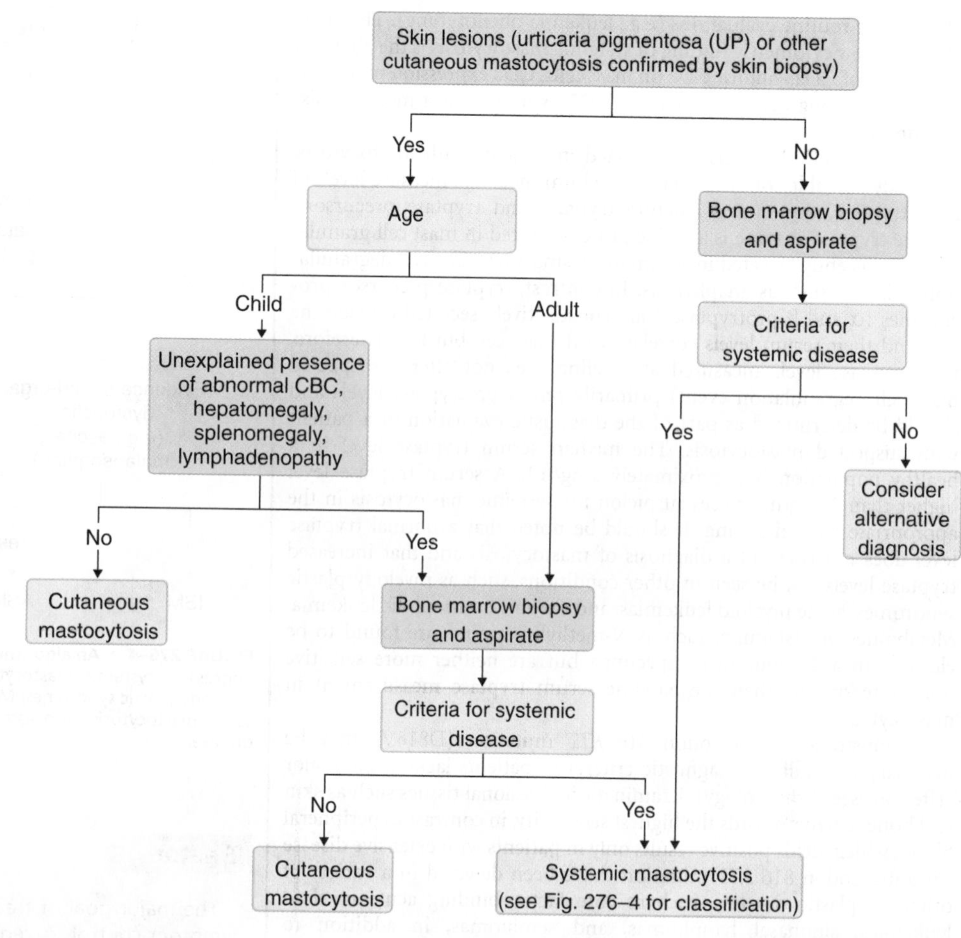

FIGURE 276–2 • Suggested diagnostic algorithm for mastocytosis. CBC = complete blood count.

FIGURE 276–3 • Diagnostic findings in the bone marrow biopsy and aspirate. A, Characteristic mast cell aggregates on tryptase staining (major criterion) in biopsy section (arrow). **B,** Mast cells with atypical spindle shapes in aspirate smear (arrow).

A

B

terion with at least one minor criterion, or demonstration of three minor criteria in the absence of the major criterion, is needed to establish a diagnosis of systemic mastocytosis and distinguish it from reactive mast cell hyperplasia. The major diagnostic criterion is the presence of multifocal, dense aggregates of 15 or more mast cells in bone marrow or other extracutaneous tissue biopsy sections (Fig. 276–3A). Such clusters are frequently observed around blood vessels and next to bone trabeculae in bone marrow biopsies. Immunohistochemical staining for tryptase is the recommended method for visualization of mast cells. Routine hematoxylin and eosin or metachromatic stains such as toluidine blue are not sufficiently sensitive to demonstrate subtle mast cell infiltrates or abnormal morphologic features of mast cells within the infiltrates in decalcified bone marrow biopsy sections.

Mast cell morphology in bone marrow provides important clues to the diagnosis of systemic mastocytosis. Normal bone marrow mast cells are round cells with a centrally located, round to oval nucleus; a low nucleus-to-cytoplasm ratio; and heavy granulation. They are observed singly in an interstitial distribution in healthy marrow, without any significant clustering. In contrast, bone marrow mast cells in systemic mastocytosis often display atypical morphology, such as an elongated (spindle) shape, hypogranularity, and an eccentric or lobulated nucleus (see Fig. 276–3B). These atypical mast cells are usually observed in close association with bone marrow spicules in the aspirate smear. Mast cells in mast cell leukemia (MCL) may be very sparsely granulated.

Flow cytometric analysis of the mast cells in a bone marrow aspirate, when performed appropriately, is a very sensitive diagnostic aid. Mast cells are identified in flow cytometric dot plots as cells highly expressing CD117 (Kit) that are also positive for surface IgE but negative for CD34. These staining characteristics allow the differentiation of mast cells from a more abundant CD117-positive bone marrow cell population, including hematopoietic progenitor cells that are intermediately positive for CD117 and CD34 but negative for surface IgE. The mean percentage of mast cells in a healthy bone marrow aspirate is approximately 0.02%, and it does not exceed 1% in most patients with mastocytosis. Therefore, to visualize the mast cell population correctly, the total cell numbers analyzed by flow cytometry should be significantly higher than those in other, more routine evaluations (e.g., leukemia phenotyping). The characteristic flow cytometric finding of systemic mastocytosis is the aberrant expression of CD25 and/or CD2 on mast cells. CD2 expression may show variability among patients, whereas CD25 expression is a more consistent finding.

Serum tryptase level may be elevated in patients with mastocytosis. Currently available commercial tryptase immunoassays measure levels of total tryptase, the sum of mature tryptase and tryptase precursors. Mature tryptase enzyme is a serine protease stored in mast cell granules and is transiently elevated in serum or plasma after mast cell degranulation episodes such as anaphylaxis. In contrast, tryptase precursor proenzymes (α and β protryptases) are constitutively secreted outside the cell, and their serum levels correlate with mast cell burden. Therefore, total tryptase levels measured at baseline (i.e., not after a suspected mast cell degranulation event) primarily reflect protryptase levels and should be determined as part of the diagnostic evaluation of a patient with suspected mastocytosis. The median serum tryptase level in a healthy population is approximately 5 ng/mL. A serum tryptase level higher than 20 ng/mL raises suspicion for systemic mastocytosis in the appropriate clinical setting. It should be noted that a normal tryptase level does not rule out a diagnosis of mastocytosis and that increased tryptase levels can be seen in other conditions, such as myelodysplastic syndromes, acute myeloid leukemias, and chronic eosinophilic leukemia. Metabolites of histamine, such as *N*-methylhistamine, are found to be elevated in a 24-hour urine specimen but are neither more sensitive nor more specific than the baseline serum tryptase measurement in mastocytosis.

Demonstration of a codon 816 *KIT* mutation (D816V) may be necessary to fulfill the diagnostic criteria in patients lacking the major criterion (see Pathobiology). Examination of lesional tissues such as skin and bone marrow affords the highest sensitivity, in contrast to peripheral blood, which yields positive results only in patients with extensive disease variants. Codon 816 *KIT* mutations have been detected in a variety of other neoplastic diseases, such as core factor–binding acute myeloid leukemias, sinonasal lymphomas, and seminomas, in addition to mastocytosis.

World Health Organization Disease Categories

Each patient diagnosed with mastocytosis should be assigned a category of disease according to the WHO classification (see Table 276–1). *Cutaneous mastocytosis* in the absence of bone marrow and internal organ involvement is the most common category in patients with pediatric-onset disease.

Systemic mastocytosis is divided into the categories of indolent systemic mastocytosis, systemic mastocytosis with associated clonal hematologic non–mast cell lineage disease (SM-AHNMD), aggressive systemic mastocytosis, and MCL. An algorithm for classification of systemic mastocytosis is presented in Figure 276–4. *Indolent systemic mastocytosis* is the most common category in adults. Patients in this category usually do not have a decreased life expectancy due to the mast cell disease, although they experience symptoms related to release of mast cell mediators. Indolent systemic mastocytosis follows a persistent course, and progression to a more advanced category is unusual. *SM-AHNMD* is the second most common category in adults, and a non–mast cell hematologic disease is usually diagnosed at the time that the diagnosis of mastocytosis is made. Therefore, bone marrow biopsy and aspirate specimens should be carefully evaluated for the presence of other hematologic disease in every patient with newly diagnosed systemic mastocytosis. *Aggressive systemic mastocytosis* is a rare category characterized by the presence of organ dysfunction resulting from destructive mast cell infiltration. Aggressive systemic mastocytosis may involve the hematopoietic, gastrointestinal, and skeletal systems in the form of cytopenias, hypersplenism, malabsorption with weight loss, hepatomegaly with portal hypertension and ascites, and large osteolytic lesions with pathologic fractures. MCL is characterized by 10% or more mast cells in the peripheral circulation or 20% or more mast cells in bone marrow aspirate smears, or both. To diagnose MCL, the mast cell percentage in bone marrow aspirate smears should be assessed in an area of the slide that is sufficiently distant from the spicules. Typical diagnostic features of MCL include a diffuse bone marrow infiltration with atypical immature mast cells and significantly elevated serum tryptase levels. *Mast cell sarcoma* and *extracutaneous mastocytoma* are rare diagnoses characterized by malignant and benign solid mast cell collections respectively.

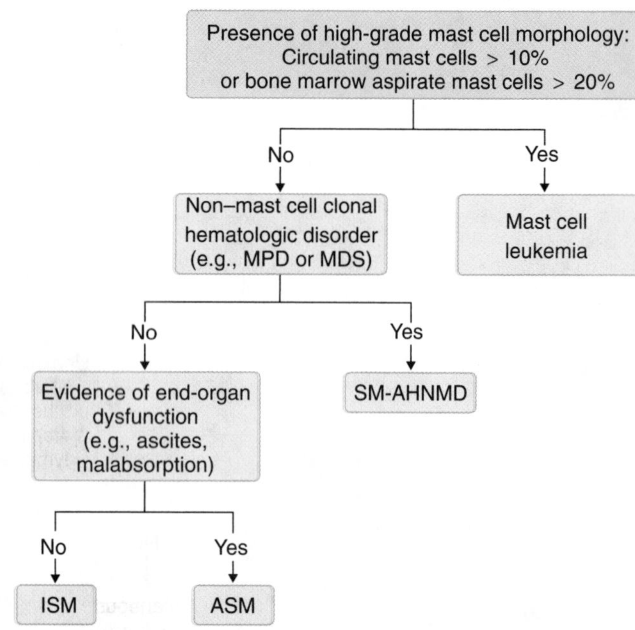

FIGURE 276–4 • An algorithm for classification of systemic mastocytosis. ASM, aggressive systemic mastocytosis; ISM, indolent systemic mastocytosis; MDS, myelodysplastic syndromes; MPD, myeloproliferative disorders; SM-AHNMD, systemic mastocytosis with associated clonal hematologic non–mast cell lineage disease.

Treatment

The major goal of treatment for all categories of mastocytosis is symptom control. A reduction in mast cell numbers is considered only in disease categories with a poor prognosis (i.e., SM-AHNMD, aggressive systemic mastocytosis, MCL, and mast cell sarcoma). Current treatment modalities have not been shown to change the natural course of the disease.

Medical Therapy

Pruritus in mastocytosis usually responds to scheduled doses of H_1 antihistamines such as fexofenadine and/or cetirizine. Sedating antihistamines such as hydroxyzine or diphenhydramine may be used before bedtime. Photochemotherapy (oral psoralen plus ultraviolet A) may be helpful in patients with refractory pruritus; it results in symptomatic improvement and temporary fading of the pigmented skin lesions in up to 50% of the patients. The side effects of phototherapy, including increased risk of skin cancer, should be taken into account when this treatment is considered.

H_2 antihistamines such as ranitidine or famotidine are usually prescribed as a first-line treatment for patients with gastrointestinal complaints such as heartburn, nausea, and abdominal pain. Proton pump inhibitors may be added in patients whose abdominal symptoms are refractory to H_2 antihistamines. Oral cromolyn sodium, at a dose of 200 mg four times daily, has been effective in reducing abdominal pain, diarrhea, nausea, vomiting, and pruritus in various studies, although the beneficial effects are variable among patients. Finally, low to moderate doses of systemic glucocorticoids can be beneficial in unusual cases of aggressive mastocytosis presenting with recalcitrant diarrhea associated with malabsorption or hepatomegaly with ascites.

Cysteinyl leukotrienes, such as LTC_4, that are produced after mast cell activation are thought to contribute to symptoms in mastocytosis. Therefore, drugs targeting the synthesis or receptor binding of leukotrienes are usually added to the treatment regimens of patients who derive suboptimal relief of itching and abdominal pain from histamine receptor–blocking therapy. However, there have been no controlled studies evaluating the clinical efficacy of this class of drugs in patients with mastocytosis.

Self-administered epinephrine should be prescribed to patients who have a history of hypotensive episodes resulting in presyncope

Rx

or syncope from acute mast cell degranulation. These episodes should be treated like systemic anaphylaxis (see Chapter 274).

Ancillary and Other Therapies

Avoidance of the triggers of mast cell degranulation is an important adjunct to the pharmacologic treatment of symptoms. These show remarkable individual variation among patients (see Pathobiology), and the individual medical history can be helpful in identifying such triggers. General anesthesia and surgery impose an additional risk to patients with mastocytosis, because several agents that are used perioperatively such as muscle relaxants, opioid analgesics, and NSAIDs, can induce acute mast cell degranulation. Prior surgical and anesthesia records should be obtained if available, and an appropriate strategy for the anesthetic management of the patient should be determined, with close communication involving the patient, anesthesiologist, surgeon, and an allergist.

Cytoreductive therapy, considered in aggressive disease variants associated with poor prognosis, has yielded disappointing results thus far. Approaches to cytoreductive treatment of mastocytosis have included interferon (IFN)-α2b and the nucleoside analog 2-chlorodeoxyadenosine (2-CDA). IFN-α2b (0.5 to 5 million units, three to five times per week), alone or with prednisone, has been reported to partially improve clinical and laboratory abnormalities in approximately 50% of patients with aggressive systemic mastocytosis, patients with osteoporosis and pathologic fractures, and patients with recalcitrant recurrent anaphylaxis, although complete histopathologic and molecular remissions appear to be rare. IFN-α is difficult to tolerate because of its many side effects, including flu-like symptoms, bone pain, and depression. A regimen of 2-CDA (0.10 to 0.14 mg/kg/day for 5 days, repeated at intervals of 4 to 8 weeks) has been reported to result in partial and transient responses in patients with advanced categories of disease in case reports and small series. MCL usually is treated with polychemotherapy as acute myeloid leukemia, although a successful treatment regimen has not yet been identified.

Non–mast cell clonal hematologic disorders associated with mastocytosis should be treated according to the standard-of-care guidelines for that disorder, regardless of the presence of mastocytosis. Bone marrow transplantation has yielded generally disappointing results for the treatment of mast cell disease, although occasional cases resulting in complete remission have been reported.

Rx

Recent availability of tyrosine kinase inhibitors has generated interest in use of these agents as investigational therapies targeting the mutated Kit protein with constitutively increased activity in mastocytosis. The currently available tyrosine kinase inhibitor imatinib does not inhibit D816V *KIT* and therefore is not predicted to be effective in patients with mastocytosis, with the exception of rare cases without this mutation. Newer kinase inhibitors with potential to inhibit the mutated *KIT* gene product are currently in clinical development.

Prognosis

The prognosis for mastocytosis varies by the category of disease. At least 50% of patients with pediatric-onset cutaneous mastocytosis have complete resolution of the disease by adolescence, and the rest of those patients experience improvement or fading of the skin lesions. Indolent systemic mastocytosis is a persistent disease but has a good prognosis without a decrease in life expectancy, and progression to a more aggressive disease category is rare. Factors associated with poorer prognosis have been reported as the absence of urticaria pigmentosa, older age at onset of symptoms, elevated serum lactate dehydrogenase or alkaline phosphatase, thrombocytopenia, anemia, peripheral blood smear abnormalities, and detectability of the D816V *KIT* mutation in peripheral blood. The prognosis for SM-AHNMD is determined by the prognosis for the associated hematologic disorder. Aggressive systemic mastocytosis and MCL have poor prognoses, with median survival times of approximately less than 3 years and less than 1 year, respectively.

SUGGESTED READINGS

Akin C, Metcalfe DD: Systemic mastocytosis. Annu Rev Med 2004;55:419. *A concise review.*

Akin C, Metcalfe DD: The biology of Kit in disease and the application of pharmacogenetics. J Allergy Clin Immunol 2004;114:13. *A review on potential use of tyrosine kinase inhibitors based on mutations in KIT.*

Barbie DA, Deangelo DJ: Systemic mastocytosis: Current classification and novel therapeutic options. Clin Adv Hematol Oncol 2006;4:768–775. *A review of classification and molecular targeted therapies.*

Valent P, Akin C, Sperr W, et al: Mastocytosis: Pathology, genetics, and current options for therapy. Leuk Lymphoma 2005;46:35. *Detailed review incorporating the latest findings in pathology of mastocytosis and treatment options.*

Section XXII

Rheumatic Disease

Cecil Medicine 23

277 APPROACH TO THE PATIENT WITH RHEUMATIC DISEASE

William P. Arend and George V. Lawry

Diseases of the musculoskeletal system are common and may be both disabling and costly. This chapter provides an approach to the evaluation of patients with rheumatic diseases by outlining the components necessary for identifying the patient's problems, formulating a diagnosis, and initiating treatment.

Musculoskeletal disorders may manifest as acute, subacute, or chronic problems. Pain and interference with daily activities are what bring the patient to a physician and determine the impact of the condition. A general medical approach to the patient with rheumatic complaints is paramount, with particular reliance on an accurate history and a thoughtful physical examination. Usually, only limited additional testing is required to diagnosis most musculoskeletal disorders, but in some instances assessment with a number of laboratory analyses, imaging studies, and other disciplines may be necessary.

Pathobiology

Categories of Musculoskeletal Diseases

Musculoskeletal diseases can be practically classified into nine categories, defined by the predominately affected tissues (Table 277–1). At each point in the evaluation (history, physical examination, and laboratory testing), it is important to ask what tissues are involved. Recognition of the pattern of predominant tissue involvement can direct attention toward the disease primarily associated with that tissue. Before consideration of clinical approaches to the evaluation of patients with musculoskeletal problems, it is useful to first review the anatomy and pathophysiology of the affected structures.

Anatomy

The structures that may be involved in musculoskeletal diseases are shown in Figure 277–1A. Foremost is the joint cavity. The lining membrane, known as the *synovium*, consists of a thin layer of macrophages (type A cells) and fibroblasts (type B cells) with a sublining of rich, vascular, loose connective tissue. Hyaline cartilage overlies the bony end plates and provides a cushion to joint motion. The cartilage has high water content and obtains its nutrition solely from the synovial fluid, which is derived from the synovium primarily as an ultrafiltrate of plasma. The synovium also secretes specialized molecules into the synovial fluid, such as hyaluronic acid. An intact bony end plate is required to support the cartilage. The joint capsule and ligaments provide further support and blend with the periosteum. Periarticular anatomy is equally important and includes the tendons, bursae, and muscles associated with each joint.

Pathophysiology

The etiology of musculoskeletal problems is usually inflammatory, metabolic, degenerative, tumor, or some combination thereof. The disorders associated with musculoskeletal tissues are summarized in Table 277–1 and Figure 277–1B. Synovial inflammatory disorders, such as rheumatoid arthritis (RA), begin in the synovium and secondarily damage the cartilage, joint capsule, and bone. Inflammation at entheses, the insertion sites of tendons or ligaments on bone, is characteristic of the spondyloarthropathies, such as ankylosing spondylitis. Crystal deposition disorders, such as gout or pseudogout, may also cause articular inflammation. Infections primarily involve the joint cavity (septic arthritis) or bone (osteomyelitis). The noninflammatory, degenerative disease osteoarthritis (OA) begins in the cartilage and leads to cartilage loss, subchondral new bone formation, and marginal bony overgrowth. Cartilage loss may also occur secondarily to synovial inflammation or trauma. Osteonecrosis of bone may be associated with secondary cartilage damage after collapse of the bony end plate. Inflammatory diseases of the muscle usually manifest with painless proximal weakness. Periarticular inflammation may involve tendons or bursae, and these structures are common causes of pain and stiffness, often misinterpreted as arising from the joint itself. Lastly, the common clinical problem of fibromyalgia is characterized by soft tissue and joint pain with local tenderness in specific points but without objective evidence of inflammation or swelling.

Diagnosis

History

Demography

An appreciation of the age, gender, and personal history of the patient is helpful, including marital status, occupation, and psychosocial factors.

Age

The age of the patient is the first step in considering a differential diagnosis. For example, arthritis is a major manifestation of hemophilia with onset during childhood. The term *juvenile RA* refers to three different forms of arthritis with onset before the age of 16 years. In young adults, inflammatory and septic arthritic conditions may be seen, but OA is exceptional. The onset of RA is often in the middle years, whereas the elderly are more prone to OA. Arthritis in the elderly is often assumed to be degenerative, when in fact the patient may have an inflammatory process such as polymyalgia rheumatica, RA, or systemic lupus erythematosus (SLE).

Gender

RA and other autoimmune diseases are more common in women, whereas ankylosing spondylitis and the other spondyloarthropathies associated with the human leukocyte antigen HLA-B27 are more common in men. Gouty arthritis is more common in men and rarely attacks women before menopause.

Occupation and Recreation

Occupation and recreational activities are also important because of associated physical and psychological stresses. The clinician should inquire about the patient's job to determine how demanding it is. Occupational factors such as repetitive joint trauma may contribute to the development of OA in susceptible individuals. Musculoskeletal symptoms may also be associated with jogging or with trauma from sports activities.

Family History

It is important to obtain a complete family history, because autoimmune diseases and gout occur with an increased incidence in families.

Onset and Evolution of Symptoms

Knowledge of the pattern of onset, location, and evolution of musculoskeletal symptoms is essential for accurate diagnosis. The development of symptoms over hours to days is characteristic of *acute arthritis* and usually represents an inflammatory or traumatic process. The persistence of symptoms for more than 6 weeks is considered *chronic arthritis,* whereas an intermediate duration of days to weeks is referred to as *subacute arthritis.* Musculoskeletal pain can be further characterized using the mnemonic "OPQRST" where O = onset, P = precipitating (and ameliorating) factors, Q = quality, R = radiation, S = severity, and T = timing. The most common symptom of musculoskeletal disease is pain; a diagnostic approach to the evaluation of patients presenting with musculoskeletal pain is presented in Figure 277–2.

Pattern of Joint Involvement

The distribution of joint involvement is one of the most essential aspects of diagnosis of musculoskeletal diseases. Monoarthritis describes symptoms in a single joint; oligoarthritis (or pauciarthritis), symptoms in two to four joints; and polyarthritis, involvement of five or more joints. Arthritis in an extremity is called *peripheral joint disease,* whereas spinal involvement is termed *axial disease.* It is important to elicit a history of symmetrical versus asymmetrical peripheral joint disease. The predominant involvement of the small joints of the hands and feet or of large joints such as the shoulder, hip, and knee also has diagnostic importance.

A critical feature in clinical diagnosis is the distinction between arthralgia (subjective joint pain) and arthritis (objective joint swelling, deformity, or impaired function). Objective findings on physical examination must be found for a diagnosis of "arthritis" to be made.

Inflammatory versus Noninflammatory Conditions

An important initial step in the evaluation of musculoskeletal symptoms is the differentiation of inflammatory versus noninflammatory disease. A history of warmth and erythema over a joint suggests inflammatory disease. Morning stiffness lasting longer than 60 minutes, a "gel"

TABLE 277–1 CLASSIFICATION OF MUSCULOSKELETAL DISEASES

Category	Prototypes	Useful Tests	Treatments
Synovitis	Rheumatoid arthritis Autoimmune diseases	Rheumatoid factor, ESR Antinuclear antibody test	DMARDs and biologic agents Prednisone and immunosuppressive drugs
Enthesopathy	Ankylosing spondylitis and spondyloarthropathies	Sacroiliac radiographs	NSAIDs, MTX, and biologic agents
Crystal-induced synovitis	Gout CPPD (pseudogout)	Joint fluid crystal examination Radiographic chondrocalcinosis	NSAIDs NSAIDs
Joint space disease	Septic arthritis	Joint fluid culture	Antibiotics
Cartilage degeneration	Osteoarthritis	Radiographs of affected area	NSAIDs, analgesics, and physical therapy
Osteoarticular disease	Osteonecrosis	Radiographs, magnetic resonance imaging	Core decompression or prosthetic joint replacement
Inflammatory myopathy	Polymyositis Dermatomyositis Inclusion body myositis	Muscle enzymes, electromyography, muscle biopsy	Corticosteroids and immunosuppressive drugs
Local and regional conditions	Tendonitis or bursitis	Aspirate bursa if infection is suspected	Local injections
General conditions	Polymyalgia rheumatica Fibromyalgia	Elevated ESR Normal ESR	Corticosteroids Aerobic exercise, stretches, and sleep medications

Biologic agents = anti-tumor necrosis factor (anti-TNF) drugs and others; CPPD = calcium pyrophosphate dehydrate disease; DMARDs = disease-modifying anti-rheumatic drugs; ESR = erythrocyte sedimentation rate; MTX = methotrexate; NSAIDs = nonsteroidal anti-inflammatory drugs.

phenomenon (stiffness after rest that is more than transient), and improvement in pain and stiffness with activity all suggest the presence of inflammatory disease. In contrast, minimal morning stiffness and worsening pain with activity suggest noninflammatory joint disease.

Extra-articular and Systemic Features

A careful history may reveal important systemic and extra-articular manifestations, including fever, fatigue, weakness, dry eyes, ocular inflammation, pulmonary symptoms, or Raynaud's phenomenon. The finding of musculoskeletal complaints in the setting of systemic symptoms and multiorgan involvement strongly suggests the possibility of a diffuse connective tissue disease such as SLE.

Functional Disability Indices

A number of self-report questionnaires such as the Stanford Health Assessment Questionnaire, Functional Disability Index, and Arthritis Impact Measurement Scales, or modifications of these, have been developed for ongoing evaluation of patients with arthritis. These instruments document patient-reported functional status with results comparable to those of traditional physician-reported measures of joint disease activity, such as tender joint count, or to a radiographic joint erosion score and erythrocyte sedimentation rate.

Physical Examination

Essential Concepts

The physical examination includes a record of the patient's gait and posture as well as examination of the spine and skeletal muscles. The joints shown in Figure 277–3 should be examined systematically, region by region, with a side-to side comparison to determine whether any are inflamed or damaged. The pattern of joint involvement, whether symmetrical, axial, or peripheral, should be recorded using the diagram. The abnormalities detected in each joint should be recorded as deformity, tenderness, erythema, swelling, and altered range of motion (ROM) to allow comparison between the same or different examiners over time.

A screening musculoskeletal examination (a rapid assessment of structure and function) and a general musculoskeletal examination (a more comprehensive assessment of joint swelling and arthritis) are demonstrated in the online material accompanying this text. The following sections are drawn from this video material.

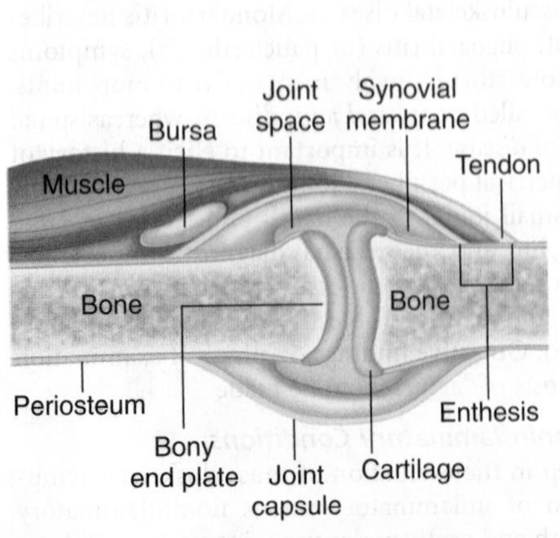

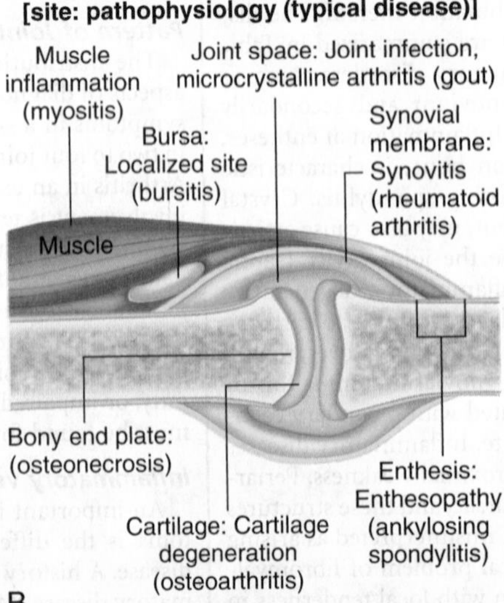

FIGURE 277–1 • Structures involved in musculoskeletal diseases. A, Anatomic structures of the musculoskeletal system. **B,** Location of rheumatic disease processes.

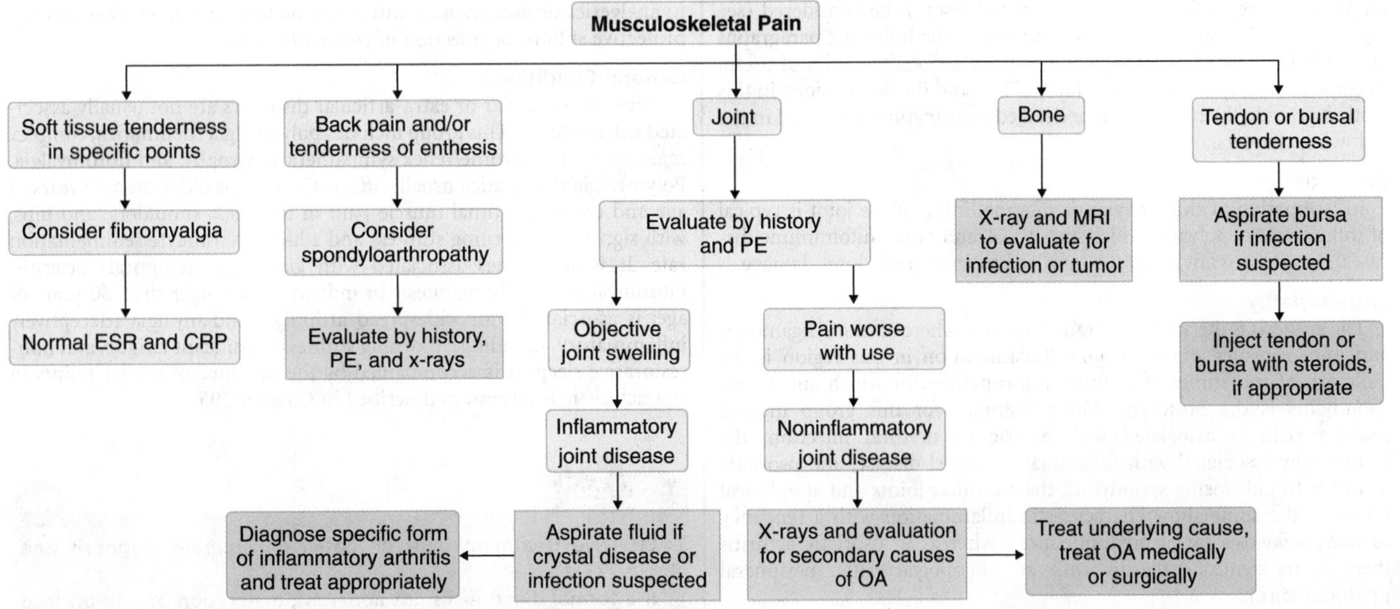

FIGURE 277–2 • Diagnostic approach to musculoskeletal pain. CRP = C-reactive protein; ESR = erythrocyte sedimentation rate; MRI = magnetic resonance imaging; OA = osteoarthritis; PE = physical examination.

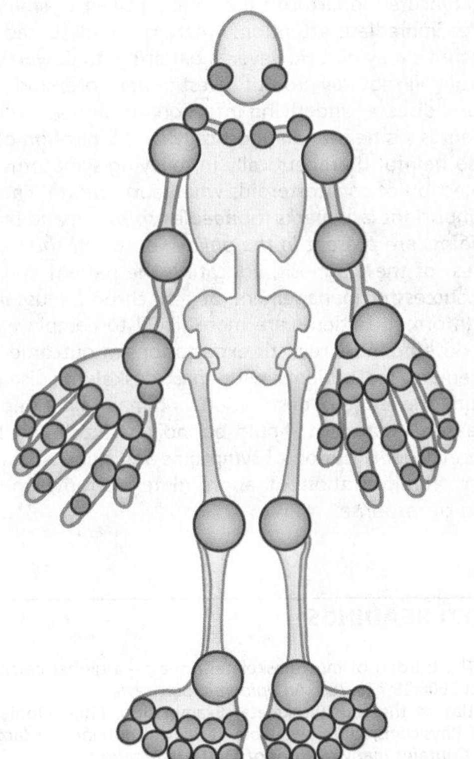

FIGURE 277–3 • A pictorial method for recording joint disease activity or destruction. The sketch can be used on a printed form or rubber stamp to chart which joints are active or deformed at the time of each assessment. (Courtesy of Dr. Hugh A. Smythe, Toronto.)

Examination Components

There are four essential steps in musculoskeletal physical examination.

Inspection

Inspect for asymmetry, deformity, erythema, and swelling.

Palpation

Palpate for tenderness, warmth, synovial thickening and effusion, bony hypertrophy, and crepitus.

Range of Motion

Take the joint through passive or active ROM (or a combination of both).

Special Testing

Perform an assessment of supporting structures (such as ligaments and tendons) or for conditions particular to a single region (such as Tinel's sign at the wrist for detection of carpal tunnel syndrome).

Objective Joint Findings

A careful examination is critical in distinguishing articular from periarticular conditions.

Joint tenderness alone is insufficient for diagnosis and must be correlated with the finding of an objective, visible, or palpable abnormality for a diagnosis of arthritis to be made. Joint redness (erythema) depends on the acuteness and severity of the underlying inflammation, and its presence may suggest the possibility of infection or crystalline arthritis. Joint warmth also depends on the acuteness of the underlying inflammation. Joint swelling is a definitive sign of arthritis and may be caused by either a joint effusion (excess synovial fluid) or an inflamed and swollen synovial membrane (synovitis). Bony hypertrophy around a joint (osteophytic swelling) is characteristic of osteoarthritis. Crepitus refers to a continuous grating sensation that is felt by the examiner's hand during joint motion. Fine or velvety crepitus may denote chronic proliferative synovitis, whereas coarse crepitus may indicate either roughening of the cartilage surface or complete loss of hyaline cartilage. Joint damage and deformity are usually signs of prior arthritis or injury (ligamentous laxity, joint subluxation, tendon rupture, or contracture).

Range of Motion

Both active and passive ROM are important in assessing joint function. Active ROM is patient-initiated movement of the joint; it tests integrated function and requires intact innervation and muscle and tendon function, as well as joint mobility. Passive ROM is examiner-initiated movement of a joint; it tests only joint mobility. The combined use of passive and active ROM minimizes the need for patient instruction and maximizes the speed and efficiency of the examination. Whenever joint motion is anticipated to be painful, it is best to first observe active ROM, to appreciate the degree of pain and dysfunction, before gently attempting passive ROM.

Extra-articular Findings

Because many rheumatic diseases are multisystem disorders, physical examination may document the presence of important extra-articular features. In RA, for example, these include subcutaneous nodules, digital vasculitis, and other systemic features as described in Chapter 285.

Classification

Clinical evaluation enables the establishment of which anatomic structures are inflamed, which are damaged, and how function is impaired. Nine types of rheumatic involvement can be identified as a framework for various diagnostic possibilities or hypotheses to be considered (see Fig. 277–1B). The nine categories presented in the following paragraphs are listed in Table 277–1 along with typical diseases, examples of useful diagnostic tests, and treatments. Table 277–1 and the descriptions in this section provide the basis for more detailed information contained in the following chapters.

Synovitis

Inflammation of the synovial membrane lining of the joint is typical of inflammatory polyarthritides such as RA and other autoimmune diseases. Persistent synovitis in RA may lead to irreversible joint damage.

Enthesopathy

The enthesis is the anatomic transition zone where tendons, ligaments, and joint capsules attach to bone. Inflammation in this region is the hallmark of the family of spondyloarthropathies, of which ankylosing spondylitis is the prototype. Other members of this group include reactive arthritis associated with enteric or urethral infection, the arthropathy associated with inflammatory bowel disease, and psoriatic arthritis. In ankylosing spondylitis, the sacroiliac joints and apophyseal joints of the spine show characteristic inflammation with a tendency to bony ankylosis (axial predominance), whereas in psoriatic arthritis there is frequently enthesitis with an oligopolyarthritis (peripheral predominance).

Crystal-Induced Synovitis

Crystals of monosodium urate (gout), calcium pyrophosphate (pseudogout), or hydroxyapatite are capable of inducing an acute inflammatory reaction in both synovial fluid and synovium. Acute crystalline arthritis usually affects only one or at most a few joints at a time. Joint aspiration and synovial fluid analysis for crystals using polarized light microscopy establish the diagnosis. Calcium pyrophosphate deposition disease (CPPD) is often associated with the radiologic appearance of chondrocalcinosis of hyaline cartilage.

Joint Space Disease

Septic arthritis may develop from hematogenous spread of microorganisms into the joint space, through local extension from adjacent soft tissues or by joint penetration. Joint infections are usually associated with intense pain even at rest, and the diagnosis is confirmed by joint aspiration with Gram stain and culture of the synovial fluid. A joint prosthesis increases susceptibility to infection in that joint. Blood in the joint space, known as *hemarthrosis*, may result from microfractures, coagulopathy, or tumor.

Cartilage Degeneration

OA is defined as loss of articular cartilage with a bony response leading to the formation of osteophytes. Primary OA is thought to be caused by biochemical abnormalities in the cartilage that predispose to microfissures in the surface and subsequent degeneration of the cartilage. Secondary OA may develop as a consequence of inflammatory conditions such as RA, ankylosing spondylitis, septic arthritis, and CPPD. Previous trauma and joint hypermobility are other mechanical factors that may predispose to OA.

Osteoarticular Disease

Osteopenia/osteoporosis may complicate many rheumatic conditions and are dealt with in Chapter 264. Osteonecrosis, which results from collapse of the bony end plate due to vascular insufficiency, causes secondary crushing and fragmentation of the overlying articular cartilage. Osteonecrosis may be idiopathic or associated with systemic conditions such as sickle cell disease or liver disease; it may occur after treatment with high-dose corticosteroids. Inflammation of the periosteum, known as *periostitis*, may be associated with hypertrophic pulmonary osteoarthropathy and clubbing. This syndrome may be a clue to underlying lung cancer.

Inflammatory Myopathy

Inflammation and (usually painless) weakness of the proximal skeletal muscles are characteristic of inflammatory myopathies: polymyositis, dermatomyositis, and inclusion body myositis. Elevated creatine kinase levels, electromyographic abnormalities, and characteristic histologic abnormalities on muscle biopsy are present in inflammatory myopathies.

Local and Regional Conditions

Nonarticular disorders such as tendonitis, bursitis, and neck and low-back strains are very common regional problems. They usually respond to analgesics or nonsteroidal anti-inflammatory drugs, physical therapy, protective splints, or injection of corticosteroids.

General Conditions

These nonarticular or extra-articular disorders are not usually associated with arthritis. This group includes polymyalgia rheumatica, complex regional pain syndrome/reflex sympathetic dystrophy, and fibromyalgia. Polymyalgia rheumatica usually affects Caucasians older than 50 years of age and causes proximal muscle pain in the neck, shoulders, and hips, with significant morning stiffness and a high erythrocyte sedimentation rate. It is sometimes associated with giant cell (temporal) arteritis. Fibromyalgia usually manifests in individuals younger than 50 years of age; is associated with widespread arthralgia and myalgia (deceptively inflammatory-sounding), morning stiffness, significant fatigue, and nonrestorative sleep. It is accompanied by the presence of tender points in characteristic locations, as described in Chapter 295.

Treatment

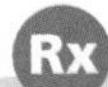

Effective treatment must be based on accurate diagnosis (see Table 277–1).

If a formal diagnosis is not apparent, generation of a prioritized problem list can be very helpful in suggesting a differential diagnosis and creating an initial management strategy. The acuteness and severity of presentation dictate whether immediate intervention is required or further observation is more appropriate. For example, an acute monarthritis (possible septic or crystalline arthritis) requires immediate attention, whereas a widespread smoldering polyarthritis may not. However, a patient with polyarthritis who is systemically ill requires prompt investigation to exclude a diffuse autoimmune disease, underlying infection, or hidden malignancy.

Arthrocentesis is helpful diagnostically, and aspiration of synovial fluid is also helpful therapeutically in relieving symptoms and permitting injection of corticosteroids when appropriate. *Photographs showing important landmarks for needle aspiration and injection of common joints are present in the online version of this text.*

Regardless of the diagnosis, educating the patient and family is crucial to successful management of any chronic musculoskeletal problem. Informed patients are more likely to comply with treatment and develop more realistic expectations of outcome. The goal of management for patients with musculoskeletal diseases is to control pain, prevent joint destruction, and maintain independence. For this reason, treatment should be individualized and based on early, accurate identification of symptoms and signs, a firm diagnosis, prompt administration of appropriate therapy, and vigilant monitoring of response.

SUGGESTED READINGS

Brooks PM: The burden of musculoskeletal disease—a global perspective. Clin Rheumatol 2006;25:778–781. *An epidemiologic review.*

Moore G: Atlas of the Musculoskeletal Examination. Philadelphia, American College of Physicians, 2003. Available at www.acponline.org (accessed June 26, 2006). *Contains many pictures of joint examination.*

Thomsen TW, Shen S, Shaffer RW, et al: Videos in clinical medicine. Arthrocentesis of the knee. N Engl J Med 2006;354:e19. *An excellent instructional video.*

278 LABORATORY TESTING IN THE RHEUMATIC DISEASES

David S. Pisetsky

The rheumatic diseases are a heterogeneous group of conditions that result from diverse pathophysiologic mechanisms and involve the musculoskeletal system as well as other organs. These conditions range from mild, diffuse joint and muscle pain to severe life-threatening kidney failure and stroke. Although the rheumatic diseases have many origins, immune disturbances resulting in local and systemic inflammation are frequently the underlying cause. The approach to diagnosis therefore entails a wide variety of laboratory tests to assess functional disturbances of individual organs and their relationship to inflammation and autoimmunity.

Laboratory testing in patients with rheumatic disease has two main purposes. The first is diagnostic, and the second is prognostic. Some tests are useful in both contexts, but others have different performance characteristics related to their specificity and pattern of expression during disease. Prognostic tests provide critical information to help distinguish activity that is reversible from damage that is fixed and irreversible. In general, the assessment of damage relies on specific tests of end-organ function or structure rather than process markers. Distinguishing activity from damage is very important in the management of rheumatic diseases, especially with respect to the use of therapies associated with toxicity.

MARKERS OF INFLAMMATION

For many patients, the initial goal of evaluation is to determine the presence of inflammation. Inflammation is the body's response to injury and is characterized by a cascade of cellular and molecular events that arise irrespective of stimulus or locale. The immediate response to inflammatory stimuli is termed the *acute phase response* and comprises a set of proteins produced primarily in the liver in response to cytokines such as interleukin-6 (IL-6), tumor necrosis factor-α (TNF-α), and IL-1. These cytokines are produced by macrophages and dendritic cells after stimulation of pattern recognition receptors called toll-like receptors (TLRs); TLRs recognize bacterial and viral products as well as molecules from damaged cells and trigger innate immunity. Many proteins in the acute phase response show dramatic increases in concentration, although some show a reduction. Because the levels of these proteins can increase hundreds to thousands of times in magnitude, they provide a sensitive and powerful set of markers for inflammation, whether induced by infection, trauma, or autoimmunity.

Of the proteins stimulated during the acute phase response, C-reactive protein (CRP) has received the most attention as a marker of inflammation in both rheumatic and nonrheumatic disease. CRP is a member of the pentraxin family; although its function is not fully known, its ability to bind to phosphocholine suggests a scavenger function to eliminate bacterial products or damaged cells and attenuate the consequences of infection or tissue injury. Other molecules, such as serum amyloid protein (SAP), fibrinogen, and complement, also show marked elevations during the acute phase response, signifying a broad-based effort at host defense.

The CRP level provides a very useful measure of inflammation and can convey information for categorization of a clinical process (e.g., inflammatory versus noninflammatory arthritis) as well as assessment of disease activity or prognosis (e.g., activity of rheumatoid arthritis [RA] or likelihood of erosion). The advantage of measuring CRP in the blood, rather than cytokines, is that the protein levels are much higher. Furthermore, CRP levels remain elevated for a longer period (days) than cytokines do; the latter may appear only transiently in the blood and thereby evade detection.

Another simple laboratory text reflecting the acute phase response is the erythrocyte sedimentation rate (ESR). In this test, commonly called the sed rate, anticoagulated blood is drawn into a long, thin tube and allowed to settle under the influence of gravity for 1 hour. The distance the blood falls depends on a number of factors, including the concentration of serum proteins such as immunoglobulins and fibrinogen, an acute phase reactant. The sedimentation rate is nonspecific with respect to disease association and also depends on age and gender. The upper limits of normal vary between women and men.

Other simple laboratory tests point to an acute phase response. For example, patients with inflammation frequently have a leukocytosis or thrombocytosis, most likely reflecting the action of cytokines and other mediators, including glucocorticoids, during this process. With chronic inflammation, anemia of chronic disease can also occur, with the hematocrit in conjunction with the white blood cell and platelet counts pointing to the presence of an inflammatory process. In systemic lupus erythematosus (SLE), lymphopenia, thrombocytopenia, and low CRP values often characterize active disease, with the discordance between laboratory and clinical findings a clue to diagnosis.

LABORATORY EVALUATION OF MUSCULOSKELETAL DISEASE

The most common presentation of musculoskeletal disease is pain in and around a joint in association with functional impairment. Collectively, diseases causing joint symptoms are called arthritis, implying inflammation. The extent of inflammation in these diseases varies markedly, however, with some forms such as osteoarthritis showing scant evidence of inflammation either locally or systemically.

Arthritis results from many different diseases and occurs in various patterns defined by the number and size of joints affected, symmetry, and involvement of the axial as well as peripheral joints. For each pattern (e.g., chronic polyarthritis), a key issue in diagnosis concerns its place in the spectrum of inflammatory versus noninflammatory arthritis. Furthermore, although many diseases can cause arthritis, their prevalence varies enormously, with osteoarthritis or degenerative joint disease being the most common form of noninflammatory arthritis and RA the most common form of inflammatory arthritis.

The differential diagnosis of arthritis is based on a comprehensive history and physical examination to assess symptoms suggesting inflammation (e.g., morning stiffness and fatigue), the presence of synovitis, and results of laboratory tests indicative of an inflammatory process. Of these tests, the ESR and CRP are nonspecific indicators of inflammation. Two autoantibody tests, rheumatoid factor (RF) and antibodies to citrullinated proteins, provide more specific diagnostic information. Given the demographics of inflammatory arthritis, testing for antinuclear antibodies is often part of this evaluation as well.

Rheumatoid Factor

RF comprises a family of specificities that bind to the immunoglobulin G (IgG) molecule. These RFs target primarily the constant region or Fc portion of IgG, reacting with antigenic determinants that are most likely conformational in origin. IgM RFs are the most abundant of these antibodies and have been easiest to measure, using agglutination assays with red blood cells or latex beads coated with IgG. More recently, enzyme-linked immunosorbent assays (ELISA) and nephelometry have been used to detect RFs.

RFs occur in approximately 80% of patients with RA and represent a criterion for the classification or diagnosis of this disease. Furthermore, high levels of RFs are often associated with a worse prognosis, the occurrence of erosion as measured by radiographs, and deformity. Despite these associations, RFs occur in sera of patients with a wide range of autoimmune and inflammatory diseases as well as in normal individuals, especially with age. The frequent occurrence of RFs may reflect their etiology and role in innate immune responses to promote the binding of IgG antigen by Fc cross-linking.

Antibodies to Citrullinated Proteins

Antibodies to citrullinated proteins are another set of autoantibody specificities that are important in the diagnosis of RA. Citrulline is a post-translational modification of the amino acid arginine that results from deimidation. This chemical reaction is catalyzed by the enzyme peptidylarginine deiminase (PAD) and may occur in the setting of inflammation; the function of this modification is unknown. Citrullination can affect many different proteins, creating antigenic sites on proteins that include keratin, fibrinogen, and filaggrin. This antibody system can be detected by Western blotting, ELISA, or cellular immunofluorescence.

Although antibodies are directed to citrullinated residues on intact proteins, they can be conveniently measured using synthetic peptides containing citrulline. Among these synthetic antigens, a citrulline-containing protein with a cyclic structure provides sensitive and specific assays in an ELISA format. Antibodies directed to this type of antigen are known as anti-CCP (cyclic citrullinated peptide) and can be formally distinguished from antibodies to the citrullinated proteins themselves (ACPA, or anti-citrullinated protein antibodies). The term anti-CCP is commonly used for these specificities, although it is formally synonymous with ACPA.

Anti-CCP antibodies are highly associated with RA. They occur in 60 to 70% of patients with RA and uncommonly in those with other forms of inflammatory arthritis, making their presence important in diagnosis. Significantly, anti-CCP antibodies can occur before the onset of other signs and symptoms of RA, suggesting utility for screening of at-risk patients and for diagnosis in the earliest stage of disease to allow initiation of therapy.

Joint Fluid Analysis

Analysis of joint fluid can provide decisive data in the evaluation of arthritis and, in some instances, a definitive diagnosis. This analysis is essential in the setting of acute monoarthritis to investigate the possibility of infection; for chronic forms of arthritis, joint fluid should be analyzed if there is uncertainty about the diagnosis and involvement of one joint out of proportion to others. Joint aspiration is a sterile procedure performed with a local anesthetic. Although fluid can be analyzed by tests to assess viscosity and mucin content, the cell count, examination of crystals, and stains and cultures to evaluate infection are the most informative.

On the basis of cell counts, joint fluids can be categorized into four main types: noninflammatory, inflammatory, septic, and hemorrhagic. A noninflammatory fluid has fewer than 2000 cells/mm^3 with mononuclear cell predominance. An inflammatory fluid has more than 2000 cells/mm^3, with 50,000 cells/mm^3 frequently used as the upper limit for this type of fluid. In an inflammatory fluid, polymorphonuclear cells predominate. A septic fluid is an inflammatory fluid in which culture or staining for microorganisms demonstrates infection. Suspicion of infection is especially high for fluids with cell counts greater than 50,000/mm^3. However, crystal-induced arthritis can produce cell counts of this magnitude, and an infected fluid can have counts below this level. Hemorrhagic fluids have red cell predominance that can approximate that of blood.

In the setting of an acute monoarthritis, crystal-induced disease is much more common than infection, with the presence of crystals demonstrated by polarization microscopy. With this technique, monosodium urate crystals in gout appear needle-shaped and are negatively birefringent. In contrast, calcium pyrophosphate dihydrate crystals in pseudogout are rhomboidal in shape and are weakly positively birefringent. Infection can coexist with crystal-induced disease, necessitating microbiologic evaluation even when crystals are found. Hemorrhagic fluids can also result from infection, although their presence suggests malignancy or trauma. Figure 278–1 provides an algorithm for the analysis of joint fluid.

Depending on the clinical findings and the results of initial laboratory testing, other studies may be performed to investigate less common diagnostic possibilities such as metabolic disease or malignancy. The laboratory evaluation of inflammatory arthritis may also include serologic tests for infections such as Lyme disease, human immunodeficiency virus (HIV) infection, or hepatitis.

LABORATORY EVALUATION OF SYSTEMIC INFLAMMATORY DISEASE

Among rheumatic diseases, some are characterized by severe systemic inflammation that can cause organ-threatening and life-threatening manifestations. These diseases can have arthritis as a component and presenting complaint, although the prominence of extra-articular manifestations, especially as they develop over time and involve organs such as the kidney, points to their systemic nature. These diseases can be categorized on the basis of clinical, serologic, and pathologic findings, with the presence of vasculitis, irrespective of blood vessel size, providing a unifying feature in disease classification.

The terms connective tissue disease (CTD) and collagen vascular disease are both used to denote a group of diseases that includes RA, SLE, Sjögren's syndrome, polymyositis, dermatomyositis, and progressive systemic sclerosis. Diseases in this group can share common or overlapping clinical features, especially early in their course, when their presentations may be similar. In this stage of disease, the condition may be called undifferentiated CTD, with serologic markers sometimes predictive of the eventual diagnosis.

Antinuclear Antibodies

The expression of antibodies to components of the cell nucleus (antinuclear antibodies, or ANAs) is characteristic of CTD and is essentially invariable in patients with SLE. These antibodies target a host of nuclear macromolecules, including DNA, RNA, and proteins as well as complexes of proteins with nucleic acid. These antigens are ubiquitously expressed in cells and subserve critical processes related to chromosomal structure, cell division, transcription, and translation. The basis for the antigenicity of these molecules is unknown, although DNA and RNA both have intrinsic immunologic activities and can stimulate cytokine production and inflammation when outside the cell.

ANAs are measured primarily by immunofluorescence assays in which sera are incubated with tissue culture cells (e.g., Hep2 cells) fixed to a glass slide. Antibody binding is revealed by fluorescence microscopy after incubation of the slide with a fluoresceinated anti-immunoglobulin reagent. Results are reported in terms of the pattern of fluorescence as well as the end-point titer of sera at which fluorescence can be observed. The patterns of binding differ depending on the location of the particular macromolecular target, although a few patterns predominate. These patterns include homogeneous, rim, nucleolar, and speckled; in addition, ANA tests can detect antibodies to cytoplasmic antigens. Despite some disease associations, these patterns do not have diagnostic significance. Table 278–1 presents a list of major ANAs with their pattern and disease associations.

A major limitation in the assays of ANA concerns the frequency of positive reactivity in the sera of otherwise normal individuals who lack evidence of a CTD. The sera of as many as 5% of normal individuals express reactivity in the ANA test. The basis of this reactivity is not fully understood, although it may reflect a predisposition to autoimmunity that is manifest in ANA production in the absence of other immunopathologic disturbances for the complete development of a CTD. Because ANA testing is often performed to evaluate nonspecific complaints such as arthralgias, fatigue, and fever, a positive test must be interpreted with

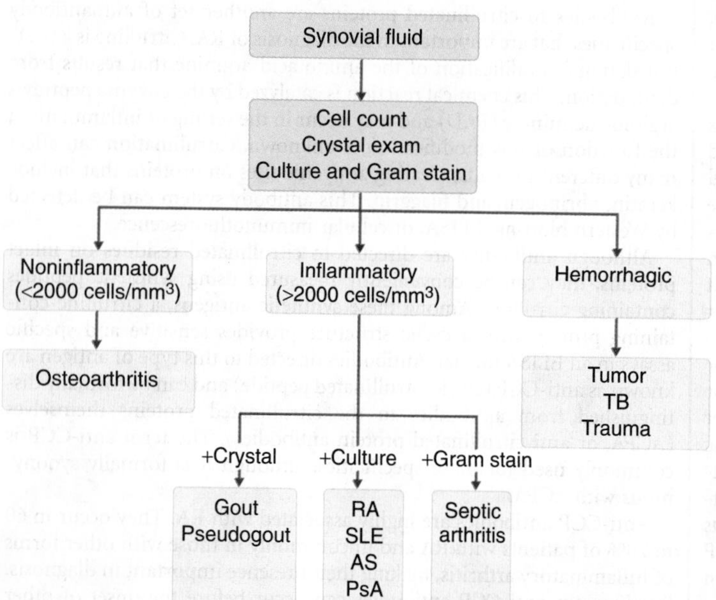

FIGURE 278–1 • Algorithm for analysis of joint fluid. Examples of inflammatory arthritis are indicated, although many conditions can produce these findings. AS = ankylosing spondylitis; PsA = psoriatic arthritis; RA = rheumatoid arthritis; SLE = systemic lupus erythematosus; TB = tuberculosis.

TABLE 278–1 SELECTED ANTINUCLEAR ANTIBODIES AND RHEUMATIC DISEASES

Pattern	Antibody	Antigen	Disease Association
Homogeneous	Anti-histone	Histones H1, H2A, H2B, H3, H4	Drug-induced lupus (>95%)
Rim	Anti-double-stranded DNA	Double-stranded DNA snRNP proteins	SLE (50%)
Speckled	Anti-Sm	snRNP proteins	SLE (30%)
	Anti-U1-RNP	U1 snRNP proteins	SLE (30%); MCTD (>95%)
	Anti-Ro (SS-A)	Two proteins complexed to small RNAs Y1–Y5	SLE (30%); Sjögren's syndrome (70–80%)
	Anti-La (SS-B)	Single protein plus RNA polymerase III transcript	SLE (15%); Sjögren's syndrome (50–70%)
	Anti-Ku	DNA binding protein	SLE (10%)
	Anti-SCL-70	DNA topoisomerase I	PSS (40–70%); CREST (10–20%)
Nucleolar	Anti-PM-Scl	Nucleolar protein complex	PSS (3%); PM (8%)
	Anti-Mi-2	Nuclear protein complex	DM (15–20%)
	Anti-RNA polymerase	Subunits of RNA polymerase I	PSS (4%)
Dividing cell	Anticentromere	Centromere/kinetocore protein	CREST (80%); PSS (30%)
	Anti-proliferating cell nuclear antigen	Auxiliary protein of DNA polymerase δ	SLE (3%)
Cytoplasmic	Anti-Jo-1	Histidyl tRNA synthetase	PM/DM (18–25%)
	Anti-PL-7	Threonyl tRNA synthetase	PM/DM (3%)
	Anti-PL-12	Alanyl tRNA synthetase	PM (4%)
	Anti-SRP	Signal recognition particle	SLE (10%)
	Anti-ribosomal P	Large ribosomal subunit	PM/DM (3%)

CREST = calcinosis, Raynaud's phenomenon, esophageal dysmotility, sclerodactyly, and telangiectasia; DM = dermatomyositis; MCTD = mixed connective tissue disease; PM = polymyositis; PSS = progressive systemic sclerosis (diffuse scleroderma); SLE = systemic lupus erythematosus; snRNP = small nuclear ribonucleoprotein.

caution and not used as proof of a CTD in the absence of correlative clinical or laboratory findings.

Because of detailed biochemical studies, the molecular identity of many ANAs is now known, allowing for the development of specific immunochemical assays using a variety of technologies. These tests can be performed individually, although multiplex assays provide simultaneous assessment of multiple specificities. Among those assays, only a few are performed routinely because of their value for diagnosis and prognosis. For several CTDs, diagnosis can be readily determined from clinical findings or other laboratory tests. In these instances, the ANA determination provides confirmatory information as well as clues for the occurrence of certain clinical manifestations.

Antibodies to DNA

Antibodies to DNA (anti-DNA) are serologic markers of SLE and represent a criterion in the classification of patients with this disease. These antibodies bind sites on both single-stranded (ss) and double-stranded (ds) DNA, although anti-dsDNA are more specific for SLE and therefore routinely measured. Although these antibodies can bind free DNA, DNA in the cell occurs in association with histones to form a structure called the nucleosome, with DNA wrapped around a histone core. Anti-DNA may therefore be considered a subset of antibodies to nucleosomes, with nucleosomes probably being the driving antigen for this response.

In clinical practice, the measurement of anti-DNA is an important element in the evaluation of patients with a broad array of clinical complaints, given the heterogeneity and multisystemic nature of SLE. Anti-DNA determinations, in addition to their value in diagnosis, also convey prognostic information and an index of disease activity. The association with disease activity appears strongest with glomerulonephritis, most likely because of the role of DNA–anti-DNA immune complexes in immunopathogenesis. The association of anti-DNA with other disease manifestations is less certain, limiting the use of this marker as a measure of overall disease activity.

Several different immunochemical approaches can be used to detect anti-DNA antibodies, although solid-phase ELISA assays are convenient and sensitive and eliminate the need for radioactivity. The assays vary in regard to the spectrum of anti-DNA detected, and results between assays may not correlate. Nevertheless, for each assay, the dynamic range for testing is very large. With treatment and disease quiescence, anti-DNA antibodies may essentially disappear; with flare, levels may increase dramatically. This property distinguishes anti-DNA from other ANAs in SLE, levels of which tend to be more consistent over time.

As is the case for other ANAs, the appearance of anti-DNA in the serum may precede other manifestations of SLE, suggesting vigilance if these antibodies are present in patients who have symptoms that suggest a CTD but lack other evidence to establish a firm diagnosis.

Other Antinuclear Antibodies

Anti-Sm and anti-RNP are related specificities that commonly occur together in the sera of patients with SLE, a phenomenon called linkage. These antibodies bind proteins on subcellular particles called snRNPs (small nuclear ribonucleoproteins) that are composed of a set of proteins and uridine-rich RNAs. Anti-Sm and anti-RNP differ in protein specificity and in the ability to cause immunoprecipitation of the bound RNA molecules.

Anti-Sm antibodies occur only in patients with SLE and represent a serologic marker in disease classification. In contrast, anti-RNP can appear in the sera of patients with other clinical presentations and, in the absence of anti-Sm, may characterize patients with overlapping CTD features, so-called mixed CTD. In SLE, the frequencies of anti-Sm and anti-RNP vary among racial and ethnic groups, although a clear association with particular clinical manifestations has not been established.

Anti-Ro and anti-La, another set of linked ANAs, are directed to protein–RNA complexes that are involved in cellular metabolism of RNA. These antibodies are expressed more widely in patients with CTD and appear in the sera of patients with SLE, RA, and Sjögren's syndrome, among others. Assessment of these antibodies is important because of their association with the neonatal lupus syndrome, which results from the transplacental passage of antibodies and causes congenital heart block as well as rash in the neonate.

Although ANAs are directed to ubiquitous antigens, they nevertheless are expressed in disease-specific patterns and may show association with particular organ-specific manifestations. These associations include anti-ribosomal P with central nervous systemic involvement in SLE, antibodies to DNA topoisomerase 1 (anti-SCL-70) with progressive systemic sclerosis (diffuse scleroderma), antibodies to centromeres with CREST syndrome, and antibodies to histidyl tRNA synthetase (anti-Jo-1) with interstitial lung disease in scleroderma. The basis for the associations is unclear, although they may reflect cross-reactivity to a tissue-specific antigen or unexpected expression of a nuclear antigen on a differentiated cell to promote tissue-specific injury.

Antibodies to Phospholipids

Originally defined by their effects on in vitro clotting tests, antibodies to phospholipids (APLs) are associated with in vivo thrombosis. Patients with these antibodies display a clinical condition, termed the antiphospholipid antibody syndrome, that is characterized by arterial or venous thrombosis, thrombocytopenia, and first-trimester spontaneous abortions. This syndrome may occur by itself or in the context of SLE, where it may contribute to the acceleration of atherosclerosis, premature stroke, and myocardial infarction.

The serology of APLs, also known as lupus anticoagulants, is complicated related to their antigenic targets as well as heterogeneity. Of phospholipids, cardiolipin is a common antigen for these assessments. Although they are designated as antibodies to cardiolipin or phospholipids, these antibodies may be directed to the protein β_2-glycoprotein 1; in the format of an ELISA, this protein may bind to phospholipids to create antigenic sites. Importantly, patients with this syndrome may lack antibodies to phospholipids when measured in these assays, although levels of these antibodies can vary over time.

Adjunctive tests involve tests directed at inhibition of in vitro clotting (e.g., activated partial thromboplastin time, dilute Russell's viper venom time), recognizing the discordancy between in vivo thrombosis and in vitro anticoagulation. The mechanism by which antibodies to phospholipids and other clotting factors induce thrombosis in vivo is unknown, although they may interact with the surface of cells (e.g., endothelium) and with soluble clotting factors to promote a prothrombotic state.

Complement

Assessment of the complement system provides valuable information in diseases in which immune complex deposition may promote inflammation and tissue injury (see Chapter 47). This system involves a large number of proteins which function in enzyme cascades to generate degradation products that amplify immunologic reactions and promote the destruction or removal of foreign organisms as well as damaged cells. In the setting of SLE and in certain forms of vasculitis and glomerulonephritis, immune complexes activate complement to promote local inflammation. This activation can be measured in terms of the total complement level in the blood by functional assays of hemolytic activity; by measurement of individual complement components such as C3 and C4, whose levels are reduced by cleavage during activation; by measurement of split products of cleaved complement components; and by measurement of complement fragments bound to red blood cells during complement activation.

Proteins of the complement system are acute phase reactants and can increase with inflammation, including active disease. Correspondingly, low levels may reflect inherited complement deficiency rather than consumption; genetic deficiency of C1q, for example, is highly associated with SLE.

Anti-neutrophil Cytoplasmic Antibodies

Anti-neutrophil cytoplasmic antibodies (ANCAs) are autoantibodies that react to determinants in the neutrophil and occur prominently in patients with certain forms of necrotizing vasculitis or rapidly progressive glomerulonephritis. Two main forms of ANCA have been distinguished on the basis of the target antigens and pattern of immunofluorescence staining of fixed neutrophils: PR3-ANCA (C-ANCA), which reacts with proteinase-3 (PR3), and MPO-ANCA (P-ANCA), which reacts with myeloperoxidase (MPO). By immunofluorescence, PR3-ANCA shows staining in the cytoplasm; staining by MPO-ANCA localizes in the perinuclear area. ANCAs to other proteins have also been identified, but these may also occur in conditions other than vasculitis.

In the evaluation of severe, multisystem inflammatory disease, ANCA testing is necessary to distinguish possible etiologies. PR3-ANCA occurs commonly in patients with Wegener's granulomatosis, whereas MPO-ANCA marks the course of vasculitis caused by microscopic polyangiitis, polyarteritis nodosum, and Churg-Strauss disease, among others. In patients with ANCA-associated glomerulonephritis, the kidney lacks evidence of immune deposits, as indicated by the lack of staining for immunoglobulins or complement. Kidney disease of this kind is termed pauci-immune glomerulonephritis. Although ANCA testing is useful in initial diagnosis, its role for assessing disease activity is less certain. Occasionally, in patients who are desperately ill and cannot tolerate a lung or kidney biopsy, the presence of an ANCA can be used as preliminary evidence for diagnosis to allow the initiation of immunosuppressive therapy.

Cryoglobulins

Cryoglobulins are serum immunoglobulins that precipitate in the cold and promote the pathogenesis of systemic inflammatory disease through tissue deposition. The presence of a cryoglobulin is detected by allowing blood, collected warm, to remain cool at 2° to 4° C for one or more days. After centrifugation, the amount of cryoprecipitate is measured and expressed as a cryocrit. Subsequent analysis of the cryoprecipitate by immunochemical assays allows determination of its components. Cryoglobulins can be classified into three main types on the basis of their composition: (1) single or type I; (2) mixed, type II; and (3) mixed, type III. A type I cryoglobulin consists of a monoclonal immunoglobulin that precipitates in the cold. A mixed-type cryoglobulin contains RFs bound to polyclonal IgG to form an immune complex. In type II cryoglobulins, the IgM RF is monoclonal, and in type III the IgM RF is polyclonal.

Type I cryoglobulins occur in patients with lymphoproliferative disorders such as Waldenström's macroglobulinemia, multiple myeloma, or chronic lymphocytic lymphoma. In contrast, patients with mixed cryoglobulins can present with a wide range of signs and symptoms resulting from vasculitis. These manifestations include purpura (a sign of leukocytoclastic vasculitis), weakness, arthritis, and neuropathy and comprise a syndrome known as essential mixed cryoglobulinemia. Most patients with this condition have infection with hepatitis C virus, with viral components present in the complexes. These patients have serologic evidence of this infection as well as manifestations attributable to the underlying liver disease. As in the case of other CTDs and systemic inflammatory diseases, the evaluation of patients with essential mixed cryoglobulinemia demands attention to the entire patient and the impact of disease on multiple organs.

SUGGESTED READINGS

Linnik MD, Hu JZ, Heilbrunn KR, et al: Relationship between anti-double-stranded DNA antibodies and exacerbation of renal disease in patients with systemic lupus erythematosus. Arthritis Rheum 2005;52:1129–1137. *Increases in anti-DNA antibodies were associated with flares of renal disease.*

Manzi S, Navratil JS, Ruffing MJ, et al: Measurement of erythrocyte C4d and complement receptor 1 in systemic lupus erythematosus. Arthritis Rheum 2004;50:3596–3604. *A novel assay to measure complement fragments on red blood cells, providing a marker for disease activity in SLE.*

Scofield RH: Autoantibodies as predictors of disease. Lancet 2004;363:1544–1546. *A clinical review.*

Van Galen FA, Linn-Rasker SP, van Venrooij WJ, et al: Autoantibodies to cyclic citrullinated peptides predict progression to rheumatoid arthritis in patients with undifferentiated arthritis: A prospective cohort study. Arthritis Rheum 2004;50:709–715. *A prospective study showing the value of an anti-CCP testing in the diagnosis of early undifferentiated arthritis.*

279 IMAGING STUDIES IN THE RHEUMATIC DISEASES

Lynne S. Steinbach

Imaging in the rheumatic diseases is essential to diagnosis and assessment of the progression of arthropathy. The mainstay for imaging has always been the radiograph. This continues to be the case, because radiographs provide a relatively low-cost baseline evaluation of the bone, joint, and soft tissue. Frequently, the information provided is adequate for diagnosis and treatment. Other imaging modalities, such as magnetic resonance imaging (MRI), computed tomography (CT), ultrasonography, and bone scintigraphy, can aid in characterization and follow-up of rheumatic disease. This chapter discusses the various imaging options for evaluation of rheumatic disease and describes their capabilities and appropriate use.

RADIOGRAPHY

Radiography uses an x-ray source that emits radiation, which penetrates the body to produce the image on a photographic plate. An x-ray generator, image detector, and image processor are needed. The radiology technician who obtains the images must be knowledgeable about the equipment and patient positioning in order to obtain adequate radiographs. The physician who reads the radiograph is responsible for the quality of the study.

The radiographic image represents a map of radiation attenuation through various tissues along the course of the x-ray beam. A white structure such as bone attenuates more radiation than a darker structure such as cartilage, muscle, or joint effusion. An analog detector with a film cassette has been used to image the body for more than a century.

Digital radiography is being increasingly used for imaging. It employs a photostimulated phosphor imaging plate and an image reader–writer that processes the latent image information. When the plate absorbs x-rays, the energy is converted to light energy by fluorescence, with the intensity of light being proportional to the energy absorbed by the phosphor. The stimulated light is used to create a digital image. This is transferred to x-ray film or to a picture archiving system (PACS) that is utilized for viewing by the clinician. Digital images have advantages over conventional radiography in that they can be manipulated by the technologist or by the clinician at the PACS station for contrast and brightness as well as window width and level. Magnification and quantification are also possible. The images can be easily stored and retrieved from a server.

The radiograph is the initial imaging technique used for evaluation of arthropathy. Radiographs are affordable, easily available and render images of the joint with high spatial resolution. Frequently, a radiograph is all that is needed to assess joint damage. Radiographs demonstrate joint changes with high resolution down to approximately 0.05 mm. No other imaging study is able to accomplish this degree of spatial resolution. The radiograph can provide detailed evaluation of osseous cortex. Features such as joint space narrowing, erosion, subluxation, calcification, new bone formation, subchondral cyst formation, subchondral sclerosis, and soft tissue swelling can be evaluated on radiographs (Fig. 279–1).

Radiographs should be obtained with at least two views of the involved bone at 90-degree angles to each other to detect and characterize abnormalities such as erosion, effusion, soft tissue swelling, subluxation, dislocation, and fracture. Standard views usually consist of a frontal and a lateral view, but occasionally oblique and special views are needed, particularly when assessing the elbow, wrist, fingers, ankle, foot, toes, pelvis, or sacroiliac joints. Weight-bearing views of joints may be of value for assessing joint space narrowing, particularly in the knee. Although there is no universal consensus on routine views for the various joints, recommended screening views are listed in Table 279–1.

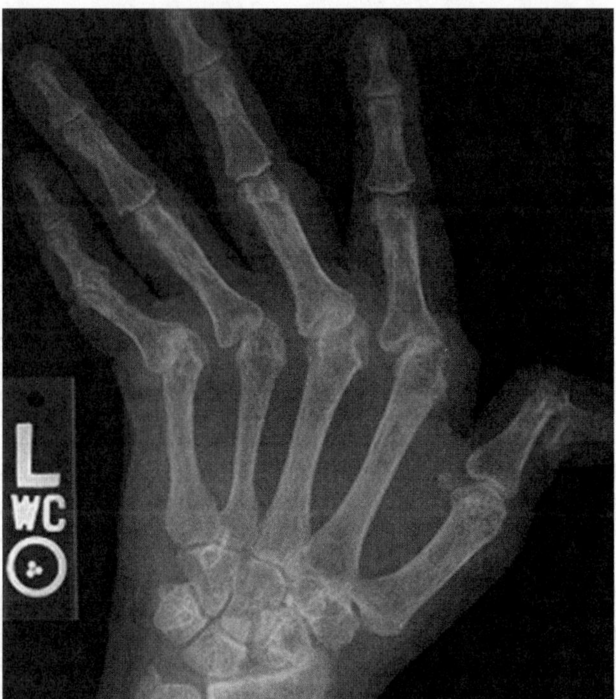

FIGURE 279–1 • Rheumatoid arthritis is demonstrated on a posteroanterior radiograph of a hand. Findings include joint space narrowing at the radiocarpal and metacarpophalangeal (MCP) joints, with subluxation of the MCP joints and the interphalangeal joint of the thumb, as well as erosions of the metacarpal heads and proximal interphalangeal (PIP) joints.

Because they have poor contrast resolution, radiographs do not reveal all aspects of arthropathy. Unlike MRI, radiography lacks the ability to show early cartilage loss and erosion, especially in the larger joints. Soft tissue pathology and muscle abnormalities cannot be assessed on radiography, as they can with MRI. Radiographs also are not as sensitive for evaluating activity of the disease. Other imaging techniques (discussed later) have these advantages and are considered complimentary to radiographs in the assessment of arthropathy.

Fluoroscopy, which employs x-ray imaging in real time, is a quick and precise method for needle placement during aspirations and injections, particularly for joints that are deep or complex and difficult to enter with the blind technique, such as the hip, shoulder, and sacroiliac joints. It can also be used to evaluate joint motion and stress. Videotaping of joint motion is useful for recording the kinematics of the joint. Because of the high dose of radiation, fluoroscopic time must be kept to a minimum. CT and ultrasonography are other imaging methods that are helpful for joint aspiration and injection (see later discussion).

Radiography transmits ionizing radiation to the patient and to medical personnel. The risk associated with this radiation, which includes carcinogenesis and genetic damage, is small but cumulative. A radiograph delivers between 0.1 to 2.0 millisieverts (mSv) to the tissue, depending on the type of tissue in the radiation path. This is less than the amount from bone scintigraphy, which tends to deliver 5 mSv, or CT, which can produce doses up to 15 mSv. The risk of cancer is estimated to be approximately 4% per Sievert by the U.S. National Academy of Sciences Committee on the Biological Effects of Ionizing Radiation. Radiation risk can be minimized with proper safety measures. The principle of the ALARA (as low reasonably achievable) dose should always be applied when using ionizing radiation. This is especially important in children and pregnant women. The number of images in one study and the frequency of follow-up studies must be prudently monitored without compromising evaluation of the joint. Appropriate collimation of the x-ray beam and reduction of fluoroscopy time should be enforced. Lead shielding of gonads and thyroid tissue is mandatory if these structures are not in the path of the body part being imaged.

MAGNETIC RESONANCE IMAGING

The demands of imaging are increased in this age of effective therapy to halt the progression of arthropathy. Over the last two decades, MRI has become the imaging modality of choice for evaluation of joint soft tissue, marrow structures, and muscle pathology, because it provides high-contrast resolution that enables the differentiation of various soft tissues from each other. Abnormal joint structures usually display different signal intensities than their normal counterparts. Morphologic changes resulting from destruction of tissue by the arthropathy and muscle inflammation are also identified.

MRI applies a strong magnetic field with radiofrequency pulses that pass through the various body tissues to produce different signal intensities. Each soft tissue structure contains unique properties that give it a characteristic signal intensity based on the proton density, T1 relaxation time, and spin density of the tissue. Various pulse sequences can be used to evaluate the joint; discussion of these pulse sequences is beyond the scope of this chapter.

Many factors can influence spatial resolution and thus the quality of the MRI. These include field strength and coil selection. Most imaging is performed on high-field superconducting magnets. Permanent or resistive magnets are also in use at lower field strengths. Field strength is measured in tesla (T). In general, the higher the field strength, the better the signal from the tissue and the shorter the imaging time.

Five types of magnets are used for clinical imaging of joints: ultra-high-field (3.0 T), high-field (1.0 to 2.0 T), midfield (0.3 to 1.0 T), low-field (less than 0.1 to 0.2 T), and ultra-low-field (less than 0.1 T). Most scanners operate between 0.3 and 1.5 T. Open scanners are less confining for claustrophobic patients but usually are not available at the high field range (above 1.0 T) that provides increased resolution. At the current time, 3.0 T scanners are proliferating in clinical and hospital settings. These ultra-high-field scanners offer the highest spatial resolution and are being increasingly used for imaging of small joints and cartilage.

TABLE 279–1 ROUTINE RADIOGRAPHIC SCREENING VIEWS OF THE SKELETON

UPPER EXTREMITY	
Fingers	PA, lateral (separate fingers)
Hand	PA, oblique, lateral
Wrist	PA, lateral (both with neutral positioning); ballcatcher oblique view is useful for inflammatory arthritis
Forearm	AP, lateral
Elbow	AP (supinated), lateral (90° flexed), oblique as needed
Humerus	AP, lateral
Glenohumeral joint	AP internal and external rotation (axillary, Grashey, or transthoracic view)
Acromioclavicular joint	AP, 15 degrees cephalad AP (bilateral weight-holding if dislocation)
Sternum	AP, oblique AP (also Hobbs view or lordotic view)
LOWER EXTREMITY	
Hip	AP internal rotation, frog-leg lateral (or cross-table)
Femur	AP, lateral
Knee, arthritis	PA flexed and AP weight-bearing views, lateral
Knee, patellofemoral joint	Merchant view (45° flexion)
Tibia/fibula	AP, lateral
Ankle	AP, lateral, mortise
Foot	AP, lateral, medial oblique (simulated weight-bearing lateral for foot alignment abnormality)
Subtalar joint	Lateral, Harris-Beath view
Calcaneus	Lateral, AP craniocaudal angulated view
Toes	AP, lateral, AP oblique
AXIAL SKELETON	
Cervical spine	AP, lateral, open mouth (odontoid); swimmer's view for lower cervical spine, oblique or pillar views for facet joints
Thoracic spine	AP, lateral; swimmer's view for upper thoracic spine
Lumbar spine	AP, lateral; oblique for pars interarticularis, flexion/extension laterals for subluxation
Sacrum	30° cephalad angulated AP, lateral
Coccyx	10° caudal angulated AP, lateral
Sacroiliac joints	30° cephalad angulated AP
Pelvis	AP; Judet views and/or inlet/outlet views for pelvic ring fractures

Modified from Lee JHE: Imaging modalities. *In* Johnson T, Steinbach L (eds): Essentials of Musculoskeletal Imaging. Rosemont, IL, American Academy of Orthopaedic Surgeons, 2004, p 6.

Coils, electrical devices that can generate or detect a magnetic field, are also important for proper joint imaging. They are placed over the body region of interest, keeping the field of view as low as possible, and improve spatial resolution. Many types of coils are available from various manufacturers for different joint sizes and configurations, including shoulder, extremity, wrist, and flex coils. Phased array coils use several coils in one component, allowing for a larger field of view; these are often used in spine imaging.

The widely used contrast agent for magnetic resonance (MR) studies is a neutral, hydrophilic salt of the gadolinium chelate, gadolinium diethylenetriamine-penta acetate (Gd-DTPA). Gadolinium can be injected intravenously or directly into the joint. Intravenous injection (indirect MR arthrography) carries the contrast agent in the vascular system to areas of hyperemia and inflammation. It is recommended for assessment of synovial activity for inflammatory joint processes. Gadolinium is taken up by inflamed synovium and is able to demonstrate thickened pannus. The slope of the curve of time versus signal intensity is useful for showing inflammatory activity and is commonly employed in research and clinical trials. Injection of dilute gadolinium into the joint (direct MR arthrography) is helpful for outlining structures to determine if there is morphologic damage. This technique is particularly effective for visualization of small structures, such as the labrum of the hip or shoulder, if there is no joint effusion. It is also helpful for demonstrating breakdown of soft tissue structures that normally prevent communication between joint compartments, such as the rotator cuff, triangular fibrocartilage of the wrist, and ligaments in the various joints.

With special regard to rheumatic disease, MRI demonstrates joint effusion, intra-articular masses, synovitis, damage to hyaline and fibrocartilage, tendons, ligaments, bone, muscle, and surrounding soft tissue (Fig. 279–2). MRI is sensitive for marrow abnormalities such as reactive edema and erosion from arthritis, although it can be nonspecific, and infectious processes can have a similar appearance. Hemosiderin has a characteristic low signal intensity on MRI, which allows for characterization of arthropathies such as pigmented villonodular synovitis and hemophilia. MRI is useful for early detection of osteonecrosis, particularly when radiographs are normal. It is also used to evaluate the spine for disc disease, nerve root compression, and inflammatory changes.

Disadvantages of MRI include the facts that it is more costly than CT and other imaging modalities and that it can be claustrophobic. Calcification is not easily identified, and radiographs or CT scans are often complementary in this regard. MRI is contraindicated in patients who have certain devices implanted into their tissues. These include cochlear implants, some heart valves, cardiac pacemakers, and spinal implants. Metal implants, such as joint prostheses and spinal hardware, are not contraindicated for MRI. Although metallic devices can cause some distortion of the image, newer materials such as cobalt-chrome cause less artifact. Various imaging parameters can also be adjusted to improve the visibility of tissues surrounding metallic devices, allowing for diagnostic interpretation.

ULTRASONOGRAPHY

In ultrasound imaging, sound waves are pulsed through tissues to obtain an image that can localize and characterize pathology. Through the years, resolution has increased markedly. Portable scanners are also being used, especially by nonradiologists. These units are less expensive. They are adequate for injections and for detection of fluid collections and tenosynovitis, but they do not provide the detailed anatomy of their high-end counterparts.

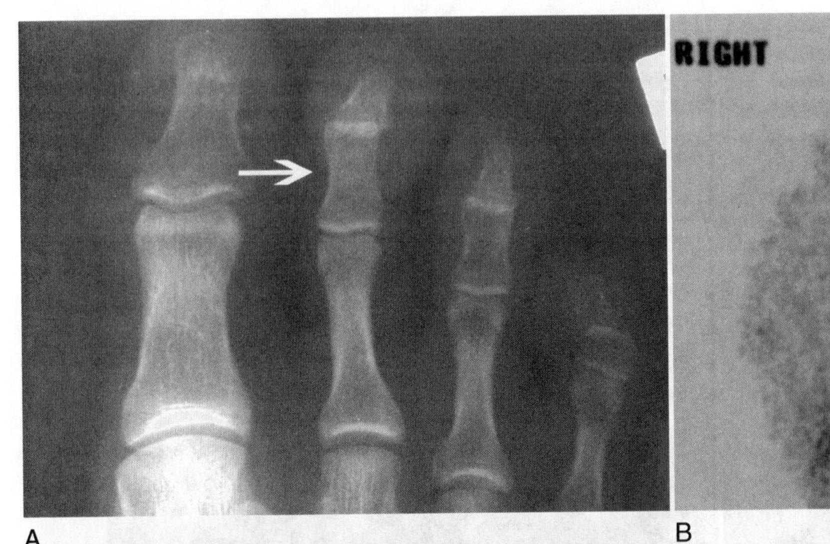
A

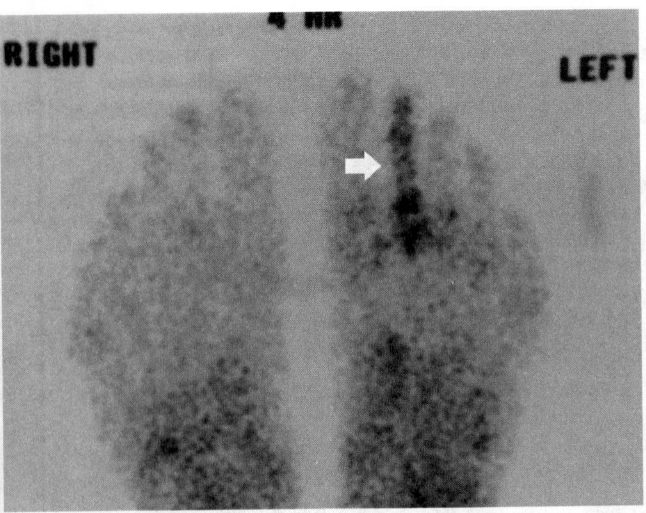

B

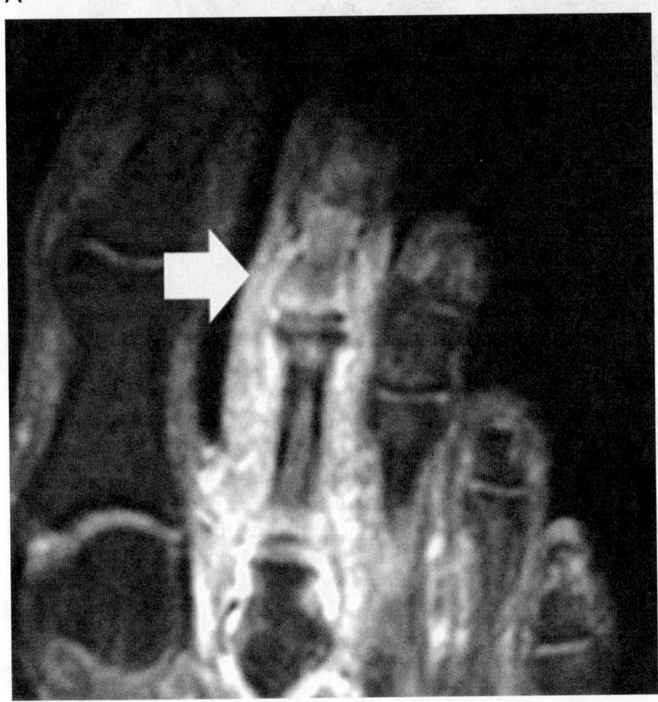
C

FIGURE 279–2 • Sausage digit in psoriatic arthritis demonstrated by radiography, scintigraphy, and magnetic resonance imaging. A, Anteroposterior radiograph of the forefoot demonstrates soft tissue swelling of the second toe without obvious bone involvement (arrow). **B,** There is increased tracer uptake of Tc^{99m}-MDP in the entire second toe, from the metacarpophalangeal joint to the distal phalanx on the bone scan, suggesting osteitis and soft tissue inflammation. **C,** A coronal fat-suppressed T1-weighted magnetic resonance image of the second toe obtained after intravenous gadolinium administration reveals high-signal-intensity uptake in the bone and surrounding soft tissues, consistent with osteitis and soft tissue inflammation.

Ultrasound provides a less expensive, noninvasive method to visualize joint structures such as tendons, ligaments, fibrocartilage, muscles, and soft tissue masses without the use of ionizing radiation. Areas of pain and swelling can be scanned in real time with the opposite side for comparison. Fluid within tendon sheaths can be easily assessed. Fluid, blood, pus, and mucin in ganglia, cysts, bursae, hematomas, seromas, and abscesses can be differentiated from solid masses based on echogenicity (Fig. 279–3). Areas around metallic hardware or other implants are easily assessed for such masses without the artifact that might limit MRI or CT evaluation.

Hypervascularity is a component of inflammatory joint disease and angiofibroblastic response in tendons that can be assessed by Doppler imaging, a sonographic method that assesses vascular flow. This information can be used for diagnosis and assessment of therapeutic response and to identify locations for injections of anesthetic agents or steroids.

Ultrasound can demonstrate dynamic properties of tendons and other structures. The real-time capability allows for identification of subluxation and impingement, pinpointing causes of pain with certain movements. Ultrasonography is a quick and inexpensive method to perform accurate aspirations and injections of joints and soft tissue structures such as tendon sheaths and bursae. Areas of hydroxyapatite crystal deposition disease can be aspirated and injected.

Ultrasound is an operator-dependent technique with a steep learning curve. It can be time-consuming for the operator scanning the patient. Some important joint structures are in sonographically inaccessible areas, such as those obscured by bone. This includes portions of the menisci and the cruciate ligaments of the knee, the labra of the hip and shoulder, and some portions of hyaline cartilage that are more easily seen with MRI. Sonography does not allow for evaluation of bone marrow pathology or global assessment of a joint, but it can be helpful for targeted diagnostic problems, as outlined earlier.

COMPUTED TOMOGRAPHY

CT employs an x-ray source with multiple detectors housed in a circular gantry that rotates 360 degrees around the patient, who lies on a table surrounded by the gantry. The computer processes the data that is displayed tomographically and in multiple planes with thin slices. A three-dimensional reconstruction of the body part can be rendered. This allows for analysis of regions with complex anatomy, such as the pelvis, hip, and spine. These images can be rotated and sometimes made into a plastic model for surgical planning. Newer CT scanners have increased numbers of detectors and are able to image more quickly and with thinner slices. They employ spiral or helical scanning through continuous rotation of

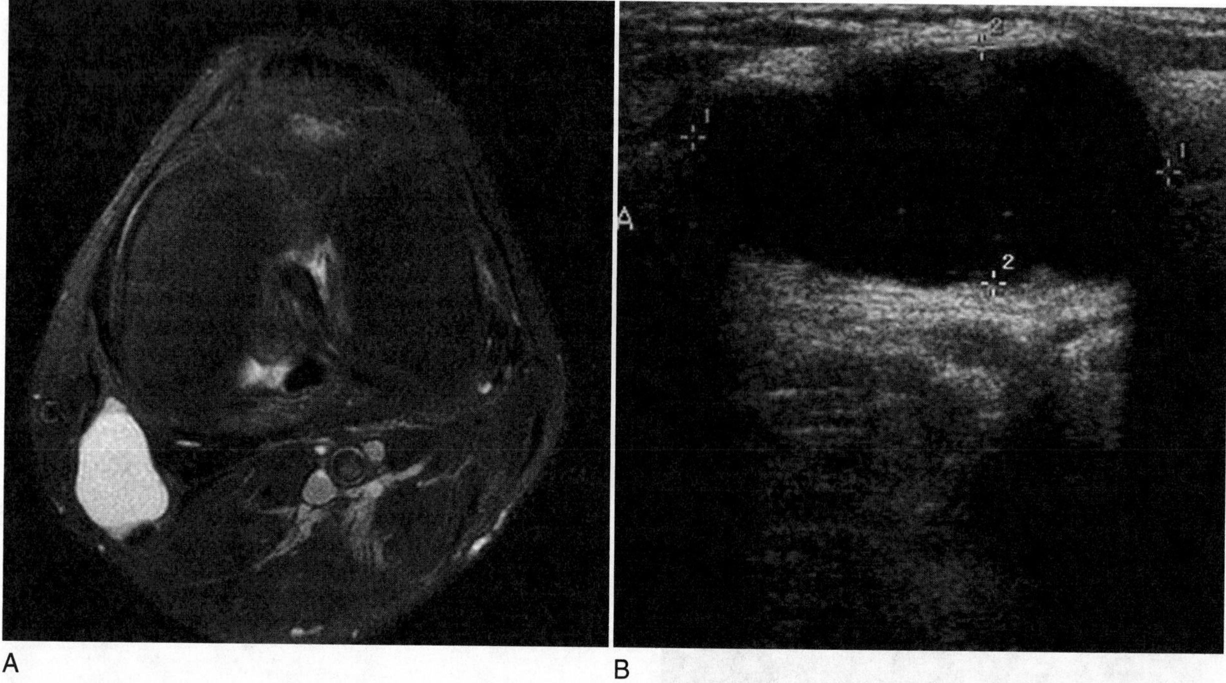

FIGURE 279–3 • Knee ganglion demonstrated by magnetic resonance imaging and ultrasonography. A, A fat-suppressed T2-weighted axial magnetic resonance image of the knee demonstrates a high-signal-intensity mass in the posterior aspect of the knee. Without intravenous gadolinium to show the enhancement pattern, it is difficult to determine whether the mass is cystic or solid. **B,** An ultrasound image demonstrates that the mass is hypoechoic, a finding consistent with a ganglion.

the x-ray source and the detectors while the patient moves on the table through the gantry.

CT is useful for evaluating vertebral alignment and fractures as well as abnormalities of the flat bones and pelvis. Complex fractures are best evaluated with CT. Joints that are difficult to assess on radiographs, including the sacroiliac, temporomandibular, wrist, and sternoclavicular joints, are well seen with CT. However, internal derangement of these joints is better appreciated on MRI, which provides better soft tissue contrast.

There are many different iodinated contrast agents that can be injected intravenously to enhance the CT study. The contrast has higher attenuation and spreads hematogenously to areas of increased vascularity and inflammation. MRI with gadolinium is the preferred method for demonstrating pannus and joint inflammation and for characterizing a soft tissue mass, but CT with contrast can be used to determine whether the mass is cystic or solid in patients in whom MRI is contraindicated, such as those subject to claustrophobia and those with aneurysm clips or cardiac pacemakers. Ultrasonography can also be used for this purpose. Fluid collections such as abscesses, seromas, bursae, and ganglia are identified on all three imaging modalities.

CT arthrography may also be performed. This is useful when MRI is contraindicated. Intra-articular injection of iodinated contrast material or room air, or both, coats the joint structures and can be useful for visualization of small and large cartilage defects, fibrocartilage, tendon and ligament tears, and ossified and cartilaginous bodies.

One must keep in mind that the radiation dose from CT is high, especially with the newer scanners. Repeated imaging with CT or a request for CT in a child or pregnant woman must be carefully considered in terms of risk versus benefit. Algorithms to reduce tissue dose are used for children and other vulnerable patients. The resulting images are of lower resolution but usually provide adequate information for diagnosis.

ARTHROGRAPHY

Arthrography involves the intra-articular placement of a needle, followed by aspiration of joint fluid and injection of a contrast agent to enhance imaging. It is often performed to exclude the possibility of infection in patients with hip pain or in those patients with total joint prostheses. It is also used occasionally to determine whether there is a full-thickness tear of the rotator cuff, triangular fibrocartilage and ligaments of the wrist, or collateral ligaments of the elbow and ankle, although MRI has replaced conventional arthrography for this indication in most centers.

Arthrography can be combined with MRI or CT to better evaluate the internal structures through joint distention and contrast-coating of structures along the articular surface, such as the labrum, ligaments, and capsule. This is discussed in the sections on individual imaging modalities.

SCINTIGRAPHY

Scintigraphy employs detectors in the form of a gamma camera that can identify decay of intravenously injected radioactive isotopes. Bone scintigraphy is used to identify sites of activity in the rheumatic diseases. The bone scan employs 99m technetium methylene diphosphate (Tc^{99m}-MDP) as the radioactive tracer. The isotope moves to areas of high bone turnover and vascular flow as well as areas of calcium or bone deposition. Three-phase bone scans are obtained at various intervals after injection. Images are obtained at three time points: the early vascular phase, the intermediate blood pool phase, and the late phase. Each phase allows for further characterization of the disease process. Abnormal tracer uptake is seen in areas of inflammation, infection, neoplasm, osteonecrosis, and fracture (see Fig. 279–3). The scan is most useful for identifying the location of lesions within the skeleton, but it is nonspecific. Further imaging of the abnormal areas is often necessary to characterize the pathology.

SUGGESTED READINGS

Adler RS, Finzel KC: The complementary roles of MR imaging and ultrasound of tendons. Radiol Clin North Am 2005;43:771–807. *Provides indications and features of ultrasound and MRI for tendon evaluation.*

American College of Rheumatology Extremity Magnetic Resonance Imaging Task Force: Extremity magnetic resonance imaging in rheumatoid arthritis: Report of the American College of Rheumatology Extremity Magnetic Resonance Imaging Task Force. Arthritis Rheum 2006;54:1034–1047. *A comprehensive review.*

Cooper G, Lutz GE, Adler RS: Ultrasound-guided aspiration of symptomatic rotator cuff calcific tendonitis. Am J Phys Med Rehabil 2005;84:81. *Describes technique for aspiration of calcific tendonitis using ultrasound.*

Gupta KB, Duryea J, Weissman BN: Radiographic evaluation of osteoarthritis. Radiol Clin North Am 2004;42:11–42. *Comprehensive review.*
Ostergaard M, Ejbjerg B: Magnetic resonance imaging of the synovium in rheumatoid arthritis. Semin Musculoskel Radiol 2004;8:287–299. *Provides current knowledge on MRI for assessment of the synovium in RA.*

280 CONNECTIVE TISSUE STRUCTURE AND FUNCTION

Richard F. Loeser

Connective tissue forms the architectural framework of the musculoskeletal system and serves as a scaffold that supports various organs and tissues. Many important structures within the body are composed primarily of connective tissue (Table 280–1). For example, articular cartilage is made up exclusively of a specialized dense connective tissue without blood vessels, nerves, or lymphatics. Tendons, ligaments, intervertebral discs, and fascia are structures also consisting of dense connective tissue, although of a different composition from cartilage. Bone contains both dense and loose connective tissue; the latter provides support for bone marrow cells and helps to fill the space within the bone cavity. Adipose tissue is also often considered to be a specialized connective tissue that has both metabolic and structural functions.

Articular joints are formed by several common types of connective tissue, including muscle, bone, tendon, ligament, cartilage, meniscus, and synovium, which function as a unit during joint movement. These tissues demonstrate distinct characteristics when imaged by magnetic resonance because of their unique cellular and matrix composition (Fig. 280–1). In this type of image, tissues with a greater water content, such as adipose tissue and cartilage, appear lighter than very dense tissues, such as the subchondral bone, which appear dark.

Despite their diversity, what connective tissues have in common is that they contain cells, usually of mesodermal origin, that have an abundant extracellular matrix. The cells within a particular connective tissue control the composition of the extracellular matrix, which, in turn, determines the physical properties of the tissue. The many types of connective tissue cells range from fibroblasts, which are present in the connective tissue found in skin, synovium, tendons, ligaments, and fascia, to more specialized cells such as chondrocytes and osteoblasts, which are found in cartilage and bone, respectively (see Table 280-1). Basement membranes are a more special form of connective tissue in that they are produced by epithelial and endothelial cells, rather than by mesenchymal cells. The connective tissue matrix consists of an intricate mixture of proteins and other macromolecules, which are responsible for the unique function of each particular type of connective tissue (Fig. 280–2). Connective tissues that must withstand high tensile loads, such as tendons, have a high content of collagen fibers, whereas tissues that must resist compression, such as cartilage, have a high content of proteoglycans.

Because of the wide distribution of connective tissues within the human body, diseases that affect connective tissue cells or extracellular matrix proteins often have systemic effects. These connective tissue disorders can be divided into three general types: those that arise from a mutation within a gene encoding a connective tissue protein (e.g., Marfan syndrome); those that are the result of an inflammatory, sometimes autoimmune, process centered in connective tissues (e.g., rheumatoid arthritis); and those that are the result of a degenerative type of process often associated with aging (e.g., osteoarthritis). A basic understanding of the composition of the various connective tissues and of the way in which this composition relates to structure and function is important for understanding the clinical presentation, as well as management, of the spectrum of musculoskeletal and connective tissue disorders.

CONNECTIVE TISSUE PROTEINS AND MACROMOLECULES

Each different type of connective tissue has a unique composition based on the amount and specific forms of extracellular matrix proteins and macromolecules. The extracellular matrix components can be grouped into families that include the collagens, proteoglycans, elastins, and other noncollagenous glycoproteins. These extracellular matrix components not only provide the scaffolding that forms the tissue, but also, importantly, create an information-rich environment that provides

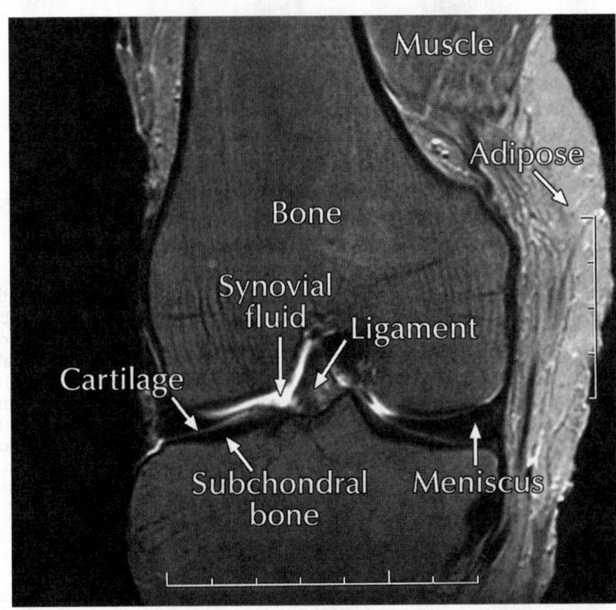

FIGURE 280–1 • Magnetic resonance image of a knee joint demonstrating the diversity of connective tissue structures. The image was obtained with a 1.5 Tesla magnet using a fast spin-echo T2-weighted imaging protocol. Tissues with a higher water content, such as adipose and articular cartilage, appear lighter, as does the synovial fluid. The subchondral bone is dark because of a high mineral and low water content and can be seen just below the very thin layer of articular cartilage. (Courtesy of Dr. Carol Muehleman, Rush Medical College, Chicago.)

TABLE 280–1 DIVERSITY OF CONNECTIVE TISSUE–CONTAINING STRUCTURES

Structure	Function	Cells	Key Matrix Components
Adipose tissue	Energy storage, organprotection	Adipocytes, fibroblasts	Fine reticular fibers
Basement membrane	Support and filtration barrier	Epithelial and endothelial cells	Type IV collagen, laminin
Bone	Skeletal support, blood cell production, mineral storage	Osteoblasts, osteoclasts, osteocytes	Type I collagen, osteocalcin, bone sialoprotein, hydroxyapatite
Cartilage	Allows joint motion, transmits loads	Chondrocytes	Type II collagen, aggrecan
Dermis	Support and resiliency	Fibroblasts	Type I collagen, elastin
Ligament	Connects bone to bone	Fibroblasts	Type I collagen, small proteoglycans
Tendon	Connects muscle to bone	Fibroblasts	Type I collagen, small proteoglycans
Stroma	Support of organs	Fibroblasts, organ specific cells	Type I, VI collagen, fibronectin
Synovium	Joint lining, produces synovial fluid	Fibroblasts, macrophages	Type I, III collagen
Vessel wall	Structural support of blood vessels	Vascular smooth muscle cells	Type III collagen, elastin

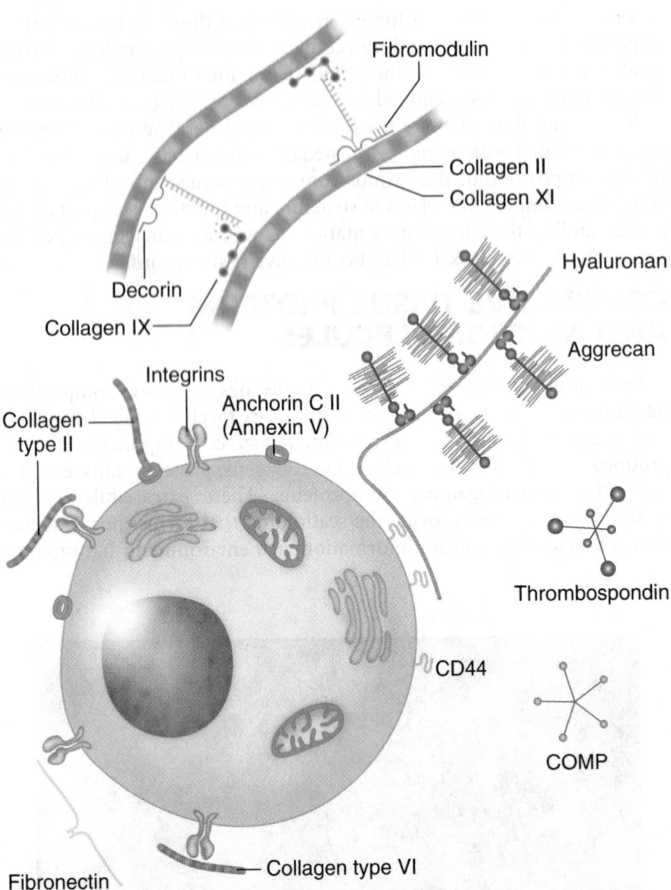

FIGURE 280–2 • Model of extracellular matrix proteins and their interaction with each other and with matrix receptors on a chondrocyte. Decorin, fibromodulin, and types IX and XI collagen all interact with type II collagen and regulate collagen fiber assembly and structure. Types II and VI collagen bind matrix receptors called integrins. Type II collagen can also bind to anchorin CII, whereas fibronectin binds to integrins. A large proteoglycan aggregate forms when multiple aggrecan molecules bind to a long strand of hyaluronic acid, which, in turn, is anchored to the cell by CD44. Additional matrix proteins shown include thrombospondin and cartilage oligomeric protein (COMP). (Adapted from Knudson W, Loeser RF: CD44 and integrin matrix receptors participate in cartilage homeostasis. Cell Mol Life Sci 2002;59:36–44.)

external cues to the connective tissue cells. Intracellular signaling, initiated through the interaction of extracellular matrix components with cell surface receptors, regulates certain important processes, including cell growth, differentiation, and survival and remodeling of the matrix. The integrins, named for their ability to integrate the extracellular matrix with intracellular cytoskeletal components, are a large and important family of cell surface receptors that recognize and bind some different extracellular matrix proteins initiating intracellular signaling (see Fig. 280–2). The signals generated by extracellular matrix proteins are integrated with signals generated by soluble mediators, also present in the matrix, including growth factors and cytokines. In normally functioning connective tissues, the cells, extracellular matrix proteins, and soluble mediators all work beautifully in concert to maintain the tissue and to adapt the tissue to meet changes in physical or biomechanical demands.

Collagens

Collagen is a major component of the extracellular matrix and is the most abundant protein in the body; it accounts for about 25 to 30% of the total protein mass. Collagens are triple-helical proteins formed when three polypeptide chains, called α chains, wind around each other to form a collagen molecule (Fig. 280–3). The α chains are rich in the amino acids proline and glycine, which are important in forming the helical conformation of the polypeptide chain. Because of its ring structure, proline stabilizes the helix. Glycine, the smallest of the amino acids, is spaced at every third position in the chain such that it occupies the tightly spaced inside portions of the triple helix. Mutations that result in the substitution of a much larger amino acid for glycine can severely disrupt the triple helical structure. Post-translational modifications, including hydroxylation of specific proline and lysine residues, occur during the processing of the collagen molecules; these modifications are important in stabilizing the collagen structure and in forming interchain and intrachain cross-links.

More than 30 collagen genes code for the collagen α chains. α chains specific for each collagen type combine to form at least 19 different collagens. The types of collagen can be grouped by structure and function (Table 280–2). In the fibrillar collagens (collagen types I, II, III, V, and XI), individual collagen molecules are packed in a staggered and ordered fashion to form a collagen fibril, which has a characteristic banding pattern when observed by high-power microscopy. Fibril formation occurs outside the cell after the N-terminal and C-terminal propeptides present on procollagen molecules are proteolytically removed to form

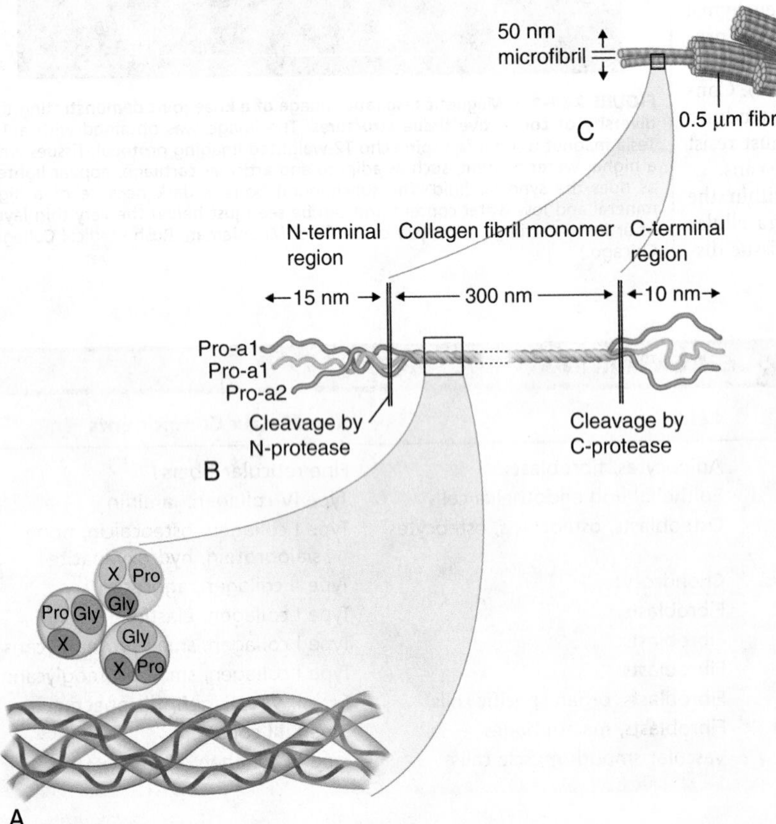

FIGURE 280–3 • Collagen structure. Three α chains (in this case, two procollagen α_1 chains and one procollagen α_2 chain) containing a high content of the amino acids glycine (Gly) and proline (Pro) wind together to form a triple helical collagen molecule (**A**). After secretion from the cell, the N-terminal and C-terminal ends are removed by proteases to form a collagen fibril monomer (**B**). Monomers are assembled to form a microfibril, which, in turn, is assembled into fibrils; finally, multiple fibrils form a complete collagen fiber (**C**).

TABLE 280–2 CONNECTIVE TISSUE COLLAGENS

Collagen Type	Chains	Molecules	Tissue Distribution	Selected Diseases from Mutations
FIBRILLAR COLLAGENS				
I	$\alpha_1(I)$ $\alpha_2(I)$	$[\alpha_1(I)]_2\alpha_2(I)$ $[\alpha_1(I)]_3$	Skin, bone, tendon, organ capsules, arteries	Osteogenesis imperfecta, Ehlers-Danlos type VIIA
II	$\alpha_1(II)$	$[\alpha_1(II)]_3$	Cartilage, vitreous humor	Stickler's syndrome, osteoarthritis
III	$\alpha_1(III)$	$[\alpha_1(III)]_3$	Skin, vessels, uterus	Ehlers-Danlos type IV, aortic aneurysms
V	$\alpha_1(V)$ $\alpha_2(V)$ $\alpha_3(V)$	$[\alpha_1(V)]_3$ $[\alpha_1(V)]_2\alpha_2(V)$ $\alpha_1(V)\alpha_2(V)\alpha_3(V)$	Skin, vessels, placenta, chorion, uterus	
XI	$\alpha_1(XI)$, $\alpha_2(XI)$	$\alpha_1(XI)\alpha_2(XI)\alpha 1(II)$	Cartilage	
BASEMENT MEMBRANE COLLAGENS				
IV	α_1-$\alpha_5(IV)$	$[\alpha_1(IV)]_2\alpha_2(IV)$	Basement membranes	Alport's syndrome, porencephaly
FIBRIL-ASSOCIATED COLLAGENS WITH INTERRUPTED TRIPLE HELIXES (FACIT)				
IX	α_1-$\alpha_3(IX)$	$\alpha_1(IX)\alpha_2(IX)\alpha_3(IX)$	Cartilage, intervertebral discs	Degenerative disc disease, osteoarthritis
XII	$\alpha_1(XII)$	$[\alpha_1(XII)]_3$	Tendons, ligaments, other soft tissues	
XIV	$\alpha_1(XIV)$		Ubiquitous	
NETWORK-FORMING COLLAGENS				
VIII	$\alpha_1(VIII)$, $\alpha_2(VIII)$		Cornea, vessels	
X	$\alpha_1(X)$	$[\alpha_1(X)]_3$	Growth plate cartilage	Spondylometaphyseal dysplasia
LONG-CHAIN, ANCHORING-FIBRIL COLLAGEN WITH INTERRUPTED TRIPLE HELIX				
VII	$\alpha_1(VII)$	$[\alpha_1(VII)]_3$	Anchoring fibrils	Epidermolysis bullosa
OTHERS				
VI	α_1-$\alpha 3(VI)$	$\alpha_1(VI)\alpha_2(VI)\alpha_3(VI)$	Cartilage, stroma	
XIII	$\alpha_1(XIII)$		Skin, gut	

mature collagen. The fibrils, in turn, are packed together to form fibers. Further cross-linking of collagen fibrils strengthens the structure. These rather stiff, ropelike structures provide the tensile strength for connective tissues. The fibril-associated collagens (collagen types IX, XII, XIV) help to form and stabilize the collagen fibrils. Unlike the fibrillar collagens, this group of collagens contains regions where the triple helical structure is interrupted, and this can result in a bend in the collagen molecule, hence the name *fibril-associated collagens with interrupted triple helixes.* Type IV collagen is the classic basement membrane collagen that forms in aggregates to provide structural support to the basement membrane.

The type and amount of collagen found in a particular connective tissue are important contributors to tissue function. Tissues such as bone, tendon, and cartilage, which must withstand high biomechanical loads, are packed with large amounts of long fibrillar collagens, primarily type I collagen in bone and tendons and type II collagen in cartilage. The loose connective tissues, such as basement membranes and organ stroma, experience much less mechanical force but require a matrix that allows more rapid diffusion of molecules and so contain a higher content of aggregating or anchoring types of collagen and less fibrillar collagen. Recent work correlating mutations in particular collagen genes with disease phenotypes in humans and studies of phenotype after gene disruption in transgenic mice have added to our knowledge of collagen function (see Table 280–2). Some examples include "brittle-bone disease" or osteogenesis imperfecta resulting from type I collagen mutations, severe premature osteoarthritis from type II collagen mutations, and fragile blood vessel and visceral walls in Ehlers-Danlos syndrome type IV from mutations in type III collagen. Excess collagen production can also disrupt tissue function, usually by causing tissue fibrosis as seen in scleroderma. Finally, fragile connective tissues can result from inadequate collagen production and cross-linking, as occurs in scurvy from vitamin C deficiency. Vitamin C (ascorbic acid) serves as a cofactor for the hydroxylation reaction necessary to modify specific prolyl and lysyl residues in procollagen and a deficiency in ascorbic acid reduces collagen secretion, stability, and cross-linking.

Proteoglycans

These matrix macromolecules consist of a protein core to which short oligosaccharides and longer chains of glycosaminoglycans are covalently attached. The large variety of proteoglycans is based on the types and lengths of glycosaminoglycans as well as the sequence and length of the protein core. Chondroitin sulfate, keratan sulfate, heparan sulfate, and dermatan sulfate are four different forms of glycosaminoglycans that consist of repeating disaccharide units. The sulfates present on the glycosaminoglycans create a highly negatively charged environment that is hydrophilic. Thus, connective tissues that contain large amounts of proteoglycans also contain relatively large amounts of water bound to the proteoglycans. In addition to water, proteoglycans bind cationic proteins, which, in some cases include growth factors resulting in a mechanism by which tissues can store growth factors in the matrix.

Aggrecan is a very large (molecular weight >200,000 kD) proteoglycan found in cartilage that contains a protein core of more than 2000 amino acids to which are attached approximately 100 long chondroitin sulfate chains, approximately 30 shorter keratan sulfate chains, and approximately 50 short oligosaccharides. Decorin, biglycan, fibromodulin, and lumican are examples of small proteoglycans that have much shorter protein cores (30 to 60 kD) and fewer glycosaminoglycan side chains. These small proteoglycans interact with collagen and function to regulate the formation of collagen fibrils and help to stabilize the collagen network (see Fig. 280–2). Although their functions are not completely understood, they also likely have other roles because of their ability to bind matrix molecules, in addition to collagen, and as a result of their affinity for growth factors.

Hyaluronic acid is a nonsulfated glycosaminoglycan that is synthesized in very long linear polymer strands. Hyaluronic acid is produced by chondrocytes and by synovial cells and is a major component contributing to the viscosity of the synovial fluid. Unlike the other glycosaminoglycans, hyaluronic acid is not attached to a protein core and so is not directly used to form proteoglycans. In cartilage, however, strands of hyaluronic acid bind aggrecan molecules through a non-covalent interaction with a globular portion of the N-terminus of the aggrecan core protein and a second small protein called *link protein*. The resulting macromolecular complex containing 100 or more aggrecan molecules linked to each long strand of hyaluronic acid forms a gel-like substance in cartilage as a result of its high sugar and water content.

The proteoglycan aggregates provide articular cartilage with resiliency. When cartilage is compressed during joint loading, water is pushed out from the proteoglycans, and the negative charges on the glycosaminoglycans become closer; this helps to resist further compression through charge repulsion. When the load is released, water is drawn back to the proteoglycans, and the result is fluid flow responsible for part of the biomechanical stimulation of the cells. The fluid flow also helps to move nutrients through the tissue, a feature that is particularly important for articular cartilage, a connective tissue that depends on diffusion from the synovial fluid for most of its nutrition. The network of collagen fibers that surrounds aggrecan prevents the proteoglycans from swelling beyond a certain size, thus creating a swelling pressure in cartilage that also helps to resist compression.

Noncollagenous Fibrillar Proteins

Elastic fibers are composed of elastin and proteins, often referred to as *microfibrils*, such as fibrillin, because their fibrils are much smaller than the classic collagen fibrils. Elastic fibers must withstand repeated stretching and deformation and must be capable of returning to a relaxed state. Tropoelastin is the precursor to elastin and is synthesized by several cell types, including vascular smooth muscle cells and dermal fibroblasts, where it contributes to the elasticity of the blood vessel wall and skin, respectively. Elastin also plays a similar role in the lung. Elastin, like collagen, forms interchain and intrachain cross-links that help to stabilize and strengthen the elastic fibers, although the stiffness of the elastin fibers is less than that of the collagen fibers. Many of the cross-links in elastin are formed through the hydroxylation of two unique amino acids found in tropoelastin, desmosine and isodesmosine. Fibrillin is found in several elastic tissues and is particularly abundant in the aorta, the suspensory ligament of the lens, and the periosteum. Fibrillin was a little-known protein until investigators discovered that fibrillin mutations are the cause of most cases of Marfan's syndrome.

Noncollagenous Glycoproteins

Along with the proteoglycans, the many other noncollagenous matrix glycoproteins found in connective tissues form much of what is sometimes described as the *ground substance* in histologic terms. This rather inert-sounding description should in no way be taken to suggest that these matrix components simply fill in or hold the tissue together. Rather, these proteins participate actively in creating the information-rich environment described earlier. Proteins in this group include fibronectin, vitronectin, osteopontin, laminin, and thrombospondin. Fibronectin is found in most connective tissues throughout the body. Laminin is particularly prominent in basement membranes, and osteopontin is found in greater amounts in cartilage and bone. All these proteins bind to cells through specific cell surface receptors to promote attachment of cells to the matrix. The proteins also interact with other matrix proteins, such as collagen and proteoglycans, to integrate the cells further with the extracellular matrix. Through the interactions with cell receptors and other matrix proteins, the noncollagenous glycoproteins function in regulating tissue morphogenesis as well as in tissue repair and remodeling. They also appear to play a role in other diverse processes, including tumor growth and metastasis.

Other Matrix Proteins

Many other matrix proteins present in connective tissues, such as tenascin, osteonectin, the matrilins, matrix Gla protein, and osteocalcin, are less completely understood but are probably no less important. Matrix Gla protein and osteocalcin are both found in bone, whereas matrix Gla protein is also present in cartilage and other soft tissues, including blood vessel walls. Both proteins require reduced vitamin K as a cofactor for a post-translational carboxylation reaction important to the cation binding properties of the proteins. Inhibition of vitamin K reduction by the drug warfarin interferes with this reaction, as it does for the coagulation factors. Warfarin is contraindicated in pregnancy because it has been shown to cause embryopathy, which includes abnormalities in skeletal formation likely secondary to effects on matrix Gla protein and/or osteocalcin.

Extracellular Matrix Protein Receptors

Connective tissue cells use several different types of cell surface receptors to bind extracellular matrix proteins. The major types of receptors include integrins, CD44, discoidin domain receptors (DDRs), and proteoglycan family receptors such as the syndecans (Table 280–3). CD44 is expressed by several different connective tissue cell types as well as by nonconnective tissue cells such as lymphocytes. On connective tissue cells, CD44 is the principal receptor for hyaluronan. CD44 binding of hyaluronan is particularly important in forming a gel-like pericellular coat found around certain connective tissue cells such as chondrocytes. DDR1 and DDR2 are receptor tyrosine kinases found on epithelial and mesenchymal cells. DDR1 can bind types I through VI and type VIII collagen, whereas DDR2 is activated only by fibrillar collagens. Syndecans contain a transmembrane protein core to which heparan sulfate proteoglycans are attached to the extracellular domain. The proteoglycans bind growth factors such as fibroblast growth factor. Syndecans also appear to interact with integrins and may modulate integrin function.

The integrins represent the largest family of cell surface matrix receptors and have been found to be the primary receptors for many matrix proteins, including collagens, fibronectin, laminin, vitronectin, osteopontin, and thrombospondin (see Table 280–3). Integrins are heterodimeric transmembrane proteins consisting of one α and one β subunit. More than 20 known integrins are formed by 14 types of α subunits and at least nine types of β subunits. The two major subfamilies of integrins function in mediating interactions between cells and extracel-

TABLE 280–3 CELL-SURFACE RECEPTORS FOR EXTRACELLULAR MATRIX COMPONENTS

Receptor	Ligands
CD 44	Hyaluronan
Syndecan (1–4)	Tenascin, fibronectin, fibroblast growth factor (FGF)
Discoidin domain receptors 1, 2	Collagen
Integrins	
$\alpha1\beta1$	Collagen, laminin, cartilage matrix protein
$\alpha2\beta1$	Collagen, laminin, chondroadherin
$\alpha3\beta1$	Laminin, fibronectin, collagen, epiligrin
$\alpha4\beta1$	Fibronectin, VCAM-1
$\alpha5\beta1$	Fibronectin
$\alpha6\beta1$	Laminin
$\alpha7\beta1$	Laminin
$\alpha8\beta1$	Tenascin, nephronectin, fibronectin, vitronectin
$\alpha9\beta1$	Laminin, collagen, tenascin
$\alpha10\beta1$	Collagen
$\alpha v\beta1$	Fibronectin, vitronectin
$\alpha v\beta3$	Vitronectin, fibrinogen, osteopontin, fibronectin, thrombospondin
$\alpha v\beta5$	Vitronectin, fibronectin
$\alpha v\beta6$	Fibronectin, tenascin
$\alpha v\beta8$	Vitronectin, laminin, collagen, fibronectin

lular matrix proteins. These are the β1 subfamily and the αv subfamily. The specificity of extracellular matrix protein binding is determined by both the α and the β subunit, although more than one integrin type can bind to the same matrix protein, often at different sites within the protein. For example, the α1β1, α2β1, α3β1, and α10β1 integrins are all capable of binding collagen, whereas α3β1, α4β1, α5β1, and αvβ3 integrins can all bind fibronectin. In addition, each type of integrin can bind more than one different type of extracellular matrix protein; for example, αvβ3 can bind vitronectin, osteopontin, or fibronectin.

Each connective tissue cell expresses a combination of integrins that is regulated, at least in part, by the mix of proteins present in the extracellular matrix. In addition, integrin expression and affinity for matrix ligands can change in response to cues from the matrix, including stimulation by growth factors and cytokines. The exact function of each particular integrin is currently a topic of investigation by numerous research laboratories. Research in bone has found that the αvβ3 integrin present on osteoclasts plays an important role in the ability of these cells to resorb bone. For this reason, chemical inhibitors of αvβ3 are being tested in early clinical trials for the treatment of osteoporosis.

Binding of extracellular matrix proteins to integrins activates certain signal transduction pathways that regulate cell responses to the matrix, including changes in gene expression. Signaling complexes are formed at sites, often referred to as *focal adhesions,* where close contact is made between the integrins and the extracellular matrix. The signaling complexes include activation of several different pathways involving tyrosine and serine-threonine kinases, phosphoinositide, and arachidonic acid, as well inducing ion fluxes. Accompanying, and intimately tied to, activation of cell signaling are changes in the organization of the cytoskeleton. In this way, integrins can mediate processes that require changes in cytoarchitecture such as cell migration and wound repair. Integrins also provide signals necessary to promote cell survival in cells that require attachment to a matrix to survive. Given the diverse roles of integrins in mediating events important to connective tissue development, repair, and remodeling, studies of integrin function should provide important new information needed to understand connective tissue in health and disease.

SPECIALIZED CONNECTIVE TISSUE STRUCTURES

Cartilage

Cartilage consists of several different types, including hyaline, elastic, and fibrocartilage. Hyaline cartilage includes articular cartilage, which is present at the ends of bones (see Fig. 280–1) and is responsible for the normal smooth gliding motion of the joints. Elastic cartilage, which is more flexible than hyaline cartilage, is found in the external ear and epiglottis. Fibrocartilage is found in the menisci and in ligaments at the site of insertion to bone or where tendons wrap around a bony pulley. Cartilage contains only one cell type, the chondrocyte, which is responsible for the synthesis and breakdown of the cartilage matrix. Very little to no cell division occurs in normal adult cartilage, and so the resident chondrocytes must maintain the tissue for the lifetime of the individual.

The extracellular matrix is very abundant in cartilage, where the cells make up only about 2 to 5% of the volume of the tissue. The matrix contains large amounts of type II collagen and the large aggregating proteoglycan aggrecan (see Fig. 280–2). The high aggrecan content is accompanied by a high water content, thus making cartilage about 70 to 80% water. Articular cartilage must resist compressive forces that occur during joint loading, and so the proteoglycan content is appropriately high. In the superficial region of cartilage, the collagen fibers are arranged parallel to the surface of the tissue to withstand the shear forces occurring at the joint surface during movement. The surface of cartilage is very smooth, with an extremely low coefficient of friction (less than that of ice on ice), which is critical for providing smooth and rapid joint movements. A protein called *superficial zone protein,* produced by chondrocytes and synovial cells, appears to be important for this function. When cartilage is damaged, normal movement is impaired, but pain usually does not result because of the lack of a nerve supply in cartilage. Pain, which occurs during the development of arthritis, results from pathologic lesions in other tissues such as bone, synovium, and the joint capsule.

Tendons and Ligaments

Tendons connect muscle to bone, and ligaments connect bone to bone. Both are composed of connective tissue that must withstand the high tensile loads occurring during movement. Tendons transmit the force from muscle contraction to bone, and the result is movement. Ligaments serve to stabilize joints, thereby allowing for a certain degree and direction of movement but resisting excessive displacement between bones. Tendon and ligament fibroblasts are responsible for synthesis and maintenance of the matrix. Tendons and ligaments contain a very high content of type I collagen, which is found in long and densely packed parallel fibers. The noncollagenous proteins include proteoglycans such as decorin and biglycan, which are much smaller than the aggrecan found in cartilage, a feature that gives them a comparatively reduced water content.

Synovium

The synovium lines diarthrodial joints and is composed of loose connective tissue. In most places within normal joints, the surface area of synovium is only a few cell layers thick. Unlike cartilage, synovium contains blood vessels, lymphatics, and nerves. It is the major source of nutrients for the cartilage and produces many of the major constituents found in the synovial fluid (see Fig. 280–1), including hyaluronic acid. The two types of cells in the synovial matrix are fibroblasts (sometimes called type B synovial cells) and macrophages (type A cells). The synovial fibroblasts are responsible for matrix protein production. The macrophages are responsible for removing cell debris and any microorganisms that could gain entrance. The synovium is a major site of inflammation in arthritic diseases, where it becomes thickened by proliferation of resident cells and by an influx of inflammatory cells from the circulation. In inflammatory arthritis, activated synovial fibroblasts produce enzymes, including the matrix metalloproteinases (MMPs), which degrade joint structures, whereas inflammatory cells produce cytokines, such as tumor necrosis factor-α and interleukin-1 among others, which stimulate MMP production and drive the inflammatory process.

Intervertebral Discs

The intervertebral discs, which assist in movement and provide flexibility to the spine, have distinct regions consisting of the inner nucleus pulposus and an outer fibrotic rim, the annulus, along with an intermediate area between the two. Blood vessels are present in the outer region of the annulus but not in the nucleus pulposus, which must obtain its nutrients by diffusion. The annulus contains denser connective tissue to provide structural support, whereas the nucleus pulposus has a higher water content and is more gel-like. Discs contain both types I and II collagen along with proteoglycans, including aggrecan, found predominately in the nucleus pulposus. The cells in this region more closely resemble chondrocytes, whereas those in the outer fibrotic regions are more similar to fibroblasts. By adulthood, very few cells are present in the nucleus pulposus. This scarcity, along with the changes associated with aging discussed in the next section, make discs very susceptible to degeneration, with an inability to repair damaged matrix.

CHANGES IN CONNECTIVE TISSUES ASSOCIATED WITH AGING

Aging has an important impact on both the structure and function of connective tissues. General age-related changes in connective tissue cells include reductions in mitogenic response and synthetic capacity, likely the result of a diminished cellular response to growth factor stimulation. In the extracellular matrix, modified and, in some cases, degraded matrix components accumulate. The matrix changes appear to decrease the capacity of aging connective tissues to resist tensile forces and to reduce resiliency. Age-related changes in elastin contribute to a loss in tissue elasticity. These changes make connective tissues more susceptible to injury and less capable of repairing damage and in this way contribute to age-associated conditions.

Evidence is mounting that age-related nonenzymatic glycation occurs in the collagen found in several different connective tissue structures, including cartilage, tendons, ligaments, and intervertebral discs. Because collagen has such a long half-life (estimated to be >100 years for type II collagen in cartilage), the progressive accumulation of collagen contains advanced glycation end products, which, in turn, can form intrachain and interchain cross-links that stiffen the collagen fibers. Increased collagen stiffness may contribute to the reduced flexibility noted in ligaments and tendons with age. Although the collagen is stiffer with age, it appears to be less able to resist tensile forces and so could be characterized as being more brittle.

Changes in proteoglycan size and sulfation also occur with age. These changes result in a reduced capacity for binding water, which contributes to an age-related decrease in hydration of connective tissues. Decreases in water content with age have been measured in articular cartilage and in intervertebral discs. Reduced hydration makes the tissues less able to respond to compression. The decreased water content of the discs, along with increased collagen cross-linking from nonenzymatic glycation, may explain why disc herniations are less common in older adults but disc degeneration is more common. Less is known about age-related changes in matrix proteins other than fibrillar collagen and the large proteoglycans. Fibronectin increases in some connective tissues with age, but the consequences of this change are not known.

CONNECTIVE TISSUE DEGRADATION

Connective tissues need to repair and remodel in response to injury, growth, and changes in the biomechanical demands at specific tissue sites. Repair and remodeling of connective tissues require that some components of the tissue be removed and replaced with new components. Healing of wounds in the skin also requires migration of cells into the damaged area, and cell migration is facilitated by matrix degradation. To accomplish these tasks, a set of enzymes capable of degrading extracellular matrix proteins is required (Table 280–4). These enzymes are produced by connective tissue cells and are released, where they act locally to degrade specific matrix components. In certain disease states (e.g., osteoarthritis and rheumatoid arthritis) excess production of matrix-degrading enzymes occurs and overwhelms the capacity of the cells to replace the lost matrix components; the results are net tissue destruction and loss.

The largest family of matrix-degrading enzymes, the MMP family, consists of enzymes that share functional domains, require zinc for activity, and are active at neutral pH. The MMPs either are released into the extracellular matrix or, in some cases, such as the membrane-type MMPs, are directly anchored to the cell. MMP-1, MMP-8, and MMP-13 are collagenases, which are the primary enzymes capable of degrading native collagen, whereas MMP-2 and MMP-9 are gelatinases, which degrade denatured collagen. MMP-3, MMP-10, and MMP-11 are stromelysins responsible for degrading noncollagen proteins such as proteoglycans and fibronectin, whereas MMP-12 functions as an elastase. The membrane-type MMPs can serve to activate other MMPs at the cell surface. More recently discovered members of the MMP family include the ADAMs (*a disintegrin and a metalloproteinase*) and the ADAMTSs (*a disintegrin and a metalloproteinase with a thrombospondin motif*). Enzymes of the ADAMS family are localized to the cell surface, at least in part through the disintegrin domain. ADAM-17 is also known as TACE (tumor necrosis factor-α–converting enzyme) because of its ability to cleave tumor necrosis factor-α to an active form. Finally, the ADAMTSs utilize the thrombospondin motif to interact with proteoglycans, which can serve as substrates for these enzymes. ADAMTS-4 and ADAMTS-5 are aggrecanases that have been shown to cleave the large proteoglycan aggrecan. Studies have suggested that ADAMTS-5 may play an important role in matrix degradation in osteoarthritis.

The MMPs are normally kept in an inactive state by a propeptide region that interacts with the zinc moiety at the active site. Cleavage of the propeptide by other MMPs or members of other protease families results in the release of active enzyme. Further control of MMP activity is provided by specific inhibitors of MMPs present in the extracellular matrix, including the tissue inhibitors of metalloproteinases. The expression of MMPs and tissue inhibitors of metalloproteinases is regulated at the transcriptional level by cytokines, growth factors, and matrix components, including, in some cases, fragments of proteins degraded by MMPs providing for a feedback loop during matrix remodeling.

Other matrix-degrading enzymes are the serine proteases, which include plasmin and elastase, the aspartic proteases, which include pepsin and cathepsin D, and the cysteine proteases, including papain and cathepsins B, C, K, L, and S. Plasmin, the cleavage product of plasminogen, can cleave MMP propeptides and can result in MMP activation. Elastase, often a product of neutrophils, can degrade elastin and some fibrillar col-

TABLE 280–4 MATRIX-DEGRADING ENZYMES

Proteinase	Substrates
MATRIX METALLOPROTEINASES (MMPs)	
MMP-1, MMP-8, MMP-13 (collagenase 1, 2, 3)	Fibrillar collagens, fibronectin, aggrecan
MMP-3, MMP-10, MMP-11 (stromelysin 1, 2, 3)	Proteoglycan, procollagenase, fibronectin
MMP-2, MMP-9 (gelatinase A, B)	Denatured collagen, aggrecan, fibronectin
MMP-7 (matrilysin)	Proenzymes, fibronectin, other matrix proteins
MMP-12 (macrophage elastase)	Elastin, fibronectin, laminin
MMP-14, MMP-15, MMP-16, MMP-17 (MT1-MT4-MMP)	Procollagenase
ADAM-17 (TACE)	Tumor necrosis factor-α
ADAMTS-4, ADAMTS-5 (aggrecanase 1, 2)	Aggrecan
SERINE PROTEASES	
Plasmin	Fibrin, pro-MMPs
Plasminogen activators	Plasminogen
Neutrophil elastase	Elastin
CYSTEINE PROTEASES	
Cathepsin K	Type I collagen
Cathepsin B	Broad specificity
ASPARTATE PROTEASES	
Cathepsin D	Aggrecan, denatured collagen
Pepsin	Broad specificity

ADAM = a disintegrin and a metalloproteinase; ADAMTS = a disintegrin and a metalloproteinase with a thrombospondin motif; MT-MMP = membrane type-MMP; TACE = tumor necrosis factor-α–converting enzyme.
Adapted from Mort JS, Poole AR: Mediators of inflammation, tissue destruction, and repair. D. Proteases and their inhibitors. *In* Klippel JH (ed): Primer on the Rheumatic Diseases, 12th ed. Atlanta, Arthritis Foundation, 2001, pp 72–81.

lagens. Cathepsin K has been recognized as a key mediator of bone resorption, where it functions to cleave collagen under the acidic conditions found at the osteoclast ruffled border. As with the MMPs, production and secretion of these proteases are controlled by signals from growth factors, cytokines, and matrix components. Thus, a fine and intricate balance connective tissues controls the integrity of the tissue and the response to injury. This balance is disturbed in disease states that cause connective tissue destruction.

Research advances that have improved our knowledge of the biology of connective tissue are being applied in the design of new therapies. We are witnessing the emergence of anticytokine therapies, such as anti–tumor necrosis factor-α and antagonists to interleukin-1 aimed not only at reducing inflammation in connective tissues but also at halting tissue destruction. Growth factors capable of stimulating repair are being studied for treatment of chronic wounds, nonhealing bone defects, and cartilage lesions. Small molecule inhibitors of MMPs and other matrix-degrading enzymes are in development and early testing. Finally, advances in tissue engineering should make it possible to reconstruct or replace many damaged connective tissue structures. Undifferentiated mesenchymal precursor cells found in the bone marrow and some connective tissues, including adipose tissue, can be induced in vitro to differentiate into cells capable of producing bone, cartilage, muscle, or adipose tissue, depending on culture conditions. These exciting advances will certainly lead to better treatments for the many common conditions affecting connective tissues.

SUGGESTED READINGS

Baroni SS, Santillo M, Bevilacqua F, et al: Stimulatory autoantibodies to the PDGF receptor in systemic sclerosis. N Engl J Med 2006;354:2667–2676. *Stimulatory autoantibodies against PDGF receptor have a causal role in the pathogenesis of systemic sclerosis.*

Bornstein P, Sage EH: Matricellular proteins: Extracellular modulators of cell function. Curr Opin Cell Biol 2002;14:608–616. *A review of the extracellular matrix proteins that mediate interactions between the cell and the matrix.*

Kresse H, Schonherr E: Proteoglycans of the extracellular matrix and growth control. J Cell Physiol 2001;189:266–274. *Describes the mechanisms by which proteoglycans regulate cellular functions, including interactions with growth factors.*

Sakkas LI, Chikanza IC, Platsoucas CD: Mechanisms of disease: The role of immune cells in the pathogenesis of systemic sclerosis. Nat Clin Pract Rheumatol 2006;2:679–685. *Review of the immune mechanisms involved in the pathogenesis of scleroderma.*

Stamenkovic I: Extracellular matrix remodeling: the role of matrix metalloproteinases. J Pathol 2003;200:448–464. *Review of the MMP family of matrix-degrading enzymes and their involvement in processes that involve remodeling of connective tissue extracellular matrix.*

Wehrle-Haller B, Imhof BA: Integrin-dependent pathologies. J Pathol 2003;200:481–487. *Review of integrin structure and function and conditions discovered to result from integrin defects.*

281 INHERITED DISEASES OF CONNECTIVE TISSUE

Reed E. Pyeritz

MUCOPOLYSACCHARIDOSES

Definition

Proteoglycans are ubiquitous components of the extracellular matrix (ECM) and the surfaces of cells, and they are among the largest and most complex of human molecules. Proteoglycans consist of a protein core to which are covalently bound glycosaminoglycans (GAG; formerly called mucopolysaccharides) of several types: dermatan sulfate, heparan sulfate, keratan sulfate, and chondroitin sulfate. These four polymeric molecules are cleaved from their protein core in lysosomes; then they, plus hyaluronan (a GAG lacking a protein core), are catabolized further in lysosomes in a stepwise fashion by more than a dozen enzymes. Genetic defects in any one of these enzymes lead to the accumulation of GAG metabolites in lysosomes, with profound disruption of cellular physiology. The phenotypes resulting from deficiencies of these catabolic enzymes are termed *mucopolysaccharidoses* (MPSs) and are classified into seven types (Table 281–1). Several additional storage disorders, termed *mucolipidoses* (MLs), are caused by a genetic defect in post-translational modification of lysosomal enzymes and share features with the MPS.

Epidemiology

All MPS disorders are rare, each with an incidence of 1 or fewer cases per 100,000 births, and are without ethnic predilection.

Pathobiology

With the exception of MPS II (Hunter's syndrome), which is X-linked, each of these disorders is autosomal recessive. All MPSs are caused by deficiency of a single lysosomal enzyme responsible for a specific step in GAG metabolism. Catabolism of GAG proceeds normally until the step requiring the defective enzyme, where further normal metabolism halts. Although a minor degree of nonspecific breakdown occurs, resulting in urinary excretion of cleaved GAG that can be useful diagnostically, the accumulation of GAG within lysosomes of cells of mesenchymal origin, endothelium, and, in most cases, neurons causes widespread, progressive cellular dysfunction and clinical effects. Lysosomal enzymes are targeted to lysosomes by posttranslational addition of mannose 6-phosphate. Deficiency of the phosphotransferase that catalyzes the first step in this reaction results in an inability to catabolize any GAG molecules. The catabolic enzymes, which normally would be transported into lysosomes, instead are secreted from the cell and are found in unusually high concentrations in plasma, providing one diagnostic test for ML.

Section XXII Rheumatology

Pathology

All pathologic manifestations of MPS and ML disorders worsen with age, and some are present from early developmental stages. Gross anatomic hallmarks are hepatosplenomegaly, marked skeletal alterations (termed *dysostosis multiplex*) that result in short stature and thoracic cage deformity, thickening and narrowing of airways and arteries, and coarsening of facial features. Although mental retardation is a prominent feature of some of these conditions, the brain may show only ventriculomegaly secondary to communicating hydrocephalus. On microscopy, mesenchymal cells show a cytoplasm full of apparently empty vacuoles; these are lysosomes from which GAG has been removed by fixation. Cells cultured from patients show greatly enlarged lysosomes filled with granular material. In the severe form of ML, dense inclusions are present, which gave rise to the common name, *I-cell disease.*

Clinical Manifestations

Each of the disorders in Table 281–1 shows a wide spectrum of clinical severity. This wide spectrum has led to a classification that gives the impression of separate disorders within some of the MPS and ML types, but these represent the apparent ends of the continuum. Some of the disorders result in death by adolescence (Hurler syndrome, severe Hunter syndrome, ML II), whereas others are commonly compatible with survival to adulthood. The latter group of disorders is emphasized here.

The milder end of the MPS I spectrum, Scheie's syndrome, may not be diagnosed until adulthood; patients present with stiffened joints, corneal clouding and glaucoma, carpal tunnel syndrome, and aortic valvular disease. Stature and intelligence are not affected. The main health risks are valvular involvement, thickening of meninges that can produce a myelopathy, and thickening of the upper airways that can produce obstructive symptoms and sleep apnea.

The milder form of MPS II, Hunter's syndrome, is distinctive because it is X-linked (affecting males almost exclusively), and the cornea shows little overt clouding. Cervical myelopathy, obstructive airway disease, and cor pulmonale are important concerns. A combined conductive-neurosensory hearing loss is common.

Neither MPS IV (Morquio's syndrome) nor MPS VI (Maroteaux-Lamy syndrome) affects intelligence. Both syndromes often are associated with severe skeletal changes, which are distinct radiographically but produce similar problems of kyphoscoliosis, pectus carinatum, restrictive lung disease, severe short stature, and joint degeneration. Cervical myelopathy

TABLE 281–1 MUCOPOLYSACCHARIDOSES AND MUCOLIPIDOSES

Type	Eponym or Common Name	Clinical Features	Inheritance	OMIM*	Enzymatic Defect
MPS IH	Hurler's syndrome	DM and short stature; MR; corneal clouding; HS; heart disease; death in childhood	AR	252800	α-L-iduronidase
MPS IS	Scheie's syndrome	Coarse facies; stiff joints, corneal clouding; aortic valve disease; normal intelligence and lifespan	AR	252800	α-L-iduronidase
MPS II	Hunter's syndrome	Severe form: coarse facies, DM and short stature, HS; MR; no corneal clouding; death by late adolescence Mild form: coarse facies, short stature; normal intelligence; survival to adulthood	XL	309900	Iduronate sulfatase
MPS IIIA	Sanfilippo's A	Severe MR and hyperactivity; mild somatic changes	AR	252900	Heparan *N*-sulfatase
MPS IIIB	Sanfilippo's B	Same as MPS IIIA	AR	252920	α-*N*-acetylglucosaminidase
MPS IIIC	Sanfilippo's C	Same as MPS IIIA	AR	252930	Acetyl-coenzyme A: α-glucosaminide acetyltransferase
MPS IIID	Sanfilippo's D	Same as MPS IIIA	AR	252940	*N*-acetylglucosamine 6-sulfatase
MPS IVA	Morquio's A	Short stature and distinct skeletal dysplasia with odontoid hypoplasia and myelopathy; corneal clouding; normal intelligence; valvular heart disease	AR	253000	Galactose 6-sulfatase
MPS IVB	Morquio's B	Same as MPS IVA	AR	253010	β-Galactosidase
MPS VI	Maroteaux-Lamy	DM and short stature; corneal clouding; normal intelligence; aortic stenosis; leukocyte inclusions; hydrocephalus in severe form	AR	253200	*N*-acetylgalactosamine
MPS VII	Sly's syndrome	DM; HS; widely variable, including MR	AR	253220	β-Glucuronidase
MPS IX	—	Short stature; periarticular soft tissue masses	AR	601492	Hyaluronidase
ML II	I-cell disease	Similar to but more severe than MPS IH but with cellular inclusions; no mucopolysacchariduria	AR	252500	UDP-*N*-acetylglucosamine: lysosomal enzyme *N*-acetylglucosaminyl-1-phosphotransferase
ML III	Pseudo-Hurler polydystrophy	Short stature and mild DM; stiff joints, arthropathy, coarse facies; variable but mild MR; survival to adulthood	AR	252500	Same as ML II

*Entries in Online Mendelian Inheritance in Man, OMIM. Bethesda, MD, National Center for Biotechnology Information, National Library of Medicine. Available at: www.ncbi.nlm.nih.gov/omim/ (accessed Feb 28, 2007).
AR = autosomal recessive; DM = dysostosis multiplex; HS = hepatosplenomegaly; MR = mental retardation; XL = X-linked.

resulting from a thickened dura is common to both disorders and is accentuated by odontoid hypoplasia in MPS IV. Thickening of the aortic and mitral valves may produce severe dysfunction necessitating their replacement. General anesthesia is especially hazardous because of the narrow upper and middle airways and cervical instability.

Patients with ML III (pseudo-Hurler polydystrophy) resemble patients with MPS VI but often have mild-to-moderate mental retardation. Aortic regurgitation is common.

Diagnosis

Differential Diagnosis

Diagnosis of these conditions is difficult in the young child, before most of the clinical features have progressed, but should be considered in any person with hepatosplenomegaly and coarsening of the facial features. Evaluation requires a pedigree analysis, skeletal radiographic survey, echocardiogram, and analysis of the urine for excretion of GAGs. Often the specific MPS is evident from radiographs, the presence or absence of corneal clouding, and the pattern of mucopolysacchariduria. Enzymatic analysis of leukocytes confirms the diagnosis. Patients with MLs do not show mucopolysacchariduria but have marked elevation of all the GAG catabolic lysosomal enzymes in plasma.

Treatment

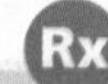

Ventriculoperitoneal shunting is necessary if intracranial pressure is elevated. Close attention to hearing and visual problems is essential throughout life. Many adults with MPS or ML require surgery for carpal tunnel. Cardiovascular surgery for valvular or coronary disease may be necessary. All use of anesthesia is high risk because of the narrow airways and, in the case of MPS IV, atlantoaxial instability. For patients who remain ambulatory, selective joint replacement can be beneficial. Because of the morbidity associated with thoracic cage deformity, consideration should be given to stabilizing the spinal deformity before it becomes severe.

Replacement of the deficient enzyme via intravenous infusion is being studied for most of the MPS disorders. Laronidase (Aldurazyme) has been approved in the United States for treatment of MPS I. An infusion every 2 weeks for 1 year in adolescent and adult patients resulted in substantial reduction in hepatosplenomegaly and modest improvement in pulmonary function, sleep apnea, and joint mobility. Whether early institution of therapy in young children modulates mental retardation in the Hurler variant

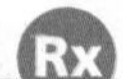

of MPS I is uncertain. Galsulfase (Naglazyme) has been approved for the treatment of MPS VI, in which somatic rather than neurologic problems predominate. Bone marrow transplantation has been attempted in many of the MPS disorders, with mixed success. The earlier transplantation occurs, the better the outcome in terms of somatic problems, but prevention of mental retardation has not occurred.

MARFAN SYNDROME

Definition

Marfan syndrome is an autosomal dominant, pleiotropic disorder caused by defects in the principal component of the extracellular microfibril, the large glycoprotein fibrillin-1. The disease manifestations occur in multiple systems, especially the eye, skeleton, heart, aorta, lung, and integument. Notable features include dislocation of the ocular lens, tall stature with particularly long limbs and digits, deformity of the thoracic cage from pectus carinatum or excavatum with abnormal curvature of the spine, mitral and tricuspid valve prolapse, dilation of the sinuses of Valsalva and predisposition to aortic dissection, spontaneous pneumothorax, abnormal skin stretch marks, hernias, and dural ectasia. If untreated, patients often die before 30 or 40 years of age from aortic dissection or congestive heart failure.

Epidemiology

Marfan syndrome is a common mendelian disorder, with an estimated incidence of about 1 per 5000 births. Marfan syndrome is found throughout the world, without ethnic or geographic predilection.

Pathobiology

Pathogenesis

Mutations in *FBN1,* which maps to human chromosome 15q21.1 and encodes fibrillin-1, cause Marfan syndrome and related connective tissue disorders. More than 800 distinct mutations have been found, and few occur in more than one family. Patients are heterozygous for mutations in *FBN1,* leading to autosomal dominant inheritance. Extracellular microfibrils are polymers of many fibrillin-1 molecules and are ubiquitous in the ECM of most tissues. Latent transforming growth factor-β (TGF-β) binding protein, which keeps the cytokine inactive, bears striking homology to regions of fibrillin. Abnormalities of either the quality or the quantity of microfibrils disrupt normal signaling by TGF-β, especially during embryonic development and postnatal growth. Recent studies in mice engineered to harbor human mutations in *FBN1* showed that excessive TGF-β signaling causes abnormal lung septation (the precursor to pneumothorax), mitral valve prolapse, muscular hypoplasia, and aortic dilatation. This fundamental shift in understanding of the pathogenesis of Marfan syndrome has suggested novel therapies, such as with small molecules that affect the activity of TGF-β.

The features of Marfan syndrome are highly variable, even among relatives who share the same mutation in *FBN1.* This variability persists after accounting for the effects of age. Men tend to be affected more severely, for unclear reasons.

Pathology

The features of Marfan syndrome are age dependent. Some severely affected infants have flagrant features and often die of mitral regurgitation and heart failure despite aggressive management. At the other end of the clinical spectrum, Marfan syndrome merges with several related disorders, and patients may not come to medical attention, let alone receive a definitive diagnosis, until adulthood.

None of the gross or microscopic pathologic changes is specific for Marfan syndrome. The medial degeneration of the aortic wall, characterized by disarray and fragmentation of the elastic fibers and increased proteoglycan (often inappropriately termed *cystic medial necrosis*) also can be seen in other disorders and in older people with hypertension. Aortic dissection usually begins just superior to the aortic valve (type A) and often progresses to the bifurcation. Death usually results from retrograde dissection and hemopericardium. About 10% of dissections begin in the descending thoracic aorta (type B).

Clinical Manifestations

The lens tends to be displaced superiorly, and usually the zonules remain intact. The retina is at increased risk of detachment, especially in patients who are highly myopic. Tubular bones overgrow, accounting for the disproportionate tall stature (dolichostenomelia), long digits (arachnodactyly), and sternal deformity. Ligaments may be lax, causing scoliosis and joint hypermobility. Alternatively, congenital contractures are common, especially of the elbows and digits. The palate typically is highly arched, and the dentition can be crowded and maloccluded. Mitral valve prolapse occurs in about 80% of cases, and the valve leaflets become progressively thickened (myxomatous on histopathology). The mitral annulus may dilate and calcify. Aortic root dilation begins in the sinuses of Valsalva and progresses with age, albeit at highly variable rates. Most males with Marfan syndrome have an aortic root dimension above the upper limit of normal for their body surface area by adolescence. Some females show a slower progression and may have a root diameter near the upper limit of normal well into adulthood. The dilation usually does not involve the distal ascending aorta. Spontaneous pneumothorax, resulting from rupture of apical blebs, occurs in about 5% of patients. Stretch marks (striae atrophicae) occur over areas of flexural stress, such as the shoulders, breasts, and lower back. The neural canal in the lumbosacral region is enlarged in most people with Marfan syndrome; this may be visible on plain radiographs, especially if the neuroforamina are widened. Imaging by computed tomography or magnetic resonance imaging is diagnostic and should be used in patients with back pain and radicular symptoms. Large anterior meningoceles in the pelvis are a severe manifestation of dural ectasia. Simple cysts in the liver and kidneys are common, increase with age, and seldom cause clinical problems.

Diagnosis

Differential Diagnosis

The conditions that overlap clinically and genetically with Marfan syndrome include familial aortic aneurysm, familial ectopia lentis, MASS phenotype (which includes many families with mitral valve prolapse syndrome), and Loeys-Dietz syndrome. Most of these conditions are diagnosed clinically, so differentiating among them is arbitrary. A careful family history is essential to this process. Molecular genetic testing has a limited role. However, if the mutation in *FBN1* is known in a family, analysis of DNA can be used effectively for presymptomatic or prenatal diagnosis. Loeys-Dietz syndrome, which is associated with generalized arterial tortuosity and susceptibility to dissection, is caused by mutation in either of two receptors for TGF-β, *TGFBR1* and *TGFBR2,* and molecular analysis is clinically available.

A question of Marfan syndrome arises most commonly in the tall, lanky adolescent who has several minor skeletal features, nearsightedness, and athletic desires. A detailed ophthalmologic examination with full pupillary dilation and a transthoracic echocardiogram are essential components in the evaluation. If these tests are negative and no one in the family has a history of Marfan syndrome or aortic dissection, the patient probably can be reassured.

Treatment

Life expectancy in Marfan syndrome has improved markedly, to the point that many patients can expect survival to advanced years. All patients should be seen at least annually by a physician who manages the overall care. Most patients require annual ophthalmologic and cardiologic consultation and orthopedic consultation as required by specific problems. A number of studies, but only one randomized clinical trial [1], support the prophylactic use of β-adrenergic blockade from an early age to slow the rate of aortic

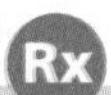

root dilation and protect against aortic dissection. Prophylactic surgical repair of the aortic root has had the greatest beneficial impact. The composite graft, involving a prosthetic valve in a Dacron tube and implantation of the coronary ostia into the graft, was the first approach to produce markedly improved survival in these patients. More recently, replacement of the aneurysm and preservation of the native aortic valve have shown promise. For the adult, aortic root surgery should be recommended when the maximal aortic diameter reaches 50 mm, and a strong family history of aortic dissection should prompt earlier repair.

EHLERS-DANLOS SYNDROMES

Definition

The Ehlers-Danlos syndromes (EDSs) are clinically variable and genetically heterogeneous. Diagnoses still are based largely on the bedside examination, and the classification scheme and diagnostic criteria have been revised recently. The unifying themes among these disorders are fragility of tissues, joint hypermobility, and skin hyperextensibility.

Epidemiology

No accurate data exist, but an incidence of about 1 in 5000 births is a reasonable estimate of how many individuals qualify for one of the EDS diagnoses. Each type represents something of a clinical spectrum, with the mild end merging with what might be considered normal variation. Just as the diagnostic criteria are arbitrary, so would be any determination of prevalence based on phenotypic criteria. The extent to which normal variation in joint hypermobility, skin elasticity, and tissue fragility represents genetic variation at loci that encode collagen or other ECM genes requires considerable research.

Pathobiology

Pathogenesis

Defects in collagen and other proteins in the ECM of various tissues underlie all forms of EDS that have been elucidated so far. The specific genetic mutations occur in a variety of genes, with the effect of altering the structure, synthesis, post-translational modifications, or stability of the collagens involved. The known molecular defects are listed in Table 281–2.

Pathology

Few findings in the routine pathologic evaluation distinguish among the various types of EDS or even distinguish individual types from normal. Thickness of the dermis is decreased in some forms, especially the vascular type, and the walls of arteries are reduced in thickness in this type. By electron microscopy, the classic, hypermobile, and kyphoscoliotic types have abnormal collagen fibers, especially when viewed in cross section (variable and often increased fiber diameter with an irregular outline). In the vascular type, some patients have dilated endoplasmic reticulum consistent with aberrant secretion of type III collagen molecules.

TABLE 281–2 EHLERS-DANLOS SYNDROMES

Type	Former Name	Clinical Features*	Inheritance	OMIM†	Molecular Defect
Classic	EDS I and II	Joint hypermobility; skin hyperextensibility; atrophic scars; smooth, velvety skin; subcutaneous spheroids	AD	130000 130010	Structure of type V collagen ?*COL5A1, COL5A2*
Hypermobility	EDS III	Joint hypermobility; some skin hyperextensibility, with or without smooth,velvety texture	AD AR	130020 225320	? Tenascin-X *(TNX)*
Vascular	EDS IV	Thin skin; easy bruising; pinched nose; acrogeria; rupture of large-caliber and medium-caliber arteries, uterus, and large bowel	AD	130050 (225350) (225360)	Deficient type III collagen *(COL3A1)*
Kyphoscoliotic	EDS VI	Joint hypermobility; congenital, progressive rupture; scoliosis; scleral fragility with globe rupture; tissue fragility, aortic dilation, MVP	AR	225400	Deficiency of lysyl hydroxylase
Arthrochalasis	EDS VII A and B	Joint hypermobility, severe, with subluxations, congenital hip dislocation; skin hyperextensibility; tissue fragility	AD	130060	No cleavage of amino terminus of type I procollagen due to mutations in *COL1A1* or *COL1A2*
Dermatosparaxis	EDS VII C	Severe skin fragility; decreased skin elasticity, easy bruising; hernias; premature rupture of fetal membranes	AR	225410	No cleavage of amino terminus of type I procollagen due to deficiency of peptidase
Unclassified types	EDS V EDS VIII EDS X EDS XI EDS IX EDS, progeroid form	Classic features Classic features and periodontal disease Mild classic features, MVP Joint instability Classic features; occipital horns Classic features and premature aging	XL AD ? AD XL AR	305200 130080 225310 147900 309400 130700	? ? ? ? Allelic to Menkes' syndrome Deficiency of galactosyltransferase I

*Listed in order of diagnostic importance.
†Entries in Online Mendelian Inheritance in Man, OMIM. Bethesda, MD, National Center for Biotechnology Information, National Library of Medicine. Available at: www.ncbi.nlm.nih.gov/omim/ (accessed Feb 28, 2007).
AD = autosomal dominant; AR = autosomal recessive; EDS = Ehlers-Danlos syndrome; MVP = mitral valve prolapse; XL = X-linked.

Clinical Manifestations

The major and minor features of each EDS are detailed in Table 281–2. Infants with classic EDS often are born prematurely by 4 to 8 weeks because of rupture of fetal membranes. Diagnosis of the vascular and kyphoscoliotic types is important because of their cardiovascular features. The vascular type, previously termed *EDS IV*, is characterized by a troublesome tendency toward spontaneous rupture of large arteries and hollow organs, especially the colon and uterus. Because these events carry considerable morbidity, life expectancy is reduced, on average, by more than half. During pregnancy, women with this form of EDS are especially vulnerable to rupture of major arteries and the uterus. In the kyphoscoliotic type, aortic root dilation and aortic regurgitation can develop. Patients with most forms of EDS are prone to develop mitral valve prolapse, and progression to mitral regurgitation occurs more often than in the common form of mitral valve prolapse.

Diagnosis

Differential Diagnosis

By carefully adherence to the clinical features shown in Table 281–2 and judicious use of laboratory tests, the various defined types of EDS can be differentiated. Many specific non-EDS syndromes need to be excluded. The kyphoscoliotic type of EDS in infants shares some features with severe Marfan syndrome. Patients with Larsen's syndrome may resemble patients with the arthrochalasis type of EDS. The skin redundancy and loss of elasticity of the dermatosparaxis type of EDS is reminiscent of autosomal dominant cutis laxa, which is not associated with easy bruising or tissue fragility.

The most difficult decision is whether any diagnosis of EDS is warranted. Patients who have only joint hypermobility without skin changes should not be labeled with EDS; a diagnosis of familial joint hypermobility might be more appropriate. Familial joint instability involves a predisposition to dislocations of major joints that is rare in most types of EDS except for arthrochalasis.

Treatment

Rx

Management of most skin and joint problems should be conservative and preventive. Sutures need to be placed with careful attention to approximating the margins and avoiding tension; removable sutures should be left in place for twice the usual time. Most instances of joint hypermobility and pain in EDS do not require surgical treatment. Benefit often is derived from physical therapy designed to strengthen the muscles that provide support for the loose ligaments. All patients should receive genetic counseling about the mode of inheritance and their risk of having children affected with EDS. The possibility of prenatal diagnosis exists for all of the EDS types with defined molecular or biochemical defects.

The vascular type of EDS requires particular surgical care; the ruptured arteries are difficult to repair because of the pronounced vascular fragility. Rupture of the bowel is a surgical emergency. Because the risk of uterine and vascular rupture is especially high during pregnancy in women with the vascular form, affected women should be advised that there is a substantial risk of death related to pregnancy and delivery. Patients should be advised to avoid contact sports and to treat blood pressure elevations aggressively. Arteriography and arterial lines should be avoided if possible. Biochemical and genetic screening holds the potential for reassuring relatives at risk that they do not have a defect in type III collagen.

The kyphoscoliotic type of EDS may improve with large doses of ascorbic acid (1 to 4 g/day), because vitamin C is a cofactor for the enzyme that is deficient. No other metabolic or genetic therapy is effective in other forms of EDS.

OSTEOGENESIS IMPERFECTA SYNDROMES

Definition

The heterogeneous group of disorders called *osteogenesis imperfecta* (OI) includes, at one end of the severity spectrum, a type that is lethal prenatally or in the neonatal period and, at the other, such mild features that distinguishing affected individuals from the general population is difficult. The unifying feature is hereditary osteopenia (insufficient bone), with primary defects in the protein matrix in bone and other tissues. The clinical syndromes all involve osteoporosis with liability to fracture.

Epidemiology

No careful epidemiologic study has been performed, and the milder forms of type I OI merge with the phenotypes of familial osteoporosis, fracture susceptibility, and joint hypermobility found in the general population. A crude estimate of the overall prevalence of OI is 1 to 2 per 20,000 births. The neonatal lethal form (type II), which is almost always caused by a new mutation in a parental gamete, has an incidence of about 1 in 50,000 births.

Pathobiology

Pathogenesis

Patients in whom mutations have been found all have defects in the two genes that encode the procollagen chains of type I collagen, *COL1A1* and *COL1A2*. Type I collagen is composed of two α1(I) and one α2(I) procollagen chains; the mature fiber requires considerable post-translational modification, which occurs appropriately only if the three procollagen chains have intertwined to form a triple helix that is perfect and completed at the right speed. A mutation that affects formation of the triple helix, such as substitution of one of the mandatory glycine residues that occurs at every third position, also has adverse effects on the modifications that render the molecule capable of forming effective mature fibers. As a result, a single nucleotide change resulting in a missense mutation can have profound effects on the ECM and produce a severe condition. Alternatively, and at first glance paradoxically, a mutation that eliminates an entire allele, or at least production of any product capable of intertwining with normal procollagen chains, has a much milder effect on the ECM and on the severity of OI. Examples of the most common classes of mutations are shown in Table 281–3. Hundreds of mutations have been described.

Pathology

Other than the gross pathology associated with the clinical manifestations, the most characteristic pathology is a primary reduction in bone matrix with secondary undermineralization.

Clinical Manifestations

The major phenotypic features of OI are shown in Table 281–3. The most severe type is type II, followed in decreasing order by types III, IV, and I. In type II, infants either are stillborn or die soon after birth of pulmonary failure secondary to the small thorax, which usually is compromised further by myriad rib fractures. A few infants have survived for at least a few years but require enormous attention to their medical needs.

Type III OI may be confused with type II at birth, but survival alone helps make the distinction. Bony deformity is pronounced and not necessarily due to fractures. Mobility is impaired, and most patients require a wheelchair at an early age. Stature may be severely compromised. Because of progressive vertebral column deformity and rib fractures, restrictive lung disease is a common problem as patients age; many die of pulmonary complications. Basilar impression causing compression of the brain stem and the craniocervical junction can produce central sleep apnea, headache, and upper motor neuron signs.

Patients with type IV OI generally have reduced stature, some bony deformity, and abnormal teeth that are opalescent and wear easily (dentinogenesis imperfecta). As in type I OI, the tendency to fracture is highest in childhood and lessens with adolescence. A distinguishing characteristic of type IV OI is a normal scleral hue.

Type I OI is probably the most common form and is associated with a bluish or blue-gray scleral hue. People with type I OI who also have dentinogenesis imperfecta tend to have more severe skeletal problems. The risk of fracture diminishes during adulthood but reemerges as a

TABLE 281–3 OSTEOGENESIS IMPERFECTA

Type	Clinical Features	Inheritance	OMIM*	Basic Defects
I	Fractures variable in number; little deformity; stature normal or nearly so; blue sclerae; hearing loss common but not always present; DI uncommon	AD	166200	Typically, one nonfunctional *COL1A1* allele
II	Lethal in utero or shortly after birth; many fractures at birth typically involving ribs (may appear "beaded") and other long bones; little calvaria; pulmonary hypertension	AD	166210	*COL1A1* or *COL1A2:* substitution of glycyl residues; occasionally deletions of a portion of the triple-helical domain
		AR	259400	Deletion in *COL1A2* plus a nonfunctional allele
III	Fractures common, but long bones progressively deform starting in utero; stature markedly reduced; sclerae often blue but become lighter with age; DI and hearing loss common	AD	259420	One single-amino acid substitution
		AR (rare)	259440	Two mutations in *COL1A1* and/or *COL1A2* (rarely)
IV	Fractures common; stature usually reduced; bone deformity common but rarely severe; scleral hue normal to grayish; hearing loss variable; DI common	AD	166220	Point mutations in *COL1A1* or *COL1A2*
			166240	Exon skipping mutations in *COL1A2*

*Entries in Online Mendelian Inheritance in Man, OMIM. Bethesda, MD, National Center for Biotechnology Information, National Library of Medicine. Available at: www.ncbi.nlm.nih.gov/omim/ (accessed Feb 28, 2007).
AD = autosomal dominant; AR = autosomal recessive; DI = dentinogenesis imperfecta.

major concern for women after menopause. Hearing impairment in all forms of OI is common and age related, being rare before adolescence. The deficits are of either a mixed or a predominantly conductive form.

Diagnosis

Differential Diagnosis

The range of diagnostic possibilities in a person with multiple fractures largely depends on age. In infancy, the genetic conditions hypophosphatasia, severe osteochondrodysplasias (e.g., achondrogenesis and forms of spondyloepiphyseal dysplasia), and Menkes' syndrome need to be excluded when a diagnosis of type II or type III OI is considered. The radiographic features eventually become entirely diagnostic, but often the neonatologist has to arrive at a definitive answer in short order. Analysis of serum alkaline phosphatase and copper can be helpful. In childhood, the most common situation leading to consideration of a mild form of OI is child abuse. In this situation, the pattern of fracture is usually distinct, and bone mineralization should be normal if the child is the object of nonaccidental or repeated accidental trauma. Abnormal scleral hue, dentinogenesis imperfecta, and wormian bones (microfractures along the cranial sutures) all support the diagnosis of OI. The legal and child-protective systems often request exclusion of OI by analysis of collagen production from cultured skin fibroblasts.

In older children, the disorder idiopathic juvenile osteoporosis should be considered in any patient seen initially with repeated fractures. Occasionally, studies of skin fibroblasts are needed to document whether a defect in type I collagen (which would be characteristic of OI) is present. Many osteochondrodysplasias are associated with short stature, skeletal deformity, and a tendency to fracture. Pyknodysostosis and osteopetrosis are associated with sclerotic bones rather than osteoporotic ones. In adulthood, early-onset osteoporosis may be confused with OI. Mutations in type I collagen also cause familial osteoporosis, and the skeletal phenotypes merge; patients with true OI may have scleral, hearing, or dental abnormalities and a positive family history.

Treatment

Rx

Management of the skeletal complications largely depends on orthopedic, physical, and occupational therapy approaches. Although no medical treatment has yet been demonstrated to improve the quality of the bone, studies of mesenchymal stem cell transplantation and bisphosphonates are under way. The long-term goals are for the patient to maintain function and independence as an individual. These goals can be advanced in some patients by judicious use of intramedullary rods in the long bones of the legs; if mobility and especially ambulation can be maintained, the demineralization associated with inactivity can be avoided.

Unaffected parents of a child with OI and all affected individuals should have genetic counseling. For the parents of a child with type II OI, the possibility of germinal mosaicism (which has been well documented in this condition) should not be overlooked. If one parent has a "new" mutation in one of the type I procollagen genes and multiple gonadal cells carry this mutation, the risk of recurrence in future children is not negligible. If the mutation in the affected child can be defined, the risk of recurrence can be quantified (through molecular analysis of sperm) if the mutation arose in the father.

PSEUDOXANTHOMA ELASTICUM

Definition

Pseudoxanthoma elasticum (PXE) is a heritable disorder of connective tissue with pleiotropic manifestations wherever elastic fibers are found but primarily in the skin, eye, and vasculature. Life expectancy is reduced, on average, because of a predisposition to myocardial infarction and gastrointestinal hemorrhage.

Epidemiology

The exact frequency of PXE is unknown, but it is probably underdiagnosed. Rough approximations suggest a prevalence of 1 in 25,000 to 100,000 births. Males and females are equally affected, although women are more likely to seek medical attention out of concern for the skin changes.

Pathobiology

Pathogenesis

In most families, PXE occurs as an autosomal recessive trait, which means, given relatively small sibships, that many patients will have no affected relatives. Apparent autosomal dominant inheritance may reflect expression in occasional heterozygotes. The gene for PXE maps to human chromosome 16 and encodes one of the adenosine triphosphate (ATP)-binding cassette transporters *(ABCC6)*. Because of the prominent histopathologic feature of calcification of elastic tissue, this gene may be important in calcium homeostasis. It is unclear, however, whether calcification is a primary or a secondary phenomenon in PXE.

Pathology

The hallmark of PXE, and an important diagnostic clue, is the histopathologic finding of hyperproliferated elastic fibers in the mid-dermis; these fibers become fragmented, clumped, and calcified. An arteriolar sclerosis develops in the media of muscular arteries and arterioles; the lumen may become progressively and concentrically narrowed. Alternatively, microaneurysms can form. Thickening of the endocardium, especially the atrial endocardium, develops in some patients. In the eye, Bruch's membrane becomes calcified and fragmented.

Clinical Manifestations

Because of the pleiotropic nature of PXE, the diagnosis initially may be suspected by any of a variety of clinicians, especially dermatologists, ophthalmologists, cardiologists, and gastroenterologists. The condition gains its name from the dermatologic feature of yellowish papules that appear at areas of flexural stress, especially the neck, groin, and popliteal and cubital fossae; in periumbilical regions; and on the buccal mucosa. The appearance of affected skin has been likened to that of a "plucked chicken." Over time, affected areas coalesce and become thickened.

Changes in the eye begin as a generalized, subtle, mottled pattern in the retina (peau d'orange) and progress to the characteristic angioid streaks. The latter changes are not specific for PXE and can be seen in diabetes mellitus, sickle cell disease, and a variety of other conditions. Streaks represent breaks in Bruch's membrane, an elastic lamina that lies between the retinal vasculature and the choroid. Spontaneous hemorrhages, especially those involving the macula, lead to progressive visual loss.

Involvement of arteries of various calibers produces problems because of occlusion and hemorrhage. The lifetime risk of serious gastrointestinal hemorrhage from any site, but especially the stomach, is about 10%. Hypertension is relatively common, in part because of involvement of the renal vasculature. Progressive occlusion of peripheral arteries leads to absence of pulses; acral ischemia is rare because of the development of collaterals. The risk for stroke, myocardial infarction, abdominal angina, and intermittent claudication is increased independent of other risk factors.

Diagnosis

Differential Diagnosis

An acquired form of PXE has been reported and is also of unclear etiology. This form is difficult to differentiate from a sporadic case potentially caused by a new mutation or by heterozygosity in the parents, but it tends to affect only the skin. As suggested by the name, the cutaneous features of PXE need to be differentiated from those of true xanthoma, which results from a disorder of lipid metabolism. The dermatologic manifestations need to be differentiated from those of Miescher's elastoma, elastic tissue nevi (Buschke-Ollendorff syndrome), and solar elastosis.

Treatment

Rx

No cure for or means of preventing PXE is known. In many instances, careful attention to the ocular features by a retinal specialist experienced in PXE can delay but not prevent loss of vision. The risk of gastrointestinal hemorrhage suggests that patients should avoid gastric irritants such as aspirin, nonsteroidal anti-inflammatory drugs, and excessive alcohol. Stool should be checked regularly for occult blood, and angiography may be necessary to detect the source of bleeding. All standard risk factors for atherosclerosis should be managed aggressively. Complaints of chest pain should prompt a rigorous investigation for coronary artery disease. Angioplasty has not been reported to be effective, and the coronary lesions tend to be

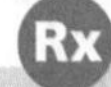

diffuse. Coronary artery bypass graft surgery has been performed, but long-term results have not been reported. It may be theoretically advantageous to use vein grafts rather than the internal mammary artery for bypass. The excessive wrinkling and pseudoxanthoma in exposed areas can be ameliorated by plastic surgery.

Future Directions

Each of these disorders poses special considerations in clinical diagnosis, utility of molecular testing, genetic counseling, and management. For the storage disorders, the clinical utility of enzyme replacement therapy is actively being pursued by several pharmaceutical companies. For several of the other conditions, somatic stem cell therapy offers some promise but is years away from routine clinical use. In Marfan syndrome, clinical trials of drugs that modulate activity of TGF-β are being planned. Considerable progress will be made over the next few years in delineating the milder ranges of the phenotypes in Marfan syndrome, OI, and EDS. Molecular testing will have an increasing role in specific circumstances, especially as the costs of screening large genes for mutations decreases. Additionally, close medical management for individuals detected as being at heightened risk for cardiovascular, skeletal, and ocular complications will remain a mainstay.

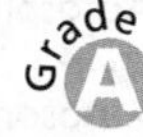

1. Shores J, Berger KR, Murphy EA, Pyeritz RE: Chronic β-adrenergic blockade protects the aorta in the Marfan syndrome: A prospective, randomized trial of propranolol. N Engl J Med 1994;330:1335–1341.

SUGGESTED READINGS

Barnes AM, Chang W, Morello R, et al: Deficiency of cartilage-associated protein in recessive lethal osteogenesis imperfecta. N Engl J Med 2006;355:2757–2764. *Describes patients with severe osteogenesis imperfecta who were found to have a recessive condition resulting in CRTAP deficiency.*

Gott VL, Greene PS, Alejo DE, et al: Surgery for ascending aortic disease in Marfan patients: A multi-center study. N Engl J Med 1999;340:1307–1313. *Follow-up of almost 700 patients documents the good long-term outcome of prophylactic repair of the dilated aortic root.*

Judge DP, Dietz HC: Marfan's syndrome. Lancet 2005;366:1965–1976. *An excellent review of Marfan syndrome.*

Le Saux O, Beck K, Sachsinger C, et al: A spectrum of *ABCC6* mutations is responsible for pseudoxanthoma elasticum. Am J Hum Genet 2001;69:749–764. *An extensive array of changes in the gene encoding a protein in a family of ATP-binding cassette transporters.*

Loeys BL, Chen J, Neptune ER, et al: A syndrome of altered cardiovascular, craniofacial, neurocognitive and skeletal development caused by mutations in TGFBR1 or TGFBR2. Nat Genet 2005;37:275–281. *A variety of conditions that have arterial fragility as a common feature and that were once confused with Marfan syndrome are now being defined by mutations in cellular receptors for the cytokine TGF-β.*

Mao J-R, Bristow J: The Ehlers-Danlos syndrome: On beyond collagen. J Clin Invest 2001;107:1063–1069. *How mutations in specific genes affect the extracellular matrix and produce complex phenotypes such as EDS.*

Miller DC: Valve-sparing aortic root replacement in patients with the Marfan syndrome. J Thorac Cardiovasc Surg 2003;125:773–778. *A critical review of the various approaches to preserving the native aortic valve while replacing the dilated proximal ascending aorta.*

Pyeritz RE: Marfan syndrome and other disorders of fibrillin. *In* Rimoin DL, Connor JM, Pyeritz RE, Korf BR (eds): Principles and Practice of Medical Genetics, 5th ed. Edinburgh, Churchill Livingstone, 2007, p 3579. *A review of the clinical, pathologic, and molecular aspects of Marfan syndrome and related disorders.*

Rauch F, Plotkin H, Zeitlin L, Glorieux FH: Bone mass, size, and density in children and adolescents with osteogenesis imperfecta: Effect of intravenous pamidronate therapy. J Bone Miner Res 2003;18:610–614. *Compared with historical controls, children and adolescents who received an average of 4 years of treatment had significantly higher bone mass, size, and density; those most severely affected at baseline had the greatest improvement.*

Shi Y, Terry SF, Terry PF, et al: Development of a rapid, reliable genetic test of pseudoxanthoma elasticum. J Mol Diagn 2007;9:105–112. *Describes a new and reliable genetic assay to assist in diagnosis of PXE, differential diagnosis of PXE-like conditions, and study of PXE genetics.*

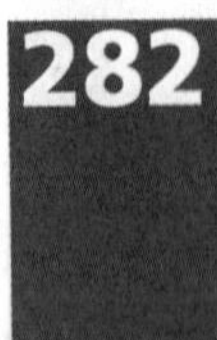

282 THE SYSTEMIC AUTOINFLAMMATORY DISEASES

Daniel L. Kastner

Definition

The systemic autoinflammatory diseases (Table 282–1) are a group of illnesses characterized by seemingly unprovoked inflammation, without evidence of high-titer autoantibodies or antigen-specific T cells, thus distinguishing them from the more classic autoimmune diseases. The first conditions recognized as autoinflammatory were the hereditary periodic fevers, a group of mendelian disorders characterized by episodic or fluctuating degrees of fever and localized inflammation. The scope of autoinflammatory disease has been broadened to include other heritable illnesses, including disorders in which purulent or granulomatous inflammation predominates. Inherited disorders of the complement system may also be placed under the autoinflammatory rubric (Chapter 47). In addition, in numerous autoinflammatory conditions, some of which present in childhood and others later in life, genetic factors play a less prominent etiologic role. Recent advances in the genetics and pathophysiology of the inherited autoinflammatory diseases suggest that these conditions are inborn errors of innate immunity, the phylogenetically more primitive part of the immune system that utilizes germline membrane and intracellular receptors expressed in granulocytes and macrophages to mount the body's first line of defense against pathogens.

TABLE 282–1 THE SYSTEMIC AUTOINFLAMMATORY DISEASES: A PARTIAL LISTING

Inherited Autoinflammatory Diseases	Inheritance/Etiology	Genes or Risk Factors	OMIM*
HEREDITARY PERIODIC FEVER SYNDROMES			
Familial Mediterranean fever (FMF)	Autosomal recessive	*MEFV*†	249100
Tumor necrosis factor receptor–associated periodic syndrome (TRAPS)	Autosomal dominant	*TNFRSF1A*†	142680
Hyperimmunoglobulinemia D with periodic fever syndrome (HIDS)	Autosomal recessive	*MVK*†	260920
Familial cold autoinflammatory syndrome (FCAS)	Autosomal dominant	*CIAS1/NALP3/PYPAF1*†	120100
Muckle-Wells syndrome (MWS)	Autosomal dominant	*CIAS1/NALP3/PYPAF1*†	191900
Neonatal-onset multisystem inflammatory disease (NOMID)/chronic infantile neurologic cutaneous and articular (CINCA) syndrome	Sporadic, autosomal dominant	*CIAS1/NALP3/PYPAF1*†	607115
GRANULOMATOUS DISORDERS			
Granulomatous inflammatory arthritis, dermatitis, and uveitis (Blau's syndrome)	Autosomal dominant	*NOD2/CARD15*†	186580
Early-onset sarcoidosis	Sporadic, autosomal dominant	*NOD2/CARD15*†	609464
Crohn's disease	Complex inheritance	*NOD2/CARD15*†	266600
PYOGENIC DISORDERS			
Syndrome of pyogenic arthritis with pyoderma gangrenosum and acne (PAPA)	Autosomal dominant	*PSTPIP1*†	604416
Chronic recurrent multifocal osteomyelitis (CRMO)	Sporadic, autosomal recessive	*LPIN2*†, when associated with congenital dyserythropoietic anemia (Majeed's syndrome)	259680
COMPLEMENT DISORDERS			
Hereditary angioedema	Autosomal dominant	*C1NH*	106100
Hemolytic-uremic syndrome	Autosomal dominant, sporadic	HF1 (complement factor H)	235400
Age-related macular degeneration	Complex inheritance	HF1 (complement factor H)	603075
OTHER AUTOINFLAMMATORY SYNDROMES			
Syndrome of periodic fever with aphthous stomatitis, pharyngitis, and cervical adenopathy (PFAPA)	Idiopathic	—	—
Systemic-onset juvenile idiopathic arthritis (SOJIA)	Complex inheritance	Interleukin-6, *MIF* polymorphisms	604302
Adult-onset Still's disease	Idiopathic	—	—
Behçet's disease	Complex inheritance	HLA-B51	109650
Synovitis, acne, pustulosis, hyperostosis, and osteitis syndrome (SAPHO)	Idiopathic	—	—
Crystalline arthropathies	Complex inheritance	—	—

*Online Mendelian Inheritance in Man, an online catalog of genetic disorders available at http://www.ncbi.nlm.nih.gov/entrez/query.fcgi?db=OMIM.
†An updated listing of disease-associated mutations is available online at http://fmf.igh.cnrs.fr/infevers/.

HEREDITARY PERIODIC FEVER SYNDROMES

Familial Mediterranean Fever

Definition

Familial Mediterranean fever (FMF) is a recessively inherited illness that typically manifests with 12- to 72-hour episodes of fever and localized serosal, synovial, or cutaneous inflammation. Between attacks, patients usually feel completely well, although biochemical evidence of inflammation may remain, and some patients eventually develop systemic amyloidosis. Before the identification of the causative gene, FMF was defined purely clinically, and clinical features remain an important part of the diagnosis, because some patients with typical disease have only one, or sometimes no, demonstrable mutation in *MEFV*, the only known causative gene.

Epidemiology

FMF is most common in individuals of Jewish, Arab, Armenian, Turkish, and Italian ancestry. The frequency of asymptomatic carriers of a single *MEFV* mutation in these populations is as high as 1:5, a finding suggesting a selective advantage for heterozygotes. With genetic testing, FMF is now frequently recognized both in Ashkenazi (Eastern European) and non-Ashkenazi Jewish populations, as well as in Mediterranean populations previously not thought to be at risk. Mutation-positive individuals with typical symptoms have been documented worldwide. FMF usually manifests in childhood, sometimes even in infancy, although approximately 10% of patients experience their first attack as adults, and infrequently FMF first occurs in persons who are more than 40 years old.

Pathobiology

MEFV, the gene for FMF, was identified by positional cloning in 1997, and it encodes a 781–amino acid protein denoted pyrin (or marenostrin) that is expressed in granulocytes, monocytes, and dendritic cells, as well as in peritoneal, synovial, and dermal fibroblasts. The N-terminal 92 amino acids of pyrin are the prototype for a motif, the PYRIN domain, that is involved in protein-protein interactions, and that defines a family of more than 20 human proteins, including pyrin itself, involved in the regulation of cytokine production (particularly the interleukin-1 [IL-1] family), nuclear factor kappa B (NF-κB) activation, and apoptosis. More than 70 FMF-associated mutations in pyrin have been identified, many of which reside in the C-terminal domain encoded by exon 10 of *MEFV*.

Clinical Manifestations

Episodes of FMF are usually more properly termed recurrent than periodic, and some patients associate attacks with psychological stress or physical exertion. Nevertheless, women of childbearing age sometimes experience their attacks with menses, with remissions during pregnancy. Some patients are unaware of fever during their attacks, but it is almost always observed when sought.

Serosal involvement in FMF is usually peritoneal or pleural. Abdominal attacks are the most frequent, and they may vary from mild discomfort to frank peritonitis, with boardlike rigidity, direct and rebound tenderness, and air-fluid levels on upright films of the abdomen. Regardless of the severity of the abdominal attack, constipation is much more common than diarrhea. When a laparotomy or laparoscopy is performed during an attack, a small amount of sterile exudate rich in polymorphonuclear leukocytes is found. Except for serosal inflammation, the appendix is normal. Repeated abdominal attacks may cause peritoneal adhesions, but ascites is rare. Pleurisy, usually unilateral, may accompany abdominal pain, or it may occur as an independent attack. Physical findings, if present, may include diminished breath sounds and a friction rub, whereas radiographs may show a small effusion or atelectasis. With multiple attacks, pleural thickening may develop. Symptomatic nonuremic pericardial involvement in FMF, although reported, is unusual.

Most typically, in adults the arthritis of FMF manifests as monoarticular involvement of the knee, hip, or ankle, and attacks of arthritis may persist for up to 1 week at a time. In children, oligoarticular or polyarticular joint involvement may also occur. Large joint effusions are sometimes present, and the synovial fluid may have as many as 100,000 leukocytes/mm^3. In approximately 5% of patients who are not treated with prophylactic colchicine, chronic arthritis (usually of the hip or knee) also may develop, often necessitating joint replacement surgery. Regardless of colchicine treatment or a particular human leukocyte antigen (HLA-B27) status, some patients with FMF develop sacroiliitis. Arthralgia without frank arthritis is common in FMF.

Cutaneous manifestations in FMF tend to be less common than serosal or synovial involvement. The characteristic skin lesion of FMF is erysipeloid erythema, a painful, demarcated erythematous area most often seen on the lower leg, ankle, or dorsum of the foot. This rash may occur independently, or it may accompany an episode of arthritis. Histologically, one sees a mixed perivascular cellular infiltrate. Other acute manifestations of FMF include unilateral scrotal inflammation (the tunica vaginalis is an embryologic remnant of the peritoneal membrane) and myalgia, either with fever or, especially in children, without fever and induced by vigorous exercise. Various forms of vasculitis have also been associated with FMF; Henoch-Schönlein purpura occurs in approximately 5% of children with FMF, and less frequently polyarteritis nodosum is seen.

Complications

Before the widespread use of colchicine prophylaxis, systemic AA amyloidosis was a frequent complication of FMF, and it is caused by the ectopic deposition of a misfolded fragment of serum amyloid A (SAA), an acute phase reactant, in the gastrointestinal tract, kidneys, spleen, lung, testes, and adrenals. Malabsorption and nephrotic proteinuria leading to renal failure are the most common manifestations of AA amyloidosis; cardiomyopathy, neuropathy, and arthropathy are rare. Several risk factors have been identified, including late diagnosis of FMF, colchicine noncompliance, male gender, and specific genotypes of *MEFV* and the *SAA* gene. Amyloidosis in FMF is less common in the United States than in the Middle East. Abdominal fat aspirates are much less sensitive than rectal or renal biopsy in detecting the amyloidosis of FMF. The latter procedure may be preferred, because of the increasing recognition of non-amyloid glomerular disease in FMF. With early diagnosis, aggressive suppression of the acute phase response with colchicine or adjunctive agents may bring about improvement, but for patients with renal failure, early renal transplantation is preferred.

Diagnosis

To establish the genetic diagnosis of FMF, two mutations in *MEFV*, in *trans*, should be identified. Nevertheless, the interpretation of genetic testing is complicated by complex alleles consisting of various combinations of mutations in *cis*, as well as by the observations that as many as one third of patients with clinically typical FMF have only one demonstrable mutation in *MEFV*, and a few patients with typical disease have no identifiable *MEFV* mutations. These latter two findings suggest that, under some circumstances, one *MEFV* mutation may be sufficient for symptoms, and/or additional genes for FMF exist.

For these reasons, clinical data remain an essential part of the diagnosis of FMF, and genetic testing plays an adjunctive role in settings where clinical experience is limited. Clinical criteria emphasize attack duration (12 to 72 hours), recurrence of symptoms (three or more episodes), documented fever (rectal temperature >38° C), painful manifestations in the abdomen, chest, joints, or skin, and the absence of other causative factors. The differential diagnosis includes the other hereditary periodic fever syndromes (Table 282–2), as well as other conditions specific to the clinical setting. For patients with recurrent abdominal pain, considerations include gynecologic disorders, porphyria (Chapter 229) (which can be distinguished by hypertension during attacks, dominant inheritance, and urine porphyrins), and hereditary angioedema (Chapter 273) (which usually does not cause fever). Still's disease in children (systemic-onset juvenile idiopathic arthritis) and adults is also considered in the differential diagnosis, and it can be distinguished by the pattern of fever

TABLE 282–2 CLINICAL FEATURES OF THE HEREDITARY PERIODIC FEVER SYNDROMES

Clinical Feature	FMF	TRAPS	HIDS	FCAS	MWS	NOMID/CINCA
Typical ethnicity	Arab, Armenian, Italian, Jewish, Turkish	Any ethnicity	Dutch, other North European	European	European	Any
Attack duration	12–72 hr	Days to weeks	3–7 days	12–24 hr	1–2 days	Continuous, with flares
Abdominal attacks	Sterile peritonitis, constipation	Sterile peritonitis, diarrhea or constipation	Severe pain, vomiting, diarrhea, rarely peritonitis	Nausea	Abdominal pain	Not common
Pleural attacks	Common	Common	Rare	Not seen	Rare	Rare
Joint/bone involvement	Monoarthritis, rarely protracted arthritis in knee or hip	Arthritis in large joints, arthralgia	Arthralgia, symmetric polyarthritis	Polyarthralgia	Polyarthralgia, oligoarthritis, clubbing	Epiphyseal overgrowth, contractures, intermittent or chronic arthritis, clubbing
Skin rash	Erysipeloid erythema on lower leg, ankle, foot	Migratory rash, underlying myalgia	Diffuse maculopapular rash, urticaria	Cold-induced urticarial rash	Urticaria-like rash	Urticaria-like rash
Lymphatic	Splenomegaly, occasional lymphadenopathy	Splenomegaly, occasional lymphadenopathy	Cervical adenopathy in children	Not seen	Rare	Hepatosplenomegaly, adenopathy
Neurologic	Aseptic meningitis?	Controversial	Headache	Headache	Sensorineural deafness	Sensorineural deafness, chronic aseptic meningitis, mental retardation, headache
Ophthalmologic involvement	Rare	Conjunctivitis, periorbital edema, rarely uveitis	Uncommon	Conjunctivitis	Conjunctivitis, episcleritis	Uveitis, conjunctivitis, progressive vision loss
Vasculitis	Henoch-Schönlein purpura (HSP), polyarteritis nodosa	HSP, lymphocytic vasculitis	Cutaneous vasculitis common, rarely HSP	Not seen	Not seen	Occasional
Systemic amyloidosis	Risk depends on *MEFV* and *SAA* genotypes; more common in Middle East	Occurs in ~10%; risk increased with cysteine mutations	Rare	Rare	Occurs in ~25%	May develop in some, usually in adulthood

FCAS = familial cold autoinflammatory syndrome; FMF = familial Mediterranean fever; HIDS = hyperimmunoglobulinemia D with periodic fever syndrome; MWS = Muckle-Wells syndrome; NOMID/CINCA = neonatal-onset multisystem inflammatory disease/chronic infantile neurologic cutaneous and articular syndrome; TRAPS = tumor necrosis factor receptor–associated periodic syndrome.

(intermittent quotidian in Still's disease versus discrete episodes in FMF), the pattern of arthritis (chronic polyarthritis versus intermittent monoarthritis), the characteristic skin involvement (evanescent rash versus erysipeloid erythema), and the presence of lymphadenopathy (more common in Still's disease). The syndrome of periodic fever with aphthous stomatitis, pharyngitis, and cervical adenopathy is probably the most common cause of unexplained recurrent fever in children and is also in the differential diagnosis. In patients presenting primarily with recurrent monoarthritis, joint aspiration for cultures and crystals may aid in excluding bacterial and crystalline arthritis, respectively.

Treatment Rx

The mainstay of therapy for FMF is daily oral colchicine, which has been shown to prevent both acute attacks of FMF and the development of systemic amyloidosis. Colchicine probably works by several mechanisms, including its effects on leukocyte adhesion and cytokine production. In adults, the therapeutic dose is 1.2 to 1.8 mg/day, and nearly 90% of patients note significant improvement at this dose. The major side effects are gastrointestinal, and they can usually be minimized by gradually increasing the dosage and by avoidance of milk products in patients who develop lactose intolerance. Most experts continue to prescribe colchicine to patients during pregnancy, with the recommendation of amniocentesis to exclude the possible slight increase in risk of trisomy 21. Use of colchicine in lactating women is considered safe. Intravenous colchicine should be used with extreme caution, if at all, in FMF, because fatal toxicity has been reported in patients already receiving oral colchicine who are given the drug intravenously. Cytokine inhibitors are investigational in patients who are poorly responsive to colchicine or who cannot tolerate therapeutic doses.

Tumor Necrosis Factor Receptor–Associated Periodic Syndrome

Definition

Worldwide, the tumor necrosis factor (TNF) receptor–associated periodic syndrome (TRAPS) is the second most frequently diagnosed hereditary periodic fever syndrome, behind FMF. TRAPS is defined by recurrent episodes of fever and localized inflammation, in many ways resembling FMF but differing in key details noted later, and caused by mutations in the 55-kD receptor for TNF (TNFRSF1A, TNFR1, p55, CD120a). Whereas a positive genetic test is not necessary to make the diagnosis of FMF, the diagnosis of TRAPS specifically requires the identification of a TNF receptor mutation. One of the first well-characterized families with what later was defined as TRAPS was of Irish ancestry, and the condition had been termed familial Hibernian fever to emphasize the ethnic background and clinical differences from FMF. However, with the discovery of TNF receptor mutations in families of other ancestry, the ethnically more neutral TRAPS nomenclature was proposed.

Pathobiology

The p55 TNF receptor is composed of four cysteine-rich extracellular domains, a transmembrane region, and an intracellular death domain. To date, all of the more than 50 mutations described are in the extracellular domains, and approximately half are missense substitutions of cysteine residues that abolish highly conserved disulfide bonds. The initial description of TRAPS documented a defect in activation-induced ectodomain cleavage of the p55 receptor in patients with the C52F *TNFRSF1A* mutation, possibly leading to a defect in homeostasis by impaired downregulation of membrane receptor and diminished shedding of potentially antagonistic soluble receptor molecules. More recent studies indicate a more complex pathogenetic picture, because not all mutant receptors exhibit this shedding defect. Additional mechanisms by which p55 mutations may lead to autoinflammation include impaired leukocyte apoptosis and impaired intracellular receptor trafficking, with possible constitutive activation of NF-κB by intracellular aggregates of mutant receptors.

Diagnosis

Although genetic testing is necessary for the diagnosis of TRAPS, certain clinical clues help to distinguish TRAPS from FMF. These include ethnicity (FMF is predominantly seen in Mediterranean and Middle Eastern populations, whereas TRAPS has a more widespread distribution), mode of inheritance (autosomal recessive in FMF, dominant in TRAPS), and duration of attacks, which tends to be longer in TRAPS and sometimes approaches continuous symptoms. The rash of FMF is typically erysipeloid erythema on the lower extremity, whereas patients with TRAPS often have a distinctive erythematous rash, often with underlying myalgia, which may migrate on the trunk or centrifugally on the extremities. Ocular involvement, with periorbital edema, conjunctivitis, and occasionally even uveitis, is observed in TRAPS but not in FMF. Finally, whereas colchicine is much more effective than corticosteroids in FMF, the opposite is true in TRAPS. Nevertheless, aside from the difference in duration and susceptibility to pharmacologic intervention, the abdominal, pleural, synovial, and even scrotal manifestations of the two diseases are rather similar. The usual age of onset for TRAPS is also in childhood, and systemic AA amyloidosis is seen in about 10% of untreated patients with TRAPS. As in FMF, life expectancy in TRAPS is normal in patients with cases not complicated by amyloidosis.

As noted earlier, the diagnosis of TRAPS is established by the identification of *TNFRSF1A* mutations in the appropriate clinical setting. One variant, the substitution of glutamine for arginine at residue 92 (R92Q), is present in more than 1% of whites and may be associated with a broader spectrum of symptoms than typically seen in TRAPS, including early inflammatory arthritis or, in some cases, no symptoms at all. The substitution of lysine for proline at residue 46 (P46L) is common among African American patients with TRAPS and is associated with a receptor shedding defect, but it is also seen among healthy African American controls. These findings establish a "gray zone" for the diagnosis of TRAPS and emphasize the potential role of polymorphisms in the periodic fever genes in other more common phenotypes.

Treatment Rx

The treatment of TRAPS depends on the frequency and severity of attacks. Patients with relatively infrequent, mild episodes may respond to nonsteroidal anti-inflammatory drugs. Patients with more severe attacks that occur infrequently may be treated with corticosteroids, although increasing doses may be required as the episodes become more frequent, and toxicities may become limiting. For patients with severe attacks occurring once a month or more frequently, treatment with etanercept, the soluble p75 TNF receptor:Fc fusion protein, may be warranted. More recently, a few patients with TRAPS have been observed who have not responded to TNF inhibition but have responded to anakinra, the IL-1 receptor antagonist.

Hyperimmunoglobulinemia D with Periodic Fever Syndrome

Epidemiology

Hyperimmunoglobulinemia D with periodic fever syndrome (HIDS) was first described in 1984 as an FMF-like illness seen in six patients of Dutch ancestry. Besides the difference in ethnicity, a key distinction was the observation of extremely high levels of immunoglobulin D (IgD) in the serum of the Dutch patients, thus prompting the HIDS nomenclature. HIDS is now recognized in a broader ethnic distribution, although northern Europeans still predominate. Overall, HIDS is still quite rare.

Pathobiology

Family studies documented autosomal recessive inheritance. In 1999, patients with HIDS were found to have mutations in *MVK*, which encodes the mevalonate kinase enzyme involved in the biosynthesis of cholesterol and nonsterol isoprenes. Enzyme activity in patients is markedly reduced, although not absent.

The elevated IgD levels seen in HIDS appear to be an epiphenomenon. They do not correlate with disease severity, either among patients or in a given patient over time, although IgD may contribute to the release of proinflammatory cytokines in vitro. Moreover, modest elevations of IgD are seen in several inflammatory conditions, including chronic infections, and can be observed in other hereditary periodic fever syndromes. Moreover, some patients (particularly young children) with typical recurrent fevers and *MVK* mutations have normal serum IgD levels. Current data suggest that isoprenoid deficiency may play a more important pathogenic role in the pathophysiology of HIDS. In vitro studies suggest that isoprenoid deficiency may lead to excessive IL-1β production, and increased body temperature can further decrease mevalonate kinase enzymatic activity, thereby setting in place a vicious circle in which infection or immunizations could precipitate HIDS attacks.

Clinical Manifestations

One of the well-recognized clinical characteristics of HIDS is the provocation of attacks by immunizations. Other distinguishing clinical features include a very early age of onset (average age, 6 months), a duration of attacks intermediate between FMF and TRAPS (3 to 7 days), prominent cervical lymphadenopathy during attacks, polyarticular joint involvement, a diffuse maculopapular rash, the predominance of diarrhea over constipation with abdominal attacks, and the infrequency of pleuritic attacks or systemic amyloidosis.

Diagnosis

The diagnosis of HIDS is made in three possible ways: documenting elevated serum IgD levels; identifying two mutations in *MVK;* or documenting elevated levels of mevalonic acid, the substrate for mevalonate kinase, in the urine during attacks. In patients in whom all three are found, the diagnosis is straightforward. In patients who have genetic and/or biochemical abnormalities without an elevated IgD, the term *Dutch-type periodic fever* has been proposed, although the significance of an elevated IgD without biochemical or genetic findings remains uncertain.

Treatment and Prognosis Rx

Nonsteroidal anti-inflammatory drugs or corticosteroids are sometimes useful in the treatment of the arthritic manifestations of HIDS. Colchicine is generally not effective in HIDS. Numerous agents are investigational in HIDS, including the statins, TNF inhibitors, and the IL-1 receptor antagonist. Patients with HIDS have a normal lifespan, and attacks may become somewhat less frequent in adulthood.

CIAS1-Associated Periodic Syndromes: The Cryopyrinopathies

Three rare recurrent febrile disorders usually beginning early in life have been associated with mutations in *CIAS1,* the gene encoding a protein variously named cryopyrin, NALP3, PYPAF1, or CATERPILLER 1.1. The least severe clinical phenotype is familial cold autoinflammatory syndrome (FCAS, formerly called familial cold urticaria), which is dominantly inherited and is notable for day-long attacks of chills, fever, headache, diffuse urticarial skin rash, arthralgia, and conjunctivitis, precipitated by generalized cold exposure. Amyloidosis is rare in FCAS. Of intermediate severity is the Muckle-Wells syndrome (MWS), also dominantly inherited, in which 1- to 2-day episodes of chills, fever, urticarial rash, limb pain, and arthritis occur independently of cold exposure. Sensorineural hearing loss is common in MWS, and systemic amyloidosis may also occur. The most severe *CIAS1*-associated phenotype is neonatal-onset multisystem inflammatory disease (NOMID), known in Europe as chronic infantile neurologic cutaneous and articular (CINCA) syndrome. It is usually sporadic, because of reduced reproductive fitness among most affected individuals. Fever and constitutional symptoms occur almost daily often from birth, with generalized urticarial skin rash, a peculiar arthropathy characterized by epiphyseal overgrowth of the long bones, and central nervous system involvement that includes chronic aseptic meningitis, uveitis, and cochlear inflammation, which may lead to mental retardation, blindness, and deafness. In all three cryopyrinopathies, the rash is not true urticaria because there is a neutrophilic rather than a mast cell infiltrate and serum histamine levels are normal.

The protein mutated in all three disorders is a critical component of a newly recognized macromolecular complex termed the *inflammasome,* which serves as an intracellular scaffold for processing of IL-1β from its 31-kD precursor form to the biologically active 17-kD form. Cryopyrin (NALP3) is so-named because it has an amino-terminal PYRIN domain, and thus it bears a structural and functional relationship with the protein mutated in FMF. Disease-associated cryopyrin mutations are thought to decrease the threshold for inflammasome activation, thereby increasing IL-1β production. In vitro studies also suggest a role for cryopyrin/NALP3 in NF-κB activation.

Because there are patients with FCAS, MWS, and NOMID/CINCA without demonstrable *CIAS1* mutations, these diagnoses remain clinical, although genetic testing does serve as a valuable adjunct and has greatly increased recognition of all three conditions. In addition, overlap syndromes that intermediate between FCAS and MWS and between MWS and NOMID/CINCA have been reported.

Data indicate that IL-1 blockade with anakinra, the IL-1 receptor antagonist, appears effective in controlling fever and acute phase reactants in all three cryopyrinopathies. Moreover, in a large series completed at the National Institutes of Health, anakinra markedly decreased central nervous system inflammation in NOMID/CINCA. Such data suggest that the major biologic effect of cryopyrin/NALP3 in humans is mediated through IL-1β, rather than by other distinct inflammatory pathways.

OTHER INHERITED SYSTEMIC AUTOINFLAMMATORY DISEASES

Syndrome of Pyogenic Arthritis with Pyoderma Gangrenosum and Acne

The syndrome of pyogenic arthritis with pyoderma gangrenosum and acne (PAPA) is a rare, dominantly inherited autoinflammatory disease characterized by intermittent episodes of sterile pyogenic arthritis, pyoderma gangrenosum, and severe cystic acne. It is caused by mutations in proline-serine-threonine phosphatase interacting protein 1 (PSTPIP1), also known as CD2BP1. PSTPIP1 is a cytoskeletal protein that interacts with certain other proteins involved in the immune response, including CD2, the Wiskott-Aldrich syndrome protein (WASP), a phosphatase denoted PTP-PEST, and pyrin, the FMF protein. PAPA mutations abrogate the binding of PSTPIP1 to PTP-PEST, thereby leading to hyperphosphorylation of PSTPIP1 and increased binding to pyrin. Both in patients and in cell lines, this finding is associated with markedly increased IL-1β production. Early in life, PAPA tends to present with monoarticular or pauciarticular pyogenic arthritis, sometimes induced by trauma. In the absence of treatment, arthritis may progress to severe joint damage and ankylosis. As patients reach puberty, skin manifestations begin to predominate, including disfiguring cystic acne. Pathergy may also develop, and extensive pyoderma gangrenosum may require opiates for pain control. The diagnosis of PAPA syndrome is made by documenting *PSTPIP1* mutations in the appropriate clinical setting. High doses of corticosteroids have been used in PAPA, with varying success, and patients with arthritis sometimes require aspiration, intra-articular corticosteroids, or open drainage. Newer investigational approaches for PAPA syndrome focus on the use of targeted cytokine inhibitors.

Granulomatous Inflammatory Arthritis, Dermatitis, and Uveitis (Blau's Syndrome)

Blau's syndrome is a rare, dominantly inherited illness characterized by the following features: early-onset granulomatous synovitis often complicated by cyst formation and camptodactyly (flexion contractures of the fingers and toes); granulomatous anterior and posterior uveitis sometimes causing retinal detachment, glaucoma, cataracts, and blindness; and an intermittent papular rash with noncaseating granulomas. Lung or other visceral involvement is generally not present. However, visceral involvement of the liver and spleen is observed in early-onset sarcoidosis (Chapter 95), which is phenotypically quite similar to Blau's syndrome. Both Blau's syndrome and some cases of early-onset sarcoidosis are caused by mutations in *NOD2/CARD15*. Distinct variants of *NOD2//CARD15* have been associated with susceptibility to Crohn's disease, which is manifested by granulomatous inflammation of the gastrointestinal tract. The protein encoded by this gene is thought to be an intracellular sensor of bacterial products. Crohn's disease–associated mutations in the ligand-binding leucine-rich repeat region of the protein may require bacterial contact in the gastrointestinal tract to cause inflammation, whereas Blau's syndrome mutations in the nucleotide binding domain may lead to constitutive extraintestinal inflammation. Topical and systemic corticosteroids are currently the mainstay of treatment of Blau's syndrome.

SUGGESTED READINGS

El-Shanti H, Majeed HA, El-Khateeb M: Familial Mediterranean fever in Arabs. Lancet 2006;367:1016–1024. *Review of the clinical and molecular aspects of FMF in Arabs.*

Hoffman HM, Rosengren S, Boyle DL, et al: Prevention of cold-associated acute inflammation in familial cold autoinflammatory syndrome by interleukin-1 receptor antagonist. Lancet 2005;364:1779–1785. *Demonstration of the efficacy of anakinra in FCAS in an experimental cold-challenge, indicating a central role for IL-1β in this disorder.*

Lidar M, Yaqubov M, Zaks N, et al: The prodrome: A prominent yet overlooked pre-attack manifestation of familial Mediterranean fever. J Rheumatol 2006;33:1089–1092. *A prodromal period heralding attacks is a newly defined and reliable FMF manifestation that reproducibly predicts attacks and may therefore help with prevention of attacks.*

Martinon F, Petrelli V, Mayor A, et al: Gout-associated uric acid crystals activate the NALP3 inflammasome. Nature 2006;440:237–240. *Evidence extending the concept of autoinflammatory diseases to the crystalline arthropathies.*

Stojanov S, Kastner DL: Familial autoinflammatory diseases: Genetics, pathogenesis, and treatment. Curr Opin Rheumatol 2005;17:586–599. *An update of recent literature.*

283 OSTEOARTHRITIS

Nancy E. Lane and Thomas J. Schnitzer

Definition

Osteoarthritis (OA) is a disorder of diarthrodial joints that is characterized clinically by pain and functional limitations, radiographically by osteophytes and joint space narrowing, and histopathologically by alterations in cartilage and subchondral bone integrity. OA is the most common of all joint diseases, and its importance derives from its economic impact, in terms of both productivity (single greatest cause of days lost from work) and cost of treatment (chronic use of analgesics and anti-inflammatory drugs). Although the etiology of OA is still not clearly understood, it has been shown to be a family of disorders with cartilage as a target organ in which biomechanical factors play a central role and risk factors such as age, weight, and occupation are also of major importance. Because there is currently no treatment to prevent or ameliorate the basic disease process, medical treatment is aimed primarily at relieving pain and improving joint function, with orthopedic intervention largely reserved for those situations that cannot be controlled with more conservative therapy.

Epidemiology

OA is by far the most common joint disorder, one of the most common chronic diseases in the elderly, and a leading cause of disability. Because OA can be defined both radiographically and clinically, with little correlation between the two, the prevalence of this condition has been variously estimated in epidemiologic studies. Using radiographic criteria, the prevalence of the joint findings of OA steadily increases, from less than 2% in women younger than 45 years of age, to 30% in those aged 45 to 64 years, and to 68% in those older than 65 years of age. Prevalence in men is slightly higher in the younger age groups (before 45 years of age), whereas women are affected more commonly at ages older than 55 years, except for disease of the hip.

The pattern of joint involvement in OA is strikingly affected by age, gender, previous joint injury, and occupational history. Before age 55, there is little difference in joint pattern between men and women. In older men, hip OA is more common, whereas older women tend to have more involvement of the proximal interphalangeal (PIP) joints and the base of the thumb (first carpometacarpal [CMC] joint). Joints subjected to repeated trauma or overuse demonstrate a higher prevalence of OA. Cotton and mill workers have increased OA of the hand and involved fingers; miners and warehouse workers who bend, squat, and lift heavy loads frequently demonstrate increased knee and spine involvement; and pneumatic drill workers experience increased elbow and wrist disease.

Racial and genetic factors are also important in OA prevalence and pattern. Chinese, Jamaican blacks, South African blacks, and Asian Indians have a lower incidence of OA of the hip than whites do, whereas Japanese have an increased incidence, apparently related to the more frequent occurrence of congenital hip dysplasia. Black women have a higher prevalence of knee OA than white women but a lower prevalence of involvement of the distal interphalangeal (DIP) joints of the hand (Heberden's nodes). Involvement of the DIP joints of the hands is particularly common in women and is often found to have a familial pattern of inheritance, with the female relatives of the proband having similar joint findings with a twofold to fivefold increased prevalence.

Large cohort studies of subjects with radiographic evidence of OA report a significant genetic contribution to the disorder. A heritable component of OA is reported from family and twin studies to be between 60 and 65%, and the genetic predisposition appears to differ by OA site. Single nucleotide polymorphisms in genes that code for structural proteins in the extracellular matrix (e.g., collagen type II), or hormones and growth factors that influence cartilage and bone metabolism (vitamin D receptor, estrogen receptor α, insulin-like growth factor-1, and frizzled-related protein), have been reported to increase the risk of OA in weight-bearing joints.

Modifiable risk factors for OA also have been identified in recent studies. Increased weight is the most significant independent predictor of both incidence and progression of OA in weight-bearing joints, and weight reduction has been shown to reduce the development and progression of knee OA. Certain types of high-impact repetitive activities are associated with an increased risk for development of OA in the stressed joint (see earlier discussion), whereas other activities are not. In particular, there appears to be an increased risk of knee OA in elite, highly competitive runners, but no increased prevalence in participants in low-impact activities such as marathon running. However, this difference may be the result of a self-selection process, in which those individuals who experience knee pain are unable to continue the activity. Smoking and osteoporosis have both been shown to be negatively associated with OA, but the explanations for these associations are unknown.

Pathobiology

Pathology

The hallmarks of OA on gross or arthroscopic examination are focal ulcerated areas of cartilage exposing underlying eburnated (ivory-appearing) bone that occur at the load-bearing areas of the joint surface, as well as juxta-articular osteophytes that grow at the joint margins. These states represent the end stage of a continuum, and OA is a pathologic process. At its earliest stage, it manifests as softening of the cartilage surface, progressing to fibrillation of the surface layers, loss of cartilage thickness, development of clefts into the depth of cartilage, and eventual loss of cartilage integrity with release of shards of cartilage. Bone participates in this process as well, with reactive changes (bony subchondral sclerosis) underlying the areas of cartilage loss, development of subchondral bone cysts that may communicate with the joint space and expand into geodes, and marginal osteophytes (new cartilage and bone growth) at non–weight-bearing areas.

The earliest histologic changes reveal loss of extracellular cartilage matrix, loss of chondrocytes in the surface layers of articular cartilage, and reactive changes in the deeper chondrocytes manifested by cellular division and "cloning" in an apparent attempt at repair. Later, there is progressive loss of chondrocytes at all levels, with marked thinning of the cartilage matrix and, in some instances, development of fibrocartilage in place of lost hyaline articular cartilage. The surrounding synovium is largely unaffected, although in later disease cartilage fragments may incite focal inflammatory lesions without the progressive and destructive pannus seen in typical inflammatory arthropathies.

Pathogenesis

Articular cartilage serves two major functions: (1) to permit nearly frictionless joint motion; and (2) to act as a "shock absorber" and transmit loads across joint surfaces to the surrounding tissues. The requisite properties of elasticity and high tensile strength are imparted by proteoglycans and collagen of the extracellular matrix, which comprise more than 90% of the cartilage macromolecules. The proteoglycan elements of the matrix are actively metabolized and turned over, with a half-life of weeks. The highly negatively charged sulfated glycosaminoglycan components of the proteoglycans impart the elastic properties to cartilage. The collagen component of cartilage matrix is characterized by a unique structure (type II collagen) that provides the tensile strength and tightly constrains the proteoglycan molecules in a three-dimensional framework. The collagen fibers are covalently linked by other matrix molecules, which are believed to provide the "glue" to hold the matrix intact. Collagen itself is metabolized very slowly (half-life of many years) in the normal state.

In OA, there is an initial phase in which chondrocyte metabolic activity is upregulated (enhanced proteoglycan synthesis), followed by eventual chondrocyte loss (apoptosis). The reason for failure of repair is unclear but may relate to the inability to re-form, once it is disrupted, the three-dimensional architecture of cartilage in mature individuals.

Degradation of collagen and proteoglycans in OA is carried out by proteolytic enzymes (metalloproteinases [MMPs]) that are synthesized by and released from the chondrocytes themselves. A number of cytokines and other mediators of inflammation, including interleukin-1β (IL-1β), tumor necrosis factor-α, IL-6, IL-8, nitric oxide (NO), and prostaglandins, can be produced by the chondrocyte and act within the cartilage to promote a catabolic state by activating MMPs. The subsequent activation of these potent enzymes overwhelms the natural matrix defenses and ultimately results in collagen breakdown and proteoglycan cleavage. Fragments from these molecules are then released into the synovial fluid and enter the circulation, where they provide "markers" of degradation and can be used as a means to detect and measure disease activity.

The factors responsible for activating chondrocytes to release MMPs are currently being elucidated. However, those conditions that cause biomechanical alteration of cartilage are known to lead to OA: joint injury; abnormal joint loading due to neuropathic changes (Charcot joint); ligamentous damage (anterior cruciate ligament [ACL]) or meniscus injuries; altered joint surface congruity, as in dysplasias or malalignment or joint laxity; and muscle atrophy in the elderly. A number of metabolic conditions are known to predispose to the early onset of OA, including ochronosis with the deposition of homogentisic acid and hemochromatosis with the deposition of iron. Gene defects affecting matrix structures might be expected to lead to OA, but thus far genetic factors have been shown to play a role only in the development of dysplasias with secondary OA. The pathogenetic mechanisms and feedback loops associated with structural damage to the cartilage structure and associated alteration in chondrocyte function are demonstrated in Figure 283–1.

Clinical Manifestations

The initial stages of the OA disease process are clinically silent, which explains the high prevalence of radiographic and pathologic signs of OA in clinically asymptomatic patients. Even in later stages of OA, there is a poor correlation between clinical symptoms and alterations in cartilage and bone integrity, defined arthroscopically or by indirect imaging techniques (radiography, magnetic resonance imaging [MRI]). The factors or events that make the OA disease process clinically apparent are unknown but are likely to be heterogeneous in nature and invoke changes within the synovium, bone, and surrounding supporting structures (muscle, ligaments) that produce pain. Pain does not derive from cartilage itself, a tissue without any innervation.

Pain is the predominant symptom that prompts the diagnosis of OA; often only one joint is involved initially, with others becoming painful subsequently. The pain of OA is most often described as a deep ache, accompanied frequently by joint stiffness after periods of inactivity (on arising in the morning or after sitting). Pain is aggravated by use of the involved joints, may radiate, and may be referred to surrounding structures. In the early stages of the disease, pain is commonly relieved by rest. With more severe disease, pain may be persistent, interfering with normal function and preventing sleep, even with medical management. Even in severe disease, however, systemic manifestations such as fever, weight loss, anemia, and elevated erythrocyte sedimentation rate (ESR) are not present.

The joints most commonly involved in OA are the metatarsophalangeal (MTP) joint of the great toe (hallux valgus or "bunion"); the PIP and DIP joints of the fingers, the CMC joint of the thumb, hips, knees, and the lumbar and cervical spine (Fig. 283–2). Other joints, even major weight-bearing joints such as the ankle, are typically spared unless involved in secondary forms of OA (Table 283–1). On physical examination, the joints may demonstrate tenderness, crepitus, and a

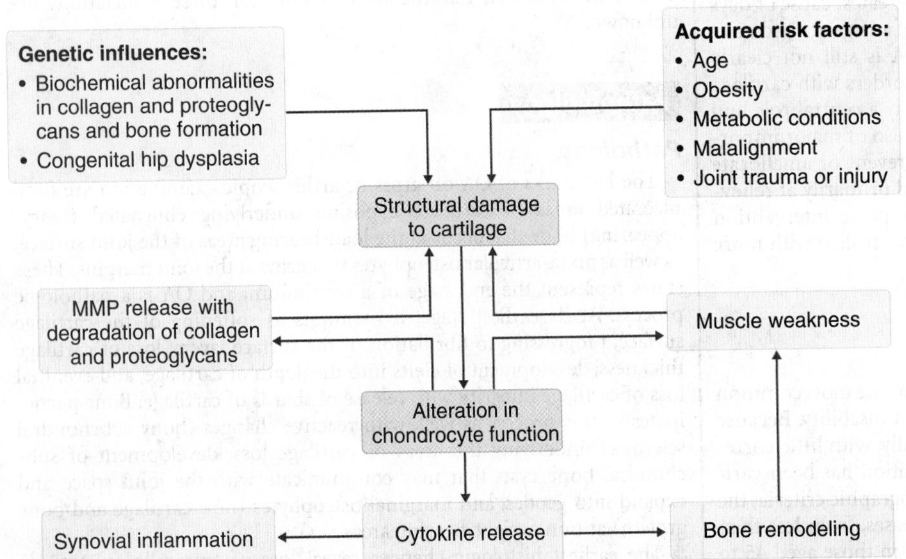

FIGURE 283–1 • Summary of the pathophysiology of osteoarthritis with emphases on structural damage to the cartilage and alteration in chondrocyte function. MMP = metalloproteinase.

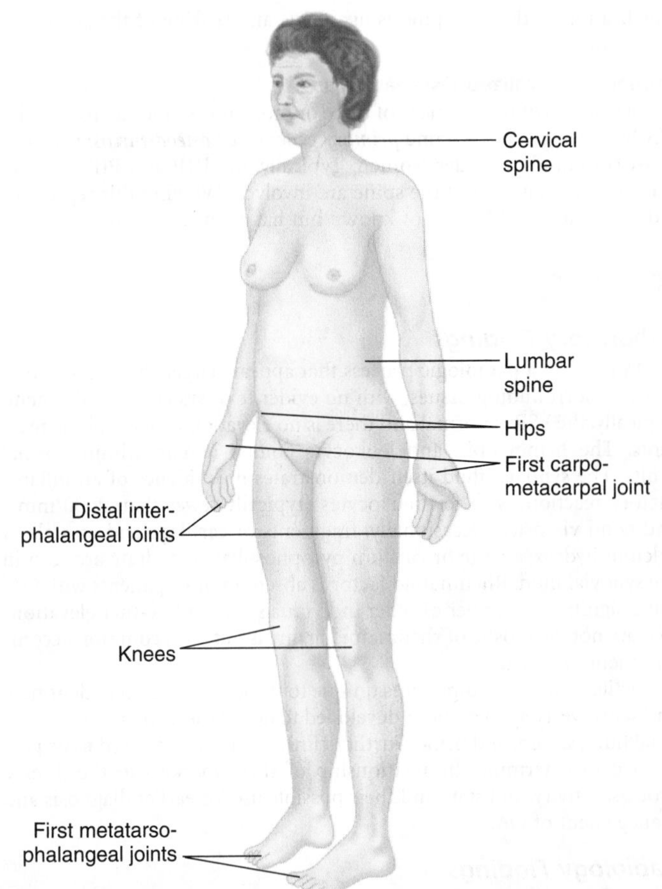

FIGURE 283–2 • Joints commonly affected by osteoarthritis.

limited range of motion. Joint swelling may be caused by an accompanying synovial effusion or by bony enlargement and the presence of osteophytes. Joint instability is seen only in severe disease or after internal derangement of the knee with disruption of one or more of the major supporting structures (e.g., ACL, medial collateral ligament). Patients with far-advanced disease exhibit gross deformity, with subluxation of the involved joints. Although OA is thought to be a uniformly progressive disease that invariably leads to joint replacement, this is not the case. The disease appears to stabilize in many patients, with no worsening of signs or symptoms, and there may be actual improvement in some patients.

Specific Joint Involvement

Hand

Firm, slowly progressive bony enlargements of the DIP joints are called Heberden's nodes and represent marginal osteophytic spurs (Fig. 283–3). Occasionally, the onset of symptoms in the hand is acute, with sudden redness and tenderness in the involved joint. These changes can lead to deformity, with lateral and flexor deviation at these joints. A related disorder, erosive OA, is associated with repetitive episodes of acute symptoms and is differentiated by the additional finding of erosive changes on radiographs of the involved joints and a tendency to bony ankylosis. A genetic basis for Heberden's nodes appears to exist, the condition demonstrating a distinct female-dominant familial tendency (women are affected 10 times more commonly than men).

Changes similar to those in the DIP joints occur in the PIP joints and are termed Bouchard's nodes (see Fig. 283–2). The only other hand joint to be commonly involved is the CMC joint of the thumb. Patients often complain of pain on use of the thumb, as in wringing out clothes (washerwoman's hands) or grasping objects such as screwdrivers and doorknobs. The condition leads to a squared appearance of the base of the hand.

Knee

Idiopathic knee OA is a leading cause of painful ambulation and is more common in women than in men. The medial compartment of the

TABLE 283–1 ETIOLOGIC CLASSIFICATION OF OSTEOARTHRITIS

Idiopathic (primary)
Localized
Hands: Heberden's nodes, erosive interphalangeal arthropathy
Feet: hallux valgus, hammer toes; talonavicular
Knees: medial, lateral, patellofemoral compartments
Hips: sites of cartilage loss—eccentric (superior), concentric (axial, medial), diffuse, and femoral osteophytes
Spine: zygapophyseal joints, intervertebral discs (spondylosis); ligaments (e.g., disseminated idiopathic skeletal hyperostosis) with osteophytes as most common radiographic findings
Other single sites: shoulder, temporomandibular joints, carpometacarpal joints
Generalized—includes three or more areas listed above
Mineral deposition diseases
Calcium pyrophosphate deposition disease
Hydroxyapatite arthropathy
Destructive disease (e.g., Milwaukee shoulder)
Secondary
Posttraumatic
Congenital or developmental
Legg-Calvé-Perthes hip dislocation
Epiphyseal dysplasias
Articular cartilage disorders associated with a gene deficiency (e.g., association with type II procollagen gene mutation)
Disturbed local tissue structure by primary disease (e.g., ischemic necrosis, tophaceous gout, hyperparathyroid cysts, Paget's disease, rheumatoid arthritis, osteopetrosis, osteochondritis)
Miscellaneous additional diseases
Endocrine: diabetes mellitus, acromegaly, hypothyroidism
Metabolic: hemochromatosis, ochronosis, Gaucher's disease
Neuropathic arthropathies
Miscellaneous: frostbite, Kashin-Beck disease, caisson disease
Mechanical: obesity, unequal lower extremity length; valgus/varus deformities, ligamentous laxity (including associations with type I procollagen gene mutations of Ehlers-Danlos syndrome)

Compiled in part by Osteoarthritis Diagnostic Criteria Committee, American Rheumatism Association, 1983.

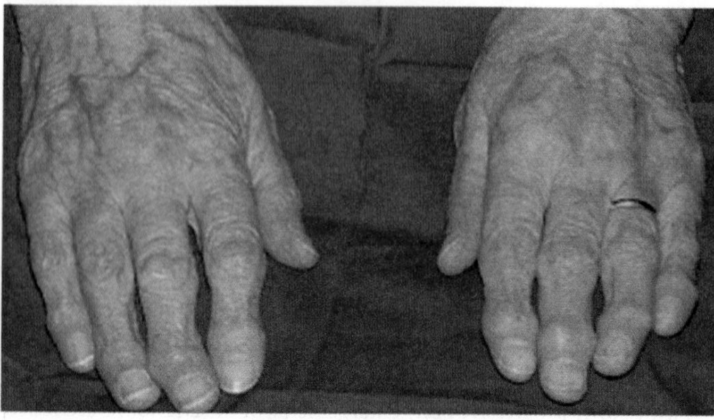

FIGURE 283–3 • Typical hand deformities in osteoarthritis. Heberden's nodes are seen on the distal interphalangeal joints, and Bouchard's nodes are at the proximal interphalangeal joints. (From Forbes CD, Jackson WF: Color Atlas and Text of Clinical Medicine, 3rd ed. London, Mosby, 2003.)

femorotibial joint space is most commonly affected, resulting in varus deformity (bow legs). Lateral compartment disease may lead to valgus deformity (knock-knee). Patellofemoral disease is also common and may represent a substantial portion of knee pathology in patients presenting with knee pain. It is important to exclude other causes of knee pain, such as internal derangements of the knee (e.g., meniscal tears, ligament tears) that may lead to secondary knee OA; soft tissue sprains; bursal inflammation; and Baker's cysts (which may coexist with knee OA). In young women, the possibility of chondromalacia patellae should always be considered. Its cause is not known; it is almost always self-limited and is not thought to lead to OA. In idiopathic knee OA, physical examination of the involved joint often elicits crepitation of the tibiofemoral joint, pain, and decreased range of motion. Effusions are not infrequently present but are often small and may be difficult to appreciate.

Hip

Although congenital (Legg-Calvé-Perthes disease) and developmental (slipped femoral capital epiphysis) abnormalities have long been implicated in secondary hip OA, most cases of primary hip OA are now believed to be the consequence of mild dysplasia of the femoral head and/or acetabulum resulting in incongruity of the articulating surfaces. With use of the joint, there is progressive cartilage degeneration and secondary bony productive changes typical of OA. Pain is usually referred to the groin, with anterior thigh and knee symptoms occasionally predominant. Many patients presenting with pain in their "hip" may have referred pain from degenerative disc disease or OA of the lumbar spine. The earliest physical finding in hip OA is loss of internal rotation; with progressive disease, range of motion is limited further in all directions, the affected leg shortens and significant functional limitation occurs, often necessitating surgery.

Foot

The first MTP joint is the primary joint involved with associated bony swelling and deformity (bunion). Significantly more common in women than men, these changes have been attributed to abnormal stresses imposed on the joint by footwear. In extreme cases, the joint space may be destroyed, leading to a condition known as hallux rigidus, which may interfere with normal ambulation and necessitate surgical correction.

Spine

Technically, OA of the spine relates strictly to changes in synovial-lined joints (apophyseal and uncovertebral joints) that can lead to localized pain as well as irritation of adjacent nerve roots with referred pain in the form of radiculopathy. Nerve root compression resulting from apophyseal joint subluxation, prolapse of an intervertebral disc, or osteophytic spurring may occur, and the patient may present with muscle weakness, hyporeflexia, and paresthesia or hypesthesia. In the cervical region, spinal involvement can lead to cord impingement with long tract signs, or it may affect the vertebral artery, producing insufficiency of the posterior circulation with associated symptoms. OA of the spine should be differentiated from diffuse skeletal hyperostosis, in which there is marked calcification of the paraspinous ligaments and sparing of the arthrodial spinal joints.

Primary Generalized Osteoarthritis

The pattern of involvement of three or more joints or joint groups with OA has been given the name *primary generalized osteoarthritis;* it is seen most commonly in older women. Typically, the DIP and PIP joints of the hand, the knees, and the spine are involved. Whether this represents a distinct subset of OA is not known but has been suggested.

Diagnosis

Laboratory Findings

OA involves a pathologic process that appears largely limited to cartilage and surrounding tissues, with no evidence of systemic involvement. Typically, the ESR is normal and there is no elevation of acute phase reactants. The hemoglobin and leukocyte counts remain within normal limits. The synovial fluid itself demonstrates no evidence of an inflammatory reaction, with few leukocytes (typically fewer than 2000/mm^3) and good viscosity. Occasionally, fragments of cartilage and crystals of calcium hydroxyapatite or calcium pyrophosphate dihydrate are seen in the synovial fluid. Rheumatoid factor is absent in most patients with OA, but a significant number of older individuals exhibit low-titer elevations that are not diagnostic of rheumatoid arthritis but are a common accompaniment of aging.

Cartilage matrix components unique to the joints have been identified, and sensitive assays have been developed to detect these "markers" in synovial fluid, serum, and urine. Further clinical correlations need to be performed to determine the relationship of these markers to the disease process, activity, and state and their possible use for earlier diagnosis and management of OA.

Radiology Findings

Pathognomonic findings of OA on plain radiography include the presence of osteophytes at the margins of involved joints, associated joint space narrowing representing areas of cartilage thinning or loss, and evidence of bony reaction marked by subchondral sclerosis and bone cysts in more progressive disease. Some patients may lack one or more of these findings.

Radiography has been shown to be insensitive to the pathologic processes occurring in the cartilage. Many patients exhibit normal radiographs with destructive cartilage changes documented by arthroscopy. However, performing a weight-bearing knee radiograph with the knee flexed to 20 degrees allows a more reliable assessment of joint space narrowing, and repeat radiographs in this view can be used to assess changes in joint space narrowing over time.

Imaging

Other techniques have been developed with greater potential sensitivity to detect cartilage change. In particular, MRI has the advantage of demonstrating cartilage as a positive image and has been used widely to document major cartilage injuries such as meniscal tears. Further refinement of this technology will enhance the resolution and increase the sensitivity to detect changes in hydration, which mark the earliest cartilage abnormalities in OA. It is anticipated that such capability will be important in the future for assessing disease progression and the efficacy of therapeutic interventions.

Other technologies being developed to evaluate the OA joint include scintigraphy and ultrasonography.

Treatment

People with OA seek pain relief and improved physical function. Because at this time there is no known therapy in humans that affects the basic disease process (i.e., to inhibit cartilage degradation or enhance synthesis), medical therapy has focused on providing symptomatic relief. Largely because of ease of administration and acceptance by patients, an unwarranted reliance has been placed on pharmacologic intervention, particularly nonsteroidal anti-inflammatory drugs (NSAIDs), as initial therapy, at the expense

Rx

of physical measures that have less morbidity and may provide longer-term benefit. The American College of Rheumatology has recently formulated evidence-based guidelines for progressive, stepwise treatment of patients with knee and hip OA that incorporate this approach.

Physical Measures

Although often overlooked, physical therapy and exercise programs provide important benefit and should be prescribed as baseline therapy for all patients with OA. Muscle atrophy commonly accompanies OA. Because muscles serve to reduce load on cartilage, maintaining muscle function is crucial for cartilage integrity and pain reduction. Both muscle strength and range of motion can be improved with appropriate physical therapy. Isometric exercises are preferred to isotonic ones, because they place less stress on the involved joint.

Heat and cold are both used, with varying effectiveness, to provide symptomatic relief to patients with OA and as an important adjunct to physical therapy regimens. Transcutaneous nerve stimulation, particularly to relieve back pain, and acupuncture are effective in some patients and sometimes may provide an alternative to pharmacologic intervention.

Periods of rest throughout the day may be an important adjunct in the routine of patients with OA. Reduction in joint loading, either by rest or by appropriate use of a cane, often permits increased periods of activity with reduced pain. Use of cushioned shoes (commercial running or walking shoes) also may ameliorate lower extremity joint symptoms. Back pain may be reduced by muscle-strengthening exercises and by a well-fitted brace. However, the fitted brace should be used only intermittently, to prevent abdominal and paraspinal muscle atrophy.

Medical Therapy

Symptomatic relief of joint pain in patients with OA may be achieved with simple analgesic agents such as acetaminophen (Table 283–2). Particularly in elderly patients with decreased renal reserve and an increased incidence of upper gastrointestinal bleeding, acetaminophen and other simple analgesics should be the drugs of initial choice. If inflammation is present (erosive OA) or symptoms are not well controlled with simple analgesics, NSAIDs are generally more effective. 1

A newer class of NSAIDs, the cyclooxygenase-2 (COX2) inhibitors, inhibit inflammatory-mediated production of prostaglandins (COX2 mediated) but permit constitutive prostaglandin production (COX1 mediated). Although they produce less gastrointestinal toxicity than traditional nonselective NSAIDs, they have been associated with an increase in cardiovascular risk, a property that may be shared with nonselective NSAIDs as well. Therefore, only one selective COX2 inhibitor, celecoxib, is being marketed in the United States. COX2 inhibitors may be preferred to nonselective NSAIDs, particularly in patients at high risk for gastrointestinal side effects, but each patient should be carefully informed of the cardiovascular risks associated with this class of medications. 2,3

Oral glucosamine and chondroitin are referred to as "nutriceuticals"; their use has been shown in some, but not all, randomized clinical trials to reduce pain in subjects with knee OA. The time to onset of pain relief, as well as the magnitude of this response, have not been well characterized. Studies are still underway to determine whether these nutriceuticals alter the structural deterioration of the knee joint in OA.

Controlled studies of intra-articular steroid injections have demonstrated safety and benefit when injections were given every 3 months for up to 2 years. 4 Intra-articular injections of steroids should not be repeated more than three or four times per year in any given joint because of the possibility of potentiating cartilage breakdown. Systemic use of steroids has no place in the treatment of OA. Intra-articular hyaluronate can improve joint symptoms and appears to be effective in subgroups of knee OA subjects. 5

Topical treatment with capsaicin, a substance-P inhibitor, has been shown to relieve localized pain in some patients with OA. The development of agents that can stimulate cartilage synthesis or prevent degradation is actively being pursued and may provide the next generation of agents used to treat OA.

Surgical Therapy

Joint replacement surgery has been the single biggest advance in the treatment of OA in the past half-century. Patients for whom optimal medical management has failed, who continue to have pain that interferes with sleep or activity or have significant limitations of joint function, are candidates for an operation. Those individuals with altered limb alignment and early OA of a hip or knee may benefit from osteotomy. Most patients have more advanced disease and require total joint replacement. Ideal candidates for total joint arthroplasty exhibit well-maintained muscle strength and should be older than 60 years of age. Younger patients are discouraged from undergoing joint replacement because of the small but real incidence of long-term failure of joint implants, mainly due to loosening. Revision arthroplasty is possible but has a higher failure rate and can be avoided by delaying the initial arthroplasty as long as possible and putting less load on the replaced joint.

Arthroscopic surgery is useful for removing loose bodies and repairing intrinsic defects of the knee, and in shoulder (rotator cuff) and ankle disease. Arthroscopic lavage (flushing of saline to remove cartilage debris) in patients with knee OA may provide pain relief. Abrasion arthroplasty (chondroplasty) has been widely used in patients with knee OA, but no data exist to demonstrate its efficacy, and it cannot be recommended currently.

TABLE 283–2 RECOMMENDATIONS FOR PHARMACOLOGIC MANAGEMENT OF OSTEOARTHRITIS OF THE HIP AND KNEE*

ORAL
Acetaminophen
Nonselective NSAID plus misoprostol or a proton pump inhibitor†
COX2-selective inhibitor
Nonacetylated salicylate
Other pure analgesics
Glucosamine and/or chondroitin sulfate
Tramadol
Opioids
INTRA-ARTICULAR
Glucocorticoids
Hyaluronan
TOPICAL
Capsaicin
Methylsalicylate

*The choice of pharmacologic therapy should be individualized for each patient.
†Misoprostol and proton pump inhibitors may be used in patients who are at increased risk for upper gastrointestinal adverse events. COX2 = cyclooxygenase-2; NSAID = nonsteroidal anti-inflammatory drug.
From the American College of Rheumatology Subcommittee on Osteoarthritis Guidelines. Arthritis Rheum 2003;43:1905–1915.

Future Directions

In the next few years, the focus of OA treatment will most likely change from use of only analgesic agents to agents that may alter the course of the disease. These future drugs may include MMP inhibitors, cartilage growth factors, NO inhibitors, or agents that can prevent chondrocyte apoptosis. In addition, research is currently being carried out involving biosynthetic cartilage replacement and improved materials for total joint replacement. Therefore, the future holds promise not only to slow the joint degeneration in OA but possibly also to reverse it.

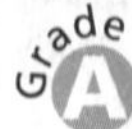

1. Towheed TE, Maxwell L, Judd MG, et al: Acetaminophen for osteoarthritis. Cochrane Database Syst Rev 2006;1:CD004257.
2. Geba GP, Weaver AL, Polis AB, et al: Efficacy of rofecoxib, celecoxib, and acetaminophen in osteoarthritis of the knee: A randomized trial. Vioxx, Acetaminophen, Celecoxib Trial (VACT) Group. JAMA 2001;283:64–71.
3. Day R, Morrison B, Luza A, et al: A randomized trial of the efficacy and tolerability of the COX-2 inhibitor rofecoxib versus ibuprofen in patients with osteoarthritis. Rofecoxib/Ibuprofen Comparator Study Group. Arch Intern Med 2000;160:1781–1787.
4. Raynauld JP, Buckland-Wright C, Ward R, et al: Safety and efficacy of long-term intraarticular steroid injections in osteoarthritis of the knee: A randomized, double-blind, placebo-controlled trial. Arthritis Rheum 2003;48:370–377.
5. Altman R, Moskowitz R: Intra-articular sodium hyaluronate (Hyalgan) in the treatment of patients with osteoarthritis of the knee: A randomized clinical trial. Hyalgan Study Group. J Rheumatol 1998;25:2203–2212.

SUGGESTED READINGS

American College of Rheumatology Subcommittee on Osteoarthritis Guidelines: Recommendations for the medical management of OA of the hip and knee. Arthritis Rheum 2000;43:1905–1915. *Consensus guidelines.*

Brosseau L, MacLeay L, Robinson V, et al: Intensity of exercise for the treatment of osteoarthritis. Cochrane Database Syst Rev 2003;(2):CD004259. *High-intensity and low-intensity aerobic exercise are equally effective in improving functional status and osteoarthritis of the knee.*

Clegg DO, Reda DJ, Harris CL, et al: Glucosamine, chondroitin sulfate, and the two in combination for painful knee osteoarthritis. N Engl J Med 2006;354:795–808. *No benefit was demonstrated alone or in combination.*

Felson DT: Osteoarthritis of the knee. N Engl J Med 2006;354:841–848. *An excellent review of osteoarthritis.*

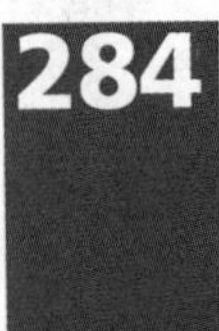

284 BURSITIS, TENDINITIS, AND OTHER PERIARTICULAR DISORDERS, AND SPORTS MEDICINE

Joseph J. Biundo

Definition

An entire array of painful and sometimes disabling musculoskeletal syndromes exist which are not articular in origin but arise from tendons and bursae. These conditions are referred to by various names, in addition to tendinitis and bursitis, including the terms nonarticular rheumatism, soft tissue diseases, regional rheumatic pain syndromes, overuse syndromes, and repetitive use syndromes (Tables 284–1 and 284–2). These entities are often ignored, misdiagnosed as arthritis, or attributed to the aging process; awareness of the existence of these conditions and knowledge of basic musculoskeletal anatomy (Figs. 284–1 and 284–2) are the fundamental requirements for diagnosis. This knowledge is coupled with brief but specific physical diagnosis techniques, which must surpass the inadequate mantra of "no clubbing, cyanosis, or edema," so often recorded by clinicians in the musculoskeletal physical examination. The accurate diagnosis and successful treatment of these conditions is gratifying to the clinician, because many people can be relieved of their chronic painful syndromes.

Various terms regarding tendon injuries are used and may be confusing. The main term used is *tendinitis. Tendinosis* has been proposed as the correct terminology, because there are degenerative changes in the tendon but very few inflammatory cells. In addition, fatty mucoid degeneration and hyaline features occur in these tendon syndromes. These tendon conditions are described by some as a *tendinopathy,* because use of this term avoids the need to decide whether inflammation is a factor. Also, tendons may *rupture* or *tear,* partially or completely. The term *tendon insufficiency* is used when the tendon is stretched or is partially or

TABLE 284–1 MUSCULOSKELETAL CONDITIONS BY ETIOLOGY

Tendinitis	Tendon Rupture	Bursitis
Rotator cuff	Rotator cuff	Subacromial
Bicipital	Bicipital	Olecranon
Volar flexor	Quadriceps	Trochanteric
de Quervain's	Patellar	Ischial
Patellar	Posterior tibialis	Iliopsoas
Posterior tibialis	Achilles	Pes anserine
Achilles		Prepatellar
Epicondylitis		Retrocalcaneal

TABLE 284–2 TENDINITIS AND BURSITIS CONDITIONS BY REGION

SHOULDER
Rotator cuff tendinitis
Rotator cuff tear
Bicipital tendinitis
Subacromial bursitis
Adhesive capsulitis
ELBOW
Olecranon bursitis
Medial epicondylitis
Lateral epicondylitis
WRIST AND HAND
de Quervain's tenosynovitis
Volar flexor tenosynovitis
Ganglion
HIP
Trochanteric bursitis
Iliopsoas bursitis
Ischial bursitis
Coccydynia
KNEE
Prepatellar bursitis
Pes anserine bursitis
Popliteal cyst (Baker's cyst)
Patellar tendinitis
Patellar/quadriceps tendon tear
ANKLE AND FOOT
Achilles tendinitis
Achilles tendon tear
Posterior tibial tendinitis
Posterior tibial tendon tear
Retrocalcaneal bursitis
Plantar fasciitis

even completely torn. The terms *tenosynovitis* and *peritendinitis* refer to an inflammatory response of the tenosynovium or peritendon, respectively.

Tendon syndromes are basically "overuse" injuries. Tendinitis may occur when the tendon repeatedly bears more load than it can withstand. This may result from excessively high loads across normal tendons or from normal loads across degenerated tendons. In addition to load and

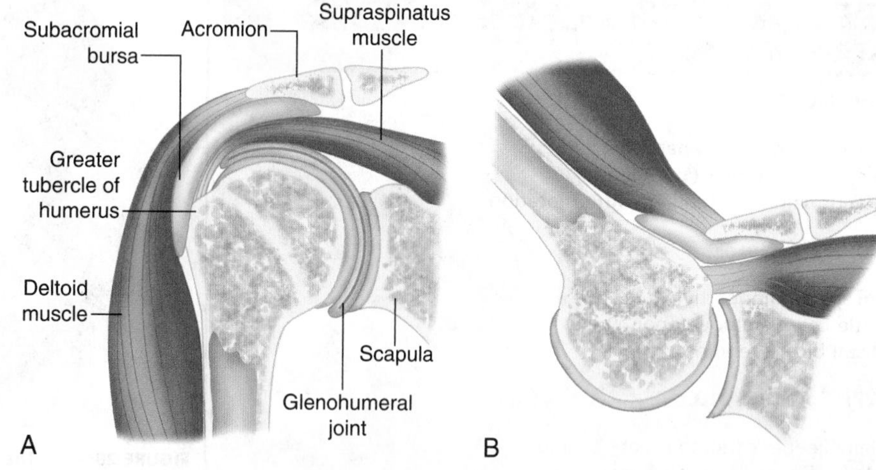

FIGURE 284–1 • Relationship of subacromial bursa (shown in blue) to supraspinatus muscle and acromion process. A, In the position of adduction of the humerus. To show this bursa more clearly, the synovial membrane of the glenohumeral joint is not shown in blue. **B,** In the position of abduction of the humerus, the acromion impinges on the subacromial bursa and the insertion of the supraspinatus tendon. (From Polley HF, Hunder GG [eds]: Rheumatologic Interviewing and Physical Examination of the Joints, 2nd ed. Philadelphia, WB Saunders, 1978, p 65.)

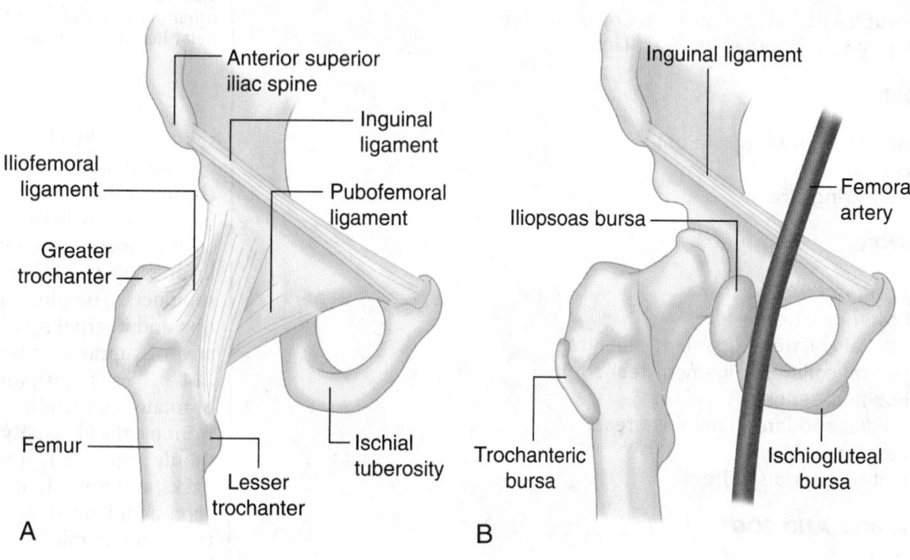

FIGURE 284–2 • Musculoskeletal anatomy of the hip. A, Anterior aspect of the hip joint and bony structures. **B,** Relationship of the distended iliopsoas, trochanteric, and ischiogluteal bursae (shown in blue) to the hip joint and adjacent structures. (From Polley HF, Hunder GG [eds]: Rheumatologic Interviewing and Physical Examination of the Joints, 2nd ed. Philadelphia, WB Saunders, 1978, p 183.)

repetitiveness, tendon changes resulting from immobility and from aging may play a role, as may the use of certain medications such as floxins and corticosteroids

Bursae are closed sacs that are lined by a synovial membrane and serve as a cushion. They are located between tendon and bone, tendon and tendon, or bone and skin and allow smooth gliding between these structures. A bursa, which normally has a small of amount of bursal fluid, can become inflamed from trauma or overuse, or become infected, producing a bursitis. When this occurs, some swelling and pain of the bursa may be present.

Epidemiology

The incidence of the nonarticular syndromes of bursitis and tendinitis is high. They are more common than both rheumatoid arthritis (RA) and systemic lupus erythematosus (SLE). (SLE is even less common than RA.) For example, the incidence of shoulder pain, largely due to rotator cuff tendinitis and rotator cuff tear, was about 20% in an elderly population older than 70 years of age.

Diagnosis

A precise history is needed to identify the conditions present, and more than one syndrome can occur concomitantly. A working knowledge of regional anatomy and an approach that uses a regional differential diagnosis will help in obtaining a specific diagnosis. A complete neuromusculoskeletal examination should be performed, emphasizing careful palpation, passive range of motion (ROM), and active ROM alone or sometimes with resistance. Systemic and infectious causes must be considered. Diagnostic ultrasonography and magnetic resonance imaging (MRI) are sometimes useful in confirming a diagnosis.

Treatment

Treatment of tendinitis and bursitis includes use of nonsteroidal anti-inflammatory drugs (NSAIDs), relative rest of the injured site, stretching and strengthening exercises, friction massage, use of modalities (heat, ice, and ultrasound), splinting, corticosteroid injections, and surgery. A comprehensive management of these regional syndromes should be undertaken, rather than relying on oral medications alone. The causative aspects should be evaluated, and activity modification should be advised as needed. The goals of therapeutic exercise are to increase flexibility by stretching, increase muscle strength by resistive exercises, and improve muscle endurance by some repetitive regimen. Caution should be exerted in performing corticosteroid injections; the injections should not be placed into the tendon proper, but rather into the peritendinous sheath. The injection should be placed beneath the subcutaneous tissue, to avoid skin and subcutaneous fat atrophy, and injections should not be given too frequently, to avoid the possibility of weakening and rupture of the tendon. The accuracy of injections may be improved with concomitant use of diagnostic ultrasonography to assist with determining the correct needle site. Also, fluoroscopically guided injections can be used to increase accuracy.

TABLE 284–3 ADDITIONAL CONDITIONS THAT ARE SPORTS RELATED

SHOULDER
Acromioclavicular separation
Glenoid labial tear (SLAP lesion)
Glenohumeral instability with dislocation
ELBOW
Triceps tendinopathy
Little League elbow (apophysitis)
Distal biceps tendinitis
WRIST AND HAND
Gamekeeper's thumb (skier's thumb)
Mallet finger (baseball finger)
Extensor carpi ulnaris tendinitis
Rupture of flexor digitorum profundus tendon
Injury to triangular fibrocartilage
HIP
Adductor strain (groin pull)
Hip pointer
Hamstring strain
KNEE
Anterior cruciate tear
Posterior cruciate tear
Medial collateral ligament teat/strain
Lateral collateral ligament tear/strain
Popliteal tendinitis
Medial and lateral meniscal tears
Patellar tendinitis
Iliotibial band syndrome
ANKLE AND FOOT
Ankle sprain
Turf toe
Stress fracture

SPORTS MEDICINE INJURIES

An overlap exists between commonly occurring conditions of tendinitis and bursitis and those attributed to sports injuries (Table 284–3). For example, lateral epicondylitis, frequently referred to as tennis elbow, occurs more commonly secondary to non–sports-related causes. In contradistinction, iliotibial band syndrome is usually related to sports. Other entities that occur more often in relation to sports include ligamentous knee injuries, patellar tendinitis, ankle sprains, turf toe, and acromioclavicular separations. It is important in both categories to know the anatomy and biomechanics of the condition, so as to better diagnose and treat the problem. Sports-related injuries are helped with the classic RICE treatment, consisting of *r*est, *i*ce, *c*ompression, and *e*levation. Often, anti-inflammatory and analgesic drugs are used. However, there is less use of corticosteroid injections in athletic injuries than in routine cases of tendinitis and bursitis.

DISORDERS OF THE SHOULDER REGION

Shoulder pain is one of the most common musculoskeletal complaints in people older than 40 years of age. In younger people, athletic injuries are a frequent source of such pain. Rotator cuff tendinitis, or impingement syndrome, is the most common cause of shoulder pain. Tendinitis (and not bursitis) is the primary cause of pain, but secondary involvement of the subacromial bursa occurs in some cases. The condition may be acute or chronic and may or may not be associated with calcific deposits within the tendon. The key finding is pain in the rotator cuff on active abduction, especially between 60 and 120 degrees, and sometimes when lowering the arm. In more severe cases, pain may begin on initial abduction and continue throughout the ROM. Typically, chronic rotator cuff tendinitis manifests as an ache in the shoulder, usually over the lateral deltoid, and occurs with various movements, especially abduction and internal rotation. Other symptoms include difficulty in dressing oneself and night pain due to difficulty in positioning the shoulders. The physical findings include pain and loss of active abduction and internal rotation, less pain on passive motion, tenderness of the area of supraspinatus insertion, and a positive impingement sign (Fig. 284–3, Neer's sign), which is pain occurring in forced flexion. The causes of rotator cuff tendinitis are multifactorial, but relative overuse, especially from overhead activity causing impingement of the rotator cuff, is commonly implicated. Treatment consists of rest and modalities such as hot packs, ultrasound, or cold applications, with specific ROM exercises as soon as tolerated. NSAIDs are often beneficial, but the most frequent treatment is injection of a depot corticosteroid into the subacromial bursa, the floor of which is contiguous with the rotator cuff.

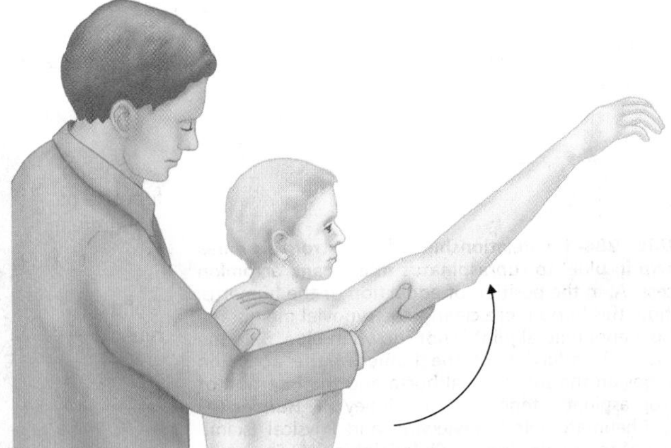

FIGURE 284–3 • The impingement sign is elicited by forced forward elevation of the arm. Pain results as the greater tuberosity impinges on the acromion. The examiner's hand prevents scapular rotation. This maneuver may be positive in other periarticular disorders. (From Neer CS II: Impingement lesions. Clin Orthop Relat Res 1983;173:70–77.)

In a rotator cuff tear, an acute tear after trauma is usually easily recognized. The trauma may be superimposed on an already degenerative and possibly even partially torn cuff. In cases of trauma resulting in a ruptured cuff, fracture of the humeral head and dislocation of the joint should also be considered. However, most patients with a tear recall no trauma. In these cases, degeneration of the rotator cuff occurs gradually, resulting ultimately in a complete tear. Rotator cuff tears are classified as small (1 cm or less), medium (1 to 3 cm), large (3 to 5 cm), or massive (greater than 5 cm). Shoulder pain, weakness on abduction, and loss of motion occur in varying degrees, ranging from severe pain and mild weakness to no pain and marked weakness. A positive drop-arm sign with inability to actively maintain 90 degrees of passive shoulder abduction may be present in patients with large or massive tears. Small complete tears and incomplete tears of the rotator cuff are treated conservatively with rest, physical therapy, and NSAIDs. Although its role has not yet been established by careful studies, a subacromial injection of a corticosteroid may relieve pain. Surgical repair is indicated in younger patients.

Bicipital tendinitis is manifested by pain, most often in the anterior region of the shoulder and occasionally more diffusely. The pain may be acute but is usually chronic and is related to impingement of the biceps tendon by the acromion. Tenosynovitis of the long head of the biceps is present, and the tendon may be frayed and fibrotic. Palpation over the bicipital groove reveals localized tenderness. The patient's response should be compared with the response to palpation of the opposite side (i.e., tendon with normal tenderness). Pain may be reproduced over the bicipital tendon in some cases by supination of the forearm against resistance (Yergason's sign), shoulder flexion against resistance (Speed test), or extension of the shoulder. Treatment of bicipital tendinitis consists of rest, hot packs, ultrasound, and, as pain subsides, passive and then active ROM exercises. NSAIDs may be helpful, and occasionally a small amount of corticosteroid carefully injected into the tendon sheath may be of benefit. Rupture of the biceps tendon can occur at the superior edge of the bicipital groove, producing a characteristic bulbous enlargement of the lateral half of the muscle belly.

Adhesive capsulitis (frozen shoulder) is associated with generalized pain and tenderness and severe loss of active and passive motion in all planes. It is rare before 40 years of age but may occur secondary to any type of shoulder problem. However, not every stiff and painful shoulder is necessarily adhesive capsulitis. Inflammatory arthritis and diabetes can cause adhesive capsulitis. Additional factors such as immobility, low pain threshold, depression, and neglect or improper initial treatment also favor the development of a frozen shoulder. Many cases, however, are idiopathic. The joint capsule adheres to the anatomic neck, and the axillary fold binds to itself, causing restricted motion. The capsule becomes thickened and contracted. Arthrography can help confirm this diagnosis by showing a decrease in volume of the shoulder joint capsule. Oral steroids improve pain and range of motion in the short term, [1] but a frozen shoulder is probably best treated with a comprehensive program involving NSAIDs and corticosteroid injections into the glenohumeral joint and the subacromial bursa. Physical therapy consists of ice packs, ultrasound, transcutaneous electrical nerve stimulation, and gentle ROM exercises, beginning with pendulum exercises and wall climbing with the fingers and progressing to active ROM and strengthening exercises.

DISORDERS OF THE ELBOW REGION

Olecranon bursitis occurs frequently and involves the subcutaneous olecranon bursa, either secondary to trauma or as an idiopathic condition. The bursa is characteristically swollen and tender on pressure, but pain may be minimal and usually no motion is lost. Aspiration may yield clear or blood-tinged fluid with a low viscosity, or grossly hemorrhagic fluid. Inflammatory olecranon bursitis may be caused by gout, RA, or calcium pyrophosphate deposition disease, and infection can also cause a bursitis. Aspiration alone and protection from trauma are usually sufficient to resolve the condition. A small dose of corticosteroid may be injected into the bursa. With septic olecranon bursitis, localized erythema is the major clue. Heat, pain, and a positive culture are also frequently present.

Lateral epicondylitis, or tennis elbow, is a common condition in those who overuse their arms. Localized tenderness directly over or slightly anterior to the lateral epicondyle is the hallmark of this disorder. Pain may occur during handshakes, while lifting a briefcase, or with other similar activities. Probably fewer than 10% of patients actually acquire lateral epicondylitis through playing tennis. Job and recreational activities, including gardening and athletics, are the usual causes. Pathologically, the condition consists of degeneration of the common extensor tendon, particularly of the extensor carpi radialis brevis tendon. Treatment is aimed at altering activities and preventing overuse of the forearm musculature. Ice packs, heat, and NSAIDs are of some benefit. A forearm brace can also be used. A local corticosteroid injection with a 25-gauge needle over the lateral epicondyle often produces satisfactory initial relief. Isometric strengthening is important as the initial part of a rehabilitation program.

Medial epicondylitis, or golfer's elbow, which mainly involves the flexor carpi radialis, is less common and less disabling than lateral epicondylitis. Local pain and tenderness over the medial epicondyle are present, and resistance to wrist flexion exacerbates the pain.

DISORDERS OF THE WRIST AND HAND

A ganglion is a cystic swelling that arises from a joint or tendon sheath and occurs most commonly over the dorsum of the wrist. It is synovial lined and contains thick, jelly-like fluid. Ganglia apparently develop secondary to trauma or prolonged wrist extension. Usually, the only symptom is swelling, but occasionally a large ganglion produces discomfort on wrist extension.

De Quervain's tenosynovitis may result from repetitive activity that involves pinching with the thumb while moving the wrist. The symptoms are pain, tenderness, and occasionally swelling over the radial styloid. Pathologic findings include inflammation and narrowing of the tendon sheath around the abductor pollicis longus and extensor pollicis brevis. A positive Finkelstein test result is usually seen: pain increases when the thumb is folded across the palm and the fingers are flexed over the thumb as the examiner passively deviates the wrist toward the ulnar side. However, this test may also be positive in patients with osteoarthritis

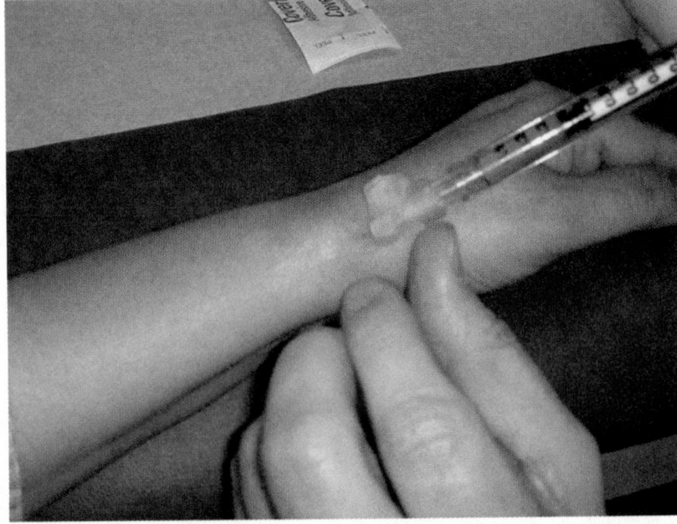

FIGURE 284–4 • Injection of de Quervain's tenosynovitis.

(OA) of the first carpometacarpal (CMC) joint and must be differentiated from this common condition. Treatment involves splinting, local corticosteroid injection (Fig. 284–4), and NSAIDs as indicated. Rarely, surgical removal of the inflamed tenosynovium is needed.

Volar flexor tenosynovitis consists of inflammation of the tendon sheaths of the flexor digitorum superficialis and flexor digitorum profundus tendons in the palm. It is extremely common but often unrecognized. Pain in the palm is felt on finger flexion, but in some cases the pain radiates to the proximal interphalangeal (PIP) and metacarpophalangeal (MCP) joints on the dorsal side, misleading the examiner. The diagnosis is made by palpation and identification of localized tenderness and swelling of the volar tendon sheaths. The middle and index fingers are most commonly involved, but the ring and little fingers can also be affected. Often a nodule composed of fibrous tissue can be palpated in the palm just proximal to the MCP joint on the volar side. The nodule interferes with the normal tendon gliding and can cause a triggering or locking, which may be intermittent and may produce an uncomfortable sensation. Similar involvement can occur at the flexor tendon of the thumb. The most common cause is overuse trauma of the hands from gripping with increased pull on the flexor tendons. It may be part of inflammatory conditions, such as RA, psoriatic arthritis, or apatite crystal deposition disease. It is seen frequently in conjunction with OA of the hands. Injection of a long-acting steroid into the tendon sheath usually relieves the problem, although surgery on the tendon sheath may be needed in unremitting cases.

Gamekeeper's thumb (skier's thumb) is caused by trauma to the thumb resulting in instability of the first MCP joint. This instability is due to laxity or rupture of the ulnar collateral ligament. It is treated by immobilization, but surgical repair may be necessary.

Avulsion of flexor digitorum profundus (jersey finger) may occur due to trauma, usually in football, when a player grabs onto a jersey. The distal phalanx, usually the fourth, is hyperextended while the digitorum profundus is contracting maximally. The avulsion of the tendon results in an inability to flex the distal phalanx of that digit. Surgery is required to correct the problem.

DISORDERS OF THE HIP REGION

Although trochanteric bursitis is common, it frequently goes undiagnosed. It occurs predominantly in middle-aged to elderly people, and somewhat more often in women than in men. The main symptom is aching over the trochanteric area and lateral thigh. Walking, various movements, and lying on the involved hip may intensify the pain. Onset may be acute, but more often it is gradual, with symptoms lasting for months. In chronic cases, the patient may fail to adequately locate or describe the pain, or the physician may fail to note the symptoms or interpret them correctly. Occasionally, the pain has a pseudoradiculopathic quality, radiating down the lateral aspect of the thigh. In a few cases, the pain is so severe that the patient cannot walk and complains of diffuse pain of the entire thigh. The best way to diagnose trochanteric bursitis is to palpate over the trochanteric area and elicit point tenderness. In addi-

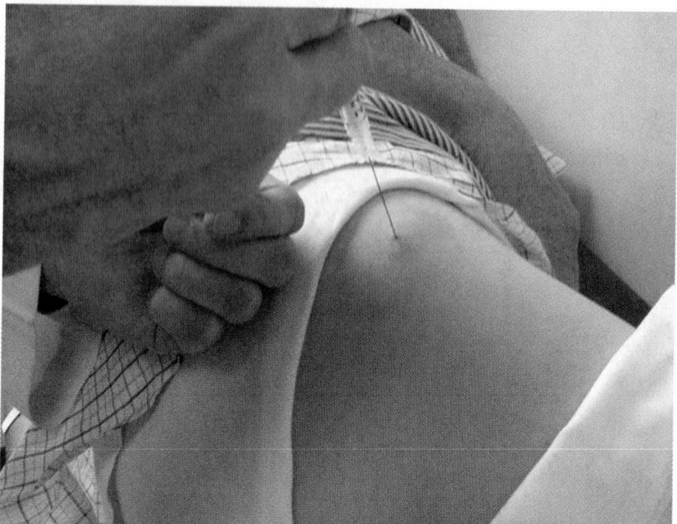

FIGURE 284–5 • Injection of trochanteric bursitis.

tion to specific pain on deep pressure over the trochanter, other tender points may be noted throughout the lateral aspect of the thigh muscle. Pain may be worse with external rotation and abduction against resistance. Although bursitis is usually described as the principal problem, the condition may actually arise at the insertions of the gluteus maximus and gluteus medius tendons. Local trauma and degeneration play a role in the pathogenesis. Conditions that may contribute to trochanteric bursitis, apparently by adding stress to the area, include OA of the lumbar spine or of the hip, leg-length discrepancy, and scoliosis. Treatment consists of local injection of depot corticosteroid using a 22-gauge, 3.5-inch needle to ensure that the bursal area is reached (Fig. 284–5). NSAIDs, weight loss, and strengthening and stretching of the gluteus medius muscle and iliotibial band help in management.

Coccydynia is manifested by pain in the coccyx area when pressure is applied to the area. This most notably occurs on sitting. The patient squirms from buttock to buttock to relieve the pressure and consequent pain, and often chooses to sit on a cushion. The symptoms may be chronic and severe. The condition may relate to a fall on the coccyx, dropping to a hard chair when sitting, or some related trauma to the coccyx. However, at times no obvious cause can be detected. Women are much more frequently affected, perhaps because the lordosis that often occurs in women exposes the coccyx to more trauma. The diagnosis is confirmed by finding localized tenderness over the coccyx on palpation. A plain x-ray can be obtained to exclude a fracture or dislocation of the coccyx. Treatment with a local injection of a long-acting corticosteroid and 2 mL of a 2% lidocaine solution is usually very effective. The exact nature of the pathology of coccydynia has not been studied, but it is presumed to be a bone bruise.

In iliopsoas bursitis, groin and anterior thigh pain are present and worsen on passive hip hyperextension and sometimes on flexion, especially with resistance. Tenderness is palpable over an involved bursa. The patient may hold the hip in flexion and external rotation to eliminate pain and may limp to prevent hyperextension of the hip. The iliopsoas bursa lies behind the iliopsoas muscle, anterior to the hip joint and lateral to the femoral vessels. It communicates with the hip in 15% of cases. The diagnosis is more apparent if a cystic mass is seen (about 30% of the cases); however, other causes of cystic swelling in the femoral area must first be excluded. A bursal mass can cause femoral venous obstruction or femoral nerve compression. As with most cases of bursitis, acute or recurrent trauma and inflammatory conditions such as RA may lead to iliopsoas bursitis (also called iliopectineal bursitis). The diagnosis is confirmed by plain x-ray with injection of a contrast medium into the bursa, or by computed tomography or MRI. Iliopsoas bursitis usually responds to conservative treatment including corticosteroid injections. With recurrent involvement, excision of the bursa may be necessary.

Ischial or ischiogluteal bursitis is caused by trauma or by prolonged sitting on hard surfaces, as evidenced by the name, "weaver's bottom." Pain is often exquisite when sitting or lying down. Because the ischiogluteal bursa is located superficial to the ischial tuberosity and separates the gluteus maximus from the tuberosity, the pain may radiate down the back of the thigh. Point tenderness over the ischial tuberosity is present. Use of cushions and local injection of a corticosteroid are helpful.

DISORDERS OF THE KNEE REGION

Anserine bursitis is seen predominantly in overweight, middle-aged to elderly women with large legs and OA of the knees. The symptoms are pain and tenderness over the medial aspect of the knee about 2 inches below the joint margin with the pain worsened by climbing stairs. The pes anserinus (Latin for "goose foot") is composed of the conjoined tendons of the sartorius, gracilis, and semitendinosus muscles. The bursa extends between the tendons and the tibial collateral ligament. The diagnosis is made by eliciting exquisite tenderness over the bursa. Anserine bursitis is often overlooked, because it frequently occurs concomitantly with OA of the knee, which, when present, is the assumed cause of pain; however, in some cases of dual involvement, anserine bursitis is the principal source of pain. The treatment is rest, stretching of the adductor and quadriceps muscles, and a corticosteroid injection into the bursa.

Prepatellar bursitis is manifested as a swelling superficial to the kneecap and results from trauma such as frequent kneeling, leading to the name "housemaid's knee." The prepatellar bursa lies anterior to the lower half of the patella and the upper half of the patellar ligament. The pain is generally slight unless pressure is applied directly over the bursa. The infrapatellar bursa, which lies between the patellar ligament and the tibia, is also subject to trauma and swelling. Chronic prepatellar bursitis can be treated by protecting the knee from the irritating trauma.

Patellar tendinitis (jumper's knee) is seen predominately in athletes engaging in activities such as repetitive running, jumping, or kicking. Pain and tenderness are present over the patellar tendon.

Iliotibial band syndrome is manifested by lateral knee pain caused by friction between the iliotibial band and the lateral femoral condyle. It is an overuse injury and is seen in runners, cyclists, and other athletes performing repetitive knee flexion activities.

Popliteal cysts, also known as Baker's cysts, are not uncommon, and the clinician should be well aware of the possibility of their dissection or rupture. A cystic swelling behind the knee with mild or no discomfort can be the only initial finding. With further distention of the cyst, however, a greater awareness and discomfort is experienced, particularly on full flexion or extension. The cyst is best seen when the patient is standing and examined from behind. Any knee disease having a synovial effusion can develop into a popliteal cyst. Popliteal cysts are most common secondary to RA, OA, or internal derangements of the knee. There are a few reported cases secondary to gout and Reiter's syndrome. A syndrome of pseudothrombophlebitis may occur as a result of cyst dissection into the calf or actual rupture of the cyst. Findings include diffuse swelling of the calf, pain, and sometimes erythema and edema of the ankle. An ultrasound or arthrogram of the knee confirms both the cyst and the possible dissection or rupture. A cyst related to an inflammatory arthritis is treated by injection of a depot corticosteroid into the knee joint, and possibly into the cyst itself, which usually resolves the problem. If the cyst results from OA or an internal derangement of the knee, surgical repair of the underlying joint lesion is usually necessary to prevent a recurrence of the cyst.

In the knee area tendon ruptures may occur, and quadriceps tendon rupture is involved about 50% of the time; otherwise, patellar tendon rupture occurs. Quadriceps tendon rupture is generally caused by sudden violent contractions of the quadriceps muscle when the knee is flexed. A hemarthrosis of the knee joint may follow. Patients with chronic renal failure, RA, hyperparathyroidism, or gout and SLE patients taking steroids have been reported to have spontaneous ruptures of the quadriceps tendon. The patient experiences a sudden sharp pain and cannot extend the leg. Radiographic studies may show a high-riding patella. The tendon is usually found to be degenerated, and surgical repair is often indicated. Rupture of the patellar tendon has been associated with a specific episode of trauma, repetitive trauma from sporting activities, and systemic diseases.

DISORDERS OF THE ANKLE AND FOOT REGION

Achilles tendinitis usually results from trauma, athletic overactivity, or improperly fitting shoes with a stiff heel counter, but it can also be caused by inflammatory conditions such as ankylosing spondylitis, Reiter's syndrome, gout, RA, and calcium pyrophosphate dihydrate crystal deposition disease. Pain, swelling, and tenderness occur over the Achilles tendon at its attachment and in the area proximal to the attachment. Crepitus on motion and pain on dorsiflexion may be present. Management includes NSAIDs, rest, shoe corrections, heel lift, gentle stretching, and sometimes a splint with slight plantar flexion. The Achilles tendon is vulnerable to rupture when involved with tendinitis, and treatment with a corticosteroid injection could increase this possibility.

Achilles tendon rupture is well known and occurs with a sudden onset of pain during forced dorsiflexion. An audible snap may be heard, followed by difficulty in walking and standing on toes. Swelling and edema over the area usually develop. Diagnosis can be made with the Thompson test, in which the patient kneels on a chair with the feet extending over the edge and the examiner squeezes the calf and pushes toward the knee. Normally this produces plantar flexion, but in a ruptured tendon no plantar flexion occurs. Achilles tendon rupture is usually occurs during athletic events or with trauma from jumps or falls. The tendon is more prone to tear in people with preexisting Achilles tendon disease and in those taking corticosteroids. Orthopedic consultation should be obtained, and immobilization or surgery may be selected, depending on the situation.

Plantar fasciitis, which is seen primarily in persons between 40 and 60 years of age, is characterized by pain in the plantar area of the heel. The onset may be gradual, or it may occur with trauma or overuse from some activity, such as athletics, prolonged walking, using improper shoes, or striking the heel with some force. Plantar fasciitis may be idiopathic; it also is likely to be present in younger patients with spondyloarthritis. The pain characteristically occurs in the morning on arising and is most severe for the first few steps. After an initial improvement, the pain may worsen later in the day, especially after prolonged standing or walking. The pain is burning, aching, and occasionally lancinating. Palpation typically reveals tenderness anteromedially on the medial calcaneal tubercle at the origin of the plantar fascia. Treatment includes relative rest with a reduction in stressful activities, NSAIDs, use of heel pad or heel cup orthosis, arch support, and stretching of the heel cord and plantar fascia. A local corticosteroid injection, using a 25-gauge needle, is often of help.

In posterior tibial tendinitis, pain and tenderness occur just posterior to the medial malleolus; it can be caused by trauma, excessive pronation, RA, or spondyloarthropathy. Extension and flexion may be normal, but pain is present on resisted inversion or passive eversion. The discomfort is usually worse after athletic activity, and swelling and localized tenderness may be present. Treatment usually includes rest, NSAIDs, and possibly a local injection of corticosteroid. Immobilization with a splint is sometimes needed.

Posterior tibialis tendon rupture, which is not commonly recognized, is a cause of progressive flat foot. It can result from trauma, chronic tendon degeneration, or RA. An insidious onset of pain and tenderness may be noted along the course of the tendon just distal to the medial malleolus, along with swelling medial to the hind foot. The unilateral deformity of hind foot valgus and forefoot abduction is an important finding. The forefoot abduction can best be seen from behind; more toes are seen from this position than would be seen normally. The result of the single heel rise test is positive when the patient is unable to rise onto the ball of the affected foot while the contralateral foot is off the floor. Treatment usually includes rest, NSAIDs, and possibly a local injection of corticosteroid. Immobilization with a splint is sometimes needed.

Manifestations of retrocalcaneal bursitis include pain at the back of the heel, tenderness of the area anterior to the Achilles tendon, and pain on dorsiflexion. Local swelling is present, with bulging on the medial and lateral aspects of the tendon. Retrocalcaneal bursitis, also called sub-Achilles bursitis, may coexist with Achilles tendinitis, and distinguishing the two is sometimes difficult. This condition may be secondary to RA, spondylitis, a reactive arthritis, gout, or trauma.

Turf toe is an injury of the big toe originally described during play on artificial turf. It results from hyperextension of the first metatarsophaleangeal (MTP) joint when a fixed, dorsiflexed foot is forced into the ground. The plantar capsular ligament may be sprained or torn.

Stress fracture is also known as march fracture or fatigue fracture, because it was associated with spontaneous fracture after long marches in army recruits. Pain, swelling, tenderness, and occasionally erythema develop over the metatarsal area, usually without any clear history of trauma. On questioning, however, the episode of spontaneous pain related to onset of the fracture can be identified in some cases. The neck of the second metatarsal bone is most frequently involved, but the third metatarsal is also a site of fracture. Aside from prolonged marching, other athletic events with overactivity, including jogging, are common causes. Stress fractures may be seen in patients with RA and in the elderly. The difficulty in diagnosing stress fractures is that the initial radiographs usually show no abnormalities or, at most, only a faint fracture line. A repeat radiograph several weeks later shows healing with callus formation. Bone scans aid the early diagnosis of stress fractures by showing an increase in uptake over the fracture site. Usually these fractures heal spontaneously, and rest and strapping of the foot are helpful. Occasionally, a cast is needed.

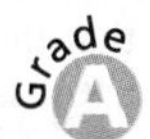

1. Buchbinder R, Green S, Youd JM, et al: Oral steroids for adhesive capsulitis. Cochrane Database Syst Rev 2006;4:CD006189.

SUGGESTED READINGS

Alvarez-Nemegyei J, Canoso JJ: Evidence-based soft tissue rheumatology: Epicondylitis and hand stenosing tendinopathy. J Clin Rheumatol 2004;10:33–40. *A practical clinical review.*

Alvarez-Nemegyei J, Canoso JJ: Evidence-based soft tissue rheumatology III: Trochanteric bursitis. J Clin Rheumatol 2004;10:102–106. *A practical clinical review.*

Alvarez-Nemegyei J, Canoso JJ: Evidence-based soft tissue rheumatology V: Plantar talalgia. J Clin Rheumatol 2004;10:259–262. *A practical clinical review.*

Burkhart SS: A 26-year-old woman with shoulder pain. JAMA 2000;284:1559–1567. *An excellent review of the differential diagnosis and management of a patient who presents with shoulder pain.*

D'Agostino MA, Ayral X, Baron G, et al: Impact of ultrasound imaging on local corticosteroid injections of symptomatic ankle, hind-, and mid-foot in chronic inflammatory diseases. Arthritis Care Res 2005;53:284–293. *Ultrasound improves diagnostic accuracy and guides more effective injections.*

Dixit S, Difiori JP, Burton M: Management of patellofemoral pain syndrome. Am Fam Phys 2007;75:192–202. *A review.*

Gomoll AH, Katz, JN, Warner JJ, et al: Rotator cuff disorders: Recognition and management among patients with shoulder pain. Arthritis Rheum 2004;50:3751–3761. *A comprehensive overview.*

Wilder RP, Sethi S: Overuse injuries: Tendinopathies, stress fractures, compartment syndrome, and shin splints. Clin Sports Med 2004;23:55–81. *A clinical review.*

285 RHEUMATOID ARTHRITIS

James R. O'Dell

Definition

Rheumatoid arthritis (RA) is a chronic systemic inflammatory disease of unknown etiology that primarily targets synovial tissues. It is relatively common, with a prevalence of approximately 0.8% in adults all over the world. RA shortens survival and significantly affects quality of life in most patients. Essentially all patients exhibit some systemic features such as fatigue, low-grade fevers, anemia, and elevations of acute phase reactants (erythrocyte sedimentation rate [ESR] or C-reactive protein [CRP]). Despite these features, the primary target of RA is the synovium, and this is responsible for most of the protean clinical features. Synovial tissues proliferate in an uncontrolled fashion, resulting in excess fluid production, destruction of cartilage, erosion of marginal bone, and damage to tendons and ligaments.

In the last decade, the landscape of treatment of RA has changed dramatically. Current therapies result in substantial clinical benefit for most patients, particularly with early diagnosis and treatment with an appropriate disease-modifying antirheumatic drug (DMARD).

Epidemiology

RA is present all over the world, with a remarkably consistent prevalence of 0.5 to 1% of adults, with some differences in certain population groups. For reasons that are still unclear, the prevalence in women is two or three times greater than in men. RA can occur at any age, but onset before the age of 45 years in men is uncommon. The relatively few, well-done inception cohorts that are available suggest that the yearly incidence of RA is approximately 40 per 100,000 for women, and about half that for men. These figures vary significantly based on the age of the cohort. The best available data suggest that the incidence of RA in women increases with age until approximately 45 years of age, then reaches a plateau. The incidence rate is much lower in young men, approximately one third that of women, but increases steadily with age and approaches that of women in the over-65 age group. Because the incidence of RA increases or is stable with age and RA is a lifelong disease, the prevalence of RA increases with each decade. Recent data strongly suggest that the incidence of RA, particularly rheumatoid factor (RF)-negative RA, is decreasing. The reasons for this are unclear, but, if elucidated, they could provide valuable insights into the etiology and pathogenesis of RA and might allow the implementation of strategies to prevent onset of the clinical disease.

RA has a significant genetic component; therefore, it is not surprising that RA is reportedly very unusual in certain populations very common in others. Most notably, cohorts have been described in rural Nigeria in which no individuals are affected with RA; in contrast, a prevalence of RA of 5% has been found in some studies of Chippewa, Yakima, and Inuit Native American tribes.

Genetics

Genetics plays a significant role in determining both the risk of developing RA and the severity of the disease. Twin studies reveal a concordance rate for RA that averages 15 to 20% for monozygotic twins and approximately 5% for dizygotic twins. These data in monozygotic twins simultaneously reveal both the significance of genetic factors and the fact that they are clearly not the only important factor, or else the concordance rate would approach unity.

The association of certain human leukocyte antigen (HLA) alleles, specifically HLA-DR4, with an increased risk of developing RA and of having more severe disease has long been recognized. It is now known that this association is explained by a particular amino acid sequence in the third hypervariable region on the DRβ1 chain. HLA-DR molecules are present on the surface of antigen-presenting cells and allow T cells to recognize antigen in the context of DR. Hypervariable regions on the DR molecule are particularly important for antigen recognition. Table 285–1 details the amino acid sequence of several DRβ1 chains that are associated with RA and some that are not. The amino acid sequence associated with RA has been called the "shared epitope" or the "at-risk allele." It has been shown by a number of investigators that patients with the shared epitope have more severe RA and more extra-articular manifestations than those who are negative for the shared epitope. Furthermore, individuals with two copies of the shared epitope, particularly those with HLA-DR4, have a further increased risk for the development of severe RA. This association with a particular antigen recognition site may ultimately aid understanding of the antigen or antigens that are important for triggering RA. Recently, proteins in which arginine has been converted to citrulline were shown to be bound with greater avidity by the shared epitope. Conversely, others have suggested that perhaps patients develop RA because the shared epitope prevents recognition of certain arthritogenic antigens. The importance of certain DRβ1 types in RA supports the concept that T cells are integrally involved in the pathogenesis.

Population-based studies have suggested that only about one third of the genetic risk for RA is explained by genes located in the HLA region. Large studies of siblings concordant for RA have suggested that ultimately multiple genes will be identified that are important for the development of RA. Recently, a functional polymorphism for the gene that encodes intracellular protein tyrosine phosphatase nonreceptor 22 (*PTPN22*) has been reproducibly associated with RA and with a number of other autoimmune diseases, including type 1 diabetes, systemic lupus erythematosus, Graves' disease, and Hashimoto's thyroiditis.

The shared epitope is present in approximately 25% of the Caucasian population, but the chance of developing RA among individuals who carry this allele is only about 1 in 25. Therefore, this test has little or no clinical utility. In addition to genetics, a number of other factors have been associated with the incidence, and in some cases the severity, of RA, including estrogen use (protective), smoking, silica exposure, and coffee consumption.

Etiology

The use of oral contraceptives has been associated with a decrease in the incidence of RA; because the effect seems to be strongest for oral contraceptives that have high estrogen content, it is postulated that estrogen is responsible for this protective effect. Studies that have tried to address the question of postmenopausal estrogen use and its effect on RA have yielded conflicting results.

TABLE 285–1 HLA ASSOCIATIONS WITH RHEUMATOID ARTHRITIS (RA)

HLA Types (Alleles) and Methods of Detection			Third Hypervariable Region Amino Acid Sequences					
Alloantisera (DR)	**MLC (Dw)**	**DNA (DRβ1)**	**70**	**71**	**72**	**73**	**74**	**Most Common Ethnic Groups**
ASSOCIATED WITH RA								
DR4	Dw4	*0401	Q	K	R	A	A	Whites (western Europe)
DR4	Dw14	*0404	·	R	·	·	·	Whites (western Europe)
DR4	Dw15	*0405	·	R	·	·	·	Japanese, Chinese
DR1	Dw1	*0101	·	R	·	·	·	Asian Indians, Israelis
DR6 (14)	Dw16	*1402	·	R	·	·	·	Yakima Native Americans
DR10	—	*1001	R	R	·	·	·	Spanish, Greeks, Israelis
NOT ASSOCIATED WITH RA								
DR4	Dw10	*0402	D	E	·	·	·	Whites (eastern Europe)
DR4	Dw13	*0403	·	R	·	·	E	Polynesians
DR2	Dw2	*1501	D	A	·	·	·	Whites
DR3	Dw3	*0301	·	·	·	G	R	Whites

A = alanine; D = aspartic acid; E = glutamic acid; HLA = human leukocyte antigen; K = lysine; MLC = mixed leukocyte cultures; Q = glutamine; R = arginine; · = the same amino acid in that position as for DRB1*0401.

Smoking has been associated with a significant increase in the risk of developing RA. This association is particularly strong in men with RF-positive disease and those who have antibodies to cyclic citrullinated peptides (CCPs). Recently, investigators in Europe have reported that coffee consumption is a risk factor for developing RA; investigators in North America have suggested that this risk may be limited to decaffeinated coffee.

RA appears to require the complex interaction of genetic and environmental factors with the immune system, and ultimately in the synovial tissues throughout the body (Fig. 285–1). RA clearly has a significant genetic component, but only about 1 in 25 whites with the so-called shared epitope develop RA. Furthermore, even if one monozygotic twin has RA, there is only approximately a 1 in 6 chance that the other twin will develop the same disease. Clearly, other factors, in addition to genetics, are active in precipitating or triggering RA. Triggers for RA have long been the target of active research. Purported triggers have included bacteria *(Mycobacteria, Streptococcus, Mycoplasma, Escherichia coli, Helicobacter pylori)*, viruses (rubella, Epstein-Barr virus, parvovirus), superantigens, and many others.

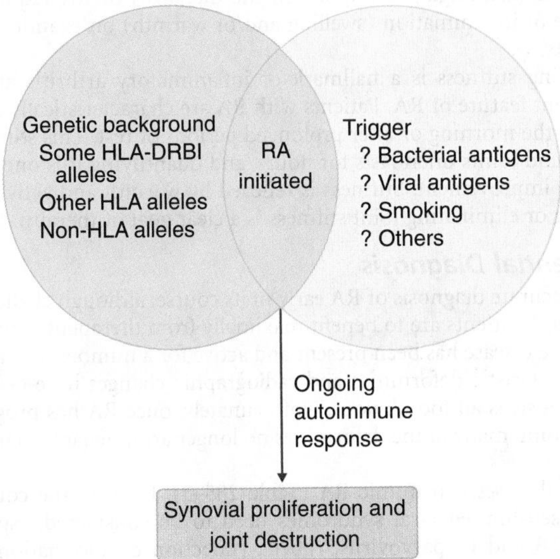

FIGURE 285–1 • Initiation of rheumatoid arthritis (RA). HLA = human leukocyte antigen.

Pathogenesis

Rheumatic fever, reactive arthritis (formerly known as Reiter's syndrome), and, more recently, Lyme arthritis are examples of arthritic syndromes for which infectious triggers have clearly been demonstrated, but these triggering agents are often difficult or impossible to isolate at the time when the arthritic syndromes occur. Many other examples exist in animal models of arthritis, including syndromes induced by mycobacteria and streptococci. Reactive arthritis is perhaps the most relevant example for RA. Reactive arthritis has clearly been shown to occur when any one of a myriad of different but specific infectious triggers is presented to a specific location in the body (the gastrointestinal or genitourinary tract) of individuals with a certain genetic background, in most cases HLA-B27. Additionally, in this syndrome, the age and gender of the individual and hence the maturity of the immune system may be critical for the development of this syndrome, which occurs primarily between the ages of 15 and 40 years in males. Once unraveled, the pathophysiology of RA is likely to be similarly complex.

Despite the absence of clear evidence linking any infectious agent to RA, it is widely believed that ultimately an important triggering role will be elucidated for infectious or other environmental agents. Once a trigger or triggers for RA are identified, strategies for prevention can be addressed, but this information may not help individuals with established disease. Possibly infections involving the innate immune system are causative in an early subclinical phase of the rheumatoid disease process, with the agents being absent once clinical disease develops.

Pathology

The synovial tissues are the primary target of the autoimmune inflammatory process that is RA; why this is true remains elusive. Once RA is initiated, the synovial tissues throughout the body become the site of a complex interaction of T cells, B cells, macrophages, and synovial cells (Fig. 285–2). The resultant proliferation of the synovial tissues (synovitis) causes the production of excessive amounts of synovial fluid and the infiltration of pannus into adjacent bone and cartilage. Synovitis results in the destruction of cartilage and bone and in stretching or rupture of the joint capsule as well as tendons and ligaments. In patients, these effects are manifested by the deformities (see Figs. 285–4 and 285–8) and disabilities that make up the clinical picture that is RA.

The relative roles of the cellular versus the humoral immune system in the initiation and perpetuation of RA are much debated; both appear to

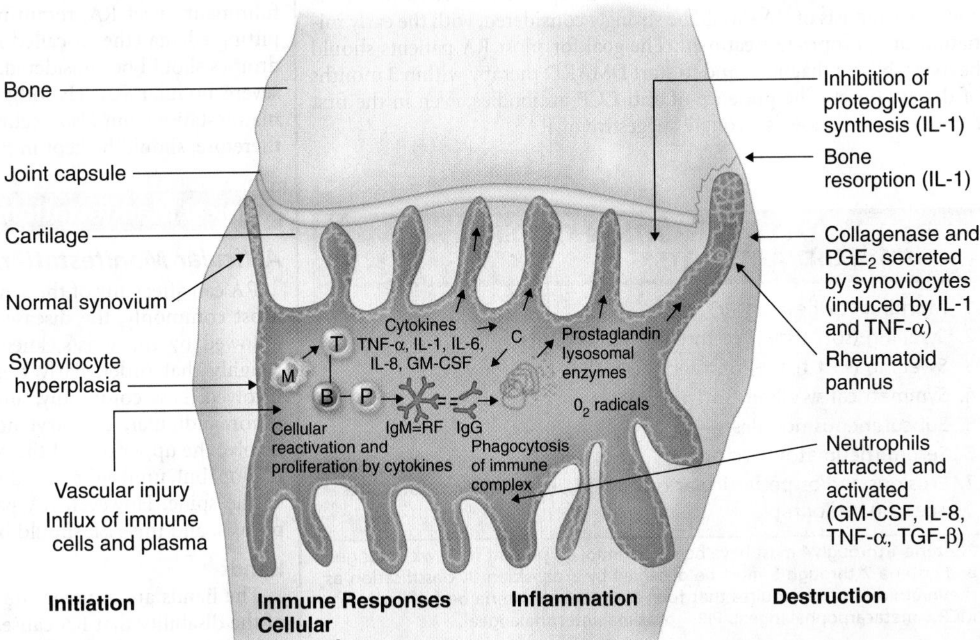

FIGURE 285–2 • Events involved in the pathogenesis of rheumatoid synovitis (progressing from left to right). B = B lymphocyte; C = complement; GM-CSF = granulocyte-macrophage colony-stimulating factor; IgG, IgM = immunoglobulin G, M; IL = interleukin; M = macrophage; P = plasma cell; PGE_2 = prostaglandin E_2; RF = rheumatoid factor; T = T lymphocyte; TGF-β = transforming growth factor-β; TNF-α = tumor necrosis factor-α.

be important. Most likely, the mechanisms of initiation of the disease process are different from those that perpetuate the chronic disease. T cells, particularly of the activated T_H1 type, appear to predominate in synovial tissues. These T cells, presumably activated by some yet unknown antigen presented by macrophages, B cells, or synoviocytes in the context of DR, secrete cytokines that drive further synovial proliferation. It is believed by many that, although RA may initially be triggered by exogenous antigen, the process, once initiated, may be perpetuated by autoantigens. Macrophage-derived cytokines, particularly interleukin-1 (IL-1) and tumor necrosis factor-α (TNF-α), play central roles in this ongoing inflammatory process. As definitive proof, biologic products directed against these cytokines have shown significant efficacy in the treatment of RA.

The humoral immune system also plays a role. RF has long been a serologic marker of RA and is well known to correlate with more severe disease, including erosions of bone, and with the presence of extra-articular features. The reason why RF is produced in excess and the exact role that it plays remain elusive. RF production may increase complement activation and result in the release of lysosomal enzymes, kinins, and oxygen-free radicals. Antibodies to CCP have been shown to have a high specificity (93 to 98%) for RA, although their sensitivity for RA with currently available assays is only about 70%. Furthermore, both RF and anti-CCP antibodies have been shown to be present in the serum of patients years before they develop clinically apparent RA, and both also correlate with more aggressive erosive disease.

Diagnosis

All current treatment paradigms for RA stress the early and aggressive use of DMARDs. Therefore, the importance of accurate early diagnosis of RA cannot be overemphasized. However, there is no one single finding on physical examination or laboratory testing that is pathognomonic of RA. Instead, the diagnosis of RA requires a collection of historical and physical features, as well as an alert and informed clinician.

Classification

Table 285–2 lists the classification criteria for RA; although they are not designed specifically for the purpose of diagnosis, these criteria are widely used as a diagnostic aid. The first five criteria are all clinical; in other words, they are established by physical examination or by talking with the patient. Only the last two criteria require laboratory tests or radiographs. The first four criteria must be present for at least 6 weeks before a diagnosis of RA can be made. This caveat is necessary because a host of conditions, including many viral-related syndromes, can cause self-limited polyarthritis syndromes that look identical to RA, including at times the presence of RF. Such conditions usually last only 2 to 3 weeks. Therefore, inflammatory arthritis that present for at least 6 weeks should not be considered a postviral condition, except for parvovirus arthritis, and the diagnosis of RA should be strongly considered, with the early initiation of appropriate treatment. The goal for most RA patients should be to establish a diagnosis and to start DMARD therapy within 3 months of disease onset. The presence of anti-CCP antibodies, even in the first few weeks of disease, is strongly suggestive of RA.

TABLE 285–2 CLASSIFICATION CRITERIA FOR RHEUMATOID ARTHRITIS*

1. Morning stiffness (≥1 hr)
2. Swelling (soft tissue) of three or more joints
3. Swelling (soft tissue) of hand joints (PIP, MCP, or wrist)
4. Symmetrical swelling (soft tissue)
5. Subcutaneous nodules
6. Serum rheumatoid factor
7. Erosions and/or periarticular osteopenia in hand or wrist joints seen on radiograph

*Criteria 1 through 4 must have been continuously present for 6 wk or longer, and criteria 2 through 5 must be observed by a physician. A classification as rheumatoid arthritis requires that four of the seven criteria be fulfilled.
MCP = metacarpophalangeal; PIP = proximal interphalangeal.

Clinical Course

Although the presentation is variable, most patients with RA have an insidious onset of pain, stiffness, and/or swelling in multiple joints over the course of weeks to months. Systemic features such as fatigue, low-grade fevers, and weight loss may accompany the joint manifestations of RA. Less commonly, the onset can be fulminant, occurring almost overnight, or patients may have persistent monoarthritis or oligoarthritis for prolonged periods before manifesting the more typical pattern of joint involvement. Rarely, patients present with extra-articular features of RA before the joint problems occur.

The distribution of involved joints is a critical clue to the underlying diagnosis. The joints that are involved in patients with RA at presentation are also variable; typically, the symptoms start in the small joints of the hands (the proximal interphalangeal [PIP] and metacarpophalangeal [MCP] joints) and in the toes (metatarsophalangeal [MTP] joints). Importantly, RA usually spares the distal interphalangeal (DIP) joints and the small joints of the toes (Fig. 285–3). If DIP involvement is a prominent finding, a different diagnosis should be considered (e.g., osteoarthritis, psoriatic arthritis). Later, RA moves, or some would say "metastasizes," to larger joints: wrists, knees, elbows, ankles, hips, and shoulders (roughly in that order). Although the patient's history of joint symptoms (arthralgia) is important, the diagnosis of RA requires the presence of inflammation (swelling and/or warmth) on examination of the joints.

Morning stiffness is a hallmark of inflammatory arthritis and is a prominent feature of RA. Patients with RA are characteristically at their worst in the morning or after prolonged periods of rest. This stiffness in and around joints often lasts for hours, and quantifying it is one way to measure improvement. Stiffness is relieved by warmth and activity, and reducing or eliminating joint stiffness is a clear goal of therapy.

Differential Diagnosis

The accurate diagnosis of RA early in its course, although challenging, is critical if patients are to benefit maximally from therapeutic intervention. Once disease has been present and active for a number of years and the characteristic deformities and radiographic changes have occurred, the diagnosis is all too obvious. Unfortunately, once RA has progressed to that point, many of the deformities no longer are amenable to medical therapy.

Many diseases can mimic RA (Table 285–3). Early in the course of disease, self-limited viral syndromes need to be considered, especially hepatitis B and C, parvovirus, rubella (infection or vaccination), and Epstein-Barr virus. At any time, systemic lupus erythematosus, psoriatic arthritis, and reactive arthritis may present diagnostic challenges. In the case of these three mimics, a targeted history and examination to elucidate their associated clinical features, such as rashes, oral ulcers, nail changes, dactylitis, urethritis, and renal, pulmonary, gastrointestinal, or ophthalmologic problems, is critical. Especially in elderly patients with fulminant-onset RA, remitting RF-negative symmetrical synovitis with pitting edema (the so-called RS3PE syndrome) and paraneoplastic syndromes should be considered. Chronic tophaceous gout may also mimic severe nodular RA. Hypothyroidism not only causes many rheumatic manifestations but also occurs commonly in conjunction with RA and, therefore, should be kept in mind.

Clinical Manifestations

Articular Manifestations

RA can affect any of the synovial (diarthrodial) joints (see Fig. 285–3). Most commonly, the disease starts in the MCP, PIP, and MTP joints, followed by the wrists, knees, elbows, ankles, hips, and shoulders in roughly that order. Early treatment helps limit the number of joints involved. Less commonly, and usually later, RA may involve the temporomandibular, cricoarytenoid, and sternoclavicular joints. RA may involve the upper part of the cervical spine, particularly the C1–C2 articulation, but, unlike the spondyloarthropathies, it does not involve the rest of the spine. However, RA patients are at an increased risk for osteoporosis, and this risk should be considered and dealt with early.

Hands

The hands are a major site of involvement, and a significant portion of the disability that RA causes is because of damage and dysfunction of the hands. Typical early disease starts with swelling of the PIPs and MCPs.

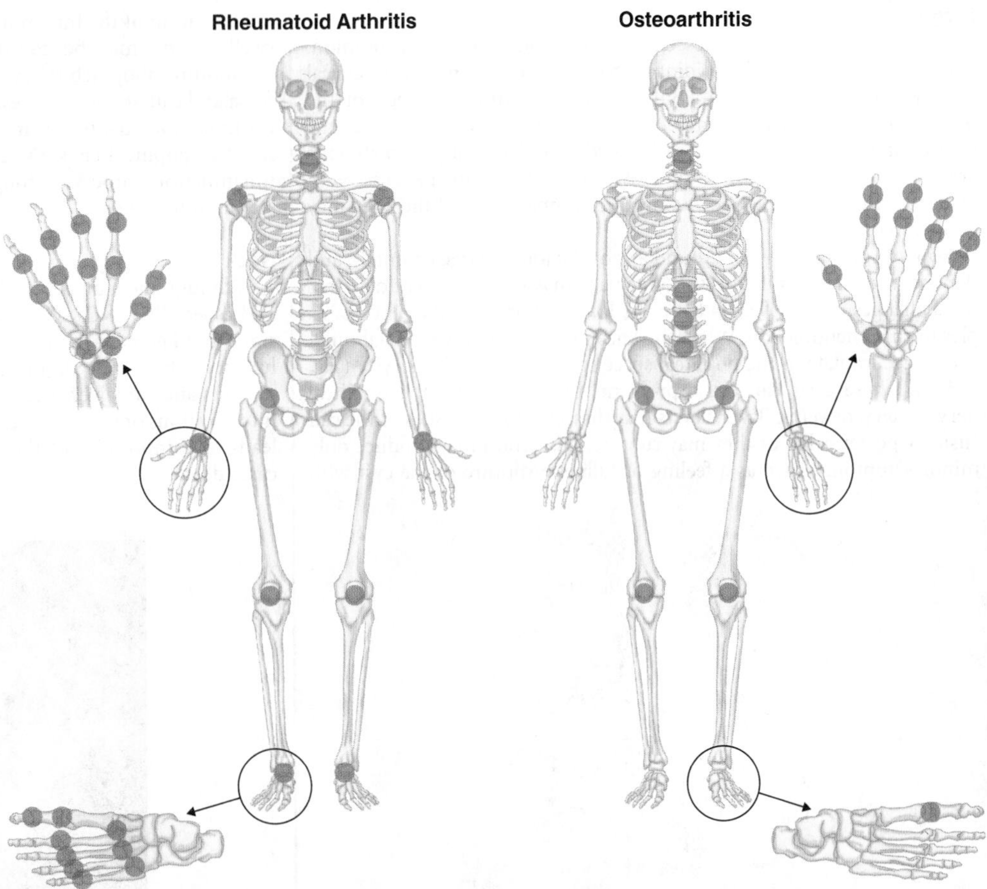

FIGURE 285–3 • Distribution of involved joints in the two most common forms of arthritis—rheumatoid arthritis and osteoarthritis. Dark circles are shown over the involved joint areas.

TABLE 285–3 DIFFERENTIAL DIAGNOSIS OF RHEUMATOID ARTHRITIS

Disorder	Subcutaneous Nodules	Rheumatoid Factor
Viral arthritis (hepatitis B and C, parvovirus, rubella, others)	−	±
Bacterial endocarditis	±	+
Rheumatic fever	+	−
Sarcoidosis	+	+
Reactive arthritis	−	−
Psoriatic arthritis	−	−
Systemic lupus erythematosus	±	+
Primary Sjögren's syndrome	−	+
Chronic tophus gout	+	−
Calcium pyrophosphate disease	−	−
Polymyalgia rheumatica	−	−
Osteoarthritis (erosive)	−	−

− = not present; + = frequently present; ± = occasionally present.

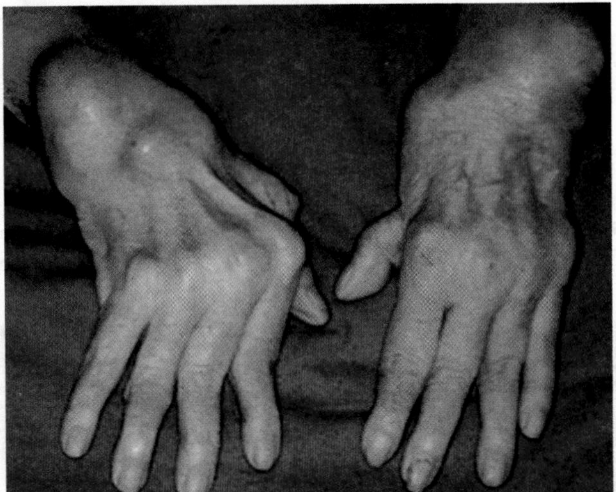

FIGURE 285–4 • Severe advanced rheumatoid arthritis of the hands. There is massive tendon swelling over the dorsal surface of both wrists, severe muscle wasting, ulnar deviation of the metacarpophalangeal joints, and swan-neck deformity of the fingers. (From Forbes CD, Jackson WF: Color Atlas and Text of Clinical Medicine, 3rd ed. London, Mosby, 2003.)

The DIP joints are rarely involved; significant involvement of the DIP joints should suggest the possibility of a different diagnosis. Figure 285–4 illustrates the classic ulnar deviation and swan-neck deformities (hyperextension of the PIP joints) that are commonly seen in late, more established disease. Boutonniere (or buttonhole) deformities also occur as a result of hyperextension of the MCP joints. If the clinical disease remains active, hand function deteriorates. Sudden loss of function of individual fingers may occur as a result of tendon rupture, which requires the expertise of a carefully selected hand surgeon to repair.

Feet

Feet, particularly the MTP joints, are involved early in most patients with RA. Radiographic erosions occur at least as early in the feet as in the hands. Subluxation of the toes is common and leads to the dual problem of breakdown of the skin with ulcers on the top of the toes and painful ambulation due to loss of the cushioning pads that usually protect the heads of the MTP joints.

Wrists

The wrist joints are involved in most patients with RA; radial deviation is the rule, and patients with severe involvement may progress to volar subluxation. Even early in the course of the disease, synovial proliferation in and around the wrists may compress the median nerve, causing carpal tunnel syndrome (Fig. 285–5). Later, this synovial proliferation may invade tendons and lead to rupture.

Large Joints

Involvement of knees, ankles, elbows, hips, and shoulders is common. Characteristically, the whole joint surface is involved in a symmetrical fashion. Therefore, RA is not only symmetrical from one side of the body to the other but also symmetrical within the individual joint. In the case of the knee (Fig. 285–6A), the medial and lateral compartments are both severely narrowed in RA; in contrast, in patients with osteoarthritis (see Fig. 285–6B), only one compartment of the knee may be involved.

Synovial cysts may occur around any of the joints (large or small), and they occasionally manifest as soft, fluctuant masses that present diagnostic challenges. Synovial cysts from the knee are perhaps the best examples of this phenomenon. When the knee produces excess synovial fluid, it may accumulate in the popliteal space (popliteal or Baker's cyst) (Fig. 285–7). These cysts can cause problems by pressing on the popliteal nerve, artery, or veins. Baker's cysts may dissect into the tissues of the calf (usually posteriorly), or they may rupture. Dissection may produce only minor symptoms, such as a feeling of fullness; rupture of the cyst with extravasation of the inflammatory content produces significant pain and swelling and may be confused with thrombophlebitis, the so-called pseudothrombophlebitis syndrome. Ultrasonography of the popliteal fossa and calf are useful to establish the correct diagnosis and to rule out thrombophlebitis, which may be precipitated by popliteal cysts. Treatment of popliteal (Baker's) cysts should be directed at interrupting the inflammatory process through an intra-articular injection of corticosteroid into the knee.

Neck

Although most of the axial skeleton is spared in RA, the cervical spine and especially the C1–C2 articulation is commonly involved. Bony erosions and ligament damage can occur in this area and may lead to subluxation (Fig. 285–8). Most often, subluxation at C1–C2 is minor; patients and caregivers need only be cautious and avoid forcing the neck into positions of flexion. Occasionally, subluxation at C1–C2 is severe and leads to compromise of the cervical cord with symptoms and in some cases death.

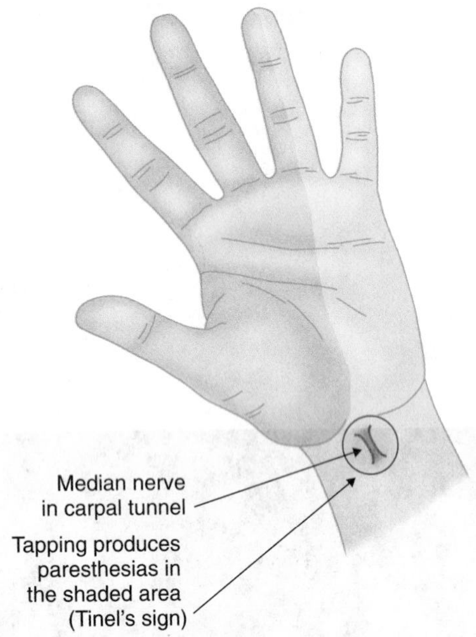

FIGURE 285–5 • Carpal tunnel syndrome. Distribution of pain and/or paresthesias (shaded area) when the median nerve is compressed by swelling in the wrist (carpal tunnel).

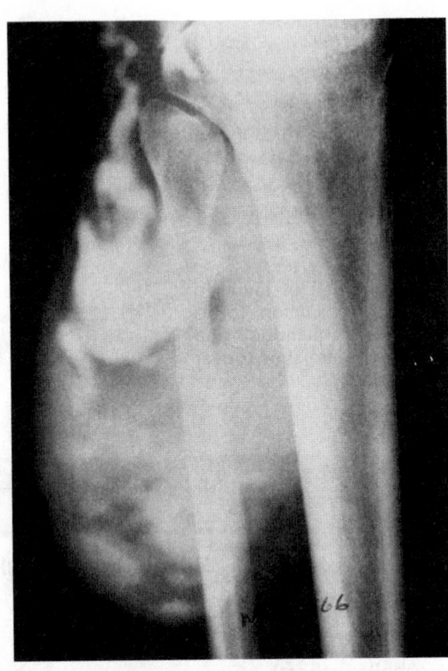

FIGURE 285–7 • Arthrogram with a radiocontrast agent injected into the knee. The dye flows into the popliteal space and through a narrow channel into a large synovial cyst (Baker's cyst) that has dissected into the soft tissue of the calf.

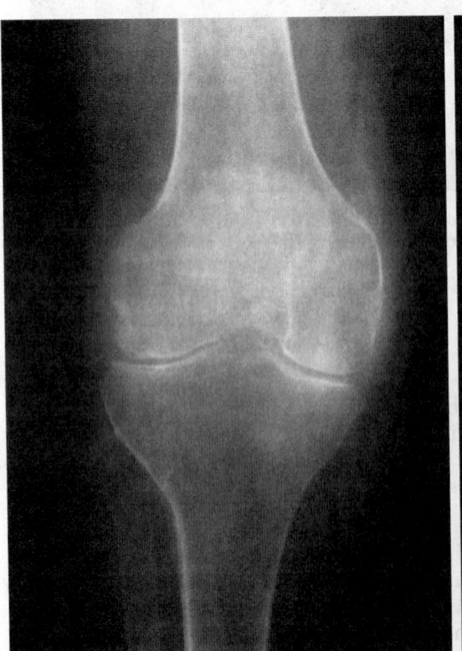

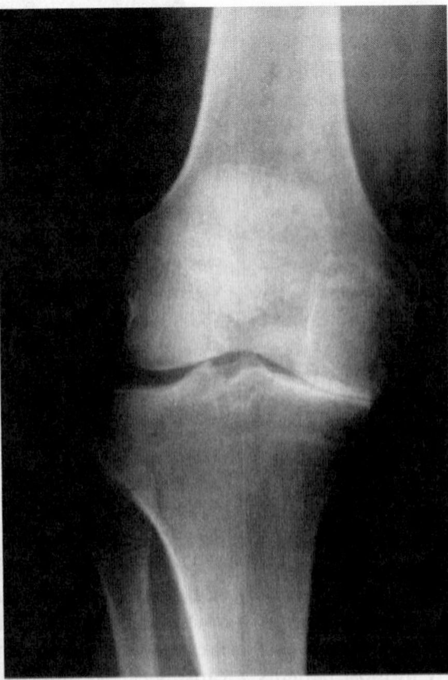

FIGURE 285–6 • Radiographs of the knees in the two most common forms of arthritis—rheumatoid arthritis and osteoarthritis. A, Severe involvement in rheumatoid arthritis, with almost complete symmetrical loss of joint space in both the medial and the lateral compartment, but with little subchondral sclerosis or osteophyte formation. **B,** Typical osteoarthritis, with severe, near-total loss of joint space of one compartment and a normal or actually increased joint space of the other compartment. Note also the significant subchondral sclerosis in the involved area, typical of osteoarthritis.

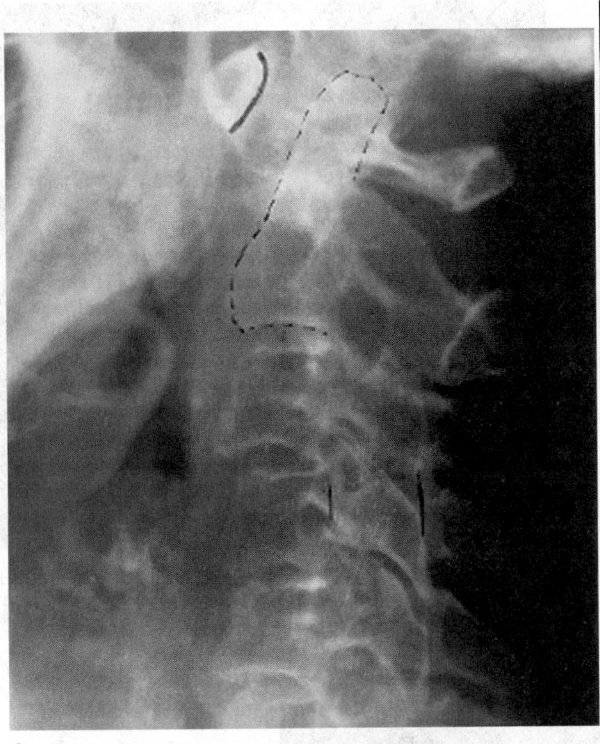

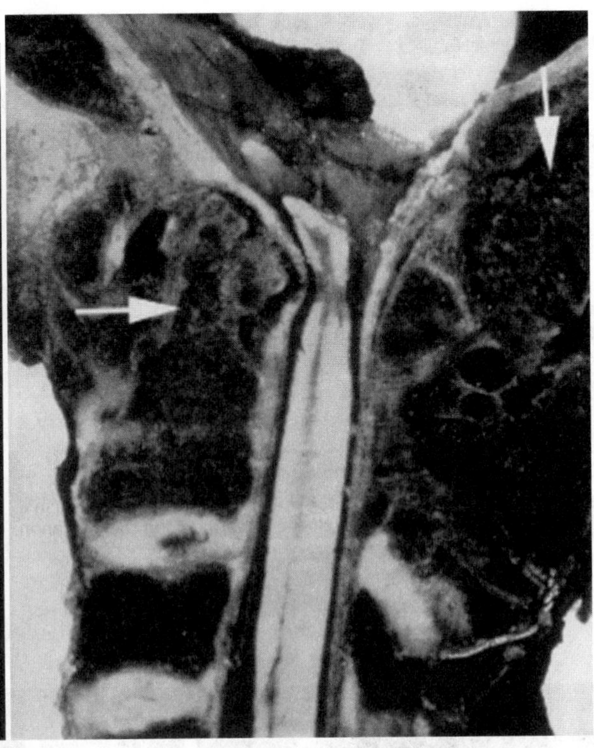

FIGURE 285–8 • Subluxation of the cervical spine in patients with rheumatoid arthritis. A, In a lateral radiograph of the cervical spine, the body of C2 and its odontoid process are outlined by the broken lines, and the posterior aspect of the anterior segment of C1 is indicated by a solid line. Normally, a space of only 2 to 3 mm separates C1 from C2. The space between C1 and the odontoid of C2 is markedly increased, indicative of subluxation of C1 and C2. **B,** Lateral view of a pathologic specimen from a patient who died of C1–C2 subluxation. The horizontal arrow shows the odontoid process that subluxed posteriorly, severely compressing and almost severing the cord. The vertical arrow shows a bone graft that had been put in place posteriorly in an attempt to prevent subluxation. Below the arrow, a nonhealing area is present through the bone graft, and inferior to that a wire fixation suture is still in place.

Other Joints

Wherever synovial tissue exists, RA can cause problems. The temporomandibular, cricoarytenoid, and sternoclavicular joints are examples of other joints that may be involved in RA. The cricoarytenoid joint is responsible for abduction and adduction of the vocal cords. Involvement of this joint may lead to a feeling of fullness in the throat, to hoarseness, and, rarely, when the cords are essentially fused in a closed position, to a syndrome of acute respiratory distress with or without stridor. In this latter situation, emergent tracheotomy may be life-saving.

Extra-articular Manifestations

Systemic features of RA such as fatigue, weight loss, and low-grade fevers occur frequently. As with all the other extra-articular features, they are more common in those patients who possess RF (Table 285–4).

TABLE 285–4 EXTRA-ARTICULAR MANIFESTATIONS OF RHEUMATOID ARTHRITIS

Skin	Nodules, fragility, vasculitis, pyoderma gangrenosum
Heart	Pericarditis, premature atherosclerosis, vasculitis, valve disease, and valve ring nodules
Lung	Pleural effusions, interstitial lung disease, bronchiolitis obliterans, rheumatoid nodules, vasculitis
Eye	Keratoconjunctivitis sicca, episcleritis, scleritis, scleromalacia perforans, peripheral ulcerative keratopathy
Neurologic	Entrapment neuropathy, cervical myelopathy, mononeuritis multiplex (vasculitis), peripheral neuropathy
Hematopoietic	Anemia, thrombocytosis, lymphadenopathy, Felty's syndrome
Kidney	Amyloidosis, vasculitis
Bone	Osteopenia

Skin

Subcutaneous nodules are seen in approximately one fourth of patients with RA, almost exclusively in those who are RF positive. Patients with nodules who are RF negative should be carefully scrutinized for a different diagnosis, such as chronic tophaceous gout. Nodules may occur almost anywhere (e.g., lungs, heart, eye), but most commonly they occur subcutaneously on extensor surfaces (particularly the forearms) (Fig. 285–9), over joints, or over pressure points. They are firm on examination, usually are not tender, have a characteristic histologic picture, and are thought to be triggered by small vessel vasculitis. A syndrome of increased nodulosis, despite good control of the disease, has been described with methotrexate therapy (Fig. 285–10).

Small vessel vasculitis, manifested as digital infarcts or leukocytoclastic vasculitis, may occur in RA (Fig. 285–11) and should prompt more aggressive DMARD treatment. A vasculitis of small and medium arteries that is indistinguishable from polyarteritis nodosa also can be seen and requires aggressive systemic therapy. Finally, pyoderma gangrenosum occurs with increased frequency in association with RA.

Cardiac Involvement

Cardiac involvement directly related to RA is uncommon; however, patients with RA have a significantly increased morbidity and mortality from coronary artery disease. The reasons are not clear, but chronic inflammation, some of the medications used to treat RA, and a sedentary lifestyle all may be significant risk factors. Pericardial effusions are common in RA (50% by echocardiography) but usually are asymptomatic. Rarely, long-standing pericardial disease may result in a fibrinous pericarditis, and patients may present clinically with constrictive pericarditis. Uncommonly, rheumatoid nodules occur in the conduction system and cause heart block.

Pulmonary Manifestations

Pulmonary manifestations of RA include pleural effusions, rheumatoid nodules, and parenchymal lung disease. Pleural effusions occur more commonly in men and are usually small and asymptomatic. Of interest,

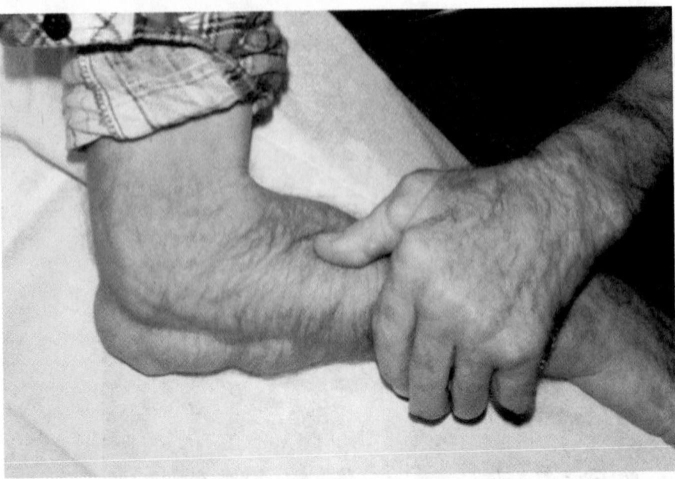

FIGURE 285–9 • **Rheumatoid nodules.** Large rheumatoid nodules are seen in a classic location along the extensor surface of the forearm and in the olecranon bursa.

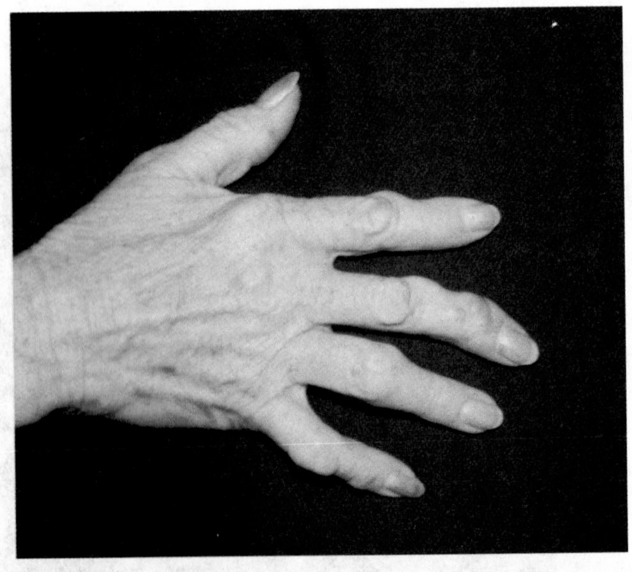

FIGURE 285–10 • **Rheumatoid nodulosis.** In this patient, multiple rheumatoid nodules are present over joints. In some cases, nodules may dominate the clinical picture. Rarely, this may be seen as a side effect of methotrexate therapy.

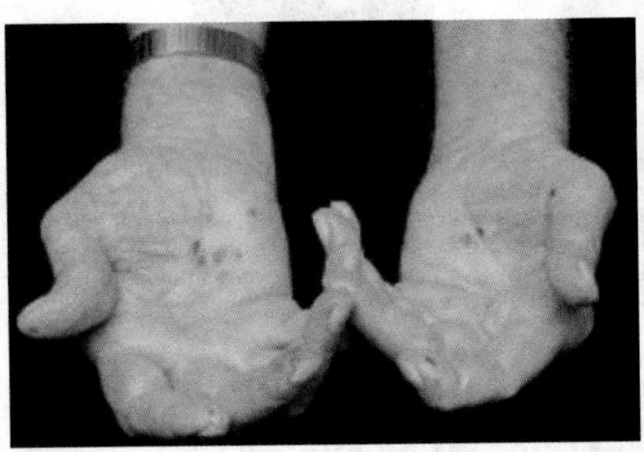

A

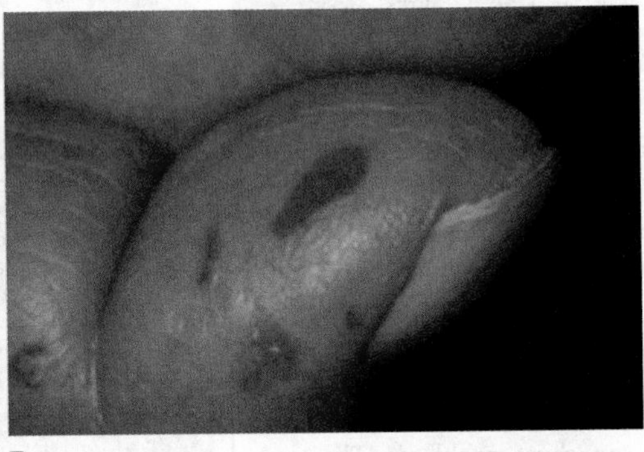

B

FIGURE 285–11 • **Small vessel vasculitis. A and B,** Rheumatoid vasculitis with small brown infarcts of palms and fingers in chronic rheumatoid arthritis. (Courtesy of Dr. Martin Lidsky, Houston, TX.)

pleural fluid in RA is characterized by low levels of glucose and low pH and, therefore, may at times be confused with empyema. Rheumatoid nodules may occur in the lung, especially in men (Fig. 285–12); these are usually solid but may calcify, cavitate, or become infected. Rarely, pulmonary nodules rupture and produce a pneumothorax. If RA patients are exposed to coal dust, diffuse nodular densities may occur (Caplan's syndrome). Differentiating rheumatoid nodules from lung cancer can be problematic, particularly if the lesion is solitary. Therefore, the presence of pulmonary nodules in a patient with RA should precipitate an aggressive diagnostic evaluation.

Diffuse interstitial fibrosis occurs in RA and may progress to a honeycomb appearance on radiography with increasing dyspnea. Rarely, bronchiolitis obliterans can be seen with or without organizing pneumonia. Bronchiolitis obliterans carries a poor prognosis and may occur more often in association with D-penicillamine or gold therapy.

Ophthalmologic Manifestations

The most common manifestation of RA in the eye is keratoconjunctivitis sicca (dry eyes) from secondary Sjögren's syndrome. Patients may have associated xerostomia (dry mouth), parotid gland swelling, or, occasionally, lymphadenopathy. Scleritis can also occur and may be painful, with progression to thinning of the sclera (with deep pigment showing through on physical examination). Scleritis may progress to perforation of the orbit (scleromalacia perforans). Rarely, tendonitis of the superior oblique muscles can result in double vision (Brown's syndrome).

Neurologic Manifestations

Peripheral nerve entrapment syndromes, including carpal tunnel syndrome (median nerve at the wrist) and tarsal tunnel syndrome (anterior tibial nerve at the ankle), are common in RA. Vasculitis can lead to mononeuritis multiplex and a host of additional neurologic problems. Subluxations at C1–C2 may produce myelopathy (see Fig. 285–8).

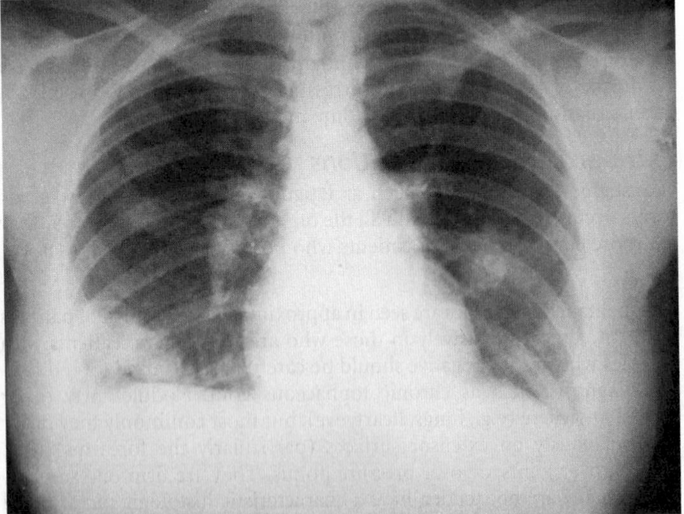

FIGURE 285–12 • **Rheumatoid nodules in the lung.** Chest radiograph demonstrates discrete rheumatoid nodules in both right and left lower lobes. (Courtesy of Dr. Martin Lidsky, Houston, TX.)

Rheumatoid nodules in the CNS have been described but are rare and usually asymptomatic.

Felty's Syndrome

Felty's syndrome is the triad of RA, splenomegaly, and neutropenia. This complication is seen in patients with severe, RF-positive disease and may be accompanied by hepatomegaly, thrombocytopenia, lymphadenopathy, and fevers. Most patients with Felty's syndrome do not require special therapy; instead, treatment should be directed toward their severe RA. If severe neutropenia exists (fewer than 500 cells/μL) and is accompanied by recurrent bacterial infections or chronic, nonhealing leg ulcers, splenectomy may be indicated.

Some patients with RA, who were previously thought to have Felty's syndrome, have peripheral white blood cell counts dominated by large granular lymphocytes with almost complete absence of neutrophils. This condition is known as the *large granular lymphocyte syndrome* and is thought to be a variant of T-cell leukemia. In the setting of RA, this syndrome has a good prognosis, with the neutropenia often responding dramatically to methotrexate therapy.

Laboratory Findings

Historically, the most characteristic laboratory abnormality in RA is the presence of RF, which is found in approximately 80% of patients. RF was first described in the 1930s and is an antibody that recognizes immunoglobulin G as its antigen. The presence of RF is strongly associated with more severe articular disease as well as with essentially all of the extra-articular features previously discussed. Importantly, RF is seen in association with many diseases other than RA, particularly in disease processes that provide chronic stimulation of the immune system (see Table 285–3). Anti-CCP antibodies found in approximately 70% of patients with RA have a high specificity (93 to 98%), are often present before clinical disease is diagnosed, and are associated with aggressive erosive disease. RA is associated with many other autoantibodies, including antinuclear antibodies (approximately 30% of patients) and antineutrophil cytoplasmic antibodies, particularly of the perinuclear type (approximately 30% of patients).

Most patients with RA have an anemia of chronic disease. The degree of anemia is proportional to the activity of the disease, and therapy that controls the disease will normalize the hemoglobin levels; rarely, erythropoietin administration may be indicated. Thrombocytosis is common, with platelet counts returning to normal as the inflammation is controlled. Acute phase reactants, ESR, and CRP levels also parallel the activity of the disease, and their persistent elevation portends a poor prognosis, in terms of both joint destruction and mortality. White blood cell counts may be elevated, normal, or, in the case of Felty's syndrome, profoundly depressed. Eosinophilia is present in some patients with RA.

Synovial fluid in RA is characterized by white blood cell counts in the range of 5000 to 100,000/mm^3, with approximately two thirds of the cells being polymorphonuclear leukocytes. There are no synovial fluid findings that are pathognomonic of RA.

Treatment

Rx

General Measures

RA is a lifelong disease process that has no known cure; the diagnosis is made based on clinical criteria, and many different options exist for treatment. All of these factors magnify the importance of the patient–physician relationship and place a premium on the art rather than the science of medicine. Optimal care for patients with RA requires effective ongoing interactions between primary care physicians and rheumatologists, and in some cases physical therapists, occupational therapists, and orthopedic surgeons. Because of the serious nature of the disease, the rapid introduction of new treatments, and the need for expertise in monitoring these therapies, all patients with RA should be monitored by a rheumatologist.

The goal of therapy is disease remission (Table 285–5). If RA is treated early, remission is possible in 20 to 40% of patients. However, remissions require the ongoing use of medications and even then are not always durable. Some combination of nonsteroidal anti-inflammatory drugs (NSAIDs), steroids, and DMARDs is necessary in most patients. In many, or perhaps most, patients with RA, combinations of different DMARDs (conventional and biologic) are necessary for optimal control. Therapy should be escalated rapidly to ensure maximal suppression of disease while minimizing toxicity and expense. Patients with RA should be educated about their disease and its treatment. In most cases, patients should have an opportunity to spend time with physical therapists and occupational therapists to learn about range-of-motion exercises, joint protection, and assistive devices.

TABLE 285–5 KEYS TO OPTIMIZE OUTCOME OF TREATMENT OF RA

Early, accurate diagnosis
Early DMARD therapy
Strive for remission in all patients
Monitor carefully for treatment toxicities
Consider and treat comorbid conditions*

*Important comorbid conditions include cardiovascular disease, increased susceptibility to infections, and osteoporosis.
DMARD = disease-modifying antirheumatic drug; RA = rheumatoid arthritis.

Rx

Medical Therapy

In the treatment of RA, three types of medical therapies are used: NSAIDs, glucocorticoids, and DMARDs (both conventional and biologic). Initial combination therapy appears to be preferred over monotherapy. 1

Nonsteroidal Anti-inflammatory Drugs

NSAIDs are important for the symptomatic relief they provide to RA patients; however, they play only a minor role in altering the underlying disease process. Therefore, NSAIDs should rarely, if ever, be used to treat RA without the concomitant use of DMARDs. Many clinicians waste valuable time switching from one NSAID to another before starting DMARD therapy.

Much has been written about the gastrointestinal toxicity of NSAIDs, and these concerns are particularly relevant to RA patients, who often have significant risk factors including age and concomitant steroid use. Therefore, cyclooxygenase-2 (COX2)-selective agents have been a popular choice for patients with RA. The recent evidence linking these agents to increased cardiovascular toxicity has been particularly troubling for patients with RA, who are already at high risk for myocardial infarction. Therefore, if COX2-selective agents are used, they should be kept at a low dose. Consideration should be given to low-dose aspirin prophylaxis in RA, but this may increase the gastrointestinal toxicity of NSAIDs. The use of concomitant misoprostol or proton pump inhibitors should be considered in all patients with RA who are taking NSAIDs. Additionally, the potential for NSAIDs to decrease renal blood flow and to increase blood pressure should be kept in mind.

Glucocorticoids

Glucocorticoids have had a significant role in the treatment of RA for more than half a century. Indeed, RA was chosen as the first disease to be treated with this new therapy, partly because it was thought that RA was a disease of glucocorticoid deficiency (an issue that remains unresolved). As was the case with the first patient treated in 1948, glucocorticoids are dramatically and rapidly effective in patients with RA. Not only are glucocorticoids useful for symptomatic improvement, but they significantly decrease the radiographic progression of RA. However, the toxicities of long-term therapy are extensive and potentially devastating. Therefore, the optimal use of these drugs requires an understanding of several principles (Table 285–6).

Glucocorticoids remain among the most potent anti-inflammatory treatments available; for this reason and because of their rapid onset of action, they are ideally suited to help control the inflammation in RA while the much slower-acting DMARDs are starting to work. Prednisone, the most commonly used glucocorticoid, should rarely be used in doses higher than 10 mg/day to treat the stiffness and articular manifestations of RA. This dose should be slowly tapered to the lowest effective dose, and the concomitant DMARD therapy should be adjusted to make this possible. Glucocorticoids should rarely, if ever, be used to treat RA without concomitant DMARD therapy. The paradigm is to shut off inflammation rapidly with glucocorticoids and then to taper them as the DMARD is taking effect ("bridge therapy"). In all patients receiving glucocorticoids, strong measure should be taken to prevent osteoporosis. Bisphosphonates have been shown to be particularly effective in this regard.

Rx

Higher doses of glucocorticoids may be necessary to treat extra-articular manifestations, especially vasculitis and scleritis.

Disease-Modifying Antirheumatic Drugs

DMARDs are a group of medications that have the ability to greatly inhibit the disease process in the synovium and modify or change the disabling potential of RA. In most cases, these drugs have the ability to halt or slow the radiographic progression of RA.

Conventional DMARDs

Included in this group of medications are methotrexate, sulfasalazine (Azulfidine), gold, antimalarials (Plaquenil and others), leflunomide (Arava), azathioprine (Imuran), and minocycline. It is critically important that clinicians and patients understand that conventional DMARDs take 2 to 6 months to exert their maximal effect, and all require some monitoring (Table 285–7). Therefore, other measures such as glucocorticoid therapy may be needed to control the disease while these medications are starting to work.

All of these DMARDs have been shown to be effective in treating both early and more advanced RA that remains active. Until additional research elucidates factors that allow selection of the best initial therapy for each patient, the choice will depend on patient and physician concerns about toxicity and monitoring issues, as well as the activity of disease and comorbid conditions. The critical factor is not which DMARD to start first but getting the DMARD therapy started early in the disease process.

METHOTREXATE. Methotrexate is the preferred DMARD of most rheumatologists, in part because patients have a more durable response, and because, with correct monitoring, serious toxicities are rare. Methotrexate is dramatically effective in slowing radiographic progression and is usually given orally in doses ranging from 5 to 25 mg/week as a single dose. This once-a-week administration is worthy of emphasis; prior experience with daily therapy in psoriasis has demonstrated the importance of allowing the liver time to recover between doses. Oral absorption of methotrexate is variable; subcutaneous injections of methotrexate may be effective if oral treatment is not. Side effects of methotrexate include oral ulcers, nausea, hepatotoxicity, bone marrow suppression, and pneumonitis. With the exception of pneumonitis, these toxicities respond to dose adjustments. Monitoring of blood counts and liver blood tests (albumin and aspartate aminotransaminase [SGOT] or alanine aminotransferase [SGPT]) should be done every 4 to 8 weeks, with dosage adjustments as needed. Renal function is critical for clearance of methotrexate; previously stable patients may experience severe toxicities when renal function deteriorates. Pneumonitis, although rare, is less predictable and can be fatal, particularly if the methotrexate is not stopped or is restarted. Folic acid, 1 to 4 mg/day, can significantly decrease most methotrexate toxicities without apparent loss of efficacy. If methotrexate alone does not sufficiently control disease, it is combined with other DMARDs. Methotrexate in combination with virtually any of the other DMARDs (conventional or biologic) has been shown to be more effective than either drug alone. 2

LEFLUNOMIDE. Leflunomide, a pyrimidine antagonist, has a very long half-life and is most commonly started at 10 to 20 mg/day orally. A loading dose of 100 mg/day for 3 days was previously recommended, but because it increases diarrhea, the most common toxic effect of this drug, loading treatment is no longer advocated. Diarrhea responds to dose reduction, and doses of leflunomide of 10 to 20 mg three to five times per week are frequently used. Also, because of its long half-life and its teratogenic potential, women wishing to become pregnant who have previously received leflunomide, even if therapy was stopped years ago, should have blood levels drawn. If toxicity occurs or if pregnancy is being considered, leflunomide can be rapidly eliminated from the body by treatment with cholestyramine. Laboratory monitoring for hematologic and hepatic toxicity should be done during treatment with leflunomide, as recommend for methotrexate.

ANTIMALARIAL DRUGS. The antimalarial drugs hydroxychloroquine (Plaquenil) and chloroquine are frequently used for the treatment of RA. They have the least toxicity of any of the DMARDs and do not require monitoring of blood tests. Yearly monitoring by an ophthalmologist is recommended to detect any signs of retinal toxicity (rare). Hydroxychloroquine is the most commonly used preparation and is given orally at 200 to 400 mg/day. These drugs are frequently used in combination with other DMARDs, particularly methotrexate. 2

SULFASALAZINE. Sulfasalazine has been the most commonly used DMARD in Europe. It is an effective treatment when given in doses of 1 to 3 g/day. Monitoring of blood counts, particularly white blood cell counts, in the first 6 months is recommended.

MINOCYCLINE. Minocycline, 100 mg twice daily, has been shown to be an effective treatment for RA, particularly when used in early, RF-positive disease. Chronic therapy (longer than 2 years) with minocycline may lead to cutaneous hyperpigmentation.

GOLD. Gold, the oldest DMARD, when given intramuscularly, remains an extremely effective therapy for a small percentage of patients. It is less commonly used because of its slow onset of action,

TABLE 285–6 GUIDELINES FOR USE OF GLUCOCORTICOIDS

Avoid use of glucocorticoids without DMARDs
Prednisone >10 mg/day is rarely indicated for articular disease
Taper to the lowest effective dose
Use as "bridge therapy" until DMARD therapy is effective
Remember prophylaxis against osteoporosis

DMARD = disease-modifying antirheumatic drug.

TABLE 285–7 CAVEATS FOR MONITORING DMARD THERAPIES*

Medication	Caveats
Prednisone	Use as bridge to effective DMARD therapy, prophylaxis for osteoporosis? (see Table 285–6)
Hydroxychloroquine	Keep dosage lower than 6.5 mg/kg/day; yearly eye checkup by ophthalmologist
Sulfasalazine	CBC for neutropenia, initially every month, then every 6 mo
Methotrexate	CBC and SGOT/SGPT every 4–8 wk; many toxicities respond to folic acid or small dose reduction; if pneumonitis, stop and do not restart; decreasing renal function may precipitate toxicities; absolute contraindication in pregnancy
Leflunomide	CBC and SGOT/SGPT evert 4–8 wk; long half-life may require cholestyramine washout; absolute contraindication in pregnancy
TNF inhibitors	If fevers or infectious symptoms of any kind, stop until symptoms resolve; aggressively work-up and treat possible infections; may precipitate congestive heart failure, demyelinating syndromes, or lupus-like syndromes

CBC = compete blood count; DMARD = disease-modifying antirheumatic drug; SGOT = serum glutamate oxaloacetate transaminase (aspartate aminotransferase); SGPT = serum glutamate pyruvate transaminase (alanine aminotransferase); TNF = tumor necrosis factor.
*Patients receiving DMARDs, both conventional and biologic, should be monitored by a rheumatologist.

Rx

need for intramuscular administration, frequent monitoring required (complete blood count and urinalysis), and frequent toxicities. Toxicities include skin rashes, bone marrow suppression, and proteinuria.

Biologic DMARDs

Recent research has continued to elucidate the central role that cytokines, most notably TNF-α and IL-1, play in the pathophysiology of RA. This has led directly to the development and clinical use of biologic agents directed against TNF-α1 (etanercept [3] [Enbrel], infliximab [4] [Remicade], adalimumab [5] [Humira]) and IL-1 (anakinra [Kineret]). Two other biologicals have recently been approved: rituximab (Rituxan) and abatacept (Orencia). All RA patients receiving biologic therapies should be monitored by a rheumatologist, and their physicians should be aware of the risk for infections that are often atypical. Currently, biologic agents should not be used in combination with each other, because all studies to date have shown a significant increase in infections.

ANTI-TNF-α DRUGS. This category of drugs includes etanercept, a recombinant TNF receptor fusion protein that is administered by subcutaneous injection at 50 mg once weekly. Infliximab is a mouse/human chimeric monoclonal antibody against TNF-α that is given intravenously (3 to 10 mg/kg) every 4 to 8 weeks. Adalimumab is a human monoclonal antibody against TNF-α that is given subcutaneously at 40 mg every other week. All three anti-TNF agents have been shown to be highly effective against both clinical symptoms and radiographic progression of RA, particularly when used in combination with methotrexate. A rapid onset of action (days to weeks) is apparent and is a significant advantage that these treatments have over conventional DMARDs. Current disadvantages include cost and long-term toxicities, in particular infections (especially tuberculosis and others), and malignancies, [6] as well as heart failure, rare demyelinating, and autoimmune syndromes.

ANAKINRA. Anakinra, a recombinant human IL-1 receptor antagonist, is given subcutaneously at 100 mg/day. It has been shown to be effective against signs and symptoms of RA as well as radiographic progression. Its onset of action is somewhat slower and less dramatic than that of the TNF inhibitors. Toxicities include injection site reactions and pneumonia (especially in patients with asthma).

RITUXIMAB. Rituximab is a chimeric monoclonal antibody that targets CD20+ B cells and is given intravenously in two infusions of 500 to 1000 mg spaced two weeks apart. This results in marked reductions in circulating B cells for 6 to 12 months and significant clinical responses. The need for and timing of further courses is determined by the patient's ongoing response. Rituximab has been used for years to treat B cell lymphoma.

ABATACEPT. Abatacept is made by genetically fusing the external domain of human CTLA4 to the heavy-chain of human IgG1 and binds both CD80 and CD86 on antigen presenting cells thus inhibiting T cells from receiving their second signal via CD28. It is administered intravenously 10 mg/kg on days 1, 15, 30 and then monthly.

Treatment of Underlying Conditions

Optimal care of patients with RA requires recognition of the associated comorbid conditions, including an increased risk of cardiovascular death, osteoporosis, infections (especially pneumonia), and certain cancers.

Cardiovascular Disease

Increasingly, cardiovascular disease is being recognized as the cause of much of the excess mortality in RA. A number of factors contribute to this mortality, including sedentary lifestyle, glucocorticoid therapy, and treatments that increase homocysteine levels, such as methotrexate and sulfasalazine. However, recently a strong association between chronic inflammation and cardiovascular disease was identified, and it is likely that this may be the most significant factor. Therapies that control RA earlier and better can be expected to decrease cardiovascular morbidity and mortality. Clinicians should consider RA a risk factor for cardiovascular disease and should aggressively address other cardiovascular risk factors in their rheumatoid patients.

Rx

Osteoporosis

Osteoporosis is common in patients with RA, and early treatment results in long-term dividends. Patients with RA are at an increased risk for infections, and some forms of treatment further increase this risk. Patients should be cautioned to seek medical attention early for even minor symptoms suggestive of infection, especially if receiving anti-TNF therapy. All patients with RA should receive a pneumococcal vaccine at appropriate intervals and yearly influenza vaccinations. Finally, patients with RA have an increased risk of lymphoma. Occasionally, B-cell lymphomas are associated with immunosuppression and regress after immunosuppression is discontinued. RA patients have significantly decreased risk (odds ratio, 0.2) of developing colon cancer. This is thought to be secondary to chronic inhibition of COX by NSAIDs.

Prognosis

Until recently, RA was thought to be a relatively benign disease. It is now clear that, once established, RA is a lifelong progressive disease that produces significant morbidity in most patients and premature mortality in many. Long-term studies have found that 50% of patients with RA have had to stop working after 10 years (approximately 10 times the average rate). Patients who are RF or anti-CCP positive and those who are positive for the shared epitope have a worse prognosis with more erosions and more extra-articular disease (see Table 285–4). Once deformities are found on examination or erosions on radiography, the damage is largely irreversible. It has been clearly shown that erosions occur in most patients in the first 1 to 2 years and that the rate of radiographic damage can be affected by early therapy. Therefore, early DMARD therapy is critical. Although limited long-term data are available, the current information strongly suggests that patients have the opportunity to benefit greatly if the newer principles of therapy are practiced.

Future Directions

Significant advances in the effective treatment of RA have come from an understanding of the cytokine imbalance that accompanies this disease. Much research is focused on the further development of biologic products to modulate this balance. Biologic therapies that modulate B-cell and T-cell function have been shown to be effective in the treatment of RA and may soon be approved for use. There remains a critical need for a cytokine thermostat that would allow titration of the desired cytokine balance to control disease without altering critical immune functions.

Even with existing therapies, there are many different effective options for patients with RA. The challenge to the clinician is to pick the right option for each patient. Few data are currently available to aid in this choice, and the establishment of parameters, genetic or otherwise, that would allow selection of the best initial option for each patient would be a major breakthrough. Finally, elucidation of the trigger or triggers for RA may allow the development of strategies to prevent onset of the clinical disease.

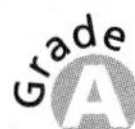

1. Goekoop-Ruiterman YP, de Vries-Bouwstra JK, Allaart CF, et al: Comparison of treatment strategies in early rheumatoid arthritis: A randomized trial. Ann Intern Med 2007;146:406–415.
2. O'Dell JR, Haire CE, Erickson N, et al: Treatment of rheumatoid arthritis with methotrexate alone, sulfasalazine and hydroxychloroquine, or a combination of all three medications. N Engl J Med 1996;334:1287–1291.
3. Bathon JM, Martin RW, Fleischmann RM, et al: A comparison of etanercept and methotrexate in patients with early rheumatoid arthritis. N Engl J Med 2000;343:1586–1593.
4. Lipsky PE, Van der Heijde D, St. Clair EW, et al: Infliximab and methotrexate in the treatment of rheumatoid arthritis. N Engl J Med 2000;243:1594–1602.
5. Weinblatt ME, Keystone EC, Furst DE, et al: Adalimumab, a fully human anti-tumor necrosis factor alpha monoclonal antibody, for the treatment of rheumatoid arthritis in patients taking concomitant methotrexate: The ARMADA trial. Arthritis Rheum 2003;38: 35–45.

6. Bongartz T, Sutton AJ, Sweeting MJ, et al: Anti-TNF antibody therapy in rheumatoid arthritis and the risk of serious infections and malignancies: Systematic review and meta-analysis of rare harmful effects in randomized controlled trials. JAMA 2006; 295:2275–2285.

SUGGESTED READINGS

Ranganath UK, Furst DE: Disease-modifying antirheumatic drug use in the elderly rheumatoid arthritis patient. Rheum Dis Clin North Am 2007;33:197–217. *A practical review.*

Scott DL, Kingsley GH: Tumor necrosis factor inhibitors for rheumatoid arthritis. N Engl J Med 2006;355:704–712. *An excellent overview of tumor necrosis factor inhibitors for rheumatoid arthritis.*

286 THE SPONDYLOARTHROPATHIES

Robert D. Inman

Definition

The spondyloarthropathies (SpAs) encompass a group of clinical syndromes that are linked in terms of disease manifestations and genetic susceptibility. The clinical subsets most commonly recognized are ankylosing spondylitis (AS), reactive arthritis (ReA), psoriatic arthritis (PsA), and enteropathic arthritis (EA) (Fig. 286–1). In addition, a sizable population of patients do not fit into one of these distinct diagnostic categories but share some of the common clinical features described in this chapter. The syndrome associated with this subset is termed undifferentiated spondyloarthropathy (USpA), which over time may evolve into a classic pattern such as AS but may remain in an undifferentiated pattern in long follow-up studies.

Pathobiology

Family studies in which there are multiple individuals with SpA have emphasized some of the common features between the four distinct subsets just mentioned. The impression from such studies is that there is a shared common path of immunogenetic susceptibility on which further genetic and environmental influences lead to characteristic clinical subsets. Thus, if EA occurs in such a family, in another family it may be PsA. In this sense, the SpAs seem to "breed true." It should be recognized, however, that some distinct clinical features can be very restricted in their manifestations (e.g., guttate psoriasis and keratodermia blennorrhagica), thus making simple discrimination sometimes difficult.

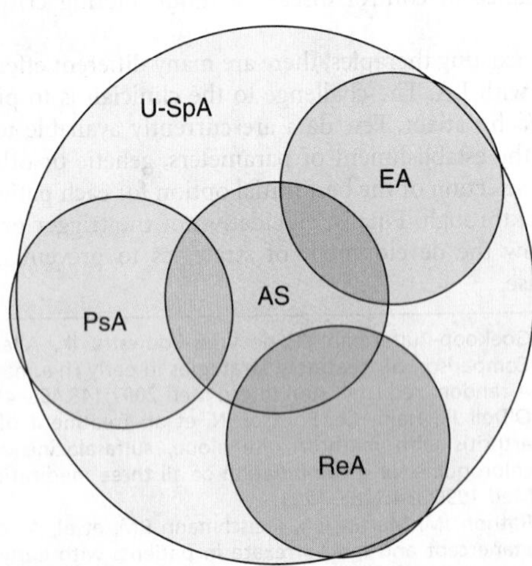

FIGURE 286–1 • Schematic relationships among the different spondyloarthropathy (SpA) subsets. Ankylosing spondylitis (AS), considered the classic SpA, encompasses the essential features of this family of diseases. AS may overlap with psoriatic arthritis (PsA), enteropathic arthritis (EA), or reactive arthritis (ReA). There are many patients with clinical features of SpA who do not meet diagnostic criteria for the four defined subsets. Such cases are termed undifferentiated SpA (U-SpA).

Clinical Manifestations

There are several common features in the family of SpAs that at once link them and serve to distinguish them from the other major contributor to chronic polyarthritis, rheumatoid arthritis (RA) (Chapter 285). The SpAs have a strong predilection for the spine, in particular the sacroiliac joints. There is a shared tendency for new bone formation at sites of chronic inflammation, with joint ankylosis as a consequence. When peripheral arthritis occurs, it is commonly lower extremity and asymmetrical. There is a predilection for sites of tendon insertion into bone (entheses), so enthesitis becomes one of the most specific clinical manifestations of the SpAs. Theories postulating the basis for this target organ involvement have invoked biomechanical factors, innervation, local vascularity, and bone marrow–derived inflammatory mediators, but the precise mechanism for this relationship remains incompletely defined. Whatever the reason, inflammation in the enthesis and contiguous subchondral bone is a characteristic feature of this arthritis, and the appearance of this inflammation on magnetic resonance imaging (MRI) is distinct enough to lead some investigators to use such imaging for diagnostic purposes.

Predilection for ocular inflammation, particularly acute anterior uveitis, is a common feature of all SpA subsets. Indeed, some investigators consider anterior uveitis to be a feature of SpAs in its own right because it may occur in the same susceptible populations of patients even in the absence of joint involvement and may have a unique genetic predisposition. Finally, all SpA subsets have an association with the class I human leukocyte antigen (HLA) allele B27, with the strength of the association varying somewhat between them.

Diagnosis

Increasingly, diagnostic criteria (Table 286–1) are being used that emphasize the common clinical features, namely, inflammatory spinal pain or asymmetrical, lower extremity synovitis. Several distinct features differentiate the SpAs from RA, the other main contributor to the differential diagnosis of chronic polyarthritis (Table 286–2). These features include sex predilection, HLA association, pattern of joint involvement, and the presence of rheumatoid factor, which becomes the serologic distinction between seropositive disease (RA) and seronegative disease (SpAs).

At the level of joint histopathology, sites of chronic inflammation in RA are associated with erosions, but in the SpAs such sites are associated

TABLE 286–1 EUROPEAN SPONDYLOARTHROPATHY STUDY GROUP CRITERIA FOR SPONDYLOARTHROPATHY

Inflammatory spinal pain
OR
Synovitis (asymmetrical or predominantly in the lower limb)
PLUS
Any one of the following:
Positive family history
Psoriasis
Inflammatory bowel disease
Urethritis, cervicitis, or acute diarrhea within 1 month before arthritis
Alternating buttock pain
Enthesopathy
Sacroiliitis

TABLE 286–2 CONTRAST OF RHEUMATOID ARTHRITIS AND SPONDYLOARTHROPATHY

Feature	Rheumatoid Arthritis	Ankylosing Spondylitis	Enteropathic Arthritis	Psoriatic Arthritis	Reactive Arthritis
Male-female ratio	1:3	3:1	1:1	1:1	10:1
HLA association	DR4	B27	B27(axial)	B27(axial)	B27
Joint pattern	Symmetrical, peripheral	Axial	Axial and peripheral	Axial and asymmetrical peripheral	Axial and asymmetrical peripheral
Sacroiliac	0	Symmetrical	Symmetrical	Asymmetrical	Asymmetrical
Syndesmophyte	0	Smooth, marginal	Smooth, marginal	Coarse, nonmarginal	Coarse, nonmarginal
Eye	Scleritis	Iritis	+/–	0	Iritis and conjunctivitis
Skin	Vasculitis	0	0	Psoriasis	Keratoderma
Rheumatoid factor	>80%	0	0	0	0

HLA = human leukocyte antigen.

with new bone formation. This distinction suggests a fundamental difference in the cytokine profile in the microenvironment of the joint, and although there is some evidence that SpAs reflect more of a type 2 T-helper cell (T_H2) cytokine profile as opposed to the T_H1 profile of RA, this issue has not been resolved and the mediators of neo-ossification await identification. Synovial histopathology in SpA is characterized by abundant neutrophils, macrophages, and hypervascularity, whereas in RA the prominent features are lymphoid aggregates, dendritic cells, lining cell hyperplasia, and citrullinated proteins.

Treatment

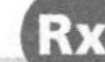

General Measures

The SpA group of diseases necessitates a global approach to management in which education of patients is the cornerstone. With the typical onset during young adulthood and with a male preponderance, these patients may express significant frustration or depression if their acute arthritis evolves into a chronic course that may significantly impair their functional capabilities and quality of life. A clinician managing patients with SpA should be aware that these psychosocial aspects of the disease are an important part of the burden of illness. Similarly, there may be important implications for the workplace, particularly if the job demands significant bending or twisting.

Exercise is an important part of the treatment plan for patients with AS. Generally, high-impact sports should be avoided, whereas swimming is an ideal exercise. Stretching to maintain mobility and maintenance of posture should be emphasized, and an experienced physiotherapist can greatly assist in instructing patients in daily exercises. Long car trips and air travel should include periodic stretching. Sleep position should emphasize a straight back position rather than one curled on the side. Deep breathing exercises and avoidance of cigarettes should be stressed.

One key area of concern for patients is prognosis because the SpAs, particularly ReA, often occur in young, active individuals for whom athletic activity is a priority. There is general recognition that ReA has a greater propensity for chronicity than was previously appreciated, and this should temper an overly optimistic projection on the natural history of the disease. At a 5-year follow-up of a cohort of patients with point source *Salmonella*-induced ReA, two thirds continued to have subjective complaints and one third demonstrated objective changes in their joints. The variability in prognosis for the large group of patients falling into the diagnostic category of USpA is perplexing for patients in this category. At present, there is a lack of reliable predictors of progression in patients with this heterogeneous cluster of articular and extra-articular features.

Rx

Medical Therapy

Nonsteroidal Anti-inflammatory Drugs

In general, joint inflammation improves significantly after the introduction of nonsteroidal anti-inflammatory drugs (NSAIDs), the exception being salicylates, which seem less effective in control of pain and stiffness. Indomethacin and diclofenac, up to 200 mg daily in divided doses, are generally well tolerated in this population of patients. These agents have to be used with caution in EA because of concern about exacerbating the underlying inflammatory bowel disease. In the case of AS, the goal with anti-inflammatory treatment is to achieve sufficient control of pain and stiffness to allow an active, sustained program of exercise and physical activity that maintains posture in addition to improvements in quality of life. Whether NSAIDs have disease-modifying capability has not been definitively resolved.

Corticosteroids

The response to the commonly used intra-articular steroid injection of peripheral joints in patients with SpA is often neither as dramatic nor as sustained as in patients with RA. Corticosteroid injection into the sacroiliac joints is usually performed under imaging guidance (fluoroscopy or computed tomography [CT]). One study observed that such injections gave a good response in 79% of 24 patients and that the improvement could persist for many months. Systemic corticosteroids (either orally or via an intravenous bolus protocol) have been used for severe symptomatic flares, but controlled trials to validate effectiveness are lacking. The goal should be prompt tapering of the dose when symptomatic control is achieved. The recognition that osteoporosis (Chapter 264) is a significant problem in AS provides further impetus to use corticosteroids sparingly. Topical steroids are usually effective for treatment of the mucous membrane and skin manifestations of reactive arthritis (ReA). For uveitis, topical corticosteroid eye drops are an integral component of management, and treatment should be monitored jointly with an ophthalmologist.

Sulfasalazine

Randomized, placebo-controlled trials have provided evidence to support some role for sulfasalazine (SSZ), particularly in PsA. 1 Three 36-week, randomized, double-blind multicenter studies of patients with AS, PsA, or ReA, respectively, were undertaken to compare SSZ (2 g/day) with placebo in each case. The different response rates in the placebo arms of these trials highlight the variability in clinical course of the SpAs. An analysis of these studies with SSZ stratified the patients into those having axial or peripheral disease. In patients with only axial disease, response criteria were met equally in the SSZ group and the placebo group. In the patients with peripheral arthritis, responses were seen in 59% of the SSZ group and 43% of the placebo group ($P < .0005$).

Rx

These findings are useful in guiding selection of patients for SSZ treatment options.

Methotrexate

Concurrent with the widespread use of methotrexate (MTX) in patients with RA, there has been increasing use of MTX in patients with SpA. Generally, responses have been good, particularly for peripheral joint disease, but few controlled trials have been conducted to substantiate these clinical impressions. There is no evidence that MTX changes the course of axial diseases in AS. Experience with long-term MTX therapy in 38 patients with PsA has been reported, and despite an improvement in joint count, there was no evidence of slowing of radiographic progression. Long-term follow-up may be required to resolve whether MTX has a joint-sparing effect in PsA.

Other Disease-Modifying Agents

There have been several therapeutic approaches to control of PsA, including chloroquine, intramuscular gold, and cyclosporine, all of which show some clinical efficacy, but long-term studies are needed to evaluate them more comprehensively. The response of SpA patients to SSZ may be attributable to the antibiotic moiety of this compound (sulfapyridine) or to the anti-inflammatory moiety (5-aminosalicylic acid [5-ASA]). A study reported that of SpA patients who had been taking SSZ and were then switched to 5-ASA, most maintained their response profile, thus supporting the notion that 5-ASA may be the active moiety in SSZ. An open study of intravenous pamidronate for refractory AS showed significant improvement in disease activity scores; this agent is under investigation at several centers.

Antibiotic Therapy

The current concept of the pathogenesis of ReA postulates that a bacterial infection, usually gastrointestinal (GI) or genitourinary (GU), is the triggering event in an immunogenetically susceptible host. For the other SpAs there is less compelling evidence to implicate infection in a causal role. It is sound clinical practice to treat any culture-proven chlamydial urethritis in conjunction with treatment of the sexual partner. For this indication, azithromycin, 1 g as a single dose, is as effective as doxycycline, 100 mg twice a day for 7 days. The role of antibiotics in the management of SpA has been controversial. An earlier retrospective review concluded that 37% of episodes of urethritis not treated with anti-*Chlamydia* agents were associated with subsequent ReA whereas only 10% of such episodes when treated with tetracycline progressed to ReA. In a 3-month, double-blind, placebo-controlled study of chronic ReA, lymecycline significantly decreased the duration of illness in patients with *Chlamydia*-induced ReA but not in patients with ReA triggered by enteric pathogens. Two controlled trials of ciprofloxacin demonstrated no significant difference from placebo in ReA and undifferentiated oligoarthritis. Ciprofloxacin was not effective in *Yersinia-* or *Salmonella*-induced ReA, but there was a trend toward response in *Chlamydia*-induced ReA. A recent study examining azithromycin in the treatment of SpA found no convincing evidence of disease-modifying potential. 2

Anti–Tumor Necrosis Factor Therapy

The role of immunomodulatory cytokines in the pathogenesis of SpA has been controversial. Some studies have implicated as an AS susceptibility marker a genetic polymorphism associated with relative impairment of tumor necrosis factor-α (TNF-α) production, but not all studies have supported this notion. Despite the uncertainties about the role of pro-inflammatory cytokines in AS, some of the newer biologic agents such as monoclonal antibodies to TNF-α (infliximab and adalimumab) or the soluble TNF receptor (etanercept) have been used in the treatment of SpA. 3 At present, the three anti-TNF agents have been shown to be effective in short-term trials of AS and PsA. 4 These studies have generally reported a prompt response in clinical outcome measures, as well as laboratory indicators of inflammation, and MRI evaluations have shown improvement in local inflammation in the sacroiliac joints and spine. The anti-TNF treatments have been well tolerated with no significant incidence of serious adverse events, but patients appear to relapse when treatment is discontinued. Experience with longer-term treatment intervals with anti-TNF agents (>2 years) has been encouraging in the persistence of the therapeutic effect and the infrequency of late adverse events. Whether anti-TNF treatments can alter the progressive ankylosis of this disease over the long course of the disease awaits further study. The significant improvements seen on MRI provide rational hope that these agents may alter the long-term outcomes of AS, both structurally and functionally.

GENETIC SUSCEPTIBILITY

HLA-B27

Definition

The major histocompatibility complex (MHC), on the short arm of chromosome 6 in humans, is one of the most polymorphic regions of the human genome (Chapter 43). This is particularly so for the B locus, which constitutes part of the class I MHC genes in this complex. More than 200 different alleles have been detected at this locus, of which B27 is just 1. As with all HLA alleles, there is codominant expression of B locus genes such that most individuals who are "B27 positive" are heterozygous for the B locus. There appears to be little clinical or prognostic significance associated with the less common homozygous B27 state. The conventional role of class I HLA antigens is to present a processed peptide to the T-cell receptor of a specific $CD8^+$ cytotoxic T cell, thereby initiating an immune response against the pathogen from which that peptide was derived by intracellular proteolysis and processing. This function places the HLA antigens in a critical role in host defense against pathogens, and it is the heterogeneity of cellular immune responses that is alleged to be an advantage for a species (such as humans) with an extensive polymorphism region of the genome. This idea has led to the concept that infectious diseases have driven allelic polymorphisms in the MHC. Such a hypothesis postulates a selective advantage in the extensive peptide-binding capabilities conferred by different alleles of the B locus, but there may also be disadvantages.

Epidemiology

It is clear that HLA is strongly associated with the SpAs, yet the prevalence of HLA-B27 varies widely in different racial and ethnic clusters around the world. It is virtually absent in aboriginal populations in Australia, occurs in 1% of the population in Japan, in 7% in northern European countries, and in 50% in some of the native tribes in western Canada. The environmental-genetic interaction that may account for the expansion or restriction of this gene in human populations is unknown, but some evidence indicates that B27 may confer more effective host response to some viruses. There is a practical impact of this variability for the clinician. Because the relative risk conferred by a gene reflects the prevalence of the gene in the affected individuals versus the prevalence of the gene in the normal population, the relative risk for SpAs is higher in a population in which the gene is uncommon (e.g., Japan) than in a population in which B27 is more common (e.g., Scandinavia). In the North American white population, the prevalence of the gene is approximately 7%. Thus, there is a 7% "false-positive" rate if one is attempting to use the gene as a diagnostic marker to decipher the cause of chronic back pain in an unselected population of patients. On the other hand, 90% of patients with AS are B27 positive, so there is a 10% "false-negative" rate in the use of the test diagnostically. The key factor is pretest probability. In a patient with chronic back pain that is clearly inflammatory in character, the addition of B27 positivity combines to strengthen the likelihood of AS accounting for the back problem. The presence of distinctive extra-articular features (such as uveitis) further increases this likelihood.

It had been held that the prevalence of AS in various parts of the globe closely parallels the prevalence of B27 in that population, and in general this pattern is valid. What has introduced complexity into this concept has been the recognition that there is not just one B27 but in fact more than 24 subtypes of B27 (ranging from B*2701 to B*2724 at present). In terms of the evolution of molecular variability, B*2705 is regarded as the primordial subtype with variability developing over time on the basis of alterations in genomic DNA. The amino acid substitutions occurring as a result are generally reflected in the peptide-binding cleft of the B27 molecule, thus supporting the argument that there has been a functional change concurrent with the structural change. This notion has been bolstered by the observation that some subtypes, notably B*2706 and B*2709, do not seem to confer increased susceptibility to the development of AS. As an extension of genetic epidemiology, this observation has led to a search for "arthritogenic peptides" that can be presented by the disease-associated subtypes such as B*2705 and B*2704 but not by the non–disease-associated subtypes. To date, no simple peptide-susceptibility relationship has been demonstrated, but this is an important clue to the pathogenic role of B27, and studies are ongoing to explore this relationship.

Other approaches have also been taken to define the mechanism whereby B27 confers disease susceptibility in addition to that of uniquely presenting an arthritogenic peptide to T cells. According to the theory of molecular mimicry, an autoimmune response can ensue after an infection if the immune response against the pathogen cross-reacts with host antigens. There is a degree of sequence homology between B27 and several candidate gram-negative enteric bacteria and there is evidence for cross-reacting monoclonal antibodies, but the significance of such homology for disease pathogenesis remains unresolved. It has also been argued that B27 is distinctive in its propensity to misfold in the endoplasmic reticulum, which may induce a pro-inflammatory cascade called the unfolded protein response. Furthermore, B27 may have a distinct tendency to form heavy chain homodimers at the cell surface, and the possible consequences of this change for the immune response are under investigation. There has also been investigation into alteration of primary host-pathogen interactions, such as modulation of invasion, intracellular replication, and pathogen clearance, but no definitive allele-specific relationships have been demonstrated in these studies, although this topic remains an area of active study. In B27 transgenic rats, the spontaneous development of pathology strikingly similar to human SpAs has supported the notion that B27 itself is the critical genetic factor in disease pathogenesis. These animals demonstrate pathology similar to that of Crohn's disease in the GI tract, spondylitis, peripheral arthritis, uveitis, and psoriasiform skin and nail changes. Of interest, if such animals are raised in a germ-free environment, there is a marked reduction in joint and gut disease, thus implying a dynamic interrelationship between microbial triggers and background host genes that seems to recapitulate the situation seen clinically.

Genome-wide screening studies of multiplex families with SpAs, particularly AS, are ongoing in several countries in order to identify other important genes that are involved in predisposing to these diseases. Several candidate loci have been identified, although considerable variability between different studies is apparent. The common observation, however, is that the strongest association of SpAs is with the HLA complex, so at least in familial AS, B27 may to a certain extent be necessary, if not sufficient to confer disease susceptibility. There are estimates of an additional four to nine genes acting in concert with B27; their identity remains a topic of active investigation. MRI studies in asymptomatic B27-positive individuals indicate that there is a much higher prevalence of sacroiliitis than previously recognized, and studies are continuing to define that prevalence and indeed the prevalence of SpAs in the general population. Some investigators have concluded that SpAs are as common as RA in the population.

CLINICAL SUBSETS OF THE SPONDYLOARTHROPATHIES

Ankylosing Spondylitis

Epidemiology

AS is the most common inflammatory disorder of the axial skeleton. The following is a useful rule of thumb: AS occurs in 0.2% of the general population, in 2% of the B27-positive population, and in 20% of B27-positive individuals with an affected family member. There is a male preponderance in the disease, with the male-to-female ratio ranging from 2.5:1 to 5:1; however, recent epidemiologic studies have found less female involvement than these estimates. The basis for the gender bias is not resolved. It is held, however, that AS is under-recognized in women, perhaps because of milder axial disease and a more delayed disease onset, but alternative diagnoses of pelvic and low back pain in women may hinder clinician awareness of the disease in female patients.

Clinical Manifestations

AS typically begins in young adulthood, but symptoms may arise in adolescence or earlier. Up to 15% of children with juvenile chronic polyarthritis are classified as having juvenile AS. Such children may have a pauciarticular pattern, with a predilection for the tarsal joints and frequently minimal axial complaints. During the adolescent years there is an increasing prevalence of radiographic sacroiliitis, with a significant proportion of patients manifesting this feature by the end of the teenage years. At the other end of the age spectrum, a small number of patients with late-onset AS may have sacroiliitis and oligoarthritis. The axial involvement and asymmetrical lower extremity involvement may serve to differentiate such patients from those with late-onset RA, although clinically there may be overlapping features. Recent studies indicate that long-term functional disability may be more marked in juvenile-onset AS than in adult-onset AS.

The classical manifestation of AS is the onset of low back pain that persists for more than 3 months, is accompanied by early morning stiffness, and is typically improved by exercise (Table 286–3). An extensive discussion of the differential diagnosis of low back pain is presented in Chapter 423. Some investigators would also include a response to NSAID therapy as a feature further differentiating AS from mechanical low back pain. Back pain that awakens the patient from sleep is often a clue to inflammatory back pain that may have previously been misdiagnosed as the pain of degenerative disc disease, the latter being the much more common cause of low back pain in the population at large. The pain typically occurs in the region of the sacroiliac joints, with or without slight radiation to the buttock area. Midthoracic pain and cervical pain, particularly at night, are less common but strongly suggest inflammatory back pain when they occur. Fatigue is also a suggestive symptom and is often highlighted by these patients because the typical young male patient sets a high functional norm in terms of sports and recreation. If the inflammation is inadequately controlled, there is increasing stiffness, which may persist most of the day, as well as progressive loss of mobility and flexibility.

Peripheral oligoarthritis is seen in up to 30% of patients with AS. Typically, it is an asymmetrical oligoarthritis with a predilection for the

TABLE 286–3 MODIFIED NEW YORK CRITERIA FOR ANKYLOSING SPONDYLITIS (1984)

CLINICAL CRITERIA
Low back pain and stiffness for more than 3 months that improve with exercise but are not relieved by rest
Limitation of motion of the lumbar spine in both the sagittal and frontal planes
Limitation of chest expansion
RADIOLOGIC CRITERIA
Sacroiliitis: grade ≥2 bilateral *or* grade 3 or 4 unilateral
GRADING
Definite AS if the radiologic criterion is associated with at least one clinical variable
Probable AS if
The three clinical criteria are present
The radiologic criterion is present without the clinical criteria

AS = ankylosing spondylitis.

lower extremities. It is important to ask about concurrent or previous tendinitis (e.g., Achilles tendinitis) or heel pain (e.g., plantar fasciitis) because either may reflect an enthesitis that is part of the clinical picture. Involvement of the hip can occur at any point in the course of AS and can follow a course to joint destruction. A hip flexion contracture on this basis may contribute to increasing stoop on standing and walking, which may otherwise be attributed to spinal involvement in the disease.

Extra-articular features primarily involve the eye. Ocular involvement may occur in up to 40% of AS patients, most typically acute anterior uveitis (iritis). The uveitis is often manifested by a slight impairment in visual acuity, and photophobia and eye pain may accompany the uveitis. Typically, it is unilateral and recurrent. Uncommon manifestations include aortic insufficiency, cardiac conduction defects, and pulmonary fibrosis.

Diagnosis

Physical Examination

Physical examination of the spine characteristically indicates restricted movement, which in the early stages may reflect paraspinal muscle spasm in part but late in the course reflects ankylosis of the zygapophyseal joints and syndesmophyte bridging of the vertebral bodies. Forward flexion is restricted and can be monitored by measuring the finger-to-floor distance on bending forward. Schober's test is used to measure mobility in the lower part of the back: with the patient standing upright, a 10-cm span is marked from the fifth lumbar vertebra upward. On maximal forward flexion, the distance between the marks is remeasured. With normal spinal mobility the flexed distance should register as 15 cm, or an increment of 5 cm. Thoracic involvement is measured in chest expansion, with the chest circumference, at maximum inspiration, being more than 5 cm greater than the circumference at maximal expiration. Changes in cervical mobility can be measured as the occiput-to-wall distance, with the patient's heels against the wall and the patient attempting to touch the back of the head to the wall. Inflammation in the sacroiliac joint may be reflected by joint line tenderness to direct pressure or by the Fabere or Gaenslen maneuver. In the former, the patient lies supine while the examiner flexes and externally rotates the hip. In the latter, the examiner extends the hip by letting the leg dangle off the side of the examining table. In both cases, stress is placed on the sacroiliac joint and may reproduce the back pain if it derives from this site.

Laboratory Findings

Laboratory tests in the evaluation of inflammatory back pain are relatively nonspecific. The erythrocyte sedimentation rate and C-reactive protein are typically elevated, but normal levels do not exclude inflammatory back pain, and the degree of elevation is typically less than would be seen in acute RA. The anemia of chronic disease may be observed if the condition is long-standing. Serum immunoglobulin A levels may be elevated, but autoantibodies are notable for their absence. HLA-B27 is rarely the definitive factor for diagnosis, and the false-positive and false-negative rates have already been discussed, but in the setting of characteristic back symptoms, the test has reasonably high sensitivity and specificity.

Imaging

Radiographic assessment is important for confirmation of disease, but early in the course of the disease there may be no radiographic changes in the sacroiliac joints. If the clinician has a high index of suspicion in such cases, the use of a bone scan, CT scan, or especially MRI may improve the sensitivity of the plain radiograph. Views of the sacroiliac joints should be requested because the obliquity of the joint renders it difficult to assess on a routine anteroposterior pelvic radiograph. The classic findings are bilateral changes in the sacroiliac joints (Fig. 286–2). Abnormalities include erosions in the joint line, pseudowidening, subchondral sclerosis, and finally, ankylosis reflected as complete bony replacement of the sacroiliac joints.

Radiographs of the spine may reveal squaring of the vertebral bodies (loss of the normal anterior concavity of the lumbar vertebra) and "shiny corners" (subchondral sclerosis at the upper edge of the vertebral body), both being manifestations of enthesitis. Syndesmophytes, which represent marginal bridging of the vertebrae (Figs. 286–3 and 286–4), eventually develop and make the diagnosis clear. Because ankylosis of the apophyseal joints may occur without syndesmophyte formation, it is important to assess the posterior joints on the lateral lumbosacral spine views, as well as the anterior margin of the vertebrae. Eventually, the changes may result in a "bamboo spine," so called because the bridging syndesmophytes can mimic the appearance of bamboo. It is now appreciated that osteoporosis is a significant feature of AS, probably reflecting both the local chronic inflammation and the abnormal biomechanical loading of the vertebrae as the disease progresses.

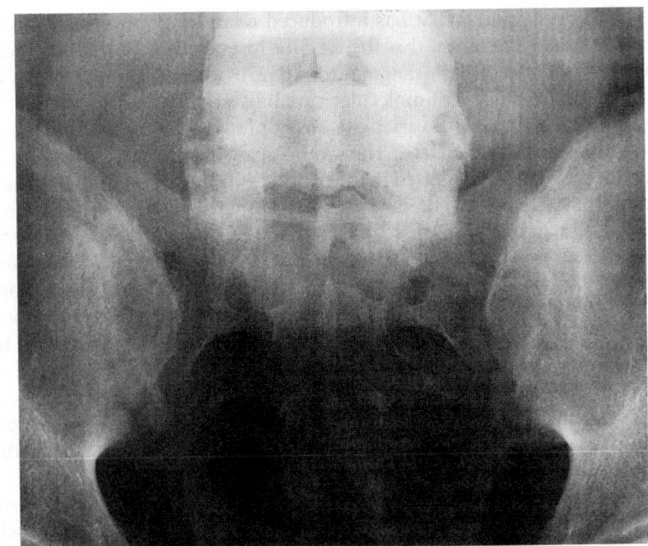

FIGURE 286–2 • Bilaterally symmetrical sacroiliitis in ankylosing spondylitis.

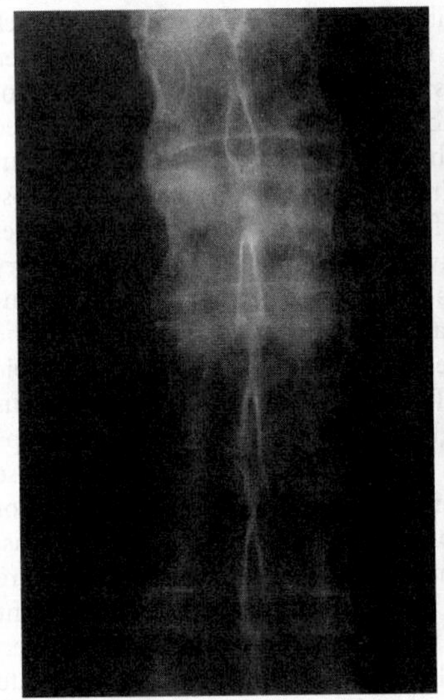

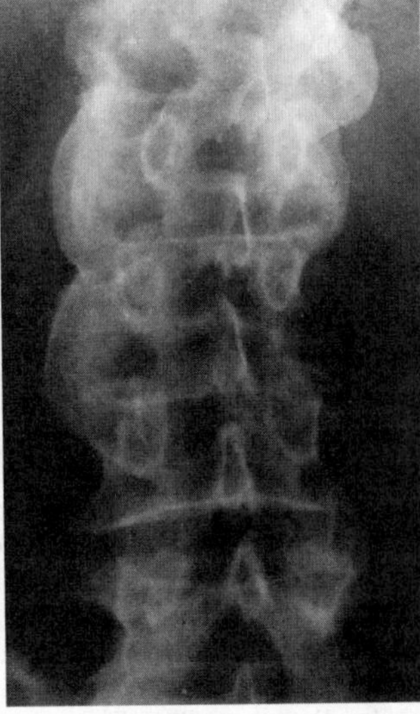

FIGURE 286–3 • Left, Lumbar spondylitis in ankylosing spondylitis with symmetrical, marginal bridging syndesmophytes and calcification of the spinal ligament. Right, The bulky, nonmarginal, asymmetrical syndesmophytes of reactive arthritis with lumbar spondylitis.

Differential Diagnosis

The differential diagnosis of AS includes the other SpAs; osteitis condensans ilii; diffuse idiopathic skeletal hyperostosis; the syndrome of synovitis, acne, pustulosis, hyperostosis, and osteomyelitis (SAPHO); and some induced hyperostotic states (vitamin A intoxication, fluorosis). New bone formation occurs in degenerative disc disease, but the bulky, horizontal appearance of osteophytes is easily distinguished from that of syndesmophytes, and narrowing of the disc space is not a feature of AS.

The clinical course and severity of AS are highly variable. Inflammatory back pain and stiffness dominate the picture in the early stages, whereas chronic pain and deformity may develop over time. In both

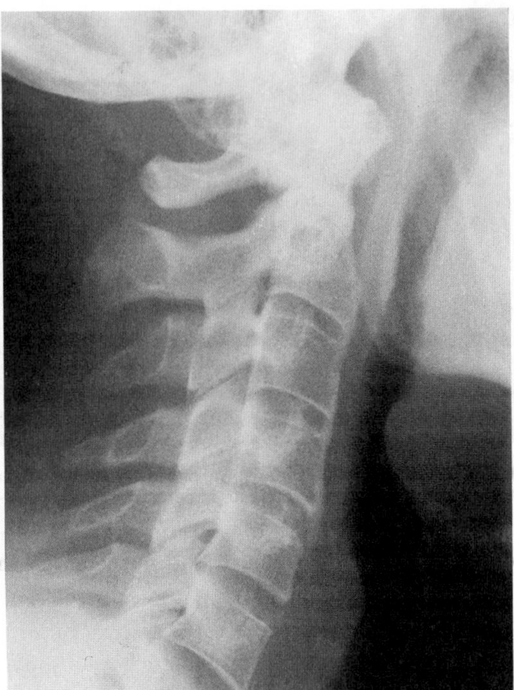

FIGURE 286–4 • A 34-year-old man who had ankylosing spondylitis for 9 years and neck pain. Radiographs demonstrate narrowing of the C2-C3 apophyseal joints posteriorly and anterior bridging marginal syndesmophytes extending from C2 to C5.

early and late phases of the disease there may be a significant impact of work disability on quality of life. In only a minority of patients may the full-blown picture of a bamboo spine eventually develop, but at present there are few variables that can reliably aid in prognosticating the course. In AS patients in whom new, refractory spinal pain develops, an intervertebral fracture should be considered and may occur after minimal trauma.

Additional late complications may include cauda equina syndrome, osteoporotic compression fractures, spondylodiscitis, and restrictive lung disease.

Reactive Arthritis

Definition

ReA is an aseptic arthritis that occurs subsequent to an extra-articular infection, most typically of the GI or GU tract. In the former, the key pathogens are *Salmonella typhimurium, Yersinia enterocolitica, Shigella flexneri*, and *Campylobacter jejuni*. For the latter, *Chlamydia trachomatis* is the most common offender.

Epidemiology

The true incidence and prevalence of ReA are not well defined. In epidemics involving *Salmonella* (Chapter 329) or *Yersinia* (Chapter 333), it is estimated that ReA develops in 2 to 7% of infected individuals but in as many as 20% of B27-positive infected individuals. In such epidemic studies, B27 confers risk not only for the onset of arthritis but also for axial involvement and chronicity. The variability in the rate of ReA is determined by the heterogeneity of the cohorts reported, which introduces confounding variables of different genetic backgrounds in the population and different species of pathogens. Even in the setting of an epidemic point source outbreak, the inoculum varies widely among the exposed individuals, and the genetic makeup of the population at risk (e.g., the prevalence of B27) may differ greatly between different studies. Case ascertainment and relative risk are even more difficult to determine for post-*Chlamydia* ReA. Young adults in the United States have a high prevalence of asymptomatic *Chlamydia* carriage in the GU tract, and establishing a causal link between *Chlamydia* and synovitis can be difficult. Nevertheless, it is with *Chlamydia* that ReA has been most intensively studied.

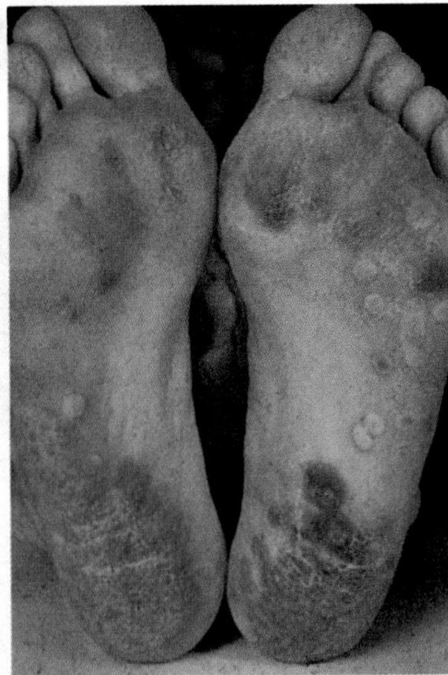

FIGURE 286–5 • Keratoderma blennorrhagicum of the feet in reactive arthritis.

Pathobiology

Although immunofluorescence studies have identified bacterial antigens in the joints of patients with ReA after both GI and GU infections, it is primarily in post-*Chlamydia* ReA that polymerase chain reaction results on synovial tissues have most consistently been positive, thus suggesting that viable *Chlamydia* may persist in the joints of such patients, albeit in a metabolically altered state.

Typically, the arthritis has its onset 1 to 3 weeks after the GI or GU infection, but the temporal details are often difficult to define precisely.

Although the definition of aseptic arthritis after an extra-articular infection may include a broader range of pathogens (e.g., *Chlamydia pneumoniae*), sites of infection (e.g., streptococcal pharyngitis), and types of infections (e.g., *Giardia* infections of the GI tract), these clinical scenarios have not generally been included in the ReA diagnosis. They lack the other associated clinical features of the SpA group of diseases, and they lack an association with B27.

Diagnosis

The pattern of joint involvement in ReA is one of asymmetrical oligoarthritis with a predilection for the lower extremity, a pattern shared by most SpA syndromes. Enthesitis may arise as Achilles tendonitis or plantar fasciitis. Dactylitis, arising as a sausage digit, may also be seen. Dactylitis is the net result of inflammatory changes affecting the joint capsule, entheses, periarticular structures, and periosteal bone. Sacroiliitis may be seen in the acute phase, but radiographic changes are seen largely in the patients with a more chronic course.

When ReA is accompanied by certain extra-articular features such as urethritis, conjunctivitis, or mucocutaneous lesions, the term *Reiter's syndrome* has been applied historically, but this term is not used any more. The urethritis may be manifested as dysuria or discharge and the rash as circinate balanitis, which appears as vesicles or shallow ulcerations on the glans penis. Painless lingual or oral ulcerations may also be seen. The fact that the cervicitis may be less symptomatic may in part account for the underdiagnosis in women. The classic skin manifestation of ReA is keratoderma blennorrhagicum, a painless papulosquamous eruption on the palms or soles (Fig. 286–5). Occasional nail dystrophy with pitting and onycholysis or subungual keratosis can be seen. The conjunctivitis can be bilateral and painful, in contrast to the acute anterior uveitis that can also be seen in this setting, which tends to be painless and unilateral.

Radiographic findings in ReA can be seen in the involved peripheral joints, with soft tissue swelling and juxta-articular osteopenia being the early findings. Areas of periostitis and new bone formation may develop in peripheral joints. When sacroiliac changes are seen, they are typically asymmetrical, in contrast to the symmetrical pattern seen in AS

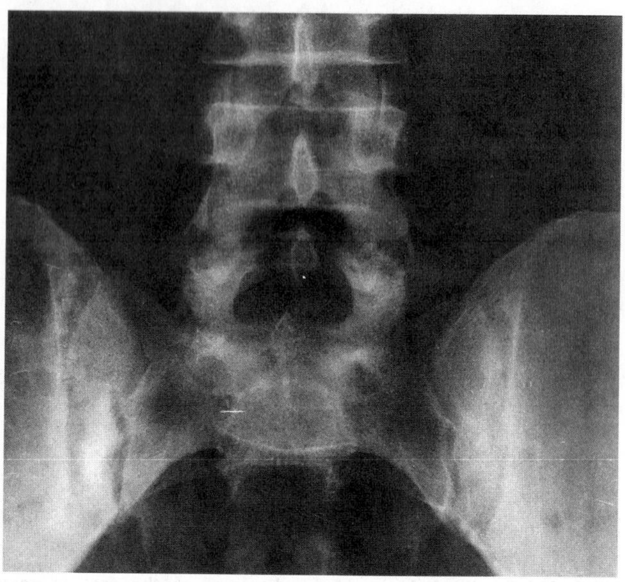

FIGURE 286–6 • Bilaterally asymmetrical sacroiliitis in reactive arthritis. Erosions, pseudowidening, and ileal sclerosis are present.

(Fig. 286–6). In the chronic phase, syndesmophytes may develop, but they are described as bulky, nonmarginal, often asymmetrical formations that differ from the classic syndesmophytes of AS. The frequency with which AS can evolve into bona fide AS has not been resolved definitively.

Differential Diagnosis

The most important differential diagnosis for such reactive arthropathies is septic arthritis. Both *Yersinia* and *Salmonella* can induce septic arthritis, so an appropriate culture of synovial fluid should precede the diagnosis of ReA whenever possible. The course of ReA is variable, and few prognostic markers are available for the clinician to predict the course in any individual case. The majority of patients have an initial episode lasting 2 to 3 months, but synovitis may persist for a year or longer. In one 5-year follow-up of a point source cohort of post-*Salmonella* ReA, 20% of patients had ongoing inflammatory joint disease at this time, and some degree of functional disability was observed in 30% of patients 5 years after the onset of disease.

Reactive Arthritis and Human Immunodeficiency Virus

An aggressive form of SpA may be seen in patients who are concomitantly infected with human immunodeficiency virus (HIV) (Chapter 409). There is no increased frequency of ReA in patients infected with HIV, but HIV may alter the course of these arthropathies, with a tendency for a more aggressive and more refractory course of joint disease. Aggressive skin and joint disease may be seen in patients in whom PsA develops in the setting of HIV infection. Most North American patients with the HIV-ReA constellation are B27 positive, but studies of comparable patients in Africa have found a sizable B27-negative component in such groups of patients. The arthritis in these patients falls into two clinical patterns: (1) an additive, asymmetrical polyarthritis or (2) an intermittent oligoarthritis that most commonly affects the lower extremities. Enthesitis, fasciitis, conjunctivitis, and urethritis can all be seen in such patients. Sacroiliitis can occur, although extensive spinal syndesmophyte formation is not common.

Psoriatic Arthritis

Epidemiology

PsA develops in 5 to 7% of patients with psoriasis. Although most cases arise in patients with established cutaneous disease, some patients (particularly children) have arthritis that antedates the appearance of the skin lesions. Although the extent of psoriatic skin disease correlates poorly with the development of arthritis, the risk for PsA increases with a family history of SpA. The age at onset can range from 30 to 55 years, with an equal predilection for women and men. Psoriatic spondylitis has a slight male preponderance.

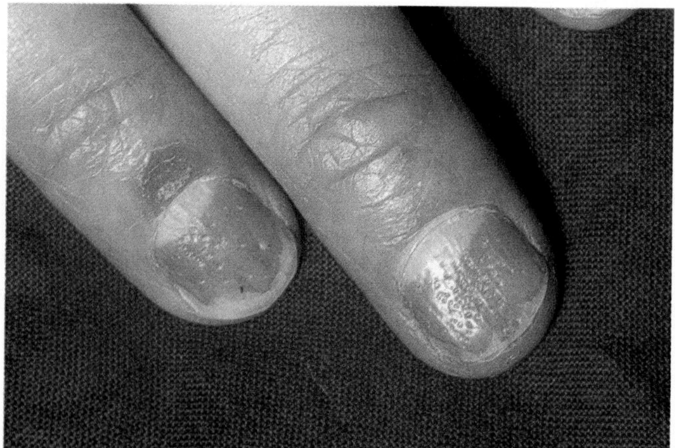

FIGURE 286–7 • Nail pitting in psoriasis. The pits are more discrete and regular compared with pits affecting the nail plate in dermatitis.

Pathobiology

The genetic associations with PsA are complex. Psoriasis itself is associated with HLA-B13, HLA-B16, HLA-B17, and HLA-Cw6. By contrast, HLA-B39 and HLA-B27 have been associated with sacroiliitis and axial involvement. No etiologic agent has been proved in PsA, although some investigators have proposed that the disease process represents ReA in response to cutaneous bacteria. The histopathology of the synovitis of PsA is comparable to that of the other SpAs, with the absence of local production of immunoglobulin and rheumatoid factor being differentiating features from RA. There is the potential for aggressive osteolysis, fibrous ankylosis, and heterotopic new bone formation to occur in PsA. As mentioned earlier, the coexistence of HIV and PsA seems to set the stage for an aggressive course of joint destruction in some patients.

Diagnosis

PsA has a variable manifestation and disease course, but several clinical patterns have been identified in prospectively monitored cohorts of patients. The clinical subsets are not mutually exclusive, nor are they static over time. The most common form, in which 30 to 50% of patients are affected, is an asymmetrical oligoarthritis that may involve both large and small joints. Dactylitis, arising as sausage digits, can be seen in fingers and toes and actually represents an enthesitis. In the second subset there is selective targeting of the distal interphalangeal joints, seen in 10 to 15% of patients. These changes are strongly associated with nail dystrophy, of which the features are onycholysis, subungual keratosis, pitting, and oil drop–like staining (Fig. 286–7). The third subset (15 to 30% of patients) has a symmetrical polyarthritis that mimics RA in many ways except for the absence of rheumatoid nodules and rheumatoid factor. The fourth clinical variant is psoriatic spondylitis, which occurs in 20% of patients; 50% of such patients are B27 positive. Finally, arthritis mutilans (5% of patients) is a destructive, erosive arthritis that affects large and small joints. It can be associated with marked deformities and significant disability.

Radiographic changes in PsA involve soft tissue swelling (particularly in the case of dactylitis), erosions, and periostitis. Axial involvement may lead to the appearance of asymmetrical sacroiliitis with syndesmophytes that are bulky, asymmetrical, and nonmarginal. The classic “pencil-in-cup” deformity may be seen in patients with distal interphalangeal joint disease or arthritis mutilans. Acro-osteolysis is noted in a minority of patients and reflects an aggressive erosive process.

Differential Diagnosis

The diagnosis of PsA depends on finding the typical skin or nail changes in association with one of the articular variants described previously. The differential for the skin lesions can include seborrheic dermatitis, dyshidrotic eczema, fungal infection, keratodermia blennorrhagica, and palmoplantar pustulosis.

TABLE 286–4 ENTEROPATHIC ARTHRITIS

Feature	Peripheral Arthritis	Sacroiliitis, Spondylitis
CROHN'S DISEASE AND ARTHRITIS		
Frequency in CD	10–20%	2–7%
HLA-B27 associated	No	Yes
Pattern	Transient, symmetrical	Chronic
Course	Related to activity of CD	Unrelated to activity of CD
Effect of surgery	Remission of arthritis uncommon	No effect
Effect of anti-TNF therapy	Effective	Effective
ULCERATIVE COLITIS AND ARTHRITIS		
Frequency in UC	5–10%	2–7%
HLA-B27 associated	No	Yes
Pattern	Transient	Chronic
Course	(More common in pancolitis than proctitis) Related to activity of UC	Unrelated
Effect of surgery	Remission of arthritis	No effect

CD = Crohn's disease; HLA = human leukocyte antigen; TNF = tumor necrosis factor; UC = ulcerative colitis.

Enteropathic Arthritis

Definition

EA refers to the arthritis associated with Crohn's disease (CD) or ulcerative colitis (UC) (Chapter 145) (Table 286–4).

Pathobiology

All extra-enteric manifestations, including arthritis, occur more commonly in CD than in UC. Peripheral arthritis occurs in 10 to 20% of CD patients and in 2 to 7% of UC patients. This pattern of arthritis occurs more commonly in patients with other extra-enteric features (e.g., erythema nodosum, iritis). It is typically an inflammatory, nonerosive polyarthritis, predominantly of large joints. In general, the clinical activity of the peripheral arthritis parallels the activity of the gut inflammation, and measures that control the GI disease usually control the joint disease concomitantly. The peripheral arthritis of EA is not associated with B27.

In contrast, the sacroiliitis or spondylitis of EA follows a pattern in which the joint inflammation waxes and wanes independently of the bowel inflammation. Axial disease occurs in 2 to 7% of CD patients and 2 to 7% of UC patients. HLA-B27 is found in 50% of patients with axial arthritis. The course tends to be chronic, as opposed to the transient course of peripheral arthritis.

The association of bowel inflammation and arthritis is supported by ileocolonoscopic studies in which subclinical inflammation of the bowel covering the entire spectrum of the SpAs has been demonstrated. Histologic evaluation demonstrates that changes of acute ileitis are seen in postdysenteric ReA whereas chronic inflammatory changes are more likely to be seen in patients with AS. As mentioned earlier, the abnormalities in the bowel of B27 transgenic rats have strong similarity to lesions of CD, and a germ-free environment minimizes inflammatory changes in both the gut and the joints. This finding argues that altered bowel permeability, with enhanced bacteremia or antigenemia, may provide the link in both cases.

Diagnosis

It is important to recognize that the musculoskeletal features of EA may precede any GI symptoms or signs. Conversely, the diarrhea preceding the onset of peripheral or axial arthritis in a young patient could as likely represent a food-borne pathogen (such as *Salmonella* or *Yersinia*) with secondary ReA as inflammatory bowel disease and accompanying EA. In the initial assessment of such a patient, it is important to carry out careful and complete stool cultures. If the GI symptoms persist, diagnostic colonoscopy is often required to resolve the issue.

Undifferentiated Spondyloarthropathy

Despite careful clinical and radiographic assessment, there are still a substantial number of patients who do not fall easily into one of the classic diagnostic subsets of SpA outlined previously. These patients are often defined as having USpA with peripheral enthesitis, with asymmetrical arthritis or sacroiliitis, or with iritis in the absence of identifiable antecedent infection or concurrent inflammatory bowel disease or psoriasis. The natural history of USpA has not been well defined, and case heterogeneity and diagnostic dilemmas plague a systematic or multicenter approach to the problem. When the clinical course has been examined, a number of such patients finally meet the diagnostic criteria for AS, but many remain with a distinct USpA pattern for prolonged periods.

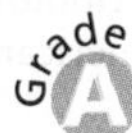

1. Clegg DO, Reda DJ, Abdellatif M: Comparison of sulfasalazine and placebo for the treatment of axial and peripheral articular manifestations of the seronegative spondyloarthropathies. Arthritis Rheum 1999;42:2325–2329.
2. Kvien TK, Gaston JS, Bardin T, et al: Three month treatment of reactive arthritis with azithromycin: A EULAR double blind, placebo controlled study. Ann Rheum Dis 2005;63:1113–1119.
3. Braun J, Brandt J, Listing J, et al: Treatment of active ankylosing spondylitis with infliximab: A randomized controlled multicenter trial. Lancet 2002;359:1187–1193.
4. Gorman JD, Sack KE, Davis JC Jr: Treatment of ankylosing spondylitis by inhibition of tumor necrosis factor alpha. N Engl J Med 2002;346:1349–1356.

SUGGESTED READINGS

Anandarajah AP, Ritchlin CT: Etanercept in psoriatic arthritis. Expert Opin Biol Ther 2003;3:169–177. *This therapy is also effective in psoriatic arthritis.*

Braun J, Davis J, Dougados M, et al: First update of the International ASAS Consensus Statement for the use of anti-TNF agents in patients with ankylosing spondylitis. Ann Rheum Dis 2006;65:316–320. *A consensus statement.*

Braun J, Sieper J, Breban M, et al: Anti TNF-α therapy for ankylosing spondylitis: International experience. Ann Rheum Dis 2002;61:51–60. *Describes anti-TNF agents, which have dramatically changed the therapeutic landscape in the spondyloarthropathies.*

Flores D, Marquez J, Garza M, et al: Reactive arthritis: Newer developments. Rheum Dis Clin North Am 2003;29:37–59. *An overview of causes and treatments.*

Kavanaugh AF, Ritchlin CT, GRAPPA Treatment Guideline Committee: Systematic review of treatments for psoriatic arthritis: An evidence-based approach and basis for treatment guidelines. J Rheumatol 2006;33:1417–1421. *A systematic approach for the treatment of psoriatic arthritis.*

Kim TH, Uhn WS, Inman RD: Pathogenesis of ankylosing spondylitis and reactive arthritis. Curr Opin Rheumatol 2005;17:400–405. *A careful review.*

Zochling J, van der Heijde D, Burgos-Vargas R, et al: ASAS/EULAR recommendations for the management of ankylosing spondylitis. Ann Rheum Dis 2006;65:442–452. *A consensus guideline.*

287 SYSTEMIC LUPUS ERYTHEMATOSUS

Mary K. Crow

Definition

Systemic lupus erythematosus (SLE) is a multisystemic autoimmune disease that results from immune system–mediated tissue damage. Manifestations of SLE can involve the skin, joints, kidney, central nervous system, cardiovascular system, serosal membranes, and the hematologic and immune systems. The disease is highly heterogeneous, with individual patients manifesting variable combinations of clinical features. In most patients with SLE the disease is characterized by a waxing and waning clinical course, although some demonstrate a pattern of chronic activity. The molecular triggers of the disease are not known, but the pathogenesis is understood to involve the production of autoantibodies exhibiting multiple specificities, with reactivity with nucleic acid–binding proteins being a common feature. Immune complexes, along with immune system cells and soluble mediators, generate inflammation and tissue damage. Therapeutic approaches generally involve immunosuppression.

Epidemiology

A notable feature of SLE is that it occurs much more frequently in females than in males. Like Hashimoto's thyroiditis and Sjögren's syndrome, the female-to-male ratio is approximately 8:1 to 9:1 in adults, and most cases are diagnosed between the ages of 15 and 44 years. Between puberty and menopause, the female-to-male ratio may be as high as 15:1. In children and women older than 55, the ratio is closer to 2:1. The prevalence of SLE is estimated to be approximately 124 per 100,000 in the United States, and the incidence of new cases is 1.8 to 7.6 per 100,000 per year. The prevalence, severity, and characteristics of disease differ in different ethnic groups, with SLE being three to four times more frequent in the African American than in the white population. The severity of disease is also greater in Hispanics than in whites, although data for Hispanic populations are less abundant. Asians may also have a higher prevalence of disease than whites. Recent studies of lupus in minority populations indicate that socioeconomic factors are major contributors to the increased prevalence and severity of disease in African Americans and Hispanics.

Pathobiology

Current understanding of lupus pathogenesis incorporates roles for genetic susceptibility based on a threshold model involving multiple genes; environmental triggers, including microbial infection, sunlight, and certain drugs; and altered immune system function. Recent advances in immunology have focused attention on the mechanisms that account for innate immune system activation. At least some of the genetic and environmental contributions to lupus are likely to promote innate immune system activation and subsequent autoimmunity. Others may contribute to inflammation and tissue damage.

Murine models have proved useful in identifying genes that could contribute to lupus susceptibility or define patterns of disease. Production of autoantibodies characteristic of SLE and development of nephritis and accelerated death have been demonstrated in numerous murine strains in which immune system genes have been modified. In most cases, no alterations have been noted in the homologous human genes. The ease of induction of lupus-like disease in murine models suggests that there are numerous possible pathogenic paths that might lead to the clinical manifestations of lupus. It is not known which of these molecular pathways are responsible for human SLE.

Genetics

An important role for a genetic contribution to lupus susceptibility in humans is suggested by the high concordance of disease in monozygotic twins (14 to 57%). Genes that might account for increased lupus susceptibility or severity include those encoding components of the complement pathway, including C1q, C2, and C4A (Table 287–1). Impaired production of these early complement components may decrease the clearance of apoptotic cells, thereby augment the pool of available autoantigens, or decrease the solubility of immune complexes. Polymorphic variants in the interferon regulatory factor 5 *(IRF5)* and *Tyk2* genes, both involved in activation of the type I interferon pathway, have been associated with a diagnosis of SLE in some populations, although altered expression or function of the associated gene products has not yet been demonstrated. Association of SLE with the major histocompatibility complex (MHC) class II alleles HLA-DR2 and HLA-DR3 has been documented in many studies and is most striking in patients expressing particular autoantibody specificities. Polymorphisms in the Fc receptor genes *FCGR2A* and *FCGR3A* have been associated with SLE nephritis, possibly based on altered clearance of immune complexes. Variants of the *PDCD1* and *PTPN22* genes, which encode proteins that negatively regulate T-cell activation, are also associated with SLE in some populations. Genetic variants of tumor necrosis factor (TNF) and possibly other cytokine genes may alter immune effector function and inflammatory responses. The available data suggest that a common theme among the genes that have been associated with lupus is that they confer either increased activation or impaired regulation of the innate or adaptive immune responses.

TABLE 287–1 CANDIDATE GENES ASSOCIATED WITH SYSTEMIC LUPUS ERYTHEMATOSUS

Gene	Protein
C1QA, B, and *C*	Complement component C1q
C2	Complement component
C4A and *C4B*	Complement component C4
CRP	C-reactive protein
FCGR2A	Activating FcγRIIA
FCGR3A	Activating FcγRIIIA
FCGR2B	Inhibitory FcγRIIb
IRF5	Interferon regulatory factor 5
TYK2	Tyrosine kinase 2
MBL	Mannose-binding lectin
MCP-1	Monocyte chemoattractant protein 1
DRB11501	MHC class II (DR2)
DRB10301	MHC class II (DR3)
PDCD1	Programmed cell death 1
PTPN22	Protein (lymphoid) tyrosine kinase N22
TNF	Tumor necrosis factor

MHC = major histocompatibility complex.

Environmental Triggers

Several classes of potential environmental triggers for lupus have been studied. Although the female preponderance of SLE implies a role for hormonal factors in the disease, recent concepts describe a possible contribution of epigenetic modification or dosage effects of the X chromosome rather than hormonal effects per se as accounting for at least some of the sex skewing. A role for microbial triggers, particularly virus infection, has been postulated for many years, consistent with the constitutional symptoms that often characterize the earliest stage of the disease. Epstein-Barr virus has garnered particular interest among investigators because the frequency of previous infection in SLE patients is significantly higher than in the general population (99 vs. 94%). Evidence of exposure to other viruses, including cytomegalovirus, is equivalent between SLE patients and healthy control subjects. Ultraviolet light exposure is a well-described trigger of lupus flares. Possible mechanisms that account for this observation include DNA damage and induction of apoptosis of skin cells, which results in concentration of nucleic acids and associated proteins in cell membrane blebs and increased availability of these self-antigens for processing by antigen-presenting cells. Recent data also support an association between current tobacco use and anti–double-stranded DNA antibodies and lupus disease activity. Certain drugs, including procainamide and hydralazine, can induce a lupus-like syndrome, but the symptoms usually abate after discontinuing use of the drug. These agents may promote demethylation of DNA, thereby increasing the availability of immunostimulatory DNA. Sulfa antibiotics have been reported to induce lupus flare in some patients. Administration of recombinant interferon-α to patients with hematologic malignancies or hepatitis C infection has been associated with induction of a lupus-like syndrome. In addition, anti-TNF agents have induced lupus autoantibodies and occasionally clinical lupus in patients with rheumatoid arthritis.

Immunologic Triggers

Genetic and environmental factors that increase the probability of development of SLE are likely to act on the immune system to induce autoimmunity and consequent tissue inflammation and damage. In addition to mechanisms that increase the availability of self-antigens, such as ultraviolet light, altered expression of gene products that mediate or regulate apoptosis, or impaired clearance of apoptotic debris, generalized activation of the immune system contributes to autoimmunity in lupus. In parallel with the events that account for effective immune responses directed at exogenous microbes, the autoimmunity that occurs in SLE patients is likely to require activation of both innate and adaptive immune responses. The innate immune response is first activated by common molecular patterns expressed on the microbe and results in augmented antigen-presenting cell capacity and successful generation of an antigen-specific adaptive immune response. The recent description of the Toll-like receptor (TLR) family of pattern recognition receptors has provided new understanding of the mechanisms through which the innate immune system is activated by exogenous and endogenous stimuli and has led to new understanding of the important role that adjuvant-like factors that stimulate the innate immune response play in inducing a successful adaptive immune response.

Type I Interferon

Recent comprehensive studies of gene expression in peripheral blood mononuclear cells of SLE patients via microarray technology have demonstrated that activation of genes regulated by type I interferon is a common feature of patients with active disease and may represent innate immune system activation. Interferon-α is gaining attention as a soluble mediator that may be responsible for many of the immunologic alterations that have been observed in SLE and is identified as a potential therapeutic target. Immune complexes containing DNA or RNA are postulated to contribute to the production of type I interferon in SLE. Demethylated CpG-rich DNA or RNA associated with nucleic acid–binding proteins can activate plasmacytoid dendritic cells and other immune system cells through TLRs and thereby result in the production of type I interferon (interferon-α or -β) and other proinflammatory cytokines (Fig. 287–1). Numerous effects of type I interferon on immune system function are consistent with the altered immune responses observed in SLE patients, including maturation of dendritic cells, increased immunoglobulin class switching to mature immunoglobulin isotypes (IgG and IgA), and induction of soluble mediators that increase B-cell differentiation and inflammatory responses, such as B-lymphocyte stimulator (BLyS) and interferon-γ. Induction of an immunostimulatory microenvironment by interferon-α may support the development of a humoral immune response directed at self-antigens, particularly intracellular particles that contain nucleic acids and nucleic acid–binding proteins. It is not known why some individuals initiate immune system activation directed at self-antigens and others do not.

Autoantibodies

The most characteristic lupus autoantibodies target intracellular particles containing both nucleic acid and nucleic acid–binding proteins. Understanding the significance of induction of these particular autoantibody specificities may provide clues to the etiology of SLE. A recent analysis of the spectrum of autoantibodies present in the sera of individuals in whom SLE is later diagnosed has suggested that autoantibodies reactive with certain RNA-binding proteins, including the Ro protein, occur early in the preclinical stage of the disease, along with a positive antinuclear antibody (ANA) test. These are followed by anti-DNA

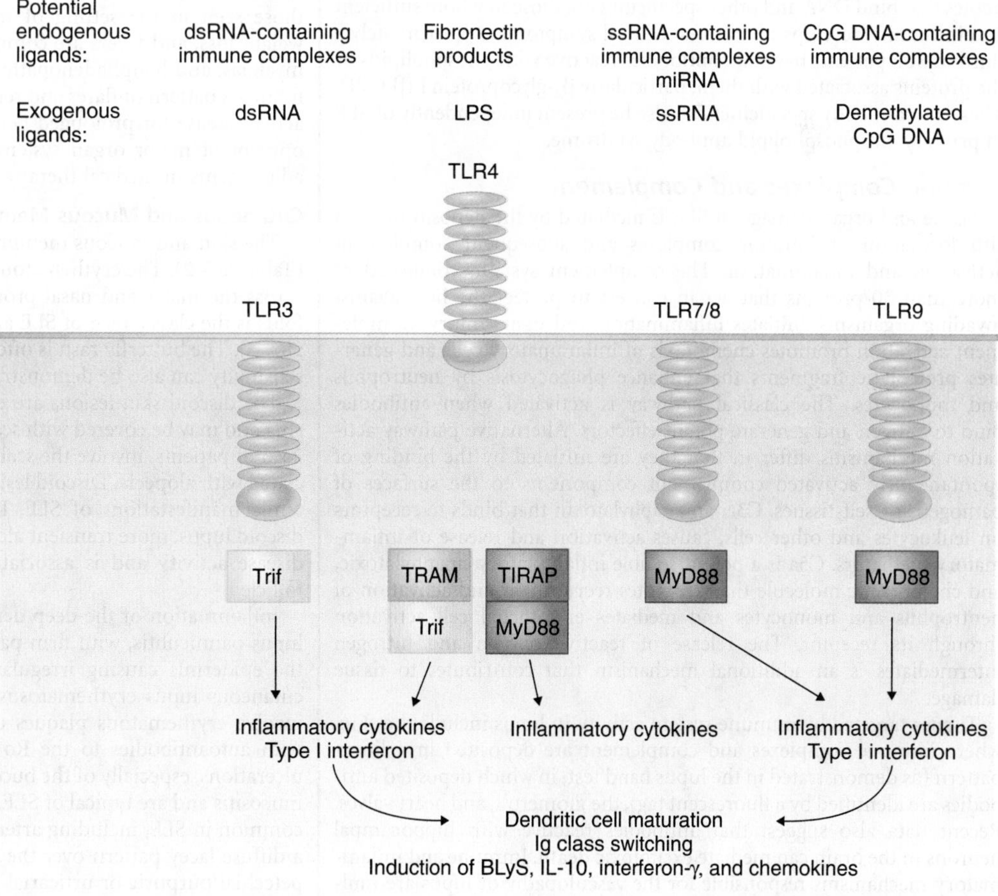

FIGURE 287–1 • Model for induction of innate immune system activation in systemic lupus erythematosus. Both exogenous and endogenous stimuli can induce Toll-like receptor (TLR) activation and thereby result in new gene transcription. Among potential endogenous ligands are immune complexes containing DNA or RNA or matrix-derived components. TLR ligands trigger the activation of intracellular adaptors, including TIR domain–containing adapter-inducing interferon-β (Trif), Trif-related adaptor molecule (TRAM), TIR domain–containing adapter protein (TIRAP), or myeloid differentiation primary response protein 88 (MyD88), and induce transcription of type I interferons or inflammatory cytokines. Type I interferons mediate diverse effects on immune system cells, including maturation of dendritic cells, increased immunoglobulin (Ig) class switching, and induction of cytokines that promote autoimmunity and inflammation, including B-lymphocyte stimulator (BLyS), interleukin-10 (IL-10), interferon-γ, and chemokines. LPS = lipopolysaccharide.

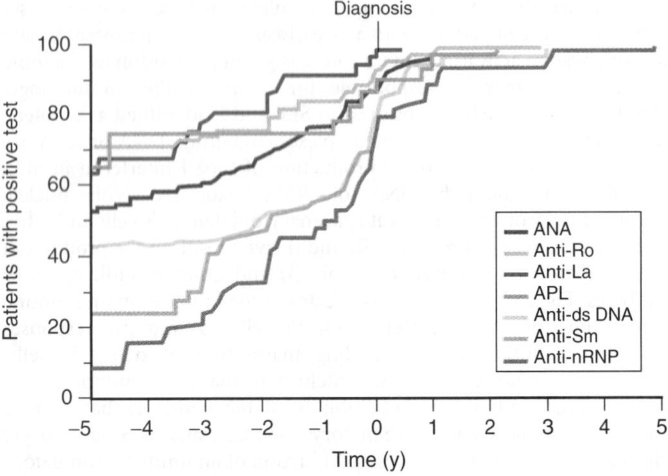

FIGURE 287–2 • Proportion of patients with positive antibody tests relative to the time of diagnosis or appearance of the first clinical manifestation of systemic lupus erythematosus (SLE). For each autoantibody, the proportion of patients testing positive relative to the time of diagnosis or to the time of appearance of the first clinical criterion was assessed. In analyses of the time from antibody development to the diagnosis of SLE, antinuclear antibodies (ANAs) appeared significantly earlier than anti-Sm antibodies ($Z = 3.22$, $P < .001$) and antinuclear ribonucleoprotein (anti-nRNP) antibodies ($Z = 4.18$, $P < .001$), but not significantly earlier than anti-Ro, anti-La, antiphospholipid (APL), or anti–double-stranded DNA antibodies (anti-dsDNA). (From Arbuckle MR, McClain MT, Rubertone MV, et al: Development of autoantibodies before the clinical onset of systemic lupus erythematosus. N Engl J Med 2003;349:16.)

antibodies and, finally, by the development of antibodies specific for the spliceosomal proteins Smith (Sm) and ribonucleoprotein (RNP) at approximately the time of diagnosis (Fig. 287–2). These observations suggest that individuals who demonstrate progression from a narrow focus of humoral immunity on proteins associated with RNA to antibodies that bind DNA and other specificities are those in whom sufficient autoimmunity develops to manifest clinical symptoms. Approximately a third of SLE patients have autoantibodies reactive with phospholipids or the proteins associated with them, particularly β_2-glycoprotein I (β_2GPI). These autoantibody specificities can also be present independently of SLE in primary antiphospholipid antibody syndrome.

Immune Complexes and Complement

Tissue and organ damage in SLE is mediated by the deposition or in situ formation of immune complexes and subsequent complement activation and inflammation. The complement system, composed of more than 30 proteins that act in concert to protect the host against invading organisms, initiates inflammation and tissue injury. Complement activation promotes chemotaxis of inflammatory cells and generates proteolytic fragments that enhance phagocytosis by neutrophils and monocytes. The classical pathway is activated when antibodies bind to antigen and generate potent effectors. Alternative pathway activation mechanisms differ in that they are initiated by the binding of spontaneously activated complement components to the surfaces of pathogens or self-tissues. C3a, an anaphylatoxin that binds to receptors on leukocytes and other cells, causes activation and release of inflammatory mediators. C5a is a potent soluble inflammatory, anaphylatoxic, and chemotactic molecule that promotes recruitment and activation of neutrophils and monocytes and mediates endothelial cell activation through its receptor. The release of reactive oxygen and nitrogen intermediates is an additional mechanism that contributes to tissue damage.

Tissues targeted by immune system activity in lupus include the skin, where immune complexes and complement are deposited in a linear pattern (as demonstrated in the lupus band test, in which deposited antibodies are identified by a fluorescent tag), the glomeruli, and heart valves. Recent data also suggest that antibodies reactive with hippocampal neurons in the brain can mediate excitotoxic death. Immune and inflammatory mechanisms responsible for the vasculopathy of lupus are multifactorial and not clearly defined. Microvascular damage is observed in splenic arteries and is characterized by the typical "onionskin" pattern of concentric connective tissue deposition. In addition to vascular damage mediated by inflammation, thrombosis, including microthrombi, contributes to ischemia and cell necrosis in the brain and other organs.

TABLE 287–2 CLINICAL MANIFESTATIONS OF SYSTEMIC LUPUS ERYTHEMATOSUS

Manifestation	Approximate Frequency (%)
Cutaneous	88
Arthritis/arthralgias	76
Neuropsychiatric	66
Pleurisy/pericarditis	63
Anemia	57
Raynaud's phenomenon	44
Vasculitis	43
Atherosclerosis	37
Nephritis	31
Thrombocytopenia	30
Sensorimotor neuropathy	28
Cardiac valvar disease	18
Pulmonary alveolar hemorrhage	12
Pancreatitis	10
Myositis	5
Myocarditis	5

Clinical Manifestations

Symptoms and Signs

Constitutional Symptoms

SLE is a disease that involves virtually all components of the immune system and can be accompanied by constitutional symptoms similar to those seen in the setting of microbial infection. Fatigue, headaches, weight loss, and fevers are common, along with generalized arthralgias, myalgias, and lymphadenopathy. The level of activity of lupus typically follows a pattern of flares and remissions, although some patients sustain active disease for prolonged periods. Careful monitoring for the development of major organ system disease is important to ensure timely adjustments in medical therapy.

Cutaneous and Mucous Membranes

The skin and mucous membranes are affected in most lupus patients (Table 287–2). The erythematous facial rash with a butterfly distribution across the malar and nasal prominences and sparing of the nasolabial folds is the classic rash of SLE and is seen in 30 to 60% of patients (Fig. 287–3). The butterfly rash is often triggered by sun exposure, but photosensitivity can also be demonstrated diffusely in other areas of the body.

The discoid skin lesions are erythematous plaques with central scarring and may be covered with scale. These lesions are often seen in about 25% of patients, involve the scalp or the face and ears, and may be associated with alopecia. Discoid lesions can be present in the absence of systemic manifestations of SLE. In addition to the scarring alopecia of discoid lupus, more transient alopecia may be a clinical sign of increased disease activity and is associated with apoptosis of cells in the hair follicle.

Inflammation of the deep dermis and subcutaneous fat can result in lupus panniculitis, with firm painful nodules that sometimes adhere to the epidermis causing irregularities in the superficial skin. Subacute cutaneous lupus erythematosus is seen in sun-exposed areas and can involve erythematous plaques or psoriasiform lesions. It is associated with autoantibodies to the Ro (SSA) RNA–binding protein. Mucosal ulcerations, especially of the buccal mucosa and upper palate, result from mucositis and are typical of SLE. Manifestations of vasculopathy are also common in SLE, including arteriolar spasm or infarcts in the nail folds, a diffuse lacey pattern over the skin described as livedo reticularis, and petechial/purpuric or urticarial lesions on the extremities. Vasculopathy in SLE is often associated with the presence of antiphospholipid antibodies.

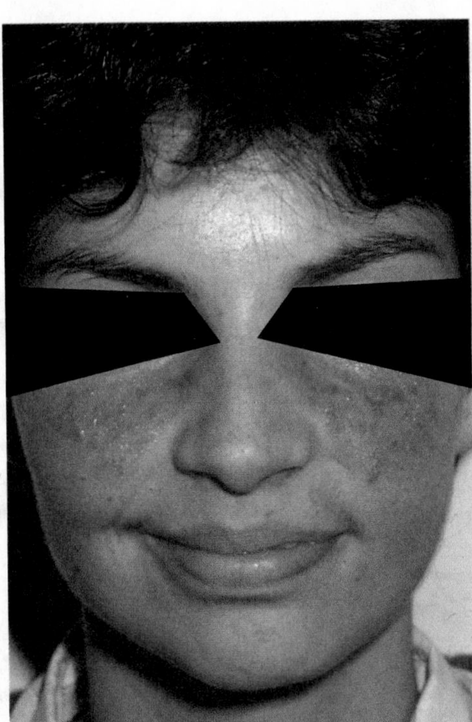

FIGURE 287–3 • Malar rash in a patient with systemic lupus erythematosus. Note that the rash does not cross the nasolabial fold. (From Gladman DD, Urowitz MB: Systematic lupus erythematosus: Clinical features. *In* Klippel JH, Dieppe PA [eds]: Rheumatology, 2nd ed. London, Mosby, 1998.)

Musculoskeletal System

Arthralgias and nonerosive arthritis are among the most common clinical features of SLE and are experienced by more than 85% of patients. The proximal interphalangeal and metacarpophalangeal joints of the hand are most commonly symptomatic, along with the knees and wrists. In some patients (about 10%), deformities resulting from damage to periarticular tissue can occur, a condition termed *Jaccoud's arthropathy.* The heavy use of corticosteroids in many lupus patients can be accompanied by the development of osteoporosis, including osteoporotic fractures, or osteonecrosis, most commonly of the hips, although the underlying vasculopathy can also contribute to joint damage.

Inflammation of the muscles with elevated creatine phosphokinase can occur rarely in SLE, and myopathy may be observed as a consequence of corticosteroid therapy. Fibromyalgia, characterized by painful trigger points at characteristic locations, commonly accompanies SLE and can contribute to fatigue and depression.

Renal System

Kidney involvement in SLE is common, with 74% of patients being affected at some time in the course of disease, and is a poor prognostic indicator. Renal pathology is generally attributed to the deposition of circulating immune complexes or in situ formation of these complexes in glomeruli and results in the activation of complement and subsequent recruitment of inflammatory cells. In addition to glomerular inflammation, necrosis, and scarring, renal pathology is characterized by vascular lesions, including thrombotic microangiopathy and extraglomerular vasculitis, and tubulointerstitial disease, including tubular atrophy and interstitial fibrosis. Hypertension may be a consequence of significant renal involvement.

Most cases of lupus nephritis present a complex immunopathologic picture, but in general, the pattern of renal disease reflects the site of deposition of immunoglobulins and the quality of the effector mechanisms that they induce. Mesangial deposition of immunoglobulin induces mesangial cell proliferation and is associated with microscopic hematuria and mild proteinuria (Fig. 287–4). Subendothelial deposition of immune complexes results in proliferative and exudative inflammation, together with hematuria, mild to moderate proteinuria, and a reduced glomerular filtration rate. Subepithelial deposition of immune complexes adjacent to podocytes and along the glomerular basement membrane can result in membranous nephritis with nephrotic-range proteinuria. In addition, antiphospholipid antibodies may support the development of thrombotic or inflammatory vascular renal lesions within or external to glomeruli.

Evaluation of renal disease in SLE includes urinalysis with microscopic analysis of urine sediment, serum blood urea nitrogen and creatinine, and 24-hour urine collection for protein and creatinine clearance. Low serum albumin would be consistent with persistent proteinuria and membranous glomerulonephritis (GN), whereas red and white blood cell casts in the urinary sediment suggest proliferative GN. Although a renal biopsy is usually performed only when the result may influence therapeutic decisions, pathologic classification of the features of renal disease can provide prognostic information.

A World Health Organization classification of lupus nephritis lesions was first published in 1975 with subsequent revisions. These classifications were reviewed and rigorously reexamined recently and resulted in publication of the International Society of Nephrology and Renal Pathology Society classification criteria for lupus GN (Table 287–3). Class I and II GN involves mesangial deposition of immune complexes (class I without and class II with mesangial hypercellularity), class III describes focal GN involving <50% of total glomeruli, class IV includes diffuse GN involving 50% or more of glomeruli, class V designates membranous lupus nephritis, and class VI is characterized by advanced sclerotic lesions. Classes III and IV have subdivisions for active and sclerotic lesions, and class IV also has subdivisions for segmental and global involvement. Pathologic diagnosis should include descriptions of tubulointerstitial and vascular disease, as well as glomerular involvement.

The prognosis of class I and II disease is usually good, whereas class IV, the most common form of lupus nephritis, has the worst prognosis, particularly when the serum creatinine level is elevated at the time of diagnosis. Class V nephritis occurs in 10 to 20% of patients, and the implication for long-term disease outcome depends on the degree of proteinuria, with mild proteinuria having a good prognosis and nephrotic syndrome with chronic edema having a more negative prognosis. It should be noted that renal veins can occasionally become involved with thrombosis, which then contributes to nephrotic syndrome. This complication can be evaluated by renal ultrasound.

Cardiovascular System

Pericarditis and valve nodules were among the first clinical manifestations described in SLE. It is only recently that the extent of premature atherosclerotic disease has been well documented. Pericarditis is the most common cardiac manifestation, but it is sometimes recognized only on imaging studies or at autopsy. It is a component of the generalized serositis that is often a feature of SLE and is associated with local autoantibodies and immune complexes. Pericarditis is usually manifested as substernal chest pain that is improved by bending forward and can be exacerbated by inspiration or coughing. The symptoms and effusions associated with pericarditis are quite responsive to moderate-dose (20 to 30 mg/day of prednisone) corticosteroid treatment.

Structural valve abnormalities in SLE range from the sterile nodules originally described by Libman and Sacks to nonspecific valve thickening. The nodules are immobile and usually located on the atrial side of the mitral valve and sometimes on the arterial side of the aortic valve. Right-sided lesions are very rare. These structural changes may in some cases result in valvar regurgitation. Although valve nodules are detected in the majority of patients with SLE at autopsy, clinically significant valvar heart disease is much less common (1 to 18%). The verrucous valvar lesions of Libman and Sacks are most likely inflammatory in nature and may be associated with the presence of antiphospholipid antibodies.

Premature and accelerated atherosclerosis is increasingly recognized as being prevalent in lupus patients, and preclinical atherosclerotic carotid plaque has been documented in 37% of SLE patients as opposed to 15% of age- and sex-matched controls. Traditional cardiovascular risk factors apply, but the diagnosis of SLE is itself a significant risk factor for premature atherosclerosis. Although the lupus-specific mechanisms that confer additional risk for atherosclerosis have not been defined, it is likely that chronic inflammation associated with immune system activation contributes to the accumulation of vascular damage. Mortality from atherosclerosis may be up to 10 times greater in patients with SLE than in age- and sex-matched controls.

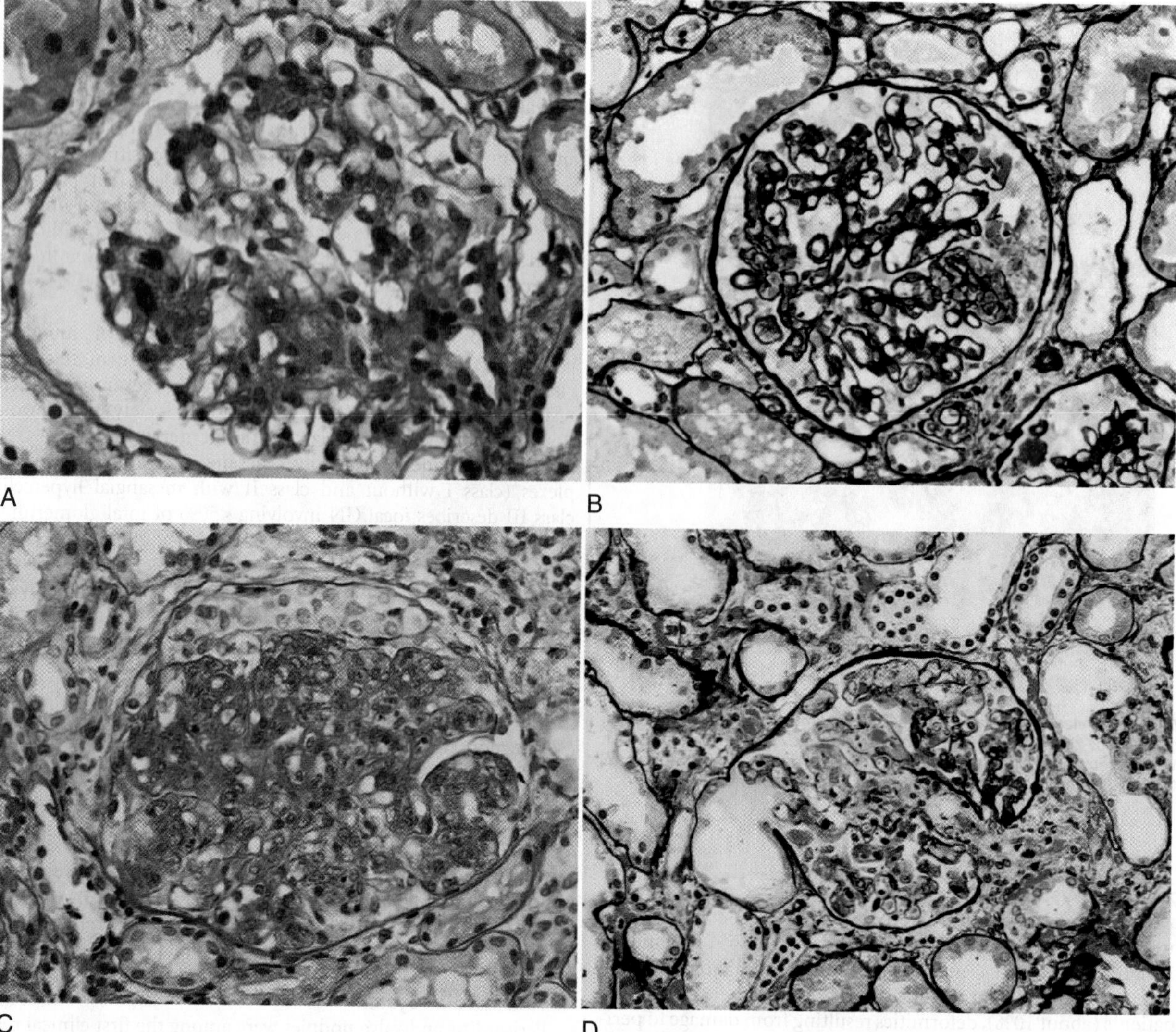

FIGURE 287–4 • Histopathology of lupus nephritis. A, Lupus nephritis class II. A light micrograph of a glomerulus shows mild mesangial hypercellularity (periodic acid–Schiff). **B,** Lupus nephritis class III (A). Light micrograph showing a glomerulus with segmental endocapillary hypercellularity, mesangial hypercellularity, capillary wall thickening, and early segmental capillary necrosis (methenamine silver). **C,** Lupus nephritis class IV-G (A/C). A glomerulus manifests global endocapillary proliferation, leukocyte influx and apoptotic bodies, double contours, crescent formation with tubular transformation, early sclerosis, and disruption of Bowman's capsule (periodic acid–Schiff). **D,** Thrombotic microangiopathy in a patient with systemic lupus erythematosus and circulating anticoagulant. A glomerulus shows severe capillary and arteriolar thrombosis, endothelial cell swelling and necrosis, neutrophil influx, and stasis of erythrocytes. No signs of immune deposits were found (methenamine silver). (From Wenning JJ, D'Agati VD, Schwartz MM, et al: The classification of glomerulonephritis in systemic lupus erythematosus revisited. J Am Soc Nephrol 2004;15:241.)

Though not specific to SLE, Raynaud's phenomenon, characterized by episodic vasospasm and occlusion of the digital arteries in response to cold and emotional stress, is a feature in up to 60% of SLE patients and contributes to pain and sometimes necrosis of the distal ends of extremities. The character of the digits classically changes from pallor to cyanosis and then to rubor as vascular perfusion becomes impaired. In addition, small arteries, arterioles, and capillaries can be affected by vasculitis and fibrinoid necrosis with clinical manifestations that include periungual telangiectases, abdominal pain, and neuropsychiatric symptoms.

Pulmonary System

Pleuritis is the most frequent manifestation of pulmonary involvement in SLE and occurs in about 30% of patients at some point in their disease course. Pleuritis is characterized by pain on respiration and by exudative effusions. Parenchymal disease is less common but may be based on several distinct mechanisms, including pneumonitis in the absence of documented infection and sometimes involving alveolar hemorrhage (in up to 12% of patients), pulmonary embolism secondary to peripheral thrombosis, or pulmonary hypertension with increased pulmonary resistance and impaired diffusing capacity.

Neuropsychiatric Involvement

Clinical features of SLE that involve the nervous system include both neurologic and psychiatric manifestations. The central and peripheral nervous systems can be affected by the disease. The American College of Rheumatology has identified 19 neuropsychiatric syndromes that can be associated with SLE, and validation of these neuropsychiatric findings has been substantiated in several independent studies (Table 247–4). The most common manifestations that are probably attributable to SLE cerebritis include cognitive dysfunction, present in 17 to 66% of SLE patients; psychosis or mood disorder, the former reported in up to 8% of patients; cerebrovascular disease in 5 to 18% of patients; and seizures, present in 6 to 51% of patients. Headaches are also common. Because none of these central nervous system manifestations are found exclusively in SLE, it can be difficult to be certain that a neuropsychiatric complaint or symptom can be attributed to SLE.

Evaluation of neuropsychiatric lupus depends on a careful clinical history and physical and laboratory examination and, in some cases, imaging studies and analysis of cerebrospinal fluid to rule out infection. Magnetic resonance imaging is useful for detecting intracranial abnormalities, which are seen in 19 to 70% of patients and include white matter lesions, cerebral infarction, venous sinus thrombosis, and sometimes atrophy. More sophisticated imaging techniques such as magnetic resonance angiography and magnetic resonance spectroscopy can be used to assess cerebral blood flow or neuronal metabolism.

Cranial nerve and ocular involvement, most likely based on vasculopathy and focal ischemia, can sometimes affect vision. Ocular

TABLE 287–3 INTERNATIONAL SOCIETY OF NEPHROLOGY/RENAL PATHOLOGY SOCIETY 2003 CLASSIFICATION OF LUPUS NEPHRITIS

Class I	**Minimal mesangial lupus nephritis** Normal glomeruli by light microscopy, but mesangial immune deposits by immunofluorescence
Class II	**Mesangial proliferative lupus nephritis** Purely mesangial hypercellularity of any degree or mesangial matrix expansion by light microscopy, with mesangial immune deposits. May be a few isolated subepithelial or subendothelial deposits visible by immunofluorescence or electron microscopy, but not by light microscopy
Class III	**Focal lupus nephritis*** Active or inactive focal, segmental, or global endocapillary or extracapillary glomerulonephritis involving <50% of all glomeruli, typically with focal subendothelial immune deposits, with or without mesangial alterations
Class III (A)	Active lesions: focal proliferative lupus nephritis
Class III (A/C)	Active and chronic lesions: focal proliferative and sclerosing lupus nephritis
Class III (C)	Chronic inactive lesions with glomerular scars: focal sclerosing lupus nephritis
Class IV	**Diffuse lupus nephritis†** Active or inactive diffuse, segmental or global endocapillary or extracapillary glomerulonephritis Involving ≥50% of all glomeruli, typically with diffuse subendothelial immune deposits, with or without mesangial alterations. This class is divided into diffuse segmental (IV-S) lupus nephritis when ≥50% of the involved glomeruli have segmental lesions and into diffuse global (IV-G) lupus nephritis when ≥50% of the involved glomeruli have global lesions. Segmental is defined as a glomerular lesion that involves less than half of the glomerular tuft. This class includes cases with diffuse wire loop deposits but with little or no glomerular proliferation
Class IV-S (A)	Active lesions: diffuse segmental proliferative lupus nephritis
Class IV-G (A)	Active lesions: diffuse global proliferative lupus nephritis
Class IV-S (A/C)	Active and chronic lesions: diffuse segmental proliferative and sclerosing lupus nephritis
	Active and chronic lesions: diffuse global proliferative and sclerosing lupus nephritis
Class IV-S (C)	Chronic inactive lesions with scars: diffuse segmental sclerosing lupus nephritis
Class IV-G (C)	Chronic inactive lesions with scars: diffuse global sclerosing lupus nephritis
Class V	**Membranous lupus nephritis** Global or segmental subepithelial immune deposits or their morphologic sequelae by light microscopy and by immunofluorescence or electron microscopy, with or without mesangial alterations Class V lupus nephritis may occur in combination with class III or IV, in which case both will be diagnosed Class V lupus nephritis shows advanced sclerosis
Class VI	**Advanced sclerosis lupus nephritis** ≥90% of glomeruli globally sclerosed without residual activity

*Indicate the proportion of glomeruli with active and with sclerotic lesions.
†Indicate the proportion of glomeruli with fibrinoid necrosis and/or cellular crescents.
From Weening JJ, D'Agati VD, Schwartz MM, et al: The classification of glomerulonephritis in systemic lupus erythematosus revisited. J Am Soc Nephrol 2004;15:241.

TABLE 287–4 NEUROPSYCHIATRIC SYNDROMES OBSERVED IN SYSTEMIC LUPUS ERYTHEMATOSUS

CENTRAL NERVOUS SYSTEM

Aseptic meningitis
Cerebrovascular disease
Demyelinating syndrome
Headache (including migraine and benign intracranial hypertension)
Movement disorder (chorea)
Myelopathy
Seizure disorders
Acute confusional state
Anxiety disorder
Cognitive dysfunction
Mood disorder
Psychosis

PERIPHERAL NERVOUS SYSTEM

Acute inflammatory demyelinating polyradiculoneuropathy (Guillain-Barré syndrome)
Autonomic disorder
Mononeuropathy, single/multiplex
Myasthenia gravis
Neuropathy, cranial
Plexopathy
Polyneuropathy

From The American College of Rheumatology nomenclature and case definitions for neuropsychiatric lupus syndromes. Arthritis Rheum 1999;42:599–608.

examination of the retina can reveal cotton-wool spots as a result of retinal ischemia or necrosis. Though rare, transverse myelopathy, frequently associated with antiphospholipid antibodies, can have devastating consequences, including paraplegia. Sensorimotor neuropathies, often asymmetrical, are more common (up to 28%) and are based on damage to small nerve fibers with vasculopathy in the small arteries that supply the nerve fibers.

As is the case with lupus nephritis, the pathophysiologic mechanisms that account for the neuropsychiatric manifestations of SLE are diverse and complex. Recent data suggest that autoantibodies cross-reactive with neuronal cell surface glutamate receptors and DNA may mediate excitotoxic death of neurons. The hypothesis that these autoantibodies are associated with altered cognitive functioning is being addressed in murine models, and parallel studies in lupus patients are under way. Antibodies directed against ribosomal P protein have also been associated with neuropsychiatric lupus, and antiphospholipid antibodies can contribute to a procoagulant state, vascular thrombosis, and cerebral ischemia. Cerebral vasculopathy has been clearly demonstrated by angiographic and pathologic studies. Noninflammatory small vessel vasculopathy is the most common lesion and can be associated with microinfarcts. Inflammatory mediators, including the cytokines interleukin-6 and interferon-α, and matrix metalloproteinases may also contribute to the neuropsychiatric manifestations of SLE.

Gastrointestinal System

Though uncommon, vasculitis of the gastrointestinal tract or mesentery can result in pain and bowel necrosis. Less common than pleuritis and pericarditis, peritonitis can be manifested as peritoneal effusion and abdominal pain. Pancreatitis occurs in less than 10% of patients but may also be due to vascular pathology. Lupoid hepatitis, a syndrome that was named for the presence of positive ANAs in patients with chronic active hepatitis, is a misnomer because elevated transaminases are only rarely seen in lupus patients.

Lymphadenopathy

About a third of SLE patients demonstrate diffuse lymphadenopathy at some time during the course of their disease. The nodes are often nontender, and lymphoma is sometimes considered in the differential diagnosis. Biopsy usually reveals follicular hyperplasia, although some histopathologic findings appear similar to the histiocytic necrotizing lymphadenitis that is a feature of Kikuchi's disease, a self-limited syndrome characterized by fever and lymphadenopathy. Recent multicenter studies have determined the frequency of malignancies in patients with SLE and have found a significant increase in hematologic malignancies, particularly non-Hodgkin's lymphoma. Splenomegaly is sometimes seen in SLE and is characterized by a classic "onionskin" histology that appears as concentric circles of collagen matrix surrounding splenic arteries and arterioles.

Hematologic System

In addition to autoantibody specificities that are fairly specific for SLE (anti-DNA, anti-Sm), antibodies that target each of the cellular blood elements are also common. Anemia is present in about 50% of patients and is multifactorial. It can be associated with a positive Coombs test or microangiopathic hemolysis or reflect chronic disease (normochromic, normocytic). Leukopenia, particularly lymphopenia, is observed, with the lymphocyte count decreasing in the setting of increased disease activity. Antibodies that bind to lymphocytes and neutrophils have been described, and an increased tendency for lymphocytes to undergo spontaneous apoptosis may contribute to lymphopenia. Idiopathic thrombocytopenic purpura can be an early manifestation of SLE, and thrombocytopenia, induced by antiplatelet antibodies, can sometimes lead to a life-threatening risk for hemorrhage. Antibodies to clotting factors can also occur and contribute to impaired clot formation and hemorrhage.

Lupus Pregnancy and Neonatal Lupus

Whether pregnancy increases the likelihood of lupus exacerbation has been debated, with different data on this point presented by different investigators. However, abundant data indicate that patients with SLE have worse fetal outcomes than healthy individuals do. Gestational hypertension, fetal growth restriction, and fetal distress are increased in patients with SLE and may lead to fetal loss or premature delivery. Preeclampsia can contribute to a poor outcome in both the mother and fetus and can be difficult to distinguish from a lupus flare associated with lupus nephritis.

Neonatal lupus is a distinct entity that can occur in infants of mothers with or without a diagnosis of SLE. The syndrome is characterized by cutaneous lesions and congenital heart block in the infant and the presence of antibodies to the Ro (SSA) or La (SSB) RNA–binding proteins (or both) in the mother. Mortality in babies with a congenital heart block is 15 to 31%. Deposition of anti-Ro IgG in the fetal heart, indicative of transplacental transfer of maternal autoantibody, and dense connective tissue encompassing the conduction system have been demonstrated in autopsy specimens. Prenatal testing of lupus mothers for the presence of anti-Ro and anti-La antibodies is appropriate, and careful monitoring with fetal echocardiography starting at week 16 of pregnancy can detect conduction defects. Fluorinated corticosteroids such as dexamethasone have been effective in reversing heart block in some cases.

Antiphospholipid Antibody Syndrome

Antiphospholipid antibodies represent a distinct class of autoantibodies that are seen in about a third of SLE patients but can also be present in individuals who do not carry a diagnosis of SLE. Although these antibodies were initially thought to be specific for phospholipids exposed in cell membranes, particularly after "flipping" of the membranes of apoptotic cells, extensive data support their primary reactivity with phospholipid-binding proteins, particularly β_2GPI. Whether in primary antiphospholipid syndrome or in SLE, antiphospholipid antibodies have been associated with venous and arterial thromboses. In addition to vascular thromboses, clinical manifestations of antiphospholipid syndrome include thrombotic microangiopathic glomerular disease, cardiac valve lesions, livedo reticularis, thrombocytopenia, hemolytic anemia, and central nervous system disease. Recent data indicate that these autoantibodies can contribute to fetal loss and growth restriction by binding to the placenta, activating the complement system, and inducing inflammation. Catastrophic antiphospholipid syndrome, triggered by the acute onset of multisystemic (three or more organs) thrombosis, is resistant to anticoagulation treatment and is fatal in approximately 50% of cases.

Diagnosis

Classification

Criteria for the classification of patients with SLE for the purpose of clinical studies were developed by the American College of Rheumatology, with the most recent full revision published in 1982 and an update published in 1997 (Table 287–5). The criteria include 11 features that encompass manifestations of skin and mucosal involvement, arthritis, serositis, renal disorder, neurologic disorder, hematologic disorder, immunologic disorder, and an abnormal titer in the ANA test, with at least four criteria required for classification as SLE. ANA has low specificity but strengthens the sensitivity of the criteria because as it is positive in virtually all lupus patients. These criteria are not intended for use as diagnostic criteria because more than 50% of patients with SLE do not meet four criteria at any point in time, although all do meet these criteria at some point during the course of the disease. The criteria are useful in reminding the clinician of the most characteristic features of SLE, but a careful history with detailed review of systems and triggering factors, as well as a family history, is essential in raising suspicion of a diagnosis of SLE. Because drugs can trigger a lupus-like syndrome, a careful drug history should be taken. At the onset of clinical symptoms, the diagnosis of SLE can be uncertain because many of the systemic manifestations of lupus can mimic other conditions, particularly viral infections or malignancy, and only some of the typical clinical symptoms may be expressed at one point in time. Important features of SLE that should be borne in mind are its multisystemic nature and characteristic serology. The differential diagnosis of SLE includes other rheumatic disorders, such as rheumatoid arthritis or vasculitis; infections, including gonococcal arthritis, parvovirus B19, and mononucleosis; inflammatory bowel disease; thrombotic thrombocytopenic purpura; drug reactions; and malignancies, particularly lymphoma.

Laboratory Findings

Laboratory tests can be very helpful in supporting the diagnosis of SLE. All cellular elements of blood can be affected in lupus, so the complete blood count is an essential test that aids in diagnosis and management. A prolonged partial thromboplastin time can indicate the presence of

TABLE 287–5 UPDATE OF THE 1982 REVISED CRITERIA FOR CLASSIFICATION OF SYSTEMIC LUPUS ERYTHEMATOSUS

Criterion*	Definition
1. Malar rash	Fixed erythema, flat or raised, over the malar eminences that tends to spare the nasolabial folds
2. Discoid rash	Erythematous raised patches with adherent keratotic scaling and follicular plugging; atrophic scarring may occur in older lesions
3. Photosensitivity	Rash as a result of unusual reaction to sunlight, by history or physician observation
4. Oral ulcers	Oral or nasopharyngeal ulceration, usually painless, observed by a physician
5. Arthritis	Nonerosive arthritis involving 2 or more peripheral joints and characterized by tenderness, swelling, or effusion
6. Serositis	A. Pleuritis—convincing history of pleuritic pain or rubbing heard by a physician or evidence of pleural effusion *or* B. Pericarditis—documented by electrocardiography, a rub, or evidence of pericardial effusion
7. Renal disorder	A. Persistent proteinuria greater than 0.5 g/day or greater than 3+ if quantitation is not performed *or* B. Cellular casts—may be red cell, hemoglobin, granular, tubular, or mixed
8. Neurologic disorder	A. Seizures—in the absence of offending drugs or known metabolic derangements; e.g., uremia, ketoacidosis, or electrolyte imbalance *or* B. Psychosis—in the absence of offending drugs or known metabolic derangements, e.g., uremia, ketoacidosis, or electrolyte imbalance
9. Hematologic disorder	A. Hemolytic anemia—with reticulocytosis *or* B. Leukopenia—less than 4000/mm^3 total on 2 or more occasions *or* C. Lymphopenia—less than 1500/mm^3 on 2 or more occasions *or* D. Thrombocytopenia—less than 100,000/mm^3 in the absence of offending drugs
10. Immunologic disorder	A. Deleted in 1997 update B. Anti-DNA: antibody to native DNA in abnormal titer *or* C. Anti-Sm: presence of antibody to Sm nuclear antigen *or* D. Positive finding of antiphospholipid antibodies based on (1) an abnormal serum level of IgG or IgM anticardiolipin antibodies, (2) a positive test for lupus anticoagulant using a standard method, or (3) a false-positive serologic test for syphilis known to be positive for at least 6 months and confirmed by *Treponema pallidum* immobilization or the fluorescent treponemal antibody absorption test (modified in the 1997 update)
11. Antinuclear antibody	An abnormal titer of antinuclear antibody by immunofluorescence or an equivalent assay at any point in time and in the absence of drugs known to be associated with "drug-induced lupus" syndrome

*The proposed classification is based on 11 criteria. For the purpose of identifying patients in clinical studies, a person shall be said to have systemic lupus erythematosus if any 4 or more of the 11 criteria are present, serially or simultaneously, during any interval of observation.
From Tan EM, Cohen AS, Fries JF, et al: The 1982 revised criteria for the classification of systemic lupus erythematosus. Arthritis Rheum 1982;25:1271.

pathogenic antiphospholipid antibodies. These antibodies are also associated with a false-positive result in the serologic test for syphilis, an observation that is mainly of historical interest. Urinalysis with microscopic evaluation is another essential laboratory test in view of the frequency of proteinuria in lupus and the significant morbidity associated with GN. In addition to protein, red blood cells, white blood cells, and cellular casts suggest active glomerular disease.

The erythrocyte sedimentation rate, although a very nonspecific indicator of systemic inflammation, is often monitored and in many patients can provide an indication of disease activity. Interestingly, C-reactive protein, an acute phase reactant, is relatively uninformative in SLE because it is often low in comparison to an erythrocyte sedimentation rate performed on the same occasion.

Assaying and monitoring characteristic lupus serologic tests can strongly support the diagnosis of SLE and, in some cases, can assist in the assessment of disease activity. The ANA test is positive in virtually all patients and does not need to be repeated once it has been documented to be positive (Table 287–6). Anti–double-stranded DNA antibodies are common in SLE, and some studies have found that monitoring their titer can be useful in assessing the activity of lupus nephritis. Autoantibodies specific for proteins that associate with nucleic acids in intracellular particles are present in many patients and can provide support for a diagnosis of SLE. Anti-Sm antibodies are highly specific for SLE and, along with anti-RNP antibodies, react with the spliceosome particle. Anti-Ro (SSA) and anti-La (SSB) antibodies are specific for proteins in an RNA-containing particle and are common in patients with Sjögren's syndrome and in mothers of babies with neonatal lupus, as well as being a feature of SLE. It is useful to document the presence of anti-Sm, anti-RNP, anti-Ro, and anti-La antibodies when the diagnosis of SLE is being made, but the titers of these autoantibodies are not helpful in monitoring disease activity.

TABLE 287–6 AUTOANTIBODIES ASSOCIATED WITH SYSTEMIC LUPUS ERYTHEMATOSUS

Target Antigen	Approximate Frequency
Nuclear antigens	99
dsDNA	70
Sm	38
RNP (U1-RNP)	33
Ro (SSA)	49
La (SSB)	35
Phospholipids	21
Ribosomal P	10

Proteins of the complement system are activated by immune complexes, such as those that form in patients with SLE. The activation products that result from enzymatic cleavage of the complement components promote inflammation directly, by binding to cell surface receptors on mononuclear phagocytes, and indirectly, by acting as chemotactic agents to recruit inflammatory cells. Decreased levels of two of the more stable complement components, C3 and C4, are typically measured in serum, and decreased C3 and C4 levels are often indicators of enhanced consumption and increased disease activity. Some laboratories also use a functional measure of total hemolytic complement activity (CH_{50}).

It is the global picture provided by a careful history, physical examination, and blood, urine, and serologic data that together support a diagnosis of SLE. It should be recognized that there is considerable heterogeneity among patients and that different combinations of clinical features will characterize any one individual. As is the case with many systemic diseases, infection and some malignancies may have a similar picture and should be included in the differential until the diagnosis of SLE is secure.

Treatment

Although current knowledge of genetic risk factors for SLE is not sufficient to predict those in whom the disease will develop, once the diagnosis has been made, regular counseling and education are fundamental to the treatment of SLE patients. Patients should be advised to avoid known triggers of disease exacerbation, such as ultraviolet light or sulfa antibiotics, and be instructed regarding the need for adequate rest. Pregnancy should be undertaken with caution and with careful monitoring. Lupus patients can be informed that recent data indicate that oral contraceptive agents do not contribute to disease exacerbations and that estrogen replacement therapy for symptoms of menopause has been associated with only a modest increase in mild disease flares, but not with severe flares. [1, 2]

Conventional Medical Therapy

Clinical manifestations of lupus that do not involve major organ systems can often be managed with nonsteroidal anti-inflammatory drugs, low-dose corticosteroids, and antimalarials. Corticosteroids are immunosuppressive agents that modulate many functions of lymphocytes and monocytes, including the production of pro-inflammatory cytokines. Oral prednisone in doses ranging from 5 to 30 mg daily is effective in treating constitutional symptoms, arthralgias, pericarditis and pleuritis, and skin disease. Topical corticosteroids are sometimes applied to cutaneous lesions. For more serious disease, particularly active nephritis, central nervous system disease, or systemic vasculitis, prednisone at 60 mg daily or 1 g of intravenous methylprednisolone administered daily for 3 days can often gain control of disease activity. Though effective, corticosteroids also have toxicities that add to the morbidity associated with lupus. The broad immunosuppression mediated by these drugs contributes to the susceptibility to infection that is an inherent feature of SLE. Osteonecrosis, osteoporotic fractures, posterior subcapsular cataracts, diabetes, myopathy, hypertension, hypoadrenalism, and emotional disturbance are additional deleterious effects of corticosteroids.

Antimalarial agents, most commonly hydroxychloroquine administered at 200 to 400 mg/day, have long been used to control skin involvement and arthralgias. An important Canadian study demonstrating an increased frequency of disease flare in patients who discontinued hydroxychloroquine contributed to its recent use in lupus for a broader range of clinical manifestations. [3] Hydroxychloroquine has been associated with a decreased incidence of thrombosis, a mechanism that could affect vasculopathy and end-organ damage. An additional potential mechanism of action implicates the TLR pathway, which is responsible for activation of the innate immune response. The effects of antimalarial agents on acidification of the intracellular vesicles where TLRs associate with their ligands may inhibit immune cell activation mediated by stimulatory nucleic acids. Antimalarials are well tolerated. Because they can rarely cause eye toxicity, ophthalmologic examinations should precede initiation of therapy and take place every 6 to 12 months.

In addition to controlling autoimmunity and inflammation in SLE, it is essential to adequately control hypertension when it occurs. In patients with a history of thrombosis, who will usually have antiphospholipid antibodies, warfarin is recommended, although the intensity of anticoagulation is still controversial and may depend on whether the thromboses are venous or arterial.

Immunosuppressive Agents

Alkylating Agents

Approximately 33% of lupus patients receive cytotoxic therapy during the course of their disease. Cyclophosphamide is a cytotoxic agent that has been one of the more reliable and studied treatments for severe organ system manifestations of lupus, particularly lupus nephritis and central nervous system involvement. Studies performed at the National Institutes of Health in the 1980s led to recommendations of a standard regimen of cyclophosphamide, 0.5 to 1.0 g/m^2 body surface area administered intravenously monthly for 6 months, followed by quarterly doses through 2 years. Cyclophosphamide is usually given together with oral prednisone in tapering doses or sometimes together with pulse methylprednisolone. [4] Although this regimen is often effective in controlling GN, overall patient survival has not been demonstrated to be increased, and cyclophosphamide is associated with significant toxicity, including cytopenia, infection, gonadal failure, and malignancy. Recent clinical studies have included modified immunosuppressive regimens, such as a 6-month induction followed by maintenance with less toxic immunosuppressive agents, including azathioprine or mycophenolate mofetil (MMF). Cyclophosphamide is relatively contraindicated in pregnant women.

Purine Synthesis Inhibitors

Azathioprine has been used for the treatment of lupus nephritis and as a steroid-sparing agent in SLE for many years. Azathioprine inhibits DNA synthesis and has recently been shown to inhibit key signaling pathways in T lymphocytes. Azathioprine is commonly dosed at 2 to 3 mg/kg/day administered as a tablet. Toxicities of azathioprine target the bone marrow and result in cytopenias, as well as the liver and occasionally result in transaminitis, and its use is rarely associated with non-Hodgkin's lymphoma. It has been used safely in pregnant women.

MMF is an inhibitor that binds to the isoform of inosine monophosphate dehydrogenase that mediates purine synthesis in activated lymphocytes. It has a good track record of utility in inhibiting allograft rejection. Recent clinical trials have compared MMF with intravenous cyclophosphamide for induction therapy in lupus nephritis; the results indicated as good or better efficacy of MMF as cyclophosphamide in patients with membranoproliferative or membranous GN. As noted, MMF may also be useful for maintenance treatment of lupus nephritis after induction with cyclophosphamide.

Methotrexate

Methotrexate is a folate antagonist that is commonly used in rheumatoid arthritis. A double-blind, randomized, placebo-controlled trial of oral methotrexate (15 to 25 mg/week for 6 months) in SLE controlled disease and allowed tapering of prednisone. [5] The most responsive clinical manifestations were cutaneous and articular.

Ancillary and Other Therapies

Intravenous Gamma Globulin

Although positive data from controlled trials of intravenous gamma globulin are not available, case reports and clinical experience indicate that administration of pooled IgG fractions can sometimes be efficacious in gaining control of lupus disease activity that is refractory to other therapies. A common regimen is 2 g/kg in divided doses over a 3- to 5-day period. Several mechanisms have been proposed for this therapy, including blockade of Fc receptors, modulation of lymphocyte function through Fc receptors, increased catabolism of pathogenic immunoglobulin, and actions of the anti-idiotype antibody that is a component of the administered IgG.

Plasmapheresis

Removal of pathogenic antibodies and immune complexes is the goal of plasmapheresis, but there are scant data supporting the utility of this therapy. Nonetheless, plasmapheresis has been occasionally useful in lupus patients with life-threatening complications in which the clinical manifestations can be clearly attributed to pathogenic autoantibodies. In particular, plasmapheresis has been effective in cases of thrombotic thrombocytopenic purpura associated with SLE.

Therapies under Investigation

Biologic therapies are being investigated at present in clinical trials. Several of these agents hold promise for more specific tar-

Rx

geting of the most relevant cells and mediators that are responsible for autoantibody production or inflammation in lupus. CTLA4-Ig is a soluble inhibitor of the interaction between CD80 or CD86 on antigen-presenting cells and CD28 on T lymphocytes. Interruption of this pathway blocks full activation of T cells after ligation of the T-cell antigen receptor by antigenic peptide associated with MHC class II molecules. This approach not only inhibits T-cell activation but also abrogates the T-cell–mediated activation of B cells and antibody production. Several agents are being tested for their capacity to effectively target B lymphocytes. Rituxan, a monoclonal antibody specific for the cell surface B-cell molecule CD20, is approved for use in B-cell lymphomas and has been used in some patients with SLE who are poorly responsive to other therapies. Rituxan depletes B cells, often for many months, and may limit T-cell activation by eliminating activated B cells that can serve as antigen-presenting cells. Efficacy and toxicity data are not yet sufficient to allow a comprehensive assessment of the utility of this treatment in SLE. A monoclonal antibody that targets the BLyS molecule is also being studied. Anti-BLyS blocks a B-cell survival signal and may reduce the production of pathogenic autoantibodies. Additional biologic approaches to modulating immune system activation in SLE include inhibitors of cytokines such as interleukin-6. Anti-TNF agents, commonly used in patients with rheumatoid arthritis, have been tried in SLE in small studies. Similar to the effects observed with the use of methotrexate, another common therapy for rheumatoid arthritis, anti-TNF therapies may be most helpful for the treatment of lupus patients who have a significant arthritis component of their disease.

Autologous hematopoietic stem cell infusion has been used in some SLE patients refractory to other therapies. This approach has been selectively used after myeloablation, and a recent report described 48 patients who underwent nonmyeloablative hematopoietic stem cell transplantation for refractory active disease. In this approach, a conditioning regimen uses escalating doses of cyclophosphamide along with antithymocyte globulin to eliminate activated and memory lymphocytes that are presumed to mediate autoimmunity and disease. In this nonrandomized protocol with a mean follow-up of 29 months, the probability of disease-free survival at 5 years after transplantation was 50%. Treatment-related mortality was 4%. This approach may be promising for some patients in whom the disease is life-threatening, but the data can be viewed only as preliminary at this time.

Future Directions

Recent advances in basic immunology, together with detailed molecular and clinical characterization of cohorts of SLE patients, have directed attention to the role that adjuvant-like factors play in activating the innate immune response through TLRs. The primary triggers of that response are not known, but abundant data support production of type I interferon as an important consequence of immune activation that has an impact on many aspects of lymphocyte function, probably including induction of self-antigen–specific immune responses. In addition to the biologic therapies currently under study that target T and B lymphocytes, future therapies may be designed that can inhibit TLR activation, signaling components downstream from TLRs, or type I interferon itself. Recognition that the complement system is an essential contributor to inflammation triggered by antiphospholipid antibodies, as well as by immune complexes, provides additional targets that might be inhibited therapeutically and limit tissue damage. Continued investigation of the genetic and environmental factors that contribute to disease susceptibility may permit identification of individuals at risk for the development of SLE and may elucidate the primary stimuli that lead to autoimmunity.

Prognosis

Although survival of patients with a diagnosis of SLE is good, lupus remains a disease that is potentially fatal. SLE demonstrates a bimodal pattern of death, with deaths within the first year attributable to active lupus and infection and late deaths attributable to atherosclerotic heart disease. Recent cohort studies have estimated 5-year survival rates greater than 90%, with improvement in medical management probably contributing to improved outcomes as opposed to earlier studies, and 85% survival rates at 10 years. However, once a diagnosis of SLE has been made, prolonged remission is rare. Of 702 patients registered in a lupus clinic in Canada, 6.5% achieved complete remission (score of 0 on the SLE Disease Activity Index), and only 1.7% maintained remission for at least 5 years with no treatment. The presence of any permanent organ damage within the first year after a diagnosis of SLE is associated with poorer survival at 10 years (a 75 vs. 95% rate in those without permanent organ damage). Regarding renal outcome, an elevated level of serum creatinine at the time of diagnosis has been correlated with an adverse outcome.

Recent studies of minority populations in the United States have indicated that predictors of high lupus disease activity include Hispanic Texan and African American ethnicities, lack of health insurance, and poor social support. African admixture and anti–double-stranded DNA antibodies also predicted high levels of disease activity, as did previous disease activity.

Data from a multicenter study of nearly 10,000 patients has supported an increased risk for hematologic malignancies in SLE patients, particularly non-Hodgkin's lymphoma. Prognostic factors for an adverse fetal outcome in pregnant lupus mothers are maternal renal disease and hypertension.

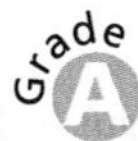

1. Petri M, Kim MY, Kalunian KC, et al: Combined oral contraceptives in women with systemic lupus erythematosus. N Engl J Med 2005;353:2550–2558.
2. Buyon JP, Petri MA, Kim MY, et al: The effect of combined estrogen and progesterone hormone replacement therapy on disease activity in systemic lupus erythematosus: A randomized trial. Ann Intern Med 2005;142:953–962.
3. The Canadian Hydroxychloroquine Study Group: A randomized study of the effect of withdrawing hydroxychloroquine sulphate in systemic lupus erythematosus. N Engl J Med 1991;324:150–154.
4. Illei GG, Austin HA, Crane M, et al: Combination therapy with pulse cyclophosphamide plus pulse methylprednisolone improves long-term renal outcome without adding toxicity in patients with lupus nephritis. Ann Intern Med 2001;135:248–257.
5. Carneiro JR, Sato EI: Double blind, randomized, placebo controlled clinical trial of methotrexate in systemic lupus erythematosus. J Rheumatol 1999;26:1275–1279.

SUGGESTED READINGS

Alarcon GS, Calvo-Alen J, McGwin G, et al: Systemic lupus erythematosus in a multiethnic cohort: LUMINA XXXV. Predictive factors of high disease activity over time. Ann Rheum Dis 2006;65:1168–1174. *Socioeconomic/demographic and behavioral/psychological variables are important mediators of high levels of disease activity in SLE over its course.*

Arbuckle MR, McClain MT, Rubertone MV, et al: Development of autoantibodies before the clinical onset of systemic lupus erythematosus. N Engl J Med 2003;349:1526–1533. *The appearance of autoantibodies in patients with SLE tends to follow a predictable course, with a progressive accumulation of specific autoantibodies before the onset of SLE.*

Bernatsky S, Boivin JF, Joseph L, et al: Mortality in systemic lupus erythematosus. Arthritis Rheum 2006;54:2550–2557. *Overall SMR was 2.4 in this large international cohort.*

Burt RK, Traynor A, Statkute L, et al: Nonmyeloablative hematopoietic stem cell transplantation for systemic lupus erythematosus. JAMA 2006;295:527–535. *In treatment-refractory SLE, autologous nonmyeloablative HSCT ameliorates disease activity, improves serologic markers, and stabilizes or reverses organ dysfunction.*

Contreras G, Pardo V, Leclercq B, et al: Sequential therapies for proliferative lupus nephritis. N Engl J Med 2004;350:971–980. *Short-term therapy with intravenous cyclophosphamide followed by maintenance therapy with mycophenolate mofetil or azathioprine appears to be more efficacious and safer than long-term therapy with intravenous cyclophosphamide.*

D'Cruz DP, Khamashta MA, Hughes GR: Systemic lupus erythematosus. Lancet 2007;369:587–596. *A clinical review.*

Ginzler EM, Dooley MA, Aranow C, et al: Mycophenolate mofetil or intravenous cyclophosphamide for lupus nephritis. N Engl J Med 2005;353:2219–2228. *Mycophenolate mofetil was more effective than intravenous cyclophosphamide in inducing remission of lupus nephritis and had a more favorable safety profile.*

Hanly G: Neuropsychiatric lupus. Rheum Dis Clin North Am 2005;31:273–298. *Review of literature.*

Roman MJ, Shanker BA, Davis A, et al: Prevalence and correlates of accelerated atherosclerosis in systemic lupus erythematosus. N Engl J Med 2003;349: 2399–2406. *Case-control study of atherosclerotic carotid plaque.*

Urowitz MB, Feletar M, Bruce IN, et al: Prolonged remission in systemic lupus erythematosus. J Rheumatol 2005;32:1467–1472. *Describes the frequency of prolonged remission in SLE, with strict criteria for remission, and defines disease characteristics and the prognosis of patients achieving this state.*

288 SCLERODERMA (SYSTEMIC SCLEROSIS)

Fredrick M. Wigley

Definition

Scleroderma (systemic sclerosis) is a chronic systemic disease that targets the skin, lungs, heart, gastrointestinal tract, kidneys, and musculoskeletal system. The disorder is characterized pathologically by three features: (1) tissue fibrosis, (2) a proliferative and occlusive vasculopathy of small blood vessels, and (3) a specific autoimmune response associated with autoantibodies. Because thickening of the skin is the most prominent clinical feature, *scleroderma* ("hard skin") has become the most popular name for this disease.

Classification

Scleroderma is classified into two major subsets that are distinguished by the extent of skin thickening: (1) limited and (2) diffuse cutaneous scleroderma (Tables 288–1 and 288–2). Patients with diffuse disease have widespread skin involvement, including areas proximal to the elbows or knees and/or the trunk. In limited scleroderma, the skin changes are restricted to the face, neck, and areas distal to the elbows and/or knees, sparing the trunk. The CREST syndrome (an acronym for subcutaneous *c*alcinosis, *R*aynaud's phenomenon, *e*sophageal dysfunction, *s*clerodactyly [scleroderma limited to the fingers], and *t*elangiectasia) is a form of limited scleroderma associated with anticentromere antibodies. Patients with limited scleroderma usually have a more benign disease course than do patients with diffuse cutaneous disease. A diagnosis of scleroderma may be suspected if a patient presents with definite Raynaud's phenomenon associated with findings of nail-fold capillary abnormalities typically seen in scleroderma, and/or scleroderma specific autoantibodies, even in the absence of the usual skin changes.

Overlap Syndromes

Overlap syndromes, defined as features of two or more rheumatic diseases occurring in the same patient, frequently include findings suggestive of scleroderma. The most common overlap syndromes involve scleroderma with inflammatory polymyositis, Sjögren's syndrome, or symmetrical polyarthritis. Mixed connective tissue disease (MCTD) is an overlap syndrome with features of scleroderma, polymyositis, lupus-like rashes, and rheumatoid-like polyarthritis. Patients with MCTD have a specific antibody response to ribonuclear protein (anti-U1snRNP). The features of scleroderma that may develop in MCTD include Raynaud's phenomenon, puffy fingers or sclerodactyly, esophageal dysmotility, and interstitial lung disease or pulmonary arterial hypertension (PHTN).

Localized Scleroderma

Localized scleroderma is a nonsystemic skin disease that is primarily seen in children. The most common form of localized scleroderma is an isolated circular patch of thickened skin, called *plaque morphea.* Multiple morphea lesions *(generalized morphea)* can occur (Fig. 288–1), and the lesions occasionally coalesce, mimicking the skin changes of systemic sclerosis. A linear pattern of several plaques *(linear morphea)* is often seen. Occasionally, the morphea lesions appear to be nodular and resemble keloids *(keloid morphea);* rarely, subepidermal bullae form, and inactive morphea may appear as flat areas of hyperpigmented skin. Active plaque morphea lesions are enlarging, geographic lesions with raised violaceous borders and ivory-white sclerotic centers. Infiltration of the dermis with lymphocytes and collagen deposition is seen in the morphea lesion.

Localized scleroderma can also manifest as a linear streak *(linear scleroderma)* that crosses dermatomes and is associated with tracking of fibrosis from the skin into deeper tissues, including muscle and fascia. In severe cases, linear scleroderma causes dramatic growth deformities of bone and supporting tissues in the affected regions. Linear scleroderma that affects the face or scalp and is associated with atrophy of muscle, underlying bone, and, rarely, brain tissue is called *en coup de sabre* ("sword stroke") lesion. Progressive hemifacial atrophy (Parry-Romberg syndrome) causes atrophy of subcutaneous tissue, muscle, and bone without skin fibrosis. Eosinophilic fascitis with deep subcutaneous sclerosis can be seen in association with morphea lesions. Although localized scleroderma may be disfiguring and disabling, it is generally a self-limited process not associated with a systemic illness. An aggressive and disabling pansclerotic morphea is reported that has a progressive course despite treatment. Patients with localized scleroderma have antinuclear antibodies most often directed against histone of chromatin or nucleosomes, suggesting the presence of a specific underlying autoimmune process.

TABLE 288–1 CHARACTERISTICS OF SUBSETS OF SCLERODERMA

DIFFUSE SCLERODERMA
Widespread skin thickening involving distal and proximal body
Rapid onset (within 1yr) of skin and other features after appearance of Raynaud's phenomenon
Significant visceral involvement including heart, lungs, gastrointestinal tract, or kidneys
High scores on disability and organ damage indices secondary to extensive fibrosis of tissues
Poor prognostic signs include later age at onset, male gender, African American or Native American race, presence of large pericardial effusion, tendon friction rubs
Associated with antinuclear antibodies and the absence of anticentromere antibody
Highly variable disease course but overall poorer prognosis with 10-yr survival rate of 40–60%
LIMITED SCLERODERMA
Limited to no skin thickening
Interval of several years or slow progression of disease from onset of Raynaud's phenomenon
Late visceral disease with unique features of isolated pulmonary hypertension and digital amputations secondary to severe ischemic vascular disease
CREST is a variant of limited scleroderma
Associated with primary biliary cirrhosis
Associated with anticentromere antibody
Relatively good prognosis with 10-yr survival rate of >70%

TABLE 288–2 CRITERIA AND CLASSIFICATION FOR SCLERODERMA (SYSTEMIC SCLEROSIS)

Classification	Criteria
Definite scleroderma	Scleroderma skin changes proximal to the MCP or MTP joints *OR* two of the following: (1) sclerodactyly (scleroderma limited to the fingers); (2) digital pitting scars or loss of finger pad; (3) bibasilar pulmonary fibrosis
Diffuse cutaneous scleroderma	Scleroderma skin changes above the elbows or knees and/or on the trunk (abdomen or chest)
Limited cutaneous scleroderma	Scleroderma skin changes distal to the elbows or knees and above the clavicles
CREST syndrome	Three or more of the following: subcutaneous calcinosis, *R*aynaud's phenomenon, esophageal dysfunction, sclerodactyly, and telangiectasia
Overlap syndromes	Diffuse or limited scleroderma plus typical features of one or more other CTD or autoimmune diseases
MCTD	Features of scleroderma, SLE, polymyositis, rheumatoid arthritis, and the presence of anti-U1snRNP
Systemic sclerosis sine scleroderma	Systemic features without skin involvement
Undifferentiated CTD	Features of scleroderma but no clinical or laboratory findings sufficient to make a definite diagnosis
Localized scleroderma	Asymmetric plaques of fibrotic skin without systemic disease
Morphea	Limited (single plaque); generalized (multiple plaques)
Linear scleroderma	Longitudinal fibrotic bands
Nodular scleroderma	Keloid-like nodules
Progressive hemifacial atrophy	Atrophy of subcutaneous tissue, muscle, and bone without skin fibrosis

CTD = connective tissue disease; MCP = metacarpophalangeal; MCTD = mixed connective tissue disease; MTP = metatarsophalangeal; SLE = systemic lupus erythematosus.

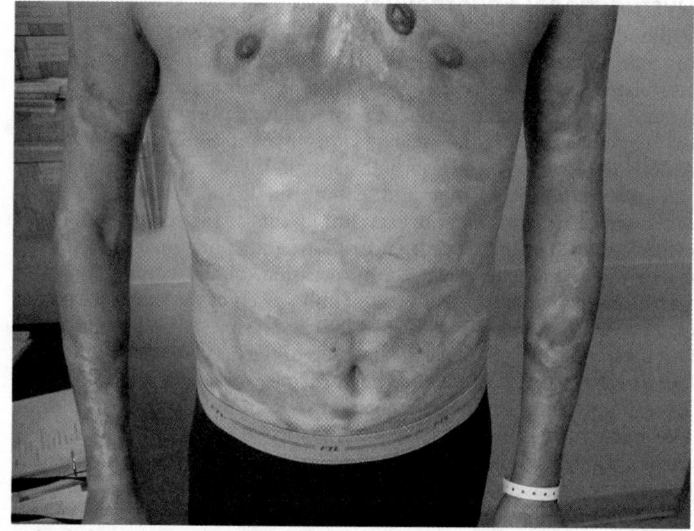

FIGURE 288–1 • Morphea. Generalized plaque morphea with multiple sclerotic skin lesions on the trunk and arms.

Epidemiology

Etiology

Autoimmune, genetic, hormonal, and environmental factors may all play a role in the development of scleroderma. The presence of disease-specific autoantibodies (e.g., anti-topoisomerase in the diffuse form, anticentromere in the limited form) and evidence of activated immune cells in tissues place scleroderma in the family of autoimmune disorders. Furthermore, autoimmune diseases such as systemic lupus erythematosus, rheumatoid arthritis, and Hashimoto's thyroiditis are frequently evident in the family members of scleroderma patients. Scleroderma-like skin changes are seen in patients with chronic graft-versus-host disease, providing evidence that activated immune cells can cause tissue fibrosis similar to scleroderma. Scleroderma is most likely a complex multigenetic disease that is influenced by environmental and epigenetic factors. Familial aggregation is rare (2%), and monozygotic twins are usually discordant for disease. Although no clear human leukocyte antigen association with scleroderma is defined, genealogic data suggest that Oklahoma Choctaw Native Americans with scleroderma inherited a common haplotype, making them susceptible to the disease. Hormonal influence on the disease is suggested by the fact that women are more likely than men to develop scleroderma, as is also true for other autoimmune diseases. Finally, environmental factors may trigger the disease in susceptible hosts. For example, silica exposure among miners has been associated with typical scleroderma. Certain chemical exposures (e.g., vinyl chloride, organic solvents) can cause scleroderma-like reactions.

Incidence and Prevalence

Scleroderma is a rare disease, with an incidence of approximately 20 per 1 million population per year and a prevalence of 100 to 300 per 1 million population. The average age at onset is between 35 and 50 years, and it is more common among women (3:1 to 7:1 female-to-male ratio). Although the disease is well described in the elderly, it is uncommon for it to manifest before 25 years of age, particularly the CREST variant. Scleroderma is found in all races and in various geographic areas. Urban to rural differences in occurrence are not apparent. The prevalence of scleroderma is higher among Native Americans, and it appears to be more severe in expression among both African Americans and Native Americans.

Raynaud's phenomenon occurs in 3 to 15% of the general population. It is more common among females (3:1 to 4:1) and is likely to begin before 20 years of age. During cold exposure (particularly during shifting temperatures and in the winter months), attacks of Raynaud's phenomenon increase in frequency and intensity.

Progressive restrictive pulmonary disease occurs in 20 to 30% of patients and is more likely to occur in patients with diffuse scleroderma, those of African American ethnicity, and those with antibodies to topoisomerase I (Scl-70 antibodies).

Natural History

The natural history of this disease is variable, but scleroderma is typically a chronic disease that evolves over many months or years. Scleroderma tends to be a monophasic disease that rarely relapses (approximately 5%) after remitting. The initial phase manifests with active inflammation that is associated with progressive fibrosis of the skin and other organs; the disease activity lasts from several months to several years. As disease activity remits, patients encounter a variety of complications resulting from skin and internal organ fibrosis. The degree of skin involvement predicts the subsequent course of events (see Table 288–1). Patients with diffuse scleroderma (arms, legs, and trunk) have a worse prognosis than those with limited scleroderma (distal arms and legs only). Patients with limited disease have normal life expectancies, with the exception of those who develop severe isolated PHTN (10 to 15%).

In contrast to patients with limited scleroderma, those with diffuse scleroderma have a rapid progression of skin disease over several months to involve the fingers, hands, arms, trunk, and legs with thickened, immobile skin. In concert with skin disease, patients with diffuse scleroderma frequently develop signs of pulmonary, musculoskeletal, gastrointestinal, cardiac, and renal dysfunction, some of which may lead to organ failure or death. Cardiac, pulmonary, and renal involvement and the presence of anti-topoisomerase I antibodies are important determinants of mortality. The aggregate experience from the United States, Europe, and Japan reveals that men have a higher risk of mortality than women.

Pathobiology and Pathogenesis

Although the pathologic process leading to scleroderma is not entirely understood, it is clear that activation of an autoimmune process is linked to a widespread vasculopathy of medium and small arteries and variable degrees of skin and internal organ fibrosis. Excess extracellular matrix deposition causes decreased flexibility of the skin and malfunction of the affected organ. This fibrotic reaction results from excessive production of collagen and other extracellular molecules secreted by activated tissue fibroblasts. Most evidence suggests that the tissue fibroblast is an innocent bystander, activated by pro-fibrotic cytokines made during other biologic events. For example, cytokines made by activated T cells or other immune or inflammatory cells (e.g., macrophages, mast cells, platelets) activate fibroblasts (Fig. 288–2). Platelet-derived growth factor (which is released by activated platelets), transforming growth factor-β, (TGF-β), connective tissue growth factor (CTGF), interleukin-4 (IL-4), and IL-1 are examples of pro-fibrotic cytokines implicated in scleroderma. The altered phenotype of scleroderma fibroblasts that makes them high producers of collagen may be acquired by activation of an autocrine signaling pathway. Altered regulation of TGF-β signaling may cause development of abnormal matrix production or clonal selection of highly activated tissue fibroblast populations. Finally, fibroblasts may be activated by tissue hypoxia or oxygen radicals produced during the ischemia-reperfusion events associated with the vascular disease of scleroderma.

Vascular Insult

A vasculopathy of small and medium arteries is a fundamental pathologic finding in scleroderma (see Fig. 288–2). Histologic examination of the arteries of affected organs demonstrates endothelial disruption, intimal proliferation, excessive collagen deposition, and overabundant extracellular matrix, all of which narrow the vessel lumen. The microvascular injury in scleroderma is characterized by vasoconstriction, endothelial cell activation, neointimal proliferative changes, platelet activation, and perivascular collagen deposition. Dysregulated angiogenesis is also clinically apparent, with some patients demonstrating numerous cutaneous and mucosal telangiectasias and markedly abnormal nail-fold capillaries. The initiating factors or cause of the vascular insult in scleroderma remains unknown. However, one of the normal compensatory mechanisms to tissue injury is new vessel formation, or angiogenesis. Defects in local or systemic mediators of angiogenesis could exacerbate critical tissue ischemia, leading to the characteristic pathologic changes observed in scleroderma tissues, such as aberrant vascular remodeling, tissue fibrosis, and consequent tissue damage leading to end-organ dysfunction. Recent studies demonstrated a defect in circulating stem cells in scleroderma, suggesting an inability to generate cellular precursors needed for vascular repair.

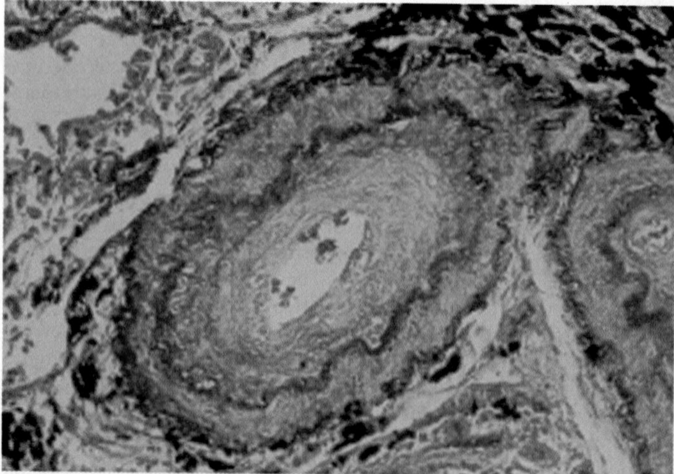

FIGURE 288–2 • Slide of small artery in the lung of a patient with scleroderma. Marked proliferation of the intimal layer of the vessel narrows the lumen and alters local blood flow. Endothelial cell dysfunction is also known to occur.

Raynaud's Phenomenon

Raynaud's phenomenon (episodic color changes of the skin triggered by cold exposure or emotional stress) is an almost universal symptom of scleroderma. Raynaud's phenomenon occurs early in the disease process, sometimes years before the diagnosis is suspected. The universality of Raynaud's phenomenon in scleroderma suggests that vascular perturbation is an early event in the pathogenesis of the disease. Although the cause of this abnormality remains unknown, blood vessels in patients with scleroderma are overly sensitive to cold temperatures and other sympathetic stimuli. In vitro studies of cutaneous vessels from patients with scleroderma showed a 300-fold increase in α_2-adrenergic smooth muscle activity compared with the level in normal vessels. Evidence from studies with animal tissue demonstrates that the adrenergic receptor subtype α2C is upregulated during cold exposure or hypoxia. Therefore, cold temperatures and repeated bouts of vasospasm with tissue ischemia could theoretically "sensitize" the vessels to circulating catecholamines.

Dysfunctional Endothelium

Blood vessels in scleroderma also show evidence of endothelial cell dysfunction, including defects in the control of intravascular coagulation and platelet activation, enhanced trafficking of inflammatory cells into tissues, and increased production of inflammatory mediators (e.g., oxygen radicals, cytokines) and regulators of angiogenesis. Dysfunctional endothelium can also cause an imbalance in the secretion of important vasoconstrictors (e.g., increased endothelin-1) or vasodilators (e.g., decreased nitric oxide and prostacyclin). Events of ischemia-reperfusion, evidenced by the clinical occurrence of Raynaud's phenomenon, are associated with cutaneous ulcers or, on occasion, digital amputation. The microvascular dysfunction affects not only vessels in the skin but also the arteries in all of the organs targeted in scleroderma. Episodic vasospasm and disease of the endomyocardial vessels of the heart cause contraction-band necrosis, or focal areas of fibrosis that can result in arrhythmias or a cardiomyopathy and heart failure. Vasospasm of the small arteries of the kidneys may be associated with severe hypertension, renal infarction, and, occasionally, renal failure. Pulmonary hypertension is a consequence of intrinsic disease of the pulmonary arteries. Gastrointestinal dysfunction is also thought to be secondary to small artery disease in the vessels supplying the esophagus and lower gastrointestinal tract coupled with neuromuscular abnormalities.

Immune Response

Immune activation is evident in scleroderma, but it is unknown whether autoimmunity is an initiating event or a biologic process that amplifies the disease after tissue injury and production of autoantigens. T cells (both $CD4^+$ and $CD8^+$) are activated; infiltrate the skin, lung, and other tissues early in the disease process; and produce pro-fibrotic cytokines (e.g., TGF-β, IL-4) that can activate tissue fibroblasts. T cells can also release mediators that injure blood vessels or alter their function. Accumulating data indicate that naïve autoreactive T cells are available to bind to newly exposed self-antigens. Cryptic epitopes of autoantigens can be exposed to autoreactive T cells during apoptotic cell death, thus triggering an autoimmune process. In vitro studies demonstrate that granzyme B derived from T cells can cleave scleroderma-specific autoantigens into fragments that reveal cryptic epitopes. Fragmentation of scleroderma autoantigens by reactive oxygen species (ROS) has also been demonstrated. Interesting new data suggest that granzyme B released during an autoimmune response may also cleave and activate other proteins involved in vascular and tissue damage.

The immune response in scleroderma is driven by self-antigens and is T cell dependent, and there is evidence that activated B cells are also present in the tissues. Serologic alterations are present early in the disease,

TABLE 288–3 AUTOANTIGENS IN SCLERODERMA

Autoantigen	Description
Topoisomerase I (SCL-70/TOPO1)	25–40% of patients with diffuse scleroderma; associated with severe lung disease; seen more frequently in blacks than in whites
Centromere (ACA)	55–96% of patients with the CREST syndrome; targets CENP-B (100%) and CENP-C (50%); associated with severe Raynaud's phenomenon with digital amputations and seen in 10% of patients with biliary cirrhosis; presence of ACA and presence of anti-TOPO1 are mutually exclusive
RNA polymerase I, II, and III	4–20% of patients; associated with diffuse skin disease, renal involvement, and less lung or muscle disease
Fibrillarin (U3snRNP)	8–10% of patients; high frequency in blacks and Native Americans; associated with muscle and cardiopulmonary disease
Th/To RNP (endoribonuclease)	10% of patients with limited scleroderma with increased risk of pulmonary hypertension and pulmonary fibrosis
Nor-90 (nucleolus organizer protein)	Rare
PM-Scl	A nucleolar complex; associated with inflammatory muscle disease in scleroderma
Nucleolin	Rare
U1snRNP (U1 RNA and polypeptides)	Associated with the overlap syndrome mixed connective tissue disease
B-23 (nucleophosmin)	A nucleolar phosphoprotein; associated with pulmonary hypertension and overlap syndrome

with a positive antinuclear antibody test observed in more than 90% of patients, and the presence of disease-specific autoantibodies is almost uniform (Table 288–3). In diffuse scleroderma, autoantibodies are directed against topoisomerase I (formerly called Scl-70) as well as fibrillarin and RNA polymerases I, II, and III. In the CREST syndrome, the antibodies are directed against centromere structures (CENP-A through CENP-C). African Americans are more likely to have diffuse skin disease with pulmonary fibrosis associated with anti-topoisomerase antibodies, whereas Caucasian Americans present more commonly with limited scleroderma and anticentromere antibodies.

Genetic Contributions

Although genetic contributions to scleroderma are suggested by certain class II major histocompatibility complex (MHC) alleles and their associations with specific scleroderma autoantibodies, no clear genetic locus or defect has been discovered. Genetic studies of scleroderma in large populations are difficult because of low disease prevalence, uncommon familial aggregation, and heterogeneous clinical expression of disease. Like other autoimmune diseases, scleroderma is complex, and it is likely that more than one genetic locus contributes to disease susceptibility.

Summary

The pathogenesis of scleroderma is a complex biologic process orchestrated by multiple genes that involves autoimmune-mediated inflammation followed by tissue fibrosis. Activated T and B cells and acute inflammation are predominant in the early phase of the disease. These immune cells propagate vascular or tissue fibrosis by the secretion of pro-inflammatory and pro-fibrotic cytokines. The late stages of the disease are characterized by varying degrees of disability and organ failure caused by established microvascular disease, tissue ischemia, and associated tissue fibrosis.

Clinical Manifestations

Raynaud's Phenomenon

In scleroderma, Raynaud's phenomenon and digital ischemia are the clinical manifestations of both fixed structural vascular disease and abnormal regulation of local blood flow. The intima of small and medium vessels is thickened with an increase in collagen content, causing a loss of vessel flexibility and obliteration of its lumen. Despite significant vascular disease, there remains sufficient vascular reserve to provide adequate blood flow and nutrition during periods of rest and in a warm ambient temperature. Digital pitting with loss of fingertip tissue and small, painful, superficial ulcerations are common and are usually secondary to disease in the small arteries and arterioles of the skin. Large, deep ulceration of the distal finger is a consequence of larger vessel (e.g., digital artery) occlusion associated with severe vasospasm. The latter event usually manifests as a sharp demarcation of the distal digit with intense, localized pain secondary to ischemia. Failure to reverse these events may lead to loss of the whole digit or limb with deep tissue infarction.

Skin Involvement

The most overt clinical manifestation of scleroderma, particularly in patients with diffuse disease, is cutaneous fibrosis. Some patients have scleroderma without any skin fibrosis (approximately 5% of cases) or with only limited skin changes. Cutaneous involvement in scleroderma begins with an edematous phase that is associated with an active inflammatory process. This phase persists for several weeks to months and is characterized by nonpitting edema of the affected limbs, erythema of the skin, and intense pruritus (Fig. 288–3A). The edematous phase eventually gives way to a fibrotic stage, which may last months or years. Excessive collagen and other extracellular material in the dermis thickens the skin, making it inflexible and causing dysfunction of skin appendages. Sweating is decreased, and hair growth on the involved area ceases. In the late stages of disease, atrophy and permanent contractures develop (see Fig. 288–3B). Patients with diffuse cutaneous scleroderma develop masked facies, small oral apertures, and vertical furrowing of the perioral skin (Fig. 288–4). As the gums atrophy and facial skin tightens, the teeth appear more prominent. Flexion contractures of fingers, wrists, and elbows often appear secondary to dermal sclerosis and fibrosis with tissue atrophy of underlying tissues. Ulceration of the skin is a late complication. Hypopigmentation and hyperpigmentation of the skin ("salt-and-pepper" appearance) may accompany the fibrotic reaction of the skin, particularly on the face, arms, and trunk. A general tanning of the skin is also common. In the late stages of the disease, the skin begins to repair and can either return to normal texture or, in the most severely affected areas (e.g., fingers and hands), become thin and atrophic or bound down to the underlying tissues. In the early active stage of diffuse scleroderma, pruritus can be one of the most distressing symptoms. Antihistamines, analgesics, and cyclic antidepressants are often used but usually are only partially effective. Drying of the skin surface results from loss of natural oils due to damage to exocrine structures; this causes pruritus and then repetitive skin trauma from scratching. Ulceration and secondary tissue infection may result. Ischemic ankle ulceration occurs in a subset of patients secondary to scleroderma microvascular disease.

Telangiectasias of the skin appear as erythematous spots that blanch on pressure and are a manifestation of abnormal dilated capillaries. Telangiectasias on the face, fingers, palms, and mucous membranes are

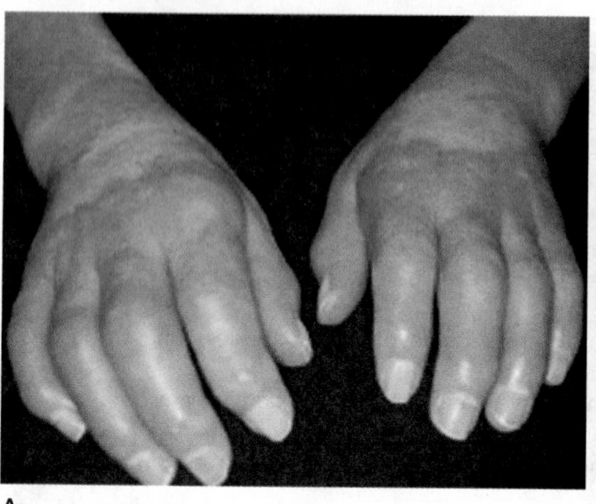
A

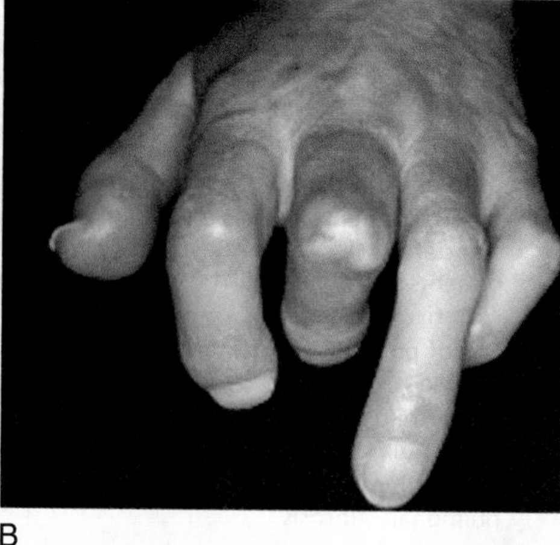
B

FIGURE 288–3 • Scleroderma involving the hands. A, Edematous phase with diffuse swelling of fingers. **B,** Atrophic phase with contracture and thickening sclerodactyly (thick skin over the fingers).

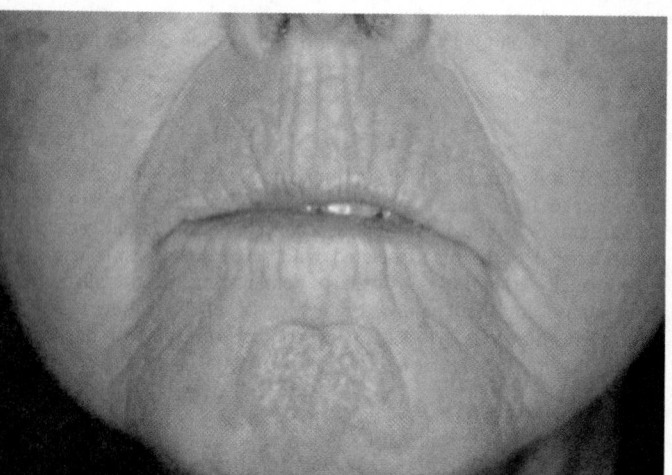

FIGURE 288–4 • Facial features in scleroderma. Note the vertical lines or furrowing around the mouth in this patient with diffuse scleroderma.

prominent in the CREST syndrome (Fig. 288–5) and may resemble Osler-Weber-Rendu disease (hereditary hemorrhagic telangiectasia). Nail-fold capillary abnormalities can be viewed using microscopy after applying immersion oil to the skin surface. In early scleroderma, the nail-fold capillaries appear enlarged. In later stages of scleroderma, the nail-fold capillaries are attenuated and irregular.

Gastrointestinal Involvement

Almost every patient with scleroderma has symptoms or signs of gastrointestinal disease. Patients may complain that chewing is difficult because of decreased facial flexibility, a decreased oral aperture, or dry mucous membranes. Poor dental health may result from difficulty with routine dental care or loss of normal amounts of saliva. Upper pharyngeal function is usually normal, but dysphagia resulting from esophageal disease sometimes mimics neuromuscular disease. Approximately 90% of patients have symptoms of esophageal disease. Heartburn, regurgitation, or dysphagia for pills and solids (more than liquids) is caused by the loss of normal smooth muscle function and dysmotility of the lower two thirds of the esophagus. Pathologic studies demonstrate atrophy of the circular smooth muscle layer of the distal esophagus in the absence of significant fibrosis. If untreated, gastrointestinal reflux may lead to esophagitis, bleeding, esophageal strictures, and/or Barrett's esophagus. The severity of symptoms may not accurately reflect the seriousness of the esophageal disease.

Bloating, abdominal distention, diarrhea, and constipation are common complaints caused by dysmotility of the small and large bowel. Sluggish or atonic bowel function allows bacterial overgrowth to result in serious diarrhea with malabsorption, weakness, and progressive loss of weight. Recurrent bouts of pseudo-obstruction are one of the most serious bowel problems in scleroderma. These episodes are sometimes mistaken for surgical emergencies. Pseudo-obstruction is the manifestation of profound loss of bowel smooth muscle function causing regions of dysmotility. Pneumatosis cystoides intestinalis sometimes complicates scleroderma of the bowel when gas leaks into the diseased intestinal wall and tracks into the mesentery of the gut or the peritoneal cavity, mimicking a bowel perforation. Asymptomatic large-mouthed diverticula, pathognomonic of scleroderma, also result from fibrosis and atrophy of the bowel wall. Volvulus, stricture, or perforation are uncommon complications of severe bowel involvement. Incontinence of stool is common and results from dysfunction of both upper and lower rectal sphincters.

Pulmonary Involvement

The most common symptom of scleroderma lung disease is dyspnea in the absence of chest pain. Nonproductive cough is a late manifestation. Active fibrosing alveolitis may be asymptomatic and undetectable by chest radiography. Patients with mild or moderate PHTN often exhibit no symptoms or only nonspecific symptoms, or they may have only minimal shortness of breath on exertion. Lung injury in scleroderma results from one of two processes: (1) fibrosing alveolitis (leading to restrictive lung disease) or (2) obliterative vasculopathy of medium and small pulmonary vessels (associated in some cases with PHTN). Both interstitial fibrosis and pulmonary vascular disease are present to some degree in most patients. However, interstitial lung disease is more characteristic of diffuse scleroderma, and isolated PHTN is more closely associated with limited disease. Obstructive airway disease and pleural reactions are uncommon in scleroderma. Spontaneous pneumothorax, adult respiratory distress syndrome, and pulmonary hemorrhage are reported rarely.

Cardiac Involvement

Cardiac disease is a major problem in scleroderma. There are diverse clinical presentations, including pericardial involvement, conduction abnormalities and arrhythmias, and myocardial disease with heart failure. The presence of cardiac involvement is often clinically silent and may not be appreciated until late in the stages of the disease.

Renal Involvement

Mild proteinuria without loss of renal function or evidence of glomerular disease is the most common sign of renal disease in scleroderma. Approximately 10% of patients with diffuse scleroderma, usually within the first 2 years after disease onset, have a renal crisis that mimics malignant hypertension, with rapidly progressive renal failure secondary to microvascular disease, vasospasm, and tissue ischemia.

Musculoskeletal Involvement

Musculoskeletal symptoms are almost always present in scleroderma and are often the initial symptom of the disease. The most common symptoms are pain, stiffness, and diffuse muscular discomfort that mimics a flulike syndrome. The pain is more intense around joints, including the fingers, wrists, elbows, shoulders, knees, and ankles, yet inflammatory signs of synovitis are infrequent. A sense of weakness in the muscles of the hands, arms, and legs can be subtle or profound. On physical examination, a coarse rub can be palpated or auscultated over

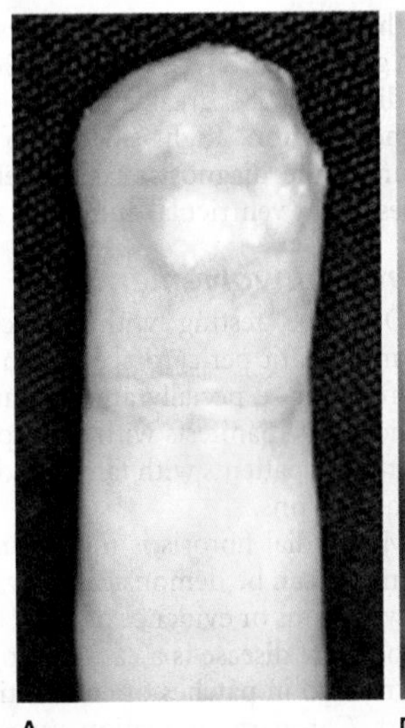

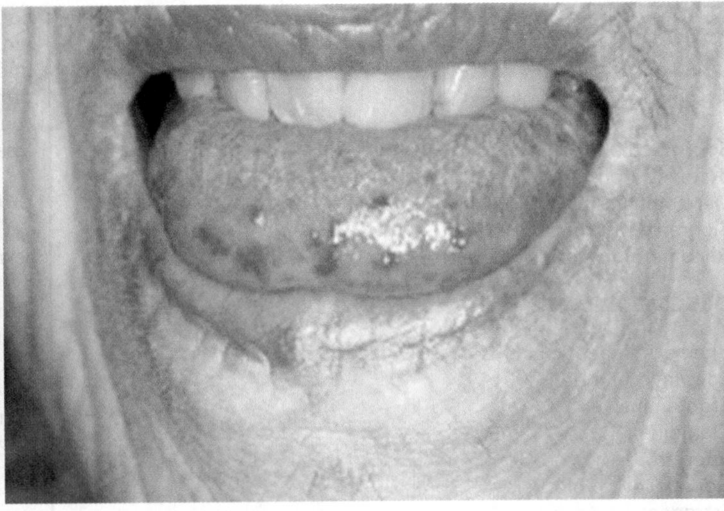

FIGURE 288–5 • Features of CREST syndrome. A, Subcutaneous calcinosis on tip of finger. **B,** Telangiectasia on mucous membrane and tongue.

the wrists, knees, or ankles. These "tendon friction rubs" are secondary to fibrin deposition and fibrosis in the tissues. They occur almost exclusively in diffuse scleroderma, and their presence is predictive of a poor overall prognosis.

Other Symptoms and Signs

Dry eyes (keratoconjunctivitis sicca) and/or dry mucous membranes (xerostomia) occur in 25% of patients. Minor lip biopsy can demonstrate fibrosis or the lymphocytic infiltration typical of Sjögren's syndrome. The central nervous system is generally spared in scleroderma, but unilateral or bilateral trigeminal neuralgia is known to occur. Carpal tunnel syndrome can complicate diffuse scleroderma, but other forms of peripheral neuropathy are uncommon. Autoimmune hepatitis and biliary cirrhosis are reported in patients with the CREST syndrome. Abnormal thyroid function in scleroderma is frequent (approximately 20%), particularly in limited scleroderma, and is associated with thyroid tissue fibrosis. Avascular necrosis of carpal bones of the wrist can occur secondary to the peripheral vascular disease. An inflammatory polyarthritis that mimics rheumatoid arthritis is seen in a subset of patients. Most data suggest normal fertility in patients with scleroderma, but there is an increased risk during pregnancy of hypertension, scleroderma renal crisis, or premature fetal loss. Sexual performance is often affected significantly, particularly in patients with diffuse disease. Impotence among male patients is common and results from local fibrosis and neurovascular disease.

Psychosocial aspects are most important and are often overlooked. Scleroderma is a disfiguring disease that alters virtually every aspect of the patient's life. The chronic nature of the disease and the threat of death have significant psychological impacts on the patient. Evidence suggests that depression in patients with scleroderma is related more to the patient's personality, the degree of pain, and social support than to disease severity. Body image dissatisfaction is a significant concern and should be assessed routinely. Pain, depression, and distress about disfigurement are common and may respond to psychological interventions.

Diagnosis

The early symptoms of scleroderma, unexplained fatigue, arthralgia, myalgia, and the new onset of Raynaud's phenomenon are nonspecific and mimic other rheumatic diseases such as systemic lupus erythematosus, polymyositis, rheumatoid arthritis, and Sjögren's syndrome. Some patients ultimately diagnosed with scleroderma defy classification at the time of presentation. These patients' conditions are best classified as "undifferentiated connective tissue disease" with features of scleroderma.

The presence of severe Raynaud's phenomenon with digital ulcers, nail-fold capillary changes, gastrointestinal symptoms (e.g., esophageal reflux), and cutaneous changes begin to distinguish scleroderma from other rheumatic diseases. The diagnosis of Raynaud's phenomenon is based on clinical criteria. The patient must give a history of excessive cold sensitivity and recurrent events of sharply demarcated pallor and/or cyanosis of the skin of the digits. Although a number of methods exist to quantitate attacks of Raynaud's phenomenon objectively, no test is considered practical or reproducible enough to replace the clinical criteria in diagnosis. Distinguishing primary Raynaud's phenomenon from that associated with an underlying disorder is frequently challenging. Primary Raynaud's phenomenon occurs when no disease process is associated with the events. Young age at onset (less than 30 years), symmetrical manifestation of symptoms, mild to moderate severity and no association with tissue gangrene, normal nail-fold capillary examination, and a negative antinuclear antibody (ANA) titer are all indicative of primary Raynaud's phenomenon. Secondary Raynaud's phenomenon occurs in a variety of settings, including connective tissues diseases (e.g., scleroderma, systemic lupus erythematosus, MCTD), occupational trauma (e.g., hypothenar hammer syndrome), the use of certain drugs, disorders that alter normal flow properties of blood, and other conditions that damage vessels (Table 288–4). The presence of intense Raynaud's attacks, especially when accompanied by skin gangrene or ulceration, warrants a thorough diagnostic evaluation for secondary causes.

Gastrointestinal Involvement

A barium swallow and a cine-esophagogram are both sensitive tests for esophageal strictures. However, direct measurement of esophageal motility via esophageal manometry may be needed if the cause of symptoms is not clear. Direct endoscopy may be appropriate to rule out Barrett's esophagus. These studies are indicated in patients who do not respond as expected to an aggressive antireflux program with a proton pump inhibitor.

Pulmonary Involvement

Pulmonary function testing is the most sensitive method for detecting early lung dysfunction, but results may be normal during the early phase of active disease. Eventually, lung function testing is abnormal in more than 60% of patients. Isolated low diffusing capacity and reduced lung volume are the most common findings in early disease. A major challenge is to accurately gauge the activity of alveolitis. Activity can be defined by serial pulmonary function testing, by high-resolution computed tomography (HRCT), or by analysis of cell counts from bronchoalveolar lavage (BAL) fluid. The presence on HRCT scan of some fibrosis and a "ground glass" appearance of the lung parenchyma is associated with a subsequent decline in lung function. Patients with an excessive percentage of neutrophils or eosinophils (more than 3%) on BAL tend to have worsening lung function over several months, whereas those with normal BAL findings usually do not show progressive worsening.

Physical findings may be absent in early PHTN, and chest radiographs are usually nondiagnostic. There are risk factors that should make the physician more suspicious of the presence of PHTN, including a diagnosis a connective tissue disease, especially limited scleroderma; a late age at onset of scleroderma; progressive decline in the diffusing capacity on pulmonary function testing; and the presence of certain autoantibodies, including anticentromere, anti-B23, anti-U3RNP, anti-U1RNP, or anti-

TABLE 288–4 CONDITIONS ASSOCIATED WITH RAYNAUD'S PHENOMENON

RHEUMATIC DISEASES
Scleroderma (95%)
Systemic lupus erythematosus (30–40%)
Dermatomyositis and polymyositis (30%)
Sjögren's syndrome (30%)
Rheumatoid arthritis (controversial)
DRUGS/CHEMICALS
Chemotherapeutic agents
Polyvinyl chloride
Ergotamines
Clonidine
Interferons
Nonselective β-blockers
Estrogen
AGENTS EXPECTED TO AGGRAVATE RAYNAUD'S PHENOMENON
Nicotine
Narcotics
Sympathomimetic agents
Cyclosporin
Cocaine
TRAUMA OR INJURY TO DIGITAL HAND VESSELS
Frostbite
Repetitive occupational stress
Thenar hammer syndrome
Thoracic outlet syndrome
CONDITIONS CAUSING ARTERIAL DISEASE
Vasculitis
Atherosclerosis
Thromboangiitis obliterans
Emboli disease
OTHER
Hypothyroidism
Malignancy
Migraine headaches
POEMS syndrome
Prinzmetal's angina
Cryoproteinemias
Cold agglutinins
Reflex sympathetic dystrophy
Carpal tunnel syndrome

POEMS = Polyneuropathy, organomegaly, endocrinopathy, monoclonal gammopathy, and skin changes.

Th/To. Rapidly progressive severe PHTN manifests more often as isolated PHTN in patients with limited scleroderma. Detection of PHTN by bedside examination is difficult until it has progressed to an advanced stage; therefore, it is recommended that echocardiography, a noninvasive method of detecting mild to moderate PHTN, be used as a screening tool. A survey of echocardiography in 691 patients with scleroderma found that 15.3% had mild PHTN (mean pulmonary artery pressure, 35 to 45 mm Hg), 6.9% had moderate PHTN (46 to 55 mm Hg), and 11.1% had severe PHTN (greater than 55 mm Hg). Echocardiography and pulmonary function testing appear to be adequate for identifying patients with advanced PHTN, but there are few data showing the reliability of these techniques in patients with clinically silent scleroderma lung disease. Echocardiography-estimated right ventricular systolic pressure (RVSP) showed a moderate positive correlation ($r^2 = 0.44, P < .005$) with both mean pulmonary artery pressure and invasively determined tricuspid gradient. In a recent study, 97% of patients with an echocardiographic finding of RVSP greater than 45 mm Hg were found to have PHTN at catheterization. Right-sided heart catheterization is recommended to confirm the diagnosis, exclude elevated left heart filling pressure, and assess right ventricular function, a critical determinant of outcome.

Cardiac Involvement

Objective testing with echocardiography can often demonstrate asymptomatic pericardial effusion or evidence of left ventricular diastolic dysfunction, especially among patients with diffuse scleroderma. Acute pericarditis manifests with chest pain, fever, and dyspnea in a small percentage of patients with tamponade or constrictive pericarditis, both rare complications.

Myocardial fibrosis is the hallmark of cardiac involvement in scleroderma; it can be demonstrated by endomyocardial biopsy in the absence of symptoms or evidence of heart dysfunction. A late consequence of this myocardial disease is a cardiomyopathy and heart failure. The fibrosis is distributed in patches of contraction band necrosis on both sides of the heart. Coronary circulation vasospasm has been demonstrated during attacks of cold-induced Raynaud's phenomenon. This suggests that myocardial fibrosis is associated with reversible vasospasm of the coronary circulation and repeated bouts of ischemia-reperfusion injury.

Renal Involvement

The presence of antibody to RNA polymerase III and diffuse skin disease increase the risk for a scleroderma renal disease. A renal crisis is also associated with the use of corticosteroids or can be precipitated in situations that compromise renal blood flow (e.g., dehydration). Studies demonstrate high levels of serum renin associated with vasospasm and intrinsic renal vessel disease. Neither microscopic urinary findings nor baseline serum renin levels are predictors of a renal crisis. Any degree of hypertension (blood pressure equal to or greater than 140/90 mm Hg) in a patient with scleroderma should be urgently evaluated, because a renal crisis is potentially reversible with appropriate management. New anemia or thrombocytopenia, with or without hypertension, also should alert the physician to scleroderma kidney disease. Microangiopathic hemolytic anemia and thrombocytopenia can accompany scleroderma renal crisis. Other causes of renal disease always need to be considered, especially in patients with limited scleroderma, significant proteinuria, or abnormal sediment on urinalysis. Cases of scleroderma with lupus nephritis or antineutrophilic cytoplasmic antibody (ANCA)-related crescentric glomerulonephritis have been reported.

Muscle Involvement

The muscle disease of scleroderma may be multifactorial. Weakness is often caused by muscle atrophy secondary to the inflexibility of fibrotic skin and lack of normal exercise. It can also occur because of malnutrition resulting from scleroderma bowel disease. Muscle weakness in scleroderma may be secondary to direct muscle disease. In diffuse scleroderma, fibrosis can extend into the striated muscle, causing muscle atrophy and clinical weakness. Approximately 5 to 10% of scleroderma patients have an inflammatory muscle disease that can follow the same course as polymyositis or other forms of idiopathic inflammatory myopathy. In some patients with severe polymyositis, myocarditis can occur with heart failure.

Differential Diagnosis

A number of disorders mimic scleroderma. *Scleredema* is characterized by thick, indurated skin that begins on the trunk, especially over the upper back and shoulders, and can spread to arms, legs, and face. Scleredema can be a transient condition occurring after infection or a more persistent disorder associated with insulin-dependent diabetes. Eosinophilic fasciitis, also called diffuse fasciitis with eosinophilia, Shulman's syndrome, fasciitis-panniculitis syndrome, can also mimic scleroderma. *Eosinophilic fasciitis* is more common in males and manifests as a progressive stiffening of the arms, legs, and trunk. Inflammation and fibrosis within fascia create puckering of the skin (Fig. 288–6) and deep venous tracks (the "groove sign"). Because the inflammatory process is deep to cutaneous tissues, skin can be pinched readily in eosinophilic fasciitis, in contrast to the thickened skin involved in scleroderma. *Scleromyxedema* (papular mucinosis) closely mimics the cutaneous manifestations of scleroderma (Fig. 288–7). Patients are usually

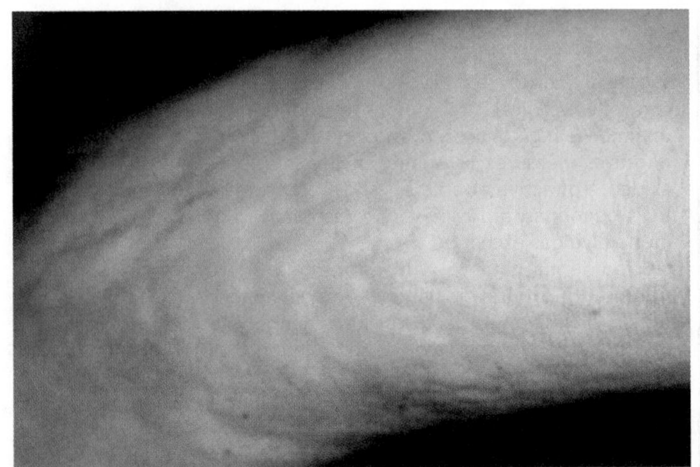

FIGURE 288–6 • Eosinophilic fasciitis. Photograph of the arm of a patient with eosmorphic fasciitis, demonstrating puckering of skin of the upper arm due to inflammation, increased collagen, and overabundant extracellular matrix in the fasciae.

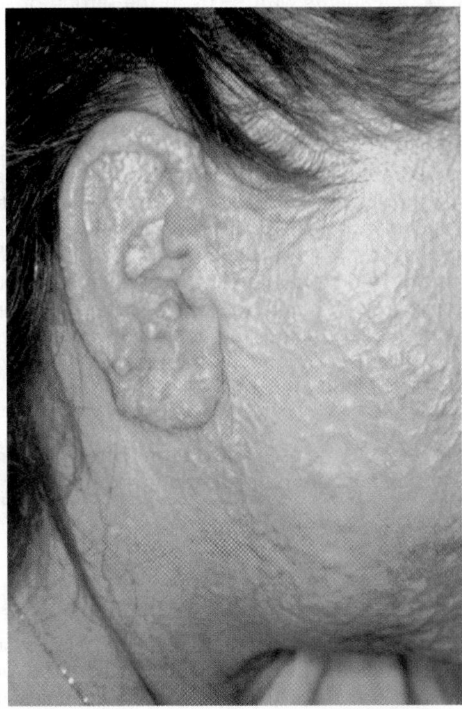

FIGURE 288–7 • Scleromyxedema. Photograph of the face of a patient with scleromyxedema (papular mucinosis) demonstrating thickened skin with cobblestone-like appearance.

between 30 and 70 years of age and have an associated paraproteinemia that consists of immunoglobulin G with λ light chains. Scleromyxedema can respond rapidly to treatment with intravenous gamma globulin. *Nephrogenic fibrosing dermopathy* (NFD) is a newly described fibrosing process seen in patients with end-stage renal failure, usually patients who are receiving chronic dialysis or who have recently undergone renal transplantation. This disorder is characterized by thickened, hardened skin with brawny hyperpigmentation and raised plaques, followed by loss of limb function due to contractures secondary to subacute and chronic fibrosis of the skin, fasciae, and muscles. By routine microscopy, the findings range from a very subtle proliferation of dermal fibroblasts in early lesions to a florid proliferation of fibroblasts and dendritic cells in fully developed cases.

Scleroderma-like skin changes have been reported in a number of other disorders, including the carcinoid syndrome, chronic graft-versus-host disease, porphyria cutanea tarda, POEMS syndrome (*p*olyneuropathy, *o*rganomegaly, *e*ndocrinopathy, *m*onoclonal gammopathy, and *s*cleroderma-like skin changes), bleomycin exposure, Werner's syndrome, and phenylketonuria. Eosinophilia-myalgia syndrome and toxic oil syndrome are toxin-induced disorders that have scleroderma-like features.

Treatment

No drug or treatment is proved effective in altering the underlying disease process in scleroderma. However, organ-specific therapy is helpful to reduce morbidity and improve quality of life. Examples include proton pump inhibitors for esophageal reflux disease, angiotensin-converting enzyme (ACE) inhibitors for scleroderma renal crisis, and epoprostenol, endothelin inhibitors, iloprost, or sildenafil for pulmonary hypertension. A multicenter placebo-controlled trial demonstrated that daily oral cyclophosphamide is helpful in active lung disease, stabilizing lung function and improving quality-of-life outcomes.

Patients with limited scleroderma are less likely to have life-threatening internal organ disease; therefore, aggressive disease-modifying treatment should be directed primarily to patients with diffuse scleroderma. If a disease-modifying agent is to be effective, it should be used during the early, inflammatory stage of the disease, before irreversible sclerosis is established. The natural course of the scleroderma is highly variable, with many patients having a mild expression of the disease. Spontaneous remission of the skin disease is almost uniformly seen after months of activity. Strategy for treatment has included antifibrotic agents, anti-inflammatory drugs, immunosuppressive therapy, vascular drugs, and a variety of agents without clear mechanisms of action. D-Penicillamine, colchicine, minocycline, potassium para-aminobenzoate, interferon, antithymocyte globulin, cyclosporin, tacrolimus (FK-506), dimethyl sulfoxide, relaxin, photopheresis, oral tolerance therapy, thalidomide, and corticosteroids have all been reported to be beneficial for scleroderma, but either evidence of clear benefit is lacking or a clinical trial with control subjects has negated initial enthusiasm.

The most popular approach in the management of early active diffuse scleroderma is to use immunosuppressive therapy (e.g., methotrexate, mycophenolate mofetil, cyclophosphamide). Low-dose weekly methotrexate may control myositis or inflammatory arthritis, but good evidence that it prevents or reverses skin or other organ fibrosis is lacking. New approaches that are being investigated include immune ablative therapy with high-dose cyclophosphamide, intravenous gamma globulin, autologous bone marrow transplantation, inhibitors of pro-fibrotic cytokines (e.g., TGF-β or CTGF antagonist), halofuginone, tyrosine kinase inhibitors, sirolimus, and long-term prostaglandin therapy. The long list of agents under study underscores the fact that no single strategy has proved satisfactory. Disease modification therapy is best done in the setting of specialized centers and research protocols.

Raynaud's Phenomenon

The most important therapeutic intervention for Raynaud's phenomenon is the maintenance of warmth. A warm ambient temperature reduces the frequency and severity of Raynaud's phenomenon. All patients with Raynaud's phenomenon must understand that clothing should be layered and loose-fitting, with the goal of maintaining a warm core body temperature, not just warmth of the affected extremities. Avoidance of aggravating factors, including smoking, sympathomimetic drugs (e.g., preparations for the common cold), nonselective β-blockers (e.g., propranolol), and narcotics is also crucial. Biofeedback alone is not helpful for Raynaud's phenomenon. Drug therapy for Raynaud's phenomenon includes oral or systemic vasodilators, antiplatelet agents, and antioxidants. The calcium-channel blockers are first-line therapy for severe Raynaud's phenomenon. Short-acting nifedipine administered three times per day reduces the severity of attacks and the number of ischemic digital ulcers. Sustained-release calcium-channel blockers have become popular (e.g., nifedipine, amlodipine, diltiazem) because of ease of administration and general safety. Although the calcium-channel blockers are the agents most likely to be effective, a host of other vasodilators have been used, including nitrates

Rx

(topical and oral) and sympatholytic agents (prazosin, phenoxybenzamine, and others). Combinations of agents are tried in refractory cases, but this strategy is generally disappointing.

Intravenous vasodilating prostaglandins (prostaglandin E_1, epoprostenol, iloprost) reduce the severity and frequency of Raynaud's attacks and are most helpful during periods of sustained critical ischemia. Oral prostaglandins, drugs that enhance nitric oxide (e.g., sildenafil), inhibitors of endothelin, blockers of serotonin uptake (e.g. fluoxetine), inhibitors of Rho-kinase, and selective α-adrenergic receptor antagonists are other experimental approaches to the problem. Patients with critical digital ischemia should be hospitalized to reduce activity, maintain warmth, and permit the rapid initiation of vasodilator therapy. Antiplatelet therapy with low-dose aspirin may be useful, but its benefit is unproven. Heparinization may be considered during acute ischemic crises of the digits, but chronic anticoagulation in scleroderma is not recommended. Chemical sympathectomy of the affected digit, performed by local infiltration with either lidocaine or bupivacaine, may provide immediate relief. For refractory cases, a surgical approach to sympathectomy can be considered. Local (at the level of the digit) rather than proximal surgical sympathectomy is preferred and is considered safe and effective. However, thoracic sympathectomy performed by videothoracoscopic technique is now used and is thought to reduce the morbidity associated with cervical sympathectomy. Studies on long-term responses to sympathectomy suggest that Raynaud's attacks eventually recur. Ischemic digital lesions should be treated with topical antibiotics and daily cleansing with soap and water. Digits that progress to dry gangrene should be permitted to undergo autoamputation. Surgical amputation is best performed only for intractable pain or deep tissue infection.

Specific Treatment Scenarios

Gastrointestinal

Education about standard nondrug antireflux measures is critical. Patients often do well by eating frequent, smaller meals; avoiding meals for several hours before bedtime; and eliminating foods that aggravate symptoms (e.g., spicy sauces). Treatment of esophagitis by suppression of gastric acid with histamine 2 (H_2)-blockers has been disappointing in scleroderma. However, protein pump inhibitors (e.g., omeprazole, lansoprazole) can be effective and usually need to be used long term. A prokinetic drug (metoclopramide, domperidone, erythromycin, tegaserod) should be added if symptoms of dysphagia or endoscopic findings of esophagitis are present despite the use of effective acid suppression. A prokinetic drug such as metoclopramide is more effective in early disease and if gastroparesis is present, but it is less likely to help in later, advanced esophageal dysfunction. Delayed gastric emptying often causes early satiety, aggravation of gastroesophageal reflux disease, anorexia, or the sensation of bloating. Occasionally, dilatation of the gastric microvasculature gives the mucosa a "watermelon stomach" appearance on endoscopy. Laser therapy may be necessary to control bleeding from these abnormal vessels.

Bowel

Management of symptoms of dysmotility of the bowel includes the use of cyclic antibiotics and prokinetic drugs. Total parenteral nutrition may be necessary for patients who have severe scleroderma-related bowel disease without response to other medical therapy.

Skin

Treatment of skin involvement is best done with frequent topical application of an emollient, periodic cleansing with soap and water, and application of topical antibiotics to any traumatic skin ulcerations. Despite evidence of active inflammation in the edematous phase, systemic corticosteroids do not appear to be effective.

Pulmonary

Pulmonary disease has become one of the most difficult to treat end-organ manifestations of scleroderma. It is associated with significant morbidity and has become the leading cause of mortality in this disease. If alveolitis is present, treatment with immunosuppressive drugs (e.g., cyclophosphamide) is indicated. A placebo-controlled clinical trial demonstrated that daily oral cyclophosphamide (2 mg/kg) prevents progressive decline in lung function and improves measures of quality of life in scleroderma patients with evidence of active alveolitis. [1] The outcome of untreated alveolitis is pulmonary fibrosis, severe restrictive ventilatory defects, and ineffective gas exchange.

Scleroderma patients with established PHTN rarely demonstrate significant acute reversibility, and fewer than 2% experience a sustained clinical response to calcium-channel blockers. Several other drugs that target the vascular remodeling of PHTN are now available. Oral therapy is recommended for moderate to severe PHTN (New York Heart Association clinical class II or III), whereas continuous infusion of a prostacyclin analog (epoprostenol, treprostinil or iloprost) via a centrally placed intravenous line is used for severe cases or after failure of oral therapy. Oral agents include endothelin receptor inhibitors (bosentan, ambrisentan, sitaxsentan) and phosphodiesterase type 5 inhibitors (sildenafil). Aerosolized prostaglandins (iloprost) are also now available for severe PHTN. The role of combination therapy (e.g., bosentan and sildenafil) for refractory cases is yet to be determined. The prognosis for scleroderma patients with severe PHTN with or without pulmonary fibrosis remains poor. Patients with PHTN in the setting of severe lung fibrosis are less likely to respond to any vasodilator therapy. Lung transplantation is a viable option for selected patients with progressive, severe PHTN.

Renal

Patients with scleroderma renal crisis who progress to renal failure and dialysis can recover renal function after months of therapy. Successful renal transplantation has been performed in patients with scleroderma, with evidence of graft survival at 3 years in about 60% and an overall definite survival benefit. The key to successful therapy is early detection and rapid intervention, with aggressive control of the hypertension by ACE inhibitors. Those patients presenting with a serum creatinine level of 3.0 mg/dL or higher have a poor prognosis. Some patients continue to have progressive renal failure despite control of blood pressure.

Musculoskeletal

Musculoskeletal symptoms in scleroderma often fail to respond to traditional anti-inflammatory medications.

Prognosis

The prognosis for patients with diffuse scleroderma may be improving. Estimates have suggested that the 5-year survival rate has improved from between 60 and 70% to more than 80%, and the 10-year survival rate from between 40 and 50% to 60%. Patients with limited scleroderma usually have a normal survival time, unless severe PHTN is present. PHTN is a leading cause of morbidity and mortality in patients with scleroderma. Recent surveys suggest that between 12 and 28% of patients with scleroderma have PHTN, and in those with severe disease the 2-year life expectancy is only 50%. Although pericardial disease may be present without symptoms, the presence of a large pericardial effusion is associated with a poor overall prognosis. Patients with diffuse cutaneous scleroderma and skeletal muscle inflammation (polymyositis) are particularly prone to develop severe cardiomyopathy and therefore have a particularly poor prognosis.

Before the discovery of ACE inhibitors, hypertensive renal crisis had an almost uniform fatal outcome. In contrast, patients treated with ACE inhibitors have a good outcome 60% of the time, and death or end-stage renal disease is now much less common.

Patients with later age at onset, diffuse skin disease, presence of tendon friction rubs, and anti-topoisomerase antibody have a worse prognosis.

Future Directions

Major studies are underway to better define clinical and biologic markers of disease activity in scleroderma. Early detection of active disease will allow prevention of disease progression by the use of new therapeutic agents, including immunosuppressive agents, vasoactive drugs (e.g., prostaglandins), and biologic agents (e.g., monoclonal autoantibodies against TGF-β). Continued investigations into the biologic processes causing scleroderma should further clarify the roles of fibroblasts, the immune system, and blood vessels in the disease.

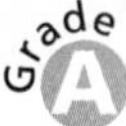

1. Tashkin DP, Elashoff R, Clements PJ, et al: Cyclophosphamide versus placebo in scleroderma lung disease. N Engl J Med 2006;22:2655–2666.

SUGGESTED READINGS

Cepeda EJ, Reveille JD: Autoantibodies in systemic sclerosis and fibrosing syndromes: Clinical indications and relevance. Curr Opin Rheumatol 2004;16:723–732. *Autoantibodies provide valuable prognostic information.*

Charles C, Clements, P, Furst DE: Systemic sclerosis: Hypothesis-driven treatment strategies. Lancet 2006;367:1683–1691. *Review of current treatment strategies in scleroderma.*

Ebert E: Esophageal disease in scleroderma. J Clin Gastroenterol 2006;40:769–775. *Comprehensive review of the manifestations and treatment of scleroderma-associated esophageal disease.*

Flavahan NA, Flavahan S, Mitra S, Chotani MA: The vasculopathy of Raynaud's phenomenon and scleroderma. Rheum Dis Clin North Am 2003;29:275–291, vi. *New information about the mechanisms of the vascular disease in scleroderma.*

Harris ML, Rosen A: Autoimmunity in scleroderma: The origin, pathogenetic role, and clinical significance of autoantibodies. Curr Opin Rheumatol 2003;15:778–784. *A review of the autoimmune process in scleroderma.*

Herrick AL: Pathogenesis of Raynaud's phenomenon. Rheumatology (Oxf) 2005;44:587–596. Epub 2005 Mar 1. *Comprehensive review of current insight into the causes of Raynaud's phenomenon.*

Ioannidis JP, Vlachoyiannopoulos PG, Haidich AB, et al: Mortality in systemic sclerosis: An international meta-analysis of individual patient data. Am J Med 2005;118:2–10. *There is a nearly twofold increased risk of mortality.*

Sakkas LI, Platsoucas CD: Is systemic sclerosis an antigen-driven T cell disease? Arthritis Rheum 2004;50:1721–1733. *A review of the evidence supporting the role of T cells in scleroderma.*

Wigley FM: Clinical practice: Raynaud's phenomenon. N Engl J Med 2002;347:1001–1008. *A practical review, based on a case discussion.*

Wigley FM, Lima JA, Mayes M, et al: The prevalence of undiagnosed pulmonary arterial hypertension in subjects with connective tissue disease at the secondary health care level of community-based rheumatologists (the UNCOVER study). Arthritis Rheum 2005;52:2125–2132. *The prevalence was about 13%.*

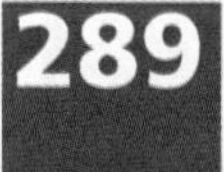

289 SJÖGREN'S SYNDROME

Stanley Naguwa and M. Eric Gershwin

Definition

Sjögren's syndrome (SS) is an autoimmune disease characterized by immune-mediated destruction of exocrine glands, particularly salivary and lacrimal glands, with secondary development of keratoconjunctivitis and xerostomia. Primary and secondary forms of SS have been defined. Primary SS occurs in the absence of a connective tissue disease; secondary SS occurs most commonly in association with a systemic connective tissue disorder, particularly rheumatoid arthritis but also systemic sclerosis, systemic lupus erythematosus, and polymyositis.

Epidemiology

SS was first described in detail in 1933, but in fact there is an earlier description in 1892, termed Mikulicz's syndrome. For more than three decades after the 1933 description, SS was considered a relatively uncommon diagnosis of older women. However, more recent data, obtained by use of standardized criteria, suggest that SS may affect 0.5 to 2% of women. The incidence of SS increases with age, and SS is virtually absent in children. Nearly 2% of women older than 60 years have features of primary SS, particularly dry eyes and dry mouth. Other exocrine glands also can be affected with subsequent development of pancreatic dysfunction, vaginal dryness, and dry cough. SS occurs in 10 to 25% of patients with systemic lupus erythematosus (Chapter 287) and 30 to 50% of patients with rheumatoid arthritis (Chapter 285).

Pathobiology

Multiple viral agents have been incriminated as etiologic factors for either the development or modulation of SS; these include Epstein-Barr virus, retroviruses, and coxsackieviruses, but in all cases, the data remain controversial. SS does have a strong immunogenetic basis, however, and it was one of the first autoimmune diseases associated with specific major histocompatibility complex genes. Several genetic alleles have been described to occur more commonly in patients with SS, particularly human leukocyte antigen (HLA) class II antigens. As with other autoimmune diseases, the specific HLA gene association varies according to the ethnic background of the individual. The responsible mechanisms are unknown, and more extensive studies are required to map class II genes precisely, particularly in the DQB1 first hypervariable region.

The significance of anti-Ro and -La antibodies in SS is speculative. These antibodies are found deposited in the salivary glands of affected patients. The Ro proteins colocalize to the blebs of apoptotic cells and may become an immune target or function as a primary immunogen. Nonetheless, serum levels of antibodies to Ro and La do not correlate with disease activity. A pathologic role of anti-Ro antibodies has been described because their passive transfer in pregnancy leads to neonatal congenital heart block. In fetuses of mothers with anti-Ro antibodies and heart block, therapy with dexamethasone, which readily passes the placenta, is preferred to prednisone.

Clinical Manifestations

The differential diagnosis of xerophthalmia (dry eyes) and xerostomia (dry mouth) is noted in Table 289–1; presentation is most common in women in their 30s to 50s. Dry mouth leads to difficulty in swallowing, recurrent dental infections, pain on eating salty or spicy foods, and difficulty in talking. In many patients, impairment of fluid secretion within the nasal and throat passage predisposes to oral thrush. Dry eyes result in complaints of ocular itching, a sense of grittiness, and an exaggerated sensitivity to ocular insults such as smoke. Other upper and lower respiratory symptoms also are secondary to dryness and include a nonproductive cough and occasionally tracheobronchitis.

Classically, SS is manifested by a painless enlargement of salivary glands, generally beginning unilaterally. This enlargement may be dramatic and cyclic in nature and is generally absent in patients with

TABLE 289–1 DIFFERENTIAL DIAGNOSIS OF DRY EYES AND MOUTH
Aging
Diabetes mellitus
Hepatitis C
Acquired immunodeficiency syndrome (AIDS)
Parkinson's disease
Head and neck radiation therapy
Sarcoidosis
Graft-versus-host disease
Medications
Antidepressants
Antihistamines
Antipsychotics
Incontinence medications
Isotretinoin
Diuretics

TABLE 289–2 SYMPTOMS OF SJÖGREN'S SYNDROME SECONDARY TO EXOCRINE GLAND DYSFUNCTION

EYE (XEROPHTHALMIA)

Burning
Blurring
Foreign body sensation
Photosensitivity

ORAL (XEROSTOMIA)

Burning (especially with atypical thrush)
Difficulty chewing
Dysphonia
Inability to "spit"
Increased dental caries
Nocturnal awakening to drink water
Pain with "spicy" and salty food (e.g., mustard)
Sialadenitis

NOSE, THROAT

Difficulty swallowing (especially dry foods)
Epistaxis, dry nares
Hoarseness

CARDIOPULMONARY

Tracheobronchitis, including a dry cough

GENITOURINARY

Dyspareunia
Dysuria
Vaginal dryness

SKIN

Xerosis

coincidental rheumatoid arthritis. The symptoms of SS develop insidiously, and often the diagnosis is not considered for several years because the complaints of sicca are attributed to medications (e.g., antihistamines, antidepressants), a dry environment, or aging. The neurologic components of SS include peripheral and cranial neuropathies and a multiple sclerosis "look-alike" central nervous system disease. Skin manifestations include palpable or nonpalpable purpura, papules, urticarial lesions, and annular lesions. Xerosis is frequently found on examination. A nonerosive arthritis, polyarthralgia, and Raynaud's phenomena are typically seen in SS. In addition to tracheobronchitis, lung involvement in SS may include bronchiectasis, interstitial pneumonitis, and fibrosis. Smoking is an additional major risk factor for pulmonary disease in patients with SS. Renal involvement may include interstitial nephritis, renal tubular acidosis, and hyposthenuria with glomerulonephritis, a more recently recognized problem. Autoimmune liver disease and pancreatitis are seen occasionally.

The classic exocrine symptoms of SS are listed in Table 289–2, but SS theoretically can affect all major organ systems (Table 289–3). Patients initially may present only with extraglandular symptoms, especially a nonerosive rheumatoid factor–positive arthritis. In addition, as a component of the inflammatory process and proinflammatory cytokine release, patients may manifest chronic fatigue and low-grade fevers. Finally, B-cell lymphoma has been described as a secondary event in SS. The incidence of lymphoma in SS varies among studies and may depend on local referral patterns (selection bias); lymphoma develops in approximately 5% of patients.

Laboratory Findings

The most commonly used test for the diagnosis of SS is Schirmer's test, performed without anesthetic eye drops, measuring the wetting of standardized tear test strips that are applied between the eyeball and the lateral inferior lid. Salivary flow and labial salivary biopsy are also commonly used for diagnosis. Patients with SS have antinuclear antibodies of either homogeneous or speckled patterns (80 to 90% frequency), antibodies to Ro (SSA; 60 to 75% frequency) and La (SSB; 40% frequency), presence of rheumatoid factor (70 to 90% frequency), mixed cryoglobulin with rheumatoid factor activity (type II; <5%), and antibodies to centromere (<5%). The presence of mixed cryoglobulinemia suggests hepatitis C infection; these complexes contain rheumatoid factor, hepatitis C antigen, and complement. Antibodies to mitochondria likewise have been described in SS but are found reliably only in patients with coexistent primary biliary cirrhosis. It has been reported that patients with SS develop antibodies to three new autoantigens called IFI16, KLHL12, and KLHL7. These autoantigens represent a family of transcription regula-

TABLE 289–3 EXTRAGLANDULAR MANIFESTATIONS OF PRIMARY SJÖGREN'S SYNDROME

CONSTITUTIONAL SYMPTOMS

Fatigue
Low-grade fever

SKIN AND VASCULAR

Small vessel vasculitis
Raynaud's phenomenon
Photosensitivity reactions similar to subacute cutaneous systemic lupus erythematosus
Xerosis

UPPER AND LOWER AIRWAYS

Pyogenic sialadenitis or parotitis
Interstitial pneumonitis or fibrosis
Chronic bronchitis
Bronchiectasis
Bronchiolitis obliterans with organizing pneumonia
Pseudolymphoma with intrapulmonary nodules
Chronic obstructive pulmonary disease

MUSCULOSKELETAL

Polyarthralgia, polyarthritis
Myopathy, polymyositis

RENAL

Type I renal tubular acidosis
Tubular interstitial nephritis
Hyposthenuria
Glomerulonephritis

NEUROLOGIC

Peripheral motor sensory neuropathy
Multiple sclerosis–like focal lesions
Transient ischemic attacks, including cerebrovascular accident
Cognitive dysfunction
Spinal cord dysfunction, including transverse myelitis

GASTROINTESTINAL

Hepatomegaly
Primary biliary cirrhosis

ENDOCRINE

Hashimoto's thyroiditis with possible hypothyroidism
Other endocrine dysfunctions secondary to autoimmune endocrinopathy

NEOPLASIA

Lymphadenopathy, pseudolymphoma, lymphoma

tors; KLHL12 and KLHL7 are kelch-like proteins of unknown physiologic function. Although diagnostic tests for these autoantigens are not widely available, we believe they will become important biomarkers for the clinical diagnosis of SS.

Patients with SS exhibit a dramatic polyclonal B-cell activation. Several other autoantibodies have been described with variable frequencies, including antibodies to carbonic anhydrase, α-fodrin, proteosomal subunits, and the muscarinic M3 receptor; the last-mentioned protein is found on salivary glands and may explain glandular dysfunction in SS. There also is evidence for altered B-cell differentiation. An SS-like disorder develops in mice transgenic for BAFF (a member of the tumor necrosis factor-α superfamily that regulates B-cell proliferation). Anemia (including autoimmune hemolytic anemia), leukopenia, and thrombocytopenia occur in SS and are most commonly found in patients with chronic disease.

The serious immune system abnormalities in SS include lymphadenopathy, pseudolymphoma, and lymphoma. The transition from a rheumatoid factor–positive, polyclonal gammopathy to a rheumatoid factor–negative, oligoclonal or monoclonal gammopathy augurs a change from a benign to a malignant process. This process can be enhanced if the $V_\kappa 3b$-related and the G6 ($V_H 1$-related) idiotypes are present. On histologic examination, the intense lymphoid infiltration includes germinal centers in the exocrine glands; the intense lymphocytic infiltrate is predominantly $CD4^+$ T-cell TCRαβ CD45RO cells. Finally, the degree of inflammation seems to be associated with a $T_H 1$ response with striking production of interferon-γ, interleukin-2, and interleukin-10. The development of severe histologic changes may be a prodrome of lymphoma. The migration of mononuclear cells to exocrine glands is mediated by chemokines and their cognate receptors, particularly macrophage inflammatory protein 1 (MIP-1) and RANTES.

Diagnosis

Diagnostic Criteria

The diagnostic criteria of SS continue to evolve, but revised American-European classification criteria are currently employed (Table 289–4 and Fig. 289–1). These criteria cannot be employed if the patient has compounding medical problems including preexisting lymphoma, acquired

TABLE 289–4 CLASSIFICATION CRITERIA FOR SJÖGREN'S SYNDROME

I. OCULAR SYMPTOMS

A positive response to at least one of the three selected questions:
1. Have you had daily, persistent, troublesome dry eyes for more than 3 months?
2. Do you have a recurrent sensation of sand or gravel in the eyes?
3. Do you use tear substitutes more than three times a day?

II. ORAL SYMPTOMS

A positive response to at least one of the three selected questions:
1. Have you had a daily feeling of dry mouth for more than 3 months?
2. Have you had recurrent or persistently swollen salivary glands as an adult?
3. Do you frequently drink liquids to aid in swallowing dry food?

III. OCULAR SIGNS

Objective evidence of ocular involvement defined as a positive result in at least one of the following two tests:
1. Schirmer's test (≤5 mm in 5 minutes)*
2. Rose bengal score (≥4 according to van Bijsterveld scoring system)

IV. HISTOPATHOLOGY

A focus score ≥1 in a minor salivary gland biopsy specimen. (A focus is defined as an agglomerate of at least 50 mononuclear cells; the focus score is defined by the number of foci in 4 mm^2 of glandular tissue.)

V. SALIVARY GLAND INVOLVEMENT

Objective evidence of salivary gland involvement defined by a positive result in at least one of the following three diagnostic tests:
1. Salivary scintigraphy
2. Parotid sialography
3. Unstimulated salivary flow (≤1.5 mL in 15 minutes)*

VI. AUTOANTIBODIES

Presence in the serum of the following autoantibodies:
1. Antibodies to Ro (SSA) or La (SSB) antigens, or both

RULES FOR CLASSIFICATION

In patients without any potentially associated disease, primary SS is diagnosed if
1. 4 of 6 criteria are met but including IV or VI
2. 3 of 4 of criteria III, IV, V, VI

For secondary SS criteria, I or II plus any 2 of criteria III, IV, V should be met.

EXCLUSION CRITERIA

Preexisting lymphoma, acquired immunodeficiency syndrome, sarcoidosis, graft-versus-host disease, past head and neck radiation treatment, use of anticholinergic drugs, and hepatitis C

*Because it has been shown that this test may be reduced in normal subjects older than 60 years, it should be excluded from the criteria or not considered indicative for a diagnosis of Sjögren's syndrome in elderly subjects.

From Vitali C, Bombardieri S, Johnsson R, et al: Classification criteria for Sjögren's syndrome: A revised version of the European criteria proposed by the American-European Consensus Group. Ann Rheum Dis 2002;61:554–558.

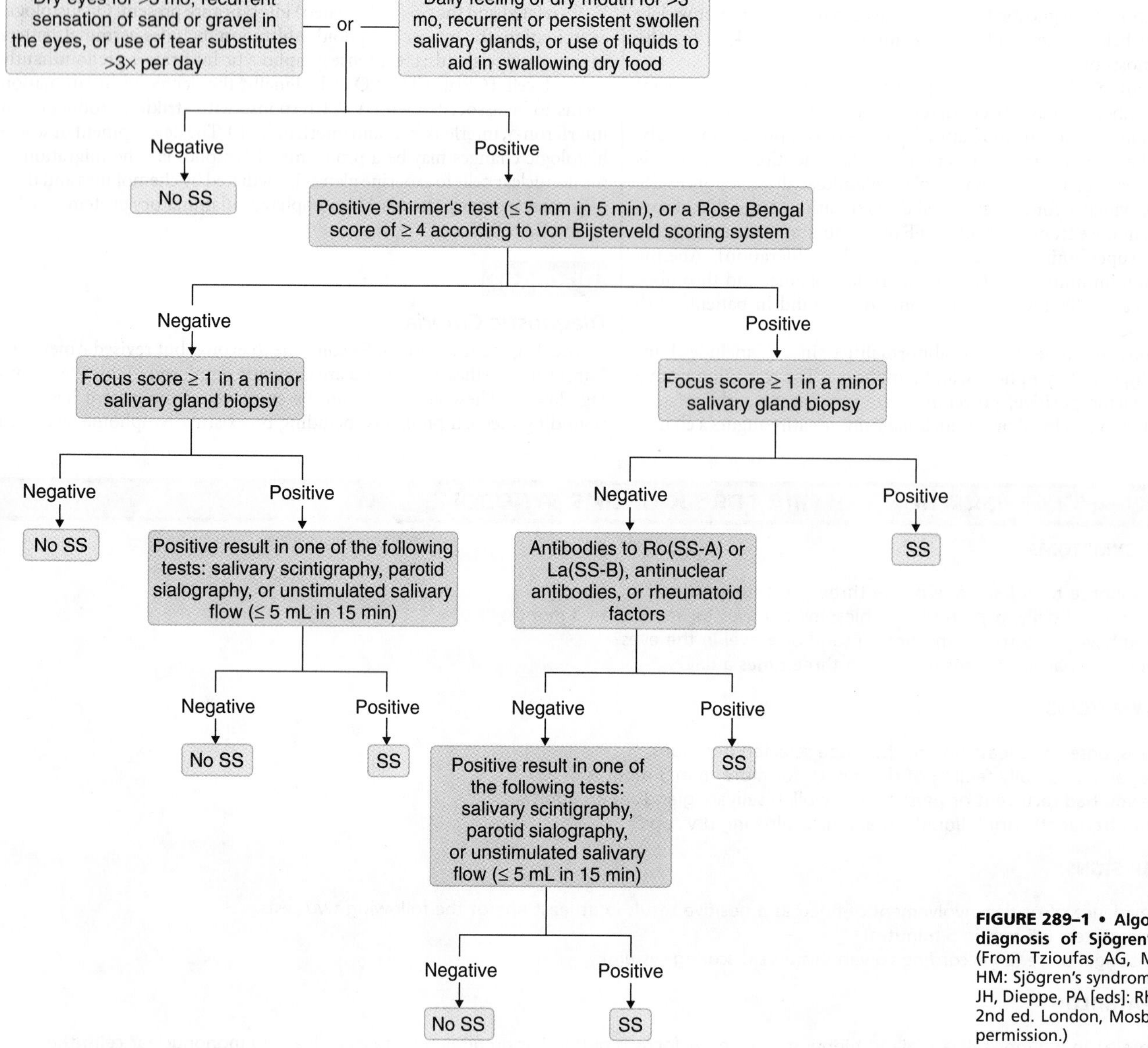

FIGURE 289–1 • Algorithm for the diagnosis of Sjögren's syndrome. (From Tzioufas AG, Moutsopoulos HM: Sjögren's syndromes. *In* Klippel JH, Dieppe, PA [eds]: Rheumatology, 2nd ed. London, Mosby, 1998, with permission.)

immunodeficiency syndrome, sarcoidosis, graft-versus-host disease, past head and neck irradiation, use of anticholinergic drugs, and hepatitis C, diseases commonly included in the differential diagnosis. A Sjögren's-like disorder is associated with graft-versus-host disease and diffuse infiltrative lymphocytosis syndrome. The diagnosis of graft-versus-host disease is clinically obvious on the basis of the history. Diffuse infiltrative lymphocytosis syndrome occurs more commonly in males in the absence of the unique autoantibody profile of SS. The classification criteria are helpful in distinguishing between SS and sicca syndrome secondary to medications. An abnormal finding on lip biopsy and the presence of autoantibodies suggest a systemic autoimmune disease. SS is more commonly associated with several other autoimmune diseases including Hashimoto's thyroiditis, primary biliary cirrhosis, chronic active hepatitis, celiac sprue, myasthenia gravis, and pernicious anemia.

Treatment

Rx

The primary treatment of SS is to minimize discomfort by use of substitutes for the dysfunctional exocrine secretions (e.g., artificial tears, artificial saliva, increased oral fluids, ocular lubricants, vaginal lubricants). Ocular steroids are not recommended because they predispose to serious secondary infections. Goggles and punctal occlusion also are used to slow the loss of tears. Oral pilocarpine and cevimeline may stimulate functional exocrine glands and improve symptoms, but the response varies greatly among patients. The appearance of thrush warrants prompt treatment because it severely aggravates oral symptoms; nystatin is generally effective for this complication. Finally, regular dental examinations and oral hygiene are crucial for reducing subsequent oral health issues (i.e., caries and periodontal disease associated with xerostomia). Tumor necrosis factor-α inhibitors have proved largely disappointing. The use of rituximab has been reported to be beneficial in SS-associated lymphoma. Multiple other biologic agents are under development.

Extraglandular manifestations of SS also are managed in a symptomatic fashion. Treatment of arthritis includes nonsteroidal anti-inflammatory drugs, prednisone, hydroxychloroquine, methotrexate, and tumor necrosis factor-α inhibitors. Constitutional symptoms are treated with hydroxychloroquine or prednisone. Inflammatory organ system disease (involving the lung, liver, neurologic system, hematologic system, and kidney) is treated individually with prednisone, methotrexate, azathioprine, or tumor necrosis factor-α inhibitors. Careful surveillance for infectious complications and neoplasia is crucial because the risk of both is increased in SS. Intravenous immunoglobulin has been suggested as a treatment of SS, but there is no evidence to support its use. The mortality of patients with SS has been estimated to be 2.7-fold greater than that of a control population.

Future Directions

It is ironic that although much has been learned about the effector mechanisms of SS, little is known about the inductive mechanisms. It is likely that future therapy will focus on interrupting the inflammatory pathways without ever understanding how the disease begins. If the latency time for development of an autoimmune disease is measured in years, it will be extremely difficult to identify the etiologic agents involved. Future work will focus on specific cytokines, chemokines, and their cognate receptor interactions in efforts to block the exocrine gland destruction. It is also likely that more specific therapy for the anti-Ro–mediated complete heart block of newborns will be developed, again focusing on abrogation of effector inflammatory pathways. Finally, it is anticipated that newer biologic agents will directly influence effector mechanisms, but they will probably be effective only if they are given to patients early in the disease course.

SUGGESTED READINGS

Fox RI: Sjögren's syndrome. Lancet 2005;366:321–331. *A detailed review.*

Garcia-Carrasco M, Fuentes-Alexandro S, Escarcega RO, et al: Pathophysiology of Sjögren's syndrome. Arch Med Res 2006;37:921–932. *Comprehensive review of what we know of the pathophysiology of the disease.*

Hansen A, Lipsky PE, Dorner T: Immunopathogenesis of primary Sjögren's syndrome: Implications for disease management and therapy. Curr Opin Rheumatol 2005;17:558–565. *Overview of the mechanisms of disease.*

Locht H, Pelck R, Manthorpe R: Clinical manifestations correlated to the prevalence of autoantibodies in a large (n = 321) cohort of patients with primary Sjögren's syndrome. A comparison of patients initially diagnosed according to the Copenhagen classification criteria with the American-European consensus criteria. Autoimmun Rev 2005;4:276–281. *A detailed analysis of a large cohort.*

Venables PJ: Management of patients presenting with Sjögren's syndrome. Best Pract Res Clin Rheumatol 2006;20:791–807. *Comprehensive review of the management of the disease.*

290 POLYMYOSITIS AND DERMATOMYOSITIS

Frederick W. Miller

Definition

Polymyositis and dermatomyositis are the most common forms of a family of acquired, systemic, connective tissue diseases, known as the idiopathic inflammatory myopathies, characterized by the clinical and pathologic effects of chronic muscle inflammation of unknown cause. Other forms of idiopathic inflammatory myopathy include inclusion body myositis and myositis seen in association with cancer or with other connective tissue diseases (such as scleroderma, systemic lupus erythematosus, and rheumatoid arthritis) as a myositis overlap syndrome. The idiopathic inflammatory myopathies, also known as the myositis syndromes, are diagnosed on the basis of a combination of clinical, laboratory, and pathologic findings (Table 290–1).

Epidemiology

Polymyositis and dermatomyositis are rare disorders described more than a century ago in Europe; they are now known to be worldwide in distribution and are likely to be increasing in frequency. The estimated annual incidence ranges from 5 to 10 per million, and estimated prevalence is 50 to 110 per million. Polymyositis and dermatomyositis peak in prevalence in childhood (7 to 15 years) and in midlife (30 to 50 years), whereas the malignancy-associated forms and inclusion body myositis are more common after 50 years of age. Current studies suggest, however, that the prevalence, frequency of clinical forms, and risk factors for development of the idiopathic inflammatory myopathies are likely to differ in different parts of the world. There is an approximately 3:1 female predominance in all forms except inclusion body myositis, in which the female-to-male ratio is inverted (approximately 1:3). Certain ethnic groups, including persons of African or Latino descent, may be at increased risk for idiopathic inflammatory myopathies with poorer outcomes compared with those of European ancestry. Anecdotal clusterings of polymyositis and dermatomyositis onset in time and space suggest strong environmental influences, but the specific agents involved remain elusive.

TABLE 290–1 CRITERIA FOR THE DIAGNOSIS OF POLYMYOSITIS AND DERMATOMYOSITIS AFTER EXCLUSION OF ALL OTHER FORMS OF MYOPATHY*

1. Symmetric, often progressive, proximal muscle weakness
2. Characteristic electromyographic triad
   - Short-duration, small, low-amplitude polyphasic potentials
   - Fibrillation potentials, seen even at rest
   - Bizarre high-frequency repetitive discharges
3. Elevations of serum activities of myositis-associated enzymes
   - Creatine kinase
   - Aldolase
   - Lactate dehydrogenase
   - Transaminases—aspartate transaminase and alanine transaminase
4. Evidence of chronic inflammation in muscle biopsy specimen
   - Necrosis of type I and type II muscle fibers
   - Degeneration and regeneration of myofibers with variation in myofiber size
   - Focal collections of interstitial or perivascular mononuclear cells
5. Characteristic rashes of dermatomyositis
   - Scaly erythematous palpable eruptions over the metacarpophalangeal or interphalangeal joints, knees, elbows, or medial malleoli (Gottron's papules)
   - Scaly erythematous macules over the metacarpophalangeal or interphalangeal joints, knees, elbows, or medial malleoli (Gottron's sign)
   - Periorbital purplish discoloration (heliotrope rash)

*Criteria originally proposed by Bohan and Peter in 1975:
Definite disease: for polymyositis, all of the first four criteria; for dermatomyositis, any three of the first four criteria plus the rash.
Probable disease: for polymyositis, any three of the first four criteria; for dermatomyositis, any two of the first four criteria plus the rash.
Possible disease: for polymyositis, any two of the first four criteria; for dermatomyositis, any one of the first four criteria plus the rash.

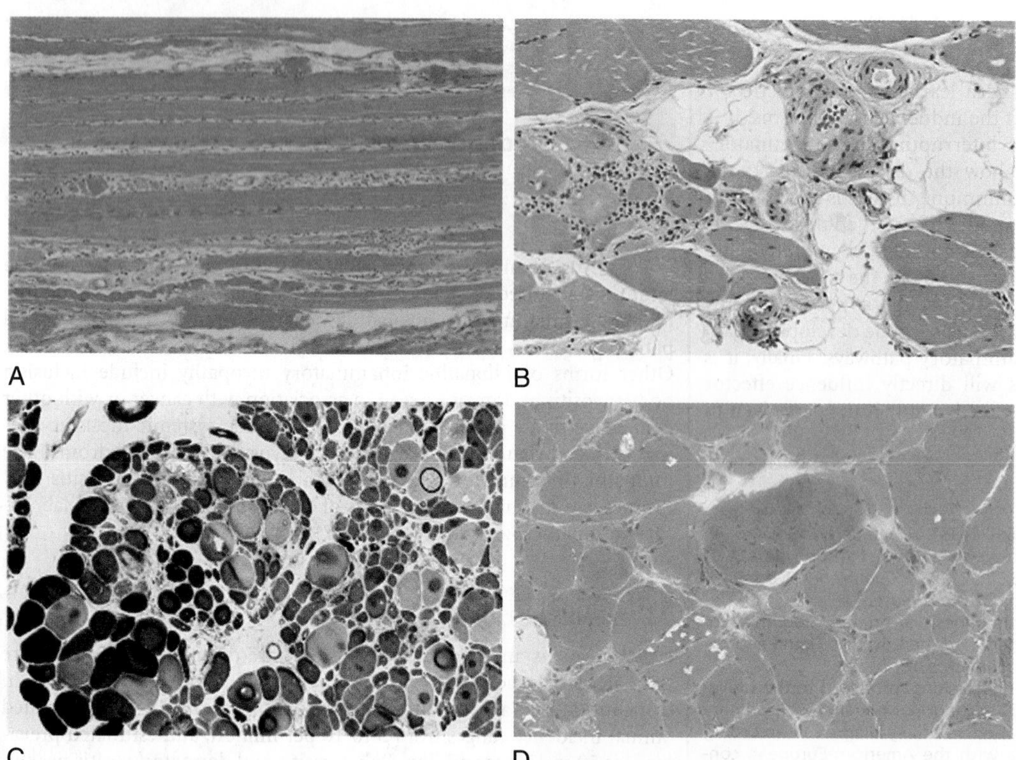

FIGURE 290–1 • Pathologic changes in myositis by light microscopy. A and B, Longitudinal and cross-sectional views of inflammatory myopathy show variation in cell size, necrosis, regeneration, and inflammation (hematoxylin and eosin stain). **C,** Perifascicular atrophy in dermatomyositis (ATPase stain). **D,** Red-rimmed inclusions, marked cell size variation, and relatively sparse inflammation in inclusion body myositis (trichrome stain). (Photographs courtesy of Dr. J. Nelson and Dr. L. Love. From Klippel JH, Dieppe PA: Rheumatology, 2nd ed. London, Mosby, 1998, with permission.)

Pathobiology

An immune-mediated component to the myositis syndromes is suggested by (1) the inflammatory process, (2) the frequent finding of autoantibodies and other immune abnormalities, (3) the overlap with autoimmune diseases such as systemic lupus erythematosus in some patients, (4) the immunogenetic risk factors, and (5) the clinical response to anti-inflammatory agents. Nonetheless, by definition, the pathogeneses remain unknown. Many lines of evidence suggest that chronic immune activation in genetically susceptible individuals, after exposure to environmental triggers, plays a pivotal role in the development of idiopathic inflammatory myopathies.

The pathologic change in the muscle, skin, and other affected tissues is characterized by focal collections of mononuclear cells. Lymphocytes are the most common cells in the infiltrates, but macrophages, plasma cells, basophils, and neutrophils are sometimes present. In certain variants, eosinophils (eosinophilic myositis) or granulomas (granulomatous myositis) predominate. The muscle cells (myocytes) show evidence of necrosis with degeneration and regeneration (Fig. 290–1), and there is often increased connective tissue or fibrosis in the interstitial areas around the myocytes.

Immunohistochemical and other studies implicate different pathogeneses in the various forms of myositis. In polymyositis and inclusion body myositis, the pathologic change suggests a cytotoxic T lymphocyte–mediated process with $CD8^+$ T cells surrounding and invading otherwise normal-appearing myocytes in endomysial areas. In dermatomyositis, however, the infiltrate is predominantly composed of B lymphocytes and $CD4^+$ helper T cells in perimysial areas around the fascicles and small blood vessels. Blood vessel pathology with endothelial cell damage from complement deposition and atrophy of the myofibers at the periphery of the fascicle (called perifascicular atrophy and caused by the more tenuous blood supply in this area) are also characteristic findings in dermatomyositis. Inclusion body myositis differs from polymyositis and dermatomyositis by the presence of characteristic reddish inclusions and vacuoles, rimmed by purple granules, inside the myocytes as demonstrated in trichrome-stained frozen muscle sections. Additional features of inclusion body myositis include frequent endomysial fibrosis, amyloid deposition, marked variation in myofiber diameter, and characteristic intranuclear and intracytoplasmic filamentous tubules seen on electron microscopy.

Autoantibodies are found in more than 90% of patients with polymyositis and dermatomyositis, although it remains unclear what role, if any, they play in pathogenesis. The most frequent of these are antinuclear antibodies, but many others are commonly seen, including rheumatoid factor, anti-U1RNP, anti-La, anti-Ro, anti-PM/Scl, and anti-Ku autoantibodies. None of these are diagnostic for polymyositis or dermatomyositis, but if present, they do assist in distinguishing the idiopathic inflammatory myopathies from the other forms of myopathy. About one third of patients with idiopathic inflammatory myopathy have autoantibodies that are diagnostic, known as myositis-specific autoantibodies. The most common of these are antisynthetase autoantibodies (and the most common antisynthetases are anti–Jo-1 autoantibodies), anti–signal recognition particle autoantibodies, and anti–Mi-2 autoantibodies that are directed against a nuclear helicase. Each of these autoantibodies is strongly associated with a distinct clinical presentation, response to therapy, and prognosis, suggesting that each autoantibody may be representative of a truly different myositis syndrome (Table 290–2). The myositis-specific autoantibodies are available commercially but need not be obtained in all patients. They may be particularly useful in the diagnosis of perplexing cases or in predicting prognosis.

As is the case for other autoimmune conditions, polymyositis and dermatomyositis are complex disorders whose etiologies are likely to involve the interaction of multiple genetic and environmental risk factors. The strongest genetic risk factors identified to date are the polymorphic genes known as human leukocyte antigen (HLA) genes that regulate the immune responses in the major histocompatibility complex. In those of European descent, the ancestral HLA haplotype containing A1, B8, DRB1*0301, and DQA1*0501 alleles is most strongly associated with all forms of myositis. The major clinical and autoantibody groups, however, each have additional HLA risk and protective alleles. In other ethnic groups, though, such as Koreans and Mesoamericans, HLA genes are not risk factors. In these ethnic groups, alleles of the genes encoding immunoglobulin proteins, which regulate levels of antibody responses to infectious agents and are known as GM and KM loci, are the major genetic risk factors for polymyositis and dermatomyositis. Alleles of other polymorphic genes, including those that regulate cytokine responses to environmental exposures, such as tumor necrosis factor-α and interleukin-1 receptor antagonist alleles, have recently been associated with the childhood myositis syndromes. The environmental triggers for polymyositis and dermatomyositis are not known, but selected viral and bacterial infections as well as certain drugs, dietary supplements,

TABLE 290–2 CLASSIFICATIONS OF THE IDIOPATHIC INFLAMMATORY MYOPATHIES

Classification Group	Associated Clinical Features	Severity of Myositis	Response of Myositis to Therapy	Prognosis (5-Yr Survival)
CLINICAL GROUPS				
Polymyositis	None of the features below	Variable	Variable	Moderate (~80%)
Dermatomyositis	Gottron's papules or heliotrope rash	Mild to moderate	Good	Moderate (~85%)
Connective tissue myositis	Overlap with other connective tissue diseases	Mild	Excellent	Good (~90%)
Cancer-associated myositis	Cancer diagnosed within 2 years of idiopathic inflammatory myopathy	Variable	Moderate to poor	Poor, secondary to cancer (~60%)
Juvenile myositis	Diagnosis before 18 years of age Dermatomyositis >> polymyositis Subcutaneous calcifications Gastrointestinal vasculitis	Variable	Moderate to good	Good (>95%)
Inclusion body myositis	Insidious onset in older white men Distal involvement, atrophy, and asymmetrical weakness Poor response to therapy	Mild but progressive	Poor	Few deaths, but significant morbidity (>85%)
SEROLOGIC GROUPS				
Antisynthetases	Acute onset in polymyositis or dermatomyositis Interstitial lung disease, fever, dyspnea on exertion, arthritis, mechanic's hands, Raynaud's phenomena	Moderate to severe	Moderate, but flares with taper	Poor (~75%)
Anti–signal recognition particle	Acute onset in black female Palpitations, cardiac disease, severe weakness No rash (clinically polymyositis)	Severe	Poor	Very poor (~30%)
Anti–Mi-2	Classic dermatomyositis "V" and "shawl" rashes, cuticular changes	Mild	Good	Good (>95%)

vaccines, medical implants, and occupational exposures have been implicated in case reports and in some epidemiologic studies. In the first worldwide study of myositis, global surface ultraviolet light intensity was found to correlate with the proportion of dermatomyositis compared with polymyositis cases at the referral centers in the study.

Clinical Manifestations

Myositis may present acutely, subacutely, or insidiously, and patients can have single or multiple episodic attacks or persistent disease activity. The idiopathic inflammatory myopathies may be divided into groups on the basis of clinical-pathologic or serologic features, and each of these groups has characteristic clinical and prognostic associations (see Table 290–2). Therefore, the manner in which the disease presents can suggest the form of idiopathic inflammatory myopathy present. For example, an acute, severe onset of polymyositis with pulmonary fibrosis may herald a difficult course with persistent disease, as is often seen in patients with anti–Jo-1 autoantibodies. In contrast, a slowly progressive onset associated with proximal and distal weakness and thigh muscle atrophy in an older man suggests inclusion body myositis.

Symmetric, proximal muscle weakness is present in most cases and results in difficulty arising from chairs, getting out of cars, reaching overhead, or combing hair. Many patients also report generalized fatigue or muscle pain. Patients with dermatomyositis can present with a variety of photosensitive rashes over the face, chest, and hands. Gottron's papules are raised, often scaly, palpable lesions overlying an erythematous base on extensor surfaces such as the metacarpophalangeal and proximal interphalangeal joints, elbows, and knees; these are virtually pathognomonic for dermatomyositis. Other characteristic rashes of dermatomyositis are Gottron's sign (macules in a distribution similar to Gottron's papules) and a characteristic purplish rash over and sometimes surrounding the upper eyelids known as the heliotrope rash. Patients may also develop a rash in the V of the neck (V sign) or in the distribution of a shawl (shawl sign). A roughening, scaling, and erythematous fissuring of the palmar and lateral aspects of the fingers, known as mechanic's hands, may be seen in patients with either polymyositis or dermatomyositis. On occasion, patients may develop classic dermatomyositis rashes without apparent muscle weakness or elevated muscle enzymes in a syndrome called dermatomyositis sine myositis. Some of these individuals, however, have subclinical myositis, as demonstrated by magnetic resonance imaging studies of muscle or muscle biopsy, whereas clinical myositis develops over time in others. Children with dermatomyositis are particularly at risk for the development of subcutaneous calcifications and occasionally present with intestinal vasculitis.

Although the patient and physician often focus on skeletal muscle involvement in these conditions, the idiopathic inflammatory myopathies are systemic diseases with frequent extramuscular manifestations that can become the most troubling aspects of the patient's disease (Table 290–3). Patients may suffer from arthralgias and arthritis, a variety of skin disorders, and general symptoms such as fatigue, weight loss, Raynaud's phenomenon, or fever. The gastrointestinal, pulmonary, and cardiac systems may also be involved, which can both complicate therapy and adversely affect prognosis. The development of these extramuscular manifestations may precede or follow the development of the myositis, and their severity may be independent of the degree of myositis.

Diagnosis

Muscle pain and weakness are frequent patient complaints arising from many causes. These can be the result of intrinsic muscle diseases (myopathies), disorders of the nerves innervating the muscle (neuropathies), or the effects of drugs, toxins, or infectious agents. All these entities must be carefully considered and excluded to allow the diagnosis of polymyositis or dermatomyositis (Table 290–4). A careful medical and family history, exposure history, complete physical examination, and directed laboratory testing with electromyography and muscle biopsy

TABLE 290–3 EXTRAMUSCULAR MANIFESTATIONS OF POLYMYOSITIS AND DERMATOMYOSITIS

General
- Fatigue
- Malaise
- Weight loss
- Raynaud's syndrome

Musculoskeletal
- Arthralgias, usually symmetrical and involving the hand joints
- Nonerosive polyarthritis, usually symmetrical and involving the hand joints
- Deforming arthropathy of hand joints
- Carpal tunnel syndrome
- Osteopenia and osteoporosis

Cutaneous
- Characteristic dermatomyositis rashes: Gottron's papules, Gottron's sign, heliotrope rash
- Other rashes: V-sign and shawl-sign rashes; linear extensor erythema; roughening, scaling, and erythematous fissuring of the palmar and lateral aspects of the fingers (mechanic's hands)
- Photosensitivity
- Periungual abnormalities including telangiectasias and cuticular overgrowth
- Irregular indurated plaques over the fingers with mucin accumulation in the dermis
- Subcutaneous and intradermal calcification, which may ulcerate with secondary infection
- Vasculitis with infarcts and digital ulcers
- Subcutaneous inflammation (panniculitis)
- Alopecia

Gastrointestinal
- Abnormal pharyngeal and cricopharyngeal function, often leading to dysphonia
- Esophageal dysphagia with occasional nasal regurgitation or aspiration
- Delayed gastric emptying and reflux
- Dysmotility of the small and large intestines sometimes leading to chronic abdominal pain
- Malabsorption
- Vasculitis with infarcts and necrosis of the bowel

Pulmonary
- Ventilatory insufficiency due to respiratory muscle weakness
- Atelectasis
- Aspiration pneumonia
- Interstitial lung disease (pulmonary fibrosis)
- Pulmonary hypertension
- Drug-related pneumonitis
- Opportunistic infections in immunocompromised patients

Cardiac
- Myocarditis with arrhythmias and congestive failure
- Cardiomyopathy
- Cor pulmonale
- Rare pericarditis and pericardial effusions

should reveal the cause of muscle weakness in most cases. Given that the pathologic changes of muscle in idiopathic inflammatory myopathy are often focal and not evenly distributed, magnetic resonance imaging of the muscle can be useful to identify where inflammation is present and to increase the yield of muscle biopsy.

Population-based studies have confirmed a two- to three-fold increased relative risk of a variety of cancers in roughly equal distribution to those in the population within 2 years of the development of dermatomyositis and to a lesser extent in polymyositis and inclusion body myositis. Patients with myositis at onset should therefore be carefully assessed for malignant neoplasms, especially cancers for which they have other risk factors. The cancer work-up should be directed and include a thorough history for any changes in habits that might suggest a neoplasm, careful physical examinations and screening rectal examinations, fecal occult blood tests, urinalysis, blood chemistry studies, chest radiograph,

TABLE 290–4 DIFFERENTIAL DIAGNOSIS OF IDIOPATHIC INFLAMMATORY MYOPATHY

Drug- and toxin-induced myopathies
- Corticosteroids
- Ethanol
- Lipid-lowering agents (HMG-CoA reductase inhibitors and fibrates)
- D-Penicillamine
- Colchicine
- Cocaine
- Cyclosporine
- Ipecac
- Chloroquine, hydroxychloroquine
- Zidovudine (AZT)
- L-Tryptophan (eosinophilia-myalgia syndrome)

Endocrine diseases
- Hypothyroidism
- Hyperthyroidism
- Acromegaly
- Diabetes mellitus

Neurologic disorders
- Amyotrophic lateral sclerosis
- Myasthenia gravis
- Eaton-Lambert syndrome
- Multiple sclerosis
- Guillain-Barré syndrome
- Motor neuron disease

Other immunologic or connective tissue diseases
- Hypereosinophilic syndrome
- Polyarteritis nodosa and other forms of vasculitis
- Polymyalgia rheumatica
- Still's disease
- Rheumatoid arthritis
- Systemic lupus erythematosus
- Systemic sclerosis
- Tendinitis and overuse syndromes

Acquired metabolic abnormalities
- Hypokalemia
- Hypercalcemia
- Hypocalcemia

Inherited metabolic myopathies
- Acid maltase deficiency
- Phosphorylase deficiency (McArdle's disease)
- Lipid metabolic defects (primary and secondary carnitine deficiency)
- Palmityltransferase deficiency
- Phosphofructokinase deficiency

Mitochondrial myopathies
- Mitochondrial encephalomyopathy, lactic acidosis, stroke (MELAS)
- Neuropathy ataxia, retinitis pigmentosa (NARP)
- Myoclonic epilepsy, ragged red fibers (MERRFs)
- Kearns-Sayre syndrome

Inherited muscle structural protein defects (muscular dystrophies)
- Duchenne's and Becker's dystrophies
- Fascioscapulohumeral dystrophy
- Dysferlinopathies and other limb girdle dystrophies
- Myotonic dystrophy
- Other dystrophies

Infectious myopathies
- Bacterial (pyomyositis, gangrene, Lyme disease)
- Parasitic (trichinosis, toxoplasmosis, sarcosporidiosis, trypanosomiasis)
- Fungal (candidiasis, cryptococcosis, sporotrichosis, actinomycosis, histoplasmosis)
- Viral (influenza, adenovirus, coxsackievirus, echovirus, Epstein-Barr virus, retroviruses including human immunodeficiency virus and human T-lymphotropic viruses 1 and 2, hepatitis B and C viruses)

and prostate-specific antigen testing in men. Women should undergo serial gynecologic examinations, Papanicolaou's stain, and CA-125 testing. Physicians should have a low threshold for performing pelvic ultrasonography or computed tomography to exclude ovarian cancer given its frequency in women with dermatomyositis. Any abnormalities in these initial studies should be followed by appropriate investigations to conclusively exclude malignant disease.

Treatment

Therapy for polymyositis and dermatomyositis is directed at decreasing inflammation in target tissues, relieving symptoms, and rebuilding endurance and muscle strength. Corticosteroids are the initial and primary therapy for these diseases. Several factors are important in determining corticosteroid responses. These are, in addition to the patient's clinical and serologic groups, an adequate initial dose (at least 1 mg/kg/day of prednisone or equivalent), the continuation of prednisone until or after the serum creatine kinase activity normalizes, and a slow rate of prednisone tapering (approximately 10 mg/month or about 15% of the existing dose per month). High-dose intravenous corticosteroids (1 g/day for 3 days) and additional immunosuppressive therapy are probably useful as initial treatments in severe cases or those in poor prognostic groups.

There is no consensus on the best treatment of corticosteroid-resistant patients. Oral methotrexate (7.5 to 20 mg weekly, depending on disease severity and body weight) and azathioprine (50 to 150 mg daily, depending on disease severity and body weight) are the major therapeutic options used in practice, but intravenous immune globulin, [1] cyclosporin A, tacrolimus, mycophenolate mofetil, cyclophosphamide, anti–tumor necrosis factor agents, anti–B cell agents such as rituximab, or combinations of these may also be beneficial in difficult cases. With the exception of the use of topical corticosteroids, hydroxychloroquine, and sunscreens for the treatment of the dermatomyositis rash, no specific treatment other than therapy for the underlying myositis is known to improve the systemic manifestations of the idiopathic inflammatory myopathy. Rehabilitation and physical therapy are important in maintaining range of motion and preventing contractures during active disease. Exercise probably improves strength and endurance when it is initiated in a graded way during periods of disease control.

The treatment of inclusion body myositis is controversial. Retrospective reviews of corticosteroid and cytotoxic therapy as well as several prospective trials suggest that the rate of deterioration may be decreased or stabilized and strength improved by treating patients with inclusion body myositis with evidence of active myositis. [2] Physical therapy, however, plays the most important role in longer term care for inclusion body myositis.

Prognosis

The prognosis of polymyositis and dermatomyositis is poorly studied, but current information suggests that each clinical and serologic group may differ in response to therapy and outcome (see Table 290–2). Patients with myositis who also have another connective tissue disease (the overlap group) tend to have the mildest myositis, best clinical responses, and fewest exacerbations of myositis over time. Patients with dermatomyositis have more severe disease, followed by patients with polymyositis. Patients with inclusion body myositis do not respond to therapy as well as do patients in the other clinical groups. The serologic groups are also different in their disease courses and prognosis. Patients with anti–Mi-2 autoantibodies tend to have mild myositis with good responses to therapy and few disease exacerbations with tapering of therapy. Patients with antisynthetase autoantibody have more severe disease, moderate therapeutic responses, but frequent exacerbations with tapering of therapy. As a group, patients with anti–signal recognition particle autoantibodies have the most acute onset and the most severe myositis, with the least response to therapy and the most persistent disease.

Any patient with an unexpectedly unresponsive or perplexing clinical course, however, should be reevaluated for possible misdiagnosis or the development of another cause of muscle weakness.

Future Directions

Given the current incurable nature of the myositis syndromes and the poor outcomes in many patients, future directions are likely to be focused on improved classification criteria to separate the idiopathic inflammatory myopathies from dystrophies and metabolic myopathies through the use of molecular genetic and immunologic information. A more complete understanding of the pathogenesis of these disorders may result in more focused therapies. Because these complex diseases probably arise from interactions of genetic and environmental risk factors, defining these elements may provide insight into the mechanisms of development of myositis. This knowledge could possibly allow the future prevention of some myositis cases by avoidance of certain environmental exposures in genetically susceptible individuals or by gene therapy.

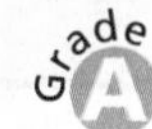

1. Dalakas MC, Illa I, Dambrosia JM, et al: A controlled trial of high-dose intravenous immune globulin infusions as treatment for dermatomyositis. N Engl J Med 1993;329:1993–2000.
2. Leff RL, Miller FW, Hicks J, et al: The treatment of inclusion body myositis: A retrospective review and a randomized, prospective trial of immunosuppressive therapy. Medicine (Baltimore) 1993; 72:225–235.

SUGGESTED READINGS

Buchbinder R, Forbes A, Hall S, et al: Incidence of malignant disease in biopsy-proven inflammatory myopathy. A population-based cohort study. Ann Intern Med 2001;134:1087–1095. *Solid epidemiologic support for increased cancers in dermatomyositis, polymyositis, and inclusion body myositis, with dermatomyositis having the highest cancer risk.*

Callen JP, Wortmann RL: Dermatomyositis. Clin Dermatol 2006;24:363–373. *Comprehensive review.*

Choy E, Hoogendijk J, Lecky B, Winer J: Immunosuppressant and immunomodulatory treatment for dermatomyositis and polymyositis. Cochrane Database Syst Rev 2005;3:CD003643. *A useful review of therapeutic trials in polymyositis and dermatomyositis.*

Nirmalananthan N, Holton JL, Hanna MG: Is it really myositis? A consideration of the differential diagnosis. Curr Opin Rheumatol 2004;16:684–691. *A comprehensive and clinically useful summary of the differential diagnosis of myositis.*

Rider LG, Giannini EH, Brunner HI, et al: International consensus on preliminary definitions of improvement in adult and juvenile myositis. Arthritis Rheum 2004;50:2281–2290. *The first validated comprehensive measures of clinical improvement in myositis by a combination of clinical and laboratory findings.*

291 THE SYSTEMIC VASCULITIDES

John H. Stone

Definition

The vasculitides are a heterogeneous group of disorders linked by the common finding of destructive inflammation within blood vessel walls. On the basis of current classification schemes, approximately 20 different forms of primary vasculitis are recognized (Table 291–1).

Classification

Classification by Vessel Size

The etiology of most forms of vasculitis remains unknown. Because of major gaps in understanding of the pathophysiologic process, the most valid basis for classification of the vasculitides is the size of the predominant blood vessels involved. The vasculitides are categorized initially by whether the vessels affected are large, medium, or small (see Table 291–1). Within individual cases, there is frequently overlap in the size of the blood vessels affected.

Additional Considerations in Classification

Several other considerations are relevant to the classification of vasculitis (Table 291–2). These are (1) age, gender, and ethnic background of the patient; (2) tropism for particular organs; (3) presence or absence of granulomatous inflammation; (4) participation of immune complexes in the pathophysiologic process; and (5) detection of characteristic autoantibodies in the patients' serum, such as antineutrophil cytoplasmic antibodies (ANCAs).

The organ tropisms of these disorders are illustrated by the following examples. Whereas Henoch-Schönlein purpura typically affects the skin, joints, kidneys, and gastrointestinal tract, Wegener's granulomatosis classically involves the upper airways, lungs, and kidneys. In contrast to both of these, Cogan's syndrome involves the eyes, the audiovestibular apparatus of the inner ear, and the large arteries (in 10 to 15% of cases). The granulomatous features of some forms of vasculitis resemble fungal and mycobacterial infections or the inflammation induced by the presence of a foreign body, suggesting a role for chronic antigenic stimulation.

Immune complexes are essential to the pathophysiologic mechanism of some forms of small- and medium-vessel vasculitis. Complexes of immunoglobulin (Ig) A1 are found in Henoch-Schönlein purpura. Immune complexes consisting of IgG, IgM, complement components, and the hepatitis C virion characterize most cases of mixed cryoglobulinemia. In contrast, "pauci-immune" types of small- and medium-vessel vasculitis, such as Wegener's granulomatosis and microscopic polyangiitis, have little immunoglobulin or complement deposition within diseased tissues. Many but not all patients with pauci-immune forms of vasculitis are ANCA positive.

TABLE 291–1 CLASSIFICATION SCHEME OF VASCULITIDES ACCORDING TO SIZE OF PREDOMINANT BLOOD VESSELS INVOLVED

Predominantly large-vessel vasculitides
- Takayasu's arteritis
- Giant cell arteritis
- Cogan's syndrome
- Behçet's disease*

Predominantly medium-vessel vasculitides
- Classic polyarteritis nodosa
- Cutaneous polyarteritis nodosa
- Rheumatoid vasculitis†
- Buerger's disease
- Kawasaki's disease
- Primary angiitis of the central nervous system

Predominantly small-vessel vasculitides
- Immune complex mediated
  - Cutaneous leukocytoclastic angiitis ("hypersensitivity" vasculitis)
  - Henoch-Schönlein purpura
  - Urticarial vasculitis
  - Cryoglobulinemia†
  - Erythema elevatum diutinum
- "ANCA-associated" disorders
  - Wegener's granulomatosis†
  - Microscopic polyangiitis†
  - Churg-Strauss syndrome†
- Miscellaneous small-vessel vasculitides
  - Connective tissue disorders†
  - Paraneoplastic diseases
  - Infection
  - Inflammatory bowel disease

*May involve small, medium, and large blood vessels.
†Frequent overlap of involvement of small and medium-sized blood vessels.
ANCA = antineutrophil cytoplasmic antibody.

Epidemiology

The epidemiologic features of individual forms of systemic vasculitis vary tremendously by geography (Table 291–3). This may reflect genetic influences, variation in environmental exposures, and other unknown disease risk factors. For example, whereas Behçet's disease is rare in North Americans, affecting only 1 person in approximately 300,000, this condition is several hundred times more common among inhabitants of countries bordering the ancient Silk Route. Similarly, although Takayasu's arteritis is rare in the United States—on the order of 3 new cases per million people per year—this disease is reportedly the most common cause of renal artery stenosis in India, where the incidence may be as high as 200 to 300 per million per year.

Age is an important consideration in the epidemiology of vasculitis. Eighty percent of patients with Kawasaki's disease are younger than 5 years of age. In contrast, giant cell arteritis virtually never occurs in patients younger than 50 years, and the mean age of patients with this disease is 72 years. Age may also have an impact on disease severity and outcome. In Henoch-Schönlein purpura, the overwhelming majority of cases in children (who represent 90% of all cases) have self-limited

TABLE 291–2 CONSIDERATIONS IN THE CLASSIFICATION OF SYSTEMIC VASCULITIS

Size of predominant blood vessels affected
Epidemiologic features
- Age
- Gender
- Ethnic background

Pattern of organ involvement
Pathologic features
- Granulomatous inflammation
- Immune complex deposition vs. "pauci-immune" histopathology

Presence of ANCA in serum

ANCA = antineutrophil cytoplasmic antibody.

TABLE 291–3 EPIDEMIOLOGY OF SELECTED VASCULITIDES

Disease	United States	Elsewhere	Age, Gender, and Ethnic Predispositions
Giant cell arteritis	Incidence: 240/million (Olmsted County, MN)	220–270/million (Scandinavian countries)	Age >50 yr, mean age 72 yr; females 3:1; northern European ancestry
Takayasu's arteritis	Incidence: 3/million	200–300/million (India)	Age <40 yr; females 9:1; Asian
Behçet's disease	Prevalence: 3/million	3000/million (Turkey)	Silk Route countries
Polyarteritis nodosa	Incidence: 7/million	7/million (Spain)	Slight male predominance
Kawasaki's disease	Incidence: 100/million*	900/million (Japan)	Children of Asian ancestry
Wegener's granulomatosis	Incidence: 4/million	8.5/million (United Kingdom)	Whites >> blacks

*Among children younger than 5 years.
From Gonzalez-Gay MA, Garica-Porrua C: Epidemiology of the vasculitides. Rheum Clin North Am 2001;27:729–749.

courses, resolving within several weeks. In adults, however, Henoch-Schönlein purpura has a higher likelihood of chronicity and a greater likelihood of a poor renal outcome.

The distribution of gender varies across many forms of vasculitis. Buerger's disease is the only form of vasculitis with a striking male predominance. The greater prevalence of smoking among males in most societies probably explains this predilection. In contrast, Takayasu's arteritis has an overwhelming tendency to occur in females (a 9:1 female-to-male ratio). The pauci-immune forms of vasculitis, such as Wegener's granulomatosis, microscopic polyangiitis, and Churg-Strauss syndrome, occur in males and females with approximately equal frequencies.

The strongest link between any single gene and vasculitis is the association of HLA-B51 with Behçet's disease. In Behçet's disease, 80% of Asian patients have the HLA-B51 gene. The prevalence of HLA-B51 is significantly higher among patients with Behçet's disease in Japan than among nondisease control subjects (55% versus less than 15%). Among the sporadic cases of Behçet's disease involving whites in the United States, however, HLA-B51 occurs in less than 15% of cases.

With the exception of Buerger's disease and smoking, no true associations between disease and environmental or occupational exposures have been confirmed. Associations have also been reported but not confirmed between exposures to silica and some types of pauci-immune vasculitis. Studies of potential associations between exposures of any type and vasculitis, however, are complicated frequently by difficulties in obtaining reliable measurements of the levels of the relevant exposure, the likelihood of recall bias among patients who are diagnosed with vasculitis, and the choice of appropriate control groups.

Pathobiology

Table 291–4 illustrates the pathologic characteristics of selected forms of vasculitis. Specific pathologic features are discussed in the subsections on each disease. The type of inflammatory cell infiltrate in vasculitis is independent of the size of blood vessels involved. Mixed cell infiltrates in vasculitis are the rule rather than the exception, and histopathologic patterns of vasculitis may include leukocytoclasis (degranulation and destruction of neutrophils within blood vessel walls), granulomatous findings (with or without giant cells), lymphoplasmacytic infiltrates, varying degrees of eosinophilic infiltration, necrosis, and combinations of all of these findings.

Individual forms of vasculitis may demonstrate more than one set of histopathologic findings. To some degree, variations from case to case within the same diagnosis are dictated by the duration of the process at the time of biopsy. For example, giant cell arteritis may be associated with a lymphocytic infiltrate in the media and adventitia in some cases but also with a panarteritis characterized by granulomatous inflammation, giant cell formation, and intimal proliferation in others. Conversely, the same inflammatory pattern may occur in several types of disease. Leukocytoclastic vasculitis may be observed by light microscopy in such disparate disorders as medication-induced cutaneous leukocytoclastic angiitis, Henoch-Schönlein purpura, and Wegener's granulomatosis. Distinction among these disorders may be facilitated by histologic findings on biopsy, particularly through the performance of immunofluorescence studies, but it often requires rigorous clinicopathologic correlation.

Pathophysiology

Regardless of the size of the predominant blood vessels involved, some pathophysiologic mechanisms are common to many different forms of vasculitis. Immune complex deposition, for example, is present in several types of vasculitis that involve both medium-sized and small blood vessels. In this section, the general concepts related to the pathogenesis of large-vessel vasculitides are discussed separately from those of medium- and small-vessel vasculitides.

Large-Vessel Vasculitides

The pathologic process in large-vessel vasculitis appears to begin in the adventitia. Here, in both Takayasu's arteritis and giant cell arteritis, abundant numbers of activated T lymphocytes are found within inflamed arterial walls, centering on the adventitia. In Takayasu's arteritis, most of these T cells appear to be of the $CD8^+$ subtype. Current evidence suggests that the cytotoxic functions of these cells, mediated by perforin and granzyme B, contribute to smooth muscle cell damage in this disease. $CD4^+$ T-cell responses in Takayasu's arteritis have not been well defined.

In giant cell arteritis, much evidence now suggests an antigen-driven disease with the site of immunologic recognition events being the adventitia. $CD4^+$ T cells that secrete interferon-γ appear to be recruited to the adventitia by a specific antigen, the identity of which remains unknown. Both the T cells that orchestrate the transmural inflammation and the inciting antigens are theorized to reach the adventitia through the vasa vasorum. Subsequently, T-cell signals from the adventitia stimulate macrophages and multinucleated giant cells to elaborate an array of downstream mediators, such as metalloproteinase and platelet-derived growth factor. The results of this inflammatory cascade are granulomatous inflammation, fibrinoid necrosis, destruction of the internal elastic lamina, arterial wall hyperplasia, smooth muscle cell proliferation, intimal thickening, vascular occlusion, and, in some cases, weakening of the vessel wall leading to dilation and aneurysm formation.

TABLE 291–4 PATHOLOGIC CHARACTERISTICS OF SELECTED FORMS OF VASCULITIS

	Takayasu's Arteritis	Polyarteritis Nodosa	Wegener's Granulomatosis	Churg-Strauss Syndrome	Henoch-Schönlein Purpura	Cutaneous Leukocytoclastic Angiitis
Vessels involved	Elastic (large) or muscle (medium-sized) arteries	Medium-sized and small muscle arteries	Small arteries and veins; sometimes medium-sized vessels	Small arteries and veins; sometimes medium-sized vessels	Capillaries, venules, and arterioles	Capillaries, venules, and arterioles
Organ involvement	Aorta, aortic arch and major branches, and pulmonary arteries	Skin, peripheral nerve, gastrointestinal tract, and other viscera	Upper respiratory tract, lungs, kidneys, skin, eyes	Upper respiratory tract, lungs, heart, peripheral nerves	Skin, joints, gastrointestinal tract, kidneys	Skin, joints
Type of vasculitis and inflammatory cells	Granulomatous with some giant cells; fibrosis in chronic stages	Necrotizing, with mixed cellular infiltrate	Necrotizing or granulomatous (or both); mixed cellular infiltrate plus occasional eosinophils	Necrotizing or granulomatous (or both); prominent eosinophils and other mixed infiltrate	Leukocytoclastic, with some lymphocytes and variable eosinophils IgA deposits in affected tissues	Leukocytoclastic, with occasional eosinophils

Medium- and Small-Vessel Vasculitides

Several different pathophysiologic mechanisms are operative among the medium- and small-vessel vasculitides. In many cases, the mechanisms outlined in the following sections overlap.

Immune Complex–Mediated Vascular Injury

Immune complex–mediated tissue injury does not produce a single clinical syndrome but rather applies to many forms of vasculitis and overlaps with injuries caused by other immune mechanisms. Numerous variables influence the nature of immune complex–mediated injury, including the physical properties of the complexes (e.g., size), the ability of the immune complexes to activate complement, the antigen-to-antibody ratio, and the hemodynamic features of specific vascular beds. Immune complexes participate in the pathophysiologic process of some forms of both medium- and small-vessel vasculitis, including polyarteritis nodosa, cryoglobulinemia, Henoch-Schönlein purpura, cutaneous leukocytoclastic angiitis, and rheumatoid vasculitis.

Hepatitis B virus (HBV) surface antigen–antibody complexes are present in the circulation of patients with HBV-associated polyarteritis nodosa. Moreover, deposits of HBV surface antigen, immunoglobulin, and complement are found in the vasculitic lesions of muscle arteries, dermal capillaries, glomeruli, and vasa nervorum. In cryoglobulinemia associated with hepatitis C virus (HCV), anti-HCV antibodies and HCV RNA are detected in cryoprecipitates from the serum as well as in dermal and renal lesions.

Role of ANCAs

ANCAs are directed against antigens that reside within the primary granules of neutrophils and monocytes. Two types of ANCA are relevant to vasculitis: (1) those directed against proteinase 3 (PR3), known as PR3-ANCA; and (2) those directed against myeloperoxidase (MPO), termed MPO-ANCA. ANCAs interact with cytokines, neutrophils, monocytes, and other elements of the immune system to amplify ongoing inflammation in certain forms of vasculitis. However, evidence for a primary role of ANCAs in the etiology of human disease associated with pauci-immune vasculitis is still absent.

The three types of vasculitis often associated with ANCAs are Wegener's granulomatosis, microscopic polyangiitis, and Churg-Strauss syndrome. Wegener's granulomatosis is typically associated with PR3-ANCA, which cause a cytoplasmic (C-ANCA) pattern of staining on immunofluorescence testing of serum. In a minority of Wegener's granulomatosis cases, however, patients have MPO-ANCA, which cause perinuclear (P-ANCA) staining on immunofluorescence testing. Between 60 and 90% of all patients with Wegener's granulomatosis are ANCA positive. Seventy percent of patients with microscopic polyangiitis have ANCAs, typically MPO-ANCA. Only about 50% of patients with Churg-Strauss syndrome are ANCA positive, with a slight tendency toward anti-MPO antibodies. One striking and still unexplained feature of ANCA-associated vasculitis is that patients virtually never have antibodies to both PR3 and MPO.

In Wegener's granulomatosis, abnormal cytokine regulation interacts with the production of ANCA to fuel the inflammatory response. T_H1 cytokines such as interferon-γ, interleukin-12, and tumor necrosis factor (TNF) appear to play important roles. Under the direction of interleukin-12, $CD4^+$ T cells from patients with Wegener's granulomatosis produce elevated levels of TNF, and peripheral blood mononuclear cells secrete increased amounts of interferon-γ. Serum levels of soluble receptors for TNF are elevated in patients with active Wegener's granulomatosis and normalize with the induction of remission. In vitro priming of activated neutrophils with TNF markedly enhances the ability of ANCA to stimulate neutrophil degranulation. Despite the strong rationale for anti-TNF strategies in Wegener's granulomatosis, however, a randomized trial of etanercept showed no efficacy in the maintenance of disease remissions. More current investigational approaches to therapy include B-cell depletion.

Superantigen Model

The degree of immune activation in Kawasaki's disease and the acute but generally self-limited nature of this illness imply a potential role for superantigens. Superantigens are proteins produced by microbial pathogens (e.g., *Staphylococcus aureus* or *Streptococcus* species) that are capable of stimulating large populations of T cells in an unrestricted, class II major histocompatibility complex (MHC)–dependent manner. Superantigens bind directly to conserved amino acid residues outside the antigen-binding groove on class II MHC molecules, thereby selectively stimulating T cells that express particular β-chain variable gene segments. Through the binding of this MHC-superantigen complex to its cognate T-cell receptors, as many as 20% of circulating lymphocytes may become activated, leading to a potentially enormous outpouring of cytokines. With regard to the etiology of Kawasaki's disease, substantial attention has focused on toxic shock syndrome toxin 1, an exotoxin produced by *S. aureus*. Superantigens have also been postulated to play roles in the susceptibility to disease flares in Wegener's granulomatosis. Nasal carriage of *S. aureus* and superantigens associated with these organisms has been linked to a greater likelihood of disease flares in some studies.

Antiendothelial Cell Antibodies

Antiendothelial cell antibodies can induce endothelial cell injury and lysis through either complement-mediated cytotoxicity or antibody-dependent cellular cytotoxicity. Both of these mechanisms have been demonstrated to cause endothelial injury in in vitro assays employing sera from patients with systemic vasculitis. The ability of these antibodies to damage endothelial cells is an appealing argument for their potential role in forms of vasculitis in which the endothelium is the focus of the inflammation (as opposed to the more external vessel wall layers). However, the true relevance of antiendothelial cell antibodies to human disease and their importance within the larger context of other disease mechanisms remain unclear.

Systemic Vasculitis and Infection

Since the 1970s, persistent HBV infection has been linked to some cases of polyarteritis nodosa. During the 1990s, firm links were established between HCV infections and 90% of the cases of essential mixed cryoglobulinemia. These strong relationships between two known viruses and clinical vasculitis syndromes, as well as animal models of vasculitis associated with viral infections (e.g., the induction of large-vessel arteritis in laboratory mice by gammaherpesvirus 68), heighten the likelihood that similar mechanisms are operative in other forms of vasculitis in humans.

Clinical Manifestations

Large-Vessel Vasculitides

Takayasu's Arteritis

Takayasu's arteritis has a predilection for the aorta and its major branches. In contrast to atherosclerosis, which is characterized by focal, irregular lesions, the lesions of Takayasu's arteritis are long, smooth, tapered stenoses (Fig. 291–1A); the most commonly involved arteries are the subclavian and innominate arteries. Because of its ability to obliterate peripheral pulses (particularly in the upper extremities), Takayasu's arteritis has been termed "pulseless disease." Exuberant collateral circulation tends to develop in response to the narrowing of major arteries, making the loss of digits or limbs from ischemia extremely rare. The pulmonary circulation is involved in approximately 50% of cases of Takayasu's arteritis.

Patients with severe narrowing of the aortic arch vessels supplying the head may develop Takayasu's retinopathy, a hypotension retinopathy leading to neovascularization. In contrast, patients with prolonged hypertension associated with renal artery stenosis demonstrate the classic ocular features of hypertension: copper wiring and multiple retinal infarctions. Takayasu's arteritis involvement of the ascending aorta may lead to aortic dilation, aortic regurgitation, aneurysm formation, and aortic rupture (Fig. 291–1B). Takayasu's arteritis may also cause intrinsic cardiac disease, including cardiomyopathy and valvar dysfunction secondary to valvulitis.

The cornerstone of treatment of Takayasu's arteritis is corticosteroids. For patients with marked symptoms and signs of an inflammatory phase, prednisone (1 mg/kg/day) is usually effective in controlling the disease. This dose should be tapered within 8 to 12 weeks to less than 20 mg/day and ultimately to less than 10 mg/day as a maintenance dose. In patients with Takayasu's arteritis that is refractory to moderate doses of corticosteroids, methotrexate (up to 25 mg/week) and mycophenolate mofetil (1500 mg twice daily) may be useful.

Cogan's Syndrome

The combination of inflammatory eye disease and vestibuloauditory dysfunction is the sine qua non of Cogan's syndrome. In addition to inflammatory disease of the eyes and ears, up to 15% of patients with Cogan's syndrome have vasculitis involving medium-sized to large blood

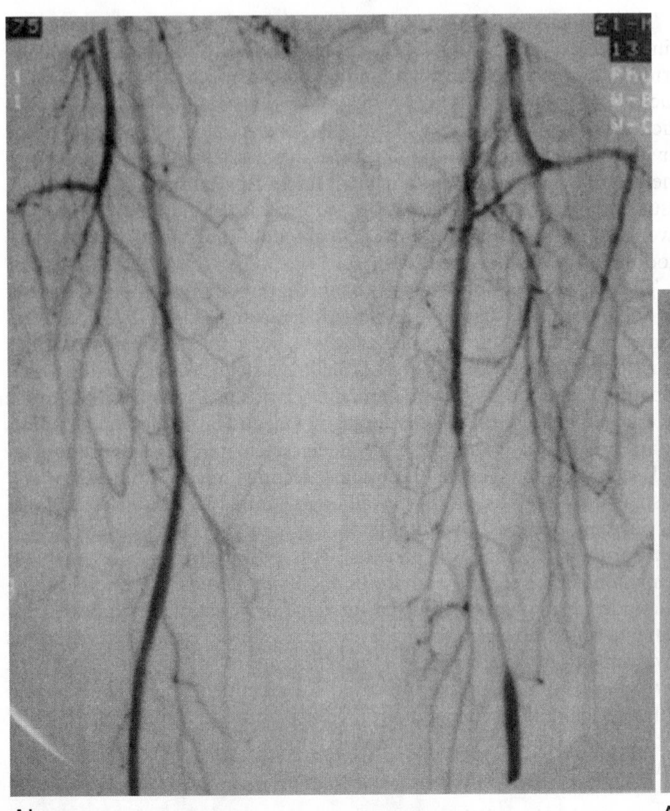
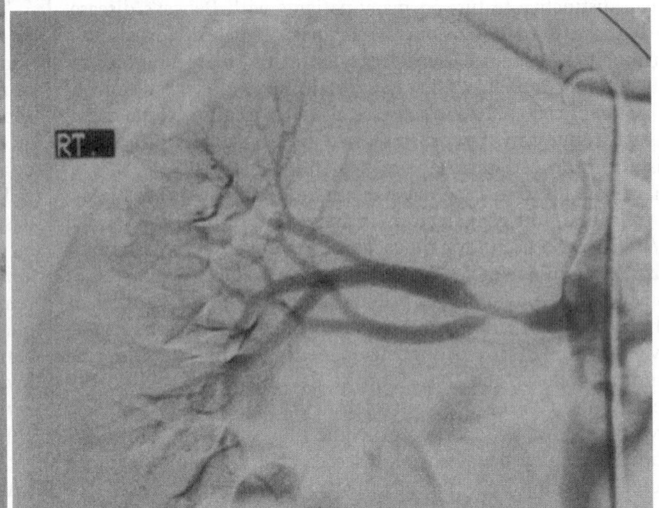

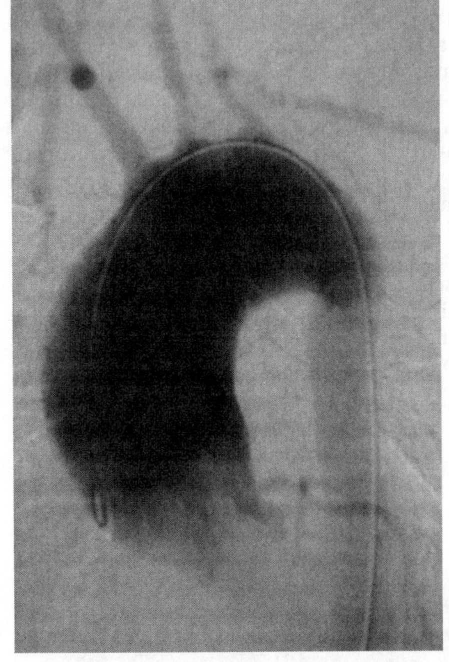

FIGURE 291–1 • Large-vessel disease in Takayasu's arteritis. A, Long, smooth tapering in the left common femoral artery (i) and the right renal artery (ii). **B,** Dilation of the ascending aorta. Aortic regurgitation necessitated an aortic valve replacement and replacement of the ascending aorta with a Gore-Tex graft.

vessels. Although the ocular manifestations vary, the classic presentation is the combination of interstitial keratitis and sensorineural hearing loss. Cogan's syndrome may appear first in either the eyes or the ears. Although intervals as long as 1 to 2 years have been described between the start of disease in one organ and the appearance of disease in the other, the time between disease manifestations in these organs is usually only a matter of months. The vascular disease in Cogan's syndrome resembles Takayasu's arteritis. Medium- and large-vessel arteritis may lead to a host of complications in patients with Cogan's syndrome, including aortitis, aortic regurgitation, coronary artery inflammation, mesenteric vasculitis, limb claudication, and other manifestations. Interstitial keratitis generally responds well to topical corticosteroid therapy. Rapidly progressive sensorineural hearing loss requires early, aggressive therapy with high doses of systemic corticosteroids. Cytotoxic agents may be added for patients with suboptimal responses to corticosteroids who still have salvageable hearing. For many patients with Cogan's syndrome, the prognosis for the retention of functional hearing during the long term is poor. Many become candidates for cochlear implants.

Behçet's Disease

Behçet's disease may affect small, medium, and large vessels, in either the venous or the arterial circulation. The most typical lesions in Behçet's disease are mucocutaneous, reflecting the involvement of small blood vessels. The triad of recurrent mouth ulcers, genital ulcers, and eye inflammation is the classic presentation. The criteria for diagnosis of the International Study Group for Behçet's Disease consist of one required manifestation—recurrent oral ulceration—plus at least two of the following: recurrent genital ulceration, characteristic eye or skin lesions, or a pathergy reaction. However, the spectrum of Behçet's disease encompasses many disease manifestations not included in these criteria. Large-vessel complications of Behçet's disease may include aneurysms in the pulmonary and systemic arterial systems. Venous complications include deep venous, vena caval, portohepatic vein, and cerebral sinus thromboses. Pathergy—the development of pustules at the sites of sterile needle pricks—is a distinctive feature in many patients with Behçet's disease, particularly those of Turkish origin. The arthritis of Behçet's disease is a nondeforming, oligoarticular, asymmetrical arthritis of large joints. Gastrointestinal lesions in Behçet's disease typically consist of ulcerations of the distal ileum or cecum. Crohn's disease, which can cause genital ulcers as well as gastrointestinal tract disease, may be particularly difficult to distinguish from Behçet's disease.

Colchicine (up to 1.5 to 2 mg/day) is sometimes effective for the treatment of mild oral and genital ulcers in Behçet's disease. Thalidomide (100 mg/day) is also useful for mucocutaneous disease manifestations. Severe disease in any organ system almost always requires high doses of prednisone (e.g., 1 mg/kg/day). Cyclophosphamide (2 mg/kg/day) or chlorambucil (0.2 mg/kg/day, increased as tolerated) is indicated for the most severe forms of uveitis or meningoencephalitis. Azathioprine (2 mg/kg/day), cyclosporine (3 to 5 mg/kg/day in two divided doses), methotrexate (up to 25 mg/week), interferon alfa (3 million to 5 million units three times a week), and pentoxifylline (300 mg three times/day) have also been employed in Behçet's disease. TNF inhibitors have not been studied in randomized trials of patients with Behçet's disease.

Medium-Vessel Vasculitides

Polyarteritis Nodosa

First described in 1866 by Kussmaul and Maier, polyarteritis nodosa was the only widely recognized form of vasculitis for decades. The 1994 International Consensus Conference on the Nomenclature of Systemic Vasculitides defined classic polyarteritis nodosa as necrotizing inflammation of medium-sized or small arteries that spares the smallest blood vessels (arterioles, venules, and capillaries). Polyarteritis nodosa has a striking predilection for certain organs, particularly the skin, peripheral nerves, gastrointestinal tract, and kidneys.

Polyarteritis nodosa usually begins with nonspecific symptoms that may include malaise, fatigue, fever, myalgias, and arthralgias. Overt signs of vasculitis may not occur until weeks or months after onset of the first symptoms. Skin lesions of polyarteritis nodosa include livedo reticularis, subcutaneous nodules, ulcers, and digital gangrene. A majority of patients with polyarteritis nodosa (>80% in some series) have vasculitic neuropathy, typically in the pattern of a mononeuritis multiplex.

The classic gastrointestinal manifestation of polyarteritis nodosa is "intestinal angina," the occurrence of postprandial abdominal pain. Polyarteritis nodosa can also affect individual gastrointestinal tract organs, such as the gallbladder or appendix, presenting as cholecystitis or appendicitis. The typical renal manifestation of polyarteritis nodosa is vasculitic involvement of the medium-sized intrarenal arteries, leading to renin-mediated hypertension and renal infarctions. Cardiac lesions, which usually remain subclinical, may lead to myocardial infarction or congestive heart failure. For reasons that are not understood, polyarteritis nodosa usually spares the lungs.

The diagnosis of polyarteritis nodosa requires either a tissue biopsy or an angiogram that demonstrates microaneurysms (Fig. 291–2). Simultaneous nerve and muscle biopsies (e.g., sural nerve and gastrocnemius muscle) are of high yield if there is a clinical suspicion of vasculitic neuropathy. The pathologic changes in polyarteritis nodosa are limited to the arterial circulation; the lesions are segmental and favor the branch points of arteries. In gross pathologic specimens, aneurysmal bulges of the arterial wall may be visible. Histologic sections reveal infiltration and destruction of the blood vessel wall by inflammatory cells, accompanied by fibrinoid necrosis. Granulomatous inflammation is absent.

Approximately half of patients with polyarteritis nodosa achieve remissions or cures with high doses of corticosteroids alone. Cyclophosphamide (2 mg/kg/day, adjusted for renal dysfunction) is indicated for patients whose disease is refractory to corticosteroids or who have serious involvement of major organs. In recent years, therapeutic regimens involving lamivudine have improved the treatment of HBV-associated polyarteritis nodosa substantially. Because of increasing use of the HBV vaccine, less than 10% of polyarteritis nodosa cases now are associated with HBV infections.

Rheumatoid Vasculitis

Rheumatoid vasculitis is a severe complication of rheumatoid arthritis that sometimes occurs in patients with long-standing, erosive disease. The typical patient has a history of seropositive disease, rheumatoid nodules, and arthritis that is no longer active. Risk factors for rheumatoid vasculitis include male gender; a high titer of rheumatoid factor; history of erosive, destructive arthritis; presence of rheumatoid nodules; history of extra-articular disease features (e.g., scleritis, pericarditis); occurrence of Felty's syndrome; and possibly possession of the HLA-DRB1*04 allele. Rheumatoid vasculitis closely mimics polyarteritis nodosa and usually requires treatment with cyclophosphamide and prednisone. In addition to the polyarteritis nodosa–like form of rheumatoid vasculitis, a milder form of vasculitis exists in rheumatoid arthritis. This benign form typically leads to minor nail bed infarctions but does not herald the onset of systemic vasculitis and does not require additional treatment beyond that required for the underlying arthritis.

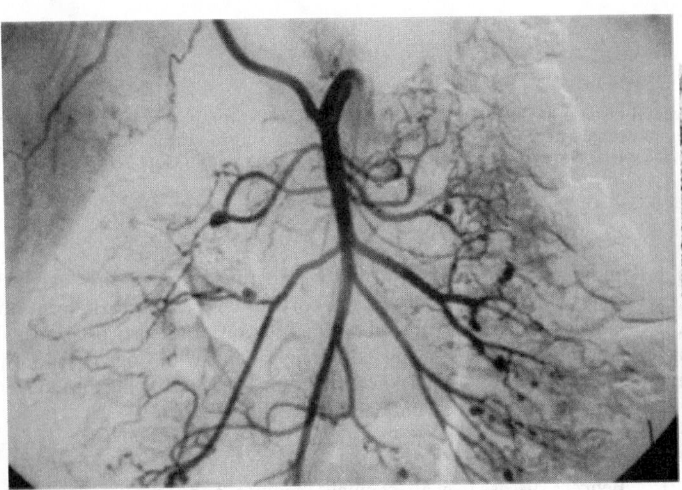

A

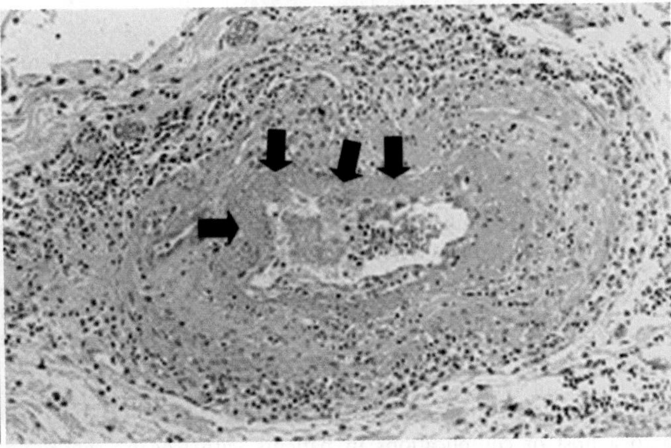

B

FIGURE 291–2 • Vasculitis of medium-sized arteries in polyarteritis nodosa. A, Mesenteric angiogram showing numerous aneurysms in medium-sized arteries. **B,** Fibrinoid necrosis in a jejunal artery from a patient who required surgical resection of necrotic bowel.

Buerger's Disease

Buerger's disease, also known as thromboangiitis obliterans, has a remarkably strong yet poorly understood association with cigarette smoking. Buerger's disease does not occur in the absence of exposure to tobacco. The vessels affected by Buerger's disease are the distal, medium-sized arteries and veins, particularly vessels at the levels of the ankles and wrists. The disease is characterized by thrombotic obliterations that begin distally and proceed proximally. Buerger's disease tends to be segmental in nature, involving 5- to 10-cm lengths of blood vessels. Arterial obliteration leads to the development of collateral vessels with a "corkscrew" appearance on angiography. Vascular occlusion in Buerger's disease often leads to the loss of digits and, if smoking persists, to loss of larger amounts of tissue (e.g., hands or feet). Despite the intense involvement of the extremities in Buerger's disease, internal organ disease almost never occurs.

Complete abstinence from tobacco is essential to the treatment of Buerger's disease. Failure to stop smoking is associated with a dramatic increase in the risk of limb loss by amputation. No other therapeutic interventions, including corticosteroids and anticoagulation, have dramatic effects on Buerger's disease.

Kawasaki's Disease

Kawasaki's disease occurs exclusively in young children. Because of its striking mucocutaneous findings and lymphadenopathy, Kawasaki's disease is also known as mucocutaneous lymph node syndrome. Features of Kawasaki's disease include high fevers, cervical adenopathy, conjunctival congestion, buccal erythema, prominence of the tongue papillae ("strawberry tongue"), polymorphous truncal rash, erythema of the palms and soles, and desquamation of skin from the fingertips occurring days to weeks into the illness. In its acuity and severity, Kawasaki's disease resembles toxic shock syndrome and scarlet fever, both of which are mediated by superantigens (see Pathophysiology).

In a small number of patients with Kawasaki's disease, panvasculitis in the coronary vessels leads to acute cardiac complications. Coronary arteritis leads to narrowing of the vessel lumen by the migration of myointimal cells from the media through the fragmented internal elastic lamina. Direct complications include aneurysmal dilation and thrombosis of the coronary arteries, leading to myocardial infarction and possibly to death (in 1 to 2% of patients with Kawasaki's disease during the acute illness). Late mortality from myocardial infarction may occur from the thrombosis of coronary artery aneurysms formed during the initial inflammatory stage.

The recommended therapeutic regimen in Kawasaki's disease is the combination of intravenous immune globulin (IVIG; 400 mg/kg/day on 4 consecutive days) and acetylsalicylic acid (100 mg/kg/day, lowered to 3 to 5 mg/kg/day after resolution of the fever). IVIG prevents the formation of coronary aneurysms in most cases. Corticosteroids are reserved for salvage therapy in patients whose treatment with IVIG and acetylsalicylic acid has failed.

Vasculitis of the Central Nervous System

Central nervous system (CNS) vasculitis includes two major categories of disease: (1) true CNS vasculitis, also known as primary angiitis of the CNS (PACNS), and (2) "benign" angiopathy of the CNS (BACNS). BACNS should be regarded as a vasculopathy, not a true vasculitis. Both PACNS and BACNS are syndromes that have many potential causes.

Primary Angiitis of the Central Nervous System

Patients with PACNS may manifest the triad of headache, encephalopathy, and multifocal strokes that the disorder develops in a subacute fashion. The first symptom is usually headache, often severe and sometimes associated with nausea and vomiting. If they are not treated, almost all patients eventually develop lethargy, confusion, and memory loss. Some patients develop multifocal strokes, seizures, evidence of increased intracranial pressure, or myelopathy. The results of routine laboratory tests (e.g., the erythrocyte sedimentation rate) are often normal in PACNS. Lumbar puncture demonstrates abnormalities of the cerebrospinal fluid in approximately 80% of cases, usually a modest monocytosis and elevated protein.

The classic abnormality on angiography in PACNS is the "string of beads" pattern produced by segmental arterial narrowing alternating with dilations. Vascular occlusions, collateral formation, and prolonged circulation time may also be seen. However, no angiographic pattern is pathognomonic, and there is a significant tendency to overdiagnose "vasculitis" on angiographic grounds alone. Other disorders, particularly those that cause vasospasm, can produce identical angiographic abnormalities. Angiograms are falsely negative in about 35% of patients with PACNS. Magnetic resonance imaging is more sensitive than computed tomography in the evaluation of possible CNS vasculitis. Typical findings are infarctions in more than one vascular territory. Hemorrhagic lesions and mass lesions also occur.

Biopsies in patients with PACNS should be directed toward radiologically evident lesions. The yield of biopsy procedures may be increased by sampling the leptomeninges as well at the underlying cortex. Histopathologic specimens of the leptomeninges and cortex in PACNS show vasculitis of the small and medium-sized arteries. Prednisone and cyclophosphamide are appropriate for treatment of patients who have abnormal findings on brain biopsy. Treatment courses of 6 to 12 months are recommended.

Benign Angiopathy of the Central Nervous System

An increasing number of cases of CNS "vasculitis" are reported in which the diagnosis is based on angiography alone, without the performance of a brain biopsy. Patients diagnosed in this fashion differ from biopsy-confirmed cases in that 80% are women, the onset of their symptoms is comparatively abrupt, their neurologic signs are less severe (encephalopathy is less common), and their lumbar punctures are normal. The term *benign* may be misleading, however, because strokes and significant neurologic dysfunction sometimes occur in BACNS. Yet patients with BACNS are less likely than those with PACNS to require cyclophosphamide or prolonged treatment with corticosteroids.

In three fourths of the patients, brain magnetic resonance imaging detects abnormalities. The typical angiographic findings in BACNS—vascular narrowing and beading—are generally indistinguishable from those of PACNS and conditions that mimic PACNS. The most distinctive angiographic feature of BACNS is that the abnormalities are completely reversible, usually within 4 to 8 weeks. Thus, these abnormalities are believed to reflect vasospasm rather than true vasculitis. In the evaluation of patients with potential BACNS, the essential diagnostic step is often repeated CNS angiography at 4 to 8 weeks. Angiographic abnormalities due to BACNS should resolve in this interval.

Prednisone alone (beginning at 1 mg/kg/day) is adequate therapy for some patients with BACNS. The corticosteroids can be tapered during 3 to 6 months. Calcium-channel blockers have been added in attempts to reduce vasospasm. Cytotoxic therapy is not indicated in BACNS.

Small-Vessel Vasculitides

Wegener's Granulomatosis

Classic Wegener's granulomatosis involves the upper respiratory tract, the lungs, and the kidneys. Distinctive features may also occur in the eyes, ears, and other organs. The three pathologic hallmarks of Wegener's granulomatosis are (1) granulomatous inflammation in the upper or lower respiratory tract, (2) necrotizing vasculitis affecting arteries or veins, and (3) segmental glomerulonephritis, associated with necrosis and thrombosis of capillary loops, with or without granulomatous lesions.

Approximately 90% of patients with Wegener's granulomatosis have nasal involvement, including crusting, bleeding, and obstruction. Cartilaginous inflammation may lead to nasal septal perforation and collapse of the nasal bridge ("saddle nose" deformity). Erosive sinus disease and subglottic stenosis (narrowing of the trachea just below the vocal cords) are highly characteristic of Wegener's granulomatosis.

Two principal forms of ear disease, conductive and sensorineural hearing loss, are typical of Wegener's granulomatosis. Conductive hearing loss, caused by middle ear disease, is more common. Orbital masses ("pseudotumors" that develop behind the eye), scleritis, and peripheral ulcerative keratitis are the most dangerous ocular lesions of Wegener's granulomatosis, but uveitis, episcleritis, and conjunctivitis also occur. The clinical manifestations of Wegener's granulomatosis in the lung range from asymptomatic nodules to fulminant alveolar hemorrhage. The most common radiographic findings are pulmonary infiltrates and nodules. The infiltrates, which may wax and wane, are often misdiagnosed initially as pneumonia. Nodules are usually multiple and bilateral and often result in cavitation.

Renal involvement is the most ominous clinical manifestation of Wegener's granulomatosis. The clinical presentation of renal disease in Wegener's granulomatosis is that of rapidly progressive

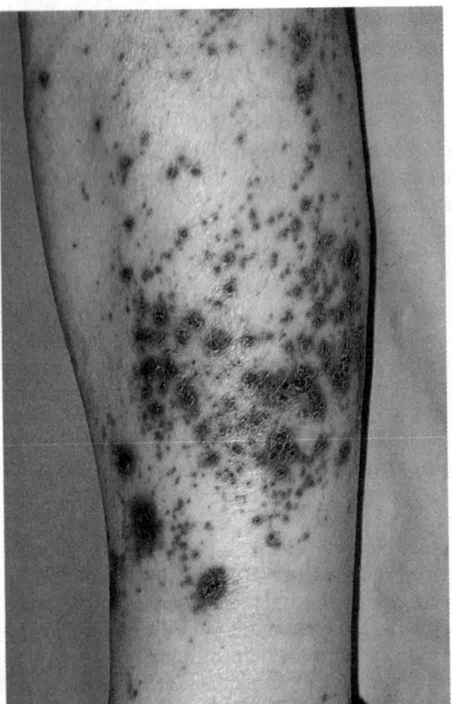

FIGURE 291–3 • Cutaneous small-vessel vasculitis showing palpable purpuric lesions with necrosis and crusting. In this patient, very rarely, the trigger was extensive crusted scabies.

glomerulonephritis: hematuria, red blood cell casts, and proteinuria (usually non-nephrotic). Without appropriate therapy, end-stage renal disease may ensue within days to weeks.

Sixty percent of patients with Wegener's granulomatosis have musculoskeletal symptoms during their disease courses. The presenting complaint is frequently arthralgias or arthritis. Splinter hemorrhages, digital ischemia, and digital gangrene may occur in Wegener's granulomatosis. Skin lesions in Wegener's granulomatosis include the full panoply of lesions associated with cutaneous vasculitis, including purpura (Fig. 291–3). Cutaneous nodules over the extensor surfaces of joints, particularly the elbow, may mimic rheumatoid nodules. Meningeal inflammation, presenting with headaches, cranial neuropathies, and a clinical picture compatible with chronic meningitis, is perhaps the most common CNS manifestation of Wegener's granulomatosis. Mononeuritis multiplex may affect the peripheral nervous system. Finally, patients with Wegener's granulomatosis are now known to be at increased risk for venous thrombotic events (deep venous thromboses and pulmonary emboli), with an incidence rate up to seven times higher than that of patients with systemic lupus erythematosus.

Wegener's granulomatosis is the prototype of conditions associated with ANCA. Positive results of immunofluorescence tests for ANCA in either the cytoplasmic or perinuclear pattern should be confirmed by enzyme immunoassays for antibodies to either PR3 or MPO. An ANCA-negative assay sample does not preclude the diagnosis of Wegener's granulomatosis because a substantial minority of patients (between 15 and 40% overall) lack these antibodies. Furthermore, ANCA titers do not correlate reliably with disease activity. Titers of ANCA usually decline after the institution of immunosuppressive therapy but do not always become negative. Despite advances in ANCA testing techniques, the cornerstone of diagnosis in Wegener's granulomatosis remains the correlation of typical clinical features with histopathologic patterns.

Manifestations of Wegener's granulomatosis that constitute immediate threats either to the function of a vital organ or to the patient's life require urgent treatment with both a cytotoxic agent (usually cyclophosphamide, 2 mg/kg orally daily) and high doses of corticosteroids (1 mg/kg orally daily, tapered during 6 to 12 months). Limited forms of Wegener's granulomatosis may respond to the combination of methotrexate (up to 25 mg/week) and corticosteroids. Methotrexate is not appropriate for first-line treatment of patients with severe involvement of the kidney, lung, or other vital organs. The first randomized, placebo-controlled trial in Wegener's granulomatosis in the United States—a comparison of etanercept in addition to standard therapy with standard therapy alone—demonstrated no benefit of specific TNF inhibition for the maintenance of disease remissions. A more recent investigational approach centers on B-cell depletion.

Microscopic Polyangiitis

Microscopic polyangiitis is characterized by (1) nongranulomatous, necrotizing vasculitis with few or no immune deposits, (2) involvement of small (and possibly medium-sized) blood vessels in the arterial or venous circulation, and (3) tropism for the kidneys and lungs. Many cases of small-vessel vasculitis once regarded as polyarteritis nodosa are now classified more properly as microscopic polyangiitis. In contrast to polyarteritis nodosa, an ANCA-negative disorder, 70% of microscopic polyangiitis patients are ANCA positive. Thus, microscopic polyangiitis is often considered to fall within a spectrum of "ANCA-associated" vasculitis. The ANCAs in microscopic polyangiitis are usually directed against MPO and cause a perinuclear pattern of staining on immunofluorescence testing (P-ANCA). Other components of the ANCA-associated vasculitis spectrum include Wegener's granulomatosis, the Churg-Strauss syndrome, and renal-limited vasculitis.

Microscopic polyangiitis is commonly implicated in pulmonary-renal syndromes. A dominant feature of microscopic polyangiitis is necrotizing glomerulonephritis, which occurs in nearly 80% of patients. Glomerulonephritis leads to crescent formation, red blood cell cast formation within the renal tubules, and red blood cell casts in the urinary sediment. Without prompt treatment, rapidly progressive glomerulonephritis leads to irreversible renal damage. Pulmonary capillaritis may lead rapidly to life-threatening alveolar hemorrhage. Glomerulonephritis (79%), weight loss (73%), mononeuritis multiplex (58%), and fever (55%) are the most common disease manifestations of microscopic polyangiitis. Upper respiratory tract symptoms in microscopic polyangiitis are much milder than those associated with Wegener's granulomatosis.

The approach to the treatment of microscopic polyangiitis is similar to the treatment of Wegener's granulomatosis. Some evidence indicates, however, that microscopic polyangiitis may be treated effectively and more safely with intravenous cyclophosphamide dosed intermittently (e.g., 750 mg/m^2 of body surface area every month) than with the daily cyclophosphamide regimen preferred for Wegener's granulomatosis. Cyclophosphamide may be continued for 6 to 12 months or replaced by methotrexate or azathioprine at an earlier time once the disease has clearly entered remission.

Churg-Strauss Syndrome

Churg-Strauss syndrome is an eosinophil-rich form of granulomatous inflammation that involves the respiratory tract and other organs. The disease is associated with necrotizing vasculitis of small to medium-sized vessels. Two hallmarks of Churg-Strauss syndrome are asthma and eosinophilia. Several phases of Churg-Strauss syndrome are described as follows:

- a prodromal phase, characterized by the presence of allergic disease (typically asthma or allergic rhinitis), which may last months to many years;
- an eosinophilia–tissue infiltration phase, in which remarkably high peripheral eosinophilia may occur and tissue infiltration by eosinophils is observed in the lung, gastrointestinal tract, and other tissues; and
- a vasculitic phase, in which systemic necrotizing vasculitis afflicts a wide range of organs, ranging from the heart and lungs to peripheral nerves and skin.

Churg-Strauss syndrome must be distinguished from a group of hypereosinophilic disorders: Löffler's syndrome, the hypereosinophil syndrome, eosinophilic gastroenteritis, chronic eosinophilic pneumonia, and eosinophilic leukemia. The two phenomena of leukotriene antagonist use and the occurrence of Churg-Strauss syndrome are probably related more to the reduction in corticosteroid dose afforded by leukotriene antagonists (and the resultant unmasking of latent Churg-Strauss syndrome) than to any truly causal relationship. Patients with mild disease may be treated with prednisone. Those with evidence of neurologic, cardiac, renal, or gastrointestinal involvement should be treated with cyclophosphamide in addition to corticosteroids. Although clinical remissions may be obtained in more than 90% of patients with Churg-Strauss syndrome, disease recurrences are seen in 25%. In most cases, relapses are heralded by the return of eosinophilia. Approximately 50% of cases of Churg-Strauss syndrome are associated with ANCA, usually MPO-ANCA, but the percentage may be higher among untreated patients.

Henoch-Schönlein Purpura

Henoch-Schönlein purpura (HSP) is characterized by non-thrombocytopenic purpura, arthritis, abdominal pain, and glomerulonephritis. The histopathologic findings are those of a leukocytoclastic vasculitis with IgA deposition. HSP can develop at any age, but 80 to 90% of the cases occur in children. Although the cause is unknown, the disease's seasonal variation and the fact that two thirds of patients with HSP experience antecedent acute upper respiratory illnesses suggest an infectious trigger. The diagnosis of HSP can be confirmed only by demonstration of IgA deposition within and around blood vessel walls.

The classic HSP patient presents with the acute onset of fever, palpable purpura on the lower extremities and buttocks, abdominal pain, arthritis, and hematuria. The clinician must be alert to the possibility of HSP even when only parts of the syndrome are present. In some patients, the cutaneous involvement takes the form of maculopapular lesions, blisters, and ulcers. HSP causes arthralgias or arthritis in large joints, especially the knees and ankles and, to a lesser degree, the wrists and elbows. Migratory patterns are typical. The abdominal pain is often colicky and may worsen after eating. Some patients experience nausea, vomiting, and upper or lower gastrointestinal bleeding. Gastrointestinal disease and arthritis may precede the onset of purpura, leading to diagnostic confusion and occasionally to exploratory abdominal surgery to exclude an acute abdomen. In contrast, glomerulonephritis almost always follows the appearance of skin disease. Approximately 60% of patients have elevated levels of serum IgA. Although there are two subclasses of IgA, HSP is associated with increases only in IgA1.

Most patients with HSP, especially children, have a self-limited disease that lasts an average of 4 weeks. Corticosteroids ameliorate the joint and gastrointestinal symptoms in most cases and improve the cutaneous manifestations in some. The efficacy of corticosteroids in the glomerulonephritis of HSP is controversial. Uncontrolled studies suggest that high-dose methylprednisolone, followed by oral prednisone combined with azathioprine or cyclophosphamide, may be useful in severe glomerulonephritis associated with HSP.

Cutaneous Leukocytoclastic Angiitis

Cutaneous leukocytoclastic angiitis has also been termed hypersensitivity vasculitis. Cutaneous leukocytoclastic angiitis is the preferred name because no hypersensitivity or allergy is evident in many cases. Histories of exposure to new medications or to infections may be elicited, however, and immune complex deposition is central to the pathophysiologic process. Although it is occasionally associated with synovitis, other signs of systemic involvement are absent.

The skin lesions in cutaneous leukocytoclastic angiitis occur in "crops" because of identical timing in an exposure to the inciting antigen. The lesions typically occur first in dependent regions, such as the lower extremities or buttocks. The rash may be asymptomatic but is usually accompanied by burning or tingling sensations. A wide array of skin lesions may occur, including palpable purpura, papules, urticaria-angioedema, erythema multiforme, vesicles, pustules, necrosis, and (rarely) ulcers. Most cases of cutaneous leukocytoclastic angiitis with clearly identified precipitants resolve during 1 to 4 weeks, often with some residual hyperpigmentation. A subset of patients, however, has recurrent disease that remains confined to the skin and requires prolonged therapy.

Keys to the management of cutaneous leukocytoclastic angiitis include (1) exclusion of any underlying form of vasculitis that may cause subclinical involvement of other organs and (2) removal of any agent (e.g., a medication) that may have triggered the vasculitis. For patients in whom a precipitant can be identified, removal of the offending agent usually leads to resolution of the vasculitis within days to weeks. The type, intensity, and duration of drug therapy are based on the degree of disease severity. Mild cases may be treated simply with leg elevation and the administration of nonsteroidal anti-inflammatory agents (and/or H_1 antihistamines). For persistent disease not associated with cutaneous gangrene, colchicine, hydroxychloroquine, or dapsone may be tried. For severe cases, immunosuppressive agents may be indicated, generally beginning with corticosteroids. Azathioprine is commonly used as a steroid-sparing agent.

Urticarial Vasculitis

At least three subtypes of urticarial vasculitis are known: (1) normocomplementemic, a form that is generally idiopathic and benign (which may be viewed as a manifestation of cutaneous leukocytoclastic angiitis); (2) hypocomplementemic, a form that is often associated with a systemic inflammatory disease; and (3) hypocomplementemic urticarial vasculitis syndrome (HUVS), a potentially severe condition usually associated with autoantibodies to the collagen-like region of C1q. Most patients with the hypocomplementemic subtype have an underlying systemic disorder, such as systemic lupus erythematosus or Sjögren's syndrome. Many HUVS patients have C1q "precipitins," that is, IgG autoantibodies to the collagen-like region of C1q. The role of anti-C1q antibodies in disease pathogenesis remains unclear.

The lesions of urticarial vasculitis must be distinguished from the far more common chronic idiopathic urticaria. Unlike idiopathic urticaria, the lesions of urticarial vasculitis last more than 48 hours, often have a purpuric component (i.e., they do not blanch), and resolve with postinflammatory hyperpigmentation. In urticarial vasculitis, lesions associated with vasculitis are often accompanied by stinging or burning. Urticarial vasculitis affects the capillaries and postcapillary venules, showing leukocytoclastic vasculitis on light microscopy. Immunofluorescence reveals both immunoglobulin and complement deposition in or around blood vessels of the upper dermis or the dermoepidermal junction.

Patients with urticarial vasculitis whose serum complement levels remain normal during attacks often have self-limited disease and require little therapy. Other cases, especially HUVS, may cause life-threatening involvement of the lungs or other organs and require periods of intensive immunosuppression. Treatment decisions in HUVS must be individualized according to the patient's clinical status.

Cryoglobulinemia

Cryoglobulins are antibodies that precipitate from serum under conditions of cold and resolubilize on rewarming. Cryoglobulins are classified into types I, II, and III on the basis of whether monoclonality and rheumatoid factor activity (the ability to bind to the Fc portion of IgG) are present. Type I cryoglobulins, which are monoclonal but lack rheumatoid factor activity, are associated with certain hematopoietic malignant neoplasms and often lead to hyperviscosity rather than to vasculitis. In contrast, type II and type III cryoglobulins may be associated with systemic vasculitis involving small (and often medium-sized) blood vessels. Vasculitis results from the deposition of cryoglobulin-containing immune complexes in blood vessel walls and the activation of complement.

Cryoglobulin types II and III are termed mixed cryoglobulins because they consist of both IgG and IgM antibodies. The IgM components in both type II and type III cryoglobulinemia possess rheumatoid factor activity (i.e., assays for rheumatoid factor are positive). Whereas the IgM component in type II cryoglobulin is monoclonal, the IgM in type III cryoglobulin is polyclonal. Ninety percent of patients with vasculitis secondary to mixed cryoglobulins are hypocomplementemic, with C4 levels characteristically more depressed than C3. Infection with HCV accounts for at least 80% of the vasculitis cases associated with mixed cryoglobulins.

The optimal therapy for most cases of cryoglobulinemic vasculitis is the successful treatment of the underlying HCV infection. For cryoglobulinemic patients with relatively mild disease (e.g., frequent purpuric lesions, shallow cutaneous ulcers), pegylated interferon alfa-2b (1 μg/kg/week) combined with ribavirin (1000 to 1200 mg/day) may be effective. For patients with mononeuritis multiplex or other manifestations of severe disease, corticosteroids and cyclophosphamide are required. Plasmapheresis may be a useful adjunctive therapy.

Diagnosis

Differential Diagnosis

The major categories of diseases that can mimic vasculitis are displayed in Table 291–5. Certain features of a patient's case should raise the diagnostic suspicion for vasculitis. First, most cases of vasculitis do not begin suddenly but rather unfold subacutely during weeks or months. Second, pain is usually a prominent feature of vasculitis, resulting from arthritis or arthralgias, myalgias, headaches, neuropathy, testicular infarction, digital ischemia, sinusitis, otalgia, back pain (caused by aortic inflammation), postprandial abdominal pain (caused by mesenteric vasculitis), or other disease manifestations. Third, signs of inflammation, such as fever, rash, weight loss, and elevated acute phase reactants, are highly characteristic. These signs of inflammation are frequently so apparent that many patients undergo empirical treatment with antibiotics for infections

TABLE 291–5 MAJOR DISEASE CATEGORIES IN THE DIFFERENTIAL DIAGNOSIS OF VASCULITIDES

Other forms of vasculitis
Simultaneous occurrence of common medical problems in the same patient
Infections
Bacterial, viral, mycobacterial, fungal
Occlusive processes
Hypercoagulable states
Atheroembolic disease
Malignant neoplasms
Lymphoma (including lymphomatoid granulomatosis)
Castleman's disease
Amyloidosis
Paraproteinemias
Connective tissue disorders
Systemic lupus erythematosus, mixed connective tissue disease
Systemic sclerosis
Rheumatoid arthritis
Miscellaneous
Atrial myxoma
Calciphylaxis
Fibromuscular dysplasia
Neutrophilic dermatoses
Pyoderma gangrenosum
Sarcoidosis

before the correct diagnosis is made. Finally, multiorgan system involvement is the rule in vasculitis. Cases of systemic vasculitis in which problems are isolated to individual organs are exceptional.

Ideally, the diagnosis of vasculitis is established through biopsy of an involved organ. Diagnoses based on angiography alone have many potential pitfalls. Angiographic findings that are "consistent with vasculitis" must be interpreted in the proper context. A diverse array of other diseases, ranging from atherosclerosis to vasospasm to pheochromocytoma, may mimic the angiographic appearance of vasculitis. Systemic vasculitis is frequently mimicked by two or more common medical problems or treatment complications occurring simultaneously in the same patient. Finally, high on the differential diagnosis of any individual form of vasculitis are other forms of vasculitis. For example, digital ischemia and splinter hemorrhages may be secondary to idiopathic polyarteritis nodosa. They may also be caused by polyarteritis nodosa associated with HBV infection, Wegener's granulomatosis, cryoglobulinemia, microscopic polyangiitis, Churg-Strauss syndrome, Buerger's disease, or some other form of vasculitis. Because the appropriate interventions for these conditions vary widely, careful distinction among these potential etiologies is essential.

Treatment

Rx

The intensity of treatment in patients with vasculitis must be guided by the degree of disease activity. Specifically, the treatment of vasculitis should be predicated not only on abnormal laboratory test results but also on clear evidence of active disease. In addition, the intensity of treatment must be adapted to the type of vasculitis. Whereas giant cell arteritis responds to high doses of corticosteroids in essentially all cases, for example, Wegener's granulomatosis nearly always requires an additional agent (usually either cyclophosphamide or methotrexate) for disease control to be obtained. In contrast, despite the dramatic fashion in which they sometimes present, most cases of Henoch-Schönlein purpura and cutaneous leukocytoclastic angiitis require no immunosuppressive treatment at all.

Conventional therapies such as corticosteroids, immunomodulating agents, and cytotoxic drugs induce remissions and control vasculitis in most cases. Moreover, in some cases—a variable percentage, depending on the type of vasculitis—the disease is curable. Unfortunately, the treatments of vasculitis have enormous potential for toxicity. Regular monitoring of patients' bone marrow, renal, and hepatic function is essential to avoid treatment-induced toxicity. Prophylaxis against opportunistic infections, particularly *Pneumocystis* pneumonia, is an important part of many vasculitis treatment regimens. During the tapering of immunosuppressive medications, disease flares are common in many forms of vasculitis.

A common error is treating patients with high doses of immunosuppressive agents for too long. The most appropriate use of medications such as cyclophosphamide and corticosteroids is to induce remission as quickly as possible with early, aggressive treatment regimens and then to convert patients to safer treatments for the maintenance of remission.

Prognosis

Assuming that the diagnosis is made before the patient has become catastrophically ill, the prognosis in systemic vasculitis is determined largely by the answers to four questions:

1. Was the diagnosis established before the occurrence of major, irreversible organ damage?
2. Was aggressive (but appropriately dosed) treatment begun in a timely fashion?
3. Was there careful monitoring during treatment, and were specific steps taken to avoid drug-induced toxicity (e.g., opportunistic infection)?
4. Were the potentially toxic medications that induced remission stopped at an appropriate juncture and replaced with less dangerous medications (or was treatment stopped altogether)?

For most forms of vasculitis, the factors that determine long-term, drug-free remissions remain poorly understood. The likelihood of achieving sustained remissions off all medications (or cures) varies according to the specific type of vasculitis.

Future Directions

Compelling laboratory and spontaneously occurring animal models of disease, combined with the known associations among HBV, HCV, and vasculitis in humans, suggest that additional links between infection and systemic vasculitis may be established in the future. Ongoing studies in Wegener's granulomatosis and cryoglobulinemia will also elucidate genetic risk factors for these and other forms of vasculitis. Important strides have been made in the description of cytokine and chemokine pathways that are operative in vascular inflammation, but relevant anti-cytokine interventions remain to be defined for clinical therapies. B-cell depletion is a promising approach for ANCA-associated vasculitides and possibly other vasculitis subtypes. Genetic, functional genomic, and proteomic studies specific to vasculitis are likely to elucidate important disease mechanisms and to identify new potential targets for therapy. Finally, multicenter collaborations among vasculitis investigators, established only in the past few years, will enhance the ability to study large numbers of patients with vasculitis to test new treatments in rigorous clinical trials.

SUGGESTED READINGS

Cacoub P, Saadoun D, Limal N, et al: PEGylated interferon alfa-2b and ribavirin treatment in patients with hepatitis C virus–related systemic vasculitis. Arthritis Rheum 2005;52:911–915. *Treatment with PEG–interferon alfa-2b plus ribavirin can achieve a complete clinical response in most patients with hepatitis C virus–related cryoglobulinemic vasculitis. Complete response correlates with viral eradication.*

Cooper LT, Tse MT, Mikhail MA, et al: Long-term survival and amputation risk in thromboangiitis obliterans (Buerger's disease). J Am Coll Cardiol 2004; 44:2410–2411. *Avoidance of digital or limb amputation in Buerger's diseases is closely linked to smoking cessation.*

Frankel SK, Cosgrove GP, Fischer A, et al: Update in the diagnosis and management of pulmonary vasculitis. Chest 2006;129:452–465. *Comprehensive review.*

Jayne D, Rasmussen N, Andrassy K, et al: A randomized trial of maintenance therapy for vasculitis associated with antineutrophil cytoplasmic autoantibodies. N Engl J Med 2003;349:36–44. *Azathioprine following 3 to 6 months of treatment with cyclophosphamide in the treatment of ANCA-associated vasculitis is as effective as 12 full months of cyclophosphamide in sustaining remissions at 18 months, provided patients remain on low doses of corticosteroids.*

Merkel PA, Lo GH, Holbrook JT, et al: Brief communication: High incidence of venous thrombotic events among patients with Wegener granulomatosis: The Wegener's Clinical Occurrence of Thrombosis (WeCLOT) Study. Ann Intern Med 2005;142:620–626. *Patients enrolled in the Wegener's Granulomatosis Etanercept Trial had a risk of venous thrombotic events seven times higher than that of lupus patients.*

Newburger JW, Sleeper LA, McCrindle BW, et al: Randomized trial of pulsed corticosteroid therrapy for primary treatment of Kawasaki disease. N Engl J Med 2007;356:663–675. *Pulsed corticosteroids had no additional benefit over conventional therapy.*

Noth I, Strek ME, Leff AR: Churg-Strauss syndrome. Lancet 2003;361:587–594. *Review of pathology, diagnosis, and treatment.*

Saleh A, Stone JH: Classification and diagnostic criteria in systemic vasculitis. Best Pract Res Clin Rheumatol 2005;19:209–221. *Review of the current approach to classification of the vasculitides (validated diagnostic criteria remain elusive for most of these conditions).*

Seo P, Stone JH: The antineutrophil cytoplasmic antibody–associated vasculitides. Am J Med 2004;117:39–50. *Comprehensive review of the clinical features, pathology, radiology, and treatment approaches to ANCA-associated vasculitis.*

Wegener's Granulomatosis Etanercept Trial (WGET) Research Group: Etanercept plus standard therapy in Wegener's granulomatosis. N Engl J Med 2005;352: 351–361. *Emphasizes the lack of efficiency of anti-TNF therapy.*

Weyand CM, Goronzy JJ: Medium- and large-vessel vasculitis. N Engl J Med 2003;349:160–169. *A focus on the current understanding of pathophysiology of the large-vessel vasculitides.*

292 POLYMYALGIA RHEUMATICA AND TEMPORAL ARTERITIS

Stephen A. Paget and Robert F. Spiera

Definition

Polymyalgia rheumatica (PMR) and temporal arteritis, also called giant cell arteritis (GCA), are companion systemic inflammatory disorders of unknown etiology that represent a spectrum from severe proximal aches and pains and constitutional symptoms to an occlusive granulomatous vasculitis of medium and large vessels that can lead to permanent blindness or other organ and tissue damage. These disorders occur primarily in patients older than 50 years, in women more than in men; they are propagated by antigen-driven, cell-mediated (T_H1) immune mechanisms that may be associated with specific genetic markers and are highly responsive to corticosteroids.

Epidemiology

In the United States, the average annual incidence of PMR is 52.5 per 100,000 patients aged 50 years and older and increases with age. The prevalence is about 0.5 to 0.7%. Internationally, the frequency varies according to country, with the highest rates occurring in the Scandinavian countries. The incidence and prevalence of GCA are approximately one third those of PMR.

Pathobiology

The etiology of PMR and GCA is unknown, but both demonstrate familial aggregation and have a genetic association with human leukocyte antigen (HLA)-DR4 and a demonstrated sequence polymorphism encoded within the hypervariable region of the HLA-DRβ1*04 gene. Disease in genetically predisposed patients may be triggered by environmental factors such as viruses or internal antigens such as elastin, and their inflammatory manifestations are directed by specific patterns of cell-mediated, T_H1-associated cytokines. The cytokine production by the mononuclear cells in the involved tissues appears to influence the clinical phenotype. Cytokine profiles characterized in temporal artery biopsy specimens obtained from patients with PMR and GCA differ. GCA tissue contains the T-lymphocyte products interferon-γ and interleukin (IL)–2 and the macrophage products IL-1β, IL-6, and transforming growth factor-β. In PMR vascular tissue, transcripts are found for transforming growth factor-β, IL-1, and IL-2 but not for interferon-γ. Patients with GCA who present with fever of unknown origin and who do *not* have ischemic symptoms, such as visual loss, have low interferon-γ levels. Arteries that express high interferon-γ levels typically have multinucleated giant cells present; these cells remove debris and secrete cytokines that stimulate intimal hyperplasia and lead to angiogenesis.

The adventitia is considered the immunologic center in the pathogenesis of GCA. Macrophages and T lymphocytes enter the vessel wall through the vasa vasorum with the aid of adhesion molecules and come into contact with an inciting antigen. Here, it is likely that clonal proliferation of $CD4^+$ T cells is triggered by the presentation of unknown antigens by antigen-presenting cells. The activated CD4 cells produce interferon-γ that attracts macrophages to the arterial wall. Some of these macrophages fuse at the intima-media to form multinucleated giant cells. These cells produce vascular endothelial growth factor, which triggers neovascularization both in the intima-media junction and at the level of the vasa vasorum, sprouting from the adventitia to the media. The subsequent immunologic events lead to a characteristic topography of mononuclear cells throughout the vessel wall. Products of the giant cells and macrophages at the intima-media junction include collagenase and nitric oxide, both of which probably contribute to tissue damage. The pathologic impact of cytokines leads not only to the characteristic medial damage but also to the significant intimal hyperplasia that eventually, if it is not treated, may cause luminal narrowing and tissue ischemia.

In GCA, a transmural (involving all layers of the vessel), inflammatory infiltrate, comprising predominantly mononuclear cells and commonly with giant cells, is found in the superficial temporal arteries as well as in other large and medium-sized arteries. In elderly patients, fragmentation of the internal elastica is characteristic and helps differentiate this vascular lesion from that of atherosclerosis. Often, macrophages containing fragments of elastic tissue are found at the intima-media junction, the histologic center of the inflammatory process. As mentioned earlier, immunochemical techniques demonstrate differing patterns of cells and their proinflammatory and profibrotic products in the adventitia, media, and intima. Intimal proliferation may be prominent and lead to luminal narrowing. Fibrinoid necrosis, a common histologic feature in polyarteritis nodosa, is not seen in GCA.

In PMR, mononuclear cell inflammation can be found not only in the proximal joints, such as the shoulders, but also in the surrounding tendons, bursae, and soft tissues consistent with enthesitis. Although muscle pains may be present, no muscle inflammation is found.

Clinical Manifestations

PMR and GCA are systemic inflammatory disorders that occur primarily in patients older than 50 years, in women more than in men (2:1), and in whites. PMR and GCA are particularly uncommon in African Americans.

Shared characteristics of the two disorders include significant cytokine-driven constitutional symptoms, such as fever, fatigue, and weight loss, as well as a markedly elevated erythrocyte sedimentation rate (ESR), anemia, and thrombocytosis. The musculoskeletal hallmark of PMR is proximal, severe, and symmetrical morning and even day-long stiffness, soreness, and pain in the shoulder, neck, and pelvic girdles. Fifty percent of patients with GCA share this characteristic proximal pain syndrome. Carpal tunnel syndrome and hand and knee synovitis may be seen in patients with PMR, but the overall presentation remains predominantly proximal, as opposed to rheumatoid arthritis, in which distal synovitis dominates. Whereas patients with PMR may appear to have proximal muscle weakness, this is invariably due to pain and not muscle inflammation (Table 292–1).

Specific signs and symptoms of GCA are best appreciated in their anatomic and physiologic contexts. GCA preferentially affects certain blood vessels, including the branches of the external carotid artery, the ophthalmic artery and particularly its posterior ciliary branches, and the large arteries that arise from the aortic arch and abdominal aorta. Headache and scalp pain are probably the most frequent symptoms,

TABLE 292–1 GIANT CELL ARTERITIS: CLINICAL FEATURES

INFLAMMATORY

Polymyalgia rheumatica
Constitutional symptoms
  Fever
  Weight loss
  Fatigue
Laboratory abnormalities
  Hematologic: anemia, thrombocytosis
  Elevated sedimentation rate, C-reactive protein

ISCHEMIC

Ocular
  Diplopia
  Amaurosis fugax
  Fixed vision loss
  Complete blindness
Cranial symptoms
  Headache
  Jaw claudication
  Scalp tenderness
  Scalp or lingual necrosis (rare)
Cerebrovascular accidents
Large-vessel disease
  Leg or arm claudication
  Diminished pulses; blood pressure asymmetry
  Aortic aneurysms

LATE COMPLICATIONS

Aortic aneurysms
  Thoracic aorta
  Abdominal aorta
Corticosteroid complications
  Osteoporosis
  Fractures
  Cataracts

occurring in 50 to 75% of patients. Headache is often the first manifestation of GCA and is described as boring, severe, and constant, unresponsive to simple pain medications and persisting through the night. Classically, patients complain of persistent and prominent temporal headaches, but occipital pains can also occur. Ear, pinna, or parotid gland pain may occur secondary to involvement of the posterior auricular artery. Jaw claudication and pain due to masseter muscle ischemia on chewing occur in 50% of patients. Lingual and maxillary artery involvement can lead to jaw or tongue pain on chewing or talking. The superficial temporal artery may become tortuous, prominent, nodular, or tender, but these findings are not invariable, and an abnormal temporal artery may be found on biopsy in vessels that appear normal.

Fixed or intermittent symptoms related to vasculitic involvement of the ophthalmic arteries and its branches are the most dreaded in this illness and demand immediate therapeutic intervention. These symptoms are related to vascular narrowing due to both active inflammation and endothelial injury–derived vasospasm. Decreased vision secondary to arteritis is the most common serious consequence of GCA, occurring in 20 to 50% of patients who present to ophthalmologists. It is the presenting symptom in 60% of patients with GCA who develop visual loss. A careful history of most patients who present with "sudden" visual loss reveals that preceding headache, constitutional symptoms, and PMR occurred in approximately 40% of patients. Even the evolution of the visual loss was often staggered with amaurosis fugax in 10% and a partial field defect progressing to complete blindness during days. If GCA remains untreated, the second eye may become involved within 1 to 2 weeks. The posterior ciliary arteries are the most frequently involved; thus, anterior ischemic optic neuropathy is the most common lesion, which can be easily defined by an ophthalmologist. Occlusion of the central retinal artery and its branches is uncommon; thus, exudates, hemorrhages, and frank vasculitis are infrequent. Five percent of patients with GCA may present with diplopia or ptosis, which may precede visual loss. The final visual abnormality can be a composite of many ischemic events occurring together in the optic nerve, the extraocular muscles, the chiasm, and the brain itself. Because GCA primarily involves arteries that contain elastica and the elastic lamina is lost as vessels pierce the dura, intracerebral lesions such as strokes are uncommon but not unheard of.

Large artery involvement most commonly presents as arm or leg claudication; rarer manifestations are stroke, subclavian steal syndrome, intestinal infarction, and symptomatic aortic aneurysm. Thus, a subclinical arteritis can exist and demands long-term monitoring.

Steroid-treated PMR and GCA are self-limited illnesses lasting 1 to 2 years in most patients. However, a subgroup of patients with both disorders can have active inflammatory disease as manifested by persistent symptoms and blood test signs of active inflammation for 7 to 10 years. Of note is the fact that thoracic aneurysms with giant cells in the tissue can develop as long as 15 years after the diagnosis, successful treatment, and discontinuation of steroids. Indeed, the incidence of thoracic and aortic aneurysms is markedly higher in patients with prior history of presumably successfully treated GCA than in age-matched control subjects. Conversely, in studies of repaired aortic aneurysms, pathologic findings consistent with GCA have been found in approximately 2% of specimens from individuals without previously recognized or suspected arteritis. In most studies, survival in PMR and GCA is similar to that of unaffected persons of the same age. However, one study did show that survival was decreased in a group of patients with GCA that had permanent visual loss and required more than 10 mg of prednisone per day at 6 months. This probably supports the experience that the morbidity and mortality are caused by steroid-related treatment complications in this high-risk, elderly group of patients possessing many comorbid conditions.

Diagnosis

The diagnoses of PMR and GCA are based on clinical facts, with supporting but not diagnostic aid obtained from laboratory tests and temporal artery biopsy (Fig. 292–1). No physician should await an abnormal finding on temporal artery biopsy or demand the presence of an elevated ESR before making the definitive diagnosis of GCA in the setting of a characteristic clinical picture. This said, the laboratory hallmark of PMR and GCA is an elevation in IL-6–stimulated acute phase reactants such as the ESR and the C-reactive protein. The ESR is usually in excess of 50 mm/hr and may exceed 100 mm/hr. An ESR in the low 20s or 30s, however, does not exclude a diagnosis of PMR or GCA if other characteristic clinical features are present and especially if the patient is already taking steroids.

Normocytic, normochromic anemia and thrombocytosis occur in approximately 50% of patients with both disorders and are excellent guides to the state of inflammation. In both PMR and GCA, the frequency of rheumatoid factor, antinuclear antibody, complement levels, monoclonal proteins, and cryoglobulins is not higher than in age-matched control subjects. Alkaline phosphatase activity may be elevated in one third of patients, primarily with GCA. Although these tests are not indicated in PMR and GCA, muscle enzymes and electromyography are normal, and muscle biopsy shows type II fiber atrophy but no inflammation.

Superficial Temporal Artery Assessment

Temporal artery tenderness, nodularity, and diminished pulsation are typical findings on physical examination in a patient with GCA. Color duplex ultrasonography has been used as an adjunctive noninvasive diagnostic tool in GCA. A hypoechoic halo around the superficial temporal artery has been reported in 73% of patients with biopsy-proven GCA. The halo, representing edema in the arterial wall, was observed bilaterally in a significant subset of patients and disappeared in a mean of 16 days after the initiation of steroids. The presence of the halo had a sensitivity of 73% and was 100% specific for GCA in one study. Other groups have been unable to replicate this experience, however, finding Doppler ultrasonography to be no more sensitive or specific than physical examination in patients thought to have the disease. [^{18}F]Fluorodeoxyglucose–positron emission tomography may be helpful in identifying large-vessel inflammation suggestive of GCA, but it is not helpful in

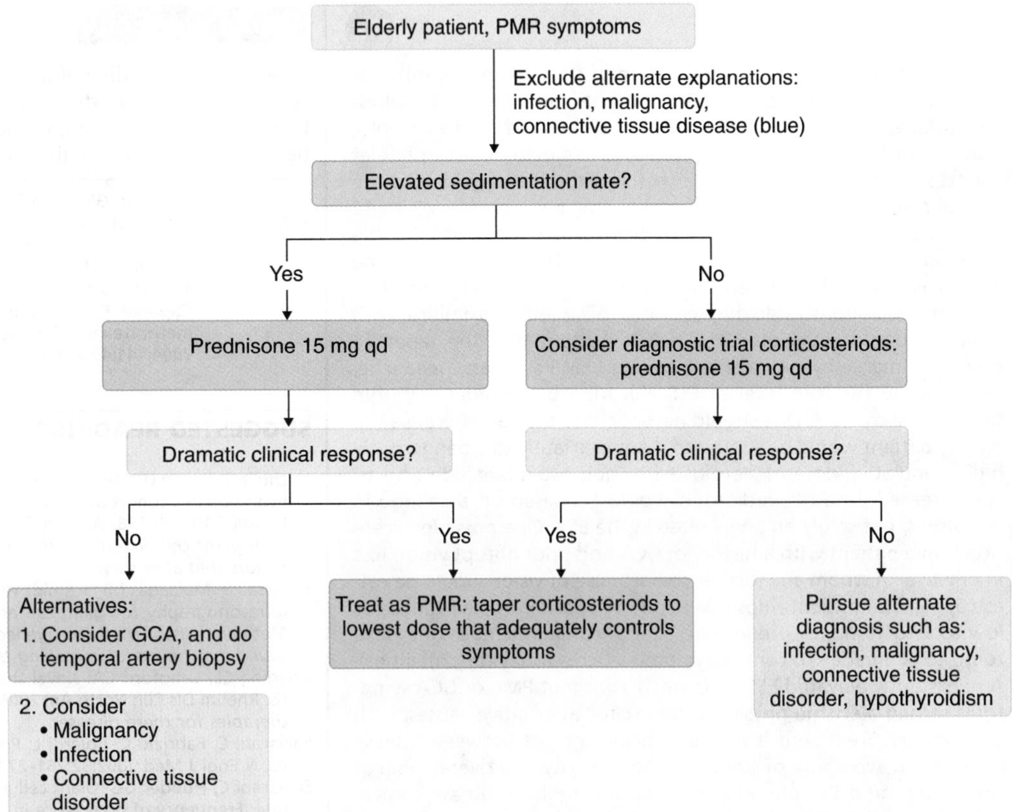

FIGURE 292–1 • Diagnostic algorithm for polymyalgia rheumatica (PMR). GCA = giant cell arteritis.

assessing the temporal arteries themselves given their relatively small size and high background uptake in that area. Temporal artery biopsy remains the diagnostic "gold standard" in GCA, and given the relatively easy accessibility of the artery and potentially significant morbidity of therapy in GCA, histologic confirmation is favored in most cases.

Although temporal artery biopsy continues to be an important diagnostic test for the presence of GCA, a few caveats must be stated. First, in a patient in whom the clinical diagnosis is likely, treatment with steroids should be instituted immediately without waiting for the biopsy results. Second, because of the skipped nature of the pathologic inflammatory lesions in the vessel wall, as many as 20 to 30% of biopsy specimens may be normal despite an overwhelming diagnostic likelihood of GCA. However, because the biopsy is helpful in confirming the diagnosis of GCA, in which high doses of steroids are employed, the following guidelines are given. Patients with pure PMR and no GCA signs or symptoms do *not* need a biopsy. However, because 10% of these patients may develop such clinical manifestations of GCA within the next year, they should be told to report such symptoms immediately. When GCA is likely, an outpatient biopsy should be performed on the symptomatic side of the head, preferably including inflamed areas with tenderness or nodularity and incorporating 2 to 3 cm of vessel. Multiple sections should be requested because of the segmental nature of the disease process. Some rheumatologists routinely perform bilateral biopsies, which may increase the likelihood of obtaining an abnormal finding by up to 5%, whereas others perform a contralateral biopsy if the first specimen is normal. Diagnostic biopsy findings continue to be present for as long as 2 to 4 weeks after the clinical diagnosis is made and steroid treatment instituted.

Differential Diagnosis

The systemic nature of these disorders and the fact that they occur in the elderly demand careful diagnostic scrutiny to avoid missing a malignant neoplasm or major infection and possibly treating patients inappropriately with high-dose steroids. This is true in PMR because there is no diagnostic test and in GCA because the GCA biopsy finding may be normal in the face of active, vision-threatening vasculitis. Infections that must be considered and ruled out if clinically appropriate include tuberculosis, endocarditis, and hepatitis B and C. Malignant neoplasms such as lymphoma and multiple myeloma may mimic PMR, and an age-appropriate cancer evaluation is always indicated in this age group. Autoimmune disorders such as elderly-onset rheumatoid arthritis and systemic lupus erythematosus as well as dermatomyositis and other types of vasculitis must be considered in the differential diagnosis and sorted out by employing clinical information and serologic testing. There is support for the concept that elderly-onset rheumatoid arthritis is the same disorder as PMR with negative rheumatoid factor, a more proximal focus of joint inflammation, and a good response to low-dose prednisone. The distinction may be semantic, as neither disorder tends to evolve into an erosive arthritis. A more protracted clinical course, however, is often seen in patients in whom distal synovitis is a prominent feature, and those patients are classified as having elderly-onset rheumatoid arthritis. PMR and GCA should always be thought of in the setting of a fever of unknown origin because symptoms and signs can be occult or the history incomplete.

Treatment

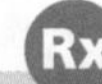

Both PMR and GCA are highly responsive to corticosteroids, and this medication is the preferred treatment choice. This response is so characteristic that an immediate and dramatic improvement in PMR and GCA symptoms within 1 to 3 days after steroid institution supports the diagnosis. Conversely, a lack of rapid and significant improvement in signs, symptoms, and function within 5 to 7 days should be considered a major point against the diagnosis. The physician should then consider an alternative diagnosis (e.g., tumor or infection) or the presence of GCA in PMR patients that might demand a higher steroid dose. Because the inflammatory set point of the two disorders is different, different doses of steroids are employed at the onset of treatment. Whereas PMR usually responds to 15 mg of prednisone daily, GCA usually requires 60 to 80 mg of prednisone per day in divided doses or higher doses if organ or tissue damage is present or threatened. In GCA, if visual symptoms are present as a fixed loss or amaurosis fugax, the patient often should be treated with high-dose intravenous methylprednisolone with doses ranging from 40 mg every 8 hours to 1 g/day for 3 days, followed by high-dose oral steroids in divided doses.

Rx

Within 2 to 3 days after the institution of steroids, most symptoms of PMR or GCA clear rapidly and patients describe a miraculous improvement. The steroid dose is then maintained for 2 to 3 weeks, during which the ESR, C-reactive protein, hemoglobin, and platelet counts normalize. Steroid taper is then instituted and guided by the clinical response. In PMR, taper is commonly by 1 mg every 7 to 10 days; in GCA, taper is by 5 to 10 mg every 7 to 10 days. In GCA, the use of alternate-day corticosteroid regimens to minimize steroid side effects is generally not recommended as randomized controlled trials have demonstrated higher rates of treatment failure with alternate-day dosing schedules. It is important that the taper be guided primarily by clinical findings (e.g., PMR stiffness, headache, fatigue) and that the level of ESR elevation be considered within that clinical context. One should never "chase the ESR" because the elderly patient would be subjected inappropriately to a dangerously high cumulative dose of steroids with their attendant side effects. An increased dose of prednisone should be based on a change in symptoms, not solely on an increase in the ESR. One possible exception is in a patient with a history of GCA and prior abrupt vision loss in one eye, in whom any further compromise of vision would be catastrophic. The effective dose demanded for a flare often can be as low as 5 to 10 mg of prednisone, and uncommonly does one have to go to 60 mg/day to control symptoms (e.g., visual abnormalities). A persistently elevated ESR (>50 mm/hr) without PMR or GCA symptoms should alert the physician to look for alternative causes, such as infection. Treatment is a careful balancing act between disease control and avoidance of steroid-related toxicity. The overall goal of the patient and the physician is to attain the best disease control with the lowest dose of steroids. In most patients, prednisone can be tapered safely in 1 to 2 years. However, other patients may need to take low doses of steroids for 2 years or more. The higher the initial dose and cumulative dose, the greater the likelihood that the patient will develop a major steroid side effect such as sepsis, osteoporosis, osteonecrosis, diabetes, emotional lability, or myopathy. Appropriate immunizations, osteoporosis regimens (calcium, vitamin D, and bisphosphonates), and metabolic monitoring are mandatory in all patients prescribed chronic steroid therapy.

The major feared outcome in GCA is ischemic complications of the disease, most often vision loss or, less frequently, cerebrovascular accidents. Vision loss is usually irreversible, and although it is uncommon once the diagnosis is suspected and glucocorticoid therapy is instituted, it can occur early in the course of treatment. Aspirin is known to be protective against ischemic events in patients with atherosclerosis and has anti-inflammatory effects in inflamed blood vessels including inhibition of interferon-γ. Low-dose aspirin (100 mg daily) has been shown in a retrospective study to be protective against ischemic complications in GCA. In most patients, adjunctive therapy with low-dose aspirin should be considered unless there is a strong contraindication to its use.

Alternative immunosuppressive agents have been tested in both PMR and GCA patients in an attempt to "spare steroids" and to control the inflammatory state. Studies examining the efficacy of methotrexate in GCA have yielded mixed results, with the largest, most recent study showing no incremental benefit from combined therapy. [1] In PMR, however, methotrexate has been shown to afford a benefit in terms of steroid sparing and possibly reducing numbers of flares. [2] The magnitude of the benefit appears modest, and at present, methotrexate is not routinely used in the management of either disease. In individual patients with refractory disease or excessive corticosteroid morbidities, however, addition of weekly rheumatoid arthritis–type doses of methotrexate (7.5 to 20 mg/week) or azathioprine (2 mg/kg/day) is employed in some instances.

Tumor necrosis factor inhibition has been of interest as a potential therapeutic strategy in GCA and PMR. Tumor necrosis factor has been demonstrated in inflamed arteries of patients with GCA, and inhibition of this cytokine has been shown to be of clinical benefit in other inflammatory granulomatous disorders, such as Crohn's disease. Randomized controlled trials of infliximab in GCA and PMR, however, have failed to demonstrate benefit in terms of preventing relapses or affording a steroid-sparing benefit.

Section XXII Rheumatology

Future Directions

Better understanding of the disease-causing roles of immunologically active cells and their cytokine products, along with genetics and correlations with clinical subsets, will lead to more focused treatment modalities, and the avoidance of the need for long-term treatment with steroids.

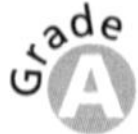

1. Hoffman GS, Cid MC, Hellmann DB, et al; International Network for the Study of Systemic Vasculitides: A multicenter, randomized, double-blind, placebo-controlled trial of adjuvant methotrexate treatment for giant cell arteritis. Arthritis Rheum 2002;46:1309–1318.
2. Caporali R, Cimmino MA, Ferraccioli G, et al: Prednisone plus methotrexate for polymyalgia rheumatica. Ann Intern Med 2004;141:493–500.

SUGGESTED READINGS

Hachulla E, Boivin U, Pasturel-Michon A-L, et al: Prognostic factors and long-term evolution in a cohort of 133 patients with giant cell arteritis. Clin Exp Rheumatol 2001;19:171–176. *An excellent clinical study of a large cohort of patients with giant cell arteritis, with a focus on their clinical courses, relapses, and factors that alter survival.*

Karassa FB, Matsaqas MI, Schmidt WA, et al: Meta-analysis: Test performance of ultrasonography for giant-call arteritis. Ann Intern Med 2005;142:359–369. *Meta-analysis of the heterogeneous literature available showing that ultrasound may be useful in making this diagnosis.*

Koening CL, Langford CA: Novel therapeutic strategies for large vessel vasculitis. Rheum Dis Clin North Am 2006;32:173–186. *Comprehensive review of new therapies for these diseases.*

Salvarani C, Fabrizio C, Boiardi L: Polymyalgia rheumatica and giant-cell arteritis. N Engl J Med 2002;32:261–271. *A comprehensive review.*

Salvarani C, Hunder GG: Giant cell arteritis with low erythrocyte sedimentation rate: Frequency of occurrence in a population-based study. Arthritis Care Res 2001;45:140–145. *Giant cell arteritis is a clinical diagnosis and should be considered in classic patients even if the sedimentation rate is normal; an important reminder from the Mayo Clinic.*

Schmidt WA, Gromnica-Ihle E: What is the best approach to diagnosing large-vessel vasculitis? Best Pract Res Clin Rheumatol 2005;19:223–242. *A review of the modalities available to diagnose large vessel vasculitis.*

293 INFECTIONS OF BURSAE, JOINTS, AND BONES

Luis R. Espinoza

INFECTION OF BURSAE

Septic Bursitis

Definition

Septic bursitis is a common clinical disorder that usually affects superficial bursae more frequently than deep bursae. Superficial bursae (present in subcutaneous tissue) such as the olecranon, prepatellar, and infrapatellar bursae are more commonly involved, whereas deep bursae such as the subacromial, trochanteric, iliopsoas, and retrocalcaneal bursae are rarely affected.

Epidemiology

The minimum population annual incidence of olecranon septic bursitis, the most commonly affected bursa, has been calculated to be 10 per 100,000. Data for other bursae are not available.

Pathobiology

Most cases of septic bursitis are accounted for by direct transcutaneous bacterial seeding secondary to trauma, including the intrabursal administration of corticosteroids for the treatment of aseptic bursitis. Other causes include hematogenous spread, preexisting bursa involvement such as gout and rheumatoid arthritis (RA), diabetes mellitus, alcoholism, iatrogenic sources, and immunocompromised states, especially for deep septic bursitis.

Clinical Manifestations

Characteristic findings include painful swelling with erythema of the overlying skin, increased warmth of the bursal sac, and normal joint range of motion. Peribursal cellulitis and evidence of cutaneous injury, usually in the form of excoriation or crust formation, are frequently present. Systemic findings such as fever, leukocytosis, and elevated C-reactive protein (CRP) may be present, depending on the severity of the illness.

Diagnosis

Septic bursitis should be suspected in any patient exhibiting the clinical picture described, but a positive bursal fluid culture is mandatory for a definite diagnosis. Analysis of bursal fluid assists in the diagnosis, although the inflammatory response is not as intense as that seen in joints. The median leukocyte count is 13,500/mm^3 with a range of less than 2000 to more than 100,000/mm^3. Frankly purulent or bloody fluid (or both) may be found in approximately 10% of cases. More than 90% of the white blood cells (WBCs) present are usually polymorphonuclear (PMN) leukocytes. Gram-stained smears of bursal fluid from patients with culture-proven septic bursitis are positive in approximately 50%.

Staphylococcus aureus (Chapter 310) is the most common pathogen and is responsible for more than 85% of cases of septic bursitis. Other gram-positive organisms such as *Staphylococcus epidermidis,* group A β-hemolytic streptococci, and less commonly, enterococci and diphtheroids may also be present. Gram-negative infections are rare, but *Brucella abortus, Escherichia coli, Campylobacter jejuni,* and more rarely others have also been described. Septic bursitis secondary to mycobacteria, spirochetes, fungi, and algae have likewise been rarely described.

Imaging studies, including magnetic resonance imaging (MRI), can be very helpful in delineating the extent of bursal involvement, but they do not differentiate septic from aseptic bursitis.

Differential Diagnosis

Nonseptic bursitis and septic or inflammatory arthritis should always be considered in the differential diagnosis of a painful, swollen, red bursa. Preservation of joint range of motion rules out intrinsic joint involvement, although in some patients (<20%) exhibiting severe involvement, joint range of motion may be compromised.

Treatment

Rx

Generally, management of septic bursitis can be accomplished in an ambulatory setting. However, in the presence of an underlying immunocompromised state, insulin-dependent diabetes mellitus, or involvement of the prepatellar bursa, hospitalization for intravenous antibiotic therapy is indicated.

The choice of antibiotics should be guided by bursal fluid analysis, as well as by any comorbid conditions present. In the absence of comorbid conditions, oral dicloxacillin, 2 g/day, can be started and maintained for at least 10 to 14 days or until after a negative culture is obtained. Longer therapy may be needed for cases of longer duration before initiation of therapy. Intravenous therapy with oxacillin, 12 g/day, a cephalosporin, or in penicillin-allergic individuals, vancomycin for up to 7 days, followed by oral antibiotics for another 1 to 2 weeks, may be initiated in hospitalized patients. Daily bursa aspiration is necessary for an optimal therapeutic response. Surgical intervention is indicated if the bursa cannot be drained adequately, if a foreign body is present, or for débridement of necrotic tissue.

The presence of bursitis refractory to antibiotic therapy, particularly with negative cultures, should raise suspicion of mycobacterial or fungal bursitis.

Prognosis

The prognosis is excellent in most patients. Morbidity (sinus tract formation, osteomyelitis, bacteremia, or septicemia) is very low and mortality is nonexistent. Caution should be exerted, however, in avoiding aspiration of a joint if the overlying bursa or skin (or both) is affected with either bursitis or cellulitis.

INFECTION OF JOINTS

Septic Arthritis

Definition

Infectious or septic arthritis is an inflammatory process of the joint space secondary to invasion of microorganisms. The ensuing inflammatory reaction leads to the development of pain, swelling, redness, limitation of joint motion, and eventually, joint destruction and disability if not properly treated.

Nongonococcal Septic Arthritis

Epidemiology

The incidence of septic arthritis in the general population both in the United States and in the United Kingdom is reported to be between 2 and 8.4 cases per 100,000 person years. Nongonococcal septic arthritis (NGSA) is more common in children than adults and affects males more commonly than females.

Pathobiology

Any microorganism, including bacteria, fungi, viruses, and protozoa, can invade joints; however, the overwhelming majority (>90%) of cases of septic arthritis are caused by pyogenic bacteria (i.e., staphylococci, streptococci; Table 293–1). Hematogenous spread to the joint space as a result of bacteremia is the most common cause of septic arthritis. Other less common routes include trauma, contiguous osteomyelitis, cellulitis, abscesses, tenosynovitis, septic bursitis, and much more rarely, direct inoculation during diagnostic or therapeutic arthrocentesis or arthroscopy (0.002 to 0.007% and 0.04 to 0.4%, respectively).

Once viable bacteria or their products, or both, enter the joint space, ingress of PMN and mononuclear leukocytes into the joint space results in the release of proteolytic enzymes, such as metalloproteinases and other collagen-degrading enzymes, as well as the release of pro-inflammatory cytokines, such as tumor necrosis factor-α (TNF-α) and interleukin-1. If left untreated or not properly treated, these inflammatory mediators will induce synovial membrane proliferation, granulation tissue, neovascularization, and eventually, cartilage and bone destruction.

Risk Factors

Known risk factors for the development of septic arthritis include diabetes mellitus, immunodeficiency states such as human immunodeficiency virus (HIV) infection and immunosuppressive therapy, preexistent joint damage (especially RA), old age, skin infection, intravenous drug use, indwelling intravenous catheters, malignancy, prosthetic joints, and much less commonly, tissue allograft reconstruction surgery. A predisposition to septic arthritis is also associated with the use of biologic therapy such as infliximab, etanercept, and adalimumab, which target TNF-α for the treatment of RA, Crohn's disease, and spondyloarthropathies.

Clinical Manifestations

The onset of NGSA is usually acute and in approximately 80% of cases is typically monarticular. Pain and limitation of joint motion are seen in more than 90% of cases. Any joint can be affected, although the knee joint followed by the hip and ankle are most commonly affected. Involvement of the sacroiliac, costochondral, or sternoclavicular joints is more commonly seen in patients with debilitating conditions and in intravenous drug users. Constitutional complaints, particularly fever with temperatures up to 102 to 103° F, malaise, anorexia, and less commonly, chills,

TABLE 293–1 MICROORGANISMS RESPONSIBLE FOR ACUTE SEPTIC ARTHRITIS AND ACUTE AND CHRONIC OSTEOMYELITIS

Septic Arthritis

Microorganism	Frequency (%)
Gram-positive	60–90
Staphylococcus aureus	50–70
Group A, B, C streptococci	15–30
Staphylococcus epidermidis	6–20
Streptococcus pneumoniae	1–3
Enterococcus sp	<1
Corynebacterium sp	<1
Gram-negative	5–25
Salmonella sp	
Pseudomonas aeruginosa	
Escherichia coli	
Klebsiella pneumoniae	
Enterobacter sp	
Kingella kingae	
Haemophilus influenzae	<1–3*
Anaerobes	1–2
Fusobacterium sp	
Bacteroides fragilis	
Miscellaneous	<5
Mycoplasma	
Mycobacterium sp	
Fungi	
Viruses	
Algae	

Osteomyelitis: Acute and Chronic

Microorganism	Frequency (%)
Gram-positive	80–90
Staphylococcus aureus	60–80
Group A, B, C streptococci	10–20
Staphylococcus epidermidis	10–15
Streptococcus pneumoniae	<1
Enterococcus sp	1–2
Corynebacterium sp	1–2
Gram-negative	5–20
Salmonella sp	
Enterobacter sp	
Pseudomonas aeruginosa	
Brucella sp	
Pasteurella multocida	
Bartonella henselae	
Propionibacterium sp	
Anaerobes	
Bacteroides sp	
Miscellaneous	5–7
Mycobacteria sp	
Fungi (candidiasis, coccidioidommycosis, blastomycosis, histoplasmosis	

*Children.

are seen in up to 80% of patients within the first 48 to 72 hours of onset. On physical examination, the affected joints can be extremely painful, red, warm, and swollen; a large effusion may be present, and these joints virtually always exhibit a marked decrease in active and passive range of motion. However, these findings may be masked in patients who are severely ill, have RA, or are receiving corticosteroids or immunosuppressive agents, including TNF-α inhibitors. Polyarthritis usually occurs in patients with RA, systemic lupus erythematosus, or underlying immunosuppressive states and carries a worse prognosis with a greater degree of permanent loss of joint function and a mortality rate of approximately 30%.

Diagnosis

Septic arthritis should be highly suspected in the presence of an appropriate clinical picture and positive imaging and synovial fluid findings. The "gold standard," however, is identification of the causative microorganism by synovial fluid culture.

Arthrocentesis is mandatory in patients with joint effusion. All fluid aspirated should be sent for Gram stain, aerobic and anaerobic bacterial culture, and cell count with a leukocyte differential. The synovial fluid cell count is usually between 40,000 and 50,000/mm^3 and can be frankly purulent with a predominance (>80%) of PMN cells. Glucose, protein, and lactate levels are not very helpful and for the most part are nonspecific. The yield of organisms from joint fluid culture in untreated patients may reach 90%. Gram stain is positive in approximately 50% of patients. The erythrocyte sedimentation rate (ESR), CRP, and peripheral blood WBC count are elevated in most patients, and the latter two may be helpful in monitoring the clinical response to therapy. A persistently elevated CRP or WBC count, or both, may imply persistence of joint infection. Plain radiographs are seldom useful early in the disease and generally show soft tissue swelling. Loss of articular cartilage and the presence of bone erosion imply a more aggressive process. More sophisticated imaging studies such as computed tomography (CT) or MRI are not cost-effective for the average patient but can be very helpful in patients suspected of having deep-seated joint infections, such as sacroiliac or facet joint involvement, and in determining the presence of coexisting osteomyelitis.

Differential Diagnosis

A number of arthritides, particularly gout and pseudogout, can exhibit an identical clinical picture to that of septic arthritis. Other diseases included in the differential diagnosis are reactive arthritis, psoriatic arthritis, and less commonly, RA and rheumatic fever.

Treatment

Immediate institution of an appropriate antibiotic, drainage of the purulent joint fluid, and if present, débridement of periarticular osteomyelitis are all essential in the management of septic arthritis. Even so, treatment of septic arthritis remains unsatisfactory, with high morbidity and mortality rates that have remained unchanged over the past 20 years. Antibiotics should be given to all patients suspected of having septic arthritis, even before the results of bacteriologic studies become available. Any delay in the initiation of antibiotic therapy may result in significant cartilage loss and functional limitation of the affected joint, especially in children. The initial selection of antibiotics should be based on the results of Gram stain of joint fluid or other body fluids or secretions. If no microorganisms are identified, empirical treatment should be initiated, with the age, risk factors, and clinical picture of the patient taken into consideration. Normal individuals should be treated initially for infections with gram-positive organisms (*S. aureus*), whereas broad-spectrum antibiotics are indicated if gram-negative organisms are suspected, such as in debilitated, severely ill, and immunocompromised individuals. Once culture results become available, antibiotics can be changed if indicated. A 3- to 4-week course of treatment (1 week of parenteral followed by oral anti-

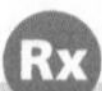

biotics) is currently the norm for most patients. Parenteral, not intra-articular therapy with either a β-lactamase–resistant penicillin or a first-generation cephalosporin should initially be given. Vancomycin should be used to treat methicillin-resistant *S. aureus* infection. Infection with gram-negative organisms should be treated with a third-generation cephalosporin such as cefotaxime or ceftriaxone or with an aminoglycoside. Septic arthritis of prosthetic joints should be treated by long-term administration of oral antibiotics. The use of linezolid, the first of a new class of antibiotics, the oxazolidinones, has been shown to be effective for chronic bone and joint infections secondary to methicillin-resistant staphylococci and enterococci.

Most patients with NGSA require closed-needle or arthroscopic aspiration (or both) on a daily basis or as often as necessary. Surgical drainage is indicated for deep-seated joints (including the hip, shoulder, and sacroiliac), where loculated effusions or contiguous osteomyelitis may be present. Joint immobilization is not indicated except early in patients with incapacitating pain or after surgical drainage. Polymerase chain reaction (PCR) analysis of synovial fluid may be used to monitor for the presence of bacterial DNA, the absence of which may assist in the decision to discontinue treatment (Fig. 293–1).

Prognosis

The outcome of NGSA depends on the underlying risk factors present, with greater morbidity and mortality in patients with polyarthritis and severe immunosuppressive states.

Gonococcal Arthritis

Epidemiology

Neisseria gonorrhoeae (Chapter 322) is the most common cause of septic arthritis in the United States, particularly in young, sexually active individuals. Women are affected two to three times as often as men. The number of cases of gonorrhea decreased by 72% between 1975 and 1997, and this change correlated with an important decrease in disseminated gonococcal infection (DGI) and arthritis. However, the reported rate of gonococcal arthritis has increased by 9.2% between 1997 and 1999 and now stands at 133.2 cases per 100,000 per year. Arthritis occurs in approximately 50% of patients with DGI, and it is always preceded by mucosal infection with *N. gonorrhoeae.* The infection frequently involves the endocervix or urethra but may also affect the pharynx and rectum and may or may not be symptomatic. The risk for gonococcal dissemination after a mucosal infection depends on the patient's immunologic status and the virulence of the microorganism.

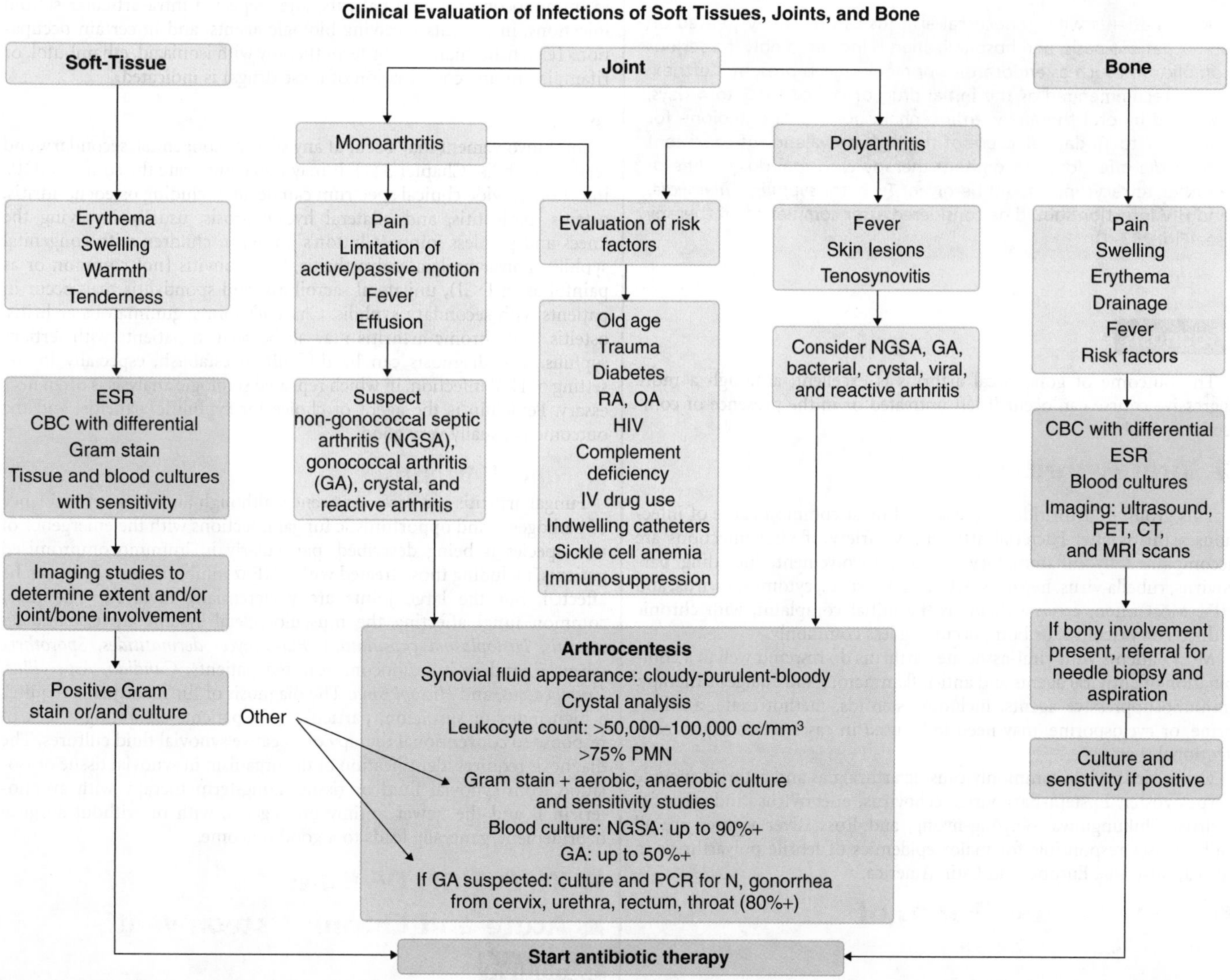

Clinical Evaluation of Infections of Soft Tissues, Joints, and Bone

Soft-Tissue
- Erythema / Swelling / Warmth / Tenderness
- ESR / CBC with differential / Gram stain / Tissue and blood cultures with sensitivity
- Imaging studies to determine extent and/or joint/bone involvement
- Positive Gram stain or/and culture → Start antibiotic therapy

Joint
- Monoarthritis
  - Pain / Limitation of active/passive motion / Fever / Effusion
  - Suspect non-gonococcal septic arthritis (NGSA), gonococcal arthritis (GA), crystal, and reactive arthritis → Arthrocentesis
- Evaluation of risk factors
  - Old age / Trauma / Diabetes / RA, OA / HIV / Complement deficiency / IV drug use / Indwelling catheters / Sickle cell anemia / Immunosuppression
- Polyarthritis
  - Fever / Skin lesions / Tenosynovitis
  - Consider NGSA, GA, bacterial, crystal, viral, and reactive arthritis → Arthrocentesis

Arthrocentesis
- Synovial fluid appearance: cloudy-purulent-bloody
- Crystal analysis
- Leukocyte count: >50,000–100,000 cc/mm³
- >75% PMN
- Gram stain + aerobic, anaerobic culture and sensitivity studies
- Blood culture: NGSA: up to 90%+
- GA: up to 50%+
- If GA suspected: culture and PCR for N, gonorrhea from cervix, urethra, rectum, throat (80%+)

Other (from Positive Gram stain or/and culture) → Gram stain + aerobic, anaerobic culture and sensitivity studies; GA: up to 50%+

Arthrocentesis → Start antibiotic therapy

Bone
- Pain / Swelling / Erythema / Drainage / Fever / Risk factors
- CBC with differential / ESR / Blood cultures / Imaging: ultrasound, PET, CT, and MRI scans
- If bony involvement present, referral for needle biopsy and aspiration
- Culture and senstivity if positive → Start antibiotic therapy

Start antibiotic therapy

FIGURE 293–1 • Investigation and management of soft tissue, joint, and bone septic involvement. CBC = complete blood count; CT = computed tomography; ESR = erythrocyte sedimentation rate; HIV = human immunodeficiency virus; IV = intravenous; MRI = magnetic resonance imaging; OA = osteoarthritis; PCR = polymerase chain reaction; PET = positron emission tomography; PMN = polymorphonuclear leukocyte; RA = rheumatoid arthritis.

Clinical Manifestations

Gonococcal arthritis is manifested as two distinct clinical syndromes. The first is the dermatitis-arthritis syndrome, in which bacteremia, fever, polyarthralgia, tenosynovitis (usually of the hands and fingers), and multiple maculopapular, vesicular, pustular, or necrotic skin lesions develop after dissemination from mucosal surfaces such as the cervix, urethra, or rectum. Rash may be observed in any region, including the palms. Asymmetrical arthritis is common, with the knee, elbow, wrist, metacarpophalangeal, and ankle joints most frequently being involved. This clinical picture is seen in approximately 60 to 70% of patients with DGI. The second syndrome—septic arthritis affecting one or a few joints or frank polyarthritis—may be seen in the absence of skin involvement and is clinically indistinguishable from other forms of septic arthritis.

Diagnosis

N. gonorrhoeae is isolated in 20 to 30% of patients with the dermatitis-arthritis syndrome and in 50% of patients with monarthritis. PCR may be helpful to distinguish DGI from other inflammatory arthritides, especially reactive arthritis. The presence of a positive culture from the genitourinary tract or, much less frequently, from the rectum or pharynx can be very helpful in establishing a diagnosis in patients with a negative synovial fluid culture.

Treatment

Rx

Most patients with gonococcal arthritis can be safely treated on an outpatient basis, and hospitalization is indicated only if a serious complication such as endocarditis or meningitis is present. Ceftriaxone is recommended as the initial drug of choice for 2 to 4 days, followed by oral therapy with a cephalosporin or a quinolone for another 7 to 10 days. Because of the high prevalence of coexistent *Chlamydia* infection, concomitant therapy with oral doxycycline or another tetracycline should be given. Tests for syphilis, *Chlamydia*, and HIV infection should be considered after completion of therapy (see Fig. 293–1).

Prognosis

The outcome of gonococcal arthritis is excellent, although a more aggressive course can occur if left untreated or in the presence of coinfection with HIV.

Viral Arthritis

This group of arthritides is the second most common cause of infectious arthritis after bacterial arthritis. A variety of viral infections are accompanied by inflammatory articular involvement, including parvovirus, rubella virus, hepatitis B, C, and A viruses, cytomegalovirus, and HIV. Most often, acute arthritis is the initial complaint, with chronic arthritis or vasculitis, or both, occurring less commonly.

Most patients with viral-associated arthritis do respond well to a combination of antiviral agents and anti-inflammatory and analgesic therapy. Immunosuppressive agents, including steroids, methotrexate, azathioprine, or cyclosporine, may need to be used in cases refractory to conventional therapy.

Other viruses less commonly causing arthralgias and arthritis include herpes zoster, Epstein-Barr virus, echovirus, adenovirus, and coxsackievirus. Chikungunya, o'nyong-nyong, and Ross River viruses are all alphaviruses responsible for major epidemics of febrile polyarthritis in Africa, Australia, Europe, and Latin America.

Miscellaneous Forms of Infectious Arthritis

Mycoplasma Arthritis

Mycoplasma hominis–induced (Chapter 338) monarthritis or oligoarthritis is relatively common in children and immunocompromised patients, including transplant recipients, particularly in individuals with agammaglobulinemia. The clinical features are identical to other bacterial forms of septic arthritis, but prolonged (often lasting 6 weeks to 6 months) antibiotic treatment with doxycycline or other tetracyclines, clindamycin, lincomycin, and fluoroquinolones is often necessary. The outcome is generally good.

Lyme Disease

Arthritis is the most common clinical manifestation of late (persistent) or stage 3 Lyme disease (Chapter 342). The knee joint is involved in almost all cases. Symmetrical or RA-like joint involvement in association with HLA-DR4 responds poorly to antibiotics. Laboratory diagnosis is based on serologic techniques. Treatment with appropriate antibiotics is effective in most patients with the correct diagnosis. Identified risk factors leading to failure of antibiotic treatment include older age and previous administration of intra-articular steroids.

Tuberculous Arthritis

Both pulmonary and extrapulmonary tuberculosis (Chapter 345) has exhibited a resurgence in the past 10 years. Two major reasons are the HIV pandemic and the increasing use of biologic agents such as inhibitors of TNF-α in patients with RA, Crohn's disease, psoriatic arthritis, and ankylosing spondylitis. Active pulmonary involvement is often not detected, but the purified protein derivative skin test is usually positive. Direct histologic evidence and culture of synovial fluid or membrane (or both) are required for diagnosis, particularly in patients with chronic monarthritis or oligoarthritis of the large joints such as the knees, hips, or ankles and in patients unresponsive to conventional therapy. Joint involvement with atypical *Mycobacterium* infection should be considered in immunocompromised patients, after repeated intra-articular steroid injections, in patients receiving biologic agents, and in certain occupations (e.g., fisherman). Long-term therapy with isoniazid, ethambutol, or rifampin (or any combination of these drugs) is indicated.

Syphilis

Joint involvement may occur at any stage of congenital, secondary, and tertiary syphilis (Chapter 341). It may also complicate the course of HIV infection. A wide clinical spectrum can occur, including osteochondritis, osteitis, periostitis, and bilateral hydrarthrosis, usually involving the knees and painless joints (Clutton's joints) in children with congenital syphilis. Polyarthralgia, polyarthritis, tenosynovitis (not common or as painful as in DGI), unilateral sacroiliitis, and spondylitis may occur in patients with secondary syphilis. Charcot's joints, gummatous arthritis, osteitis, and chronic arthritis may all be seen in patients with tertiary syphilis. The diagnosis can be difficult to establish, especially in the setting of HIV infection, in which repeated serologic analysis is often necessary. Penicillin is the agent of choice for syphilitic arthritis, and the outcome is usually very good.

Fungal Arthritis

Fungal arthritis is a rare occurrence, although an increased incidence of pathogenic and opportunistic fungal infections with the emergence of new species is being described, particularly in immunocompromised patients, including those treated with TNF-α inhibitors. Any joint can be affected, but the large joints are preferentially involved. The most common fungi affecting the musculoskeletal system are *Coccidioides immitis, Histoplasma capsulatum, Blastomyces dermatitides, Sporothrix schenckii,* and in immunocompromised patients, *Candida, Aspergillus, Cryptococcus,* and *Histoplasma.* The diagnosis of fungal arthritis requires a high index of suspicion, particularly in patients exhibiting a lack of response to conventional therapy or negative synovial fluid cultures. The diagnosis requires identification of the organism in synovial tissue or isolation from synovial fluid or tissue. Long-term therapy with amphotericin B and the newer antimycotic agents, with or without surgical débridement, generally leads to a good outcome.

INFECTION OF BONE

Acute and Chronic Osteomyelitis

Definition

Osteomyelitis is an inflammatory process that affects any portion of the bone, leads to destruction, and is caused by infectious microorganisms. Acute osteomyelitis is characterized by an inflammatory process that develops over a period of several weeks, usually 4 to 6, whereas the chronic form is a long-standing infection of bone that develops over a span of months or, less often, years.

Epidemiology

The epidemiology of acute osteomyelitis is well characterized. It is more common in males, especially of lower socioeconomic status, and it varies among geographic areas. In contrast, the epidemiology of chronic osteomyelitis is less well characterized, except in diabetics, in whom a foot problem will eventually develop in an estimated 15% or more during their lifetime. In a small, but important proportion of diabetic patients, limb amputation may be required.

Pathobiology

S. aureus is the most commonly isolated pathogen in both acute and chronic osteomyelitis. Streptococci are the second most common group of microorganisms involved. In diabetic foot infections, aerobic microorganisms such as *S. aureus, S. epidermidis,* enterococci, other streptococci, and *Corynebacterium* sp and anaerobic microorganisms such as *Peptostreptococcus* sp are most commonly involved. In osteomyelitis secondary to puncture wounds in the foot, *Pseudomonas aeruginosa* is identified frequently and is associated with wearing sneakers. *Salmonella* is associated with sickle cell disease. Other less common causes include a variety of fungi, mycobacteria, brucellae, actinomycetes, and parasites.

Hematogenous spread, especially in children and elderly individuals, is the most common mechanism associated with bone infection, although trauma, surgery, and implantation of joint prosthetics are also recognized. Diabetes patients are at an increased risk for osteomyelitis secondary to the metabolic consequences of the disease, ischemia of bone and soft tissue, and the presence of peripheral motor, sensory, and autonomic neuropathy.

Risk Factors

Several factors, both extracellular and cell associated, elaborated by pathogenic microorganisms greatly contribute to their virulence. Factors that promote adhesion (adhesins) to extracellular matrix proteins play a key role in the initiation of osteomyelitis. Other factors promote resistance to host defense mechanisms (protein A, toxins, and capsular polysaccharides), whereas exotoxins attack host cells or degrade components of the extracellular matrix to promote invasion or tissue penetration by microorganisms. In addition, *S. aureus* strains possess other virulence factors, including factors that promote its endocytic uptake by epithelial or endothelial cells. Once inside the cell, these bacteria may remain in a metabolically altered state and can even change morphology, the so-called small-colony variants, which may explain their persistence in bones.

Staphylococci and some gram-negative organisms can also form biofilms, which are difficult to treat with antimicrobial agents. This resistance of biofilms is mediated by a number of factors, including low metabolic rates, adaptive stress responses, and downregulated rates of cell division of the deeply embedded microbes.

Finally, bone resorption and necrosis are a direct result of the release of inflammatory mediators such as prostaglandins, growth factors, and cytokines such as TNF-α from activated monocytes and osteoclasts.

Pathology

The inflammatory process in bone is influenced by the microorganisms present; by the nature of the cell infiltrate resulting in the release of inflammatory mediators, such as prostaglandins, growth factors, and cytokines; and by the rigid nature of bone. Inflammation of bone leads to increased intramedullary pressure, compression of sinuses and capillaries in the marrow, and eventually ischemia with infarction or bone necrosis. Reactive hyperemia present at the edge of the infarction is associated with increased osteoclastic activity. Segments of bone devoid of blood supply can separate to form sequestra that are retained within the overall bone structure and might continue to harbor bacteria despite antimicrobial therapy.

Clinical Manifestations

Acute Osteomyelitis

The clinical picture of acute osteomyelitis evolves over a period of several days or a few weeks, and it may be difficult to distinguish from acute septic arthritis. Soft tissue swelling, redness, and warmth occur late in osteomyelitis. Early signs in children, particularly infants, are an inability to move the affected limb and pain on passive motion. The presence of these findings in association with an acute febrile illness should lead one to a high suspicion of skeletal infection. Most radiographs do not show evidence of infection until at least 10 to 14 days after the onset, but soft tissue swelling may be an early finding.

Chronic Osteomyelitis

The clinical picture of chronic osteomyelitis depends on the site and risk factors involved. Chronic osteomyelitis in long bones usually occurs as a result of trauma and less often is due to hematogenous spread. Patients generally exhibit malaise, anorexia, weight loss, fever, and night sweats and often complain of persistent pain and drainage through sinus tracts. Because of the chronicity of the process and the difficulty in eradicating the responsible microorganism, there is persisting inflammation leading to necrosis, sequestra, and the formation of sinus tracts. Septic arthritis, pathologic fracture, septicemia, and amyloidosis are potential complications.

Back pain is the most common complaint of patients with vertebral osteomyelitis. The pain is worse at night, increased by activity, and relieved by rest. Osteomyelitis associated with an infected prosthesis, especially of the hip, is a common and challenging disorder. The risk for infection is highest during the first 2 years after implantation but persists at lower levels for the lifespan of the prosthesis. Reported infection rates for hip and knee replacements are 0.5 to 3% and 1 to 2%, respectively, and this risk rises if the joint fails mechanically. Most patients experience little or no fever and have a painful, unstable joint on examination or radiography, most commonly within the first few years after implantation. It is difficult to distinguish mechanical from septic loosening, and a positive culture of fluid or tissue (including histopathology) is required for diagnosis. *S. aureus* or coagulase-negative staphylococci are responsible for the majority of the bacteria cultured from infected prosthetic joints.

Osteomyelitis should also be highly suspected in diabetes patients with soft tissue inflammation or skin ulcerations in the feet that are present for at least a week. The patient may be afebrile and without significant pain, but physical examination reveals redness and swelling. MRI is the most useful procedure in early infection, and changes noted on plain radiographs are a late finding. Microbiologic diagnosis is best made by bone biopsy. *S. aureus* is the predominant microorganism in diabetic foot infections, but other gram-positive or gram-negative aerobic or anaerobic bacteria must also be considered.

Diagnosis

Osteomyelitis should be considered in a patient with an appropriate history and physical examination findings and confirmed by relevant radiographic and microbiologic testing. A high index of suspicion also is required (see Fig. 293–1).

Acute Osteomyelitis

In children and infants, limping or pain in a limb should always raise suspicion of osteomyelitis. The ESR and CRP are elevated in most patients (>90%), but normal values do not rule out the diagnosis. Blood cultures are positive in approximately 50% of patients. Plain radiographs are necessary at both initial evaluation and follow-up and show soft tissue swelling, narrowing or widening of the joint space, bone destruction, and periosteal reaction. It should be kept in mind that it usually takes 10 to 14 days to destroy 50% of the bone. Ultrasonography can be useful for early diagnosis in acute osteomyelitis or for detection of a purulent collection in soft tissue.

Both CT and MRI, as well as positron emission tomography (PET) with ^{18}F-fluoro-D-deoxyglucose (FDG) combined with CT, can be very helpful to delineate the presence of sequestra or soft tissue involvement, confirm the diagnosis, and assist in the planning of surgery. The "gold standard" test, however, is identification of the microorganism in cultures of material obtained by needle aspiration from the infected area. Whenever bone biopsies are performed, the samples should be processed for aerobic and anaerobic cultures. Samples should also be collected for mycobacterial and fungal cultures, especially if routine bacteriologic cultures are negative. Tissue specimens obtained for histopathology are likewise important because the presence of more than five neutrophils per high-power field indicates infection with a sensitivity of 43 to 84% and a specificity of 93 to 97%. Visualization of granulomatous lesions with positive Ziehl-Nielsen staining is indicative of mycobacterial infection, although it should be confirmed by culture.

Differential Diagnosis

Chronic recurrent multifocal osteomyelitis (CRMO) and SAPHO (synovitis, acne, pustulosis, hyperostosis, and osteitis) syndrome are two conditions that may be difficult to distinguish from osteomyelitis. Both CRMO and SAPHO syndrome, however, are benign disorders, more commonly seen in girls (CRMO) and young adults (SAPHO). These disorders are accompanied by skeletal lesions that affect both the metaphyses and other bones such as the clavicle, pelvis, and spine, but bone cultures are negative.

Other bone conditions such as histiocytosis X (eosinophilic granuloma), Gaucher's disease, and Ewing's sarcoma may also be rarely confused with osteomyelitis, but bone culture should assist in the diagnosis.

Treatment

Acute Osteomyelitis

A combined antimicrobial and surgical approach should be considered in all cases of acute osteomyelitis, although surgery is not usually required. The choice of initial antibiotic can be inferred from the results of Gram-stained specimens and modified if necessary after the results of culture become available. Most patients can be treated for a minimum of 3 weeks for infections caused by staphylococci or gram-negative bacilli. Longer periods of therapy may be required if the clinical response is slow or if the ESR remains elevated. Oral antibiotics can be considered after a short course of parenteral therapy, provided that the organism is well characterized and sensitive and the patient and family are compliant.

Rx

Chronic Osteomyelitis

Chronic osteomyelitis generally requires antibiotics and surgical intervention. Oftentimes, cure can be achieved with little antibiotic treatment, provided that necrotic bone and foreign material are removed.

Surgery for chronic osteomyelitis, including diabetic foot infection, is aimed at the removal of sequestra and resection of scarred and infected bone and soft tissue. In vertebral osteomyelitis, surgery is undertaken to relieve compression of the spinal cord or to drain epidural or paravertebral abscesses and to improve spinal stability. The basic approach in prosthetic joint infection is to remove the device, followed by débridement of bone and soft tissue, along with the administration of parenteral antibiotic therapy for 4 to 6 weeks before reconstruction is carried out.

Single-agent antimicrobial therapy is usually adequate for the treatment of chronic osteomyelitis, except for infections of prosthetic joints, for which a combination of antimicrobials, including rifampicin, is commonly used. As a general principle, intravenous antibiotic therapy should be given for 4 to 6 weeks.

Because the most common infecting organism in chronic osteomyelitis is *S. aureus,* benzylpenicillin, 12 to 20 million U daily, is the drug of choice for penicillin-sensitive organisms. Alternative antibiotics include cefazolin, 1 g every 6 hours, clindamycin, 600 mg every 6 hours, or vancomycin, 1 g every 12 hours. For methicillin-sensitive *S. aureus* infections, nafcillin, 1 or 1.5 g every 4 to 6 hours, or cefazolin, 2 g every 8 hours, is the drug of choice. Other alternatives include second-generation cephalosporins, such as cefuroxime, cefamandole, clindamycin, vancomycin, ciprofloxacin, or levofloxacin, in combination with rifampicin. For methicillin-resistant *S. aureus,* the drug of choice is vancomycin, 1 g every 12 hours, or teicoplanin, 400 mg every 24 hours (first day every 24 hours). Rifampin or rifampin plus gentamicin has been used in addition to vancomycin. Linezolid can also be used.

Therapy for osteomyelitis secondary to gram-negative microorganisms is based on sensitivities of the infecting pathogen.

In mixed infections with aerobic and anaerobic microorganisms, ampicillin-sulbactam, 2 to 3 g every 6 to 8 hours, is the drug of choice, and as alternative, imipenem, 500 mg every 6 hours, can be given. Outpatient parenteral therapy followed by long-term oral therapy should be considered in patients with chronic osteomyelitis after initial inpatient parenteral therapy (Table 293–2).

TABLE 293–2 ANTIBIOTIC THERAPY FOR SELECTED MICROORGANISMS IN SEPTIC ARTHRITIS* AND OSTEOMYELITIS†

Microorganism	Agent of Choice	Alternative
Staphylococcus aureus (methicillin sensitive)	Oxacillin or nafcillin, 2 g IV q6h	Cefazolin, vancomycin
Staphylococcus aureus (methicillin resistant)	Vancomycin, 1 g IV q12h	Gentamicin or trimethoprim-sulfamethoxazole plus rifampin, linezolid
Group A or B β-hemolytic streptococci and *Streptococcus pneumoniae*	Penicillin G, 10–20 million units IV daily	Clindamycin, vancomycin, erythromycin, cefazolin, linezolid
Enterococci	Ampicillin, 2 g IV q4h	Vancomycin, linezolid if vancomycin resistant
Neisseria gonorrhoeae	Ceftriaxone, 1 g IM or IV qd, followed by oral cefixime, 400 mg bid, or ciprofloxacin, 500 mg bid × 7–10 days. If penicillin sensitive, use penicillin G, ampicillin, or amoxicillin with probenecid	If allergic to β-lactams, ciprofloxacin, 500 mg IV q12h, or spectinomycin (also if pregnant), 2 g IM q12h, followed by oral therapy ×7 days
Enteric gram-negative bacilli	Ciprofloxacin, 400–750 mg IV q12h	Ceftriaxone, levofloxacin
Pseudomonas aeruginosa	Ciprofloxacin, 400 mg IV q12h	Piperacillin plus aminoglycoside
Bacteroides sp	Clindamycin, 600 mg IV q6h	Imipenem, metronidazole, ampicillin
Mixed infection (aerobic and anaerobic microorganisms)	Ampicillin-sulbactam, 2–3 g q6–8h	Imipenem, levofloxacin plus metronidazole

*Treatment should last at least 3 weeks—1 week of intravenous therapy followed by oral therapy.
†Treatment should last a minimum of 4 to 6 weeks and may last up to 24 months in patients with prosthetic joint infection or diabetic infection.

Prognosis

Outcomes in patients with acute osteomyelitis are very good without the development of chronic osteomyelitis. In contrast, both the morbidity and mortality associated with chronic osteomyelitis are high, especially in diabetics.

Future Directions

The development of more rapid, sensitive, and specific techniques such as PCR and DNA analysis should allow better and prompt identification of offending microorganisms in bursa, joint, and bone infection. Moreover, the development of newer antibiotics useful in the treatment of resistant microorganisms should lead to a better outcome. Finally, refinement of imaging techniques such as CT, MRI, and PET scanning should eventually allow distinction between sterile inflammation and infection.

SUGGESTED READINGS

Ayral X: Arthroscopy and joint lavage. Best Pract Res Clin Rheumatol 2005;19:401–415. *Review of the role of arthroscopy and joint lavage in the management of septic arthritis.*

Berendt T, Byren J: Bone and joint infection. Clin Med 2004;4:510–518. *Review of bone and joint infection.*

Garcia-DeLaTorre I: Advances in the management of septic arthritis. Infect Dis Clin North Am 2006;20:773–788. *Excellent review of septic arthritis.*

Kapoor A, Page S, Lavalley M, et al: Magnetic resonance imaging for diagnosing foot osteomyelitis: A meta-analysis. Arch Intern Med 2007;167:125–132. *MRI can be used to rule in or out osteomyelitis of the foot and ankle, and its performance was superior to that of technetium 99m bone scanning.*

Lazzarini L, Lipsky BA, Mader JT: Antibiotic treatment of osteomyelitis: What have we learned from 30 years of clinical trial? Int J Infect Dis 2005;9:127–138. *Comprehensive review of antibiotic use in osteomyelitis.*

Lew DP, Waldrogel FA: Osteomyelitis. Lancet 2004;364:369–379. *Comprehensive review of a complex issue.*

Lipsky DA: International consensus group on diagnosing and treating the infected diabetic foot. Diabetes Metab Res Rev 2004;1:568–577. *Review of a difficult condition.*

Ross JJ, Hu LT: Septic arthritis of the pubic symphysis: Review of 100 cases. Medicine (Baltimore) 2003;82:340–345. *Review of risk factors, clinical features, and management of this not uncommon condition.*

Schett G, Hera KP, Graninger W, et al: *Listeria*-associated arthritis in a patient undergoing etanercept therapy: Case report and review of the literature. J Clin Microbiol 2005;43:2537–2541. *Report illustrating the emergence of musculoskeletal septic complications during the course of therapy with TNF-α inhibitors.*

Zimmerli W, Trampuz A, Ochsner PE: Current concepts: Prosthetic-joint infections. N Engl J Med 2004;351:1645–1654. *A comprehensive review.*

294 CRYSTAL DEPOSITION DISEASES

Robert Terkeltaub

Supersaturation of body fluids with a variety of solutes may result in the deposition of different forms of crystals and calculi. Pathologic crystallization can be a clinical problem not only within extracellular fluids (e.g., biliary tract and urinary tract calculi) but also within the matrix of certain connective tissues (e.g., arterial wall calcification in atherosclerosis). In gout, systemic elevation of uric acid promotes deposition of the monosodium salt of uric acid at stereotypical locations, including the synovium and cartilage of peripheral joints, the olecranon bursa, and the helix of the ear. The loose avascular connective tissue of articular cartilage is particularly susceptible to calcification with aging in idiopathic chondrocalcinosis, with osteoarthritis, and with an intra-articular excess of inorganic pyrophosphate (PP_i) in these conditions and certain metabolic disorders. This chapter discusses crystal deposition diseases that are predominantly manifested as joint disease (with the principal focus on gout, calcium pyrophosphate dihydrate [CPPD] crystal deposition disease, hydroxyapatite [HA] crystal deposition, and the articular manifestations of oxalate crystal deposition).

GOUT AND HYPERURICEMIA

Definition

The term *gout* refers to heterogeneous disorders resulting from tissue deposition of monosodium urate crystals or crystallization of uric acid in the urinary tract. Fundamental to the development of gout is a substantial increase in total body uric acid stores, as reflected in the metabolic disorder hyperuricemia. The definition of hyperuricemia is a serum uric acid level at least 2 SD above the norm established by individual laboratories according to gender. Serum urate levels rise with puberty, and then in females, they remain relatively stable overall until menopause, at which time concentrations begin to rise in association with loss of the ability of estrogen to promote renal excretion of uric acid. Typically, hyperuricemia is defined as a serum uric acid level greater than 7.0 mg/dL in adult men and 6.0 mg/dL in premenopausal women.

Epidemiology

Gout is predominantly an idiopathic or multifactorial disease of adult men, with a peak incidence in the fifth decade. Gout rarely occurs in men before adolescence or in women before menopause. The disease is common. In 1986, the prevalence of self-reported gout in America was 13.6 per 1000 men and 6.4 per 1000 women. The prevalence has increased over the past few decades in countries that have an improving standard of living. Its prevalence in persons of Pacific Islander ethnic extraction appears to be substantially higher than in white individuals. In association with increased longevity, the frequency of metabolic syndrome, and the common use of hyperuricemia-promoting thiazide diuretics, the prevalence of gout in the United States is also rising in both aging men and women, particularly in association with chronic renal insufficiency. Dietary and lifestyle risk factors for the development of gout in men include a relatively high intake of meat, seafood, and beer, with a protective effect in men associated with relatively high intake of low-fat dairy products. [1,2]

Hyperuricemia can be documented in at least 5% of asymptomatic Americans on at least one occasion during adulthood. The duration and magnitude of hyperuricemia directly correlate with risk for the development of gout. However, in only a minority of individuals with sustained hyperuricemia does clinical gout eventually develop, partly because increases in serum urate levels are relatively mild (i.e., serum urate less than 9.0 mg/dL) in most individuals or occur transiently in response to dietary and pharmacologic changes. Therefore, asymptomatic hyperuricemia without gout is not a disease.

Pathobiology

Uric acid is normally produced as an end product of the degradation of purine compounds (Fig. 294–1). However, the solubility of the principal physiologic salt of uric acid, monosodium urate, in connective tissues is normally close to 7 mg/dL at 37° C, and urate solubility declines progressively at cooler temperatures such as those in distal peripheral joints. Thus, in humans, "normal" serum urate concentrations provide only a narrow safety margin for urate crystal deposition. Human beings, like other high mammals, lack uric acid oxidase (uricase), which oxidizes uric acid to the more soluble compound allantoin. Significantly, not only do genetically engineered uricase knockout mice demonstrate a marked increase in levels of serum urate (from ≈1.0 to 11.0 mg/dL), but severe uric acid nephrolithiasis with compromise of renal function in early life also develops.

Miscible total body urate stores are approximately 1.2 g (range, 800 to 1600 mg) in healthy men and about half this value in healthy women. Significantly, urate synthesis averages around 750 mg/day in men, and dietary purine intake stimulates additional uric acid production. Gastrointestinal elimination of uric acid via bacterial urate oxidation in the gut can remove a few hundred milligrams of uric acid daily, but this elimination pathway has limited potential for adaptive increases in capacity. Renal urate excretion in normal adult men ingesting a purine-free diet averages approximately 400 mg/day, with the normal range being between 250 and 750 mg/day with a typical Western diet. Renal urate excretion can increase substantially in adaptation to increased uric acid generation. However, physiologic limits to renal elimination of uric acid

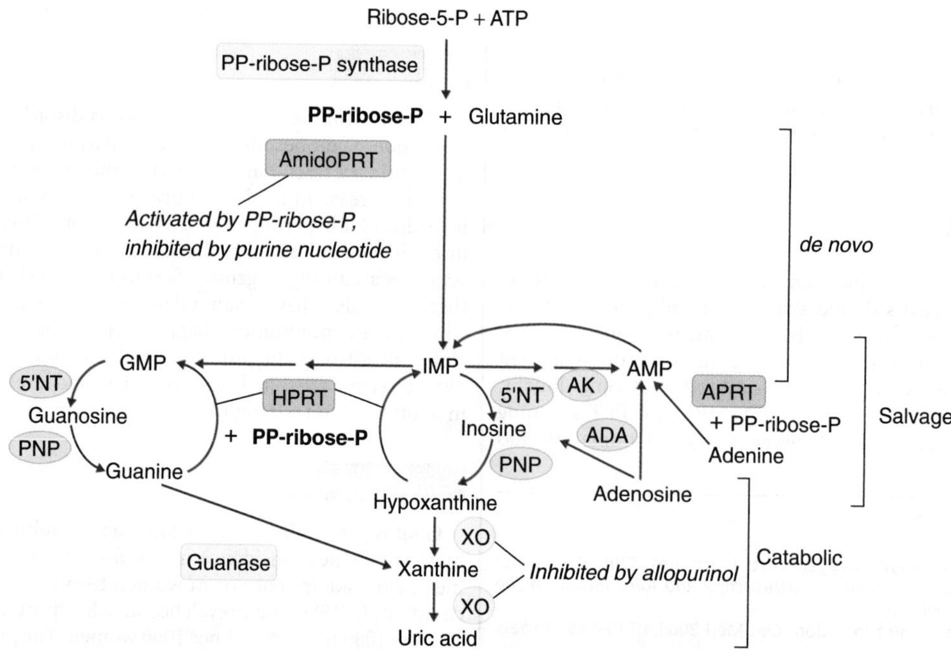

FIGURE 294–1 • Intracellular purine metabolism and generation of uric acid. The synthesis of purine nucleotides involves closely regulated biochemical pathways, termed "de novo" and "salvage." In the de novo pathway, a purine ring is synthesized from small-molecule precursors and sequentially added to a ribose-phosphate backbone donated by 5-phosphoribosyl 1-pyrophosphate (PP-ribose-P). The first reaction of the de novo pathway is catalyzed by amidophosphoribosyltransferase (AmidoPRT). This reaction is the main site of pathway regulation via antagonistic interaction involving inhibition by relatively abundant purine nucleotide products and activation by PP-ribose-P, which is normally relatively sparse. At inosine monophosphate (IMP), the pathway branches and gives rise to adenosine monophosphate (AMP) and guanosine monophosphate (GMP) and their derivatives. Control of purine nucleotide production also occurs at distal points in the pathways governing the formation of adenylate and guanylate derivatives. In the salvage pathway, the preformed purine bases hypoxanthine, guanine, and adenine, derived from turnover of IMP, GMP, and AMP, are directly condensed with PP-ribose-P by hypoxanthine-guanine phosphoribosyltransferase (HGPRT) and adenine phosphoribosyltransferase (APRT). Factors that govern the relationship between rates of purine base salvage and purine synthesis include the availability of PP-ribose-P and concentrations of the nucleotide products common to both pathways. The catabolic steps that generate uric acid from nucleic acids and free purine nucleotides involve degradation to hypoxanthine and xanthine through purine nucleoside intermediates. Some of the hypoxanthine formed by nucleotide turnover is diverted to the liver and metabolized in sequential reactions catalyzed by xanthine oxidase (XO) to uric acid; the remainder is salvaged by HGRPT. Operation of the salvage pathway reduces de novo pathway activity because HGRPT and APRT have greater affinity for PPRP than amidoPRT does inasmuch as base salvage lowers the concentration of PP-ribose-P and the nucleotide end products of the HRPT and APRT reactions directly inhibit AmidoPRT. Clinically, inherited mutations or regulatory defects of PP-ribose-P synthetase related to superactivity of this enzyme are associated with hyperuricemia. Deficiency of HGPRT promotes hyperuricemia via enhanced conversion of hypoxanthine and guanine to uric acid and a compensatory increase in de novo pathway activity because of reduced formation of inhibitory nucleotides and increased availability of PP-ribose-P for the AmidoPRT reaction. Increased net ATP breakdown can cause hyperuricemia by enhancing the production of XO substrates and by releasing inhibition of AmidoPRT. Hyperuricemia associated with net ATP catabolism in muscle and liver may occur acutely in certain conditions (including severe hypoxia and tissue ischemia and hereditary fructose intolerance) (see Table 294–1) and chronically in association with excessive alcohol consumption, which places increased demands on hepatocellular ATP stores for metabolism of alcohol. Therapeutically, allopurinol, by blocking XO-catalyzed generation of uric acid, enhances salvage of hypoxanthine, thus further inhibiting de novo activity. This action reduces purine excretion more than expected from inhibition of uric acid formation alone. ADA = adenosine deaminase; AK = adenosine kinase; 5′NT = 5′-nucleotidase; PNP = purine nucleoside phosphorylase.

constrain the capacity of this urate removal pathway, and excessive uric acid filtration is nephrotoxic, as discussed later. Therefore, the majority of total body urate stores is normally turned over daily, thus providing a narrow physiologic window for urate balance with the potential for substantial expansion of total body urate stores.

Multiple social, environmental, and genetic factors influence uric acid formation and removal. Familial occurrence of gout is reported in approximately 20% of affected patients. Family and twin studies suggest that both hyperuricemia and renal handling of uric acid are polygenic traits. In a given individual, single and combined disorders of uric acid formation and excretion can be responsible for hyperuricemia and gout (Table 294–1). A minority of patients with gout have urate overproduction alone as the primary abnormality. The most common defect identifiable in patients with gout is renal underexcretion of urate via an undefined mechanism. Recent cloning of the key renal urate reabsorption transporter URAT1 may help in elucidating the molecular basis for this common observation.

Abnormal Renal Handling of Urate

Almost all plasma urate is filtered at the glomerulus, with more than 95% of the filtered load undergoing proximal tubular (presecretory) reabsorption. The major effector of proximal tubular reabsorption of urate is URAT1, an organic anion exchanger expressed at the apical membrane of proximal tubule epithelial cells that faces the tubule lumen. URAT1-induced urate reabsorption is stimulated by intracellular organic anions, including lactate. The capacity of estrogen to suppress URAT1 expression plays a central role in the uricosuric effects of estrogen that normally suppress serum urate levels in premenopausal women. The balance between proximal tubular secretion and reabsorption of filtered urate ultimately determines net renal uric acid excretion. A decreased glomerular filtration rate, heredity, and the effects of hydration, a variety of organic acids, including lactate and ketoacids, certain drugs, and exogenous toxins such as lead on tubular handling of uric acid can all impair renal excretion of uric acid (see Table 294–1). Alcohol decreases uric acid excretion via elevated lactic acid production. Among the offending pharmacologic agents are diuretics, cyclosporine, pyrazinamide, and low-dose acetylsalicylic acid (see Table 294–1). Patients with gout tend to have a relatively high incidence of other diseases that predispose to renal insufficiency, including hypertension, which can increase tubular urate reabsorption even in patients not treated with thiazide diuretics. A substantial fraction of patients with both hyperuricemia and primary gout have metabolic syndrome, in which insulin resistance is a central factor in the renal reabsorption of not only sodium, bicarbonate, and chloride but also uric acid. The impairment of urinary alkalinization in metabolic syndrome may be a factor in the elevated prevalence of uric acid urolithiasis in subjects with hyperuricemia.

Increased Urate Production

The pathways by which uric acid is generated in the metabolism of purine nucleotides are illustrated in Figure 294–1. In addition, the legend to Figure 294–1 summarizes the clinical implications of disordered activity of the uric acid synthetic pathways and the therapeutic mechanisms of action of xanthine oxidase inhibitors such as allopurinol. Between 10 and 20% of patients with gout produce excessive uric acid. In approxi-

TABLE 294–1 HYPERURICEMIA: CAUSES AND CLASSIFICATION*

A. Uric acid overproduction
  1. Primary hyperuricemia
     Idiopathic
     HGPRT deficiency (partial and complete)
     PRPP synthetase superactivity
  2. Secondary hyperuricemia
     Excessive dietary purine intake
     Increased nucleotide turnover (e.g., myeloproliferative and lymphoproliferative disorders, hemolytic diseases, psoriasis, and Paget's disease of bone)
     Accelerated ATP degradation
        Ethanol abuse
        Glycogen storage diseases (types I, III, V, VII)
        Fructose ingestion, hereditary fructose intolerance
        Hypoxemia and tissue underperfusion
        Severe muscle exertion
        ? Hypertriglyceridemia (via metabolism of excess acetate)
B. Uric acid underexcretion
  1. Primary hyperuricemia
     Idiopathic (influenced by gender and ethnicity)
     Familial juvenile hyperuricemic nephropathy
  2. Secondary hyperuricemia
     Diminished glomerular filtration rate
     Enhanced tubular urate reabsorption
        Dehydration
        Diuretics
        Insulin resistance (metabolic syndrome)
     Inhibition of tubular urate secretion
        Competitive anions (e.g., keto and lactic acidosis)
     Mechanism incompletely defined
        Hypertension
        Hyperparathyroidism
        Hypothyroidism
        Certain drugs (e.g., cyclosporine, pyrazinamide, ethambutol, and low-dose salicylates)
        Lead toxicity with nephropathy

*Increased uric acid production and diminished uric acid excretion by the kidney, alone or in combination, promote hyperuricemia in patients with gout. Classification of patients with gout by the mechanism or mechanisms causing hyperuricemia helps in directing the diagnosis of unsuspected, underlying disorders and is useful in guiding therapy. This table provides such a classification scheme in which primary hyperuricemia refers to inherently disordered uric acid metabolism not associated with a distinct acquired disorder such as ethanol abuse or diuretic therapy.
ATP = adenosine triphosphate; HGPRT = hypoxanthine-guanine phosphoribosyltransferase; PRPP = phosphoribosylpyrophosphate.

mately 10% of patients with gout, an excess of uric acid production can readily be documented by the excretion of more than 800 to 1000 mg/day of uric acid in a 24-hour urine collection (while ingesting a typical Western diet). Alcohol consumption is a particularly common factor in promoting hyperuricemia by increasing both uric acid production and renal urate reabsorption (see Table 294–1, Fig. 294–1). The high content of the readily absorbable dietary purine guanosine in beer and alcohol-induced accelerated hepatic breakdown of adenosine triphosphate (ATP) both promote increased uric acid production. Overproduction of uric acid also occurs commonly in several acquired and genetic disorders that are characterized by excessive rates of cell and therefore nucleic acid turnover (see Table 294–1). Inherited derangements in mechanisms regulating purine nucleotide synthesis (see Fig. 294–1, Table 294–1) account for a tiny fraction of patients with urate overproduction.

Pathogenesis

Tissue Deposition of Urate Crystals and Inflammatory Disease in Gout

Tophaceous deposits of urate crystals and the morphology of individual urate crystals are seen in Figures 294–2 and 294–3, respectively. Tophi commonly develop in osteoarthritic interphalangeal joints, thus suggesting roles of connective tissue matrix structure and turnover in urate crystal deposition. The predilection for marked urate crystal deposition in the first metatarsophalangeal (MTP) joint may also relate to repetitive minor trauma at that site. Microscopic tophaceous deposits of urate crystals are often present in the synovial membrane at the time of the first gouty attack and may also be detected within cartilage. Abrupt rises and declines in serum urate levels, as stimulated by diuretic and alcohol use and initiation of therapy with antihyperuricemic drugs, may promote the release of urate crystals from tophi via changes in packing of crystals in tophaceous deposits. Free urate crystals have considerable pro-inflammatory potential via the ability to activate synovial lining cells and leukocytes, induce activation of the membrane attack complex of complement, and trigger certain other inflammatory cascades. Yet in some individuals with gout, urate crystals can be found in asymptomatic MTP and knee joints that have never been involved in an acute attack or in noninflamed joints between acute attacks of gout at these sites. These findings reinforce that urate deposition in tissues can be asymptomatic.

Urate crystals activate cells in large part via recognition at the plasma membrane mediated by the toll-like receptors TLR2 and TLR4 and by TLR-mediated signal transduction pathways that promote activation of the nuclear factor kappa β (NF-κB) transcription factor. Urate crystals induce the cellular release of nitric oxide; cyclooxygenase (COX)- and lipoxygenase-derived metabolites of arachidonic acid; cytokines, including tumor necrosis factor-α, interleukin-1, and CXCL8; and certain matrix metalloproteinases. The ingress of neutrophils into the joint is central in triggering acute gouty arthritis, and effects on neutrophil-endothelial interaction probably represent a major locus for the prophylactic and therapeutic effects of colchicine. CXCL8 and closely related chemokines that bind CXCR2 (including CXCL1) appear to be critical in initiating and perpetuating neutrophil ingress in acute gouty inflammation. The acute gouty attack is often spontaneously self-limited by 7 to 10 days, probably mediated by an altered balance between pro- and anti-inflammatory mediators (e.g., transforming growth factor -β [TGF-β]) in the joint. However, low-grade synovitis may persist in affected joints. Inflammatory mechanisms in gout, especially in untreated disease, can lead to chronic synovial proliferation, cartilage loss, and bone erosion.

Clinical Manifestations

Gout is classically manifested as recurrent attacks of acute arthritis characterized by often excruciatingly painful articular and periarticular inflammation, including erythema and edema of the skin that can mimic bacterial cellulitis. Acute gouty arthritis is typically monarticular or oligoarticular. Stereotypical involvement of the first MTP joint is termed *podagra*. Acute polyarticular gout can also occur, particularly in the elderly and in transplant patients taking cyclosporine. This manifestation can be associated with substantial systemic leukocytosis and temperature elevation mimicking sepsis. Chronic gouty inflammation and proliferative, erosive arthritis in gout can also mimic rheumatoid arthritis.

Gouty tophi (see Fig. 294–2) can involve not only the synovium and cartilage of joints but also subchondral bone and soft tissues, including the olecranon bursa, the first MTP joint bursa, and the helix of the ear. Olecranon bursitis may occur in association with gout, but tophi in the olecranon bursa often remain clinically quiescent. Uric acid urolithiasis is a common manifestation of gout, particularly in acid urine. Excessive excretion of uric acid in the urinary tract also promotes calcium oxalate urolithiasis. Interstitial nephropathy, characterized by the deposition of monosodium urate in the renal medulla at physiologic pH, is currently a rare manifestation of gout, largely because of advances in recognition and treatment of gout and hypertension.

Onset of gout (with or without tophaceous crystal deposits) in early adulthood and a high incidence of uric acid urinary tract stones constitute the common clinical phenotype in both partial deficiency of hypoxanthine-guanine phosphoribosyltransferase (HGPRT) and milder forms of superactivity of 5-phosphoribosyl 1-pyrophosphate (PP-ribose-P) synthetase. Severe HGPRT deficiency is associated with spasticity, choreoathetosis, mental retardation, and self-mutilation (Lesch-Nyhan syndrome). In some subjects, regulatory defects in PP-ribose-P synthetase are accompanied by sensorineural deafness and neurodevelopmental defects. The genes for both HGPRT and PP-ribose-P synthetase are X-linked. Thus, homozygous males are affected, and postmenopausal

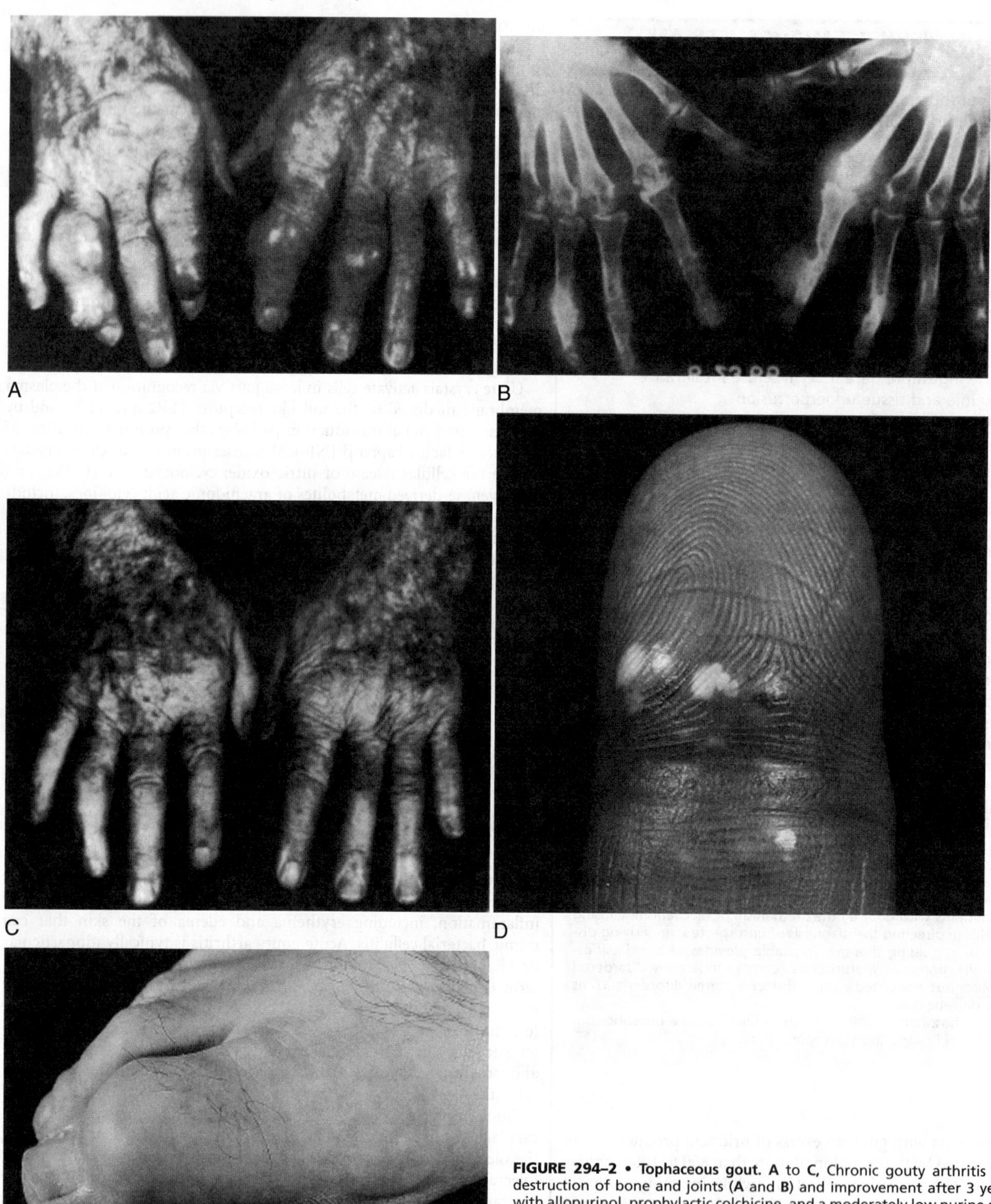

FIGURE 294–2 • Tophaceous gout. A to **C,** Chronic gouty arthritis with tophaceous destruction of bone and joints (**A** and **B**) and improvement after 3 years of treatment with allopurinol, prophylactic colchicine, and a moderately low purine diet (**C**). **D,** Tophaceous deposits in the digital pad of a 28-year-old man with systemic lupus erythematosus under treatment with diuretics. A single attack of gout had occurred 2 years earlier. **E,** Tophaceous enlargement of the great toe in a 44-year-old man with a 4-year history of recurrent gouty arthritis.

gout and urinary tract stones can occur as the phenotype of carrier females. Hyperuricemia in prepubertal boys always suggests the need to determine whether one of these enzymatic defects is the etiology.

Diagnosis

The combination of the classic picture of acute gouty arthritis described earlier, or urolithiasis, and evidence of past or current hyperuricemia is highly suggestive of gout. Importantly, the serum uric acid level may fluctuate and is often normal at the time of an acute gout attack. The synovial fluid in acute gout typically demonstrates leukocytosis and other nonspecific features of joint inflammation. The ability of gout to mimic septic arthritis and vice versa is noteworthy, and free and intracellular urate crystals (or CPPD crystals) are sometimes found as a secondary effect of inflammation in septic joints. Thus, the diagnostic importance of arthrocentesis with adequate synovial fluid crystal analysis and, in many instances, concomitant exclusion of joint infection is emphasized (Fig. 294–4). As illustrated in Figure 294–3, urate crystals (needle-shaped, brightly negatively birefringent crystals, many of them within neutrophils) can be identified by compensated polarized light microscopy of wet preparations of synovial fluid in the vast majority of

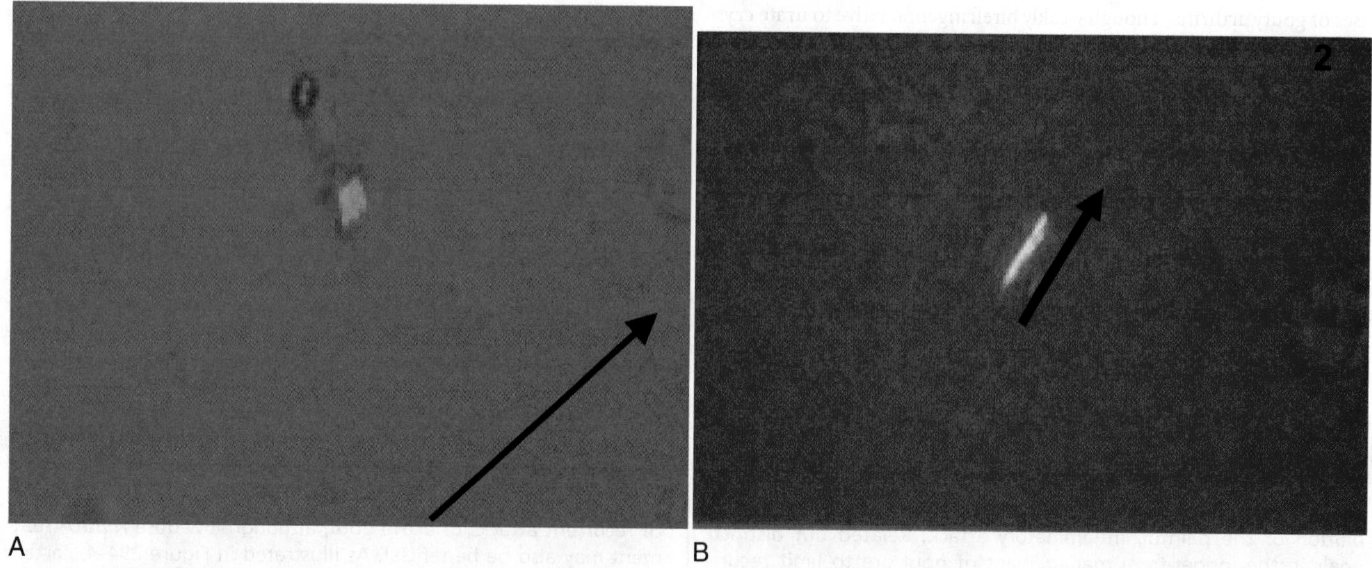

FIGURE 294–3 • Comparison of calcium pyrophosphate dihydrate (CPPD) and monosodium urate crystals identified under compensated polarized light microscopy of synovial fluid. CPPD crystals **(A)** and monosodium urate crystals **(B)** are shown as identified in wet preparations of synovial fluid by compensated polarized light microscopy. Both crystal types are found within leukocytes, and both can be extracellular, as also shown for CPPD crystals here. CPPD crystals are weakly birefringent and more variable in shape, with rhomboid, square, or rodlike structures that can resemble urate crystals. Urate crystals are uniformly needle shaped and more brightly birefringent than CPPD crystals are. The arrows indicate the axis of slow rotation of light of the first-order red plate compensator used in compensated polarized light microscopy. Urate crystals are negatively birefringent (i.e., yellow when the long axis of the crystal is parallel to the red plate compensator axis and blue when the long axis of the crystal is perpendicular to the compensator axis). CPPD crystals are positively birefringent (i.e., blue when the long axis of the crystal is parallel to the axis of slow rotation of light of the red plate compensator and yellow when the long axis of the crystal is perpendicular to the axis of the compensator), as seen for the two CPPD crystals in **A.** These findings indicate the need for compensated polarized light microscopy to both identify urate and CPPD crystals and to accurately distinguish between these crystal types. (**A,** Available at *http://www.emedicine.com/med/topic1938.htm,* accessed March 6, 2006. **B,** ACR Clinical Slide Collection on the Rheumatic Diseases. American College of Rheumatology, 1998.)

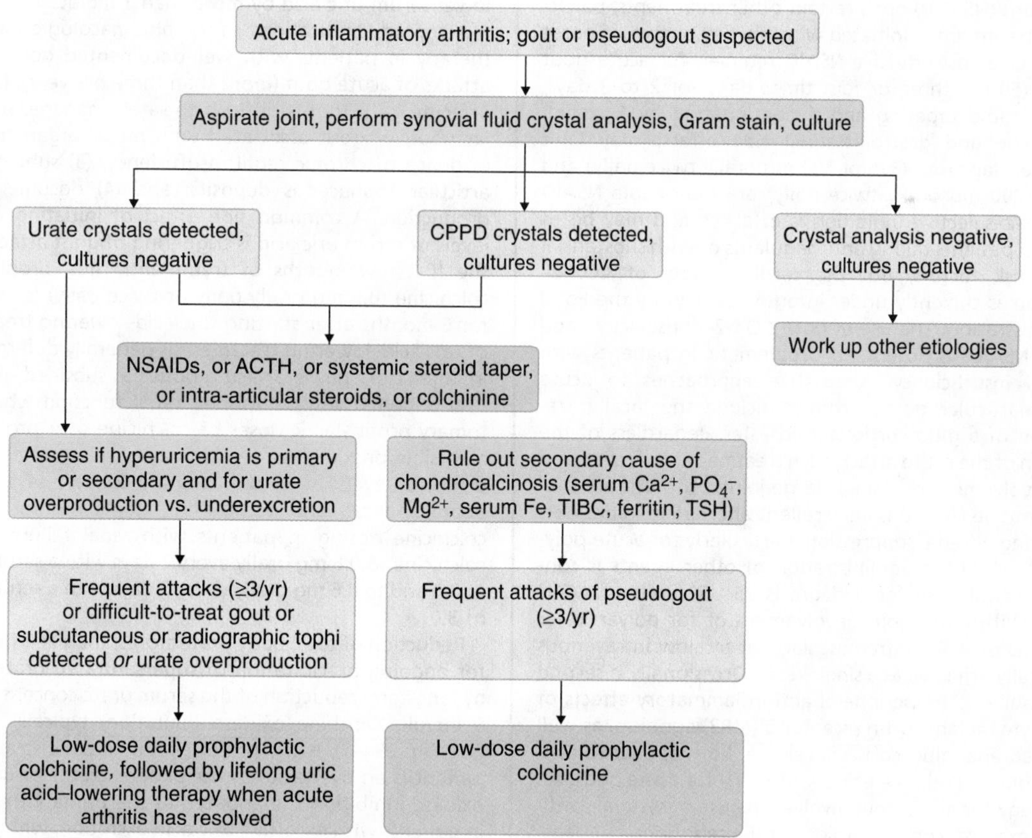

FIGURE 294–4 • Algorithm for the clinical approach to acute gouty arthritis and pseudogout. In this scheme, central emphasis is placed on the diagnostic importance of arthrocentesis and synovial fluid analysis. ACTH = adrenocorticotropic hormone; CPPD = calcium pyrophosphate dihydrate; NSAIDs = nonsteroidal anti-inflammatory drugs; TIBC = total iron-binding capacity; TSH = thyroid-stimulating hormone.

cases of gouty arthritis. Though weakly birefringent relative to urate crystals and often rhomboid in shape, CPPD crystals (see Fig. 294–3) can be rod shaped and intracellular and thereby resemble urate crystals. Thus, the use of compensated polarized light microscopy is essential to exclude positively birefringent CPPD crystals. Other investigations of diagnostic value that can also assist in management decisions include measurement of levels of 24-hour uric acid excretion and the use of radiographs to detect classic tophaceous changes of articular gout. Certain radiographic findings in gout, such as sharply marginated bone erosions with overhanging edges, are clearly distinct from the radiographic findings in CPPD deposition disease and rheumatoid arthritis. Measurement of 24-hour urinary uric acid in subjects with intact renal function and no clear cause for hyperuricemia is valuable to identify subjects with uric acid overproduction.

Treatment

Rx

The principal goal of therapy for acute gout is rapid and safe resolution of the painful, inflammatory attack. Related but distinct goals in the longer-term management of gout are to limit recurrences of acute gouty arthritis, prevent the disabling tissue consequences of monosodium urate crystal deposition and urolithiasis, and recognize and appropriately treat medical conditions commonly associated with gout (e.g., hypertension, obesity, hyperlipidemia, alcohol abuse, chronic renal insufficiency, and possibly hypothyroidism). Xanthine oxidase inhibitors, exemplified by allopurinol, or in carefully selected patients, uricosurics, exemplified by probenecid, are used to reduce serum urate levels. These antihyperuricemic agents do not have intrinsic anti-inflammatory properties.

Acute Gouty Arthritis

Acute gouty arthritis generally responds well to nonsteroidal anti-inflammatory drugs (NSAIDs) or to certain other treatments, particularly when the treatment is initiated within a day or two of onset (see Fig. 294–4). One cost-effective NSAID regimen for acute gout is indomethacin (50 mg three or four times daily for 2 to 3 days, with subsequent rapid tapering and discontinuation by 1 week). However, headache and gastrointestinal side effects may limit indomethacin use. Naproxen (375 or 500 mg orally twice daily) and sulindac (150 or 200 mg orally twice daily) are reasonable NSAID alternatives. COX-2–selective inhibition is effective and may be of particular value in patients taking anticoagulants or with substantial gastrointestinal risk factors, but the cardiac safety of COX-2–selective inhibitors is currently under intensive review by the Food and Drug Administration. The use of both COX-2–nonselective and COX-2–selective NSAIDs is potentially problematic in patients with significant renal insufficiency. Alternative approaches to acute therapy for monarticular gouty arthritis include the local intra-articular injection of a glucocorticosteroid ester. Regardless of the previous duration of the acute attack, such treatment is effective and pragmatic for involvement of a single large joint. Synthetic adrenocorticotropic hormone (ACTH) is an excellent alternative in patients without preexisting adrenal suppression, particularly for acute polyarticular gout or when the administration of other agents is contraindicated. A typical dose for podagra is 25 USP units of ACTH subcutaneously. With larger joint involvement or for polyarticular gout, 40 USP units of ACTH intramuscularly or by slow intravenous infusion is generally effective as a single dose. Occasionally, a second dose may be required. The peripheral anti-inflammatory effects of ACTH via leukocyte melanocortin receptor 3 (MR3) agonism, as well as induction of adrenal glucocorticoid release, both appear to contribute to the rapid and reliable efficacy of ACTH for acute gout. An alternative strategy for acute gout involves the use of systemic anti-inflammatory doses of corticosteroids (oral prednisone, at least 30 mg/day to start, with a typical regimen being 60 mg/day with a steady taper over a 14-day period). Alternatively, a short course of intravenous methylprednisolone at up to double these prednisone doses is effective in severe cases.

Colchicine at low doses (e.g., 0.6 mg twice daily with normal renal and hepatic function) is a useful adjunct to NSAIDs, ACTH, and corticosteroids for the treatment of severe or refractory acute attacks of gout and may help prevent clinical rebound on discontinuation of the primary anti-inflammatory treatment. 1 To abort early recurrences of acute gouty arthritis, patients can also be instructed to initiate therapy with either low-dose oral colchicine (e.g., 0.6 mg once every hour for up to 3 hours) or an NSAID at the first premonition or symptom of an impending episode. The use of larger doses of oral colchicine as a primary modality for acute gouty arthritis has fallen out of favor because the therapeutic benefit-toxicity ratio is most often inferior for colchicine relative to NSAIDs, glucocorticoids, and ACTH. In general, the use of intravenous colchicine is not advisable. Potentially fatal marrow suppression may occur even with low doses (less than 2 mg) of intravenous colchicine in patients with renal insufficiency and hepatobiliary disease, particularly in older subjects.

Treatment between Gouty Attacks (Interval Therapy) and for Chronic Gout and Hyperuricemia

Colchicine (0.6 mg once or twice daily) is effective for prophylaxis of recurrent attacks of acute gout, although low-dose NSAID treatment may also be beneficial. As illustrated in Figure 294–4, certain findings support the institution of uric acid–lowering therapy for gout. Importantly, antihyperuricemic therapy in gout is potentially toxic and requires lifelong continuation. Thus, the therapeutic aims and the potential benefit-risk ratio of treatment should be weighed on a case-by-case basis. In some individuals, the serum urate concentration can be successfully normalized without antihyperuricemic drugs by cessation of alcohol, substitution of another class of antihypertensive agent for a thiazide in antihypertensive treatment, or better control of obesity. Low-carbohydrate weight reduction diets specifically tailored to treat metabolic syndrome may be of value to substantially diminish hyperuricemia in this condition. However, purine-restricted diets are generally unpalatable and typically fail to lower serum uric acid by more than 1 mg/dL.

Accepted indications for pharmacologic antihyperuricemic therapy in patients with well-documented gout are (1) frequent attacks of acute gout (more than three per year); (2) the occurrence of acute gout that is difficult to safely manage, such as polyarticular gout, or gout associated with major organ transplantation or evidence of chronic renal insufficiency; (3) subcutaneous or intra-articular tophaceous deposits; and (4) documented urate overproduction. A common side effect of initiating therapy to lower levels of serum uric acid is triggering of gout attacks, particularly in the first few months of treatment. Thus, prophylactic low-dose colchicine (0.6 mg orally daily or twice daily) is typically continued for 6 months after starting uric acid–lowering treatment. Initiation of uric acid–lowering treatment is generally deferred until after the inflammatory phase of acute gout has subsided.

In patients with diminished renal function who are taking customary prophylactic doses of colchicine over prolonged periods, a reversible proximal myopathy may develop, often accompanied by elevated levels of serum creatine kinase; severe bone marrow depression can also occur. Thus, guidelines for safe prophylactic colchicine dosing in patients with renal failure include reducing colchicine to 0.6 mg orally every 2 days with a serum creatinine level of 2.0 and to 0.6 mg orally every 3 days with a serum creatinine level of 3.0.

Reduction of total body urate stores, the size of tophi, and the risk for ongoing precipitation of supersaturated urate is best achieved by long-term reduction of the serum urate concentration to less than 6 mg/dL. Xanthine oxidase inhibition, typically using allopurinol (see Fig. 294–1), is the preferred therapeutic strategy, whether the patient is an overproducer or underexcretor of uric acid. Xanthine oxidase inhibition is mandated as the primary therapeutic strategy in patients with excessive uric acid excretion, with a previous history of uric acid stones, or with renal insufficiency. Minor hypersensitivity reactions to allopurinol, including pruritus and dermatitis, are common. Approximately half of patients with such minor reactions can be successfully desensitized to allopurinol, and more than half can be successfully treated with oxypurinol, the major active metabolite of allopurinol. Severe cutaneous adverse reactions to allopurinol are strongly linked to HLA-B5801 in the Han Chinese.

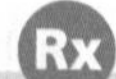

Adverse effects with allopurinol are potentially more dangerous and occur more often than with uricosuric drugs. For example, allopurinol hepatotoxicity can be severe. The allopurinol hypersensitivity syndrome, which typically consists of fever, eosinophilia, dermatitis, elevation of hepatic enzymes, renal failure, and vasculitis, has a mortality rate of approximately 20%. The risk for allopurinol hypersensitivity is greatly augmented in patients with diminished renal function. Therefore, such subjects should be treated with an initial allopurinol dose adjusted downward from the usual dose of 300 mg/day in a manner proportional to the impairment in creatinine clearance.

Uricosuric drugs such as probenecid (and benzbromarone, a potentially hepatotoxic drug that is not currently available in the United States) increase renal clearance of uric acid in a manner that depends on inhibition of URAT1-mediated tubular reabsorption. Probenecid is effective as a first-line agent for patients with gout associated with urinary uric acid underexcretion and intact renal function without a history of urolithiasis. As such, probenecid can serve as an alternative to xanthine oxidase inhibitors in carefully selected patients. Febuxostat, a nonpurine inhibitor of xanthine oxidase, is more effective than allopurinol at lowering uric acid levels but not at reducing flares of gout. [2] A moderate uricosuric effect, specific within the drug class, has been described for the angiotensin type 1 receptor blocker losartan, as well as for fenofibrate and atorvastatin. Clinical value of the urate-lowering effects of losartan, fenofibrate, and atorvastatin is not well established for use of these agents either alone or in synergy with primary antihyperuricemic agents.

Acute, massive uric acid precipitation within renal tubules can be catastrophic in patients undergoing cytotoxic chemotherapy for certain malignancies, and thus prophylactic use of allopurinol is required. However, in the population at large, hyperuricemia alone is not related to the development of clinically significant renal disease. The cause of asymptomatic hyperuricemia should be diagnostically considered, but treatment of asymptomatic hyperuricemia is not indicated unless there is evidence of chronic uric acid overproduction.

Prognosis

Recognition of gout is important because the disease frequently leads to painful and destructive arthropathy and urolithiasis and because gout is associated with a variety of potentially serious medical conditions. However, the inflammatory manifestations of gout are most often satisfactorily managed, and treatment of hyperuricemia is most often effective in preventing and reversing many of the long-term consequences of the disease.

Future Directions

Further clinical development of uric acid–lowering drug alternatives to allopurinol and the current generation of uricosuric drugs should assist in the treatment of refractory patients with gout. Patients with gout in association with renal failure and hypersensitivity to allopurinol can be difficult to manage successfully. Limited-term infusion of recombinant uric acid oxidase is also under investigation for reduction of the tophus burden in selected patients with severe tophaceous gout refractory to other agents. However, the immunogenicity of uricase and the oxidative stress precipitated by uricase-catalyzed hydrogen peroxide generation impose significant limits on safe and effective use of uricase.

CARTILAGE CALCIFICATION: CPPD CRYSTAL DEPOSITION DISEASE AND ARTICULAR HYDROXYAPATITE CRYSTAL DEPOSITION

Definition

The calcium-containing crystals deposited in the pericellular matrix of cartilage are often in the form of CPPD, a disorder termed chondrocalcinosis, pyrophosphate arthropathy, and when associated with acute arthritis, pseudogout. Crystals of the basic calcium phosphate (BCP) HA, the mineral phase deposited in growth cartilage and in bone, may also be deposited in articular cartilage. Deposition of HA and closely related BCP crystals in periarticular structures and in loci other than cartilage, such as the rotator cuff and subacromial bursa of the shoulder (calcific tendonitis and bursitis), can also be manifested as painful inflammatory conditions.

Epidemiology

Radiographic and autopsy studies have indicated that knee chondrocalcinosis is present in approximately 15% of 65-year-olds and more than 50% of those 85 years or older. Most elderly individuals with CPPD deposition disease in the United States have a primary (idiopathic) disorder. Studies of synovial fluid and cartilage specimens from patients with osteoarthritis have suggested that HA crystalline material is frequently present, often in conjunction with CPPD crystals. Both CPPD and HA crystals are commonly present within articular cartilage in the late stages of osteoarthritis.

Pathobiology

Articular cartilage, unlike growth plate cartilage, is specialized to not undergo matrix calcification. However, certain features of growth cartilage chondrocyte differentiation shared by chondrocytes in degenerative and aging cartilage (including foci of proliferation, hypertrophy, and apoptosis) appear to stimulate articular chondrocalcinosis. The ability of chondrocytes to mineralize their pericellular matrix also depends on the concentrations of calcium, inorganic phosphate (P_i), and PP_i, and the solubility products of these solutes. In addition, mineralization of matrix by chondrocytes depends on certain alterations in the extracellular matrix and other promineralizing factors, including activation of the tissue transglutaminase TG2 and the tissue form of factor XIII transglutaminase. In aging and osteoarthritic cartilage, the activity of PP_i-generating nucleoside triphosphate pyrophosphohydrolase (NPP) isoenzymes, including NPP1, as well as PP_i generation and expression by chondrocytes of the PP_i transporter ANKH, is markedly increased (Fig. 294–5). Other factors that promote extracellular PP_i excess in chondrocalcinosis in aging and osteoarthritic cartilage include altered chondrocyte sensitivity to TGF-β and resistance to insulin-like growth factor I (IGF-I), which in normal chondrocytes act as potent and mutually antagonistic stimulatory and inhibitory factors, respectively, for extracellular PP_i levels.

ANKH stimulates the intracellular-to-extracellular movement of PP_i and thereby promotes increased extracellular PP_i levels. Several mutations in the gene for ANKH (Fig. 294–6) have been causally implicated in chromosome 5p–linked autosomal dominant familial chondrocalcinosis, which is typically manifested as severe articular CPPD crystal deposition and degenerative arthropathy before 30 years of age. Homozygosity for a mutation in the ANKH 5′-untranslated region is linked to approximately 4% of cases of sporadic chondrocalcinosis associated with aging. Chondrocyte ATP depletion via mitochondrial dysfunction from oxidative stress in aging and osteoarthritic cartilage also appears to play a role in enhanced PP_i production, driven in part by ATP salvage via NPP activity and catalyzed partly by the NPP isoenzyme NPP1.

Depending on the cartilage PP_i concentration, ATP concentration, and the level of activity of P_i-generating ATPases and pyrophosphatases (which also degrade PP_i), CPPD or HA crystal formation (or both) may be promoted (see Fig. 294–6). It does not appear that all HA crystalline deposits in cartilage are directly made by chondrocytes in osteoarthritis. Some of the HA crystalline material in osteoarthritic cartilage is derived from bone shards embedded in cartilage and some from the extracellular matrix immediately surrounding chondrocytes.

Several metabolic disorders associated with CPPD crystal deposition disease (Table 294–2) may help induce chondrocalcinosis, in part by promoting intra-articular PP_i excess. Such disorders include genetic deficiency of the PP_i-degrading enzyme tissue-nonspecific alkaline phosphatase in hypophosphatasia, acquired tissue excess of the pyrophosphatase inhibitor iron in hemochromatosis, and deficiency of the pyrophosphatase cofactor magnesium in hypomagnesemia.

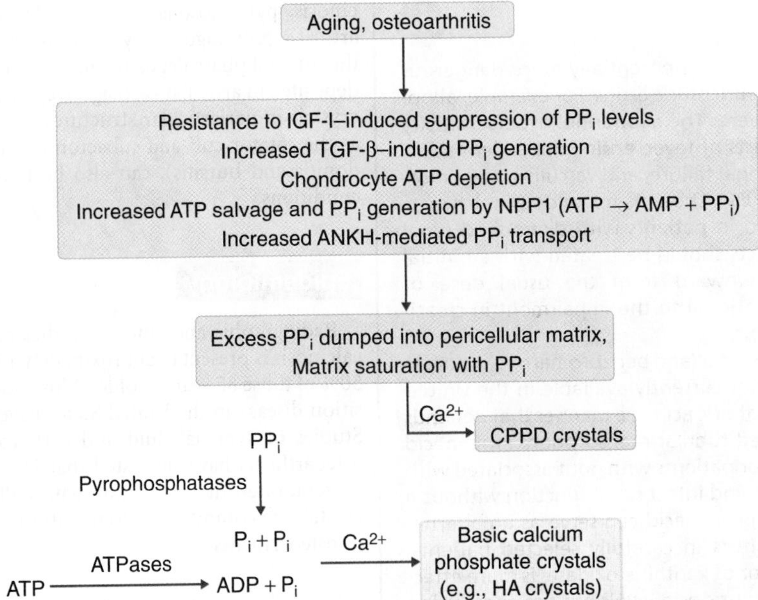

FIGURE 294–5 • Proposed inorganic pyrophosphate (PP_i)-dependent mechanisms stimulating calcium pyrophosphate dihydrate (CPPD) and hydroxyapatite (HA) crystal deposition in aging and osteoarthritis: roles of adenosine triphosphate (ATP) and PP_i metabolism and inorganic phosphate (P_i) generation in cartilage calcification. In this model, discussed in the text, excess PP_i generation in cartilage, in idiopathic CPPD deposition disease of aging, and in osteoarthritic cartilage is mediated in part by altered chondrocyte sensitivity to transforming growth factor-β (TGFbeta) and resistance to insulin growth factor type I (IGF-I), which in normal chondrocytes act as potent and mutually antagonistic stimulatory and inhibitory factors, respectively, of extracellular PP_i levels. Chondrocyte ATP depletion via mitochondrial dysfunction from redox stress also appears to play a role in enhanced PP_i production, driven in part by ATP salvage via nucleoside phosphodiesterase pyrophosphatase (NPP) activity and catalyzed partly by the NPP isoenzyme NPP1. In idiopathic chondrocalcinosis of aging, mean cartilage PP_i and NPP levels average double the normal levels. Increased intracellular-to-extracellular PP_i transport by increased expression and/or "gain of function" of the chondrocyte multiple-pass transmembrane protein ANKH also factors into the extracellular PP_i excess in osteoarthritis, idiopathic chondrocalcinosis in aging, and certain forms of autosomal dominant familial chondrocalcinosis linked to specific ANKH mutations (see Fig. 294–6). NPP1 and ANKH are both upregulated in osteoarthritic cartilage and in chondrocalcinosis cartilage in vivo. Depending on the extracellular availability of substrate PP_i and the activity of pyrophosphatases, the availability of substrate ATP and the activity of ATPases, and other factors such as substantial local Mg^{2+} concentrations, HA crystal deposition, as opposed to CPPD deposition, may be stimulated in this model. ADP = adenosine diphosphate; AMP = adenosine monophosphate.

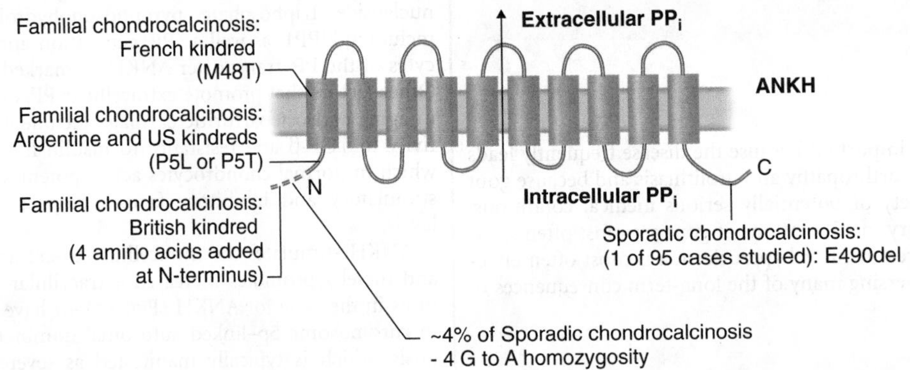

FIGURE 294–6 • Model of the structure of the multiple-pass transmembrane protein ANKH involved in inorganic pyrophosphate (PP_i) transport and schematic of described mutants of ANKH associated with chondrocalcinosis. This figure schematizes the multiple-pass transmembrane protein structure of ANKH, which appears to function in PP_i transport from the cytoplasm to the extracellular space. Distinct mutations in ANKH promote distinct phenotypes. The figure summarizes sites of known ANKH gene mutations associated with chromosome 5p–linked autosomal dominant familial chondrocalcinosis (calcium pyrophosphate dihydrate [CPPD] crystal deposition disease). The figure also illustrates an ANKH C-terminal deletion mutation identified in 1 of 95 subjects studied with "sporadic" chondrocalcinosis. In addition, the figure illustrates the -4-base pair G-to-A transition in the 5′-untranslated region of ANKH, homozygosity for which has been linked to "sporadic "chondrocalcinosis in approximately 4% of aged subjects. It has been proposed that some of the described ANKH mutations linked to human chondrocalcinosis promote chronic low-grade extracellular PP_i excess via either increased ANKH expression in chondrocytes or increased "leakiness" of ANKH for PP_i, thereby ultimately stimulating CPPD crystal formation.

Chondrocalcinosis secondary to hyperparathyroidism appears to be mediated not only by hypercalcemia but also by the ability of excess parathyroid hormone (PTH) to activate and alter the differentiation of articular chondrocytes, which normally express PTH/PTH-related peptide (PTHrP) receptors.

CPPD and HA crystals can stimulate both chondrocytes and intra-articular leukocytes. Polymorphonuclear leukocytes can traffic to the synovium, promote the expression of connective tissue–degrading enzymes, and trigger inflammation, thereby contributing to cartilage degradation and worsening of osteoarthritis. Many of the same basic mechanisms described earlier for gout mediate the inflammatory manifestations associated with CPPD and HA crystal deposition.

Clinical Manifestations

The clinical findings and primary and secondary etiologic factors associated with CPPD deposition disease are summarized in Table 294–2. As in gout, acute attacks of severely painful inflammatory synovitis (pseudogout) in patients with CPPD deposition disease can be provoked by minor trauma or intercurrent medical or surgical illness. Leukocyte counts in synovial fluid are substantially elevated, and intraleukocytic CPPD crystals are most often detectable by compensated polarized light microscopy in pseudogout (see Fig. 294–3). Patients with CPPD disease can have episodes of hemarthrosis, often post-traumatic and in the

TABLE 294–2 CPPD CRYSTAL DEPOSITION DISEASE: COMMON CAUSES AND CLINICAL FINDINGS

CAUSES OF CPPD CRYSTAL DEPOSITION DISEASE

High prevalence:
- Idiopathic in association with aging (most frequent)
- Complication of established osteoarthritis
- Long-term consequence of mechanical joint trauma or knee meniscectomy

Lower prevalence:
- Familial
- Associated with systemic metabolic disease (hyperparathyroidism, hemochromatosis, hypomagnesemia, myxedematous hypothyroidism, or ochronosis)

COMMON CLINICAL FINDINGS IN PATIENTS WITH CPPD CRYSTAL DEPOSITION DISEASE

- Asymptomatic or incidental finding (e.g., asymptomatic knee fibrocartilage chondrocalcinosis)
- Recurrent acute inflammatory monarticular arthritis ("pseudogout") (e.g., knee or wrist)
- Chronic degenerative arthritis ("pseudo-osteoarthritis" or "pseudo–neuropathic arthritis")
- Chronic symmetrical inflammatory polyarthritis ("pseudo–rheumatoid arthritis")
- Recurrent acute hemarthrosis
- Carpal tunnel syndrome
- Ligamentum flavum involvement (has the potential to cause spinal canal stenosis and myelopathy)

CPPD = calcium pyrophosphate dihydrate.

knee. Some patients with CPPD deposition disease demonstrate "pseudorheumatoid" arthritic joints that reflect local synovial and periarticular tenosynovial proliferation. Ingestion of not only CPPD but also HA crystals by synovial lining cells and lysosomal catabolism of such ingested crystals stimulate synovial proliferation, in part via solubilization of the crystalline calcium.

CPPD deposition disease can be manifested as a chronic degenerative arthropathy that commonly affects certain joints that are usually spared in primary osteoarthritis (e.g., the MCP joints, wrists, elbows, and glenohumeral joints). Concentrated CPPD crystal deposition can also occur in tendons, ligaments, bursae, and occasionally bone. CPPD deposits in tendons (e.g., Achilles, triceps, and obturator tendons) are usually fine and linear on radiologic examination. CPPD deposits within the ligamentum flavum can be sizable and progress to cause canal stenosis and myelopathy. Similarly, carpal tunnel syndrome can be promoted by CPPD deposits in tendons, as well as in wrist synovium.

Familial CPPD deposition disease has been described in certain countries and ethnic groups, including kindreds from Spain, Czechoslovakia, Holland, France, England, Germany, Sweden, Israel, the United States, Canada, Chile, and Japan. In an English kindred with CPPD disease, recurrent childhood seizures were strongly associated with the later development of CPPD deposition disease. Familial chondrocalcinosis may be more prevalent in Spain. It has been proposed that a mutation originating in Spain may have spread across Europe and into South America along military and trade routes highly traveled in the 17th century. The pattern of inheritance and the clinical features of familial CPPD deposition disease are variable. Some families manifest early-onset polyarthritis, which can include ankylosing intervertebral and sacroiliac joint disease, but in others, a late-onset chondrocalcinosis occurs that is difficult to distinguish from common, idiopathic CPPD deposition disease. Not all cases of increased predisposition to CPPD disease are linked to inherited mutations in the gene for ANKH.

Unlike urate and CPPD crystal deposition, acute synovitis caused by HA crystal deposition is unusual. However, acute inflammatory syndromes, including pseudopodagra, may occur in association with periarticular HA crystal deposition in tendons, ligaments, and soft tissues, as seen in certain post-traumatic conditions and the systemic autoimmune diseases scleroderma and dermatomyositis. Shoulder rotator cuff tendonitis and subacromial bursitis associated with HA are common. A distinctive noninflammatory syndrome of rotator cuff tear and marked cartilage degeneration associated with abundant intra-articular HA and related BCP crystalline material has also been described. In this entity (termed *cuff tear arthropathy* or *Milwaukee shoulder syndrome*), the crystal deposition may function as a significant etiopathogenic factor.

Diagnosis

Because CPPD deposition disease can imitate several other conditions (see Table 294–2), a precise diagnosis is essential. Idiopathic CPPD deposition disease of aging is the most common form of the disease. Diagnosis of CPPD deposition disease before the age of 50, particularly if CPPD deposition is widespread, should prompt consideration of a metabolic or familial disorder (see Table 294–2). The demonstrable presence of CPPD crystals in synovial fluid or in tissues via compensated polarized light microscopy (see Fig. 294–3) (as discussed earlier for gout vs. pseudogout) is definitive evidence of the disease. The appearance and number of CPPD crystals can change with storage. The clinician must be careful to examine relatively fresh specimens collected in vials free of calcium-chelating anticoagulants.

Laboratory Evaluation

A thorough laboratory evaluation of a patient with newly diagnosed CPPD deposition disease routinely includes the determination of serum levels of calcium, phosphorus, magnesium, alkaline phosphatase, ferritin, iron and total iron-binding capacity, and thyroid-stimulating hormone. Patients with arthritis who are suspected of having CPPD deposition disease can be adequately screened radiographically by obtaining an anteroposterior view of each knee, an anteroposterior view of the pelvis (to detect symphysis pubis involvement), and posteroanterior views of both hands, including visualization of both wrists. Chondrocalcinosis, typically seen as linear calcific deposits, may or may not be detectable by x-ray screening of these areas in patients with CPPD deposition disease. Radiographic evidence other than chondrocalcinosis may point to the correct diagnosis, including subchondral cyst formation, scaphoid-lunate widening in the wrist secondary to ligamentous degeneration, and patellofemoral joint space narrowing (often isolated, with the patella "wrapped around" the femur).

Radiologic Evaluation

HA crystal deposition may be detected via radiographic evidence of calcifications. Unlike urate and CPPD crystals, HA crystals are nonbirefringent. HA crystals stain with alizarin red and may be visualized as globules within cells in synovial fluid. However, specialized techniques, including transmission electron microscopy, may be needed to confirm HA crystal deposition.

Treatment

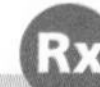

No specific treatment is available for idiopathic CPPD deposition disease, unlike the case for CPPD deposition secondary to certain metabolic disorders (e.g., hyperparathyroidism or hypomagnesemic conditions). The potential benefits of prevention of cartilage degeneration with appropriate treatment of secondary causes of established CPPD deposition disease are unclear because the ability to detect chondrocalcinosis on plain radiography is usually indicative of advanced deposition of CPPD crystals and significant replacement of cartilage matrix.

Episodes of pseudogout generally respond to NSAIDs or intra-articular steroids, or both, though sometimes more slowly than in gout. ACTH and systemic glucocorticosteroids, also given as described earlier for acute gout, are effective in most cases of acute pseudogout. The response to colchicine is less consistent than that generally seen in acute gout, but pseudogout episodes can be diminished in frequency by low-dose daily oral colchicine prophylaxis, as used for gouty arthritis.

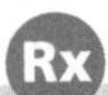

NSAIDs and local steroid injection are effective treatment options for HA crystal–associated calcific tendonitis and subacromial bursitis. Ultrasound as a therapeutic modality promotes short-term clinical improvement and helps stimulate the dissolution of calcific deposits of HA in the rotator cuff.

Prognosis

Only a small fraction of patients with CPPD deposition disease have prolonged, recurring polyarticular inflammation. Progressive degenerative arthropathy is more common. Although CPPD deposition disease appears to be a common and significant public health problem in the elderly, the "disease impact" and the long-term course of CPPD-associated degenerative arthropathy in an unselected population have not been extensively evaluated.

Future Directions

The potential to develop therapies based on new molecular targets has been raised by the recent identification of specific molecular mediators of cartilage calcification, including NPP1, ANKH, and the tissue transglutaminase TG2, a direct inducer of hypertrophic differentiation of chondrocytes that mediates calcification in response to certain inflammatory cytokines upregulated in osteoarthritic cartilage.

OXALATE CRYSTAL DEPOSITION AND JOINT DISEASE

Joint tissues are one of the sites of deposition of oxalate crystals in patients with primary hyperoxaluria and in patients with secondary hyperoxalemia and dialysis-dependent renal failure. Articular and periarticular clinical manifestations of oxalate crystal deposition include chondrocalcinosis, acute and chronic arthritis (typically symmetrical and involving the small joints of the hands, but sometimes affecting large joints), flexor tenosynovitis, ligamentum flavum involvement, and inflammatory manifestations caused by skin and vascular deposits of oxalate crystals. A high index of clinical suspicion is important for diagnosis, which can be confirmed by crystal analysis of tissue specimens and synovial fluid. The classic shape of oxalate crystals is bipyramidal (like a postal envelope), and they are associated with strong positive birefringence. However, oxalate crystals are commonly polymorphic and can mimic HA and CPPD crystals in appearance.

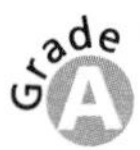

1. Schlesinger N, Schumacher R, Catton M, et al: Colchicine for acute gout. Cochrane Database Syst Rev 2006(4):CD006190.
2. Becker MA, Schumacher HR Jr, Wortmann RL, et al: Febuxostat compared with allopurinol in patients with hyperuricemia and gout. N Engl J Med 2005;353:2450–2461.

SUGGESTED READINGS

Bieber JD, Terkeltaub RA: Gout: On the brink of novel therapeutic options for an ancient disease. Arthritis Rheum 2004;50:2400–2414. *A detailed review of recent changes in gout epidemiology and clinically relevant advances in the pathogenesis of dysregulated renal urate handling and gouty inflammation.*

Choi HK, Atkinson K, Karlson EW, et al: Alcohol intake and risk of incident gout in men: A prospective study. Lancet 2004;363:1277–1281. *Alcohol intake is strongly associated with the risk of gout.*

Choi HK, Atkinson K, Karlson EW, et al: Purine-rich foods, dairy and protein intake, and the risk of gout in men. N Engl J Med 2004;350:1093–103. *High intake of meat and seafood is associated with the risk of gout.*

Choi HK, Mount DB, Reginato AM, et al: Pathogenesis of gout. Ann Intern Med 2005;143:499–516. *A review.*

Keith MP, Gilliland WR: Updates in the management of gout. Am J Med 2007;120:221–224. *A management update.*

Maldonado I, Prasad V, Reginato AJ: Oxalate crystal deposition disease. Curr Rheumatol Rep 2002;4:257–264. *A valuable review of the etiology and clinical manifestations of oxalate crystal deposition.*

Pay S, Terkeltaub R: Calcium pyrophosphate dihydrate and hydroxyapatite crystal deposition in the joint: New developments relevant to the clinician. Curr Rheum Rep 2003;5:235–243. *An extensive review of the pathogenesis of calcific crystal deposition in aging and osteoarthritic articular cartilage.*

Terkeltaub R: Clinical practice: Gout. N Engl J Med 2003;349:1647–1655. *A thorough review of the practical management of hyperuricemia and gouty inflammation.*

Zhang Y, Brown MA: Genetic studies of chondrocalcinosis. Curr Opin Rheumatol 2005;17:330–335. *A review of familial chondrocalcinosis and the role of ANKH mutations in the disease.*

295 FIBROMYALGIA AND CHRONIC FATIGUE SYNDROME

Robert M. Bennett

Fibromyalgia (FM) and chronic fatigue syndrome (CFS) are multisymptomatic syndromes defined respectively by the core features of chronic widespread pain and chronic unexplained fatigue. The 1990 American College of Rheumatology classification criteria for FM are universally used in diagnosing FM (Table 295–1). The 1994 Centers for Disease Control and Prevention (CDC) definition is the most widely used diagnostic criteria for CFS (see Table 295–1). According to these definitions, FM and CFS are separate entities, but in practice there is a large overlap, with many patients being given both labels. Myofascial pain is a universal experience that is usually self-limited; when it becomes persistent, it may accentuate and perpetuate the experience of chronic fatigue and FM.

FIBROMYALGIA

Epidemiology

Chronic musculoskeletal pain is commonly encountered in the general population with an estimated prevalence of about 35%. It is subdivided into chronic regional pain, with a prevalence of about 25%, and chronic widespread pain, with a prevalence of about 10%.

FM is considered to be a subset of chronic widespread pain and has a prevalence of about 2% in women and 0.5% in men. There is a steady increase in FM with age, with about 12% of women in their 60s being affected. Chronic musculoskeletal pain is associated with a reduction in overall health status, and FM patients have more impairment than do patients with chronic widespread pain or chronic regional pain. The prevalence of FM in the medical setting is much greater, with about 20 to 30% of the rheumatology visits in the United States made for FM.

Pathobiology

There is persuasive evidence that FM pain results from abnormal sensory processing within the central nervous system. This is commonly referred to as *central sensitization* and results from amplification of peripheral sensory stimuli. The magnification of peripheral sensory input is readily visualized as increased activity in somatosensory areas of the brain on magnetic resonance imaging in FM subjects versus healthy controls. Central sensitization is the result of a persistent neuronal hyperexcitability that continues long after the original sensitizing input has waned. The pathophysiology of this phenomenon is based, in part, on temporal summation of neural impulses. This occurs when pain fibers (unmyelinated C) are repetitively stimulated at a rate greater than one impulse every 3 seconds. At a biochemical level, such stimulation results in depolarization of *N*-methyl-D-aspartate (NMDA) receptors, which causes transcriptional changes that affect pain processing. Experimentally, this has been demonstrated in FM patients after repetitive thermal stimulation of the skin and after intramuscular electrical stimulation. Thus, persistent pain input may eventually give rise to central sensitization in some individuals, probably based at least in part on a genetic predisposition.

The frequent development of FM from focal pain states, such as in rheumatoid arthritis, post-traumatic injuries, and endometriosis, is thought to depend on temporal summation. However, the occurrence of FM in relation to persistent psychological stressors and infections cannot

TABLE 295–1 COMPARISON OF CLASSIFICATION CRITERIA FOR FIBROMYALGIA AND CHRONIC FATIGUE SYNDROME

	Fibromyalgia	Chronic Fatigue Syndrome
Primary symptom	Persistent unexplained widespread pain of ≥3 months' duration Widespread is defined as pain in ≥3 quadrants of the body, plus pain in an axial distribution such as the neck, the front of the chest, the thoracic spine, or the low part of the back	Unexplained persistent or relapsing chronic fatigue that is of new or definite onset (has not been lifelong); is not the result of ongoing exertion; is not substantially alleviated by rest; and results in a substantial reduction in previous levels of occupational, educational, social, or personal activities
Secondary features	None	Concurrent occurrence of 4 or more of the following symptoms, all of which must have persisted or recurred during 6 or more consecutive months of illness and must not have predated the fatigue: Sore throat Tender cervical or axillary lymph nodes Muscle pain Multijoint pain without swelling or redness Headaches of a new type, pattern, or severity Unrefreshing sleep Postexertional malaise lasting >24 hours
Physical examination	The finding of ≥11 of 18 designated tender points examined at a palpation pressure of 4 kg	None
Exclusionary diagnoses	None	Any active medical condition that may explain the presence of chronic fatigue Any previous condition that might explain fatigue and that is still ongoing Any past or current diagnosis of a major depressive disorder with psychotic or melancholic features, bipolar affective disorders, schizophrenia disorders, delusional disorders, dementias, anorexia nervosa, bulimia, substance abuse within 2 years before onset, severe obesity

be readily explained by temporal summation. FM developing in these settings is now thought to involve the activation of glial cells by cytokines, chemokines, and other neuronal activators. Several studies have reported elevated blood levels of interleukin-8 and a two- to three-fold increase in central nervous system substance P and nerve growth factor in patients with FM.

There is increasing evidence that a descending pain system from the midbrain to the dorsal horn is important in modulating transmission of nerve impulses to the brain. Activation of the nuclei in the midbrain involved in this system occurs in response to opioids, endorphins, emotions, and the placebo response. This modulation may upregulate or downregulate sensory processing and in part underlies the influence of the psyche on the pain experience. Several studies have shown reduced thalamic blood flow in FM subjects. This finding is in accord with other chronic pain states and is postulated to be associated with loss of the tonic disinhibition of thalamic activity that normally downregulates sensory impulses reaching the somatosensory cortex.

Understanding of the biologic basis for central sensitization has provided an explanation for the common association of FM with conditions such as irritable bowel syndrome, overactive bladder, multiple chemical hypersensitivity, and chronic daily headaches.

Other common symptoms in FM such as fatigue and cognitive dysfunction cannot currently be understood in terms of central sensitization. These symptoms are the principal features of CFS, and their pathobiologic basis remains ill defined.

Clinical Manifestations

Signs and Symptoms

Pain

The core *symptom* of FM is chronic widespread pain and stiffness. Characteristically, the pain is described as a constant dull ache that is worsened by muscle overactivity. FM-related pain is usually perceived as arising from muscle; however, many patients also report joint pain but have no objective evidence of arthritis.

Fatigue

Easy fatigability from physical exertion, mental exertion, and psychological stressors is typical of FM. Patients with CFS have many similarities with FM patients; about 75% of patients meeting the diagnostic criteria for CFS also meet criteria for the diagnosis of FM.

Disordered Sleep

FM patients have nonrestorative sleep. Even if they sleep continuously for 8 to 10 hours, they awake feeling tired. Many exhibit an alpha-delta electroencephalographic pattern that would explain their never achieving the restorative stages 3 and 4 of non–rapid eye movement sleep. A poor night's sleep is often followed by worsening of FM symptoms the next day.

Cognitive Dysfunction

Cognitive dysfunction is a prominent complaint of many FM patients. They commonly describe difficulties with short-term memory, concentration, logical analysis, and motivation. Recent studies have documented defects in working memory and verbal fluency.

Psychological Distress

Having a chronic painful disorder for which there is currently no generally accepted cure often produces an existential crisis. Approximately 30% of FM patients have significant depression at any given time, and about 60% have a lifetime prevalence of depressive illness. Although psychiatric disorders are common in FM patients, they do not seem to be intrinsically related to the pathophysiology of FM; effective treatment of depression with a selective serotonin re-uptake inhibitor (SSRI) does not eliminate FM pain. However, FM and depression show familial clustering suggestive of an underlying genetic susceptibility.

History

Initiation and Maintenance of Fibromyalgia

FM seldom emerges "out of the blue." Many patients relate an acute injury, repetitive workload, persistent stress, infections, and toxins to its onset. It is not uncommon for a regional pain state to evolve into FM. FM is commonly found as an accompaniment of other painful disorders,

TABLE 295–2 MAJOR ISSUES IN THE MANAGEMENT OF PATIENTS WITH FIBROMYALGIA
Education
Pain
Fatigue
Sleep
Psychological distress
Deconditioning
Endocrine dysfunction
Associated disorders

such as rheumatoid arthritis, low back pain, systemic lupus erythematosus, Sjögren's syndrome, inflammatory bowel disease, endometriosis, and osteoarthritis. There is increasing evidence that FM is a common occurrence in victims of post-traumatic stress disorder; for instance, both FM and CFS were common diagnoses after Operation Desert Storm in 1991.

Diagnosis

The diagnosis of FM is usually based on the 1990 classification criteria recommended by the American College of Rheumatology (ACR) (see Table 295–1).

The following are the locations of the nine paired tender points:

Occiput: bilateral, at the suboccipital muscle insertions
Low cervical: bilateral, at the anterior aspects of the intertransverse spaces at C5–C7
Trapezius: bilateral, at the midpoint of the upper border
Supraspinatus: bilateral, at the origins, above the scapular spine near the medial border
Second rib: bilateral, at the second costochondral junctions just lateral to the junctions on the upper surfaces
Lateral epicondyle: bilateral, 2 cm distal to the epicondyles
Gluteal: bilateral, in the upper outer quadrants of the buttocks in the anterior fold of muscle
Greater trochanter: bilateral, posterior to the trochanteric prominence
Knee: bilateral, at the medial fat pad proximal to the joint line

FM is not a diagnosis of exclusion; thus, laboratory tests and imaging studies play no role in establishing the diagnosis according to the 1990 ACR criteria, although they are often indicated in the evaluation of accompanying peripheral pain generators.

Treatment

Successful management of FM requires a thorough analysis in terms of the biopsychosocial model of disease. The major management issues that require attention are listed in Table 295–2.

Education

There is evidence that higher educational attainment is associated with a better prognosis in many chronic disorders, such as FM. Education has a positive effect through cognitive behavioral strategies, such as goal setting and reassessment of priorities. Educated patients are more likely to take an active role in self-management.

Pain

In considering the management of pain in FM, it is logical to focus on the major sites of pain processing, namely, peripheral pain generation and central pain pathways. There is no specific tissue pathology, at least in peripheral tissues, that is characteristic of FM. However, once the central nervous system is sensitized, not only are peripheral pain generators perceived as being more painful, but they also prolong and amplify the central neuroplastic changes. Thus, a critical first component of treating FM pain is to identify and effectively treat all peripheral pain generators, which commonly include peripheral arthritis, axial arthritis, spinal stenosis, myofascial trigger points, neuropathic pain, vascular headaches, visceral pain (e.g., irritable bowel syndrome, overactive bladder), postsurgical pain, and pelvic pain syndromes (e.g., endometriosis).

Management of central sensitization is typically initiated with heterocyclic antidepressant (HCA) medications such as amitriptyline, trazodone, or nortriptyline. Highly selective SSRIs such as fluoxetine exhibit a modest pain benefit in some FM patients. There is some evidence that antidepressant medications with balanced re-uptake inhibition of serotonin and norepinephrine (e.g., venlafaxine, duloxetine, milnacipran) are more effective in treating FM pain. [1,2] Importantly, the mechanism of action of these drugs is independent of any antidepressant effect and results from upregulation of the descending pain system that originates in the brain stem and uses serotonin and norepinephrine as neurotransmitters at dorsal horn synapses. Tizanidine, an α_2-adrenergic agonist, activates this descending pain system and is proving useful as an adjuvant pain medication. Anticonvulsant medications such as gabapentin, pregabalin, and topiramate are increasingly being used in FM and other chronic pain states; they inhibit the presynaptic release of glutamate and thus modulate the activation of NMDA receptors. [3] Blocking NMDA receptors with ketamine or dextromethorphan (or both) has reduced FM pain in an experimental setting, but no controlled trials have been conducted. Randomized controlled trials of acupuncture have yielded conflicting results.

Opioids are often used in the treatment of FM, but long-term trials are lacking. They should not be the first choice of analgesia; however, they should not be withheld if less powerful analgesics have failed. Tramadol (both Ultram and Ultracet) has proved useful in reducing FM pain in two controlled trials. [4] Tramadol is a weak opioid agonist that also inhibits the re-uptake of serotonin and norepinephrine at the level of the dorsal horn. It is metabolized by CYP2D6, as are many antidepressant medications. FM patients who are taking tramadol or any of several antidepressants that are eliminated by CYP2D6 are at risk for the development of a serotonin syndrome. Thus, careful review of concomitant medications is an important prerequisite in the prescription of new medications, especially in difficult-to-treat patients who are often taking multiple medications.

Fatigue

A search for a treatable cause of fatigue is always indicated (Table 295–3). Common treatable causes of chronic fatigue in FM patients are (1) inappropriate dosing of medications, (2) depression, (3) aerobic deconditioning, (3) primary sleep disorder (e.g., sleep apnea), (4) nonrestorative sleep, (5) a coexisting inflammatory disorder, and (6) neurally mediated hypotension. As in CFS, the underlying cause of *primary* fatigue in FM is not known.

Sleep

Low-dose HCAs are the mainstay of sleep pharmacotherapy in FM patients. Some patients cannot tolerate HCAs because of unacceptable levels of daytime drowsiness or weight gain. In these patients, short-acting benzodiazepine-like medications such as zolpidem, zapelon, and eszopiclone may be beneficial. About 25% of male and 15% of female FM patients have sleep apnea that usually requires treatment with continuous positive airway pressure or surgery. By far the most common sleep disorder in FM patients is restless leg syndrome/periodic limb movement disorder. Treatment is with dopamine agonists such as L-dopa/carbidopa (Sinemet), pramipexole (Mirapex), or ropinirole (Requip).

Psychological Distress

Stressors related to psychosocial/economic and health issues often develop in FM patients. Psychological intervention in terms of improving the internal locus of control and more effective problem

TABLE 295–3 DIFFERENTIAL DIAGNOSIS OF CHRONIC FATIGUE

CHRONIC INFECTIONS	**CHRONIC INFLAMMATORY DISORDERS**
Hepatitis C Lyme disease Parasitic infections Fungal infections Tuberculosis Human immunodeficiency virus	Rheumatoid arthritis Systemic lupus erythematosus Sjögren's syndrome Polymyositis/dermatomyositis Vasculitis Sarcoidosis
SLEEP DISORDERS	**CARDIOPULMONARY**
Sleep apnea Restless leg syndrome Circadian rhythm disorder Alpha-delta sleep Narcolepsy/parasomnias Gastroesophageal reflux	Congestive heart failure Neurally mediated hypotension Postural orthostatic tachycardia syndrome Pulmonary hypertension Chronic obstructive pulmonary disease Persistent atrial fibrillation and other arrhythmias
ENDOCRINE/METABOLIC DISORDERS	**GASTROINTESTINAL**
Addison's disease Cushing's syndrome Poorly controlled diabetes Thyroid (hyperthyroidism, hypothyroidism, and Hashimoto's thyroiditis) Hemochromatosis Diabetes insipidus	Celiac disease Inflammatory bowel disease Autoimmune hepatitis
	MALIGNANCY
	Lymphoma Other occult malignancies
GENERAL MEDICAL DISORDERS	**NEUROLOGIC DISORDERS**
Anemia (any cause) Chronic renal/hepatic failure Morbid obesity (body mass index >40) Malnutrition Medication side effects	Multiple sclerosis Myasthenia gravis Muscular dystrophies Metabolic myopathies
TOXINS	**LIFESTYLE DYSFUNCTIONS**
Chronic carbon monoxide poisoning Heavy metal poisoning Pesticide poisoning Organic solvent poisoning	Chronic overwork Persistent unresolved stress Inadequate exercise Drug/alcohol dependency
PSYCHOLOGICAL	
Persistent stress Mood disorders (depression/anxiety/bipolar) Schizophrenia Personality disorder Post-traumatic stress disorder Anorexia nervosa/bulimia Early dementia	

Rx

solving is important in such patients. Cognitive-behavioral therapy is particularly well suited to effect these changes. 5 Although antidepressant medications are commonly used in the treatment of pain and disordered sleep in FM patients, the doses are often suboptimal for treating depressive illness.

Deconditioning

A carefully graded program of aerobic conditioning and stretching is a critical component of an effective FM treatment program. 6 The benefits of exercise are based on good scientific evidence, but exercise may also be deleterious. Overtraining results in a syndrome of chronic fatigue, reduced performance, depression, impaired hormonal stress responses, increased susceptibility to muscle damage, and infections. In general, exercise needs to be added to the program *after* some control of pain, sleep, and depression has been achieved.

Endocrine Dysfunction

There is no good evidence that FM is primarily due to an endocrine disorder. However, common problems such as hypothyroidism and menopausal symptoms often aggravate pain and fatigue, and appropriate replacement therapy is frequently worth a trial.

Prognosis

FM symptoms usually persist for many years. However, patients seen in the community rather than tertiary care centers have been reported to have a 24% remission rate after 2 years. The consequences of pain, fatigue, and cognitive dysfunction negatively influence the sustained performance of physical and mental tasks. Everyday activities take longer for FM patients, who need more time to get started in the morning and often require extra rest periods during the day. A survey of FM patients seen in academic centers reported that 70% perceived themselves as being disabled and 16% were receiving Social Security benefits.

CHRONIC FATIGUE SYNDROME

Epidemiology

Fatigue is a common symptom; indeed, some 50% of individuals report "feeling fatigued" in population surveys. Fatigue is one of the most common problems reported to primary care doctors.

In many cases fatigue is self-limited or the causes are self-evident (e.g., insufficient rest, a medical illness, depression, or insomnia). On the other hand, the prevalence of CFS has varied from 0.006 to 3.0% in various population surveys. CFS is diagnosed predominantly in women aged 30 to 45 years.

Pathobiology

The cause of CFS remains poorly defined. Older theories suggesting that it was the result of chronic infection or untreated depression have proved unfounded. Although many CFS patients complain of nonrestorative sleep, polysomnographic studies have been inconclusive. The similarity between CFS and early Addison's disease has prompted numerous neuroendocrine studies. They have failed to show a clinically treatable endocrine deficiency, although subtle changes in the hypothalamic-pituitary-adrenal response to acute stressors is found in about 30% of patients. A similar proportion of CFS patients have abnormal results on tilt-table testing with evidence of autonomic dysfunction in terms of neurally mediated hypotension or postural orthostatic tachycardia syndrome. This may be of relevance in a subpopulation of patients, but treatment with fludrocortisone was of no benefit in one large placebo-controlled study. Many studies have suggested a low level of immune stimulation in CFS, the most common abnormalities being reduced natural killer cell function and increased numbers of cytotoxic T cells. However, these findings are not diagnostically useful, and clinical improvement has not been associated with any significant change in immune markers. Extensive psychological testing in CFS patients has failed to reveal a common psychiatric denominator. Nevertheless, it is generally accepted, as in FM and other chronic illnesses, that psychosocial distress and maladaptive coping strategies play a role in symptom attribution and perpetuation.

Clinical Manifestations

The chief complaint of patients in whom CFS is diagnosed is an abrupt onset of debilitating fatigue that causes significant impairment in daily activities, work ability, and social relationships. Typically, these patients report excellent health status just before the onset of fatigue, which is often preceded by a flulike prodrome. Symptoms suggestive of an infectious etiology include low-grade fever, drenching night sweats, tender cervical lymph nodes, sore throat, myalgias, and headaches. As in FM, many CFS patients complain of generalized musculoskeletal pain, cognitive dysfunction, irritable bowel syndrome, temporomandibular pain disorders, nonrestorative sleep, and multiple chemical sensitivities.

Diagnosis

Current diagnosis of CFS is based on the recommendations of the 1994 international CFS study group (see Table 295–1). This revision added the minor criteria of postexercise fatigue and cognitive dysfunction to the original 1988 CDC working case definition. Unlike the definition of FM, there are no physical findings in the CFS criteria. Furthermore, the definition of FM contains no exclusionary criteria, whereas the definition of CFS excludes patients with fatiguing medical disorders, melancholic depression, psychotic disorders, substance abuse, and severe obesity (body mass index >40). Because CFS is not a diagnosis of exclusion, it is important to systematically evaluate the patient for treatable causes of fatigue (see Table 295–3).

Treatment

Rx

In general, management of CFS follows the general management guidelines for FM. Patients with presumed CFS should have a general medical work-up to exclude treatable causes of fatigue (e.g., hypothyroidism or anemia), and consideration should be given to more specialized studies such as polysomnography and tilt-table testing in selected cases. Currently, there is no generally accepted pharmacologic intervention for patients with CFS. Antidepressants (HCAs and SSRIs) are of minimal benefit, although two studies have reported modest benefit with the use of monoamine oxidase inhibitors in patients with significant vegetative symptoms. Inconsistent benefits have been described with fludrocortisone and low-dose corticosteroids. The mainstay of treating CFS is to engage the patient in a gently graded program of aerobic exercise. [7] Many, but not all, will benefit from a short program of cognitive behavioral therapy to correct dysfunctional thought patterns and misattributions. [8] Management of pain and psychological distress in CFS is the same as for FM.

MYOFASCIAL PAIN

Pain arising from muscle is a universal human experience. In most instances it is due to muscle *macrotrauma* (i.e., a muscle tear or sprain) or muscle *microtrauma* (i.e., injury at the sarcomere level resulting from repetitive muscle use or overexertion). After appropriate rest, the pain usually dissipates over a period of a few days to weeks. In some cases, a persistent pain focus develops that has the characteristics of a myofascial trigger point. This diagnosis should be considered if the patient complains of focal pain that is aggravated by muscle use or psychological stressors that cause increased muscle tension.

A myofascial trigger point is a well-defined point of focal tenderness within a muscle. Palpation usually reveals a ropelike induration referred to as a "taut band." In many instances, firm palpation of this area causes pain in a referred distribution that reproduces the patient's symptoms. Importantly, referred pain from a trigger point does not follow a nerve root distribution (i.e., it is not dermatomal). Trigger points frequently cause dysfunction in terms of a restriction in range of movement and weakness; the involved muscle or muscles often demonstrate easy fatigability (Table 295–4).

The pathophysiologic basis for the trigger point phenomena is not fully understood. Electromyographic recordings from trigger points show spontaneous low-voltage activity resembling end plate spike potentials. In normal muscle, depolarization of the motor end plate initiates the release of calcium ions from the sarcoplasmic reticulum, which in turn results in activation of the myosin-actin contractile elements ("contraction coupling"). It is thought that the areas of electrical hyperexcitability in trigger points result from a nonphysiologic focal contraction caused by an influx of calcium ions into the damaged sarcomeres. If this process

TABLE 295–4 DIAGNOSTIC FEATURES OF A MYOFASCIAL TRIGGER POINT

Focal area of tenderness on palpation of the involved muscle
Reproduction of the pain complaint by trigger point palpation and/or injection
Palpation reveals induration of the adjacent muscle (the "taut band")
Restricted range of movement in the involved muscle
Pseudoweakness of the involved muscle

is not "switched off," excessive utilization of adenosine triphosphate may result in a focal energy crisis in the injured muscle and thus perpetuate the problem.

Factors commonly cited as predisposing to trigger point formation include deconditioning, poor posture, repetitive mechanical stress, mechanical imbalance (e.g., leg length inequality), joint disorders, and nonrestorative sleep. The muscle pain experienced by FM patients is often the result of pain originating from myofascial trigger points and amplified by central sensitization. It is hypothesized that myofascial pain is an important "peripheral pain generator" that may, in some FM patients, perpetuate and accentuate the process of central sensitization.

Treatment

Management of myofascial trigger points is based on the following principles:

Postural and Ergonomic

An important issue in the effective management of myofascial pain syndromes is correction of predisposing factors (see earlier). These factors interfere with the ability of the muscle to fully recover and are the most common reason for treatment failure.

Stretching

Restoration of a muscle to its full stretch length breaks the link between the energy crisis and contraction of injured sarcomeres (see earlier). Commonly used stretching techniques include spray and stretch with ethyl chloride, acupressure, postisometric relaxation, and deep stroking massage.

Strengthening

Muscles harboring trigger points usually become weak because of the inhibitory effects of pain. A program of slowly progressive strengthening is essential to restore full function and minimize the risk for recurrence and perpetuation of satellite trigger points.

Trigger Point Injections

Needling the myofascial trigger point with a "peppering technique" often provides a worthwhile and long-lasting benefit. Although dry needling is effective, the use of a local anesthetic (1% lidocaine or 1% procaine) helps confirm the accuracy of the injection and provides immediate relief. Validation of the accuracy of the injection is suggested by the patient's report that the pain is reproduced on entry of the needle into the trigger point; in superficial muscles a local twitch response may be observed, and this provides further evidence of an accurate injection. Successful elimination of the trigger point generally results in relaxation of the taut band. There is no evidence that the injection of corticosteroids provides any added benefit. Botulinum toxin injections are of reported benefit, but not obviously superior to local anesthetics. [9]

Medications

Treatment of myofascial trigger points is mainly nonpharmacologic. Nonsteroidal anti-inflammatory drugs and other analgesics often provide moderate symptomatic relief. As in FM, drugs that modulate pain at the central level are a useful adjunct in difficult-to-treat patients, especially if central sensitization is suspected.

Future Directions

Both FM and CFS represent a major challenge to modern medicine in understanding a constellation of common and sometimes disabling symptoms that originate within the central nervous system but cannot be explained in terms of a classic psychological disorder. The central sensitization demonstrated in FM patients has provided important insight into the physiologic basis for the complaint of widespread pain, but no such breakthrough has occurred in the comprehensive understanding of fatigue in either FM or CFS. Current research suggests that both these conditions have a genetic predisposition that interacts with environmental insults such as infections, trauma, myofascial foci, and persistent psychological stressors. One common denominator actively being explored in both conditions is activation of glial cells within the central nervous system by cytokines and chemokines. Both these disorders are prime examples of the need to integrate the classic biomedical model of disease with psychosocial influences (i.e., the biopsychosocial model of disease). The challenge that faces investigators in the 21st century is to discern how mental processes can influence and interact with environmental stressors, acting on a genetic background, to change the expression of genes involved in pain processing and fatigue. It is unlikely that the answer to this conundrum will be found in the direct-line approach, as envisaged in Koch's postulates and the infectious disease paradigm of illness. More likely the solution will entail a circuitous route that involves multiple branching pathways with difficult-to-resolve uncertainties about whether the latest finding is the "cause" or a "cause of the cause," and so on.

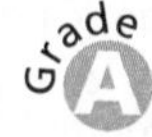

1. Arnold LM, Lu Y, Crofford LJ, et al: A double-blind, multicenter trial comparing duloxetine with placebo in the treatment of fibromyalgia patients with or without major depressive disorder. Arthritis Rheum 2004;50:2974–2984.
2. Vitton O, Gendreau M, Gendreau J, et al: A double-blind placebo-controlled trial of milnacipran in the treatment of fibromyalgia. Hum Psychopharmacol 2004;19(Suppl. 1):S27–S35.
3. Crofford LJ, Rowbotham MC, Mease PJ, et al: Pregabalin for the treatment of fibromyalgia syndrome: Results of a randomized, double-blind, placebo-controlled trial. Arthritis Rheum 2005;52: 1264–1273.
4. Bennett RM, Kamin M, Karim R, Rosenthal N: Tramadol and acetaminophen combination tablets in the treatment of fibromyalgia pain: A double-blind, randomized, placebo-controlled study. Am J Med 2003;114:537–545.
5. Thieme K, Gromnica-Ihle E, Flor H: Operant behavioral treatment of fibromyalgia: A controlled study. Arthritis Rheum 2003;49: 314–320.
6. Busch A, Schachter CL, Peloso PM, et al: Exercise for treating fibromyalgia syndrome. Cochrane Database Syst Rev 2002;(3): CD003786. *Supervised aerobic exercise training has beneficial effects on physical capacity and fibromyalgia symptoms.*
7. Moss-Morris R, Sharon C, Tobin R, Baldi JC: A randomized controlled graded exercise trial for chronic fatigue syndrome: Outcomes and mechanisms of change. J Health Psychol 2005; 10:245–259.
8. Bazelmans E, Prins JB, Lulofs R, et al: Cognitive behaviour group therapy for chronic fatigue syndrome: A non-randomised waiting list controlled study. Psychother Psychosom 2005;74:218–224.
9. Kamanli A, Kaya A, Ardicoglu O, et al: Comparison of lidocaine injection, botulinum toxin injection, and dry needling to trigger points in myofascial pain syndrome. Rheumatol Int 2005;25: 604–611.

SUGGESTED READINGS

Borg-Stein J, Simons DG: Focused review: Myofascial pain. Arch Phys Med Rehabil 2002;83(3 Suppl. 1):S40–S49. *A practical review of diagnosis and treatment.*

Cairns R, Hotopf M: A systematic review describing the prognosis of chronic fatigue syndrome. Occup Med (Lond) 2005;55:20–31. *A review of 25 studies showing that recovery from treated chronic fatigue syndrome is rare.*

Goldenberg DL, Burckhardt C, Crofford L: Management of fibromyalgia syndrome. JAMA 2004;292:2388–2395. *Practical suggestions for treatment.*

Prins JB, van der Meer JW, Bleijenberg G: Chronic fatigue syndrome. Lancet 2006;367:346–355. *A comprehensive review.*

296 THE AMYLOIDOSES

Joel N. Buxbaum

Definition

The amyloidoses, a subset of a larger class of diseases produced by the aggregation of misfolded proteins, are characterized by extracellular deposits of the aggregated protein. The deposits are usually at a distance from the site of synthesis and ultimately compromise function of the target organ. Kidney involvement, seen in several forms of amyloidosis (Table 296–1), is manifested by proteinuria progressing to nephrotic

TABLE 296–1 CHEMICAL CLASSIFICATION OF HUMAN AMYLOID

Amyloid Protein	Precursor*	Clinical Syndromes	Involved Tissues
AA	(Apo)serum AA	Chronic inflammation, familial Mediterranean fever, familial amyloid nephropathy with urticaria and deafness, tumors, Muckle-Wells syndrome	Kidney, liver, spleen
AL	Ig light chain, κ or λ	Primary/myeloma associated	Kidney, heart, peripheral nerve, tongue, bone marrow
AH	Ig heavy chain	Primary/myeloma associated	Kidney heart, peripheral nerve, tongue, bone marrow
ATTR	Transthyretin	Familial amyloidotic polyneuropathy, familial amyloidotic cardiomyopathy, senile systemic (cardiac) amyloid	Peripheral and autonomic nerves, heart, kidney
AApoAI	Apolipoprotein A-I	Familial amyloidotic polyneuropathy	Heart, skin, larynx, vessels, liver, kidney, nerve
AApoAII	Apolipoprotein A-II	Familial nephropathy	Kidney
AApoAIV	Apolipoprotein A-IV	Sporadic, aging associated	Vessels
AGel	Gelsolin	Finnish corneal lattice dystrophy with cranial neuropathy	Cornea, cranial and peripheral nerves, kidney
ACys	Cystatin C	Hereditary cerebral hemorrhage with amyloid	Cranial vessels
Aβ	Aβ protein precursor (AβPP)	Alzheimer's disease, aging	Central nervous system
$A\beta_2M$	β_2-Microglobulin	Dialysis-related amyloid	Synovium, carpal tunnel, tongue
APrP	Prion protein	Creutzfeldt-Jakob disease, Gerstmann-Sträussler-Scheinker disease, fatal familial insomnia	Central nervous system
ABri*	*BRI* gene product	Familial neurodegeneration	Central nervous system, blood vessels
ACal	Procalcitonin	Medullary thyroid carcinoma	Thyroid
AANF	Atrial natriuretic factor	Atrial amyloid of aging	Atria
AIAPP	Islet amyloid polypeptide	Senile amyloid of the pancreas	Pancreas
ALys	Lysozyme	Ostertag renal amyloid	Kidney, liver, salivary glands
AFib	Fibrinogen α chain	Hereditary renal amyloid	Kidney
APin	AOaap	Odontogenic tumor	Pindborg tumors
Ack	Cytokeratins	Cutaneous	Skin
Apro	Prolactin	Aging pituitary, prolactinomas	Pituitary
AIns	Insulin	Iatrogenic	Pancreas
ALac	Lactoferrin	Corneal deposition	Cornea
Amed	Lactadherin	Atherosclerosis	Aorta
AKer	Keratoepithelin	Familial corneal deposition	Cornea
ASeml	Semenogelin	Sporadic, aging	Seminal vesicle
Atau	Tau	Alzheimer's disease, aging, other cerebral conditions	Brain

*ADan is from the same gene as ABri and has an identical N-terminal sequence. ADan is therefore not included in the nomenclature as a separate protein. From Westermark, P, Benson MD, Buxbaum JN, et al: Amyloid: Toward terminology clarification. Report from the Nomenclature Committee of the International Society of Amyloidosis. Amyloid 2007, in press.

syndrome, renal failure, or both. Cardiac deposits result in congestive heart failure, arrhythmias, or anginal syndromes. Peripheral nerve infiltration produces symptomatic neuropathy, whereas central nervous system deposition may produce dementia or cerebral hemorrhage when the deposits are primarily vascular.

Amyloid deposits are identified in pathologic specimens by their homogeneous appearance when stained with hematoxylin and eosin; they have a discrete fibrillar ultrastructure on electron microscopy. The deposits bind the dye Congo red, thereby yielding positive birefringence when viewed with polarized light. They also bind metachromatic dyes such as thioflavine T and S; however, the latter is less specific than the interaction with Congo red. These properties are those of the major fibrillar component because fibrils isolated from tissue by low–ionic strength extraction show the same characteristics. The deposits also contain a set of accessory molecules that can be detected by staining with specific antibodies. Such molecules include the serum amyloid P component, apolipoprotein E, and the heparan sulfate proteoglycan perlecan. In other disorders of protein conformation, notably Huntington's and Parkinson's diseases, the aggregates are predominantly intracellular with nuclear or nuclear and cytoplasmic inclusions. These aggregates do not generally stain with Congo red. Tissue deposits in intracellular or extracellular nonamyloid aggregation diseases have not been shown to contain the same accessory molecules.

Epidemiology

Current data indicate that the most common form of systemic amyloidosis worldwide is amyloid A (AA) secondary to either infectious or noninfectious inflammation. In the United States, light chain amyloid (AL) is the form most commonly seen clinically, but recent autopsy studies suggest that late-onset deposition of transthyretin amyloid (ATTR) in the heart is more common, particularly in African Americans. ATTR has been reported to occur in 2% of autopsies in individuals older than 60 years, a frequency far higher than that of AL in autopsy or death certificate studies. In some geographic areas, notably the northern coastal region of Portugal, several districts in northern Sweden, and the Arao and Nagano prefectures in Japan, familial amyloidotic polyneuropathy (FAP) secondary to a mutation in the transthyretin gene is the most common amyloid seen in clinical practice.

Amyloid, derived from β_2-microglobulin (β_2M), is deposited in periarticular soft tissues, the carpal tunnel, the skeleton, and rarely, the tongue of patients undergoing long-term hemodialysis. The mechanism is unclear. It may represent a combination of the membrane pore size being too small to allow passage of the β_2M dimer and a reactive process involving macrophage activation. After 15 years of dialysis, virtually all patients show some evidence of $A\beta_2M$ deposition with symptoms related to nerve compression and joint immobilization secondary to synovial deposition.

The amyloid proteins derived from normal-sequence islet amyloid polypeptide (IAPP) and Aβ are seen with increasing frequency in the elderly, although the true incidence of either amyloid protein is unknown. Aβ deposition or toxic molecules generated in the course of its aggregation are clearly involved in the pathogenesis of Alzheimer's disease (AD). Although IAPP deposition in the pancreas does not initiate glucose intolerance, it may play a role in the gradual loss of beta cells involved in the progression of type 2 diabetes in the elderly.

Pathobiology

More than 20 proteins form clinically relevant amyloid deposits (see Table 296–1). The precursors appear to have no common amino acid sequences. The dominant structural feature of the deposited fibril, regardless of the precursor, is the β-pleated sheet. In vitro studies of many of the precursors have begun to elucidate the steps involved in the aggregation process leading to amyloid deposits. In each case, a critical early event appears to be the formation of a misfolded monomer that may be facilitated by structural change secondary to a mutation. When there is no mutation, amyloid deposition may result from increased precursor concentration as a result of increased synthesis (AA) or an expanded clone of precursor-producing cells (AL), a decrease in the normal process of degradative proteolytic cleavage, or abnormal cleavage of a normal protein, any or all of which increase the absolute amount of misfolded conformer. In the case of the prion diseases, other mechanisms may be operating that have not yet been elucidated.

Clinical Manifestations

The clinical features and course of the systemic amyloidoses are a function of the site and rate of deposition. Each protein seems to have a characteristic hierarchy of tissue deposition. The kidney is the most frequent site of deposition in both AL and AA, is common in some ATTR mutants, and is the only site in some of the hereditary amyloidoses. The most common finding is proteinuria, with the full nephrotic syndrome found in many cases. Renal tubular acidosis may also occur early. Without effective treatment, the course is one of progressive renal failure. In some cases, the initial manifestation is renal failure. Complications of renal failure are a frequent cause of death, regardless of the nature of the precursor producing the renal disease.

Cardiac deposition is common in AL, with approximately 20% of patients having arrhythmias or congestive heart failure as an initial manifestation. Many of the mutant ATTRs also have cardiac infiltration as the dominant clinical feature (familial amyloidotic cardiomyopathy). Myocardial deposition of wild-type ATTR in the elderly (senile systemic amyloidosis) is probably the most common form of amyloid heart disease. Whatever the precursor, ventricular myocardial deposition leads to diastolic dysfunction, congestive heart failure, and a variety of arrhythmias, including atrial standstill, atrial fibrillation, complete heart block, and sudden death, presumably related to ventricular irritability or abnormalities in autonomic control. Cardiac ATTR appears to progress at a far slower rate than that related to AL deposition, presumably as a function of the concentration of the amyloidogenic precursor.

The diagnosis of cardiac amyloid can be suspected on the basis of low voltage on the electrocardiogram and characteristic echocardiographic features, including ventricular septal thickening and an increase in the E/A ratio (*e*arly atrial to ventricular flow/flow related to *a*trial contraction) consistent with ventricular noncompliance. There is also distortion of the normal relationship between left ventricular mass (as determined by echocardiography) and left ventricular voltage on the electrocardiogram. Frequently, cardiac binding of technetium 99 is noted during the course of a soft tissue computed tomography (CT) scan in a patient with amyloid. Even though the finding is not sensitive, its occurrence should raise one's level of suspicion and suggest further investigation. The definitive diagnostic test is endomyocardial biopsy with specific analysis by Congo red staining and the detection of known amyloid precursors by immunohistochemical or immuno-electron microscopic techniques.

Approximately 10% of patients with AA disease have cardiac involvement. In most of these individuals, the coronary and intramyocardial vessels are affected, with angina pectoris or myocardial infarction being the initial manifestation of the disease.

Peripheral neuropathy is seen in FAP, with mutant ATTR, and in AL disease. The symptoms are usually sensorimotor and can result in painless ulcerations or Charcot joints. Dysesthesias are a troubling symptom in some patients. FAP patients also have striking autonomic involvement. This is frequently the most disabling feature of the entire FAP symptom complex.

Though not a true polyneuropathy, carpal tunnel syndrome may be seen in patients with AL, FAP, and dialysis-related amyloid. Only a small proportion of all patients with isolated carpal tunnel syndrome have amyloid deposition. In most cases, the protein is transthyretin, frequently with no evidence of disease elsewhere.

Hepatic and splenic deposition is common in AL and AA, but clinical consequences are uncommon. Visceral infiltration presents a risk in closed liver biopsy, in which hepatic rupture or excessive bleeding has been reported. Coagulopathies occur in AL. Severe factor X deficiency has been related to sequestration of the protein by fibrils, but recent reports have suggested that this might not be the entire explanation. Nonetheless, because of the vascular fragility related to deposition within vessel walls, bleeding may be severe in these patients and therefore coagulation parameters should be monitored regularly.

Diagnosis

Specific organ involvement can be determined by a variety of diagnostic techniques, including CT scans, echocardiograms, peripheral nerve conduction studies, renal sonograms, and biochemical assays of liver function. Attribution of the dysfunction to amyloid deposition and the nature of the precursor can be made only by appropriate examination of involved tissue (Fig. 296–1). Staining with Congo red with examination under polarized and fluorescent light to reveal the characteristic birefringence and fluorescence, followed by more detailed immunohistochemical analysis with antibodies to specific precursors, allows a definitive diagnosis in almost all cases. Examination of an involved organ with these techniques has great sensitivity, as well as specificity, and yields a diagnosis in more than 90% of cases. Errors in tissue handling or staining, particularly related to antibody specificity, are the most common causes of diagnostic failure. Tissue sampling in early disease, when involvement may be patchy, may also lead to false-negative results. In some circumstances, notably early FAP or monoclonal immunoglobulin deposition disease, nonamyloid tissue aggregates stain with specific antiprecursor antibodies and do not bind Congo red. This finding implies the presence of a nonamyloidotic, but nonetheless pathogenic precursor state.

Diagnosis of the amyloidoses has been facilitated by the development of relatively benign methods of tissue sampling. Rectal biopsy and subcutaneous fat aspiration are safe and efficient means of obtaining tissue for pathologic examination. Labial gland and gastric biopsies are also useful but have not yet been widely used in the United States. Samples obtained by any of these techniques can be stained with Congo red and identified with specific antiprecursor antibodies. A combination of rectal biopsy and subcutaneous fat aspiration has a diagnostic yield greater than 80%. In the absence of technical mishaps, biopsy of a clinically involved organ (notably the liver or kidney) gives a diagnosis in more than 90% of cases. A summary of results from current sampling procedures is listed in Table 296–2.

Treatment

Rx

The critical step in the treatment of any of the amyloidoses is accurate recognition of the precursor. Even though the nature of the precursor allows identification of the primary pathologic process, effective specific treatments are not yet available for most of the individual amyloidoses, so it is possible to mistreat an individual patient. The Hippocratic caveat "above all do no harm" is particularly applicable in this set of disorders. For example, cardiac involvement by AL or late-onset ATTR deposition may have identical clinical features at the time of initial evaluation, including the presence of a coincidental monoclonal immunoglobulin in individuals with ATTR

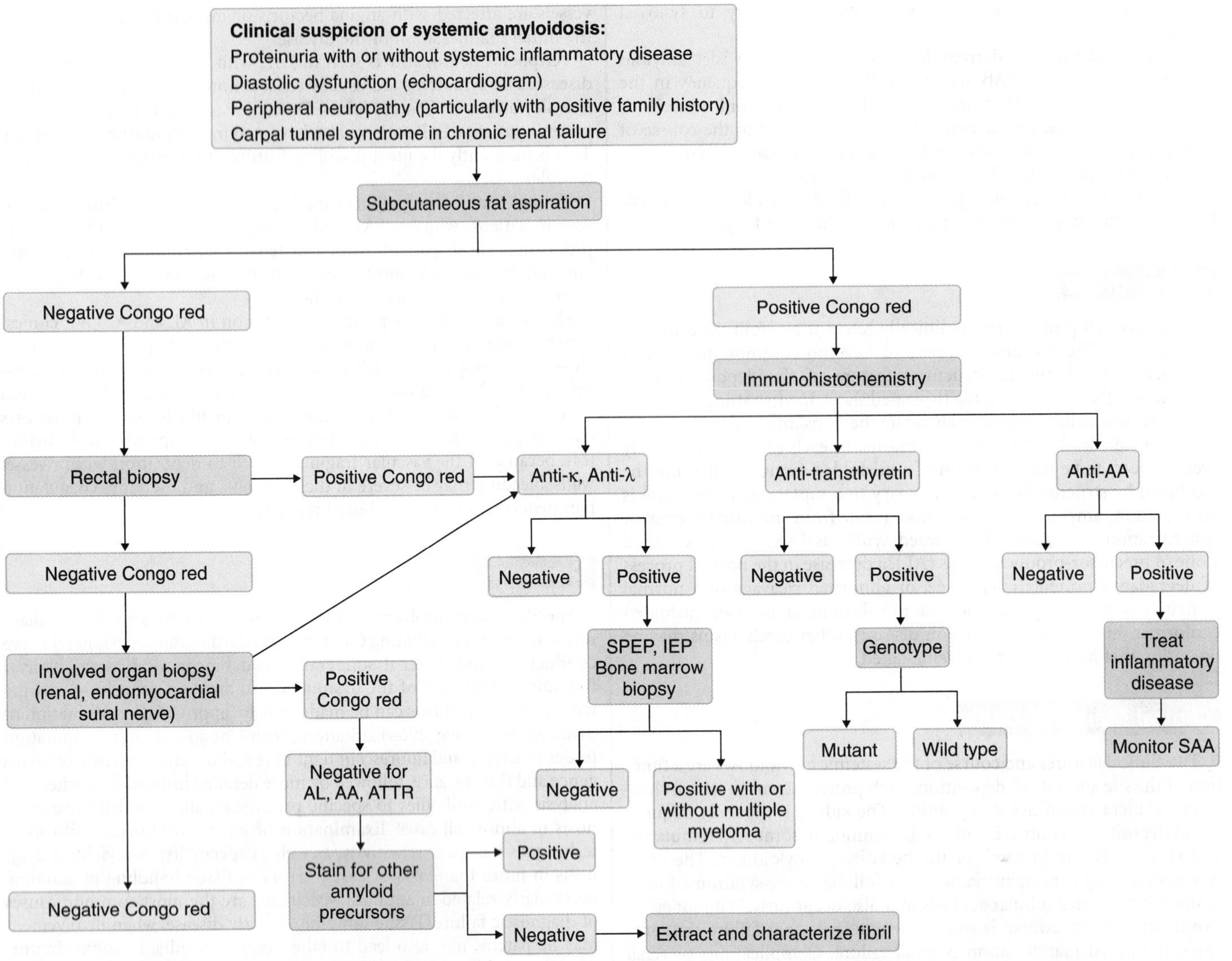

Clinical suspicion of systemic amyloidosis:
Proteinuria with or without systemic inflammatory disease
Diastolic dysfunction (echocardiogram)
Peripheral neuropathy (particularly with positive family history)
Carpal tunnel syndrome in chronic renal failure

Subcutaneous fat aspiration

Negative Congo red
Positive Congo red
Immunohistochemistry
Rectal biopsy
Positive Congo red
Anti-κ, Anti-λ
Anti-transthyretin
Anti-AA
Negative Congo red
Negative
Positive
Negative
Positive
Negative
Positive
SPEP, IEP
Bone marrow biopsy
Genotype
Treat inflammatory disease
Involved organ biopsy (renal, endomyocardial sural nerve)
Positive Congo red
Mutant
Wild type
Monitor SAA
Negative for AL, AA, ATTR
Negative
Positive with or without multiple myeloma
Stain for other amyloid precursors
Positive
Negative Congo red
Negative
Extract and characterize fibril

FIGURE 296–1 • Approach to a patient with possible systemic amyloidosis. AA = amyloid A; AL = light chain amyloid; ATTR = transthyretin amyloid; IEP = immunoelectrophoresis; SAA = serum amyloid A; SPEP = serum protein electrophoresis.

TABLE 296–2 DIAGNOSTIC YIELD OF TISSUE SAMPLING PROCEDURES IN THE MAJOR AMYLOIDOSES

Tissue	AL	AA	ATTR
Subcutaneous fat aspiration*	541/689 (79%)	56/91[†] (62%)	58/71 (82%)
Rectal biopsy*	146/194 (75%)	54/65 (83%)	—
Bone marrow biopsy	221/394 (56%)	12/26 (46%)	—
Stomach and small bowel biopsy	19/23 (83%)	15/16 (94%)	—
Labial salivary gland biopsy	13/16 (81%)	13/14 (93%)	—

*Neither subcutaneous fat aspiration nor rectal biopsy is useful in $A\beta_2$-microglobulin.
[†]The results of subcutaneous fat aspiration in AA amyloid do not include patients with familial Mediterranean fever, who are not generally positive from this site.
AA = amyloid A; AL = amyloid light chain; ATTR = transthyretin amyloid.

disease. Whereas the supportive treatment of both conditions is identical (i.e., loop diuretics and avoidance of digoxin and calcium-channel blocking agents), the use of potentially toxic antineoplastic therapy is appropriate only in AL. Thus, immunohistologic identification of the deposited protein as immunoglobulin light chain or ATTR derived is critical for adequate care.

Once the nature of the protein is definitively established, institution of protein-specific therapies, to the extent that they exist, can be initiated. AL, as either the primary disease or in association with

multiple myeloma, is treated as a clonal disorder of plasma cells (Chapter 198). In randomized controlled trials, a combination of melphalan and prednisone prolonged survival after diagnosis. Colchicine alone or added to the melphalan/prednisone regimen had no effect. High-intensity chemotherapy with stem cell replacement is currently being extensively used in the treatment of myeloma. Data thus far suggest that this treatment may be effective in AL patients without significant cardiac involvement. However, studies examining outcomes to date indicate that the

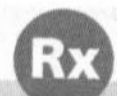

patients who appear to benefit might be the group that would do well anyway, even with less aggressive treatment.

Because AA occurs in the course of a variety of inflammatory diseases, the primary goal of any treatment is to suppress the inflammatory process. There is an increasing amount of data indicating that more aggressive treatment of both adult and juvenile rheumatoid arthritis, particularly with tumor necrosis factor inhibitors, is associated with a lower frequency of amyloid renal disease. In some cases there has been demonstrable improvement in clinical parameters of already established renal amyloidosis. In addition, suppression of the inflammatory episodes of familial Mediterranean fever with colchicine prevents the development of renal AA, formerly the main cause of death in these patients. It appears that reduction plus maintenance of the serum AA level at less than 10 mg/mL is sufficient to allow absorption of the deposits. If the renal failure does not resolve, renal transplantation, after adequate suppression of inflammation, can be effective treatment.

Treatment of the amyloidoses related to mutations in the transthyretin gene is accomplished by a crude form of gene therapy in which patients receive a liver transplant containing two normal transthyretin alleles. Progression of the disease is arrested in most instances. Post-transplant functional status is related to the degree of nutritional and visceral compromise present at the time of transplantation. For reasons that are unclear, cardiac involvement in patients with mutations other than transthyretin Val30Met responds poorly to liver transplantation, and combined heart and liver transplantation may be a more effective procedure.

There has been some progress toward prevention of the β_2M amyloidosis associated with dialysis. Even though data regarding the frequency of deposition with different dialysis membranes are not yet available, there is a suggestion that high-flux dialysis and close attention to the quality of the dialysate reduce the frequency of this form of amyloidosis.

A variety of agents have been used to specifically scan for amyloid deposits as a way to measure therapeutic response. The longest experience has been with iodinated serum amyloid P. Liver, spleen, renal, and adrenal deposits of amyloid are well visualized by this technique, although it has not been consistently useful in cardiac scanning. Labeled aprotinin seems to have better affinity for cardiac deposits. The usefulness of this technique in primary diagnosis has not yet been established, but in patients with a positive initial scan, a reduction in binding of the agent has been associated with clinical response. Neither of these technologies is currently available in the United States.

Supportive measures include antibiotics when indicated, careful fluid management and diuresis for congestive heart failure and the edema of nephrotic syndrome, dialysis, and renal transplantation for end-stage renal disease. Nutritional status should be maintained with supplements if necessary.

Future Directions

Despite its increasing use, high-intensity chemotherapy with stem cell autotransplantation for AL is still experimental and is best carried out in a center experienced in both supportive therapy for amyloidosis and transplantation as part of a research protocol. It is likely that the indications and benefits of this treatment modality will not become clear in the absence of a randomized prospective study. Response to therapy can be monitored by following the level of free monoclonal light chains in serum. In FAP, a variety of compounds have been shown to inhibit transthyretin fibril formation in vitro and represent potential effective therapeutic agents. Some of these compounds should reach clinical trial status over the next few years, perhaps obviating or reducing the need for liver transplantation. In β_2M amyloidosis, current studies of high-flux dialysis and the role of different dialysis membranes should provide conclusive data regarding prevention of deposition.

An anionic sulfonate compound that has been shown to be very effective in the prevention of AA deposition in a murine inflammatory model is now in late phase II clinical trials in patients with AA. A similar compound designed to cross the blood-brain barrier is in an earlier phase of development for AD.

One of the most striking, potentially therapeutic interventions reported to date involves administering antibodies specific for the Aβ fibril precursor to mice with experimental AD pathology related to the presence of a human AD-associated Aβ transgene. Deposits were cleared with some improvement in neurologic function. A trial of active immunization in humans was aborted after meningoencephalitis developed in some of the participants; however, a trial of passive immunization is currently in progress. Based on these findings, similar immunologic approaches to other forms of systemic amyloidosis are being carried out in various experimental models.

SUGGESTED READINGS

Benson MD: Ostertag revisited: The inherited systemic amyloidoses without neuropathy. Amyloid 2005;12:75–87. *A review of the less common hereditary amyloidoses, thus omitting the transthyretin-related disorders.*

Falk RH: Diagnosis and management of the cardiac amyloidoses. Circulation 2005;112:2047–2060. *Current views on the clinical approach to the cardiac amyloidoses.*

Fernandez-Nebro A, Tomero E, Ortiz-Santamaria V, et al: Treatment of rheumatic inflammatory disease in 25 patients with secondary amyloidosis using tumor necrosis factor alpha antagonists. Am J Med 2005;118:552–556. *The results of aggressive anti-inflammatory treatment of inflammatory joint disease when amyloidosis is already present.*

Gershoni-Baruch R, Brik R, Zacks N, et al: The contribution of genotypes at the MEFV and SAA1 loci to amyloidosis and disease severity in patients with familial Mediterranean fever. Arthritis Rheum 2003;48:1149–1155. *A genotype-phenotype correlation.*

Gertz, MA, Lacy MQ, Dispenzieri A, et al: Amyloidosis. Best Pract Res Clin Haematol 2005;18:709–727. *A review from a major center with emphasis on AL.*

Gillmore JD, Lovat LB, Persey MR, et al: Amyloid load and clinical outcome in AA amyloidosis in relation to circulating concentration of serum amyloid A protein. Lancet 2001;358:24–29. *An excellent study of how the Centre for Amyloidosis and Acute Phase Proteins (UK) monitors their patients with AA.*

Hazenberg BPC, van Rijswijk MH: Where has secondary amyloid gone? Ann Rheum Dis 2000;59:577–579. *A review discussing the apparent decrease in AA secondary to systemic inflammatory diseases.*

Lachmann HJ, Gallimore R, Gillmore JD, et al: Outcome in systemic AL amyloidosis in relation to changes in concentration of circulating free immunoglobulin light chains following chemotherapy. Br J Haematol 2003;122:78–84. *A major center validates the use of circulating amyloid precursor as a monitor for therapeutic response.*

Mumford AD, O'Donnell J, Gillmore JD, et al: Bleeding symptoms and coagulation abnormalities in 337 patients with AL-amyloidosis. Br J Haematol 2000;110:454–460. *Coagulation abnormalities in AL, a comprehensive analysis.*

Poullos PD, Stollman N: Gastrointestinal amyloidosis: Approach to treatment. Curr Treat Options Gastroenterol 2003;6:17–25. *Emphasizes symptom-directed therapy.*

Shah KB, Inoue Y, Mehra MR: Amyloidosis and the heart: A comprehensive review. Arch Intern Med 2006;166:1805–1813. *A review.*

Skinner M, Sanchorawala V, Seldin DC, et al: High-dose melphalan and autologous stem-cell transplantation in patients with AL amyloidosis: An 8-year study. Ann Intern Med 2004;140:85–93. *Selected patients had hematologic remission, improved 5-year survival, and reversal of amyloid-related disease with these therapies.*

297 SYSTEMIC DISEASES IN WHICH ARTHRITIS IS A FEATURE

Sterling G. West

Arthritis, arthralgias, and myalgias can be significant features of several systemic diseases and may be the presenting symptoms for some of these disorders (Table 297–1). Appropriate evaluation of these musculoskeletal symptoms, including selected laboratory tests and radiographs, provide clues for the earlier diagnosis of these diseases. Brief descriptions of the arthritic manifestations for some of these sys-

TABLE 297–1 SYSTEMIC DISEASES ASSOCIATED WITH ARTHRITIS

Disease	Test*
GASTROINTESTINAL DISEASES	
Hemochromatosis	Iron studies, radiographs, *HFE gene*
Autoimmune hepatitis	Liver-associated enzymes, *ASMA*
Primary biliary cirrhosis	Alkaline phosphatase, *antimitochondrial Ab*
Pancreatitis-arthritis syndrome	Lipase, amylase, *abdominal CT scan*
Whipple's disease	*PCR for* Tropheryma whippelii *DNA*
Gluten-sensitive enteropathy	*Antitransglutaminase antibody, small bowel biopsy*
Inflammatory bowel disease	Stool guaiac, *colonoscopy*
Hepatitis B/hepatitis C	Liver-associated enzymes, *hepatitis serology*
Intestinal bypass arthritis	*Cryoglobulins*
HEMATOLOGIC DISORDERS	
Hemophilia	PTT, *factor VIII and IX levels*
Hemoglobinopathies	CBC, *hemoglobin electrophoresis*
Hypogammaglobulinemia	Low total protein, *SPEP, immunoglobulins*
Plasma cell dyscrasias	High total protein, *SPEP, UPEP, IEF*
ENDOCRINE DISORDERS	
Diabetes mellitus	Glucose, *hemoglobin A_{1c}*
Thyroid disorders	TSH, *thyroxine*
Parathyroid disorders	Calcium, phosphorus, *PTH*
Acromegaly	Radiographs, *growth hormone*
Hyperlipoproteinemia	Lipid panel
Paget's disease	Alkaline phosphatase, radiographs, *bone scan*
MALIGNANT DISORDERS	
Hypertrophic osteoarthropathy	Radiographs (hands, wrists, chest)
Leukemia and lymphoma	CBC, LDH, *bone marrow/tissue biopsy*
Carcinomatous polyarthritis	*Cancer screen*
Palmar fasciitis and arthritis	*CA-125, pelvic CT scan*
OTHER DISEASES	
Multicentric reticulohistiocytosis	Radiographs, *skin/synovial biopsy*
Sarcoidosis	Chest radiograph, *ACE level, tissue biopsy*
Relapsing polychondritis	*Cartilage biopsy*
Cystic fibrosis	Chest radiograph, *sweat chloride*
Pigmented villonodular synovitis	Synovial fluid analysis, *MRI, synovial biopsy*
Systemic infections	Cultures, serologies (RPR, HIV, parvovirus)

*Tests listed are common laboratory tests and radiographs that are frequently ordered; this information should provide a clue that a systemic disease is a possible cause of the patient's musculoskeletal symptoms. These tests, coupled with the history and physical examination, should be followed by more specific serologies and biopsies (listed in italics) to confirm the diagnosis.
Ab = antibody; ACE = angiotensin-converting enzyme; ASMA = anti–smooth muscle antibody; CBC = complete blood cell count; CT = computed tomography; HIV = human immunodeficiency virus; IEF = immunoelectrophoresis; LDH = lactate dehydrogenase; MRI = magnetic resonance imaging; PCR = polymerase chain reaction; PTH = parathyroid hormone; PTT = partial thromboplastin time; RPR = rapid plasmin reagin; SPEP = serum protein electrophoresis; TSH = thyroid-stimulating hormone; UPEP = urine protein electrophoresis.

temic disorders follow; more detailed discussion of each entity is found in other chapters devoted to these diseases. Because of the rarity of many of these diseases, evidence-based treatments with Food and Drug Administration–approved medications are lacking.

HEMOCHROMATOSIS

Joint involvement occurs in 40 to 75% of patients with hereditary hemochromatosis (Chapter 231). The metacarpophalangeal (MCP) joints (especially second and third MCP joints), wrists, knees, hips, shoulders, and ankles are most often involved in a symmetrical pattern. The arthropathy resembles osteoarthritis with joint swelling resulting from bone enlargement but is separated clinically by involvement of atypical joints, such as MCP joints, wrists, and ankles. Radiographs show joint space narrowing, subchondral cysts, sclerosis, and osteophytes that are hook-like at the MCP joints. Chondrocalcinosis is present in up to 50% of patients. It is typically asymptomatic but in some patients leads to attacks of acute inflammatory synovitis (pseudogout), which may result in the misdiagnosis of rheumatoid arthritis (RA). The prevalence of overt arthritis increases with age, and it may be only minimally symptomatic when the disease arises in other organs. However, it is not uncommon for articular pain to be the initial presenting complaint. Consequently, all patients (especially male) presenting with premature osteoarthritis occurring in atypical joints, especially MCP joints and wrists, should be screened for hereditary hemochromatosis with iron studies. The mechanism whereby iron causes arthritis is unclear but may be related to hemosiderin deposits in the synovial membrane and chondrocytes activating degradative enzymes. Treatment is symptomatic with nonsteroidal anti-inflammatory drugs (NSAIDs) and, when severe, total joint arthroplasties. Phlebotomy for iron removal does not alter the course of the arthritis. Additional rheumatic manifestations in patients with hemochromatosis include osteoporosis related to hypogonadotropic hypogonadism and osteomalacia related to vitamin D deficiency when liver disease is severe.

AUTOIMMUNE HEPATITIS

Patients with type I autoimmune hepatitis (Chapter 152) may present with a syndrome resembling systemic lupus erythematosus (SLE). Patients with the early-onset subset are frequently young and female, with complaints of polyarthralgia and occasionally fever. Laboratory examination may show leukopenia, a positive antinuclear antibody (70 to 90%), elevated erythrocyte sedimentation rate, polyclonal gammopathy, and elevated liver-associated enzymes. Antibodies against double-stranded DNA are usually not seen, whereas antibodies against the smooth muscle antigen (F1 actin) support the diagnosis. Joint radiographs show soft tissue swelling without erosions or deformity. Joint pain resolves with corticosteroid therapy for the liver disease.

PRIMARY BILIARY CIRRHOSIS

Up to 50% of patients with primary biliary cirrhosis (Chapter 159) have other autoimmune disorders including RA, Sjögren's syndrome, limited scleroderma, and autoimmune thyroiditis. In addition to antimitochondrial antibodies, rheumatoid factor, antinuclear, and anticentromere antibodies are often present. More than 10% of patients with primary biliary cirrhosis have a symmetrical or asymmetric small joint inflammatory arthritis. Unlike RA, it can involve distal interphalangeal joints and is rarely erosive or deforming. Other musculoskeletal manifestations include osteomalacia related to vitamin D deficiency, osteoporosis related to renal tubular acidosis, and hypertrophic osteoarthropathy associated with liver disease.

WHIPPLE'S DISEASE

An inflammatory arthritis occurs in 60 to 90% of patients with Whipple's disease (Chapter 143) and may precede other clinical manifestations by years. The joint involvement is typically an intermittent, migratory oligoarthritis affecting large more than small joints or spine, lasting from several hours to days. The synovial fluid is inflammatory with a predominance of mononuclear cells. Subcutaneous nodules are occasionally seen, contributing to an erroneous diagnosis of rheumatic fever or RA. However, patients consistently test negative for rheumatoid factor and antinuclear antibodies. Synovial biopsies show rod-shaped bacilli on electron microscopy, which have been identified as *Tropheryma whippelii*. Diagnosis can now be made by polymerase chain reaction to detect DNA of the organism in peripheral blood, cerebrospinal and synovial fluid, or tissue biopsy specimens. Typically, the arthritis does not cause radiographic changes or deformities. Prolonged antibiotic therapy results in resolution of musculoskeletal as well as other symptoms of this disease.

GLUTEN-SENSITIVE ENTEROPATHY (CELIAC DISEASE)

A monoarthritis, oligoarthritis, or symmetrical polyarthritis occurs in 25% of adults with celiac disease. It may precede the enteropathic symptoms by months to years. Large joints such as knees and ankles, more than hips and shoulders, are most commonly involved. Axial involvement is reported. The arthritis does not cause deformities or radiographic changes and resolves with a gluten-free diet in 40 to 50% of cases. Another musculoskeletal manifestation is osteomalacia related to vitamin D malabsorption, which may mimic diffuse fibromyalgia.

PANCREATIC-ARTHRITIS SYNDROME

Pancreatic panniculitis is a systemic syndrome occurring in some patients with pancreatic acinar cell carcinoma and less commonly in patients with pancreatitis or hematologic malignancies. This syndrome is characterized by tender, red nodules usually on the extremities, which are frequently misdiagnosed as erythema nodosum but on biopsy are areas of lobular panniculitis with fat necrosis. Arthritis occurs in 60% of patients and usually involves the ankles and knees. Synovial fluid is typically noninflammatory and creamy in color. It contains multiple lipid droplets because of necrosis of fat in the synovial membrane. Other manifestations include osteolytic lesions from bone marrow fat necrosis, pleuropericarditis, fever, and eosinophilia. The prominent fat necrosis is due to release of lipase, amylase, and trypsin from the diseased pancreas. Another musculoskeletal manifestation resulting from pancreatic disease is osteomalacia from vitamin D deficiency related to malabsorption from insufficiency of the pancreas.

HEMOPHILIA

Hemophilia A (factor VIII deficiency) and hemophilia B (factor IX deficiency) (Chapter 180) are associated with hemarthrosis. Almost all patients with factor levels less than 1% of normal experience recurrent hemarthroses spontaneously or after minor trauma. Large joints are most commonly involved. Intramuscular hemorrhage can also occur. Recurrent hemarthrosis can lead to proliferative synovitis and cartilage degradation, resulting in both erosive and degenerative changes on radiographs. Physical examination shows bone enlargement, crepitus, atrophic muscles, and joint contractures. Treatment of acute monoarthritis is with factor replacement to achieve a level of 30% or greater, given at the first sign of joint swelling. Patients with fever (temperature >38° C) or who fail to respond to factor replacement need joint aspiration to rule out septic arthritis, which occurs with an increased incidence in hemophilia. Chronic arthritis is treated with NSAIDs that do not inhibit platelet function, arthroscopic synovectomy for chronic synovitis, and total joint arthroplasty for end-stage joint disease.

HEMOGLOBINOPATHIES

Patients with sickle cell anemia (S-S) (Chapter 167) or the heterozygous state of sickle β-thalassemia, sickle-C (S-C), and sickle-D (S-D) disease frequently experience polyarthralgia. Local sickling of cells leads to obstruction of the microcirculation and to bone infarctions. Patients most commonly experience painful crises causing chest, back, and joint pain. A painful large joint arthritis (usually knees) often with noninflammatory synovial effusions lasting days to 2 to 3 weeks can also occur. Bone infarcts in the metaphyses of bones are commonly found on joint radiographs. Vertebral bodies have a characteristic central cup-like indentation ("codfish vertebrae"). Femoral and humeral head osteonecrosis can occur in up to 33% of S-S and S-C cases. Because of splenic dysfunction, septic arthritis and osteomyelitis (50% caused by *Salmonella*) have been associated with sickle cell disease. In adults, gout has been reported, whereas in children younger than 2 years an acute, painful, nonpitting swelling of the hands and feet (hand-foot syndrome) associated with fever and leukocytosis may be the first manifestation of sickle cell anemia. Treatment includes intravenous hydration, oxygen, and analgesics. In patients with β-thalassemia major (Cooley's anemia), significant expansion of bone marrow develops as a result of increased erythroid precursors, leading to osteoporosis and microfractures that affect primarily the lower extremities.

HYPOGAMMAGLOBULINEMIA

Patients with congenital X-linked hypogammaglobulinemia (Bruton's disease) or acquired common variable immunodeficiency (CVID) can develop a nonerosive, noninfectious large joint oligoarthritis that responds to intravenous gamma globulin therapy. However, septic arthritis caused by common pathogens or *Mycoplasma* can also occur and must be rigorously excluded. In adults with acquired CVID, autoimmune conditions are common (22%) including autoimmune cytopenias, RA, and pernicious anemia. Selective immunoglobulin A (IgA) deficiency is associated with various rheumatic manifestations, including positive autoantibodies, in the absence of clinical disease. Systemic autoimmune disorders, including SLE and juvenile RA as well as others, and organ-specific autoimmune disorders, such as type 1 diabetes mellitus and myasthenia gravis, also occur in IgA-deficient individuals.

DIABETES MELLITUS

Diabetic stiff hand syndrome of limited joint mobility (diabetic cheiroarthropathy) occurs in over 30% of patients with long-standing, poorly controlled type 1 or type 2 diabetes mellitus (DM) (Chapters 247 and 248). Patients present with the insidious development of flexion contractures and thickened skin of the fingers, which may be confused with scleroderma. These changes may be due to excess glycosylation of tendinous structures and accumulation of sugar alcohols producing excess water content in the skin, leading to increased stiffness. As a result of the inability to extend the fingers fully, the "prayer sign" is observed on physical examination. Unlike diabetic stiff hand syndrome, Dupuytren's contractures are due to a chronic thickening of the palmar aponeurosis causing flexion deformities of the third and fourth digits. It is the most frequent musculoskeletal complication, occurring in over 20% of type 2 diabetics. A less common manifestation includes Charcot, or neuropathic, joints, occurring in less than 1% of all patients with long-standing diabetes. All patients have a diabetic peripheral neuropathy and most commonly present with painless swelling of the feet caused by destruction most commonly of the tarsometatarsal joints. Deformities can occur with midtarsal collapse ("rocker bottom" feet), predisposing to ulceration and infection of the skin over desensate bone prominences. Radiographs are diagnostic, and treatment should include supportive footwear and protected weight bearing.

Unlike the Charcot joint, diabetic osteolysis and diabetic amyotrophy are unique to diabetes. The osteolysis is characterized by resorption of the distal metatarsal bone and proximal phalanges of the feet, giving radiographs a characteristic "licked candy" appearance. Pain is variable and treatment conservative because the process may terminate on its own. Diabetic amyotrophy is a lumbar polyradiculopathy (L2-L4) that arises with severe pain, dysesthesias, and rapid atrophy of the proximal muscles of one or both thighs. Carpal tunnel syndrome (25%), adhesive capsulitis of the shoulder (frozen shoulder), flexor tenosynovitis (trigger finger) of the hands, diffuse idiopathic skeletal hyperostosis, osteopenia (type 1 DM), diabetic muscle infarction usually of the thigh, osteomyelitis of the foot, and septic joints are all musculoskeletal conditions that occur with increased frequency in diabetic patients. Aggressive control of the blood glucose helps prevent some of these musculoskeletal complications.

THYROID DISORDERS

Musculoskeletal symptoms occur in 33% of patients with clinical hypothyroidism (thyroid-stimulating hormone levels >20 μU/mL) (Chapter 244). Patients can present with carpal tunnel syndrome, Raynaud's phenomenon, or muscle aching and stiffness similar to fibromyalgia and polymyalgia rheumatica. Patients with severe hypothyroidism can experience a noninflammatory myopathy with proximal muscle weakness and elevated creatine kinase, which may be confused clinically with polymyositis. Similarly, myxedematous patients can develop a symmetrical arthropathy of the large joints, especially the knees, associated with noninflammatory synovial fluid with increased viscosity. The association of hypothyroidism with chondrocalcinosis is controversial, but clearly patients initiating treatment with thyroid replacement can experience an acute attack of pseudogout. Patients with hyperthyroidism can develop proximal myopathy (70%), adhesive capsulitis of the shoulder (10%), osteoporosis, or thyroid acropachy. Thyroid acropachy occurs in less than 1% of patients with Graves' disease and consists of soft tissue swelling of the hands, digital clubbing, and periostitis, particularly involving the metacarpal and phalangeal bone shafts. Pain is usually mild, radiographs are characteristic, and there is no effective therapy. Patients with autoimmune thyroid disease have an increased prevalence of positive antinuclear antibodies and an increased association with systemic connective tissue disease such as Sjögren's syndrome.

PARATHYROID DISORDERS

Primary hyperparathyroidism can arise with osteoporosis and fractures or with chondrocalcinosis and episodes of acute pseudogout. In severe hyperparathyroidism, which is rare, vague myalgias and arthralgias resembling fibromyalgia; a reversible, painless, proximal myopathy with normal creatine kinase; and osteitis fibrosa cystica with bone pain can be seen. Osteitis fibrosa cystica occurs primarily in patients with secondary hyperparathyroidism associated with renal failure and has a characteristic appearance radiographically with subperiosteal resorption on the radial side of the phalanges, small erosions in the hands and distal clavicles, and discrete lytic bone lesions (brown tumors). Ectopic calcifications, joint laxity, and tendon ruptures have also been reported in patients with severe hyperparathyroidism. Hypoparathyroidism has also been associated with a myopathy and ectopic calcifications. Patients with type Ia pseudohypoparathyroidism and pseudo-pseudohypoparathyroidism have a shortened fourth metacarpal bone bilaterally.

ACROMEGALY

Up to 75% of patients with acromegaly (Chapter 242) develop an atypical form of osteoarthritis. The knees, shoulders, hips, and lumbosacral and cervical spine are the most frequently symptomatic areas, although the hands reveal the most characteristic radiographic changes. Carpal tunnel syndrome (50%), Raynaud's phenomenon (33%), and proximal muscle weakness with normal creatine kinase can also occur.

HYPERLIPOPROTEINEMIA

Type IIa familial hyperlipidemia is associated with tendinous and tuberous-osseous xanthomas as well as episodic Achilles tendinitis. An acute, migratory inflammatory arthritis persisting up to a month and resembling rheumatic fever occurs in up to 50% of patients. Large more than small joints are predominantly affected. In addition, a self-limited, acute monoarticular or oligoarticular arthritis involving the knee or ankle can occur. Patients with type III familial hyperlipoproteinemia can develop tendon and bone xanthomas. Patients with human immunodeficiency virus (HIV) infection taking protease inhibitor drugs can develop dyslipidemia leading to tendon xanthomas. In all hyperlipidemias, gout must be excluded before ascribing the symptoms to hyperlipoproteinemia. Therapy with NSAIDs and treatment of the underlying lipid disorder should be pursued. Notably, some of the therapies used to treat hyperlipidemia can cause musculoskeletal symptoms including hyperuricemia and gout from nicotinic acid and myalgias with or without elevated creatine kinase from statin therapy.

PAGET'S DISEASE

Paget's disease (Chapter 268) can cause bone pain and deformity. An elevated bone-specific alkaline phosphatase and characteristic radiographic changes can help make the diagnosis. Joint pain caused by secondary osteoarthritis in areas of involvement of bone from Paget's disease most commonly occurs in the hip, knee, or vertebrae. Spinal stenosis from Paget's disease of the spine has been reported.

HYPERTROPHIC OSTEOARTHROPATHY

Hypertrophic osteoarthropathy is a syndrome that includes clubbing of the fingers and toes, periostitis of long bones (distal tibia, femur, and radius), and arthritis. Hypertrophic osteoarthropathy is classified into primary (hereditary) and secondary forms. Between 80 and 90% of secondary hypertrophic osteoarthropathy is associated with non–small cell lung cancer. Other causes include other neoplasms (mesothelioma), chronic pulmonary infections, congenital heart disease, cirrhosis, HIV infection, and inflammatory bowel disease. Patients with secondary hypertrophic osteoarthropathy can present with acute, severe, burning bone pain and a noninflammatory arthritis caused by periarticular periostitis. Pain is accentuated by dependency of the limbs. Pitting edema, warmth, and tenderness of the legs and forearms can be seen. Radiographs show diagnostic changes of periosteal elevation or new bone formation, or both, along the distal ends of long bones. Therapy is symptomatic, and hypertrophic osteoarthropathy resolves with successful treatment of the underlying primary disease.

LEUKEMIA AND LYMPHOMA

Leukemia can arise as a symmetrical or migratory polyarthritis, monoarthritis (rare), back pain (10%), or nocturnal bone pain. Articular manifestations occur in 14 to 50% of children and 4 to 16% of adults with acute leukemia and can precede the diagnosis by months. Joint pain is attributed to leukemic synovial infiltration and usually involves the ankle or knee but can be polyarticular, resembling juvenile or adult RA. The joint pain is disproportionally more severe than the clinical findings. Synovial effusions are uncommon, and evidence of leukemic cells in the synovial fluid is rare. Bone pain occurs in up to 50% and is more common in the lower extremities. The peripheral white blood cell count may be normal initially, but lactate dehydrogenase is always elevated, frequently to very high levels. Radiographs are normal in 50%. The musculoskeletal symptoms are poorly responsive to NSAIDs but can resolve with successful therapy of the leukemia. Musculoskeletal symptoms occur in 25% of patients with non-Hodgkin's lymphoma. Nocturnal bone pain is the most common presenting musculoskeletal complaint. A seronegative monoarthritis or polyarthritis can occur and should be suspected in patients with severe constitutional symptoms or lymphadenopathy out of proportion to the degree of arthritis. Patients with T-cell lymphoma may occasionally develop a chronic, nonerosive polyarthritis with erythroderma.

CARCINOMATOUS POLYARTHRITIS

Polyarthritis can rarely be the presenting manifestation of an occult malignancy. It may precede the discovery of the malignancy by several months. Breast, colon, lung, ovarian, and lymphoproliferative malignancies are the most commonly associated cancers. Clinical features suggesting carcinomatous polyarthritis include explosive onset of a rheumatoid factor–negative, asymmetric polyarthritis predominantly involving the lower extremities and sparing the hands and wrists in a patient older than 60 years. Polymyalgia rheumatica and RA must be excluded. Treatment of the underlying malignancy results in improvement of the arthritis.

PALMAR FASCIITIS AND ARTHRITIS SYNDROME

Ovarian carcinoma is the most common malignancy found in patients with palmar fasciitis and arthritis. Patients present with a severe painful and symmetrical inflammatory polyarthritis and fasciitis causing contractures primarily of the hands and less commonly the feet. Patients may have vasomotor instability causing diagnostic confusion with reflex sympathetic dystrophy syndrome or RA. This syndrome portends a poor prognosis because it typically manifests after tumor metastasis. Response to treatment is poor, although clinical improvement can be seen with successful eradication of the underlying tumor.

MULTICENTRIC RETICULOHISTIOCYTOSIS

Multicentric reticulohistiocytosis (MRH) is a chronic, symmetrical, inflammatory polyarthritis, most commonly affecting the hands and cervical spine. It may resemble RA but can be differentiated by its prominent distal interphalangeal joint synovitis. Joint involvement remits and relapses initially but in 50% of cases worsens into a severely deforming arthritis mutilans. Firm, nonpruritic, reddish-brown or yellow papulonodular lesions ("coral beads") that wax and wane occur around the nail beds and on the face, hands, ears, and other areas predominantly above the waist. The skin lesions have a diagnostic histology. However, in 50 to 66% of patients, these diagnostic nodules follow the onset of arthritis by months to years. Additional associations include xanthelasma (33%) and malignancies of various types (25%), which may precede or follow the onset of MRH. MRH usually remits spontaneously in 8 to 10 years but often leaves permanent cutaneous and joint damage. Treatment may include cytotoxic therapy if the arthritis is aggressive. Anti–tumor necrosis factor α (TNF-α) therapy has been reported to be beneficial in resistant cases.

SARCOIDOSIS

Joint manifestations including arthritis, periarthritis, and arthralgias occur in 2 to 38% of patients with sarcoidosis (Chapter 95). Rheumatic involvement is divided into acute and chronic types. The first consists of the triad of arthritis, erythema nodosum, and hilar adenopathy on chest radiograph (Löfgren's syndrome), which may be accompanied by fever. Arthritis arises most often in the knees and ankles, and periarticular pain can be severe. Treatment is with NSAIDs or colchicine, or both, and symptoms usually remit spontaneously over several weeks. The less common type of joint involvement in sarcoidosis consists of synovitis that accompanies the slower onset, more chronic, and systemic form of sarcoidosis. The joint involvement may be polyarthritis, oligoarthritis, or monoarthritis of the small or large joints and is typically nondestructive but in some cases can be aggressive. Dactylitis resulting from sarcoid bone and soft tissue involvement can occur. In contrast to the acute type, chronic sarcoid arthropathy is characterized by inflammatory synovial fluid and histologic granulomas on synovial biopsy. Treatment consists of NSAIDs, low-dose corticosteroids, hydroxychloroquine, and methotrexate or azathioprine. In refractory cases, anti–TNF-α therapy has been successful. Other musculoskeletal manifestations include lytic or sclerotic bone lesions and a myopathy.

RELAPSING POLYCHONDRITIS

Relapsing polychondritis is an uncommon multisystem disorder characterized by recurrent episodes of inflammation of cartilaginous tissues. Patients with relapsing polychondritis typically present with sudden onset of pain and erythema involving the cartilage of the external ear, larynx or trachea, or nose. A nonerosive, seronegative polyarthritis or oligoarthritis affecting small, large, or costochondral joints (23 to 47%); ocular inflammation including episcleritis or scleritis; and audiovestibular disturbances may also be presenting symptoms. The arthritis is typically acute, migratory, and episodic but rarely can become chronic. Tenosynovitis is also common. Relapsing polychondritis is presumably due to a cell-mediated immune response against cartilage components; biopsies showing acute and chronic inflammation destroying cartilage support the diagnosis. Late sequelae of relapsing polychondritis include deformity of the pinnae or nose, reduced vision or hearing, tracheal narrowing or collapse, and aortic insufficiency resulting from aortic ring dilatation as well as other cardiovascular abnormalities. Patients with relapsing polychondritis frequently have associated coexisting diseases, such as systemic vasculitis, various connective tissue diseases (e.g., RA), myelodysplastic syndromes and other cancers, and thyroid disease. Treatment depends on the severity of the presentation and whether major organs are involved. Mild episodes of inflammation are treated with NSAIDs, colchicine, dapsone, and low-dose corticosteroids. Life-threatening or organ-threatening complications are treated with high-dose corticosteroids and immunosuppressive agents, such as methotrexate or cyclophosphamide.

CYSTIC FIBROSIS

In up to 10% of patients with cystic fibrosis, an episodic, nondestructive, inflammatory oligoarthritis develops, most commonly involving the fingers and lower extremity joints. This arthritis is thought to be due to immune complex deposition caused by chronic lung infections. Attacks last for a few days and may be associated with fever and painful nodular skin lesions and purpura. Other musculoskeletal manifestations include osteoporosis and osteomalacia related to malabsorption and, more rarely, hypertrophic osteoarthropathy and a small vessel vasculitis.

PIGMENTED VILLONODULAR SYNOVITIS

Pigmented villonodular synovitis occurs most commonly in the third and fourth decades of life. It is characterized by the onset of unilateral pain and swelling of a joint, typically the knee. Unusually, a tendon, bursae, or another joint can be involved. The synovial fluid is characteristically brown or hemorrhagic, and radiographs may show soft tissue swelling, osteolysis, subchondral cysts, and bone erosions. Pigmented villonodular synovitis is a nonmalignant condition that is diagnosed by synovial biopsy. Microscopic examination reveals a characteristic histology including marked synovial cell hyperplasia and subsynovial invasion by masses of polygonal cells, multinucleated giant cells, and lipid-filled macrophages. Hemosiderin deposits are between and within cells and have a characteristic appearance on magnetic resonance imaging scans that can define the extent of this synovial tumor. The treatment for pigmented villonodular synovitis is synovectomy.

Future Directions

With the advances being made in immunology and genetics, there will be an increased understanding of the pathogenesis of many of these diseases. Treatments such as immunomodulating biologic agents or cartilage-preserving therapy with metalloproteinase inhibitors will be developed on the basis of new discoveries elucidating the etiology of these unusual disorders.

SUGGESTED READINGS

Fenollar F, Puechal X, Raoult D: Medical progress: Whipple's disease. N Engl J Med 2007;356:55–66. *Discusses the pathophysiology, clinical manifestations, and diagnostic considerations of this disease and treatment options for it.*

Gergely P Jr, Poor G: Relapsing polychondritis. Best Pract Res Clin Rheumatol 2004;18:723–738. *Review of clinical manifestations, diagnosis, and therapy.*

Jordan JM: Arthritis in hemochromatosis or iron storage disease. Curr Opin Rheumatol 2004;16:62–66. *A concise review.*

Orchard T, Wordsworth P: Enteropathic arthritis. Rheum Dis Clin North Am 2003;29:513–530. *A comprehensive review.*

Smith LL, Burnet SP, McNeil JD: Musculoskeletal manifestations of diabetes mellitus. Br J Sports Med 2003;37:30–35. *Good glucose control appears to improve or prevent rheumatic conditions.*

Torralba KD, Quismorio FP Jr: Sarcoid arthritis: A review of clinical features, pathology, and therapy. Sarcoidosis Vasc Diffuse Lung Dis 2003;20:95–103. *An updated review on the spectrum and treatment of joint and bone involvement in sarcoidosis.*

298 MULTIFOCAL FIBROSCLEROSIS

Wilmer L. Sibbitt, Jr.

Definition

Idiopathic multifocal fibrosclerosis (IMF) is an inflammatory disease characterized by the development of inflammatory pseudotumors; it results in some combination of retroperitoneal fibrosis, mediastinal fibrosis, orbital pseudotumor, Dupuytren's contracture, lymphoid hyperplasia, Peyronie's disease, vasculitis, thyroiditis, primary biliary cirrhosis, testicular fibrosis, and pachymeningitis. Retroperitoneal fibrosis (Ormond's disease) is a subset of IMF and is characterized by fibrosis of the retroperitoneum that entraps and distorts retroperitoneal structures, including the great vessels, ureters, nerves, kidneys, and biliary tree.

Epidemiology

IMF is a rare condition with a prevalence estimated at less than 20 per 100,000 and an incidence of less than 3 per 100,000 per year. However, in relevant populations with predisposing conditions, these figures are considerably higher. For example, methysergide is associated with an incidence of IMF at the rate of 1 case in 5000 users per year. The mean age at diagnosis is 56 years, and the male-to-female ratio is 3:1. The cumulative actuarial survival rate is 86% at 1 year and 78% at 2 years.

Pathobiology

The histopathology of IMF is characterized by multifocal fibrosis, granulation tissue, B cells, helper T cells, large numbers of spindle-shaped cells expressing macrophage markers, and activated fibroblasts. T-cell receptor gene rearrangements have been reported as having a 40% association with HLA-B27, but these associations have not been proved. Degenerative and inflammatory diseases of the aorta (atherosclerosis, aortitis, inherited diseases of collagen, trauma, infection, aortic aneurysm) shed inflammatory lipids and oxidized lipoproteins through the aortic adventitia into the retroperitoneum, thereby resulting in an intense inflammatory process in which cytokines, including platelet-derived growth factor and connective tissue growth factor, have been implicated. Thus, the presence of IMF should trigger an evaluation for aortic disease. Confounding syndromes, including lymphoma, crystal-storing histiocytosis, immunocytoma, neuroblastoma, diffuse retroperitoneal carcinoma (pancreatic, scirrhous gastric, prostate, ovarian, renal, uterine cervix, carcinoid), Wegener's granulomatosis, xanthogranulomatous pyelonephritis, chronic pyelonephritis, tuberculosis, guinea worm infestation, sarcoidosis, and aortic graft infection, should be excluded by appropriate imaging, biopsy, aspiration, or serologic tests, or any combination. Secondary retroperitoneal fibrosis can be caused by drugs and toxins (methysergide, methyldopa, levodopa, ergot, bromocriptine, pergolide, asbestos, fluoropyrimidine), aortic aneurysm, malignant tumors (metastatic carcinomas, carcinoid, lymphoma), retroperitoneal injury (hemorrhage, infection, radiation, surgery, stenting, angioplasty), autoimmune disease, Erdheim-Chester disease, tuberculosis, sarcoidosis, biliary tract disease, gonorrhea, and ascending lymphangitis.

Clinical Manifestations

IMF is commonly manifested as (1) isolated retroperitoneal fibrosis; (2) retroperitoneal, mesenteric, pulmonary, and periarticular fibrosis accompanied by subcutaneous panniculitis; (3) a triad of sclerosing cholangitis, retroperitoneal fibrosis, and Riedel's thyroiditis; and (4) other less common combinations. The retroperitoneal form of IMF is typically manifested as (1) ill-defined pain in the lower part of the abdomen, lumbosacral region, or flank; (2) visceral obstruction resulting in vomiting, diarrhea, or dehydration; (3) hydronephrosis and renal insufficiency; (4) severe peripheral edema and venous varicosities; or (5) claudication, pain, dysesthesias, weakness, or spasticity resulting from nerve entrapment and epidural cord compression. Pulmonary emboli, deep venous thrombosis, and obstruction of the bowel, bladder, or bronchi can occur. Mediastinal fibrosis may result in a lymphoma-like mass and superior vena cava syndrome with edema and venous dilation of the arms, neck, and head. Extrahepatic portal vein obstruction, portal hypertension, esophageal varices, and uveitis may occur. A definitive diagnosis should be undertaken rapidly and therapy seriously considered.

Diagnosis

Computed tomography (CT), magnetic resonance imaging (MRI), and urography with appropriate contrast demonstrate a retroperitoneal inflammatory reaction; obstruction of the ureters, great vessels, biliary tree, or pancreatic ducts; or the presence of diffuse or discrete unifocal or multifocal retroperitoneal masses. Fibrosis may extend into the root of the mesentery, the bladder, and peribronchial areas and result in traction, distortion, and obstruction of the gut, urethra, and bronchi. Indium 111–labeled leukocyte and gallium radionuclide scans and ^{18}F-fluorodeoxyglucose positron emission tomography are useful to exclude abscesses, demonstrate inflammatory processes, and monitor disease activity. The presence of autoimmune diseases, drug use, and toxin exposure should be excluded by appropriate history and serologic testing. After suspicious masses are identified, biopsy is usually essential to confirm the diagnosis and to exclude confounding conditions, especially neoplasia and infection. Biopsy may be guided by CT, ultrasound, mediastinoscopy, laparoscopy, or retroperitoneal exploration and can often be accomplished by percutaneous needle biopsy.

Treatment Rx

All recommendations for prevention and treatment of IMF are based on relatively small series and case reports. The most important therapy or prevention of IMF is removal of the cause, most commonly an offending drug. Otherwise, treatment of IMF is largely empirical but may be necessary because the disease is often progressive and fatal. Nonsurgical therapies include high-dose oral corticosteroids, pulse methylprednisolone, penicillamine, azathioprine, cyclophosphamide, and cyclosporine, all of which have had some success. Tamoxifen has been used as primary therapy on a limited basis with some success and very little toxicity. Lifelong anticoagulation is required for patients with large vein involvement and associated deep venous thrombosis. Surgical interventions include lysis of fibrotic masses and stenting of ureteral, biliary, venous, and arterial obstructions. Surgical repair or stenting of an abdominal aortic aneurysm may be either an exacerbating or ameliorating factor for IMF; thus, therapy for aneurysm must be individualized.

Future Directions

The inflammatory and cytokine networks that are triggered by drugs, crystals, or anatomic changes associated with IMF are poorly understood and parallel those of other fibrotic diseases. Animal models of IMF need to be developed and validated. National registries and interinstitutional cooperative studies are also necessary to support basic and clinical research in this rare disease. New treatments to prevent cellular inflammation and biologic-derived therapies directed at individual cytokines may be applicable in therapy for IMF. Antilipid agents, especially the statins, may have some effect in halting the local dissemination of cholesterol crystals from atherosclerotic aortas, thus preventing IMF. New interventional modalities, including transcutaneous biopsy, retroperitoneoscopy, intravascular and intraureteral stenting, and angioplasty and arterioplasty performed together, may also be helpful in treating IMF.

SUGGESTED READINGS

Vaglio A, Buzio C: Chronic periaortitis: A spectrum of diseases. Curr Opin Rheumatol 2005;17:34–40. *An excellent review of this disorder.*

Vaglio A, Salvarani C, Buzio C: Retroperitoneal fibrosis. Lancet 2006;367:241–251. *A comprehensive review.*

van Bommel EF, Hendriksz TR, Huiskes AW, et al: Tamoxifen therapy for non-malignant retroperitoneal fibrosis. Ann Intern Med 2006;144:101–106. *Small observational study suggesting tamoxifen may be a therapeutic option.*

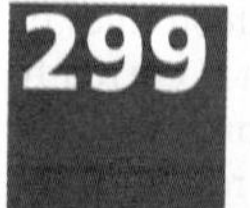

299 SURGICAL TREATMENT OF JOINT DISEASES

Victor M. Goldberg and Matthew J. Kraay

Epidemiology

Based on data from the Centers for Disease Control and Prevention in 2005, nearly one in three adults in the United States is affected with arthritis, and arthritis and other rheumatic conditions are the leading cause of disability in Americans. Health care expenses for the treatment of arthritis and other related chronic joint disorders in the United States are estimated to be more than $116 billion annually. As our population ages, the impact of these problems on our society will continue to increase steadily. In 2003, approximately 418,000 total knee replacements and more than 220,000 hip replacements were performed in the United States. This number appears to be increasing at a rate of 11% for knee replacement and 2.5% for hip replacement per year.

Pathobiology

Osteoarthrosis, whether primary or secondary, is the most common arthritic disorder of the joints. Asymmetrical articular cartilage loss with subchondral sclerosis, osteophyte formation, angular deformity, progressive loss of motion, and the usual absence of synovitis is the typical clinical manifestation. The pathogenesis and medical treatment of osteoarthrosis are addressed elsewhere in this text (Chapter 283).

Inflammatory arthropathies, with rheumatoid arthritis as the prototype, are immunologic disorders that initially involve the synovial tissues lining the joint capsule (Chapter 285). Cytokines and a variety of potent inflammatory mediators liberated by the uncontrolled synovitis of rheumatoid arthritis result in often rapid, progressive destruction of articular cartilage. Early in the course of the disease, medical therapies are directed toward control of this synovitis to prevent the occurrence of articular damage. Surgical synovectomy can be helpful in controlling inflammatory synovitis in the rare patient in whom aggressive medical management fails. Because of the systemic nature of these diseases, polyarticular involvement is frequent in most inflammatory forms of arthritis, and extra-articular manifestations can occur. The end result of uncontrolled synovitis is end-stage arthritis, which can be difficult to distinguish from osteoarthrosis.

Arthritis can also develop secondary to a diverse variety of other causes, including trauma (intra-articular fractures, blunt osteochondral injury, ligament and meniscal injury), metabolic disorders (gout, chondrocalcinosis, Paget's disease, acromegaly), bleeding disorders (hemophilia), and circulatory disorders of bone (avascular necrosis). The various surgical options for treatment of these joint disorders are reviewed in this chapter. Surgical indications and options vary according to the condition (Table 299–1).

SURGICAL THERAPY

Arthrodesis

With the refinement in total joint replacement over the last 30 years, the indications for joint fusion or arthrodesis are limited. Arthrodesis involves surgical removal of articular cartilage from both sides of the joint and immobilization (either externally or internally) until the adjacent

TABLE 299–1 OPERATIVE TREATMENT OPTIONS FOR ARTHRITIS

Type of Arthritis	Affected Joint	Favored Surgical Options
Osteoarthritis	Knee, hip, shoulder	Arthroscopic débridement Osteotomy (hip, knee) Arthrodesis Arthroplasty
	Interphalangeal, wrist	Synovectomy Arthrodesis
	Ankle	Arthroscopy Arthrodesis Arthroplasty (infrequently)
	Elbow	Arthroscopy for loose bodies Arthroplasty
Rheumatoid and other inflammatory arthritides	Knee, hip, shoulder	Arthroscopic synovectomy Arthroplasty
	Wrist	Arthroscopic synovectomy Arthrodesis Arthroplasty (infrequently)
	Ankle	Arthrodesis Arthroplasty (more often)
	Elbow	Arthroscopic synovectomy

bones fuse together. Arthrodesis of the large joints of the body (hip, knee, and shoulder) is rarely indicated except in extremely young, active patients, in whom total joint replacement will not be expected to last for a major portion of their lives and who would, as a result, probably require multiple revisions during their lifetime.

In addition to concern regarding the durability of joint replacement implants, total joint replacement requires adequate motor (both muscular and neurologic) function and good soft tissue coverage to allow primary wound healing and prevent infection of the implant. However, this is not a prerequisite for arthrodesis, and in patients who do not meet these criteria for total joint replacement, arthrodesis is a preferred treatment option. These younger patients have often suffered major previous joint trauma with resultant traumatic arthrosis, soft tissue deficiencies, or neurologic deficits that would compromise the outcome of a joint replacement procedure. Although the functional outcome of arthrodesis of the hip, knee, or shoulder is inferior to that of total joint replacement, it is a durable solution that provides reliable pain relief for these complex joint problems in young, high-demand patients. With the development of more durable joint replacement implants and with the more widespread use of total joint replacement in an increasingly younger patient population, fewer patients and surgeons are willing to accept the limitations and disability associated with arthrodesis of the hip, knee, and shoulder. Arthrodesis of the hip, if properly performed, can be converted to a total hip arthroplasty 20 to 25 years later with a good result anticipated. Because of the significant disability associated with arthrodesis of the knee, it is rarely used except as a salvage procedure in patients with multiple failed total knee replacements, especially when associated with infection.

Arthrodesis is a reliable, durable, and frequently used treatment option for patients with arthritis involving the small joints of the body, for which successful joint replacement implants are not available. The small joints of the carpus, tarsus (including the subtalar joint), and the interphalangeal joints of the hands and feet affected by arthritis of any etiology can be reliably treated by joint arthrodesis. Although the results of total joint replacement of the wrist (radiocarpal joint) and ankle are improved with the use of newer implant designs, arthrodesis of these joints still remains the primary choice because of a long history of clinical success and the shortcomings of earlier total wrist and total ankle implant designs.

Osteotomy

Osteotomy is a rarely used, but important joint-preserving surgical option for patients with early arthrosis and other joint conditions associated with limb malalignment or joint malformation from variety of causes. In a patient with valgus or varus deformity of the knee, developmental dysplasia of the hip, or malunion of a fracture involving a weight-bearing long bone (i.e., femur or tibia), the associated alterations in joint biomechanics result in articular cartilage overloading and will frequently lead to secondary osteoarthrosis if unrecognized and untreated. The underlying goal of any osteotomy, therefore, is normalization of the altered joint biomechanics and loading by realignment of the limb or correction of the articular deformity. Osteotomies are thus not indicated for patients with inflammatory joint disorders such as rheumatoid arthritis and its variants. In these patients, inflammatory synovitis and not altered joint biomechanics is responsible for the progressive joint deterioration.

The joint most commonly treated by osteotomy is the knee. Normally, the mechanical axis of the lower extremity (defined as a straight line drawn from the center of the femoral head to the center of the ankle) passes through the approximate center of the knee joint. Ideally, this arrangement results in approximately equal loading between the medial and lateral tibiofemoral compartments of the knee joint. In patients with subtle valgus ("knock-knee") or varus ("bow-legged") deformities, early osteoarthrosis, or previous joint injury or those with a variety of other conditions resulting in joint or limb deformity, the mechanical axis of the limb deviates away from the center of the knee joint with resultant relative overloading of one compartment of the knee. As the deformity progresses with time, a vicious cycle of unloading of one compartment and overloading of the opposite compartment ensues with progressive mechanical overloading of the articular cartilage and the development of secondary osteoarthrosis.

If recognized early before severe tibiofemoral articular cartilage narrowing and deformity occur, realignment osteotomy of the knee can result in significant pain relief, a slower progression of joint degeneration, and a delay in the eventual need for a total knee replacement. Because osteotomy does not result in regeneration or replacement of worn articular cartilage, pain relief may be incomplete or relatively short-lived in comparison to total knee replacement. However, osteotomy does avoid the risks and limitations associated with total knee replacement and is therefore best suited for a younger, more active patient with noninflammatory unicompartmental arthrosis who is a less than ideal candidate for total knee replacement.

In the more common patient with varus deformity, the osteotomy is typically performed at the level of the proximal end of the tibia, whereas in a patient with a valgus deformity, it is typically performed at the level of the distal end of the femur. Rigid fixation with plates and screws allows early range of motion after osteotomy performed at either location. In patients with malunion of previous extra-articular fractures, corrective osteotomies can potentially eliminate the need for joint replacement if performed early before significant joint degeneration is initiated.

Osteotomies for disorders of the hip joint are an area of intense current interest in orthopedics. Although the relationship of developmental dysplasia of the hip to secondary osteoarthrosis is well established, more subtle degrees of acetabular dysplasia and combined femoroacetabular deformity, which are not readily apparent on routine plain radiographs, have recently been recognized to be associated with secondary arthrosis of the hip. These dysplasias of the acetabulum result in incomplete "coverage" of the femoral head by the acetabulum, with the end result being reduced contact area between the femoral head and the acetabulum, increased joint load per unit area, and mechanical overloading of the articular cartilage of the hip. Although a wide variety of osteotomies of both the pelvis and femur have been proposed in the past, it is currently generally agreed that most of the deformity responsible for secondary arthrosis of the hip occurs in the acetabulum. As a result, most osteotomies of the hip performed today involve correction of the abnormal periacetabular anatomy responsible for this type of secondary arthrosis of the hip. Although these complicated joint-preserving surgical procedures are typically performed only in large referral centers, early recognition and treatment can eliminate the need for hip replacement in younger patients with these potentially correctable deformities.

Arthroscopy and Joint Débridement

Arthroscopic surgery is the most commonly performed surgical procedure in the United States. Most of these procedures are performed for joint problems related to trauma to the menisci of the knee or labral structures in the hip or shoulder, as well as for problems related to the articular cartilage or ligamentous support structures of the involved joint (Fig. 299–1). If neglected, injuries to these structures may predispose to post-traumatic or secondary osteoarthrosis.

The potential benefits of arthroscopy for the treatment of established arthritis are limited. Although some symptomatic short-term relief may be gained from joint lavage performed at the time of arthroscopy, arthroscopic (or open) joint "débridement" alone does nothing to address the primary problem of articular cartilage degeneration associated with osteoarthrosis. The principal reason for this is the avascular nature of hyaline cartilage and the resultant limited ability of articular cartilage to heal after injury. Techniques that include drilling or "microfracture" through full-thickness articular defects into subchondral bone to allow vascular ingrowth into the defect may promote limited healing with hyaline-like fibrocartilage. This hyaline-like repair cartilage, however, is not as durable as normal healthy hyaline articular cartilage.

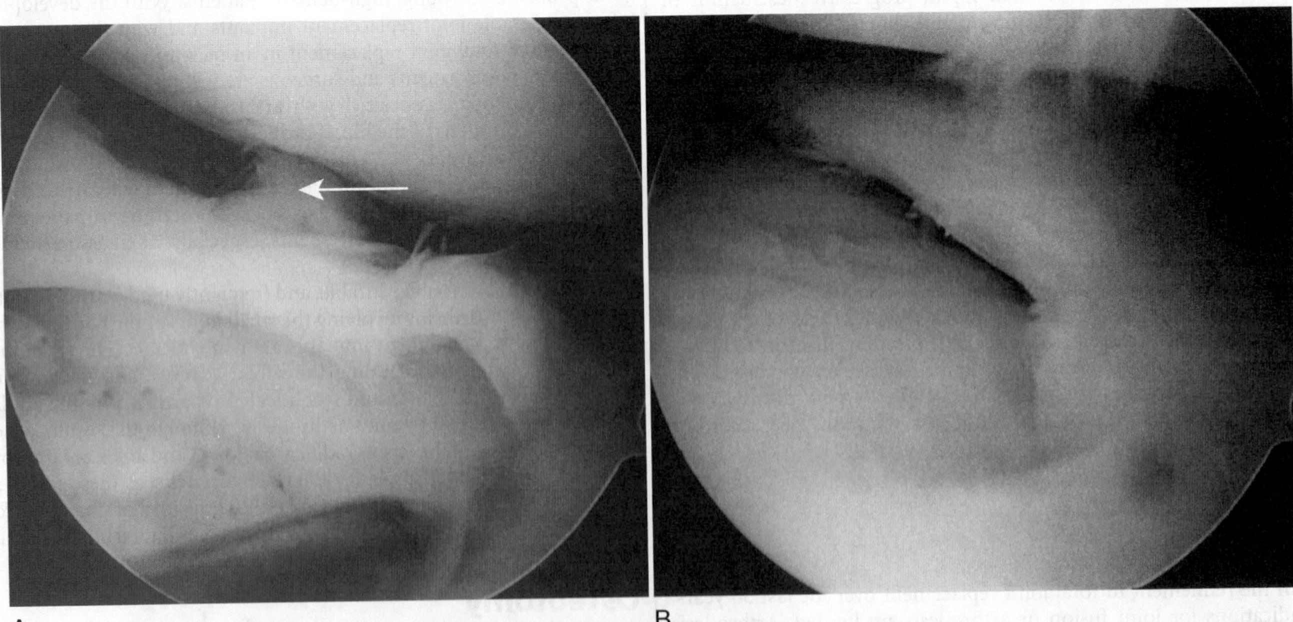

FIGURE 299–1 • Arthroscopic surgery. A degenerative medial meniscal tear is viewed before **(A)** and after **(B)** arthroscopic resection. The arrow in **A** indicates the site of the tear.

So-called mechanical symptoms such as "catching," "locking," and "giving way" or "buckling" associated with meniscal or labral tears, osteocartilaginous loose bodies, and unstable flaps of damaged articular cartilage can frequently be relieved by arthroscopic débridement, which may be beneficial despite the presence of arthritis in the joint. Symptoms of an arthritic nature are not typically relieved by arthroscopic surgery and are best treated by one of the other techniques described in this chapter.

Recently, the role of femoral neck impingement on the anterior acetabular rim has been recognized to be a potential cause of secondary osteoarthrosis of the hip. This condition is frequently associated with tearing of the acetabular labrum and a complex, combined deformity of the acetabulum and femoral neck. Preliminary results of treatment by arthroscopic débridement of the labral tear and recontouring or "osteoplasty" of the femoral neck are encouraging.

In patients with inflammatory arthritis, such as rheumatoid arthritis, or other conditions associated with prominent synovitis (e.g., hemophilia), arthroscopic synovectomy may be helpful in reducing pain and joint effusions and slowing the progression of inflammatory arthropathy in the involved joint. Patients with limited joint space loss and with refractory synovitis of 6 months' duration that persists despite maximal medical therapy are potential candidates for synovectomy. Depending on the specific joint involved, synovectomy can be performed either arthroscopically or by open arthrotomy.

Total Joint Arthroplasty

Total hip replacement and total knee replacement are two of the most reliable and predictable interventions in all of medicine. Despite their safety and efficacy, total joint arthroplasty should be considered the last rather than the first treatment option for patients with end-stage arthritis of the hip and knee. Other causes of the patient's pain should be considered because pain referred from the back can easily be confused for pain associated with arthritis of the hip or knee and pain from an arthritic hip can occasionally be referred to the knee. Obviously, successful medical and especially surgical treatment requires accurate diagnosis and localization of the patient's pain. Though less commonly performed, total joint replacement of other joints such as the shoulder also work well but should be considered treatments of last resort.

Consideration of total joint replacement should be undertaken seriously only after a reasonable attempt at nonoperative management has been completed and determined to be unsuccessful. Because these health problems are not life-threatening and are considered elective surgical procedures, patients should be in reasonable health and medically fit for these procedures. Thorough medical evaluation with attention to assessment and minimization of perioperative medical and anesthetic risk is recommended. Major perioperative concerns include cardiac, respiratory, and vascular status, along with infection and prophylaxis for thromboembolism. The condition of the patient's teeth and skin and urinary tract problems can contribute to a perioperative infection that could result in a disastrous periprosthetic infection after surgery, and thus these issues should be addressed preoperatively.

As the population ages, the definition of the "appropriate patient" for total joint replacement surgery continues to evolve. In general, there is no set upper age limit for potential candidates for joint replacement, and the decision is perhaps best based on the patient's degree of disability, general medical condition, and "physiologic age." Despite improvement in implant design, materials, and surgical techniques, total joint arthroplasty should still be expected to have a finite lifespan, and as a result, biologic and joint-preserving procedures are preferred for younger, more active patients.

Minimally Invasive Total Joint Replacement

In the past several years, considerable interest has been directed toward the possibility of performing joint replacement through "minimally invasive" surgical approaches. The goal of these minimally invasive approaches is a reduction in postoperative pain, enhanced perioperative rehabilitation, and earlier return to normal activities after surgery. In particular circumstances, standard surgical approaches have simply been shortened or modified, or innovative new approaches have been developed. With certain of these approaches, limited visualization within the surgical field has resulted in a higher rate of perioperative complications. Computer-assisted surgical navigation shows promise in allowing total joint replacement to be performed more accurately, especially when done through a minimally invasive surgical approach. As of this time, the safety and efficacy of these minimally invasive approaches have not yet been established, and our understanding of the potential risks and benefits of minimally invasive total joint replacement and computer-assisted surgical navigation is incomplete.

Total Hip Replacement

Total hip arthroplasty is a commonly performed procedure for the treatment of end-stage arthritis of the hip caused by a variety of disorders, including osteoarthrosis, rheumatoid arthritis, avascular necrosis, ankylosing spondylitis and other forms of spondyloarthropathy, and post-traumatic arthrosis. Resurfacing of the worn, arthritic "ball and socket" hip joint with a "ball and socket" prosthetic hip joint results in dramatic pain relief and improvement in ambulation, function, and quality of life in the overwhelming majority of patients (Fig. 299–2).

Conventional total hip arthroplasty involves removal of the arthritic cartilage from the socket or acetabulum, as well as removal of the arthritic femoral head and a portion of the femoral neck. An acetabular component made of metal with a plastic, ceramic, or metal bearing surface liner inserted without cement or a plastic component inserted into the prepared acetabulum with acrylic bone cement is used to resurface the acetabulum. Soft cancellous bone in the proximal end of the femur is removed, and a stem designed to fit within the intramedullary canal of the femur, with a ball on the end to articulate with the acetabular com-

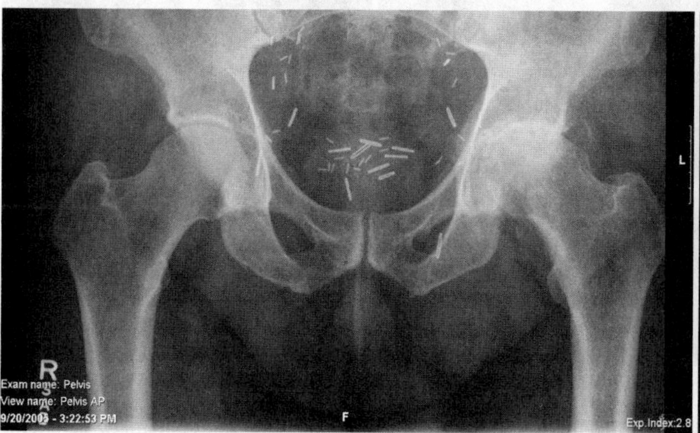

A

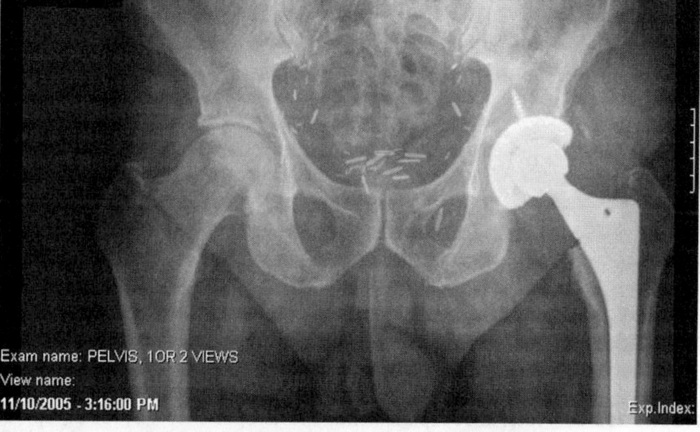

B

FIGURE 299–2 • Total hip arthroplasty. A, Anteroposterior (AP) pelvic radiograph in a patient with significant osteoarthrosis of the left hip. The left hip joint space is completely obliterated, whereas the right hip joint space is well maintained with minimal narrowing. **B,** AP view of the pelvis after cementless left total hip arthroplasty.

ponent, is secured inside the canal by tight press-fit or by grouting it in place with acrylic bone cement.

Implant designs, materials, and surgical techniques for total hip replacement have undergone extensive change since their introduction in the United States in 1969. With standard perioperative prophylaxis, the expected incidence of periprosthetic infection should be less than 1%. The development of modern implant alloys and materials has essentially eliminated the risk for implant breakage. Using contemporary designs, materials, and surgical techniques, implant survival rates of 98 to 99% at 10 years and 90 to 95% at 15 to 20 years can be expected with either cemented or uncemented methods of implant fixation.

Refinement of total hip replacement over the past 30 years has been and continues to be an ongoing process. The major focus over the past decade and a half has been directed toward reduction of bearing surface wear and the biologic reaction to this periprosthetic wear debris or "osteolysis." This osteolytic reaction to particulate wear debris is a major cause of implant loosening. To address the long-term issues of wear and osteolysis, "alternative bearing surfaces" such as cross-linked polyethylene, ceramic-on-ceramic, and metal-on-metal bearing surfaces have been introduced within the last several years. Although the early results of these new materials are promising, long-term follow-up is necessary to determine whether these new bearing surfaces provide a significant reduction in wear over conventional polyethylene, which has been used almost exclusively in the past.

Total Knee Replacement and Unicompartmental Knee Replacement

Like total hip arthroplasty, total knee arthroplasty is a commonly performed procedure for the treatment of end-stage arthritis of the knee as a result of a variety of degenerative joint disorders (Fig. 299–3). The total knee arthroplasty designs currently in use typically require removal of a thin layer of subchondral bone and the overlying arthritic cartilage, followed by anatomic resurfacing all three compartments of the knee with a metal implant and polyethylene bearing surface. Collateral ligaments are retained for stability, although either one or both of the cruciate ligaments are excised and their functions substituted for by the implant. Implants are typically fixed to the underlying bone with acrylic bone cement, but cementless fixation of porous-coated implants is occasionally used in young, active, heavy patients, who are at high risk for failure of cemented fixation.

Like total hip arthroplasty, pain relief is typically excellent after a well-performed total knee replacement. Patient motivation and active participation in postoperative rehabilitation are even more critical after total knee replacement to maximize recovery of range of motion and strength after surgery. Although the perioperative medical and anesthetic risks are somewhat increased and the rehabilitation is somewhat more difficult, simultaneous bilateral total knee replacement is convenient for many patients and can still be performed safely in healthy, motivated patients who are willing to accept the associated risks.

Implant designs, materials, and surgical techniques for total knee replacement have undergone extensive refinement since their introduction in the United States in the early 1970s. Current implant designs and sophisticated surgical instrumentation provide close restoration of normal knee range of motion, function, and kinematics. Restoration of normal anatomy and mechanical alignment of the limb after surgery has been identified to be an important determinant of implant survival and outcome after total knee replacement. With the use of contemporary designs, materials, and surgical techniques, implant survival rates of 98 to 99% at 10 years and 90 to 95% at 15 to 20 years can be expected after total knee replacement, just as with total hip arthroplasty. With standard perioperative prophylaxis, the expected incidence of periprosthetic infection should be less than 1 to 2%. Similar to total hip replacement, the development of modern implant alloys and materials has essentially eliminated the possibility of implant breakage after total knee replacement.

Considerable interest has recently been directed toward unicompartmental arthroplasty of the knee (Fig. 299–4). Improved results of newer unicompartmental knee replacement designs and the ability to perform these procedures through a "minimally invasive" surgical approach make this option appealing for the occasional patient with isolated unicompartmental tibiofemoral arthritis. Ideal patients for unicompartmental knee replacement should have noninflammatory arthrosis, mild valgus or varus angular deformities, reasonable range of motion, stable collateral and cruciate ligaments, and most important, absence of significant arthrosis in the patellofemoral and opposite tibiofemoral compartments. Patients with significant arthrosis in the patellofemoral compartment or opposite tibiofemoral compartment are at risk of having incomplete and disappointing pain relief immediately after surgery or experiencing progression of arthrosis in the unresurfaced compartments of the knee within a few years of unicompartmental knee replacement surgery. Most of these latter patients are best served by total knee replacement because

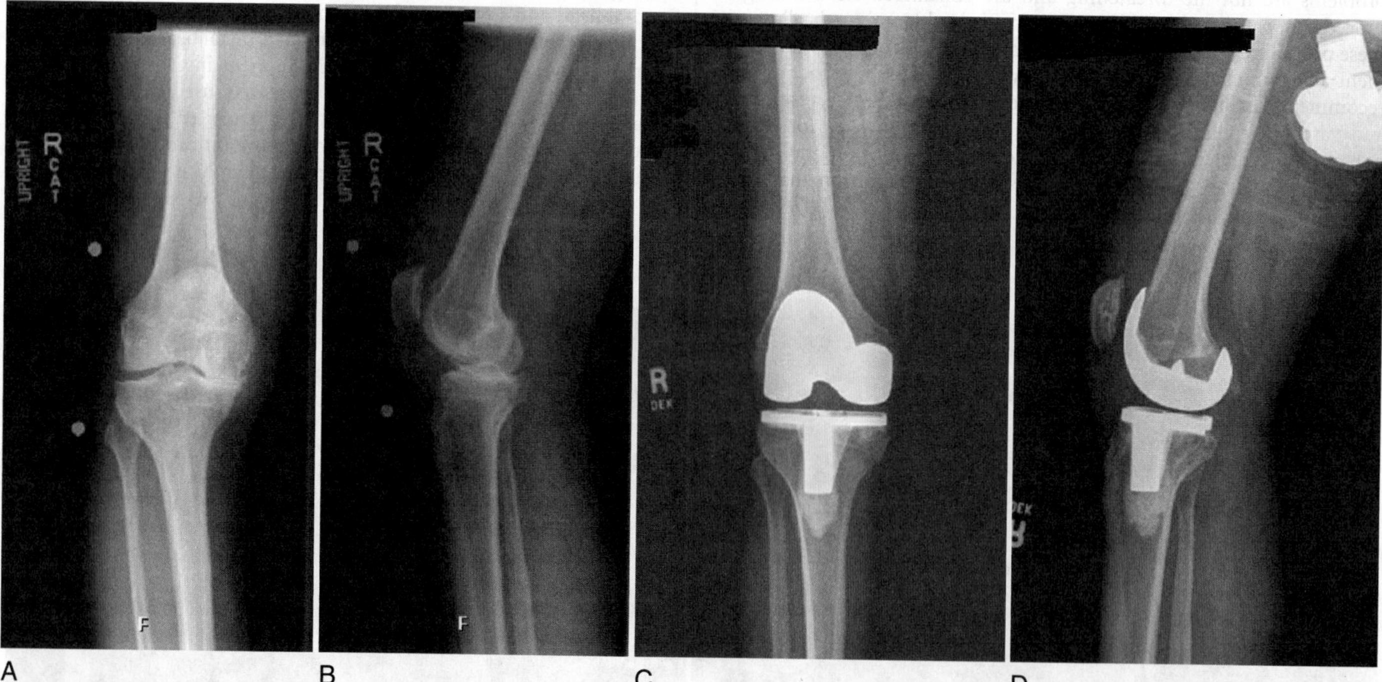

FIGURE 299–3 • Total knee replacement. A, Anteroposterior (AP) radiograph of a patient with osteoarthrosis of the right knee and varus deformity. Significant medial tibiofemoral compartment joint space narrowing with a normal lateral compartment is apparent on this view. **B,** Lateral knee radiograph of the same patient. Significant involvement of the patellofemoral compartment with osteophytes on the articular surface of the patella and in the trochlear groove of the distal end of the femur is apparent in this view. **C,** AP radiograph of the same patient after right total knee replacement. All three compartments (medial, lateral, and patellofemoral) of the knee are resurfaced with a total knee replacement. **D,** Lateral radiograph of the same patient after total knee replacement. Note the resurfacing of the arthritic trochlear groove and articular surface of the patella.

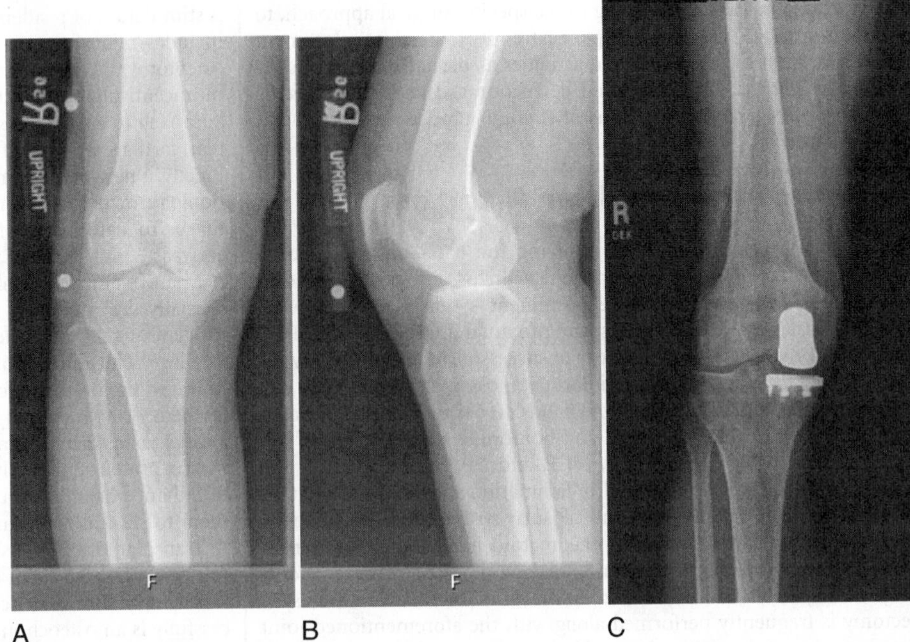

FIGURE 299–4 • Unicompartmental knee arthroplasty. A, Anteroposterior (AP) radiograph of a patient with medial compartment osteoarthrosis. Note the normal lateral compartment and mild varus deformity. **B,** Lateral radiograph of same patient with minimal arthritic changes in the patellofemoral compartment. The patient's symptoms and arthritis are exclusively localized to the medial compartment only, thus making him a good candidate for medial unicompartmental knee arthroplasty. **C,** AP radiograph of the same patient after medial unicompartmental knee replacement. Unlike total knee replacement, the opposite lateral tibiofemoral and patellofemoral compartments are not resurfaced.

it provides more reliable and durable pain relief than unicompartmental knee replacement does. Unicompartmental knee arthroplasty preserves the anterior and posterior cruciate ligaments, which is probably responsible for the improved range of motion, more physiologic function, and outcome more like that of a normal knee in comparison to a total knee replacement. Patients with unicompartmental knee replacement performed via a minimally invasive surgical approach do appear to have more rapid recovery, easier rehabilitation, and slightly more normal function than patients undergoing conventional total knee replacement do. For many patients, unicompartmental knee replacement may be considered the first step toward a total knee replacement and is perhaps best suited for a 40- to 60-year-old patient deemed too young for a total knee replacement and too old for a knee osteotomy.

Total Shoulder Replacement

In comparison to total hip and total knee replacement, total shoulder replacement is an uncommonly performed procedure. As a result of the non–weight-bearing nature of the shoulder joint, arthritis in the shoulder is perhaps more easily tolerated than arthritis of the hip or knee. However, in view of the importance of the shoulder in positioning the hand in space and in attending to activities of daily living, arthritis of the shoulder, especially when associated with significant limitation of range of motion, can be quite disabling. Shoulder replacement surgery is a safe and reliable treatment of end-stage arthritis of the shoulder. Either total shoulder arthroplasty or partial shoulder "hemiarthroplasty" can be performed.

Similar to the "ball and socket" hip joint, total shoulder replacement involves resurfacing of the arthritic glenoid surface with a polyethylene prosthetic glenoid and resurfacing of the humeral head with a metal ball attached to an intramedullary stem inserted into the humerus. More complete and lasting pain relief is likely with a total shoulder replacement than with hemiarthroplasty; however, loosening of the glenoid component is a concern, especially in more active patients. In this latter situation, hemiarthroplasty may be more durable and preferred over total shoulder replacement. Postoperative physical therapy is important to optimize recovery of range of motion after surgery. Postoperative pain relief is generally excellent with shoulder arthroplasty.

The ultimate functional outcome after shoulder replacement surgery depends on a variety of factors, including preoperative range of motion, status of the patient's rotator cuff, the patient's motivation, and quality of the postoperative physical therapy. In patients with unreconstructible rotator cuff tears associated with rotator cuff arthropathy, postoperative range of motion, functional outcome, and pain relief are typically disappointing with conventional total shoulder replacement or hemiarthroplasty. Improved function and range of motion have been reported with a new "reverse ball and socket" shoulder prosthesis, although long-term outcome data are not yet available for this device.

Total Elbow Replacement

Though rarely performed, total elbow arthroplasty can be a gratifying procedure for patients with end-stage inflammatory arthritis and a limited number of other conditions affecting the elbow. Inflammatory arthritis of the elbow can result in serious functional impairment and limitation of activities of daily living, especially if associated with significant arthritis of the ipsilateral wrist, hand, and shoulder. When compared with other joint replacements, total elbow replacement has a relatively high rate of infection and loosening. Careful patient selection and meticulous surgical technique are essential to minimize the risk for these complications. Total elbow replacement should be restricted to use in low-demand patients with inflammatory arthritis or elderly patients with unreconstructible supracondylar fractures or nonunion of the elbow. Active patients with osteoarthrosis or post-traumatic arthrosis of the elbow have an unacceptable incidence of loosening, and total elbow replacement is thus contraindicated in these patients.

Total Ankle Replacement

Until recently, total ankle replacement was a procedure of historical interest only. Because of a high rate of loosening and mechanical failure of earlier ankle prostheses, ankle arthrodesis has become the preferred treatment for end-stage arthritis of the ankle, regardless of etiology. Early results of total ankle arthroplasty with recent implant designs appear to be significantly improved over those obtained with implants of the past. As of this time, total ankle replacement should be limited to low-demand patients with inflammatory arthritis. Further clinical evaluation is necessary to more accurately establish the durability of total ankle replacement and the appropriateness of its use in more active patients with osteoarthrosis and post-traumatic arthrosis of the ankle.

Activities after Total Joint Replacement

Because of concern regarding implant wear, mechanical failure, and prosthetic loosening from the underlying bone, it seems prudent that patients with total joint replacements should exercise a reasonable degree of caution regarding their activities after surgery. Although most surgeons allow return to unlimited low-impact activities, patients should, in general, avoid high-impact and joint-overloading activities such as running, jumping, and heavy lifting. Walking, biking, swimming, water exercises, low-impact aerobics, cross-country skiing, golf, and doubles tennis are acceptable low-impact activities for patients after total joint replacement. Patients with total hip replacement may have certain positional restrictions, varied according to the specific surgical approach, to prevent dislocation. Patients with upper extremity total joint replacement may need to limit overhead use and activities associated with pounding and forceful impact. Patients should be encouraged to discuss specific limitations and activity restrictions after total joint replacement with their surgeons.

Surgery of the Hand for Arthritis

Surgical treatment of arthritis involving the hand deserves special consideration. Patients with rheumatoid arthritis and other forms of inflammatory arthritis often have prominent synovitis of the wrist, metacarpophalangeal (MCP) joints, and proximal interphalangeal (PIP) joints. When medical management is unsuccessful in controlling synovitis in these locations, progressive joint space loss and characteristic secondary deformities of the rheumatoid hand can occur, such as ulnar drift of the MCP joints and swan neck and boutonnière deformities of the fingers. Synovectomy of the wrist, MCP, and PIP joints can slow the progress of joint deterioration and inflammation-mediated attenuation of the periarticular ligamentous and capsular structures responsible for the characteristic deformities of a rheumatoid hand. Because extensor and, less frequently, flexor tendon tenosynovitis often occurs concurrently with synovitis of the adjacent small joints of the hand, tenosynovectomy is frequently performed along with the aforementioned joint procedures. In patients with advanced inflammatory arthritis of the MCP and PIP joints, silicone implant arthroplasty with concurrent extensor tendon realignment and capsular reconstruction of the involved joints can be performed. Significant arthritis of the distal interphalangeal joints, regardless of etiology, is best treated with arthrodesis.

Patients with osteoarthrosis and traumatic arthritis place higher stress and demands on their hands than do patients with rheumatoid arthritis. As a result, although implant arthroplasty of the wrist and hand are acceptable options for patients with rheumatoid arthritis, these devices are, in general, not durable enough for use in patients with osteoarthrosis or traumatic arthritis. In the wrist, several common injury patterns result in associated characteristic patterns of post-traumatic arthrosis. A variety of limited intercarpal fusions have been described to maintain wrist motion while simultaneously eliminating pain from the intercarpal joints affected by arthritis.

Osteoarthrosis of the carpometacarpal (CMC) joint of the thumb is a common finding in patients with previous local trauma to the base of the thumb or with a history of repetitive occupational stress to their hands. Early in this process, attenuation of the capsular ligaments of the thumb CMC joint with resultant instability of the joint occurs. Ligamentous reconstruction and stabilization of the joint can prevent the development of arthrosis of the basilar joint of the thumb, if performed early. If advanced arthrosis of the CMC joint is present, ligamentous stabilization plus interpositional arthroplasty using allograft or autograft tendon is a preferred treatment option. The MCP joints of the thumb and index finger are subject to considerable force during normal use and hand grasping in patients with osteoarthrosis of these joints. Consequently, arthrodesis of the thumb and index finger MCP joints is preferred over implant arthroplasty in these high-demand patients.

Restoration of Articular Cartilage

This chapter has discussed the use of prosthetic devices as a treatment approach to arthritic problems of articular cartilage. The results of total joint arthroplasty are excellent. However, because of an increasing number of younger patients with articular cartilage defects, major emphasis has been placed on the use of biologic treatments to restore articular cartilage. Articular cartilage is a unique tissue with significant limitations for repair or regeneration. It is avascular, so the normal inflammatory response is not seen. Chondrocytes, the cells in cartilage, have a limited capacity to respond to injury, and the tissue structure is sufficiently complex that it is difficult for chondrocytes to reproduce. To provide a long-term functional outcome for any biologic treatment of articular cartilage loss, regeneration of the tissue with cells and matrix identical to its original state is necessary. This goal has never been accomplished in an adult; however, some data indicate that complete spontaneous repair of partial-thickness defects of articular cartilage is possible in the fetal environment.

A number of strategies can be used to restore articular cartilage. One is stimulation of resident articular cartilage to repair itself. This approach includes microfracture to stimulate marrow in the subchondral bone, osteotomy, the use of growth factors with or without artificial matrices, nutraceuticals, and intra-articular hyaluronate treatments. The other approach to cartilage repair is transplantation of tissue, including articular cartilage grafts, soft tissue grafts, and cells alone or with a matrix. Finally, a new field is emerging, tissue engineering, in which a combination of growth factors, matrices, and cells are used to repair articular cartilage. To date, most of these outcomes, though clinically satisfactory early, are unpredictable in the long term.

Microfracture or multiple perforations into subchondral bone with specially designed awls is intended to provide an increased number of progenitor cells from the subchondral marrow to synthesize new hyaline cartilage. The clinical follow-up of these patients has been encouraging; however, no long-term or randomized controlled studies have been performed. Growth factors have been used to stimulate resident cartilage in animal experimentation. One recent study using recombinant bone matrix protein-2 in adult rabbits demonstrated the capacity of this factor to enhance healing of a full-thickness defect. Application of this treatment to clinical problems remains in the future.

Transplantation of osteochondral grafts has been performed to treat full-thickness defects of articular cartilage for a number of decades with satisfactory clinical outcomes. One tissue graft that has been used successfully is an osteochondral autograft. These grafts are removed by specially designed instruments from non–weight-bearing portions of the knee joint and are transplanted into full-thickness defects on the weight-bearing surface of the knee joint. The clinical results have been good to excellent in almost 90% of patients. Hyaline cartilage is usually seen at follow-up arthroscopy; however, host-graft integration is generally incomplete. This treatment approach is most effective for small lesions of the distal femoral condyle.

Another approach to transplantation has been the use of fresh or frozen osteochondral allografts for large lesions. Long-term patient follow-up has demonstrated early allograft survival and good to excellent results in 95% of patients. However, with further long-term assessment of patients, the satisfactory results have diminished to 66%. Two other approaches to tissue transplantation are autologous periosteal or perichondral grafting, although experimental and clinical studies indicate limited regeneration of the normal zones of articular cartilage by hyaline cartilage.

Cell-based therapies for cartilage repair involving the use of autologous chondrocytes have recently been introduced. Autologous cartilage implantation was first reported in 1994 and has developed into a major treatment modality for large full-thickness chondral injuries. The treatment includes harvesting of autologous chondrocytes from non–weight-bearing surfaces, culturing them in an in vitro environment to expand their numbers, and reinjecting them under a periosteal flap into the osteochondral defect. Follow-up has been reported in the first 100 patients who received autologous cartilage implants. The overall clinical outcomes are excellent or good in 80% of patients. Repeat arthroscopies have demonstrated hyaline cartilage in the defects.

A newer treatment approach is tissue engineering—an interdisciplinary field that merges the principles of engineering and life sciences to generate biologic substitutes for the restoration of tissues or organs. Cells and a biodegradable matrix used as a carrier with or without growth factors have been combined to repair articular cartilage defects. The cell source has been autologous chondrocytes grown on scaffolding in an in vitro supportive environment. Early follow-up indicates that more than 90% of patients have functional improvement and pain relief.

The application of tissue engineering in orthopedics has great possibilities for future treatment modalities intended for the reconstruction of articular cartilage and other musculoskeletal tissue. However, there are significant hurdles to overcome, including technical, regulatory, and commercial challenges, before this technology can generally be applied to clinical problems.

COMPLICATIONS

Infection

Infection is a devastating complication of joint replacement surgery, primarily because successful eradication of deep periprosthetic infection frequently necessitates a complex two-stage course of treatment consisting of implant removal, a prolonged course of parenteral antibiotics, and delayed reimplantation of a new joint prosthesis. Infection can occur at the time of surgery by inoculation of the open surgical wound or years later by hematogenous seeding of a well-functioning joint prosthesis from a bacterial infection at a remote site. Patients with diabetes mellitus, rheumatoid arthritis, psoriatic arthritis, or previous joint surgery, as well as immunosuppressed patients currently receiving corticosteroids or other immunosuppressive medications, are at significantly higher than normal risk for both perioperative and late hematogenous infection.

Appropriate use of prophylactic parenteral antibiotics administered within 1 hour of skin incision and continued for 24 hours postoperatively is the single most important factor in the prevention of perioperative infection after total joint replacement. Other methods, including the use of laminar flow or ultraclean ventilation systems, body exhaust isolation suits, iodophor-impregnated adherent skin barrier drapes, and limitation of unnecessary operating room traffic, can also result in a reduced incidence of infection after total joint replacement surgery.

Late hematogenous seeding of a successful total joint replacement can occur years after surgery. Patients with a total joint replacement should be advised to seek prompt medical attention in the event of a suspected bacterial infection at any site. Urinary tract infections, periodontal and dental disease, skin conditions (especially psoriasis and venous stasis ulcers) resulting in secondary cellulitis, and respiratory infections are common sources of late periprosthetic joint infections. Prompt diagnosis and appropriate treatment of remote bacterial infection will reduce the risk for bacteremic seeding of the replaced joint. The American Academy of Orthopaedic Surgeons and the American Dental Association have developed guidelines for the use of periprocedural antibiotics in all patients with total joint replacements. The high-risk patients mentioned earlier should receive prophylactic antibiotics before dental procedures associated with a risk for bacteremia. Consideration should also be given to the use of periprocedural antibiotics in total joint replacement patients undergoing other invasive medical procedures (e.g., urologic) associated with a risk for bacteremia.

Thromboembolic Disease

Thromboembolic disease is a potentially life-threatening complication of major lower extremity total joint replacement. Without appropriate prophylaxis, the incidence of deep venous thrombosis in patients undergoing total hip and knee replacements may be as high as 50 to 70%, and the incidence of fatal pulmonary embolism may as high as 1 to 3%. Fortunately, changes in surgical practice (relatively rapid postoperative ambulation) and widespread acceptance of the importance of routine perioperative prophylaxis for thromboembolic disease have reduced the incidence of this dreaded complication in this high-risk patient population. Although the ideal prophylactic regimen and optimal duration of perioperative prophylaxis are unknown, several strategies appear to be safe and effective.

Warfarin administered to achieve a target international normalized ratio of 2.0 to 2.5, low-molecular-weight heparin, and fondaparinux all appear to be effective and relatively safe in the prevention of venous thromboembolic disease in patients undergoing total hip or knee arthroplasty. Although warfarin is more cumbersome to use and has a delayed onset of action in comparison to its alternatives, bleeding complications appear to be less common with warfarin than with low-molecular-weight heparin or fondaparinux. Administration of perioperative anticoagulants or antithrombotic agents to total joint replacement patients after surgery is associated with a definite risk for wound hematoma formation, which can result in wound-healing problems, deep infection, fibrosis, and neurologic injury with a possible need for additional surgery. Sequential pneumatic compressive devices and plantar plexus foot pumps are not associated with bleeding complications but have not been as extensively evaluated as pharmacologic methods of prophylaxis. Variable patient compliance with these mechanical devices is a concern, and they may best be used as an adjunctive measure in an extremely high-risk patient with a past history of venous thromboembolic disease who is undergoing total hip or knee replacement.

Controversy exists regarding the duration of prophylaxis for thromboembolism after total hip or knee replacement. Patients are clearly at increased risk for venous thrombosis for a variable period after surgery; however, the exact time when the risk for prophylaxis outweighs the risk for venous thrombosis is unknown. Because the typical hospital stay for patients undergoing total hip and knee replacement in the United States is currently between 3 and 5 days, clearly patients require prophylaxis for a variable time after hospital discharge. Though unknown, prophylaxis may be needed for as long as 10 to 14 days in patients after total knee replacement and for 28 to 35 days in patients undergoing total hip replacement.

Dislocation

Total hip arthroplasty using typical implant designs and materials warrants the use of a prosthetic femoral head or ball that is considerably smaller than the normal femoral head. These geometric design factors and the need for an incision through the strong capsular ligaments of the hip joint at the time of total hip arthroplasty result in some obligatory limitations in range of motion of the hip after surgery. Restoration of leg length, the lever arm of the hip abductor muscles, and version or rotational alignment of the total hip replacement components by implant selection and intraoperative positioning is also an important determinant of stability. Although patients typically achieve a functional amount of motion postoperatively and have few positional restrictions after surgery, occasionally the limits of motion of a total hip replacement can be exceeded and result in dislocation. Patient education and understanding of the limitations of total hip replacement, especially regarding the potential for dislocation and range-of-motion restrictions, can help minimize the occurrence of this complication. Unique patient anatomic factors, surgical factors, and patient compliance with these restrictions can contribute to the development of recurrent dislocation, which can be frustrating and difficult for both the patient and surgeon.

Leg Length Discrepancy

Leg length discrepancy can occur after total hip arthroplasty. Typically, patients with hip arthritis have some relative shortening of the operative leg because of loss of articular cartilage associated with the arthritic process. The biomechanics of the hip is improved with resultant minimization of limp and optimization of gait and stability of the joint if premorbid leg length is restored after total hip replacement. Exact restoration of leg length is difficult, however, because of inherent inaccuracies in intraoperative leg length measurement and the inherent relative instability of the prosthetic hip in comparison to the normal hip. Slight lengthening of the leg at the time of surgery is often necessary to minimize the risk for dislocation, although patients can typically accommodate to a slight difference in leg length. Determination of the actual leg length discrepancy can be difficult because other factors such as degenerative scoliosis of the spine and contractures and angular deformities of the hip and knees can result in apparent, but not true leg length discrepancies.

SUGGESTED READINGS

Greenwald AS: Current concepts in joint replacement. Orthopedics 2006;29:757–759. *A review.*

McLaughlin MA, Orosz GM, Magaziner J, et al: Preoperative status and risk of complications in patients with hip fracture. J Gen Intern Med 2006;21:219–225. *An uncorrected major abnormality before surgery or on admission was associated with nearly a threefold increase in postoperative complications.*

Quintana JM, Escobar A, Arostegui I, et al: Health-related quality of life and appropriateness of knee or hip joint replacement. Arch Intern Med 2006;166:220–226. *The use of explicit appropriateness criteria for surgery were associated with better quality of life outcomes.*

Scopp J, Mandelbaum B: A treatment algorithm for the management of articular cartilage defects in the treatment of unicompartmental arthritis of the knee. Orthop Clin North Am 2005;36:419–426. *A practical approach.*

Section XXIII

Infectious Diseases

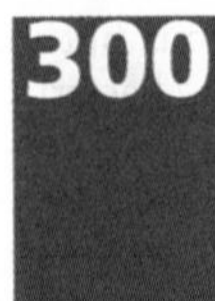

INTRODUCTION TO MICROBIAL DISEASE: HOST-PATHOGEN INTERACTIONS

W. Michael Scheld

Infectious diseases have profoundly influenced the course of human history. The "black death" (caused by *Yersinia pestis*) changed the social structure of medieval Europe, in the process eliminating approximately a third of the population. The outcomes of military campaigns have been altered by outbreaks of diseases such as dysentery and typhus. Examples include Napoleon's retreat from Russia after typhus did more damage to his army than the opposition forces did, the decision by the French to sell the Louisiana territory after the death of French soldiers from yellow fever in Cuba and the gulf coast, and the introduction of smallpox to the non-immune population of the New World by Europeans, thus facilitating the "conquest" and the dawn of the colonial age. Malaria influenced the geographic and racial pattern and distribution of hemoglobins and erythrocyte antigens in Africa. The development of *Plasmodium falciparum* is inhibited by the presence of hemoglobin S, and Duffy blood group–negative erythrocytes are resistant to infection with *Plasmodium vivax.* Thus, populations with these erythrocyte factors are found in areas where malaria is common.

Infections are a major cause of morbidity and mortality in the world. Of the approximately 53 million deaths worldwide in 2002, at least a third were due to infectious diseases. In the United States, pneumonia is the fifth leading cause of death overall and the most common cause of death related to infection. In addition, invasive disease caused by *Streptococcus pneumoniae* and community-acquired pneumonia overall have increased in incidence over the past decade. Acquired immunodeficiency syndrome (AIDS) threatens to disrupt the social fabric in many countries of Africa and is severely distressing the health care system in the United States and other parts of the world. The year 2006 marked the 25th "anniversary" of the AIDS epidemic. Approximately 40 million people worldwide are currently infected with human immunodeficiency virus (HIV), and since 1981 approximately 25 million have died. AIDS is now the leading cause of death in sub-Saharan Africa.

Infection may be defined as multiplication of microbes (e.g., from viruses to multicellular parasites) in the tissues of the host. The host may or may not be symptomatic. For example, HIV infection may cause no overt signs or symptoms of illness for years. The definition of infection should also include instances of multiplication of microbes on the surface or in the lumen of the host that cause signs and symptoms of illness or disease. For example, toxin-producing strains of *Escherichia coli* may multiply in the gut and cause a diarrheal illness without invading tissues. Microbes can cause diseases without actually coming in contact with the host by virtue of toxin production. *Clostridium botulinum* may grow in certain improperly processed foods and produce a toxin that can be lethal on ingestion. A relatively trivial infection such as that caused by *Clostridium tetani* in a small puncture wound can cause devastating illness because of a toxin released from the organism growing in tissues. It has now become apparent that multiple virulence factors of microorganisms may be carried in tandem on so-called pathogenicity islands of the genome.

We live in a virtual sea of microorganisms, and all our body surfaces have indigenous bacterial flora. This normal flora actually protects us from infection. Reduction of gut colonization increases susceptibility to infection by pathogens such as *Salmonella enteritidis* serovar *typhimurium.* Bacteria that constitute the normal flora are thought to exert their protective effect by several mechanisms: (1) utilizing nutrients and occupying an ecologic niche, thus competing with pathogens; (2) producing antibacterial substances that inhibit the growth of pathogens; and (3) inducing host immunity that is cross-reactive and effective against pathogens. These conclusions appear to be oversimplistic, however. For example, colonization of the gastrointestinal tract with *Bacteroides fragilis* expressing an immunodominant bacterial polysaccharide, through dendritic cell activation and induction of a T_H1-mediated response, leads to a splenic response characterized by normal numbers of $CD4^+$ T cells, lymphoid architecture, and systemic lymphocytic expansion. Thus, a single bacterial molecule in our gut is necessary to make us "immunologically fit." In addition to the normal flora, transient colonization may be seen with known or potential pathogens. This may be a special problem in hospitalized patients because it can lead to nosocomial infection (Chapter 304).

Only a small proportion of microbial species may be considered to be primary or professional pathogens, and even among these species a relatively small number of clones have been shown to cause disease (Chapter 309). For example, epidemic meningococcal meningitis and meningococcemia are due to a small number of clones of *Neisseria meningitidis,* and the worldwide explosion of penicillin-resistant *S. pneumoniae* can be traced to a few clones originating in South Africa and Spain. This observation supports the concept that pathogenic organisms are highly adapted to the pathogenic state and have developed characteristics that enable them to be transmitted, attach to surfaces, invade tissue, avoid host defenses, and thus cause disease. In contrast, opportunistic pathogens cause disease principally in impaired hosts, and these organisms, which may be harmless members of normal flora in healthy persons, can act as virulent invaders in patients with severe defects in host defense mechanisms. Although opportunistic infection has traditionally been viewed as exploitation of a weakened host through physiologic stress or immunocompromise (or both) by relatively "avirulent" pathogens, this is an oversimplification. For example, *Pseudomonas aeruginosa* recognizes host immune activation, specifically by binding interferon-γ to a cell surface protein, OprF, which in turn, through a quorum-sensing signaling system, leads to the overexpression of virulence determinants such as PA-I (lecA) and pyocyanin. Thus, bacteria have developed a "contingency system" that recognizes immunologic pertubations in the host and counters this response by expression of virulence factors.

Pathogenic organisms may be acquired by several routes. Direct contact has been implicated in the acquisition of staphylococcal disease. Airborne spread, usually by droplet nuclei, occurs in respiratory diseases such as influenza and in severe acute respiratory syndrome (SARS). Contaminated water is the usual vehicle in *Giardia* infection and typhoid fever. Foodborne toxic illnesses may be caused by extracellular toxins produced by *Clostridium perfringens* and *Staphylococcus aureus.* Blood and blood products may be vectors for transmitting hepatitis B and C viruses, as well as HIV. Sexual transmission is also important for these agents and for a variety of pathogens, including *Treponema pallidum* (syphilis), *Neisseria gonorrhoeae* (gonorrhea), and *Chlamydia trachomatis* (nonspecific urethritis). The fetus may be infected in utero, and the infection may be devastating if the agent is rubella virus or cytomegalovirus. Arthropod vectors may be important, as illustrated by mosquitoes for malaria and dengue, ticks for Lyme disease and ehrlichiosis, and lice for typhus.

Pathogens are able to cause disease because of a finely tuned array of adaptations, including the ability to attach to appropriate cells, often mediated by specialized structures such as the pili on gram-negative rods. Microbes such as *Shigella* species have the ability to invade cells and cause damage. Toxins may act at a distance or may intoxicate only infected cells. Pathogens have the ability to thwart host defenses by a variety of ingenious maneuvers. The antiphagocytic coat of the pneumococcus is an example. Organisms may change their surface antigen display at an astonishingly rapid rate to outmaneuver the host immune system. Examples include influenza virus and trypanosomes. Certain pathogens have the ability to inhibit the respiratory burst of phagocytes *(Toxoplasma gondii),* and others can destroy phagocytic cells that have engulfed them (e.g., *Streptococcus pyogenes*). The environment plays an important role in infection, both in transmission and in the ability of the host to combat the invader. The humidity and temperature of air may affect the infectivity of airborne pathogens. The sanitary state of food and water, woefully lacking in many areas of the developing world, is an important factor in the acquisition of enteric pathogens, one of the major causes of mortality and morbidity, such as physical and mental developmental delay leading to poor performance in school and other consequences. The malaria associated with the "bad air" of swamps is, in fact, due to the mosquitoes, but the environmental association was appropriate. The nutritional status of the host is clearly a significant factor in certain infectious diseases. It is likely that micronutrient deficiency contributes to the invasion and multiplication of certain pathogens. Establishment of infection is a complicated interplay of factors involving the microbe, the host, and the environment.

Host reaction to infection may result in illness. For example, previous infection with *Campylobacter jejuni* is responsible for about 40% of cases of Guillain-Barré syndrome. The mechanism is thought to be the production of antibodies against *C. jejuni* lipopolysaccharides that cross-react with gangliosides in peripheral nerves. Similarly, much of the damage resulting from meningitis is due to the host's response to invading bacterial pathogens.

With unusual exceptions, infectious diseases are often treatable and curable. Thus, it is important to make an accurate etiologic diagnosis and institute appropriate therapy promptly. In acute infections such as pneumonia, meningitis, or sepsis, rapid institution of therapy may be lifesaving, and thus a presumptive etiologic diagnosis should be established before a definitive diagnosis. This presumptive diagnosis is based on the history, physical examination, epidemiology of illness in the community, and rapid techniques such as microscopic examination of appropriate Gram-stained specimens. Antimicrobial therapy can then be instituted for the presumptive etiologic agents, but it must be reevaluated as more definitive diagnostic information becomes available.

The study as well as understanding of infectious diseases is a dynamic process. A number of factors or themes of current interest contribute to this conclusion, including the following:

1. *Emerging infections.* The most obvious is AIDS, but scores of pathogens, new diseases, and new syndromes have been described in the past 2 decades. West Nile virus is now firmly entrenched in the Western Hemisphere. Since 2002, several new pathogens have been described, including a human metapneumovirus responsible for upper and lower respiratory tract infections and perhaps occasional asthma in both children and adults. A novel coronavirus is associated with SARS, a new worldwide epidemic of atypical pneumonia first described in March 2003, and H5N1 influenza has emerged in Far East Asia. A roundworm associated with raccoons that can cause fatal encephalitis is now evident. The second report from the Institute of Medicine on emerging infections (February 2003) has shaped the framework for a response by the Centers for Disease Control and Prevention and other agencies.
2. *Genomics.* The exact sequence of the genome of more than 200 pathogens relevant to humans has been determined in less than a decade. This new information, in concert with genomic information from multicellular organisms such as the *Anopheles* mosquito, offers significant promise for the development of new therapies and vaccines. Careful analysis of the genomes of pathogens will continue to yield important information on the pathogenesis of infection. For example, genome sequencing of group A streptococci, collected over time with relevant robust clinical information, has detected the acquisition of new determinants (often by prophage) responsible for increased virulence resulting in toxic shock syndrome or necrotizing fasciitis, or both.
3. *Genetic factors altering susceptibility to infection and the response to infectious diseases.* This field, though in its infancy, promises new and significant information relevant to the wide variety of responses to infectious diseases in humans. For example, an overvigorous response with generation of tumor necrosis factor-α may accentuate the development of cerebral complications in falciparum malaria. Analysis of single-nucleotide polymorphisms of the human genome will lead to an enhanced understanding of two fundamental issues in infectious diseases: why invasive, overt disease develops in only a small fraction of individuals colonized with a given microbe and why infections are more severe in some people than in others.
4. *Antimicrobial resistance.* It is perhaps surprising (if not frightening) that the development of new antimicrobial agents has slowed despite the burgeoning problem of antimicrobial resistance. This disconnect has been the focus of meetings among the pharmaceutical industry, the Infectious Diseases Society of America, and the Food and Drug Administration (FDA). Multiresistant pneumococci, vancomycin resistance in *S. aureus,* the exploding epidemic of community-associated methicillin-resistant *S. aureus* (CA-MRSA), and vancomycin-resistant enterococci are just a few examples among many that have emerged.
5. *The role of infectious agents in chronic diseases.* Many so-called idiopathic diseases may in fact have an infectious basis. A list of conditions for which there is some evidence (but not conclusive evidence) includes diabetes, atherosclerosis, acute leukemia, collagen vascular diseases, and inflammatory bowel disease. Detection of "uncultivatable" microorganisms by newer techniques, such as 16S RNA analysis, may uncover agents responsible for "noninfectious" diseases or suggest a role in conditions that are considered infectious but in which the pathogen or pathogens are controversial (e.g., bacterial vaginosis). In addition, we know that hepatitis C virus, human papillomavirus (HPV), and *Helicobacter pylori* cause human cancers. Indeed, a vaccine for HPV recently approved by the FDA has been shown in clinical trials to be highly effective in reducing the incidence of cervical cancer.
6. *New therapies.* The number of antivirals has more than quadrupled in the last 15 years. Furthermore, immunotherapy or adjunctive agents hold promise for the treatment of various diseases. Examples include activated protein C (drotrecogin-α) for severe sepsis and septic shock and, perhaps, interleukin-2 in the treatment of advanced AIDS.
7. *Bioterrorism.* The anthrax attacks of late 2001 in the eastern United States have brought this issue to the attention of politicians, public health authorities, physicians in general, and the public. Experts within and outside the discipline of infectious diseases have been struggling with smallpox vaccination policies. A vaccine with considerable adverse effects is to be used in military personnel and health care workers in a setting in which the natural disease does not exist. This is a unique experiment. The consequences are not insignificant because the actual risk for a deliberate smallpox event is unknown at present. The benefit of smallpox vaccination in this setting is not measurable in absence of the disease, whereas the adverse effects are readily measurable and may lead to reluctance of the public to accept vaccination against other pathogens. This would be an unfortunate outcome because vaccination to prevent infection is probably the greatest achievement of medical science.

SUGGESTED READINGS

de Jong MD, Simmons CP, Thanh TT, et al: Fatal outcome of human influenza A (H5N1) is associated with high viral load and hypercytokinemia. Nat Med 2006;12:1203–1207. *Fatal H5N1 infection ("bird flu") in humans is associated with a high viral load and the resultant intense pro-inflammatory response.*

Mazmanian SK, Liu C-H, Tzianabos AO, et al: An immunomodulatory molecule of symbiotic bacteria directs maturation of the host immune system. Cell 2005;122:107–118. *A single bacterial molecule from a gut symbiont,* Bacillus fragilis *polysaccharide, elicits a wide variety of responses essential for immune homeostasis.*

Schroder NWJ, Schumann RR: Single nucleotide polymorphisms of Toll-like receptors and susceptibility to infectious disease. Lancet Infect Dis 2005;5:156–164. *A thorough review of this burgeoning field.*

Van Belkum A: Staphylococcal colonization and infection: Homeostasis versus disbalance of human (innate) immunity and bacterial virulence. Curr Opin Infect Dis 2006;19:339–344. *A complete discussion of staphylococcal invasion procedures and innate immune system evasion strategies.*

PRINCIPLES OF ANTI-INFECTIVE THERAPY

George M. Eliopoulos

Among the pharmaceutical agents used in the treatment of human disease, antimicrobial agents are distinctive because they target invading microorganisms rather than abnormal human cellular functions. As a result, to select an appropriate antimicrobial regimen it is necessary to consider both the activity of the agent against the known or suspected pathogen and the effects that the antimicrobial agent may have on the individual under treatment. Although the term "anti-infective agent" can be used more broadly to include substances that ameliorate infection by altering virulence of the pathogen or modulating the host's response to infection, for purposes of this chapter, "anti-infective agent" and "antimicrobial agent" will be used interchangeably to refer to drugs used to inhibit the growth of microbial pathogens. This chapter will focus primarily on agents directed against bacterial pathogens, although many parallels can be drawn to the use of antimicrobial agents for the treatment of fungal, viral, or parasitic infections.

Natural substances have been used since antiquity to treat infections, and even today research continues to identify active antimicrobial compounds within these products. However, on the time scale of human history, the modern antibiotic era is short. Only 25 years or so separates the introduction of penicillin for general clinical use in the mid-1940s and the first walk on the moon in 1969. In the decades since, the numerous antimicrobial agents developed for human use have saved countless lives, as well as led to amazing advances in cancer chemotherapy, organ transplantation, and implant surgery that have improved and extended the lives of many others. Unfortunately, over time, resistance to available antibiotics has become widespread among many common bacterial pathogens, thus making selection of appropriate antimicrobial regimens ever more challenging and threatening to thrust an unfortunate few once again into the preantibiotic era.

SELECTING ANTIMICROBIAL THERAPY TARGETING THE PATHOGEN

Empirical Antimicrobial Therapy

In most instances, selection of initial antimicrobial therapy proceeds empirically, before a causative organism is identified or tested for susceptibility to antimicrobial agents. The clinician's first decision is whether a patient's symptoms are likely to represent infection. Fever may result from neoplastic, rheumatologic, or other noninfectious processes and does not necessarily imply the presence of infection. Noninfectious causes of fever such as deep vein thrombophlebitis, drug reaction, or vasculitis may pose just as great a risk to the patient as infection and must not be overlooked.

Additional symptoms and signs and laboratory or radiographic data will usually help define more clearly whether infection is likely and, if so, help localize the organ systems involved. This information allows an initial prediction about organisms likely to be involved. For example, if the initial data cause one to suspect a diagnosis of community-acquired pneumonia in a previously healthy person who does not have unusual exposure, *Streptococcus pneumoniae* and atypical bacteria such as *Mycoplasma pneumoniae* or *Chlamydophila pneumoniae* would appear prominently on the list of potential pathogens to be targeted in selecting antimicrobial therapy. Examination of a Gram-stained slide of expectorated sputum may provide valuable information. The prominent appearance of gram-positive cocci in clusters, for example, would alert the clinician to the possible presence of *Staphylococcus aureus,* some strains of which are now methicillin resistant.

Guidance regarding probable pathogens for site-specific infections and the susceptibility of these organisms to antimicrobial agents is available from a number of sources. In some cases, the susceptibility of suspected pathogens can be predicted with a high degree of certainty. For example, isolates of *Streptococcus pyogenes* remain uniformly susceptible to penicillin G. In other instances, resistance has emerged to antimicrobials previously considered to have been highly active against a species. Rates of resistance to trimethoprim-sulfamethoxazole or even to fluoroquinolones among isolates of *Escherichia coli* are now substantial in some centers. Resistance rates for a given organism may vary widely by region, by health care institution, or even by patient care area within a hospital. For this reason, access to periodically updated, cumulative antibiotic susceptibility profile data specific to an institution can be very important. Typically presented in tabular form, these "antibiograms" show the percentage of recently isolated bacterial pathogens (grouped by genus or species) that proved "susceptible" to the antibiotics tested and can help guide the selection of appropriate regimens for empirical therapy at that practice site.

There is mounting evidence that selection of an appropriate regimen (i.e., one that contains an antimicrobial that can be expected to inhibit the causative pathogen at the site of infection) plus prompt application of that agent for empirical treatment of serious infection results in improved clinical outcomes, especially in the critical care setting. Published guidelines for the treatment of community-acquired pneumonia strive for administration of the first dose of appropriate antimicrobial therapy while the patient is still in the emergency room.

Whenever possible, samples of purulent exudates, blood, or other body fluids suspected to be infected should be obtained for culture before starting antimicrobial therapy. The results of such cultures can be used to direct subsequent definitive treatment based on identification and susceptibility of the microorganisms detected. At times, this principle must be overridden. For example, when bacterial meningitis is suspected, antibiotic therapy (often with adjunctive corticosteroids) must not be delayed when a lumbar puncture cannot be performed promptly to obtain material for culture. In such instances, blood samples taken for culture before the administration of antibiotics will often reveal the causative organism, or the pathogen may grow from spinal fluid even if lumbar puncture is delayed.

Definitive Antimicrobial Therapy

Identification of the causative microorganism and determination of its susceptibility to available drugs serve as the basis for optimizing regimens for definitive antimicrobial therapy. Often, antibiotics used for empirical therapy will be appropriate for definitive therapy and can be continued. At other times, identification and susceptibility test results will allow switch to a narrower spectrum, better tolerated, or less expensive antimicrobial. In some instances, testing results will dictate the need to broaden the spectrum of an anti-infective regimen by adding or substituting agents active against pathogens inadequately targeted by the initial empirical regimen.

In almost all cases it is desirable to test the susceptibility of an infecting organism directly to antimicrobials that may be useful. To extend the example cited earlier, although it is not necessary to test the susceptibility of *S. pyogenes* to penicillin G, some isolates are resistant to macrolide antibiotics (e.g., erythromycin, azithromycin) and other drugs, so testing of alternative agents might be useful for patients who are intolerant of β-lactam antibiotics. Even when the activity of certain antimicrobials can be predicted with great confidence, susceptibility testing is still useful. For example, surveillance studies that have examined hundreds of isolates predict that vancomycin or linezolid would inhibit virtually all *S. aureus* strains recovered from clinical specimens. On statistical grounds, testing these agents would thus not seem warranted; however, rare isolates resistant to these agents have now been encountered, and it would be advantageous to detect such isolates for both therapeutic and epidemiologic purposes. Demonstrating susceptibility to commonly used agents other than vancomycin or linezolid in this example also makes possible the design of potentially less expensive or more convenient regimens. By avoiding intensive use of only one or two drug classes, clinicians can potentially minimize selective pressure for resistance to these valuable antimicrobials.

For most bacterial pathogens, resistance to commonly used agents is sufficiently frequent that testing of antimicrobials considered for definitive therapy is essential. This observation is especially evident for gram-negative bacteria. Organisms of the family Enterobacteriaceae resistant to multiple antibiotics are isolated with sufficient frequency, even among outpatients, that susceptibility to agents previously considered to be broadly active, including third-generation cephalosporins, fluoroquinolones, and aminoglycosides, can no longer be ensured. Even more challenging problems of drug resistance are encountered among isolates of species such as *Pseudomonas aeruginosa, Acinetobacter baumannii,* and *Stenotrophomonas maltophilia.*

Susceptibility Testing

Several methods are available for determining the susceptibility of a bacterial isolate to antimicrobial agents that might be considered for therapy. Tests used in clinical microbiology laboratories today are variations of three methods: serial dilution, disc diffusion, and gradient diffusion. The minimal inhibitory concentration (MIC) represents the lowest concentration of an antimicrobial tested that inhibits growth of the microorganism in test media.

In the dilution method, the antimicrobial is diluted in broth or agar to span a range of (usually) two-fold decreasing concentrations, and the medium is then inoculated with a standardized number of organisms. After incubation for a specified period (usually 16 to 24 hours) at 35 to 37° C, the series of dilution tubes or microtiter wells (for broth dilution) or agar plates (for agar dilution) is examined for growth in comparison to that on control media containing no antibiotic. Thus, the MIC is determined by direct inspection as the lowest concentration that prevents turbidity of the broth or colony formation on agar. Modifications of this method permit automation of many steps in the process, thereby permitting greater efficiency in test performance.

In the disc diffusion method, paper discs impregnated with a standardized amount of the antimicrobial are placed on an agar plate, the surface of which has been seeded with the bacterium to be tested. During incubation, the antimicrobial diffuses from the disc into the surrounding agar and inhibits growth of the seeded organism in a concentration-dependent manner. After a specified period of incubation, the zone of growth inhibition around the disc is measured. By this method, the MIC is not determined directly. Instead, relying on accumulated data correlating inhibition zones with MICs, the measured zone is used to predict the susceptibility of the organism to the drug tested.

The gradient diffusion method is similar to the disc diffusion method, except that instead of using a round paper disc impregnated with a single concentration of the antimicrobial, this test uses a strip impregnated with the antimicrobial applied in a concentration gradient along its length. The strip is laid on the surface of an agar plate that has been inoculated with a suspension of the organism to be tested, and the plate is then incubated. By visually inspecting where the zone of growth inhibition on the agar surface intersects the strip (which is marked at intervals corresponding to MIC equivalents), it is possible to determine an MIC value directly.

To perform and interpret the results of susceptibility studies, it is necessary to identify the organism to be tested. The nature of the organism determines which antibiotics are appropriate for testing. For example, microdilution panels designed for testing gram-positive bacteria would contain agents such as oxacillin and vancomycin, which would be irrelevant for gram-negative bacteria. In addition, identification of the microorganism allows selection of the appropriate interpretive criteria to determine whether an organism is "susceptible," "intermediate," or "resistant" to an antimicrobial based on measurement of the MIC or inhibition zone diameter. To illustrate this point, consider that an enterococcus is determined to be susceptible to penicillin if the MIC is less than or equal to 8 μg/mL, whereas for viridans group streptococci, the corresponding breakpoint for susceptibility to penicillin is an MIC of 0.12 μg/mL. Thus, knowledge that the MIC of a gram-positive coccus growing in short chains is 2 μg/mL does not allow interpretation of whether it is susceptible to penicillin unless the organism has been identified.

Additional tests are sometimes required to allow full assessment of susceptibility to an antimicrobial. For oxacillin-susceptible *S. aureus,* a test for penicillinase production is performed by the laboratory to assess susceptibility to penicillin G. For erythromycin-resistant, clindamycin-susceptible *S. aureus,* the laboratory may perform a supplementary D-zone test before reporting the clindamycin result. A positive D-zone test (i.e., the inhibition zone around a clindamycin disc is blunted in proximity to an erythromycin disc) predicts the presence of *erm* genes. These genes, which code for ribosomal methylases that have the potential to confer resistance to clindamycin, are often not expressed because clindamycin is a poor inducer of this resistance trait (in contrast to erythromycin, which is a good inducer). However, mutations allowing constitutive production of methylase can be selected during treatment, thereby resulting in the emergence of clindamycin resistance and an increased risk of clinical failure when this drug is used to treat serious staphylococcal infections caused by strains with the *erm* gene.

For *E. coli* or *Klebsiella* species, growth on screening concentrations of certain β-lactams prompts testing for the presence of extended-spectrum β-lactamases (ESBLs). When the presence of ESBLs is predicted by such testing, susceptibility interpretations for various cephalosporins are overridden to "resistant," irrespective of direct test results for those agents, because "susceptible" results for these agents can be misleading.

In principle, tests for the presence of resistance genes or their products, or both, can be used in place of phenotypic resistance testing. Such methods have the potential to provide answers more rapidly than with the usual susceptibility tests of growth inhibition, which generally require several hours of incubation. However, at present, these tests have not been widely adopted, with the exception of testing for methicillin resistance by detection of the *mecA* gene or its product, penicillin-binding protein 2a.

Bactericidal Activity

In some circumstances, an antimicrobial regimen that kills pathogenic microorganisms would be preferable to an alternative regimen that only inhibits growth of the pathogen. Bactericidal activity is desirable in the treatment of endocarditis or meningitis; in these infections, bacteriostatic agents have generally performed poorly, possibly because of inadequate host responses to infection at these sites. Tests to measure the bactericidal activity of an antibiotic in vitro have been developed. They can be viewed as modifications of the broth dilution test used to determine MICs, in which samples are removed at various times and plated onto antibiotic-free media. Incubation of these antibiotic-free plates allows bacteria that have been inhibited in the presence of the antibiotic, but not killed by it, to grow once the antibiotic is removed. If there is no growth, the bacteria have been killed, and a minimum bactericidal concentration can be determined.

Another test of bactericidal activity is the time-kill curve method. Here, aliquots of a broth culture exposed to a specific concentration of the antibiotic are removed at indicated times during incubation and plated onto antibiotic-free media to determine counts of viable bacteria. Bactericidal activity is usually defined as a 99.9% reduction in the number of viable colony-forming units (CFU) relative to the inoculum density at a specified incubation time, which is usually 20 to 24 hours.

Despite the theoretical benefit of determining the bactericidal activity of an antibiotic or drug regimen, these tests are rarely used in clinical care because of several factors, including (1) the labor-intensive nature of the tests, (2) the potential for discordant results from the various methods and criteria for determining bactericidal activity, and (3) imperfect correlation between bactericidal activity measured in vitro and clinical outcomes observed.

SELECTING ANTIMICROBIAL THERAPY APPROPRIATE TO THE INFECTION AND PATIENT

Nature of the Infection

Determination that a pathogenic microorganism is susceptible to an antibiotic in vitro does not ensure that treatment with that drug will result in a successful clinical outcome. The antimicrobial must reach the site of infection in adequate concentration, generally assumed to be some multiple of the MIC, and must demonstrate activity in the infection milieu. For some infections and antimicrobials, these requirements cannot easily be met.

A number of antimicrobials fail to penetrate sufficiently well into cerebrospinal fluid to permit their use for the treatment of bacterial meningitis in adults. First-generation cephalosporins or aminoglycosides given intravenously do not enter the subarachnoid space well enough to allow their use as primary agents for treatment of this disease. Aminoglycosides have been administered by intrathecal or intraventricular instillation when needed for the treatment of gram-negative meningitis, but the availability of newer β-lactams with broad activity, high potency, and reasonable penetration represents a major advance.

In other situations, antimicrobials may penetrate to the site of infection, only to be inactivated by local factors. For example, daptomycin is inactivated by interaction with pulmonary surfactant, so this antibiotic is not indicated for the treatment of bronchopneumonia, even though it is highly active against *S. pneumoniae* isolates in vitro. Antibiotics can also be inactivated by cellular debris or macromolecules present within abscesses or exhibit reduced potency at the low pH and reduced oxygen tensions prevailing at these sites. Aminoglycosides, clindamycin, and erythromycin, for example, are all less active at acid pH than at neutral or alkaline pH, whereas aminoglycoside transport into bacterial cells requires aerobic conditions. Finally, high densities of microorganisms within abscesses may elaborate sufficiently high concentrations of β-lactamases to inactivate some relatively labile β-lactam antibiotics. All these factors provide a rationale for drainage of large abscesses as an adjunct to antimicrobial therapy.

Bacterial infections associated with foreign bodies such as artificial joints, cardiac pacemakers, or prosthetic heart valves can be particularly difficult to eradicate without removing the foreign material. The reasons for this observation are not completely understood but relate, at least in part, to the presence of biofilm, which is composed of bacteria embedded within the extracellular matrices and is adherent to the foreign material. It was once believed that the extracellular matrix prevented antibiotics from reaching the embedded bacteria and that this mechanism explained the difficulty in eradicating biofilm-associated bacteria. More recent work has shown that antibiotic penetration is only minimally retarded by the extracellular material. Instead, bacteria recovered from biofilms are metabolically different from and less susceptible to antimicrobial agents than planktonic cells (i.e., those freely suspended in liquid medium) of the same organism are. Rifampin is often added to antimicrobial regimens for the treatment of infections involving prosthetic material. This antibiotic, which is an inhibitor of RNA polymerase, rapidly penetrates into biofilms and demonstrates relatively similar activity against both biofilm-associated and planktonic cells of a susceptible organism. However, because resistance to rifampin emerges rapidly, it is not used as a single agent in these circumstances but rather must be combined with a second active drug to minimize the risk that resistance to rifampin will emerge. Despite such approaches, many infections involving implanted devices prove refractory to antimicrobial therapy alone and require removal of the foreign material for eradication.

Host Factors

After considering the nature of the infection and the antimicrobials determined in vitro to be active against a bacterial isolate (or likely to be active against probable pathogens when an isolate is not yet available), the ultimate choice of an antimicrobial regimen must take into account a number of additional patient-specific factors, some examples of which are illustrated in the following paragraphs.

Allergies

It is imperative to obtain a history of previous allergic reactions to antimicrobial agents. Some reactions are by nature so severe and potentially life-threatening that one must avoid using the same agent or drugs within the same class for which cross-reactivity is likely to occur. Examples of such reactions include an immediate hypersensitivity reaction to penicillin (e.g., hives, lip swelling, laryngeal edema, circulatory collapse) or a mucocutaneous bullous eruption from a sulfonamide (e.g., Stevens-Johnson syndrome).

In cases in which the allergic reaction has been mild, such as a faint self-limited rash in a patient receiving penicillin, the clinician may elect to use a related antimicrobial, such as a cephalosporin, when the probability of cross-sensitivity and the risk for a severe adverse outcome, were a reaction to occur, are both assessed to be low. In these instances, careful monitoring of the patient for adverse reactions is essential. Rarely, for patients with significant allergy to a potentially life-saving antimicrobial agent for which no alternative exists, desensitization of the patient to the antimicrobial is attempted so that the agent can be used. For example, desensitization protocols are available for penicillin and for trimethoprim-sulfamethoxazole. Because of the risks involved, these procedures may need to be performed in intensive care unit settings where maximum resources for resuscitation are available if necessary.

Pregnancy

A number of antimicrobial agents have the potential to cause fetal harm if administered to a pregnant woman. For example, tetracyclines can cause tooth discoloration and hypoplasia of dental enamel and are thus avoided in pregnant women and young children. Streptomycin given during pregnancy can cross the placenta, and evidence of eighth nerve toxicity has been reported. Evidence of fetal harm has been noted with the antiretroviral agent efavirenz, a non-nucleoside reverse transcriptase inhibitor. In this case, teratogenicity was reported in primates and neural tube defects were seen in a few children exposed in utero. A few other antimicrobials are labeled by the Food and Drug Administration (FDA) as pregnancy category D (evidence of human risk) or are absolutely contraindicated because of fetal harm. Many more antimicrobials, however, are assigned to category C, where potential for risk to the fetus exists based on animal studies. When designing antimicrobial regimens, the possibility of pregnancy should be considered in any woman of child-bearing age so that the risks of candidate agents can be individually reviewed and the safest possible therapy selected.

It should also be noted that many antibiotics used to treat lactating women can be found in breast milk. Thus, it may be necessary to suspend breast-feeding during antimicrobial treatment if exposure of the infant to the drug must be avoided.

Pregnant women may be particularly susceptible to certain antimicrobial-associated toxicities. Deaths resulting from hepatic failure have been described in pregnant women receiving large doses of tetracycline. Potentially life-threatening hepatic steatosis has been observed in patients treated with a combination of the antiretroviral agents didanosine plus stavudine; pregnant women may be especially vulnerable to this toxic effect.

Age

For reasons discussed earlier, tetracycline antibiotics are avoided in children during tooth development to prevent discoloration and enamel hypoplasia of the permanent teeth. Because fluoroquinolone antimicrobials have been shown to produce erosion of cartilage and arthropathy in juvenile animals, they represent another example of antimicrobials that have been avoided in children when alternative agents are available. Recently, however, ciprofloxacin has received limited pediatric indications (for complicated urinary tract infection/pyelonephritis and for treatment after inhalational exposure to anthrax). Musculoskeletal complaints appear to be more frequent in children treated with ciprofloxacin than with comparator antimicrobials.

Pediatric dosing regimens differ from those appropriate for adults. Some agents, such as linezolid, are eliminated much more rapidly in young children (excluding preterm neonates) than in older children and adults, so higher doses are required. At the extremes of age, dosing of antibiotics may require modification. In premature infants and neonates, renal function has not yet reached full capacity and drug elimination may be delayed. Similarly, hepatic clearance activity is not fully developed in the very young, which has led to cardiovascular collapse and fatalities resulting from the accumulation of toxic levels of chloramphenicol. Absorption of oral antimicrobials may also be age dependent if their absorption is dependent on gastric pH. The gastric pH of young children is higher than that of adults, and achlorhydria resulting in higher gastric pH is more common in adults older than 60 than in younger adults. Thus, in young children and older adults, the absorption of oral drugs that are unstable in acid, such as penicillin G, may be higher than that in younger adults. On the other hand, antimicrobials such as ketoconazole require gastric acid for absorption and may be less bioavailable in persons with reduced gastric acid production.

As adults age, both renal function and muscle mass may decline, and such decline can result in an overestimation of renal elimination capacity from serum creatinine alone. A subtle decline in renal function and alterations in body composition (which may affect drug distribution) can result in altered pharmacokinetic disposition of antimicrobials in the aged. For recently developed antimicrobials, pharmacokinetic characteristics in older individuals are described in the FDA-approved drug label. Although the serum concentrations of several drugs may be somewhat higher in older individuals, differences are not usually of sufficient magnitude to warrant dosage adjustments based on age alone.

A curious association of rash with age and sex has been noted during development of the fluoroquinolone antimicrobial gemifloxacin. In clinical studies, rash was more common in young women than in men and older women, thus suggesting that there may be hormonal influences on the risk for development of rash. For the new ketolide antibiotic telithromycin, transient blurring of vision and difficulty focusing have been described during clinical studies. This side effect was seen more commonly in persons younger than 40 years and may relate to alterations in visual accommodation, which is usually more robust in the younger population.

Renal and Hepatic Function

Renal or hepatobiliary excretion, or both, are the major routes of elimination for antimicrobial agents. Relatively few antibacterial agents can be administered without dosage adjustment in patients with renal dysfunction. Included among these drugs are nafcillin, ceftriaxone, doxycycline, azithromycin, and linezolid. Although linezolid exposure is not significantly altered, microbiologically inactive metabolites of the compound do accumulate in end-stage renal disease; what, if any effect this has is unknown.

At the other extreme, a number of antimicrobial agents require major dosage adjustments in the presence of renal dysfunction. The dosing interval for ceftazidime, usually administered every 8 hours in patients with normal renal function, is extended to once every 48 hours in persons with creatinine clearance below 10 mL/min. Vancomycin is also administered at substantially increased dosing intervals in those with end-stage renal disease, sometimes as infrequently as once weekly. However, because of the increased efficiency of newer hemodialysis membranes in removing vancomycin, dosing is usually based on measured serum drug concentrations and may be required as frequently as each dialysis session.

In some instances, clearance of the antimicrobial agent is not affected by renal dysfunction, but excipients may accumulate with the potential for toxic effects. For example, clearance of the antifungal agent voriconazole is not dependent on renal function. However, the intravenous preparation of this antimicrobial contains the solubilizing agent sulfobutyl ether β-cyclodextrin, which does accumulate in the presence of renal insufficiency. With renal dysfunction the intravenous preparation should not be used, but the oral formulation, which does not contain β-cyclodextrin, can be administered. Amprenavir oral solution is another example of a formulation that is contraindicated in patients with renal failure, even though the antiretroviral itself is cleared by nonrenal mechanisms. In this case, the oral solution contains large amounts of propylene glycol, which can accumulate to toxic levels in patients with renal dysfunction.

A number of other antimicrobials potentially accumulate in the presence of severe liver disease, with the possibility of an increased risk for adverse events. Examples of antimicrobials requiring dose adjustments for various levels of hepatic insufficiency include metronidazole, chloramphenicol, tigecycline, caspofungin, and voriconazole. For ceftriaxone, dosage adjustments or careful monitoring may be required in patients with both hepatic and renal dysfunction. Several of the newer antimicrobials, such as daptomycin, linezolid, and micafungin, have not been studied sufficiently to determine whether dosing modifications are required in patients with severe liver disease.

Drug-Drug Interactions

One of the most important considerations in the selection of an appropriate antimicrobial regimen is to determine whether the drug or drugs will interact with other medications that the patient is taking. Some drug-drug interactions can have severe or even fatal consequences. There are too many potential interactions to list comprehensively, but some examples are provided in this section. Fortunately, resources are now available that allow the clinician to check for potential drug-drug interactions when an antimicrobial agent is ordered.

A large number of antimicrobials are eliminated via cytochrome P-450 pathways. As a result, they may interfere with the elimination of other drugs cleared by these pathways and lead to their accumulation to potentially dangerous levels. Several macrolide antibacterials, some fluoroquinolones, and human immunodeficiency virus (HIV) protease inhibitors are among the most likely antimicrobials to inhibit the clearance of other drugs. For example, use of the protease inhibitor nelfinavir is contraindicated with several drugs, including the antiarrhythmics amiodarone and quinidine, ergot derivatives, the neuroleptic drug pimozide, and certain sedative/hypnotic agents. Macrolides may result in increased levels of 3-hydroxy-3-methylglutaryl coenzyme A (HMG-CoA) reductase inhibitors, which can lead to rhabdomyolysis. Quinupristin-dalfopristin is not itself eliminated by the cytochrome P-450 system, but this drug does inhibit the elimination of various agents cleared by this pathway, including cyclosporine, midazolam, nifedipine, and others.

In contrast, administration of rifampin induces the cytochrome P-450 system and may enhance the clearance of other drugs, some of which have narrow therapeutic windows. This may result in a number of important effects, including reduced effectiveness of oral contraceptives and increasing warfarin requirements to maintain desired levels of anticoagulation. It is very important to remember these potential interactions not only when starting rifampin therapy but also when *stopping* treatment. When rifampin is stopped, unless the previously increased dose of warfarin is adjusted downward accordingly, over-anticoagulation and possibly serious bleeding can occur.

A number of other drug interactions have been described. Linezolid has weak monoamine oxidase inhibitor activity. As such, it has the potential to enhance the hypertensive effect of adrenergic agonists and has been associated with the development of serotonin syndrome in patients taking selective serotonin re-uptake inhibitors (SSRIs). Patients with this syndrome can exhibit a number of signs and symptoms, including fever, tachycardia, tremulousness, agitation, confusion, clonus, and others, occasionally with fatal results. Serotonin syndrome has been described in patients taking linezolid together with drugs other than SSRIs and could in principle occur when linezolid is combined with any of a large number of agents that increase serotonin concentrations in the central nervous system.

Other Host Factors

Several additional host factors may influence the choice of a suitable antimicrobial regimen. Some antimicrobials have the potential to induce hemolysis in persons with glucose-6-phosphate dehydrogenase deficiency. Among the drugs that should be avoided in these individuals are primaquine, nitrofurantoin, and various sulfonamides.

Coexisting diseases should also be taken into account. Use of fluoroquinolones such as gatifloxacin has been associated with abnormalities in glucose homeostasis. Although it would be desirable to avoid hyperglycemia or hypoglycemia in anyone, patients with diabetes mellitus might be disproportionately affected by such events. Hyperkalemia has been observed in patients with renal insufficiency during treatment with trimethoprim-sulfamethoxazole because trimethoprim blocks renal potassium excretion in the distal tubule. Because of the common occurrence of renal disease in persons with diabetes mellitus, it is best to avoid or limit the use of potentially nephrotoxic agents such as aminoglycosides in this population, if possible.

Several examples can be cited in which the occupation of the patient could play a role in selection of a treatment regimen. Antibiotics that can cause transient (minocycline) or permanent (streptomycin) dizziness or unsteadiness may create hazardous situations in those whose occupations require excellent balance. Antimicrobial agents with potential to cause photosensitivity, such as tetracyclines, fluoroquinolones, trimethoprim, and sulfonamides, may be problematic in persons with high levels of sustained sun exposure during outdoor employment or other activities.

ANTIMICROBIAL COMBINATIONS

It is very common for hospitalized patients to receive more than one antimicrobial agent simultaneously. The rationale for using antimicrobials in combination is not always clearly defined, and there are a number of potential disadvantages to combination therapy. The basis for using combination therapy is considered in this section.

Possible Reasons for Using Combination Antimicrobial Therapy

Clinical indications for using combination antimicrobial therapy fall into one of five categories. Two of these categories (empirical therapy and polymicrobial infections) relate to maximizing the likelihood that at least one agent of the combination will be active against known or suspected pathogens. The other three reasons for using combinations (minimizing toxicity, preventing the emergence of resistance, and obtaining synergistic inhibition or killing) attempt to exploit unique advantages of the combinations as compared with any component drug alone.

Broad Coverage during Empirical Therapy

A common reason for using more than one antimicrobial in hospitalized patients is to provide broad coverage against potential pathogens and to maximize the likelihood of delivering an active antimicrobial agent as quickly as possible to seriously ill patients. When the pathogen is unknown, the choice of antimicrobials will often include an agent broadly active against gram-positive bacteria, including methicillin-resistant *S. aureus* (MRSA), such as vancomycin, as well as an agent active against aerobic or facultative gram-negative bacteria. Selection of the latter will be strongly influenced by local patterns of antimicrobial resistance specific to the institution and might include an extended-spectrum cephalosporin, an aminoglycoside, a fluoroquinolone, a β-lactam–β-lactamase inhibitor drug, or a carbapenem. The latter two choices would also provide activity against gram-negative anaerobes if desired, such as for an intra-abdominal infection. Alternatively, one could add an agent such as metronidazole to provide anaerobic activity. In some situations, for patients who are not severely ill, a β-lactam might be used empirically as monotherapy when MRSA or other β-lactam–resistant gram-positive organisms are deemed unlikely pathogens.

Because of the high frequency of antibiotic resistance in *Pseudomonas aeruginosa* isolates, in settings in which *P. aeruginosa* is encountered frequently, empirical use of two agents with antipseudomonal activity could be justified to maximize the likelihood that at least one of the agents will inhibit the organism.

Combination therapy is widely used in the initial treatment of hospitalized patients with community-acquired pneumonia. Commonly used regimens include a third-generation cephalosporin such as ceftriaxone with a macrolide or fluoroquinolone. The cephalosporin provides antimicrobial activity against *S. pneumoniae, Haemophilus influenzae, Moraxella catarrhalis,* and several other "typical" bacterial pathogens associated with community-acquired pneumonia, with the notable exception of MRSA, which can sometimes cause pneumonia in outpatients. The macrolide—azithromycin is commonly used—or the fluoroquinolone inhibits "atypical" bacteria that cause pneumonia, including *M. pneumoniae, C. pneumoniae,* and *Legionella* sp. Although fluoroquinolones approved for respiratory tract infections are likely to cover most or all of the organisms targeted by the cephalosporin, isolates of *S. pneumoniae* resistant to fluoroquinolones do exist, so many clinicians prefer the extra security of combination therapy in patients with severe pneumonia requiring hospitalization.

Treatment of Documented Polymicrobial Infections

For many infections from which two or more pathogens are recovered, it is possible to provide adequate coverage with a single, broadly active antimicrobial agent. Switching to a single agent reduces exposure of the patient to potential antibiotic toxicities, is usually more convenient for nursing, and may be less expensive. For some patients, susceptibility profiles or allergy to broad spectrum agents justifies the use of antibiotic combinations for treatment of polymicrobial infections.

Attempts to Reduce Toxicity

It is theoretically possible to use two or more drugs of different classes, with additive antimicrobial activities and independent toxicities, each at relatively low doses to achieve sufficient potency while avoiding toxicity. However, there are no instances in current bacterial therapy in which the approach of using submaximal doses of multiple agents is predictably effective in accomplishing this goal. This does not exclude the possibility that in isolated instances a successful response may be attained when drugs with marginal activity are combined. In antifungal therapy, combinations of antifungal agents can potentially improve the clinical response when poor results are noted with the usual doses of individual drugs and toxicities preclude further dose escalation of a single agent.

Preventing the Emergence of Drug Resistance

Antimicrobial use in the treatment of tuberculosis provides the paradigm for using combination drugs in an attempt to prevent the emergence of resistance to any one agent. The basis for this approach is that if resistance to two different agents occurs by independent mechanisms, the probability of resistance developing to both drugs will be the product of the probability of resistance to each drug, which is likely to be very low, so resistance should not emerge. For example, if the frequency of resistance to drug A is 10^{-6} and that of resistance to drug B is 10^{-7}, resistance to both drugs should be encountered no more frequently than once in 10^{13} colonies.

Similar reasoning has justified the use of combination regimens when rifampin is required for the treatment of nonmycobacterial infections. Rifampin is not used alone (with rare exceptions, such as brief courses for eradication of meningococcal carriage) because resistance to this agent emerges quickly. As mentioned earlier, rifampin is particularly useful in the treatment of infections related to foreign devices because of its activity against biofilm-associated bacteria. In such use, it is combined with another active antimicrobial, such as vancomycin for coagulase-negative staphylococcal prosthetic valve endocarditis (usually with a brief course of gentamicin as well to reduce the bacterial inoculum further at the beginning of therapy) or a fluoroquinolone for orthopedic device–related infections.

It has been more difficult to show unequivocally that combination therapy provides protection against the emergence of resistance to antimicrobial drugs in other situations, including infections caused by *P. aeruginosa* or *Enterobacter* sp. There are two plausible explanations why combinations may not prevent resistance predictably. First, there may be differential penetration of the two antimicrobials to an infected site or differences in activity at the site of infection. Thus, a more readily penetrating agent may be left relatively unprotected in a privileged site of infection. Second, for many commonly encountered bacteria, resistance mechanisms against unrelated antimicrobial classes may not be truly independent. Some bacterial efflux pumps recognize chemically unrelated substrates, so upregulation of pump activity may confer resistance to several classes of antimicrobials. In other instances there may be coordinated upregulation of efflux mechanisms and downregulation of outer membrane protein channels (porins), again potentially conferring resistance simultaneously to two or more antimicrobial classes.

Use of Combinations to Attain Synergism

Decades ago, the surprising benefits of using penicillin and streptomycin together for the treatment of enterococcal endocarditis were discovered empirically. Penicillin alone usually inhibits but does not kill enterococci, and failure rates were high when penicillin G was used alone to treat enterococcal endocarditis. Streptomycin has no significant activity against enterococci at clinically relevant concentrations. However, the combination results in bactericidal synergism in vitro and high cure rates in patients with enterococcal endocarditis. Detailed studies of this phenomenon demonstrated that in the presence of a cell wall–active antibiotic, uptake of the aminoglycoside into the bacterial cell increases substantially. Unfortunately, increasing rates of high-level resistance to streptomycin (MIC >2000 μg/mL) or to gentamicin (MIC >500 μg/mL), or both, has nullified the benefit of such combinations against a substantial number of enterococcal isolates today. An example of bactericidal synergism between vancomycin and gentamicin against an *Enterococcus* isolate is illustrated in Figure 301–1A.

Since the early demonstrations of synergistic killing of enterococci, combinations of cell wall–active agents plus aminoglycosides have been shown to achieve synergistic killing against a broad range of gram-positive and gram-negative bacteria when tested in vitro. Modest clinical benefits were shown when short courses of gentamicin were added to nafcillin for the treatment of *S. aureus* endocarditis. Against strains of viridans streptococci that are relatively insensitive to penicillin, the addition of an aminoglycoside for the first 2 weeks of a 4-week course of penicillin G is believed to result in a higher likelihood of cure.

Once considered important in the treatment of gram-negative bacterial infections, especially in immunocompromised (e.g., neutropenic) patients, the clinical value of a synergistic combination of a cell wall–active agent and an aminoglycoside has been difficult to prove in recent experience. To a large extent, the introduction of agents with very potent

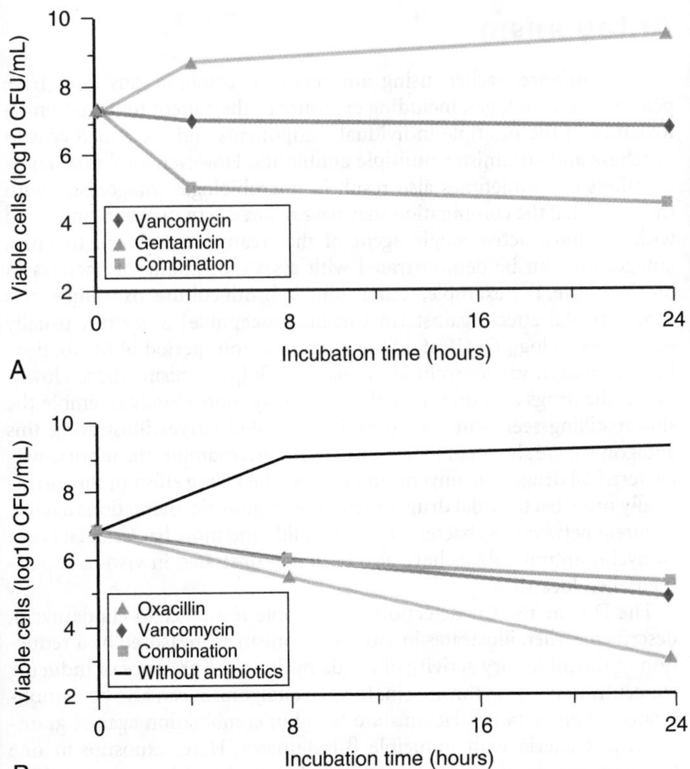

FIGURE 301–1 • Bactericidal synergism and antagonism. A, Bactericidal synergism between vancomycin (diamonds) and gentamicin (triangles) against an isolate of *Enterococcus* sp. Killing by the combination (squares) is substantially greater than by each agent alone. **B,** Antagonism of the bactericidal activity of oxacillin (triangles) against an isolate of *Staphylococcus aureus* by the more slowly bactericidal agent vancomycin (diamonds). Killing by the combination (squares) is less than that by oxacillin alone. Growth in the absence of antibiotics is shown by the solid line without markers. CFU = colony-forming units.

activity against gram-negative bacteria has diminished interest in and the perceived value of synergistic combinations. Nevertheless, there is some evidence that administering two or more active drugs for empirical therapy may achieve a better outcome than possible with a single active agent for *P. aeruginosa* infections, especially in neutropenic patients. Soon after the introduction of ciprofloxacin, high rates of inhibitory synergism against *P. aeruginosa* were demonstrated in vitro when antipseudomonal β-lactams were combined with this fluoroquinolone. In recent years, however, an increasing proportion of isolates have become resistant to fluoroquinolones, as well as to antipseudomonal β-lactams. Although resistance does not preclude the possibility of synergistic interactions, it is unlikely that such positive interactions would occur as frequently today as was documented 2 decades ago.

The combination of sulfamethoxazole with trimethoprim, agents that block sequential steps in folic acid synthesis, can also achieve bactericidal (or bacteriostatic) synergism against a number of important gram-positive and gram-negative pathogens. This agent has been available for more than 30 years and still enjoys wide use. Quinupristin and dalfopristin are streptogramin antibiotics that display inhibitory activity against gram-positive organisms. Combining these two agents results in bactericidal synergism against organisms susceptible to both. Quinupristin-dalfopristin is provided as a 30:70 mixture of the two components and is approved for the treatment of staphylococcal or streptococcal complicated skin and skin structure infections and for infections caused by vancomycin-resistant enterococci that are associated with bacteremia.

β-Lactam–β-lactamase inhibitor antimicrobials represent another example of synergistic combinations. Four drugs of this category are currently marketed in the United States: amoxicillin-clavulanate, ampicillin-sulbactam, ticarcillin-clavulanate, and piperacillin-tazobactam. The β-lactamase inhibitors themselves, clavulanic acid, sulbactam, and tazobactam, are devoid of significant antimicrobial activity, with rare exceptions. However, by inhibiting the common β-lactamases that are sensitive to these agents, the inhibitors restore the activity of the hydrolyzable penicillins against many target pathogens elaborating these enzymes.

Antagonism

As mentioned earlier, using antimicrobial combinations does have possible disadvantages, including exposure of the patient to the potential toxicities of the multiple individual components and the added cost to purchase and administer multiple antibiotics. However, antibiotic combinations can sometimes also result in microbiologic antagonism, with the result that the combination may have *reduced* activity when compared with the most active single agent of the treatment regimen. In vitro, antagonism can be demonstrated with assays for killing of bacteria in broth culture. For example, tested alone in broth culture, oxacillin exerts a bactericidal effect against (methicillin-susceptible) *S. aureus*, usually defined as ≥3 $\log_{10}$ CFU/mL killing over a 24-hour period of incubation. In such assays, vancomycin alone tends to kill organisms more slowly. When the drugs are combined, the result may more closely resemble the slower killing seen with vancomycin. Time-kill curves illustrating this antagonism are shown in Figure 301–1B. In this example, the more slowly bactericidal drug, vancomycin, antagonizes the killing effect of the intrinsically more bactericidal drug, oxacillin. Antagonistic interactions against *S. aureus* between less bactericidal (linezolid) and more bactericidal (vancomycin) antimicrobials have also been demonstrated in vivo in experimental endocarditis.

The D-zone test for detection of inducible resistance to clindamycin, described earlier, illustrates in vitro antagonism as measured by a reduction of the inhibitory activity of clindamycin in the presence of inducing concentrations of erythromycin. In vitro antagonism can also be demonstrated when certain β-lactams are tested in combination against gram-negative bacteria with inducible β-lactamases. Here, exposure to one β-lactam can de-repress the synthesis of inducible β-lactamases, which then degrade the second antibiotic.

The most striking example of clinically important antagonism emerged from studies on the treatment of bacterial meningitis. In 1951, Lepper and Dowling reported pneumococcal meningitis mortality rates of 21% in patients treated with penicillin alone. For patients who also received chlortetracycline, the mortality rate was greatly increased at 79%. In this case, inhibition of bacterial growth by the bacteriostatic agent (chlortetracycline) is believed to have compromised the bactericidal activity of penicillin, which is greatest against actively growing bacteria.

Nevertheless, it is uncommon to encounter clinically apparent antagonism between antibiotics in the patient care setting, in part because offending combinations such as the ones described in the preceding paragraphs are not very likely to be used in routine clinical care today. However, if in desperation unusual antimicrobial combinations are used increasingly against isolates exhibiting multiple drug resistance, it is possible that clinically relevant antagonism will be encountered more often in the future. Antagonism of bactericidal activities may also be difficult to detect in clinical practice because most common infections (with the exception of endocarditis and meningitis) do not unequivocally benefit from bactericidal therapy. As long as one agent maintains inhibitory activity, it is unlikely that failure resulting from antagonism will be observed.

CONSIDERATIONS IN ANTIMICROBIAL ADMINISTRATION

Route of Administration

In almost all instances, antimicrobial therapy for infections of mild to moderate severity that are usually treated in the outpatient setting can be undertaken with oral agents. There are notable exceptions, such as the use of intramuscular injections of procaine penicillin for the treatment of syphilis or ceftriaxone for the treatment of otitis media or gonorrhea caused by strains resistant to oral agents.

Drugs such as levofloxacin and linezolid demonstrate virtually complete bioavailability when administered by the oral route in persons with normally functioning gastrointestinal tracts and can be used by this route as an alternative to intravenous therapy in many patients with more serious infections. Even for these well-absorbed antimicrobials, however, treatment of seriously ill patients in the hospital is often initiated with intravenous formulations because of the uncertainty of gastrointestinal tract function under conditions of hemodynamic instability.

Antimicrobial therapy can be administered by other routes, including topical administration for the treatment of infected skin lesions (e.g., mupirocin ointment) and intravaginal administration for candidiasis (e.g., azole creams) or for bacterial vaginosis (e.g., metronidazole gel). Topical administration *onto* the eye is used to treat conjunctivitis or as adjunctive therapy for deeper infections or *into* the globe itself as a component of regimens for the treatment of endophthalmitis. Infections associated with peritoneal dialysis are frequently treated by intraperitoneal instillation of antimicrobials admixed with the dialysis solution. Rarely, direct administration into the thecal space or into the cerebral ventricles is necessary for the treatment of meningitis when the required antimicrobials do not achieve adequate concentrations in cerebrospinal fluid after systemic administration. Vancomycin, almost always given orally but occasionally directly into the intestine, is used for the intraluminal treatment of *Clostridium difficile*–associated diarrhea.

The availability of protocols for the outpatient use of long venous catheters, whether inserted centrally or peripherally, has made it possible to administer antimicrobial therapy increasingly outside the hospital for agents that are not well absorbed after oral administration. Thus, many patients who require long-term antibiotic treatment for infections such as endocarditis, osteomyelitis, neuroborreliosis, and other conditions can be treated as outpatients after an initial period of hospitalization that may be required for full assessment of the infection, initiation of therapy, and stabilization of the medical condition. In addition to monitoring for adverse effects from the antibiotic itself, patients treated via indwelling intravenous devices also require close observation for complications related to the catheter, such as thrombophlebitis, entry site infections, or line-related blood stream infections.

Pharmacodynamic Considerations

In recent years, the scientific basis for selection of dosing regimens has extended well beyond empirical dosing strategies designed primarily from the pharmacokinetic characteristics of antimicrobial agents. Pharmacodynamic considerations relate the time course of antibiotic concentrations after dosing with the observed antimicrobial effects against likely pathogens and with the potential adverse effects of the agent.

Studies of the pharmacokinetic and pharmacodynamic properties of antimicrobial agents allow prediction of their activities with various dosing regimens. For β-lactam antibiotics, the time that the concentration of free drug (i.e., the non–protein-bound fraction) exceeds the MIC of the pathogen best relates to antimicrobial effectiveness in animal models. This provides the rationale for the frequent dosing schedules of β-lactams with short half-lives, such as penicillin G and the antistaphylococcal penicillins.

In contrast, the aminoglycosides and fluoroquinolones demonstrate concentration-dependent killing of bacteria. For these drugs, animal models show that either the ratio of "peak concentration to MIC" or "area under the 24-hour drug concentration curve (AUC) to MIC" would better predict effectiveness. With these agents, less frequent, higher dosing would be expected to be optimal. For the aminoglycosides, less frequent dosing may also allow more time for washout of the drug from the kidney, thus potentially minimizing the risk for nephrotoxicity; however, the advantages of this approach are not striking.

For vancomycin, the most important index for clinical success is less clear. Although killing by vancomycin is not generally concentration dependent, some data point to the importance of AUC/MIC or even peak/MIC ratios. For this drug, it may be more important to maintain adequate trough serum concentrations when treating serious infections. For daptomycin, the adoption of once-daily dosing largely mitigated the muscle toxicity that had been seen earlier with more frequent dosing and allowed development of this agent for serious gram-positive infections.

MONITORING ANTIMICROBIAL CONCENTRATIONS

From a practical point of view, there are few situations in which assays to determine concentrations of antimicrobials in blood or body fluids are readily available. Commercial assays for measurement of serum aminoglycoside concentrations are available and, because of the great potential for toxicity of these agents, are used frequently to detect excessively high trough concentrations, which may either predispose to or result from nephrotoxicity. Commercial assays to measure vancomycin concentrations are also widely available, although their usefulness for routine care has been debated. In most cases, adequate dosing can be derived from standard nomograms based on estimates of creatinine clearance. It may be prudent to monitor serum concentrations of vancomycin in patients with unstable renal function, undergoing hemodialysis, at the extremes of body composition, or with particularly serious infections in which high concentrations may be desirable. In some young adults, clearance of vancomycin may be so great that unexpectedly low concentrations result with the usual dosing regimens.

In rare cases, standard doses of other antimicrobials may result in unacceptably low concentrations. Therapeutic drug monitoring (measurement of trough concentrations) has been advocated during treatment of HIV infection in highly select circumstances, such as when significant drug-drug interactions are unavoidable; when absorption or elimination cannot be adequately predicted because of gastrointestinal, hepatic, or renal abnormalities; in pregnancy; or when there is an unanticipated failure to respond.

ADMINISTRATIVE ASPECTS RELATING TO ANTIMICROBIAL THERAPY

Formularies

In most practice settings today, the choice of antimicrobials is constrained in some way. For example, in hospitals and other facilities, institutional formularies may limit the choice of antimicrobial agents available, require special approval for the use of selected agents, or both. Such policies can in principle enhance efficiency by avoiding the need to stock and dispense multiple agents with very similar antimicrobial activities, minimize costs by allowing purchase of the most cost-effective alternatives, and have the potential to increase patient safety by allowing clinical personnel to become familiar with a manageable number of agents. In the outpatient setting, where the assignment of oral drugs to various tiers of coverage and copayments by health insurers is common practice, there may be dramatic financial benefits or disincentives to the patient for prescription of specific agents. In both health care settings, the practitioner must become familiar with the options available to patients under these constraints.

Interchangeability

It is important to remember that although two antimicrobials may have antimicrobial spectra that are so similar that only one need be represented on an inpatient or outpatient formulary, it is not always safe to assume that the activity of either agent will be predicted perfectly by susceptibility to the other. For example, for most bacterial species the percentage of isolates susceptible to meropenem and to imipenem will be roughly comparable. However, there are differences in mechanisms of resistance to these two carbapenems, so it is possible that a specific strain will be susceptible to one but resistant to the other. For serious infections, even when two drugs are considered interchangeable, the antimicrobial used should be the one for which susceptibility testing was performed, and vice versa.

Impact on the Institutional Environment

In contrast to other medications that almost always affect only the patient receiving treatment, antimicrobial use can have a significant impact on the institutional environment as well. As a result, it is sometimes necessary or desirable to manage the use of antimicrobial agents on an administrative level to avoid selective pressure leading to the spread of antibiotic resistance. Within institutions, antimicrobial-resistant organisms not only threaten the patient treated with the antimicrobial but can also be transmitted to other vulnerable persons, including those who have not been exposed to the drug.

Faced with the increasing incidence of vancomycin-resistant enterococcal isolates causing infection and colonization in U.S. hospitals, recommendations were presented at a national level in 1995 by the Hospital Infection Control Practices Advisory Committee for the prudent use of vancomycin in health care settings. Temporary constraints on the use of certain antibiotics may also be imposed by institutions to deal with an immediate resistance problem. For example, hospitals attempting to control infections caused by ESBL-producing isolates of *Klebsiella pneumoniae* may place strict limits on the use of cephalosporin antibiotics. Although this approach can be very successful, declines in cephalosporin-resistant *K. pneumoniae* may be accompanied by increases in resistance to the alternative antibiotics used, a phenomenon that illustrates the challenges of attempting to influence institutional resistance rates by policies intended to modify antibiotic use.

SUGGESTED READINGS

Bryskier A (ed): Antimicrobial Agents. Antibacterials and Antifungals. Washington, DC, ASM Press, 2005. *A comprehensive compendium of antimicrobial drugs, their properties, and clinical uses.*

Finberg RW, Moellering RC, Tally FP, et al: The importance of bactericidal drugs: Future directions in infectious diseases. Clin Infect Dis 2004;39:1314–1320. *An expert panel reviewed the roles of bactericidal versus bacteriostatic antibiotics in clinical practice.*

Gilbert DN, Moellering RC Jr, Eliopoulos GM, Sande MA (eds): The Sanford Guide to Antimicrobial Therapy, 36th ed. Sperryville, VA, Antimicrobial Therapy, 2006. *General information for selecting and properly using antimicrobials in clinical care.*

Goossens H, Ferech M, Coenen S, et al: Comparison of outpatient systemic antibacterial use in 2004 in the United States and 27 European countries. Clin Infect Dis 2007;44:1091–1095. *Antibiotic use in the United States is higher than in most European countries.*

Gruchalla RS, Pirmohamed M: Antibiotic allergy. N Engl J Med 2006;354:601–609. *The authors describe strategies to assess patients with a history of antibiotic allergy.*

Hooper DC: Efflux pumps and nosocomial antibiotic resistance: A primer for hospital epidemiologists. Clin Infect Dis 2005;40:1811–1817. *A review of how drug efflux pumps contribute to multiple antibiotic resistance.*

Nahum GG, Kennedy DL: Antibiotic use in pregnancy and lactation. What is and is not known about teratogenic and toxic risks. Obstet Gynecol 2006; 107:1120–1138. *Authors review the pharmacokinetics of selected antibiotics in pregnancy and risks associated with their use.*

Paul M, Silbiger I, Grozinsky S, et al: Beta-lactam antibiotic monotherapy versus beta-lactam–aminoglycoside antibiotic combination therapy for sepsis. Cochrane Database Syst Rev 2005;25:CD003344. *Meta-analysis showed no difference in all-cause mortality in patients with sepsis, including that caused by* P. aeruginosa.

Rybak MJ: The pharmacokinetic and pharmacodynamic properties of vancomycin. Clin Infect Dis 2006;42(Suppl. 1):S35–S39. *Review of vancomycin pharmacodynamics.*

Safdar N, Handelsman J, Maki DG: Does combination antimicrobial therapy reduce mortality in gram-negative bacteremia? A meta-analysis. Lancet Infect Dis 2004;4:519–527. *Combination therapy did not offer a survival advantage except for* P. aeruginosa *infection.*

The choice of antibacterial drugs. Med Lett Drugs Ther 2001;43:69–78. *A practical overview.*

302 APPROACH TO FEVER OR SUSPECTED INFECTION IN THE NORMAL HOST

James Leggett

Infectious diseases remain the most common cause of mortality worldwide and have profoundly influenced our individual physiology and the course of history of our civilizations. Although infectious diseases were thought to be on the verge of being conquered in the 1960s, much focus is now on "emerging" infectious diseases caused by new pathogens, reemergence of previously controlled infections, and new recognition of the infectious etiology of disease previously ascribed to other causes.

We are constantly exposed to microorganisms via our environment, our skin, or our mucosal membranes. Most microorganisms are adapted to niches in the environment that make them avirulent to us. Pathogens in a normal host are relatively few, and most of the time exposure results in only transient or stable colonization. Infection is defined as invasion of a pathogen that triggers an immune response, whether the infection is asymptomatic or symptomatic. Manifestations of infection are protean and due as much to our immune response as to attributes of the particular pathogen.

The inflammatory response that accompanies infection is usually marked by fever. Fever is a tightly controlled elevation in body temperature above the normal range in response to a central nervous system change in the set point. Defining normal body temperature is somewhat problematic because it is dependent on both physiology and methodology. Normal oral temperature in 99% of the population ranges from 36.0 to 37.7° C, with a circadian variation of 1° C or more between the morning nadir and the evening peak. Mean oral temperature in healthy adults is 36.8 ± 0.4° C, with women exhibiting slightly higher values (36.9 vs. 36.7° C). In menstruating women, morning temperatures may rise by 0.6° C with ovulation and remain higher until menses occur. Measured rectal temperatures are 0.4° C higher than oral and 0.8° C higher than aural (tympanic membrane) temperatures. However, considerable individual variability exists. Clinicians generally define significant fever as a temperature higher than 38.3° C (101.0° F). Despite historical claims, fever patterns do not appear to be especially helpful in establishing a specific diagnosis.

The vast majority of acute febrile illnesses lasting less than 2 weeks have an infectious etiology. These infections occur predominantly where body surfaces interact with the environment, such as the upper and lower respiratory tracts, gastrointestinal and genitourinary systems, and the skin. The majority of these acute respiratory and gastrointestinal infections are viral in nature. As the duration of the febrile illness lengthens beyond 3 weeks, other inflammatory illnesses enter more prominently into the differential diagnosis. Most chronic febrile illnesses are not caused by infection.

PATHOBIOLOGY OF INFECTION AND FEVER

Infection ensues only when a pathogen overcomes both nonspecific innate and specific adaptive humoral and cellular immune responses. The normal indigenous microflora, host physical barriers (e.g., skin, mucous membranes, cilia), and soluble factors (e.g., cytokines, complement) provide an important barricade to pathogen invasion. Disruption of these barriers, which provide a first line of defense, permits invasion of pathogens. The acute phase response triggered by such disruption provides direct antimicrobial activity and prompts the development of adaptive immunity mediated by lymphocytes and macrophages. This inflammatory response plays an important role in containing infection. Unfortunately, an exaggerated response may worsen the clinical condition. It is the neutrophil response that causes the damage seen in septic arthritis and the unchecked immune response that precipitates the systemic inflammatory response syndrome.

Fever has been recognized as an important sign of infection since ancient times. Body temperature is regulated both physiologically and behaviorally. Basal metabolic processes, governed especially by thyroid hormones but also by catecholamines and growth hormone, are responsible for the normal resting body temperature. Moderate activity increases thermogenesis and results in transiently increased temperature until heat-dissipating processes are engaged. Each 1° F increase in temperature results in a 7% increase in the basal metabolic rate. Vaporization from the lungs and skin accounts for a third of basal body heat loss and as much as all heat loss at ambient dry temperatures above 36° C. Thermogenesis may be increased up to 80% by hyperthyroidism and decreased as much as 50% by hypothyroidism. The elderly show a decrease in basal metabolism, with an average 0.5° C lower body temperature, as well as blunted responses to thermogenetic stimuli.

The hypothalamus contains temperature-sensitive neurons that have receptors for pro-inflammatory and anti-inflammatory cytokines, which are continuously balanced to maintain a homeothermic set point. When body temperature becomes elevated, cutaneous vasodilation and sweating occur, and people may reduce activity and seek a cooler environment. Inversely, low body temperature is increased by shivering, piloerection, cutaneous vasoconstriction, adding clothes, and seeking a warmer environment. In a febrile illness, symptoms may be due to the underlying disease or the fever itself. Malaise is the rule, and many febrile patients experience myalgia secondary to the muscle contractions used to generate temperature elevation. Although it has been thought that the back and thigh pain related to rigors suggests bacteremia, any febrile stimulus may produce such symptoms. The chill associated with rigors may be related to the surface vasoconstriction that accompanies the increase in core temperature.

Fever is a complex physiologic process involving metabolic and immunologic responses (Fig. 302–1). Exogenous pyrogens cause fever largely through mediation of endogenous pro-inflammatory pyrogenic cytokines produced by phagocytic leukocytes, including interleukin-1 (IL-1), IL-2, IL-6, tumor necrosis factor-α, and interferon-γ. These cytokines stimulate the immune responses of T and B cells, macrophages, and polymorphonuclear leukocytes. They appear to act via a common mechanism involving the induction of prostaglandin synthesis. Feedback inhibitory responses are mediated by adrenocorticotropic hormone, arginine vasopressin, serotonin, dopamine, and other homeostatic mechanisms, thus emphasizing the orchestrated nature of fever production and response to infection. These thermoregulatory mechanisms rarely allow fevers to exceed 41° C (106° F). Temperatures exceeding 41° C are often due to drug-induced imbalance in these mechanisms and may cause direct cellular damage.

Failure of fever to develop during severe bacterial infection has, in some studies, been associated with higher morbidity and mortality. Whether this is due to absence of fever per se or associated conditions such as chronic renal failure or corticosteroid use has not been determined. Favorable effects of fever on host-microbe interactions are suggested by inhibited multiplication of some pathogens such as *Streptococcus pneumoniae* and *Treponema pallidum*, reduced proliferation of pathogens in the presence of hypoferremia, augmented complement-mediated lysis, and increased neutrophil entry into inflammatory sites. Temperature-pulse dissociation, in which there is relative bradycardia as compared with the usual increase in pulse of about 10 beats/min/1° F, has been described in typhoid fever, leptospirosis, brucellosis, and drug-induced fever, for unclear reasons.

No laboratory abnormalities accompany typical benign acute viral infections. Leukocytosis of various lineages is usually seen in other infections in immunocompetent adults. Neutrophilia is the norm in most acute infections, whatever the etiology. The elderly, though not mounting a neutrophilic response, generally display bandemia during an acute bacterial infection. Neutropenia may be seen in rickettsial, severe viral, and overwhelming bacterial infections. Eosinophilia is typical of invasive helminthic and some protozoal infections. Lymphocytosis may accompany many viral and rickettsial infections and is common during

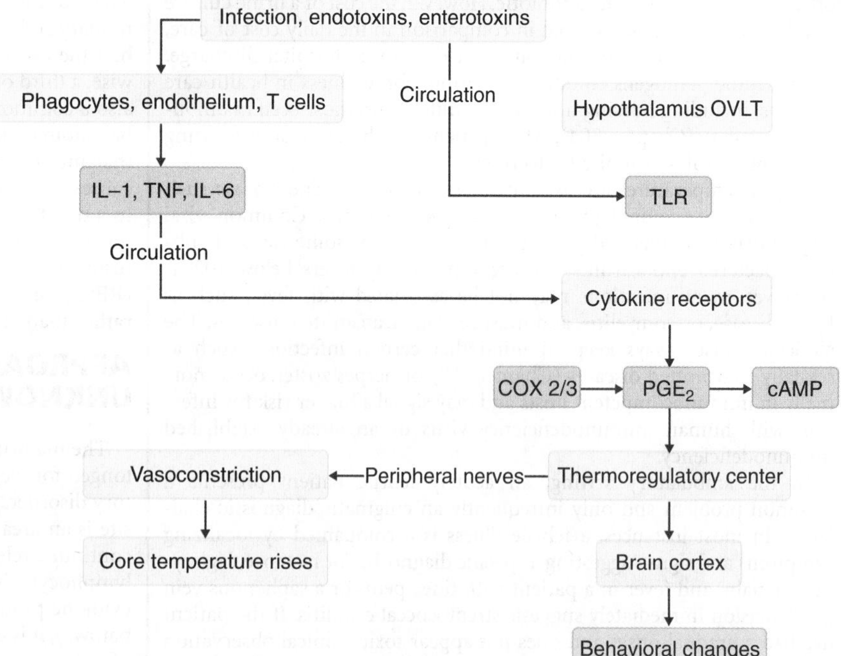

FIGURE 302–1 • Pathways leading to the production of fever in bacterial infection, whether local or systemic. Bacteria release cell wall products such as peptidoglycans and endotoxin, as well as enterotoxins, that bind to toll-like receptors (TLRs) on phagocytes (neutrophils, macrophages) and endothelial cells. As a result, pyrogenic cytokines such as interleukin-1 (IL-1) and IL-6 or tumor necrosis factor-α (TNF-α) are released into the circulation and bind to cytokine receptors in the hypothalamic organum vasculosum laminae terminalis (OVLT). Bacterial products may also directly bind to TLRs on the OVLT. Activation of TLRs and cytokine receptors induces cyclooxygenase-2 (COX-2), which leads to the production of prostaglandin E_2 (PGE_2) and results in the release of cyclic adenosine monophosphate (cAMP) in the brain. This, in turn, triggers neurons in the thermoregulatory center to raise the hypothalamic thermostatic set point. In addition, neuronal signals to the cortex prompt behavioral changes to conserve heat (e.g., posturing, clothing). The hypothalamus also triggers sympathetic peripheral efferent nerves that constrict peripheral blood vessels and conserve central heat until hypothalamic PGE_2 levels fall.

convalescence from acute bacterial infection. Monocytosis may be seen in tuberculosis. Virtually all infections have an impact on the erythroid system, but given the long half-life of erythrocytes, only chronic infections or other inflammatory diseases usually result in anemia. Few acute infections rapidly produce anemia. For instance, *Helicobacter pylori* may induce a bleeding ulcer, *Plasmodium falciparum* may directly lyse erythrocytes, overwhelming bacterial infections associated with disseminated intravascular coagulopathy may cause hemolytic anemia, and *Mycoplasma pneumoniae* may induce immunologically mediated hemolysis.

APPROACH TO FEBRILE ILLNESS IN OUTPATIENTS AND INPATIENTS

Infectious disease epidemiology depends on the interaction between pathogens, susceptible hosts, and environmental conditions allowing exposure. Most infections are transmitted horizontally between people via contact (e.g., hands, fomites), a common vehicle (e.g., food, water), air (e.g., tuberculosis), or vectors (e.g., mosquitoes). Evaluation of a patient with a known or possible infection should determine whether the condition might be due to a transmissible agent, its source, recent travel, whether there are secondary causes, and what measures need to be taken to contact health department officials and prevent additional infections.

The age of a patient influences which illnesses should be considered. Natural exposure or immunization generally limits certain illnesses to children and adolescents, such as rubeola, rubella, or varicella. Waning of immunity may likewise lead to pertussis in young adults or reactivation of tuberculosis in the elderly. Other physiologic effects of aging, such as impaired bladder emptying, lead to increased rates of urinary tract infection in the elderly.

A patient's occupation and travel history should be noted. An abattoir worker would more likely have been exposed to *Brucella* (Chapter 331) than someone with another occupation. Indiana residents would more likely be infected with histoplasmosis (Chapter 353), whereas those from the Southwest desert may have coccidioidomycosis (Chapter 354) in a similar febrile illness. Many other illnesses are likewise directly related to specific geographic exposure, with varying incubation times before their onset. Typhoid fever should be manifested within a few weeks, whereas amebic liver abscess might take months to cause symptoms after return of a traveler from endemic areas (Table 302–1). The Centers for Disease Control and Prevention website and many others provide more specific information about prevalent infections in all parts of the globe (available at *http://www.cdc.gov*).

Many travelers return home with fever occurring after a variable incubation time, generally with other symptoms and signs as well. The first

TABLE 302–1 SELECTED EXAMPLES OF FEVER AND RECENT TRAVEL

	Incubation Period	
Disease	**<2–3 wk**	**>3–4 wk**
COMMON		
Diarrhea	+	
Entamebic liver abscess		+
Enteric fever	+	
Malaria	+	+
Pulmonary tuberculosis		+
Viral hepatitis		+
LESS COMMON		
Brucellosis		+
Ehrlichiosis	+	
Leptospirosis	+	
Schistosomiasis		+
Viral (hemorrhagic, encephalitic)	+	
Visceral leishmaniasis		+

consideration in evaluating such a patient is that an infection that might just as easily have been acquired without travel is more likely the cause of the illness. Once such routine infections have been ruled out, the differential diagnosis should include infections related to travel, whether within a region of the country or abroad (Chapter 308). For example, prompt evaluation of patients who have traveled to malaria-endemic areas should be undertaken and blood tests performed to determine the presence of parasites. It is not simply international travel that requires knowledge about the geography of diseases, but also travel to parts of the United States where there are geographically focal infections (e.g., ehrlichiosis, Colorado Tick Fever, hantavirus) and Europe (e.g., visceral leishmaniasis, tick-borne encephalitis).

The setting in which a febrile illness occurs influences both the diagnostic approach and the differential diagnosis. In the ambulatory arena, with a generally healthy febrile patient, the clinician should not necessarily pursue a diagnosis as aggressively as with a hospitalized or chronically ill patient. Empirical treatment of a presumed urinary tract infection is warranted for an outpatient, where the cost of a culture is often more than that of the antibiotic. However, the cost of a urine culture in a hospital setting is minimal in comparison to the daily cost of care, and accurately identifying the pathogen may speed hospital discharge. Likewise, the pathogens commonly causing febrile illness in health care facilities, including nursing homes, may differ from those seen in ambulatory settings (Chapter 304). Most patients in the ambulatory setting have noncritical, self-limited infections.

Higher temperatures are usually due to invasive visceral disease such as community-acquired pneumonia or pyelonephritis. Common viral respiratory infections and gastroenteritis, as well as some cases of subacute bacterial endocarditis, are accompanied by fevers below 102° F. Moreover, many infections may not be associated with fever, such as Lyme disease, osteomyelitis, and most sexually transmitted diseases. The clinician must always keep in mind that certain infections, such as sexually transmitted diseases (Chapter 307) or herpes zoster, occur normally in immunocompetent hosts and may signal a higher risk for infection with human immunodeficiency virus or an already established immunodeficiency.

In the ambulatory setting, an acutely febrile patient presents a common problem and only infrequently an enigmatic diagnostic challenge. In most instances, a febrile illness is accompanied by localizing symptoms and signs suggesting a specific diagnosis. For instance, leg erythema, pain, and fever in a patient with tinea pedis or a saphenous vein graft incision immediately suggests streptococcal cellulitis. If the patient has had a gradual onset and does not appear toxic, clinical observation and follow-up are all that are required. A toxic patient generally exhibits tachycardia, tachypnea, and apprehension or confusion accompanying localized findings. If the patient appears toxic, several clinically focused diagnostic studies should be performed immediately and the patient considered for hospitalization. When a patient has fever and only nonspecific constitutional symptoms, it may be more difficult to address the problem in a single, ambulatory clinic visit. A balance between observation and investigation of serious illness must be undertaken in such a situation.

Fever and leukocytosis are probably the main clinical parameters for evaluating potential infections in hospitalized patients. However, about 10% of nosocomial bacteremias occur without fever, and health care–associated infections occur without fever in a substantial proportion of patients who are elderly or have significant comorbid conditions. Most cases of hospital-associated fever represent nosocomial infection, which typically involves the lower respiratory tract, urinary tract, or surgical wounds (Table 302–2) (Chapter 304). Some important causes of nosocomial fever may not be accompanied by easily discernible localizing symptoms or signs. Antibiotic-induced colitis secondary to *Clostridium difficile* is increasing in prevalence and may be characterized by little or no diarrhea. It is probably the most common cause of a leukemoid reaction in hospitalized patients. Other intra-abdominal processes involving the hepatobiliary system, bowel infarction, viscus perforation, or abscesses may have little in the way of localizing symptoms or signs.

Given the greater severity of illness and comorbid conditions in intensive care unit (ICU) patients, it is logical that fever and infection are more frequent in the ICU than elsewhere. Infection has recently been found to be present in more than 80% of febrile ICU patients, although both infectious and noninfectious causes of fever may coexist. Indeed, ischemia or devitalization of tissue provokes an inflammatory response similar to that prompted by infection. About half of patients with acute myocardial infarction will have a temperature between 38.0 and 38.5° C within 2 to 3 days of their infarction. Patients with deep venous thrombosis and pulmonary embolism have a temperature in a similar range in approximately half the cases, most commonly in the first 3 days after diagnosis. Likewise, a third or more of patients with strokes demonstrate fever, which is also a common consequence of subarachnoid hemorrhage and subdural hematoma. The fever in such cases may result from damage to the hypothalamus or pulmonary aspiration secondary to obtundation. Iatrogenic causes of fever should be considered. Fever and chills may be seen in up to a quarter of patients receiving platelet transfusions, although the frequency is much less with other blood products. Platelet-associated transfusion infections are also more common than those of red blood cell (RBCs), presumably because of storage of platelets at room temperature rather than at 4° C, as for RBCs.

APPROACH TO FEVER OF UNKNOWN ORIGIN

The majority of febrile illnesses are short lived, but fever may be prolonged for weeks or months as part of an infectious disease, inflammatory disorder, or occult neoplasm. When fever is caused by infection, the site is an area not easily controlled by host defenses, thereby leading to continued release of inflammatory cytokines. Likewise, macrophage and lymphocyte involvement in inflammatory disorders causes persistent cytokine production, as do certain neoplasms. Given this final common pathway, it is easy to understand that the majority of cases of classic fever of unknown origin (FUO) are found in these three broad categories. Two other categories round out the bulk of FUO illnesses: miscellaneous illness and cases in which fever remains undiagnosed (Table 302–3). The proportion of patients reported in each category varies with geographic locale, the age of patients included, the duration of the fever, whether patients are immunocompromised, and the decade in which the study was performed. As more effective methods of diagnosing viral and bacterial infections have become available and as improved serologic studies to detect collagen vascular disorders have emerged, as well as better imaging techniques to detect occult malignancies, the proportion of

TABLE 302–2 SELECTED CAUSES OF HOSPITAL-ASSOCIATED FEVER

Common	Less Common
INFECTIOUS	**INFECTIOUS**
Clostridium difficile enterocolitis	Biliary tract disease
Pneumonia	Endometritis
Surgical wound	Intra-abdominal abscess
Urinary tract	Mediastinitis
Vascular catheter	Sinusitis
NONINFECTIOUS	**NONINFECTIOUS**
Drug-induced fever	Adrenal insufficiency
Hematoma	Gout
Immediate postoperative state	Myocardial infarction
Transfusion reaction	Organ infarction
Venous thromboembolism	Pancreatitis

TABLE 302–3 FREQUENCY OF SELECTED CHRONIC FEBRILE ILLNESSES

Infection, 25–50%	Malignancy, 20–30%	Collagen Vascular Disease, 15–30%	Miscellaneous, 10–20%	Undiagnosed, 10–30%
Cytomegalovirus	Carcinomatosis	Polyarteritis nodosa	Drug-induced fever	
Endocarditis	Leukemia	Rheumatoid arthritis	Granulomatous hepatitis	
Intra-abdominal	Local tumor	Still's disease	Inflammatory bowel disease	
Mycoses	Lymphoma	Systemic lupus erythematosus	Pancreatitis	
Occult abscess		Temporal arteritis	Pulmonary embolism	
Tuberculosis				

patients with FUO in the latter two categories of miscellaneous and undiagnosed has now increased up to about a third of the total in developed countries. The longer a febrile illness persists without a diagnosis or appropriate therapy, the less likely it is to be due to an infection. In one study, only 6% of patients who had persistent FUO beyond 6 months were found to have infection.

Bacterial species, particularly *Mycobacterium tuberculosis,* make up the largest category of infections that cause prolonged FUO. *M. tuberculosis* and other bacterial pathogens causing FUO have adapted to survive intracellularly or frequently change their surface antigens so that they are not readily eradicated by host defenses. Other infections causing FUO are localized in cryptic abscesses, especially intra-abdominally, or reside on heart valves where the inflammatory response is blunted. Persistent viral infections constitute a small and shrinking subset of patients with FUO because modern techniques more readily detect infection with Epstein-Barr virus, cytomegalovirus, and others. Among pathogens likely to be characterized initially by fever alone, cytomegalovirus, Epstein-Barr virus, and malaria are more common than psittacosis, Q fever, or Rocky Mountain spotted fever.

Malignancy may result in persistent fever by producing inflammatory cytokines, undergoing necrosis, or being accompanied by a complicating infection. The most common malignancies manifested as FUO are lymphomas and leukemias (especially nonlymphocytic leukemias) when the peripheral smear is nondiagnostic. The classic solid tumor causing FUO is renal cell carcinoma. Inflammatory processes such as collagen vascular disorders may lead to tissue inflammation, which produces fever as a prominent feature of the illness. In a recent series, adult Still's disease was the leading rheumatologic disorder manifested as FUO. Temporal arteritis and polymyalgia rheumatica are seen almost exclusively in patients older than 50 years. Systemic lupus erythematosus is still an occasional cause of FUO, especially if manifested in atypical fashion.

The miscellaneous category of FUO includes several disparate categories of disease. Granulomatous diseases such as granulomatous hepatitis, Crohn's disease, or sarcoidosis may incite cellular immune responses that result in fever. Granulomatous hepatitis was present in up to 6% of National Institutes of Health cases with fever lasting longer than 6 months. Chronic pancreatitis may occasionally cause FUO, as may recurrent pulmonary embolism. Drug-induced fever is a potential cause of FUO, especially in patients without exanthema or with eosinophilia.

Drug-induced fever (Table 302–4) may be the only manifestation of an adverse drug event in up to 5% of cases of drug hypersensitivity. Recognizing drug-induced fever is important clinically to avoid extra tests, additional therapy, and prolonged hospitalization. The mechanisms by which drugs incite fever are not well understood in many cases. These events may result from hypersensitivity reactions, altered thermoregulatory homeostasis directly related either to drug administration or to the pharmacologic action of a drug, or an idiosyncratic reaction. Hypersensitivity reactions are usually accompanied by an exanthem or enanthem and hepatic, renal, or pulmonary dysfunction, in addition to fever. However, fever may be the only manifestation of hypersensitivity. Antimicrobial agents appear to be the most common cause of drug-induced fever and are responsible for approximately a third of episodes in some studies. β-Lactams and sulfonamides account for most cases because they are among the most frequently administered antimicrobials. Anticonvulsants are also common causes of drug-induced fever secondary to hypersensitivity reactions. Allopurinol less commonly causes such a reaction and is usually accompanied by other manifestations of hypersensitivity. Altered thermoregulation is possible with a variety of drugs, including those with anticholinergic activity such as phenothiazines and tricyclic antidepressants. Sympathomimetic agents such as amphetamines and cocaine may also cause fever. Drug administration itself may cause fever if the vehicle of the drug is contaminated with exogenous pyrogens or chemical phlebitis occurs. Some drugs appear to have intrinsic pyrogenic properties, such as amphotericin B and bleomycin. Others cause fever as a result of their pharmacologic activity, such as interferon-α or IL-2. The parallel case for antibiotics occurs with rapid lysis of spirochetes or other bacteria, known as the Jarisch-Herxheimer reaction. Idiosyncratic drug-induced febrile reactions include malignant hyperthermia, neuroleptic malignant syndrome, and serotonin syndrome. Drugs implicated in these reactions include inhaled anesthetic agents, central nervous system dopamine-depleting agents, and serotonin re-uptake inhibitors, among others. Drug-induced fever is usually a diagnosis of exclusion. Neither the duration of drug exposure before the onset of fever, the clinical appearance of the patient, nor the pattern of the fever is particularly useful. Elimination of a single drug at a time, beginning with the one most likely to be implicated, is the usual means of identifying the causative agent. The fever will abate once the drug has been eliminated from the body, usually within 3 to 4 days of discontinuing use of the drug. Proof of causation requires re-exposure to the offending agent, which is rarely necessary and seldom done.

TABLE 302–4 SELECTED AGENTS ASSOCIATED WITH DRUG-INDUCED FEVER

Common	Less Common
ANTIMICROBIAL	
Amphotericin B β-Lactams Sulfonamides	Clindamycin Fluoroquinolones Rifampin
CARDIOVASCULAR	
Procainamide Quinidine	Diltiazem Hydralazine
CENTRAL NERVOUS SYSTEM	
Carbamazepine Phenytoin	Haloperidol Serotonin re-uptake inhibitors
MISCELLANEOUS	
Bleomycin Interferon-α Interleukin-2	Allopurinol Cimetidine Halothane

SYNDROMIC APPROACH: FEVER AND RASH

A syndromic approach is valuable in narrowing the multitude of possible causes in a patient with a suspected infection. Two approaches must be juxtaposed in this evaluation, and both are key in recognizing patterns. On the one hand, the clinician must be aware of the differential diagnosis of a particular type of lesion observed and, on the other hand, must be aware of the constellation of findings produced by individual pathogens. Unfortunately, because of the variety of manifestations possible and the often overlapping symptoms and signs, neither alone suffices, and both remain key elements in arriving at probable diagnoses. Moreover, fever and associated findings such as exanthem, lymphadenopathy, or jaundice may be due to noninfectious systemic diseases, as well as infectious ones. For instance, leukocytoclastic vasculitis and fever may be found in meningococcemia, Rocky Mountain spotted fever, and hepatitis C, but they may also be seen in noninfectious inflammatory diseases. Likewise, fever and adenopathy may be due to lymphoma, as well as cat-scratch disease.

A recognizable exanthem may lead to immediate recognition of a particular pathogen, but there is often a larger differential diagnosis that must be entertained. The clinician must recognize the type or types of skin lesions present, the distribution of the exanthem, and the chronologic progression with respect to the onset of fever and other symptoms (Table 302–5). Morphologic variations in skin lesions help in the differential diagnosis. Maculopapular exanthems are frequently seen in viral illness, hypersensitivity drug reactions, and immune complex–mediated diseases. Some of the most common viral causes include the many enteroviruses, but similar lesions may also be seen with hepatitis B and West Nile viruses, as well as some cases of parvovirus B19 infection in adults. Erythema multiforme, a subset of maculopapular exanthem, appears to result from various viral infections or drug eruptions. It may have a spectrum of disease that goes from benign to the life-threatening Stevens-Johnson syndrome/toxic epidermal necrolysis complex. Herpes simplex virus is perhaps the most common cause of erythema multiforme. Although drugs are the major precipitating factor for the

TABLE 302–5 SELECTED INFECTIONS WITH FEVER AND RASH

Etiology	Macules, Papules	Vesicles, Bullae	Petechiae, Purpura
BACTERIA			
Borrelia burgdorferi	+ (ECM)*		
Capnocytophaga canimorsus			+
Neisseria gonorrhoeae	+		+
Neisseria meningitidis			+
Rickettsia rickettsii	+		+
Treponema pallidum	+ (secondary)		
Vibrio vulnificus		+	
FUNGI AND MYCOBACTERIA			
Disseminated disease	+ (nodular)		
PROTOZOA			
Plasmodium falciparum			+
VIRUSES			
Adenovirus	+		+
Enteroviruses	+	+	+
Epstein-Barr	+		+
Hemorrhagic fever			+
Hepatitis B	+		+
Herpes		+	
HIV	+		

ECM = erythema chronicum migrans.

Stevens-Johnson syndrome/toxic epidermal necrolysis complex, *M. pneumoniae* has been associated with it as well. Evolution of the cutaneous findings over time may give clues to the etiology; for example, initial blanching, erythematous, maculopapular lesions may later evolve into petechiae, as seen in meningococcemia, Rocky Mountain spotted fever, and dengue. Secondary syphilis may be manifested by a multitude of morphologic skin lesions. Sometimes many different manifestations may occur simultaneously in the same patient. Most vesiculobullous skin exanthema are immunologically mediated. The few infections that manifest these eruptions include herpes simplex and varicella-zoster viruses and enteroviruses such as echovirus and coxsackievirus. The poxviruses, which may also cause such exanthema, are much more rare or associated with bioterrorism. Pustules, or vesicles containing leukocytes, are usually associated with psoriasis or infections with *Pseudomonas, Staphylococcus,* or *Neisseria.* Bullous exanthema in the presence of sepsis suggest severe streptococcal cellulitis or necrotizing fasciitis, staphylococcal impetigo, or *Vibrio* infections.

Petechial and purpuric eruptions are due to extravasation of RBCs and should always call into question a potentially serious illness. The most common pathogens creating such lesions include *Neisseria meningitidis, Rickettsia,* and *Capnocytophaga canimorsus,* but these eruptions may be seen with a variety of other pathogens, including *Staphylococcus aureus,* group B streptococci, and other gram-negative bacilli. A petechial exanthem may also be seen with enteroviruses and viral hemorrhagic fevers. The most common causes of petechiae not attributable to infections include thrombocytopenia and vasculitis.

The presence of fever and rash involving the palms and soles allows considerable narrowing of the differential diagnosis (Table 302–6). In addition to the diffuse erythema with illnesses such as toxic shock syndrome, illnesses such as Rocky Mountain spotted fever, secondary syphilis, hand-foot-mouth disease, *Neisseria* infections, and rat-bite fever should be considered in patients with maculopapular exanthema involving these areas.

Nodular skin lesions may be both noninfectious, as seen in malignancy or with certain drugs (e.g., sulfonamides), and infectious, as seen in a variety of inflammatory diseases. Atypical mycobacteria and disseminated fungi often produce skin nodules. The nodules of erythema nodosum are usually multiple and located pretibially, but they may be solitary or occur on other parts of the body. They do not typically suppurate and heal without scarring. Infectious agents are the most likely cause of erythema nodosum. Diffuse erythema may be seen with scarlet fever, toxic shock syndrome, Kawasaki's disease, Stevens-Johnson syndrome, and toxic epidermal necrolysis, with desquamation occurring late in all these syndromes. Sweet's syndrome, a febrile neutrophilic dermatosis, represents a hypersensitivity reaction often preceded by an upper respiratory tract infection. Typically, patients have fever and leukocytosis, as well as a variety of other symptoms, and Sweet's syndrome is a diagnosis of exclusion.

TABLE 302–6 FEVER AND RASH INVOLVING THE PALMS AND SOLES

Erythema multiforme
Hand-foot-and-mouth disease
Neisseria infection
Rocky Mountain spotted fever
Streptobacillus moniliformis infection
Subacute bacterial endocarditis
Syphilis (secondary)
Toxic shock syndrome
Varicella-zoster infection

SYNDROMIC APPROACH: FEVER AND MUSCULOSKELETAL COMPLAINTS

Septic arthritis is generally and osteomyelitis is often accompanied by fever and localized tenderness, swelling, or erythema. Septic bacterial arthritis in adults is usually manifested acutely and involves a single large joint such as the knee, hip, or shoulder, unless directly inoculated by trauma or surgery. Septic oligoarthritis may be seen with endocarditis and rat-bite fever. Disseminated gonococcal disease is the usual cause of arthritis involving small joints of the wrist, ankle, and digits, often with

TABLE 302–7 COMMON CAUSES OF FEVER AND LYMPHADENOPATHY

Regional	Generalized
CERVICAL	Brucellosis
Epstein-Barr virus	Cytomegalovirus
Streptococci	Epstein-Barr virus
Tuberculosis	Human immunodeficiency virus
Viral upper respiratory tract infection	Lymphoma
PERIPHERAL	Sarcoidosis
Bartonella henselae	Syphilis (secondary)
Herpesviruses	Toxoplasmosis
Lymphoma	Viral hepatitis
Metastatic cancer	
Sporotrichosis	
Streptococci	
INGUINAL	
Chancroid	
Herpes	
Lymphogranuloma venereum	
Syphilis (primary)	

tenosynovitis. Acute or subacute polyarthritis may be seen in several viral diseases, including parvovirus B19 and hepatitis B, or in Lyme disease, but it is more typical of immunologic disorders. Rheumatologic diseases generally have more subacute manifestations with more symmetrical polyarthritis. Hematogenous osteomyelitis in adults frequently involves the vertebrae and is almost always initiated by discitis with symmetrical involvement of adjacent vertebrae (as opposed to malignant metastasis, which is asymmetrical and does not involve the disc).

Myositis secondary to clostridia, streptococci, *Aeromonas,* or mixed aerobic/anaerobic infections usually causes an acutely septic picture with painful, edematous involvement of the limb or torso. Pyomyositis frequently involves deep muscles such as the psoas or gluteus and is due to *S. aureus* or gastrointestinal flora. Diffuse myositis may be seen with leptospirosis or toxoplasmosis, and rhabdomyolysis occurs with a variety of viral infections.

SYNDROMIC APPROACH: FEVER AND LYMPHADENOPATHY OR HEPATOSPLENOMEGALY

Fever and lymphadenopathy may suggest a variety of illnesses, both infectious and noninfectious (Table 302–7). Lymphadenopathy may be regional or generalized. Local enlargement can occur with either a local infection or some systemic illnesses (e.g., posterior cervical lymphadenopathy with Epstein-Barr virus and other viral illnesses). Generalized lymphadenopathy usually suggests a systemic disorder, which may itself be either infectious or noninfectious. Although the combination of fever and lymphadenopathy secondary to infection is especially common during childhood, it is also frequently seen in adults. As in other syndromes, acute versus chronic adenopathy tilts the diagnosis toward different broad categories of illness. In the latter, histopathologic evaluation of enlarged lymph nodes may point to a particular diagnosis. For instance, toxoplasmosis or cat-scratch disease may be easily differentiated from mycobacterial disease or sarcoidosis.

Fever and hepatosplenomegaly may provide an important clue to the cause of a febrile illness, which is typically either an infection or malignancy arising from bone marrow or the reticuloendothelial system. Jaundice may also serve to limit the differential diagnosis (Table 302–8). Aside from the viral hepatitides and other diseases primarily affecting the liver, many pathogens producing sepsis may cause hyperbilirubinemia.

TABLE 302–8 COMMON CAUSES OF FEVER AND JAUNDICE

Bacterial sepsis
Cholangitis
Hepatic abscesses
Leptospirosis
Malaria
Viral hepatitis
Yellow fever

INITIAL MANAGEMENT OF SUSPECTED INFECTION IN THE AMBULATORY SETTING

An acutely febrile patient in the ambulatory setting presents a common, but often demanding problem in diagnosis. In most cases the history and physical examination will reveal diagnostic clues and may guide decisions about diagnostic studies or therapy. A more difficult problem is faced when fever occurs without localizing symptoms or is accompanied only by nonspecific symptoms such as malaise or anorexia. Fortunately, such acute undifferentiated febrile illnesses are mostly benign and resolve spontaneously within 1 or 2 weeks without a specific diagnosis having been made. In such cases, no further evaluation beyond the initial visit is warranted. If symptoms persist, the history and physical examination should be repeated to look for previously unsought clues and new physical findings. Laboratory studies might need to be initiated.

In patients with a cough illness of less than 3 weeks' duration, evaluation should focus on ruling out serious illness. Normal vital signs and a chest examination effectively rule out most cases of pneumonia. Such cough illness is caused by viral pathogens in more than 90% of cases. Not only are antibiotics ineffective in such patients, but antimicrobial therapy does not prevent bacterial complications such as pneumonia. The presence of sputum and its characteristics are not helpful in distinguishing bacterial from viral infections. Initial management should include avoidance of cigarette smoke and consideration of bronchodilators, oral liquids, or steam (from a shower or bath) to loosen secretions and antipyretics and antitussives for symptomatic relief. Adults with prolonged coughing lasting beyond 3 weeks or with recurrent episodes should be evaluated for reactive airway disease, smoking, postnasal drip, gastroesophageal reflux, angiotensin-converting enzyme inhibitor–induced cough, environmental exposure, bronchiectasis, or even malignancy. Infections rarely causing prolonged cough include *Bordetella pertussis, M. pneumoniae,* and *Chlamydia pneumoniae.* Clinicians in this case should obtain a chest radiograph, treat for exacerbation of chronic obstructive pulmonary disease (fever, leukocytosis, and purulent sputum) if present, treat a confirmed bacterial infection, and direct therapy to a specific underlying cause or other causes.

Symptoms and signs of pharyngitis include fever, tonsillar exudates, tender anterior cervical lymph nodes, and the absence of cough. If fewer than two of these criteria are present, a patient should be managed as though viral pharyngitis were the cause. With two or more of these criteria, one should consider obtaining a rapid streptococcal antigen test. Because of the low incidence of streptococcal infection and acute rheumatic fever in adults, a negative rapid test alone is sufficient to rule out infection with *Streptococcus pyogenes.* If, on the other hand, the antigen test is positive, the patient may be managed with a β-lactam if not allergic. Ninety percent of cases of pharyngitis in adults are viral in origin. Symptomatic treatment includes avoidance of cigarette smoke, gargling with dilute salt water, antipyretics, and throat lozenges as necessary.

In a patient with symptoms of upper respiratory tract infection and a mucopurulent nasal discharge of less than 10 days' duration, it is important to remember that purulent nasal secretions do not predict bacterial infection. Most cases of acute rhinosinusitis seen in the outpatient setting are caused by uncomplicated upper respiratory viral infection, for which antimicrobial therapy does not improve the symptoms or prevent complications. If symptoms have been present for more than 10 days without improvement or if there are specific symptoms of sinusitis of any duration (purulent nasal discharge lasting 3 to 4 days, unilateral facial pain and pressure, maxillary toothache, or worsening of symptoms after initial improvement), amoxicillin or another β-lactam should be considered, with other antimicrobial classes used in a penicillin-allergic patient. A higher dose of amoxicillin should be used when a patient has risk factors for drug-resistant *S. pneumoniae* or is in a geographic area where the prevalence of such resistance is known to be high.

Community-acquired pneumonia should be suspected in patients with newly acquired lower respiratory tract symptoms such as cough, sputum production, or dyspnea, especially if accompanied by fever and altered breath sounds. A chest radiograph should be performed to confirm the diagnosis. The initial site of where to care for the patient is the most important immediate decision and involves assessment of any preexisting conditions that can compromise the safety of ambulatory care alone, determination of the risk class of the patient, and clinical judgment. Outpatient care generally suffices for patients younger than 50 years with no cardiopulmonary disease, no comorbid conditions (including malignancy, heart failure, diabetes, hospitalization within the last year), and no physical examination findings such as altered mental status, pulse of 125/min or greater, or respiratory rate of 30/min or greater. Initial clinical approaches vary according to geography, with many clinical advisory committees in the United States suggesting a macrolide and their counterparts in Europe more commonly suggesting a prescription of amoxicillin empirically. Fluoroquinolones should be used for outpatients only when the patient has failed first-line therapy or has known allergy to a first-line agent.

Skin and soft tissue infections are caused for the most part by streptococcal species, a minority being due to *S. aureus* and rarely other bacteria whose presence may be suggested by epidemiologic considerations (e.g., swimming in fresh water, where *Aeromonas* may become the pathogen). Pain may be present for 12 hours or more before skin discoloration is noted. A furuncle or abscess formation should prompt consideration of *S. aureus* and, rarely, *Streptococcus milleri.* Incision and drainage may be all that is necessary for skin abscess, although the rapidly expanding, virulent community-acquired methicillin-resistant *S. aureus* phenotype may in addition require antimicrobial therapy. Septic bursitis is nearly always due to *S. aureus,* and the infected bursa should be aspirated and drained in addition to using antibiotics.

Gastrointestinal infections may be due to ingested toxin, viruses, or less commonly, bacteria with or without associated toxin production. The appropriate approach depends on considerations related to the epidemiologic setting, such as improper food storage, travel abroad, or contact with another ill person. As noted earlier, symptoms of cystitis in a young, sexually active woman may be treated with empirical antibiotics, but when fever and flank pain are present and the patient is nauseated, consideration of a brief hospital admission or an initial intravenous dose of antibiotics may be necessary. The possibility of pelvic inflammatory disease should also be entertained.

In the initial evaluation of a patient with a more chronic, persistent fever, a careful history plus physical examination plays a major role in providing important diagnostic clues directing further investigation. The initial goal is to characterize the illness accurately, in addition to eliciting important host and epidemiologic factors. A careful review of systems is necessary to understand the extent of involvement of various organ systems, as well as to note previous medical conditions. The examination should be broader than for an acute febrile illness with localizing symptoms and signs. Laboratory tests may also play a more important role in guiding further investigation. Repeat evaluations are the norm rather than the exception in these cases.

INITIAL MANAGEMENT OF SUSPECTED NOSOCOMIAL INFECTION

Determination of the nature of a febrile illness in hospitalized patients must take into account the host, the setting, and the timing of recent trauma or type and duration of surgery, in addition to the general approach taken for ambulatory patients. A classic mnemonic may come in handy to help guide the evaluation. The six W's of this mnemonic indicate "wind, water, wound, walk, wonder drug, and what we did." "Wind" refers to fever within the first 24 hours of surgery, when it is unusual to have an infection. A fever at this time has often been thought to be related to the anesthetic agent or to surgical trauma. The only bacteria believed to cause significant infections within 24 hours of surgery are *S. pyogenes* and *Clostridium* sp, both of which are unusual in the typical hospital patient. "Water" refers to a urinary tract infection occurring after the third day of urinary catheterization. Because nearly all nosocomial urinary tract infections occur in patients with indwelling urinary catheters or in those who have undergone urologic instrumentation, urinalysis or culture (or both) should be performed routinely only in febrile patients with such risk factors. On the other hand, there is a high prevalence of bacteriuria in patients who have been catheterized for 3 days or longer, and there is a relatively low incidence of true infection attributable to bacteriuria. "Wound" infections commonly occur about 5 to 7 days postoperatively, whether they are surface wounds or complications of dehiscence of gastrointestinal anastomoses. Some of the highest rates of skin and soft tissue infections in the National Nosocomial Infection Surveillance database are seen with gastrointestinal procedures. Toxin-producing *C. difficile* is the only significant nosocomial gastrointestinal infection seen in hospitalized patients, so a routine bacterial culture is not necessary. "Walk" refers to possible pulmonary embolism in someone who has not received appropriate prophylaxis or who is otherwise at risk for thrombosis. Fever induced by a "wonder drug" is typically seen after approximately 7 to 10 days of use if the patient does not already have an allergy to that medication, in which case it recurs immediately. An exception to this rule is sulfamethoxazole, in which approximately half of hypersensitivity reactions occur within 3 days of initiation. Finally, "what we did" alerts the clinician to the possibility of an iatrogenic infection such as intravenous catheter–related bacteremia.

In conclusion, the initial management of patients with febrile illnesses requires responses to several questions. First, is the illness more likely to be infectious or more likely to be related to some other process? Excessive antibiotic use in instances in which they are not warranted, such as for viral infections or collagen vascular disease, may cause an adverse reaction in addition to contributing to a worldwide increase in antimicrobial resistance. On the other hand, an empirical antibiotic is appropriate in many instances of fever and localizing signs of bacterial infection. Second, the clinician must rapidly assess the severity of the illness and whether it is likely to cause significant organ damage or even death. In a febrile patient who has signs of sepsis, the clinician must quickly decide which specific therapy is indicated because delay in initiation of antimicrobial therapy has been correlated with increased morbidity and mortality. Finally, the clinician needs to determine whether supportive care alone, including antipyretic therapy, is adequate. Of note, fever is not usually harmful, and antipyretics may confuse the clinical picture by dampening it, although their anti-inflammatory effects are often beneficial.

SUGGESTED READINGS

Bottieau E, Clerinx J, Schrooten W, et al: Etiology and outcome of fever after a stay in the tropics. Arch Intern Med 2006;166:1642–1648. Plasmodium falciparum *malaria was the leading cause of mortality.*

Mandell GL, Bennett JE, Dolin R (eds): Principles and Practice of Infectious Diseases, 6th ed. Philadelphia, Elsevier, 2005. *A comprehensive textbook.*

Mourad O, Palda V, Detsky AS: A comprehensive evidence-based approach to fever of unknown origin. Arch Intern Med 2003;163:545–551. *A systematic review of FUO publications from 1966 to 2000.*

303 APPROACH TO FEVER AND SUSPECTED INFECTION IN THE COMPROMISED HOST

Lowell S. Young

Definition

A compromised host may be defined as a patient with either an inborn or acquired impairment in the ability to resist infection. This term is used almost synonymously with "immunocompromised host," which implies a defect in either innate or adaptive immunity. Although there are non-immune conditions in which an abnormality in host response has been described, such as severe trauma or burns, for working purposes a defect in immune response is assumed to be part of the susceptibility of a "compromised" patient to infection. The spectrum of patients included in this large group varies from those with neoplastic diseases (particularly hematologic disorders such as leukemia and lymphoma), recipients of organ transplants treated with intense immune suppression to prevent graft rejection, and patients with collagen vascular, autoimmune, or hypersensitivity disorders who are treated with medications that can blunt the immune response. New medications that have very specific targets in suppressing the immune response (such as cytokine pathways mediating inflammation) have been applied to management of organ grafts and extended to inflammatory disorders of the skin, joints, and bowel; such patients may thus have acquired (but potentially reversible) defects in cell-mediated immunity and are susceptible to diseases such as tuberculosis or reactivated fungal infection (e.g., histoplasmosis). Some individuals are born with congenital immunodeficiencies such as defects in white cell killing, neutrophil locomotion, or antibody production and are clearly more susceptible to infection. Subtle congenital defects such as abnormalities in receptors for the host cytokine response have broadened the definition of host susceptibility. Management of individuals with the acquired immunodeficiency syndrome (AIDS) caused by human immunodeficiency virus type 1 (HIV-1), not recognized until 2 decades ago, is discussed in Chapters 407 through 417.

Recognizing that a large group of compromised patients are those with hematologic disorders or neoplasia, Table 303–1 is an attempt to relate defects in host response with examples of disease and pharmacologic intervention that can lead to similar defects. The absolute number of phagocytic cells belonging to the neutrophil or polymorphonuclear leukocyte series may be reduced or the function of these cells impaired. Neutrophils respond to acute infection. Severe qualitative impairment in function (e.g., the killing defect of chronic granulomatous disease) or quantitative impairment, such as in acute blastic leukemia, where the cells are abnormal in morphology and function and only a small proportion of normally functioning cells circulate, is associated with a marked increase in susceptibility to bacterial infection. Another component of the population of phagocytic cells includes circulating monocytes and tissue macrophages and the fixed mononuclear cells of the reticuloendothelial system. These cells collaborate with helper T cells in defense against pathogens that can survive intracellularly, such as mycobacteria, fungi, and some viruses and parasites. There may be quantitative defects in humoral factors that are critical in host defense, such as circulating IgG and IgM antibodies, secretory IgA antibodies, and components of the complement cascade that can directly lyse some bacteria and viruses. Host defenses are often collaborative; for example, the interaction of anti–cell wall antibodies with bacteria facilitates uptake or opsonization of pathogens by white blood cells.

It must be remembered that therapeutic intervention with a growing number of medications can impair the function of leukocytes and depress antibody production. Combination therapies with cytotoxic and immunosuppressive medications of multiple classes can exacerbate a preexisting immune defect and result in a markedly enhanced risk for infection.

Diagnosis

Approach to the Compromised Patient

The onset of fever in a compromised patient can be an ominous development, and depending on the nature and magnitude of the impaired host defenses, a febrile response can herald the onset of a life-threatening systemic infection. If fever is accompanied by neutropenia, as exemplified by circulating neutrophil counts of less than 1000/mm^3, the risk for bacterial infection is real and increases proportionally with the decline in neutrophil count. The most common definition of significant neutropenia is a level lower than 500 cells/mm^3, whereas profound neutropenia is recognized at a neutrophil concentration less than 100 cells/mm^3. The risk for documented bacteremia is at least 20% in patients with profound neutropenia. Intense immune suppression with corticosteroids and therapies that can blunt T-cell-mediated immunity can still predispose to overwhelming bacterial infections, even with normal circulating neutrophil counts. The chronicity of the defect or the tempo at which critical components of host defense are impaired clearly affects the judgment to initiate diagnostic studies and empirical therapy. For instance, in treatment of acute leukemia, a total neutrophil count that declines by half on each successive day indicates that total white cell production has been ablated and profound neutropenia is very likely to ensue. The duration of significant neutropenia is also a risk factor for disseminated bacterial or fungal disease, with the risk for such infection increasing by each successive week in which white cell counts are less than 500 cells/mm^3.

Clinical Evaluation

For practical purposes, fever is defined as an oral temperature in excess of 38.3° C or 101° F for 1 hour or more in the absence of an obvious cause (Fig. 303–1). When such temperature elevation in a compromised host is accompanied by evidence of sepsis syndrome, as manifested by elevations in the heart or respiratory rate, a decrease in oxygenation to less than 92% O_2 saturation (room air), or hematologic abnormalities with a white cell count exceeding 12,000 cells/mm^3 or less than 4000 cells/mm^3, empirical treatment should strongly be considered after laboratory studies are initiated. A significantly low neutrophil count (<500 cells/mm^3) or a high band percentage (in excess of 10%), or both, in the presence of fever are compelling points that support the initiation of empirical therapy. The presence of hypotension (systolic blood pressure <90 mm Hg) mandates the start of treatment within minutes.

Although fever is the hallmark of infection, it is not specific for the presence of an infectious process. The converse of fever, hypothermia (−1.5° C or more), should also alert clinicians to the presence of infection. The development of fever may be a result of multiple causes, including medications, reaction to blood components, or graft-versus-host

TABLE 303–1 IMMUNE DEFECTS PRESENT IN HEMATOLOGIC DISORDERS

Host Defect	Disease	Pharmacologic Therapy Causing a Similar Defect*
Impaired phagocytic function	Acute leukemia	Corticosteroids (high dose)
Phagocyte mobilization	"Lazy leukocyte" syndrome	Alkylating agents
Neutropenia	Aplastic anemia Acute leukemia	Corticosteroids Antimetabolites
Impaired cell-mediated immunity	Hodgkin's disease	Antilymphocyte globulin Corticosteroids Cyclosporine Anti-TNF antibody, TNF receptor antagonist Tacrolimus
Decreased antibody levels	Multiple myeloma Chronic lymphocytic leukemia	Alkylating agents Antimetabolites

*Ionizing radiation in sufficient dose will suppress all components of the host response.
TNF = tumor necrosis factor.

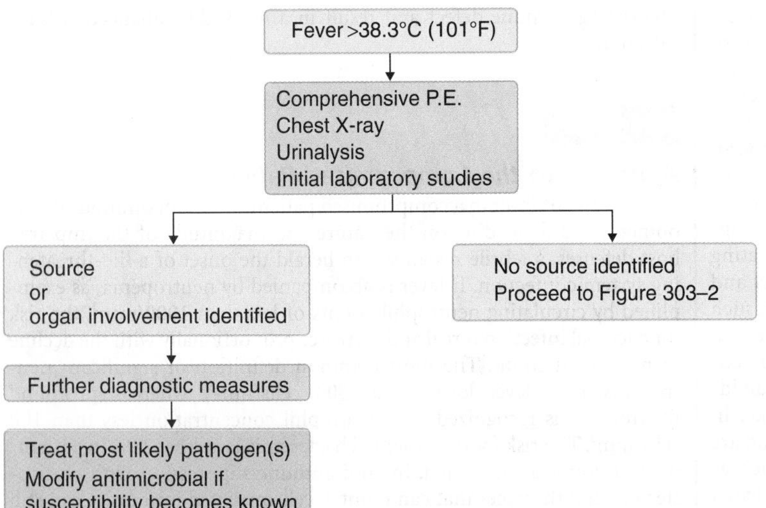

FIGURE 303–1 • Clinical evaluation of fever in the compromised host. P.E. = physical examination.

disease in a transplant recipient. The fundamental principle is that infection should be suspected as the most likely cause of fever in a compromised host, and depending on the overall immune status of the host, urgent measures to diagnose and treat infection should be promptly initiated while evaluating the patient and determining the most likely cause of the fever. Patients who are severely compromised and subjected to repeated courses of treatment aimed at the underlying disease, such as a patient with hematologic malignancy, will probably have multiple episodes of fever during prolonged hospitalization. Each episode requires comprehensive assessment; after a documented infection it should not be assumed that a subsequent episode of fever is caused by the same recrudescent pathogen.

The onset of fever should trigger a prompt and thorough bedside evaluation of the patient. Beginning with examination of the head and neck, there should be a specific examination for evidence of central nervous system (CNS) infection, as well as a general evaluation of mental status. The oropharynx must be examined for evidence of pharyngitis and gum inflammation and the anterior and posterior aspects of the lungs for evidence of an abnormality in breathing or an airway abnormality. Complete examination of the heart should take place coincident with a thorough examination of all lung fields. In addition to palpation of the abdomen and the costovertebral angles, auscultation of the abdomen for quality of bowel movements should be undertaken. The perirectal area and the entire integument should be examined. Pelvic examination in a female patient is not mandatory unless symptoms are pointing toward involvement of the genital structures. If a patient has a foreign body in place such as an intravenous or intra-arterial catheter, it should be carefully examined, as well as the surrounding tissue for signs of pain and redness, and blood should be drawn through all catheter channels for culture. Additionally, confirmation of blood stream infection should be sought by drawing venous blood for culture from another distal, noncatheterized site. Thus, at least two sets of blood cultures are recommended: one drawn through each of the vascular catheter channels and another from a venous site. Laboratory studies should be undertaken, with emphasis placed on procedures that can yield prompt results, such as Gram stain of body fluids, exudates, or aspirates. Routine blood work should include a complete blood count with differential, serum creatinine, and screening liver function studies. A chest radiograph should be part of the initial evaluation, as well as routine urinalysis. If the patient has any findings pointing toward the CNS or a change in mental status, lumbar puncture is included in the initial evaluation (except, perhaps, in an extremely thrombocytopenic patient, in whom platelet transfusions are advised before attempted lumbar puncture). Cerebrospinal fluid (CSF) should be examined for leukocytes, glucose, protein, and cryptococcal antigen and should be Gram stained and cultured. In the presence of signs of increased intracranial pressure, CNS imaging (computed tomography [CT], magnetic resonance imaging [MRI]) should first be undertaken. Suspicion of cryptococcal (Chapter 357) or *Aspergillus* (Chapter 360) infection should lead to serum antigen testing for these entities; the cryptococcal antigen test on CSF and serum is more reliable, whereas false-positive *Aspergillus* (galactomannan) antigen test results are seen in patients treated with piperacillin or tazobactam.

Differential Diagnosis

Table 303–2 summarizes some of the major clinical syndromes and the causative microbial agents that may be responsible for the clinical pattern. This categorization is simplistic in its anatomic localization of symptoms; nonetheless, if the signs and symptoms of infection can be localized to a specific anatomic site, the differential diagnosis is simplified and prudent anticipation of the most likely pathogens is possible.

Central Nervous System

Both gram-positive and gram-negative bacteria (including anaerobes) can cause a brain abscess or meningitis. *Listeria monocytogenes* is a common cause of meningitis in a compromised host. This pathogen is a gram-positive pleomorphic bacillus that may be difficult to identify on routine Gram stains of CSF. Encapsulated bacteria such as pneumococci and staphylococci can cause metastatic CNS disease and meningitis. In patients with impaired cell-mediated immunity, such as Hodgkin's disease or AIDS, *Cryptococcus neoformans* is also a leading cause of CNS infection. Although cryptococci (Chapter 357) are usually the most common fungal pathogens of the brain, *Candida, Aspergillus,* and other molds can invade the CNS. The herpesviruses include herpes simplex, cytomegalovirus, and Epstein-Barr virus, and involvement of the CNS by these viruses results in meningoencephalitis. Infection of the CSF with HIV-1 can cause CNS reactive pleocytosis. Reactivated or quiescent CNS syphilis should also be considered in patients with severe immunologic impairment.

Respiratory Tract

The lungs are a challenging site in evaluating fever in a compromised patient because detection of abnormalities is easy but obtaining lung secretions or infected tissues can be difficult. Pneumonia should be suspected in a patient who has respiratory symptoms as manifested by cough, shortness of breath, chest pain, and hypoxia. In the early stages of pneumonitis, routine chest radiographs may be negative, whereas more expensive imaging procedures such as computed axial tomography may reveal pulmonary infiltrates or abscesses. Both community-acquired pathogens such as pneumococci and *Haemophilus influenzae* can cause lobar or diffuse pneumonia. Gram-negative bacilli can cause pneumonia of a necrotizing type in severely neutropenic patients. All patients who are receiving ventilator support are at risk for secondary gram-negative bacillary pneumonia or staphylococcal pneumonia. Clusters of outbreaks of *Legionella pneumophila* infection have occurred in immunocompromised patients maintained in dialysis, transplant, or intensive care units; these outbreaks reflect institutional environmental contamination.

Opportunistic fungi appear to be increasing causes of lung infection in severely compromised patients. A travel history is essential in a compromised patient who has evidence of lung disease; epidemic mycoses such as blastomycosis, coccidioidomycosis, and histoplasmosis may be manifested as acute pneumonia after recent exposure, but more typically, initial exposure in a normal host leads to containment of an initial focus of fungal lung disease. After immune suppression, the primary focus can be the source of reactivated disease. *Candida* species, in contrast, are uncommon primary lung pathogens. Although *Candida* species

TABLE 303–2 INFECTIOUS DISEASE SYNDROMES AND ETIOLOGIC AGENTS IN COMPROMISED HOSTS

Pattern of Involvement	Bacteria	Fungi	Viruses	Parasites
Disseminated disease with skin lesions (vasculitis, abscesses, or papules)	*Staphylococcus aureus* *Pseudomonas aeruginosa* *Aeromonas hydrophila* Other gram-negative bacteria *Nocardia* Noncholera vibrios Mycobacteria	*Candida* sp *Aspergillus* *Histoplasma* *Zygomycetes* *Sporothrix schenckii* *Pseudallescheria* *Trichosporon* sp Other molds	Herpes simplex Varicella-zoster	
Diffuse pneumonia*	Any gram-negative or gram-positive bacteria, including *Legionella, Nocardia,* and *Mycobacterium* *Chlamydia*	*Aspergillus* *Candida* *Zygomycetes* sp Other molds *Pneumocystis jiroveci*	Herpes simplex Varicella-zoster Cytomegalovirus Influenza Adenovirus Measles Respiratory syncytial virus	*Toxoplasma gondii* *Strongyloides stercoralis*
Central nervous system infection, meningoencephalitis, possibly brain abscess	*Listeria monocytogenes* *Nocardia* *S. aureus* *P. aeruginosa* *Mycobacterium tuberculosis*	*Cryptococcus neoformans* *Aspergillus fumigatus* *Zygomycetes* *Candida* sp	Varicella-zoster Herpes simplex	*Toxoplasma gondii*
Oroesophageal syndromes	Anaerobes Aerobes: streptococci and gram-negative rods, particularly *P. aeruginosa*	*Candida* *Aspergillus*	Herpes simplex Cytomegalovirus	
Diarrhea	*Clostridium difficile* *Salmonella* *Shigella* *Campylobacter*		Adenovirus Coxsackievirus Rotavirus	*Cryptosporidium* *Giardia lamblia* *Isospora belli* *Microsporidia*

*Consider also underlying disease, radiation, and drug reactions.

commonly colonize indwelling vascular and urinary catheters, candidal pneumonia is unusual in the absence of systemic candidiasis. Systemic candidiasis usually originates from the gastrointestinal or genitourinary tract if not secondary to vascular catheter dissemination. *Pneumocystis* (now referred to as *P. jiroveci*) has been reclassified as a fungus on the basis of DNA sequencing, which most closely matches that of yeasts. Though traditionally associated with an "interstitial pattern" of lung infiltration, *Pneumocystis* pneumonia can be manifested as local consolidation or pulmonary nodules. The molds, which include *Aspergillus,* Zygomycetes, and now some more unusual forms such as *Pseudallescheria boydii* and *Scedosporium apiospermum,* are difficult to treat. These infections may be accompanied by chest pain and occasionally hemoptysis. From an initial focus, *Aspergillus* infection can spread through the pulmonary vasculature, which sets the stage for pulmonary infarction. After infarction, the necrotic lung tissue retracts to yield the radiologic image of a cavity. Pulmonary involvement is primary with tuberculosis but may be secondary with nontuberculous mycobacteria such as *Mycobacterium avium,* which usually originates from the gastrointestinal tract.

Viral infections that involve the lung are difficult to diagnose in immunocompromised patients. It has long been recognized that measles (Chapter 390), varicella-zoster (Chapter 398), and respiratory syncytial virus (Chapter 385) can complicate immunosuppression, but added to this list would be the adenoviruses (Chapter 388) and reactivated cytomegalovirus (Chapter 399). The latter can appear almost indistinguishable from *Pneumocystis* pneumonia and may be coexistent.

Diarrheal Syndromes

There are multiple causes of diarrhea in a compromised host, including conventional enteric pathogens such as *Salmonella* (Chapter 329), *Shigella* (Chapter 330), and *Campylobacter* (Chapter 326), but particularly in a patient who has been in the hospital and receiving multiple courses of antibiotic treatment, *Clostridium difficile* is a common occurrence. *C. difficile* diarrhea should be suspected in patients who had received a course of antibiotics as long as a month previously. Two acid-fast staining parasites are *Isospora belli* and *Cryptosporidium,* and they are associated with predisposing impairments in cell-mediated immunity. More recently recognized are the microsporidians. *Giardia lamblia* is classically associated with hypogammaglobulinemia. Individuals who have received long courses of chemotherapy, radiation, and antibiotics commonly experience *Candida* mucosal overgrowth in the mouth and esophagus. Herpes simplex virus and cytomegalovirus can cause symptoms identical to those of *Candida* esophagitis. Thus, dysphagia and even an abnormal barium swallow study should not be conclusively attributed to *Candida* infection, but endoscopy is required for diagnosis of *Candida* esophagitis. In severely neutropenic patients, anaerobic streptococci and gram-negative pathogens such as *Pseudomonas aeruginosa* can cause severe mucositis/pharyngitis. In cancer patients, these organisms take advantage of the cytotoxic effects of chemotherapy, which promotes sloughing of mucosal surfaces and subsequently predisposes to microbial overgrowth.

Cutaneous Syndromes

Cutaneous abnormalities can provide a clue to bacteremia, and aspiration and culture of suspicious lesions can be as valuable as a blood culture. Ascending streptococcal or staphylococcal cellulitis can occur in both immunocompromised and normal patients. Metastatic abscesses are a well-recognized part of the *Staphylococcus aureus* bacteremia syndrome. Necrotizing vasculitis is classically associated with *P. aeruginosa* infections (the cutaneous lesion of ecthyma gangrenosum is an erythematous, indurated target or "bull's eye" lesion with an area of central necrosis that can appear in crops). However, other gram-negative endotoxin-producing bacteria have been associated with similar cutaneous lesions. Fungal pathogens such as *Aspergillus* and *Candida* can cause comparable metastatic cutaneous lesions. The important approach to patients should be to use such suspicious lesions as an opportunity for enhancing diagnosis through aspiration, biopsy, and culture after careful skin preparation. Results may be available faster than with blood cultures.

Treatment

Rx

Initial Antibiotic Therapy

Progression of infection can occur rapidly in compromised hosts. The choice of antimicrobial regimen should be tailored to the experience of the institution in dealing with specific types of underlying conditions (Fig. 303–2). Thus, knowledge of the most common types of blood stream and nosocomial infection for the specific institution and unit of care within the institution could be a helpful factor in influencing the choice of drugs; for example, a high incidence of problem pathogens such as methicillin-resistant *S. aureus,* vancomycin-resistant enterococci, or multidrug-resistant gram-negative bacilli should affect the choice of initial regimens. Overall, gram-positive bacteremias outnumber gram-negative blood stream infections in compromised hosts, as they now do in most nosocomial infection surveys. However, a large proportion of such infections are due to coagulase-negative staphylococci, which are not associated with high case-fatality ratios. Indwelling vascular catheter use is so prevalent that such devices may be left in place while empirical therapy is initiated. If fever persists and clinical or culture evidence points to the vascular catheter as the source of infection, catheter removal should be strongly considered unless there are compelling reasons that prevent selection of an alternative catheter site. Evidence of subcutaneous tunnel infection (pain and redness along the subcutaneous tract of the catheter) or infection in and around devices such as an indwelling intravenous port usually makes removal of the device necessary. Other indications for catheter or device removal are the presence of obstruction to flow and evidence of septic emboli originating from the catheter. Catheter infections caused by *S. aureus,* fungi, gram-negative bacilli, and nontuberculous mycobacteria are not usually successfully treated in situ by antimicrobial therapy; catheters should be removed after identification of the offending microorganism.

Despite the appearance of fever and evidence of sepsis syndrome, it is important to distinguish, particularly in neutropenic patients, individuals who fall into low-risk and high-risk categories. Individuals considered to be in the low-risk category are those who are hemodynamically stable and have an underlying disorder such as a solid tumor being treated with chemotherapy; the duration of significant neutropenia in such patients is likely to be less than a week. If febrile but clinically stable, these individuals may be managed with oral therapy, for instance, the combination of a fluoroquinolone such as ciprofloxacin in combination with amoxicillin-clavulanate or levofloxacin alone. 1 Some patients in low-risk categories may be managed as outpatients, with the understanding that medical providers can be reached quickly if clinical conditions worsen.

No single broad-spectrum antibacterial regimen is applicable to all institutions. Choices must be based on local experience and antimicrobial resistance patterns demonstrated among the most frequent blood stream pathogens. The major choices involve the decision to use vancomycin initially in high-risk patients (out of clinical concern for gram-positive infection) and whether multidrug, broad-spectrum antibacterial coverage is required for treatment of the suspected gram-negative bacillary component of the initial infectious process. Monotherapy with third-generation cephalosporins such as ceftazidime or cefepime has its advocates, but in the decade and a half since these compounds have become generally available, an increased incidence of resistance among gram-positive pathogens (particularly *S. aureus*) has become a major factor in treatment decisions. In some centers the most predictably effective broad-spectrum monotherapeutic regimen consists of a carbapenem such as imipenem or meropenem. The most popular two-drug combination regimens include an aminoglycoside plus a β-lactam agent (e.g., an antipseudomonal penicillin, third-generation cephalosporin, carbapenem, plus either gentamicin, amikacin, or tobramycin). If a regimen that spares aminoglycoside use is desired (out of consideration for potential aminoglycoside toxicity), vancomycin plus an antipseudomonal penicillin, vancomycin plus a broad-spectrum cephalosporin, or vancomycin plus a carbapenem can be considered. Therapy should always be delivered intravenously in high- risk patients, as exemplified by those with severe neutropenia and hematologic malignancy, transplant recipients, and patients receiving large doses of corticosteroids (e.g., prednisone doses exceeding 60 mg/day).

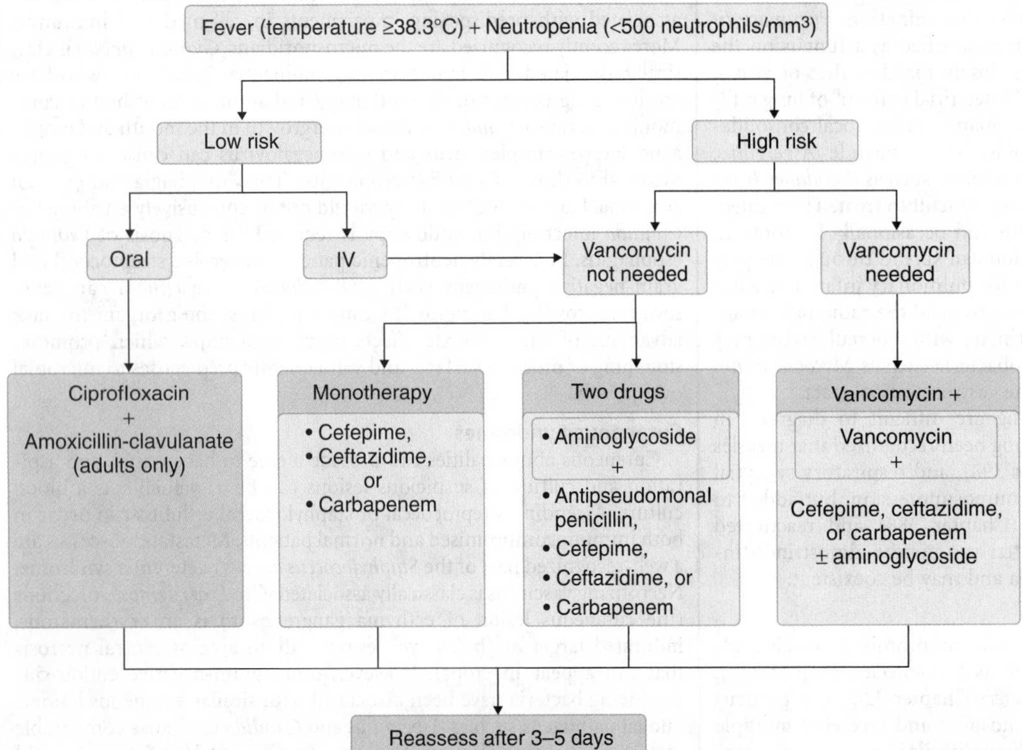

FIGURE 303–2 • Algorithm for the initial management of febrile neutropenic patients. (Reproduced with permission from Hughes WT, Armstrong D, Bodey GP, et al: 2002 Guidelines for the use of antimicrobial agents in neutropenic patients with cancer. Clin Infect Dis 2002;34:730–751.)

Rx

The Initial Five Days

Treatment of neutropenic patients with broad-spectrum intravenous antibiotics can result in defervescence within the first 5 days; prompt defervescence on the first day may create doubt about the original indication for empirical therapy, and clinical judgment should prevail. It must be borne in mind that some patients with microbiologically proven bacterial infection who are receiving adequate treatment may require 5 days or more of antimicrobial therapy before defervescence occurs. If the cause of fever is determined by culture within 3 to 5 days, treatment can be tailored to the safest, narrow-spectrum, most cost-effective regimen—provided that the neutrophil count is higher than 100 cells/mm^3. (If the neutrophil count remains very low, the initial successful regimen should probably be maintained.) If the patient was initially treated with vancomycin and no confirmatory cultures supporting continued vancomycin use are obtained after 3 days (e.g., no coagulase-negative staphylococci from blood or methicillin-resistant *S. aureus*), intravenous vancomycin therapy should be discontinued. During the first 5 days patients should still be carefully examined on at least a daily basis. Alterations or modifications in therapy during this first 5 days appear to be justified if patients are deteriorating. If patients are stable yet still febrile during a period of prolonged and severe neutropenia, clinical judgment must be used in deciding whether to maintain the initial regimen or switch to an alternative regimen. If patients become afebrile after 3 to 5 days of antibacterial treatment but cultures are negative, some authorities recommend continuing the broad-spectrum intravenous coverage until recovery of the neutrophil count. This, however, may not be practical for patients with leukemia in blastic crisis or refractory aplastic anemia, in whom periods of aplasia lasting weeks or more are common. Others believe that a switch to oral treatment is justifiable (e.g., a fluoroquinolone possibly paired with a β-lactam) if the patient becomes afebrile and appears to be clinically stable. If the patient remains afebrile and there is rapid improvement in the underlying condition, such as recovery of the circulating neutrophil count to higher than 500 cells/mm^3, total discontinuation of treatment is an option after 5 to 7 days. If the neutrophil count recovers to above 500/mm^3 and fever persists, it is a matter of clinical judgment to continue antimicrobial therapy while a search for the cause of the fever is continued.

In a patient with persistent fever after 72 hours or longer in whom no focus of infection or organism has been identified despite comprehensive cultures, other diagnostic tests may suggest that the patient may be experiencing a nonbacterial infection, has a resistant bacterial infection, is slow to respond to the initial regimen, may have a superinfection, is being treated with antimicrobial regimens that achieve inadequate serum and tissue concentrations, or may be experiencing a hypersensitivity reaction. To ensure adequacy of therapy, serum concentrations of important agents such as vancomycin and aminoglycosides should be measured at least once and preferably twice weekly. Noninfectious causes of persistent fever include hematomas, pulmonary emboli, splenic infarcts, and underlying malignancy. Infection around an intravascular catheter should always be considered, but routine catheter removal without evidence pointing to the catheter as the source of the infection may be a low-yield approach in achieving defervescence.

Issues Relating to Augmented Gram-Positive Coverage

During the last 2 decades, major changes have occurred in the epidemiology of infection in tertiary care hospitals and those specializing in cancer treatment or organ transplantation. Besides the upsurge in gram-positive staphylococcal (coagulase-negative) infections related to the use of indwelling vascular catheters, some institutions face problems with vancomycin-resistant enterococci, and many hospitals are dealing with the problem of methicillin-resistant *S. aureus* of both community and nosocomial origin (Chapter 304). Some of these *S. aureus* isolates show reduced vancomycin susceptibility. Well-principled efforts at decreasing vancomycin use are being implemented to reduce selection pressure that favors the emergence of vancomycin resistance. Several studies, albeit more than a decade old, indicate that initial vancomycin use ("front loading") is not warranted in the routine management of febrile neutropenic patients; the implication has been that coagulase-negative staphylococcal infections are sufficiently indolent that there is time to identify the pathogen and use more specific therapy at the time that blood cultures become positive. Still, institutions may be facing problems with particularly virulent viridans streptococci that show relative resistance to penicillin-type agents. With the prevalence of methicillin-resistant *S. aureus* exceeding 50% in some communities and hospitals, the initial use of vancomycin may be justified until the results of cultures are available. Alternatives to vancomycin as coverage for resistant gram-positive pathogens include other glycopeptides, daptomycin, quinupristin/dalfopristin, linezolid, and tigecycline. For all of these vancomycin alternatives, published experience in compromised hosts is very limited. As soon as the susceptibility pattern of identified gram-positive pathogens is known and vancomycin or the alternative agents are not thought to be needed, it seems prudent that vancomycin or the alternative anti–gram-positive agent be discontinued.

Persisting Fever in Compromised Hosts

Persistence of fever in a compromised host whose underlying condition has not improved despite broad-spectrum empirical antibacterial therapy is a major challenge. Management from this point on is controversial, particularly treatment of cancer patients with severe neutropenia or subjects with bone marrow failure syndromes (Fig. 303–3). In a large percentage of patients, sometimes exceeding the majority, no pathogen is identified after 4 to 7 days of broad antibacterial treatment. Options range from discontinuation of all antibiotics, continuation of antibacterial therapy, and initiation of additional empirical therapy, including broad-spectrum antifungal treatment. For instance, if an initial regimen of a broad-spectrum β-lactam with or without vancomycin has been unsuccessful in bringing about defervescence, one option is the addition of an aminoglycoside to broaden coverage and possibly obtain a synergistic effect against the putative pathogen. Changing from one aminoglycoside to another or from one cephalosporin to another may occasionally make a difference, depending on resistance patterns at a specific institution. Nonetheless, the focus in recent investigations has been on adding empirical broad-spectrum antifungal therapy to a "failing" regimen of antibacterial agents (i.e., one that has not succeeded in achieving defervescence).

Studies that are decades old have shown that abrupt discontinuation of antibacterial coverage in febrile neutropenic cancer

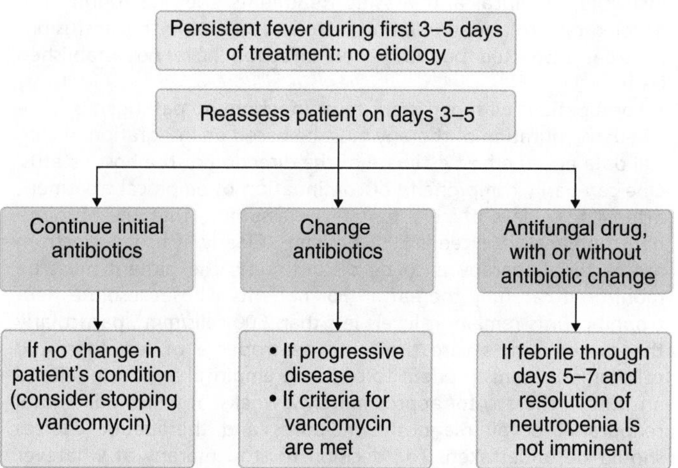

FIGURE 303–3 • Guide to treatment of patients who have persistent fever after 3 to 5 days of treatment and for whom the cause of the fever is not found. (Reproduced with permission from Hughes WT, Armstrong D, Bodey GP, et al: 2002 Guidelines for the use of antimicrobial agents in neutropenic patients with cancer. Clin Infect Dis 2002;34:730–751.)

Rx

patients leads to rebound catastrophic consequences, including shock and death. Persistent use of broad-spectrum antibiotics led to fungal superinfection in almost a third of patients, whereas initiation of empirical amphotericin B at 7 days (added to broad-spectrum antibacterials) led to more rapid defervescence and only rare fungal superinfection. Amphotericin B has well-recognized toxicities, and more recently there have been studies in which empirical voriconazole, lipid formulations of amphotericin B, and caspofungin have been added to antibacterial regimens in patients with persistent febrile neutropenia, usually after at least 4 days of broad-spectrum antibacterial exposure. 2 Still, the great majority of patients treated with empirical antifungal therapy added to antibacterial coverage have not been proved to have a documented fungal infection or occult bacterial infection (or both), and more precise methods for diagnosing the cause of persistent fever in these febrile neutropenic patients are an unmet need. Of the antifungal choices available to the clinician, voriconazole, caspofungin, or an equivalent of these azole and echinocandin compounds that may be available seem to be prudent choices based on available trials. Lipid formulations of amphotericin B remain an alternative, but nephrotoxicity, electrolyte imbalance, and infusion-related disorders still occur more often than with the azole or echinocandin alternatives.

Approaches involving the use of empirical antifungal therapy (see Fig. 303–3) are strongly supported if there is clinical evidence of fungal disease, including

1. Isolation of *Candida* species from the urine of a patient who does not have an indwelling urinary catheter
2. Isolation of fungi from discrete skin lesions
3. Appearance and progression of lung infiltrates on radiograph, CT, or MRI in the face of broad-spectrum antibacterial coverage
4. Appearance of ocular lesions suggesting *Candida* endophthalmitis (which is admittedly rare in a severely neutropenic subject)

Duration of Antibacterial Therapy and Other Treatments

The simplest recommendation is to treat documented pathogens until the signs and symptoms of infection subside. On the other hand, persistently compromised hosts may remain febrile for weeks without identification of the cause. Noninfectious causes of fever, such as an uncontrolled neoplasm in a cancer patient or graft-versus-host disease in a transplant patient, require clinical/laboratory confirmation. The use of antiviral drugs on an empirical basis has no justification, but search for a herpesvirus-related cause of fever, particularly cytomegalovirus, is justified with both serologic and nucleic acid detection techniques because specific treatments for herpesvirus (Chapter 397) and cytomegalovirus (Chapter 399) are available. Empirical antiparasitic treatments and the routine use of leukocyte colony-stimulating factors or granulocyte transfusions to treat suspected but unproven infection have no established basis.

For a patient with persistent fever in whom no pathogen is identified, the duration of therapy must be based on integration of clinical data and the best estimate of the direction of the host's status. One can easily comprehend discontinuation of empirical treatment after 4 to 7 days of persistent fever, assuming that the absolute neutrophil count exceeds 500 cells/mm^3. Clearly, if broad-spectrum antibacterial therapy is to be discontinued, the patient must be monitored carefully thereafter. For patients whose absolute neutrophil counts remain at levels less than 500 cells/mm^3, particularly the subset with severe profound neutropenia of less than 100 cells/mm^3, it seems prudent to continue empirical antibacterial and antifungal therapy for approximately 2 weeks, at which point total reappraisal of all diagnostic measures and therapeutic choices should be undertaken. The decision to stop therapy at whatever arbitrary interval (recognizing that there are no well-controlled studies available for patients treated for more than 2 weeks with empirical antibacterial and subsequent antifungal agents) may be justified if the patient's condition is stable.

Rx

Prophylactic Agents and Considerations after Defervescence

This issue is controversial, and approaches to this problem must be based on a comprehensive understanding of the patient's underlying disease and the likelihood of further treatment. For patients undergoing remission, induction and maintenance chemotherapy for their leukemia and antibiotic prophylaxis with agents such as trimethoprim-sulfamethoxazole are well founded for the specific prophylaxis of *Pneumocystis* pneumonia. This form of prophylaxis may also prevent *Listeria* infection.

Numerous studies have indicated that fluoroquinolone agents can reduce the incidence of fever in leukemic patients and those undergoing allogeneic hematopoietic stem cell transplantation. Nonetheless, the use of quinolone prophylaxis, such as with ciprofloxacin, has been discouraged because of failure to demonstrate improvement in overall patient survival. A documented reduction in the number of febrile episodes and gram-negative infections has been reported in many studies. Concern about selection for increasing quinolone resistance is a negative factor. Some studies indicate less total antibiotic use in patients given quinolone prophylaxis, and when quinolone prophylaxis has been given on outpatient basis to solid tumor patients (i.e., "low risk"), the incidence of hospitalization has been reduced. Thus, the benefits may be in terms of economic considerations rather than a survival benefit. Increasing resistance to quinolone antibiotics should cause such routine prophylaxis practices to be regularly reassessed.

Azole prophylaxis for systemic fungal infections has been supported in patients undergoing allogeneic hematopoietic stem cell transplantation because there is evidence showing increased survival. Antiviral prophylaxis with acyclovir or ganciclovir also appears to be warranted for patients undergoing allogeneic hematopoietic stem cell transplantation.

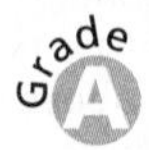

1. Bucaneve G, Micozzi A, Menichetti F, et al: Levofloxacin to prevent bacterial infection in patients with cancer and neutropenia. N Engl J Med 2005;353:977–987.
2. Walsh TJ, Teppler H, Donowitz GR, et al: Caspofungin versus liposomal amphotericin B for empirical antifungal therapy in patients with persistent fever and neutropenia. N Engl J Med 2004;351:1391–1402.

SUGGESTED READINGS

Hughes WT, Armstrong D, Bodey GP, et al: 2002 Guidelines for the use of antimicrobial agents in neutropenic patients with cancer. Clin Infect Dis 2002;34:730–751. *Consensus recommendations.*

Viscoli C, Varnier O, Machetti M: Infections in patients with febrile neutropenia: Epidemiology, microbiology, and risk stratification. Clin Infect Dis 2005;40:S240–S245. *A clinical review.*

304 PREVENTION AND CONTROL OF HOSPITAL-ACQUIRED INFECTIONS

David K. Henderson and Neil Fishman

Health care–associated infections, often referred to as *nosocomial* (from the Greek word *nosocomium,* meaning hospital), have been traditionally defined as infections that occur after hospital admission and that were neither present nor incubating at the time of admission. Because the site of health care delivery and management has increasingly shifted to the ambulatory setting, the relevance of traditional "hospital-associated" infections has diminished. An increasing number of patients are intermittently exposed to the health care environment and may become colonized or infected with health care–associated pathogens without ever being admitted to the hospital and thus may acquire "health care–associated" infections before admission. For example, patients may have received ablative chemotherapy for a stem cell transplant and then be seen only as outpatients until substantial medical problems occur, including infections. Similarly, an increasing number of patients who have malignancies are being treated in "day hospital" settings and may never get admitted unless problems occur with respect to their care, including health care–associated infections.

Additionally, some health care–associated infections become manifested after hospital discharge. Delayed manifestations of these infections usually occur within days of discharge but may occasionally not become clinically apparent for months or even years. Development of these infections is dependent on the incubation period of the particular infection, the individual immunologic response to the infection, and the various specific risk factors for the infection. For example, operative insertion of prosthetic devices (such as joints) can impair the immune response to infection and allow an insidious infection to continue developing and finally be manifested months after insertion of the device. Similarly, hepatitis B or C infection acquired during surgery often does not become evident for weeks to months after discharge. Health care–related infections are associated with increased patient morbidity and mortality, substantial inconvenience for the patient and institution, and striking increases in the cost of care that are primarily absorbed by the institution in which they occur.

HISTORY

The earliest European hospitals were established in the Middle Ages and bore little resemblance to modern hospitals in either form or function. These primitive institutions were generally thought of as places where patients who had intractable diseases could be cared for until they died. Because most patients in that era died of infections, many of which were transmissible, contagion occurred commonly in hospitals. Crowding was so extreme in these institutions that hospital beds were sometimes used for multiple patients and beds often had to be used in shifts. Such intense physical proximity allowed for effective transmission of organisms between patients and resulted in high rates of infection among those who did not die rapidly of their underlying diseases. According to some 19th century reports, surgery was almost always followed by infection, and 60% of limb amputations resulted in fatal infections. These squalid conditions led to early hospitals being called "pest houses."

The discovery plus clinical application of antibacterial agents such as sulfa and penicillin during the 1930s and 1940s was heralded as a medical miracle and resulted in lower rates of surgical infection. These momentous discoveries were followed, however, by the development of antimicrobial resistance to these new agents and the subsequent development of health care–associated infections caused by bacteria resistant to the new antibiotics. The first isolate of penicillin-resistant *Staphylococcus aureus* (PRSA) was noted at the time of discovery of penicillin, even before its widespread clinical use. Within a relatively short period, some hospitals reached epidemic rates of PRSA, thus rendering the new wonder drug powerless. Giving penicillin to patients who had penicillin-resistant infections had no effect. A pandemic of PRSA nosocomial infections led to national and international meetings, which in turn led to a consensus that required the creation of hospital infection control programs. The absence of effective antimicrobial therapy led to the realization that such infections might not always be curable and that prevention might thus be a more important intervention.

Other life-saving medical advancements were similarly associated with new types of lethal infections, such as catheter-related blood stream infection, prosthetic valve infection (endocarditis), and ventilator-associated pneumonia. In the 1970s, gram-negative bacillary infection became a somewhat more common cause of health care–associated infection, but infection with gram-positive cocci became predominant again in the 1980s. In the 1980s, *S. aureus* and coagulase-negative staphylococci displayed increasing frequencies of resistance to new agents that had been developed to combat resistance, such as methicillin and other β-lactam antibiotics. In the 1990s, vancomycin-resistant enterococci (VRE) emerged as a frequent cause of health care-associated infection, particularly in seriously immunocompromised patients. Advancements in medical science during these decades allowed prolongation of life for patients who had sustained severe trauma and other severe illnesses. Advances in chemotherapy and immunosuppression permitted successful and life-prolonging therapy for previously untreatable neoplastic and autoimmune diseases; however, impairment of the immune system resulting from these aggressive therapies also made these patients highly susceptible to common and uncommon health care–associated infections.

IMPORTANCE OF HEALTH CARE–ASSOCIATED INFECTIONS

The literature from the 1970s suggests that six to eight health care–associated infections occurred for every 100 patients admitted to the hospital. Although the number of patients admitted to hospitals in the United States was subsequently reduced by about 10 to 15% during the 1990s in an effort to contain health care costs, the number of health care–associated infections remained essentially unchanged. Because of the decrease in hospital admissions, the rate of health care–associated infections actually increased. The number and rates of these infections increased in great measure because the most severely ill patients continued to be admitted. Because of both their underlying disease states and the aggressive and invasive therapies used to manage their illnesses, seriously ill patients often have the highest risks for health care–associated infections. For a variety of reasons, discussed in more detail later, the numbers and types of antimicrobial-resistant organisms continued to increase, and these antibiotic-resistant infections have spread with facility throughout health care institutions. During the 1990s the Centers for Disease Control and Prevention (CDC) estimated that the number of deaths directly or indirectly related to health care–associated infections increased from 80,000 to 88,000 annually.

Health care–associated infections are important because they cause additional inconvenience, suffering, and mortality for patients. Furthermore, these infections prolong hospitalization and significantly increase the cost of care, thus having a significant adverse impact on the health care system. The increased cost related to health care–associated infections also presents substantial burdens for third-party payers, as well as for the members of society who ultimately pay the bill for health care. The National Foundation for Infectious Diseases has estimated the cost of nosocomial infections with resistant organisms to be 4.0 to 4.5 billion dollars annually. Both the mildest infections (e.g., urinary tract infections) and the most severe infections (e.g., septic shock) are associated with unnecessary increases in cost and inconvenience for patients. Moreover, in the era of prospective payment plans, third-party payers will not reimburse for approximately 95% of the cost of nosocomial infections. For a variety of reasons, then, health care institutions must focus on prevention of these infections, not only to increase patient survival and satisfaction but also to save money.

The attributable cost of nosocomial infections relates in part to prolonged duration of intensive care unit (ICU) or total hospital stays and in part to costs associated with the management of specific infections (e.g., additional diagnostic tests, antimicrobial therapy, personal protective equipment for isolation, and sometimes surgery). Studies have demonstrated that nosocomial blood stream infections result in a 7-day prolongation of hospitalization associated with $40,890 in additional cost for surviving ICU patients and an attributable mortality rate as high as 30%. Generally, surgical site infections result in prolongation of hospitalization for an additional week. Infections after coronary artery bypass surgery result in prolonged stay and extra cost ranging from $14,211 to $20,103, depending on the method used to ascribe cost. Health care–associated pneumonia usually occurs in patients who have been receiving mechanical ventilation and often results in 7 or more excess days in the hospital, frequently in the ICU. These patients often require ventilator support and expensive antimicrobial agents. Cases of health care–associated pneumonia result in increases in cost similar to those incurred by blood stream and surgical site infections (Table 304–1).

Urinary tract infection, the most frequent and least severe health care–related infection, has been associated with a 3-day increase in length of stay in two large case-control studies from different countries. Cost estimates varied between the two countries, but the study in the United States estimated a median additional cost per infection of $3803 (in 1992 U.S. dollars). Although urinary tract infections are generally milder infections, they can cause more severe illness when infection ascends to the kidney or when secondary blood stream infection occurs. Blood stream infection secondary to urinary tract infection is associated with a crude case-fatality rate of 13 to 30%.

TABLE 304–1 RATE AND IMPACT OF NOSOCOMIAL INFECTIONS IN ACUTE CARE HOSPITALS

Site	No. of Infections/ 100 Admissions	% of All NIs	Direct COD	Extra Days	% of NI Extra Days
Urinary tract	2.5	30	<1%	1–3	15
Surgical site	1.4	15	1–2%	7	23
Lung	1.4	15	5–10%	7	23
Blood stream					
Primary	1.4	15	3%	7	23
Secondary	0.3	3	25%	10	5
Others	2.2	24	<1%	2	11

COD = cause of death; NI = nosocomial infection.

RESERVOIRS AND TRANSMISSION OF HEALTH CARE–ASSOCIATED INFECTIONS

Health care–associated infections occur for a wide variety of reasons and are caused by a broad spectrum of pathogens. In some cases (particularly in instances in which patients are severely immunocompromised by disease or treatment), a microbe that would rarely produce an infection may colonize and ultimately infect a hospitalized patient. Hospitalization and the diagnostic and therapeutic interventions associated with hospitalization may provide access to some normally protected parts of the body (e.g., insertion of a percutaneous catheter through the skin provides a portal of entry into the blood stream). Other pathogens that cause these infections are not present in or on the host at the time of hospital admission but colonize the host after admission (frequently after spending just 24 hours in the hospital). After variable periods of colonization, these health care–associated pathogens may produce active infections. Because many patients become colonized or infected with health care–associated pathogens, spread from one patient to another in a health care institution may occur by direct contact between patients, by contact with contaminated environmental surfaces, and perhaps most commonly, by the contaminated hands, clothing, or equipment of health care providers. Health care workers move from patient to patient and, in the absence of appropriate hand hygiene, may easily transmit hospital pathogens. Recent studies have found that health care workers, on average, follow hand hygiene recommendations after only 40% of patient contacts that should prompt the use of hand hygiene. Nurses and allied health professionals comply more often than physicians do, but no category of health care provider achieves rates of compliance greater than 70%. Poorest compliance has been observed in areas at highest risk for transmission, such as the ICU, where the number, types, and immediacy of invasive interventions are the highest and where, unfortunately, patients at the highest risk for adverse outcomes of these infections are often housed.

ANTIBIOTIC-RESISTANT INFECTIONS

No discussion of health care–associated infections during the last half-century would be complete without a thorough discussion of infections caused by antibiotic-resistant microorganisms, as well as strategies to prevent transmission of these organisms. Resistant microorganisms became a significant problem in health care institutions within only a few years after the introduction of antibiotics for clinical therapy. Infections caused by antibiotic-resistant organisms are important because they are generally associated with prolonged illnesses, longer hospital stays, increased risk for death, and greater cost to the health care system than infections caused by antibiotic-susceptible strains of the same species. Antimicrobial resistance to new agents occurs rapidly and is often identified within months of the introduction of a new antimicrobial agent into the pharmacologic armamentarium (Table 304–2). Resistance is often first identified in hospitals and later in the general community. PRSA emerged in just this fashion. For some antibiotics (e.g., vancomycin), resistance did not appear until 3 decades after its introduction. VRE first appeared in the mid-1980s. The organism seems to have different origins in the United States and Europe. In the United States, emergence of resistance is thought to be due to clinical overuse of vancomycin, but in Europe, it is attributed to the use of a related compound (avoparcin) as a nutritional supplement and growth enhancer in farm animals.

TABLE 304–2 ANTIBIOTIC DISCOVERY AND DEVELOPMENT OF RESISTANCE

Antibiotic	Discovery	Clinical Use	Resistance Identified
Penicillin	1940	1943	1940
Streptomycin	1944	1947	1947
Tetracycline	1948	1952	1956
Erythromycin	1952	1955	1956
Vancomycin	1956	1972	1987
Gentamicin	1963	1967	1970

Two predominant risk factors have been identified for infection with antibiotic-resistant pathogens in hospitals: the volume of antimicrobial agents (especially broad-spectrum agents) used in the institution and spread from patient to patient in an institution (frequently via health care providers). The reason that the prevalence of antibiotic-resistant pathogens has grown so rapidly in hospitals was perhaps most clearly explained by Charles Darwin, who noted that nature selects the strain or species most suited to survive within each environment. Because up to half of all patients in U.S. hospitals and almost all patients in ICUs receive antibiotics, a microbe that is resistant to currently administered antimicrobials has a selective advantage to survive, proliferate, and spread. For some combinations of microbe and antibiotic, the probability of a spontaneous mutation to resistance to that particular drug is so high that giving that drug alone for infections caused by that microbe invariably results in antimicrobial resistance. Two prime examples of the risk for development of resistance when using a single agent are tuberculosis and human immunodeficiency virus (HIV) infection.

For example, the risk of mutation to isoniazid resistance among *Mycobacterium tuberculosis* isolates is so high that monotherapy for active tuberculosis with isoniazid results in the development of resistance in 70% of patients. For other combinations of microbes and antibiotics, however, the probability of a spontaneous mutation to resistance is much lower, and administration of that drug alone does not result in an increased risk for resistance of that microbe to that drug. The latter pattern is true for combinations such as enterococci and vancomycin or *S. aureus* and methicillin, which correspond to two of the most frequent antibiotic-resistant infections in U.S. hospitals. The pattern mentioned earlier (i.e., that large proportions of hospital patients are taking antibiotics and that microbes are routinely transported from patient to patient) has resulted in a steadily growing prevalence of antibiotic-resistant pathogens such as methicillin-resistant *S. aureus* (MRSA) and VRE inside U.S. hospitals (Fig. 304–1).

Widespread and sometimes injudicious use of antibiotics along with the ready transmission of bacteria between patients in the hospital has resulted in an alarming trend in the emergence of antimicrobial-resistant organisms. Figure 304–1 illustrates the most recent data reported by the National Nosocomial Infection Surveillance (NNIS) program run by the CDC. Not only are both gram-positive and gram-negative organisms

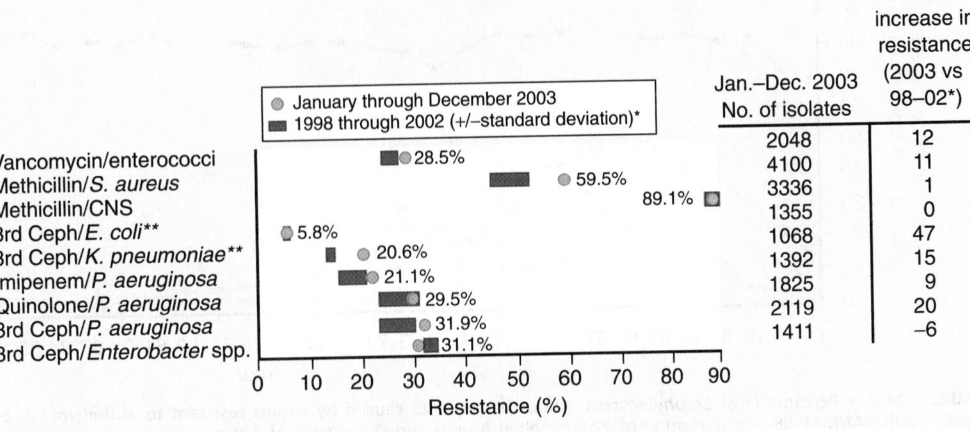

FIGURE 304–1 • Selected antimicrobial-resistant pathogens associated with nosocomial infections in intensive care unit patients and comparison of resistance rates from January through December 2003 with 1998 through 2002, CDC/NNIS system. (From Cardo D, National Nosocomial Infections Study Team of the Division of Healthcare Quality Promotion, National Center for Infectious Diseases, Centers for Disease Control and Prevention: National Nosocomial Infectious Surveillance (NNIS) system report, data summary from January 1992 through June 2004, issued October 2004. Am J Infect Control 2004;32:470–485.)

becoming increasingly resistant to available agents, but many bacteria are also acquiring genes that render them resistant to multiple antibiotics (i.e., multidrug-resistant organisms).

GENERAL STRATEGIES EFFECTIVE IN PREVENTING SPREAD OF RESISTANCE IN HOSPITALS

Antibiotic Stewardship

Many experts believe that improving or shortening the duration of antibiotic use (or both) may be among the most cost-effective means of controlling antibiotic-resistant infections. Bacteria naturally acquire chromosomal mutations or, in other instances, acquire genetic material from other bacteria that confer resistance to antibacterial drugs. Subsequent survival of the resistant organisms depends on a number of factors. Extensive use of antimicrobial agents can promote selective pressure for the survival of resistant pathogens. The risk of emergence of antimicrobial resistance increases markedly after the administration of antibiotics for just 7 days. Thus, inappropriate or unnecessarily prolonged use of antimicrobial agents can select for antimicrobial-resistant isolates. Such strains can colonize and cause infection and can be transmitted between patients.

Several prospective studies have documented a clear association between the use of antimicrobial agents and colonization or infection with resistant organisms in health care institutions, including an association with the use of broad-spectrum agents. In many studies, other interventions were implemented at the same time as restriction of antibiotic use, thus making interpretation of the relative importance of antibiotic restriction problematic. Antibiotic stewardship may be a more effective means of preventing the emergence of resistance in certain organisms (such as gram-negative bacteria), whereas prevention of transmission may be the more important intervention for others (such as MRSA).

Hand Hygiene

Proper use of hand hygiene clearly reduces nosocomial transmission of resistant organisms. Adherence to hand hygiene recommendations is associated with a reduced risk for health care cross-contamination, and failure to perform appropriate hand hygiene is generally considered to be the leading cause of patient-to-staff-to-patient transmission of health care–associated infections. Hands that are visibly dirty or contaminated should be washed with soap and water, and hands that are not visibly soiled should be decontaminated with an alcohol-based hand rub before contacting patients or engaging in clinical procedures. Similarly, health care workers should use an alcohol-based rub after contacting patients' intact or nonintact skin, mucous membranes, or body fluids. Finally, hand hygiene should be used after removing gloves and after any contact with inanimate objects or medical equipment in the vicinity of patients. Alcohol-based hand hygiene products have been demonstrated to be superior to soap and water for general hand hygiene. These products are rapidly bactericidal, are easier to use, do not require a sink, save time, and are less irritating to the skin than handwashing with soap and water. However, soap and water appears to be the preferable mode of hand hygiene when providing care for patients with *Clostridium difficile*–associated disease.

Staffing Strategies

Cohorting care means having staff dedicated solely to providing care for patients known to be infected or colonized with resistant pathogens. When cohorting, staff do not cross-cover both infected/colonized and noncolonized patients. In an outbreak setting, keeping infected and colonized patients separate from uninfected and uncolonized patients, as well as managing them with separate staff, provides a powerful mechanism to prevent transmission. Understaffing clearly contributes to the spread of resistant organisms, particularly in epidemic settings. An association among understaffing, patient overcrowding, and the spread of infectious diseases has been established in several studies.

Decreasing Hospital and Intensive Care Unit Stay

Decreasing the length or the frequency of hospital stay, or both, as well as the length and frequency of stay in critical care units, has been suggested to be an effective mechanism to decrease the risk for spread of resistant organisms, and the results from a number of clinical studies provide support for this concept. Several studies conducted over the past 10 years provide evidence that shortening the hospital or ICU stay decrease rates of infection with resistant organisms.

Microbiologic Surveillance

Although interventions aimed at controlling institutional use of antimicrobials have been associated with modest control of resistance, their success has been far from uniform. Some experts argue for aggressively identifying colonized patients (i.e., an important reservoir for institutional spread), by performing prospective surveillance cultures, and then implementing contact isolation precautions to limit opportunity for transmission. This latter strategy has been shown to decrease the spread of resistant pathogens, in some instances even in the absence of antibiotic control measures (Fig. 304–2). The relative efficacy of these interventions—antimicrobial stewardship versus aggressive identification and isolation—probably varies from organism to organism, if not from institution to institution.

A controversial issue in the health care epidemiology community is whether to use aggressive microbiologic surveillance (termed active surveillance) as an intervention in an attempt to minimize transmission of resistant microorganisms. By microbiologically screening all patients admitted to a health care setting, one can prospectively identify those who are colonized or infected with these organisms. Such patients can then be managed aggressively with isolation precautions, cohorting, or even attempts at decolonization. Active surveillance is labor-intensive and costly, and from a practical standpoint only specific organisms can be targeted. Conversely, active surveillance is likely to identify problematic

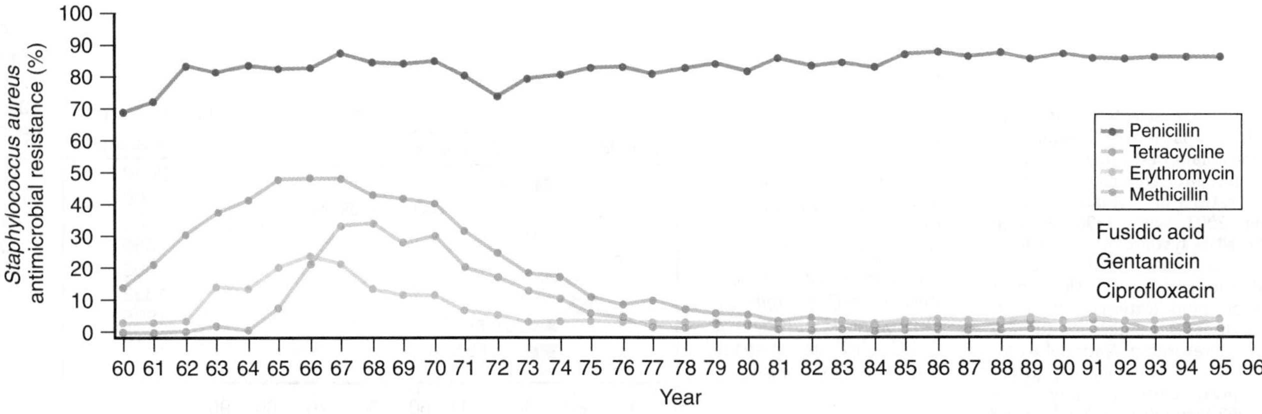

FIGURE 304–2 • Percentage of *Staphylococcus aureus* bacteremias caused by strains resistant to antimicrobials in Danish hospitals from 1960 to 1995. (From Bager F [ed]: DANMAP 98—Consumption of Antimicrobial Agents and Occurrence of Antimicrobial Resistance in Bacteria from Food Animals, Food, and Humans in Denmark. Copenhagen, Danish Zoonosis Centre, 1999.)

pathogens sooner and thus enable measures to be taken to prevent their spread within the health care environment. Many experts believe that tight control is reasonably important to prevent cross-contamination with multiply resistant organisms. To date, no studies have definitively demonstrated the efficacy of this strategy as an independent intervention. Similar to the investigations of antimicrobial stewardship interventions, although some studies have demonstrated a benefit of prospective surveillance cultures, virtually all of them introduced several infection control interventions simultaneously. Because of the simultaneous use of several strategies, one simply cannot determine which of the interventions were actually beneficial.

Some European and Scandinavian countries have implemented policies of restrictive antibiotic use and aggressive surveillance. The Netherlands uses both an aggressive surveillance approach for the prevention of MRSA transmission, as well as a policy of restrictive antibiotic use. In the Netherlands, prospective surveillance cultures of all admissions are performed, strict barrier precautions are required for patients who carry the identified resistant organisms, temporary furloughs are provided for colonized health care workers, and hospital wards—and sometimes even entire institutions—are closed when the prevalence starts to rise. As an example of the efficacy of this approach, the prevalence of staphylococcal isolates resistant to methicillin and causing infection in the Netherlands is currently less than 2%. Similar approaches have been used in Denmark (see Fig. 304–2). Many U.S. hospitals have not implemented the aggressive surveillance approach because of the cost of both the microbiologic procedures and the requisite isolation gear.

Contact Isolation

Most major infection control guidelines for multiply resistant organisms recommend some kind of isolation for patients who harbor these organisms; the category of isolation most frequently used is contact isolation. In studies in which contact isolation has been used as part of a program designed to limit the spread of resistant pathogens, the overall approach has been reasonably effective. However, as previously discussed, contact isolation has typically been implemented concurrently with other (usually several) infection control measures. Therefore, attributing the benefit to one intervention is not generally possible. Using contact isolation as an infection control strategy does have a downside. Recent studies have found that isolated patients were far more likely to experience adverse events during their hospitalizations and were less likely to have narrative notes from physicians or nurses in their charts. Additionally, isolated patients in this study were substantially more likely than controls to experience failure of supportive care, including falls, pressure ulcers, and fluid and electrolyte imbalances. Thus, the potential benefits associated with the use of isolation in an attempt to limit spread of resistant pathogens must be evaluated in the context of the potential adverse impact on patient care.

Antibiotic Cycling

Antibiotic cycling—that is, rotating or cycling the use of different antimicrobials or antimicrobial combinations over time—has been advocated as a possible approach to limiting resistance in health care institutions. To date, the data are quite limited and somewhat contradictory about this approach. Furthermore, this approach has been studied only in the ICU setting and may not be generalizable throughout the health care institution. In short, the verdict is not yet in concerning the relative efficacy of this approach.

Combinations of Strategies

Based on mathematical modeling, strategies that might be expected to be effective in preventing or reducing the prevalence of resistant bacteria in hospitals include reducing antibiotic use, decreasing the length of hospital stays (i.e., increasing patient turnover), and instituting infection control measures to disrupt the spread of bacteria. These infection control measures include restriction of contact between patients and health care workers carrying resistant bacteria, improved hand hygiene, and the use of personal protective equipment (e.g., gloves, masks, protective eyewear or face shields, and gowns). These models also suggest that an important byproduct of these interventions is that interdictions that reduce transmission of all bacteria within a hospital will disproportionately reduce the prevalence of colonization with resistant bacteria. These interventional strategies based on mathematical models need to be subjected to empirical testing to confirm their veracity and utility in clinical settings.

At a more pragmatic level, educating the staff about the epidemiology, pathogenesis, and general routes of transmission of resistant bacteria within the hospital environment, as well as the role that antibiotic use plays in the emergence and spread of bacterial resistance, is of paramount importance. Staff knowledge is required both to understand the rationale for interventions and to encourage compliance with infection control measures.

CATEGORIES OF HEALTH CARE–ASSOCIATED INFECTIONS

Urinary Tract Infections

Nosocomial urinary tract infection usually follows instrumentation of the urinary tract, most often with a catheter. Infection occurs in about 1% of individuals who undergo a single in-and-out catheterization. For patients who have an indwelling urinary catheter, the risk of infection remains relatively constant at about 3 to 6% per catheter day (higher for female than for male patients and increased by manipulation of the catheter). After 10 to 14 days, about half of catheterized patients have bacteriuria. Thus, infection develops at some point in virtually all patients who have long-dwelling urinary catheters. Because enteric flora are the usual cause of urinary tract infection and because diarrhea predisposes to contamination of the catheter-urethra interface, diarrhea is an independent risk factor for catheter-associated urinary tract infection. Urinary tract infections account for between 30 and 40% of all health care–associated infections.

According to data from the CDC's NNIS, the pathogens most frequently responsible for health care–associated urinary tract infections are (in order of decreasing relative frequency) *Escherichia coli, Enterococcus* species, *P. aeruginosa*, *Candida* species, *Klebsiella pneumoniae*, *Enterobacter* species, *Proteus mirabilis*, coagulase-negative staphylococci, other fungi, *Citrobacter* species, and *S. aureus*. Studies of preventive measures have confirmed the efficacy of closed drainage systems and antiseptic-impregnated (i.e., silver alloy) urinary catheters for preventing health care–associated urinary tract infections.

Pneumonia

Infection of the pulmonary parenchyma can occur after the aspiration of either microbe-laden secretions from the upper respiratory tract or regurgitated gastric contents. Infection at a distant site in the body, such as *S. aureus* infection of a central venous catheter or an arteriovenous fistula used for hemodialysis, can sometimes result in hematogenously spread septic pulmonary emboli, which in turn can produce infection in the pulmonary parenchyma (often with a radiographically distinct pattern of multiple diffuse expanding pneumatoceles throughout the lungs). Another rare source of health care–associated pneumonia is direct inhalation of a microbe from the air. Examples of microbes that usually cause pneumonia by inhalation include *M. tuberculosis* and *Aspergillus fumigatus*. Infection with the former occurs by contagion via small-particle droplet nuclei from a coughing patient. These droplet nuclei float in the air for hours and may infect patients several rooms away, although those closer to the coughing patient are at greater risk. Infection with *A. fumigatus* occurs by inhalation of its spores, which may be liberated from the surface of almost any organic material on which it can grow (e.g., an orange). These spores are virtually ubiquitous and may be present in both outdoor and indoor air. *Legionella* infection was originally thought to result from inhalation, but it may occur more frequently after the aspiration of *Legionella*-contaminated potable water. Viruses such as respiratory syncytial virus, parainfluenza virus, and adenovirus have also been described as causes of health care–associated pneumonia, particularly in severely immunocompromised patients.

Most patients who acquire nosocomial pneumonia have been maintained on mechanical ventilators in an ICU. The most frequent microbial agents causing these kinds of health care–associated pulmonary infections, according to NNIS data, are *S. aureus*, *P. aeruginosa*, *Enterobacter* species, *K. pneumoniae*, and *E. coli* (in decreasing order of relative frequency). Rates of pneumonia in mechanically ventilated patients range from 6 to 30%, with a risk of 1 to 3% per day of intubation and mechanical ventilation. A number of factors influence the risk for nosocomial pneumonia in these patients. In a critically ill, supine, ventilated patient, oropharyngeal secretions pool in the oropharynx and subglottic space above the tracheal tube cuff and form a reservoir of contaminated secretions. These secretions often get aspirated into the pulmonary parenchyma along the endotracheal tube. Using a device that provides continual subglottic suction to prevent pooling of these secretions has been associated with lower rates of clinical aspiration and early ventilator-associated pneumonia (defined as pneumonia occurring within 3 to 5 days of intubation).

The inner lumen of an endotracheal tube rapidly becomes covered with a biofilm containing high concentrations of microorganisms. Pieces of this biofilm (carrying large numbers of bacteria) can be inoculated directly into the lower respiratory tract, either by ventilatory flow or by inserting devices through the tube (such as might occur during suctioning or therapeutic bronchoscopy). These pieces of biofilm can seed the pulmonary parenchyma with microorganisms and serve as a nidus for ongoing infection.

The use of either continuous or intermittent enteral feeding also increases gastric pH and, at least in some studies, has been associated with an 80% risk for gram-negative colonization of the stomach. Conversely, maintenance of adequate nutritional status is clearly associated with a reduced risk for ventilator-associated pneumonia, and enteral nutrition is clearly the route of choice for supplementing the nutritional status of these patients.

Abnormal elevation of gastric pH related to the patient's underlying disease or to the use of histamine type 2 (H_2) blockers, proton pump inhibitors, or antacid therapy is associated with an increased risk for infection because of the resulting microbial overgrowth in stomach fluids. When these fluids are regurgitated and aspirated, they may rapidly produce pneumonia because of the large bacterial inocula involved. Use of sucralfate, which does not affect gastric pH as substantially as H_2-blockers or proton pump inhibitors do, to prevent stress ulceration during mechanical ventilation has been associated with lower rates of nosocomial pneumonia in some studies; however, other studies have suggested that this agent may not be as effective in preventing gastrointestinal bleeding as H_2-blockers are.

Aspiration of gastric contents occurs four times more frequently when the patient is in the supine position than when the head of the patient's bed is elevated at a 45-degree angle. Studies have demonstrated that isolation of the same organisms from the stomach, pharynx, and endobronchial samples occurs extremely uncommonly in semirecumbent patients when compared with patients placed in the supine position. Nonetheless, gastric reflux occurs frequently, irrespective of body position, in mechanically ventilated patients who have nasogastric tubes.

Selective digestive tract decontamination with antibiotics (e.g., swabbed onto the teeth as a paste or squirted into the stomach via a nasogastric tube, or both) has also been shown to result in significantly lower health care–associated pneumonia rates, but this approach has not generally been used in the United States because of potential for the rapid development of antimicrobial resistance among the gut flora in these patients. However, good oral hygiene does help prevent health care–associated pneumonia without introducing the risk of antimicrobial resistance.

Surgical Site Infections

Historically, surgical site infection was almost inevitable because of the inhospitable environment in early hospitals. Today, the reverse is true for "clean," elective procedures (e.g., coronary bypass graft or total hip replacement). A large majority of such operations are not complicated by infection because of the use of strict aseptic technique (i.e., antiseptic preparation of the surgeon's hands and the patient's skin), the use of sterile barriers (e.g., surgical gown and gloves), timely administration of prophylactic antibiotics before (and when appropriate, additional doses during) the procedure, and sterilization of surgical instruments used for the procedure. Despite these major improvements, infections still do occur. In the 21st century the occurrence of these infections is most highly dependent on the technical skills of the surgeon and the presence of comorbid conditions in the patient who is undergoing the procedure.

The most frequent microbial pathogens causing surgical site infections (according to NNIS data) are, in decreasing order of relative frequency, *S. aureus;* coagulase-negative staphylococci; enterococci; gram-negative bacilli such as *E. coli*, *Enterobacter*, *Klebsiella*, and *Serratia;* and *Candida*.

Both surgery-related and patient-related factors contribute to the risk for surgical site infections. Despite equivalent provision of care and preventive measures, differences in postoperative infection rates can still occur for a variety of reasons. A higher prevalence of comorbid conditions in patients being referred for care (i.e., obesity, diabetes mellitus, severe peripheral vascular disease) inevitably results in higher surgical site infection rates. A variety of factors related to the technical aspects of surgery also influence the risk for infection. For example, the presence of dead space and the presence of dead tissue in the wound (e.g., as might occur through the excessive use of electrocautery) are both associated with an increased risk for infection. Other technical factors also influence this risk; for example, shaving to remove hair the day before the operation is associated with higher infection risk than is using clippers to remove hair within the hour before the operation.

The timing of antimicrobial prophylaxis is an important variable for surgical site infections. Making certain that agents with the appropriate antimicrobial spectrum are administered in time to ensure adequate blood levels of the drug or drugs at the time of scalpel entry into the skin and that adequate levels are maintained throughout the procedures is key to the success of perioperative prophylaxis. Antibiotics should be administered within 1 hour before incision to guarantee adequate serum levels and should be redosed if the procedure lasts longer than 4 hours. Finally, antibiotics administered for prophylaxis should not be continued for longer than 24 hours after the procedure and frequently are not required at all postoperatively.

Patients who have intrinsically contaminated wounds (e.g., a ruptured appendix) have a much higher risk for intra-abdominal infection, despite modern preventive measures, primarily because high-inoculum microbial exposure occurs and infection may already be established before surgery begins. Gut decontamination before surgery remains an important, effective option to reduce the risk for postoperative infection in some settings. For example, elective colon surgery after appropriate antimicrobial prophylaxis and mechanical cleansing is associated with much lower infection rates.

Serum glucose control has also been shown to decrease the risk for surgical site infections. Finally, surgical infection rates can also be reduced by providing information about postoperative infectious complications to the surgeons.

Blood Stream Infections

Blood stream infections may result from primary infection within the cardiovascular system (e.g., from an infected vascular catheter) or be secondary to a local infection in another organ (e.g., *E. coli* infection of the urinary tract). Approximately 80% of health care–associated blood stream infections are primary, and the overwhelming preponderance of them are due to vascular catheter infections. Approximately 20% are secondary to infections in other organs. According to NNIS data, the most frequent microbial causes of primary blood stream infection in the past decade have been (in decreasing order of frequency) coagulase-negative staphylococci, *S. aureus*, enterococci, *Candida*, and gram-negative bacilli such as *Enterobacter*. Although coagulase-negative staphylococci definitely do cause such infections, a large proportion of blood cultures growing this organism actually represent contamination and not true infection. By contrast, *S. aureus* and *Candida* are more virulent and associated with a much higher probability of true blood stream infection.

Microorganisms can reach the circulation via three separate pathways associated with the use of intravascular catheters. Organisms can reach the blood stream by colonizing the catheter insertion site and subsequently moving along the catheter through the tissues; by colonizing hubs, junctions, and other connectors and gaining access to the system when these sites are manipulated; and through intrinsic or extrinsic contamination of the infusion fluid.

Catheter-related blood stream infection most frequently begins with colonization of the catheter. Because vascular catheters are usually placed through the patient's skin, most such colonizing microbes come from the patient's resident skin flora. Studies using electron microscopy have shown that microbial contamination of catheters is virtually universal from the first day after insertion. Organisms migrate from skin along the insertion tract by capillary action. Colonization often occurs at time of insertion but may also take place days afterward. Initially, organisms colonize along the external surface of the catheter. By contrast, after 10 days of placement, ultrastructural studies demonstrate an increasing relative frequency of intraluminal contamination, and most long-term catheters appear to become colonized and produce blood stream infection by the intraluminal route. Colonization is facilitated by the formation of a fibrin sheath around the catheter as a result of platelet deposition and is also facilitated by organism-produced biofilm.

The reason that all vascular catheters do not uniformly result in clinical infection relates to the body's innate immune response and its ability to kill microbial invaders and limit their growth and spread. Because most colonizing and infecting flora come from the patient's skin, use of antiseptics to prepare the site before catheter insertion and every few days thereafter to decrease the microbial burden has been a successful strategy for decreasing the risk for infection. In several clinical trials, chlorhexidine gluconate skin preparation has been shown to reduce the risk for catheter colonization significantly when compared with alcohol or povidone-iodine preparation of the skin. Although most such trials were designed to have statistical power only to be able to detect a reduction in catheter colonization, two of the studies demonstrated significant reductions in catheter-related blood stream infections as well. The use of maximal barriers to create a large sterile field during catheter insertion has also been shown to decrease the risk for infection.

A number of other factors, such as the type of dressing, the composition of the catheter, the number of lumens, and the type of intravenous administration system used, all influence the risk for catheter-associated primary blood stream infection. Either cotton gauze dressings covered by tape or semipermeable transparent membrane dressings can be used to protect the insertion site; however, the cutaneous microbial burden increases substantially underneath the semipermeable dressing. Conversely, the semipermeable dressing requires less frequent changes/manipulations and anchors the device in place more securely than gauze and tape dressing does. A recent study and a subsequent meta-analysis showed the two dressings to be equivalent with respect to infection rate and local complications. Once again, preparation of the site with chlorhexidine gluconate during dressing changes also decreases the infection rate. However, gauze dressings may be preferable if the insertion site is oozing. Several catheter characteristics or properties have been suggested to be associated with an increased risk for catheter-associated infection. For example, catheters made of stiff materials traumatize the vascular endothelium and move around in the insertion site—both facilitating colonization. Larger-bore catheters are also probably associated with increased risk for colonization and infection. Finally, the manner in which catheters are used may influence the risk for infection. In critically ill patients, for example, pulmonary artery catheters are frequently repositioned to obtain accurate readings (increasing local endothelial trauma, as well as the likelihood for catheter colonization).

Health care–related factors also contribute to the risk for catheter-associated primary blood stream infection. For example, antimicrobial therapy may alter the patient's skin flora, thereby facilitating colonization with an aggressive pathogen. Furthermore, health care workers who do not practice appropriate hand hygiene may inadvertently colonize a patient's catheter insertion site with health care–associated pathogens (e.g., MRSA). Manipulating the intravascular delivery system (e.g., to reposition the catheter, obtain a blood sample, administer medications) also increases the likelihood of catheter colonization. Techniques used for insertion and maintenance of catheters likewise influence the risk for infection. Inserting central venous catheters with less than maximal sterile barriers increases the risk for infection. The site chosen for insertion of a central venous catheter also influences the risk; insertion into the femoral vein is associated with a greater risk for colonization and infection than is insertion into either the subclavian or internal jugular vein. Although guidelines from the Healthcare Infection Control Practices Advisory Committee have recently recommended the subclavian route of insertion over the internal jugular approach, the data that support this recommendation are quite limited.

One approach to attempt to reduce the risk for catheter-associated infections has been to bond antimicrobial substances (antiseptics or antimicrobial agents) to the catheter. A catheter impregnated with antiseptic (chlorhexidine–silver sulfadiazine) reduced both colonization and blood stream infection by nearly 50%. Antibiotic-coated catheters (e.g., minocycline-rifampin–coated catheters) may be associated with even greater risk reduction. Minocycline-rifampin catheters are coated on both the internal and external surfaces of the catheters, whereas first-generation chlorhexidine–silver sulfadiazine catheters were coated only on their external surfaces. Preliminary studies have demonstrated that the efficacy of minocycline-rifampin catheters may be prolonged when compared with the first-generation chlorhexidine–silver sulfadiazine–coated catheters. The second-generation chlorhexidine–silver sulfadiazine catheters are coated on both the internal and external surfaces but have not yet been compared with minocycline-rifampin–coated catheters. Antimicrobial agent–coated catheters are associated with at least a theoretical risk for the development of antimicrobial resistance to the agents coating the catheters, although such resistance has not yet been documented in studies including hundreds of patients.

Recently, studies have demonstrated that the use of needleless administration systems also contributes to the risk for intravascular device–associated infections. When these devices were initially marketed, they had two primary goals—health care worker safety and device patency. They were not intended to reduce infection rates. Unfortunately, some recent studies suggest that these devices actually increase the risk for infection. The care and use practices of staff who are unfamiliar with these systems often do not follow the manufacturer's recommendations. Staff may not disinfect the device properly, or the device may be intrinsically difficult to disinfect. Nonetheless, several studies have documented increased risk for health care–related primary blood stream infections associated with the use of these devices.

Prevention of primary blood stream infections should be an important focus for all health care institutions. Recently, the Institute for Healthcare Improvement (IHI) advocated bundling five infection prevention strategies—each of which is known to be independently effective—to prevent primary blood stream infections. The five techniques are effective hand hygiene; maximal barrier precautions at insertion; cutaneous antisepsis with chlorhexidine; optimal insertion site selection; and daily review of the necessity for maintaining the catheter, with prompt removal when it is no longer needed. Recently, the Joint Commission on

Accreditation of Healthcare Organizations (JCAHO) has adopted the IHI recommendation and requires implementation of these five strategies as a standard for continued accreditation.

Other Nosocomial Infections

During a national study of nosocomial infections conducted by the CDC in the 1970s, only about 6% of recognized infections did not involve the four main body sites listed earlier (see Table 304–1); currently, about 25% of all infections acquired in hospitals conducting hospital-wide surveillance are of this miscellaneous type. This category includes gastrointestinal infections caused by organisms such as *C. difficile*, rotavirus, and *Salmonella;* viral infections caused by varicella, influenza, and respiratory syncytial virus; and candidal infections of the mouth, esophagus, and vagina. *C. difficile*–associated diarrhea and enterocolitis are of particular concern because of the emergence of a new, highly virulent strain associated with epidemic spread in the United States. This strain, which was previously quite uncommon, has variations in its toxin genes and is distinguishable, at least in part, by its increased resistance to fluoroquinolones. The highly virulent strain has emerged as an increasingly common cause of health care–associated epidemics.

INFECTION CONTROL PROGRAMS

Formal infection control programs did not exist in most hospitals until the 1970s. These programs were introduced into U.S. hospitals at that time, based on recommendations from the CDC, the American Hospital Association (AHA), and JCAHO. The primary rationale for the creation of these programs was to attempt to control antibiotic-resistant infections, which had soared out of control in most hospitals during the 1950s and 1960s.

As hospitals began to implement such programs, the CDC conducted a national study of the effectiveness of these efforts titled the Study of the Efficacy of Nosocomial Infection Control (SENIC). The largest study of infection control ever conducted, SENIC used a probability sample of general hospitals nationwide, determined nosocomial infection rates, and assessed predictors in multivariate analysis. The size and intensity of work by the infection control program were found to predict infection rates. The most important predictors of success in decreasing health care–associated infection rates were (in decreasing order of importance) the intensity of surveillance, the intensity of control measures, the ratio of infection control practitioners to number of patient beds, the presence of a trained hospital epidemiologist on staff, and provision of surgical site infection rates to surgeons. The most effective programs (i.e., those with all these predictors) experienced a 32% relative reduction in the nosocomial infection rate in comparison to hospitals that did not have infection control programs.

Although programs vary from institution to institution, depending on the needs and resources available, most programs share certain essential functions, among which are surveillance for health care–associated infections; investigation of outbreaks, problematic trends, or distinctive or unusual infections; and education of staff about the epidemiology, pathogenesis, and prevention of health care–associated infections. In addition, hospital epidemiology programs work closely with other professionals in the health care setting who share similar interests. Specifically, infection control programs routinely form working partnerships with the clinical medical and nursing staffs, the infectious diseases service, the occupational medicine service, clinical microbiology, and the hospital safety program. The work of each of these services is complementary to the hospital epidemiology program. Communication among these groups is essential for success of the program.

The most likely reason that surveillance for nosocomial infections was important in SENIC is straightforward. By understanding what is happening microbiologically in an institution, specific control measures can be fashioned to intervene and thereby limit outbreaks and reduce high endemic rates of infection.

Initially, many hospitals implemented continual hospital-wide surveillance. Because some infections appeared to be more important than others in analyses from the SENIC database in terms of prolongation of stay and extra cost and because interhospital comparison of crude hospital rates was thought to be difficult given the differences in severity of underlying illness in patients admitted to hospitals of different types in different regions, some authorities advocated targeted surveillance programs with a focus on the most significant problems for each hospital. Even though such a strategy does allow an institution to focus its efforts on its most pressing problem, the strategy may also cause institutions to overlook significant problems. For instance, outbreaks in ICUs may be missed for months in hospitals targeting only surgical site infections.

Over the past 2 decades many hospitals were downsized in terms of both patient admissions and health care personnel to cut costs; because infection control programs were not viewed as revenue generating, they were often cut as well. Even when they were not reduced in size, these programs often had to assume additional duties that were not part of their original focus. For example, new Occupational Safety and Health Administration (OSHA) requirements to protect health care workers from infection with blood-borne pathogens required orientation and annual retraining of all health care workers, as well as the development and annual review of exposure control plans for all hospital units and departments. Similar requirements were enacted by OSHA to protect health care workers from nosocomial tuberculosis. These activities clearly relate to infection control and were thus usually assigned to infection control programs. Because they were unfunded mandates, however, the requirements for added work were usually given to infection control programs with no added resources. Infection control programs in U.S. hospitals are often underfunded and undermanned. A recent consensus report from the CDC, JCAHO, AHA, and a variety of other agencies and national societies concluded that infection control is more difficult in the hospital now than it was during the 1970s and 1980s when SENIC was conducted. That consensus report also concluded that more than one infection control practitioner per every 250 hospital beds (the ratio found to be essential by SENIC) is needed to do an effective job of controlling infections. This report has had limited impact, however, because many hospitals continue to reduce support for infection control activities and others are now requiring infection control personnel to work on other adverse effects associated with health care (e.g., prescribing errors, patient falls), thus again increasing the infection control program workload without increasing program resources.

OCCUPATIONAL/NOSOCOMIAL INFECTIONS IN HEALTH CARE WORKERS

Nosocomial infection can affect health care workers as well as patients. Health care workers in facilities that pay limited attention to the rising prevalence of colonization of patients with antibiotic-resistant pathogens are more likely to become colonized at a higher rate than the general population. Casually contagious viral infections such as influenza, varicella, rubella, and measles occur more frequently in health care workers because they are exposed to sick people in the community, as well as to patients who are not always recognized and placed on appropriate isolation precautions. Several infectious diseases are worthy of more detailed consideration with respect to occupational exposure and infection, among which are hepatitis B, hepatitis C, HIV, and tuberculosis.

Occupational Risk for Human Immunodeficiency Virus Infection

The risk for acquiring HIV infection from a patient in the health care setting is small. Fewer than 75 documented occupational infections with HIV have occurred in more than 5 million health care workers in the United States during the $2\frac{1}{2}$ decades since acquired immunodeficiency syndrome (AIDS) and HIV entered the health care workplace. The routine use of universal/standard infection control precautions, development and implementation of safer devices and other engineered controls, and education and training of staff have all contributed to additional risk reduction.

A multinational case-control study conducted by the CDC and collaborators showed that deep percutaneous injuries, visibly bloody sharp instruments, devices that had been used in blood vessels, and exposure to source patients who had end-stage HIV disease (i.e., who died within 2 months after exposure—presumably a surrogate marker for high viral burden) were independent predictors of HIV transmission. In this study, administration of postexposure antiretroviral chemoprophylaxis with zidovudine was associated with an almost 80% relative reduction in the risk for infection in multivariate analysis. This finding led to a U.S. Public Health Service recommendation for the routine administration of postexposure chemoprophylaxis after occupational exposure to HIV. The CDC updates its recommended guidelines for the use of postexposure antiretroviral prophylaxis periodically, with the most recent of these recommendations published in fall 2005.

Because the long-term consequences of taking antiretroviral agents for a month are unknown and because significant adverse effects such as nausea, vomiting, and diarrhea develop in more than 70% of health care workers who take these agents for postexposure prophylaxis, they should not be administered casually or unnecessarily. Institutions should have defined protocols for determining whether an exposure has occurred, for encouraging reporting of exposures, and for facilitating access to antiretroviral agents when they are needed.

Occupational Risk for Hepatitis

Before development of the hepatitis B vaccine, hepatitis B represented the largest occupational risk to health care providers who were exposed to blood in the health care workplace. Standard precautions and OSHA requirements to offer free hepatitis B vaccine to health care workers have resulted in a dramatic decrease in hepatitis B infection in health care workers. However, approximately 10% of those vaccinated do not respond to vaccine, and some workers decline to be vaccinated because of concerns about side effects. Studies have shown the vaccine to be safe, and compliance has probably increased with dissemination of this information.

No vaccine is available as yet for hepatitis C, the most common blood-borne viral infection and the most frequent indication for severe chronic liver disease requiring liver transplantation in the United States. A recent open trial of early interferon therapy for acute hepatitis C virus (HCV) infection, as well as a recent National Institutes of Health consensus conference, documented higher cure rates for patients treated for acute hepatitis C than had been demonstrated for the treatment of established chronic infection. Although no formal recommendations have been issued for the management of health care workers who sustain occupational exposure to HCV, one approach is to monitor the health care worker by polymerase chain reaction (PCR) for HCV RNA. Those who become PCR positive are then monitored for a brief period to make certain that the PCR findings are reproducible and to see whether individuals can clear their infections immunologically (which is thought to occur in as many as 50% of cases). Those who do not clear their infections spontaneously can be treated for acute hepatitis infection as described earlier.

Occupational Risk for Tuberculosis

Rates of tuberculosis in the United States declined for more than a century, and this decline was accelerated in the 1950s in association with the discovery and clinical use of effective antituberculous therapy. In 1985, tuberculosis rates once again began to increase and continued to do so until 1992. Epidemiologic analysis of the increase suggested that increased immigration of persons with tuberculosis and the expanding pool of immunocompromised patients produced by the HIV epidemic were the two predominant factors influencing this increase. The increase in case rates was compounded by a simultaneous, marked increase in resistance to antituberculous agents among isolates during this period as well.

Both these factors contributed substantially to health care–associated tuberculosis outbreaks in New York, New Jersey, and Florida. Major factors contributing to these outbreaks included (1) inadequate administrative controls (e.g., index of suspicion for the diagnosis, policies for placing patients in appropriate isolation, policies requiring that isolation patients remain in isolation), (2) inadequate engineering controls (i.e., lack of appropriate negative-pressure ventilation rooms for the isolation of patients with possible or known tuberculosis), and (3) inadequate use of personal protective equipment (e.g., respirators). These outbreaks resulted in the development of new CDC recommendations and OSHA requirements mandating administrative and engineering controls, as well as a program of respirator fit testing, annual or semiannual purified protein derivative testing, and regular retraining regarding tuberculosis. Tuberculosis case rates and health care–associated spread of tuberculosis were controlled before these guidelines were issued, thus leaving the question of the relative importance of respirators and respirator fit testing to the overall tuberculosis control effort in health care institutions unanswered. Since 1992, the rate of tuberculosis has steadily decreased in the United States, and nosocomial outbreaks have been reported much less frequently.

SUGGESTED READINGS

Boyce JM, Cookson B, Christiansen K, et al: Methicillin-resistant *Staphylococcus aureus.* Lancet Infect Dis 2005;5:653–663. *A comprehensive overview.*

Crum NF, Lee RU, Thornton SA, et al: Fifteen-year study of the changing epidemiology of methicillin-resistant *Staphylococcus aureus.* Am J Med 2006;119:943–951. *Evidence for a rapid increase in the incidence of MRSA infections since 2002.*

Dellit TH, Owens RC, McGowan JE Jr, et al: Infectious Diseases Society of America and the Society for Healthcare Epidemiology of America guidelines for developing an institutional program to enhance antimicrobial stewardship. Clin Infect Dis 2007;44:159–177. *Outlines a framework for developing an evidence-based program.*

Fishman N: Antimicrobial stewardship. Am J Med 2006;119:S53–S61. *A review of strategies to prevent and limit antimicrobial resistance.*

Panlilio AL, Cardo DM, Grohskopf LA, et al: Updated U.S. Public Health Service guidelines for the management of occupational exposures to HIV and recommendations for postexposure prophylaxis. MMWR Recomm Rep 2005; 54(RR-9):1–17. *Consensus guidelines.*

Pronovost P, Needham D, Berenholtz S, et al: An intervention to decrease catheter-related bloodstream infections in the ICU. N Engl J Med 2006;355:2725–2732. *There was a sustained decline in the rate of catheter-related infections following an evidence-based intervention.*

Segers P, Speekenbrink RG, Ubbink DT, et al: Prevention of nosocomial infection in cardiac surgery by decontamination of the nasopharynx and oropharynx with chlorhexidine gluconate: A randomized controlled trial. JAMA 2006;296:2460–2466. *Use of chlorhexidine was associated with a decreased incidence of postoperative infections, including those of the lower respiratory tract and wound.*

305 APPROACH TO THE PATIENT WITH SUSPECTED ENTERIC INFECTION

Herbert L. DuPont

Epidemiology

Enteric infections are second only to respiratory tract infections as common medical problems. In certain populations, enteric infections are hyperendemic: poorly nourished infants living in developing tropical countries showing excessive rates of mortality, infants in certain daycare centers, residents of custodial institutions for the mentally retarded, patients with advanced immunosuppression, and visitors from industrialized areas to developing regions with "travelers' diarrhea."

Etiology

In approaching a patient with an enteric infection, epidemiologic (Table 305–1) and clinical features (Table 305–2) are used to identify the type of etiologic agent responsible for illness and to develop a plan for evaluation (Table 305–3) and management (Table 305–4).

Recent travel to mountainous regions or recreational lakes of North America should raise the suspicion of infection caused by *Giardia lamblia.* When diarrhea occurs during or after travel to a developing tropical region, a bacterial enteropathogen should be suspected. The leading causes of travelers' diarrhea worldwide are the diarrheogenic *Escherichia coli:* enterotoxigenic *E. coli* (ETEC) and enteroaggregative *E. coli* (EAEC). The invasive bacteria (*Shigella, Salmonella,* and *Campylobacter*) cause diarrhea among travelers to all regions but are more common in Asia, where ciprofloxacin-resistant *Campylobacter* is of special importance. Travel to Russia, particularly St. Petersburg, is associated with an increased risk of infection by *Cryptosporidium parvum* and *G. lamblia* because there the protozoa can be found in drinking water. Infection with *Cyclospora* should be suspected when persistent or recurrent diarrhea follows travel to Nepal, Haiti, and Peru.

TABLE 305–1 EPIDEMIOLOGIC FEATURES IMPORTANT IN DETERMINING POTENTIAL CAUSE OF ENTERIC INFECTION IN A PERSON OR PERSONS WITH DIARRHEA

Epidemiologic Feature	Etiologic Agent to Suspect
Travel to mountainous areas of North America	*Giardia lamblia*
Travel to Russia (especially St. Petersburg)	*Cryptosporidium, G. lamblia*
Travel to Nepal	*Cyclospora*
Travel to the developing tropical/semitropical world from an industrialized region	Enterotoxigenic *Escherichia coli*, enteroaggregative *E. coli, Shigella, Campylobacter, Salmonella*, other bacterial causes, *G. lamblia, Cyclospora, Cryptosporidium*, and noroviruses (e.g., Norwalk)
Presence of associated cases (an outbreak)	Use incubation period and clinical features (see Table 305–2) to determine probable cause
Antibiotic, chemotherapy, or proton pump inhibitor use in the past 2 mo, particularly with a history of recent or current hospitalization	*Clostridium difficile*
Contact with daycare centers	Any enteropathogen, often the low-dose organisms: *G. lamblia, Cryptosporidium, Shigella*, or viral pathogens
Homosexual male	Any organism spread by fecal-oral route; in those with proctitis suspect *Neisseria gonorrhoeae, Chlamydia trachomatis*, herpes simplex, or *Treponema pallidum*
Immunosuppressed person	Any agent, especially *Cryptosporidium*, microsporidia, *Cyclospora, Isospora, Shigella, Salmonella, Campylobacter jejuni, C. difficile, Mycobacterium avium-intracellulare*, herpes simplex virus, and cytomegalovirus
Recent or current cruise ship travel	Norovirus

TABLE 305–2 CLINICAL FEATURES IN THE PERSON WITH ENTERIC INFECTION

Clinical Syndrome	Etiologic Agents Suspected	Special Considerations
Sustained fever often with systemic toxicity (enteric or typhoid fever)	*Salmonella typhi*, nontyphoid *Salmonella, Campylobacter, Shigella, Yersinia enterocolitica*	Stool and blood cultures; empirical antibiotics generally indicated
Acute watery (secretory) diarrhea	Any agent. Consider *Vibrio cholerae* (if water losses are major), enterotoxigenic or enteroaggregative *Escherichia coli, Shigella, Salmonella, Campylobacter jejuni*, viral or parasitic protozoal pathogen	Fluid and electrolyte therapy crucial for recovery in dehydration
Recurrent vomiting (gastroenteritis)	Viral agents (rotavirus or norovirus, e.g., Norwalk virus) or preformed toxin (*Staphylococcus aureus* or *Bacillus cereus*)	In case of an outbreak, incubation period suggests the etiology
Bloody diarrhea (dysentery)	*Shigella, C. jejuni, Salmonella*, Shiga toxin–producing *E. coli* (e.g., O157:H7) or invasive *E. coli, Aeromonas hydrophilia*, noncholera *Vibrio, Yersinia enterocolitica, Entamoeba histolytica*, or inflammatory bowel disease	Stool culture and occasionally parasite examination important to determining cause; hemolytic uremic syndrome may complicate diarrheal disease caused by *E. coli* O157:H7 or *Shigella dysenteriae*
Diarrhea lasting ≥2 wk (persistent diarrhea)	*Giardia lamblia* and other protozoal parasites, bacterial overgrowth, bacterial diarrhea, lactase deficiency, Brainerd's diarrhea, postinfectious irritable bowel syndrome (PI-IBS), unmasked inflammatory bowel disease, or celiac sprue	Stool culture and parasite examination indicated; empirical anti-*Giardia* therapy may be useful; remove milk from diet; raw milk or untreated (well or surface) water consumption or international travel not responding to antimicrobial therapy suggests the possibility of Brainerd's diarrhea or PI-IBS

A specific food or water vehicle cannot be suspected unless multiple cases of illness with a common exposure occur. All too frequently, persons assume the last food consumed before an illness is responsible for the symptoms. The highly variable incubation period for diarrheal disease, which may as short as 2 hours after eating a food for preformed toxins to a week or even longer for low-dose bacterial infections, makes the determination of a specific food or beverage in a single case of illness impossible. When an outbreak of diarrhea results in multiple cases, a category of etiology can often be determined by calculating the incubation period after looking at timing of the common exposure. Short incubation periods are associated with food poisoning associated with enterotoxins (2 to 7 hours for cases caused by *Staphylococcus aureus*, 2 to 4 hours

TABLE 305–3 LABORATORY TESTS AND PROCEDURES USEFUL IN THE DIAGNOSIS OF INFECTIOUS DIARRHEA

Specific Test or Procedure	When Indicated	Clinical Significance
Fecal leukocyte test	For moderate to severe cases	Indicates diffuse colonic inflammation, often with diarrhea caused by *Shigella*, *Salmonella*, *Campylobacter*, or *Clostridium difficile*
Fecal lactoferrin	For moderate to severe cases to help identify inflammatory forms of enteric infection, to utilize in health care–associated diarrhea to help determine whether *C. difficile* toxin test should be performed	More sensitive test than fecal leukocytes and picks up less striking degrees of inflammation seen in enteroaggregative *Escherichia coli* (EAEC) and *C. difficile* diarrhea
C. difficile toxins A and B	Diarrhea associated with use of antibiotics, chemotherapy, or proton pump inhibitors, especially associated with current or recent hospitalization	Most sensitive tests are culture and tissue culture assay; most specific tests are enzyme immunoassay for toxins A and B; least useful is latex agglutination test
Stool culture for *Shigella*, *Salmonella*, and *Campylobacter*	Moderate to severe diarrhea and when stools are positive for inflammatory markers or contain gross blood and mucus (dysentery)	The three principal invasive bacteria are the only ones routinely sought by most laboratories.
Specialized stool culture for vibrios; or *E. coli* O157:H7, and other Shiga toxin–producing *E. coli*	For cases of profuse watery diarrhea in cholera-endemic areas; or in outbreaks of diarrhea especially associated with dysenteric illness	Cholera cases may need aggressive fluid therapy. Outbreaks of dysenteric diarrhea should be evaluated for Shiga toxin–producing *E. coli*.
Parasite examination: (1) trichome stain; (2) acid-fast stain for *Cyclospora*, *Cryptosporidium;* or (3) enzyme immunoassay (EIA) for *Giardia*, *Cryptosporidium*, and *E. histolytica*	In any patient with persistent diarrhea and when diarrhea follows visits to mountainous or recreational lakes in North America, Nepal, Haiti, Peru, or Russia (particularly St. Petersburg)	If microscopic evaluation is performed, experience of the laboratory personnel is important. The commercially available EIAs are sensitive tests.
Esophagogastroduodenoscopy and flexible sigmoidoscopy	Persistent diarrhea in patients without evidence of cause of illness	Identified cause of diarrhea is treated; without diagnosis, subjects may be treated symptomatically

TABLE 305–4 THERAPY AND PREVENTION OF INFECTIOUS DIARRHEA

Therapeutic Option	Indication	Pharmacologic Agent
Oral fluid and electrolyte therapy	For infants, elderly persons, and anyone with profuse watery diarrhea	Soups, soft drinks, and saltine crackers are sufficient; formal oral rehydration treatment may be needed with dehydrating forms of diarrhea.
Diet	In all forms of diarrhea to facilitate enterocyte renewal and recovery	Soups and broth, saltine crackers, steamed vegetables, baked or broiled meats
Nonspecific therapy	For temporary (≤48 hr) control of diarrhea in older children and adults without evidence of severe diarrhea caused by an invasive or inflammatory bacterial or parasitic pathogen	Loperamide is the most effective symptomatic treatment and decreases number of stools passed by 60%, bismuth subsalicylate is much less effective and reduces number of stools by 40%; new antisecretory agents are being developed.
Empirical antibacterial drugs	Enteric fever with toxicity Febrile dysenteric diarrhea Travelers' diarrhea	Fluoroquinolones for 7–10 days Fluoroquinolone or azithromycin for 3 days Rifaximin for 3 days, fluoroquinolone or azithromycin for 1–3 days
Specific antibacterial therapy	Shigellosis, campylobacteriosis, cholera	See Chapters 331, 327, 326
Antiparasitic drugs	Giardiasis, amebiasis, cryptosporidiosis, cyclosporiasis	See Chapters 373, 374, 376
Prophylaxis in travelers' diarrhea	Persons traveling to developing areas on tight schedules, those with history of prior illness, and those interested in prophylaxis	Rifaximin 200 mg twice a day with meals while in a high-risk region

for *Bacillus cereus* enterotoxin food poisoning). Longer incubation periods (usually 12 to 48 hours) are associated with most cases of intestinal infection.

The clinical expression of diarrheal illness gives clues to the etiologic agent (see Table 305–2). In the patient with diarrhea who is receiving or has recently completed a course of an antimicrobial drug, a proton pump inhibitor, or an anticancer drug, particularly with recent or current hospitalization, *Clostridium difficile* should be suspected. The number of patients with *C. difficile* diarrhea or colitis in the community is increasing. When a person has close contact with an infant or infants attending a daycare center, a number of low-dose pathogens found in this setting (e.g., *Giardia, Cryptosporidium, Shigella,* or viral pathogens) should be suspected. Because of sexual practices, some homosexual males may show high rates of enteric infection acquired through fecal-oral contamination, often associated with infection by multiple pathogens, or the practice of receptive anal intercourse may lead to proctitis related to sexually transmitted organisms. When persons experience advanced acquired immunodeficiency syndrome (AIDS) or other forms of severe immunodeficiency associated with metastatic malignancy or chronic use of immunosuppressive drugs, depressed intestinal immunity may lead to enteric infection with a variety of parasitic, bacterial, or viral pathogens (see Table 305–1).

Enteric infection syndromes may be divided into at least five groups on the basis of the clinical presentation: (1) febrile systemic disease (enteric fever), (2) acute watery diarrhea (secretory diarrhea), (3) recurrent vomiting as the primary manifestation of enteric disease (gastroenteritis), (4) passage of many small-volume stools containing blood and mucus (dysentery), and (5) diarrhea lasting 2 weeks or longer (persistent diarrhea). Table 305–2 lists the major syndromes along with the expected cause.

Norwalk virus has become the major cause of foodborne gastroenteritis and is an identified cause of waterborne enteric disease in the United States. *Campylobacter* is the most common reportable bacterial enteropathogen in industrialized countries and is the most important definable cause of Guillain-Barré syndrome, often resulting in severe disease requiring assisted ventilation, intensive care unit confinement, and permanent neurologic sequelae. *E. coli* O157:H7 and other Shiga toxin–producing *E. coli* are important causes of foodborne and waterborne colitis complicated by hemolytic-uremic syndrome in children and occasionally in elderly persons.

Diagnosis

Laboratory Findings

Laboratory tests (Fig. 305–1 and Table 305–3) can be useful and are of particular value in the more severely ill patients when subjects are forced by their illness to alter activities or are totally disabled and confined to bed or when many patients are afflicted during an outbreak. In each of these situations, the laboratory may help establish cause and allow development of a proper plan of treatment (see Table 305–4). Useful laboratory tests include procedures looking for fecal inflammatory markers such as microscopic detection of fecal leukocytes or the more sensitive, commercially available test fecal lactoferrin. These tests are particularly helpful to suggest the presence of the invasive bacterial pathogens *Shigella, Salmonella,* and *Campylobacter* or the noninvasive but inflammatory *C. difficile.* Stool culture is performed in more severe cases of sporadic diarrhea and in disease outbreaks and is carried out with blood culture in a patient with fever and systemic toxicity. Other indications for stool culture are the presence of dysentery (passage of grossly bloody

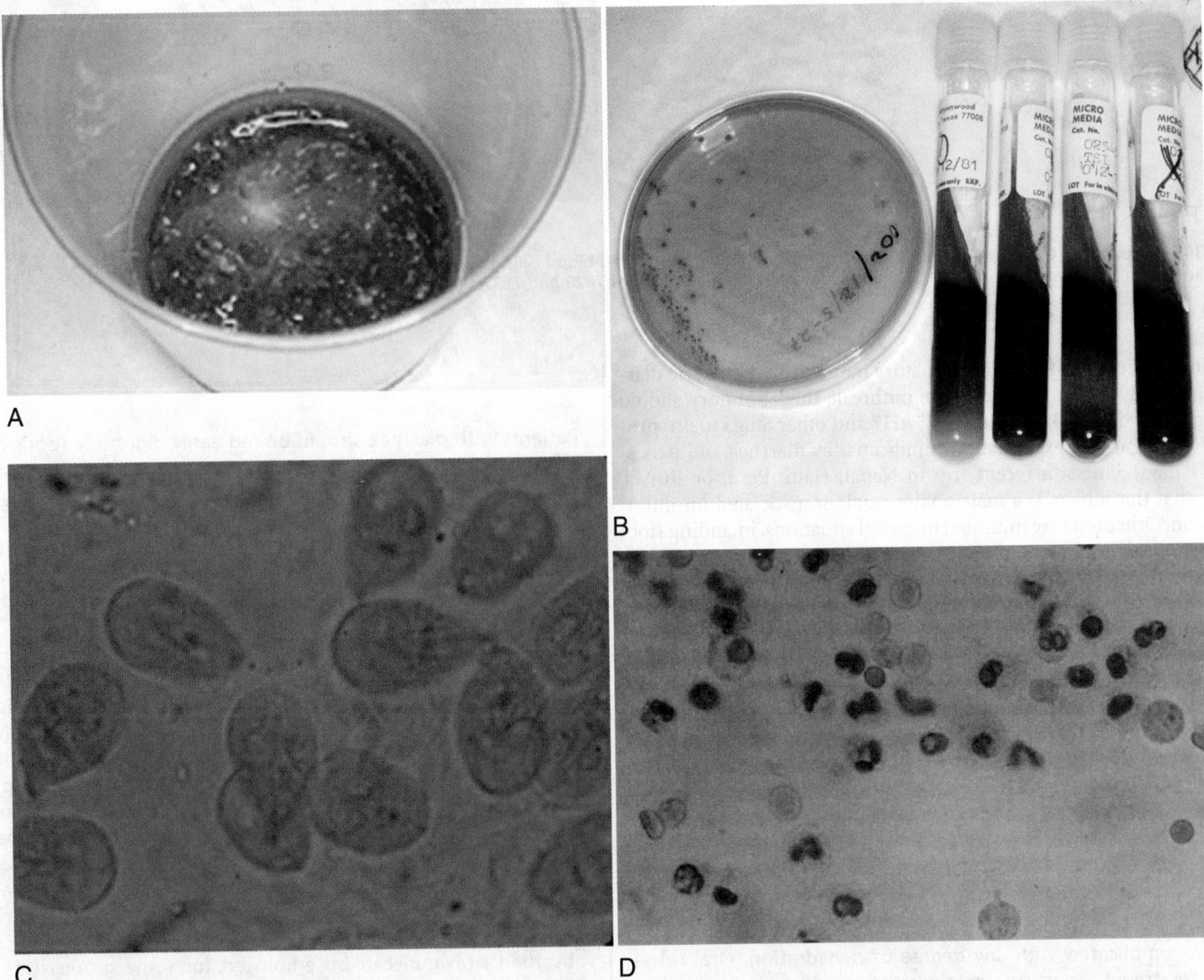

FIGURE 305–1 • Laboratory tests to diagnose cause of diarrhea. A, Dysenteric stool. **B,** Stool culture and biochemical tests confirm *Salmonella.* **C,** *Giardia* trophozoites. **D,** Many leukocytes in diffuse colonic inflammation.

Continued

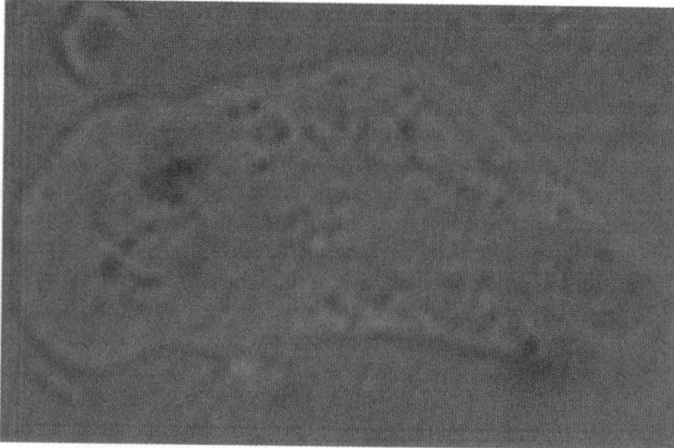

E

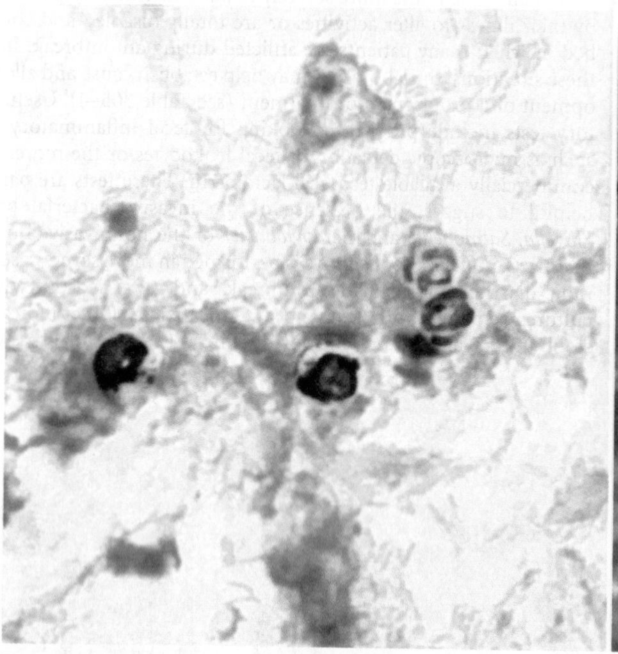

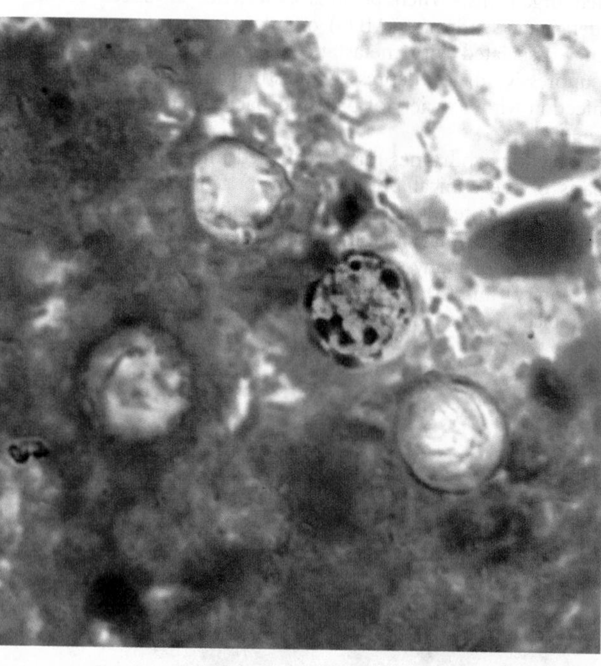

F

FIGURE 305–1, cont'd • **E,** *Entamoeba histolytica* trophozoite with ingested red blood cells. **F,** Oocysts of *Cryptosporidium* (left) and *Cyclospora* (right). (From the CDC Public Health Information Library, http://phil.cdc.gov/phil/home.asp, images 7829 and 7827.

stools) and the finding of fecal inflammatory markers. In dysenteric diarrhea, particularly in the presence of an outbreak, the laboratory should also be instructed to look for *E. coli* O157:H7 and other Shiga toxin–producing *E. coli.* Parasite examination is indicated by diarrhea and persistent (≥14 days) illness; a recent trip to Nepal, Haiti, Peru, or Russia; evidence that the subject is a male homosexual; or associated immunosuppression. Other tests are indicated in special situations, including stool culture for *Vibrio cholerae* in a patient with severe watery diarrhea with excessive fluid losses in a cholera-endemic area and culture for *Mycobacterium avian-intracellulare*, herpes simplex, and cytomegalovirus in those with immunosuppression. For patients with persistent diarrhea without an etiologic diagnosis when routine tests are employed, endoscopy-esophagogastroduodenoscopy and flexible sigmoidoscopy may be indicated in attempting to determine the cause of illness.

Treatment

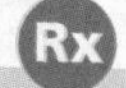

Treatment of diarrhea should be tailored to the clinical syndrome. Oral rehydration treatment with fluids and electrolytes is used in acute watery diarrhea and gastroenteritis and in all forms of enteric infection complicated with any degree of dehydration. Oral rehydration treatment is particularly important in infants; it can be lifesaving in developing countries for infants with severe diarrhea.

Rx

Patients with diarrhea should be fed easily digestible foods to facilitate enterocyte renewal and to speed up disease recovery. In afebrile, nondysenteric diarrhea, symptomatic drugs may allow older children and adults with illness to return earlier to school or work. Loperamide is the most active drug for improvement of symptoms. Bismuth subsalicylate can reduce diarrhea and is mildly effective in reducing nausea and vomiting associated with viral gastroenteritis.

For enteric fever, febrile dysenteric disease, and moderate to severe cases of travelers' diarrhea, empirical antimicrobial therapy is indicated (see Table 305–4). For outbreaks of dysenteric diarrhea, particularly in children in whom fever is not significant, antibacterial and antimotility drugs should be initially withheld while the etiology of the outbreak is being established in order to prevent patients infected by Shiga toxin–producing *E. coli* from being predisposed to hemolytic-uremic syndrome. For bacterial and parasitic pathogen-specific diarrhea, antimicrobial therapy is often advised (see other chapters in the text for specific treatments). Because of the importance of diarrhea when persons travel from industrialized regions to developing countries, prophylaxis with the orally poorly absorbed rifaximin can be employed for some groups (see Table 305–4), with protection rates exceeding 70%, although this practice is not routinely recommended for most travelers.

TABLE 305–5 NONINFECTIOUS CAUSES OF DIARRHEA

Running	Small bowel bacterial overgrowth
Fecal impaction	Systemic mastocytosis and eosinophilic gastroenteritis
Drugs and laxatives	Tropical sprue
Enteral feeding	Celiac sprue
Irradiation	Dermatitis herpetiformis
Pancreatic insufficiency	Whipple's disease
Intestinal lymphangiectasia	Thyrotoxicosis
Foods (especially dietetic)	Adrenal insufficiency
Cirrhosis and biliary obstruction	Factitious
Diabetic diarrhea	Inflammatory bowel disease
Alcoholism	Food allergy
Collagenous colitis	Carcinoid
VIPoma	Villous adenoma
Ischemic bowel disease	Stress with autonomic stimulation
Irritable bowel syndrome	

In sporadic cases of acute or persistent diarrhea, infectious agents are not always responsible. Table 305–5 offers a partial list of the noninfectious causes of diarrhea that should be considered.

SUGGESTED READINGS

DuPont HL: Travelers' diarrhea: Antimicrobial therapy and chemoprevention. Nat Clin Pract Gastroenterol Hepatol 2005;2:191–198. *A practical approach.*

DuPont HL: What's new in enteric infectious diseases at home and abroad. Curr Opin Infect Dis 2005;18:407–412. *Review, including recent trends.*

Thielman NM, Guerrant RL: Clinical practice. Acute infectious diarrhea. N Engl J Med 2004;350:38–47. *Comprehensive review.*

306 APPROACH TO THE PATIENT WITH URINARY TRACT INFECTION

S. Ragnar Norrby

Definition

This chapter addresses bacterial and fungal infections of the normally sterile urine, including asymptomatic bacteriuria, cystitis, pyelonephritis, and urosepsis. Urethritis caused by *Chlamydia trachomatis, Ureaplasma urealyticum,* or *Neisseria gonorrhoeae* and prostatitis and renal tuberculosis are addressed elsewhere in this text.

In the 1950s, Kass studied patients with or without bacterial colonization of the bladder urine. He defined *significant bacteriuria* as 10^5 or more colony-forming units (CFUs, where 1 CFU is one or more bacterial cells forming a colony when growing on an agar plate) per milliliter in two consecutive samples of midstream urine (i.e., urine obtained during voiding, discarding the first and last urine portions). This definition has been updated, and significant bacteriuria has been redefined to optimize the sensitivity and specificity of the diagnostic tests. In women with symptoms of uncomplicated cystitis, significant bacteriuria is now defined as 10^2 or more CFU/mL midstream urine plus pyuria (≥5 leukocytes/mm^3 of urine). In women with uncomplicated pyelonephritis and men with urinary tract infections (UTIs), significant bacteriuria is defined as 10^4 CFU/mL plus pyuria. In patients with complicated UTIs, the definition is 10^5 or more CFU/mL with or without pyuria.

Classification

It is clinically important to classify UTIs by type of infection, presence or absence of symptoms, tendency to recur, and presence or absence of complicating factors (Table 306–1). Recurrent infections can be subdivided into reinfections caused by new bacterial strains and relapses caused by the same strains that caused the preceding infections. Complicating factors are host factors facilitating establishment and maintenance of bacteriuria or worsening the prognosis of UTIs engaging the kidneys. The most common ones are listed in Table 306–2.

TABLE 306–1 CLASSIFICATION OF URINARY TRACT INFECTIONS

CLASSIFICATION BY TYPES OF UTIs	
Type of UTI	Cystitis Pyelonephritis Asymptomatic bacteriuria
Symptoms	Symptomatic Asymptomatic
Recurrences	Sporadic (≤1 UTI/6 mo and ≤2 UTIs/yr) Recurrent (≥2 UTIs/6 mo or ≥3 UTIs/yr) Relapse Reinfection
Complicating factors	Uncomplicated Complicated (see text)

UTI, urinary tract infection.

TABLE 306–2 HOST FACTORS COMPLICATING BACTERIURIA

Outcome	Factors
Facilitated establishment and maintenance of bacteriuria	Residual bladder urine after voiding Physiologic Neurogenic bladder Prostate hyperplasia/tumor Turbulent urethral urine flow Strictures Foreign bodies Catheters Calculi Tumors Atrophic vaginal mucosa after menopause Vesicoureteral reflux Anatomic defects Pregnancy
Worse prognosis of urinary tract infections involving the kidneys	Childhood pyelonephritis Diabetic nephropathy Malignant hypertension Chronic pyelonephritis

Epidemiology

Worldwide, at least 150 million cases of symptomatic UTIs occur each year. Because many UTI patients have recurrent infections, the number of individuals who have UTIs each year is lower than the number of cases.

In general, 90% of the patients have cystitis and 10% pyelonephritis. The infections are sporadic in about 75% of the patients and recurrent in 25%. About 2% have complicated infections related to factors that increase the risk of establishment and maintenance of bacteriuria. These patients typically have frequently recurring UTIs. If factors that may increase the severity of a renal infection are included, the frequency of complicated infections is about 8%.

UTIs are somewhat more common in very young boys than in very young girls because of the higher frequency of urethral malformations in boys. Later in childhood, symptomatic UTI is more common in girls, who also more frequently have asymptomatic bacteriuria. In most cases, this is due to the short urethra but may also be the result of sexual abuse. Symptomatic UTIs are most common in sexually active women. In young men, bacterial UTIs are rare and often the result of underlying infections of the prostate. In elderly people, both symptomatic UTIs and asymptomatic bacteriuria are common. In women, that is often the result of an atrophic vaginal mucosa, and in men, a consequence of prostate hyperplasia or prostate cancer.

UTI is also the most common type of hospital-acquired infection because of the frequent use of bladder catheters.

Pathobiology

In a majority of patients, UTIs are the result of colonization of the urine with fecal bacteria, which grow aerobically. Growth of anaerobic bacteria, such as *Bacteroides fragilis,* in the urine indicates a communication between the intestines and the urinary tract. That is seen in rare cases of fistulas between the intestines and the renal tract and following reconstructive surgery in the urinary tract, which involves the intestines. Growth of fungi in the urine may be seen in patients with bladder catheters and in immunocompromised patients with hematologic dissemination of *Candida* spp from infections at other sites.

In women, bacteria colonize the periurethral area, from which they reach the distal part of the urethra. Atrophic vaginal mucosa after menopause with altered vaginal flora and diaphragms and spermicides in sexually active women are factors that increase the risk of colonization with large numbers of uropathogenic bacteria. Sexual intercourse results in increased numbers of bacteria in the periurethral area of the vagina and the distal part of the urethra, increasing the risk of bacteriuria.

In the normal male urethra, the distance between the end of the urethra and the bladder is too long to allow ascending transport of bacteria to the bladder. Therefore, bacteriuria in men should always be considered an abnormal finding, and men cannot have uncomplicated infections. However, transport of bacteria to the bladder urine through the male urethra is possible when there is turbulent urine flow, such as with a stricture or obstruction of the urethra, as a result of prostatic hyperplasia, and when the patient has a bladder catheter.

The female urethra is short and allows transport of bacteria to the bladder in healthy individuals. With many uropathogens, such transport is facilitated by adherence of the bacteria to urethral epithelial cells. Bacterial cells, such as *Escherichia coli* strains causing uncomplicated pyelonephritis, have fimbriae that adhere to -D-Gal-4-β-D-Gal receptors (the P blood group) on the mucosal cells in the urethra and the ureters, thus facilitating establishment of bacteriuria and further transport to the kidneys. Such adhesion stimulates mucosal cells to release cytokines such as interleukin-6, which causes fever and increases in C-reactive protein, and interleukin-8, which mobilizes leukocytes. Individuals who lack the receptors for the bacterial adhesions (those who do not have the P blood group) are less likely to have acute pyelonephritis. In patients with complicated UTIs, bacterial adhesion seems to be of less importance. The role in the pathogenesis of UTIs of other bacterial virulence factors, such as the O and K antigens of *E. coli,* is less well known.

When bacteria have reached the bladder, establishment of bacteriuria is facilitated by incomplete bladder emptying. Even with residual urine volumes as low as 10 mL, which are not uncommon in healthy individuals, bacterial growth in the urine may be established. Pyelonephritis results from ascending bacteriuria from the bladder through the ureter to the renal pelvis and the renal parenchyma. This transport may be facilitated by host factors such as anatomic defects of the ureters or the kidneys, vesicoureteral reflux, or, in patients without anatomic defects, adhesion to the ureter mucosa. About one third of patients with pyelonephritis are also bacteremic.

In rare cases, bacteriuria and funguria may result from hematogenous dissemination of bacteria to the kidneys causing a renal abscess. The primary focus of the infection is usually an infection at a site outside the renal tract, such as endocarditis.

Patients with asymptomatic bacteriuria frequently harbor organisms that are less virulent than those causing symptomatic infections. Such organisms are often killed by normal human plasma or serum ("serum bactericidal effect"). Patients with persistent asymptomatic bacteriuria may be protected from symptomatic UTIs by large numbers of less virulent bacteria ($\geq 10^6$ CFU/mL) in the urine. However, in pregnant women and in patients with type 2 diabetes, asymptomatic bacteriuria is a strong predictor of subsequent symptomatic infections. Pyelonephritis is common during pregnancy because vesicoureteral reflux often occurs during the last two trimesters. In children and adults, asymptomatic bacteriuria may be a sign of underlying urinary tract malformations.

Bladder catheterization leads to bacteriuria or funguria in all patients who have had their catheters for more than 1 week. Formation of a biofilm on the catheter surfaces facilitates growth of microorganisms. Urosepsis, resulting from dissemination of bacteria from the urine to the blood in a patient with bacteriuria, is often the consequence of removal or change of a bladder catheter during the preceding 24 to 48 hours. This risk is further increased if the catheter has been in place for more than 1 week when the softener in the plastic material of the catheter is eluted, rendering the catheter stiff. The urethral mucosa may also be damaged by crystals that form on the catheter surface.

Etiology

The microbiologic etiology of a UTI depends on several factors. Table 306–3 summarizes the most common findings. In all types of UTI, *E. coli* is the dominating bacterial species, causing up to 85% of all symptomatic UTIs in women with community-acquired, sporadic, uncomplicated infections. In most countries, the second most common species causing such infections is *Staphylococcus saprophyticus,* which, at least in Northern Europe, has a pronounced seasonal pattern, accounting for up to 40% of all uncomplicated cases of cystitis and pyelonephritis in July and August and virtually no infections in January and February. In patients

TABLE 306–3 MICROBIAL ETIOLOGY OF URINARY TRACT INFECTIONS

Organisms	Clinical Characteristics
GRAM-NEGATIVE BACTERIA	
Escherichia coli	Typical
Klebsiella pneumoniae	Often reinfection
Enterobacter spp	Often reinfection and/or health care–associated infection*
Proteus spp	May indicate tumor or calculi
Providencia stuartii	Often reinfection and/or health care–associated infection*
Morganella morganii	Often reinfection and/or health care–associated infection*
Serratia marcescens	Often health care–associated infection*
Acinetobacter baumannii	Often health care–associated infection*
Burkholderia spp	Often health care–associated infection*
Pseudomonas aeruginosa	Often health care–associated infection*
Stenotrophomonas maltophilia	Often health care–associated infection*
GRAM-POSITIVE BACTERIA	
Staphylococcus saprophyticus	Most common during summer
Staphylococcus aureus	May indicate focus outside the genitourinary tract
Enterococcus spp	Often reinfection
Other gram-positive bacteria	In most cases contaminants
FUNGI	
Candida spp	May indicate focus outside the genitourinary tract

*Includes hospital and nursing home care.

with recurrent infections, species such as *Enterococcus faecalis, Enterococcus faecium, Klebsiella* spp, *Proteus* spp, *Providencia stuartii,* and *Morganella morganii* become more common. In patients with very frequent recurrences or bladder catheters, especially in hospital and nursing home settings where antimicrobials are frequently used, *Pseudomonas aeruginosa, Acinetobacter baumannii, Serratia marcescens,* and *Stenotrophomonas maltophilia* are important organisms. In such patients, *E. coli* accounts for less than 50% of the infections. Findings of *Proteus mirabilis* or other *Proteus* spp may indicate that the patient has renal calculi or a tumor because these organisms grow in an alkaline environment. Calculi in the renal pelvis, ureter, or bladder may also be formed as a result of growth of ammonia-producing organisms such as *Proteus* spp. Because *Proteus* spp are common in the male preputial flora, the finding of such organisms in a voided urine sample from uncircumcised men or young boys could represent contamination and not bacteriuria.

Clinical Manifestations

Typical symptoms of cystitis, pyelonephritis, and urosepsis are listed in Table 306–4. Onset of cystitis is rapid, and symptoms develop over less than 24 hours. It is clinically often impossible to differentiate between cystitis and urethritis caused by chlamydia, *Ureaplasma,* or gonococci, especially when there is no urethral discharge. Fever is unusual among patients with cystitis. In sexually active women, cystitis commonly occurs 24 to 48 hours after intercourse, especially if the practice of postcoital bladder emptying has not been followed. Cystitis patients normally have symptoms for 3 to 5 days. Antimicrobial therapy does not markedly reduce the duration, and bacteriuria may persist after treatment.

Pyelonephritis also has a rapid onset with or without preceding cystitis symptoms. About one third of the patients develop bacteremia. The typical loin pain, resulting from inflammation and edema of the renal parenchyma, may be masked by intake of analgesic drugs such as acetaminophen, which may also reduce the fever. An important differential diagnosis is renal calculi, which may result in a similar location of the pain but normally without fever. Also, patients with appendicitis and cholecystitis can present with loin pains similar to those in a patient with right-sided pyelonephritis.

Urosepsis is a life-threatening condition caused by dissemination of bacteria from the urine in a patient with bacteriuria. The most common reason for urosepsis is withdrawal (and sometimes insertion) of a bladder catheter. Thus, uroseptic patients do not always have renal infection.

Diagnosis

Laboratory Findings

The hallmark of the types of UTIs dealt with here is demonstration of bacteriuria in a urine sample that has been incubated in the bladder for at least 2 hours to allow growth of bacteria. The most reliable result is obtained if the sample is taken by suprapubic aspiration, a technique frequently used in infants but rarely in older children and adults. It is superior to sampling by bladder catheterization, which carries a risk of about 2% for introduction of bacteria into the bladder and subsequent iatrogenic bacteriuria. The normal procedure for quantitative cultures is to collect a midstream urine sample. This requires that the patient is well informed about the sampling procedures. Men should withdraw the foreskin and women should keep the labia apart. Washing of the genital tract before sampling is not recommended. During voiding, the first and the last parts of the urine should not be sampled. After sampling, the urine should be chilled (but not frozen) to prevent growth during transportation to the laboratory. At the laboratory, the sample is streaked onto agar plates using a loop, which delivers a known amount of urine. The result is obtained after incubation overnight and allows determination of the bacterial species present in the sample and the number of organisms per milliliter of urine. The presence of more than one species in a sample usually indicates defective sampling procedures and contamination.

A simplified quantitative urine culture can be obtained outside the microbiologic laboratory by using a dip slide. With that technique, a plastic slide with agar media on both surfaces is dipped in the urine sample or the urine sample is poured over the slide's surfaces. After overnight culture at room temperature or in a simple incubator, the culture allows highly reliable quantification of bacteriuria. Because gram-negative, but not gram-positive, bacteria grow on both sides of the slide, the method also allows quick classification. However, if determination of the species or the antimicrobial sensitivity pattern is required, the dip slide must be transported to a regular laboratory. The dip slide is most suitable for use in outpatient settings, especially when laboratories are locally unavailable.

All culture techniques require overnight incubation. For screening of bacteriuria, a nitrite test can be used. It is a stick test that demonstrates the presence of nitrite in the urine. Gram-negative bacteria, with the exception of *P. aeruginosa,* metabolize nitrate to nitrite, which can be demonstrated by a color reaction on a paper stick. Gram-positive bacteria and fungi do not metabolize nitrate. The technique is rapid (<1 minute) and inexpensive. It has a high degree of specificity but is rather insensitive because it does not detect infections caused by gram-positive organisms. Thus, it is not suitable for use in patients with recurrent infections (in whom enterococcal etiology is common) or when the frequency of *S. saprophyticus* infections is high.

Pyuria should be demonstrated in patients with UTIs. This is best done by staining uncentrifuged urine and counting leukocytes in a Bürker chamber. The second best technique is to use a leukocyte esterase stick test, which is highly sensitive and allows a crude quantification of pyuria. The previously used routine technique, to count leukocytes in the sediment obtained after centrifugation of a urine sample, is imprecise and is not recommended. Persistent pyuria with negative routine bacteriologic cultures should lead to a suspicion of renal tuberculosis, and a sample should be obtained for direct microscopy and culture for *Mycobacterium tuberculosis.*

Blood cultures should be obtained in all patients with suspected pyelonephritis or urosepsis. It is recommended that at least two cultures be obtained.

Imaging

Radiography and ultrasound examination are normally not helpful in the acute phase of a suspected pyelonephritis unless there is a suspicion of a blockage of the urine flow, which may indicate formation of a renal abscess. When the patient has recovered, such investigations are recommended in patients with recurrent infections to exclude complicating factors. Normally, a simple pyelography or ultrasound examination is performed. For diagnosis of vesicoureteral reflux, special radiographic techniques are used.

Differential Diagnosis

Although clinical manifestations should lead to a relatively clear differentiation of acute cystitis and acute pyelonephritis, it is often difficult to diagnose the latter. Laboratory tests may offer some help and should be used. Patients with acute pyelonephritis but not those with acute cystitis have increased values of C-reactive protein in blood. That acute phase parameter increases rapidly in patients with acute pyelonephritis. It is also a useful test for determination of response to therapy and diagnosis of recurrences. Erythrocyte sedimentation rate, on the other hand, is a less useful test because it takes several days to increase in a patient

TABLE 306–4 CLINICAL SYMPTOMS OF URINARY TRACT INFECTIONS

Type of Urinary Tract Infection	Typical Symptoms
Cystitis	Frequent voiding Burning during and after voiding Suprapubic pain Hematuria and/or cloudy urine
Pyelonephritis	Fever Chills Flank pains Cystitis symptoms (may be absent)
Urosepsis	Fever Chills Septic shock

with acute pyelonephritis. In patients with acute pyelonephritis, leukocyte casts can often be demonstrated in urine sediment. When a patient with suspected acute pyelonephritis has become afebrile, the diagnosis can be supported by testing urine osmolality, which is markedly reduced for at least 1 month after the onset of symptoms. Although not routinely indicated, the osmolality of urine is checked in a sample of urine obtained after 12 hours of fasting and no fluid intake or 1 to 8 hours after intramuscular or subcutaneous injection of a small dose of desmopressin, a vasopressin analogue. Urine osmolality in individuals with normal renal concentration ability is 850 to 1000 mOsm/L and varies with age. Demonstration of antibody-coated bacteria in the urine is neither a sensitive nor a specific method to diagnose pyelonephritis and is no longer recommended.

Treatment

Rx

All symptomatic UTIs should be treated. The purpose of early treatment of cystitis is to reduce the risk of progression to pyelonephritis. Treatment does not affect the duration of symptoms, which is 3 to 4 days. In patients with pyelonephritis, early treatment is important to reduce the duration of symptoms, eliminate microorganisms from the renal parenchyma, and reduce the risk of dissemination to the blood.

Because verification of the microbial etiology and determination of the susceptibility to antimicrobial drugs take at least 1 and often more than 2 days, initial treatment is empirical. The best guide is the antimicrobial susceptibility pattern of organisms obtained from comparable patients. For example, if the patient is a woman with a sporadic uncomplicated cystitis or pyelonephritis, antimicrobial susceptibility patterns generated from outpatients with sporadic UTIs are the appropriate reference. If, on the other hand, the patient is hospitalized and has a hospital-associated pyelonephritis, susceptibility patterns generated from samples collected in the hospital, preferably in the department or ward where the patient acquired the infection, are the appropriate reference. Large national or international surveillance studies have limited value for decisions on choice of antimicrobial treatment for individual patients. Susceptibility patterns developed from large reference laboratories may overestimate antimicrobial resistance because patients with uncomplicated infections are less likely to have cultures.

Cystitis

Table 306–5 lists possible choices for antimicrobial treatment of cystitis. Ideally, the antimicrobial should be excreted renally to achieve high concentrations in the renal parenchyma and in the urine. The safety profile is also important because cystitis is common and is associated with low mortality. The treatment time varies with type of antimicrobial. Trimethoprim, trimethoprim-sulfamethoxazole, and fluoroquinolones are effective treatments and reduce the number of uropathogenic bacteria in the periurethral flora and the fecal flora; 3 days of therapy are recommended. β-Lactam antimicrobials and nitrofurantoin generally have shorter elimination times and do not affect the periurethral and fecal flora; 5 to 7 days of treatment are required to eliminate bacteriuria in most patients. Single-dose treatment is recommended only for a high dose of trimethoprim-sulfamethoxazole and for fosfomycin (which is licensed only for single-dose treatment). Although these single-dose regimens may seem preferable to treatment for several days, 3-day regimens seem to have the best acceptance among patients. When patients have recurrent or complicated cystitis, treatment duration should be at least 7 days. 1

Fluoroquinolones are not recommended for routine use in sporadic cystitis, although many of them have well-documented efficacy when used at relatively low doses for 3 days or even as a high single dose. The reason is that widespread use in cystitis patients is likely to lead to overuse and emergence of resistance.

Patients with frequently recurring cystitis can benefit from early self-treatment if they are well informed and compliant. If treatment is started very shortly after the onset of symptoms, a 3-day course or even a single dose of antimicrobial gives rapid relief of symptoms.

TABLE 306–5 ANTIMICROBIALS USED FOR TREATMENT OF CYSTITIS

Antimicrobial	Dose and Duration
Trimethoprim	100–150 mg q12h for 3 days
Trimethoprim/sulfamethoxazole	80/400 mg q12h for 3 days or 320/1600 mg single dose
Nitrofurantoin	50 mg q8h for 5–7 days
Amoxicillin/clavulanic acid	250 mg (amoxicillin dose) q8h for 5–7 days
Cefuroxime axetil	250 mg q8h for 5–7 days
Cefpodoxime proxetil	200 mg q8h for 5–7 days
Cefixime	400 mg qd for 5–7 days
Ceftibuten	400 mg qd for 5–7 days
Cefprozil	250 mg qd for 5–7 days
Norfloxacin*	200 mg q12h for 7 days
Ciprofloxacin*	100 mg q12h for 7 days
Levofloxacin*	250 mg qd for 7 days
Fosfomycin	400 mg single dose

*Should be reserved for recurrent and/or complicated cystitis.
Note: Doses are those for adults with normal renal function. The need for dose reductions because of renal impairment related to infections in the kidneys, other renal diseases, or advanced age should always be considered.

Rx

Pyelonephritis

For antimicrobial treatment of pyelonephritis, the primary decision should be whether the patient needs initial treatment with a parenteral antimicrobial or whether oral treatment alone will suffice. Table 306–6 lists antimicrobials suitable for treatment of pyelonephritis. Oral formulations of penicillins or cephalosporins should be used only after initial treatment with parenteral therapy. When treatment is started with a parenteral drug, transition to oral treatment is normally possible after 24 to 48 hours unless the patient does not improve. The recommended treatment time is still 14 days, although recent information indicates that in patients with uncomplicated pyelonephritis treatment for 7 days may suffice.

Only fluoroquinolones and trimethoprim-sulfamethoxazole can be used for initial oral treatment of pyelonephritis if the patient's general condition allows it. Because both of these alternatives are unsuitable for use in pregnant women, pyelonephritis during pregnancy should be treated with a parenteral antimicrobial, preferably a cephalosporin, followed by oral step-down therapy.

Bacteriuria

Bacteriuria in patients with catheters should not be treated unless the patient is febrile or has other evidence of systemic infection. Administration of antimicrobials to catheterized patients with asymptomatic bacteriuria inevitably results in selection of multiresistant and difficult-to-treat organisms.

Urosepsis

In patients with suspected urosepsis, antimicrobial treatment must start as early as possible. Antimicrobials should be given intravenously. Antimicrobials recommended for injectable treatment of pyelonephritis should be used. Previous antimicrobial treatment should always be sought in patients with urosepsis because such treatment may have resulted in selection of resistant organisms. A relatively new etiology of urosepsis is vancomycin-resistant enterococci (*Enterococcus faecium or Enterococcus faecalis*), which usually occurs in immunocompromised patients.

Funguria

Funguria can be treated with fluconazole 400 mg once daily for 1 day followed by 200 mg once daily for 7 to 14 days. Funguria in

TABLE 306–6 ANTIMICROBIALS USED FOR TREATMENT OF PYELONEPHRITIS

Route of Administration and Antimicrobial	Dosage	Comments
INJECTABLE		
Cefepime	2 g q12h	Health care–associated infections*
Cefotaxime	1 g q12h	Community-acquired infections
Ceftazidime	1 g q12h	Health care–associated infections*
Ceftriaxone	2 g qd	Community-acquired infections
Cefuroxime	750 mg q8h	Community-acquired infections
Amikacin	15 mg/kg qd	Monitor renal function
Gentamicin	4.5 mg/kg qd	Monitor renal function
Netilmicin	4.5 mg/kg qd	Monitor renal function
Tobramycin	4.5 mg/kg qd	Monitor renal function
Ciprofloxacin	200 mg q12h	
Levofloxacin	250 mg qd	
Trimethoprim/sulfamethoxazole	160/800 mg q12h	Community-acquired infections
ORAL		
Amoxicillin/clavulanic acid	500 mg (amoxicillin dose) q8h	Only step-down therapy
Cefuroxime axetil	250 mg q12h	Only step-down therapy
Cefpodoxime proxetil	200 mg q8h	Only step-down therapy
Cefixime	400 mg qd	Only step-down therapy
Ceftibuten	400 mg qd	Only step-down therapy
Cefprozil	250 mg qd	Only step-down therapy
Norfloxacin	400 mg q12h	
Ciprofloxacin	100 mg q12h	
Levofloxacin	250 mg qd	

*Includes hospital and nursing home care.
Note: Doses are those for adults with normal renal function. The need for dose reductions because of renal impairment related to infections in the kidneys, other renal diseases, or advanced age should always be considered.

catheterized patients should be treated only when there is a symptomatic UTI.

Follow-up

Patients with sporadic, uncomplicated cystitis do not require follow-up. Patients with symptomatic recurrences, pyelonephritis, or complicated UTI should be observed. Table 306–7 lists some examinations that may be considered. Follow-up cultures are important because bacteriuria may persist and cause renal damage in afebrile pyelonephritis patients. The decision process for upper (pyelonephritis) and lower (cystitis) UTIs appears in Table 306–8.

TABLE 306–7 FOLLOW-UP PROCEDURES IN PATIENTS WITH URINARY TRACT INFECTIONS OTHER THAN SPORADIC CYSTITIS

Procedure	Recommendation
Urine culture	All patients with pyelonephritis, complicated infections, or frequent recurrences; 4–5 days and 3–4 weeks after treatment
Pyuria test	Always together with urine cultures
C-reactive protein	4–5 days and 3–4 weeks after treatment of pyelonephritis
Radiography or ultrasonography	After pyelonephritis to exclude scars from childhood infections in patients with recurrent infections to exclude complications
Serum creatinine	Before treatment in elderly; 3–4 weeks after treatment in patients with pyelonephritis
Urine osmolality	Verification of suspected pyelonephritis

Prevention

There are well-known measures that markedly reduce the risk of recurrences of UTIs. The most important one is to recommend that sexually active women urinate shortly after sexual intercourse. In doing so, they wash out the increased number of bacteria in the distal urethra. Another useful suggestion is to recommend double or triple voiding to patients with recurrent UTIs. This means that the patient should make extra efforts to empty the bladder at each urination. The volume of residual urine is then decreased. Increased fluid intake was previously advocated, probably because of the risk of crystalluria with older sulfonamides. There are no obvious benefits with excessive diuresis.

Antimicrobial prophylaxis of UTIs is today used with considerable restrictions. 2 One group in which it is still recommended is pregnant women with asymptomatic bacteriuria. As a consequence of that, screening for bacteriuria at regular intervals during pregnancy is recommended. Another group in which screening of bacteriuria and prophylaxis have been proposed is patients with diabetes mellitus, especially those with type 2.

Prophylaxis is sometimes used in patients with frequently recurring UTIs, especially when there are no defined, treatable complications. In such patients, one daily dose of nitrofurantoin 50 to 100 mg or trimethoprim 150 to 200 mg, taken at bedtime, is recommended.

Antimicrobial prophylaxis should not be used in catheterized patients because it results in selection of microbes resistant to the antimicrobial used.

In postmenopausal women with atrophic vaginal mucosa and recurrent symptomatic UTIs, replacement therapy with estriol orally or vaginally should be considered. Such treatment restores a premenopausal vaginal and periurethral normal microbial flora and, subsequently, reduces the incidence of symptomatic UTIs.

TABLE 306–8 DECISION PROCESS FOR UPPER (PYELONEPHRITIS) AND LOWER (CYSTITIS) URINARY TRACT INFECTIONS

	Cystitis	Pyelonephritis
SIGNS AND SYMPTOMS		
Fever	No	Yes
Dysuria	Yes	May be present
Frequency	Yes	May be present
Flank pain	No	Yes
DIAGNOSIS		
Pyuria	Yes	Yes
Nitrite test	Normally positive	Normally positive
Bacteriuria	Yes	Yes
C-reactive protein	Normal	Increased
Blood cultures	Negative	Positive in ~30%
TREATMENT		
First line	Trimethoprim or trimethoprim-sulfamethoxazole for 3 days	Fluoroquinolone or trimethoprim-sulfamethoxazole for 2 wk orally
Second line	Fluoroquinolone for 3 days or cephalosporin for 5–7 days	Injectable cephalosporin until afebrile followed by oral step-down for total of 2 wk
Pregnant women	Nitrofurantoin or cephalosporin for 5–7 days	Injectable cephalosporin until afebrile followed by oral cephalosporin for 2 wk

Prognosis

The prognoses of uncomplicated cystitis and pyelonephritis are generally good unless urosepsis occurs. Secondary morbidity is rare.

In patients with complications such as renal scars from childhood pyelonephritis, chronic pyelonephritis or glomerulonephritis, or other chronic renal diseases, acute pyelonephritis may lead to further reduction of renal function. As mentioned earlier, infections with *Proteus* spp or other ammonia-producing organisms may lead to formation of calculi or worsening of existing ones.

Patients with urosepsis have a poor prognosis, with fatality rates of about 30% or higher. Factors increasing the risk of death are high age and underlying diseases but also inadequate choice of antimicrobial treatment. It has been demonstrated that in patients with sepsis caused by gram-negative bacteria, the death rate increases drastically if the organisms are resistant to the empirical treatment given.

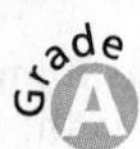

1. Milo G, Katchman EA, Paul M, et al: Duration of antibacterial treatment for uncomplicated urinary tract infection in women. Cochrane Database Syst Rev 2005;(2):CD004682.
2. Albert X, Huertas I, Pereiro II, et al: Antimicrobials for preventing recurrent urinary tract infection in non-pregnant women. Cochrane Database Syst Rev 2004;(3):CD001209.

SUGGESTED READINGS

Car J: Urinary tract infections in women: Diagnosis and management in primary care. BMJ 2006;332:94–97. *Overview of outpatient diagnosis and treatment of urinary tract infections.*

Fihn SD: Clinical practice. Acute uncomplicated urinary tract infection in women. N Engl J Med 2003;349:259–266. *A practical overview.*

Hooton TM, Scholes D, Stapleton AE, et al: A prospective study of asymptomatic bacteriuria in sexually active young women. N Engl J Med 2000;343:992–997. *Asymptomatic bacteriuria in young women is common, rarely persistent, but predictive of subsequent symptomatic infection.*

Nicolle LE: Urinary tract infection in diabetes. Curr Opin Infect Dis 2005;18:49–53. *Overview, with emphasis on issues specific to diabetic patients.*

307 APPROACH TO THE PATIENT WITH A SEXUALLY TRANSMITTED DISEASE

Michael F. Rein

SEXUALLY TRANSMITTED DISEASES

Definition

The sexually transmitted diseases (STDs) are diverse infections caused by biologically dissimilar microbial agents. They are grouped together because sexual contact plays a statistically and clinically significant role in their overall epidemiology.

Epidemiology

The STDs remain common infections. Many of the most important are not reported, and their incidence and prevalence are poorly defined. Even among the reportable STDs (e.g., gonorrhea, chancroid, syphilis, lymphogranuloma venereum, donovanosis, human immunodeficiency virus [HIV]), there is considerable underreporting. Chancroid (Chapter 324) is principally seen in major urban areas, especially among sex workers. The incidence of syphilis (Chapter 340) declined to 2.2 per 100,000 in the United States in 2000, but it has been increasing since then, principally among men who have sex with men. Seroepidemiologic studies suggest that approximately 20% of the U.S. population is infected with herpes simplex virus type 2 (HSV-2) (Chapter 397), but most newly acquired genital infections, particularly among younger people, are now due to HSV-1. At any given point in time, an estimated 20 million people in the United States have human papillomavirus (HPV) infections (Chapter 396) that can be transmitted to others, and every year about 5.5 million people acquire a genital HPV infection.

Pathobiology

The contribution of sexual transmission to the incidence of these infections varies; it plays a major role in the transmission of gonorrhea and chlamydial infection, a far less significant role for hepatitis C, and a very small role in vulvovaginal candidiasis. For some conditions, such as bacterial vaginosis, the role of sexual transmission remains incompletely defined.

The causative microorganisms depend on sexual contact for transmission for several reasons: (1) many of them, such as *Treponema pallidum* and *Trichomonas vaginalis,* have limited environmental survival and are susceptible to drying; (2) only limited sites can be infected by some (e.g., *Neisseria gonorrhoeae* and *Chlamydia trachomatis* can produce primary infection at only certain mucosal surfaces); and (3) lesions containing microorganisms in numbers adequate to transmit disease frequently occur only at the anatomic sites used for sexual contact.

Although sexual contact is not the exclusive means of transmission for any of these agents, recognizing an infection as sexually transmitted has profound clinical significance. First, one can immediately identify a group at very high risk for the STD, namely the sexual partners of patients in whom a diagnosis has been made. Obviously, not all sexual partners are at equal risk. Some have had only a single sexual contact, whereas others may be in a regular sexual relationship. Specific sexual practices, including anatomic sites of contact and the use of various contraceptives, influence the likelihood of transmission. Transmission is also influenced by the concentration of microorganisms in lesions or body fluids, which varies during the course of most infections. Finally, there are individual variations in susceptibility that remain incompletely defined. For example, prior infection with HSV-1 reduces the likelihood that an exposed individual will become infected with HSV-2.

Diagnosis and Coprevalence

A second consequence of sexual transmissibility is *coprevalence.* High-risk sexual behaviors increase the likelihood of acquiring each of the STDs and, thus, a patient presenting with one sexually transmitted condition should be screened carefully for others, including infection with HIV (Chapter 407). The coprevalence of gonococcal and chlamydial infection is so high that patients diagnosed with gonorrhea are routinely treated for chlamydial infection as well. In addition to epidemiologic coprevalence, a number of STDs have been shown to increase the risk of acquiring HIV. Genital inflammation appears to increase the rate of HIV synthesis, and ulcerative or inflammatory processes may serve as a portal of entry for the virus.

Sexual contact includes the full range of heterosexual or homosexual behavior, including genital, oral-genital, oral-anal, and genital-anal contact. The anatomic sites at which one should seek evidence of infection are guided by the sexual practices involved, and a complete, nonjudgmental sexual history is an essential part of the evaluation.

Treatment

Rx

The high prevalence of some conditions among sexual partners has led to the principle of *epidemiologic treatment,* which is a cornerstone of the management of STDs. Epidemiologic treatment is provided on the basis of statistical risk rather than on the basis of a specific diagnosis. Sexual partners of patients with some infections (denoted by an asterisk in Table 307–1) should be treated at the time of initial presentation.

Finally, STDs are best managed when sexual partners are treated simultaneously, meaning that all have completed treatment before unprotected sexual contact is resumed. When one cares for a patient with an STD, one is always obliged to consider other people, who may be either the source of the patient's infection or secondary cases to whom the infection has been spread. For this reason, establishing a microbiologic diagnosis and cooperating with health department case reporting and partner assistance protocol requirements are essential.

Management of sexually transmitted infections is complicated by their frequent lack of symptoms. Most women with gonococcal or chlamydial infection are asymptomatic or have symptoms that do not persuade them to seek medical attention. Only about 20% of patients with genital herpes have classical clinical findings and know that they are infected. HPV is another "hidden epidemic." It may be the most common STD among young, sexually active people.

Prevention

STDs are preventable. The Centers for Disease Control and Prevention recommends five strategies as the foundation for an effective prevention program: (1) education and counseling of persons at risk to motivate adoption of safer sexual behavior; (2) identification of asymptomatic infected persons and symptomatic persons unlikely to seek diagnostic and treatment services; (3) rapid and effective diagnosis and treatment of infected persons; (4) evaluation, treatment, and counseling of exposed sexual partners; and (5) preexposure vaccination of persons at risk for vaccine-preventable STDs.

Abstinence/Monogamy

Abstaining from sexual intercourse or being in a long-term, mutually monogamous relationship with an uninfected partner is the most reliable way to prevent STDs. Abstinence should be recommended during treatment for an STD and for anyone who wants to avoid STDs and unintended pregnancy. Both partners should be tested for STDs, including HIV, before initiating sexual intercourse.

Condoms

When used consistently and correctly, male latex condoms are effective in preventing the sexual transmission of HIV infection and can reduce the risk for other STDs (i.e., gonorrhea, chlamydia, and trichomoniasis). However, because condoms do not cover all exposed areas, they are likely to be more effective in preventing infections transmitted by fluids from mucosal surfaces (e.g., gonorrhea, chlamydial infection, trichomoniasis, and HIV) than in preventing those transmitted by skin-to-skin contact (e.g., HSV, HPV, syphilis, and chancroid). Male condom failure usually results from inconsistent or incorrect use rather than condom breakage. Nonlatex condoms (i.e., those made of polyurethane or other synthetic material) can be substituted for persons with latex allergy. Less information is available to demonstrate the effect of female condoms on the incidence of STDs, although some promising data suggest that when they are used consistently and correctly, protection is afforded.

Counseling

Interactive counseling, some video presentations, peer groups, and other formats that emphasize correct condom use have reduced the incidence of subsequent infections among STD clinic patients and adolescents. [1] Randomized controlled trials demonstrate that structured risk reduction counseling can reduce the incidence of infections by 25 to 40% among some STD clinic populations. [2]

Outreach to Possibly Infected Persons

Outreach to partners of those with STDs is one strategy to promote access to diagnosis and treatment. Clinicians can facilitate this process, alone or in collaboration with state and local health agencies. A newer approach gaining support is to target the social networks in which the patient operates, not just the persons who are identified contacts. Another is to ask the infected patient to deliver therapy to contacts and others at risk. Regardless of the method of outreach, accurate identification, treatment of infected persons and their partners, and timely reporting that adheres to state requirements are core components of a successful program. When in doubt about reporting requirements and methods, clinicians should seek advice from their local or state STD programs.

Preexposure Vaccination

Preexposure vaccination is one of the most effective methods for preventing transmission of certain STDs. For example, because hepatitis B virus infection is frequently sexually transmitted, hepatitis B vaccination is recommended for all unvaccinated persons being evaluated for an STD. In addition, hepatitis A vaccine is currently licensed and is recommended for men who have sex with men and illegal drug users (both injection and noninjection). Vaccines for HPV are now available, and vaccines to prevent other STDs may emerge in the next several years.

TABLE 307–1 SEXUALLY TRANSMITTED AGENTS AND THEIR SYNDROMES

Microorganism	Syndromes
BACTERIA	
*Neisseria gonorrhoeae**	Urethritis, cervicitis, bartholinitis, proctitis, pharyngitis, salpingitis, epididymitis, conjunctivitis, perihepatitis, arthritis, dermatitis, endocarditis, meningitis, amniotic infection syndrome
Gardnerella vaginalis and many other organisms	Bacterial vaginosis†
*Treponema pallidum**	Syphilis (multiple clinical syndromes)
*Haemophilus ducreyi**	Chancroid
Calymmatobacterium granulomatis	Granuloma inguinale (donovanosis)
Shigella species	Enteritis in men who have sex with men
Campylobacter species	Enteritis in men who have sex with men
Group B *Streptococcus*	Neonatal sepsis and meningitis
CHLAMYDIAE	
*Chlamydia trachomatis**	Nongonococcal urethritis, purulent hypertrophic cervicitis, epididymitis, salpingitis, conjunctivitis, trachoma, pneumonia, perihepatitis, lymphogranuloma venereum, Reiter's syndrome
MYCOPLASMAS	
*Ureaplasma urealyticum**	Nongonococcal urethritis, ? premature rupture of membranes and abortion
Mycoplasma hominis	Postpartum fever, pelvic inflammatory disease
Mycoplasma genitalium	Nongonococcal urethritis
VIRUSES	
Herpes simplex virus (HSV)	Genital herpes, proctitis, meningitis, disseminated infection in neonates
Hepatitis A virus	Hepatitis in men who have sex with men
Hepatitis B virus	Hepatitis, periarteritis nodosa, hepatoma; especially prevalent in men who have sex with men
Hepatitis C virus	Hepatitis, cryoglobulinemia
Cytomegalovirus	Congenital infection (birth defects, infant mortality, mental deficiency, hearing loss), mononucleosis syndrome
Human papillomavirus (HPV)	Condyloma acuminatum, cervical and perianal warts, cervical, vulvar, and penile cancer
Molluscum contagiosum virus	Molluscum contagiosum
Human immunodeficiency virus (HIV)	Acquired immunodeficiency syndrome and related illnesses
PROTOZOA	
*Trichomonas vaginalis**	Trichomonal vaginitis, occasional urethritis
Entamoeba histolytica	Enteritis in men who have sex with men
Giardia lamblia	Enteritis in men who have sex with men
FUNGI	
Candida albicans	Vaginitis, balanitis
ECTOPARASITES	
*Phthirus pubis**	Pubic lice infestation
*Sarcoptes scabiei**	Scabies

*Epidemiologic treatment of sexual partners is recommended.
†Sexual transmission plays an undefined role.

Section XXIII Infectious Diseases

COMMON SYNDROMES

Urethritis

Definition

Urethritis, arising as some combination of urethral discharge and dysuria, is usually caused by one or more sexually transmitted organisms (Table 307–2). Nonsexually transmitted urethritis is seen most commonly in men with underlying diseases such as diabetes.

Diagnosis

Urethritis is diagnosed when one or more of the following are demonstrated: (1) mucopurulent or purulent urethral discharge, (2) Gram stain of urethral secretions demonstrating 5 or more leukocytes per oil immersion microscopic field, or (3) a positive leukocyte esterase test on first-void urine or microscopic examination of first-void urine demonstrating 10 or more leukocytes per high-power field. The Gram stain of urethral discharge is the preferred rapid diagnostic test for documenting both urethritis and the presence or absence of gonococcal infection. Gonococcal infection (Chapter 322) is established by documenting the presence of leukocytes containing intracellular gram-negative diplococci. The presence of these organisms identifies a case of gonococcal urethritis but does not rule out the possibility of coincidental infection with *Chlamydia* (Chapter 339) or another cause of nongonococcal urethritis (NGU). In the absence of identifiable gonococci, the diagnosis of NGU is reliably made. If no discharge is expressed from the meatus, urethral material should be obtained by inserting a calcium alginate swab into the urethra to the depth of about 4 to 5 cm. The swab may be rotated during removal, and the material thus collected is transferred to a microscope slide by rolling the swab along the glass.

TABLE 307–2 CAUSES OF NONGONOCOCCAL URETHRITIS

SEXUALLY TRANSMITTED

Chlamydia trachomatis (15–50%)
Ureaplasma urealyticum (10–40%)
Mycoplasma genitalium (30%??)
Trichomonas vaginalis (1–17%)
Herpes simplex virus (primary) (?%)

NOT SEXUALLY TRANSMITTED

Gram-negative rods
Adenovirus
Microsporidia (in acquired immunodeficiency syndrome)
Neisseria meningitidis
Streptococcus pneumoniae
Staphylococcus saprophyticus??
Haemophilus species??
Bacteroides ureolyticus??

Testing to determine the specific etiology of urethritis is recommended because both chlamydial infection and gonorrhea are conditions that are reportable to health departments, and a specific diagnosis may enhance partner notification and improve compliance with treatment, especially in the exposed partner. If diagnostic tools are unavailable, patients should be treated for both infections. Nucleic acid amplification tests enable detection of *N. gonorrhoeae* and *C. trachomatis* on all specimens. These tests are more sensitive than traditional culture techniques for *C. trachomatis* and are the preferred method for the detection of this organism.

Treatment

Rx

Treatment should be initiated as soon as possible after diagnosis. Single-dose regimens have the advantage of improved adherence and direct observation. To improve compliance, the medication should be provided on site where feasible.

Unfortunately, *N. gonorrhoeae* has become resistant to many antimicrobials such as the fluoroquinolones. This is particularly true of infections acquired in the Pacific Rim and the West Coast of the United States or among men who have sex with men. Current therapy is described in Chapter 322. Appropriate treatments for NGU are listed in Table 307–3. Azithromycin and doxycycline are equally effective choices for most patients. 3 The diagnosis of either gonococcal urethritis or NGU calls for the epidemiologic treatment of female and male sexual partners. Treatment is usually highly effective, but some patients return with persistent symptoms. The clinician must first document the persistence of urethritis by identifying leukocytes on the Gram stain of urethral material. A careful sexual history can help exclude the possibility of reinfection. Treatment failures related to antimicrobial resistance are not rare, and in these cases an alternative antimicrobial regimen should be tried. *T. vaginalis* resists all of the standard antibacterial therapies for NGU but is usually susceptible to metronidazole or tinidazole. NGU that has failed to respond to a tetracycline should be treated with metronidazole in combination with either a macrolide/azalide or a fluoroquinolone. Patients in whom initial treatment with a macrolide/azalide or a fluoroquinolone fails should be treated with metronidazole. Women with urethritis usually present with some combination of dysuria and pyuria. This condition must be differentiated from bacterial cystitis. Because the symptoms of sexually transmitted urethritis often respond to therapies directed against classical uropathogens, the clinician must maintain a high index of suspicion for STD, especially in the setting of frequently recurring lower urinary tract symptoms, which may result from reinfection by an untreated sexual partner.

TABLE 307–3 SYNDROMIC TREATMENT OF NONGONOCOCCAL URETHRITIS

Drug	Dose	Comments
Doxycycline	100 mg PO bid for 7 days	
Azithromycin	1000 mg as a single oral dose	
Minocycline	100 mg PO qhs for 7 nights	
Ofloxacin	300 mg PO bid for 7 days	
Levofloxacin	500 mg PO qd for 7 days	
Erythromycin	500 mg PO qid ×7	
Tetracycline hydrochloride	500 mg PO qid ×7 *or* 250 mg PO qid ×14 days	
Clindamycin	450 mg PO tid for 10 days	If known to be chlamydial
Sulfisoxazole	500 mg PO qid for 10 days	If known to be chlamydial. Trimethoprim-sulfamethoxazole has no advantage

From Lau C, Qureshi AK: Azithromycin versus doxycycline for genital chlamydial infections: A meta-analysis of randomized clinical trials. Sex Transm Dis 2002;29:497–502.

Genital Ulcers

The differential diagnosis of genital ulcer disease is difficult, and the relative frequency of specific etiologies varies geographically. Genital infection with HSV (Chapter 397) is the most common cause of genital ulcer disease in the United States.

Genital herpes usually develops after an incubation period of 3 to 13 days and arises initially as clustered vesicles on an erythematous base. The vesicles become somewhat pustular and then rupture to form shallow, painful ulcers, which may coalesce. The ulcers heal by crusting over, and the process is usually completed in about 2 to 3 weeks with initial infection. Recurrences proceed through the same stages but generally last only about 5 to 7 days. Local paresthesias may precede the appearance of recurrent lesions. Only about 20% of infected individuals manifest the classical presentation, 60% have relatively atypical symptoms, and 20% are completely asymptomatic, although they shed the virus intermittently. Most people acquiring genital herpes do so from individuals who do not realize they are infected. Asymptomatic individuals and those with recurrence who are currently asymptomatic appear to shed virus approximately 3 to 4% of the time, and so they pose a risk to sexual partners.

Chancroid, infection with *Hemophilus ducreyi* (Chapter 324), produces ragged, dirty ulcers and tender inguinal lymphadenopathy, which may be fluctuant. Unlike the lesions of HSV, these are likely to vary in size.

The primary ulcerative lesion of syphilis (Chapter 340), the chancre, is palpably indurated and is usually painless.

In several studies, multiple organisms have been identified in a single ulcerative lesion. Molecular techniques have superseded cultures for diagnosis.

Genital Warts

HPV infection (Chapter 396) is usually asymptomatic but some patients develop visible genital warts. These are usually painless soft, moist, pink, or flesh-colored swellings that vary in shape and can be raised or flat, single or multiple, small or large, and sometimes cauliflower shaped. They occur in the vulva, vagina, and anus; on the cervix; and on the penis, scrotum, groin, or thigh. Genital warts are diagnosed by visual inspection.

Lower Genital Tract Infections in Women

Infections of the female genitourinary tract produce several syndromes with overlapping symptoms (dysuria, vaginal discharge, vulvar irritation), but a diagnosis can usually be established after a careful history, examination, and a few simple laboratory tests. The initial approach depends on the primary anatomic site of infection—urinary tract, endocervix, or vagina. In the adult, the columnar epithelium of the endocervix is susceptible to infection with *N. gonorrhoeae, C. trachomatis,* or HSV, and the vagina is susceptible to infection with *Candida albicans, Trichomonas vaginalis,* or the syndrome of bacterial vaginosis. Women with urethritis or cystitis often recognize dysuria as "internal," whereas it is often perceived as "external" by women with vulvovaginitis. Cervicitis is diagnosed on physical examination; the cervix may be red or friable, and cervical discharge, normally clear, may be mucopurulent. The cervix may appear completely normal in women with cervical infection. Vaginitis is associated with an increased vaginal discharge that may differ from its normal microfloccular appearance.

Vaginal Infections

Although there is considerable clinical overlap, a specific diagnosis can be made in most women with vaginal infections.

Bacterial Vaginosis

Bacterial vaginosis (BV) is the most common vaginal infection in the United States. Affected women are often minimally symptomatic but may note mild vaginal discharge, vaginal odor (often increased after coitus), and a relative absence of vaginal discomfort. The normal vagina contains hydrogen peroxide–producing lactobacilli such as *Lactobacillus crispatus* and *Lactobacillus jensenii,* which defend the vagina against a number of pathogens. *Lactobacillus acidophilus* is rarely found in the normal vagina, which probably explains the failure of yogurt as a preventative or remedy. BV apparently begins with the disappearance of the normal vaginal flora and its replacement with *Gardnerella vaginalis* and many other species of bacteria. The precise mechanism causing this shift in vaginal flora is poorly understood. The discharge is homogeneous and may contain bubbles. Vaginal pH is elevated above the normal 4.0 to 4.5. Adding 10% KOH to the vaginal discharge on the microscope slide or in the speculum elicits an amine-like, fishy odor, yielding a positive "whiff test" because of the elaboration of amines by the anaerobic flora. Examination of vaginal material as a wet mount reveals the absence of bacilli and their replacement with clumps of coccobacilli. Some vaginal epithelial cells are coated with coccobacilli, which may obscure their edges (clue cells). Relatively few polymorphonuclear leukocytes (PMNs) are observed, and large numbers of leukocytes in the wet mount of a woman with BV suggest a coincident infection, possibly trichomoniasis or cervicitis.

BV is not a benign infection. It is associated with an increased rate of upper tract infection (endometritis, salpingitis) and with several complications of pregnancy, including premature rupture of the membranes and premature delivery. Treatment is generally directed against the anaerobic flora and consists of metronidazole 500 mg orally twice daily for 7 days or clindamycin 300 mg orally twice daily for 7 days. Vaginal preparations of these two medications are also available but may be less effective in some situations. Unfortunately, the relapse rate, even in the absence of sexual exposure, is about 30%. Simultaneously treating male sexual partners, who are always asymptomatic, confers no therapeutic advantage. Recurrence is common and the precise contribution of sexual contact is unclear, but clinicians making this diagnosis should evaluate patients for STDs.

Vulvovaginal candidiasis is also common and is seen more frequently in women taking antibiotics or using oral contraceptives. The role of sexual transmission is quite limited. Affected women usually complain of vulvar itching and discomfort and may or may not notice an accompanying discharge. The vagina usually maintains normal numbers of lactobacilli, and the vaginal pH is therefore usually normal, which is very helpful in discriminating between candidiasis and other vaginal infections. The labia and vaginal walls may be quite erythematous. Although classically described as "curdy," the discharge of candidiasis is frequently loose and distinguished from other discharges only with difficulty. Vaginal material may be treated with 10% KOH to destroy other cellular elements and make the fungi easier to observe. Wet mount, however, has a sensitivity of only about 50%, and a woman with classical presentation should be treated even if fungal elements are not observed.

A wide range of topical antifungal medications is available, and these drugs are approximately equally effective. The cure rate with some single-dose therapies appears lower than that with longer regimens. Fluconazole administered as a single oral dose of 150 mg is highly effective. Infection with yeasts other than *Candida albicans* may require longer therapy. Recurrent vulvovaginal candidiasis is a problem for many women, and optimal management has not been defined. Elimination of predisposing factors is important.

Vaginal infection with *T. vaginalis* has become less common in the United States, possibly because of the use of metronidazole in the sexually active population to treat BV. Infected women usually complain of discharge, which may be yellow or green, and vulvar irritation. There may be internal or external dysuria. The vaginal walls are red, and the vagina contains an excessive yellow or green discharge displaying large bubbles. The exocervix may also be inflamed. Vaginal pH is elevated, but the whiff test is often negative. Wet mount reveals large numbers of PMNs, and motile protozoa, about the same size as PMNs, are recognized in about two thirds of cases. Therapy for trichomoniasis is described in Chapter 374. Organisms resistant to metronidazole are encountered with increasing frequency.

Upper Genital Tract Infections in Women

Salpingitis is an important clinical problem, resulting in considerable morbidity to the estimated 250,000 to 500,000 women affected annually in the United States.

N. gonorrhoeae or *C. trachomatis* can ascend from the cervix into the uterine cavity, producing endometritis, and thence to the fallopian tubes, causing salpingitis. Chlamydial salpingitis may be mild, and patients may not seek medical attention. Some intrauterine devices have been associated with an increased risk of salpingitis, and some data support douching as a predisposing factor. Anaerobic bacteria and mycoplasmas are also thought to play a role, particularly in chronic or recurrent disease.

Finding adnexal tenderness on bimanual examination makes the clinical diagnosis of salpingitis. Cervical tenderness, fever, leukocytosis, and an elevated sedimentation rate are sometimes observed. The clinical diagnosis is confirmed laparoscopically in only about 70% of cases. Vaginal ultrasonography or computed tomography is often helpful in defining the cause of pelvic pain syndromes.

Involuntary infertility complicates approximately 15% of initial attacks of salpingitis and about 75% after three or more attacks. Ectopic pregnancy and tubo-ovarian abscess are additional complications.

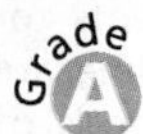

1. Ward DJ, Rowe B, Pattison H, et al: Reducing the risk of sexually transmitted infections in genitourinary medicine clinic patients: A systematic review and meta-analysis of behavioural interventions. Sex Transm Infect 2005;81:386–393.
2. Gottlieb SL, Douglas JM Jr, Foster M, et al, Project RESPECT Study Group: Incidence of herpes simplex virus type 2 infection in 5 sexually transmitted disease (STD) clinics and the effect of HIV/STD risk-reduction counseling. J Infect Dis 2004;190:1059–1067.
3. Lau CY, Qureshi AK: Azithromycin versus doxycycline for genital chlamydial infections: A meta-analysis of randomized clinical trials. Sex Transm Dis 2002;29:497–502.

SUGGESTED READINGS

Centers for Disease Control and Prevention: Sexually Transmitted Disease Treatment Guidelines, 2006. MMWR 2006;55(No. RR-11):1–94. *The classic reference, recently updated.*

Eckert LO: Acute vulvovaginitis. N Engl J Med 2006;355:1244–1252. *A comprehensive review.*

Fredricks DN, Fiedler TL, Marrazo JM: Molecular identification of bacteria associated with bacterial vaginosis. N Engl J Med 2005;353:1899–1911. *Molecular techniques permit the identification of large numbers of unculturable bacteria.*

Golden MR, Whittington WL, Handsfield HH, et al: Effect of expedited treatment of sex partners on recurrent or persistent gonorrhea or chlamydial infection. N Engl J Med 2005;352:676–685. *Demonstrates effectiveness.*

Low N, Broutet N, Adu-Sarkodie Y, et al: Global control of sexually transmitted infections. Lancet 2006;368:2001–2016. *Details an approach to control sexually transmitted infections other than HIV.*

APPROACH TO THE PATIENT BEFORE AND AFTER TRAVEL

Paul Arguin

According to the World Tourism Organization, approximately 700 million international trips are taken each year. This estimate includes travel to and from developed and developing countries and exotic vacation destinations, as well as travel for business, government, or humanitarian activities in remote areas of the world. International travelers encompass a wide variety of unique subsets, including children, the elderly, the immunocompromised, missionaries, military personnel, immigrants, and refugees. In addition, a recent survey showed that 23% of international travelers from the United States reported having some chronic illness, including heart disease, diabetes, and cancer. Some of these subsets of travelers may be particularly vulnerable to certain problems while traveling and may require more specialized counseling. In fact, first- and second-generation immigrants to developed countries who return to their countries of origin to visit friends and relatives have some of the highest risk for acquiring infectious diseases during travel.

PRETRAVEL HEALTH CARE AND RISK ASSESSMENT

Destination country–based recommendations are not applicable to everyone. To determine the best health advice for prospective travelers, travel health advice needs to be tailored both to the individual and to the itinerary. Thus, the practice of travel medicine has become a new specialty; its practitioners include primarily physicians in internal medicine, primary care, family medicine, pediatrics, emergency medicine, and occupational health, as well as nurses. These health care providers review the entire itinerary with the traveler to optimally characterize potential risks and exposures along the route. These risks are dependent on the destination city, the style of travel, the length of stay, the altitude of the destination, and the season of travel. The underlying health of the traveler is also important. Previous and current medical problems must be considered, as well as potential immunodeficiency, current prescription and over-the-counter medications, previous vaccinations, and pregnancy. It is essential to determine whether the traveler has medical conditions that would affect the ability to complete the planned itinerary or would alter any prophylactic measures.

PREVENTION AND RISK REDUCTION

Based on assessment of the risk, travelers should be advised about and provided with appropriate vaccinations, medications for prevention or self-treatment of certain diseases such as malaria and travelers' diarrhea, and prevention counseling about behavioral modifications that can help reduce the risk for injuries, infections, and other adverse health events. Specific advice should include information on hand washing. Hand washing is one of the most important practices in preventing illness from infections at home and while traveling. Travelers should wash their hands often with soap and water or an alcohol-based hand rub to remove potentially infectious material from the skin and help prevent transmission of diseases. Finally, all travelers should be given some guidance about common over-the-counter items (in addition to their prescription medications) that they should remember to carry with them in their travel health kit: pain relievers and antipyretics, cold and motion sickness medicines, antacids, laxatives, sunscreen, and insect repellent. Unless security regulations demand it, travelers should be told to keep these kits with them at all times and not to place them in checked baggage.

Some primary care providers are comfortable in giving some pretravel health advice and are encouraged to learn the basics. However, patients who have more complicated travel itineraries or multiple medical problems should be referred to a travel health specialist. International travelers should contact health care providers who provide pretravel health advice at least 4 to 6 weeks before departure to obtain vaccinations and prophylactic medications. Travel to developed countries (e.g., United States, Canada, Australia, New Zealand, Japan, and western Europe) involves lower risk than travel to developing countries. Travelers visiting urban tourist areas and staying in first-class accommodations may also have a lower risk for exposure to infectious diseases. Thus, additional vaccines and protective measures may be recommended for the more adventuresome travelers.

After their pretravel visit but before departure, travelers should continue to assess both their health status and the conditions at their destination. It is advisable for persons to postpone travel if they are not feeling well, particularly if they have febrile illnesses. By delaying travel, persons who are ill avoid potential emergencies and are courteous toward other travelers who may not wish to be exposed to someone with a transmissible illness. Travelers should be aware of the occurrence of any disease outbreaks, natural disasters, political unrest, or other major events at their international destinations. Current travel notices on diseases of international concern are posted on the Travelers' Health home page on the Centers for Disease Control and Prevention (CDC) website at *www.cdc.gov/travel.*

Injury Prevention

Most international travel health guidelines concentrate on the prevention of exotic infectious diseases. However, injuries, especially those caused by motor vehicle accidents, are the leading cause of preventable mortality among travelers. Trauma from motor vehicle accidents accounts for 21 to 26% of travel-associated deaths. Accidents tend to occur more frequently at dusk, in poor weather conditions, at crossroads, while speeding, while passing other drivers, and when the participants are impaired by alcohol consumption. Other factors such as failure to use safety measures, including seat belts and helmets, contribute not only to increased accidents but also to increased injuries. Travelers should always try to choose safe vehicles equipped with seat belts and use them. If their vehicle has only two wheels, they should always wear a helmet.

Protection against Mosquitoes and Other Arthropods

In addition to being nuisances, the bites of mosquitoes and other arthropods such as ticks can transmit a variety of infectious diseases, many of which are associated with specific travel itineraries (e.g., malaria, dengue fever, Japanese encephalitis, and African tick bite fever). Thus, no matter where they travel, patients should be counseled on avoidance of arthropod bites. Health care providers should remind travelers of some commonsense prevention tips, such as wearing long sleeves and pants, sleeping under a mosquito net if not in air-conditioned quarters, and using appropriate insect repellents.

For the prevention of malaria, the CDC recommends as the repellent of choice an insect repellent with DEET (*N,N*-diethyl-*m*-toluamide) in concentrations up to 50% for both adults and children. Lower concentrations are also effective but may not last as long, thus necessitating more frequent reapplication. An additional skin-based repellent is now available in the United States that contains picaridin (KBR 3023). Picaridin may be used if a DEET-containing repellent is not acceptable to the user. However, much less information is available on how effective picaridin is at protecting against all of the types of mosquitoes that transmit malaria. In addition, because the percentage of picaridin available in the United States is low, this repellent may protect against bites for only 1 to 4 hours. Products containing higher concentrations of picaridin are available in other countries. To avoid overexposure to the repellents, these products should be applied only to exposed skin, not under the clothing. They should not be applied to mucous membranes or sprayed in enclosed spaces. Parents should also apply the repellent to young children rather than allowing them to do it themselves. In addition, certain insect repellents, such as those containing permethrin, are recommended for use on clothing, shoes, bed nets, and camping gear. Permethrin-treated clothing repels and kills ticks, mosquitoes, and other arthropods and retains this effect after repeated laundering, but it should be reapplied after every five washings.

Immunizations

Immunizations for international travel can be categorized as routine, recommended, and required (Table 308–1). Routine vaccinations are childhood and adult vaccinations recommended for all persons regardless of travel. Recommended vaccinations are those that are prescribed according to the traveler's risk for infection. Required vaccinations are

TABLE 308–1 VACCINATIONS THAT MAY BE INDICATED FOR TRAVELERS*

Vaccine	Indication
ROUTINE VACCINES: RECOMMENDED REGARDLESS OF TRAVEL	
Tetanus and diphtheria toxoid (TD)	Every 10 years; substituting a tetanus and diphtheria toxoid and acellular pertussis (TDaP) booster once for the next TD booster is now recommended as well
Measles, mumps, and rubella (MMR)	Two documented doses if born after 1956
Varicella	Evidence of previous infection or vaccination
Pertussis	
Pneumococcal vaccine	Older/chronically ill persons if not already appropriately vaccinated
RECOMMENDED VACCINES: PRESCRIBED IF TRAVEL POSES AN EXPOSURE RISK	
Hepatitis A	First dose at least 4 weeks before travel to developing countries; second dose 6–12 months later
Hepatitis B	Three dose series for those with indications or at risk for exposure
Influenza	Travel at any time during the year, especially to tropical latitudes
Japanese encephalitis	Travel to rural southern and eastern Asia with extensive outdoor exposure
Meningococcal disease	Travel to the sub-Saharan meningitis belt during the dry season or to areas experiencing outbreaks
Poliomyelitis	Single adult booster for travel to countries where disease is present or where outbreaks have recently occurred
Rabies	Travel to countries where rabies is common and exposure to animals is anticipated
Typhoid fever	Travel to developing countries
Yellow fever	Travel to yellow fever–endemic zones in sub-Saharan Africa and South America, unless contraindicated (older age, thymus disease)
REQUIRED VACCINES: REQUIRED BY INTERNATIONAL HEALTH REGULATIONS OR SPECIFIC COUNTRIES TO CROSS INTERNATIONAL BORDERS	
Meningococcal vaccine	Travel to Saudi Arabia during Hajj and Umrah pilgrimages
Yellow fever	Travel to countries where vaccination is required by international health regulations or the country's regulations unless waived for medical contraindications by an official vaccine provider; primary dose at least 10 days before departure, administered by a World Health Organization Yellow Fever Vaccinating Center and documented on the international certificate of vaccination to be carried by the traveler

*Vaccine recommendations continue to evolve, so always check *www.cdc.gov/travel* for the most current advice for travelers and other information about indications, contraindications, dosing, and side effects.

those needed to cross international borders, as required by international health regulations or specific countries. The specifics of vaccine administration are provided in package inserts and should be consulted before giving any vaccine. It is the responsibility of the health care provider to ensure that travelers are not allergic to any of the vaccine components. Multiple vaccines may be given at the same time at different sites, depending on patient tolerance. Live-virus vaccines should be administered simultaneously or at a 4-week interval to avoid immune interference.

Routine Immunizations

A consultation before travel is an excellent opportunity to update routine immunizations, especially because adults are often not up to date on these. The CDC recommends that most adults have a tetanus and diphtheria toxoid (TD) booster vaccine every 10 years; have two recorded doses of measles, mumps, and rubella (MMR) vaccine (if born after 1956); and have evidence of previous varicella infection or vaccination. New recommendations have recently been issued for pertussis vaccination in adults: to be given as tetanus toxoid, reduced diphtheria toxoid, and acellular pertussis vaccine, adsorbed (TDaP), in place of the next booster dose of TD vaccine. Finally, the pretravel visit is also a great opportunity to provide pneumococcal vaccine to older or chronically ill patients who have not received it from their primary care providers.

Recommended Immunizations

Hepatitis A

Hepatitis A, transmitted through contaminated food or water or intimate contact with another infected person, is one of the most frequently reported vaccine-preventable, travel-related illnesses. The risk for infection is approximately 300 per 100,000 travelers per month in tourist areas in developing countries, and the risk is five to seven times higher for backpackers and those traveling off the usual tourist routes. Though not usually fatal, acute hepatitis A infection can result in weeks of lost work time and early repatriation of travelers. The hepatitis A vaccine is indicated for most travelers to the developing world unless they are known to be immune. Ideally, a single dose should be administered at least 4 weeks before travel, although many people will have a sufficient immune response by 2 weeks. A second dose 6 to 12 months later increases that protection to long term. Before the introduction of hepatitis A vaccine, immune globulin injections were used to provide short-term protection against hepatitis A. They are still recommended for children younger than 1 year and in persons without sufficient lead time for vaccination before travel.

Hepatitis B

Hepatitis B is transmitted through infected blood and body fluids, has a case-fatality rate of 1%, and can result in chronic infection in up to 10% of adults. Recent data have shown that almost a quarter of international travelers have pretravel indications for hepatitis B vaccine, including occupational risk for exposure to blood and body fluids or a history of a recent sexually transmitted disease. Almost 10% of travelers experience exposures that would be categorized as high risk for hepatitis B infection during travel. However, less than a third of persons who should be immunized against hepatitis B receive the full three-dose series before travel. Travelers should be advised to avoid behavior that is high risk for the acquisition of hepatitis B, although it is clear that it is difficult to identify travelers at risk during the pretravel encounter. Those with indications should receive the three-dose series. The usual schedule for this vaccine is a dose at 0, 1, and 6 months, which is often difficult to complete for last-minute travelers. There are also non–Food and Drug Administration–approved accelerated schedules, with doses at 0, 7, and 21 days. The CDC recommends that persons who receive vaccinations on an accelerated schedule also receive a booster dose 6 months after the start of the series to promote long-term immunity. A combination vaccine that provides protection against hepatitis A and B infections is also available.

Influenza

Recent surveillance data suggest that travelers are at risk for influenza infection throughout the year, particularly in the tropical latitudes. Thus, all travelers, especially those at high risk for complications, should be considered candidates for influenza vaccination.

Japanese Encephalitis

Japanese encephalitis is transmitted by infected mosquitoes in rural parts of southern and eastern Asia. Travelers to endemic areas who will have extensive rural outdoor exposure, such as campers and hikers, should consider receiving this three-dose vaccination series and be very vigilant in their mosquito avoidance measures.

Meningococcal Disease

The sub-Saharan African "meningitis belt," which extends from Mali to Ethiopia, experiences increased rates of transmission of *Neisseria meningitidis* regularly during the dry season, which is usually December through June. Travelers to an area where there is an ongoing outbreak of meningococcal disease and those traveling to the "meningitis belt" of sub-Saharan Africa during the dry season should receive one of the two quadrivalent (A, C, Y, and W-135) meningococcal vaccines that are currently available: the polysaccharide and the conjugate vaccine.

Poliomyelitis

The global polio eradication effort has reduced the number of countries with ongoing transmission to just a few, specifically, Afghanistan, Pakistan, India, Nigeria, and Egypt. However, occasional outbreaks of polio still occur in countries that had previously eradicated it. A single adult booster for polio is recommended for travel to all of these countries.

Rabies

Rabies is a fatal disease transmitted by the bite of infected mammals; however, effective prevention strategies are available. The three-dose preexposure vaccination series is indicated for persons with a higher likelihood of encountering animals such as stray dogs in countries where both rabies transmission is known to occur and access to antirabies biologics, including human rabies immune globulin and cell culture–produced vaccines, may not be available. Travelers who will be spending extended periods outdoors, such as hikers, spelunkers, and small children, are examples of persons who may be at higher risk for rabies. Health care providers should counsel travelers on appropriate behavior around stray, wild, or domesticated animals not known to be vaccinated against rabies to try to prevent rabies exposure. Travelers should always avoid contact with these animals and not feed or pet them. In the event of an animal bite, all travelers should be instructed to seek appropriate rabies postexposure prophylaxis. Previously unimmunized persons will need to receive the full postexposure regimen, including vaccine and rabies immune globulin. It is important to realize that persons who received the preexposure series still need two booster doses of rabies vaccine if they are bitten by a rabid animal. Health care providers should be strongly discouraged from deviating from these established preexposure and postexposure regimens in an attempt to reduce costs or for the convenience of the traveling patient.

Typhoid Fever

Annually in the world, 22 million cases of typhoid fever result in 200,000 deaths. In the United States, approximately 400 travel-associated cases are reported each year, mostly among travelers visiting friends and relatives and returning from their home countries. Although typhoid fever is a treatable bacterial infection, prevention is preferable because of increasing rates of antibiotic resistance. Travelers to certain developing countries should be vaccinated against typhoid fever with either of the two types of typhoid vaccine: the live oral vaccine (Ty21a) and the inactivated injectable vaccine (Vi capsular polysaccharide).

Yellow Fever

Yellow fever is transmitted by the bite of infected mosquitoes in sub-Saharan Africa and tropical South America, where it is endemic and intermittently epidemic. All persons traveling to the yellow fever–endemic zones without contraindications should be vaccinated with the live viral vaccine. In rare but severe instances, yellow fever–like syndromes develop from the attenuated live vaccine virus; these adverse events are characterized as either viscerotropic disease or neurotropic disease. Being older than 60 years and having a history of thymus disease have been identified as independent risk factors for development of one of these severe, but rare adverse events. Persons with contraindications should reconsider their travel itinerary. If they choose to travel to yellow fever–endemic areas despite contraindications, they should be very vigilant in their mosquito avoidance measures.

Required Immunizations

Meningococcal Meningitis

Vaccination against meningococcal disease is not a requirement for entry into any country except Saudi Arabia for travelers to Mecca during the annual Hajj and Umrah pilgrimage.

Yellow Fever

In addition to vaccination for protection of the traveler, yellow fever vaccine may be required by some countries as a condition of entry, as outlined in the International Health Regulations. These are mostly countries where yellow fever does not occur, but competent mosquitoes are present that could transmit the virus. Vaccination becomes valid for the purpose of entry 10 days after primary inoculation, and it must be administered at an approved World Health Organization Yellow Fever Vaccinating Center. Receipt of the vaccine must be documented on an international certificate of vaccination that should be carried with the passport. A national registry of such providers in the United States is available on the CDC website at *http://www2.ncid.cdc.gov/travel/yellowfever/*. Persons for whom the vaccine is contraindicated should be issued a vaccination waiver letter bearing the official yellow fever vaccine provider stamp.

Malaria Protection

As many as 30,000 travelers from industrialized countries acquire malaria annually. From 1985 through 2002, 11,896 cases of malaria in U.S. civilians were reported to the CDC, including 76 fatalities. The CDC also maintains a country-by-country listing, often with regional- or sub-country-level recommendations for malaria prevention. All travelers to malaria-endemic countries should be counseled to avoid mosquito bites by the appropriate use of repellents and mosquito nets. All travelers to malaria-endemic areas should also correctly and consistently take their antimalarial chemoprophylaxis. Depending on the destination, there are usually several medication options so that travelers who may not have tolerated one type of medication in the past because of unpleasant side effects can still be prescribed one of the others. For travel to areas of risk where chloroquine-resistant malaria has *not* been reported, chloroquine is recommended for prophylaxis. For areas with chloroquine resistance, the CDC currently recommends mefloquine, doxycycline, or the combination of atovaquone and proguanil as equal alternatives. The choice of one or the other is usually based on the side effects, cost, and duration of the trip.

Travelers should also be warned about trying to acquire malaria medications while overseas, either for reasons of cost or for convenience. Medicines with similar-sounding names, such as Malarone, Malasone, or Maloprim, do not contain the same active ingredients. In addition, one study of malaria medicines produced and sold overseas demonstrated that 36% of the medicines either contained smaller amounts or none of the active ingredient stated on the box. Travelers should also be counseled to be alert for symptoms consistent with malaria after returning and to seek prompt evaluation and treatment if indicated.

Travelers' Diarrhea

A diarrheal illness develops in about 50% of travelers to developing countries, with an average duration, if untreated, of approximately 4 days. All travelers should be instructed on ways to avoid illnesses transmitted through food and water. Although diarrheal illness is sometimes very difficult to avoid, travelers should be taught when possible to make safer choices to reduce the chance of acquiring a food-borne or waterborne illness. They should avoid tap water or ice made with tap water in favor of beverages that have been boiled or placed in sealed containers, such as bottled water or carbonated items. Selecting foods freshly prepared rather than eating from communal vessels or buffets is also a safer choice.

Frequently, despite the best efforts, diarrhea occurs and travelers should be taught how to appropriately manage the situation by drinking abundant fluids to avoid dehydration and by trying to manage symptoms with over-the-counter medications such as bismuth subsalicylate or loperamide. The current standard of care also includes prescribing an antibiotic for the traveler to carry—not to take to prevent diarrhea—but rather to have readily available for use when needed to treat a moderate to severe case of diarrhea acquired while traveling. Fluoroquinolone antibiotics are generally used for self-treatment of diarrhea, although azithromycin is now also being used for travel to areas with high rates of antibiotic resistance (e.g., parts of Southeast Asia) and for treatment of children and pregnant women.

POST-TRAVEL CARE

Travelers may be exposed to a variety of pathogens and risks, both exotic and mundane. Approximately half of all travelers will experience some health problems while traveling. Overall, during international travel, 5 to 8% of travelers seek medical attention, some requiring emergency medical evacuation. Health care providers who see returned travelers should be aware that most ailments diagnosed during the post-travel period are not necessarily travel related. However, providers should also be able to recognize important syndromes in returned travelers that may be travel related and require prompt treatment or referral for definitive management. A thorough history, including a review of the travel itinerary and specific exposures (e.g., insect bites, unprotected sexual contact, and consumption of untreated water), is an essential first step. The most frequent health problems in ill returned travelers are chronic diarrhea, rashes, and respiratory infections. Although gastrointestinal ailments are the most frequent problem, fever is the most serious. Fever in a traveler who has recently returned from a malaria-endemic region should be immediately evaluated so that antimalarial treatment can be initiated rapidly if indicated. Finally, certain long-term travelers should be evaluated by a travel or tropical medicine specialist when they return to screen for conditions that may be asymptomatic, such as schistosomiasis or strongyloidiasis.

SUGGESTED READINGS

Bottieau E, Clerinx J, Schrooten W, et al: Etiology and outcome of fever after a stay in the tropics. Arch Intern Med 2006;166:1642–1648. *Clinical observation over a five-year period determined that imported fever is highly destination-specific.*

Centers for Disease Control and Prevention: Health information for international travel, 2005–2006. Atlanta, US Department of Health and Human Services, Public Health Service, 2005. *Also known as "the Yellow Book," this text is updated and published every 2 years and is considered the "gold standard" source of prevention guidelines for international travelers' health.*

Centers for Disease Control and Prevention: Travelers' health website. *www.cdc.gov/travel. An up-to-date source of travel health information searchable by disease and geographic region, as well as timely travel-related notices such as information on disease outbreaks or vaccine shortages.*

Freedman DO, Weld LH, Lozarsky PE, et al: Spectrum of disease and relation to place of exposure among ill returned travelers. N Engl J Med 2006;354:119–130. *Travel destinations are associated with the probability of the diagnosis of certain diseases.*

Hill DR, Ericsson CD, Pearson RD, et al. for the Practice Guidelines Committee of the Infectious Diseases Society of America: The practice of travel medicine: Guidelines by the Infectious Diseases Society of America. Clin Infect Dis 2006;43:1499–1539. *Consensus guidelines.*

309 ANTIBACTERIAL THERAPY

William A. Craig

In the 60 to 70 years since the introduction of sulfonamides and penicillin, a large array of antibacterial agents have been developed for the treatment and prevention of infectious diseases. This modern era of antibacterial chemotherapy has had a significant impact in reducing the morbidity and mortality from infections. It has also been successful in reducing infectious complications associated with surgery, trauma, and organ transplantation. The broad use of antibacterials in modern medicine has not been problem free, however. These drugs or their metabolites can occasionally produce untoward reactions either directly or through interaction with other drugs. Antibacterial agents also provide selective pressure for the emergence of resistance. Despite the availability of a large number of drugs, the emergence of multiply resistant pneumococci, staphylococci, enterococci, *Pseudomonas aeruginosa,* and *Mycobacterium tuberculosis* demonstrates the need for additional antibacterials, especially those with new mechanisms of action.

MECHANISMS OF ACTION

The clinical success of antibacterials is due to their selective in vivo toxicity in that they primarily kill or inhibit the growth of microorganisms without inflicting harm on the host. This action is accomplished by attacking targets unique to bacteria or more susceptible to inhibition in bacteria than in human cells. The peptidoglycan cell wall is unique to bacteria and has been a very successful target for the development of many β-lactam and glycopeptide antibiotics. The bacterial ribosome is smaller than the mammalian ribosome and has much greater affinity for aminoglycosides, macrolides, clindamycin, and tetracyclines. Bacteria must synthesize dihydrofolate, whereas mammalian cells can form dihydrofolate from dietary sources. The enzymes involved in this synthesis are inhibited by sulfonamides. The bacterial dihydrofolate reductase enzyme, which converts dihydrofolate to the active tetrahydrofolate, binds trimethoprim about 55,000 times more avidly than the mammalian enzyme does. The site and mechanism of action of major classes of antibacterial agents are listed in Table 309–1.

Antibacterials that only inhibit bacterial growth are called *bacteriostatic,* whereas those that kill bacteria over an 18- to 24-hour period are called *bactericidal.* Occasionally, the mechanism of bacterial killing is different from the mechanism of bacterial inhibition for some antibacterials. For most bacteria, inhibition of cell wall synthesis by the penicillins indirectly activates bacterial enzymes (murein hydrolases) that cause killing by cell lysis. Combinations of drugs can produce antibacterial effects that are greater than the sum of the individual antimicrobial activities, a relationship called *synergism.* For example, penicillin, ampicillin, and vancomycin can enhance bacterial uptake of aminoglycosides, thereby resulting in bactericidal synergism against enterococci. The sequential inhibition of multiple steps in a biosynthetic pathway, such as inhibition of folic acid synthesis by a sulfonamide and trimethoprim, can also result in synergism.

FACTORS INFLUENCING ANTIBACTERIAL SELECTION

Infecting Organism and Susceptibility Testing

Effective therapy is dependent on identifying the causative pathogen from appropriate cultures, from Gram stain of biologic samples (sputum, pus, etc.), or on the basis of clinical findings. Because therapy is often required before culture and susceptibility test results are known, the clinician must be able to formulate the probable organisms for the site and severity of infection and the underlying diseases in the patient. Knowledge of local susceptibility patterns for various antibacterials helps the clinician decide whether initial therapy should address the possibility of resistant organisms, such as penicillin-resistant *Streptococcus pneumoniae* and methicillin-resistant *Staphylococcus aureus* (MRSA). Modifications in therapy can be made once culture and susceptibility test results are known. The final antimicrobial regimen should be as targeted as possible.

The standard method for measuring antimicrobial activity in vitro is determination of the *minimal inhibitory concentration* (MIC) and the *minimal bactericidal concentration* (MBC). By definition, the MIC is the lowest concentration of drug that prevents visible bacterial growth over an 18- to 24-hour incubation period. The MBC is the lowest concentration that kills 99.9% of the organisms over the same period. MIC values and qualitative tests, such as the disc diffusion method, are used to classify organisms as *susceptible, intermediate,* or *resistant* by using standards established by the Clinical and Laboratory Standards Institute. Many laboratories use automated techniques to report MIC values routinely. MBC determinations are reserved for infections in which bactericidal activity is required. An organism that is not killed by an antibiotic that generally kills that species is said to be tolerant, which is usually defined as an MBC greater than 16 times the MIC.

Antimicrobial Resistance

Antimicrobial resistance has become a major limitation to the continued success of antibacterial chemotherapy. The mechanisms of resistance

TABLE 309–1 MECHANISMS OF ACTION OF ANTIBACTERIAL AGENTS

Agent	Site of Action	Effect	Cidal	Static
β-Lactams (penicillins, cephalosporins, carbapenems, and aztreonam)	Cell wall: penicillin-binding proteins	Inhibit cross-linking of peptidoglycan (transpeptidation), impair cell wall synthesis	+	Occasionally (enterococci)
Vancomycin, teicoplanin, dalbavancin, and telavancin	Cell wall: terminal D-alanyl-D-alanine of pentapeptide peptidoglycan precursor	Inhibit polymerization of disaccharide precursors to peptidoglycan (transglycosylation), impair cell wall synthesis	+	Occasionally (enterococci)
Daptomycin	Cell membrane	Rapid depolarization of membrane potential	+	Occasionally (enterococci)
Aminoglycosides	Protein synthesis: 30S ribosome subunit	Inhibit peptide elongation, cause misreading of genetic code, inhibit protein synthesis	+	
Tetracyclines and glycylcyclines	Protein synthesis: 30S ribosome subunit	Inhibit binding of transfer RNA, inhibit protein synthesis	Occasionally	+
Chloramphenicol	Protein synthesis: 50S ribosome subunit	Block attachment of aminoacyl transfer RNA, inhibit protein synthesis	Occasionally	+
Macrolides, azalides, and ketolides	Protein synthesis: 50S ribosome subunit	Block transfer of amino acids to peptide chain, inhibit protein synthesis	Occasionally	+
Clindamycin	Protein synthesis: 50S ribosome subunit	Blocks transfer of amino acids to peptide chain, inhibits protein synthesis	Occasionally	+
Quinupristin-dalfopristin	Protein synthesis: 50S ribosome subunit	Blocks extrusion of peptide chains, inhibits protein synthesis	+	+ (with quinupristin resistance)
Linezolid	Protein synthesis: 50S ribosome subunit	Blocks formation of the 70S initiation complex, inhibits protein synthesis	Occasionally	+
Rifampin	Nucleic acid synthesis: B subunit of DNA-dependent RNA polymerase	Inhibits RNA synthesis	+	
Metronidazole	Nucleic acid synthesis	Damages nucleic acids, inhibits DNA synthesis	+	
Quinolones	Nucleic acid synthesis: DNA gyrase and topoisomerase IV	Impair supercoiling of DNA, prevent decatenation of DNA molecules after replication, inhibit DNA synthesis	+	
Sulfonamides	Folic acid synthesis: dihydropteroate synthetase	Competitive inhibition of synthesis of dihydrofolate from p-aminobenzoic acid, pteroate, and glutamic acid	Occasionally (when used with trimethoprim)	+
Trimethoprim	Folic acid synthesis: dihydrofolate reductase	Inhibits reduction of dihydrofolate to tetrahydrofolic acid	Occasionally (when used with sulfonamide)	+

are varied and include alteration of the drug's target, decreased permeability of the outer cell membrane, active drug efflux from the bacterial cell, and drug inactivation (Table 309–2). An increasing number of organisms have multiple mechanisms of resistance. The genes that account for these resistance mechanisms are acquired by mutations of existing DNA or acquisition of new DNA. New genes mediating resistance are usually spread from organism to organism by plasmids through conjugation, transduction, or transformation. Some resistance genes are linked to transposons, which can move between plasmids and chromosomes. Expression of resistance genes can be constantly functional or induced by exposure to antimicrobial agents. The ability of bacteria to share various resistance genes accounts for the remarkable speed at which some resistance mechanisms spread.

Alteration of the target site is a major mechanism of resistance and can occur by different mechanisms. For example, most resistance to rifampin in mycobacteria is due to altered amino acids in the β-subunit of the polymerase enzyme as the result of gene mutations. On the other hand, methicillin resistance in staphylococci is due to acquisition of the chromosomal gene (*mecA*) that encodes for penicillin-binding protein 2a, which has very low affinity for penicillins. Finally, enzymatic modification of the target site can reduce drug affinity; methylation of the 23S rRNA of the 50S ribosome leads to resistance to macrolides, clindamycin, and streptogramin B.

One of the most common mechanisms of antimicrobial resistance is enzymatic inactivation of the drug. Enzymatic cleavage of the β-lactam ring by β-lactamases is the primary reason for resistance to the penicillins. The genes for these enzymes can be on the chromosome or on plasmids and transposons. In staphylococci, the enzymes are secreted into the surrounding milieu. In contrast, β-lactamases in gram-negative bacilli are secreted into the periplasmic space between the inner and outer cell membrane. Some of the common enzymes in gram-negative bacilli are TEM-1, TEM-2, SHV-1, and PSE-1. These enzymes inactivate

TABLE 309–2 MECHANISMS OF ANTIBACTERIAL RESISTANCE

Antibacterial Agent	Mechanism	Representative Organism
β-Lactams (penicillins, cephalosporins, carbapenems, aztreonam)	Altered target (penicillin-binding proteins)	Methicillin-resistant *Staphylococcus aureus* (MRSA), penicillin-resistant *Streptococcus pneumoniae, Enterococcus faecium*
	Reduced permeability	*Enterobacter* species, *Pseudomonas aeruginosa*
	Enhanced efflux	*P. aeruginosa*
	β-Lactamases	*S. aureus,* Enterobacteriaceae (includes ESBLs), *Haemophilus influenzae, Moraxella catarrhalis, Neisseria gonorrhoeae, Enterococcus faecalis*
Aminoglycosides	Inactivating enzymes (acetylation, adenylation, phosphorylation)	*S. aureus,* enterococci, *P. aeruginosa,* Enterobacteriaceae
	Reduced permeability	Enterobacteriaceae, *P. aeruginosa,* enterococci
	Enhanced efflux	*P. aeruginosa*
	Decreased ribosomal binding	*S. aureus, E. faecalis,* mycobacteria (streptomycin)
Chloramphenicol	Enhanced efflux	*H. influenzae*
	Reduced permeability	Enterobacteriaceae
	Inactivating enzyme (acetylation)	*S. aureus, S. pneumoniae,* enterococci, Enterobacteriaceae
Daptomycin	Altered target	*S. aureus*
Glycyclcyclines	Enhanced efflux	Enterobacteriaceae, especially *Proteus*
Macrolides, clindamycin, ketolide, quinupristin	Altered target (methylation of ribosomal RNA)	*S. aureus, S. pneumoniae* (not ketolide), streptococci, *Bacteroides fragilis*
	Enhanced efflux (not clindamycin or ketolide)	*S. pneumoniae,* streptococci
	Reduced permeability	Enterobacteriaceae
	Inactivating enzymes	*Escherichia coli, Klebsiella pneumoniae, S. aureus*
Linezolid	Altered target	Enterococci, *S. aureus*
Quinolones	Altered target (DNA gyrase, topoisomerase IV)	Enterobacteriaceae, *S. aureus*
	Reduced permeability	Enterobacteriaceae, *P. aeruginosa*
	Enhanced efflux	*E. coli, P. aeruginosa*
Tetracyclines	Altered target (ribosome)	*N. gonorrhoeae,* streptococci
	Enhanced efflux	*E. coli, S. pneumoniae*
	Reduced permeability	Enterobacteriaceae
	Drug inactivation	*B. fragilis*
Rifampin	Altered target (β-subunit of polymerase)	*E. coli, S. aureus*
Sulfonamides, trimethoprim	Altered target (dihydropteroate synthetase or dihydrofolate reductase)	Enterobacteriaceae, *Moraxella catarrhalis*
	Enhanced *p*-aminobenzoic acid production	*S. aureus, N. gonorrhoeae*
	Reduced permeability	*P. aeruginosa,* Enterobacteriaceae
Vancomycin	Altered target (peptidoglycan precursor–binding site)	*E. faecium, E. faecalis, S. aureus*

ESBLs = extended-spectrum β-lactamases.

penicillins and some cephalosporins, but not the cephamycins (cefoxitin and cefotetan) and third-generation cephalosporins. However, mutations in the genes of these enzymes have created modified enzymes called extended-spectrum β-lactamases, primarily in *Klebsiella* species and *E. coli,* that are capable of destroying the third-generation cephalosporins. Some of the newer metalloenzymes are also capable of inactivating carbapenems. All these enzymes tend to be susceptible to inhibition by the so-called β-lactamase inhibitors (clavulanic acid, sulbactam, and tazobactam).

Other β-lactamases are produced at low levels in *P. aeruginosa, Enterobacter* sp, *Citrobacter freundii, Serratia* sp, and some other gram-negative bacilli. However, high levels of these β-lactamases can be induced or stably de-repressed, thereby resulting in resistance to penicillin/β-lactamase inhibitor combinations and most cephalosporins. These AmpC β-lactamases have also spread to *Klebsiella pneumoniae* and *E. coli.* Carbapenems, on the other hand, are not inactivated by these β-lactamases.

Decreased permeability of the outer cell membrane of gram-negative bacilli is a common mechanism of intrinsic resistance to antimicrobials. The permeability of the outer membrane is due to special proteins called *porins,* which form specific channels through the outer membrane. Mutational change of the porin proteins in the channel that carbapenems use to cross the outer cell membrane has resulted in resistance in *P. aeruginosa.* However, much of what was attributed to decreased permeability in the past is now explained by the presence of efflux pumps. Such pumps have been found in an increasing variety of organisms. Efflux is the major mechanism for macrolide resistance in pneumococci in North America.

Pharmacokinetic Considerations

The goal of antibacterial activity is to provide adequate, but nontoxic concentrations of drug at the site of infection for a sufficient period to aid in eradication of the infecting pathogen. Knowledge of the major pharmacokinetic properties of antibacterial agents (summarized in Table 309–3) is essential for their proper use. Capillaries with pores that readily allow the passage of antibacterials supply most tissues in the body. Thus, the therapeutic drug concentrations achieved in serum are usually achieved at most extracellular sites of infection. Antibacterials even penetrate into abscesses, but other factors such as slow bacterial growth and low pH often necessitate surgical drainage for maximum efficacy. Prosthetic joints and other foreign bodies can also provide the environment

TABLE 309–3 DOSAGE REGIMEN, PHARMACOKINETICS, AND ADJUSTMENT IN PATIENTS WITH HEPATIC AND RENAL FAILURE

Class/Agent	Dose,* Systemic Infection	Oral Formulation	Peak Serum Concentration (mg/mL)	Protein Binding (%)	Normal Serum Half-Life (hr)	Hepatic Failure	Renal Failure	Serum Levels Affected by Dialysis
AMINOGLYCOSIDES								
Amikacin	5 mg/kg q8h or 15 mg/kg q24h	—	35	0	2–3	No	Major	Yes (H, P)
Gentamicin	1.7 mg/kg q8h or 5 mg/kg q24h	—	7	0	2–3	No	Major	Yes (H, P)
Netilmicin	1.7 mg/kg q8h or 5 mg/kg q24h	—	7	0	2–3	No	Major	Yes (H, P)
Tobramycin	1.7 mg/kg q8h or 5 mg/kg q24h	—	7	0	2–3	No	Major	Yes (H, P)
ANTITUBERCULOUS AGENTS								
Ethambutol	15 mg/kg q24h (PO)	Yes	2	10	3.3	No	Major	Yes (H, P)
Isoniazid	5 mg/kg or 300 mg q24h (PO)	Yes	4.5	10	3	Yes	Major	Yes (H, P)
Pyrazinamide	10 mg/kg q8h (PO)	Yes	12	—	10	Yes	Yes	Yes (H)
Rifampin	10 mg/kg or 600 mg q24h (PO)	Yes	7	70	3	Yes	Minor	No (H)
CARBAPENEMS								
Ertapenem	1–2 g q24h	—	155	95	4–5	Unknown	Yes	Yes (H)
Imipenem	0.5–1 g q6h	—	40	15	1	No	Avoid	Yes (H)
Meropenem	0.5–2 g q8–12h	—	50	<10	1	No	Yes	Yes (H)
FIRST-GENERATION CEPHALOSPORINS								
Cefadroxil	1000 mg q12h (PO)	Yes	16	20	1.5	No	Yes	Yes (H)
Cefazolin	0.5–2 g q8h	—	180	80	2	No	Major	Yes (H) No (P)
Cephalexin	500 mg q6h (PO)	Yes	18	15	1	No	Yes	Yes (H, P)
Cephradine	500 mg q6h	Yes†	140	10	1.3	No	Yes	Yes (H, P)
SECOND-GENERATION CEPHALOSPORINS								
Cefaclor	500 mg q8h (PO)	Yes†	10	25	0.8	No	Yes	Yes (H)
Cefoxitin	1–2 g q6–8h	—	220	70	0.8	No	Yes	Yes (H) No (P)
Cefprozil	500 mg q12h (PO)	Yes	10	35	1.4	No	Yes	Yes (H)
Cefuroxime	1 g q8h	—	100	50	1.5	No	Yes	Yes (H, P)
Cefuroxime axetil	500 mg q12h (PO)	Yes	9	50	1.5	No	Yes	Yes (H, P)
THIRD-GENERATION CEPHALOSPORINS								
Cefdinir	300 mg q12h (PO)	Yes	2	65	1.7	Unknown	Minor	Yes (H)
Cefditoren pivoxil	400 mg q12h (PO)	Yes	4	88	1.6	No	Yes	Yes (H)
Cefixime	400 mg q24h (PO)	Yes	3–5	67	3	No	Yes	No (H, P)
Cefotaxime	1g q8h	—	200	50	1.5	Minor	Minor	Yes (H) No (P)
Cefpodoxime proxetil	200–400 mg q12h (PO)	Yes	3	25	2.5	No	Yes	Yes (H)
Ceftazidime	1 g q8h	—	160	60	2	No	Major	Yes (H, P)
Ceftibuten	400 mg q24h (PO)	Yes	15	65	2.5	Unknown	Yes	Yes (H)
Ceftizoxime	1 g q6–8h	—	130	30	1.3	No	Major	Yes (H) No (P)
Ceftriaxone	1–2 g q12–24h	—	250	90	8	No	No	No (H)

Continued

Section XXIII Infectious Diseases

TABLE 309–3 DOSAGE REGIMEN, PHARMACOKINETICS, AND ADJUSTMENT IN PATIENTS WITH HEPATIC AND RENAL FAILURE—cont'd

Class/Agent	Dose,* Systemic Infection	Oral Formulation	Peak Serum Concentration (mg/mL)	Protein Binding (%)	Normal Serum Half-Life (hr)	Hepatic Failure	Renal Failure	Serum Levels Affected by Dialysis
FOURTH-GENERATION CEPHALOSPORINS								
Cefepime	1 g q8h	—	193	20	2	No	Yes	Yes (H, P)
PENICILLINS								
Amoxicillin	500 mg q8h (PO)	Yes	10	20	1	No	Yes	Yes (H) No (P)
Ampicillin	1 g q6h	Yes†	200	20	1	No	Yes	Yes (H) No (P)
Indanyl carbenicillin	500 mg q6h (PO)	Yes	6	50	1	Minor	Major	Yes (H, P)
Cloxacillin	500 mg q6h (PO)	Yes†	9	95	0.5	No	No	No (H, P)
Dicloxacillin	500 mg q6h (PO)	Yes†	18	97	0.5	No	No	No (H, P)
Nafcillin	1–2 g q4–6h	—	160	90	0.5	Yes	No	No (H, P)
Oxacillin	1–2 g q4–6h	—	200	90	0.5	Yes	No	Yes (H, P)
Penicillin G	3–4 million units q4–6h	Yes†	60	60	0.5	No	Yes	Yes (H) No (P)
Penicillin V	500 mg q6h (PO)	Yes	5	80	1	No	No	Yes (H) No (P)
Piperacillin/ tazobactam	3.375–4.5 g q6–8h	—	240	50	1	Minor	Minor	Yes (H)
Ticarcillin/ clavulanate	3.1 g q4–8h	—	220	50	1	Minor	Major	Yes (H, P)
QUINOLONES								
Ciprofloxacin	500–750 mg q12h (PO)	Yes†	2–3	30	4	No	Minor	No (H, P)
Gemifloxacin	320 mg q24h (PO)	Yes	1.6	60–70	7	No	Minor	No (H, P)
Levofloxacin	250–750 mg q24h (PO)	Yes	6–9	25	7	No	Yes	NO (H, P)
Moxifloxacin	400 mg q24h (PO)	Yes	4–5	50	10	No—minor	No	NO (H, P)
TETRACYCLINES-GLYCYLCYCLINES								
Doxycycline	100 mg q12–24h (PO)	Yes	1.5–2.1	93	15–20	Avoid	No	No (H, P)
Minocycline	100 mg q12–24h (PO)	Yes	2.2	75	15	No	Avoid	No (H, P)
Tetracycline	500 mg q6h (PO)	Yes†	4	50	7	Avoid	Avoid	No (H, P)
Tigecycline	100 mg, then 50 mg q12h	—	0.6–0.9	70	37–38	Minor	No	No (H, P)
SULFONAMIDES								
Sulfadiazine	15 mg/kg q6h	Yes	30	50	3	Avoid	Avoid	Unknown
Sulfamethoxazole	0.5–1 g q6–8h (PO)	Yes	100	50	9	Avoid	Major	Yes (H) No (P)
Trimethoprim (with sulfamethoxazole)	3–5 mg/kg q6–8h (IV) (based on trimethoprim component)	Yes	3–9	60	10	No	Avoid	Yes (H) No (P)
MACROLIDES-LINCOSAMIDES-KETOLIDES								
Azithromycin	500 mg first dose, followed by 250 mg q24h (PO)	Yes†	0.4	25	12–50	Unknown	No	No (H, P)
Clarithromycin	500 mg q12h (PO)	Yes	2–3	70	7	No	Minor	Yes (H) No (P)
Clindamycin	0.3–0.4 g q6–8h	Yes	15	90	2.5	Minor	No	No (H, P)
Erythromycin	500 mg q6h (PO)	Yes†	1.8	70	2	Minor	No	No (H, P)
Telithromycin	800 mg q24h (PO)	Yes	2	65	10	No	No	No (H)

TABLE 309–3 DOSAGE REGIMEN, PHARMACOKINETICS, AND ADJUSTMENT IN PATIENTS WITH HEPATIC AND RENAL FAILURE—cont'd

Class/Agent	Dose,* Systemic Infection	Oral Formulation	Peak Serum Concentration (mg/mL)	Protein Binding (%)	Normal Serum Half-Life (hr)	Hepatic Failure	Renal Failure	Serum Levels Affected by Dialysis
OTHER AGENTS								
Aztreonam	1g q8h	—	250	60	2.	No	Major	Yes (H, P)
Chloramphenicol	0.25–1 g q6h	Yes	8–14	60	1.5	Minor	No	Yes (H) No (P)
Daptomycin	4–6 mg/kg q24h	—	58–100	90	8–9	No	Minor	No (H, P)
Linezolid	600 mg q12h	Yes	18	30	5	No—minor	No	Yes (H)
Metronidazole	500 mg q6h	Yes	25	20	8	Yes	No	Yes (H) No (P)
Nitrofurantoin	100 mg q6h (PO)	Yes	Nil	60	0.3	No	Avoid	Yes (H)
Quinupristin/dalfopristin (30:70)	7.5 mg/kg q8–12h	—	3.2/8‡	90/30	3/1‡	Minor	No	No (P)
Spectinomycin	2 g/m/24 hr	—	100	0	2	No	Avoid	Unknown
Vancomycin	15 mg/kg q12h	Yes§	35	10	6	No	Major	No (H, P)

*Dose in milligrams per kilogram body weight at hour interval and/or oral dose in milligrams in patients with normal renal function; all doses are parenteral unless specified PO.
†Significant decrease or delay in absorption when administered with food.
‡Includes parent compound and active metabolites.
§Oral vancomycin is not absorbed; it is used for intraluminal therapy only.
H = hemodialysis; P = peritoneal dialysis.

for biofilm formation, which can protect organisms from many antibacterials. Drugs that are eliminated primarily by the kidney provide high urine concentrations for the treatment of urinary tract infections. Nitrofurantoin, however, provides low and ineffective urinary concentrations in patients with renal impairment. Biliary excretion can enhance efficacy in biliary tract infections, but bile levels of antibacterials are markedly reduced in the presence of biliary tract obstruction. Penetration of drugs into respiratory secretions, such as epithelial lining fluid, cannot be readily predicted from serum concentrations and is an important determinant of the outcome of antibacterial therapy for pneumonia.

Antibacterial concentrations inside cells and tissues supplied by capillaries without pores, such as the central nervous system and the vitreous humor of the eye, are dependent more on the lipid solubility of the drug than on its pharmacokinetics in serum. For example, rifampin, macrolides, and fluoroquinolones provide high intracellular concentrations and activity against intracellular pathogens such as mycobacteria and *Legionella pneumophila.* Metronidazole, rifampin, and chloramphenicol are lipid-soluble drugs that provide adequate cerebrospinal fluid (CSF) penetration in the absence of meningeal inflammation. Inflammation can enhance the influx of many β-lactam antibiotics into the CSF and reduce active efflux of the same drugs from the CSF by the choroid-plexus pump. The aminoglycosides and first-generation cephalosporins are examples of drugs with marginal or inadequate CSF penetration, even with inflammation.

Parenteral administration is preferred for serious infections and those that require high dosages, such as endocarditis and meningitis. Certain antibacterials with high oral bioavailability make oral dosing an acceptable alternative to parenteral therapy for some moderately severe infections. For example, the fluoroquinolones are effective orally for the treatment of osteomyelitis. With impaired renal function, the dose or frequency of administration of an antimicrobial may need to be reduced. Any drug that is excreted primarily unchanged in urine requires downward adjustment in proportion to the decrease in renal function. Similar modifications are necessary in hepatic impairment for antimicrobials with major hepatic metabolism or biliary excretion. The usual dosage regimens for the various antibacterials and the need for dosage modification in patients with renal and hepatic impairment are listed in Table 309–3.

Pharmacodynamic Considerations

Pharmacodynamics is concerned with the relationship between drug concentrations and the time course of antimicrobial activity. The MIC and MBC are good indicators of the potency of an antibiotic, but they provide minimal information about the time course of antimicrobial activity. Parameters such as rate of killing with increasing concentrations and persistent effects (e.g., postantibiotic effect) are much better predictors of the time course of antimicrobial activity. For the aminoglycosides, fluoroquinolones, and daptomycin, bacterial killing is concentration dependent. The higher the drug concentration, the faster and more extensive the rate of killing. Thus, the peak level and the amount of drug, as reflected by the area under the concentration-versus-time curve (AUC) in serum, are important predictors of the efficacy of fluoroquinolones and aminoglycosides. Peak/MIC levels of 8 to 10 are required for high response rates with aminoglycosides. This has led to once-daily dosing of these drugs. This form of dosing can also lessen the frequency or the rate at which nephrotoxicity develops.

Bacterial killing by β-lactam antibiotics, in contrast, is slower and shows little dependence on drug concentration. The duration of time that drug concentrations exceed the MIC is the important predictor of efficacy for these drugs. Serum concentrations need to exceed the MIC for 40 to 50% of the dosing interval to achieve high rates of bacterial eradication in acute otitis media, acute maxillary sinusitis, and pneumonia.

Persistent effects, such as the postantibiotic effect, are potentially important for determining the frequency of dosing regimens. The postantibiotic effect refers to persistent suppression of bacterial growth after antibiotic exposure and when drug concentrations fall below the MIC. Antibacterials such as the aminoglycosides produce prolonged postantibiotic effects with gram-negative bacilli. This provides additional rationale for the once-daily administration of large doses of these drugs. On the other hand, β-lactam antibiotics produce very short or no postantibiotic effects with most bacteria. The frequency of dosing with these drugs largely depends on the elimination half-life of the drug. For example, ceftriaxone has a half-life of about 8 hours and is usually administered once daily, whereas most of the penicillins have half-lives of 30 to 60 minutes and are administered every 4 to 6 hours. Continuous intravenous infusion of β-lactam antibiotics, especially those with rapid half-lives, can allow serum concentrations to constantly exceed the MIC, even with lower daily total doses of drug.

Protein binding of antibacterials to serum proteins can have important pharmacodynamic effects. First, protein binding reduces the activity of antibacterials; it is only the free drug fraction that has antimicrobial activity at any point in time. Thus, the important determinants of in vivo antimicrobial activity are the free peak concentration, the AUC of free drug, and the time above MIC for free drug. Protein binding can also affect the elimination of some antibacterials. For example, the high protein binding of ceftriaxone and ertapenem slows the filtration of these drugs by the kidney and significantly extends the duration of their elimination half-life. Because of their long half-life, ceftriaxone and ertapenem still provide free drug serum concentrations that exceed the MIC of most respiratory pathogens with only once-daily dosing.

Patient-Related Considerations

Antibiotic choice is also dependent on patient characteristics and the site of infection. Recent exposure to an antibiotic, as well as residence in an intensive care unit, nursing home, or daycare center, increases the risk for antimicrobial resistance. Tetracyclines are not used in children because they bind and discolor developing permanent teeth. Quinolones are currently avoided in children because of the theoretical risk of cartilage damage. Both these drugs are also excreted in breast milk and could pose a risk to neonates and infants. Most antimicrobials administered to pregnant women cross the placenta and expose the fetus. Certain drugs, such as trimethoprim and rifampin, are not recommended in pregnancy because they are teratogens in animals. Antimicrobials recommended in pregnancy are the β-lactams, including penicillin/β-lactamase inhibitor combinations, and erythromycin. For many sites of infection, a bacteriostatic antibiotic is as effective as a bactericidal drug because the body's host defenses (neutrophils, macrophages, antibodies) kill and eliminate the infecting pathogen. However, endocarditis, meningitis, and osteomyelitis are infections that occur in areas of impaired host defenses. Bactericidal drugs are required for effective treatment of these infections. Patients with neutropenia or significant defects in neutrophil function should also receive bactericidal drugs.

ANTIBACTERIAL COMBINATIONS

The major reason for using drugs in combination is to enhance antimicrobial activity. As stated earlier, the addition of an aminoglycoside to penicillin improves the killing effect against most enterococci. This combination also improves efficacy for enterococcal endocarditis over penicillin monotherapy. Antibacterial combinations are also used to treat mixed infections, to broaden coverage in infections of unknown cause, and to prevent the selection of resistant organisms. Tuberculosis is the primary infection in which drug combinations have successfully prevented the emergence of resistant organisms. Drug combinations have had variable success in preventing resistance in gram-negative bacilli, such as *P. aeruginosa.* The major concerns with antimicrobial combinations are the added cost and increased risk for side effects. In addition, the combination of bacteriostatic and bactericidal drugs can produce antagonism, as was observed with the use of penicillin plus tetracycline for pneumococcal meningitis.

INDIVIDUAL AGENTS

Table 309–4 lists the agents of choice and some of the alternative antibacterials recommended for treatment of infections caused by specific bacteria. Table 309–5 gives more detailed information on the activity of specific antimicrobial agents against multiple pathogenic organisms that commonly cause infections.

β-Lactams

The β-lactam antibiotics are the most commonly used antimicrobial agents because of their high potency, low incidence of serious adverse reactions, and proven effectiveness. Penicillin G is still the drug of choice for most streptococcal infections, meningococcal infections, actinomycosis, rat-bite fever, *Pasteurella multocida* infections, periodontal infections, and syphilis. Although penicillin G is effective for many anaerobic infections of the lung, clindamycin appears to be more effective in cases of lung abscess. Benzathine and procaine salts of penicillin G are relatively insoluble preparations that are absorbed slowly from intramuscular injection sites. However, serum concentrations of benzathine penicillin are so low that this preparation is used only for highly susceptible organisms, as with syphilis and streptococcal pharyngitis, and for prophylaxis against rheumatic fever.

Penicillinase-resistant penicillins (nafcillin and oxacillin and the oral agents cloxacillin and dicloxacillin) remain the drugs of choice for infections caused by methicillin-susceptible *S. aureus.* However, the increasing incidence of methicillin-resistant strains (MRSA) has forced many clinicians to use vancomycin or other MRSA-active antimicrobials for initial empirical therapy until susceptibility results are known. Ampicillin is the preferred agent over penicillin G for enterococcal and *Listeria* infections. Amoxicillin is the most potent β-lactam antibiotic against *S. pneumoniae* and is a common initial choice for the treatment of acute otitis media and acute bacterial sinusitis. Ampicillin and amoxicillin are active against certain gram-negative bacteria, including *E. coli, Proteus mirabilis, Shigella, Salmonella,* and *Haemophilus influenzae.* Their use for *Salmonella* infections, *Shigella* infections, and urinary tract infections has been reduced by the appearance of resistant strains.

Even greater activity against gram-negative bacteria, including many strains of *P. aeruginosa,* is obtained with ticarcillin and piperacillin. Piperacillin is more potent than ticarcillin against *P. aeruginosa,* but this higher potency has not resulted in any major increase in clinical efficacy.

Clavulanic acid, sulbactam, and tazobactam are potent, irreversible inhibitors of the β-lactamases of staphylococci, *Bacteroides fragilis, Klebsiella,* and most of the common plasmid-mediated enzymes found in *H. influenzae, E. coli,* and other gram-negative bacteria. They do not inhibit the chromosomal β-lactamases produced by *Enterobacter, Citrobacter, Serratia,* and *Pseudomonas.* Sulbactam and tazobactam also have direct activity against *Acinetobacter calcoaceticus.* Amoxicillin plus clavulanic acid and ampicillin plus sulbactam have been useful for upper and lower respiratory tract infections, staphylococcal and streptococcal skin infections, and bite wound infections. Ticarcillin plus clavulanic acid and piperacillin plus tazobactam have provided effective therapy for nosocomial pneumonia, intra-abdominal infections, and severe skin and soft tissue infections. The combination of ticarcillin plus clavulanic acid is also active against many *Stenotrophomonas maltophilia* strains.

The first-generation cephalosporins are active against staphylococci, most streptococci, *E. coli, K. pneumoniae,* and *P. mirabilis.* However, these drugs are used primarily as an alternative to penicillin for staphylococcal and streptococcal infections and surgical prophylaxis. The second-generation cephalosporins can be divided into two groups. The cephamycins (cefoxitin, cefotetan, and cefmetazole) have increased activity against *B. fragilis* and are used primarily for the prevention and treatment of mixed aerobic and anaerobic infections. The remaining second-generation cephalosporins include many oral and parenteral agents with increased activity against *H. influenzae,* including β-lactamase–producing strains. These drugs are used as alternative agents for upper and lower respiratory tract infections. The third-generation cephalosporins are 10 to 100 times more potent against enteric bacteria than the earlier generations of cephalosporins are. Ceftriaxone and cefotaxime provide adequate CSF concentrations in the presence of inflammation and are commonly used for bacterial meningitis. Cefoperazone and ceftriaxone are excreted extensively into bile. Ceftazidime has good activity against *P. aeruginosa.* Cefepime, a fourth-generation cephalosporin, combines the activity of first- and third-generation drugs. These drugs are used for a variety of serious gram-negative bacillary infections.

The carbapenems (imipenem, meropenem, and ertapenem) have a broader spectrum of activity than any other antimicrobial agent. When administered alone, imipenem is inactivated in the kidney by a dehydropeptidase enzyme found along renal tubular cells, thereby resulting in low urine levels and nephrotoxicity. The addition of cilastatin, which blocks the activity of this enzyme, eliminates the nephrotoxicity and produces high urine levels. Meropenem and ertapenem are much less susceptible to such inactivation and do not require cilastatin in the commercial product. Aztreonam, the only available monobactam, is active solely against aerobic gram-negative bacteria. An advantage of aztreonam is that it does not appear to cause cross-reactivity in patients with allergic reactions to other β-lactams.

TABLE 309–4 ANTIBACTERIAL DRUGS OF CHOICE FOR SELECTED BACTERIA

Infecting Organism	Agent of Choice*	Alternative Agent†
GRAM-POSITIVE COCCI		
Staphylococcus aureus/coagulase-negative staphylococci		
Non–penicillinase producing	Penicillin G or V	Cephalosporin,‡ vancomycin, clindamycin, erythromycin
Penicillinase producing	Nafcillin, oxacillin	Cephalosporin,‡ vancomycin, clindamycin, carbapenem, penicillin/β-lactamase inhibitor combination, daptomycin
Methicillin resistant§	Vancomycin	Trimethoprim-sulfamethoxazole, minocycline, daptomycin, linezolid, tigecycline, clindamycin
β-Hemolytic streptococci (groups A, B, C, G)	Penicillin G or V	Cephalosporin,‡ erythromycin, clindamycin, vancomycin
Viridans streptococci	Penicillin G	Cephalosporin, vancomycin, erythromycin
Streptococcus bovis		
Enterococci§		
Uncomplicated urinary tract infection	Ampicillin, amoxicillin	Nitrofurantoin, quinolone¶
Moderately severe wound infection	Ampicillin	Penicillin G, vancomycin
Serious infection: endocarditis or meningitis	Ampicillin plus gentamicin or streptomycin	Vancomycin plus gentamicin or streptomycin (test for high-level aminoglycoside resistance)
Streptococcus pneumoniae§		
Pneumonia, upper respiratory tract infection	Penicillin G, amoxicillin	Cephalosporin, macrolide, clindamycin, quinolone,¶ vancomycin
Meningitis	Ceftriaxone, cefotaxime	Ceftriaxone plus vancomycin ± rifampin, vancomycin + rifampin, penicillin G if MIC <0.1 µg/mL
GRAM-NEGATIVE COCCI		
Neisseria gonorrhoeae	Ceftriaxone, cefixime	Second- or other third-generation cephalosporin,** quinolones, spectinomycin, trimethoprim-sulfamethoxazole, azithromycin
Neisseria meningitidis	Penicillin G	Third-generation cephalosporin,** chloramphenicol, sulfonamide (if susceptible)
Moraxella catarrhalis	Trimethoprim-sulfamethoxazole	Amoxicillin-clavulanate, third-generation cephalosporin,** cefuroxime, clarithromycin
GRAM-POSITIVE BACILLI		
Bacillus anthracis (anthrax)	Ciprofloxacin, doxycycline	Clindamycin, levofloxacin
Corynebacterium diphtheriae	Erythromycin	Clindamycin, penicillin G
Corynebacterium sp	Vancomycin	Penicillin G + gentamicin
Listeria monocytogenes	Ampicillin or penicillin G ± gentamicin	Trimethoprim-sulfamethoxazole, vancomycin, doxycycline
Clostridium perfringens	Penicillin G	Metronidazole, doxycycline, chloramphenicol, imipenem
Clostridium difficile	Metronidazole	Vancomycin (oral only), bacitracin
GRAM-NEGATIVE BACILLI‡		
Acinetobacter sp	Imipenem/meropenem ± gentamicin	Quinolone, aminoglycoside, tigecycline
Bordetella pertussis (pertussis)	Erythromycin	Trimethoprim-sulfamethoxazole, ampicillin
Brucella sp (brucellosis)	Doxycycline + gentamicin or streptomycin	Rifampin + doxycycline or quinolone, gentamicin+ trimethoprim-sulfamethoxazole
Campylobacter fetus sp *jejuni*	Erythromycin, quinolone¶	Tetracycline
Enterobacter sp	Carbapenem,** cefepime	Quinolone,¶ third-generation cephalosporin,** aminoglycoside, trimethoprim-sulfamethoxazole
Eikenella corrodens	Penicillin G, ampicillin	Trimethoprim-sulfamethoxazole, tetracycline, cefoxitin, third-generation cephalosporin**
Escherichia coli		
Uncomplicated urinary tract infection	Trimethoprim-sulfamethoxazole	Quinolone, ampicillin, cephalosporins, trimethoprim, tetracycline
Systemic infection	Third-generation cephalosporin**	Aminoglycoside, quinolone, penicillin/β-lactamase inhibitor, aztreonam, trimethoprim-sulfamethoxazole, carbapenem
Helicobacter pylori	Omeprazole + amoxicillin+ clarithromycin	Bismuth subsalicylate + metronidazole + tetracycline or amoxicillin, bismuth subsalicylate + tetracycline + clarithromycin
Francisella tularensis (tularemia)	Streptomycin, gentamicin	Doxycycline, ciprofloxacin, chloramphenicol

Continued

TABLE 309–4 ANTIBACTERIAL DRUGS OF CHOICE FOR SELECTED BACTERIA—cont'd

Infecting Organism	Agent of Choice*	Alternative Agent†
Haemophilus influenzae		
Meningitis, bacteremia	Ceftriaxone, cefotaxime	Meropenem, ampicillin (if β-lactamase negative)
Other infection	Ampicillin-sulbactam, amoxicillin-clavulanate	Trimethoprim-sulfamethoxazole, cefuroxime, quinolone, third-generation cephalosporin**
Haemophilus ducreyi (chancroid)	Ceftriaxone	Azithromycin, erythromycin, amoxicillin-clavulanate, ciprofloxacin
Klebsiella pneumoniae/ oxytoca	Third-generation cephalosporin**	Quinolone, penicillin/β-lactamase inhibitor; carbapenem, aztreonam, aminoglycosides
Legionella pneumophila	Quinolone¶ ± rifampin	Erythromycin ± rifampin
Nocardia asteroides	Sulfonamides (high dose)	Trimethoprim-sulfamethoxazole, minocycline, carbapenem, linezolid
Pasteurella multocida	Penicillin G	Tetracycline, amoxicillin-clavulanate, third-generation cephalosporin**
Proteus mirabilis	Ampicillin	Cephalosporin,** trimethoprim-sulfamethoxazole
Proteus (indole positive)	Third-generation cephalosporin	Carbapenem, aminoglycoside, trimethoprim-sulfamethoxazole, quinolone¶
Salmonella sp	Quinolone, ceftriaxone	Chloramphenicol, trimethoprim-sulfamethoxazole
Serratia marcescens	Third-generation cephalosporin**	Carbapenem, quinolone,¶ aztreonam, aminoglycoside
Shigella sp	Quinolone¶	Trimethoprim-sulfamethoxazole, azithromycin
Stenotrophomonas maltophilia	Trimethoprim-sulfamethoxazole	Ticarcillin-clavulanate, ceftazidime, doxycycline
Pseudomonas aeruginosa		
Urinary tract infection	Quinolone,¶ piperacillin-tazobactam, ticarcillin-clavulanate	Aminoglycoside,†† ceftazidime, carbapenem, aztreonam
Pneumonia, bacteremia	Ceftazidime, cefepime or piperacillin-tazobactam + aminoglycoside††	Imipenem, meropenem, or aztreonam + aminoglycoside††; antipseudomonal β-lactam + ciprofloxacin or levofloxacin
Vibrio vulnificus	Doxycycline + ceftazidime	Cefotaxime, quinolone
Yersinia pestis (plague)	Streptomycin, gentamicin	Doxycycline, chloramphenicol
ANAEROBIC GRAM-NEGATIVE		
Bacteroides fragilis group	Metronidazole	Clindamycin, cefoxitin, carbapenem, penicillin/β-lactamase inhibitor

*Dose and route of administration vary depending on the severity and site of infection and host characteristics (organ dysfunction, immune function).
†The list of alternative agents is not fully inclusive; confirm susceptibility in vitro.
‡First-generation cephalosporin preferred (cephradine, cephalexin, cefazolin).
§Must test susceptibility; resistant strains are increasingly frequent.
¶Ciprofloxacin, levofloxacin, or moxifloxacin (or for urinary tract infection, norfloxacin).
¶Penicillin-resistant *S. pneumoniae* susceptible to gemifloxacin, levofloxacin, and moxifloxacin.
**Third-generation cephalosporins for this indication include ceftriaxone, cefotaxime, and ceftizoxime.
††Aminoglycosides for this indication include gentamicin, tobramycin, netilmicin, and amikacin.
MIC = minimal inhibitory concentration.

Aminoglycosides

Streptomycin, kanamycin, neomycin, gentamicin, and tobramycin are naturally occurring aminoglycosides, whereas amikacin and netilmicin are semisynthetic derivatives developed for their activity against resistant strains. The aminoglycosides are active primarily against aerobic gram-negative bacilli. Tobramycin is the most active agent against *P. aeruginosa*, whereas amikacin shows the least resistance. Despite their potential for toxicity, they are recommended for use in combination with broad-spectrum β-lactams for serious gram-negative bacillary infections. In combination with β-lactams, gentamicin and streptomycin exhibit synergism against staphylococci, streptococci, and enterococci unless the bacteria show high-level aminoglycoside resistance. Such combinations have improved the efficacy or shortened the duration of therapy for endocarditis and bacteremia caused by gram-positive cocci.

Streptomycin is still a useful agent for tuberculosis, tularemia, plague, and brucellosis (in combination with a tetracycline). Neomycin is used orally (to reduce bowel organisms) or topically. Spectinomycin, which is not an aminoglycoside but does contain an aminocyclitol ring, is only occasionally used to treat gonorrhea, especially β-lactamase–producing strains.

Quinolones

The quinolones are synthetic compounds consisting of nalidixic acid and its fluorinated derivatives. Several quinolones (enoxacin, grepafloxacin, lomefloxacin, sparfloxacin, and trovafloxacin) have been withdrawn or are used infrequently because of adverse reactions. Ciprofloxacin is the most potent quinolone against *P. aeruginosa* and other gram-negative bacilli. The newer fluoroquinolones (gemifloxacin, levofloxacin, moxifloxacin) are slightly less active than ciprofloxacin against gram-negative bacilli, but they have increased activity against gram-positive cocci. Many quinolones are active against intracellular pathogens, such as mycobacteria, *Chlamydia*, and *Legionella.* Their efficacy has also been documented in a variety of gastrointestinal infections, including traveler's diarrhea and bacterial gastroenteritis.

Macrolides, Tetracyclines, Ketolides, and Clindamycin

The macrolides, especially clarithromycin and azithromycin, and the tetracyclines are broad-spectrum agents with activity against many

Text continued on p. 2165.

TABLE 309–5 ACTIVITY OF MAJOR ANTIBACTERIALS AGAINST SELECTED ORGANISMS[a]

	Streptococci	*Streptococcus pneumoniae*[b]	Enterococci[c]	*Staphylococcus aureus* (MSSA)	*Staphylococcus aureus* (MRSA)	Coagulase-Negative Staphylococci[d]	*Listeria monocytogenes*	*Neisseria gonorrhoeae*
Penicillin G	+	+	+	±	0	0	+	±
Oxacillin[f]	+	±	0	+	0	±	0	0
Ampicillin[g]	+	+	+	0	0	0	+	±
Ampicillin-sulbactam[g]	+	+	+	+	0	±	+	+
Ticarcillin-clavulanate	+	±	+	+	0	±	+	+
Piperacillin-tazobactam	+	+	+	+	0	±	+	+
Cefazolin[h]	+	±	0	+	0	±	0	±
Cefoxitin[i]	+	±	0	±	0	±	0	+
Cefuroxime	+	+	0	+	0	±	0	+
Ceftriaxone	+	+	0	+	0	±	0	+
Ceftazidime	+	±	0	±	0	±	0	+
Cefepime	+	+	0	+	0	±	0	+
Cephalexin[h]	+	±	0	+	0	±	0	+
Cefixime	+	±	0	0	0	0	0	0
Cefpodoxime proxetil	+	+	0	+	0	±	0	+
Imipenem[j]	+	+	±	+	0	±	+	+
Aztreonam	0	0	0	0	0	0	0	+
Vancomycin	+	+	+	+	+	+	±	0
Daptomycin	+	+	+	+	+	+	0	0
Linezolid	+	+	+	+	+	+	+	ND
Gentamicin[k]	C/S	0	C/S	C/S	±	C/S	C/S	0
Ciprofloxacin	±	±	±	±	0	±	±	+
Levofloxacin[l]	+	+	±	+	0	±	±	+
Clindamycin	+	+	0	+	0	±	0	0
Clarithromycin[m]	+	+	0	±	0	±	ND	+
Erythromycin	+	+	0	±	0	±	±	±
Doxycycline[n]	±	±	0	±	0	0	±	0
Tigecycline	+	+	+	+	+	+	0	+
Metronidazole	0	0	0	0	0	0	0	0
Trimethoprim-sulfamethoxazole	+	+	0	+	±	±	+	±
Chloramphenicol	+	+	0	±	0	0	±	+
Rifampin[o]	+	C/S	±	C/S	C/S	C/S	C/S	+

Continued

TABLE 309–5 ACTIVITY OF MAJOR ANTIBACTERIALS AGAINST SELECTED ORGANISMS[a]—cont'd

	Neisseria meningitidis	*Moraxella catarrhalis*	*Haemophilus influenzae*	*Escherichia coli*	*Enterobacter* sp	*Klebsiella* sp	*Proteus mirabilis*	*Salmonella* sp
Penicillin G	+	0	0	0	0	0	±	0
Oxacillin[f]	0	0	0	0	0	0	0	0
Ampicillin[g]	+	0	±	±	0	0	+	+
Ampicillin-sulbactam[g]	+	+	+	+	±	+	+	+
Ticarcillin-clavulanate	+	+	+	+	±	+	+	+
Piperacillin-tazobactam	+	+	+	+	±	+	+	+
Cefazolin[h]	0	+	0	+	0	+	+	0
Cefoxitin[i]	+	+	+	+	±	+	+	+
Cefuroxime	+	+	+	+	±	+	+	+
Ceftriaxone	+	+	+	+	±	+	+	+
Ceftazidime	+	+	+	+	±	+	+	+
Cefepime	+	+	+	+	+	+	+	+
Cephalexin[h]	0	±	±	+	0	+	+	0
Cefixime	+	+	+	+	0	+	+	+
Cefpodoxime proxetil	+	+	+	+	0	+	+	+
Imipenem[j]	+	+	+	+	+	+	+	+
Aztreonam	+	+	+	+	±	+	+	+
Vancomycin	0	ND	ND	0	0	0	0	0
Daptomycin	0	0	0	0	0	0	0	0
Linezolid	ND	+	+	0	0	0	0	0
Gentamicin[k]	0	+	+	+	+	+	+	0
Ciprofloxacin	+	+	+	+	+	+	+	+
Levofloxacin[l]	+	+	+	+	+	+	+	+
Clindamycin	0	0	0	0	0	0	0	0
Clarithromycin[m]	+	+	+	0	0	0	0	0
Erythromycin	+	+	±	0	0	0	0	0
Doxycycline[n]	+	+	+	±	0	0	0	0
Tigecycline	0	+	±	±	±	0	±	0
Metronidazole	0	0	0	0	0	0	0	0
Trimethoprim-sulfamethoxazole	±	+	+	+	±	+	+	+
Chloramphenicol	+	+	+	+	0	±	+	+
Rifampin[o]	+	+	+	0	0	0	0	ND

	Serratia sp	*Shigella* sp	*Acinetobacter* sp	*Pseudomonas aeruginosa*	*Stenotrophomonas maltophilia*	*Pasteurella multocida*	*Legionella* sp
Penicillin G	0	0	0	0	0	+	0
Oxacillin[f]	0	0	0	0	0	0	0
Ampicillin[g]	0	±	0	0	0	+	0
Ampicillin-sulbactam[g]	0	±	0	0	0	+	0
Ticarcillin-clavulanate	+	+	+	+	±	+	0
Piperacillin-tazobactam	±	+	+	+	±	+	0
Cefazolin[h]	0	0	0	0	0	+	0
Cefoxitin[i]	+	+	0	0	0	+	0
Cefuroxime	0	+	0	0	0	+	0
Ceftriaxone	+	+	±	0	0	+	0
Ceftazidime	+	+	±	+	±	+	0
Cefepime	+	+	±	+	0	ND	0
Cephalexin[h]	0	0	0	0	0	0	0
Cefixime	0	+	0	0	0	+	0
Cefpodoxime proxetil	0	+	0	0	0	ND	0
Imipenem[j]	+	+	+	+	0	+	ND
Aztreonam	+	+	0	+	0	+	0
Vancomycin	0	0	0	0	0	0	0
Daptomycin	0	0	0	0	0	0	0
Linezolid	0	0	0	0	0	ND	ND
Gentamicin[k]	+	ND	±	+	0	0	0
Ciprofloxacin	+	+	±	+	0	+	+
Levofloxacin[l]	+	+	±	±	0	+	+
Clindamycin	0	0	0	0	0	0	0
Clarithromycin[m]	0	0	0	0	0	ND	+
Erythromycin	0	0	0	0	0	0	+
Doxycycline[n]	0	0	0	0	0	+	+
Tigecycline	±	0	±	0	0	0	±
Metronidazole	0	0	0	0	0	0	0
Trimethoprim-sulfamethoxazole	+	+	0	0	+	±	+
Chloramphenicol	0	0	0	0	+	+	ND
Rifampin[o]	0	ND	0	0	ND	ND	C/S

Continued

TABLE 309–5 ACTIVITY OF MAJOR ANTIBACTERIALS AGAINST SELECTED ORGANISMS[a]—cont'd

	Chlamydia sp	*Mycoplasma pneumoniae*	*Rickettsia* sp	*Bacteroides fragilis* group[e]	*Clostridium* sp	*Prevotella*	*Actinomyces* sp
Penicillin G	0	0	0	0	+	+	+
Oxacillin[f]	0	0	0	0	0	0	0
Ampicillin[g]	0	0	0	0	+	+	+
Ampicillin-sulbactam[g]	0	0	0	+	+	+	+
Ticarcillin-clavulanate	0	0	0	+	+	+	+
Piperacillin-tazobactam	0	0	0	+	+	+	+
Cefazolin[h]	0	0	0	0	0	±	+
Cefoxitin[i]	0	0	0	±	+	+	+
Cefuroxime	0	0	0	0	+	+	+
Ceftriaxone	0	0	0	0	+	+	+
Ceftazidime	0	0	0	0	+	+	+
Cefepime	0	0	0	0	ND	ND	NC
Cephalexin[h]	0	0	0	0	ND	+	+
Cefixime	0	0	0	0	0	+	ND
Cefpodoxime proxetil	0	0	0	0	ND	ND	ND
Imipenem[j]	0	0	0	+	+	+	+
Aztreonam	0	0	0	0	0	0	0
Vancomycin	0	0	0	0	+	0	±
Daptomycin	0	0	0	0	=	0	0
Linezolid	ND	+	ND	0	+	+	ND
Gentamicin[k]	0	0	0	0	0	0	0
Ciprofloxacin	+	+	+	0	0	0	ND
Levofloxacin[l]	+	+	ND	0	0	0	ND
Clindamycin	ND	0	0	+	+	+	+
Clarithromycin[m]	+	+	ND	0	+	+	+
Erythromycin	+	+	±	0	+	+	+
Doxycycline[n]	+	+	+	0	±	+	±
Tigecycline	=	=	±	±	+	+	±
Metronidazole	0	0	0	+	+	+	0
Trimethoprim-sulfamethoxazole	0+	0	0	ND	ND	ND	ND
Chloramphenicol	+	+	+	+	+	+	+
Rifampin[o]	+	ND	±	+	+	+	ND

[a]Activity estimate is based on both in vitro susceptibility and clinical efficacy, where available. Activity against aerobic gram-negative bacilli can vary markedly between studies.
[b]Full resistance to penicillin is increasingly prevalent; resistance to first- and second-generation cephalosporins parallels that to penicillin.
[c]*Enterococcus faecium* is intrinsically more resistant than *Enterococcus faecalis;* resistance to penicillin, ampicillin, vancomycin, and aminoglycosides (high level) is becoming increasingly frequent.
[d]Many nosocomially acquired strains are methicillin resistant.
[e]Some of the *Bacillus fragilis* group (*B. thetaiotaomicron, B. distasonis, B. ovatus, B. vulgatus*) are more resistant than *B. fragilis.*
[f]Similar activity for methicillin, nafcillin, cloxacillin, and dicloxacillin.
[g]Similar activity for amoxicillin and amoxicillin-clavulanate.
[h]Similar activity for other first-generation cephalosporins.
[i]Similar activity for cefoxitin and cefmetazole.
[j]Similar activity to other carbapenems, except that ertapenem is not active against *Pseudomonas aeruginosa.*
[k]Similar activity against gram-negative bacilli for tobramycin and netilmicin; resistance of gram-negative bacilli is less frequent to amikacin.
[l]Similar activity for gatifloxacin and moxifloxacin.
[m]Similar activity for azithromycin.
[n]Similar activity for other tetracyclines.
[o]Broad spectrum of activity, but resistance emerges rapidly; limit use to combination therapy or eradication of meningococcal and *Haemophilus influenzae* pharyngeal carriage.
0 = uniformly or frequently resistant; + = usually susceptible; ± = variable susceptibility; C/S = used in combination or for synergy; ND = insufficient or no data; MRSA = methicillin-resistant *S. aureus;* MSSA = methicillin-susceptible *S. aureus.*

TABLE 309–6 ADVERSE EFFECTS OF ANTIBACTERIAL AGENTS*

	Target—Manifestation					
Agent	**General**	**Skin**	**GI Tract**	**Blood Cells**	**Kidney**	**Nervous System**	**Other**
Penicillin	Hypersensitivity, anaphylaxis, serum sickness	Rash, urticaria, erythema multiforme	Diarrhea (ampicillin, amoxicillin-clavulanate), hepatitis (oxacillin)	Coombs-positive hemolytic anemia Impaired platelet function (ticarcillin), leukopenia, thrombocytopenia	Nephritis (methicillin), hypokalemia (carboxy- and ureido-penicillins)	Seizures, twitching (high doses, renal failure)	Inactivates aminoglycosides when admixed; possible with concurrent therapy in renal failure
Cephalosporins	Serum sickness (cefaclor), hypersensitivity, anaphylaxis (rare)	Rash, urticaria	Diarrhea (cefoperazone), hepatic dysfunction, precipitates in bile (ceftriaxone), mild increase in LFTs	Neutropenia, increased prothrombin time—bleeding (due to MTT side chain), impaired platelet function (moxalactam), positive Coombs test	Enhance aminoglycoside toxicity, acute renal failure (rare), interstitial nephritis		Disulfiram-like reaction with alcohol use (MTT side chain)
Carbapenems	Hypersensitivity	Rash, urticaria, erythema multiforme	Vomiting with rapid infusion (imipenem) Abnormal LFTs	Bone marrow suppression, positive Coombs test	Renal dysfunction	Seizures, myoclonus	
Aminoglycosides	Fever	Rash			Reversible renal failure	Irreversible vestibular toxicity and/or auditory damage, muscular blockade (with anesthetics and myasthenia gravis)	
Vancomycin	Allergy, fever	Rash		Leukopenia, thrombocytopenia	Nephrotoxic with aminoglycoside	Decreased hearing, neuropathy	Histamine release with flushing and hypotension (infusion <1 hr—antihistamines prevent)
Quinolones	Headache, allergy, anaphylaxis (rare)	Rash (gemifloxacin), urticaria, photosensitivity (lomefloxacin)	GI distress, abnormal LFTs			Dizziness, insomnia, nervousness, tremors, visual changes, seizures	Tendon rupture, arthropathy in young animals

Continued

TABLE 309–6 ADVERSE EFFECTS OF ANTIBACTERIAL AGENTS*—cont'd

	Target—Manifestation						
Agent	**General**	**Skin**	**GI Tract**	**Blood Cells**	**Kidney**	**Nervous System**	**Other**
Sulfonamides	Hypersensitivity, anaphylaxis, serum sickness fever	Rash, Stevens-Johnson syndrome, photosensitivity	Hepatitis	Hemolysis (G6PD deficiency), agranulocytosis, marrow suppression	Crystalluria	Neuropathy	Vasculitis
Trimethoprim with/without sulfamethoxazole	Fever	Rash, erythema multiforme, Stevens-Johnson syndrome, TEN	Hepatitis, pancreatitis	Marrow suppression	Hyperkalemia, acute renal failure		
Chloramphenicol	Fever			Marrow suppression (dose related), aplastic anemia		Optic neuritis, neuropathy	Circulatory collapse (gray baby syndrome—neonate)
Tetracyclines	Hypersensitivity	Photosensitization (doxycycline, demeclocycline)	GI discomfort, hepatotoxicity in azotemia or pregnancy		Antianabolic aggravation of azotemia (except doxycycline)	Vertigo (minocycline)	Deposition in bone (dysplasia) and teeth (staining)
Macrolides	Fever	Rash	GI discomfort, cholestatic jaundice (erythromycin estolate)			Reversible decreased hearing	Phlebitis (IV erythromycin), metallic taste (clarithromycin)
Clindamycin	Fever	Rash	Diarrhea, pseudomembranous colitis				
Metronidazole	Headache, hypersensitivity		Nausea, metallic taste, pancreatitis	Leukopenia		Peripheral neuropathy, ataxia	Mutagenic, carcinogenic in rodents, disulfiram-like reaction with alcohol

*Not all reactions are listed; check other sources for unusual reactions. Reactions to sulfonamides are not repeated.
GI = gastrointestinal; G6PD = glucose-6-phosphate dehydrogenase; LFTs = liver function tests; MTT = methylthiotetrazole ring; TEN = toxic epidermal necrolysis.

respiratory pathogens. These drugs are recommended for outpatient management of community-acquired pneumonia. However, resistance to macrolides and tetracyclines is increasing in *S. pneumoniae*. Telithromycin, the first ketolide antibacterial, is active against pneumococci resistant to most other drugs. Clindamycin is used for anaerobic infections and as an alternative agent for mild to moderate streptococcal and staphylococcal infections. The tetracyclines are useful drugs for a variety of sexually transmitted diseases, such as nongonococcal urethritis, granuloma inguinale, and lymphogranuloma venereum, and for rickettsial infections, Lyme disease, and brucellosis (with streptomycin or rifampin). Tigecycline, the first glycylcycline, is active against most strains resistant to tetracycline because of tetracycline-specific efflux or ribosomal protection.

Vancomycin, Quinupristin-Dalfopristin, Daptomycin, and Linezolid

Vancomycin is active against most gram-positive bacteria, including MRSA, *Staphylococcus epidermidis, Clostridium difficile,* and enterococci. The increased use of vancomycin over the past decade has contributed to the emergence of vancomycin-resistant enterococci. Quinupristin-dalfopristin, linezolid, and daptomycin are recently approved drugs with activity against vancomycin-resistant enterococci; quinupristin-dalfopristin is active only against *Enterococcus faecium*. Linezolid, which has high oral bioavailability, and daptomycin are active against MRSA.

DURATION OF THERAPY

Just like initial antibacterial selection, the optimal duration of therapy depends on a variety of drug, pharmacodynamic, and infection site characteristics. Single doses of ceftriaxone, cefixime, and a fluoroquinolone are highly effective for superficial mucosal infections such as uncomplicated gonorrhea. Fluoroquinolones and trimethoprim-sulfamethoxazole exhibit optimal efficacy for urinary tract infections with 3 days of therapy. Longer courses are required with nitrofurantoin and β-lactams to provide similar efficacy. Short courses of therapy (5 days) are being used with fluoroquinolones and ketolides for respiratory tract infections because of their concentration-dependent killing. On the other hand, infections in which bacteria are growing slowly, such as endocarditis and osteomyelitis, require longer 4- to 6-week courses of therapy. Patients with impaired host defenses also usually receive longer courses of therapy.

ADVERSE REACTIONS AND DRUG-DRUG INTERACTIONS

Most adverse reactions with antibacterial therapy are mild and quickly resolve when the causative agent is discontinued. The major adverse reactions observed with various classes of antimicrobials are outlined in Table 309–6. Adverse reactions can also result from interactions between drugs that increase or decrease elimination, alter protein binding, or enhance drug toxicity. For example, amphotericin B, cyclosporine, and vancomycin can increase the risk for aminoglycoside nephrotoxicity. Some drugs that are metabolized by the hepatic and intestinal microsomal cytochrome P-450 (CYP) enzymes are inhibitors of the enzyme, as well as substrates. For example, rifampin and rifabutin induce CYP3A enzymes, which increase the clearance of many drugs such as corticosteroids, cyclosporine, phenytoin, warfarin, simvastatin, oral contraceptives, quinidine, β-blockers, and protease inhibitors. The same protease inhibitors can inhibit the clearance of rifabutin by these enzymes and thereby result in higher toxic concentrations of rifabutin.

FAILURE OF ANTIBACTERIAL THERAPY

Persistent fever or symptoms of infection during antibacterial therapy always require reassessment of the initial antibiotic selection and dosage regimen, review of microbiologic data and susceptibility results, and even new culture data to look for the emergence of resistance or superinfection. Other causes of antibacterial failure include (1) an obstructed drainage system, (2) an undrained abscess or infected fluid collection, (3) persistence of a foreign body or nonviable tissue (e.g., sequestra), (4) drug fever, and (5) suboptimal drug concentration because of drug interactions or poor oral bioavailability.

SUGGESTED READINGS

Craig WA: Basic pharmacodynamics of antibacterials with clinical applications to the use of β-lactams, glycopeptides, and linezolid. Infect Dis Clin North Am 2003;17:479–501. *A review of the basic concepts of the pharmacodynamics of antibacterials with an emphasis on the β-lactams, glycopeptides, and linezolid.*

Fishman N: Antimicrobial stewardship. Am J Med 2006;119(6 Suppl 1):S53–S61. *Appropriate drug selection and dose usage is an important component of a strategy to limit antibiotic resistance.*

Gilbert DN, Moellering RC Jr, Sande MA: The Sanford Guide to Antimicrobial Therapy 2006. Hyde Park, VT, Antimicrobial Therapy, 2006. *A detailed pocket guide to antimicrobial use that is updated and published annually.*

Jacoby GA, Munoz-Price LS: The new β-lactamases. N Engl J Med 2005;352: 380–391. *A review of the new β-lactamase enzymes and their molecular epidemiology.*

Kaye KS, Engemann JJ, Fraimow HS, Abrutyn E: Pathogens resistant to antimicrobial agents; epidemiology, molecular mechanisms and clinical management. Infect Dis Clin North Am 2004;18:467–511. *A discussion of the epidemiology and molecular mechanisms of antimicrobial resistance.*

Kucers A, Crowe SM, Grayson ML, Hoy JF (eds): The Use of Antibiotics: A Clinical Review of Antibacterial, Antifungal and Antiviral Drugs, 5th ed. Oxford, Butterworth-Heinemann, 1997. *The latest edition of an extensively referenced textbook on antimicrobial agents.*

Li XZ, Nikaido H: Efflux-mediated drug resistance in bacteria. Drugs 2004;64:159–204. *A detailed discussion of efflux as a mechanism for resistance to antibacterials.*

Samore MH, Bateman K, Alder SC, et al: Clinical decision support and appropriateness of antimicrobial prescribing: a randomized trial. JAMA 2005; 294:2305–2314. *Clinical decision support systems implemented in rural primary care settings reduced overall antimicrobial use and improved appropriateness of antimicrobial selection for acute respiratory tract infections.*

310 STAPHYLOCOCCAL INFECTIONS

Gordon L. Archer

Definition

Staphylococcus aureus has been recognized as one of the most important and lethal human bacterial pathogens since the beginning of the 20th century. Until the antibiotic era, more than 80% of patients whose blood grew *S. aureus* died; most of those had been healthy, with no underlying disease. Although infections caused by coagulase-positive *S. aureus* were generally known to be potentially lethal, coagulase-negative staphylococci had been dismissed as avirulent skin commensals incapable of causing human disease. However, since the mid-1980s, coagulase-negative staphylococcal infections have emerged as one of the major complications of medical progress. They are currently the pathogens most commonly isolated from infections of indwelling foreign devices and are the leading cause of hospital-acquired bacteremias in U.S. hospitals. This ascendancy of staphylococci as preeminent nosocomial pathogens has also been associated with an increase in the proportion of these isolates that are resistant to β-lactam and other antimicrobial agents (methicillin-resistant staphylococci). As a cause for additional concern, since 2000, methicillin-resistant *S. aureus* (MRSA) has been found increasingly as the cause of community-acquired *S. aureus* infections. If the trend continues, we may be forced to revisit the serious staphylococcal infections of the preantibiotic era that textbooks have long since relegated to medical history.

Physiology

The name *Staphylococcus* means "bunch of grapes" and describes the clusters and clumps of gram-positive cocci seen on Gram staining of both infected material and organisms recovered from culture bottles and agar plates. Staphylococci produce catalase, breaking down hydrogen peroxide to H_2O and O_2; streptococci do not. This is the definitive test for separating the two genera of gram-positive cocci. Staphylococci are nonmotile and are facultative anaerobes. The latter characteristic predicts that these organisms should grow equally well in both aerobic and

TABLE 310–1 STAPHYLOCOCCAL SPECIES FOUND ON HUMAN SKIN AND MUCOUS MEMBRANES

Coagulase-Positive	Coagulase-Negative	
S. aureus	*S. epidermidis*	*S. cohnii*
	S. saprophyticus	*S. xylosus*
	S. haemolyticus	*S. auricularis*
	S. warneri	*S. simulans*
	S. capitis	*S. schleiferi*
	S. hominis	*S. lugdunensis*
	S. saccharolyticus	*S. caprae*
		S. pasteuri

anaerobic media. The coagulase test identifies the exoenzyme produced by *S. aureus* that interacts with a prothrombin-like plasma factor, converting fibrinogen to fibrin and causing plasma to clot. This test traditionally separates the pathogenic species, *S. aureus,* from the numerous nonpathogenic staphylococci, collectively referred to as coagulase-negative staphylococci.

S. aureus is a homogeneous species, as determined by biochemical testing and nucleic acid analysis, whereas coagulase-negative staphylococci are sufficiently varied to be assigned to numerous species. Coagulase-negative staphylococci are found as normal skin flora on all mammals, and 31 distinct species are currently recognized. Of these, 15 species colonize the cornified squamous epithelium and mucous membranes of humans. Each species has a unique niche on the body, but *Staphylococcus epidermidis* is the predominant species. Some laboratories report specific species of coagulase-negative staphylococci to clinicians, and a list of the most prevalent human pathogenic species is shown in Table 310–1. Because only 60 to 70% of coagulase-negative species identified from specimens processed by the clinical laboratory are *S. epidermidis,* it is not correct to refer to coagulase-negative staphylococci as "*S. epidermidis.*" However, with the exception of *Staphylococcus saprophyticus,* the clinical implications of all coagulase-negative staphylococci are similar, and routine species identification of these organisms is mainly useful for epidemiologic investigation.

The complete DNA sequence of both the *S. aureus* and *S. epidermidis* genomes has been determined and is publicly available. These data should prove to be invaluable for molecular typing, for understanding the virulence of these bacteria, and for devising vaccines for disease prevention.

Resistance

Resistance to β-lactam antibiotics is mediated by the production of penicillinase, a drug-inactivating enzyme, and by the production of a new, drug-insensitive target. The penicillinase is narrow spectrum and only mediates resistance to penicillins. However, the gene, *mecA,* that encodes a drug-insensitive target called penicillin binding protein 2a (PBP2a) mediates resistance to all β-lactam antibiotics. The earliest resistance detected that was mediated by this gene was to the semisynthetic penicillin, methicillin. Even though this antibiotic is no longer available, the resistance mediated by this gene is still called methicillin resistance. It is currently detected in the clinical laboratory by resistance to the semisynthetic penicillin, oxacillin, by the production of PBP2a, or in rare instances by polymerase chain reaction amplification of the *mecA* gene. The methicillin resistance phenotype is important because many isolates resistant to β-lactam antibiotics mediated by PBP2a are also multiresistant to other antistaphylococcal antimicrobials (Table 310–2).

TABLE 310–2 ANTIMICROBIAL AGENTS EFFECTIVE FOR TREATING *STAPHYLOCOCCUS AUREUS* INFECTIONS

	Resistance*	
Agents	Hospital Acquired	Community Acquired
Penicillin G	>90	>90
Antistaphylococcal penicillins and cephalosporins	50	10–30
Erythromycin	60	20
Clindamycin	60	20
Sulfamethoxazole-trimethoprim	20	S
Tetracycline	20	10
Minocycline	S	S
Doxycycline	S	S
Quinupristin/Dalfopristin (Synercid)	S†	S
Linezolid	S	S
Rifampin	S	S
Gentamicin	30	S
Quinolones	60	S
Vancomycin	S	S
Daptomycin	S	S
Tigecycline	S	S

*Numbers are percentage of isolates from patients with hospital-acquired or community-acquired infections resistant to each agent; S = >95% susceptible.
†Resistance is common to quinupristin but most isolates retain susceptibility to dalfopristin. Susceptibility to one member of this combination but not the other renders the drug bacteriostatic.

Epidemiology

S. aureus is carried asymptomatically on the mucous membranes in the anterior nares, nasopharynx, vagina, and/or perianal area in 20 to 40% of healthy adults. Carriage can be transient, lasting hours to days, intermittent, lasting weeks to months, and recurring or chronic, persisting for months to years despite attempts at eradication. Intact cornified squamous epithelium does not support intermittent or chronic carriage of *S. aureus* for reasons that are not clear but may involve bacteriostatic skin lipids, the absence of *S. aureus*-specific receptors, or interference by colonizing coagulase-negative staphylococci. However, transient hand carriage clearly occurs and is an important means of exchange between patients and hospital personnel. Certain conditions markedly increase skin and nasal carriage of *S. aureus.* These include a variety of acute and chronic skin conditions, most prominently burn injuries, atopic dermatitis, eczema, psoriasis, and decubitus ulcers. In addition, needle use by persons with insulin-dependent diabetes and intravenous drug users has been associated with increased *S. aureus* carriage. Some health care workers have been found to have a higher prevalence of nasal colonization than individuals not involved with patients or hospitals, and patients receiving long-term hemodialysis and those with the acquired immunodeficiency syndrome (AIDS) have a higher than expected colonization rate.

S. aureus is extremely hardy and can survive drying, extremes of environmental temperature, wide ranges of pH, and high salt levels. It can therefore survive in the hospital on inanimate objects such as pillows, sheets, and blood pressure cuffs (called fomites) for some time. Fomite carriage is suspected to be a major means of transmission during outbreaks of community-acquired MRSA infections among members of athletic teams. However, the major reservoir of *S. aureus,* in both hospitals and nature, is humans. *S. aureus* infections result when patients become infected with the same strain with which they are colonized (autoinoculation). A study found that 82% of patients who had *S. aureus* bacteremia carried the identical strain, as determined by molecular typing, in both their blood and nares. Autoinoculation accounts for most hemodialysis shunt and peritoneal dialysis catheter infections, for infective endocarditis in intravenous drug abusers, for both individuals and families who suffer from recurrent staphylococcal furunculosis, and for sternal wound infections after cardiovascular surgery. Eradicating nasal carriage in patients by using topical mupirocin ointment has been shown to reduce the incidence of shunt infections in patients receiving hemodialysis and in those with recurrent furunculosis.

Coagulase-negative staphylococci colonizing the skin and mucous membranes of hospitalized patients and some hospital personnel are usually more resistant to antimicrobial agents than are staphylococci found on the skin of outpatients or hospital personnel not working on inpatient units. Antimicrobial use selects more resistant organisms on patients' skin and creates a huge hospital reservoir for multiple-antibiotic–resistant coagulase-negative staphylococci that can be transferred among patients, can be acquired by hospital personnel, and may eventually be inoculated into wounds in association with implanted, indwelling foreign devices.

Pathobiology

S. aureus causes disease syndromes by two different mechanisms. The organism can become locally or systemically invasive by producing molecules that thwart host defense mechanisms, or it can elaborate toxins that cause disease without the need for the organism itself to invade tissue (toxinoses).

Local Infection

The hallmark of the localized staphylococcal infection is an *abscess,* a walled-off lesion consisting of central necrosis and liquefaction and containing cellular debris and multiplying bacteria surrounded by a layer of fibrin and intact phagocytic cells. The abscess may be superficial, occurring in skin (furuncle), or deep, present in organs (carbuncle), as a result of bacteremic dissemination. Intact cornified squamous epithelium is normally a barrier to both colonization and infection by *S. aureus,* and even injecting virulent organisms into the skin causes infection only if a foreign body (e.g., suture) is also present. Sera from adults contain both heat-labile and heat-stable opsonins (complement and specific antibody) that are highly efficient at mediating the phagocytosis and killing of *S. aureus* by neutrophils.

Because humoral immunity and opsonophagocytosis are the body's major defense against pyogenic microorganisms such as *S. aureus,* most individuals are well equipped to resist infection. The role of neutrophils and opsonophagocytosis as the primary antistaphylococcal host defenses is illustrated by patients with neutrophil defects (Chapters 175 and 303) who have an increase in *S. aureus* infection. These include defects in intracellular killing (chronic granulomatous disease and Chédiak-Higashi syndrome) and impaired neutrophil chemotaxis and humoral immunity (Job's syndrome). When the balance is tipped in favor of the organism, *S. aureus* possesses certain factors that may produce an abscess and promote the organism's survival inside the lesion. Although no single factor has been shown to be the major abscess-forming virulence factor, and mutants deficient in each of the factors have been recovered from full-blown infections, the general feeling is that, because most of these factors differentiate the pathogenic (*S. aureus*) from the nonpathogenic (coagulase-negative staphylococci) members of the genus, they probably play some coordinate role in initiating and maintaining infection. Table 310–3 outlines *S. aureus* factors that may contribute to the establishment of local infections.

TABLE 310–3 *STAPHYLOCOCCUS AUREUS* FACTORS THAT MAY PROMOTE LOCAL INFECTIONS BY THWARTING HOST DEFENSE

Factor	Proposed Mechanisms for Interfering with Host Defense
Coagulase	Prevents neutrophil access to infection site
Microcapsule	Inhibits phagocytosis
Protein A	Inhibits immunoglobulin G–mediated opsonization (binds Fc fragment)
Clumping factor (fibrinogen receptor)	Inhibits opsonization (fibrin coating)
Catalase	Interferes with intracellular killing
Proteases, nuclease, lipase, and cytolysins (α, β, and δ)	Liquefaction necrosis and phagocyte dysfunction
Leucocidin and gamma toxin	Neutrophil cytolysis
Fatty acid metabolizing enzyme	Inactivates bactericidal lipids

Disseminated Infection

A small percentage of local infections progresses to dissemination, in which *S. aureus* gains access to the blood. Dissemination is characterized by *bacteremia* and *metastatic infection.* The factors leading to dissemination and the type and appearance of local infections that are more likely to disseminate are not known.

S. aureus produces such enzymes as *staphylokinase* (a fibrinolysin), *hyaluronidase,* and various *proteases* that may enable it to escape the abscess, invade tissue, and eventually enter the blood. Once it is in the blood, the most lethal immediate consequence is *sepsis* or *septic shock* (Chapter 109). This syndrome is mediated chiefly by *enterotoxins* and *toxic shock syndrome toxin* (TSST-1), all of which contain similar motifs (superantigens) that enable them to bind to T cells and macrophages, thus stimulating the production of such sepsis-associated cytokines as interleukin-1, tumor necrosis factor, and interleukin-6. All *S. aureus* isolates probably contain a gene for one of the many genotypes of enterotoxin or TSST-1. Toxins that form pores in eukaryotic membranes may also contribute to sepsis and overwhelming lethal infection. Pore-forming toxins include α-toxin and the leukocidins (γ-hemolysin, leukocidin, and Panton-Valentine leukocidin).

One of the target cells for bacteremic *S. aureus* is the endothelial cell. Organisms adhere to and are internalized by endothelial cells, where, by releasing cytolysins, the bacteria can disrupt the endothelial cell layer and invade underlying tissue. *S. aureus* can also exist inside intact endothelial cells. The ability of the organisms to survive inside phagocytes and endothelial cells may explain their propensity to cause recurrent and refractory bacteremia despite seemingly appropriate therapy.

Toxinoses

S. aureus produces three toxins, or classes of toxin, that produce specific syndromes without a need for the organism itself to invade and disseminate. *Staphylococcal food poisoning* occurs when a preformed, heat-stable *enterotoxin* is ingested and interacts with parasympathetic ganglia in the stomach, producing vomiting. At least 17 closely related toxin genotypes can all produce the characteristic symptoms. *Staphylococcal scalded skin syndrome (Ritter's or Lyell's syndrome)* results from the production of *exfoliative toxin* by *S. aureus* isolates that colonize or infect the skin of newborns. The characteristic exfoliation of the superficial stratum granulosum layer of the epidermis results from the action of the toxin on desmosomes that hold the cells of this skin layer together. Two exfoliating serotypes, A and B, are recognized. *Toxic shock syndrome* associated with tampon use in young women is the result of entrance of TSST-1 into the blood through the vagina and is produced by one of several closely related clones of *S. aureus* that colonize the mucosa.

Clinical Manifestations

Staphylococcus aureus *Infections*

Skin and Soft Tissue Infections

The most common *S. aureus* infections are *folliculitis* and the *furuncle,* or boil (Table 310–4). These infections involve a single hair follicle or a localized area of the epidermis and dermis. Although most *S. aureus* furuncles do not cause systemic symptoms, those on the face should be treated aggressively because of their potential to migrate to the brain by means of the venous circulation. Furuncles can coalesce and spread through deeper skin layers or can extend down to and along a fascial plane, causing a much more extensive and serious infection called a *carbuncle.* Carbuncles are most common over the upper back and back of the neck, where they can form multiple draining sinuses; bacteremia occurs in approximately one fourth of patients. A boil or furuncle may also be called a *skin abscess* if it becomes large but remains circumscribed, confined to one area, and fluctuant. A nonlocalized *S. aureus* skin infection is called *cellulitis* and may resemble the skin infections caused by *Streptococcus pyogenes,* the most common cause of cellulitis (Chapter 312). *S. aureus* cellulitis can also lead to bacteremia, thereby proving the staphylococcal origin of some of these infections. *S. aureus* cellulitis is

TABLE 310–4 INFECTIONS CAUSED BY *STAPHYCOCCUS AUREUS*

Common or Usual Etiologic Pathogen	Less Common Etiologic Pathogen	Uncommon or Rare Etiologic Pathogen
Furuncle or skin abscess	Cellulitis	
Bullous impetigo	Hospital-acquired pneumonia	
Surgical wound infection		Ascending urinary tract infection
Hospital-acquired bacteremia	Brain abscess	
	Empyema	Meningitis
Bacterial endocarditis	Necrotizing fasciitis	Enterocolitis
Hematogenous osteomyelitis	Community-acquired (necrotizing) pneumonia	
Septic arthritis		
Pyomyositis		
Renal carbuncle		
Scalded skin syndrome		
Toxic shock syndrome		
Food-borne gastroenteritis (short incubation)		
Botryomycosis		
Paraspinous or epidural abscess		

particularly common in individuals with preexisting chronic skin disease such as stasis dermatitis and diabetic, trophic, or decubitus ulcers. Adults can also develop a form of impetigo called *bullous impetigo.* The lesions are characterized by erythema with a crusty surface and small or large bullous lesions. The bullae are attributed to the elaboration of exfoliative toxin and are the localized, adult equivalent of the scalded skin syndrome seen in infants. Infections caused by community-acquired MRSA are predominantly skin infections, particularly furunculosis, but a serious deep tissue infection, *necrotizing fasciitis,* has been described in some patients infected with these organisms.

The most common health care–associated *S. aureus* skin and soft tissue infection is the *wound infection,* in which wounds at surgical or catheter exit sites are contaminated with *S. aureus,* become erythematous, and drain purulent or serosanguineous fluid. *S. aureus* is the most common and most serious cause of hospital-acquired wound infections, and it leads to local, deep-wound infections and systemic, metastatic infections related to bacteremia.

Recurrent furunculosis can occur in members of families, usually because of persistent nasal or perineal carriage in family members with autoinoculation of skin by scratching. The infections are commonly superficial and without systemic symptoms but are painful and annoying. Interruption is not possible until the nasal carrier state is eradicated in all family members. Although most individuals with recurrent furunculosis have normal immune systems, a condition called *Job syndrome* (Chapter 175) is recognized in individuals with recurrent *S. aureus* furunculosis. In addition to recurrent furunculosis, patients have high levels of serum immunoglobulin E, neutrophil chemotactic defects, and a generalized disorder of immunoregulation. Adults with this syndrome usually not only describe a long history of recurrent skin infections since childhood but also often have had recurrent sinopulmonary infections.

Pleuropulmonary Infections

S. aureus is an uncommon cause of pneumonia in otherwise healthy, nonhospitalized adults; it accounts for less than 10% of community-acquired pneumonia. However, following influenza A infections, the risk of *S. aureus* pneumonia is increased. Chest radiographs of patients with community-acquired *S. aureus* pneumonia may show abscesses and thin-walled cysts, resembling the pneumatoceles seen in infants. Necrotizing pneumonia has also been seen among small numbers of patients, predominantly children, infected with strains of community-acquired MRSA. Panton-Valentine leukocidin has been implicated as an important marker of virulence in these strains.

In contrast to its role in community-acquired pneumonia, *S. aureus* is a prominent cause of nosocomial pneumonia, particularly in intubated patients receiving mechanical ventilation. Cultures of specimens from intubated patients obtained by techniques designed to minimize contamination of the specimens by organisms colonizing the upper airway have shown *S. aureus* in up to one third of patients. Pneumonia in ventilator-dependent patients is a particularly lethal event, with one fourth to one half of the patients dying as a direct result of their pulmonary infection. Nothing seems to distinguish the radiographic appearance of nosocomial *S. aureus* pneumonia from that of pneumonia caused by other nosocomial pathogens. *S. aureus* bacteremia related solely to nosocomial pneumonia is uncommon.

Septic pulmonary emboli in patients with right-sided *S. aureus* endocarditis (see later) can also manifest as primary pneumonia. However, these patients all have *S. aureus* bacteremia and usually have discrete lesions in multiple lobes, often accompanied by hemoptysis and chest pain.

S. aureus is cultured from the pleural space in up to 15% of adults with empyema, but it is found in pure culture in fewer than 10%. The incidence of *S. aureus* as a cause of empyema seems to have decreased overall since the mid-1980s, but it is still a prominent etiologic pathogen in patients with nosocomial empyema.

Endocarditis

The extensive database provided by the International Collaboration on Endocarditis has established that *S. aureus* has replaced streptococci as the number 1 cause of endocarditis worldwide (Chapter 76). Two different and distinct populations have endocarditis caused by *S. aureus;* these are compared in Table 310–5. One group consists of older patients with underlying diseases who have primarily left-sided endocarditis and have a high mortality rate (20 to 30%). Approximately half of these patients experience heart failure, half have central nervous system manifestations, and 40 to 50% have had either a skin infection or an intravenous catheter as the presumed portal of entry. Although patients with left-sided *S. aureus* endocarditis can present acutely, with symptoms compatible with the sepsis syndrome, and *S. aureus* can infect previously normal valves, most patients have had more subacute symptoms of fever, malaise, and fatigue for 1 to 2 weeks, and three fourths have evidence by history or echocardiography of previously damaged or abnormal valves. Increasing proportions of patients in this category (almost half in one series) have infected cardiac valves as a result of a hospital-onset bacteremia. Patients with nosocomial *S. aureus* endocarditis may be infected with MRSA.

The second population in which *S. aureus* endocarditis develops consists of those who inject illicit drugs intravenously. These individuals are younger, are healthier, usually have no known valvular heart disease, and have infections of the tricuspid valve in 80 to 90% of cases. The patient, not the intravenous drug, is the source of the infecting organism. The major presenting symptoms in these patients are those of septic pulmonary emboli. The chest film typically shows multiple nodular infiltrates in various lobes that often cavitate and occasionally form pneumatoceles. Most of these patients have pure right-sided endocarditis and only rarely have any peripheral left-sided manifestations. However, a murmur of tricuspid insufficiency is heard in less than half

TABLE 310–5 *STAPHYCOCCUS AUREUS* ENDOCARDITIS IN DIFFERENT POPULATIONS OF PATIENTS

Characteristics of Patients and Disease	IV Drug Abusers	Persons Who Are Not IV Drug Abusers
Mean age (yr)	30	50
Underlying disease	No	Yes
Portal of *Staphylococcus aureus* entry	Skin (IV injection)	Skin (infection or IV catheter)
Valves involved	Tricuspid	Mitral, aortic
Preexisting valve abnormality	No	Yes or no
Presentation	Chest pain, fever, hemoptysis	Fever, fatigue, malaise; sepsis (less common)
Peripheral manifestations	Septic pulmonary emboli	Skin manifestations; central nervous system abnormalities; metastatic infection in bone, kidney, and spleen
Heart failure	Rare	Common
Mortality	<5%	20–30%
Treatment duration	2–3 wk	4-6 wk

IV = intravenous.

the cases. The mortality rate is extremely low for these patients, usually only 2 to 5%, but recurrence is relatively common, given the individuals' proclivity for continued drug abuse.

Bacteremia

S. aureus is second only to coagulase-negative staphylococci as a cause of hospital-acquired bacteremia. The usual source of nosocomial bacteremia is intravenous catheters. The consequences of nosocomial bacteremia are usually only fever and malaise, but they can include endocarditis, osteomyelitis, metastatic abscesses in various organs, and death from overwhelming sepsis. Treatment must be prolonged, to eradicate the organism from tissues and organs. Bacteremia caused by *S. aureus* is usually continuous and high grade, with the organism grown from all cultures of blood drawn over a period of time even if no endocarditis or infected foreign body is present. Furthermore, bacteremia may persist for several days even with appropriate therapy and removal of an infected catheter (complicated bacteremia). This persistence is believed to result from the organism's ability to survive host phagocytic defense and to be sequestered inside cells.

In contrast to that of nosocomial *S. aureus* bacteremia, the source of community-acquired bacteremia is often obscure. It may originate from a skin infection, an intravenous injection of illicit drugs, or an infected focus in the heart or at a peripheral site. In all patients with community-acquired *S. aureus* bacteremia, a diligent search should be made for an infected source. If none is found, patients should be treated as if they have endocarditis.

Osteomyelitis

S. aureus is the most common cause of acute hematogenous osteomyelitis (Chapter 293). Most cases occur in children, but adults are also at risk, particularly those who have had *S. aureus* bacteremia. Children have osteomyelitis almost exclusively in long bones; one third to half of adult cases occur in the lumbar or thoracic vertebrae. Vertebral osteomyelitis results when *S. aureus* initially seeds the intervertebral disc space and then spreads from the disc space to involve contiguous vertebrae. A paraspinous or epidural abscess frequently occurs as an extension of the initial intervertebral focus. Patients present with fever and back pain and may have neurologic symptoms from spinal cord compression. Radiographs typically show narrowing of one or more intervertebral disc spaces with collapse of adjacent vertebrae. A magnetic resonance imaging scan is particularly helpful in defining the extent of vertebral osteomyelitis. Long bones may be involved after hematogenous dissemination of *S. aureus,* but osteomyelitis in these locations is more typically the result of contiguous spread from an infected decubitus trophic ulcer, or traumatic wound. One of the most common causes of *S. aureus* osteomyelitis of the foot bones is infection of ulcers in diabetic patients with vascular disease. Occasionally, hardware used to repair long-bone fractures becomes infected with *S. aureus.* These infections are particularly refractory to therapy without removal of the foreign body.

Septic Arthritis

S. aureus is a common cause of acute septic arthritis (Chapter 293). Unlike in children, *S. aureus* septic arthritis in adults typically occurs in joints that have previously been damaged by a chronic inflammatory arthritis or osteoarthritis, in joints that have been violated by needle aspiration, injection, or surgery, or in joints that contain a prosthetic device. Occasionally, an otherwise normal joint is seeded by the hematogenous route, or the joint space is invaded from a contiguous focus of osteomyelitis. These infections need to be differentiated from other causes of acute monarticular arthritis such as gout and gonococcal infection. In all cases of septic arthritis, arthrocentesis should be performed before therapy is begun so a specific microbial diagnosis can be made. *S. aureus* pyarthrosis can be present with relatively little systemic toxicity in patients with chronic inflammatory arthritis who take large doses of anti-inflammatory medication; this condition may be particularly difficult to diagnose. One unique form of *S. aureus* septic arthritis involves infection of the sternoclavicular joint and is usually seen in intravenous drug users or in patients who have had subclavian intravenous catheters.

Genitourinary Tract Infections

The most important *S. aureus* infections of the genitourinary tract are those that result from hematogenous dissemination. These include microabscesses, renal carbuncles, and perinephric abscesses. The presence of *S. aureus* in the urine is either the result of contamination asymptomatically colonized in the vagina and/or perianal area or an indication that the kidney has been infected during an episode of *S. aureus* bacteremia. The absence of cells in the urine should suggest contamination. If *S. aureus* is repeatedly cultured from urine or present in the urine together with pyuria or hematuria, the patient should be evaluated for bacteremia, for a deep focus that could have caused disseminated infection, and for an intrarenal or perinephric abscess. The presence of *S. aureus* in the urine should *never* be assumed to be secondary to a lower urinary tract infection.

Central Nervous System Infections

Although brain abscess and meningitis can be caused by *S. aureus,* they are relatively rare. Fewer than 10% of cases of meningitis and 20 to 30% of cases of brain abscess are caused by *S. aureus.* They are usually the result of metastatic seeding as a result of bacteremia from an identified focus, direct inoculation after trauma or a neurosurgical procedure, or infection of an indwelling foreign body, such as a ventricular shunt. The prognosis of patients infected as a result of metastatic seeding is particularly poor, with a mortality rate of 30 to 50%. The one infection associated with the central nervous system that is almost always caused by *S. aureus* is a paraspinous or epidural abscess, usually secondary to vertebral osteomyelitis.

Pyomyositis

Infection of the large skeletal muscles is the result of *S. aureus* in more than 80% of cases. It is prevalent in tropical countries, hence the name "tropical pyomyositis," but it is being increasingly described in temperate climates. Patients in tropical countries are usually adults who have no underlying disease and who present with fever, pain, and swelling in the involved muscle, but without evidence of local inflammation. Diagnosis is made by needle aspiration of pus. Because eosinophilia is common in patients in tropical countries who have pyomyositis, parasites are believed to have a role in the pathogenesis of this disease. Pyomyositis in temperate climates arises in much the same manner but more often is seen in children or in adults with underlying diseases, particularly those who have AIDS. It is associated with muscle trauma in more than half of patients and more frequently involves more than one noncontiguous muscle group.

Toxinoses

Staphylococcal scalded skin syndrome is usually a disease of neonates and is caused by the action of the exfoliative toxins A and B. This syndrome results from *S. aureus* colonization or local infection, usually of the umbilical stump, and causes generalized desquamation of the superficial granulosum cell layer of the epidermis. The adult equivalent is bullous impetigo, associated with localized skin involvement, but adult cases of more generalized desquamation have been described. It is important to differentiate staphylococcal scalded skin syndrome from toxic epidermal necrolysis. The *toxic shock syndrome* was initially described in young, menstruating women and was associated with tampon use in women vaginally colonized with *S. aureus* that produced TSST-I. However, the number of tampon-associated cases has decreased markedly. Most cases are now secondary to *S. aureus* infections of skin or other sites, and the etiologic toxin is often one of the enterotoxins rather than TSST-I. The criteria for the diagnosis of staphylococcal toxic shock syndrome are shown in Table 310–6. Staphylococcal toxic shock syndrome is associated with relatively low mortality and is a true toxinosis; bacteremia is rare.

Gastroenteritis or *staphylococcal food poisoning* is the result of ingesting preformed staphylococcal enterotoxin. Enterotoxin-producing *S. aureus* are inoculated into food by a colonized or infected food handler. If the food sits at room temperature before being cooked, the organism multiplies and produces toxin. Subsequent cooking does not inactivate the heat-stable toxin, and ingestion produces symptoms predominantly of vomiting after a short (2- to 8-hour) incubation period.

TABLE 310–6 DIAGNOSTIC CRITERIA FOR STAPHYLOCOCCAL TOXIC SHOCK SYNDROME

1. Fever (usually >38.9° C or 102° F)
2. Rash (resembling diffuse macular erythroderma, sunburn, or scarlet fever)
3. Desquamation, 1 to 2 weeks after onset of illness, particularly of palms and soles
4. Hypotension (systolic blood pressure <90 mm Hg or orthostatic syncope)
5. Involvement of three or more of the following organ systems: gastrointestinal (nausea and vomiting), muscular (myalgias), mucous membrane (hyperemia), renal, hepatic, hematologic (↓platelets), central nervous system, or pulmonary (adult respiratory distress syndrome)
6. *Staphylococcal aureus* infection or mucosal colonization

Miscellaneous Infections

The older literature describes "botryomycosis," a chronic *S. aureus* infection of skin, lung, or bone that produces granules resembling those seen in actinomycosis, and "enterocolitis," a necrotizing infection of bowel in surgical patients associated with sheets of organisms seen on Gram staining of stool. These infections are rarely seen today. The recent increase of MRSA infections in the community has prompted the description of infections that were thought to be rarely caused by *S. aureus.* These include necrotizing pneumonia, necrotizing fasciitis, and the Waterhouse-Fredrickson syndrome.

Community-Acquired Methicillin-Resistant *Staphylococcus Aureus*

Beginning in the late 1990s worldwide, patients were described who were infected with MRSA but who had no health care contact. Many of these patients were children, were members of indigenous populations, and were remote from medical care. In addition, outbreaks were described in the United States among members of athletic teams who shared towels, among prison inmates, and among male homosexuals. Many of these isolates from disparate sources were closely related genetically and were distinct from nosocomial MRSA in other ways: infections were largely confined to the skin (furunculosis), isolates were not multiresistant but were susceptible to most antibiotics except β-lactams, nasal carriage of outbreak strains was difficult to document, and all carried the gene for Panton-Valentine leukocidin. These community-acquired MRSA infections have continued to spread in the United States, particularly in the pediatric population, and offer new challenges to outpatient treatment of skin and soft tissue infections. The contrast between hospital-acquired and community-acquired MRSA is summarized in Table 310–7.

Coagulase-Negative Staphylococcal Infections

The major infections caused by coagulase-negative staphylococci are hospital acquired and involve indwelling foreign devices (Table 310–8). In general, coagulase-negative staphylococci are of low virulence

TABLE 310–8 CHARACTERISTICS OF COAGULASE-NEGATIVE STAPHYLOCOCCAL INFECTIONS

1. Associated with health care
2. Caused by *S. epidermidis* (70–80%)
3. Resistant to multiple antimicrobial agents (>80% methicillin resistant)
4. Involving indwelling foreign devices (e.g., catheters, prosthetic heart valves and joints, vascular grafts, central nervous system shunts)
5. Often exhibiting a long latent period between device contamination and clinical presentation

TABLE 310–7 HEALTH CARE–ASSOCIATED VERSUS COMMUNITY-ACQUIRED* METHICILLIN RESISTANT *STAPHYLOCOCCUS AUREUS*

	Nosocomial MRSA	Community-Acquired MRSA
Typical infection	Catheter-associated bacteremia; wound infection	Skin infection (furunculosis); rare necrotizing pneumonia
Infected population	Hospitalized patients	Children, native populations, athletic teams, prison inmates, male homosexuals
Antimicrobial susceptibility	Resistant to multiple antimicrobials	Resistant to β-lactam and macrolide antimicrobials; increasing resistance to fluoroquinolones
Unique virulence genes	None unique (many and varied)	Panton-Valentine leukocidin
Strain genetics	Multiple clones	A few unique clones
Prevalence	~50% of nosocomial *Staphylococcus aureus*	8 to 20% of community-acquired *Staphylococcus aureus;* highly geographically variable

*Community-acquired also called community-associated. Defined as MRSA infections in individuals with no health care contact.
MRSA = methicillin-resistant *Staphylococcus aureus.*

and rarely cause metastatic infections, even though they are the most common causes of hospital-acquired bacteremia. Bacteremia is usually the result of intravascular catheter or other invasive device infection. However, coagulase-negative staphylococci can be lethal when they infect prosthetic cardiac valves. They are the most common causes of prosthetic valve endocarditis and usually arise in the first year after surgery, presumably after inoculation into the area of the sewing ring during valve implantation. Valve dysfunction results from dehiscence or obstruction of the valve orifice, and most patients require surgery for cure.

The exceptions to infections described in Table 310–8 are those caused by *S. saprophyticus*. This organism is second only to *Escherichia coli* as a cause of ascending urinary tract infections in young, sexually active outpatient women, and it is implicated in 15 to 20% of cases in this population (Chapter 306). In addition, low colony counts of this staphylococcal species have been recovered from urine obtained by suprapubic aspiration in some women with the anterior urethral syndrome or symptomatic abacteriuria.

Diagnosis

The diagnosis of staphylococcal infections requires that the organism be seen on Gram staining of an infected specimen and be grown on artificial media, preferably in pure culture. Although various tests for serum antibody to *S. aureus* antigens (e.g., teichoic acid antibody) have been evaluated for their ability to differentiate serious, deep-seated infection from trivial infections or self-limited bacteremia, none has proved to have a sensitivity or specificity sufficient to warrant its use as a basis for making clinical decisions. Newer tests, based on polymerase chain reaction amplification of genomic DNA, are available that can speed identification of staphylococci, methicillin resistance, and other characteristics of specific isolates. At present, these tests complement but do not replace culture-based methods.

Because coagulase-negative staphylococci are the most common contaminants of any culture obtained by crossing skin, it is important that multiple cultures grow the same organism before a diagnosis of true bacteremia or invasive infection is made. This is a major reason for obtaining blood culture samples from two different sites and avoiding drawing blood through intravenous catheters, the hub of which may be contaminated. Even when both cultures grow coagulase-negative staphylococci, true bacteremia may not be present, and additional studies to demonstrate strain identity may be useful. The most discriminatory test currently available is the generation of genomic DNA fingerprints by pulsed field gel electrophoresis.

Determining the susceptibility to β-lactam and other antimicrobial agents is essential in the treatment of bacteremia and other serious staphylococcal infections. Standard susceptibility tests are the foundation for this, with some caveats. β-Lactam antibiotics should not be used to treat a staphylococcal infection if laboratory tests indicate that the isolate is resistant to methicillin, even if tests indicate apparent susceptibility to these agents. When a patient is not responding to nafcillin or similar drugs, additional tests should be done to exclude the possibility of heterotypic methicillin resistance, which is sometime missed on initial tests. Occasionally, small colony variants appear in laboratory cultures. These organisms have various mutations that slow their growth in the laboratory but may increase their intracellular survival in the patient, especially in indolent and recurrent infections such as chronic osteomyelitis. Prolonged treatment and specific drug combinations may be required for cure.

Treatment

Rx

Antimicrobial agents effective for treating *S. aureus* infections are listed in Table 310–2. Treatment of hospital-acquired infections is difficult because resistance to many of these agents is common. Methicillin-resistant isolates are *cross-resistant* to *all β-lactams* (penicillins, cephalosporins, and carbapenems [imipenem and meropenem]) and are usually also resistant to at least three additional classes of antimicrobial agents (multiresistant). In most areas, 40 to 50% of nosocomial *S. aureus* isolates are methicillin resistant and multiresistant, and more than 70% of nosocomial coagulase-negative staphylococci are methicillin resistant and multiresistant. Empirical treatment should be selected on the basis of local susceptibility patterns, but in most areas, infections caused by nosocomial coagulase-negative staphylococci are usually treated with vancomycin. Vancomycin is the mainstay of therapy for most nosocomial infections caused by methicillin-resistant organisms. To increase the bactericidal activity needed to treat endocarditis, complicated bacteremia, and metastatic infections caused by *S. aureus*, some recommendations suggest combining vancomycin with an aminoglycoside or rifampin, or using the newer agent, daptomycin. Less serious nonbacteremic infections could be treated with bacteriostatic agents such as a tetracycline, sulfamethoxazole-trimethoprim, linezolid, or others.

Reports of a few patients in the United States and in several other countries who have been infected with *S. aureus* and coagulase-negative staphylococci with significantly reduced susceptibilities to vancomycin portend a worrisome trend. Treatment of these infections with vancomycin is usually unsuccessful. More recently, *S. aureus* highly resistant to vancomycin has been recovered from a few patients. These isolates acquired vancomycin resistance genes from enterococci, probably through plasmid-mediated transfer. Therefore, the potential exists for these genes to become more widely disseminated among *S. aureus*, to increase the number of resistant isolates, and to decrease the utility of vancomycin even further.

Another disturbing trend is the increase in outpatient infections caused by MRSA. Many of these infections are in patients who have had recent exposure to a health care or extended care facility, but some infections are truly community acquired, occurring in patients with no obvious health care association. These isolates are usually not multiresistant but resistant only to β-lactam and macrolide antibiotics, although the number of isolates resistant to fluoroquinolones is increasing.

Treating staphylococcal infections usually consists of administering antimicrobial agents, draining abscesses either surgically or through a catheter, and removing foreign bodies. The duration of therapy is usually 1 to 2 weeks for localized, drained infections not associated with bacteremia or a foreign body. In general, infections can rarely be cured if the foreign material is left in place. Infections requiring more specialized therapeutic decisions are discussed in the next two paragraphs.

Bacteremia and Endocarditis

For *S. aureus*, all patients with community-acquired bacteremia who have evidence of a metastatic infection or who have no obvious source for bacteremia should be treated as if they have endocarditis. The search for metastatic infection must be thorough (including an ophthalmologic examination) and should be repeated throughout the clinical course. For intravenous drug abusers with right-sided endocarditis, treatment consists of 2 to 3 weeks of an antistaphylococcal penicillin (nafcillin or oxacillin) or vancomycin plus gentamicin for the entire treatment period; for left-sided endocarditis, it consists of 4 to 6 weeks of an antistaphylococcal penicillin or vancomycin, with gentamicin for the first week (Chapter 76). However, in patients with *S. aureus* bacteremia acquired in the hospital from a removable focus (usually an intravascular catheter), the decision becomes more difficult. The patients whose fever and bacteremia resolve within 3 days after removing the infected focus, those who have no complications or evidence of metastatic infection, and those who have no abnormality of cardiac valves can receive 2 weeks of therapy. All other patients with nosocomial bacteremia who do not meet all the exclusions should be treated as if they have endocarditis.

Osteomyelitis

Patients with *S. aureus* osteomyelitis require a minimum of 6 weeks of therapy, with the initial 2 to 4 weeks of treatment parenteral. Therapy for osteomyelitis of long bones is often unsuccessful if sequestra are left in place.

Prevention

Preventing hospital-acquired infections is accomplished by paying attention to tenets of infection control (Chapter 304) including handwashing and regloving between patients, as well as strict adherence to aseptic technique when creating or caring for any kind of wound. Patients undergoing procedures that may result in wound or implanted device infections should also receive prophylactic antibiotics before and during the procedure.

Patients with recurrent *S. aureus* infections of skin, catheters, or dialysis shunts should have their nares cultured and, if they are *S. aureus* carriers, should be treated with regimens designed to reduce bacterial carriage. Systemic antimicrobial regimens (e.g., with rifampin, trimethoprim-sulfamethoxazole, minocycline, or a fluoroquinolone) have variable clinical efficacy and are often complicated by the emergence of resistance (actually, some older studies have shown that rifampin and minocycline were very successful at eradicating carriage in the short term, but recolonization and/or resistance occurred fairly quickly). Topical decolonization regimens with mupirocin, alone or in combination with chlorhexidine-based products, is a more promising approach, although mupirocin resistance can also emerge in settings in which this regimen is often used. Various approaches to development of an antistaphylococcal vaccine have provided some protection in animal models, but no product has been proven to be effective in humans.

Future Directions

Elucidation of the staphylococcal genome and advances in understanding gene regulation and mechanisms of infection provide exciting opportunities to expand our armamentarium against this formidable foe. In addition to exploring new targets for conventional antimicrobial drug discovery and development, strategies that interfere with adhesion, expression of virulence factors, or the action of virulence factors are under active investigation.

SUGGESTED READINGS

Fowler VG, Boucher H, Corey GR, et al: Daptomycin versus standard therapy for bacteremia and endocarditis caused by *Staphylococcus aureus*. N Engl J Med 2006;355:653–665. *Randomized comparison shows 2.4% more patients receiving 6 mg per kg of body weight intravenously of daptomycin achieved a successful outcome 42 days after therapy began than those on standard therapy.*

Fowler VG Jr, Miro JM, Hoen B, et al: *Staphylococcus aureus* endocarditis: A consequence of medical progress. JAMA 2005;293:3012–3021. *One of the most recent contributions of the International Collaboration on Endocarditis—Prospective Cohort Study group that documents* S. aureus *as the most common cause of endocarditis worldwide and most cases as health care associated.*

Fowler VG Jr, Olsen MK, Corey GR, et al: Clinical identifiers of complicated *Staphylococcus aureus* bacteremia. Arch Intern Med 2003;163:2066–2072. *A helpful scheme for deciding when bacteremia is likely to lead to complications.*

Fridken SK, Hageman JC, Morrison M, et al: Methicillin-resistant *Staphylococcus aureus* disease in three communities. N Engl J Med 2005;352:436–444. *An excellent description of the epidemiology and presentation of community-associated MRSA in three geographically dispersed communities.*

Grundmann H, Aires-de-Sousa M, Boyce J, et al: Emergence and resurgence of methicillin-resistant *Staphylococcus aureus* as a public-health threat. Lancet 2006;368:874–885. *Emphasizes the current threat.*

Miller LG, Perdreau-Remington F, Rieg G, et al: Necrotizing fasciitis caused by community-associated methicillin-resistant *Staphylococcus aureus* in Los Angeles. N Engl J Med 2005;352:1445–1453. *This is an emerging clinical entity that should influence empirical treatment choices.*

Moran GJ, Krishnadasan A, Gorwitz RJ, et al: Methicillin-resistant *S. aureus* infections among patients in the emergency department. N Engl J Med 2006;355:666–674. *In 11 US cities, MRSA was the most common identifiable cause of skin and soft-tissue infections among patients presenting to the emergency department.*

Moreillon P, Que YA, Glausner MP: *Staphylococcus aureus* (including staphylococcal toxic shock) *In* Mandell RD, Bennett JE (eds): Principles and Practices of Infectious Diseases, 6th ed. New York, Churchill Livingstone, 2005, pp 2321–2351. *A comprehensive and detailed description of* S. aureus *biology and clinical manifestations.*

Von Eiff C, Becker K, Machka K, et al: Nasal carriage as a source of Staphylococcus aureus bacteremia. N Engl J Med 2001;344:11–16. *The best study done to date documenting the importance of autoinfection in the pathogenesis of serious* S. aureus *infections.*

311 PNEUMOCOCCAL PNEUMONIA

Lionel A. Mandell

Definition

The term *pneumococcal pneumonia* refers to infection of the pulmonary parenchyma and its associated structures by *Streptococcus pneumoniae.* The estimated 500,000 cases that occur annually in the United States result in approximately 50,000 deaths.

The Pathogen

S. pneumoniae is a gram-positive coccus that typically grows in pairs or short chains. Careful examination of the diplococcal form reveals slightly tapered ends that give rise to its "lancet-shaped" appearance. It is a facultative anaerobe that grows best on blood agar plates in a 5% carbon dioxide ambient environment. The colonies are typically surrounded by a greenish zone of hemolysis resulting from degradation of hemoglobin by a pneumococcal toxin. The organism can be distinguished from other streptococci by its susceptibility to ethyl hydrocuprein (optochin) and bile solubility.

The surface of the pneumococcus consists of a capsule and a cell wall. The capsule, which helps prevent phagocytosis, is composed of polysaccharides that define the 90 pneumococcal serotypes. The cell wall is a dynamic structure composed of more than a dozen distinct glycopeptides.

Epidemiology

The pneumococcus causes about two thirds of cases of community-acquired pneumonia and is responsible for a corresponding percentage of deaths; it can cause hospital-acquired pneumonia as well. The false impression that *S. pneumoniae* is uncommon has arisen because at least a third of patients with community-acquired pneumonia are unable to produce sputum and, even if they do, often provide an inadequate sample. Moreover, if the patient has recently taken just one dose of a drug to which the pneumococcus is susceptible, it may not be possible to isolate.

The ecologic niche of the pneumococcus is the nasopharynx, and up to 80% of infants and 20% of healthy adults may be colonized. This process may begin within the first few days of life and appears to be inversely related to age. Simultaneous colonization with more than one capsular type has been reported, and it appears that asymptomatic colonization is an immunizing experience because homologous anticapsular antibodies may be demonstrated in individuals after colonization with a specific serotype.

A particular serotype may colonize the nasopharynx for varying periods, but the average duration in infants is 7 weeks. Carriage rates are highest during the late fall, winter, and early spring. Although each of the 90 serotypes is potentially pathogenic, the most frequently encountered are types 3, 4, 6, 7, 9, 12, 14, 18, 19, and 23.

Person-to-person transmission results from close interpersonal contact. Although pneumococcal pneumonia is typically a sporadic illness, epidemics can occur in crowded settings such as daycare centers, barracks, nursing homes, or prisons.

The incidence of pneumococcal pneumonia is about 18 per 100,000 per year. For persons 5 years or younger and 75 years or older, rates are about 23 and 35.8 per 100,000, respectively. For pneumococcal bacteremia, the incidence is about 7.5 per 100,000 per year and increases with age; the case-fatality rate is 21%.

Risk factors for pneumococcal pneumonia include dementia, seizure disorders, heart failure, cerebrovascular disease, chronic obstructive pulmonary disease, human immunodeficiency virus (HIV) infection, previous viral respiratory illness, alcoholism, malnutrition, diabetes, cirrhosis, and renal insufficiency.

Certain ethnic groups such as Native Americans, particularly Alaskan natives, and Australian aboriginals, appear to be particularly susceptible to invasive pneumococcal infection. Any individual who has a defect in IgG synthesis (Chapter 271) or phagocyte function (Chapter 175) or who has undergone splenectomy is also at increased risk for invasive pneumococcal infection.

TABLE 311–1 PREDISPOSING FACTORS FOR PNEUMOCOCCAL PNEUMONIA

Increased exposure to *Streptococcus pneumoniae*
Prison
Military barracks
Daycare centers
Shelters for the homeless
Decreased host defenses
Complement deficiency
Antibody deficiency
Functional or anatomic asplenia
Decreased numbers or function of phagocytes
Specific disease entities
Multiple myeloma
Lymphoma
Chronic lymphocytic leukemia
Human immunodeficiency virus infection
Respiratory/pulmonary problems
Chronic obstructive pulmonary disease
Smoker
Allergies
Previous viral infection

Pathobiology

Pneumonia is the result of a breakdown in the interplay between colonizer and host. In pneumococcal pneumonia, the microorganism first colonizes the nasopharynx in a process that depends on the lectin-like interaction between bacterial surface proteins and host cell carbohydrate. Aspiration of small amounts of oropharyngeal contents occurs in deep sleep, even in normal individuals, but if the oropharyngeal material includes pneumococcal serotypes associated with invasive infection and if normal clearance mechanisms fail, the colonizers may become pathogens. The risk for infection is increased by any process or condition that exposes the host to the pathogen, that allows oropharyngeal secretions to bypass upper airway defenses, or that interferes with the host's ability to ingest and kill the pneumococci (Table 311–1).

Although the cellular and molecular mechanisms have not been completely elucidated, it appears that aspirated pneumococci adhere to type II cells in the alveolus if they are not cleared by normal defense mechanisms. Attachment to resting cells is mediated by two classes of glycoconjugates, but local inflammatory mediators upregulate host cell receptors, such as those for platelet-activating factor (PAF), and provide a site of attachment for the bacteria. This interaction between PAF receptor and pathogen seems to be an important step in internalization of the bacteria by means of an endocytic vacuole and may promote invasion.

Once in the lung, the pneumococci are able to activate complement and stimulate the cytokine response. Initially, the alveoli fill with fluid exudate (Fig. 311–1), which allows the infection to spread to adjacent uninfected alveoli. In healthy lungs, polymorphonuclear leukocytes (PMNs) constitute less than 1 to 2% of alveolar cells and normally reside in the interstitial areas of the lung and in adjacent capillaries. Recruitment of PMNs into alveoli depends on the generation of chemoattractants necessary for the directed migration of neutrophils.

The pneumococcal polysaccharides of the bacterial capsule help the organism resist phagocytosis, and absence of anticapsular antibody limits the ability to opsonize and ingest pathogens. Ultimately, the signs and symptoms of disease are due both to the pathogens themselves and to the body's response to them. The bacterial cytotoxin pneumolysin and pneumococcal cell wall components, such as teichoic acid and peptidoglycan, are able to induce a variety of effects that initiate and then enhance the inflammatory response, thereby resulting in the various signs and symptoms of pneumonia.

The effects of pneumococcal infection are ultimately manifested as changes in lung mechanics secondary to reductions in lung volumes and lung compliance, as well as gas exchange problems resulting from intrapulmonary shunting and subsequent arterial hypoxemia. If severe enough, death may ensue.

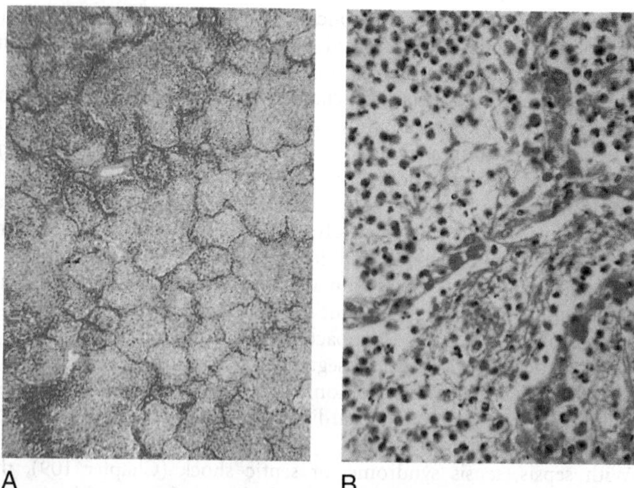

FIGURE 311–1 • Pneumonia. A, Low-power magnification (× 100) of hematoxylin and eosin (H&E) stain of tissue section from left lower lobe of lung. Note intact alveolar walls and alveoli filled with edema and thick cellular exudates. **B,** Higher magnification (× 500) H&E stain of same section shown in **A.** Note heavy infiltrate of polymorphonuclear cells and intact alveolar walls.

Antibiotic Resistance

The phenotypic expression of antibiotic resistance corresponds to genetic alterations resulting either from horizontal acquisition of foreign genetic information or from mutations in the microbial genome. In the case of *S. pneumoniae,* resistance may be acquired by direct DNA incorporation and remodeling from closely related oral commensal bacteria by the process of natural transformation. Pneumococcal resistance to β-lactams such as penicillin is due solely to the presence of low-affinity penicillin-binding proteins (PBPs). The PBPs themselves are trans and carboxypeptidase enzymes that are involved in bacterial cell wall synthesis and represent the primary sites of action for the penicillins and other β-lactam drugs.

Resistance to macrolides, in contrast, can occur through multiple mechanisms, including target site modification or an efflux pump. Target site modification is caused by a ribosomal methylase encoded by the *ermB* gene. A change in 23S rRNA mediated by this gene can result in resistance to macrolides, lincosamides, and streptogramin B–type antibiotics (MLS_B phenotype). The efflux mechanism is encoded by the *mefA* gene, which results in an M phenotype. The former is typically associated with high-level resistance with minimum inhibitory concentrations (MICs) of 64 μg/mL or higher, whereas the latter is usually associated with low-level resistance with MICs of 1 to 32 μg/mL. These two mechanisms account for approximately 45 and 55%, respectively, of resistant isolates. Some pneumococcal isolates have been found with both the *erm* and *mef* gene, but the exact significance of such a finding is unknown.

Resistance to fluoroquinolones may be mediated by changes in one or both target sites (topoisomerase II and IV), which usually results from mutations in the *gyrA* and *parC* genes, respectively. An efflux pump may have a role as well.

Clinical Manifestations

The clinical features of pneumococcal pneumonia depend on factors such as whether the patient is immunocompetent or immunosuppressed, the severity of illness, and whether the patient has taken antibiotics. Temperatures can vary from 101° F to higher than 103° F (38 to 39.5° C), can be accompanied by chills and rigors, and are usually associated with a tachycardic response. A cough, typically productive of purulent and occasionally blood-tinged sputum, is often present, and as many as 46% of patients report chest pain. About 20% have gastrointestinal symptoms such as nausea, vomiting, or diarrhea. In the elderly, symptoms and signs may be more subtle. For example, older patients may have predominantly confusion, so the physician must have a high level of suspicion.

On examination, the patient is often listless and may be cyanotic. The respiratory rate is increased; if pleuritic pain is marked, the patient may be splinting the affected side. Dullness to percussion over a lung segment suggests consolidation, whereas a flat percussion note is typically associated with a pleural effusion. Breath sounds may be "distant" if there is an overlying effusion, but they are bronchial in nature if the underlying lung is consolidated. Rales may be noted. If the patient has pleurisy without much pleural fluid, a friction rub may be heard.

No radiographic appearance is characteristic of pneumococcal pneumonia (Chapter 97). Typically, however, involvement is limited to one or more segments within a single lobe. Involvement is unilateral approximately 80% of the time, and the presence of cavitation or lung abscess is uncommon. Forty-five percent of patients have an associated pleural effusion, but only 15% have an effusion of sufficient size to warrant drainage (>10 mm on lateral decubitus views).

Patients with lobar consolidation are more likely to be bacteremic, but there are no consistently significant differences in the radiologic manifestations of bacteremic and nonbacteremic pneumococcal pneumonia, and even patients with a small subsegmental opacity can have bacteremia. Bacteremic pneumococcal pneumonia may seed distant sites and cause meningitis (Chapter 437), endocarditis (Chapter 76), or septic arthritis (Chapter 293).

With sepsis, sepsis syndrome, or septic shock (Chapter 109), the patient may be hypotensive, and the findings of organ failure vary depending on the target organ involved. For example, oliguria, anuria, and acidosis suggest renal failure; myocardial impairment suggests heart failure; and jaundice is consistent with hepatic failure. Systemic activation of coagulation together with consumption of clotting proteins can result in simultaneous clotting and bleeding (Chapter 181). In some cases, peripheral gangrene and purpura fulminans may be seen.

Diagnosis

Despite extensive testing, even in university medical centers, a specific etiologic agent is not found in half or more of patients with community-acquired pneumonia. The history, physical examination, chest radiograph, sputum Gram stain, and blood and sputum cultures are insensitive and lack specificity, whereas more invasive methods (e.g., endotracheal aspirate, bronchoscopy techniques, pleural fluid aspiration, and lung biopsy) require special expertise and are infrequently indicated. As a general rule, routine diagnostic tests to identify a pathogen are optional for outpatients with community-acquired pneumonia, but more extensive testing is recommended for hospitalized patients (Table 311–2).

Ultimately, the diagnosis should be based on suggestive clinical features plus a chest radiograph with or without corroborating microbiologic data. Because *S. pneumoniae* is the most common etiologic agent of community-acquired pneumonia, virtually any recommended treatment regimen must provide adequate coverage for it, so documentation of its presence has little or no effect on ultimate clinical outcomes. From the point of view of epidemiology and antimicrobial susceptibility, however, documentation of a pathogen is desirable.

The sputum Gram stain is a relatively simple and inexpensive procedure to document the presence of certain pathogens. The adequacy of the specimen is based on the relative number of PMNs and squamous epithelial cells (SECs). There should be at least 25 PMNs and less than 10 SECs per low-power field (×100 magnification). The sensitivity of sputum Gram stain for *S. pneumoniae* is 55%, whereas the specificity is higher than 80%. Unfortunately, approximately 30% of patients overall are unable to produce an appropriate sputum sample. In the elderly, this figure reaches almost 70%. If grading criteria are used to assess the quality of sputum, only 40% at best are rated as being of good quality, so a maximum of 28% (40% of 70%) are good-quality specimens. Sputum cultures are neither sensitive nor specific, particularly when dealing with relatively fastidious pathogens such as *S. pneumoniae.*

Blood cultures are positive in only 5 to 14% of patients with community-acquired pneumonia. If patients have taken a previous dose of antibiotic, culture results are even less useful. As a result, sputum Gram stain, sputum culture, and blood cultures are generally recommended only in patients with selected clinical indications (see Table 311–2). In patients with severe community-acquired pneumonia, an expectorated sputum sample should be replaced by an endotracheal aspirate sample if the patient is intubated.

Pneumococcus can also be detected by polymerase chain reaction, but this relatively sensitive and very specific technique is currently limited to research laboratories. Pneumococcal capsular polysaccharide can be detected in urine and by a variety of techniques, and this approach may occasionally be helpful for diagnosis after antibiotic therapy has been started. Detection of antibody to pneumococcal polysaccharide is not useful.

TABLE 311–2 INDICATIONS FOR MORE EXTENSIVE DIAGNOSTIC TESTING

Intensive care unit admission for community-acquired pneumonia
Failure of outpatient treatment
Radiographic appearance of cavities on initial evaluation
Infection resulting in neutropenia
Alcohol abuse
Chronic severe liver disease
Severe chronic obstructive lung disease
Asplenia (anatomic or functional)
Recent travel (within 2 weeks)
Positive rapid *Legionella* or pneumococcal urinary antigen test
Pleural effusion

Prevention

Polysaccharide Vaccine

A polysaccharide vaccine contains 25 µg of each of the 23 capsular polysaccharides that account for 90% of invasive infections (Chapter 16). Polysaccharide vaccines stimulate B-cell responses, thereby resulting in type-specific antibody production that enhances ingestion and killing of the pathogens by phagocytes. The antigens, however, are T cell independent and therefore do not result in long-lasting immunity. Two types of polysaccharide vaccine have been available—Pneumovax (Merck) and Pnu-Imune (Lederle).

The effectiveness of the pneumococcal polysaccharide vaccine ranges from 56 to 81%. It is not effective in immunocompromised patients, such as those with sickle cell disease, chronic renal failure, immunoglobulin deficiency, Hodgkin's disease, non-Hodgkin's lymphoma, leukemia, and multiple myeloma. It is also not effective in preventing nonbacteremic pneumonia. The vaccine is recommended for (1) persons 65 years or older; (2) persons 2 to 64 years old with chronic illnesses such as cardiovascular disease, chronic pulmonary disease (not asthma), diabetes mellitus, alcoholism, chronic liver disease, or cerebrospinal fluid leaks; (3) persons 2 to 64 years old with functional or anatomic asplenia; and (4) persons 2 to 64 years old living in special environments or social settings (Alaskan natives, certain Native American populations, residents of long-term care facilities).

Although the effectiveness of the vaccine is less in these subgroups, the following immunocompromised patients 2 years or older should also be immunized: (1) persons with HIV infection, leukemia, lymphoma, or Hodgkin's disease and (2) those with multiple myeloma, generalized malignancy, chronic renal failure, nephrotic syndrome, or organ or bone marrow transplants and individuals being treated with immunosuppressive chemotherapy, including steroids.

The lack of an anamnestic response with polysaccharide vaccines means that antibody levels decrease over time and revaccination is required. Although the exact timing is unclear, most experts suggest revaccination at 5 years. For immunocompetent persons 65 years or older, a second dose is suggested if the patient was given the first vaccine 5 years earlier at an age younger than 65 years. For persons 2 to 64 years of age with asplenia, a single revaccination is suggested 5 years after the initial dose if the patient is older than 10 years. However, if the patient is younger than 10 years, revaccination should be given 3 years after the first dose. For immunocompromised patients, revaccination should be given 5 years after the first dose if the patient is older than 10 years and 3 years after the first dose if the patient is younger than 10 years.

Conjugated Vaccine

A seven-valent pneumococcal conjugate vaccine (Prevenar, Wyeth-Lederle) has also been approved for use. The basis of this newer vaccine is that pneumococcal polysaccharide is conjugated to a carrier protein, thereby producing T-cell-dependent antigens, which results in long-term immunologic memory. In this case, the carrier protein is CRM 197, which is similar to diphtheria toxoid. The seven serotypes (4, 6B, 9V, 14, 18C, 19F, 23F) are found most commonly in children and account for approximately 80% of invasive infections in children younger than 6 years. As well as interfering with the spread of resistant pneumococcal serotypes, the conjugate vaccine may help decrease resistance because of its effect on antibiotic use and lessening of antibiotic selection pressure.

The pneumococcal conjugate vaccine should be given to infants at 2, 4, 6, and 12 to 15 months of age. Older, previously unvaccinated infants should be given the vaccine at 7 to 11 months (two doses at least 4 weeks apart) and a third dose at 12 months or older; the second and third doses should be separated by at least 2 months. Children 12 to 23 months old should receive two doses at least 2 months apart. Children 2 to 9 years old should receive one dose. Children in high-risk groups should be given two doses at least 2 months apart.

High-risk groups include patients with HIV infection, immunocompromised states, chronic illnesses such as nephrotic syndrome, chronic pulmonary and symptomatic heart conditions, and patients with sickle cell disease and anatomic or functional asplenia. At this point, there are no indications for revaccination.

Treatment

Rx

Empirical therapy is often begun for community-acquired pneumonia (Chapter 97; Table 311–3). If pneumococcal infection can be documented, antibiotic therapy can be targeted to this agent alone.

Treatment Regimens

Directed Therapy against Known *S. pneumoniae*

S. pneumoniae can be treated with a number of antimicrobials, including various β-lactams, macrolides, and selected fluoroquinolones (Table 311–4). Unfortunately, resistance has been described for virtually all these agents. The National Committee for Clinical Laboratory Standards (NCCLS) defines strains with MICs to penicillin of less than 0.06 μg/mL as sensitive, 0.1 to 1.0 μg/mL as intermediate, and 2 μg/mL or higher as resistant. Multidrug-resistant pathogens, which are resistant to three or more antimicrobial agents with different mechanisms of action, have been seen in a number of countries. Risk factors for drug-resistant pneumococcal infection include recent antimicrobial therapy, age younger than 2 years or older than 65 years, attendance at a daycare center, recent hospitalization, and HIV infection.

If a good-quality Gram stain of sputum reveals sheets of PMNs with lancet-shaped gram-positive diplococci as the only organism, if the patient has no risk factors for infection with resistant *S. pneumoniae,* and if the patient is not living in an area endemic for penicillin-resistant *S. pneumoniae,* it is reasonable to initiate treatment with penicillin G, 2.4 million U/day. For outpatients, oral therapy is usually given in the form of amoxicillin, 500 mg orally three times daily. For infection with *S. pneumoniae* with penicillin MICs of up to 1 μg/mL, penicillin is still an appropriate agent. For strains with penicillin MICs of 2 to 4 μg/mL, data regarding efficacy are conflicting, and higher doses may be better. If the patient is allergic to penicillin, a macrolide such as azithromycin (500 mg on day 1, then 250 mg/day) or clarithromycin (500 mg twice daily) may be used. Five days is the minimum recommended duration of treatment of community-acquired pneumonia that is not complicated, severe, or associated with bacteremia.

For patients who are hospitalized because of community-acquired pneumonia, higher doses of parenteral antibiotics are generally used: penicillin in the range of 12 million U (2 to 3 million every 4 hours) or ampicillin, 4 g/day (1 g every 6 hours). Third-generation cephalosporins such as ceftriaxone (1 to 2 g every 24 hours) and cefotaxime (1 to 2 g every 8 hours) are other alternatives.

The patient can be switched to an oral regimen when cough and shortness of breath are improving, the white blood cell count is normalizing, and oral intake and gastrointestinal tract absorption are adequate. Febrile patients are frequently treated outside the hospital, so absence of a fever is not a prerequisite for switching to an oral regimen.

TABLE 311–3 RECOMMENDED EMPIRICAL ANTIBIOTICS FOR COMMUNITY-ACQUIRED PNEUMONIA

OUTPATIENTS

1. Previously healthy and no use of antimicrobials within the previous 3 months: A macrolide (azithromycin, clarithromycin, or erythromycin) *or* doxycycline
2. Presence of comorbid conditions or use of antimicrobials within the previous 3 months (in which case an alternative from a different class should be selected):
   Respiratory fluoroquinolone, moxifloxacin, gemifloxacin, levofloxacin (750 mg)
   β-Lactam *plus* a macrolide (high-dose amoxicillin, e.g., 1 g tid, or amoxicillin-clavulanate, 2 gm bid, is preferred; alternatives include ceftriaxone, cefpodoxime, cefuroxime; doxycycline is an alternative to the macrolide)
3. In regions with a high rate (>25%) of "high-level" (MIC >16 μg/mL) macrolide-resistant *S. pneumoniae,* consider the use of alternative agents listed above in 2

INPATIENTS, NON-ICU

1. Respiratory fluoroquinolone
2. β-Lactam *plus* a macrolide (preferred β-lactam agents include cefotaxime, ceftriaxone, ampicillin; ertapenem in selected patients; with doxycycline as an alternative to the macrolide; respiratory fluoroquinolone should be used for penicillin-allergic patients)

INPATIENTS, ICU

A β-lactam (cefotaxime, ceftriaxone, ampicillin-sulbactam) *plus* either azithromycin *or* a respiratory fluoroquinolone (for penicillin-allergic patients, a respiratory fluoroquinolone and aztreonam are recommended)

SPECIAL CONCERNS

If *Pseudomonas* is a consideration, an antipneumococcal, antipseudomonal β-lactam (piperacillin/tazobactam, cefepime, imipenem, meropenem) plus either ciprofloxacin or levofloxacin (750-mg dose)
or
The above β-lactam plus an aminoglycoside and either azithromycin or an antipneumococcal fluoroquinolone
or
For penicillin-allergic patients, aztreonam plus an aminoglycoside and either a respiratory fluoroquinolone or a macrolide
If CA-MRSA is a consideration, add linezolid or vancomycin

CA-MRSA = community-acquired methicillin-resistant *Staphylococcus aureus;* ICU = intensive care unit; MIC, minimum inhibitory concentration.

Rx

Empirical Treatment

For patients in whom *S. pneumoniae* cannot be documented as the cause of community-acquired pneumonia, an empirical antibiotic regimen is recommended (see Table 311–3) to cover the range of organisms that may cause the syndrome (Chapter 97). Initial coverage need not be broadened to cover every conceivable organism. 1

TABLE 311–4 ANTIMICROBIAL DOSES AND FREQUENCY OF ADMINISTRATION

Antimicrobial	Dose and Route	Frequency
MACROLIDE		
Azithromycin	500 mg × 1 then 250 mg PO	q24h
Clarithromycin	500 mg PO	q12h
Erythromycin	500 mg PO	q6h
TETRACYCLINE		
Doxycycline	100 mg PO	q12h
FLUOROQUINOLONE		
Moxifloxacin	400 mg PO or IV	q24h
Gemifloxacin	320 mg PO	q24h
Levofloxacin	750 mg PO or IV	q24h
Ciprofloxacin	400 mg IV	q12h
β-LACTAMS		
Amoxicillin	1 g PO	q8h
Amoxicillin-clavulanate	2 g PO	q12h
Ampicillin-sulbactam	2 g IV	q6h
Aztreonam	2 g IV	q8–12h
Cefepime	1–2 g	q12h
Cefixime	400 mg PO	q12h
Cefotaxime	1–2 g IV	q8h
Ceftriaxone	1–2 g IV	q24h
Cefpodoxime	100–200 mg	q12h
Cefuroxime	500 mg PO	q12h
Ertapenem	1 g IV	q24h
Imipenem	500 mg IV	q6h
Meropenem	1 g IV	q8h
Piperacillin-tazobactam	3.375 g IV	q6h
AMINOGLYCOSIDE		
Amikacin	15 mg/kg	OD or ÷ 2 q12h
Gentamicin	1.7 mg/kg	OD or ÷ 3 q8h
Tobramycin	1.7 mg/kg	OD or ÷ 3 q8h
MISCELLANEOUS		
Linezolid	600 mg PO or IV	q12h
Vancomycin	0.75–1 g IV	q12h

OD = once daily.

Rx

For those admitted to a regular hospital floor, either a β-lactam (such as a third-generation cephalosporin) plus a macrolide or a fluoroquinolone alone should be used (Chapter 97). The fluoroquinolones offer logistic and financial benefits because they permit once-daily dosing with a single drug. It should be noted, however, that resistance to fluoroquinolones has already been well documented, and misuse of these drugs may result in widespread resistance.

For patients treated in the intensive care unit, a fluoroquinolone or macrolide in combination with a β-lactam is suggested if *Pseudomonas aeruginosa* is not a concern (Chapter 97). If it is, an antipneumococcal, antipseudomonal β-lactam plus ciprofloxacin or levofloxacin is recommended. Monotherapy with a fluoroquinolone for severe community-acquired pneumonia is to be discouraged.

Prognosis

In an otherwise well, relatively young patient with no comorbid conditions and with mild to moderate infection, the elevated temperature and white blood cell count usually resolve by days 2 to 4 and 4, respectively. The patient looks and feels better within a few days, but it is important to keep in mind that even in patients younger than 50 years, only 60% will have resolved radiologically by 1 month. In patients older than 50 years or those with more severe infection or chronic obstructive pulmonary disease, only 25% may clear radiographically by 1 month.

A patient who fails to respond or deteriorates after initial treatment must be carefully reassessed with a detailed review of the history and treatment course, plus appropriate radiographic studies and cultures. If the diagnosis is incorrect, other infectious causes of pneumonia such as *Haemophilus influenzae* (Chapter 323) or the atypical agents (Chapter 97) must be considered. Noninfectious illnesses that may account for the clinical and radiographic findings must also be considered: heart failure (Chapter 57), pulmonary embolism (Chapter 99), neoplasm (Chapter 201), radiation injury (Chapter 18), drug reaction (Chapter 275), and inflammatory lung disease, to name a few. If the original diagnosis was correct, metastatic infection, lung abscess (Chapter 98) or empyema, and unsuspected drug resistance must be considered. Drug factors such as errors in selection, dose, or route of administration are possible explanations, especially in patients who receive oral medication.

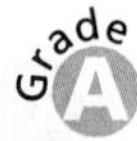

1. Shefet D, Robenshtok E, Paul M, et al: Empirical atypical coverage for inpatients with community-acquired pneumonia: Systematic review of randomized controlled trials. Arch Intern Med 2005;165:1992–2000.

SUGGESTED READINGS

File T: *Streptococcus pneumoniae* and community-acquired pneumonia: A cause for concern. Am J Med 2004;117(3A):39S–50S. *An excellent overview of the importance of* S. pneumoniae *as a cause of CAP.*

Lujan M, Gallego M, Rello J: Optimal therapy for severe pneumococcal community-acquired pneumonia. Intensive Care Med 2006;32:971–980. *Cefotaxime, ceftriaxone, and high-dose amoxicillin are generally successful.*

Mandell L: Antimicrobial resistance and treatment of community-acquired pneumonia. Clin Chest Med 2005;26:57–64. *A discussion of the significance of antimicrobial resistance and the treatment of CAP, including pneumococcal pneumonia.*

Mandell LM, Wunderink RG, Anzueto A, et al: IDSA/ATS Consensus Guidelines on the management of community-acquired pneumonia in adults. Clin Infect Dis 2007;44, Supplement 2:S27–S72. *Consensus guidelines.*

Shorr AF: Preventing pneumonia: The role of pneumococcal and influenza vaccines. Clin Chest Med 2005;26:123–134. *An excellent overview of vaccine issues as they pertain to* S. pneumoniae *and influenza virus.*

312 STREPTOCOCCAL INFECTIONS

Dennis L. Stevens

Definition

Streptococci are gram-positive globular or coccoid bacteria that grow in chains. Streptococci colonize the skin and mucous membranes of animals, do not produce catalase, and may be aerobic, anaerobic, or facultative. Streptococci require complex media containing blood products for optimal growth. On blood agar plates, streptococci may cause complete (β-), incomplete (α-), or no (γ-) hemolysis. Hemolytic streptococci can be classified into types A through O on the basis of acid-extractable carbohydrate antigens of cell wall material. The recent development of rapid latex agglutination kits provides even small clinical laboratories with the means to identify streptococci according to Lancefield group. Bacitracin susceptibility, bile esculin hydrolysis, and the CAMP (Christie-

Atkins-Munch-Peterson) test (flame-type synergistic hemolysis on a *Staphylococcus aureus* blood agar streak) are useful presumptive tests for classifying groups A, D, and B streptococci, respectively. Modern schemes of classification of hemolytic and nonhemolytic streptococci use complex biochemical and genetic techniques.

GROUP A STREPTOCOCCAL INFECTIONS

Epidemiology

The concept of group A streptococcus as a pure human pathogen is supported by the following observations: (1) natural group A streptococcus infection in animals is rare; (2) laboratory animals are not useful models of streptococcal pharyngitis, scarlet fever, erysipelas, rheumatic fever, or poststreptococcal glomerulonephritis; (3) the inoculum needed to cause infection in laboratory animals is orders of magnitude greater than that estimated to cause infection in humans; and (4) streptococci have developed highly sophisticated defensive molecules that bind, inactivate, or destroy human immune response molecules (e.g., immunoglobulin G antibody and complement [C5a]).

All group A streptococcal infections have the highest incidence in children younger than 10 years. The asymptomatic prevalence is also higher (15 to 20%) in children than in adults (≤5%). Age is not the only factor; crowded conditions in temperate climates during the winter months are also associated with epidemics of pharyngitis in school children as well as in military recruits. Impetigo is most common in children aged 2 to 5 and may occur year round in tropical areas but largely in the summer in temperate climates. Similarly, 90% of cases of scarlet fever occur in children 2 to 8 years old, and, like pharyngitis, scarlet fever is most common in temperate regions during winter. An epidemic of scarlet fever that occurred on the Danish Faeroe Islands several decades after the illness had disappeared affected all age groups, a finding suggesting that other factors, such as the lack of protective antibody against scarlatina toxin or the introduction of a new strain, rather than age, predisposes individuals to clinical illness.

In contrast to pharyngitis, impetigo, and scarlet fever, bacteremia has had the highest age-specific attack rate in elderly people and in neonates. Between 1986 and 1988, the prevalence of bacteremia increased 800 to 1000% in adolescents and adults in Western countries. Although some of this increase is attributable to intravenous drug abuse and puerperal sepsis, most of the increase results from cases of streptococcal toxic shock syndrome, in which a defined portal of entry is not apparent in 50% of cases.

Human mucous membranes and skin serve as the natural reservoirs of *Streptococcus pyogenes*. Pharyngeal and cutaneous acquisition is by person-to-person spread through aerosolized microdroplets or by direct contact, respectively. Epidemics of pharyngitis and scarlet fever have also occurred after the consumption of contaminated, nonpasteurized milk or food. Epidemics of impetigo have been reported, particularly in tropical areas, in daycare centers, and among underprivileged children. Group A streptococcal infections in hospitalized patients occur during childbirth (puerperal sepsis), in times of war (epidemic gangrene), and during surgical convalescence (surgical wound infection, surgical scarlet fever) or as a result of burns (burn wound sepsis). Thus, in most clinical streptococcal infections, the modes of transmission and portal of entry are easily ascertained, with the exception of toxic shock syndrome, as noted earlier.

Pathobiology

Adherence of streptococci to the mucosal epithelium is necessary but not sufficient to cause disease in all cases inasmuch as prolonged asymptomatic carriage is well documented. Complex interactions between host epithelium and streptococcal factors such as M protein, lipoteichoic acid, and fimbriae are necessary for adherence. Fibronectin binding protein (protein F) also contributes to adherence because protein F–deficient mutants are incapable of binding to epithelial cells. Protein F is upregulated by oxygen and is decreased in anaerobic conditions.

Within the tissues, streptococci may impede opsonophagocytosis by virtue of a hyaluronic acid capsule, a C5a peptidase that destroys or inactivates complement-derived chemoattractants and opsonins, or by immunoglobulin binding protein. Expression of M protein in the absence of type-specific antibody also protects the organism from phagocytosis by polymorphonuclear leukocytes and monocytes. In tissues, streptolysin O secreted in high concentration destroys approaching phagocytes. Distal to the focus of infection, lower concentrations of streptolysin O stimulate polymorphonuclear leukocyte adhesion to endothelial cells, thus effectively preventing continued granulocyte migration and promoting vascular damage. In a nonimmune host, streptolysin O, streptococcal pyrogenic exotoxins (SPE A, B, C, MF, and SSA), and other streptococcal components stimulate host cells to produce tumor necrosis factor (TNF) and interleukin-1 (IL-1), cytokines that mediate hypotension, stimulate leukostasis, and eventually result in shock, microvascular injury, multi-organ failure, and, if excessive, death. A unique feature of the pyrogenic exotoxins and some M protein fragments is their ability to interact with certain V_β regions of the T-cell receptor in the absence of classical antigen processing by antigen-presenting cells (Fig. 312–1). This interaction results in massive clonal proliferation of T lymphocytes and release of both monokines and lymphokines. SPE type B, a cysteine protease, may play a role in the pathogenesis of necrotizing fasciitis and shock through its ability to cleave pre–IL-1β into active IL-1β, its activation of endogenous metalloproteases, and its cleavage of high-molecular-weight kinino-

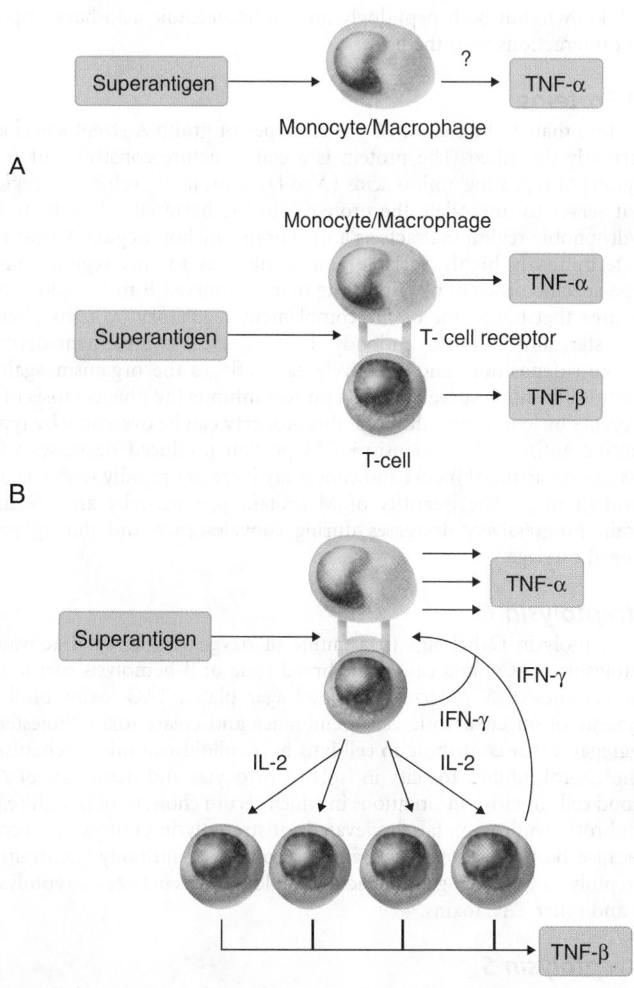

FIGURE 312–1 • Superantigen-induced production of tumor necrosis factor-α (TNF-α) and lymphotoxin (TNF-β) by peripheral blood mononuclear cells. A, Superantigens induce human monocytes to produce TNF-α; however, it is unclear whether such production results solely from direct stimulation of the monocyte by the superantigen. **B,** In mixed mononuclear cell populations, superantigens stimulate TNF-α synthesis in monocytes and, by binding to specific V_β regions of the T-cell receptor, induce the synthesis of lymphotoxin (TNF-β) from T cells. **C,** The T-cell response to superantigen stimulation includes the production of interleukin-2 (IL-2), which results in clonal proliferation with concordant production of interferon-γ (IFN-γ) and TNF-β. IFN-γ can then amplify monocyte synthesis of TNF-α, IL-1, and IL-6. (From Stevens DL, Bryant AE, Hackett SP: Sepsis syndromes and toxic shock syndromes: Concepts in pathogenesis and a perspective of future strategy. Curr Opin Infect Dis 1993;6:374–383.)

gen into bradykinin. Thus, in streptococcal toxic shock syndrome, lymphokines (TNF-β, interferon-γ, and IL-2), monokines (TNF-α, IL-1, and IL-6), and bradykinin may be crucial in the mediation of shock and organ failure.

Pathophysiology

Capsule

Some strains of *S. pyogenes* possess capsules of hyaluronic acid and form large mucoid colonies on blood agar. Luxuriant production of M protein may also impart mucoid colony morphology, and this trait has been associated with M-18 strains. An operon promoter sequence is the key element in both the constitutive and dynamic regulation of hyaluronic acid synthesis in group A streptococci, and its activity is increased during ideal growth conditions and log-phase growth. It plays an important role in pharyngitis, soft tissue infection, and invasive disease by binding to CD44 on epithelial cells and by serving as an antiphagocytic factor.

Cell Wall

The cell wall is composed of a peptidoglycan backbone with integral lipoteichoic acid components. The function of lipoteichoic acid is not well known, but both peptidoglycan and lipoteichoic acid have important interactions with the host.

M Proteins

More than 150 different M protein types of group A streptococci are currently described. The protein is a coil structure consisting of four regions of repeating amino acids (A to D), a proline/glycine-rich region that serves to intercalate the protein into the bacterial cell wall, and a hydrophobic region that acts as a membrane anchor. Region A near the N terminus is highly variable, and antibodies to this region confer type-specific protection. Within the more conserved B to D regions lies an area that binds one of the complement regulatory proteins (factor H), sterically inhibits antibody binding and complement-derived opsonin deposition, and effectively camouflages the organism against humoral immune surveillance. M protein inhibits the phagocytosis of *S. pyogenes* by leukocytes, although this property can be overcome by type-specific antisera. The quantity of M protein produced decreases with passage on artificial media and conversely increases rapidly with passage through mice. The quantity of M protein produced by an infecting strain progressively decreases during convalescence and during prolonged carriage.

Streptolysin O

Streptolysin O belongs to a family of oxygen-labile, thiol-activated cytolysins (TACs) and causes the broad zone of β-hemolysis surrounding colonies of *S. pyogenes* on blood agar plates. TAC toxins bind to cholesterol on eukaryotic cell membranes and create toxin-cholesterol aggregates that contribute to cell lysis by a colloid-osmotic mechanism. Cholesterol inhibits toxicity in isolated myocytes and hemolysis of red blood cells in vitro. In situations in which serum cholesterol is high (e.g., nephrotic syndrome), falsely elevated antistreptolysin O titers may occur because both cholesterol and antistreptolysin O antibody "neutralize" streptolysin O. Striking amino acid homology exists between streptolysin O and other TAC toxins.

Streptolysin S

Streptolysin S is a cell-associated hemolysin that does not diffuse into agar media. Purification and characterization of this protein have been difficult, and its role in pathogenesis may be in direct or contact cytotoxicity. Streptolysin S has been cloned and shown to be a lantibiotic whose synthesis is controlled by seven genes.

Deoxyribonucleases A, B, C, and D

Expression of deoxyribonucleases (DNases) in vivo elicits the production of anti-DNase antibody following both pharyngeal and skin infection; this response is most true for DNase B with group A streptococci. DNases may also contribute to cytokine production, although their importance in pathogenesis has not been established.

This extracellular enzyme hydrolyzes hyaluronic acid in deeper tissues, thereby facilitating the spread of infection along fascial planes. Antihyaluronidase titers rise following *S. pyogenes* infections, especially those involving the skin.

Pyrogenic Exotoxins

SPE types A, B, and C, also called scarlatina toxin and erythrogenic toxins, induce lymphocyte blastogenesis, potentiate endotoxin-induced shock, induce fever, suppress antibody synthesis, and act as superantigens. Identification of these three different types of SPEs may in part explain why some individuals may have multiple attacks of scarlet fever. The gene for pyrogenic exotoxin A *(speA)* is transmitted by bacteriophages, and stable production depends on lysogenic conversion in a manner analogous to diphtheria toxin production by *Corynebacterium diphtheriae.* Control of SPE A production is not yet understood, although the quantity of SPE A produced varies dramatically from decade to decade. Historically, strains producing SPE A have been associated with severe cases of scarlet fever and, more recently, with streptococcal toxic shock syndrome. Although all strains of group A streptococci are endowed with genes for SPE B *(speB),* as with SPE A, the quantity of toxin produced varies greatly.

Pyrogenic exotoxin type C (SPE C), like SPE A, is bacteriophage mediated, and expression is likewise highly variable. Mild cases of scarlet fever in England and the United States have been associated with SPE C–positive strains. Numerous other pyrogenic exotoxins, including streptococcal superantigen (SPE SSA) and mitogenic factor (SPE MF), have been described, and their roles in pathogenesis are being studied.

Nicotine Adenine Dinucleotidase

Studies have demonstrated a high association of nicotine adenine dinucleotidase production among strains isolated from patients with invasive group A streptococcal infections. Nicotine adenine dinucleotidase impairs neutrophil chemotaxis and alters respiratory burst activity.

Clinical Manifestations

Pharyngitis and the Asymptomatic Carrier

Patients with streptococcal pharyngitis have an abrupt onset of sore throat, submandibular adenopathy, fever, and chilliness but not usually frank rigors. Cough and hoarseness are rare, but pain on swallowing is characteristic. The uvula is edematous, tonsils are hypertrophied, and the pharynx is erythematous with exudate that may be punctate or confluent (Fig. 312–2). Acute pharyngitis is sufficient to induce antibody against M protein, streptolysin O, DNase, hyaluronidase, and, if present, pyrogenic exotoxins. Depending on the infecting strain, pharyngitis may progress to scarlet fever, bacteremia, suppurative head and neck infections, rheumatic fever, poststreptococcal glomerulonephritis, or streptococcal toxic shock syndrome. Pharyngitis is usually self-limited, and pain,

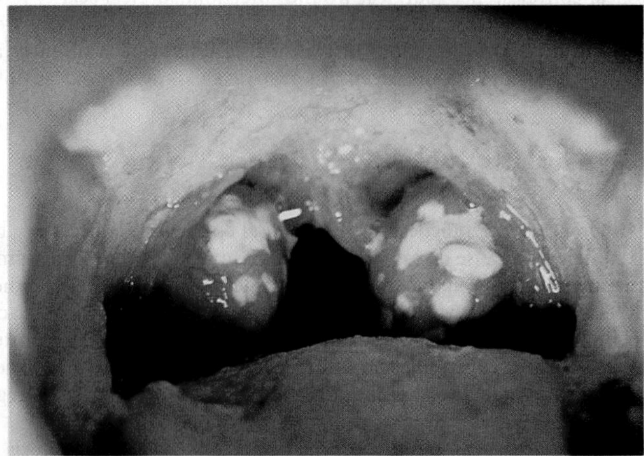

FIGURE 312–2 • Acute streptococcal pharyngitis. Pus is present in the tonsillar crypts, and some palatal petechiae are seen. (From Forbes CD, Jackson WF: Color Atlas and Text of Clinical Medicine, 3rd ed. London, Mosby, 2003.)

Section XXIII Infectious Diseases

swelling, and fever resolve spontaneously in 3 to 4 days even without treatment.

Guideline recommendations exist for the selective use of throat cultures, but antibiotic treatment based only on positive rapid test or throat culture results can reduce unnecessary use of antibiotics for treatment of pharyngitis. Definitive diagnosis is difficult when it is based only on clinical parameters, especially in infants, in whom rhinorrhea may be the dominant manifestation. Even in older children with all the preceding physical findings, the correct clinical diagnosis is made in only 75% of patients. Absence of any one of the classic signs greatly reduces the specificity. Rapid antigen detection tests in the office setting have a sensitivity and specificity of 40 to 90%. A recommended approach in clinical practice is to obtain two throat swab samples from the posterior of the pharynx or tonsillar surface. A rapid streptococcal test is performed on the first sample, and if it is positive, the patient is treated with antimicrobials and the second swab is discarded. If the rapid streptococcal test is negative, the second sample is sent for culture, and treatment is withheld pending a positive culture.

Scarlet Fever

During the past 30 to 40 years, outbreaks of scarlet fever in the Western world have been notably mild, and the illness has been referred to as "pharyngitis with a rash" or "benign scarlet fever." In contrast, in the latter half of the 19th century, mortalities of 25 to 35% were common in the United States, Western Europe, and Scandinavia. The fatal or malignant forms of scarlet fever have been described as either septic or toxic. *Septic scarlet fever* refers to the development of local invasion of the soft tissues of the neck and complications such as upper airway obstruction, otitis media with perforation, meningitis, mastoiditis, invasion of the jugular vein or carotid artery, and bronchopneumonia. *Toxic scarlet fever* is rare today, but historically, severe sore throat, marked fever, delirium, skin rash, and painful cervical lymph nodes initially developed. In severe toxic cases, temperatures of 107° F, pulses of 130 to 160 beats per minute, severe headache, delirium, convulsions, little if any skin rash, and death within 24 hours were common. These cases occurred before the advent of antimicrobials, antipyretics, and anticonvulsants, and sudden deaths were the result of uncontrolled seizures and hyperpyrexia. In contrast, children with septic scarlet fever had prolonged courses and succumbed 2 to 3 weeks after the onset of pharyngitis. Complications of streptococcal pharyngitis and malignant forms of scarlet fever have been less common in the antimicrobial era. Even before antimicrobials became available, necrotizing fasciitis and myositis were not described in association with scarlet fever.

Erysipelas

Erysipelas is caused exclusively by *S. pyogenes* and is characterized by an abrupt onset of fiery red swelling of the face or extremities. Distinctive features are well-defined margins, particularly along the nasolabial fold, scarlet or salmon-red rash, rapid progression, and intense pain. Flaccid bullae may develop during the second to third day, yet extension to deeper soft tissues is rare. Surgical débridement is not necessary, and treatment with penicillin is effective. Swelling may progress despite treatment, although fever, pain, and the intense redness diminish. Desquamation of the involved skin occurs 5 to 10 days into the illness. Infants and elderly adults are most commonly afflicted.

Streptococcal Pyoderma (Impetigo Contagiosa)

Impetigo is most common in patients with poor hygiene or malnutrition. Colonization of the unbroken skin occurs first, and then intradermal inoculation is usually initiated by minor abrasions or insect bites. Single or multiple thick-crusted, golden-yellow lesions develop within 10 to 14 days. Penicillin orally or parenterally and bacitracin or mupirocin topically are effective treatments for impetigo, and they also reduce the transmission of streptococci to susceptible individuals. None of these treatments, including penicillin, prevents poststreptococcal glomerulonephritis. In recent times, *Staphylococcus aureus,* including the methicillin-resistant strain (MRSA), has been implicated in 50% of cases of impetigo.

Cellulitis

Group A streptococcus is the most common cause of cellulitis; however, alternative diagnoses may be obvious when cellulitis is associated with a primary focus such as an abscess or boil *(Staphylococcus aureus),* dog bite *(Capnocytophaga),* cat bite *(Pasteurella multocida),* freshwater injury *(Aeromonas hydrophila),* seawater injury *(Vibrio vulnificus),* and so on (Chapters 310 and 321). Clinical clues to diagnosis are important because aspiration of the leading edge or punch biopsy yields a causative organism in only 15 and 40% of cases, respectively. Patients with lymphedema of any cause such as lymphoma, filariasis, or sequelae of regional lymph node dissection (as in mastectomy or carcinoma of the prostate) are predisposed to streptococcal cellulitis, as are patients with chronic venous stasis. Recurrent saphenous vein donor site cellulitis has been attributed to group A, C, or G streptococci. Group A streptococci may invade the epidermis and subcutaneous tissue and may cause local swelling, erythema, and pain. The skin becomes indurated and, unlike the brilliant redness of erysipelas, is pinkish with indistinct borders. Streptococcal cellulitis responds quickly to penicillin, although when staphylococcus is of concern, nafcillin or oxacillin may be a better choice. If fever, pain, or swelling increases, if bluish or violet bullae or discoloration appears, or if signs of systemic toxicity develop, a deeper infection such as necrotizing fasciitis or myositis should be considered (see later). When an elevated serum creatine phosphokinase level suggests deeper infection, prompt surgical inspection and débridement should be performed.

Lymphangitis

Cutaneous infection with bright red streaks ascending proximally is invariably the result of group A streptococcus. Prompt parenteral antimicrobial treatment is mandatory because bacteremia and systemic toxicity develop rapidly when streptococci reach the blood stream through the thoracic duct.

Necrotizing Fasciitis

Necrotizing fasciitis, originally called "streptococcal gangrene," is a deep-seated infection of the subcutaneous tissue that results in progressive destruction of fascia and fat but may spare the skin itself. Subsequently, *necrotizing fasciitis* has become the preferred term because *Clostridium perfringens, Clostridium septicum,* and *Staphylococcus aureus* can produce a similar pathologic process. Infection may begin at the site of trivial or inapparent trauma. Within the initial 24 hours, swelling, heat, erythema, and tenderness develop and rapidly spread proximally and distally from the original focus. During the next 24 to 48 hours, the erythema darkens, changing from red to purple and then to blue, and blisters and bullae form that contain clear yellow fluid. On the fourth or fifth day, the purple areas become frankly gangrenous. From the seventh to the tenth days, the line of demarcation becomes sharply defined, and the dead skin begins to reveal extensive necrosis of the subcutaneous tissue. Patients become increasingly prostrated and emaciated, and they may become unresponsive, mentally cloudy, or delirious. Aggressive fasciotomy and débridement ("bear claw fasciotomy") and irrigations with Dakin's solution achieved mortality rates as low as 20% even before antimicrobials were available. Since 1989, the mortality rate of necrotizing fasciitis despite antimicrobials, surgical débridement, and intensive care unit treatment has become higher than that reported by Meleney in 1924, probably because of the increased virulence of streptococci (see Streptococcal Toxic Shock Syndrome later).

Myositis

Historically, streptococcal myositis has been an extremely uncommon infection; only 21 cases were documented from 1900 to 1985. More recently, the prevalence of streptococcal myositis has increased in the United States, Norway, and Sweden. Translocation of streptococci from the pharynx to the deep site of trauma (muscle) must occur hematogenously. Symptomatic pharyngitis or penetrating trauma is uncommon. Severe pain may be the only symptom, and swelling and erythema may be the only signs of infection. In some cases, a single muscle group is involved; however, because patients are frequently bacteremic, multiple sites of myositis or abscess can occur. Distinguishing streptococcal myositis from spontaneous gas gangrene caused by *C. perfringens* or *C. septicum* may be difficult, although the presence of crepitus or gas in the tissue would favor clostridial infection. Myositis is easily distinguished from necrotizing fasciitis anatomically by surgical exploration or incisional biopsy, although the clinical features of both conditions overlap. In fact, many cases of necrotizing fasciitis have associated myositis and myonecrosis. In published reports, the case-fatality rate of necrotizing fasciitis is between 20 and 50%, whereas that of streptococcal myositis is between 80 and 100%. Aggressive surgical débridement is extremely important because of the poor efficacy of penicillin described in human cases as well as in experimental models of streptococcal myositis (see the later discussion of antimicrobial efficacy).

Pneumonia

Pneumonia caused by group A streptococcus historically has been most common in women in the second and third decades of life in association with large pleural effusions and empyema that develop rapidly. Chest tube drainage of empyema is necessary even though multiple loculations and fibrinous effusions resulting in restrictive lung disease complicate management. Prolonged penicillin therapy, thoracoscopy, and decortication of the pleura may be necessary to prevent adhesive pleuritis, fibrosis, and subsequent restrictive lung disease. Recently, group A streptococcal pneumonia has been associated with streptococcal toxic shock syndrome and has a high mortality.

Streptococcal Toxic Shock Syndrome

In the late 1980s, invasive group A streptococcal infections occurred in North America and Europe in previously healthy individuals of all age groups. This illness is associated with bacteremia, deep soft tissue infection, shock, multiorgan failure, and death in 30% of cases. Although streptococcal toxic shock syndrome occurs sporadically, minor epidemics have been reported. Most patients have either a viral-like prodrome, a history of minor trauma, insect bites, burns, cuts, recent surgery, or varicella infection. The prodrome may result from a viral illness predisposing to toxic shock syndrome, or these vague early symptoms may be related to the evolving infection. In approximately 50% of cases associated with necrotizing fasciitis, the infection begins deep in the soft tissue at a site of minor trauma that frequently did not result in a break in the skin. The abrupt onset of severe pain is a common initial symptom of streptococcal toxic shock syndrome (Table 312–1). The pain most commonly involves an extremity but may also mimic peritonitis, pelvic inflammatory disease, acute myocardial infarction, or pericarditis. Treatment with nonsteroidal anti-inflammatory agents may mask the initial symptoms or may predispose the patient to more severe complications such as shock.

Fever is the most common initial sign, although some patients have profound hypothermia secondary to shock (see Table 312–1). Confusion is present in more than half the patients and may progress to coma or combativeness. On admission, 80% of patients have tachycardia, and more than half have systolic blood pressure lower than 110 mm Hg. Of those patients with normal blood pressure on admission, most become hypotensive within 4 hours. Soft tissue infection evolves to necrotizing fasciitis or myositis in 50 to 70% of patients, and these conditions require emergency surgical débridement, fasciotomy, or amputation. An ominous sign is progression of soft tissue swelling to violaceous or bluish vesicles or bullae. Many other clinical pictures may be associated with streptococcal toxic shock syndrome including endophthalmitis, myositis, perihepatitis, peritonitis, myocarditis, meningitis, septic arthritis, and overwhelming sepsis. Patients with shock and multiorgan failure without signs or symptoms of local infections have a worse prognosis because definitive diagnosis and surgical débridement may be delayed.

Hemoglobinuria is present and serum creatinine is elevated in most patients at the time of admission. Serum albumin concentrations are moderately low (3.3 g/dL) on admission but drop progressively over 48 to 72 hours. Hypocalcemia, including ionized hypocalcemia, is detectable early in the hospital course. The serum creatinine phosphokinase level is a useful and rapid test to detect deeper soft tissue infections such as necrotizing fasciitis or myositis.

The initial hematologic studies demonstrate only mild leukocytosis but a dramatic left shift (43% of white blood cells may be band forms, metamyelocytes, and myelocytes). The mean platelet count is normal on admission. However, it may drop rapidly by 48 hours, even in the absence of criteria for disseminated intravascular coagulopathy.

Shock is apparent early in the course, and fluid management is complicated by profound capillary leak. Adult respiratory distress syndrome occurs frequently (55%), and renal dysfunction that precedes hypotension in many patients may progress despite treatment. In patients who survive, serum creatinine levels return to normal within 4 to 6 weeks, but many patients require dialysis in the interim. Overall, 30 to 60% of patients die despite aggressive treatment including intravenous fluids, colloid, pressors, mechanical ventilation, and surgical interventions such as fasciotomy, débridement, exploratory laparotomy, intraocular aspiration, amputation, and hysterectomy.

Group A streptococcus is isolated from blood in 60% of cases and from deep tissue specimens in 95% of cases. M types 1, 3, 12, and 28 are the most common strains isolated but account for only 60 to 70% of the isolates; the remaining isolates are a wide variety of M typable and nontypable strains. Pyrogenic exotoxin A or B has been found in isolates from the majority of patients with severe infection, although the quantities of these toxins that are produced in vitro vary widely. Infections in Norway, Sweden, and Great Britain have been primarily the result of M type 1 strains that produce pyrogenic exotoxin B. Other novel pyrogenic exo-

TABLE 312–1 CLINICAL AND LABORATORY FEATURES OF STREPTOCOCCAL TOXIC SHOCK SYNDROME

SYMPTOMS

Viral-like prodrome
Severe pain
Confusion
Nausea
Chills

SIGNS

Fever
Soft tissue swelling and tenderness
Tachycardia
Tachypnea
Hypotension

LABORATORY FINDINGS

HEMATOLOGIC TESTS
Marked left shift
Red cell hemolysis
Thrombocytopenia

CHEMISTRY TESTS
Azotemia
Hypocalcemia
Hypoalbuminemia
Creatine phosphokinase elevation

URINALYSIS
Hematuria

BLOOD GASES
Hypoxia
Acidosis

RADIOGRAPHIC FINDINGS

ARDS
Soft tissue swelling

COMPLICATIONS

Profound hypotension
ARDS
Renal failure
Liver failure
Necrotizing soft tissue infections
Bacteremia
Death (30%)

ARDS = adult respiratory distress syndrome.

toxins are also being described and may explain the recently enhanced virulence of group A streptococcus.

Nonsuppurative Complications

The nonsuppurative complications of streptococcal disease are acute rheumatic fever and acute glomerulonephritis. These conditions are discussed in Chapters 313 and 122, respectively.

Treatment

Rx

During epidemics, particularly when rheumatic fever or post-streptococcal glomerulonephritis is prevalent, treatment of asymptomatic carriers may be necessary. Studies by the U.S. military have shown that monthly injections of benzathine penicillin greatly reduce the incidence of streptococcal pharyngitis and rheumatic fever in young soldiers living in crowded conditions.

Erythromycin resistance of *S. pyogenes* is currently 4% in Western countries. However, in Japan in 1974, the rate reached 72%, and reports of high level resistance have emanated from Scandinavia (100%) and more recently from Pittsburgh, Pennsylvania (>75%). Increased resistance has been proportional to erythromycin usage in each geographic area. Sulfonamide resistance is currently reported in less than 1% of group A streptococcal isolates.

The recommended antimicrobial therapies for group A streptococcal diseases are shown in Table 312–2. Resistance to penicillin has not been described, yet in some settings a lack of in vivo efficacy is seen despite in vitro susceptibility to penicillin. Three mechanisms may explain this lack of efficacy.

1. *β-lactamase production by coinfecting organisms.* Penicillin failure in pharyngitis, tonsillitis, or mixed infections may result from inactivation of penicillin in situ by β-lactamases produced by co-colonizing organisms such as *Bacteroides fragilis, Haemophilus influenzae*, or *Staphylococcus aureus*. For example, the failure rate of penicillin treatment of group A streptococcal pharyngitis may approach 25%, and if such patients are treated with a second course of penicillin, the failure rate may approach 80%, perhaps because of selection of β-lactamase–producing bacteria. In contrast, cure rates of 90% have been achieved when treatment consisted of amoxicillin plus clavulanate or clindamycin.
2. *Genotypic tolerance.* Genotypic tolerance to penicillin may also contribute to penicillin's lack of efficacy in tonsillitis or pharyngitis. In fact, penicillin-tolerant strains have also caused epidemics of pharyngitis. Tolerant strains demonstrate a slower rate of growth, a slower rate of bacterial killing by penicillin, and an absence of β-lactam–induced cell lysis. The role of tolerance in antimicrobial treatment failure is not fully understood.
3. *Inoculum effect.* Studies in animals infected with group A streptococcus demonstrate that penicillin is effective only if it is given early or if small numbers of streptococci are used to initiate infection. It is likely that streptococci are not in a logarithmic phase of growth when the clinical diagnosis of necrotizing fasciitis or myositis is made. Penicillin is most effective against streptococci in log-phase growth, a stage in their life cycle when five penicillin binding proteins are expressed. Conversely, during the stationary phase, the two penicillin binding proteins with the greatest affinity for penicillin are absent.

Clindamycin is superior to penicillin in experimental necrotizing infections. In addition, retrospective clinical studies have substantiated the greater efficacy of clindamycin compared with penicillin in patients with invasive streptococcal infections. Clindamycin's greater efficacy could be the result of its ability to suppress M protein and toxin synthesis, its longer post-antimicrobial effect, an indifference to the in vivo inoculum effect, or its effects on the host's immune system such as suppression of TNF synthesis.

Patients with streptococcal toxic shock syndrome require intensive care monitoring, aggressive fluid replacement, ventilator support, and dialysis, as well as surgical consultation and rapid administration of antimicrobials. Transfusion may be necessary in patients with bacteremia as a result of intravascular hemolysis caused by streptolysin O and S. Because of diffuse capillary leak, albumin levels may drop to 1 g/dL or less, and this change should prompt infusion of colloid. Intravenous gamma-globulin has been shown to reduce mortality in some studies and case reports; however, there is little quality assurance regarding specific antitoxin titers in various batches. More studies are needed, but if gamma-globulin were to be used, it would need to be given promptly to patients with intractable hypotension and organ dysfunction.

TABLE 312–2 ANTIMICROBIAL THERAPY FOR GROUP A STREPTOCOCCAL INFECTIONS

Condition	Route	Doses
PHARYNGITIS AND IMPETIGO		
Benzathine penicillin	IM	1.2 million U (>27 kg)
Penicillin G (or V)	PO	200,000 U qid for 10 days
Erythromycin	PO	40 mg/kg/day (up to 1 g/day)
RECURRENT STREPTOCOCCAL PHARYNGITIS/TONSILLITIS		
Same as above, *or*		
Ampicillin plus clavulanic acid	PO	20–40 mg/kg/day
Oral cephalosporin		Check *PDR*
Clindamycin	PO	10 mg/kg/day
Cellulitis and erysipelas		
Penicillin G or V	PO	200,000 U qid for 10 days
Dicloxacillin*	PO	500 mg qid for 10 days (adults)
NECROTIZING FASCIITIS/MYOSITIS/STREPTOCOCCAL TOXIC SHOCK SYNDROME		
Clindamycin	IV	1,800–2,100 mg/day (adults)
Penicillin	IV	2 million U q4h (adults)
PROPHYLAXIS FOR RHEUMATIC FEVER (CHAPTER 313)		

*Alternative to penicillin if *Staphylococcus aureus* is of concern. Cephalosporins could be used; however, most (except ceftriaxone) have less activity than penicillin G against streptococci.
IM = intramuscular; IV = intravenous; PDR = *Physicians' Desk Reference*; PO = oral.

NON–GROUP A STREPTOCOCCAL INFECTIONS

Group B streptococci are the most common cause of neonatal pneumonia, sepsis, and meningitis in the United States and western Europe (Table 312–3). The incidence is 1.8 to 3.2 cases per 1000 live births.

Clinical Manifestations

Streptococcus agalactiae

Streptococcus agalactiae (group B streptococci) colonizes the vagina, gastrointestinal tract, and occasionally the upper respiratory tract of normal humans. These organisms are recognized as gray-white colonies, slightly larger than group A streptococci, but with a narrower zone of hemolysis. They are resistant to bacitracin, do not hydrolyze bile esculin,

TABLE 312–3 NON–GROUP A STREPTOCOCCAL INFECTIONS

Organism	Lancefield Group	Type of Infection	Therapy
S. agalactiae	B	Neonatal sepsis Postpartum sepsis Septic arthritis Soft tissue infection Osteomyelitis	Ampicillin or penicillin
Enterococcus faecalis/ faecium	D	Endocarditis Bacteremia Urinary tract infection Abscesses, gastrointestinal infection	Chapter 314
S. milleri	A, C, F, G, and nontypable	Abscesses Bacteremia	Penicillin
S. bovis	D	Bacteremia Abscesses	Penicillin
S. equi	C	Bacteremia Cellulitis Pharyngitis	Penicillin
S. canis	G	Bacteremia Cellulitis Pharyngitis	Penicillin
"Viridans"	Nontypable		
S. salivarius		Nonpathogenic	
S. mutans		Endocarditis Caries	Penicillin
S. sanguis		Endocarditis	Penicillin
S. mitior		Endocarditis	Penicillin

demonstrate a positive CAMP (Christie, Atkins, and Munch-Petersen) test, and hydrolyze sodium hippurate. Definitive identification is made with group-specific antiserum or commercial kits that use agglutination end points. The polysaccharide capsule is the prime virulence factor in group B streptococci and is instrumental in the evasion of phagocytosis. Currently, six different capsular polysaccharide types of group B are recognized and are designated Ia, Ib, II, III, IV, and V. Immunity results from the development of opsonic type-specific antibody.

Diagnosis

Preterm infants born to mothers with premature rupture of membranes who are colonized with group B streptococci are at highest risk for early-onset pneumonia and sepsis. The mean time of onset is 20 hours, and symptoms are respiratory distress, apnea, fever, and hypothermia. Ascent of the streptococcus from the vagina to the amniotic cavity causes amnionitis. Infants may aspirate streptococci either from the birth canal during parturition or from amniotic fluid in utero. Radiographic evidence of pneumonia and or hyaline membrane disease is present in 40% of neonates with infection, and meningitis occurs in 30 to 40% of cases. Type III group B streptococcus causes most cases of meningitis.

Late-onset neonatal sepsis occurs 7 to 90 days post partum, with symptoms of fever, poor feeding, lethargy, and irritability. Bacteremia is common, and meningitis occurs in 80% of cases.

Adults with group B infections include postpartum women and patients with peripheral vascular disease, diabetes, or malignant disease. Soft tissue infection, septic arthritis, and osteomyelitis are the most common findings.

Treatment

Although penicillin is the treatment of choice, in practice many neonates are treated empirically with ampicillin (300 to 400 mg/kg/day) plus gentamicin. When the diagnosis is established, penicillin should be given, at 200 to 500,000 U/kg/day. Adults should receive 10 to 12 million U/day of penicillin for bacteremia, soft tissue infection, or osteomyelitis, but the dose should be increased to 18 to 24 million U/day for meningitis. Vancomycin and a first-generation cephalosporin are alternatives for penicillin-allergic patients. Intrapartum administration of ampicillin to women colonized with group B streptococcus who also had premature labor or prolonged rupture of membranes prevents group B neonatal sepsis. Infants should continue to receive ampicillin for 36 hours post partum. It is imperative that women during the third trimester be screened for risk factors for premature labor, and those at high risk should undergo culturing for streptococci. Women in labor who have not had such studies could be screened with a rapid antigen detection kit, even though the false-negative rate may be 10 to 30%. Passive immunization with intravenous immune globulin or active immunization with multivalent polysaccharide vaccine shows promise and is probably the best approach to prevent neonatal sepsis as well as postpartum infection of the mother.

Enterococcus faecalis and *Enterococcus faecium*

These gram-positive, facultatively anaerobic bacteria are usually nonhemolytic but may demonstrate α- or β-hemolysis. Enterococci were previously classified as group D streptococci because they hydrolyze bile esculin and possess the group D antigen. On the basis of nucleic acid hybridization studies, they are now designated *Enterococcus*. Enterococci are commonly isolated from the stool, urine, and sites of intra-abdominal and lower extremity infection. Enterococci cause subacute bacterial endocarditis and have become an important cause of health care–associated infection, not because of increased virulence but because of antimicrobial resistance (Chapter 314).

Streptococcus bovis

Streptococcus bovis is also a cause of subacute bacterial endocarditis and bacteremia in patients with underlying gastrointestinal or malignant disease. Unlike the enterococcus, it remains highly sensitive to penicillin.

Groups C and G Streptococci

These organisms may be isolated from the throats of both humans and dogs, produce streptolysin O, and resemble group A in colony morphology and spectrum of clinical disease. Before rapid identification tests were developed, many infections caused by groups C and G streptococci were mistakenly attributed to group A, such as pharyngitis, cellulitis, skin and wound infections, endocarditis, meningitis, osteomyelitis, and arthritis. Rheumatic fever following group C or G infection has not been described. These strains also cause recurrent cellulitis at the saphenous vein donor site in patients who have undergone coronary artery bypass graft surgery. Both organisms are susceptible to penicillin, erythromycin, vancomycin, and clindamycin.

Streptococcus milleri

Streptococcus milleri bacteria are usually β-hemolytic but may also be nonhemolytic or α-hemolytic and produce minute colonies on blood agar plates. They normally colonize the oropharynx, upper gastrointestinal tract, and appendix. Infections are most commonly related to contiguous abscess formation such as a tooth abscess or periappendiceal abscess. Primary bacteremia with or without endocarditis and metastatic abscesses of the brain, lung, bone, joints, liver, and spleen are characteristic of *S. milleri*.

SUGGESTED READINGS

Bisno AL, Brito MO, Collins CM: Molecular basis of group A streptococcal virulence. Lancet Infect Dis 2003;3:191–200. *Reviews surface proteins, extracellular toxins, and molecular epidemiology.*

Bisno AL, Gerber MA, Gwaltney JM Jr, et al: Practice guidelines for the diagnosis and management of group A streptococcal pharyngitis: Infectious Diseases Society of America. Clin Infect Dis 2002;35:113–125.

Darenberg J, Ihendyane N, Sjolin J, et al, Streptlg Study Group: Intravenous immunoglobulin G therapy in streptococcal toxic shock syndrome: A European randomized, double-blind, placebo-controlled trial. Clin Infect Dis 2003; 37:333–340. *Suggestions but not proof of benefit.*

Humair JP, Revaz SA, Bovier P, et al: Management of acute pharyngitis in adults: Reliability of rapid streptococcal tests and clinical findings. Arch Intern Med 2006;166:640–644. *RSAT had high sensitivity (91%) and specificity (95%) for streptococcal pharyngitis, leading to nearly optimal treatment (94%) and antibiotic prescription (37%), with minimal antibiotic overuse (3%) and underuse (3%).*

Malhotra-Kumar S, Lammens C, Coenen S, et al: Effect of azithromycin and clarithromycin therapy on pharyngeal carriage of macrolide-resistant streptococci in healthy volunteers: A randomised, double-blind, placebo-controlled study. Lancet 2007;369:482–490. *Both macrolides significantly increased the proportion of macrolide-resistant streptococci compared with the placebo at all points studied.*

McIsaac WJ, Kellner JD, Aufricht P, et al: Empirical validation of guidelines for the management of pharyngitis in children and adults. JAMA 2004;291:1587–1595 (erratum in JAMA 2005;294:2700). *Recommendations from two guidelines (those of the Infectious Diseases Society of America and of the American College of Physicians-American Society of Internal Medicine/American Academy of Family Physicians/US Centers for Disease Control and Prevention) were compared with rapid testing alone, a clinical prediction rule, and treatment for positive throat culture results only. Throat culture of all adults or those selected on the basis of a clinical prediction rule had the highest sensitivity and specificity.*

Neuner JM, Hamel MB, Phillips RS, et al: Diagnosis and management of adults with pharyngitis: A cost-effectiveness analysis. Ann Intern Med 2003;139: 113–122. *Observation, culture, and two rapid antigen test strategies for diagnostic testing and treatment in adults have very similar effectiveness and costs, but culture is the least expensive and most effective strategy when the prevalence of streptococcal pharyngitis is approximately 10%.*

Nielsen HU, Kolmos HJ, Frimodt-Moller N: Beta-hemolytic streptococcal bacteremia: A review of 241 cases. Scand J Infect Dis 2002;34:483–486. *In bacteremic patients with erysipelas, mortality increased from 8 to 50% when bullae were observed.*

Stevens DL: Streptococcal toxic shock syndrome. Clin Microbiol Infect 2002;8:133–136. *Overview emphasizing that early diagnosis remains a problem and aggressive surgery often cannot be avoided.*

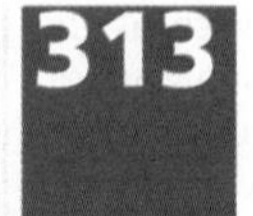

313 RHEUMATIC FEVER

Alan L. Bisno

Definition

Rheumatic fever is an inflammatory disease that occurs as a delayed, nonsuppurative sequela of upper respiratory tract infection with group A streptococci. Its clinical manifestations include polyarthritis, carditis, subcutaneous nodules, erythema marginatum, and chorea in varying combinations. In its classic form, the disorder is acute, febrile, and largely self-limited. However, damage to heart valves may be chronic and progressive and cause cardiac disability or death many years after the initial episode.

Etiology

The development of acute rheumatic fever requires antecedent infection with a specific organism—the group A streptococcus—at a specific body site—the upper respiratory tract. Cutaneous streptococcal infection, a precursor of poststreptococcal acute glomerulonephritis, has never been shown to cause rheumatic fever.

Individual strains of group A streptococci vary in their rheumatogenic potential. In discrete epidemics of acute rheumatic fever in the United States, a limited number of group A streptococcal serotypes tend to predominate (e.g., 3, 5, 18, 24), and the infecting organisms are often heavily encapsulated, as evidenced by their growth as mucoid colonies on blood agar plates.

Epidemiology

The epidemiology of acute rheumatic fever mirrors that of streptococcal pharyngitis. The peak age of incidence is 5 to 15 years, but both primary and recurrent cases occur in adults. Acute rheumatic fever is rare in children younger than 4 years, a fact that has led some observers to speculate that repetitive streptococcal infections are necessary to "prime" the host for the disease. No clear-cut gender predilection has been observed, although certain manifestations, such as Sydenham's chorea and mitral stenosis, are more likely to develop in female patients.

The frequency with which acute rheumatic fever develops after untreated group A streptococcal upper respiratory tract infection differs with the prevalence of highly rheumatogenic strains in the population and the epidemiologic circumstances. In the years after World War II, careful prospective studies were conducted among personnel in military camps suffering from outbreaks of streptococcal infection; acute rheumatic fever developed in approximately 3% of untreated patients. Among children with endemic exposure, attack rates are usually less than 1%. The magnitude of the antistreptolysin O titer increase, persistence of the infecting organism in the pharynx, and clinically severe exudative pharyngitis are associated with a higher risk of rheumatic fever; however, one third or more of cases occur after streptococcal infections that are mild or asymptomatic.

Patients with a history of acute rheumatic fever are susceptible to recurrent attacks after an immunologically significant streptococcal infection. In one long-term prospective study of subjects with a history of rheumatic fever, one of every five documented streptococcal infections gave rise to a recurrence of the disease. The risk of recurrence is greater in patients with preexisting rheumatic heart disease and in those experiencing symptomatic throat infections; the risk declines with advancing age and with increasing interval since the most recent rheumatic attack. Nevertheless, rheumatic patients remain at increased risk well into adult life.

Rheumatic fever occurs in all parts of the world, without any racial predisposition. In temperate climates, acute rheumatic fever peaks in the cooler months of the year, particularly in the winter and early spring. The major environmental factor favoring occurrence appears to be crowding, as in military barracks or similar closed institutions and large households. Crowding favors interpersonal spread of group A streptococci and perhaps enhances streptococcal virulence by frequent human passage.

Acute rheumatic fever is common in developing areas such as the Middle East, the Indian subcontinent, and many nations of Africa. Extremely high acute rheumatic fever attack rates occur among indigenous populations such as the Maori of New Zealand and the Australian aborigines. In striking contrast, the incidence of acute rheumatic fever and the prevalence of rheumatic heart disease have declined both in North America and in western Europe during the 20th century. Rates of fewer than 2 per 100,000 schoolchildren are typical, especially in affluent suburbs. The higher incidence rates reported for blacks than for whites appear to be due to socioeconomic rather than to genetic factors.

The mid-1980s, however, witnessed some startling developments in the epidemiology of acute rheumatic fever in the United States. Outbreaks of the disease were reported from many communities. The largest was in Salt Lake City, Utah, and environs, where more than 500 cases occurred between 1985 and 2001. Equally surprising was that in many of these outbreaks, the victims were predominantly white, middle-class children dwelling in the suburbs. At the same time, epidemics of acute rheumatic fever occurred in military training bases in Missouri and California. Group A streptococci recovered from patients with acute rheumatic fever, their families, and the community and from training camp surveys were generally highly mucoid and belonged to well-established rheumatogenic serotypes (e.g., serotypes 3 and 18). These outbreaks demonstrate that reemergence of rheumatic fever does occur and that appropriate treatment of underlying streptococcal pharyngitis is essential.

Pathobiology

The mechanism by which group A streptococci elicit the connective tissue inflammatory response that constitutes acute rheumatic fever remains unknown. Various theories have been advanced, including toxic effects of streptococcal products such as streptolysins O and S, inflammation mediated by antigen-antibody complexes or streptococcal superantigens, and "autoimmune" phenomena induced by the similarity of certain streptococcal and human tissue antigens (molecular mimicry).

Most authorities currently favor the theory that the tissue damage in acute rheumatic fever is mediated by the host's own immunologic responses to the antecedent streptococcal infection. This theory is rendered more credible by the demonstration of numerous examples of antigenic similarity between somatic constituents of group A streptococci and human tissues, including heart, synovium, and neurons of the basal ganglia of the brain. Taken together, these immunologic cross-reactions could account for most of the manifestations of acute rheumatic fever.

Patients with acute rheumatic fever have, on average, higher titers of antibodies to streptococcal extracellular and somatic antigens than do patients with uncomplicated streptococcal infections. Data relating to cellular immunity are more limited. Patients with acute rheumatic fever exhibit an exaggerated cellular reactivity to streptococcal cell membrane antigens, as demonstrated by in vitro inhibition of migration of peripheral blood lymphocytes. During active rheumatic carditis, both the number of helper (CD4) lymphocytes and the ratio of CD4 to CD8 cells are increased in heart valves and peripheral blood.

Several observations suggest that development of rheumatic fever may be modulated, at least in part, by the specific genetic constitution of the host. These observations include the tendency of rheumatic fever to affect more than one member of a given family, the fact that acute rheumatic fever develops in only a small percentage of all individuals experiencing an immunologically significant streptococcal infection, the tendency of rheumatic individuals to experience recurrent attacks, and the propensity of rheumatic subjects to exhibit exaggerated immunologic responses to streptococcal antigens. To date, however, no consistent associations have been demonstrated between specific class I or class II human leukocyte antigens (HLAs) and susceptibility to acute rheumatic fever. A unique non-HLA alloantigen has been found to be strongly expressed on the B cells of virtually all patients with acute rheumatic fever but in less than 20% of controls.

Pathophysiology

Acute rheumatic fever is characterized by exudative and proliferative inflammatory lesions in connective tissue, especially connective tissue of the heart, joints, and subcutaneous tissue. The early lesions consist of edema of the ground substance, fragmentation of collagen fibers, cellular infiltration, and fibrinoid degeneration. In the heart, diffuse degeneration and even necrosis of muscle cells may be observed. At a slightly later stage, focal perivascular inflammatory lesions develop. These so-called Aschoff's nodules, considered virtually pathognomonic of rheumatic fever, consist of a central area of fibrinoid surrounded by lymphocytes, plasma cells, and large basophilic cells, some of them multinucleate. Many of these cells have elongated nuclei with a distinctive chromatin pattern, sometimes called caterpillar or owl-eye nuclei, depending on their orientation in microscopic cross section. Cells containing these nuclei are called Anichkov's myocytes, even though most authorities believe them to be of mesenchymal origin.

Cardiac findings may include pericarditis, myocarditis, and endocarditis. Foci of coronary arteritis may also be observed. A thickened and roughened area (MacCallum's patch) is frequently present in the left atrium above the posterior leaflet of the mitral valve. Valvar lesions appear early as small verrucae along the line of closure (Fig. 313–1). Later, as healing occurs, the valves may become thickened and deformed, the chordae shortened, and the commissures fused. These changes result in valvar stenosis or insufficiency. The mitral valve is involved most commonly, followed by the aortic, the tricuspid, and very rarely the pulmonic valves.

On pathologic examination, the arthritis of acute rheumatic fever is characterized by a fibrinous exudate and sterile effusion without erosion of the joint surfaces or pannus formation. The subcutaneous nodules have many histologic features in common with Aschoff's nodules and consist of central zones of fibrinoid necrosis surrounded by histiocytes, fibroblasts, occasional lymphocytes, and rare polymorphonuclear cells. Inflammation of the smaller arteries and arterioles may occur throughout the body. Despite pathologic evidence of diffuse vasculitis, aneurysms and thrombosis are not typical features of acute rheumatic fever.

Clinical Manifestations

Rheumatic fever may involve a number of different organ systems, most notably the heart, joints, skin, subcutaneous tissue, and central nervous system, and the clinical picture is variable (Table 313–1). Five clinical features of the disease are so characteristic that they are recognized as major manifestations according to the revised Jones criteria (see

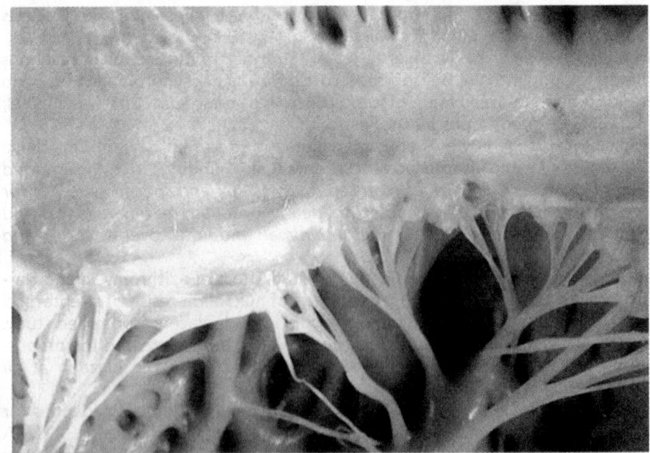

FIGURE 313–1 • Multiple verrucous vegetations along the line of mitral valve closure in a fatal case of acute rheumatic fever. (From Virmani R, Farb A, Burke AP, Narula J: Pathology of acute rheumatic fever. *In* Narula J, Virmani R, Reddy KS, Tandon R [eds]: Rheumatic Fever. Washington, DC, American Registry of Pathology, 1999.)

TABLE 313–1 THE MANY FACES OF ACUTE RHEUMATIC FEVER: POSSIBLE FEATURES

High fever, prostration, crippling polyarthritis
Lassitude, tachycardia, new cardiac murmurs
Acute pericarditis
Fulminant heart failure
Sydenham's chorea without fever or toxicity
Acute abdominal pain mimicking appendicitis
Varying combinations of the above

later) for the diagnosis of acute rheumatic fever: carditis, polyarthritis, chorea, subcutaneous nodules, and erythema marginatum. Other nonspecific findings, including arthralgia, fever, and certain laboratory findings, have been designated minor manifestations.

The latent period between the antecedent streptococcal infection and the onset of symptoms of acute rheumatic fever averages 19 days and ranges between 1 and 5 weeks. When acute polyarthritis is the initial complaint, the onset is often abrupt and may be marked by high fever and toxicity. If isolated carditis is the initial manifestation, the onset may be insidious or even subclinical. Between these two extremes, diverse gradations exist in the initial features of acute rheumatic fever (see Table 313–1). In most attacks, fever and joint involvement are the earliest clinical manifestations, although they may occasionally be preceded by abdominal pain localized to the periumbilical or infraumbilical areas. At times, the location and severity of the pain as well as fleeting signs of peritoneal inflammation may lead to a misdiagnosis of acute appendicitis. Carditis, if it is to appear, usually does so within the initial 3 weeks of the illness. In contrast, chorea tends to occur later in the disease course, sometimes after all other manifestations have subsided. Chorea and polyarthritis rarely occur simultaneously. Epistaxis may be a feature of acute rheumatic fever occurring both at the onset and throughout the acute phase of the illness; it may be severe.

The incidence of major manifestations varies in reported series. Overall, however, arthritis occurs in approximately 75% of initial attacks of acute rheumatic fever, carditis in 40 to 50%, chorea in 15%, and subcutaneous nodules and erythema marginatum in less than 10%. The frequency of individual manifestations varies with age. Carditis is more frequent in the youngest age groups and is relatively uncommon in initial attacks occurring in adults. Chorea occurs primarily in persons between the age of 5 years and puberty. It is seen more frequently in female patients and virtually never occurs in adult men. Thus, the majority of acute rheumatic fever attacks occurring in adults are manifested primarily by arthritis.

Arthritis

Joint involvement ranges from arthralgia alone to acute, disabling arthritis characterized by swelling, warmth, erythema, severe limitation of motion, and exquisite tenderness to pressure. The larger joints of the extremities are usually involved, most frequently the knees and ankles but also the wrists and elbows. The hips and small joints of the hands and feet are affected occasionally. Involvement of shoulders and lumbosacral, cervical, sternoclavicular, and temporomandibular joints occurs in a relatively small percentage of cases. The synovial fluid contains thousands of white blood cells, with a marked preponderance of polymorphonuclear leukocytes; bacterial cultures are sterile. Characteristically, the articular involvement in acute rheumatic fever assumes a pattern of migratory polyarthritis. Migratory does not mean that inflammation in one joint disappears before the next is attacked. Rather, a number of joints are affected in succession, and the periods of involvement overlap. Inflammation in one joint may subside while another is becoming symptomatic, so the process seems to migrate from joint to joint. In untreated cases, as many as 16 joints may be affected, and arthritis develops in more than six joints in about half the patients. This classic migratory pattern is not invariable, however; in some cases, the pattern may be additive, persisting in several joints simultaneously. When effective anti-inflammatory therapy is administered early in the course of the disease, the involvement not infrequently remains monarticular or pauciarticular.

In most instances, inflammation in any one joint begins to subside spontaneously within a week, and the total duration of involvement is no more than 2 or 3 weeks. The entire bout of polyarthritis rarely lasts more than 4 weeks and resolves completely, with no residual joint damage. Some authors have described the rare occurrence of Jaccoud's arthritis, so-called chronic post–rheumatic fever arthropathy of the metacarpophalangeal joints, after repetitive bouts of rheumatic polyarthritis. This entity is not a true arthritis but a form of periarticular fibrosis; its relationship to rheumatic fever remains unresolved.

Carditis

Rheumatic fever may involve the endocardium, myocardium, and pericardium (Table 313–2), and thus the disease is capable of inducing a true pancarditis. Carditis is the most important manifestation of acute rheumatic fever because it is the only one that can cause significant permanent organ damage or death. Although the clinical picture may at times be fulminant, it is more frequently mild or even asymptomatic and may escape notice in the absence of more obvious associated findings, such as arthritis and chorea. The diagnosis of carditis requires the presence of one of the following four manifestations: organic cardiac murmurs not previously present, cardiomegaly, pericarditis, or congestive heart failure. In practice, the characteristic murmurs of acute rheumatic fever are almost always present in cases of rheumatic carditis, unless the ability to hear them is obscured (e.g., loud pericardial friction rub, large pericardial effusion, low cardiac output, severe tachycardia). The diagnosis of carditis should be made with caution in the absence of one of the following three murmurs: apical systolic, apical mid-diastolic, and basal diastolic. Such murmurs, if they are destined to develop, do so usually within the first week and almost always within the first 3 weeks of illness. (An exception to this rule may occur in patients with "pure" chorea; see later.)

TABLE 313–2 CLINICAL MANIFESTATIONS OF CARDITIS IN ACUTE RHEUMATIC FEVER

Murmurs*
Apical systolic
Apical mid-diastolic (Carey Coombs murmur)
Basal diastolic
Pericarditis
Cardiomegaly
Congestive heart failure

*At least one of the characteristic murmurs is almost always present in acute rheumatic carditis.

Certain patients with acute rheumatic fever have echocardiographic evidence of valvar regurgitation in the absence of an audible murmur. Although valvar regurgitation can also be detected in normal individuals by two-dimensional echo-Doppler and color flow Doppler techniques, criteria for discriminating physiologic from pathologic regurgitation have been proposed by experienced investigators. At present, so-called echocarditis is not considered diagnostic of rheumatic carditis for the purpose of fulfilling the Jones criteria, and its prognostic significance remains uncertain. The issue, however, remains controversial.

A number of different rhythm disturbances may occur during the course of acute rheumatic fever. By far the most common is first-degree atrioventricular block. Second- and third-degree heart block, nodal rhythm, and premature contractions may also be observed; atrial fibrillation, on the other hand, is usually a feature of chronic rather than acute rheumatic involvement. Conduction disturbances do not in themselves indicate acute carditis, and their presence or absence is unrelated to the subsequent development of rheumatic heart disease.

Echocardiographic studies have demonstrated that in the absence of preexisting rheumatic valvar disease, patients with acute rheumatic fever and congestive heart failure have preserved left ventricular systolic function but mitral or aortic regurgitation or both. Thus, the etiology of heart failure appears to be valvar dilation and not myocarditis.

In cases of acute rheumatic fever with severe carditis, areas of patchy pneumonitis are sometimes seen. Many observers believe that these pulmonary infiltrates represent a specific rheumatic pneumonia. The case is difficult to prove, however, because of the confusion induced by such confounding clinical entities as pulmonary edema, pulmonary embolization, superimposed bacterial pneumonia, and acute respiratory distress syndrome in these severely ill and toxic patients.

Sydenham's Chorea (Chorea Minor, St. Vitus' Dance)

This neurologic syndrome occurs after a latent period that is variable but on average longer than that associated with the other manifestations of acute rheumatic fever. It frequently occurs in "pure" form, either unaccompanied by other major manifestations or, after a latent period of several months, when all other evidence of acute rheumatic activity has subsided. In some cases of pure chorea, echocardiographic evidence of subclinical valvar regurgitation may be present. Chorea is characterized by rapid, purposeless, involuntary movements, most noticeable in the extremities and face. The arms and legs flail about in erratic, jerky, uncoordinated movements that may sometimes be unilateral (hemichorea). Facial tics, grimaces, grins, and contortions are evident. The speech is usually slurred or jerky. The tongue, when protruded, retracts involuntarily, and asynchronous contractions of lingual muscles produce a "bag of worms" appearance. The involuntary motions disappear during sleep and may be partially suppressed by rest, sedation, or volition.

Patients with chorea display generalized muscle weakness and an inability to maintain a tetanic muscle contraction. Thus, when the patient is asked to squeeze the examiner's fingers, a squeezing and relaxing motion occurs that has been described as milkmaid's grip. The knee jerk may have a pendular quality. No cranial nerve or pyramidal involvement occurs, and sensory modalities are unaffected. The electroencephalogram may display abnormal slow wave activity.

Emotional lability is characteristic of Sydenham's chorea and may often precede other neurologic manifestations, with teachers and parents left puzzled over apparently inexplicable personality changes. Recent interest has focused on the possibility that in a certain subgroup of children, obsessive-compulsive disorder or tic disorders may be triggered by streptococcal infections. Studies of this putative but unproven association, known as post-streptococcal autoimmune neuropsychiatric disorders associated with streptococci (PANDAS), are continuing.

Subcutaneous Nodules

These nodules are firm, painless subcutaneous lesions that vary in size from a few millimeters to approximately 2 cm. The skin overlying them is freely movable and not inflamed. The lesions tend to occur in crops over bone surfaces or prominences and over tendons. Sites of predilection include the extensor surfaces of the elbows, knees, and wrists; the occiput; and the spinous processes of the thoracic and lumbar vertebrae (Fig. 313–2). Nodules are virtually never the sole major manifestation of acute rheumatic fever; they almost always appear in association with carditis, and the cardiac involvement in such cases tends to be clinically severe. Nodules ordinarily do not appear until at least 3 weeks after the onset of an attack and persist for several weeks. They may appear in repeated crops in patients with protracted carditis. Similar nodules may be seen in systemic lupus erythematosus and in rheumatoid arthritis. Subcutaneous nodules in the latter disease are larger and more persistent than those in rheumatic fever.

Erythema Marginatum

The rash begins as an erythematous macule or papule and then extends outward while the skin in the center returns to normal. Adjacent lesions coalesce and form circinate or serpiginous patterns. The lesions may be raised or flat, are neither pruritic nor indurated, and blanch on pressure. They vary greatly in size and appear mostly on the trunk and proximal parts of the extremities, with the face being spared. The lesions are evanescent, migrating from place to place, at times changing before the observer's eyes, and leaving no residual scarring. The erythema may be brought out by applying heat. Individual lesions may come and go in minutes to hours, but the process may go on intermittently for weeks to months uninfluenced by anti-inflammatory therapy. Its persistence is not necessarily an adverse prognostic sign. In most cases, erythema marginatum is accompanied by carditis; it also tends to be associated with subcutaneous nodules.

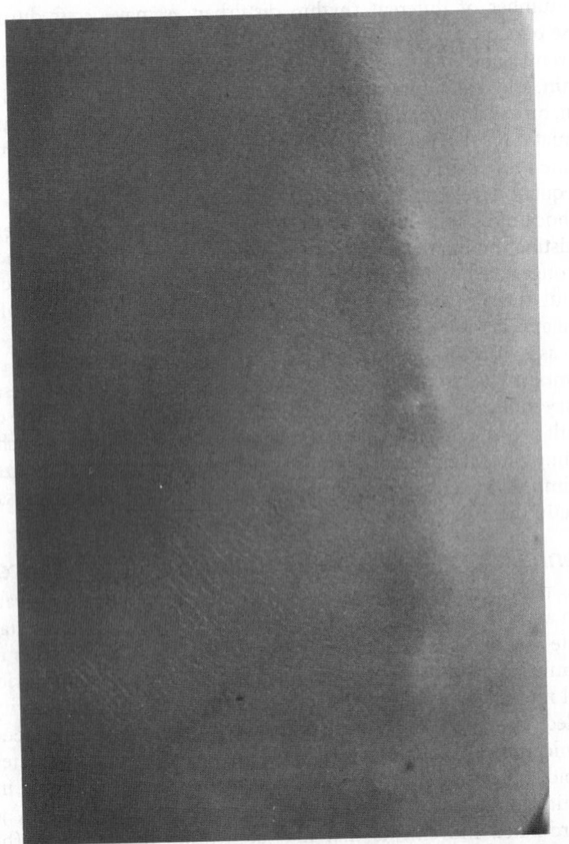

FIGURE 313–2 • Subcutaneous nodules over spinous processes on the back of a patient with acute rheumatic carditis. (Courtesy of S. Levine, MD.)

Diagnosis

No single laboratory test is diagnostic of acute rheumatic fever. Usually, leukocytosis with an increase in the proportion of polymorphonuclear leukocytes is observed. A mild to moderate normocytic, normochromic anemia is the rule. Evidence of acute inflammation is prominent, including elevated serum levels of C-reactive protein and elevation of the erythrocyte sedimentation rate. An exception is pure chorea, which may appear after indices of inflammation have returned to normal.

The urine may contain protein, white cells, and red cells. Biopsy studies have revealed a variety of renal abnormalities, but the classic proliferative glomerular abnormalities that characterize post-streptococcal acute glomerulonephritis occur rarely in acute rheumatic fever. Electrocardiographic and radiographic studies may reveal evidence of rhythm disturbances, pericarditis, or congestive heart failure. Two-dimensional echo-Doppler and color flow Doppler echocardiography may document valvar dysfunction and pericardial effusion.

The major laboratory contribution to the diagnosis of acute rheumatic fever is the documentation of recent group A streptococcal infection. Throat culture should always be performed but is positive in only a minority of cases. The low rate of culture positivity remains unexplained, although it may be due in part to the time lapse of several weeks between the onset of the pharyngeal infection and the throat culture. The serum titer of antistreptolysin O is elevated in 80% or more of patients with acute rheumatic fever. If two streptococcal antibody tests (e.g., antistreptolysin O and anti–DNase B) are performed, an elevated titer of at least one is found in 90% of patients with acute rheumatic fever. The definition of an elevated titer varies, depending on the test used, the patient's age, and the geographic locale. At times, serial sampling may detect an increasing titer of streptococcal antibodies in patients seen early in the course of a rheumatic attack.

Differential Diagnosis

Although acute rheumatic fever is readily recognized in individuals with multiple major manifestations or in epidemic circumstances, the disease may be extraordinarily difficult to diagnose with confidence at other times because of the variability of its clinical features, the frequency with which only a single major manifestation is detected, and the fact that no definitive diagnostic laboratory test is available. Nevertheless, precise diagnosis is especially important in this disease because of the need to advise the patient about prolonged antimicrobial prophylaxis (see later). The diagnostic criteria of T. Duckett Jones, initially proposed in 1944 and subsequently modified by committees of the American Heart Association, attempt to minimize overdiagnosis and underdiagnosis (Table 313–3). The most recent (1992) revision specifies that the guidelines are designed to assist in the diagnosis of the initial attack of acute rheumatic fever, but they are also applicable to patients presenting with recurrent polyarthritis or chorea. Two major manifestations or one major and two minor manifestations indicate a high probability of acute rheumatic fever if supporting evidence of recent streptococcal infection is present. Although a positive throat culture or rapid antigen test for group A streptococci technically satisfies this requirement, streptococcal carriage rates as high as 15% may occur among school-aged children during the fall and winter. Elevated titers of antibodies to streptococcal extracellular products, although not diagnostic of acute rheumatic fever, do indicate a recent, immunologically significant streptococcal infection.

The modified Jones criteria are only guidelines. They are most difficult to apply confidently when polyarthritis is the single major manifestation. Under such circumstances, the diagnosis of acute rheumatic fever should be made only after the exclusion of other causes of polyarthritis, such as

TABLE 313–3 GUIDELINES FOR DIAGNOSIS OF THE INITIAL ATTACK OF RHEUMATIC FEVER (JONES CRITERIA, UPDATED 1992)*

Major Manifestations	Minor Manifestations	Supporting Evidence of Antecedent Group A Streptococcal Infections
Carditis	Clinical findings	Positive throat culture or rapid streptococcal antigen test
Polyarthritis	Arthralgia	
Chorea	Fever	
Erythema marginatum	Laboratory findings	Elevated or rising streptococcal antibody titer
Subcutaneous nodules	↑Acute phase reactants	
	↑Erythrocyte sedimentation rate	
	↑C-reactive protein	
	Prolonged PR interval	

*If supported by evidence of preceding group A streptococcal infection, the presence of two major manifestations or one major and two minor manifestations indicates a high probability of acute rheumatic fever.
From Special Writing Group of the Committee on Rheumatic Fever, Endocarditis, and Kawasaki Disease of the Council on Cardiovascular Disease in the Young of the American Heart Association: Guidelines for the diagnosis of rheumatic fever. Jones criteria, 1992 update. JAMA 1992;268:2069–2073, with permission. Copyright, 1992, American Medical Association.

rheumatoid arthritis, Still's disease, Lyme disease, viral arthritides (e.g., rubella, hepatitis B), the early prepurpuric phase of Henoch-Schönlein purpura, and septic arthritis including gonococcal arthritis. As experience grows, the echocardiographic demonstration of valvar insufficiency (by use of strict criteria to differentiate physiologic regurgitation) may help clarify the diagnosis in some cases. Echocardiography is of established value in the evaluation and management of acute and chronic rheumatic heart disease.

Some patients have been described as manifesting polyarthritis that is atypical in time of onset and duration, does not respond dramatically to salicylate therapy, and is unassociated with other clinical features of acute rheumatic fever. Such individuals have on occasion been categorized as having "post-streptococcal reactive arthritis." The existence of this entity as a distinct syndrome, however, and its relationship to rheumatic fever remain uncertain. Pending further clarification, such individuals should be considered to have acute rheumatic fever if they fulfill the Jones criteria and alternative diagnoses have been excluded.

Serum sickness is frequently a serious consideration, particularly if the patient has received penicillin or other antibiotics for a preceding respiratory infection. Systemic lupus erythematosus, sickle cell hemoglobinopathies, and infective endocarditis may involve the joints and the heart. Other differential diagnostic considerations include congenital heart lesions, viral and idiopathic forms of myocarditis and pericarditis, and functional heart murmurs. Nonfamilial forms of chorea have been described in systemic lupus erythematosus, rarely in association with the use of birth control pills, and in patients with neoplasms involving the basal ganglia. The involuntary jerks of Gilles de la Tourette syndrome may be confused with chorea. It remains uncertain how often episodes of chorea occurring during pregnancy (chorea gravidarum) represent attacks of rheumatic fever. Other disorders that may at times be confused with acute rheumatic fever are gout, sarcoidosis, Hodgkin's disease, and acute leukemia.

In certain circumstances, acute rheumatic fever can be diagnosed even when the guidelines set forth in Table 313–3 have not been met, provided that alternative diagnoses are excluded. Because of the long latent period between the antecedent streptococcal infection and the appearance of the neurologic abnormalities in some patients with Sydenham's chorea, evidence of inflammation encompassed in the minor manifestations may no longer be present, and previously elevated antibody titers may have declined to normal. A similar situation occasionally occurs in patients with indolent carditis, who may not come to medical attention until a prolonged period after the onset of the disease.

Treatment

Rx

Antibiotics neither modify the course of a rheumatic attack nor influence the subsequent development of carditis. Nevertheless, it is conventional to give a course of antibiotics designed to eradicate any rheumatogenic group A streptococci remaining in the tonsils and pharynx to prevent spread of the organism to close contacts. The recommended regimens are those conventionally used for the treatment of acute streptococcal pharyngitis (Chapter 312). Benzathine penicillin G is preferred in non–penicillin-allergic patients. After completion of this therapy, continuous antistreptococcal prophylaxis should commence (see later discussion).

Treatment with anti-inflammatory agents is effective in suppressing many of the signs and symptoms of acute rheumatic fever. [1] These agents do not "cure" the disease, nor do they prevent the subsequent evolution of rheumatic heart disease. They should be avoided in mild or equivocal cases because by suppressing the clinical manifestations, they may obscure the diagnosis. The two drugs most widely used are aspirin and corticosteroids. Aspirin is used in patients with acute polyarthritis, as long as carditis is either absent or mild and no evidence of congestive heart failure is found. Aspirin is effective in decreasing fever, toxicity, and joint inflammation. It should be given in a dosage of 90 to 100 mg/kg/day in children and 6 to 8 g/day in adults administered in equally divided doses every 4 hours for the initial 24 to 36 hours; thereafter, it may be given in four doses during waking hours. Maintenance of a salicylate level of 25 mg/dL is usually satisfactory. The incidence of nausea and vomiting may be minimized by starting somewhat below the optimal dosage level and gradually increasing during a few days. The patient should be observed for evidence of significant gastrointestinal bleeding and for signs and symptoms of salicylism (e.g., hyperpnea, tinnitus). After 1 to 2 weeks, the dosage is reduced to 60 to 70 mg/kg/day for an additional 6 weeks. These dosage schedules represent general guidelines only. The precise aspirin dose must be determined by the patient's clinical response, blood salicylate levels, and tolerance of the drug.

Corticosteroids are generally reserved for patients who have severe carditis manifested by congestive heart failure, who are unable to tolerate large doses of salicylates, or whose signs and symptoms are inadequately suppressed by aspirin. As with aspirin, the dosage must be individualized. Prednisone, 40 to 60 mg/day in divided doses, may be used initially. After 2 to 3 weeks, it should be withdrawn slowly during an additional 3-week period. In cases of fulminating carditis with profound heart failure, intravenous corticosteroids may be used, and emergent valve replacement may at times be life-saving. As for other patients receiving corticosteroids, the physician should be alert to problems such as gastrointestinal bleeding, sodium and water retention, and impaired glucose tolerance. Suppression of the pituitary-adrenal axis or the host immune system is a potential problem but not ordinarily a major one during this relatively short course of treatment. Although nonsteroidal anti-inflammatory drugs would appear a reasonable alternative for patients who do not tolerate salicylates but do not require

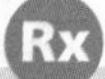

corticosteroids, there is a paucity of data on the use of these agents in acute rheumatic fever. Two small studies, one using naproxen and one tolmetin, reported nonsteroidal anti-inflammatory drugs equivalent to aspirin in efficacy with fewer side effects. Further experience with these agents is required before specific recommendations can be made.

After cessation of anti-inflammatory therapy, clinical or laboratory evidence of acute rheumatic fever may reappear. Such therapeutic "rebounds" occur more frequently after corticosteroid therapy than after treatment with aspirin. They may be minimized by prolonging salicylate therapy for 9 to 12 weeks and, when corticosteroids have been required, by continuing aspirin for a month after corticosteroid use has been discontinued. Congestive heart failure is managed by conventional measures but with the recognition that in patients without preexisting rheumatic heart disease, myocardial function is usually well preserved (see earlier discussion). If digitalis is used, the potential risk of drug-induced arrhythmias in patients with active myocarditis must be kept in mind. Patients with Sydenham's chorea require a quiet environment. Corticosteroids and sedatives such as phenobarbital or diazepam may be helpful. Trials of plasmapheresis and intravenous immune globulin in the management of severe and intractable chorea are currently in progress.

TABLE 313–4 SECONDARY PREVENTION OF RHEUMATIC FEVER (PREVENTION OF RECURRENT ATTACKS)

Agent	Dose	Mode
Benzathine penicillin G	1,200,000 U every 4 wk* *or*	Intramuscular
Penicillin V	250 mg twice daily *or*	Oral
Sulfadiazine	0.5 g once daily for patients ≤ 27 kg (60 lb)	Oral
	1.0 g once daily for patients > 27 kg (60 lb)	
For individuals allergic to penicillin and sulfadiazine		
Erythromycin	250 mg twice daily	Oral

*In high-risk situations, administration every 3 weeks is justified and recommended.

From Dajani A, Taubert K, Ferrieri P, et al: Treatment of acute streptococcal pharyngitis and prevention of rheumatic fever: A statement for health professionals. Committee on Rheumatic Fever, Endocarditis, and Kawasaki Disease of the Council on Cardiovascular Disease in the Young, the American Heart Association. Pediatrics 1995;96:758. Copyright American Academy of Pediatrics.

TABLE 313–5 DURATION OF SECONDARY RHEUMATIC FEVER PROPHYLAXIS

Category	Duration
Rheumatic fever with carditis and residual heart disease (persistent valvar disease*)	At least 10 yr since last episode and at least until age 40 yr, sometimes lifelong prophylaxis
Rheumatic fever with carditis but no residual heart disease (no valvar disease*)	10 yr or well into adulthood, whichever is longer
Rheumatic fever without carditis	5 yr or until age 21 yr, whichever is longer

*Clinical or echocardiographic evidence.

From Dajani A, Taubert K, Ferrieri P, et al: Treatment of acute streptococcal pharyngitis and prevention of rheumatic fever: A statement for health professionals. Committee on Rheumatic Fever, Endocarditis, and Kawasaki Disease of the Council on Cardiovascular Disease in the Young, the American Heart Association. Pediatrics 1995;96:758. Copyright American Academy of Pediatrics.

Prevention

Primary prevention of acute rheumatic fever consists of accurate diagnosis and appropriate treatment of streptococcal sore throat (Chapter 312). Although straightforward in theory, primary prevention is often frustratingly difficult to achieve. In many of the densely populated indigent communities in which the risk of acute rheumatic fever is greatest, children with self-limited illnesses such as sore throats may never come to medical attention, and throat culture services are usually unavailable to aid in diagnosis. Moreover, in one third or more of cases, acute rheumatic fever may arise after a clinically unapparent streptococcal infection.

Perhaps the most effective strategy for avoiding the mortality and chronic cardiac disability associated with acute rheumatic fever is that of secondary prevention. This strategy focuses on the group of persons who have already suffered a rheumatic attack and who experience a high rate of recurrence after an immunologically significant streptococcal upper respiratory tract infection. Recurrent attacks tend to be mimetic in nature, so patients who have suffered carditis with their previous attack are likely to have repetitive cardiac involvement and progressive cardiac damage. However, carditis with recurrent attacks of acute rheumatic fever may develop even in patients who experienced only arthritis or chorea in their initial attack; thus, all patients who have experienced a documented attack of acute rheumatic fever should receive continuous antimicrobial prophylaxis to prevent either symptomatic or asymptomatic streptococcal infections. The specific regimens to be used are indicated in Table 313–4. The most effective of these regimens is intramuscular benzathine penicillin G. 2 Rheumatic recurrences are unusual in compliant patients receiving an injection every 4 weeks. In areas of the world where the incidence of acute rheumatic fever and the risk of recurrence are high, however, injections every 3 weeks provide more complete protection.

The total duration of intramuscular or oral rheumatic fever prophylaxis remains unresolved. The risk of rheumatic recurrence is known to diminish with increasing age and increasing interval since the most recent rheumatic attack. Patients who escape carditis during their initial attack are less likely to experience rheumatic recurrences and are less susceptible to the development of carditis if a recurrence does ensue. These facts suggest that prophylaxis need not be perpetual for all rheumatic subjects. Recommendations of the American Heart Association for the duration of secondary prophylaxis are listed in Table 313–5. The decision to remove a rheumatic subject from continuous prophylaxis should be an individualized one based on the physician's assessment of the risk and probable consequences of recurrence and taken with the patient's informed consent. Particular care should be taken with those at high risk of streptococcal acquisition (e.g., parents of schoolchildren, schoolteachers, military recruits, nurses, pediatricians, and residents of areas with a high incidence of acute rheumatic fever). Patients taken off prophylaxis must be instructed to return immediately for medical follow-up whenever symptoms of pharyngitis occur.

Patients with rheumatic valvar heart disease must receive prophylaxis designed to avoid bacterial endocarditis whenever they undergo dental or surgical procedures likely to evoke bacteremia. Such prophylaxis is not necessary in a rheumatic subject who is free of residual heart disease. Regimens to prevent endocarditis (Chapter 76) are different from those prescribed for preventing acute rheumatic fever, and the fact that a patient is receiving rheumatic fever prophylaxis does not exempt that patient from endocarditis prophylaxis. This concept is a frequent point of confusion not only among patients but among physicians and dentists as well.

Prognosis

The average duration of an untreated attack of acute rheumatic fever is approximately 3 months. The duration tends to be longer, up to 6 months, in patients with severe carditis. Less than 5% of patients have continuing rheumatic activity for longer than 6 months. In a few of these patients, the disease is limited to chorea and is otherwise benign. Other patients exhibit evidence of persistent inflammatory activity, including arthritis, carditis, and subcutaneous nodules. "Chronic rheumatic fever" occurs more frequently in patients who have had one or more previous attacks; cardiac involvement in chronic rheumatic fever tends to be frequent and severe.

Congestive heart failure occurring in patients without preexisting rheumatic heart disease is not due to myocarditis per se but rather to inflammatory valvulitis and annular dilation, accompanied in more severe cases by chordal elongation and mitral valve leaflet prolapse. Death from intractable congestive failure during the acute phase of acute rheumatic fever is rare. Once the acute attack has subsided, the only long-term sequela is that of rheumatic heart disease, manifested primarily by scarring or calcification of the mitral and aortic valves (Chapter 75) and leading to insufficiency or stenosis. The prognosis from a cardiac standpoint is related to the clinical findings when the patient is initially seen. In one large study, for example, 347 patients were examined during an acute rheumatic attack and again 10 years later. Among patients who had been free of carditis during their acute attack, only 6% had residual heart disease on follow-up. Patients with mild carditis during their acute attack (i.e., apical systolic murmur without pericarditis or heart failure) had a relatively good prognosis in that only approximately 30% had heart murmurs 10 years later. About 40% of subjects with apical or basal diastolic murmurs and 70% of subjects with heart failure or pericarditis during their acute attacks had residual rheumatic heart disease. The prognosis was worse in patients with preexisting rheumatic heart disease and in those who had experienced recurrent attacks of acute rheumatic fever in the 10-year interval.

These data indicate that patients in whom carditis does not develop during an acute attack and who are protected from recurrences of acute rheumatic fever are unlikely to suffer from rheumatic heart disease. Patients with pure chorea represent an exception to this rule. Some patients who have no evidence of carditis when they are initially examined may have rheumatic valvar disease on prolonged follow-up. Although the explanation for this phenomenon is unknown, it is conceivable that in view of the long latent period associated with chorea, signs of carditis might have been present earlier but subsided by the time that the neurologic abnormality became evident. Moreover, echocardiographic studies have detected subclinical valvulitis in some of these patients.

Once the acute attack has subsided completely, the patient's subsequent level of physical activity depends on cardiac status. Patients without residual heart disease may resume full and unrestricted activity. It is important that patients not be subjected to unwarranted invalidism because of either their own inaccurate perceptions of the nature of the rheumatic process or those of parents, teachers, or employers.

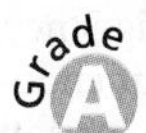

1. Cilliers AM, Manyemba J, Saloojee H: Anti-inflammatory treatment for carditis in acute rheumatic fever. Cochrane Database Syst Rev 2003;2:CD003176.
2. Manyemba J, Mayosi BM: Intramuscular penicillin is more effective than oral penicillin in secondary prevention of rheumatic fever—a systematic review. S Afr Med J 2003;93:212–218.

SUGGESTED READINGS

Carapetis JR, McDonald M, Wilson NJ: Acute rheumatic fever. Lancet 2005; 366:155–168. *A comprehensive review.*

Cunningham MW: Autoimmunity and molecular mimicry in the pathogenesis of post-streptococcal heart disease. Front Biosci 2003;8:s533–s543. *A review of current concepts of rheumatic fever pathogenesis by a leading investigator in this field.*

Gentles TL, Colan SD, Wilson NJ, et al: Left ventricular mechanics before and after acute rheumatic fever: Contractile dysfunction is closely related to valve regurgitation. J Am Coll Cardiol 2001;37:201–207. *A study characterizing left ventricular mechanics in acute rheumatic fever and defining the factors contributing to myocardial damage during and after the acute attack.*

Ravisha MS, Tullu MS, Kamat JR: Rheumatic fever and rheumatic heart disease: Clinical profile of 550 cases in India. Arch Med Res 2003;34:382–387. *This analysis documents the clinical manifestations in the initial attack of rheumatic fever in 550 patients studied during 31 years.*

Veasy LG, Tani LY, Daly JA, et al: Temporal association of the appearance of mucoid strains of *Streptococcus pyogenes* with a continuing high incidence of rheumatic fever in Utah. Pediatrics 2004;113(pt 1):e168–e172. *Evidence of the importance of rheumatogenic streptococcal strains in the pathogenesis of acute rheumatic fever.*

314 ENTEROCOCCAL INFECTIONS

Eli N. Perencevich and Trish M. Perl

Definition

Enterococci, formerly called group D streptococci, are endogenous human flora that have often been considered pathogens with low virulence. However, over the past 2 decades they have emerged as increasingly important health care–acquired (nosocomial) pathogens. This emergence is predominately due to their inherent resistance to commonly used antimicrobials, acquisition of high-level resistance to vancomycin, persistence in the environment, and transmission from patient to patient via the contaminated hands of health care workers. The emergence of vancomycin-resistant enterococci (VRE) has limited the therapeutic options in confirmed enterococcal infections and in empirical treatment of infections in severely ill hospitalized patients. Ten to 30% of enterococcal isolates from hospitalized patients are now reported to be highly resistant to vancomycin. Recently, there have been several reported cases of vancomycin-resistant *Staphylococcus aureus* (VRSA). In each case, the *Staphylococcus* is believed to have acquired a vancomycin resistance gene (vanA) from a VRE isolate that colonized the same VRSA-infected patient. Such acquisition highlights the fact that resistance in one species can have an impact on the evolution of resistance in another pathogenic species and that failure to control one species can have a negative impact on patient outcomes in those infected with other bacteria.

Enterococci are common residents of the human gastrointestinal tract and the female genitourinary tract and act as opportunistic pathogens in severely ill patients. They are known to cause urinary tract infections (UTIs), intra-abdominal abscesses, bacteremia, endocarditis, and less commonly, osteoarticular infections and meningitis.

The Pathogen

Members of the genus *Enterococcus* were classified within group D of the genus *Streptococcus.* However, in the past 25 years they have been reclassified on the basis of new molecular and genetic analyses. Enterococci are catalase-negative gram-positive cocci that can appear singly or in pairs of short chains. They are facultative anaerobes that grow optimally at 35° C in broth containing 6.5% NaCl and hydrolyze esculin in the presence of 40% bile salts (bile-esculin medium). Demonstration of group D antigen may assist in the identification of enterococci; however, it is not a particularly sensitive test because the antigen is present in about 80% of enterococcal strains. *Enterococcus faecalis,* the most common cause of enterococcal infection in humans, is the causative agent for 80 to 90% of enterococcal infections, followed by *Enterococcus faecium,* which is found in 5 to 10% of infections. *Enterococcus casseliflavus* and *Enterococcus raffinosus* have been reported in clustered infections. Other *Enterococcus* species reported to cause infections in humans include *E. avium, E. cecorum, E. dispar, E. durans, E. gallinarum, E. gilvus, E. hirae, E. mundtii,* and *E. pallens.*

Epidemiology

The proportion of infections caused by enterococci in hospitalized patients has been increasing over the past several decades. Overall, UTIs are the most common clinical condition attributable to enterococci. *Enterococcus* species are now the second most common isolate from UTIs in hospitalized patients; they cause 14 to 16% of these infections in North

America and can be involved in both complicated and uncomplicated UTI. Enterococci are the third or fourth most common cause of nosocomial blood stream infections and are involved in approximately 5 to 15% of all cases of infective endocarditis. Overall, they are the second most common nosocomial pathogen in the United States.

Enterococci are part of the normal human gut flora, and infections in both hospitalized and nonhospitalized patients can arise from an endogenous source. However, most infections are acquired in the hospital and appear to result from an exogenous source, which means that transmission from the environment, another patient, or the hands of a health care worker has occurred before infection. Nearly all infections are preceded by some period of colonization, and although infection does not develop in most colonized patients, they are still able to shed and transmit bacteria to other hospitalized patients. Increasingly, hospitalized patients, if they are colonized or infected with an *Enterococcus* species, tend to have a strain resistant to vancomycin (i.e., VRE).

VRE were first reported in Europe in 1986. Since the mid-1990s the proportion of enterococcal strains resistant to vancomycin has risen steadily. Approximately 10 to 30% of hospital isolates are now resistant to vancomycin. According to the National Nosocomial Infections Surveillance System of the Centers for Disease Control and Prevention, the proportion of nosocomial enterococcal infections in intensive care unit (ICU) patients that were VRE in 2003 was 28.5%, a 12% increase over the preceding 5-year period. There are several genotypes and phenotypes for acquired vancomycin resistance, with vanA and vanB being the most common operons found in clinical isolates. vanA encodes high-level resistance to vancomycin and teicoplanin and is carried on a transposon usually found on a plasmid that is transferable to other gram-positive cocci, including *S. aureus.* vanB encodes variable resistance to vancomycin but not teicoplanin.

The epidemiology of VRE differs between Europe and North America. In Europe, VRE are often detected in farm animals, probably because of use of the antibiotic avoparcin in animal feeds until it was banned in 1997. The proportion of VRE among enterococcal clinical isolates in hospitalized Europeans has historically been lower than in the United States; however, these rates are increasing. In the United States, avoparcin was never used in animal feeds, and therefore VRE are not usually found in farm animals or healthy humans. In contrast, the proportion of enterococcal isolates resistant to vancomycin is higher in U.S. hospitals than in European hospitals.

The most common mode of nosocomial transmission of VRE is patient-to-patient cross-transmission by the hands of health care workers who become transiently colonized with the organism. Enterococci with genetic relatedness by pulsed-field gel electrophoresis have been cultured on the hands of health care workers caring for infected patients. A study in a U.S. hospital's medical ICU found that the number of patients already colonized with VRE in a defined geographic area ("colonization pressure") was the most significant variable in predicting new acquisition of VRE. This finding was significant in that it highlights the important role that patient-to-patient transmission has had in the emergence of VRE. Similarly, a study involving hemodialysis patients found that the only significant predictor of VRE colonization was hospitalization in the previous year, thus suggesting the importance of nosocomial transmission in the acquisition of VRE, and a study in hospitalized patients recently admitted to non-ICU wards found that the most sensitive factor for predicting VRE colonization on surveillance culture was previous admission to an acute care hospital in the past year. Importantly, once colonized with VRE, patients may harbor the strain in their gastrointestinal tract for years.

Apart from preexisting gastrointestinal colonization, risk factors for enterococcal infection, particularly VRE infection, include severe underlying conditions such as renal failure, previous solid organ or bone marrow transplantation, solid and hematologic malignancy, diabetes mellitus, and neutropenia. Other factors associated with infection include previous surgical or gastrointestinal procedure, the presence of a vascular or urinary indwelling catheter, hospital factors such as location in the ICU or oncology ward, proximity to colonized patients, prolonged length of hospitalization, and recent antimicrobial exposure.

Numerous epidemiologic investigations have revealed that most classes of antimicrobials have been associated with VRE infections. In particular, the use of vancomycin and cephalosporins has been linked to acquisition of VRE. However, the observational nature of these studies, including the difficulty in controlling for preexisting comorbid conditions and the underlying severity of illness, makes measuring the attributable impact of a particular antibiotic on acquisition of VRE difficult. Antimicrobial agents with antianaerobic activity seem to be associated with increased risk for stool colonization by VRE.

Pathobiology

Enterococci are commensals that colonize the human gastrointestinal and female genital tracts. Although they are not as intrinsically virulent as other gram-positive pathogens, under certain conditions the commensal relationship is disrupted and serious infections occur. Several adhesion factors, including aggregation substance, have been identified that allow binding to epithelial surfaces and enhance the colonization ability of enterococci. The ability to adhere to heart valves and urinary tract epithelium enables enterococci to cause endocarditis and UTIs. Enterococci are also known to secrete potential virulence factors, including cytolysin/hemolysin, which is a bacterial toxin that is produced in a higher proportion of infecting strains than in stool-colonizing strains. Infecting strains also possess the ability of intestinal translocation, although the exact mechanisms of this process have yet to be determined. To this point, little is known about the host defense mechanisms in enterococcal infections. In addition, the exact role of capsular polysaccharides in colonization or infection is unknown. Strains have been shown to survive within phagocytic cells, yet it is unclear whether such survival represents successful host defense or evasion by enterococci. The inherent resistance to multiple antimicrobials that enterococci possess enhances their ability to survive and multiply in the many hospitalized patients treated with broad-spectrum antimicrobials.

Clinical Manifestations

There are no specific clinical manifestations to help distinguish enterococcal infections from those caused by other bacteria. Enterococci are not thought to cause lower respiratory tract infections or ventilator-associated pneumonia and, if found in these settings, probably represent colonization and not infection.

Urinary Tract Infections

UTIs are the most frequent type of infection caused by enterococci. Most infections are nosocomial in origin and include uncomplicated cystitis, pyelonephritis, prostatitis, and perinephric abscess. These infections are typically secondary to urinary catheterization or instrumentation. In contrast to nosocomial UTI, enterococci cause less than 5% of uncomplicated cases of cystitis or pyelonephritis in otherwise healthy nonhospitalized women. Patients with diabetes mellitus appear to be at increased risk for enterococcal UTI. Bacteremia is only infrequently associated with enterococcal UTI.

Bacteremia

The incidence of bacteremia caused by enterococci continues to increase. Specific risk factors include prolonged hospitalization, preexisting urethral catheters or intravascular lines, recent surgery, malignancy, neutropenia, and biliary pathology. Secondary bacteremia without endocarditis usually arises from the urinary tract, hepatobiliary tract, or soft tissue infection. Bacteremia secondary to an intra-abdominal source carries a high mortality rate. Risk factors for VRE bacteremia parallel those mentioned earlier but additionally include severe preexisting comorbid conditions such as hematologic malignancy, infection with human immunodeficiency virus, chronic renal insufficiency, liver transplantation, and previous exposure to broad-spectrum antimicrobials, including those with antianaerobic activity such as clindamycin or metronidazole. Enterococcal bacteremia is frequently polymicrobial, and the clinical picture is often influenced by whether enterococci are isolated alone or with other bacteria. When enterococci are the sole organisms isolated, the course is typically indolent, and fever is frequently the only sign. In contrast, polymicrobial bacteremia is more severe and often manifested as shock or disseminated intravascular coagulation. VRE bacteremia is associated with higher mortality rates than bacteremia with vancomycin-susceptible strains, and treatment with an appropriate antibiotic within the first 48 hours has been associated with improved outcomes.

Endocarditis

Enterococci, particularly *E. faecalis,* are an increasingly frequent cause of endocarditis, even though most enterococcal bacteremias are not complicated by endocarditis. The disease occurs most often in older patients, with a male preponderance. Most cases appear to arise in the community; however, nosocomial cases do occur. Patients with preexisting valvar heart disease, including prosthetic valves, are at highest risk, yet many patients lack underlying heart disease. Enterococci more commonly cause left-sided endocarditis with a mitral valve predominance. The clinical picture most closely resembles subacute bacterial endocarditis, similar to viridans streptococci, with many patients having symptoms for weeks or months before seeking medical care.

Intra-abdominal Infections

In intra-abdominal infections, enterococci are often detected in mixed culture. These infections typically arise from a hepatobiliary source, including postoperative infection in liver transplants, and are complicated by secondary bacteremia.

Skin and Soft Tissue Infections

Enterococci rarely cause cellulitis or other soft tissue infections alone but are often isolated in mixed surgical site infections, diabetic foot infections, and decubitus ulcers along with other gram-negative bacilli, gram-positive cocci, and anaerobic bacteria. Their clinical significance in these situations has not been adequately quantified. Enterococci are not thought to be primary pathogens in chronic osteomyelitis. When they are identified, it is believed that they may represent solely superinfection, and thus adequate therapy may not require antibiotics directed at enterococcal eradication.

Diagnosis

Diagnosis of an enterococcal infection is made by isolating the organism through culture of a sterile site, such as blood or urine. The diagnosis and differential diagnosis of specific conditions are the same as discussed for UTIs (Chapter 306) and endocarditis (Chapter 76).

Treatment

Rx

Therapy for enterococcal infections is complicated by the fact that strains exhibit inherent resistance to many commonly used antibiotics, including cephalosporins. In fact, even when enterococci appear to be susceptible to trimethoprim-sulfamethoxazole in vitro, it should not be used for therapy because clinical failures have been reported secondary to the ability of enterococci to utilize exogenous folate. Recently, isolation of *E. faecium* strains with intrinsic resistance to penicillins has been increasing. Importantly, *E. faecalis* is intrinsically resistant to quinupristin/dalfopristin; therefore, these antibiotics should not be used in therapy for infections caused by this species. However, most *E. faecalis* strains remain susceptible to ampicillin, in contrast to most *E. faecium* strains, which are resistant to ampicillin. In addition, enterococci have acquired resistance to a wide-range of antibiotic classes, including aminoglycosides, β-lactams, fluoroquinolones, lincosamides, macrolides, oxazolidinones (linezolid), quinupristin/dalfopristin, rifampin, tetracyclines, and vancomycin. Thus, effective directed therapy for any severe enterococcal infection requires susceptibility testing by experienced microbiology laboratories with therapy adjusted according to results of culture. Optimal therapy for most infections includes intravenous ampicillin, penicillin, or vancomycin. Given the resistance or tolerance to cell wall–targeting antibiotics, including penicillins and vancomycin, standard therapy with these antibiotics, except for UTIs, should include the addition of an aminoglycoside (streptomycin or gentamicin). This strategy of two-drug therapy has been associated with improved outcomes. If VRE strains are known to be susceptible, potential therapy for these infections includes linezolid, quinupristin/dalfopristin, and the newly Food and Drug Administration–approved daptomycin. There have already been reports of the emergence of resistance in enterococcal strains to all three of these newer antibiotics. Quinupristin/dalfopristin is associated with myalgias and arthralgias, and linezolid is associated with bone marrow suppression, including thrombocytopenia, and both have only bacteriostatic activity against the enterococci. Given the complexity of enterococcal infections, an infectious disease consultation should be considered for therapeutic guidance.

Urinary Tract Infections

A single agent can generally be used to treat enterococcal UTIs, including ampicillin (1 g every 6 hours), amoxicillin (500 mg every 8 hours), or intravenous vancomycin (1 g every 12 hours). Vancomycin is typically reserved for penicillin-allergic patients or if the strain has high-level penicillin resistance. β-Lactam/β-lactamase inhibitor combinations are usually reserved for polymicrobial infections. Nitrofurantoin is also occasionally used because most strains remain susceptible. Duration is dependent on whether the UTI is complicated.

Bacteremia without Endocarditis

Many cases of enterococcal bacteremia are transient or self-limited, yet antibiotic therapy with penicillin or ampicillin has been shown to improve outcomes. Unlike endocarditis therapy, it is not known whether patients benefit from combination therapy (penicillin, ampicillin, or vancomycin plus an aminoglycoside), except perhaps when an indwelling intravascular catheter is present. In the setting of an indwelling intravascular catheter, removal of the catheter should be considered.

Endocarditis

Combination therapy (intravenous penicillin, ampicillin, or vancomycin plus an aminoglycoside) is the standard therapy for enterococcal endocarditis. Doses and durations can be found in Chapter 76. The duration of therapy is typically 4 weeks, with a 6-week duration used in patients who have had prolonged symptoms before seeking therapy, prosthetic valve infection, or relapse after initial treatment. If the causative enterococcal strain is highly resistant to both gentamicin and streptomycin aminoglycosides, alternative agents or durations, or both, must be explored, and surgery to excise infected valves should be considered. Optimal therapy for VRE strains that are resistant to ampicillin is not known but includes combination therapy under the guidance of an infectious disease consultant. Several newly approved agents, including quinupristin/dalfopristin, linezolid, and daptomycin, could be considered if the strain is found to be susceptible. VRE endocarditis may require early surgery because outcomes with antibiotic therapy can be poor. Careful microbiologic and clinical assessment of all patients with enterococcal endocarditis and VRE in particular is helpful in deciding when surgery is necessary. If repeated blood cultures remain positive for more than 7 days during medical therapy or other signs of uncontrolled infection (persistent fever or leukocytosis) are present, surgical repair of the valve or valve replacement should be considered early in the treatment course if there are no absolute contraindications to surgery.

Primary Prevention

At this point, the concept of an enterococcal vaccine is purely theoretical. Although high-risk groups such as ICU patients have been identified, their period of risk is short, which suggests that targeting these patients with active immunization may not be effective. Thus, optimal methods of prevention are currently directed at preventing incident colonization in high-risk hospitalized patients. Nearly all enterococcal infections, including VRE infections, are preceded by colonization, and although infections do not develop in most colonized patients, they are still able to shed and transmit bacteria to other hospitalized patients. At least with VRE, a colonization-to-infection ratio of 10:1 has been reported, which suggests that for every one clinical infection in an ICU, there may be 10 colonized patients lurking undetected in the unit. Thus, the unrecognized colonized patients represent the target population for infection control efforts such as active surveillance. Active surveillance programs use perianal surveillance swabs to detect previously unrecognized, colonized patients and isolate them to prevent further transmission. In May 2003, the Society of Healthcare Epidemiology of America published guidelines for preventing nosocomial transmission of multidrug-resistant *Enterococcus.* The main recommendation was that surveillance cultures are indicated at the time of hospital admission for patients at high risk for carriage of VRE and that colonized patients should be placed in contact isolation. Isolation typically entails private rooms, dedicated equipment such as stethoscopes, and gloves and gowns for all patient contact. However, no final recommendation regarding what represents a "high-risk" group was given. Some hospitals do use active surveillance in the ICU and other wards with a high prevalence of VRE, although overall adoption of this strategy has been hindered by the perceived high cost of surveillance programs and lack of available randomized control trial data. Studies have shown that infection control methods that seek to isolate only patients with past or recent infections detect only a small proportion of patients requiring isolation and are largely ineffective for that reason.

Prognosis

Apart from enterococcal endocarditis, the mortality attributable to enterococcal infections is difficult to quantify because of the predilection of enterococci to infect patients with preexisting comorbid conditions and high levels of illness severity. In addition, the impact of vancomycin resistance on underlying mortality is uncertain. A recent meta-analysis reported that the odds of dying of a VRE blood stream infection were 2.5 times higher than dying of an infection caused by susceptible enterococci. The unadjusted mortality in patients with susceptible enterococcal bacteremia was 20%. It is unclear why resistance is associated with higher mortality, although it is thought that a delay in adequate empirical therapy may play a role. In addition, most studies that examined the clinical impact of resistance in enterococci were completed before the availability of newer antimicrobials with activity against VRE. Enterococcal bacteremia is also associated with prolonged hospitalization and added costs when compared with similar patients without enterococcal bacteremia.

SUGGESTED READINGS

Chang S, Sievert DM, Hageman JC, et al: Infection with vancomycin-resistant *Staphylococcus aureus* containing the vanA resistance gene. N Engl J Med 2003;348:1342–1347. *A complete description of the first ever case of vancomycin-resistant* Staphylococcus aureus.

Diaz Granados CA, Zimmer SM, Klein M, Jernigan JA: Comparison of mortality associated with vancomycin-resistant and vancomycin-susceptible enterococcal bloodstream infections: A meta-analysis. Clin Infect Dis 2005;41:327–333. *A thorough analysis of the mortality impact of vancomycin resistance in enterococci.*

Kauffman CA: Therapeutic and preventive options for the management of vancomycin-resistant enterococcal infections. J Antimicrob Chemother 2003;51(Suppl. 3):iii23–iii30. *A thorough overview of the treatment options for vancomycin-resistant enterococcal infections.*

McDonald JR, Olaison L, Anderson DJ, et al: Enterococcal endocarditis: 107 cases from the international collaboration on endocarditis merged database. Am J Med 2005;118:759–766. *Enterococcal native valve endocarditis has a distinctive clinical picture with a good prognosis.*

Muto CA, Jernigan JA, Ostrowsky BE, et al: SHEA guideline for preventing nosocomial transmission of multidrug-resistant strains of *Staphylococcus aureus* and enterococcus. Infect Control Hosp Epidemiol 2003;24:362–386. *An important guideline and review of the prevention measures that are particularly important for hospital epidemiologists, critical care specialists, and hospitalists.*

Vernon MO, Hayden MK, Trick WE, et al: Chlorhexidine gluconate to cleanse patients in a medical intensive care unit: the effectiveness of source control to reduce the bioburden of vancomycin-resistant enterococci. Arch Intern Med 2006;166:306–312. *The incidence of VRE acquisition was 26 colonizations per 1000 patient-days in the soap and water bath group compared to 9 per 1000 patient-days in the group that was cleansed with chlorhexidine-saturated cloths.*

315 DIPHTHERIA AND OTHER CORYNEBACTERIA INFECTIONS

Roland W. Sutter

DIPHTHERIA

Definition

Diphtheria is an acute infectious disease caused by *Corynebacterium diphtheriae,* a gram-positive bacillus. The organism primarily infects the respiratory tract, where it causes tonsillopharyngitis or laryngitis, or both (typically with a pseudomembrane), as well as the skin, where it is responsible for a variety of indolent lesions. If the infecting strain produces exotoxin, myocarditis and neuritis may ensue.

The Pathogen

C. diphtheriae is a member of a group of aerobic, nonmotile, unencapsulated, nonsporulating, pleomorphic gram-positive bacilli. Its name comes from the Greek *korynee* (meaning "club"), which describes the shape of the organism on stained smears with one end usually being wider, and *diphtheria* (meaning "leather hide"), for the characteristic adherent membrane. The genus *Corynebacterium* is characterized by bacilli that line up in parallel groups and bend when dividing to create "Chinese character" arrangements. Both nontoxigenic and toxigenic *C. diphtheria* strains exist. Toxigenicity is conferred when a nontoxigenic organism is infected with a beta-phage carrying the gene for the toxin (*tox*). *C. diphtheriae* has three biotypes—*gravis, mitis,* and *intermedius*—that are distinguished by colonial morphology and varying biochemical and hemolytic reactions. Strains may be distinguished for epidemiologic purposes by molecular techniques. *Corynebacterium ulcerans* can also produce classic diphtheria, including local respiratory tract and distal toxic complications.

Epidemiology

Humans are the only natural reservoir of *C. diphtheriae,* although the organism has occasionally been isolated from a variety of domestic and other animals. Spread occurs in close-contact settings through respiratory droplets or by direct contact with respiratory secretions or skin lesions. The organism survives for weeks and possibly months on environmental surfaces and in dust, and fomite transmission may occur. The majority of nasopharyngeal *C. diphtheriae* infections result in asymptomatic carriage, with clinical disease developing in only about one in seven individuals. However, asymptomatic carriers are important in maintaining transmission.

Diphtheria immunization protects against disease but does not prevent carriage. In the prevaccine era, respiratory disease dominated in temperate climates, with a fall/winter peak in incidence. Most individuals acquired natural immunity by the midteen years. Cutaneous disease is the predominant form of the disease in tropical countries, but over the past 2 decades, outbreaks of this form of diphtheria have occurred in the United States and Europe, typically in homeless and alcoholic inner-city adults.

Vaccination with diphtheria toxoid (formalin-treated toxin) was introduced in the 1920s. Immunization of children in an era when the majority of older individuals had natural immunity resulted in a dramatic drop in the incidence of diphtheria and an even more rapid decline in the proportion of toxigenic strains isolated, presumably because the selective advantage of the *tox* gene—promotion of greater replication and spread of the organism—is lost in an immune host. In most Western countries, toxigenic *C. diphtheriae* has virtually been eliminated. In the United States, reported cases fell from 147,991 in 1920, to 15,536 in 1940, to a total of 40 cases from 1980 to 1993. The absence of reported diphtheria cases in the United States in recent years, however, does not indicate that circulation of toxigenic *C. diphtheriae* has ceased. Investigations in a Northern Plains Indian community in North Dakota and First Nations communities in Ontario, Canada, suggested that *C. diphtheriae* strains might have circulated independently for more than 2 decades in these communities despite the absence of reported respiratory diphtheria cases.

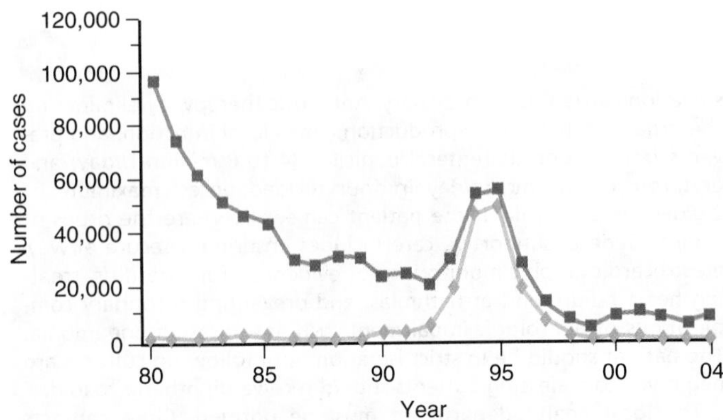

FIGURE 315–1 • **Reported diphtheria cases, worldwide and by European Region of the World Health Organization, 1980–2004.** ■ = total cases worldwide; ◆ = cases in European region of WHO. (Data from the World Health Organization.)

Vaccine-induced immunity to diphtheria wanes with time, and there is a growing cohort of individuals with no natural diphtheria immunity. Serosurveys indicate that 20 to 60% of adults in industrialized countries have diphtheria antitoxin levels below minimal protective levels. A level of 0.01 IU/mL from an in vitro neutralization assay, the "gold standard" test, is considered the lower limit of protection. As long as a high proportion of the population remains susceptible, the danger of reintroduction or reemergence of toxigenic strains exists.

Since 1990 there has been a major resurgence of diphtheria in several countries of the former Soviet Union. In Russia, the number of reported cases rose from 593 in 1989 to 39,582 in 1994, with over two thirds of cases occurring in adults. Large-scale campaigns of mass administration of diphtheria toxoid to virtually the entire population in the affected new independent states of the former Soviet Union have since led to significant decreases in the incidence of diphtheria, from a peak of 50,449 cases in 1995, to 7197 cases in 1997, to pre-resurgence levels by the late 1990s (Fig. 315–1).

Pathobiology

In classic respiratory diphtheria, *C. diphtheriae* colonizes the mucosal surface of the nasopharynx and multiplies locally without blood stream invasion. Released toxin causes local tissue necrosis with the formation of a tough, adherent pseudomembrane composed of a mixture of fibrin, dead cells, and bacteria. The membrane usually begins on the tonsils or posterior of the pharynx. In more severe cases, it spreads by progressively extending over the pharyngeal wall, fauces, and soft palate and into the larynx, which may result in respiratory obstruction. Toxin entering the blood stream causes tissue damage at distant sites, particularly the heart (myocarditis), nerves (demyelination), and kidney (tubular necrosis). Nontoxigenic strains may cause mild local respiratory disease, sometimes including a membrane.

Diphtheria toxin is an extremely potent inhibitor of protein synthesis, and the estimated human lethal dose is 0.1 mg/kg. The extent of toxin absorption varies with the site of infection, being much less from the skin or nose than from the pharynx.

Clinical Manifestations

Respiratory Diphtheria

Infection limited to the anterior nares is manifested as a chronic serosanguineous or seropurulent discharge without fever or significant toxicity. A whitish membrane may be observed on the septum. The faucial (pharyngeal) form is most common. After an incubation period of 1 to 7 days, the illness begins with a sore throat, malaise, and mild to moderate fever. Initially there is mild pharyngeal erythema, usually followed by progressive formation of a whitish tonsillar exudate, which over a period of 24 to 48 hours changes into a grayish membrane that is tightly adherent and bleeds on attempted removal. In more severe cases, the patient appears toxic and the membrane is more extensive. Cervical adenopathy and soft tissue edema may occur and result in the typical bull neck appearance and stridor. Laryngeal involvement, which may develop on its own or as a result of membrane extension from the nasopharynx, is manifested as hoarseness, stridor, and dyspnea.

The likelihood of toxic complications depends primarily on the interval between disease onset and administration of antitoxin. The severity of disease at initial evaluation closely predicts the likelihood of a severe clinical course, complications, and death. Myocarditis typically occurs in the first or second week after the onset of respiratory symptoms and develops either suddenly or insidiously with signs of low cardiac output and congestive failure. Conduction disturbances, which may occur without other signs of myocarditis, include ST-T wave abnormalities, arrhythmias, and heart block. Neurologic impairment is manifested as cranial nerve palsies and peripheral neuritis. Palatal or pharyngeal paralysis (or both) occurs during the acute phase; peripheral neuritis, symmetrical and predominantly motor, occurs 2 to 12 weeks after onset of the disease. Motor deficit may range from minor proximal weakness to complete paralysis. Complete recovery is the rule. In fulminant, sometimes called "hypertoxic," diphtheria, toxic circulatory collapse with hemorrhagic features occurs.

Cutaneous Diphtheria

Cutaneous diphtheria lesions are classically indolent, deep, punched-out ulcers that may have a grayish-white membrane. However, the lesions may be indistinguishable from impetigo, or *C. diphtheriae* may infect chronic dermatoses such as stasis dermatitis. Coinfection with *Streptococcus pyogenes* or *Staphylococcus aureus,* or both, occurs frequently. Toxic complications of cutaneous diphtheria are rare.

Diagnosis

The decision to initiate therapy should be based on clinical grounds because delayed treatment, especially delays in antitoxin administration, is associated with worse outcomes. A high index of suspicion is required. Specimens for culture should be taken from beneath the membrane, from the nasopharynx, and from any suspicious skin lesions. Because special media are required, the laboratory should be alerted to the concern about diphtheria. *C. diphtheriae* is best isolated on selective media that inhibit the growth of other nasopharyngeal organisms; one containing potassium tellurite is generally used. Based on colonial morphology and Gram stain appearance, a presumptive diagnosis may be possible within 18 to 24 hours. Cultures may be negative if the patient previously received antibiotics. Toxigenicity testing should be performed on all *C. diphtheriae* isolates. Because both nontoxigenic and toxigenic strains may be isolated from the same patient, more than one colony should be tested. Traditional methods include guinea pig inoculation and the Elek test, in which the isolate and appropriate controls are streaked on a culture plate in which a filter strip soaked with antitoxin has been embedded; toxin production is confirmed by an immunoprecipitation line in the agar. Polymerase chain reaction may allow both detection of the organism and determination of toxigenicity.

Differential Diagnosis

The differential diagnosis includes streptococcal and viral tonsillopharyngitis, infectious mononucleosis, Vincent's angina, candidiasis, and acute epiglottitis. A history of travel to a region with endemic diphtheria or a history of contact with a recent immigrant from such an area increases the possibility of diphtheria, as does a pre-antitoxin treatment serum antitoxin level of less than 0.01 IU/mL.

Treatment

The goals of treatment are to neutralize the toxin rapidly, eliminate the infecting organism, provide supportive care, and prevent further transmission (Table 315–1). The mainstay of therapy is equine diphtheria antitoxin. Because only unbound toxin can be neutralized, treatment should commence as soon as the diagnosis is suspected, and each day of delay in administration increases the likelihood of a fatal outcome. A single dose ranging in quantity from 20,000 units for localized tonsillar diphtheria up to 100,000 units is given for extensive disease with severe toxicity. Antitoxin may be administered intramuscularly or intravenously; particularly for more severe cases, the intravenous route is preferred. Tests for sensitivity to antitoxin should be performed before administering it and desen-

TABLE 315–1 GOALS AND PROPOSED INTERVENTIONS FOR THE MANAGEMENT OF SUSPECTED DIPHTHERIA CASES

Goals	Proposed Interventions
Neutralize toxin as soon as possible to reduce severe complications, including death	After a presumptive diagnosis of diphtheria, immediately obtain and administer antitoxin, initiate antimicrobial treatment, and arrange for appropriate supportive care
Prevent further spread of *C. diphtheriae* to close contacts, including hospital staff	Isolate the patient; strictly observe respiratory barrier procedures Notify the health department Review the vaccination status of the family and other close contacts, and initiate postexposure prophylaxis
Confirm the diagnosis	Collect appropriate specimens for culture (alert the laboratory to ensure that it can prepare specific culture media)
Induce long-term protection against *C. diphtheriae* in case and close contacts	Complete the primary series with diphtheria toxoid as needed

sitization carried out if necessary. Antibiotic therapy, by eliminating the organism, halts toxin production, limits local infection, and prevents transmission. Parenteral penicillin (4 to 6 million U/day) and erythromycin (40 mg/kg/day in four divided doses; maximum of 2 g/day, usually orally if the patient can swallow) are the drugs of choice. General supportive care includes ensuring a secure airway, electrocardiographic monitoring for evidence of myocarditis, treating heart failure and arrhythmias, and preventing secondary complications of neurologic impairment such as aspiration pneumonia. The patient should be in strict isolation until follow-up cultures are negative. Convalescing patients should receive diphtheria toxoid.

The local health department must be notified. Close contacts should have cultures performed and be administered prophylactic antibiotics. A positive culture in a contact may confirm the diagnosis if the patient is culture negative. All contacts without full primary immunization and a booster within the preceding 5 years should receive diphtheria toxoid. Because manufacturers in the United States discontinued diphtheria antitoxin production, no licensed product is available. However, diphtheria antitoxin for the therapeutic purposes can be obtained from the Centers for Disease Control and Prevention (CDC), which distributes an European-produced antitoxin (Pasteur Merieux, Lyon, France) under an Investigational New Drug protocol.

Prevention

Immunization with diphtheria toxoid is the only effective means of primary prevention. The primary series is four doses of diphtheria toxoid (given with tetanus toxoid and pertussis vaccine) at 2, 4, 6, and 15 to 18 months; a preschool booster dose is given at 4 to 6 years of age. There-

TABLE 315–2 CORYNEBACTERIA AND RELATED ORGANISMS ASSOCIATED WITH HUMAN DISEASE

Site of Infection	Pathogen	Clinical Syndrome	Comment
Respiratory tract	*C. diphtheriae*	Classic diphtheria	
	C. ulcerans	Diphtheria	Zoonotic infection May produce diphtheria toxin
	C. pseudodiphtheriticum	Pharyngitis Rarely, pneumonia in patients with advanced AIDS	
	Arcanobacterium haemolyticum	Pharyngitis, tonsillar abscess, rash	Clinically indistinguishable from streptococcal pharyngitis
Skin and soft tissue	*C. pseudotuberculosis*	Granulomatous lymphadenitis	Zoonotic infection, especially in sheep; occupational risk for veterinarians and butchers
	C. minutissimum	Erythrasma	
	C. kroppenstedtii	Granulomatous breast abscess	
Genitourinary tract	*C. glucuronolyticum*	Urinary tract infection in men; chronic prostatitis	
	C. urealyticum *C. riegelli*	Chronic and recurrent urinary tract infection Encrusted cystitis	More common in the elderly, chronically ill, immunosuppressed patients, and those with indwelling catheters
Health care–associated infections	*C. jeikeium* and less commonly many others, including *C. amycolatum, C. striatum,* and *C. urealyticum*	Catheter- and device-associated infections Postprocedure wound and soft tissue infections Prosthetic valve joint infections Nosocomial pneumonia Cerebrospinal fluid shunt infections	*C. jeikeium* is the most common corynebacterial pathogen in hospitals and causes severe infections in immunosuppressed patients and those with indwelling devices

after, boosters should be given as part of the adolescent immunization visit (i.e., between 11 and 13 years of age), followed by doses administered every 10 years. Since 2005, the CDC recommends the routine use of tetanus toxoid, reduced diphtheria toxoid, and acellular pertussis vaccine, adsorbed (Tdap), in adolescents 11 to 18 years of age in place of tetanus and diphtheria toxoid (Td) vaccines. In addition, the CDC recommends routine use of a single dose of Tdap for adults 19 to 64 years of age to replace the next booster dose of Td.

Prognosis

Diphtheria, at the beginning of the 21st century, remains a serious disease associated with a high case-fatality rate. In the United States, the diphtheria case-fatality rate has remained virtually unchanged (between 5% and 10%) over recent decades.

OTHER CORYNEBACTERIUM SPECIES

Corynebacteria other than *C. diptheriae* are ubiquitous in the environment and are among the normal flora colonizing humans and animals. The pathogenic potential of many of these organisms was not appreciated in the past, but many are now known to be associated with specific and often serious infectious diseases, especially in immunosuppressed, chronically ill, and hospitalized patients (Table 315–2). In general, these organisms remain susceptible to vancomycin, but resistance to other classes of antimicrobials is not uncommon and varies among species.

SUGGESTED READINGS

Efstratiou A, Engler KH, Mazurova IK, et al: Current approaches to the laboratory diagnosis of diphtheria. J Infect Dis 2000;181 Suppl 1:S138–145. *A review of the diagnostic options.*

Marston CK, Jamieson F, Cahoon F, et al: Persistence of a distinct *Corynebacterium diphtheriae* clonal group within two communities in the United States and Canada where diphtheria is endemic. J Clin Microbiol 2001;39:1586–1590. *Evidence for persistence of endemic transmission of C. diphtheriae over 2 decades in Native American communities in the United States and Canada.*

Vitek CR: Diphtheria. Curr Top Microbiol Immunol 2006;304:71–94. *A comprehensive review.*

Wharton M, Dittman S, Strebel PM, et al (eds): Control of epidemic diphtheria in the Newly Independent States of the former Soviet Union, 1990–1998. J Infect Dis 2000;181(Suppl. 1):S1–S248. *Diphtheria outbreaks (and control measures) in newly independent states are summarized in detail, as well as findings of research studies to understand the reasons for these outbreaks.*

316 LISTERIOSIS

Bennett Lorber

Definition

Listeriosis is a foodborne infection caused by the gram-positive bacillus *Listeria monocytogenes.* Most patients have impaired cell-mediated immunity and are seen with life-threatening bacteremia or meningitis, although a mild, self-limited, febrile gastroenteritis in healthy persons also occurs.

The Pathogen

Widely distributed in nature, *L. monocytogenes* may be found in soil, on vegetation, and in the stool of healthy mammals, including humans. It causes disease in animals, especially herd animals, and in humans. The organism has been isolated from many foods, including raw vegetables, raw milk, fish, poultry, and meat.

Epidemiology

Ingestion of contaminated foods appears to be the source of most human infection. Outbreaks have been documented in association with coleslaw, milk, soft cheese, pâté, ready-to-eat pork products, deli counter meats, smoked fish, and butter. Sporadic cases have been traced to contaminated cheese, milk, deli counter meats, turkey frankfurters, and alfalfa tablets. Molecular epidemiologic tools such as pulsed-field gel electrophoresis are an important tool when tracking outbreaks.

Information on annual incidence comes from active surveillance studies performed by the Centers for Disease Control and Prevention. Although the annual incidence of listeriosis decreased by 44% between 1989 and 1993, possibly related to more stringent regulations in the food processing industry, it has since remained stable at approximately 5 cases per million population and accounts for 1500 to 2500 cases per year in the United States and about 400 deaths. Neonates and adults older than 50 years have the highest infection rates. Pregnant women make up 30% of all cases. Adults at increased risk for invasive listeriosis (bacteremia, meningitis) include those who have hematologic malignancy, advanced acquired immunodeficiency syndrome (AIDS), a solid organ transplant, or iron overload and anyone treated with corticosteroids or an anti–tumor necrosis factor agent. However, as many as a fourth of all invasive listeriosis cases occur in apparently healthy persons, particularly those older than 60 years.

Pathobiology

L. monocytogenes enters the human body through the intestine, most often after the ingestion of contaminated food. The bacterium induces its own uptake by gastrointestinal cells and macrophages. Within the host cell the bacterium is enclosed in a phagolysosome, but through the production of an exotoxin called listeriolysin O, it destroys the phagolysosome membrane and gains access to the cytoplasm. All pathogenic strains of *L. monocytogenes* produce listeriolysin O, the major virulence factor. Listeriae actively divide in the cytoplasm, migrate to the periphery of the cell by polymerization of host cell actin, and then push out the cell membrane to form pseudopods, which are taken up by adjacent host cells. The bacteria move from cell to cell in this fashion and repeat their life cycle.

After invasion through the gastrointestinal tract, listeriae may disseminate hematogenously to any body site but show a particular tropism for the central nervous system (CNS).

Immunity to listerial infection is handled through the cell-mediated arm of the immune system; persons with abnormalities solely of humoral immunity or leukocytes are not at increased risk for infection.

Clinical Manifestations

The incubation period for invasive listeriosis (time from ingestion of contaminated food to illness) averages about 30 days. Invasive listeriosis in an immunocompromised adult is most often manifested as bacteremia without an obvious focus. In such cases, patients have nonspecific complaints such as fever, malaise, myalgias, and back pain. Bacteremia is the form of invasive listeriosis that complicates pregnancy; CNS infection is extremely rare in the absence of other risk factors. Listeriosis during pregnancy may lead to spontaneous abortion or neonatal sepsis, but early antimicrobial therapy may result in the birth of a healthy child. Endocarditis with *L. monocytogenes* can occur on both native and prosthetic valves and carries a high rate of septic complications. Endocarditis, but not bacteremia per se, may be a clue to underlying colon cancer; colonoscopy should be considered in all cases of listerial endocarditis.

Persons in whom *L. monocytogenes* bacteremia develops may progress to CNS infection, most commonly manifested as meningitis. *Listeria* has a predilection for infecting brain tissue, as well as the meninges, and unlike other common bacterial causes of meningitis, it not infrequently causes encephalitis or brain abscess. Brain abscess as a result of infection by *L. monocytogenes* exhibits unusual features when compared with other bacteria: listerial brain abscess coexists with bacteremia in nearly all cases and with meningitis in a fourth; in addition, abscesses are often subcortical.

L. monocytogenes is the most common cause of bacterial meningitis in patients with lymphomas, organ transplant recipients, and patients treated with corticosteroids for any reason. Affected persons usually have the classic acute symptoms of meningitis but may also have a subacute disease course more characteristic of tuberculous meningitis. Most have a stiff neck, but 15 to 20% may not. Focal neurologic findings, including ataxia, tremors, myoclonus, and seizures, may be seen consistent with the tropism of *Listeria* for brain parenchyma. Cerebrospinal fluid (CSF) glucose is normal in more than 60% of cases. Gram stain of CSF reveals *L. monocytogenes* in only about 40% of cases, and even when seen, the organisms may be mistaken for pneumococci.

Listerial rhombencephalitis is an unusual form of listerial encephalitis involving the brain stem, similar to the unique zoonotic listerial infection known as circling disease of sheep. Unlike other listerial CNS infections, rhombencephalitis usually occurs in healthy adults. The typical clinical picture is one of a biphasic illness with a prodrome of fever, headache, nausea, and vomiting lasting about 4 days, followed by the abrupt onset of asymmetrical cranial nerve deficits, cerebellar signs, and hemiparesis or hemisensory deficits, or both. Respiratory failure develops in about 40% of patients. Nuchal rigidity is present in about half, and CSF findings are only mildly abnormal, with a positive CSF culture in about 40%. Almost two thirds of patients are bacteremic. Magnetic resonance imaging is superior to computed tomography for demonstrating rhombencephalitis. Mortality is high, and serious sequelae are common in survivors.

Localized infection may occur after hematogenous seeding (e.g., liver abscess, septic arthritis) or, rarely, after direct inoculation (e.g., conjunctivitis, cellulitis).

Well-documented reports of food-borne outbreaks have demonstrated that ingestion of *L. monocytogenes* in a sufficiently large inoculum can result in a self-limited illness consisting of fever, chills, diarrhea, abdominal cramps, and sometimes nausea and vomiting. Symptoms follow exposure by 1 to 2 days and last for about 2 days.

Diagnosis

Differential Diagnosis

Clinical situations in which a diagnosis of listeriosis should be considered include (1) neonatal sepsis or meningitis; (2) meningitis or parenchymal brain infection in patients with hematologic malignancies, AIDS, organ transplantation, or corticosteroid immunosuppression; (3) meningitis or parenchymal brain infection in adults older than 50 years; (4) simultaneous infection of the meninges and brain parenchyma; (5) subcortical brain abscess; (6) fever during pregnancy, particularly in the third trimester; (7) blood, CSF, or other normally sterile specimen reported to have "diphtheroids" on Gram stain or culture; and (8) food-borne outbreak of febrile gastroenteritis when routine cultures fail to identify a pathogen. The differential diagnosis of listerial CNS infection includes the more common causes of bacterial meningitis and brain abscess; indolent listerial meningitis or rhombencephalitis may mimic CNS tuberculosis.

Laboratory Findings

The diagnosis of listeriosis is best made by routine bacterial culture of specimens from usually sterile sites such as blood or CSF. The laboratory must exercise caution because *L. monocytogenes* may be mistaken for diphtheroids, streptococci, enterococci, or *Haemophilus influenzae.* Stool culture is recommended only when routine stool cultures are negative in the setting of an outbreak of gastroenteritis; many people have enteric colonization with *L. monocytogenes* without invasive disease. The laboratory must be advised that listerial infection is suspected because the organism is unlikely to be identified with routine stool culture media.

Serologic testing (antibody to listeriolysin O) is not useful in invasive disease but may be helpful in the retrospective identification of outbreaks of food-borne febrile gastroenteritis when routine cultures are negative.

Prevention

Guidelines for preventing listeriosis are similar to those for preventing other food-borne illnesses. In general, one should thoroughly cook raw food from animal sources, wash raw vegetables thoroughly before eating, keep uncooked meats separate from vegetables and from cooked and ready-to-eat foods, avoid raw (unpasteurized) milk or foods made from raw milk, and wash hands, knives, and cutting boards after each handling of uncooked foods.

People at high risk for listeriosis may choose to avoid soft cheeses such as feta, Brie, Camembert, blue-veined, and Mexican-style cheese such as queso fresco. Hard cheeses, processed cheeses, cream cheese, cottage cheese, and yogurt are safe. Leftover foods or ready-to-eat foods such as hot dogs should be cooked until steaming hot. It is best to avoid foods from delicatessen counters, such as prepared salads, meats, and cheeses, or at least to reheat cold cuts thoroughly until they are steaming hot before eating.

Listeriosis is effectively prevented by trimethoprim-sulfamethoxazole given as *Pneumocystis* prophylaxis to organ transplant recipients or to individuals infected with human immunodeficiency virus. In areas with a high prevalence of AIDS, the widespread use of trimethoprim-sulfamethoxazole for *Pneumocystis* prophylaxis appears to have resulted in a marked decline in nonperinatal listeriosis.

Second episodes of neonatal listerial infection are virtually unheard of, and intrapartum antibiotics are not recommended for women with a history of perinatal listeriosis.

Except from infected mother to fetus, human-to-human transmission of listeriosis does not occur; patients do not need to be isolated.

Treatment

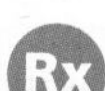

Recommendations for the treatment of infection with *L. monocytogenes* derive from in vitro data, animal models, and clinical experience with small numbers of patients; no controlled trials have been performed to prove the efficacy of one drug over another. Many antimicrobials show in vitro activity against *L. monocytogenes. Clinical utility is more relevant than in vitro susceptibility test results because cephalosporins and other drugs to which the bacterium appears to be susceptible are inadequate to treat infection.*

Twenty percent of cases of bacterial meningitis in those older than 50 years are due to *L. monocytogenes.* Therefore, empirical therapy for bacterial meningitis in all adults older than 50 years should include either ampicillin or trimethoprim-sulfamethoxazole, especially in the absence of associated pneumonia, otitis, sinusitis, or endocarditis that would suggest a cause other than *L. monocytogenes.* Cephalosporins, commonly used in the treatment of bacterial meningitis, should not be used alone when *Listeria* is a diagnostic consideration.

Ampicillin is generally considered the drug of choice for treating confirmed cases of listeriosis. In cases of meningitis and endocarditis and in patients with severely impaired T-cell function, most authorities recommend the addition of gentamicin to ampicillin for synergy based on in vitro testing and animal models. For meningitis, therapy should be continued for at least 3 weeks; bacteremic patients without CNS involvement may be treated for 2 weeks. Endocarditis and brain abscess should be treated for at least 6 weeks. Meningitis doses should be used to treat all cases of invasive listeriosis, even in the absence of CNS or CSF abnormalities.

In patients with penicillin hypersensitivity, trimethoprim-sulfamethoxazole is the preferred agent. It is bactericidal and appears to be as effective as the combination of ampicillin and gentamicin. Drugs that should be avoided because of treatment failure and relapse include cephalosporins, chloramphenicol, tetracycline, and erythromycin.

Corticosteroids appear to be important adjunctive agents in treating the most common forms of bacterial meningitis. Their role in the treatment of listerial CNS infection is unknown.

Iron is a virulence factor for *L. monocytogenes,* and clinically, iron overload states are risk factors for listerial infection. Therefore, in patients with listeriosis and iron deficiency, it may be prudent to withhold iron replacement until antimicrobial therapy is complete.

Prognosis

Listeria meningitis carries a mortality of about 25%; mortality is higher in those with underlying malignancy. Mortality from brain abscess and endocarditis is about 50%; survivors of brain abscess commonly have significant neurologic residua.

SUGGESTED READINGS

Brouwer MC, van de Beek D, Heckenberg SG, et al: Community-acquired *Listeria monocytogenes* meningitis in adults. Clin Infect Dis 2006;43:1233–1238. *Review of Listeria meningitis.*

Dussurget O, Pizarro-Cerda J, Cossart P: Molecular determinants of *Listeria monocytogenes* virulence. Annu Rev Microbiol 2004;58:587–610. *A detailed review of the molecular biology of this unique pathogen.*

MacDonald PDM, Whitwam RE, Boggs JD, et al: Outbreak of listeriosis among Mexican immigrants as a result of consumption of illicitly produced Mexican-style cheese. Clin Infect Dis 2005;40:677–682. *Description of an outbreak due to an unpasteurized milk product and a reminder of the importance of educating all pregnant women about food safety.*

Mylonakis E, Paliou M, Hohmann EL, et al: Listeriosis during pregnancy: A case series and review of 222 cases. Medicine (Baltimore) 2002;81:260–269. *A comprehensive review of listeriosis in this important risk group.*

Ooi ST, Lorber B: Gastroenteritis due to *Listeria monocytogenes.* Clin Infect Dis 2005;40:1327–1332. *A comprehensive review.*

Varma JK, Samuel MC, Marcus R, et al: *Listeria monocytogenes* infection from foods prepared in a commercial establishment: A case-control study of potential sources of sporadic illness in the United States. Clin Infect Dis 2007;44:521–528. *Epidemiologic data on the possible sources of foodborne Listeria cases.*

317 ANTHRAX

Daniel R. Lucey

Definition

Anthrax is caused by *Bacillus anthracis*, a spore-forming, gram-positive rod that is aerobic or facultatively anaerobic. The name comes from the Greek word for "coal," a reference to the black eschar that eventually forms in the cutaneous form of anthrax. Anthrax is primarily a disease of animals, but it has also been developed in past decades by some nations as a biowarfare weapon and was used by one or more unidentified persons as a bioterrorist weapon in 2001 in the United States. Historical names that reflect the zoonotic nature of most human anthrax infections include "woolsorter's disease" and "ragpicker's disease."

The Pathogen

The bacterium is a large (1 to 1.5 by 3 to 5 μg), gram-positive rod. It has a "ground-glass appearance" of growth on sheep blood agar, with 2- to 5-mm, nonhemolytic, tenacious ("beaten egg white") colonies after 15 to 24 hours of culture; oval, central to subterminal spores; and a capsule that can be visualized by India ink staining and that may also be seen in smears of blood or cerebrospinal fluid.

Epidemiology

Human infection with *B. anthracis* is usually linked to a zoonotic source such as goats, sheep, cattle, antelope, kudu, pigs, horses, zebu, and other animals. Animal-related products that can transmit the infection include meat, wool, hides, bones, and hair. Soil contaminated with spores that can persist for many years is also a source of infection. The spores can infect humans or animals, after which they germinate into the vegetative form of the bacteria and then cause clinical disease.

Classically, two closely related strains of anthrax (A and B) have been described by analysis of six genomic and two plasmid-encoded variable tandem repeat regions. The group A strain is located worldwide and is linked to the international trade and domestication of livestock, whereas the group B strain is restricted largely to southern Africa. In addition, however, in January 2006 a new strain of *B. anthracis* was reported from nonhuman primates in Côte d'Ivoire and Cameroon.

The World Health Organization makes available online an extensive global epidemiology database for anthrax and offers guidelines on epidemiologic and ecologic control issues in both humans and animals. From 1900 to 2005, at least 82 cases of inhalation anthrax were reported in detail in the worldwide medical literature, including 18 from the United States diagnosed before 1977 with naturally acquired disease. Many of these 18 patients had environmental exposure to spores, such as in goat hair–processing plants in New England. In 2006, the first patient with naturally acquired inhalational anthrax in the United States in 30 years was hospitalized in Pennsylvania; the source was dried African animal hides used in making drums.

Recent clinical experience with inhalational anthrax in the United States is primarily related to events in 2001 when 11 persons were infected after spores were sent in letters that arrived in several locations, including Florida, New York, New Jersey, Washington, DC, and Virginia (Chapter 19). A previous attempt to use anthrax as a bioterrorist weapon, by releasing it from a Tokyo rooftop in 1993, failed to cause any human illness.

In 1979, accidental release of anthrax from a military facility in Sverdlovsk (now Ekaterinberg), Russia, resulted in the deaths of many dozens of humans and animals. Eventually, epidemiologic and clinical data revealed that the deaths followed the probable airborne path ("plume") of the anthrax spores downwind from the military facility. At autopsy, 50% of 42 patients who died had anthrax meningitis in addition to inhalational anthrax.

Some of the largest outbreaks of anthrax in humans have involved the cutaneous form. For example, an estimated 10,000 human infections with cutaneous anthrax occurred in Zimbabwe from 1979 to 1985, primarily attributed to human exposure to an outbreak in cattle that had not been vaccinated against anthrax. In the United States, bioterrorism via anthrax in mailed letters caused 11 cases of cutaneous anthrax in addition to the 11 inhalational cases.

Notably, *B. anthracis* is not transmitted from person to person through the air. There is, however, evidence of spores being able to reaerosolize under some experimental indoor and outdoor conditions.

Pathobiology

The major virulence factors of *B. anthracis* include its two binary toxins, "edema factor" (EF) and "lethal factor" (LF), and its antiphagocytic poly-D-glutamic acid capsule. Both EF and LF must first bind a third anthrax toxin component," protective antigen" (PA), to bind to a cellular "anthrax toxin receptor" (ATR). For example, edema toxin consists of EF bound to PA (EF-PA binary toxin), and lethal toxin consists of LF bound to PA (LF-PA binary toxin). EF, LF, and PA are all encoded on one plasmid ("pX-01"), and the immune system–evading, antiphagocytic capsule is encoded on a second plasmid ("pX-02").

The pathogenesis of anthrax is linked to its two binary toxins. Two cellular receptors serve as the ATR: tumor endothelial marker 8 (TEM8) and capillary morphogenesis protein 2 (CMG2). Once the PA component of the edema toxin and lethal toxin binds to a cellular receptor, the toxin complex can enter the target cell, first going into the acidic endosome and then the cytosol.

EF is a calmodulin-dependent, adenylate cyclase enzyme that catalyzes excessive production of cyclic adenosine monophosphate from adenosine triphosphate and results in water and calcium dysregulation, which is manifested as the characteristic edema of anthrax (sometimes described as "gelatinous"). Edema toxin is also reported to impair the function of polymorphonuclear leukocytes.

LF is a zinc-dependent metalloproteinase that impairs the immune system by interfering with the function of macrophages and other antigen-presenting cells, such as dendritic cells, that are essential to normal T-cell function. Dendritic cell function is inhibited by blockade of costimulatory molecules that are required for the presentation of antigen to T-cells, such as CD40, CD80, and CD86, and by blockade of the activation of cytokines that help prime naïve T-cells, such as interleukin-12.

The primary mechanism of action of lethal toxin is to inhibit the mitogen-activated protein kinase ("MAP kinase") intracellular signal transduction pathway. Lethal toxin is linked to excessive production of inflammatory cytokines and dyregulation of the cytokine network, possibly leading to a "cytokine storm" that contributes to rapid multiorgan clinical failure, shock, and death. Lethal toxin is also reported to impair platelets, again by inhibiting MAP kinase pathways, such as p38 MAP kinase. In addition, lethal toxin can impair human whole blood clotting in vitro. Thus, lethal toxin may contribute in several ways to the striking bleeding diathesis, including bleeding into lymph nodes, the pleural space, the meninges, the intestines, and ascitic fluid.

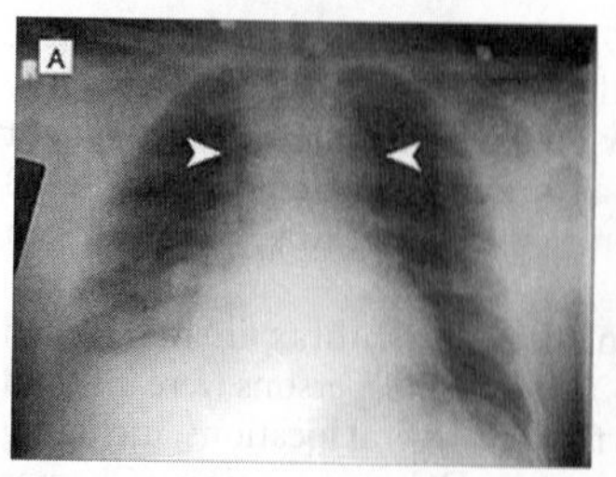

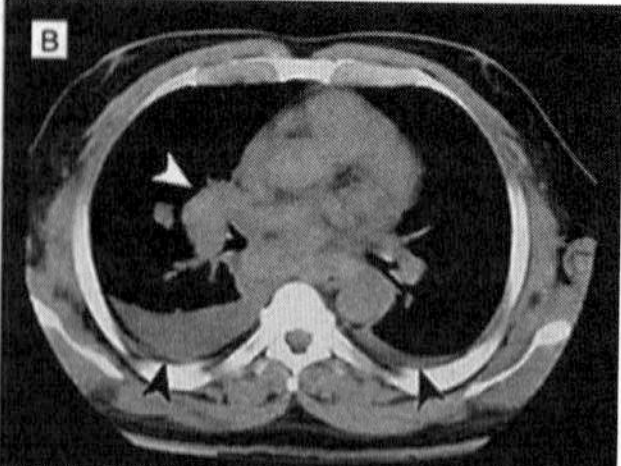

FIGURE 317–1 • Clinical features of anthrax. A, A portable chest radiograph in a 56-year-old man with inhalational anthrax depicts a widened mediastinum (arrowheads), bilateral hilar fullness, right pleural effusion, and bilateral perihilar air space disease. **B,** A non–contrast-enhanced spiral computed tomography scan depicts an enlarged and hyperdense right hilar lymph node (white arrowhead), bilateral pleural effusions (black arrowheads), and edema of mediastinal fat. (From Mayer TA, Bersoff-Matcha S, et al: Clinical presentation of inhalational anthrax following bioterrorism exposure. JAMA 2001;286:2549–2543.)

Clinical Manifestations

Four major clinical manifestations of anthrax infection—inhalational, cutaneous, gastrointestinal, and meningeal—are related to the three routes by which *B. anthracis* can enter the body: inhalation, ingestion, or via the skin.

Inhalational anthrax typically causes mediastinal adenopathy that results in mediastinal widening (Fig. 317–1), as well as pleural effusions that are often bloody, can expand rapidly, recur if drained by thoracentesis rather than by chest tube, and can be rapidly fatal if not treated with multiple antibiotics and pleural drainage. In 2005, a new clinical staging system for inhalational anthrax (Table 317–1) added an "intermediate-progressive stage" based on clinical, microbiologic, and radiologic information acquired from the 11 patients in 2001. Radiography demonstrated either pulmonary infiltrates or consolidation in 8 of the 11 patients. The incubation period of inhalational anthrax is generally 3 to 14 days, with a range of 2 to 43 days in humans. In all six of the patients who survived the anthrax attacks in 2001, anthrax was diagnosed during the "intermediate-progressive stage," and prompt therapy prevented progression of disease beyond this stage.

Cutaneous anthrax is the most common form of the disease (95%). The incubation period is usually 1 to 12 days. Cutaneous anthrax typically progresses from a papule that is pruritic, to a central vesicular or bullous lesion with surrounding nonpitting edema, and finally to a necrotic and hemorrhagic central lesion that evolves into the classic painless black eschar with surrounding edema (Fig. 317–2). This sequence of progressive cutaneous lesions can still occur even if appropriate antibiotics are given, and total resolution can take up to 2 months. The differential diagnosis includes brown recluse spider bites (which typically cause a painful lesion unlike the painless anthrax lesion; Chapter 380), cutaneous leishmaniasis (Chapter 369), plague (Chapter 333), tularemia (Chapter 332), typhus (Chapter 348), and warfarin (Coumadin) or heparin necrosis (Chapter 35), among others.

Gastrointestinal anthrax can be divided into an oropharyngeal form and an intestinal form. Extremely rare in the United States, gastrointestinal anthrax in other nations is often linked to consumption of the meat of infected animals, thereby suggesting that the vegetative form of the bacteria can cause gastrointestinal disease in humans. The oropharyngeal form is accompanied by painful cervical adenopathy and fever. The incubation period ranges from 2 to 144 hours. Oral lesions can ulcerate and progress to cause a white pseudomembrane, hoarseness, and dysphagia. Three phases of intestinal disease have been noted: an initial prodromal phase with fever, malaise, and syncope; a second progressive phase with abdominal pain, nausea, vomiting, abdominal distention, ascites, and severe weakness; and a fulminant third phase with suddenly increasing abdominal girth and expanding ascites, paroxysmal abdominal pain, and shock.

Anthrax meningoencephalitis can occur in association with inhalational, cutaneous, or gastrointestinal anthrax, and in rare cases it occurs without a known portal of entry. Anthrax meningitis is nearly always fatal. Cerebral edema, parenchymal brain hemorrhages, vasculitis, and subarachnoid hemorrhages can be seen.

TABLE 317–1 CLINICAL STAGING SYSTEM FOR INHALATIONAL ANTHRAX

I. EARLY-PRODROMAL STAGE

Nonspecific illness sometimes described as "flulike" and including any of the following: fever, cough, headache, chills, nausea, chest pain, or abdominal pain. Laboratory tests and radiographs are nondiagnostic. The prognosis for cure is good with appropriate therapy, but the diagnosis is difficult to confirm acutely in this stage.

II. INTERMEDIATE-PROGRESSIVE STAGE

Any of the following findings are defining inclusion criteria for this stage:
1. Positive blood cultures (typically positive in <24 hours)
2. Mediastinal adenopathy
3. Pleural effusions: bloody, often large, require drainage, and may recur

Findings in this stage may include high fever, dyspnea, confusion or syncope, or increasing nausea and vomiting. Exclusion criteria for this stage include:
1. Meningitis
2. Respiratory failure requiring intubation and mechanical ventilation or
3. Shock

Importantly, patients in this "intermediate-progressive" stage can still be cured with appropriate antibiotics *and* drainage of pleural effusions by thoracentesis and/or chest tube to reduce the adverse mechanical effect on respiration by large-volume effusions and to remove potentially toxin-producing *Bacillus anthracis* from the pleural space.

III. LATE-FULMINANT STAGE

Inclusion criteria include any one of the following findings:
1. Meningitis
2. Respiratory failure requiring intubation and mechanical ventilation
3. Shock: end-organ hypoperfusion

Findings in this stage may also include any of those from previous stages, so there are no exclusion criteria. The probability of survival is lowest in this stage. Novel therapeutics that safely and effectively neutralize anthrax toxin may be needed to increase survival.

Diagnosis

Most importantly, if anthrax is suspected, blood should be obtained immediately for culture before any antibiotics are started; patients with inhalation anthrax will grow the typical large, gram-positive rods in less than 24 hours. Surprisingly, even one dose of an effective antibiotic can sterilize the blood cultures. Nasal cultures should not be performed as a clinical diagnostic test for individual patients but might be useful as part of an epidemiologic investigation. If the initial culture is suggestive, three additional tests that should be performed in a biosafety cabinet are motility (nonmotile), catalase (positive), and hemolysis (negative). If these characteristics are found, *B. anthracis* is suspected but not proved until a sample is sent to a reference laboratory where polymerase chain reaction can identify *B. anthracis* and gamma-phage lysis of the encapsulated bacteria can provide confirmation. In addition, the Anthrax Quick ELISA (enzyme-linked immunosorbent assay) test can detect the eventual presence of antibodies to anthrax in blood.

A non–contrast-enhanced computed tomography scan can be a valuable adjunctive diagnostic tool for inhalational anthrax and is better than chest radiography for demonstrating the characteristic hyperattenuating mediastinal adenopathy and pleural effusions seen with inhalational anthrax. The hyperattenuation is consistent with bleeding into the lymph nodes and thus is helpful in distinguishing anthrax from tularemia (Chapter 332), histoplasmosis (Chapter 353), tuberculosis (Chapter 345),

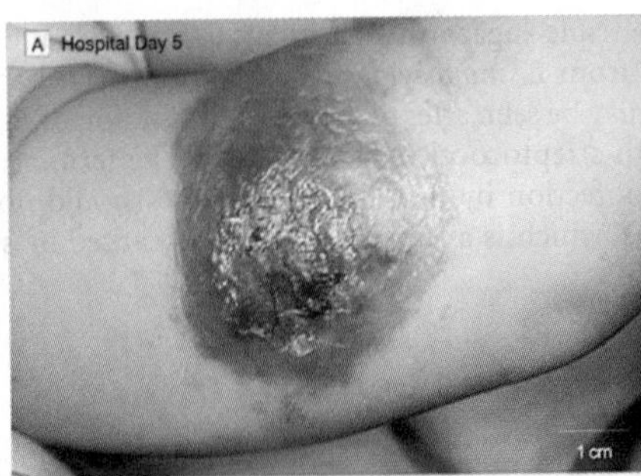

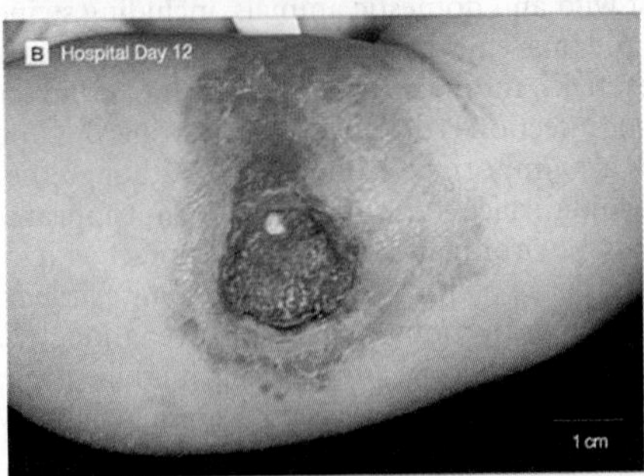

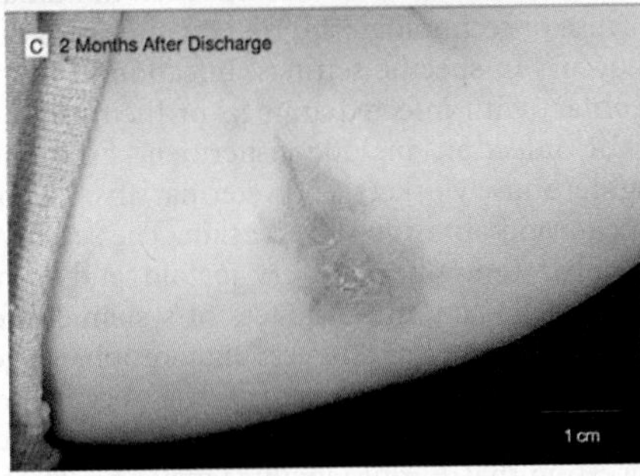

FIGURE 317-2 • The lesion of cutaneous anthrax. (From Freedman A, Freedman A, Afonja O, et al: Cutaneous anthrax associated with micro-angiopathic hemolytic anemia and coagulopathy in a 7-month-old infant. JAMA 2002; 287:869–874.)

sarcoidosis (Chapter 95), and most other causes of hilar or mediastinal adenopathy.

Anthrax meningitis is typically bloody and neutrophilic. Large gram-positive rods distinguish it from other causes of gram-positive rod meningitis, such as the smaller *Listeria monocytogenes* (Chapter 316).

Prevention

Clinical anthrax can be prevented by preexposure vaccination or by postexposure antibiotic prophylaxis. The current Food and Drug Administration (FDA)-licensed anthrax vaccine contains PA as the vaccine antigen and alum as an adjuvant. It requires six shots over an 18-month period when given before exposure. In contrast, postexposure prophylaxis, which is an off-label use of this same vaccine and thus needs an Investigational New Drug (IND) protocol, requires only three shots given over a 1-month period. This vaccine is in limited supply and is dedicated primarily to use by the military, so it is not available for routine use by civilian populations.

Antibiotics that are approved by the FDA for postexposure prophylaxis include ciprofloxacin, doxycycline, and procaine penicillin G, as well as levofloxacin for adults at least 18 years of age. In addition, in certain situations (children, pregnant women, and breast-feeding mothers), the Centers for Disease Control and Prevention (CDC) has advised that amoxicillin is another option for postexposure prophylaxis. Either doxycycline or ciprofloxacin is recommended by the CDC for initial prophylaxis when the antibiotic susceptibility of an anthrax strain is unknown. The CDC website on anthrax (available at *http://www.bt.cdc.gov/agent/anthrax*) is the best source for detailed recommendations regarding the choice of antibiotics, doses, and durations for both prevention and treatment of anthrax. Recommendations currently include either ciprofloxacin, 500 mg orally every 12 hours, or doxycycline, 100 mg orally every 12 hours, for a total of 60 days. Levofloxacin has the potential for once-daily 500 mg dosing, but safety data beyond 28 consecutive days in adults are very limited, and recommendations from the CDC have not yet been made.

Prevention of anthrax secondary to bioterrorism remains a priority. Evolving approaches for detecting and responding to any future bioterrorism attacks with anthrax include the Biowatch System and the Autonomous Detection Systems. The "Cities Readiness Initiative" was initially described on the CDC website in June 2004 as a program for multiple U.S. cities and metropolitan areas to help prepare them for large-scale public health emergencies, including bioterrorism attacks (e.g., with aerosolized anthrax or another organism). Large volumes of medical supplies, including but not limited to antibiotics, could be delivered rapidly from the Strategic National Stockpile to one or multiple locations across the nation, followed by local and regional distribution.

Treatment

Treatment of clinical anthrax includes antibiotics and, in the case of inhalational anthrax, pleural fluid drainage. The CDC recommendations for treatment include a multidrug regimen with either ciprofloxacin (400 mg intravenously every 12 hours) or doxycycline (100 mg intravenously every 12 hours) plus one or more additional antimicrobials for inhalational or gastrointestinal anthrax: rifampicin, vancomycin, penicillin, ampicillin, chloramphenicol, imipenem, clindamycin, or clarithromycin. Penicillin (or ampicillin) should not be used as a single agent in the initial therapy for inhalational anthrax because of the risk that resistance will develop. A detailed algorithm for the management of cutaneous anthrax is posted on the website of the American Academy of Dermatology (available at *www.aad.org/professionals/educationcme/bioterrorism/CutaneousAnthrax.htm*). Initial treatment of suspected anthrax meningitis should be combination therapy with a fluoroquinolone given intravenously and one or two other antibiotics that penetrate well into the central nervous system and are active against *B. anthracis,* such as penicillin, ampicillin, meropenem, vancomycin, or rifampicin.

If persons are potentially exposed to aerosolized anthrax spores, they should also receive three doses of anthrax vaccine at 0, 2, and 4 weeks under an FDA IND protocol, according to recommendations made by the CDC in 2004. Although only limited supplies of the current generation of anthrax vaccine exist, an additional stockpile of the next-generation anthrax vaccine, made with a recombinant PA, has been ordered via the U.S. Bioshield program. Postexposure anthrax vaccination might permit a shorter course of antibiotics by stimulating protective immunity faster than the infection itself can.

A 60-day course of antibiotic therapy is recommended for inhalational anthrax because of concern that residual spores may germinate into vegetative bacteria if antibiotic therapy is stopped sooner. When clinically appropriate, intravenous therapy can be changed to oral therapy, and multiple antibiotics might be reduced to only ciprofloxacin or doxycycline. Cutaneous anthrax is usually treated for 7 to 10 days rather than 60 days if inhaled spores are not an issue.

Adjunctive corticosteroids have been used historically for anthrax meningitis and for severe airway compromise caused by cutaneous anthrax of the neck. However, steroids have not been shown in a randomized clinical trial to be beneficial in any clinical forms of anthrax.

Another critical treatment modality for inhalational anthrax is pleural drainage via chest tube or by thoracentesis initially performed when the patient is still in the intermediate-progressive stage, if possible.

Prognosis

The inhalational anthrax of all six patients who survived the attacks of 2001 was diagnosed during the "intermediate-progressive stage," and prompt therapy prevented progression beyond this stage. The 45% case-fatality rate in 2001 was much improved over the 88% rate seen in the

United States from 1900 to 1976. Survival is more likely in patients who undergo pleural drainage, receive multidrug antibiotic regimens, do not require intubation or tracheotomy, and do not progress to anthrax meningoencephalitis. The mortality from cutaneous anthrax is approximately 20% if untreated, including patients in whom upper airway compression develops from a lesion on the neck or in whom secondary bacteremic anthrax meningitis develops.

Future Directions

Research is ongoing in an attempt to develop a commercially available, clinically validated, rapid test for the diagnosis of infection with *B. anthracis,* either before symptoms start, in the early-prodromal stage of the illness, or in later clinical stages if the patient may have received antibiotics before blood or cerebrospinal fluid was obtained for culture. In the future, anthrax antitoxins, such as anthrax immune globulin and multiple other candidate antitoxins, could become available if needed through FDA regulatory mechanisms such as the IND and Emergency Use Authorization systems. Such anthrax toxin inhibitors, in conjunction with antibiotics, could be particularly useful in treating patients who have progressed beyond the early-prodromal stage. In addition, antitoxin could be useful in the setting of infection with an engineered form of multidrug-resistant (MDR) anthrax. Currently, however, the best hope for the treatment of MDR anthrax is to find one or more licensed or investigational antibiotics to which such an MDR anthrax organism is still susceptible. New anthrax vaccines are also being tested.

SUGGESTED READINGS

CDC website on anthrax: Available at http://www.bt.cdc.gov/agent/anthrax. *Comprehensive and regularly updated with antibiotic doses and durations.*

Holty J-E, Bravata DM, Liu H, et al: Systematic review: A century of inhalational anthrax cases from 1900 to 2005. Ann Intern Med 2006;144:270–280. *Review of 82 patients with inhalational anthrax over a 105-year period.*

Infectious Disease Society of America (IDSA): Anthrax: Current, comprehensive information on pathogenesis, microbiology, epidemiology, diagnosis, treatment, and prophylaxis. Infectious Disease Society of America (IDSA) website: Available at www.cidrap.umn.edu/idsa/bt/anthrax/biofacts/anthraxfactsheet.html. *Detailed and updated online source.*

Lucey DR: An improved clinical staging system for inhalational anthrax. Clinicians' Biosecurity Network, 8 November 2005. Available at http://www.upmc-cbn.org/. *Presents a new clinical staging system.*

Sejvar JJ, Tenover FC, Stephens DS: Management of anthrax meningitis. Lancet Infect Dis 2005;5:287–295. Available at http://infection.thelancet.com. *Most recent and thorough review of anthrax meningitis.*

Vietri NJ, Purcell BK, Lawler JV, et al: Short-course postexposure antibiotic prophylaxis combined with vaccination protects against experimental anthrax. Proc Natl Acad Sci U S A 2006;103:7813–7816. *Rhesus macaques exposed to anthrax spores by aerosol were more likely to survive if they received the licensed anthrax vaccine plus antibiotics after exposure.*

318 *ERYSIPELOTHRIX* INFECTIONS

Annette C. Reboli

Definition

Erysipelothrix rhusiopathiae causes three well-defined patterns of human infection: (1) erysipeloid, a cellulitis of the fingers and hands (also known as whale finger or pork finger), which is the most common manifestation of infection with *E. rhusiopathiae;* (2) a diffuse cutaneous form; and (3) a bacteremic form, with or without cutaneous involvement, usually complicated by endocarditis.

The Pathogen

E. rhusiopathiae is a thin, pleomorphic, nonsporulating, microaerophilic gram-positive rod. It may be confused with other gram-positive bacillary organisms, in particular, *Listeria monocytogenes* and *Corynebacterium* species. It can be differentiated from *L. monocytogenes* by its lack of motility, lack of catalase and coagulase production, and resistance to neomycin. Most strains of *E. rhusiopathiae* produce hydrogen sulfide on triple sugar iron agar slants, a feature that distinguishes *E. rhusiopathiae* from *L. monocytogenes* and from corynebacteria. Because α-hemolysis may be seen after 48 hours of incubation of *E. rhusiopathiae,* confusion with streptococci may also occur. The term *erysipeloid* refers to cutaneous infection by *E. rhusiopathiae* and should not be confused with erysipelas, which is a superficial cellulitis caused by streptococci or staphylococci.

Epidemiology

E. rhusiopathiae is found worldwide as a commensal or as a pathogen in a variety of wild and domestic animals, including swine, sheep, cattle, horses, dogs, rodents, chickens, ducks, turkeys, penguins, and parrots, as well as in flies, ticks, mites, and lice. The greatest commercial impact of *E. rhusiopathiae* infection is due to disease in swine, but infection of sheep and poultry is also important economically. Although the organism colonizes the mucoid surface slime of fish, it does not appear to cause disease in these animals. Environmental surfaces in contact with infected animals or their products are potential sources of *E. rhusiopathiae.* It can persist for prolonged periods in contaminated soil. Even though *E. rhusiopathiae* is resistant to smoking, salting, and pickling, it is killed within 15 minutes by heating to 55° C and by several commercially available home disinfectants.

Although the incidence of cutaneous infection in humans seems to be decreasing because of technologic advances in animal industries, human infection still occurs in specific settings. Infection in humans is usually the result of contact with infected animals or their products. Persons at greatest risk for infection include fishermen, fishmongers, farmers, butchers, slaughterhouse workers, and veterinarians. The organism gains entry through cuts and abrasions on the skin. The seasonal incidence of erysipeloid parallels that of swine erysipeloid and is highest in the summer and early fall. The rare instances of systemic infection that do not have an occupational link suggest that oropharyngeal or gastrointestinal colonization with the organism may occur. Erysipeloid and erysipeloid with bacteremia have been reported rarely after cat and dog bites, thus suggesting that *E. rhusiopathiae* may be part of the oral flora of these animals.

Pathobiology

The virulence of *E. rhusiopathiae* is associated, at least in part, with resistance to phagocytosis by polymorphonuclear leukocytes. This antiphagocytic ability results from its possession of a capsule. In the absence of specific antibodies, *E. rhusiopathiae* evades phagocytosis, but even if phagocytized, it is able to replicate intracellularly in these cells. The enzyme neuraminidase may also be a virulence factor.

Clinical Manifestations

Because of its mode of acquisition (contact with infected animals or their products, with organisms inoculating abrasions on the skin), lesions are usually confined to the fingers and hands. A well-defined, slightly elevated, violaceous lesion accompanied by a very painful, throbbing, burning, or itching sensation develops within 2 to 7 days of traumatic dermal inoculation. The infected area is swollen. Vesicles may be present, but suppuration is absent. The lesion spreads slowly to other fingers but rarely involves the fingertips or the skin above the wrist. As the lesion spreads peripherally, the central area clears. Systemic signs and symptoms are rare. There may be sterile arthritis of an adjacent joint. Regional lymphadenopathy or lymphadenitis occurs in about 20% of cases, and low-grade fever develops in approximately 10%. Lesions usually resolve within 3 weeks without treatment. Relapse occurs in 1% of cases.

The diffuse cutaneous form is rare. The cutaneous lesion progresses proximally from the site of inoculation or appears at remote areas. Patients often have fever and arthralgias, but blood cultures are generally negative.

Systemic infection with *Erysipelothrix* is uncommon. Approximately 70 cases of bacteremia have been reported; most of the patients had endocarditis, and all but two cases involved native valves. In 60% of cases, infection developed on apparently normal heart valves. One third of patients had an antecedent or concurrent skin lesion of erysipeloid. The clinical manifestations of endocarditis secondary to *E. rhusiopathiae* and other microorganisms are similar. *E. rhusiopathiae* endocarditis correlates highly with occupation, exhibits a tropism for the aortic valve, affects more males than females, and is associated with high mortality. Cases of *E. rhusiopathiae* endocarditis have been complicated by paravalvar and myocardial abscess formation, cerebral emboli, and acute renal failure. A few cases of systemic infection have occurred in immunocompromised hosts, although a third had a history of ethanol abuse. There has been a suggestion that *E. rhusiopathiae* bacteremia without endocarditis occurs more frequently than was previously believed and that bacteremia may be occurring with increased frequency in immunocompromised patients whereas endocarditis usually occurs in immunocompetent patients. Focal infections, including brain abscess, osteomyelitis, septic arthritis, necrotizing fasciitis, and peritonitis, have been reported. Some of these infections were complications of bacteremia. Septic arthritis has occurred after arthroscopic reconstruction of the anterior cruciate ligament. Peritonitis has complicated peritoneal dialysis.

Diagnosis

E. rhusiopathiae grows on routine laboratory media. Because *E. rhusiopathiae* is located only in deeper parts of the skin in cases of erysipeloid, biopsy of the entire thickness of the dermis from the edge of the lesion yields maximum recovery of the organism. Routine blood culture techniques are adequate for growth and isolation of the organism in suspected cases of bacteremia or endocarditis. Various selective media have been used to improve the isolation of *E. rhusiopathiae* from contaminated specimens. Molecular techniques such as polymerase chain reaction with primers specific for *E. rhusiopathiae* have been developed and may improve the efficiency of detection and identification.

Treatment

Rx

Most isolates of *E. rhusiopathiae* are susceptible to penicillin, cephalosporins, imipenem, clindamycin, ciprofloxacin, and ofloxacin. Some resistance has been observed with erythromycin, tetracycline, and chloramphenicol. *E. rhusiopathiae* is resistant to vancomycin, aminoglycosides, trimethoprim-sulfamethoxazole, and sulfonamides. Penicillin G is the treatment of choice. Uncomplicated cutaneous lesions generally respond well to a 5- to 7-day course of oral penicillin. Treatment hastens healing, although relapse may still occur. Bacteremia should be treated with intravenous penicillin; cases of endocarditis should be treated with 12 to 20 million U of penicillin G daily or ceftriaxone, 1 g daily for 4 to 6 weeks. Cephalosporins are an alternative in an penicillin-allergic patient. The use of quinolones, in particular, ofloxacin or ciprofloxacin, may be considered for *Erysipelothrix* infections when the patient is allergic to β-lactams. Valve replacement may be necessary in patients with endocarditis. Vaccines are available for commercial use in animals only.

Prevention

Proper cleaning and disinfection of work surfaces and attention to hygienic work practices, including the use of gloves and hand hygiene, reduce the risk for infection.

SUGGESTED READINGS

Brooke CJ, Riley TV: *Erysipelothrix rhusiopathiae:* Bacteriology, epidemiology and clinical manifestations of an occupational pathogen. J Med Microbiol 1999;48:789–799. *A comprehensive review including recent advances in molecular approaches to diagnosis and understanding of taxonomy and pathogenesis.*

Fidalgo SG, Riley TV: Detection of *Erysipelothrix rhusiopathiae* in clinical and environmental samples. Methods Mol Biol 2004;268:199–205. *A review of diagnostic methods with an emphasis on polymerase chain reaction.*

Nassar IM, de la Llana R, Garrido P, Martinez-Sanz R: Mitro-aortic infective endocarditis produced by *Erysipelothrix rhusiopathiae:* Case report and review of the literature. J Heart Valve Dis 2005;14:320–324. *A review of clinical features of cases of endocarditis.*

Robson JM, McDougall R, van der Valk S, et al: *Erysipelothrix rhusiopathiae:* An uncommon but ever present zoonosis. Pathology 1998;30:391–394. *Clinical manifestations, pathologic findings, and treatment are reviewed.*

Shimoji Y: Pathogenicity of *Erysipelothrix rhusiopathiae:* Virulence factors and protective immunity. Microbes Infect 2000;2:965–972. *Recent advances in our understanding of pathogenicity and protective immunity are discussed.*

319 CLOSTRIDIAL INFECTIONS

John G. Bartlett

CLOSTRIDIAL MYONECROSIS

Definition

Clostridial gas gangrene is myonecrosis caused by toxins elaborated by *Clostridium* species, primarily *C. perfrigens* and less often by *C. septicum, C. novyi, C. histolyticum, C. bifermentans,* and *C. fallax.*

Epidemiology

Gas gangrene has historically been a complication of battlefield injuries. The incidence associated with war wounds was 5% in World War I, 0.7% in World War II, 0.2% in the Korean War, and 0.02% in the Vietnam War. The estimated annual number of cases in the United States is about 1000 per year. Traumatic injuries account for about 50% of cases and postoperative complications for 30% of cases, and approximately 20% are "spontaneous" or nontraumatic. Among trauma cases, vehicular accidents account for 70% of infections, and the remaining develop in patients after crush injuries, industrial accidents, gunshot wounds, and burns. Minor injuries that can result in secondary clostridial infections include puncture wounds, intramuscular injections, simple lacerations, and subcutaneous injections, especially with epinephrine. Postoperative infections are most frequently associated with surgery on the appendix, biliary tract, or intestine.

Pathobiology

Clostridia are widely distributed in nature and can be cultured from nearly all soil samples, from environmental sites, including the hospital, and from the human intestine. One review of 187,936 open traumatic wounds reported that 3.8% were contaminated by clostridia but the frequency of gas gangrene was very low. A critical factor is the physiologic state of the wound with conditions that support germination and toxin production by toxigenic clostridia. Particularly critical are a low oxidation-reduction potential, hypoxia, appropriate substrates, and calcium ions. The probability of infection is substantially increased by devitalized muscle and the presence of foreign material such as dirt. *C. perfringens* elaborates at least 12 recognized toxins; especially important and possibly essential is the α-toxin of *C. perfringens* type A, which produces myonecrosis and histologic features of gas gangrene after intramuscular injection in experimental animals. This toxin possesses phosphonolipase and sphingomyelinase activity that causes cell death.

Clinical Manifestations

Initial symptoms usually occur 1 to 4 days after the precipitating event, although the range may be from 8 hours to 3 weeks. The initial symptom is pain that is often sudden and severe at the site of surgery or trauma. The involved skin has intense edema and is initially pale before progressing to a bronze or magenta color, followed by the formation of bullae. The bullae contain fluid that may be clear or hemorrhagic. The discharge has an odor that is described as "foul-sweet."

Circulatory collapse is common and may reflect the effect of α-toxin, which suppresses cardiac contractility. About 15% of patients have bacteremia that is usually complicated by rapid hemolysis with a dramatic drop in the hematocrit, which may decrease to 0%. Common complications include jaundice, hypotension, hepatic failure, and renal failure. The renal failure is often due to hemoglobulinuria and myoglobulinuria but may also be due to acute tubular necrosis from hypotension. The hypotension often does not respond to a fluid challenge because it is generally due to direct suppression of cardiac contractility by α-toxin. Despite the severity of the illness, the patient's mental status is usually remarkably good until very late-stage disease.

Surgical intervention shows necrotic muscle that does not contract with stimulation. Deeper dissection reveals beefy red necrotic muscle that becomes black and extremely friable in the late stages. There is a watery, brownish discharge that seeps through wounds and has the characteristic odor.

Uterine gas gangrene, which was frequently seen after septic abortions, is now rare but may complicate normal delivery, amniocentesis, cesarean section, or abortion. The onset is usually sudden with fever, tachycardia, hypotension, renal failure, and jaundice. Radiography may show gas in the uterine wall. The urine is often "port wine" in color as a result of hemoglobulinuria, and there is often jaundice because of massive intravascular hemolysis. The usual causes are *C. perfringens* or *C. sordellii.*

Spontaneous myonecrosis, which is a variant of gas gangrene, occurs in the absence of trauma. One distinctive association is colon cancer or neutropenic enterocolitis. This infection is also seen with acute leukemia and is most common with chemotherapy for solid tumors and after stem cell transplantation. The usual portals of entry are the terminal ileum, cecum, and ascending colon, hence the term "typhlitis." Some patients have cyclic neutropenia. The usual manifestation is a necrotizing infection in an extremity or in the abdominal wall accompanied by hypotension and renal failure. Examination shows spreading crepitations with rapid clinical deterioration over a period of hours, and imaging reveals gas. The most common pathogens are *C. perfringens* and *C. septicum,* but a more benign form is found with *C. tertium.*

Diagnosis

The diagnosis of gas gangrene is usually based on a constellation of characteristic clinical features, including myonecrosis, shock, and renal failure. The patient typically complains of very severe pain. Early recognition is important because early institution of treatment may strongly influence the prognosis. The diagnosis is established by examination of the muscle, which shows the putrid discharge, the characteristic bullae, and crepitations. Gram stain demonstrates abundant gram-positive bacilli and no inflammatory cells. Histopathologic examination of the lesion shows myonecrosis without polymorphonuclear leukocytes, a finding that is remarkably different from most soft tissue infections, which do not feature necrosis and have abundant inflammatory cells. Gas is present in the tissue and may be detected by physical examination, radiography, or other method of imaging. Conditions that are often confused with gas gangrene include gas-forming cellulitis, streptococcal myonecrosis, and necrotizing fasciitis (Table 319–1).

Prevention

The basic principles of prevention are adequate management of traumatic wounds—establishing adequate drainage, removing foreign bodies, draining hematomas, and ensuring good hemostasis.

Treatment

Rx

The most important facet of treatment is prompt surgical débridement. Many or most cases require extensive, often mutilating surgery. Penicillin and clindamycin are recommended but will rarely be adequate without radical surgery, except in patients with neutropenic enterocolitis, who may often be managed with antibiotics. The rationale for penicillin combined with clindamycin is that some strains of clostridia are resistant to clindamycin, but clindamycin is probably the superior drug for reducing toxin formation at subtherapeutic doses. Other antibiotics that are generally effective include metronidazole, chloramphenicol, and tetracyclines. The use of hyperbaric oxygen is controversial, in part because the therapeutic trials are either of poor quality or not convincing.

Prognosis

Factors associated with a poor prognosis include elderly age, location on the trunk, association with severe underlying disease, leukopenia, renal failure, hemolysis, and shock. The best results are seen in young patients with involvement of a single extremity. Management plays an important role, particularly the use of early and aggressive surgery, as well as antibiotics. The overall mortality rate of patients with traumatic gas gangrene in tertiary centers is about 25%.

CLOSTRIDIUM DIFFICILE–ASSOCIATED DIARRHEA AND COLITIS

Definition and Pathogen

C. difficile–associated diarrhea or colitis is defined as otherwise unexplained diarrhea or colitis associated with a positive test for *C. difficile* toxin A or toxin B. *C. difficile* is a spore-forming organism that survives well in nature and is widely distributed in the environment.

Epidemiology

Three well-characterized risk factors are antibiotic use, advanced stage, and stay in an acute or chronic care facility. It is most common in bathroom facilities and rooms of patients with *C. difficile*–associated diarrhea and on the hands of health care workers who care for them. About 3%

TABLE 319–1 DIFFERENTIAL DIAGNOSIS OF GAS GANGRENE

	Gas Gangrene	Gas-Forming Cellulitis	Streptococcal Myonecrosis	Necrotizing Fasciitis
Preceding event	Trauma	Trauma	Trauma	Diabetes trauma
Incubation period	1–4 days	>3 days	3–4 days	1–4 days
Pathogen	Clostridia	Clostridia	*Streptococcus pyogenes*	Anaerobes
Toxicity	Severe	Minimal	Moderate	Moderate
Skin appearance	Tense, bullae	Swollen	Edema	Bullae
Gas	Usually	Abundant	No	Usually
Muscle involvement	Yes	No	Yes	No
Drainage	Foul and dark	Thin, dark, foul	Pus	Dishwater foul
Gram stain	GPB, no PMNs	PMNs, GPB	PMNs, GPC	Mixed flora
Surgery	Extensive	Débridement	Excision	Fillet

GPB = gram-positive bacilli; GPC = gram-positive cocci; PMNs = polymorphonuclear leukocytes.

of healthy adults harbor *C. difficile* as a component of their colonic flora, but the frequency is 20 to 40% in hospitalized patients and increases with the duration of hospitalization. Nearly all antibiotics have been implicated, but the most common are clindamycin, the cephalosporins, and the fluoroquinolones. This disease is rare in children despite frequent exposure to antibiotics, but the risk increases with increasing age and is both most common and most severe in persons older than 65 years. Many hospitals and chronic care facilities have epidemics, which require stringent infection control policies, sometimes augmented by programs to control the use of implicated antibiotics.

Pathobiology

Factors contributing to the pathogenesis of *C. difficile*–associated diarrhea and colitis include (1) a source of the organism, presumably the host's normal flora or an environmental source; (2) altered intestinal flora as a result of antibiotic exposure; (3) toxin production, which occurs with rapid growth of the vegetative forms of toxigenic strains; and (4) host-related susceptibility such as age and possibly immunologic naïveté. The toxins implicated in this complication are designated A and B. Most strains of *C. difficile* are toxigenic and produce both toxins under identical culture conditions, although occasional strains produce toxin B without toxin A and there is variation in the amount of toxins produced. Toxin B is a potent cytotoxin that causes nonlethal disruption of actin microfilaments of the cytoskeleton. Toxin A causes similar cytotoxic changes but is much less potent in tissue culture assays; it causes neutrophilic infiltration and severe mucosal damage in intestinal loops of various rodents. Some strains exhibit deletion of an 18–base pair gene designated *tcdC* that is responsible for downregulation of toxin A and B production. Some strains also produce "binary toxin," which is related to the ι-toxin of *C. perfringens* type E. *C. difficile*–associated enteric disease is mediated by toxin, and the assumption is that disruption of the flora induced by antibiotic exposure results in conversion of *C. difficile* spores to the vegetative forms, which produce both toxin A and B. The toxins appear to account for most or all of the biologic effects.

Clinical Manifestations

C. difficile is like nearly all other enteric pathogens in that it causes a wide spectrum of clinical symptoms ranging from asymptomatic carriage of *C. difficile* toxins with no clinical consequences to severe and sometimes life-threatening colitis complicated by major fluid losses and systemic complications. Many patients simply have "nuisance diarrhea" that resolves when the implicated drug is discontinued. Others with more characteristic features of colitis have substantial fluid losses combined with fever, cramps, fecal leukocytes, and leukocytosis.

A protein-losing enteropathy may cause hypoalbuminemia, sometimes progressing to anasarca. Leukocytosis is common and sometimes reaches leukemoid levels of 30,000 to 60,000/mm^3 or higher. Factors that usually indicate severe or late-stage disease include toxic megacolon, a leukemoid reaction, high fever, severe fluid losses, hypoalbuminemia, and renal failure.

Diagnosis

The diagnosis should be suspected in any patient who has otherwise unexplained diarrhea in association with antibiotic use, although only about 20% of patients in this category actually have evidence of *C. difficile*. Factors that more specifically suggest this diagnosis include evidence of colitis (cramps, fever, leukocytosis, fecal leukocytes), hypoalbuminemia, toxic megacolon, pseudomembranes on colonoscopy, imaging showing toxic megacolon, or exposure to high-risk antibiotics, including clindamycin, cephalosporins, or fluoroquinolones.

Colitis may be seen by endoscopy or imaging such as computed tomography. The most characteristic form of colitis is pseudomembranous colitis, which is almost always due to *C. difficile*. The disease is nearly always restricted to the colon.

The standard test to establish the diagnosis is an assay to detect toxin A or toxin A plus toxin B. The latter is preferred because about 1 to 3% of strains produce toxin B but not toxin A. The most common laboratory method is an enzyme immunoassay (EIA), but its sensitivity is only 60 to 80%, so repeat tests are often necessary, and some patients require empirical treatment when tests are negative but clinical features are compelling. The standard cytotoxin assay is more sensitive than EIA but has the disadvantages of a 24- to 48-hour delay and requirement for tissue culture facilities that are not always readily available in clinical laboratories. Some laboratories test for the presence of *C. difficile* instead of the toxin, but this approach substantially reduces specificity because many people, especially in hospitals, are colonized but do not exhibit toxin production. A third approach used by some laboratories is to culture for *C. difficile* or test for "common antigen," which is a marker for *C. difficile*, as screening tests and then test for toxin in those who are positive.

The differential diagnosis includes patients who have an alternative enteric pathogen that causes colitis, antibiotic-associated diarrhea, ischemic colitis, or idiopathic inflammatory bowel disease. For patients with antibiotic-associated diarrhea and no evidence of colitis, the cause of the diarrhea with a negative *C. difficile* toxin assay is not usually defined but is commonly attributed to disturbances in colonic flora with resulting colitis because of failure to metabolize carbohydrates or bile acids, or both.

Prevention

The two principles of prevention are avoidance of unnecessary use of antibiotics, particularly those that are implicated in this disease, and infection control. Patients with this disease should be in single rooms with bathroom facilities if possible. Careful attention needs to be paid to handwashing with soap and water, and rooms of patients with this disease should be cleaned with a sporicidal agent at discharge. In epidemics, it may be necessary to restrain using antibiotics that account for the majority of cases.

Treatment

Rx

Standard treatment is discontinuation of the implicated antibiotic, supportive care, and avoidance of antiperistaltic agents. These measures alone often result in resolution of symptoms in patients who are not seriously ill. When antimicrobials are needed, the only drug that has been proved efficacious in a placebo-controlled trial is oral vancomycin, 125 mg four times daily. 1 The alternative is metronidazole, which provides response rates comparable to those of vancomycin, is much less expensive, and avoids the concern about vancomycin-resistant enterococcus. One approach is to use vancomycin in patients who are seriously ill and to substitute it for metronidazole if there is a delayed response. The anticipated response with either of these two drugs is rapid defervescence with gradual normalization of bowel habits by day 5 to 8 of treatment. Failure to respond often means that the disease has progressed too far or an alternative condition is accounting for the symptoms.

Other antibiotic options include oral fusidic acid, teicoplanin, and bacitracin. Another approach is to use agents that bind *C. difficile* toxins (e.g., cholestyramine) or to attempt to replace the normal flora (e.g., oral lactobacillus). However, there is no evidence that these options are as good as vancomycin or metronidazole. For patients who have severe and progressive disease despite standard therapy, there may be an indication for colectomy. About 20% of patients given either vancomycin or metronidazole have recurrence of symptoms when treatment is stopped because of the persistence of *C. difficile* spores or acquisition of a new strain. Treatment is readministration of either vancomycin or metronidazole.

Prognosis

The majority of patients respond to simple withdrawal of the implicated antibiotic combined with a single course of metronidazole or vancomycin. Some patients with progressive disease eventually require colectomy or intensive care. The attributable mortality rate is as high as 16%, and the majority of lethal cases occur in patients older than 65 years. Some patients have multiple relapses that require repeated courses of antibiotics, usually metronidazole or vancomycin.

BOTULISM

Definition

Botulism is a severe neuroparalytic disease caused by botulinum toxin produced by clostridial species, usually *Clostridium botulinum.*

The Pathogen

C. botulinum is a gram-positive, spore-forming obligate anaerobe that is widely distributed in nature and frequently found in soil, marine environments, and agricultural products. Each strain produces one of seven immunologically distinct toxins designated by the letters A to G. Related clostridial species, including *Clostridium baratii* and *Clostridium butyricum,* may produce botulinum toxin as well. All these neurotoxins produce the same syndrome, and the causes of disease in humans are types A, B, and E, with rare cases involving type F.

Epidemiology

Six categories of botulism have substantially different epidemiologic characteristics, but generally similar clinical features.

Food-borne botulism is the most common form of botulism in the world but is second to infant botulism in the United States, with 2 to 30 cases occurring per year. Foods most frequently implicated are home processed, and most cases are sporadic (single cases) or involve two to three people in the "outbreak." Type A is the predominant form in the West, and type B predominates in the East. Alaska has the highest rate of any state, approximately 27% of all U.S. cases; it is often associated with nontraditional fermentation methods to prepare marine food. Meat and meat products are most frequently implicated in Europe, where the predominant toxin type is B. In China, the most frequent vehicle is a vegetable product, and type A predominates.

Wound botulism, first described in 1943, usually involves toxin types A or B, reflecting their presence in soil, and generally results from traumatic wounds. Outbreaks have also been related to "skin popping" with contaminated black tar heroin (Chapter 32).

Infant botulism, which is the most frequently recognized form in the United States, results from production of botulinum toxin in the intestine after colonization in children aged 1 to 9 months. The source of *C. botulinum* is sometimes honey but is usually never identified. Nearly all cases are type A or B. The disease spectrum shows considerable variation, but the most commonly recognized form is the "floppy baby syndrome," characterized by lethargy, diminished sucking, weakness, feeble cry, and decreased spontaneous activity with loss of head control.

Inhalation botulism is a category A form of bioterrorism, which indicates that it is one of the top six agents in terms of probability for use as a bioweapon. The presumed mechanism would be contamination of food, a water supply, or a commercial beverage. Iraqi officials admitted to having 10,000 L of concentrated botulinum toxin for use as bioweapons after the Persian Gulf War. It is estimated that a point source aerosol release of the toxin could incapacitate or kill 10% of people within a 0.5-km radius.

Iatrogenic botulism results from the use of botulinum toxin for cosmetic or therapeutic purposes. Doses for cosmetic treatment are far too low for systemic disease, but the use of unlicensed products with high concentrations of botulinum toxin can cause systemic symptoms. Higher doses used for the management of muscle movement disorders have caused occasional cases with systemic botulism-like symptoms.

Adult intestinal botulism results from intestinal colonization by *C. botulism* with in situ production of botulinum toxin. The pathophysiology is similar to that of infant botulism but differs from foodborne botulism, which is characterized by the ingestion of preformed toxin, although there may be some overlap. This form of botulism is rare in adults and most often seen in patients with anatomic or functional abnormalities of the intestines, sometimes augmented by antibiotics.

Pathobiology

Toxins are absorbed from the intestine (ingested preformed toxin or in situ production in the intestine), inhaled (aerosol from bioterrorism), or absorbed from cutaneous sources (wound or iatrogenic). The toxin is disseminated by the systemic circulation and causes neurotoxicity by binding presynaptic motor neuron terminals and blocking acetylcholine transmission across the neuromuscular junction, thereby causing flaccid paralysis. The estimated lethal doses of purified botulinum toxin A for a 70-kg human are 0.09 to 0.15 μg when given intravenously, 0.8 to 0.9 μg when inhaled, and 70 μg when given orally.

Clinical Manifestations

All symptoms reflect absorption of botulinum toxin from the gut, lung, or wound; the toxin does not penetrate intact skin. Clinical symptoms consist of highly distinctive symmetrical cranial nerve palsies, followed by a symmetrical descending flaccid paralysis. Prominently involved cranial nerves III, IV, and VI cause blurred vision and diplopia; involvement of cranial nerve VII causes the characteristic expressionless facies and dysphagia; and involvement of cranial nerve IX causes dysarthria. Thus, the initial symptoms include the "four Ds": diplopia, dysphonia, dysarthria, and dysphagia. These findings are followed by a descending symmetrical paralysis of voluntary muscles. Neurologic examination shows bilateral sixth cranial nerve paresis, ptosis, dilated pupils with a sluggish reaction, diminished gag reflex, and then descending involvement of motor neurons, including the muscles of respiration. The most common cause of death is respiratory failure. Deep tendon reflexes are diminished or absent. Mentation remains clear, vital signs are normal, and the neurologic findings are symmetrical. The tempo of the disease and the extent of paralysis in the absence of treatment are highly variable. The symptoms may be restricted to a few cranial nerves, or there may be complete paralysis of all voluntary muscles. Progression may occur over a period of hours or days. Variations in tempo and extent of neurologic deficit depend on the inoculum size of botulinum toxin.

Diagnosis

Botulism should be suspected in patients with an acute flaccid paralysis, particularly in the presence of bilateral sixth cranial nerve dysfunction, associated neurologic findings, and a 3- to 5-day food history indicating consumption of home-canned foods. The finding of two or more cases that are epidemiologically linked is virtually diagnostic because all other syndromes that resemble botulism are rare and sporadic. Exposure of injection drug users to black tar heroin and the possibility of bioterrorism are other sources of epidemics. With bioterrorism, the epidemiology may reflect a common geographic source exposure such as a local water supply or aerosolized toxin, but it may also be widely distributed as with a contaminated milk supply.

Standard laboratory tests for suspected food-borne botulism include analysis of serum, stool, gastric contents, or food for botulinum toxin and analysis of stool or food for *C. botulinum.* Toxin assays should be performed before treatment with antitoxin. With wound botulism, the diagnosis is established by recovery of *C. botulinum* from wound cultures or detection of toxin in serum. With suspected inhalation botulism, diagnostic specimens include gastric fluid, stool, and serum. The toxin assays are generally available only at public health laboratories. The standard is mouse bioassay for detection and quantification of toxin; the toxin is quantified by the mouse intraperitoneal lethal dose in 50% of mice ($MIPLD_{50}$). Toxin type is determined by type-specific antibody neutralization. In general, adult patients with clinical evidence of botulism show detectable toxin in sera in a third of cases and toxin in stool in a third of cases; the organism is recovered from stool in about 60%.

The differential diagnosis includes myasthenia gravis (Chapter 448), Guillain-Barré syndrome (Chapter 446), tick paralysis, cerebrovascular accident (Chapter 422), trichinosis (Chapter 378), Lambert Eaton syndrome (Chapter 448), hypocalcemia (Chapter 266), hypermagnesemia (Chapter 120), organophosphate poisoning (Chapter 111), atropine poisoning (Chapter 111), and paralytic poisoning by shellfish or puffer fish (Chapter 382). Electromyography using repetitive stimulation at 20 to 50 Hz often distinguishes among causes of flaccid paralysis. Electromyography shows a diminished amplitude of muscle action potentials with a single supramaximal stimulus and facilitation of action potentials with paired or repetitive stimuli. The results of cerebrospinal fluid analysis and cranial imaging are normal in botulism.

Prevention

The disease may be prevented by destruction of spores in the original food source, by inhibition of germination, or by destruction of preformed toxin.

1. *Destruction of spores* with heat or irradiation: Spores of types A and B survive boiling for several hours, especially at high altitudes such as in Colorado. Spores are destroyed if kept at 120° C for 30 minutes in pressure cookers. Spores of type E are more heat labile and are killed by heating at 80° C for 30 minutes. Modern industrial canning ("retort canning") predictably kills botulinum spores.
2. *Germination* may be inhibited by reducing the pH, refrigerating, freezing, drying, or adding inhibitory substances such as salt, sugar, or sodium nitrate.
3. *Preformed toxin* may be inactivated by heating at 85° C for 5 minutes.

Treatment

Rx

Clinicians who suspect botulism should (1) immediately seek clinical consultation, (2) notify public health authorities, and (3) give antitoxin. The agency to contact in the United States is the public health authorities (state health department or Centers for Disease Control and Prevention 24-hour emergency service at 770-488-7100); similar public health agencies would be contacted in other countries. Treatment consists of supportive care and passive immunization with botulinum antitoxin.

The standard treatment of adults is trivalent antitoxin if the toxin type is not known or type-specific antitoxin for types A, B, or E; the standard dose is one vial (5500 to 8500 IU) diluted 1:10 in saline and delivered by slow intravenous infusion. An experimental heptavalent vaccine (A to G) from the U.S. Army may be available for unusual types associated with bioterrorism. The antitoxin should be given as early as possible and should not be delayed while awaiting microbiologic results. This treatment will not reverse paralysis or neutralize toxin already bound to nerve endings, but it will neutralize unbound toxin in the circulation to prevent progression. The antitoxin is horse serum, which is associated with anaphylaxis in 2% and other hypersensitivity reactions in 9% of patients when larger doses are used; patients should be given small doses to screen for reaction before the full dose.

Respiratory failure is a major risk, and patients must be monitored carefully with liberal use of ventilatory support. The requirement for mechanical ventilation varies from about 20% in adults with foodborne disease to 60% with infant botulism. Other forms of supportive care include enteral or parenteral feeding and positioning in the reverse Trendelenburg position.

Toxin may be removed from the gastrointestinal tract by gastric lavage, cathartics, and enemas early in the course. Antibiotic treatment is unnecessary except for wound botulism. Infants should be given the orphan drug intravenous human botulism immune globulin (Human) (BIG-IV) as a single intravenous infusion of 50 mg/kg. 2

Prognosis

The case-fatality rate for untreated food-borne botulism was 60 to 70%, but it is currently about 6%. Infant botulism in the United States now causes a mortality rate of less than 1%; use of human antitoxin has reduced the median duration of hospitalization from 6 to 3 weeks. 2 Patients who survive any form of botulism generally have complete recovery.

TETANUS

Definition

Tetanus is a neurologic syndrome caused by a neurotoxin elaborated at the site of injury by *Clostridium tetani*.

The Pathogen

C. tetani is an anaerobic, gram-positive, slender motile bacillus. The sporulated form has a characteristic drumstick or tennis racket shape with a terminal spore. The vegetative form produces tetanospasmin, a protein neurotoxin with a molecular weight of approximately 151 kD, including a heavy chain (100 kD) that binds neuronal cells and a light chain that blocks release of neurotransmitters.

Epidemiology

C. tetani can be found in 2 to 23% of soil samples, with the highest yield in cultivated land and the lowest yield in virgin soil. The organism can also be found in stool from a variety of animals, house dust, operating rooms, and contaminated heroin.

Tetanus is most common in warm climates and in highly cultivated rural areas. The greatest problem occurs in resource-limited countries because of poor immunization standards and unhygienic practices. An example is the practice of dressing the umbilical stump with animal dung or "dusting powder," a local dried clay sold for cosmetic purposes, after childbirth by unimmunized mothers. It is estimated that the annual toll from neonatal tetanus in developing countries is 400,000, mostly secondary to tetanus neonatorum (see later). In the United States, 50 to 70 cases are reported annually, and almost all occur in unimmunized or inadequately immunized persons. A review of 110 cases of tetanus from 1989 to 1990 in the United States showed that 86 (78%) were associated with an acute injury, 10 (9%) were complications of chronic wounds, and 5 (5%) represented complications of injection drug use. There was 1 case of neonatal tetanus, and 10 (9%) had no recognized portal of entry. The age of these patients was near 60 years in 58% and younger than 20 years in 6%; this age distribution reflects the impact of waning immunity with aging.

Pathobiology

Tetanospasmin ranks with botulism toxin as the most potent known microbial toxin; 1 mg is capable of killing 50 to 70 million mice. Clinical tetanus requires a source of the organism, local tissue conditions that promote toxin production, and immunologic naïveté. The usual portals of entry are traumatic wounds, surgical wounds, subcutaneous injection sites, burns, skin ulcers, infected umbilical cords, and otitis media with perforation of the tympanic membrane. The spores are ubiquitous in the environment, and most cases reflect contamination from exogenous sources, although endogenous infection is conceivable in occasional cases that follow intestinal surgery. Important factors at the site of injury are necrotic tissue, suppuration, and the presence of a foreign body, all of which are responsible for a reduction in the local oxidation-reduction potential, thus promoting reversion of spores to the vegetative forms that produce tetanospasmin.

Tetanospasmin binds the peripheral nerve terminals and is then carried intra-axonally within membrane-bound vesicles to spinal neurons at a transport rate of approximately 75 to 250 mm/day. On reaching the perikarya of the motor neurons, the light chain passes to the presynaptic terminals, where it blocks the release of neurotransmitters, including glycine, which is the neurotransmitter used by group 1A inhibitory afferent motor neurons. Loss of the inhibitory influence results in unrestrained firing with sustained muscular contraction. In severe cases, involvement of the sympathetic chain causes autonomic dysfunction. Binding of the toxin is irreversible, so recovery requires the generation of new axon terminals.

Clinical Manifestations

Forms of tetanus include generalized, localized, cephalic, and neonatal.

Generalized tetanus, which is the most common form of tetanus, accounts for 85 to 90% of reported cases in the United States. The extent of the associated trauma varies from a rather trivial injury that may be forgotten by the patient to a severe, contaminated crush injury. The usual incubation period is 7 to 21 days, depending largely on the distance of the site of injury from the central nervous system. The "onset period" refers to the time from the first clinical symptoms of tetanus to the first generalized spasm. An incubation period of less than 9 days and an onset period of less than 48 hours appear to be associated with more severe symptoms.

Generalized tetanus is characterized by a persistent tonic spasm with brief exacerbations. The neck and jaw are almost always involved, with trismus grimacing resulting in the appearance of "risus sardonicus."

Trismus is the initial complaint in 75% of cases, so the patient is often initially seen by a dentist or oral surgeon. Other early features include irritability, restlessness, diaphoresis, and dysphagia with hydrophobia and drooling. Persistent spasm of the back musculature may cause opisthotonos. These early manifestations reflect involvement of the bulbar and paraspinous muscles, possibly because they are innervated by the shortest axons. Waves of opisthotonos are highly characteristic of the disease. With progression, all muscles contract, with stronger muscles overtaking the weaker muscles such that involvement of the extremities causes painful flexion and adduction of the arms, clenched fists, and extension of the legs. Noise or tactile stimuli may precipitate spasms and generalized convulsions, which may also occur spontaneously. Involvement of the autonomic nervous system may result in severe arrhythmias, blood pressure oscillation, profound diaphoresis, hyperthermia, rhabdomyolysis, laryngeal spasm, and urinary retention. In most cases, the patient remains lucid and afebrile. The condition may progress for 2 weeks despite antitoxin therapy because of the time required for intra-axonal toxin transport. Complications include convulsions, fractures from sustained contractions, pulmonary emboli, bacterial infections, and dehydration.

Localized tetanus, which refers to involvement of the extremity from a contaminated wound, shows considerable variation in severity. In mild cases, patients may simply have weakness of the involved extremity, presumably limited by partial immunity. In more severe cases, there are intense, painful spasms that usually progress to generalized tetanus. This relatively unusual form of tetanus has an excellent prognosis for survival.

Cephalic tetanus generally follows a head injury or occurs with *C. tetani* infection of the middle ear. Clinical symptoms consist of isolated or combined dysfunction of the cranial motor nerves, most frequently the seventh cranial nerve. This dysfunction may remain localized or progress to generalized tetanus. Cephalic tetanus is a relatively unusual form of tetanus, but the incubation period is only 1 or 2 days, and the prognosis for survival is usually poor.

Tetanus neonatorum, which refers to generalized tetanus resulting from *C. tetani* infection in neonates, occurs primarily in underdeveloped countries, where it accounts for up to half of all neonatal deaths. The usual cause is the use of animal dung or "dusting powder" to dress the umbilical cord in newborns of unimmunized mothers. The usual incubation period after birth is 3 to 10 days, and it is sometimes referred to as "disease of the seventh day," reflecting the average incubation period. The child typically shows irritability, facial grimacing, and severe spasms with touch. The mortality rate exceeds 70%.

Diagnosis

The diagnosis of tetanus is usually based on clinical observations. The putative agent, *C. tetani,* is infrequently recovered with culture of the wound. A confirmed history of immunization or a serum antitoxin level greater than 0.01 U/dL makes tetanus unlikely, but exceptions have been reported. Results of cerebrospinal fluid analysis are entirely normal, and the electroencephalogram generally shows a sleep pattern. Diagnostic testing is not usually necessary except in cases lacking an identified portal of entry. The differential diagnosis depends on the dominant clinical features and includes dystonic reactions as a result of neuroleptic toxicity (Chapter 111), meningitis (Chapter 437), dental abscess (Chapter 451), seizure disorder (Chapter 426), subarachnoid hemorrhage (Chapter 432), hypocalcemic or alkalotic tetany (Chapter 266), alcohol withdrawal (Chapter 31), and strychnine poisoning (Chapter 111). Strychnine also antagonizes glycine, and strychnine poisoning is the only condition that truly mimics tetanus. Strychnine levels in blood and urine establish the diagnosis. Dystonic reactions may resemble tetanus and are distinguished by rapid response to anticholinergic agents.

Prevention

Tetanus is a disease of medical neglect. Immunization (Chapter 16) is virtually 100% effective, so nearly all cases of tetanus occur in unimmunized or inadequately immunized individuals. The Immunization Practices Advisory Committee recommends active immunization of infants and children with DPT (diphtheria and tetanus toxoids and pertussis adsorbed) at 2 months, 4 months, 6 months, 15 months, and 4 to 6 years. Tetanus toxoid is a highly effective antigen, and protective levels of serum antitoxin in persons who complete the primary series persist for at least 10 years. Td (tetanus and diphtheria toxoids adsorbed for adult use) is recommended every 10 years at mid-decade ages (15 years, 25 years, 35 years, etc.). This recommendation is commonly neglected, as demonstrated by serosurveys showing that 40% of persons older than 60 years in the United States lack protective levels of tetanus antitoxin. The recommended primary immunization series for unimmunized persons older than 7 years is Td at time 0, 4 to 8 weeks, 6 to 12 months after the second dose, and then every 10 years. Nearly all states now require DPT immunization for school enrollment. About 95% of tetanus cases in the United States occur in persons who have not received the primary series of tetanus toxoid. Immunization of childbearing women confers protection for their infants through transplacental maternal antibody. [3]

Prevention of tetanus after injury (Table 319–2) requires appropriate wound management, assurance of adequate immunity, and consideration of antibiotic prophylaxis. The aim of surgery is to eliminate necrotic tissue, purulent collections, and foreign bodies that promote the environmental conditions necessary for spore germination. Passive immunization with tetanus immune globulin (TIG) is recommended only for "tetanus-prone" wounds in patients with inadequate or unknown primary immunization status. The definition of *tetanus prone* depends on the interval between injury and treatment, the degree of contamination, the extent of devitalized tissue or foreign bodies within the site of injury, and the depth of injury. Antimicrobial agents such as penicillin, erythromycin, or metronidazole may be given to inhibit replication of the vegetative forms of *C. tetani,* but immunization and wound cleansing are considered more important.

TABLE 319–2 GUIDELINES FOR TETANUS PROPHYLAXIS IN WOUND MANAGEMENT

History of Adsorbed Tetanus Toxoid	Clean and Minor Wounds		Other Wounds*	
NO. OF DOSES	Td	TIG	Td	TIG
Unknown or <3	Yes	No	Yes	Yes
≧3 Doses†	Yes if >10 years since the last dose	No	Yes if >5 years since the last dose	No

*Wounds contaminated with dirt, stool, soil, and so forth; puncture wounds; avulsions; missile wounds, crush injuries, burns, and frostbite.
†If only three doses of toxoid have been administered, a fourth should be given.
Td = tetanus and diphtheria toxoids adsorbed; TIG = tetanus immune globulin.

Treatment

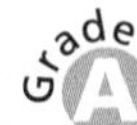

Patients with tetanus require intensive care with particular attention to respiratory support, treatment with benzodiazepines, autonomic nervous system support, passive and active immunization, surgical débridement, and antibiotics directed against *C. tetani.* There may be clinical progression for about 2 weeks despite antitoxin treatment because of the time required to complete transport of toxin. The severity of disease may be reduced by partial immunity, so some patients have mild disease with minimal mortality, whereas others have mortality rates as high as 60% despite expert care.

Supportive Care

It is most important to assess airway function. Many patients require endotracheal intubation with benzodiazepine sedation and neuromuscular blockade; a tracheostomy should be placed if the endotracheal tube causes spasms. A nasal feeding tube is usually required for nutritional support.

Control of Muscle Spasms

Benzodiazepines have become the mainstay of therapy to control spasms and provide sedation. The most extensively studied is diazepam given in 5-mg increments; lorazepam and midazolam are equally effective. Patients with tetanus may have high tolerance for the sedation effects of these drugs and require exceptionally high doses. When tetanus symptoms resolve, the drugs must be tapered over at least a 2-week period to prevent withdrawal reactions. If control of spasms cannot be achieved by benzodiazepines, long-term neuromuscular blockade is performed with vecuronium (6 to 8 mg/hr).

Passive Immunization

Human TIG should be given as soon as possible to neutralize toxin that has not entered neurons. The usual dose is 500 IU intramuscularly. Higher doses or intrathecal administration does not appear to be more effective. An alternative to TIG is pooled intravenous immunoglobulin. Equine TIG is equally effective, but the rate of allergic reactions is high because of the equine source; this preparation should no longer be used except in underdeveloped countries, where cost dictates such medical decisions.

Active Immunization

The standard three-dose schedule of immunization with tetanus toxoid should be given at an injection site separate from that used for immunoglobulin.

Antibiotic Therapy

C. tetani is susceptible in vitro to penicillins, cephalosporins, imipenem, macrolides, metronidazole, and tetracyclines. Clinical studies favor the use of metronidazole, which should be given in an intravenous dose of 2 g/day for 7 to 10 days.

Autonomic Nervous System Dysfunction

This complication generally reflects excessive catecholamine release and is usually treated with labetalol (0.25 to 1.0 mg/min) for blood pressure control. Other treatments of hypertension include morphine by continuous infusion, magnesium sulfate infusion, or epidural blockade of the renal nerves. Hypotension may require norepinephrine infusion. Bradycardia may require a pacemaker.

Surgery

Any wounds should be appropriately débrided.

Prognosis

The overall mortality rate for generalized tetanus is 20 to 25%, even in modern medical facilities with extensive resources. Patients with moderate or severe generalized tetanus generally require treatment for 3 to 6 weeks. The highest mortality rates are at the extremes of age. The most frequent cause of death is pneumonia, but many patients have no obvious findings at autopsy, thus suggesting that death was directly due to the neurotoxin. Patients who recover usually recover completely.

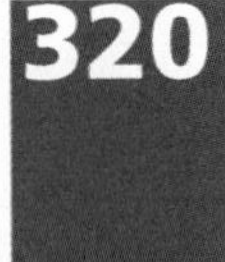

1. Keighley MR, Burdon DW, Arabi Y, et al: Randomized controlled trial of vancomycin for pseudomembranous colitis and postoperative diarrhea. BMJ 1978;16:1667–1669.
2. Arnon SS, Schechter R, Maslanka SE, et al: Human botulism immune globulin for the treatment of infant botulism. N Engl J Med 2006;354:462–471.
3. Vaccines for women to prevent neonatal tetanus. Cochrane Database Syst Rev 2005;19:CD00259.

SUGGESTED READINGS

Bartlett J: The new epidemic of *Clostridium difficile*–associated enteric disease. Ann Intern Med 2006;145:758–764. *A narrative review.*

Buoza E, Burillo A, Munoz P: Antimicrobial therapy of *Clostridium difficile*–associated diarrhea. Med Clin North Am 2006;90:1141–1163. *Review of the treatment options for this important disease.*

Cloud J, Kelly CP: Update on *Clostridium difficile*–associated disease. Curr Opin Gastroenterol 2007;23:4–9. *Comprehensive review.*

McDonald LC, Kittgore GE, Thompson A, et al: An epidemic, toxin gene–variant strain of *Clostridium difficile*. N Engl J Med 2005;353:2433–2441. *An epidemic that emphasized many key aspects of this disease.*

Rhee P, Nunley MK, Demetriades D, et al: Tetanus and trauma: A review and recommendations. J Trauma 2005;58:1082–1088. *The recommendation is toxoid only for those not immunized in the past 10 years, and there is no urgency to give it.*

Sobel J: Botulism. Clin Infect Dis 2005;41:1167–1173. *A comprehensive review.*

320 DISEASES CAUSED BY NON–SPORE-FORMING ANAEROBIC BACTERIA

Ellie J. C. Goldstein

Definition

Anaerobic bacteria are the predominant indigenous, normal flora of the human body, including the skin and the oral, gastrointestinal, and vaginal mucosa (Fig. 320–1; Table 320–1).

The Pathogens

Taxonomic advances have led to the reclassification of many anaerobic species (Table 320–2). The term "*Bacteroides*" is reserved for species of the *Bacteroides fragilis* group. What were previously considered "oral" *Bacteroides* and "pigmented" *Bacteroides* species have been reclassified as *Prevotella* (saccharolytic, pigmented species), *Porphyromonas* (asaccharolytic species), and other genera. Organisms that are capnophilic and not true anaerobes are often more related to *Campylobacter, Capnocytophaga,* and other genera. In addition, many new genera and several new species have been created to accommodate pathogens such as *Bilophila wadsworthia, Sutterella wadsworthensis,* and *Anaerobiospirillum thomasii.*

Epidemiology

Although these organisms perform beneficial functions, they are also consummate opportunistic pathogens that can cause serious infections, typically in combination with aerobic bacteria. Because the flora of these infections is often complex and culture results may be delayed, knowledge of the usual flora at the location of infection is an indispensable guide for selecting and instituting empirical antimicrobial therapy.

Pathobiology

Anaerobic bacteria range from those that die with very brief exposure to oxygen and are usually isolated only in normal flora studies to those that can survive on the surface of a fresh agar plate even in the presence of atmospheric oxygen (e.g., *B. fragilis*). Most anaerobes require an environment with a low oxidation-reduction potential (eH gradient), which can be accomplished in association with low pH, tissue destruction,

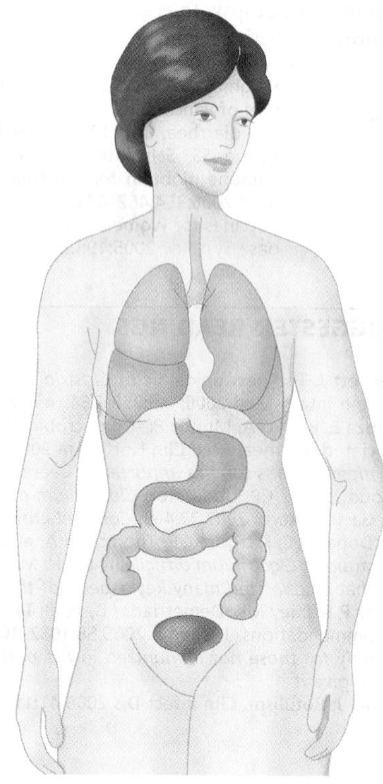

FIGURE 320–1 • Anaerobes as predominant normal microflora of the human body by general anatomic location. (Adapted from Finegold SM, Sutter VL: Diagnosis and Management of Anaerobic Infections. Kalamazoo, MI, Upjohn, 1976. Copyright by Dr. Finegold.)

byproducts from aerobic bacterial metabolism, or low oxygen content. Though not true anaerobes, some organisms such as microaerophilic streptococci and other capnophilic or hard-to-grow organisms are sometimes lumped together with anaerobes because of their fastidious nature. Some genera such as *Lactobacillus* and *Actinomyces* contain both aerobic and anaerobic species.

Anaerobic bacteria possess a variety of virulence factors that differ among species (Table 320–3).

Clinical Manifestations

Bacteremia

Transient anaerobic bacteremia occurs in approximately 85% of patients immediately after dental cleaning or manipulation. More than 200 cases of endocarditis from anaerobes are reported annually in the United States, usually in association with anatomic abnormalities or damaged cardiac valves (Chapter 76). The majority of anaerobic bacteremias are intermittent and associated with serious intra-abdominal or female genital tract infections, whereas a significant minority are associated with skin and soft tissue infections, often near the fecal stream. Overall, about 10% of bacteremias are due to anaerobes, and anaerobes are the sole isolates in 80% of such infections. *B. fragilis* group bacteremia is associated with an attributable mortality rate of 19% and a 16-day increase in length of hospital stay.

Head and Neck

Dental infections (Chapter 451) associated with a variety of oral anaerobic bacteria include periodontal disease, gingivitis, acute necrotizing ulcerative gingivitis, localized juvenile periodontitis, adult periodontitis, pericoronitis, endodontitis, dental abscess, and postextraction infection. Peritonsillar abscess (Chapter 455) is a deep-seated and potentially life-threatening complication of acute tonsillitis. It may extend into the various potential spaces of the neck or even the mediastinum and cause jugular vein thrombosis. Anaerobes may be isolated in more than 50% of such cases, usually in mixed culture with aerobes. Other regional infections include cervicofacial actinomycosis (Chapter 350), Ludwig's angina, *Fusobacterium necrophorum* sepsis with metastatic infection (Lemierre's syndrome), and neck space infections. Although their acute counterparts are generally infections caused by aerobes, chronic sinusitis (Chapter 452) and chronic otitis media (Chapter 452) often involve anaerobic bacteria of the normal oral flora.

TABLE 320–1 LOCATION OF VARIOUS GROUPS OF NONSPORULATING ANAEROBES AS NORMAL MICROFLORA IN HUMANS

	Location			
Organism	**Skin**	**Oral/Respiratory**	**Gastrointestinal Tract**	**Genitourinary Tract**
Actinomyces		+		
Bacteroides		+	+	
Eubacterium		+	+	
Fusobacterium		+	+	
Lactobacillus			+	+
Peptostreptococcus	+	+	+	+
Porphyromonas		+	+	
Prevotella		+	+	
Propionibacterium	+			
Veillonella		+	+	

TABLE 320–2 TAXONOMY OF ANAEROBIC BACTERIA

Current Name	Synonym/Comment
Bacteroides fragilis	
Bacteroides caccae	
Bacteroides distasonis	
Bacteroides merdae	
Bacteroides nordii	New species
Bacteroides salyersi	New species
Bacteroides goldsteinii	New species
Bacteroides eggerthii	*Bacteroides fragilis* group
Bacteroides stercoralis	
Bacteroides ovatus	
Bacteroides thetaiotaomicron	
Bacteroides vulgatus	
Bacteroides uniformis	
Campylobacter gracilis	*Bacteroides gracilis*
Bacteroides ureolyticus	New species
Bacteroides tectus	New species
Chlorochromatium finegoldii	New species
Prevotella bivia	*Bacteroides bivius*
Prevotella buccae	*Bacteroides buccae (ruminicola)*
Prevotella dentalis	*Mitsuokella dentalis, Hallella sergens*
Prevotella disiens	*Bacteroides disiens*
Porphyromonas somerae	*Prevotella levii*–like (PELO)
Prevotella nigrescens	*Prevotella intermedia*
Prevotella melaninogenica	*Bacteroides melaninogenicus*
Prevotella oralis	*Bacteroides oralis*
Prevotella oris	*Bacteroides oris*
Prevotella tancerae	New species
Porphyromonas asaccharolytica	*Bacteroides asaccharolyticus*
Porphyromonas uenosis	New species
Porphyromonas forsythus	*Bacteroides forsythus*
Porphyromonas gingivalis	*Bacteroides gingivalis*
Porphyromonas salivosa	*Bacteroides salivosus*
Fusobacterium canefelinum	New species
Fusobacterium necrophorum	
Fusobacterium ulcerans	New species
Anaerobiospirillum thomasii	New species
Bilophila wadsworthia	New species
Sutterella wadsworthensis	New species
Tannerella forsythensis	*Bacteroides forsythus*
Bacteroides tectium	New species
Prevotella tannerae	New species
Bacteroides zoogleoformens	New species

TABLE 320–3 POTENTIAL VIRULENCE FACTORS IN VARIOUS ANAEROBES

Factor	Species
ADHESION	
Capsule	*Bacteroides fragilis* group, *Prevotella melaninogenica*
Pili/fimbriae	*B. fragilis* group *Porphyromonas gingivalis*
Hemagglutinin	*P. gingivalis*
Lectin	*Fusobacterium nucleatum*
INVASION/TISSUE DAMAGE	
Proteases	*Fusobacterium necrophorum* *Bacteroides* species *Porphyromonas* species
Hemolysins	Many species
Endotoxin	*B. fragilis*
Fibrinolysin	*B. fragilis* group *Porphyromonas* species
Heparinase	*B. fragilis* group *Porphyromonas* species
Neuraminidase	*B. fragilis* group *Porphyromonas* species
ANTIPHAGOCYTIC	
Capsule	*B. fragilis* group *P. gingivalis*
Lipopolysaccharide	*B. fragilis* group *F. necrophorum, P. gingivalis*
Metabolic products	Most anaerobes
TOXINS	
Endotoxin	*B. fragilis* *F. necrophorum*
Enterotoxin	*B. fragilis*

Adapted from Duerden BI: Virulence factors in anaerobes. Clin Infect Dis 1994;18(Suppl. 4):253.

Pulmonary

Anaerobic bacteria are the predominant normal flora of the oral cavity and upper respiratory tract, and most pneumonias are due to aspiration of indigenous oral flora (Chapter 97). Aspiration of oral flora may be a result of altered consciousness, dysphagia, or mechanical devices such as intubation equipment. Poor oral hygiene is associated with an increased anaerobic bacterial burden, and the presence of aerobes or necrotic tissue lowers pH, which in turn facilitates the growth of anaerobes. Anaerobes are involved in 90% of patients with community-acquired aspiration pneumonia, and in many cases they may be the sole pathogens. Anaerobes can be isolated in 35% of patients with nosocomial aspiration pneumonia. If the anaerobic component of aspiration pneumonia is not treated, the anaerobes can cause a persistent abscess (Chapter 98).

Management requires good pulmonary toilet and antimicrobial therapy. For mild to moderate aspiration pneumonia, intravenous clindamycin is generally as good an empirical therapy as more expensive alternatives such as β-lactam/β-lactamase inhibitor combinations and carbapenems. 1

Intra-abdominal

Anaerobes outnumber aerobes by 1000:1 in the large intestine, so it is not surprising that they play an important role in almost all intra-abdominal infections. Most visceral abscesses (e.g., hepatic; Chapter 152), chronic cholecystitis (Chapter 159), perforated and gangrenous appendicitis (Chapter 145), postoperative wound infections and abscesses, diverticulitis (Chapter 145), and any infection associated with fecal contamination of the abdominal cavity involve both aerobes and anaerobes. *B. fragilis* group members are especially important pathogens because they are encapsulated and resist phagocytosis, are often resistant to many commonly used antibiotics, and promote abscess formation. They may also be associated with concomitant bacteremia and sepsis. Effective antimicrobials include moxifloxacin, 2 piperacillin-tazobactam, tigecycline, 3 and carbapenems (ertapenem, imipenem, and meropenem). 4

Diarrhea

Enterotoxin-producing strains of *B. fragilis* can cause diarrhea and may be associated with bacteremia. *A. thomasii*, a motile gram-negative spiral bacterium with bipolar flagella, has been isolated from the feces of asymptomatic dogs and cats and has been transmitted from them to humans. It may also be associated with bacteremia.

TABLE 320–4 OBSTETRIC-GYNECOLOGIC INFECTIONS THAT COMMONLY INVOLVE ANAEROBES

Abscesses
Pelvic
Vulvovaginal
Vaginal cuff
Tubo-ovarian
Bartholin's gland
Skene's gland
Endometritis
Myometritis
Parametritis
Pelvic cellulitis
Pelvic thrombophlebitis
Bacterial vaginosis
Salpingitis
Chorioamnionitis
Intrauterine device–associated infection
Pelvic actinomycosis
Postabortal sepsis

TABLE 320–5 CLUES TO THE PRESENCE OF ANAEROBIC INFECTION

Infection in proximity to a mucous membrane
Foul odor from a discharge or wound
Gas or crepitus in a tissue
Infection associated with necrotic tissue or malignancy
Gram stain morphology consistent with anaerobes
"Sulfur" granules (actinomycosis)
Infection after a human or animal bite
Dental infection
Infection after abdominal or pelvic surgery
No growth on routine bacterial culture (especially if Gram stain shows organisms)
Fistulous tracts
Any abscess
Typical clinical picture of gas gangrene or necrotizing fasciitis
Failure to respond to drugs not active against anaerobes (e.g., trimethoprim-sulfamethoxazole, aminoglycosides, older quinolones)

Adapted from Finegold SM: Anaerobic Bacteria in Human Disease. New York, Academic Press, 1977, p 42.

Obstetric-Gynecologic

A variety of obstetric-gynecologic diseases involve anaerobes (Table 320–4). Bacterial vaginosis, which has been linked to a perturbation in the normal anaerobic vaginal flora, accounts for 45% of all cases of vaginitis. Bacterial vaginosis is present in approximately 20% of college women and up to 45% of women attending sexually transmitted disease clinics; it can be diagnosed by the presence of a foul, gelatinous vaginal discharge, a vaginal pH higher than 4.5, the presence of "clue cells," and a fishy amine odor after 10% KOH is added to vaginal secretions. Bacterial vaginosis has also been associated with preterm labor or delivery, chorioamnionitis, low birthweight, postpartum endometritis, vaginal cuff cellulitis, and postabortal pelvic inflammatory disease. Bacterial vaginosis can increase the risk of infection with human immunodeficiency virus type 1 and the development of other sexually transmitted diseases (Chapter 307). Culture of tubo-ovarian abscess, a complication of chronic pelvic inflammatory disease (Chapter 307), grows anaerobes in up to 85% of cases.

Skin and Soft Tissue

Diabetes

An infected fetid foot is the most frequent infectious reason why diabetics are hospitalized (Chapter 247). Anaerobes are present in more than 50% of these infections and are more often associated with vascular insufficiency, tissue necrosis, and amputation. Anaerobic infections are more common in patients with fever, long-standing wounds, crepitus, foul odor, abscess, or previous antimicrobial therapy.

Bites

Anaerobes, which are part of the oral flora of the biting animal, are present in approximately 65% of animal bite wound infections (Chapter 349), especially those that are more severe or associated with tissue necrosis or abscess formation. Most are penicillin/ampicillin susceptible. *Pasteurella multocida, Staphylococcus intermedius, Staphylococcus aureus,* and streptococci should also be considered potential pathogens.

Human bites, both occlusional and clenched fist injuries, tend to be more serious than animal bites. Anaerobes, which can be isolated from 55% of human bite wounds, are frequently β-lactamase producing and penicillin resistant. Septic arthritis and osteomyelitis can also result from human bite wounds. *Eikenella corrodens,* streptococci, *S. aureus,* and *Haemophilus* species must also be considered as potential pathogens when choosing empirical antimicrobial therapy.

Gangrene

Gangrene, which indicates necrosis, most often of skin and subcutaneous tissue, is frequently rapidly progressive. Types of infectious gangrene, which may sometimes be indistinguishable on a clinical basis, include the following:

1. *Gas gangrene,* which can incidentally involve other anaerobes besides *Clostridium perfringens* (Chapter 319) and other clostridia.
2. *Progressive bacterial synergistic gangrene* often involves microaerophilic streptococci and peptostreptococci, as well as aerobic bacteria such as *S. aureus* and Enterobacteriaceae.
3. *Synergistic necrotizing cellulitis* involves a mix of aerobic and anaerobic bacteria, including *B. fragilis* and peptostreptococci, especially in diabetic patients. The cellulitis is markedly painful, crepitus may be present, and the discharge has a foul odor.
4. *Fournier's gangrene,* which is a serious infection of the scrotum or perineum, starts with scrotal pain and erythema and then progresses rapidly to necrosis and gangrene, which can lead to sloughing of tissue. It is more often seen in diabetics and can be associated with trauma.

Diagnosis

Anaerobic infections should be suspected in a number of specific clinical scenarios (Table 320–5). An appropriately collected microbiologic specimen (Table 320–6) is critical for accurate diagnosis.

Treatment

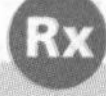

General principles of treatment (Table 320–7) include appropriate antimicrobial therapy coupled with prompt drainage and surgical débridement. The various clinically important anaerobes can be characterized by reasonably predictable susceptibility patterns to antimicrobial agents (Table 320–8), but culture and sensitivity results should ultimately guide therapy.

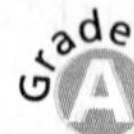

1. Kadowaki M, Demura Y, Mizuno S, et al: Reappraisal of clindamycin IV monotherapy for treatment of mild-to-moderate aspiration pneumonia in elderly patients. Chest 2005;127:1276–1282.
2. Malangoni MA, Song J, Herrington J, et al: Randomized controlled trial of moxifloxacin compared with piperacillin-tazobactam and amoxicillin-clavulanate for the treatment of complicated intra-abdominal infections. Ann Surg 2006;244:204–211.
3. Babinchak T, Ellis-Grosse E, Dartois N, et al: The efficacy and safety of tigecycline for the treatment of complicated intra-abdominal infections: Analysis of pooled clinical trial data. Clin Infect Dis 2005;41:(Suppl. 5):S354–S367.
4. Solomkin JS, Yellin AE, Rotstein OD, et al: Ertapenem versus piperacillin/tazobactam in the treatment of complicated intra-abdominal infections. Ann Surg 2003;237:235–245.

TABLE 320–6 SPECIMENS ACCEPTABLE FOR ANAEROBIC CULTURE

ACCEPTABLE

Any aspirate: abscess, joint, lung, empyema, suprapubic (urine), brain, myringotomy, percutaneous abdominal, or pelvic
Tissue biopsy
Cellulitis after débridement of superficial debris
Bile
Surgical specimen (not contaminated with normal flora)
Transtracheal aspirate of sputum
Culdocentesis fluid
Antral sinus puncture
Deep gingival pocket

UNACCEPTABLE

Sputum
Voided urine
Nasal discharge
Feces/diarrhea
Vaginal discharge
Superficial wounds
Mucous membrane

TABLE 320–7 GENERAL PRINCIPLES OF THERAPY FOR ANAEROBIC INFECTIONS

Elimination of dead space
Débridement
Drainage
Irrigation
Provision of adequate circulation when possible
Removal of foreign bodies
Antimicrobials
- Activity against most likely pathogen(s): location dependent, normal flora considered
- Absorption, appropriate route of administration
- Penetration into site of infection
- Dosage appropriate for local tissue levels, body mass of patient, renal and liver function
- Duration appropriate for condition
- Susceptibility testing of isolate to guide specific therapy

TABLE 320–8 ANTIMICROBIAL SUSCEPTIBILITY PATTERNS FOR ANAEROBIC BACTERIA*

	Drug							
Bacteria	**Penicillin**	**β-Lactamase†**	**Cefoxitin**	**Cefotetan**	**Imipenem, Meropenem, Ertapenem**	**Moxifloxacin**	**Clindamycin**	**Metronidazole**
Bacteroides fragilis	–	+	+	+	+	+	V	+
Bacteroides thetaiotaomicron	–	+	V	V	+	V	V	+
B. fragilis group, other	–	+	V	V	+	+	V	+
Prevotella species	V	+	+	+	+	+	+	+
Fusobacterium nucleatum	V	+	+	+	+	V	+	+
Fusobacterium necrophorum	+	+	+	+	+	V	+	+
Porphyromonas species	+	+	+	+	+	+	+	+
Peptostreptococcus	+	+	+	+	+	+	+	V
Propionibacterium acnes	+	+	+	+	+	+	+	–
Veillonella	+	+	+	+	+	+	+	+
Actinomyces	+	+	+	+	+	+	+	–

*Based on a variety of in vitro susceptibility studies from different laboratories and using different techniques.
†β-Lactamase inhibitor–β-lactam combination (e.g., ticarcillin/clavulanate, ampicillin/sulbactam, piperacillin/tazobactam).
+ = Susceptible; – = resistant; V = variable.

SUGGESTED READINGS

Austin MN, Beigi RH, Meyn LA, et al: Microbiological response to treatment of bacterial vaginosis with topical clindamycin or metronidazole. J Clin Microbiol 2005;43:4492–4497. *Metronidazole may be the preferred therapy.*

Goldstein EJC, Snydman DR: Intra-abdominal infections: Review of the bacteriology, antimicrobial susceptibility and the role of ertapenem in their therapy. J Antimicrob Chemother 2004;53(Suppl. 2):ii29–ii36. *A clinical review.*

Hecht DW: Prevalence of antibiotic resistance in anaerobic bacteria: Worrisome developments. Clin Infect Dis 2004;39:92–97. *Emphasizes the importance of testing an organism's sensitivity to potential antibiotic therapies.*

Miki T, Kuwahara T, Nakayama H: Simultaneous detection of *Bacteriodes fragilis* group species by leuB-directed PCR. J Med Invest 2005;52:101–108. *LeuB-directed PCR using BacLBF and BacLBR is a useful for rapid diagnosis of Bacteroides infection.*

Stein GE, Goldstein EJ: Fluoroquinolones and anaerobes. Clin Infect Dis 2006;42:1598–1607. *A clinical review.*

321 MENINGOCOCCAL INFECTIONS

Michael A. Apicella

Definition

Meningococcal infections are a major cause of mortality and morbidity in developed and developing nations. *Neisseria meningitidis* is the causative agent in meningococcal infections. It is associated with enormous epidemics in developing countries and has become the most common cause of bacterial meningitis in American children since the use of the *Haemophilus influenzae* type b protein–capsular polysaccharide conjugate vaccine in infants dramatically reduced the incidence of meningitis caused by that organism. Because the meningococcal vaccine has limited effectiveness in the group at greatest risk for infection, children younger than 2 years, meningococcal infection is still a major problem worldwide. The devastating nature of systemic meningococcal infection makes it imperative that preventive measures be developed to control this disease fully. In addition, an effective vaccine against meningococcal serogroup B infection has not been developed. Until this goal is realized, it is crucial that the clinician recognize and be able to treat the infection successfully as early as possible in its course to ensure an outcome with minimum mortality and morbidity.

The Pathogen

N. meningitidis is a gram-negative diplococcus. Meningococci are considered a fastidious species, and media containing appropriate supplementation must be used to ensure reliable growth from clinical samples. The use of selective media such as Thayer-Martin medium has allowed isolation of the organism from sites such as the nasopharynx that contain diverse background flora. The organism grows best between 35 and 37° C in an atmosphere of 5% carbon dioxide. The organism does not grow below 32° C or above 41° C. Laboratory confirmation of the presence of the organism depends on the metabolism of glucose and maltose with production of acid but not gas.

Thirteen serologically distinct encapsulated forms have been implicated in infection, and their immunochemical differences are the basis for assigning encapsulated meningococci to serogroups. Over 98% of cases are caused by five serogroups: A, B, C, W135, and Y. Nonencapsulated strains are frequently identified as carrier strains in nasopharyngeal cultures during endemic periods but have not been isolated from body fluids of patients with systemic meningococcal disease. Meningococci can also be serotyped on the basis of antigenic differences in their outer membrane proteins and lipopolysaccharides. These serotypes have become important in studies of the epidemiology of infection and in the development of new vaccines.

Epidemiology

Endemic Infection

N. meningitidis can cause endemic and epidemic infection. At present, meningococcal infection is endemic in the United States, with approximately 2500 cases per year (case rate approximately 1 in 10^5 total population) reported to the Centers for Disease Control and Prevention (CDC). The case-fatality rate is approximately 12%. Disease rates in children younger than age 2 are approximately 10 times higher than in the overall population. Seasonal variation occurs, with the highest attack rates in February and March and the lowest in September. The male/female ratio of patients is approximately 1. The predominant serogroups causing infection in the United States currently are B, C, and Y.

Epidemic Infection

The epidemic form of meningococcal disease was first described in medical journals in Geneva in 1807, 80 years before the causative organism was identified by Weichselbaum.

Before World War II, periodic epidemics of meningococcal infection ravaged American cities. These were caused primarily by the serogroup A meningococcus. With improving standards of living, these epidemics have abated in this country and infection related to serogroup A has virtually disappeared.

Large-scale epidemics still occur with deadly frequency in Africa, parts of Asia, South America, and the countries of the former Soviet Union. These epidemics are most commonly caused by the serogroup A meningococcus and occasionally by the serogroup C meningococcus. In an area appropriately named the "meningitis belt" because it crosses the waist of sub-Saharan Africa, epidemics of meningococcal infection occur every 7 to 10 years. The case rate during these epidemics can be as high as 1 in 1000 total population. Case rates in children younger than age 2 can be 1 in 100 and may be due to particularly virulent clones of meningitis serogroup A. Over the past 10 years, outbreaks of infection due to W135 have occurred in Asia, Europe, and Africa.

In the developed nations of Western Europe, epidemics caused by serogroup B meningococcus have occurred over the past decade. Norway suffered such an epidemic with case rates of 1 in 10,000 individuals. A high attack rate was seen among teenagers in this epidemic.

Etiology

The reason for the epidemic spread of the meningococcus is not known. The organism is considered a respiratory pathogen, and spread is most likely by the aerosol route. It is clear that the high attack rates seen in the less well-developed countries are in part due to poverty and the consequences of crowding, poor sanitation, and malnutrition. Factors such as herd immunity and specific virulence factors associated with "epidemic strains" have been implicated as factors in the rapid spread of infection in these situations. From studies of an epidemic in central and east Africa, clonal analysis indicated that the epidemic strain had arisen in central Asia almost 7 years before the African epidemic. It had spread through northern India and Pakistan to Saudi Arabia and then with pilgrims from Mecca to Africa. A number of American pilgrims returning from Mecca at that time were found to have nasopharynx colonization with this epidemic strain.

Predisposition to meningococcal infection has been associated with preceding respiratory tract infection, particularly influenza. In one study of an epidemic limited to American schoolchildren traveling on the same school bus, it was shown that school absenteeism was higher during the 3 weeks before the outbreak than at any time in the preceding 3 years. This suggests a particularly severe outbreak of respiratory illness. The five children who developed meningococcal sepsis all complained of influenza-like symptoms before the meningococcal disease. On the basis of serologic analysis, a case-control study revealed that children in this population who complained of respiratory tract symptoms had B/Ann Arbor1/86 influenza. These data add to evidence suggesting that influenzal respiratory infection predisposes to meningococcal disease.

Epidemic infections in American military recruit camps were a major problem before the introduction of vaccination. Throughout the 19th century, the unique susceptibility of military recruits was attested to by the clinical descriptions of this infection that can be found in the records of the Crimean and American civil wars. Since the introduction of vaccination of all recruits in 1972 with a tetravalent vaccine containing serogroup A, C, Y, and W135 polysaccharides, epidemics have not occurred.

Pathobiology

The meningococcus has a narrow environmental niche. It is a strict human pathogen that has been isolated only from human mucosal surfaces or body fluids. A number of factors contribute to the ability of the organism to colonize and cause infection. The meningococcus has a typical gram-negative cell wall containing lipopolysaccharide or endotoxin, which is the primary toxin. Meningococci express pili (attachment organelles), which are important in adhesion to nasopharyngeal epithelial cells. Meningococci can express polysaccharide capsules, which are important virulence factors.

The molecular pathogenesis of meningococcal infection is beginning to be understood. Figure 321–1A outlines schematically the process involved in mucosal invasion, and Figure 321–1B shows the factors associated with the generation of the shock state and disseminated intravascular coagulopathy (DIC). The pathogenesis of *N. meningitidis* begins with colonization of the nasopharyngeal surface, which is essential for the evolution to systemic infection. The only exceptions are the rare occurrences in which *N. meningitidis* is inadvertently inoculated parenterally, in the laboratory or in the clinical setting. Infection of the nasopharynx occurs by inhalation of aerosolized particles containing meningococci, which penetrate the mucous layer and adhere to the mucosal upper airway epithelium. The pili act as long-range attachment organelles that bind to a receptor on the human cell surface and enhance attachment. Outer membrane surface proteins such as the class V proteins (opa and opc) also play a role in attachment and may be important in defining the tissue specificity of the organism. Lipo-oligosaccharide phase variation appears to play a role in the adherence process. Only unencapsulated meningococci enter epithelial cells, and capsular biosynthesis has been shown to stop as the meningococcus enters the epithelial cell.

On contact with the epithelial cell, the meningococcus initiates cytoskeletal changes within the epithelial cell, and a process that resembles receptor-mediated endocytosis incorporates the bacteria into vacuoles.

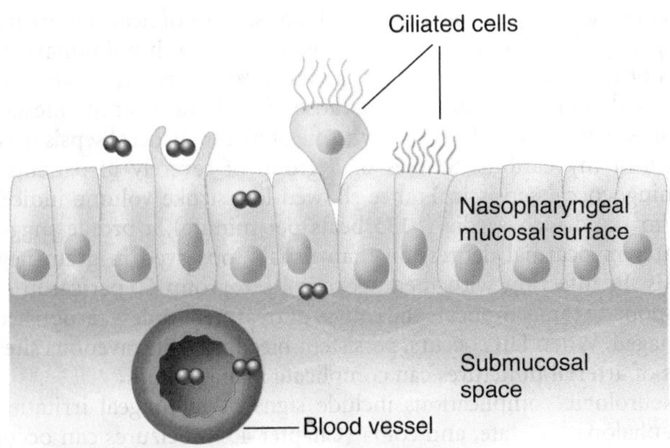

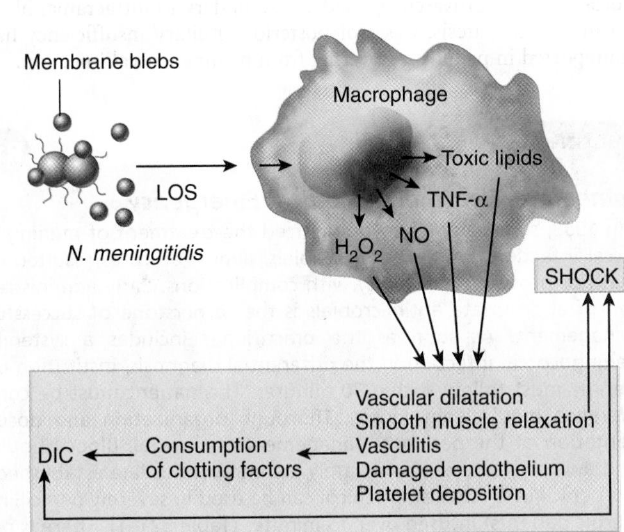

FIGURE 321–1 • A, Schematic representation of nasopharyngeal invasion by the meningococcus. The process involves attachment to the surface of nonciliated cells by meningococcal pili. Short-range attachment factors (meningococcal surface components) are probably involved in the endocytotic engulfment process as microvilli of the nasopharyngeal cell surround the organism. The nonciliated cells through which the organisms transmigrate do not appear to sustain damage. By contrast, the ciliated mucosal cells die and are extruded from the mucosal surface. Meningococcal lipo-oligosaccharide, peptidoglycan, and possibly other toxins are thought to be responsible for this cytolytic activity. Organisms in the submucosal space then have access to entry into capillaries and arterioles and can invade the vascular system. **B,** The rapid doubling time of the meningococcus and its ability to shed large amounts of endotoxin by a process called blebbing rapidly lead to a high-grade septic state with shock. Endotoxin (lipo-oligosaccharide, or LOS) interacts with macrophages to release cytokines, vasoactive lipids (prostaglandins), and free radicals such as H_2O_2, O^-, and NO. These substances damage vascular endothelium, resulting in platelet deposition and vasculitis. This leads to vascular disruption and the petechiae and ecchymoses that are frequently seen during meningococcal infection. Clotting factors are consumed, and disseminated intravascular coagulopathy (DIC) ensues, which is an ominous consequence of delayed treatment. Occasionally, the intravascular clotting can lead to occlusion of major arterial vessels in the extremities, requiring amputation. The most dire consequence of all these vascular effects is Waterhouse-Friderichsen syndrome, which is multiorgan failure caused by shock and hemorrhagic diathesis. (**A,** Data from Stephens DS: Gonococcal and meningococcal pathogenesis as defined by human cell, cell culture, and organ culture assays. Clin Microbiol Rev 1989;2:S104–S111; **B,** Data from Brandtzaeg P, Ovstebo R, Kierulf P: Compartmentalization of lipopolysaccharide production correlates with clinical presentation in meningococcal disease. J Infect Dis 1992;166:650–652.)

The factors allowing the survival of the organism within the epithelial cell vacuole are now being elucidated. *Neisseria* type 2 immunoglobulin A1 (IgA1) protease cleaves lysosome-associated membrane protein 1 and promotes survival of bacteria within epithelial cells. The meningococci are transported within the vacuole to the basolateral surface of the cell and released into the submucosal space, where they enter capillaries and arterioles. In the absence of specific antibody, the capsular polysaccharide provides an antiphagocytic barrier that protects the organism against normal host clearing mechanisms.

The rapid doubling time of the meningococcus and its ability to shed large amounts of endotoxin by a process called blebbing rapidly lead to a high-grade septic state with shock. Endotoxin and cytokine levels in meningococcal sepsis have been measured, and high tumor necrosis factor-α and interferon-γ levels have been shown to correlate with a poor prognosis. Endotoxin interacts with macrophages to release cytokines, vasoactive lipids, and free radicals such as H_2O_2, O^-, and NO. These substances damage vascular endothelium, resulting in platelet deposition and vasculitis. This process leads to vascular disruption and the petechiae and ecchymoses that are frequently seen during meningococcal infection. It is responsible for consumption of clotting factors and DICs, which are an ominous consequence of delayed treatment. Occasionally, the intravascular clotting can lead to occlusion of major arterial vessels in the extremities, necessitating amputation. The most dire consequence of all of these vascular effects is Waterhouse-Friderichsen syndrome, with multiorgan failure related to shock and hemorrhagic diathesis. There may be a genetic predisposition to the development of septic shock. Studies have suggested that variations in the plasminogen activator inhibitor 1 gene may influence the development of septic shock but not the probability of contracting meningococcal disease.

The propensity of the meningococcus to invade the central nervous system (CNS) and cause meningitis is poorly understood. The organism probably gains entry through the arachnoid villi. The release of endotoxin and peptidoglycan in the cerebrospinal fluid (CSF) evokes inflammatory factors that are chemoattractive for polymorphonuclear leukocytes (PMNs). Enzymes released by PMNs intensify the meningeal inflammation, leading to increased cerebrovascular permeability and brain edema.

Diagnosis

The laboratory diagnosis of systemic meningococcal infection is based on the isolation of the *N. meningitidis* from blood cultures, CSF, or other affected tissues. Blood cultures are positive in 60 to 80% of untreated patients, whereas CSF cultures are positive in 50 to 70%. Gram stain analysis of CSF requires a skilled, patient observer, but it can provide diagnostic results rapidly. Gram staining of the CSF can be useful as a rapid diagnostic tool, especially in patients with meningococcal meningitis. Approximately 50% of these patients have a positive Gram stain. In cases of meningococcemia without overt meningitis, the CSF Gram stain is positive in less than 25% of patients. Gram stain analysis of punch biopsy or needle aspiration samples of hemorrhagic skin lesions in meningococcal sepsis without clinical evidence of meningitis can lead to rapid diagnosis in up to 70% of cases. The tinctorial results for punch biopsy specimens were not affected by antimicrobials because Gram staining gave positive results up to 45 hours after the start of antimicrobial therapy. Cultures of these biopsy specimens or aspirates were also useful diagnostically for as long as 13 hours after the institution of antimicrobial therapy. Detection of meningococcal capsular polysaccharide in CSF can also be used as a method for rapid diagnosis. The test is most sensitive for the A and C polysaccharides and considerably less sensitive for serogroup B polysaccharide. In meningococcemia without clinically apparent meningitis, the antigen detection methods can be negative despite profound sepsis. The polymerase chain reaction has been found to be a rapid method for making the diagnosis of CSF infection. Studies in Great Britain during a meningococcal meningitis outbreak indicated its value in establishing the diagnosis in spite of antimicrobial therapy prior to hospitalization.

Clinical Manifestations

The Carrier State

There are several different meningococcal infection syndromes. The nasopharyngeal carrier state is considered an active infection because some individuals have symptomatic pharyngitis and rises in serologic titers to the infecting organism. A recent study indicated that a transmissible bacteriophage may be responsible for the differences between benign carrier strains and invasive disease-causing strains. The phage, which is of the filamentous family, excises from the chromosome and is secreted by the type IV pilin secretin. This element, by spreading among the population, may promote the development of new epidemic clones of *N. meningitidis* that are capable of disturbing the normal commensal relationship with humans and causing invasive disease. It is likely that all cases of acute systemic meningococcal infection are preceded by recent nasopharyngeal colonization, but most carriers remain asymptomatic. Studies have shown that the carrier state can persist for long periods of time, with about 5% of the population carrying the meningococcus in the nasopharynx during endemic periods. The majority of these isolates are unencapsulated. During epidemics, the carrier rate can rise to over 30% of the population, with the majority of individuals carrying the epidemic strains in the nasopharynx.

In a study of an epidemic among military recruits, nasopharyngeal colonization by the meningococcal strain responsible for the epidemic resulted in a 40% incidence of systemic infection if the person colonized also lacked bactericidal antibodies to the epidemic strain. This study confirmed the role of nasopharyngeal carriage as the source of systemic infection and the importance of serum antibody in protection against systemic meningococcal infection.

Meningitis and Meningococcemia

Acute systemic infection can be manifest clinically by three syndromes: meningitis, meningitis with meningococcemia, and meningococcemia without obvious signs of meningitis. Typically, an otherwise healthy patient has sudden onset of fever, nausea, vomiting, headache, decreased ability to concentrate, and myalgia. The patient frequently tells the physician that this is the sickest he or she has ever felt. Many have a feeling of impending death. In children, the infection is rare in those younger than 6 months because of protection by placentally transferred antibodies. Because children younger than 2 years cannot relate many symptoms, sudden onset of fever, leukocytosis, and lethargy are important signs. Initially, the physical examination may not reveal specific evidence of meningococcal disease. The pharyngitis sometimes associated with nasopharyngeal carriage can be misdiagnosed as streptococcal infection. This diagnosis frequently results in treatment with low-dose penicillin, which has little effect on the emerging meningococcal sepsis. Alternatively, the patient may be diagnosed with influenza because of complaints of fever, chills, and myalgia. In general, patients with meningococcal infection are considerably sicker on presentation than the majority of patients with streptococcal or viral infections. The vital signs show a low blood pressure with an elevated pulse rate. Diaphoresis is common. In such patients, an intensive search for petechiae should be mounted (Fig. 321–2). A complete examination of the skin with the patient completely undressed is essential. The physical examination should include provocative tests of meningeal irritability, the Kernig and Brudzinski signs. It must be remembered that patients with meningococcemia may not necessarily have meningeal signs, but 50 to 80% have petechiae on presentation. The mucosal surfaces of the soft palate and ocular and palpebral conjunctiva must also be examined for petechiae.

The infection can progress rapidly. Depending on the presentation of the patient, a critical situation can occur quickly. Profound shock with a DIC is the most ominous development in these patients. Coagulopathy, defined as a partial thromboplastin time of more than 50 seconds or a fibrinogen concentration less than 150 μg/dL, is a predictor of a poor prognosis. A number of studies have demonstrated that myocardial dysfunction can occur in meningococcal sepsis. Signs of heart failure including gallop rhythms and congestive heart failure with pulmonary edema are not uncommon. In one large series, 15% of pediatric patients were admitted to intensive care units because of cardiovascular manifestations. Approximately 25% of patients who die of meningococcal sepsis have evidence of myocarditis. Studies of a group of severely ill patients with meningococcal sepsis in France showed low stroke volume indices (29 mL/m^2) and tachycardia (>135 beats per minute), a profile suggesting greater myocardial depression than usually observed in gram-negative sepsis. In infection with meningococcal serogroup C, pericarditis with tamponade can complicate the course of treatment unless recognized and managed. When DIC occurs, persistent bleeding at intravenous sites and sites of arterial punctures can complicate management.

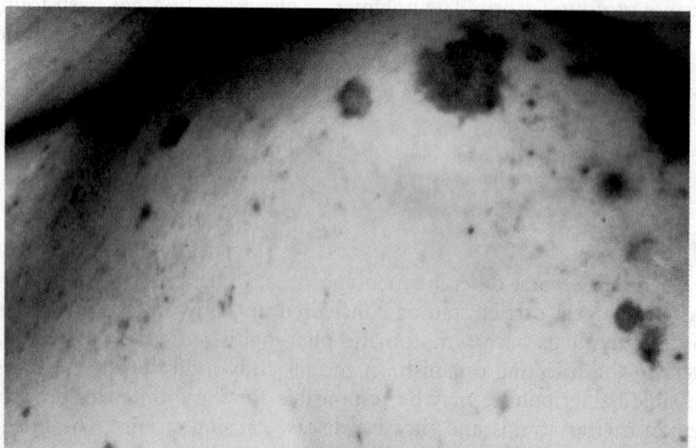

FIGURE 321–2 • A patient with advanced meningococcemia who has multiple petechiae and ecchymoses on the shoulders, chest, and arm.

Neurologic complications include signs of meningeal irritation, an encephalopathic state, and coma (Chapter 437). Seizures can occur but are less common than in other forms of bacterial meningitis. In general, patients surviving meningococcal CNS infection have remarkably few sequelae, but cerebrovascular accidents secondary to intracranial bleeding can lead to paresis. Cases of posterior pituitary insufficiency have been reported in patients recovering from meningococcal infection.

Treatment

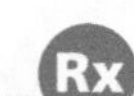

Immediate Treatment: Medical Emergency

In 1933, sulfonamides revolutionized the treatment of meningococcal infection. Before antimicrobials, almost all cases resulted in death or profound morbidity with complications. Early administration of appropriate antimicrobials is the cornerstone of successful management. As soon as the practitioner includes a systemic meningococcal infection in the differential diagnosis, institution of therapy must follow within 30 minutes. The patient must be considered a medical emergency. Thorough organization and documentation of the patient's management are crucial. Blood should be drawn for cultures immediately, an intravenous line established, and penicillin G (chloramphenicol can be used in severely penicillin-allergic patients) infused over 15 minutes (Table 321–1). There is no evidence that release of endotoxin that may occur after antimicrobial administration adversely affects outcome. This should not be a reason to delay the onset of therapy. Antimicrobial administration should not be delayed while waiting for the spinal tap to be done. If the spinal tap is obtained within 45 minutes of the antimicrobials, there is limited reduction in positive CSF cultures and no modification of the CSF cytology or hypoglycorrhachia. In two studies in Great Britain, it was shown that the administration, before hospitalization, of high-dose penicillin to patients suspected of having meningococcal infection greatly reduced morbidity and mortality.

Treatment after Stabilization: The Intensive Care Unit

Patients with meningococcal sepsis frequently have multisystem involvement. If the patient is not at a tertiary care hospital, transfer of the stabilized patient to such a facility should be considered. The patient should be cared for in an intensive care situation with continuous monitoring and careful management of fluids and electrolytes. Because of fluid loss related to fever and the increased vascular permeability, fluids, electrolytes, and colloid should be administered and blood pressure, urine output, and cardiac function monitored. A number of studies indicate that meningococcal sepsis

TABLE 321–1 ANTIMICROBIAL MANAGEMENT OF SYSTEMIC MENINGOCOCCAL INFECTION

Antimicrobial	Dose
Penicillin G	300,000 units/kg/day IV, up to 24 million units/day
Ampicillin	150–200 mg/kg/day IV, up to 12 g/day
Ceftriaxone	2 g/day IV
Chloramphenicol	For use in penicillin-allergic patients, 100 mg/kg/day IV, up to 4 g/day

Rx

is associated with cardiac failure; thus, attention must be paid to cardiac status during the sepsis and shock state. Studies measuring release of cardiac troponin as an index of cardiac cell death demonstrated significant increases in 62% of infected children 24 hours after the diagnosis of meningococcal disease. Treatment of heart failure may be indicated. Vasoactive agents such as dopamine may be necessary to maintain blood pressure and tissue perfusion.

Clotting Parameters

Because DIC occurs frequently, monitoring of clotting parameters such as platelets, fibrinogen, and fibrin split products is a crucial part of management. Correction of this problem is a key to survival and reduced morbidity and may require the advice of one skilled in management of bleeding disorders. Studies have shown that the use of fresh frozen plasma may negatively influence outcome in systemic meningococcal disease. Careful consideration should be given before the administration of such products to these patients. Studies have suggested that exchange transfusion may improve the survival rate of patients with fulminant meningococcal sepsis. The beneficial effect is most likely not based on the elimination of endotoxin. Promising results have been obtained in patients with meningococcal sepsis using a truncated version of recombinantly produced bactericidal/permeability-increasing protein (rBPI). This product is undergoing testing in patients and is not available for general use.

Skin Necrosis

One of the most serious causes of morbidity in fulminant meningococcal sepsis is skin necrosis with loss of distal digits and limbs. Epidural sympathetic blockade may prove useful in preserving the lower extremities of such patients. Skin necrosis can be managed by débridement, grafting, and nutritional support after the patient's condition has been stabilized.

Resistance

In the early 1950s, penicillin became the drug of choice for treatment of systemic meningococcal infections. It has remained the cornerstone of therapy since that time. The meningococcus is sensitive to a wide range of antimicrobials, including third-generation cephalosporins and quinolones. Ampicillin is equivalent to penicillin G and can be used if there is uncertainty about the etiologic diagnosis at the time when therapy is instituted. Reports from southern Europe (primarily Spain and Greece) of the isolation of penicillin-resistant meningococci could have ominous consequences if epidemics involving these organisms occur. In Spain, the prevalence of *N. meningitidis* isolates that are moderately susceptible to penicillin and ampicillin has increased to almost 50% of isolates. These strains do not produce β-lactamase. In these strains, the basis of meningococcal resistance to penicillin is alterations in a group of inner membrane enzymes, the penicillin-binding proteins (PBPs), which are responsible for cell wall synthesis. Specifically, alterations in PBP-2 result in decreased affinity of binding of penicillin and ampicillin to these enzymes. Third-generation cephalosporins are usually effective against organisms that are resistant on this basis. However, careful antimicrobial sensitivity testing should be performed to ensure that this is the case because some third-generation cephalosporins may also not bind efficiently to these modified PBPs. Studies have demonstrated that disc diffusion methods can still be used to analyze such strains, although plate dilution methods are preferred. Sulfonamide-resistant meningococci are still common in the United States; hence, sulfonamides should not be used in treatment of acute infections.

Complications

Complement Deficiency and Meningococcal Sepsis

Individuals with deficiencies in complement components appear to be uniquely susceptible to meningococcal infection. In properdin-deficient patients, fulminant meningococcal sepsis is a frequent cause of death. Families of such individuals should be investigated for a history of sudden septic death in relatives. Such families should be observed closely and undergo vaccination with the tetravalent meningococcal vaccine.

In patients with late complement component deficiencies (LCCDs), meningococcal infection occurs in older individuals (mean age, 17 years) and tends to be milder (mortality ~2%) and caused by less common serogroups (serogroup Y and W135) than occur in the general population. Patients with LCCDs respond normally to meningococcal capsular polysaccharide vaccine with the development of antibodies that are functional in both complement-dependent bactericidal assays and opsonophagocytic assays. These patients have a more rapid decline in capsular antibody than is seen in normal individuals. These studies suggest that patients with LCCDs are critically dependent on capsular antibody for protection against meningococcal disease. Vaccination, probably on a recurrent basis, is an important component in the prevention of meningococcal disease in patients with LCCDs.

Chronic Meningococcemia

Chronic meningococcal sepsis, which is indistinguishable from the gonococcal dermatitis-arthritis syndrome, can occur. These patients have typical painful skin lesions usually on the extremities, with migratory polyarthritis and tenosynovitis. This form of meningococcal sepsis can persist for weeks if untreated. It responds promptly to antimicrobial therapy.

Respiratory Tract Infection

Pneumonia related to *N. meningitidis* has been reported since the 1930s. In one study of community-acquired infections in Finland, *N. meningitidis* was implicated as the etiologic agent in 6% of such infections. Epidemic pneumonia caused by serogroup Y strains has occurred at a military training center. The patients presented with chills, chest pain, and cough. Rales and fever occurred in almost all patients. Infections in these men were frequently multilobar (40%). The incidence of sepsis associated with these infections is quite low, and the diagnosis is usually made with sputum or endotracheal aspirates. There was no mortality in these patients, and all responded well to treatment with penicillin.

Meningococcal Pericarditis

Pericarditis is usually associated with infections by *N. meningitidis* serogroup C. It has been associated with meningococcemia and reported as an isolated syndrome. Patients can present with chest pain and signs of tamponade, but relatively asymptomatic disease can occur with detection made by ultrasonography. Treatment with antimicrobials and removal of the pericardial fluid usually result in a successful outcome. Pericarditis can occur in patients convalescing from meningococcal sepsis. It should be considered if fever and shortness of breath on minimal exertion occur when the patient is recovering from meningococcal sepsis. Echocardiography provides a rapid diagnosis of this complication of infection. In convalescent patients, antimicrobial therapy should be continued and pericardiocentesis may be indicated. There is no evidence that corticosteroids or anti-inflammatory agents have a role in management.

Meningococcal Urethritis

Meningococci have been isolated from the urethra and can cause clinical urethritis. In one study of more than 5000 urethral cultures from homosexual men, the isolation rate was 0.2% compared with 4.7% for *Neisseria gonorrhoeae* in the same population. Eight of these patients had symptomatic urethritis. In the same study, there were no isolates among almost 9000 urethral cultures from heterosexual males or almost 16,000 cervical cultures. This study strongly suggested that there is an association between orogenital sex and urethral acquisition of the meningococcus. Meningococcal urethritis has been managed successfully with penicillin or tetracycline therapy, or both.

Prevention

Eradication of the carrier state in intimate contacts of index cases with chemoprophylaxis is an effective way to prevent secondary cases and it an important prevention effort in the United States and other countries with sporadic cases and rare outbreaks. Use of short-term antimicrobial therapy (one to two doses) can achieve long-term (3- to 4-week) eradication of the meningococcus from the nasopharynx. However, success is dependent on use of the correct antimicrobial regimen. Penicillin, penicillin derivatives, and first- and second-generation cephalosporins are not effective for prophylaxis because eradication of the meningococcus is not achieved during the short courses of therapy. Rifampin and ceftriaxone are effective agents for prophylaxis (Table 321–2). Quinolone derivatives are also effective for chemoprophylaxis.

Antimicrobials

Intimate contacts of cases are at 100- to 1000-fold increased risk for acquiring meningococcal infection. Close contacts include household members, daycare center contacts, college roommates, and anyone directly exposed to the patient's oral secretions (e.g., through kissing, mouth-to-mouth resuscitation, endotracheal intubation, or endotracheal tube management). Such individuals should be told about the increased risk, monitored closely for emergence of coprimary cases (cases that arise within 48 hours of the primary case), and given chemoprophylaxis to prevent secondary cases of infection. Hospital personnel who provide routine care for patients with meningococcal disease are not at increased risk for acquisition of infection. Studies have shown that individuals seated in proximity to an index case of meningococcal infection on prolonged airline flights (over 8 hours) may be at high risk for acquiring carriage and possibly disease. The recommendation has been made that antimicrobial chemoprophylaxis should be considered for passengers seated next to an index case patient.

Isolation

Isolation of case patients in hospitals is a common practice. It can be limited to respiratory isolation and terminated 24 hours after institution of appropriate antimicrobial therapy.

Vaccination

The ability of the meningococcal capsular polysaccharides to evoke a protective immune response is the basis for the meningococcal vaccines. An effective tetravalent capsular polysaccharide vaccine (containing A, C, Y, and W135 polysaccharide) was first made available for the prevention of meningococcal infections in individuals older than 2 years in the 1970s.

A principal drawback of the polysaccharide vaccine is the lack of immunogenicity in children younger than 2 years. This has limited widespread application of the current vaccine in countries with recurrent epidemic infections. Children younger than age 2 respond poorly to polysaccharides for reasons that are not clearly understood. Successes in vaccinating young children with *H. influenzae* polysaccharide conjugated to proteins suggested that a similar strategy might be useful for meningococcal polysaccharides, and a meningococcal tetravalent conjugate vaccine has been licensed in the United States. This tetravalent conjugate vaccine is immunogenic in children age 2 to 11 and produces high-titer bactericidal antibodies against *N. meningitidis* serogroup A, C, Y, and W135 strains. It is the recommended vaccine for this age group. Adults are still recommended to receive the tetravalent meningococcal polysaccharide vaccine but can be given the conjugate vaccine if the polysaccharide vaccine is unavailable. Studies of the efficacy of the tetravalent conjugate vaccine in children age 3 months to 2 years are not complete, and no recommendation for its use has been made in this age group.

Vaccine (conjugated and nonconjugated) should be administered to all intimate contacts of index cases at the start of chemoprophylaxis according to the preceding recommendations. The meningococcal polysaccharide vaccine has been used effectively in the U.S. military and in aborting epidemics caused by serogroup strains represented in the vaccine. In addition, because of an elevated risk of meningococcal disease, it is now recommended that college freshmen who live in dormitories be immunized with the tetravalent polysaccharide vaccine. Adolescents are now advised to receive the vaccine before high school entry as the most effective means of protection. The lack of an antigen capable of eliciting protection against meningococcal serogroup B infection is a problem. The serogroup B polysaccharide is a poor immunogen even in adults, perhaps because it resembles self-antigens. Vaccine development for serogroup B strains has focused on other meningococcal subcapsular surface antigens (proteins and possibly lipopolysaccharide). These vaccines are based on serotypical protein antigens, and the vaccine must be tailored to the serotype of the specific meningococcal strain causing the epidemic. A noncapsular serogroup B vaccine has been tested in an epidemic in Brazil, and the results indicate that the vaccine was effective in children older than 2 years.

TABLE 321–2 CHEMOPROPHYLAXIS AND IMMUNOPROPHYLAXIS FOR PREVENTION OF MENINGOCOCCAL INFECTION

CHEMOPROPHYLAXIS

Antimicrobial	Dose
Rifampin	Adults who are not pregnant, 600 mg PO q12h for 2 days. Children >1 mo, 5 mg/kg PO; <1 mo, 10 mg/kg PO q12h for 2 days
Ceftriaxone	Single 250 mg IM dose for adults, single 125 mg IM dose for children <15 years of age
Ciprofloxacin	Adults who are not pregnant, 500 mg as a single PO dose. Limited experience in children <18

IMMUNOPROPHYLAXIS

Adults: Monovalent A, monovalent C, bivalent A-C, or quadrivalent A, C, Y, and W135 vaccine is administered once by volume according to manufacturer. Amount of polysaccharide delivered is usually 50 µg. Vaccination should be considered an adjunct to antimicrobial chemoprophylaxis for household or intimate contacts of meningococcal disease cases when appropriate serogroups are causing disease. If the conjugate vaccine is unavailable, the tetravalent conjugate can be used.

Children age 2 to 11 years: Meningococcal tetravalent conjugate vaccine, single dose according to manufacturer.

Prognosis

Prognosis can vary depending on the presentation of the patient, the skill and completeness of the physician, and the nature of the facility. At tertiary care hospitals during endemic periods of infection, mortalities as low as 8% have been reported. Patients who present with meningococcemia alone tend to have a higher mortality (up to 20%). Early recognition and early empirical treatment probably reduce mortality.

SUGGESTED READINGS

Bilukha O: Prevention and control of meningococcal disease. MMWR Recomm Rep 2005;54(RR-07):1–21. *Describes the recommendations for the meningococcal tetravalent conjugate and polysaccharide vaccines.*

Bruce MG, Rosenstein NE, Capparella JM, et al: Risk factors for meningococcal disease in college students. JAMA 2001;286:688–693. *Analysis of risk of meningococcal disease in college students and recommendations for vaccination.*

Conterno LO, Silva Filho CR, Ruggeberg JU, et al: Conjugate vaccines for preventing meningococcal C meningitis and septicaemia. Cochrane Database Syst Rev 2006;3:CD001834. *The meningococcal serogroup C conjugate vaccine appears to be safe and immunogenic.*

Fraser A, Gafter-Gvili A, Paul M, et al: Antibiotics for preventing meningococcal infections. Cochrane Database Syst Rev 2006;(4):CD004785. *Rifampin, ciprofloxacin, and ceftriaxone are effective, but rifampin in an outbreak setting might lead to resistance.*

Gardner P: Prevention of meningococcal disease. N Engl J Med 2006;355: 1466–1473. *A clinical review.*

Kvalsvig AJ, Unsworth DJ: The immunopathogenesis of meningococcal disease. J Clin Pathol 2003;56:417–422. *Description of the immune response to meningococcal disease and how individual variation determines susceptibility.*

Nathan N, Borel T, Djibo A, et al: Ceftriaxone as effective as long-acting chloramphenicol in short-course treatment of meningococcal meningitis during epidemics: A randomised non-inferiority study. Lancet 2005;366:308–313. *This study from Africa favors ceftriaxone.*

Richardson DC, Louie L, Louie M, et al: Evaluation of a rapid PCR assay for diagnosis of meningococcal meningitis. J Clin Microbiol 2003;41:3851–3853. *Sensitivity was 97% and specificity was 99.6%.*

Rosenstein NE, Perkins BA, Stephens DS, et al: Meningococcal disease. N Engl J Med 2001;344:1378–1388. *Comprehensive review of meningococcal infections.*

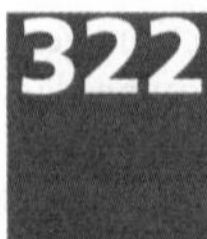

GONOCOCCAL INFECTIONS

H. Hunter Handsfield and P. Frederick Sparling

Definition

Neisseria gonorrhoeae is a sexually transmitted organism that primarily infects the columnar epithelia of mucosal surfaces and causes urethritis in men and endocervicitis and urethritis in women. Other sites of primary infection include the rectum, pharynx, and conjunctiva, and vulvovaginitis can occur in prepubertal girls. The most common complication is acute salpingitis, or pelvic inflammatory disease, which can lead to infertility and ectopic pregnancy. Other complications are epididymitis, posterior urethritis, urethral stricture, Bartholin gland abscess, and perihepatitis. Bacteremia may occur, with production of characteristic cutaneous lesions, arthritis, and rarely endocarditis or meningitis. Neonatal conjunctivitis (ophthalmia neonatorum) was formerly a common cause of blindness.

The Pathogen

N. gonorrhoeae is a gram-negative, aerobic diplococcus that produces cytochrome oxidase. Many strains require an atmosphere containing 3 to 10% CO_2 for optimal growth, and the organism grows best on media with added starch, which blocks the inhibitory effect of the fatty acids present in agar. Growth is less rapid than that of most bacteria that compose the normal flora of the genitourinary tract, rectum, or pharynx, so selective media that incorporate antibiotics to inhibit the growth of competing bacteria are required for optimal isolation by culture. The gonococcus metabolizes glucose but not maltose, sucrose, or lactose, the historic basis for differentiation from *Neisseria meningitidis, Branhamella (Moraxella)* sp, and nonpathogenic *Neisseria* sp.

When propagated on agar-containing media, *N. gonorrhoeae* forms colonies of varied morphology known as phase variation. Small, cohesive colonies dominate in the first one or two passages, contain organisms with pili (filamentous projections of the organism's outer membrane), and retain virulence when inoculated into human volunteers. The larger colonies that come to predominate after unselective passage contain nonpiliated gonococci and have limited infectivity for human volunteers. Gonococci propagated in the laboratory also undergo rapid variation in the antigenic type of pili expressed, which probably contributes to prolonged infection without treatment and to the susceptibility of persons to acquire repeat infections.

Gonococcal strains can be phenotypically distinguished on the basis of antigenic differences in outer membrane proteins (serotyping) and according to genetically determined nutritional requirements of the organism for specific amino acids and nucleotides (auxotyping). More recently, genetic techniques such as rapid DNA sequencing of the porin gene are replacing the older phenotypic methods in applied epidemiology studies.

Epidemiology

Gonorrhea is the second most commonly reported infectious disease in the United States, after genital infection with *Chlamydia trachomatis.* About 330,000 cases were reported in 2004, an incidence of 114 cases per 100,000 population, but the true incidence is probably twice as high. The incidence declined dramatically in most industrialized countries from the 1970s to the mid-1990s, but the rate has declined only slightly in the United States since 1997. The incidence of gonorrhea is lowest in western Europe, but the disease remains epidemic in eastern Europe, much of Africa, the Indian subcontinent, and parts of Asia and South America.

The epidemiology of gonorrhea varies widely among geographic areas and populations. In the United States, as many as 5% of persons at risk, or up to 20% of persons attending some public sexually transmitted disease (STD) clinics, may be infected at any time, but the prevalence is lower than 1% in most clinical venues. The highest incidence occurs in young (15 to 30 years of age), single persons of low socioeconomic and educational attainment, in inner city residents, and in some rural settings, especially in the Southeast. The incidence of reported gonorrhea is 20-fold higher in African Americans than in whites; rates in persons of Hispanic or Native American ethnicity are 2-fold and 4-fold higher than in whites, respectively, whereas the reported incidence is 30% lower in persons of Asian or Pacific Island ancestry than in whites. The differences between racial and ethnic groups are reflections of differing sex partner network structures, socioeconomic attainment, education, and access to health care. Persons of lower socioeconomic status selectively attend public clinics, where reporting is more complete than in the private sector, but this bias accounts for only a small part of the observed differences among population groups.

The incidence of gonorrhea is several times higher in men who have sex with men (MSM) than in women and heterosexual men. Rates of gonorrhea and other STDs rose dramatically among MSM in the United States and other industrialized countries from 1997 to 2005, in association with behavioral changes that followed improved antiretroviral therapy and survival of persons infected with human immunodeficiency virus (HIV).

The likelihood that a woman will acquire gonorrhea from a man with urethral infection is approximately 50% per episode of unprotected vaginal intercourse, whereas the transmission risk from female to male averages 20 to 30% per exposure. Transmission rates for other exposures have not been quantified, but anal intercourse is clearly a relatively efficient mode of transmission. Transmission by fellatio also occurs frequently, especially from the insertive to the receptive partner, and pharyngeal gonococcal infection is especially common in MSM. Both transmission and acquisition of gonorrhea by cunnilingus appear to be rare. Gonococci die rapidly on drying, and with the exception of occasional acquisition by laboratory personnel working with the organism, nonsexual transmission does not occur in adults. Perinatal transmission causing neonatal ophthalmitis or pharyngeal infection is now rare.

The large majority of urethral infections in men cause overt, symptomatic urethritis, with no more than a small percentage of asymptomatic infections. By contrast, up to 70% of infections in women cause no symptoms or mild ones that do not lead to a health care visit. The proportion of persons with urethral or cervical infection who remain asymptomatic depends in large part on the local prevalence of particular strains of *N. gonorrhoeae* that selectively cause subclinical infection. Most rectal and pharyngeal gonococcal infections are asymptomatic. Because many persons with genital discharge, pain, or other symptoms spontaneously cease sexual activity, gonorrhea and other STDs are selectively transmitted by people with subclinical infections.

Pathobiology

Pili help gonococci attach to mucosal surfaces by binding to the host cell receptor CD46. Attachment is also mediated by a family of outer membrane proteins designated opacity proteins, which bind to either CD66 or heparin-like molecules on host cells. Attachment and invasion of host epithelium are influenced by antigenic variations in pili and opacity proteins and by variations in the core sugars of lipo-oligosaccharide components of the organism's outer membrane. These variations also help the host to evade the immune response. Typical urethral infections result in prominent inflammation, probably as a result of the release of toxic lipo-oligosaccharide and peptidoglycan fragments, as well as the release of chemotactic factors that attract neutrophilic leukocytes. The reasons that some gonococcal strains selectively cause asymptomatic genital infection are poorly understood, but this propensity may be related to differences in the ability of the organism to bind complement-regulatory proteins that downregulate the production of chemotactic peptides.

In the preantibiotic era, gonorrhea usually persisted for 2 to 3 months before host defenses eradicated the infection. These defenses include serum opsonic and bactericidal antibodies, as well as mucosal antibodies of the IgG and IgA classes. All gonococci produce IgA1 protease, an enzyme that inactivates the major class of secretory IgA, thereby perhaps contributing to the persistence of mucosal infection. Gonococcal opacity proteins also appear to downregulate the immune response, which possibly accounts for the observed paucity of mucosal antibodies after natural infection.

Serum bactericidal antibodies are important in preventing bacteremia, as indicated by the increased likelihood of disseminated infection in persons infected with strains resistant to normal serum bactericidal activity. In addition, persons with homozygous deficiency of one of the complement components C6, C7, C8, or C9, which results in diminished serum bactericidal activity without alteration in serum opsonic activity, are particularly prone to gonococcemia and to meningococcal meningitis and bacteremia.

Clinical Manifestations

Gonococcal infections can result in a number of specific clinical syndromes, each of which has its own manifestations, differential diagnosis, and recommended evaluation.

Diagnosis

Microscopy

Microscopy of a Gram-stained smear is positive when polymorphonuclear neutrophils are observed to contain intracellular gram-negative diplococci of typical morphology (Fig. 322–1). Gram-stained smears are 90 to 98% sensitive in the diagnosis of symptomatic gonococcal urethritis in men and have a specificity of greater than 95%, so confirmation by culture or another test is optional. However, the sensitivity is only about 50% for cervical or rectal infection and for asymptomatic urethral gonorrhea. Although Gram stain is often considered highly specific for such infections, the actual performance varies with the skill and experience of the examiner, and rectal and cervical smears are unreliable in many clinical settings. Smears are both insensitive and nonspecific for pharyngeal gonococcal infection and are not recommended.

Culture

Isolation of *N. gonorrhoeae* by culture, generally using antibiotic-containing selective media, is the historic mainstay of the diagnosis of gonorrhea. Ideally, growth media should be inoculated directly and placed promptly into a humid atmosphere with increased carbon dioxide, such as a candle extinction jar. However, standard transport systems (e.g., Culturette) are acceptable if specimens are kept moist, not refrigerated, and processed within 6 hours. When testing specimens not likely to be colonized by competing flora (e.g., synovial fluid), nonselective chocolate agar should be used.

Nucleic Acid Amplification Tests

In many settings, culture is being supplanted by nucleic acid amplification tests (NAATs), including tests based on polymerase chain reaction, transcription-mediated amplification, and DNA strand displacement. The NAATs for *N. gonorrhoeae* are no more sensitive than culture, and they are more expensive and do not preserve an isolate for antimicrobial susceptibility testing. However, some NAATs retain excellent sensitivity when used to test voided urine or self-obtained vaginal swabs and offer more convenient specimen management than culture does. Combination assays for *N. gonorrhoeae* and *C. trachomatis* may facilitate screening for both STDs in some settings. Specificity is excellent, and one NAAT that tests for both organisms (Aptima Combo II) retained a positive predictive value greater than 95% in a population with only a 0.5% prevalence of gonorrhea. The currently available NAATs have been approved only for testing genital specimens or urine, although preliminary data suggest that some tests perform well on rectal swab specimens. No NAAT is yet approved or recommended for the diagnosis of pharyngeal gonococcal infection.

Older nonculture tests, based on nonamplified DNA probe technology or immunochemical detection of gonococcal antigens, are substantially less sensitive and probably less specific than culture or the NAATs, and they cannot be used to test urine or anatomic sites other than the urethra or cervix. These tests have little clinical use today and are no longer recommended.

SPECIFIC CLINICAL SYNDROMES

Urogenital Gonorrhea in Males

Clinical Manifestations

Gonococcal urethritis in men ("clap") is typically characterized by purulent urethral discharge and dysuria. The usual incubation period is 2 to 6 days. A small minority of men who acquire urethral infection, generally estimated at 1 to 10% and varying with the auxotype/serotype class of the infecting strain, remain asymptomatic.

Physical examination typically reveals purulent urethral exudate (Fig. 322–2), usually apparent spontaneously but sometimes expressed only by compression of the urethra. Erythema of the meatus is sometimes present. Nongonococcal urethritis (Chapter 307) is typically characterized by less copious and less purulent discharge, and meatal erythema is uncommon, except in occasional cases caused by herpes simplex virus or adenoviruses.

Diagnosis

The diagnosis of gonococcal urethritis is usually suspected clinically, confirmed preliminarily by a Gram-stained smear showing leukocytes with intracellular gram-negative diplococci (see Fig. 322–1), and made definitively when *N. gonorrhoeae* is identified by culture or, increasingly, NAAT.

Prognosis

Acute epididymitis, though uncommon, probably remains the most frequent complication of gonococcal urethritis, but more common causes of epididymitis are *C. trachomatis* or, in men older than 35 years,

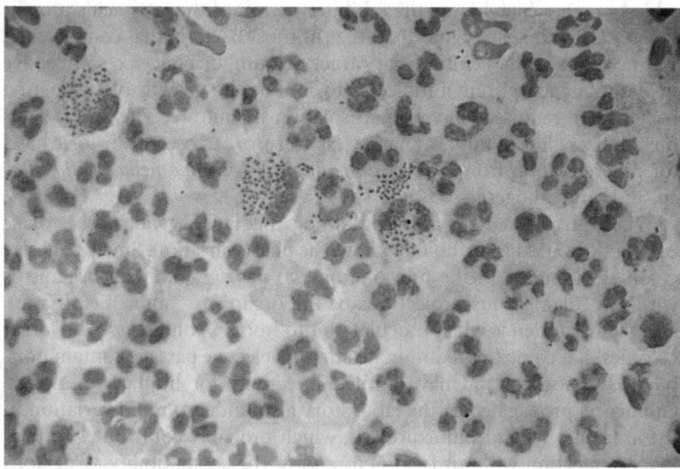

FIGURE 322–1 • Photomicrograph revealing the histopathology in an acute case of gonococcal urethritis with Gram stain technique. This slide is used to demonstrate the nonrandom distribution of gonococci among polymorphonuclear neutrophils. Note that there are both intracellular and extracellular bacteria in the field of view.

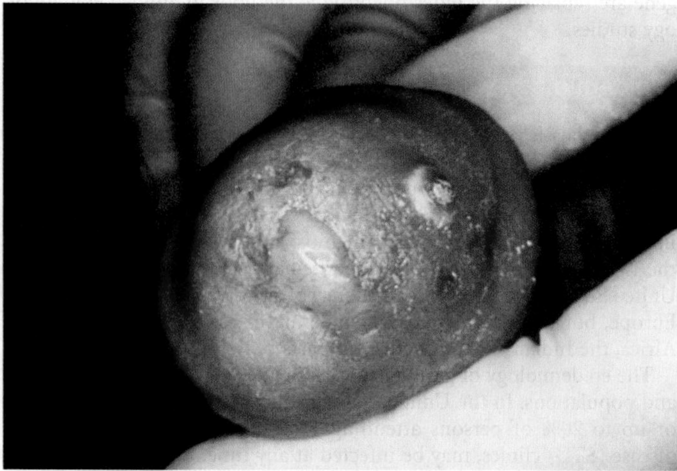

FIGURE 322–2 • Male with a purulent penile discharge from gonorrhea and an overlying penile pyodermal lesion. Pyoderma involves the formation of a purulent skin lesion, as in this case located on the glans penis and overlying the sexually transmitted disease gonorrhea.

Section XXIII Infectious Diseases

Escherichia coli and other uropathogens. Epididymitis is usually accompanied by unilateral testicular pain and swelling, often with fever. Posterior urethritis or prostatitis, typically manifested as pelvic or perineal pain and urinary retention, was once fairly common but is now rare. Urethral stricture was also formerly a common complication but is presently rare. Even in the preantibiotic era, many strictures attributed to gonorrhea may have resulted from the use of caustic treatment regimens, including urethral irrigation with antiseptic solutions such as silver nitrate or potassium permanganate.

Lower Genital Tract Gonorrhea in Females

Clinical Manifestations

The primary site of infection in women is the endocervical canal, and *N. gonorrhoeae* is isolated from the cervix in 85 to 90% of women with gonorrhea. When symptoms are present, the dominant ones are vaginal discharge and abnormal vaginal bleeding, typically manifested as scant intermenstrual bleeding, often after intercourse, or enhanced bleeding during menses (metrorrhagia). Dysuria is also frequent, and *N. gonorrhoeae* can be isolated from the urethra in up to 80% of women with gonorrhea, although the urethra is rarely the only infected site, except in women who have had hysterectomies.

Findings on physical examination may be normal, but many women have evidence of cervicitis with purulent or mucopurulent exudate and often edema and easily induced bleeding (e.g., with gentle swabbing, sometimes mistakenly called "friability") in an area of endocervical ectopy. Many women with gonorrhea have simultaneous bacterial vaginosis or trichomonal vaginitis with abnormal vaginal discharge (Chapter 307). However, gonorrhea itself does not cause vaginitis because *N. gonorrhoeae* does not infect the estrogen-influenced, glycogen-rich squamous vaginal epithelium of sexually mature women. In uncomplicated infection, purulent exudate can sometimes be expressed from a Bartholin gland duct, near the vaginal introitus laterally, or from Skene's glands, adjacent to the urethral meatus.

Diagnosis

Microbiologic diagnosis usually rests on identification of *N. gonorrhoeae* in cervical secretions by culture or NAAT; Gram-stained smears are insensitive and little used.

Prognosis

A Bartholin gland abscess, which is an uncommon complication, is manifested as a tender introital mass and may involve superinfection with facultative and anaerobic bacteria. Gonococcal ophthalmia is occasionally seen in adults, generally as a result of autoinoculation in persons with anogenital gonorrhea; it is accompanied by acute, purulent conjunctivitis that can result in corneal ulceration if not treated promptly.

Pelvic Inflammatory Disease

Clinical Manifestations

The most common complication of gonorrhea is acute salpingitis, often in association with endometritis, a combination collectively termed pelvic inflammatory disease (PID), which is estimated to occur in 10 to 20% of infected women. *C. trachomatis* (Chapter 339) is the dominant cause of PID in the United States, but gonorrhea remains a common cause, and *Mycoplasma genitalium* (Chapter 338) may cause some cases. Regardless of the initiating infection, several other vaginal organisms, such as *Mycoplasma hominis* and various facultative and anaerobic gram-positive and gram-negative bacteria, are often implicated as copathogens. Low abdominal pain is the dominant symptom; fever and other systemic manifestations such as malaise and anorexia are common. Vaginal discharge or other symptoms of lower genital tract infection are frequently present, but their absence does not exclude the diagnosis of PID.

Examination usually discloses low abdominal tenderness, cervical motion tenderness, and bilateral adnexal tenderness, sometimes with a palpable mass. Most women have signs of cervicitis or bacterial vaginosis. In a small proportion of cases, the abdominal or adnexal signs may be unilateral and cause confusion with appendicitis (Chapter 145), ectopic pregnancy, and other conditions. Right upper quadrant abdominal tenderness is sometimes present and due to Fitz-Hugh–Curtis syndrome, in which intra-abdominal extension of infection results in perihepatitis, which can mimic acute cholecystitis or viral hepatitis. Sometimes perihepatitis occurs in the absence of other abdominal or pelvic findings of typical PID, perhaps especially when caused by *C. trachomatis*. Severe PID may be accompanied by signs of generalized peritonitis.

Diagnosis

Laboratory studies often show elevation of the white blood cell count and erythrocyte sedimentation rate. However, these tests are frequently normal, and they are more useful in judging clinical severity than serving as diagnostic criteria.

The clinical diagnosis of PID is inexact. When laparoscopy showing visible salpingitis is used as the definitive test, the clinical diagnosis of PID is both insensitive and nonspecific; that is, many cases of PID lack the classic signs and symptoms, and some women with clinically typical PID have no laparoscopic abnormality. Histologic evidence of endometritis or plasma cells on endocervical biopsy, which can be performed by an aspiration technique with little pain or morbidity, has been used as a research tool and promoted as a useful aid to diagnosis but is not in widespread use in clinical settings. Because the consequences of untreated PID may be severe, the U.S. Centers for Disease Control and Prevention (CDC) recommends that all sexually active women with uterine or adnexal tenderness and cervical motion tenderness be treated for possible PID if no other cause is readily apparent.

Prognosis

Fallopian tube scarring secondary to PID often results in infertility or ectopic pregnancy, and previous gonococcal and chlamydial infections are among the most common antecedents of both complications. The incidence of tubal infertility has been estimated at 15% after one episode of PID and up to 50% after three attacks. The incidence of ectopic pregnancy is increased up to 10-fold in women with previous salpingitis. However, most cases of tubal infertility and ectopic pregnancy attributable to STDs occur in women with neither a previous diagnosis of PID nor past symptoms suggestive of pelvic infection, thus indicating that subclinical infection—usually with *C. trachomatis* but perhaps with *N. gonorrhoeae* as well—can result in tubal scarring. Chronic pelvic pain, sometimes of disabling severity, is also a common consequence of PID. Each episode of PID, whether due to *N. gonorrhoeae*, *C. trachomatis*, or neither of these organisms, significantly increases the risk for recurrent salpingitis. Many recurrent cases are associated with neither chlamydial infection nor gonorrhea; the initial infection may alter tubal clearance mechanisms or other defenses against ascending infection by normal vaginal bacteria.

Rectal Infection

Clinical Manifestations

Gonococcal infection of the rectum is common in women and in MSM. In women, infection is acquired either through perineal contamination with cervicovaginal secretions or by anal intercourse; the latter is the exclusive route of infection in MSM. In women with cervical gonorrhea and in MSM with gonorrhea at any anatomic site, about 40% have rectal infection. Most infections are subclinical, but symptomatic proctitis is occasionally manifested as varying combinations of anal pruritus, mucopurulent discharge (often characterized by the patient as "mucus" coating feces), pain, tenesmus, and bleeding. Symptomatic proctitis seems to be more common in MSM than in women with rectal gonorrhea, which suggests that the size of the infecting inoculum or the trauma of anal intercourse may contribute to the clinical manifestations.

Diagnosis

Diagnosis of rectal gonorrhea depends on identification of *N. gonorrhoeae* by culture or, increasingly, by NAAT. The Gram-stained smear is insensitive and nonspecific. The differential diagnosis of symptomatic proctitis includes other traditional STDs, (e.g., herpes, syphilis, and chlamydial infection, including lymphogranuloma venereum; Chapter 307), as well as ulcerative colitis, Crohn's colitis, anal fissure, rectal lacerations, and proctocolitis caused by *Shigella, Campylobacter, Yersinia enterocolitica,* and other enteric pathogens.

Pharyngeal Infection

Clinical Manifestations

Pharyngeal gonococcal infection results from orogenital exposure, is more efficiently acquired by fellatio than by cunnilingus, and is typically found in about 5% of heterosexual men, 5 to 10% of women, and 10 to 20% of MSM with gonorrhea. Asymptomatic infection is the rule, although rare cases may exhibit exudative pharyngitis and cervical lymphadenopathy. Isolated pharyngeal infection is rare, complications are infrequent, and most cases resolve spontaneously within a few weeks or in response to therapy for genital or rectal infection. For these reasons, testing persons at risk for pharyngeal gonococcal infection is optional, although most providers routinely test MSM. Culture is the only recommended test.

Gonorrhea in Children

Gonococcal conjunctivitis may develop in infants born to mothers with gonorrhea, a condition termed *ophthalmia neonatorum.* Formerly a common cause of blindness, gonococcal ophthalmia is now rare in industrialized countries because of both improved control of gonorrhea and routine use of neonatal ocular prophylaxis with topical antibiotics or 1% silver nitrate. Neonates may also acquire pharyngeal or rectal infection and, rarely, gonococcal pneumonia or sepsis. Neonatal vaginal infection is uncommon because under the influence of maternal estrogen, the glycogen-rich squamous epithelium of the neonatal vagina is resistant to gonococcal infection, just as *N. gonorrhoeae* does not cause vaginitis in sexually mature women. Beyond the neonatal period, purulent vaginitis is the most common manifestation of gonorrhea or chlamydial infection in girls, and rectal or pharyngeal infection is the most common manifestation in prepubertal boys. Most cases are acquired through sexual abuse, but occasional cases in young children may be acquired from fomites or by nonsexual personal exposure in crowded conditions, perhaps especially in tropical climates. Culture is the test of choice for all cases of childhood gonorrhea.

Disseminated Gonococcal Infection

Clinical Manifestations

Disseminated gonococcal infection is usually manifested by various combinations of polyarticular tenosynovitis, dermatitis secondary to focal septic embolization, and septic arthritis. Disseminated gonococcal infection has been estimated to occur in 1 to 3% of adults with gonorrhea, but the risk depends on the likelihood of infection with particular strains of *N. gonorrhoeae* and is probably well under 1% in most geographic areas. Women may be somewhat more susceptible to disseminated gonococcal infection than men, and onset often occurs in association with menstruation. Severity varies from a mild illness with slight joint discomfort, few skin lesions, and little or no fever to a fulminant illness with overt polyarthritis, innumerable skin lesions, high fever, and prostration. Many persons with disseminated gonococcal infection have no symptoms of genital gonorrhea because certain strains of *N. gonorrhoeae* are prone both to disseminate and cause subclinical genital infection.

Early in the course of disseminated gonococcal infection, the main symptoms are polyarthralgias, skin lesions, and fever (arthritis-dermatitis syndrome). Axial skeletal involvement is uncommon, a feature that can help differentiate disseminated gonococcal infection from reactive arthritis (Chapter 286). The arthritis-dermatitis syndrome often subsides spontaneously, or it may evolve over a period of several days into a second stage of overt septic arthritis with purulent synovial fluid, usually involving only one or two joints. Sequential evolution from arthritis-dermatitis syndrome is often not observed, so some patients are initially seen with septic arthritis. The knee, ankle, elbow, and wrist are most commonly affected, but any joint may be involved.

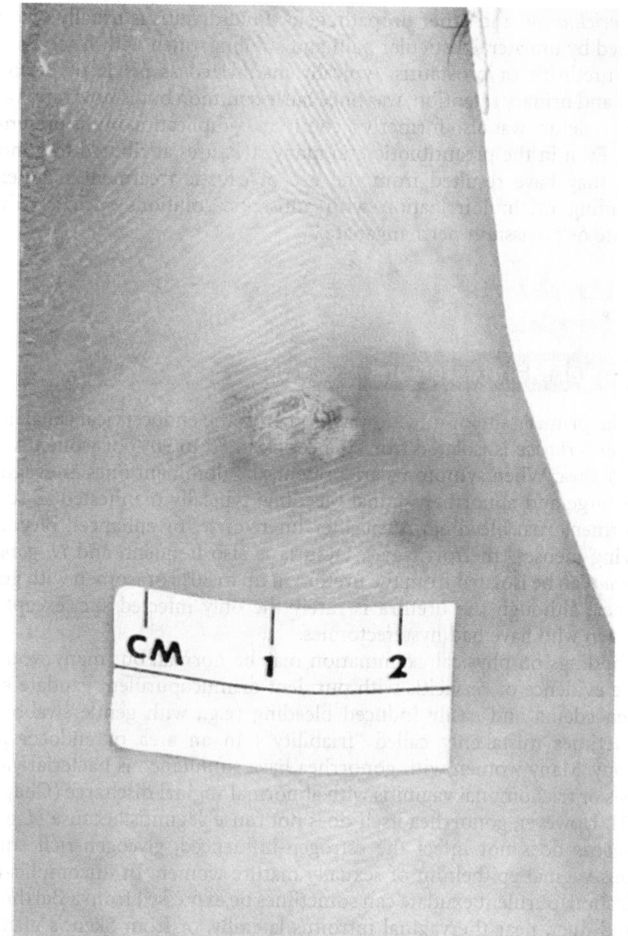

FIGURE 322–3 • Cutaneous gonococcal lesion secondary to disseminated *Neisseria gonorrhoeae* bacterial infection. Though a sexually transmitted disease, if gonorrhea is allowed to go untreated, the *N. gonorrhoeae* bacteria responsible for the infection can become disseminated throughout the body and form lesions in extragenital locations.

Physical examination of patients with arthritis-dermatitis syndrome generally reveals tenosynovitis of two or more joints, most commonly the wrists, ankles, hands, and feet and less commonly the knees or elbows. Skin lesions are usually few in number (typically 5 to 30) and are generally limited to the extremities. Individual lesions tend to evolve over several days from papules to pustules (Fig. 322–3), often with a hemorrhagic component, and then to dry eschars, and lesions at various stages may be present simultaneously. Bullae, petechiae, or overtly necrotic lesions that mimic ecthyma gangrenosum are occasionally seen. Although other conditions (e.g., bacterial endocarditis, meningococcemia) can cause similar lesions, the rash is sufficiently typical that it should strongly suggest disseminated gonococcal infection when seen in a sexually active young person. In patients with septic gonococcal arthritis, findings on physical examination are typical for that syndrome and consist of joint swelling, warmth, and often overlying erythema, usually with overt synovial effusion. Skin lesions are frequently absent, or healing lesions may be observed.

Diagnosis

Blood cultures are often positive for *N. gonorrhoeae* during the arthritis-dermatitis syndrome, but bacteremia is intermittent, so several cultures should be obtained to maximize the likelihood of isolation. The main clinical manifestations appear to be caused directly by bacteremic dissemination of the organism. The leukocyte count is generally elevated but may be normal. The leukocyte count in synovial fluid, when obtained, is usually less than 20,000/mm^3 and culture is negative. Cultures of skin lesions are generally negative despite demonstrable gonococci by fluorescent antibody; it seems likely that NAATs may be positive, but no data have been reported. Liver function tests often show elevations in aminotransferase levels suggestive of mild hepatitis. Circulating immune complexes are sometimes present but are most likely not responsible for the clinical manifestations. In patients with septic gonococcal arthritis, synovial fluid typically contains at least 40,000 leukocytes/mm^3, and *N. gonorrhoeae* can generally be isolated by culture; blood cultures are usually negative. Regardless of the clinical stage, gonococci can generally be identified at one or more mucosal sites by culture or NAAT.

Sexually active young persons with arthritis, tenosynovitis, or papulopustular skin lesions should be tested for *N. gonorrhoeae* at all potentially exposed anatomic sites. The diagnosis of disseminated gonococcal infection is secure when gonococci are identified by culture or NAAT from the blood, a skin lesion, or synovial fluid but is often made presumptively when genital, rectal, or pharyngeal gonorrhea is present in a patient with a typical clinical syndrome that responds promptly to antibiotics.

The differential diagnosis includes reactive arthritis (Chapter 286), meningococcemia (Chapter 321), other kinds of septic arthritis (Chapter 293), rheumatoid arthritis (Chapter 285), systemic lupus erythematosus (Chapter 287), and other rheumatologic conditions and infectious diseases. Reactive arthritis, often triggered by sexually acquired chlamydial infection, is the principal consideration in young adults. The skin lesions of the two conditions, when present, are generally distinct and often pathognomonic for one syndrome or the other. In addition, conjunctivitis and involvement of the axial skeleton (e.g., sacroiliitis) are common in Reiter's syndrome and infrequent in disseminated gonococcal infection.

Prognosis

Rare manifestations of disseminated gonococcal infection include bacterial endocarditis, meningitis, and myocarditis. Gonococcal endocarditis usually involves the aortic valve and often progresses rapidly with valve destruction and heart failure. Many cases of arthritis-dermatitis syndrome may resolve spontaneously, but untreated septic arthritis can lead to contiguous osteomyelitis or joint destruction.

Prevention

Control of gonorrhea depends on prompt diagnosis and effective treatment of infected persons, screening of sexually active women in settings where gonorrhea is prevalent, treatment of patients' partners, and rescreening. Asymptomatic MSM in many settings, including many HIV-infected men, remain sexually active and at high risk for gonorrhea and other STDs and should be tested periodically for rectal and pharyngeal gonococcal infection and for other STDs. The value of screening asymptomatic males for urethral infection (by NAAT of urine) is uncertain; the yield is low in most settings.

Public education and personal counseling of persons with or at risk for gonorrhea should emphasize the effectiveness of mutual monogamy, selection of partners at low risk, and except in mutually exclusive relationships, the use of condoms or other barrier methods. Every patient with gonorrhea should be counseled about risks for HIV infection and should be tested for HIV, *C. trachomatis*, and syphilis. Because accurate epidemiologic data are essential to generate and maintain resources for prevention and control of STDs, all cases of gonorrhea, chlamydial infection, syphilis, and HIV infection should be promptly reported to the health department in accordance with local laws. Ultimate control of gonorrhea may require immunization, but no effective vaccine is on the horizon despite intensive research for 3 decades.

Treatment

Rx

Antimicrobial Susceptibility

Gonococci with chromosomal or plasmid-borne mutations that confer relative or absolute resistance to the penicillins, tetracyclines, and sulfonamides are prevalent worldwide, and none of these drugs remains acceptable as empirical therapy anywhere in the world. The prevalence of β-lactamase (penicillinase) plasmids, which confer absolute resistance to penicillin, ampicillin, and amoxicillin, varies from about 10% of gonococci in the United States and western Europe to almost 50% in some developing countries. Strains with relative resistance to some but not all cephalosporins are common in parts of Japan, and ongoing surveillance for cephalosporin remains a high priority in all areas. All gonococci were highly susceptible to the fluoroquinolones when these drugs were first introduced, but resistant strains are now widespread. Clinicians who treat patients for gonorrhea and other STDs should keep abreast of regional trends in resistance and be alert to modified therapeutic recommendations.*

Principles of Treatment

Gonorrhea almost always responds to single-dose treatment with an appropriate antibiotic. Because of the need to curtail transmission, therapy is usually selected on the basis of clinical or epidemiologic suspicion, before the diagnosis is microbiologically confirmed. Even when *N. gonorrhoeae* is isolated by culture, antimicrobial susceptibility testing is not generally performed. Accordingly, routine treatment is dictated by local or regional patterns of antimicrobial susceptibility, without knowledge of susceptibility in individual patients. However, susceptibility testing should be used to guide the treatment of gonococcal septic arthritis, endocarditis, or other serious complications.

In North America, 5 to 10% of MSM, 10 to 20% of heterosexual men, and 20 to 40% of women with gonorrhea are also infected with *C. trachomatis,* so routine treatment of chlamydial infection is advised in addition to specific therapy for gonorrhea. At one time it was considered important that gonorrhea therapy be effective against syphilis, but incubating or active syphilis is now uncommon in persons with gonorrhea, and widespread treatment of gonorrhea with antibiotics inactive against *Treponema pallidum* does not influence the incidence of syphilis in the population.

Treatment Regimens

Ceftriaxone, 125 mg intramuscularly, or an oral cephalosporin such as cefixime, 400 mg, or cefpodoxime, 400 mg, should be given for uncomplicated gonorrhea (Table 322–1). 1 The distribution of cefixime was recently halted in the United States, but reintroduction may occur. Cefuroxime, 1.0 g, is also an option but might be slightly less effective than other regimens for gonococcal urethritis. Cefpodoxime and cefuroxime are probably less effective than ceftriaxone and cefixime against pharyngeal gonococcal infection.

Single-dose oral therapy with ciprofloxacin, ofloxacin, or levofloxacin is highly effective for genital, rectal, or pharyngeal infection by susceptible strains but should not be used to treat gonorrhea in MSM or infection acquired outside the United States or in geographic areas where fluoroquinolone-resistant strains are prevalent.* Other fluoroquinolones would probably be effective, but most have not been studied for efficacy against gonorrhea or have no advantage over the recommended regimens. Spectinomycin can be used in the rare circumstance when neither a cephalosporin nor a fluoroquinolone can be given, most commonly for the treatment of pregnant woman with allergy to β-lactam antibiotics.

Directly observed therapy is recommended. When persons with bacterial STDs are given prescriptions, many fail to take the drug properly or even to fill the prescription. All persons with gonorrhea should be routinely treated with an oral regimen active against *C. trachomatis,* usually azithromycin in a single dose of 1 g or doxycycline, 100 mg twice daily for 7 days. 1

Women with acute PID should be treated with antibiotics active against *N. gonorrhoeae, C. trachomatis,* and a broad range of facultative and anaerobic pathogens, regardless of whether gonococcal or chlamydial infection is documented. Recommended oral regimens are levofloxacin (500 mg once daily) or ofloxacin (400 mg twice daily) plus metronidazole (500 mg twice daily) for 14 days; however, some experts consider metronidazole optional. 1 Alternatively, patients may be given a single dose of one of the parenteral cephalosporins, such as ceftriaxone (250 mg intramuscularly) or cefoxitin (2 g intramuscularly), followed by doxycycline (100 mg twice daily), with or without metronidazole (500 mg twice daily), for 14 days. For hospitalized patients or others who require parenteral

*In early 2007, the CDC recommended that fluoroquinolones no longer be used in the United States as routine treatment for any patient with uncomplicated gonorrhea.

Section XXIII Infectious Diseases

TABLE 322–1 ANTIBIOTIC REGIMENS RECOMMENDED FOR UNCOMPLICATED GONORRHEA IN ADULTS IN THE UNITED STATES*

Regimens of Choice	Alternative Regimens
INITIAL SINGLE-DOSE THERAPY	
Ceftriaxone, 125 mg IM†	Cefpodoxime, 400 mg PO‡
Cefixime, 400 mg PO§	Cefuroxime, 1 g PO¶
Ciprofloxacin, 500 mg PO¶	Ceftizoxime, 500 mg IM
Ofloxacin, 400 mg PO¶	Cefotaxime, 500 mg IM
Levofloxacin, 250 mg PO¶	Gatifloxacin, 400 mg PO¶
	Lomefloxacin, 400 mg PO¶
	Spectinomycin, 2 g IM**
	Azithromycin, 2 g PO
FOLLOW-UP THERAPY (IF CHLAMYDIAL INFECTION NOT RULED OUT)	
Azithromycin, 1 g PO in a single dose *or*	
Doxycycline, 100 mg PO twice daily for 7 days††	

*Author's recommendations, modified from the Centers for Disease Control and Prevention sexually transmitted diseases treatment guidelines, 2002.
†The smallest marketed dose of ceftriaxone is 250 mg; therefore some clinicians administer the entire 250 mg. It may be reconstituted in 1% lidocaine to reduce injection pain.
‡A 200-mg dose is approved by the U.S. Food and Drug Administration, but confirmatory data have not been published, and efficacy for rectal and pharyngeal infections is uncertain. Pharmacokinetic considerations favor the 400-mg dose.
§Oral regimen of choice, but not available in the United States.
¶May have lower efficacy for male urethral infection than for cervical gonorrhea in women.
¶In early 2007, the CDC recommended that fluoroquinolones no longer be used in the United States as routine treatment for any patient with uncomplicated gonorrhea.
**Spectinomycin is ineffective against pharyngeal gonococcal infection.
††Another tetracycline may be substituted in therapeutically equivalent dosage, such as tetracycline HCl, 500 mg four times daily, or minocycline, 100 mg PO twice daily.

therapy, the CDC recommends intravenous cefotetan or cefoxitin plus doxycycline orally or parenteral therapy with clindamycin plus gentamicin. Other options include intravenous levofloxacin or ofloxacin, with or without metronidazole, and intravenous ampicillin/sulbactam plus doxycycline orally. For all of these regimens, parenteral therapy is continued until improvement is observed, after which oral therapy is prescribed to complete 14 days' total treatment. [1]

Most persons with disseminated gonococcal infection should be hospitalized and treated with a parenteral third-generation cephalosporin such as ceftriaxone, cefotaxime, or ceftizoxime or with ciprofloxacin, ofloxacin, or levofloxacin if the infecting strain is known to be sensitive. Joint irrigation or drainage appears not to be necessary for septic arthritis, although repeated aspiration of synovial fluid may speed clinical improvement. Oral treatment (e.g., cefixime, cefpodoxime, or a fluoroquinolone) can usually be substituted after improvement begins and then continued to complete 7 days' therapy. More prolonged parenteral treatment and higher doses are indicated for the treatment of gonococcal meningitis or endocarditis, although modern data are lacking. Gonococcal epididymitis, bartholinitis, and other localized complications should generally be treated for 7 to 14 days with drugs active against both *N. gonorrhoeae* and *C. trachomatis*. Gonococcal conjunctivitis in adults can be managed with a single dose of ceftriaxone, 1 g intramuscularly, optionally with saline lavage.

Management of Sex Partners

Failure to ensure treatment of patients' sex partners contributes to continued transmission of gonorrhea and often results in reinfection of the index case. Most persons with genital discharge, lesions, or dysuria cease sexual activity and seek treatment, so gonorrhea and other STDs are selectively transmitted by persons with subclinical infection or with ignored symptoms. This fact explains the necessity of taking active steps to ensure treatment of patients' sex partners; many persons from whom patients acquired their infections are unlikely to seek care spontaneously. For gonorrhea, all partners in the preceding 1 to 2 months should be treated. Except for syphilis and, increasingly, HIV infection, few health departments in the United States routinely have sufficient resources to contact the sex partners of persons with STD, and the responsibility to ensure that partners are treated lies jointly with the patient and the clinician. The partners or persons with gonorrhea should undergo diagnostic testing for gonorrhea, chlamydial infection, syphilis, and HIV infection, but antibiotics active against *N. gonorrhoeae* and *C. trachomatis* should be administered without awaiting the results of diagnostic tests.

When partner referral is not likely to be successful, the CDC and other authorities advise expedited partner therapy (EPT), whereby partners are treated without professional counseling or clinical evaluation. EPT may be accomplished by writing a prescription for the partner or by giving the patient extra drug to share with one or more partners. Three randomized controlled trials found that EPT was superior to standard partner referral in preventing persistent or recurrent gonorrhea or chlamydial infection, resulted in more partners receiving treatment, and reduced the likelihood that patients would resume sex with untreated partners. [2]

Follow-up

The recommended regimens cure 96 to 100% of uncomplicated genital or rectal gonorrhea caused by susceptible strains, and retesting of infected patients to ensure resolution ("test of cure") is not recommended unless therapeutic compliance is unlikely or circumstances require treatment with a suboptimal regimen. [1] When test of cure is indicated, culture may be performed a week after treatment is completed, but retesting by NAAT should be delayed until at least 2 weeks after treatment to reduce the possibility of detecting persistent gonococcal DNA despite eradication of viable organisms.

Although test of cure per se is not generally advised, rescreening is recommended. Rescreening is retesting 3 to 6 months after treatment to detect reinfection and occasional cases of persistent infection. Studies show that 10 to 20% of both men and women with gonorrhea or chlamydial infection once again have positive tests within a few months, regardless of whether they believe that their sex partners were treated. Therefore, rescreening is indicated for all women and heterosexual men with either gonorrhea or chlamydial infection. [1,2] Using urine or vaginal swab testing by NAAT, rescreening can be accomplished without directly examining the patient and even without an office visit if specimen transport can be arranged. Persons with gonorrhea should be retested for both *N. gonorrhoeae* and *C. trachomatis;* in most settings, those with chlamydial infection need not be retested for *N. gonorrhoeae*. Rescreening has not been evaluated in MSM but is probably wise.

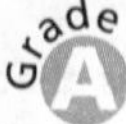

1. Centers for Disease Control and Prevention: Sexually transmitted diseases treatment guidelines, 2006. MMWR Recomm Rep 2006;55(RR-11):1–93.
2. Golden MR, Whittington WL, Handsfield HH, et al: Effect of expedited treatment of sex partners on recurrent or persistent gonorrhea or chlamydial infection. N Engl J Med 2005;352: 676–685.

SUGGESTED READINGS

Cook RL, Hutchinson SL, Østergaard L, et al: Systematic review: Noninvasive testing for *Chlamydia trachomatis* and *Neisseria gonorrhoeae*. Ann Intern Med 2005;142:914–925. *Review of nucleic acid amplification tests and their performance in testing urine in lieu of urethral or cervical swabs.*

Ghanem KG, Giles JA, Zenilman JM: Fluoroquinolone-resistant *Neisseria gonorrhoeae;* the inevitable epidemic. Infect Dis Clin North Am 2005;19:351–365. *Documents the worldwide evolution and spread of resistant gonococci.*

Newman LM, Moran JS, Workowski KA, et al: Update on the management of gonorrhea in adults in the United States. Clin Infect Dis 2007;44:S84–101. *A comprehensive review.*

323 HAEMOPHILUS AND MORAXELLA INFECTIONS

Michael S. Simberkoff

HAEMOPHILUS INFECTIONS

Definition

The name *Haemophilus* is derived from the Greek nouns *haima,* meaning "blood," and *philos,* meaning "lover." *Haemophilus* species primarily infect the respiratory tract, skin, or mucous membranes of humans. From these sites, organisms can invade and cause bacteremia, meningitis, epiglottitis, endocarditis, septic arthritis, or cellulitis.

The Pathogen

Haemophilus species are small, nonmotile, aerobic or facultative anaerobic, pleomorphic, gram-negative bacilli. The prototype of this genus, *Haemophilus influenzae,* was originally recovered from patients with influenza by Pfeiffer in 1893, and it was considered the cause of that disease for many years. Primary isolation of *Haemophilus* species is best accomplished on chocolate agar medium in a CO_2-enriched atmosphere.

Epidemiology

The precise prevalence and incidence of *H. influenzae* infections are unknown. This organism can be detected in the nasopharynx of both children and adults. Between 3 and 5% of infants harbor *H. influenzae* type b in their nasopharynx. Nontypable *H. influenzae* can be detected in nasopharyngeal cultures of more than 70% of young children, but infection occurs in only a small proportion of colonized patients. However, the risk for infection in nonimmune household contacts of a patient with invasive *H. influenzae* disease is approximately 600-fold greater than the risk in the age-adjusted general population.

H. influenzae type b was the most common cause of meningitis in young children before effective vaccines were introduced in the 1980s. Vaccination has had a dramatic impact on the incidence of infection in this group. In a population-based study in Atlanta over a 1-year period, invasive *H. influenzae* disease occurred in only 5.6 per 100,000 children and 1.7 per 100,000 adults. Forty of the 47 strains associated with invasive disease from adult patients in this study were serotyped. Twenty of these isolates (50%) were *H. influenzae* type b, 19 (47.5%) were nontypable, and 1 (2.5%) was type f.

Patients with human immunodeficiency virus (HIV) infection are at increased risk for *H. influenzae* infection. Rates of invasive *H. influenzae* infection in men aged 20 to 49 with HIV infection and acquired immunodeficiency syndrome (AIDS) were 14.6 and 79.2 per 100,000, respectively. The majority of these infections were caused by nontypable *H. influenzae* strains, although in a second study, 10 of 15 bacteremic *H. influenzae* type b infections observed in adults occurred in patients at risk for HIV infection, and AIDS was documented in 7 of these patients.

Other factors also increase the risk for *H. influenzae* infection, including globulin deficiencies, sickle cell disease, splenectomy, malignancy, pregnancy, cerebrospinal fluid (CSF) leaks, head trauma, alcoholism, chronic obstructive pulmonary disease (COPD), and race. Eskimo, Navajo, and Apache children have *H. influenzae* type b infection rates that are significantly greater than those in comparable non-native populations. In addition, daycare attendance, crowding, the presence of siblings, prior hospitalizations, and previous otitis media have been shown to increase the risk for *H. influenzae* type b disease in young children, whereas breast-feeding decreases this risk.

Pathobiology

H. influenzae consists of encapsulated (typable) and nonencapsulated (nontypable) forms. The former are responsible for most of the invasive infections in children and acute epiglottitis in both children and adults, whereas the latter cause respiratory mucosal infections, conjunctivitis, female genital tract infections, and invasive disease in adults. The capsules of *H. influenzae* consist of polysaccharide antigens. Six capsular serotypes (a through f) exist and are important virulence factors that inhibit opsonization, clearance, and intracellular killing of the organisms. *H. influenzae* type b, formerly the most common cause of meningitis in infancy and childhood worldwide, contains a pentose capsular polysaccharide consisting of polyribosyl ribitol phosphate (PRP). Other serotypes contain hexose polysaccharides. *H. influenzae* type b is more virulent than other serotypes, probably because it is highly resistant to clearance once bacteremia has been initiated.

Fimbriae are important virulence factors that enhance the adherence of *H. influenzae* to mucosal surfaces. Both typable and nontypable *H. influenzae* isolates contain fimbriae. The lipo-oligosaccharides (LOSs) of *H. influenzae* also contribute to their virulence. LOSs appear to play a crucial role in facilitating the survival of *H. influenzae* on mucosal surfaces within the nasopharynx and in initiating invasive disease (blood stream invasion) from these sites.

Outer membrane proteins (OMPs) also serve as virulence factors in *H. influenzae* disease. At least 15 different *H. influenzae* OMPs have been identified. One of these (P2, 39 to 40 kD) functions as a porin, and others are associated with iron binding. Successful scavenging of iron within the human host is crucial for multiplication of *H. influenzae.*

Antibodies have been recognized for decades as an important part of host defenses against *H. influenzae* diseases. The classic studies of Fothergill and Wright in 1933 demonstrated that most cases of *H. influenzae* meningitis occur in young children after they lose passively acquired maternal antibodies and before active humoral immunity to the organism develops. These protective antibodies function primarily to opsonize and facilitate *H. influenzae* clearance rather than to kill virulent organisms directly.

Complement is also an essential component of host defenses against some *H. influenzae* diseases. Children with congenital deficiencies of C2, C3, and factor I have an increased incidence of *H. influenzae* infections. Patients who lack a functional spleen or who have undergone splenectomy also are at risk for the development of overwhelming infection with *H. influenzae* type b.

Clinical Manifestations

Meningitis

H. influenzae meningitis commonly occurs in children younger than 5 years and in adults with a history of skull trauma or CSF leaks. *H. influenzae* type b strains cause the overwhelming majority of these cases. A review of 493 episodes of acute bacterial meningitis in adults over a 27-year period showed that 19 cases (4%) were due to *H. influenzae.*

H. influenzae meningitis is clinically indistinguishable from other forms of acute bacterial meningitis. Most patients with *H. influenzae* meningitis have CSF white blood cell counts greater than 1000/mm^3 and hypoglycorrhachia. CSF Gram stain shows pleomorphic gram-negative bacilli in 60 to 70% of untreated cases. In some patients, however, the bipolar staining may result in a mistaken diagnosis of pneumococcal meningitis. Thus, Gram stain is neither sensitive nor specific for diagnosing *H. influenzae* meningitis.

A diagnosis of *H. influenzae* type b meningitis can be rapidly and reliably established by detecting PRP capsular antigens in CSF. The diagnosis can be established in most cases even when antibiotics have been given before CSF is obtained. Other serotypes (most commonly type f) can also cause meningitis in adults. Therefore, serologic tests for type b antigen in CSF cannot be relied on to rule out *H. influenzae* meningitis in all cases.

Epiglottitis

H. influenzae type b is the most common cause of acute epiglottitis in both children and adults. Epiglottitis is a life-threatening infection in children that usually occurs in those younger than 5 years. The symptoms are fever, drooling, dysphagia, and respiratory distress or stridor, which appear over the course of hours. In adults, fever, sore throat, dysphagia, and odynophagia occur. Cervical tenderness and lymphadenopathy can be found at all ages. Laryngoscopy demonstrates a swollen, cherry-red epiglottis. However, this procedure should be avoided or undertaken only by experts because it may precipitate acute airway obstruction and thus make emergency tracheotomy necessary. A lateral radiograph of the neck more safely confirms the diagnosis of acute epiglottitis. The patient must be maintained in an upright position during this procedure, however, to avoid additional compromise of the airway. The etiology is usually established by blood culture. Cultures of the pharynx and other mucosal surfaces are less useful because *H. influenzae* may be part of the normal flora. One review suggests that although vaccination has effectively reduced the incidence of this disease in children, it may be increasing in adults.

Pneumonia

H. influenzae is a common cause of pneumonia in both children and adults. These organisms can also cause nosocomial infections, including ventilator-associated pneumonia. The clinical features of *H. influenzae* pneumonia include fever, cough, and signs and radiographic findings of lobar consolidation. Parapneumonic effusions or empyema occur commonly in patients with *H. influenzae* pneumonia. Gram-negative bacilli in sputum suggest the diagnosis, but isolation of *H. influenzae* from sputum culture alone is inadequate to prove an etiology because of the high frequency with which this organism colonizes the respiratory tract. A diagnosis can be established by isolating *H. influenzae* from either blood or pleural fluid. Most isolates are nontypable.

Tracheobronchitis

Tracheobronchitis is a condition characterized by fever, cough, and purulent sputum that occurs in the absence of radiographic infiltrates suggestive of pneumonia. It frequently develops in patients with known chronic lung disease. Blood cultures are rarely positive. A combination of pleomorphic gram-negative bacilli predominating in purulent sputum, antibody titers to *H. influenzae* that rise after infection, and a response, at least transiently, to treatment of *H. influenzae* infection strongly suggests this diagnosis.

Sinusitis

H. influenzae and *Streptococcus pneumoniae* are the most frequent bacterial isolates from antral punctures or surgical specimens of patients with acute purulent sinusitis. Most *H. influenzae* isolates are nontypable. Although patients may respond initially to treatment directed against *H. influenzae,* the response is transient if the sinus obstruction is not relieved. *H. influenzae* is not an important pathogen in patients with chronic sinusitis.

Otitis Media

H. influenzae is the most frequent cause of otitis media in young children. Approximately 90% of the *H. influenzae* isolates obtained by tympanocentesis are nontypable; *H. influenzae* type b causes most of the remaining 10% of infections. Patients with otitis media may have ear pain or exhibit irritability. Drainage can be present. An inflamed, opaque, bulging, or perforated tympanic membrane is usually demonstrated. The etiology can be proved by Gram stain and culture of purulent fluid obtained by tympanocentesis. Otitis caused by *H. influenzae* type b may occur in association with bacteremia and meningitis.

Cellulitis

H. influenzae type b is the cause of 5 to 15% of cases of cellulitis in young children. Most of the infections occur on the face or neck. *H. influenzae* cellulitis is often described as causing a distinctive blue or violaceous discoloration of the skin. However, the fever, erythema, and tenderness observed may not be distinguishable from those due to other causes. The diagnosis is established by culture of blood or tissue aspirates from the involved area, or both.

Bacteremia without a Primary Focus of Infection

H. influenzae causes primary bacteremia in both children and adults. In infants or children, occult meningitis or epiglottitis can be present. Rigorous clinical and laboratory evaluation is essential to avoid missing diagnoses of life-threatening focal infections in these patients. In adults, primary *H. influenzae* type b bacteremia often occurs in those with underlying diseases such as lymphoma, leukemia, or alcoholism.

Obstetric and Gynecologic Infection

Pregnancy is associated with a significant risk for *H. influenzae* infection. In the Atlanta study, 7 of 47 adult *H. influenzae* invasive infections occurred in pregnant women. Nontypable *H. influenzae* is also an important cause of tubo-ovarian abscess and salpingitis in women.

Pericarditis

H. influenzae type b is an important cause of primary bacterial pericarditis in children. It rarely causes this infection in adults; however, pericarditis can occur in association with pneumonia, probably as a result of contiguous spread of the infection.

Endocarditis

H. influenzae is a very unusual cause of endocarditis in view of the frequency with which invasive disease occurs. Most infections occur in patients with preexisting valvar heart disease. Because of its slow initial growth in blood culture media, diagnosis of this infection may be delayed or missed. Patients with *H. influenzae* endocarditis are at high risk for arterial embolic phenomena.

Septic Arthritis

H. influenzae type b is a common cause of septic arthritis in young children; it is rare in adults. *H. influenzae* type b arthritis is clinically indistinguishable from other causes of pyogenic arthritis.

Purulent Conjunctivitis and Brazilian Purpuric Fever

H. influenzae, biogroup *aegyptius* (Koch-Weeks bacillus), causes epidemic purulent conjunctivitis in children. This disease commonly occurs in hot climates or in the summer season.

The infection is characterized by conjunctival erythema, edema, mucopurulent exudate, and varying discomfort in the eyes. An unusually virulent clone of *H. influenzae,* biogroup *aegyptius,* causes an invasive infection called Brazilian purpuric fever, which is characterized by petechial or purpuric skin lesions and vascular collapse; it occurs days to weeks after an initial episode of conjunctivitis in infants and children younger than 10 years.

Treatment

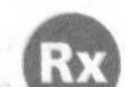

Third-generation cephalosporins are considered the treatment of choice for serious *H. influenzae* infections, such as meningitis or epiglottitis. Treatment with ceftriaxone (adult dose: 1 to 2 g intravenously every 12 hours) or cefotaxime (adult dose: 2 g intravenously every 6 hours) should be started in patients with proven or suspected *H. influenzae* infection, and it should be continued at least until full susceptibility data are available.

Ampicillin was effective treatment of all *H. influenzae* infections until the mid-1970s. Since the first reports of ampicillin-resistant *H. influenzae* isolates in 1972, however, the prevalence of resistance has increased dramatically. Most resistance is due to a plasmid-mediated, R-factor enzyme (TEM-1), β-lactamase, which can be detected rapidly in the laboratory. A small number of isolates, however, have altered penicillin binding proteins that have decreased binding affinity to penicillin and other β-lactam antibiotics. As a consequence, the isolates may be resistant to some cephalosporins, such as cefaclor, cefamandole, and cefuroxime, in addition to ampicillin. Therefore, patients with proven or suspected *H. influenzae* infections should not be treated with ampicillin or second-generation cephalosporins until susceptibility to these antibiotics has been proved. Chloramphenicol resistance also occurs in *H. influenzae;* an inactivating enzyme, chloramphenicol acetyltransferase, causes resistance. A small number of *H. influenzae* isolates are resistant to both ampicillin and chloramphenicol.

Oral antibiotics are commonly used to treat tracheobronchitis in patients with COPD and otitis media in children, in whom *H. influenzae* isolates are common. Because of resistance, ampicillin and amoxicillin cannot be recommended for the more serious of these infections unless the susceptibility of isolates is known. Most *H. influenzae* isolates are susceptible to amoxicillin-clavulanate. They

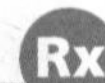

are also susceptible to azithromycin and clarithromycin, the newer macrolide antibiotics. Fluoroquinolones, such as ciprofloxacin, ofloxacin, levofloxacin, and gatifloxacin, are active against these organisms. Trimethoprim-sulfamethoxazole is also effective for most isolates.

Prevention

The first *H. influenzae* type b vaccines were licensed for use in the United States in 1985. They contained purified PRP antigens. However, postlicensing studies of PRP vaccines in the United States showed variable efficacy. The PRP vaccines elicit a type 2, thymus-independent B-cell response, generate few (if any) memory B cells, and fail to stimulate a response in neonates and infants.

Protein-conjugated PRP vaccines were developed to overcome the problem of lack of immune response in the most susceptible infants and some young children. Several are now licensed for use in infants. At present, protein-conjugated PRP vaccines are recommended for use in all infants older than 2 months but not earlier than 6 weeks of age. Recent studies have shown that protein-conjugated vaccines are effective in diverse populations, including adults with COPD.

Antibiotic prophylaxis should be used for nonimmunized household or daycare contacts of a patient with invasive *H. influenzae* type b disease. Rifampin is the treatment of choice. It should be given in a dosage of 10 mg/kg once daily for 4 days to neonates younger than 1 month, 20 mg/kg (up to a maximum of 600 mg) once daily for 4 days to older children, and 600 mg/day for 4 days to adults.

Other *Haemophilus* Species

H. parainfluenzae can be found as part of the normal flora of the mouth and pharynx (Table 323–1). It is a rare cause of meningitis in children and an even rarer cause of meningitis in adults. It may cause dental infections or dental abscesses. Cases of brain abscess, epidural abscess, liver abscess, osteomyelitis, pneumonia, empyema, epiglottitis, peritonitis, septic arthritis, and septicemia have been reported to be caused by this organism. *H. parainfluenzae* also causes subacute endocarditis, often in young adults. *Haemophilus* species are responsible for approximately 1% of cases of infective endocarditis in non–drug-abusing patients. *H. parainfluenzae, H. aphrophilus,* and *H. paraphrophilus* are the species most frequently recovered from these patients. *H. parainfluenzae* forms bulky vegetations on heart valves. Arterial embolization is common in patients with *H. parainfluenzae* endocarditis. Most isolates are sensitive to ampicillin, but some produce β-lactamases.

TABLE 323–1 SITES OF COLONIZATION AND INFECTIONS BY *HAEMOPHILUS INFLUENZAE*

Species	Normal Flora	Associated Diseases
H. influenzae	Nasopharynx Upper respiratory tract	Meningitis Epiglottitis Sinusitis Otitis Pneumonia Cellulitis Arthritis Osteomyelitis Obstetric infections Endocarditis
H. influenzae type b *aegyptius*	No	Purulent conjunctivitis Brazilian purpuric fever

MORAXELLA INFECTIONS

Definition

Moraxella species are organisms named for Victor Morax, a Swiss ophthalmologist who isolated and described the organism now known as *Moraxella lacunata. Moraxella* species are associated with a variety of infections, the most common of which is exacerbation of chronic bronchitis by *Moraxella catarrhalis.*

The Pathogen

Moraxella organisms are small, gram-negative bacteria that grow well on blood or chocolate agar. They are catalase and oxidase positive. These small diplococci are morphologically difficult to distinguish from *Neisseria*. Some *Moraxella* species are gram-negative bacilli.

M. catarrhalis is the most important pathogen of this genus (Table 323–2).

Pathobiology

The organism is isolated exclusively from humans and is found predominantly in the respiratory tract. *M. catarrhalis* adheres to mucosal cells with the aid of pili. Infection is believed to result from contiguous spread of the organism from sites of colonization, possibly as a result of the introduction of new, more virulent strains to which the host lacks immunity.

Clinical Manifestations

M. catarrhalis is associated with exacerbations of chronic bronchitis. Studies indicate that this organism can be isolated from 0.2 to 8.1% of the sputum aspirates of patients with this disease. It is the third most common pathogen isolated from these patients behind *S. pneumoniae* and *H. influenzae.*

M. catarrhalis can cause pneumonia, particularly in elderly patients with COPD and other underlying conditions such as diabetes mellitus. Sir William Osler is believed to have died as a result of *M. catarrhalis* pneumonia. Cases of bacteremic pneumonia have been reported. In addition, *M. catarrhalis* can cause nosocomial pneumonia with evidence of patient-to-patient spread of the organism.

M. catarrhalis is a common cause of otitis media in young children. Microbiologic studies indicate that this organism is present in approximately 15% of the aspirates from such patients. The organism also causes sinusitis and is a rare cause of bacteremia in children and adults.

Serious infections with other *Moraxella* species are uncommon. However, these organisms are associated with chronic conjunctivitis. Furthermore, case reports have documented the rare occurrence of invasive infections, including bacteremia, endocarditis, arthritis, pericarditis, and meningitis. The latter may occur in patients with complement deficiency.

TABLE 323–2 SITES OF COLONIZATION AND INFECTION BY *MORAXELLA* SPECIES

Species	Normal Flora	Associated Diseases
M. catarrhalis	Oral cavity and upper respiratory tract	Chronic bronchitis exacerbation Otitis media Pneumonia Sinusitis Bacteremia, endocarditis Arthritis, osteomyelitis, epiglottitis, etc. (all extremely rare)
M. lacunata	Upper respiratory tract	Chronic conjunctivitis
Other *Moraxella*	Upper respiratory tract	Rare cases of bacteremia, endocarditis, arthritis, meningitis

Treatment

Rx

Oral antibiotics are sufficient for the treatment of most *M. catarrhalis* infections. Inducible β-lactamases are present in many isolates. Therefore, treatment with a β-lactamase–stable antibiotic such as amoxicillin-clavulanate (usual adult dose: 500 mg every 12 hours), a cephalosporin (e.g., cefaclor, usual adult dose: 500 mg every 8 hours), or a non–β-lactam antibiotic such as trimethoprim-sulfamethoxazole (usual adult dose: 1 double-strength tablet every 12 hours) should be initiated pending susceptibility test results.

SUGGESTED READINGS

Foxwell AR, Cripps AW, Dear KB: *Haemophilus influenzae* oral whole cell vaccination for preventing acute exacerbations of chronic bronchitis. Cochrane Database Syst Rev 2006;(4):CD001958. *Although larger trials are needed, vaccinating patients with recurrent exacerbations of chronic bronchitis in the autumn may reduce the number and severity of exacerbations over the following winter.*

Ioannidis JPA, Worthington M, Griffiths JK, Snydman DR: Spectrum and significance of bacteremia due to *Moraxella catarrhalis.* Clin Infect Dis 1995;21:390–397. *A review of 58 cases of* M. catarrhalis *bacteremia; bacteremia most commonly occurred in elderly patients with pneumonia, and the prognosis was worse for those with endocarditis and immunologic deficiency.*

Myotte JM: Nursing home–acquired pneumonia: Update on treatment options. Drugs Aging 2006;23:377–390. *An excellent review, including a discussion on H. influenzae.*

Sethi S, Evan N, Grant BJ, et al: New strains of bacteria and exacerbations of chronic obstructive pulmonary disease. N Engl J Med 2002;347:465–471. *In 81 patients with COPD, nontypable* H. influenzae *and* M. catarrhalis *were the most commonly isolated bacterial pathogens. Molecular typing of the isolates showed a highly significant association between exacerbations of chronic bronchitis and acquisition of new* M. catarrhalis *strains.*

Shah RK, Roberson DW, Jones DT: Epiglottitis in the *Hemophilus influenzae* type B vaccine era: Changing trends. Laryngoscope 2004;114:557–560. *Hemophilus remains an important cause of epiglottitis even in the vaccination era.*

Tristram S, Jacobs MR, Appelbaum PC: Antimicrobial resistance in *Haemophilus influenzae*. Clin Microbiol Rev 2007;20:368–389. *A review of antimicrobial resistance in H. influenzae.*

324 CHANCROID

Edward W. Hook III

Definition

The Pathogen

Chancroid is a sexually transmitted infection caused by *Haemophilus ducreyi,* which is a small gram-negative bacillus with rounded ends that typically forms chains or parallel aggregates in lesions. Though originally thought to be closely related to other *Haemophilus* species, rRNA studies suggest that it is a member of the family Pasteurellaceae.

Epidemiology

The World Health Organization estimates the annual global incidence of the infection to be about 6 million cases, but it is an uncommon disease in the United States, with about 30 to 50 cases annually. As for other genital ulcer diseases, chancroid is associated with an increased risk for infection with human immunodeficiency virus (HIV). The majority of reported cases occur in men. There are strong epidemiologic links between chancroid and prostitution, but it is quite likely that chancroid has been underdiagnosed in women in the past. The usual incubation period is 2 to 5 days, but it may be up to 14 days. In one outbreak, the incubation period averaged nearly 2 weeks in women.

Clinical Manifestations

Although the clinical manifestations of chancroid are quite variable, the classic initial finding is an inflammatory macule that then becomes a vesicle-pustule and finally progresses to become a sharply circumscribed, somewhat ragged and undermined painful ulcer (Fig. 324–1). The ulcer base is moist and may be covered with a grayish necrotic exudate. Removal of the exudate reveals purulent granulation tissue. Lesions are typically single with surrounding cutaneous erythema, but they may be multiple, possibly because of autoinoculation of nearby tissues. Lesions in men usually occur on the penile shaft or glans. In women, lesions may occur on the cervix, vagina, vulva, or perianal area. Lesions occasionally occur on or spread to the abdomen, thigh, breast, fingers, or lips. Intraoral lesions are uncommon. Inguinal adenopathy is noted in 50% of patients, approximately two thirds of whom have unilateral adenopathy. Systemic symptoms are rare.

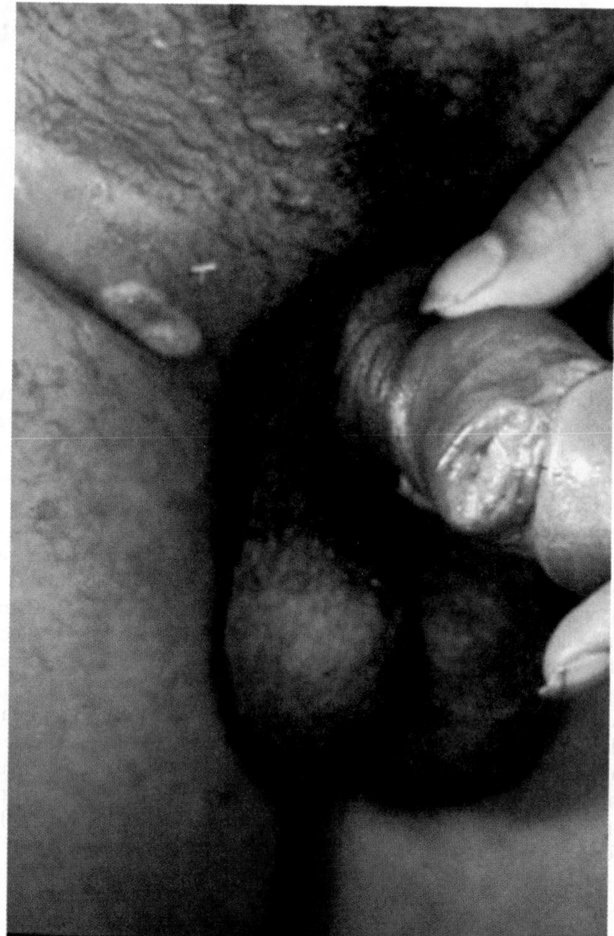

FIGURE 324–1 • A typical chancroid lesion with a genital ulcer and an involved regional lymph node. (Reproduced with permission from Herpes-Coldsores.com. Available at http://www.herpes-coldsores.com/std/chancroid_pictures.htm. Accessed September 8, 2006.)

When chancroid is manifested as a transient genital ulcer followed by significant inguinal adenopathy, it may be difficult to distinguish from lymphogranuloma venereum. Other uncommon clinical variants include the phagedenic type of ulcer with secondary superinfection and rapid tissue destruction; giant chancroid, characterized by a very large single ulcer; serpiginous ulcer, characterized by rapidly spreading, indolent, shallow ulcers on the groin or the thigh; and a follicular type with multiple small ulcers in a perifollicular distribution.

Diagnosis

Definitive diagnosis requires either morphologic demonstration of typical organisms in the lesions or demonstration of *H. ducreyi* by culture or polymerase chain reaction (PCR) assays. Most commonly, however, the disease is diagnosed clinically and treated without a definitive diagnosis. PCR assays for the diagnosis of chancroid have been developed and found to be more sensitive than culture but are research tools that are not currently available commercially.

Under optimal conditions, positive cultures can be obtained from the lesion in up to 80% of cases. After necrotic debris is removed from the ulcer with physiologic saline, the base and edges of the ulcer should be swabbed with a cotton-tipped swab and inoculated directly onto the culture plate if possible; swabs may be put into Amies transport medium if culture plates are not immediately available. Smears obtained from the undermined edges should be gently rolled onto a slide. Typical organisms are seen in 50 to 80% of cases. Organisms may also be obtained by aspirating the inguinal nodes. Nodes should be aspirated by placing the needle through normal skin to avoid the formation of fistulous tracts. There is no commercially available serologic test for chancroid.

Differential Diagnosis

The differential diagnosis (Chapter 308) includes syphilis (Chapter 340), herpes genitalis (Chapter 397), lymphogranuloma venereum (Chapter 339), traumatic ulcers, and granuloma inguinale (Chapter 337). Of these, the most commonly confused are syphilis and genital herpes. Simultaneous infection with multiple pathogens is relatively common. Outpatients with suspected chancroid should have a culture or other test for herpes simplex virus, a serologic test for syphilis, and preferably, a darkfield examination as well.

Treatment

Rx

The preferred therapeutic regimens are a single intramuscular dose of ceftriaxone, 250 mg; ciprofloxacin, 500 mg orally twice daily for 3 days; a single 1-g dose of azithromycin given orally; or erythromycin, 500 mg orally three times daily for 7 days. Nodes should not be incised.

No recent large therapeutic trials of chancroid therapy have been performed, and resistance may be emerging to the recommended regimens. In addition, persons infected with HIV or uncircumcised males may not respond well to therapy. Hence, reexamination is recommended at 3 to 7 days; symptoms should improve by day 3 and objective improvement should be apparent by day 7 after therapy. Serologic testing for HIV is recommended in all patients treated for possible chancroid. All regular sexual partners should be examined and treated with a similar regimen.

Prevention

No vaccine is available. Use of a condom is presumably helpful. There are no data regarding the efficacy of antibiotic prophylaxis, but most experts recommend prophylactic therapy for persons sexually exposed to chancroid in the preceding 10 days.

SUGGESTED READINGS

Bauer ME, Townsend CA, Ronald AR, et al: Localization of *Haemophilus ducreyi* in naturally acquired chancroidal ulcers. Microbes Infect 2006;8:2465–2468. *The organism is found mainly in the granulocytic infiltrate of the ulcer.*

Centers for Disease Control and Prevention; Sexually transmitted diseases treatment guidelines, 2006. MMWR 2006;55(RR-11):1–94. *Current treatment and management recommendations for chancroid.*

Hoyo C, Hoffman I, Moser BK et al: Improving the accuracy of syndromic diagnosis of genital ulcer disease in Malawi. Sex Transm Dis 2005;32:231–237. *Describes the relative sensitivities of different diagnostic tests for chancroid and recent temporal trends in an endemic setting.*

Sehgal VN, Srivastava G: Chancroid: Contemporary appraisal. Int J Dermatol 2003;42:182–190. *A detailed review.*

325 CHOLERA AND OTHER *VIBRIO* INFECTIONS

Eduardo Gotuzzo and Carlos Seas

CHOLERA

Definition

Cholera is a feared epidemic diarrheal disease caused by *Vibrio cholerae* serogroup O1 and, since 1992, by the new serogroup O139. The disease is characterized by acute watery diarrhea. In its more severe form, a person may be severely dehydrated and in hypovolemic shock; the patient may die in a matter of a few hours after contracting the infection if treatment is not provided. Cholera is endemic today in Africa and Asia, and cases are also reported from Latin America, North America, and Europe. Seven pandemics have been registered in history since 1816; the most recent has lasted more than 4 decades since its recognition in Indonesia in 1961.

The Pathogen

V. cholerae is a curved gram-negative bacillus that belongs to the family Vibrionaceae and shares common characteristics with the family Enterobacteriaceae. *V. cholerae* O1 can be classified into three serotypes according to the presence of somatic antigens and into two biotypes, classic and El Tor, according to specific phenotypic characteristics. There is no evidence of different clinical spectra among the three serotypes of *V. cholerae.* The classic biotype, responsible for the first six pandemics of cholera, causes an approximately equal number of symptomatic and asymptomatic cases, whereas the El Tor biotype causes more asymptomatic infections. The classic biotype is confined to the south of Bangladesh, and the El Tor biotype is responsible for the current pandemic. The O139 serogroup is composed of a variety of genetically diverse strains, both toxigenic and nontoxigenic; it is genetically closer to El Tor *V. cholerae.*

Epidemiology

Cholera has both a predisposition to cause epidemics with pandemic potential and an ability to remain endemic in all affected areas. People of all ages are at risk to contract the infection in epidemic settings, whereas children older than 2 years are mainly affected in endemic areas. *V. cholerae* lives in riverine, brackish, and estuarine ecosystems, where both O1 and non-O1 strains coexist, with non-O1 and nontoxigenic O1 strains predominating over toxigenic O1 strains. In its natural environment, *V. cholerae* lives attached to algae or to crustacean shells and copepods, with which it coexists in a symbiotic manner. Several conditions, such as temperature, salinity, and availability of nutrients, determine the survival of *V. cholerae;* when these conditions are adverse, vibrios survive in a viable, but nonculturable state. More recent data suggest that cholera phages modulate the abundance of *V. cholerae* in the environment and determine the beginning and end of epidemics. Phages may also play a role in the emergence of new *V. cholerae* serogroups by transferring genetic material to nontoxigenic strains.

From its aquatic environment, *V. cholerae* is introduced to humans through contamination of water sources and food. Once humans are infected, very high attack rates may take place, particularly in previously naïve populations. Acquisition of the disease by drinking contaminated water from rivers, ponds, lakes, and even tube well sources has been documented. Drinking unboiled water, introducing hands into containers used to store drinking water, drinking beverages from street vendors, drinking beverages to which contaminated ice has been added, and drinking water outside the home are risk factors; these factors contributed to the acquisition of cholera during the large Peruvian epidemic of 1991. Drinking boiled water, acidic beverages, and carbonated water, as well as using narrow-necked vessels for storing water, are protective measures. Epidemics of cholera associated with the ingestion of leftover rice, raw fish, cooked crabs, seafood, raw oysters, and fresh vegetables and fruits have been documented. Person-to-person transmission is less likely to occur because a large inoculum is necessary to transmit disease.

Epidemics of cholera tend to occur during the hot season. Factors affecting climate change and climate variability have an impact on the incidence of cholera. The El Niño-southern oscillation (ENSO), a periodic phenomenon representative of global climate variability, affects the transmission of cholera and vector-borne diseases. ENSO causes warming of normally cool waters in the Pacific coastline of Peru, thereby promoting phytoplankton bloom, zooplankton bloom, and *V. cholerae* proliferation.

Some host factors are important in the transmission of cholera. The chronic gastritis associated with *H. pylori* predisposes to cholera by inducing hypochlorhydria, which reduces the ability of the stomach to contain the infection. An unexplained predisposition toward severe disease in persons with the O blood group has been observed in Asia and more recently in Latin America. Thus, complex associations among climatic, seasonal, bacterial, and human factors affect cholera transmission. Although for the most part developing countries are affected by cholera, several developed countries such as the United States, Canada, and Australia have reported indigenous and imported cases. Fifty-six countries officially reported 101,383 cases to the World Health Organization in 2004, with 2345 deaths; 94% of these cases were reported from Africa. Figure 325–1 shows the world distribution of cholera in 2004.

Pathobiology

V. cholerae O1 and O139 cause clinical disease by secreting an enterotoxin that promotes the secretion of fluids and electrolytes by the small intestine. The infectious dose of bacteria varies with the vehicle. When water is the vehicle, more bacteria are needed to cause disease (10^3 to 10^6), but when the vehicle is food, lower amounts are needed (10^2 to 10^4). The incubation period varies from 12 to 72 hours. Cholera toxin (CTX) has two subunits, the pentamer B subunit and a monomer A subunit. The B subunits allow binding of the toxin to a specific receptor, a ganglioside (GM_1) located on the surface of the cells lining the mucosa along the intestine of humans and certain suckling mammals. The active, or A, subunit has two components, A1 and A2, linked by a disulfide bond. Activation of adenylate cyclase by the A1 component results in an increase in cyclic adenosine monophosphate, which blocks the absorption of sodium and chloride by microvilli and promotes the secretion of chloride and water by crypt cells. These events lead to the production of watery diarrhea with electrolyte concentrations similar to that of plasma, as shown in Table 325–1. A few other toxins have been isolated from pathogenic *V. cholerae,* but their roles in genesis of the disease are less clear.

The genetic material of *V. cholerae* O1 El Tor is included in two circular chromosomes, the larger containing 3 megabases and the smaller containing 1.07 megabases. The main virulence genes are *ctx*A and *ctx*B, which encode for CTX subunits A and B, respectively, and *tcp*A, which codes for toxin coregulated pilus. Regulation of expression of these genes is complex. Recent data suggest that vibrios are able to upregulate the expression of CTX in response to intestinal fluid components, as well as in the presence of certain environmental factors. Genes unique to El Tor *V. cholerae* may encode for specific features that allow this biotype to better survive in the environment, as well as to be more infectious to humans.

Clinical Manifestations

Cholera is characterized by watery diarrhea and dehydration, which ranges from mild to severe and life-threatening. Patients with mild dehydration cannot be differentiated from those infected by other enteric pathogens causing watery diarrhea. On the other hand, patients with severe dehydration secondary to cholera are easy to identify in that their stools have the appearance of rice water and no other clinical illness produces such severe dehydration as quickly (in a matter of a few hours) as cholera. Onset of the disease is abrupt and characterized by watery diarrhea, vomiting, generalized cramps, and oliguria. Physical examination shows a feeble pulse, fever is rarely present, patients look anxious and restless, the eyes are very sunken, mucous membranes are dry, the skin has lost its elasticity and when pinched retracts very slowly, the voice is almost nonaudible, and intestinal sounds are prominent. Although watery diarrhea is the hallmark of cholera, some patients do not have diarrhea but instead have abdominal distention and ileus, a relatively rare type of cholera called cholera "sicca."

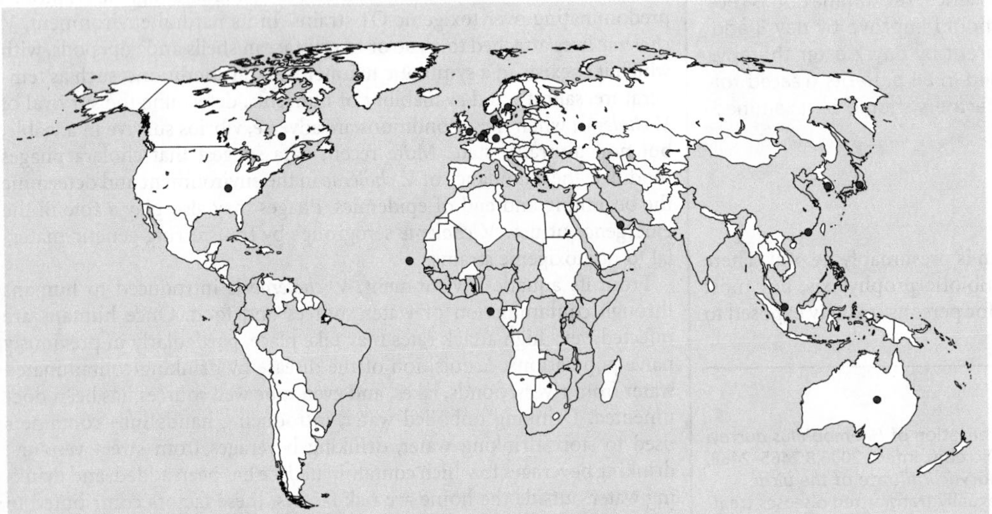

FIGURE 325–1 • World distribution of cholera in 2004 based on reports to the World Health Organization. The colored areas represent countries that reported cholera cases to the World Health Organization; the dots represent countries that reported imported cases. (Reprinted with permission, World Health Organization: Cholera, 2004. Weekly Epidemiol Rec 2005; 80[31]:261–268.)

TABLE 325–1 ELECTROLYTE COMPOSITION OF CHOLERA STOOLS AND SOLUTIONS RECOMMENDED FOR TREATMENT

	Na^+	Cl^-	K^+	HCO_3^-	Glucose	Osmolarity
Stools of adults with severe cholera	130	100	20	44		
Intravenous lactated Ringer's solution	130	109	4	28*	0	271
Intravenous normal saline	154	154	0	0	0	308
Standard oral rehydration solution promoted by the WHO	90	80	20	10†	111	311
Reduced-osmolarity oral rehydration solution promoted by the WHO	75	65	20	10†	75	245
Rice-based oral rehydration solution	90	80	20	10†		270

Glucose, electrolyte concentration, and osmolarity are in the unit mmol/L.
*Lactated Ringer's solution contains citrate instead of bicarbonate.
†Bicarbonate is replaced by trisodium citrate.
WHO = Word Health Organization.
Modified with permission from Seas C, DuPont HL, Valdez LM, et al: Practical guidelines for the treatment of cholera. Drugs 1996;51:966–973.

Laboratory findings in patients with severe dehydration consist of an increase in packed cell volume, serum specific gravity, and total protein; azotemia; metabolic acidosis with a high anion gap; normal or low serum potassium levels; and normal or slightly low sodium and chloride levels. The calcium and magnesium content in plasma is high as a result of hemoconcentration. Leukocytosis is observed in patients with severe cholera. Hyperglycemia caused by high concentrations of epinephrine, glucagon, and cortisol stimulated by hypovolemia is more commonly seen than hypoglycemia. Acute renal failure is the most severe complication of cholera. Incidence rates of 10.6 cases per 1000 were reported in Peru during the first months of the 1991 epidemic. Patients with acute renal failure almost always have a history of improper rehydration. Cholera in pregnant women carries a bad prognosis. Pregnant women have more severe clinical illness, especially when the disease is acquired at the end of the pregnancy. Fetal loss occurs in as many as 50% of these pregnancies. Cholera in the elderly also carries a bad prognosis because of an increase in complications, particularly acute renal failure, severe metabolic acidosis, and pulmonary edema.

Diagnosis

Chaotic movement under darkfield microscopy and a high number of bacteria in a stool sample from patients with diarrhea are characteristic of *V. cholerae* infection. Specific antisera against the serotype block the movement of vibrios and allow confirmation of the diagnosis. Under epidemic conditions, observing bacteria with a darting movement in a stool sample from a suspected patient under darkfield microscopy is adequate to make the diagnosis. Definitive confirmation requires isolation of the bacterium in culture. Specific medium is needed to isolate *V. cholerae* from stool. High sensitivity and specificity have been reported more with DNA amplification by polymerase chain reaction for detection of vibrios in stool and environmental samples.

Treatment Rx

The objectives of therapy are to restore the fluid losses caused by diarrhea and vomiting, correct the metabolic acidosis, restore potassium deficits, and replace continuous fluid losses. Treatment of patients with milder forms of dehydration is easy, but treatment of patients with severe dehydration requires experience and proper training. The intravenous route should be restricted to patients with some dehydration who do not tolerate the oral route, those who purge more than 10 to 20 mL/kg/hr, and all patients with severe dehydration. Rehydration should be accomplished in two phases: the rehydration phase and the maintenance phase. The purpose of the rehydration phase is to restore normal hydration status, and it should last no more than 4 hours. Intravenous fluids should be infused at a rate of 50 to 100 mL/kg/hr in severely dehydrated patients. Lactated Ringer's solution is preferred, but other solutions may be used as well (see Table 325–1). All signs of dehydration should have disappeared and the patient should pass urine at a rate of 0.5 mL/kg/hr or greater after finishing the rehydration phase. The maintenance phase follows immediately. During this phase the objective is to maintain normal hydration status by replacing ongoing losses. The oral route is preferred during this phase, and the use of oral rehydration solutions is highly recommended. Oral rehydration therapy uses the principle of common transportation of solutes, electrolytes, and water by the intestine not affected by the cholera toxin. People with diarrhea can undergo successful rehydration with simple solutions containing glucose and electrolytes. The World Health Organization recommends an oral rehydration solution with reduced osmolarity (245 mOsm/L) to treat all diarrheal diseases. This solution contains lower sodium than the standard oral rehydration solution promoted since 1975 (75 vs. 90 mEq/L). Use of this low-osmolarity solution in cholera patients offers no clinical benefit over the standard solution but causes hyponatremia and polyuria and may potentially induce neurologic complications. The addition of L-histidine to rice-based oral rehydration solutions has recently been shown to reduce the volume and duration of diarrhea and the unscheduled use of intravenous therapy in adult cholera patients. [2] Patients without severe dehydration who tolerate the

TABLE 325–2 RECOMMENDATIONS FOR TREATING CHOLERA PATIENTS

1. Determine the degree of dehydration on arrival.
2. Rehydrate the patient in two phases:
   Rehydration phase—lasts 2–4 hours
   Maintenance phase—lasts until the end of the diarrheal episode
3. Register and periodically review input and output in predesigned charts.
4. Use the intravenous route in the following situations:
   In all severely dehydrated patients, in whom the speed of the infusion varies from 50–100 mL/kg/hr
   Patients with some dehydration unable to tolerate the oral route
   Patients with high stool output (>10 mL/kg/hr) during the maintenance phase
5. Use oral rehydration solutions, glucose or rice based, during the maintenance phase to match ongoing losses. Volumes of 800–1000 mL/hr are usually required. Low-osmolarity solutions are not recommended.
6. Start an oral antimicrobial agent in patients with severe cholera when full rehydration has been achieved and oral tolerance is confirmed. Single-dose doxycycline, 300 mg, is the preferred regimen. Erythromycin or a quinolone is a suitable alternative.
7. Discharge patients only if oral tolerance is adequate (≥1000 mL/hr), urine output is ≥40 mL/hr, and stool volume is low (≤400 mL/hr).

Modified with permission from Seas C, DuPont HL, Valdez LM, et al: Practical guidelines for the treatment of cholera. Drugs 1996;51:966–973.

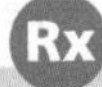

oral route can be rehydrated with oral rehydration solutions exclusively and discharged promptly from the health center. Recommendations for treating cholera patients are shown in Table 325–2. Treatment of cholera caused by O139 *V. cholerae* is the same as described earlier.

Antimicrobial agents are not life-saving and always need to be accompanied by fluid therapy. Effective antibiotics in patients with severe dehydration decrease the duration of diarrhea and the volume of stool by nearly half. Oral tetracycline and doxycycline are the agents of choice in areas of the globe where sensitive strains predominate. A single dose of doxycycline (300 mg) is the preferred regimen. Pregnant women can be treated with erythromycin or furazolidone. Because of the emergence of resistance to tetracyclines and other antimicrobials in many endemic areas, the quinolones and, more recently, azithromycin have been tested in clinical trials. A single-dose regimen of azithromycin (20 mg/kg) showed comparable clinical and bacteriologic results to a 3-day regimen with erythromycin in children [2] and now appears to be preferred over ciprofloxacin in adults. [3] Antimotilty agents such as loperamide or diphenoxylate, adsorbents, analgesics, and antiemetics are not recommended. Antisecretory drugs, including racecadotril, an encephalinase inhibitor, are not useful in patients with severe cholera. Chemoprophylaxis of household contacts of cholera cases is not routinely recommended.

Prevention

Access to potable water and ensuring proper management of excreta to avoid contamination of other water sources are important measures to reduce cholera transmission. Alternative ways to prevent cholera transmission are necessary in developing countries. Water can be made safer to drink by boiling, adding chlorine, or filtering it with cloth made of cotton. An inability to implement these measures to curtail cholera transmission has prompted a search for vaccines. An ideal vaccine against cholera should elicit a fast and long-lasting immune response with minimal side effects. Parenteral vaccines are no longer recommended. Two oral vaccines, the two-dose regimen of the inactivated vaccine WC-BS (whole cell plus B subunit) and a single dose of the live attenuated

CVD 103-HgR vaccine, have been extensively tested in epidemic settings and in field trials in endemic areas. Although the WC-BS vaccine showed good short-term protective efficacy (85% at 6 months), the results at 3 and 5 years were less impressive (60%), particularly in children. A large effectiveness study in Mozambique confirmed the high short-term protection against cholera (80%) by this vaccine, especially against severe dehydration (90%). Additionally, reanalysis of data on this vaccine in field trials has shown that it may also confer herd protection in the unvaccinated population. A large field trial of the live attenuated vaccine showed no protective efficacy. Indications for the use of currently available cholera vaccines include travel to endemic areas and situations in which high attack rates of cholera are expected, such as after environmental disasters, in refugee camps, and in urban slums in highly endemic areas.

Prognosis

Patients with severe cholera left untreated or improperly treated carry a poor prognosis, with mortality rates higher than 50%. Case-fatality rates during epidemics may be reduced to values below 1% even in disaster situations, provided that adequate access to health care centers and proper management of patients can be ensured. In contrast, figures higher than 10% have been reported in epidemic settings when patients had no access to health care or received improper treatment.

OTHER *VIBRIO* INFECTIONS

Noncholera vibrios have worldwide distribution and coexist in environments in which *V. cholerae* lives. They cause a spectrum of clinical syndromes, including acute diarrhea, soft tissue infections, and sepsis, especially in immunocompromised hosts. In the United States, about 400 cases of noncholeragenic *Vibrio* illnesses were reported each year during the period 2000 to 2004. The most frequently reported *Vibrio* species were *V. parahaemolyticus, V. vulnificus,* and nontoxigenic *V. cholerae. Vibrio* illnesses in the United States are seasonal and peak during the summer (Fig. 325–2). The incubation period for noncholeragenic *Vibrio* infection is usually 12 to 72 hours but can be as long as 1 week.

Nontoxigenic *V. cholerae* causes gastroenteritis, but unlike toxigenic *V. cholerae* O1 or O139, nontoxigenic *V. cholerae* does not cause epidemics. Illness ranges in severity from mild diarrhea to severe watery diarrhea. Fever and bloody diarrhea are unusual, but immunocompromised persons and those with liver disease can experience a more severe illness, including fever, chills, and septic shock.

V. parahaemolyticus lives in marine environments and is a source of intestinal illness associated with the ingestion of contaminated shellfish. Certain serovars have shown pandemic spread (O3 : K6 and O4 : K68). It is not well known how this vibrio causes infection in humans, but the clinical illness may mimic cholera, although the vast majority of cases are milder and self-limited forms of acute watery diarrhea. Acute dysentery is reported rarely.

In the United States, *V. parahemolyticus* and *V. vulnificus,* as well as other noncholeragenic vibrios, caused skin and soft tissue infections in victims and responders affected by the Gulf Coast hurricane disasters in fall 2005. *V. parahaemolyticus* wound infections are generally less severe than those caused by *V. vulnificus.* However, in persons with liver disease or immunocompromising conditions, fatal infections can occur.

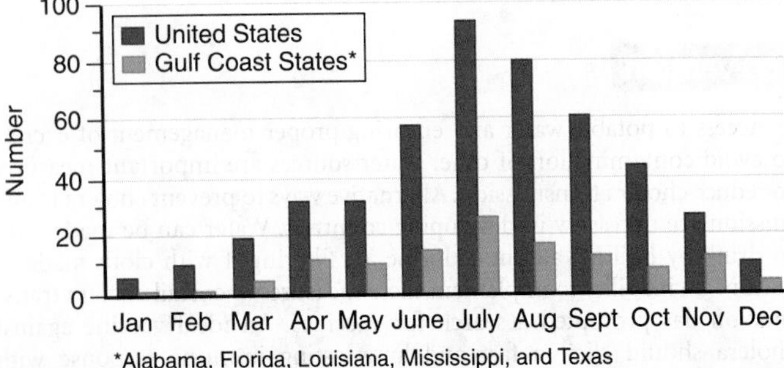

FIGURE 325–2 • Cases of noncholeragenic *Vibrio* infection, 2000 to 2004, United States. (Vibrio Illnesses after Hurricane Katrina—multiple states, August–September 2005. MMWR Morb Mortal Wkly Rep 2005;54(37):928–931.)

V. vulnificus is associated with wound infections in persons in contact with contaminated water, as well as with primary sepsis in immunocompromised hosts. Wound infections follow trauma and are characterized by rapid progression of skin and soft tissue involvement, with necrosis and bulla formation in the more severe cases. Fever, chills, and sepsis syndrome may rapidly ensure. Primary sepsis with bacteremia and metastatic lesions on the skin, characterized by disseminated erythematous lesions that may evolve to necrotic lesions, is a distinctive clinical manifestation in patients with chronic liver illnesses, those who are addicted to alcohol, and patients with blood disorders such as thalassemia. A history of seafood ingestion, usually oysters, is typical. Patients are acutely ill with high fever and need to be managed aggressively with fluid resuscitation, surgical débridement, general supportive care, and antibiotic coverage. An intravenous combination of cefotaxime, 2 g four times a day, plus doxycycline, 100 mg two times a day, is recommended. This combination is synergistic in vitro. Alternative antimicrobials are ceftazidime and ciprofloxacin.

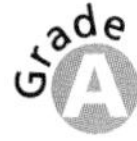

1. Rabbani GH, Sack DA, Ahmed S, et al: Antidiarrheal effects of L-histidine–supplemented rice-based oral rehydration solution in the treatment of male adults with severe cholera in Bangladesh: A double-blind, randomized trial. J Infect Dis 2005;191:1507–1514.
2. Khan WA, Saha D, Rahman A, et al: Comparison of single-dose azithromycin and 12-dose, 3-day erythromycin for childhood cholera: A randomised, double-blind trial. Lancet 2002;360: 1722–1727.
3. Saha D, Karim MM, Khan WA, et al: Single-dose azithromycin for the treatment of cholera in adults. N Engl J Med 2006;354: 2452–2462.

SUGGESTED READINGS

Ansaruzzaman M, Lucas M, Deen JL: Pandemic serovars (O3:K6 and O4:K68) of *Vibrio parahaemolyticus* associated with diarrhea in Mozambique: Spread of the pandemic into the African continent. J Clin Microbiol 2005; 43:2559–2562. *Detailed description of the spread of pandemic serovars in Africa.*

Centers for Disease Control and Prevention (CDC): *Vibrio* illnesses after Hurricane Katrina—Multiple states, August–September 2005. MMWR Morb Mortal Wkly Rep 2005;54(37):928–931. *Documents emergence in the United States.*

Haq SM, Dayal HH: Chronic liver disease and consumption of raw oysters: A potentially lethal combination. A review of *Vibrio vulnificus* septicemia. Am J Gastroenterol 2005;100:1195–1199. *A review of primary sepsis by* V. vulnificus.

Hill DR, Ford L, Lalloo DG: Oral cholera vaccines: Use in clinical practice. Lancet Infect Dis 2006;6:361–373. *Review of the efficacy of and indications for cholera vaccination.*

Lucas ME, Deen JL, von Seidlein L, et al: Effectiveness of mass oral vaccination in Beira, Mozambique. N Engl J Med 2005;352:757–767. *Mass oral vaccination confers 80% protection against cholera and 90% protection against severe dehydration.*

Sack DA, Sack RB, Nair GB, et al: Cholera. Lancet 2004;363:223–233. *A comprehensive review.*

Thompson FL, Klose KE, AVIB Group: Vibrio 2005: The first international conference on the biology of vibrios. J Bacteriol 2006;188:4592–4596. *Overview of the biology and classification of vibrio organisms.*

326 *CAMPYLOBACTER* INFECTIONS

Ban Mishu Allos and Martin J. Blaser

Definition

Campylobacter jejuni is one of the most commonly recognized bacterial causes of diarrhea in developed nations. More than 95% of campylobacters isolated in developed countries are *C. jejuni* or *C. coli.* However, other *Campylobacter* species are also associated with human disease.

The Pathogen

Campylobacters are motile, curved, gram-negative rods that are found in domestic and wild animals—especially poultry—all over the world. *C. jejuni* is microaerophilic, requires 3 to 15% oxygen for growth, and is oxidase and catalase positive. It grows best at 42° C; however, other *Campylobacter* species that may also be pathogenic grow best at 37° C.

Epidemiology

C. jejuni infections are endemic in young children in developing nations, where they may be isolated in up to 20% of children younger than 5 years with diarrhea. In developed nations, *Campylobacter* infections are among the most common bacterial causes of diarrhea in children and adults, but the incidence of *C. jejuni* infection in the United States fell by more than 30% from 21.7 per 100,000 population in 1998 to 12.9 in 2003. The actual burden of disease caused by *Campylobacter* is probably much higher because even active surveillance systems substantially under-report the true incidence of infection. Epidemiologic studies have estimated that more than 2 million people in the United States are infected with *C. jejuni* each year. Similarly high rates of infection are observed in Europe. In the United States, Europe, and Australia, *C. jejuni* infections show a substantial peak in warmer months. Such seasonality is not observed in tropical developing countries, perhaps because of the absence of extreme temperature variations.

The incidence of *Campylobacter* infections is highest in early childhood—an epidemiologic feature common to many food-borne bacterial pathogens. However, in the United States and other industrialized countries, the incidence of *Campylobacter* infections peaks again in early adulthood. The incidence of infection is also higher in men, a gender difference most pronounced in young adults.

Most human *C. jejuni* infections occur sporadically, with only a tiny fraction occurring as part of outbreaks. The dominant source of sporadic infections in both developed and developing countries is consumption or handling of poultry. Other sources of transmission in developed nations include foreign travel, contact with pets and other animals, contaminated drinking water, and consumption of unpasteurized milk. Cross-contamination within a kitchen (e.g., use of the same utensils or cutting boards to prepare uncooked chicken and to chop fruit) has led to a variety of foods being implicated as sources of human *C. jejuni* infection. In contrast to sporadic infections, the most common source of *C. jejuni* outbreaks is unpasteurized milk; occasionally, large waterborne outbreaks occur. Transmission of *C. jejuni* infection from ill food handlers is uncommon. Even in households in which an individual has culture-proven *C. jejuni* gastroenteritis, secondary transmission to other family members is unusual.

Pathobiology

Persons become infected with *C. jejuni* as a result of orally ingesting the organism, usually in food or water. Factors that affect whether *Campylobacter* infection leads to illness include the dose of bacteria ingested, the virulence of the organism, and the specific immunity of the host to the ingested organism. The minimum number of bacteria needed to cause illness varies between people, but it may be quite low, especially in water; because *C. jejuni* is susceptible to gastric acidity, ingestion of very few organisms may cause illness if gastric pH is elevated as a result of illness or medication. The median incubation period is 2 to 4 days, although it may range from 1 to 7 days.

In early infection, *C. jejuni* multiplies in the bile-rich upper intestines; subsequently, tissue injury is seen in the jejunum, ileum, and colon. Gross inspection of the bowel shows a diffuse, bloody, edematous enteritis. Microscopic examination shows an inflammatory infiltrate consisting of neutrophils, mononuclear cells, and eosinophils in the lamina propria. The mucosal epithelium is ulcerated, and crypt abscesses may be seen. The pathologic appearance is nonspecific and may mimic ulcerative colitis or Crohn's disease.

Invasion of the epithelium by *C. jejuni* appears to be central to its pathogenesis, and many factors influence how *C. jejuni* adheres to and invades intestinal tissues. A superficial conserved antigen, PEB1, appears to be a major adhesin and is a target of the immune response to *C. jejuni* infection. Other factors that contribute to *C. jejuni's* invasiveness and pathogenicity, which may be encoded by a virulence plasmid, include type IV secretion systems and mechanisms that disrupt microtubules in host cells. Glycolipids and glycoproteins on the surface of *C. jejuni* are important in the organism's survival in the intestinal lumen and in pathogenesis because they have an impact on cell-to-cell interactions, as well as the host's immune response to infection. *C. jejuni* may produce extracellular toxins, but their role in pathogenesis has not been confirmed, with the possible exception of the cytoskeletal distending toxin (cdt), which may facilitate intracellular activities that lead to apoptosis.

Regardless of the organism's virulence, host factors are pivotal in affecting the clinical outcome of infection. In healthy volunteers fed a fixed dose of a single *C. jejuni* strain, a spectrum of illnesses develop. Patients infected with *C. jejuni* excrete the organism in feces for 2 to 3 weeks. In developing nations, where the level of immunity to *C. jejuni* is higher because of recurrent exposure, the period of convalescent excretion of *C. jejuni* is shorter.

After recovery from *Campylobacter* infection, at least short-term immunity develops. The decreasing illness-to-infection ratio with age seen in developing nations also suggests that individuals are acquiring immunity. Specific IgA, IgG, and IgM antibodies in serum and IgA antibodies in intestinal secretions develop in patients infected with *C. jejuni.* Patients with congenital or acquired hypogammaglobulinemia are at risk for severe or recurrent *C. jejuni* infections. Because the incidence of *C. jejuni* infection is markedly higher in persons infected with human immunodeficiency virus (HIV), cell-mediated immunity might also play a role in preventing and terminating infection.

Clinical Manifestations

The clinical consequences of *Campylobacter* infection range from complete absence of symptoms to fulminant sepsis and death. In most cases, however, illnesses are brief and do not require hospitalization. In developed nations, detection of *C. jejuni* in the stool of asymptomatic persons is rare. However, in developing nations, where infections are endemic and recurrent infections occur frequently, asymptomatic infections are more common. In both developing and developed nations, persons infected with *C. jejuni* typically contract a diarrheal illness that resolves within a week. The case-fatality rate associated with this infection is low, about 0.05 deaths per 1000 infections.

The gastroenteritis that is caused by infection with *C. jejuni* is clinically indistinguishable from that caused by other bacterial enteric pathogens, such as *Salmonella* (Chapter 329), *Shigella* (Chapter 330), or *Escherichia coli* O:157H7 (Chapter 327). The most common symptoms are diarrhea, malaise, fever, and abdominal pain (Table 326–1). Most patients with *C. jejuni* gastroenteritis experience at least 1 day with 10 or more stools; the diarrhea may be loose, watery, or bloody. Nausea is reported by some patients, but vomiting is less common. More than half the patients describe subjective fever. The abdominal cramping may be severe and is sometimes the predominant symptom. Although in most patients the symptoms resolve within 7 days, symptoms may persist in 10 to 20% of patients, and another 5 to 10% may experience a relapse.

Almost regardless of the nature of the symptoms, fecal leukocytes are found in 75% of infected patients; gross or occult blood is seen in 50%. Peripheral white blood cell counts may be elevated, but liver function test results, the hematocrit, and serum electrolytes are usually normal. Sigmoidoscopic examination reveals diffuse colonic inflammation, which is nonspecific.

TABLE 326–1 CLINICAL FEATURES OF CAMPYLOBACTER ENTERITIS DERIVED FROM OUTBREAKS IN WHICH MORE THAN 50 PATIENTS WERE INFECTED

Symptom	Median Frequency (%)	Range (%)
Fever	52	6–75
Diarrhea	85	52–100
Headache	47	6–69
Abdominal pain	80	56–99
Myalgia	37	28–59
Vomiting	11	1–42
Blood in feces	13	0.5–32

Modified from Skirrow MB, Blaser MJ: Clinical aspects of *Campylobacter* infection. *In* Nachamkin I, Blaser MJ (eds): *Campylobacter,* 2nd ed. Washington, DC, ASM Press, 2000, pp 69–88.

Local complications of *C. jejuni* gastroenteritis are rare. In its most severe form, infection may lead to massive gastrointestinal hemorrhage or toxic megacolon. Infection of the biliary tract may result in obstructive hepatitis, cholecystitis (Chapter 159), or pancreatitis (Chapter 147). Other reported local complications include peritonitis (Chapter 145), splenic rupture, and exacerbations of inflammatory colitis. Bacteremia is detected in 1.5 per 1000 intestinal infections, with higher rates in persons who are immunocompromised or elderly, but transient bacteremia may be more common because blood cultures are infrequently obtained in patients with diarrhea and the bacteria are killed rapidly by normal human serum. Other extraintestinal complications such as meningitis, endocarditis, osteomyelitis, and purulent arthritis are rare.

Guillain-Barré syndrome (Chapter 436), which is a postinfectious complication of *C. jejuni* infection, occurs about once in every 2000 infections; between 30 and 50% of all cases may be triggered by a preceding *C. jejuni* infection. Because the onset of neurologic symptoms occurs about 1 to 3 weeks after the onset of gastrointestinal symptoms, cross-reactivity between antibodies formed against the lipopolysaccharide and capsule of *C. jejuni* and proteins in peripheral nerve myelin or other glycolipids in peripheral nerves is probably the cause. Certain *C. jejuni* serotypes (O type 19, O type 41) are over-represented in patients in whom Guillain-Barre syndrome develops after culture-documented *C. jejuni* infection. Other postinfectious complications of *C. jejuni* infection include reactive arthritis (seen mostly in persons with HLA-B27 histocompatibility antigens), uveitis, hemolytic-uremic syndrome, erythema nodosum, encephalitis, carditis, and hemolytic anemia.

Diagnosis

The diagnosis of *C. jejuni* infection should be considered in any patient with an acute febrile diarrheal illness. The diagnosis is established by culturing the organism from stool or tissue. Primary isolation of *Campylobacter* species from blood may take up to 14 days.

The presence of curved gram-negative rods on a Gram stain of stool is specific but only 50 to 75% sensitive for detecting *C. jejuni*. Examination of fecal specimens by darkfield microscopy is useful if done within 2 hours of passage; the characteristic darting motility of *Campylobacter* provides a presumptive diagnosis. Serum serologic studies and polymerase chain reaction of stool are currently available only as research tools.

Differential Diagnosis

In patients with acute colitis and bloody diarrhea, especially those whose symptoms last longer than 1 week, *Campylobacter* enteritis may be mistaken for ulcerative colitis or Crohn's disease (Chapter 144). In such cases, it is critical to exclude infectious colitis before starting immunosuppressive therapy. In patients with severe abdominal pain, appendicitis may be suspected and unnecessary appendectomy may result (Chapter 145).

Prevention

Because the most common source of transmission of *C. jejuni* infection to humans in developed countries is by consumption and handling of poultry, interrupting this route of infection will probably have the greatest effect on reducing the burden of disease caused by *Campylobacter.* The nearly universal colonization of poultry flocks with *C. jejuni* makes eradication of the organism in chickens unlikely, but improvements in slaughtering plants appear to be reducing the level of contamination of products reaching humans. For the consumer, careful food preparation methods are critical; chicken must be cooked thoroughly. To avoid cross-contamination in the kitchen, cutting boards, knives, and other utensils used to prepare raw chicken should be washed with hot soapy water before being used to prepare foods eaten uncooked such as fruits or vegetables. Person-to-person transmission of *Campylobacter* is not common; nevertheless, all persons with diarrhea, especially those who handle food, should wash their hands after using the bathroom. Travelers and campers should be cautioned against drinking untreated water. Many outbreaks of *C. jejuni* infection might also be avoided if persons abstain from drinking unpasteurized milk. Antibiotic prophylaxis for travelers is not advised.

Treatment

As is true for most patients with infectious or noninfectious diarrhea, the most important principle of treatment of *Campylobacter* gastroenteritis is restoration of proper hydration and electrolyte balance, typically with oral fluids (Chapter 305). Occasionally, intravenous fluids are needed, especially in elderly patients or young children. Most *C. jejuni* infections are self-limited and resolve without specific antibiotic treatment. Furthermore, treatment with antibiotics shortens the duration of illness by <48 hours. [1] Prompt antimicrobial therapy is indicated for patients with high fever (>38.5° C), prolonged illness (>1 week), bloody stools, or worsening symptoms or for those who have relapsed. Antimicrobial treatment is also warranted in the elderly, infants, pregnant women, and persons who are immunocompromised, including those infected with HIV.

The antibiotic of choice for the treatment of *C. jejuni* gastroenteritis is erythromycin (500 mg twice daily for 5 days); azithromycin and clarithromycin are equally effective but considerably more expensive. One concern with erythromycin, which is primarily metabolized by CYP3A4, is the risk of sudden cardiac death. The risk is increased fivefold when erythromycin is given with medications that inhibit CYP3A4. [2] In patients taking one or more of these medications, azithromycin may be substituted for erythromycin.

Fluoroquinolones, carbapenems, aminoglycosides, and clindamycin may also be effective, but resistance to quinolones is now common in many parts of the world. In general, rates of resistance to ampicillin, amoxicillin, and cephalosporins are too high for them to be useful in the treatment of *C. jejuni* infections.

Critically ill or septic persons with *Campylobacter* infection may benefit from imipenem or aminoglycosides, agents to which campylobacters are exquisitely susceptible, with resistance rates consistently less than 1%. In contrast, persons with persistent or relapsing infection, especially those who are immunocompromised, may require prolonged use (sometimes months) of antibiotics. In the absence of continuing sepsis, oral agents may be used.

OTHER *CAMPYLOBACTER* SPECIES

Campylobacter fetus may cause systemic and diarrheal illnesses in compromised hosts and diarrheal illnesses in normal hosts. Most *C. fetus* strains, unlike *C. jejuni,* are not susceptible to the lethal effect of normal human serum because they possess a protein capsule (S layer). In immunocompromised persons, *C. fetus* can cause extraintestinal illnesses such as bacteremia, vascular infections, and meningitis. *C. fetus* infection may also cause perinatal infection and fetal loss. Prolonged treatment with erythromycin plus either imipenem, meropenem, an aminoglycoside, or a third-generation cephalosporin is indicated for serious *C. fetus* infections.

Campylobacter upsaliensis may cause acute or chronic diarrhea in healthy or immunocompromised persons. The organism is frequently isolated from dogs with diarrhea, which could be a source for transmission to humans. Some *C. upsaliensis* strains are resistant to erythromycin, but most are susceptible to fluoroquinolones, doxycycline, third-generation cephalosporins, and amoxicillin-clavulanate.

Campylobacter hyointestinalis was first recognized as a cause of proliferative enteritis in swine; *Campylobacter lari* is most often cultured from gulls and other birds. Both organisms have now been identified as rare causes of watery diarrhea and abdominal cramping in immunocompetent children and adults. Most infected patients do not require antimicrobial therapy; all isolates studied in vitro have been susceptible to erythromycin.

Helicobacter cinaedi and *Helicobacter fennelliae,* once called "*Campylobacter*-like organisms," are causes of proctocolitis or enterocolitis and have also been reported to cause bacteremia in immunocompromised patients. The organisms are frequently resistant to erythromycin; fluoroquinolones are considered the treatment of choice in patients who require antimicrobial therapy. The organisms are also susceptible to third-generation cephalosporins, aminoglycosides, and carbapenems.

Other *Campylobacter* or related species that have rarely been associated with human illness include *C. mucosalis, C. doylei, C. curvus, C. concisus, C. rectus, C. helveticus, Arcobacter butzleri,* and *Arcobacter cryaerophila.* Illnesses include diarrhea and localized infections, presumably as a result of transient bacteremia from intestinal sources.

Prognosis

Even in critically ill patients, 1 week of therapy is generally sufficient to eradicate infection.

Campylobacter infections in HIV-positive patients may be more severe, persist, recur, and be antibiotic resistant. More severe and extraintestinal illness is also more likely to occur in patients with acquired or congenital hypogammaglobulinemia. Most *C. jejuni* gastrointestinal infections in pregnant women are mild and self-limited, with no severe consequences for the mother or baby. However, if bacteremia develops in the mother, placental infection and fetal death may ensue. Infection during the third trimester can also cause neonatal sepsis and death if the woman is excreting *Campylobacter* in her stool at the time of delivery.

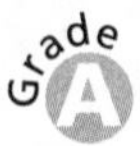

1. Ternhag A, Asikainen T, Giesecke J, Ekdahl K: A meta-analysis on the effects of antibiotic treatment on duration of symptoms caused by infectioin with *Campylobacter* species. Clin Infect Dis 2007;44:696–700.
2. Ray WA, Muway KT, Meredith S, et al: Oral erythromycin and the risk of sudden death from cardiac causes. N Engl J Med 2004; 351:1089.

SUGGESTED READINGS

Gibreel A, Taylor DE: Macrolide resistance in *Campylobacter jejuni* and *Campylobacter coli.* J Antimicrob Chemother 2006;58:243–255. *Use of macrolides in veterinary medicine has promoted a point mutation that confers resistance.*

Moore JE, Barton MD, Blair IS, et al: The epidemiology of antibiotic resistance in *Campylobacter.* Microbes Infect 2006;8:1955–1966. *Update on resistance to fluoroquinolones and macrolides.*

Yuki Nikoga M: Bacterial infections in Guillain-Barré and Fisher syndromes. Curr Opin Neurol 2006;19:451–457. *Emphasizes the role of* Campylobacter.

327 *ESCHERICHIA* ENTERIC INFECTIONS

Richard L. Guerrant

Definition

Escherichia coli, which is the predominant aerobic coliform species in the normal colon, can be an enteric pathogen and cause intestinal disease, usually diarrhea. The diarrhea associated with *E. coli* may be watery, inflammatory, or bloody, depending on the organism's genetic codes for virulence traits, such as enterotoxigenic, enteroinvasive, enterohemorrhagic, enteropathogenic, or enteroadherent. Each of these categories can be further defined by the type of enterotoxin (e.g., the cholera-like heat-labile toxin [LT] or the heat-stable toxin [ST]) or adherence (e.g., localized and effacing, aggregative, or diffuse) that it causes. Enterotoxigenic *E. coli* (ETEC) is a major bacterial cause of morbidity and mortality from diarrhea on a global scale, particularly among children in tropical, developing areas and in travelers. Enteroaggregative *E. coli* (EAEC) also appear to be a common cause of traveler's diarrhea, as well as persistent diarrhea and malnutrition in children. Taken together, the various types of *E. coli* diarrhea not only constitute the major category of bacterial enteric pathogens but also illustrate the many ways that enteric pathogens can cause disease.

The Pathogen

E. coli is a small catalase-positive, oxidase-negative, gram-negative bacillus in the family Enterobacteriaceae. It characteristically reduces nitrates, ferments glucose and usually lactose, and is either motile (with peritrichate flagella) or nonmotile. It gives a positive methyl red reaction and negative reactions with Voges-Proskauer, urease, phenylalanine deaminase, and citrate agents. *E. coli* is the predominant facultative gram-negative bacillus in the intestinal tract of humans and other mammals. As with other gram-negative organisms, the lipopolysaccharide cell wall contains lipid A and 2-keto-3-deoxyoctanate, a core glycolipid that has been used to develop vaccines that provide cross-protection against systemic infections with other gram-negative organisms. Smooth (S) forms of *E. coli* have O-specific carbohydrate chains attached to this core glycolipid to provide 173 O serogroups, as well as at least 56 heat-labile protein flagellar (H) antigens, by which strains are currently serotyped. Historically, some 80 variably heat-labile capsular (K) antigens have also been described (L, B, and A), not including the numerous adherence, enterotoxin, cytotoxin, and invasiveness factors that may be gained or lost by a particular serotype because they are characteristically encoded on transmissible genetic elements such as plasmids or bacteriophages. Consequently, this common inhabitant of the normal human intestinal tract becomes a pathogen when it houses one or more specific traits contributing to its colonization and virulence in the intestinal tract. Other traits such as the O and H serogroup may also be important for certain enteropathogenic and enteroinvasive organisms. For reasons that remain obscure, only a few O serogroups tend to predominate in the normal human colon (O groups 1, 2, 4, 6, 7, 8, 18, 25, 45, 75, and 81), whereas others (Table 327–1) tend to be associated with specific virulence traits and thus different types of pathogenesis in the intestine. The O antigens of invasive *E. coli* often cross-react with various *Shigella* species, which further suggests that in addition to the 140-Md plasmid, serotype has a role in pathogenesis.

At least three different types of *E. coli* enterotoxins may cause intestinal secretion (ETEC), others are enteroinvasive (EIEC), and still others cause food-borne hemorrhagic colitis (EHEC) and produce *Shiga*-like toxin (SLT) (see Table 327–1). By comparison, the classically recognized enteropathogenic *E. coli* (EPEC) serotypes are neither enterotoxigenic nor invasive, but rather attach and efface the epithelium. Still other types of enteroadherent *E. coli* exhibit aggregating (EAggEC) or diffuse adherence (DAEC) traits and may be associated with prolonged diarrhea in children in tropical, developing areas and in patients infected with human immunodeficiency virus (HIV).

Epidemiology

Enteric *E. coli* infections are essentially acquired by the fecal-oral route and thus primarily reflect a human reservoir for most recognized types of EPEC. ETEC is also an important veterinary pathogen, especially in calves and piglets. However, the attachment traits of animal strains are different from those that infect humans.

The infectious doses of ETEC, EIEC, and EAggEC have been determined in volunteers to be 10^6 to 10^{10}, numbers that usually require multiplication in contaminated food or water vehicles for their transmission. Heavy contamination with ETEC has been documented in foods prepared in homes and restaurants and by street vendors, as well as in drinking water in many tropical areas, and contaminated water and food probably represent the major sources of their acquisition, primarily in warm or wet seasons. In the United States, a large waterborne outbreak of diarrhea at a popular national park was caused by ETEC, and a widespread outbreak of EIEC enteritis was traced to consumption of French Camembert cheese. Bloody, noninflammatory diarrhea has increasingly been associated with EHEC (O157:H7 and others) from eating undercooked hamburgers or from ingestion of contaminated unpasteurized apple juice, spinach, or seed sprouts. EHEC infections are especially alarming because they are increasing in frequency and may cause hemolytic-uremic syndrome (Chapter 179), which can be fatal despite antimicrobial therapy, which in some instances may actually induce phage and toxin production. Occasional nosocomial outbreaks of ETEC and EPEC serotypes have also occurred in hospitalized infants in the United States and other industrialized countries.

As with most diarrheal illnesses, the highest age-specific attack rates of ETEC infections are found in young children, especially at the time of weaning, when ETEC accounts for 15 to 50% of illnesses. Like immunologically inexperienced young children, a traveler visiting tropical areas has a 30 to 50% chance of acquiring travelers' diarrhea (Chapters 143 and 305) over a 2- to 3-week stay unless untreated water or ice and uncooked foods such as salads are strictly avoided. The most commonly recognized pathogen associated with travelers' diarrhea in most tropical areas of the world is ETEC that produces either the STa, LT, or both enterotoxins. A close second to ETEC as a cause of traveler's diarrhea is EAEC, now reported in 19 to 33% of cases in travelers to India or Mexico.

Of potential immunologic significance is the continued occurrence of symptomatic infections with *E. coli* that produce the less immunogenic STa in adult residents of tropical or other areas endemic for ETEC infection. In contrast, adult residents in endemic areas often carry LT-producing *E. coli* asymptomatically, thus suggesting that they may be protected from symptoms, if not from colonization.

TABLE 327–1 DIFFERENT TYPES OF ENTERIC ESCHERICHIA COLI INFECTIONS

Type	Mechanism	Predominant O Serogroups	Genetic Code	Detection	Clinical Syndromes
ENTEROTOXIGENIC *E. COLI* (ETEC)					
1. Cholera-like, heat-labile toxin (LT)	Activates intestinal adenylate cyclase	6, 8, 11, 15, 20, 25, 27, 63, 80, 85, 139	Plasmid	ELISA, RIA, PIH, CHO, Y1 cells, 18-hr loops, gene probe	Watery diarrhea, travelers' diarrhea
2. Heat-stable toxin (STa: STh or STp)	Activates intestinal guanylate cyclase	12, 78, 115, 148, 149, 153, 155, 166, 167	Plasmid (transposon)	ELISA, RIA, suckling mice, 6-hr loops, gene probes	Watery diarrhea, travelers' diarrhea
3. Heat-stable toxin (STb)	? Not cyclic adenosine or guanosine monophosphate		Plasmid	Piglet loops, gene probe	?
ENTEROINVASIVE *E. COLI*					
4. Enteroinvasive *E. coli* (EIEC)	Cell invasion and spread	11, 28ac, 29, 124, 136, 144, 147, 152, 164, 167	Plasmid (140Md, pWR110)	Sereny test, gene probe, (lys⁻, NM, often lactose⁻)	Inflammatory dysentery
ENTEROHEMORRHAGIC *E. COLI*					
5. Enterohemorrhagic (EHEC)	Shiga-like toxin(s) (SLT) and adhesin fimbriae	26, 39, 113, 121, 128, 139, 145, 157, occ 55, 111	Phage(s) and adhesin plasmid(s)	ELISA for SLT, serotype, HeLa, Vero cells, sorbitol, agar, SLT or *eae* gene probes	Bloody noninflammatory diarrhea; hemolytic-uremic syndrome
ENTEROPATHOGENIC *E. COLI*					
6. Focal attaching and effacing (EPEC)	Attach, then efface the mucosa	55, 111, 119, 125, 126, 127, 128, 142, 158,	Plasmid (60Md, pMAR2) + chromosomal (*esp, eae,* and *tir*)	Serotype, focal HEp2 adhesion, gene probes for *EAF* or *eae*	Infantile diarrhea
ENTEROADHERENT *E. COLI*					
7. Enteroaggregating *E. coli* (EAggEC)	Colonize; toxins (EAST, EALT)	3, 15, 44, 51, 77, 78, 91	Plasmid	HEp2 cell adherence; AA probe	Persistent diarrhea
8. Diffusely adherent *E. coli* (DAEC)	Colonize (F 1845 fimbriate adhesin)	75 (F 1845), 15 (57-1), ? (189)	Chromosomal/ plasmid	HEp2 cell adherence; DA gene probe	Persistent diarrhea in children >18 mo old

AA = aggregated adherence; CHO = Chinese hamster ovary cell; DA = diffuse adherence; ELISA = enzyme-linked immunosorbent assay; NM = nonmotile; PIH = passive immune hemolysis; RIA = radioimmunoassay.

Limited data on invasive *E. coli* suggest that infectious doses are relatively high. As with ETEC infections, such large numbers have readily been spread in food with high attack rates. EPEC has been recognized primarily in urban areas, especially among hospitalized infants in their first year of life, with apparent cross-infection in hospital nurseries. Although sporadic cases still occur, nosocomial outbreaks of EPEC diarrhea during the summer appear to have become less common and less severe in industrialized countries in the last few decades. EAEC increasingly appears to be an important cause of persistent diarrhea and malnutrition, especially in children in tropical areas and in patients with HIV infection.

Pathobiology

The pathogenesis of enteric *E. coli* infection begins with ingestion of the organism in contaminated food or water, which then faces the normal gastric acid barrier. Both ETEC and EIEC appear to be sensitive to gastric acid; neutralization of gastric acid reduces the infectious dose by 100- to 1000-fold. Ingestion is followed by an incubation period of 2 to 7 days, during which colonization of the involved part of the intestinal tract, toxin production, and invasion or other disruption of cell function take place. For example, colonization by ETEC in the upper portion of the small bowel involves one of at least five major colonization factor antigen groups (which are fimbriate or fibrillar protein structures on the surface of the organism). The colonization fimbriae bind the organism to cell surface receptors in the upper part of the small bowel, where the enterotoxin is delivered to reduce normal absorption and cause net electrolyte and water secretion. LT, with a molecular weight of about 86,000, has a binding and active subunit that like cholera toxin, binds to a monosialoganglioside (GM_1) receptor. Also like cholera toxin, the active subunit adenosine diphosphate ribosylates the regulatory subunit of adenylate cyclase to activate adenylate cyclase. The consequently increased chloride secretion and reduced sodium absorption combine to cause net isotonic electrolyte loss that must be replaced to prevent severe dehydration, hypotension, and their potential consequences. Other strains produce the heat-stable toxin (STa), which is a much smaller molecule of 18 to 19 amino acids and activates intestinal particulate guanylate cyclase. Like cyclic adenosine monophosphate, the cyclic guanosine monophosphate thus formed also causes net secretion. The roles of other enterotoxins such as LTII, EAST, EIET, and others seen in ETEC, EAggEC, and EIEC, respectively, are unclear at present. Both the colonization traits and production of enterotoxin are encoded on transmissible plasmids. Besides the complications of dehydration, the only significant pathologic change is depletion of mucus from intestinal goblet cells.

Other *E. coli,* often of certain serogroups (see Table 327–1), have the capacity, analogous to *Shigella,* to invade and multiply in epithelial cells, cause conjunctivitis in guinea pigs (Sereny test), and produce inflammatory colitis and dysenteric or bloody diarrhea. As seen with shigellosis, a striking inflammatory response occurs, with numerous polymorphonuclear leukocytes in stool. The colon shows patchy, acute inflammation in the mucosa and submucosa with focal denuding of the surface epithelium, usually without deeper invasion or systemic spread. Although epithelial cell invasiveness in both EIEC and *Shigella* appears to be encoded on a large 120- to 140-Md plasmid, several chromosomal determinants, including the O antigen, are crucial for full invasive virulence.

Classically recognized EPEC serotypes often fail to produce known enterotoxins or to be invasive. Nevertheless, they are well-established causes of infantile diarrhea and exhibit a remarkable array of chromosomal- and plasmid-encoded traits that orchestrate their initial attachment and subsequent effacement of the brush border epithelium. The majority of classically recognized EPEC serotypes, such as O55 and O111, exhibit both plasmid-encoded localized adherence to epithelial cells and chromosomally mediated attachment and effacement of the microvilli. There is also villous atrophy, mucosal thinning, inflammation in the lamina propria, and variable crypt cell hyperplasia. These morphologic changes are associated with a reduction in mucosal brush border enzymes and may contribute to the impaired absorptive function and diarrhea.

EHEC, most notably serotype O157:H7 but also serogroups O26, 39, and others, are associated with food-borne outbreaks of bloody, usually nonfebrile noninflammatory diarrhea and hemolytic-uremic syndrome. These organisms produce SLTs that may be responsible for the characteristic colonic mucosal disruption and hemorrhage, as well as the complication of hemolytic-uremic syndrome. The mechanisms by which EAEC (which adhere in an aggregative pattern to the mucosa and produce heat-stable and heat-labile "toxins"), DAEC, or colonization alone may cause diarrhea remain unclear at present.

Clinical Manifestations

The most common clinical manifestation of enteric *E. coli* infections is the watery diarrhea that characterizes ETEC infections, particularly in young children and travelers to tropical or developing areas. Diarrhea may range from mild to severe and cholera-like; it may be life threatening, especially in small children and elderly patients, who are particularly prone to dehydration, undernutrition, and electrolyte imbalance (especially hypokalemia and acidosis).

The incubation period (2 to 7 days) varies inversely with the size of the inoculum. Characteristic symptoms include malaise, abdominal cramping, anorexia, and watery diarrhea, occasionally associated with nausea, vomiting, or low-grade fever. The illness is generally self-limited to 1 to 5 days and rarely extends beyond 10 days or 2 weeks. Infections with *E. coli* that produce both ST and LT or ST alone may be more severe than those caused by only LT-producing *E. coli.* The persistence of impaired mucosal absorptive capacity for 1 to 3 weeks may further compound the cycle of malnutrition that complicates diarrheal illnesses in children in developing, tropical areas.

Infection with EIEC is characterized by inflammatory colitis, often with abdominal pain, high fever, tenesmus, and bloody or dysenteric diarrhea, essentially like that seen with *Shigella,* to which this organism is closely related. The incubation period is usually 1 to 3 days, with the duration generally self-limited to 7 to 10 days.

Outbreaks of EPEC infection in newborn nurseries have ranged from mild transient diarrhea to severe and rapidly fatal diarrheal illnesses, especially in premature or otherwise compromised infants. The more severe illnesses appear to have been more common in industrialized countries before 1950. However, more recent outbreaks and sporadic cases are well documented.

Hemorrhagic colitis associated with the SLT-producing *E. coli* (EHEC) O157:H7, O26:H11, and others is characterized by grossly bloody diarrhea, often with remarkably little fever or inflammatory exudate in stool. Although this diarrheal illnesses is self-limited, potentially fatal hemolytic-uremic syndrome or thrombotic thrombocytopenic purpura subsequently develops in a significant number of children and adults. Outbreaks of hemorrhagic colitis secondary to EHEC in nursing homes or other institutions may be common and quite severe. The incubation period in two outbreaks has been 3 to 4 days (range, 1 to 7 days), and the illness is characteristically self-limited to 5 to 12 days (mean, 7.8 days).

EAEC has been associated with persistent diarrhea and malnutrition in children in developing areas, in HIV-positive patients, and in travelers who experience diarrhea (especially those genetically predisposed to greater inflammatory responses). DAEC has also been associated with diarrhea in children older than 18 months.

Diagnosis

With the exception of EHEC (which should be sought by enzyme-linked immunosorbent assay or testing for SLT and sorbitol-negative EHEC O157:H7 in all patients with bloody diarrhea), definitive etiologic diagnosis of *E. coli* diarrhea requires documentation of a specific virulence trait—such as enterotoxin, invasiveness, enteroadherence—or serotype, which requires specialized immunologic, tissue culture, animal bioassay, or gene probes that are usually available only in research and reference laboratories. Other than for EHEC, such tests are rarely cost-effective or clinically indicated, except in outbreak or research situations. Fortunately, a probable diagnosis can often be suspected by the clinical and epidemiologic setting.

Sigmoidoscopy, which is rarely indicated, generally reveals only moderately hyperemic mucosa, and barium enema may reveal a thumbprint pattern of submucosal edema in the ascending and transverse colon. Some patients have superficial ulceration with mild neutrophil infiltration in the edematous submucosa.

Differential Diagnosis

Numerous other causes of diarrhea must be considered, depending on the clinical circumstances (Chapters 143 and 305). For example, self-limited, noninflammatory diarrhea in tropical, developing areas is most likely due to ETEC, rotaviruses (young children), or noroviruses (older children and adults) (Chapter 403). Noninflammatory diarrhea in older children or younger adults in the winter months in temperate areas is more likely to be due to Noroviruses. *Vibrio* infections (Chapter 325) are common in areas endemic for cholera or in any coastal area where inadequately cooked seafood may be eaten. If noninflammatory diarrhea persists, especially with weight loss, other possibilities include *Giardia lamblia* (Chapter 372), *Cryptosporidium* (Chapter 371), *Cyclospora* (Chapter 374), and microsporidial infection (Chapter 374). In outbreaks of food poisoning, *Staphylococcus aureus* (Chapter 310), *Clostridium perfringens* (Chapter 319), and *Bacillus cereus* (Chapter 317) should be considered.

Inflammatory colitis with high fever and tenesmus, as well as leukocytes, mucus, and blood in the stool, may well be due to EIEC but should prompt a stool culture for more common invasive pathogens such as *Campylobacter jejuni* (Chapter 326), *Shigella* (Chapter 330), and *Salmonella* (Chapter 329) or even EAEC, *Clostridium difficile* (Chapter 319), *Yersinia enterocolitica* (Chapter 333), or noncholera *Vibrio* (Chapter 325). On the other hand, bloody diarrhea without high fever and with few, if any fecal leukocytes (or minimal or no fecal lactoferrin elevation) should prompt consideration of SLT-producing EHEC such as strain O157:H7. *E. coli* O157:H7 is often suspected as a sorbitol-negative *E. coli,* which then requires further study for serotype or SLT production; testing for SLT directly is also needed to document EHEC strains other than O157:H7.

Prevention

Prevention of many *E. coli* enteric infections is ultimately related to basic economic development, adequate sanitary facilities, and sufficient availability of safe water. In the interim, especially in areas where adequate water supplies and sanitary facilities are not available, measures such as breast-feeding for at least 6 to 12 months and handwashing reduce the likelihood of acquiring *E. coli* enteric infections. Travelers to developing or tropical areas should avoid drinking untreated or unboiled water or ice and eating uncooked fruits or vegetables that may have been "freshened" with highly contaminated water. Although a number of antimicrobial agents are effective over short periods when taken prophylactically, their effectiveness is sharply limited by rapidly emerging resistance to antimicrobial drugs, as well as by the potential side effects of their indiscriminate, widespread use. For example, tetracycline resistance among ETEC is common, and resistance to trimethoprim-sulfamethoxazole and even some quinolones is rapidly emerging around the world. EHEC infections can largely be prevented by adequately cooking beef, especially hamburger, and by careful handwashing and other hygienic measures in daycare centers and nursing homes. Finally, developing toxoid or colonization factor vaccines holds considerable promise for prevention of ETEC diarrhea.

Treatment

As with all diarrheal illnesses, the primary treatment is replacement and maintenance of water and electrolytes, usually with a simple oral rehydration solution that uses the intact, sodium-coupled glucose or amino acid absorption (or both) to replace fluid losses (Chapter 325). Oral rehydration solution should be given ad libitum with free water, and in breast-fed infants, continued breast-feeding and early refeeding can compensate for the nutritional losses.

Because most *E. coli* diarrhea is self-limited, the role of antimicrobial agents is debated and remains of secondary importance to rehydration. In areas where ETEC remains sensitive, early initiation of sulfamethoxazole-trimethoprim, tetracycline, or a quinolone antibiotic may reduce a 3- to 5-day illness to a 1- to 2-day illness if the agent is started with the first loose stool in travelers to endemic, tropical areas (Chapter 329). The use of antimotility agents should be tempered by the potential added risk of worsening or prolonging inflammatory diarrheas and increasing the risk for hemolytic-uremic syndrome (Chapter 179) with EHEC infections and their lack of effectiveness in reducing fluid loss, even though abdominal cramping and overt diarrhea may be temporarily reduced. Bismuth subsalicylate may reduce symptoms in travelers' diarrhea but should be used with caution to avoid toxic doses of salicylate. Because of the potential severity of the disease in infants, some use neomycin, 100 mg/kg/day orally divided into three or four daily doses for 5 days, for documented EPEC infections in neonates.

Prognosis

The overall prognosis of the various types of *E. coli* diarrhea is generally excellent if they are adequately treated. However, the impact of *E. coli* and other common diarrheas on mortality and morbidity (particularly with repeated infections compounding malnutrition in young children) remains one of the major health problems on a global scale. The potentially serious complication of hemolytic-uremic syndrome (Chapter 126) may follow EHEC infection.

SUGGESTED READINGS

Jiang ZD, Okhuysen PC, Guo DC, et al: Genetic susceptibility to enteroaggregative *Escherichia coli* diarrhea: Polymorphism in the interleukin-8 promoter region. J Infect Dis 2003;188:506–511. *Seminal report of a clear, common genetic determinant of EAEC diarrhea in travelers.*

Kaper JB, Nataro JP, Mobley HL: Pathogenic *Escherichia coli.* Nat Rev Microbiol 2004;2:123–140. *Overview of major pathogenic mechanisms of* E. coli *diarrhea.*

Nataro JP, Mai V, Johnson J: Diarrheogenic *Escherichia coli* infection in Baltimore, Maryland and New Haven, Connecticut. Clin Infect Dis 2006;43;408–410 *ECAC is a common cause of diarrhea not due to a more obvious agent.*

Spears KJ, Rose AJ, Gally DK: A comparison of enteropathogenic and enterohaemorrhagic *Escherichia coli* pathogenesis. FEMS Microbiol Lett 2006;255:181–202. *EHEC infections express Shiga toxins; EPEC infections are overt pathogens.*

328 *PSEUDOMONAS* AND RELATED GRAM-NEGATIVE BACILLARY INFECTIONS

Gerald B. Pier

Definition

The *Pseudomonas*-related group of organisms comprises a set of gram-negative rods, including *Pseudomonas aeruginosa,* the most commonly encountered human pathogen in the family Pseudomonadaceae. Also included in this group are relatively low-virulence, uncommon pathogens such as members of the genus *Burkholderia* and *Stenotrophomonas* and two highly pathogenic species, *Burkholderia mallei* and *Burkholderia pseudomallei,* which can cause serious infections in the limited parts of the world where they occur naturally. On occasion, some non–*P. aeruginosa* organisms in the genus *Pseudomonas* or the related genus *Ralstonia* cause human infection, although such infection is almost always due to improper contamination of a medication or a device used to treat humans.

The Pathogen

P. aeruginosa is readily identified as a gram-negative, straight or slightly curved rod with a length ranging from 1 to 3 μm and a width of 0.5 to 1.0 μm. Major morphologic characteristics on laboratory media include production of pigments, notably a soluble blue phenazine pigment called pyocyanin. Some strains produce red or black colonies because of the synthesis of pigments termed pyorubin and pyomelanin, respectively. Another diffusible yellow-green to yellow-brown pigment produced by *P. aeruginosa* is called pyoverdin, which when produced along with pyocyanin, gives rise to a typical green to green-blue colony on solid media. The name *aeruginosa* stems from the green-blue hue seen within colonies of many clinical isolates.

Epidemiology

In adult clinical medicine, *P. aeruginosa* is primarily encountered as a nosocomial pathogen. However, as cystic fibrosis (CF) patients survive longer and their medical care as adults is increasingly shifted away from pediatric providers, treatment of chronic *P. aeruginosa* CF lung disease by adult practitioners is becoming more common. This organism is able to survive in environments that have only minimal nutritional components. Within the hospital, *P. aeruginosa* can colonize moist surfaces of the axilla, ear, and perineum and is also isolated from other moist, inanimate environments, including water in sinks and drains, toilets, and showers. Pathogenic strains have likewise been isolated from the water used for flowers in patients' rooms. Hospital equipment that comes in contact with water, such as mops, respiratory ventilators, cleaning solutions, and food and food processing machines, can be sources of *P. aeruginosa.*

Infections with *P. aeruginosa* have remained relatively constant in terms of incidence and tissue sites of occurrence over the past 30 years, as tracked by the National Nosocomial Infections Surveillance System. Data from medical intensive care units during the surveillance period 1992 to 1997 indicated that *P. aeruginosa* caused about 3% of blood stream infections; 21% of pneumonias (making it the most frequently isolated nosocomial pathogen from the lungs); 10% of urinary tract infections (fourth most common pathogen); 13% of eye, ear, nose, and throat pathogens (third most common); and 5% of cardiovascular infections.

Though much less of a problem than nosocomial infection, community-acquired *P. aeruginosa* infection does occur in certain settings, and such infection is often associated with exposure to moist environments. *P. aeruginosa* infections in the community are related to the use of hot tubs, whirlpools, swimming pools, and other types of baths, as well as the use of contact lenses, particularly the extended-wear variety. It is also a cause of otitis externa. Puncture wounds through tennis shoes can give rise to serious *P. aeruginosa* infection. *P. aeruginosa* endophthalmitis after surgery or eye trauma can result in serious visual compromise, and *P. aeruginosa* endocarditis is frequently found in injection drug users.

Pathogenesis

Host Factors in Pathogenesis

Because the major manifestations of *P. aeruginosa* infection are nosocomial diseases, chronic lung infection in CF, and contact lens–associated ulcerative keratitis, it is clear that the primary determinant of the pathogenic potential of *P. aeruginosa* virulence factors is actually the health status of the human host. For example, in burn and wound infections, *P. aeruginosa* is able to take advantage of dead or poorly perfused tissue, grow in this site, and eventually achieve a density in the wound sufficient to allow it to seed the blood at levels that overwhelm host innate immunity. Loss of mucosal barrier function, such as occurs in the tracheobronchial tree of mechanically ventilated patients, is another host condition that allows *P. aeruginosa* to potentially become a major pathogen. Usually, the normal bacterial flora in the gastrointestinal tract and oropharynx provides stiff competition for pathogens by preventing colonization and growth, but disruption of this flora by antibiotic treatment can allow an organism such as *P. aeruginosa* to colonize a mucosal surface. Compromises to host function, such as entrapment of foreign organisms in mucus that are normally cleared by peristalsis in the gastrointestinal tract, by mucociliary clearance in the respiratory tract, and by urination in the genitourinary tract, are also host conditions associated with colonization and subsequent infection by *P. aeruginosa*.

The panoply of cytokines and chemokines that humans can produce in response to infection, with their additive, synergistic and complementary, and antagonistic effects, makes it difficult to ascribe a role in resistance to *P. aeruginosa* infection to a single cytokine. Consistent with this conclusion are numerous reports, mostly from studies in transgenic mice, implicating some cytokines and chemokines as key elements in both resistance and enhancement of pathology related to *P. aeruginosa* infection. Among these substances are interleukin-1 (IL-1), tumor necrosis factor-α, IL-4, IL-6, IL-9, IL-10, IL-18, transforming growth factor-β, and nitric oxide.

Although all known monocytic, granulocytic, and lymphocytic cell types have shown some effect in having an impact on *P. aeruginosa* infection in both human and experimental animal infections, it is overwhelmingly clear that the major cellular mediators of resistance to *P. aeruginosa* infection are polymorphonuclear leukocytes (PMNs). Even though the incidence of serious *P. aeruginosa* infection in neutropenic hosts seems to have declined in the past 10 to 15 years when compared with the incidence in the 1970s, neutropenia in humans is still a major risk factor for *P. aeruginosa* infection. Animal studies completely confirm that neutropenia dramatically increases susceptibility to *P. aeruginosa* infection, with the lethal dose after experimental challenge being reduced by as much as 1 million– to 10 million–fold.

Epithelial cells, particularly in the lung, are among the first cell types to encounter *P. aeruginosa* after exposure. Principally through studies directed at elucidating why CF patients are so commonly infected with *P. aeruginosa* (>80% of patients are infected by 15 to 20 years of age), a lot has been learned about the role of epithelial cells in orchestrating innate immunity to *P. aeruginosa* infection. The major challenge has been to correlate the genetic defect leading to the synthesis of either no cystic fibrosis transmembrane conductance regulator (CFTR) protein or dysfunctional CFTR to the pathogenesis of *P. aeruginosa* infection. Lack of functional CFTR compromises the host's ability to respond rapidly to *P. aeruginosa* with a protective inflammatory response involving such diverse factors as epithelial uptake of bacteria via binding to CFTR, which in turn leads to rapid cytokine responses and PMN infiltration to protect against further bacterial spread within the bronchial mucosa. Delays in these responses could underlie the ability of *P. aeruginosa* to survive in the CF lung and ultimately lead to destructive inflammation.

Bacterial Factors in Pathogenesis

P. aeruginosa is a fascinating bacterial pathogen to study and a formidable pathogen for humans because of the multitude, diversity, and complexity of its virulence factors. Virtually all major classes of bacterial virulence systems are found in this organism (Table 328–1), including exotoxins, endotoxins, type III secreted toxins, pili, flagella, proteases, phospholipases, iron-binding proteins, exopolysaccharides, the ability to form biofilms, and elaboration of toxic small molecules such as pyocyanins. The potential of *P. aeruginosa* to causes infection in virtually any body site is probably due to the array of factors that it can call on from its large genome to establish itself at a specific site and use a wide variety of nutrients for growth, along with the ability to produce a panoply of factors to counteract host defenses.

When initially colonizing a host, *P. aeruginosa* encounters a rich array of innate and acquired immune factors that usually mediate high levels of resistance to infection. Bacterial factors produced to counter host defenses include expression of long O-side chains on bacterial lipopolysaccharide to prevent lysis by complement and production of a variety of proteases that can inactivate host immune effectors and kill immune effector cells, as well as degrade tissue components, thereby allowing the organism to advance the infectious process. The best studied proteases of *P. aeruginosa* are elastolytic proteases encoded by the *lasA* (LasA protease) and *lasB* (elastase) genes, alkaline protease, and protease IV.

P. aeruginosa uses typical siderophore systems to acquire iron, specifically involving factors referred to as pyoverdin and pyochelin. Pyoverdin is secreted, scavenges iron from mammalian sources, and brings it back to the cell in the form of ferripyoverdin by binding to the FpvA bacterial membrane receptor. Pyochelin binds to the bacterial ferric pyochelin receptor encoded by the *fptA* gene.

One major cellular toxin produced by *P. aeruginosa* is exotoxin A, an adenosine diphosphate–ribosylating toxin with activity very similar to that of diphtheria toxin. Purified exotoxin A is lethal to experimental animals in small doses, its production is affected by iron levels, and it has been used in a variety of settings as a chimeric protein fused to growth factors or targeting antibodies to produce potential clinical benefit by destroying aberrant cells in settings such as autoimmune disease and cancer.

Strains of *P. aeruginosa* can induce hemolysis of red blood cells as a result of the production of PlcHR, a hemolytic phospholipase C. A second, nonhemolytic phospholipase C, PlcN, is also made by *P. aeruginosa* strains. Type III secretion systems are highly conserved features of bacterial pathogens, including *P. aeruginosa.* This system allows direct injection of bacterial toxins into eukaryotic cells, which disrupts cellular trafficking by inhibiting the actin cytoskeleton and also by affecting protein synthesis. For *P. aeruginosa,* clinical isolates expressing type III toxins are isolated significantly more frequently from patients who have poor clinical outcomes, including mortality in acutely infected patients. Four major effector proteins are known: ExoS, ExoT, ExoU, and ExoY. The apparatus for injection is formed as a complex structure on the bacterial surface that is composed of five proteins, PcrG, PcrV, PcrH, PopB, and PopD, encoded in the chromosomal pcrGVH-popBD operon.

Extensive cellular injury occurs during *P. aeruginosa* infection, particularly in the lung, and involves both epithelial and endothelial cells. Some of this damage is mediated by pyocyanin, which damages cells by producing reactive oxygen species such as hydrogen peroxide and superoxide. *P. aeruginosa* resists the effects of these antibacterial molecules by limiting the redox cycling of pyocyanin and producing three catalases (KatA, KatB, and KatC) and two superoxide dismutases—one using manganese as a cofactor and the other using iron.

As bacterial counts increase in a tissue, the organisms reach a critical mass that is thought to allow them to effectively communicate with each other through the system of quorum sensing (QS). For *P. aeruginosa* three

TABLE 328–1 VIRULENCE FACTORS FOR *PSEUDOMONAS AERUGINOSA*

Location or Class	Example(s)	Activity/Effects on Host
Cell surface	Alginate	Antiphagocytic/resist opsonic killing
	LPS	Endotoxic/antiphagocytic/avoid preformed antibody to previously encountered O antigens
	Pili	Twitching motility, biofilm formation, adherence to host tissues
	Flagella	Motility, biofilm formation, adherence to host tissues and mucin components
	Injection of type III secretion factors	PcrG, PcrV, PcrH, PopB, and PopD proteins form injection bridge for type III effectors
Outer membrane	Siderophore receptors	Provides iron for microbial growth and survival
	Efflux pumps	Removes antibiotics
Type III secretion	ExoS, ExoT, ExoU, Exo Y	Intoxicates cells (ExoS/ExoT); cytotoxic (ExoU), disrupts actin cytoskeleton
Secreted proteases	LasA protease, LasB elastase, alkaline protease, protease IV	Degrade host immune effectors (antibody, complement, etc.), degrade matrix proteins
Iron acquisition	Pyoverdin, pyochelin	Scavenge iron from the host for bacterial use
Secreted toxins	Exotoxin A, leukocidin, phospholipases, hemolysins, rhamnolipid	Inhibit protein synthesis, kill leukocytes, hemolysis of red cells, degrade host cell surface glycolipids
Secreted oxidative factors	Pyocyanin, ferripyochelin	Produces reactive oxygen species: H_2O_2; O_2^-
		Inflammatory, disrupts epithelial cell function
Quorum sensing	LasR/LasI, RhlR/RhlI, PQS	Biofilm formation, regulation of virulence factor secretion

LPS = lipopolysaccharide; PQS = *Pseudomonas* quinolone signal.

major, interrelated QS systems are known to date, designated the las, rhl, and *Pseudomonas* quinolone system (PQS). The molecular mediators of the QS system are known as autoinducers because of their self-regulatory effects on bacterial responses to the environment. These three systems, along with some other regulatory factors, have a complex interaction in the context of regulation of gene transcription and production of virulence factors.

Another major bacterial phenotype regulated by the QS system is the formation of *P. aeruginosa* biofilms, a well-studied area but with some important limitations in terms of applicability to clinical infection and disease. The extensive use of implantable devices in modern medicine has certainly led to the appreciation that structured bacterial communities known as biofilms can form on these devices and contribute to infection. In addition, in chronic infections such as osteomyelitis or CF lung infection, it is thought that biofilms play an important role in pathogenesis. Although impressive microscopic and artistic renditions of *P. aeruginosa* biofilms formed in vitro have been published, these structured communities are not really observed in infected tissues, notably the CF lung. Rather, microcolonies or aggregates of bacteria are present, and these microcolonies contain not only bacterial factors but also host factors, including host DNA, mucus, actin, and probably other products from dead and dying bacterial and host cells. How these in vivo microcolonies are actually related to the QS-controlled biofilms studied in vitro on abiotic surfaces is still unclear and doubtful in many investigators' minds.

Clinical Manifestations

Bacteremia

The clinical manifestations of *P. aeruginosa* blood stream infection are rarely different from those of bacteremia in general. Patients are usually febrile, but more severely ill patients in shock may be hypothermic. The only point differentiating this entity from other causes of gram-negative sepsis may be the occurrence of distinctive skin lesions known as ecthyma gangrenosum, which occur almost exclusively in markedly neutropenic patients. These small, painful, reddish, maculopapular, well-circumscribed lesions have a geographic margin and begin pink, darken to purple, and finally become black and necrotic. Histopathology indicates that the lesions are caused by vascular invasion after bacteremia and are teeming with bacteria.

Acute Pneumonia

The respiratory tract remains the most frequent site of infection by *P. aeruginosa*. This organism ranks either first or second in most lists as the causative pathogen in ventilator-associated pneumonia (VAP). However, much debate centers on the actual role of the organism in VAP because the conclusion that *P. aeruginosa* plays a major role in VAP is based on results of cultures of endotracheal tube aspirates. Frequently, these culture results represent nothing more than nonpathogenic colonization of the tracheobronchial tree, formation of an innocuous biofilm on the endotracheal tube, or simple tracheobronchitis. In the absence of radiologic evidence of pneumonia, the question remains whether *P. aeruginosa* is causing anything more than purulence in tracheobronchial secretions (i.e., tracheobronchitis). At the current time there is an emerging consensus that an invasive procedure such as bronchoalveolar lavage or protected brush sampling of the distal airways should be used to obtain material for quantitative culture of the lung to substantiate the occurrence of *P. aeruginosa* pneumonia.

Chronic Respiratory Tract Infections

P. aeruginosa is responsible for chronic infections of the airways associated with a number of underlying or predisposing conditions, the most prevalent being CF, which is found predominantly in white populations. A description and management of *P. aeruginosa* infection in patients with CF can be found in Chapter 89. A somewhat similar state of chronic colonization beginning early in childhood is seen in some Asian populations in a disease of unknown etiology called chronic or diffuse panbronchiolitis. The disease is most often described in Japan but is not restricted to that country. However, not unlike CF, there is a chronic relapsing infection by *P. aeruginosa* that is characterized by increased sputum production, fever, and focal lung infiltrates. Strains of *P. aeruginosa* isolated from these patients also undergo the same type of mucoid conversion as do strains from patients with CF, which reflects overproduction of an exopolysaccharide termed alginate, a clear pathogenic factor in chronic CF lung disease.

Bone and Joint Infections

P. aeruginosa is not a frequent cause of bone or joint infections. These infections result from at least three different mechanisms: bacteremia, direct inoculation into bone, or spread from contiguous infection. Bacteremia secondary to either injection of contaminated illicit drugs or infective endocarditis in the addict population has been well documented to cause vertebral osteomyelitis and sternoclavicular joint arthritis. The clinical manifestation of vertebral *P. aeruginosa* osteomyelitis is more indolent than that of staphylococcal osteomyelitis. The duration of symptoms in the addict population with vertebral osteomyelitis is from weeks to months. Fever is not uniformly present but, when present, tends to be low grade. Sternoclavicular septic arthritis from *P. aeruginosa* is seen almost exclusively in intravenous drug addicts. It may occur with or without endocarditis, but a primary site of infection is often not found.

Pseudomonas osteomyelitis of the foot most often follows puncture wounds through sneakers. The organism has been found between the rubber sole layers of sneakers in many cases. Most of these cases are reported in children, but it is also seen in adults. The main manifestation is pain in the foot, and there may be superficial cellulitis around the puncture wound and tenderness on deep palpation of the wound.

Central Nervous System Infections

Primary central nervous system infections by *P. aeruginosa* are a relative rarity. Involvement is almost always secondary to a surgical procedure or head trauma and is occasionally noted after bacteremia. The entities seen most often are postoperative or post-traumatic meningitis and occasionally subdural or epidural infections resulting from initial contamination of access areas. Brain abscess secondary to embolic disease from endocarditis has also been described in intravenous drug addicts. The cerebrospinal fluid profile of *P. aeruginosa* meningitis is no different from that of pyogenic meningitis. Other forms of *P. aeruginosa* central nervous system infection, such as brain abscesses and epidural and subdural empyema, generally require surgical drainage in addition to antibiotics.

Eye Infections

Eye infections by *P. aeruginosa* occur from direct inoculation into tissue as a result of trauma or surface injury caused by contact lenses. Keratitis is the most frequent type of disease seen, and its association with contact lens wear, especially extended-wear lenses, is well established. However, any form of trauma may predispose to this type of infection, including surgery and burns. Keratitis can be slowly or rapidly progressive, but the classic description is that of disease progressing over a 48-hour period and leading to involvement of the entire cornea with opacification and sometimes perforation. *P. aeruginosa* keratitis should be considered a medical emergency because of the rapidity with which it can progress and lead to loss of sight.

P. aeruginosa endophthalmitis is one of the most feared of *P. aeruginosa* infections. Loss of sight or very much reduced visual acuity is the most common outcome of these infections. This entity may result from penetrating injuries, surgery, perforation of a corneal ulcer, or seeding from bacteremia. The disease is fulminant, with severe pain, chemosis, decreased visual acuity, anterior uveitis, vitreous involvement, and panophthalmitis. *P. aeruginosa* also causes a number of uncommon eye infections, including orbital cellulitis in neutropenic patients and gangrene necrosis of the eyelids, both of which result from bacteremia.

Ear Infections

P. aeruginosa ear infections vary from the mild swimmer's ear, to chronic persistent draining ears, to serious life-threatening infections that lead to neurologic sequelae or even death. Swimmer's ear is commonly seen in children and results from infection of moist macerated skin of the external ear canal. The source of the organism is likely to be the swimming pool if underchlorinated. The natural history of most of these cases is resolution without sequelae, but chronic drainage occurs in some patients. Systemic symptoms such as fever develop in a small minority of patients. The diagnosis is made easily as long as there is a high index of suspicion, which there should be in diabetics and patients with acquired immunodeficiency syndrome.

Another poorly understood form of *P. aeruginosa* ear infection is a chronic middle ear drainage called chronic suppurative otitis media. *P. aeruginosa* is isolated from a large percentage of these draining middle ears. Often it is in mixed culture, but in about 30% of cases it is the sole organism isolated from aerobic cultures. The pathogenesis of this condition is unclear. It is possible that it begins with external otitis similar to swimmer's ear, with subsequent middle ear involvement followed by chronic mastoiditis.

Urinary Tract Infections

P. aeruginosa urinary tract infections generally occur as a complication of the presence of a foreign body such as a stone, stent, or catheter in the urinary tract or an obstruction within the genitourinary system or after instrumentation or surgery on the urinary tract. Paraplegic patients are at high risk for *P. aeruginosa* urinary tract infections, and frequent use of antibiotics in this setting may select for *P. aeruginosa.* Not withstanding the relationship between obstructive lesions and *P. aeruginosa* urinary tract infections, there have been descriptions of *P. aeruginosa* urinary tract infections in outpatient children without stones or evident obstruction. One of the most important aspects of *P. aeruginosa* urinary tract infections is the observation that it frequently serves as the nidus for *P. aeruginosa* bacteremia by ascending infection.

Skin and Soft Tissue Infections, Including Burns

P. aeruginosa causes ecthyma gangrenosum in neutropenic patients, an entity described earlier in this chapter. Secondary infection of chronic skin ulcers or burns (see later) can also occur. Maceration of normal skin, such as from soaking in a hot tub, can lead to superficial infection. Folliculitis and other papular or vesicular lesions attributed to *P. aeruginosa,* collectively called dermatitis, have now been extensively described. Multiple outbreaks have been linked to whirlpools, spas, and swimming pools. Thus, control of growth of this organism in the home or recreational environment by proper antibacterial treatment of water is essential, comparable to the control commonly practiced in hospitals.

Burn wound infections by *P. aeruginosa* constituted one of the most significant problems caused by this organism during the 1960s and 1970s. A specific clinical picture of sepsis, with high colony counts of *P. aeruginosa* exceeding 10^5 organisms per gram of tissue, was the defining feature. Patients generally had a picture of progressive formation of a black necrotic eschar and sepsis, with or without bacteremia. The occurrence of *P. aeruginosa* burn wound sepsis does not appear to be as frequent as reported in the past, when as many as 10% of burn patients had *P. aeruginosa* sepsis. The diagnosis may be made by blood culture or by the pathognomonic clinical picture of an expanding burn lesion caused by infection with *P. aeruginosa.* Clinicians usually rely on isolation of *P. aeruginosa* from wounds or blood along with the finding of sepsis in diagnosing burn wound sepsis secondary to *P. aeruginosa.*

Endovascular Infections

P. aeruginosa may cause endovascular infections, including infective endocarditis. In intravenous drug addicts, the source is generally contaminated paraphernalia or illicit drugs. This organism has also been reported to cause prosthetic valve endocarditis. Outbreaks of *P. aeruginosa* endocarditis on native heart valves have been described in drug addicts residing in particular cities, probably resulting from local contamination of illicit drugs. The manifestations of *P. aeruginosa* endocarditis resemble other forms of acute endocarditis in addicts except that it appears to be more indolent than *Staphylococcus aureus* endocarditis.

P. aeruginosa Infections in Febrile Neutropenia

P. aeruginosa infections during febrile neutropenia occupy a historical place as the organism against which empirical coverage must always be included. Currently, the organism does not appear to be as common in neutropenic patients as it once was. However, the importance of *P. aeruginosa* infection in neutropenic patients has not diminished simply because when it does cause bacteremia, mortality is likely to be high if not appropriately treated by empirical therapy. Additionally, in some parts of the world, *P. aeruginosa* continues to be a significant problem in neutropenic patients in that it is responsible for the largest proportion of infections caused by a single organism. The historical clinical syndromes in febrile neutropenic patients were bacteremia, pneumonia, and soft tissue infections mainly manifested as ecthyma gangrenosum.

Uncommon P. aeruginosa Infections

In addition to the entities just described, *P. aeruginosa* can cause a number of infrequently seen syndromes, including noma neonatorum, a necrotizing mucosal and perianal infection of newborns, toe web infections (especially in the tropics), and the "green nail syndrome" caused by *P. aeruginosa* paronychia as a result of frequent submersion of the hands in water. In the last entity the green discoloration results from diffusion of pyocyanin into the nail bed.

Treatment

Rx

Treatment of Bacteremia

Removal of an infected vascular catheter may be needed to control device-related bacteremia. The standard of care for *P. aeruginosa* bacteremia is usually an effective β-lactam antibiotic combined with an aminoglycoside. Monotherapy with an aminoglycoside has generally resulted in very poor outcomes. There have been at least four studies, none of which have been prospective, double-blinded studies, indicating that *P. aeruginosa* bacteremia has the same outcome when treated with a single antipseudomonal β-lactam or such an agent combined with an aminoglycoside. Overall, none of the dogmas concerning the appropriate therapy for *P. aeruginosa* bacteremia can be considered to be established by blinded, controlled clinical studies.

Depending on the antibiotic susceptibility of *P. aeruginosa* isolates routinely found in a specific setting, one of the following regimens would be appropriate for *P. aeruginosa* bacteremia, pending return of susceptibility testing results. Adult, nonazotemic patients may be given ceftazidime, 2 g intravenously every 8 hours, cefepime, 2 g intravenously every 12 hours, meropenem, 1 g every 8 hours, or imipenem, 0.5 g every 6 hours. Aztreonam, 1.5 g to 2.0 g every 6 to 8 hours, has been used for patients with serious β-lactam allergy. If piperacillin-tazobactam is used empirically, the lack of contribution by tazobactam to the antipseudomonal activity of piperacillin may make the usual dose of 3.375 g every 6 hours inadequate, so 4.5 g every 6 hours or the addition of amikacin, 15 mg/kg every 24 hours, may be preferred. The addition of an aminoglycoside to the other regimens is perhaps less critical and probably depends on the level of resistance to β-lactam antibiotics seen in any given institution. At the current time, the highest levels of susceptibility are to amikacin in most regions of the world.

Treatment of Pneumonia

Therapy for *P. aeruginosa* pneumonia has not been determined by rigorous studies. As with bacteremia, high failure rates were seen when aminoglycosides were used as single agents. The drugs of choice for *P. aeruginosa* pneumonia would appear to be similar to those mentioned earlier for bacteremia. A strong case cannot be made for inclusion of the aminoglycoside component for fully susceptible organisms, given the evidence that aminoglycosides are not optimally active in the lungs at concentrations normally used for intravenous administration. Aerosolized aminoglycoside might provide adequate drug levels in the tracheobronchial tree, but there is no reason to believe that the drug would penetrate into the consolidated lung. The usually recommended drug is tobramycin, 300 mg inhaled daily. Patients with nosocomial pneumonia may have *P. aeruginosa* isolates resistant to many of the usual drugs, a problem that appears to be getting progressively worse.

Diffuse panbronchiolitis patients respond clinically to antipseudomonal therapy, but the organism is not eradicated. Significant advances have, however, been made in its management with the long-term use of macrolides, a class of drugs that have no antibacterial activity against *P. aeruginosa* but are thought to suppress the inflammatory response and perhaps suppress production of *P. aeruginosa* virulence factors. The most commonly used agents have been clarithromycin and azithromycin.

Treatment of Other Infections

With the exception of osteomyelitis after puncture wounds, which occurs mainly in children, antibiotic therapy for other *P. aeruginosa* infections is difficult. The choices are single-drug therapy with an antipseudomonal β-lactam antibiotic or ciprofloxacin. However, it should be noted that *P. aeruginosa* resistance to ciprofloxacin has increased dramatically worldwide and may preclude its use in many cases.

For treatment of meningitis, the general principles involved in the treatment of this infection apply, that is, the need for high doses of bactericidal agents to attain high levels within cerebrospinal fluid. The agent with which there is some published experience for *P. aeruginosa* meningitis is ceftazidime, but other antipseudomonal β-lactam agents that achieve high cerebrospinal fluid concentrations, such as cefepime and meropenem, have also been used successfully.

The usual therapy for keratitis is topical antibiotics. Fortified aminoglycoside preparations or fluoroquinolones are recommended. In cases in which involvement is extensive, ceftazidime or gentamicin may be given by subconjunctival injection.

Therapy for endophthalmitis includes both systemic antibiotics at high doses to achieve better concentrations in the eye and intravitreal antibiotics. Ceftazidime has been the most frequently used antibiotic for this entity, but little is written about outcomes. Its penetration into the vitreous is excellent. Aminoglycosides are also injected subconjunctivally and by intraocular routes and sometimes given intravenously. Adjunctive surgery is generally performed to remove infected vitreous.

Management of otitis externa involves the use of topical antibiotic agents (otic solutions). Aminoglycoside-containing solutions are the most frequently used. Recurrences are frequent and can lead to chronically draining ears that may require more intensive topical therapy.

Treatment of malignant external otitis has undergone significant changes since it was first described by Chandler in 1960. At the current time, the approach appears to be débridement of the ear canal, including any necrotic tissue cartilage and adjacent bone, rather than extensive bony débridement or facial nerve decompression. Treatment with a single agent, usually ceftazidime or ciprofloxacin, has been successful.

Most *P. aeruginosa* urinary tract infections fit into the category of complicated urinary tract infections, where therapy is more prolonged than the usual course recommended for cystitis. There are no real comparative data on proper therapies. Foley catheters, stents, or stones should be removed if possible to prevent relapse. Generally, 7 to 10 days of antibiotic treatment will suffice, with up to 2 weeks for pyelonephritis. Antipseudomonal β-lactams, ciprofloxacin, levofloxacin, gatifloxacin, and aminoglycosides given once daily are all equally acceptable, given their normally high levels of urinary excretion. Alternative antibiotics that may be used for oral treatment of *P. aeruginosa* urinary tract infections include doxycycline, to which many strains are sensitive; in cases of multiple antibiotic resistance or in patients with very low urinary output, bladder irrigation with 0.25% acetic acid may be useful. Relapse is common, and it may not be due to antibiotic resistance but to host factors.

Management of *P. aeruginosa*–infected burn wounds is both surgical and medical. Extensive débridement of colonized eschar or necrotic tissue is required. The general principle is to reduce the organism count, which would probably diminish the sepsis response, but importantly this would reduce the risk of resistance developing during therapy given the extremely high microbial burden of such wounds. At the current time, true burn wound sepsis secondary to *P. aeruginosa* is probably best managed with a combination of antibiotics.

For treatment of *P. aeruginosa* infections in febrile, neutropenic patients, antipseudomonal β-lactams such as cefepime, ceftazidime, or a carbapenem can be used either alone or in combination with an aminoglycoside. Alternatively, an antipseudomonal penicillin such as piperacillin can be used in combination with an aminoglycoside if so preferred.

Antibiotic Resistance and Antibiotic Therapy for Multiresistant Pseudomonas Infections

P. aeruginosa strains that occur worldwide and carry multiple resistance determinants that mediate β-lactam multiresistance, along with fluoroquinolone and aminoglycoside resistance, have emerged as significant causes of infection. The medical community is now turning to drugs such as colistin and polymyxin, which were discarded decades ago but are now being considered as antimicrobials for the "21st century." Alternative approaches to the management of multiresistant *P. aeruginosa* began some time ago because of the complexity of management of such organisms in patients with CF. Colistin (polymyxin E) is used intravenously, not withstanding its toxicity. Use of this agent—or the related peptide antibiotic polymyxin

B—is now rapidly becoming the therapy of choice of last resort in non-CF patients infected with multiresistant *P. aeruginosa*. The dose of either agent needs to be adjusted for renal insufficiency. One recommended schedule for colistin is as follows: for patients with creatinine clearance greater than 20 mL/min, 75 to 100% of the daily dose given in two divided doses; for creatinine clearance of 5 to 20 mL/min, 50% of the daily dose given in two divided doses; and for creatinine clearance less than 5 mL/min, 30% of the daily dose given in two divided doses every 12 to 18 hours.

Infections Caused by Organisms at One Time Classified As Pseudomonads

Most of these infections are due to members of the genus *Burkholderia,* including *B. cenocepacia,* a complex of about 10 related species previously referred to as genomovars that are phenotypically similar but distinguished primarily by nucleic acid sequences, and by *B. mallei* and *B. pseudomallei,* causes of glanders and melioidosis, respectively. Infections caused by members of the genus *Ralstonia* and non–*P. aeruginosa* pseudomonads such as *P. fluorescens* are generally rare and often iatrogenically induced by accidental contamination of solutions or medications delivered to patients. *Stenotrophomonas maltophilia* is an uncommon cause of a variety of diseases and often occurs as part of a polymicrobial infection; it can be involved in pneumonia, endocarditis, bacteremia, and urinary tract infections. This organism is generally resistant to many types of common antibiotics used for *P. aeruginosa* but is often sensitive to trimethoprim-sulfamethoxazole, ticarcillin-clavulanate, many fluoroquinolones, and rifampin.

Organisms in the *B. cenocepacia* complex are usually pathogenic for immunocompromised hosts and individuals with long-standing underlying serious disease. It infects the lungs of about 4% of CF patients, most commonly after many years of tissue destruction from chronic *P. aeruginosa* infection. Some strains of *B. cenocepacia* are known to cause precipitous deterioration in the clinical condition of CF patients who acquire these hypervirulent strains and, though relatively rare, can still cause focal outbreaks in CF centers. Outside of CF, *B. cenocepacia* infection can be acquired from either hospital surfaces or sources or brought in from outside the hospital because of its ubiquity in the environment. As with *P. aeruginosa, B. cenocepacia* is found in moist or water-based environments. Pseudobacteremia caused by contamination of blood culture bottles has to be suspected when *B. cenocepacia* organisms are reported. Treatment of *B. cenocepacia* infections can be highly problematic because the organisms are at times naturally resistant to almost all commonly used antibiotics. Nonetheless, combinations of meropenem with ciprofloxacin and tobramycin appear to be successful, and in CF patients with β-lactam hypersensitivity, meropenem monotherapy has been effective. In vitro susceptibility profiles can be used to guide initial therapy.

Melioidosis from *B. pseudomallei* can occur in humans and animals and is endemic in parts of Southeast Asia and northern Australia. Findings range from asymptomatic infection to localized skin infections, chronic lung infection, and even fulminant septicemia with multiple organ failure. *B. pseudomallei* infections can occur in individuals who have recently traveled to endemic areas and is also a category B bioterrorism agent. Infection with *B. pseudomallei* can remain latent for long periods and then become reactivated, so lack of recent exposure or travel to an infected area may be insufficient to exclude a diagnosis of melioidosis. Underlying conditions such as diabetes, excessive alcohol consumption, and renal disease are found in more than half of such patients. Initial intensive therapy for 10 to 14 days can include ceftazidime, meropenem, or imipenem, to which trimethoprim-sulfamethoxazole can be added. For eradication therapy, 3 months or more of trimethoprim-sulfamethoxazole with or without doxycycline is used.

Glanders, caused by *B. mallei,* is primarily a disease of horses and is thus an occupational risk for those who come in contact with these animals. Glanders has been eliminated from enzootic foci in most countries, but some pockets remain in South America, Asia, Africa, and the Middle East. A history of contact with horses or similar species such as donkeys in one of these areas is consistent with a diagnosis of glanders. Incubation periods can be short (1 to 2 days after inhalation) or up to a few months, and as with *B. pseudomallei,* latent foci can be reactivated years after primary exposure. Clinical manifestations include an acute febrile illness and necrosis in the tracheobronchial tree accompanied by mucopurulent discharge from the eyes, nose, or lips. Systemic infections along with lymphadenopathy, respiratory tract involvement, and skin lesions are also manifestations of this disease. Untreated, the infection is lethal within 10 to 14 days. Antibiotic susceptibility and treatment are similar to that for *B. pseudomallei,* although newer macrolides appear to be effective against glanders, but they are not effective against melioidosis, as is gentamicin. *B. mallei* is also a category B bioterrorism agent and was used during World War 1 by German agents to infect and incapacitate horses in the United States, Europe, and Argentina.

SUGGESTED READINGS

Bonomo RA, Szabo D: Mechanisms of multidrug resistance in *Achinetobacter* species and *Pseudomonas aeruginosa*. Clin Infect Dis 2006;43:S49–S56. *Comprehensive review of the mechisms of multidrug resistance in these pathogens.*

Hauser AR, Sriram P: Severe *Pseudomonas aeruginosa* infections. Tackling the conundrum of drug resistance. Postgrad Med 2005;117:41–48. *Approach to drug-resistant infections.*

Klibanov OM, Raasch RH, Rublein JC: Single versus combined antibiotic therapy for gram-negative infections. Ann Pharmacother 2004;38:332–337. *Identifies situations in which monotherapy is a safe alternative.*

Rossolini GM, Mantengoli E: Treatment and control of severe infections caused by multiresistant *Pseudomonas aeruginosa.* Clin Microbiol Infect 2005; 11(Suppl. 4):17–32. *A practical overview.*

329 *SALMONELLA* INFECTIONS (INCLUDING TYPHOID FEVER)

Keith S. Kaye and Donald Kaye

Definition

Salmonella, a genus of the family Enterobacteriaceae, can cause an asymptomatic intestinal carrier state or clinical disease in both humans and animals. One classification system puts all salmonellae that infect humans into one species, *Salmonella choleraesuis,* or more commonly, the species name *Salmonella enterica,* which includes more than 2000 serotypes. Each serotype designation then follows the species name (e.g., *S. choleraesuis* serotype *typhimurium* or *S. enterica* serotype *typhi*). The more commonly used, less cumbersome system, which is used in this chapter, defines each serotype as simply *Salmonella* followed by the serotype name (e.g., *S. typhimurium* or *S. typhi*).

The Pathogen

Salmonellae are motile, gram-negative, non–spore-forming bacilli. They are differentiated from other Enterobacteriaceae by biochemical tests. They ferment glucose, maltose, and mannitol but not lactose or sucrose. They reduce nitrates and do not produce cytochrome oxidase. Almost all salmonellae produce acid and gas with fermentation. Exceptions to the rules that are helpful in identification are the following: *S. typhi* does not produce gas, and *S. gallinarum-pullorum* is nonmotile. As another confounding exception, lactose-fermenting strains of salmonellae have been isolated.

Salmonellae can be differentiated into more than 2000 serotypes (serovars) by their somatic (O) antigens, which are composed of lipopolysaccharides and are part of the cell wall, and by their flagellar (H) and capsular (Vi) antigens. There are six serogroups based on O antigens: A, B, C1, C2, D, and E. Some of the important serovars and their groups are *S. typhi* (group D), *S. choleraesuis* (group C1), *S. typhimurium* (group B), and *S. enteritidis* (group D). *S. enteritidis* and *S. typhimurium* are the most common causes of human disease and together represent almost 50% of human isolates. Other common isolates are *S. heidelberg, S. hadar, S. newport, S. agona, S. montevideo, S. oranienburg, S. meunchen,* and *S. thompson.*

Epidemiology

S. typhi, S. paratyphi A, S. schottmuelleri (S. paratyphi B), S. hirschfeldii (S. paratyphi C), and *S. sendai* are either solely or almost exclusively pathogens in humans, and human-to-human transmission is important. As a result of modern sewage and water treatment facilities, typhoid fever and paratyphoid fever have become rare in developed countries but remain a problem in countries without adequate sanitation and a safe water supply. There are usually fewer than 500 cases of typhoid fever each year in the United States, mainly acquired abroad, as compared with an estimated 16 million cases elsewhere in the world. Most cases of *Salmonella* infection occurring in the United States are sporadic rather than related to outbreaks. However, when an infection occurs, other members of the household also tend to have positive stool cultures. It has been estimated that 1 to 2 million cases of *Salmonella* infection occur each year in the United States. A disproportionate number of infections occur in July through October, probably related to warm weather. *Salmonella* infections are most common in infants and children younger than 5 years.

Epidemiologic tracing of *Salmonella* outbreaks has been accomplished by phenotypic methods (e.g., antibiotic susceptibility), bacteriophage typing, plasmid analysis, ribotyping, polymerase chain reaction (PCR)-based techniques, pulsed-field gel electrophoresis, and other methods.

Resistance

Salmonellae have become increasingly resistant to antibiotics, usually by acquiring resistance transfer factors (e.g., plasmid mediated). It is believed that much of the resistance has been associated with the widespread use of antimicrobial agents in farm animals. A multidrug-resistant strain of *S. typhimurium* (definitive type 104 [DT 104]) has emerged as an important cause of infection in the world and is responsible for about 40% of infections caused by *S. typhimurium* in the United States. These salmonellae are resistant to ampicillin, chloramphenicol, streptomycin, sulfonamides, and tetracycline. In addition, resistance to fluoroquinolones worldwide has been increasing, particularly in Asia.

Etiology

Salmonellae are transmitted by the ingestion of fecally contaminated food or water. The source of contamination is feces from an acute case or from an asymptomatic fecal carrier.

Contaminated Animal Products

The remaining serovars of salmonellae are widely spread in the animal kingdom, and salmonellae have been isolated from virtually all species, including birds, mammals, reptiles, amphibians, and insects. *Salmonella* infection in humans usually occurs from ingesting contaminated animal food products, most often eggs, poultry, and meat. Eggs usually become contaminated from feces on the surface of the egg shell, with small cracks allowing entry into the egg. However, infection of the ovary allows primary incorporation of salmonellae into the egg. Furthermore, salmonellae can penetrate the intact shell of an egg. Animal and poultry carcasses, which are occasionally contaminated, become widely contaminated at the slaughterhouse, with salmonellae spread from carcass to carcass, usually on the carcass surface. *S. choleraesuis* is associated with pig products and *S. dublin* with cattle and consumption of unpasteurized milk from cattle. During the past 25 years, *S. enteritidis* outbreaks related to eggs have increased dramatically. Salmonellae may survive cooking at relatively low temperatures in the center of eggs or cooked turkeys, or food may be contaminated after cooking from kitchen utensils or from the hands of food preparers who handle raw food. Multiplication of organisms can then occur if the food is not refrigerated. Any food can become contaminated by feces, and outbreaks have occurred from contaminated cheese, ice cream, vegetables, fruit, juice, and alfalfa sprouts.

Contaminated Food and Water

Contamination by Pets

Salmonella infections have been acquired after contamination of food or water with the feces of pet turtles, chicks, ducks, birds, dogs, cats, and many other species. These pets become infected from their food.

Contamination by Humans

Salmonella infection can also be acquired by eating food or, less commonly, by drinking water contaminated by human carriers who have not adequately washed their hands. Infection has been spread by the fecal-oral route in children, by contaminated enema and fiberoptic instruments, by diagnostic and therapeutic preparations made from animal or insect products (e.g., pancreatic extract, carmine dye), and from intentional contamination of restaurant salad bars. Men who have sex with men are prone to fecal-oral infection. Outbreaks of salmonellosis occur in institutionalized patients, who are probably more prone to the development of *Salmonella* infections for three reasons. First, within institutionalized populations there is an increased prevalence of underlying diseases that decrease host defense mechanisms against salmonellae, such as disorders of gastric acidity and intestinal motility; second, the use of antimicrobial agents reduces the normal, protective intestinal flora; and third, institutional food prepared in bulk is more likely to be contaminated than individually prepared meals. Outbreaks in nurseries and in the elderly in nursing homes are associated with the highest mortality rates (i.e., >5%).

Pathobiology

After the ingestion of organisms, the likelihood of infection developing, as well as the severity of infection, is related to the dose and virulence of the *Salmonella* strain and the status of host defense mechanisms. Large inocula such as 10^5 to 10^7 bacteria are usually required to produce clinical infection in a normal host. Smaller inocula are less likely to result in infection and more likely to produce a transient intestinal carrier state. Gastric acid serves as a host defense mechanism by killing many of the ingested organisms, and intestinal motility is probably also a host defense mechanism. In the absence of or a decrease in gastric acidity (as in infants and the elderly; after gastrectomy, vagotomy, or gastroenterostomy; or with drugs that reduce gastric acidity) and with decreased intestinal motility (as with antimotility drugs), much smaller inocula can produce infection, and the infection tends to be more severe.

Water-borne outbreaks of *Salmonella* infection tend to be caused by smaller inocula of organisms than food-borne outbreaks do. In water-borne outbreaks, as compared with food-borne outbreaks, typhoid fever can occur after longer incubation periods, and the attack rate is lower.

Administration of antimicrobial agents before the ingestion of salmonellae can markedly reduce the size of the inoculum needed to produce infection, presumably by reducing the concentration of protective bowel flora.

Although any *Salmonella* serotype can produce any of the *Salmonella* syndromes (transient asymptomatic carrier state, enterocolitis, enteric fever, bacteremia, and chronic carrier state), each serotype tends to be associated with certain syndromes much more frequently than others. For example, *S. anatum* usually causes asymptomatic intestinal infection, whereas *S. typhimurium* generally causes enterocolitis. *S. choleraesuis* is more likely to produce bacteremia (often with metastatic infection) than asymptomatic infection or enterocolitis, and some serotypes such as *S. typhi* and *S. paratyphi* are most likely to cause enteric fever, as well as the chronic carrier state. Fortunately, most *Salmonella* serotypes are of relatively low pathogenicity for humans; therefore, although food products are commonly contaminated, large outbreaks occur only when more virulent serotypes are involved.

To produce infection, invasion must occur across the mucosa of the intestine. When the organisms reach the lamina propria, an influx of polymorphonuclear leukocytes serves as a host defense mechanism to prevent invasion of the lymphatics. Certain serotypes seem more able than others to invade the lymphatics and subsequently produce bacteremia (e.g., *S. choleraesuis* and *S. dublin,* which commonly produce bacteremia after intestinal infection). Both the small intestine and colon are involved in the inflammatory process.

With *S. typhi* and other causes of enteric fever, salmonellae invade the mononuclear phagocytes in Peyer's patches in the ileum and mesenteric lymph nodes, multiply intracellularly, and are carried through the lymphatic system and blood stream to the liver, spleen, bone marrow, and other parts of the reticuloendothelial system. Once in the reticuloendothelial system, they multiply intracellularly in mononuclear phagocytes and produce the systemic manifestations of enteric fever. The onset of fever is associated with bacteremia and release of cytokines (e.g., tumor necrosis factor and interleukins) from mononuclear phagocytes. Ulcerations over Peyer's patches are responsible for the intestinal manifestations of enteric fever such as pain, perforation, and bleeding.

In *Salmonella* enterocolitis, the organisms remain localized in the intestinal mucosa and diarrhea results from the inflammation produced by polymorphonuclear leukocytes. In addition, watery stools may occur, apparently the result of secretion of water and electrolytes by small intestinal epithelial cells in response to an enterotoxin secreted by some of the *Salmonella* strains or in response to tissue mediators of inflammation.

Patients with diseases that impair host defense mechanisms seem to have an increased frequency of severe *Salmonella* infection. For many years, a striking association has been recognized between diseases producing hemolysis and *Salmonella* bacteremia. Specifically, *Salmonella* bacteremia is common in patients with sickle cell disorders, malaria, and bartonellosis. In fact, because of the frequency of *Salmonella* bacteremia in sickle cell diseases and the underlying bone disease in these patients to which salmonellae localize, these organisms are the most common cause of osteomyelitis in patients with sickle cell disorders. Prolonged *Salmonella* bacteremia occurs in patients with hepatosplenic schistosomiasis, probably related to localization on and in the intravascular schistosomes. Patients with lymphoma and leukemia are also more prone to the development of *Salmonella* bacteremia. A markedly increased frequency and severity of *Salmonella* infections in general have been observed in patients with acquired immunodeficiency syndrome (AIDS). For example, prolonged and recurrent refractory *Salmonella* bacteremia occurs in these patients. Other risk factors that increase the frequency and severity of *Salmonella* infection are extremes of age, immunocompromised states (e.g., from immunosuppressive agents), and probably diabetes.

Clinical Manifestations

Asymptomatic Intestinal Carrier State

The asymptomatic intestinal carrier state may result from inapparent infection (which is the most common form of *Salmonella* infection) or may follow clinical disease (in which case the patient becomes a convalescent carrier). The carrier state is usually self-limited to several weeks to months, with the incidence of positive stool cultures rapidly decreasing over time. By 1 year, far less than 1% of carriers still have positive stools. The major exception is with *S. typhi;* about 3% of those infected excrete the organism for life. Women and older men are those most likely to become chronic carriers of *S. typhi*, related to the presence of biliary tract disease, especially calculi. A patient who has had salmonellae in stool for 1 year (chronic carrier) is likely to become a lifelong carrier with the reservoir in the biliary tree, usually in calculi in the gallbladder. Patients with *Schistosoma haematobium* infections are predisposed to become chronic urinary carriers of salmonellae.

Enterocolitis

After an incubation period, which is usually 12 to 48 hours, the illness starts suddenly with crampy abdominal pain and diarrhea. A chill is common. Although occasional patients have nausea and vomit once or twice, the vomiting is not usually persistent. The diarrhea may be watery and of large or small volume. Stools may contain mucus and are occasionally bloody. Polymorphonuclear leukocytes are present in the stool. Diarrhea may be mild or may be severe with up to 20 to 30 stools a day. Fever is present in most patients, whose temperature may reach 40° C (104° F) or higher. The abdomen is tender to palpation. Transient bacteremia may occur and is most commonly seen in infants, the elderly, and patients with impaired host defense mechanisms.

Symptoms generally improve over a period of days, with fever lasting no more than 2 to 3 days and diarrhea no more than 5 to 7 days. However, these symptoms may occasionally persist for up to 14 days. More severe disease is seen with malnutrition, inflammatory bowel disease, and AIDS. Reactive arthritis may follow enterocolitis in up to 7% of cases. It is especially frequent in those with the HLA-B27 phenotype.

Enteric Fever

Enteric fever is produced by *S. typhi* (typhoid fever) or occasionally by a serotype other than *S. typhi* (most often *S. paratyphi A, S. schottmuelleri*, or *S. hirschfeldii*). On occasion, it may immediately follow classic enterocolitis caused by the same organism. The syndrome is characterized by prolonged sustained fever, relative bradycardia, splenomegaly, rose spots, and leukopenia. The enteric fever produced by serotypes of salmonellae other than *S. typhi* is usually milder than typhoid fever, and the chronic carrier state follows less commonly than after typhoid fever.

Therapy aborts the course of the disease. The following is a description of untreated illness. After an incubation period of 5 to 21 days (generally 7 to 14 days), fever and malaise develop, often associated with cough. A small proportion of patients may have diarrhea during the incubation period. The fever tends to rise in stepwise fashion over the first few days to a week and then becomes sustained, usually at 39.4 to 40° C (103 to 104° F) or higher. Relative bradycardia is seen in up to half of the patients. Apathy, confusion, delirium, and even psychosis may occur. Abdominal distention, pain, and tenderness may occur in the first week and be associated with diarrhea or constipation; these symptoms are generally more pronounced during the second week of fever. Most patients will have abdominal tenderness during the course of the illness.

In about 30% of patients, rose spots develop on the abdomen or chest (or both) toward the end of the first week or during the second week of fever. These spots are faint salmon-colored maculopapular lesions that are subtle and difficult to see, particularly in dark-skinned patients. Salmonellae can be cultured from punch biopsies of these lesions. Hepatosplenomegaly occurs in about half the patients. Leukopenia and neutropenia are seen in about 20%. Abnormal liver function test results are common.

After 2 weeks of illness, the severe complications of intestinal hemorrhage or perforation related to necrosis of Peyer's patches may be observed in about 5% of patients. These perforations may require surgical as well as medical therapy and may occur even in a patient treated with antibiotics. Intestinal perforation is the leading cause of death from enteric fever.

The illness usually resolves by the end of the fourth week in an untreated patient. Relapse may occur in untreated as well as treated patients, but the illness is milder than the original episode.

Rarely, some of the following complications may occur: pancreatitis, cholecystitis, infective endocarditis, pneumonia, hepatic or splenic abscess, orchitis, or focal infection at virtually any site.

Bacteremia

Patients with the syndrome of *Salmonella* bacteremia usually complain of fever and chills lasting days to weeks. Gastrointestinal symptoms are unusual, but in some patients the syndrome of *Salmonella* bacteremia follows classic enterocolitis. Other symptoms are nonspecific, such as malaise, anorexia, and weight loss. Metastatic infection of bones, joints, aneurysms (particularly of the abdominal aorta), meninges (mainly in infants), pericardium, pleural space, lungs, heart valves, cysts, uterine myomas, malignancies, and other sites is common, and symptoms may be related to the site of metastatic infection. Stool cultures are often negative for salmonellae, but blood cultures are positive.

Although any *Salmonella* serotype can produce the syndrome of bacteremia, *S. choleraesuis* and *S. dublin* are most likely to cause this syndrome; more than 50% of *S. choleraesuis* infections are bacteremic.

Salmonella bacteremia occurs with increased frequency in infants and the elderly and in patients with diseases associated with hemolysis (e.g., sickle cell diseases, malaria, and bartonellosis), lymphoma, leukemia, disseminated histoplasmosis, and perhaps systemic lupus erythematosus. Localization to bone is common in patients with sickle cell diseases.

Prolonged *Salmonella* bacteremia lasting for months occurs in patients with hepatosplenic schistosomiasis. In patients with AIDS, recurrent, relapsing *Salmonella* bacteremia may develop that may be difficult to cure with antibiotics.

Diagnosis

Although *Salmonella* enterocolitis is an invasive disease, the differential diagnosis includes all causes of acute diarrhea, including invasive bacteria such as *Campylobacter jejuni, Shigella* species, invasive *Escherichia coli, Yersinia enterocolitica,* and *Vibrio parahaemolyticus;* toxigenic bacteria such as *Vibrio cholerae,* enterotoxigenic *E. coli,* enterohemorrhagic *E. coli* (e.g., *E. coli* O157 : H7), *Staphylococcus aureus, Bacillus cereus, Clostridium perfringens,* and *Clostridium difficile;* viruses; and protozoa such as *Entamoeba histolytica, Giardia lamblia,* and *Cryptosporidium* species. Invasive bacterial causes of diarrhea, enterohemorrhagic *E. coli,* and *C. difficile* infection are also associated with polymorphonuclear leukocytes in stool, whereas bacterial toxigenic causes (other than *C. difficile* and enterohemorrhagic *E. coli*), viruses, and protozoa are generally not. The bacterial toxigenic causes of diarrhea other than *C. difficile* and enterohemorrhagic *E. coli* do not produce fever.

Stool culture is definitive for the diagnosis of *Salmonella* enterocolitis, but by the time that the results of stool culture are available, most patients are recovering. A stained smear of the stool usually demonstrates polymorphonuclear leukocytes. Serologic studies are of little clinical value in *Salmonella* enterocolitis, but they may be of use in epidemiologic studies.

The differential diagnosis of *Salmonella* bacteremia includes all acute infectious and noninfectious causes of fever, including bacteremia caused by other organisms. The diagnosis is proved by isolation of the microorganism from blood or a site of localization.

The differential diagnosis of enteric fever is very broad and depends in part on the area of the world in which the infection was acquired. All causes of sustained fever are in the differential diagnosis, including infective endocarditis, miliary tuberculosis, brucellosis, tularemia, *Mycoplasma pneumoniae* infection, rickettsial infections, and viral infections such as infectious mononucleosis. Depending on the site of acquisition, diseases such as malaria, amebic abscess of the liver, and visceral leishmaniasis enter into the differential diagnosis.

The diagnosis of enteric fever is best proved by isolation of the microorganism from blood, stool, or bone marrow. During the first week of illness, blood cultures are positive in about 90% of patients, but culture positivity decreases over the next 2 weeks to less than 50% during the third week of illness. Stool cultures are usually negative during the first week but by the third week are generally positive. Bone marrow cultures give the highest yield, with up to 95% being positive, and should be obtained in suspected cases with negative blood cultures. Bone marrow cultures may be positive even after several days of antimicrobial treatment, when blood cultures have become negative. Urine cultures and cultures of punch biopsies of rose spots may also be positive. The string test to obtain samples of bile from the duodenum has also yielded positive cultures.

The peripheral leukocyte count is usually normal, but leukopenia, which occurs in about 20%, may be suggestive of enteric fever. Fecal leukocytes are generally present.

The Widal and other serologic tests that detect serum antibodies against *S. typhi* are not very useful clinically because of false-negative and false-positive results. PCR and other molecular techniques are not widely available and are not standardized.

Treatment

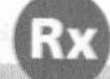

Enterocolitis

The primary approach to treatment of *Salmonella* enterocolitis is fluid and electrolyte replacement. Drugs with antiperistaltic effects such as loperamide or diphenoxylate with atropine can relieve cramps but should be used sparingly because they can prolong the diarrhea.

Salmonella enterocolitis is self-limited, and antimicrobial therapy is not usually indicated. Furthermore, antibiotic therapy has been reported to have little effect on the clinical course and, in some studies, has prolonged the duration that salmonellae are excreted in stool. In addition, most patients are improving by the time that salmonellae or other bacterial pathogens are isolated from stool.

The fluoroquinolones are active against virtually all bacterial pathogens that cause diarrhea (including salmonellae), except for *C. difficile* and many *Campylobacter* organisms. Thus, it is reasonable to use the fluoroquinolones for patients with suspected or known *Salmonella* enterocolitis who are severely ill and suspected of being bacteremic. The threshold for antimicrobial treatment is also decreased in those who are at increased risk for severe illness (e.g., infants, the elderly, patients with sickle cell disease, and immunosuppressed individuals). As an example, in adults, ciprofloxacin, 500 mg every 12 hours orally or 400 mg every 12 hours intravenously for 3 to 5 days or until defervescence, has been widely used. A third-generation cephalosporin such as ceftriaxone is an alternative. In the presence of gross bloody diarrhea, antimicrobial therapy should be withheld until the possibility of *E. coli* O157:H7 infection has been eliminated because antibiotic therapy may increase the frequency of development of hemolytic-uremic syndrome.

Other agents, such as amoxicillin and trimethoprim-sulfamethoxazole, have also been widely used in severely ill adults. However, many strains of *Salmonella* are now resistant to these agents.

Enteric Fever

For many years, chloramphenicol was the drug of choice for the treatment of patients with enteric fever and still is in some developing countries because of low cost. However, in countries where cost is not the major consideration, other agents have largely replaced chloramphenicol because they are probably more effective and do not have the serious bone marrow toxicity of chloramphenicol.

The fluoroquinolones have emerged as the agents of choice for the treatment of enteric fever for several reasons. They are available orally and have high bioavailability, they concentrate in bile and the bowel, and they often retain activity against multidrug-resistant strains of *S. typhi* and other causes of enteric fever. Most importantly, the fluoroquinolones have proved to be effective in the treatment of enteric fever, even with short courses (e.g., 3 to 7 days). Cure rates exceed 95%, and relapse and chronic fecal carriage after therapy are uncommon. Ciprofloxacin (500 mg orally twice a day) or ofloxacin (400 mg orally twice a day) for 7 to 14 days is the treatment of choice for enteric fever. If a patient cannot tolerate oral therapy, the fluoroquinolones can be administered intravenously. Reduced susceptibility to nalidixic acid has been found in strains of *S. typhi* in some developing countries and has been associated with failure of fluoroquinolone treatment. All isolates should be tested in vitro against nalidixic acid, as well as against the fluoroquinolone to be used. If fluoroquinolone resistance is suspected or demonstrated, a third-generation cephalosporin (e.g., intravenous ceftriaxone) is indicated.

Third-generation cephalosporins such as ceftriaxone (intravenously) are reliable agents for the treatment of enteric fever. Ceftriaxone dosed at 1 to 2 g every 12 to 24 hours for adults and 75 mg/kg daily for children given intravenously or intramuscularly for 10 to 14 days results in cure rates of 95%. Resistance to ceftriaxone has been described in clinical strains of *S. typhi,* although this occurs rarely.

Alternative therapies that have been used for the treatment of typhoid fever are chloramphenicol, ampicillin, trimethoprim-sulfamethoxazole, and azithromycin. The chloramphenicol dose is 50 mg/kg/day orally divided into four doses. Chloramphenicol can be given intravenously at the same dose if oral therapy is not possible.

Ampicillin (25 mg/kg intravenously every 6 hours) and trimethoprim-sulfamethoxazole (4/20 mg/kg intravenously or orally every 12 hours) given for 10 to 14 days are other alternative therapies. However, because of the dissemination and spread of multidrug-resistant strains, these agents, as well as chloramphenicol, are not reliable first-line therapies. More recently, azithromycin (10 mg/kg/day orally for 7 days) has been shown to be effective in the treatment of multidrug-resistant strains.

Patients often require supportive care with intravenous saline, correction of electrolyte and acid-base disturbances, and in the setting of intestinal bleeding, blood transfusion. If perforation is suspected, abdominal imaging should be performed to evaluate for free air. If perforation seems likely, laparotomy should be performed as soon as possible to repair the perforation. In the setting of

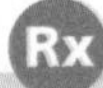

perforation, antimicrobial therapy should be broadened to cover bowel flora.

Steroid therapy has shown to be beneficial in some patients with severe enteric fever and coma, delirium, or shock. Dexamethasone is administered at doses of 3 mg/kg initially, followed by 1 mg/kg every 6 hours for 48 hours. Steroids can mask the signs and symptoms of abdominal perforation and should not be continued for more than 48 hours. Salicylates should be avoided.

Relapses of typhoid fever should be treated with the same antimicrobial regimen as the initial attack.

Bacteremia

The agents of choice to treat *Salmonella* bacteremia are the fluoroquinolones, such as ciprofloxacin, and the third-generation cephalosporins, such as ceftriaxone. Typical doses are ciprofloxacin, 400 mg every 12 hours intravenously, and ceftriaxone, 1 to 2 g every 12 to 24 hours intravenously. When the salmonellae are known to be susceptible, ampicillin, 1 to 2 g intravenously every 4 to 6 hours, or trimethoprim-sulfamethoxazole, 8 mg/kg/day of the trimethoprim component intravenously, can be used. Chloramphenicol is an additional option. Antimicrobial susceptibility testing is necessary because of the emergence of infections caused by salmonellae resistant to fluoroquinolones or third-generation cephalosporins.

In cases of sustained bacteremia, the possibility of endovascular infection should be investigated. For transient bacteremia or bacteremia without localization, therapy is continued for 7 to 14 days. With localization to bone, aneurysms, heart valves, and various other sites, antimicrobial therapy should be given for much longer periods (e.g., 6 weeks). Surgical drainage, removal of foreign bodies, or resection of an aneurysm is often necessary to cure localized infection.

Curing schistosomiasis in patients with *Salmonella* bacteremia may cure the bacteremia. Patients with AIDS tend to relapse repeatedly after treatment courses for *Salmonella* bacteremia. Long-term suppressive therapy has been recommended by some.

Carriers

Chronic carriers (i.e., >1 year) of salmonellae other than *S. typhi* are rare. Stools of convalescent carriers spontaneously become negative over a period of weeks to months, and no therapy should be given. The rare chronic carrier of non–*S. typhi* serotypes (usually infected with *S. paratyphi A, S. schottmuelleri,* or *S. hirschfeldii*) may be treated with amoxicillin, trimethoprim-sulfamethoxazole, or a fluoroquinolone in the doses listed later for 4 to 6 weeks. Patients who experience relapse usually have gallbladder disease (most often calculi) and will not be cured with antimicrobial therapy alone. Cholecystectomy plus antimicrobial therapy may cure these patients, but it is doubtful that the carrier state per se is a sufficient indication for cholecystectomy.

Chronic fecal carriers of *S. typhi* can be treated for 4 to 6 weeks with amoxicillin at doses of 100 mg/kg/day in three to four divided doses, plus probenecid, 30 mg/kg/day in divided doses. Trimethoprim-sulfamethoxazole (160/800 mg twice daily) and ciprofloxacin (750 mg twice daily) are other options. Patients with persistent urinary carriage and *S. haematobium* infection should be treated with praziquantel before eradication of *S. typhi* is attempted. For patients with persistent carriage and anatomic abnormalities (such as gallstones), cholecystectomy combined with antimicrobial therapy is often necessary. For patients with persistent carriage despite adequate antimicrobial therapy and without an identifiable anatomic abnormality, chronic suppressive therapy may be considered. It should be noted that chronic carriers who do not prepare food and who practice adequate personal hygiene do not usually constitute a public health hazard. Therefore, after institution of appropriate personal hygienic precautions, in the absence of evidence of a chronic carrier infecting others, cholecystectomy is probably not indicated to eradicate the carrier state.

Prevention

Salmonella infection is best prevented by properly managing the water supply and sewage disposal, cooking and refrigerating foods, pasteurizing milk and milk products, and handwashing before preparing foods. Careful handwashing after handling animals and uncooked animal products is also important for preventing *Salmonella* infection caused by organisms other than *S. typhi* and *S. paratyphi*. Persons traveling to developing countries should avoid consuming untreated water, including ice, raw vegetables, and fruits. Food should be cooked or peeled and drinks should be boiled, carbonated, or commercially bottled. Despite these precautions, because of the widespread presence of salmonellae in the animal kingdom, it is unlikely that the frequency of *Salmonella* infections will be significantly diminished.

There is no vaccine for *Salmonella* infection other than that for *S. typhi*. Travelers should be vaccinated before going to areas that are endemic for typhoid fever. Two vaccines are available in the United States. One is the typhoid Vi polysaccharide vaccine, which is administered as a single intramuscular injection (0.5 mL or 25 µg), with booster doses given every 2 to 3 years if needed. This vaccine is licensed for persons older than 2 years because children younger than 2 years do not respond reliably with antibody production.

The other licensed typhoid fever vaccine is the live oral attenuated Ty21a vaccine. This vaccine is safe, and revaccination is necessary every 5 years if indicated. The Ty21a vaccine is given as one capsule every other day for a total of four capsules and is licensed for persons older than 6 years. It should not be used in the immunocompromised or persons receiving antibiotics. Both these vaccines confer greater than 75% protective efficacy. These two vaccines have replaced the inactivated whole cell vaccines, which have high rates of adverse effects and reactogenicity.

A newer Vi polysaccharide conjugate vaccine, Vi-rEPA (a conjugate of the Vi polysaccharide of *S. typhi* and a nontoxic recombinant of *Pseudomonas aeruginosa*), has been demonstrated to elicit protective efficacy of approximately 90% in children 2 to 5 years old, but use in children younger than 2 years has not been studied. A live attenuated oral vaccine, M01ZH09, is also being developed.

Vaccines afford only partial immunity to typhoid fever. Persons who have been vaccinated should still restrict their diet to avoid potentially contaminated food and fluids. When cases of imported typhoid in the United States are identified, the local health department should be informed and will monitor stool cultures. Cases of typhoid fever that are acquired in the United States are typically investigated by the public health department to identify potential sources and chronic carriers.

Prognosis

Mortality in patients with *Salmonella* enterocolitis is rare; infants and the elderly are at greatest risk, with death occurring as a result of dehydration and electrolyte imbalance. Mortality from *Salmonella* bacteremia is not uncommon and is most likely to occur in the very young, the very old, and the immunocompromised. *S. choleraesuis* bacteremia has the highest mortality rate (20 to 30% if untreated) of any *Salmonella* serotype.

Before the advent of antibiotic therapy, typhoid fever had a mortality rate of 15 to 20%. This rate has been reduced to less than 1% in industrialized countries. However, the mortality rate remains as high as 30 to 50% in some areas of developing countries. In a treated patient, the temperature usually returns to normal after 3 to 5 days of therapy.

In the preantibiotic era, 5 to 10% of patients who recovered from typhoid fever had relapses. Relapses continued to occur in 10 to 15% of patients treated with chloramphenicol, ampicillin, and trimethoprim-sulfamethoxazole but seemed to be much less frequent in those treated with ceftriaxone and fluoroquinolones (<5%). Intestinal bleeding or perforation occurs in about 5% of patients. With perforation, mortality rates of 10 to 30% have been reported. Up to 3% of patients recovering from *S. typhi* infection become chronic fecal carriers.

SUGGESTED READINGS

Bhan MK, Bahl R, Bhatnagar S, et al: Typhoid and paratyphoid fever. Lancet 2005;366:749–762. *A comprehensive review of typhoid and paratyphoid fever.*

Centers for Disease Control and Prevention: Outbreak of multidrug-resistant *Salmonella typhimurium* associated with rodents purchased at retail pet stores—

United States, December 2003–October 2004. MMWR Morb Mortal Wkly Rep 2005;54:429–433. *A report of an outbreak of salmonellosis related to pet hamsters.*

Huang DB, DuPont HL: Problem pathogens: Extra-intestinal complications of *Salmonella enterica* serotype *typhi* infection. Lancet Infect Dis 2005;5:341–348. *A review of the involvement of extraintestinal sites in typhoid fever.*

Su LH, Chiu CH, Chu C, Ou JT: Antimicrobial resistance in nontyphoid *Salmonella* serotypes: A global challenge. Clin Infect Dis 2004;39:546–551. *A review of the emerging problems with antimicrobial resistance of* Salmonella.

Swanson SJ, Snider C, Braden CR, et al: Multidrug-resistant *Salmonella enterica* serotype *typhimurium* associated with pet rodents. N Engl J Med 2007;356:21–28. *Pet rodents probably are an underrecognized source of human Salmonella.*

Thaver D, Zaidi AK, Critchley J, et al: Fluoroquinolones for treating typhoid and paratyphoid fever (enteric fever). Cochrane Database Syst Rev 2005;(2): CD004530. *Fluoroquinolones have emerged as the agent of choice for the treatment of enteric fever.*

von Seidlein LV: The need for another typhoid fever vaccine. J Infect Dis 2005;192:357–359. *A review of available typhoid vaccines and vaccines under development.*

330 SHIGELLOSIS

Marcia B. Goldberg

Definition

Shigellosis ("bacillary dysentery") is an acute infectious colitis that involves predominantly the rectosigmoid colon. Clinical disease is characterized by diarrhea that is frequently grossly bloody, abdominal cramping, tenesmus, and fever.

The Pathogen

The etiologic agents of shigellosis are enteric gram-negative bacilli of the family Enterobacteriaceae and the genus *Shigella.*

Epidemiology

Each year in the United States, shigellae are estimated to cause 450,000 cases of diarrhea, with approximately 5 cases reported per 100,000 individuals. The number of reported cases is a gross underestimation of the prevalence of disease because most cases do not result in medical evaluation with diagnostic stool culture. Worldwide, shigellae are an important cause of diarrhea and dysentery. They are classified into four species, *Shigella dysenteriae* 1 (group A), *Shigella sonnei* (group D), *Shigella flexneri* (group B), and *Shigella boydii* (group C), that are distinguished by antigenic and biochemical characteristics. In industrialized countries, the majority of infections are due to *S. sonnei,* with the remainder being due to *S. flexneri;* in developing countries, *S. dysenteriae* 1 is also a frequent cause of illness. Disease caused by *S. boydii* is rare.

Humans are the only natural reservoir of *Shigella* sp. Infection occurs after the ingestion of as few as 10 to 100 organisms, whereas for most other enteric pathogens, the minimum inoculum is at least 2 orders of magnitude higher. Consequently, unlike most other enteric pathogens, intermediate replication of *Shigella* in contaminated food or water is not required for the inoculum to be sufficient to cause disease. In 80% of cases, spread is thought to be directly from person to person via the fecal-oral route. In the remainder, spread is thought to be via contaminated water or food; the frequency of spread by contaminated water or food appears to be increasing. Several common-source outbreaks have been traced to raw vegetables or cold salads, such as potato or macaroni salad, thought to be contaminated by a food handler who was infected with *Shigella* or at a food preparation facility with substandard hygiene. Several common-source outbreaks have occurred on cruise ships.

Infection by *Shigella* sp is most prevalent in young children, with more than half of all cases in the United States occurring in children younger than 4 years. As a result of the low infectious inoculum, transmission occurs readily under conditions of crowding or suboptimal hygiene, such as daycare centers or institutional living situations, and the secondary infection rate among family members is near 20%. As for many food- and water-transmitted enteric infectious diseases, disease is more common in late summer and early fall.

Pathobiology

Shigellae are nonflagellated organisms that cause disease by entering into and spreading through the colonic epithelium. The bacteria induce their own uptake into epithelial cells, reside within the cytoplasm of these cells, and use cellular factors to spread directly into adjacent cells. Initial uptake by *Shigella* is frequently by colonic microfold cells (M cells), which overlie lymphoid follicles present throughout the intestine. Consequently, *Shigella*-induced ulcerations are often found to overlie lymphoid follicles in the rectosigmoid colon. When taken up by macrophages, shigellae induce cellular apoptosis, thereby leading to death of infected macrophages. The process of entry and spread of *Shigella* induces the release of host pro-inflammatory mediators, and an intense acute inflammatory response develops.

Most of the *Shigella* proteins that mediate these events are encoded on a large virulence plasmid that is found in all pathogenic shigellae, the presence of which distinguishes *Shigella* sp from the genetically similar organism *Escherichia coli.* Critical to pathogenesis is a 32-kilobase virulence plasmid locus that encodes the structural components of a specialized secretion apparatus. This secretion apparatus enables extracellular bacteria in proximity to mammalian cells to introduce bacterial effector proteins directly into the cytoplasm of these cells. A subset of these effector proteins, also encoded on the virulence plasmid, induce changes in the cellular actin cytoskeleton that lead to cellular uptake of the bacterium. Others effectors induce the cellular inflammatory response that enhances the process of infection. In addition, depending on the species, proteins that contribute to virulence are also encoded on one to several chromosomal loci. *S. dysenteriae* 1 is the only species of *Shigella* that carries the genetic locus encoding Stx toxin (formerly designated Shiga toxin), although all species encode at least one other less pathogenic enterotoxin.

Clinical Manifestations

Disease caused by shigellae is characterized by frequent small-volume diarrhea that is often grossly bloody and may contain mucus, as well as by abdominal cramping, tenesmus, and fevers to 101° F or higher. Symptoms develop an average of 3 days (range, 1 to 7 days) after ingestion of the organism (Table 330–1). The patient may be toxic appearing, with hyperactive bowel sounds and abdominal tenderness, particularly in the left lower quadrant. Untreated, the disease is typically self-limited, and resolution of symptoms occurs within 7 days.

Laboratory values may show a marked leukocytosis with the appearance of immature forms. Metabolic abnormalities may also be present. The diagnosis is made by culture of fresh stool, which is generally positive for the organism during the acute phase of infection. Later during infection, the organism may be cultured from material obtained from rectal ulcerations by sigmoidoscopy or colonoscopy. Plating the freshly passed stool as soon as possible after excretion increases the yield from stool culture. Nevertheless, a single stool culture is only 67% sensitive; sensitivity increases if stool cultures are obtained on 3 consecutive days. Identification of the organism from stool culture is routine in most clinical microbiology laboratories. Shigellae enter the blood stream only rarely; therefore, blood cultures are positive in less than 5% of patients.

Detection of leukocytes in a methylene blue–stained preparation of stool is highly suggestive of infection by shigellae, nontyphoidal salmonellae, *Campylobacter* sp, or *Yersinia* sp and is not found in infections with enteroviruses or enterotoxigenic bacteria. Methylene blue analysis involves placing a small amount of fresh stool on a glass slide, adding 2 drops of methylene blue, covering with a coverslip, and examining microscopically.

TABLE 330–1 CLINICAL SYNDROMES AND COMPLICATIONS IN SHIGELLOSIS

Stage	Time of Appearance after Onset of Illness	Symptoms and Signs	Pathology and Pathogenesis
Prodrome	Earliest	Fever, chills, myalgias, anorexia	None or early colitis
Nonspecific diarrhea	0–3 days	Fever, abdominal cramps, loose stool, watery diarrhea, tenesmus	Rectosigmoid colitis with mucosal ulceration, fecal leukocytes
Dysentery	1–8 days	Frequent stools containing blood and mucus, abdominal tenderness, tenesmus, rectal prolapse	Colitis, which may extend to the proximal portion of the colon, crypt abscesses
Acute complications	3–10 days	Dehydration, seizures, bacteremia, leukemoid reaction, intestinal obstruction	Severe colitis, terminal ileitis
Additional acute complications of infection with *Shigella dysenteriae* 1	3–10 days	Toxic megacolon, hemolytic-uremic syndrome	Severe colitis, expression of Stx toxin
Postinfectious syndromes	1–3 weeks	Reactive arthritis, with or without urethritis and conjunctivitis	Reactive inflammation, most common with the HLA-B27 haplotype

Metabolic abnormalities are common, although because stool volume is low, severe dehydration is unusual. Other complications include bacteremia (4% of cases) and, in the setting of severe colonic disease, intestinal obstruction (2.5% of cases) (see Table 330–1). In infection with *S. dysenteriae* 1, toxic megacolon occurs in 3% of cases, and hemolytic-uremic syndrome occurs rarely. Hemolytic-uremic syndrome is caused by Stx toxin, which is expressed by *S. dysenteriae* 1 and by enterohemorrhagic *E. coli;* in the United States, enterohemorrhagic *E. coli* is a much more common cause of this complication. Reactive arthritis is a rare complication that can occur alone or in conjunction with urethritis and conjunctivitis. It develops 1 to 2 weeks after infection. Seventy percent of patients in whom postinfectious reactive arthritis develops are of the HLA-B27 haplotype. In children, additional complications include seizures (5% of cases), which generally occur in the setting of high fever and metabolic abnormalities, and rectal prolapse.

Diagnosis

In patients with fever, abdominal cramps, and diarrhea, the differential diagnosis includes infectious enteritis secondary to *Campylobacter* sp, nontyphoidal *Salmonella* sp, *Yersinia* sp, or *Entamoeba histolytica;* toxin-mediated colitis secondary to toxin-producing *Clostridium difficile;* and inflammatory bowel disease. The diarrhea associated with *Campylobacter* sp is generally profuse and watery, whereas that caused by *Shigella* is small in volume and frequent. Grossly bloody stool is present in most cases of *Shigella* diarrhea, 30% of cases of *Campylobacter* diarrhea, and only rarely in cases of nontyphoidal *Salmonella* diarrhea. The abdominal tenderness that accompanies *Yersinia* enteritis is generally localized to the right lower quadrant, whereas that accompanying *Shigella* enteritis is generally localized to the left lower quadrant. In addition, vomiting is frequently present in *Yersinia* enteritis but rare in *Shigella* enteritis. *C. difficile* colitis usually occurs during or immediately after the administration of antibiotics for another reason. In the absence of fever and the presence of grossly bloody stool, infection by enterohemorrhagic *E. coli* should be considered. While awaiting definitive culture data, a presumptive diagnosis can often be made on clinical grounds.

In the clinical microbiology laboratory, colonies of *Shigella* are readily distinguished from *Campylobacter* sp, *Yersinia* sp, and enterohemorrhagic *E. coli*, but not from *Salmonella* sp, by their growth as lactose-negative colonies on standard indicator media. Additional biochemical tests allow distinction of *Shigella* from *Salmonella* sp. The diagnosis is generally made 48 to 72 hours from the time that the stool cultures are plated. If stool cultures are negative but symptoms persist beyond 5 to 7 days, inflammatory bowel disease should be considered.

Treatment

Rx

Because the infectious inoculum for *Shigella* is only 10 to 100 organisms, it is readily spread from person to person. Moreover, after resolution of symptoms, asymptomatic shedding of the organism occurs for up to 6 weeks in a percentage of convalescent individuals. Therefore, public health guidelines recommend that anyone with a stool culture positive for *Shigella* be treated with a course of antibiotics, even if the individual's symptoms have resolved.

Initiation of antibiotics early in the course of clinical disease reduces the duration of fever and diarrhea by an average of 2 days. Therefore, when *Shigella* is suspected, it is appropriate to begin antibiotics as soon as stool is obtained for culture while awaiting the results of culture. The only exception is when enterohemorrhagic *E. coli* is in the differential diagnosis (see Diagnosis) because with infection by enterohemorrhagic *E. coli,* the administration of trimethoprim-sulfamethoxazole or a β-lactam antibiotic increases the risk for hemolytic-uremic syndrome, a serious and life-threatening complication of this disease. It is at present unclear whether all groups of antibiotics or only a subset of antibiotics increase the risk for hemolytic-uremic syndrome in this setting.

Antimicrobial resistance among *Shigella* isolates is an increasing problem. In the United States, the most recent nationwide susceptibility data, compiled by the National Antimicrobial Resistance Monitoring System for Enteric Bacteria for the period 1999 to 2002, found 78% of isolates resistant to ampicillin, 46% resistant to trimethoprim-sulfamethoxazole, and 38% resistant to both. Though not currently a significant problem in the United States, resistance to fluoroquinolones occurs occasionally among isolates from the Asian subcontinent and Southeast Asia. In view of the increased incidence of antimicrobial resistance, obtaining stool for culture and susceptibility testing of these isolates is important, particularly for infections that might have been acquired in Asia.

Given the observed patterns of antibiotic resistance, if susceptibility of the isolate is unknown, the antibiotic of choice for adults is a fluoroquinolone, such as ciprofloxacin, 500 mg orally twice daily, or levofloxacin, 500 mg/day orally for 3 to 5 days. After oral administration, fluoroquinolones achieve high concentrations in stool and serum and will treat other possible causes of infectious diarrhea, including nontyphoidal *Salmonella* and *Campylobacter* sp, which is particularly useful if the cause is unknown at initiation of therapy. A shorter course of a fluoroquinolone, consisting of one or two

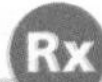

doses only, has been effective in some cases but should not be used for *S. dysenteriae* 1, which requires a full 5-day course. For patients in whom fluoroquinolones should be avoided, azithromycin, 500 mg orally once, then 250 mg/day orally for 4 days, is an effective alternative treatment. If the isolate is known to be susceptible to trimethoprim-sulfamethoxazole or ampicillin, trimethoprim-sulfamethoxazole, 160/800 mg twice daily, or ampicillin, 500 mg orally four times daily for 3 days, is an effective alternative treatment. Ampicillin is preferable to amoxicillin because ampicillin is less rapidly absorbed from the gastrointestinal tract and thereby achieves higher levels in the intestinal lumen. For immunocompromised patients, the course of therapy should be extended to 7 to 10 days. Because of poor efficacy in some studies, oral cephalosporins should not be used as first-line therapy in adults.

For children, if susceptibility of the isolate is unknown, effective oral antibiotics include azithromycin or a fluoroquinolone such as ciprofloxacin. If the child is ill enough to require hospitalization, parenteral ceftriaxone is effective and appropriate. Oral cephalosporins should not be used because some studies indicate limited effectiveness. In infants younger than 1 year, fluoroquinolones should be avoided because of the difficulty of assessing for the rare complication of arthropathy, but in older children a short course is reasonable. In one study, resolution of diarrhea and clearance of *Shigella* from stool occurred more rapidly after treatment with azithromycin than after treatment with oral cefixime. [1] If the isolate is known to be susceptible to trimethoprim-sulfamethoxazole or ampicillin or if the case is part of an outbreak (e.g., at a daycare center) in which another isolate is known to be susceptible to one of these agents, treatment with oral trimethoprim-sulfamethoxazole or ampicillin is effective.

Symptoms generally resolve within 3 to 5 days of initiation of therapy. In the vast majority of cases, treatment leads to cure and clearing of the organism from stool. For certain individuals, particularly those who are food handlers, HIV positive, or elderly or who work in child care, schools, or health care, repeat stool culture should be performed to ensure eradication of the organism. If symptoms do not resolve, one should consider other causes, including inflammatory bowel disease, the manifestations of which can mimic those of shigellosis.

It is unknown whether treatment decreases the incidence of reactive arthritis and its associated illnesses or, in the case of *S. dysenteriae* 1 infection, Stx-mediated hemolytic-uremic syndrome. In enterohemorrhagic *E. coli* infection, the risk for hemolytic-uremic syndrome is increased by treatment with certain antibiotics. There is reason to believe that the same may not hold true for *S. dysenteriae* 1 infection because expression of Stx toxin is under distinct regulatory control in this organism; however, at present there are no data available on this issue.

Because most cases of *Shigella* are acquired by fecal-oral spread, the key to prevention of disease is good personal hygiene. If *Shigella* organisms contaminate hands, washing with warm water and soap will kill them, and those that contaminate dry inert objects survive poorly. Currently, approximately 20% of cases are acquired by the ingestion of contaminated water or food, and this percentage appears to be increasing. Prevention of infection from these sources involves appropriate refrigeration of foods, washing of fresh fruit and vegetables, and adequate cooking or heating of prepared foods and meat.

Daycare center outbreaks are particularly difficult to control. Recommendations for control of these outbreaks include implementation of strict handwashing guidelines, exclusion of infected children from the facility until they recover, and cohorting of convalescent children in a separate room until their stool cultures are negative.

No effective vaccine against *Shigella* is available in the United States currently. Certain candidate vaccines have been shown to protect against infection with a single serotype of *Shigella*, but no multivalent vaccine has yet been proved to be effective. Rifaximin, a nonabsorbable antibiotic, can prevent shigellosis after experimental challenge. [2]

Prognosis

The prognosis is good, with rare cases not responding to antibiotics or experiencing spontaneous resolution of symptoms. If symptoms do not resolve, repeat culture and susceptibility testing are appropriate to verify *Shigella* as the etiologic agent and to ensure that the isolate is susceptible to the antibiotic that is being administered. Forty-one serotypes of *Shigella* exist, approximately 5 of which cause the majority of human infections. Because natural immunity is serotype specific, reinfection with an organism of the same serotype is unusual, but new infection with an organism of another serotype can occur.

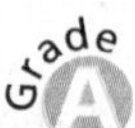

1. Basualdo W, Arbo A: Randomized comparison of azithromycin versus cefixime for treatment of shigellosis in children. Pediatr Infect Dis J 2003;22:374–377.
2. Taylor DN, McKenzie R, Durbin A, et al: Rifaximin, a nonabsorbed oral antibiotic, prevents shigellosis after experimental challenge. Clin Infect Dis 2006;42:1283–1288.

SUGGESTED READINGS

Aragon TJ, Vugia DJ, Shallow D, et al: Case-control study of shigellosis in San Francisco: The role of sexual transmission and HIV infection. Clin Infect Dis 2007;44:327–334. *Among homosexual men, shigellosis is predominantly a sexually transmitted disease, with direct oral-anal contact conferring the highest risk.*

Centers for Disease Control and Prevention (CDC): National Antimicrobial Resistance Monitoring System for Enteric Bacteria. Available at http://www.cdc.gov/narms/. *An online resource on the prevalence of resistance of enteric bacterial pathogens to various antibiotics.*

Centers for Disease Control and Prevention (CDC): Preliminary FoodNet data on the incidence of infection with pathogens transmitted commonly through food—10 states, United States, 2005. MMWR Morb Mortal Wkly Rep 2006;55(14):392–395. *An overview of the epidemiology of diseases caused by enteric pathogens commonly transmitted by food in the United States.*

Gore JI, Surawicz C: Severe acute diarrhea. Gastroenterol Clin North Am 2003;32:1249–1267. *A comprehensive review of acute diarrhea.*

Gupta A, Polyak CS, Bishop RD, et al: Laboratory-confirmed shigellosis in the United States, 1989–2002: Epidemiologic trends and patterns. Clin Infect Dis 2004;38:1372–1377. *An overview of the epidemiology of* Shigella *infection in the United States.*

Klein EJ, Boster DR, Stapp JR, et al: Diarrhea etiology in a children's hospital emergency department: A prospective cohort study. Clin Infect Dis 2006;43:807–813. *The epidemiology of diarrhea in children treated in an emergency department in the United States.*

331 BRUCELLOSIS

Robert A. Salata

Definition

Bacteria of the genus *Brucella* cause disease with protean manifestations. Infection is transmitted to humans from animals as a consequence of occupational exposure or ingestion of contaminated milk products. Despite the attempt to institute effective control measures, brucellosis remains a significant health and economic burden in many countries.

The Pathogen

Brucellae are slow-growing, small, aerobic, nonmotile, nonencapsulated, non–spore-forming, gram-negative coccobacilli. *Brucella abortus, Brucella suis, Brucella melitensis,* and *Brucella canis* are known to infect humans and are typed on the basis of biochemical, metabolic, and immunologic criteria. DNA hybridization analysis shows a high degree of homology between strains.

Epidemiology

Etiology

There are differences in virulence among the four species. *B. abortus,* with a reservoir in cattle, is usually associated with mild to moderate sporadic disease; suppurative or disabling complications are rare. *B. suis* infection, resulting from swine contact, is often associated with destructive, suppurative lesions and may have a prolonged course. *B. melitensis*, with a reservoir in sheep and goats, may cause severe, acute disease and disabling complications. *B. canis*, spread to humans from infected dogs, causes disease with an insidious onset, frequent relapse, and a chronic course that is indistinguishable from that of infection related to *B. abortus*. Studies indicate that there are two new species, *Brucella pinnipediae and Brucella cetaceae*, related to seals and cetaceans, respectively. Two cases of human marine-associated *Brucella* spp infection have been reported.

Incidence and Prevalence

More than 500,000 cases of brucellosis are reported yearly to the World Health Organization from 100 countries. *B. melitensis* infection accounts for the majority of cases, distributed primarily in the Mediterranean region (particularly Spain and Greece), Latin America, the Arabian Gulf, and the Indian subcontinent. *B. abortus* infection occurs worldwide but has been effectively eradicated in several European countries, Japan, and Israel. *B. suis* occurs mainly in the midwestern United States, South America, and Southeast Asia, whereas *B. canis* infection is most common in North America, South America, Japan, and Central Europe. Identification of the *Brucella* species recovered in humans can provide clues to the likely source of infection.

In animals, brucellosis is a chronic infection that persists for life. In association with effective control programs in animals, human brucellosis has decreased dramatically in the United States, from over 6000 cases in 1947 to fewer than 200 cases per year since 1980. States reporting the greatest number of cases include Texas, California, Virginia, and Florida. In North America, brucellosis occurs mainly in spring and summer and is most common in men, usually related to occupational exposure.

Brucella infection in the United States occurs mostly through direct contact with animals or their secretions in high-risk groups, including slaughterhouse workers, farmers and dairymen, veterinarians, travelers to endemic areas, and laboratory workers handling the organisms. More than one half of reported cases occur in the meat-processing industry, particularly in the kill areas, where infection is spread through abraded or lacerated skin and the conjunctiva, possibly by aerosolization, and rarely by ingestion of infected tissue. Many cases of *B. abortus* infection in veterinarians have accidentally resulted from the strain 19 vaccine used to immunize cattle. *B. melitensis* infection, transmitted through the ingestion of goat's milk cheese, has been seen in U.S. travelers to and immigrants from Mexico. Brucellosis contracted abroad may not become symptomatic until the patient returns to the United States. Although persons with human immunodeficiency virus (HIV) infection are at risk for intracellular pathogens, the clinical manifestations of brucellosis in HIV-infected and noninfected individuals are similar in the few cases reported.

Brucellosis in children accounts for only 3 to 10% of all reported cases worldwide, is common in endemic areas (may account for 20 to 25% of cases), and is often a mild, self-limited process. Infection occurs most frequently in school-aged children and in familial outbreaks. No convincing evidence exists to associate *Brucella* infection with abortion in humans.

Pathobiology

Pathogenesis

After penetrating the epithelial cells of human skin, conjunctiva, pharynx, or lung, *Brucella* organisms initially induce an exuberant polymorphonuclear neutrophil response in the submucosa. After ingestion of organisms by neutrophils and tissue macrophages, spread to regional lymph nodes occurs. If host defenses within the lymph nodes are overwhelmed, bacteremia follows. The usual incubation period between infection and bacteremia is 1½ to 3 weeks. Bacteremia is accompanied by phagocytosis of free *Brucella* organisms by neutrophils and localization of bacteria primarily to the spleen, liver, and bone marrow, with the formation of granulomas.

If the inoculum is large and the patient receives no treatment, large granulomas may form, suppurate, and serve as a source of persistent bacteremia with the potential for multiorgan spread. The primary virulence factor of *Brucella* appears to be cell wall lipopolysaccharide.

Both virulent and attenuated strains of *Brucella* are readily phagocytized by neutrophils after opsonization with normal human serum. Whole bacteria and extracts of *Brucella* species may inhibit neutrophil oxidative burst activity and degranulation. Intracellular killing of ingested bacteria has been demonstrated with *B. abortus* but not *B. melitensis;* this may explain differences in pathogenicity between these species. The major cell wall antigen and virulence factor of *Brucella* is the smooth lipopolysaccharide (S-LPS), containing A and M antigens, which also dominates antibody production.

Immunity

Humoral factors may be important in the host defense against *Brucella*. Even in the absence of specific agglutinating antibody, normal human serum is bactericidal for *Brucella* organisms; *B. abortus* is more susceptible to serum lysis than *B. melitensis*. The intracellular location within macrophages of the organism may provide a means for the bacteria to escape the lethal effects of serum. Specific serum agglutinating antibody has opsonic activity but does not correlate with the development of protective immunity.

A role for mononuclear phagocytes and cell-mediated immunity in brucellosis has been demonstrated. Protection against *Brucella* infection in animals is associated with preceding infection with *Listeria monocytogenes* or *Mycobacterium tuberculosis*, both of which stimulate cell-mediated immune mechanisms. Skin testing with *Brucella* proteins elicits a typical delayed hypersensitivity response in infected individuals. Macrophages, activated with T helper 1–type cytokines (e.g., interferon-γ, tumor necrosis factor-α, interleukin-1, and interleukin-12), kill *Brucella*.

Clinical Manifestations

Clinically, human brucellosis may be conveniently, but arbitrarily, divided into subclinical illness, acute or subacute disease, localized disease and complications, relapsing infection, and chronic disease (Table 331–1).

Subclinical Illness

Detected only by serologic testing, asymptomatic or clinically unrecognized human brucellosis often occurs in high-risk groups, including slaughterhouse workers, farmers, and veterinarians. More than 50% of abattoir workers and up to 33% of veterinarians have high anti-*Brucella* antibody titers but no history of recognized clinical infection. Children in endemic areas frequently have subclinical illness.

Acute and Subacute Disease

After an incubation period of several weeks or months, acute brucellosis may occur as a mild, transient illness (with *B. abortus* or *B. canis*) or as an explosive, toxic illness with the potential for multiple complications (with *B. melitensis*). Approximately 50% of patients have an abrupt onset over days, whereas the remainder has an insidious onset over weeks. Symptoms in brucellosis are protean and nonspecific. More than 90% of patients experience malaise, chills, sweats, fatigue, and weakness. More than 50% of patients have myalgias, anorexia, and weight loss. Fewer patients complain of arthralgias, cough, testicular pain, dysuria, ocular pain, or visual blurring. Likewise, few localizing physical signs are apparent. Fever, with temperatures often greater than 39.4° C (103° F), occurs in 95% of patients. An undulating or intermittent fever pattern is unusual. A relative pulse temperature deficit may occur. Splenomegaly is present in 10 to 15%, and lymphadenopathy occurs in up to 14% (axillary, cervical, and supraclavicular locations are most frequent, related to hand wound or oropharyngeal routes of infection); hepatomegaly is less frequent. Other laboratory findings in acute or subacute disease may include mild anemia, lymphopenia or neutropenia (especially with bacteremia), lymphocytosis, thrombocytopenia, or (rarely) pancytopenia. The majority of infected individuals recover completely without sequelae if the diagnosis is appropriately made and prompt therapy is initiated.

Localized Disease and Complications

Brucella organisms may localize in almost any organ but most commonly localize in bone, joints, central nervous system (CNS), heart, lung, spleen, testes, liver, gallbladder, kidney, prostate, and skin. Localized disease may occur simultaneously at multiple sites. Localized complications most often appear in association with a more chronic course of illness, although complications may occur with acute disease caused by *B. melitensis* or *B. suis*. In the United States, localized disease is most frequently related to *B. suis*.

TABLE 331–1 CLINICAL CLASSIFICATION OF HUMAN BRUCELLOSIS

	Duration of Symptoms before Diagnosis	Major Symptoms and Signs	Diagnosis	Comments
Subclinical		Asymptomatic	Positive (low titer) serology, negative cultures	Occurs in abattoir workers, farmers, and veterinarians
Acute and subacute	Up to 2–3 mo and 3 mo to 1 yr	Malaise, chills, sweats, fatigue, headache, anorexia, arthralgias, fever, splenomegaly, lymphadenopathy, hepatomegaly	Positive serology, positive blood or bone marrow cultures	Presentation can be mild, self-limited *(B. abortus)* or fulminant with severe complications *(B. melitensis)*
Localized	Occurs with acute or chronic untreated disease	Related to involved organs	Positive serology, positive cultures in specific tissues	Bone/joint, genitourinary, hepatosplenic involvement most common
Relapsing	2–3 mo after initial episode	Same as acute illness but may have higher fever, more fatigue, weakness, chills, and sweats	Positive serology, positive cultures	May be extremely difficult to distinguish relapse from reinfection
Chronic	Longer than 1 yr	Nonspecific presentation but neuropsychiatric symptoms and low-grade fever most common	Low titer or negative serology, negative cultures	Most controversial classification; localized disease may be associated

Relapsing Infection

Up to 10% of patients with brucellosis experience relapses after antimicrobial therapy. Relapses occur usually 3 to 6 months after completion of therapy but may be seen up to 2 years after treatment. Relapses are associated frequently with antimicrobial resistance as well as the intracellular location of the organisms, which protects the bacteria from certain antibiotics and host defense mechanisms. Relapsing infection is difficult to distinguish from reinfection in high-risk groups with continued exposure. Studies have shown that relapses are associated with inappropriate or insufficient antimicrobial therapy, positive blood cultures on initial presentation, and an acute onset of disease.

Chronic Disease

Disease with a duration of more than 1 year has been called chronic brucellosis. A majority of patients classified as having chronic brucellosis really have persistent disease caused by inadequate treatment of the initial episode, or they have focal disease in bone, liver, or spleen. About 20% of patients diagnosed as having chronic brucellosis complain of persistent fatigue, malaise, and depression; in many aspects this condition resembles the chronic fatigue syndrome. These symptoms frequently are not associated with clinical, microbiologic, or serologic evidence of active infection and may represent a preexisting psychoneurosis.

Diagnosis

Culture

Many more common illnesses mimic the clinical presentation of brucellosis. The most conclusive means of establishing the diagnosis of brucellosis is by positive cultures from normally sterile body fluids or tissues. Rates of positive cultures have ranged from 15 to 90% depending on the methods employed and specimen type. The culture of *Brucella* organisms is potentially hazardous to laboratory personnel.

In acute brucellosis, positive blood cultures are obtained in 10 to 30% of cases (as high as 85% with *B. melitensis*). Blood culture positivity decreases with increasing duration of illness. With *B. melitensis* infection, bone marrow cultures are of higher yield than blood cultures. Blood processed in radiometric detection or isolator systems may yield positive cultures in less than 10 days. With localized brucellosis (e.g., lymph nodes, spleen, liver, or skeletal system), cultures of purulent material or tissues usually yield *Brucella* organisms. Culture of cerebrospinal fluid is positive in 45% of patients with meningitis. Antibody against *Brucella* may be demonstrated in cerebrospinal fluid by enzyme-linked immunosorbent assay (ELISA).

Standard Tube Agglutination

Most patients mount significant serologic responses to *Brucella* infections. The most frequently used test is the standard tube agglutination (STA) test, measuring antibody to *B. abortus* antigen. A four-fold or greater rise in titer to 1 : 160 or higher is considered significant. A presumptive case is one in which the agglutination titer is positive (1:160) in single or serial specimens, with symptoms consistent with brucellosis. By 3 weeks of illness, more than 97% of patients demonstrate serologic evidence of infection. This test equally detects antibodies to *B. abortus, B. suis,* and *B. melitensis* but not to *B. canis.* Serologic confirmation of *B. canis* infection requires *B. canis* or *Brucella ovis* antigen. Despite adequate antibiotic treatment, significant STA titers can persist for up to 2 years in 5 to 7% of cases. Because the STA titer may remain elevated, it is not useful in differentiating relapsing infection from other febrile illnesses in patients with past *Brucella* infections. Individuals with subclinical infection may demonstrate significant STA titers. In chronic localized brucellosis, STA titers may appear absent or low owing to a prozone phenomenon. This prozone effect appears to be related to the presence of immunoglobulin G (IgG) or immunoglobulin A (IgA) blocking antibodies; it can be eliminated if dilutions are carried out to at least 1:1280. False-positive STA titers related to immunologic cross-reactivity have been associated with *Brucella* skin testing, cholera vaccination, or infections with *Vibrio cholerae, Francisella tularensis,* or *Yersinia enterocolitica.*

Other Tests

Immunoglobulin M (IgM) is the major agglutinating antibody formed in the first few weeks after infection with *Brucella* organisms; thereafter, IgG levels also rise. The STA test measures both IgM and IgG. With prompt and adequate therapy, IgG antibody levels usually become undetectable after 6 to 12 months. If therapy is given, the patients who develop persistent *Brucella* infection usually maintain elevated IgG agglutinins. Certain newer antibody tests, including an ELISA, are more sensitive and specific than the STA; these methods are becoming more widely employed. Preliminary studies for diagnosis of brucellosis using the polymerase chain reaction with random or selected primers of blood and other fluids or tissues have been promising, but additional evaluation is necessary and access to this diagnostic technology is still limited.

TABLE 331–2 TREATMENT FOR BRUCELLOSIS

	Treatment	Comments
Acute		
With no endocarditis or central nervous system involvement	Doxycycline (200 mg/day) plus rifampin (600 to 900 mg/day) for 6 wk	Treatment of choice by World Health Organization; widely used; low rate of relapse; intramuscular administration of streptomycin may be difficult
	or Tetracycline (2 g/day) for 6 wk plus streptomycin (1 g/day) or gentamicin for 3 wk. *Alternative agents:* chloramphenicol, fluoroquinolones, trimethoprim-sulfamethoxazole, imipenem	Combination therapy still preferred; fluoroquinolones plus rifampin an alternative
In children	Trimethoprim-sulfamethoxazole plus rifampin	
Central nervous system	Doxycycline plus rifampin and trimethoprim-sulfamethoxazole	Third-generation cephalosporin can be substituted if susceptible in vitro
Localized	Surgically drain abscesses plus antimicrobial therapy for ≥6 wk	
Brucella endocarditis	Bactericidal drugs; early valve replacement may be necessary	Possible aortic valve destruction and/or major arterial emboli

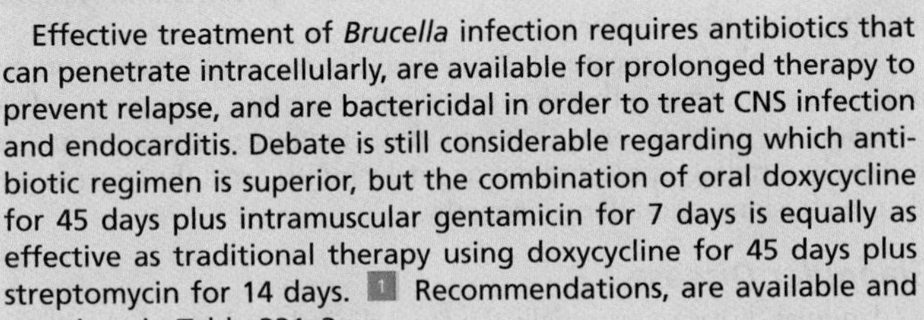

Treatment

Rx

Effective treatment of *Brucella* infection requires antibiotics that can penetrate intracellularly, are available for prolonged therapy to prevent relapse, and are bactericidal in order to treat CNS infection and endocarditis. Debate is still considerable regarding which antibiotic regimen is superior, but the combination of oral doxycycline for 45 days plus intramuscular gentamicin for 7 days is equally as effective as traditional therapy using doxycycline for 45 days plus streptomycin for 14 days. [1] Recommendations, are available and are given in Table 331–2.

Prevention

The control of human brucellosis is related directly to prevention programs in domestic animals and avoiding unpasteurized milk and milk products. In slaughterhouses, important means of prevention include careful wound dressing, protective glasses and clothing, prohibition of raw meat ingestion, and the use of previously infected (immune) individuals in high-risk areas.

Prognosis

Brucellosis appropriately treated within the first month of symptom onset is curable. Acute brucellosis often produces severe weakness and fatigue, and patients are frequently unable to work for up to 2 months. Immunity to reinfection follows initial *Brucella* infection in the majority of individuals. With early antimicrobial therapy, cases of chronic brucellosis or localized disease and complications are rare. Of patients who die of brucellosis, 84% have endocarditis involving a previously abnormal aortic valve, often associated with severe congestive heart failure.

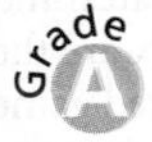

1. Hasanjani Roushan MR, Mohraz M, Hajiahmadi M, et al: Efficacy of gentamicin plus doxycycline versus streptomycin plus doxycycline in the treatment of brucellosis in humans. Clin Infect Dis 2006;42:1075–1080.

SUGGESTED READINGS

Elfaki MG, Uz-Zaman T, Al-Hokail AA, Nakeeb SM: Detection of *Brucella* DNA in sera from patients with brucellosis by polymerase chain reaction. Diagn Microbiol Infect Dis 2005;53:1–7. *Demonstrates the rapid and accurate use of PCR for* B. melitensis *infection.*

Pappas G, Akritidis N, Bosilkovski M, et al: Brucellosis. N Engl J Med 2005;352:2325–2336. *An excellent review.*

Pappas G, Solera J, Akritidis N, Tsianos E: New approaches to the antibiotic treatment of brucellosis. Int J Antimicrob Agents 2005;26:101–105. *Reviews traditional and new antimicrobial regimens utilized in the treatment of brucellosis.*

332 TULAREMIA AND OTHER *FRANCISELLA* INFECTIONS

William Schaffner

Definition

Tularemia is an infectious zoonosis caused by a small aerobic pleomorphic gram-negative bacillus, *Francisella tularensis.* Many animal species may harbor the organism, most prominently rabbits, squirrels, and muskrats. Humans acquire the infection through various means: direct contact with infected animal tissues, ingestion of contaminated water or meat, the bite of an infected tick or deer fly, or breathing an aerosol of bacteria. Although *F. tularensis* is highly infectious and is a well-recognized risk to laboratory personnel manipulating culture plates of the organism, it is a paradox that the illness is not communicable from person to person.

The original description of a typhoidal disease after the ingestion of hare meat was made in Japan in 1837. In the United States in 1906, McCoy was alert to the possibility of outbreaks of bubonic plague after the large earthquake in San Francisco when he came on a plaguelike illness in ground squirrels. His persistent efforts culminated in the first isolation of the responsible organism, which he named *Bacterium tularense* after Tulare County, California, where he had found the ill squirrels. Edward Francis subsequently established that deer flies could transmit the infection from animals to humans and provided detailed descriptions of its clinical manifestations. In recognition, the genus name of the organism was changed to *Francisella.* Colloquially, the disease is often referred to as "rabbit fever" or "deer fly fever."

The Pathogen

The organism occurs in two major subspecies (biovars). *F. tularensis* biovar *tularensis* (type A) is more virulent in animals and humans, has distinctive biochemical reactions (it produces acid from glycerol and has citrulline ureidase activity), and is the common North American biovar. In contrast, *F. tularensis* biovar *holarctica* (type B) is less virulent and occurs commonly in Europe and Asia. Type B is most frequently isolated from rodent species, including muskrats *(Ondatra zibethicus),* mice *(Mus musculus),* beaver *(Castor canadensis),* voles (*Microtus* sp), and water voles *(Arvicola terrestris),* and has been associated with an outbreak of infection in wild-caught prairie dogs. Specific virulence factors for *F. tularensis* have not been identified.

Epidemiology

Tularemia has been reported in the United States, Canada, Mexico, Japan, and Europe, particularly Scandinavia. It has not been reported in the United Kingdom or the Southern Hemisphere. In the United States, reported cases have diminished during the second half of the 20th century from a high of 2291 cases in 1939 to the approximately 125 cases reported annually at present. Tularemia has occurred in all the continental states, but four states account for 56% of reported cases: Arkansas, Missouri, Oklahoma, and South Dakota. The island of Martha's Vineyard off the coast of Massachusetts is also a focus of tularemia.

In the United States, tularemia is usually acquired from tick bites or from contact with infected animals, especially rabbits. Tick-associated cases now constitute the majority and occur during the summer. The most common vectors in the United States are the wood tick *(Dermacentor andersoni),* the dog tick *(Dermacentor variabilis),* and the Lone Star tick *(Amblyomma americanum).* A smaller peak of autumn-winter cases is a consequence of rabbit hunting when hunters skin and eviscerate their game. Public health education materials directed at hunters to reduce the hazard of handling wild animals have contributed to the reduction of tularemia in hunters. Mosquitoes are the common vectors in northern Europe. Occasional individuals acquire infection from the bite of an infected animal or, more likely, from the bite of an animal whose mouth was contaminated from recently eating a diseased animal. The latter probably explains most instances of cat bite tularemia.

Males experience a higher incidence of disease than females do in all age groups, probably as a consequence of their greater exposure to outdoor and animal-related activity and less use of protective measures against tick bites. Persons in all age groups are affected, with children 5 to 14 years of age and older adults most prominently represented. In the United States, American Indians/Alaska natives experience the highest annual incidence (0.5 per 100,000); whites have a lower risk (0.04 per 100,000) and African Americans and Asians/Pacific Islanders the lowest occurrence of tularemia (≤0.01 per 100,000).

Although tularemia is usually a sporadic infection, outbreaks of disease have been traced to laboratory exposure, contaminated ground water, muskrat handling, lawn mowing, and brush cutting. In the latter, primary pneumonic tularemia apparently occurred when the affected individuals created an environmental aerosol by mowing grass and brush that had been contaminated with *F. tularensis* excreted in the urine and feces of infected rodents. The organism can survive in water, mud, and straw for weeks to months.

Recently, interest in tularemia has been enhanced because of its potential use as a bioterrorist agent. Its high infectivity (as few as 10 organisms have induced pneumonic disease), ease of dissemination, and difficulty in rapidly diagnosing acute illness are characteristics that merit its inclusion among threat agents. Thus, tularemia is a disease that is immediately reportable to local public health authorities. Unusual patterns of disease will be investigated for both conventional and bioterrorist sources.

Pathobiology

F. tularensis can infect humans through several portals of entry, including the skin, mucous membranes, and the gastrointestinal and respiratory tracts. It requires intracellular residence and can multiply within macrophages and other cells. After inoculation into the skin and subcutaneous tissue, local bacterial multiplication occurs and evokes a suppurative necrotic reaction characterized by an initial polymorphonuclear response followed by an influx of macrophages and lymphocytes. These suppurative lesions evolve into granulomas. Bacteremia can occur both early and late during this process. The infection can disseminate to the lymph nodes, liver, spleen, lungs, and pleura. Viable *F. tularensis* can persist in tissues for long periods and contribute to the tendency to relapse after treatment.

Clinical Manifestations

Classically, the clinical manifestations of tularemia have been separated into six categories: ulceroglandular, glandular, oculoglandular, typhoidal, oropharyngeal, and pneumonic. Although this classification has historic roots, it ought not be used rigidly because many patients have features of several types. The course of illness is determined by the portal of entry, the degree of systemic involvement, and the dose and virulence of the infecting strain of *F. tularensis.*

The general features of tularemia are similar regardless of the portal of entry. After exposure, the usual incubation period is 3 to 5 days (range, 1 to 21 days). The disease begins abruptly with the onset of fever (≥101° F), chills, malaise, and headache. Myalgia, vomiting, sore throat, and abdominal pain can also occur. Almost half the patients have a pulse rate that is substantially slower than would be anticipated from the height of the fever ("pulse-temperature dissociation"). The fever may abate somewhat after 1 to 3 days, only to recur and continue along with other symptoms for 2 to 3 weeks. Untreated, weight loss, easy fatigue, and lymphadenopathy may persist for weeks longer.

Ulceroglandular Disease

Ulceroglandular disease is the form of the infection most readily recognized by most physicians. Along with fever and other constitutional symptoms, the patient calls attention to tender, swollen lymph nodes that drain an inoculation site. The nodes are usually axillary or inguinal, and a local lesion appears concurrently or just 1 or 2 days before or after the lymphadenopathy. The lesions at the site of inoculation begin as small, red, tender, or painful papules that progress to pustules and then undergo necrosis to produce an ulcer with sharp, somewhat elevated edges and a flat base that becomes black. Untreated, the ulcers heal over a period of weeks and leave a scar. Tick-induced infections produce lesions on the trunk, about the waist, and in the perineum along with the expected local adenopathy. Children typically have occipital and cervical adenopathy from tick bites on the neck and in the hair. Animal exposure often produces lesions on the hands and forearms. Lesions may be multiple. Because the organisms evoke a localized granulomatous response, frank lymphangitis does not occur in uncomplicated tularemia, but an occasional patient manifests a chain of nodules in "sporotrichoid" fashion along the lymphatic drainage.

Patients with such apparently "localized" disease often have symptoms and findings indicating that they actually have a more widespread infection. Sore throat with or without an erythematous pharynx occurs, as well as chest radiographic findings of patchy infiltrates in the lower lobes, pleural effusions, and hilar adenopathy.

Glandular Disease

Glandular disease is essentially the same clinical syndrome but without the local lesion. Thus, the patient has fever, constitutional symptoms, and lymphadenopathy. The local lesion may have been on a part of the body where it was not seen, or it may have been small and already healed when the patient sought medical care. It accounts only for 3 to 20% of cases. Typhoidal disease does not show evidence of lymphadenopathy and is essentially characterized by fever of unknown etiology. These illnesses evade diagnosis unless the physician specifically considers the possibility of tularemia and inquires about tick or animal exposure. Occasionally, the diagnosis is made fortuitously when a positive blood culture is reported.

Oculoglandular Disease

Oculoglandular disease is rare (<5% of cases) and occurs when the conjunctival sac is the portal of entry via an aerosol, splash, or contaminated fingers. It is almost always unilateral and can have a dramatic manifestation with inflamed, swollen eyelids, chemosis, and painful conjunctivitis. The palpebral conjunctiva often shows small yellow nodules and ulcers, counterparts to the skin lesions of ulceroglandular disease. The affected regional lymph nodes are those of the head and neck.

Oropharyngeal Disease

Oropharyngeal disease is also uncommon in the United States and occurs when the mucous membranes of the mouth and pharynx are the portal of entry. Contaminated water or food (inadequately cooked game meat) is the source. Painful exudative pharyngitis and tonsillitis, pharyngeal ulcers, and swollen retropharyngeal and cervical lymph nodes are seen.

Pneumonic Disease

Although other tularemic syndromes may have pneumonia as an aspect of the total illness, *pneumonic tularemia* refers to an illness that is manifested as a distinctive pneumonia. It accounts for about 10% of reported cases and occurs from inhalational exposure. It is the form of the disease that would be the consequence of a bioterrorist event. In addition to fever and malaise, patients may have a dry cough, substernal discomfort, pleural pain, dyspnea, and sore throat. These pulmonary symptoms may not be very prominent in the context of the systemic illness. Hemoptysis is unlikely. The results of physical examination reflect the extent and distribution of the pneumonic process, which may range from barely evident to frank consolidation with pleural effusion. Radiographic findings range from modest peribronchial infiltrates early in the illness to distinctive bronchopneumonia with effusion. Hilar adenopathy is present in more than a third of cases. Sputum examination is not helpful. Pleural effusions generally contain more than 1000 lymphocytes per cubic millimeter. Gram stains are negative and pleural biopsies may occasionally contain granuloma, thus inviting confusion with tuberculosis. Without a suggestive history of tick or animal exposure, patients with tularemic pneumonia may be considered to have poorly responding community-acquired pneumonia. Fluoroquinolone antibiotics have commonly been used as empirical therapy in this circumstance to treat some patients with undiagnosed tularemia pneumonia.

Diagnosis

The diagnosis of tularemia usually involves serologic testing with tube agglutination or microagglutination techniques. Antibody concentrations do not reach diagnostic levels until after the 11th day of illness. A single acute titer of 1:160 is considered presumptive; a confirmed diagnosis requires a fourfold rise in titer between acute and convalescent specimens. Titers of both IgM and IgG antibodies may remain elevated for many years after the illness.

Differential Diagnosis

The differential diagnosis of patients with tularemia is substantial. The local lesions can be confused with cat-scratch disease, brown recluse spider bites, *Mycobacterium marinum* infection, herpes simplex infection, and even syphilis and chancroid when the lesions are in the perineum or on the penis. Pneumonic tularemia resembles common community-acquired pneumonia, as well as less common infections such as psittacosis, legionellosis, and Q fever. The glandular and typhoidal forms can resemble typhoid fever, brucellosis, ehrlichiosis, and other illnesses accompanied by nonspecific fevers.

Routine laboratory studies do not provide specific results. Leukocyte counts may be within normal limits or elevated; thrombocytopenia, elevated liver enzymes, and sterile pyuria occur with some frequency. *F. tularensis* may be isolated from blood cultures and tissue specimens when media containing cysteine are used. Laboratory personnel should be notified when tularemia is suspected so that appropriate media can be used and also to ensure that safeguards are in place to protect against the production of hazardous aerosols.

Treatment

Rx

Because tularemia is a relatively uncommon disease, therapeutic recommendations are based on a combination of in vitro studies and accumulated clinical experience. The preferred antimicrobials are streptomycin or gentamicin, either for 10 days. Streptomycin is given as 1 g intramuscularly twice daily. Gentamicin may be more readily available and is administered at 5 mg/kg intramuscularly or intravenously once daily. Both chloramphenicol and the tetracyclines have been used in the past to treat tularemia; however, use of both of these bacteriostatic agents has resulted in higher rates of relapse than with streptomycin or gentamicin treatment. Because chloramphenicol may produce bone marrow toxicity, it is rarely used today. Doxycycline is administered at 100 mg intravenously twice daily for 14 days. In recent years, ciprofloxacin has been used successfully in a growing number of patients; it is given at 400 mg intravenously twice daily for 10 days. Both these drugs may be switched to oral administration in the same doses as soon as tolerated by the patient.

Primary Prevention

Prevention of tularemia entails minimizing exposure to ticks and avoidance of direct exposure to wild animals. Tick protection includes clothing that extends to the wrists and ankles, regular inspection for attached ticks, and the use of insect repellents containing diethyltoluamide (DEET). Gloves should be worn when skinning and dressing game animals, especially rabbits, and all wild rabbit and other game meats should be cooked thoroughly.

A live, attenuated vaccine has been used in the past to provide some protection to researchers working with *F. tularensis*. The vaccine is not available commercially.

Prognosis

Before treatment became available, acute tularemia often lasted as long as a month with several subsequent months of debility. Mortality approached 10%. When appropriately diagnosed and treated, the mortality from tularemia is now 1% or less.

SUGGESTED READINGS

Eliasson H, Broman T, Forsman M, et al: Tularemia: Current epidemiology and disease management. Infect Dis Clin North Am 2006;20:289–311. *A comprehensive review.*

Ellis J, Oyston PCF, Green M, Titball RW: Tularemia. Clin Microbiol Rev 2002;15:631–646. *A comprehensive introduction to pathogenesis.*

Feldman KA, Enscore RE, Lathrop SL, et al: An outbreak of primary pneumonic tularemia on Martha's Vineyard. N Engl J Med 2001;345:1601–1606. *A clever and rigorous public health investigation of an unexpected outbreak of a rare disease.*

Griffin KF, Oyston PC, Titball RW, et al: *Francisella tularensis* vaccines. FEMS Immunol Med Microbiol 2007;49:315–323. *A review of vaccine research.*

Haristoy X, Lozniewski A, Tram C, et al: *Francisella tularensis* bacteremia. J Clin Microbiol 2003;41:2774–2776. *An excellent example of the precision of modern molecular diagnostic methods.*

Oyston PCF, Sjostedt A, Titball RW: Tularaemia: Bioterrorism defence renews interest in *Francisella tularensis*. Nat Rev Microbiol 2004;2:967–978. *Tularemia in an ominous new light.*

333 PLAGUE AND OTHER *YERSINIA* INFECTIONS

Kenneth L. Gage

The genus *Yersinia* currently contains 11 species, only 3 of which are known to be significant human pathogens (*Y. pestis, Y. enterocolitica,* and *Y. pseudotuberculosis*). The remaining species (*Y. aldovae, Y. bercovieri, Y. frederiksenii, Y. intermedia, Y. kristensenii, Y. mollaretii, Y. rohdei,* and *Y. ruckeri*) are normally considered to be nonpathogenic. Although these minor yersiniae have been identified primarily from environmental samples, they have occasionally been recovered from patient isolates, thus suggesting possible roles as human pathogens.

YERSINIA PESTIS

Definition

Plague is a highly fatal, flea-borne disease that is best known as the cause of the Black Death of the Middle Ages. Its etiologic agent, *Y. pestis,* is a gram-negative coccobacillus belonging to the family Enterobacteriaceae.

The Pathogen

Y. pestis is microaerophilic, nonmotile, and nonsporulating; can exist as a facultative intracellular pathogen; and exhibits bipolar staining with Wayson, Giemsa, or Wright stains (Fig. 333–1). It is fragile outside its hosts or vectors but can be grown within 24 to 48 hours on a variety of bacteriologic media at temperatures ranging from 4 to 40° C. *Y. pestis* lacks a true capsule but has a carbohydrate-protein envelope referred to as the capsular or fraction 1 antigen. Production of this antigen occurs only at temperatures above 33° C. Wild-type strains typically bear three plasmids with sizes of approximately 100 to 110 kilobases (kb), 70 to 75 kb, and 9.5 kb (19 kb if present as a dimer). Although only one serotype is thought to exist, strains can be classified into biotypes. The three classic biotypes (antiqua, mediaevalis, and orientalis) differ in their ability to ferment glycerol and reduce nitrates. All three biotypes occur in Asia, which is generally accepted as the site where plague first evolved. Two biotypes exist in Africa (antiqua and orientalis), but only the orientalis biotype occurs in the Americas. Although these three biotypes have historical and biogeographic significance, all are highly virulent and appear to cause virtually identical signs and symptoms in humans. Recently, a fourth biotype (microtus), which is purportedly nonpathogenic for humans, has been reported from east-central Asia. More modern typing methods, including ribotyping, multiple-locus variable-number tandem repeat assays, and single-nucleotide polymorphism analysis, are useful for molecular epidemiology studies, identification of probable environmental sources of human infection, and phylogenetic analysis.

Epidemiology

Y. pestis is maintained in nature through transmission cycles involving certain rodent species and their fleas, which act as vectors. Although other mammals often become infected with *Y. pestis* and occasionally succumb to plague, the only nonrodent species thought to be important as hosts for infecting vector fleas are some species of rabbits and hares, the steppe pika of central Asia, and the house shrew of southeastern Asia and Madagascar. Rodent-consuming carnivores and raptors might also play indirect roles in spreading plague by transporting infected rodent fleas from one area to another.

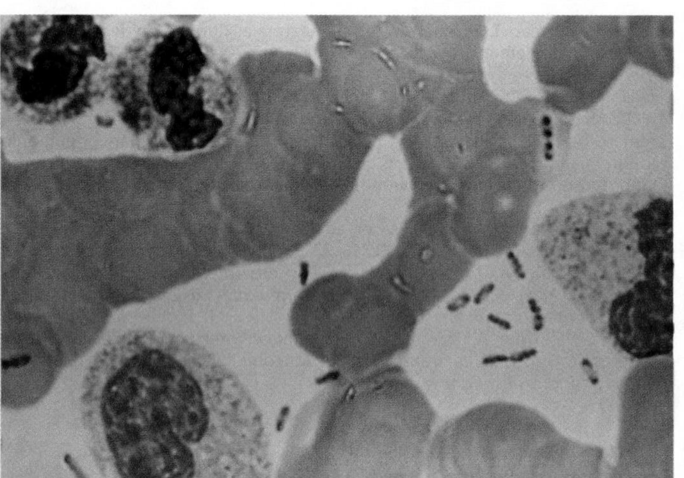

FIGURE 333–1 • Wayson-stained blood smear from a fatal case of human septicemic plague. (Courtesy of Centers for Disease Control and Prevention archives.)

Foci of *Y. pestis* infection occur in rodent populations in many regions of Asia, Africa, and the Americas, although only about 2500 human cases were reported each year to the World Health Organization in the years 1989 to 2003. Most of these cases occurred in Madagascar and other countries in the African region (81.5% of the total). Asian countries reported 14.2% of the total cases; only 4.3% were reported from countries in the Americas, including the United States. Since 1970, evidence of *Y. pestis* infection has been identified in animals or their fleas in 17 western states, and human cases have been identified in 13 of these states (Fig. 333–2).

Humans most frequently acquire plague as a result of being bitten by infectious fleas. On a worldwide basis, the risk of flea bite exposure is highest in poverty-stricken areas that are situated near natural plague foci and have large infestations of commensal rats (*Rattus* sp) heavily infested with fleas, particularly the oriental rat flea (*Xenopsylla cheopis*). *X. cheopis* readily feeds on humans and is an efficient vector of *Y. pestis* to people, as well as rats. Persons are most likely to be bitten by infectious *X. cheopis* when plague epizootics cause massive mortality among susceptible rats, thereby forcing these fleas to seek new hosts. Currently, certain regions of central and southern Africa (including Madagascar), southeastern Asia and India, and a few areas in South America remain at high risk for rat-associated plague outbreaks. The spread of rat-associated plague from one region to another, perhaps by natural movement of rats or transport of these animals along with trade goods, poses the threat that major epidemics will occur in large rat-infested cities. The appearance of bubonic cases acquired via flea bite in large cities also greatly increases the threat that pneumonic plague will develop in untreated bubonic cases and that the infection will spread to others through coughing and expulsion of infectious respiratory droplets (primary pneumonic plague). Though rare in the United States, primary pneumonic plague still poses a threat in developing countries, with outbreaks occurring in the past 15 years in

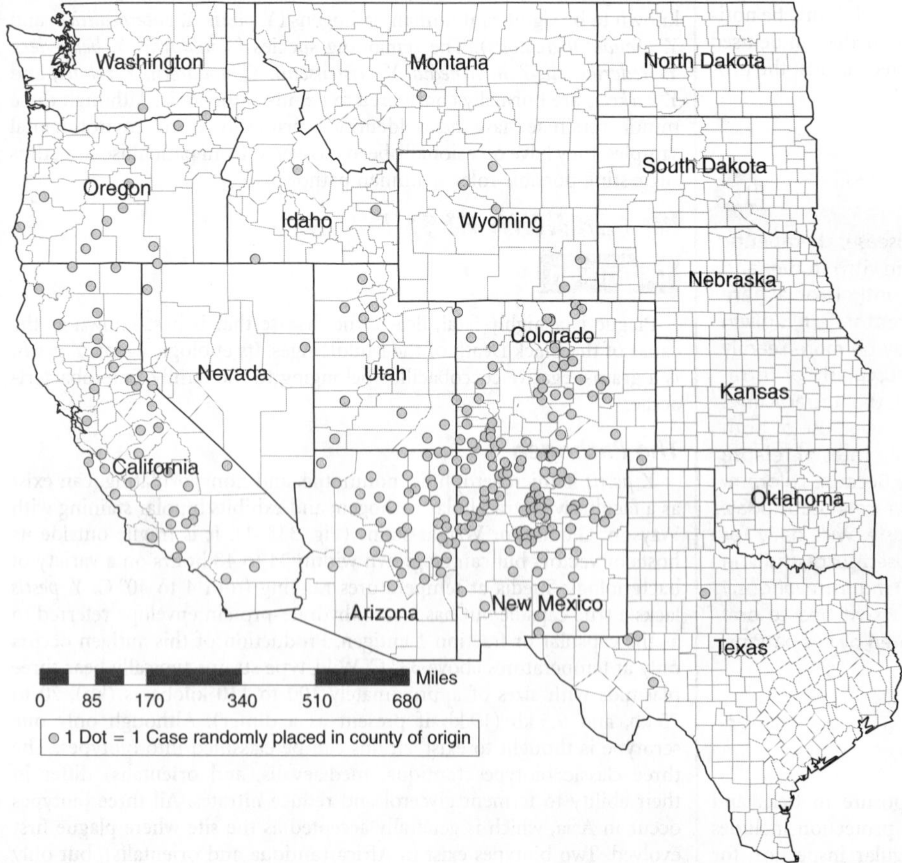

FIGURE 333–2 • Distribution of human plague cases in the United States. Case points were randomly placed within counties where exposures occurred to indicate the general distribution and clustering of cases by region. (Courtesy of John Montenieri, Centers for Disease Control and Prevention.)

India, Ecuador, Madagascar, and probably the Democratic Republic of Congo.

At present, rat-associated plague poses little risk to persons in the United States, with the last cases being reported in 1925. Since that time, most cases have occurred as a result of being bitten by infectious wild rodent fleas (79% in one case series), although a significant number (19%) were also exposed while handling *Y. pestis*–infected animals, including rabbits, domestic cats, wild rodents, and wild carnivores. These direct contact exposures occurred primarily in persons who had been bitten or scratched by infected cats or had skinned infectious rabbits or rodents for meat or certain wild carnivores for their fur. The risk of exposure to infectious wild rodent fleas or animals is typically greatest when epizootics cause high mortality in certain rodent species in the western United States, particularly ground squirrels, prairie dogs, wood rats, and chipmunks. Epizootics appear to progress most rapidly during late spring to early fall, an interval when human cases also peak, probably because these are the periods of greatest flea vector activity. The few human cases reported during the winter months are typically acquired through direct contact with infected animals, and affected individuals have a history of hunting or trapping wild animals or handling domestic cats. The exposure sites for most U.S. cases are peridomestic environments, with smaller numbers of exposures occurring during recreational activities such as hunting or camping. Occupational exposure has also rarely occurred among veterinary staff, biologists, and trappers. Rarely, primary pneumonic plague has been acquired in the United States through inhalation of infectious materials (2% of cases) by means of close face-to-face contact with *Y. pestis*–infected cats that had oral lesions or signs of plague pneumonia, including cough.

Recently, concern has been raised that plague could be used as an agent of bioterrorism (Chapter 19). In most projected scenarios, bioterrorists would spread plague in an aerosol form, potentially resulting in numerous primary pneumonic cases, high mortality, and widespread panic, especially if the *Y. pestis* strains released have been engineered to be resistant to antimicrobial agents commonly used to treat plague.

Pathobiology

Few bacteria can rival the pathogenicity of *Y. pestis* for humans. *Y. pestis* usually enters the body at the site of a flea bite or perhaps as a result of contact between abraded or cut skin and blood or other body fluids from a *Y. pestis*–infected animal. On entering the body, plague bacteria come under attack by host phagocytes and other host defenses. The ability to escape from these defenses and disseminate to regional lymph nodes depends in part on a protease (Pla) that helps degrade fibrin clots and promote the production of excess plasmin that can affect inflammatory exudates, break down extracellular proteins and basement membranes, and reduce levels of chemoattractants, possibly because of inhibition of interleukin-8 production at the site of initial infection. Another virulence factor, YopM, is one of many *Yersinia* outer proteins, or Yops, encoded by genes on the midsized (70 to 75 kb) plasmid of *Y. pestis.* Although most other Yops are degraded by the Pla protease, YopM is resistant to its activity and probably aids in the dissemination of *Y. pestis* by competing with platelets for thrombin, a factor that not only reduces clotting but also inhibits activation of platelets, thereby lowering local inflammatory responses and promoting the dissemination of *Y. pestis* to regional lymph nodes. Initial invasion and dispersal to regional lymph nodes also depend on the ability of *Y. pestis* to survive for at least brief periods in host phagocytes. Survival in such environments is promoted by other Yops that work in concert with a type III secretory apparatus to deliver into host phagocytes those Yops that act as intracellular effectors. These effector Yops disturb the cytoskeletal dynamics of phagocytic cells and block their production of pro-inflammatory cytokines. Affected phagocytes are rendered incapable of killing the invading *Y. pestis,* thereby allowing this bacterium to survive extracellularly in lymphoid tissues. Survival of *Y. pestis* in mammalian hosts also depends on its ability to acquire sufficient quantities of iron for growth. The most important means of iron uptake in *Y. pestis* is a siderophore (yersiniabactin) system that can effectively compete with host iron-binding molecules for this essential nutrient. Although the ability of *Y. pestis* to resist host phagocytic killing and survive intracellularly in phagocytes is thought to be particularly important during the early stages of infection, plague bacteria also express a glycoprotein capsular antigen (caf1 or fraction 1 antigen) that confers resistance to phagocytosis. Expression of caf1 is temperature dependent, being repressed at the cooler temperatures found in the flea vector and upregulated at mammalian host body temperatures.

Infected lymph nodes, termed buboes, can appear edematous and congested early in the course of illness but exhibit little evidence of inflammatory infiltrates or vascular injury. These buboes represent the most obvious manifestation of the lymphatic system's efforts to arrest the spread of *Y. pestis,* and within a few days after infection they contain massive numbers of *Y. pestis* and heavy neutrophil infiltrates, which causes them to swell to the size of a hen's egg and become surrounded by serous fluid. As illness progresses, hemorrhagic necrosis and vascular damage in the node become apparent; some nodes spontaneously rupture, and abscesses appear. Although *Y. pestis* can be present in small quantities in blood samples taken relatively early in the course of infection, large quantities of plague bacteria usually appear in the blood of patients with bubonic plague only after the lymph node defenses are overwhelmed.

As the bacteria escape from the node and proliferate in blood, patients with bubonic plague begin to exhibit evidence of plague septicemia (secondary septicemic plague). Patients with inadequately treated septicemic plague can experience widespread and overwhelming destruction of tissues as *Y. pestis* spreads to various organs, eventually resulting in their failure. Patients who die of plague often experience diffuse interstitial myocarditis, cardiac dilation, diffuse hemorrhagic splenic necrosis, renal glomeruli containing fibrin thrombi, and multifocal necrosis in the liver. Disseminated intravascular coagulation can lead to thrombosis within capillaries, vascular necrosis, ecchymoses, acral gangrene, and cutaneous, mucosal, and serosal petechiae. In a small proportion of cases, septicemia occurs in the absence of buboes or other signs of localized infection, a condition referred to as primary septicemic plague. Septicemic plague can also occur secondarily to primary pneumonic plague.

Rarely, plague can be acquired through the inhalation of infectious respiratory droplets or other materials. These patients with primary pneumonic plague typically experience a rapidly progressing lung infection that is at first lobular, then lobar, and finally multilobar, with large numbers of *Y. pestis* being present in the alveoli and pulmonary secretions of affected sites. Pneumonic plague can also occur secondarily to bubonic or primary septicemic plague. In these instances, *Y. pestis* invades the lungs in a diffuse manner, with most bacilli appearing in interstitial spaces. The most common pathologic findings are edema, diffuse pulmonary congestion, limited neutrophilic infiltration, and hemorrhagic necrosis. Cavitation and liquefaction necrosis can also occur and result in scarring of the lungs, particularly at sites of consolidation.

Clinical Manifestations

The three most commonly observed forms of plague (listed in order of decreasing occurrence) are bubonic, septicemic, and pneumonic. Unusual manifestations of plague include meningitis and pharyngitis. In rare instances, *Y. pestis* has also been inoculated through the conjunctiva, thereby resulting in oculoglandular plague. The incubation period is 2 to 6 days for bubonic plague and 1 to 3 days for primary pneumonic plague.

The characteristic swollen and tender lymph nodes (buboes) of bubonic plague usually appear in the node or nodes located closest to the site of initial infection (Fig. 333–3). Most cases of bubonic plague in the United States are thought to be acquired from flea bites on the legs, as indicated by the appearance of inguinal or femoral lymph node involvement on the side where the flea bite initially occurred. Axillary buboes also commonly occur, often indicating handling of an infected animal or other flea-infested object. Cervical buboes are much less commonly observed in the United States than in many developing countries, perhaps because persons in the latter are more likely to sleep on dirt floors in flea-infested huts, thus increasing the chance that they will be bitten about the head and neck by infectious fleas. Rarely, a skin lesion will appear at the site of an infectious flea bite or other source of inoculation.

Symptoms of bubonic plague include fever, chills, myalgia, arthralgia, headache, malaise, and prostration. Untreated patients with bubonic plague become increasingly toxic, remain febrile, and experience tachycardia, agitation, confusion, delirium, and convulsions.

Septicemic plague is manifested as a rapidly progressive, overwhelming endotoxemia. Patients often complain of gastrointestinal symptoms,

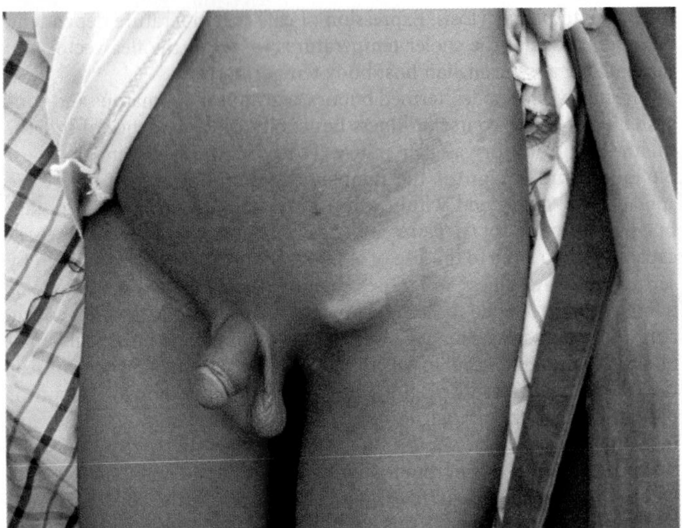

FIGURE 333–3 • Young Malagasy boy with a bubo. (Courtesy of Brook Yockey, Centers for Disease Control and Prevention.)

including nausea, vomiting, diarrhea, and abdominal plain. Disseminated intravascular coagulation can also occur with the appearance of petechiae, ecchymoses, bleeding, and ischemia in the tips of the extremities. Later-stage septicemic patients are likely to experience refractory hypotension, renal shutdown, obtundation, and other signs of shock. Patients with late-stage septicemic plague can also exhibit adult respiratory distress syndrome (Chapter 105), which has occasionally been confused with hantaviral pulmonary syndrome (Chapter 349) in the American Southwest. Because septicemic plague is likely to be fulminant and fatal, favorable outcomes depend on rapid diagnosis and prompt treatment with appropriate antimicrobials.

Pneumonic plague can be accompanied by fever, cough, chest discomfort that becomes increasingly painful, tachycardia, dyspnea, bacteria-laden sputum, chills, fever, headache, achiness, weakness, and dizziness. As the illness progresses, patients can also experience increasing respiratory distress, hemoptysis, cardiopulmonary insufficiency, and circulatory collapse. Patients with primary pneumonic plague in the early stages of illness can have signs of localized pulmonary involvement, beginning in a single lung and rapidly progressing to segmental consolidation and later bronchopneumonia, with death ensuing within 24 hours of the onset of symptoms. Localized infection is unlikely to be observed in the lungs of patients with secondary pneumonic plague because the lung tissues are infected initially through circulatory spread, which results in a diffuse interstitial pneumonitis. The appearance of sputum also differs between primary and secondary pneumonic plague, being watery or mucoid, frothy, and perhaps tinged with blood in primary pneumonic cases but scanter, thicker, and more tenacious in secondary pneumonic cases.

Diagnosis

Plague fatalities are typically related to delays in seeking treatment or misdiagnosis. The differential diagnosis of plague in its various clinical forms includes staphylococcal (Chapter 310) or streptococcal adenitis (Chapter 312) or pneumonia (Chapter 97); cat-scratch disease (Chapter 336); tularemia (Chapter 332); chancroid (Chapter 324); acute filarial lymphadenitis (Chapter 388); mycobacterial infection (Chapter 346); septicemia caused by other bacteria; meningococcemia; bacterial endocarditis; mycoplasmal pneumonia and other community-acquired pneumonias (Chapter 97); legionnaires' disease (Chapter 335); Q fever; influenzal pneumonitis (Chapter 92); hantaviral pulmonary syndrome (Chapter 349); viral pneumonia caused by respiratory syncytial virus (Chapter 385), cytomegalovirus (Chapter 399), or other viruses; and strangulated inguinal hernia.

Laboratory confirmation relies on bacterial culture accompanied by specific bacteriophage lysis tests or detection of a four-fold rise in antibody titer to the *Y. pestis* F1 capsular antigen over a period of 2 to 4 weeks. Although the procedures for obtaining a confirmed laboratory diagnosis of *Y. pestis* infection are relatively simple, confirmation can be delayed because the relevant expertise and reagents are often limited to a few public health or reference laboratories. Because cases of plague can rapidly progress to a life-threatening illness and culture of *Y. pestis* on bacteriologic media can also require 48 or more hours before colonies become visible, it is essential that patients suspected of having plague receive appropriate antimicrobial therapy immediately after samples have been taken. Direct fluorescent antibody assays can be used to identify *Y. pestis* bacteria in bubo aspirates, sputum samples, and tracheal washes; this procedure requires about 1 hour and provides strong presumptive evidence of infection. A presumptive diagnosis can also be obtained rapidly by detecting *Y. pestis* DNA in polymerase chain reaction (PCR) assays or *Y. pestis*–specific antigens in immunologic assays, but these tests are not widely available. Preferred laboratory samples include blood, serum, bubo aspirates, tracheal washes, and swabs of skin lesions or pharyngeal mucosa. Cerebrospinal fluid can also be collected from patients in whom plague meningitis is suspected.

Prevention

No commercially available plague vaccine exists in the United States. Newer recombinant vaccines designed to stimulate immune responses to the F1 and V antigens of *Y. pestis* are undergoing clinical trials and have yielded promising results but are unlikely to be available in the near future.

Human plague risk can be reduced through the implementation of effective surveillance programs to rapidly identify human cases and threatening epizootics. When appropriate, affected areas can be treated with insecticides to reduce the risk for flea bite exposure. Appropriate steps should be taken to reduce the amount of food and shelter available to rodents. In rare instances, rodenticides can be used to reduce host numbers, but their use is not recommended before the implementation of effective flea control measures. Persons living in or visiting areas endemic for plague should also avoid sick or dead animals and use insect repellents to reduce the risk for infectious flea bites. Dogs and cats should be prevented from roaming freely in rodent-infested areas, and these animals should be treated with flea control agents that safely and effectively kill fleas. Although most dogs appear somewhat resistant to plague, cats are highly susceptible, often experience severe illness, and can serve as sources of infection for their owners or veterinary staff. Cats that roam outside in endemic areas and suddenly become seriously ill should be taken to a veterinarian for evaluation.

Persons with pneumonic plague should be held in respiratory isolation for at least 48 hours after the initiation of appropriate antimicrobial therapy, and persons caring for such patients should follow respiratory droplet precautions (mask, gloves, gown, eye protection). Although human-to-human transmission has not been reported in the United States for many decades, rare cases of primary pneumonic plague have occurred after face-to-face contact with infected cats that had oral lesions or symptoms of pneumonic plague. Veterinary staff from plague-enzootic areas should take appropriate precautions (mask, gloves, gown, eye protection) when handling sick cats with illnesses suggestive of plague.

Prophylactic antimicrobial therapy is generally recommended for persons with possible plague exposure only in relatively high-risk situations, such as after close contact with pneumonic plague patients, handling of *Y. pestis*–infected animals, or being bitten by rodent fleas in an area with a recent history of epizootic activity. The most recently recommended prophylactic antimicrobials are doxycycline and ciprofloxacin (Table 333–1).

Treatment

The most commonly recommended agent for treating plague is streptomycin (Table 333–1), but a recently completed randomized trial in Tanzania concluded that gentamicin and doxycycline were effective for treating plague in adults and children and caused few adverse responses. [1] A recent review of human cases treated in New Mexico also strongly suggested that gentamicin is effective and can be substituted for streptomycin. Tetracyclines are effective for

TABLE 333–1 WORKING GROUP RECOMMENDATIONS FOR TREATMENT OF PATIENTS WITH PNEUMONIC PLAGUE IN CONTAINED AND MASS CASUALTY SETTINGS AND FOR POSTEXPOSURE PROPHYLAXIS*

Patient Category	Recommended Therapy
CONTAINED CASUALTY SETTING	
Adults	Preferred choices Streptomycin, 1 g IM twice daily Gentamicin, 5 mg/kg IM or IV once daily or 2-mg/kg loading dose followed by 1.7 mg/kg IM or IV 3 times daily Alternative choices Doxycycline, 100 mg IV twice daily or 200 mg IV once daily Ciprofloxacin, 400 mg IV twice daily† Chloramphenicol, 25 mg/kg IV 4 times daily‡
Children§	Preferred choices Streptomycin, 15 mg/kg IM twice daily (maximum daily dose, 2 g) Gentamicin, 2.5 mg/kg IM or IV 3 times daily¶ Alternative choices Doxycycline If ≥45 kg, give adult dosage If <45 kg, give 2.2 mg/kg IV twice daily (maximum, 200 mg/day) Ciprofloxacin, 15 mg/kg IV twice daily† Chloramphenicol, 25 mg/kg IV 4 times daily‡
Pregnant women¶	Preferred choice Gentamicin, 5 mg/kg IM or IV once daily or 2-mg/kg loading dose followed by 1.7 mg/kg IM or IV 3 times daily‖ Alternative choices Doxycycline, 100 mg IV twice daily or 200 mg IV once daily Ciprofloxacin, 400 mg IV twice daily†
MASS CASUALTY SETTING AND POSTEXPOSURE PROPHYLAXIS**	
Adults	Preferred choices Doxycycline, 100 mg orally twice daily†† Ciprofloxacin, 500 mg orally twice daily† Alternative choice Chloramphenicol, 25 mg/kg orally 4 times daily‡‡
Children§	Preferred choices Doxycycline†† If ≥45 kg, give adult dosage If <45 kg, give 2.2 mg/kg orally twice daily Ciprofloxacin, 20 mg/kg orally twice daily Alternative choice Chloramphenicol, 25 mg/kg orally 4 times daily‡‡
Pregnant women¶	Preferred choices Doxycycline, 100 mg orally twice daily†† Ciprofloxacin, 500 mg orally twice daily Alternative choice Chloramphenicol, 25 mg/kg orally 4 times daily‡‡

*These are consensus recommendations of the Working Group on Civilian Biodefense and are not necessarily approved by the Food and Drug Administration. One antimicrobial agent should be selected. Therapy should be continued for 10 days. Oral therapy should be substituted when the patient's condition improves.
†Other fluoroquinolones can be substituted at doses appropriate for age. The ciprofloxacin dosage should not exceed 1 g/day in children.
‡The concentration should be maintained between 5 and 20 µg/mL. Concentrations greater than 25 µg/mL can cause reversible bone marrow suppression.
§In children, the ciprofloxacin dose should not exceed 1 g/day, and the chloramphenicol dose should not exceed 4 g/day. Children younger than 2 years should not receive chloramphenicol.
¶Aminoglycosides must be adjusted according to renal function. Evidence suggests that gentamicin, 5 mg/kg IM or IV once daily, would be efficacious in children, although this is not yet widely accepted in clinical practice. Neonates up to 1 week of age and premature infants should receive gentamicin, 2.5 mg/kg IV twice daily.
‖In neonates, a gentamicin loading dose of 4 mg/kg should be given initially.
**The duration of treatment of plague in a mass casualty setting is 10 days. The duration of postexposure prophylaxis to prevent plague infection is 7 days.
††Tetracycline could be substituted for doxycycline.
‡‡Children younger than 2 years should not receive chloramphenicol. An oral formulation is available only outside the United States.
Adapted from Inglesby TV, Dennis DT, Henderson DA, et al: Plague as a biological weapon: Medical and public health management. Working Group on Civilian Biodefense. JAMA 2000;283:2281–2290.

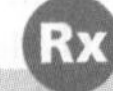

treating uncomplicated cases of bubonic plague, and chloramphenicol is believed to be effective, particularly for plague meningitis. Although antimicrobial resistance is not believed to be a problem in the United States, strains resistant to tetracyclines and other agents have been described occasionally, and resistance to streptomycin and chloramphenicol may also occur. The occasional persistence of *Y. pestis* in necrotic or partially necrotic tissues emphasizes the importance of adequately excising these tissues.

Prognosis

Patients with uncomplicated bubonic plague respond quickly to appropriate antimicrobial therapy and typically defervesce, with relief from most other systemic manifestations within 2 to 5 days. Large buboes can remain swollen, however, for more than a week after the *Y. pestis* infection has been eliminated, and some patients require many weeks of convalescence before feeling fully recovered. In rare instances, ischemic necrosis in septicemic cases has resulted in the amputation of digits.

ENTEROPATHOGENIC YERSINIAE

Definition

Y. enterocolitica and *Y. pseudotuberculosis* differ significantly from *Y. pestis* in that they are enteropathogenic, rarely cause death, and are spread via the fecal-oral route. Like *Y. pestis,* both of these bacteria are gram-negative members of the family Enterobacteriaceae.

The Pathogens

Y. enterocolitica is genetically quite distinct from *Y. pseudotuberculosis* and *Y. pestis;* the plague bacterium is thought to have arisen as a recent clone of *Y. pseudotuberculosis,* and the chromosomal DNA of these two species is extremely similar. All three species share an approximately

70-kb plasmid that encodes for various proteins (Yops) that are key virulence factors. Unlike *Y. pestis,* the enteropathogenic yersiniae are urease positive and motile at temperatures lower than 30° C. *Y. pseudotuberculosis* is rhamnose positive, thereby distinguishing it from the closely related *Y. pestis* and the more distantly related *Y. enterocolitica.* The enteropathogenic yersiniae are genetically more diverse than the more recently evolved plague bacterium. *Y. enterocolitica* contains 6 biogroups and more than 50 serogroups, whereas *Y. pseudotuberculosis* has been classified into six distinct serogroups (O groups 1 to 6).

Epidemiology

Enteropathogenic yersiniae are transmitted via the fecal-oral route, and successful infection of hosts requires large doses of bacteria (median infective dose of 10^8 to 10^9 bacteria). Typical sources of infection include consumption of contaminated foods such as dairy products or inadequately cooked meat. Both *Y. enterocolitica* and *Y. pseudotuberculosis* can survive and proliferate slowly at refrigerator temperatures. Though far less common, person-to-person transmission has been reported, as has transmission via blood transfusion. Pigs, rodents, rabbits, sheep, goats, cattle, horses, dogs, cats, and sometimes birds serve as reservoirs for these yersiniae. Most hosts act as asymptomatic carriers, but a few human cases have been associated with handling sick animals. Symptomatic patients shed large amounts of yersiniae for as long as 2 to 3 weeks. Untreated, infected persons can become carriers and shed for 2 to 3 months.

Yersiniosis is a reportable disease in many countries. Most cases result from *Y. enterocolitica* infection, and this agent reportedly accounts for 1 to 3% of all cases of acute enteritis in some areas. The overall annual incidence rate is about 0.9 cases per 100,000 persons in the United States, but the incidence rates vary among ethnic groups, being highest in African Americans (3.2 cases per 100,000) and lower in Asian Americans (1.5 cases per 100,000), Hispanics (0.6 cases per 100,000), and whites (0.4 cases per 100,000). The highest incidence occurs in African American infants (141.9 cases per 100,000). Regardless of ethnicity, the incidence decreases with age. High rates among African American populations have been associated with home preparations of chitterlings made from contaminated pork intestines.

Y. enterocolitica serotypes O:3, O:8, O:9, and O:5,27 have been associated with human disease. Serotype O:3 predominates in most countries and is found most commonly in swine. Serotype O:9 has been isolated from sheep, cows, and goats. Although serotype O:8 infections appear to be decreasing in incidence in the United States, they are becoming increasingly important in Japan, Italy, and France. In Europe, most cases involve serotype O:3 infections, although a few are associated with serotypes O:9 and O:5,27. Biotype 1A appears to be nonpathogenic, and biotype 5 has been isolated only from hares. Strains pathogenic in humans are esculin, salicin, and pyrazinamidase negative.

Y. pseudotuberculosis has been isolated from rodents, cattle, sheep, cats, dogs, and birds. It occurs worldwide but is most common in northern Europe and Asia, including Japan. O group 1, 2, and 3 strains are associated with human disease, with most cases being attributed to O:1 or O:2 strains. Infected animals serve as chronic carriers and sources for infecting water and food such as meat and dairy products. Some cases have been associated with handling kittens and puppies. A recent outbreak of *Y. pseudotuberculosis* O:3 in Finland was traced to eating iceberg lettuce. A large Canadian outbreak was associated with milk that had been pasteurized but nevertheless became contaminated. Outbreaks in the former Soviet Union have been associated with the consumption of root vegetables that were stored underground for winter consumption and presumably became contaminated with rodent excreta containing *Y. pseudotuberculosis.*

Pathobiology

On reaching the ileum, *Y. enterocolitica* adheres to the mucosa, where intracellular infections in Peyer's patches, mucosal cells, and macrophages can occur. Invasion of the ileal mucosa is favored by the presence of invasin, an outer membrane protein, and a 17-kD surface factor (Ail). An inflammatory response causes abdominal pain and diarrhea, as well as ulcerative ileitis, mesenteric adenitis, and necrosis within Peyer's patches. If the regional defenses are breached, the bacteria can disseminate and cause sepsis and hepatic and splenic abscesses. Polyarthritis can also occur later in the course of illness, particularly in human leukocyte antigen B27 (HLA-B27)–positive individuals.

Like *Y. pestis,* the enteropathogenic yersiniae attack host lymphoid tissues. Invasion of these tissues and resistance against host defenses depend on possession of an approximately 70-kb plasmid that bears genes encoding for various Yops and the so-called V antigen. The products of this plasmid work in concert to inhibit phagocytosis and reduce inflammation, thereby suppressing the host immune response and favoring persistence of these microbes.

Once *Y. enterocolitica* and *Y. pseudotuberculosis* become established in the lymph nodes, they can resist phagocytosis, which allows them to replicate extracellularly and form aggregates in the nodes. The ability to acquire host iron can be a significant factor contributing to the virulence of *Y. enterocolitica* strains. O:8 serotypes, which are virulent for mice, have the *irp2* (iron repressible 2) gene that encodes for a pair of high-molecular-weight outer membrane proteins, whereas the mouse avirulent O:3 and O:9 serotypes lack *irp2.* O:3 and O:9 serotypes typically remained confined to the guts of their hosts, except in situations in which iron overload is present or patients are being treated with an iron chelator.

Patients with reactive arthritis are more likely to have fewer gastrointestinal symptoms, lower T-cell proliferative responses to *Yersinia* antigens, lower initial IgM responses, higher and more persistent IgG and IgA responses, and increased levels of IgA with a secretory component. *Yersinia*-specific antibody responses are also more likely to persist in patients with reactive arthritis than in patients who experience uncomplicated gastrointestinal disease. *Yersinia* antigens thought to contribute to reactive arthritis include Yops and released proteins, which stimulate host CD4 cells, and heat shock protein 60, which has been hypothesized to work in conjunction with other antigens to modulate the host immune response. Evidence exists that hosts can maintain chronic *Y. enterocolitica* infections for years after the initial infection, a factor that may induce the inflammation associated with reactive arthritis.

Clinical Manifestations

After an incubation period of about 3 to 7 days, a gastroenteritis typically develops that can be difficult to distinguish from *Salmonella* (Chapter 329) or *Campylobacter* (Chapter 326) gastroenteritis (Chapter 134). The most common clinical syndromes associated with *Y. enterocolitica* infection are acute enteritis with fever, diarrhea, vomiting, right lower quadrant pain suggestive of appendicitis (Chapter 145), erythema nodosum, and reactive arthritis. Other common symptoms include associated pharyngitis, rash, joint pain, and headache. Stool examination reveals leukocytes or erythrocytes, and a fourth of patients experience bloody diarrhea.

Y. pseudotuberculosis infections are most commonly manifested as acute mesenteric adenitis with diarrhea, fever, vomiting, and bloody stools.

Enterocolitis is most likely to occur in younger children, but older children more frequently experience acute terminal ileitis, mesenteric adenitis, and systemic disease. Pseudoappendicitis has been reported in patients with mesenteric lymphadenitis. Sepsis is uncommon and most likely to occur in persons with underlying conditions such as diabetes mellitus, cirrhosis, immunosuppression, older age, and hemochromatosis. Splenic abscesses, meningitis, or endocarditis can develop in septic patients, and mortality can approach 50%. Erythema nodosum is identified in about a third of all patients and 10% of adults.

Diagnosis

Yersiniosis should be suspected in patients with abdominal pain and fever, especially if living in endemic areas. Diagnosis is best accomplished by isolation of the bacterium from stool, blood, or other appropriate samples. Recovery of *Y. enterocolitica* and *Y. pseudotuberculosis* from clinical and environmental samples can be greatly complicated by the presence of other bacteria that are likely to predominate. The preferred selective agar for isolation from stool specimens is CIN (cefsulodin-irgasan-novobiocin) agar prepared with relatively low cefsulodin concentrations. Isolation of yersiniae is also helped by culture at 25 to 30° C, which results in better growth than when cultures are kept at 35° C and favors growth of the more cold-tolerant yersiniae over other bacteria that require higher temperatures. Once obtained, isolates can be confirmed as enteropathogenic *Yersinia* by biochemical tests. Biotyping and serotyping, which are often available only in research or reference laboratories, can provide useful epidemiologic information. Isolation difficulties and the reported low sensitivity (about 10^3 to 10^6 colony-forming units per gram of sample) of current isolation techniques have led some to suggest that PCR or other DNA-based methods are likely to result in more rapid and sensitive detection of these bacteria.

Tube or microagglutination tests can identify antibodies to the pathogenic *Y. enterocolitica* serogroups O:3, O:9, O:5,27, and O:8, but cross-reactivity can be a problem, particularly between *Y. enterocolitica* O:9 and *Brucella* species. PCR for O-genotyping of *Y. pseudotuberculosis* could eventually replace traditional serotyping methods. Immunologically mediated *Yersinia* illnesses, including reactive arthritis, are associated with the production of IgA antibodies that can be detected by enzyme-linked immunosorbent assay or immunoblotting. IgG antibodies can persist for many years, but persistence of IgA antibodies for more than a few months could indicate a chronic *Yersinia* infection.

Prevention

Prevention depends on measures intended to protect persons from contact with contaminated environments, foods, and wastes: using proper sewage disposal methods, protecting water supplies from contamination with human or animal wastes, following appropriate procedures for animal husbandry and slaughtering, thoroughly cooking meats (especially pork), avoiding long-term storage of meats at 39° F, and consuming only pasteurized milk. Individuals should thoroughly wash their hands after handling potentially contaminated pork or other foods. Diarrheic persons should not work in food-handling areas, care for young children, or work with patients, and hospital staff should follow enteric precautions. Vaccines are not available.

Treatment

Rx

Antibiotics have not been shown to improve the course of uncomplicated enterocolitis or mesenteric adenitis, and the use of antimicrobial therapy is not recommended for intestinal forms of the disease. Such therapy is, however, recommended for immunocompromised patients, patients with septicemia, and those with systemic disease or extraintestinal foci of infection. It should be noted that in vitro susceptibility does not necessarily indicate efficacy in vivo.

Broad-spectrum cephalosporins, sometimes accompanied by aminoglycosides, have been used with successful outcomes in patients with extraintestinal forms of yersiniosis, including septicemia. Ciprofloxacin, cefotaxime, and ceftriaxone are considered the most effective agents for treating *Y. enterocolitica* serogroup O:3 infection. In addition, *Y. enterocolitica* serogroup O:3 and O:9 isolates possess chromosomally determined β-lactamases that can confer resistance to ampicillin, carbenicillin, and cephalothin. Although serogroup O:8 strains, which produce type A β-lactamase, show resistance to the latter two agents, they are susceptible to ampicillin. It has yet to be determined whether antimicrobial therapy is useful for treating immunologically mediated forms of yersinial illness, including reactive arthritis.

Prognosis

Cases of *Y. enterocolitica* enteritis are generally mild and self-limited after a 2- to 3-week course of illness. Sequelae most commonly include reactive arthritis and erythema nodosum. Reiter's syndrome, glomerulonephritis, and myocarditis have also been reported, particularly with serogroup O:3, biotype 4, phage type 8 infections. Other sequelae include endocarditis, pericarditis, and osteitis. *Y. enterocolitica*–induced reactive arthritis, which can appear 1 to 3 weeks after infection, is oligoarticular, asymmetrical, and peripheral; it occurs most frequently in the lower limbs and eventually resolves over a period of a few weeks to months. HLA-B27–positive patients are more likely to experience severe and prolonged arthritis.

Y. pseudotuberculosis infections are also generally mild and self-limited. Reported complications include erythema nodosum, iritis, Reiter's syndrome, arthritis, and nephritis.

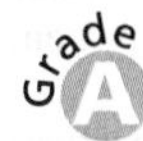

1. Mwengee W, Butler T, Mgema S, et al: Treatment of plague with gentamicin or doxycycline in a randomized trial in Tanzania. Clin Infect Dis 2006;42:614–621.

SUGGESTED READINGS

Boulanger LL, Ettestad P, Fogarty JD, et al: Gentamicin and tetracyclines for the treatment of human plague: Review of 75 cases in New Mexico, 1985–1999. Clin Infect Dis 2004;38:663–669. *A case-based review.*

Koirala J: Plague: Disease, management and recognition of act of terrorism. Infect Dis Clin North Am 2006;20:273–287. *A comprehensive review.*

Perdikogianni C, Galanakis E, Michalakis M, et al: *Yersinia enterocolitica* infection mimicking surgical conditions. Pediatr Surg Int 2006,22:589–592. *A review of 71 cases.*

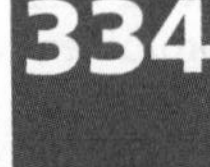

334 WHOOPING COUGH AND OTHER *BORDETELLA* INFECTIONS

Erik L. Hewlett

Definition

Whooping cough, or pertussis, is an acute respiratory illness caused by infection with *Bordetella pertussis* or related members of the genus, especially *Bordetella parapertussis.* The infection can be both endemic and epidemic in a population, and the organism is highly contagious, with spread primarily by large respiratory droplets generated by coughing or sneezing. It is not solely a pediatric illness, and the greatest increases in incidence in recent years have been in adolescents and adults. Although death is rare except in infants, in whom mortality approaches 1% in the United States, worldwide, almost 300,000 people are believed to die of pertussis each year.

The Pathogen

There are now at least eight species of *Bordetella,* but *B. pertussis, B. parapertussis,* and *B. bronchiseptica* (primarily a veterinary pathogen) are most likely to cause respiratory infections in humans. Recently identified *Bordetella* species such as *B. holmesii* and *B. trematum* have been associated with bacteremia and wound infections. The organisms are gram-negative, coccobacillary in shape, and particularly small relative to other gram-negatives. *B. pertussis* was first isolated by Bordet and Gengou in 1906, and the medium used for culture (Bordet-Gengou agar) still bears their names.

Epidemiology

Historically, pertussis was considered a childhood illness and immunity was believed to be lifelong. Hence the disease has not gotten much attention in adult medicine. Furthermore, with the extensive use of pertussis vaccines in the United States and other parts of the world, pertussis was thought to be "controlled" and no longer a problem. However, in 2004, 25,827 cases of pertussis were reported in the United States, the highest number since 1959. Approximately 60% of these cases occurred in adolescents and adults. In fact, seroepidemiologic data suggest that 25% of adolescents and adults with a cough greater than 1 week in duration have pertussis. The disease is endemic in the United States, but epidemics occur every 3 to 4 years.

B. pertussis is highly contagious, with spread believed to be primarily by large droplets. Even though there is no classic "carrier" state, as recognized for many infectious organisms, the organism can be cultured for a brief time even when exposed individuals remain asymptomatic. Although these subjects could, in theory, spread the organism, it is unlikely that they do so to any great extent because they are not coughing. Dissemination in a community is often due to symptomatic adolescents, who spread the organism during school attendance and social events. Health care personnel are also important sources of transmission, and health care–associated outbreaks can affect both vulnerable patients and their care providers.

Before the use of pertussis vaccines most people contracted pertussis during childhood. Immunity after clinical illness is not lifelong, but continued exposure in the population in the prevaccine era allowed individuals to maintain immunity with limited clinical disease. After the introduction of whole-cell pertussis vaccine in the 1940s for infants and children only, there was a marked reduction of disease in the population, particularly in the 1- to 6-year-old group.

Pathobiology

Although *B. pertussis* and related organisms produce a number of interesting toxins and pertussis has been described as a "toxin-mediated" disease, there is not a clear pathophysiologic link between the known virulence factors and clinical manifestations of disease. The infection is localized to the respiratory tract, with organisms adhering to the cilia of ciliated epithelial cells. There is damage to respiratory epithelial cells, some of which are lost from the mucosa. Mucous secretion is prominent, especially during later stages of the illness. Intracellular *B. pertussis* organisms have been demonstrated both in vitro and in samples collected from patients, but the significance of these observations remains unknown. It is not an obligate intracellular organism.

The toxins and adhesins are important both for their potential role in pathogenesis of disease and for their use as antigens in acellular pertussis vaccines. Filamentous hemagglutinin (FHA), pertactin, and fimbriae are adhesins that are components of some of the acellular vaccines, but all currently available vaccines include pertussis toxin (PT). In addition to being an adhesin, FHA has been shown to contain an RGD (arginine-glycine-asparagine–containing sequence) site, interact with the integrin CD11b/CD18 (also known as CR3 or Mac-1), and modulate the functions of cells in the host immune system. PT is a member of the family of adenosine diphosphate–ribosylating toxins that includes cholera toxin and diphtheria toxin, and it has as its intracellular target several guanosine triphosphate–binding proteins such as $G_{i\alpha}$. Although PT causes lymphocytosis and enhances insulin secretion, its target cell or cells and its contribution to the clinical manifestations of pertussis are still a mystery. *Bordetella* also possess an adenylate cyclase (AC) toxin, which is a bacterial AC that enters host cells to produce supraphysiologic levels of cyclic adenosine monophosphate (cAMP). AC toxin acts against phagocytic cells, such as polymorphonuclear leukocytes and alveolar macrophages, whose antibacterial functions are inhibited by the increased cAMP. Additional "toxins" have been identified by virtue of their activities in vitro or in animals, including the tracheal cytotoxin, BrkA, tracheal colonization factor, and heat-labile or dermonecrotic toxin. The relationship of these toxins to disease remains ill defined.

Clinical Manifestations

Although the paroxysmal cough that is classic for pertussis is striking and unforgettable, not all patients experience the typical cough. Infants may have apnea as an early manifestation and only sometimes does the usual cough develop subsequently.

Incubation Period

After exposure to a patient with active pertussis (typically by way of aerosol from coughing), an individual will experience an onset of symptoms after 1 to almost 3 weeks. This relatively long incubation period makes it difficult to track transmission and increases the time necessary for intervention and institution of control measures.

Catarrhal Phase

Importantly, the symptoms that initiate the catarrhal phase (rhinorrhea, increased lacrimation, conjunctival injection, and sometimes low-grade fever) are nonspecific and not ones that suggest pertussis, except in the setting of an ongoing hospital or community outbreak. This phase, which can last as little as a few days or as long as a week, is often associated with the onset of nonproductive cough.

Paroxysmal Phase

It is not until a patient makes the transition to the paroxysmal phase and begins to manifest the typical cough that one is likely to consider the diagnosis of pertussis. This striking cough consists of a series of uncontrollable expirations, followed by gasping inhalation, which depending on the airway anatomy, is responsible for the "whooping" sound. Whoop is more frequent in children than adults. It is not uncommon for each episode of coughing to be associated with cyanosis and end with gagging and vomiting, which in an infant can result in dehydration and malnutrition. The paroxysmal stage can last up to 4 weeks, and the development of fever or worsening pulmonary function during this time should suggest the possibility of secondary pneumonia. Eighty percent or more of adolescents and adults with pertussis have paroxysmal cough, but the frequency of whoop and post-tussive vomiting in this population is quite variable. In addition, during the paroxysmal stage, adults experience symptoms not described in children, such as a scratchy throat, other pharyngeal symptoms, and episodes of sweating.

Convalescent Phase

A reduction in the frequency and severity of coughing attacks marks the transition to the convalescent phase, which can last several months. It is during this time that adults present to the health care system with "chronic cough" and may be evaluated for conditions such as asthma, tuberculosis, other chronic lung diseases, malignancies, and gastroesophageal reflux. After the coughing spells have ended, patients may have return of the paroxysmal cough in conjunction with an unrelated upper respiratory illness; this is often incorrectly interpreted as recurrence of pertussis. Eighty percent of adults with pertussis have an illness of at least 3 weeks' duration, and 27% are still coughing after 90 days.

Complications

In infants and children younger than 5 years, hospitalization is common, 5 to 10% have pneumonia, nearly 1 in 100 infants experiences seizures, and encephalopathy is seen in 0.1%. Pertussis pneumonia in infants and small children can be complicated by pulmonary hypertension. Adolescents and adults have these same complications with lower frequency, but adults can experience other problems associated with underlying medical conditions. For example, there are anecdotal reports of cough syncope, herniated intervertebral disc, sudden-onset hearing loss, angina episodes, and carotid artery dissection.

Diagnosis

Several methods can be used to detect *B. pertussis*, its products, and the host response to them, but each has its limitations. Culture is the "gold standard" (specificity approaching 100% in symptomatic patients), but even with the use of specialized transport medium and a careful, interested laboratory, recovery rates are often less than 50% and are completely dependent on the duration of illness and whether antimicrobial treatment has been initiated before specimen collection. Polymerase chain reaction (PCR)-based diagnostic tests are much more sensitive than culture and can remain positive for several days into antimicrobial treatment. In addition, appropriately designed PCR assays identify and distinguish between *B. pertussis, B. parapertussis,* and *B. bronchiseptica.* There have been, however, several apparent "outbreaks" of pertussis that were later found to represent false-positive PCR results. Detection of serum antibodies to products of *B. pertussis* can be used to identify patients during infection, but care must be taken to distinguish an acute response from residual antibodies to vaccine antigens.

In view of the limitations in resources and equipment for diagnosis of pertussis, the World Health Organization has established a clinical case definition: 21 or more days of paroxysmal coughing with laboratory confirmation or epidemiologic linkage. Though useful for clinical trials, it is now clear that this definition results in cases of lesser severity or shorter duration being missed.

Treatment

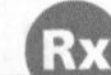

Supportive Therapy

Because infants and young children have the highest risk for complications and death, supportive therapy is often the most important component of their medical care. Close observation (preferably in the hospital) is essential to ensure adequate feeding, oxygenation, and hydration to minimize complications in this age group. None of the pharmacologic interventions that have been tested for amelioration of cough and other symptoms have been found to be effective.

Antimicrobial Agents

There are two purposes for the use of antimicrobials in a patient with pertussis: first, to eliminate the causative organism and reduce transmission and, second, to limit the course of illness in a treated patient by eliminating the infection. Because individuals can remain culture positive and potentially transmit *B. pertussis* for several weeks after the onset of symptoms, it is appropriate to treat patients who are seen within that time frame. Symptomatic relief from antimicrobials is controversial, but it is certainly possible only when treatment is started within the first week of symptoms.

The recommendation of the Centers for Disease Control and Prevention for the treatment of pertussis in adults is azithromycin (500 mg on day 1, followed by 250 mg/day on days 2 to 5), clarithromycin (1 g/day in two divided doses for 7 days), or erythromycin (2 g/day in four divided doses for 14 days) or trimethoprim-sulfamethoxazole (trimethoprim, 320 mg/day, sulfamethoxazole, 1600 mg/day, in two divided doses for 14 days). [1] Treatment with erythromycin for 7 days has now been shown to be as effective as 14 days. The newer macrolides (azithromycin [2] and clarithromycin) are better tolerated, though more expensive.

Prevention

Chemoprophylaxis

Chemoprophylaxis with the aforementioned antimicrobial agents is an important mechanism for controlling outbreaks in hospitals or the community. This approach is effective when initiated before the onset of symptoms and is recommended for individuals exposed within the preceding 3 weeks, high-risk persons with underlying health problems, particularly infants, or those who might have occupational or other contact with susceptible hosts.

Immunization

Attempts to make a vaccine started soon after isolation of *B. pertussis* in the early 1900s, and a killed, whole-cell vaccine was introduced into general use in the late 1940s. Use of that product had a dramatic effect on the incidence of pertussis, with the number of reported cases in the United States falling from more than 200,000 annually to less than 2000 in 1980. In the 1970s and 1980s, with lower rates of pertussis, there was increasing recognition of the adverse events associated with the whole-cell product and public concern for the development of a safer vaccine. The more highly purified acellular pertussis vaccines were designed and are in use today.

Current acellular pertussis vaccines, which contain one or more purified protein antigens (all contain PT and other combinations of FHA, pertactin, and fimbriae types 2 and 3), are administered to infants and children up to the age of 6 years. They have been established to be safe and efficacious and cause significantly fewer adverse reactions than the whole-cell vaccines do. In recognition of the significant incidence of pertussis in adolescents and adults and their role in transmission to infants and small children, several vaccines are now licensed for administration to these age groups. Use of these vaccines is now routinely recommended to boost immunity in adolescents 11 to 18 years old who completed the recommended childhood vaccination series. An important group for whom adult booster immunization is not yet available is pregnant women, who can acquire *B. pertussis* and transmit it to their neonates.

Future work will be directed at improving and standardizing diagnostic methods and increasing vaccine coverage to include pregnant women and other adults.

Prognosis

Most patients will eventually clear *B. pertussis,* even without antimicrobial treatment. In addition, antimicrobials are of limited effectiveness in altering the course of the illness, unless started before the paroxysmal phase.

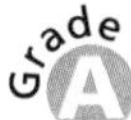

1. Centers for Disease Control and Prevention: Recommended antimicrobial agents for the treatment and post-exposure prophylaxis of pertussis: 2005 CDC guidelines. MMWR Recomm Rep 2005;54(RR-14):1–16.
2. Langley JM, Halperin SA, Boucher FD, et al: Azithromycin is as effective and better tolerated than erythromycin estolate for treatment of pertussis. Pediatrics 2004;111:e96–e101.

SUGGESTED READINGS

Centers for Disease Control and Prevention: Health Topic: Pertussis. Available at http://www.cdc.gov/doc.do/id/0900f3ec80228696. Accessed April 2007. *Extensive compilation of recommendations on all aspects of pertussis from both the National Immunization Program and the National Center for Infectious Diseases.*

Crowcroft NS, Pebody RG: Recent developments in pertussis. Lancet 2006;367: 1926–1936. *A comprehensive review.*

Halperin S: The control of pertussis—2007 and beyond. N Engl J Med 2007;356:110–113. *A concise overview.*

Hewlett EL, Edwards KM: Pertussis—not just for kids! N Engl J Med 2005;32:1215–1222. *Recent summary of clinical pertussis with emphasis on disease in adolescents and adults.*

Mattoo S, Cherry JD: Molecular pathogenesis, epidemiology, and clinical manifestations of respiratory infections due to *Bordetella pertussis* and other *Bordetella* subspecies. Clin Microbiol Rev 2005;18:326–382. *Comprehensive review of the pathophysiology, epidemiology, and clinical diseases of* Bordetella.

Ward JI, Cherry JD, Chang S-J, et al: Efficacy of an acellular pertussis vaccine among adolescents and adults. N Engl J Med 2005;353:1555–1563. *Data illustrating the efficacy of acellular pertussis vaccine in adolescent and adult populations.*

335 *LEGIONELLA* INFECTIONS

Paul H. Edelstein

Definition

Legionellosis is the term used to describe infections caused by bacteria of the genus *Legionella.* The most important of these diseases is pneumonia, called *legionnaires' disease.* Either as part of legionnaires' disease or distinct from it, legionellae may cause infections elsewhere in the body, usually in the form of abscesses. Pontiac fever, which is a self-limited mild febrile illness, is assumed to be caused by legionellae, although this assumption is unproven.

Legionnaires' disease was initially recognized when it caused epidemic pneumonia among members of the American Legion attending a convention in Philadelphia in 1976; this outbreak resulted in 34 deaths and 221 cases of pneumonia. Charles McDade and William Shepard of the U.S. Centers for Disease Control and Prevention determined that the disease was caused by an ostensibly newly discovered bacterium, which was named *Legionella pneumophila* (Fig. 335–1). In retrospect, the first documented epidemic of legionnaires' disease occurred in a meat-packing plant in Minnesota in 1957, and the first recorded isolation of the bacterium took place in 1943.

The Pathogen

More than 50 *Legionella* species have been recognized to date. About half of them have been isolated from patients with legionnaires' disease, and about half have been isolated only from the environment. The *Legionella* species that most commonly cause disease are *L. pneumophila, L. micdadei, L. bozemanae, L. dumoffii,* and *L. longbeachae.* Sixteen serogroups are recognized for *L. pneumophila,* and several other species

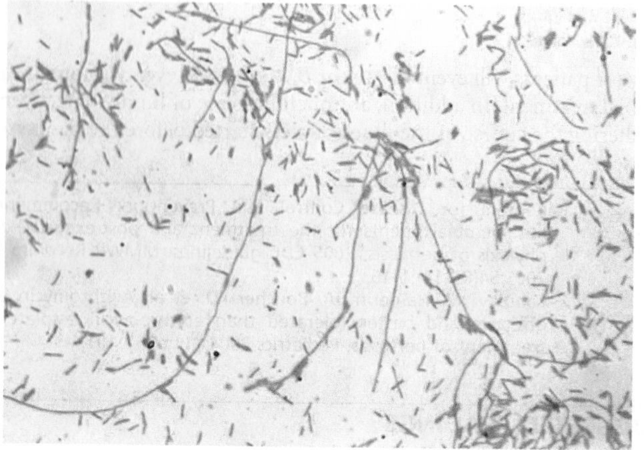

FIGURE 335–1 • *Legionella pneumophila*. Gram-stained micrograph of *L. pneumophila* bacteria growing in culture shows chains and solitary gram-negative bacilli.

contain up to two serogroups. *L. pneumophila* serogroup 1 causes 70 to 90% of cases of legionnaires' disease in nonimmunocompromised individuals. *L. micdadei* is probably the second most common cause of legionnaires' disease and frequently causes legionnaires' disease in immunocompromised patients. All *Legionella* species other than *L. pneumophila* infect mainly immunocompromised patients, with the exception of *L. longbeachae*, a common cause of community-acquired legionnaires' disease in Australia.

Legionellae are small, gram-negative, obligately aerobic bacilli that require complex growth media because of an absolute nutritional requirement for L-cysteine. Optimum growth occurs on buffered charcoal-yeast extract medium but not on conventional bacteriologic media. Their usual habitat is natural and treated waters such as lakes, ponds, and tap water. Legionellae are found in the highest concentration in warm water, especially in water heaters, hot water plumbing fixtures, and cooling towers. They appear to be obligate or facultative parasites of freshwater amebae such as *Hartmannella* and *Acanthamoeba*. Humans are very likely accidental hosts of these bacteria.

A large number of bacterial virulence genes have been identified in *L. pneumophila*, almost all of which control the ability of the bacterium to grow within macrophages. The most important of these virulence genes appear to be the *dot/icm* group.

Epidemiology

Legionnaires' disease occurs worldwide but is primarily a disease found in technically advanced countries. Case reports from underdeveloped countries are rare, perhaps because of limited diagnostic facilities and also perhaps because of the infrequent use of air conditioning and complex plumbing systems. Normal children rarely acquire this disease. Major risk factors for the acquisition of legionnaires' disease are presented in Table 335–1. Legionnaires' disease is an uncommon disease in patients with acquired immunodeficiency syndrome, although they are at increased risk of acquiring the disease. Men contract legionnaires' disease about twice as often as women, although this difference did not hold true for several epidemics of legionnaires' disease. There is emerging evidence that Toll-like receptors (TLRs), which are part of the innate immune system, play a role in human susceptibility to legionnaires' disease. For example, people with TLR-5 mutations may be more susceptible to the disease and those with TLR-4 mutations less susceptible. No good evidence exists for person-to-person spread of legionnaires' disease.

An estimated 8000 to 18,000 cases occur each year in the United States, but only 2 to 10% are reported. Most cases are sporadic; 23% are nosocomial and 10 to 20% can be linked to outbreaks. Outbreaks of the disease have occurred among hotel guests, cruise ship guests, hospital inpatients and outpatients, office building workers, and factory workers. People with occupational water exposure appear to have little, if any increased risk for acquisition of disease.

TABLE 335–1 RISK FACTORS FOR LEGIONNAIRES' DISEASE

ALTERED LOCAL AND SYSTEMIC HOST DEFENSES
Glucocorticosteroid administration or Cushing's disease (5–10)*
Cytotoxic chemotherapy (5)
Cigarette smoking (2–10)
Diabetes (2)
Male gender or age older than 50 years (>2)
Acquired immunodeficiency syndrome (40)
Immune suppressive therapy for solid organ transplantation (>2)
Chronic heart or lung disease (>1)
Renal failure requiring dialysis (20)
Lung or hematologic cancer (especially hairy cell leukemia) (7–20)
INCREASED CHANCE OF EXPOSURE TO ENVIRONMENTAL *LEGIONELLA* BACTERIA
Recent travel away from home (2)
Use of domestic well water (2)
Recent plumbing work in home or at work (2)
Exposure to poorly maintained hot tub spas
Hospitalization

*Numbers in parentheses represent the approximate relative risk of acquiring legionnaires' disease over that for someone without the risk, where estimates are available.

From 1 to 5% of all community-onset pneumonias requiring hospitalization in adults are due to legionnaires' disease. Hospital-onset infections are associated with exposure to contaminated water in the form of an aerosol or in some cases via microaspiration.

Pontiac fever has been recognized primarily as an epidemic illness, with attack rates in excess of 90%. It has been noted to occur in office and factory workers and in recreational bathers using spa or whirlpool-type baths. The disease very likely has a sporadic form, but the lack of specific diagnostic tests makes diagnosis of this form very difficult.

Pathobiology

Legionnaires' disease is acquired by inhaling aerosolized water containing *Legionella* organisms or possibly by pulmonary aspiration of contaminated water. The contaminated aerosols are derived from humidifiers, shower heads, whirlpool baths, decorative fountains, respiratory therapy equipment, industrial cooling water, cooling towers, and other sources of warm water. Aerosols formed by contaminated water in plumbing systems and in cooling towers are the most common sources of infection. Inhaled organisms undergo phagocytosis by pulmonary alveolar macrophages, which are unable to kill the bacteria. The bacteria multiply within the phagosome. Eventually, the multiplying bacteria kill the macrophage, either by inducing apoptosis or by cytotoxicity, and are released extracellularly. The intracellular infection cycle is reinitiated in another macrophage. Continuing bacterial multiplication and consequent lung damage produce symptoms 2 to 10 days after the initiation of infection. Bacterial uptake and multiplication are curtailed by the action of cytokines (e.g., interferon-γ) produced by macrophages and lymphocytes. Natural killer and lymphokine-activated killer cells probably lyse infected macrophages and thereby abort the intracellular infection cycle. The role of polymorphonuclear phagocytes is unclear, although they probably have some part in eliminating bacteria, especially after activation by interleukin-2 and tumor necrosis factor. Antibody appears to have little function in host immunity or defense, whereas T lymphocytes play a major role in the immune process. The actual mechanism of pulmonary damage is not well understood and could be due to bacterial toxins, immune reactions to infection, or both. The bacteria may spread to extrapulmonary sites via the lymphatic system and blood stream; they are probably transported in blood by infected blood mononuclear cells. The mechanism whereby the pneumonia exerts systemic effects is unknown, but it could be the result of disseminated bacterial infection, the effect of toxin, or production of host factors such as tumor necrosis factor. Specific pathologic changes are found only in the lung in the vast majority of fatal cases of legionnaires' disease. Intense inflammation is present in alveoli, alveolar ducts, respiratory bronchioles, and alveolar septa. The inflammatory process consists of bacteria, polymorphonuclear leukocytes, and macrophages. On occasion, pleuritis, pleural empyema, pericarditis, and cavitary lung disease are found. Very rarely, abscess formation occurs outside the chest cavity.

The pathogenesis and cause of Pontiac fever are a mystery. Inhalation of water contaminated with many different types of bacteria, including *Legionella* species, produces the disease. The incubation period of the disease, 12 to 36 hours, is too short to allow bacterial infection and multiplication. It is possible that bacterial or fungal toxins present in the water produce this illness, as has been hypothesized for a closely related disease, "humidifier fever." Recently, high levels of bacterial endotoxin in water have been demonstrated at sites causing Pontiac fever. Another possibility is an immune response to one or more of the multiple microorganisms found in the water. Antibody to *Legionella* species found in contaminated water is present in some disease victims, but it is unclear what this immune response means.

Clinical Manifestations

Legionnaires' disease is manifested as a febrile systemic illness with pneumonia. Several prospective and retrospective studies of patients with different types of pneumonia have shown that legionnaires' disease has few, if any characteristic clinical features and that it cannot be clinically distinguished from pneumococcal pneumonia. However, clinical observations during epidemics of legionnaires' disease have often documented characteristic clinical findings. It is probable that the spectrum of clinical findings is wide, ranging from a "typical" form of legionnaires' disease to one indistinguishable from other causes of pneumonia. This chapter describes the "typical" form of legionnaires' disease, which in reality may be present in a minority of patients. A prodromal illness consisting of malaise, low-grade fever, and anorexia may develop several days before the onset of more severe symptoms. Myalgia, extreme fatigue, and high temperature then develop. Gastrointestinal complaints are common and include generalized or localized abdominal pain, nausea, vomiting, and diarrhea; the diarrhea is generally watery and not dehydrating. Recurrent rigors and prostration may occur. Symptoms referable to the respiratory tract may not develop until later. It is this paucity of respiratory tract symptoms, despite evidence of a systemic febrile illness, that can either be a clue to diagnosis or mislead clinicians. When the patient is pressed for details regarding symptoms, a history of a nonproductive cough or one productive of nonpurulent, sometimes bloody secretions is usually obtained. Production of large amounts of grossly purulent sputum is unusual. Pleuritic chest pain, sometimes in concert with hemoptysis, may occur and can mislead the clinician into considering pulmonary infarction. Mental confusion is commonly reported in some series; obtundation, seizures, and focal neurologic findings may occur less frequently.

Fever is almost uniformly present in cases of legionnaires' disease, although short (days) afebrile periods have been reported in some immunosuppressed patients with *L. micdadei* pneumonia. Chest examination early in the disease may reveal only scattered rales or evidence of pleural effusion. However, later in the course, most patients have the classic findings of consolidating pneumonia. Abdominal examination may reveal generalized or local tenderness and, in rare cases, evidence of peritonitis. Splenomegaly is uncommon. No rash is associated with this disease, except that caused by other factors such as drug therapy. Clinically significant extrapulmonary infection in patients with legionnaires' disease is quite rare, but sinusitis, pericarditis, prosthetic valve endocarditis, peritonitis, dialysis shunt infections, and abscess formation in a variety of tissues and organs have been reported.

Pontiac fever is a nonfatal influenza-like disease, with symptoms of myalgia, fever, headache, and malaise occurring in 60 to 90% of patients. Arthralgia occurs with variable frequency, as do cough, anorexia, and abdominal pain. The illness generally is not sufficiently severe or long in duration to cause most patients to seek medical attention. Not much is known about its physical findings early in the disease; findings after 3 to 5 days of illness are generally normal except for fever and possibly tachypnea. Pneumonia does not occur. The illness lasts about 3 to 5 days, although some patients may have persistent fatigue or nonfocal neurologic complaints for weeks to months afterward.

Diagnosis

The results of multiple nonspecific laboratory tests may be abnormal in patients with legionnaires' disease. These abnormal findings include proteinuria, pyuria, hematuria, leukocytosis, leukopenia, and thrombocytopenia. Disseminated intravascular coagulation may be seen in patients with respiratory failure caused by legionnaires' disease. Hyponatremia, hypophosphatemia, hyperbilirubinemia, and elevated serum alanine transaminase, serum aspartate transaminase, and alkaline phosphatase concentrations may also be found. Elevation of creatine kinase (MM isoenzyme) is common, and myoglobinuria and renal failure develop in some patients. Cerebrospinal fluid is usually normal, although rare patients may have 25 to 100 white blood cells per microliter of cerebrospinal fluid.

Legionnaires' disease can be diagnosed by specific laboratory tests (Table 335–2). The most sensitive test for *L. pneumophila* serogroup 1

TABLE 335–2 SPECIFIC DIAGNOSTIC TESTS FOR *LEGIONELLA*

Type	Suitable Specimens	Sensitivity* (%)	Specificity (%)	Notes
Culture	Sputum, lung, pleural fluid, blood, abscess contents	—	100	Use of special and selective media required; 3–5 days required for growth
Immunofluorescent microscopy	Sputum, lung, pleural fluid, abscess contents	25–75	95–99.9	Species-specific monoclonal antibody available; not helpful for diagnosis of all species; highest specificity for *L. pneumophila;* relative low specificity for other species; 2–3 hr required for testing
Urine antigen detection	Urine	90–95	99.9	Useful only for detection of *L. pneumophila* serogroup 1, the most common cause of legionnaires' disease; 2–3 hr required for testing; may be positive despite antimicrobial therapy
Antibody	Serum	60–70	90–99	Requires testing of paired specimens; seroconversion may not occur until 2–3 mo after infection; most specific for *L. pneumophila* serogroup 1; cross-reactions with antibodies to many other bacteria

*Sensitivity versus culture. Culture is the most sensitive diagnostic technique, but its absolute sensitivity is unknown; reasonable estimates are 50 to 90%. Urinary antigen detection is more sensitive than culture in some circumstances; absolute sensitivity is about 50% in epidemics.

infection is urinary antigen determination. For all other *Legionella* species, the most sensitive and specific test is culture of respiratory tract secretions, such as sputum (Fig. 335–2). Because the infecting type cannot be determined a priori, both urine and culture tests should be performed for maximum sensitivity. Sputum culture for *Legionella* should be performed on every patient suspected of having this disease. Serologic testing is more useful to epidemiologists than to clinicians because of cross-reactions with antibodies to unrelated organisms. Molecular amplification tests, such as polymerase chain reaction (PCR), are used in some research and public health laboratories and produce reliable results, although there are also reports of unreliable or insensitive PCR tests. A recently available commercial PCR assay may prove to be very useful for diagnosis, but this has yet to be proved conclusively. No laboratory test currently available is 100% accurate for the diagnosis of legionnaires' disease. In particular, a negative urine antigen test does not reliably exclude legionnaires' disease when the pretest probability is high; the negative predictive value is approximately 85% when the pretest probability of disease is 25% or greater, but around 97% if the pretest probability is 5% or less. Thus, empirical therapy must be considered in appropriate clinical settings, regardless of negative laboratory test results.

Legionnaires' disease causes alveolar-filling infiltrates that usually eventuate in consolidation. Interstitial infiltrates are rare, although they may occur early in the course of disease and then progress to consolidating infiltrates. The infiltrates may be unilateral or bilateral and can spread very quickly to involve the entire lung. Pleural effusion, generally small in volume, occurs commonly and may be the sole abnormal radiographic finding in early disease.

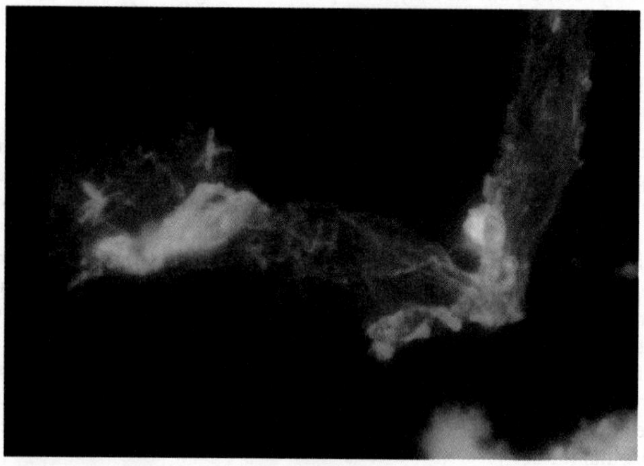

The diagnosis of Pontiac fever is based on demonstration of legionellae in water to which the patient was exposed, significant increases in antibody to the isolated *Legionella* species, and a clinical course compatible with this diagnosis. To be certain about the diagnosis of Pontiac fever, it is almost always necessary to perform extensive studies of unaffected people and their environments because recovery of legionnellae from water and elevated antibodies to *Legionella* are relatively common events. Thus, it is nearly impossible to diagnose nonepidemic cases of Pontiac fever specifically.

FIGURE 335–2 • Diagnosis of *Legionella pneumophila*. The indirect fluorescent antibody test was positive for *L. pneumophila* in the sputum of a patient with legionnaire's disease. (From CDC PHIL.)

Differential Diagnosis

The differential diagnosis of legionnaires' disease is broad because the disease is usually manifested as a nonspecific pneumonia. Mycoplasmal pneumonia is generally much less severe and causes significant respiratory system complaints. Pneumococcal pneumonia, in contrast to legionnaires' disease, is generally responsive to penicillin. Psittacosis and Q fever can have clinical features quite similar to those of legionnaires' disease.

Treatment

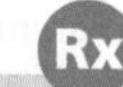

Optimal therapy for patients with community-acquired pneumonia remains controversial, and no survival advantage has been shown when treatment of "atypical pneumonia" is included in the regimen. However, in a recent meta-analysis, treatment of atypical pneumonia was associated with improved clinical outcome when the patient had legionnaires' disease. [1] Empirical treatment of patients hospitalized with community-acquired pneumonia should include coverage for *Legionella* (Chapter 97). Azithromycin or levofloxacin is the drug of choice for this disease, except for mild cases in nonimmunocompromised patients, in whom erythromycin or doxycycline may be used (Table 335–3). Intravenous drug therapy should be given until clinical improvement is seen, which usually occurs in 2 to 4 days. Afterward, oral drug therapy is continued. Mild cases of legionnaires' disease can be treated with oral therapy exclusively. Fluoroquinolone antimicrobials (especially levofloxacin, but also ciprofloxacin or moxifloxacin) and azithromycin are more effective than erythromycin or doxycycline in experimental laboratory studies. Levofloxacin is preferred for organ transplant patients because of its very high activity in experimental legionnaires' disease

TABLE 335–3 ANTIMICROBIAL DRUG THERAPY FOR LEGIONNAIRES' DISEASE

Patient Type	Disease Severity*	First Choices	Dosage	Alternatives	Dosage
Normal host	Mild to moderate	Erythromycin† *or*	500 mg IV, 500 mg PO, each 4 times daily; 14 days	Levofloxacin†‡ *or*	500 mg IV or PO once daily; 7–10 days
		Doxycycline *or*	200 mg IV or PO once daily; 14 days		
		Azithromycin†	500 mg IV or PO once daily; 3 days	Clarithromycin	500 mg PO twice daily *or* 1 g (extended release) once daily; 14 days
	Severe	Levofloxacin†‡	500 mg IV or PO once daily; 7–10 days	Azithromycin†	Same dosage as above; 5 days
Immunosuppressed	Any type	Levofloxacin†‡	Same as above	Azithromycin†	Same dosages as above; 5–7 days

*Severe disease is that causing respiratory failure, bilateral pneumonia, or rapidly worsening pulmonary infiltrates or the presence of at least two of the following three: blood urea nitrogen 30 mg/dL or greater (11 mmol/L), diastolic blood pressure lower than 60 mm Hg, or respiratory rate higher than 30/min.
†Approved by the Food and Drug Administration for the treatment of legionnaires' disease.
‡Acceptable alternatives include ciprofloxacin, 400 mg twice daily intravenously or 500 mg twice daily orally (the dose for severe disease is 750 mg orally twice daily or 400 mg intravenously every 8 hours), and moxifloxacin, 400 mg once daily intravenously or orally for 7 to 14 days.

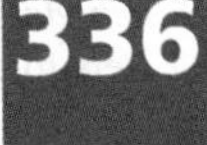

and lack of interference with cyclosporine levels. In addition, most immunocompromised patients and most patients with severe legionnaires' disease should receive levofloxacin or azithromycin rather than erythromycin. Because of its potent activity in experimental legionnaires' disease, many clinicians add rifampin to an erythromycin or doxycycline regimen for the treatment of severe cases of legionnaires' disease; however, no clinical data have indicated the superiority of such combination therapy. The availability of newer and more active drugs makes such combination therapy unnecessary, and there is no good clinical or laboratory evidence that combinations of levofloxacin and azithromycin are superior to either drug alone or that the addition of rifampin to either drug is of benefit. Penicillins, cephalosporins (first, second, and third generation), and aminoglycosides are ineffective for the treatment of legionnaires' disease. In fact, failure of pneumonia to respond to these agents should prompt consideration of legionnaires' disease and perhaps initiation of specific anti-*Legionella* therapy. No effective therapy for Pontiac fever is known.

Prevention

The most important principle for preventing *Legionella* infection is to eliminate exposure to environmental water sources that harbor the organism. Proper cooling tower maintenance, whirlpool and spa cleaning and disinfection, and potable water disinfection are important. Hospitals very often have complex water systems, and thorough assessment of the entire system and remediation are indicated if a nosocomial outbreak is suspected. Isolation precautions are not warranted because person-to-person transmission does not occur.

Prognosis

Most patients with legionnaires' disease respond within 2 to 4 days to specific antimicrobial therapy. The symptoms clearing most rapidly are rigors, mental confusion, myalgia, anorexia, fatigue, and abdominal complaints. Fever may persist for a week after the initiation of therapy but starts a downward trend within a few days. Despite this clinical evidence of improvement, other findings may falsely imply disease progression, such as evidence of increased pulmonary consolidation on physical examination and radiography. A period of weeks to months is required for resolution of the pulmonary infiltrates. Patients with respiratory failure have a relatively poor prognosis and tend to have a much slower response to therapy. The majority of previously healthy people recover from untreated legionnaires' disease after 7 to 10 days of severe illness; those who do not recover die of progressive respiratory and multisystem failure. The fatality rate of untreated legionnaires' disease is about 3 to 30% in nonimmunosuppressed patients, about 40% in most nosocomial infections, and up to 80% in immunocompromised patients.

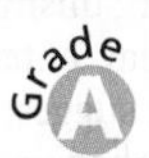

1. Shefet D, Robenshtock E, Paul M, Leibovici L: Empiric antibiotic coverage of atypical pathogens for community acquired pneumonia in hospitalized adults. Cochrane Database Syst Rev 2005;2:CD004418.

SUGGESTED READINGS

Cunha BA: The atypical pneumonias: Clinical diagnosis and importance. Clin Microbiol Infect 2006;Suppl 3:12–24. *A review of the atypical pneumonias.*

Fields BS, Benson RF, Besser RE: *Legionella* and legionnaires' disease: 25 years of investigation. Clin Microbiol Rev 2002;15:506–526. *Comprehensive description of epidemiologic and clinical trends.*

Garcia-Vidal C, Carratala J: Current clinical management of legionnaires' diseae. Expert Rev Anti Infect Ther 2006;4:995–1004. *An excellent review of the management of legionnaires' disease.*

Pedro-Botet L, Yu VL: *Legionella:* Macrolides or quinolones? Clin Microbiol Infect 2006;Suppl 3:25–30. *A review of the ongoing debate of macrolides or quinolones for* Legionella.

336 DISEASE CAUSED BY *BARTONELLA* SPECIES

Craig J. Hoesley and David A. Relman

Definition

The genus *Bartonella* includes at least 24 species or subspecies, but only 10 (*B. henselae, B. quintana, B. bacilliformis, B. elizabethae, B. clarridgeiae, B. vinsonii* subsp *berkhoffii, B. vinsonii* subsp *arupensis, B. washoensis, B. koehlerae,* and *B. grahamii*) have been implicated in human disease. During recent years, an increasing number of distinct *Bartonella* taxa have been identified, particularly in animals, and members of this genus, extended by unification with the genera *Rochalimaea* and *Grahamella* (Fig. 336–1), are considered emerging pathogens in humans.

Three major histologic varieties of disease are attributed to *Bartonella* infection: vasculoproliferative disease, endovascular disease with primary bacteremia, and granulomatous disease. Examples of vasculoproliferative disease include bacillary angiomatosis and peliosis caused by *B. henselae* or *B. quintana,* and verruga peruana, which is a manifestation of chronic *B. bacilliformis* infection. Bacteremia may occur during any form of bartonellosis; however, it is convenient to consider the specific disorders of the endovascular compartment in which bacteremia is a dominant feature separately: trench fever (caused by *B. quintana*), infective endocarditis (caused by *B. henselae, B. quintana, B. elizabethae, B. vinsonii* subsp *berkhoffii,* and *B. koehlerae*), and Oroya fever (caused by *B. bacilliformis*). *B. henselae* also causes the granulomatous disorder known as cat-scratch disease, which primarily affects the lymph nodes but can sometimes cause systemic complications. *B. clarridgeiae* has been implicated as a cause of cat-scratch disease in a small number of individuals, and *B. grahamii* DNA was detected in the aqueous humor of a single patient with neuroretinitis.

The state of host immune competence plays an important role in determining which of these disparate forms of pathology become manifested during *Bartonella* infection. For example, *B. henselae* usually causes bacillary angiomatosis in immunocompromised individuals and cat-scratch disease in immunocompetent hosts. Genetic differences between *Bartonella* species or strains may also account for differences in tissue tropism, pathogenicity, and host response. *B. quintana* and *B. henselae* are equally likely to cause the cutaneous lesions of bacillary angiomatosis, but *B. quintana* is more likely to induce subcutaneous or osseous lesions, whereas *B. henselae* is almost exclusively implicated in disease of the liver, spleen, and lymph nodes.

B. henselae and *B. quintana* have each been cultivated directly from and detected in tissues affected by bacillary angiomatosis, as well as a variant form of pathology, bacillary peliosis.

Vasculoproliferative Disease

B. henselae is responsible for cases of bacillary angiomatosis-peliosis associated with cat exposure, and *B. quintana* is responsible for cases in

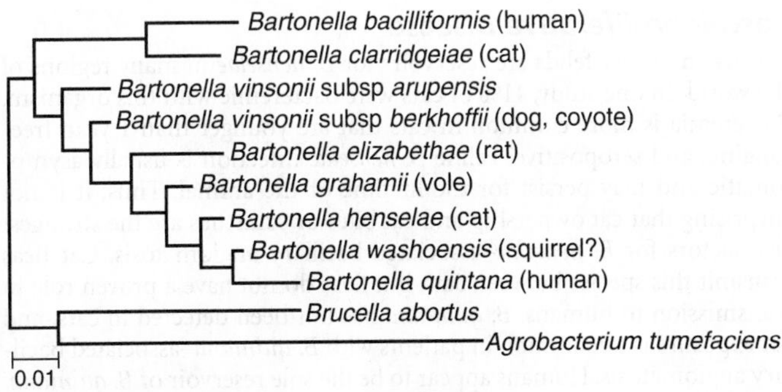

FIGURE 336–1 • Phylogenetic relationships among some of the α-proteobacteria, including the *Bartonella* species pathogenic for humans, based on small-subunit ribosomal RNA sequence analysis. Many of these organisms are endosymbiotic and may have evolved in close association with insects or plants. The primary reservoirs for the *Bartonella* species are indicated in parentheses after their names, if known. The scale bar indicates 0.01 nucleotide substitutions.

impoverished, homeless individuals infested by lice. Certain *B. henselae* genotypes appear to be more capable than others of causing hepatosplenic disease.

Classic bartonellosis (*B. bacilliformis* infection; Carrión's disease) is a sandfly-borne disorder characterized by two well-defined clinical stages: Oroya fever and verruga peruana, the second of which is accompanied by vascular proliferative lesions similar to those of bacillary angiomatosis.

Bacteremic Disease

Trench fever was first described during World War I, when more than 1 million soldiers were affected by this disorder. Trench fever has also been called 5-day or quintan fever, shinbone fever, shank fever, and His-Werner disease and has primarily been recognized during war-related epidemics. In 1961 the organism was isolated from infected lice and human blood and assigned to the genus *Rochalimaea* as *R. quintana.* The agent was renamed *B. quintana* in 1993. *B. quintana, B. henselae, B. elizabethae, B. koehlerae,* and *B. vinsonii* subsp *berkhoffii* have all been associated with endocarditis in humans. *B. vinsonii* subsp *arupensis* has been identified in a cattle rancher with fever and bacteremia; the reservoir for this pathogen is thought to be the mouse. *B. washoensis* was identified in a single patient with fever, bacteremia, and myocarditis; the reservoir for this pathogen is believed to be the ground squirrel.

Granulomatous Disease

In 1983, small pleomorphic, weakly gram-negative, but strongly argyrophilic bacilli were first described in tissues involved in cat-scratch disease. Eighty-four to 88% of patients who meet traditional diagnostic criteria for cat-scratch disease (see later) demonstrate a significant elevation in serum immunoglobulin G (IgG) antibodies directed against *B. henselae,* whereas approximately 20% of asymptomatic cat owners and 4 to 6% of the general population have elevated titers. In addition, *B. henselae* DNA and antigens can be detected in tissues from these patients with polymerase chain reaction (PCR) and in situ immunohistochemistry. *B. henselae* has also been cultivated from the blood and tissues of patients with cat-scratch disease. In a small number of cases, *B. clarridgeiae* is believed to be the causative agent of cat-scratch disease.

The Pathogens

B. henselae is a slightly curved, small (0.5 × 1 to 2 μm), self-aggregating, gram-negative bacillus that is capable of twitching motility. Optimal growth occurs on enriched media supplemented with 5% sheep or rabbit blood at 35° C in a 5 to 10% CO_2 humidified atmosphere. Colonies become visible after 9 to 21 days of primary culture (two different morphologies) and after 3 to 5 days on subsequent laboratory passage. *B. quintana* grows under similar conditions and has been recovered particularly effectively after cocultivation with endothelial cell monolayers. *B. bacilliformis* grows preferentially at 25 to 30° C. Species identification requires specific antisera, cellular fatty acid analysis, or DNA sequence analysis.

Epidemiology

Vasculoproliferative Disease

Cats and other felids are reservoirs for *B. henselae* in many regions of the world. In one study, 41% of cats were bacteremic with this organism. Bacteremia is more common in cats that are younger than 1 year, free-ranging, and seropositive. Feline *B. henselae* infection is usually asymptomatic and may persist for the lifetime of the animal. Thus, it is not surprising that cat ownership and cat bites or scratches are the strongest risk factors for *B. henselae*–associated bacillary angiomatosis. Cat fleas transmit this species between cats, but fleas do not have a proven role in transmission to humans. *B. quintana* has not been detected in cats, and cat exposure is uncommon in patients with *B. quintana*–associated bacillary angiomatosis. Humans appear to be the sole reservoir of *B. quintana,* and the human body louse, *Pediculus humanus,* serves as the transmission vector. The microorganism has been found in saliva, feces, and material regurgitated by lice. Direct human-to-human transmission has not been demonstrated. Risk factors for *B. quintana*–associated disease include homelessness, low economic status, and louse infestation. Approximately 90% of patients with bacillary angiomatosis-peliosis are coinfected with human immunodeficiency virus (HIV) or are immunocompromised by another mechanism.

B. bacilliformis infection is restricted to the habitat of its principal vector, the sandfly, *Phlebotomus verrucarum.* The sandfly breeds and transmits the infection in river valleys of the Andes Mountains at altitudes between 2500 and 9000 ft. Humans are the only known reservoir of the microorganism. Convalescent individuals may have low-grade bacteremia for months to years after infection, and *B. bacilliformis* may be recovered from 5 to 10% of apparently healthy persons in an endemic area. These carriers represent the greatest epidemiologic threat.

Bacteremic Disease

Trench fever and *B. quintana* have a worldwide distribution; disease occurs sporadically in endemic sites, such as eastern Europe, Russia, and Mexico. Epidemic disease was described during World Wars I and II in Europe. In the 1990s, temporal and geographic clusters of endemic disease were recognized for the first time among urban homeless populations in the United States and western Europe. In one study, 20% of attendees at an inner-city clinic in Seattle had elevated antibody titers to *B. quintana.* In a separate study in France, 30% of homeless persons seeking care in hospital emergency departments were seropositive for *B. quintana* and 14% were bacteremic.

Bartonella species account for approximately 3% of all cases of infective endocarditis and a significant portion of "culture-negative" endocarditis cases in both immunocompetent and immunocompromised hosts. *B. henselae* has been incriminated in 5% of cases of fever of unknown origin in children.

Granulomatous Disease

Cat-scratch disease affects approximately 22,000 persons in the United States per year. The highest incidence of the disease occurs in the 5- to 14-year-old age group and in the South, where cat fleas are most prevalent and *B. henselae* infection of cats is most common. The disease generally occurs in the summer and autumn. A history of a cat scratch or bite is elicited in approximately 75% of patients. Less than 5% of cases of cat-scratch disease belong to a family cluster; however, small clusters of disease with neurologic complications have been noted.

Pathobiology

Vasculoproliferative Disease

The lesions of bacillary angiomatosis assume diverse macroscopic appearances, including an erythematous, polypoid or papular, cutaneous, or mucosal pattern; deeply erythematous and indurated dermal plaques; and subcutaneous or visceral nodules. In all of these lesions, a distinctive lobular proliferation of capillaries is seen within a fibrous stroma. Hematoxylin-eosin staining reveals granular amphophilic material in the interstitium between vessels. This and other microscopic features distinguish bacillary angiomatosis from Kaposi's sarcoma. The amphophilic material corresponds to clumps of extracellular bacteria, which are best seen with the Warthin-Starry silver stain or by electron microscopy. Bacillary peliosis, which is a histologically variant form of bacillary angiomatosis, is characterized by blood-filled cystic spaces, fibromyxoid stroma, and inflammatory cells; it is almost always associated with *B. henselae* and occurs most often within the liver and spleen. The pathogenesis of bacillary angiomatosis includes early blood-borne dissemination of organisms throughout the body. The bartonellae readily attach to and may enter erythrocytes; persistence within the intravascular compartment suggests bacterial mechanisms for avoidance of opsonization and host phagocytosis. In humans, infection of the endothelium with *B. bacilliformis, B. henselae,* or *B. quintana* can lead to marked vasoproliferation manifested as benign vascular tumors. Host immunosuppression appears to be a prerequisite for vascular tumor formation (e.g., bacillary angiomatosis, peliosis, hepatitis) by *B. henselae* and *B. quintana.*

After inoculation by the sandfly, *B. bacilliformis* invades erythrocytes and endothelial cells. In most untreated patients who survive the acute hemolytic anemia (Oroya fever stage), the chronic cutaneous lesions of verruga peruana eventually develop. The partial state of immunosuppression occurring at the end of the Oroya fever stage of infection allows for the development of hemangiomatous nodules, which consist of proliferating small vessels infiltrated by lymphocytes and macrophages. Verruga may also occur in viscera, bones, and the central nervous system.

Bacteremic Disease

The pathology and pathogenesis of trench fever are not well characterized. In contrast to the angioproliferation seen with bacillary angiomatosis, biopsy specimens of skin lesions from patients with trench fever reveal perivascular lymphocytic infiltration; bacteria are not seen within vascular endothelial cells, but intraerythrocytic *B. quintana* has been visualized in peripheral blood smears of homeless persons with or without clinical symptoms. *Bartonella* endocarditis usually occurs in persons with preexisting valvar disease (most often the aortic valve) and leads to further valve destruction. Electron microscopy reveals intracellular and extracellular clusters of bacteria in valve tissue. In Oroya fever, erythrocyte parasitization results in increased fragility of red blood cells and increased phagocytosis by the reticuloendothelial system. In severe cases, as many as 90% of circulating erythrocytes may be parasitized. Peripheral blood smears reveal a normochromic macrocytosis and striking polychromasia, Howell-Jolly bodies, Cabot's rings, and nucleated erythrocytes. The Coombs test and other assays for red blood cell agglutinins and hemolysins are generally negative. Cells of the reticuloendothelial system may contain intracellular organisms, presumably as a result of erythrophagocytosis. Reactive hyperplasia of lymphatic tissue is common.

Granulomatous Disease

Histologic changes in lymph nodes evolve over a period of months in patients with cat-scratch disease. Follicular hyperplasia and hypertrophy, sinus histiocytosis, and B-cell proliferation are followed by granuloma formation and later by neutrophilic infiltration with central or stellate necrosis and surrounding palisades of histiocytes. Microabscesses are common. Bacilli are best visualized with the Warthin-Starry silver impregnation stain early in the course of the disease.

Clinical Manifestations

Vasculoproliferative Disease

Bacillary angiomatosis is most often associated with tender cutaneous or subcutaneous lesions. Mucosal lesions are also common. Lesions of bacillary angiomatosis may be indistinguishable from those of Kaposi's sarcoma. The lesions may be solitary or multiple, red, purple, or flesh-colored dome-shaped papules, nodules, polypoid tumors, or plaques. With age the lesions may ulcerate, form a crust, or develop a collarette of scale. Subcutaneous lesions sometimes erode underlying bone; this finding should raise suspicion of bacillary angiomatosis. In an undetermined percentage of cases, visceral bacillary angiomatosis-peliosis occurs, sometimes in the absence of cutaneous disease. Visceral involvement may be asymptomatic or, as in disseminated cutaneous disease, may be associated with fever, chills, malaise, and anorexia. The liver, spleen, and internal lymph nodes appear to be the most frequent sites of extracutaneous disease. Biliary obstruction has resulted from external compression of periportal lymph nodes. Other sites affected by bacillary angiomatosis include bone marrow, lung, and brain. In general, cases of bacillary angiomatosis and peliosis are less frequent in the current era of more potent HIV-specific therapies.

Verruga peruana develops after a latent period of weeks to months following the resolution of acute *B. bacilliformis* infection in untreated patients. This disorder is characterized by 1- to 2-cm hemangiomatous nodules that typically evolve over a period of 1 to 2 months in crops on exposed skin but also on mucous membranes and within internal organs. The lesions are usually nontender and may vary morphologically, sometimes appearing as ulcers or as secondarily infected pustules. The verruga may persist for months to years in untreated patients.

Bacteremic Disease

The incubation period for trench fever ranges from 4 to 35 days. In human volunteers the average duration is 22 days. Clinical manifestations vary from a febrile illness of 4 to 5 days' duration in some patients to a severe illness with prolonged fever in others. In the classic descriptions of more severe disease, infected persons experience three to five febrile paroxysms, each lasting approximately 5 days (quintan or 5-day fever). A syndrome of continuous fever lasting 2 to 6 weeks has also been noted. In addition to fever and chills, symptoms of trench fever include malaise, anorexia, night sweats, headache with retro-orbital pain, and severe bone pain in the neck, back, and lower extremities, especially the tibia (shin-bone fever). Conjunctival injection, hepatosplenomegaly, mild to moderate leukocytosis, and an erythematous maculopapular truncal rash occur in most patients. Symptoms and signs are typically most severe during the initial febrile period. Subsequent attacks are milder, with the exception of persistent, severe bone pain. Irregular episodes of remission and late relapses have been reported. Specific antibodies to *B. quintana* appear within several weeks of primary infection, but they are not fully protective because reinfection has been documented within 3 to 6 months of the initial illness.

The clinical manifestations of *Bartonella* endocarditis are similar to those of more typical forms of infective endocarditis. *B. henselae, B. quintana, B. elizabethae, B. koehlerae,* and *B. vinsonii* subsp *berkhoffii* have all been reported to cause infective endocarditis. The majority of patients have fever with a temperature higher than 38° C, and approximately 40% manifest embolic phenomena. Echocardiography typically reveals valvar (predominantly aortic) vegetation.

Signs of sepsis or localized (granulomatous or angioproliferative) disease are uncommon in cases of *B. henselae* or *B. quintana* bacteremia. Fever, headache, myalgias, and arthralgias may persist or recur over a period of weeks to months despite therapy. Homeless persons with *B. quintana* bacteremia are more likely to have been exposed to lice, have headaches and severe leg pain, and have lower platelet counts than homeless people who have no serologic evidence of exposure to *B. quintana* and no bacteremia. In some cases, *B. henselae* bacteremia has been associated with lymphocytic meningitis.

Within 2 to 6 weeks after the bite of an infected sandfly, Oroya fever, characterized by the insidious onset of myalgias and low-grade fever and followed by high fever, headache, and painful muscles and joints, develops in a nonimmune host. Pallor, hepatomegaly, cardiac murmur, and jaundice are common. Tender lymphadenopathy is also common, but splenomegaly is rare. Erythrocyte counts decrease rapidly within a few days and may fall as low as 1 million/mm^3. Some patients have a febrile crisis, followed by rapid resolution of symptoms and signs, increased erythropoiesis, and gradual reduction of fever. Recurrence of fever after initial improvement suggests secondary infection. Salmonellosis is an especially important complication of acute *B. bacilliformis*–associated disease in South America and may reflect transient immunosuppression. In addition, malaria, amebiasis, and tuberculosis appear to be more common in these patients.

Granulomatous Disease

After an incubation period of 3 to 10 days, an erythematous papule develops at the inoculation site in more than 50% of patients in whom cat-scratch disease is later diagnosed. These lesions may form a crust or become pustular, with spontaneous resolution in 1 to 3 weeks. Within a few weeks of inoculation, regional lymphadenopathy becomes apparent; usually a lymph node in the axillary or neck region is found to be enlarged and tender (Table 336–1). Low-grade fever, malaise, anorexia, and nausea each occur in a minority of patients. In a typical case of cat-scratch disease, lymph nodes remain enlarged for at least 2 to 4 months. Infrequently, inoculation of the eye results in a granulomatous conjunctival lesion and preauricular adenopathy, a condition known as the

TABLE 336–1 SELECTED CLINICAL FEATURES OF CLASSIC CAT-SCRATCH DISEASE

Feature	Percentage of Cases
Site of lymphadenopathy	
Axilla	25–52
Neck	26–39
Groin	7–18
Elbow	2–13
Preauricular region	5–7
Single-node involvement	43–85
Lymphadenopathy only	48–51
Fever	31–48
Splenomegaly	11–12
Hospitalization	9–17

oculoglandular syndrome of Parinaud (affecting 4 to 6% of patients with cat-scratch disease).

Severe or systemic non-neurologic manifestations, including persistent fever, weight loss, splenomegaly, diffuse papular rash, erythema nodosum, pleuritis, splenic abscess, central lymphadenopathy, osteolytic lesions, hepatitis, and thrombocytopenic purpura, are reported in 2% of patients with cat-scratch disease. Neurologic complications develop in an additional 2% of patients with cat-scratch disease. Encephalopathy or encephalitis is most common and is manifested by seizures and confusion; other findings include radiculitis, meningitis, cranial neuritis, neuroretinitis, and cerebral arteritis. Neurologic complications occur 2 to 3 weeks after onset of the initial illness. Spontaneous, complete resolution is the rule in these cases.

Diagnosis

Vasculoproliferative Disease

The diagnosis of both bacillary angiomatosis and cat-scratch disease rests on tissue examination and serologic tests in a compatible clinical setting. The histology typical of bacillary angiomatosis in hematoxylin-eosin–stained tissue is suggestive of the diagnosis. Warthin-Starry stains usually confirm this diagnosis (i.e., revealing clumps of small, pleomorphic bacilli). Commercial laboratories, as well as the Centers for Disease Control and Prevention, offer an immunofluorescent or enzyme-linked immunosorbent assay for serum IgG antibodies directed against *B. henselae, B. quintana,* and *B. elizabethae.* Most assays cannot reliably distinguish among humoral responses to each of these species. Cultivation of *Bartonella* species and detection of specific DNA sequences by PCR or antigens by immunohistochemical methods are more specialized procedures that are not available at most clinical microbiology laboratories. Kaposi's sarcoma is the most important entity confused with bacillary angiomatosis. Visual detection of bacilli distinguishes the latter from the former. Lytic bone lesions in an HIV-infected individual should raise the possibility of bacillary angiomatosis.

Bacteremic Disease

Bartonella species are slow growing and fastidious, but they can be cultivated on blood-enriched media or in the presence of endothelial cells (see earlier). Formation of colonies on an agar surface directly from an infected clinical specimen may require more than 21 days of incubation and subculturing on freshly prepared media. Acridine orange staining procedures and lysis centrifugation culture methods enhance the detection and recovery, respectively, of *Bartonella* species from blood specimens. Serologic methods may aid in the diagnosis of *Bartonella* bacteremic disease. The serologic cross-reactivity of *Chlamydia* and *Bartonella* species may present a diagnostic problem because both groups of microorganisms must be considered in patients with culture-negative endocarditis. PCR assays have also proved successful in identifying *Bartonella* species on resected heart valve tissue.

The differential diagnosis of trench fever includes epidemic (louse-borne) typhus (Chapter 348), which occurs under similar demographic circumstances and shares the same vector *(P. humanus)* as trench fever, endemic (murine) typhus, ehrlichiosis (Chapter 348), Q fever (Chapter 348), Rocky Mountain spotted fever (Chapter 348), relapsing fever (Chapter 343), Lyme disease (Chapter 342), malaria (Chapter 366), and plague (Chapter 333). Local disease endemicity or a history of body louse infestation should raise clinical suspicion of trench fever.

The diagnosis of Oroya fever is made by examining a peripheral blood smear or by serology. Bacilli may be seen within red blood cells as single organisms or in pairs or clusters. With Giemsa staining, the bacilli appear as 0.3- to 1.5-μm pleomorphic red-purple rods.

Granulomatous Disease

Cat-scratch disease is diagnosed most often by examination of Warthin-Starry silver–stained tissue or by using serologic methods. The differential diagnosis for localized cat-scratch disease may include pyogenic lymphadenitis, mycobacterial infection (Chapter 345), tularemia (Chapter 332), brucellosis (Chapter 331), lymphogranuloma venereum (Chapter 339), syphilis (Chapter 340), fungal disease, toxoplasmosis (Chapter 370), and Epstein-Barr virus (Chapter 400) or cytomegalovirus infection (Chapter 399).

TABLE 336–2 TREATMENT SUGGESTIONS

SEVERE CAT-SCRATCH DISEASE*	
Doxycycline plus	100 mg bid
rifampin or	300 mg bid
azithromycin	500 mg/day × 1 day, then 250 mg/day × 4 days
BACILLARY ANGIOMATOSIS-PELIOSIS OR *BARTONELLA* BACTEREMIA†	
Erythromycin or	250–500 mg qid
doxycycline plus	100 mg bid
rifampin (severe disease)	300 mg bid
Consider the addition of an aminoglycoside	

*Therapy should be continued for at least 14 days.
†Treat patients with bacillary angiomatosis-peliosis for at least 8 weeks, patients with *Bartonella* bacteremia for 2 to 4 weeks, and patients with *Bartonella* endocarditis for at least 6 weeks.

Treatment

Rx

Because there are few data from prospective randomized studies, retrospective or empirical clinical observations offer the primary basis for the suggested approaches (Table 336–2). Antibiotic susceptibility testing has demonstrated that *Bartonella* species are frequently susceptible in vitro to a variety of classes of antimicrobial agents, including β-lactams, tetracyclines, macrolides, aminoglycosides, rifampin, and fluoroquinolones. Unfortunately, the minimum inhibitory concentrations derived in laboratory testing do not consistently correlate with in vivo efficacy. Corticosteroids are not recommended for any of these diseases.

Vasculoproliferative Disease

All forms of *Bartonella*-associated vasculoproliferative disease warrant antimicrobial treatment. Based on empirical observations, the treatment of choice for bacillary angiomatosis-peliosis is either erythromycin, 500 mg every 6 hours, or doxycycline, 100 mg every 12 hours. Azithromycin and clarithromycin are alternative therapies. Patients who are severely ill or unable to absorb oral medications should be treated with intravenous formulations. Rifampin could be added to the regimen for patients in the former category. Because disease relapse is otherwise so common in these immunocompromised hosts, patients should be treated for at least 8 weeks. Verruga lesions do not respond consistently to antimicrobial agents, but more than 80% of patients with the eruptive phase of bartonellosis have reported a good response to rifampin, and about 50% have a modest response to streptomycin.

Bacteremic Disease

The same drugs and doses used for bacillary angiomatosis-peliosis are recommended for primary bacteremias despite the fact that some immunocompetent hosts with *B. quintana* bacteremia clear their infection spontaneously. All patients should be evaluated for endocarditis. Treatment should be continued for at least 6 weeks in patients with endocarditis and probably for 4 weeks in patients without endocarditis. Rifampin should be added to the regimen for the treatment of endocarditis. Aminoglycoside administration for at least 2 weeks appears to be an important component of antibiotic treatment regimens. Close monitoring of hemodynamics is essential because historically, the majority of endocarditis patients have ultimately required valve repair or replacement, perhaps related to delay in diagnosis in many instances. Patients with trench fever usually respond rapidly to antibiotic therapy, with resolution of fever and other symptoms within 1 to 2 days. Relapses in treated patients have been well described.

In patients with Oroya fever, clinical observations suggest that penicillin, chloramphenicol, tetracycline, and streptomycin are effective. Chloramphenicol at a dose of 2 to 4 g/day for 7 or more days

Rx

is the therapy of choice because of the frequent association of *Salmonella* infection in endemic regions. After the institution of therapy, fever generally disappears within 2 to 3 days, although blood smears may remain positive for some time.

Granulomatous Disease

Most patients with cat-scratch disease do not require more than symptomatic support. A fluctuant or suppurative lymph node may benefit from needle aspiration. Antibiotic therapy should be reserved for immunocompromised individuals or those with evidence of severe or systemic disease. It remains unclear what constitutes the most useful agents in this setting. Doxycycline plus rifampin may be effective, but well-controlled data are lacking. A randomized, placebo-controlled study suggests that a 5-day course of azithromycin speeds resolution of cat-scratch lymphadenopathy. [1]

Prognosis

Vasculoproliferative disease generally responds to antimicrobial treatment, but verruga lesions refractory to antimicrobial therapy may require surgical resection. In patients with endocarditis, about 90% require valve surgery despite antibiotic therapy, and the mortality rate is close to 30%. Historically, mortality in untreated Oroya fever approached 50% as a result of both acute hemolytic anemia and secondary infections, but the mortality rate is now only about 9%; after resolution of the febrile hemolytic anemia, immunity develops, and relapses or reinfections are unusual. Cat-scratch disease usually resolves without treatment in immunocompetent patients and responds well to therapy in immunocompromised patients.

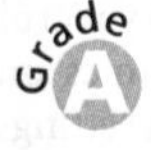

1. Bass JW, Freitas BC, Freitas AD, et al: Prospective randomized double blind placebo-controlled evaluation of azithromycin for treatment of cat-scratch disease. Pediatr Infect Dis J 1998;17: 1059–1061.

SUGGESTED READINGS

Chomel BB, Boulouis HJ, Maruyama S, et al: *Bartonella* spp. in pets and effect on human health. Emerg Infect Dis 2006;12:389–394. *A practical overview.*

Dehio C: *Bartonella*–host-cell interactions and vascular tumour formation. Nat Rev Microbiol 2005;3:621–631. *Overview of* Bartonella *pathogenesis and virulence factors.*

Foucault C, Brouqui P, Raoult D: *Bartonella quintana* characteristics and clinical management. Emerg Infect Dis 2006;12:217–223. *Review of the history, ecology, and biology of this organism.*

Maguina C, Garcia PJ, Gotuzzo E, et al: Bartonellosis (Carrión's disease) in the modern era. Clin Infect Dis 2001;33:772–779. *Describes the clinical manifestations and treatment of acute (Oroya fever) and chronic (eruptive) bartonellosis in 145 symptomatic patients.*

Rolain JM, Brouqui P, Koehler JE, et al: Recommendations for treatment of human infections caused by *Bartonella* species. Antimicrob Agents Chemother 2004;48:1921–1933. *Review of in vitro susceptibility data and clinical experience in the treatment of* Bartonella *infections, with emphasis on* B. henselae *and* B. quintana.

337 GRANULOMA INGUINALE (DONOVANOSIS)

Edward W. Hook III

Definition

Granuloma inguinale, also known as donovanosis, is a slowly progressive ulcerative disease that involves principally the skin and subcutaneous tissues of the genital, inguinal, and anal regions.

The Pathogen

The causative organism is *Klebsiella granulomatis* (formerly *Calymmatobacterium granulomatis*). The organism is challenging to cultivate but can be grown in yolk sacs, and successful cell culture has been reported from laboratories in South Africa and Australia. Successful culture has in turn permitted the development of polymerase chain reaction (PCR) assays for research purposes. It appears to be a facultative intracellular parasite.

Epidemiology

The organism is primarily transmitted sexually but can probably be transmitted by nonsexual contact as well. Multiple sexual contacts with an infected partner seem to be necessary for transmission of infection. The disease is uncommon in the United States, with fewer than 100 recorded cases annually. Historically, however, it is more common in certain other areas of the world, including India, Papua New Guinea, Southern Africa, and parts of Australia. Even in these endemic areas, the limited data available suggest that the disease may be becoming less common.

Clinical Manifestations

The initial lesion usually appears as a subcutaneous nodule that erodes through the surface and develops into a beefy, elevated granulomatous lesion (Fig. 337–1). The lesion is painless and unassociated with systemic symptoms. Secondary bacterial infection may cause a necrotic painful ulcerative lesion that may be rapidly destructive. A cicatricial form may also occur with a depigmented elevated area of keloid-like scar containing scattered islands of granulomatous tissue. Genital lesions are commonly associated with pseudobuboes in the inguinal region; these swellings are not usually due to involvement of the inguinal lymph nodes but rather to granulomatous involvement of subcutaneous tissue. Metastatic infection of bones or other viscera is occasionally seen. Clinical experience suggests that secondary carcinomas may be a complication of granuloma inguinale.

Diagnosis

The diagnosis is made by demonstrating intracellular "Donovan bodies" in histiocytes or other mononuclear cells from lesion scrapings or biopsy samples. Wright stain and Giemsa stain of fresh impression smears or unfixed biopsy specimens usually demonstrates the bacilli relatively easily, although multiple biopsies may be necessary in chronic cases. Histologic examination of biopsy specimens shows mononuclear cells with some infiltration by polymorphonuclear leukocytes but no giant cells. In infected lesions, *K. granulomatis* is found primarily in histiocytes or other mononuclear cells. Cell culture and PCR methods have

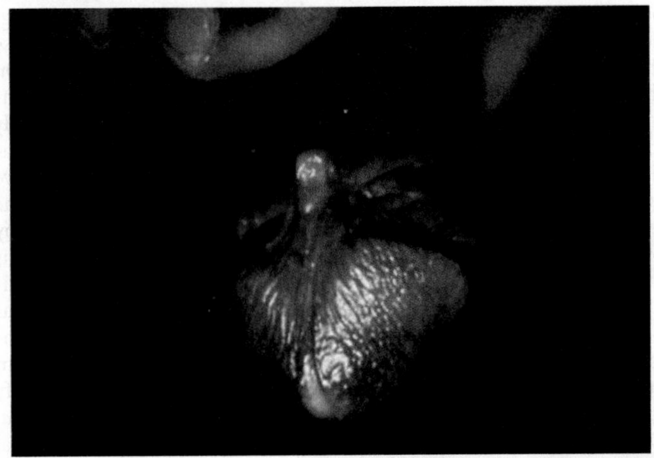

FIGURE 337–1 • Typical primary lesion of granuloma inguinale. (Reproduced with permission from Herpes-Coldsores.com. Available at http://www.herpes-coldsores.com/std/lymphogranuloma_pictures.htm. Accessed September 8, 2006.)

been described but are primarily research tools. A serologic test has been devised but is not clinically available.

Differential Diagnosis

The differential diagnosis (Chapter 307) includes tumor, chancroid (Chapter 324), lymphogranuloma venereum (Chapter 339), syphilis (Chapter 340), and other ulcerative granulomatous diseases. Chancroid is usually differentiated by its irregular undermined borders, which are not seen in the usual cases of granuloma inguinale. Darkfield examination and serologic tests should help distinguish syphilis. Biopsy of lesions may be necessary to distinguish granuloma inguinale from certain tumors.

Treatment

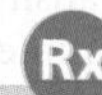

Recommended treatment consists of azithromycin, 1.0 g weekly, ciprofloxacin, 750 mg twice daily, or erythromycin base, 500 mg four times daily. Trimethoprim-sulfamethoxazole, one double-strength tablet twice daily, is also effective. An aminoglycoside (e.g., gentamicin, 1 mg/kg intravenously every 8 hours) may be added if these regimens do not result in clinical improvement within the first few days of therapy. Treatment should be administered for at least 3 weeks and until lesions are completely healed. Patients should be monitored for at least several weeks after treatment is discontinued because of the possibility of relapse. Although the risk of communicability appears to be low, sexual contacts should also be examined; at present, treatment of contacts is not indicated in the absence of clinically evident disease.

SUGGESTED READINGS

Lupi O, Madkan V, Tyring SK: Tropical dermatology: Bacterial tropical disease. J Am Acad Dermatol 2006;54:559–578. *Useful overview and differential diagnosis.*

O'Farrell N: Donovanosis. Sex Transm Infect 2002;78:452–457. *A comprehensive review.*

338 *MYCOPLASMA* INFECTIONS

Stephen G. Baum

Definition

Mycoplasma organisms of the class Mollicutes are ubiquitous as pathogens and colonizing agents in the plant, animal, and insect kingdoms. They represent the smallest known free-living forms, but because they have fastidious growth requirements, they are difficult to culture. On the other hand, the presence of several species of *Mycoplasma* as commensals in animals and on human oral and genital mucosa has frequently in the past resulted in contamination of cell cultures. Such contamination has in turn led to the false implication of mycoplasmas as causative agents in many human diseases, both trivial and life threatening. Of the human diseases proved to be due to mycoplasmas, pneumonia caused by *Mycoplasma pneumoniae* is by far the most clinically important. This infection constitutes a significant proportion of cases previously classified as "atypical pneumonia," a nonspecific term for patchy pneumonias that do not, in general, respond to β-lactam antibiotics and have etiologic agents that are not easily cultured or visible on Gram stain. The term atypical pneumonia persists despite our increasing ability to identify specific etiologic agents such as viruses, *Legionella*, and *Chlamydia*. Other proven *Mycoplasma* infections include those in the urogenital tract caused by *Ureaplasma urealyticum* and *Mycoplasma hominis*, wound infections by *M. hominis*, and overwhelming systemic infection in immunocompromised patients caused by *Mycoplasma fermentans* (*incognitus* strain).

The Pathogen

In tissue culture mycoplasmas are intracellular, but in vivo, infection is primarily extracellular and affects epithelial cells and their organelles such as cilia. Because of the low fatality of most *Mycoplasma* infections, there is little human pathologic material. Inoculation onto animal tracheal organ cultures is followed by ciliary damage and desquamation of surface epithelium. This latter effect is probably responsible for the hacking cough in *Mycoplasma* respiratory infection.

Mycoplasmas are active in stimulating several components of the immune system. They can act as polyclonal T-cell and B-cell activators and can cause capping of lymphocytes. Macrophages can also be stimulated by some mycoplasmas in vitro. *M. pneumoniae* is capable of inducing several cytokines, including granulocyte-macrophage colony-stimulating factor and interferon, as well as several pro-inflammatory interleukins.

Epidemiology

M. pneumoniae infection is spread person to person by respiratory droplets produced by coughing. Relatively close association with the index case appears to be required. The disease is usually introduced into families by a young child, and in some studies most of the adults who were infected were the parents of young children. As opposed to most viral respiratory infections, which are clinically manifested 1 to 3 days after infection, *Mycoplasma* has an incubation period of 2 to 3 weeks. The shorter incubation period seen in experimentally induced infections may have resulted from the use of large inocula to induce disease. Therefore, a careful history showing several weeks between cases within a family may give an important clue regarding mycoplasmal etiology. Organisms can be cultured from the sputum of infected individuals for weeks to months after clinically efficacious treatment, and the effect of treatment of an index case on subsequent transmission to family members is unclear.

Most cases of *Mycoplasma* respiratory infection occur singly or as family outbreaks. However, in closed populations such as military recruit camps and boarding schools, *Mycoplasma* can cause mini-epidemics and may be responsible for 25 to 75% of cases of pneumonia in such settings. Serologically based epidemiologic studies have documented the high incidence of *Mycoplasma* respiratory infection throughout the world. In the United States, it is estimated that each year at least one case of *Mycoplasma* pneumonia occurs for every 1000 persons, or more than 2 million cases annually. The incidence of *Mycoplasma* nonpneumonic respiratory infection may be 10 to 20 times greater. The highest attack rates are in individuals 5 to 20 years old, but *M. pneumoniae* infection can occur at any age and may cause particularly severe disease in neonates.

As opposed to viral respiratory infections that peak in winter in temperate climates, a few studies have reported a peak incidence of *M. pneumoniae* outbreaks in the fall. This is not surprising given the age-related incidence and the fact that late summer and fall represent the time of return to school. Most surveys, however, show little or no seasonal predominance in sporadic cases. There is an age-related relationship of upper versus lower respiratory tract infection caused by *M. pneumoniae*. In children younger than 3 years, primarily upper respiratory tract infection develops, whereas in those 5 to 20 years old, bronchitis and pneumonia tend to occur. In older adults, pneumonia predominates.

The prevalence and incidence of clinical urogenital disease caused by *U. urealyticum*, *M. hominis*, and *Mycoplasma genitalium* are much less well documented (Table 338–1). These organisms are rarely cultured outside the realm of clinical studies, and they exist as clinically unapparent commensals of the genitourinary tract. Diseases attributed to *Ureaplasma* include urinary tract infection with and without calculus formation. The organism has been implicated as a cause of low birth-weight in neonates. *M. hominis* is a common genitourinary and oral commensal as well and has been documented as a cause of endometritis and postpartum fever.

M. hominis has also caused sternal wound infection after cardiothoracic surgery and has been implicated in arthritis in immunocompromised patients. *Mycoplasma salivarium* may be involved in periodontal disease and *M. genitalium* in some cases of nongonococcal urethritis and vaginitis. *M. fermentans*, *incognitus* strain, was identified about 2 decades ago as an infectious agent in immunocompromised patients, in whom it causes overwhelming multisystem involvement.

TABLE 338–1 SITES AND INFECTIONS RELATED TO HUMAN MYCOPLASMAS

Subgroup	Sites of Isolation	Diseases	Occurrence
M. hominis	GU tract (F > M)	Cervicitis, vaginitis, ?prostatitis	Common
	Conjunctivae (neonate)	Conjunctivitis	
	Blood (peripartum)	Peripartum sepsis	
	Surgical wounds, joints	Sternotomy infection, arthritis (immunocompromised)	
M. orale	Oropharynx	?	Common
M. pneumoniae	Respiratory tract	URI, pneumonia	Common
M. salivarium	Oropharynx, gingiva	?Periodontal disease	Common
M. fermentans	GU tract, blood, tissues	Multisystem disease in AIDS	Uncommon
M. genitalium	GU tract	Urethritis	Uncommon
Ureaplasma urealyticum	GU tract	Urethritis, upper GU infection	Common

AIDS = acquired immunodeficiency syndrome; F = female; GU = genitourinary; M = male; URI = upper respiratory tract infection.

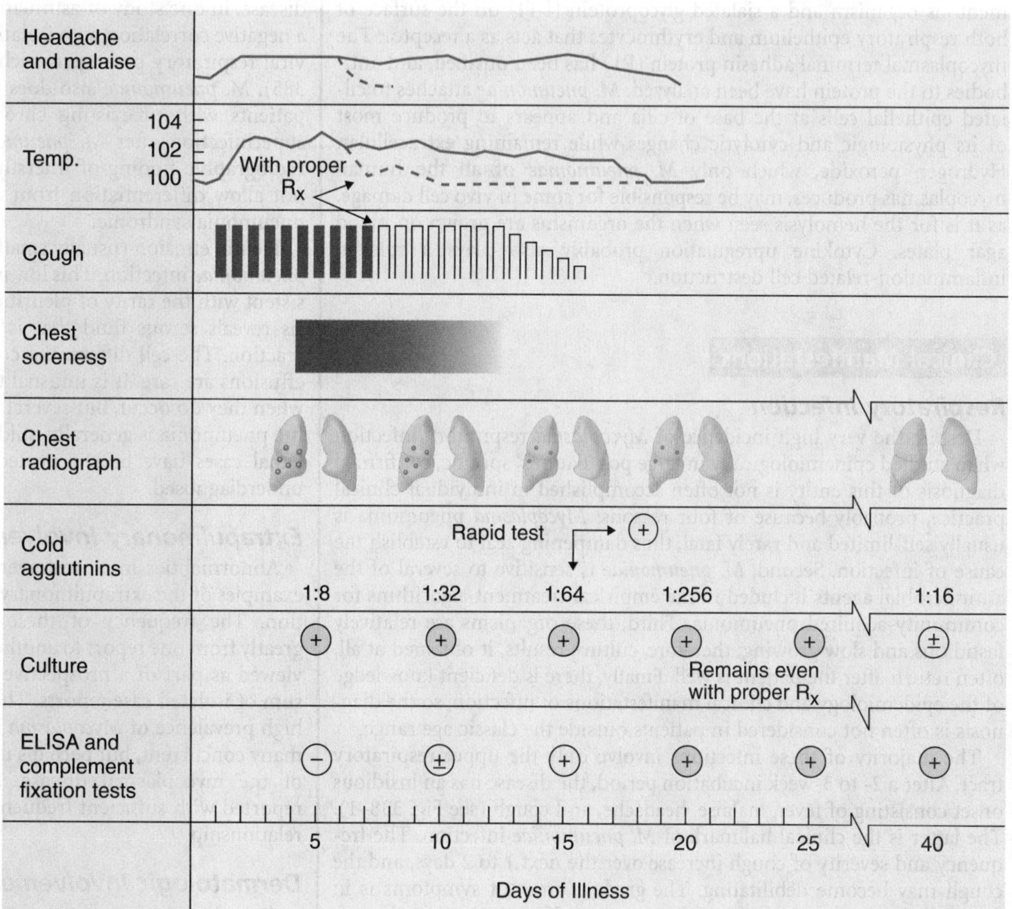

FIGURE 338–1 • Major clinical and laboratory manifestations of mycoplasmal pneumonia. ELISA = enzyme-linked immunosorbent assay. (Adapted from Baum SG: Mycoplasmal infections. *In* Wyngaarden JB, Smith LH Jr [eds]: Cecil Textbook of Medicine, 17th ed. Philadelphia, Saunders, 1985, p 1506.)

Pathobiology

In the course of *M. pneumoniae* infection, some patients will produce cold agglutinins. These oligoclonal M-type immunoglobulins (IgM) cross-react with "I" antigens, one of the blood group antigens common to almost all mature human erythrocytes, and high titers may cause hemolysis (presumably as a result of complement-activated, Coombs-positive erythrocyte destruction) and may lead to some of the complications described in the Clinical Manifestations section. Like other IgM antibodies, the *Mycoplasma*-induced cold agglutinins develop early in the disease (7 to 10 days) and are therefore often present by the time that the patient seeks medical attention. The titer of these agglutinins peaks at 2 to 3 weeks and they persist for 2 to 3 months (Fig. 338–1).

Several theories about factors triggering the formation of cold agglutinins in *Mycoplasma* pneumonia have been proposed. One is that the organism alters the I antigen such that it is made antigenic to the patient. The hydrogen peroxide elaborated by *M. pneumoniae* could be responsible for this alteration. One study has indicated that the I antigen in a sialated state may serve as a receptor for *M. pneumoniae* and that the cold agglutinins are directed at the modified receptor. Other studies indicate that the cold agglutinins are directed at mycoplasmal substructures themselves and merely cross-react with the I antigen (altered or native) on red cells. Given their apparent target, these antibodies could either contribute to cytolysis and exacerbate infection or interfere with cell-to-cell spread by blocking or disrupting the cell receptor for the mycoplasma. High titers of cold agglutinins have also been associated with hemolysis, presumably as a result of activation of complement-mediated erythrocyte destruction. The direct Coombs test is positive in many of these patients. Although clinically significant hemolysis is uncommon, subclinical levels of red cell destruction are common.

Because of two fortunate aspects of *Mycoplasma* pneumonia—its relatively low severity and low mortality—there is relatively little information on pathologic findings in this disease, and knowledge rests on relatively few specimens. Sickle cell disease, sickle-related hemoglobinopathies, and hypogammaglobulinemia predispose to increased severity and to mortality. Some of the available pathologic data may therefore be influenced by the pathophysiology of these underlying conditions. When deaths have occurred, they have been in patients with diffuse pneumonia, adult respiratory distress syndrome, thromboembolism, and disseminated intravascular coagulopathy.

In nonfatal cases in which lung biopsy was performed, the inflammatory process primarily involved the trachea, bronchioles, and peribronchial tissue. The lumen of the respiratory tree was filled with purulent exudate rich in polymorphonuclear leukocytes. The lining of the bronchial and bronchiolar walls showed metaplastic cells, and the walls themselves were infiltrated with monocytic elements, especially plasma cells. There was widening of the peribronchial septa and hyperplasia of type II pneumocytes.

Several characteristics of *M. pneumoniae* probably play a direct role in the respiratory pathogenicity of this organism. The first is the relatively great affinity of *M. pneumoniae* for respiratory epithelial cells. Attachment appears to be between a terminal organelle at one end of the filamentous organism and a sialated glycoprotein (I-FI) on the surface of both respiratory epithelium and erythrocytes that acts as a receptor. The mycoplasmal terminal adhesin protein (P1) has been purified, and antibodies to the protein have been analyzed. *M. pneumoniae* attaches to ciliated epithelial cells at the base of cilia and appears to produce most of its physiologic and cytolytic changes while remaining extracellular. Hydrogen peroxide, which only *M. pneumoniae* of all the human mycoplasmas produces, may be responsible for some in vivo cell damage, as it is for the hemolysis seen when the organisms are grown on blood agar plates. Cytokine upregulation probably also plays a role in inflammation-related cell destruction.

Clinical Manifestations

Respiratory Infection

Despite the very high incidence of *Mycoplasma* respiratory infection when studied epidemiologically in large populations, specific, confirmed diagnosis of this entity is not often accomplished in individual clinical practice, probably because of four reasons: *Mycoplasma* pneumonia is usually self-limited and rarely fatal, thus dampening zeal to establish the cause of infection. Second, *M. pneumoniae* is sensitive to several of the antimicrobial agents included in the empirical treatment algorithms for community-acquired pneumonia. Third, these organisms are relatively fastidious and slow growing; therefore, culture results, if obtained at all, often return after the patient is well. Finally, there is deficient knowledge of the epidemiology and clinical manifestations of infection, so the diagnosis is often not considered in patients outside the classic age range.

The majority of these infections involve only the upper respiratory tract. After a 2- to 3-week incubation period, the disease has an insidious onset consisting of fever, malaise, headache, and cough (see Fig. 338–1). The latter is the clinical hallmark of *M. pneumoniae* infection. The frequency and severity of cough increase over the next 1 to 2 days, and the cough may become debilitating. The gradual onset of symptoms is in contradistinction to the often fulminant manifestation of respiratory infection caused by influenza virus or adenovirus.

In 5 to 10% of patients, depending somewhat on age, the infection progresses to tracheobronchitis or pneumonia. In these cases, the original manifestations persist and the cough becomes more severe. It is usually relatively nonproductive but may yield white or occasionally blood-flecked sputum. Gram staining of this sputum reveals inflammatory cells but no predominant bacterial species (part of the definition of atypical pneumonia). With continued cough, parasternal chest soreness may develop as a result of muscle strain, but true pleuritic pain is unusual. Fever is usually at the level of 101 to 102° F and may be associated with chilly sensations. As opposed to pneumonia caused by *Streptococcus pneumoniae* (Chapter 314), that caused by *M. pneumoniae* rarely produces true shaking chills. In comparison to influenza, which can also be manifested as an atypical pneumonia syndrome, myalgias and gastrointestinal complaints of nausea and vomiting are unusual. Diarrhea, sometimes a concomitant of adenoviral or *Legionella* pneumonia, is uncommon in *Mycoplasma* infection.

On physical examination, the general appearance is that of a patient who is not terribly ill. In fact, this disease is the paradigm of the term *walking pneumonia.* The pharynx may be injected and erythematous, usually without the marked cervical adenopathy seen with group A streptococcal pharyngitis. *M. pneumoniae* is not a common cause of isolated pharyngitis in the pediatric or adult population. Much has been made of the finding of bullous myringitis in this disease. This abnormality was associated with experimentally induced *M. pneumoniae* infection in about 20% of volunteers. However, true bullous myringitis in naturally occurring *Mycoplasma* disease is rare. In a study involving a pediatric population, otitis was rarely associated with isolation of *Mycoplasma* and, on the contrary, was often associated with bacterial and viral upper respiratory tract pathogens. The important synthesis of these data is that the absence of myringitis, bullous or otherwise, should not dissuade one from a diagnosis of *Mycoplasma* pneumonia.

Examination of the chest in patients with *Mycoplasma* pneumonia is often unrevealing, even in patients with severe, productive cough. There may be no auscultative or percussive findings, or only minimal rales may be present. The disparity between physical findings and radiographic evidence of pneumonia in this condition may be the greatest of any of the atypical pneumonia syndromes. Although wheezing can occur in this disease, in one study of asthmatic patients the presence of wheezing had a negative correlation with isolation of *M. pneumoniae,* as compared with viral respiratory pathogens such as respiratory syncytial virus (Chapter 385). *M. pneumoniae* also does not seem to be a common pathogen in patients with preexisting chronic obstructive lung disease. Bacterial superinfection after *M. pneumoniae* respiratory infection is rare. The radiographic finding of interstitial or patchy alveolar pneumonia does not allow differentiation from any of the other causes of the atypical pneumonia syndrome.

Pleural effusion (usually small) occurs in 5 to 20% of patients with *M. pneumoniae* infection. This low incidence of pleural inflammation is consistent with the rarity of pleuritic pain. If effusion is present, thoracentesis reveals serous fluid that is exudative with minimal inflammatory reaction. The cell differential count in the fluid is variable, and bloody effusions are rare. It is unusual to isolate *M. pneumoniae* from effusions when they do occur, but several reports of such isolation exist. Although the pneumonia is generally mild and self-limited, fulminant, severe, and lethal cases have been reported in normal young adults and may be underdiagnosed.

Extrapulmonary Involvement

Abnormalities in almost every organ system have been described as examples of the extrapulmonary manifestations of *M. pneumoniae* infection. The frequency of these extrapulmonary manifestations varies greatly from one report to another, and they are much less common when viewed as part of a prospective epidemiologic study rather than as the sum of isolated case reports. The lesson from this appears to be that the high prevalence of *Mycoplasma* infection predisposes to the reporting of many concurrent, but perhaps unrelated events as though they were part of the mycoplasmal disease. Several clinical syndromes have been reported with sufficient frequency to provide some support for a causal relationship.

Dermatologic Involvement

A wide variety of transient dermatologic conditions have been reported in conjunction with *Mycoplasma* pneumonia, including macular, morbilliform, and papulovesicular eruptions, as well as erythema nodosum and urticaria. Again, the variety and high incidence of these rashes in the absence of *Mycoplasma* infection make it difficult to define the relationships, if any, among these occurrences. Furthermore, the role that concurrent antibiotic therapy plays in development of the exanthems seen during *M. pneumoniae* infection is unknown. One skin condition that occurs often enough in concert with *M. pneumoniae* infection to provide some basis for relatedness is erythema multiforme major, or Stevens-Johnson syndrome (Fig. 338–2). This rash has been reported in up to 7% of patients with *Mycoplasma* pneumonia and consists of erythematous vesicles, plaques, and bullae involving the skin, with particular localization at mucocutaneous junctions. The conjunctivae may also be involved, as may organs of the gastrointestinal and genitourinary tracts and the joints. Stevens-Johnson syndrome has been associated in isolated cases with many other infections, including some that can be manifested as atypical pneumonia syndrome. Such infections include legionnaires' pneumonia, adenovirus respiratory-conjunctivitis syndrome, and influenza B infection. However, among possible associations

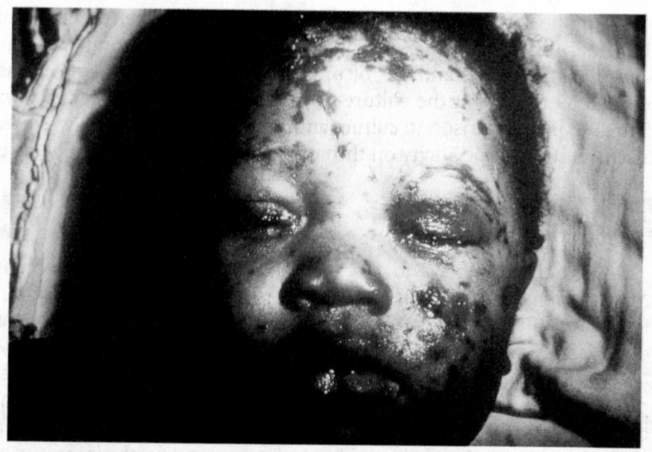

FIGURE 338–2 • Stevens-Johnson syndrome in a child with *Mycoplasma* pneumonia. (From Baum SG: *Mycoplasma pneumoniae* and atypical pneumonia. *In* Mandell GL, Bennett JE, Dolin R [eds]: Mandell, Douglas, and Bennett's Principles and Practice of Infectious Diseases, 6th ed. Philadelphia, Churchill Livingstone, 2005, p 2274.)

of Stevens-Johnson syndrome with infectious diseases, the association with *M. pneumoniae* infection is by far the most common. This complication tends to occur in younger patients with *Mycoplasma* pneumonia and has a definite male preponderance (2:1 to 4:1).

The pathogenesis of this syndrome in any of the diseases in which it occurs is unclear. It has long been supposed that immunity plays a major role, but several reports have noted culture of *M. pneumoniae* from the lesions. The relationship to the level of cold agglutinins in this disease is variable. It has been suggested that the development of Stevens-Johnson syndrome may be the result of augmented sensitivity to antibiotics in the presence of *M. pneumoniae* infection, but erythema multiforme major develops in some patients in the absence of previous or concurrent antibiotic therapy. Most patients clear the lesions in 1 to 2 weeks without scarring unless impetiginization supervenes.

Raynaud's syndrome, a transient reversible vasospasm of the digits that develops on exposure to cold, is not technically a dermatologic syndrome; however, it is manifested in the skin. This phenomenon occurs in many people, usually women, without any association with infection. It has been reported in patients with acute *Mycoplasma* pneumonia, regardless of whether these patients manifested this syndrome before infection. Although the pathophysiology of this condition in *M. pneumoniae* infection is unclear, it may be related to the in vivo action of cold agglutinins (see Diagnosis, later). Other vascular complications reported in *M. pneumoniae* infection include internal carotid artery occlusion and cerebral infarction.

Cardiac Complications

Cardiac abnormalities are the second most commonly reported extrapulmonary manifestations of *M. pneumoniae* infection. Most studies have involved hospitalized patients, so the true incidence of cardiac effects may be underestimated. Signs and symptoms suggesting involvement of the heart are arrhythmia, congestive failure, chest pain, and electrocardiographic abnormalities, particularly conduction defects. One report suggests that a loud third heart sound may be the only clue to cardiac involvement. Although cardiac abnormalities have been reported in as many as 10% of cases of *M. pneumoniae* infection, other reports indicate a much lower prevalence. Cardiac complications are more common with increasing age. They prolong illness but have rarely led to death. The mechanism of heart damage is unknown, but *M. pneumoniae* has been isolated from the pericardial fluid of at least one patient.

Neurologic Complications

Proof of involvement of the central nervous system in *Mycoplasma* pneumonia is somewhat tenuous. Aseptic meningitis and meningoencephalitis, transverse myelitis, brain stem dysfunction, Guillain-Barré syndrome, and peripheral neuropathy have all been reported. In aggregate, these central nervous system manifestations occur no more frequently than 1 per 1000 patients. Cerebrospinal fluid findings in these cases are variable, but cellular response is usually minimal, with slightly elevated protein and normal to slightly depressed glucose. Most often, diagnosis of *Mycoplasma*-related central nervous system involvement is made by exclusion of other causes, the presence of an antecedent or intercurrent respiratory illness, and a rise in antibody titer to *M. pneumoniae* in serum. Occasionally, *Mycoplasma*-specific antibodies have been demonstrated in cerebrospinal fluid, but these titers have paralleled serum antibody titers. Neurologic complications are usually reversible; however, mortality in patients with central nervous system involvement is higher than that in patients without such involvement. Although *M. pneumoniae* has been isolated from a few of these patients, polymerase chain reaction failed to detect *M. pneumoniae* DNA in the cerebrospinal fluid of 11 patients deemed to have *M. pneumoniae*–related central nervous system disease on serologic grounds. Therefore, immune mechanisms of neural damage have been suggested. Some mycoplasmas elaborate a neurotoxin, but this has not been described for *M. pneumoniae.*

Musculoskeletal, Renal, and Hematopoietic Complications

Polyarthralgias are common in *Mycoplasma* pneumonia, but monoarticular or migratory arthritis is rare. Although immune mechanisms have been postulated for this complication, there have been a few reports of isolation of *M. pneumoniae* from joint fluid. Several of the cases of frank arthritis have been reported in patients with hypogammaglobulinemia. Nonhuman mycoplasmas probably cause arthropathy in several animal species.

Renal complications associated with immune complex deposition and high-titer cold agglutinins have been reported. There are several case reports of *M. pneumoniae*–associated aplastic anemia.

Conditions Leading to Increased Susceptibility

Several reports have emphasized the unusually high severity of *M. pneumoniae* infection in patients with sickle cell disease or sickle-related hemoglobinopathies (Chapter 167). Large pleural effusions and marked respiratory distress may develop in these patients. Functional asplenia and its attendant opsonization deficiencies may contribute to overwhelming infection with *M. pneumoniae,* as they do with *S. pneumoniae* infection. Some patients with sickle cell disease and *M. pneumoniae* infection in whom extremely high cold agglutinin titers develop may experience digital necrosis, as they do with *S. pneumoniae.* A hypothesis on pathogenesis is given in the discussion on cold agglutinins in the section Diagnosis. Children with immune deficiency syndromes have been the subjects of case reports of *M. pneumoniae* infection. Because *Mycoplasma* infections are so common in normal children, the contribution of the immune deficiency is unclear. *M. pneumoniae* is not a very common opportunistic agent in patients with acquired immunodeficiency syndrome, but another mycoplasma, *M. fermentans* (*incognitus* strain), has been identified in these patients. Unusually severe but nonlethal *M. pneumoniae* infection has also been reported in children with Down syndrome.

Diagnosis

The diagnosis of *Mycoplasma* pneumonia is made primarily on clinical grounds. The organism can be grown in cell-free media, but most hospital diagnostic laboratories are not prepared to culture mycoplasmas. In the course of *M. pneumoniae* infection, several classes of antibody are produced. Some of these fulfill the desired role of antibody production—neutralization of the agent—and others appear to be autoantibodies. The latter include agglutinins to lung, brain, cardiolipins, and smooth muscle. The best studied of these autoagglutinins are the cold isohemagglutinins described in 1943 by Finland and colleagues in 50 to 70% of patients with Eaton agent (later, *Mycoplasma*) pneumonia. These agglutinins were found to be capable of clumping erythrocytes at 4° C. Agglutination was reversible by warming the serum-erythrocyte mixture to 37° C and, unlike hemagglutination by myxoviruses and paramyxoviruses, was repeatable with the same sample, thus indicating that receptor-destroying enzyme (neuraminidase) played no role in the dissociation at 37° C.

Although a cold agglutination phenomenon is not unique to patients with *Mycoplasma* pneumonia and even though demonstrable cold agglutinins never develop in many patients with *Mycoplasma* pneumonia, this assay has remained a common confirmatory test for this disease. In the diagnostic laboratory, cold agglutinins are demonstrated by combining the patient's serum and type O erythrocytes (to avoid A-B incompatibility). The mixture is incubated at 4° C for several minutes, and the presence or absence of hemagglutination (macroscopic red cell clumping) is noted. If positive, the patient's serum is serially diluted and the test is repeated. The highest dilution causing hemagglutination at 4° C is reported as the cold agglutinin titer. A titer of 1:32 or greater is highly suggestive of infection with *M. pneumoniae.* Other diseases that can give rise to cold agglutinins are mononucleosis caused by Epstein-Barr virus (anti-i), cytomegalovirus (anti-I), some other viral diseases, and lymphoma.

The results of this test as performed in a laboratory will not be available for at least a day and in some cases a week, but a rapid version can be done at the bedside. In this test, 1 mL of the patient's blood is drawn into a tube containing anticoagulant. The type of tube used to collect specimens for prothrombin determination is preferred. Before cooling, examination shows a smooth coating of the tube by red cells. The blood is cooled to 4° C by placing it on liquid ice or in a standard refrigerator. After several minutes, the tube is examined for the presence of macroscopic erythrocyte agglutination. The tube is then rewarmed to 37° C in an incubator or by exposure to body heat and re-examined. The agglutination should dissociate at 37° C, and the appearance of the tube is again as before cooling. This temperature-associated agglutination and dissociation can be repeated many times on the same sample. A positive result in the "bedside" test correlates with a laboratory titer of 1:64 or greater and is therefore less sensitive than the laboratory test. It can be accomplished in minutes, however, and if positive, it is highly suggestive of *Mycoplasma*-related cold agglutination. The presence of cold agglutinins can also artifactually give rise to macrocytic indices secondary to in vitro clumping of erythrocytes, as measured by the Coulter counter method. In this case, the red cell distribution width would be high, indicative of heterogeneity in measured red cell size.

M. pneumoniae infection leads to the production of complement-fixing antibodies as well. These antibodies arise early in the disease (2 to 3 weeks) and persist for 2 to 3 months. Antibody production of both IgG and IgA classes plays a part in protection against the disease. However, second cases of *M. pneumoniae* infection have been reported in apparently immunocompetent individuals.

Laboratory confirmation of *M. pneumoniae* infection has depended on demonstration of cold agglutinins or complement-fixing antibodies. The former, though appearing relatively early in the disease, are both insensitive and nonspecific indicators of *M. pneumoniae* infection. Complement-fixing antibodies, although far more specific, do not arise early enough in infection to be helpful in guiding diagnostic and therapeutic decisions. They are useful primarily in epidemiologic studies or to provide intellectual satisfaction in having made a good clinical diagnosis.

Culture of *M. pneumoniae* is an elaborate and time-consuming procedure that requires 1 to 2 weeks and the use of specialized media. Rapid diagnostic tests with high sensitivity and specificity for *M. pneumoniae* are being developed. These assays fall into three categories: detection of *M. pneumoniae*–specific immunoglobulins in serum and detection of *M. pneumoniae*–specific antigens or mycoplasmal nucleotide sequences directly in clinical specimens. An enzyme-linked immunoassay has been developed to detect IgM and IgG directed against *M. pneumoniae.* Both immunoglobulins were chosen as targets of the assay because adults with *M. pneumoniae* infection may elaborate only an IgG response. The enzyme immunoassay has a specificity higher than 99% and a sensitivity of 98%. Specificity was retained but sensitivity dropped to only 46% when IgG alone was the target. This test may be negative early (less than 7 to 10 days) into infection and does not provide the desired confirmation soon enough to guide initial therapy in many cases.

Detection of *M. pneumoniae* antigens directly in sputum specimens has been accomplished with the use of an antigen capture indirect enzyme immunoassay. The specificity of the assay was high, the reagents reacting only with *M. pneumoniae* and *M. genitalium.* Sensitivity was also relatively high (91%) when the assay was used on sputum and nasopharyngeal aspirates from patients who were shown either by culture or serologically to have *M. pneumoniae* infection.

Detection of *M. pneumoniae*–specific nucleotide sequences directly in clinical material has been accomplished with the use of test kits developed commercially and in house by large reference laboratories. The test, which can be completed in 2 hours, uses radioiodine-labeled DNA complementary to *M. pneumoniae* ribosomal RNA. When compared with culture as the "gold standard" of proven infection, the nucleotide assay detected 89 to 95% of the culture-positive specimens; its specificity was 85 to 89% in comparison to culture and serology when sputum was used; its sensitivity and specificity on throat washings were considerably lower.

Treatment

Despite the number and variety of tests for the rapid diagnosis of *M. pneumoniae* infection, most cases are encountered in the ambulatory setting, and institution of antimicrobial therapy remains empirical and based on clinical recognition of the syndrome.

Antimicrobial therapy is not necessary for mycoplasmal upper respiratory tract infection, and the mycoplasmal etiology of this syndrome probably most often goes undiagnosed. The pneumonia caused by *Mycoplasma* is self-limited and not life threatening in most cases. However, treatment with effective antimicrobials can shorten the duration of illness and, by reducing cough and the number of organisms per unit volume of sputum, can perhaps reduce the spread of infection to contacts.

As would be predicted by the lack of a cell wall, *M. pneumoniae* is unaffected by treatment with β-lactam antibiotics such as the penicillins and cephalosporins. Aminoglycosides are effective in vitro but have not been evaluated for efficacy in vivo. The mainstays of treatment of *M. pneumoniae* respiratory tract infection are macrolides and tetracyclines. Use of either of these antimicrobials significantly shortens the duration of illness. The radiographic findings may take a week or longer to resolve, even with appropriate therapy (see Fig. 338–1), and organisms may continue to be culturable from sputum for several weeks after a complete course of clinically effective treatment. This may be a result of the fact that although *M. pneumoniae* causes respiratory disease as an extracellular parasite, it has the capacity to reside intracellularly as well, thus making it difficult to eradicate the organism in vivo as opposed to cell cultures. The effect of therapy on extrapulmonary manifestations is unknown. *M. hominis* is not sensitive to erythromycin.

Although the tetracyclines are very active against *M. pneumoniae,* their use is precluded in young children because of adverse effects of the drug on developing teeth and bones. On the other hand, erythromycin is poorly tolerated by many people because of its gastrointestinal side effects, including nausea, vomiting, abdominal pain, and diarrhea. Erythromycin also raises theophylline levels, a consideration in the few asthmatic patients who may still be taking this drug.

Because of the adverse effects of erythromycin and tetracycline, there is considerable interest in the antimycoplasmal efficacy of other agents. Doxycycline is somewhat better tolerated than tetracycline and can be administered in two daily doses rather than three. In vitro, doxycycline is as effective as tetracycline against *M. pneumoniae* but, again, is contraindicated in young children.

Several other classes of antimicrobials have been found to have significant in vitro and in vivo activity against *M. pneumoniae* and other *Mycoplasma* species, including the fluoroquinolones, broad-spectrum macrolides (azithromycin, clarithromycin), ketolides (telithromycin), and streptogramins (quinupristin-dalfopristin). There are no good data on the optimal duration of therapy needed to minimize carriage and relapse with these agents.

The macrolides are more active in vitro than the tetracyclines are. Fluoroquinolones have adequate activity for treatment of these infections. They are more active than the tetracyclines but are at least 100 times less active than the macrolides. However, quinolones are also relatively contraindicated in children because of their adverse effects on weight-bearing joints in young animals. The streptogramins are also less active than the macrolides but more active than the tetracyclines. There is a significant cost differential in the use of these drugs. The newer macrolides and quinolones are 50 to 60 times more expensive than the tetracyclines and 6 to 10 times more costly than erythromycin. No erythromycin-resistant strains of *M. pneumoniae* have been found. Taking all this into account, recommended therapy would include doxycycline, 100 mg every 12 hours in older children and adults, or azithromycin, 500 mg

on day 1 and then 250 mg every 24 hours. The usual duration of therapy is 7 to 14 days; shorter courses may lead to relapse. *M. hominis* is not sensitive to macrolides, but it is sensitive to the other antimicrobials recommended for *M. pneumoniae* infection.

Prevention

Because of outbreaks of *M. pneumoniae* respiratory infection among military recruits, there was for a time great enthusiasm and activity to produce a vaccine to protect against this organism. The vaccines did induce specific antibody responses, but protection was limited to no more than 50% of vaccine recipients. Live vaccines using attenuated wild-type and temperature-sensitive mutant mycoplasmas have proved no more effective. In one study, volunteers who received vaccine but did not mount an antibody response had more severe disease when rechallenged with wild-type *Mycoplasma* than did nonvaccinated personnel.

Although *M. pneumoniae* continues to be perhaps the leading cause of atypical pneumonia syndrome in closed populations, the enthusiasm for development of a vaccine for this disease appears to have waned. Vaccine development technology involving DNA expression library immunization has proved successful in animal studies with nonhuman mycoplasmas. These methods may breathe new life into *M. pneumoniae* vaccine development.

Secondary Prevention

Examination of the effects of prophylactic antibiotic use in family members exposed to *Mycoplasma* has shown a decrease in clinical disease in these patients, but seroconversion was not prevented. A study showed that azithromycin prophylaxis, given as a 500-mg loading dose and 250 mg/day on days 2 through 5, significantly reduced the secondary attack rate of *M. pneumoniae* infection in a long-term care facility.

SUGGESTED READINGS

Braun GS, Wagner KS, Huttner BD, et al: *Mycoplasma pneumoniae*: Usual suspect and unsecured diagnosis in the acute setting. J Emerg Med 2006;30:371–375. *A review of the disease presentation, complications, diagnostic means, and therapeutic options of* Mycoplasma pneumoniae.

Daxboeck F: *Mycoplasma pneumoniae* central nervous system infections. Curr Opin Neurol 2006;19:374–378. Mycoplasma pneumoniae *and its relationship to central nervous system infections.*

Daxboeck F, Krause R, Wensich C: Laboratory diagnosis of *Mycoplasma pneumoniae* infection. Clin Microbiol Infect 2003;9:263–273. *A comprehensive review of the laboratory diagnosis.*

Puljiz I, Kuzman I, Dakovic-Rode O, et al: *Chalmydia pneumoniae* and *Mycoplasma pneumoniae* pneumonia: Comparison of clinical, epidemiological characteristics and laboratory profiles. Epidemiol Infect 2006;134:548–555. *A comparison of the clinical presentation of CAP caused by* M. pneumoniae *from* C. pneumoniae.

339 DISEASES CAUSED BY CHLAMYDIAE

Robert C. Brunham

Chlamydiae are obligate intracellular bacteria whose biosynthetic defects in intermediate metabolism and energy generation cause them to be absolutely dependent on a eukaryotic host cell for growth and replication. They are common human infectious agents and produce much disability, although little mortality.

Definition

Genome analysis demonstrates that pathogenic and environmental chlamydiae are a unique monophyletic bacterial group that last shared a common ancestor more than 700 million years ago. The many virulence mechanisms found in modern pathogenic chlamydiae are also found in environmental chlamydiae, thus suggesting that ancient chlamydiae evolved these mechanisms for the exploitation of eukaryotic cells. Radical revision to chlamydial taxonomy has been proposed but not yet widely accepted; currently, chlamydiae are composed of four species (Table 339–1).

TABLE 339–1 CLASSIFICATION OF BIOLOGIC VARIANTS (BIOVARS) AND SEROLOGIC VARIANTS (SEROVARS) OF THE GENUS *CHLAMYDIA*

	Biovar	Serovar
C. trachomatis	Trachoma	12
	Lymphogranuloma venereum	3
	Mouse pneumonitis	1
C. pneumoniae	TWAR	1
C. psittaci	Birds, mammals	Unknown, multiple
C. pecorum	Ruminants	Unknown, multiple

TWAR = Taiwan acute respiratory strain of *C. pneumoniae.*

The Pathogen

The chlamydial bacterial cell has a gram-negative cell wall structure consisting of an outer membrane and an inner cytoplasmic membrane. No peptidoglycan layer is found within the periplasmic space separating these two layers. The outer membrane is rich in protein and composed of a single major outer membrane protein (MOMP; 40 kD) and two minor outer membrane–associated proteins (60 and 12.5 kD). All three proteins are extraordinarily rich in the amino acid cysteine, and intermolecular and intramolecular disulfide bonding produces a supramolecular protein complex that confers structural rigidity to the bacterial cell, analogous to the role played by peptidoglycan in other bacteria. Within *Chlamydia trachomatis,* MOMP variation determines the serologic types that characterize the individual serovars. Polymorphic membrane proteins are also found on the surface of the chlamydial cell, but their role in pathogenesis is undefined. Like other gram-negative bacteria, the chlamydial outer membrane additionally contains lipopolysaccharide (LPS). Chlamydial LPS is a rough type without *O*-saccharides and is composed of a trisaccharide of 3-deoxy-D-manno-octulosonic acid in a unique 2.8 linkage.

Chlamydiae share a common and distinctive developmental cycle (Fig. 339–1). The chlamydial genome is small, with *C. trachomatis* containing 894 protein-coding genes and *C. pneumoniae* containing 1052 genes. Most strains of *C. trachomatis* also contain a 7-kilobase (kb) cryptic plasmid; some strains of *Chlamydia pneumoniae* contain a 4-kb phage. Chlamydiae absolutely depend on host cells to obtain nutrients from the extracellular environment and convert them into forms that they can use, and they are virtually unique in being able to transport phosphorylated compounds found in the host cell cytoplasm.

Pathobiology

Macrophages appear to be the principal host cells for *Chlymadia psittaci* and *C. trachomatis* lymphogranuloma venereum (LGV) biovars. The columnar epithelial cells found in mucous membranes are the usual host cells for the *C. trachomatis* trachoma biovar and for *C. pneumoniae.* Host cell tropism correlates with the type of inflammation elicited by chlamydiae. The LGV biovar and *C. psittaci* produce granulomatous inflammation characteristic of delayed hypersensitivity reactions. The trachoma biovar produces neutrophilic exudate during acute infection and submucosal mononuclear infiltration with lymphoid follicle formation during later stages of infection.

Despite the wide spectrum in tissue tropism and disease phenotype, all *C. trachomatis* genomes are remarkably similar in gene content and gene order. Genomic correlates for tissue tropism and disease phenotype include small differences in the tryptophan synthase and cytotoxin genes. Invasive strains of LGV also produce a phosphorylation pattern of host cell proteins that is different from the pattern found in noninvasive mucosal strains of trachoma and urogenital isolates. Overall, these findings suggest that small genetic differences in chlamydiae produce large changes in the clinical expression of disease.

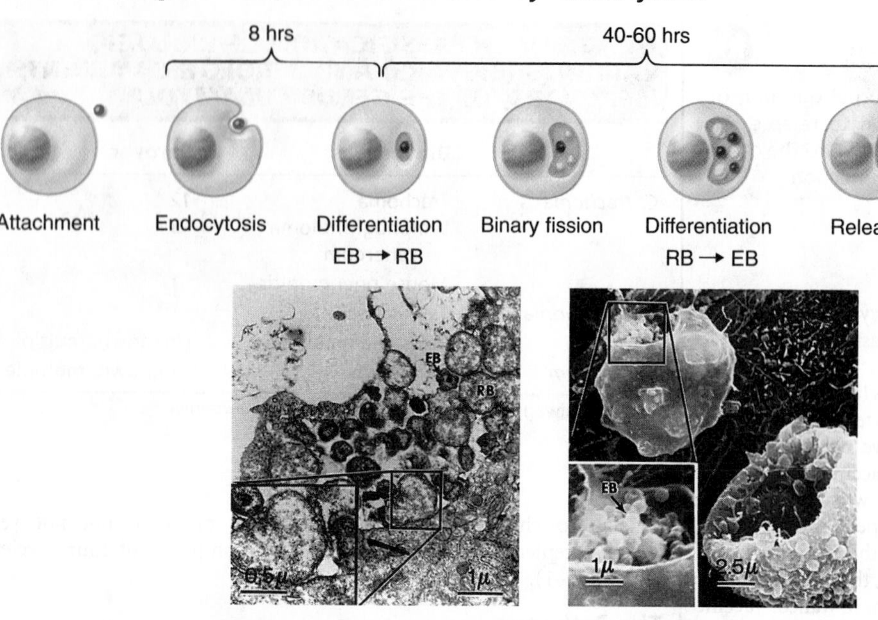

FIGURE 339–1 • The top panel schematically shows the developmental cycle common to all chlamydiae. The red circles represent elementary bodies (EBs), and the blue circles represent reticulate bodies (RBs). Chlamydiae infect eukaryotic cells through multiple attachment mechanisms, best understood for *Chlamydia trachomatis.* A trimolecular complex with a secreted heparan sulfate–like glycosaminoglycan synthesized by *C. trachomatis* acts as a bridge between ligands on the chlamydial EB and the eukaryotic cell surface. Different mechanisms exist in different chlamydial species, which may explain their distinct tropism. After attachment, EBs enter the cell within a membrane-bound vacuole that remains unfused with lysosomes. EBs reorganize into RBs and asynchronously replicate 8 to 12 times with a doubling time of 2 to 3 hours. At the conclusion of the growth cycle, RBs differentiate back to EBs, and each inclusion yields 100 to 1000 new infectious EBs. The bottom left panel, a transmission electron micrograph taken 40 hours after infection, shows the large RBs and the smaller EBs, which have a condensed nucleoid structure within their cytoplasm. The bottom right panel, a scanning electron micrograph taken 60 hours after infection, shows a membrane-bound vacuole containing many EBs exiting from an infected HeLa cell.

TABLE 339–2 MAJOR DISEASES CAUSED BY *CHLAMYDIA* AND CARDINAL EPIDEMIOLOGIC FEATURES

	Disease	Host Reservoir	Transmission Route	Epidemiologic Periodicity
C. trachomatis	Trachoma	Children	Fomites/flies	Endemic
	Urethritis/cervicitis	Sexually active teenagers and adults	Direct sexual contact	
	Epididymitis/salpingitis	Sexually active teenagers and adults	Direct sexual contact	
	Lymphogranuloma venereum	Sexually active teenagers and adults	Direct sexual contact	
	Inclusion conjunctivitis	Infected pregnant mothers	Direct perinatal contact	
	Infant pneumonia	Infected pregnant mothers	Direct perinatal contact	
C. psittaci	Atypical pneumonia	Birds	Aerosol	Epidemic
	Culture-negative endocarditis			
C. pneumoniae	Bronchitis	Humans	Respiratory droplet	Epidemic and endemic
	Atypical pneumonia			

Chlamydiae elicit both humoral and cellular immune responses. *C. trachomatis* elicits secretory IgA and circulatory IgM and IgG antibodies. Serum antibodies commonly recognize chlamydial LPS as detected in the complement fixation assay. *C. trachomatis* infection also elicits antibodies to MOMP as detected by the microimmunofluorescence assay. Women with reproductive sequelae such as tubal infertility or ectopic pregnancy from *C. trachomatis* infection often have antibody to the heat shock protein 60 of chlamydiae.

Because chlamydiae produce intracellular infection, T-cell–mediated immune responses are prominent. HLA-restricted $CD4^+$ and $CD8^+$ T-cell responses occur. $CD4^+$ T_H1 activation with interferon-γ secretion correlates with immunity, and $CD4^+$ T-cell secretion of interleukin-10 correlates with susceptibility to infection. $CD8^+$ T-cell responses occur, but their role in resistance or immunopathogenesis is unclear.

Chlamydial infection persists even after the development of an adaptive immune response, which suggests that the organism has evolved strategies for immune evasion. In the absence of antimicrobial treatment, approximately 50% of women with sexually acquired *C. trachomatis* infection remain persistently infected at 1 year and 10% at 3 years. Persistent infection or episodes of reinfection appear to elicit the immune mechanisms that cause tissue injury. Infection of previously exposed tissue results in an accelerated and intensified inflammatory response, and tissue destruction appears to be directly correlated with the intensity of inflammation. This is best elucidated for *C. trachomatis* ocular infection. Inflammatory and scarring (cicatricial) trachoma are diseases of reinfection, and the more intense the inflammatory response, the more prominent the late fibrotic response. Thus, the mechanism of host injury with *C. trachomatis* infection is thought to be mediated by cellular immune responses. Additionally, host cells infected by chlamydiae release pro-inflammatory chemokines and cytokines, which may cause tissue damage during persistent infection.

CHLAMYDIAL DISEASES

Table 339–2 lists the most frequent chlamydial diseases.

Chlamydia trachomatis

The major diseases caused by *C. trachomatis* are trachoma produced by serovars A, B, Ba, and C; sexually and perinatally transmitted diseases caused by serovars D through K; and sexually transmitted LGV caused by serovars L_1, L_2, and L_3. Trachoma and LGV are primarily diseases in developing areas of the world (although LGV is emerging in some populations of homosexual men in developed countries), whereas sexually and perinatally transmitted chlamydial infections are distributed globally. Trachoma and sexually/perinatally transmitted chlamydial infections are restricted to the mucosal surfaces of the body, and LGV is a systemic infection, principally of the lymphoid system.

Trachoma

Epidemiology

Trachoma is a distinctive ocular disease caused by specific serovars of *C. trachomatis*. An estimated 150 million people worldwide, most of whom are young children, are afflicted with trachoma. Trachoma is especially common in poor areas of sub-Saharan Africa. It is a major public health problem because scarring subsequently develops in 1 to 5% of infected individuals; scarring deforms the eyelid, causes inward turning of the eyelashes (entropion), and results in corneal abrasion (trichiasis). Over time, corneal damage results in blindness. Trachoma is the most common preventable cause of blindness and currently affects an estimated 6 million people. Most of these individuals are middle-aged and older adults. Active trachoma often occurs within the first 1 to 2 years of life and recurs during childhood until 10 to 15 years of age. Among children, the frequency of face washing, access to water, sharing a sleeping room with an affected individual, and the intensity of eye-seeking fly exposure are important risk factors for trachoma. Active trachoma can also occur in adults, especially in mothers caring for young children with active disease. Trichiasis is related to repeated intense trachoma episodes in childhood, is more common in women than in men, and occurs in families.

The *C. trachomatis* serovars that produce trachoma are spread by direct contact with contaminated fomites such as washcloths or eye-seeking flies. Perinatal exposure to *C. trachomatis* from maternal genital tract infection is not important in transmitting trachoma.

Clinical Manifestations

Trachoma is a chronic follicular conjunctivitis that causes macroscopically visible lymphoid follicles to form in the submucosa. They are especially apparent along the upper tarsal plate. The bulbar conjunctiva is minimally involved. Limited mucoid ocular discharge occurs; preauricular lymphadenopathy is rare and, if present, suggests other diagnoses such as adenovirus infection. Superficial vascularization and lymphocytic infiltration (pannus) develop in the cornea. Epidemic bacterial conjunctivitis secondary to *Haemophilus influenzae* can supervene on trachoma and cause a marked purulent conjunctivitis involving the bulbar conjunctiva. Bacterial conjunctivitis worsens the trachoma inflammatory damage. Tarsal conjunctival scarring deforms the eyelid structure and produces entropion and trichiasis in adulthood. Eventually, the corneal epithelium is eroded, and bacterial keratitis occurs. The cornea subsequently heals with opacification, thereby resulting in blindness.

Diagnosis

Trachoma is most often a clinical diagnosis and is made if two of the following findings are observed: lymphoid follicles along the upper tarsal plate, lymphoid follicles (or Herbert's pits) along the corneal limbus, linear conjunctival scarring, and corneal pannus. Because most cases of trachoma occur in remote areas of the developing world without access to laboratory testing, the majority of cases are diagnosed clinically. When laboratories are available, isolation of *C. trachomatis* in cell culture provides definitive proof of the diagnosis. Culture is most often positive in young children with active disease and is rarely positive in adults with late scarring disease. Even in young children with active disease, culture is positive in only a third to half of cases. Nonculture tests such as direct immunofluorescent detection of elementary bodies (EBs) with monoclonal antibody or detection of chlamydial antigen by enzyme-linked immunosorbent assay (ELISA) are more frequently positive than cultures. Detecting chlamydial DNA by polymerase chain reaction (PCR) is the most sensitive diagnostic test, with about 70 to 80% of children with active trachoma testing positive. Few adults with late cicatricial disease are found to have positive tests for chlamydial EBs, antigen, or DNA.

Treatment

Rx

Active trachoma in children can be treated with the topical ocular application of tetracycline or erythromycin ointment for 21 to 60 days. Because extraocular *C. trachomatis* infection of the nasopharynx and gastrointestinal tract is relatively common during childhood trachoma, oral antibiotics such as erythromycin may be preferred. Single-dose oral azithromycin (20 mg/kg) (maximum of 1 g) is as effective as 6 weeks of topical tetracycline.

Prevention

In 1998, the World Health Organization recommended that all countries in which trachoma is endemic take steps to eliminate blinding trachoma by the year 2020 by using the integrated SAFE strategy: surgery, antimicrobials, facial cleanliness, and environmental improvement. For those at imminent risk for blindness, a simple surgical intervention that can be performed by trained nurses prevents the eyelashes from abrading the cornea and reduces progression to blindness. Patients with complicated or recurrent cases still require specialized care.

Antimicrobial treatment is used to eliminate infection and prevent transmission. Mass therapy for young school-aged children has a temporary impact on the prevalence of trachoma. Mathematical models suggest that repeated biannual mass antimicrobial administration may be able to eliminate trachoma from endemic areas. Mass treatment of all members of a community with azithromycin has dramatically reduced the prevalence of infection for up to 2 years without an increase in antimicrobial resistance. Of concern, recent experience suggests that communities may exhibit enhanced susceptibility to re-introduction of trachoma following mass treatment, perhaps due to effects on herd immunity. Facial cleanliness to keep the area around the eyes clear of secretions helps reduce the risk of transmission through contact with fingers and flies.

Environmental improvement includes measures to reduce the number of eye-seeking flies in the community and improve general sanitation and access to clean water. The prevalence of trachoma in a community responds dramatically to socioeconomic development.

Sexually and Perinatally Transmitted Chlamydial Infections

Epidemiology

C. trachomatis is the most prevalent sexually transmitted bacterial infection in the United States. More than 3 million chlamydial infections occur annually, and prevalence rates are highest in sexually active adolescent females. The prevalence is higher in inner-city areas in individuals of lower socioeconomic status and in minority ethnic groups such as African Americans in the United States and Native Americans in Canada. In the United States, the direct and indirect costs of chlamydial disease exceed $2.4 billion annually. From a global perspective, the estimated 90 million infections that occur each year are a major cause of the total disease burden and morbidity because of effects on the reproductive health of women and because infection facilitates the transmission of human immunodeficiency virus and promotes the development of human papilloma virus–induced cervical cancer.

Clinical Manifestations

Urethritis

C. trachomatis causes 30 to 40% of cases of nongonococcal urethritis (NGU) in men, and an estimated 40 to 60% of urethral chlamydial infections are symptomatic with NGU. NGU is characterized by complaints of mild urethral discharge, urethral discomfort, and mild dysuria. On examination, a mild to moderate, clear or cloudy urethral exudate can be detected. Often, it is best observed in the morning before voiding. Sometimes, urethral discharge is apparent only on "milking" the urethra from the base of the penis to the glans. Gram stain of urethral exudate demonstrates five or more polymorphonuclear leukocytes per 1000× field and no gram-negative intracellular diplococci. Asymptomatic urethral infection is common with *C. trachomatis* infection and can be recognized by the urinary leukocyte esterase test on unspun first-void urine.

C. trachomatis urethral infection also occurs in women, in whom it produces an acute urethral syndrome characterized by dysuria and pyuria (more than five white blood cells per 1000× field). The diagnosis should be suspected in women with pyuria but negative cultures for uropathogens. Urinary frequency and urgency are usually absent. Mild urethral exudate may be observed during pelvic examination when the urethra is compressed against the pubic ramus.

Epididymitis

In some men with urethral chlamydial infection (an estimated 1 to 3%), infection spreads from the urethra to the epididymis and causes unilateral testicular pain, scrotal erythema and tenderness, or swelling over the epididymis. Epididymitis associated with urethritis is most commonly due to *C. trachomatis* or *Neisseria gonorrhoeae* (Chapter 321). In men younger than 35 years, *C. trachomatis* is the principal cause of epididymitis. (In men older than 35 years, complicated urinary tract infection with uropathogens is more commonly the cause of epididymitis.)

Reactive Arthritis

Reactive arthritis can complicate chlamydial infection (Chapter 285). About 50% of men with nondiarrheal reactive arthritis have urethral *C. trachomatis* infection. It is estimated that reactive arthritis develops in approximately 1% of men with chlamydial urethritis.

Mucopurulent Cervicitis

As with NGU, *C. trachomatis* causes 40 to 50% of cases of mucopurulent cervicitis. Twenty to 50% of women with cervical chlamydial infection have mucopurulent cervicitis. Women with mucopurulent cervicitis may complain of mucoid vaginal discharge. Unless concurrent infection with other pathogens is present, the vaginal discharge lacks odor, and vulvar pruritus does not occur. Mucopurulent cervicitis is best recognized during vaginal speculum examination with the cervix fully exposed and well illuminated. There is a yellow or cloudy mucoid discharge from the cervix, although the color may be better appreciated on the tip of a cotton swab than in situ. Gram stain of endocervical mucus shows more than 10 polymorphonuclear leukocytes per 1000× field. Often, a red area of columnar epithelium is visible on the face of the cervix (ectopy). The area is erythematous and edematous and bleeds easily when touched with a cotton-tipped swab.

Endometritis and Salpingitis

C. trachomatis infection can spread from the cervix to the endometrium and produce endometritis and to the fallopian tubes and produce salpingitis. Spread occurs in 10 to 40% of women with cervical chlamydial infection. If *C. trachomatis* spreads to the endometrium after therapeutic or postvaginal delivery, it can produce late-onset postpartum or postabortal endometritis. More commonly, chlamydial infection spreads spontaneously to the upper reproductive tract. Although endometritis and salpingitis can occur subclinically, clinically patent disease includes the following features: subacute onset of low abdominal pain during menses or during the first 2 weeks of the menstrual cycle, pain during sexual intercourse (dyspareunia), and prolonged menses or intermenstrual vaginal bleeding. Fever is not a common feature of *C. trachomatis* endometritis or salpingitis.

Infant Inclusion Conjunctivitis and Pneumonia

Perinatally transmitted *C. trachomatis* infection is an important health problem for infants. More than 60% of infants perinatally exposed to *C. trachomatis* acquire infection. Clinically patent disease occurs in about 75% of infected infants. Inclusion conjunctivitis of the newborn develops in one in three exposed infants and a distinctive pneumonia syndrome in about one in six. Because 5 to 20% of pregnant women in the United States have *C. trachomatis* cervical infection, the morbidity from perinatally transmitted chlamydial infection is substantial.

The distinctive pneumonia syndrome has a subacute onset in infants between 1 and 4 months of age. The natural history of the illness is protracted, and importantly, fever is absent. The cardinal clinical characteristic is a distinctive staccato cough reminiscent of pertussis but without the whoop or post-tussive vomiting. Hematologic examination consistently shows eosinophilia and hypergammaglobulinemia.

Lymphogranuloma Venereum

LGV is the result of sexually transmitted infection with *C. trachomatis* serovars L_1, L_2, or L_3. It is a systemic infection that involves lymphoid tissue. LGV is most common in sub-Saharan Africa, although accurate statistics are lacking. LGV is rare in the United States, with a few hundred cases reported annually. Since 2004, outbreaks of LGV have been reported in homosexual men in Europe and Canada, where it has produced a distinctive proctitis and inguinal lymphadenopathy syndrome.

The *C. trachomatis* serovars that produce LGV are much more invasive than other *C. trachomatis* serovars. Similar to diseases caused by other *C. trachomatis* serovars, LGV produces acute disease and late fibrotic complications. Among heterosexuals, primary LGV infection produces an evanescent and rarely observed genital ulcer 2 to 3 weeks after exposure. The ulcer spontaneously heals, and 2 to 4 weeks later painful bilateral inguinal lymphadenopathy develops, often associated with signs of systemic infection such as fever, headache, arthralgias, leukocytosis, and hypergammaglobulinemia. In the absence of treatment, LGV spontaneously heals, sometimes leaving lymphatic scarring. Late fibrotic complications of LGV include genital elephantiasis, strictures, and fistulas of the penis, urethra, and rectum.

In women and men, rectal infection with *C. trachomatis* L_1, L_2, or L_3 strains produces a severe febrile proctocolitis illness. Patients complain of frequent painful defecation (tenesmus) with urgency and, less commonly, mucopurulent bloody discharge in stool. Biopsy of rectal mucosa shows submucosal granulomas, crypt abscesses, and diffuse mononuclear cell inflammation. The clinical, endoscopic, and histopathologic findings can mimic Crohn's disease of the rectum.

Diagnosis

Empirical treatment of *C. trachomatis* infection should be initiated when a specific chlamydial syndrome is recognized. However, definitive diagnosis of *C. trachomatis* infection depends on laboratory identification of the organism. Laboratory diagnosis confirms the clinical diagnosis, assists in managing contacts of infected cases, and detects asymptomatic but infectious individuals. Screening women for *C. trachomatis* has been demonstrated to reduce the incidence of acute salpingitis, as well as prevent pelvic inflammatory disease.

The "gold standard" for diagnosing *C. trachomatis* infection is isolation of the organism in cell culture. The development of culture-independent technologies to identify *C. trachomatis* infection was an important advancement. Culture-independent tests detect (1) *C. trachomatis* EBs in mucosal exudate by fluorescent-labeled monoclonal antibody, (2) antigen (mainly LPS) in extracted mucosal exudate by ELISA, (3) plasmid DNA by direct probing, and (4) chlamydial DNA by PCR amplification. The relative sensitivity of these tests is as follows: cell culture or PCR (capable of detecting a single EB) is more sensitive than LPS antigen detection by ELISA (lower limit of detection, $\approx 10^3$ EBs), which is more sensitive than chromosomal or plasmid DNA probe detection (lower limit of detection, $\approx 10^3$ to 10^4 EBs). Because many chlamydial infections such as NGU, salpingitis, and trachoma are characterized by low numbers of organisms, PCR amplification–based tests are preferred. At present, the higher costs of these tests limit their widespread use, and antigen- or probe-based tests remain the most commonly used tests. Interpreting a positive ELISA test for chlamydia antigen can be difficult in situations in which the prevalence of *C. trachomatis* is low (<5%) because such tests typically have false-positive rates of 1 to 3%. When the test is used to screen individuals from a low-prevalence population, the predictive value of positive tests is very low. Clinicians should verify positive antigen ELISA tests with a second *C. trachomatis* diagnostic test based on a different method if the risk of a false-positive test could result in adverse medical, social, or legal consequences.

Serology is infrequently used to diagnose *C. trachomatis* infection, except in two circumstances: specific *C. trachomatis* IgM antibody at a titer of 1:32 or more is useful to diagnose the infant pneumonia syndrome, and a complement fixation antibody titer of 1:64 or more suggests LGV.

Treatment

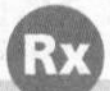

C. trachomatis is uniformly susceptible to tetracyclines, macrolides, and sulfonamides. Recent data also suggest that selected quinolones (ofloxacin and levofloxacin) are useful in treating *C. trachomatis* infection.

The recommended treatment of uncomplicated *C. trachomatis* urethritis and mucopurulent cervicitis is doxycycline (100 mg orally twice daily for 7 days) or azithromycin (1 g orally in a single dose), although azithromycin is substantially more expensive than doxycycline. Alternative treatment regimens include erythromycin base (500 mg orally four times a day for 7 days), erythromycin succinate (800 mg orally four times a day for 7 days), ofloxacin (300 mg orally twice daily for 7 days), or levofloxacin (500 mg orally once a day for 7 days). *C. trachomatis* epididymitis and endometritis/salpingitis should be treated for 10 to 14 days. LGV should be treated for 3 weeks.

Sexual partners and parents of infants infected with *C. trachomatis* should be evaluated, tested, and empirically treated. Sexual contacts within the preceding 30 to 60 days should be seen. Epidemiologic treatment, in which individuals with *C. trachomatis* infection are offered medication to give to their sexual partners or in which clinicians provide medication to contacts without a clinical examination, may reduce the risk for persistent or recurrent chlamydial infection.

Chlamydia pneumoniae

In 1986, a new chlamydial pathogen that causes respiratory illness—*C. pneumoniae*—was recognized. Genome analysis demonstrates that *C. pneumoniae* is a separate species more closely related to *C. psittaci* than to *C. trachomatis.* Pneumonia and bronchitis are the most frequently identified illnesses caused by *C. pneumoniae.* Emerging evidence suggests that *C. pneumoniae* may contribute to atherosclerosis.

Epidemiology

More than 50% of adults in the United States and other developed countries are seropositive. Most seroconversion occurs during childhood, with rates of 6 to 9% per year for the age group 5 to 14. Many seroconversions occur subclinically. *C. pneumoniae* causes both endemic and epidemic atypical pneumonia syndromes. In Seattle, the average annual endemic incidence of *C. pneumoniae* pneumonia was 1.2 per 1000 population. Approximately 10% of pneumonia illnesses were attributed to *C. pneumoniae.* Periods of increased incidence were observed at 3- to 4-year cycles. This organism also produces epidemics of atypical pneumonia in closed populations such as military recruits, university students, and the institutionalized elderly. Patient-to-patient transmission appears to involve respiratory droplet spread with an average case-to-case interval of 1 month. Both diseased and asymptomatically infected individuals transmit infection.

Clinical Manifestations

Even though most acute infections are seen in children, the majority of *C. pneumoniae* disease occurs in adults, especially the elderly. It causes an afebrile, usually relatively mild pneumonia. Extrapulmonary findings are not prominent. Nonproductive cough with sore throat and hoarseness is characteristic. The time from onset of illness to clinical manifestations is long. On auscultation, localized crackles are often heard. Chest radiography shows pneumonitis, most often evident as a single subsegmental lesion. Hematologic studies show a normal leukocyte count but a high erythrocyte sedimentation rate.

C. pneumoniae also causes bronchitis and sinusitis. Bronchitis is often subacute in onset and lasts several days or weeks. Some patients with bronchitis unexpectedly have pneumonia on radiography. Sinusitis is frequently demonstrated by sinus percussion tenderness. Isolated pharyngitis is rarely attributable to *C. pneumoniae* infection, but when pharyngitis, sinusitis, and bronchitis are observed in association with pneumonia, *C. pneumoniae* is a probable cause.

Diagnosis

Serology, isolation, and nonculture detection are the primary methods for laboratory diagnosis of *C. pneumoniae* infection. The indirect microimmunofluorescent test for *C. pneumoniae* antibodies remains the best method for laboratory diagnosis. Isolation of *C. pneumoniae* in cell culture (HL cell line) is successful in 50 to 75% of cases of serologically confirmed infections but is technically demanding. PCR of *C. pneumoniae*–specific DNA is about 25% more sensitive than culture and will probably become the diagnostic test of choice. At present, no effective diagnostic method for *C. pneumoniae* is commercially available.

Treatment

Rx

C. pneumoniae is susceptible to tetracycline and macrolides but not sulfonamides. The clinical response to treatment is not usually dramatic. Recommended regimens include tetracycline or erythromycin base, 500 mg orally four times a day for 10 to l4 days.

Association with Atherosclerosis

Four lines of evidence suggest that *C. pneumoniae* may cause atherosclerosis and plaque instability. Seroepidemiologic studies have shown an excess prevalence of *C. pneumoniae* antibodies in patients with atherosclerosis as opposed to controls. *C. pneumoniae* has been isolated from atherosclerotic plaque on several occasions and has been identified in plaque by nonculture tests in more than 50% of cases. *C. pneumoniae* infection in hyperlipidemic animal models causes atherosclerosis. However, large-scale randomized clinical trials have failed to show that antimicrobial treatment of *C. pneumoniae* alters the risk for cardiovascular disease events in individuals with established atherosclerosis. Antibiotics are not recommenced for secondary prevention of cardiovascular disease caused by atherosclerosis.

Chlamydia psittaci

Epidemiology

C. psittaci is the least common chlamydial infection but remains reportable because it produces common-source outbreaks of serious disease often related to infected imported birds. *C. psittaci* is a heterogeneous chlamydial species that naturally infects a variety of nonhuman mammals and birds. *C. psittaci* strains appear to be host specific, and most human psittacosis infections are linked to bird and not mammal exposure. One hundred to 200 cases of psittacosis are reported annually in the United States, with no apparent periodicity. The annual incidence has been stable for the past 15 years. Psittacine birds (parrots, parakeets, and budgerigars) are most commonly implicated as source contacts, although human cases have been traced to contact with pigeons, ducks, turkeys, chickens, and other birds. Among infected birds, *C. psittaci* is present in nasal and cloacal secretions, guano, and feathers. Psittacosis in birds is a mild illness manifested by ruffled feathers and anorexia. Recovered and asymptomatically infected birds can shed the organism for months.

Transmission to humans is by the aerosol route to the respiratory tract. The infectious inoculum is probably very small, and brief contact with a contaminated environment can result in transmission. Person-to-person spread of *C. psittaci* rarely occurs.

Clinical Manifestations

Psittacosis is a systemic infection of the reticuloendothelial system and the interstitium and alveoli of the lung. Seven to 14 days after aerosol exposure, an abrupt febrile illness begins with shaking chills and a fever as high as 40° C. Headache, myalgias, and arthralgias can be disabling. Cough appears early in the illness but is usually nonproductive. Auscultation may be normal or show bilateral crackles. Chest radiographs show single or multiple localized bronchopneumonic patches. Clinically, psittacosis can resemble legionnaires' disease. In distinction to *C. pneumoniae* pneumonia, psittacosis is more severe with high fever and absent or minimal upper respiratory complaints.

Extrapulmonary findings are usual with psittacosis, and myalgias can mislead the clinician to suspect meningitis or pyelonephritis. Fulminant psittacosis can produce meningoencephalitis, hepatitis, and a faint macular rash (Horder's spots) resembling the rose spots of typhoid fever. Like typhoid fever, psittacosis may cause abdominal pain, diarrhea, constipation, and splenomegaly. Endocarditis develops in occasional patients, especially with underlying valvar heart disease, and *C. psittaci* is a recognized, if rare cause of culture-negative endocarditis. Untreated psittacosis can be fatal, but most patients recover slowly after an illness lasting 10 to 21 days.

Diagnosis

The diagnosis can be established by isolating the organism in cell culture or by serology. Because laboratory-acquired *C. psittaci* infections are well documented, isolation by cell culture is discouraged and serology is the preferred test method. If culture is attempted, it is essential to contain the specimen in a biosafety cabinet for processing. Blood and respiratory secretions can be used to isolate the organism during acute disease. Psittacosis is most readily diagnosed by demonstrating a rising titer of complement-fixing antibody in serum. Acute and 3- to 6-week convalescent sera should be tested.

Treatment

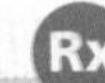

C. psittaci is susceptible to tetracyclines and macrolides but resistant to sulfonamides. Tetracycline has had the greatest clinical use. Psittacosis is the most gratifying of all chlamydial diseases to treat. Defervescence and marked symptomatic relief of systemic signs occur within 24 to 48 hours after starting tetracycline, 500 mg four times a day, or doxycycline, 100 mg twice a day. Treatment should be continued for 10 to 21 days.

Prevention

Epidemic psittacosis is preventable by quarantining and giving all imported psittacine birds tetracycline. Prevention of psittacosis acquired from nonpsittacine birds is more problematic and will remain a continuing source of human infection. No vaccine is commercially available.

The burden of ocular, genital, and respiratory diseases and perhaps chronic cardiovascular, musculoskeletal, and neurologic diseases caused by *Chlamydia* presents a major global health challenge. Effective prophylactic or therapeutic vaccines could have a tremendous impact on protecting people of all ages from the consequences of this ubiquitous pathogen. Progress in genomic sequencing and understanding the immunopathogenesis of disease is accelerating, but for now, long-lasting protective immunity remains elusive. Success will depend in part on the development of new vaccine delivery systems that exploit DNA and plasmid expression systems, viral vectors, adjuvants, and other promising approaches. Even more challenging will be the development of delivery systems that efficiently provide access to vaccines among people in global communities that lack the infrastructure and access to care.

SUGGESTED READINGS

Atik B, Thanh TT, Luong VQ, et al: Impact of annual targeted treatment on infectious trachoma and susceptibility to reinfection. JAMA 2006;296:1488–1497. *Increasing reinfection rates suggest that treatment may interrupt the duration of infection required for developing immunity, increasing the number of individuals susceptible to reinfection.*

Golden MR, Wittington WLH, Handsfield HH, et al: Effect of expedited treatment of sex partners on recurrent or persistent gonorrhea or chlamydial infection. N Engl J Med 2005;352:676–685. *A randomized controlled trial showing the beneficial effect of expedited treatment of sexual partners on recurrent or persistent gonorrhea or chlamydial infection.*

Miller KE: Diagnosis and treatment of *Chlamydia trachomatis* infection. Am Fam Physician 2006;73:1411–1416. *An excellent review of* Chlamydia trachomatis *infection.*

Mariotti SP: New steps toward eliminating blinding trachoma. N Engl J Med 2004;351:2004–2007. *A review of blinding trachoma and the comprehensive World Health Organization program to prevent it.*

Molano M, Meyer CJLM, Weiderpass E, et al: The natural course of *Chlamydia trachomatis* infection in asymptomatic Colombian women: A 5-year follow-up study. J Infect Dis 2005;191:907–916. *An unique study of the natural history of untreated cervical chlamydial infection showing that 5 to 10% of women remain persistently infected after 3 to 5 years of follow-up.*

Peipert JF: Genital chlamydial infections. N Engl J Med 2003;349:2424–2430. *A succinct overview of the clinical aspects of sexuality transmitted* C. trachomatis *infection.*

340 SYPHILIS

Edward W. Hook III

Definition

Syphilis, which is a chronic infectious disease caused by the bacterium *Treponema pallidum*, is usually acquired by sexual contact with another infected individual. Syphilis is remarkable among infectious diseases in its large variety of clinical manifestations. It progresses, if untreated, through primary, secondary, and tertiary stages. The early stages (i.e., primary and secondary) are infectious. Spontaneous healing of early lesions occurs, followed by a long latent period. In about 30% of untreated patients, late disease of the heart, central nervous system (CNS), or other organs may develop years after initial infection. Although the disease is less common now than previously, it remains a challenge to clinicians because of its protean manifestations, and it is of interest to biologists because of the prolonged, tenuous balance between the host and the invading spirochete.

The Pathogen

The causative agent of syphilis, *T. pallidum*, is closely related to other pathogenic spirochetes (Chapter 341), including those causing yaws (*T. pallidum* subspecies *pertenue*) and pinta (*Treponema carateum*). *T. pallidum* is a thin, helical bacterium approximately 0.15 μm wide and 6 to 15 μm long. The organism has 6 to 14 spirals and is tapered on either end. It is too thin to be seen by ordinary Gram stain but can be visualized in wet mounts by darkfield microscopy or in fixed specimens by silver stain or fluorescent antibody methods.

Unlike most bacteria, which have protein-rich outer membranes, the *T. pallidum* outer membrane appears to be composed of predominantly phospholipids with few surface-exposed proteins. It has been hypothesized that because of this structure, syphilis can progress despite a brisk antibody response to non–surface-exposed internal antigens. Between the outer membrane and the peptidoglycan cell wall are six axial fibrils. The axial fibrils are attached three at each end and overlap in the center of the organism. They are structurally and biochemically similar to flagella and are in part responsible for motility of the organism.

It is possible to culture *T. pallidum*, but sustained in vitro cultivation is not yet possible and yields are very low. Culture is of limited use in research but of no use in clinical practice. All isolates studied have been susceptible to penicillin and are similar antigenically. The only known natural hosts for *T. pallidum* are humans and certain monkeys and higher apes.

Epidemiology

Syphilis, with the exception of congenital syphilis, is acquired almost exclusively by intimate contact with the infectious lesions of primary or secondary syphilis (e.g., chancres, mucous patches, condylomata lata). Disease is usually acquired through sexual intercourse, including anogenital and orogenital intercourse. Health care workers have sometimes been infected during unsuspecting examination of patients with infectious lesions. Infection by contact with fomites is extremely uncommon.

Syphilis is most common in large cities and in young, sexually active individuals. The highest rate is found in men between the ages 30 and 45 years, an age that is considerably older than for gonorrhea and chlamydial infection. In recent years, about 80% of the 3139 U.S. counties reported no cases of primary or secondary syphilis, and just 20 locales accounted for about 50% of all reported infections. The disease is most prevalent in the Southeast.

Syphilis spares no class, race, or group but is more prevalent in the United States among persons living on the margins of society. U.S. syphilis rates are about six-fold greater in African Americans than in non-Hispanic whites (about 9 vs. 1.6 cases per 100,000 people). Increased numbers of different sexual partners and perhaps indiscriminate choice of partners increase the risk of acquiring sexually transmitted disease (Chapter 307). Patients with primary and secondary syphilis name on average nearly three different sexual contacts within the previous 90 days. A traditional cornerstone of control of syphilis has been epidemiologic investigation and treatment of sexual contacts of patients with primary or secondary lesions and patients with early latent disease. As syphilis has become associated with drug use and anonymous sex, epidemiologic investigations have become less efficacious.

The incidence of syphilis has generally declined worldwide for more than 100 years, with the exception of periods of war or social upheaval. With the introduction of penicillin, there was a rapid decline in primary and secondary syphilis to annual rates of approximately 4 cases per 100,000 people in 1957. This decline was followed by reductions in federal expenditure for syphilis control, which resulted in a subsequent resurgence of infectious primary and secondary syphilis in the United States in which peaks of more than 12 cases per 100,000 people were attained several times in the period from 1965 through the mid-1990s. Because many cases of syphilis are not reported, the true incidence is much higher.

Over the past 40 years in the United States, syphilis epidemics have occurred serially in at least three population subgroups. In the 1970s and 1980s, men who had sex with other men accounted for a disproportionate number of the total cases of infectious syphilis. Similar trends occurred in other countries. After a period of decline, U.S. syphilis rates nearly doubled from 1986 to 1990, with 50,578 cases reported in 1990 in an epidemic disproportionately affecting multiracial heterosexual men and women and occurring contemporaneously with an epidemic of crack cocaine use. After 1990, syphilis rates again declined, and in 2001, there were 6103 cases of primary and secondary syphilis reported, one of the lowest numbers since 1959. The epidemic of the late 1980s probably also contributed to the spread of human immunodeficiency virus (HIV) infection (see Syphilis-HIV Interactions) and to dramatic increases in the rate of congenital syphilis. Since 2000, syphilis rates have again begun to increase in men, especially men infected with HIV, but not in women.

Patients with clinically evident late syphilis, particularly those with cardiovascular or gummatous syphilis, are becoming less common, perhaps as a result of the effectiveness of penicillin therapy for early syphilis. However, surveys indicate that there are still significant numbers of patients with untreated neurologic syphilis, especially in older age groups.

Natural Course of Untreated Syphilis

The incubation period from the time of exposure to development of the primary lesion averages approximately 21 days (range, 10 to 90 days). Initially, a painless papule develops at the site of inoculation and soon breaks down to form a clean-based ulcer, the chancre, with raised, indurated margins. The chancre persists for 2 to 6 weeks and then heals spontaneously. Several weeks later, a secondary stage characterized by low-grade fever, headache, malaise, generalized lymphadenopathy, and a mucocutaneous rash typically develops. There may be involvement of visceral organs. The secondary eruption may occur while the primary chancre is still healing or several months after disappearance of the chancre. Secondary lesions also heal spontaneously within 2 to 6 weeks, and the infection then enters latency. In more than 20% of patients with untreated latent syphilis, relapsing lesions later develop, similar to those of the secondary stage; rarely, the relapse takes the form of recurrence of the primary chancre. In the era before antibiotics, late, destructive tertiary lesions involving one or more of the eyes, the CNS, the heart, or other organs, including the skin, eventually developed in about a third of untreated patients. These lesions may occur in a few years to as late as 25 years after infection.

The incidence of late complications of untreated syphilis is currently unknown but seems to be less than seen previously. Cases of gumma are now so rare as to be reportable.

Pathobiology

T. pallidum may penetrate through normal mucosal membranes and through minor abrasions on epithelial surfaces. In experimental rabbit syphilis, spirochetes can be found in the lymphatic system within 30 minutes of inoculation and are detected in blood shortly thereafter. There have been a few instances of transfusion syphilis in humans resulting from use of blood from a donor who was in the incubation stage of the disease. The first lesions appear at the site of primary inoculation. In laboratory animals, there is an inverse relationship between the number of treponemes inoculated and the time required for development of the primary cutaneous lesion. The minimal number of treponemes needed to establish infection is not known but may be as low as one treponeme. Multiplication of organisms is slow, with a division time in rabbits of approximately 33 hours. The slow growth of treponemes in humans probably accounts in part for the protracted nature of the illness and for the relatively long incubation period.

Syphilis is a systemic disease from the onset. Treponemes are capable of specific attachment to host cells, but it is not known whether attachment results in damage to host cells. Most treponemes are found in the intercellular spaces, but they are occasionally seen within phagocytic cells. However, there is no evidence of prolonged intracellular survival of treponemes. *T. pallidum* is not known to produce toxins.

The primary pathologic lesion of syphilis is a focal endarteritis with an increase in adventitial cells, endothelial proliferation, and the presence of an inflammatory cuff around affected vessels. Lymphocytes, plasma cells, and monocytes predominate in the inflammatory lesion, and polymorphonuclear cells are seen in some cases. The vessel lumen is frequently obliterated. With healing, there is considerable fibrosis. Treponemes may be seen in most early lesions of syphilis and in some of the late lesions, such as the meningoencephalitis of general paresis.

Granulomatous reaction is common in secondary and late syphilis. The granulomas are histologically nonspecific, and cases of syphilis have been incorrectly diagnosed as sarcoidosis or other granulomatous diseases. Human inoculation studies suggest that the pathogenesis of the gumma, which is a granulomatous lesion, involves hypersensitivity to small numbers of virulent treponemes introduced into a previously sensitized host.

Intracutaneous inoculation of partially purified antigens of *T. pallidum* into patients with syphilis in various stages has shown that delayed cellular hypersensitivity develops only late in secondary syphilis but is uniformly present in latent syphilis. There may be temporary hyporesponsiveness of lymphocytes from patients with primary and secondary syphilis to treponemal antigens. It is possible that the unusual waxing and waning of lesions in early syphilis depend on the balance between the development of effective cellular immunity and suppression of thymus-derived lymphocyte function.

The host also responds to infection with the production of numerous antibodies; in some instances, circulating immune complexes may be formed as well. For example, nephrotic syndrome has been recognized occasionally in secondary syphilis, and renal biopsy specimens from such patients have shown membranous glomerulonephritis characterized by focal subepithelial basement membrane deposits containing immunoglobulin G (IgG), C3, and treponemal antibody.

Clinical Manifestations

Primary Syphilis

The typical lesion of primary syphilis, the chancre, is a painless, clean-based, indurated ulcer (Fig. 340–1A). The chancre starts as a papule, but then superficial erosion results in ulceration. The borders of the ulcer are raised, firm, and indurated. Occasionally, secondary infections change the appearance and cause a painful lesion. Most chancres are single, but multiple ulcers are sometimes seen, particularly when skin folds are apposed (i.e., kissing chancres). An untreated chancre heals in several weeks and

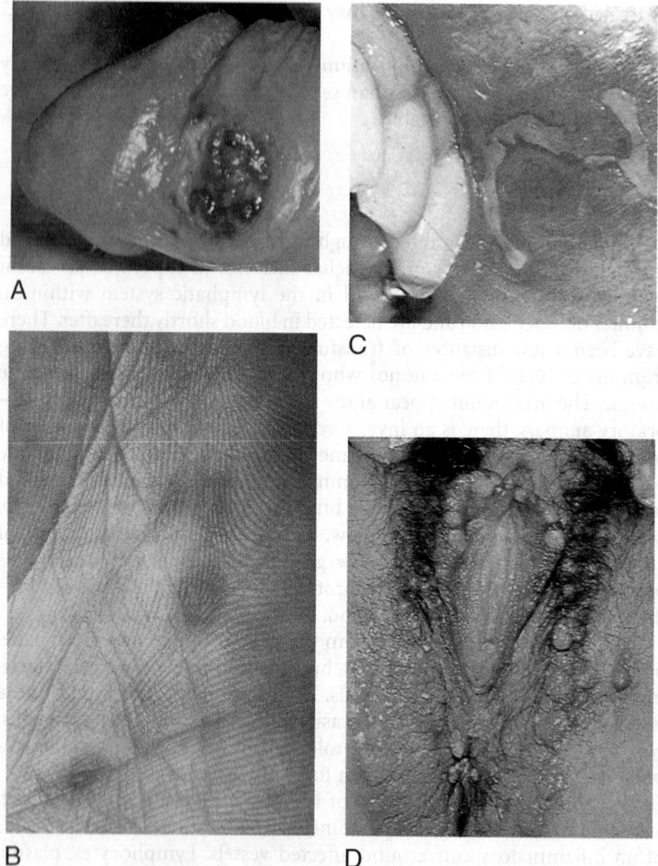

FIGURE 340–1 • Syphilis lesions. A, Chancre in primary syphilis. **B,** Palmar lesions of a coppery color in secondary syphilis. **C,** Mucous patch in secondary syphilis. **D,** Condylomata lata in secondary syphilis. **(A, C, and D,** From Forbes CD, Jackson WF: Color Atlas and Text of Clinical Medicine, 3rd ed. London, Mosby, 2003; **B,** From Habif TP, Cambell JI, Quitadamo MJ, et al: Skin Disease: Diagnosis and Treatment. St Louis, Mosby, 2001.)

leaves a faint scar. The chancre is usually associated with regional adenopathy, which may be unilateral or bilateral. The regional nodes are movable, discrete, and rubbery. If the chancre occurs in the cervix or the rectum, the affected regional iliac nodes are not palpable.

Chancres may occur at any site of potential inoculation by direct contact, with most occurring in anogenital locations. Chancres may also be seen in the pharynx, on the tongue, around the lips, on the fingers, on the nipples, and in other diverse areas. The morphology depends in part on the area of the body in which they occur and on the host's immune response. Chancres in previously infected individuals may be small and remain papular. Chancres of the finger may appear more erosive and can be quite painful. Chancres of the anal canal may be missed in men who have sex with men unless a careful examination is undertaken.

Secondary Syphilis

Between 4 and 8 weeks after appearance of the primary chancre, signs and symptoms of secondary syphilis typically develop. Symptoms may include malaise, fever, headache, sore throat, and other systemic complaints. Most patients have generalized lymphadenopathy, including involvement of the epitrochlear nodes. Approximately 30% of patients have evidence of a healing chancre, although many patients, disproportionately including men who have sex with men and women, give no history of a primary lesion.

At least 80% of patients with secondary syphilis have cutaneous or mucocutaneous lesions at some point in their illness. The diagnosis is generally first suspected on the basis of the cutaneous eruption. The rash is often minimally symptomatic, and many patients with late syphilis do not recall primary or secondary lesions. The rashes are quite varied in appearance but have certain characteristic features. The lesions are usually widespread, are symmetrical in distribution, and are frequently pink, coppery, or dusky red (particularly the earliest macular lesions). They are generally nonpruritic, although occasional exceptions have been reported, and they are rarely vesicular or bullous in adults. They are indurated, except for the very earliest macular lesions, and frequently have a superficial scale (i.e., papulosquamous lesions). The lesions tend to be polymorphic and rounded, and on healing they may leave residual pigmentation or depigmentation. They may be quite faint and difficult to visualize, particularly on dark-skinned individuals.

The earliest pink macular lesions are typically seen on the margins of the ribs or the sides of the trunk, with later spread to the rest of the body. The face is often spared, except around the mouth. Subsequently, a papular rash appears that is usually generalized but is quite marked on the palms and soles (see Fig. 340–1B). These rashes are often associated with superficial scale and may be hyperpigmented. When the rash occurs on the face, it may be pustular and resemble acne vulgaris. Occasionally, the scale may be so great that it resembles psoriasis. Ulceration may occur and produce lesions resembling ecthyma. In malnourished or debilitated patients, extensive and destructive ulcerative lesions with a heaped-up crust may occur, the so-called rupial lesions. Lesions around the hair follicles may result in patchy alopecia of the beard or scalp.

Ringed or annular lesions may occur, especially around the face and particularly on dark-skinned individuals. A lesion at the angle of the mouth or the corner of the nose may have a central linear erosion, the so-called split papule.

The palate and pharynx may be inflamed. In approximately 30% of secondary syphilis patients, so-called mucous patches (see Fig. 349–1C) develop; these slightly raised, oval areas are covered by a grayish white membrane that when raised, reveals a pink base that does not bleed. These lesions may be seen on the genitalia, in the mouth, or on the tongue and, like condylomata lata, are highly infectious.

In warm, moist areas such as the perineum, large, pale, flat-topped papules may coalesce to form condylomata lata (see Fig. 340–1D). Papules may also be seen in the axilla and rarely occur in a generalized form. They are extremely infectious. These papules are not to be confused with the common venereal warts (i.e., condylomata acuminata), which are small, often multiple, and more sharply raised than condylomata lata.

Other manifestations of secondary syphilis include hepatitis, which has been reported in up to 10% of patients in some series. Jaundice is rare, but an elevated alkaline phosphatase level is common. Liver biopsy reveals small areas of focal necrosis and mononuclear infiltrate or periportal vasculitis. Spirochetes can often be visualized with silver stains. Periostitis with widespread lytic lesions of bone has been reported occasionally; bone scanning appears to be a sensitive test for early syphilitic osteitis. An immune complex type of nephropathy with transient nephrotic syndrome has been documented rarely. There may be iritis or an anterior uveitis. Between 10 and 30% of patients have pleocytosis in cerebrospinal fluid (CSF), but symptomatic meningitis is seen in less than 1% of patients. Symptomatic gastritis may occur.

Relapsing Syphilis

After resolution of primary or secondary syphilis skin lesions, 20 to 30% of patients experience cutaneous recurrences. Recurrent lesions may be fewer or more firmly indurated than the initial lesions and, like the typical lesions of primary or secondary syphilis, are infectious for exposed sexual partners.

Latent Syphilis

By definition, latent syphilis is the stage in which there are no clinical signs of syphilis and the CSF is normal. Latency, which begins with passing of the first attack of secondary syphilis and may last for a lifetime thereafter, is usually detected by reactive serologic tests for syphilis (see Diagnosis). Congenital syphilis must also be excluded before the diagnosis of latent syphilis can be made. Patients may or may not have a clinical history of earlier primary or secondary syphilis.

Latency has been divided into two stages, early and late latency. Most infectious relapses occur in the first year, and epidemiologic evidence shows that the most infectious period is during the first year of infection. Early latency in the United States is therefore defined as the first year after resolution of the primary or secondary lesions or as a newly reactive serologic test for syphilis in an otherwise asymptomatic individual who has had a negative serologic test within the preceding year. Late latent syphilis is ordinarily not infectious, except for a pregnant woman, who may transmit infection to her fetus after many years. Most latent syphilis diagnosed at the present time is most accurately called latent syphilis of unknown duration and should be treated in the same manner as late latent syphilis (see later).

TABLE 340–1 NEWLY DIAGNOSED TERTIARY SYPHILIS IN 105 PATIENTS IN DENMARK, 1961–1970

Type of Tertiary Syphilis	No. Observed*
Neurosyphilis	72
Asymptomatic	45
Tabes dorsalis	11
General paresis	13
Meningovascular	1
Optic atrophy	2
Cardiovascular syphilis	44
Aortic insufficiency	16
Aortic aneurysm	13
Uncomplicated aortitis†	15
Late benign syphilis (gumma)	4

*Some patients had more than one form of late syphilis.
†Autopsy diagnoses only.

Late Syphilis

Late syphilis (Table 340–1) is usually slowly progressive, although certain neurologic syndromes may have a sudden onset because of endarteritis and CNS thrombosis. Late syphilis is not infectious through sexual contact. Any organ of the body may be involved, but three main types of disease can be distinguished: late benign (gummatous), cardiovascular, and neurosyphilis.

Late Benign Syphilis

In the penicillin era, gummas are rare. They typically develop 1 to 10 years after the initial infection and may involve any part of the body. Although gummas may be very destructive, they respond rapidly to treatment and are therefore relatively benign. Histologically, the gumma is a granuloma.

Gummas may be solitary or multiple and most often come to medical attention as space-occupying lesions. They are usually asymmetrical and are often grouped. Gummas may start as a superficial nodule or as a deeper lesion that breaks down to form punched-out ulcers. They are ordinarily indolent, slowly progressive, and indurated on palpation. There is often central healing with an atrophic scar surrounded by hyperpigmented borders. Cutaneous gummas may resemble other chronic granulomatous ulcerative lesions caused by tuberculosis, sarcoidosis, leprosy, and other deep fungal infections. Precise histologic diagnosis may not be possible. However, syphilitic gummas are the only such lesions to heal dramatically with penicillin therapy.

Gummas may also involve deep visceral organs, particularly the respiratory tract, gastrointestinal tract, and bones. In addition, they may involve the larynx or the pulmonary parenchyma. Gummas of the stomach may masquerade as carcinoma of the stomach or lymphoma. Gummas of the liver were once the most common form of visceral syphilis and were often manifested as hepatosplenomegaly and anemia and occasionally as fever and jaundice. Skeletal gummas typically produce lesions in the long bones, skull, and clavicle; a characteristic symptom is nocturnal pain. Radiologic abnormalities, when present, include periostitis and lytic or sclerotic, destructive osteitis.

Cardiovascular Syphilis

The primary cardiovascular complications of syphilis are aortic insufficiency (Chapter 75) and aortic aneurysm (Chapter 78), usually of the ascending aorta. Less commonly, other large arteries may be affected, and involvement of the coronary ostia rarely results in coronary insufficiency (Chapter 75). All these complications are caused by obliterative endarteritis of the vasa vasorum with resultant damage to the intima and media of the great vessels. This damage results in dilation of the ascending aorta, but the valve cusps remain normal. An aneurysm is occasionally manifested as a pulsating mass bulging through the anterior chest wall. Syphilitic aortitis may also involve the descending aorta proximal to the renal arteries.

Cardiovascular syphilis usually begins within 5 to 10 years of initial infection but may not be manifested clinically until 20 to 30 years later. Cardiovascular syphilis does not occur after congenital infection—a phenomenon that remains unexplained.

Asymptomatic aortitis is best diagnosed by visualizing linear calcifications in the wall of the ascending aorta by radiography. The signs of syphilitic aortic insufficiency are the same as for aortic insufficiency of other causes. In aortic insufficiency resulting from dilation of the aortic ring, the decrescendo murmur is often loudest along the right sternal margin. Syphilitic aneurysms may be fusiform but are more typically saccular and do not lead to aortic dissection. Between 10 and 20% of patients with cardiovascular syphilis have coexistent neurosyphilis.

Neurosyphilis

CNS involvement occurs throughout the natural history of syphilis. Neurosyphilis may be divided into five groups: asymptomatic, syphilitic meningitis, meningovascular syphilis, tabes dorsalis, and general paresis. Asymptomatic neurosyphilis may occur at any time, whereas syphilitic meningitis is most common during the secondary stage of infection. Meningovascular syphilis, tabes dorsalis, and general paresis are typically manifestations of late syphilis. The divisions are not absolute, and overlap between syndromes is typical. Current cases of neurosyphilis are more likely than heretofore to be variants of the classic syndromes, possibly as a result of the use of antimicrobial agents for other diseases.

Syphilitic Meningitis

Acute to subacute aseptic meningitis may occur at any time after the primary stage but usually within the first year of infection. It frequently involves the base of the brain and may result in unilateral or bilateral cranial nerve palsies. Mild aseptic meningitis may be relatively common in patients with early syphilis, but severe disease occurs in only about 1.5% of untreated patients.

Meningovascular Syphilis

Some patients have sufficient endarteritis and perivascular inflammation to result in cerebrovascular thrombosis and infarction, generally 5 to 10 years after the initial infection. Patients frequently have associated aseptic meningitis. Most cerebrovascular accidents are not caused by syphilitic arteritis, even in patients with a reactive serologic test result for syphilis. However, syphilis should be considered a potential cause in young patients with a history of syphilis and without other causes for cerebrovascular accidents.

Tabes Dorsalis

Tabes dorsalis, which appears to be far less common than in the prepenicillin era, is a slowly progressive, degenerative disease that involves the posterior columns and posterior roots of the spinal cord and results in progressive loss of peripheral reflexes, impairment of vibration and position sense, and progressive ataxia. There may be chronic destructive changes in the large joints of the affected limbs in far-advanced cases (i.e., Charcot's joints). Incontinence of the bladder and impotence are common. Sudden and severely painful crises of uncertain origin are a characteristic part of the syndrome. These features most typically involve the lower extremities but may occur at any site. Severe, sharp abdominal pains may lead to exploratory surgery. These attacks may be triggered by exposure to cold or other stresses or may arise with no obvious precipitating cause.

Optic atrophy is seen in 20% of cases. In 90% of patients, the pupils are bilaterally small and fail to constrict further in response to light but do respond normally to accommodation (i.e., Argyll Robertson pupils).

The onset of tabes dorsalis is usually first noticed 20 to 30 years after the initial infection. Its cause is unclear, and spirochetes cannot be demonstrated in the posterior column or dorsal root.

General Paresis

This form of neurosyphilis is a chronic meningoencephalitis resulting in gradually progressive loss of cortical function. It typically occurs 10 to 20 years after the initial infection. Pathologically, there is a perivascular and meningeal chronic inflammatory reaction with thickening of the meninges, granular ependymitis, degeneration of the cortical parenchyma, and abundant spirochetes in tissues. In the United States, first admissions to mental hospitals because of syphilitic psychosis declined from 7694 in 1940 to 154 in 1968, the last year for which definite figures are available.

In its early stages, general paresis results in nonspecific symptoms such as irritability, fatigability, headaches, forgetfulness, and personality changes. Later, there is impaired memory, defective judgment, lack of insight, confusion, and often depression or marked elation. Patients may be delusional, and seizures sometimes occur. There may also be loss of other cortical functions, including paralysis or aphasia.

Physical signs are primarily those of the altered mental status. Cranial nerve palsies are uncommon, and optic atrophy is rare. The complete Argyll Robertson pupil is also uncommon, but irregular or otherwise abnormal pupils are not infrequent. Peripheral reflexes are often somewhat increased.

Syphilis-HIV Interactions

Syphilis, like other genital ulcer diseases, is associated with a three- to five-fold increased risk for acquisition of HIV infection. Presumably, genital ulcers act as portals of entry through which HIV may more readily infect exposed individuals. As a result, HIV serologic testing 3 months after diagnosis is recommended for all patients in whom syphilis is diagnosed. Conversely, in individuals with HIV infection who acquire syphilis, the natural history of the infection may be modified. HIV-infected syphilis patients are somewhat more likely than non–HIV-infected patients to be seen initially with secondary syphilis. HIV-infected, secondary syphilis patients are also more likely than HIV-negative, secondary syphilis patients to have coexistent chancres, thus suggesting that healing of chancres is delayed or the appearance of secondary manifestations is accelerated in the presence of HIV coinfection.

Congenital Syphilis

Congenital syphilis results from transplacental, hematogenous spread of syphilis from the mother to the fetus. The incidence of congenital syphilis diagnoses in the United States fell below 1000 per year for the first time in 1975, and fewer than 500 cases occurred per year until 1988, when the epidemic of syphilis in adults led to parallel increases in congenital infections. From 1990 through 1993, more than 3000 new cases of congenital syphilis were reported each year. A Venereal Disease Research Laboratory (VDRL) test should be performed in all expectant mothers at the beginning of pregnancy and should be repeated near the end of pregnancy in women living in areas where syphilis is relatively common.

The risk for fetal infection is greatest in the early stages of untreated maternal syphilis and declines slowly thereafter, but the mother may infect her fetus during at least the first 5 years of her infection. Adequate treatment of the mother before the 16th week of pregnancy usually prevents clinical illness in the neonate. Later treatment may not prevent late sequelae of the disease in the child. Untreated maternal infection may result in stillbirth, neonatal death, prematurity, or syndromes of early or late congenital syphilis in surviving infants.

Manifestations of early congenital syphilis are often seen in the perinatal period but may not develop until the infant has been discharged from the hospital. The disease resembles secondary syphilis in adults except that the rash may be vesicular or bullous. The child often has rhinitis, hepatosplenomegaly, hemolytic anemia, jaundice, and pseudoparalysis (i.e., immobility of one or more extremities) as a result of painful osteochondritis. There may be thrombocytopenia and leukocytosis. The early stages of congenital syphilis must be differentiated from congenital rubella, cytomegalovirus infection, toxoplasmosis, bacterial sepsis, and other diseases.

Late congenital syphilis is defined as congenital syphilis diagnosed after more than 2 years' duration. The disease may remain latent with no manifestation of late damage. Cardiovascular alterations have not been observed in patients with congenital syphilis. Neurologic manifestations are common and may include eighth cranial nerve deafness and interstitial keratitis. Periostitis may result in prominent frontal bones of the skull, depression of the bridge of the nose (i.e., saddle nose), poor development of the maxilla, and anterior bowing of the tibias (i.e., saber shins). There may be late-onset arthritis of the knees (i.e., Clutton's joints). The permanent dentition may show characteristic abnormalities known as Hutchinson's teeth; the upper central incisors are widely spaced, centrally notched, and tapered in the manner of a screwdriver. The molars may show multiple, poorly developed cusps (i.e., mulberry molars).

Diagnosis

Darkfield Examination

The most definitive means of making a diagnosis is finding spirochetes of typical morphology and motility in lesions of early acquired or congenital syphilis. Darkfield examination is often positive in cases of primary syphilis and in patients with the moist mucosal lesions of secondary and congenital syphilis. The result may occasionally be positive for aspirates of lymph nodes in secondary syphilis. False-negative results may occur in primary syphilis because of patient application of soaps, antiseptics, or other compounds toxic to *T. pallidum* to lesions. A single negative result is therefore insufficient to exclude syphilis. For high-risk individuals (e.g., drug users, homosexually active men), it is appropriate to treat presumptively based on suspicious lesions after performing serologic tests. Confusion may also arise because of the presence of spirochetes morphologically indistinguishable from *T. pallidum* organisms in the mouth, particularly around the gingival margins.

To perform a darkfield examination, the surface of the suspected ulcerative lesion should be cleaned with saline solution and gauze without producing bleeding. Squeezing of the lesion (with gloves on) may help produce serous fluid, which can be picked up on a glass slide, covered with a coverslip, and examined with the darkfield microscope. Living *T. pallidum* organisms demonstrate gradual motion to and fro, rotational movement around the long axis, and rather sudden 90-degree flexing near the center of the organism. Because most physicians do not have the proper equipment and are not familiar with darkfield microscopy techniques, public health authorities can be called for assistance. *T. pallidum* may also be demonstrated in biopsy or pathologic specimens by fluorescent antibody stains or by silver stains.

Serologic Tests

Two basic types of serologic tests (Table 340–2) are widely used to diagnose infection with *T. pallidum:* (1) nontreponemal tests that detect antibodies reactive with diphosphatidylglycerol (cardiolipin), which is a normal component of many tissues, and (2) specific treponemal antibodies.

Nontreponemal Tests

The standard tests to detect anticardiolipin antibody are the VDRL and rapid plasma reagin (RPR) tests, which are slide flocculation tests. The VDRL and RPR are readily quantified, so they are the tests of choice for monitoring patients' responses to treatment. The relative proportion of patients with a false-positive VDRL result depends on the prevalence of syphilis in the community; the lower the prevalence of syphilis, the higher the proportion of reactive VDRL test results from nonsyphilitic causes.

The VDRL test begins to turn positive about 1 week after onset of the chancre, but only about two thirds of patients with primary syphilis have a positive test, so a nonreactive VDRL test does not exclude primary syphilis, particularly if the lesion is less than 1 week old. The VDRL test result is positive in 99% of patients with secondary syphilis (Table 340–3). Patients with advanced HIV infection may have negative test results, and some patients have such high titers of antibody that they are in antibody excess; dilution of their serum will paradoxically result in conversion of a negative to a positive test result, the prozone reaction. VDRL reactivity tends to diminish in later stages of syphilis, and only about 70% of patients with cardiovascular or neurosyphilis have positive VDRL test results.

TABLE 340–2 SEROLOGIC TESTS FOR SYPHILIS

Type	Use
NONTREPONEMAL (ANTICARDIOLIPIN) ANTIBODIES	
VDRL (slide flocculation)	Screening, quantitation, after response to treatment
RPR (circle card) (agglutination)	Screening
SPECIFIC TREPONEMAL ANTIBODIES	
FTA-ABS (immunofluorescence with absorbed serum)	Confirmatory, diagnostic, not for routine screening
TP-PA (microhemagglutination)	Similar to FTA-ABS but can be quantified and automated

FTA-ABS = fluorescent treponemal antibody absorption test; TP-PA = *Treponema pallidum*—particle agglutination; RPR = rapid plasma regain test; VDRL = Venereal Disease Research Laboratory.

TABLE 340-3 FREQUENCY OF POSITIVE SEROLOGIC TESTS IN UNTREATED SYPHILIS

Stage	VDRL (%)	FTA-ABS (%)	TP-PA (%)
Primary	70	85	50–60
Secondary	99	100	100
Latent or late	70	98	98

FTA-ABS = fluorescent treponemal antibody absorption test; TP-PA = *Treponema pallidum*—particle agglutination; VDRL = Venereal Disease Research Laboratory.

The *quantitative titer* of the VDRL or RPR test is somewhat useful in diagnosis and quite useful for monitoring therapeutic response. The titer is reported as the highest dilution that gives a positive response. Most patients with secondary syphilis have titers of at least 1:16. Most patients with false-positive VDRL test results have titers of less than 1:8. No single titer is in itself diagnostic. Significant rises (four-fold or greater) in paired sera, however, strongly indicate acute syphilis.

Treponemal Tests

In the fluorescent treponemal antibody absorption (FTA-ABS) test, the patient's serum is first absorbed with extracts of nonpathogenic cultivable treponemes to remove cross-reacting treponemal antibodies, then with *T. pallidum,* and finally with fluorescein-conjugated antihuman antibody. Agglutination of particles to which *T. pallidum* antigens have been fixed is the basis of the *T. pallidum* particle agglutination (TP-PA) test.

The FTA-ABS test is best used as a confirmatory test to verify that persons with reactive nontreponemal tests have antibodies to *T. pallidum.* It is somewhat more difficult to perform than the VDRL test and cannot be easily quantified. It is sensitive and has a high degree of specificity in that it is reactive in only approximately 1% of normal individuals. It is reactive in 85% of patients with primary syphilis, 99% with secondary syphilis, and at least 95% with late syphilis. It may therefore be the only test with a positive result in patients with cardiovascular or neurologic syphilis. For patients with late syphilis, the FTA-ABS test often remains reactive for life despite adequate therapy. The FTA-ABS test is reported in terms of relative brilliance of fluorescence, from borderline to 4 plus, and most laboratories report only tests with 2 plus or greater reactivity as positive. For patients lacking historical or clinical evidence of syphilis but with a reactive FTA-ABS test result, the FTA-ABS test should be repeated. Use of another treponemal test such as the TP-PA test may be helpful in problem cases. The TP-PA test is slightly less sensitive than the VDRL or FTA-ABS test in primary syphilis. Its sensitivity and specificity are otherwise nearly identical to those of the FTA-ABS test.

Enzyme-linked immunoassays (EIAs) for detection of antitreponemal antibodies use cloned *T. pallidum* antigens generated from bacterial expression systems. EIA serologic tests permit screening of large numbers of sera and have performance characteristics (sensitivity, specificity, predictive values) similar to those of other treponemal tests. Persons with syphilis diagnosed by treponemal antigen EIAs should be tested with quantitative nontreponemal tests such as the VDRL for confirmation and to permit use of these tests for evaluation of the subsequent response to therapy.

Differential Diagnosis

The differential diagnosis of a genital ulcer (Chapter 307) includes genital herpes (Chapter 397), chancroid (Chapter 324), lymphogranuloma venereum (Chapter 339), and a number of other ulcerative processes. Classically, herpetic ulcers are multiple, painful, superficial, and if seen early, vesicular. However, atypical manifestations may be indistinguishable from a syphilitic chancre. Genital herpes is orders of magnitude more common than syphilis. As a result, genital herpes is now the most common cause of a "typical chancre" in North America. Syphilitic chancres may also be coinfected with herpes simplex virus in about 15% of cases. The ulcers of chancroid are usually painful, often multiple, and frequently exudative and nonindurated. Lymphogranuloma venereum may produce a small, papular lesion associated with regional adenopathy. Other conditions that must be distinguished include granuloma inguinale (Chapter 337), drug eruptions, carcinoma, superficial fungal infections (Chapter 464), traumatic lesions, and lichen planus (Chapter 464). Final distinction in most cases is made on the basis of darkfield examination, which is positive only in syphilis.

The differential diagnosis of the skin lesions of secondary syphilis (Chapter 464) includes pityriasis rosea, which can be differentiated by the occurrence of lesions along lines of skin cleavage and frequently by the presence of a herald patch. Drug eruptions, acute febrile exanthems, psoriasis, lichen planus, scabies, and other diseases must also be considered in some cases. A mucous patch may superficially resemble oral candidiasis (i.e., thrush). Infectious mononucleosis (Chapter 400) may appear very similar to secondary syphilis, with sore throat, generalized adenopathy, hepatitis, and a generalized rash. Hepatitis (Chapter 151) may also cause confusion.

False-Positive Serologic Test Results for Syphilis

The VDRL or RPR test will be reactive in patients with other treponemal diseases, such as pinta, yaws, and endemic syphilis (Chapter 341). These tests may also be falsely reactive in persons who do not have treponemal infections based on a negative clinical history or negative results on serum FTA-ABS or other treponemal tests.

Acute (<6 months) false-positive VDRL test results occur with low frequency in patients with atypical pneumonia, malaria, and other bacterial or viral infections and may occur after smallpox or other vaccinations as well. Chronic false-positive VDRL test results (persisting >6 months) are relatively common in patients with autoimmune disorders such as systemic lupus erythematosus (SLE; Chapter 287), in parenteral drug users, in HIV-infected patients, in patients with leprosy, and in aged persons. Between 8 and 20% of patients with SLE have false-positive VDRL test results, and the false-positive result may develop many years before the onset of other manifestations of the disease. A chronic false-positive VDRL test result in female patients 20 years or younger carries a significant risk for the future development of SLE, thyroiditis, or other autoimmune disorders. As many as a third of parenteral drug users have false-positive VDRL test results. More than 1% of persons 70 years old and 10% of those older than 80 also have low-titer, false-positive VDRL test results. Most false-positive VDRL tests have a titer of less than 1:8, although a few patients with lymphoma and other diseases have very high-titer, false-positive VDRL test results.

There is also an increased incidence of false-positive FTA-ABS results in SLE and other chronic inflammatory diseases associated with hyperglobulinemia, including rheumatoid arthritis and biliary cirrhosis. Occasionally, reproducible positive FTA-ABS results are obtained in patients with no clinical or historical evidence of syphilis and no evidence of diseases typically associated with false-positive FTA-ABS results. If in doubt and if the patient is not allergic to penicillin, it is often prudent to treat such patients for possible syphilis.

Neurosyphilis

Asymptomatic neurosyphilis is diagnosed when there are CSF abnormalities, such as lymphocytic pleocytosis, protein elevation, or a reactive VDRL test result in a syphilis patient in the absence of signs and symptoms of neurologic disease. Although numerous other processes may cause CSF pleocytosis or protein elevations, false-positive CSF VDRL test results are rare in the absence of a traumatic tap. If the CSF is normal 2 or more years after the initial infection, a positive CSF finding is not likely to develop later. Routine lumbar punctures for examining CSF are not indicated in early syphilis unless the patient is known to have HIV infection. Although a nonreactive CSF FTA-ABS result may be useful to rule out the diagnosis, no diagnosis of asymptomatic (or symptomatic) neurosyphilis should be based solely on the CSF FTA-ABS test.

In syphilitic meningitis, the CSF shows a lymphocytic pleocytosis with increased protein and usually normal glucose concentrations. The CSF VDRL test is nearly always reactive. Rarely, the CSF glucose concentration is decreased. Without treatment, syphilitic meningitis generally resolves, similar to the course of other manifestations of early syphilis. This syndrome can mimic tuberculous or fungal meningitis or nonpurulent meningitis of various causes.

In tabes dorsalis, the VDRL test for serum is nonreactive in as many as 30 to 40% of patients, and 10 to 20% of patients (even before the advent of penicillin) have normal CSF VDRL results. The FTA-ABS test for serum is nearly always reactive.

In general paresis, the CSF is nearly always abnormal, with lymphocytic pleocytosis and an increased total protein concentration. The VDRL test is usually reactive for CSF and serum.

Congenital Syphilis

Because many infants with congenital syphilis are clinically normal at birth but serious, symptomatic disease may develop some weeks later, it is important to determine whether a newborn with a reactive VDRL or FTA-ABS test result has passively transferred maternal antibody or is actively infected. If the mother has been adequately treated for syphilis during pregnancy and the infant is clinically normal at birth, one option is to monitor the infant carefully by serial examinations and VDRL titers. If the reactive VDRL result for the infant is caused by passively transferred maternal antibody, the titer will fall markedly in the first 2 months of life; a rising titer indicates active disease and the need for treatment. However, the risk of failure of proper follow-up of VDRL-positive, but clinically normal neonates makes immediate, empirical administration of effective therapy an attractive alternative.

Prevention

All patients with syphilis should be reported to public health authorities. In the absence of an effective vaccine, control of syphilis depends on finding and treating persons with infectious lesions of primary and secondary syphilis before they can further transmit the disease and on finding and treating persons with incubating syphilis before infectious lesions develop. All patients with early syphilis (primary, secondary, or early latent) should be carefully interviewed by qualified persons to determine the nature of their recent sex contacts. Approximately 16% of the named recent contacts of patients with early syphilis are found to have active, untreated syphilis on examination, and a similar proportion of individuals named as suspects or associates also have active syphilis.

Treatment of sexual contacts of patients with early syphilis with 2.4 million U of benzathine penicillin G intramuscularly is recommended even if the contacts are clinically and serologically normal on examination because syphilis eventually develops in 30% of clinically normal individuals named as contacts of persons with infectious lesions of syphilis within the previous 30 days if untreated. In general, preventive treatment is given to all sexual contacts in the past 90 days, although nearly all cases of syphilis in contacts develop within 60 days of exposure.

Treatment

T. pallidum is inhibited by less than 0.01 μg/mL of penicillin G. Because treponemes divide slowly and penicillin acts only on dividing cells, it is necessary to maintain serum levels of penicillin for many days (Table 340–4).

Early Infectious Syphilis

Early syphilis (<1 year) may be treated with a single injection of 2.4 million U of benzathine penicillin G, which provides low, but effective, serum levels for more than 2 weeks and cures approximately 95% of patients. [1] It is not necessary to examine CSF at this stage because penicillin prevents the later development of neurosyphilis.

Persons with other sexually transmitted diseases may have also been exposed to syphilis at the time that they became infected. Treatment with a single dose of β-lactam antibiotics (penicillins, cephalosporins), which provide relatively high serum levels for a brief period, is ineffective in established early syphilis but is curative if the disease is still in the incubating stage. The ceftriaxone regimen useful for gonorrhea (Chapter 322) is probably curative for incubating syphilis, but careful follow-up is indicated if there is reason to suspect exposure to syphilis in a patient treated for gonorrhea with ceftriaxone. Single-dose therapy with 2.0 g of azithromycin administered orally has been as effective as benzathine penicillin therapy in several studies of early syphilis, [2] but treatment failures have been reported in persons with coexistent HIV infection. Currently, azithromycin should not be used for the treatment of early syphilis unless close follow-up can be ensured.

For patients allergic to penicillin, 100 mg of doxycycline orally twice daily for 14 days is recommended. Particularly careful follow-up is necessary for patients treated with drugs other than penicillin because patients may not be fully compliant with these prolonged courses of oral therapy and these regimens have been less fully evaluated clinically. Ceftriaxone, given in doses of 500 mg to 1.0 g intramuscularly daily for 10 days, may be effective but has been studied only in small numbers of patients with syphilis. Quinolone antibiotics have essentially no effect on syphilis.

TABLE 340–4 PENICILLIN TREATMENT PRACTICE FOR SYPHILIS AS RECOMMENDED BY THE U.S. PUBLIC HEALTH SERVICE

	Dosage and Administration*	
Indications for Syphilis Therapy†	**Benzathine Penicillin G**	**Aqueous Benzylpenicillin G or Procaine Penicillin G**
Primary, secondary, and early latent syphilis (<1 year); epidemiologic treatment	Total of 2.4 million U; single IM dose of two injections of 1.2 million U in one session	Total of 4.8 million U IM in doses of 600,000 U daily for 8 consecutive days
Late latent (>1 year) or when CSF was not examined in "latency"; cardiovascular syphilis, late benign (cutaneous, osseous, visceral gumma)	Total of 7.2 million U IM in doses of 2.4 million U at 7-day intervals over a 21-day period	Total of 9 million U IM in doses of 600,000 U daily over a 15-day period
Symptomatic or asymptomatic neurosyphilis	2 to 4 million U of aqueous (crystalline) penicillin G IV every 4 hours for at least 10 days	2 to 4 million U procaine penicillin IM daily and probenecid, 500 mg orally four times daily, for 10–14 days
Congenital		
Infants	CSF normal: Total of 500,000 U/kg IM in a single or divided dose at one session	CSF abnormal: Total of 50,000 U/kg/day IM for 10 consecutive days‡
Older children	CSF normal: Same as for early congenital syphilis, up to 2.4 million U	CSF abnormal: 200,000–300,000 U/kg/day aqueous crystalline penicillin IV for 10–14 days

*Individual doses can be divided for injection in each buttock to minimize discomfort.
†In *pregnancy*, treatment depends on the stage of syphilis.
‡For aqueous penicillin, give in two divided intravenous doses per day; for procaine penicillin, give as one daily dose intramuscularly.
CSF = cerebrospinal fluid.

Section XXIII Infectious Diseases

Rx

Syphilis of More than 1 Year's Duration

Prolonged therapy with intramuscular injections of 2.4 million U of benzathine penicillin G weekly for 3 weeks is recommended for treatment of late latent syphilis and latent syphilis of unknown duration. Limited evidence suggests that treating latent syphilis with a total dose of 7.2 million U of benzathine penicillin over a 3-week period is curative, even if the patient has asymptomatic neurosyphilis. However, because of the possible lack of efficacy of benzathine penicillin in some patients with CNS syphilis, it is preferable to examine the CSF in most patients with latent syphilis to exclude asymptomatic neurosyphilis, particularly in HIV-positive patients, in whom the prevalence of asymptomatic neurosyphilis is higher. Alternatively, a lumbar puncture may be performed at the conclusion of the follow-up period (2 years); if the CSF is normal, the patient can be reassured that neurosyphilis will not develop.

Larger doses of penicillin are recommended for persons with proven neurosyphilis (Table 340–4). General paresis responds well to penicillin therapy if administered early, although progressive neurologic decline may develop in as many as a third of treated patients in later years. Carbamazepine in doses of 400 to 800 mg/day has been reported to treat the lightning pains effectively. Published studies show that a total of 6.0 to 9.0 million U of penicillin G results in a satisfactory clinical response in approximately 90% of patients with neurosyphilis who do not have HIV infection. There are anecdotal reports of increased treatment failures in patients with concomitant HIV infection, and there is considerable rationale to treat with intravenous penicillin G (20 million U/day for at least 10 days). Therapy for neurosyphilis can result in increased CSF pleocytosis for 7 to 10 days after starting treatment and may transiently convert a normal CSF to abnormal.

Although there is no evidence that therapy with antimicrobial drugs is clinically beneficial in patients with cardiovascular syphilis, treatment is recommended to prevent further progression of disease and because approximately 15% of patients with cardiovascular syphilis have associated neurosyphilis. If patients are allergic to penicillin, it is mandatory that the CSF be examined before therapy is undertaken; if the CSF is abnormal, desensitization to penicillin is generally recommended. With a normal CSF, tetracycline (500 mg orally four time a day) or doxycycline (100 mg orally two times a day) taken for 4 weeks is probably effective.

Syphilis in Pregnancy

Because of the risk to the fetus, evaluation and treatment of a VDRL-positive patient must be rapid, particularly for patients first seen in the later stages of pregnancy. If a confirmatory FTA-ABS test is positive and the patient has not been treated, penicillin should be administered in doses appropriate for early or late syphilis, as outlined earlier. For penicillin-allergic patients, penicillin desensitization is preferred; patients should not be treated with tetracycline or erythromycin because of toxicity (tetracycline) or lack of efficacy (erythromycin). For patients who are VDRL positive but FTA-ABS negative and who have no clinical signs of syphilis, treatment may be withheld; a quantitative VDRL test and another FTA-ABS test should be repeated in 4 weeks. If the VDRL titer has risen by four-fold or more or if clinical signs of syphilis have developed, the patient should be treated. If after repeat examination the diagnosis remains equivocal, the patient should be treated to prevent possible disease in the neonate. After treatment, a quantitative VDRL titer should be monitored monthly; if it rises four-fold, the patient should be treated a second time.

Congenital Syphilis

Proper treatment of the mother usually prevents active congenital syphilis in the neonate. However, infected infants may be clinically normal at birth, and the infant may be seronegative if the mother's infection was acquired late in pregnancy. The infant should be treated at birth if the mother has received no or inadequate treatment or has been treated with drugs other than penicillin, if the mother has not yet responded to possibly effective therapy, or if the infant cannot be carefully monitored for several months after birth. The infant's CSF should be examined before treatment. If the CSF is normal, the child may be treated with a single intramuscular injection of 50,000 U/kg (up to 2.4 million U) of benzathine penicillin G. If the CSF is abnormal, the infant should be treated with 50,000 U/kg of aqueous penicillin G given intramuscularly or intravenously twice daily for a minimum of 10 days. Alternatively, a single daily intramuscular injection of 50,000 U/kg of procaine penicillin may be given for 10 days. Antimicrobial agents other than penicillin are not recommended for treating congenital syphilis.

Jarisch-Herxheimer Reactions

Up to 60% of patients with early syphilis and a significant proportion of patients with later stages of syphilis experience a transient febrile reaction after therapy for syphilis. The pathogenesis is unclear, but it may be caused by liberation of antigens from spirochetes.

This reaction usually occurs in the first few hours after therapy, peaks at 6 to 8 hours, and disappears within 12 to 24 hours of therapy. Occasionally, Herxheimer reactions are mistaken for allergic reactions to syphilis therapy. Temperature elevation is usually low grade, and there is often associated myalgia, headache, and malaise. The skin lesions of secondary syphilis are frequently exacerbated during the Herxheimer reaction, and cutaneous lesions that were not visible may become visible. The reaction is generally of no clinical significance and in most cases may be treated with salicylates. Corticosteroids have been used to prevent adverse effects of the Herxheimer reaction, but there is no evidence that they are clinically beneficial (other than reducing fever) or necessary. Institution of treatment with small doses of penicillin does not prevent the Herxheimer reaction.

Prognosis

Follow-up Examinations

All HIV-seronegative patients with early or congenital syphilis should return for quantitative VDRL titers and clinical examination 6 and 12 months after treatment. For HIV-positive patients, serologic tests should be repeated at 1, 2, 3, 6, 9, and 12 months. Patients with late latent syphilis should also be examined 24 months after therapy; if CSF was not examined before therapy, a lumbar puncture should be done before discharge to rule out inadequately treated asymptomatic neurosyphilis.

In about 85% of patients with early (i.e., primary, secondary, or early latent) syphilis, quantitative VDRL titers decline two or more dilutions (four-fold) by 6 and 12 months after therapy. Prolonged reactive VDRL test results are associated with higher initial VDRL titers, prolonged infection, more advanced stage (primary < secondary < early latent), or repeated infection. Chronic, low-titer VDRL reactivity after therapy is much more common in cases of late syphilis and should not be viewed with alarm. The FTA-ABS test may remain positive for years despite adequate therapy. A four-fold or greater rise in VDRL titer after therapy is sufficient evidence for repeat treatment. Patients with treated early syphilis are susceptible to reinfection, and many clinical and serologic relapses after therapy are probably reinfections. As such, they represent failures of proper epidemiologic case finding and preventive therapy for the patient's sexual contacts.

Patients with neurosyphilis should be monitored with serologic tests for at least 3 years and with repeat CSF examinations at 6-month intervals. CSF pleocytosis is the first abnormality to disappear, but cell counts may not be normal for 1 to 2 years. Elevated CSF protein levels fall still more slowly, followed by a change in the positive CSF VDRL test, which may take years to become negative. It is not known whether high-dose intravenous penicillin therapy accelerates the return of CSF to normal. Rising CSF cell counts, protein, and VDRL titer obtained at follow-up are an indication for repeat treatment.

Antibiotic therapy should ultimately cure essentially all patients with early or secondary syphilis, although treatment failures may occur in patients with concomitant HIV infection. In tabes dorsalis, penicillin usually arrests progression but does not reverse the symptoms. Meningovascular syphilis generally responds well, except for residual damage resulting from ischemic infarcts.

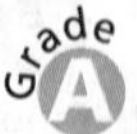

1. Rolfs RT, Joesoef MR, Hendershot EF, et al: A randomized trial of enhanced therapy for early syphilis in patients with and without human immunodeficiency virus infection. N Engl J Med 1997;337:307–314.
2. Riedner G, Rusizoka M, Todd J, et al: Single-dose azithromycin versus penicillin G benzathine for the treatment of early syphilis. N Engl J Med 2005;353:1236–1244.

SUGGESTED READINGS

Centers for Disease Control and Prevention: Sexually transmitted diseases treatment guidelines, 2006. MMWR Recomm Rep 2006;55:(RR-11):1–94. *Current guidelines for treatment of STDs, including syphilis.*

Doroshenko A, Sherrard J, Pollard AJ: Syphilis in pregnancy and the neonatal period. Int J STD AIDS 2006;17:221–227. *A practical review.*

Golden MR, Marra CM, Holmes KK: Update on syphilis: Resurgence of an old problem. JAMA 2003;290:1510–1514. *A brief overview.*

Lukehart SA, Godornes C, Molini BJ, et al: Macrolide resistance in *Treponema pallidum* in the United States and Ireland. N Engl J Med 2004;351:154–158. *A ribosomal mutation for resistance to azithromycin is present in more than 10% of* T. pallidum *isolates from syphilis patients, especially HIV-positive patients.*

341 NONSYPHILITIC TREPONEMATOSES

Edward W. Hook III

Definition

The nonsyphilitic treponematoses (yaws, endemic syphilis [previously known as bejel], and pinta) are the spirochetal diseases caused by *Treponema pallidum* subspecies (yaws and endemic syphilis) or a closely related organism, *Treponema carateum* (pinta). Like syphilis, the nonsyphilitic treponematoses are usually transmitted through direct contact with an infectious cutaneous or mucosal lesion. The natural history of the nonsyphilitic treponematoses likewise has a number of similarities to syphilis (Chapter 340).

The Pathogen

Yaws is caused by *T. pallidum* subspecies *pertenue,* pinta is caused by *T. carateum,* and endemic syphilis is caused by *T. pallidum* subspecies *endemicum.* The *T. pallidum* subspecies causing nonsyphilitic treponematosis is closely related to *T. pallidum* subspecies *pallidum,* which causes venereal syphilis; there is a high degree of DNA homology, and they share unique pathogen-restricted antigens. Like *T. pallidum,* these treponemes are spirochetal bacteria with helical structures and measure about 0.2 μg in diameter and 10 μg in length. They are visible by darkfield microscopy but cannot be cultivated for prolonged periods in vitro.

Epidemiology

Yaws is prevalent in moist, humid regions, including rural areas of tropical Africa, the Americas, Southeast Asia, and Oceania. The highest incidence occurs in children between 2 and 5 years of age. Endemic syphilis occurs in more arid climates, including Africa, in eastern Mediterranean countries, on the Arabian peninsula, in central Asia, and in Australia. Pinta occurs in rural areas of tropical Central and South America and affects mostly older children and adolescents. Humans are the only known carriers of the nonsyphilitic treponematoses. The spirochete enters the skin only after it is broken, as by a scratch or insect bite. Transmission is believed to occur by contacting the skin directly or indirectly by contaminated hands or fomites and is facilitated by conditions of poor personal hygiene and crowding.

Pathobiology

Primary nodular or ulcerative lesions typically develop at sites of inoculation after an incubation period of several weeks. Untreated primary lesions serve as a source for local spread through scratching or for hematogenous dissemination, which gives rise to a secondary stage of infection characterized by the development of widespread manifestations involving the skin, lymph nodes, and bone or cartilage. Without therapy, the primary and secondary manifestations of infections resolve and the infection becomes latent, although periodic recurrent secondary manifestations may occur for several years. A proportion of persons with longstanding untreated infection are at risk for late sequelae, which may include bony deformity, destruction of nasal cartilage, or chronic skin changes. Unlike syphilis, the nonsyphilitic treponematoses are primarily diseases of children, are not congenitally transmitted across the placenta, and do not invade the central nervous system.

Clinical Manifestations

Yaws, the most common nonsyphilitic treponematosis, produces a skin papule at the inoculation site after an incubation period of 3 to 4 weeks. The most common sites are the legs and buttocks. The papule enlarges, ulcerates, and forms a serous crust from which treponemes can be recovered. Regional lymphadenitis may accompany the papule, which heals spontaneously within 6 months. A generalized secondary rash occurs before or after the initial lesion heals, and these rashes are also papular and often covered with brown crusts. Relapsing crops of lesions can occur. Papillomas may result, and the plantar surfaces of the feet are involved with hyperkeratotic lesions. Periostitis of the long bones leads to tenderness, and fever may be present. Relapsing lesions of early yaws may occur over a period of several years and result in chronic ulcerations and destructive gummatous lesions affecting the skin and bones.

Endemic syphilis produces patches on the mucous membranes of the oral cavity and pharynx and can cause split papules at the mucocutaneous junction of the oral angles. Anal, genital, and other intertriginous skin areas can be affected by lesions that resemble secondary syphilis. Regional lymphadenitis is common, and generalized rashes are rare. Healing of these early lesions is followed by latency manifested as seropositivity or by late lesions that resemble gummatous tertiary syphilis. Lesions include nodular ulcers of the skin, deformities of bones, and ulcerative lesions that can perforate the palate.

Pinta starts similarly as a cutaneous papule with regional lymphadenitis and is followed by a generalized maculopapular eruption. One to 3 years after healing of the initial lesion, large hyperpigmented macules that are brown or blue develop and subsequently lose their pigment and become white. The time required for lesions to pass through these stages varies, so the same patient may have coexisting areas of increased pigment and loss of pigment.

Diagnosis

Clinical diagnosis is difficult, with skin lesions of the endemic treponematoses resembling other cutaneous processes, including impetigo (Chapter 465), cutaneous fungal infections (Chapter 464), and other diseases. By darkfield microscopy, the causative spirochetes from early skin lesions can be observed directly. Spirochetes have also been demonstrated in lymph node aspirates. There is no specific test for any of the nonsyphilitic treponematoses, but serologic tests for syphilis detect cross-reacting antibodies in these diseases. The Venereal Disease Research Laboratory (VDRL) test and the fluorescent treponemal antibody absorption test each give positive results if serum is obtained at least 2 weeks after the lesions initially appear.

Prevention

The prevalence of these diseases was reduced in the 1950s by mass penicillin treatment campaigns in areas where they were prevalent. The World Health Organization treated about 53 million cases of yaws and 350,000 cases of pinta in the 1950s with good results. These campaigns, however, were not adequate to eradicate the disease, and in recent years the prevalence of yaws has again increased. Current estimates suggest that worldwide as many as 2.5 million persons are infected, 75% of whom are younger than 15 years. Although penicillin is effective for prevention of infection in exposed persons, it has been suggested that reduction in transmission requires improvements in sanitation and the economic standards of people living in endemic areas.

Treatment and Prognosis

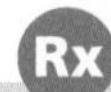

Single-dose, long-acting benzathine penicillin G given as 1.2 million units intramuscularly is the preferred treatment in patients with early lesions. For patients with late manifestations, this therapy should be repeated twice at approximately 7-day intervals. The early lesions heal rapidly, and most seropositive cases convert to seronegative status. Late destructive lesions take longer to show improvement.

SUGGESTED READINGS

Antal GM, Lukehart SA, Meheus AZ: The endemic treponematoses. Microbes Infect 2002;4:83–94. *Review with clinical descriptions and discussion of genetic differences among the* T. pallidum *subspecies.*

Bora D, Dhariwal AC, Lal S: Yaws and its eradication in India. J Commun Dis 2005;37:1–11. *Description of a recent effective eradication program.*

Farnsworth N, Rosen T: Endemic treponematosis: Review and update. Clin Dermatol 2006;24:181–190. *A clinical review.*

342 LYME DISEASE

Stephen E. Malawista and Linda K. Bockenstedt

Definition

Lyme disease is a tick-borne, inflammatory disorder caused by the spirochete *Borrelia burgdorferi.* Its clinical hallmark is an early expanding skin lesion, called *erythema migrans* (EM), which may be followed weeks to months later by neurologic, cardiac, or joint abnormalities. Signs and symptoms may refer to any of these four systems alone or in combination. All stages of Lyme disease may respond to antimicrobials, but response to treatment of early disease is the most efficient.

Epidemiology

The Pathogen

Although cases of the illness are concentrated in certain endemic areas, foci of Lyme disease are widely distributed within the United States, Europe, and Asia.

Lyme arthritis was recognized in November 1975 because of unusual geographic clustering of children with inflammatory arthropathy in the region of Lyme, Connecticut. It soon became clear that this was a multisystem disorder *(Lyme disease)* occurring at any age, in both sexes, and often preceded by a characteristic expanding skin lesion, EM. In Europe, EM had been associated with the bite of the sheep tick, *Ixodes ricinus,* and with tick-borne meningopolyneuritis. In the Lyme region, a closely related deer tick, *Ixodes scapularis,* was implicated as the principal disease vector on epidemiologic grounds. In 1982, Burgdorfer and associates isolated a spirochete, now called *B. burgdorferi,* from *I. scapularis* and linked it serologically to patients with Lyme disease. It was then soon recovered from patients' specimens.

Incidence and Prevalence

Although Lyme disease is widespread, there are three distinct foci in the United States: the Northeast from southern Maine to Maryland, the upper Midwest, and the West in California and Oregon. More than 90% of reported cases come from just nine states: New York, Pennsylvania, New Jersey, Massachusetts, Connecticut, Wisconsin, Maryland, Minnesota, and Delaware. However, the illness has been reported in 49 states and the District of Columbia as well as across Europe and Asia. The earliest known cases in the United States occurred on Cape Cod, Massachusetts, in 1962 and in Lyme, Connecticut, in 1965; annual cases now number about 24,000. Onset of illness is generally between May 1 and November 30, with the peak in June and July.

Lyme disease accounts for more than 90% of reported vector-borne infectious diseases in the United States. Its primary vectors are tiny, hard-shelled ixodid ticks, often overlooked by patients. Major foci of disease correspond to the distribution of *I. scapularis* (Northeast, Midwest), *Ixodes pacificus* (West), *I. ricinus* (Europe), and *Ixodes persulcatus* (Eurasia, Asia). Seasonal variation in infection incidence correlates with the peak questing period for nymphal ticks, the primary vector for transmission to humans; in the Northeast, this period spans May through September. Preferred hosts for *I. scapularis* larvae and nymphs are white-footed mice, the main reservoir for spirochetes; for adults, it is the white-tailed deer, in whose fur they mate. Because deer are not competent reservoirs for *B. burgdorferi* and the spirochete is not passed transovarially from adult tick to egg, passage of *B. burgdorferi* between small rodents and ticks maintains the pathogen in nature, whereas deer facilitate tick survival. A less successful transmission cycle involving the dusky footed wood rat has been described in California.

The rising incidence of Lyme disease in the United States may be explained by multiple factors, including an increase in the numbers of ixodid ticks, the outward migration of residential areas into previously rural woodlands (habitats favored by ixodid ticks and their hosts), an exploding deer population, and increased recognition.

In areas in which Lyme disease is endemic, the prevalence of *B. burgdorferi* in nymphal *I. scapularis* ranges from about 20% to more than 60% (for *I. pacificus,* 1 to 2%), but rates of human infection after tick bite are much lower. The organism has been isolated or a specific antibody found in the blood and tissues of a wide variety of large and small animals, including domestic dogs and birds. Indiscriminate feeding on a variety of animals by *I. scapularis* nymphs may favor the spread of infection.

Pathobiology

Pathogenesis

Recovery of *B. burgdorferi* is straightforward from the tick but difficult from the patient—except from the leading border of EM lesions—in part because of a relative paucity of organisms in tissue and fluid specimens from the latter. Nevertheless, rare positive cultures are reported at all stages of the illness—from blood (early), secondary annular lesions, meningitic cerebrospinal fluid (CSF), heart biopsies, joint fluid, ligament, and in one case even a late skin lesion, *acrodermatitis chronica atrophicans,* that had been present for 10 years. Spirochetes have been identified by silver stain or by immunofluorescence in some histologic sections of EM and rarely in secondary annular lesions, synovium, brain, eye, heart, striated muscle, ligament, liver, spleen, kidney, and bone marrow.

From these data, combined with the clinical and epidemiologic features of Lyme disease, the following pathogenetic sequence is likely. *B. burgdorferi* is transmitted to the skin of the host by the tick vector but usually only after about 48 hours of engorgement. After establishing local infection in the skin, the organism can migrate as early as 3 days or as late as several weeks outward in the skin (EM), spread in lymph (i.e., regional adenopathy), or disseminate in blood. Disease is primarily detected in the nervous system, joints, heart, or other skin sites (i.e., secondary annular lesions); other organs may manifest disease but generally not in the absence of more classical signs of Lyme disease. Maternal-fetal transmission is distinctly uncommon. Although organisms are hard to find in later stages of untreated Lyme disease, persistent live spirochetes or their undegraded antigens are believed to be driving the illness throughout its course. Evidence for this interpretation includes the responsiveness of most patients to antimicrobials, the rare sightings of spirochetes in affected tissues, the variable recovery from affected tissues and fluids of spirochetal DNA amplified by the polymerase chain reaction (PCR), and an expansion of the antibody response to additional spirochetal antigens over time. If live spirochetes persist, it is not clear how they occasionally remain out of harm's way in the presence of antimicrobial therapy and the body's usual phagocytic and other immune clearance mechanisms.

Pathophysiology

B. burgdorferi is an organism that lives primarily in extracellular tissues; no intracellular stage of this organism has been confirmed, despite the rare sighting of spirochetes passing through cells. Mechanisms to evade phagocyte recognition, specific antibody, and complement have been identified. These include diminished expression of lipoproteins during host adaptation for persistence and antigenic variation, particularly as mediated by *vlsE* genes. *B. burgdorferi* also possess a family of *erp* genes, whose protein products bind host factor H and inhibit complement-mediated lysis. Autoimmune mechanisms have been proposed, although not proved, in the propagation of prolonged (i.e., chronic) Lyme arthritis, which in any case typically affects only a single joint and generally resolves within 4 years.

B. burgdorferi does not destroy tissue directly. During the innate immune response (i.e., before antibodies have developed), the spirochete's surface lipoproteins can mediate inflammation through Toll-like receptors and activate monocytes, macrophages, synovial lining cells, natural killer cells, B cells, and complement, resulting in the elaboration of a host of proinflammatory materials. The spirochetes adhere to extracellular matrix proteins, to endothelial cells (and penetrate endothelial monolayers), and to neural glycolipid. They can induce the production of cross-reactive antibodies and of specific immune B and T lymphocytes that may be associated histologically with endarteritic, microvascular occlusive changes (e.g., in nervous tissue, hearts, joints), but it is not clear that these phenomena persist in the absence of live spirochetes or their antigens.

At disease onset (i.e., EM), almost all patients have evidence of circulating immune complexes, although detection of these is not relevant to diagnosis. Early immunoglobulin M (IgM) against *B. burgdorferi* arises from innate B cells that produce antibody in the absence of T cell help. Later, follicular B cells produce IgM and, with engagement of T-cell helper function, IgG. The strength of adaptive T- and B-cell responses increases as disease progresses and is especially apparent with signs of disseminated infection when neurologic, cardiac, or joint involvement is present. As infection progresses beyond 6 weeks, serum IgM levels usually (not always) return to normal, but *B. burgdorferi*–specific IgG is elevated. Mononuclear cells from peripheral blood increase their antigen-specific proliferative response as the disease progresses, but the greatest reactivity to antigen is seen in cells from diseased sites, such as inflamed joints. Biopsy of involved joints reveals a proliferative synovium, often replete with lymphocytes and plasma cells that are presumably capable of producing immunoglobulin locally. An initially disseminated, immune-mediated inflammatory disorder becomes in some patients localized and propagated in joints.

In addition to factors related to the pathogenicity of specific isolates of *B. burgdorferi*, the immunogenetic makeup of the host may play a role in whether infected individuals can rid themselves of spirochetes, their antigens, or their effects. In this regard, patients with treatment-resistant chronic arthritis have been reported to have an increased frequency of human leukocyte antigen HLA-DRB1*0401 or related alleles.

Clinical Manifestations

Lyme disease is conveniently divided into three, overlapping clinical stages that reflect the establishment of *B. burgdorferi* infection in the skin (early localized infection), its dissemination (acute disseminated disease), and persistence in select tissues (late disease). Seroconversion can occur in asymptomatic individuals.

Early Manifestations

EM, the unique clinical marker for Lyme disease, is recognized in 80% or more of patients. It begins as a red macule or papule at the site where the tick vector, usually long gone, had engorged. As the area of redness expands to about 15 cm (range, 3 to 68 cm), there is often partial central clearing. The outer borders are red, generally flat, and without scaling. The centers are occasionally red and indurated, even vesicular or necrotic. Variations may occur, such as multiple rings. The thigh, groin, and axilla are particularly common sites. The lesion is warm to touch but not often sore, and it is easily missed if out of sight. Routine histologic findings are nonspecific: a heavy dermal infiltrate of mononuclear cells, without epidermal change except at the site of the tick bite.

Within days of the onset of EM, one fourth or fewer patients in the United States develop multiple annular secondary lesions (more did so in the initial study) (Table 342–1). These lesions, from which spirochetes have been cultured, represent clear evidence of dissemination. They resemble EM itself but are generally smaller, migrate less, and lack indurated centers. Individual lesions may come and go, and their borders sometimes merge. Other occasional skin lesions are mentioned in Table 342–1. Benign lymphocytoma cutis has been reported in Europe. In the United States, EM and secondary lesions fade in 3 to 4 weeks (range is 1 day to 14 months), but fading takes longer on average in Europe. In untreated patients, they may recur.

Skin involvement is often accompanied by musculoskeletal influenza-like symptoms: malaise and fatigue, headache, fever and chills, myalgia, and arthralgia (Table 342–2). Even without EM, this syndrome in summer and in an endemic area for Lyme disease is grounds for treatment. Some patients have evidence of meningeal irritation or mild encephalopathy (e.g., episodic attacks of excruciating headache and neck pain, stiffness, or pressure) that typically lasts only for hours at this stage of the illness and have no CSF pleocytosis or objective neurologic deficit. Except for fatigue and lethargy, which are often constant, the early signs

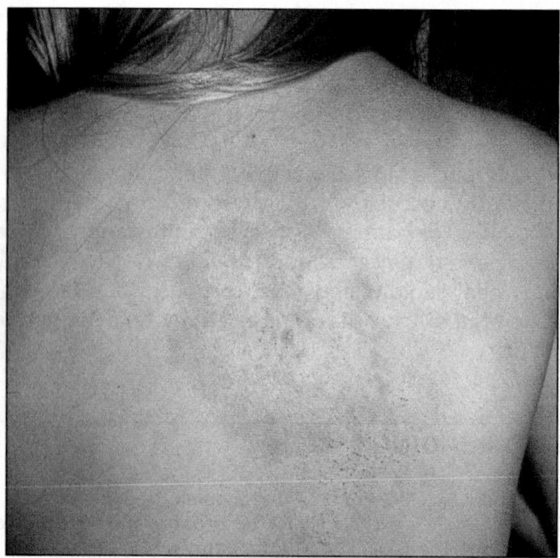

FIGURE 342–1 • Erythema migrans (EM) is the major dermatologic manifestation of Lyme disease. (Courtesy of Michael O. Murphy, MD.)

TABLE 342–1 EARLY SIGNS OF LYME DISEASE IN A STUDY OF 314 PATIENTS

Signs	No. of Patients (%)
Erythema migrans	314 (100)*
Multiple annular lesions	150 (48)
Lymphadenopathy	
Regional	128 (41)
Generalized	63 (20)
Pain on neck flexion	52 (17)
Malar rash	41 (13)
Erythematous throat	38 (12)
Conjunctivitis	35 (11)
Right upper quadrant tenderness	24 (8)
Splenomegaly	18 (6)
Hepatomegaly	16 (5)
Muscle tenderness	12 (4)
Periorbital edema	10 (3)
Evanescent skin lesions	8 (3)
Abdominal tenderness	6 (2)
Testicular swelling	2 (1)

*Erythema migrans was required for inclusion in this study.
From Steere AC, Bartenhagen NH, Craft JE, et al: The early clinical manifestations of Lyme disease. Ann Intern Med 1983;99:76–82.

TABLE 342-2 EARLY SYMPTOMS OF LYME DISEASE IN A STUDY OF 314 PATIENTS

Symptoms	No. of Patients (%)
Malaise, fatigue, and lethargy	251 (80)
Headache	200 (64)
Fever and chills	185 (59)
Stiff neck	151 (48)
Arthralgias	150 (48)
Myalgias	135 (43)
Backache	81 (26)
Anorexia	73 (23)
Sore throat	53 (17)
Nausea	53 (17)
Dysesthesia	35 (11)
Vomiting	32 (10)
Abdominal pain	24 (8)
Photophobia	19 (6)
Hand stiffness	16 (5)
Dizziness	15 (5)
Cough	15 (5)
Chest pain	12 (4)
Ear pain	12 (4)
Diarrhea	6 (2)

From Steere AC, Bartenhagen NH, Craft JE, et al: The early clinical manifestations of Lyme disease. Ann Intern Med 1983;99:76–82.

and symptoms are typically intermittent and changing. For example, a patient may have meningitic attacks for several days, a few days of improvement, and then the onset of migratory musculoskeletal pain. The pain may involve joints (generally without swelling), tendons, bursa, muscle, and bone. The pain tends to affect only one or two sites at a time and to last a few hours to several days in a given location. The various associated symptoms may occur several days before EM (or without it) and last for months (especially fatigue and lethargy) after the skin lesions have disappeared.

Disseminated Infection

Neurologic Involvement

Within several weeks to months of the onset of illness, about 15% of untreated patients develop frank neurologic abnormalities occurring in various combinations including meningitis, encephalitis, cranial neuritis (including bilateral facial palsy), motor and sensory radiculoneuritis, or mononeuritis multiplex. The usual pattern is fluctuating meningoencephalitis with superimposed cranial nerve (particularly facial) palsy and peripheral radiculoneuropathy, but Bell's-like palsy may occur alone. At this point, patients with meningitic symptoms have a lymphocytic pleocytosis (about 100 cells/mm^3) in the CSF and sometimes diffuse slowing on an electroencephalogram. However, the neck is rarely stiff except in extreme flexion; Kernig's and Brudzinski's signs are absent. Neurologic abnormalities typically last for months but usually resolve completely.

Cardiac Involvement

Weeks to months after onset, about 8% of patients develop cardiac involvement. The most common abnormality is fluctuating degrees of atrioventricular block (i.e., first-degree, Wenckebach, or complete heart block). Some patients have evidence of more diffuse cardiac involvement, including electrocardiographic changes compatible with acute myopericarditis, radionuclide evidence of mild left ventricular dysfunction, or, rarely, cardiomegaly. None has had heart murmurs. Cardiac involvement is usually brief (3 days to 6 weeks), but it may recur.

Arthritis

Weeks to as long as 2 years after the onset of illness, about 60% of patients develop frank arthritis, usually characterized by intermittent attacks of asymmetric joint swelling and pain primarily in large joints, especially the knee, one or two joints at a time. Affected knees are commonly more swollen than painful, often hot, and rarely red; Baker's cysts may form and rupture early. Occasionally small joints may be affected, but symmetrical polyarthritis is distinctly rare. Attacks of arthritis, which generally last weeks to months, typically recur for several years and decrease in frequency with time. Fatigue is common with active joint involvement, but fever or other systemic symptoms at this stage are unusual. Joint fluid white blood cell counts vary from 500 to 110,000 cells/mm^3, with an average of about 25,000 cells/mm^3, mostly polymorphonuclear leukocytes. Total protein ranges from 3 to 8 g/dL. The C3 and C4 levels are generally greater than one third and glucose levels usually more than two thirds that of serum. Rheumatoid factor and antinuclear antibody are absent.

In about 10% of patients with arthritis, involvement in large joints may be prolonged (>1 year), occasionally with pannus formation and erosion of cartilage and bone. Synovial biopsy findings may mimic those of rheumatoid arthritis: surface deposits of fibrin, villous hypertrophy, vascular proliferation, and a heavy infiltration of mononuclear cells. There may be an obliterative endarteritis and (rarely) demonstrable spirochetes. *B. burgdorferi* stimulate mononuclear cells to produce cytokines (e.g., interleukin-1, tumor necrosis factor-α, interleukin-6), and elevated concentrations of inflammatory cytokines have been found in synovial fluid. In one patient with chronic Lyme arthritis, synovium grown in tissue culture produced large amounts of collagenase and prostaglandin E_2. In Lyme disease, the joint fluid cell counts, immune reactants (except for rheumatoid factor), synovial histology, amounts of synovial enzymes released, and occasionally the destruction of cartilage and bone may be similar to those in rheumatoid arthritis. The major difference is that prolonged Lyme arthritis typically resolves in time.

Other late findings (years) associated with this infection include a chronic skin lesion—*acrodermatitis chronica atrophicans*—well known in Europe but still rare in the United States. The examiner sees violaceous infiltrated plaques or nodules, especially on extensor surfaces, that eventually become atrophic. Uncommon, late, chronic neurologic disease includes transverse myelitis, diffuse sensory axonal neuropathy, and demyelinating lesions of the central nervous system (CNS). Mild memory impairment, subtle mood changes, and chronic fatigue states may also occur.

Diagnosis

Laboratory Findings

The diagnosis of Lyme disease is based on recognizing clinical features of the illness in a patient with a history of possible exposure to the causative organism.

The most common nonspecific laboratory abnormalities, particularly early in the illness, are a high erythrocyte sedimentation rate, an elevated serum IgM level, and increased serum levels of aspartate transaminase. The enzyme levels generally return to normal within several weeks. Patients may be mildly anemic early in the illness and occasionally have elevated white blood cell counts with shifts to the left in the differential count. A few patients have had microscopic hematuria, sometimes with mild proteinuria (dipstick); values for creatinine and blood urea nitrogen have been normal. Throughout the illness, serum C3 and C4 levels are generally normal or elevated. Rheumatoid factor and antinuclear antibodies are usually absent.

Culture

Culture of *B. burgdorferi* from patients is definitive but has rarely been successful, except from skin biopsy specimens. The organism can be isolated from blood in a significant minority of patients with systemic manifestations of early disease; it grows very slowly. Special tissue staining techniques generally have a low yield and are not readily available.

Antibody Tests

Enzyme-Linked Immunosorbent Assay

Determination of specific antibody titers, usually performed by enzyme-linked immunosorbent assay (ELISA), is the most helpful adjunctive diagnostic test for Lyme disease. In serum, specific IgM antibody titers against *B. burgdorferi* usually reach a peak between the third and sixth weeks after the onset of disease; specific IgG antibody titers rise more slowly and are generally highest months later when arthritis is

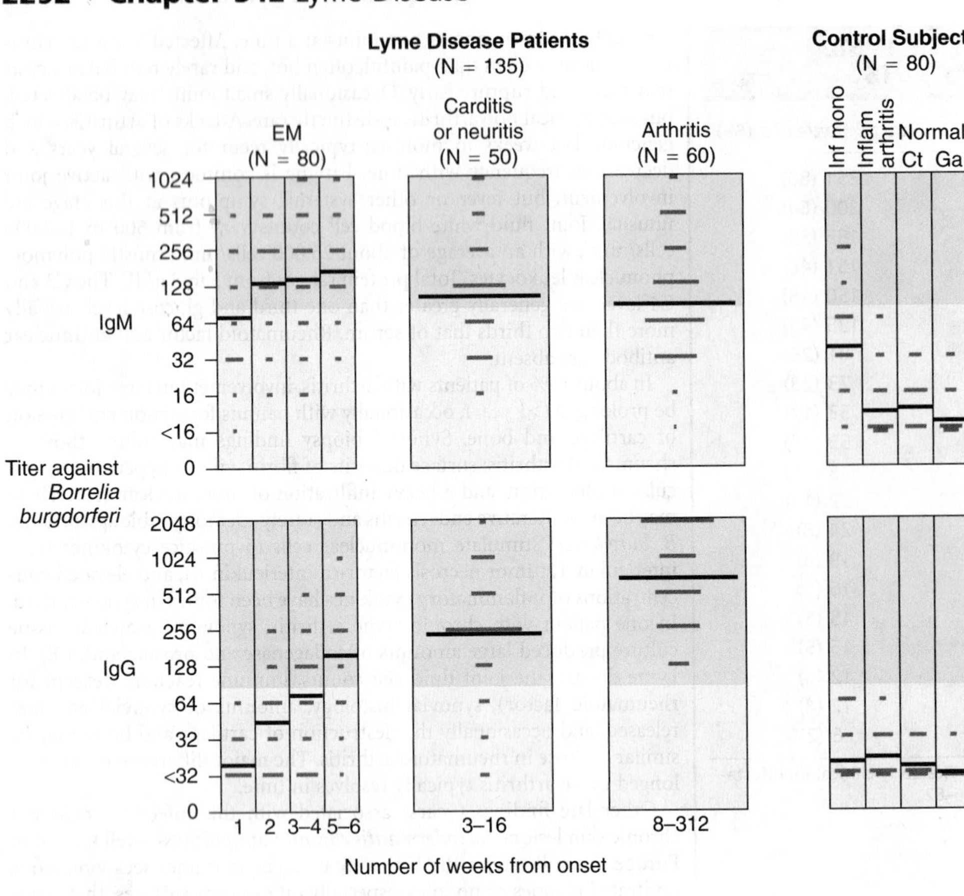

FIGURE 342–2 • Antibody titers against *Borrelia burgdorferi*. Antibody titers are shown in serum samples from 135 patients with different clinical manifestations of Lyme disease and from 80 control subjects with infectious mononucleosis, inflammatory arthritis, or no disease (titers determined by indirect immunofluorescence). The black bar shows the geometric mean titer for each group; the *yellow* shaded areas indicate the range of values generally observed in control subjects. Notice that all patients with Lyme arthritis have elevated immunoglobulin G antibody titers. (Adapted from Steere AC, Grodzicki RL, Kornblatt AN, et al: The spirochetal etiology of Lyme disease. N Engl J Med 1983;308: 733–740. Copyright 1983 Massachusetts Medical Society.)

present (Fig. 342–2). Individuals with untreated Lyme disease of more than 6 weeks' duration can be expected to have elevated levels of specific antibodies. However, the tests employed are not standardized, and results from different commercial laboratories may vary, especially for borderline elevations. Most individuals with established Lyme arthritis have elevated specific IgG titers. This finding makes antibody titers against *B. burgdorferi* particularly useful in differentiating Lyme disease from other rheumatic syndromes, especially when EM is missed, forgotten, or absent. Antibodies may cross-react with other spirochetes, including *Treponema pallidum*, but patients with Lyme disease do not have positive Venereal Disease Research Laboratory (VDRL) test results. The C6 peptide ELISA, based on a constant region of the VlsE protein, may be more sensitive than the standard ELISA for detecting early infection and is useful to distinguish infection-induced antibodies in patients who have been vaccinated against Lyme disease.

Western Blot

Western blots are important for confirmation of positive ELISA results but should not be routinely performed when the ELISA is negative. Early in infection, when IgM antibodies are prevalent, reactivity to two of three bands (23, 39, and 41 kD) constitutes a positive Western blot. When symptoms have been present for more than 6 weeks, only IgG reactivity should be considered to support the diagnosis. Reactivity to 5 out of 10 bands constitutes a positive IgG immunoblot: 18, 21, 28, 39 (BmpA), 41 (Fla), 45, 58, 66, and 93 kD (Fig. 342–3).

Polymerase Chain Reaction

Another test of diagnostic interest uses the PCR to detect spirochetal DNA in host material. Although this powerful tool is notorious for false-positive results when not performed under the most stringent conditions, it can be very useful when properly done, particularly in cases of Lyme arthritis, in which synovial fluid from most untreated patients is positive.

Differential Diagnosis

EM is the unique herald lesion of Lyme disease. When it is present in its classical form, there is little else that may be confused with it. However, some patients are not aware of having had EM, and in others, its appearance is not always characteristic. Secondary lesions may suggest *erythema*

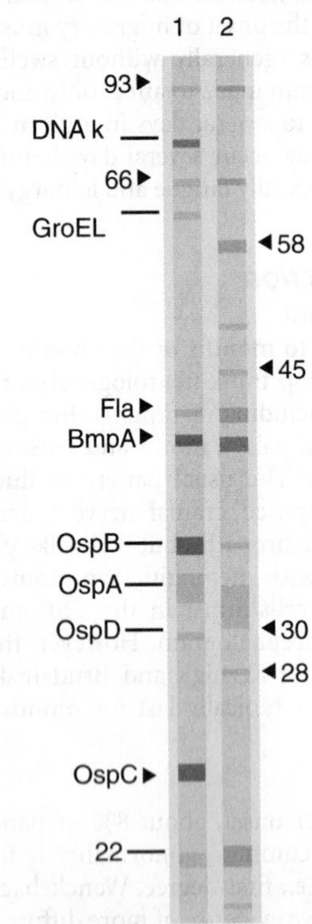

FIGURE 342–3 • Example of immunoblot calibration. Lane 1, monoclonal antibodies defining selected antigens of *Borrelia burgdorferi* strain B31 separated in a linear sodium dodecyl sulfate–polyacrylamide gel electrophoresis (SDS-PAGE) gel. Lane 2, human serum immunoglobulin G reactive with the 10 antigens scored in the currently recommended criteria for blot interpretation. Arrowheads adjacent to lanes 1 and 2 mark the bands recommended for scoring; lines on the left of lane 1 indicate other calibrating antibodies. Molecular masses are in kilodaltons. (From the Centers for Disease Control and Prevention.)

multiforme, but blistering, mucosal lesions and involvement of the palms and soles are not features of Lyme disease. Malar rash may suggest systemic lupus erythematosus; an urticarial rash suggests hepatitis B infection or serum sickness. Evanescent blotches and circles may resemble *erythema marginatum,* but those of Lyme disease do not expand.

An EM-like rash has been associated with the bite of the lone star tick, *Amblyomma americanum,* and is due to infection with a noncultivable spirochete, *Borrelia lonestari.* Patients with this southern tick–associated rash illness (STARI) are seronegative for Lyme disease. The illness follows the distribution of *Amblyomma americanum* in the southeast and south central states.

Early musculoskeletal influenza-like symptoms may be misinterpreted, especially when EM is absent or missed or is not the first manifestation. In patients with particularly severe constitutional symptoms, the physician should consider possible concomitant infection with two other agents transmitted by the same tick: *Anaplasma phagocytophilum,* which causes the rickettsia-like disorder human granulocytic ehrlichiosis (watch for leukopenia, thrombocytopenia, elevated transaminases, occasional inclusions in granulocytes) (Chapter 348), or *Babesia microti,* which results in the malaria-like disorder babesiosis (occasional inclusions in erythrocytes) (Chapter 374).

Severe headache and stiff neck may resemble symptoms of other forms of aseptic meningitis; abdominal symptoms, those of hepatitis; and generalized tender lymphadenopathy and splenomegaly, those of infectious mononucleosis. As in mononucleosis, fatigue in Lyme disease may be a major and persistent complaint. However, initial presentations of an isolated chronic fatigue syndrome or of fibromyalgia-like complaints (e.g., diffuse aching, trigger points, sleep disturbance) are not characteristic of Lyme disease.

In later stages, Lyme disease may mimic other immune-mediated disorders. Like rheumatic fever, Lyme disease may be associated with sore throat followed by migratory polyarthritis (more often, polyarthralgias) and carditis but have no evidence of valvular involvement or of a preceding streptococcal infection. Migratory pain in tendons and joints may also suggest disseminated gonococcal disease. An isolated facial weakness may mimic Bell's-like palsy of other causes. Late neurologic involvement may suggest multiple sclerosis (i.e., transverse myelitis), Guillain-Barré syndrome (i.e., symmetrical peripheral neuropathy), primary psychosis, or brain tumor. In adults with Lyme arthritis, the large knee effusions can resemble those in reactive arthritis, and the occasional symmetrical polyarthritis may mimic rheumatoid arthritis. In children, the attacks of arthritis, although generally shorter, may be identical to those seen in the oligoarticular form of juvenile rheumatoid arthritis but without iridocyclitis.

Treatment

Rx

The major goal of therapy in Lyme disease is to eradicate the causative organism. Like other spirochetal diseases, Lyme disease is most responsive to antimicrobials early in its course. Treatment regimens have evolved over time on the basis of controlled clinical data and clinical experience. Because of the difficulty in proving that bacteria have been eradicated and the common persistence of some symptoms long after treatment, the end point of antimicrobial therapy is not always clear. However, prolonged courses of antimicrobials beyond those outlined in Table 342–3 are of no proven benefit. The treatment regimens presented here represent guidelines that will no doubt be further refined in time.

Early Lyme Disease

If patients are treated early with oral antimicrobials, EM typically resolves promptly, and major later sequelae (i.e., myocarditis, meningoencephalitis, or recurrent arthritis) usually do not occur. Prompt treatment is therefore important, even though such patients may be susceptible to reinfection. Antimicrobial choices and doses are listed in Table 342–3; doxycycline or amoxicillin is favored. Doxycycline is the drug of choice if concomitant human granulocytic ehrlichiosis, which does not respond to the penicillins, is suspected.

About 10% of patients with early Lyme disease experience a Jarisch-Herxheimer–like reaction (i.e., higher fever, redder rash, or greater pain) during the first 24 hours of antimicrobial therapy.

TABLE 342–3 RECOMMENDATIONS FOR ANTIMICROBIAL TREATMENT OF LYME DISEASE IN ADULTS*

EARLY LYME DISEASE[†]
Doxycycline, 100 mg, PO twice daily for 10–21 days
Amoxicillin, 500 mg, PO three times daily for 14–21 days
Cefuroxime axetil, 500 mg, PO twice daily for 14–21 days
If intolerant to all of the preceding drugs, select macrolides can be given[#]
NEUROLOGIC MANIFESTATIONS
Bell's-like palsy alone
Oral regimens of doxycycline or amoxicillin may suffice
Other neurologic abnormalities
Ceftriaxone, 2 g, IV daily for 10–28 days
Cefotaxime, 2 g, IV every 8 hr for 10–28 days
Penicillin G, 20 million units, IV daily (in six divided doses) for 10–28 days
If intolerant to all of the preceding drugs: doxycycline, 100–200 mg, PO twice daily (oral or intravenous) for 30 days[‡]
ARTHRITIS[§]
Oral regimens of doxycycline, amoxicillin, or cefuroxime axetil for 28 days
For arthritis that fails to improve or for recurrent joint swelling after oral therapy, repeat 28-day oral therapy, or intravenous therapy with ceftriaxone, 2 g daily, or other parenteral antibiotics (cefotaxime or penicillin G) for 14–28 days
CARDITIS[¶]
Without advanced atrioventricular block:
Oral regimens with doxycycline or amoxicillin
With advanced atrioventricular block:
Parenteral regimens as for neurologic disease for 14–21 days
PREGNANCY
Standard therapy for a given stage of disease, but avoid doxycycline and clarithromycin
TICK BITES
Rarely employ a single dose of doxycycline, 200 mg

*These are guidelines to be modified by new findings and to be applied always with close attention to the clinical context of individual patients.

[†]Without neurologic, cardiac, or joint involvement. For early Lyme disease, limited to a single erythema migrans lesion, 10 days is sufficient. Fluoroquinolones are not effective against *Borrelia burgdorferi.*

[#]Azithromycin (500 mg PO daily for 7–10 days), clarithromycin (1500 PO twice daily for 14–21 days if the patient is not pregnant), or erythromycin (500 mg PO four times daily for 14–21 days).

[‡]No published experience in the United States; may be ineffective for late neuroborreliosis.

[§]An oral regimen should be selected if there is no neurologic involvement.

[¶]Oral regimens have been reserved for mild carditis limited to first-degree heart block with PR ≤0.30 seconds and normal ventricular function.

Adapted from Wormser GP, Dattwyler RJ, Shapiro ED, et al: The clinical assessment, treatment, and prevention of Lyme disease, human granulocytic anaplasmosis, and babesiosis: Clinical practice guidelines by the Infectious Diseases Society of America. Clin Infect Dis 2006;43:1089–1134.

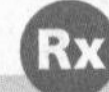

Whichever drug is given, 30 to 50% of patients have brief (hours to days) recurrent episodes of headache, musculoskeletal pain, and fatigue that may continue for extended periods. The cause of these symptoms is unclear; they may result from the immune response to undegraded spirochetal antigens. It is clear, however, that the risk of delayed resolution is greatest in individuals with disseminated manifestations of infection (i.e., multiple skin lesions, headache,

Rx

fever, lymphadenopathy, or Bell's-like palsy) before the institution of antimicrobials. In a randomized, double-blind, placebo-controlled study, extending treatment with doxycycline from 10 to 20 days or adding one dose of ceftriaxone at the start of a 10-day course of doxycycline did not enhance therapeutic efficacy in patients with EM. [1] In all groups, objective evidence of treatment failure was extremely rare.

Acute Disseminated Disease

Intravenous therapy is generally recommended for acute disseminated Lyme disease with neurologic involvement (except Bell's palsy). Ceftriaxone (2 g/day for 10 to 28 days) has largely replaced intravenous penicillin G (20 million units each day in six divided doses for 10 to 28 days) because its once-daily administration schedule is amenable to outpatient therapy and it has improved penetration of the cerebrospinal fluid compared with penicillin. Headache and stiff neck usually begin to subside by the second day of therapy and disappear by 7 to 10 days; motor deficits and radicular pain frequently resolve over 7 to 8 weeks but do not require longer antimicrobial courses. Intravenous penicillin and cefotaxime have been found equally effective for the treatment of acute neurologic Lyme disease (meningitis or radiculitis) in a group of patients studied in Germany. One study demonstrated that 3 weeks of oral doxycycline was equally effective for acute disseminated disease, excluding meningitis. For Bell's-like palsy alone, oral regimens may suffice.

Mild carditis responds within days to oral therapy. Recovery from carditis was the rule even in the era before antimicrobials, but untreated patients are at high risk for later manifestations of Lyme disease. Prednisone (40 to 60 mg/day in divided doses) has in the past seemed to hasten resolution of high-grade heart block, but the physician should hesitate to institute glucocorticoids during antimicrobial administration because they may impede eradication of infecting organisms. If second- or third-degree heart block is present, the patient should be admitted to the hospital for cardiac monitoring and intravenous antimicrobials; temporary pacing is occasionally required for complete heart block.

Late Lyme Disease

Lyme arthritis has been successfully treated with oral and parenteral antimicrobials, but failures occur with any regimen chosen. Unless CNS involvement coexists, first-line treatment with 1 or 2 months of doxycycline (100 mg twice each day) or amoxicillin (500 mg three times each day) is recommended. Most patients respond, although complete response can be delayed 3 months or longer after therapy is completed, and some patients may develop neurologic disease later. During treatment, the affected joint should be kept at rest and effusions drained by needle aspiration as for any infected joint. In patients in whom one or more courses of antimicrobials fail, arthroscopic synovectomy appears to cure most of the patients. Even without antimicrobial or surgical treatment, persistent Lyme arthritis tends to resolve within several years.

Recommended therapy for the later neurologic complications of Lyme disease is like that for earlier neurologic disease but generally for the full 28 days (see Table 342–3). Recovery from chronic involvement may be slow. The frequency of subtle, chronic encephalopathy and peripheral neuropathy is debated. These entities, when suspected, should be carefully documented through neurologic, neuropsychological, and electrophysiologic testing before antimicrobial therapy is instituted. The infiltrative lesions of *acrodermatitis chronica atrophicans* are usually cured by 30 days of penicillin V (1 g three times each day) or of doxycycline (100 mg twice each day).

Pregnancy

Recommended therapy for a given stage of disease during pregnancy differs from that for nonpregnant patients only in the avoidance of doxycycline. Because the spirochetes that cause relapsing fever and syphilis can cross the placenta, there has been concern regarding this possibility in Lyme disease. Maternal-fetal transmission of *B. burgdorferi* resulting in neonatal death or stillbirth has been reported in rare instances in which symptomatic, early Lyme disease occurred early in pregnancy and was untreated or inadequately treated. In follow-up studies conducted by the Centers for Disease Control and Prevention, maternal Lyme disease was not directly implicated as a cause of fetal malformations. There have been no cases of fetal infection occurring when the recommended antimicrobial regimens for Lyme disease have been used during pregnancy. Women acquiring the illness during pregnancy should be reassured that most infants born to women in these circumstances have been entirely well.

Post-Lyme Syndrome

After recommended courses of antimicrobials for Lyme disease, some patients have persistent fatigue, myalgias, arthralgias without arthritis, dysesthesias or paresthesias, or mood and memory disturbances, with or without seropositive results for *B. burgdorferi*. Some of these individuals have been treated with extended courses of antimicrobials, sometimes with reported relief during their administration. However, in a placebo-controlled study of such individuals, those who received intravenous ceftriaxone (2 g/day for 30 days) followed by oral doxycycline (200 mg/day for 60 days) did no better symptomatically than the placebo control group. [2] Prolonged treatment with antimicrobials is not benign and cannot be recommended in patients without objective evidence of persistent infection. Supportive therapy is indicated.

Prevention

Tick Bites

A single 200-mg dose of doxycycline given within 72 hours of a bite by *I. scapularis* can prevent the development of Lyme disease. However, the attack rate among bitten but untreated control subjects in the hyperendemic area where the relevant study was done was only 3.2% (i.e., 96.8% of untreated subjects did not develop Lyme disease). Prophylaxis may be most reasonable when the tick is a nymphal deer tick that is at least partially engorged with blood, with flat ticks not having had time to transmit disease, and in a region where the incidence of Lyme disease is high. Otherwise, tick bites may be observed for development of EM and patients cautioned regarding the common associated symptoms of early Lyme disease. A watched tick bite allows very early treatment of EM in the few patients in whom it develops, and this is the stage of disease most amenable to therapy.

Vaccination

A marketed vaccine against Lyme disease based on one of the outer surface proteins (OspA) of *B. burgdorferi* appeared to be safe and effective but was withdrawn by the manufacturer because of limited demand.

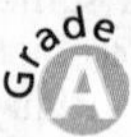

1. Wormser GP, Ramanathan R, Nowakowski JM, et al: Duration of antibiotic therapy for early Lyme disease. Ann Intern Med 2003; 138:769–704.
2. Klempner MS, Hu LT, Evans J, et al: Two controlled trials of antibiotic treatment in patients with persistent symptoms and a history of Lyme disease. N Engl J Med 2001;345:85–92.

SUGGESTED READINGS

Hayes EB, Piesman J: How can we prevent Lyme disease? N Engl J Med 2003;348:2424–2430. *A comprehensive overview of prevention strategies in light of the demise of the Lyme disease vaccine.*

Wormser GP: Clinical practice. Early Lyme disease. N Engl J Med 2006;354:2794–2801. *A clinical review.*

Wormser GP, Dattwyler RJ, Shapiro ED, et al: The clinical assessment, treatment, and prevention of Lyme disease, human granulocytic anaplasmosis, and babesiosis: Clinical practice guidelines by the Infectious Diseases Society of America. Clin Infect Dis 2006;43:1089–1134. *Includes doses and durations of recommended therapy for the treatment and prevention of Lyme disease.*

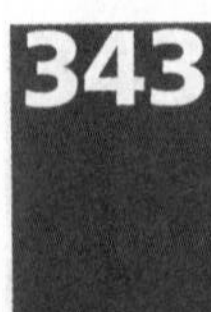

RELAPSING FEVER AND OTHER *BORRELIA* INFECTIONS

William A. Petri, Jr.

Definition

Relapsing fever is a spirochetal infection with bacteria of the genus *Borrelia*. There are two modes of transmission: epidemic louse-borne and endemic tick-borne relapsing fever.

The Pathogen

Borrelia are motile spirochetes that measure 0.5 µm in diameter and 5 to 40 µm in length. They are aerophilic and require long-chain fatty acids for growth. Louse-borne relapsing fever is caused by *Borrelia recurrentis*. Tick-borne relapsing fever organisms are named after their tick vector and include the closely related species *Borrelia duttonii* (Old World) and *Borrelia hermsii, Borrelia turicatae,* and *Borrelia parkeri* (North America).

Epidemiology

Tick-borne endemic relapsing fever occurs throughout the world and is transmitted to humans by *Ornithodoros* soft ticks. The ticks become infected by feeding on wild rodents (including mice, rats, squirrels, and chipmunks), which serve as natural reservoirs for the organisms. In the United States, relapsing fever is limited to humid, mountainous areas of the West at altitudes of 1500 to 8000 ft where the tick vector *Ornithodoros hermsii* resides in forests of ponderosa pine and Douglas fir trees. A key diagnostic clue has been a history of sleeping in rodent-infested rustic cabins in western U.S. national parks. In Tanzania, where house infestation with *Ornithodoros* tick vectors can be very high, relapsing fever was identified in 11% of children seen at a clinic with fever.

The Pathogen

Louse-borne epidemic relapsing fever is caused by *B. recurrentis* and is carried from person to person by the human body louse *(Pediculus humanus)*. There is no animal reservoir. The spirochete lives in the louse hemolymph; infection is transmitted to humans when the louse is crushed on human skin and infective spirochetes penetrate the skin or mucous membranes. Epidemics have occurred during famines and at wartime when breakdown in sanitation favors the transmission of body lice. Louse-borne disease remains endemic in central and east Africa (Ethiopia, Somalia, Chad, and the Sudan) and in the South American Andes (Bolivia and Peru).

Pathobiology

Borrelia infection begins in the skin at the site of the louse or tick bite and is followed by rapid dissemination of the spirochetes through the blood stream. Spirochetes are visible on Wright-stained peripheral blood smears during the initial febrile episode and during each febrile relapse in most patients. Clearance of spirochetes from the blood is associated with the production of serotype-specific immune sera; anti-*Borrelia* antibodies have been shown in animal models to be the major mechanism of immune clearance of infection.

Relapses are associated with cyclic antigenic variation in the variable major proteins (VMPs), which are the abundant outer membrane proteins of the spirochete that carry the serotype-specific epitopes. Antigenic variation is the consequence of recombination events occurring between VMP genes at silent and expression sites on linear plasmids. A single *B. hermsii* bacterium may produce as many as 40 distinct serotypes. Because spirochetes undergo one or several antigenic phases during infection, no specific or standard procedure has been developed for routine serodiagnosis of relapsing fever.

Clinical Manifestations

An abrupt onset of fever to 38.5 to 40° C (>39° C in most patients), headache, myalgias, and shaking chills characterizes the onset of illness. Cough, nausea and vomiting, and fatigue are less frequent complaints. Signs include fever, tachycardia, lethargy or confusion, conjunctival injection, and epistaxis. Hepatosplenomegaly, jaundice, and often a truncal petechial rash are common signs in louse-borne relapsing fever. Untreated louse-borne disease lasts 6 days, and relapses occur once after an afebrile period of 9 days. The initial illness of tick-borne relapsing fever lasts about 4 days without antibiotic treatment, with an average of two relapses (each after an average 10-day afebrile period) before the diagnosis is made.

Relapsing fever in pregnancy results in miscarriage in a third of patients. Neonatal infection by both the tick- and louse-borne forms is accompanied by jaundice, hepatosplenomegaly, and often sepsis and hemorrhage. Fever and hepatosplenomegaly are also common signs in children.

Diagnosis

The diagnosis should be considered in patients with fever who are returning from a stay in cabins in the mountainous and high-elevation areas of the western United States. Only a few patients will remember tick exposure because *O. hermsii* is a night feeder, has a painless bite, and remains attached for only 15 minutes. Internationally, relapsing fever can occur sporadically wherever dwellings are infected with *Ornithodoros* ticks, as well as in epidemics with louse-borne disease.

Because the number of organisms in blood is extremely high, the diagnosis is most often made by direct visualization of the organism on a blood smear, although the diagnosis can also be made with polymerase chain reaction and serodiagnostic tests. Spirochetes can be demonstrated on peripheral blood smears taken during febrile episodes in 70% of patients. Because of their characteristic locomotion, spirochetes can be readily detected by direct visualization of thick blood films under low-power microscopy. Culture of the organism requires a special medium and is not practical in a clinical laboratory setting. The white blood cell count is generally normal, but platelet counts less than 50,000/mm^3 occur in up to 90% of cases of louse-borne disease. Prothrombin and partial thromboplastin times are often prolonged. In louse-borne disease, elevations in liver function test results (serum transaminases and bilirubin) and blood urea nitrogen are common. Urinalysis may reveal proteinuria and microscopic hematuria.

Treatment

Rx

A single 500-mg dose of tetracycline may be as effective as longer treatments in clearing the spirochetemia of louse-borne disease, although many physicians still treat with 500 mg of tetracycline every 6 hours for 5 to 10 days. Erythromycin is also effective and should be used in pregnant women and children younger than 7 years (in whom tetracyclines can stain the permanent teeth). Penicillin treatment has been reported to clear the spirochetemia more slowly than tetracycline does.

The Jarisch-Herxheimer reaction (typically characterized by a rise in body temperature of 1° C, rigors, a rise in blood pressure followed by a fall, and transient leukopenia) occurs 2 to 3 hours after treatment in many patients with louse-borne disease, less commonly in tick-borne disease, and should be anticipated and managed supportively. Deaths as a result of shock from the Jarisch-Herxheimer reaction occur rarely. The Jarisch-Herxheimer reaction has been associated with accelerated phagocytosis of spirochetes by neutrophils and transient elevations in tumor necrosis factor-α (TNF-α), interleukin-6 (IL-6), IL-8, and IL-10. In small numbers of patients with louse-borne relapsing fever, anti–TNF-α antibodies have been effective at prevention.

Prevention

Prevention of louse-borne relapsing fever requires both delousing and antibiotic treatment, as well as removal of structural flaws in cabins and other residences so that rodents cannot nest in or around them.

Prognosis

Epidemics of louse-borne relapsing fever have been reported, with mortality rates approaching 40%; mortality from tick-borne disease is less than 5%. Autopsies of patients with louse-borne disease have documented intracranial hemorrhage, brain edema, bronchopneumonia, hepatic necrosis, and splenic infarcts.

SUGGESTED READINGS

Brahim H, Perrier-Gros-Claude J, Postic D, et al: Identifying relapsing fever *Borrelia*, Senegal. Emerg Infect Dis 2005;11:474–475. *Polymerase chain reaction was used to test blood samples from 7750 patients submitted for the suspected diagnosis of malaria, with spirochete infection diagnosed in 33.*

Dworkin MS, Shoemaker PC, Fritz CL, et al: Epidemiology of tick-borne relapsing fever in the United States. Am J Trop Med Hyg 2002;66:753–758. *Four hundred fifty cases of tick-borne relapsing fever from 1770 through 2000 in the Northwest are reviewed with an emphasis on clinical complications, serodiagnosis, epidemiology, entomology, and geographic distribution.*

Kisinza WN, McCall PJ, Mitani H: A newly identified tick-borne *Borrelia* species and relapsing fever in Tanzania. Lancet 2003;362:1283–1284. *A species characterized by PCR analysis.*

Paul WS, Maupin G, Scott-Wright AO, et al: Outbreak of tick-borne relapsing fever at the north rim of the Grand Canyon: Evidence for effectiveness of preventive measures. Am J Trop Med Hyg 2002;66:71–75. *Review of effective prevention.*

Rich SM, Sawyer SA, Barbour AG: Antigen polymorphism in *Borrelia hermsii*, a clonal pathogenic bacterium. Proc Natl Acad Sci U S A 2001;98:15038–15043. *Describes molecular mechanisms underlying the generation of polymorphism in the surface lipoprotein alleles.*

Roscoe C, Epperly T: Tick-borne relapsing fever. Am Fam Physician 2005;72: 2039–2044. *A clinical review.*

Schwan TG, Policastro PF, Miller Z, et al: Tick-borne relapsing fever caused by *Borrelia hermsii*, Montana. Emerg Infect Dis 2003;9:1151–1154. *Describes the first cases of tick-borne relapsing fever in Montana.*

344 LEPTOSPIROSIS

Albert I. Ko

Definition

Leptospirosis, which is a major zoonotic health problem in developing countries, has been recognized as an emerging infectious disease in developed countries. Infection with *Leptospira* spirochetes occurs during contact with animal reservoirs or an environment contaminated with their urine. The clinical course of leptospirosis ranges from a mild acute febrile illness to life-threatening manifestations such as Weil's disease, which consists of the triad of jaundice, acute renal failure, and bleeding. Leptospirosis has also been recognized as an important cause of severe pulmonary hemorrhage syndrome worldwide.

The Pathogen

The etiologic agent, which can be identified by darkfield microscopy or silver staining procedures, is a motile spirochete 6 to 20 μm in length and 0.1 μm in diameter (Fig. 344–1). Leptospires are obligate aerobes whose relatively large genome (two chromosomes of 4.3 megabase and 350 kilobase) reflects its ability to adapt to external and host environments. *Leptospira* are classified into 17 species and genomospecies, 11 of which (*L. interrogans, L. kirschneri, L. noguchii, L. weillii, L. borgspetersenі, L. santarosai, L. fanei, L. inadai, L. broomii, L. alexandrii*, and genomospecies 1) are pathogenic. Serologic classification provides more useful epidemiologic information because serogroups and serovars, of which there are more than 25 and 250, respectively, are associated with specific animal reservoirs.

Epidemiology

Leptospirosis has a worldwide distribution because of the broad spectrum of animal reservoirs, including domestic and wild rodents, dogs, pigs, cattle, and sheep. Leptospires colonize the renal tubules, are excreted in urine, and survive for weeks to months in the environment. Transmission to humans occurs when leptospires penetrate the skin or mucous membranes during contact with contaminated water, soil, or vegetation. Abrasions in the skin facilitate entry of the pathogen. Direct contact with urine and tissues is an important mode of transmission in risk groups such as abattoir workers and veterinarians. Ingestion of contaminated food, inhalation of droplet aerosols, or swallowing contaminated water, as found during a 1998 outbreak among triathletes, occasionally causes infection. Humans are accidental hosts and do not serve as reservoirs because sufficient concentrations of viable organisms are not excreted in urine. Rare human-to-human transmission is associated with transplacental infection and breast-feeding.

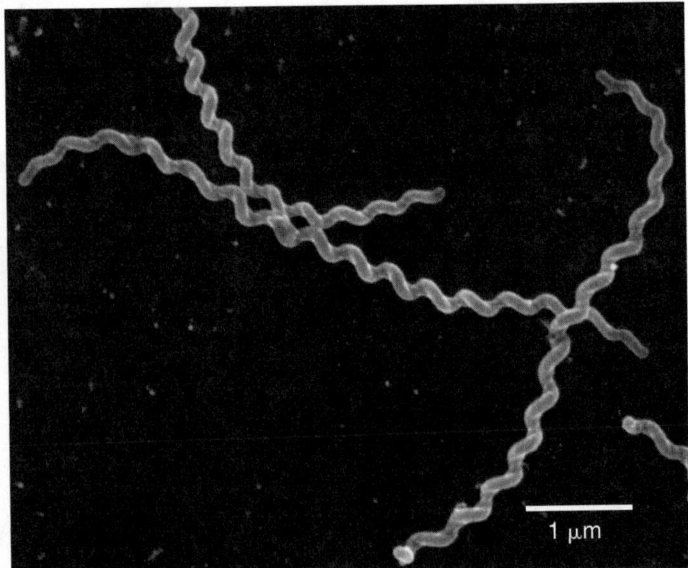

FIGURE 344–1 • Scanning electron micrograph of *Leptospira interrogans* serovar *copenhageni*. Original magnification, 17,000; bar = 1 μm.

Leptospirosis is a major public health problem in developing countries, where it is an endemic disease among subsistence farmers, sharecroppers, and livestock herders. Furthermore, it is the cause of large epidemics in urban slums, where inadequate sanitation favors rodent-borne transmission. Although leptospirosis has traditionally been a sporadic occupation-related disease in developed countries, it has emerged to become a health problem associated with travel, water sports, and recreation (white water rafting, swimming). Outbreaks frequently follow natural disasters, heavy seasonal rainfall, and flooding, as seen during the aftermath of hurricanes in the Caribbean and monsoons in Mumbai. Leptospirosis may also be an under-recognized problem in U.S. inner cities inasmuch as sporadic cases have been reported in this setting.

Pathobiology

Leptospires disseminate rapidly to all tissues shortly after infection by means of direct tissue penetration and hematogenous spread. Symptoms develop 5 to 14 days after exposure, although the incubation period may vary from 2 to 30 days. Leptospires are cleared from the blood stream by agglutinating antibodies, whose titers rise at the end of early-phase "leptospiremic" illness. The late-phase immunopathogenic process is responsible for the severe manifestations of the disease. *Leptospira* lipopolysaccharide and lipopeptides are potent stimulators of pro-inflammatory cytokines such as tumor necrosis factor-α, and these cytokines produce a septic shock–like picture. Damage to the vascular endothelium, which is a hallmark of severe leptospirosis, causes capillary leakage, hemorrhage, and in a subset of cases, vasculitis. Unlike gram-negative sepsis, systemic infection does not cause disseminated intravascular coagulation. The pronounced disturbances in hepatic and renal function are believed to be due to the toxic effects of products released from killed organisms because pathologic examination of tissues reveals mild inflammatory cell infiltrates and sparse intact leptospires. Although the immune response eventually eliminates the pathogen, leptospires may persist for prolonged periods in immunoprivileged sites, such as the anterior chamber of the eye and the renal tubules, and then may be shed in urine weeks after resolution of the illness.

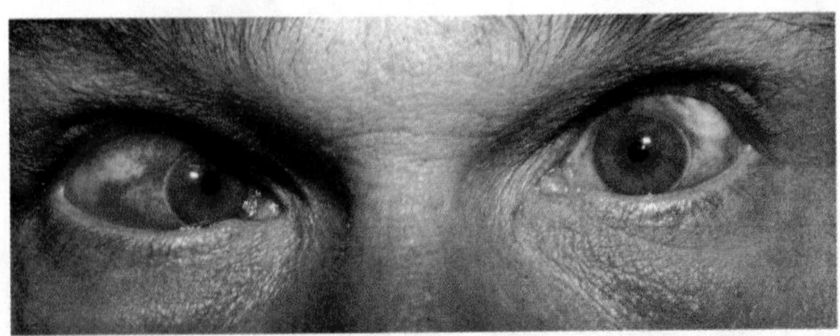

FIGURE 344–2 • Conjunctival suffusion in a patient with Weil's disease. Conjunctival suffusion, a pathognomonic sign for leptospirosis, is best seen along the right upper palpebral border, above the subconjunctival hemorrhage. (Courtesy of Antonio Seguro and Paulo Marotto, Hospital Emílio Ribas and Universidade de São Paulo.)

Clinical Manifestations

The clinical findings in early-phase leptospirosis (initial 3 to 7 days of illness) are nonspecific. The onset of high fever (38 to 40° C), myalgias, and headache (retro-orbital and frontal) may be abrupt and accompanied by symptoms of nausea, vomiting, abdominal pain, diarrhea, cough, and photophobia. Muscle tenderness is pronounced, especially in the calves and lumbar region; if muscle tenderness involves the abdominal wall musculature, it can mimic the symptoms of an acute abdomen. Rash, which occurs in 10 to 20% of patients, has erythematous macular, papular, urticarial, or purpuric components distributed in a truncal or pretibial ("Fort Bragg fever") pattern. Hepatomegaly, splenomegaly, and lymphadenopathy are less common (<20%) findings. Conjunctival suffusion, which is a pathognomonic symptom seen in about 30% of patients, develops toward the end of early-phase illness and is characterized by hyperemia of the conjunctival vessels along the palpebral fissures and chemosis (Fig. 344–2).

A minority (5 to 15%) of patients progress to severe late-phase disease. Jaundice is a poor prognostic sign because acute renal failure and hemorrhage are frequently associated complications (Weil's disease). Anicteric leptospirosis tends to be a milder late-phase finding characterized by prolonged fever and aseptic meningitis. Life-threatening complications are hypotension, hemorrhage, and renal and respiratory failure.

Leptospirosis causes nonoliguric, hypokalemic renal insufficiency, with impaired proximal sodium reabsorption, increased distal sodium delivery, and potassium wasting. As volume loss progresses, oliguric renal insufficiency develops as a result of prerenal azotemia and acute tubular necrosis. Cardiac rhythm disturbances, precipitated by electrolyte imbalance, uremia, and pericarditis, are observed in 20 to 40% of patients and include atrial fibrillation, first-degree atrioventricular block, and alterations in ventricular repolarization.

Severe thrombocytopenia and anemia secondary to hemolysis or blood loss are observed in up to 30% of patients. The prothrombin and partial thromboplastin times remain normal or are only mildly elevated. Leptospirosis is now recognized as an important cause of severe pulmonary hemorrhage syndrome. Acute respiratory distress syndrome, which is a prominent feature of this manifestation, can also occur in the absence of documented bleeding. In addition to pulmonary hemorrhage, massive spontaneous gastrointestinal bleeding is a major cause of death. Other late-phase findings include diffuse or focal interstitial pneumonitis and pneumonia, myocarditis, pancreatitis, and rhabdomyolysis.

Aseptic meningitis, which is the most frequent neurologic manifestation, is characterized by cerebrospinal fluid pleocytosis with early neutrophilic and late mononuclear cell predominance. Leptospirosis has also been reported to cause encephalitis, cerebral hemorrhage and arteritis (Moyamoya disease), transverse myelitis, and cranial (Bell's palsy) and peripheral neuropathies.

Diagnosis

Few clinical or laboratory findings differentiate early-phase leptospirosis from other causes of an acute febrile illness associated with myalgias and headache. Conjunctival suffusion is a highly specific, but insensitive clinical finding. The white blood cell count may be mildly elevated or normal in early-phase illness.

Severe leptospirosis is often recognized by the classic manifestations of Weil's disease, but severe complications may occur in anicteric disease. Furthermore, aseptic meningitis and uveitis may develop in patients with icteric leptospirosis, manifestations classically associated with anicteric disease.

Laboratory confirmation of leptospirosis is based on the presence of a four-fold rise in antibody titer in the microagglutination test (MAT) or isolation of pathogenic leptospires from a normally sterile site. However, these standard diagnostic methods provide only retrospective confirmation of the disease. MAT requires acute- and convalescent-phase sera and is performed routinely in few reference laboratories worldwide. A positive MAT titer (1:100 or greater) from a single acute-phase sample provides suggestive evidence of leptospirosis but must be interpreted with caution in areas of high endemic transmission. Isolation of *Leptospira* requires specific media (Ellinghausen-McCullough-Johnson-Harris or Fletcher medium) and may take more than 4 weeks to identify a positive culture. Commercial anti–whole *Leptospira* immunoglobulin M (IgM) detection kits in enzyme-linked immunosorbent assays or rapid formats are used to provide presumptive confirmation of leptospirosis. However, sensitivity is low (39 to 72%) during acute-phase illness. Polymerase chain reaction–based diagnostic methods have been developed, but their use has been limited to reference laboratory settings.

Differential Diagnosis

Leptospirosis is frequently confused with dengue (Chapter 404) or malaria (Chapter 366) in regions where these diseases are endemic. Severe leptospirosis must be differentiated from other causes of acute jaundice and acute renal failure, such as viral hepatitis; typhoid fever; rickettsial disease; hantavirus-associated hemorrhagic fever renal syndrome and pulmonary syndrome; gram-negative sepsis; endocarditis; and autoimmune disorders. Icteric leptospirosis is associated with elevated serum conjugated bilirubin concentrations and can be differentiated from viral hepatitis by the findings of elevated serum creatine phosphokinase and mild elevations (<400 U/L) in aminotransaminases. The finding of moderate to severe hypokalemia is useful in distinguishing leptospirosis from other infectious causes of acute renal failure.

Treatment

Rx

Antimicrobial therapy is efficacious for early and severe late-phase leptospirosis. Mild leptospirosis is treated with oral doxycycline (100 mg twice a day) or ampicillin or amoxicillin (500 mg every 8 hours). Severe leptospirosis is treated with intravenous penicillin (1.5 million U every 6 hours). Intravenous ceftriaxone (1 g once a day) and cefotaxime (1 g every 6 hours) have equivalent efficacy as penicillin for severe leptospirosis. 

Other antimicrobial agents may have potential therapeutic use, although at present their efficacy is unproven. *Leptospira* organisms are susceptible in vitro to chloramphenicol and to quinolone and macrolide agents. Azithromycin and clarithromycin are efficacious in experimental animals. The duration of antimicrobial therapy is usually 7 days. Although patients require monitoring for Jarisch-Herxheimer reactions during initiation of antimicrobial therapy, this complication is less frequently observed than with other spirochetal infections.

Reducing mortality from severe leptospirosis requires prompt triage of high-risk patients and aggressive supportive care for hypotension, renal and respiratory distress, and hemorrhage. Patients with nonoliguric hypokalemic renal insufficiency have a better overall prognosis and can be treated by volume and potassium repletion. Timely initiation of dialysis is critical to prevent mortality from oliguric renal insufficiency. Continuous hemofiltration is more effective than peritoneal dialysis in treating infection-associated acute renal failure.

Prevention

Prevention of leptospirosis is based on controlling animal reservoirs, interrupting transmission routes, and preventing disease in humans. Control measures that target defined animal populations, such as dogs, pigs, and cattle, are highly effective. Immunization of domestic animals and livestock may reduce carriage and transmission to humans. Chemical pesticides and environmental control of the habitats of domestic rodent reservoirs are important, but difficult to implement, especially in urban slum settings. Control of sylvatic reservoirs is often not feasible. When possible, environmental sources of transmission can be decontaminated with hypochlorite solution and isolated. Protective clothing such as gloves and boots reduces the risk for occupational exposure. Although infection after exposure to human urine has not been documented, precautions need to be taken when handling patients' secretions.

Doxycycline chemoprophylaxis (200 mg orally per week) is efficacious in preventing clinical disease but not in reducing infection rates in endemic areas. [3] Doxycycline (100 mg orally twice a day for 3 to 7 days) or amoxicillin can be used for postexposure prophylaxis, although the efficacy of these regimens has been not been evaluated. Bacterin-based vaccines have been used for high-risk groups in several countries and in mass immunization campaigns in Cuba and China; at present, however, the effectiveness and safety of these vaccines is uncertain.

Prognosis

Although leptospirosis is usually a self-limited illness, mortality is high in patients with severe disease manifestations. Case-fatality rates in patients with Weil's disease and severe pulmonary hemorrhage syndrome are 5 to 40% and higher than 50%, respectively. Prognostic predictors for death are older age (>40 years), oliguria, respiratory insufficiency, pulmonary hemorrhage, cardiac arrhythmias, and altered mental status. Follow-up of patients has found that hepatic and renal function typically returns to baseline levels within 1 month and 6 months, respectively, after acute illness. However, unilateral or bilateral uveitis characterized by iritis, iridocyclitis, and chorioretinitis may develop up to 18 months after systemic illness and persist for years.

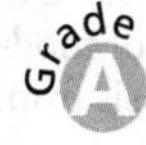

1. Panaphut T, Domrongkitchaiporn S, Vibhagool A, et al: Ceftriaxone compared with sodium penicillin G for treatment of severe leptospirosis. Clin Infect Dis 2003;36:1507–1513.
2. Suputtamongkol Y, Niwattayakul K, Suttinont C, et al: An open, randomized, controlled trial of penicillin, doxycycline, and cefotaxime for patients with severe leptospirosis. Clin Infect Dis 2004; 39:1417–1424.
3. Seghal SC, Suqunan AP, Murhekar MV, et al: Randomized controlled trial of doxycycline prophylaxis against leptospirosis in an endemic area. Int J Antimicrob Agents 2000;13:249–255.

SUGGESTED READINGS

Dolhnikoff M, Mauad T, Bethlem EP, Carvalho CR: Leptospiral pneumonias. Curr Opin Pulm Med 2007;13:230–235. *Review of the pathophysiology and clinical manifestations of leptospiral pneumonias.*

Griffith ME, Hospenthal DR, Murray CK: Antimicrobial therapy of leptospirosis. Curr Opin Infect Dis 2006;19:533–537. *Complete review of the current treatment options for leptospirosis.*

McBride AJA, Athanazio DA, Reis MG, et al: Leptospirosis. Curr Opin Infect Dis 2005;18:376–386. *Focuses on current diagnosis and treatment.*

Ricaldi JN, Vinetz JM: Leptospirosis in the tropics and in travelers. Curr Infect Dis Rep 2006;8:51–58. *A comprehensive review.*

345 TUBERCULOSIS

Michael D. Iseman

Definition

Tuberculosis is an infectious disease caused by *Mycobacterium tuberculosis.* Characteristic features include patient-to-patient airborne transmission, a prolonged latency period between the initial infection and overt disease, a granulomatous response associated with intense tissue inflammation and damage, and prominent pulmonary disease, although many other organs can be involved as well.

The Pathogen

Mycobacteria are small, rod-shaped, aerobic, non–spore-forming bacilli. The genus *Mycobacterium* contains a group of organisms so closely related that they are referred to as the "tuberculosis complex": *M. tuberculosis, M. bovis, M. canetti, M. africanum,* and *M. microti.* However, given the singular epidemiologic, clinical, public health, and therapeutic considerations associated with *M. tuberculosis,* the term *tuberculosis* should be reserved exclusively for infection or disease caused by this organism. Disease caused by other organisms of this genus should be referred to as "mycobacteriosis due to *M. x*" and not as "atypical tuberculosis" or "tuberculosis due to . . ." (Chapter 346).

Organisms of the genus *Mycobacterium* are found variably in the environment, predominately in soil and water. However, *M. tuberculosis* has become so adapted to the human body that it has no natural reservoirs in nature other than infected/diseased persons. Although disease caused by strains of *M. tuberculosis* has been reported rarely in primates, elephants, and other mammals, the presumption is that the infection was originally introduced into the animals by humans.

Mycobacterial cell walls contain high concentrations of lipids or waxes, which makes them resistant to standard staining techniques. They can be induced to take up a dye such as carbol fuchsin by imposing alkalinity or by heating. After dye absorption, they are resistant to the potent decolorizing agent acid-alcohol, a trait that provides the basis of the reference to acid-fast bacilli (AFB).

M. tuberculosis and most of the other mycobacteria grow quite slowly; their replication time in most media is approximately 18 to 24 hours. Readily discernible colonies typically do not appear on solid media for 2.5 to 5 week, so there has been great interest in rapid, novel techniques to indicate the presence, species, and drug susceptibility of mycobacteria, including *M. tuberculosis.*

Epidemiology

Globally, tuberculosis is one of the leading infectious causes of adult mortality. Most tuberculosis cases occur because of late reactivation of the vestigial lesions of primary infection in the lungs or in extrapulmonary sites. Rapid progression to overt disease occurs in a minority of newly infected persons who cannot mount sufficient immune responses. Groups at high risk include children from infancy through 4 years of age, the infirm elderly, and immunocompromised subjects, including patients with acquired immunodeficiency syndrome (AIDS), organ transplant recipients, and other patients who are immunosuppressed by malnutrition, illnesses, or chemotherapy. Recently, treatment of rheumatologic disease and inflammatory bowel disease with anti–tumor necrosis factor-α (anti–TNF-α) antibody therapy has been associated with reactivation tuberculosis.

Worldwide

The World Health Organization (WHO) estimates that approximately a third of the world's population is latently infected with *M. tuberculosis.* From this pool, 8 to 10 million new active cases emerge per year, and the WHO estimates that roughly 50% are communicable forms of pulmonary disease. Regions in the world where the infection and disease are most prevalent include the Pacific Rim nations, Asia, the Indian subcontinent, sub-Saharan Africa, Latin America, Russia, and the former Soviet Republics. Because of delayed, inadequate, or unavailable therapy, 2 to 3 million persons die annually; the WHO estimates that more than a fourth of preventable deaths in developing nations are attributable to tuberculosis.

United States

The United States has a considerably lower prevalence of infection, with recent Centers for Disease Control and Prevention (CDC) estimates suggesting that only 4 to 6% of the population (10 to 15 million persons) harbor latent infections. Case rates in the United States fell consistently from 1953 to 1984, but there was a substantial upsurge in 1985 to 1992. Elements feeding this increase included human immunodeficiency virus (HIV) infection, immigration, and most significantly, deterioration of the public health infrastructure. After treatment programs were strengthened and measures were taken to reduce nosocomial transmission, case rates dropped from 10.5 per 100,000 in 1992 to 4.9 per 100,000 in 2004, with an all-time low of 14,571 cases in 2004.

Among Americans of color, tuberculosis is largely a disease of young adults, with the peak incidence between the ages of 25 and 44 years. By comparison, the peak age in whites is 70 years and older, presumably because of reactivation of latent infections from early in life. In 2004, 53% of U.S. tuberculosis cases occurred in immigrants, and nearly another 30% occurred in U.S.-born minority populations. When compared with the 2004 case rate for the white population in the United States (1.3 cases per 100,000 persons per year), the relative risks were 8.3 for African Americans, 7.5 for Hispanic Americans, and 20 for Asian/Pacific Islanders. Within these three groups, foreign-born individuals accounted for 27% of cases in African Americans, 74% of cases in Hispanics, and 95% of cases in Asian/Pacific Islanders. The case rate for foreign-born persons (25.3) is now 10-fold higher than that for persons born in the United States. Major sources of these cases include Mexico, the Philippines, Southeast Asia, the Caribbean, and Latin America.

Human Immunodeficiency Virus Infection and Acquired Immunodeficiency Syndrome

HIV infection and AIDS have contributed to the rising case rates of tuberculosis through three broad pathways. First, individuals with latent tuberculosis infection who acquire HIV infection are at much greater risk of reactivation as their immune capacity diminishes. Second, persons with HIV infection or AIDS may well be at higher risk of acquiring new tuberculosis infections, probably because of biologic factors (e.g., impaired defenses) and situational factors (e.g., more time spent in high-risk, congregate environments, including hospitals). Third, young adults with HIV infection and active tuberculosis transmit tuberculosis to people with whom they reside. The upsurge in tuberculosis cases in the United States since 1985 has presumably been linked to the HIV epidemic, although full quantification of the association is not possible because of incomplete serologic testing. However, there can be no question that HIV/AIDS is playing a major role in rising case rates in many regions of the world, including sub-Saharan Africa, Russia, and Southeast Asia.

Transmission

Infection is spread almost exclusively by aerosolization of contaminated respiratory secretions. Patients with *cavitary* lung disease are particularly infectious because their sputum contains relatively greater numbers of bacilli and they cough frequently.

For infection to occur, bacilli must be delivered to the distal air spaces of the lung (the alveoli), where they are not subject to mucociliary clearance. To reach the alveoli, the bacilli must be suspended in very fine units that behave as the air itself. These units are the dehydrated residuals of finer particles generated by high-velocity exhalational maneuvers; cough-inducing procedures such as bronchoscopy or endotracheal intubation are particularly likely to generate infectious aerosols. These droplet nuclei are calculated to be 0.5 to 3 μm in diameter, may remain suspended in room air for many hours, and when inhaled, can traverse the airways to reach the alveoli.

Although patients with cavitary tuberculosis expectorate massive numbers of bacilli, the probability of generating infectious particles is relatively low. Household contacts of patients with extensive pulmonary disease who have had productive coughs for weeks or months before diagnosis have, on average, less than a 50% chance of being infected. The usual case of pulmonary tuberculosis has a low order of infectiousness when compared with an airborne disease such as measles. However, uncommon cases demonstrate extremely high rates of transmission; specific factors in these instances have not been clearly elucidated.

Transmission also occurs via aerosols generated by débridement or by dressing changes of skin or soft tissue abscesses caused by *M. tuberculosis*. Tissue agitation associated with autopsies and direct inoculation into soft tissues from contaminated instruments or bone fragments have also been reported. Fomites do not play a significant role in transmission.

Pathobiology

The natural history and various clinical syndromes of tuberculosis are intimately related to host defenses. Tubercle bacilli do not elaborate classic toxins; rather, the inflammation and tissue injury that characterize the disease are mediated by products elaborated by the host during the immune response to infection.

To initiate infection, the tubercle bacillus must be taken up by phagocytic cells within the body. When an immunologically naive alveolar macrophage engulfs a tubercle bacillus, it initially provides a nurturing environment within its phagosome in which the bacilli survive and replicate. Indeed, part of the pathogenic strategy of the tubercle bacillus is the ability to prevent fusion of the phagosome with the lysosome. However, the infected phagocytic cells release substances that attract a variety of immune effector cells, including peripheral blood monocyte-derived dendritic cells and T lymphocytes. The dendritic cells, which are the primary antigen-presenting cells, participate in both the local inflammatory process and, after migration to regional lymph nodes, initiation of the more comprehensive immune process. Recent studies suggest a significant role for Toll-like receptors in the innate defenses against tuberculosis.

In normal, otherwise healthy adults, the host initially prevails in more than 95% of cases. However, this initial encounter typically extends over a few weeks to several months, during which the bacillary population has proliferated massively and undergone various degrees of dissemination. Tissues that are most heavily seeded during this bacillemia, such as the apices of the lungs, the kidneys, bones, meninges, or other extrapulmonary sites, are common foci for subsequent *reactivation tuberculosis*. Through complex interactions involving mononuclear phagocytes and various T-cell subsets, host defenses are enhanced. This *cell-mediated immunity* is related to but not identical with *delayed-type hypersensitivity*. Delayed-type hypersensitivity is associated with development of the tuberculin reaction, an indurated response 48 to 96 hours after the intradermal injection of tuberculosis protein antigens (e.g., purified protein derivative [PPD]). Skin test reactivity typically appears 4 to 6 weeks after infection, although intervals up to 20 weeks have been reported. It is not known what percentage of newly infected subjects fail to develop delayed-type hypersensitivity, but up to 20% of adults with active tuberculosis do not react to the PPD.

As these defenses gain momentum, involution of the numerous disseminated granulomatous foci occurs in the lungs, lymph nodes, and scattered sites. Typically, all that remains overtly to mark this encounter is the tuberculin skin test reactivity. In a minority of cases, a small, single residual site of the primary infection (i.e., Ghon focus) appears in the lung parenchyma; occasionally, this focus is accompanied by calcifications of the ipsilateral hilar nodes. In some patients, fibronodular shadowing also develops in one or both lung apices (i.e., Simon foci), presumably as the residua of subclinical disease at these sites. This dormant, asymptomatic, noninfectious state is known as latent tuberculous infection.

Tubercle bacilli undergo spontaneous mutations that confer resistance to the various antituberculosis medications. These mutations occur at predictable frequencies, usually in the range of 1 in 10^5 to 10^8 replications, and they are unlinked, thus resulting in resistance to only one drug or drug category. In cavitary tuberculosis, the population of bacilli is so great that small numbers of mycobacteria exist that are resistant to each of the standard medications. However, because the mutations are unlinked, there is an extremely low probability of spontaneous resistance to two or more drugs by a single bacillus.

Clinical Manifestations

Because the primary infection results in bacillemic dissemination, tuberculosis can involve extrathoracic as well as pulmonary or pleural sites. Hosts with more competent immunity tend to have disease limited to their lungs or other single sites, whereas hosts with less robust defenses have multifocal or disseminated disease.

Excluding patients with HIV infection, about 80% of adults have exclusively pulmonary parenchymal disease, 15% have disease at extrapulmonary sites, and approximately 5% have simultaneously active disease at intrathoracic and extrathoracic locations. Although most patients complain of feeling "feverish," a substantial proportion do not have fever when measured.

Pulmonary Disease

Classic symptoms include cough, fever, and sweating. Cough is nearly universal; typically, it is initially dry but then progresses with increasing volumes of purulent secretions and the variable appearance of blood streaking or gross hemoptysis. Feverishness is common as the disease advances, and actual temperatures range from subnormal to extreme elevations. Sweating, including drenching night sweats, is typical. Other common complaints include malaise, fatigue, weight loss, nonpleuritic chest pain, and dyspnea.

Signs may be limited until the disease is in advanced stages. Fever with peaks as high as 40 to 41° C, typically occurring in the evening, develops in patients with various forms and stages of tuberculosis. Localized rales are early findings, coarse rhonchi evolve as secretions become more voluminous and tenacious, and signs of lung consolidation are rarely heard. Wheezing or regionally diminished breath sounds, or both, may be heard in patients with peribronchial or endobronchial airway narrowing. Nevertheless, some patients with fairly extensive radiographic abnormalities may have minimal or no adventitious sounds on auscultation.

Extrapulmonary Tuberculosis

Extrapulmonary tuberculosis occurs in roughly a sixth of HIV-negative adults with active disease in the United States. The most common sites are lymphatic, genitourinary, bone, joint, central nervous system, gastrointestinal, and pericardial (Table 345–1). Eye involvement, though unusual, is virtually pathognomonic (Fig. 345–1).

The severe wasting seen with advanced pulmonary disease (i.e., consumption) rarely accompanies extrapulmonary tuberculosis. Feverishness occurs with more extensive disease, prominently including miliary, pleural, and genitourinary disease.

Diagnosis

The tuberculin skin test reaction is falsely negative in 20 to 25% of otherwise immunocompetent normal adults at the time of diagnosis. The clinician should not be diverted from considering the diagnosis by

TABLE 345–1 COMMON FORMS OF EXTRAPULMONARY TUBERCULOSIS IN PATIENTS WITHOUT HIV INFECTION

Organ System*	Relatively High-Risk Groups	Common Clinical Manifestations	Diagnosis	Management
Lymphatic	Youngsters and young adults; F > M, Asian and Indian females at higher risk	Unilateral, cervical; painless; sinus tracts late	Excisional biopsy with culture; PPD usually positive	May respond slowly to medication; rarely may require excision
Pleural	Young adults with primary infection; older adults with reactivation disease	May be acute *or* indolent; severe pleurisy or asymptomatic	Lymphatic exudate; AFB smear usually negative; biopsy with culture gives best yield	Usually responds well to medication; rarely needs tube thoracostomy drainage
Genitourinary	Rare in young; more frequent in females, foreign born, and Native Americans	May involve the kidneys, ureters, bladder, testes, epididymis, uterus, fallopian tubes	Culture urine; biopsy and culture masses and uterine scrapings	Usually responds well to medication; beware of early or late obstructive uropathy
Bone or joint	More common in elderly, although seen in all ages	Lumbar and low dorsal spine common in older patients; high dorsal in young; weight-bearing bones and joints	Needle biopsy and aspiration for spinal lesions; synovial biopsy and culture for joints	Débride and stabilize spine; try to avoid fusing joints
Disseminated	Most frequent in very young or old, blacks, and Native Americans	Chest x-ray film abnormalities may lag; progressive fever and inanition; PPD negative in 50%	Smears and cultures of involved fluids, organs, and mesothelia; smear and culture of urine	Early therapy vital; corticosteroids of uncertain value
Meninges or CNS	Most common in infants/children with XPTB; higher risk for Hispanic Americans, blacks, and Native Americans	Three stages; early, fever, headache, and malaise; later, confusion, obtundation, seizures, and coma	Lumbar puncture: ↑ protein and cells, ↓ glucose, ↑ pressure; smears rarely positive; special tests (see text)	Prognosis related to stage; corticosteroids indicated in most cases; drugs must penetrate CNS
Peritoneal or gastrointestinal	Increases with age; higher risk in minorities	Mainly mesothelial, but ileal involvement may resemble Crohn's disease; abdominal swelling and vague pain common	Laparoscopic biopsy ideal; smear and culture ascites; stool cultures may be useful	Beware of adhesions and obstruction; corticosteroids may be useful
Pericardial	Rare in children; more common in blacks	Acute pain rare; cough, dyspnea, and vague discomfort	Widened cardiac silhouette; left pleural effusion; ECG low voltage and chronic ST-T wave changes; ↓ heart sounds, rubs rare	Corticosteroids: ↓ effusion, improve performance; may reduce late adhesive complications; pericardiectomy for tamponade

*In persons without HIV infection, roughly 15 to 16% of cases of tuberculosis are manifested as extrapulmonary involvement. Lymphatic and pleural diseases are the most common forms.

AFB = acid-fast bacilli; CNS = central nervous system; ECG = electrocardiogram; PPD = purified protein derivative test; XPTB = extrapulmonary tuberculosis.

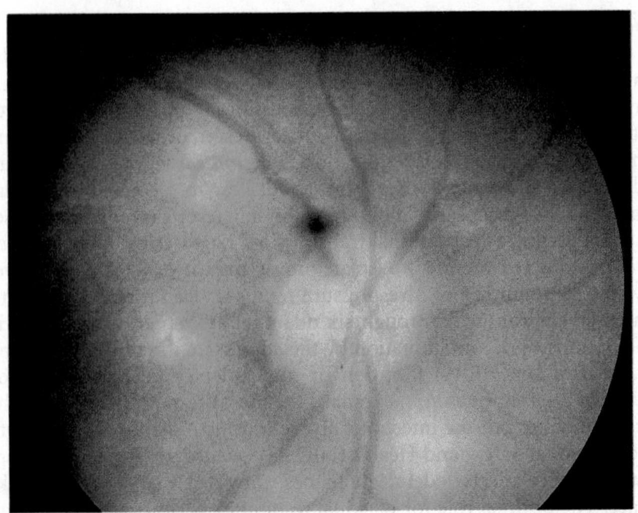

FIGURE 345–1 • Choroidal tubercles in acute miliary tuberculosis. This appearance is virtually diagnostic, so it is essential to examine the fundi of any patient in whom miliary tuberculosis is a possibility. (From Forbes CD, Jackson WF: Color Atlas and Text of Clinical Medicine, 3rd ed. London, Mosby, 2003.)

nonreactive tuberculin skin test results or lack of fever in patients with other typical features of tuberculosis.

Interferon-γ release assays of whole blood or mononuclear cells after stimulation by selected mycobacterial antigens appear to be more sensitive and specific than the tuberculin skin test. One assay has been approved for use in the United States, but clinical adoption of this assay will depend on its technical demands and expense.

The chest radiograph is central to the diagnosis of pulmonary tuberculosis. Upper lung zone fibronodular shadowing involving one or both apices is seen in most cases. As these lesions advance, they enlarge and become fluffy or softly marginated; the lesions coalesce, and cavitation devolves as intense local inflammation produces necrosis and sloughing of lung tissue. The most common sites involved in reactivation adult tuberculosis are, in descending order, the posterior and apical segments of the right upper lobe, the apical-posterior segment of the left upper lobe, and the superior segments of the lower lobes. Lower zone disease is seen at initial evaluation in less than 15% of HIV-negative adults; it is seen somewhat more commonly in diabetics and patients with prominent peribronchial and endobronchial involvement. Pleural effusions or hilar adenopathy is uncommon in adults with reactivation-type pulmonary disease.

Sputum smears and cultures are the most specific components of diagnosis. Some contemporary laboratories still use the classic acid-fast stains (i.e., Ziehl-Neelsen or Kinyoun); however, most use a modified acid-fast method, auramine O, a dye that fluoresces when excited by ultraviolet light. With this fluorochrome technique, the mycobacteria are more easily discernible (i.e., bright yellow on an inky black background) than with the older methods (i.e., red on a blue and white background). The finding of AFB on microscopic examination of respiratory secretions associated with suitable clinical, epidemiologic, and radiographic findings is highly suggestive of tuberculosis. However, microscopy is not specific because other pathogenic mycobacteria may be found in sputum. The test is not very sensitive; the likelihood of positive smears depends heavily on the extent of pulmonary involvement. With readily visible cavities and no previous treatment, it is rare to have negative sputum results on microscopy. However, with noncavitary fibronodular or miliary patterns on chest films, negative microscopic results are common. Overall, 50 to 60% of patients with culture-positive pulmonary tuberculosis have AFB smear–positive sputum. Cultures are the "gold standard" for diagnosis; however, current methods typically entail 3 to 6 weeks to cultivate and identify species. More rapid cultivation and identification techniques that use liquid media or radiometric, molecular biologic, or chromatographic methods have reduced the required time substantially. Nucleic acid amplification techniques potentially offer a diagnosis in 1 to 2 days; these tests are particularly useful in differentiating tuberculosis from environmental mycobacterioses such as *Mycobacterium avium* complex. The diagnosis is occasionally made on the basis of symptoms, radiographic findings, and response to empirical therapy *without* culture confirmation. Because of the clinical importance of resistance to first-line drugs, susceptibility testing on all initial *M. tuberculosis* isolates is recommended.

Extrapulmonary Tuberculosis

Diagnosis of extrapulmonary tuberculosis is often problematic because of the relative paucity of bacilli. Histopathologic analysis of involved tissues typically shows giant cell granulomas with caseating necrosis and few, if any demonstrable AFB. Analysis of mesothelial effusions (i.e., pleural, peritoneal, or pericardial) characteristically reveals a lymphocyte-rich exudate with low concentrations of glucose; however, the *initial* inflammatory response in these spaces may be predominantly polymorphonuclear leukocytes. An elevated level of adenosine deaminase in pleural or peritoneal fluid is highly sensitive and specific for tuberculosis. Cerebrospinal fluid (CSF) findings in meningitis (Chapter 437) begin with a modest leukocytosis that shift from polymorphonuclear to lymphocyte dominance; leukocyte counts typically range from 50 to 300 cells/mL. The CSF protein concentration is generally moderately elevated. Glucose levels are progressively depressed in relation to the degree of leukocytosis.

Persons with Human Immunodeficiency Virus Infection or Acquired Immunodeficiency Syndrome

Early in the course of HIV infection, the clinical manifestations of tuberculosis are quite similar to those in normal hosts. However, with the progressive reduction in the $CD4^+$ lymphocyte population, several major changes ensue: (1) a steady reduction in the proportion who react significantly to tuberculin skin testing, reaching a nadir of 10 to 20% of reactors among those with advanced AIDS; (2) substantially greater extrapulmonary involvement, reaching a 60 to 80% prevalence of extrapulmonary tuberculosis, including exotic manifestations such as diffuse lymphadenitis, cutaneous disease, or disseminated multiorgan involvement; and (3) changing patterns of disease on chest radiography, evolving from classic upper zone fibronodular, cavitary disease to lower zone, nondescript pneumonic patterns, infrequent cavity formation, interstitial or miliary shadowing, very prominent hilar or paratracheal adenopathy, and substantial pleural effusions.

Prevention

Modalities to control tuberculosis include treatment of latent infection to prevent active clinical disease, bacille Calmette-Guérin (BCG) vaccination, and measures to limit nosocomial spread.

Treatment of Latent Infection: Preventive Therapy

Because most cases of tuberculosis in the United States arise from endogenous reactivation of latent infection acquired remotely in time, chemotherapy given to persons harboring such infections is an efficient prevention strategy. In a series of randomized, placebo-controlled studies conducted decades ago, treatment of latent tuberculosis infection reduced morbidity by 70% in the year of treatment and by 54% in the post-treatment years. Even higher rates of protection ranging from 70 to 90% with 6- and 12-month treatment, respectively, were shown in a large trial in eastern Europe.

Indications for Treatment of Latent Tuberculosis Infection

The recommendations focus on persons who are deemed to be at relatively higher risk for the development of active disease (see Table 345–4). A recently noted risk factor is the TNF-α–modifying therapy used for rheumatoid arthritis (Chapter 285), inflammatory bowel disease (Chapter 144), and psoriasis (Chapter 464). Among patients in whom anti–TNF-α agents are to be used, careful pretreatment evaluation for latent tuberculosis should be conducted. If the tuberculin test is reactive (≥5 mm) *or* if epidemiologic risk factors suggest a high likelihood of previous tuberculosis infection (known exposure, country of origin, employment, etc.), treatment of latent tuberculosis should be initiated before commencing the anti–TNF-α agent.

In most instances, the tuberculin skin test is the key method to identify latent infection; in some instances, however, therapy may be recommended despite nonreactivity. Because of the shortcomings of the tuberculin test, tests based on the release of interferon-γ after ex vivo exposure of blood to mycobacterial antigens are being studied. Preliminary data suggest comparable or better sensitivity, improved specificity, and the potential to distinguish reactivity as a result of tuberculosis from that engendered by BCG or environmental mycobacteria.

Special Considerations in the Treatment of Latent Infection

HIV infection is the most potent risk factor for endogenous reactivation. Persons with positive HIV serologic results or strong epidemiologic or clinical markers for HIV risk should be assigned very high priority for treatment of latent tuberculosis infection. In addition to protecting the individual patient from tuberculosis, such treatment may extend survival by ameliorating the accelerated progression of HIV infection seen with active tuberculosis and may prevent transmission to other, very vulnerable HIV-infected persons (e.g., in shared health care, social, or residential environments).

Others patients requiring particular attention are foreign-born persons from high-risk nations, notably Mexico, the Philippines, Vietnam, India, China, Haiti, and Korea. Immigrants from these and other endemic regions, particularly newly arrived immigrants, should be screened and, if found to be infected, considered for treatment of latent tuberculosis infection.

Regimen Options for Treatment of Latent Infection

Nine months of isoniazid (INH) therapy is the standard for all subjects, with 6 months as an acceptable option. An alternative is a 4-month rifampin regimen, which is associated with fewer side effects, lower rates of hepatitis, less frequent interruptions, and higher completion rates. Rifampin alone should not be given to persons with AIDS because of the risk of acquired drug resistance.

Monitoring for Compliance and Toxicity

Patients receiving treatment of latent tuberculosis infection should be seen periodically to promote adherence to the treatment regimen and survey for signs or symptoms of drug toxicity. Intermittent directly observed preventive therapy is not widely feasible; however, it may be applicable in selected circumstances, such as for prisoners, especially those with HIV infection, or for recently infected infants or children in households where reliable treatment is unlikely.

The major toxicity of INH, rifampin, and pyrazinamide is hepatitis, which may prove fatal if therapy is continued into the period at which symptoms and gross chemical derangements occur. It is therefore important that initial education alert the patient or responsible family members (or both) to the early manifestations of liver injury (i.e., anorexia, nausea, malaise, loss of taste for cigarettes, and dark urine) and provide instructions to stop therapy and report promptly for evaluation. Patients should also have monthly communication with a health care worker, directly if possible but by telephone as an alternative, to inquire about their health and to reiterate the education. Biochemical monitoring of liver chemistry parameters is not routinely indicated. If patients report symptoms, liver function tests should be performed immediately, and even modest derangements are grounds for halting therapy. Unless there was major toxicity, the same drug may be reinstituted later or an alternative regimen can be attempted.

Bacille Calmette-Guérin Vaccination

BCG is a live vaccine prepared from an attenuated strain of *M. bovis*. It has been used widely around the world, but its efficacy and utility are debated. The performance of various strains of BCG given to different populations over time has ranged from 80% protection to paradoxical detrimental effects (e.g., more tuberculosis in those receiving the vaccine). A meta-analysis of published BCG studies indicated that vaccinations offered an overall 50% protective effect, with higher levels of protection against meningeal or disseminated tuberculosis. However, studies have shown that the efficacy of BCG diminishes in populations near the equator. Although the calculated protection in this meta-analysis reached statistical significance, no explanation was offered for the failure to show efficacy in recent large trials conducted in India and Malawi.

Because BCG is presumed to work by conferring immunity to tuberculosis in persons not previously infected, it is not appropriate for widespread use in the United States, where most cases arise in those already infected with *M. tuberculosis*.

Limiting Nosocomial Transmission

Substantial microepidemics of tuberculosis have been documented in various institutions, including hospitals, clinics, residential facilities, and prisons. To prevent institutional transmission, the CDC have advocated a three-tiered system: administrative measures, environmental programs, and personal respiratory protection. *Administrative measures* include educational programs to alert staff about how to recognize and isolate possible active cases early. Staff tuberculin skin testing is required to assess the risk for intra-institutional transmission. *Engineering or environmental programs* are intended to isolate proven or suspected cases effectively by placing them in negative-pressure rooms and diluting the air in the patients' environment through six or more air changes per hour, with the options of decontamination by the adjunctive use of high-efficiency particulate air (HEPA) filtration or ultraviolet germicidal irradiation. *Personal respiratory protection* entails the use of respirators that can theoretically filter out the infectious droplet nuclei. A National Institute for Occupational Safety and Health (NIOSH) category N95 personal respiratory device meets federal guidelines, provided that fit testing takes place. The optimal role for personal respirators is controversial. Perhaps the most suitable role is to protect health care workers who have unavoidable exposure to smear-positive patients during cough-inducing procedures such as bronchoscopy or intubation. Use in other circumstances depends on the source case and environmental factors. The regulations regarding mandated use of these devices are under review. For considerations of public health concerns and regulatory oversight, all institutions that may be involved in caring for tuberculosis patients should have an active program to limit the hazard of nosocomial transmission to health care workers and other patients or clients.

Treatment

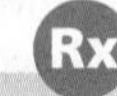

Because of the hazard of casual, airborne transmission of infection and the potentially morbid or lethal consequences for those to whom the infection is transmitted, there is a singular public health mandate that *persons with communicable tuberculosis must be treated or quarantined.* The guidelines of the American Thoracic Society (ATS), CDC, and Infectious Disease Society of America (IDSA) explicitly state that "the responsibility for successful treatment is clearly assigned to the public health program or private provider, *not* the patient. It is strongly recommended that the initial treatment strategy utilize patient-centered case management with an adherence plan that emphasizes direct observation of therapy." U.S. public health policy throughout the 20th century empowered governmental representatives to quarantine patients with potentially lethal infectious diseases. In the case of tuberculosis, modern chemotherapy has effectively become a chemical quarantine; nonadherence to treatment may be seen as breaching this quarantine. Because of the consequences of inadequate or incomplete treatment, directly observed therapy (DOT) to prevent noncompliance has become a standard rather than an exceptional or punitive protocol (see the later section on nonadherence).

Indications for Commencing Treatment

Because it often takes 3 to 8 weeks to culture and identify species, treatment of most patients is initiated before a definitive diagnosis is established. The diagnosis is usually based on an amalgam of historical and epidemiologic features; radiographic, tissue, or fluid analysis; and microscopic findings. Initiation of empirical therapy for patients with potentially rapid, life-threatening conditions, such as central nervous system or miliary disease, generally entails a low threshold of suspicion; however, care should be taken to obtain optimal diagnostic specimens before commencing medication to avoid suppression of growth in paucibacillary material by the chemotherapy.

Principles of Multidrug Treatment

Patients with active tuberculosis should receive multiple agents to accelerate bacterial clearance and, more crucially, to prevent the emergence of drug-resistant mutants, which can significantly and permanently compromise the treatment outcome. According to the

Rx

principle of multidrug therapy, INH-resistant mutants are killed by rifampin, and rifampin-resistant mutants are killed by INH. Early in treatment, when the mycobacterial burden is greatest, at least two effective agents must be used.

If patients are nonadherent and stop taking one of their medications without knowledge of the clinician, unopposed mutant bacilli may proliferate, thereby resulting in treatment failure or relapse associated with acquired drug resistance. When this process occurs serially, multidrug resistance is created. Such organisms can be transmitted to other persons and give rise to initial drug-resistant tuberculosis.

In addition to combating drug resistance, multidrug regimens can shorten the required duration of treatment through unique contributions by the various agents. A regimen of INH and ethambutol requires 18 months to cure the typical case of pulmonary tuberculosis. Adding rifampin to INH reduces the duration to 9 months, and when an initial 2-month phase of pyrazinamide is added to INH and rifampin, cure occurs in 6 months.

Choice of Regimen

Because of concern over the prevalence of drug resistance, current recommendations advocate a four-drug regimen (Table 345–2) with specific doses (Table 345–3) for most cases of known or suspected tuberculosis. INH and rifampin are the central agents of any regimen because of their superior bactericidal activity and low toxicity. Pyrazinamide has special utility in promoting rapid, early reduction of the bacillary burden; in drug-susceptible cases, it needs to be given only for the initial 2 months to produce this effect. Ethambutol is useful primarily to protect against the emergence of drug resistance in cases with unknown initial susceptibility patterns and large mycobacterial burdens. Ethambutol may be terminated if susceptibility is reported or continued throughout the duration of treatment if resistance is present. Streptomycin, a parenteral agent, is now used infrequently because of problems with regularly administering intramuscular injections; however, for patients with very extensive tuberculosis, streptomycin may accelerate the initial bactericidal activity. Rifapentine, which is a long-acting, potent form of rifamycin, has been used mainly in once-weekly, continuation-phase regimens. Recent trials using INH and rifapentine in once-weekly schedules during the continuation phase of treatment (months 3 to 6) of active infection demonstrated overall failure and relapse rates slightly higher than those with INH and rifampin given twice or three times weekly in the comparator arms. [1,2] Hence, administration of INH and rifapentine in the continuation phase of therapy is advocated only for patients who have noncavitary lung disease and whose sputum smears are negative after 8 to 9 weeks of treatment. Because of the possible risk of acquired resistance to the rifamycins, rifapentine is not indicated for patients with AIDS. Rifabutin, a long-acting rifamycin, does not induce the hepatic cytochrome P-450 pathways to the same extent as rifampin does and is therefore useful for simultaneous treatment of tuberculosis and antiretroviral therapy for AIDS.

In practice, clinicians should review every proven or suspected case and consider individual modifications or exemptions to the standard four-drug regimen. For example, in an elderly patient with remote exposure to tuberculosis in the era before chemotherapy, with no recent contacts, and with no history of tuberculosis, medical treatment may reasonably be started with a three-drug (i.e., INH, rifampin, and ethambutol) regimen because of the very low likelihood of drug resistance, the poor tolerance to pyrazinamide in the

TABLE 345–2 RECOMMENDED TREATMENT REGIMENS FOR TUBERCULOSIS IN THE UNITED STATES

Regimen	Medications	Total Duration	Comments
ATS/CDC*	INH and RIF daily for 6 mo; PZA daily and SM or EMB daily for 2 mo	6 mo	Add SM or EMB in areas or patients at risk for initial drug resistance. Stop PZA, EMB, or SM after 2 mo if strain susceptible; continue or modify regimen if resistance present
Denver	INH, RIF, PZA, and SM daily for 2 wk, then twice weekly for 6 wk. Follow with INH and RIF twice weekly for 18 wk. Note: All intermittent regimens must be given as DOT	6 mo	EMB has replaced SM in most cases. Stop PZA and EMB at 8 wk if strain is susceptible; continue through 6 mo if there is initial INH resistance; 24 wk of twice-weekly therapy facilitates DOT
Hong Kong	INH, RIF, PZA, and SM or EMB thrice weekly for 6 mo (may stop PZA, SM, or EMB after 2 mo). Note: All intermittent regimens must be given as DOT	6 mo	All intermittent. If strain is susceptible, may stop PZA and SM or EMB after 2 mo. If there is INH resistance, stop INH and the add fourth drug (EMB or SM)
Arkansas	INH and RIF daily for 1 mo, then INH and RIF twice weekly for 8 mo	9 mo	This regimen should only be used in populations with a very low prevalence of drug resistance. Initial therapy should probably include a third drug until drug susceptibility is reported. Although this regimen is self-administered in Arkansas, authorities strongly recommend DOT for all intermittent regimens
CDC trial 22	INH, RIF, PZA, and EMB for 2 mo; may be given daily, per the Denver regimen, or per the Hong Kong regimen; then INH and rifapentine once weekly for 4 mo (not for persons with AIDS)	6 mo	Rifapentine is a potent and long-acting rifamycin. In trials comparing once-weekly INH and rifapentine with twice-weekly INH and RIF, the rifapentine regimen performed slightly less well and hence is recommended only for patients with noncavitary lung disease and negative sputum smears at 2 mo of therapy

*The ATS and CDC advocate initial four-drug therapy for cases in communities with a background prevalence of initial drug resistance of 4% or greater. If susceptibility has been demonstrated or if resistance is deemed very unlikely, initial three-drug regimens may be used.
AIDS = acquired immunodeficiency syndrome; ATS = American Thoracic Society; CDC = Centers for Disease Control and Prevention; DOT = directly observed therapy; EMB = ethambutol; INH = isoniazid; PZA = pyrazinamide; RIF = rifampin; SM = streptomycin.

TABLE 345–3 DOSAGE, TOXICITY, AND SPECIAL CONSIDERATIONS FOR STANDARD ANTITUBERCULOSIS MEDICATIONS

Drug	Daily Dosage	Usual Adult Dose, Thrice/ Twice Weekly	Toxicity	Special Considerations	Comments
Isoniazid (INH)	300 mg PO	600 mg II 900 mg	Hepatitis, neuritis, mood/cognition, lupus reaction	Pregnancy: safe Liver disease: caution Renal impairment: ↓ dose if severe	Monitor liver function test results monthly in most patients; clinically significant interactions with phenytoin and antifungal agents (azoles)
Rifampin (RIF)*	600 mg PO 450 mg in persons <50 kg body weight	600 mg II (same)	Hepatitis, thrombopenia, nephritis, flu syndrome	Pregnancy: acceptable Liver disease: caution Renal impairment: safe	Key: multiple, profound drug interactions possible (see later); turns urine and fluids red
Rifapentine (RPT)	Not recommended	Not recommended (600 mg PO once weekly)	Similar to RIF	Similar to RIF	The primary role for RPT is in *once-weekly* continuation therapy given with INH. Not indicated for persons with AIDS
Rifabutin (RBU)	150–300 mg/kg PO	300 mg II (same)	Similar to RIF; modestly more neutropenia and thrombopenia than with RIF	Similar to RIF	The primary role for RBU is for tuberculosis in persons with AIDS to lessen drug-drug interactions
Pyrazinamide (PZA)	20–30 mg/kg PO	30–40 mg/kg II 40–50 mg/kg	Hepatitis, arthralgias, and arthritis from hyperuricemia, gastrointestinal distress, rash	Pregnancy: unknown (avoid) Liver disease: caution Renal impairment: caution	Urate levels always rise; do not treat or stop PZA unless unmanageable gout develops
Ethambutol (EMB)	15–20 mg/kg PO	30–35 mg/kg II 40–50 mg/kg	Optic neuritis, gastrointestinal distress, rare peripheral neuritis	Pregnancy: safe Liver disease: safe Renal impairment: ↓ dose/ frequency	Monitor visual acuity and color vision regularly
Streptomycin (SM)	12–15 mg/kg IM	15 mg/kg II (same)	Vestibular and auditory, cation depletion	Pregnancy: high-risk (avoid) Liver disease: safe Renal impairment: ↓ dose/ frequency	Reduce dose and/or frequency in case of renal impairment

*Rifampin drug interactions have been reported with antiretroviral agents, including protease inhibitors and non-nucleoside reverse transcriptase inhibitors, oral contraceptives, anticoagulants, methadone, corticosteroids, estrogen replacement, calcium-channel blockers, β-blockers, cyclosporine, antifungal agents (azoles), phenytoin, theophylline, sulfonylureas, haloperidol, and others (see *Physicians' Desk Reference*).

Rx

elderly, and a low risk of absconding or abandoning treatment. In contrast, an individual who gives a history of previous antituberculosis therapy or comes from a household in which there has been prior multidrug-resistant (MDR) tuberculosis may receive an empirically expanded regimen, including the standard four oral agents plus a fluoroquinolone and amikacin.

Specific Treatment Issues

Acquired Immunodeficiency Syndrome

Treatment of tuberculosis in persons with AIDS is similar to standard therapy. Particular issues of concern are drug-drug interactions among the antituberculosis agents and the various antiretroviral medications or drugs given for other opportunistic infections, the

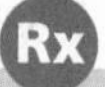

immune reconstitution syndrome in which antiretroviral therapy restores the host's capacity to mount an inflammatory response, and the potential for malabsorption of medications because of various AIDS-related enteropathies.

Rifampin, by inducing hepatic cytochrome P-450 pathways, causes accelerated elimination of most protease inhibitors and non-nucleoside reverse transcriptase inhibitors, as well as antifungal azoles and other drugs. Conversely, the various antiretroviral drugs may result in accelerated elimination or retarded catabolism of the antituberculosis agents. Given the potentially severe consequences of these interactions, including treatment failure, acquired drug resistance, and toxicity related to both categories of therapy, simultaneous antituberculosis and antiretroviral therapy should be undertaken only in specialized centers or with skilled consultative support.

Section XXIII Infectious Diseases

Rx

Contemporary information on the extensive list of drug-drug interactions is available at *www.atsjournals.org.*

As antiretroviral therapy restores $CD4^+$ lymphocyte levels and reconstitutes immune function, patients may experience increased symptoms or other manifestations from preexisting infections such as tuberculosis. Examples include higher fever, worsening of infiltrates or effusions seen on chest radiographs, and enlarging lymph nodes. Patients may be particularly troubled by enlarging central nervous system lesions or pericardial disease, where deterioration might be lethal. Up to a third of patients who have AIDS and tuberculosis and who receive antiretroviral therapy experience such paradoxical worsening. Delaying the initiation of antiretroviral therapy until several months of tuberculosis treatment has been completed lessens the likelihood and severity of the reactions but does not obviate the risk. Most patients can be managed through the reactions, but antiretroviral therapy may be terminated or steroids given for several weeks (or both) in an attempt to lessen the inflammatory reaction in severe cases.

Current guidelines in HIV-positive patients recommend 6 months of treatment but that therapy be extended for patients who are slow to respond. Because effective antiretroviral therapy extends survival for persons with HIV infection, it is possible that more post-treatment tuberculosis relapses will be seen. Positive sputum cultures after 2 months of therapy are a useful marker of patients at higher risk for failure or relapse. In such patients, therapy should be extended to 9 months' total duration. Reassessment to exclude malabsorption or cryptic noncompliance is also appropriate, and persons with AIDS should be given high priority for DOT.

Central Nervous System Disease

Smaller, nonionized molecules such as INH and pyrazinamide cross the blood-brain barrier well, even in the absence of gross inflammation. Rifampin crosses less well, although therapeutic effects are seen. CSF levels of ethambutol are significantly lower than those in serum, and its use in meningitis is less well established. Streptomycin and the other aminoglycoside antibiotics are large, complex, ionically charged molecules; they are active early in the presence of inflammation but lose their efficacy as the inflammation subsides.

Combating Nonadherence with Directly Observed Intermittent Chemotherapy

Treatment given intermittently, twice or three times weekly, is generally comparable in efficacy to daily treatment. These intermittent schedules make it practical for patients to come to treatment centers or have visits by outreach workers at home or in shelters, schools, or work sites to observe ingestion or to administer medications. Most reported regimens begin with a daily phase of therapy and switch to an intermittent schedule after 1 or 2 months. However, effective treatment can entail a brief (2-week) initial daily phase or be intermittent (three times weekly) throughout. The ATS/CDC guidelines now regard DOT as standard practice that should be available in all communities or regions of the United States. Clinicians may elect to have patients self-administer treatment but, in so doing, assume responsibility for any consequences of nonadherence.

Clinicians' Errors Contributing to Acquired Drug Resistance

Among the more common errors that contribute to the evolution of multidrug resistance are failure to recognize and cope with nonadherence in a timely manner, failure to identify an individual at high risk for preexisting drug resistance that results in the use of an inadequate initial regimen, and adding a single drug to a failing regimen.

Monitoring for and Coping with Drug Toxicity

In the general population, significant reactions requiring transient or permanent discontinuation of one or more drugs develop in about 5% of patients receiving a typical three- or four-drug regimen (Table 345–4). Vague gastrointestinal complaints are relatively common, but most patients can tolerate these drugs. Oral medications must not be taken with meals, antacids, or H_2-receptor blockers, all of which may substantially reduce absorption.

TABLE 345–4 HIGH-RISK CANDIDATES FOR INFECTION PREVENTIVE THERAPY

Candidates for the treatment of latent infection or preventive therapy are persons at high risk for tuberculosis. Some persons with latent tuberculosis infection are at relatively great risk for the development of active disease. The degree of tuberculin skin test reactivity used to identify such persons varies with epidemiologic and biologic factors. The recommended duration of therapy is 9 months of isoniazid for most candidates. The 2000 American Thoracic Society and Centers for Disease Control and Prevention guidelines identified various alternative regimens, including 6 months of isoniazid (INH), 4 months of rifampin (RIF), and 2 or 3 months of RIF and pyrazinamide (PZA) twice weekly or daily. [Because of the risk for severe, even lethal hepatitis, recommendations for the RIF/PZA regimen have been withdrawn]

Certain groups within the infected population are at greater risk than others and should receive high priority for preventive therapy. In the United States, persons with any of the following six risk factors should be considered candidates for preventive therapy, regardless of age, if they have not previously been treated:

1. Persons (≥5-mm tuberculin skin test reaction) with human immunodeficiency virus (HIV) infection and persons with risk factors for HIV infection whose HIV infection status is unknown but who are suspected of having HIV infection
2. Close contacts of persons with newly diagnosed infectious tuberculosis (≥5 mm) and tuberculin-negative (<5 mm) children and adolescents who have been close contacts of infectious persons within the past 3 months are candidates for preventive therapy until a repeat tuberculin skin test is performed 12 weeks after contact with the infectious source
3. Recent converters, as indicated by a tuberculin skin test (≥10-mm increase within a 2-year period)
4. Persons (≥5 mm) with abnormal chest radiographs showing fibrotic lesions that probably represent old healed tuberculosis
5. Intravenous drug users (≥10 mm) known to be HIV seronegative
6. Persons (≥10 mm) with medical conditions that have been reported to increase the risk for tuberculosis. Tumor necrosis factor-α–modifying agents such as infliximab or etanercept appear to be potent risk factors for reactivation of tuberculosis (see text)

In the absence of any of the previous risk factors, persons younger than 35 years in the following high-incidence groups are appropriate candidates for preventive therapy if their reaction to a tuberculin skin test is ≥10 mm:

1. Foreign-born persons from high-prevalence countries
2. Medically underserved, low-income populations, including high-risk racial or ethnic minority populations, especially blacks, Hispanic Americans, and Native Americans
3. Residents of facilities for long-term care (e.g., correctional institutions, nursing homes, mental institutions)

Public health officials should be alert for additional high-risk populations in their communities. For example, through a review of cases reported in the community over a period of several years, health officials may use geographic or sociodemographic factors to identify groups that should be targeted for intervention. Screening and preventive therapy programs should be initiated and promoted within these populations based on an analysis of cases and infection in the community. To the extent possible, members of high-risk groups and their health care providers should be involved in the design, implementation, and evaluation of these programs. Staff of facilities in which an individual with disease would pose a risk to large numbers of susceptible persons (e.g., correctional institutions, nursing homes, mental institutions, other health care facilities, schools, child care facilities) may also be considered for preventive therapy if the tuberculin reaction is a ≥10-mm induration

Adults should have baseline measurement of liver function; complete blood counts, including platelets; measurement of uric acid (if pyrazinamide is included); and evaluation of vision, including acuity and color discrimination (if ethambutol is used). These tests can identify preexisting problems and enable comparison with data from subsequent testing. Monitoring during therapy is generally by clinical assessment. Patients receiving DOT should be queried regularly for any perceived adverse effects, and patients who self-administer drugs should be seen monthly and instructed regarding prompt reporting of possible adverse effects.

Duration of Treatment and Post-treatment Surveillance

A 6-month regimen consisting of INH and rifampin supplemented by an initial 2-month phase of pyrazinamide is regarded as sufficient and curative for most cases caused by drug-susceptible strains. However, guidelines now recommend sputum cultures after the first 2 months of therapy because of significantly higher risks for failure and relapse in patients who remain culture positive at this juncture. Patients who have cavitary disease and whose 2-month culture is still positive should be treated for a total of 9 months. If these three agents cannot be used, the duration of treatment may be prolonged (see Table 345–4). Other situations in which therapy may be extended beyond 6 months include the following:

HUMAN IMMUNODEFICIENCY VIRUS INFECTION OR ACQUIRED IMMUNODEFICIENCY SYNDROME. Although no well-controlled studies have demonstrated the superiority of longer therapy, some clinicians fear that impaired immunity may place these patients at higher risk for relapse.

FAR-ADVANCED CAVITARY LUNG DISEASE WITH A DELAYED CLINICAL RESPONSE OR SPUTUM CONVERSION. About 85 to 90% of patients become culture negative by 2 months of treatment; for patients who remain positive longer than this, treatment for a total of 9 months is recommended.

IRREGULAR, INTERRUPTED THERAPY. If patients fail to attend 10% or more of DOT encounters or are otherwise deemed to have been significantly noncompliant with treatment, extended treatment is prudent. Approaches to determine the need for extended therapy are described in the 2003 ATS/CDC/IDSA guidelines.

MILIARY OR MENINGEAL CASES. Because of the concern that such patients may be less competent hosts and because of the implications of recurrent disease, therapy may be extended to 9 to 12 months.

Indications for Corticosteroid Therapy

Corticosteroids can reduce acute inflammation and limit delayed fibrotic complications in HIV-negative patients. Acute reductions in inflammation with significant benefits in survival have been demonstrated in patients with meningitis. [3] In patients with less advanced disease, there may be reduced post-treatment sequelae. Neither the optimal agent nor the preferred dose has been identified. Prednisone at 1 mg/kg and dexamethasone at 0.3 mg/kg body weight have been used; it should be noted that rifampin will significantly reduce the bioavailability of steroids. Less well proven are the benefits of steroid therapy for pleural, pericardial, peritoneal, miliary, or extensive pulmonary disease, although salutary effects may occur in individual cases. High-dose corticosteroids may impair immune responses, but there is no evidence that they adversely affect the outcome of treatment when given for 4 to 8 weeks to patients who are receiving adequate chemotherapy.

Adrenal insufficiency secondary to tuberculous destruction is now uncommon. However, in patients with marginal cortisol production, rifampin may precipitate hypocorticism by accelerating the catabolism of endogenous steroids.

Drug-Resistant Tuberculosis

During the past decade, drug resistance in the United States has dropped considerably. In 1991, the overall prevalence of drug resistance was 14.2%. INH resistance was most common; it occurred in 8.2% of new cases and 21.5% of previously treated cases. Resistance to INH and rifampin (i.e., MDR tuberculosis) occurred in 3.5% of cases. By the year 2003, the rate of drug resistance to INH was 7.9% in patients not previously treated, with rates of 4.6% for American-born and 10.6% for foreign-born patients. The rate of resistance to both INH and rifampin was 0.9% overall, with rates of 0.6% for American-born and 1.2% for foreign-born patients. In patients previously treated, resistance rates in 2003 were considerably higher: the rate of resistance to INH was 12.6% overall, with rates of 7.1% for American-born and 17.6% for foreign-born patients. The multidrug resistance rate for patients with previous tuberculosis was 3.6% overall, with rates of 1.3% for American-born and 5.8% for foreign-born patients.

MDR tuberculosis is of particular importance because of the profoundly increased risk for treatment failure, further acquired resistance, and nosocomial transmission. MDR tuberculosis may be associated with resistance to other first-line drugs, which further compromises treatment prospects. The most significant aspect of MDR tuberculosis is resistance to rifampin because it is this drug, not INH, that is central to short-duration therapy.

Patients with suspected MDR tuberculosis (i.e., those with previous treatment, with recent exposure to an MDR case, or from extremely high-risk areas) should be considered for initially extended empirical regimens, especially if they have extensive lung disease or perilous extrapulmonary forms such as miliary or meningeal disease. For patients with proven MDR tuberculosis, it is important to use at least four drugs to which the organisms are susceptible, usually three oral agents and one injectable agent. Patients should receive prompt, expert consultation and have the highest priority for DOT. For patients with high-level (five or six drugs) resistance, resectional surgery may be a useful adjunct. Preventive therapy or treatment of latent infection in contacts of persons with MDR tuberculosis is problematic; the only agents widely regarded as appropriate are INH and rifampin, although moxifloxacin has also been used for this purpose.

Contact Investigation

Clinicians must realize that their responsibilities are not complete when they have established the diagnosis and initiated chemotherapy for a patient. Tuberculosis is a reportable disease in all U.S. communities and states; clinicians are obligated to notify public health authorities promptly of all cases of proven or *suspected* tuberculosis. Contact investigation of the home, workplace, school, or other congregate facilities may reveal other active cases or newly infected persons who are at substantial risk for tuberculosis. Priority must be given to cases in which infants or HIV-positive patients have been exposed because of their compressed incubation periods for potentially lethal forms of tuberculosis. Treatment of latent infection in infected contacts is a highly efficient means of curtailing tuberculosis morbidity. Weekly administration of the combination of rifapentine and isoniazid is effective and well tolerated in this setting. [4]

Prognosis

Contemporary antituberculous regimens involving INH and rifampin for 6 months and pyrazinamide for the initial 2 months result in 96 to 99% durable cure rates for HIV-negative patients with drug-susceptible tuberculosis. Most recurrences occur within 2 years and are associated with the same drug susceptibility profile as before treatment began. Current guidelines do not compel post-treatment surveillance. Instead, patients should be instructed to return after treatment when there are changes in their clinical status; suitable tests, including sputum analysis, chest radiographs, or other studies, should be performed if symptoms or signs appear.

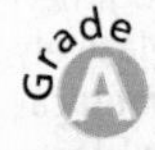

1. Tam CM, Chan SL, Lam CW, et al: Rifapentine and isoniazid in the continuation phase of treating pulmonary tuberculosis: Initial report. Am J Respir Crit Care Med 1998;157:1726–1733.
2. Tuberculosis Trials Consortium: Rifapentine and isoniazid once a week versus rifampicin and isoniazid twice a week for treatment

of drug-susceptible pulmonary tuberculosis in HIV-negative patients: A randomised clinical trial. Lancet 2002;360:528–535.
3. Thwaites GE, Bang ND, Dung, et al: Dexamethasone for the treatment of tuberculous meningitis in adolescents and adults. N Engl J Med 2004;351:1741–1751.
4. Schechter M, Zajdenverg R, Falco G, et al: Weekly rifapentine/isoniazid or daily rifampin/pyrazinamide for latent tuberculosis in household contacts. Am J Respir Crit Care 2006;173:922–926.

SUGGESTED READINGS

Blumberg HM, Leonard MK Jr, Jasmer RM: Update on the treatment of tuberculosis and latent tuberculosis infection. JAMA 2005;293:2776–2784. *A clinical review.*

Campbell IA, Bah-Sow O: Pulmonary tuberculosis: Diagnosis and treatment. BMJ 2006;332:1194–1197. *A concise review.*

Johnson R, Streicher FM, Louw RF, et al: Drug resistance in *Mycobacterium tuberculosis*. Curr Issues Mol Biol 2006;8:97–111. *A careful overview.*

Lee JY, Choi HJ, Park IN, et al: Comparison of two commercial interferon-gamma assays for diagnosing *Mycobacterium tuberculosis* infection. Eur Respir J 2006; 28:24–30. *Demonstrates the accuracy of these new assays.*

Menzies D, Dion M-J, Rabinovitch B, et al: Treatment completion and costs of a randomized trial of rifampin for 4 months versus isoniazid for 9 months. Am J Respir Crit Care Med 2004:170:445–449. *Experience in Montreal indicates that rifampin alone is a well-accepted and efficient means for treatment of latent tuberculosis infection.*

Riquelme A, Calvo M, Salech F, et al: Value of adenosine deaminase (ADA) in ascetic fluid for the diagnosis of tuberculous peritonitis: A meta-analysis. J Clin Gastroenterol 2006;40:705–710. *A level >39 IU/L had very high sensitivity and specificity.*

Trunz BB, Fine P, Dye C: Effect of BCG vaccination on childhood tuberculous, meningitis, and miliary tuberculosis worldwide: A meta-analysis and assessment of cost-effectiveness. Lancet 2006;367:1173–1180. *BCG vaccination is highly cost-effective.*

346 THE NONTUBERCULOUS MYCOBACTERIA

Steven M. Holland

Definition

Nontuberculous mycobacteria generally include the growing number of mycobacteria other than *Mycobacterium tuberculosis* and its close relatives and *Mycobacterium leprae*. Other names that have been used include "atypical mycobacteria," "mycobacteria other than tuberculosis," and "environmental mycobacteria." The number of nontuberculous mycobacteria is growing rapidly as a result of the advent of DNA sequence typing for determining criteria for speciation. Accordingly, the number of species of nontuberculous mycobacteria has doubled to more than 100 in the last decade and will continue to increase for the near future.

The Pathogens

Identification of any mycobacteria requires that the appropriate tests be thought of ahead of time and be performed because routine microbiologic testing does not identify mycobacteria. Nontuberculous mycobacteria are typically first detected on acid-fast smears of sputum or other body fluids. When levels of organisms are high, mycobacteria may be seen on Gram stain as gram-positive beaded rods, but this finding is unreliable. The first step in identification is to request the appropriate smear (acid-fast or fluorochrome) and culture. Nontuberculous mycobacteria are broadly differentiated into rapidly growing (<7 days) and slowly growing (>7 days) forms. Tuberculosis, by contrast, typically takes 2 or more weeks to grow. Formation of pigment in light (photochromogens) or dark (scotochromogens) and lack of pigment (nonchromogens) have also been used to help categorize nontuberculous mycobacteria. In contrast, tuberculosis is beige, rough, dry, and flat. Current diagnoses use biochemical, nucleic acid, or cell wall composition on high-performance liquid chromatography for speciation (Table 346–1). For purposes of diagnosis, prognosis, and therapy, identification of nontuberculous mycobacteria should be taken to the species level.

TABLE 346–1 COMMON NONTUBERCULOUS MYCOBACTERIA

Organism	Disease
RAPIDLY GROWING NONTUBERCULOUS MYCOBACTERIA	
M. abscessus	Lung, disseminated, lymph node
M. chelonae	Skin
M. fortuitum	Line infections, lung
M. smegmatis	Almost never disease associated
SLOWLY GROWING NONTUBERCULOUS MYCOBACTERIA	
M. avium complex	Lung, disseminated, lymph node
M. kansasii	Lung
M. marinum	Skin, tendons (fish tank granuloma)
M. xenopi	Lung
M. simiae	Lung
M. szulgai	Lung
M. malmoense	Lung
M. scrofulaceum	Lymph node
M. haemophilum	Disseminated, skin
M. genevense	Disseminated
M. ulcerans	Skin (Buruli ulcer; toxin producing)
M. neoarum	Disseminated
M. celatum	Disseminated
M. gordonae	Almost never causes disease
M. terrae complex	Disseminated

Epidemiology

As a group, the nontuberculous mycobacteria are ubiquitous in soil and water and are often found in certain animals, but they rarely cause disease in humans. There are no known instances of human-to-human transmission of nontuberculous mycobacteria. Because these infections are not reported to health agencies and their identification is sometimes problematic, reliable data on incidence and prevalence are lacking. In the United States, however, isolates of nontuberculous mycobacteria have exceeded those for tuberculosis for many years. In patients with cystic fibrosis (Chapter 89), for example, rates of clinical nontuberculous mycobacterial infection range from 3 to 15%, but even more patients harbor the organism; however, differentiating active disease from commensal harboring of the organism remains problematic. Other patient groups, such as those with bronchiectasis, also have elevated rates of nontuberculous mycobacterial infection, but the rates are undefined. The bulk of nontuberculous mycobacterial disease in North America is due to *Mycobacterium kansasii*, *Mycobacterium avium* complex (MAC), and *Mycobacterium abscessus*.

Pathobiology

Because exposure is essentially universal and disease is rare, normal host defenses against nontuberculous mycobacteria must be highly effective. Therefore, otherwise healthy individuals in whom disease develops may have specific susceptibility factors that permit these infections to become established, multiply, and cause disease.

With the advent of human immunodeficiency virus (HIV) infection, $CD4^+$ T lymphocytes have been identified as key effectors against nontuberculous mycobacteria. Much of the genetic basis of susceptibility to disseminated nontuberculous mycobacterial infection outside HIV infection has been found to be due to specific mutations in the interferon-γ (IFN-γ)/interleukin-12 (IL-12) synthesis and response pathways. However, only about 50% of disseminated cases unassociated with HIV infection have a genetic diagnosis, and genetic causes of predisposition to nontuberculous mycobacterial lung disease are still very few.

Mycobacteria are typically phagocytosed by macrophages, which respond with production of IL-12, a heterodimer composed of p35 and p40 moieties that together comprise IL-12p70 (Fig. 346–1). IL-12 activates T lymphocytes and natural killer cells through binding to its

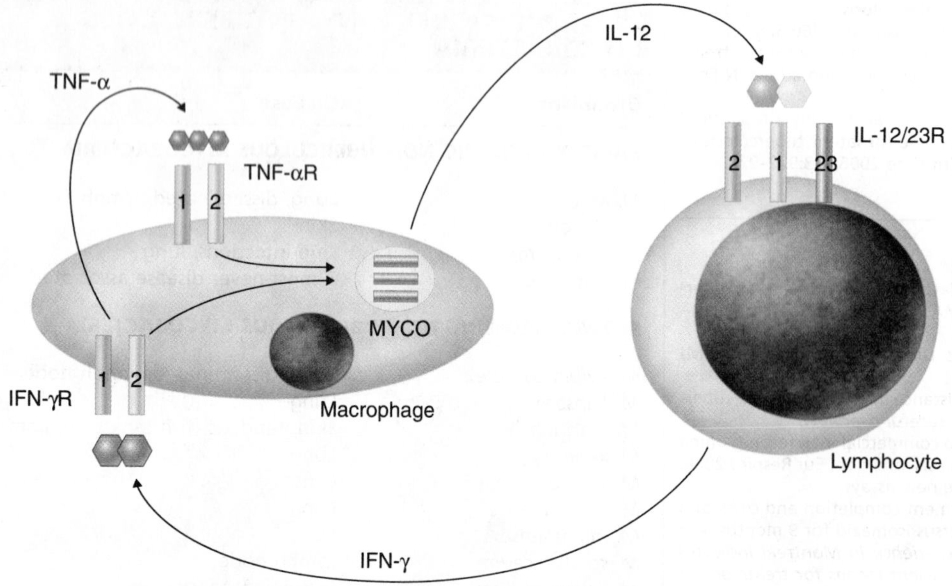

FIGURE 346–1 • Schematization of the critical cytokine interactions between infected macrophages and T and natural killer lymphocytes. Organisms (MYCO) infect macrophages, which release heterodimeric interleukin-12 (IL-12). This acts on the IL-12/23 receptor complex and leads to the production of homodimeric interferon-γ (IFN-γ). IFN-γ acts on its receptor to stimulate the production of tumor necrosis factor-α (TNF-α) and kill intracellular organisms such as mycobacteria, salmonellae, and some fungi. Homotrimeric TNF-α acts on its own receptor and also contributes to killing of intracellular infections. Both IFN-γ and TNF-α lead to upregulation of IL-12. TNF-α–blocking antibodies work either by blocking the ligand (infliximab, adalimumab) or by providing soluble receptor (etanercept). Mutations in both chains of IFN-γR, IL-12p40, IL-12Rβ1, and signal elements for IFN-γR and TNF-αR have been identified through their predisposition to mycobacterial infections.

receptor (composed of IL-12Rβ1 and IL-12Rβ2/IL-23R) and results in phosphorylation of STAT4. IL-12 stimulation leads to secretion of IFN-γ, which activates neutrophils and macrophages to produce reactive oxidants and increase major histocompatibility complex and Fc receptors. IFN-γ signals through its receptor (composed of IFN-γR1 and IFN-γR2), thereby leading to phosphorylation of STAT1, which in turn regulates IFN-γ–responsive genes such as IL-12 and tumor necrosis factor-α (TNF-α). Therefore, the positive feedback loop between IFN-γ and IL-12/IL-23 is pivotal in the immune response to mycobacteria and other intracellular infections. The advent of potent TNF-α inhibitors, such as infliximab, adalimumab, and etanercept, has provided the ability to neutralize this critical cytokine, which has occasionally resulted in mycobacterial and fungal infections.

Clinical Manifestations

Disseminated Disease

Disseminated nontuberculous mycobacterial disease secondary to MAC infection used to occur commonly in the setting of advanced acquired immunodeficiency syndrome but is now uncommon in North America because of MAC prophylaxis and improved treatment of HIV infection. The portal of entry was the bowel, with spread to bone marrow and the blood stream. Rapidly growing mycobacteria such as *Mycobacterium fortuitum* sometimes infect deep indwelling lines. The severe disseminated infection seen with immune defects is typically associated with malaise, fever, and weight loss, and it is often accompanied by organomegaly and lymphadenopathy. Disseminated (two or more organ) involvement in a child without an underlying iatrogenic cause should prompt an investigation of the IFN-γ/IL-12 pathway. Nontuberculous mycobacterial osteomyelitis is especially common with dominant negative mutations in IFN-γR1. A male with conical or peg teeth or an abnormal hair pattern and disseminated nontuberculous mycobacterial infection should be evaluated for defects in the pathway that activates nuclear factor κB. Some patients with disseminated, rapidly growing infections (predominantly *M. abscessus*) have high-titer autoantibodies to IFN-γ.

Pulmonary Disease

Lung disease caused by nontuberculous mycobacteria is by far the most common form of the infection in North America. Predisposing factors include underlying lung disease, such as bronchiectasis (Chapter 90), pneumoconiosis (Chapter 93), chronic obstructive pulmonary disease (Chapter 88), and cystic fibrosis. The manifestations of *M. kansasii* can be very similar to tuberculosis (Chapter 345) and consist of hemoptysis, chest pain, and cavitary lung disease. MAC infection most commonly occurs in women in their sixth or seventh decade who have had months to years of nagging intermittent cough and fatigue, with or without sputum production or chest pain. Bronchiectasis and nontuberculous mycobacterial infection often coexist and progress in tandem, thus making causality difficult to determine. When compared with male smokers with upper lobe cavitary disease, who tend to carry the very same single strain of MAC indefinitely, nonsmoking females with nodular bronchiectasis tend to carry several strains simultaneously and change them over the course of their disease process. Patients with pulmonary alveolar proteinosis (Chapter 91) are prone to pulmonary nontuberculous mycobacterial and *Nocardia* infections. Esophageal motility disorders, such as achalasia (Chapter 140), have been associated with pulmonary disease, especially that caused by the rapidly growing nontuberculous mycobacteria such as *M. abscessus.*

Cervical Lymph Nodes

Isolated cervical lymphadenopathy, most frequently caused by MAC, is the most common form of nontuberculous mycobacterial infection in young children in North America. The organism is generally MAC, but other nontuberculous mycobacteria can also cause disease. The cervical swelling is often firm and relatively painless with a paucity of systemic signs. Because the differential diagnosis of painless adenopathy includes malignancy, many of these infections are inadvertently diagnosed at biopsy. Local fistulas usually resolve completely with resection or antibiotic therapy, or both.

Skin and Soft Tissue Disease

Mycobacterium marinum causes skin infections, usually papules or ulcers, associated with water exposure and is known "fish tank granuloma." Numerous outbreaks of skin infections caused by rapidly growing mycobacteria (especially *M. abscessus, M. fortuitum,* and *M. chelonae*) have been due to skin contamination from instruments used for surgical procedures (especially cosmetic surgery), injections, and other procedures. These infections are typically accompanied by painful, erythematous, draining subcutaneous nodules, usually without associated fever or systemic symptoms.

Diagnosis

With the continued decline in cases of tuberculosis, nontuberculous mycobacteria are now the most common mycobacteria isolated from humans in North America. The conventional tuberculin skin test (purified protein derivative [PPD]) evokes a cell-mediated response to secreted mycobacterial antigens. Unfortunately, the PPD test does not differentiate well between nontuberculous mycobacterial and tuberculosis infection, although large PPD reactions (>15 mm) more commonly signify tuberculosis. With the progressive decline in active tuberculosis in the United States, nontuberculous mycobacteria are likely to account for significant proportions of PPD reactivity.

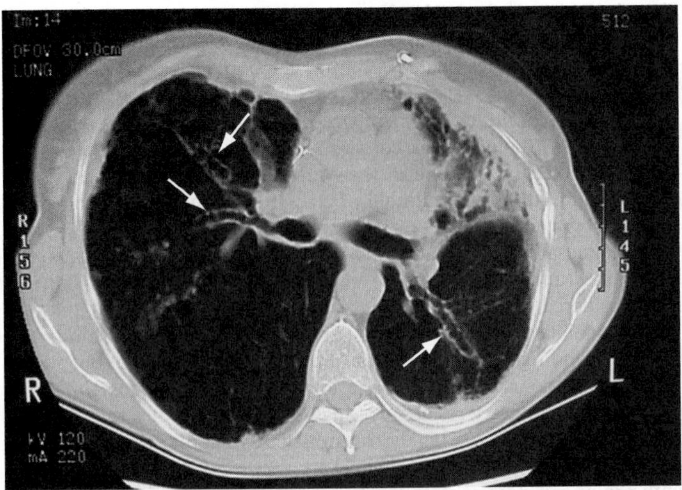

FIGURE 346–2 • Chest computed tomography in a patient with severe pulmonary *Mycobacterium abscessus* infection. Arrows indicate bronchiectasis. Note the extensive left upper lobe destruction and diffuse pleural reaction. In addition, the left lung is smaller than the right as a result of extensive loss of lung parenchyma.

Isolation of nontuberculous mycobacteria from blood specimens is clear evidence of disease. However, because the slow-growing nontuberculous mycobacteria typically do not grow well in routine blood culture media, the diagnosis must be suspected. Isolation of nontuberculous mycobacteria from a biopsy specimen is strong evidence of infection, but cases of laboratory contamination do occur. Identification of organisms on stained section of biopsy material confirms the authenticity of the culture. Some unusual nontuberculous mycobacteria require lower incubation temperatures or special additives for growth.

The radiographic appearance of nontuberculous mycobacterial disease in the lung ranges from normal to nodules, bronchiectasis, air space disease, and extensive cavity formation, similar to that seen in tuberculosis (Fig. 346–2). Isolation of nontuberculous mycobacteria from respiratory samples presents special problems in both sensitivity and specificity. *Mycobacterium gordonae* is often recovered from respiratory samples and is almost never thought to be a real pathogen. Many patients, especially those with bronchiectasis, will occasionally have nontuberculous mycobacteria recovered from sputum culture without such mycobacteria being seen on smear. Specific criteria for definitive diagnosis of nontuberculous mycobacterial lung disease exist for MAC, *M. abscessus,* and *M. kansasii,* but they are probably good guidelines for other nontuberculous mycobacteria as well. A positive diagnosis requires that two of three sputum samples grow nontuberculous mycobacteria, regardless of smear findings; a positive bronchoscopic alveolar sample, regardless of smear findings; or a biopsy of pulmonary parenchyma with granulomatous inflammation or mycobacteria found on section and nontuberculous mycobacteria on culture.

Once isolated, identification of nontuberculous mycobacteria is important because it will determine the broad class of antimycobacterial therapy to be used. Many laboratories now use DNA probes to identify MAC, *M. gordonae,* and *M. kansasii.* Drug susceptibility testing is of limited and largely unproven value, although clarithromycin susceptibility testing for MAC and rifampin susceptibility testing for *M. kansasii* are indicated. Initial isolates of MAC that have not been exposed to macrolides are almost always susceptible to macrolides. Any nontuberculous mycobacteria that have resisted a course of antimicrobials should probably be tested for antibiotic susceptibility as well.

Prevention

Prophylaxis of MAC disease in patients infected with HIV is started when the $CD4^+$ T-lymphocyte count is less than 50 cells/μL. Azithromycin, 1200 mg weekly, clarithromycin, 1000 mg daily, or rifabutin, 300 mg daily, are effective.

Treatment

Rx

It is rarely an emergency to initiate treatment of nontuberculous mycobacterial infections, which are relatively slow-growing, chronic infections that evolve over a period of weeks to years, not hours to days. Therefore, empirical therapy is not usually needed, and identification of the species is advisable before starting complex, often poorly tolerated, and potentially toxic regimens. Similar to the case with tuberculosis, single-drug therapy is almost always associated with the emergence of antimicrobial resistance and is strongly discouraged.

MAC infection often requires complex multidrug therapy, the foundation of which is a macrolide (clarithromycin or azithromycin), ethambutol, and a rifamycin (rifampin or rifabutin). For disseminated nontuberculous mycobacterial disease in HIV-infected patients, the use of rifamycins poses special problems of drug interactions with protease inhibitors. For pulmonary MAC disease, three-times-weekly administration of drugs has been used successfully. The duration of therapy is prolonged, generally for 12 months after culture conversion, typically for a total of at least 18 months. Other drugs with activity against MAC include aminoglycosides, fluoroquinolones, and clofazimine.

M. kansasii lung disease is similar to tuberculosis in many ways and is also effectively treated with isoniazid (300 mg/day), rifampin (600 mg/day), and ethambutol (15 mg/kg/day). Treatment should continue until cultures have been negative for at least 1 year. Other drugs with very high activity against *M. kansasii* include clarithromycin, fluoroquinolones, and aminoglycosides.

Rapidly growing mycobacteria pose special therapeutic problems. Extrapulmonary disease in an immune competent host is usually due to inoculation (e.g., surgery, injections, trauma) or line infection and is often treated successfully with a macrolide and another drug (based on in vitro susceptibility), along with removal of the offending focus. By comparison, pulmonary disease, especially that caused by *M. abscessus,* is extremely difficult to cure, although repeated courses of treatment are usually effective in reducing the infectious burden and symptoms. Therapy generally includes a macrolide along with an intravenous agent such as amikacin, a carbapenem, cefoxitin, or tigecycline. Other oral agents used according to in vitro susceptibility testing and tolerance include fluoroquinolones, doxycycline, or linezolid.

Treatment of the other nontuberculous mycobacteria is less well defined, but macrolides and aminoglycosides are usually effective, with other agents added as indicated. Expert consultation is strongly encouraged for difficult or unusual nontuberculous mycobacterial infections.

Prognosis

The effect of nontuberculous mycobacterial infection on longevity is closely tied to the underlying condition (e.g., IFN-γ/IL-12 pathway defect, cystic fibrosis). With no or inadequate treatment, symptoms are intrusive, and the infections can lead to fatal complications, including overwhelming infection or severe lung destruction.

SUGGESTED READINGS

Dailloux M, Abalain ML, Laurain C, et al: Respiratory infections associated with nontuberculous mycobacteria in non-HIV patients. Eur Respir J 2006;28: 1211–1215. *Large multicenter retrospective description of nontuberculous infections in HIV-negative patients.*

Field SK, Cowie RL: Lung disease due to the more common nontuberculous mycobacteria. Chest 2006;129:1653–1672. *A practical review.*

Griffith DE, Aksamit T, Brown-Elliot BA, et al: American Thoracic Society: Diagnosis, treatment and prevention of nontuberculous mycobacterial diseases. Am J Respir Crit Care Med 2007;175:367–416. *The consensus statement on laboratory, clinical, and therapeutic aspects.*

Wallis RS, Broder MS, Wong JY, et al: Granulomatous infectious diseases associated with tumor necrosis factor antagonists. Clin Infect Dis 2004;38: 1261–1265. *Review of the infectious complications of TNF-α inhibitors.*

LEPROSY (HANSEN'S DISEASE)

Joel D. Ernst

Definition

Leprosy (Hansen's disease) is a chronic infection caused by *Mycobacterium leprae*, an acid-fast, slowly growing bacterium that cannot yet be cultured in vitro. Leprosy is found worldwide, although nine countries of high prevalence currently account for more than 80% of reported cases. The primary manifestations of infection with *M. leprae* occur in the skin and peripheral nerves. The skin lesions of leprosy are classically hypopigmented, hypoesthetic or anesthetic, and nonpruritic. Peripheral nerves can be damaged by direct infection with *M. leprae* or by the patient's immune response to the infection; the result is loss of sensation and motor function. Additional morbidity is due to peripheral nerve dysfunction, including painless traumatic and burn injuries, secondary bacterial infections, and muscle atrophy and contractures. Leprosy per se is not a cause of death, but the debility associated with leprosy contributes to the severity of poverty and the likelihood of death from malnutrition or other infections. Despite the low transmissibility of *M. leprae* and the ability of multiple-drug therapy to cure leprosy, it remains a stigmatized disease that can pose a challenge to diagnosis and therapy.

The Pathogen

M. leprae is an acid-fast bacillus that contains a mycolic acid–rich cell wall and a single membrane. Despite nearly 150 years of effort, *M. leprae* remains uncultivatible in vitro. For biochemical and structural characterization, *M. leprae* can be grown in large quantities in nine-banded armadillos *(Dasypus novemcinctus)*, and inoculation of the footpads of athymic mice allows semiquantitation of viable bacilli.

The genome of *M. leprae* consists of 3,268,203 base pairs (bp), as compared with the *Mycobacterium tuberculosis* genome of 4,411,529 bp, and the functional genome (the number of expressed genes) of *M. leprae* is approximately 60% smaller than that of *M. tuberculosis.* Because *M. leprae* and *M. tuberculosis* probably evolved from a common mycobacterial ancestor, *M. leprae* appears to have lost approximately 2000 genes since this divergence, which has left it dependent on highly specialized ecologic niches for its survival. Among the genes that are lacking in *M. leprae* are those of the *mbt* complex, whose products are involved in bacterial acquisition of iron. *M. leprae* also lacks many of the genes for lipid biosynthesis and modification that are characteristic of *M. tuberculosis.* The genome sequence has also allowed a directed approach to identifying four "strains" of *M. leprae* from geographically diverse sources.

Epidemiology

Leprosy is found worldwide, although endemic leprosy is absent from northern Europe, where it was present in epidemic form as recently as the 19th century. The global prevalence of leprosy is about 285,000 known cases, and the current incidence is about 400,000. By definition of the World Health Organization (WHO) Strategic Plan for the Elimination of Leprosy, a newly diagnosed patient who has been treated with multidrug therapy is removed from the prevalence registry, which explains the lower prevalence than incidence of this chronic infection. Since initiation of the WHO Strategic Plan (whose goal is to eliminate leprosy as a public health problem, i.e., a prevalence of <1 in 10,000 in all regions), an estimated 14 million people have been cured of leprosy.

The success of multidrug therapy notwithstanding, leprosy remains a public health problem in six countries in Africa, two in Southeast Asia (India and Nepal), and one in the Americas (Brazil). India and Brazil currently have the largest number of cases. Although domestic transmission of leprosy is extremely rare in the United States, 95 cases of leprosy were diagnosed in 2003, including cases in immigrants from India, the Philippines, and Mexico. Because leprosy is not highly transmissible, it is not considered a disease of travelers other than immigrants.

The inability to culture *M. leprae* in vitro has been a major hindrance to understanding the modes of transmission and reservoirs of the organism. Observational studies reveal a low frequency of leprosy in casual travelers or temporary residents of high-incidence regions, thus indicating that *M. leprae* is not highly transmissible. In addition, even in areas of high incidence, clusters of leprosy are rare outside families or others with prolonged close contact. It is believed that transmission of *M. leprae* commonly occurs through the respiratory route because nasal secretions of people with lepromatous leprosy may contain 10^7 viable bacilli per milliliter. In addition, transmission of *M. leprae* is thought to occur through contact with contaminated soil, although soil has not been found to be a reservoir for the bacilli.

Pathobiology

Immunology

There is an inverse correlation between the number of lymphocytes and the number of acid-fast bacteria present in skin lesions. "Tuberculoid" lesions have abundant lymphocytes, well-formed granulomas, and few bacteria (hence this form of leprosy is also termed paucibacillary). In contrast, "lepromatous" lesions have very few lymphocytes, poorly organized or no granulomas, and large numbers of bacteria (also termed multibacillary leprosy). Between these polar extremes are intermediate forms that represent a continuum of the histopathologic and bacteriologic findings, termed "borderline tuberculoid," "borderline," and "borderline lepromatous" (Fig. 347–1). In addition to correlating with the number of bacteria in individual lesions, the polar forms of leprosy correlate with the total number of skin lesions in an individual patient: tuberculoid leprosy exhibits few (less than five) lesions, whereas lepromatous leprosy is characterized by multiple lesions (five or more, up to hundreds).

Leprosy provides a paradigm for the effect of the cellular immune response to a bacterial pathogen on the clinical manifestations of the infection. Individuals in whom a T helper-1 (T_H1)-based immune response (characterized by antigen-specific T cells that produce interferon-γ, lymphotoxin, or interleukin-2 [IL-2] and no IL-4 or IL-5) develops to *M. leprae* exhibit few skin lesions and few bacteria within the lesions (paucibacillary leprosy). In contrast, people in whom a T_H2 immune response develops (T cells that produce little interferon-γ, lymphotoxin, or IL-2 but do produce IL-4, IL-5, and IL-13) have larger numbers of skin lesions and large numbers of bacteria within their lesions (multibacillary leprosy). The primary determinant of the differential immune response to *M. leprae* is incompletely understood, although substantial evidence indicates that host genetic polymorphisms contribute to the likelihood of paucibacillary versus multibacillary leprosy.

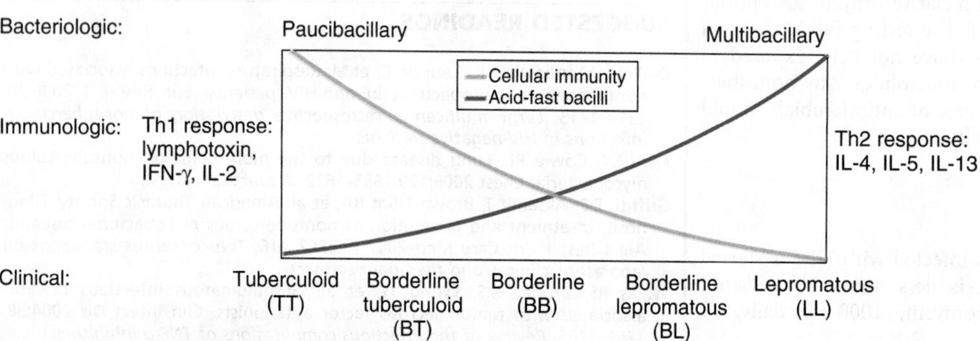

FIGURE 347–1 • Bacteriologic, immunologic, and clinical spectrum of leprosy. Tuberculoid (paucibacillary) leprosy is characterized by a T_H1 immune response and few or no detectable bacilli in biopsy specimens of skin lesions or smears of skin slits. At the opposite pole of the spectrum, lepromatous (multibacillary) leprosy is accompanied by a T_H2 immune response, numerous skin lesions, and numerous acid-fast bacilli on skin biopsies or smears. The intermediate forms can be classified according to their resemblance to tuberculoid or lepromatous leprosy. IFN = interferon; IL = interleukin.

A major determinant of T_H1 differentiation is IL-12. Expression of IL-12 is approximately 10-fold higher in tuberculoid lesions than in lepromatous lesions, although peripheral blood monocytes and monocyte-derived dendritic cells from patients with lepromatous leprosy and tuberculoid leprosy produce similar amounts of IL-12 in response to a lipopeptide derived from *M. leprae.* Lipopeptide stimulation of IL-12 production is mediated by Toll-like receptors 1 (TLR1) and 2 (TLR2), and expression of TLR1 and TLR2 is higher in lesions of tuberculoid than lepromatous leprosy. Deficient expression of TLR2 in lepromatous lesions may be secondary to higher expression of leukocyte immunoglobulin receptors, especially LIR-7, whose stimulation decreases TLR expression.

Pathogenesis of Nerve Damage

Peripheral nerve damage, which is the most important consequence of infection with *M. leprae,* occurs in all forms of leprosy and underlies nearly all the morbid complications of the infection. *M. leprae* invades Schwann cells, the glial cells of peripheral nerves. Schwann cells form a functional unit with peripheral nerve axons and are surrounded by a basal lamina containing laminin-2, a neural-specific extracellular matrix protein. The G domain of laminin-2 can bind simultaneously to *M. leprae* and to the Schwann cell laminin receptor α-dystroglycan, which promotes high-affinity binding of *M. leprae* to Schwann cells by using laminin-2 as a bridging molecule. Laminin-2 interacts with at least two distinct molecules on the surface of *M. leprae,* a 21-kD protein and phenolic glycolipid-1 (PGL-1); either can mediate internalization by Schwann cells. Once *M. leprae* or its PGL-1 is bound and internalized by Schwann cells, it can cause direct demyelination of peripheral nerves in the absence of an immune response. *M. leprae*–mediated demyelination occurs without early cell death or toxicity, although Schwann cells and neurons can die by apoptosis later after infection. In addition, dead *M. leprae* or PGL-1 shed from live or dying *M. leprae* can mediate peripheral nerve demyelination and may contribute to the ongoing nerve damage that can follow initiation of chemotherapy. In addition to PGL-1–mediated demyelination, an *M. leprae* 19-kD lipoprotein can mediate Schwann cell apoptosis in vitro, and apoptotic Schwann cells can be found in human leprosy lesions. These mechanisms are probably responsible for the nerve damage in multibacillary leprosy.

In addition to direct damage to peripheral nerves by *M. leprae,* the immune response in leprosy also contributes to nerve damage, especially in paucibacillary (tuberculoid) leprosy, in which the bacteria or PGL-1 (or both) are present in insufficient quantity to cause widespread nerve damage, and in reversal reactions, where inflammation is particularly prominent. Several distinct immunologic mechanisms probably contribute to the nerve damage in leprosy. Pro-inflammatory cytokines such as tumor necrosis factor-α (TNF-α), IL-1β, and interferon-γ are especially prominent in lesions during reversal reactions, when marked and irreversible nerve damage can occur. Because these molecules can contribute to inflammatory tissue damage and can induce apoptosis of Schwann cells in vitro, it is likely that these mediators play an active role in nerve damage. Reversal reactions are also characterized by an increase in the number of $CD4^+$ T lymphocytes in lesions, and at least some of these $CD4^+$ cells exhibit a cytotoxic phenotype and kill *M. leprae*–infected Schwann cells through antigen- and major histocompatibility complex class II–dependent secretion of cytotoxic granule contents. Whether these mechanisms of nerve damage occur in chronic tuberculoid leprosy is not established, but similar cytokines and T lymphocytes are found in tuberculoid lesions.

Genetics

Cases of leprosy cluster in families, partly because of shared environments and similar exposure, but also probably because of genetic determinants of susceptibility. Genetic loci whose allelic variants are related to altered susceptibility to infection with *M. leprae* include *NRAMP1, TNF,* and two closely linked and coregulated genes, *PARK2* and *PACRG.* NRAMP1 and TNF are expressed by macrophages, and quantitative or temporal differences in their expression may account for differences in innate susceptibility to infection. PARK2 and PACRG are widely expressed, including expression in macrophages and Schwann cells, and were discovered by linkage analysis of families with leprosy in Vietnam and Brazil. The roles of PARK2 and PACRG in the biology of leprosy remain to be determined. Genes with polymorphisms associated with a predisposition to distinct clinical forms of leprosy (i.e., lepromatous vs. tuberculoid) include HLA-DRB1*1501 and HLA-DRB1*1502, NRAMP1, TNF, IL-10, and TAP2. In contrast, variants in the T_H2 cytokine gene cluster on chromosome 5q31 have not been associated with a predisposition to lepromatous leprosy.

Clinical Manifestations

The most common manifestations of leprosy involve the skin and peripheral nerves and are determined by the polarity of the disease: paucibacillary (tuberculoid) or multibacillary (lepromatous). The onset of leprosy is usually insidious. Depending on the form of leprosy, numbness may be an initial complaint or finding, and skin lesions may become apparent only months or years later. The classification of leprosy as tuberculoid, lepromatous, or one of the borderline forms is based on the combination of clinical examination, the number of bacteria seen on skin slit smears or skin biopsy specimens, and the histologic appearance. Because the nature of the potential complications and the specific course of chemotherapy are determined by the form of leprosy, accurate diagnosis and classification are essential.

Tuberculoid Leprosy

Tuberculoid leprosy is characterized by the presence of fewer than five skin lesions, which are typically hypopigmented or erythematous macules with raised erythematous borders and an atrophic center (Fig. 347–2). The skin lesions in tuberculoid leprosy are usually hypoesthetic or anesthetic; when multiple lesions are present, their distribution is asymmetrical. The skin lesions may be large and are most commonly found on the face, trunk, or extremities; however, they are not found in the axillae, groin, or perineum or on the scalp, presumably because of the preference of *M. leprae* for temperatures lower than 37° C.

Local peripheral nerve involvement is common in tuberculoid leprosy and is asymmetrical. In addition to hypoesthesia or anesthesia of the skin lesions, nerve involvement in tuberculoid leprosy is manifested as enlargement or tenderness (or both) of the peripheral nerves that serve the region of the skin lesions. Superficial nerves such as the ulnar, superficial peroneal, or greater auricular nerves may be visibly enlarged, depending on the location of the skin lesions. Functional complications of nerve involvement, such as muscle atrophy and contractures, may be present at the time of diagnosis of tuberculoid leprosy. Tuberculoid leprosy is a stable form; it does not convert to the borderline or lepromatous forms.

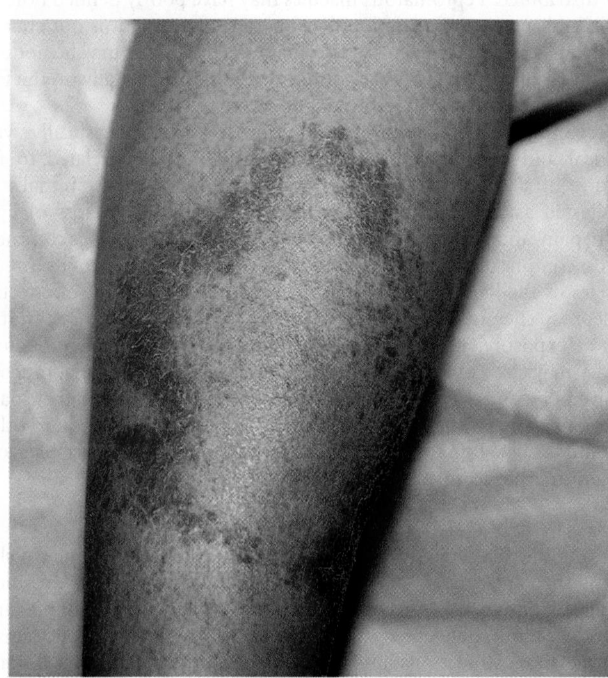

FIGURE 347–2 • Tuberculoid leprosy. A single large lesion with irregular, raised, erythematous borders and a depressed, hypopigmented center is shown. (From Hansen disease [leprosy]. *In* James WD, Berger TG, Elston DM [eds]: Andrews Diseases of the Skin, 10th ed. Philadelphia, Elsevier, 2006.)

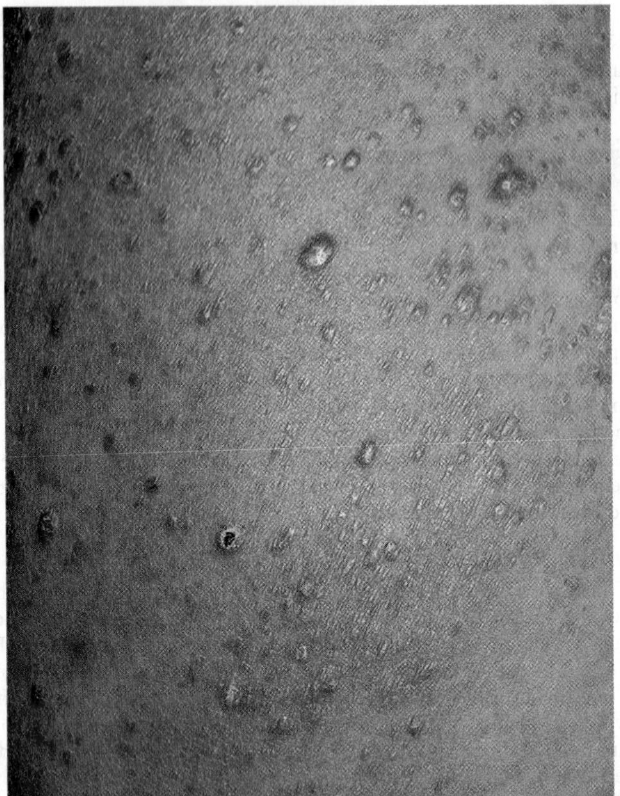

FIGURE 347–3 • Lepromatous leprosy. Numerous papules and nodules are apparent. Lepromatous macules have ill-defined borders, with normal sensation usually maintained. (From Hansen disease [leprosy]. *In* James WD, Berger TG, Elston DM [eds]: Andrews Diseases of the Skin, 10th ed. Philadelphia, Elsevier, 2006.)

Lepromatous Leprosy

Lepromatous leprosy is characterized by multiple skin lesions that are smaller than those observed in tuberculoid leprosy (Fig. 347–3). Although the sites of skin lesions are similar to those of tuberculoid leprosy, the multiple lesions of lepromatous leprosy are often symmetrically distributed. Lepromatous macules may have poorly defined borders and exhibit no loss of sensation; local nerve enlargement is not characteristic. In addition to macules, lepromatous skin lesions may be nodules or plaques, or they may diffusely infiltrate the skin, especially on the face (which may cause loss of eyebrows and "leonine facies").

Nerve involvement in lepromatous leprosy is characteristically symmetrical and exhibits a stocking-glove distribution, unrelated to the location of skin lesions. Peripheral nerve involvement may initially be manifested as loss of temperature sensation, followed by loss of light touch, pain, and deep pressure sense. In addition, dysesthesia is common. Motor complications, including muscle weakness and atrophy of the muscles of the hands, feet, and face, develop in the absence of effective antileprosy chemotherapy. Involvement of the facial nerve may result in corneal exposure, ulceration, and blindness. People with lepromatous leprosy may also have prominent rhinorrhea as a result of nasal mucosal involvement, and they may shed large numbers of *M. leprae* in their nasal secretions—one of the major sources of bacilli for transmission to other individuals. Like tuberculoid leprosy, lepromatous leprosy is stable; conversion to other forms does not occur.

Borderline Forms of Leprosy

Borderline tuberculoid leprosy is characterized by the presence of skin lesions that are similar to those of tuberculoid leprosy but are more numerous and may be accompanied by satellite lesions around large lesions. In borderline leprosy, the skin lesions are numerous but remain asymmetrical. The lesions are usually plaques rather than macules and exhibit satellite lesions. Nerve involvement in borderline leprosy is manifested as thickening or tenderness of local nerves, but the skin lesions retain sensation. Borderline lepromatous leprosy is characterized by numerous symmetrical small macules, papules, plaques, and nodules, but not the diffuse skin infiltration found in full-blown lepromatous leprosy. Unlike tuberculoid and lepromatous leprosy, the borderline forms are unstable and progress to the lepromatous form over time unless effective treatment is provided. Reactional states, including both reversal reactions and downgrading reactions, occur in people with borderline forms of leprosy.

Reactional States

People with leprosy who may otherwise avoid care may exhibit acute reactional symptoms and signs. This form is what physicians in developed countries may encounter in acute care settings.

Type 1 reactions, which are mediated by cellular immune responses to *M. leprae* antigens in skin lesions and nerves, occur in people with borderline tuberculoid, borderline, and borderline lepromatous leprosy. Type 1 reactions are frequently accompanied by worsening of peripheral nerve manifestations and may result in permanent nerve damage; they should be considered medical emergencies. Reversal reactions, which are type 1 reactions that occur after initiation of chemotherapy for leprosy or human immunodeficiency virus (HIV) infection, are associated with enhanced T_H1 immune responses that develop in people with a large burden of *M. leprae;* they are most severe in those with borderline lepromatous leprosy. Downgrading reactions occur in association with the transition of borderline disease toward the lepromatous form. Although the immune mechanisms that underlie reversal reactions and downgrading reactions are believed to be distinct, their clinical manifestations are indistinguishable. Type 1 reactions may have an acute or insidious onset, and they are characterized by inflammation of preexisting skin and nerve lesions. Skin lesions, which become erythematous and edematous, may also become tender and thereby resemble cellulitis, but type 1 reactions are not accompanied by fever or other systemic symptoms or signs. Increased expression of TNF has been found in lesions during type 1 reactions and may contribute to the clinical and functional consequences.

Type 2 reactions, also known as erythema nodosum leprosum (ENL), occur in people with borderline lepromatous and lepromatous leprosy and are mediated by immune complexes rather than cellular immune responses. Type 2 reactions, which occur most often after initiation of antileprosy chemotherapy or during pregnancy, are generally accompanied by fever and arthralgias. Additional signs of systemic inflammatory disease may appear, including hepatosplenomegaly, lymphadenopathy, arthritis, nephritis, keratitis, and iritis. The skin lesions of ENL resemble those of classic erythema nodosum (Chapter 466), with widely distributed erythematous dermal and subcutaneous nodules whose location is unrelated to the leprosy lesions. Biopsy of ENL lesions show leukocytoclastic vasculitis.

Leprosy and Human Immunodeficiency Virus

$CD4^+$ T-cell–mediated immunity is essential for control of *M. leprae,* and the extent of T_H1 immunity determines whether an individual will have tuberculoid or lepromatous leprosy. However, coinfection with HIV and depletion of $CD4^+$ T lymphocytes does not affect the rate of progression of leprosy, nor does it cause conversion of tuberculoid leprosy to the lepromatous form. In contrast, type 1 reversal reactions may accompany immune reconstitution subsequent to initiation of effective combination antiretroviral therapy for HIV infection. The manifestations of these reversal reactions are similar to those observed in people who are not infected with HIV.

Diagnosis

The diagnosis of leprosy should be considered in any patient with a complex of skin and peripheral nerve manifestations, especially those who have lived in countries where leprosy is endemic. Although leprosy is a chronic infection, its acute complications require prompt diagnosis and therapy to prevent irreversible peripheral nerve damage. It is also important to classify a patient's disease as tuberculoid, lepromatous, or one of the specific borderline forms because correct classification is necessary for selecting optimal therapy and anticipating potential reactional states. Because *M. leprae* cannot be cultured in vitro and there is currently no serologic test or other diagnostic biomarker for leprosy, diagnosis and classification of leprosy depend on the combination of clinical examination, histopathologic evaluation, and acid-fast staining of skin slits or biopsy specimens.

Clinical Examination

Examination of an individual with possible or confirmed leprosy must include evaluation and documentation of the number, location, and characteristics of skin lesions. In addition to descriptions of the skin lesions, accurate classification of leprosy depends on whether the lesions are distributed symmetrically and whether they are hypoesthetic or anesthetic. The examination must also include a search for enlarged and tender peripheral nerves, the presence of sensory deficits (especially temperature sensation and pain) and skin ulcerations, and the nature and distribution of motor deficits, muscle atrophy, and contractures. Because some medications used for the treatment of leprosy are contraindicated in pregnancy, women of childbearing age should be evaluated for pregnancy.

Skin Smears and Biopsies

In developing countries, classification of multibacillary or paucibacillary leprosy is made by the combination of clinical examination and bacterial counts as determined on acid-fast–stained smears made from skin slits of lesions and skin from cool areas of the body, such as the earlobes. In developed countries, skin biopsies are usually performed instead of skin slits. Skin specimens should be obtained from the active border of lesions and should include subcutaneous tissue. On hematoxylin-eosin staining, tuberculoid leprosy is characterized by granulomas with giant cells, aggregates of epithelioid macrophages that are neither vacuolated nor foamy, and lymphocytes at the periphery. Although granulomas may be found in other skin diseases, selective destruction of nerve trunks and perineural fibrosis are specific features of leprosy. Acid-fast stains (preferably done with the Fite procedure) show rare or undetectable bacilli in tuberculoid leprosy. Lesions of lepromatous leprosy show poorly organized granulomas without giant cells or lymphocytes; macrophages are foamy and lipid laden. Acid-fast staining of lepromatous leprosy lesions reveals abundant bacilli that usually appear in large clumps ("globi"). The borderline forms of leprosy exhibit less well organized granulomas, with fewer giant cells and lymphocytes but more foamy macrophages and acid-fast bacilli as the spectrum varies from borderline tuberculoid to borderline lepromatous.

Specialized immunohistochemistry stains, such as for $CD4^+$ T lymphocytes or cytokine expression, are useful in research studies but are not currently used for the diagnosis or classification of leprosy. Polymerase chain reaction amplification of *M. leprae* genomic DNA from skin slits or skin biopsy specimens, though often productive, has not yet contributed to enhanced sensitivity or specificity of diagnosis or classification.

Diagnosis of Reactional States

The diagnosis of type 1 reactions is based on clinical findings in a patient with borderline tuberculoid, borderline, or borderline lepromatous leprosy and acute inflammation of preexisting skin lesions, with or without worsening of nerve lesions. Type 1 reactions are not accompanied by systemic findings such as fever or arthritis. At highest risk for type 1 reactions are patients who have recently initiated antileprosy chemotherapy, although type 1 reactions can occur spontaneously. Diagnosis of a type 2 reaction (ENL) is also based on clinical findings of new erythematous subcutaneous or dermal nodules in a patient with borderline lepromatous or lepromatous leprosy. There are currently no diagnostic tests or biomarkers for ENL, and skin biopsy will not distinguish ENL from classic erythema nodosum.

Treatment

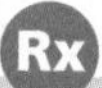

Agents to Treat Leprosy

The first-line antimicrobial agents for leprosy are dapsone and rifampin. Clofazimine, minocycline, certain fluoroquinolones, and clarithromycin are also useful in specific contexts, including drug intolerance or resistance.

Dapsone is inexpensive and well tolerated, has a long serum half-life (≈28 hours), and is safe for use during pregnancy. Glucose-6-phosphate dehydrogenase (G6PD)-deficient individuals are susceptible to dapsone-induced methemoglobinemia and hemolysis, and all patients should be screened for G6PD deficiency before starting dapsone. Patients with mild G6PD deficiency (the African type, caused by mutations that lead to instability of the enzyme) can begin dapsone at 25 mg/day but require close monitoring for anemia. Dapsone can also cause bone marrow suppression and profound neutropenia. Other rare adverse effects of dapsone include hepatitis, cholestatic jaundice, and a syndrome characterized by exfoliative dermatitis, generalized lymphadenopathy, fever, and hepatosplenomegaly.

Rifampin, which is the most bactericidal drug against *M. leprae*, is well absorbed after oral administration and has a serum half-life of approximately 3 hours. Rifampin should never be used as monotherapy because resistance can develop with single point mutations in its target, RNA polymerase II. Because rifampin is bactericidal and rapid release of components from dead bacteria can have pro-inflammatory effects, some experts withhold rifampin during active reversal reactions. Adverse effects of rifampin include maculopapular rash, hepatotoxicity, a flulike syndrome (most frequent with intermittent therapy), and orange discoloration of tears, urine, saliva, and sweat. Thrombocytopenia occurs occasionally but is not usually severe. Rifampin also induces metabolism and decreases serum concentrations of other drugs, including antiretroviral protease inhibitors and non-nucleoside reverse transcriptase inhibitors, methadone, and oral contraceptives. Rifampin decreases serum concentrations of dapsone, but this effect is not clinically significant with a dapsone dose of 100 mg/day.

Clofazimine is a lipophilic dye that is bacteriostatic against *M. leprae*. It has a very long (≈70 days) half-life and appears to have anti-inflammatory activity, as well as direct bacteriostatic activity. Because of its anti-inflammatory activity, clofazimine is useful in the treatment of type 1 reactional states. Clofazimine is generally well tolerated; its major side effect is discoloration of the skin, which occurs in nearly all clofazimine-treated patients. The skin discoloration can range from reddish tan to bluish black and can be blotchy, but it is reversible within 6 to 12 months of discontinuing use of the drug. In chronic reactional patients maintained on high doses of clofazimine (200 to 300 mg/day), enteropathy with crampy abdominal pain, mild nausea or diarrhea (or both), and even bowel obstruction can develop.

Regimens to Treat Leprosy

Chemotherapy for leprosy involves the use of multiple drugs to optimize the rate of cure and prevent the emergence of drug resistance. The regimen currently recommended in the United States for paucibacillary leprosy consists of dapsone, 100 mg, and rifampin, 600 mg, both given daily for 12 months. The recommended regimen for multibacillary leprosy is dapsone, 100 mg, plus rifampin, 600 mg, and clofazimine, 50 mg, each given daily for 24 months (available at *http://bphc.hrsa.gov/nhdp/default.htm*). In resource-limited countries, where the burden of leprosy is highest, the WHO regimen for paucibacillary leprosy is dapsone, 100 mg daily, plus rifampin, 600 mg once a month, for 6 months. The WHO regimen for multibacillary leprosy is dapsone, 100 mg daily, plus rifampin, 600 mg once a month, plus cofazimine, 50 mg daily, plus an additional dose of clofazimine, 300 mg once a month (available at *http://www.who.int/lep/disease/disease.htm*). The monthly doses of rifampin and clofazimine should be administered under supervision.

Response to Therapy

Response to effective therapy for leprosy is seen clinically as flattening and resolution of the papules, nodules, or plaques, with or without improvement in nerve function. Clinical improvement may begin within the first months of therapy, but resolution of skin lesions is often delayed as long as 1 to 2 years after completion of therapy. Quantitation of the bacillary load to assess response to treatment is cumbersome, semiquantitative, and not recommended.

Patients who have been adequately treated may experience worsening of nerve and skin symptoms, perhaps because of a late reversal reaction or relapsed leprosy. If skin specimens do not reveal acid-fast organisms, a therapeutic trial of corticosteroids, which will ameliorate the symptoms of reversal reactions but not those of relapsed leprosy, can help make the distinction and assist in choos-

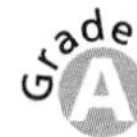

ing subsequent therapy. Patients who experience relapse after treatment of paucibacillary disease should be treated for multibacillary disease because the most likely cause of relapse is previous multibacillary disease that was misclassified. Patients with multibacillary disease who relapse should be retreated with a regimen containing dapsone and rifampin, with the addition of at least two drugs that were not used in the initial treatment regimen, unless susceptibility testing is available and confirms that the organisms remain susceptible to dapsone and rifampin. The choices among additional drugs include minocycline, moxifloxacin, and clarithromycin. Relapsed multibacillary patients may benefit from lifelong maintenance therapy after completing 2 years of a salvage regimen. Because susceptibility testing cannot be performed with direct in vitro assays, the mouse footpad assay has been used, but it is becoming less available. The alternative approach to determining susceptibility by sequencing the targets of dapsone and rifampin (*folP1* and *rpoB*, respectively) offers promise but has not yet been rigorously tested.

Treatment of Reactional States

Type 1 reactions may develop before, during, or several years after completing antileprosy chemotherapy. Type 1 reactions that involve worsening of nerve symptoms and findings are medical emergencies because permanent nerve damage can occur. Type 1 reactions usually respond to prednisone at a daily dose of 60 to 80 mg, which can be tapered slowly once symptoms are controlled. Type 1 reactions can also respond to high-dose clofazimine (200 to 300 mg/day), although reactions with worsening nerve symptoms should be treated initially with prednisone. Patients who have type 1 reactions that occur before or during antileprosy chemotherapy and whose reactions include nerve involvement should have rifampin withheld until the worsened nerve symptoms resolve because release of proinflammatory components from dying bacteria may contribute to inflammation and nerve damage. Dapsone and clofazimine should be continued during treatment of type 1 reactions.

The treatment of choice for severe type 2 reactions (ENL) is thalidomide, except in pregnant or potentially pregnant women. Thalidomide requires that patients and the prescribing physician be enrolled in the System for Thalidomide Education and Prescribing Safety (STEPS) program to avoid the drug's teratogenic effects. The mechanism of action of thalidomide is incompletely understood but is likely to include inhibition of TNF. The dose of thalidomide for ENL varies, depending on the severity of the reaction. In patients with ENL and high fever, frank arthritis, and large subcutaneous plaques, up to 100 mg four times daily may be required to achieve a clinical response. Once a clinical response is achieved, the dose of thalidomide may be tapered to a maintenance dose of 50 to 100 mg given once daily at night (because thalidomide is sedating). For milder cases of ENL, 50 to 100 mg per night may be sufficient to achieve and maintain control. ENL in women of childbearing age and thalidomide-unresponsive cases may respond to corticosteroids. Antileprosy chemotherapy, including rifampin, should be continued in patients with ENL.

Other Therapy

Nerve damage in leprosy, which can result in muscle atrophy, contractures, and autoamputation, is a major cause of debility. Supportive care, reconstructive surgery, physical and occupational therapy, and rehabilitation can be extremely valuable in allowing patients to achieve and maintain optimal function.

Prevention

There is currently no effective specific vaccine for leprosy, but several trials have observed a partial protective effect of bacille Calmette-Guérin vaccination. 1 It is likely that improved understanding of transmission of *M. leprae* will be generated by the use of DNA-based strain typing, so better preventive measures are likely to become available in the near future.

Prognosis

Multidrug chemotherapy cures a high proportion of people with paucibacillary and multibacillary leprosy. The currently recommended regimens provide high rates of response, with relapse rates of approximately 0.1% per year in paucibacillary cases and up to 5% per year in multibacillary cases. Some cases of paucibacillary leprosy may enter remission or even self-cure, but all cases of multibacillary leprosy are progressive. Because of its efficacy and low toxicity, multidrug chemotherapy should be used in all people in whom leprosy is diagnosed to minimize long-term morbidity.

1. Cunha SS, Rodrigues LC, Pedrosa V, et al: Neonatal BCG protection against leprosy: A study of Manaus, Brazilian Amazon. Lepr Rev 2004;75:357–366.

SUGGESTED READINGS

Bakker M, Hatla M, Kwenang A, et al: Risk factors for developing leprosy—a population-based cohort in Indonesia. Lepr Rev 2006;77:48–61. *Patients who were seropositive or PCR positive were at highest risk.*

Britton WJ, Lockwood DN: Leprosy. Lancet 2004;363:1209–1219. *An authoritative review with extensive references.*

Moet FJ, Meima A, Oskam L, et al: Risk factors for the development of clinical leprosy among contacts and their relevance for targeted interventions. Lepr Rev 2004;75:310–326. *Interventions should be aimed at close contacts inside and outside the home.*

Monot M, Honore N, Garnier T, et al: On the origin of leprosy. Science 2005;308:1040–1042. *Analysis and identification of sequence variants of* M. leprae *and their use to determine the global spread of leprosy.*

348 RICKETTSIOSES

Didier Raoult

Definition

Rickettsioses are emerging infectious diseases. Because of better diagnostic tools and changes in tick exposure, many new rickettsial diseases have been described in the past 15 years. Three families of diseases are grouped under this name: rickettsioses, ehrlichioses, and Q fever.

The Pathogens

The agents of rickettsial diseases (formerly grouped in the order Rickettsiales) are small gram-negative bacteria that grow within eukaryotic cells. They have never been grown in axenic media thus far and for culture require living hosts such as cell cultures, embryonated eggs, or susceptible animals. With the exception of *Rickettsia prowazekii*, the agent of epidemic typhus, these bacteria infect humans incidentally and are mainly animal pathogens. On the basis of molecular phylogeny, the bacteria causing rickettsial diseases have been reclassified into three phyla (Table 348–1).

Because of their difficult growth in vitro, the main diagnostic tool for rickettsioses is serology. Serologic evaluation is frequently hampered by late positivity and cross-reactivity. The development of direct staining in blood smears or skin biopsy samples, as well as polymerase chain reaction (PCR) amplification of DNA in blood samples or biopsy specimens, has considerably helped identification at the species level and led to the description of emerging pathogens.

■ RICKETTSIOSES (DISEASES CAUSED BY *RICKETTSIA* SPECIES AND *ORIENTIA TSUTSUGAMUSCHI*)

Definition

Rickettsia sp are small gram-negative bacteria that multiply free in the cytoplasm of their host cells. The target cells in humans are endothelial cells, and vasculitis is the most prominent clinical manifestation. These bacteria invade cells by phagocytosis and escape the phagosome vacuole.

TABLE 348–1 GENETIC CLASSIFICATION OF RICKETTSIALES

	Genus	Group	Species	Subspecies	First Year of Isolation or Discovery
Rickettsiae	*Rickettsia*	Typhus	*R. prowazekii*		1916
			R. typhi		1920
		Spotted fever	*R. conorii*	*conorii*	1932
				israeli	1974
				caspia	1991
				indica	2001
			R. rickettsii		1919
			R. sibirica	*sibirica*	1946
				mongolitimonae	1996
			R. slovaca		1997
			R. honei		1991
			R. japonica		1992
			R. parkeri		2003
			R. massiliae		2006
			R. monacencis		2007
			R. heilonjanghensis		1998
			R. aeschlimannii		2001
			R. helvetica		2000
			R. australis		1950
			R. felis		2001
			R. akari		1946
	Orientia	Scrub typhus	*O. tsutsugamushi*		1920
Ehrlichiae	*Ehrlichia*		*E. chaffeensis*		1991
			E. ewingii		1999
			E. canis		1996
	Anaplasma		*A. phagocytophilum*		1992
	Neorickettsia		*N. sennetsu*		1957
	Wolbachia		*W. pipientis*		2001
Coxiellae			*C. burnetii*		1931

The genome of *Rickettsia* is small, between 1.1 and 1.6 Mb, and there are no mobile genetic elements. These bacteria have four (typhus group) or five outer membrane proteins of the surface cell antigen family, including rOmpA (lacking in typhus group) and rOmpB. These proteins are major antigens that help identify the rickettsial species, and their encoding genes are used for amplification and sequencing for diagnostic or taxonomic purposes. Among rickettsiae, two subgroups, the typhus group (TG) and the spotted fever group (SFG), were identified on the basis of growth conditions and antigenicity. A specific group antigen, determined to be lipopolysaccharide, has been identified. The optimal growth temperature is 37° C for TG and 32 to 35° C for SFG. The complete genome sequencing of *R. prowazekii* (from the typhus group) showed that it is mainly a subset of *Rickettsia conorii* (a member of the spotted fever group).

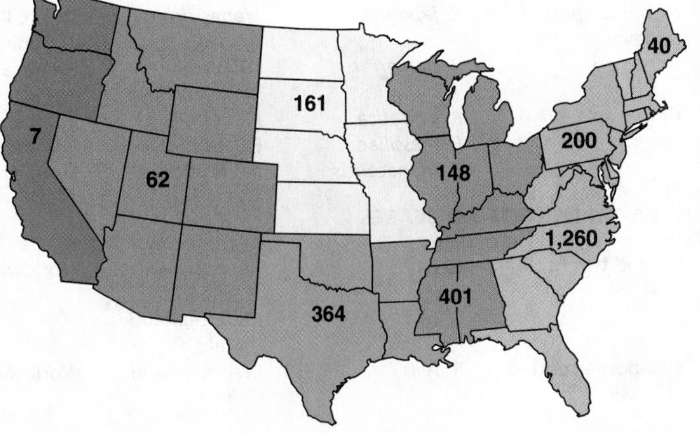

FIGURE 348–1 • Number of reported cases of Rocky Mountain spotted fever by region, 1994 to 1998.

Tick-Borne Rickettsioses

Rocky Mountain Spotted Fever

Epidemiology

Rocky Mountain spotted fever (RMSF), the most severe of the rickettsioses, is caused by *Rickettsia rickettsii* (Table 348–2). It is the major tick-transmitted rickettsiosis recognized in America, with *Rickettsiae africae* in the West Indies and *Rickettsia parkeri* in southern states. It was described first in the 19th century in the western United States. RMSF is prevalent in at least 44 states in the United States (Fig. 348–1) and in Central and South America (Argentina, Brazil, Colombia, Costa Rica, Mexico, and Panama).

Rickettsia is transmitted transovarially to tick progeny from one generation to the next. The infecting ticks are mainly *Dermacentor andersoni* (a wood tick) in the western United States; *Dermacentor variabilis* (the American dog tick) in the East, the Midwest, and the South; and *Rhipicephalus sanguineus* in Arizona. In Central and South America, *Amblyomma cajennense* is the major vector. Humans are infected through infected saliva after a tick bite. The duration of attachment is critical in any tick-borne rickettsiosis, and transmission is unlikely when the tick feeds for less than 20 hours. The tick bite is painless and frequently unnoticed. Rarely, an eschar at the site of the tick bite is observed in RMSF. The epidemiology of RMSF undergoes largely unexplained yearly variations. This temporal repartition is determined by tick activity and human encounter. More than 500 cases occur each year, and over 90% are reported from April to September. The disease is more prevalent in children younger than 10 years.

Clinical Manifestations

Two to 14 days after the tick bite, fever and headaches appear. The fever is high (temperature >102° F) and associated with nonspecific symptoms, including malaise, myalgias, nausea, vomiting, anorexia, and diarrhea. At

TABLE 348–2 RICKETTSIAL DISEASES IN HUMAN BEINGS

Disease	Organism	Arthropod Host	Geographic Area	Rash	Eschar Tache Noire	Regional Lymph Node	High Fever	Fatality Rate
TICK-TRANSMITTED SPOTTED FEVERS								
Rocky Mountain spotted fever	*R. rickettsii*	*Dermacentor andersoni* *Dermacentor variabilis* *Rhipicephalus sanguineus* *Amblyomma cajennense*	America (North, Central, and South)	Yes, may be purpuric	Very rare	No	Yes	High
Mediterranean spotted fever Astrachan fever, Israeli spotted fever	*R. conorii*	*Rhipicephalus sanguineus*	Mediterranean, India, Caspian Sea, Africa	Yes, papular may be purpuric	Yes	No	Yes	Moderate
African tick bite fever	*R. africae*	*Amblyomma hebraum* *Amblyomma variegatum*	Sub-Saharan Africa, West Indies	Yes, half of cases may be vesicular	Yes (frequently multiple)	Yes	No	Low
Queensland tick typhus	*R. australis*	*Ixodes holocyclus*	Eastern Australia	Yes, may be vesicular	Yes	?	Yes	Moderate
Siberian tick typhus	*R. sibirica*	*Dermacentor nuttallii*	Siberia, China, Mongolia	Yes	Yes	No	Yes	Low
Tick-borne lymphadenopathy (TIBOLA)	*R. slovaca*	*Dermacentor marginatus* *Dermacentor reticulatus*	Europe, Pakistan	Very rare	Yes, may be erythematous	Yes (painful)	No	Low
Lymphangitis-associated rickettsiosis (LAR)	*R. sibirica mongolitimonae*	*Hyalomma asiaticum*	Mongolia, Africa, Europe	Yes	Yes	Yes	Yes	Low
Unnamed	*R. aeschlimannii*	*Hyalomma sp.*	Mediterranean, Africa	Yes	Yes	Yes	Yes	Unknown
Flinders Island spotted fever	*R. honei*	*Ixodes granulosus*	Flinders Island, eastern Australia	Yes	Yes	Yes	Yes	Low
Japanese spotted fever	*R. japonica*	*Ixodes ricinus*	Japan, Korea (China?)	Yes	Yes	No	Yes	Low
Unnamed	*R. parkeri*	*Amblyomma maculatum*	America	Yes	Yes	No	Yes	
Unnamed	*R. helvetica*	*Ixodes ricinus*	Europe, Asia	No	Yes	No	No	
	R. massiliae	RH. *sanguineus*	Europe, USA	Yes	Yes	No	Yes	Unknown
	R. monacencis	*Ixodes ricinus*	Europe	Yes	Yes	No	Yes	Unknown
FLEA-TRANSMITTED DISEASES								
Murine typhus	*R. typhi*	*Xenopsylla cheopis* *Ctenocephalides felis*	Worldwide	Yes	No	No	Yes	Low
Flea-borne spotted fever	*R. felis*	*Ctenocephalides felis*	Worldwide	Sometimes	Sometimes	Unknown	Yes	Unknown
LOUSE-TRANSMITTED DISEASE								
Epidemic typhus	*R. prowazekii*	*Pediculus humanus corporis* *Arnblyomma* ticks(?)	Worldwide	Yes	No	No	Yes	High
American sylvatic typhus	*R. prowazekii*	Flying squirrel ectoparasites	United States	Yes	No	No	Yes	Low
Brill-Zinsser disease (relapse of epidemic typhus)	*R. prowazekii*		Worldwide	Yes, could lack	No	No	No	Low
MITE-TRANSMITTED DISEASE								
Rickettsialpox	*R. akari*	*Liponyssoides sanguineus*	Worldwide	Yes, vesicular	Yes	Yes	Yes	Low
Scrub typhus	*Orientia tsutsugamushi*	*Leptotrombidium* sp (chiggers)	Central and eastern Asia Australia	Yes	Yes	Yes	Yes	High, may relapse

this stage, RMSF is not frequently diagnosed, but during the "tick season," patients with high fever who live in or have a history of travel to an endemic location and, possibly, a history of tick bite should be considered as possibly having RMSF.

The most characteristic feature is a rash. However, the classic triad of fever, headache, and rash is present in only 44% of confirmed cases. Rash is found in 14% of cases on the first day of disease and in less than 50% in the first 3 days. The rash is macular; it appears first on the ankles and wrists and then generalizes. Spots are 1 to 5 mm in diameter and can evolve from pink to purpuric. A rash can appear later or even not at all; Rocky Mountain "spotless" fever represented 34% of cases in a series from the Centers for Disease Control and Prevention (CDC). Involvement of the palms and soles theoretically differentiates the typhus diseases (in which it is absent) from the spotted fevers.

Untreated patients worsen progressively. The disease is associated in various degrees with general manifestations related to vascular inflammation and increased vascular permeability and with multiple organ involvement that can lead to multiple organ dysfunction syndrome (MODS). In severe forms, patients suffer from edema, hypovolemia, hypoalbuminemia, and hypotension leading to shock. In very severe cases, necrosis and gangrene of the extremities occur. In some instances, noncardiogenic pulmonary edema develops; pulmonary involvement leading to respiratory distress can cause death. Renal failure can result either from hypovolemia and shock and be reversible or from acute tubular necrosis and require hemodialysis. The usual neurologic symptoms are confusion, lethargy, and stupor. In severe cases, delirium, coma, and seizures are observed. Cerebrospinal fluid (CSF) sampling exhibits meningitis in a third of cases; generally, a few monocyte cells (10 to 100) are observed, along with increased protein but normal glucose levels. Heart involvement can cause arrhythmia. Liver involvement is manifested as an increase in transaminases in a third of patients and jaundice in 8%. Jaundice can also reflect hemolysis. Intestinal tract involvement is manifested as abdominal pain, diarrhea, vomiting, and severe bleeding (upper gastrointestinal hemorrhage can cause death). Ocular involvement consists of conjunctivitis and retinal abnormalities, including hemorrhages, papilledema, and arterial occlusion.

The blood cell count shows a normal number of white blood cells but often immature myeloid cells. Thrombocytopenia is observed in 30 to 50% of cases and may be marked in severe cases. Anemia develops in 30% of patients. Coagulopathy with decreases in clotting factors (including fibrinogen) and prolonged coagulation times may contribute to bleeding; albuminemia may be low and proteins of the acute phase response increased (C-reactive protein, ferritin, fibrinogen). Hyponatremia and hypocalcemia may be noted and correlate with severity, as with an increase in creatininemia. Increased concentrations of serum enzymes such as aminotransferases (aspartate [AST] and alanine aminotransferase [ALT]), lactate dehydrogenase (LDH), and creatine phosphokinase usually reflect the severity of organ involvement, including the lung, heart, and liver and multifocal rhabdomyolysis.

Diagnosis

The diagnosis of RMSF should be based on clinical and epidemiologic findings and lead to early use of doxycycline. The most important clue is unexplained fever in a patient with a history of tick exposure in an endemic area. When a rash is present, RMSF should be suspected and the patient treated accordingly unless another cause is demonstrated. The differential diagnosis includes other rickettsioses (such as these caused by *R. parkeri* in southeastern states), meningococcemia, enterovirus infections, typhoid, leptospirosis, ehrlichiosis, gonococcemia, toxic shock syndrome, syphilis, rubella, measles, and the Kawasaki syndrome. Drug hypersensitivity, especially after antimicrobial use for febrile illness, is sometimes confused with RMSF.

The main diagnostic test relies on serology, and treatment should never be delayed to obtain diagnostic confirmation. Criteria for laboratory confirmation include a fourfold or greater change in antibody titer determined by serology (measured by immunofluorescence assay [IFA], complement fixation, or latex agglutination) or direct detection of the bacterium by demonstration of specific antigens by immunodetection, genomic amplification by PCR, or culture. A biopsy specimen of a skin lesion is the best sample for this purpose. Culture of *Rickettsia* takes 3 to 7 days and is restricted to specialized laboratories. It is performed on cell lines such as Vero, L929, or HEL cells. Immunodetection by IFA or immunohistochemistry is sensitive and specific. It can be performed with frozen or fixed and paraffin-embedded material and allows retrospective diagnosis. PCR amplification and identification give promising results in rickettsioses in general but have not been properly evaluated for diagnosis of RMSF. Skin biopsy and direct detection in removed ticks yield the best results because blood contains inhibitors and only few copies of rickettsial DNA.

Two serum samples should be tested (early and convalescent). The early serum is usually negative because patients seroconvert between the 7th and 15th days. IFA is highly sensitive and specific. A cutoff value of 1/64 for total immunoglobulin and 1/32 for IgM antibodies is required for diagnosis. The latex agglutination cutoff is 1/64 or 1/128. Cross-reactive antibodies have been reported with infections caused by other rickettsioses, *Ehrlichia, Bartonella, Legionella,* and *Proteus.* False positives, including IgM, may be observed when rheumatoid factor is present in serum and in patients with viral infection generating nonspecific B-lymphocyte proliferation (cytomegalovirus, Epstein-Barr virus). Complement fixation (which lacks sensitivity) and the Weil-Felix test (using antibodies that cross-react with *Proteus* strains) should not be used.

Treatment

Rx

The prognosis for patients with RMSF depends on the timing of antimicrobial treatment. Doxycycline saves patients with RMSF. The recommended dose is 100 mg two times a day, and treatment should be continued for at least 3 days after the fever resolves. Oral treatment is effective, but in patients with gastric intolerance or coma, the intravenous route is advised. Several antimicrobials are effective in vitro against *R. rickettsii,* including fluoroquinolones, rifampin, and new macrolide antimicrobials (but not erythromycin), but lack of clinical experience precludes their use for RMSF. β-Lactam antimicrobials, aminoglycosides, and cotrimoxazole are not effective.

Severely ill patients should be treated in intensive care units and fluid administration carefully monitored. Mechanical ventilation is used in case of respiratory distress, hemodialysis in patients with renal insufficiency, and antiseizure drugs in patients with seizures. Anemia and coagulation abnormalities may also be corrected. For patients with gangrene of the extremities, amputation may be necessary. Glucocorticoids have not proved useful.

Prevention

Prevention is based on avoidance of tick bites by using repellents or protective garments, or both. Apply repellents to discourage tick attachment. Repellents containing permethrin can be sprayed on boots and clothing and will last for several days. Repellents containing DEET (*N,N*-diethyl-*m*-toluamide) can be applied to the skin but will last only a few hours before reapplication is necessary. It is also useful to check for ticks after exposure. Careful examination of the scalp, groin, and axillae is recommended. The tick can be removed by forceps and the skin should be disinfected (Fig. 348–2).

Prognosis

The evolution of RMSF depends strongly on the timing of diagnosis and antimicrobial treatment. The current fatality rate is 2.4% on the basis

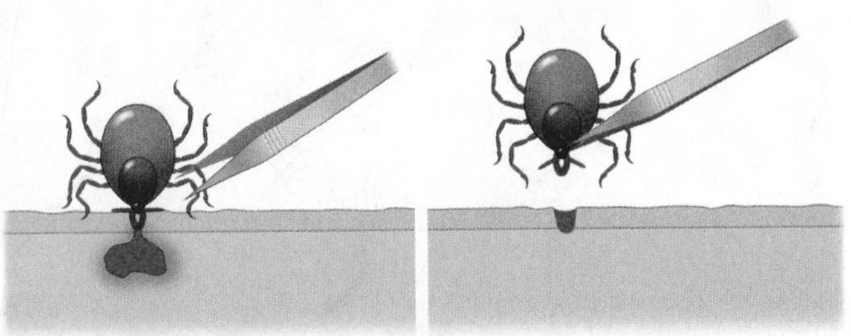

FIGURE 348–2 • Tick removal technique.

of a 4-year national survey in the United States (27 deaths were attributable to RMSF during this period). No significant difference in outcome was observed between blacks and whites, but the case-fatality rate was highest in people older than 70 years (9%). Patients with glucose-6-phosphate dehydrogenase (G6PD) deficiency were more susceptible to severe infection. Chloramphenicol was associated with a poorer outcome than treatment with doxycycline was. Usually, recovery from RMSF is complete, but neurologic sequelae can remain, and amputation of extremities may be necessary after gangrene.

Other Tick-Borne Rickettsioses

Epidemiology

As with other tick-transmitted diseases, rickettsioses have a limited geographic distribution that is determined mainly by the tick vector ecology (Fig. 348–3). *R. parkeri* has recently been identified in the United States and South America. In Europe, *R. conorii* is found around the Mediterranean and Caspian seas (Astrakhan serotype), *Rickettsia slovaca* and possibly *Rickettsia helvetica* in western and central Europe, and *Rickettsia sibirica mongolitimonae* in France and Greece. Elsewhere, a number of specific agents of rickettsial disease have been identified (see Table 348–2).

Clinical Manifestations

R. conorii comprises different, but closely related subspecies. Many names are given to the infection caused by *R. conorii:* Mediterranean spotted fever (MSF), boutonneuse fever, Marseilles fever, Kenya tick typhus (caused by the subspecies *R. conorii conorii*), Astrakhan fever (caused by *R. conorii caspia*), Israeli spotted fever (caused by *R. conorii israeli*), and Indian tick typhus (caused by *R. conorii indica*). *R. conorii* is closely related to *R. rickettsii,* with which it shares many common antigens that generate cross-reactive antibodies. MSF resembles RMSF but has several specificities. The spontaneous evolution is milder, but a fatality rate of 1.5 to 2.5% in hospitalized patients is still observed. A malignant form of the disease that includes purpuric rash, shock, and MODS has been described in alcoholic, diabetic, human immunodeficiency virus (HIV)-infected, and old or debilitated patients. The typical clinical manifestation is that of a patient with fever, a rash, and a tache noire (i.e., a black eschar at the site of the tick bite). A tache noire is found in 50 to 80% of cases. Multiple lesions do not occur because the dog tick vector, *R. sanguineus,* seldom bites humans. The rash is frequently clearly papular, which led to one of the names of the disease, boutonneuse fever. Israeli tick bite fever and Astrakhan fever appear to be milder than typical MSF, and tache noire is usually lacking.

R. africae, which causes African tick bite fever, may be responsible for most of the rickettsioses worldwide. It is transmitted by African ticks, *Amblyomma hebraeum* and *Amblyomma africanum.* These ticks are often infected; as many as 60% can harbor *R. africae.* They usually feed on ungulates but attack human beings in groups and cause a high prevalence of infection in rural Africa (60% of tested patients exhibit antibodies) and in travelers. The tick attacks typically generate clusters of cases in Safari tourists. The disease differs from MSF in that it is much milder, fever is frequently absent, a rash is observed in only half the patients, and the rash may be vesicular (which has never been reported in confirmed MSF). Moreover, several taches noires are frequently observed. They are prevalently found on the lower limbs and often associated with draining lymphadenopathy in the groin.

Japanese spotted fever (caused by *Rickettsia japonica*) and Siberian tick typhus (caused by *R. sibirica*) resemble MSF. Infections caused by *R. sibirica mongolitimonae* resemble MSF but in some cases exhibit specific clinical features, including a tache noire, groin lymphadenopathy, and lymphangitis joining these two lesions. The disease has been recently been named lymphangitis-associated rickettsiosis. *Rickettsia australis* (Queensland tick typhus) and *Rickettsia honei* (Flinders Island spotted fever) cause diseases resembling MSF, but their rash can be vesicular.

R. slovaca causes a disease apparently common in Europe (Hungary, France, Spain). Its tick vectors, *Dermacentor marginatus* and *Dermacentor reticulatus,* preferentially bite in cold months and bite the scalp because they prefer hairy prey. In contrast to other tick-borne rickettsioses, the disease is more prevalent in children and women. It is rarely exanthematic; the typical clinical picture consists of an erythematous skin lesion at the site of the tick bite on the scalp that ranges from 2 to 8 cm in diameter and a draining neck lymphadenopathy (which may be painful). Rarely, patients may exhibit fever and a rash. Deep postinfectious asthenia and residual alopecia at the site of the tick bite can be observed. The occurrence of this rickettsiosis without rash may stimulate research on other new rickettsial diseases with only localized manifestations.

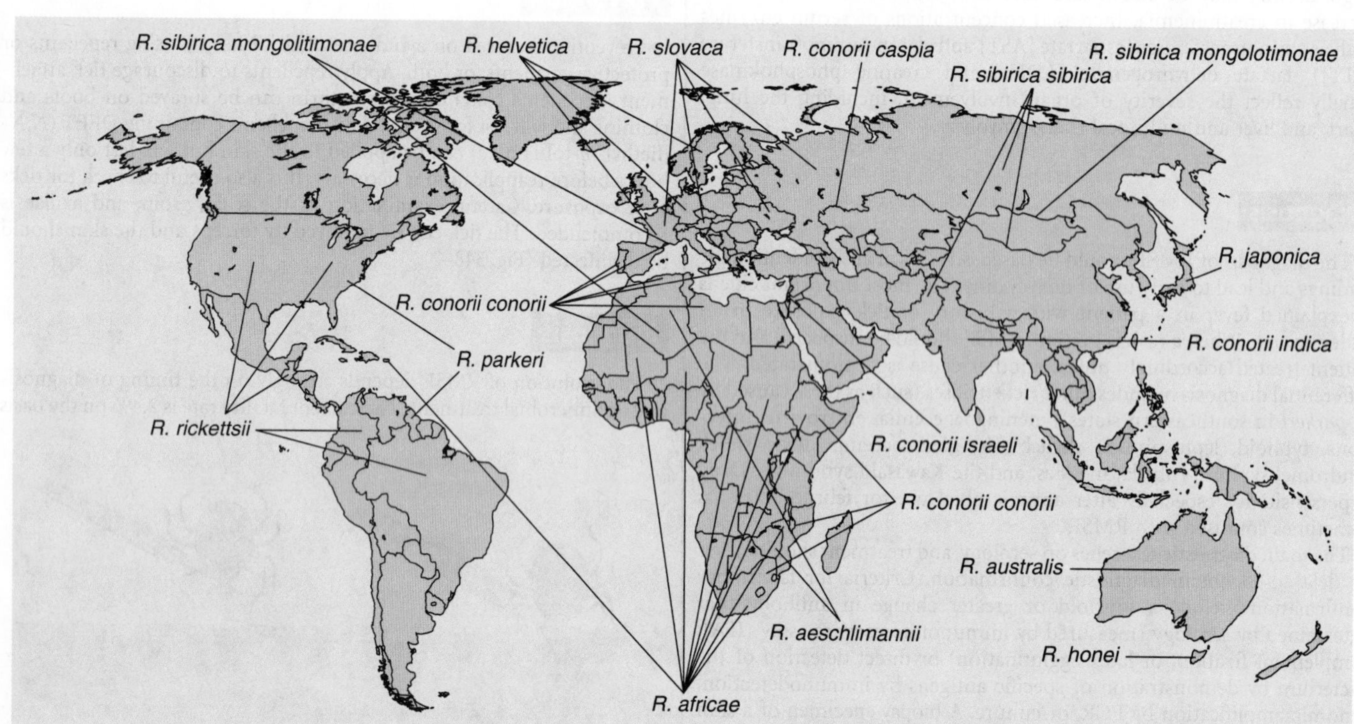

FIGURE 348–3 • Geographic repartition of tick-borne rickettsioses.

Diagnosis

The diagnosis of other tick-borne rickettsioses is similar to that of RMSF, mainly by serology (IFA; see earlier). An exception is *R. slovaca* infection, in which the serologic response is weak, possibly because of its lack of general infection; in this case PCR of a skin lesion or a lymph node aspirate is the best solution. In *R. africae* infection, the serologic response occurs later than in RMSF and MSF, and late serum samples are therefore recommended.

Treatment

Rx

Doxycycline (100 mg twice daily for adults or 4.4 mg/kg body weight per day in two divided doses for children under 45.4 kg [100 lb]) is the drug of choice for treatment. A single day of therapy usually suffices, but in adults with more severe disease, it should be administered until the patient is afebrile for 24 hours. In pregnant women, josamycin, a macrolide antimicrobial, has proved efficient at a dose of 3 g daily for 7 days for MSF; quinolones and newer macrolide antimicrobials give results comparable to those of doxycycline but with longer regimens.

Flea-Transmitted Diseases

Fleas can harbor two rickettsial species. *Rickettsia typhi*, the agent of murine typhus, and *Rickettsia felis*, the agent of flea-borne spotted fever. Both rickettsiae can be transmitted transovarially in the flea. Vectors are *Xenopsylla cheopis* and *Pulex irritans*, but also *Ctenocephalides felis*, a cat flea. Rats, cats, opossums, and dogs can propagate infected fleas. These reservoirs and vectors are distributed worldwide, and thus these diseases have a global distribution. Fleas can be infected by both species at the same time.

Murine Typhus

Definition

Maxcey distinguished murine typhus, or endemic typhus, from epidemic typhus in 1926. Fleas are usually infected by *R. typhi* when feeding on apparently healthy rats that have blood-borne infection. Humans and other mammals are infected through autoinoculation by scratching a fleabite that is contaminated with feces from an infected flea. Murine typhus, because of its cycle, is more prevalent in hot and humid areas, when rats proliferate.

Epidemiology

In the United States, 50 to 100 cases are reported yearly, mainly in southern California and southern Texas. In California, a transmission cycle involving opossums and cat fleas has been demonstrated.

Clinical Manifestations

Based on studies of infected volunteers, the incubation period is generally 8 to 16 days. The disease begins with abrupt fever, nausea, vomiting, myalgias, arthralgias, and headache. A rash is observed in 40 to 50% of patients about 6 days after the onset. It is detected even less frequently in patients with dark skin. The rash begins as pink maculae that can evolve to be maculopapular. It is often discrete, starting in the axilla; it generalizes to the trunk but does not usually involve the face, palms, and soles. In severe cases it can become purpuric. The most frequently involved organ is the lung. A third of patients have a cough, and in a fourth a nonspecific interstitial pneumonia develops that is sometimes associated with a pleural effusion. In severe forms, respiratory failure occurs. In patients with severe disease, neurologic symptoms range from confusion and stupor to coma and seizures. Cerebral hemorrhages may occur. Digestive involvement can be manifested as vomiting, abdominal pains, jaundice, and in severe cases, hematemesis.

The white blood cell count shows leukopenia and then hyperleukocytosis. Thrombocytopenia can be noted as well as anemia, specifically when hemolysis is observed (frequently in patients with G6PD deficiency). A moderate increase in serum liver enzymes is common. In patients with severe disease, hyponatremia and hypoalbuminemia are observed.

Diagnosis

The diagnosis is based mainly on serology (IFA) with titers similar to those of RMSF. Serologically, *R. typhi* cross-reacts with *R. prowazekii*; it can be differentiated either by comparing titers (two dilutions or more if IgG and IgM titers are discriminative) or by cross-adsorption. In this technique, the serum is absorbed with either antigen and then retested, and the causative agent is that removing antibodies to both bacteria. Skin biopsies and blood samples for culture and PCR may be valuable.

Treatment

Treatment is the same as that for RMSF.

Prognosis

The prognosis is usually favorable, but 10% of patients require intensive care and 1% die. Older patients and those with G6PD deficiency or chronic debilitating conditions are at higher risk.

Flea-Borne Spotted Fever Caused by Rickettsia felis

R. felis is mainly transmitted transovarially. This is a new, incompletely defined disease. The bacterium is found in fleas in the Americas, Asia, Europe, Africa, and New Zealand. Seven cases were reported from Texas, Mexico, Brazil, France, and Germany. Reported cases all exhibited fever, a rash in six of seven cases, and inoculation eschar in some cases. The diagnosis can be based on serologic evaluation using specific *R. felis* antigen or PCR of blood or skin biopsy samples. Treatment has not been established, but the bacterium is highly susceptible to doxycycline and resistant to erythromycin.

Louse and Mite Infections

Epidemic Louse-Borne Typhus

Epidemiology

The human body louse lives in clothes and multiplies rapidly when cold weather and lack of hygiene allow it to. The body louse transmits three bacterial diseases: trench fever (caused by *Bartonella quintana*), relapsing fever (caused by *Borrelia recurrentis*), and exanthematic typhus (caused by *R. prowazekii*). The name *typhus* is derived from the Greek *tuphos*, which describes the neurologic condition associated with this disease and with typhoid. The body louse is prevalent during war, in poor countries, and in the homeless population of rich countries, including the United States and Europe. A 100,000-person outbreak of typhus was reported during the civil war in Burundi in 1997, and cases were reported in Russia, Peru, the United States, Algeria, and France in the 1990s. Ch. Nicolle, who received the Nobel Prize for this discovery, demonstrated the role of the louse in transmission in 1909. Louse-transmitted diseases killed more people than weapons did during central and eastern European wars in the 19th and 20th centuries.

The epidemiology of *R. prowazekii* is mainly related to humans as reservoirs and lice as vectors. In the United States, the eastern flying squirrel *(Glaucomys volans volans)* is also a reservoir, and its fleas, lice, and mites can be infected.

R. prowazekii has also been found in *Amblyomma* ticks, but their role is not known. The louse is infected when feeding on blood, which it does five times a day. *R. prowazekii* multiplies in the gut of the louse and is released in feces; after a few days, it destroys intestinal epithelium, which causes bright red blood to spread from the gut (typhus was also named the red louse disease). The patient is usually contaminated by infected feces (in which *R. prowazekii* survives for weeks), through aerosols, or by skin autoinoculation after scratching. Patients who recover from typhus may harbor the bacterium in a dormant form and suffer relapses under stressful conditions years later; this relapsing form is called Brill-Zinsser disease. During the relapse, a bacteremia occurs that may allow the start of a new outbreak if lice bite the patient.

Clinical Manifestations

Typhus begins abruptly with fever, headaches, and myalgias, which may have led to the crouched posture termed "sutama" in the largest recent outbreak in Burundi. Cough and neurologic signs (stupor, confusion, or coma) are common. A rash is observed in 20 to 80% of patients, depending on the population studied; it is probably commonly observed on dark skin. It generally starts in the axilla and then spreads. The rash is usually macular but can be papular or purpuric in severe cases. In some cases, diarrhea and jaundice are reported. Splenomegaly is infrequently found. In severe cases, shock occurs and the fatality rate is 20 to 30%. Leukopenia, thrombocytopenia, and anemia may be noted, as well as an increase in serum hepatic enzymes.

Sylvatic typhus in the United States is caused by an *R. prowazekii* variant and is a milder disease. The most prominent clinical features are neurologic. Few cases have been described and nearly all occurred in areas where the eastern flying squirrel is found, east of the Mississippi.

Brill-Zinsser disease is hard to diagnose because rash is rare and recent exposure to lice can be lacking. Interviewing the patient may reveal prior exposure to lice, associated or not with a diagnosis of typhus in previous years. The disease is mild and the prognosis is good.

Diagnosis

The diagnosis of typhus should be considered when grouped cases of high fever with confusion are observed in patients exposed to lice. The most common diagnostic error is to attribute the findings to typhoid, which can have fatal consequences because the antimicrobials typically prescribed for that condition (β-lactams, cotrimoxazole, and quinolones) are ineffective treatment of typhus. In tropical countries, typhus is frequently confused with malaria, hemorrhagic fever, and dengue. In people with lice, it can be confused with trench fever and relapsing fever, but treatment for both can be prescribed.

The diagnosis of typhus should be clinical because the fatality rate is high and the treatment safe and efficient. Any outbreak of unexplained fever in unhygienic environments may suggest typhus, including outbreaks during civil wars (such as in Algeria, Rwanda, and Burundi), during social collapses (such as in Russia and Ukraine), in jails (such as in Rwanda and Burundi), and in chronically poor and cold countries. The diagnosis is based mainly on serology, in which there is cross-reaction with *R. typhi* (see earlier). When the investigation is performed under difficult field conditions, a drop of blood applied on filter paper and sent to a reference laboratory is valuable for serologic testing. Culture and PCR are helpful and can be performed with a skin biopsy sample or blood. Lice are good diagnostic tools because they can be tested even when dry and can be sent in closed containers without specific temperature conditions.

Treatment

Rx

Treatment of typhus is extremely simple, cheap, and effective: 200 mg of doxycycline orally in two divided doses is life-saving. Comatose patients should be treated parenterally. In allergic patients, chloramphenicol is the only known alternative, prescribed at a dose of 2 g/day for 10 days. There is no current vaccination, and the fight against lice is the major prevention strategy. Because lice are fragile, changing and boiling clothes are efficient. When this is not possible, insecticide (primarily permethrin) or invermectin orally should be used.

Scrub Typhus (Orientia tsutsugamushi)

Epidemiology

Scrub typhus is transmitted by the bite of trombiculid mite larvae infected by *O. tsutsugamushi.* These mites, also named chiggers, are vertically infected through their mother. Scrub typhus distribution is limited to a triangle extending between northern Japan, eastern Australia, and eastern Russia and includes the Far East, China, and the Indian subcontinent. All together, 1 billion people may be exposed. Seasonality is determined by the emergence of larvae. In temperate zones, it occurs mainly in autumn and to a lesser extent in spring. *O. tsutsugamushi* species have a wide heterogenicity that may allow the definition of several species, but currently a single species is recognized with many serotypes. The more frequent are Kato, Karp, Gilliam, and Kawasaki.

Clinical Manifestations

The disease occurs in patients exposed to rural or urban foci of scrub typhus after a delay of 10 or more days. The onset is usually sudden and includes fever, headache, and myalgias. Attentive examination may reveal an inoculation eschar at the site of the mite bite and tender draining lymph nodes. Generalized lymphadenopathy and rash may be observed. The symptoms vary according to organ involvement. Neuromeningeal symptoms are relatively common. Severe forms can be manifested as septic shock.

Leukopenia, thrombocytopenia, and increased levels of hepatic enzymes can occur. Evolution depends on the hosts and strains, and the fatality rate ranges from 0 to 30%. Scrub typhus is not more severe in HIV-infected patients, and surprisingly, HIV suppressive factors appear to be produced during infection. Relapses may occur in this disease.

Diagnosis

Diagnosis may be difficult. Because the clinical features are frequently not specific, epidemiologic factors are critical. A diagnosis of infectious mononucleosis has erroneously been made in patients with scrub typhus. The bacterium can be detected by culture (in cells or mice) or by PCR in blood and biopsy specimens. Serologically, the technique first used was agglutination of *Proteus mirabilis* serotype OXK in the Weil-Felix reaction. This test lacks sensitivity and specificity and should be replaced by IFA or enzyme-linked immunosorbent assay tests using the three or four major serotypes.

Treatment

Chloramphenicol was the mainstay of treatment for many years, but now doxycycline is recommended. Single-day treatment with doxycycline is followed by relapses, and even repeated treatment for 2 days at a 7-day interval does not prevent all relapses. Hence, the currently recommended regimen is doxycycline, 100 mg orally twice a day, for 7 days. Cases resistant to doxycycline have been reported, and rifampin (600 mg orally daily) is a reasonable alternative. Prophylaxis is based on the use of repellents.

Rickettsialpox (Rickettsia akari)

Epidemiology

Rickettsialpox was first described in New York City, where it is still prevalent, by a general practitioner in 1946. *R. akari*, the causal agent, is transmitted by the bite of the mouse mite *(Liponyssoides sanguineus).* Its prevalence is probably underestimated; an active search revealed 13 cases in a New York hospital in the 1980s. Cases have been reported in Arizona, Utah, and Ohio. After the terrorist attacks of 9/11/01, cases of black skin eschars were investigated as possible anthrax in New York but were in fact rickettsialpox. High seroprevalence was reported among intravenous drug users in Baltimore. Cases have also been reported from Russia, Ukraine, Slovenia, and Korea.

Clinical Manifestations

Ten days after the mite bite, the beginning of the illness is marked by fever, headache, and myalgia. Careful examination reveals an inoculation eschar and a draining lymphadenopathy that could be mistaken for cutaneous anthrax. Two to 6 days later, a rash appears and comprises 5 to 40 macular, then papular and vesicular spots. This aspect led to the name of the disease. It is frequently mistaken for chickenpox. The disease is usually mild.

Diagnosis

The diagnosis can be made by serologic testing with IFA. Specific antigens react with high titer, but antibodies to other rickettsia may be detected. The diagnosis may also be made on skin specimens by culture, immunodetection, or PCR.

Treatment

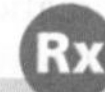

The prescription of doxycycline is highly efficient in these patients. Prevention is based on the control of mice.

EHRLICHIOSES AND ANAPLASMOSES

Definition

The first ehrlichial infection diagnosed in human beings was reported in Japan in the late 1950s in patients with mononucleosis. In retrospect, the outbreak was found to be attributable to the ingestion of local raw fish (gray mullet) parasitized by *Ehrlichia*-infected worms.

The index case of modern ehrlichiosis was reported in the United States in 1987. The patient died of fever, presumably acquired after a tick bite in Arkansas, despite receiving chloramphenicol. The patient had several initially confusing diagnostic features: on blood smears, morulae in polymorphonuclear (PMN) cells were seen, and antibodies to *Ehrlichia canis,* a pathogen of dogs but not humans, were detected. He was then thought to have *Ehrlichia chaffeensis,* but this bacterium infects monocytes, not PMN cells. A diagnosis of *Anaplasma phagocytophila* (or human granulocytic *Ehrlichia* [HGE]), was considered, but the tick vector of this disease is absent in Arkansas. The most likely diagnosis is currently believed to be infection with *Ehrlichia ewingii,* an agent transmitted by *Amblyomma americanum* that is prevalent in Arkansas, infects PMN cells, and cross-reacts with *E. canis,* although it typically affects immunocompromised hosts. This case illustrates the progress in knowledge on ehrlichioses and how difficult it is to conclude the etiology of an atypical infection definitively on the basis of serology alone.

All *Ehrlichia* pathogenic for humans except *E. ewingii* can be cultured. The ehrlichiae have been reclassified into four genera, mainly on the basis of 16S ribosomal RNA–derived phylogenetic analysis. Two are the tick-associated genera *Ehrlichia* and *Anaplasma* (*A. phagocytophila,* or the HGE agent that was formerly named *Ehrlichia phagocytophila*). One is a helminth-associated genus, *Neorickettsia,* including *N. sennetsu* (formerly *Rickettsia sennetsu,* then *Ehrlichia sennetsu*). The fourth is *Wolbachia pipientis,* a bacterium associated with arthropods (insects, crustaceans, and acarids) and helminth worms (mainly filaria). These organisms elicit cross-reactive antibodies.

Ehrlichiae multiply exclusively in vacuoles of their eukaryotic cell host, where they form clusters known as morulae. The vacuoles are derived from phagosomes and help the organism escape bactericidal lysosomal fusion. In humans, ehrlichiae are associated with monocytes (*E. chaffeensis, E. canis, N. sennetsu*) or PMN cells (*A. phagocytophila, E. ewingii*).

Ehrlichioses can be acquired through tick bites, by ingesting nematodes via contaminated water or animals (fish, snails), or as a consequence of filariasis.

American Human Monocytic Ehrlichiosis *(Ehrlichia chaffeensis)*

Epidemiology

Human monocytic ehrlichiosis (HME) is caused by *E. chaffeensis.* This organism has been isolated or identified by PCR only in the United States, mainly in the southeastern, south central, and mid-Atlantic states and California (Table 348–3). Many publications report the presence of antibodies to *E. chaffeensis* in Europe, Asia, and Africa. However, because of the cross-reactions among *Ehrlichia,* these findings do not allow one to infer an extension of the distribution of *E. chaffeensis.* In the United States, the American tick *A. americanum* (Lone Star tick) is the vector and the white-tailed deer is the main mammalian reservoir. Immature ticks are infected by blood while feeding on persistently bacteremic reservoirs. *E. chaffeensis* is transmitted trans-stadially in the tick and infects its next host (deer or human) during its next blood meal. The disease epidemiology reflects the tick habitat and activity, with most cases being contracted in the southern United States, in rural areas, and from April to September. In highly endemic areas, the incidence can reach 100 cases per 100,000 inhabitants. The severity is age dependent, which may explain the lower incidence reported in children. Males are more often affected than females, with a sex ratio of 4:1.

Clinical Manifestations

The incubation lasts for 7 to 10 days after an identified tick exposure in 80% of cases. Patients have fever, headache, malaise, nausea, and anorexia. Untreated patients worsen and may require intensive care. Digestive tract involvement consisting of nausea, vomiting, diarrhea, and abdominal pains is common. Central nervous system infection is manifested in many forms from confusion to coma. A rash is observed in a third of cases and lymphadenopathy in a fourth. In severe forms, sepsis syndrome and MODS may occur.

The white blood cell count typically shows leukopenia, caused by both lymphopenia and neutropenia. Thrombocytopenia is also frequently noticed; anemia may appear later. Coagulopathy may be observed in severe forms. Increases in serum enzymes, including AST, ALT, and LDH, may reflect organ involvement, as does creatininemia. CSF examination in patients with neurologic symptoms reveals pleocytosis and increased protein levels. Cells may be monocytic or PMN. The prognosis depends on early antimicrobial treatment, but the fatality rate is still high at 2.5%. In persons coinfected with HIV it may be most severe; in one series, 6 of 13 patients died.

Diagnosis

The diagnosis of HME should be considered in patients with a history of tick exposure and unexplained fever. HME resembles RMSF, but rash

TABLE 348–3 EHRLICHIOSES

Disease	Agent	Vector	Geographic Repartition
American monocytic ehrlichiosis	*Ehrlichia chaffeensis*	*Amblyomma americanum*	South central, southeastern, mid-Atlantic coastal states
Human granulocytic ehrlichiosis	*Anaplasma phagocytophila*	*Ixodes ricinus* *Ixodes scapularis*	Europe Northeast, upper Midwest, northern California
E. ewingii	*Ehrlichia ewingii*	*Amblyomma americanum*	South central, southeastern, mid-Atlantic coastal states
Japanese monocytic ehrlichiosis	*Neorickettsia sennetsu*	Helminth of the gray mullet?	Japan
E. canis	*Ehrlichia canis*	*Rhipicephalus sanguineus*	Venezuela

is less frequent. Later in the disease it can be misdiagnosed as anything that causes severe sepsis.

Leukopenia associated with thrombocytopenia and an increase in liver enzyme levels may establish the etiology. Careful examination of blood and CSF smears may help identify typical morulae. Treatment should be started in any suspected case. The diagnosis can be confirmed by culture in specialized laboratories using a canine cell line, DH82. However, PCR is more practical; confirmatory PCR using a second target gene is useful. Most cases are currently diagnosed serologically by a fourfold or greater increase in antibody titer or by seroconversion. The reference technique is IFA. A single titer of 25 is indicative of the diagnosis. There are cross-reactive antibodies among *Ehrlichia* species and with *A. phagocytophila.* Western blotting may be valuable to distinguish among these bacteria.

Treatment

Rx

Doxycycline (100 mg twice daily for adults) is the drug of choice for patients with ehrlichiosis. The optimal duration of therapy has not been established, but current regimens recommend continuation of treatment for at least 3 days after the fever subsides and until evidence of clinical improvement, for a minimum total course of 5 to 7 days. Severe or complicated disease may require longer treatment courses. Because tetracyclines are contraindicated in pregnancy, rifampin has been used successfully in a limited number of pregnant women with documented HGE.

Human Granulocytic Ehrlichiosis *(Anaplasma phagocytophila)*

Epidemiology

A. phagocytophila was identified in ungulates in the 1930s as an agent causing chronic neutropenia and consequent superinfections. The first human case was recognized in 1990. The disease is found in America and in Europe (Fig. 348–4). It is transmitted by *Ixodes scapularis* (eastern North America), *Ixodes pacificus* (western North America), *Ixodes ricinus* (Europe), and *Ixodes persulcatus* (Asia), the vectors of Lyme disease, and its epidemiology is similar. Coinfection with the two diseases may occur. The temporal distribution of the disease parallels that of nymph tick activity, with two peaks in spring and autumn. Ticks are born free of *Ehrlichia* and are infected while feeding on bacteremic small mammals. Deer play a major role as hosts of adult ticks and reservoirs. In highly endemic areas, the incidence can reach 50 per 100,000 inhabitants per year. The mean age of diagnosed patients is high, and males are more frequently infected than females, with a sex ratio of 3:1.

Clinical Manifestations

The incubation time is usually between 7 and 10 days, and 80% of patients report a history of tick exposure. Many infections may be asymptomatic or too mild to require a diagnostic procedure. The disease frequently begins abruptly, with fever, headache, malaise, and myalgias that may be particularly severe. Rash is found in less than 10% of cases. Visceral involvement may be observed and includes digestive symptoms such as nausea, vomiting, and diarrhea. Neurologic symptoms may include confusion, meningitis, and meningoencephalitis.

The evolution of the disease is favorable in most cases, even without specific therapy, but in some patients the disease may evolve to septic shock. Patients with underlying diseases are more at risk of dying. Most deaths are the consequence of *Ehrlichia*-induced immunosuppression, and patients may experience invasive aspergillosis, candidiasis, cryptococcosis, and herpes esophagitis.

Diagnosis

Laboratory findings consist of the association of thrombocytopenia and leukopenia (lymphopenia and/or neutropenia). An increase in serum transaminases is also frequent. The diagnosis can be made by careful examination of blood smears for morulae within PMN cells. Culture from blood is possible in appropriate cells (HL-60), and PCR is useful as for HME. Most cases are diagnosed by serologic testing with IFA, which is comparable to that in HME (see earlier).

Treatment

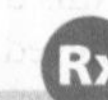

Treatment is also similar to that for HME except that *A. phagocytophila* is susceptible to fluoroquinolones in vitro, but these drugs have not been tested in patients.

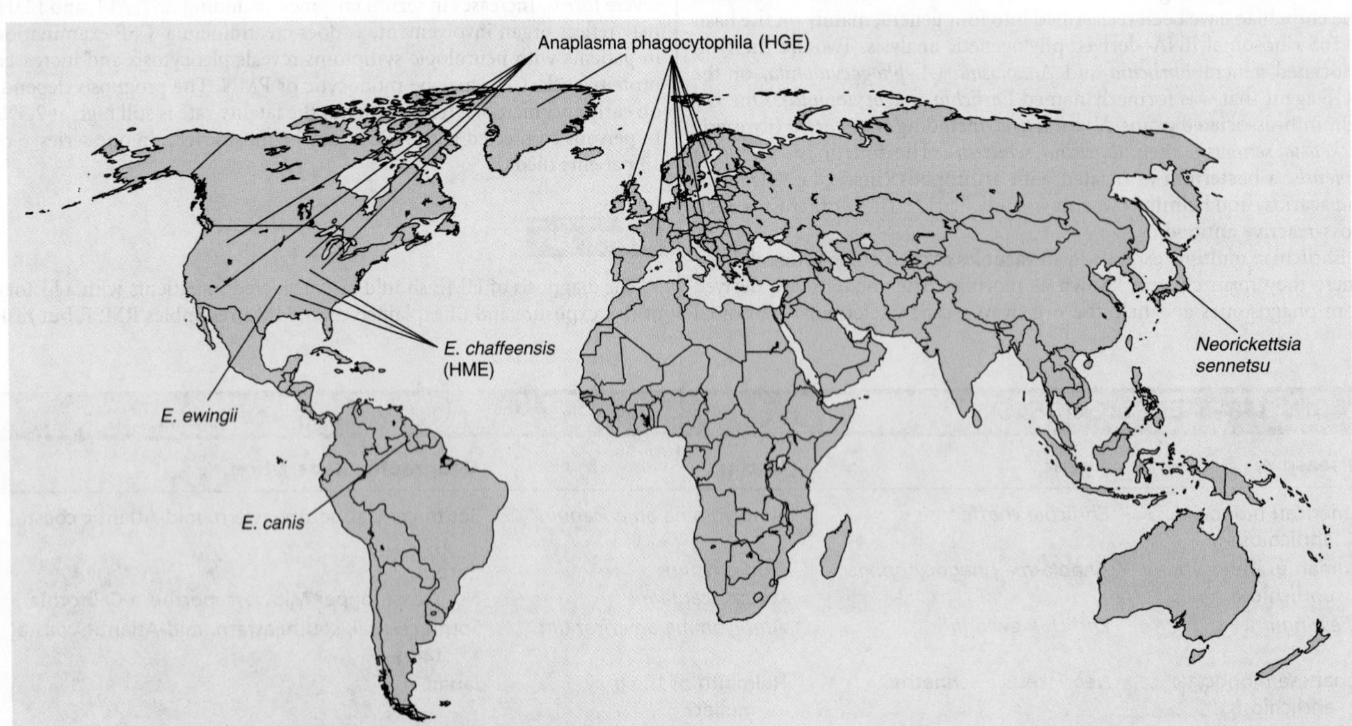

FIGURE 348–4 • Geographic repartition of ehrlichioses. HGE = human granulocytic ehrlichiosis; HME = human monocytic ehrlichiosis.

Ehrlichia ewingii

Canine granulocytic ehrlichiosis, reported in the United States in 1972, is caused by *E. ewingii.* This bacterium was characterized by amplification and sequencing of the 16S ribosomal RNA gene. The vector of *E. ewingii* is *A. americanum,* which also transmits *E. chaffeensis.* Among 60 cases of ehrlichiosis in Missouri in 1999, 4 were caused by *E. ewingii;* 4 other cases have been reported since by the CDC. The disease was prevalent in immunocompromised hosts (seven of eight) coinfected with HIV or receiving immunosuppressive drugs. Patients who report tick exposure are noted to have fever, thrombocytopenia, leukopenia, and various symptoms, including meningitis. Morulae may be seen on blood smears in PMN cells. The evolution in reported cases was good; patients responded dramatically to doxycycline. Patients have antibodies to *E. chaffeensis,* and PCR has been shown to be useful when applied to blood samples. This diagnosis should be considered when ehrlichiosis is suspected in immunocompromised patients exposed to *A. americanum* ticks.

Ehrlichia canis

Canine monocytic ehrlichiosis was reported first in Algeria in the 1930s. It is caused by *E. canis* and transmitted by the dog tick *R. sanguineus.* This tick is found worldwide and is prevalent in temperate and hot areas. In 1996, a single case of infection was reported in an asymptomatic man from Venezuela who owned an infected dog. Recently, cases have been reported in patients in South America.

Wolbachia Species

Wolbachia bacteria are endosymbionts of arthropods and nematodes. They were known to be present in filarial worms, but it was later shown that they may play a role in human disease. These bacteria manipulate the fertility of their host. Eradication of *Wolbachia* in filaria may lead to infertility and stop the microfilaria from spreading. This effect was demonstrated by field treatment with doxycycline in patients with onchocerciasis. The patients improved when treated with this drug, which is effective on *Wolbachia* and subsequently on the worm's fertility but not on the worm itself. In 2001 it was shown that the adverse reactions observed after treatment of lymphatic filariasis may be caused by the release of *Wolbachia* from destroyed worms. Some authors suggested that eradicating *Wolbachia* before the anthelmintic prescription would avoid these reactions.

Q FEVER

Definition

Q fever is a worldwide zoonosis caused by *Coxiella burnetii.* The name Q fever is derived from "query" to emphasize the surprising aspect of the disease first described in Queensland, Australia, in 1935 by Derrick. The infection in humans is variable in its severity, clinical expression, and natural course (i.e., acute or chronic). It is considered by the CDC to be a potential agent of bioterrorism. Ungulates and pets are the major sources of human infection.

The Pathogen

C. burnetii is a gram-negative bacterium that naturally infects its host's monocytes. It multiplies in an acidic vacuole. Strains are heterogeneous genetically and antigenically and are associated with acute infections of variable severity. *C. burnetii* in vitro generates a deleted, avirulent mutant also named phase II. This mutant exhibits diagnostic antigens that are useful because they are more reactive during acute infection.

C. burnetii is incompletely eliminated after acute infection in immunocompromised hosts and patients with cardiac valve lesions. *C. burnetii* continues to multiply despite high levels of antibodies and causes chronic infection. In patients with endocarditis, the level of interleukin-10 (an immunosuppressive cytokine) is elevated and monocytes are unable to control *C. burnetii* growth. Control of the disease in acute Q fever is associated with the constitution of a granuloma.

Epidemiology

C. burnetii infects a wide range of animals, including mammals, birds, and ticks. Ungulates and pets (cats and dogs) are the most common source of the disease. Mammals are infected through aerosols and may shed *Coxiella* in feces, urine, milk, and birth products. Humans are usually infected by aerosols or less frequently by exposure to milk products. Interhuman infections through sexual intercourse, during delivery, or by blood transfusion have been reported. *Coxiella* survives in the environment and can be spread far by the wind. In the past few years, major outbreaks were related to sheep and goats. The disease is partly seasonal and related to lambing time. The current geographic repartition is largely unknown. Males have more severe disease but are not more often exposed to Q fever, and middle-aged people are more frequently affected and hospitalized.

Clinical Manifestations

After contamination by *C. burnetii,* 60% of patients seroconvert without apparent disease, 38% experience a self-limited disease, and only 2% require diagnostic evaluation. Months to years after the primary infection, a chronic infection associated with an immunocompromised situation, a cardiac valve lesion, or a vascular prosthesis or aneurysm develops in 0.2 to 0.5% of patients.

Patients with diagnosed acute infection may have a variety of symptoms (Table 348–4). Isolated prolonged fever was observed in 14% of more than 1000 patients. Pneumonia was found in 37% and was the only symptom in 17%. This percentage may vary according to the place of study and reach 90% of diagnosed cases. Some cases may be associated with respiratory distress. Hepatitis is found in 60% of patients and is the sole manifestation in 40%. The association of fever and a moderate

TABLE 348–4 SITUATIONS THAT SHOULD PROMPT SEROLOGIC TESTING FOR Q FEVER

ACUTE Q FEVER (PHASE II ANTIGEN AND IgG ≥200 AND IgM ≥50)
Fever in a patient in contact with ungulates
Unexplained prolonged fever (>7 days)
Granulomatous hepatitis
Fever and thrombocytopenia
Meningoencephalitis
Myocarditis
Erythema nodosum
Fever during pregnancy
Fever in a patient in contact with a parturient pet
Unexplained atypical pneumonia
Fever and an increase in transaminases (2–5 times the normal level)
Aseptic meningitis
Guillain-Barré syndrome
Pericarditis
Spontaneous abortion
CHRONIC Q FEVER (PHASE I ANTIGEN AND IgG ≥800 AND IgA ≥100)
Blood culture–negative endocarditis
Patient with a valvulopathy and unexplained
Fever
Weight loss
Fatigue
Increased erythrocyte sedimentation rate
Increased transaminases
Thrombocytopenia
Patient with unusually rapid degradation of a prosthetic valve
Fever in a patient with a vascular aneurysm or prosthesis
Aseptic osteomyelitis
Chronic pericarditis
Multiple spontaneous abortions

increase in transaminases is an important clue. Some hepatitides, specifically in middle-aged men, are associated with an inflammatory syndrome and autoantibodies and may be resistant to antimicrobial treatment. Liver biopsy, when performed, exhibits granulomas that may be typified by a lipid vacuole and surrounded by a fibrinoid ring in the form of a doughnut. Less frequently, in 1.5% of cases, patients exhibit a rash. Patients can have specific neurologic manifestations such as meningitis, encephalitis, meningoencephalitis, or peripheral neuropathy. In 1 to 2% of cases, patients have cardiovascular manifestations such as pericarditis or more rarely myocarditis.

Evolution is usually favorable even without treatment, except in special hosts. In pregnant women, symptomatic or not, Q fever compromises the pregnancy. When infected during the first trimester, the patient usually aborts spontaneously. When the patient is infected later, the disease can result in fetal death or prematurity, or the outcome may be normal. Chronic uterine infection may develop in half the patients infected during pregnancy, and they may later experience multiple spontaneous abortions. Thirty to 50% of patients with heart valve or vascular lesions may experience chronic endocarditis within 2 years. This evolution is not prevented by regular treatment.

Patients with Q fever endocarditis have a chronic infection with low-grade fever, progressive degradation of valve function, and progressive heart failure. Fever is intermittent, and vegetations are frequently absent on cardiac echocardiography. Endocarditis is therefore not frequently considered in the initial differential diagnosis. If not diagnosed, the disease progressively worsens and emboli (mainly cerebral) may be observed, as well as renal insufficiency, splenomegaly, and hepatomegaly. Digital clubbing may also be seen. The main clue to the diagnosis in a patient with a valvulopathy is unexplained sickness (unexplained fatigue, weight loss, fever), a biologic abnormality (leukopenia, increased erythrocyte sedimentation rate, thrombocytopenia, increase in hepatic enzymes), or rapid degradation of a prosthetic valve. Chronic osteomyelitis, hepatitis, and infection of an aneurysm and vascular prosthesis have been reported.

Leukopenia may be observed; thrombocytopenia is frequent, as are increases in hepatic enzymes. Circulating anticoagulant associated with antiphospholipid antibodies may be observed, as may anti–smooth muscle antibodies. During endocarditis, antinuclear antibodies, microhematuria, and rheumatoid factor are frequently found.

Diagnosis

The diagnosis is based mainly on serology (see Table 348–4). Direct detection by culture and PCR or immunochemistry in valve, liver, or blood samples is also useful, but serologic evaluation by IFA is the best method. Two antigens (phase I and phase II) can be tested. Acute Q fever is diagnosed when seroconversion or a fourfold increase is obtained with phase II antigen. A single serum test exhibiting IgG antibodies of 200 or greater and IgM of 50 or greater against phase II is also diagnostic. During chronic Q fever, antibodies are at higher titer and directed against both phase I and phase II. IgG against phase I at a titer of 800 or 1600 is diagnostic of chronic infection, as is IgA at 100 or greater. Serology is useful for follow-up of patients with acute Q fever and underlying disease and those with treated chronic Q fever.

Treatment

Rx

Treatment is easy during acute Q fever. Doxycycline is the most efficient antimicrobial, and it should be prescribed for 2 weeks. Some patients with hepatitis do not respond well because of an excessive immune response. They rapidly improve with a short course of glucocorticoids. In pregnant women, cotrimoxazole during the entire pregnancy may decrease the chance of an unfavorable outcome. As for endocarditis, bactericidal treatment is necessary. In vitro, antimicrobial efficacy is impaired by the low pH of the vacuole in which *C. burnetii* resides. Hydroxychloroquine increases the pH of this vacuole and restores the bactericidal effect of doxycycline. In patients with endocarditis, the recommended treatment is a combination of doxycycline (200 mg daily) and hydroxychloroquine (600 mg/day, then adjusted to reach a 1-mg/mL plasma concentration). This regimen is prescribed for 18 to 36 months according to serologic results. We recently observed that a more rapid favorable outcome was obtained with doxycycline serum levels higher than 5 μg/mL. Some strains may be resistant to doxycycline, and new macrolides may be an alternative. The major problem with this treatment is photosensitivity; sun exposure should be avoided. An alternative treatment is a combination of doxycycline and ofloxacin for 3 or more years.

Prevention

Prevention is based on veterinary control in animals. A vaccine is currently available in Australia.

SUGGESTED READINGS

Bakken JS, Dumler JS: Clinical diagnosis and treatment of human granulocytotropic anaplasmosis. Ann NY Acad Sci 2006;1078:236–247. *An overview of the diagnosis and treatment of human granulocytotropic anaplasmosis.*

Lacz NL, Schwartz RA, Kapila R: Rocky Mountain spotted fever. J Eur Acad Dermatol Venereol 2006;20:411–417. *A comprehensive review.*

Masters EJ, Olson GS, Weiner SJ, et al: Rocky Mountain spotted fever: A clinician's dilemma. Arch Intern Med 2003;163:769–774. *Treatment with doxycycline must be based on clinical suspicion even in the absence of a petechial rash or history of a known tick bite.*

Maurin M, Bakken JS, Dumler JS: Antimicrobial susceptibilities of *Anaplasma (Ehrlichia) phagocytophilum* strains from various geographic areas in the United States. Antimicrob Agents Chemother 2003;47:413–415. *Doxycycline, rifampin, and levofloxacin are recommended.*

Parker NR, Barralet JH, Bell AM, et al: Q fever. Lancet 2006;367:679–688. *A comprehensive review.*

Parola P, Raoult D: Ticks and tickborne bacterial diseases in humans: An emerging infectious threat. Clin Infect Dis 2001;32:897–928. *A review of ticks as reservoirs and vectors of infectious diseases.*

Parola P, Raoult D: Tropical rickettsioses. Clin Dermatol 2006;24:191–200. *An overview of scrub typhus, murine typhus, and epidemic typhus as well as an update on the emerging tropical rickettsioses.*

Rolain JM, Boulos A, Mallet MN, Raoult D: Correlation between ratio of serum doxycycline concentration to MIC and rapid decline of antibody levels during treatment of Q fever endocarditis. Antimicrob Agents Chemother 2005; 49:2673–2676. *The latest study on treatment on Q fever endocarditis.*

349 ZOONOSES

Stuart Levin

Definition

Zoonoses are most simply defined as human infections derived from animals. Approximately 200 different infectious agents, many of them rare, cause disease in humans and fulfill the definition of a zoonosis. The more than 50 million dogs in the United States facilitate the transmission of over 50 infectious agents and cause more than 1 million bite injuries each year. There is an even greater number of cats in the United States, and more than 40 infectious diseases have been transmitted by them. In addition, the list of exotic pets, including ferrets, monkeys, and reptiles, continues to grow. Almost all arthropod-transmitted infectious agents in the United States are due to either ticks or mosquitoes, with ticks being the more common villain and Lyme disease (Chapter 342) being the most common arthropod-transmitted infectious disease in the United States.

Epidemiology

The risk of contracting a zoonosis is increased by direct animal contact; in meat handlers, poachers, hunters, exotic animal smugglers, and inter-

Section XXIII Infectious Diseases

national travelers; by exposure to and inhalation of infectious air particles; by insect bites, contact with previously infected human blood products, and contact with and ingestion of infectious agents transmitted by animal-contaminated water; and by insufficiently cooked meat, eggs, dairy products, fish, and shellfish. Raw shellfish, which are the "garbage filters" of the ocean, can transmit at least 25 different infectious or toxic illnesses to humans. Ticks not infrequently introduce more than one pathogen while feeding; Lyme disease (Chapter 342), ehrlichiosis (Chapter 348), and babesiosis (Chapter 374) can all be transmitted by a single tick bite. Threats from mosquito bites include malaria (Chapter 366) and West Nile virus (Chapter 405). Farmers, pet owners, hunters, laboratory researchers, cave explorers, hikers, and veterinarians, among others, are at higher risk for a zoonosis than the general population is. Infectious agents transmitted by these routes from animal sources essentially include members of all microbial classes: viruses, bacteria, fungi, and parasites. Immunocompromised hosts such as splenectomized patients, transplant recipients, patients with acquired immunodeficiency syndrome (AIDS), and pregnant women and their fetuses are at higher risk for clinical disease when exposed to these various infectious agents.

As the world shrinks, warms, flattens, and remains in conflict, new infectious diseases seem inevitable, and previously rare ones are seen in unexpected places (Table 349–1) because of global warming trends, human intrusion into previously underexplored or never-explored sites, world travel, and an increasing threat of biologic terrorism or warfare.

Clinical Manifestations

Zoonoses can be manifested as a variety of clinical syndromes, including respiratory disease (Table 349–2), central nervous system disease (Table 349–3), and rash or skin lesions (Table 349–4).

Emerging zoonotic infectious diseases include Nipah virus and Hendra virus encephalitis (Chapter 439), Hantavirus pneumonia (Chapter 97), the coronavirus that causes severe acute respiratory syndrome (SARS; Chapter 97), the 3-year coast-to-coast spread of West Nile encephalitis in the United States, the monkeypox (Chapter 395) outbreak in the upper Midwest from pet prairie dogs, the identification of at least 8 to 10 new tick-borne rickettsial spotted fever rickettsioses worldwide, and the flea-borne *Rickettsia felis* in California (Chapter 348). Avian or "bird flu" (H5N1; Chapter 387), SARS, monkeypox, and West Nile fever have recently exposed the smallness of our world village. Nevertheless, zoonoses remain a less frequent cause of fever in travelers (Chapter 308) than the well-known gastrointestinal and pulmonary pathogens.

Diagnosis

Non–animal-associated environment- or travel-related infectious diseases can be confused with zoonoses. The vast majority of clinical diseases caused by *Legionella pneumophila, Plasmodium falciparum, Entamoeba histolytica, Giardia lamblia, Burkholderia pseudomallei, Chromobacterium violaceum, Aeromonas hydrophila,* and airborne fungi such as *Blastomyces dermatitidis, Coccidioides immitis,* and *Histoplasma capsulatum* are acquired through environmental exposure and are only rarely related to animal hosts. *Sporothrix schenckii,* almost always an environmentally acquired pathogen stemming from vegetation injuries, has also been transmitted from cats with draining cutaneous ulcers to owners and animal handlers. Histoplasmosis has been acquired by explorers (spelunkers) in caves contaminated by bat guano. Other non-infectious toxin-induced diseases acquired from animals and insects, such as tick paralysis and the fish toxin illnesses (Chapter 382), do not represent zoonoses.

Unfortunately, some descriptive disease titles can be misleading to clinicians and can thus interfere with considering the correct diagnosis. The transmission of tick-borne Rocky Mountain spotted fever actually occurs much more commonly in the southeastern United States than in the Rocky Mountains and has even occurred in the middle of New York City. Urban New York City continues as a major source of rickettsialpox

TABLE 349–1 NEWER ZOONOSES IN THE UNITED STATES

Disease*	Infectious Agent	Clinical Information	Vector/Acquisition	See Chapter
Ehrlichiosis, monocytic	*Ehrlichia chaffeensis*	Fever, myalgia, leukopenia, monocyte inclusions not often seen, maculopapular rash	*Amblyomma* (Lone Star) tick bite	348
Human granulocytic anaplasmosis (HGE)	*Anaplasma phagocytophilium*	Fever, myalgia, leukopenia, granulocyte inclusions often seen on blood smear	*Ixodes* (deer) tick bite	348
"Flu syndrome"	*Ehrlichia ewingii*	Immunocompromised host—fever, myalgia	*Amblyomma*	348
Cat-scratch disease	*Bartonella* species	Cervical lymphadenopathy in normal hosts and cutaneous and hepatic angiomatosis in AIDS patients	Cat scratch or bite	336
Hemorrhagic diarrhea	Enterohemorrhagic *Escherichia coli* O157:H7 (other species)	Rectal bleeding, dysentery, hemolytic-uremic syndrome	Contaminated, undercooked meat	327
Hantavirus pulmonary syndrome (HPV)	Hantavirus—Sin Nombre	Noncardiac pulmonary edema, elevated hematocrit	Fomites of wild rodents	404
Cryptosporidium diarrhea	*Cryptosporidium parvum*	Prolonged watery diarrhea	Contaminated water—cattle and sheep	371
Dysentery	*Campylobacter jejuni*	Dysentery, Reiter's syndrome, Guillain-Barré syndrome	Contaminated chicken	326
Pyogenic skin ulcer	*Capnocytophaga canimorsus*	Sepsis, skin infection	Dog bites	
West Nile fever encephalitis	West Nile virus	Encephalitis, myelitis, Guillain-Barré syndrome	Mosquito bite, birds	405, 406
SARS	Coronavirus	Severe lower respiratory tract infection	Civet cat (presumed)	389

*See table of contents and index to locate a more detailed discussion of each disease.
AIDS = acquired immunodeficiency syndrome; SARS = severe acute respiratory syndrome.

TABLE 349–2 RESPIRATORY TRACT ZOONOSES

Disease*	Microorganism†	Clinical Syndrome	Reservoir and/or Vector	See Chapter
Psittacosis‡	*Chlamydia psittaci*	Pneumonia, often severe	Aerosols from parrots, ducks, turkeys	339
Q fever	*Coxiella burnetii*	Pneumonia, hepatitis, or myocarditis	Airborne from soil contaminated by sheep, goats, and cats, particularly if parturient	348
Tularemia	*Francisella tularensis*	Cutaneous ulcer and regional node, pneumonia and hilar node; pleural effusion	Rabbit contact (winter) and tick bites	332
Plague	*Yersinia pestis*	Inguinal nodes, bubonic plague (basilar pneumonia develops in 10%); hilar node enlargement	Fleas from prairie dogs, rock squirrels, rats	333
Hantavirus syndrome	*Hantavirus*	Upper respiratory to lower respiratory to adult respiratory distress syndrome to death	Deer mouse fomites: urine, feces, saliva	404
Rhodococcus pneumonia	*Rhodococcus equi*	Pneumonia often cavitates in patients with AIDS and other immunosuppressed patients	Horse manure, soil	
Mycoplasma arginini pneumonia	*Mycoplasma arginini*	Pneumonia, sepsis, neutropenia	Sheep, goats	338
Foot-and-mouth disease	*Aphthovirus*	Nonspecific upper respiratory tract infection, oral vesicles	Cloven-footed mammals	402
Whooping cough	*Bordetella bronchiseptica*	Pneumonia, bronchitis, whooping cough	Dogs	334
Histoplasmosis	*Histoplasma capsulatum*	Pneumonia or fever of unknown origin	Bats	353
Anthrax	*Bacillus anthracis*	Mediastinal widening, CT scan pneumonia often absent	Herbivores	317
Glanders	*Burkholderia mallei*	Pneumonia, erosive tracheobronchitis	Horses, mules	328

*See table of contents and index to locate a more detailed discussion of each disease.
†Because of the fastidious nature of some organisms, the rapid development of diagnostic tools, and the risk that some agents pose to laboratory workers, we recommend that a clinical microbiologist be consulted if these agents are considered in a patient's differential diagnosis.
‡Occurs in more than 1000 animal species.
AIDS = acquired immunodeficiency syndrome; CT = computed tomography.

TABLE 349–3 CENTRAL NERVOUS SYSTEM INFECTION: ZOONOSES

Disease*	Organism	Clinical Syndrome and Diagnosis	Acquisition	See Chapter
Listeriosis	*Listeria monocytogenes*	Purulent meningitis during pregnancy, in patients older than 65 yr, and in neonates; immunosuppressed	Unpasteurized cheese and other dairy products; cattle, goats	316
Leptospirosis	*Leptospira interrogans*	Aseptic meningitis, hepatorenal syndrome	Asymptomatic dogs, cattle; common water source	344
Herpes B encephalitis	Cercopithecine herpesvirus (herpes B virus)	Diffuse, progressive encephalitis	*Macaca* monkey bites or scratches	397
Lyme disease	*Borrelia burgdorferi*	Lymphocytic meningitis, motor-sensory neuropathy, facial palsy	Acquired from tick bites	342
Lymphocytic choriomeningitis	Lymphocytic choriomeningitis virus	Lymphocytic meningitis, occasionally with pneumonia	Inhalation of mouse secretions: urine, feces, saliva	439
Mosquito-borne encephalitis, United States	Eastern, Western equine encephalitis; St. Louis, California encephalitis; West Nile virus	Diffuse encephalitis, least severe; California encephalitis, most severe; Eastern equine encephalitis	Mosquito-borne from horses, birds	439
Rabies encephalitis	Rabies virus	Almost always fatal; encephalitis	Bites from dogs, skunks, bats, raccoons, foxes	441
Toxoplasmosis	*Toxoplasma gondii*	CNS, multiple brain masses, AIDS patient	Cat feces or ingestion of undercooked lamb or pork	370

TABLE 349–3 CENTRAL NERVOUS SYSTEM INFECTION: ZOONOSES—cont'd

Disease*	Organism	Clinical Syndrome and Diagnosis	Acquisition	See Chapter
Cerebral cysticercosis	*Taenia solium*	Epilepsy, CNS cysts, eosinophilic meningitis, hydrocephalus	Fecal-oral; contamination of food with pork tapeworm eggs	375
New-variant Creutzfeldt-Jakob disease	Prion (proteinaceous infectious particle)	Dementia, ataxia, and myoclonus	Beef from cattle fed scraps from contaminated sheep carcasses	442
Nipah virus	Paramyxovirus	Acute encephalitis, death	Pig contact	439
Hendra virus	Paramyxovirus	Pneumonitis, encephalitis	Horses, fruit bats	439

*See table of contents and index to locate a more detailed discussion of each disease.
AIDS = acquired immunodeficiency syndrome; CNS = central nervous system.

TABLE 349–4 RASH OR SKIN NODULE-ULCER: ZOONOSES

Disease*	Microorganism†	Clinical Information And Diagnosis	Reservoir and/or Vector	See Chapter
Ehrlichiosis	*Ehrlichia chaffeensis* (monocytic)	Macular rash (seen in less than a third of patients), central distribution; in south central United States	Tick bite	349
Leptospirosis	*Leptospira interrogans*	Central macular rash in 20%, with occasional enanthem, conjunctival suffusion, hepatorenal syndrome	Urine-contaminated water; dogs, cattle	344
Lyme disease	*Borrelia burgdorferi*	Primary lesion is erythema migrans; 40% have multiple lesions	Mouse reservoir—tick bite	342
Rocky Mountain spotted fever	*Rickettsia rickettsii*	Acral or peripheral distribution of maculopapular to hemorrhagic rash to gangrenous lesions—no eschar	Tick bite	348, 406
Typhus (epidemic)	*Rickettsia prowazekii*	Central distribution, macular rash (can be hemorrhagic)	Flying squirrel fleas or fomites	348
Scabies	*Sarcoptes scabiei*	Pruritic macules on trunk; skin burrow	Dogs—close contact. Up to a third of asymptomatic dogs have mite infection	380
Flea bite dermatitis	*Pulex irritans*	Pruritic papules, urticarial vesicles; fleas found on pets or in the environment	Fleas on dogs	380
Cat-scratch disease	*Bartonella* species	Bacillary angiomatosis, peliosis hepatitis, cervical adenopathy, subacute bacterial endocarditis, and fever of unknown origin	Cat scratch or bite	336
Tularemia	*Francisella tularensis*	Ulcer and node, typhoidal syndrome, pneumonia	Rabbit contact and tick bite	332
Anthrax	*Bacillus anthracis*	Painless, edematous, nonpurulent ulcer, mediastinitis	Herbivore, infected animal product	317
Rickettsialpox	*Rickettsia akari*	Fever, rash, eschar (multiple)	Mouse mite	348
"Spotted fever *Rickettsia*"	*Rickettsia conorii, Rickettsia africae*—8 others, all continents	Tache noire (eschar)—usually multiple with *R. africae*	Tick	348
Monkeypox	Orthopoxvirus	Multiple maculopustular lesions with lymphadenopathy	Prairie dog pet—USA, African rodents	395
Erysipeloid	*Erysipelothrix rhusiopathiae*	Red, tender, swollen finger; subacute bacterial endocarditis	Skin pricked while cleaning fish, domestic meat animals	318

*See table of contents and index to locate a more detailed discussion of each disease.
†Because of the fastidious nature of some organisms, the rapid development of diagnostic tools, and the risk that some agents pose to laboratory workers, we recommend that a clinical microbiologist be consulted if these agents are considered in a patient's differential diagnosis.

(Chapter 348), where it was first described 60 years ago. Vegetarians and other strict non–pork-eating persons have been seriously infected with the pig tapeworm *Taenia solium* (Chapter 375) as a result of fecal contamination of food from unsuspected infected human food-handling sources. Human influenza A (Chapter 387), until recently, was not generally considered a zoonosis; however, interspecies spread and mixing of swine, avian, and human influenza viruses can occur in unique geographic areas, such as southern China, where dense concentrations of ducks, pigs, and people cohabit. Viral incubation of the three influenza species in the pig with reassortment of antigens and subsequent spread of virulent "new" influenza strains to humans can lead to massive influenza pandemics that in sheer number (billions) surpass any past epidemics of smallpox or plague. The recent species jump from chicken to human of the highly fatal to humans H5N1 "bird flu" is another example of this risk. In a similar manner, the initial infections with human immunodeficiency virus type 1 (HIV-1) almost definitely began as zoonoses transmitted as simian immunodeficiency viruses from chimpanzees and mangabey primates to humans. As with influenza, the subsequent 60 million and counting cases of HIV no longer require an animal reservoir for continuing transmission.

Leprosy (Chapter 347), an illness of biblical notoriety transmitted from human to human, is endemic in at least three animal species, including the armadillo. This animal has rarely been implicated in transmission of this disease to humans in the United States.

Despite the large number of zoonoses described, clinicians evaluating an individual patient usually need consider only a limited number of historical details to arrive at an appropriate differential diagnosis:

1. Questions regarding direct contact with animals or animal products, animal bites, arthropod exposure, and food ingestion may offer clues to the correct cause.
2. Consideration must be given to a patient's travel history; a number of zoonoses are quite limited in geographic distribution.
3. Details about occupational and recreational high-risk activities must be ascertained.
4. The patient's clinical manifestation (course and organ involvement) is used to focus on the most likely cause and disease considerations simultaneously (see Tables 349–2, 349–3, and 349–4). Additional lists of zoonotic agents can be generated for the differential diagnoses of arthritis, jaundice, diarrhea, sepsis, shock, renal failure, fever of unknown origin, and endocarditis.
5. Though neither specific nor sensitive, the inoculation nodule (eschar, tache noire, chancre, necrotic ulcer), with or without fever, rash, or local lymphadenopathy, is the only general physical examination clue that might alert the physician to a zoonosis when the history does not.

Treatment

Rx

The approach to treatment of the various zoonoses is presented in their respective chapters.

Prevention

Guidelines have been published to help prevent nosocomial transmission of zoonotic diseases. Preventive measures to decrease infection in compromised hosts include routine immunization of pets, neutering pets, using caution when handling pet fomites, rigorous handwashing practices, and avoiding the ingestion of undercooked meat, fish, shellfish, and eggs.

Isolation is recommended for anthrax, Andes hantavirus disease, herpes B, monkeypox, Q fever, rabies, plague, and the hemorrhagic fever illnesses caused by Argentine, Bolivian, Crimean-Congo, Ebola, Lassa, and Marburg viruses.

Prognosis

The prognosis of zoonoses vary widely, but a number have very high case-fatality rates (Table 349–5).

TABLE 349–5 HIGHLY FATAL ZOONOSES

Disease*	Fatality Rate (%)
Creutzfeldt-Jakob disease (new variant)	100
Rabies	100
Anthrax inhalational	80–90
Herpes simiae†	50–75
Ebola virus	70
Eastern equine encephalitis	50–70
Hantavirus pulmonary syndrome, United States‡	60
Yellow fever§	20–50
Lassa fever§	15–25
Plague†	50–80
Rocky Mountain spotted fever†	20–60
East African sleeping sickness†	20–30
Anthrax—cutaneous†	20
Tularemia—pneumonic†	30–60
Tularemia—cutaneous	2–10
Visceral leishmaniasis†	5–25
Louse-borne relapsing fever†	5–40

*See table of contents and index to locate a more detailed discussion of each disease.
†Fatality rate if untreated.
‡Case mortality of hospitalized patients.
§If jaundiced.

SUGGESTED READINGS

Ackerman GA: It is hard to predict the future: The evolving nature of threats and vulnerabilities. Rev Sci Tech 2006;25:353–360. *Overview of the threat to human health.*

Bender JB, Hueston W, Osterholm M: Recent animal disease outbreaks and their impact on human populations. J Agromed 2006;11:5–15. *Diseases in people exposed to animals may represent index cases of zoonoses.*

Kahn LH: Confronting zoonoses, linking human and veterinary medicine. Emerg Infect Dis 2006;12:556–561. *Suggests benefits of closer links between human and veterinary medicine.*

350 ACTINOMYCOSIS

Itzhak Brook

Definition

Actinomycosis is an uncommon, chronic bacterial infection that induces both suppurative and granulomatous inflammation. Localized swelling with suppuration, abscess formation, tissue fibrosis, and draining sinuses characterizes this disease. The infection spreads contiguously and often forms draining sinuses that extrude characteristic, but not pathognomonic "sulfur granules." Infections of the oral and cervicofacial regions are most common, but any site in the body can be infected, including the thoracic region, abdominopelvic region, and the central nervous system (CNS). Musculoskeletal and disseminated disease is rare but does occur.

The Pathogen

Actinomycetes of the genera *Actinomyces, Propionibacterium,* or *Bifidobacterium* act as the principal pathogens. However, 98 to 99% of actinomycoses are caused by non–spore-forming anaerobic or microaerophilic bacterial species of the genus *Actinomyces,* family Actinomycetaceae, order Actinomycetales. Of the 30 *Actinomyces* species, 8 may cause disease in humans: the strictly anaerobic *A. israelii, A. gerencseniae* (formerly known as *A. israelii* serotype II), *A. odontolyticus, A. naeslundii, A. meyeri, A. viscosus, A. pyogenes,* and *A. georgiae. A. israelii* is the most common species causing human disease. *Propionibacterium propionicum* (formerly known as *Arachnia propionica*) and *Bifidobacterium dentium* (formerly known as *Actinomyces eriksonii*) are also associated with clinically indistinguishable infection. The organisms are filamentous, branching, gram-positive, pleomorphic, non–spore-forming, non–acid-fast anaerobic or microaerophilic bacilli. *Actinomyces* organisms are fastidious bacteria that require enriched culture media; 6 to 10% ambient CO_2 may aid in their growth, which takes 3 to 10 or more days in culture. Characteristically, *Actinomyces* species appear as "molar tooth" colonies on agar or as "bread crumb" colonies suspended in broth media. They are prokaryotes with cell walls that contain both muramic acid and diaminopimelic acid. Most actinomycotic infections are polymicrobial and involve other aerobic and anaerobic bacteria. The most common co-isolates depend on the infection site and are *Actinobacillus actinomycetemcomitans, Eikenella corrodens, Bacteroides, Fusobacterium, Capnocytophaga,* aerobic and anaerobic streptococci, *Staphylococcus,* and Enterobacteriaceae.

Epidemiology

Actinomyces species are members of the endogenous mucous membrane flora in the oral cavity, gastrointestinal tract, bronchi, and female genital tract. No external environmental reservoir such as soil or straw has been documented, nor has person-to-person transmission of pathogenic *Actinomyces* species been demonstrated. Although infection can occur in all age groups, it is rarely seen in children or patients older than 60 years. Most cases are encountered in individuals in the middle decades of life. A male-to-female infection ratio of 3:1 is reported in most series. The explanation for this ratio is the higher prevalence of poor oral hygiene and oral trauma in men. The annual reported incidence in the United States is fewer than 100 cases. However, because of the fastidious nature of the organism, many cases are undiagnosed and the true incidence is probably much higher.

Pathobiology

Actinomyces species are agents of low pathogenicity and require disruption of the mucosal barrier to cause disease. Actinomycosis usually occurs in immunocompetent persons but may afflict persons with diminished host defenses. Oral and cervicofacial diseases are commonly associated with dental caries and extractions, gingivitis and gingival trauma, infection in erupting secondary teeth, chronic tonsillitis, otitis or mastoiditis, diabetes mellitus, immunosuppression, malnutrition, and local tissue damage caused by surgery, neoplastic disease, or irradiation. Pulmonary infections generally arise after aspiration of oropharyngeal or gastrointestinal secretions. Gastrointestinal infection frequently follows loss of mucosal integrity, such as with surgery, appendicitis, diverticulitis, trauma, or foreign bodies. The use of intrauterine contraceptive devices (IUDs) increases risk for the development of actinomycosis of the female genital tract. Other predisposing factors are steroid use, immunosuppression, and human immunodeficiency virus infection.

Other bacterial species that are frequently copathogens with *Actinomyces* species may assist in the spread of infection by inhibiting host defenses and reducing local oxygen tension. Once the organism is established locally, it may spread to surrounding tissues in a progressive manner. The infection tends to spread without regard for anatomic barriers, including fascial planes and lymphatic channels. The end result is a chronic, indurated, suppurative infection (usually with draining sinuses and fibrosis, especially in pelvic and abdominal infection). The fibrotic walls of the mass before suppuration are "wooden" in nature and may be confused with a neoplasm. Hematogenous spread can be fulminant but is rare.

Actinomyces species grow in microscopic or macroscopic clusters of tangled filaments surrounded by neutrophils. Plasma cells and multinucleated giant cells are often observed with lesions, as may large macrophages with foamy cytoplasm around purulent centers. When visible, these clusters are pale yellow and exude through sinus tracts; they are called "sulfur granules" (originally called "Drusen"). These granules (1 to 2 mm in diameter) are made of aggregates of organisms and contain calcium phosphate. A central purulent loculation surrounds the granules. Their centers have a basophilic staining property, with eosinophilic rays terminating in pear-shaped "clubs." One to six granules can be present per loculation, and up to 50 loculations can be present in a lesion. Multicenter giant cells can be seen as well.

Clinical Manifestations

Cervicofacial

Cervicofacial infection is the most common manifestation of actinomycosis. This infection is generally odontogenic in origin and evolves as a chronic or subacute painless or painful soft tissue swelling or mass involving the submandibular or paramandibular region. However, the submental and retromandibular spaces, temporomandibular joint, and cheek can be involved. The swelling may have a ligneous consistency caused by tissue fibrosis. Depending on the composition of the concomitant synergistic flora, the onset of actinomycosis may be acute, subacute, or chronic. When *Staphylococcus aureus* or β-hemolytic streptococci are involved, an acute painful abscess or a phlegmatous cellulitis may be the initial manifestation. The chronic form of the disease is characterized by painless infiltration and induration that generally progress to form multiple abscesses and draining sinus tracts discharging pus that may contain sulfur granules in up to 25% of instances. Periapical infection, trismus, fever, pain, and leukocytosis may be present. The infection can extend to the carotid artery, tongue, sinuses, ears, mastoid orbit, salivary glands, pharynx, masseter muscle, thyroid, larynx, trachea, or thorax. Bone (most commonly the mandible) may be invaded from the adjacent soft tissue and result in periostitis or osteomyelitis. Cervical spine or cranial bone infection may lead to subdural empyema and invasion of the CNS. The differential diagnosis includes tuberculosis (scrofula), fungal infections, nocardiosis, suppurative infections by other organisms, and neoplasms.

Thoracic

Thoracic actinomycosis is an indolent, slowly progressive process involving the pulmonary parenchyma and pleural space. This form accounts for 15 to 30% of actinomycosis cases and is caused by aspiration of infective material from the oropharynx, as well as rarely after esophageal perforation, by extension into the mediastinum from the neck, by spread from an abdominal site, or by hematogenous spread to the lung. Infection spreads from a pneumonic focus across lung fissures to involve the pleura and the chest wall, with eventual fistula formation and drainage containing sulfur granules (Fig. 350–1). The mediastinum, pericardium, and myocardium can also rarely be affected. Granules are seldom present in sputum. The incidence of this complication, as well as the destruction of thoracic vertebrae and adjacent ribs, has declined in the antimicrobial era.

The complaints of patients with thoracic actinomycosis are nonspecific. The most common are chest pain, a productive cough, dyspnea, weight loss, and fever. Anemia, mild leukocytosis, and an elevated sedimentation rate are relatively common. There is often a history of underlying lung disease, and patients are rarely initially seen in an early stage of infection. The pulmonary lesion is either a mass lesion or pneumonitis and may resemble tuberculosis, especially when cavity formation occurs, or blastomycosis, which may destroy ribs posteriorly but rarely forms sinuses. Nocardiosis, bronchogenic carcinoma, cryptococcosis, aspiration pneumonia, pulmonary infection, and lymphoma can also mimic thoracic actinomycosis. Pleural thickening, effusion, or emphysema is common.

Abdominal

Abdominal actinomycosis is a chronic, localized inflammatory process that can occur weeks, months, or years after the integrity of the gastrointestinal mucosa is breached by surgery. Acute appendicitis with perforation, perforated colonic diverticulitis, and emergency surgery for trauma to the lower intestinal tract are among the predisposing factors. Occasionally, abdominal actinomycosis may develop without previous trauma or surgery. The ileocecal region is involved most frequently (usually after appendicitis with perforation) with the formation of a mass lesion. The infection extends slowly to contiguous organs, especially the liver, and may involve retroperitoneal tissues, the spine, or the abdominal wall. Hepatic, renal, or splenic dissemination is an uncommon complication. Persistent draining sinuses may form, and those involving the perianal region can simulate Crohn's disease or tuberculosis. The extensive fibrosis of actinomycotic lesions, recognized by the examiner as a mass, often suggests tumor. A frequent finding on computed tomography (CT) is an infiltrative mass with dense inhomogeneous contrast medium enhancement. Constitutional symptoms and signs are nonspecific, the

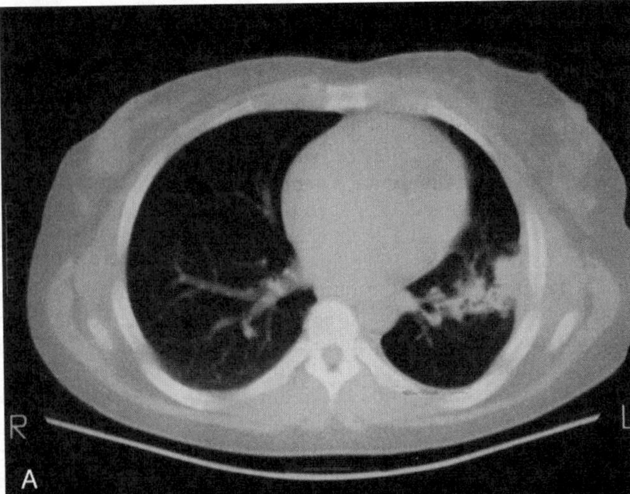

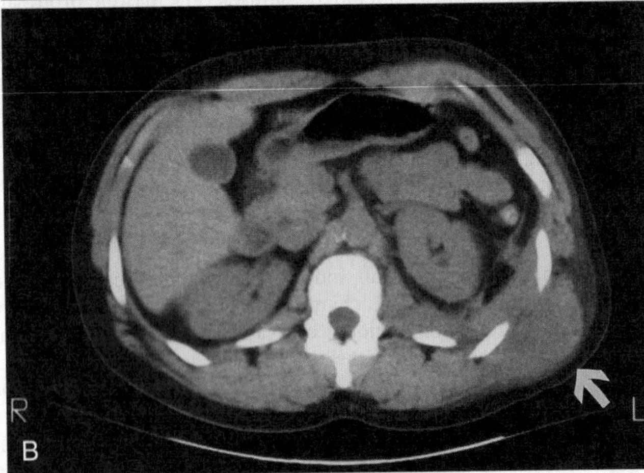

FIGURE 350–1 • Thoracic computed tomography scan of a 43-year-old woman with pulmonary actinomycosis. There is consolidation of the lung with pleural thickening adjacent to the parenchymal disease **(A)**. Abscess extended into the left breast and inferiorly to the costophrenic sulcus, to the retroperitoneum, and into the lateral abdominal wall **(B)** (arrow).

most common being fever, diarrhea or constipation, weight loss, nausea, vomiting, pain, and sensation of a mass.

Pelvic

Pelvic infection is observed in patients with prolonged use of IUDs, usually for longer than 2 years. Pelvic actinomycosis may also occur from extension of intestinal infection, commonly from indolent ileocecal disease. Manifestations of infection may range from a chronic vaginal discharge to pelvic inflammatory disease with tubo-ovarian abscesses or pseudomalignant masses. Patients generally have abnormal vaginal bleeding or discharge, abdominal or pelvic pain, menorrhagia, fever, and weight loss.

Endometritis is the earlier form of the infection, followed by tubo-ovarian abscesses. Extension to the uterus, bladder, rectal area, abdominal wall, peritoneum, pelvic bones, thorax, and systemic circulation can also occur.

Central Nervous System

Infections of the CNS are very rare and generally manifested as single or multiple encapsulated brain abscesses that appear as ring-enhancing lesions with a thick wall that may be irregular or nodular on contrast CT scans. There are no features that readily distinguish actinomycosis from other brain abscesses. Rarely, solid nodular or mass lesions termed actinomycetomas or actinomycotic granulomas are found. Headache and focal neurologic signs are the most common finding. Most actinomycotic infections of the CNS are seeded hematogenously from a distant primary site, but direct extension of cervicofacial disease also occurs. Sinus formation is not a characteristic of CNS disease. The rare meningitis caused by *Actinomyces* is chronic and basilar in location, and the pleocytosis is usually lymphocytic. Thus, it may be misdiagnosed as tuberculous meningitis.

Diagnosis

A combination of appropriate microbiologic and pathologic studies are essential for proper diagnosis. A high index of suspicion should be communicated to the microbiology diagnostic laboratory, along with material from draining sinuses, from deep-needle aspiration, or from biopsy specimens. It is important to avoid antimicrobial therapy before obtaining a specimen. Anaerobic culture is required, and no selective media are available to restrict overgrowth of the slow-growing *Actinomyces* by associated microflora. The presence, in pus or tissue specimens, of non–acid-fast, gram-positive organisms with filamentous branching is very suggestive of the diagnosis. The characteristic morphology of sulfur granules and the presence of gram-positive organisms within are helpful. In tissue sections stained with hematoxylin-eosin, sulfur granules are round or oval basophilic masses with a radiating arrangement of eosinophilic terminal "clubs." However, *Actinomyces* species are infrequently visible in sections stained with hematoxylin-eosin; visualization is facilitated by special stains such as Gomori methenamine silver, *p*-aminosalicylic acid, McCallen-Goodpasture, and Brown-Benn. Multiple biopsy sections from different tissue levels are recommended to improve the histopathologic diagnosis. The granules must be distinguished from similar structures that are sometimes produced in infections caused by *Nocardia, Monosporium, Cephalosporium, Staphylococcus* (botryomycosis), and others. *Actinomyces* and *Arachnia* can generally be differentiated from other gram-positive anaerobes by means of their growth rate (slow), by catalase production (negative, except for *A. viscosus*), and by gas-liquid chromatographic detection of the acetic, lactic, and succinic acids produced in peptone-yeast-glucose broth. Direct fluorescent antibody conjugates and immunofluorescence testing can be used but are not readily available to clinical microbiology laboratories.

Imaging methods such as conventional radiography, CT, and magnetic resonance imaging do not provide a specific diagnosis but allow more accurate definition of the dimensions and extension of the infection.

Treatment

Prolonged antimicrobial therapy (i.e., 6 to 12 months) has typically been recommended for patients with all clinical forms of actinomycosis to prevent disease recrudescence. However, individualization of courses of therapy is recommended because the duration of treatment depends on the initial burden of disease, the site of infection, and the clinical and radiologic response. Adequate drainage is indicated if abscesses are present.

Penicillin G is the drug of choice for treating an infection caused by any of the *Actinomyces*. It is given in high dosage over a prolonged period because the infection has a tendency to recur. Most deep-seated infections can be expected to respond to intravenous penicillin G, 10 to 20 million U/day given for 2 to 6 weeks, followed by an oral phenoxypenicillin in a dosage of 2 to 4 g/day. A few additional weeks of oral penicillin therapy may suffice for uncomplicated cervicofacial disease; complicated cases and extensive pulmonary or abdominal disease may require treatment for 12 to 18 months. Little evidence exists of acquired resistance to penicillin G by *Actinomyces* during prolonged therapy. Alternative first-line antibiotics include tetracycline, erythromycin, chloramphenicol, and clindamycin. First-generation cephalosporins, ceftriaxone, and imipenem have also been used successfully. Metronidazole, aminoglycosides, and antifungal drugs are not active against these organisms. In vitro antimicrobial susceptibility testing of *Actinomyces* is difficult, and the results may not be predictive of antimicrobial effect in vivo.

The need to use combination antimicrobial therapy to attack microorganisms that are isolated in association with *Actinomyces* has not been established. However, because many of these organisms are known pathogens, treatment is usually appropriate, especially with lower abdominal infections. Surgical removal of infected tissue may also be necessary in some cases, especially if extensive necrotic tissue or fistulas are present, if malignancy cannot be

Rx

excluded, and if large abscesses cannot be drained by percutaneous aspiration. When well-defined IUD-related symptoms and Papanicolaou smears demonstrate *Actinomyces* by specific fluorescent-labeled antibody, the IUD should be removed. Antimicrobial administration for a 2-week period may be indicated. More serious infections require prolonged therapy.

Prognosis

The availability of antimicrobial treatment has greatly improved the prognosis for all forms of actinomycosis. At present, cure rates are high and neither deformity nor death is common.

SUGGESTED READINGS

Oostman O, Smego RA: Cervicofacial actinomycosis: Diagnosis and management. Curr Infect Dis Rep 2005;7:170–174. *A practical overview.*

Wagenlehner FM, Mohren B, Naber KG, Mannl HF: Abdominal actinomycosis. Clin Microbiol Infect 2003;9:881–885. *A clinical review.*

Yildiz O, Doganay M: Actinomycoses and *Nocardia* pulmonary infections. Curr Opin Pulm Med 2006;12:228–234. *Clinical review of pulmonary actinomycosis infection.*

351 NOCARDIOSIS

Frederick S. Southwick

Definition

Nocardiosis refers to infections caused by *Nocardia* species. *Nocardia* most commonly causes pneumonia, but it also can infect the central nervous system (CNS) and skin. Less commonly this organism can disseminate throughout the body. These infections usually occur in patients with defective immunity.

The Pathogen

Nocardia species are thin, aerobic, gram-positive bacilli that form branching filaments. The bacteria stain irregularly and appear beaded on Gram stain. Speciation of *Nocardia* has been problematic. The original classification was based on the ability of *Nocardia* to use specific nutrients and to decompose substrates such as adenine, casein, urea, gelatin, and xanthine. However, gene sequencing and DNA-DNA hybridization have now defined the true taxonomy. The species called *Nocardia asteroides* was previously reported to be the most common cause of human disease, but the majority of these bacteria were misidentified by today's standards. The number of *Nocardia* species causing human disease is large and includes *N. abscessus, N. brevicatena/paucivorans* complex, *N. nova* complex, *N. transvalensis* complex, *N. farcinica, N. asteroides* complex, *N. brasiliensis,* and *N. pseudobrasiliensis.* Species have similar morphologic characteristics but differ in their antimicrobial susceptibility.

Epidemiology

Nocardia species are ubiquitous and primarily originate in soil. Despite being found throughout the environment, they rarely cause symptomatic infection in humans. Because nocardiosis is not a reportable disease, the frequency of this disease is unknown. However, the annual incidence has been estimated to be approximately 0.4 case per 100,000 persons. The risk for symptomatic *Nocardia* infection is greatly increased in individuals who are immunocompromised (incidence estimated to be more than 1000-fold higher), including patients who are receiving immunosuppressive agents after bone marrow or solid organ transplantation and patients with acquired immunodeficiency syndrome (AIDS) (especially when the $CD4^+$ T-lymphocyte count drops below 100). The increased use of potent anti-inflammatory agents such as corticosteroids and anti–tumor necrosis factor-α antibody (infliximab) for inflammatory bowel disease, lupus erythematosus, and rheumatoid arthritis is likely to increase the incidence of nocardiosis further. Cancer, Cushing's disease, chronic granulomatous disease, and dysgammaglobulinemia also increase the risk for nocardiosis. Finally, patients with chronic pulmonary disorders, particularly alveolar proteinosis, are more susceptible to this infection. In approximately a third of patients with nocardiosis, no predisposing condition can be identified.

Pathobiology

Most *Nocardia* species gain entry to the host via the respiratory tract or, less commonly, by skin inoculation. Invading bacteria illicit a neutrophil response that inhibits growth but does not kill the organism. The bacteria are phagocytosed by neutrophils and macrophages and become enclosed in a membrane-bound phagolysosome. In this closed environment neutrophils and macrophages are able to kill many species of bacteria by synthesizing superoxide and hydrogen peroxide. However, *Nocardia* is able to survive in this hostile environment by producing superoxide dismutase, an enzyme that inactivates these toxic oxygen byproducts. In addition, *Nocardia* species produce a mycolic acid, called cord factor, that inhibits the fusion of lysosomes with the phagolysomal compartment, thereby preventing toxic proteases and other antibacterial products from reaching the intracellular bacteria. In addition to neutrophils and macrophages, cell-mediated immunity and humoral immunity play roles in protecting the host against *Nocardia* invasion, thus explaining the wide range of immunocompromised patients who are at increased risk for contracting nocardiosis.

Clinical Manifestations

Nocardiosis has no pathognomonic characteristics, and delays in diagnosis are common. Failure of a pulmonary or skin infection to respond to conventional antibiotic therapy should raise the possibility of infection by *Nocardia.* Nocardiosis should always be considered in an immunocompromised patient.

Pulmonary Nocardiosis

Pulmonary infection develops in approximately two thirds of patients with nocardiosis. Pulmonary disease is generally subacute in onset, mimics fungal or mycobacterial infection, and is most commonly misdiagnosed as tuberculosis. The most common complaints are a persistent cough producing purulent sputum, fever, anorexia, and weight loss. Less commonly, patients may report pleuritic chest pain and dyspnea. Hemoptysis is rare but can develop in patients with large cavitary lesions. Acute onset of pneumonia has occasionally been reported in an immunocompromised host.

Central Nervous System Infection

CNS infection develops in approximately a third of patients with nocardiosis. Multilocular brain abscess is the most common CNS manifestation and is usually caused by transient bacterial dissemination from the lung. Lesions can occur in any region of the brain, and symptoms depend on location. Headache is the usual initial complaint and is frequently localized to the site of the abscess. Patients may also have neurologic deficits, as well as seizures. In AIDS patients, brain abscess is often accompanied by an abnormal chest radiograph, whereas in other patients chest x-ray abnormalities may not be present. The combined finding of a lung nodule on chest radiography plus a ring-enhancing CNS lesion is frequently mistaken for metastatic lung carcinoma. Other diagnoses that should be considered when an immunocompromised host has both a lung and CNS focus are disseminated aspergillosis and toxoplasmosis. Meningitis is a less common CNS manifestation and is often associated with brain abscess (40% of meningitis cases). Meningitis is generally subacute to chronic in onset and is characterized by fever, stiff neck, and generalized headache. Cerebrospinal fluid cultures are frequently negative, and patients fail to respond completely to empirical antibiotic therapy.

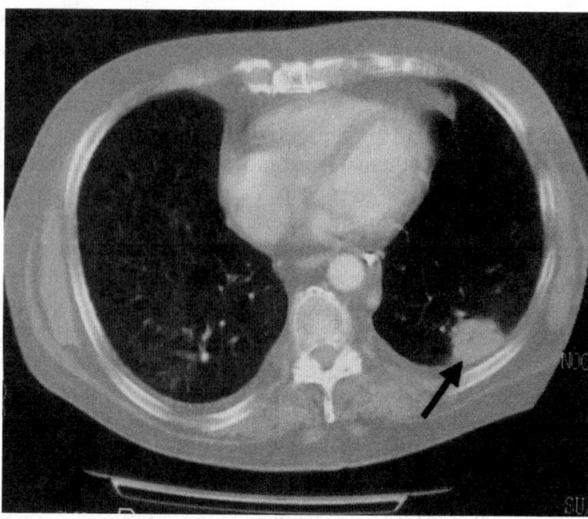

FIGURE 351–1 • Chest computed tomography showing a peripheral nodular lung lesion (arrow) caused by *Nocardia* infection.

Cutaneous Infection

Skin infection is usually caused by *N. brasiliensis* and generally follows a break in the skin that is contaminated by soil. Cutaneous disease has been reported in association with trauma, postoperative wounds, insect bites, thorn bush scratches, and even a cat scratch. Initially, a pustule or moderately erythematous, nonfluctuant nodule develops at the site of inoculation. Erythema can extend along the lymphatic system and is associated with tender lymphadenopathy. This form of cutaneous infection has been termed lymphocutaneous or sporotrichoid disease. Similar skin manifestations are seen with other causes, including cat-scratch disease, tularemia, *Mycobacterium marinum,* and sporotrichosis. In an immunocompromised host, disseminated infection may be manifested by multiple erythematous raised nodules and is an ominous finding. In tropical regions of South and Central America, *Nocardia* species can cause ulcerations and large tumor-like lesions called mycetomas that are usually found on the lower part of the legs.

Diagnosis

Radiology

In pulmonary disease, chest x-ray findings are variable, with pulmonary nodules or mass lesions most often being seen. Less frequently, consolidation, cavitary lesions with air-fluid levels, interstitial infiltrates, and pleural effusions are found. Chest computed tomography (CT) often demonstrates areas of low attenuation within consolidations, multiple nodules, and chest wall extension of the infection (Fig. 351–1). AIDS patients are more likely to have multiple pulmonary nodules, cavitary lesions, and upper lobe infiltrates. In some patients the infiltrate may resolve, particularly those with normal immune function. However, a brain abscess may develop several months later as a consequence of transient dissemination. In CNS infection, CT or magnetic resonance imaging with contrast usually demonstrates one or more ring-enhancing lesions (Fig. 351–2). *Nocardia* brain abscess are more commonly multiloculated; otherwise, the radiologic findings are similar to other bacterial causes of brain abscess.

Histopathology

Invasive procedures are generally required for specific diagnosis. For pulmonary infection, bronchoscopy with transbronchial biopsy or skinny-needle biopsy is recommended. For brain abscess, CT-guided needle aspiration is the diagnostic procedure of choice. Histopathology usually reveals an acute inflammatory response with a predominance of neutrophils. Micronodular abscesses with minimal capsular formation are commonly found. Gram stain or Brown-Brenn stains reveal gram-positive beaded, branching forms. The morphology is identical to that of *Actinomyces* sp; however, the high lipid content of its cell wall often renders *Nocardia* sp modified acid-fast positive, whereas *Actinomyces* sp are modified acid-fast negative. However, acid fastness may be variable when staining *Nocardia* colonies from cultures and is unreliable for direct clinical samples.

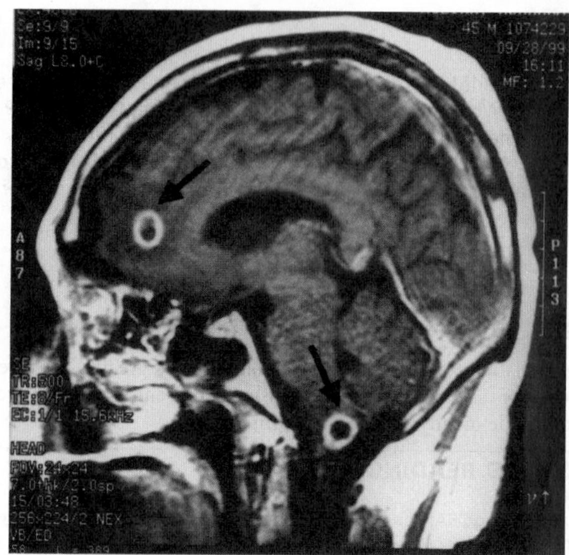

FIGURE 351–2 • Multiple, gadolinium-enhanced brain lesions (arrows) caused by *Nocardia* infection.

Culture

Isolation of the organism on culture provides a definitive diagnosis for needle aspirate samples from a brain abscess and a presumptive diagnosis when grown from respiratory and cutaneous samples. *Nocardia* sp grow best under aerobic conditions with 5 to 10% carbon dioxide. Because the organism grows slowly on blood agar, with 3 to 5 days needed to form colonies, if other organisms are present in the culture sample (sputum and skin samples), they can overgrow and mask the presence of *Nocardia.* Furthermore, many gram-negative bacteria inhibit this organism's growth. Therefore, it is important to notify the clinical laboratory if *Nocardia* is suspected to allow the use of selective media and prolonged incubation. Because increasing numbers of *Nocardia* sp have been shown to be resistant to sulfonamides, antimicrobial susceptibility testing should always be performed to guide the choice of antibiotics.

Treatment

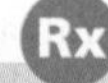

Sulfonamides remain the treatment of choice for pulmonary and cutaneous disease. Trimethoprim-sulfamethoxazole given orally or intravenously at a dose of 5 to 10 mg/kg/day of the trimethoprim component given two to four times per day is a common adult regimen. When patients with disseminated or CNS *Nocardia,* or both, are treated with sulfonamides alone, survival rates have been less than 50%. One of the most common species to cause disseminated disease, *N. farcinica,* is also one the most common *Nocardia* sp to be resistant to sulfonamides. In these more serious conditions, combination therapy is generally recommended, the exact regimen being guided by antibiotic susceptibility testing. One recommended empirical regimen is trimethoprim-sulfamethoxazole at the aforementioned dose or intravenously, amikacin (7.5 mg/kg every 12 hours), and either ceftriaxone (2 g twice daily) or imipenem (500 mg every 6 hours). Linezolid, 600 mg twice a day, has been used successfully in a small number of CNS infections. However, because prolonged therapy with this agent can lead to bone marrow toxicity, weekly monitoring of peripheral cell counts is warranted. Recently, the newer fluoroquinolones moxifloxacin and gatifloxacin (400 mg/day orally recommended for both agents) have been shown to have activity against several strains of *Nocardia,* including *N. farcinica* and *N. brasiliensis,* and these agents may prove be useful in patients who cannot tolerate sulfonamides. Minocycline (100 mg orally twice daily) and amoxicillin-clavulanate (875/125 mg orally twice daily) are other potentially effective alternative treatments of *Nocardia* infection. Because of the intracellular nature of *Nocardia* and slow rates of bacterial growth, antibiotic treatment for 6 to 12

Rx

months in an immunocompromised host and 4 to 6 months in a normal host is usually required to prevent relapse.

In addition to antimicrobial treatment, for patients with brain abscess or subcutaneous abscesses, surgical drainage is required for cure.

Prognosis

The overall mortality for nocardiosis is approximately 25%. In otherwise healthy individuals, pulmonary nocardiosis has a better prognosis (15% mortality). The survival rate is worse in patients with bacteremia, patients with acute infection (symptoms for less than 3 weeks), patients receiving corticosteroids or cytotoxic agents, organ transplant recipients, patients with disseminated disease involving two or more noncontiguous organs, and patients with meningitis.

SUGGESTED READINGS

Brown-Elliott BA, Brown JM, Conville PS, Wallace RJ: Clinical and laboratory features of *Nocardia* spp. based on current molecular taxonomy. Clin Microbiol Rev 2006;19:259–282. *An up-to-date review of the speciation of Nocardia. Also discusses clinical manifestations and antibiotic treatment.*

Hitti W, Wolff M: Two cases of multidrug-resistant *Nocardia farcinica* infection in immunosuppressed patients and implications for empiric therapy. Eur J Clin Microbiol Infect Dis 2005;24:142–144. *Describes two patients with disseminated infection caused by* N. farcinica *resistant to sulfonamides. In severe* Nocardia *infection, initial empirical treatment with amikacin and imipenem should be considered.*

Lederman ER, Crum NF: A case series and focused review of nocardiosis: Clinical and microbiologic aspects. Medicine (Baltimore) 2004;83:300–313. *Reviews the many clinical manifestations of nocardiosis in adults.*

352 SYSTEMIC ANTIFUNGAL AGENTS

David A. Stevens

AMPHOTERICIN B–BASED PREPARATIONS

Mechanism of Action

The structures of systemic antifungal agents are shown in Figure 352–1. Amphotericin B is a lipophilic molecule that exerts its antifungal effect by insertion into the fungal cytoplasmic membrane. Amphotericin B causes membrane permeability to increase, and the subsequent loss of intracellular molecules impairs fungal viability. Its onset of action is rapid. Amphotericin B also has effects on oxidation that may enhance antifungal activity.

Spectrum of Activity and Mechanisms of Resistance

Amphotericin B is active against most fungi, and its spectrum of activity is not influenced by the choice of formulation. When resistance occurs, it is generally attributed to reductions in ergosterol biosynthesis and synthesis of alternative sterols that lessen the ability of amphotericin B to interact with the fungal membrane. Primary resistance is common for *Aspergillus terreus, Scedosporium apiospermum, Scedosporium prolificans,* and *Trichosporon beigelii.* Among the *Candida* species, primary resistance is noted at meaningful frequencies most often for *Candida lusitaniae.* The development of resistance in isolates of normally susceptible species is uncommon. In studies, the principal pharmacodynamic driver of the in vivo response has been the ratio of the peak achieved serum concentration to the minimal inhibitory concentration (MIC).

Available Formulations

Four amphotericin B formulations are commercially available: amphotericin B deoxycholate (ABD) and three lipid-associated formulations (amphotericin B colloidal dispersion, amphotericin B lipid complex, and liposomal amphotericin B). In an attempt to produce lower-cost lipid-associated formulations, some reports have advocated mixing ABD with a parenteral fat emulsion. Although less nephrotoxicity has been observed in adults with this preparation at a dose of 1 mg/kg daily than with infusions of ABD in 5% dextrose, no advantage was found in children. Serum amphotericin B concentrations were also lower with the fat emulsion, thus raising the possibility that amphotericin B was simply aggregating in the fat emulsion but the cloudiness could not be perceived in the milky-looking lipid. Use of such preparations should be reserved for investigational settings.

Amphotericin B Deoxycholate

Formulation

ABD for intravenous use is a colloidal suspension. If a filter with a 0.22-μm pore diameter is placed in the infusion line, considerable drug is removed by the filter. The addition of electrolyte will aggregate the colloids, so the solution becomes cloudy. ABD is currently available from several generic manufacturers, and significant differences have been reported and may be part of the cause of the intersubject variation in toxicity observed.

Pharmacology

Concentrations of amphotericin B in biologic fluids have usually been measured by bioassay. Most of the drug leaves the circulation promptly, with only a small percentage being excreted in urine or bile. Amphotericin B is stored in the liver and other organs; the drug appears to re-enter the circulation slowly. Blood levels are uninfluenced by hepatic or renal failure. Hemodialysis does not alter blood levels, except in an occasional patient with lipemic plasma, who may be losing drug by adherence to the dialysis membrane. Concentrations of amphotericin B in fluid from inflamed areas, such as pleura, peritoneum, joint, vitreous humor, and aqueous humor, are roughly two thirds of the nadir serum level. Amphotericin B penetrates poorly into either normal or inflamed meninges, saliva, bronchial secretions, brain, pancreas, muscle, bone, vitreous humor, or normal amniotic fluid. Urine concentrations are similar to serum concentrations. Peak serum concentrations with conventional intravenous doses are roughly 0.5 to 2.0 μg/mL and rapidly fall initially to slowly approach a plateau of roughly 0.2 to 0.5 μg/mL. The initial half-life is about 24 hours; the β-phase half-life is roughly 15 days. Serum concentrations can be detected for at least 7 weeks after the end of therapy, presumably reflecting release from cell lipids. The drug also has complex immunomodulatory properties, potentially of clinical significance.

Nephrotoxicity

ABD causes a dose-dependent decrease in the glomerular filtration rate. The direct vasoconstrictive effect of amphotericin B on afferent renal arterioles results in reduced glomerular and renal tubular blood flow. Other effects on the kidney include potassium, magnesium, and bicarbonate wasting and decreased erythropoietin production. Loss of renal function is due to destruction of renal tubular cells, disruption of tubular basement membrane, and loss of functioning nephron units. Saline loading, such as infusion of 1 L of saline before ABD, has been associated with reduced nephrotoxicity in some studies. Potassium wasting often requires supplemental oral or intravenous potassium. Renal tubular acidosis from bicarbonate wasting rarely requires base replacement, but other drugs and diseases that promote acidosis may act synergistically.

The azotemia caused by amphotericin B is often worse in patients taking other nephrotoxic drugs. Hypotension, intravascular volume depletion, and other preexisting renal disease all magnify the management problems associated with amphotericin B–induced azotemia. These toxicities are lessened by use of the lipid-associated formulations of amphotericin B.

Early in a course of therapy with ABD, azotemia may increase rapidly, often falls a little, and then stabilizes after several days. Adults with no other renal disease will have an average serum creatinine level of 2 to 3 mg/dL at therapeutic doses, and therapy should not be withheld unless the azotemia exceeds this level. Attempting to give ABD to an adult without causing azotemia will usually lead to inadequate therapy.

Other Chronic Toxicity

Nausea, anorexia, and vomiting are common, and phlebitis occurs if peripheral vein catheters are used. Normocytic normochromic anemia occurs gradually. The hematocrit rarely falls below 20 to 25% unless other causes of anemia are present. Rarely, thrombocytopenia, modest leukopenia, arrhythmias, coagulopathy, hemorrhagic enteritis, tinnitus, vertigo, encephalopathy, seizures, hemolysis, or dysesthesia of the soles of the feet may be observed.

Acute Reactions

About 30 to 45 minutes after beginning the first few ABD infusions, chills, fever, and tachypnea may develop, peak in 15 to 30 minutes, and slowly abate over a period of 2 to 4 hours. A patient with underlying cardiac or pulmonary disease may have hypoxemia. These reactions are less common in young children or patients receiving corticosteroids. Subsequent infusions at the same dose cause progressively milder reactions. Premedication with acetaminophen or the addition of hydrocortisone, 25 to 50 mg, to the infusion solution can diminish the reactions. Meperidine given early in a chill shortens the rigors but may induce nausea or emesis. Concern about this kind of reaction in an unstable patient had led some physicians to use a test dose of 1 mg given over a 15-minute period to assess the subsequent reaction over 1 hour before deciding whether the next dose should be a full therapeutic dose. Patients with rapidly progressive mycoses should receive a full therapeutic dose within 24 hours. These reactions should not be mistaken for anaphylaxis or otherwise considered a contraindication to further amphotericin B. True allergic reactions are extremely rare.

Administration

ABD is infused over a 2- to 4-hour interval. Infusions 1 hour in duration appear to be generally safe for persons who have tolerated slower infusions. Rapid infusion in patients with severely compromised renal function may lead to acute, marked hyperkalemia and ventricular fibrillation.

Patients receiving a stable daily dose may be switched to a double dose on alternate days to reduce the frequency of infusion-associated toxicity, particularly anorexia, and as a convenience for outpatient therapy. Doses higher than 1.5 mg/kg are not generally given on this schedule because the toxicity of such infusions is not well described. Continuous infusion of ABD with doses up to 2.0 mg/kg/24 hr has been described based on limited data as another strategy for reducing toxicity, but this approach is not consistent with the observation that the principal pharmacodynamic driver of efficacy for amphotericin B is the peak drug concentration.

Dosage

Daily ABD doses of 0.3 mg/kg often suffice for esophageal candidiasis. A dose of 0.5 mg/kg is appropriate for blastomycosis, disseminated histoplasmosis, and extracutaneous sporotrichosis. Patients with cryptococcal meningitis are generally given doses of 0.6 to 0.8 mg/kg; those with coccidioidomycosis may require doses of 1 mg/kg. Patients with mucormycosis or invasive aspergillosis are given daily doses of 1 to 1.5 mg/kg until improvement is clearly present. Local instillation of ABD into cerebrospinal fluid, joints, or pleura is rarely indicated. One exception is coccidioidal meningitis, which is treated with intrathecal ABD because it may produce superior results to systemic azole therapy, particularly in the long term, though with far greater toxicity. Intraocular administration for fungal endophthalmitis is occasionally used; doses of 10 μg appear to avoid retinal toxicity. Corneal baths with 1 mg/mL in sterile water are useful for fungal keratitis but are irritating.

Lipid-Associated Formulations of Amphotericin B

Lipid-associated formulations of amphotericin B (LFAB) and ABD must be infused in 5% dextrose with no electrolytes added. Infusion bottles need not be protected from light.

Pharmacology and Toxicity

The three LFAB have quite different pharmacokinetic patterns. When compared on the basis of equal mg/kg dosages, LFAB produce tissue amphotericin B concentrations that range from 90% lower to 500% higher than those noted for ABD, with the most consistent relative reduction seen in the kidney. The LFAB are typically given at mg/kg doses that are 5- to 12-fold higher than those used for ABD. All three LFAB generally require higher doses in experimental animals to achieve the same therapeutic effect as ABD.

These higher but equipotent doses are notably better tolerated than ABD, with reductions in both the frequency and severity of acute infusion-related reactions and chronic nephrotoxicity. An exception is amphotericin B colloidal dispersion, which generally shows acute infusion-related reactions similar to those for ABD.

Randomized clinical trials comparing ABD as therapy for a defined mycosis are limited to demonstrations of liposomal amphotericin B of similar efficacy for cryptococcal meningitis and greater efficacy for histoplasmosis. Randomized comparisons with ABD as therapy for persistently neutropenic and febrile cancer patients provide consistent demonstration of a generally better tolerability profile, but little data on differential antifungal effect. The aggregate open-label data efficacy rates for LFAB are similar to those for ABD. Although LFAB are notably more costly than ABD (from 10- to 60-fold more expensive), the purchase price of the compound must be balanced against the morbidity and financial cost of monitoring, treating, and managing ABD-related nephrotoxicity.

FLUCYTOSINE

Formulation and Pharmacology

Flucytosine (5-fluorocytosine) is the fluorine analogue of a normal body constituent, cytosine. Flucytosine is marketed as 250- and 500-mg capsules. Absorption from the gastrointestinal tract is rapid and complete, and approximately 90% is excreted unchanged in urine. Cerebrospinal fluid concentrations approximate 74% of simultaneous serum concentrations; flucytosine also penetrates well into aqueous humor, joints, bronchial secretions, peritoneal fluid, brain, bile, and bone. The drug is readily cleared by hemodialysis and peritoneal dialysis.

The half-life of the flucytosine in the serum of patients with normal renal function is 3 to 5 hours and higher in newborns. Abnormal hepatic function has no influence, but decreased renal function prolongs the half-life.

Mechanisms of Action and Resistance

Isolates of *Candida* species are usually susceptible, as are most isolates of *Cryptococcus neoformans*. Flucytosine is often active against isolates of *Aspergillus* and against the melanin-pigmented molds that cause chromoblastomycosis. The mechanism of flucytosine's antifungal action appears to be deamination to 5-fluorouracil and then conversion through several steps to 5-fluorodeoxyuridylic acid monophosphate, a noncompetitive inhibitor of thymidylate synthetase that interferes with DNA synthesis, or through its conversion to 5-fluouridine triphosphate, which causes aberrant transcription RNA. In studies, the principal pharmacodynamic driver of response was the proportion of the time that the blood level exceeded the MIC. Resistance may be due to loss of the cytosine permease that permits flucytosine to cross the fungal cell membrane or loss of any of the enzymes that lead to its conversion into the forms that interfere with DNA or RNA synthesis.

Administration and Dosage

Flucytosine is usually administered by mouth at 100 to 150 mg/kg/day in four divided doses. As an approximation, the total daily dose should be reduced to 75 mg/kg with a creatinine clearance of 26 to 50 mL/min and to 37 mg/kg when creatinine clearance is 13 to 25 mL/min. Ideally, the blood level should be measured in azotemic patients 2 hours after the last dose and immediately before the next dose. These values should range between 20 and 100 μg/mL. Patients requiring hemodialysis may be given a single postdialysis dose of 37.5 mg/kg. Further doses are adjusted by blood level. Reliable methods are available to assay flucytosine.

Flucytosine given alone to patients with normal renal, hematologic, and gastrointestinal function is associated with very infrequent adverse effects, including rash, diarrhea, and hepatic dysfunction. In the presence of azotemia, such as that caused by concomitant amphotericin B, leukopenia, thrombocytopenia, and enterocolitis may occur. These complications seem to be far more frequent in patients whose flucytosine blood levels attain and especially if they exceed 100 to 125 μg/mL. Patients receiving flucytosine whose renal function is changing should have their serum flucytosine concentrations determined twice per week and the leukocyte count, platelet count, alkaline phosphatase, and aminotransferase levels determined at a similar frequency. Patients in whom loose stools or dull abdominal pain suddenly develops or who have laboratory evidence consistent with flucytosine toxicity should have their flucytosine blood levels checked and consideration given to withholding therapy with the drug until the situation is clarified. Patients with bone marrow and gastrointestinal toxicity from flucytosine often tolerate the drug at reduced dosage. Uncommonly, vomiting, bowel perforation, confusion, hallucinations, headache, sedation, and euphoria have been reported. Flucytosine is contraindicated in pregnancy.

Conversion of flucytosine to 5-fluorouracil within the human body occurs in sufficient degree to be a possible explanation for toxicity to bone marrow and the gastrointestinal tract. It is likely that the drug is secreted into the gut, where flucytosine becomes deaminated by intestinal bacteria and is reabsorbed as 5-fluorouracil.

Flucytosine has a beneficial effect in patients with cryptococcosis, candidiasis, and chromoblastomycosis. It is not the drug of choice for any infection because (1) its clinical efficacy in the first two mycoses is inferior to that of amphotericin B, (2) primary drug resistance is not uncommon in *Candida* infection, and (3) secondary drug resistance is common in cryptococcosis and chromoblastomycosis.

Flucytosine and amphotericin B are at least additive in their effects in vitro and in mice. Flucytosine permits the use of a lower dose of amphotericin B to gain the same therapeutic effect, and amphotericin B prevents the emergence of secondary drug resistance. The same advantages have been confirmed in two large multicenter studies of cryptococcal meningitis.

Flucytosine is more difficult to manage in patients with diminished bone marrow reserve. Intravenous flucytosine is no longer available in the United States but is used at the same dose as the capsule formulation.

Flucytosine resistance has occurred, albeit uncommonly, during combination therapy. Use of the combination in such patients incurs the risk of toxicity without evidence that flucytosine adds to the therapeutic effect. In most laboratories, an MIC of 20 μg/mL or less is considered susceptible.

AZOLE ANTIFUNGAL AGENTS

Mechanism of Action

The azole ring confers antifungal activity on a variety of synthetic organic compounds. Methods for in vitro susceptibility testing are increasingly becoming available as standardized tools.

N-substitution of imidazoles has created a family of drugs called triazoles that have the same mechanism of action as imidazoles, a similar or broader spectrum of activity, and less effect on human sterol synthesis. Both imidazoles and triazoles inhibit 14α-demethylation of lanosterol in fungi, which leads to reduced concentrations of ergosterol, a sterol essential for a normal fungal cytoplasmic membrane. Inhibition of cytochrome P-450 (CYP) also decreases the synthesis of testosterone and glucocorticoids in mammals. In studies, the principal pharmacodynamic driver for response to the triazole antifungal agents has been the ratio of total drug exposure (area under the time-concentration curve [AUC]) to the MIC.

Newer triazoles have properties that make them preferable to ketoconazole—not only less hormonal inhibition but also fewer drug interactions, both parenteral and oral formulations, a broader spectrum, better distribution into body fluids, and less hepatotoxicity. Resistance to azoles in previously susceptible species is emerging. Resistance mechanisms include increased drug efflux and altered or increased 14α-demethylase. All agents in this class have the potential for embryotoxicity and teratogenicity and should be avoided during pregnancy.

Ketoconazole

Formulations and Pharmacology

The synthetic agent ketoconazole is available as tablets. Ketoconazole is metabolized in the liver and excreted as inactive drug in bile and, to a small extent, in urine. The drug is not removed significantly by hemodialysis or peritoneal dialysis. Decreased renal or hepatic function does not alter plasma drug levels. The initial half-life is approximately 2 hours, with a β-phase half-life of about 9 hours commencing 8 to 12 hours after ingestion.

Oral absorption of ketoconazole differs among individuals. Serious gastrointestinal disease may lead to low blood levels. Inhibitors of gastric acid secretion should not be given to patients taking ketoconazole because blood levels of the latter drug are drastically reduced. Citrus fruit juices or cola beverages administered with ketoconazole improve absorption in hypochlorhydric patients. Antacids given to patients should follow ketoconazole by 1 to 2 hours. Rifampin causes substantial lowering of ketoconazole blood levels by CYP enzyme induction. Other coadministered drugs may have their levels raised because of CYP enzyme blockade. Cyclosporine blood levels should be monitored during ketoconazole therapy because these levels usually increase. Penetration into cerebrospinal fluid is poor, even in the presence of inflammation. Low concentrations are found in vaginal secretions, saliva, and breast milk, but penetration into inflamed joints is better.

Uses

When taken as 400 mg daily, ketoconazole is effective in chronic mucocutaneous candidiasis, coccidioidomycosis, histoplasmosis, paracoccidioidomycosis, and blastomycosis in nonimmunosuppressed hosts. Therapy is continued for 6 to 12 months or longer, when the response is slow, to prevent relapse. Improvement may require weeks to months to be evident. Although the dose can be advanced to 600 or 800 mg daily in patients not responding to therapy, more evidence of increased toxicity than increased efficacy has been observed. Some patients with chromoblastomycosis and cutaneous sporotrichosis respond, but itraconazole would be preferred.

Aspergillosis does not respond to ketoconazole. Additionally, concern exists that subsequent use of amphotericin B after azoles may be antagonized. The agents of mucormycosis have all been resistant to most azoles.

Adverse Effects

The most frequent toxic effects are anorexia, nausea, and vomiting. Dividing doses above 400 mg/day has not been recommended because hormonal suppression is prolonged. Ketoconazole causes a dose-dependent depression in serum testosterone- and adrenocorticotropic hormone–stimulated cortisol response. Doses of 800 to 1200 mg/day cause a profound enough effect to have prompted trials in the treatment of Cushing's syndrome and prostatic cancer. Hypertension has been seen in a few of these high-dose patients in association with increased mineralocorticoid precursors. Gynecomastia, oligospermia, and menstrual irregularities may also develop during prolonged therapy. Allergic rash and pruritus have been noted.

Perhaps the gravest complication of ketoconazole therapy is hepatitis. Fortunately, this complication is quite rare and is estimated to appear in 1 in 15,000 exposed individuals. An asymptomatic slight elevation of transaminase levels occurs in 5 to 15% and is generally transient. Ketoconazole-associated hepatitis begins as anorexia, malaise, nausea, and vomiting. Abnormalities in either or both serum transaminase and alkaline phosphatase become increasingly profound and are soon accompanied by jaundice. Eighty percent of cases occur within the first 3 months. Progression can be swift. Patients should be instructed to discontinue ketoconazole therapy if they experience the aforementioned symptoms and to call their physician. If hepatotoxicity is suspected, serum transaminase and alkaline phosphatase levels should be measured. Rechallenge should be done with great caution. Some authorities have recommended that liver function be routinely measured periodically. This procedure does not protect a patient who has a rapid onset of hepatitis in the interval between tests but does require that all patients with abnormalities be contacted to inquire about symptoms and to arrange for repeat testing.

Itraconazole

Formulations and Pharmacology

Itraconazole is marketed as a capsule, as an oral suspension in cyclodextrin (an oligosaccharide ring), and as a solution in cyclodextrin for intravenous administration. The ring entraps the hydrophobic, water-insoluble drug. The drug is thus made soluble and is then released either at the lipid membrane of the enterocyte after oral administration or directly into tissues after intravenous administration. The solution makes possible delivery of the drug through a nasogastric tube in intubated patients and makes dosing of infants and small children more convenient. Oral absorption of the capsule is significantly enhanced by food, although absorption of the solution is best on an empty stomach. Coadministration of a cola beverage with itraconazole capsules increases absorption. Peak levels with either preparation are achieved 4 to 6 hours after a dose. Steady state is achieved only after 13 to 15 days, at which time the β-elimination half-life is about 19 to 22 hours. Absorption of the capsule is markedly depressed in bone marrow transplant recipients, probably because of hypochlorhydria, mucositis, and graft-versus-host intestinal changes, and in patients with acquired immunodeficiency syndrome (AIDS) because of enteritis, but the depressed absorption can be alleviated by using the solution.

The intravenous solution of itraconazole is given at 200 mg every 12 hours for four doses (2 days) and then at 200 mg/day. This regimen produces blood levels comparable to those achieved with 200 mg twice daily of the oral preparations. Because the cyclodextrin component is cleared by renal excretion and is nephrotoxic, use of this formulation is not recommended in patients with creatinine clearance less than 30 mL/min.

For deep mycoses, an initial itraconazole dose of 200 mg three times per day is recommended for the first 3 days to quickly give high serum and tissue levels. Hydroxyitraconazole, a metabolite of itraconazole, appears in blood in amounts roughly twice that of the parent drug and has antifungal activity and pharmacokinetics similar to those of the parent compound.

Bioassays of itraconazole give much higher concentrations than high-pressure liquid chromatography does, the difference depending on the susceptibility of the bioassay organism to hydroxyitraconazole. Concentrations of itraconazole in tissue, pus, and bronchial secretions are generally higher than plasma concentrations, but cerebrospinal fluid concentrations are usually unmeasurable, even in patients with meningitis. Ocular levels are low. Saliva concentrations persist for 8 hours after the solution and provide a possible benefit in treating oral disease or eradicating oral colonization. The drug is metabolized in the liver and excreted in feces as metabolites. Of the cyclodextrin liquid administered, less than 0.5% is absorbed. No significant amount of bioactive itraconazole appears in urine. Plasma concentrations do not increase in patients with renal insufficiency or decrease with hemodialysis. The half-life is prolonged in those with cirrhosis.

Adverse Effects

The most common adverse effect of itraconazole is dose-related nausea and abdominal discomfort, but symptoms rarely necessitate stopping therapy. Dividing the dose into twice-daily administration improves tolerance and raises blood levels. Hypokalemia and edema may occur at doses of 400 mg/day or higher. Allergic rash is seen occasionally. Itraconazole is infrequently hepatotoxic and does not suppress adrenal or testicular function at the dosages recommended. Diarrhea, nausea, and other gastrointestinal complaints are more frequent with the solution. A negative inotropic effect is rarely seen.

Drug Interactions

Blood levels of itraconazole are reduced by about half in patients taking drugs that decrease gastric acidity. Rifampin, rifabutin, isoniazid, phenytoin, carbamazepine, phenobarbital, and cisapride decrease itraconazole blood levels. Itraconazole decreases blood levels of rifampin and increases blood levels of the antihistamines terfenadine and astemizole, potentially causing polymorphic ventricular tachycardia (torsades de pointes), as well as increases levels of cisapride, warfarin, benzodiazepines, hepatic hydroxymethylglutaryl–coenzyme A reductase cholesterol-lowering agents, dihydropyridine calcium-channel blockers, digoxin, quinidine, cyclosporine, tacrolimus, methylprednisolone, human immunodeficiency virus (HIV) protease inhibitors (ritonavir, indinavir), and vinca alkaloids (vincristine, vinblastine).

Uses

Itraconazole is useful for the treatment of invasive aspergillosis, allergic bronchopulmonary aspergillosis, [1] blastomycosis, histoplasmosis, meningeal and nonmeningeal coccidioidomycosis, paracoccidioidomycosis, sporotrichosis, phaeohyphomycosis, mucosal candidiasis, ringworm, including onychomycosis, and tinea versicolor. Itraconazole is also useful for the prevention of relapse in AIDS patients with disseminated histoplasmosis. It may be useful for prophylaxis against fungal infections during neutropenia and as empirical therapy for febrile episodes in neutropenia.

Fluconazole

Formulations and Pharmacology

Fluconazole is currently available in tablets, a powder for oral suspension, and an intravenous formulation. Fluconazole is well absorbed from the gastrointestinal tract. Of the oral dose, 60 to 75% appears unchanged in urine. Oral absorption is not decreased in patients with AIDS or those taking H_2-blocking agents.

Concentrations of fluconazole in cerebrospinal fluid are approximately 70% of simultaneous blood levels, regardless of whether the meninges are inflamed, and the drug penetrates into the brain. Penetration into saliva, sputum, urine, and other body fluids is also excellent.

The half-life of fluconazole in patients with normal renal function is 27 to 34 hours and increases to 59 and 98 hours in groups with creatinine clearances of 35 and 14 mL/min, respectively. The normal dose should be reduced to 50% when creatinine clearance is reduced to 50 mL/min and to 25% when creatinine clearance is below 20 mL/min. A loading dose of twice the daily dose is recommended. Patients undergoing hemodialysis should have one daily dose after each session.

Drug Interactions

Fluconazole can cause significant increases in the blood level of phenytoin, glipizide, glyburide, tolbutamide, warfarin, rifabutin, or cyclosporine. Rifampin lowers fluconazole blood levels by about a fourth.

Side Effects

Adverse effects are uncommon. Even with chronic therapy, including doses exceeding 400 mg/day, headache, hair loss, and anorexia were the most common symptoms, whereas 10% had rises in aspartate aminotransferase levels. Alopecia is reversible, even in some instances when fluconazole is continued at lower doses. Neurotoxicity has been described after heroic doses of 2000 mg daily. Rarely, anaphylaxis after the first dose or Stevens-Johnson syndrome has been observed.

Indications

Candidiasis

Provided that patients do not have fluconazole-resistant *Candida*, fluconazole is effective for the treatment of oropharyngeal candidiasis and esophageal candidiasis. A single dose of 150 mg is approximately as effective as topical treatment of vulvovaginal candidiasis. Patients with candidemia who are not neutropenic or otherwise seriously immunosuppressed respond as well to intravenous fluconazole therapy as to amphotericin B. A study comparing fluconazole with a combination of fluconazole plus amphotericin as initial therapy for candidemia suggested that the combination might produce more rapid clearance of the blood stream. In a few patients with *Candida* endocarditis, long-term fluconazole therapy has been used to prevent relapse after amphotericin B therapy. For immunosuppressed patients and rapidly progressing or severely ill patients with deep candidiasis, amphotericin B or caspofungin would be preferred.

Cryptococcal Meningitis

Many authorities recommend amphotericin B or amphotericin B plus flucytosine for at least the first 2 weeks. Therapy can be changed to fluconazole, 400 mg daily for 2 months, if the patient has remained clinically stable. [2] The propensity of AIDS patients for relapse has led to lifelong maintenance therapy with fluconazole, 200 mg daily. Itraconazole capsules are inferior to fluconazole for maintenance therapy. Relapse because of fluconazole resistance has been rare. Fluconazole is effective for the eradication of genitourinary foci. For patients without AIDS, fluconazole is useful for those who have completed a course of amphotericin B and seem to have a high risk of relapse.

Other Mycoses

Fluconazole is useful for coccidioidal meningitis and for disseminated nonmeningeal coccidioidomycosis, but a direct comparison with itraconazole found a trend favoring itraconazole that was driven by the superior efficacy of itraconazole for skeletal infections. The two drugs were similarly efficacious for soft tissue and pulmonary infection. Cutaneous sporotrichosis, ringworm, histoplasmosis, and blastomycosis may respond, but the results are inferior to those with itraconazole. Fluconazole is not indicated for aspergillosis, mucormycosis, or scedosporiosis (pseudallescheriasis).

Prophylaxis in Neutropenic Patients

Fluconazole decreases the incidence of death from deep mycoses in bone marrow transplant recipients. All the protection afforded seemed to occur in patients with deep candidiasis. In a long-term follow-up of one study, bone marrow transplant recipients who received at least 75 days of fluconazole prophylaxis also had improved survival. Use for prophylaxis may result in shifts to less susceptible species.

Prophylaxis in Patients with AIDS

Fluconazole has reduced the incidence of oral and vulvovaginal candidiasis and cryptococcosis in patients with advanced HIV infection, but with negligible effects on other mycoses. Cost, lack of effect on survival, and the possibility of azole resistance have led the Infectious Diseases Society of America advisory committee to recommend against fluconazole prophylaxis in AIDS patients.

Voriconazole

Formulations and Pharmacology

Voriconazole is marketed as a tablet and as a solution in sulfobutyl ether β-cyclodextrin for intravenous administration. Voriconazole is cleared by hepatic metabolism, with less than 2% of the dose excreted unchanged in urine. Voriconazole exhibits significantly nonlinear pharmacokinetics because of saturation of the clearance pathways at higher doses. The principal enzyme involved in clearance is hepatic CYP2C19. This enzyme has significant genetic polymorphisms that affect the amount of metabolism of voriconazole. Despite these differences in metabolism, the plasma levels achieved overlap, and dose adjustment based on genotype or racial group is not recommended.

Standard loading dosing regimens followed by maintenance doses that are 50% of normal are recommended for individuals with mild to moderate hepatic cirrhosis. Dosage adjustments are not required for renal dysfunction, and voriconazole is not significantly cleared by hemodialysis. Because of nephrotoxicity from the cyclodextrin, the intravenous formulation should not be used in patients with creatinine clearance less than 50 mL/min.

Drug Interactions

Voriconazole has many drug interactions. Rifampin, carbamazepine, and long-acting barbiturates induce the hepatic enzymes responsible for clearance of voriconazole and reduce voriconazole levels. Voriconazole and either rifabutin or phenytoin reciprocally alter their clearance. Sirolimus levels are increased dramatically. Reduction in clearance of terfenadine, astemizole, cisapride, pimozide, and quinidine is predicted to be sufficient to place the patient at risk for QTc prolongation. Reduction in the clearance of ergot alkaloids could lead to ergotism. Cyclosporine, tacrolimus, warfarin, oral coumarins, lipid-lowering statin agents, benzodiazepines, calcium-channel blockers, sulfonylureas, and vinca alkaloids may be coadministered, but the dosage of these drugs may need to be reduced, and clinical or laboratory monitoring is suggested. Voriconazole significantly reduces the rate of clearance of omeprazole. Other interactions are possible, and any CYP inhibitors, blockers, or inducers should be considered to possibly have an interaction with voriconazole.

Side Effects

Voriconazole is generally well tolerated. The most frequently reported adverse event is a transient, reversible visual disturbance beginning approximately 30 minutes after a dose. Patients should be advised to avoid activities that require keen visual acuity while experiencing visual changes. Hallucinations and confusion have also been reported.

Indications

Aspergillosis

Voriconazole was licensed for the treatment of invasive aspergillosis on the basis of a randomized, unblinded comparative trial in which patients with invasive aspergillosis were randomized to receive initial therapy with either voriconazole or ABD. [3] After initial randomization, patients could be switched to other licensed therapies as dictated by clinical events. After 12 weeks, 53% of the patients randomized to voriconazole but only 32% of those randomized to ABD had a successful outcome.

Other Mycoses

Voriconazole is also licensed for the treatment of invasive fusariosis and scedosporiosis based on high response rates for these diseases. The drug is efficacious in esophageal candidiasis, invasive candidiasis, and refractory candidiasis. Although voriconazole has appealing features for use in prophylaxis, there has been concern about breakthrough zygomycoses with long-term use.

Posaconazole

Formulations and Pharmacology

Posaconazole is given orally as a solution and has a long terminal-phase half-life (25 to 35 hours). Absorption is unaffected by stomach pH. Bioavailability is increased by food, and drug exposure is increased when doses are divided (up to four times per day). Posaconazole is metabolized in the liver, and maximum plasma concentrations are achieved after 6 hours. At steady state, 800 mg/day produces a C_{max} of 4.2 and nadir of 3.1 μg/mL. Interpatient serum concentrations are quite variable. A scant amount of active drug appears in urine. Animal studies indicate good penetration into liver, adrenal, pancreas, and kidney tissues. No dose adjustments are needed for hepatic failure, renal failure, or hemodialysis.

Drug Interactions

Concomitant therapy with posaconazole significantly elevates levels of cyclosporine, rifabutin, phenytoin, midazolam, and tacrolimus, and posaconazole levels are decreased by cimetidine (not by pH effect), rifabutin, and phenytoin. Contraindicated drugs include terfenadine, astemizole, cisapride, pimozide, halofantrine, quinidine, and ergot alkaloids.

Side Effects

The drug has a low toxicity profile; in clinical studies the only effects greater than with placebo were dry mouth, dizziness, and constipation, and these were seen in only about 10% of recipients.

Indications

Posaconazole has a very broad spectrum of activity against molds, including many zygomycetes, a unique property among azoles. The molecular interaction with the fungal 14α-demethylase enzyme, the azole target, may be novel, thus explaining a lack of cross-resistance of many fungi, particularly aspergilli, resistant to other azoles. However, fluconazole-resistant *Candida* tends to have considerably higher posaconazole MICs. In animal models, posaconazole is approximately equipotent to ABD against aspergillosis, including central nervous system disease, superior to fluconazole against candidiasis, superior to all other agents against coccidioidomycosis, and additive to amphotericin B against *Candida albicans* or *Aspergillus* infections. Successful outcome appears to correlate with AUC/MIC or nadir drug level/MIC ratios.

The clinical results are thus far concordant with these preclinical data. Although short courses of only 400 mg daily too frequently resulted in less than durable responses in coccidioidomycosis, studies with higher doses for long durations have produced excellent results in patients failing previous therapy with other agents. Similarly, salvage therapy results for aspergillosis have been excellent, particularly with disease caused by isolates other than *Aspergillus fumigatus;* plasma levels correspond with outcome. Activity against oropharyngeal candidiasis is equivalent to that of fluconazole. Fungal brain abscesses caused by a variety of pathogens have been responsive, although results for cryptococcal meningitis are not noteworthy. Open trials against zygomycoses, including brain infections, have also shown remarkable results; *Rhizomucor* species seem less responsive. Prophylaxis studies in stem cell transplant patients with graft-versus-host disease, acute myelogenous leukemia, and myelodysplastic syndromes have shown reduction of fungal infections, particularly aspergillosis, [4] and posaconazole also appears to be superior to fluconazole or itraconazole when used as prophylaxis in patients with fever and neutropenia. [5]

ECHINOCANDIN ANTIFUNGAL AGENTS

General Features

The echinocandin antifungal agents act by inhibiting the synthesis of 1,3β-D-glucan in the fungal cell wall. In studies, the principal pharmacodynamic driver of in vivo response has been the ratio of the peak concentration achieved to the MIC. All are cyclic lipopeptides that must be given intravenously.

Echinocandins are fungicidal against all *Candida* species, including isolates resistant to other agents. Reduced activity against isolates of

Candida parapsilosis and *Candida guilliermondii* and a paradoxical effect of high concentrations permitting growth in vitro have been noted in a minority of *Candida* isolates and do not appear to be clinically relevant. All are active against *Aspergillus* species, but activity is limited to growing and dividing hyphal elements. Their activity against other fungi is variable.

Caspofungin

Formulations and Pharmacology

Caspofungin is marketed for intravenous infusion. Clearance of caspofungin is through a combination of spontaneous chemical degradation, hydrolysis, and *N*-acetylation. Dose adjustments are not required for renal function or hemodialysis. Clearance of caspofungin is modestly reduced in subjects with moderate hepatic insufficiency, and thus a dosage lower than the usual daily dose is recommended. Penetration into infected tissues appears to be good.

Drug Interactions

Caspofungin has few meaningful drug interactions. Cyclosporine coadministration increases caspofungin exposure and has been associated with increased hepatic transaminase levels, so concomitant use should be cautious. Caspofungin coadministration reduces tacrolimus exposure by approximately 20%, and dosage adjustments may be required. Rifampin reduces caspofungin blood levels by about 30%, and the daily dosage of caspofungin should be increased from 50 to 70 mg if these drugs are coadministered. Likewise, limited data with other inducers of drug clearance (efavirenz, nevirapine, phenytoin, dexamethasone, and carbamazepine) suggest that reduced caspofungin levels are possible and that an increase in the daily dose, to 70 mg, should be considered.

Side Effects

Adverse reactions with caspofungin have overall been infrequent and minor. Symptoms possibly related to histamine release during rapid infusion have been reported.

Indications

Caspofungin is indicated for the treatment of invasive candidiasis and esophageal candidiasis. [6] It is also indicated as therapy for invasive aspergillosis in patients who are refractory to or intolerant of other therapies. With activity against these two major opportunistic pathogens, use of caspofungin for empirical therapy in high-risk situations is logical and supported by clinical trials.

Micafungin

Micafungin is a newly approved echinocandin with an in vitro spectrum and properties similar to those of caspofungin and is similarly fungicidal for *Candida* species and nonfungicidal in vitro against *Aspergillus*.

Formulations and Pharmacology

Micafungin is light sensitive. After an intravenous infusion, the terminal half-life is about 15 hours. A 50-mg dose produces a C_{max} of 3.4 μg/mL. Metabolism appears to be via an *O*-methyltransferase enzyme; less than 1% is excreted in urine. The drug appears to penetrate particularly well into the lungs, liver, kidney, and gastric mucosa. It increases the phagocyte respiratory burst and interacts synergistically with phagocytes in inhibiting fungi. No adjustment for hepatic insufficiency is needed.

Drug interactions

Micafungin has fewer drug interactions than caspofungin does; there is none with cyclosporine. The interaction with amphotericin in vitro against *Aspergillus* is indifference.

Side Effects

Micafungin has had an excellent safety profile thus far. Histamine release, resulting most prominently in erythema over the body, can be avoided by slow infusion.

Indications

In addition to the activity mentioned, micafungin is also active in vitro against the endemic pathogens (tested in the mycelial form). In animal models it is active against candidiasis and aspergillosis. In clinical dose-finding studies against *Candida* esophagitis, doses of 75 to 150 mg/day were particularly effective and, against candidemia, 50 to 100 mg/day. A trial of prophylaxis in neutropenic patients with hematopoietic stem cell transplants showed efficacy at 50 mg/day.

Anidulafungin

Formulations and Pharmacology

Anidulafungin is available for intravenous use. Its half-life is 30 to 40 hours. The optimal dose of anidulafungin, at least for candidiasis, is a 200-mg loading dose followed by 100 mg/day. A 100-mg dose produces a C_{max} of 8.6 μg/mL at a T_{max} of 6 to 7 hours. It is degraded nonenzymatically in plasma and excreted by the liver. No dosage adjustment appears necessary in patients with renal or hepatic disease. Evidence from animal studies indicates excellent penetration into the lung, liver, spleen, and kidney.

Drug Interactions

Anidulafungin appears to have few drug interactions, including scant interaction with cyclosporine.

Side Effects

Side effects of anidulafungin have been uncommon in clinical trials; hypotension, hypokalemia, vomiting, constipation, nausea, and fever have been reported.

Indications

In vitro, anidulafungin has activity against all *Candida* species (although *C. parapsilosis* and *C. lusitaniae* are relatively resistant and resistance is seen in occasional isolates of *C. glabrata* and *C. guilliermondii*), *Aspergillus* (and synergy with azoles has been shown), *Coccidioides*, and *Sporothrix* isolates, and *Histoplasma* is susceptible but tolerant. Anidulafungin was effective in treating invasive candidiasis (where it was shown to be superior to fluconazole) in clinical studies, as well as in treating esophageal candidiasis (although relapse was a problem). Anidulafungin is approved by the Food and Drug Administration for use in the treatment of candidemia, intra-abdominal abscess, and peritonitis, as well as esophageal candidiasis.

COMBINATIONS AND OTHER AGENTS

Combinations of antifungal agents are increasingly being used in an effort to improve appalling response rates in some diseases and to combine drugs with different mechanisms of action. Although synergy in vitro is relatively easy to demonstrate, there are few examples of synergy in animal model studies, and the clinical advantages of the amphotericin-flucytosine combination in cryptococcosis have yet to be duplicated in other situations. [7] Immunomodulators, particularly cytokines, hold promise, but insufficient clinical data exist to determine where and how these drugs might be used. Granulocyte-macrophage colony-stimulating factor was shown to be effective in one trial when given prophylactically during induction therapy for high-risk leukemia patients.

Therapy for the various forms of tinea with systemic agents is discussed in Chapter 464. Although *Pneumocystis jiroveci (P. carinii)* is now classified among the fungi, the drugs used to treat it are principally used to treat parasitic infections (Chapter 364).

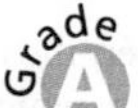

1. Stevens DA, Schwartz HJ, Lee JY, et al: A randomized trial of itraconazole in allergic bronchopulmonary aspergillosis. N Engl J Med 2000;342:756–762.
2. Van der Horst CM, Saag MS, Cloud GA, et al: National Institute of Allergy and Infectious Diseases Mycoses Study Group AIDS Clinical Trials Group: Treatment of cryptococcal meningitis associated with the acquired immunodeficiency syndrome. N Engl J Med 1997; 337:15–21.
3. Herbrecht R, Denning DW, Patterson TF, et al: Voriconazole versus amphotericin B for primary therapy of invasive aspergillosis. N Engl J Med 2002;347:408–415.
4. Ullmann AJ, Lipton JH, Vesole DH, et al: Posaconazole or fluconazole for prophylaxis in severe graft-versus-host disease. N Engl J Med 2007;356:335–347.
5. Cornely OA, Maertens J, Winston DJ, et al: Posaconazole vs. fluconazole or itraconazole prophylaxis in patients with neutropenia. N Engl J Med 2007;356:348–359.

FIGURE 352–1 • Structures of the systemic antifungal agents.

Continued

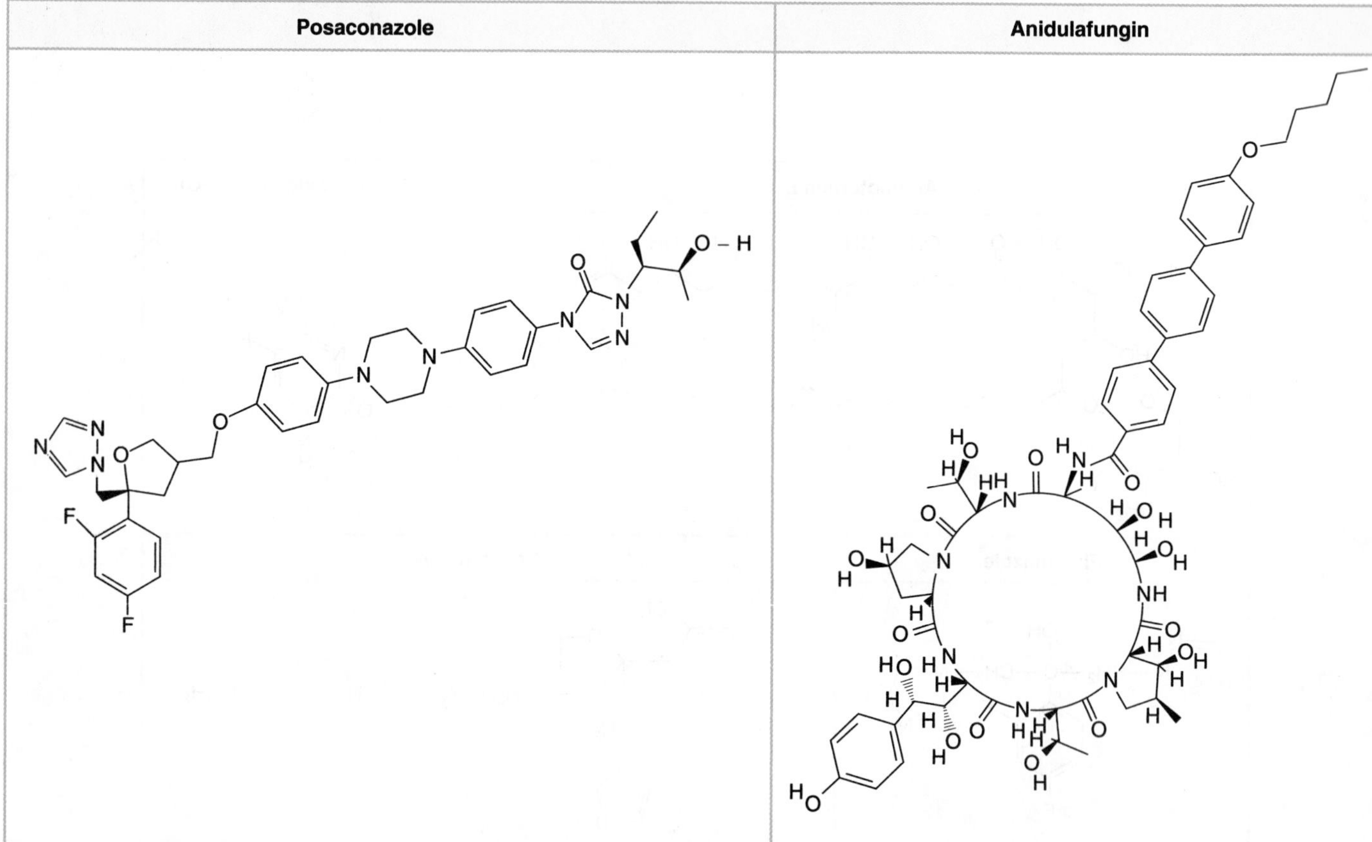

FIGURE 352–1 • Structures of the systemic antifungal agents, continued

6. Mora-Duarte J, Betts R, Rotstein R, et al: Caspofungin Invasive Candidiasis Study Group. Comparison of caspofungin and amphotericin B for invasive candidiasis. N Engl J Med 2002;347: 2020–2029.
7. Mukherjee PK, Sheehan DJ, Hitchcock CA, Ghannoum MA: Combination treatment of invasive fungal infections. Clin Microbiol Rev 2005;18:163–194.

SUGGESTED READINGS

Antoniadou A, Dupont B: Lipid formulations of amphotericin B: Where are we today? J Mycol Med 2005;15:230–238. *A review of the latest developments.*

Bennett JE: Echinocandins for candidemia in adults without neutropenia. N Engl J Med 2006;355:1154–1159. *A clinical review.*

Dixon S, McKeen E, Tabberer M, Paisley S: Economic evaluations of treatments for systemic fungal infections. Pharmacoeconomics 2004;22:421–433. *A review of the costs associated with these sometimes expensive interventions.*

Dodds Ashley ES, Lewis R, Lewis JS, et al: Pharmacology of systemic antifungal agents. Clin Infect Dis 2006;43:S28–S39. *A review of pharmacokinetics and pharmacodynamics.*

Donnelly JP, DePauw BE: Voriconazole—a new therapeutic agent with an extended spectrum of antifungal activity. Clinical Microbiol Infect 2004; 10(Suppl. 1):107–117. *A practical review.*

Leather HL, Wingard JR: Prophylaxis, empirical therapy, or pre-emptive therapy of fungal infections in immunocompromised patients: Which is better for whom? Curr Opin Infect Dis 2002;15:369–375. *A critique of various approaches to preventing opportunistic mycoses in susceptible populations.*

Loeffler J, Stevens DA: Antifungal drug resistance. Clin Infect Dis 2003; 36:S31–S41. *Delineation of how some fungi have developed evasions of our armamentarium.*

Spanakis EK, Aperis G, Mylonakis E: New agents for the treatment of fungal infections: Clinical efficacy and gaps in coverage. Clin Infect Dis 2006;43:1060–1068. *An excellent review.*

Vazquez JA, Sobel JD: Anidulafungin: A novel echinocandin. Clin Infect Dis 2006;43:215–222. *A review.*

353 HISTOPLASMOSIS

Carol A. Kauffman

Definition

Histoplasmosis is the most common endemic mycosis in the United States. Most infections are self-limited, but the organism has the ability to cause severe acute pulmonary and disseminated infection, as well as chronic pulmonary and disseminated infection.

The Pathogen

Histoplasma capsulatum var *capsulatum* is a thermally dimorphic fungus. In the environment and at temperatures lower than 35° C, it exists as a mold that produces conidia, both tuberculate macroconidia, which are helpful for identification purposes in the laboratory, and microconidia, which are probably the infectious form. In tissues and at 35 to 37° C, *H. capsulatum* transforms into tiny 2- to 4-μm oval yeasts that reproduce by budding and parasitize macrophages. African histoplasmosis is caused by a different subspecies of *H. capsulatum* (var *duboisii*) and has different disease manifestations.

Epidemiology

Histoplasmosis, though found worldwide, is primarily a disease of North and Central America. *H. capsulatum* is endemic in the Mississippi and Ohio River valleys, with extension into the St. Lawrence basin; microfoci exist in discrete isolated areas in several eastern states. Soil, caves, and abandoned buildings containing high concentrations of bird or bat guano support luxuriant growth of the organism. Every year, hundreds of thousands of individuals who live in areas endemic for *H. capsulatum* are infected. Most cases are sporadic and the exact source of exposure is unknown. Point-source outbreaks that have included as few as 4 or 5 persons and as many as 100,000 have been well described in association with disruption of soil; cleaning attics, bridges, or barns; tearing down old structures laden with guano; and spelunking.

Pathobiology

After inhalation of microconidia into the alveoli, a localized pulmonary infection ensues. Neutrophils and macrophages phagocytize the organism, now in the yeast phase; the organism is able to survive and travel within macrophages to the hilar and mediastinal lymph nodes and throughout the reticuloendothelial system by hematogenous dissemination. Such dissemination probably occurs in most persons who are infected and in normal hosts is associated with no symptoms. After several weeks, T cells specifically sensitized by *H. capsulatum* antigens activate macrophages, which are then able to kill the intracellular fungi. Histoplasmosis is a classic example of the pivotal importance of the cell-mediated immune system in containing intracellular pathogens. Not surprisingly, most patients with severe infection are those who have cellular immunodeficiencies.

The extent of disease is determined by both the number of conidia inhaled and the immune response of the host. A small inoculum can cause severe pulmonary infection or progress to acute symptomatic disseminated histoplasmosis in patients with advanced acquired immunodeficiency syndrome (AIDS) because their cell-mediated immune system is unable to contain the organism. Conversely, severe life-threatening pulmonary infection may develop in a healthy individual if a large number of conidia are inhaled, as might occur during the demolition of old buildings or while spelunking in a heavily infested cave.

Reinfection occurs in persons who previously had histoplasmosis, almost always in the setting of heavy exposure. Histoplasmosis reinfection is usually less severe than primary infection because of residual immunity induced by the initial episode. Reactivation of latent infection occurs in patients who have deficient cell-mediated immunity, as evidenced by the occurrence of histoplasmosis in persons who grew up in the endemic area but have not been back in that area for years.

Clinical Manifestations

Acute Pulmonary Histoplasmosis

Infection is asymptomatic in most people infected with *H. capsulatum*. Those who do have symptomatic pulmonary infection usually have a self-limited illness that begins several weeks after exposure and is characterized by fever, chills, fatigue, nonproductive cough, anterior chest discomfort, and myalgia. Arthritis or arthralgia, often accompanied by erythema nodosum, occurs in 5 to 10% of patients with acute pulmonary histoplasmosis. A patchy lobar or multilobe nodular infiltrate is noted on chest radiograph.

The differential diagnosis of acute pulmonary histoplasmosis includes pneumonia from *Blastomyces dermatitidis, Mycoplasma pneumoniae, Legionella* sp, and *Chlamydia pneumoniae.* When enlarged hilar or mediastinal lymph nodes are present, histoplasmosis should be strongly considered. The most difficult to differentiate is acute pulmonary blastomycosis because the endemic areas overlap, a comparable history of outdoor activities is often obtained, and radiographs show similar findings.

In patients who have experienced heavy exposure to *H. capsulatum* and in those who are immunosuppressed, acute pulmonary histoplasmosis can be life-threatening. High spiking fevers, chills, prostration, dyspnea, and cough are prominent. Chest radiographs show diffuse reticulonodular pulmonary infiltrates, and respiratory failure can occur rapidly.

Chronic Pulmonary Histoplasmosis

Chronic cavitary pulmonary histoplasmosis is a progressive, fatal form of histoplasmosis that develops almost exclusively in older patients who have chronic obstructive pulmonary disease. Symptoms include fever, fatigue, anorexia, weight loss, cough productive of purulent sputum, and hemoptysis. On chest radiograph, the usual findings are unilateral or bilateral upper lobe infiltrates with multiple cavities and extensive fibrosis in the lower lobes. Bronchopleural fistula formation and pneumothorax can occur. Chronic pulmonary histoplasmosis mimics tuberculosis, other fungal pneumonias (especially blastomycosis and sporotrichosis), and nontuberculous mycobacterial infections with regard to symptoms, signs, and radiographic findings.

Complications of Pulmonary Histoplasmosis

The mediastinal and hilar lymph nodes often calcify as the infection resolves; years later they can erode into bronchi and cause hemoptysis and expectoration of broncholiths. Granulomatous mediastinitis is an uncommon syndrome characterized by continuing inflammation and necrosis in the mediastinal lymph nodes. The enlarged nodes are readily apparent on chest radiographs, and computed tomography (CT) scans show central necrosis and impingement on adjacent structures, including the esophagus, airways, and blood vessels. Although symptoms usually resolve without treatment, obstructive syndromes can be severe and the nodes can persist for years.

Fibrosing mediastinitis is a rare, but fatal complication of histoplasmosis in which the host responds to the infection with an inappropriate excessive fibrotic response. Obstruction of the esophagus, airways, superior vena cava, or the pulmonary arteries and veins can occur with resultant progressive right heart failure and respiratory insufficiency. Mediastinal widening is seen on chest radiographs, and CT scans define the extent of invasion and obstruction of mediastinal structures.

Pericarditis is a manifestation of a local inflammatory reaction to adjacent histoplasmosis. Patients respond promptly to anti-inflammatory medications without antifungal therapy. Hemodynamic compromise, though unusual, requires drainage of pericardial fluid; only rarely has progression to constrictive pericarditis been documented.

Disseminated Histoplasmosis

Symptomatic disseminated histoplasmosis occurs mostly in immunosuppressed patients. Patients with AIDS and CD4 counts lower than 150/μL, infants, and those who have a hematologic malignancy, have received an organ transplant, or are taking corticosteroids or anti–tumor necrosis factor agents are at greatest risk for acute disseminated histoplasmosis. Symptoms and signs include chills, fever, anorexia, weight loss, hypotension, dyspnea, hepatosplenomegaly, and skin and mucous membrane lesions. Pancytopenia, diffuse pulmonary infiltrates on chest radiograph, findings of disseminated intravascular coagulation, and acute respiratory failure are common. This syndrome is indistinguishable from sepsis due to any bacterial or viral etiology. In AIDS patients, the differential diagnosis includes cytomegalovirus, disseminated *Mycobacterium avium* complex infection, and tuberculosis.

Chronic progressive disseminated histoplasmosis is a fatal form of histoplasmosis that occurs mostly in middle-aged to elderly men who have no known immunosuppressive illness. The illness is characterized by fever, night sweats, weight loss, anorexia, and fatigue. Patients appear chronically ill, hepatosplenomegaly and mucocutaneous ulcerations are common, and a small proportion have signs of adrenal insufficiency. An increased erythrocyte sedimentation rate, elevated alkaline phosphatase, pancytopenia, and diffuse reticulonodular infiltrates on chest radiographs are typical. Patients with this form of histoplasmosis often have fever of unknown origin. Miliary tuberculosis, lymphoma, and sarcoidosis must be excluded.

Involvement of almost every organ system has been reported with disseminated infection. Adrenal insufficiency must be sought in any patient who has unexplained hypotension, hyponatremia, and hyperkalemia. Abdominal CT shows markedly enlarged adrenal glands. Central nervous system involvement is manifested either as meningitis or as focal lesions seen on magnetic resonance imaging and is more common in patients with AIDS. Skin lesions, also more common in patients with AIDS, can be papular, pustular, or ulcerated. *Histoplasma* endocarditis is a rare form of disseminated infection.

Presumed Ocular Histoplasmosis

Choroiditis causing visual loss has been attributed to histoplasmosis based on residence in an area endemic for histoplasmosis and histoplasmin skin test reactivity rather than demonstration of the organism in the eye. So-called histo spots are not a manifestation of active infection of the eye with *H. capsulatum* and should not be treated with antifungal agents.

Diagnosis

The definitive diagnostic test for histoplasmosis is growth of the organism in culture. Unfortunately, *H. capsulatum* may take as long as 6 weeks to grow in vitro. Tissue samples, bronchoalveolar lavage fluid, sputum, and blood are appropriate for culture. For patients who have evidence of dissemination, blood cultures are best performed with the lysis-centrifugation (Isolator tube) system; bone marrow and liver biopsy material often yield *H. capsulatum* in the setting of dissemination. If pulmonary histoplasmosis is a diagnostic consideration, the laboratory should be informed so that a special medium that decreases the growth of commensal fungi can be used for the culture of pulmonary samples. As soon as growth of a mold has been detected, highly specific DNA probes for *H. capsulatum* allow rapid identification of the organism.

If the patient is acutely ill, tissue biopsy should be performed to search for the distinctive 2- to 4-μm oval budding yeasts, which allows a tentative diagnosis to be made as quickly as possible. Routine tissue stains do not show the tiny yeasts; biopsy material must be stained with methenamine silver or periodic acid–Schiff stains. In patients with disseminated disease, bone marrow, liver, skin, and mucocutaneous lesions usually reveal many organisms. The organisms can also be seen with Wright stain of peripheral blood from patients with acute disseminated infection. In patients with chronic pulmonary histoplasmosis or granulomatous mediastinitis, biopsy of lung or lymph nodes may reveal the organism. It is unusual to find the small yeasts of *H. capsulatum* on cytologic examination of sputum or bronchoalveolar lavage fluid.

Serology plays an important role in the diagnosis of some forms of histoplasmosis. Complement fixation (CF) assays that use two different antigens, mycelial and yeast, and immunodiffusion (ID) tests are available. The ID test is more specific than the CF test, but CF tests are more sensitive. CF antibody titers frequently remain positive at low titer for years after the infection. Serology is often the most important diagnostic test for establishing the diagnosis of acute pulmonary histoplasmosis. In this form of histoplasmosis cultures are often negative. The diagnosis can be made by a four-fold rise in CF titer, a CF titer higher than 1:32, or the appearance of an M precipitin band by ID assay. These tests are also quite useful in patients with chronic forms of pulmonary or disseminated histoplasmosis, but they are rarely useful in immunosuppressed patients, who cannot mount an antibody response. Serologic tests are less definitive in patients who have mediastinal lymphadenopathy and should always be confirmed by tissue biopsy. False-positive CF test results occur in patients with lymphoma, tuberculosis, sarcoidosis, and other fungal infections, all of which may be manifested as mediastinal masses.

An enzyme immunoassay for *H. capsulatum* polysaccharide antigen in urine and serum is extremely helpful in patients with disseminated infection. The sensitivity for antigen detection is higher in urine than in serum. Antigen levels should become undetectable with successful therapy; persistence of antigen implies active infection. Antigen assays are also helpful in patients who have acute pulmonary histoplasmosis. Almost 75% of those who have had a heavy exposure and demonstrate diffuse infiltrates will have a positive urinary antigen test. However, those with mild pulmonary involvement or chronic cavitary histoplasmosis most often have a negative antigen assay. Cross-reactivity has been noted with blastomycosis, paracoccidioidomycosis, and penicilliosis.

Skin testing with histoplasmin antigen was enormously important in defining the epidemiology of histoplasmosis, but is no longer available.

Treatment

Guidelines for the treatment of histoplasmosis have been published by the Mycoses Study Group and the Infectious Diseases Society of America. Itraconazole is the drug of choice for mild to moderate histoplasmosis, and amphotericin B is for severe, life-threatening infection. Lipid formulations of amphotericin B are as effective as standard amphotericin B. Fluconazole is less active and should be considered a second-line agent, and ketoconazole has become a second-line agent because of increased toxicity in comparison to itraconazole. The role of voriconazole and posaconazole in the treatment of histoplasmosis is not clear. The echinocandins do not appear to be effective for histoplasmosis.

Pulmonary Histoplasmosis

Treatment is not usually given for acute pulmonary histoplasmosis; many times the diagnosis is not made until after the symptoms have resolved. However, if the patient remains symptomatic after 4 weeks, therapy with itraconazole, 200 mg daily for 6 to 12 weeks, can be given. Patients who have severe outbreak-associated histoplasmosis and all immunosuppressed patients should be treated. Initial therapy with amphotericin B, 0.7 to 1 mg/kg daily, can be followed by oral itraconazole after a favorable response is noted. Antifungal therapy should be given to all patients with chronic pulmonary histoplasmosis. Itraconazole, 200 mg once or twice daily for 12 to 24 months, is preferred; if amphotericin B is used, the total dosage should be 30 to 35 mg/kg.

A trial of itraconazole for 6 to 12 months is recommended for patients with symptomatic granulomatous mediastinitis, although there are no data proving such therapy to be effective. Surgical resection of nodes causing obstructive symptoms may be beneficial. Antifungal therapy probably offers no benefit for patients with fibrosing mediastinitis. However, because of the inexorable downhill course of this illness, a several-month course of itraconazole is often tried. Surgery for this condition carries a high operative mortality rate. Intravascular stents have been used successfully in some patients with vascular obstruction.

Disseminated Histoplasmosis

All patients with symptomatic disseminated histoplasmosis should receive antifungal therapy. Patients who have only mild to moderate symptoms with acute disseminated disease and most patients with chronic progressive disseminated histoplasmosis can be treated with itraconazole, 200 mg twice daily. A total of 12 months of therapy is generally adequate, but for those with chronic progressive disease, the duration of treatment should be determined by the patient's clinical course. Patients who have AIDS should be maintained on chronic suppressive itraconazole therapy, 200 mg daily, after they receive an initial course of 12 weeks of twice-daily itraconazole. Therapy can be stopped only after their CD4 count remains higher than 200/μL for at least a year.

Immunosuppressed patients with moderately severe to severe symptoms should be treated with amphotericin B, 0.7 to 1 mg/kg daily. For most patients, therapy can be changed to itraconazole after their condition has improved and they are able to take oral medications. If it is elected to treat only with amphotericin B, the total dosage should be 35 mg/kg. For certain patients, including stem cell and solid organ transplant recipients and those taking nephrotoxic drugs or with preexisting renal failure, a lipid formulation of amphotericin B should be used.

Prognosis

Acute pulmonary histoplasmosis is usually a self-limited disease. Patients who require treatment generally respond promptly to antifungal agents. However, the response of patients with chronic cavitary pulmonary histoplasmosis is often poor, primarily because of their severe underlying pulmonary disease. Patients with disseminated histoplasmosis, even those with advanced AIDS, usually respond promptly to antifungal therapy. Older patients with chronic progressive disseminated histoplasmosis have a slower, but usually complete response to therapy.

SUGGESTED READINGS

Cano M, Hajjeh RA: The epidemiology of histoplasmosis: A review. Semin Respir Infect 2001;16:109–118. *Excellent overview of the epidemiology of histoplasmosis.*

Kauffman CA: Histoplasmosis: A clinical and laboratory update. Clin Microbiol Rev 2007;20:115–132. *An excellent review.*

Wheat LJ: Histoplasmosis: A review for clinicians from non-endemic areas. Mycoses 2006;49:274–282. *An overview in suspecting, diagnosing, and treating patients with histoplasmosis.*

Wheat LJ: Improvements in diagnosis of histoplasmosis. Expert Opin Biol Ther 2006;6:1207–1221. *A comprehensive review of histoplasmosis.*

354 COCCIDIOIDOMYCOSIS

John N. Galgiani

Definition

Coccidioidomycosis is a systemic fungal infection caused by *Coccidioides* species endemic to some deserts of the Western Hemisphere (Table 354–1).

The Pathogen

Coccidioides immitis and *Coccidioides posadasii* are dimorphic fungi that are classified as ascomycetes by ribosomal gene homology. In their vegetative state, mycelia with true septations mature to produce arthroconidia, single cells approximately 2 to 5 µm in diameter. After infection, an arthroconidium enlarges to a spherule up to 75 µm in diameter and undergoes internal septation to produce scores of endospores. When the spherules rupture, packets of endospores are released and produce more spherules in infected tissue or revert to mycelia if removed from the body.

Epidemiology

Coccidioides organisms can be recovered from the soil of the low deserts of Arizona, the Central Valley of California, parts of other states including New Mexico and Texas, and parts of Central and South America. Endemic regions follow the climatologic Sonoran life zone, which is characterized by modest rainfall, mild winters, and low humidity. Mycelia bloom beneath the surface during periods of rain, and arthroconidia develop as the earth dries. Rates of infection are highest during dry months and are accentuated when soil is disturbed by windstorms or construction equipment. Exposure to contaminated bales of cotton or other fomites can result in infection beyond the endemic regions, but this is rare. Person-to-person transmission of pulmonary infection has not been reported, and isolation precautions are unnecessary. *Coccidioides* species are listed by the Centers for Disease Control and Prevention as select agents that could be used for bioterrorism.

TABLE 354–1 COCCIDIOIDOMYCOSIS: CLINICAL CHARACTERISTICS AND TREATMENT

Characteristic	Description
Causative fungi	*Coccidioides immitis* and *Coccidioides posadasii*
Primary geographic distribution	Lower Sonoran deserts of the Western Hemisphere, including parts of Arizona, California, and New Mexico; western Texas; and parts of Central and South America
Primary route of acquisition	Respiratory (inhalation of arthroconidia)
Principal site of disease	Lungs most common; spread to skin, bones, meninges, and other viscera uncommon but serious
Opportunistic infection in compromised hosts	Diffuse pneumonia and widespread infections common in patients with T-lymphocyte defects or during high-dose corticosteroid therapy
Drug of choice for most patients	No antifungal is required for uncomplicated pneumonia; fluconazole or itraconazole for progressive forms of infection
Alternative therapy	Amphotericin B (especially with diffuse pneumonia or rapidly progressive infections), voriconazole, posaconazole

Incidence and Prevalence

In general, the annual risk for infection within the most strongly endemic areas is 3% and results in approximately 150,000 new infections. With unusually intense exposure, such as at archeology sites or during military maneuvers within endemic regions, infections can develop in the majority of persons exposed for only a matter of days. More than 60% of new infections are likely to occur in Arizona because of the rapid growth of populations in the Phoenix and Tucson areas.

Pathobiology

Inhaling a single arthroconidium to the level of the terminal bronchiole initiates virtually all coccidioidal infections. Fungal proliferation engenders both granulomatous inflammation, which is associated with intact spherules, and acute inflammation, including eosinophils, which is associated with spherule rupture. Focal pneumonia is often associated with ipsilateral hilar adenopathy, and less frequently, infection enlarges the peritracheal, supraclavicular, and cervical nodes. Lesions occurring elsewhere are the result of hematogenous dissemination, and most become apparent within 2 years of the initial infection. Although progressive dissemination occurs in less than 1% of infections, as many as 8% of persons with self-limited infection manifest asymptomatic chorioretinal scars, thus suggesting that subclinical hematogenous spread may be frequent. Within weeks after infection, durable T-cell immunity normally arrests fungal proliferation, which allows the inflammation to resolve and prevents reinfection in the future. However, control of the infection may occur without sterilizing lesions, and reactivation of dormant infection or a second infection is possible, even many years later, in patients whose cell-mediated immunity becomes deficient.

Clinical Manifestations

At least two of every three infections are detected only by finding dermal hypersensitivity to coccidioidal antigens. Those who become ill usually experience self-limited pulmonary syndromes. However, complications or progressive forms of infection that display a broad variety of manifestations and pose difficult problems in management for the clinician develop in a few patients.

Primary Pulmonary Infections

Symptoms develop within 5 to 21 days after exposure. For residents or recent visitors to southern Arizona, coccidioidomycosis accounts for approximately a third of cases of community-acquired pneumonia. Fever, weight loss, fatigue, a dry cough, and pleuritic chest pain are common, but not specific complaints. Arthralgia of multiple joints without significant effusion is also frequent and referred to as "desert rheumatism." Occasionally, skin manifestations develop, including a short-lived nonpruritic maculopapular rash, erythema multiforme, or erythema nodosum. These arthritic and dermatologic manifestations are mediated by circulating immune complexes or other immunologic phenomena rather than fungal dissemination. Radiographs of the chest may show no abnormalities or may demonstrate pulmonary infiltrates, either segmental or lobar. Hilar adenopathy is often a distinctive finding. Peripneumonic pleural effusions may occur and generally resolve without intervention, although cultures of pleural biopsies usually yield *Coccidioides* species. Eosinophilia is frequently a prominent finding in differential leukocyte counts of peripheral blood, and the erythrocyte sedimentation rate is generally elevated. Symptoms may persist for several weeks before improvement is clearly under way, and the illness, especially lassitude, may persist for months.

The primary pulmonary process produces a variety of sequelae. The most frequent is the development of a pulmonary nodule (Fig. 354–1), typically measuring 1 to 4 cm and lying within 5 cm of the hilus. Despite their harmless nature, coccidioidal nodules may engender concern because of their similarity to a malignant mass. For this reason, management usually requires percutaneous needle aspiration or resection. Another consequence of pulmonary coccidioidomycosis is cavitation of the infiltrate, which occurs in approximately 5% of cases of pneumonia. Most cavities are solitary and thin walled and reside in an upper lobe close to the pleura. Occasionally, they produce pain, hemoptysis, or adjacent infiltrates. Cavities may acquire mycetomas from either *Coccidioides*

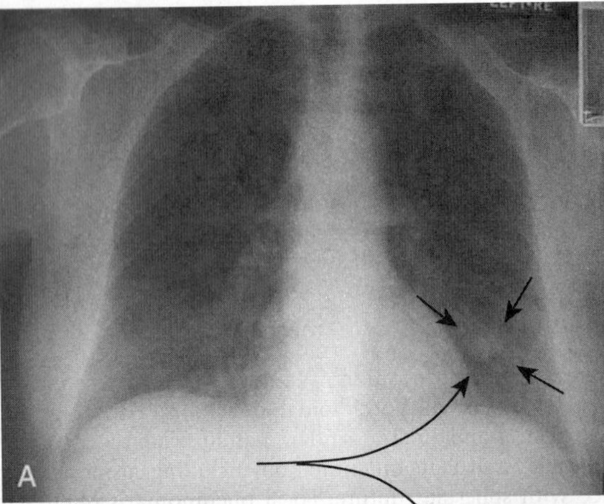

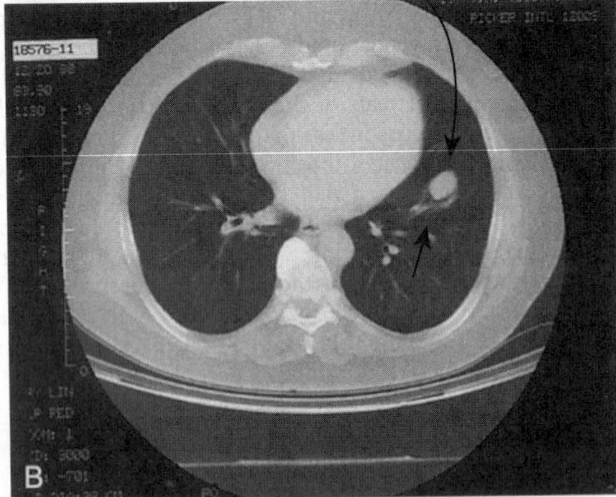

FIGURE 354–1 • Coccidioidomycosis. A, Benign nodule secondary to coccidioidomycosis (arrows). B, Computed tomography scan of the nodule shown in A (arrows).

or some other colonizing mold. Infrequently, a cavity ruptures and forms a pyopneumothorax. This is usually the first symptom of coccidioidal infection and typically occurs in otherwise healthy young men. An air-fluid level in the pleural space, detectable by roentgenography, often helps differentiate this problem from a spontaneous pneumothorax. Surgical resection of the cavity is the preferred treatment of this complication. The least common pulmonary complication is persistent fibrocavitary infection that progresses to involvement of both lungs.

Extrapulmonary Dissemination

Coccidioidomycosis in immunosuppressed patients, such as solid organ recipients, those with acquired immunodeficiency syndrome or lymphoma, or women during their third trimester of pregnancy, usually results in dissemination beyond the lungs. However, disseminated infection also occurs in some patients who have no underlying disease and do not manifest heightened susceptibility to other infections. The most common locations for disseminated lesions are the skin (cutaneous papules or subcutaneous abscesses); joints (especially the knee); bones, including the vertebrae; and the basilar meninges. Such infections may produce one or many lesions and are frequently subacute or chronic in their manifestation. In broadly immunosuppressed patients, coccidioidal infections may be more fulminant, with fungemia detectable in blood cultures and diffuse reticulonodular embolic pulmonary infiltrates. Although the kidneys and the urinary bladder are rarely involved, *Coccidioides* may be recovered from concentrated specimens of urine because of either transient fungemia or focal dissemination to the prostate. In contrast to histoplasmosis, the gastrointestinal tract is rarely involved in coccidioidomycosis.

Diagnosis

The diagnosis is firmly established by recovering *Coccidioides* species from clinical specimens. On direct examination of respiratory specimens or tissue, spherules can be seen as large structures with refractile walls and internal organization; they are also seen on hematoxylin-eosin, silver, or periodic acid–Schiff stains of histologic preparations. Gram stain does not detect spherules. In culture, mycelial growth is often evident within the first week of incubation, and DNA probing with commercially available kits allows rapid species identification. Recovery of *Coccidioides* species from patients who have only scant respiratory secretions associated with the initial pneumonia and from the cerebrospinal fluid of patients with meningitis may be difficult.

A presumptive diagnosis of coccidioidal infection is often based on detecting specific antibodies in serum. Within the first weeks of initial infections, a precipitin-type antibody is detected, usually by immunodiffusion techniques. Later, complement fixation (CF)-type antibodies generally appear. When reported quantitatively, CF antibodies are usually found to be highest in the most extensive infections and decrease in concentration in patients whose infections are controlled. An important means of diagnosing coccidioidal meningitis is by detection of CF antibodies in cerebrospinal fluid, along with other abnormalities such as leukocytosis, elevated protein concentration, or low glucose concentration.

Treatment

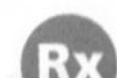

The role of antifungal therapy for primary uncomplicated infections is controversial because clinical trials have not been performed to determine whether treatment either shortens the course of symptoms or diminishes the chance of complications. However, the value of treatment is clear for patients with progressive illness. Because many coccidioidal infections are chronic in nature, treatment with oral azole antifungal agents, such as fluconazole and itraconazole, is often used for initial therapy. Responses to the two drugs are similar, but itraconazole is preferred in patients with skeletal infection. [1] Doses of these azoles are 400 mg/day or higher, and treatment is usually continued for a year or more. Responses with these agents are satisfactory in approximately two thirds of patients. Fluconazole is effective therapy for coccidioidal meningitis and has greatly reduced the number of patients treated with intrathecal amphotericin B. Unfortunately, cessation of azole therapy, especially therapy for coccidioidal meningitis, is often followed by recurrence of symptoms. Therefore, many patients may need protracted or even lifelong therapy to maintain control of disease activity. Amphotericin B remains a rational choice in patients in whom treatment with azole antifungals has failed. Daily doses range from 0.4 to 1 mg/kg, and cumulative therapy ranges from 0.5 to 3 g. Occasionally, in a patient in whom disease progression is rapid, amphotericin B may produce a more rapid therapeutic response and therefore is preferred initial therapy. Delivery of amphotericin B in liposomes or lipid complexes is also effective and generally less toxic than amphotericin B suspended with deoxycholate. In addition to selection of antifungal agents, surgical removal of necrotic tissue is often essential to control the damage from specific lesions.

Prognosis

After resolution of the initial infection, most patients maintain lifelong immunity, and infections after re-exposure are rare. However, cessation of symptoms is frequently accomplished without eradicating *Coccidioides* completely, and recurrence of the original infection up to many years after the original episode is a well-recognized risk of intercurrent profound immunosuppression. For patients in whom the initial infection cannot be resolved, the disease typically follows a protracted course. Although infection is more often debilitating than fatal, fulminant respiratory failure can occur, and if untreated, coccidioidal meningitis is nearly always fatal within 2 years.

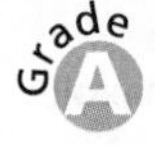

1. Galgiani JN, Catanzaro A, Cloud GA, et al: Comparison of oral fluconazole and itraconazole for progressive nonmeningeal coccidioidomycosis: A randomized, double-blind trial. Mycoses Study Group. Ann Intern Med 2000;133:676–686.

SUGGESTED READINGS

Anstead GM, Graybill JR: Coccidioidomycosis. Infect Dis Clin North Am 2006;20:621–643. *A comprehensive review focusing on treatment.*

Blair JE, Douglas DD, Mulligan DC: Early results of targeted prophylaxis for coccidioidomycosis in patients undergoing orthotopic liver transplantation within an endemic area. Transpl Infect Dis 2003;5:3–8. *Presents a protocol for managing patients undergoing solid organ transplantation with possible previous coccidioidal infection.*

Blair JE, Smilack JD, Caples SM: Coccidioidomycosis in patients with hematologic malignancies. Arch Intern Med 2005;165:113–117. *The largest case series of patients with hematologic malignancy and coccidioidomycosis.*

Crum NF, Lederman ER, Stafford CM, et al: Coccidioidomycosis: A descriptive survey of a reemerging disease. Clinical characteristics and current controversies. Medicine (Baltimore) 2004;83:149–175. *Review of the spectrum of coccidioidal infections that are seen in the military.*

Galgiani JN, Ampel NM, Blair JE, et al: Coccidioidomycosis. Clin Infect Dis 2005;41:1217–1223. *Revised consensus statement regarding current therapy for coccidioidomycosis. Accessible online at http://www.idsociety.org.*

Johnson RH, Einstein HE: Coccidioidal meningitis. Clin Infect Dis 2006;42:103–107. *A review of meningitis secondary to Coccidioides infection.*

Park BJ, Sigel K, Vaz V, et al: An epidemic of coccidioidomycosis in Arizona associated with climatic changes, 1998–2001. J Infect Dis 2005;191:1981–1987. *Analysis of factors associated with recent increases in reported coccidioidal infections in Arizona.*

355 BLASTOMYCOSIS

Carol A. Kauffman

Definition

Blastomycosis (North American blastomycosis) is an endemic mycosis that primarily causes infection of the lungs and skin and, less commonly, infection of the osteoarticular and genitourinary systems.

The Pathogen

Blastomyces dermatitidis is a thermally dimorphic fungus. In the environment in the mold phase, the organism produces conidia, which when aerosolized and inhaled cause infection. At 37° C on culture media and in tissues, the organism is a yeast that is 5 to 20 μm in diameter, has a thick refractile cell wall, and produces single broad-based buds.

Epidemiology

B. dermatitidis exists in many diverse geographic areas worldwide, but most cases of blastomycosis are reported from the south central and north central United States. The ecology of *B. dermatitidis* is not well defined, but it is likely that the natural niche is soil and decaying vegetation. Although most cases occur sporadically, several well-described outbreaks have helped define the natural habitat. The largest outbreak traced the source of *B. dermatitidis* to decaying wood and a beaver lodge on a pond in Wisconsin. The typical patient in whom blastomycosis develops is a middle-aged man who has an outdoor occupation or hobby.

Pathobiology

After the inhalation of conidia, *B. dermatitidis* transforms into the yeast phase and causes pulmonary infection. Although many patients manifest only pulmonary symptoms, others have cutaneous lesions in the absence of other organ involvement or have disseminated infection. It is likely that most patients have asymptomatic hematogenous dissemination after the initial pulmonary infection. Thus, cutaneous lesions should be viewed as a manifestation of hematogenous spread of the organism. Except in rare instances, blastomycosis is not acquired by inoculation. Cellular immunity involving T lymphocytes and macrophages is an important component of the host response to infection with *B. dermatitidis*, but neutrophils probably also play a role. Most patients with blastomycosis are healthy hosts. Patients who are immunosuppressed are more likely to have severe disease. Infection in an immunosuppressed host can occur after new exposure to *B. dermatitidis* or from reactivation of a latent focus of infection acquired years earlier.

Clinical Manifestations

Pulmonary

Most patients with acute pulmonary blastomycosis are asymptomatic or are thought to have a "viral syndrome." Patients with acute pneumonia have fever, malaise, a nonproductive cough, and a pulmonary infiltrate that shows lobar or multilobar patchy or nodular infiltrates on chest radiograph. Development of skin lesions is a strong clue for blastomycosis. Chronic pulmonary blastomycosis must be differentiated from tuberculosis, other fungal infections, and lung cancer. Fever, night sweats, weight loss, fatigue, cough, sputum production, hemoptysis, and dyspnea are commonly noted. On chest radiograph, the lesions are cavitary, nodular, fibrotic, or mass-like in appearance. Hilar and mediastinal lymphadenopathy and pleural effusions are uncommonly seen. Rarely, overwhelming pulmonary disease with acute respiratory distress syndrome occurs; it appears to be more common in older adults and immunosuppressed patients.

Disseminated Infection

Cutaneous lesions are the most common manifestation of disseminated blastomycosis. The lesions are usually well-circumscribed, painless papules, nodules, or plaques that become verrucous and develop multiple punctate draining areas in the center. Cutaneous lesions, sometimes single but more often multiple, are most common on the face and extremities but can appear anywhere. The skin lesions of blastomycosis clinically mimic those associated with nontuberculous mycobacteria, other fungal infections, mycosis fungoides, and bromide use. An uncommon manifestation, seen more often in immunocompromised patients, is the appearance of hundreds of pustular lesions that readily reveal the organism when aspirated.

Another manifestation of disseminated blastomycosis is osteoarticular involvement. Osteomyelitis can be associated with contiguous skin lesions or can appear at sites distant from cutaneous lesions. It is helpful to obtain a bone scan in all patients with disseminated blastomycosis because of the propensity of the organism to infect bone. Genitourinary involvement may be asymptomatic or associated with signs of prostatism and the presence of a nodule on digital examination. Infrequently occurring findings include laryngeal and oropharyngeal nodules; ocular lesions; central nervous system involvement, either meningitis or intracerebral mass lesions; and dissemination to the liver, spleen, and lymph nodes.

Diagnosis

The definitive diagnostic test for blastomycosis is growth of the organism from an aspirate, tissue biopsy specimen, sputum, or body fluid. Urine obtained before and after prostatic massage should be sent for fungal culture in those with disseminated blastomycosis. The mold phase takes several weeks to grow at room temperature. Once growth has occurred, the organism can be rapidly identified as *B. dermatitidis* with highly specific and sensitive DNA probes. Histopathologic examination of cutaneous or pulmonary lesions, cytologic examination of sputum, bronchoalveolar lavage fluid, or other tissue fluids, and KOH smears of sputum or purulent material from pustular lesions should be performed to look for the distinctive large, thick-walled yeast with a single broad-based bud. Identification of characteristic organisms allows a tentative diagnosis of blastomycosis and initiation of antifungal therapy before culture results are known. Standard serologic assays for blastomycosis are neither sensitive nor specific.

Treatment

Guidelines for the treatment of blastomycosis have been published by the Mycoses Study Group under the auspices of the Infectious Diseases Society of America. Many patients with acute pulmonary blastomycosis are better before the diagnosis is estab-

lished and do not need antifungal therapy. All patients with skin lesions or other manifestations of dissemination should receive systemic antifungal therapy to prevent progression of disease. Patients who have mild to moderate pulmonary or disseminated blastomycosis should be treated with itraconazole, 200 mg once or twice daily. The length of treatment is 6 to 12 months to achieve mycologic cure and prevent relapse. Fluconazole is not as effective as itraconazole. However, if the patient is unable to take itraconazole, fluconazole can be used, but the dosage should be 400 to 800 mg daily for 6 to 12 months. There are only anecdotal case reports describing the use of voriconazole for blastomycosis. The echinocandins are not active against *B. dermatitidis* and should not be used.

Patients who have severe pulmonary or disseminated blastomycosis, all patients who have central nervous system infection, and most immunosuppressed patients should be treated initially with amphotericin B. The daily dosage is 0.7 to 1 mg/kg daily. A total of 1 to 2 g can be given, or after clinical improvement has occurred, therapy can be changed to itraconazole, 200 mg twice daily, for a total of 6 to 12 months of therapy.

Prognosis

The prognosis for patients with pulmonary or disseminated blastomycosis treated with itraconazole is excellent; more than 90% are cured. If relapse does occur, a second course of itraconazole is usually successful. Most reported deaths occur in patients with overwhelming pneumonia and acute respiratory distress syndrome.

SUGGESTED READINGS

Chapman SW, Bradsher RW, Campbell GD, et al: Practice guidelines for the management of patients with blastomycosis. Clin Infect Dis 2000;30:679–683. *Consensus guidelines of the Infectious Diseases Society of America for treating blastomycosis.*

Kauffman CA: Endemic mycoses: Blastomycosis, histoplasmosis, and sporotrichosis. Infect Dis Clin North Am 2006;20:645–662. *An excellent review of endemic mycoses.*

Pappas PG: Blastomycosis. Sem Respir Crit Care Med 2004;25:113–121. *Review of the manifestations of blastomycosis.*

Watts B, Argekar P, Saint S, et al: Clinical problem-solving. Building a diagnosis from the ground up—a 49-year-old man came to the clinic with a 1-week history of suprapubic pain and fever. N Engl J Med 2007;356:1456–1462. *A clinical case presentation of a patient who is diagnosed with blastomycosis.*

356 PARACOCCIDIOIDOMYCOSIS

Carol A. Kauffman

Definition

Paracoccidioidomycosis (South American blastomycosis) is a subacute to chronic mycosis that is endemic in Central and South America. The disease is characterized primarily by pulmonary, mucous membrane, and cutaneous lesions, but disseminated disease also occurs.

The Pathogen

Paracoccidioides brasiliensis is a thermally dimorphic fungus. In the environment and at temperatures below 35° C, the organism is a mold that produces conidia (spores). In tissues and at 37° C, the organism assumes the yeast form with multiple narrow-based buds.

Epidemiology

P. brasiliensis exists only in humid areas of Central and South America. The presumed ecologic niche is in soil, but the exact conditions that favor growth of the organism have not been elucidated. The disease is most prevalent in middle-aged to elderly men from rural areas. The reason for the sexual imbalance (male-to-female ratio of 13:1) is possibly related to the inhibitory effects of estrogens on growth of the organism rather than solely environmental exposure. Although the disease classically develops later in life, it is likely that initial exposure occurs in childhood in the endemic areas. Cases seen in areas outside Central and South America have all been linked to previous residence in the endemic area.

Pathobiology

Paracoccidioidomycosis develops after the inhalation of aerosolized conidia encountered in the environment. Once in the alveoli, the mycelial phase converts to the yeast phase, a transformation noted to be inhibited by estrogens. The infection may remain localized to the lungs, although it is likely that asymptomatic hematogenous dissemination occurs during most infections. The primary host defense mechanism against *P. brasiliensis* appears to be cell-mediated immunity, but neutrophils may also play a role in host defense. The histopathologic picture includes both neutrophilic and granulomatous responses. There have been increasing reports of paracoccidioidomycosis in patients with acquired immunodeficiency syndrome (AIDS) and in other immunosuppressed patients; in these patients there is widespread dissemination, and histopathology shows poorly formed granulomas. Reactivation of latent infection acquired in childhood is the presumed pathogenesis of most cases of the chronic adult form of paracoccidioidomycosis and cases that appear years after the patient has left the endemic area.

Clinical Manifestations

Acute-Subacute (Juvenile) Paracoccidioidomycosis

This form of paracoccidioidomycosis occurs in less than 10% of patients. It is a disease of the reticuloendothelial system with widespread dissemination to the liver, spleen, lymph nodes, and bone marrow. Patients younger than 30 years typically have this manifestation of paracoccidioidomycosis; however, older adults, especially those who are immunosuppressed, can also manifest this type of rapidly progressive disease. In the most severe involvement, as seen in patients with AIDS, cutaneous lesions are common and pulmonary involvement often progresses to respiratory failure.

Chronic (Adult) Paracoccidioidomycosis

This form of paracoccidioidomycosis is seen in more than 90% of patients, most of whom are older men. The disease progresses slowly over a period of years. Pulmonary involvement is prominent and clinically mimics tuberculosis and other chronic fungal pneumonias. Radiographically, nodular, interstitial, or cavitary lesions are seen but differ from those of tuberculosis and histoplasmosis in that the infiltrates tend to be in the middle and lower lung fields rather than the apices. Most patients with the adult form of paracoccidioidomycosis also have ulcerative or nodular mucous membrane lesions, primarily in the anterior nares and oral cavity. Cutaneous lesions, particularly on the face, are also common and may be papular, nodular, ulcerative, or plaquelike. The mucocutaneous lesions must be differentiated from mucocutaneous leishmaniasis and squamous cell carcinoma. Adrenal involvement has been noted frequently in several, but not all series of the adult form of paracoccidioidomycosis.

Diagnosis

Definitive diagnosis of paracoccidioidomycosis is made by detection of *P. brasiliensis*. The organism may take as long as 4 weeks to grow. For seriously ill patients, direct examination of body fluids, sputum, or purulent material treated with KOH or histopathologic examination of tissue biopsy samples can provide a tentative diagnosis while awaiting culture results. A presumptive diagnosis can be made and therapy initiated if the characteristic yeast forms with multiple small, circumferentially attached, narrow-based daughter buds creating a distinctive morphologic picture likened to a ship's steering wheel are seen.

Immunodiffusion, counterimmunoelectrophoresis, and complement fixation assays are available in endemic areas, but there continue to be problems with sensitivity and specificity. In the United States, complement fixation and immunodiffusion assays are available through the Centers for Disease Control and Prevention.

Treatment

Rx

The drug of choice for the treatment of paracoccidioidomycosis is itraconazole (100 mg daily for 6 to 12 months), although to date, randomized clinical trials have not been large enough to draw definitive conclusions. [1] Even though ketoconazole at a dosage of 200 to 400 mg daily for 1 year is effective and certainly less expensive than itraconazole, the incidence of side effects is usually greater and there appear to be more relapses than with itraconazole. There is little experience with fluconazole, which should remain a second-line agent. Sulfonamides had been used for years for treating paracoccidioidomycosis but are less effective than the azoles. Amphotericin B is effective but rarely required, except in immunosuppressed patients with life-threatening disseminated disease. Most AIDS patients with paracoccidioidomycosis have been treated with amphotericin B as initial therapy, followed by lifelong suppressive therapy with either itraconazole or trimethoprim-sulfamethoxazole. The latter is preferred in AIDS patients because it also prevents infections with *Pneumocystis carinii* and *Toxoplasma gondii.*

Prognosis

Patients with paracoccidioidomycosis have an excellent prognosis when appropriate therapy is given. The response in patients with AIDS appears to be less successful.

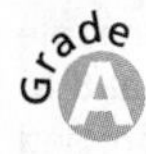

1. Menezes VM, Soares BG, Fontes CJ: Drugs for treating paracoccidioidomycosis. Cochrane Database Syst Rev 2006;2:CD004967.

SUGGESTED READINGS

Correa MM, Medoya AM, Guerrero MP, et al: Diagnosis of paracoccidioidomycosis by a dot blot assay using a recombinant *Paracoccidioides brasiliensis* p27 protein. Mycoses 2007;50:41–47. *Confirms its value in the serodiagnosis.*

Rodrigues DR, Dias-Melicio LA, Calvi SA, et al: *Paracoccidioides brasiliensis* killing by IFN-gamma, TNF-alpha and GM-CSF activated human neutrophils: Role for oxygen metabolites. Med Mycol 2007;45:27–33. *Cytokine activation is required for* P. brasiliensis *killing by human PMNs.*

Souza AS Jr, Gasparetto EL, Davaus T, et al: High resolution CT findings of 77 patients with untreated pulmonary paracoccidioidomycosis. Am J Roentgenol 2006;187:1248–1252. *Typical findings are ground-glass attenuation with nodules.*

357 CRYPTOCOCCOSIS

Carol A. Kauffman

Definition

Cryptococcosis occurs most often in persons who are immunosuppressed, especially those infected with human immunodeficiency virus (HIV). Meningitis is the most common clinical manifestation, but pulmonary and other organ involvement also occurs. *Cryptococcus neoformans* is a yeast in both the environment and in tissues. In tissues, the organism is enveloped by a large polysaccharide capsule that is a major virulence factor. In the environment, *C. neoformans* yeast cells are smaller and less encapsulated and thus more easily aerosolized and inhaled.

Pathogen and Epidemiology

There are two varieties of the species: *C. neoformans* var *neoformans* and *C. neoformans* var *gatti.* Both varieties are pathogenic and cause similar disease manifestations. *C. neoformans* var. *neoformans* accounts for most cases of human disease throughout the world. This organism has been linked to pigeons; the birds do not become infected, but rather the organism grows luxuriantly in dried pigeon excreta because of its high nitrogen content. *C. neoformans* var. *gatti* is more restricted, found mostly in subtropical and tropical areas of Australia, Southeast Asia, Africa, and the Americas. In the United States, most infections with this variety occur in California. The ecologic niche of the *gatti* variety is the eucalyptus tree. There are at least 38 other species of *Cryptococcus,* and only rarely have these non-*neoformans* isolates (*Cryptococcus laurentii* and *Cryptococcus albidus,* primarily) caused disease.

Before highly active antiretroviral therapy (HAART), cryptococcosis occurred in 5 to 10% of patients with acquired immunodeficiency syndrome (AIDS). Patients at highest risk were those with less than 50 $CD4^+$ cells/μL. Though less commonly seen now, cryptococcosis remains extremely common among AIDS patients in Africa, and in the United States it is seen almost entirely in those who have not received medical therapy or who refuse HAART. In the non-AIDS population, cryptococcosis is a frequent opportunistic infection in patients who have received an organ transplant; have been treated with corticosteroids; or have diabetes mellitus, renal failure, liver dysfunction, or chronic pulmonary disease. For some patients, the only risk factor appears to be older age. In every reported series, approximately 20% of patients have no known underlying illness.

Pathobiology

The organism is inhaled from the environment and causes pulmonary infection initially. The primary host defense at this stage is complement-dependent macrophage and neutrophil phagocytosis and killing. Natural killer cells also have the ability to kill the organism. Ultimately, however, T-cell immunity is the most important host determinant in limiting the replication of *C. neoformans.* In normal hosts, the infection remains localized to the lungs and does not cause symptomatic infection. It is likely that a few organisms exist as walled-off subpleural granulomas in many who have had pulmonary infection. If the host becomes immunosuppressed, the organism can then reactivate and disseminate to other sites. *C. neoformans* is clearly neurotropic, and the primary disease manifestation is meningoencephalitis. However, dissemination to many organs is likely, especially in those with deficient T-cell immunity.

Virulence factors for *C. neoformans* include the capsule, which requires opsonization for efficient phagocytosis, and the production of melanin, which has been shown to occur in vivo and enables the organism to resist intracellular killing. Both these factors may help explain the virulence of the organism once it has reached the central nervous system. Antibody and complement levels are low in the brain, and thus phagocytosis of the organism is minimal. Brain tissue provides high concentrations of substrates, such as catecholamines, for the phenol oxidase enzyme systems of *C. neoformans* that produce melanin, thereby aiding survival of the organism.

Clinical Manifestations

Central Nervous System Infection

The most common manifestation of cryptococcosis is central nervous system infection. The typical picture is that of a subacute to chronic meningoencephalitis. Patients usually have increasingly severe headaches over a period of several weeks. Other symptoms and signs include nuchal rigidity, lethargy, personality changes, confusion, visual abnormalities (photophobia, diplopia, decreased visual acuity, papilledema, extraocular nerve palsies), and nausea and vomiting. Less commonly, hearing loss, ataxia, and seizures occur. Fever is present in only approximately half the patients. Elderly persons with cryptococcal meningitis may have only dementia, without other neurologic findings. AIDS patients often have subtle central nervous system symptoms but usually have fever and other constitutional symptoms and rapidly manifest signs of dissemination.

Pulmonary Infection

In non–HIV-infected patients, the most common underlying risk factor for pulmonary cryptococcal infection is chronic obstructive pulmonary disease, followed by corticosteroid use and receipt of a solid organ transplant. *C. neoformans* may merely be an airway colonizer in some patients; in others, symptomatic infection, mostly manifested by fever, cough, and dyspnea, requires treatment with an antifungal agent. The typical lesion noted with pulmonary cryptococcosis is a pleural-based nodular lesion. However, patchy pneumonitis, multiple nodular lesions, cavitary lesions, masslike lesions, and diffuse pulmonary infiltrates have all been noted with pulmonary cryptococcosis. Patients with advanced HIV infection are likely to have diffuse infiltrates that can progress rapidly to acute respiratory insufficiency. Given the proclivity of *C. neoformans* to invade the central nervous system, all patients who have pulmonary cryptococcosis should undergo lumbar puncture to be certain that meningitis is not present.

Involvement of Other Organs

C. neoformans has been reported to infect most organs during the course of disseminated infection, especially in AIDS patients. Skin lesions are a prominent clue to dissemination. Papules that resemble molluscum contagiosum or an acneiform rash, nodules, ulcers, plaques, draining sinuses, and cellulitis have all been reported. Focal involvement can occur in the prostate and other genitourinary tract organs, in osteoarticular structures, in the breast, and in the eye, larynx, and other head and neck structures. The prostate, in particular, has been noted as a sanctuary from which persisting organisms can later disseminate.

Diagnosis

The diagnosis of cryptococcosis is established when the yeast is grown in culture. Appropriate specimens for culture include cerebrospinal fluid (CSF), blood, sputum, material from skin lesions, and other body fluids or tissues that appear to be infected. The organism grows in several days on most standard agar media. Most automated blood culture systems allow rapid growth of *C. neoformans*. Visualization of the capsule and performance of a few simple tests differentiate *C. neoformans* from other yeasts. Tissue biopsy shows the 5- to 10-μm yeast surrounded by the capsule. Definitive diagnosis of cryptococcosis can be made with a mucicarmine stain, which selectively stains the polysaccharide capsule a deep rose color. In CSF or other body fluids, an India ink preparation allows visualization of the budding yeast cells surrounded by the large capsule.

The latex agglutination assay for cryptococcal polysaccharide antigen (CRAG) is a highly sensitive and specific diagnostic test. CRAG is positive in CSF in almost 100% and in serum in about 75% of patients who have meningitis. In AIDS patients, serum CRAG is almost always positive and is an excellent screening tool; titers in both CSF and serum are exceptionally high because of the enormous burden of organisms. In non-AIDS, nonmeningeal, pulmonary cryptococcosis, the CRAG assay is positive in only 25 to 50% of cases. False-positive results with the CRAG assay are uncommon, generally low in titer, are more likely with serum than with CSF, and can be caused by interference with the assay by rheumatoid factor. The rare patient with *Trichosporon asahii* infection can have a positive CRAG test because of cross-reacting antigens shared by both fungi.

The CSF of patients with cryptococcal meningitis typically has an increased number of white blood cells (but rarely >500/μL), a predominance of lymphocytes (although neutrophils are sometimes prominent early in the course), elevated protein, and decreased glucose. AIDS patients most often have normal or only mildly abnormal findings as a result of their markedly defective immune response. Despite normal CSF findings in regard to cells, protein, and glucose, every AIDS patient with a headache must have a CRAG, India ink preparation, and culture performed on CSF. It is extremely important that an opening pressure be obtained when lumbar puncture is performed. Especially in AIDS patients, extremely high intracranial pressure (>350 mm H_2O) has been associated with poor outcomes and must be aggressively lowered.

All patients with cryptococcal meningitis should have a computed tomography or magnetic resonance imaging study of the brain to look for mass lesions (cryptococcomas) and to assess ventricular size. Obstructive hydrocephalus is uncommon but requires a shunting procedure to decrease the pressure. More commonly, the increased intracranial pressure with cryptococcal infection is associated with normal-sized ventricles and is due to blockage at the arachnoid villi or increased brain edema (or both), perhaps related to the osmotic effect of the polysaccharide capsule. Different methods for reducing pressure are used in this situation.

Treatment

Guidelines for the treatment of cryptococcal infection have been published by the Mycoses Study Group and the Infectious Diseases Society of America. All recent controlled treatment trials have been carried out in AIDS patients; most recommendations for treatment of non-AIDS patients have used the results obtained in AIDS patients.

Central Nervous System Infection

Early multicenter randomized trials in non-AIDS patients showed superiority of the combination of amphotericin B and flucytosine for 6 weeks over amphotericin B alone for 10 weeks. Subsequent randomized trials in the azole era have been performed only in the AIDS population. They have confirmed the benefit of flucytosine added to amphotericin B for induction therapy and have shown that initial therapy with fluconazole is not as effective as amphotericin B. [1, 2] Itraconazole is not as effective but can be used if for some reason fluconazole cannot be given. Current recommendations are to give intravenous amphotericin B (0.7 to 1 mg/kg daily) combined with oral flucytosine (100 mg/kg daily, given in four divided doses) for a minimum of 2 weeks or longer if required, until CSF cultures become negative and the patient has begun to improve. Note that the dosage of flucytosine should *not* be 150 mg/kg daily as described in the package insert because of its dose-related marrow toxicity. Therapy can then be switched to oral fluconazole (400 mg daily) for a minimum of 8 to 10 weeks. Many AIDS patients will require lifelong suppression with 200 mg fluconazole daily; others who have a sustained increase in $CD4^+$ cells above 200/μL will be able to stop maintenance therapy. [3] Suppressive therapy with fluconazole for non-AIDS patients has not been studied, but an additional 6 to 12 months of fluconazole, 200 mg daily, for immunosuppressed patients is recommended. Whether suppressive therapy should be used in "normal" hosts with cryptococcal meningitis is not clear and left to the clinician's judgment.

Open-label studies with lipid formulations of amphotericin B have been performed in AIDS patients. These agents, at daily dosages of 3 to 6 mg/kg, are as effective as amphotericin B and should be used in patients who have preexisting renal insufficiency and those at risk for nephrotoxicity. There are only a few case reports on the use of voriconazole and posaconazole for cryptococcal meningitis. The echinocandins are not active against *C. neoformans* and should not be used.

A significant observation from the AIDS treatment trials was the role of increased intracranial pressure as a cause of early death from cryptococcal meningitis. An aggressive approach to the diagnosis and treatment of increased intracranial pressure in both AIDS and non-AIDS patients is mandatory and should include daily lumbar puncture or placement of a temporary lumbar drain or ventriculostomy until the opening pressure remains lower than 190 mm H_2O. Treatment with corticosteroids, acetazolamide, or mannitol has not proved efficacious in this setting.

Pulmonary and Other Nonmeningeal Infections

Treatment of nonmeningeal cryptococcosis depends on the severity of the infection. Many patients with isolated pulmonary or other focal infections are not severely ill, and an oral azole can be used. The preferred therapy is oral fluconazole, 400 mg daily for 6 to 12 months. Itraconazole, 200 mg twice daily, is a second-line choice. For patients who are severely ill, initial therapy with intravenous amphotericin B, 0.7 mg/kg daily, and oral flucytosine, 100 mg/kg daily, is warranted for the first few weeks before switching to oral fluconazole after clinical improvement has occurred.

Prognosis

The outcome for both AIDS and non-AIDS patients with cryptococcal meningitis has improved markedly over the last decade. In the last randomized treatment trial of AIDS patients, the overall mortality was less than 10%. In non-AIDS patients, a recent large, retrospective review noted a mortality rate of 12% from cryptococcosis. Dementia in older patients may not be reversed even though mycologic cure is achieved.

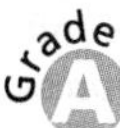

1. Van der Horst CM, Saag MS, Cloud GA, et al: Treatment of cryptococcal meningitis associated with the acquired immunodeficiency syndrome. N Engl J Med 1997;337:15–21.
2. Saag MS, Powderly WG, Cloud GA, et al: Comparison of amphotericin B with fluconazole in the treatment of acute AIDS-associated cryptococcal meningitis. N Engl J Med 1992;326:83–89.
3. Vibhagool A, Sungkanuparph S, Mootsikapun P, et al: Discontinuation of secondary prophylaxis for cryptococcal meningitis in human immunodeficiency virus–infected patients treated with highly active antiretroviral therapy: A prospective, multicenter, randomized study. Clin Infect Dis 2003;36:1329–1331.

SUGGESTED READINGS

Chayakulkeeree M, Perfect JR: Cryptococcosis. Infect Dis Clin North Am 2006;20:507–544. *Comprehensive review.*

Idnurm A, Bahn YS, Nielsen K, et al: Deciphering the model pathogenic fungus *Cryptococcus neoformans.* Nat Rev Microbiol 2005;3:753–764. *Review of the recent advances in the understanding of the pathophysiology and genetics of the organism.*

Loftus BJ, Fung E, Roncaglia P, et al: The genome of the basidiomycetous yeast and human pathogen *Cryptococcus neoformans.* Science 2005;307:1321–1324. *Description of the sequencing of the genome of this organism.*

Pappas PG, Perfect JR, Cloud GA, et al: Cryptococcosis in human immunodeficiency virus–negative patients in the era of effective azole therapy. Clin Infect Dis 2001;33:690–699. *Report on a large series of non-AIDS patients with cryptococcosis.*

358 SPOROTRICHOSIS

Carol A. Kauffman

Definition

Sporotrichosis is a subacute or chronic infection that is usually localized to cutaneous and lymphocutaneous structures, but pulmonary, osteoarticular, and disseminated infection can occur in patients who have certain underlying diseases.

The Pathogen

Sporothrix schenckii is a thermally dimorphic fungus. In the environment at temperatures lower than 35 to 37° C, the organism is a mold and produces conidia, the infectious form. In tissues and at 35 to 37° C, *S. schenckii* transforms into the yeast phase; the yeasts are 4 to 6 μm in diameter; are cigar shaped, round, or oval; and reproduce by budding.

Epidemiology

S. schenckii is found worldwide in climates ranging from temperate to tropical. The organism exists in a variety of environmental niches, including soil, sphagnum moss, hay, decaying wood, and other vegetation. Infection is seen almost entirely in persons whose vocation, avocation, or living condition brings them into contact with the organism in the environment. Landscaping activities, gardening, farming, and motor vehicle accidents have been associated with sporotrichosis. Most cases of sporotrichosis are sporadic, but outbreaks have been described. Sporotrichosis also occurs as a zoonotic infection acquired directly from infected animals, especially cats, or passively from soil by scratches or bites from animals. Inhalation of *S. schenckii* conidia occurs less commonly and results in pulmonary and rarely disseminated sporotrichosis.

Pathobiology

Infection is almost always acquired by inoculation of conidia and remains localized to the immediate and contiguous cutaneous, subcutaneous, and lymphatic structures. Some strains of *S. schenckii* grow poorly at temperatures higher than 35° C; these strains usually cause fixed cutaneous lesions without lymphatic spread. The typical host response to infection with *S. schenckii* is a mixed neutrophilic and granulomatous reaction. Antibody is not protective; T lymphocytes are important in containing infection. In individuals who have underlying illnesses that include alcoholism, diabetes mellitus, and chronic obstructive pulmonary disease, *S. schenckii* is more likely to involve osteoarticular structures and lungs. Widespread dissemination develops in persons infected with human immunodeficiency virus (HIV) but is a distinctly unusual event in normal hosts.

Clinical Manifestations

Lymphocutaneous

Days to weeks after inoculation of *S. schenckii* conidia, a papular lesion develops at the inoculation site; the lesion becomes nodular and often ulcerates. Drainage is not grossly purulent, and the lesion is not terribly painful. Similar lesions occur along the lymphatic channels proximal to the primary lesion. Verrucous or ulcerative fixed cutaneous lesions do not exhibit lymphatic extension. The differential diagnosis of lymphocutaneous sporotrichosis includes *Nocardia* infections, particularly *Nocardia brasiliensis;* atypical mycobacterial infections, especially *Mycobacterium marinum; Leishmania brasiliensis* infections; and tularemia.

Visceral and Osteoarticular

Pulmonary sporotrichosis occurs most often in middle-aged men who have chronic pulmonary disease and abuse alcohol. Fever, night sweats, weight loss, fatigue, dyspnea, cough, purulent sputum, and hemoptysis are common. Chest radiographs show unilateral or bilateral upper lobe cavities with variable amounts of fibrosis and nodular lesions. The disease mimics tuberculosis in almost all aspects. Osteoarticular sporotrichosis is found most often in middle-aged men and occurs more frequently in alcoholics. Infection may involve one or multiple joints; the joints most commonly affected are the knee, elbow, wrist, and ankle. Isolated bursitis, tenosynovitis, and nerve entrapment syndromes have been reported. Osteoarticular infection can follow local inoculation, but most patients probably have had hematogenous spread. Isolated case reports document sporotrichosis involving the pericardium, eye, perirectal tissues, larynx, breast, epididymis, spleen, liver, bone marrow, lymph nodes, and meninges. Disseminated sporotrichosis, manifested as widespread ulcerative cutaneous lesions with or without visceral involvement, is uncommon; most cases have been reported in patients with advanced HIV infection.

Diagnosis

Growth of *S. schenckii* from material aspirated from a lesion, a tissue biopsy specimen, sputum, or body fluid is the most effective method of establishing the diagnosis of sporotrichosis. Growth of the mold phase of the organism is usually evident within a few days. Histopathologic examination of biopsy material shows a mixed granulomatous and pyogenic process; however, the organisms are often present in small numbers and are frequently not visualized. Serology is not useful in the diagnosis of sporotrichosis.

Treatment

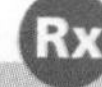

Because sporotrichosis is usually a localized subacute to chronic infection, oral antifungal agents are preferred; amphotericin B is reserved for severe visceral infections. Guidelines for the management of sporotrichosis have been published by the Mycoses Study Group and the Infectious Diseases Society of America. Itraconazole is the drug of choice for lymphocutaneous sporotrichosis. The usual dosage is 200 mg daily, and treatment should continue for several weeks after all lesions have disappeared, generally for a total of 3 to 6 months. Saturated solution of potassium iodide (SSKI) has been used to treat sporotrichosis for more than a century. The initial dose is 5 to 10 drops three times daily in water or juice, with the dose increasing over a period of several weeks to a maximum of 40 to 50

Rx

drops three times daily. SSKI has many side effects, including salivary gland swelling, metallic taste, rash, and fever; the only advantage is that it is inexpensive. Fluconazole is less effective than itraconazole but for occasional patients can be used at a dosage of 400 mg daily. Terbinafine appears to be effective for sporotrichosis, but few patients have been treated with this agent to date. Local hyperthermia, induced by a variety of different warming devices or baths, has been shown to be effective in some patients with fixed cutaneous lesions.

Osteoarticular and pulmonary sporotrichosis is usually treated with itraconazole, 200 mg twice daily for 1 to 2 years. Other azoles are less effective, and SSKI is ineffective. For a seriously ill patient with pulmonary sporotrichosis, amphotericin B, 0.7 to 1 mg/kg daily, should be used as initial therapy. After the patient has shown improvement, therapy can be changed to itraconazole. Amphotericin B is the drug of choice for disseminated sporotrichosis. Therapy can be changed to itraconazole, 200 mg twice daily, once the patient has stabilized. Patients with acquired immunodeficiency syndrome with disseminated sporotrichosis should remain on lifelong maintenance therapy with itraconazole, 200 mg daily.

Prognosis

The prognosis for patients with cutaneous and lymphocutaneous sporotrichosis is excellent. Almost all patients are cured with one course of therapy; relapses occur in only a small proportion of patients. Extracutaneous forms of sporotrichosis do not respond well to therapy, partly because of delays in diagnosis and partly because of the underlying diseases that are frequently found in those who have extracutaneous sporotrichosis. The outcome of disseminated sporotrichosis in patients with HIV infection has been especially poor.

SUGGESTED READINGS

Barros MBL, Schubach AO, Valle ACF, et al: Cat-transmitted sporotrichosis epidemic in Rio de Janeiro, Brazil: Description of a series of cases. Clin Infect Dis 2004;38:529–535. *Highlights the little-known role of cats in the spread of sporotrichosis.*

da Rosa AC, Scroferneger ML, Vettorato R, et al: Epidemiology of sporotrichosis: A study of 304 cases in Brazil. J Am Acad Dermatol 2005;52:451–459. *Interesting case series looking at the epidemiology and presentation of this infection.*

Kauffman CA: Endemic mycoses: Blastomycosis, histoplasmosis, and sporotrichosis. Infect Dis Clin North Am 2006;20:645–662. *Comprehensive clinical review.*

Ramos-e-Silva M, Vasconcelos C, Carneira S, et al: Sporotrichosis. Clin Dermatol 2007;25:181–187. *Comprehensive review.*

359 CANDIDIASIS

Carol A. Kauffman

Definition

Candidiasis encompasses a wide variety of clinical syndromes that are caused by yeasts of the genus *Candida*. Of the species that cause infection in humans, *Candida albicans* is the most common; *Candida glabrata, Candida parapsilosis,* and *Candida tropicalis* are responsible for most of the remaining infections. Organisms such as *Candida krusei, Candida lusitaniae,* and *Candida guilliermondii* are less common causes of infection.

The Pathogen

Candida species are 2- to 6-μm yeastlike organisms that reproduce by budding. Most species, with the exception of *C. glabrata,* form pseudohyphae (elongated buds that remain attached to the mother cell) and hyphae in tissues.

Candida species cause a wide spectrum of diseases ranging in severity from localized mucous membrane infection to life-threatening disseminated disease. The major determinant of the severity of infection is the host's immune response. Local infections are often related to overgrowth of *Candida* as a result of changes in the normal flora. Invasive infections that remain within an organ system, such as urinary tract infections, often occur because of local anatomic abnormalities. In an immunosuppressed host, especially a patient with neutropenia, widespread visceral dissemination is common.

Epidemiology

Candida species are part of the normal human flora of the gastrointestinal and genitourinary tracts and skin. As colonizers, *Candida* species do not cause infection unless there is a defect in host defense mechanisms or exogenous factors, such as antibiotic use, have upset the ecology of the normal flora. *C. albicans* is the species most commonly found colonizing humans; *C. glabrata* is the second most common species, and *C. tropicalis, C. parapsilosis,* and others are found less often. Changes in the species of *Candida* colonizing patients occur during hospitalization and with use of antifungal agents. *C. glabrata* and *C. krusei,* species known to be relatively and totally resistant to fluconazole, respectively, are associated with increased use of this agent in the hospital setting.

Though uncommon, acquisition of *Candida* from health care workers or from environmental sources has been noted. Most often the *Candida* species associated with transmission from contaminated fluids or devices, especially central intravenous catheters, has been *C. parapsilosis.* This species is also the most frequent colonizer of the hands of health care workers.

Candidiasis is the most common opportunistic fungal infection as a result of both the ubiquity of the organisms and the increasing number of patients with risk factors for infection with these organisms. The classic immunosuppressed host who is at risk for serious *Candida* infections is a patient who has a hematologic malignancy, is neutropenic, and has received cytotoxic agents and corticosteroids. Increasingly, however, candidiasis is an infection seen in patients who are in intensive care units (ICUs). Risk factors for the development of serious *Candida* infections in ICU patients include broad-spectrum antimicrobials, indwelling central venous catheters, previous surgical procedures, renal failure, parenteral nutrition, and high Acute Physiology and Chronic Health Evaluation (APACHE) score. Certain ICU populations, especially very low birthweight neonates and burn victims, are at even higher risk for *Candida* infection than the typical ICU patient is.

The acquired immunodeficiency syndrome (AIDS) epidemic has led to a marked increase in *Candida* infections. However, in contrast to candidiasis in the hospital setting, the primary manifestation of *Candida* infection in AIDS patients is mucocutaneous infection, especially oropharyngeal candidiasis. The development of *Candida* infection is directly related to deficient T-cell immunity as reflected by a low $CD4^+$ lymphocyte count. With appropriate antiretroviral therapy, oropharyngeal candidiasis has become an uncommon opportunistic infection that is seen almost entirely in patients with advanced human immunodeficiency virus (HIV) infection that is untreated or refractory to therapy.

Pathobiology

The usual mode of infection with *Candida* is egress from its normal niche into the blood stream or other tissues; most times the source is the gastrointestinal tract, but the skin and genitourinary tract are other sources. The primary host defense in response to this event is phagocytosis and killing by neutrophils, monocytes, and macrophages. Phagocytosis is enhanced in the presence of specific anti-*Candida* antibody and complement. Several different mechanisms are operative within neutrophils and macrophages that allow killing of yeasts. Thus, patients who are neutropenic, especially those with chemotherapy-induced disruption of the gut mucosa, are at greatest risk for invasion with *Candida* species. Once *Candida* gains access to the blood stream, widespread hematogenous dissemination is the rule. Biopsy of many different organs usually shows multiple microabscesses composed of neutrophils (in a host who has these cells), budding yeasts, and often pseudohyphae or hyphae. Over time, the lesions show a mixed neutrophilic and granulomatous response.

T-cell immunity is also an important host defense against infection with *Candida*. T-cell immunity controls *Candida* at mucosal surfaces. In contrast to those with neutropenia, patients with deficient T-cell immunity are at risk for persistent and recurrent mucocutaneous candidiasis, but invasive infection rarely develops.

Clinical Manifestations

Mucocutaneous Candidiasis

Oropharyngeal Candidiasis

Local mucous membrane and cutaneous lesions are the most common forms of *Candida* infection. Oropharyngeal candidiasis, or thrush, can be due either to local factors or to T-cell dysfunction. Local factors include the use of broad-spectrum antimicrobials or inhaled corticosteroids, xerostomia, and radiation treatment of the head and neck. Chronic atrophic candidosis, also called denture stomatitis, occurs frequently in persons who wear full upper dentures, especially those who do not remove their dentures at night.

Thrush secondary to T-cell dysfunction is most commonly seen in patients with HIV infection and is the most frequent opportunistic infection noted in patients with AIDS. The appearance of thrush in a previously healthy individual with no known risk factors should immediately raise suspicion of HIV infection.

Thrush is manifested by white plaques on the buccal mucosa, palate, oropharynx, or tongue. Scraping the lesions with a tongue depressor reveals an erythematous, nonulcerated mucosa under the plaques. Denture stomatitis is almost always manifested as a painful erythematous palate without plaques. Angular cheilitis, or perlèche, which is the presence of painful cracks at the corners of the mouth, can occur with or without thrush.

Esophagitis

Esophagitis may accompany oropharyngeal candidiasis or may occur independently of lesions in the oropharynx. Almost always the development of *Candida* esophagitis is related to immune dysfunction and not simply to local factors. Though seen most often in AIDS patients with low CD4 counts, esophagitis also occurs in patients with leukemia and others taking immunosuppressive agents. The classic symptom of *Candida* esophagitis is odynophagia localized to a discrete substernal area; in AIDS patients the differential diagnosis includes herpes simplex, cytomegalovirus, and idiopathic ulcers seen with advanced AIDS.

Vulvovaginitis

Candida vulvovaginitis is a common infection in women of childbearing age and the most frequent mucocutaneous manifestation of *Candida* infection. Risk factors include conditions associated with increased estrogen levels, such as the use of oral contraceptives and pregnancy, diabetes mellitus, therapy with corticosteroids or broad-spectrum antimicrobials, and HIV infection. Symptoms include vaginal discomfort, discharge, and vulvar pruritus. The discharge is usually curdlike, but it can also be thin and watery. The labia are erythematous and swollen, and the vaginal walls show erythema and white plaques. Although most women have only a few episodes throughout their life, a minority have frequent recurrences; in most of these patients no discrete risk factor is found, and they are presumed to have local immune dysregulation as the cause.

Cutaneous Candidiasis

Candida infection of the skin occurs mostly in the intertriginous areas or under a large pannus or pendulous breasts. The lesions are erythematous, pruritic, and frequently pustular; have a distinct border; and are almost always associated with smaller satellite lesions. The presence of satellite lesions helps distinguish candidiasis from tinea cruris or corporis. *Candida* onychomycosis results in thickened, opaque, and onycholytic nails. *Candida* can also cause paronychia, especially in those whose occupation involves frequent immersion of their hands in water.

Chronic Mucocutaneous Candidiasis

This uncommon syndrome usually begins in childhood and is characterized by recalcitrant and relapsing thrush, vaginitis, onychomycosis, and hyperkeratotic skin lesions on the face, scalp, and hands. It is thought to be due to a specific defect in the T-cell response to *Candida* antigens. Some patients have associated endocrinopathies, such as hypoparathyroidism, hypothyroidism, and hypoadrenalism.

Disseminated Infections

Candidemia

The most common manifestation of disseminated *Candida* infection is candidemia. However, candidemia merely implies the presence of *Candida* in blood but does not define the extent of visceral involvement. *Candida* obtained from a blood culture should never be considered a contaminant and should always prompt a search for the probable source and the extent of infection. Risk factors for candidemia include broad-spectrum antimicrobials, central intravenous catheters, parenteral nutrition, renal failure, surgical procedures involving the gastrointestinal tract, neutropenia, and corticosteroid therapy. The attributable mortality from candidemia approaches 40%; overall mortality is higher in the elderly and neonates.

Although candidemia is the most obvious manifestation of serious infection with *Candida* species, septic shock can occur along with invasion of multiple viscera in the absence of positive blood cultures. The clinical picture of disseminated candidiasis is indistinguishable from that caused by bacterial infection. The histologic picture characteristic of disseminated candidiasis consists of multiple microabscesses in many organs. The eyes, kidneys, liver, spleen, and brain are the most commonly infected sites, but virtually all organs have been noted to have microabscesses caused by *Candida*. Clinical clues to the diagnosis of disseminated candidiasis include the appearance of the skin and retinal lesions. The nonpainful, nonpruritic skin lesions are papular to pustular and surrounded by a zone of erythema. The eye lesions appear as distinctive white exudates in the retina; with extension into the vitreous body, the retina becomes obscured.

Endocarditis

Candida endocarditis is an uncommon and often fatal complication of candidemia. It occurs most often in intravenous drug users, patients who have prosthetic cardiac valves, and those with central venous catheters in place. Blood cultures are usually persistently positive, and echocardiography reveals large vegetations that can readily embolize to major vessels.

Chronic Disseminated Candidiasis (Hepatosplenic Candidiasis)

This syndrome almost always occurs in leukemic patients who have had an episode of neutropenia. After the neutrophil count returns to normal, fevers that are often quite high, right upper quadrant tenderness, and nausea develop. The alkaline phosphatase level is generally elevated, and distinctive punched-out lesions are seen in the liver, spleen, and sometimes the kidneys on computed tomography (CT). Biopsy of these lesions shows microabscesses that contain budding yeasts.

Focal Invasive Infections

These forms of candidiasis result from local inoculation, contiguous spread, or hematogenous spread. Hematogenous spread, which often goes undetected, is probably the most common pathogenetic mechanism. Although *Candida* infection of all organs has been reported, the most frequent focal infections are urinary tract infections, osteoarticular infections, endophthalmitis, peritonitis, and meningitis.

Urinary Tract Infections

Urinary tract infections are the most common locally invasive *Candida* infection. Candiduria is a frequent finding in patients in the hospital. Factors predisposing to candiduria include diabetes mellitus, broad-spectrum antimicrobial treatment, indwelling urinary devices, and genitourinary tract structural abnormalities. Most patients with candiduria have only bladder colonization and not infection, and most have no urinary tract symptoms. Patients with actual *Candida* infection of the bladder can have symptoms indistinguishable from those of bacterial cystitis. Those who have upper urinary tract infection can have fever, flank pain, nausea, and vomiting, similar to the symptoms seen with acute bacterial pyelonephritis. A fungus ball composed of fungal hyphae can develop at any level of the collecting system and lead to obstruction with subsequent infection.

Osteoarticular Infections

Osteoarticular infections arise secondary to hematogenous seeding or exogenous inoculation during intra-articular injection, a surgical procedure, or trauma. Vertebral osteomyelitis is probably the most common manifestation of osteoarticular candidiasis. The symptoms of back pain and fever may occur weeks after an episode of fungemia. A unique triad of face, scalp, and upper chest folliculitis, endophthalmitis, and sternoclavicular or costochondral septic arthritis has been reported to be due to *C. albicans* in drug users who inject brown heroin intravenously.

Endophthalmitis

Exogenous endophthalmitis occurs secondary to trauma or ophthalmic surgery. Most often, the procedure involved is cataract extraction with or without lens implantation, and the most common infecting species is *C. parapsilosis.* Primary infection occurs in the anterior chamber, but ultimately the posterior chamber is also involved. Endogenous *Candida* endophthalmitis results from hematogenous seeding of the choroid and retina and is one of the most serious complications of candidemia. Characteristic white exudates are visible in the retina, and with progression of the infection, vitritis occurs and the risk for loss of vision is quite high.

Peritonitis

Candida peritonitis can follow bowel surgery or perforation. Symptoms are the same as those noted in bacterial peritonitis. Usually, this type of infection is polymicrobial, and abscess formation is common. In patients maintained on continuous ambulatory peritoneal dialysis, *Candida* peritonitis generally develops as a late infection after previous episodes of bacterial peritonitis. A cloudy dialysate, abdominal pain, and fever are typically noted.

Meningitis

Acute *Candida* meningitis occurs as part of disseminated infection, especially in low-birthweight neonates. Chronic meningitis, an uncommon manifestation of candidiasis, resembles cryptococcal or tuberculous meningitis with regard to symptoms and cerebrospinal fluid findings.

Diagnosis

The diagnosis of mucocutaneous candidiasis is often made clinically. Culture is rarely indicated. Confirmation can be sought by scraping the lesions and performing either a potassium hydroxide preparation or a Gram stain to look for budding yeasts and pseudohyphae. Pseudohyphae are not always noted and are never seen in infection with *C. glabrata.* In circumstances in which disease is recurrent or unresponsive to standard therapy, lesions should be cultured to establish whether a more resistant species, such as *C. glabrata* or *C. krusei,* is the causative agent. In the event of suspected esophagitis, endoscopy should be performed; biopsy of the plaquelike lesions or ulcerations will show mucosal invasion with budding yeasts and pseudohyphae.

The diagnosis of invasive or disseminated candidiasis is more difficult. Evidence for dissemination is usually sought by culturing blood or other sterile body sites. Automated blood culture systems (BacT/ALERT by bioMerieux, Inc.; BACTEC by Becton, Dickinson and Company; and ESP by Difco Laboratories) are as sensitive as the lysis-centrifugation system for growing *Candida* from blood. However, no system is sensitive enough for clinicians to rely on blood cultures to establish the diagnosis of invasive candidiasis in all cases or to rule out candidiasis as a diagnostic possibility. In addition, 1 to 4 days is required for growth to occur; in a desperately ill patient, this delay is problematic.

The tips of intravenous catheters that have been removed should be sent for culture. However, no studies have evaluated the number of yeasts that are indicative of infection, and many physicians accept the growth of any yeast as affirming infection that requires treatment. Because osteomyelitis and other focal forms of candidiasis are generally indistinguishable from bacterial infection, biopsy should be performed for histopathologic and culture studies.

In a seriously ill patient suspected of having candidiasis, the development of pustular skin lesions or typical retinal lesions can be helpful. Budding yeasts typical of *Candida* species should be sought by smearing material from a pustule on a slide and staining it with Gram stain or by performing a biopsy of a lesion and staining the tissue section with a silver stain. All patients who are candidemic or suspected of having disseminated *Candida* infection should undergo an ophthalmologic examination to look for typical retinal lesions.

Imaging studies are invaluable for certain forms of candidiasis, especially chronic disseminated candidiasis, and can be of major help in defining the extent of infection in other types of *Candida* infection, such as urinary tract infection and endocarditis.

Candida antibody tests are of no benefit in the diagnosis of *Candida* infections. The serum β-D-glucan assay, which detects a component of the cell wall of many different fungi, may prove beneficial in the diagnosis of invasive fungal infections, including candidiasis; however, more experience is needed to verify this test's usefulness.

Treatment

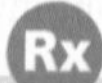

Guidelines for treatment of the various forms of candidiasis have recently been published by the Mycoses Study Group under the auspices of the Infectious Diseases Society of America. Mucocutaneous disease is obviously treated in a much different fashion from disseminated life-threatening illness. Because diagnostic tests are not sensitive, empirical therapy is indicated in some circumstances, and for patients at the highest risk for infection, antifungal prophylaxis can be used to decrease the risk for *Candida* infection.

Mucocutaneous Infections

Most mucocutaneous infections should initially be treated with local creams, solutions, troches, or suspensions. For thrush, clotrimazole troches (10 mg four or five times daily) are preferred to nystatin suspension (commonly given as "swish and swallow" four times daily). Patients with AIDS may not respond to local therapy, especially when their $CD4^+$ lymphocyte counts are low; in this situation, oral fluconazole, 100 mg daily, or itraconazole solution, 200 mg daily, should be used. Posaconazole is as effective as fluconazole acutely and more likely to result in sustained success. [1] For vaginitis, a variety of creams and vaginal tablets (miconazole, clotrimazole, and others) are effective, but many women prefer to take a single oral 150-mg fluconazole tablet. Recurrent vaginitis is a more complicated therapeutic issue and often requires chronic suppressive therapy with fluconazole. Esophagitis should always be treated with a systemically absorbed agent; the usual treatment is either 100 mg fluconazole or 200 mg itraconazole solution (not capsules) daily for 14 days.

In patients with advanced AIDS and low $CD4^+$ lymphocyte counts, who are often taking chronic suppressive therapy with fluconazole to prevent recurrent candidiasis, fluconazole-refractory disease may develop. For these patients, increasing the dosage of fluconazole or switching to itraconazole suspension or oral voriconazole should be effective. If oral tablets and solutions are no longer effective, intravenous amphotericin B, caspofungin, anidulafungin, and micafungin are alternative agents that can be used. Patients with the syndrome of chronic mucocutaneous candidiasis require lifelong suppressive therapy with oral azole agents.

Candidemia and Other Disseminated Infections

All patients with candidemia should be treated with an antifungal agent, including patients who have only one blood culture that yields *Candida* and those with a vascular catheter tip that yields *Candida.* The rationale for this recommendation relates to the high rate of metastatic foci in major organs associated with hematogenously disseminated candidiasis. Several antifungal agents can be used to treat candidemia, including fluconazole, 400 or 800 mg daily, caspofungin, 50 mg daily, anidulafungin, 100 mg daily, micafungin, 100 mg daily, voriconazole, 3 mg/kg twice daily, amphotericin B, 0.7 mg/kg daily, or a lipid formulation of amphotericin B, 3 to 5 mg/kg daily. [2] Fluconazole has generally been the preferred agent for the last decade, but caspofungin is increasingly being used, especially if the patient has previously received fluconazole or if *C. glabrata* is a common species isolated in the hospital in which the patient is receiving care. All vascular catheters should be removed because removal has been shown to help clear *Candida* from blood more quickly. Repeated blood cultures should be obtained to be certain that the fungemia has resolved, and treatment should continue for 2 weeks after the date of the first negative blood culture.

Because diagnostic tests are not sensitive, seriously ill patients who could have disseminated candidiasis may need to be treated before culture confirmation. This approach is used frequently in neutropenic patients, in whom outcomes are poor if disseminated fungal infection goes untreated. Several different antifungal agents can be used empirically, including a lipid formulation of amphotericin B, caspofungin, or voriconazole; these agents have activity against filamentous fungi, as well as *Candida* species. The other

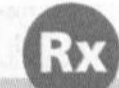

patients in whom this approach has been used are those in the ICU. However, the risk factors for candidiasis are less well defined in this group than in those who are neutropenic, and recommendations for empirical treatment have not been defined. Fluconazole is generally used because filamentous fungi are rarely noted in this setting.

Endocarditis should be treated with either standard amphotericin B or a lipid formulation of amphotericin B in combination with flucytosine. Caspofungin has also been reported to be effective for endocarditis. The infected valve should be replaced. A few patients have been reported for whom valve replacement was not an option and for whom lifelong suppression with fluconazole appeared to be effective.

Chronic disseminated candidiasis generally requires months of therapy for cure. Most patients begin therapy with a lipid formulation of amphotericin B and then are switched to fluconazole and treated until the lesions disappear on CT scan.

Focal Invasive Infections

Treatment of focal infections depends on the organ system involved. Perhaps the simplest to treat are urinary tract infections. Most patients with candiduria are not infected but merely colonized; removing the selective pressure of antimicrobials and indwelling catheters eliminates candiduria in many of these patients. For those who have an infection, oral fluconazole is the preferred treatment. Treatment should continue long enough to allow eradication of upper as well as lower tract infection; 2 weeks of 200 mg fluconazole daily is an appropriate regimen. [3] Bladder irrigation with amphotericin B should not be used because it eradicates only bladder colonization, requires that a catheter be placed into the bladder, and is associated with a high recurrence rate. It is not clear whether any of the newer antifungal agents will have a role in the treatment of urinary tract infections.

Osteoarticular infections require months of therapy; amphotericin B or caspofungin can be given initially, followed by long-term therapy with fluconazole or voriconazole. Peritonitis associated with chronic ambulatory peritoneal dialysis can be treated with amphotericin B, fluconazole, or an echinocandin, depending on the species of *Candida* causing infection. Intraperitoneal administration of amphotericin B can be extremely irritating and should not be attempted. The dialysis catheter should be removed. Meningitis should be treated initially with amphotericin B and flucytosine; patients with the more chronic form of the disease can be switched to fluconazole for a longer duration of therapy.

Treatment of *Candida* eye infections varies with the extent of ocular involvement. Lesions that are discovered early at the stage of choroidal or retinal involvement can probably be treated effectively with systemic antifungal agents (amphotericin B, caspofungin, fluconazole, or voriconazole) alone. Lesions that have extended into the vitreous body require more aggressive therapy. The best results have been obtained with pars plana vitrectomy, which also provides material for culture, injection of amphotericin B into the vitreous, and a systemic antifungal agent such as fluconazole or voriconazole. Clearly, management must be individualized and performed in concert with an ophthalmologist experienced in the treatment of this infection. Treatment of endophthalmitis associated with an intraocular lens implant requires removal of the implant, vitrectomy, and local amphotericin B injections. The use of systemic antifungal therapy is debated, but fluconazole has proved useful.

Prevention

For certain populations at highest risk for invasive fungal infection, prophylactic antifungal agents have been shown to prevent infection. The prophylactic use of fluconazole has become standard in the bone marrow transplant population, although itraconazole is also effective, [4] but in leukemic patients with neutropenia, its efficacy is not as clear-cut. Antifungal treatment is effective in preventing invasive fungal infections but not in improving survival in recipients of solid organ transplants. [5] Controversy surrounds the use of prophylactic fluconazole in ICU patients. Restricting the use of prophylaxis to those at the highest risk for disseminated candidiasis is essential to prevent widespread use of azoles with subsequent selection of resistant species. The role of new antifungal agents for prophylaxis has yet to be defined.

Prognosis

The prognosis for patients with mucocutaneous infections is excellent. The major problem occurs in AIDS patients, who continue to have recurrent infections unless their $CD4^+$ lymphocyte counts revert toward normal with antiretroviral therapy. The prognosis for focal invasive infections depends on the organ involved and the immune state of the patient. For example, although pyelonephritis may respond well to antifungal therapy, meningitis is more difficult to treat and has a poor outcome. Disseminated infection has a high mortality rate. The immune state of the host is the primary determinant of outcome. If the risk factors that led to candidemia and widespread visceral dissemination, especially neutropenia, are not corrected, the outcome is poor.

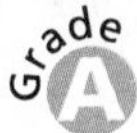

1. Vazquez JA, Skiest DJ, Nieto L, et al: A multicenter randomized trial evaluating posaconazole versus fluconazole for the treatment of oropharyngeal candidiasis in subjects with HIV/AIDS. Clin Infect Dis 2006;42:1179–1186.
2. Mora-Duarte J, Betts R, Rotstein C, et al: Comparison of caspofungin and amphotericin B for invasive candidiasis. N Engl J Med 2002;347:2020–2029.
3. Sobel JD, Kauffman CA, McKinsey D, et al: Candiduria: A randomized, double-blind study of treatment with fluconazole and placebo. Clin Infect Dis 2000;30:19–24.
4. Maertens J: Evaluating prophylaxis of invasive fungal infections in patients with hematologic malignancies. Eur J Haematol 2007;78: 275–282.
5. Playford EG, Webster AC, Sorell TC, et al: Antifungal agents for preventing fungal infections in solid organ transplant recipients. Cochrane Database Syst Rev 2004;(3):CD004291.

SUGGESTED READINGS

Bennett JE: Echinocandins for candidemia in adults without neutropenia. N Engl J Med 2006;355:1154–1159. *A clinical review.*

Garey KW, Rege M, Pai MP, et al: Time to initiation of fluconazole therapy impacts mortality in patients with candidemia: A multi-institutional study. Clin Infect Dis 2006;43:25–31. *Delay in the initiation of fluconazole in candidemic patients was associated with an increased mortality.*

Golan Y, Wolf MP, Pauker SG, et al: Empirical anti-*Candida* therapy among selected patients in the intensive care unit: A cost-effectiveness analysis. Ann Intern Med 2005;143:857–869. *Empirical fluconazole is cost-effective if the likelihood of invasive candidiasis is >2.5% and fluconazole resistance is <24%.*

Pappas PG, Rex JH, Sobel JD, et al: Guidelines for treatment of candidiasis. Clin Infect Dis 2004;38:161–189. *Consensus guidelines for treating candidiasis by the Infectious Diseases Society of American.*

ASPERGILLOSIS

David A. Stevens

Definition

Aspergillosis refers to infection with any of the species of the genus *Aspergillus.* They are in mold form in the environment, on artificial media, and when invading tissues. The clinical characteristics of aspergillosis and its treatment are summarized in Table 360–1.

The Pathogens

The most common species infecting humans are *Aspergillus fumigatus, Aspergillus flavus, Aspergillus niger,* and *Aspergillus terreus.* Some are speciated by the clinical laboratory only with difficulty, and they may be reported solely as "*Aspergillus* species or *Aspergillus* sp." Some variants or sibling species of *A. fumigatus* may be particularly drug resistant. In tissues, aspergilli may be seen as septate hyphae, dichotomously branched

TABLE 360–1 ASPERGILLOSIS: CLINICAL SUMMARY

Causative fungus	*Aspergillus* species: *A. fumigatus, A. flavus, A. niger, A. terreus*, other species
Primary geographic distribution	Ubiquitous: human habitat, soil, water, air
Primary route of acquisition	Inhalation of spores
Principal site of disease	Lung
Opportunistic infection in compromised infection hosts	Invasive form, pulmonary
Drug of choice for most patients	Voriconazole, lipid amphotericin preparations, itraconazole, amphotericin B deoxycholate, caspofungin
Alternative therapy	Combinations of antifungals

TABLE 360–2 ASPERGILLOSIS SYNDROMES

Invasive disease	Asthma
Aspergilloma (fungus ball)	Invasive airways disease
Superficial bronchial disease	Bronchocentric granulomatosis
Extrinsic allergic alveolitis	Pleural disease
Mixed forms	Local disease
Allergic bronchopulmonary disease	Endocarditis

(resembling the divergence of fingers from one another), and they may produce their characteristic conidia in tissues or artificial media, which is one way to differentiate them. If the septation can be seen, they can be differentiated from organisms of the class Zygomycetes; they may be confused with *Pseudallescheria boydii,* however, unless the characteristic terminal spores of the latter are seen.

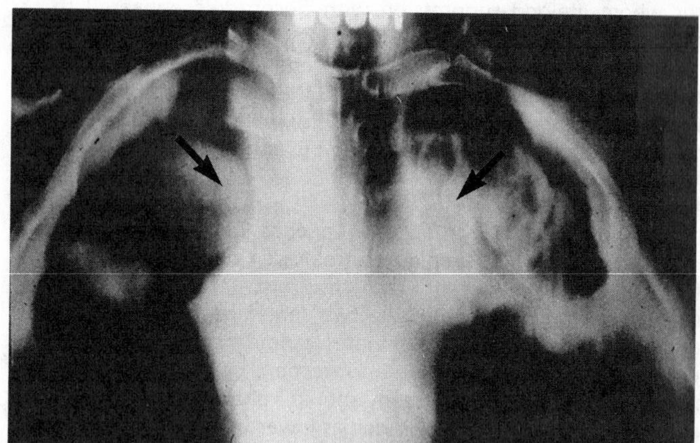

FIGURE 360–1 • Tomogram of pulmonary aspergillomas (arrows).

Epidemiology

Aspergilli are ubiquitous in the environment and have been isolated with ease from soil and air and even from swimming pools and saunas. They are associated with decaying matter and may grow at temperatures of 40 to 50° C (e.g., self-heating organic compost). The ease with which they are isolated from composting materials, silos, and the cooling canals of nuclear power plants has been an environmental and industrial concern. Aspergilli are easily isolated from houses, particularly from basements, crawl spaces, bedding, humidifiers, ventilation ducts, potted plants, and house dust; in surveys they have even been found in condiments, pasta, and marijuana samples. This pervasiveness should make it not surprising that they are sometimes found in normal expectorated sputa. Aspergilli are important pathogens of marine organisms, insects, and birds (both domesticated and wild), and they cause abortion in cattle. As they grow, they produce toxins, such as aflatoxin—one of the most potent carcinogens known—which contaminates the food chain and thus poses a risk to animals and humans. The frequency of invasive aspergillosis is rising worldwide. Their threat to hospitalized patients has been revealed in outbreaks of infection, particularly pulmonary infection in immunocompromised hosts, associated with building renovation and new construction. The suspected vector has been unfiltered air, as from inlets contaminated with bird excreta and fireproofing materials. Hospital water, which may become aerosolized during activities such as patient showering, is a newly described possible source.

Aspergillosis usually results from airborne conidia and is not contagious.

Clinical Manifestations

The main forms of clinical aspergillosis are listed in Table 360–2. *Invasive disease* is generally a problem of immunocompromised hosts, and more aggressive immunosuppression and anticancer therapy are the most important factors contributing to the rise of *Aspergillus* infections. Series have reported an incidence as high as 41% in those with acute leukemia at autopsy, and in 89% of these cases *Aspergillus* played a significant role in death of the patient. In 97% pulmonary involvement was present, and in 25% the infection was disseminated widely to various organs. Similarly, in a group of heart transplant recipients, the incidence of infection was 28%. The incidence in bone marrow transplant recipients has ranged from 5 to 20%, with a higher frequency in certain groups such as patients with graft-versus-host disease, and mortality is 68% to more than 95% in various series. *Aspergillus* is also common in lung, liver, and heart transplant recipients and other steroid-treated patients, including those with chronic obstructive pulmonary disease. It is likewise a problem in patients with neutrophil defects such as chronic granulomatous disease.

Diagnosis is difficult because aspergilli are frequently contaminants in sputum and in other cultures during handling. In patients with leukemia, *Aspergillus* is particularly associated with relapses of the malignancy, and three or four of the following factors are usually present: leukopenia, glucocorticoid therapy, cytotoxic chemotherapy, and broad-spectrum antibacterials. The classic picture is that of fever and pulmonary infiltrates or nodules, especially progressing to a cavity (generally when granulocytopenia is reversed), or wedge-shaped densities resembling infarcts. The pulmonary pathology in all these entities is that of hemorrhagic infarction and pneumonia. Pulmonary emboli are common because of the organism's tendency to invade blood vessel walls. These processes often combine to produce a "target lesion" consisting of a necrotic center surrounded by a ring of hemorrhage.

Targets of *disseminated disease* include, most commonly, the central nervous system, where abscesses are characteristic. The glucose level in cerebrospinal fluid (CSF) is normal, and cultures of CSF are negative. Mycelia invading blood vessels may produce a microangiopathic hemolytic anemia. Dissemination can result in Budd-Chiari syndrome, myocardial infarction, gastrointestinal disease, or skin lesions. Esophageal ulcers may produce gastrointestinal bleeding. Abscesses are common in the kidney, liver, and myocardium.

Endocarditis is associated with cardiac surgery and particularly with prostheses or intravenous drug abuse. Major arterial emboli occur in 83% of patients, and neurologic findings are common. Only 8% have positive blood cultures, and this positivity is usually delayed 14 to 20 days, thus contributing to the poor record of diagnosis antemortem, which is usually made on histologic examination of an embolus. Overall, the survival rate is about 5%, and these individuals have undergone valve replacement. The disease should be suspected in any patient after cardiac surgery who has endocarditis or emboli and negative blood cultures.

The typical picture of an aspergilloma is a fungus ball (i.e., matted hyphae and debris) in a cavity in an upper lobe of the lung (Fig. 360–1). It has been reported as a complication in as many as 11% of old tuberculous cavities. Patients have cough (87%), hemoptysis (81%), dyspnea (61%), weight loss (61%), fatigue (61%), chest pain (31%), or fever (25%). Sputum culture is positive in most. Patients with marked underlying lung disease, large or numerous aspergillomas, rising anti-*Aspergillus* antibody, or sarcoidosis or those who are immunocompromised do particularly poorly.

Pleural disease is associated with tuberculosis and bronchopleural fistulas. It may occur after surgery or spontaneously.

Allergic bronchopulmonary aspergillosis is generally superimposed on a background of chronic asthma or cystic fibrosis. The disease appears to be triggered in genetically susceptible individuals by specific *Aspergillus* antigens. It is characterized by episodic airway obstruction, fever, eosinophilia, mucous plugs, positive sputum cultures, the presence of grossly visible brown flecks in sputum (hyphae), transient infiltrates and parallel "tramline" or ring markings on chest radiographs, proximal bronchiectasis, upper lobe contraction, and elevated levels of total immunoglobulin G (IgG), especially when the patient is symptomatic. It is more common in agricultural areas and in the winter, presumably representing an association with stored agricultural products (especially moldy hay) and spore production. The eosinophilia is present in blood, sputum, and the lung on biopsy. The mucous plugs contain mycelia, and the plugs may be the cause of the infiltrates, with collapse and inflammation occurring peripherally, or inflammatory edema may be responsible. The parallel or ring markings are caused by thickened ectatic bronchi, and the upper lobe changes are a result of progressive apical fibrosis. The infiltrates may be nonsegmental and transient, with clinical findings of "eosinophilic pneumonia," asthma, and eosinophils in blood and sputum; alternatively, they may be segmental and associated with blocking of bronchi by plugs, and asthma and eosinophilia may be absent. A biphasic skin test response may assist in the diagnosis. A scratch test with *Aspergillus* antigens produces an immediate wheal and flare reaction that is mediated by IgE and blocked by antihistamines but not by corticosteroids. An intracutaneous test with the antigens produces a later (6 to 8 hours) reaction that is mediated by IgG antibody and complement and blocked by steroids. Similarly, bronchial challenge with the antigens can produce a biphasic response.

Extrinsic allergic alveolitis is an unusual form of *Aspergillus* lung disease that has been most frequently associated with *Aspergillus clavatus* in malt workers. A hypersensitivity pneumonitis with dyspnea and fever develops 4 hours after exposure. Diffuse micronodular infiltrates may be present at the time of symptoms. Patients have IgG precipitins and cell-mediated immune reactions against *Aspergillus* antigens, and granulomas are identified on biopsy. Eosinophilia is not a feature. The scratch test is negative, although an intradermal test produces a reaction in 4 hours, with immunoglobulins and complement present on biopsy. Bronchial challenge produces a reaction in 4 hours consisting of systemic symptoms and a restrictive defect but without airway resistance. The entity can progress to irreversible fibrosis. The same pathophysiology may be involved in episodes after massive inhalation of spores, which usually occurs in farm environments. Symptoms are present within 24 hours, and granulomas are found on biopsy.

Superficial bronchial disease, an acute or chronic bronchitis with brown-flecked sputum, *extrinsic asthma* secondary to airborne conidia, and *bronchocentric granulomatosis,* a peribronchial destructive disease with wheezing or fever and weight loss, are other important pulmonary diseases. The aspergilloma, allergic, alveolitis, and superficial forms rarely progress to invasive disease. However, more *invasive airway disease* with ulcerative, pseudomembranous, or plaquelike tracheobronchitis occurs, particularly in immunocompromised hosts, and may presage parenchymal invasion. *Chronic necrotizing pulmonary aspergillosis* generally occurs in patients with underlying lung disease or a mildly immunosuppressive condition (or both), often with features of invasive disease and aspergilloma.

Examples of *locally invasive disease* abound and are usually severe. They include invasion of burn wounds, keratitis, external otitis (particularly in the tropics), focal rhinitis (particularly in immunosuppressed or granulocytopenic hosts), sinusitis (in these hosts or after dental procedures), stomatitis, and osteomyelitis or endophthalmitis (after fungemia, trauma, or surgery). Cutaneous ulcers have been associated with the use of adhesive tape. Blood-borne disease in addicts can produce foci of dissemination that are similar to those associated with the invasive pulmonary form of the disease. A noninvasive form of sinus disease has a predominantly allergic component and eosinophilia. It is responsive to drainage and corticosteroids.

Diagnosis

Some of the modalities of diagnosis have been mentioned in connection with specific syndromes. Antibody to *Aspergillus* has been detected by a variety of techniques and with a variety of antigen preparations. Data from the more commonly reported techniques suggest a high degree of sensitivity in allergic disease or aspergillomas but a low degree of sensitivity in invasive disease. Because the frequency of false-positive reactions is low, even in the presence of other mycoses, a positive test result in cases of invasive disease may be useful. IgE and IgG antibody specific to *Aspergillus* antigens is another serodiagnostic adjunct in allergic disease. Sputum culture, though having good positive predictive value in the appropriate setting (especially a neutropenic patient, particularly if febrile), is positive in only 8 to 34% of cases, and tissue must be obtained to make the diagnosis. Prospective culturing of the nose of granulocytopenic patients has been of some value because a positive nasal culture (particularly the presence of nasal *Aspergillus* lesions) has led to the early diagnosis of concurrent pulmonary or sinus disease. However, negative nasal cultures are common in pulmonary aspergillosis. Detection of a galactomannan antigen in serum, initially studied by latex agglutination methods and later by enzyme-linked immunosorbent assay, has been useful, particularly with serial testing, in identifying invasive disease, especially with repeatedly positive results and serial monitoring, and in monitoring responses to therapy. Several causes of false-positive tests, such as other infections and some antibacterial therapy, have been documented. Other body fluids, such as CSF and urine, have been fruitful for antigen detection. In some laboratories, detection of *Aspergillus* DNA in blood by polymerase chain reaction (PCR) has demonstrated high specificity and sensitivity, and detection of glucan in serum is promising. Culture or cytology of bronchoalveolar lavage fluid and, in the appropriate population, antigen testing are also useful in the diagnosis of invasive disease. The problem with some serodiagnostic modalities is the lack of a generally available, standardized technique in the United States. The physician should know the background data (i.e., the sensitivity and specificity of the assay in the various syndromes) for the laboratory to which the specimens may be sent.

In severe disease, an aggressive, invasive approach, as well as making a tissue diagnosis early in the illness, appears to be a key to survival. In the appropriate clinical setting, such as an immunocompromised host with fever and a pulmonary infiltrate, repeated isolation of the same species in culture, particularly bronchial lavage or other endobronchial culture, correlates with invasive disease; sometimes even a single sputum culture (especially with heavy growth) may have to be the stimulus for therapy if invasive procedures cannot be performed. Negative culture results do not rule out invasive disease. Blood cultures are rarely helpful. Computed tomographic scanning of the chest done at the earliest suspicion of this diagnosis may initially reveal a lesion with peripheral haziness (i.e., the halo sign) or later reveal a lesion with an air crescent; both lesions are highly predictive of this diagnosis (Fig. 360–2). These are radiographic correlates of edema or hemorrhage and infarction that are related to the organism's vasculotropism. In these situations, a positive galactomannan assay, PCR, or glucan test is particularly helpful in prompting therapy, even if a specific microbiologic diagnosis from tissue is not possible. Computed tomography or magnetic resonance imaging is valuable in delineating sinus disease.

Treatment

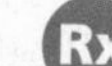

The role of granulocyte transfusions, colony-stimulating factors, or pro-inflammatory cytokines is unclear. In endocarditis, in addition to prompt, aggressive chemotherapy, valve replacement appears to be necessary. Locally invasive disease in other sites also requires systemic or local chemotherapy, particularly intravitreal therapy or nephrostomy irrigation in renal disease. Surgical excision has an important role in the invasion of bone, burn wounds, epidural abscesses, vitreal disease, sinus disease in nonimmunocompromised hosts, endocarditis, and removal of catheters for peritonitis and silk sutures for bronchial stump (postpneumonectomy) aspergillosis. Surgery may have a function in invasive pulmonary disease for which chemotherapy has failed or when disease impinges on major vascu-

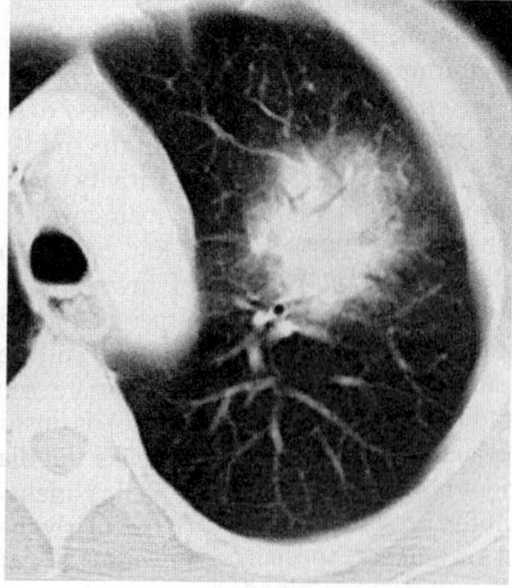

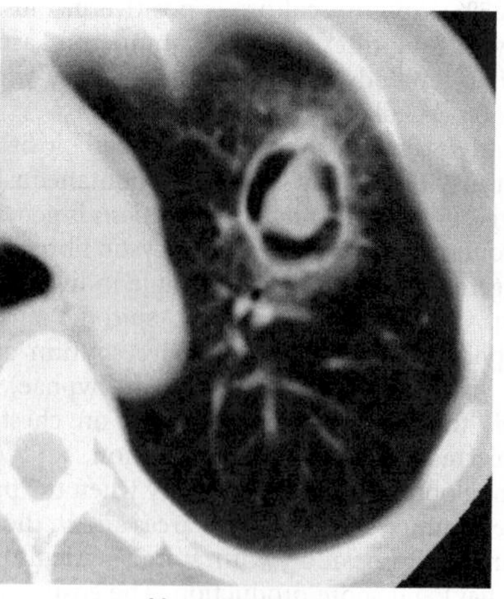

FIGURE 360–2 • Evolution of radiography of invasive aspergillosis in an immunocompromised host. D = days after the lesion is first noted.

lar structures. In pleural disease, local instillation of nystatin or amphotericin has been helpful.

In cases involving aspergilloma, there is evidence that patients with fever, cough, weight loss, malaise, and hemoptysis have an element of allergy that can be demonstrated by bronchial challenge or the presence of specific IgG and IgE. These patients symptomatically improve if given glucocorticoids. Intravenous amphotericin B therapy in patients with aspergilloma produces results no better than those with routine pulmonary toilet. Intracavitary antifungals, instilled through a catheter, are a heroic form of therapy that has been attempted in some patients.

The role of surgery for aspergilloma is controversial. Between 7 and 15% of mycetomas undergo spontaneous lysis. The overall operative mortality rate aggregated from several series is 7%, but it may be as high as 14% in some large series. The frequency of various operative complications aggregated from several series is 22%, with a range of 7 to 60%. New aspergillomas have developed after surgical successes. On the other hand, in various series, 18 to 26% of patients with adequate follow-up and treated without surgery died of disease complications, usually hemoptysis, whereas 50% had significant improvement symptomatically and radiographically. If any consensus exists, it is that surgical resection has a role in treating patients with recurrent, significant hemoptysis. Alternative temporary therapies, particularly for nonsurgical patients, are selective bronchial arterial embolization of the bleeding vessel or percutaneous instillation of antifungals. Oral itraconazole may have a role in treating chronic aspergilloma.

In allergic disease, measures that have *not* worked include hyposensitization and avoidance of sites in the environment. Cromolyn is inadequate in most patients. Aerosolized antifungals have produced remission but do not prevent recurrence. Treating the clinical disease is more complicated than the effects of drug blockade demonstrable in challenge tests. Continuous use of systemic glucocorticoids can prevent the acute infiltrates and some accompanying symptoms. Intermittent use of glucocorticoids or raising the dose in patients receiving chronic therapy can produce rapid resolution of marked symptomatic episodes; this is also indicated for patients with rising IgE or worsening spirometry readings. Bronchodilators ameliorate acute exacerbations, and leukotriene modifiers may be of benefit. The long-term beneficial effects of glucocorticoids are less clear; they are not so useful in arresting dyspnea or wheezing in the long term, and they do not prevent development of the accompanying bronchiectasis. A randomized study using oral itraconazole indicated amelioration of disease and a steroid-sparing effect. The proper approach to extrinsic alveolitis is to avoid the stimulus.

When systemic chemotherapy has been indicated, most clinical experience has been with amphotericin B in deoxycholate. Its track record is generally poor for invasive or disseminated disease in immunocompromised hosts, especially in those with cerebral or hepatic disease and in bone marrow transplant recipients. In an immunocompromised host, the drug should be used aggressively, with prompt progression to a full therapeutic dose, which should be greater than 1 mg/kg/day, if tolerated. Some species, such as *A. terreus,* may be more resistant to amphotericin. A new triazole, voriconazole, proved superior in aspergillosis therapy in a randomized trial. Prophylactic therapy may have a role in patients who have survived invasive disease and will become neutropenic again.

Itraconazole as sole therapy has produced similar response rates in invasive disease and is an alternative if the patient is reliable, can be shown to absorb the drug adequately (by monitoring serum concentrations), and is not receiving other drugs that interact with itraconazole and present management difficulties. Oral itraconazole as a continuation therapy after amphotericin is logical and appears safe. A new oral solution in cyclodextrin lessens absorption problems, and an intravenous formulation is available for patients who cannot take or absorb oral preparations.

Lipid-complexed amphotericin B given in higher doses than amphotericin B deoxycholate has also produced similar response rates in historical comparisons and is less nephrotoxic but more expensive. A new class of antifungals (echinocandins) that inhibit glucan synthesis have shown activity against *Aspergillus* in vivo, and caspofungin has been licensed on the basis of data showing responsiveness of cases refractory to conventional chemotherapy. Rifampin almost always potentiates the activity of amphotericin in vitro against aspergilli, whereas results with flucytosine are unpredictable. Animal models have shown an enhanced effect of combinations of these drugs over amphotericin alone. Clinical data to support combination therapy are limited, but given the poor record of monotherapy in invasive disease, combination therapy appears to be a logical avenue to explore, particularly if synergy in vitro can be demonstrated. Combinations of polyenes, azoles, and echinocandins are being explored. Therapy should be continued after the lesions are resolving, cultures are negative, and reversible underlying predispositions have abated. Reinstating therapy in patients who have previously responded should be considered if immunosuppression is reinstituted or if neutropenia recurs.

Prevention

Prophylaxis in susceptible patients, such as immunocompromised hosts, with intranasal, inhaled, or systemic antifungals or prophylaxis in allergic patients with inhaled or systemic antifungals is an approach to avoid disease and the need for therapy. Reducing airborne spores, such as by filtering hospital air, reducing activities that increase spore counts when the patient is in the room such as room maintenance, preventing dust, and restricting contaminated materials (e.g., potted plants), is believed to be a worthwhile effort for patients who will be transiently immunosuppressed or neutropenic.

Prognosis

In invasive disease, prompt, aggressive chemotherapy has produced superior survival statistics at some institutions, although recovery from neutropenia is a necessary accompaniment of recovery in almost every success.

SUGGESTED READINGS

Barnes PD, Marr KA: Aspergillosis: Spectrum of disease, diagnosis, and treatment. Infect Dis Clin North Am 2006;20:545–561. *A comprehensive review of the range of infections caused by* Aspergillus *species, the challenges of diagnosis, and current treatment options.*

Patterson TF, Kirkpatrick WR, White M, et al: Invasive aspergillosis. Disease spectrum, treatment practices, and outcomes. Medicine (Baltimore) 2000; 79:250–260. *Reviews sites and treatment outcomes in 595 nonrandom invasive aspergillosis cases.*

Virnig C, Bush RK: Allergic bronchopulmonary aspergillosis: A US perspective. Curr Opin Pulm Med 2007;13:67–71. *A review of allergic bronchopulmonary aspergillosis.*

361 MUCORMYCOSIS

David A. Stevens

Definition

Mucormycosis is usually an acute and rapidly developing fungal infection caused by fungi of the class Zygomycetes. In healthy hosts, these organisms seldom cause infection. However, in debilitated or immunosuppressed hosts, they commonly produce a fulminant opportunistic infection that results in marked tissue destruction. Several predisposing conditions have been identified. The infection is most commonly associated with diabetic ketoacidosis. Prolonged treatment with antimicrobials, corticosteroids, and cytotoxic drugs and, most recently, the use of deferoxamine in dialysis patients have also been associated with mucormycosis, as have severe malnutrition, hematologic malignancies, neutropenia, cytomegalovirus infection, and extensive burns.

The clinical characteristics of mucormycosis and its treatment are summarized in Table 361–1.

The Pathogens

The pathogenic zygomycetes are largely in the order Mucorales, which is related to the term for this infection, mucormycosis. Zygomycosis has also been used to refer to disease caused by organisms of the class, but this term would include diseases caused by fungi of the order Entomophthorales. The latter diseases are generally different from those caused by Mucorales organisms (i.e., largely superficial infections in tropical and subtropical areas). The Mucorales pathogens are morphologically distinct from other fungi. Their hyphae are pauciseptate, broad, and variable in size and shape. Branching of the hyphae is usually at right angles. Species of the genera *Rhizopus, Mucor,* and *Rhizomucor* are the common pathogens in this group. Other genera, including *Absidia, Cunninghamella,* and *Apophysomyces,* have also been reported to cause disease. These genera cannot be differentiated histopathologically.

TABLE 361–1 MUCORMYCOSIS: CLINICAL CHARACTERISTICS AND TREATMENT

Causative fungus	The order Mucorales; *Rhizopus, Mucor* species most common
Primary geographic distribution	Ubiquitous: air, bread, fruit, vegetables, soil, manure
Primary route of acquisition	Inhaling spores
Principal sites of disease	Rhinocerebral, pulmonary, cutaneous, gastrointestinal, disseminated, central nervous system
Opportunistic infection in compromised hosts	Pulmonary, rhinocerebral
Drug of choice for most patients	Amphotericin B
Alternative therapy	Amphotericin combined with rifampin, azoles, flucytosine; posaconazole

Further speciation requires culturing the pathogen and characterizing the isolates by their morphologic and physiologic features.

Epidemiology

Members of Mucorales are ubiquitous saprophytic fungi and are abundant in nature. They have been recovered from bread, fruits, vegetables, soil, and manure. These fungi have been isolated from the nose, stool, and sputum of healthy individuals. Various longitudinal series indicate a frequency of approximately 1% in solid organ transplants and 1 to 4% in autopsy series of patients with hematologic malignancies or allogeneic marrow transplants, and the incidence is rising. A recent upsurge in cases apparently associated with the use of voriconazole, a broad-spectrum antifungal, may be rooted in an earlier trend of an increase in cases in hematopoietic stem cell transplant patients, particularly late after transplantation and with immunosuppression for graft-versus-host disease. The disease is not transmissible from person to person. Cases appear to occur more frequently in summer or fall.

Pathobiology

There is no unifying concept of the pathogenesis of mucormycosis. In diseases of the airways (e.g., sinus, lung), the infection is presumed to originate from inhaled spores, although the lung may also be involved because of blood stream invasion. Colonization may be more common in people with diabetes. Whereas normal human serum can inhibit growth of the organisms, serum obtained from patients with diabetic ketoacidosis is not inhibitory and may even promote fungal growth, possibly because of decreased transferrin iron binding. Undefined defects in macrophages and neutrophils contribute to the loss of immunity against this infection in a susceptible host. Corticosteroids weaken normal inhibitors of spore germination in tissue. Unlike most pathogenic fungi, these can grow in the absence of oxygen. The iron chelators used in therapy for overload in dialysis patients may act as siderophores for these fungi and stimulate their growth.

Invasion, thrombosis, and necrosis are the characteristic findings in this disease. After the fungal spores have germinated at the site of infection, the hyphal elements are very aggressive and tend to invade blood vessels, nerves, lymphatics, and tissues. The infarction leads to further tissue hypoxia and acidosis, thereby resulting in a vicious cycle that enhances rapid growth and infection. The paucity of a granulomatous reaction is quite characteristic. The fungal hyphae sometimes have little or no inflammation around them.

Clinical Manifestations

Mucormycosis can be manifested as at least six distinct clinical entities, depending on the types of predisposing factors of the patient and the portal of entry of the organism.

Rhinocerebral Mucormycosis

Rhinocerebral mucormycosis, the most common manifestation, accounts for more than 75% of cases in the literature. It frequently affects poorly controlled diabetic patients who have ketoacidosis. It has also been reported in patients with hematologic malignancies who have been neutropenic for an extended period and who have received broad-spectrum antibacterial drugs or immunosuppressive therapy, in other acidotic patients, and in those with azotemia. Rhinocerebral mucormycosis can be one of the most rapidly fatal fungal diseases if left undiagnosed. Hyphae invade the paranasal sinuses and palate from the oronasal cavity. From the sinuses, especially the ethmoid sinus, the infection spreads to involve the retro-orbital region or the central nervous system (CNS). Epistaxis, severe unilateral headache, altered mental status, and eye symptoms such as lacrimation, irritation, or periorbital anesthesia are common symptoms. Examination of the nose may reveal the classic black necrotic turbinates (too often mistaken for dried blood) or perforation of the nasal septum. However, in the early stage of infection, the nasal mucosa may appear only inflamed and friable. Facial cellulitis and palatal necrosis may be seen. Early eye findings include mild proptosis, periorbital edema, decreased visual acuity, and lid swelling. In more advanced orbital involvement, exophthalmos, complete ophthalmoplegia, conjunctival hemorrhage, blindness, fixed and dilated pupil, and corneal anesthesia may be found. These conditions result from fungal invasion of the roof of the orbit and involvement of the nerves (i.e., third, fourth, and sixth cranial nerves and the ophthalmic branch of the fifth cranial nerve), muscles, and orbital vessels, a condition also known as the *orbital apex syndrome.* The infection can spread through the superior orbital fissure or cribriform plate to involve the brain. Cavernous sinus thrombosis is a frequent complication that usually results from hematogenous spread from the ophthalmic veins.

Such spread results in additional cranial nerve involvement outside the orbital apex, specifically, the trigeminal nerve ganglion and the root of the facial nerve, and leads to ipsilateral paresthesia of the face or peripheral facial palsy. Internal carotid artery thrombosis as a result of retrograde spread from the ophthalmic artery or invasion from the cavernous sinus is another late complication that leads to cerebral infarction. The middle ear may be involved by means of blood, cerebrospinal fluid (CSF), or the eustachian tube.

The radiographic manifestations are nonspecific (Fig. 361–1). Plain roentgenograms of the sinuses and orbits may reveal nodular thickening of the mucosa of multiple sinuses, usually without air-fluid levels, or spotty destruction of bone through the walls of the sinuses or into the orbit. Computed tomography or magnetic resonance imaging is useful in better defining the bone destruction and soft tissue involvement, which may be important in guiding subsequent surgical intervention. CSF findings are usually nonspecific and often normal, even in the presence of CNS involvement. Common findings are pleocytosis, with about 50% polymorphonuclear cells and slight protein elevation; hypoglycorrhachia is rare. Results of smear and culture of CSF are usually negative for fungus, even in cases with documented meningeal involvement. Several infectious diseases can produce a similar picture. Black necrotic lesions may also be seen with invasive aspergillosis and with infections by *Pseudomonas aeruginosa* or *Pseudallescheria boydii.* The only definitive method of differentiating these possibilities is by examination of tissue. Cavernous sinus thrombosis secondary to *Staphylococcus aureus* infection, as well as rhinoscleroma, aggressive orbital tumor, midline granuloma, and other fungal infections, can mimic the disease.

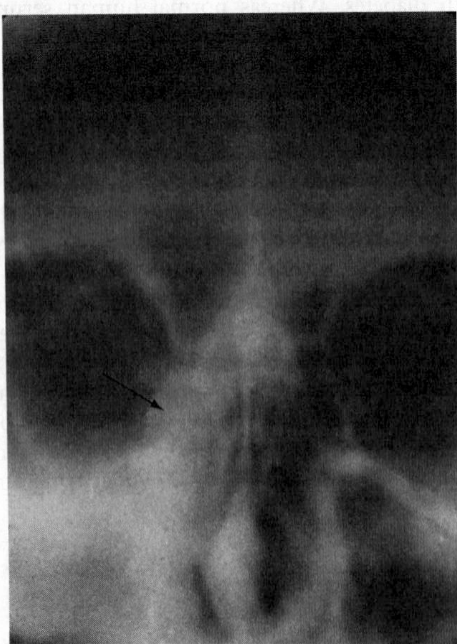

FIGURE 361–1 • Diabetic, alcoholic patient with oro-sino-rhino-orbital mucormycosis. Arrow indicates sinus.

Pulmonary Mucormycosis

Pulmonary mucormycosis usually occurs in patients with hematologic malignancies or diabetes. The clinical findings are generally acute, and patients are often profoundly ill with variable complaints of cough and fever. No pathognomonic clinical or radiographic findings exist, although multiple (>10) nodules or pleural effusions may be especially common. Sputum culture is usually negative. Antemortem diagnosis is often missed because of the acuteness of the illness, lack of consideration of the diagnosis, and need for tissue to establish the diagnosis. Renal insufficiency, metabolic acidosis, and neutropenia are associated with a worse outcome.

Invasive pulmonary aspergillosis or other mycoses, nocardiosis, other bacterial infections such as *Pseudomonas* infection, malignant invasion, hemorrhage, and pulmonary embolism or infarction may mimic the manifestations of pulmonary mucormycosis.

Cutaneous Mucormycosis

Cutaneous mucormycosis is rare and primarily a nosocomial infection in burn and trauma victims. Local infection has resulted from using contaminated elastic bandages. The involved area is erythematous and painful, with various degrees of central necrosis that can progress to gangrenous cellulitis. Skin biopsy is necessary for diagnosis. Cutaneous infection can also occur as a result of dissemination from another site of involvement. Skin and subcutaneous infections can occur in diabetics.

Gastrointestinal Mucormycosis

Gastrointestinal mucormycosis is the least common form of infection. It is seen primarily in patients suffering from intrinsic abnormalities of the gastrointestinal tract or severe malnutrition. The infection is thought to arise from fungi entering the body with food. Any part of the gastrointestinal tract is susceptible to infection, with the stomach, terminal ileum, and colon being the most common sites. Wall invasion, ischemic infarction, and ulceration are characteristic. The diagnosis is frequently made at autopsy. Gastrointestinal zygomycosis, a similar entity caused by *Basidiobolus ranarum,* generally occurs in otherwise healthy individuals and responds to surgery.

Disseminated Mucormycosis

Disseminated mucormycosis is defined as infection occurring in two or more noncontiguous organ systems. The distant sites are infected by blood stream invasion from a local site. Although any organ can be affected, the lungs and CNS are the two common sites. The outcome of this infection is almost invariably fatal.

Isolated Central Nervous System Mucormycosis

Isolated CNS mucormycosis results from hematogenous spread and is seen primarily in intravenous drug addicts.

Diagnosis

The diagnosis of any form of mucormycosis depends on direct and histologic examination of scrapings and biopsies of necrotic material. In contrast to most fungi, these organisms are readily seen in hematoxylin-eosin–stained tissue. The Gomori methenamine silver stain is usually adequate, but some special fungus stains, such as periodic acid–Schiff, do not demonstrate the organism well. However, a more rapid, but preliminary diagnosis can sometimes be made by demonstrating hyphal elements after potassium hydroxide digestion of a fresh tissue scraping. The alkali digests some of the tissue debris but not the fungus, which makes identifying the fungi easier. Swabs of discharge or abnormal tissue are not adequate and can give erroneous information. Fungal cultures are occasionally positive, but a negative culture result does not exclude the diagnosis nor make it less likely. Teasing rather than homogenization of the tissue may increase the yield of cultures. The media used for culturing these fungi should not contain cycloheximide. No skin tests or serologic methods are adequate for diagnosing mucormycosis, and blood cultures are not helpful.

Treatment

A successful outcome in treating this aggressive infection relies on early diagnosis by invasive procedures, immediate correction of the underlying predisposing condition, aggressive surgical débridement, and early systemic antifungal therapy. Endoscopic surgery has a role in early rhinocerebral cases. Amphotericin B is the principal approved drug with proven clinical efficacy, and a high therapeutic dosage (e.g., 1.0 to 1.5 mg/kg/day, if tolerated) should be achieved as soon as possible. It may be reduced to alternate-day dosing after the patient has stabilized. Typically, a cumulative dose of 2 to 5 g may be needed to achieve cure. Lipid-complexed amphotericin could enable continued aggressive therapy in a nephrotoxic patient. Although local irrigation of infected sites with amphotericin is an unproven adjunct, given the difficulty of perfusing infected areas because of the tendency to thrombosis, this measure may be useful. Similarly, potentiation of amphotericin with other drugs (e.g., rifampin, azoles, flucytosine) is of unproven benefit, but given the poor results with conventional therapy, this approach should be considered if susceptibility testing can be done in vitro with the patient's isolate to show synergy and exclude antagonism. Aside from successful use of itraconazole for basidiobolomycosis, the only apparently useful azole is posaconazole. Doses of 800 mg/day have produced response rates comparable to those with amphotericin, but the drug has been available only for oral use. Improvement of survival may necessitate repeated major surgical débridement of necrotic tissue, which can result in significant disfiguring. Hyperbaric oxygen therapy may be of some value in deterring progression. Colony-stimulating factors may accelerate neutrophil return in neutropenic patients. If the patient survives, major reconstructive surgery may be needed. Pulmonary lesions may be amenable to surgical removal.

Prognosis

Mucormycosis remains a disease with a guarded prognosis. It is difficult to ascertain the effectiveness of any therapeutic approach accurately because the disease is uncommon and there is a general bias toward reporting cases only if therapy is effective. Cases associated with cancer, marrow transplantation, or deferoxamine do particularly poorly. With the introduction of amphotericin B in 1961, it is generally accepted that the survival rate significantly improved. Rhinocerebral mucormycosis is the most common form of infection and is thought to have an overall mortality rate of about 50%. Patients in whom hemiplegia or nasal deformity develops have higher mortality rates. Pulmonary or disseminated mucormycosis frequently escapes antemortem diagnosis. Superficial infections, particularly in immunocompetent patients, can be successfully treated with débridement and antifungal therapy. Deeper cutaneous infections of the extremities generally require amputation, and when the head or trunk is involved, the condition is commonly fatal.

The most aggressive approach we can take toward this lethal disease is rapid diagnosis, correction of underlying conditions, and immediate institution of surgical débridement plus systemic and local chemotherapy.

SUGGESTED READINGS

Prabhu RM, Patel R: Mucormycosis and entomophthoromycosis: A review of the clinical manifestations, diagnosis and treatment. Clin Microbiol Infect 2004;10(Suppl.):31–47. *Recent thorough review.*

Ribes JA, Vanover-Sams CL, Baker DJ: Zygomycetes in human disease. Clin Microbiol Rev 2000;13:236–301. *Comprehensive review.*

Sridhara SR, Paragache G, Panda NK, et al: Mucormycosis in immunocompetent individuals: An increasing trend. J Otolaryngol 2005;34:402–406. *Treatment requires débridement and amphotericin B.*

362 *PNEUMOCYSTIS* PNEUMONIA

Judith E. Feinberg

Definition

It was the diagnosis of two clusters of *Pneumocystis* pneumonia in previously healthy young gay men in Los Angeles and New York that led to the recognition of acquired immunodeficiency syndrome (AIDS) as a new clinical entity in 1981. It is still the most common life-threatening opportunistic infection associated with AIDS. In the first decade of the epidemic it was the AIDS-defining illness in almost two thirds of persons infected with human immunodeficiency virus (HIV). By the latter 1990s, the dramatic successes of *Pneumocystis* prophylaxis and triple combination antiretroviral therapy changed AIDS from a lethal to a chronic disease and led to enormous declines in the incidence of *Pneumocystis* pneumonia, with a 65% decrease from 1995 to 1998. *Pneumocystis* pneumonia still occurs in those who are unaware of their HIV serostatus, lack access to care, are nonadherent to their therapy for HIV disease, or fail to respond to appropriate therapy. This condition also occurs sporadically in other immunocompromised populations, especially children with acute lymphocytic leukemia and solid organ transplant recipients.

First identified in guinea pigs by Chagas in 1909 and long thought to be a protozoan, *Pneumocystis carinii* was reclassified as a fungus and renamed *Pneumocystis jirovecii* in 2001 to honor the man who first identified the organism in humans. However, it is still commonly referred to by its original name, as is the pneumonia (PCP, for *P. carinii* pneumonia) that it causes in profoundly immunosuppressed individuals.

Moderate to severe episodes result in appreciable morbidity, and even with effective therapy, some cases are still fatal. For mild episodes, in which the fatality rate is considerably less than 5%, the diagnosis can be challenging because signs and symptoms may mimic community-acquired bacterial infections. Occasionally, the findings may be atypical. It is therefore imperative that episodes be detected when gas exchange alterations are mild and lung damage is minimal if hospitalization and mortality are to be minimized. Clinicians caring for HIV-infected patients must be aware of the various manifestations of *Pneumocystis* infection so that therapy can be initiated as early as possible.

The Pathogen

P. jirovecii is a eukaryotic microbe with morphologic features similar to those of protozoa. There are both intracystic and extracystic forms. The cysts are small and round to oval in shape, about the size of a red blood cell (5 to 8 μm), and contain four to eight nucleated sporozoites. The cysts collapse easily, which gives them a helmet or banana shape on staining. Extracystic trophozoites, 2 to 5 μm in diameter, are the most commonly seen form and are pleomorphic, often with an eccentric nucleus. Lack of growth on fungal culture media, response to the antiprotozoal drug pentamidine, and lack of response to most antifungal agents have also supported the notion that it is a protozoan. However, *P. jirovecii* has an affinity for fungal stains, is ultrastructurally similar to fungi, and is phylogenetically closely related to the Ascomycetes yeasts by molecular analysis of its 16S ribosomal RNA and mitochondrial DNA. This is not a purely academic issue. Although *Pneumocystis* does not respond to antifungal drugs such as amphotericin or azoles, β-glucan synthesis in the cyst wall is inhibited by newer antifungal agents such as the echinocandins. Because the organism cannot be reliably grown in culture, its life cycle is not fully understood; both pathogenesis and treatment studies have been conducted in various animal models.

Epidemiology and Transmission

Within the first few years of life, nearly all children have serologic evidence of exposure to *Pneumocystis.* It may cause subclinical or mild upper respiratory symptoms in healthy children, but it causes serious disease only in immunodeficient individuals. Although the organism has a worldwide distribution, cases are far more common in the United States and Europe than in less developed areas. The reasons for this distribution are unclear because *Pneumocystis* infects a broad range of wild and domestic mammals and each is host specific according to antigen studies; humans do not acquire animal species, and *P. jirovecii* cannot be studied in animal models. The environmental reservoir for human *P. jirovecii* is unknown. The pathogenesis of PCP was originally thought to be reactivation of latent infection as a result of severe immune system depression. However, few data support chronic carriage because the organism is detected neither in lung sections at autopsy of previously healthy individuals nor by polymerase chain reaction (PCR) in bronchoalveolar lavage (BAL) fluid of immunocompetent adults. Molecular typing studies have demonstrated 59 distinct strains of *P. jirovecii,* and in AIDS patients with suspected relapse or with subsequent discrete episodes, infection by a different strain has been detected. Genotypic analysis of *P. jirovecii* obtained from AIDS patients with PCP across the United States has shown that these strains have geographic differences, with the disease-causing strain being more related to those occurring in the area where patients were diagnosed than to their place of origin. Therefore, although early infection is almost ubiquitous, it may well be transient, and active disease may occur as the result of de novo acquisition or reacquisition later in life.

Even though sporadic cases are the rule, clusters and familial and nosocomial spread have been reported. These data suggest that *Pneumocystis* may be acquired by person-to-person spread, and some institutions isolate persons with *Pneumocystis* pneumonia from others at high risk for this reason. However, definitive data for person-to-person transmission are lacking.

Pathobiology

In cortisone-treated rats, inhaled *Pneumocystis* adheres to type I alveolar cells mediated by fibronectin. After several weeks, small clusters of organisms can be detected in alveolar spaces. Later, air sacs become filled with *Pneumocystis,* thus indicating that although replication is slow, proliferation is extensive in this immunosuppressed model. Histologic analysis typically shows foamy alveolar exudates consisting of degenerative *Pneumocystis* cell membranes, surfactant, host proteins, and a modest number of alveolar macrophages. As infection progresses, mononuclear cells accumulate, septal hypertrophy occurs, and interstitial edema is evident. Similar abnormalities are seen in humans.

These abnormalities result in increased alveolar-capillary permeability, which is associated with physiologic alterations: impaired gas exchange and decreases in membrane diffusing capacity, compliance, total lung capacity, and vital capacity. Soon after anti-*Pneumocystis* therapy begins, lung function may be further impaired by an inflammatory response, as evidenced by a rapid decline in oxygenation that reaches its nadir after 3 to 4 days of treatment. This inflammatory reaction appears to be mediated by tumor necrosis factor-α (TNF-α), interleukin-1 (IL-1), IL-6, and IL-8 released by alveolar macrophages. TNF-α is modulated by the β-glucan component of the cell wall, further evidence that *P. jirovecii* is a fungus.

Risk for Infection

In the rat model, depletion of T lymphocytes is the critical determinant in the development of *Pneumocystis* pneumonia. In humans, *Pneumocystis* infection occurs in association with AIDS, lymphoreticular malignancy, certain congenital immune disorders, solid organ transplantation, and therapy with cyclosporine or corticosteroids, all of which have in common varying defects in T-cell function. In patients with HIV, the risk for development of *Pneumocystis* pneumonia is directly related to a decrease in T lymphocytes with the CD4 surface phenotype. The median $CD4^+$ T-cell count is typically 50 to 70 at the time of a first episode. In the Multicenter AIDS Cohort Study, participants with 200 or fewer $CD4^+$ cells/mm^3 had a 4.9-fold increased risk for the development of PCP in the ensuing 12 months as compared with subjects with counts above 200. That *Pneumocystis* pneumonia may occur with transient dramatic declines in $CD4^+$ T-cell counts to less than 100 during primary HIV infection suggests it is the absolute number of $CD4^+$ T cells and not the stage of HIV infection that is important in determining the risk for PCP. Although more than 90% of episodes occur at total counts of less than 200, *Pneumocystis* pneumonia may occur at somewhat higher counts, especially in individuals whose $CD4^+$ T cells are declining rapidly and those with thrush and unexplained fever (>100° F for more than 2 weeks). A history of previous PCP elevates the risk for a subsequent episode, and a number of studies have also demonstrated increased risk for HIV-infected persons who have already had another AIDS-defining opportunistic infection.

Histopathology

Microscopic analysis of lung tissue from AIDS patients with *Pneumocystis* pneumonia shows a prominent eosinophilic, foamy, intra-alveolar exudate and proliferation of type II pneumocytes, but only mild interstitial inflammation. Detection of *Pneumocystis* requires special stains. Diffuse alveolar damage is common. Interstitial fibrosis is present in approximately 6% of cases, and intraluminal fibrosis occurs in almost 40%; fibrosis appears to be related to the severity of the inflammatory response and is more common in patients with multiple episodes. In contrast, acute exudative alveolar damage is unusual, and hyaline membranes have been detected in less than 5% of lung biopsy samples, but they may occasionally be so prominent that they obscure the typical eosinophilic alveolar material. Other less common abnormalities include pneumatoceles and cavities, granulomas, lymphocytic interstitial infiltrates, microcalcifications, vasculitis, and alveolar proteinosis. In patients with cavitation and pneumothorax, *Pneumocystis* invades the interstitium, and unlike typical cases, greater proportions of trophozoites are present.

Clinical Manifestations

Early recognition and treatment are imperative. Figure 362–1 shows that the risk for a fatal outcome increases progressively in patients whose room air arterial oxygen partial pressure (Pa_{O_2}) is less than 75 mm Hg and alveolar-arterial oxygen difference (A–a D_{O_2}) is 35 mm Hg or higher at initial evaluation. Because A–a D_{O_2} is the best prognostic indicator, clinicians must be familiar with both the typical and the unusual manifestations of *Pneumocystis* pneumonia so that therapy can be instituted promptly.

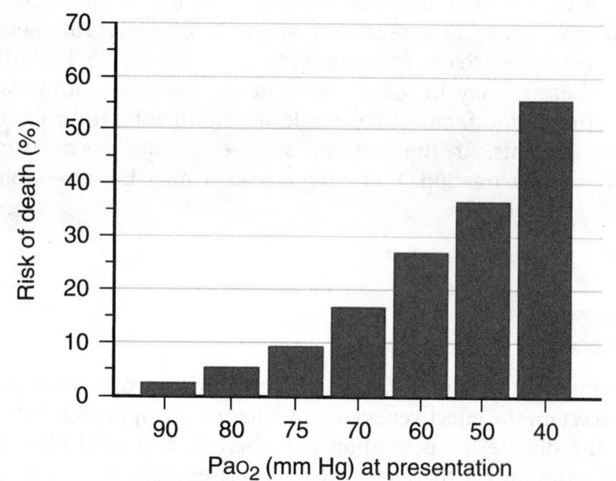

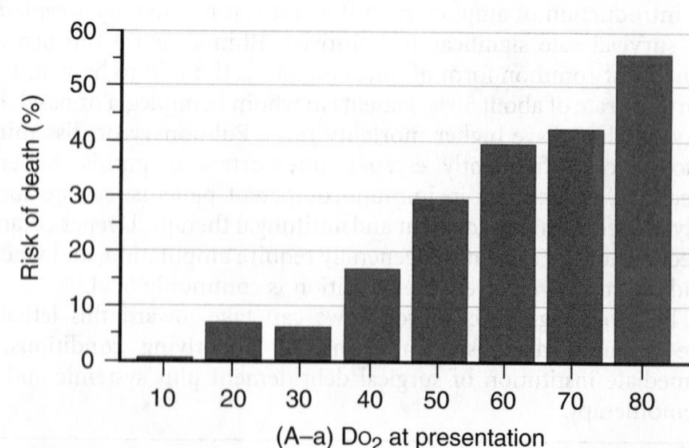

FIGURE 362–1 • Outcome of *Pneumocystis* pneumonia. A, Risk of death according to the partial pressure (Pa_{O_2}) of oxygen on room air at the time of admission to the hospital for patients receiving conventional therapies without adjunctive corticosteroids. **B,** Risk of death according to the alveolar-arterial oxygen difference (A–a D_{O_2}) on room air at the time of admission to the hospital for patients receiving conventional therapies without adjunctive corticosteroids. (Adapted from the U.S. Public Health Service: Consensus Statement on the Use of Corticosteroids As Adjunctive Therapy for *Pneumocystis* Pneumonia in the Acquired Immunodeficiency Syndrome. Available at www.cdc.gov.)

Typical Manifestation

The onset of *Pneumocystis* pneumonia in HIV-infected individuals is generally insidious and marked by slow, but steady progression of symptoms, including fever, chills, sweats, malaise, fatigue, and ultimately, exertional dyspnea. The cardinal manifestation is a hacking, typically nonproductive cough that may have been present for weeks or even months. Retrosternal chest tightness, intensified by coughing and inspiration, is also common. Fever occurs in 80 to 90%. Dyspnea develops when oxygenation is moderately to severely impaired. Patients who do not give a clear history of gradually increasing exertional dyspnea can often describe limiting their activities to avoid dyspnea when prompted. In contrast, *Pneumocystis* pneumonia in HIV-seronegative patients, such as those with lymphoreticular malignancies, is typically acute in onset with high fever and evident chest x-ray abnormalities. In one study comparing PCP in patients with and without AIDS, the median duration of symptoms was 28 days in the former versus 5 days in the latter.

Physical findings in AIDS patients are often limited and nonspecific. Tachypnea does not usually occur with mild episodes, whereas respiratory distress, use of accessory muscles, cyanosis, and frank respiratory failure may be seen in severe cases. Auscultation is frequently normal because dry ("cellophane") rales occur in only 30 to 40% of cases and are usually a late finding indicating greater severity. Occasionally, patients have wheezing or overt bronchospasm. In one report, 84% of patients had peak expiratory flow rates (PEFRs) less than 80% of predicted, with 54% of these patients responding to bronchodilator therapy as compared with those without *Pneumocystis,* of whom only 23% had a low PEFR and 3% had a response to bronchodilator therapy.

Extrapulmonary physical findings may be helpful. Oropharyngeal thrush is a nearly universal finding in AIDS patients, and facial seborrheic dermatitis is also common. Generalized adenopathy with lymph nodes larger than 1 cm is rare because patients with *Pneumocystis* usually have severe immunodeficiency with hypoplastic lymph nodes.

Atypical Manifestations

Pneumothorax and Cavitation

Pneumothorax, which can be associated with refractory bronchopleural fistulas and chronic lung cavitation, has occurred in up to 10% of episodes. Pneumothorax developed spontaneously in 20 (2%) of 1030 patients with AIDS at one medical center; 50 to 95% of these episodes were associated with active PCP. HIV-positive patients with spontaneous pneumothorax should be evaluated and treated presumptively for *Pneumocystis* pneumonia, along with lung re-expansion. Lung destruction and cavitation may appear as solitary, thin-walled cavities, regional honeycombing, blebs, or bullae; these findings are often bilateral, generally occur in the upper lobes, and precede the development of pneumothorax. Although cavitation and pneumothorax were initially associated with aerosol pentamidine prophylaxis, these complications may occur in the absence of aerosol therapy, as well as in nonsmokers, in first episodes, and in patients with previous bronchoscopy or mechanical ventilation and barotrauma.

Fever of Unknown Origin

In some AIDS patients, *Pneumocystis* pneumonia may be manifested as an occult febrile illness with minimal respiratory symptoms. Nonspecific complaints of high fever, night sweats, fatigue, and malaise are prominent. Other causes of fever of unknown origin in this population, such as occult sinusitis, cytomegalovirus retinitis, disseminated *Mycobacterium avium* infection, and endocarditis, must be excluded. Oxygen desaturation with exercise and histologic evidence of *Pneumocystis* should be sought.

Extrapulmonary Infection

Extrapulmonary infection with *Pneumocystis* may occur in 0.5 to 3.0% of patients with advanced HIV disease and was more frequently reported in the early 1990s when many patients were receiving aerosol pentamidine prophylaxis. When extrapulmonary pneumocystosis is diagnosed, more than 50% of patients have concurrent pneumonia. Nucleotide sequences of the dihydrofolate reductase (*DHFR*) gene have been detected by PCR in the blood of 5 of 11 patients with acute *Pneumocystis* pneumonia, thus suggesting that hematogenous dissemination occurs. Clinical findings depend on the location of extrapulmonary involvement, although nonspecific complaints of fever and sweats predominate. The diagnosis is complicated by the broad range of possible extrapulmonary sites, including the ear (external auditory polyps), mastoids, choroid, cutaneous lesions or digital necrosis from vasculitis, small bowel obstruction, ascites with gastric and duodenal nodules, liver, spleen, hilar or mediastinal lymphadenopathy, thyroid and parathyroid glands, thymus, kidney, heart, pancreas, central nervous system, and bone marrow, resulting in cytopenia. Some sites have been detected only at autopsy. The lymph nodes, liver, spleen, and bone marrow are the most commonly affected organs. Two extrapulmonary sites are associated with specific symptoms or signs. Thyroid involvement may be accompanied by neck pain, hyperthyroidism or hypothyroidism, and goiter, which may be multinodular or a solitary neck mass. The thyroid is usually "cold" on ^{125}I scanning, and the diagnosis is made by fine-needle aspiration. Choroiditis appears as slightly elevated, yellow-white plaques, without involvement of retinal vessels or evidence of intraocular inflammation. Identification of typical choroidal lesions may provide the first clue of disseminated infection. Although the lung is involved in nearly 90% of cases, choroiditis may be the only evidence of extrapulmonary disease. A single case of maternal-fetal transmission has been documented. Extrapulmonary disease has also been described in non-AIDS patients. Histologic analysis of affected organs shows foci of eosinophilic frothy exudates and the presence of organisms by special stains. Unlike lesions in the lung, these lesions are often calcified (punctate or rim-like) and characterized by vasculitis with frank invasion of vessel walls.

Extensive extrapulmonary infection portends a poor prognosis, frequently associated with organ failure and death, but involvement of a single extrapulmonary site often responds favorably to anti-*Pneumocystis* therapy.

Laboratory Abnormalities

Pulmonary Function Tests

Hypoxemia is the most useful marker of *Pneumocystis* pneumonia and is highly predictive of outcome. At initial evaluation, PaO_2 less than 80 mm Hg or A–a DO_2 greater than 15 mm Hg on room air is noted in more than 80% of patients.

In patients with normal or nearly normal PaO_2, A–a DO_2, and chest radiographs, graded exercise testing results in increases in A–a DO_2, and pulse oximetry readily demonstrates oxygen desaturation. Carbon monoxide diffusing capacity (DLCO) is a sensitive, but nonspecific marker. Despite the lack of specificity, DLCO values greater than 80% make *Pneumocystis* unlikely (i.e., negative predictive value >98%). In AIDS patients with asthma who have cough and hypoxemia, DLCO results should be normal when the hypoxemia is due solely to bronchospasm.

Radiographic Procedures

Routine Radiology

Chest radiographs typically show interstitial infiltrates beginning in the perihilar areas and spreading to the lower and finally to the upper lung fields in a "butterfly" pattern. The apices are usually spared. Although this is the "classic" pattern, it is neither sensitive nor specific. Alveolar patterns with air bronchograms may be superimposed on the interstitial process in more advanced infection, although alveolar infiltrates may be the initial finding in up to 10% of cases. Because *Pneumocystis* pneumonia is so common, the range of radiographic findings is very wide. In 10 to 30% of cases, the radiograph is atypical, with asymmetrical or predominantly upper lobe infiltration, especially in patients receiving aerosol pentamidine prophylaxis. Other radiographic findings include cysts, pneumatoceles, cavitation, honeycombing, pneumothorax, adenopathy (with or without calcifications), pleural effusions, abscesses, lobar or segmental consolidation, solitary parenchymal nodules, postobstructive infiltration from endobronchial nodules, and a completely normal chest radiograph. In a series of 100 patients with *Pneumocystis* pneumonia, cysts were documented in 34%, and of these, 32 had multiple cysts measuring 1.0 to 5.0 cm in diameter and occurring predominantly in the upper lobes. These cystic cavitary lesions may mimic those of tuberculosis (Fig. 362–2), and pneumothorax is not uncommon. Effusions, especially substantial ones, are rare and should raise suspicion of a concomitant pulmonary process such as tuberculosis or Kaposi's sarcoma; in two series, 15 to 18% of AIDS patients with PCP had another concurrent pulmonary condition. Patients receiving aerosol pentamidine prophylaxis are more likely to have upper lobe infiltrates, which may be due to limited aerosol deposition in the upper lobes or swifter clearance of the drug from these sites (or both). Of note, chest radiographs may be entirely normal initially in 10 to 20% of patients with documented *Pneumocystis* pneumonia.

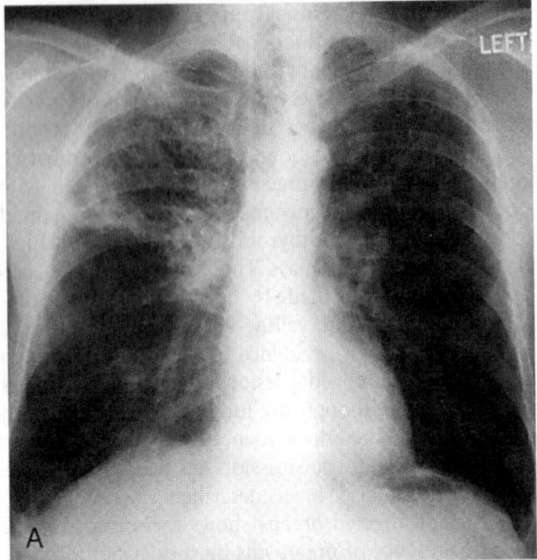

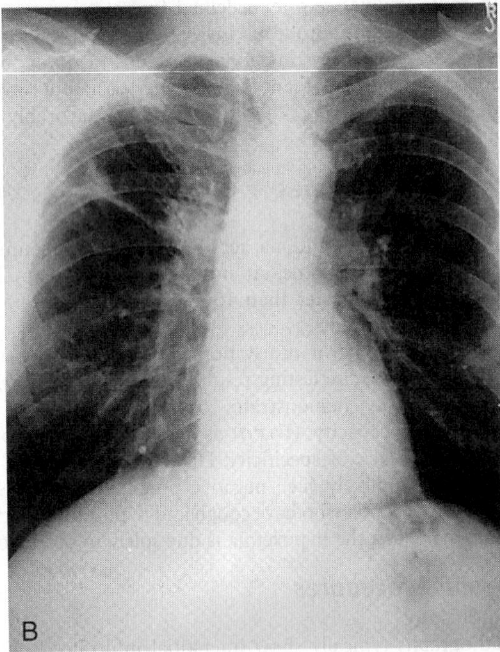

FIGURE 362–2 • Radiographic diagnosis of *Pneumocystis* pneumonia. A, This chest radiograph was obtained from a 42-year-old man with a 14-month history of chronic cough, dyspnea with minimal exertion, and 25-lb weight loss. He was treated for 8 weeks with four standard antituberculous drugs plus intravenous amikacin, but cultures for *Mycobacterium tuberculosis* remained negative. A repeat induced sputum at that time showed large numbers of *P. jirovecii* organisms. **B,** Chest radiographs from the same patient after a 3-week course of therapy with oral trimethoprim-sulfamethoxazole (15 mg/kg/day of the trimethoprim component). At the completion of therapy, the cough and dyspnea had completely subsided.

Computed Tomography

High-resolution computed tomography (HRCT) typically shows fine, diffuse alveolar consolidation with bronchial wall thickening, even when chest radiographs are normal, and less often, regional consolidation or cystic air spaces. HRCT is primarily valuable in patients who have normal chest radiographs or unsuspected extrapulmonary pneumocystosis, although there are no well-designed formal evaluations of its sensitivity and specificity. Low-attenuation lesions and calcifications in lymph nodes, spleen, liver, and kidneys may be present in patients with extrapulmonary involvement.

Other Diagnostic Approaches

Gallium-67 scanning, pre-exercise and postexercise oxygen saturation testing, and serum lactate dehydrogenase (LDH) levels were all studied extensively in the early years of the AIDS epidemic for their diagnostic utility. However, all these tests, though suggestive of PCP in the right circumstances, are nonspecific. Now that flexible fiberoptic bronchoscopy is widely available, these tests are no longer used for the diagnosis of PCP. It should be noted that LDH has been shown to have prognostic value, and levels greater than 500 IU/L at initial evaluation have been associated with an increased risk for a fatal outcome. In addition, serial tests show gradual improvement in responders.

$CD4^+$ T-Cell Counts

Typically, $CD4^+$ T-cell counts are less than 100 cells/mm^3, and more than 90% of patients have values less than 200 cells/mm^3 when *Pneumocystis* pneumonia is diagnosed.

Diagnosis

Definitive diagnosis of *Pneumocystis* pneumonia is made by demonstrating the organism in appropriate BAL, sputum, or tissue specimens. Antibody detection and PCR technology have thus far been more useful for epidemiologic studies than for diagnosis. There are a number of diagnostic modalities, and the procedure of choice depends on the expertise available, so clinicians should be familiar with the diagnostic procedures available in their locale.

Bronchoalveolar Lavage

BAL is the cornerstone of diagnosis and consistently has a sensitivity of 95 to 99%. It is the diagnostic approach of choice when induced sputum examination is negative or not available. BAL is a safe and well-tolerated procedure, even in very ill patients with low white blood cell and platelet counts. Although some patients may experience a temperature spike within 12 hours of the procedure and infiltrates at the lavage site may be seen on radiographs, they are usually transient. Though limited in availability, bilateral BAL yields a diagnosis in 94%, as compared with 84% in patients who have previously undergone unilateral BAL. The diagnostic yield is lower—only 62%—in patients who have received aerosol pentamidine and who have predominantly upper lobe disease.

Transbronchial Biopsy

Transbronchial biopsy may be particularly useful in a patient whose BAL is nondiagnostic and who is not responding to empirical therapy for *Pneumocystis* and bacterial pathogens. The yield from transbronchial biopsy approaches that of BAL if tissue is obtained without crush artifact and contains at least 25 alveoli. The risk for pneumothorax with transbronchial biopsy—9% in one review—makes BAL the more attractive initial approach. If both BAL and transbronchial biopsy are performed, diagnostic sensitivity approaches 100%. Consequently, open lung biopsy is rarely indicated.

Sputum Induction

In centers with expertise and experience in diagnosing *Pneumocystis* by staining of induced sputum, this is the safest and least expensive approach. In experienced hands, diagnostic sensitivity has been reported to be 75 to 95%. Success is dependent on the methods used to obtain and process the specimen. Expectorated sputum provides a low yield. However, pulmonary secretions obtained by ultrasonic nebulization of hypertonic saline and treated with mucolytic agents to solubilize oral debris before centrifugation can be very useful for diagnosis in experienced hands. Fluorescent staining with monoclonal antibodies for *Pneumocystis* generally produces the highest yields. Because the sensitivity is variable, a negative result for induced sputum does not exclude the diagnosis.

Identification of Pneumocystis jirovecii

Cyst Wall Stains

The standard staining procedure for identifying *Pneumocystis* when PCP was diagnosed by open lung biopsy used Gomori methenamine silver; the cyst wall stained black against a light greenish background. Although the sensitivity of this stain was greater than 95%, the procedure is demanding and takes many hours. Toluidine blue O stains the cyst purple, is more rapid, and is comparably reliable.

Non–Cyst Wall Stains

Wright-Giemsa and Diff-Quik stains are commonly used. They stain trophozoites, cyst nuclei, and intermediate forms, and they can be completed within 30 minutes. However, organisms may be missed in 10 to 15% of cases. Papanicolaou silver stains the nonspecific foam surrounding large clusters, but organisms are not readily identified. However, this methodology is quick and may be useful for screening.

Immunochemical Stains

Immunofluorescent staining with monoclonal antibody results in yields greater than 90% for BAL specimens and appears to be more sensitive for sputum samples than silver or Wright-Giemsa stains are.

Molecular Identification

Oligonucleotide probes and PCR are promising methodologies that may increase the diagnostic yield in identifying *Pneumocystis*, especially with induced sputum specimens. However, the primers investigated thus far proved to be too sensitive and have thus resulted in unacceptable false-positive rates.

Treatment

Rx

Initiating Therapy

The key to successful treatment is prompt suspicion of the diagnosis and early initiation of therapy. Because sputum induction and bronchoscopy are not generally performed after hours and the results of special stains may not be immediately available, patients with typical clinical features of *Pneumocystis* pneumonia and moderate to severe hypoxemia should be treated empirically. Such treatment does not impair the ability to make a specific diagnosis because large numbers of organisms are detectable in lung tissue and secretions for weeks after therapy is begun.

Severe Episodes

Initial therapy should be given parenterally in patients with moderate to severe impairment in oxygen exchange, as determined by a PaO_2 less than 70 mm Hg or A–a DO_2 greater than 35 mm Hg (Table 362–1). Drugs with high oral bioavailability, such as trimethoprim-sulfamethoxazole (TMP-SMX), may be erratically absorbed from the gut in subjects with severe hypoxemia. AIDS patients may have enteropathy and malabsorption even in the absence of diarrhea; consequently, drug concentrations may be subtherapeutic.

Trimethoprim-Sulfamethoxazole

The antifolate combination of TMP-SMX is the "gold standard" for treatment of *Pneumocystis* pneumonia, regardless of severity (Chapters 412 and 414). Prospective double-blind studies, each involving more than 300 patients, have confirmed that TMP-SMX is more effective than trimetrexate, atovaquone, or aerosolized pentamidine in AIDS patients with *Pneumocystis.* Its enhanced efficacy may be due to sequential blockade of key enzymes in folate synthesis—DHFR and dihydropteroate synthetase (DHPS)—as well as its broad spectrum of activity against many bacterial respiratory pathogens; 15 to 18% of patients with *Pneumocystis* pneumonia harbor a second pulmonary condition, most commonly bacterial pneumonia. TMP-SMX is therefore the therapy of choice for patients who do not have severe intolerance. Studies have shown that patients who previously experienced adverse effects are subsequently able to tolerate TMP-SMX. Although no comparably rigorous studies have compared TMP-SMX with parenteral pentamidine, TMP-SMX is associated with less serious adverse effects.

The most frequent potentially serious adverse effect of TMP-SMX is neutropenia (Table 362–2). Because this reaction is dose-dependent, a lower dose (15 mg/kg/day of the trimethoprim component) than was used at the outset of the AIDS epidemic (20 mg/kg/day) is preferred. Several controlled trials have indicated that this dose results in survival rates of 88% or greater for severe episodes, thus suggesting that it does not compromise outcomes. Other common problems include rash, nausea, and hepatitis.

Parenteral Pentamidine

Parenteral pentamidine is also highly effective. As with TMP-SMX, adverse reactions are common (see Table 362–2). In one study in which patients received a minimum of 14 days of therapy, nephrotoxicity (>1-mg/L rise in serum creatinine) developed in 64% of patients, hypotension in 27%, and hypoglycemia in 21%. Impaired renal function and hypoglycemia are dose dependent and are more likely to be seen after 2 weeks of therapy or a total dosage higher than 4 g. Hypotension generally occurs during or shortly after intravenous infusion and may last several hours, although low blood pressure may persist for several months. Infusion-related hypotension can be minimized by slow administration over a 1-hour period.

TABLE 362–1 ESTABLISHED THERAPIES FOR INITIAL TREATMENT OF *PNEUMOCYSTIS* PNEUMONIA

INTRAVENOUS THERAPY	
Trimethoprim-sulfamethoxazole	5 mg/kg of the trimethoprim component every 8 hr
Pentamidine*	4 mg/kg once daily
Trimetrexate plus leucovorin	For patients <50 kg: 1.5 mg/kg trimetrexate once daily plus leucovorin, 0.5 mg/kg IV or PO every 6 hr For patients 50–80 kg: 1.2 mg/kg trimetrexate daily plus leucovorin, 0.5/kg IV or PO every 6 hr For patients >80 kg: 1.0 mg/kg trimetrexate daily plus leucovorin, 0.8 mg/kg IV or PO every 6 hr Continue leucovorin for 72 hr after the last dose of trimetrexate
Clindamycin plus primaquine base (oral)†	600–900 mg IV every 8 hr plus 15 or 30 mg PO once daily
ORAL THERAPY	
Trimethoprim-sulfamethoxazole	2 double-strength tablets tid
Trimethoprim plus dapsone	4–5 mg/kg tid plus 100 mg once daily
Clindamycin plus primaquine base†	450–600 mg tid or qid plus 15 or 30 mg once daily
Atovaquone‡	750 mg tid
AEROSOL THERAPY	
Pentamidine	600 mg daily by the Respirgard II jet nebulizer§

*Intramuscular therapy may cause sterile abscesses and should be avoided.
†The combination is not advisable in situations in which absorption may be impaired (e.g., severe hypoxemia, vomiting, diarrhea, ileus, malabsorption) because clindamycin alone has no activity against *Pneumocystis jirovecii.*
‡Must be given with fatty food because serum concentrations are two- or three-fold lower when the drug is administered on an empty stomach.
§Administered at 50 psi and 8 L/min of oxygen.

Hypoglycemia is the most insidious reaction and occurs in 10 to 20% of AIDS patients treated with pentamidine; it results from sudden increases in serum insulin caused by lysis of pancreatic beta cells. Because of the prolonged binding of pentamidine to tissue, precipitous hypoglycemia may occur after use of the drug is discontinued, with fatal reactions reported up to 2 weeks after the last dose. When hypoglycemia is detected, pentamidine should be discontinued, and patients should be monitored closely with daily glucose measurements for several weeks.

Trimetrexate

Trimetrexate is a powerful antifolate drug that binds to the DHFR of *Pneumocystis* nearly 1500 times more avidly than trimethoprim does, and it is concentrated in the organism. Leucovorin (folinic acid) must be coadministered to protect against bone marrow toxicity. In a comparative study, trimetrexate was effective but inferior to TMP-SMX for moderate to severe episodes. [1] Treatment-limiting toxicity, particularly critical neutropenia, thrombocytopenia, and anemia, occurred significantly more often with TMP-SMX than with trimetrexate. To mimic the sequential DHFR-DHPS blockade provided by TMP-SMX, trimetrexate can be coadministered with oral dapsone,

TABLE 362–2 TOXICITIES ASSOCIATED WITH STANDARD THERAPIES FOR *PNEUMOCYSTIS* PNEUMONIA

Drug	Frequent Causes of Drug Morbidity	Infrequent Causes of Morbidity
Trimethoprim-sulfamethoxazole	Fever Morbilliform rash Nausea and vomiting Neutropenia* Thrombocytopenia† Anemia‡	Stevens-Johnson syndrome Exfoliative dermatitis Diarrhea Elevated transaminases Elevated serum creatinine Hyperkalemia Hyponatremia Renal impairment Hallucinations or agitation
Parenteral pentamidine	Fever Morbilliform rash Nausea and vomiting Renal impairment Hypoglycemia Hypotension Pancreatitis	Hypocalcemia Ventricular tachycardia/fibrillation Torsades de pointes Neutropenia Thrombocytopenia Elevated transaminases Ketoacidosis and diabetes Hypomagnesemia Myoglobinuria Hematuria
Trimetrexate plus leucovorin	Fever Neutropenia	Elevated transaminases Morbilliform rash Thrombocytopenia Mucositis
Dapsone	Fever Morbilliform rash Nausea and vomiting	Methemoglobinemia Hemolytic anemia Sulfone syndrome
Clindamycin	Fever Morbilliform rash Diarrhea	Elevated transaminases *Clostridium difficile* colitis
Primaquine	Nausea Abdominal distress Neutropenia	Methemoglobinemia Hemolytic anemia Hypertension Arrhythmias
Atovaquone	Rash	Fever Nausea and vomiting Elevated transaminases
Aerosolized pentamidine	Cough Bronchospasm Metallic taste	Contact dermatitis Morbilliform rash Hypoglycemia Pancreatitis Renal impairment

*Reduced to less than 1000 cells/μL.
†Reduced to less than 50,000 cells/μL.
‡Greater than a 2-g/dL decline.

Rx

100 mg daily (see later), although this combination has not been rigorously studied.

Adjunctive Corticosteroids

The major breakthrough in the search for more effective therapies for *Pneumocystis* has been the irrefutable evidence that mortality with severe episodes can be reduced nearly two-fold by the use of corticosteroids within 72 hours after beginning specific anti-*Pneumocystis* therapy (Table 362–3). With adjunctive corticosteroids, oxygen desaturation occurs less often, and fewer patients require mechanical ventilation. 2,3 Serious adverse consequences are uncommon, perhaps because the course is limited (21 days) and the taper is rapid; an increase in mucocutaneous herpes infections was seen in the largest study. However, adjunctive corticosteroids can be deleterious if given with empirical anti-*Pneumocystis* therapy to patients who have undiagnosed concomitant pulmonary fungal infection or tuberculosis; these patients may show initial improvement, which could delay the diagnosis and specific antimicrobial

TABLE 362–3 ADJUNCTIVE CORTICOSTEROIDS* FOR PATIENTS WITH *PNEUMOCYSTIS* PNEUMONIA AND A–a Do_2 ≥35 mm Hg OR Pao_2 ≤70 mm Hg

Drug	Dose	Treatment Days
Oral prednisone	40 mg bid	1–5
	40 mg once daily	6–10
	20 mg once daily	11–21
Intravenous methylprednisolone	30 mg bid	1–5
	30 mg once daily	6–10
	15 mg once daily	11–21

*Efficacy established only when adjunctive corticosteroids are initiated within 72 hours of starting specific treatment of *P. jirovecii* pneumonia.

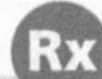

therapy for their other pulmonary condition. Corticosteroids can also aggravate and accelerate the progression of cutaneous and pulmonary Kaposi's sarcoma.

Mild Episodes

For mild episodes (Pao_2 >70 mm Hg or A–a Do_2 <35 mm Hg), management should focus on tolerable oral agents that can be used in an ambulatory setting because hospitalization is usually unnecessary and mortality rates are low (see Table 362–1). TMP-SMX is also the treatment of choice for milder episodes and is very inexpensive.

Trimethoprim-Dapsone

Trimethoprim-dapsone, like TMP-SMX, results in sequential blockade of folate synthesis in *Pneumocystis.* Dapsone, a sulfone, binds to DHPS two-fold more avidly than sulfamethoxazole does. Treatment-limiting neutropenia and transaminase elevations occur less frequently than with TMP-SMX.

Clindamycin-Primaquine

The antibacterial clindamycin and the antimalarial drug primaquine together have excellent activity against *Pneumocystis,* but neither agent is effective alone, and the mechanism of action is unclear. The combination has been effective as initial therapy for *Pneumocystis,* with response rates in the range of 90%, regardless of whether clindamycin is given intravenously or orally and whether the dose of primaquine base is 15 or 30 mg/day. Controlled trials have not established whether trimethoprim-dapsone and clindamycin-primaquine are as effective as TMP-SMX. [4, 5] In a comparative study of these three oral regimens for mild to moderate disease, the frequency of treatment-limiting adverse effects was not significantly different among the arms of the study, although the specific types of adverse effects varied. Clindamycin-primaquine was the most common cause of severe rash and anemia, whereas TMP-SMX more frequently caused neutropenia and hepatitis and trimethoprim-dapsone more often caused nausea and vomiting. Awareness of the potential common problems with each of these regimens permits better matching of *Pneumocystis* therapy to the patient's clinical status at diagnosis. The U.S. Public Health Service has not recommended adjunctive corticosteroids for mild episodes because the mortality rate is very low. However, one study indicated that there was less desaturation, better exercise tolerance, and a quicker return of elevated LDH levels to baseline with adjunctive corticosteroids for episodes of mild or moderate severity.

Atovaquone

Atovaquone is an oral hydroxynaphthoquinone originally developed as an antimalarial. It inhibits the mitochondrial electron transport necessary for the biosynthesis of pyrimidines in protozoa, but its mode of action against *Pneumocystis* is unknown. In a comparative study of atovaquone and TMP-SMX in 322 patients with mild to moderate (A–a Do_2 <45 mm Hg) *Pneumocystis* pneumonia, failure secondary to inadequate therapeutic response occurred in 31% of patients receiving atovaquone and 16% receiving TMP-SMX (P = .002). Mortality rates were also imbalanced, with 1 death in the TMP-SMX group and 11 in the atovaquone arm. Patients in whom atovaquone failed were more likely to have low plasma concentrations (<15 mg/mm) and diarrhea. Atovaquone must be given with fatty food because blood levels are two- to three-fold lower when it is taken on an empty stomach.

Echinocandins

These newer antifungals are active against *Pneumocystis* in animal models but have not been systematically tested for *Pneumocystis* infection in humans.

Monitoring Treatment

Patients with PCP should be monitored closely for response to therapy and drug toxicity. Oxygenation should be evaluated by pulse oximetry or blood gas determinations. A complete blood count, liver function tests, electrolytes, and serum creatinine should be obtained at least twice a week, and glucose levels should be checked in patients receiving pentamidine.

Outcome and Prognosis

Clinical parameters at initial evaluation that are associated with an increased risk for a fatal outcome include Pao_2 less than 70 mm Hg or A–a Do_2 greater than 35 mm Hg, diffuse alveolar damage, BAL neutrophils greater than 5%, and serum LDH above 500 IU/dL.

Changing Therapy

It can be difficult to know when therapy is failing in a specific patient. Persistence of fever or lack of improvement on chest radiographs is common, especially during the first several days of treatment. Unchanged or progressive infiltrates frequently occur even in patients who ultimately respond. Oxygenation reaches its nadir 3 to 4 days after beginning treatment. A sustained respiratory rate greater than 35 per minute and an absolute increase in room air A–a Do_2 of more than 20 mm Hg above baseline have proved to be reproducible end points for failure in clinical trials. These signs provide objective justification for changing therapy and for evaluating other possible complications in the lung. It is important to remember that another concurrent pulmonary condition exists in 15 to 18% of AIDS patients with *Pneumocystis* pneumonia, so a thorough evaluation for other entities should be undertaken in patients who are not responding to adequate therapy.

Supportive Care

Evidence suggests that the degree of alveolar damage is the most important determinant of outcome. As with adult respiratory distress syndrome, which has histologic features similar to those of severe *Pneumocystis* infection, supportive care is crucial for severely ill patients. Continuous positive airway pressure by facemask improves oxygenation in patients with tachypnea and refractory desaturation with standard masks and may mitigate the need for mechanical ventilation.

Mechanical Ventilation and Intensive Care

The mortality rate for AIDS patients undergoing mechanical ventilation in intensive care units has ranged from 30 to 50%, thus supporting the value of aggressive measures in selected patients. A low albumin level, arterial pH less than 7.35, or need for positive end-expiratory pressure greater than 10 cm H_2O after 96 hours in the intensive care unit portends a several-fold greater risk for a fatal outcome. Patients with better nutritional status and those who have less severe alveolar damage and a normal pH may benefit most from ventilatory support.

Salvage Therapy

After respiratory failure has developed, the prognosis is poor. Although there is some evidence that *Pneumocystis* can develop resistance to sulfamethoxazole as a result of mutations in the DHPS enzyme, the limited data are conflicting regarding the clinical impact of this phenomenon. Respiratory failure is thought to ensue largely from diffuse alveolar damage. Parenteral TMP-SMX, pentamidine, trimetrexate, and clindamycin-primaquine have all been evaluated for salvage in uncontrolled studies and appear to provide limited benefit. Little reason has been put forward to favor any of these agents, and no data are available to support the use of multiple concurrent therapies.

Prophylaxis

The U.S. Public Health Service recommends prophylaxis for *Pneumocystis* in patients at high risk for infection (Table 362–4). Those at highest risk include patients with previous *Pneumocystis* infection, those with fewer than 200 $CD4^+$ T cells/mm^3, and patients with thrush and a fever higher than 100° F for at least 2 weeks; a prior AIDS-defining illness may also increase the risk for *Pneumocystis* infection. TMP-SMX is the most effective form of prophylaxis. [6] In several studies, the relative hazard of *Pneumocystis* infection developing was approximately three to four times less with TMP-SMX than with aerosolized pentamidine. In controlled trials, dapsone has been comparable to aerosolized pentamidine but somewhat inferior to TMP-SMX. When combined with pyrimethamine (usually 50 mg once weekly), dapsone is also effective in preventing toxoplasmosis, as is TMP-SMX. Atovaquone and dapsone appear equally useful in sulfa-intolerant patients.

Significant immune recovery in AIDS patients is possible with potent combination antiretroviral therapy. Several studies have demonstrated

TABLE 362–4 PROPHYLACTIC THERAPIES FOR PREVENTION OF *PNEUMOCYSTIS* PNEUMONIA

Drug*	Dose or Regimen	Alternate Dose or Regimen
Trimethoprim-sulfamethoxazole	1 double-strength tablet daily	1 double-strength tablet 3 times weekly 1 single-strength tablet daily
Dapsone	100-mg tablet daily	50-mg tablet once or twice daily
Dapsone-pyrimethamine	50-mg tablet of dapsone daily plus 50-mg tablet of pyrimethamine weekly	None
Aerosolized pentamidine	300 mg monthly by the Respirgard II jet nebulizer	None
Atovaquone	1500 mg once daily	None
Primaquine-clindamycin	Unknown	None

*Patients receiving therapy for toxoplasmosis are unlikely to need additional prophylaxis for *Pneumocystis*.

that *Pneumocystis* prophylaxis may be safely discontinued in patients whose total CD4+ T-cell count has increased above 200/mm^3 for at least 3 months; [7] prophylaxis should be reintroduced if the cell count falls below 200. An associated "immune reconstitution syndrome," manifested by a marked inflammatory response and clinical worsening because of a sharp increase in CD4+ T cells, has not yet been convincingly demonstrated for *Pneumocystis* infection as it has for other common AIDS-associated opportunistic infections such as cytomegalovirus retinitis or disseminated *M. avium* complex infection.

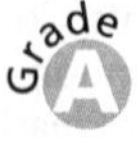

1. Sattler FR, Frame P, Davis R, et al: Trimetrexate with leucovorin versus trimethoprim-sulfamethoxazole for moderate to severe episodes of *Pneumocystis carinii* pneumonia in patients with AIDS: A prospective, controlled multicenter investigation of the AIDS Clinical Trials Protocol 029/031. J Infect Dis 1994;170:165–172.
2. Bozzette SA, Sattler FR, Chui J, et al: A controlled trial of early adjunctive treatment with corticosteroids for *Pneumocystis carinii* pneumonia in the acquired immunodeficiency syndrome. N Engl J Med 1990;323:1451–1457.
3. Briel M, Bucher HC, Boscacci R, et al: Adjunctive corticosteroids for *Pneumocystis jirovecii* pneumonia in patients with HIV infection. Cochrane Database Syst Rev 2006;CD006150.
4. Safrin S, Finkelstein DM, Feinberg J, et al: Comparison of three regimens for treatment of mild to moderate *Pneumocystis carinii* pneumonia in patients with AIDS: A double-blind, randomized trial of oral trimethoprim-sulfamethoxazole, dapsone-trimethoprim, and clindamycin-primaquine. Ann Intern Med 1996;124:792–802.
5. Toma E, Fournier S, Dumont M, et al: Clindamycin-primaquine versus trimethoprim-sulfamethoxazole as primary therapy for *Pneumocystis carinii* pneumonia in AIDS: A randomized, double blind pilot trial. Clin Infect Dis 1993;17:178–184.
6. Hardy DW, Feinberg J, Finkelstein DM, et al: A controlled trial of trimethoprim-sulfamethoxazole or aerosolized pentamidine for secondary prophylaxis of *Pneumocystis carinii* pneumonia in patients with the acquired immunodeficiency syndrome: AIDS Clinical Trials Group Protocol 021. N Engl J Med 1992;327:1842–1848.
7. Lopez Bernalde de Quiros JC, Miro JM, Pena JM, et al: A randomized trial of the discontinuation of primary and secondary prophylaxis against *Pneumocystis carinii* pneumonia after highly active antiretroviral therapy in patients with HIV infection. Grupo de Estudio del SIDA 04/98. N Engl J Med 2001;344:159–167.

SUGGESTED READINGS

Huang L, Morris A, Limper AH: An official ATS Workshop Summary: Recent advances and future directions in *Pneumocystis* pneumonia (PCP). Proc Am Thorac Soc 2006;3:655–664. *Consensus guidelines.*

Mussini C, Pezzotti P, Antinori A, et al: Discontinuation of secondary prophylaxis for *Pneumocystis carinii* pneumonia in human immunodeficiency virus–infected patients: A randomized trial by the CIOP Study Group. Clin Infect Dis 2003;36:645–651. *Patients with symptoms after discontinuation of secondary prophylaxis should be evaluated for PCP despite a high CD4 count and complete virus suppression.*

Roblot F, Le Moal G, Godet C, et al: *Pneumocystis carinii* pneumonia in patients with hematologic malignancies: A descriptive study. J Infect 2003;47:19–27. *PCP can occur with various hematologic malignancies, and its prognosis remains poor in that patient population.*

Stringer JR, Beard CB, Miller RF, et al: A new name (*Pneumocystis jirovecii*) for *Pneumocystis* from humans. Emerg Infect Dis 2002;8:891–896. *The organism that causes human PCP has been renamed.*

Thomas CF Jr, Limper AH: Current insights into the biology and pathogenesis of *Pneumocystis* pneumonia. Nat Rev Microbiol 2007;5:298–308. *Review of recent findings in the biology and pathogenesis of this infection.*

363 MYCETOMA

Dimitrios P. Kontoyiannis

Definition

Mycetoma (a tumor produced by fungi) was first described in 1842 in the Madura district of India, hence the terms "Madura foot," "maduromycosis," and "maduromycetoma." However, there is evidence of its existence as far back as the Byzantine era.

Mycetoma is a chronic, slowly progressive infection that starts in subcutaneous tissue and spreads across tissue planes to contiguous structures. The disease has a diverse etiology; the offending organism is inoculated into subcutaneous tissue by trauma typically associated with soil contamination. The hallmarks of mycetoma are the presence of "grains" that consist of colonies of the infectious organism and chronically draining sinus tracts. There is some confusion in the literature, however, because the term *pulmonary mycetoma* is used inappropriately to describe fungus balls typically caused by *Aspergillus* species that colonize a preexisting lung cavity; the term *aspergilloma* is more appropriate for this entity, the pathogenesis of which is distinctly different from that of true mycetoma.

The Pathogen

Two groups of pathogens, each of which accounts for approximately 50% of cases, cause mycetoma: (1) filamentous aerobic actinomycetes, hence the term actinomycetoma, and (2) a wide range of saprophytic soil and woody plant fungi, hence the term eumycetoma. A variety of *Nocardia* species (e.g., *Nocardia brasiliensis, Nocardia asteroides*), *Actinomadura* species (e.g., *Actinomadura pelletierii, Actinomadura madurae*), and *Streptomyces* species (e.g., *Streptomyces somaliensis*) have been reported to cause actinomycetoma. Even more numerous are the agents that cause eumycetoma, such as *Madurella* species (e.g., *Madurella mycetomatis, Madurella grisea*), probably the most prevalent mycetoma-causing fungal species worldwide, as well as *Fusarium, Acremonium, Pseudallescheria boydii, Exophiala,* and *Curvularia* species. There is controversy about whether the various dermatophytes and *Aspergillus* species can cause mycetoma. Eumycetoma is often further characterized on the basis of the color of the grains; specifically, white to yellow grain mycetomas (white piedra) are typically caused by hyalohyphomycetes (e.g., *P. boydii, Fusarium* species, *Acremonium* species), and black grain eumycetomas (black piedra) are caused by *Madurella* species and other less common fungi. However, the geographic distribution of the fungi that cause black grain eumycetoma is variable.

Epidemiology

Although mycetoma has a broad worldwide distribution, it occurs primarily in the tropical and, to a lesser extent, the temperate zones. More specifically, the infection is quite prevalent in India, Mexico, Central America, South America, the Middle East, and especially sub-Saharan Africa (the "mycetoma belt"); indigenously acquired mycetoma is sporadic in North America and Europe. However, the globalization of tourism and the increase in immigration from countries with high endemicity of mycetoma to the Western countries necessitate awareness of this entity, even in the developed world.

The relative frequency of actinomycetoma and eumycetoma differs among geographic areas. Eumycetoma is more common in India and Africa, and actinomycetoma is more common in Latin America. Furthermore, the causative agents of mycetoma differ in their geographic distribution. For example, *P. boydii* is the most common agent of mycetoma in North America, and *Actinomadura* and *Nocardia* species are predominant in Central and South America. Finally, *S. somaliensis* and *M. mycetomatis* are predominant in sub-Saharan Africa and India. The recent development of molecular typing procedures such as polymerase chain reaction–restriction fragment length polymorphism holds promise in expanding our knowledge on the environmental sources and the pathogenesis of some agents of eumycetoma such as *M. mycetomatis.*

Pathobiology

Local trauma introduces a mycetoma-causing organism into the skin and subcutaneous tissue and initiates a chain of events that leads to chronic, suppurative granulomatous inflammation, tumefaction, the formation of multiple fistulous tracts and sinuses, deep abscesses, fibrosis and scar formation, and extension to adjacent connective tissue across the lines of least resistance (fascia) and ultimately to bones, muscles, nerves, and tendon sheaths, where it leads to gross anatomic distortion of the affected site. In addition, a chronic suppurative granuloma featuring reactive fibrosis and grains (sclerotia), which is a matrix consisting of vegetative aggregates of the etiologic agents and host-derived inflammatory response, is characteristic of mycetoma in histologic sections. This infection is not contagious, however. Even though the genetics and immunopathogenesis of mycetoma are not well defined, it appears that there are differences in host susceptibility inasmuch as some affected persons have impaired or delayed hypersensitivity reactions. The lack of appropriate animal models that simulate the macroscopic features of subcutaneous human infection limits our understanding of the pathogenesis of mycetoma.

Clinical Manifestations

The clinical manifestations and natural history of mycetoma are variable and, to some degree, related to the pathogenic agent involved. For example, progression of eumycetoma is likely to be slower than that of actinomycetoma. In addition, eumycetoma lesions tend to be more confined and have less inflammation and fewer granulomas and fistulas but more fibrosis than actinomycetoma lesions do. Furthermore, male mycetoma patients predominate over female patients (5:1), and the disease is typically seen in rural areas and in persons susceptible to local trauma and contamination from soil (e.g., thorns). Hence, farmers, gardeners, wood cutters, herders, and people who work outside while barefoot are more susceptible to this infection. Not surprisingly, the foot is the most common site involved in mycetoma (Fig. 363–1), but any other part of the body, such as the hands, thighs, torso, and back of the head, may become involved. Painless nodular or papular swelling (or both) is the most common early manifestation of mycetoma and is followed by a slow evolution to painless woody induration. This infection typically runs a chronic, relentless course, sometimes spanning several decades. It is characterized by recurring, vicious cycles of suppuration, draining sinuses, bacterial superinfection, and scar formation. Old sinuses may close up but new ones may occur, and satellite lesions may be seen. Constitutional symptoms are surprisingly rare. In particular, the presence of fever indicates bacterial superinfection. Bone involvement clinically mimicking chronic osteomyelitis with osteolytic cavitary bone lesions (seen in radiographic, computed tomography [CT], or magnetic resonance imaging [MRI] studies), osteoporosis, and reactive periosteal bone formation may occur; such involvement can be substantial. However, pathologic fractures are rare. In addition, because nerves are relatively spared from involvement, neuropathic manifestations are uncommon. Inexorable limb deformity and misuse because of destruction of deeper tissues may be seen in chronic, refractory, and advanced cases. Finally, because mycetoma does not spread hematogenously, visceral dissemination is not seen. However, because lymphatic spread can occur (typical incidence of 1 to 3% but more common with actinomycetoma and especially after surgery), regional lymphadenitis may develop.

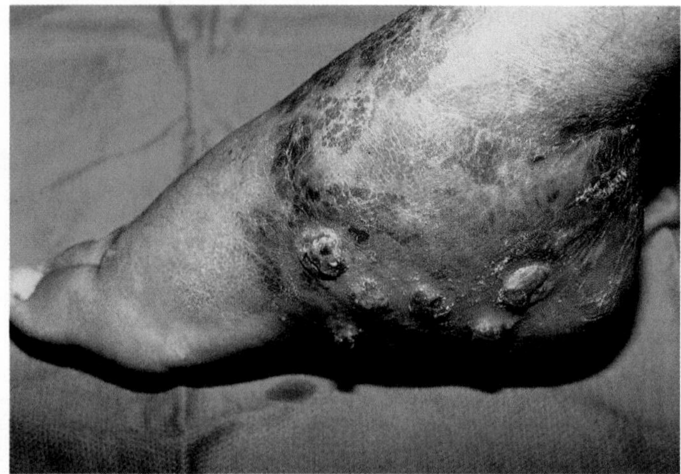

FIGURE 363–1 • Madura foot. Note the soft tissue swelling of the foot as well as multiple nodules with pustular discharge. (From Bolognia JL, Jorizzo, JL, Rapini, RP: Dermatology. New York, Mosby, 2003, p 1188.)

Diagnosis

Mycetoma, especially in its advanced forms, has a rather characteristic manifestation that facilitates diagnosis with a high degree of accuracy, especially in endemic areas. For instance, the macroscopic and microscopic appearance of grains in pus-filled draining sinuses frequently allows presumptive diagnosis of the offending pathogen. However, basing the diagnosis on the presence of grains in tissue may be difficult. Grains may be contaminated by surface bacteria or fungi. Therefore, a deep tissue biopsy specimen is ideal for staining with hematoxylin and eosin, and appropriate selective bacterial (e.g., Löwenstein-Jensen culture medium) and fungal (e.g., blood agar and modified Sabouraud dextrose agar with antibiotics) cultures and stains (Gram stain, modified Ziehl-Neelsen stain, Gomori methenamine silver, periodic acid–Schiff stain) are preferable for primary detection. The culture should be maintained for several weeks because some of the causative agents of mycetoma (e.g., *Nocardia* and *Streptomyces* species) can take 4 to 6 weeks to grow. Serologic tests for diagnosis and follow-up after therapy remain limited to only certain institutions.

Differential Diagnosis

The specific manifestations of mycetoma are sometimes confused with other rare entities. For example, mycetoma must occasionally be distinguished from chronic cutaneous fungal infections such as sporotrichosis (mycetomatous lymphatic sporotrichosis) and dermatophytic mycetoma. The latter infection, which is typically seen in Africans and sometimes called pseudomycetoma, is a painless granulomatous induration of the skin and subcutaneous tissue caused by ringworm that may be associated with grains consisting of fungi. However, unlike mycetoma, dermatophytic mycetoma is confined to the skin and subcutaneous tissue and does not spread to fasciae or bone. Similarly, chronic severe botryomycosis (typically caused by gram-positive cocci) with purulent exudates, grains, and draining sinus tracts may be confused with mycetoma; however, the presence of visceral dissemination supports a diagnosis of (severe) botryomycosis. Actinomycosis, which is caused by endogenous microaerophilic actinomycetes (part of the normal mucosa flora), also has a propensity for grains and the formation of draining sinus tracts, but unlike mycetoma, its location (e.g., neck, chest, pelvis) is rather characteristic. In addition, differentiation between mycetomas with bone involvement and chronic osteomyelitis may be difficult. Finally, in cases of mycetoma without draining sinus tracts, benign or malignant skin tumors, chronic granulomatous lesions (e.g., thorn granuloma, cutaneous tuberculosis), chromomycosis, and verrucous leishmaniasis are diagnoses that should be excluded. Unfortunately, a delay in specific diagnosis by many months or even years is not uncommon in areas with high endemicity.

Treatment

Rx

Therapy for mycetoma should be individualized. Optimal management has not been well defined, however, because the literature consists of rather heterogeneous and uncontrolled small studies. No single agent is effective against all causative agents of mycetoma. Hence, successful treatment necessitates a reliable diagnosis, differentiation between actinomycetoma and eumycetoma, assessment of the extent of the lesion, and identification of the causative agent. Specifically, the degree of tissue invasion, especially bone involvement (as determined by radiology studies), the site affected, and the specific etiologic diagnosis determine the type and intensity of therapy; in general, because of the refractoriness of eumycetoma to medical therapy, surgery plays a more prominent role. In contrast, because of the satisfactory response of actinomycetoma to medical therapy (success rate of up to 90%) and the recognized risk for lymphatic spread after surgery, chronic antibiotic administration is the mainstay of management of actinomycetoma.

For actinomycetoma, treatment consists primarily of chronic antimicrobial therapy (for at least 9 to 12 months) in conjunction with limited debulking surgery in selected cases; combination therapy is preferred. A variety of drugs (trimethoprim-sulfamethoxazole, tetracyclines, dapsone, streptomycin) have been used in different sequences and combinations according to the specific cause of actinomycetoma (e.g., trimethoprim-sulfamethoxazole with or without dapsone for *Nocardia* species or *S. somaliensis,* streptomycin with dapsone for *A. madurae*). Parenteral streptomycin is usually reserved for cases that do not respond to oral therapy. Responses to these drugs tend to occur slowly (within at least 1 month). Moreover, relapse is not uncommon, and multiple cycles of therapy may be needed for chronically recurrent disease. Side effects and compliance issues after prolonged administration of antibiotics are common problems.

For eumycetoma, however, medical therapy has produced mixed results. The best results were obtained with prolonged (9 to 12 months) use of oral imidazoles (e.g., 200 mg of ketoconazole given twice a day for *M. mycetomatis*). The experience using newer triazoles (e.g., itraconazole or voriconazole) is not as extensive or encouraging, however. In addition, intravenous amphotericin B and its lipid formulations have been used for refractory cases with rather disappointing results, which is not surprising because most eumycetoma-causing agents are resistant to amphotericin B in vitro.

The need for and extent of surgery for mycetoma depend on the etiologic agent and, more important, the extent of the lesion. Early wide-margin surgery for early localized lesions is curative. Although it is potentially curative, major disfiguring or mutilating surgery (e.g., amputation) is reserved for very advanced or refractory cases. Furthermore, primary reliance on surgery could result in recurrence or even spreading of the disease because of incomplete excision.

Prevention

Because mycetoma represents a significant, yet frequently ignored socioeconomic burden for tropical and subtropical countries, every effort at preventing mycetoma should be made. Education of persons at risk in endemic areas is crucial for prompt recognition to achieve a better outcome of this difficult-to-manage, chronic infection.

Prognosis

The prognosis for mycetoma depends on the site and degree of tissue involvement (e.g., worse with involvement of the back because of poor healing or in the presence of bone destruction) and, more important, the timeliness of the diagnosis and monitoring of recurrence and extension to other tissues, especially bone. CT and MRI are important modalities for early detection of bone involvement.

SUGGESTED READINGS

Ahmed AO, van Leeuwen W, Fahal A, et al: Mycetoma caused by *Madurella mycetomatis:* A neglected infectious burden. Lancet Infect Dis 2004;4:566–574. *Comprehensive review of the common cause of eumycetoma with emphasis on new developments in epidemiology, molecular typing, pathogenesis, in vitro susceptibility testing, and future research directions.*

Lichon V, Khachemoune A: Mycetoma: A review. Am J Clin Dermatol 2006;7:315–321. *Comprehensive review.*

364 DEMATIACEOUS FUNGAL INFECTIONS

Peter G. Pappas

Definition

Dematiaceous fungi represent a large group of fungal organisms characterized by the presence of abundant melanin in the cell wall, which gives rise to a brown-black coloration on artificial culture media. A related term, *phaeohyphomycosis,* refers broadly to infection by these pigmented fungi. The two items are often used interchangeably, but when dematiaceous fungal infections are reviewed, three distinct clinical conditions are encountered: eumycetoma (e.g., Madura foot), chromomycosis (i.e., chromoblastomycosis), and phaeohyphomycosis. This chapter focuses on the latter two entities.

The Pathogens

More than 100 dematiaceous fungi causing colonization or disease have been isolated from humans. The more common organisms and their related conditions are listed in Table 364–1. The taxonomy of the dematiaceous fungi is somewhat confusing because these agents belong to different classes, including Hyphomycetes, Ascomycetes, Basidiomycetes, Coelomycetes, and Zygomycetes. The most common agents of phaeohyphomycosis include species in the following genera: *Bipolaris, Curvularia, Exophiala, Cladophialophora, Alternaria, Exserohilum, Ochroconis, Wangiella, Phialophora,* and *Phaeoacromonium.* These agents are ubiquitous saprophytes of soil and decaying matter, and some are important plant pathogens. In tissue, these organisms exist as yeastlike cells, septated

TABLE 364–1 DEMATIACEOUS FUNGI AND ASSOCIATED CONDITIONS

Clinical Condition	Common Etiologic Agents
Chromomycosis	*Fonsecaea pedrosi* *Cladophialophora carrionii* *Phialophora verrucosa*
Cutaneous or subcutaneous condition	*Exophiala jeanselmei* *Wangiella dermatitidis* *Phialophora* sp *Bipolaris* sp *Alternaria* sp
Sinusitis	*Bipolaris* sp *Curvularia* sp *Exserohilum* sp *Alternaria* sp
Central nervous system	*Cladophialophora bantiana* *Ochroconis gallopavum* *Ramichloridium mackenziei*
Disseminated	*Wangiella dermatitidis* *Exophiala jeanselmei* *Bipolaris* sp *Ochroconis gallopavum* *Phialophora* sp

hyphae, or a combination of yeast and hyphae. Many have a histologic appearance similar to *Aspergillus* and *Fusarium* species, but they may be distinguished on the basis of positive melanin staining with the Fontana-Masson procedure.

Chromomycosis is a chronic skin and soft tissue infection that is observed most frequently in the tropics. Virtually all cases of chromomycosis are caused by three species: *Fonsecaea pedrosoi, Cladophialophora carrionii,* and *Phialophora verrucosa.* The distinctive histologic appearance is characterized by the presence of thick-walled, dark brown bodies known as *sclerotic cells* or *copper pennies,* which represent individual organisms and may be seen in clusters or as single cells. The etiologic fungi are indistinguishable on histologic examination of tissue.

Epidemiology and Pathobiology

The agents of chromomycosis and phaeohyphomycosis are found worldwide. Although there is no unique endemic area for most of these infections, some observations are relevant. Allergic fungal sinusitis associated with dematiaceous fungi appears to be more common in the southern United States. Chronic infections of the lower extremities are more commonly seen in men and in tropical areas. Chromomycosis is more prevalent in rural populations in the tropics and is hyperendemic in certain geographic areas such as Madagascar, where most infection is caused by *C. carrionii.*

Most cutaneous infections occur as a result of minor skin trauma and direct inoculation of the organism. In the nosocomial setting, infection from contaminated intravascular catheters and intravenous fluids is reported. Other risk factors include intravenous drug abuse, chronic sinusitis, freshwater immersion, and chronic corticosteroid therapy.

In the developed world, phaeohyphomycosis is an important emerging fungal infection, particularly among immunocompromised patients such as solid organ and hematopoietic stem cell transplant recipients, patients with prolonged neutropenia, and other chronically immunocompromised individuals. Phaeohyphomycosis is reported in human immunodeficiency virus–infected patients but is far less common than other opportunistic fungi. Extracutaneous invasive disease occurs in otherwise normal patients but is much less common.

Clinical Manifestations

Chromomycosis is manifested as a cutaneous or subcutaneous lesion that may range in size from a small papule to a large plaque. Lesions may remain unchanged in size and consistency for months or years, although most tend to progress in the absence of specific therapy. Single or multiple lesions may be seen, and ulceration may occur. Chronic lesions may become dry and crusted with a raised border, which may be smooth or irregular. Multiple lesions can coalesce to form larger plaques in which central scarring develops. Occasionally, lesions assume a verrucous, warty appearance. The differential diagnosis includes other fungal infections such as blastomycosis (Chapter 355), coccidioidomycosis (Chapter 354), sporotrichosis (Chapter 358), histoplasmosis (Chapter 353), and paracoccidioidomycosis (Chapter 356). Nocardiosis and cutaneous mycobacteriosis can also mimic the lesions of chromomycosis. Cutaneous lesions usually remain confined to one anatomic site, although nodular lymphangitis and autoinoculation resulting in multifocal cutaneous disease may occur. Disseminated disease involving visceral organs is rare.

Phaeohyphomycosis is associated with several well-described clinical syndromes. *Superficial* infection is characterized by tinea nigra and black piedra. Tinea nigra is a darkening of the skin caused by growth of *Phaeoannellomyces werneckii* in the stratum corneum. Black piedra is associated with the development of focal thickening on the hair shaft and results from colonization of the shaft by *Piedraia hortae. Cutaneous* phaeohyphomycosis involves deeper skin structures and results in dermatomycosis and onychomycosis; it is frequently due to agents such as *Scytalidium* and *Phyllosticta* species.

Subcutaneous phaeohyphomycosis is relatively common and may be confused with chromomycosis. Patients have discrete subcutaneous nodules or cysts that result from direct inoculation or penetrating trauma. The most common organisms are *Exophiala jeanselmei, Wangiella dermatitidis, and Phialophora* sp. *Mycotic keratitis* as a result of infection with *Curvularia, Exophiala,* and *Exserohilum* species has occurred after corneal trauma or surgery.

Foreign body–related infections are seen in patients undergoing chronic ambulatory peritoneal dialysis in whom fungal peritonitis develops and in patients with indwelling intravenous catheters.

Fungal sinusitis is commonly associated with dematiaceous fungi and can be manifested as allergic fungal sinusitis, a fungus ball (eumycetoma) in a sinus cavity, and invasive fungal sinusitis associated with extension into bone, soft tissue, and the central nervous system. This latter manifestation is indistinguishable from rhinocerebral zygomycosis or invasive *Aspergillus* sinusitis. *Bipolaris, Curvularia,* and *Alternaria* species are the most common organisms causing invasive fungal sinusitis.

Systemic phaeohyphomycosis may result from direct extension from a colonized area or dissemination from a distant source. Most patients with systemic disease have significant underlying immunosuppression, and the organisms have a proclivity for involvement of the brain, lungs, endocardium, and other visceral organs. Among patients with central nervous system disease, *Cladophialophora bantiana, Ochroconis gallopavum,* and *Ramichloridium mackenziei* are the most common etiologic agents, and the majority of these patients have no known underlying immunodeficiency.

Diagnosis

The diagnosis of phaeohyphomycosis is suggested by direct examination of a clinical specimen with a 10% potassium hydroxide preparation or special stains to demonstrate pigmentation in the cell walls of these organisms. For patients with chromomycosis, the finding of sclerotic bodies or copper pennies on skin biopsy is characteristic, and special stains are usually unnecessary. For patients with other forms of phaeohyphomycosis, the Fontana-Masson stain is useful in distinguishing organisms with significant melanin content. Culture remains the "gold standard" by which a specific etiologic diagnosis is established, and the identity of the organism is largely based on colonial and microscopic morphology. Serologic studies and molecular diagnostics are not generally available for these organisms.

Treatment

Rx

In many instances, surgical excision of a cutaneous or subcutaneous lesion is curative, although antifungal therapy is usually given in conjunction with surgery. There are limited clinical studies that have assessed the efficacy of antifungal therapy for these conditions. Historically, 5-flucytosine (5-FC, 150 mg/kg/day) has been advocated for the oral treatment of chromomycosis based on moderate in vitro activity and clinical experience. Because of limited availability, the need for prolonged therapy, and the necessity of monitoring serum levels, 5-FC is uncommonly used for this purpose. Amphotericin B has only modest in vitro activity against most of the dematiaceous fungi and is most often reserved for patients with life-threatening or disseminated disease. The triazoles, including itraconazole (200 mg orally twice daily), voriconazole (200 mg orally twice daily), and posaconazole (400 mg orally twice daily), demonstrate the best in vitro activity, although clinical studies with these agents are limited. Among the triazoles, posaconazole offers the most potential in the clinical setting based on scattered reports from patients with central nervous system infection, but comparative clinical data are not available because of the relative rarity of these infections. Terbinafine (500 mg orally twice daily) has also been used successfully for the treatment of chromomycosis and is an effective alternative to azole therapy. The length of therapy with any of the oral antifungal agents for dematiaceous fungal infections is unclear, but treatment should probably be continued for at least 6 months or until 1 month after resolution of all signs and symptoms of disease.

Prognosis

For patients with localized disease, surgical excision is important in the management of chromomycosis and phaeohyphomycosis.

SUGGESTED READINGS

Al-Abdely HM, Alkhunaizi AM, Al-Tawfiq JA, et al: Successful therapy of cerebral phaeohyphomycosis due to *Ramichloridium mackenziei* with the new triazole posaconazole. Med Mycol 2005;43:91–95. *Dramatic case report of a patient with a remarkable response to posaconazole after failure with other modalities.*

Brandt ME, Warnock DW: Epidemiology, clinical manifestations, and therapy of infections caused by dematiaceous fungi. J Chemother 2003;2(Suppl.):36–47. *Excellent recent clinical and epidemiologic review of this group of infections, though somewhat outdated concerning therapy.*

Lopez Martinez R, Mendez Tovar LJ: Chromoblastomycosis. Clin Dermatol 2007;25:188–194. *Clinical review of this subtype of dematiaceous fungal infection.*

Revankar SG: Dematiaceous fungi. Mycoses 2007;50:91–101. *Comprehensive review.*

Revankar SG: Phaeohyphomycosis. Infect Dis Clin North Am 2006;20:609–620. *Comprehensive clinical review.*

Revankar SG, Patterson JE, Sutton DA, et al: Disseminated phaeohyphomycosis: Review of an emerging mycosis. Clin Infect Dis 2002;34:467–476. *Review of disseminated disease in immunocompromised patients, this report emphasizes central nervous system, pulmonary, and other visceral involvement.*

Revankar SG, Sutton DA, Rinaldi MG: Primary central nervous system phaeohyphomycosis: A review of 101 cases. Clin Infect Dis 2004;38:206–216. *The largest and most comprehensive review of central nervous system phaeohyphomycosis, this report defines the most common pathogens, clinical manifestations, treatment, and outcome in this rare disorder.*

365 ANTIPARASITIC THERAPY

Richard D. Pearson

A number of factors, including development of the global economy, international travel, immigration, and the increased prevalence of human immunodeficiency virus/acquired immunodeficiency syndrome (HIV/AIDS) and other immunocompromising conditions have drawn attention to the importance of parasitic diseases worldwide. Although vaccines are lacking to protect against them, a number of highly effective drugs are available to treat them. This chapter provides an overview of antiparasitic chemotherapy based on taxonomic relationships. A number of generalizations emerge from this approach that help in organizing an otherwise vast amount of information.

In considering chemotherapy, it is helpful to divide parasitic infections into those caused by helminths, multicellular worms that have complex internal structures, and protozoa, single-celled organisms that multiply by cell division. Helminths are further divided into nematodes, or roundworms, which are subdivided into those that infect the gastrointestinal tract and those found within the body, and the platyhelminths, or flat worms, which are further subdivided into cestodes, or tapeworms, and trematodes, or flukes.

The protozoa are divided into those that reside under anaerobic conditions in the gastrointestinal tract or vagina and those that live aerobically in the body. The most important systemic protozoan infections are attributable to members of the Apicomplexa, which have a particular apical complex within the cell. Such infections include malaria, babesiosis, and toxoplasmosis. The other major group is the kinetoplastids, which have a specialized mitochondrial structure and cause Chagas' disease, African trypanosomiasis (sleeping sickness), and leishmaniasis.

Many of the drugs used to treat parasitic infections are not well known by physicians practicing in the United States. They are the focus of this chapter. A few of the antiparasitic drugs are active against pathogenic bacteria or fungi and are discussed elsewhere (Chapters 309 and 352). Detailed descriptions of antiparasitic drugs are available in textbooks of infectious diseases and tropical medicine. An excellent compilation of therapeutic recommendations for parasitic diseases is available in *The Medical Letter on Drugs and Therapeutics*, "Drugs for Parasitic Infections" (available at *www.medicalletter.org*).

TREATMENT OF HELMINTHS

Intestinal Roundworms (Nematodes)

The intestinal roundworms (Chapter 377) are among the world's most prevalent parasites. They are found in impoverished areas with poor sanitation. *Ascaris lumbricoides*, the hookworms, and *Trichuris trichiura* are each harbored in the gastrointestinal tracts of more than a billion people. It is not unusual for persons in impoverished areas to be infected with multiple species. Though frequently asymptomatic, infections can cause malnutrition, iron deficiency anemia, and poor performance in school or at work. *Strongyloides stercoralis* is less prevalent, but unique among intestinal roundworms in its ability to produce autoinfection. It can persist for decades and disseminate to produce hyperinfection in persons concurrently infected with human T-cell lymphotropic virus type 1 (HTLV-1) or immunocompromised by corticosteroids, neoplasm, malnutrition, or other conditions.

Albendazole has a broad spectrum of activity against intestinal roundworms. It is active against *A. lumbricoides*, the hookworms *Ancylostoma duodenale* and *Necator americanus*, and *T. trichiura*. Administered as a single 400-mg dose, it has been used successfully in mass treatment programs in developing countries. Daily doses for 3 days are recommended for those with heavy *T. trichiura* infections. Twice-daily doses of 400 mg for 7 days are used as an alternative to ivermectin for *S. stercoralis* infections, but failures can occur. Albendazole is effective in treating the pinworm *Enterobius vermicularis*, as well as cutaneous larva migrans and visceral larva migrans, which are caused by migrating stages of the intestinal helminths of animals. It is considered an alternative drug for *Trichostrongylus* species, *Trichinella spiralis*, and *Capillaria philippinensis*.

Administered twice daily at a dosage of 100 mg orally for 3 days, mebendazole has a similar spectrum of activity as albendazole against *A. lumbricoides*, the hookworms, and *T. trichiura* but it is poorly absorbed and not effective for *S. stercoralis*. Mebendazole in this regimen is more effective than a single dose of albendazole for *T. trichiura*. It is the treatment of choice for trichinosis. It kills *T. spiralis* adults and has some activity against invasive larvae. Mebendazole is also effective in treating pinworm (100 mg orally in one dose, followed by a second dose at 2 weeks).

A number of other drugs have activity against intestinal roundworms and may be indicated in specific situations. Pyrantel pamoate is a relatively safe, poorly absorbed drug with activity against the hookworms, *A. lumbricoides*, *E. vermicularis*, and *Trichostrongylus* species, but it is not effective against *T. trichiura* or *S. stercoralis*. It is administered as an oral suspension in a single 11-mg/kg dose (to a maximum of 1 g). Albendazole, mebendazole, and pyrantel pamoate have replaced a number of older anthelmintics that are more toxic, such as piperazine.

Ivermectin at an oral dose of 200 μg/kg daily for 2 days is considered the treatment of choice for *S. stercoralis*. It is also recommended for cutaneous larva migrans. It has activity against *A. lumbricoides* and *T. trichiura*, but not hookworms. Thiabendazole, which is no longer manufactured in the United States, was once the drug of choice for strongyloidiasis, but it has substantial untoward effects. Nitazoxanide (see later), which was recently approved in the United States for the treatment of giardiasis and cryptosporidiosis, has activity against a number of intestinal helminths, but its role in their treatment awaits further study.

Systemic Roundworms

Diethylcarbamazine is the drug of choice for several filarial infections (Chapter 379), including *Wuchereria bancrofti*, *Brugia malayi*, *Brugia timori*, and *Loa loa*, and for persons with tropical pulmonary eosinophilia. It promotes the host's killing of microfilariae of these species and also damages or kills the adult worms. In heavy *L. loa* infection, the rapid release of antigens can elicit encephalopathy, and apheresis or treatment with albendazole can be used first to reduce the microfilarial burden. Diethylcarbamazine is not marketed in the United States but is available from the Centers for Disease Control and Prevention (CDC) (404-639-3670, *www.cdc.gov/ncidod/srp/drugs/formulary.html*). Diethylcarbamazine is used prophylactically to prevent *L. loa* infection in endemic areas.

Ivermectin has activity against the microfilariae of *W. bancrofti*, *B. malayi*, and *L. loa*, but it does not kill the adult worms and is not recommended for them. Either albendazole or mebendazole is used for *Man-*

sonella perstans. Endosymbiotic *Wolbachia* bacteria are necessary for filarial development and provide a potential target for chemotherapy. Preliminary studies indicate that long-term therapy with doxycycline in patients with lymphatic filariasis results in loss of *Wolbachia* and a block in microfilarial production. A promising approach may be to combine chemotherapy against both *Wolbachia* and filariae. By decreasing the *Wolbachia* burden, doxycycline may diminish the systemic release of *Wolbachia* components (such as lipopolysaccharide) during subsequent standard therapy. Indeed, doxycycline may find a role before diethylcarbamazine treatment, although further studies are needed to address this issue.

Diethylcarbamazine leads to rapid killing of the microfilariae of *Onchocerca volvulus,* but it is not used for the treatment of onchocerciasis because the rapid release of *Onchocerca* antigens, as well as lipopolysaccharides derived from filaria-harbored *Wolbachia* endiosymbionts, can elicit severe systemic and ocular inflammatory reactions. Ivermectin, which is associated with much less severe reactions, is the drug of choice and is administered in a single dose of 150 μg/kg. It does not kill adult worms, but it decreases ova production. Retreatment is usually necessary at 6-to 12-month intervals. Profits from the use of ivermectin for the treatment of the dog heartworm *Dirofilaria immitis* have permitted the manufacturer to provide the drug free to persons with onchocerciasis in developing areas.

Tapeworms

Praziquantel, which has a broad spectrum of activity against tapeworms (Chapter 375) and flukes, is the drug of choice for adult tapeworms in the human intestinal tract. It is effective against *Taenia solium* (pork tapeworm), *Taenia saginata* (beef), *Diphyllobothrium latum* (fish), and *Hymenolepis nana* (dwarf) when administered as a single dose. Niclosamide, which is not absorbed, is an alternative treatment of *T. saginata* and *D. latum.* It also kills adult *T. solium,* but disintegration of the worm and release of viable ova into the intestinal lumen raise the theoretical possibility of autoinfection. Praziquantel is thus preferred. In the case of *H. nana,* a dose of 500 mg nitazoxanide daily for 3 days provides an alternative to praziquantel.

Neurocysticercosis from the larval or tissue phase of *T. solium* is a major cause of seizures and other central nervous system (CNS) abnormalities in residents of Latin America and other endemic areas and immigrants from those regions. Both albendazole and praziquantel can kill cysticerci in the brain, but indications for their use are debated. Corticosteroids should always be administered concurrently to reduce the inflammatory response to cysticercal antigens and the increase in intracranial pressure that can result. Albendazole is the drug of choice because of its favorable pharmacodynamics and is administered for 15 days at 15 mg/kg/day (max 800 mg) in two divided doses. Praziquantel is the alternative at a dose of 50 mg/kg/day in three doses for 30 days. The concurrent use of corticosteroids increases the cerebrospinal fluid (CSF) level of albendazole and decreases that of praziquantel. Albendazole is also the drug of choice for persons with echinococcosis at a dose of 400 mg twice daily for individuals greater than 60 kg and 15 mg/kg divided (max 800 mg) into two doses daily for those who weigh less than 60 kg, generally for several months. It cures more than a third of patients with *Echinococcus granulosus* cysts. It is also given to persons with echinococcal cysts before ultrasound-guided percutaneous aspiration-injection-reaspiration (PAIR) or surgery to prevent seeding of the peritoneum if cyst contents are spilled during the procedure. Albendazole is likewise used for the suppression of inoperable *Echinococcus multilocularis* disease.

Flukes (Trematodes)

Praziquantel is the drug of choice for the treatment of all forms of schistosomiasis (Chapter 376), as well as intestinal, lung, and liver flukes (Chapter 377), with the exception of *Fasciola hepatica.* For schistosomiasis, two to three doses are given in 1 day. The flukes are treated with three doses on 1 or 2 days, depending on the species. Oxamniquine is an alternative for *Schistosoma mansoni,* but it is more toxic and less effective. Higher doses of oxamniquine are recommended for the treatment of *S. mansoni* in areas of Egypt and equatorial Africa. *F. hepatica* responds to the veterinary agent triclabendazole and to bithionol, which is more toxic. Either praziquantel or albendazole can be used to treat *Clonorchis sinensis.*

Drugs Used for Helminthic Infections

Albendazole is poorly soluble in water, but it is well absorbed when administered with a fatty meal. It undergoes rapid first-pass metabolism in the liver to albendazole sulfoxide, which has excellent anthelmintic activity. The serum half-life of albendazole sulfoxide is 8 to 9 hours. Elimination of albendazole sulfoxide and other metabolites of albendazole is primarily through the kidney. Albendazole binds to tubulin in susceptible parasites, inhibits microtubule assembly, and decreases glucose absorption. It also inhibits fumarate reductase in helminths. The CSF concentration of albendazole is 40% of that in serum. Concurrent administration of dexamethasone, which is frequently administered to prevent cerebral edema in neurocysticercosis, increases serum levels by approximately 50%. Albendazole is generally well tolerated when given as a single dose for the treatment of intestinal nematode infections, although gastrointestinal discomfort may occasionally develop or patients may experience migration of adult *A. lumbricoides* from the nose or mouth or in stool. Albendazole is embryotoxic in animals and contraindicated during pregnancy. High-dose, prolonged therapy, such as that recommended for echinococcal disease, can be complicated by alopecia, bone marrow suppression, which is reversible with discontinuation of the drug, or hepatocellular injury.

Mebendazole is only slightly soluble in water and is relatively poorly absorbed from the gastrointestinal tract, which is advantageous for intestinal parasites but limits its effectiveness against tissue-dwelling helminths. Absorbed drug is metabolized in the liver and excreted in urine. Mebendazole selectively binds to helminthic tubulin, blocks its assembly into microtubules, and inhibits glucose uptake, thereby leading to depletion of glycogen stores and ultimately parasite death. Human tubulin is not affected. It is relatively well tolerated in the doses used to treat intestinal helminths. Transient abdominal pain and diarrhea occur in a small number of recipients. Mebendazole is contraindicated during pregnancy.

Ivermectin is a macrocyclic lactone produced by *Streptomyces avermitilis.* It has a broad spectrum of activity against helminths and arthropods, including *Sarcoptes scabiei,* the cause of scabies. It is well absorbed after oral administration. Ivermectin is highly protein bound, has a serum half-life of 12 hours, and accumulates in adipose tissue and the liver. It is subject to enterohepatic recirculation and ultimately eliminated in stool. Ivermectin activates the opening of gated chloride channels, which are found only in susceptible helminths and arthropods. The result is an influx of chloride ions and paralysis of the pharyngeal pumping mechanism of helminths. It is generally well tolerated.

Diethylcarbamazine, a piperazine derivative, is well absorbed orally and has a half-life of 8 hours. The parent drug and its metabolites are excreted through the kidney. Although the mechanism of action is uncertain, the piperazine moiety may result in paralysis of sensitive helminths. Diethylcarbamazine also alters the surface membranes of sensitive microfilariae, thereby resulting in destruction by the host's immune system. Side effects include those attributable directly to the drug and those that result from the release of parasite antigens, as well as lipopolysaccharides derived from filaria-harbored *Wolbachia* endiosymbionts. *Adverse effects* include nausea, vomiting, anorexia, headache, malaise, weakness, arthralgias, and rarely, acute psychotic reactions. In patients with lymphatic filariasis, localized swelling or nodules may develop along the lymphatics during treatment, or there may be transient lymphedema or hydrocele formation. Diethylcarbamazine is not used for the treatment of onchocerciasis because it rapidly kills microfilariae, which release antigens that can elicit hypotension, pruritus, fever, tachycardia, wheezing, chorioretinitis, and uveitis. This symptom complex is known as the Mazzotti reaction. Life-threatening encephalopathy has been reported in patients with heavy *L. loa* infection treated with diethylcarbamazine.

Praziquantel is well absorbed after oral administration. It undergoes extensive first-pass metabolism, and the metabolites, which are inactive, are excreted in urine. Praziquantel is approximately 80% protein bound; its serum half-life is 4 to 6 hours. It is rapidly taken up by susceptible cestodes and trematodes. Studies of the tapeworm *Hymenolepis diminuta* indicate that praziquantel causes blebs in the neck of the adult tapeworm and release of calcium from endogenous stores. This results in paralysis and expulsion of the worm from the gastrointestinal tract. In the case of schistosomes, praziquantel damages the tegument, which results in intense vacuolation and increased permeability to calcium. Adult schistosomes are paralyzed and translocated to the liver through the portal circulation. Sequestered antigens are exposed on the parasite's surface, thereby permitting binding of antibodies and phagocytes and immune destruction of the parasite. Praziquantel is an alternative to albendazole for the treatment of neurocysticercosis. Its concentration in CSF is approximately 15 to 20% of that in plasma. The concurrent administration of corticosteroids, which are necessary to decrease inflammation and edema in the brain, reduces the CSF concentration.

Praziquantel is frequently associated with mild, transient side effects, including headaches, lassitude, dizziness, nausea, vomiting, and abdominal discomfort, but they are seldom severe enough to interrupt therapy. Untoward reactions apparently caused by the release of parasite antigens have been reported in patients treated for schistosomiasis and pulmonary paragonimiasis. Increased intracranial pressure resulting from cysticercal antigens is a potentially life-threatening consequence in patients receiving praziquantel for neurocysticercosis. Corticosteroids should be administered concurrently. Praziquantel is contraindicated in persons with cysticerci in the eye or spinal cord because of the deleterious consequences of local inflammatory reactions.

TREATMENT OF PROTOZOAL DISEASES

Intestinal and Vaginal Protozoa

Several major luminal pathogens, *Entamoeba histolytica* (Chapter 373), *Giardia lamblia* (Chapter 372), and *Trichomonas vaginalis* (Chapter 374), which live in anaerobic conditions in the intestine or vagina, are susceptible to metronidazole and tinidazole. The latter has favorable pharmacodynamics and is better tolerated. Because neither metronidazole nor tinidazole reliably eradicate cysts of *E. histolytica*, a luminal agent should be used alone with them. Luminal agents include paromomycin, diloxanide furoate, and iodoquinol. Any of these agents can be used alone in persons with asymptomatic cyst excretion. Nitazoxanide, which is available in an oral formulation, can be used for the treatment of giardiasis in children. Diloxanide is not available in the United States, although a distributor can be contacted at 800-247-9767. Tetracycline is the treatment of choice for *Balantidium coli;* metronidazole and iodoquinol are considered alternatives.

Cryptosporidium, which has been responsible for major water-borne epidemics in North America and elsewhere and is an important pathogen in persons with AIDS, is resistant to most antiprotozoal drugs (Chapter 374). Nitazoxanide is effective for the treatment of cryptosporidiosis in immunocompetent persons. Unfortunately, failures are common in persons with AIDS. Trimethoprim-sulfamethoxazole, which inhibits successive steps in the folic acid pathway, is effective for the treatment of *Isospora belli* and *Cyclospora cayetanensis.* Ciprofloxacin, a fluoroquinolone antibiotic that acts on topoisomerase II, is an alternative. Finally, albendazole is effective in the treatment of intestinal, ocular, and disseminated microsporidiosis caused by *Encephalitozoon (Septata) intestinalis* and some other microsporidia in patients with AIDS, but not all microsporidia are susceptible.

Metronidazole, a nitroimidazole, is rapidly absorbed after oral administration and has a half-life of 8 hours. More than half of each dose is metabolized in the liver. The metabolites and remaining parent drug are excreted in urine. It is activated by reduction of its 5-nitro group through a sequence of intermediate steps involving microbial electron transport proteins of low redox potential. It is concentrated in anaerobic organisms and serves as an electron sink. Nausea, vomiting, diarrhea, and a metallic taste are often associated with the use of metronidazole. They are less common with the lower doses recommended for the treatment of giardiasis than with the higher doses used for amebiasis. Other untoward effects include headache, dizziness, vertigo, and numbness. Potentially severe disulfiram-like reactions occur in patients who ingest alcohol while taking metronidazole.

Tinidazole, another 5-nitroimidazole, has a similar mechanism of action and spectrum of activity as metronidazole, but more favorable pharmacodynamics and is better tolerated. It has been widely used around the world and recently gained Food and Drug Administration (FDA) approval for the treatment of giardiasis, intestinal amebiasis, and trichomoniasis in the United States. In comparison to metronidazole, it has a longer half-life, a shorter and less complicated dosing regimen, and fewer gastrointestinal side effects. It, too, can cause severe disulfiram-like reactions after alcohol ingestion.

Nitazoxanide, a 5-nitrothiazole-salicylamide derivative, has a broad spectrum of activity against protozoa and helminths. It is formulated as a liquid. Nitazoxanide is well absorbed orally and hydrolyzed to its active metabolite tizoxanide, which undergoes conjugation to tizoxanide glucuronide. The parent compound is not detectable in serum. Maximum concentrations of the metabolites are observed in 1 to 4 hours. They are both excreted in urine and bile. Tizoxanide is highly protein bound. Although the mechanism of action is uncertain, tizoxanide may inhibit pyruvate:ferredoxin oxidoreductase–dependent electron transport reactions essential to the metabolism of anaerobic organisms.

Prophylaxis and Treatment of Malaria

Malaria is a major cause of morbidity and mortality among residents of the tropics and poses a substantial risk to nonimmune travelers who visit them. Recommendations for prophylaxis and treatment depend on the infecting *Plasmodium* species and the site visited or to be visited (Chapter 366). The CDC provides updated information for countries at *www.cdc.gov/travel/* and in "Health Information for International Travel, 2005–2006."

Chloroquine, a 4-aminoquinoline, has a bitter taste but is well absorbed from the gastrointestinal tract. Its half-life, which varies among persons, averages 4 days, thus permitting once-weekly administration for prophylaxis. Approximately half the parent drug is excreted unchanged in urine and the remainder is metabolized in the liver. Its mechanism of action has been extensively studied. Chloroquine is concentrated in the hemoglobin-containing digestive vesicles of asexual intraerythrocytic parasites. It inhibits the parasite's heme polymerase that incorporates ferriprotoporphyrin type IX complexes, which are potentially toxic to the parasite, into insoluble, nontoxic, crystalline hemozoin. Chloroquine-resistant strains of *Plasmodium falciparum* actively transport chloroquine out of the intraparasitic compartment. Although this action can be blocked by calcium-channel inhibitors in vitro, chloroquine resistance has not been effectively reversed in humans. Hydroxychloroquine (Plaquenil), which is used for rheumatologic diseases, is also effective against chloroquine-sensitive *Plasmodium* species.

Chloroquine is generally well tolerated when used at the doses recommended for the prophylaxis and treatment of malaria. Side effects include headache, nausea, vomiting, blurred vision, dizziness, and fatigue. Some Africans and African Americans experience pruritus, which responds to antihistamines. Rare side effects include depigmentation of hair, exacerbation of psoriasis, blood dyscrasias, seizures, neuropsychiatric effects, and reactions in persons with porphyria. Retinal damage has occurred in persons receiving chloroquine at high doses for the treatment of rheumatologic disorders, but it has not been documented as a problem in those taking it weekly over a period of many years for malaria prophylaxis. Chloroquine has been used for chemoprophylaxis during pregnancy. Children are more sensitive to the toxic effects of chloroquine than adults are, and cardiopulmonary collapse and death have occurred after accidental overdose and in adults attempting suicide. As little as 5 g of chloroquine can be fatal unless treatment is initiated with mechanical respiration, diazepam to control seizures, and blood pressure support. An intravenous preparation of chloroquine is available outside the United States, but it must be given slowly and with great caution because of its propensity to produce respiratory depression, heart block, hypotension, cardiovascular collapse, and seizures.

Doxycycline taken daily provides effective prophylaxis against all *Plasmodium* species. Either tetracycline or doxycycline can be administered with quinine to treat acute chloroquine-resistant malaria. They do not act rapidly enough to be used alone. The tetracyclines are well absorbed after oral administration, and they are generally well tolerated. They can produce gastrointestinal symptoms. Doxycycline can also cause severe esophagitis if it does not pass through to the stomach. Consequently, it should be taken with a full glass of water, and the recipient should remain upright for an hour after ingestion. Other potential untoward effects include photosensitivity dermatitis, *Candida albicans* vaginitis, and antibiotic-associated colitis. Finally, tetracyclines should not be used in children younger than 8 years because of the potential for dental staining or in pregnant women.

Atovaquone plus ***proguanil*** (Malarone, adult tablets contain 250 mg atovaquone and 100 mg proguanil), when administered daily, is effective for prophylaxis in areas with chloroquine-resistant *P. falciparum* and for the treatment of uncomplicated cases of acute malaria. Atovaquone is a highly lipophilic compound with low aqueous solubility. Administration with food enhances its absorption two-fold. Plasma concentrations do not increase proportionately with dose. Atovaquone is highly protein bound with a half-life exceeding 60 hours. It undergoes extensive enterohepatic cycling and is eventually excreted unchanged in feces. Atovaquone selectively inhibits electron transport at the level of the cytochrome bc_1 complex, which results in collapse of mitochondrial membrane potential. It also affects pyrimidine biosynthesis, which is obligatorily coupled to electron transport in *Plasmodium* through ubiquinone/ubiquinol. Resistance develops rapidly when atovaquone is used alone to treat malaria. Atovaquone is generally well tolerated but can cause gastrointestinal side effects, including nausea, vomiting, and diarrhea, as well as rash and pruritus. Adherence to the daily regimen can be challenging for those who stay in an endemic area for a prolonged period.

Proguanil is slowly absorbed after oral administration. The serum level falls to zero within 24 hours, so it must be taken daily for prophylaxis. Its triazine metabolite cycloguanil inhibits dihydrofolate reductase in susceptible *Plasmodium* species. Resistance is well documented when proguanil is used alone. Proguanil also acts synergistically with atovaquone to collapse mitochondrial membrane potential in susceptible *Plasmodium* species. It is generally well tolerated. At higher doses it can cause nausea, vomiting, abdominal pain, and diarrhea. Hematologic effects occur rarely. The combination of atovaquone-proguanil (Malarone) is generally the best tolerated of the options for prevention of chloroquine-resistant malaria, but abdominal pain, nausea, vomiting, diarrhea, headache, pruritus, and rash may occur. Asymptomatic, transient elevations in liver enzymes have been observed with treatment doses of Malarone.

Mefloquine, a quinoline methanol compound derived from quinine, has been widely used for the prophylaxis and treatment of chloroquine-resistant *P. falciparum* malaria. Concern about neuropsychiatric toxicity and the availability of better-tolerated alternatives have limited its use in recent years. Mefloquine is available for oral administration only, and it is slowly and incompletely absorbed. It is 99% protein bound and has a variable half-life ranging from 6 to 23 days with a mean of approximately 14 days. It is metabolized and excreted slowly through bile and feces. Although its mechanism of action is uncertain, mefloquine appears to interfere with the food vacuoles of the intraerythrocytic asexual stage of the parasite.

Considerable attention has been paid to the untoward effects of mefloquine. It is reasonably well tolerated in most recipients, although it can cause transient nausea, dizziness, vivid dreams, fatigue, and lassitude. Less common but of substantial concern are neuropsychiatric reactions, including anxiety, depression, acute psychosis, and seizures. Mefloquine is therefore contraindicated in persons with a history of epilepsy or psychiatric problems. It can depress atrial-ventricular conduction and should not be used in persons taking β-blockers for cardiac indications. It also has antibacterial activity and can inactivate the live oral typhoid vaccine (*Salmonella typhi* Ty21a) if administered concurrently. Rare side effects include exfoliative erythroderma, agranulocytosis, and paresthesias. Mefloquine is not approved by the U.S. FDA for use during pregnancy or in children who weigh less than 15 kg, but it can be used in situations when the potential benefits are judged to outweigh the risks.

Primaquine, an 8-aminoquinoline, is well absorbed orally and rapidly converted to carboxyprimaquine, which has a half-life of approximately 7 days. The precise mechanism of action is unknown, but it is thought to interfere with mitochondrial function and possibly transport of vesicles in the parasite. Primaquine eradicates the hypnozoite hepatic stages of *Plasmodium vivax* and *Plasmodium ovale* species and can be used at the end of treatment or prophylaxis with other agents to prevent relapse. It can also be used daily for prophylaxis. Primaquine is generally well tolerated, although some recipients experience abdominal cramps, epigastric distress, and nausea. The major concern is hemolysis in persons with glucose-6-phosphate dehydrogenase (G6PD) deficiency. The G6PD status of the recipient should be determined before it is administered. Rarely, primaquine causes neutropenia, methemoglobinemia, hypertension, or arrhythmias. Primaquine is contraindicated during pregnancy and in breast-feeding mothers because life-threatening hemolysis may occur if the fetus or baby is G6PD deficient. Travelers should be warned not to give the drug to fellow travelers who have not been screened for G6PD deficiency.

Quinine sulfate, a cinchona alkaloid, is the oldest of the antimalarials. It has a very bitter taste. It is rapidly absorbed after oral administration and has a half-life of 16 to 18 hours in persons with malaria. The mechanism of its action is unknown, but quinine is thought to act at the level of the parasites' hemoglobin-containing digestive vesicle and may interfere with ferriprotoporphyrin IX metabolism. Quinine has the poorest therapeutic-to-toxicity ratio of any antimalarial drug. The side effects, known collectively as cinchonism, include tinnitus, decreased hearing, headache, nausea, vomiting, dysphoria, and visual disturbances. They are dose related and reversible. Quinine has also been associated with severe hypoglycemia in persons with heavy *P. falciparum* infection as a result of the utilization of glucose by the parasites and release of insulin from the pancreas. Hypoglycemia can be prevented or treated by the administration of intravenous glucose. Rare complications with quinine include massive hemolysis in patients with heavy *P. falciparum* infection resulting in hemoglobinuria and renal failure (blackwater fever), cutaneous hypersensitivity reactions, agranulocytosis, and hepatitis. Quinine can cause respiratory paralysis in persons with myasthenia gravis. It stimulates uterine contractions and can produce abortions, but it has saved the lives of many pregnant women with *P. falciparum* malaria.

Quinidine gluconate, the stereoisomer of quinine, is recommended for the intravenous treatment of patients with acute malaria who cannot take quinine or other antimalarials orally. Quinidine gluconate was once widely used for the treatment of ventricular ectopy. It has been replaced by newer antiarrhythmic agents, which has decreased its availability in many medical centers. Its side effects include prolongation of the QT interval, arrhythmias, and hypotension, particularly if it is infused too rapidly. Persons receiving intravenous quinidine should be monitored in an intensive care setting and therapy switched to oral quinine as soon as they can take medications by mouth. Where it is available, intravenous quinine dihydrochloride can be used if quinidine is not available. It, too, can produce myocardial depression, peripheral vascular collapse, respiratory depression, and death. Patients must be monitored closely during its infusion. Intravenous therapy with either drug should be terminated as soon as the patient is able to take oral drugs.

The artemisinins, including ***artesunate, artemisinin, artemether, arteether,*** and ***artelinic acid,*** are sesquiterpene lactones derived from the Chinese herbal medication for malaria, quinghaosu, which comes from the wormwood plant *Artemisia annua.* Although not available in the United States, they are increasingly used around the world for the treatment of chloroquine–resistant *P. falciparum* malaria. They are endoperoxide-containing compounds. In the presence of intraparasitic iron, they are thought to be converted into free radicals and other intermediates that alkylate specific malarial proteins and act rapidly to kill intraerythrocytic parasites. They are administered with a second antimalarial that has a different mechanism of action and longer half-life to reduce resistance. The route of administration with artemisinins varies; some are administered orally, whereas others are given intravenously, intramuscularly, or by suppository. Artemether plus lumefantrine (Coartem) is available as a fixed oral drug combination. They are rapidly cleared from the circulation. Adverse effects are infrequent and mild and include abdominal pain, diarrhea, and drug fever. Decreased reticulocytes and neutrophils and cerebellar dysfunction have been observed. Contact dermatitis has also been associated with sesquiterpene lactones. Neuropathic effects have been reported in dogs given chronic, high-dose therapy. The short half-life of the artemisinin derivatives has precluded their use for malaria prophylaxis.

Toxoplasmosis and Babesiosis

Toxoplasma gondii (Chapter 370) and *Babesia* species (Chapter 374) are other important pathogens of the phylum Apicomplexa. Pyrimethamine and sulfadiazine are recommended for the treatment of toxoplasmosis. They inhibit sequential steps in the folic acid metabolic pathway. Pyrimethamine preferentially inhibits dihydrofolate reductase in susceptible parasites. It is well absorbed orally. The major side effect is macrocytic anemia, which can be prevented by the concurrent administration of leucovorin. Sulfonamides reduce the activity of dihydropteroate synthetase and the binding of *p*-aminobenzoic acid to it. In ocular toxoplasmosis with macular involvement, corticosteroids are recommended along with anti-*Toxoplasma* chemotherapy. Clindamycin is used as an alternative to sulfadiazine. Atovaquone plus pyrimethamine is another option in sulfonamide-intolerant patients. For primary prophylaxis in AIDS patients with $CD4^+$ T-cell counts less than 100, options include trimethoprim-sulfamethoxazole, pyrimethamine with dapsone, and atovaquone with or without pyrimethamine. The macrolide spiramycin is used for the treatment of toxoplasmosis during pregnancy. Two regimens are available for the treatment of babesiosis. The greatest experience is with the combination of clindamycin and quinine, but side effects are common. Atovaquone plus azithromycin is effective and better tolerated (see Chapter 374).

TREATMENT OF CHAGAS' DISEASE, AFRICAN TRYPANOSOMIASIS, AND LEISHMANIASIS

Trypanosoma cruzi, Trypanosoma brucei rhodesiense, and *Trypanosoma brucei gambiense* pose difficult therapeutic challenges. Nifurtimox and benznidazole are used for the treatment of acute Chagas' disease (Chapter 368). Both are associated with substantial toxicity. Benznidazole has been recommended by some for the treatment of children and young adults with indeterminate-phase *T. cruzi* infection, but the percentage of those cured is debated. Neither benznidazole nor nifurtimox reverses the manifestations of chronic Chagas' disease, including cardiomyopathy and megadisease of the esophagus or intestine. However, both agents have been used to treat chronic infection in conjunction with cardiac transplantation.

Suramin, pentamidine, and melarsoprol are used for the treatment of human African trypanosomiasis (sleeping sickness) (Chapter 367). Eflornithine (difluoromethylornithine), the "resurrection drug," is effective against the hemolymphatic and CNS stages of *T. brucei gambiense* infection. It does not have activity against *T. brucei rhodesiense.* Unfortunately, eflornithine is costly, those affected by the disease live in impoverished areas, and supplies are currently very limited.

Liposomal amphotericin B (AmBisome) is the only drug approved for the treatment of visceral leishmaniasis (Chapter 369) in the United States. Amphotericin B deoxycholate is highly effective, but has more side effects. Liposomes deliver the drug to the reticuloendothelial system and are theoretically attractive because leishmaniae reside in mononuclear phagocytes. Liposomal amphotericin is also better tolerated than the parent drug. Other lipid-associated amphotericin B preparations appear to be effective but have been less extensively studied. The pentavalent antimonials, stibogluconate sodium and meglumine antimoniate, have been used for many years in developing areas. Resistance is now common in India. Miltefosine, a phosphocholine analogue that is administered orally, is effective there and under study in other areas (see later). Amphotericin B deoxycholate is an alternative.

Treatment of cutaneous leishmaniasis depends on the infecting *Leishmania* species, its propensity to cause mucosal disease, and the size and location of the skin lesion or lesions. Stibogluconate sodium (available from the CDC) and meglumine antimonite are still widely used (see later). A number of other drugs have some antileishmanial activity, including the imidazole antifungals ketoconazole, itraconazole, and fluconazole, which inhibit ergosterol biosynthesis. The imidazoles vary in their activity against different *Leishmania* species. Amphotericin B deoxycholate and pentamidine are highly effective, but more toxic alternatives. Paromomycin has been used topically with methylbenzethonium chloride in soft white paraffin for the treatment of cutaneous leishmaniasis caused by *Leishmania major.* Though not fully studied, failures have occurred with the use of both liposomal amphotericin B and miltefosine for the treatment of cutaneous leishmaniasis. Further studies are needed to define their role in the treatment of cutaneous leishmaniasis.

Benznidazole, a nitroimidazole, is used orally for the treatment of Chagas' disease in Latin America. It is administered orally for 30 to 90 days. It is frequently associated with skin reactions, dose-dependent polyneuropathy, gastrointestinal symptoms, bone marrow suppression, and psychiatric side effects. Benznidazole is not available in the United States.

Nifurtimox, a nitrofuran, is used for the treatment of Chagas' disease in the United States. Although it is no longer in production, it is available through the CDC. Nifurtimox lowers mortality from myocarditis and meningoencephalitis and shortens the duration of symptoms in acute Chagas' disease. It is administered orally for a period of 90 to 120 days. Side effects are frequent and include anorexia, vomiting, abdominal pain, weight loss, sleep disorders, paresthesias, weakness, and polyneuritis. These untoward effects are usually reversible when treatment with the drug is stopped, but they often pose a therapeutic dilemma given the long duration of treatment. Seizures, rash, and neutropenia occur rarely.

Suramin is a urea derivative that is used for treatment of the hemolymphatic stage of *T. brucei rhodesiense* infection. It is administered intravenously and is available in the United States only from the CDC. Suramin is frequently associated with side effects, including nausea, vomiting, urticarial eruptions, paresthesias, hyperesthesias, and peripheral neuropathy. Less frequent side effects are renal toxicity, blood dyscrasias, loss of consciousness, and shock.

Pentamidine isethionate, a diamidine, is used for treatment of the hemolymphatic stage of *T. brucei gambiense* infection and occasionally for the treatment of leishmaniasis, as well as for *Pneumocystis jiroveci.* Its mechanism of action remains uncharacterized. Pentamidine is usually administered intravenously. Intramuscular injections are associated with inflammation and sterile abscesses at the site of inoculation. Side effects are common and include gastrointestinal complaints, dizziness, tachycardia, flushing, and hypotension if the drug is infused too rapidly. Renal function is impaired transiently. A major concern is hypoglycemia resulting from the release of insulin from damaged pancreatic beta cells. Patients with higher pentamidine levels appear to be at greater risk. Fatalities from hypoglycemia have been reported. Insulin-dependent diabetes mellitus is an important potential long-term consequence.

Melarsoprol, a trivalent arsenical available from the CDC, is administered intravenously for the treatment of East African trypanosomiasis (*T. brucei rhodesiense*) with CNS involvement. It is also used for CNS disease caused by *T. brucei gambiense* when eflornithine is not available. Fever, abdominal pain, vomiting, arthralgias, myocardial toxicity, hypertension, albuminuria, and peripheral neuropathy are common. More importantly, allergic encephalitis characterized by headache, dizziness, mental dullness, confusion, ataxia, obtundation, and seizures develops in approximately 6% of recipients and can result in death. Cardiovascular collapse is a rare complication.

Eflornithine (***difluoromethylornithine***) can be administered orally or intravenously for all stages of West African trypanosomiasis (*T. brucei gambiense*). The ratio of its level in CSF to serum ranges from 0.09 to 0.45; the ratio is highest in patients who have the most severe CNS involvement. Most of the drug is excreted in urine. In contrast to other drugs used to treat African trypanosomiasis, eflornithine is relatively well tolerated. Flatulence, nausea, vomiting, and diarrhea can occur, but they are transient. Reversible anemia, thrombocytopenia, or neutropenia develops in some recipients. Diplopia, dizziness, or hypersensitivity reactions occur rarely.

Sodium stibogluconate and ***meglumine antimoniate,*** pentavalent antimony–containing drugs, have been widely used for the treatment of leishmaniasis. Sodium stibogluconate is available through the CDC in the United States and in Britain, whereas meglumine antimoniate is used in French-speaking areas and in Latin America. They are administered intravenously or intramuscularly on the basis of their pentavalent antimony content. The mechanism of action is uncertain, but they may function by impairing parasite glycolysis pathways. Although most patients are able to complete a full course of therapy, side effects are common and include nausea, vomiting, abdominal pain, anorexia, myalgias, arthralgias, headache, and malaise. Chemical pancreatitis is observed in many patients, and severe pancreatitis occurs in some. It is particularly common in persons with renal failure. Nonspecific ST-T wave changes are common. Less frequent side effects are elevated liver enzymes, bradycardia, leukopenia, thrombocytopenia, and anemia. Renal toxicity, myocardial damage, and shock are rare. Sudden death, possibly from arrhythmia, has been reported in persons receiving more than the recommended dose.

Miltefosine (***hexadecylphosphocholine***) is the only orally administered antileishmanial drug. It was developed initially as an antineoplastic agent. Although the precise mechanism of action is uncertain, it is known to interact with membrane constituents. It affects cell signaling pathways by inhibiting phosphokinase C and protein kinase C. It also interferes with the synthesis of glycosylphosphatidylinositol membrane anchors, which are important in leishmaniae and related kinetoplastids. Miltefosine is relatively well tolerated, but nausea, vomiting, and motion sickness occur. Elevations of transaminases, blood urea nitrogen, and creatinine have been noted but usually resolve with continuation of the drug. It is contraindicated during pregnancy.

SUGGESTED READINGS

Arguin PM, Kozarsky PE, Navin AW (eds): Health Information for International Travel, 2005–2006. Philadelphia, Mosby, 2005. Available at http://www.cdc.gov/travel/. *Recommendations for the prevention of malaria and other travel-related diseases.*

Canduri F, Perez PC, Caceres RA, et al: Protein kinases as targets for antiparasitic chemotherapy drugs. Curr Drug Targets 2007;8:389–398. *Explores this target for novel antiparasitic agents.*

Cooper PJ, Chico ME, Vaca MG, et al: Effect of albendazole treatments on the prevalence of atopy in children living in communities endemic for geohelminth parasites: A cluster-randomised trial. Lancet 2006;367:1598–1603. *There was no evidence that albendazole treatment was associated with an increase in atopy prevalence.*

Drugs for parasitic diseases. Med Lett Drugs Ther 2004;46:1–12. Available at www.medicalletter.org. *Consensus recommendations for the treatment of parasitic diseases are provided. Key articles are referenced.*

Marra F, Salzman JR, Ensom MH: Atovaquone-proguanil for prophylaxis and treatment of malaria. Ann Pharmacother 2003;37:1266–1275. *Review of the use of atovaquone-proguanil for the prophylaxis and treatment of malaria.*

Nitazoxanide (Alinia)—a new anti-protozoal agent. Med Lett Drugs Ther 2003;45:29–31. *A detailed review of nitazoxanide and its indications for the treatment of giardiasis, cryptosporidiosis, and trichomoniasis.*

Tinidazole (Tindamax)—a new anti-protozoal drug. Med Lett Drugs Ther 2004;46:70–72. *A comprehensive review of tinidazole and its indications and untoward effects written after it received FDA approval for use in the United States.*

366 MALARIA

Donald J. Krogstad

Definition

Malaria is characterized by recurrent fever and chills associated with the synchronous lysis of parasitized red blood cells. Its name is derived from the belief of the ancient Romans that malaria was caused by the bad air of the marshes surrounding Rome.

Although precise data are difficult to obtain, malaria is one of the most common infectious diseases worldwide. Several billion cases of malaria occur each year, with 2 to 3 million deaths. Most deaths are caused by *Plasmodium falciparum* infection and occur in children younger than 5 years who live in sub-Saharan Africa. One of the major unanswered questions about malaria is how plasmodia produce repetitive infections without stimulating an effective (protective) immune response.

The prevalence of malaria varies widely. It may reach 70 to 80% or more among children in hyperendemic areas during the transmission season. Its impact on the health of the developing world is enormous.

The major factors responsible for the resurgence of malaria are drug resistances: the widespread resistance of the anopheline vector to economical insecticides such as chlorophenothane (DDT) and the increasing prevalence of resistance to chloroquine and pyrimethamine-sulfadoxine (Fansidar) in *P. falciparum*, which is established in South America, Southeast Asia, and Africa.

The Pathogen

Malaria is produced by intraerythrocytic parasites of the genus *Plasmodium.* Four plasmodia produce malaria in humans: *Plasmodium falciparum, Plasmodium vivax, Plasmodium ovale,* and *Plasmodium malariae.* The severity and characteristic manifestations of malaria are governed by the infecting species, the magnitude of the parasitemia, the metabolic effects of the parasite, and the cytokines released as a result of the infection.

Epidemiology

The life cycle can be viewed as beginning with synchronous asexual replication of the erythrocytic stage of the parasite (Fig. 366–1). During

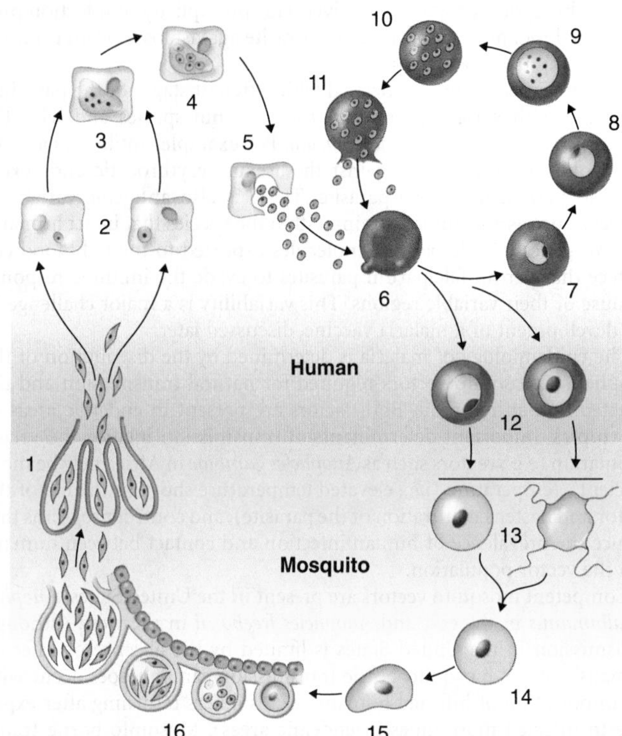

FIGURE 366–1 • Life cycle of the malaria parasite. The upper and lower halves of the diagram indicate the human and anopheline mosquito parts of the cycle, respectively. Sporozoites from the salivary gland of a female *Anopheles* mosquito are injected under the skin (1). They then travel through the blood stream to the liver (2) and mature within hepatocytes to become tissue schizonts (4). Up to 30,000 parasites are then released into the blood stream as merozoites (5) and produce symptomatic infection as they invade and destroy red blood cells. However, some parasites remain dormant in the liver as hypnozoites (2, between 1 and 3). They are the parasites that cause relapsing malaria (in *Plasmodium vivax* or *Plasmodium ovale* infection). Once within the blood stream, merozoites (5) invade red blood cells (6) and mature to the ring (7, 8), trophozoite (9), and schizont (10) asexual stages. Schizonts lyse their host red blood cells as they mature and release the next generation of merozoites (11), which invade previously uninfected red blood cells. Within the red blood cell, some parasites differentiate to sexual forms (male and female gametocytes) (12). When taken up by a female *Anopheles* mosquito, the gametocytes mature to male and female gametes, which produce zygotes (14). The zygote invades the gut of the mosquito (15) and develops into an oocyst (16). Mature oocysts produce sporozoites, which migrate to the salivary gland of the mosquito (1) and repeat the cycle. The horizontal line between 12 and 13 indicates that absence of the mosquito vector prevents natural transmission by means of this cycle. Infection by the injection of contaminated blood bypasses this constraint and permits transmission among intravenous drug addicts or to recipients of blood transfusions. (From Krogstad DJ: Blood and tissue protozoa. *In* Schaechter M, Medoff G, Eisenstein BI [eds]: Mechanisms of Microbial Diseases, 2nd ed. Baltimore, Williams & Wilkins, 1993, p 600.)

the asexual erythrocytic cycle, parasites mature from rings to trophozoites and ultimately to schizonts, which rupture the red blood cell and release merozoites that enter uninfected red blood cells via receptors such as Duffy factor in *P. vivax* infections; they then repeat the asexual cycle. In contrast, some erythrocytic parasites mature to sexual forms (gametocytes) that are ingested by the female anopheline mosquito. Within the mosquito, male and female gametocytes mature to gametes and fuse to form ookinetes that mature to zygotes, which produce the sporozoites that are infectious for humans. When an infected mosquito bites a human, sporozoites travel through the blood stream to the liver, where they enter hepatocytes and mature to tissue schizonts. Tissue schizonts then release merozoites that are infectious for red blood cells and produce the asexual erythrocytic cycle. Two of the four species that infect humans (*P. vivax* and *P. ovale*) produce dormant (hypnozoite) forms in the liver, which may mature 2 to 11 months or more after the initial infection and produce relapsing malaria.

Two characteristics of the life cycle are essential for long-term survival of the parasite: multiplicity of infection and antigenic variability. *Multiplicity of infection* is apparent at each stage of the life cycle. The mature asexual erythrocytic schizont releases 8 to 32 merozoites when it ruptures its host red blood cell, up to 10,000 sporozoites result from one zygote, and 10,000 to 30,000 merozoites are released from each tissue (exoerythrocytic) schizont in the liver. This multiplicity of infection provides a redundancy that protects the parasite against losses from immune and nonimmune host factors.

Antigenic variability is associated with different stages of the parasite's life cycle, with variability among strains within species and with the expression of *var* genes in *P. falciparum.* For example, antibodies against sporozoites are ineffective against the asexual erythrocytic and sexual (gametocyte) stages of the parasite. There is also antigenic variability between species and among strains within the species that infect humans. The *var* genes encode parasite molecules exported to the red blood cell surface that permit falciparum parasites to evade the immune response because of their variable regions. This variability is a major challenge in the development of a malaria vaccine, discussed later.

The epidemiology of malaria is determined by the distribution of the anopheline mosquito vectors required for natural transmission and the infected human reservoir. Both factors are present in endemic areas of the tropics. Important determinants of transmission include the vector population (e.g., vectors such as *Anopheles gambiae* in Africa may be more efficient), temperature (i.e., elevated temperature shortens the life of the vector and hastens maturation of the parasite), and control programs that reduce the prevalence of human infection and contact between humans and the vector population.

Competent mosquito vectors are present in the United States: *Anopheles albimanus* in the east and *Anopheles freeborni* in the west. Although transmission in the United States is limited by the absence of infected humans, natural mosquito-borne transmission can and does occur with the importation of infected humans (e.g., soldiers returning after exposure to infected mosquitoes in endemic areas). Mosquito-borne transmission (i.e., introduced malaria) occurred in the United States after World War II, the Korean War, the Vietnam War, and the arrival of refugees from Southeast Asia.

Pathobiology

Species-Dependent Factors

Malaria is a multifactorial disease that can be explained in part by the magnitude of the parasitemia. *P. falciparum* is the most lethal parasite because it can invade red blood cells of any age and produce unrestricted parasitemia involving 10^6 or more parasitized red blood cells per microliter of blood (>20% of circulating red blood cells). Conversely, *P. vivax* and *P. ovale,* which invade only young red blood cells, are limited to parasitemias less than 25,000/μL, and *P. malariae,* which invades only older red blood cells, is limited to parasitemias of less than 10,000/μL.

Host Immune Response

Because millions of people experience repetitive episodes of malaria throughout their lives in the tropics, the immune response to natural infection is inadequate by definition. The term *semi-immune* is used for residents of endemic areas who are reinfected regularly but are at reduced risk for severe or complicated malaria. The reasons for this incomplete host immune response (i.e., protection against severe disease but not against infection) are not clear but are likely to be key for the development of a successful vaccine. Although virtually all exposed persons make antibodies against the repetitive epitopes on the surface of the sporozoite and although antibodies to asexual stages reduce the magnitude of the parasitemia in children, cell-mediated responses may be essential for effective immunity. Factors potentially responsible for poor cell-mediated responses to sporozoite antigen include host immune restriction related to human leukocyte antigen (HLA) haplotype and the dependence of cellular responses on hypervariable regions downstream from the coding region.

Peripheral Sequestration of Parasitized Red Blood Cells

With maturation, red blood cells with *P. falciparum* parasites develop knobs that contain histidine-rich proteins. In vivo, these knobs adhere to endothelial cells in the peripheral microvasculature by means of receptors such as intercellular adhesion molecule type 1 (ICAM-1), thrombospondin, and CD36. This phenomenon has at least two consequences. First, it exacerbates the microvascular pathology produced by the parasite, and second, it removes mature *P. falciparum* parasites from the circulation so that only early asexual erythrocytic stages, such as rings, are seen on peripheral blood smears.

Cytokines in the Pathogenesis of Malaria

Studies suggest that cytokine release is a central factor in the pathogenesis of severe disease. Cytokines shown to be important include tumor necrosis factor (TNF). Serum levels of TNF are elevated in severe *P. falciparum* infection and correlate with complications such as cerebral malaria and death. Interferon-γ has antiparasitic activity against the exoerythrocytic stages of the parasite in the liver.

The pathology of severe malaria is that of a microvascular disease involving the brain, lung, and kidney. Postmortem examination after fatal *P. falciparum* infection demonstrates parasitized red blood cells in the capillaries and venules of the brain and other affected organs. In severe cases, acute tubular necrosis may be present, and the liver, spleen, and other sites in the reticuloendothelial system may be filled with malarial pigment from the phagocytosis of parasitized red blood cells. This predominantly microvascular pathology is consistent with the roles of sequestration and cytokine release in the pathogenesis of severe disease. In contrast, the other malarias that infect humans produce lower parasitemia, do not sequester, and are rarely fatal.

Clinical Manifestations

Fever and Chills

Most patients with malaria have recurrent fever and chills at 48-hour intervals with *P. vivax* and *P. ovale* and at 72-hour intervals with *P. malariae.* Patients with *P. falciparum* infection typically have irregular fever and chills and rarely have a regular 48-hour cycle of symptoms despite the 48-hour erythrocytic cycle of the asexual parasite.

Coma

Coma (i.e., cerebral malaria) is the most feared complication of *P. falciparum* infection and has a substantial fatality rate. Although it has been attributed to blockage of cerebral capillaries with parasitized red blood cells, hypoglycemia and the effects of cytokines such as TNF-α are important factors. Hypoglycemia in *P. falciparum* malaria may have at least three causes: glucose consumption by the massive numbers of parasites present in the blood, liver glycogen depletion in persons who have not eaten for several days before seeking medical care because they were ill with malaria, and insulin released from pancreatic beta cells by quinine or quinidine during treatment. Hypoglycemia is particularly important because it is readily treatable. Although the effects of TNF contribute to cerebral malaria, it is difficult to separate them from the magnitude of the parasitemia because the concentration of TNF correlates with the magnitude of the parasitemia.

Renal Failure

Patients with massive parasitemia may have dark urine from the free hemoglobin produced by hemolysis (blackwater fever), and renal failure may subsequently develop. Although most patients recover uneventfully, acute renal failure may occur and require dialysis similar to other causes of acute tubular necrosis.

Pulmonary Edema

Pulmonary edema also occurs in patients with high *P. falciparum* parasitemia (≈5% of circulating red blood cells). Hemodynamic measurements indicate that this is a noncardiogenic form of pulmonary edema with normal pulmonary arterial and capillary pressure. These findings and the association with high TNF levels suggest that the pathogenesis of pulmonary edema is similar in severe malaria and bacterial septicemia.

Gastrointestinal Manifestations

Diarrhea is common in children with *P. falciparum* infection. The pathogenesis of this complication is unclear, although postmortem studies of children with diarrhea have revealed parasitized red blood cells in the microvasculature of the intestine.

Diagnosis

Giemsa-Stained Thick and Thin Smears

The most direct way to diagnose malaria is to examine Giemsa-stained, thick or thin smears with oil immersion magnification (1000×). Giemsa

TABLE 366–1 MALARIA PARASITES THAT INFECT HUMANS

Plasmodium Species	Parasitemia (per μL Blood)	Complications	Morphology: Red Blood Cell Stage	Morphology: Schüffner's Dots	Morphology: Stages on Smear	Relapse from Hypnozoites	Antimalarial Resistance
P. falciparum	$\geq 10^6$	Coma (cerebral malaria) Hypoglycemia Pulmonary edema, renal failure Severe malarial anemia (<5 g Hgb/dL)	No RBC enlargement	Absent	Rings, occasional gametocytes	No	Chloroquine, mefloquine, halofantrine, pyrimethamine-sulfadoxine, plus partial resistance to quinine and quinidine
P. vivax	≤25,000	Late splenic rupture (2–3 mo)	Enlarged host RBCs	Present	All stages	Yes	Chloroquine
P. ovale	≤25,000	—	Enlarged host RBCs	Present	All stages	Yes	None known
P. malariae	≤10,000	Immune complex nephrotic syndrome	No RBC enlargement	Absent	All stages	No	None known

Hgb = hemoglobin; RBCs = red blood cells.

stain is preferable to Wright stain, especially for persons with *P. vivax* or *P. ovale* infection, because the Schüffner's dots characteristic of these species may not be visible with Wright stain. Thick smears are more sensitive than thin smears because the red blood cells have been lysed. As a result, approximately 10 times as much blood can be examined per field and therefore per unit of time. However, because the red blood cells have been lysed, it is not possible to determine the effect of the parasite on red blood cell size or the position of the parasite within the red blood cell on a thick smear (Table 366–1). Persons without previous experience reading thick smears should consider using thin smears to identify the infecting parasites. A common mistake is to require characteristic gametocytes for a diagnosis of *P. falciparum* infection. Because gametocytes require longer to develop than asexual parasites do (7 to 10 days vs. 2 days), they are not usually present in peripheral blood during initial infection, such as when nonimmune tourists or expatriates first become ill. Conversely, gametocytes are frequently present in the blood of semi-immune residents of endemic areas with few or no symptoms or asexual parasites. A second common mistake is to assume that the patient can have only one parasite species; approximately 5% of persons with malaria are infected with more than one species.

Antigen Detection

Testing for parasite antigen (e.g., parasite lactate dehydrogenase) is a potential alternative to microscopy for the diagnosis of *P. falciparum* infection, especially in nonendemic areas where skilled microscopists are rare. Potential advantages of this approach include the ability to distinguish between *P. falciparum* and *P. vivax*.

Fluorescent Staining with Acridine Orange (QBC System)

Because parasitized red blood cells are less dense, they are at the top of the red blood cell layer after centrifugation. However, parasites of all species are visualized with fluorescence microscopy because all species stain with acridine orange. For this reason it can be difficult to distinguish among species with this technique.

DNA Probes and Polymerase Chain Reaction

DNA probes and polymerase chain reaction (PCR) methods may both achieve the sensitivity of a thick smear. However, obstacles to the routine use of these methods in endemic areas include the need for nonisotopic labeling of DNA probes versus the cost of a thermocycler and consumable reagents for PCR analysis. For these reasons, neither DNA probes nor PCR is used routinely in malaria-endemic areas.

Serology (Antibody Testing)

Testing for antibodies to plasmodia is of limited value in individual patients because the decision to treat must be made in the first few hours of evaluation whereas 3 to 4 weeks may be required to develop a diagnostic rise in antibody titer. In endemic areas, most persons have antibody titers from previous infections regardless of whether they have been infected recently. Serology may be of value retrospectively in nonimmune persons (e.g., expatriate tourists) who have been treated empirically for malaria without a microscopic diagnosis. For example, a high titer of antibodies to *P. vivax* suggests that the patient had a *P. vivax* infection recently and should receive primaquine to prevent relapse, if primaquine had not been given previously.

Treatment

Successful treatment of patients with malaria depends primarily on the use of effective antimalarial drugs, but it also depends on ancillary measures as diverse as the infusion of glucose and dialysis. Monitoring of the blood glucose level during initial therapy is important because hypoglycemia is a common cause of coma and both quinine and quinidine stimulate the release of insulin directly from pancreatic beta cells. Steroids are contraindicated in cerebral malaria because they prolong the duration of coma.

The use of chloroquine for the treatment of susceptible malaria isolates (*P. vivax, P. ovale, P. malariae*, and chloroquine-susceptible *P. falciparum*) is satisfactory (Table 366–2) because chloroquine is a safe and effective antimalarial. Patients with chloroquine-resistant *P. vivax* have alternatively been treated with mefloquine or halofantrine. However, treatment of chloroquine-resistant *P. falciparum* infection is more complicated. In areas without mefloquine resistance, patients able to tolerate oral medications may be treated with oral mefloquine alone. In areas with mefloquine resistance, treatments include quinine plus pyrimethamine-sulfadoxine, doxycycline, or clindamycin; and atovaquone plus proguanil (see Table 366–2).

The major factor responsible for the resurgence of malaria is drug resistance: the widespread resistance of the anopheline vector to

TABLE 366–2 TREATMENT OF MALARIA

Drug	Dosage
CHLOROQUINE-RESISTANT *P. FALCIPARUM*	
FOR PATIENTS ABLE TO TAKE ORAL MEDICATIONS	
PO quinine	650 mg quinine sulfate q8h × 3–7 days
plus	
PO doxycycline (Vibramycin)	100 mg bid × 7 days
or plus	
PO tetracycline	250 mg qid × 7 days
or plus	
PO clindamycin	20 mg/kg/day in 3 doses × 7 days
or	
PO atovaquone	1000 mg/day atovaquone (2 Malarone tablets bid) × 3 days
plus	
Proguanil (Malarone)	400 mg/day proguanil (2 Malarone tablets per day) × 3 days
or	
PO mefloquine*	15 mg base/kg (750 mg), followed by 10 mg base/kg 500 mg (500 mg) in 8–12 hr. Can also be given as a single 1250-mg dose, though less well tolerated
or	
PO artesunate†	4 mg/kg/day × 3 days‡
plus	
PO mefloquine	25 mg base/kg (750 mg), followed by 10 mg base/kg 500 mg (500 mg) in 8–12 hr
PO lumefantine plus artemether (Coartem)†	80 mg artemether and 480 mg lumefantrine (4 tablets) at 0 and 8 hr on day 1, followed by the same doses at 0 and 8 hr on days 2 and 3 (total dose of 24 tablets for adults containing a total of 480 mg artemether and 2880 mg lumefantrine over the course)
FOR PATIENTS UNABLE TO TOLERATE ORAL MEDICATIONS	
IV quinidine	6.25 mg base/kg (10 mg gluconate salt/kg, up to a maximum of 600 mg salt) in normal saline over 1- to 2-hr period, followed by 0.125 mg base/kg (0.02 mg gluconate salt/kg)/min until parasitemia is <1% or the patient tolerates oral medications
or	
IV quinine	16.7 mg/kg base (20 mg dihydrochloride salt/kg) loading dose in D_5W over 4-hr period, followed by 8.3 mg base/kg (10 mg/kg dihydrochloride salt/kg) over 2- to 4-hr period, with the maintenance dose repeated q8h until the patient tolerates oral medications. Maximum daily dose, 1800 mg dihydrochloride salt/day
or	
IM quinine	8.3 mg base/kg (10 mg dihydrochloride salt/kg) q8h until able to take oral medications; may begin with 16.7 mg base/kg (20 mg quinine dihydrochloride salt/kg) loading dose. Divide the dose in half, and administer both into the thighs, not the buttock
or	
IM artemether†	3.2 mg/kg initially on day 0, followed by 1.6 mg/kg/day × 5–7 days‡
FOR MULTIPLY RESISTANT *P. FALCIPARUM*	
PR artesunate†	1200–1600 mg PO over 3 days‡
or	
PO artesunate†	1200–1600 mg PR × 3 days‡
plus	
PO mefloquine	750 mg, followed by 500 mg 12 hr later
CHLOROQUINE-RESISTANT *P. VIVAX*	
PO quinine	650 mg quinine sulfate q8h × 3–7 days
plus	
Doxycycline (Vibramycin)	100 mg bid × 7 days
or	
PO mefloquine	750 mg, followed by 500 mg in 8–12 hr
or	
PO chloroquine	25 mg base/kg over 3 days
plus	
PO primaquine§	2.5 mg base/kg divided into 3 doses, administered over 48-hr period
P. VIVAX, P. OVALE, P. MALARIAE,* AND CHLOROQUINE-SUSCEPTIBLE *P. FALCIPARUM	
FOR PATIENTS ABLE TO TAKE ORAL MEDICATIONS	
PO chloroquine§	10 mg base/kg = 600 mg base, followed by an additional 5 mg base/kg (maximum, 300 mg base) after 6, 24, and 48 hr (1500 mg base total = 2500 mg chloroquine phosphate salt)
FOR PATIENTS UNABLE TO TAKE ORAL MEDICATIONS	
IM chloroquine	2.5 mg base/kg IM q4h or 3.5 mg/kg q6h (total dose not to exceed 25 mg/kg base)
IV chloroquine	10 mg base/kg over 4-hr period, followed by 5 mg/kg base q12h (given in a 2-hr infusion; total dose not to exceed 25 mg base/kg)
TO PREVENT RELAPSE OF *P. VIVAX* OR *P. OVALE* INFECTION	
PO primaquine§	30 mg primaquine base (26.3 mg primaquine phosphate) daily × 14 days

Dosages are for adult dosing.
*For areas without mefloquine resistance.
†Not yet available in the United States.
‡Doses used vary among investigators for intramuscular artemether on subsequent days of treatment (after the initial 3.2-mg/kg dose) from 0.8 to 1.6 mg/kg for 4 to 7 days and for oral artesunate as 12 mg/kg over a 3- to 7-day period; for per rectum (PR) artesunate, the information available suggests that effective PR doses are likely to be approximately four times greater than oral doses.
§To prevent potentially severe hemolysis, patients should be tested for glucose-6-phosphate dehydrogenase deficiency before treatment with primaquine.
D_5W = 5% dextrose in water.

Rx

economical insecticides such as chlorophenothane (dichlorodiphenyltrichloroethane, DDT) and the increasing prevalence of resistance to chloroquine and pyrimethamine-sulfadoxine (Fansidar) in *P. falciparum,* which is established in South America, Southeast Asia, and Africa.

Antimalarial combinations with artemisinins are being used with increasing frequency to reduce the risk for resistance. Although artemisinins are used extensively in endemic areas because they are rapidly effective against resistant parasites, they are embryotoxic in rodents and have not been approved by the U.S. Food and Drug Administration. For patients who cannot tolerate oral medications, potential strategies include intravenous quinidine, intravenous quinine, intramuscular quinine, and intramuscular artemether or artesunate, which are reported to be effective without detectable neurologic toxicity. However, intravenous quinidine must be used under close monitoring and in a telemetry unit whenever possible because it has been associated with QT prolongation, hypotension, hypoglycemia, and cardiac dysrhythmias. Because quinidine gluconate can be difficult to obtain, physicians may obtain advice on potential sources by calling the CDC Malaria Hot Line at 770-488-7788 (770-488-7100 after regular hours). The general principle of parenteral treatment is to stabilize patients until they can tolerate oral medications. Oral regimens are available for multiply resistant *P. falciparum.*

Patients with *P. vivax* or *P. ovale* infection should be tested for glucose-6-phosphate dehydrogenase deficiency before treatment with primaquine, which is used for eradication of persistent hypnozoites in the liver to prevent relapse.

Prevention

Exposed nonimmune persons may reduce their risk for malaria by taking antimalarials prospectively (i.e., chemoprophylaxis), by using insect repellents and insecticide-impregnated bed nets to reduce contact with the anopheline vector, and possibly in the future by a malaria vaccine (i.e., immunoprophylaxis).

Chemoprophylaxis

Drugs used for chemoprophylaxis must be safe because they are given to healthy persons for long periods. Several have been chosen for their long serum half-lives so that they can be given infrequently. On the basis of these criteria, chloroquine is an excellent drug for chemoprophylaxis in areas without chloroquine-resistant *P. falciparum* (Table 366–3). It is the only chemoprophylactic agent known to be safe for pregnant women and does not produce retinal toxicity at the doses used for antimalarial chemoprophylaxis. Unfortunately, strains of *P. falciparum* resistant to chloroquine and to pyrimethamine-sulfadoxine are established in Southeast Asia, South America, and Africa. For areas with chloroquine-resistant *P. falciparum,* mefloquine is the recommended chemoprophylactic agent, although resistance to mefloquine is developing in Southeast Asia and South America. Doxycycline and atovaquone-proguanil are alternatives. The advantage of doxycycline is that it reduces the frequency of traveler's diarrhea; its disadvantages include the need for daily dosing, photosensitivity reactions, and yeast vaginitis. Major disadvantages of atovaquone-proguanil are its cost and the recent appearance of resistance. Because of the potential for serious hypersensitivity reactions to pyrimethamine-sulfadoxine, it is not generally recommended for chemoprophylaxis. For patients taking other medications, it is important to check for drug-drug interactions that may lower serum levels of the chemoprophylaxis agent.

Vector Control

Because of widespread *P. falciparum* drug resistance, increasing emphasis has been placed on reducing exposure to the anopheline vector. Strategies that are successful and should be considered include pyrethrin (insecticide)-impregnated bed nets and insect repellents containing diethyltoluamide (DEET) or picaridin. DDT is no longer effective in most regions of the world because of widespread mosquito resistance.

TABLE 366–3 CHEMOPROPHYLAXIS OF MALARIA*

Drug	Regimen
FOR AREAS WITH CHLOROQUINE-RESISTANT *PLASMODIUM FALCIPARUM*	
Mefloquine (Lariam)	250 mg/wk. Start 1 week before travel; continue weekly during exposure and for 4 wk after leaving the endemic area
Doxycycline	100 mg/day. Start 1 week before travel; continue daily during exposure and for 4 wk after leaving the endemic area
Atovaquone-proguanil (Malarone)	250 mg/day–100 mg/day (1 Malarone tablet) starting 1–2 days before travel; continue daily during exposure and for 1 wk after leaving the endemic area
Primaquine	30 mg daily during exposure and for 1 wk after leaving the endemic area
FOR AREAS WITHOUT CHLOROQUINE-RESISTANT *PLASMODIUM FALCIPARUM*	
Chloroquine phosphate (Aralen)	500 mg/wk (300 mg chloroquine base) starting 1 week before travel; continue during exposure and for 4 wk after leaving the endemic area

*Alternatives for areas with chloroquine-resistant *P. falciparum* include weekly chloroquine plus daily proguanil (200 mg/day; note that the chloroquine + proguanil regimen has not been approved by the Food and Drug Administration and that breakthroughs occur with some frequency in areas with chloroquine-resistant *P. falciparum*) and weekly chloroquine plus single-dose presumptive treatment as needed with pyrimethamine-sulfadoxine (Fansidar) for presumed breakthrough infection with 75 and 1500 mg of pyrimethamine and sulfadoxine (3 tablets), respectively. In the United States, updated information on malaria chemoprophylaxis may be obtained from Centers for Disease Control and Prevention (CDC) hotlines at 770-488-7788 (770-488-7100 after hours, ask to page the malaria person on call), 404-639-2888, and 404-332-4565 and from the CDC and *Medical Letter* websites at *www.cdc.gov* and *www.medletter.com*, respectively; see also Med Lett Drugs Ther 2004;46:1–12 and 2005;47:100–103.

Immunoprophylaxis—Development of a Malaria Vaccine

Although a malaria vaccine is not available, it is hoped that this goal will ultimately be achievable. Because the three major parasite stages in humans are antigenically distinct, a successful vaccine will probably need to contain at least three parasite antigens (e.g., sporozoite, merozoite, gametocyte). A recent encouraging study found efficacies of 35 and 49% for protecting children against uncomplicated and severe malaria. However, a vaccine need not be 100% effective to be valuable. For example, a vaccine that requires boosting could be quite effective for residents of endemic areas because of repetitive exposure to natural infection. Alternatively, a vaccine that limits the magnitude of parasitemia could improve the survival of nonimmune persons even if it had no effect on the incidence of infection because high parasitemia produces severe morbidity and death in nonimmune persons.

Prognosis

Most patients with *P. vivax, P. ovale,* or *P. malariae* infection respond well to chloroquine and make an uneventful recovery. Chloroquine-resistant strains of *P. vivax* have responded to treatment with mefloquine or halofantrine. For patients with *P. falciparum* infection, the quantitative parasite count is the best predictor of outcome. Patients with greater than 5% parasitemia (≈250,000 parasites/μL of blood) are at increased risk for severe and complicated malaria, including death. In addition to standard antimalarial treatment directed at the parasite (see Table 366–2), such patients may require glucose for hypoglycemia, treatment of acidosis, dialysis for renal failure, and respiratory support. The role of exchange transfusion is controversial, in part because there have been no controlled clinical trials. Oral treatment, including nasogastric administration, may be successful even in patients with severe or cerebral malaria.

SUGGESTED READINGS

Alonso P, Sacarlal J, Apnte JJ, et al: Duration of protection with RTX,S/AS02A malaria vaccine in prevention of *Plasmodium falciparum* disease in Mozambican children: Single-blind extended follow-up of a randomized clinical trial. Lancet 2005;366:2012–2018. *Encouraging evidence for 35 and 49% protection against uncomplicated and severe malaria that persists for at least 18 months in children younger than 5 years.*

Chen LH, Wilson ME, Schlagenhauf P: Prevention of malaria in long-term travelers. JAMA 2006;296:2234–2244. *Long-term travelers have a higher risk of malaria than short-term travelers, and long-term travelers underuse personal protective measures and adhere poorly to continuous chemoprophylaxis regimens.*

Greenwood BM, Bojang K, Whitty CJ, et al: Malaria. Lancet 2005;365:1487–1498. *A comprehensive review.*

Laufer MK, Thesing PC, Eddington ND, et al: Return of chloroquine antimalarial efficacy in Malawi. N Engl J Med 2006;355:1959–1966. *Randomized trial showed 99% efficacy of chloroquine among children in Malawi.*

Marx A, Pewsner D, Egger M, et al: Meta-analysis: Accuracy of rapid tests for malaria in travelers returning from endemic areas. Ann Intern Med 2005;142:836–846. *Rapid malaria tests may be a useful diagnostic adjunct to microscopy in centers without major expertise in tropical medicine although microscopy is still required for species identification and confirmation.*

Ratcliff A, Siswantoro H, Kenangalem E, et al: Two fixed-dose artemisinin combinations for drug-resistant falciparum and vivax malaria in Papua, Indonesia: An open-label randomised comparison. Lancet 2007;369:757–765. *Both combinations were safe and effective, although the dihydroartemisinin-piperaquine provided greater post-treatment prophylaxis than did artemether-lumefantrine.*

367 AFRICAN TRYPANOSOMIASIS (SLEEPING SICKNESS)

Thomas C. Quinn

Definition

Known widely as sleeping sickness, African trypanosomiasis is an acute and chronic disease caused by the flagellated protozoan parasite *Trypanosoma brucei*. The parasites are transmitted to humans through the bite of tsetse flies located in 36 countries of Africa between 15 degrees north and 15 degrees south latitude. In humans, there are two distinct forms of the disease: East African trypanosomiasis caused by *T. brucei rhodesiense* and West African trypanosomiasis caused by *T. brucei gambiense*. Although there is some clinical overlap, East African trypanosomiasis primarily causes an acute febrile illness with myocarditis and meningoencephalitis that is rapidly fatal if not treated, whereas West African trypanosomiasis is characterized as a chronic debilitating disease with mental deterioration and physical wasting (Table 367–1). A closely related variant, *T. brucei brucei*, is noninfectious for humans but causes a chronic wasting illness in cattle, called *nagana*, that has a considerable indirect effect on human nutrition in sub-Saharan Africa.

The Pathogens

Trypanosomes are motile hemoflagellates with a single undulating membrane that passes along the length of the parasite and terminates in an anterior flagellum (Fig. 367–1). Located anteriorly is a kinetoplast, an organelle containing topologically interlocked circular DNA molecules and mitochondria. In the peripheral blood of humans, trypanosomes vary in length from 10 to 40 μm. Both short, stumpy and long, slender forms can be present in a patient at the same time. The different variants of *T. brucei* cannot be distinguished morphologically but can be identified by differences in pathogenicity for certain animals, as well as differences in biochemical requirements, electrophoretic pattern of component enzymes, and DNA hybridization.

T. brucei is transmitted by the tsetse fly *Glossina*, within which it undergoes several developmental changes. When biting an infected host, trypanosomes are ingested and, within the insect's midgut, rapidly differentiate into procyclic forms with loss of their dense surface coat, which is composed of variant surface glycoprotein (VSG). After 2 to 3 weeks of multiplication within the midgut, the procyclic trypanosomes migrate to the insect's salivary glands, where they change morphologically into epimastigotes. These forms then undergo further multiplication and ultimately differentiate into metacyclic trypanosomes that are coated with characteristic VSG and are infectious to mammalian hosts. When a new host is bitten by the tsetse fly, the trypanosomes present in the salivary glands are injected into connective tissue and blood. Within the human host they divide by binary fission and undergo antigen variation, a process by which they continually change their VSGs and evade the immune system of the host. With the bite of another tsetse fly, ingestion of the parasite occurs, and the life cycle of the organism is completed (Fig. 367–2). Mechanical transmission can theoretically also occur via blood

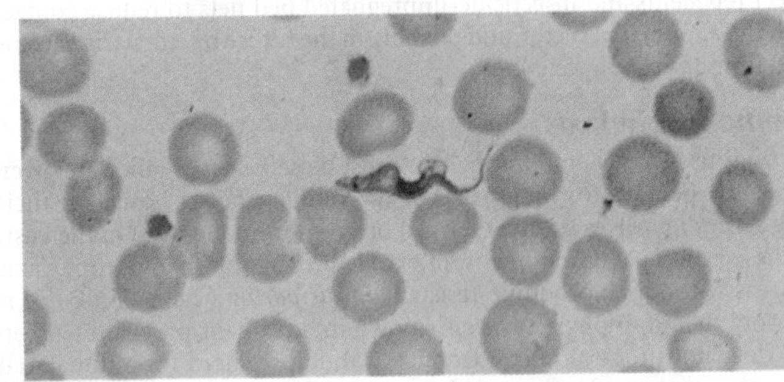

FIGURE 367–1 • *Trypanosoma rhodesiense* in peripheral blood. It has a nucleus, posterior kinetoplast, undulating membrane, and flagellum (×1500).

TABLE 367–1 COMPARISON OF GAMBIAN AND RHODESIAN SLEEPING SICKNESS

	Gambian (West African)	Rhodesian (East African)
Etiologic agent	*Trypanosoma brucei gambiense*	*Trypanosoma brucei rhodesiense*
Vector	*Glossina palpalis* or *tachinoides* (riverine tsetse)	*Glossina morsitans* (savanna tsetse)
Distribution	Western and central Africa	Eastern Africa
Reservoir	Humans (domestic animals)	Wild game
Course of infection	Slow (months–years)	Rapid (<1 yr)
Clinical features		
Lymphadenopathy	++ (Winterbottom's sign)	±
Myocarditis, heart failure	–	++
Neurologic symptoms	++	+
Disseminated intravascular coagulation	–	+
Parasitemia	Low	High

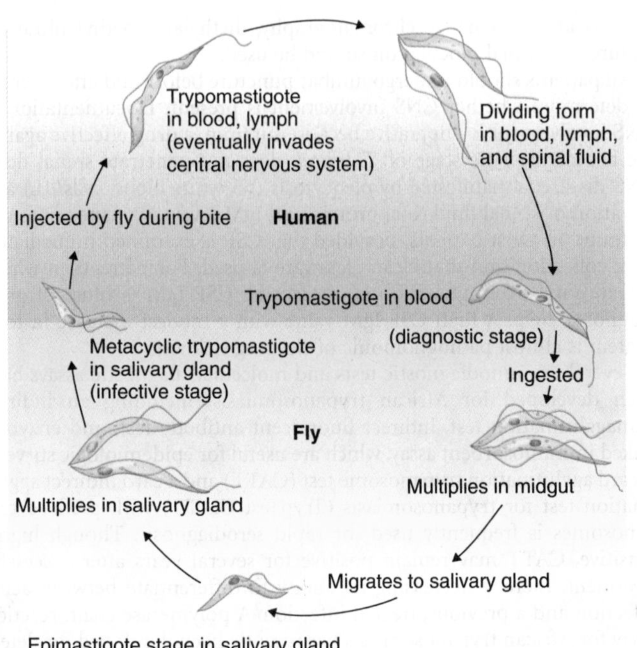

FIGURE 367–2 • Life cycle of *Trypanosoma (Trypanozoon) brucei, Trypanosoma (Trypanozoon) brucei gambiense,* and *Trypanosoma (Trypanozoon) brucei rhodesiense.*

transfusion or by interrupted biting of a tsetse fly feeding on an infectious person and directly thereafter biting an uninfected individual.

Epidemiology

It is estimated that 400,000 people are currently suffering from African trypanosomiasis, more than 100,000 Africans become infected annually, and 66,000 people die of it each year. Approximately 50 million people in 36 African countries live at risk of acquiring trypanosomiasis because of the presence of the disease and its vector, and the disease is responsible for more than 2 million disability-adjusted life years lost annually. Within recent years there has been a resurgence of African trypanosomiasis, particularly in central African countries such as Sudan, Uganda, Angola, and the Democratic Republic of the Congo, because of decreased surveillance, prophylaxis, and treatment as a result of war and civil unrest. In some areas the prevalence of African trypanosomiasis has increased 10-fold over the past decade. Approximately 4 million square miles in Africa remain unpopulated because of the presence of *T. brucei brucei* infection, which results in loss of domestic and wild animals, including cattle, waterbuck, bushbuck, and buffalo.

T. brucei gambiense occurs primarily in the western and central regions of sub-Saharan Africa. Although it primarily infects humans, there may be animal reservoirs such as pigs, dogs, and sheep. Gambian sleeping sickness is spread mainly by three species of tsetse fly: *Glossina palpalis, Glossina tachinoides,* and *Glossina fuscipes.* Distribution of these flies includes shaded areas along rivers and streams, where the conditions of temperature, darkness, and moisture are optimum.

T. brucei rhodesiense differs from *T. brucei gambiense* in that it is primarily a parasite of wild game, with humans serving only as occasional hosts. The geographic distribution of *T. brucei rhodesiense* is primarily eastern Africa from Ethiopia and eastern Uganda south to Zambia and Botswana. Rhodesian sleeping sickness is spread by tsetse flies of the *Glossina morsitans* group, including *Glossina pallidipes* and *Glossina swynnertoni.* These flies can survive in the open savanna, and Rhodesian sleeping sickness usually occurs in individuals visiting or traveling through an endemic area. Consequently, hunters, fishermen, and tourists are at risk by exposing themselves to vectors that usually feed on wild animals.

Imported African trypanosomiasis is a rare disease with only 20 to 30 cases reported to the Centers for Disease Control and Prevention over the past 2 decades. Most cases were due to *T. brucei rhodesiense* acquired by Americans who had been on safari in East Africa for a brief period. Nearly all these cases were initially misdiagnosed because of the unfamiliarity of U.S. physicians with this disease. With an increase in international travel, 20,000 Americans are now estimated to visit endemic areas yearly, and approximately 10,000 aliens enter the United States each year from countries in Africa where the infection is endemic.

Pathobiology

After the bite of a tsetse fly, trypanosomes accumulate in connective tissue, where they multiply to produce a local chancre (trypanoma). Subsequent spread of the organisms through the lymphatics results in enlargement of lymph nodes secondary to reactive plasma cell and macrophage infiltration. The trypanosomes eventually disseminate to the circulatory system, where the parasitemia usually remains at low intensity and the organisms multiply by binary fission. Systemic African trypanosomiasis without central nervous system (CNS) involvement is generally referred to as *stage I disease.*

The host's immune response plays an integral role in the pathogenesis of African sleeping sickness, although the exact nature of the immunopathogenic reactions has not been clearly defined. Trypanosomes survive by periodically altering their surface antigenic coat, thereby avoiding successful eradication by the host. Any single parasite may contain some 1000 genes for VSG that can be activated in a variety of ways and selected by the host's antibody response. Consequently, trypanosomes occur in the peripheral blood of infected individuals in waves, with each parasite wave consisting of a serologically distinct organism.

Tissue damage is induced by either toxin production or immune complex reaction with release of proteolytic enzymes. Immune complexes consisting of variant antigens of the organism and complement-fixing antibodies have been demonstrated in both the circulation and the target organs of infected patients. Production of autoantibodies is a prominent feature, and they are frequently directed against antigen components of red blood cells, brain, and heart. Thus, the host-parasite interaction can result in generalized febrile episodes, lymphadenopathy, and myocardial and pericardial inflammation, along with anemia, thrombocytopenia, disseminated intravascular coagulation, and renal disease primarily during the acute stage of the disease.

Stage II of human African trypanosomiasis involves invasion of the CNS, which occurs during the period of circulatory dissemination when trypanosomes localize in the small vessels of the CNS. Pathologic changes in the CNS are most prominent in chronic cases of Gambian sleeping sickness. The meninges are thickened and infiltrated with lymphocytes, plasma cells, and morular cells. Morular cells are modified plasma cells (20 µm in diameter) with large granular inclusions that have been shown to consist of immunoglobulin. These cells may play an important role in the local production of immunoglobulin M (IgM) in cerebrospinal fluid (CSF). Edema, hemorrhage, and granulomatous lesions are frequently present, along with thrombosis as a result of endarteritis, as well as neuronal degeneration.

African trypanosomes appear to induce a state of B-cell polyclonal activation caused either by interference with the host's T-cell control of antibody production or by a B-cell mitogen released by the parasite. Polyclonal hypergammaglobulinemia, with very high levels of IgM, is commonly seen. High levels of nonspecific heterophile antibody, rheumatoid factor, and autoantibodies are also produced. In patients with late-stage *T. brucei gambiense* disease, circulating levels of tumor necrosis factor-α and interleukin-10 are markedly elevated, but they decline after effective treatment.

Clinical Manifestations

The signs and symptoms of sleeping sickness differ according to the infecting organism (see Table 367–1). Rhodesian sleeping sickness, caused by *T. brucei rhodesiense,* is a rapid, progressive disease that often results in cardiac failure and acute neurologic manifestations. Gambian sleeping sickness, caused by *T. brucei gambiense,* is typically a more chronic illness with primarily neurologic features. However, this difference is not absolute; in some cases Gambian sleeping sickness can progress rapidly, and occasionally Rhodesian sleeping sickness may follow a more chronic course.

Gambian Sleeping Sickness

Within several days after a bite by an infected tsetse fly, a trypanosomal nodule or chancre develops, typically on the exposed parts of the body. Within a week the lesion becomes a hard, painful nodule surrounded by erythema and swelling, which persists for 1 to 2 weeks. After this incubation period, clinical features develop after systemic, lymphatic, and circulatory invasion of trypanosomes. Fever, headache, dizziness, and weakness occur in the majority of these patients. Febrile episodes may last 1 to 6 days, alternating with afebrile periods. Lymphadenopathy with prominent supraclavicular and posterior cervical enlargement is seen in more than 80% of infected individuals. Known as *Winterbottom's sign,* these enlarged lymph nodes are usually discrete, rubbery, and painless. Moderate splenomegaly may occur, and urticaria and erythematous rashes have also been observed. Electrocardiograms are often abnormal, but clinical signs of heart disease are unusual.

Six months to several years after symptoms first appear, the clinical features of this early hemolymphatic stage progress to a late meningoencephalitic stage. Behavioral and personality changes are often the first signs of CNS involvement. Later, more florid psychological changes consisting of hallucinations and delusions may occur. Reversion of sleep rhythm is characteristic, with drowsiness during the day, a feature from which the disease derives its name. Other nervous system symptoms include tremor, most characteristically of the face and lips, and hyperesthesia, which causes some patients to avoid common practices such as closing (Kerandel's sign) or locking doors (key sign). Without treatment, the patient's level of consciousness progressively deteriorates until there is lapse into stupor. Alterations in thermoregulation may lead to hypothermia or hyperthermia, and progressive neurologic alterations lead to convulsions, chorea, and athetosis. Adrenal insufficiency, hypothyroidism, and hypogonadism are frequently observed, and pituitary function tests suggest an unusual combined central (hypothalamic/pituitary) and peripheral defect in hormone secretion. CSF shows an increase in cells and protein, much of which is IgM. Free immunoglobulin light chains may be present. Most of the cells are lymphocytes, but a few are plasma cells and morular cells. Trypanosomes may also be evident within CSF.

Rhodesian Sleeping Sickness

This disease is more acute than Gambian sleeping sickness, and symptoms generally occur a few days after the victim has been bitten by a tsetse fly. Alternating periods of high fever, malaise, and headache, followed by several days of well-being, are often misinterpreted as acute malaria infection. Lymphadenopathy is not prominent in this variety of the disease, and Winterbottom's sign is usually absent. Tachycardia with arrhythmias and extrasystoles is common. Anemia, thrombocytopenia, and disseminated intravascular coagulation are generally evident within the first several weeks of infection. Liver enzyme values are often elevated, and electrocardiograms are abnormal, usually reflecting underlying myocarditis. Neurologic features are similar to those described for Gambian sleeping sickness, but they occur much earlier and with more rapid deterioration. Without treatment, the disease may result in death within a matter of weeks to months, without clear distinction into an early and late phase, as described for Gambian trypanosomiasis.

Diagnosis

Although a presumptive diagnosis of trypanosomiasis is based on clinical suspicion, a history of travel to areas where this disease is endemic, and tsetse fly exposure, confirmation of the diagnosis is based solely on the demonstration of trypanosomes. These organisms may be found in blood (see Fig. 367–1), bone marrow, centrifuged CSF, lymph node aspirates, and scrapings from the chancre. Giemsa or Wright staining of the buffy coat of centrifuged heparinized blood makes identification easier because the trypanosomes are often concentrated in the buffy coat. In one technique, referred to as the *quantitative buffy coat,* 60 μL of blood obtained by a finger prick is drawn up in a glass hematocrit tube precoated with acridine orange and anticoagulant (QBC, Becton Dickinson, Franklin Lakes, NJ). After centrifugation, the buffy coat can be examined and trypanosomes fluoresce greenish yellow, remain motile, and are easily identified. In patients with Gambian sleeping sickness, in which trypanosomes are found less frequently in blood, concentration methods such as anion exchange chromatography, diethylaminoethyl filtration, culture, or animal inoculation should be used.

All patients should undergo lumbar puncture before and after therapy to determine whether CNS involvement is present. Documentation of CNS involvement is imperative because suramin, a drug effective against the hemolymphatic stage of *T. brucei,* does not penetrate spinal fluid. CNS disease is manifested by pleocytosis (>5 white blood cells/μL) and elevation of spinal fluid total protein and IgM levels. Trypanosomes can be found in most patients, provided that CSF is examined immediately after collection and that clean glassware is used. For patients in whom trypanosomes cannot be found, measuring CSF IgM is often of great diagnostic help. A high CSF IgM value with a modest increase in total protein is almost pathognomonic of sleeping sickness.

Several immunodiagnostic tests and molecular diagnostic assays have been developed for African trypanosomiasis, including an indirect hemagglutination test, indirect fluorescent antibody test, and enzyme-linked immunosorbent assay, which are useful for epidemiologic surveys. A card agglutination trypanosome test (CATT) and a card indirect agglutination test for trypanosomiasis (TrypTest CIATT) with prefixed trypanosomes is frequently used for rapid serodiagnosis. Though highly sensitive, CATT may remain positive for several years after successful treatment, thereby decreasing its ability to differentiate between acute infection and a previous, treated infection. A polymerase chain reaction assay for African trypanosomiasis has recently been developed for detection of trypanosomal DNA in blood and CSF. Although the test is highly sensitive, its specificity for detection of active disease still needs to be determined more accurately in large clinical trials. A novel test using proteomic signature analysis has also been developed and found to have high sensitivity and specificity (100 and 98.6%, respectively). Evaluation of this test in larger clinical trials is also warranted.

Treatment

Suramin* is the drug of choice for the early hemolymphatic stage of both *T. brucei gambiense* and *T. brucei rhodesiense* infections before CNS invasion has occurred. Suramin does not cross the blood-brain barrier adequately, and it does not cure the disease once CNS invasion has occurred. The dose is 20 mg/kg of body weight given slowly intravenously up to a maximum single dose of 1 g. Suramin is freshly prepared as a 10% aqueous solution. Intramuscular injection is not advised because of local irritation and pain. Suramin binds to plasma proteins and may persist in the circulation at low concentrations for as long as 3 months. A test dose of 100 to 200 mg is given initially; if no adverse side effects are noted, full doses of the drug may be given on days 1, 3, 7, 14, and 21. A single course for an adult is usually 5 g; it should not exceed 7 g.

Suramin is a toxic drug that may result in idiosyncratic reactions in some individuals (1 in 20,000). The drug is excreted entirely by the kidneys; renal damage may result because the drug is deposited in the renal tubules. The drug should not be given to patients with preexisting renal insufficiency. Urine should be examined before administering each dose of suramin, and if proteinuria or casts are present, treatment should be stopped. Other side effects include a papular eruption, photophobia, arthralgias, peripheral neuritis, fever, and agranulocytosis.

Pentamidine isethionate* is an alternative drug for treating early hemolymphatic African trypanosomiasis, but it is much less active against *T. brucei rhodesiense* than suramin is. The dose is 4 mg/kg body weight given every other day by intramuscular injection for a total of 10 injections. Pentamidine is also ineffective for treating CNS trypanosomiasis.

The arsenical melarsoprol* is the treatment of choice for both Gambian and Rhodesian sleeping sickness once involvement of the CNS has occurred. The drug is given in three courses of 3 days each. The recommended dosage is 2 to 3.6 mg/kg/day given intravenously in three divided doses for 3 days, followed 1 week later by 3.6 mg/kg/day in three divided doses for 3 days. This latter course is then

*Available from the Centers for Disease Control and Prevention, Atlanta, GA.

Rx

repeated 10 to 21 days later. A recent trial showed similar efficacy with 10 daily injections of 2.2 mg/kg of melarsoprol instead of the standard 26-day course, although additional studies are required to examine the long-term effects from either treatment regimen. Melarsoprol is a highly toxic drug and should be administered with great care. If signs of arsenical toxicity occur, the drug should be discontinued. The most important side effects involve the CNS. A reactive encephalopathy, probably caused by release of trypanosomal antigens, may occur early in the course of treatment, and its incidence has been reported to be as high as 18%. It may develop very rapidly or insidiously and has a high mortality rate. Clinical indications of reactive encephalopathy include high fever, headache, tremor, seizures, and finally coma. It has been suggested that corticosteroids protect patients from melarsoprol encephalopathy, but this assertion has not been clearly documented.

An alternative drug for both systemic and CNS involvement by *T. brucei gambiense* infection is difluoromethylornithine (eflornithine, DFMO), a specific, irreversible inhibitor of orboxylase. In a large trial of 207 patients with late-stage *T. brucei gambiense* sleeping sickness, eflornithine was highly effective in successful treating both the hemolymphatic and CNS stages of infection. Eflornithine dramatically reduced symptoms and rapidly cleared parasites from blood and CSF, even in patients who had relapsed after melarsoprol therapy. The recommended dosage is 400 mg/kg/day given intravenously in four divided doses for 2 weeks, followed by 300 mg/kg/day given orally in four doses for 30 days. In a multicenter, randomized, controlled trial of 321 patients, a 7-day course of eflornithine was effective in the treatment of relapsing cases of Gambian trypanosomiasis but was inferior to the 14-day course for treatment of new cases. Frequent side effects include diarrhea and anemia. Unfortunately, its efficacy in patients with *T. brucei rhodesiense* infection has been quite variable, and its cost and long duration of therapy have limited its usefulness in the field. In addition, immunocompromised patients such as those with human immunodeficiency virus infection do not respond to treatment as effectively with any of the earlier mentioned agents because a normal immune response is necessary for cure. Regular follow-up with clinical examination and lumbar puncture is necessary in all patients for at least a year after treatment. New promising compounds for the treatment of African trypanosomiasis include aromatic diamidines and imidazopyridines, which are now in clinical or preclinical phases.

Control and Prevention

Measures to prevent and control African trypanosomiasis can be instituted at three different levels: surveillance and treatment, chemoprophylaxis, and vector control. Surveillance plus treatment is necessary to reduce the human reservoir of infection, particularly in areas where epidemics have occurred in the past. Pentamidine has been successfully used as a chemoprophylactic for Gambian sleeping sickness after mass screening and treatment of seropositive and trypanosomal-positive individuals, regardless of symptoms. Pentamidine is given as a single intramuscular injection of 4 mg/kg every 3 to 6 months. However, the drug is not generally recommended for mass use, and it appears to be ineffective against Rhodesian trypanosomiasis.

Vector control requires destruction of tsetse fly habitats by selective clearing of vegetation and spraying with insecticides, which are effective only temporarily. Because of the wide range of the tsetse fly, these vector control measures are not economically feasible except when it is necessary to break transmission in epidemics. For individual protection, avoidance of contact with infected tsetse flies is best achieved by the use of repellents and protective clothing.

A vaccine is not currently available because of the occurrence of antigenic variation. However, the potential for development of a vaccine has increased with progress in cultivation of *T. brucei* in vitro and analysis of the chemical structure of its variant antigens.

Prognosis

Untreated African sleeping sickness is almost invariably fatal. Many patients with early Gambian sleeping sickness may remain relatively well for months to years without treatment, but once CNS involvement has occurred, death is inevitable unless treatment is given. Death frequently results from pneumonia in Gambian sleeping sickness and from heart failure in Rhodesian sleeping sickness. Treatment with suramin in the early phase of sleeping sickness results in a cure rate of greater than 90%. CNS involvement may subsequently develop in a few patients and require further treatment. Melarsoprol achieves a parasitologic cure in at least 90% of cases of advanced disease, and many patients may recover completely. Unfortunately, some patients are left with irreversible neurologic damage. Approximately 5% of patients may die during the course of melarsoprol therapy.

SUGGESTED READINGS

Barrett MP, Burchmore RJ, Stich A, et al: The trypanosomiases. Lancet 2003;362:1469–1480. *A comprehensive review.*

Berriman M, Ghedin E, Hertz-Fowler C, et al: The genome of the African trypanosome *Trypanosoma brucei.* Science 2005;309:416–422. *The first publication of the genome of African* Trypanosoma brucei.

Bisser S, N'Siesi FX, Lejon V, et al: Equivalence trial of melarsoprol and nifurtimox monotherapy and combination therapy for the treatment of second-stage Trypanosoma brucei gambiense sleeping sickness. J Infect Dis 2007;195: 311–313. *A consecutive 10-day low-dose melarsoprol-nifurtimox combination is more effective than the standard melarsoprol regimen.*

Chappuis F, Udayraj N, Stietenroth K, et al: Eflornithine is safer than melarsoprol for the treatment of second-stage *Trypanosoma brucei gambiense* human African trypanosomiasis. Clin Infect Dis 2005;41:748–751. *A comparative trial of treatment with eflornithine for second-stage African trypanosomiasis in southern Sudan compared with melarsoprol.*

Hutchinson OC, Fevre EM, Carrington M, et al: Lessons learned from the emergence of a new *Trypanosoma brucei rhodesiense* sleeping sickness focus in Uganda. Lancet Infect Dis 2003;1:42–45. *Describes the evolution of a new epidemic of trypanosomiasis in Uganda and efforts to control it with new molecular biology techniques and successful disease control management.*

Jannin J, Cattand P: Treatment and control of human African trypanosomiasis. Curr Opin Infect Dis 2004;17:565–570. *An excellent review of recent developments and prospects for new diagnostic tools and safer drugs.*

Kennedy PGE: Human African trypanosomiasis of the CNS: Current issues and challenges. J Clin Invest 2004;113:496–504. *A review of the issues related to diagnosis and staging of CNS disease, its neuropathogenesis, and possibility of new therapies.*

Moore AC: Prospects for improving African trypanosomiasis chemotherapy. J Infect Dis 2005;191:1793–1795. *Editorial reviewing new advances in treatment.*

368 AMERICAN TRYPANOSOMIASIS (CHAGAS' DISEASE)

Franklin A. Neva

Definition

Chagas' disease, which results from infection with the protozoan parasite *Trypanosoma cruzi,* is named after the Brazilian physician Carlos Chagas, who discovered the parasite. Distinction should be made between infection caused by the parasite, as manifested by positive serologic findings, and clinical disease. Chronic disease manifestations in the form of chronic cardiomyopathy or dysfunction of the esophagus or colon (mega syndromes) develop years after initial infection.

The Pathogen

The causative agent, *T. cruzi,* is usually transmitted as a zoonosis. Various species of blood-sucking reduviid bugs become infected when they take a blood meal from animals or humans who have circulating parasites, or trypomastigotes, in blood. The ingested parasites transform into epimastigotes and multiply in the midgut of the insect vector, where

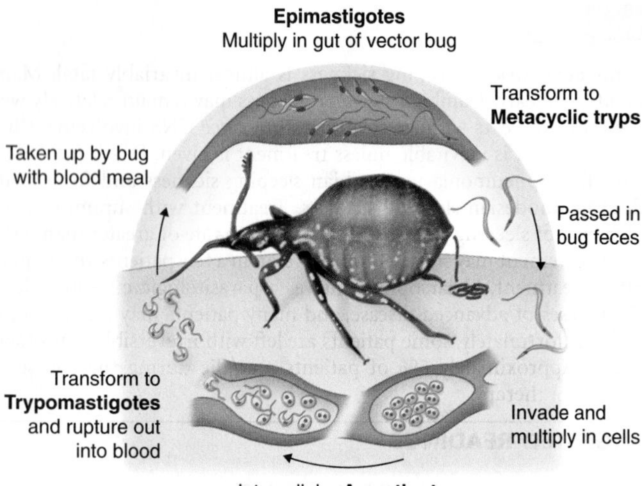

FIGURE 368–1 • Life cycle of *Trypanosoma cruzi.*

they later transform once again into metacyclic trypomastigotes in the hindgut of the bug. When the infected bug takes a subsequent blood meal, it frequently defecates during or after feeding, and the infective metacyclic forms are deposited on the skin. Transmission to a second vertebrate host occurs when the feeding puncture site or a mucous membrane is inadvertently contaminated with infective bug feces. The parasites can penetrate a variety of host cell types, within which they transform into intracellular amastigote forms. In contrast to certain other intracellular organisms, amastigotes of *T. cruzi* are not enclosed in phagolysosomes. They multiply in the cytoplasm, elongate, transform into motile trypomastigotes, and rupture out of the cells. Liberated organisms penetrate new cells or are carried into the blood stream to initiate further cycles of multiplication, preferentially in muscle cells, or are ingested by new vectors to maintain the cycle (Fig. 368–1).

Asymptomatic infected individuals with low-level parasitemia can transmit the organism via blood transfusion. Another route of transmission of the parasite is congenital infection.

Epidemiology

T. cruzi and its arthropod vectors are widely distributed from the southern United States through Mexico and Central America into South America down to central Argentina and Chile. The parasite is restricted to the Western Hemisphere. In most countries where it occurs, the parasite cycle is sylvatic; that is, it takes place in wild animals and their associated vector bugs. A peridomestic cycle occurs under conditions in which infected animals, such as opossums and rats, live close to human habitations and vector bugs invade houses to seek a blood meal. Certain species of triatomine bugs, such as *Triatoma infestans* and *Rhodnius prolixus,* have a great propensity to invade and breed in houses if suitable microenvironments are present. Cracks and holes in adobe mud huts or in crude wooden walls, thatched roofs, and household rubble provide hiding and breeding places for the bugs, which venture out at night to feed on sleeping inhabitants. Under these conditions, *T. cruzi* is transmitted from person to person—a domiciliary cycle—and Chagas' disease becomes a public health problem. Thus, human trypanosomiasis in Latin America is primarily an infection of poor rural people living in substandard housing.

The prevalence of antibodies to the parasite in human populations varies widely in different countries, as well as within regions of a country. A recent nationwide survey in Brazil found about 10% of the rural population to be infected. It is not unusual for up to half of all inhabitants in selected villages to be antibody positive. Countries with the highest incidence of both infection and disease secondary to *T. cruzi* include Brazil, Argentina, Chile, Bolivia, and Venezuela. It is estimated that in all of the Americas a total of 15 million people are infected. In many Latin American countries, positive serologic findings for *T. cruzi* constitute a social stigma; a lower socioeconomic background is implied, and employers are reluctant to hire someone in whom chronic Chagas' disease may develop later.

Considerable geographic variation exists in both the prevalence and the type of chronic disease manifestations. In Brazil, for example, cardiomyopathy and megadisease are common, and a patient often has both types of involvement. However, chagasic megaesophagus and megacolon are virtually unknown in Venezuela, Colombia, and Panama, whereas cardiomyopathy is relatively high, moderate, and low in prevalence, respectively. In general, the frequency of cardiac disease in seropositive persons in Central America and Mexico is low, even though rates of seropositivity may be substantial. Also in these countries, heart disease tends to develop later in life than in Brazil.

The situation regarding Chagas' disease in the United States is interesting because only four acute cases in persons native to the United States have been reported before 2001 despite the presence of *T. cruzi* in vector bugs, as well as in animal reservoirs. The lack of widespread transmission of *T. cruzi* to humans in this country is probably due to preference of the vectors for sylvatic habitats and their tendency to defecate late after feeding. Yet in some areas of the West, bites from aggressive and abundant reduviid bugs can be a source of annoyance and allergic reactions in suburbanites and outdoorspeople. Because of increased Hispanic immigration in recent years, sporadic cases of chronic Chagas' disease are encountered in the United States. In addition, several new cases of Chagas' disease have been reported in the United States in recipients of solid organ transplants between 2001 and 2006. In these cases, the organ donors were either immigrants from South America or traveled to an area endemic for *T. cruzi.* Because organ recipients frequently receive blood transfusions, infection can be transmitted to recipients either by transfusion or through the transplanted organs.

Pathobiology

In *acute Chagas' disease,* a local inflammatory lesion called a chagoma may develop at the site of entry of the parasite. Histologically, the chagoma shows mononuclear cell infiltration, interstitial edema, and intracellular aggregates of amastigotes in cells of subcutaneous tissue and muscle. Biopsy specimens from enlarged lymph nodes show hyperplasia, and amastigotes may be present in reticular cells. Skeletal muscle tissue from muscle biopsy specimens has shown organisms and focal inflammation. In acute cases that have a fatal outcome, there is invariably myocarditis with an enlarged heart. Microscopically, there is degeneration of cardiac muscle fibers and prominent, but patchy areas of inflammation with nests of amastigotes in the muscles. The brain and meninges may also be parasitized in acute Chagas' disease. Virtually all organs and cell types can be invaded by *T. cruzi.*

The organs primarily affected in *chronic Chagas' disease* are the heart and certain hollow viscera such as the esophagus and colon. Surprisingly, intracellular *T. cruzi* cannot usually be found in the affected organs, or a few may be demonstrable after a protracted search of many tissue sections. The heart, in patients with chronic disease who die suddenly (presumably of ventricular arrhythmias or heart block), may be normal in size or only moderately enlarged. In other patients with chronic chagasic cardiomyopathy, cardiomegaly develops and they die of intractable failure. The hearts are both hypertrophied and dilated, with thinning, especially at the apex to form a characteristic apical aneurysm. Mural thrombi, with subsequent embolization of the lungs and peripheral organs, are frequently seen. The coronary arteries are generally normal.

Microscopic findings in the heart are not specific and consist of focal mononuclear cell infiltrates, hypertrophy of cardiac fibers with patchy areas of necrosis, variable fibrosis, and edema. The components of the conduction system of the heart most often involved by inflammatory changes are the sinoatrial and atrioventricular nodes, as well as the right branch and left anterior branches of the bundle of His. Studies of these pathologic changes have indicated that they correlate well with electrocardiographic (ECG) changes during life but are diffusely scattered without specific localization to the conducting system.

When either the esophagus or the colon is affected in chronic Chagas' disease, the gross appearance is that of dilation and hypertrophy of the affected organ. The microscopic pathologic changes are disappointingly similar to those in the heart, again with no or very few organisms. However, myenteric ganglion cells are strikingly reduced in number. This type of parasympathetic denervation may also be found in other hollow viscera, such as the duodenum, ureters, or biliary tree.

The significant pathology of *congenital Chagas' disease* is chronic placentitis, with inflammatory changes and focal necrosis in the chorionic villi. Amastigotes of *T. cruzi* are found in the lesions. The presence of lesions and organisms in the placenta may be associated with abortion, stillbirth, or acute disease in the fetus. However, pregnancy may result in a normal fetus, even though placental lesions are present.

The extent and clinical significance of pathologic changes in individuals with antibodies to *T. cruzi* but without evidence of disease (i.e., the *indeterminate form*) are not yet clear. Such indeterminate cases may involve significantly reduced numbers of esophageal or colonic ganglion cells. It has been claimed that endocardial biopsy specimens from indeterminate cases have recognizable pathologic changes. In addition, in some indeterminate cases there is a chronic low level of parasitemia. Therefore, one point of view is that everyone with positive serologic findings has a continuing subclinical disease process that will become manifested with time. On the other hand, even in areas where chronic Chagas' disease is common, half or more of those with positive serology will die of causes other than Chagas' disease. In most Latin American countries, where endemicity is much lower, a positive serologic finding constitutes a relatively small risk factor for later chronic disease.

The pathogenesis of acute Chagas' disease is straightforward, but the sequence of events leading to the late manifestations of chronic cardiomyopathy or megadisease is still poorly understood. Key features of the chronic disease that must be explained include the following: (1) a latent period of up to 20 years from presumed initial infection with *T. cruzi* before manifestations of cardiomyopathy or megadisease appear; (2) no or very few intracellular parasites in the affected organs, in contrast to abundant parasites in tissues in acute cases; (3) destruction of autonomic parasympathetic ganglia (Auerbach's plexus) of the esophagus and colon; and (4) great geographic variation in the frequency and type of chronic Chagas' disease. Genetic diversity in parasite strains, including variation in animal virulence, may explain geographic differences in disease. Exaggerated immune responses to *T. cruzi* are not present in patients with chronic Chagas' disease, at least as judged by humoral antibody levels and lymphocyte proliferative responses. The autoimmunity concept of pathogenesis lost favor when the tissue reactive antibody in patients was found to be heterophile in nature. Direct cell-mediated cytotoxicity to heart muscle has also been proposed as a mechanism for the chronic disease. An even more complicated type of autoimmune response involving anti-idiotypic antibodies as T-cell antigens, as well as differential responses in antigen presentation, has also been proposed to explain chronic Chagas' disease. However, a unifying concept of the pathogenesis of chronic Chagas' disease is still lacking.

The indeterminate latent stage of infection with *T. cruzi* may be activated into a state of acute disease under conditions of severe immunosuppression. This can occur in seropositive recipients of organ transplants. In addition, reports of activation of disease are increasing, especially with brain involvement similar to that produced by *Toxoplasma,* in patients with acquired immunodeficiency syndrome (AIDS) who also have latent *T. cruzi* infection.

Clinical Manifestations

In endemic areas, first exposure to *T. cruzi* is generally subclinical and goes unnoticed. When clinical manifestations do develop in those initially exposed, the disease is an acute systemic infection. Chronic Chagas' disease, in contrast, evolves as a later sequela with specific organ involvement, but without systemic symptoms such as fever or lymphadenopathy.

Acute Chagas' Disease

Although acute Chagas' disease is most commonly seen in children, it can occur at any age, depending on the nature of exposure to the causative organism. The incubation period under natural conditions cannot be established accurately but is probably at least a week. A local area of erythema and induration (chagoma) may develop in the skin at the site of parasite entry. When infection takes place via the conjunctival route, as it frequently does, the local periorbital swelling is referred to as Romaña's sign. The chagoma is often accompanied by regional adenopathy and persists for several weeks. Other signs of acute Chagas' disease include fever, generalized lymphadenopathy, hepatosplenomegaly, and transient skin rash.

Myocarditis, accompanied by tachycardia and nonspecific ECG changes, can occur in the acute stage. Meningoencephalitis is another serious complication, particularly in very young patients. Fatal outcome in acute Chagas' disease is rare, but when it does occur, it is due to myocarditis and congestive failure or meningoencephalitis.

Signs and symptoms of acute disease gradually subside within a few weeks to several months, even without treatment. Trypanosomes, which have been demonstrable by direct microscopy in peripheral blood during the acute phase, become more difficult to find and subsequently disappear. The patient then enters the *indeterminate phase,* which is characterized by the presence of antibodies to *T. cruzi* and often also by the presence of low-level parasitemia in blood demonstrable only by special sensitive methods. This state of apparent complete recovery with positive serologic findings may continue indefinitely without further evidence of disease or sequelae. However, in a variable proportion of indeterminate cases, signs and symptoms of chronic Chagas' disease will develop years to a decade or more later. Except for epidemiologic experience from a particular geographic region, there are no laboratory or clinical indicators to predict the likelihood of future chronic disease.

Chronic Chagas' Disease

Cardiac signs and symptoms are the most common manifestations of chronic disease and are apt to begin with palpitations, dizziness, precordial discomfort, and even syncope. These findings reflect a variety of arrhythmias, including ventricular extrasystoles, bouts of tachycardia, and various degrees of heart block. Sudden death from ventricular tachycardia in an otherwise healthy young adult is not unusual. Symptoms attributable to arrhythmias may be present for a long time before cardiomegaly or evidence of cardiac failure appears. When congestive failure develops, it is predominantly right sided and is likely to lead to a fatal outcome within a few years. Peripheral emboli to the brain or other organs are frequent.

Symptomatic heart involvement in chronic disease is manifested by characteristic ECG abnormalities, often without cardiomegaly. The most common of these abnormalities is complete right bundle branch block. Other frequent ECG findings are left anterior hemiblock, ventricular extrasystoles, and even complete heart block. If heart failure is present, radiographs and echocardiograms will show generalized cardiomegaly with a reduced ejection fraction (Fig. 368–2).

Physical examination reveals only an irregular pulse, distant heart sounds, and perhaps a gallop rhythm. With failure, the heart can be very large, functional regurgitant murmurs may be heard, and there is often congestive hepatomegaly and peripheral edema.

The second most common chronic manifestation is megadisease of the esophagus or colon, most frequently the former. The symptoms are indistinguishable from those of idiopathic achalasia and include dysphagia, feeling of fullness after eating or drinking only small amounts, chest pain, and regurgitation. Aspiration with secondary pneumonia is a common complication in advanced cases, as are weight loss and cachexia. Salivary gland hypertrophy secondary to hypersalivation is sometimes seen. Esophageal cancer is reported to be more frequent in patients with chagasic megaesophagus, as with idiopathic achalasia.

Patients with chagasic megacolon suffer from chronic constipation and abdominal pain. Volvulus, obstruction, and perforation of the bowel may occur. An astonishing history of going several weeks between bowel movements has been obtained from some patients with severe megacolon. Megaesophagus and megacolon may both be present in the same patient, and cardiomyopathy can occur with either form of megadisease.

Diagnosis

For both acute and chronic Chagas' disease, a history of possible exposure to *T. cruzi* should be sought. Usual tourist travel to endemic areas is not likely to provide sufficient exposure to infected vectors. Blood transfusion or organ transplantation from a chronically infected donor can be a source of infection.

For *acute Chagas' disease,* direct microscopic examination of anticoagulated blood or a buffy coat preparation for motile trypanosomes is the most important procedure. Organisms are more difficult to find on stained thin or thick blood films, but the morphology of organisms seen on direct microscopy should be confirmed in a stained preparation. Red cells may be lysed with 0.083% NH_4Cl to concentrate parasites by

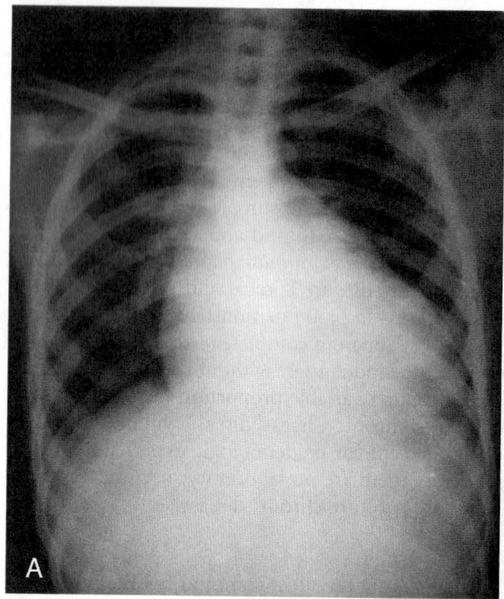

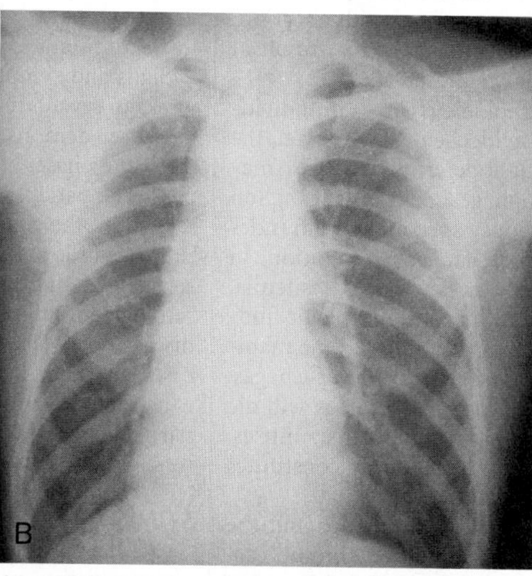

FIGURE 368–2 • Imaging of chronic Chagas' disease. A, Cardiac silhouette in a patient with chronic chagasic cardiomyopathy and heart failure. **B,** Chest radiograph showing a widened mediastinum because of a greatly dilated megaesophagus of chronic Chagas' disease.

centrifugation. If parasites cannot be found in the peripheral blood and acute disease is still suspected, blood can be cultured on Novy-MacNeal-Nicolle medium or other suitable media. Inoculation of mice with the patient's blood may sometimes result in recovery of the parasite. Biopsy of an enlarged lymph node or skeletal muscle for culture or histologic examination (or both) is another possibility.

The most sensitive technique for recovering trypanosomes from blood is a procedure referred to as xenodiagnosis. It is basically a form of blood culture involving the insect vector in which up to 40 normal, laboratory-reared reduviid bugs are allowed to feed directly on the patient or on the patient's blood through a membrane. Circulating parasites ingested by the bugs multiply in the gut and can be detected when the intestinal contents are examined 30 days later. Under experimental conditions, polymerase chain reaction techniques to demonstrate low levels of parasitemia appear promising and more sensitive than xenodiagnosis, but no standardized methods are yet available for routine use.

Serologic testing is not generally needed to diagnose acute disease. Parasite-specific immunoglobulin M (IgM) antibodies detected by immunofluorescence or direct agglutination do not become positive until 20 to 40 days after the onset of symptoms. In certain situations this delayed antibody response permits the demonstration of seroconversion. Other laboratory tests often show nonspecific changes such as lymphocytic leukocytosis, elevated sedimentation rate, or transient ECG abnormalities. Reversible cardiomegaly and even pericardial effusion may occur.

The diagnosis of *chronic Chagas' disease* requires demonstration of antibodies to *T. cruzi* in the presence of the characteristic cardiac abnormalities or megadisease, or both. Thus, except for the positive serologic findings, the diagnosis relies heavily on clinical judgment in excluding other causes of heart disease or gastrointestinal dysfunction. A positive xenodiagnosis result is strongly supportive, but not in itself diagnostic of chronic disease because patients in the indeterminate phase may have low-level parasitemia. A variety of assays for specific antibody are available, and the results of different tests are generally comparable. However, there are cross-reactions in some tests with sera from patients with leishmaniasis or syphilis, for example. Therefore, in individual cases it may be helpful to confirm the presence of antibody to specific antigens of *T. cruzi* with more sophisticated tests such as immunoblots.

Chagasic megaesophagus in the early stages shows only delayed emptying and minimal dilation on studies after a barium swallow. With more advanced disease, retention of swallowed material and esophageal dilation are progressively increased. Manometric studies show spasm of the esophageal sphincter and uncoordinated peristaltic movements. Endoscopy should be performed to rule out malignant disease. However, all these findings are indistinguishable from those of idiopathic achalasia. Barium enema with air contrast shows the dilated colon with impaired peristalsis, but other causes of colonic obstruction must be ruled out.

Differential Diagnosis

When acute Chagas' disease is symptomatic and severe, it can resemble a variety of acute systemic infections. Romaña's sign must be distinguished from other causes of unilateral orbital edema, such as reaction to an insect bite, trauma, or orbital cellulitis.

Congenital infections are virtually indistinguishable from congenital toxoplasmosis, cytomegalic inclusion disease, and syphilis.

Various cardiomyopathies, such as postpartum, alcoholic, and endomyocardial fibrosis, can resemble chronic Chagas' heart disease. Endocardial biopsy is of dubious diagnostic value because of the nonspecific pathologic changes in chagasic cardiomyopathy; it might, however, identify other causes of heart disease. The characteristic heart murmurs of rheumatic valvar disease are helpful in differentiating this entity from chagasic cardiomyopathy. The value of positive serologic findings for *T. cruzi* in the differential diagnosis of both heart disease and megadisease depends on the background prevalence of antibodies in the general population.

Treatment

Two drugs with reasonable antitrypanosomal activity are currently in use for treating Chagas' disease. One is the nitrofuran derivative nifurtimox,* which has been extensively evaluated. Nifurtimox is the only drug available in the United States for treating Chagas' disease; it is used in doses of 8 to 10 mg/kg/day in adults. Higher doses (12 to 20 mg/kg/day) are used in children. The second drug, benznidazole (5 to 7 mg/kg/day), is a nitroimidazole derivative that appears to be equal to nifurtimox in efficacy, although there is less experience with its use. The exact mechanism of antitrypanosomal action of both these drugs is not known.

The frequency of side effects from both nifurtimox and benznidazole is high; because they are administered for 60 to 90 days, drug toxicity is a serious problem. The most common adverse effect with nifurtimox is gastrointestinal intolerance, with anorexia, nausea, vomiting, and abdominal pain. Neurologic symptoms include restlessness, insomnia, disorientation, paresthesias, polyneuritis, and even seizures. Rashes can also occur. Peripheral neuropathy and bone marrow suppression have been reported with benznidazole. These side effects subside when the dosage of the drugs is reduced or treatment is stopped.

*An investigational drug that must be obtained from the Centers for Disease Control and Prevention drug service (telephone: 404-639-3670).

Rx

Because these drugs have shown effectiveness in the treatment of acute Chagas' disease, some Latin American physicians are also treating chronic and indeterminate cases. There is no evidence that the established pathologic changes associated with chronic Chagas' disease can be reversed by nifurtimox or benznidazole therapy. The question of whether drug treatment in indeterminate cases (i.e., asymptomatic patients with positive serologic findings) would prevent the development of later chronic disease is controversial. Some data suggest that low-level parasitemia, as assessed by xenodiagnosis, can be reduced or eliminated after treatment with antitrypanosomal drugs, but such studies require critical confirmation to establish their ultimate influence on the development of chronic disease, as well as risk-versus-benefit evaluation.

Treatment of patients with established chronic heart disease is supportive. Patients with frequent ventricular premature beats can benefit from antiarrhythmic drugs such as amiodarone. Cardiac pacemakers will prolong the survival of those with complete heart block. The congestive failure of chagasic cardiomyopathy is disappointingly refractory to the usual cardiotropic drugs.

More options are open for managing and treating megadisease. In the early stages of megaesophagus, pneumatic dilation of the esophageal sphincter is probably more effective than bougienage. For more advanced cases, various surgical procedures involving myotomy of the sphincter or partial resection are necessary. Early stages of megacolon can be managed by manipulating the diet and using laxatives and occasionally enemas. Sometimes an aperistaltic section of the colon can be resected in more severe cases.

Prevention

Chagas' disease could be eliminated as a serious health problem for the rural poor of Latin America by adequate housing and education. However, stark socioeconomic realities dictate another approach to control consisting mainly of the use of residual insecticides directed at domiciliary vectors. The use of benzene hexachloride, sprayed once or twice a year, has been very effective when used systematically.

Serologic testing in blood banks to avoid the use of seropositive donors is carried out in endemic areas. Another precaution is to add 1:4000 gentian violet to blood 24 hours before use to kill any trypanosomes that may be present. With the recent occurrence of several transfusion-associated cases of acute Chagas' disease in North America, the question of serologic screening of blood donors has been raised for areas of the country with large Latin American populations. The development of vaccines is still in the research stage.

Prognosis

There is now considerable evidence that if patients with acute Chagas' disease are treated with either nifurtimox or benznidazole, the extent of disease and parasitemia are usually reduced. More important, however, many patients treated in the acute phase never acquire antibodies to *T. cruzi* or do so only transiently. From this observation, plus the fact that xenodiagnosis in such treated patients is often negative, it is assumed that parasites can be eliminated and the patient cured if treated in the acute stage. However, nifurtimox is not uniformly effective in producing these results, and parasite strains from certain geographic areas (Brazil) appear to be less responsive to treatment than do strains from other countries (Argentina and Chile).

SUGGESTED READINGS

Coura José R, de Castro Solange I: A critical review on Chagas' disease chemotherapy. Mem Inst Oswaldo Cruz 2002;97:3–24. *This review, which concentrates mainly on chemotherapy for Chagas' disease, also touches on other aspects of the subject.*

Marin-Neto JA, Cunha-Neto E, Maciel BC, et al: Pathogenesis of chronic Chagas' heart disease. Circulation 2007;115:1109–1123. *Discusses the major mechanisms involved in the development of Chagas' heart disease.*

Miles MA, Feliciangeli MD, de Arias AR: American trypanosomiasis (Chagas' disease) and the role of molecular epidemiology in guiding control stategies. BMJ 2003;326:1444–1448. *Reviews advances in epidemiology of this disease.*

Pinto Dias JC: The treatment of Chagas' disease. Ann Intern Med 2006; 144:772–774. *An editorial on therapeutic options.*

Rassi A, Rassi A, Little WC, et al: Development and validation of a risk score for predicting death in Chagas' heart disease. N Engl J Med 2006;355:799–808. *Class III or VI status, cardiomegaly on CXR, LV systolic dysfunction on echo, VT on Holter and low QRS voltage predicted adverse outcomes.*

Viotti R, Vigliano C, Lococo B, et al: Long-term cardiac outcomes of treating chronic Chagas' diseases with benznidazole versus no treatment. Ann Intern Med 2006;144:724–734. *Benznidazole was associated with reduced progression of Chagas' disease.*

369 LEISHMANIASIS

Selma M. B. Jeronimo, Anastacio de Queiroz Sousa, and Richard D. Pearson

Definition

Leishmaniasis refers to the spectrum of clinical disease produced by species of the protozoan *Leishmania*, which are endemic in scattered areas on every continent except Antarctica. They are transmitted by phlebotomine sandflies. Depending on the geographic location and *Leishmania* species, various wild or domestic animals or humans serve as reservoirs. The clinical manifestations of leishmaniasis depend on the parasite's pathogenicity, which differs among species, and the genetically determined cell-mediated immune response of its human host. Leishmaniasis is truly a spectral disease. Leishmanial infections can be asymptomatic and self-resolving. Some are associated with skin lesions and result in cutaneous leishmaniasis. In a subset of patients with cutaneous leishmaniasis, there is also later involvement of the nose, mouth, or oral pharynx resulting in mucosal leishmaniasis. In visceral leishmaniasis, parasites disseminate throughout the reticuloendothelial system and involve the spleen, liver, and bone marrow. A number of other clinical variations have been described in addition to these three major syndromes.

An estimated 350 million people are at risk of acquiring leishmanial infection in focally endemic regions scattered throughout the world. The incidence of cutaneous leishmaniasis is estimated to be 1 to 1.5 million cases a year and that of visceral leishmaniasis to be 500,000 cases per year. Cutaneous leishmaniasis poses a substantial threat for settlers, residents, military personnel, and expatriates working or traveling in endemic areas of Latin America, the Middle East, and Asia. Mucosal leishmaniasis secondary to *Leishmania braziliensis* and related species is still a serious health concern for residents of Latin American countries. Visceral leishmaniasis is endemic in eastern India and Bangladesh; the Sudan, where major epidemics have occurred over the past decade in refugees; and in Latin American countries, where urban outbreaks have been reported in perimetropolitan areas of Brazil. Visceral leishmaniasis has emerged as an important opportunistic disease in persons with acquired immunodeficiency syndrome (AIDS). Finally, an epidemic of canine leishmaniasis has occurred among foxhounds in the United States, but there has been no related human infection. It is believed that the parasite has been transmitted from dog to dog and not by arthropod vectors.

The Pathogen

The *Leishmania* species that cause human disease, their geographic locations, and the clinical syndromes that they typically produce are summarized in Table 369–1. Although there are slight ultrastructural differences among species, such differences cannot be used to differentiate one from another. Speciation is available through World Health Organization reference laboratories. Further refinement of the classification system is likely in the future.

The life cycle is depicted in Figure 369–1. Leishmaniae exist in two morphologic forms. In humans and other mammals, leishmaniae are

TABLE 369–1 GEOGRAPHIC DISTRIBUTION AND CLINICAL SYNDROMES CAUSED BY *LEISHMANIA* SPECIES

Clinical Syndromes	*Leishmania* Species	Location
VISCERAL LEISHMANIASIS		
Kala-azar: generalized involvement of the reticuloendothelial system (e.g., spleen, bone marrow, liver)	*L. donovani*	Indian subcontinent, northern and eastern China, Pakistan, Nepal
	L. donovani	Sudan, Kenya, Ethiopia
	*L. infantum** *L. chagasi**	Middle East, Mediterranean littoral (e.g., Spain, southern France, Italy), Balkans, central and southwestern Asia, northern and northwestern China, northern and sub-Saharan Africa, Latin America
	L. amazonensis	Brazil
	L. tropica	Israel, India, and "viscerotropic" disease in Saudi Arabia (U.S. troops)
Post–kala-azar dermal leishmaniasis	*L. donovani*	Indian subcontinent
	L. donovani	Sudan, Kenya, Ethiopia, Somalia
OLD WORLD CUTANEOUS LEISHMANIASIS		
Single or limited number of skin lesions	*L. major*	Middle East, northwestern China, northwestern India, Pakistan, Africa
	L. tropica	Mediterranean coastal regions, Middle East, western Asiatic area, Indian subcontinent, Kenya
	L. aethiopica	Ethiopian highlands, Kenya, Yemen
	*L. infantum**	Mediterranean basin
	L. donovani	Sudan, Kenya, Ethiopia, Somalia
Diffuse cutaneous leishmaniasis	*L. aethiopica*	Ethiopian highlands, Kenya, Yemen
NEW WORLD CUTANEOUS LEISHMANIASIS		
Single or limited number of skin lesions	*L. mexicana* (chiclero ulcer)	Central America, Mexico, Texas
	L. amazonensis	Amazon basin, including Brazil and neighboring countries
	L. braziliensis	Multiple areas of Central and South America
	L. guyanensis† (forest yaws)	Guyana, Surinam, northern Amazon basin
	L. panamensis†	Panama, Costa Rica, Colombia
	L. peruviana (uta)	Peru (western Andes), Argentinean highlands
	L. lainsoni	Peru, neighboring areas
	L. pifanoi	Venezuela
	L. garnhami	Venezuela
	L. venezuelensis	Venezuela
	*L. chagasi**	Central and South America
Diffuse cutaneous leishmaniasis	*L. amazonensis*	Amazon basin, neighboring areas, Bahia and other states in Brazil
	L. pifanoi	Venezuela
	L. Mexicana	Mexico, Central America
	Leishmania sp	Dominican Republic
American mucosal leishmaniasis	*L. braziliensis* (espundia)	Multiple areas in Latin America

*Recent evidence suggests that *L. infantum* and *L. chagasi* are the same species.
†*L. guyanensis* and *L. panamensis* are closely related.
Adapted from Pearson RD, Sousa AQ: Clinical spectrum of leishmaniasis. Clin Infect Dis 1996;22:1. Data from Lainson R, Shaw JJ: Evolution, classification, and geographic distribution. *In* Peters W, Killick-Kendrick R (eds): The Leishmaniases in Biology and Medicine, vol 1. London, Academic Press, 1987, pp 1–20.

found within mononuclear phagocytes as intracellular amastigotes that are oval or round and 2 to 3 µm in diameter. They have a relatively large, eccentrically located nucleus; an internalized flagellum; and a rod-shaped specialized mitochondrial structure, the kinetoplast, which contains extranuclear DNA in catenated minicircles and maxicircles. Amastigotes are adapted for survival in phagolysosomes in macrophages at mammalian body temperature.

Female sandflies serve as vectors. They ingest amastigote-containing macrophages when they take a blood meal from an infected reservoir. Leishmaniae convert to flagellated, extracellular promastigotes in the gut of the sandfly. Promastigotes are 15 to 26 µm in length and 2 to 3 µm in width. They develop from amastigotes and multiply at ambient temperatures of 22 to 26° C. They differentiate through multiple steps to become infectious metacyclic promastigotes. The time needed for development in the gut of the sandfly varies among *Leishmania* species but is approximately 1 week. Infective metacyclic promastigotes then migrate to the proboscis and are inoculated when the sandfly attempts to take its next blood meal.

Epidemiology

A number of different sandflies can transmit leishmaniae. *Lutzomyia* species predominate in Latin America, and *Phlebotomus* species transmit *Leishmania* elsewhere in the world. Some are peridomestic and live in rubble and debris near houses or farm buildings; others thrive in thick vegetation in forest areas. Sandflies are modified pool feeders and tend to bite at night. Rodents, dogs, humans, and occasionally other animals serve as reservoirs, depending on the *Leishmania* species and the geographic location.

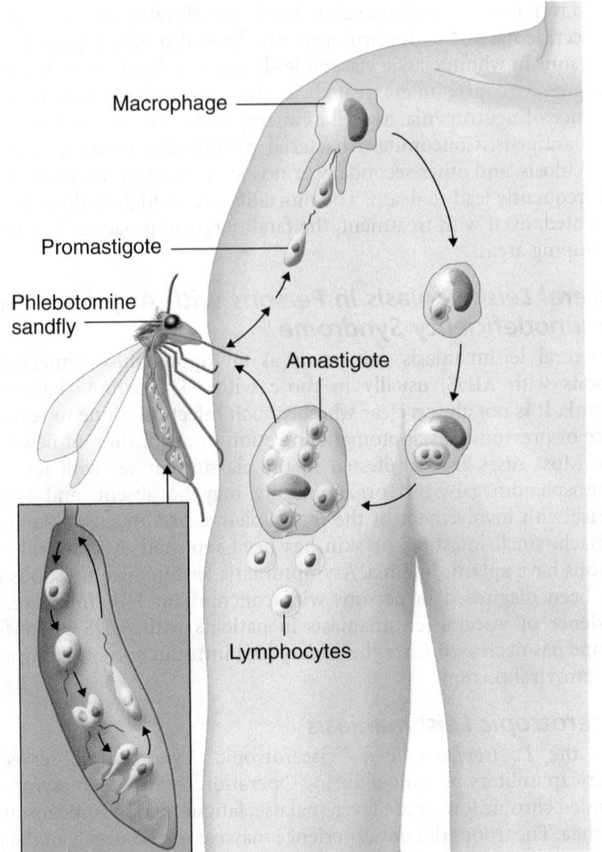

FIGURE 369–1 • Life cycle of *Leishmania*. Humans serve as the reservoir for *Leishmania donovani* in India, as depicted here. In most settings, leishmaniasis is a zoonosis with rodents or canines as reservoirs.

After inoculation, promastigotes are phagocytosed by macrophages in the skin and convert to amastigotes within them. Sandfly saliva contains factors that result in local vasodilation and enhance parasite survival. They can also elicit immune responses. Once inside a macrophage, promastigotes convert to amastigotes in phagolysosomes, multiply, and eventually spread to other macrophages.

Immunologic Characteristics

The outcome of leishmanial infection depends on the virulence characteristics of the infecting *Leishmania* species and the genetically determined, cell-mediated immune responses of its mammalian hosts. There appears to be a tenuous balance between the development of protection and disease-permissive immune elements. Studies in animal models of experimental leishmaniasis and humans with naturally acquired infection indicate that immunity is mediated by T lymphocytes. Persons immunocompromised by either human immunodeficiency virus (HIV) infection or other types of immunosuppressive disorders are more susceptible to leishmaniasis. Resolution of *Leishmania* infection and protection against reinfection correlate with the expansion of *Leishmania*-specific $CD4^+$ lymphocytes of the T-helper 1 (T_H1) type and with the secretion of interleukin-12 (IL-12) and interferon-γ in response to leishmanial antigens. Exposure to interferon-γ produced by T_H1 or $CD8^+$ lymphocytes or direct contact with *Leishmania*-specific $CD4^+$ T cells activates macrophages to kill intracellular amastigotes. The production of nitric oxide after induction of nitric oxide synthase in concert with oxygen intermediates is responsible for the microbicidal effect. Tumor necrosis factor-α (TNF-α) appears to contribute to the protective response. Once infection has resolved, humans are typically resistant to disease with the infecting *Leishmania* species unless they become immunocompromised.

The development of protective T_H1 responses is delayed or inhibited in persons with clinically apparent visceral leishmaniasis. In the case of cutaneous leishmaniasis, this occurs locally at the site of the lesion in the skin. In those with progressive visceral leishmaniasis it is generalized. Two cytokines, IL-10 and transforming growth factor-β, are thought to be important in interfering with the development of protective T_H1 responses in patients with visceral leishmaniasis. Antileishmanial antibodies are produced during infection, but they are not protective. The highest titers are observed in persons with progressive visceral leishmaniasis and large parasite burdens. Antibody titers decrease after successful treatment, when a protective cellular immune response develops.

Despite intensive study, the precise interactions among infected macrophages, dendritic cells, and lymphocyte populations and the cytokines that they produce have not yet been fully characterized. A number of factors may affect the outcome of infection. There is evidence to suggest that the size of the infecting inoculum, natural macrophage resistance factors, the sequence of the initial cytokine response, and the manner in which leishmanial antigens are presented influence the immune response and outcome of infection.

VISCERAL LEISHMANIASIS

Epidemiology

Most cases of visceral leishmaniasis (see Table 369–1) are caused by *Leishmania donovani* or *Leishmania infantum/Leishmania chagasi.* The latter two species are closely related if not identical. On occasion, *Leishmania* species predominantly associated with cutaneous disease, such as *Leishmania tropica* or *Leishmania amazonensis,* are isolated from patients with clinical visceral leishmaniasis.

Transmission of the parasite is dependent on an appropriate reservoir and sandfly vector. Other, less common modes include congenital transmission, transfusion of contaminated blood, sharing of needles by intravenous drug users, and accidental needlestick injuries in the laboratory. Recent epidemics of canine leishmaniasis have occurred among foxhound dogs in the United States. The mode of transmission seems to be dog to dog, and no insect vector has yet been identified.

More than half the world's cases of visceral leishmaniasis each year are caused by *L. donovani* in eastern India and Bangladesh. Humans are the reservoir of infection there; transmission is by anthropophilic sandflies that become infected when they feed on persons with visceral leishmaniasis or post–kala-azar dermal leishmaniasis. Disease occurs in persons of all ages.

L. donovani is also endemic in focal areas of eastern Africa in Kenya, Ethiopia, Somalia, and the Sudan, where a large epidemic occurred in refugees who were displaced into endemic regions during the past 2 decades. The reservoirs include rodents and small carnivores. Humans may serve as a reservoir during epidemics.

Visceral leishmaniasis caused by *L. infantum* occurs sporadically in southern Europe, northern Africa, the Middle East, Central Asia, and China, although cases are now rare in the latter. The disease is most common in infants, children, and immunocompromised persons with AIDS or malignancy. Canines, including domestic dogs, are reservoirs. Visceral leishmaniasis has been an important opportunistic infection among persons with AIDS in Spain, southern France, and Italy.

L. chagasi is responsible for visceral leishmaniasis in Brazil, Colombia, Venezuela, and other countries in Latin America. It occurs sporadically in endemic rural areas, but large perimetropolitan epidemics have emerged over the past decade in Brazil. Most cases occur in children younger than 10 years. The gender distribution is approximately equal in those younger than 5 years, but males predominate later in life. Domestic dogs and foxes have been incriminated as reservoirs. Family clustering suggests that humans might also serve as a reservoir during outbreaks.

In a small group of American troops in the Persian Gulf War who were infected with *L. tropica,* a species that is usually associated with cutaneous disease, a "viscerotropic" syndrome developed. These individuals had fever, malaise, and other constitutional symptoms but lacked massive hepatosplenomegaly and other manifestations of progressive visceral leishmaniasis.

Pathobiology

Infection is acquired when promastigotes are inoculated by female sandflies into an exposed area of skin. The parasites convert to amastigotes and multiply within mononuclear phagocytes. Although a cutaneous nodule or ulcer may arise, most patients in whom visceral leishmaniasis develops are unaware of the site of primary inoculation. Amastigotes subsequently disseminate via regional lymphatics and the vascular system to mononuclear phagocytes throughout the reticuloendothelial system. Most infections are asymptomatic and resolve spontaneously; only a minority progress to classic visceral leishmaniasis, known in many areas as kala-azar. There is strong evidence from animal models and humans of a genetic predisposition to the development of progressive visceral leishmaniasis. Linkage and allelic association have been demonstrated between clinical visceral leishmaniasis and the gene *SLC11A1,* which regulates macrophage activation. IL-4 polymorphism is also associated with susceptibility to visceral leishmaniasis. AIDS, malnutrition, malignancy, and other forms of immunosuppression are additionally important variables.

In persons with visceral leishmaniasis, increased numbers of mononuclear phagocytes, many containing amastigotes, are found in the liver and spleen and result in hypertrophy. The spleen often becomes massively enlarged. Splenic lymphoid follicles are replaced by parasitized mononuclear cells. Amastigote-containing mononuclear phagocytes may also be found in the liver, bone marrow, lymph nodes, and other organs. Widespread dissemination involving the intestinal tract and respiratory system occurs in some persons with concurrent AIDS.

Clinical Manifestations

The incubation period for visceral leishmaniasis is quite variable but typically ranges from 2 to 8 months. The onset is often insidious and difficult to date. The disease usually has a subacute or chronic course, but in some cases the onset is more abrupt. Symptoms include fever, malaise, anorexia, weight loss, and enlargement of the abdomen. Fever may be intermittent, remittent with twice-daily temperature spikes to 38 to 40° C, or less commonly, continuous. It is generally well tolerated. Of note, visceral leishmaniasis has developed in former residents of endemic areas who became immunocompromised years after leaving the areas.

Splenomegaly and hepatomegaly are hallmarks of classic visceral leishmaniasis. The spleen is firm and nontender and frequently becomes massively enlarged (Fig. 369–2). Lymphadenopathy is common in some geographic areas, such as the Sudan, and rare in others, such as Latin America. Wasting can be pronounced in chronic infection. Hyperpigmentation may develop in patients in India and has led to the name *kala-azar,* meaning "black fever" in Hindi. Jaundice is occasionally present. Late in visceral leishmaniasis patients may experience epistaxis, gingival bleeding, and petechiae. Edema and ascites may also develop as a result of hypoalbuminemia.

On laboratory examination, anemia, thrombocytopenia, neutropenia, and hypergammaglobulinemia are common. The anemia is usually normocytic and normochromic unless complicated by blood loss. The white blood cell count may be as low as 1000/mL; eosinopenia is common. Thrombocytopenia may be associated with evidence of bleeding. Hemophagocytosis has been observed in bone marrow specimens. The erythrocyte sedimentation rate and C-reactive protein are elevated. Levels of gamma globulin are markedly increased, at times in the range of 9 to 10 g/dL, as a consequence of polyclonal B-cell activation. Circulating immune complexes, autoantibodies, and rheumatoid factors are present in many patients. Glomerulonephritis may develop, but renal failure is rare. Liver enzyme and bilirubin levels are elevated in some. Hypertriglyceridemia and hypofibrinogenemia have also been reported.

Persons in whom classic visceral leishmaniasis develops typically have a progressive course unless treated. Severe cachexia may result. They have evidence of neutropenia, as well as anergy to *Leishmania* and eventually other antigens. Concomitant bacterial pneumonia, measles, dysentery, tuberculosis, and other secondary or nosocomial infections are common and frequently lead to death. The mortality rate is high in those who are untreated. Even with treatment, the fatality rate approaches 5 to 10% in developing areas.

Visceral Leishmaniasis in Persons with Acquired Immunodeficiency Syndrome

Visceral leishmaniasis can occur as an opportunistic infection in persons with AIDS, usually in those with $CD4^+$ counts lower than 100/mL. It is not always clear whether such infection is due to recrudescence of previously asymptomatic infection or acquisition of new infection. Most cases are manifested in the classic manner with fever and hepatosplenomegaly, but organomegaly may be absent, and atypical disease with involvement of the lungs, pleura, oral mucosa, esophagus, stomach, small intestine, or skin has been reported. A small subset of persons have aplastic anemia. Asymptomatic leishmanial infections have also been diagnosed in persons with concomitant HIV infection. The incidence of visceral leishmaniasis in patients with AIDS in southern Europe has decreased since the widespread introduction of highly active antiretroviral therapy.

Viscerotropic Leishmaniasis

In the *L. tropica*–related "viscerotropic" syndrome observed in American military personnel during Operation Desert Storm, symptoms included chronic low-grade fever, malaise, fatigue, and in some instances, diarrhea. The troops did not experience massive splenomegaly or the progressive wasting associated with classic visceral leishmaniasis.

Post–Kala-Azar Dermal Leishmaniasis

Post–kala-azar dermal leishmaniasis develops in approximately 5 to 10% of persons treated for visceral leishmaniasis in India and up to 50% of those treated in the Sudan. In Africa, the lesions appear during or shortly after treatment and persist for several months. In India, they appear up to 2 years after treatment and persist for months to as long as 20 years. The skin lesions vary from hyperpigmented macules or maculopapules to nodules (see Fig. 369–2). Lesions are frequently found on the face, trunk, and extremities and may be confused with leprosy. Macrophages containing amastigotes are found in them. Although the immunopathology is not well understood, patients with post–kala-azar dermal leishmaniasis have high serum levels of IL-10.

Persons with post–kala-azar dermal leishmaniasis are thought to serve as reservoirs of infection in areas where transmission occurs by anthroponotic sandflies. Post–kala-azar dermal leishmaniasis is not typically a feature of *L. infantum/L. chagasi* infection in Latin America, Europe, or the Middle East, but it has been reported after the treatment of persons with concurrent AIDS and visceral leishmaniasis in those areas.

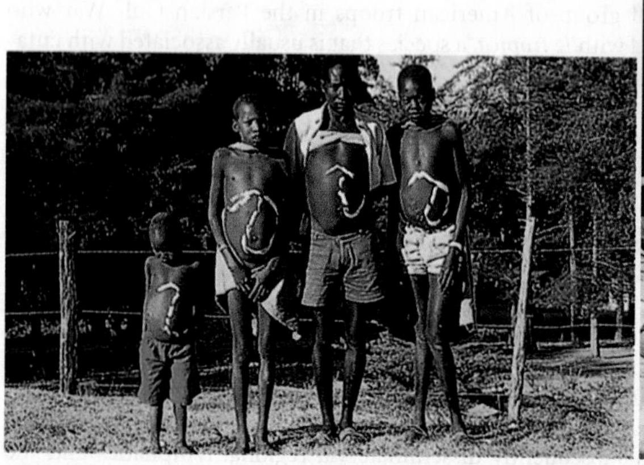

A

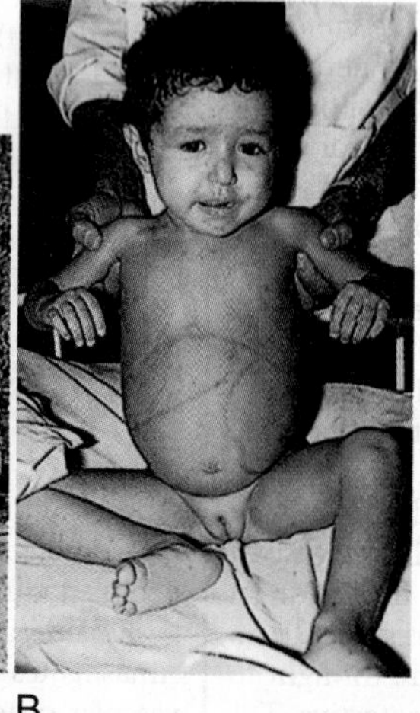

B

FIGURE 369–2 • Clinical picture of kala-azar in Kenya (A) and infantile kala-azar (B) in an infant infected in the northeast of Brazil with *Leishmania chagasi* (regarded by some to be synonymous with *L. infantu* of the Old World). (From Peter W, Pasvol G: Tropical Medicine and Parasitology, 5th ed. New York, Mosby, 2002, p 69.)

Diagnosis

A presumptive diagnosis of visceral leishmaniasis is often based on the classic clinical manifestation of fever, splenomegaly, hepatomegaly, and hematologic abnormalities in endemic areas. The diagnosis may be delayed or missed in early infection, in an immigrant or traveler returning to a nonendemic country, and in persons with concurrent AIDS and atypical features.

The diagnosis is confirmed by identifying amastigotes in tissue or by growing promastigotes in culture. Splenic aspiration results in a parasitologic diagnosis in 96 to 98% of cases. It is relatively safe when performed by an experienced physician, but significant hemorrhage can occur, particularly in patients with clotting abnormalities. Bone marrow aspiration for examination and culture is safer but less sensitive, with about 80 to 85% positivity. Alternative sites for aspiration or biopsy (or both) include the liver or lymph nodes if they are enlarged. Culture of the buffy coat can also be performed. Polymerase chain reaction (PCR)-based assays applied to blood, bone marrow, or other samples appear promising and have been shown to be more sensitive and positive in some asymptomatic patients, but they are not widely available. In patients with concurrent AIDS, amastigotes may be observed in macrophages in unexpected sites, such as bronchoalveolar lavage fluid, pleural effusions, or lesions in the oral pharynx, larynx, stomach, or intestine.

Antileishmanial antibodies are present in high titer in immunocompetent persons with visceral leishmaniasis. An enzyme-linked immunosorbent assay (ELISA) using rK39, a recombinant kinesin-related antigen, is both sensitive and specific for the diagnosis of visceral leishmaniasis. ELISAs using other leishmanial antigens, indirect immunofluorescence assays, and direct agglutination assays are also available. The sensitivity and specificity vary depending on the antigen used and the methodology. Persons with concurrent AIDS may have low titers or undetectable antileishmanial antibodies. The leishmanin skin test, also known as the *Montenegro test,* is nonreactive in persons with visceral leishmaniasis. It eventually becomes positive in the majority of patients who undergo clinically successful chemotherapy. The skin test may also be positive in otherwise healthy individuals in endemic areas who have no history of symptomatic visceral leishmaniasis. The leishmanin skin test is not approved for use in the United States but is widely used in South America.

Treatment

Rx

Liposomal amphotericin B, the only drug licensed for the treatment of visceral leishmaniasis in the United States, is highly effective and relatively well tolerated. It is theoretically attractive because liposomes deliver the drug to macrophages, the site of leishmanial infection. Liposomal amphotericin B, 3 mg/kg of body weight daily on days 1 through 5, 14, and 21, is recommended for immunocompetent persons. A higher dose and longer duration of therapy are recommended for patients with AIDS, 4 mg/kg/day on days 1 to 5, 10, 17, 24, 31, and 38. Other forms of lipid-associated amphotericin B, though less well studied, also appear to be effective. The high cost of liposomal and lipid-associated amphotericin preparation has limited their use in developing areas.

The pentavalent antimonials sodium stibogluconate (Pentostam) and meglumine antimoniate (Glucantime) have been the mainstay of therapy for visceral leishmaniasis in many areas. Unfortunately, antimony resistance is now prevalent among *L. donovani* isolates in India and is emerging in some other areas.

Stibogluconate sodium and meglumine antimoniate continue to be used in Latin America and other sites where *Leishmania* species remain sensitive. These two agents appear to have comparable efficacy and toxicity and are administered on the basis of their pentavalent antimony content. In the United States, stibogluconate sodium is available from the Centers for Disease Control and Prevention drug service. The recommended treatment course of pentavalent antimony is 20 mg/kg body weight daily for 28 days. Relapses occur and patients should be monitored closely for at least 6 months after therapy. A second course of pentavalent antimony can be used in patients who relapse. Side effects are common and more severe in the elderly and include pancreatitis, arthralgias, myalgias, nausea, vomiting, headache, liver enzyme abnormalities, leukopenia, rash, and cardiac toxicity. ST-T wave changes are common. Sudden death has occurred in patients who have received more than the recommended dose.

Recent reports from India indicate that miltefosine, a phosphocholine analogue that is administered orally, is effective for the treatment of visceral leishmaniasis and post–kala-azar dermal leishmaniasis in areas where antimony-resistant *L. donovani* is prevalent. In adults, doses of 100 mg/day (approximately 2.5 mg/kg/day) for 3 to 4 weeks have been 97% effective after 6 months. Gastrointestinal effects are common but do not usually prevent the completion of therapy. The drug is contraindicated in pregnancy. Studies now under way should determine its role in the treatment of visceral leishmaniasis elsewhere. It has not been approved by the U.S. Food and Drug Administration.

In addition, conventional amphotericin B deoxycholate (0.5 to 1 mg/kg intravenously daily for 20 days) and pentamidine are alternative drugs, but both have potentially serious side effects. Amphotericin B desoxycholate is associated with renal insufficiency, electrolyte disorders, fever, weight loss, and constitutional symptoms. Pentamidine can produce hypotension, pancreatic beta cell damage, hypoglycemia followed later by hyperglycemia, renal toxicity, and bone marrow suppression. Resistance to pentamidine has been reported from India. Paromomycin (aminosidine) has also been used parenterally in India to treat patients with pentavalent antimony-resistant *L. donovani.*

Unfortunately, persons with concurrent AIDS frequently relapse after initially successful antileishmanial chemotherapy. Secondary suppressive therapy should be considered, although the optimal drug and regimen have yet to be defined. Highly active antiretroviral therapy should be instituted to improve immune responsiveness.

CUTANEOUS AND MUCOSAL LEISHMANIASIS

Epidemiology

Leishmania species also produce a spectrum of cutaneous disease (see Table 369–1). Most common are single or a limited number of chronic ulcerative lesions (Fig. 369–3A). In the Western Hemisphere, cutaneous leishmaniasis is caused by the *Leishmania* species *L. mexicana, L. amazonensis, L. braziliensis, L. panamensis, L. guyanensis, L. peruviana, L. lainsoni,* and several other species, including dermatotropic strains of *L. chagasi.* Except for *L. peruviana* and *L. chagasi,* which are found in dogs and other canines, the reservoirs are forest rodents. The vectors are ground-dwelling or arboreal species of sandflies. Humans become infected when they enter endemic forested areas for work, recreation, or military activities. A number of cases of cutaneous leishmaniasis have been reported in North American and European travelers who visit rural areas of Belize and other Latin America countries.

L. mexicana is found in focal areas extending from Texas to Argentina. Autochthonous transmission has occurred in Texas, but the number of cases is small. *L. braziliensis* is endemic throughout Latin America and produces mucosal disease in approximately 3 to 5% of those infected in Brazil. A dermatopathic strain of *L. chagasi* has been isolated from cutaneous lesions in Central America.

Most cases of cutaneous leishmaniasis in Europe, Africa, the Middle East, India, and Asia are caused by three *Leishmania* species. *Leishmania major* is an important problem in settlers, visitors, and troops in endemic rural areas of the Middle East, Central Asia, and North Africa. Rodents are the principal reservoir. *L. tropica* is found primarily in urban areas of the Middle East, the Mediterranean littoral, India, Pakistan, and Central Asia. The reservoirs are dogs and humans. *Leishmania aethiopica* is endemic in Ethiopia, Kenya, and southwestern Africa, where hyrax are reservoirs. On occasion, either *L. donovani* or *L. infantum* is isolated from a cutaneous lesion.

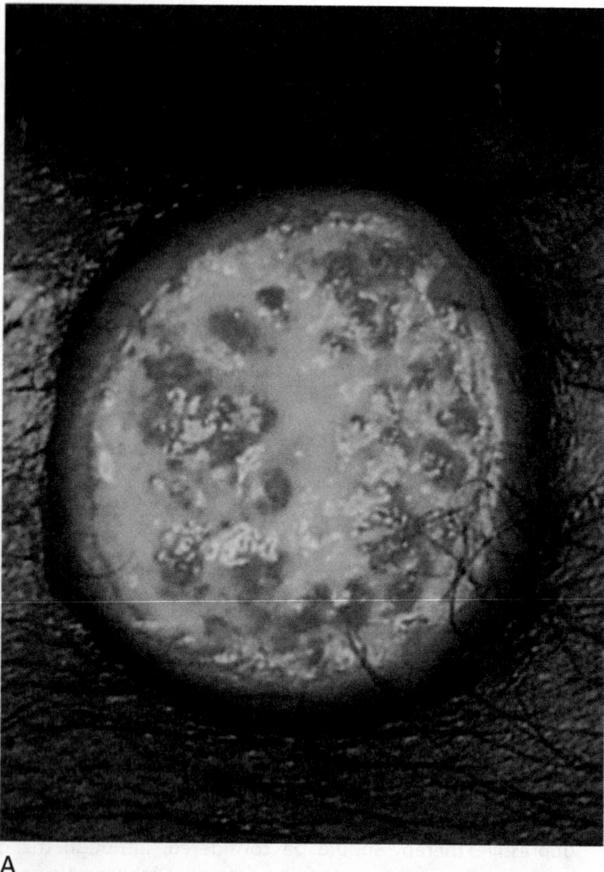

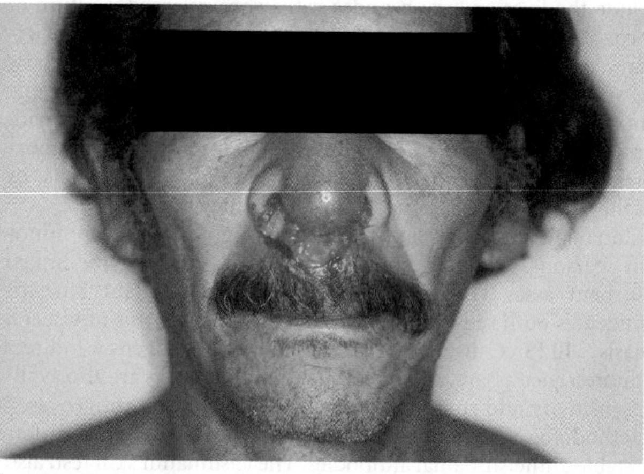

FIGURE 369–3 • Cutaneous and ulcerative leishmaniasis. A, Cutaneous leishmaniasis caused by *Leishmania braziliensis.* **B,** Brazilian patient with mucosal leishmaniasis caused by *L. braziliensis.* Note the destructive lesion involving the nose.

Pathobiology

A cutaneous lesion develops at the site where promastigotes are inoculated by sandflies. Amastigote-infected macrophages are the predominant finding early in infection as circulating monocytes home to the site. Over time, a granulomatous response develops with increasing numbers of lymphocytes, decreasing numbers of parasites, and necrosis of the skin resulting in ulceration. Histopathologic examination usually reveals acute and chronic inflammation with granulomatous changes. Peripheral blood mononuclear cells from persons with typical cutaneous leishmaniasis proliferate and produce interferon-γ in response to leishmanial antigens in vitro, and patients demonstrate delayed-type hypersensitivity responses in vivo. In the lesion there seems to be a stalemate between potentially protective and disease-enhancing immune responses. Eventually the lesion heals and leaves an atrophic scar.

The spectrum of cutaneous leishmaniasis includes several variants. One extreme is diffuse cutaneous leishmaniasis, a relatively infrequent, anergic condition characterized by disseminated nodular skin lesions that contain large numbers of amastigote-infected macrophages. These lesions do not ulcerate, protective T_H1 responses do not develop, and the syndrome persists indefinitely. Another extreme is represented by the chronic, destructive lesions observed in patients with mucosal leishmaniasis. There is evidence of a vigorous T_H1 response, decreased IL-10 production, and a low response to exogenous IL-10. The leishmanin skin test is positive. Amastigotes are usually scant, but the lesion persists.

Clinical Manifestations

Cutaneous Leishmaniasis

Cutaneous leishmaniasis may involve single or multiple lesions. The lesions are relatively heterogeneous and vary as a function of the infecting *Leishmania* species, the geographic area, and the host's immune response. Lesions are usually found on exposed areas of the skin. They typically start as erythematous papules at the site where promastigotes are inoculated, slowly increase in size, become nodular, and eventually ulcerate. Despite substantial tissue destruction, they are not generally painful. Satellite lesions may be found at or near the edges of the primary site of infection. Though variable, lesions are often characterized as "wet" or "dry." Wet lesions are covered with exudate and have raised borders (see Fig. 369–3A). They are frequently associated with superficial, secondary bacterial or fungal infections. Dry lesions have a central crust. Wet lesions are commonly associated with *L. braziliensis* and *L. major.* Dry ones are associated with *L. mexicana* and *L. tropica,* but the morphology of lesions varies widely, and substantial overlap occurs. Sometimes lesions are nodular and resemble neoplasms. On occasion, cutaneous leishmaniasis caused by *L. braziliensis, L. guyanensis,* or other species involves local lymphatics and mimics sporotrichosis. Depending on the infecting *Leishmania* species, cutaneous lesions can persist for months and, in some cases, years before they spontaneously heal and leave flat, hypopigmented, atrophic scars.

Observations in northeastern Brazil indicate that *L. braziliensis* can cause regional lymphadenopathy, fever, and constitutional symptoms before the primary cutaneous lesion or lesions become apparent. Splenomegaly occurs in some patients. These systemic findings resolve as the skin lesion develops. It has been hypothesized that *L. braziliensis* disseminates to distant mucosal sites during this early phase of infection.

Disseminated Cutaneous Leishmaniasis

Disseminated cutaneous leishmaniasis is a relatively new syndrome caused by *L. braziliensis* infection in northeastern Brazil. It is characterized by a large number of skin lesions; approximately 40% of those infected have mucosal involvement. A disseminated pattern has also been observed in persons with AIDS.

Diffuse Cutaneous Leishmaniasis

Diffuse cutaneous leishmaniasis is a rare anergic variant of cutaneous leishmaniasis. It starts as a localized papule that does not ulcerate. Satellite lesions develop (Fig. 369–4), and eventually multiple cutaneous nodules form on the face and extremities. Large numbers of amastigotes

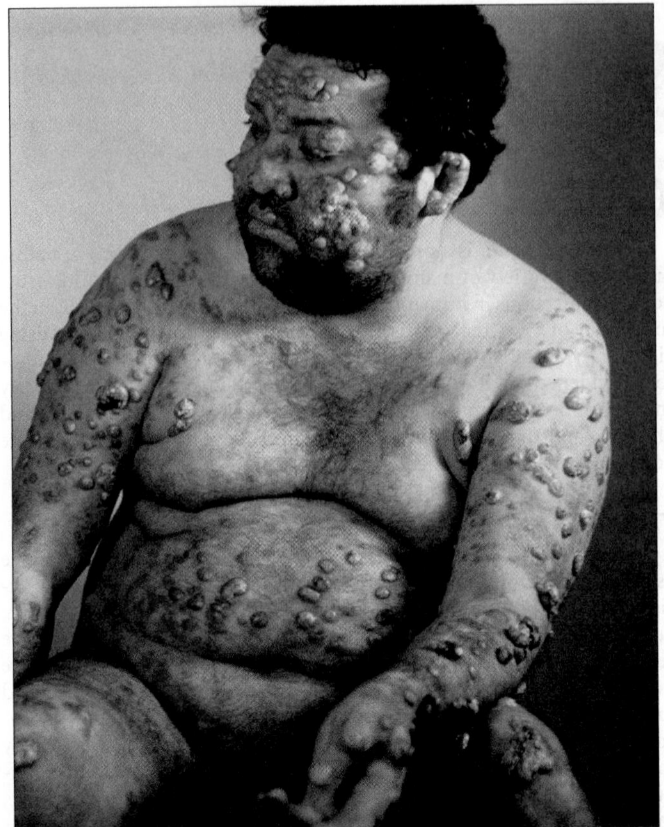

FIGURE 369–4 • Disseminated cutaneous leishmaniasis.

are present in macrophages in the skin. The disease progresses slowly and may persist for decades. The syndrome is most frequently associated with *L. aethiopica* infection in Africa and *L. amazonensis* in Latin America.

Leishmaniasis Recidivans

Leishmaniasis recidivans, typically associated with *L. tropica* infection in the Middle East, is a chronic syndrome. Skin lesions appear on exposed areas of the face or extremities and enlarge slowly. They tend to heal in the center. The lesions can persist for many years to decades. Biopsy findings reveal chronic inflammatory changes. Amastigotes are rarely seen in tissue.

American Mucosal Leishmaniasis (Espundia)

In approximately 3 to 5% of persons infected with *L. braziliensis* or related species in Latin America, mucosal lesions develop in the nose, mouth, pharynx, or larynx months to years after the primary skin ulcer heals (see Fig. 369–3B). Nasal disease typically begins with nasal inflammation and stuffiness, followed by ulceration of the mucosa. Histologically, the lesions are characterized by a chronic granulomatous response. There is destruction of the mucosa and eventually the underlying cartilage of the nasal septum or palate. The differential diagnosis of American mucosal leishmaniasis includes paracoccidioidomycosis, histoplasmosis, tertiary syphilis, tertiary yaws, sarcoidosis, Wegener's granulomatosis, angiocentric T-cell lymphoma, rhinoscleroma, and carcinoma.

Mucosal involvement is also occasionally observed in persons with visceral leishmaniasis, particularly those with concurrent AIDS. It can occur in post–kala-azar dermal leishmaniasis and, on occasion, from contiguous extension of simple cutaneous lesions or leishmaniasis recidivans.

Diagnosis

Cutaneous leishmaniasis should be considered in the differential diagnosis of any chronic, localized skin lesion in persons who have been exposed in an endemic area. The diagnosis can be confirmed parasitologically in 50 to 80% of lesions by identifying amastigotes in tissue or by growing promastigotes in culture. A biopsy sample and aspirate should be obtained from the margin of the lesion after it has been meticulously cleaned. Touch preparations are stained with a Wright-Giemsa preparation. The remaining tissue should be divided. One portion should be cultured for leishmaniae, fungi, and mycobacteria. Another should be submitted for histopathologic analysis. Species-specific PCR-based diagnostic assays are under development in research settings. Serologic tests are not diagnostic. Antileishmanial antibodies are detectable in the serum of less than half of those with parasitologically confirmed cutaneous leishmaniasis, titers are usually low, and cross-reactions occur with other organisms. The leishmanin skin test, which is not available in the United States, is positive in simple cutaneous leishmaniasis, leishmaniasis recidivans, and mucosal leishmaniasis. It is negative in patients with diffuse cutaneous leishmaniasis.

Parasites are usually scant in mucosal lesions caused by *L. braziliensis.* A positive leishmanin skin test, a history of exposure in an endemic area, and evidence of a healed cutaneous lesion allow a presumptive diagnosis.

Treatment

Rx

Small, inconspicuous, or healing skin lesions caused by *Leishmania* species that are not associated with mucosal disease can be monitored expectantly. Cutaneous lesions that are large or located in cosmetically important sites and those that are caused by *L. braziliensis* or other *Leishmania* species known to be associated with mucosal disease should be treated.

The pentavalent antimonials stibogluconate sodium and meglumine antimoniate are used for the treatment of cutaneous leishmaniasis in many situations. Full doses of 20 mg of pentavalent antimony per kilogram of body weight per day are recommended for 28 days; lower doses may favor the development of antimony resistance. Cutaneous lesions heal slowly during antimony therapy. As described earlier for visceral leishmaniasis, pentavalent antimonials are frequently associated with toxicity, and clinical failures occur.

Oral fluconazole, itraconazole, and ketoconazole have variable activity against *Leishmania* species. For example, fluconazole, 200 mg/day for 6 weeks, resulted in a response rate of 90% in American troops with cutaneous leishmaniasis caused by *L. major.* In contrast, studies in the Americas showed high failure rates in persons infected with *L. braziliensis* who were treated with imidazoles.

A number of other drugs and therapeutic approaches have been studied. Direct injection of pentavalent antimony compounds into cutaneous lesions is used in some areas. The administration of intralesional or topical human granulocyte-macrophage colony-stimulating factor with systemic pentavalent antimony has been reported to improve the cure rate and reduce the time to healing in persons with cutaneous leishmaniasis in Brazil. A topical formulation of paromomycin sulfate, methylbenzethonium chloride, and white paraffin has been used successfully to treat skin lesions caused by *L. major* in the Middle East and, to a limited degree, elsewhere. In addition, immunotherapy with killed promastigotes inoculated with bacille Calmette-Guérin has also been reported to be effective in Latin America.

Treatment of persons with mucosal leishmaniasis and diffuse cutaneous leishmaniasis is far more challenging. Therapeutic failures and relapses are common after treatment with pentavalent antimony, and long courses of therapy have been recommended. Amphotericin B deoxycholate and pentamidine are potentially effective, but toxic alternatives. Lipid-encapsulated amphotericin B and miltefosine have not yet been fully evaluated, but recent data suggest that *Leishmania* species in the New World are not as susceptible as *L. donovani* in India. The concurrent administration of pentavalent antimony with pentoxifylline or thalidomide, which decrease TNF-α production, has been reported to improve responses in patients with refractory mucosal leishmaniasis. When necessary, reconstructive surgery in persons with mucosal disease should be delayed for 6 to 12 months after chemotherapy because relapses are common and can result in a poor cosmetic outcome.

Prevention

In general, transmission of *Leishmania* species depends on the presence of a sandfly vector and appropriate reservoirs. Residual insecticide spraying has been used successfully to limit transmission by peridomestic sandflies, but it is seldom used because of emerging insect resistance and environmental concerns. Personal protective measures, including insecticide-impregnated, fine-mesh netting for sleep, insect repellents containing diethyltoluamide (DEET) applied to the skin, and permethrin-impregnated clothing, reduce the frequency of sandfly bites and the likelihood of transmission. Unfortunately, these measures are often not available for residents of endemic areas. Large-scale control programs have been carried out in areas of South America where domestic dogs are a reservoir, but their efficacy is debated. Deltamethrin-impregnated collars were shown to decrease canine anti-*Leishmania* antibody titers significantly by 50%. However, the long-term impact on transmission will depend on collar coverage and the rate of loss. Clinical observations in humans and studies of experimental animal models suggest that immunoprophylaxis should be possible. Experience with killed-promastigote vaccines is mixed. Recent studies have focused on the development of DNA, recombinant, and live attenuated vaccines, but none are currently available for human use.

SUGGESTED READINGS

Castellucci L, Cheng LH, Araujo C, et al: Familial aggregation of mucosal leishmaniasis in northeast Brazil. Am J Trop Med Hyg 2005;73:69–73. *The epidemiology and clinical manifestations of American cutaneous and mucosal leishmaniasis were characterized in a family study done in a highly endemic area of Brazil.*

Machado PR, Lessa H, Lessa M, et al: Oral pentoxifylline combined with pentavalent antimony: A randomized trial for mucosal leishmaniasis. Clin Infect Dis 2007;44:788–793. *The addition of pentoxifylline to pentavalent antimony reduces the healing time and prevents the need for further courses of pentavalent antimony.*

Murray HW, Berman JD, Davies CR, Saravia NG: Advances in leishmaniasis. Lancet 2005;366:1561–1577. *An overview of the more recent advances in leishmaniasis is presented. Its epidemiology, pathogenesis, and treatment are reviewed in detail.*

Weina PJ, Neafie RC, Wortmann G, et al: Old world leishmaniasis: An emerging infection among deployed US military and civilian workers. Clin Infect Dis 2004;39:1674–1680. *A review of infection and disease development in a naive population exposed to* Leishmania *is presented.*

Wilson ME, Jeronimo SM, Pearson RD: Immunopathogenesis of infection with the visceralizing *Leishmania* species. Microb Pathog 2005;38:147–160. *The immunopathogenesis of visceral leishmaniasis is reviewed.*

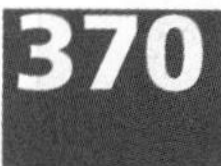

370 TOXOPLASMOSIS

Oliver Liesenfeld

Definition

Toxoplasma gondii is a protozoan parasite that is ubiquitous in nature and infects a variety of mammals and birds throughout the world. Acute acquired infections in humans are usually asymptomatic and result in the formation of cysts that persist for the life of the host without causing signs or symptoms (*Toxoplasma* infection). However, clinical or pathologic evidence of disease (i.e., toxoplasmosis) may occur, particularly in immunocompromised patients, congenitally infected fetuses and children, and those in whom chorioretinitis develops during the acute acquired or reactivated infection.

The Pathogen

There are three forms of the parasite: the tachyzoite, which is the asexual invasive form; the tissue cyst, which contains bradyzoites and persists in tissues of infected hosts during the latent phase of the infection; and the oocyst, which contains sporozoites and is produced during the sexual cycle in the intestine of members of the cat family, the definitive host. The extraintestinal asexual cycle occurs in all incidental hosts and in cats. After the ingestion of tissue cysts or oocysts, bradyzoites or sporozoites, respectively, are released into the intestinal lumen, where they invade surrounding cells, become tachyzoites, and disseminate throughout the body via blood. The *tachyzoite* (Fig. 370–1A) has a crescent shape, measures approximately 4 to 8 μm in length, requires an intracellular habitat for survival, and can infect all mammalian cells. Continued multiplication results in destruction of the host cell and release of tachyzoites, which can then infect other cells. Tachyzoites are found in tissues during the acute stage of the infection or during reactivation of the chronic infection. Freezing and thawing, desiccation, and gastric secretions kill tachyzoites. Development of immunity is associated with the disappearance of tachyzoites and formation of tissue cysts containing bradyzoites.

Tissue cysts (see Fig. 370–1B) are 10 to 200 μm in diameter and may contain up to several thousand bradyzoites, which are indiscernible from tachyzoites by light microscopy. *Bradyzoites* can be found in all organs

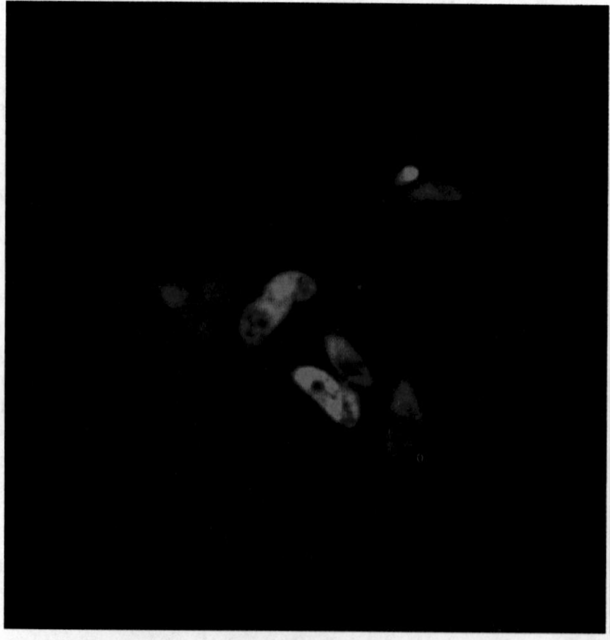

A

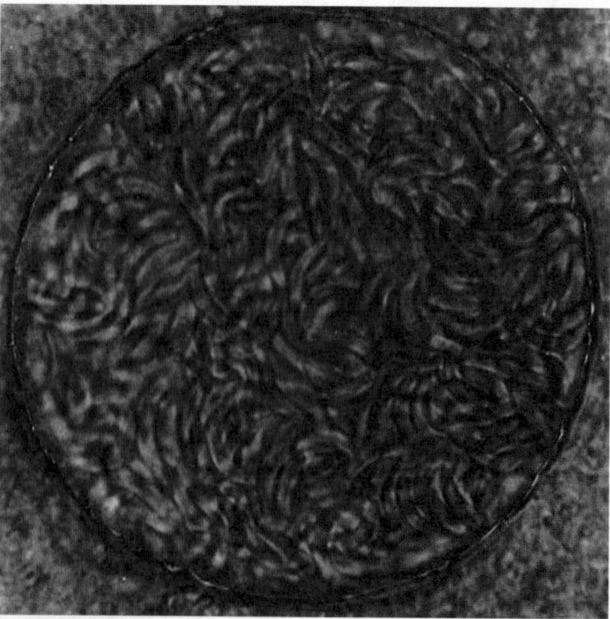

B

FIGURE 370–1 • *Toxoplasma gondii.* **A,** Tachyzoites. **B,** *T. gondii* cyst containing bradyzoites.

and are most readily observed in the central nervous system (CNS) and in myocardial, skeletal, and smooth muscle. In humans, they persist for life and most likely are the site of reactivation in immunocompromised hosts. Unlike tachyzoites, bradyzoites released from tissue cysts are relatively resistant to the digestive process of the gastrointestinal tract.

The enteroepithelial sexual cycle results in the formation of oocysts in the cat's intestine. *Oocysts* containing sporozoites are 10 to 12 μm in diameter, are excreted in feces 3 to 34 days after the cat becomes infected, and continue to be excreted for 7 to 20 days, after which excretion rarely recurs. They become infectious only after they are excreted and sporulation occurs; the duration of this process depends on environmental conditions but is usually 2 to 5 days. They may remain infectious in the environment for more than 1 year. Transmission is primarily by the oral route through the ingestion of raw or undercooked meat containing *T. gondii* cysts or through accidental ingestion of food or water contaminated with oocysts.

Virulence in laboratory mice, isoenzyme pattern analysis, restriction fragment length polymorphisms, and serotyping of polymorphic peptides have been used to differentiate strains of *T. gondii,* which can be divided into three clonal lineages designated genotypes I, II, and III. They appear to be derived from two genetically distinct ancestries by sexual recombination. The acquisition of direct oral transmission appears to be a rather recent evolutionary change that has contributed to widespread expansion of the parasite. The frequency and severity of infection with type I, II, or III strains are a focus of ongoing research.

TABLE 370–1 INCIDENCE OF CONGENITAL *TOXOPLASMA GONDII* INFECTION ACCORDING TO GESTATIONAL AGE AT TIME OF INFECTION OF THE MOTHER

Weeks of Gestation*	No. of Infected Fetuses/ Total No. of Fetuses (%)
0–2	0/100 (0)
3–6	6/384 (1.6)
7–10	9/503 (1.8)
11–14	37/511 (7.2)
15–18	49/392 (13)
19–22	44/237 (19)
23–26	30/116 (26)
27–30	7/32 (22)
31–34	4/6 (67)
Unknown	8/351 (2.3)
Total	194/2632 (7.4)

*Patients were treated with spiramycin.
From Hohlfeld P, Daffos F, Costa J-M, et al: Prenatal diagnosis of congenital toxoplasmosis with a polymerase-chain-reaction test on amniotic fluid. N Engl J Med 1994;331:695–699.

Epidemiology

In the United States, depending on geographic locale and population group, 3 to 67% of adults have serologic evidence of infection. In other parts of the world, including tropical countries and some areas of western Europe, up to 75% of adults are seropositive. The prevalence of antibodies to *T. gondii* does not differ between men and women. Transmission to humans occurs by ingestion of tissue cysts or oocysts, the transplacental route, blood product transfusion, solid organ transplantation (i.e., kidney, heart, or liver from a seropositive donor to a seronegative recipient), and laboratory accident. Outbreaks of toxoplasmosis caused by eating undercooked meat or exposure to oocysts (e.g., contaminated water) have occurred. Commercial cuts of game, lamb, and pork may contain tissue cysts that remain infectious unless the meat is frozen to −20° C or heated throughout to 66° C. The percentage of commercial cuts of meat containing tissue cysts has declined to below 5% in industrialized countries. Transmission by eating undercooked or raw meat containing tissue cysts rather than consumption of vegetables or other food products contaminated with oocysts is the main source of infection in Europe. The estimated incidence of congenital toxoplasmosis in the United States and Europe is 1 case per 1000 to 10,000 live births. Transplacental infection resulting in congenital infection can occur in immunocompetent pregnant women with recently acquired *T. gondii* infection and in immunocompromised pregnant women with reactivation of their chronic infection. The frequency of transmission to the fetus probably depends on maternal parasitemia, maturity of the placenta, and competency of the maternal immune response to *T. gondii.* Congenital transmission has been shown to vary considerably depending on the time during gestation that the mother acquired her infection (Table 370–1). The earlier the transmission to the fetus, the more severe the outcome. Approximately 85% of infants with congenital infection, especially those infected later during pregnancy, appear normal at birth. However, if untreated, as many as 85% of these children will later have signs and symptoms of the disease, in most cases chorioretinitis or delays in development. Maternal infection acquired weeks before, around the time of conception, and within the first 2 weeks of gestation does not usually result in transmission.

Toxoplasmic encephalitis (TE) in patients with acquired immunodeficiency syndrome (AIDS) and in bone marrow transplant recipients is almost always caused by reactivation of latent infection. The incidence of this disease is therefore proportional to the prevalence of *T. gondii* antibodies (i.e., latent infection) in a given population and the stage of human immunodeficiency virus (HIV) infection in the respective patients (usually a $CD4^+$ T-cell count <200 cells/μL). In the United States, *T. gondii* seroprevalence in HIV-infected individuals varies from 10 to 45%. It is estimated that TE ultimately develops in 20 to 47% of HIV-infected, *T. gondii*–seropositive patients if they are not receiving appropriate antiparasitic prophylaxis or highly active antiretroviral therapy (HAART). In a European multicenter study, the incidence of toxoplasmosis was 6%, and patients initially had encephalitis or pulmonary or disseminated disease at diagnosis; the incidence of *Toxoplasma* infection (detection of *Toxoplasma*-specific DNA in blood by polymerase chain reaction [PCR]) was 16%.

Pathobiology

Pathogenesis

After infection by the oral route, tachyzoites disseminate from the gastrointestinal tract (possibly in $CD11c^+$ dendritic cells as a Trojan horse strategy) and can invade virtually any cell or tissue, where they proliferate, infect adjoining cells, and produce necrotic foci surrounded by inflammation. In immunocompromised individuals, acute infection may result in severe damage to multiple organs. Cell-mediated immunity and humoral immunity play a crucial role in resistance against *T. gondii.* In mice, recognition of *T. gondii* and its antigens by antigen-presenting cells and the resulting interleukin-12 (IL-12) production are in part mediated by toll-like receptor 11 and chemokine receptor 5. Immune mechanisms that contribute to control of acute infection and termination of continued tissue destruction by the proliferating parasite include local and systemic activation of the helper T-cell type 1 (T_H1) response. Activation of the monocyte-macrophage system after phagocytosis of parasites leads to death of the parasite. The αβ and γδ T cells are activated, and sensitized $CD4^+$ and $CD8^+$ T cells are cytotoxic for *T. gondii*–infected cells. Proinflammatory (e.g., interferon-γ, IL-12, tumor necrosis factor-α) and regulatory (e.g., IL-10, transforming growth factor-β) cytokines exert and balance the response; interferon-γ plays the pivotal role in this immunity. *T. gondii* infection triggers the production of immunoglobulin G (IgG), IgM, IgA, and IgE antibodies against multiple *T. gondii* proteins of the surface (i.e., SAG1-4), dense granules, and micronemes. Despite a normal immune response, tissue cysts form in multiple organs. Disruption of cysts or "leakage" of bradyzoites from cysts appears to occur in normal hosts without causing disease. However, conversion into tachyzoites and replication can result in life-threatening disease in immunocompromised patients. Localized reactivation in the eye of immunocompetent children or adults may be manifested as recurrent retinochoroiditis.

Genetic regulation of susceptibility to infection has been reported in murine models of the disease. In AIDS patients, human leukocyte antigen HLA-DQ3 was found to be a genetic marker of susceptibility to the development of TE, whereas HLA-DQ1 was found to be a genetic marker of resistance to the development of TE.

Pathology

Pathologic changes vary, depending on the immune status of the individual. Histologic preparations of tissues of normal individuals rarely reveal the presence of tissue cysts; when present, they do not have a surrounding inflammatory response. However, immunocompetent adults suffering from toxoplasmic retinochoroiditis may have tachyzoites, necrosis, and mononuclear cell infiltrates in their retinas and choroids.

Histopathologic changes of toxoplasmic lymphadenitis in immunocompetent patients consist of a distinctive and usually diagnostic triad of reactive follicular hyperplasia, irregular clusters of epithelioid histiocytes that encroach on and blur the margins of germinal centers, and focal distention of sinuses with monocytoid cells. These findings reflect an immune response to infection rather than the presence of the organism, which is rarely observed.

Tissues of immunocompromised patients with toxoplasmosis exhibit, in addition to tissue cysts, foci of intracellular tachyzoite proliferation with resultant cell death, tissue necrosis, and inflammation. The inflammatory response can occur in multiple tissues and consists of lymphocytes, plasma cells, mononuclear phagocytes, and few neutrophils. It occurs most commonly in the brain, lung, heart, and gastrointestinal tract but has also been observed in the liver, spleen, pancreas, kidney, seminiferous tubules, prostate, adrenals, bone marrow, and skeletal muscle. The most frequently clinically apparent site of involvement in these patients is the CNS, which may have acute focal or diffuse meningoencephalitis with necrosis, microglial nodules, and perivascular mononuclear inflammation. These lesions are usually multiple and diffusely distributed. Tachyzoites and tissue cysts are generally found at the periphery of necrotic areas. TE has a predilection for the subcortical area of the cerebral hemispheres, basal ganglia, cerebellum, and brain stem. Some patients have a diffuse form of TE with widespread microglial nodules without abscess formation that involves the gray matter of the cerebrum, cerebellum, and brain stem. Spinal cord involvement can occur and mimic tumor. Pulmonary involvement is second in frequency only to TE in AIDS patients and is characterized by interstitial or necrotizing pneumonitis and areas of consolidation.

Clinical Manifestations

Acute Infection in Immunocompetent Patients

T. gondii infection is symptomatic in only approximately 5% of immunocompetent individuals. In these patients, toxoplasmosis is most often manifested as lymphadenopathy. Although any or all lymph node groups may be involved, cervical lymphadenopathy is most common; nodes are usually discrete, nontender, nonsuppurative, and asymptomatic. However, some patients may experience fever, myalgias, arthralgias, fatigue, headache, visual disturbances (as a result of chorioretinitis), sore throat, maculopapular rash, urticaria, hepatosplenomegaly, and rarely, pulmonary disease and myocarditis. Involvement of the retroperitoneal or mesenteric nodes may be associated with abdominal pain.

Ocular Toxoplasmosis in Immunocompetent Patients

T. gondii infection has been reported to be responsible for approximately 35% of cases of retinochoroiditis in older children and adults in the United States. Acute infection rather than a late manifestation of congenital infection is the principal cause of *T. gondii* retinochoroiditis. *T. gondii* retinochoroiditis as a reactivation of congenital infection is seen more often in children younger than 10 years. Reactivation is uncommon after the age of 40. Patients may have blurred vision, scotoma, pain, photophobia, or epiphora. Macular involvement may impair central vision. Systemic symptoms do not usually accompany ocular involvement. Ophthalmologic examination reveals multiple, yellow-white, cotton-like patches with indistinct margins located in small clusters in the posterior pole. These changes are often sufficient to make the diagnosis. Relapses of chorioretinitis are frequently associated with scarred lesions juxtaposed to the fresh lesion. Retinochoroiditis may be part of a syndrome of panuveitis; isolated anterior uveitis has not been associated with *T. gondii*. It remains to be shown whether pathology in the eye is mainly due to direct damage by the parasite or instead caused by the immune response against the parasite.

Lesions may heal spontaneously, in which case they become atrophic with whitish gray plaques and distinct margins surrounded by areas of black choroidal pigment. Lesions at different stages of development may be present simultaneously. Multiple relapses may occur in patients with congenital as well as postnatally acquired infection and may result in glaucoma and loss of vision.

Toxoplasmosis in Immunocompromised Patients

In most cases, toxoplasmosis in immunocompromised patients is the result of reactivation of latent infection. Numerous conditions that compromise the immune system have been associated with toxoplasmosis, with the highest frequencies in patients with AIDS, those with lymphoma, and other patients who are taking high-dose corticosteroids or other immunosuppressive agents for the treatment of malignancies and collagen vascular disorders or for prevention of organ transplant rejection. In patients with these conditions, toxoplasmosis may also be caused by exogenous acquisition of infection, especially in seronegative recipients of solid organ (i.e., heart) transplants from seropositive donors. If untreated, toxoplasmosis in immunocompromised patients is often rapidly progressive and fatal.

Clinical manifestations most commonly reflect involvement of the CNS, lungs, eyes, and heart. In 30 to 50% of HIV-infected, *Toxoplasma*-seropositive individuals, TE will develop if they are not receiving appropriate antiparasitic prophylaxis or HAART. TE has traditionally been the most common manifestation and, along with lymphoma, has been the most frequent cause of intracerebral mass lesions in patients with AIDS (Chapter 417); the relative incidence of TE has decreased markedly after the introduction of HAART. As a result of multifocal involvement of the CNS, clinical findings vary widely and include alterations in mental status, seizures, motor weakness, cranial nerve disorders, sensory abnormalities, cerebellar signs, meningismus, movement disorders, and neuropsychiatric manifestations. Typically, TE is characterized by focal neurologic abnormalities of subacute onset, frequently accompanied by nonfocal signs and symptoms such as headache, altered mental status, and fever. The most common focal neurologic sign is motor weakness, but patients may also experience cranial nerve abnormalities, cognitive disorders, speech disturbances, visual field defects, sensory disturbances, cerebellar signs, focal seizures, and movement disorders. Meningeal signs may be present. Analysis of cerebrospinal fluid (CSF) may detect a slight mononuclear pleocytosis, increased protein level, and normal glucose level. Although radiologic findings are not pathognomonic, the presence of multiple focal lesions in AIDS patients strongly favors the diagnosis of TE, whereas the presence of a single lesion makes lymphoma more likely. Computed tomography (CT) usually shows multiple bilateral cerebral lesions that tend to be located at the corticomedullary junction and the basal ganglia. Lesions are surrounded by edema, are generally hypodense, and show ring enhancement after intravenous contrast. CT scans tend to underestimate the number of lesions and may show a single lesion when magnetic resonance imaging (MRI) reveals two or more lesions. Because MRI is more sensitive for detecting the lesions of TE, it is the preferred radiologic method for patients with suspected TE and is of particular importance in patients with only a single lesion indicated on CT scans. The differential diagnosis of TE includes CNS lymphoma, progressive multifocal leukoencephalopathy, and infections caused by other pathogens, including viruses, fungi, and bacteria.

Toxoplasmic pneumonitis may develop in the absence of extrapulmonary disease. Its clinical and radiologic features are nonspecific and may mimic those of *Pneumocystis jirovecii* pneumonia. Patients experience fever, dyspnea, and nonproductive cough, and the chest radiograph usually shows bilateral interstitial infiltrates. Disseminated toxoplasmosis in AIDS patients has been reported to present a picture of septic shock and adult respiratory distress syndrome. Although ocular toxoplasmosis is uncommon in patients with AIDS, it is still the second most common cause of retinal infection in these individuals. Toxoplasmic chorioretinitis in AIDS patients is characterized by yellow-white areas of retinitis with fluffy borders. It should be distinguished from ocular involvement by cytomegalovirus, syphilis, herpes simplex, varicella zoster, *P. jirovecii*, fungi, and lymphoma. When compared with the lesions of cytomegalovirus retinitis, those of toxoplasmic chorioretinitis usually occur at the posterior pole, are more fluffy and edematous, have ill-defined margins, and are nonhemorrhagic. Clinical manifestations from cardiac involvement occur but are unusual. In non-AIDS immunocompromised patients, congestive heart failure, arrhythmias, and pericarditis have been reported. Toxoplasmic myocarditis can mimic heart transplant rejection.

Diagnosis

Toxoplasmosis can be diagnosed by isolation of the organism, PCR methods, demonstration of tachyzoites in tissues or body fluids by histologic or cytologic analysis, and serologic testing. Whereas direct demonstration of the parasite is often used for diagnosis of the infection in immunocompromised patients, serologic analysis is most commonly used for diagnosis in immunocompetent patients. Serologic tests for detection of *Toxoplasma* IgG and IgM antibodies are most commonly used for the diagnosis of *T. gondii* infection and toxoplasmosis. IgG antibodies can be detected with the Sabin-Feldman dye test (considered the "gold standard"), indirect fluorescent antibody, agglutination, or enzyme-linked immunosorbent assay. IgG antibodies measured by the dye test and the indirect fluorescent antibody test usually appear 1 to 2 weeks after infection, peak in 6 to 8 weeks, and gradually decline thereafter; low titers generally persist for life. The agglutination test is a sensitive and inexpensive method to screen for IgG antibodies.

Detection of IgM antibodies is frequently useful when attempting to diagnose acute infection. IgM antibodies are demonstrable as early as 5 days after infection and usually decrease after a few weeks or months. However, because IgM antibodies may persist for 1 year or longer after infection, a positive IgM antibody titer finding does not necessarily mean that the patient has recently been infected. Furthermore, many commercial serologic testing kits to detect *T. gondii* IgM antibodies give unacceptable numbers of false-positive results. The greatest value of an IgM antibody test lies in determining whether an otherwise normal individual has *not* been infected recently. A negative IgM serologic test result in immunocompetent patients virtually rules out recently acquired infection unless sera are tested so early that an antibody response has not yet developed or is not yet detectable. Correct interpretation of serologic test results is of utmost importance for the diagnosis of infection in pregnant women. For example, pregnant women may choose abortion when informed of a positive IgM test result; a negative IgM test result late in gestation may reflect the fact that the patient had not recently acquired the infection or that IgM antibodies, because of *T. gondii* infection acquired early in pregnancy, may have disappeared by that time. Testing of the avidity (i.e., functional affinity) of *Toxoplasma* IgG antibodies has proved to be an excellent tool to distinguish recent and distant infection in patients with positive IgM antibodies; the presence of high-avidity antibodies in the first trimester excludes an infection acquired during pregnancy, whereas low-avidity antibodies may persist for several months. Appropriate diagnosis and interpretation of results in pregnant women often require that a panel of tests be performed and evaluated in a reference laboratory to assist in discriminating between recent and more distant infection. Confirmatory testing in a reference laboratory has revealed that recently acquired infections had occurred in only 40% of women who had positive results in tests for IgM antibodies in commercial laboratories; 17% of these women had their pregnancies terminated when informed of the results. Communication of the results and their correct interpretation by an expert in *Toxoplasma* serologic characteristics decreased the rate of unnecessary abortions by 50% in women with positive IgM *Toxoplasma* antibody test results by commercial laboratories. Whether detection of IgA antibodies increases the accuracy of routine testing for IgG and IgM antibodies in pregnant women has not been evaluated in detail.

Definitive serologic diagnosis of acute infection requires the demonstration of seroconversion (i.e., from seronegative to seropositive). Recent infection is likely when serial specimens obtained at least 3 weeks apart and tested in parallel show a significant rise in IgG antibody titer and when IgM, IgA, or IgE antibody titers are present in conjunction with an "acute" pattern in an avidity test result.

Serologic testing in HIV-infected patients is mainly useful for identifying those at risk for the development of toxoplasmosis and in assisting physicians faced with the problem of diagnosing the cause of CNS lesions in such individuals. All HIV-positive patients should be tested for the presence of IgG antibodies. In AIDS patients with $CD4^+$ T-cell counts less than 200/μL, high IgG *Toxoplasma* antibody titers are associated with a greater likelihood of the development of TE. Serologic test findings may be misleading in chronically infected patients who receive heart or other organ transplants because these patients can have rising titers of IgG and IgM antibodies without clinical evidence of active *T. gondii* infection. Definitive diagnosis of toxoplasmosis in immunodeficient patients ultimately relies on histologic studies, isolation of the parasite, or identification of *T. gondii* DNA in body fluids or tissues. However, a presumptive diagnosis of TE in AIDS patients can be made when a compatible clinical manifestation, multiple ring-enhancing lesions on CT or MRI, and IgG *Toxoplasma* antibodies are present. HIV-infected patients who have a single lesion on MRI, are seronegative for *T. gondii* antibodies, or are not responding to specific treatment should be considered for brain biopsy.

Isolation of *T. gondii* is accomplished by inoculating blood, CSF, bronchoalveolar lavage (BAL) fluid, vitreous fluid, amniotic fluid, or tissue specimens into mice or cell culture. Mouse inoculation is more sensitive but less rapid than cell culture. Positive results obtained in isolation studies from tissue samples do not necessarily indicate acute infection because a positive result may be caused by the presence of bradyzoites (cysts), which is indicative of latent infection.

PCR has been used successfully on CSF, amniotic fluid, BAL samples, and blood to diagnose toxoplasmosis. The sensitivity of PCR on CSF ranges from 11 to 77%; PCR on blood has been successfully used primarily in patients with disseminated disease caused by *T. gondii.* PCR on amniotic fluid has been successfully used for the diagnosis of fetal infection at 18 weeks' gestation. Because of its greater sensitivity and specificity, which approach approximately 100%, rapid performance, and safety, PCR on amniotic fluid has replaced conventional prenatal diagnostic techniques, including fetal blood sampling. In addition to conventional PCR, more recently, several quantitative real-time PCR (Q-PCR) assays have been developed for measurement of *T. gondii* in amniotic fluid, placenta, aqueous humor, whole blood, CSF, and BAL fluid. Q-PCR assays may significantly improve the diagnosis of toxoplasmosis. They remain, however, in the experimental phases of development. Routine histologic and cytologic staining may not allow tachyzoites to be identified in tissue sections. An immunohistochemical method (e.g., immunoperoxidase staining) should be used to confirm their presence. The finding of multiple cysts in tissue sections near an area of inflammation and necrosis is highly suggestive of active infection. The characteristic lymph node histologic findings are often sufficient to make the diagnosis of toxoplasmic lymphadenitis.

Treatment Rx

The need for and duration of therapy depend on the clinical manifestations of toxoplasmosis and the immune status of the patient. All commonly used drug regimens target the tachyzoite stage of the parasite, but none of the drug regimens tested thus far have been proved to eradicate cysts effectively from the host. The drug combination of pyrimethamine and sulfadiazine is considered the regimen of choice and is synergistic against tachyzoites. It is not active against the tissue cyst form. For the treatment of cerebral toxoplasmosis in adults, a loading dose of 200 mg of pyrimethamine is administered orally in two divided doses on the first day. Thereafter, patients receive 50 to 75 mg/day orally; the dosage depends on the severity of the disease and the immunologic status of the patient. Sulfadiazine is administered at a dose of 1000 mg (<60 kg) to 1500 mg (>60 kg) orally four times a day. Other sulfonamides have less activity against *T. gondii.* Treatment is usually continued for 1 to 2 weeks after resolution of the signs or symptoms in other than the most severely immunocompromised patients, such as those with AIDS. Thereafter, careful follow-up observation is indicated. AIDS patients receive maintenance (secondary prophylaxis) therapy as long as their immune system has not been reconstituted by HAART. Because pyrimethamine is a folate antagonist, the most common side effect is dose-related bone marrow suppression. Patients receiving pyrimethamine should be prescribed an oral dose of 10 to 25 mg/day of folinic acid (not folic acid) and have complete blood cell and platelet counts measured twice weekly. Patients receiving sulfonamides should maintain high urinary flow to prevent crystal-induced nephrotoxicity. Other important side effects of sulfonamides are fever, rash, leukopenia, and hepatitis. In patients with side effects during sulfadiazine therapy, clindamycin is commonly used in combination with pyrimethamine. However, clindamycin therapy results in side effects such as rash and diarrhea in a significant number of patients.

Acute Infection in Immunocompetent Patients

Patients with toxoplasmic lymphadenitis do not require antimicrobial therapy unless symptoms are severe and persistent. Patients with toxoplasmic retinochoroiditis are treated with pyrimethamine, sulfadiazine, and folinic acid in most centers. The recommended dose of pyrimethamine in these cases is 50 to 75 mg/day as a single dose; the recommended dose of sulfadiazine is 1 to 1.5 g four times a day. Clindamycin, alone or in combination with pyrimethamine or sulfadiazine, has also been effective. Systemic corticosteroids are added to the regimen when chorioretinitis involves the macula, optic nerve head, or papillomacular bundle. Infections acquired after a blood transfusion or laboratory accident may be severe and should therefore be treated.

Acute Infection in Pregnant Women

Spiramycin at a dose of 3 g/day divided into three equal doses until term or until fetal infection is confirmed has been stated to reduce the incidence of fetal infection by about 60% (spiramycin is obtained from the U.S. Food and Drug Administration, 301-827-2335). If prenatal diagnosis reveals infection in the fetus, the pregnant patient should receive pyrimethamine, sulfadiazine, and folinic acid to treat the fetus. Because of potential teratogenicity, pyrimethamine should not be administered in the first trimester. If necessary, sulfadiazine may be used, but its efficacy when used alone for this purpose has not been studied.

Toxoplasmosis in Immunocompromised Patients

Immunodeficient patients with toxoplasmosis or with serologic evidence of acute *T. gondii* infection should be treated. Latent asymptomatic infection does not require treatment. In non-AIDS immunodeficient patients, therapy is usually administered for 4 to 6 weeks after all clinical evidence of toxoplasmosis has resolved. Treatment is usually based on the presumptive diagnosis of TE. Treatment of toxoplasmosis in AIDS patients has two phases: acute-stage therapy and maintenance treatment. Acute therapy should be administered for at least 6 weeks. Pyrimethamine and sulfadiazine or pyrimethamine plus clindamycin has been used with comparable results (Table 370–2). Most patients respond to these regimens, and neurologic improvement generally takes place within the first 7 days. Brain biopsy should be considered if clinical improvement does not occur during the first 10 days of treatment or if deterioration occurs during the first 7 days. Brain biopsy should also be considered at initial evaluation in AIDS patients who are seronegative for IgG antibodies to *T. gondii* and those compliant with primary prophylaxis against toxoplasmosis (see Prevention) who have focal lesions indicated by neuroimaging. Many AIDS patients do not tolerate one or the other regimen because of rash (pyrimethamine and sulfadiazine), rash and diarrhea (pyrimethamine plus clindamycin), or bone marrow suppression (pyrimethamine and sulfadiazine or pyrimethamine plus clindamycin). Atovaquone has been used in combination with pyrimethamine or sulfadiazine in patients who did not tolerate either of the latter drugs. Short courses of corticosteroids should be administered to treat mass effects attributed to focal lesions or associated cerebral edema. Anticonvulsants should be administered to patients with a history of seizures.

The mortality rate for treated patients ranges from approximately 1 to 25%. Because most AIDS patients relapse when treatment is discontinued, maintenance therapy is necessary in those patients in whom immune functions have not been reconstituted by HAART. Generally, the same drugs used for acute therapy are continued, but at lower doses (see Table 370–2). For patients who do not tolerate any of these regimens for acute-stage or maintenance therapy, the alternatives listed in Table 370–3 can be tried in combination with pyrimethamine. Recommendations regarding discontinuation of secondary prophylaxis are given in the Prevention section.

Prevention

Preventing the infection is particularly important for seronegative immunocompromised patients and pregnant women. Because the infection is acquired primarily via the oral route—through the ingestion of undercooked meat or food/water contaminated with oocysts—it is preventable in most cases. It is the responsibility of the physician to instruct patients on how to prevent infection. Recommendations include eating meat (i.e., game, lamb, pork, and beef) only if it is well cooked through-

TABLE 370–2 GUIDELINES FOR ACUTE AND MAINTENANCE THERAPY FOR TOXOPLASMIC ENCEPHALITIS IN AIDS PATIENTS

	Acute Therapy	Maintenance Therapy*
SUGGESTED REGIMENS (GRADE A EVIDENCE)		
Pyrimethamine *plus*	200-mg loading dose PO, then 50 (<60 kg of body weight) to 75 mg (>60 kg) qd	25 to 50 mg qd
Folinic acid (leucovorin)	10 to 25 mg qd PO (up to 50 mg qd)	10 to 25 mg qd
plus one of the following:		
Sulfadiazine	1000 (<60 kg) to 1500 (>60 kg) mg PO q6h	0.5 g q6h
or		
Clindamycin	600 mg PO or IV q6h	300 to 450 mg q6h
ALTERNATIVE REGIMENS† (GRADE B EVIDENCE)		
Trimethoprim-sulfamethoxazole	(5 mg TMP, 25 mg SMX)/kg PO or IV q12h	No adequate data
Atovaquone	1500 mg PO q12h with meals	
Pyrimethamine and folinic acid	As in Suggested Regimens	As in Suggested Regimens
plus one of the following:		
Atovaquone	1500 mg PO q12h with meals	750 mg q6h
Azithromycin	900 to 1200 mg qd PO	
Sulfadiazine plus:	As in Suggested Regimens	
Atovaquone	1500 mg PO q12h with meals	

*Drugs administered orally.
†Data inadequate for definitive recommendation.
Adapted from Benson CA, Kaplan JE, Masur H, et al: Treating opportunistic infections among HIV-exposed and infected children: Recommendations from CDC, the National Institutes of Health, and the Infectious Diseases Society of America. MMWR Recomm Rep 2004;55(RR-15):1–112.

TABLE 370–3 PRIMARY PROPHYLAXIS FOR TOXOPLASMOSIS IN AIDS PATIENTS*

FOR *TOXOPLASMA GONDII*–SEROPOSITIVE HIV-INFECTED INDIVIDUALS†	
SUGGESTED REGIMEN (GRADE A EVIDENCE)	
Trimethoprim-sulfamethoxazole	1 double-strength tablet daily
ALTERNATIVE REGIMENS (GRADE B EVIDENCE)	
Pyrimethamine-dapsone	Pyrimethamine, 50 mg once each week, plus dapsone, 50 mg qd, plus folinic acid (leucovorin), 25 mg qd
	Pyrimethamine, 75 mg once each week, plus dapsone, 200 mg once each week, plus folinic acid (leucovorin), 25 mg qd
Trimethoprim-sulfamethoxazole	1 single-strength tablet daily
FOR PREVENTION OF CONGENITAL TRANSMISSION OF *T. GONDII* IN SEROPOSITIVE, HIV-INFECTED PREGNANT WOMEN‡	
Spiramycin	1 g q8h

*Drugs are administered orally.
†These regimens have been reported to be effective for primary prophylaxis of toxoplasmic encephalitis in AIDS patients.
‡Although no data are available on the efficacy of prophylaxis against congenital transmission in this group of patients, we consider it prudent to recommend spiramycin because preliminary studies suggest that the transmission rate for congenital toxoplasmosis in these women is remarkably and significantly higher than in non–HIV-infected, *T. gondii*–seropositive women.
AIDS = acquired immunodeficiency syndrome; HIV = human immunodeficiency syndrome.
Adapted from Liesenfeld O, Wong SY, Remington JS: Toxoplasmosis in the setting of AIDS. *In* Merigan TC Jr, Bartlett JG, Bolognesi D (eds): Textbook of AIDS Medicine. Baltimore, Williams & Wilkins, 1999, pp 225–259; and from 2001 U.S. Public Health Service and Infectious Disease Society of America guidelines for the prevention of opportunistic infections in persons infected with HIV, November 28, 2001 (available at www.hivatis.org/guidelines/other/OIs/).

out, washing hands after touching raw meat, washing fruits and vegetables, and avoiding contact with cat feces. In an attempt to prevent congenital toxoplasmosis, routine serologic screening of pregnant women has been performed to identify fetuses at risk for becoming infected. Mandatory screening programs have been successfully implemented in France and Austria. If serologic testing should be chosen, the serologic status of pregnant women should be evaluated no later than the 10th or 12th week of gestation. Those who are seronegative should be retested at the 20th to 22nd week and then again near term.

Administering spiramycin to acutely infected pregnant women (see Treatment) was stated to reduce the incidence of congenital infection by approximately 60%. In Massachusetts and in Denmark, a secondary screening program consisting of serologic screening of all newborns (for IgG or IgM antibodies, or both) has been implemented because of the lack of feasibility of screening all pregnant women. When compared with initial clinical examination, neonatal screening showed dramatically higher sensitivity for the diagnosis of congenital infection. However, because detection of IgM antibodies in newborns is only 75% sensitive, a significant number of subclinically infected infants or infants infected in the late third trimester will be missed. Moreover, a secondary prevention program does not allow prenatal diagnosis and subsequent treatment of the fetus. Such treatment has proved to be highly effective in preventing severe fetal damage.

The high rate of relapse in patients with toxoplasmic chorioretinitis was successfully decreased by prophylactic treatment with trimethoprim-sulfamethoxazole (1 double-strength tablet every 3 days).

It seems prudent to avoid transfusions of blood products from a seropositive donor to a seronegative, immunocompromised patient when feasible. If possible, seronegative recipients should receive transplanted organs from seronegative donors. If not feasible, seronegative patients who receive organs from seropositive donors should be treated with pyrimethamine (25 mg/day) for 6 weeks.

For primary prophylaxis in *T. gondii*–seropositive, HIV-infected patients with a $CD4^+$ T-cell count of less than 200 cells/μL, administering trimethoprim-sulfamethoxazole or pyrimethamine-dapsone is indicated to prevent the development of toxoplasmosis (see Table 370–3). Discontinuation of primary prophylaxis against TE has proved safe in AIDS patients receiving HAART and demonstrating an increase in their $CD4^+$ T-cell counts to at least 200 cells/μL for at least 3 months. Secondary prophylaxis (i.e., maintenance therapy) in AIDS patients was found to be effective in the prevention of relapse of TE (see Table 370–2). Discontinuation of secondary prophylaxis against TE has proved safe in AIDS patients receiving HAART and demonstrating an increase in their $CD4^+$ T-cell counts to at least 200 cells/μL for at least 6 months.

Prognosis

Toxoplasmic lymphadenopathy is a self-limited disease, although fatigue or lymphadenopathy, or both, may persist or recur for months. Clinical illness as a result of reinfection from an exogenous source has not been reported.

SUGGESTED READINGS

Dedicoat M, Livesley N: Management of toxoplasmic encephalitis in HIV-infected adults (with an emphasis on resource-poor settings). Cochrane Database Syst Rev 2006;3:CD005420. *Bactrim appears to be an effective alternative therapy in resource-poor settings when pyrimethamine plus sulfadiazine are not available.*

Kravetz JD, Federman DG: Toxoplasmosis in pregnancy. Am J Med 2005;118:212–216. *A review with emphasis on risk factors and appropriate counseling of pregnant women.*

McLeod R, Boyer K, Karrison T, et al: Outcome of treatment for congenital toxoplasmosis, 1981–2004: The National Collaborative Chicago-Based, Congenital Toxoplasmosis Study. Clin Infect Dis 2006;42:1383–1394. *Treatment of infants who had moderate or severe neurologic disease at birth resulted in normal neurologic and/or cognitive outcomes for >72% of patients.*

Montoya JG, Liesenfeld O: Toxoplasmosis. Lancet 2004;363:1965–1976. *A comprehensive review.*

Thiebaut R, Leproust S, Chene G, et al: Effectiveness of prenatal treatment for congenital toxoplasmosis: A meta-analysis of individual patients' data. Lancet 2007;369:115–122. *A systematic review of cohort studies showing weak evidence for an association between early treatment (within 3 weeks of seroconversion) compared with treatment started after 8 or more weeks and reduced risk of congenital toxoplasmosis.*

371 CRYPTOSPORIDIOSIS

Beth D. Kirkpatrick and Cynthia L. Sears

Definition

Cryptosporidium species are intestinal protozoan parasites of the phylum Apicomplexa and are related to *Toxoplasma* and *Cyclospora.* Cryptosporidiosis is a leading cause of endemic and epidemic diarrheal disease worldwide. Two species cause most infections in humans, *Cryptosporidium parvum* and *Cryptosporidium hominis.*

Cryptosporidium was first described by Tyzzer in 1907 in the intestinal tract of mice. Human disease was recognized in 1976 and attracted interest in the early 1980s, when it was identified as a cause of chronic diarrhea in patients with acquired immunodeficiency syndrome (AIDS). Cryptosporidiosis came to public attention in 1993 as a result of the Milwaukee *C. parvum* outbreak, which affected 403,000 people, the largest recorded diarrheal disease outbreak from a public water supply in U.S. history. There is increasing recognition of outbreaks caused by contamination of food and water with *Cryptosporidium* oocysts. Fortunately, widespread use of highly active antiretroviral therapy (HAART) in patients with AIDS has decreased the impact of cryptosporidiosis in this population.

The Pathogen

The two major genotypes of *Cryptosporidium* are *C. hominis* (i.e., "human adapted," type 1) and *C. parvum* ("animal adapted," type 2).

Subspecies of *C. hominis* and *C. parvum* have been identified and are used to characterize outbreaks.

Epidemiology

Transmission of *Cryptosporidium* occurs through the fecal-oral route by the ingestion of oocysts, which are shed in very high numbers in the feces of many mammals, including humans. For example, AIDS patients with symptomatic cryptosporidiosis may shed up to 1.2 billion oocysts per day. Originally thought to be predominantly a zoonosis, transmission of *Cryptosporidium* is now thought to occur primarily through person-to-person contact or contaminated water. Transmission from environmental sources, such as food, fomites, and animals, also occurs. Polymerase chain reaction (PCR)-based molecular epidemiology data suggest 13 recognized species of *Cryptosporidium,* 10 of which have been found to infect humans. The oocysts of *C. parvum* are ubiquitous and highly infectious. Thick-walled cysts survive well in the environment and are extremely resistant to sterilizing agents, including iodine and chlorine. In the United States it is estimated that 80% of surface water and up to 26% of treated drinking water contain *C. parvum* oocysts, although in most studies the viability of oocysts has not been assessed. Studies of human volunteers have demonstrated that clinical disease may result from the ingestion of less than 10 to 500 oocysts, depending on the *C. parvum* isolate. Because of the high infectivity, secondary transmission occurs, ranging from 5% if an adult is the index case to 20% if a child is the index case. The secondary transmission rate of *C. parvum* parallels that of other highly infectious enteric organisms, such as *Shigella.*

Water-borne outbreaks of cryptosporidiosis have highlighted its epidemic potential. Attack rates during epidemics of cryptosporidiosis are as high as 62%. In addition to the magnitude of the 1993 Milwaukee outbreak, a notable 1994 Las Vegas outbreak occurred with a state-of-the-art water filtration system without signs of malfunction, thus indicating that current water treatment regulations do not consistently prevent *Cryptosporidium* water contamination. Swimming pools, lakes, and water parks have been the sources of recreational water-borne outbreaks, including a large New York "Sprayground" water park outbreak in 2005 associated with illness in approximately 3000 individuals. Food-borne outbreaks are infrequently recognized but occur because of fecal contamination of food. In 1993, 160 cases of cryptosporidiosis resulted from contamination of unpasteurized apple cider by cattle feces. Eighty-eight persons were infected in a university outbreak traced to an infected food handler. Multiple outbreaks, including daycare settings and nosocomial spread, have also been reported as a result of direct person-to-person transmission. Inapparent fecal contamination of objects also causes nosocomial disease, including one outbreak from a contaminated ice machine on a psychiatric ward. With the use of appropriate infection control precautions, however, transmission of *C. parvum* from hospitalized, human immunodeficiency virus (HIV)-infected patients to uninfected HIV-positive roommates can be prevented. Because of the technical difficulty of identifying oocysts in stool specimens and faulty commercial assays, false outbreaks have also been reported.

C. parvum is responsible for endemic acute and persistent diarrheal disease in normal hosts domestically and abroad. The prevalence of infection varies greatly from industrialized to developing countries. Among immunocompetent adults in industrialized nations, the prevalence of *C. parvum* in stool is approximately 2 to 6% and seroprevalence to oocyst antigens is 17 to 32%. In less developed countries, however, cryptosporidiosis is primarily a disease of childhood; for example, in Brazil more than 95% of children are seropositive by 5 years. Populations at increased risk for exposure and infection include veterinary workers, caregivers of infected patients, daycare workers, and travelers. In immunocompromised patients, particularly those with predominately T-cell defects, infection is more severe and protracted than in normal hosts. Before the use of HAART in patients with AIDS, *C. parvum* was the cause of 14 to 24% of cases of chronic diarrhea.

Pathobiology

Cryptosporidium has a complex life cycle that is completed entirely in a single host (monoxenous). After oocysts are ingested, excystation occurs in the upper part of the small intestine after contact with gastric acid and proteolytic enzymes. Four crescentic sporozoites are released per oocyst. Via gliding motility, sporozoites penetrate the brush border membrane of the enterocyte and rearrange host actin to reside in a distinctive intracellular but extracytoplasmic position. Sporozoites develop into trophozoites intracellularly and divide asexually to form a schizont with four to eight merozoites, which are released by rupture of the enterocyte. Some merozoites invade adjacent cells, thereby expanding the infection asexually. Others form sexual stages in host cells to produce male and female gametocytes that result in oocyst formation. It appears that 80% of oocysts are thick walled and excreted into the environment whereas 20% are thin walled and capable of initiating cycles of autoinfection. Autoinfection expands and augments infection and, if uncontrolled by host defenses, is presumed to cause persistent disease in immunocompromised hosts. The intracellular position of *C. parvum* may protect the organism from host immune defenses.

All structures contiguous to the intestine that are lined with polarized epithelial cells are at risk for infection. Infection is typically concentrated in the small bowel, with less colonic involvement. The biliary and pancreatic tracts and, very rarely, the respiratory tract may also be infected. Intestinal infection results in structural damage with villous atrophy, decreased brush border enzymes, crypt hyperplasia, and paracellular permeability, all contributing to the pathogenesis of diarrhea. Combined small and large bowel infection correlates with the severity of clinical disease in AIDS patients. A variable inflammatory infiltrate of neutrophils and mononuclear cells is found in the lamina propria.

Piglet studies of the pathophysiology of *C. parvum* infection indicate that impaired glucose-stimulated sodium and water absorption in the jejunum and ileum also contributes to malabsorptive diarrhea. Cholera-like stool losses (20 L) in some AIDS patients infected with *C. parvum* have additionally prompted the search for a possible enterotoxin. Although no specific toxin has been found, animal models show a net increase in chloride secretion mediated by prostaglandin E_2, which may be responsible in part for a secretory diarrheal response. The secretory response may be further augmented by epithelial cell secretion of pro-inflammatory cytokines, including tumor necrosis factor-α and interleukin-8.

The specific immune response to *C. parvum* in humans is incompletely understood. Severe cryptosporidiosis is found in patients with cellular or humoral immune defects, and both arms of the immune response are thought to be necessary to control infection. In humans, specific serum antibodies (IgG, IgM, and IgA) and intestinal secretory IgA are found in response to infection but have not been shown to be protective. The presence of IgG antibodies in healthy adults with previous infection confers a relative resistance to reinfection only at low oocyst doses. After reinfection of healthy adults, diarrhea recurs at the same frequency as in primary infection, although the diarrheal illness is less severe and fewer oocysts are shed. Epidemiologic data suggest that maternal antibodies may be an important defense against primary infection; breast-fed children appear to have less *C. parvum* infection before 6 months of age. Studies of cell-mediated immune responses have demonstrated a role for systemic and intraepithelial $CD4^+$ helper T cells and interferon-γ, but not $CD8^+$ cytotoxic T cells or natural killer cells, in preventing and recovering from disease. However, high levels of interferon-γ have not been shown to be helpful in controlling infection in AIDS patients.

Clinical Manifestations

Clinical manifestations of infection vary with age and immune status. Diarrhea is the predominant symptom in all groups. In otherwise healthy adults, the incubation period is 2 to 14 days, followed by the onset of watery diarrhea, which may be copious, as seen in other infectious diarrheal diseases. Diarrhea is frequently associated with abdominal cramping, nausea, flatulence, and vomiting. Symptoms are usually self-limited, with recovery in 10 to 14 days. Relapse of diarrhea can occur after 1 to 2 days of apparent recovery. Fever and other systemic signs of infection occur in about a third of immunocompetent patients (36% had fever in a Milwaukee outbreak based on clinical criteria and 57% in those with laboratory-confirmed infection), and weight loss may be prominent. In the Milwaukee outbreak, approximately 75% of otherwise healthy people with diarrhea lost a median of 10 lb. Infection with *C. parvum* may also be asymptomatic.

In developing nations, cryptosporidiosis is predominately a childhood disease and is recognized as a major cause of persistent diarrhea in these populations. As found in Peru and Brazil, children younger than 1 year appear to be at greater risk for persistent diarrhea and may suffer enhanced morbidity from other enteric infections and growth stunting after *C. parvum* infection. Malnutrition and vitamin A deficiency preceding infection are found in Haitian children with acute cryptosporidiosis. Brazilian children with cryptosporidiosis before 2 years of age have impaired functional status (i.e., physical fitness and cognitive function) 4 to 7 years after the initial infection.

In immunocompromised hosts, the severity and duration of infection are directly related to the type and degree of immunosuppression. Disease is more likely to be fulminant, persistent, and life-threatening. Excessive fluid and electrolyte loss with malabsorption can cause progressive weight loss, dehydration, and malnutrition. Although most data are derived from patients with AIDS, severe, chronic cryptosporidiosis has been found in almost all immunocompromised populations, including patients with common variable immunodeficiency, hematologic malignancies, and hypogammaglobulinemia and during chemotherapy and steroid use. Most patients have primarily T-cell defects. Reversal of the immune compromise often results in rapid cessation of the symptoms of cryptosporidiosis.

In HIV-positive patients with chronic diarrhea, intestinal cryptosporidiosis is an AIDS-defining illness. Up to 30% of this group may also have a second intestinal coinfection. Uncontrolled, persistent diarrhea is directly related to the $CD4^+$ T-cell count; patients with CD4 levels higher than 180/μL are able to recover from *C. parvum* infection, whereas those with lower CD4 counts often have chronic diarrhea with an associated poor survival of approximately 6 months. In this population, the disease fits one of four patterns: cholera-like (31%), chronic diarrhea (37%), relapsing (14%), or resolved (17%). Acalculous cholecystitis and, less frequently, sclerosing cholangitis are found in 10 to 15% of AIDS patients with cryptosporidiosis; such patients have symptoms of fever, right upper quadrant pain, and nausea. Pancreatitis and respiratory tract involvement have also been reported, although the clinical significance of the latter is unknown.

Diagnosis

Laboratory Findings

C. parvum enteric infection is diagnosed by stool examination. The classic acid-fast stain of stool with modified Ziehl-Nielsen stain demonstrates bright pink, 4- to 6-μm-diameter oocysts. Sensitivity is diminished with formed stool but is increased by techniques to concentrate oocysts. Direct immunofluorescence stains, including acridine orange and auramine-rhodamine, are often used to screen stool samples in clinical laboratories and are more sensitive than acid-fast staining, but they may not distinguish oocysts from yeast forms. Monoclonal and polyclonal antibodies to *Cryptosporidium* antigens are used in commercial enzyme-linked immunosorbent and immunofluorescent assays. These assays are costly but are rapid and easier to interpret than acid-fast–stained smears are. Their use is often favored in clinical laboratories that infrequently diagnose *Cryptosporidium.* The sensitivity of these commercially available assays is variable (66 to 100%), but their specificity is generally high (≈93%). Important to all assays, *Cryptosporidium* must be differentiated from yeast and the oocysts of *Cyclospora,* which are 8 to 10 μm in diameter and, unlike *C. parvum,* glow with ultraviolet light. Serologic methods are not useful in the diagnosis of acute disease. Diagnostic and species-specific PCR techniques are being developed. Rarely, intestinal biopsy is necessary for diagnosis. Histologic samples are stained with hematoxylin-eosin and demonstrate *C. parvum* in the brush border of intestinal epithelial cells.

Other laboratory findings are nonspecific. Signs of malabsorption may be found by measuring serum vitamin B_{12}, stool fat, or D-xylose absorption. In biliary disease, alkaline phosphate, γ-glutamyltransferase, and bilirubin levels may be increased; transaminase levels are usually normal. Ultrasound and computed tomography (CT) scans may show irregular dilation of the biliary ducts. Endoscopic retrograde cholangiopancreatography to obtain bile or tissue is the most sensitive method of diagnosing biliary disease.

Differential Diagnosis

Acute diarrhea with *C. parvum* has no distinguishing features, and the differential diagnosis varies with the patient population and the clinical setting. In patients with AIDS and persistent diarrhea, other parasitic infections such as *Microsporidia, Isospora,* and *Cyclospora* should be considered, as well as cytomegalovirus and *Mycobacterium avium.* Cryptosporidiosis should be included in the differential diagnosis of persistent diarrhea in all hosts, particularly in children of developing nations, travelers, and immunocompromised populations, and as a cause of any epidemic of diarrheal disease.

Treatment

The cornerstone of therapy is fluid replacement. For immunocompetent patients (>1 year of age), the antiparasitic agent nitazoxanide is the only treatment of cryptosporidiosis approved by the Food and Drug Administration, and it limits the duration of diarrhea and gastrointestinal symptoms associated with disease. Doses of 500 mg twice daily for 3 days are used for adults. In immunocompromised patients, reversal of the immunodeficiency may be the only effective means of eliminating the disease. Since 1996, complete resolution of established cryptosporidial diarrhea in AIDS patients has been shown after initiation of effective HAART. Chemoprophylaxis with rifampin and the macrolide clarithromycin in AIDS patients may be protective against the development of cryptosporidiosis. In a placebo-controlled trial, treatment of AIDS patients with nitazoxanide at 500 or 1000 mg twice daily for 14 days led to parasitologic cure in 63% and 67% of patients, respectively. Parasitologic cure was correlated with complete resolution of the diarrheal syndrome in 86% of the treated patients. However, parasitologic cure rates were predominantly limited to patients with $CD4^+$ T-cell counts above 50/μL, and "seriously ill" patients were excluded from the study. Paromomycin treatment of cryptosporidiosis in patients with advanced AIDS is no more effective than placebo. Paromomycin used with azithromycin to treat chronic cryptosporidiosis in patients with AIDS ($CD4^+$ T-cell count <100) dramatically reduced oocyst excretion, but not the volume of diarrheal stools. Passive oral transfer of antibody through hyperimmune bovine colostrum has had limited success in diminishing symptoms in AIDS patients with cryptosporidiosis. It is hoped that data from completion of sequencing the *C. parvum* and *C. hominis* genome (2004) will lead to rational drug development against cryptosporidiosis. For example, targeted drug development may take advantage of the new genome-based knowledge that *Cryptosporidium* lacks many critical enzymes for nutrient production and depends heavily on nutrient salvage from the host.

Prevention

Eliminating exposure to *C. parvum* oocysts is the cornerstone of preventing infection. Specific guidelines for the prevention of cryptosporidiosis in persons infected with HIV are published by the U.S. Public Health Service. Avoidance of contact with human and animal feces in water and food and through sexual practices is essential for all hosts, particularly for immunocompromised patients. Contact with newborn animals and patients with diarrhea should be minimized and handwashing emphasized.

The difficulty of eliminating *C. parvum* from public drinking water remains an important public health problem. In outbreak settings, drinking water can be considered safe when boiled for 1 minute, purified with ozone, filtered with an absolute less than 1-μm filter, or treated with reverse osmosis. Filters should meet the National Sanitation Foundation standard #53 criterion for cyst removal. Because sources differ, bottled water should not be assumed to be free of oocysts. The risk of acquiring cryptosporidiosis in tap water in non–outbreak-associated settings is unknown. No special tap water precautions are recommended for HIV-infected and immunocompromised patients.

SUGGESTED READINGS

Chen X-M, Keithly JS, Paya CV, LaRusoo NF: Cryptosporidiosis. N Engl J Med 2002;346:1723–1731. *An excellent review, well referenced.*

Leav BA, Mackay M, Ward HD: *Cryptosporidium* species: New insights and old challenges. Clin Infect Dis 2003;36:903–908. *A succinct review of the taxonomy, pathogenesis, and immunology of* Cryptosporidium *species.*

USPHS/IDSA Guidelines for the Prevention of Opportunistic Infections in Persons with HIV. Available at http://aidsinfo.nih.gov/guidelines/op_infections/OI_112801.pdf. *Consensus guidelines.*

Xiao L, Ryan U: Cryptosporidiosis: An update in molecular epidemiology. Current Opin Infect Dis 2004;17:483–490. *An update on the molecular epidemiology of* Cryptosporidium.

372 GIARDIASIS

Cynthia L. Sears

Definition

Giardia duodenalis, also known as *Giardia intestinalis* or *Giardia lamblia,* is the most common human protozoan enteric pathogen worldwide and is the only *Giardia* species infecting humans and many other mammals. It causes endemic and epidemic diarrheal illnesses, but the parasite is most often carried asymptomatically by humans.

The Pathogen

Discovered in 1681, this eukaryotic parasite has a simple life cycle alternating between trophozoite and cyst stages. The pear-shaped, flagellated trophozoites (10 to 15 μm long and 5 to 15 μm wide) contain two nuclei and resemble a "face" microscopically (Fig. 372–1). Trophozoites proliferate in the small bowel and may be identified in the liquid stools of symptomatic patients. Encystation in the jejunum yields the immediately infective cyst stage (10 to 12 μm long and 7 to 10 μm wide) identified in fecal samples (Fig. 372–2). The oval cysts are resistant to chlorine and can survive in water for up to 3 months. The hardiness of *Giardia* cysts makes this parasite one of the most frequently identified water-borne pathogens.

The taxonomy of *Giardia* species is evolving. Molecular analysis shows considerable genetic heterogeneity within *G. duodenalis* populations, with two major genetic assemblages, termed A and B. Human isolates segregate into both assemblages A and B along with other genetically related mammalian isolates, thus suggesting the potential for zoonotic transmission. At present, the relationship between genetic assemblages and clinical disease expression is uncertain.

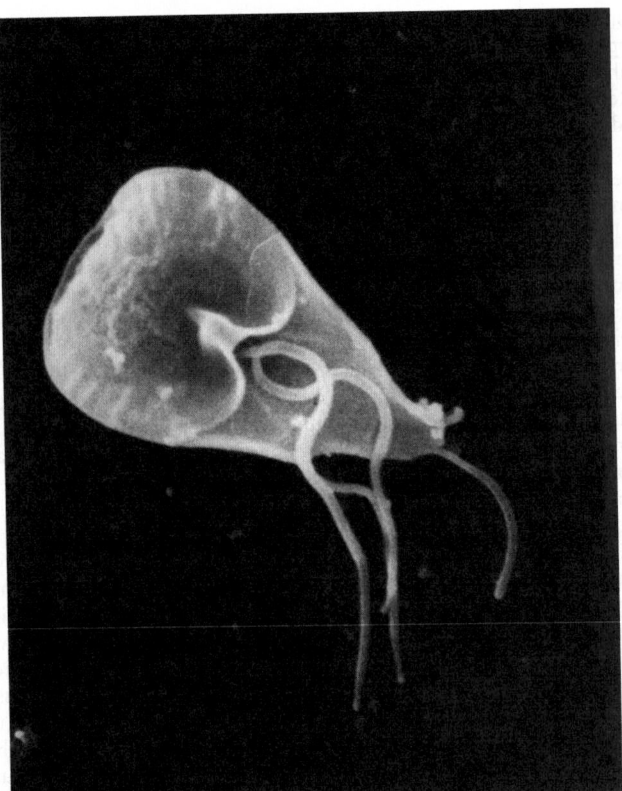

FIGURE 372–1 • *Giardia lamblia.* This scanning electron micrograph revealed some of the external ultrastructural details displayed by a flagellated *G. lamblia* protozoan parasite.

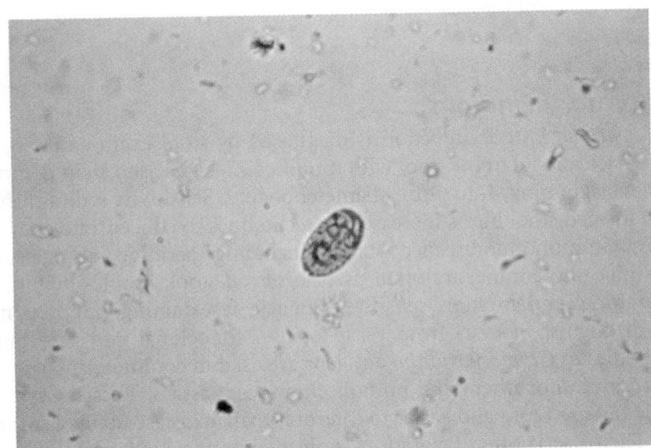

FIGURE 372–2 • *Giardia lamblia* cyst. A photomicrograph shows a *Giardia lamblia* cyst enhanced with an iodine stain.

Epidemiology

Transmission of *G. duodenalis* infection occurs directly by person to person or indirectly by ingestion of contaminated water or, less often, food. Person-to-person, fecal-oral transmission and small-scale water contamination result in endemic infection, whereas epidemic disease is recognized when food or large-scale drinking water contamination occurs. The infection is transmitted by the ingestion of as few as 10 to 100 *G. duodenalis* cysts. Persons of all age groups are susceptible to this infection, although exclusive breast-feeding may lower the risk for infection in young children; the milk antimicrobial protein lactoferrin kills *Giardia* trophozoites in vitro, and maternal immunoglobulin A (IgA) can neutralize *Giardia* antigens and provide important passive immunity to nursing infants. In the developing world, infection is nearly universal by the age of 5 years, but recurrent infections are not uncommon, thus indicating that the primary immune response to infection is incompletely protective. In the United States, infection is generally sporadic, with certain groups of individuals at higher risk, including children (particularly those attending daycare centers), male homosexuals engaging in oral-anal sexual behavior, campers and hikers (from the ingestion of untreated surface water), and international travelers. A notable association of travel to Russia (particularly St. Petersburg) with the acquisition of *G. duodenalis* infection is amply documented.

Although both T- and B-cell–mediated immune mechanisms appear necessary to eradicate infection, immunocompromised patients with hypogammaglobulinemia (e.g., common variable immunodeficiency, X-linked hypogammaglobulinemia) are primarily those at increased risk for prolonged, sometimes intractable infection. Patients infected with human immunodeficiency virus (HIV) do not generally experience more severe disease. *G. duodenalis* does not clearly exhibit enhanced virulence in patients with HIV infection or selective IgA deficiency. Individuals with selective IgA deficiency are typically relatively deficient in IgA but produce low levels of IgA that appear sufficient to promote clearance of *Giardia* infection. Similar to other enteric infections, achlorhydria or hypochlorhydria enhances the likelihood of infection, and proton pump inhibitors may increase the risk for giardiasis. Although humans are the main reservoir of *G. duodenalis* infection, genetically related species infect humans, beavers, guinea pigs, cats, and dogs, consistent with zoonotic transmission of *Giardia* infection. Surface water (e.g., streams) contaminated with cysts excreted by beavers has been linked to human infection.

Pathobiology

G. duodenalis is strictly a small bowel, noninvasive enteric pathogen. Infection is initiated by ingestion of the cyst form of the parasite, which releases two trophozoites aided by the pH and protease conditions of the upper part of the small bowel. Trophozoites firmly attach to the small bowel mucosa by means of a disc-shaped sucker on the ventral surface, aided initially by surface lectin and subsequently by contractile parasitic proteins and the negative pressure created by the parasite's beating flagella. Attachment is most often patchy and imprints the mucosa, thereby creating localized microvillus damage. A well-established sequela of this pathology is inhibition of mucosal digestive enzyme activity. In some patients, these events culminate in the onset of symptoms after an incubation period of 6 to 15 days. As trophozoites migrate distally in the small bowel, higher bile concentrations stimulate encystation and result in excretion of the environmentally resistant, but immediately infective, cyst form of the parasite.

The histopathologic response to *G. duodenalis* infection varies and imperfectly correlates with the clinical findings. In asymptomatic patients, electron microscopy often reveals evidence of ultrastructural changes in microvilli not observed by light microscopy. Surprisingly, small bowel biopsies of symptomatic patients examined by light microscopy are also usually normal but may reveal villous atrophy, crypt hyperplasia, and an inflammatory lamina propria infiltrate consisting of polymorphonuclear leukocytes, plasma cells, and lymphocytes. Lymphoid nodular hyperplasia has been associated with giardiasis and hypogammaglobulinemia.

The pathophysiology of *Giardia* infection is complex and incompletely understood. One of the unresolved puzzles is how *G. duodenalis* causes a broad spectrum of disease ranging from asymptomatic infection to acute and sometimes chronic diarrhea. Two major postulates accounting for disease variability have been proposed. First, experimental animal and human infections suggest that *Giardia* strains vary in virulence, although specific essential virulence genes have yet to be identified. *G. duodenalis* undergoes surface antigenic variation (variant-specific surface proteins [VSPs] encoded by at least 150 genes) that is most likely stimulated by the host immune response or the intestinal microenvironment. Interestingly, recent studies suggest that epigenetic mechanisms control VSP antigenic variation inasmuch as DNA rearrangement does not appear to play a role. The presence of distinct and changing VSPs by individual trophozoites in an infecting population may assist the parasites in eluding host immune responses and increase the chance for successful reinfection or development of a persistent initial infection. Second, the host response, particularly the mucosal immune response, to the parasite may vary. These postulates for disease pathogenesis are not mutually exclusive. Clarification of the host-parasite relationship will require further characterization of infecting strains by molecular approaches and correlation of these results with the clinical disease observed.

The mechanisms by which infection with *G. duodenalis* results in diarrhea appear to be multifactorial. First, documented disaccharidase deficiencies and the ultrastructural and histopathologic changes observed in association with some *G. duodenalis* infections are consistent with the clinical observation of malabsorption in infected patients. Experimental animal and in vitro epithelial cell infections also reveal increased intestinal permeability, impaired glucose and amino acid–dependent sodium absorption, and in some instances, net sodium and chloride secretion. Second, the patchy distribution of *G. duodenalis* infection in contrast to the large surface area of the small bowel and the absence of overt abnormalities in gut architecture in the majority of symptomatic individuals suggest that the parasite may secrete one or more factors that alter intestinal transport. Only limited experimental data support this hypothesis. Third, the mucosal immune response may contribute to intestinal secretion through the release, for example, of cytokines known to stimulate chloride secretion by intestinal epithelial cells.

Clinical Manifestations

Giardiasis is manifested as one of three clinical forms: the asymptomatic carrier state (accounting for most infections); acute, self-limited diarrheal illnesses; and persistent (lasting >2 weeks) or chronic (lasting >30 days), sometimes relapsing diarrhea associated with malabsorption and, in young children in the developing world, growth retardation (i.e., stunting). Diarrhea develops in about 40 to 50% of infected persons, and the majority of *Giardia* infections are self-limited, consistent with the existence of effective host defenses. Experimental studies suggest that intestinal secretory IgA, helper T lymphocytes ($CD4^+$), and interleukin-6 production are central to resolution of infection. Emerging data suggest that recurrent *G. duodenalis* infection in the first years of life is associated with poor cognitive function years later. Although disease chronicity may be associated with certain immunodeficient conditions (see earlier), immunocompetent hosts are also susceptible to protracted illness with *G. duodenalis*. Symptomatic patients experience anorexia and nausea combined with, most characteristically, explosive, watery, foul-smelling diarrhea with increased passage of gas. Only low-grade fever occurs, and the blood white cell count is normal. Leukocytes and blood are not present in feces, and even mucus in stool is rare. Nevertheless, the diarrheal illness caused by *G. duodenalis* is indistinguishable from that caused by other small bowel enteric pathogens. In those with persistent or chronic illness, malabsorption (including fats, vitamin B_{12}, and lactose) may be associated with foul-smelling, oily stools that float and prominent weight loss. Lactose intolerance may last for several weeks after successful therapy for giardiasis. Rare associations with *G. duodenalis* infection include urticaria, cholecystitis, pancreatitis, arthritis, retinal arteritis, and iridocyclitis.

Diagnosis

Demonstration of the cysts or, rarely, trophozoites of *G. duodenalis* in concentrated, stained fecal specimens is the traditional approach to diagnosis. However, diagnosis can be elusive because cyst excretion may be erratic and symptoms may begin before the organism is detectable in stool. Examination of two stools after concentration and staining for parasite forms or by direct immunofluorescence assay to detect intact organisms or an enzyme-linked immunosorbent assay to detect soluble *Giardia* stool antigens generally yields the diagnosis in more than 90% of infected individuals. The use of an "enterotest" (i.e., gelatin capsule-string test) or endoscopy to detect trophozoites in the upper part of the small bowel is rarely necessary for patient management. Polymerase chain reaction approaches remain experimental. Repeat stool examinations for "test of cure" after treatment are not necessary.

Treatment

Rx

The nitroimidazoles metronidazole and tinidazole are most often the drugs of choice and are more than 90% effective. Tinidazole offers the advantage of single-dose treatment and is approved for therapy by the U.S. Food and Drug Administration (FDA) for children (>3 years old) and adults. The adult dosage is 2 g orally, whereas the pediatric dosage is 50 mg/kg. Notable side effects include a metallic taste and gastrointestinal and central nervous system (e.g., headache, vertigo) symptoms. Rarely, transient leukopenia and neutropenia, peripheral neuropathy, and seizures have been reported. Nitazoxanide, a broadly active antiprotozoal and anthelmintic agent, is FDA approved for treatment in children (>1 year old) and adults and is available as a suspension. The dosage is 100 to 500 mg orally twice daily for 3 days for children or adults, respectively. Clinical efficacy is 80% or better. Nitazoxanide is well tolerated, with only headache, nausea, and diarrhea occurring more often with nitazoxanide treatment than with placebo. Though not approved by the FDA for giardiasis, metronidazole is frequently used at a dosage of 250 mg orally three times daily for 5 days.

Alternative therapies include furazolidone and albendazole. Furazolidone is approximately 80% effective, FDA approved, and available as a suspension. The adult dosage is 100 mg orally (1.25 to 2 mg/kg/dose four times a day for 7 to 10 days for children >1 month old) four times a day for 7 to 10 days. Furazolidone may precipitate hemolysis in patients with glucose-6-phosphate deficiency and is contraindicated in patients taking monoamine oxidase inhibitors. Albendazole, a benzimidazole, has excellent in vitro activity against *Giardia* isolates and clinical efficacy when given for 5 or more days. The dosage is 400 mg (or 15 mg/kg/day for 5 to 7 days in children) orally daily for 5 days. Gastrointestinal side effects may occur.

Treatment failures may occur with any of these standard therapies, consistent with in vivo and in vitro data, thus suggesting that strain-dependent drug resistance exists and may be induced during therapy. The nitroimidazoles and furazolidone inhibit aldehyde dehydrogenase and may precipitate a disulfiram-like reaction if taken with alcohol. None of these therapeutic alternatives are clearly safe in pregnancy, for which the poorly absorbed oral

Rx

aminoglycoside paromomycin has been suggested. Metronidazole is an alternative in pregnancy for serious cases, although its use in pregnancy remains controversial because well-controlled human studies on its safety are lacking (FDA category B). Quinacrine (mepacrine), an effective but potentially toxic therapy, is no longer available in the United States. Limited clinical data suggest that dual drug therapy offers benefit in recalcitrant infections.

Prevention

Because *G. lamblia* is transmitted by environmentally resistant cysts and does not stimulate complete protective immunity, prevention of infection requires public health measures to ensure the availability of clean water and education to promote excellent personal hygiene for interruption of the infection cycle. Boiling of water for 1 minute or treatment with two to four drops of household bleach or 0.5 mL of a 2% tincture of iodine per liter for at least 60 minutes (overnight if the water is cold) before drinking renders cysts noninfective. Although a commercial vaccine for cats and dogs is available, the antigenic variability of *G. lamblia* and the ill-defined correlates of protective immunity hinder human vaccine development for this infection.

SUGGESTED READINGS

Ali AA, Hill DR: *Giardia intestinalis.* Curr Opin Infect Dis 2003;16:453–460. *This article provides an up-to-date review of progress in the giardiasis field of study.*

Gardner TB, Hill DR: Treatment of giardiasis. Clin Microbiol Rev 2001;14:114–128. *A comprehensive review of therapeutic approaches to* Giardia *infection.*

Huang DB, White AC: An updated review on *Cryptosporidium* and *Giardia.* Gastroenterol Clin North Am 2006;35:291–314.

Roxström-Lindquist K, Palm D, et al: *Giardia* immunity—an update. Trends Parasitol 2006;22:26–31. *A current view of the immunopathogenesis of* Giardia.

Thompson RCA, Hopkins RM, Homan WL: Nomenclature and genetic groupings of *Giardia* infecting mammals. Parasitol Today 2000;16:210–213. *A clear description of the genetic complexity of* Giardia *and its impact on disease epidemiology.*

373 AMEBIASIS

Frederick L. Schuster and Carol A. Glaser

Definition

Amebiasis has been virtually synonymous with amebic dysentery for decades. With the recognition of several other human diseases caused by pathogenic amebae, the term has come to have a broader meaning and is used in this chapter to encompass all human amebic infections (Table 373–1).

The Pathogens

Entamoeba histolytica is the etiologic agent of amebic dysentery. The organism is an obligate parasite and does not occur outside the human host, except in its dormant transmissive cyst stage. Since its recognition in 1875 by Fedor Lösch in St. Petersburg, Russia, amebic dysentery was considered the sole amebic disease in humans until about 40 years ago, when an otherwise innocuous group of free-living amebae were recognized as agents of human encephalitis. They have a wide distribution in soil and water and can be found in the home environment. This group includes *Naegleria fowleri, Acanthamoeba* sp, and *Balamuthia mandrillaris.* These amebae are recognized as opportunistic or facultative parasites.

Of these several diseases, amebic dysentery is easily the most common and widespread globally, with approximately 500 million infections and an estimated 100,000 deaths each year, mainly in developing and impoverished areas of the world. With increased ease of travel and immigration, dysentery has become more of a concern in developed countries of the world, although cases remain uncommon in the United States. Cases of amebic encephalitis are much fewer in numbers, with approximately 500 since the role of amebae in the disease was first recognized in the 1960s. Their occurrence is primarily reported from countries with advanced diagnostic capabilities. Despite their low numbers, the amebic encephalitides are a concern because of the unknown risk factors and

TABLE 373–1 COMPARATIVE FEATURES OF HUMAN AMEBIC INFECTION

Ameba	Disease	Symptoms	Portal of Entry	Groups at Risk	Differential Diagnosis
Entamoeba histolytica	Amebic dysentery, hepatic and brain abscesses	Diarrhea, abdominal tenderness, fever	Fecal-oral route, venereal transmission	Residents of and travelers to endemic areas	Ulcerative colitis, diverticulitis, bacillary dysentery, carcinoma
Naegleria fowleri	Primary amebic meningoencephalitis	Headache, stiff neck, nausea, fever, changes in mental status	Nasal passages while swimming	Children and young adults exposed to amebae in water	Bacterial encephalitis
Acanthamoeba spp	Granulomatous encephalitis; systemic, cutaneous infections	Headache, stiff neck, changes in mental status	Breaks in skin, respiratory tract	Immunocompromised hosts	Viral, bacterial, fungal, and mycobacterial encephalitis
	Amebic keratitis	Pain, tearing, photophobia, blurred vision	Corneal surface	Contact lens wearers	Viral keratitis
Balamuthia mandrillaris	Granulomatous encephalitis; systemic, cutaneous, sinus infections	Headache, stiff neck, changes in mental status	Breaks in skin, respiratory tract	Immunocompromised and immunocompetent hosts	Viral, fungal, and mycobacterial infections; ADEM; toxoplasmosis; neoplasia; neurocysticercosis

prevalence, the diagnostic challenge that they present, and the lack of effective antimicrobial therapy, which has resulted in high mortality.

Acanthamoeba, in addition to being a cause of encephalitis, is also the agent of amebic keratitis. More than 3000 cases of amebic keratitis have been reported in association with corneal trauma, but mostly with contact lens use.

AMEBIC DYSENTERY

The causal agent of amebic dysentery, *E. histolytica,* exists in two different life cycle stages: the active ameba (15 to 25 μm) and the dormant cyst (10 to 20 μm). The trophic ameba is found in the human colon and the cyst is the transmissive stage passed with stool.

Epidemiology

Amebic dysentery is associated with poverty, overcrowding, and poor sanitation. It is endemic in several tropical or subtropical regions of the world but also occurs in temperate areas. Mexico and India are endemic areas, but an outbreak of dysentery occurred in 1933 in the city of Chicago at the time of the World's Fair. At present, most cases in developed countries occur in travelers to or immigrants from endemic regions.

Dormant cysts are expelled from the intestine and, as a result of poor sanitation, enter the drinking water supply. Cysts are able to survive for a period of 2 to 4 weeks in a warm, moist environment, but they are poorly equipped to survive desiccation or temperature extremes. Transmission of cysts to the human host is by the fecal-oral route. Cysts in drinking water, salad greens, or other uncooked agricultural products tainted with unclean water are carried to the colon, where they germinate and give rise to trophic amebae. The ameba stage is not infective because it is vulnerable to the low pH environment in the stomach. Spread of disease in the population can occur by asymptomatic food handlers and by homosexual men as a consequence of anal intercourse. Insects such as roaches and flies can be mechanical vectors carrying cysts to food.

Invasive amebic dysentery and extraintestinal infections are more likely to occur in males than in females, although the incidence of asymptomatic infections is the same in both sexes. Determination of the prevalence of amebiasis in populations is complicated by the existence of an *E. histolytica* look-alike, *Entamoeba dispar,* a noninvasive ameba found in the colon. Because *E. dispar* is the more widespread in distribution of the two species, it can be difficult to distinguish between carriers of *E. dispar* and asymptomatic carriers of *E. histolytica,* the latter group being a factor in the spread of dysentery.

Pathobiology

After ingestion by the host, cysts germinate in the colon, with each cyst giving rise to eight trophic amebae. Ameba membrane lectin specific for galactose aids attachment to the colonic epithelium and facilitates its colonization. The cecal and sigmoidorectal areas, where flow of intestinal content slows, are the most likely areas of colonization. An abundant supply of bacteria present in the intestinal lumen provides a food source for the amebae, and when blood vessels erode, the erythrocytes released are similarly ingested. Flask-shaped lesions develop in the intestinal lining as a result of enzyme activity (phospholipase, cysteine protease), which can lead to perforation of the colon with a mortality rate of approximately 70%. An ameboma made up of granulomatous tissue may arise from fusion of colonic lesions.

Clinical Manifestations

The clinical syndrome of *E. histolytica* infection involves noninvasive intestinal infection, invasive intestinal amebiasis, ameboma, and disseminated infection. Severity is highest in the very young or elderly, pregnant women, and those receiving steroids. The virulence of the infecting amebic strain can affect the course of disease. An incubation period of about a week to 10 days, sometimes longer, follows infection, and early symptoms may be nonspecific. Patients with noninvasive *E. histolytica* infection are either asymptomatic or have nonspecific gastrointestinal complaints such as bloating and cramps. Fulminant amebic dysentery, characterized by bloody diarrhea, abdominal tenderness, tenesmus, and mucus and bits of sloughed colonic surface in stool, occurs in about 10% of infected individuals. Fever develops in approximately a third of infections. The liver may be enlarged, even in the absence of hepatic involvement by amebae. The inflammatory response is weak, with a mild leukocytosis and a white blood cell (WBC) count of 12,000/mL or less, mainly polymorphonuclear leukocytes (PMNs). Ongoing dysentery can result in dehydration, weight loss, and malaise. The differential diagnosis includes bacillary dysentery, ulcerative colitis, diverticulitis, inflammatory bowel disease, and in the case of ameboma, carcinoma.

The liver is the most common site of involvement in extraintestinal disease, but the lungs, pericardium, skin, and brain may be involved as well. The liver becomes enlarged and tender, accompanied by abdominal pain and fever. Liver function is usually normal and not indicative of disease, and aside from an elevated alkaline phosphatase level in patients with chronic amebic liver abscess, testing is noninformative. Liver abscess, however, can occur in the absence of intestinal infection. When pulmonary amebiasis develops, it is generally the right lung that is affected. Primary cutaneous amebiasis has been reported but is rare. A cerebral abscess can develop as a result of hematogenous spread of amebae from the colon or other sites in the body to the central nervous system (CNS), where lesions in the brain are detectable by neuroimaging. Symptoms are typical of encephalitis (e.g., fever and change in mental status), but the condition is difficult to recognize and the diagnosis is usually made postmortem.

Diagnosis

Examination of stool specimens for cysts or trophic amebae has long been the standard for diagnosis of amebic dysentery. It typically involves stained smears (e. g., trichrome, hematoxylin stains) and, less often, direct microscopic examination of wet-mount fecal samples. The presence of red blood cells in amebae is diagnostic of *E. histolytica.* In its early formative stage, the cyst contains distinctive dark-staining, rod-shaped chromatoid bodies. The existence of several nonpathogenic amebae (*Entamoeba coli, Endolimax nana, Iodamoeba bütschlii*) in the human intestine and in stool can complicate diagnosis. Discrimination between *E. histolytica* and *E. dispar* is an important consideration in diagnosis, and several kits on the market can differentiate these organisms. Polymerase chain reaction can distinguish between the two species based on their respective DNA. Serology is useful as a diagnostic tool. Sonography and neuroimaging (magnetic resonance imaging and computed tomography) aid in visualizing extraintestinal abscess formations.

Prevention and Treatment

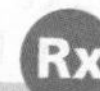

Sewage-contaminated water is the prime source of infection, and preventing contamination of water is the means for controlling amebic dysentery. Vegetables and other foodstuff that are contaminated by cyst-containing water are another vehicle of infection if eaten without cooking. Asymptomatic cyst carriers—food handlers in particular—need to be aware of the importance of handwashing after use of the toilet. Despite avoidance of possibly contaminated water, unforeseen sources of infection, particularly for tourists, can be water used to brush teeth and ice cubes made with contaminated water.

Antimicrobial therapy for the various forms of amebic dysentery is summarized in Table 373–2. With the use of effective antimicrobial agents, the prognosis for recovery from amebic dysentery, amebic colitis, and extraintestinal amebic abscesses is excellent. The presence of nonpathogenic *E. dispar* in the colon does not require antimicrobial therapy.

AMEBIC ENCEPHALITIDES

Amebae responsible for amebic encephalitis are *N. fowleri, Acanthamoeba* spp and *B. mandrillaris.* A fourth ameba, *Sappinia diploidea,* has been reported from a single case but is not thought to be of great significance.

TABLE 373–2 ANTIMICROBIAL TREATMENT OF AMEBIC INFECTIONS

Type of Infection	Antimicrobials	Dosage*
ENTAMOEBA HISTOLYTICA		
Asymptomatic cases	Iodoquinol *or*	650 mg tid for 20 days
	Paromomycin	25–35 mg/kg/day in 3 doses for 7 days
	Diloxanide furoate† (as an alternative)	500 mg tid for 10 days
Dysentery and extraintestinal disease	Metronidazole *or* Tinidazole	750 mg tid for 7–10 days 2 g qd for 5 days
Mild disease (amebic colitis; carrier status)	Metronidazole *or* Tinidazole	500–750 mg tid for 7–10 days 2 g qd for 5 days
NAEGLERIA FOWLERI		
Primary amebic meningoencephalitis	Amphotericin B, miconazole,‡ rifampin, sulfisoxazole	
ACANTHAMOEBA SPP		
Cutaneous infections	Ketoconazole, flucytosine	
Nasopharyngeal infections (sinusitis)	Pentamidine isethionate, amphotericin B, levofloxacin, flucytosine, rifampin, itraconazole	
Granulomatous encephalitis (disseminated infection)	Sulfadiazine, pyrimethamine, fluconazole	
Keratitis	Polyhexamethylene biguanide Chlorhexidine Propamidine isethionate (as Brolene§)	
BALAMUTHIA MANDRILLARIS		
Granulomatous encephalitis	No optimal treatment, but the following have been used with success: flucytosine, fluconazole, pentamidine isethionate, sulfadiazine, azithromycin/clarithromycin, trifluoperazine	

*Where treatment has been formalized (e.g., amebic dysentery), antimicrobials and adult dosages are given. Where optimal antimicrobial therapy has not been formulated, the names of drugs that have been successful in treatment are given. The clinician, however, is advised to consult the literature for specific information.
†Not available commercially in the United States.
‡Not approved by the U.S. Food and Drug administration at the time of publication.
§An over-the-counter drug available in the United Kingdom, but not approved for sale in the United States.

Naegleria fowleri

Primary amebic meningoencephalitis (PAM) is a fulminant disease caused by *N. fowleri*, a free-living ameba that is found in soil and fresh water. Its life cycle consists of a trophic ameba stage (15 to 30 μm), a cyst stage (7 to 15 μm), and a flagellate that develops from the ameboid stage. It is thermotolerant and, in vitro, can survive at temperatures up to 45° C.

Epidemiology

N. fowleri favors warm fresh water. It has been isolated from artificial and natural lakes, rivers, hot springs, inadequately chlorinated swimming pools, children's wading pools, and household water supplies. Humans are exposed to the amebae (or cysts or flagellates) while swimming, bathing, or recreating in such waters. The portal of entry is the nasal passages. Susceptible individuals are typically immunocompetent children or young adults. Transmission of ameba cysts on wind currents into the respiratory tract has been implicated in several cases of PAM, and *N. fowleri* has also been isolated from the nostrils of asymptomatic individuals. In the United States, most cases occur in the southern tier of the country, often during the warm months of the year.

Pathobiology

Once having entered the nostrils, amebae bind to the olfactory mucosa and, after penetrating into the submucosa, move along the olfactory nerve tracts, cross through the cribriform plate, and gain entrance to the brain. Rapid proliferation follows, with extensive damage to the olfactory and frontal lobes and subsequent spread to other parts of the brain, particularly the base of the brain, the brain stem, and the cerebellum. Amebae may also be found as a purulent exudate in the subarachnoid space of the meninges. Amebae in the brain parenchyma concentrate in the perivascular regions. Release of enzymes may account for their destructiveness once in the brain. Although infection is generally restricted to the CNS, myocarditis, bronchopneumonia, and splenitis have been reported.

Clinical Manifestations

The onset of symptoms is generally 2 to 5 days after exposure. Early symptoms may include changes in smell or taste followed by an abrupt onset of severe headache, persistent fever, vomiting, and lethargy. The symptoms rapidly progress to produce seizures, altered mental status, and coma. Death ensues in most cases within a week of onset.

Diagnosis

The basis for considering a diagnosis of PAM should be encephalitis with a recent history of swimming or washing in warm fresh water. Cerebrospinal fluid (CSF) findings often resemble those of bacterial meningitis and consist of an elevated WBC count (often >1000 WBCs/mL), elevated protein, and depressed glucose. The peripheral white count is often elevated. Neuroimaging may show cerebral edema. The presence of trophic amebae in fresh and unrefrigerated CSF is pathognomonic of the disease. The amebae can be mistakenly identified as WBCs but are recognizable by their anterior, eruptive pseudopod formation (Fig. 373–1). There is a prominent nucleus (≈5 μm) with a central nucleolus. In

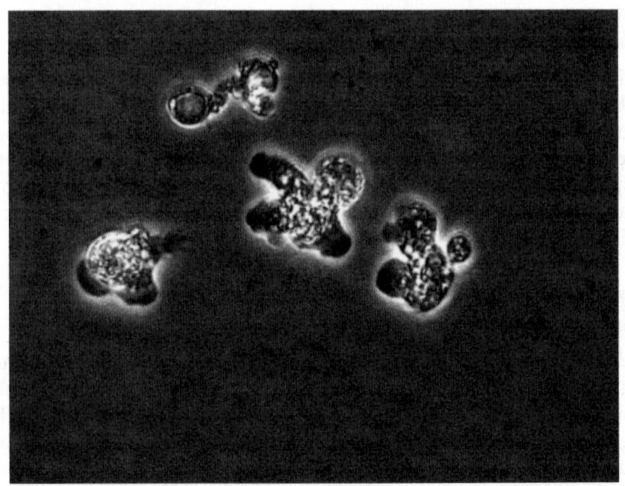

FIGURE 373–1 • *Naegleria fowleri* trophic amebae in a wet-mount preparation viewed with a phase-contrast microscope. Clear ectoplasmic, eruptive pseudopods are seen, which are characteristic of *Naegleria* amebae, as might be seen in a fresh cerebrospinal fluid preparation. The nucleus is obscured by intracellular vacuoles and granules. (From Schuster FL, Visvesvara GS: Free-living amoebae as opportunistic and non-opportunistic pathogens of humans and animals. Int J Parasitol 2004;34:1001–1027).

contrast, leukocytes move sluggishly by means of indistinct pseudopods (undulating membrane) and do not have a large nucleolus. As a confirmatory measure, amebae suspended in distilled water and observed over an approximately 1-hour period will transform into flagellates. The differential diagnosis includes bacterial meningitis. In PAM, however, the CSF is sterile.

Prevention and Treatment

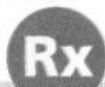

Because the etiologic agent of PAM can be isolated from many naturally or artificially warmed fresh waters, avoidance can be a problem. In the case of swimming pools, maintenance of effective chlorine levels is essential. This, however, is usually impossible to achieve in swimming areas such as natural and artificial lakes, spas, and hot springs.

Water entering the nostrils is the primary source of human infection. Thus, underwater swimming, diving, and prolonged stay in the water increase the chance for entry of amebae. Individuals in whom PAM develops are typically children or young adults, who are more likely to be more active in the water than older individuals. It is perhaps reassuring to note that of more than 2000 outbreaks of waterborne infections in the United States over a 1-year period, only 4 cases of PAM were reported. In Florida, which has had a number of cases of PAM associated with its warm lakes, the chance of infection has been estimated as 1 per 2.6 million exposures.

Although the case-fatality rate is extremely high, case reports of successful outcomes suggest that early treatment with amphotericin B (and steroids in some cases) might significantly alter the outcome (see Table 373–2).

Prognosis

The prognosis for recovery is poor. Early diagnosis and initiation of treatment are critical to successful recovery. Only about a half-dozen such recoveries with varying neurologic sequelae out of approximately 200 cases have been reported in the literature since its first recognition as a disease entity in the 1960s.

GRANULOMATOUS AMEBIC ENCEPHALITIS

Acanthamoeba spp and *B. mandrillaris* are two amebae associated with granulomatous amebic encephalitis. The disease is generally distinguished from PAM (see the previous section) by the absence of meningeal involvement, an insidious course, and granuloma formation. The latter may be absent in immunocompromised individuals as a result of an impaired adaptive immune response.

Acanthamoeba Species

Of the approximately 20 different species of *Acanthamoeba*, relatively few are associated with human infection. *Acanthamoeba* granulomatous encephalitis and *Acanthamoeba* keratitis are well-known disease entities, whereas nasopharyngeal (as sinusitis), cutaneous, and disseminated infections are less familiar. Granulomatous amebic encephalitis and disseminated infections occur almost exclusively in immunocompromised and debilitated hosts, whereas keratitis occurs in immunocompetent individuals and is associated with the use and improper care of contact lenses (see later). The ameba life cycle consists of alternating trophic ameba (15 to 30 μm) and cyst stages (10 to 15 μm). Cysts are particularly resistant to extreme conditions (desiccation, disinfectants, ultraviolet irradiation, antimicrobials, heat) and have been reported to remain viable for more than 20 years. Pathogenic species and strains are mostly thermotolerant and grow optimally at temperatures of 30°C or higher.

Epidemiology

Acanthamoeba spp have a nearly universal distribution in soil and water. They have been isolated from fresh water and seawater, tropical and arctic environments, sewage, and beach sand. In the health care setting, they have been detected in hospital showerheads and water taps, ventilators, humidifiers, hydrotherapy baths, intensive care units, and laboratory emergency eye wash stations. *Acanthamoeba* isolates have been found to harbor *Legionella* bacteria and may play a role in the spread of legionellosis and Pontiac fever, particularly in a nosocomial setting.

Infection occurs through a break in the skin that may become contaminated with soil or via the respiratory tract by cysts carried through the air on wind currents. *Acanthamoeba* is an opportunistic pathogen in that virtually all patients exhibit some loss of immunocompetence. *Acanthamoeba* infections have developed in many human immunodeficiency virus (HIV)-infected patients and those with acquired immunodeficiency syndrome (AIDS), as well as in organ transplant recipients, cancer patients undergoing chemotherapy, and persons in a debilitated state of health (e.g., alcoholics, diabetics, intravenous drug users, patients with systemic lupus erythematosus).

Pathobiology

Acanthamebiasis is a chronic disease and may have an incubation period of months before becoming clinically apparent. Amebae that gain entrance to the body through the skin or the respiratory tract are carried to the CNS hematogenously. Hemorrhagic necrotizing lesions are produced in the brain, mainly in the cerebrum, cerebellum, and brain stem, but amebae are rarely found in the CSF of patients, although *Acanthamoeba* mitochondrial DNA can be detected by the polymerase chain reaction. In the brain parenchyma, they cluster in the perivascular spaces of blood vessels. Ameba virulence factors include proteases, induction of apoptosis in host cells, and aggressive phagocytosis.

Clinical Manifestations

Acanthamebiasis affecting the CNS often runs an insidious course characterized by fever, headache, nausea, vomiting, meningismus, or any combination of these symptoms. Focal neurologic symptoms are often present. Progressive deterioration occurs and ultimately leads to death. Infection with *Acanthamoeba* can also cause widespread extracerebral disease and affect essentially any organ of the body, including the skin, lungs, and bone. Skin lesions, which can be manifested as skin papules, pustules, subcutaneous or dermal nodules, or a nonhealing ulcer, may be an isolated finding or part of disseminated disease.

Diagnosis

Antemortem diagnosis is unusual unless there is high index of suspicion. Spinal fluid from affected individuals often shows a modest CSF pleocytosis with a predominance of lymphocytes, increased protein, and low glucose. Multifocal areas of signal intensity, often with a mass effect, are seen on neuroimaging. Brain edema and hydrocephalus may also be present. Neuroimaging frequently reveals mass lesions. The differential diagnosis includes bacterial, fungal, and mycobacterial infections.

If a brain biopsy is performed, amebae can be seen on hematoxylin-eosin (H&E)-stained tissue slides, but they have been overlooked or misidentified because of lack of familiarity with their appearance. Pathologists should be alerted to the possible presence of *Acanthamoeba* in biopsy specimens. A characteristic feature of the ameba that distinguishes it from host cells is the presence of a nucleus with a large, centrally situated nucleolus. The ameba may also encyst in host tissue and produce a rounded form enclosed by a thick wall. Indirect immunofluorescent staining of tissue sections is helpful in revealing the amebae. Because the disease is chronic, the host generates an antibody response that can be demonstrated by immunofluorescent antibody staining. Immunocompromised individuals or those receiving steroids, however, may not generate antibodies against the amebae.

Prevention and Treatment

Detection of *Acanthamoeba* antibodies in many, if not most human sera suggests that individuals come in contact with the amebae either in the outdoor or in the home environment. Disease is a rarity and requires an immunocompromised status.

Few patients have recovered after acanthamebiasis. There is no optimal antimicrobial therapy for the different forms of the disease, and combinations of antimicrobials have been used empirically (see Table 373–2). Different *Acanthamoeba* strains and species may exhibit variations in drug sensitivity, including resistance, thus further complicating the course of therapy. Cysts develop in tissues, and it is not known whether they can germinate after completion of antimicrobial therapy to reactivate the disease.

Prognosis

The prognosis for recovery is poor, even with treatment. The same antimicrobial treatment that leads to recovery in some patients has failed in treating others. Early recognition of the disease can be a factor in survival. The virulence of strains of pathogenic *Acanthamoeba* differs and may also be a factor. It is worth noting that appropriate management of HIV/AIDS itself has considerably reduced acanthamebiasis as an opportunistic infection in this high-risk group of patients.

Balamuthia mandrillaris

Balamuthia is the agent of a granulomatous disease similar to acanthamebiasis. A trophic ameba stage (45 to 85 μm) and a cyst stage (10 to 30 μm) make up the life cycle of the organism. The ameba was recognized as a causal agent of encephalitis less than 20 years ago, initially from immunocompromised patients (HIV/AIDS patients, poor health), but is now most often reported from overtly immunocompetent children and, less often, adults. Cases have also been reported from primates and several other mammals, mostly in zoos. In addition to cases in the United States, cases have been reported from Mexico, South America, the Czech Republic, Portugal, Great Britain, Japan, Thailand, Canada, and Australia.

Epidemiology

There is scant information about the epidemiology of the disease. The amebae have been isolated from soil, and in the United States, several patients had exposure to soil in common: digging a drain in a backyard or working with composted soil, playing with flowerpot soil, and windblown soil while riding in a jeep or motorcycle in dusty areas. The organism is difficult to isolate and grow in vitro. Because balamuthiasis has nonspecific symptoms, it is likely that cases go unrecognized. Since its first reports in the 1990s, there have been more than 100 cases, with a significant number occurring in persons of Hispanic ethnicity.

Pathobiology

Balamuthiasis may have an incubation period as long as 2 years, and although it has an insidious course, it can occasionally develop subacutely. Other aspects of the disease are similar to those of *Acanthamoeba* encephalitis. The initial site of infection can be a break in the skin or the respiratory tract, with hematogenous spread to the CNS. Pathologic examination often shows brain edema, hemorrhage, and subacute necrotizing infiltration.

Clinical Manifestations

Balamuthia infections can have a wide range of manifestations, including headache, stiff neck, nausea, vomiting, low-grade fever, personality change, mental status change, and cranial nerve palsies. Otitis media has preceded balamuthiasis in several pediatric patients. Patients with balamuthiasis may have symptoms of a space-occupying lesion such as hemiparesis, aphasia, or seizures. Hydrocephalus has developed in several patients. In South America, the disease manifests as a rubbery-to-hard cutaneous lesion, often midfacial and involving the nose, eventually progressing to CNS disease.

Diagnosis

Most cases are diagnosed postmortem based on finding amebae in H&E-stained brain tissue. *Balamuthia* amebae are larger than *Acanthamoeba,* but otherwise the two organisms are similar in morphology. *Balamuthia* also encysts in brain tissue and produces a triple-walled structure. Nuclei may contain multiple nucleoli. Typically, the amebae are not found in CSF. CSF frequently has elevated WBC and protein levels, the latter often significantly high (>1000 mg/dL). Testing for *Balamuthia* antibody is helpful because of the long incubation period of the disease. Neuroimaging may reveal ring-enhancing lesions (Fig. 373–2) or hydrocephalus. The differential diagnosis for balamuthiasis includes neurocysticercosis, brain abscess, tumor, tuberculoma, tuberculous meningitis, acute disseminated encephalomyelitis, and viral encephalitis. For cuta-

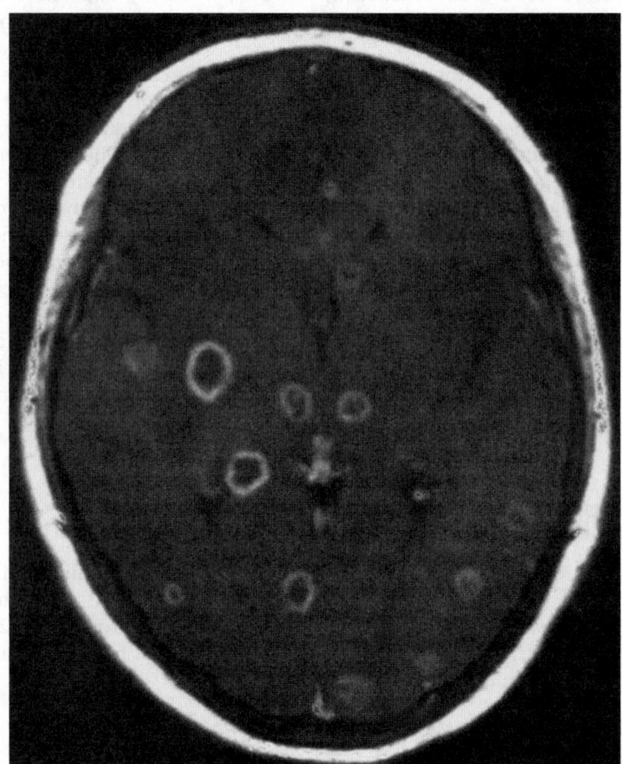

FIGURE 373–2 • Magnetic resonance image of a 12-year-old boy with a fatal case of balamuthiasis. Numerous ring-enhancing lesions are visible in the section, a feature suggestive of balamuthiasis. (Courtesy of Dr. David Michelson, Loma Linda, CA.)

neous balamuthiasis, the differentials are fungal infection, mucocutaneous leishmaniasis, cutaneous tuberculosis, leprosy, and necrotizing granulomatous vasculitis (Wegener's granulomatosis).

Prevention and Treatment

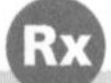

Preventive measures are uncertain because the ameba is found in soil and perhaps water. Patients include both immunocompromised and immunocompetent persons, with children making up most of the latter category.

Optimal therapy for balamuthiasis has yet to be formulated, and drug combinations have been used, with several case reports of successful outcomes. However, after having received so many different antimicrobials, it is unclear which might have worked. Successful therapy may have been associated with the combined use of flucytosine, fluconazole, pentamidine isethionate, sulfadiazine, azithromycin, or clarithromycin and a phenothiazine (see Table 373–2). In vitro drug testing against *Balamuthia* has shown efficacy for miltefosine (this drug has not been approved by the U.S. Food and Drug Administration at the time of publication), polymyxin B, colistin, promethazine, and haloperidol as amebastatic or amebicidal agents.

Prognosis

The prognosis is poor for patients with balamuthiasis, and thus far mortality is close to 100%. With early diagnosis, initiation of antimicrobial therapy may lead to improved outcomes.

ACANTHAMOEBA KERATITIS

Amebic keratitis is treated separately from the systemic *Acanthamoeba* diseases because of pronounced differences between the two: the host for amebic keratitis is immunocompetent, the disease is self-limited, and drug therapy is mostly successful with an excellent prognosis.

Epidemiology

The disease is associated with ocular trauma or the use of soft contact lenses in immunocompetent individuals. Amebic keratitis has developed as a result of injury to the corneal surface from a scratch or from a cinder blown into the eye. Most recently, cases have resulted from the overnight use of contact lenses as treatment of myopia. Improper care plus storage of contact lenses has also been a factor in infections; bacterial growth in the lens case can serve as a food source for the amebae, particularly when tap water has been used to prepare homemade ophthalmic solutions. Despite millions of users of contact lenses, only 3000 to 4000 cases have been reported.

Pathobiology

When *Acanthamoeba* infects the eye, an acute or mixed inflammatory infiltrate occurs. A dendritiform epithelial pattern is observed, followed by a ring-shaped stromal infiltrate made up of PMNs streaming toward the affected area. Amebae can burrow into the corneal stroma and encyst, thus making it difficult to eliminate them with topical antimicrobials.

Clinical Manifestations

Symptoms of amebic keratitis often start as a foreign body sensation followed by intense pain, lacrimation, photophobia, blepharospasm, conjunctivitis, and blurred vision. Usually only one eye is affected, and there have been no reports of the infection developing into encephalitis. Because the disease mimics viral (often herpes simplex virus), bacterial, or fungal keratitis, inappropriate therapy may be started and result in further growth of amebae in the eye.

Diagnosis

Corneal scrapings can be examined for amebae or cysts with the fluorescent dye calcofluor white and can also be used for isolation of *Acanthamoeba.*

Prevention and Treatment

Observing manufacturers' specifications for care of contact lenses reduces the risk of amebae colonizing the surface. The lens case must also be kept clean and free of bacterial biofilm. Tap water, when used in lens care, may carry cysts of amebae. Contact lenses should not be worn in hot tubs, which may support the growth of amebae, or while swimming.

Corneal grafting (keratoplasty) has been performed to improve vision and reduce the ameba load in the eye. Reinfection of the graft from cysts in surrounding tissue may occur and require a second keratoplasty. Amebae are more sensitive than cysts to drug therapy. The use of antimicrobials may stimulate encystment, but cysts germinate after therapy has halted. The drugs of choice in treating amebic keratitis are polyhexamethylene biguanide (PHMB) and chlorhexidine gluconate. Propamidine isethionate, another successful drug, may be used by itself or in combination with PHMB and chlorhexidine. These drugs are effective against trophic amebae and cysts. Drug therapy in its earliest stages of disease requires frequent topical application of the drugs and must be continued for 3 to 4 months. Steroids are also used to reduce inflammation. Their role is somewhat controversial because it has been reported that dexamethasone may stimulate excystation of dormant cysts and cause flare-up of the infection.

Prognosis

Before the use of PHMB and chlorhexidine in treating amebic keratitis, successful recovery was problematic, sometimes requiring enucleation. With their use, however, the prognosis is highly favorable.

SUGGESTED READINGS

Bloch KC, Schuster FL: Inability to make a premortem diagnosis of *Acanthamoeba* species infection in a patient with fatal granulomatous amebic encephalitis. J Clin Microbiol 2005;43:3003–3006. *This paper explores some of the difficulties in arriving at a diagnosis of acanthamebiasis in an immunocompromised patient.*

Haque R, Huston CD, Hughes M, et al: Amebiasis. N Engl J Med 2003;348:1565–1573. *A scholarly review.*

Schuster FL, Visvesvara GS: Free-living amoebae as opportunistic and non-opportunistic pathogens of human and animals. Int J Parasitol 2004;34:1001–1027. *An expanded review of free-living amebic infections with consideration of the biology of the free-living amebae.*

Stanley SL Jr: Amoebiasis. Lancet 2003;361:1025–1034. *A comprehensive review.*

Stauffer W, Ravdin JI: *Entamoeba histolytica:* An update. Curr Opin Infect Dis 2003;16:479–485. *A review.*

Tanyuksel M, Petri WA Jr: Laboratory diagnosis of amebiasis. Clin Microbiol Rev 2003;16:713–729. *Addresses the methods available to detect* Entamoeba histolytica.

Wells CD, Arguedas M: Amebic liver abscess. South Med J 2004;97:673–682. *Detailed review of liver abscess as an extraintestinal consequence of dysentery, with recommended antimicrobial treatment.*

374 BABESIOSIS AND OTHER PROTOZOAN DISEASES

Richard D. Pearson

BABESIOSIS

Babesiosis is a tick-borne, malaria-like disease caused by *Babesia* species that infect erythrocytes. They are important pathogens of animals around the world.

The Pathogen

Most human infections in North America are caused by *Babesia microti,* which is found in areas of coastal New England, including the barrier islands of Nantucket, Martha's Vineyard, Long Island, Block Island, and Shelter Island; New Jersey; the upper Midwest, particularly Wisconsin; and occasionally elsewhere. Sporadic human cases caused by the *Babesia* WA-1 variant have been reported from Washington and northern California and by the M0-1 variant from Missouri. Babesiosis is endemic in other areas of the world. *Babesia divergens* is responsible for most European cases.

In the northeastern United States, the major reservoir is the white-footed deer mouse *Peromyscus leucopus,* but other rodents may be involved. The vector is the deer tick *Ixodes scapularis* (*Ixodes dammini*), the same tick that transmits *Borrelia burgdorferi,* the cause of Lyme disease (Chapter 342), and human granulocytic ehrlichiosis. Concurrent cases of babesiosis and Lyme disease or ehrlichiosis have been reported. *B. divergens* in Europe is transmitted by *Ixodes ricinus.*

Babesia organisms are transmitted to humans by the nymph stage of the tick, which is 1.5 to 2.5 mm long and easily missed by the patient, or less commonly by adult ticks, which are somewhat larger. The likelihood of transmission increases with the length of time that the tick feeds on the patient. Adult *I. scapularis* feeds on deer. Although the deer do not become infected, an increase in the deer population can result in an increase in ticks and thus heighten the potential for transmission. The convergence of mice, deer, and humans is necessary for tick-borne transmission. Blood transfusions have been implicated in a limited number of cases. Congenital infection can occur but is rare.

Clinical Manifestations

Most individuals infected by ticks are unaware of the bite. The incubation period varies from 1 to 6 weeks after tick transmission and up to 9 weeks after blood transfusion. *Babesia* infections are frequently subclinical or mild and self-limited in immunocompetent persons, but they can be severe and life-threatening in splenectomized persons, the elderly, or those with acquired immunodeficiency syndrome (AIDS), pregnancy, or chronic illnesses that suppress immunity. Symptomatic patients may experience a range of flulike symptoms, including intermittent fever, sweats, chills, headache, myalgia, fatigue, anorexia and other constitutional symptoms. Fulminant cases may result in severe disease, including sepsis, disseminated intravascular coagulation, congestive heart failure, or acute respiratory distress syndrome. The proportion of infected red blood cells, or parasitemia burden, is often less than 10% in normal hosts, but significantly higher levels can be reached in splenectomized individuals. Parasitemia of greater than 10% often correlates with severe illness. Unlike malaria, there is no periodicity to the disease, and chronic infection is rare in immunocompetent hosts. Parasitemia generally persists for a few weeks to several months in untreated persons.

Diagnosis

Most cases of babesiosis occur in endemic areas of the United States between May and September. Fever is frequently the only abnormality on physical examination, but hepatomegaly or splenomegaly may be present. Erythema migrans may be observed in persons with concurrent *B. burgdorferi* infection. In Europe, *B. divergens* has been associated with the sudden onset of fulminant disease that can progress to death, which is seen mostly in splenectomized individuals.

Depending on the severity of illness, there is frequently evidence of hemolytic anemia. The white blood count may be normal or decreased, and the platelet count is often low. Liver enzymes and bilirubin can be elevated, particularly in fulminant cases. Severe cases may also be associated with gross hemoglobinuria, jaundice, congestive heart failure, or acute respiratory distress syndrome. Babesiosis is diagnosed by identifying intraerythrocytic *Babesia* species in thick and thin Giemsa-stained (Fig. 374–1) or Wright-stained blood smears. They must be differentiated from *Plasmodium falciparum* and other *Plasmodium* species, which can be accomplished by documenting a detailed travel history and confirmed morphologically. In contrast to malaria, *Babesia* species do not form hemoglobin-derived pigment. Dividing *Babesia* can form a tetrad of merozoites that appears as the characteristic "Maltese cross," but this finding is uncommon. Blood smears may be negative in patients with low levels of parasitemia. Antibodies to *B. microti* can be detected by indirect immunofluorescent assay, but the test may not readily differentiate persons with previous exposure from those with acute infection and may be negative in persons infected with the WA-1 variant on the West Coast. High titers are indicative of recent or active infection and decline over an 8- to 12-month period after resolution of disease. Inoculation of Syrian hamsters and polymerase chain reaction (PCR)-based assays have been used to diagnose cases in which the blood smears were negative.

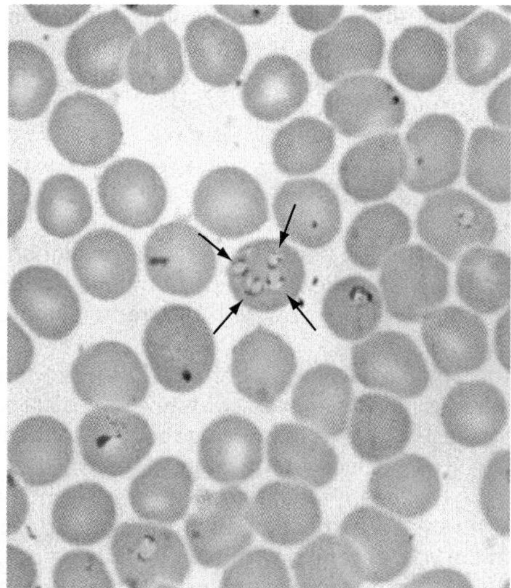

FIGURE 374–1 • A giemsa stain of a blood film from an infected human was used to identify the parasite *Babesia microti.* (*http://phil.cdc.gov/phil/home.asp. Figure #3899.*)

Treatment

Many cases of babesiosis in North America occur in immunocompetent persons and are self-limited. In adult patients who have symptoms, particularly those who are asplenic or elderly or have comorbid conditions, babesiosis has been treated with 650 mg of quinine sulfate taken orally three times daily plus either 1.2 g of clindamycin administered twice daily intravenously or 600 mg orally three times daily for 7 to 10 days. The pediatric dosage is clindamycin, 20 to 40 mg/kg/day orally in three divided doses, and quinine, 25 mg/kg/day orally, also in three divided doses. However, a high percentage of patients experience side effects with the clindamycin/quinine regimen, including tinnitus (39%), diarrhea (33%), hearing loss (28%), vertigo (17%), and rash (11%). An alternative regimen of azithromycin, 600 mg/day orally, plus atovaquone, 750 mg orally twice daily for 7 to 10 days, appears to be as effective and is better tolerated. Exchange transfusion has been used in severely ill patients with high parasitemia and should be considered for patients with parasitemia greater than 10%. Consideration should be given to evaluating patients in whom babesiosis is diagnosed for concurrent Lyme disease because of the prevalence of coinfection in North America. Immunosuppressed patients, in particular those after splenectomy, patients infected with human immunodeficiency virus (HIV), or the elderly, may require longer antibiotic courses. Resolution of disease in such individuals can be monitored clinically and confirmed by clearance of the organism on blood smear. Therapy should be initiated early in persons infected with *B. divergens* in Europe, particularly those who have been splenectomized, because rapidly increasing parasitemia can result in massive hemolysis, renal failure, and death.

TRICHOMONIASIS

Trichomonas vaginalis is among the most prevalent of all pathogenic protozoa and an important cause of vaginitis around the world. The organism is oval, approximately 10 by 15 μm wide, and has four free flagella at its anterior pole and a fifth in an undulating membrane that runs along one side of the body. *T. vaginalis* is usually spread by sexual contact. The highest incidence of infection occurs in women with multiple sexual partners and those with other sexually transmitted diseases (Chapter 306). *T. vaginalis* can also be passed from infected mothers to their newborn daughters, but it is seldom symptomatic in girls before menarche. The parasite is able to survive for some time in moist environments, and nonvenereal transmission, though uncommon, can occur. Trichomoniasis, like other sexually transmitted diseases, may increase the likelihood of transmission of HIV.

Clinical Manifestations

The incubation period for trichomoniasis is 5 to 28 days. Vaginitis with a purulent discharge is the prominent symptom and can be accompanied by vulvovaginal irritation, dyspareunia, abdominal pain, and dysuria. The discharge tends to be watery and copious, but it may be thick, yellow or green, and frothy. Patients may notice an odor, but this is more common with bacterial vaginosis. Symptoms may worsen during menstruation. Population-based studies indicate that as many as half of *T. vaginalis* infections in women are asymptomatic. On pelvic examination, there is typically inflammation of the vaginal walls. Punctate hemorrhages on the exocervix, or colpitis macularis or "strawberry cervix," are seldom visible on gross inspection, but they are observed in approximately half of all cases if colposcopy is performed. The pH of the vaginal contents is typically elevated above the normal level of 4.5, as it is in bacterial vaginosis.

T. vaginalis can frequently be isolated from the male partners of infected women. Although most men are asymptomatic, *T. vaginalis* can produce symptomatic urethritis. Urethral discharge is generally scant in these cases. Rarely, *T. vaginalis* is associated with epididymitis; superficial penile ulcerations, which are usually located under the prepuce; or involvement of the prostate.

Diagnosis

In women, vaginal and urethral secretions should be examined. *T. vaginalis* is seen in wet mounts of vaginal secretions in approximately 60% of infected women, thus confirming the diagnosis. The organisms have a twitching motion with active flagella. Polymorphonuclear leukocytes are usually present. Direct immunofluorescent antibody staining is more sensitive than wet mounts, but technically more difficult. Culture is a more sensitive method of diagnosis. Commercial kits are available, but the results are not available for 3 to 7 days. *T. vaginalis* is occasionally identified in Papanicolaou-stained smears. PCR-based assays of vaginal specimens have been sensitive and specific in preliminary studies. For men, a wet mount of material from a platinum loop scraping of the anterior urethra reveals the organism in approximately half the cases. Prostatic massage before collecting urine for *Trichomonas* culture is a more sensitive diagnostic approach. Serologic studies lack sensitivity and specificity.

Treatment

Rx

Tinidazole, a single 2-g oral dose in adults, or metronidazole, either as a single 2-g oral dose or 500 mg twice daily for 7 days, is the treatment of choice. Tinidazole is the better tolerated of the two. Sexual partners should be treated concurrently to prevent reinfection because nearly 20% of male partners are coinfected. Single-dose therapy (metronidazole or tinidazole) ensures patient compliance but can produce nausea and a metallic taste, particularly with metronidazole. Both tinidazole and metronidazole have a disulfiram-like effect, and patients who consume alcohol within 24 hours of metronidazole or 72 hours of tinidazole may experience severe nausea, vomiting, and flushing. The use of tinidazole and metronidazole is relatively contraindicated during pregnancy (given the lack of well-controlled studies during pregnancy). Treatment failures with metronidazole are uncommon but well documented. Some result from reinfection, others from poor compliance, but some are caused by metronidazole-resistant parasites. A repeat course of metronidazole (2–4 g orally daily for 7 to 14 days) may be

Rx

tried. Alternatively, tinidazole, 500 mg orally four times daily for 14 days, along with intravaginal tinidazole, 500 mg twice a day, has been effective in treating a subset of persons with metronidazole-resistant isolates. If patients remain refractory to appropriate treatment, metronidazole sensitivity can be tested by the Centers for Disease Control and Prevention (available at www.dpd.cdc.gov/dpdx/HTML/DiagnosticProcedures.htm).

CYCLOSPORIASIS

Cyclospora cayetanensis, a coccidian parasite, is acquired through the ingestion of contaminated food or water and lives within enterocytes in the small bowel. It has emerged as an important cause of gastroenteritis in tropical and subtropical areas, including Peru, Mexico, Haiti, Caribbean countries, and Nepal. Since 1990, at least 11 food-borne outbreaks affecting approximately 3600 persons have been documented in the United States and Canada among persons who have eaten contaminated raspberries imported from Guatemala, fresh basil, snow peas, or mesclun. Cyclosporiasis is occasionally diagnosed in returning international travelers.

After an incubation period of approximately 1 week, *C. cayetanensis* produces watery diarrhea, nausea, vomiting, abdominal pain, myalgias, anorexia, and fatigue. Symptoms can be prolonged (10 to 12 weeks) and associated with substantial weight loss, particularly in persons with AIDS. Infections may also be asymptomatic.

The diagnosis is confirmed by identifying *Cyclospora* in stool samples stained with modified acid-fast or modified safranin preparations. The organism appears autofluorescent in stool specimens examined by ultraviolet microscopy. PCR assays have proved to be specific, but not always sensitive. They are available only in research settings.

Treatment

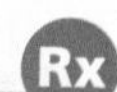

C. cayetanensis responds to treatment with 160 mg trimethoprim and 800 mg sulfamethoxazole taken twice daily for 7 to 10 days. HIV-infected patients may require an increased intensive dosing frequency of four times daily for 10 days. Chronic suppressive therapy with 160 mg trimethoprim/800 mg sulfamethoxazole three times weekly is often necessary thereafter in HIV-infected patients. Rehydration is also important.

OTHER ENTERIC PROTOZOANS

A number of other protozoa have been associated with enteric disease (Table 374–1). They are acquired through the ingestion of contaminated food or water. Some reside in the lumen of the bowel, and others invade and multiply within enterocytes. Enteric protozoa should be considered in the differential diagnosis of patients with persistent diarrhea and abdominal symptoms, particularly those with a history of recent international travel. Along with *Cryptosporidium* and *C. cayetanensis, Isospora belli* and microsporidia can cause chronic diarrhea and weight loss in persons with AIDS.

The diagnosis is typically made by identifying ova or parasites in stool. Microscopic examination should be performed by an expert because these parasites may be confused with fecal debris. Pathogenic protozoa must also be differentiated from nonpathogens such as *Entamoeba coli, Endolimax nana, Iodamoeba bütschlii, Trichomonas hominis,* and *Chilomastix mesnili.*

Treatment

Therapy includes administration of the appropriate antiprotozoal drug and rehydration as listed in Table 374–1.

TABLE 374–1 ENTERIC PROTOZOA

Organism	Epidemiology	Manifestations	Therapy*
Balantidium coli	Primarily an infection of animals, especially pigs, but also affects humans	Asymptomatic or mild and self-resolving; occasionally more severe with abdominal pain, blood, and mucus in stool	Tetracycline (500 mg qid for 10 days). Alternative: metronidazole (750 mg tid for 5 days) or iodoquinol (650 mg tid for 20 days)
Blastocystis hominis	Probably worldwide, including North America; often found concomitantly with *Giardia lamblia*	Pathogenicity is debated	The need for treatment is debated, but symptomatic improvement has been reported with metronidazole (750 mg tid for 10 days), iodoquinol (650 mg tid for 20 days), or trimethoprim-sulfamethoxazole (1 double-strength tablet bid for 7days)
Cyclospora cayetanensis†	Distribution appears to be worldwide in tropical and subtropical areas; food-borne outbreaks associated with imported raspberries from Guatemala; fresh basil, snow peas, or mesclun	Can produce severe watery diarrhea, anorexia, fatigue, weight loss lasting weeks, and prolonged disease in those with AIDS	Trimethoprim, 160 mg, and sulfamethoxazole, 800 mg, bid for 7 to 10 days; HIV-infected patients may require long-term suppressive therapy
Dientamoeba fragilis	Worldwide distribution; frequently found concomitantly with the pinworm *Enterobius vermicularis*	Often asymptomatic; diarrhea reported	Paromomycin (25–35 mg/kg body weight per day in 3 doses for 7 days), tetracycline (500 mg qid for 10 days), metronidazole (500–750 mg tid for 10 days), or iodoquinol (650 mg tid for 20 days)
Isospora belli†	Worldwide distribution, most prevalent in Latin America and Africa	Self-limited diarrhea in immunocompetent residents and travelers, but persistent, severe diarrhea in patients with AIDS	Trimethoprim, 160 mg, plus sulfamethoxazole, 800 mg, bid for 10 days; HIV-infected patients may require higher doses for longer periods, followed by long-term suppressive therapy
Microsporidia† (*Enterocytozoon bieneusi* and *Encephalitozoon intestinalis*)	Apparent worldwide distribution	AIDS patients with persistent diarrhea and wasting; self-limited cases in immunocompetent persons	Oral fumagillin (60 mg daily for 14 days) has been effective for *E. bieneusi*, but it has been associated with thrombocytopenia. Albendazole (400 mg bid for 21 days) has been effective for *E. intestinalis*. Treatment with HAART may lead to clinical response in HIV-infected patients with microsporidial diarrhea
Sarcocystis species	Common pathogens of animals; rare in humans; acquired by ingesting contaminated beef or pork	Often asymptomatic; nausea, vomiting, abdominal pain, and diarrhea may occur; eosinophilic necrotizing enteritis has been reported	No specific therapy

*Recommendations are based on Drugs for Parasitic Infections (Med Lett Drugs Ther 2004;46:1–12. Available at www. medicalletter.org). The dosages and durations are for adults.
†Associated with persistent, severe diarrhea in persons with AIDS.
AIDS = acquired immunodeficiency syndrome; HAART = highly active antiretroviral therapy; HIV = human immunodeficiency virus.

SUGGESTED READINGS

DPDx Laboratory identification of parasites of public health concern. Centers for Diseases Control and Prevention. Available at http://www.dpd.cdc.gov/dpdx/Default.htm). *Excellent review of human parasites, life cycles, clinical syndromes, and diagnostic studies.*

Drugs for parasitic diseases. Med Lett Drugs Ther 2004;46:1–12. Available at www.medicalletter.org. *Consensus recommendations for the treatment of parasitic diseases are provided. Key articles are referenced.*

Eberhard ML, Arrowood MJ: Cyclospora spp. Curr Opin Infect Dis 2002; 15:519–522. *Review of the parasitology, epidemiology, and clinical manifestations associated with* Cyclospora *sp infection.*

Hatcher JC, Greenberg PD, Antique J, Jimenez-Lucho VE: Severe babesiosis in Long Island: Review of 34 cases and their complications. Clin Infect Dis 2001; 32:1117–1125. *A series of cases characterizes the manifestations, complications, and treatment of severe* B. microti *infection.*

Herwaldt BL, McGovern PC, Gerwel MP, et al: Endemic babesiosis in another eastern state: New Jersey. Emerg Infect Dis 2003;9:184–188. *The authors provide composite data on 40 cases of babesiosis acquired in New Jersey.*

Section XXIII Infectious Diseases

Ho AY, Lopez AS, Eberhart MG, et al: Outbreak of cyclosporiasis associated with imported raspberries, Philadelphia, Pennsylvania, 2000. Emerg Infect Dis 2002;8:783–788. *The description of an outbreak of cyclosporiasis associated with imported raspberries.*

Krause PJ: Babesiosis. Med Clin North Am 2002;86:361–373. *The life cycle, epidemiology, clinical manifestations, and diagnosis of babesiosis are reviewed.*

Krieger JN: Consider diagnosis and treatment of trichomoniasis in men. Sex Transm Dis 2000;27:241–242. *An excellent summary of the clinical manifestations of trichomoniasis in men.*

Soper D: Trichomoniasis: Under control or undercontrolled? Am J Obstet Gynecol 2004;190:281–290. *An excellent review of the consequence of* Trichomonas vaginalis *infection in women.*

Tinidazole (Tindamax)—a new anti-protozoal drug. Med Lett Drugs Ther 2004;46:70–72. *A comprehensive review of tinidazole, its indications, and untoward effects written after it received FDA approval for use in the United States.*

Verdier RI, Fitzgerald DW, Johnson WD Jr, Pape JW: Trimethoprim-sulfamethoxazole compared with ciprofloxacin for treatment and prophylaxis of *Isospora belli* and *Cyclospora cayetanensis* infection in HIV-infected patients: A randomized, controlled trial. Ann Intern Med 2000;132:885–888. *Trimethoprim-sulfamethoxazole is the treatment of choice for* C. cayetanensis*; ciprofloxacin is an alternative.*

Wendel KA: Trichomoniasis: What's new? Curr Infect Dis Rep 2003;5:129–134. *An overview of diagnosis and treatment.*

Wormser GP, Dattwyler RJ, Shapiro ED, et al: The clinical assessment, treatment, and prevention of Lyme disease, human granulocytic anaplasmosis, and babesiosis: Clinical practice guidelines by the Infectious Disease Society of America. Clin Infect Dis 2006;43:1089–1134. *Evidence-based guidelines prepared by an expert panel.*

375 CESTODE INFECTIONS

Charles H. King

The eight cestode species that most commonly cause human infection are listed in Table 375–1. Although this class of parasites is often referred to collectively as tapeworms, not all cestode parasites develop into tapeworms in the human host. The key to understanding the rather broad spectrum of cestode-associated illness is to recall that these parasites divide their life cycle between two or more different animal hosts called *intermediate* and *definitive* hosts. The intermediate host harbors the immature parasite as a tissue cyst, whereas the subsequent definitive host harbors the mature parasite as a tapeworm. For a given cestode species, humans may serve as intermediate or definitive hosts.

The intermediate host is typically an insect or herbivorous (omnivorous) vertebrate that ingests parasite eggs in fecally contaminated food or water. The cestode eggs hatch into invasive oncospheres in this primary host's intestinal tract and then migrate into the host viscera or muscles to develop into immature cystic forms called cysticerci or cysticercoids (for Cyclophyllidea cestodes such as *Taenia* and *Hymenolepis*) or procercoid and plerocercoid larvae (for Pseudophyllidea cestodes such as *Diphyllobothrium*). Humans become intermediate hosts for cestode species by ingesting parasite eggs in food or water, as in echinococcosis, or rarely by direct transfer of plerocercoid larvae from animal tissues, as in sparganosis.

The *definitive* host for a cestode species is a carnivorous or omnivorous mammal that acquires infection by consuming larval cysts in the uncooked tissues of an intermediate host. On exposure to stomach acid and bile salts in the digestive tract, the larvae excyst and develop into mature tapeworms within the intestinal lumen. Adult tapeworms contain two sections: a *scolex* (or head), used to adhere to the wall of the intestine, and a *strobila,* a tapelike chain of developing segments called proglottids. The hermaphroditic proglottids produce large numbers of fertile, infectious parasite eggs that reach the environment free or enclosed within parasite segments in the host's feces. Carnivorous humans become definitive hosts by ingesting the cyst-infested meat of intermediate hosts (e.g., fish, pork, beef), after which the cysts develop into intraluminal, intestinal tapeworms.

Humans are strictly definitive hosts for the cestodes *Diphyllobothrium latum* (i.e., fish tapeworm), and *Taenia saginata* (i.e., beef tapeworm). These adult tapeworms do not enter the tissues of the human body and cause only minimal clinical symptoms. In contrast, humans are solely intermediate hosts for *Echinococcus granulosus* (hydatid cyst disease), *Echinococcus multilocularis* (alveolar cyst disease), *Taenia multiceps* (coenurosis), and *Spirometra* species. In the human body, these parasites develop as larval cysts and cause significant symptomatic tissue damage.

There are two exceptions to this rule. First, patients with *Taenia solium* infection may be infected with larval cysts (cysticercosis), adult tapeworms (i.e., pork tapeworm), or both. Second, in the case of the dwarf tapeworm *Hymenolepis nana,* complete egg to tapeworm development can take place within a single human host. *H. nana* can be transmitted directly from person to person, and internal autoinfection may substantially increase the tapeworm burden of an infected individual. For all other cestode infections, increases in parasite burden occur only by means of continued exposure to egg-contaminated or larva-infested food and water.

INTESTINAL CESTODE (TAPEWORM) INFECTIONS

Diphyllobothrium latum

Definition

D. latum tapeworms, the largest parasites that infect humans, range in length up to 10 m. Infection is acquired by the ingestion of parasite cysts in the tissues of smoked or uncooked freshwater fish (e.g., sushi, sashimi, ceviche, carpaccio). Tapeworms develop to maturity within 3 to 6 weeks after exposure and may survive for up to 20 years.

TABLE 375–1 COMMON HUMAN CESTODE INFECTIONS

Species	Stage Found in Humans	Common Name	Pathology	Therapy
Diphyllobothrium latum	Adult	Fish tapeworm	Pernicious anemia	Niclosamide Praziquantel
Hymenolepis nana	Adult	Dwarf tapeworm	Rarely symptomatic	Niclosamide Praziquantel
Taenia saginata	Adult	Beef tapeworm	Rarely symptomatic	Niclosamide Praziquantel
Taenia solium	Adult	Pork tapeworm	Rarely symptomatic	Niclosamide Praziquantel
	Larva	Cysticercosis	Brain and tissue cysts	Albendazole Praziquantel Surgery
Echinococcus granulosus	Larva	Hydatid cyst disease	Solitary tissue cysts	Surgery Albendazole
Echinococcus multilocularis	Larva	Alveolar cyst disease	Multilocular cysts	Surgery Albendazole
Taenia multiceps	Larva	Bladderworm, coenurosis	Brain and eye cysts	Surgery
Spirometra mansonoides	Larva	Sparganosis	Subcutaneous larvae	Surgery

Epidemiology

Infection is prevalent (up to 2% of local residents) in many parts of the world, and endemic foci are found in the lake or delta regions of Scandinavia, Russia, Japan, Europe, Chile, and North America. Contamination of freshwater bodies by raw sewage increases the risk for *D. latum* infection, but stable transmission may also occur because of local infection of alternative definitive hosts such as foxes, wolves, minks, and bears.

Clinical Manifestations

In most patients, *D. latum* infection produces few or no symptoms, which are typically limited to nonspecific complaints of weakness, dizziness, craving for salt, diarrhea, and intermittent abdominal discomfort. Some patients may experience vomiting, severe abdominal pain, and weight loss. In cases of multiple infections, biliary or intestinal obstruction may occur. In 1 to 2% of patients with *D. latum* infection, significant vitamin B_{12} deficiency develops and results in megaloblastic anemia or neurologic disease. Folate deficiency may also occur. Vitamin B_{12} deficiency is a consequence of extensive vitamin uptake by the worm and worm-induced interference with gastrointestinal uptake by the host despite normal gastric acidity and production of intrinsic factor. Vitamin B_{12} deficiency is most common in older individuals and is more likely to occur in those with low dietary intake of vitamins, multiple tapeworms, or a tapeworm in the proximal jejunum. In a debilitated host, nervous system complications can be quite extensive and range from peripheral neuropathy to the syndrome of subacute combined degeneration (Chapter 443).

Diagnosis

The diagnosis of *D. latum* infection is made by examination of stool for the characteristic operculated eggs, which are 65 by 45 μm in diameter. Recovery of proglottids is uncommon because of segment degeneration during intestinal transit.

Treatment

Rx

D. latum infection is treated with niclosamide or praziquantel, as summarized in Table 375–2. Severe vitamin B_{12} deficiency can be treated rapidly by parenteral vitamin injections.

Prevention

Fish tapeworm infection is prevented by avoiding the consumption of raw, smoked, pickled, or salted fish from endemic areas. Parasite cysts may be killed by cooking (>56° C for 5 minutes) or by freezing (−20° C for 24 hours).

Hymenolepis nana

Epidemiology

H. nana, or the dwarf tapeworm, is frequently found in warm, dry climates and is prevalent in southern and eastern Europe, Asia, Africa, Central and South America, Papua New Guinea, and Australia. It is the only human tapeworm that does not require an intermediate host. In the small intestine, hatching eggs release oncospheres that penetrate the villi of the mucosa. Four to 5 days later, the developed cysticercoid ruptures out of the villus, and a parasite scolex attaches to the lining of the ileum, where it matures in 10 to 12 days. Mature worms are small, 25 to 40 mm long and 1 mm wide. Autoinfection can occur internally (i.e., within the small bowel) or externally through the fecal-oral route and result in heavy infection. With time, however, a regulatory immunity to infection may develop such that *H. nana* infection can be spontaneously cleared. Intensive infection is more common in institutionalized, malnourished, or immunodeficient individuals and should be screened for during the process of international adoptions.

Clinical Manifestations

The clinical manifestations of *H. nana* vary with the intensity of infection and may include diarrhea, anorexia, abdominal pain, and pallor. A statistical association with phlyctenular keratoconjunctivitis has been observed and tentatively ascribed to the immune response to infection.

Diagnosis

The diagnosis of *H. nana* infection is made by examining stool for eggs 30 to 47 μm in diameter that have a characteristic double membrane (Fig. 375–1). Proglottids are not usually seen in stool.

Treatment

H. nana infection is treated with niclosamide or praziquantel, as outlined in Table 375–2. When compared with the treatment of other tapeworm infections, longer courses of niclosamide and

TABLE 375–2 THERAPY FOR INTESTINAL CESTODE (TAPEWORM) INFECTION

	Niclosamide	Praziquantel
Dosage		
Adults	2 g (4 tablets)	5–10 mg/kg for all age groups (25 mg/kg for *Hymenolepis nana*)
Children >34 kg	1.5 g (3 tablets)	
Children 11–34 kg	1 g (2 tablets)	
Administration	For most tapeworm species, taken as a single dose; tablets must be thoroughly chewed before swallowing to obtain a complete therapeutic effect; a 7-day course of drugs is used for *H. nana*, with reduced pediatric doses on days 2–7	Taken as a single dose for all species; may repeat after 7 days for heavy *H. nana* infection
Side effects	Nausea, vomiting, abdominal pain, diarrhea, drowsiness, dizziness, headache, pruritus	Mild but frequent, including dizziness, myalgias, nausea, vomiting, diarrhea, abdominal pain
Pregnancy	No known mutagenic effects; considered safe if indicated; because of risk for cysticercosis by autoinfection in *Taenia solium* tapeworm infection, therapy should not be delayed	

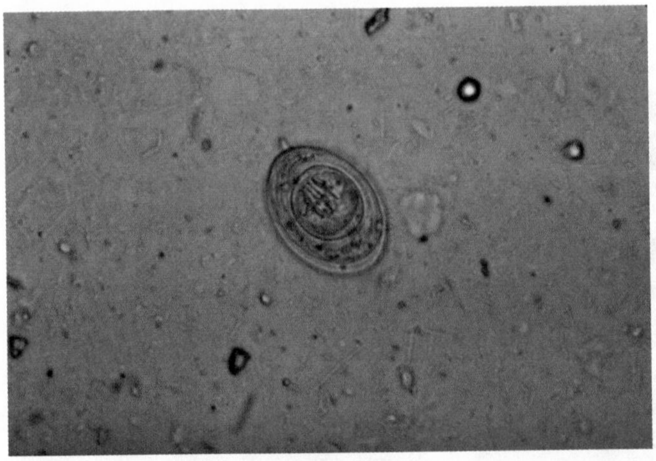

FIGURE 375–1 • Micrograph depicting an egg from a *Hymenolepis nana* tapeworm, or cestode. *H. nana* eggs are oval or subspherical in shape, 40 to 60 μm × 30 to 50 μm in size—smaller than those of *Hymenolepis diminuta*. On the inner membrane are two poles from which four to eight polar filaments spread out between its two membranes.

Rx

higher doses of praziquantel are recommended for the treatment of *H. nana* infection because of the relative resistance of larval cysticercoids to drug therapy. As a result of the potential for late emergence of worms from viable cysticercoids remaining in the ileum, heavily infected individuals should be retested for infection and retreated 10 to 14 days after initial therapy.

Prevention

Because *H. nana* is easily transmitted from person to person, sanitation and handwashing are essential to control this parasite. Mass chemotherapy may also be used to suppress endemic transmission, particularly within closed institutions.

Taenia saginata

Epidemiology

T. saginata, or the beef tapeworm, is widespread in cattle-breeding areas of the world. Endemic foci (defined as a prevalence >10%) are found in the southern Russian republics, in the Near East, and in central and eastern Africa. Infection is less common in other parts of the world but is found at prevalence rates of 0.1 to 5% in Europe, Southeast Asia, and South America. Infection is acquired by consuming cysticerci in the muscle tissue of infected cattle. The consumption of dishes such as steak tartare, "bleu" or rare steak, and undercooked shish kebab is associated with infection in North American travelers to endemic areas.

Clinical Manifestations

T. saginata infection may cause nonspecific complaints of weakness and mild abdominal discomfort in up to a third of patients. Because *T. saginata* proglottids are motile, they may cause acute abdominal symptoms by migrating into and obstructing the appendix or the pancreatic and biliary ducts. A psychologically distressing feature of infection (and often the first symptom reported by the patient) occurs when motile proglottids migrate out of the anus onto skin or clothing or when they are observed moving in feces.

Diagnosis

The diagnosis of taeniasis is most readily established by stool examination and perianal inspection for parasite proglottids and eggs. It is not possible, however, to distinguish *T. saginata* eggs from those of *T. solium* morphologically, and a definitive diagnosis of *T. saginata* infection requires pathologic examination of proglottid features or DNA-based species identification studies. In practice, because patients with *T. solium* are at risk for self-infection with cysticercosis and because medical therapy for taeniasis is both safe and highly effective, treatment of an infection by undetermined *Taenia* species should not be delayed pending speciation of the infecting tapeworm.

Treatment

Rx

Beef tapeworm infection is treated with praziquantel or niclosamide, as outlined in Table 375–2. Both medications are highly effective in eliminating infection, and no special preparation or purgation is required. After therapy, the parasite scolex is digested within the gastrointestinal tract before it is passed in feces. Although with the highly effective medications in use it is no longer necessary to collect the scolex to be assured that the parasite head has been expelled, digestive destruction of the head limits the ability to establish a species-specific clinical diagnosis for individual *Taenia* infections.

Prevention

T. saginata infection is prevented by avoiding foods containing undercooked or raw beef. As for the fish tapeworm, cooking to 56° C for 5 minutes or freezing at −20° C for 7 to 10 days destroys the infective larvae.

Taenia solium

Definition

T. solium, also known as the pork tapeworm, causes human infection in two different forms. Intestinal *T. solium* tapeworms develop in individuals who consume undercooked pork containing intermediate parasite cysts. Intermediate parasite cysts may develop within the tissues of individuals who consume parasite eggs. (This condition, called *cysticercosis*, is described in more detail in the section on tissue cestode infections.) Autoinfection, most likely through the fecal-oral route, is possible, and a single patient may harbor both an adult tapeworm and tissue cysticerci.

Epidemiology

T. solium infection is prevalent in Mexico, Central and South America, Africa, the Cape Verde Islands, southern Europe, Southeast Asia, and the Philippines. Most infections seen in the United States and Canada are found in immigrants from these endemic foci.

Clinical Manifestations

T. solium tapeworms are relatively short (3 m) but may survive for several decades once established in the human jejunum. Generally, tapeworm infections with *T. solium* produce no or minimal symptoms, which are limited to mild, nonspecific abdominal complaints. Unlike *T. saginata* proglottids, the segments of *T. solium* are nonmotile and unlikely to cause obstruction.

Diagnosis

The diagnosis of intestinal infection with *T. solium* tapeworm is made by examining the stool for eggs and proglottids. Because the eggs are morphologically indistinguishable from those of *T. saginata*, study of the proglottid or head of the tapeworms is required for species identification (Fig. 375–2). Stool samples and proglottids should be handled with care because of the risk of acquiring cysticercosis by accidental ingestion of *T. solium* eggs.

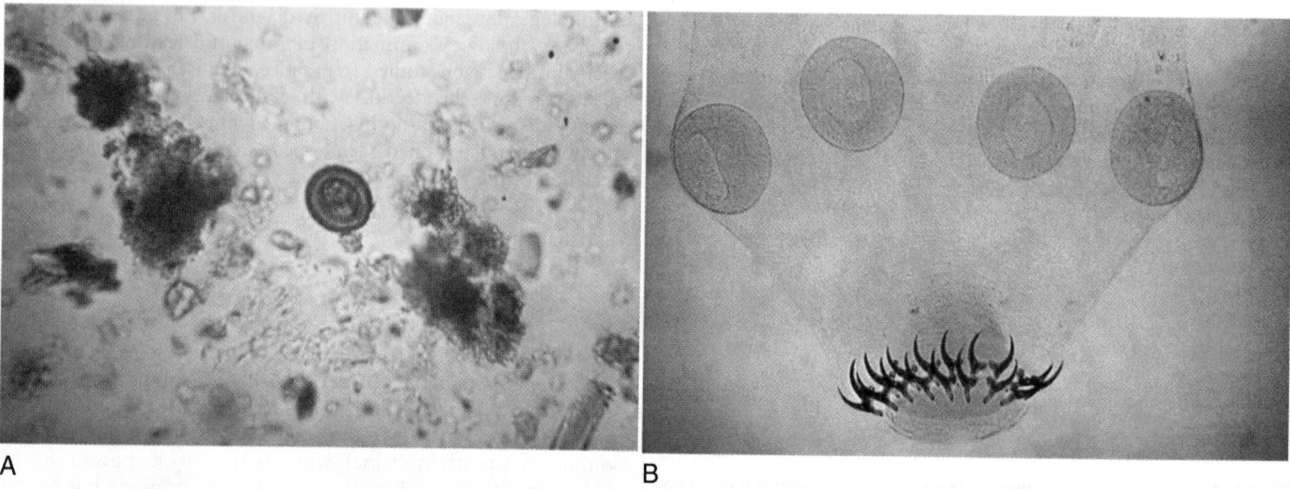

FIGURE 375–2 • *Taenia* infection. A, Micrograph depicting an egg from either a *Taenia saginata* or *Taenia solium* cestode (i.e., tapeworm). The eggs of *T. saginata* and *T. solium* are rounded or subspherical with a thick, radially striated brown shell. The diameter is 31 to 43 μm. Inside each shell is an embryonated oncosphere with six hooks. **B,** Micrograph revealing the morphology of a *T. solium* tapeworm scolex with its four suckers and two rows of hooks. In the human intestine, the cysticercus (i.e. the larval stage) develops over a period of 2 months into an adult tapeworm, which can survive for years by attaching to and residing in the small intestine with the suckers and hooks located in its head region, or scolex.

Treatment

Rx

T. solium tapeworm infection is treated with niclosamide or praziquantel, as outlined in Table 375–2. After the diagnosis is established and concurrent central nervous system (CNS) and ocular cysticercosis has been excluded, therapy should be instituted as soon as possible because of the risk for autoinfection with cysticercosis. Therapy for concurrent cysticercosis is substantially longer and more intensive than that for intestinal infection and is described later in the section on tissue cestode infection.

Other Intestinal Cestodes

Other tapeworms that occasionally infect humans include the dog tapeworm *Dipylidium caninum* and the rodent tapeworm *Hymenolepis diminuta.* These tapeworms are most common in children and are acquired by inadvertently ingesting the intermediate larval forms of these parasites in the bodies of fleas or other insects. Usually, *D. caninum* and *H. diminuta* infections produce minimal symptoms. The diagnosis is established by stool examination, and infections are readily treated with standard doses of niclosamide or praziquantel.

TISSUE CESTODE (CYST) INFECTION

Echinococcosis

Definition

Human echinococcosis causes significant morbidity and mortality in livestock-raising regions in all parts of the world. The causative agents of "hydatid" and "alveolar" cyst disease in humans are the intermediate larval forms of the tapeworms *E. granulosus* and *E. multilocularis,* respectively.

Like other cestodes, *Echinococcus* tapeworms have intermediate and definitive hosts. For *Echinococcus* species, dogs and other canines are the definitive hosts. These tapeworm-infected canines pass eggs in their feces, which contaminate the local environment. Contamination of grazing areas and foodstuff results in ingestion of eggs by intermediate hosts such as humans, sheep, goats, camels, yaks, and horses for *E. granulosus* and mice or other small rodents for *E. multilocularis.* Life cycle transmission is completed when the definitive carnivore host consumes meat or offal of the intermediate host that contains hydatid or alveolar cysts. Protoscolices within the cysts mature in the lumen of the canine gut to become adult, egg-bearing tapeworms. Because the cysts of *Echinococcus* contain a germinal layer that can produce multiple internal "daughter" cysts by asexual budding, an individual dog may become infected with dozens of tapeworms after consuming a single, large cyst. After the tapeworms mature, a heavily infected dog may contaminate 10 or more hectares of ground with infectious eggs in a week.

In most areas of the world, burial practices make humans a "dead-end" host for *Echinococcus;* human infection does not perpetuate transmission in the local ecosystem. Nevertheless, the "inadvertent" hydatid cyst disease caused by *E. granulosus* and the more aggressive alveolar cyst disease caused by *E. multilocularis* are severe or even fatal illnesses for a significant minority of infected individuals.

Epidemiology

E. granulosus is common in livestock-raising areas of developed and developing countries. Sheep- and goat-herding populations that keep dogs as pets or work animals are at highest risk for hydatid cyst disease. Until recently, hydatid disease was common in Australia, New Zealand, Argentina, Chile, Ireland, Scotland, the Basque country, the Mediterranean basin, and throughout middle Europe. Currently, the area with the highest prevalence in the world is the Turkana and Samburu region of northwestern Kenya, where domestic and feral transmission of *E. granulosus* is perpetuated among nomadic farmers by poor hygienic practices. Occasional hydatid disease transmission is also found in central Asia, Mexico, the United States, and South America.

Alveolar cyst disease caused by *E. multilocularis* is usually transmitted by wild animals such as foxes and bush dogs and is found in the arctic regions of the United States, Canada, and the former Soviet Union, as well as in rural areas of Europe and Turkey.

Clinical Manifestations

Human disease caused by *Echinococcus* species results from blood-borne invasion of the liver (50 to 70% of patients), lungs (20 to 30%), or other organs by developing parasite oncospheres. As these oncospheres mature, they grow within tissues by concentric enlargement (*E. granulosus*) or by extension through adjacent host tissues (*E. multilocularis*). At any given time, most infected individuals are asymptomatic, and it may take 5 to 20 years for a cyst to grow to sufficient size (3 to 15 cm) to cause symptoms. When present, symptoms and findings refer to the anatomic site of involvement and derive from local inflammation, secondary bacterial infection, obstruction, or a local mass effect. In hydatid cyst disease, the growing cyst becomes surrounded by a fibrous capsule formed by host immune reaction. Within this primary unilocular cyst, multiple daughter cysts, each containing an infective protoscolex, develop by asexual budding of the germinal layer. In alveolar cyst disease, the parasite cyst is not well separated from surrounding tissue, and lateral budding and malignancy-like growth (including distant metastasis of daughter cysts) may occur.

Patients with symptomatic hydatid liver cysts may complain of abdominal discomfort or a mass in the right upper quadrant. Cyst leakage into the peritoneal cavity or pleural space may be associated with fever, urticaria, or a severe anaphylactoid reaction. Invasion of the biliary system often leads to the passage of daughter cysts into the common bile duct, with clinical and chemical evidence of intermittent obstruction resembling choledocholithiasis. Individuals with symptomatic hydatid involvement of the lungs initially demonstrate cough, hemoptysis, and pleurisy. Spontaneous rupture of the cyst may lead to intrathoracic spread or to evacuation of daughter cysts through the bronchus. At lung or liver sites, bacterial superinfection may cause an acute manifestation with symptoms of sepsis. Hydatid involvement of the brain is marked by a slow-onset mass effect, hydrocephalus, and frequently, seizures. Cysts of the bone often fail to form a discrete capsule but rather cause local erosion of the cortex that results in a pathologic fracture.

Symptomatic alveolar cyst disease most frequently refers to liver involvement and is manifested as vague, mild upper quadrant and epigastric pain. Signs of hepatomegaly or obstructive jaundice may be present. Occasionally, metastatic lesions in the lung or brain are the first to cause symptoms via local inflammation or a mass effect.

Diagnosis

Laboratory evaluation may show marked eosinophilia, but this finding is inconstant (30% prevalence). In hydatid cyst disease, radiographic and ultrasonographic studies typically demonstrate characteristic large, avascular cysts containing internal structures consistent with daughter cysts. Detection of mural calcification strongly favors the diagnosis of hydatid cyst. The differential diagnosis includes hemangioma, metastatic carcinoma, and remote bacterial or amebic liver abscess. Confirmatory evidence of infection may be obtained by serology (sensitivity of 60 to 90%, depending on the test used). Serologic testing is available commercially or from the Centers for Disease Control and Prevention (CDC) through local state health departments. Until recently, it has not been recommended that closed aspiration be performed on the cyst for diagnosis because cyst leakage has the potential to initiate a severe allergic reaction and may result in the metastatic spread of daughter cysts. However, clinical series have reported successful computed tomography (CT)- or ultrasound-guided thin-needle aspiration of hydatid cysts for diagnosis. This procedure, when followed by immediate treatment to kill viable protoscolices, is rarely associated with side effects and is usually followed by regression of cysts on follow-up scans.

With alveolar cyst disease caused by *E. multilocularis,* the organism's appearance on radiographic and sonographic imaging often mimics that of hepatic carcinoma. Definitive diagnosis may require angiography or open biopsy at surgery. Precautions must be taken to prevent metastatic dissemination of daughter cysts at the time of surgery.

Treatment

Rx

Stable, asymptomatic, calcified cysts do not require specific therapy but should be monitored by serial imaging over a period of several years to ensure a benign resolution. When technically feasible, expanding, symptomatic, or infected cysts are best removed in toto at surgery, with care taken to isolate the cyst to avoid secondary spread during the procedure. Controversy has arisen over the practice of intraoperative instillation of cysticidal agents because in some patients sclerosing cholangitis has developed as a late complication of surgery when hepatic cysts communicate with the biliary system. Perioperative drug therapy alone is likely to be sufficient to prevent the spread of daughter cysts at the time of surgery. If a cysticidal agent is used during surgery, hypertonic saline (25 to 30%) or 95% ethanol appears to pose the least risk to the patient, whereas instillation of iodophor and formalin should definitely be avoided. Surgical resection should include careful closure of biliary and enteric fistulas and extensive postoperative drainage of the cyst bed to prevent fluid accumulation and secondary bacterial infection. Alveolar cyst disease may require wide resection (i.e., total lobectomy of the liver or lung or even organ transplantation) to remove all cyst material.

In many cases, symptomatic echinococcal cysts are not amenable to resection. In such cases, oral drug therapy with anthelmintics, either long-term mebendazole (40 mg/kg of body weight per day in

Rx

three divided doses for 6 to 12 months) or albendazole (400 mg twice daily for 1 to 6 months), has been recommended for cure or palliation. [1] Cure rates, particularly for difficult cases with recurrent or extrahepatic or extrapulmonary cysts, have been low (<33%), although most patients show some improvement. Because the efficacy of drug therapy is limited, it is usually necessary to tailor a combined medical-surgical approach for each patient.

A minimally invasive option, *p*ercutaneous *a*spiration, *i*njection, and *r*easpiration (PAIR procedure), performed under ultrasound or CT guidance, has been successful in controlling hydatid disease in many patients with inoperable intra-abdominal or bone cysts, although it has been less successful in patients with lung cysts. [2] During PAIR, the risk of parasite spread should be minimized by concurrent anthelmintic therapy, and immediate treatment should be available for possible allergic reactions during the procedure.

Cysticercosis

Epidemiology

Cysticercosis represents human tissue infection with the intermediate cyst forms of the pork tapeworm *T. solium.* Cysticercosis is acquired by the ingestion of *T. solium* eggs in contaminated food. The prevalence of infection is approximately 5 to 25% in endemic areas of Latin America, India, Asia, Indonesia, and parts of Africa. Because of its potentially life-threatening complications, cysticercosis has greater clinical significance than intestinal *T. solium* tapeworm infection does, particularly if cyst disease involves the CNS, eyes, heart, or other vital organs.

Clinical Manifestations

Clinical manifestations depend on the location and number of infecting cysts. Cysticerci are bladder-like, fluid-filled cysts containing an invaginated protoscolex. They are often surrounded by a dense, fibrous capsule of host origin. In infected humans, cysticerci are usually multiple, 0.5 to 2 cm in diameter, and distributed widely throughout the body. Many patients have minimal or no symptoms of infection. However, symptomatic *neurocysticercosis* (e.g., cerebral cysticercosis, eye or spinal cord involvement) requires medical attention. Because this condition may prove lethal, any neurologic, cognitive, or personality disorder in an individual from an endemic area should be considered a possible manifestation of undiagnosed neurocysticercosis. Diagnosis has been facilitated by CT and magnetic resonance imaging (MRI), both of which are highly sensitive in detecting CNS cysticerci. Patients with CNS involvement have an average of 10 cysts distributed throughout the brain and spinal cord. These cysts may be in different stages of development, with symptoms commonly arising when older cysts begin to die, lose osmoregulation, and release antigenic material that provokes a significant host inflammatory response.

In practice, neurocysticercosis may be divided into six discrete syndromes for management. In the *acute invasive* stage of cysticercosis, immediately after infection, the patient may experience fever, headache, and myalgia associated with significant peripheral eosinophilia. Heavy infection at this stage may result in a clinical picture of "cysticercal encephalitis" associated with coma and rapid deterioration. This manifestation should be treated aggressively with anti-inflammatory drugs. After cysticerci become established, *parenchymal CNS cysticercosis* (50% of cases) may be accompanied by seizures, intellectual impairment, and personality changes. Compression secondary to swelling or inflammation around the cysts may result in focal deficits, signs of cerebral edema, and hydrocephalus. Seizures may be focal (jacksonian), referring to the specific cortical locus of involvement, or may be generalized. *Subarachnoid cysticercosis* (30% of cases) is frequently associated with obstruction to flow of cerebrospinal fluid (CSF). Intracranial hypertension may be manifested as vomiting, headache, and visual disturbances. Sensorial changes may include apathy, amnesia, dementia, hallucination, and emotional disturbance. Like other forms of basilar meningitis, pericysticercal inflammation at the base of the brain may cause obstruction or vasculitis of the cerebral arteries and lead to intermittent ischemia or stroke.

Intraventricular cysticercosis (15% of cases), because of its location, is the most difficult to diagnose and treat. Symptomatic cysts are most frequent in the fourth ventricle, where they cause outflow obstruction and increased intracranial pressure without localizing signs. An aggressive variant of ventricular neurocysticercosis involves the basal cisterns. This form of cysticercosis occurs most often in young women and involves multiple, rapidly spreading cysts in the cerebrum and around the base of the brain. Whereas symptoms attributable to isolated cysts may remit, cisternal cysticercosis usually has a progressive, deteriorating course if therapy is not undertaken. Those with *spinal cysticercosis* may suffer cord compression, radiculopathy, transverse myelitis, or signs of meningitis, depending on the location of involvement. *Ocular cysticercosis* is a distinct syndrome that is manifested as eye pain, scotomas, and decreasing vision because of iridocyclitis, clouding of the vitreous, and retinal inflammation or detachment.

Diagnosis

A definitive diagnosis of cysticercosis requires examination of biopsy material obtained from a tissue cyst. However, a presumptive diagnosis may be made on the basis of a history of residence in an endemic area, the presence of characteristic radiographic findings on plain films (i.e., calcified cysts in soft tissues) or scans (i.e., low-density, enhanced, and unenhanced lesions on CT or MRI), and suggestive laboratory findings. Concomitant infection with *T. solium* tapeworm is present in about 25% of cases of neurocysticercosis. In patients with neurocysticercosis, lumbar puncture is contraindicated in the presence of increased intracranial pressure. When obtainable, CSF may show hypoglycorrhachia, elevated total protein levels, and lymphocytic and eosinophilic pleocytosis (5 to 500 cells/μL). Although serum enzyme-linked immunosorbent assay (ELISA) and immunoblot assays may prove insensitive for the detection of infection (as low as 50% in some MRI series of symptomatic patients), the CSF ELISA and immunoblot tests for specific immunoglobulin M (IgM) and IgG anticysticercal antibodies have a sensitivity of 75 to 100%. These tests are available through commercial laboratories or from the CDC (samples should be sent through state health departments). However, antiparasitic antibodies may persist long after infection, and positive IgG serology may indicate only previous *Taenia* exposure, not necessarily active disease. The differential diagnosis of neurocysticercosis includes tumor, hydatid cyst disease, vasculitis, and chronic fungal and mycobacterial infection.

Treatment

Given the high prevalence of cysticercosis in some areas of the world, it is evident that most cysticerci do not cause significant symptoms. For *symptomatic cysts outside the CNS,* the optimal therapy is surgical removal to ensure complete elimination of the cyst.

Inactive, asymptomatic neurocysticercosis does not need to be treated and should be monitored prospectively. In cases of *active neurocysticercosis,* symptomatic therapy is definitely indicated, but surgery may be risky or technically unfeasible. For most intraparenchymal brain cysts, optimal therapy involves control of seizures with anticonvulsants and reduction of cerebral inflammation with anti-inflammatory doses of corticosteroids, as needed. As shown in placebo-controlled randomized trials, specific antiparasitic therapy is not generally helpful in speeding resolution of symptoms in these patients, except possibly for reducing the frequency of seizures in some subsets of patients. [3-5] For patients with extraparenchymal neurocysticercosis (i.e., ventricular or subarachnoid disease), antiparasitic therapy may limit extension of the infection and reduce the number of complications. For such patients, antiparasitic therapy must be combined with relief of hydrocephalus through shunting, along with control of local inflammation with the use of corticosteroids. When anthelmintics are to be used, therapy with albendazole (10 to 15 mg/kg/day for 8 to 30 days) or praziquantel (50 to 100 mg/kg/day in three divided doses for 30 days) is recommended. Recommendations for drug therapy continue to evolve, however, and it is appropriate to review the latest literature before embarking on a course of drug treatment. Follow-up tomographic scanning should be repeated 1 to 3 months after therapy is stopped to ensure an adequate response. In cases of progressive disease, a repeat course of drug therapy with the alternate antiparasitic agent may be given to improve response.

Before institution of antiparasitic therapy, a careful examination should be made for eye involvement. In about 20% of treated cases, initiation of drug therapy is associated with an increased inflammatory response at the site of the cyst. Because parasite-induced ocular inflammation does not respond well to systemic anti-inflammatory agents, patients with cysticercosis of the eye (20% of cases of neurocysticercosis) should not receive drug therapy until the eye disease has been controlled surgically.

Coenurosis

A different and less common form of tissue cysticercosis may be caused by larval stages of the dog tapeworms *T. multiceps* and *Taenia serialis.* Lesions tend to be solitary and are distinguished pathologically from *T. solium* cysticerci on biopsy. Ocular involvement is common, and surgical resection is the only effective mode of therapy.

Sparganosis

Sparganosis is a tissue cestode infection caused by the plerocercoid larval stages of *Spirometra* tapeworms of cats and other carnivores. Humans may become infected by ingesting infected water fleas (*Cyclops*), by eating uncooked meat from infected animals (i.e., reptiles, birds, or mammals), or by cutaneous exposure (i.e., traditional skin or eye poultices) to uncooked, infected meat. Usually, the larva encysts within the intestinal submucosa or skin. In some cases, however, parasites may invade the eye or CNS and cause significant inflammatory pathology at the site of encystment. Occasionally, proliferation into surrounding tissue occurs by lateral budding of the parasite, called *sparganum proliferum.* The treatment of choice for sparganosis is ethanol injection or surgical removal, or both, because the limited experience with medical anthelmintic therapy has shown no beneficial effect.

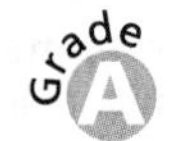

1. Keshmiri M, Baharvahdat H, Fattahi SH, et al: Albendazole versus placebo in treatment of echinococcosis. Trans R Soc Trop Med Hyg 2001;95:190–194.
2. Smego RA, Bhatti S, Khaliq AA, et al: Percutaneous aspiration-injection-reaspiration drainage plus albendazole or mebendazole for hepatic cystic echinococcosis: A meta-analysis. Clin Infect Dis 2003;37:1073–1083.
3. Salinas R, Counsell C, Prasad K, et al: Treating neurocysticercosis medically: A systematic review of randomized, controlled trials. Trop Med Int Health 1999;4:713–718.
4. Gogia S, Talukdar B, Choudhury V, et al: Neurocysticercosis in children: Clinical findings and response to albendazole therapy in a randomized, double blind, placebo-controlled trial in newly diagnosed cases. Trans R Soc Trop Med Hyg 2003;97:416–421.
5. Garcia HH, Pretell EJ, Gilman RH, et al: A trial of antiparasitic treatment to reduce the rate of seizures due to cerebral cysticercosis. N Engl J Med 2004;350:249–258.

SUGGESTED READINGS

Del Brutto OH, Roos KL, Coffey CS, et al: Meta-analysis: Cysticidal drugs for neurocysticercosis: Albendazole and praziquantel. Ann Intern Med 2006;145:43–51. *Analysis of 11 studies found that the drug therapy results in better resolution of colloidal and vesicular cysticerci, lower risk for recurrence of seizures, and reduction in rate of seizures with treatment.*

Filippou D, Tselepis D, Filippou G, et al: Advances in liver echinococcosis: Diagnosis and treatment. Clin Gastroenterol Hepatol 2007;5:152–159. *Review of recent advances in treatment.*

Garcia HH, Del Brutto OH, Nash TE, et al: New concepts in the diagnosis and management of neurocysticercosis (*Taenia solium*). Am J Trop Med Hyg 2005;72:3–9. *Summary of recent advances in serodiagnostics, imaging, and treatment approaches for different forms of neurocysticercosis.*

Maggi P, Brandonisio O, Carito V, et al: *Hymenolepis nana* parasites in adopted children. Clin Infect Dis 2005;41:571–572. *Cases highlighting the frequency and symptoms.*

Nash TE, Singh G, White AC, et al: Treatment of neurocysticersosis: Current status and future research needs. Neurology 2006;67:1120–1127. *Review of neurocysticercosis treatment.*

376 SCHISTOSOMIASIS (BILHARZIASIS)

Edgar M. Carvalho and Aldo A. M. Lima

Definition

Schistosomiasis is one of the most important parasitic diseases of humans and is a global public health problem in the developing world. The disease is caused by trematodes of the genus *Schistosoma,* and it is estimated that 300 million people are infected, another 600 million are at high risk for infection, and 20 million have debilitating disease. Mortality from schistosomiasis was estimated at 11,000 deaths per year and the burden of disease at 1.7 million disability-adjusted life years lost per year.

The Pathogen

Five major species of *Schistosoma* affect humans: *S. mansoni, S. haematobium, S. japonicum, S. intercalatum,* and *S. mekongi.* Other *Schistosoma* species that occasionally infect humans include *S. bovis, S. mathei,* and some avian schistosomes. These species differ biologically from one another and in their geographic distribution and the type of disease that they produce. The schistosomes are digenetic parasitic trematodes (Fig. 376–1). Although they are morphologically distinct, the species of *Schistosoma* that infect humans share some common factors. The large male (0.6 to 2.2 cm × 2 to 4 mm) has a ventral gynecophoric canal in which the female (1.2 to 2.6 cm × 1 to 2 mm) is held during copulation.

Epidemiology

Schistosomiasis occurs mainly in rural agricultural and periurban areas. *S. mansoni* is found in 55 countries, including the Arabian peninsula, Egypt, Libya, Sudan, most countries in sub-Saharan Africa, Brazil, Suriname, and Venezuela. *S. hematobium* is endemic in 53 countries in the Middle East and most of the African continent, including the island of Madagascar and Mauritius. *S. japonicum* is endemic in China, Indonesia, and the Philippines; it has also been reported from Thailand. *S. intercalatum* has been reported from 10 countries in Africa. *S. mekongi* is found in Cambodia and Laos.

The endemicity of schistosomiasis depends on the urban disposal of urine *(S. haematobium)* and feces *(S. mansoni, S. japonicum, S. intercalatum, S. mekongi),* the presence of suitable snail hosts, and human exposure to cercariae. The freshwater snail intermediate hosts are *Biomphalaria* sp in Africa and *Biomphalaria glabrata (Australorbis)* and *Tropicarbis* in South America and the West Indies. In some cases, the endemicity of schistosomiasis may be maintained by animal reservoirs.

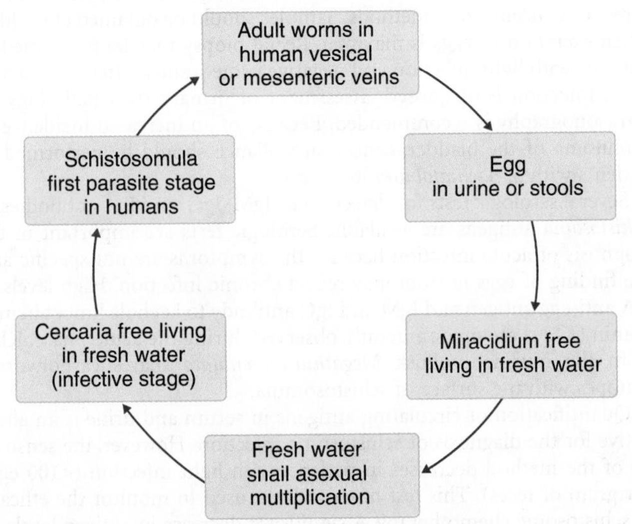

FIGURE 376–1 • Schistosome life cycle.

Such is the case with *S. japonicum,* which infects dogs and cows. Rodents, monkeys, and baboons have been found infected in nature, but the role of these animals as reservoirs does not seem to be epidemiologically important.

Etiology and Life Cycle

Adult worms live in the mesenteric veins (*S. mansoni, S. japonicum, S. mekongi,* and *S. intercalatum*) or in the venous plexus around the lower ends of the ureters and the urinary bladder *(S. haematobium).* In these sites, they start their sexual reproduction by releasing eggs. Once deposited in the host, eggs may stay in the mesenteric vein, be trapped in the intestines, escape to the intestinal lumen, and migrate by portal blood to the liver *(S. mansoni, S. japonicum).* Eggs of *S. haematobium* may be trapped in the intestines and bladder and may escape to the intestinal or bladder lumen. After being excreted with feces or urine into fresh water, the eggs hatch and release ciliated motile miracidia that penetrate into the snail intermediate host. Following asexual multiplication in the snail, the development of cercariae, the infective forms for humans, takes 4 to 7 weeks. After leaving the snails, the cercariae can survive in fresh water for almost 72 hours. When penetration of the skin in the human host occurs, the cercariae lose their tails and change into schistosomula. Schistosomula migrate to the lungs and, in about 6 weeks, mature to adult worms and descend to their final habitat. Viable eggs can be seen in excretions (i.e., stool or urine) 5 to 9 weeks after cercarial penetration. The lifespan of the worms ranges from 5 to 10 years.

Pathobiology

The pathogenesis of acute human schistosomiasis is mainly related to egg deposition and liberation of antigens of adult worms and eggs. A strong inflammatory response characterized by high levels of pro-inflammatory cytokines such as interleukin-1 (IL-1), IL-6, and tumor necrosis factor-α (TNF-α) and circulating immune complexes participate in the pathogenesis of the disease.

In chronic schistosomiasis, tissue injury is mediated by egg-induced granulomas and the subsequent appearance of fibrosis. Because the habitat of *S. mansoni, S. japonicum, S. mekongi,* and *S. intercalatum* worms is the mesenteric blood vessels, the intestines are involved primarily, and egg embolism results in secondary involvement of the liver. An association between the HLA class II allele DQB1*0201 and a greater chance for hepatosplenic involvement has been demonstrated. Moreover, IL-4 and IL-13 have been associated with granuloma formation and liver fibrosis. Enzymes and antigens released from eggs sensitize host lymphocytes, which migrate to areas of egg deposition and recruit other cell types, such as macrophages, eosinophils, and fibroblasts. The size of these granulomas and the resulting fibrosis lead to most of the chronic fibro-obstructive lesions in schistosomiasis. In the liver, the granulomas result in perisinusoidal obstruction of portal blood flow, portal hypertension, splenomegaly, esophageal varices, and portosystemic collateral circulation. Liver cell perfusion is not reduced; consequently, liver function test results remain normal for a long time.

In schistosome-infected populations, the intensity of infection increases during the first 2 decades of life as children accumulate worms and then declines. The susceptibility of younger children to infection is even more evident when intensities of reinfection are studied after the elimination of existing worms by chemotherapy. Although there is a decrease in exposure with age, the lower intensities of infection in older individuals are due in part to acquired resistance. Both T_H1 (interferon-γ) and T_H2 types of immune response, mediated by IgE, may participate in resistance to reinfection. In the *S. haematobium*–infected population, IgE increases progressively with age, and IgE antibodies directed against adult worm antigens are associated with subsequent low intensities of reinfection. Similar associations between high IgE levels or a high IgE/IgG4 ratio and resistance to reinfection have been found among Brazilian and Kenyan subjects exposed to *S. mansoni.* Evidence that a T_H1-type immune response may also be involved in the protection against *S. mansoni* comes from immunologic studies in subjects who are highly exposed to contaminated water but have negative stool examination results. In these subjects, there is evidence of higher interferon-γ production in response to *S. mansoni* membrane extract. The existence of a major codominant gene, called *SM1,* that controls the intensity of infection by *S. mansoni* has been demonstrated. The localization of *SM1* on chromosome 5q31-q33, close to several genes involved in regulation of the immune response, including those for colony-stimulating factor-1 receptor, granulocyte-macrophage colony-stimulating factor, IL-3, IL-4, IL-5, IL-13, and immune regulatory factor-1 and a locus regulating IgE levels, indicates that genetic factors are probably critical to susceptibility and resistance to schistosome infection.

Because modulation of the immune response is a characteristic of chronic schistosomiasis, *S. mansoni* infection has modified the clinical course of autoimmune and inflammatory diseases in experimental models and in humans. *S. mansoni* infection attenuates the clinical manifestations of type 1 diabetes and experimental autoimmune encephalitis in mice. In humans, *S. mansoni* attenuates the clinical manifestations of asthma and is inversely associated with the development of myelopathy related to human T-cell leukemia virus type 1 (HTLV-1) infection.

Clinical Manifestations

Clinical manifestations of schistosomiasis are divided into schistosome dermatitis, acute schistosomiasis, and chronic schistosomiasis. Schistosome dermatitis, or swimmer's itch, is seen mainly when avian cercariae penetrate the skin and are destroyed. Although this manifestation is not common in human schistosomiasis, recognition of this clinical entity is gradually expanding. Schistosome dermatitis is a sensitization phenomena because it occurs in previously exposed persons. The cercariae are destroyed in the epithelial layers of the skin. They evoke an acute inflammatory response with edema, early infiltration of neutrophils and lymphocytes, and later invasion of eosinophils. A pruritic papular rash occurs within 24 hours after the penetration of cercariae and reaches maximal intensity in 2 to 3 days.

Acute schistosomiasis occurs with the beginning of oviposition, usually 20 to 50 days after primary exposure. Though asymptomatic in endemic areas, acute schistosomiasis is becoming a frequent and major clinical problem in nonimmune individuals from urban regions who are exposed for the first time to a heavy infection in an endemic area.

The clinical syndrome (i.e., fever, chills, liver and spleen enlargement, and marked eosinophilia) originally described for *S. japonicum* infection and still common for this species is increasingly being diagnosed in Brazil in individuals with *S. mansoni* infection. Malaise, diarrhea, weight loss, cough, dyspnea, chest pain, restrictive respiratory insufficiency, and pericarditis are important findings in this phase. High levels of TNF-α and circulating immune complexes are found in the patient's serum in this phase of illness, and they correlate with the presence of abdominal pain, diarrhea, and weight loss and with respiratory and pericardial manifestations, respectively. Acute disease is not observed in individuals living in endemic areas of schistosomiasis because of modulation of the immune response by antigens or idiotypes transferred from mother to child.

In chronic schistosomiasis, abdominal pain, irregular bowel movements, and blood in the stool are the main symptoms of intestinal involvement. Colonic polyposis may occur, especially in Egypt.

Hepatosplenic involvement is the most important cause of morbidity with *S. mansoni* and *S. japonicum* infection. Patients may remain asymptomatic until the manifestation of hepatic fibrosis and portal hypertension develop. Hepatic fibrosis is caused by a granulomatous reaction to *Schistosoma* eggs that have been carried to the liver. Hepatic fibrosis in *S. mansoni* infection has been associated with the intensity of infection, genetic background, and immunologic response. Although the severity of infection is clearly linked with liver disease, the immune response, collagen deposition, and genetic factors potentiate disease in some individuals with only moderate infections or inhibit disease in others with heavy infections.

Hematemesis from bleeding esophageal or gastric varices may occur. In such cases, anemia and decreasing levels of serum albumin are observed. A few patients have severe hepatosplenic disease with decompensated liver disease. Jaundice, ascites, and liver failure are then observed. Concomitant infection by *Salmonella* species and, less extensively, other gram-negative bacteria with *S. mansoni* or *S. haematobium* leads to a picture of prolonged fever, hepatosplenomegaly, and mild leukocytosis with eosinophilia. Coinfection with *S. mansoni* and hepatitis C virus is associated with a greater chance of chronic hepatitis. Other complications associated with hepatosplenic schistosomiasis include pulmonary hypertension, glomerulonephritis, infantilism, and hypersplenism. In hospitalized adult patients with *S. japonicum* infection, cerebral schistosomiasis occurs in 1.7 to 4.3%. It may occur as early as 6 weeks after infection, and the most common sign is focal jacksonian epilepsy. Signs and symptoms of generalized encephalitis may occasionally be found. In *S. mansoni* infection, nervous system involvement is rare and mainly characterized by transverse myelitis. An association between *S. mansoni* or *S. hematobium* and human immunodeficiency virus (HIV) infection has been documented in areas where both infectious agents are found. Although the immune response of patients with schistosomiasis is altered by HIV, no clear changes regarding the degree of infection or severity of schistosomiasis have been reported.

In *S. haematobium* infection, the main system involved is the urinary tract. The acute granulomatous response to parasite eggs in the early stages causes urinary tract disease, such as urethral ulceration and bladder polyposis. In chronic disease, usually in older patients, granulomas at the lower end of the ureters obstruct urinary flow and may cause hydroureter and hydronephrosis. Bladder fibrosis and calcification are also seen in this phase. Up to 70% of infected individuals have hematuria, dysuria, or urinary frequency. Urine examination reveals proteinuria and hematuria. Radiologic findings include hydronephrosis, hydroureter, ureteral strictures, dilation or distortion, ureteral calcifications, ureterolithiasis, calcified bladder, polyps, reduction in bladder capacity, irregular contraction of the bladder wall, or a dilated bladder because of bladder neck fibrosis. An increased incidence of squamous cell carcinoma of the bladder has been reported in endemic areas of *S. haematobium* infection, but the mechanism of carcinogenesis is unknown. *S. haematobium* eggs have occasionally been found in the lungs, with subsequent focal pulmonary arteritis and pulmonary hypertension.

Diagnosis

A definitive diagnosis of schistosomiasis can be made only by finding schistosome eggs in feces, urine, or a biopsy specimen, usually from the rectum (Table 376–1). A history of contact with contaminated water and appropriate clinical manifestations are important steps in establishing the diagnosis. Because schistosome eggs may be few, concentration by sedimentation should be performed. All eggs from feces, urine, or tissues should be examined under high power to determine their viability by visualizing the activity of cilia of the excretory flame cells of the enclosed miracidium. Dead eggs may persist for a long time after successful therapy or natural death of the worms. The presence of only dead eggs does not necessarily require treatment. Because the intensity of infection is associated with morbidity, quantitative techniques are recommended. For *S. mansoni* and *S. japonicum,* the Kato-Katz thick smear method is used. Rectal biopsy may be used for those with light infection. In patients with chronic *S. mansoni* and *S. japonicum* infection and liver disease, the diagnosis is sometimes made by documentation of eggs in liver specimens. Ultrasonography allows determination of the degree of liver fibrosis. *S. mekongi* and *S. intercalatum* infection is diagnosed by examining the stool for eggs.

Urine examination for *S. haematobium* eggs can be performed by direct or concentration methods. Samples should be obtained at midday, when excretion of eggs is maximal. Rectal biopsy may be performed in patients with light infection and negative urine results. After *S. haematobium* infection is diagnosed, assessment of urinary tract pathology by ultrasonography is recommended. Because of an increased incidence of carcinoma of the bladder, cancer surveillance should be performed in patients with *S. haematobium* infection.

Several serologic tests for detection of IgM, IgG, and IgA antibodies to *Schistosoma* antigens are available. Serologic tests are important in the diagnosis of acute infection because the symptoms are not specific and the finding of eggs in stool may reflect chronic infection. High levels of IgA anti-egg antigen and IgM and IgG antibody to keyhole limpet hemocyanin (KLH) are predominantly observed during the acute phase. KLH from the murine mollusk *Megathura crenulata* shares carbohydrate epitopes with the surface of schistosomula.

Quantification of circulating antigens in serum and urine is an alternative for the diagnosis of schistosome infection. However, the sensitivity of the method decreases in patients with light infection (<100 eggs per gram of feces). This test has also been used to monitor the efficacy of schistosome chemotherapy. A significant decrease in antigen levels or negativity of the test is observed as early as 10 days after therapy.

TABLE 376–1 DIAGNOSIS OF SCHISTOSOMIASIS

Schistosome	Eggs	Diagnosis
S. haematobium	Mainly found in urine but may be found in stools or rectal biopsy specimens Eggs: 143 × 50 µm; spindle shaped: rounded anterior, conical posterior, tapering to a terminal delicate spine	Obtain urine sample at midday (when eggs are excreted); more than one sample may be needed Examine urine directly or by filtering 10 mL of urine through a Nuclepore membrane Rectal biopsy in suspected cases with normal urine Serologic testing to diagnose early or light infection
S. mansoni	Eggs: 155 × 66 µm; oval with lateral, long spine	Examine stool for eggs Use the Kato-Katz thick smear method for quantification purposes Rectal biopsy or serologic testing to diagnose stool-negative cases, particularly in lightly infected patients
S. japonicum	Found in stool; eggs: 89 × 67 µm; oval or rounded with a lateral, short, sometimes curved spine	Examine stool for eggs Kato-Katz thick smear (for quantitative assessment) Rectal biopsy for those with light infections, especially with less common manifestations (i.e., cerebral schistosomiasis)
S. mekongi	Found in stool; eggs: 60 × 32 µm; smaller than eggs of *S. japonicum*	Examine stool for eggs
S. intercalatum	Found in stool; eggs: 180 × 65 µm; terminal spine	Examine stool for eggs

Treatment

Rx

Chemotherapy is by far the major tool for control and cure of schistosomiasis. Three compounds are in use—metrifonate, oxamniquine, and praziquantel—and all three are included in the World Health Organization's list of essential drugs. Praziquantel, a pyrazinoisoquinoline derivative, is the drug of choice for the treatment of schistosomiasis for four reasons: high efficacy against all schistosome species and against cestodes, lack of serious short-term and long-term side effects, administration as a single oral dose, and competitive cost.

The standard recommended treatment consists of a single dose of 40 mg/kg for *S. mansoni, S. haematobium,* and *S. intercalatum* infection. In *S. japonicum* infection, a total dose of 60 mg/kg is recommended, split into two or three doses in a single day. *S. mekongi* may require two treatments at 60 mg/kg body weight. With these dosages, recorded cure rates are 75 to 85% for *S. haematobium,* 63 to 85% for *S. mansoni,* 80 to 90% for *S. japonicum,* 89% for *S. intercalatum,* and 60 to 80% for double infections with *S. mansoni* and *S. haematobium.* A decrease in the efficacy of praziquantel has been observed in patients coinfected with HTLV-1.

Praziquantel is well tolerated and effective in patients of all ages and for different clinical forms of schistosomiasis, including advanced hepatosplenic cases *(S. mansoni),* cerebral schistosomiasis *(S. japonicum),* and neurologic syndromes *(S. mansoni* and *S. haematobium),* possibly in association with corticosteroids. However, praziquantel has low prophylactic effect, which reduces its efficacy in areas of high transmission. There have been several reports of persistent schistosome egg shedding after treatment, thus posing concern about the emergence of drug resistance.

The effects of praziquantel on schistosomes can be summarized under three headings: muscular contraction, tegumental damage (i.e., vacuolization and blebbing), and metabolic alterations (i.e., decreased glucose uptake, lactate excretion, and glycogen content). Praziquantel's activity also depends on the immune system. Several studies have reported that praziquantel induces the exposure of worm surface antigens that may function as targets for immune responses.

The most common side effects observed with praziquantel or oxamniquine are related to the gastrointestinal tract: abdominal pain or discomfort, nausea, vomiting, anorexia, and diarrhea. These symptoms can be observed in up to 50% of patients but are usually well tolerated. Other side effects are related to the central nervous system (e.g., headache, dizziness, drowsiness) and the skin (e.g., pruritus, eruptions) or may be nonspecific (e.g., fever, fatigue). The toxicity of praziquantel is very low in animal studies, and no genotoxic risk has been reported. In general, the cumulative experience from a large number of studies allows the conclusion that praziquantel is an extremely well tolerated drug that requires minimal medical supervision and is therefore particularly suitable for mass chemotherapy programs.

Although a reduction in the intensity of infection and morbidity has been documented after mass chemotherapy, provision of clean water, use of molluscicides, and adequate sanitation should also be implemented to control the disease.

SUGGESTED READINGS

Barsoum RS: Schistosomiasis and the kidney. Semin Nephrol 2003;23:34–41. *Schistosomiasis can cause glomerulonephritis, fibrosis, calcification in the lower urinary tract, and precancerous bladder lesions.*

de Jesus AR, Silva A, Santana LB, et al: Clinical and immunologic evaluation of 31 patients with acute schistosomiasis mansoni. J Infect Dis 2002;185:98–105. *Some immune markers were associated with specific clinical manifestations.*

Fenwick A, Webster JP: Schistosomiasis: Challenges for control, treatment, and drug resistance. Curr Opin Infect Dis 2006;19:577–582. *A review that highlights the continued challenges in the treatment and prevention of this disease.*

Gryseels B, Polman K, Clerinx J, et al: Human schistosomiasis. Lancet 2006;368:1106–1118. *Overview of the disease and its treatment.*

Magnussen P: Treatment and re-treatment strategies for schistosomiasis control in different epidemiological settings: A review of 10 years' experiences. Acta Trop 2003;86:243–254. *Cheap and simple screening of urine and stool specimens can lead to effective therapy with praziquantel.*

Meltzer E, Artom G, Marva E, et al: Schistosomiasis among travelers: New aspects of an old disease. Emerg Infect Dis 2006;12:1696–1700. *Description of the diagnosis and presentation of schistosomiasis in a cohort of travelers.*

Ross AG, Vickers D, Olds GR, et al: Katayama syndrome. Lancet Infect Dis 2007;7:218–224. *Clinical review of this early manifestation of schistosomiasis infection.*

Utzinger J, Keiser J, Shuhua X, et al: Combination chemotherapy of schistosomiasis in laboratory studies and clinical trials. Antimicrob Agents Chemother 2003;47:1487–1495. *An overview of drug therapy.*

LIVER, INTESTINAL, AND LUNG FLUKE INFECTIONS

Adel A. F. Mahmoud

Definition

Parasitic flukes belong to the phylum Platyhelminthes. Clinically relevant flukes are usually grouped according to the main location of adult worms in infected humans: liver, intestinal, and lung (Table 377–1). Blood flukes, or schistosomes, are discussed in Chapter 376.

The Pathogen

Flukes are dorsoventrally flattened and are typically bilaterally symmetrical. With the exception of schistosomes, all flat worms of clinical significance are hermaphroditic. Morphologically, the body of adult worms is leaf-shaped, varies in size from 1 to 7 cm, and possesses two prominent suckers, one located anteriorly and the other ventrally. These suckers are attachment organs that help anchor adult worms in their habitat within the definitive host. During the typical life cycle of a flat worm, the organism uses two, three, or more hosts; one is the definitive host and the others are intermediate hosts. Fluke infections challenge the protective mechanisms of their definitive hosts because of their size, complex anatomic and antigenic structure, and remarkable ability to evade expulsion.

Epidemiology

The geographic distribution of liver, intestinal, and lung flukes (Table 377–2) is global. The liver flukes *Clonorchis sinensis, Opisthorchis felineus,* and *Opisthorchis viverrini* are the most prevalent. The life cycle of the different fluke infection in humans is similar. Eggs are passed in the feces or sputum of infected individuals and hatch in the aquatic outside environment. The released miracidia seek specific snail intermediate hosts, where they undergo several asexual multiplication steps that finally result in the shedding of cercariae. This stage is free living but has a limited lifespan; it has to encyst on vegetation or in the tissues of fish or crabs, where it changes into the metacercarial stage, which is infective to humans. Acquisition of infection by humans depends on ingestion of metacercariae in raw or improperly cooked aquatic plants or animals.

LIVER FLUKES

Several species of liver flukes are capable of inducing significant morbidity and mortality in humans. Opisthorchiasis and clonorchiasis are the most common of these infections.

Opisthorchiasis

Human infection is caused by *O. viverrini* or *O. felineus,* parasitic flukes of cats, dogs, and other fish-eating mammals. Human infection is acquired by ingestion of metacercariae found in the second intermediate host (e.g., cyprinoid fish, carp). The metacercariae excyst in the duodenum and migrate through the ampulla of Vater to reach their final habitat in the bile ducts. *O. viverrini* is endemic in Thailand, Laos, and Cambodia, and *O. felineus* is distributed widely in Russia and eastern and central Europe (see Table 377–2). The incidence of *O. viverrini* in northeastern Thailand has been increasing, with 90% of the population affected in specific foci.

Pathobiology and Clinical Features

Adult flukes inhabit the distal bile ducts and may occasionally be seen in the gallbladder. Most infected individuals are asymptomatic. The biliary system may show hyperplasia of ductal epithelium resulting in obstruction and bile retention. There is significant correlation between the intensity of infection and the severity of observed lesions. Because very few controlled studies have been performed in infected and uninfected populations in endemic areas, the specificity of symptoms and signs is questionable. Symptomatic infections are associated with right upper quadrant discomfort, dyspepsia, and change in bowel habits.

TABLE 377–2 GEOGRAPHIC DISTRIBUTION OF FLUKES

Fluke	Distribution
LIVER	
Opisthorchis viverrini	Thailand, Laos, Cambodia
Opisthorchis felineus	Russia, eastern and central Europe
Clonorchis sinesis	China, Japan, Korea, Taiwan, Vietnam, Hong Kong (imported fish from China)
Fasciola hepatica	United States, Europe, Africa, Asia
Fasciola gigantica	Less common: Africa, Asia, Hawaii
Dicrocoelium sp	Europe, Africa, Asia, North America
INTESTINAL	
Fasciolopsis sp	Taiwan, Thailand, Bangladesh, India, plus other Asian and Western countries
Echinostoma sp	Indonesia, Philippines, Thailand, Taiwan
Heterophyes heterophyes	Egypt, Iran, Far East, Southeast Asia
Metagonimus yokogawai	China, Japan, Korea, Taiwan
Gastrodiscoides hominis	India, Southeast Asia, Russia
LUNG	
Paragonimus sp	Asia, West Africa, Central and South America

TABLE 377–1 MAJOR LIVER, INTESTINAL, AND LUNG FLUKE INFECTIONS IN HUMANS

Infection	Causative Organisms	Second Intermediate Host	Size of Adult Fluke (mm)	Final Habitat in Humans	Size of Eggs (mm)
Opisthorchiasis	*O. viverrini* *O. felineus*	Cyprinoid fish	5–10 × 1–2	Distal bile ducts, gallbladder	28 × 16 Operculated
Clonorchiasis	*C. sinensis*	Carp fish	10–24 × 3–5	Bile and pancreatic ducts	29 × 16 Operculated
Fascioliasis	*F. hepatica* *F. gigantica*	Aquatic vegetation or water	20–30 × 13 75 × 20	Large biliary ducts	140 × 75 Inconspicuous operculum 175 × 80
Fasciolopsiasis	*F. buski*	Aquatic plants	50–75 × 8–20	Small intestine	135 × 35 Small operculum
Paragonimiasis	*P. westermani*	Freshwater and brackish water crabs	7–16 × 4–8	Lungs, brain, or abdominal organs	100 × 60 Operculated

Generalized symptoms such as decreased appetite and weight loss also have been observed. In severe cases, relapsing cholangitis and cholecystitis may occur. Associations between *O. viverrini* and cholangiocarcinoma, gallstones, and obstructive jaundice have been reported. Clinically, liver enlargement is demonstrated in most symptomatic individuals, along with imaging evidence of biliary tree disease.

Infection with *O. felineus* has a characteristic clinical course. In its acute phase (2 to 3 weeks after infection), clinical features include irregular fever, lymphadenopathy, myalgia, and eosinophilia. In chronic infections, symptoms and signs of biliary disease resemble those of *O. viverrini* infection; however, the worms may also be found in the pancreatic duct and cause manifestations related to this organ.

Clonorchiasis

C. sinensis also is frequently referred to as the Chinese or oriental liver fluke. Carnivorous animals such as dogs, cats, and rats are probably the reservoir hosts in nature. Human infection is acquired by ingestion of the second intermediate host, a freshwater carp of the family Cyprinidae. Clonorchiasis is also seen in other countries, including the United States in immigrants from endemic areas. Importation of *C. sinensis* is a risk in the international food trade.

Pathobiology and Clinical Features

The life cycle, pathologic features, and clinical manifestations of clonorchiasis are similar to those of opisthorchiasis. Adult flukes reside in the medium-sized and small bile ducts. They may also be found in the gallbladder, common bile duct, and pancreatic duct. In early infection, the pathologic features consist of edema and epithelial desquamation in bile ducts associated with an inflammatory response. Later, metaplasia and glandular proliferation occur with dilation and thickening of bile ducts. The final pathologic insult is related to marked periductal fibrosis. The specificity of symptoms attributed to clonorchiasis such as anorexia, epigastric pain, or diarrhea has been questioned in studies performed on immigrants to the United States from the Far East. In endemic areas, association with cholangitis, gallstones, and cholangiocarcinoma has been reported. Sonography or computed tomography (CT) demonstrates the pathologic changes in the liver: flukes within dilated bile ducts and periductal changes.

Fascioliasis

Human infection with the zoonotic flukes *Fasciola hepatica* and *Fasciola gigantica* is acquired by ingestion of metacercariae that are attached to various aquatic plants or through drinking water contaminated with the infective stage of the organisms. The natural hosts of fascioliasis include sheep, goats, cattle, and horses; endemic regions occur in all five continents (see Table 377–2). After the infective metacercariae are consumed, they excyst in the duodenum, penetrate its wall, and travel through the peritoneal cavity to enter the liver through its capsule. The organisms migrate into the liver parenchyma to reach their final habitat in the large bile ducts.

Pathobiology and Clinical Features

Human fascioliasis is usually associated with mild clinical features. The resulting syndromes may be conveniently divided into the *acute migratory phase,* while the organisms are finding their way through the peritoneal cavity to the liver capsule and parenchyma, and the *established phase,* which is associated with the mature flukes taking residence in the bile ducts. The acute phase is marked by fever, right upper quadrant or epigastric pain, and eosinophilia and may last 4 to 8 weeks. Stool examination during this phase is usually negative for parasite eggs. During the established phase, most infected individuals are asymptomatic. Some may complain of abdominal pain and dyspepsia. Hepatomegaly and jaundice may occur, as well as significant peripheral blood eosinophilia. Borderline changes in liver function test results also have been reported. CT of the liver may help in demonstrating hepatic lesions, including the nodular or the more characteristic linear hypodense tracks, particularly if they are located subcapsularly. In the *biliary stage,* ultrasonography may demonstrate adult flukes in the bile ducts or gallbladder.

Dicroceliasis

Human infection with *Dicrocoelium dendriticum* or *Dicrocoelium hospes* is rare. Dicroceliasis is a zoonosis in sheep, goats, deer, and other herbivores. Its life cycle is similar to that of other liver flukes, except that metacercariae encyst in ants, the second intermediate host. Humans are infected by eating metacercariae-containing ants. Most cases of dicroceliasis are asymptomatic. In those with heavy infection, vague abdominal complaints—vomiting, diarrhea or constipation, and biliary colic—have been observed.

INTESTINAL FLUKES

More than 50 species of intestinal trematodes from the Far East, Middle East, and North Africa have been reported to cause human infection; however, clinically significant disease may be encountered in infection with only a few species.

Fasciolopsiasis

The giant intestinal fluke *Fasciolopsis buski* inhabits the small intestine of pigs. Humans are infected by ingestion of raw stems, leaves, and pods of aquatic plants with encysted metacercariae. The geographic distribution is given in Table 377–2. Endemicity depends on close contact among water plants, pigs, and populations that consume raw aquatic plants.

F. buski flukes attach to the mucosa of the small intestine, particularly the duodenum and jejunum. Most infected individuals are asymptomatic. The site of attachment, however, becomes ulcerated, and a local inflammatory response follows. In cases of heavy infection, intestinal obstruction and protein-losing enteropathy have been reported. With heavy infection, abdominal pain and diarrhea may be observed along with edema and anasarca caused by hypoalbuminemia.

Echinostomiasis

Humans can be infected with any of several genera of the family Echinostomatidae. The common species are *Echinostoma ilocanum, Echinostoma malayaman,* and *Echinostoma revolutum.* Adult flukes are parasites of the small intestine of birds and mammals. Humans are occasionally infected after eating undercooked pila, other fish, and tadpoles. Mature adult worms attach to intestinal mucosa and cause ulceration and a subsequent inflammatory response. Little morbidity has been reported in association with echinostomiasis. High-intensity infection may be associated with abdominal pain and diarrhea.

Heterophyiasis

Heterophyes heterophyes infects humans, cats, dogs, and other fish-eating mammals. Infection is acquired by ingestion of fish second intermediate host, which contains metacercariae. Common fish hosts include mullet and minnow and the brackish water fish *Mugil capito.* They are usually consumed raw or salted. Metacercariae can live in salted fish for approximately 1 week. Adult *H. heterophyes* flukes attach to the mucosa of the jejunum and upper ileum and produce shallow ulcers and a mild inflammatory response. Symptomatic patients complain of gastroenterocolitis with diarrhea and tenesmus. Stools characteristically contain abundant mucus and occasionally blood.

Other Intestinal Flukes

Several other species may cause disease limited to defined geographic areas. The life cycle of *Metagonimus yokogawai* and associated disease syndromes are similar to those of *H. heterophyes,* but *M. yokogawai* may invade the mucosa of the small intestine and result in ulceration and granuloma formation. Another intestinal fluke, *Gastrodiscoides hominis,* has its final habitat in humans in the cecum. Clinically, it is believed to produce mucous diarrhea.

LUNG FLUKES

Paragonimiasis

Human infection by species of *Paragonimus* may cause considerable pulmonary or extrapulmonary morbidity in several endemic areas (see

Table 377–2). *Paragonimus* infection exists in nature in humans and carnivores. At least 10 species of *Paragonimus* are known to cause human disease; of these, *Paragonimus westermani* is most common. Infection is acquired by ingestion of metacercariae encysted in freshwater and brackish water crabs or crayfish (raw or undercooked). Infection may also be transmitted to humans through contaminated utensils used to prepare crabs or crayfish. Rarely, consumption of wild boar meat may result in transmission of immature flukes to humans, in whom they complete their development into adult worms.

Pathobiology and Clinical Features

Disease in infected humans is related to migration of young flukes from the gastrointestinal tract to their final habitat (i.e., early or acute stage) and more characteristically results when adult worms become established in the lungs or at extrapulmonary sites (i.e., late or chronic stage).

Acute paragonimiasis occurs during the 3-week period after infection. It passes unnoticed in most infected individuals. Symptoms include diarrhea, abdominal pain, fever, and malaise associated with cough, dyspnea, and night sweats. Pulmonary paragonimiasis results from invasion of the host's lungs and establishment of adult worms in cysts or abscess cavities. The lung parenchyma demonstrates hemorrhage and inflammatory response predominantly of eosinophils. Worm cysts are 1 to 2 cm in diameter and generally contain one or two worms. Pathologic changes in the remaining lung tissue may result in bronchopneumonia, bronchiectasis, fibrosis, and pleural thickening. The established pulmonary stage of paragonimiasis usually results in mild chronic cough with the production of mucoid, rusty brown sputum. Hemoptysis, which may be severe and life-threatening, occurs rarely.

Microscopic examination of sputum demonstrates necrotic tissue and parasite eggs. The results of physical examination in patients with pulmonary paragonimiasis are usually within normal limits. Chest radiography findings may be normal in 10 to 20% of cases. Typical changes in the lungs include pathway infiltrate and a ring shadow with a crescent-shaped "corona." Cystic and nodular lesions are also commonly seen. Pleural lesions, including effusion, pneumothorax, and thickening, may be encountered in approximately two thirds of infected individuals. Other imaging methods, such as CT, may better define the pulmonary abnormalities, including worm migration tracks.

Extrapulmonary paragonimiasis develops as a result of migration of maturing flukes to tissues other than the lungs or migration of adult flukes from the lungs to other tissues. It is believed that extrapulmonary paragonimiasis may be caused mainly by *Paragonimus* flukes other than *P. westermani*. The tissues most commonly affected are the brain, abdominal organs, and skin. In cerebral paragonimiasis, the clinical findings may be acute or chronic. Acute cerebral paragonimiasis is manifested as fever, headache, visual disturbances, paralysis, and generalized or focal convulsions. There may be evidence of an intracranial inflammatory process, such as papilledema, high cerebrospinal fluid pressure, and eosinophilic pleocytosis. Chronic cerebral paragonimiasis is characterized by space-occupying lesions that cause epilepsy or paralysis. Abdominal or cutaneous paragonimiasis results from invasion of the liver, spleen, or skin by maturing or adult flukes, which cause space-occupying lesions, abscesses, or migratory swellings.

MANAGEMENT OF LIVER, INTESTINAL, AND LUNG FLUKE INFECTIONS

Diagnosis

Diagnosis of human infection with liver, intestinal, or lung flukes requires knowledge of the geographic distribution of these infections, a high degree of clinical correlation of mainly nonspecific symptoms and signs with a history of possible exposure, and demonstration of peripheral blood eosinophilia. Definitive diagnosis is established by finding the characteristically shaped fluke eggs in fecal samples or sputum. In general, the sensitivity of fecal or sputum examination is enhanced by examining two or three separate specimens. Seroimmunodiagnostic tests are available for fascioliasis and paragonimiasis. They are particularly helpful in early infection, for which parasitologic diagnosis usually yields negative results.

Treatment

Rx

Chemotherapy for fluke infections has become a more effective management strategy with the introduction of praziquantel. This anthelmintic agent is orally administered. It results in cure rates of 70 to 90% and an even more remarkable decrease in egg counts. Its administration is associated with few side effects. The recommended dose of praziquantel is 75 mg/kg of body weight divided into three doses and given in 1 day. A 2-day course of praziquantel is necessary for the treatment of paragonimiasis. For fascioliasis, the drug of choice is triclabendazole, which is given orally as 10 mg/kg once or twice.

Prevention

Prevention of infection with any of these parasitic trematodes depends on proper medical advice given to individuals traveling or planning to reside in endemic areas (Chapter 308). Avoidance of ingestion of suspected intermediate hosts and proper washing, cooking, or preservation methods of such food items constitute the most effective strategy. Engaging in some of the local dietary habits in endemic areas should be discouraged. Water for drinking must be properly purified to prevent the possible transmission of *F. hepatica*. Control of parasitic trematodes in endemic areas is a much more complex challenge that involves changing long-established cultural, dietary, and sanitary habits.

With the availability of a safe broad-spectrum anthelmintic (praziquantel), chemotherapy may play a significant role in controlling infection and disease. As a long-term strategy, vaccines and socioeconomic development will be needed.

SUGGESTED READINGS

Chan HH, Lai KH, Lo GH, et al: The clinical and cholangiographic picture of hepatic clonorchiasis. J Clin Gastroenterol 2002;34:183–186. *Clinical and imaging features of clonorchiasis in endemic areas.*

Choi MS, Choi D, Choi MH, et al: Correlation between sonographic findings and infection intensity in clonorchiasis. Am J Trop Med Hyg 2005;73:1139–1144. *Sonography but not symptoms correlated with the intensity of infection.*

Choi D, Lim JH, Lee KT, et al: Cholangiocarcinoma and Clonorchis sinensis infection: A case-control study in Korea. J Hepatol 2006;44:1066–1073. *There was a clear correlation.*

Drugs for Parasitic Infections: Med Lett Drugs Ther 2004;1. *Drugs of choice and alternatives.*

Fried B, Graczyk TK, Tamang L: Food-borne intestinal trematodioses in humans. Parasitol Res 2004;93:159–170. *Detailed description of intestinal trematodes.*

Guoqing L, Xiaozhu H, Kanu S: Epidemiology and control of *Clonorchiasis sinensis* in China. Southeast Asian J Trop Med Public Health 2001;32(Suppl. 2):8–11. *A brief summary of the situation in China.*

Obara A, Nakamura-Uchiyama F, Hiromatsu K, Nawa Y: Paragonimiasis cases recently found among immigrants in Japan. Intern Med 2004;43:388–392. *The spectrum of disease in an immigrant population in Japan.*

Rana SS, Bhasin DK, Nanda M, et al: Parasitic infestations of the biliary tract. Curr Gastroenterol Rep 2007;9:156–164. *Clinical review.*

Robertson KB, Janssen WJ, Saint S, et al: Clinical problem-solving. The missing piece. N Engl J Med 2006;355:1913–1918. *Clinical case of a young man with lung fluke.*

Stauffer WM, Sellman JS, Walker PF: Biliary liver flukes (opisthorchiasis and clonorchiasis) in immigrants in the United States: Often subtle and diagnosed years after arrival. J Travel Med 2004;11:157–159. *The clinical spectrum as seen in the United States.*

378 NEMATODE INFECTIONS

James W. Kazura

NEMATODE INFECTION

Definition

Nematodes (phylum Nematoda), or roundworms, include a vast number of species of free-living and parasitic helminths. These multicellular organisms differ from unicellular bacteria and protozoa in that they have organ systems with specialized nervous, muscular, gastrointestinal, and reproductive functions. Unlike the situation pertaining to bacterial, viral, or protozoan infections, casual or a low degree of exposure to infective stages of parasitic helminths generally does not result in patent infection or pathologic manifestations. Repeated or intense exposure to a large number of infective larvae is generally required for infection to be established and disease to develop.

The Pathogens

Parasitic nematodes vary in length from several millimeters to approximately 2 m and have four larval stages and adult worms of both sexes. With the exception of *Strongyloides stercoralis* and a few other helminths of medical importance, larvae are produced after mating of sexually mature adult worms, which by themselves are incapable of multiplying in the mammalian host. The inability of adult worms to replicate has important implications for the propensity of this class of organism to establish an infection and cause disease.

Epidemiology

Nematode infections are endemic in temperate and tropical climates. They are transmitted by the fecal-oral route or by inoculation of infective larvae into the skin, either by direct contact with contaminated soil or by blood-feeding intermediate insect vectors. The prevalence of infection is greatest in circumstances conducive to the development and transmission of infective forms of the parasites, such as the overcrowded, perennially warm geographic areas with poor sanitation in many developing countries of Africa, Asia, and Latin America and economically poor areas of North America and Europe.

The epidemiology of human nematode, as well as trematode and cestode, infections has several unique features. In an endemic area most individuals have low parasite burdens, and a few harbor relatively high burdens. Persons in the latter group contribute the most substantially to transmission and are most likely to develop pathologic manifestations. Therefore, transmission in an endemic area may be decreased or interrupted by reduction of the parasite burden in a small proportion of the population.

Nematode infections of medical importance may be broadly classified as those that primarily affect the gastrointestinal tract, where adult worms become established and cause disease, and those that affect other tissues and organ systems. The former group includes hookworms *(Ancylostoma duodenale, Necator americanus)*, the roundworm *Ascaris lumbricoides*, the pinworm *Enterobius vermicularis*, and the whipworm *Trichuris trichiura*. Animal intestinal nematodes such as *Trichostrongylus* and *Anisakis* species also occasionally infect and cause disease in the gastrointestinal tract of humans. *Trichinella spiralis, Strongyloides stercoralis*, and *Angiostrongylus cantonensis* infect humans by the oral route, but disease manifestations primarily result from migration in other tissues. Nematodes that invade and cause disease in tissues outside the gastrointestinal tract include lymphatic filariae *(Wuchereria bancrofti, Brugia malayi, and Brugia timori)*, skin-dwelling *Onchocerca volvulus* and *Loa loa*, and the guinea worm, *Dracunculus medinensis*.

Intestinal Nematodes

Intestinal nematode infections include hookworm disease, ascariasis, enterobiasis, trichuriasis, and, rarely, animal nematodiases. They are prevalent in temperate and tropical areas of the world, especially those with overcrowding and poor sanitation. Intestinal nematode infections result in little morbidity in most cases, except when children in developing countries experience repeated and chronic infections. They are easily treated with albendazole, which is approved for use in the United States by the Food and Drug Administration, although the drug is classified as investigational.

HOOKWORM DISEASE

Definition

The major hookworms that infect humans are *A. duodenale* and *N. americanus. Ancylostoma ceylonicum* infection is less common and occurs primarily in the South Pacific. Animal hookworms such as *Ancylostoma braziliense* and *Uncinaria stenocephala* do not undergo full development in incidentally exposed humans. Infection occurs when exposed skin maintains contact for several minutes with soil contaminated with parasite eggs containing viable larvae. Larvae penetrate the skin and subsequently migrate to and mature in the lungs. The parasites then break into the air spaces, ascend the trachea, and are swallowed. Adult worms mature in the upper small intestine and attach to the mucosa (Fig. 378–1). Female worms release more than 10,000 eggs per day, which are passed in the stools and deposited in the soil. The prepatent period (i.e., time between infection and passing of eggs in the feces) is 40 to 105 days. Adult hookworms have a lifespan of 2 to 5 years.

Epidemiology

Hookworms infect more than 1 billion persons worldwide. The highest prevalences of infection (80 to 100%) occur in tropical and less developed countries, where environmental and socioeconomic conditions are especially favorable to transmission. These factors include warm, moist soil; lack of public sewage disposal systems; and the habit of walking barefoot. The higher prevalence of hookworm infection in children than adults results from more frequent exposure of skin to larvae in soil. Acquired resistance is minimal or does not appear to develop as a consequence of previous infection.

Pathobiology

Hookworm disease is caused primarily by gastrointestinal blood loss and attendant iron deficiency anemia. The latter correlate directly with the total worm burden. Adult worms attached to the mucosa of the upper small intestine digest ingested blood and cause focal bleeding. *A. duodenale* is estimated to cause a blood loss of 0.3 mL/day per worm; *N. americanus* induces loss of approximately 0.03 mL/day.

Clinical Manifestations

Light infections (<400 eggs/g of feces) do not cause blood loss sufficient to induce iron deficiency. However, nutritional deficiencies from

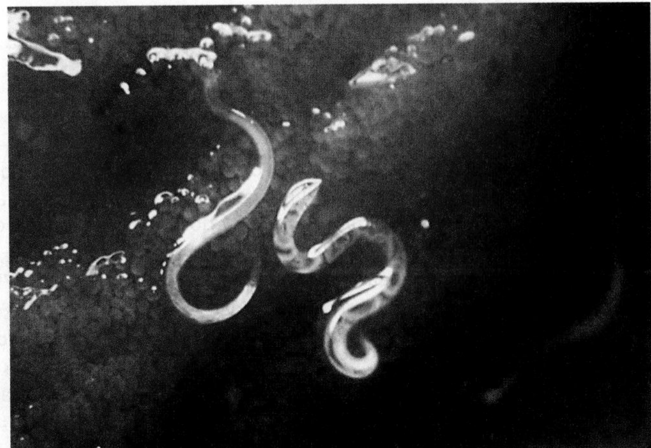

FIGURE 378–1 • Enlargement showing hookworms, *Ancylostoma caninum*, attached to the intestinal mucosa. Barely visible larvae penetrate the skin (often through bare feet), are carried to the lungs, go through the respiratory tract to the mouth, are swallowed, and eventually reach the small intestine. This journey takes about a week. (From the Centers for Disease Control and Prevention Image Bank.)

coexisting conditions that result in low iron stores (i.e., malabsorption or insufficient dietary intake in children and multiparous women) contribute significantly to morbidity. Hypoproteinemia has been reported in children with hookworm disease in less developed countries. This complication most likely results from coexisting malnutrition rather than gastrointestinal disease caused by hookworm infestation. Abdominal signs or symptoms are not caused by hookworm infection.

Pruritus at the site of larval skin penetration ("ground itch") occurs occasionally (Fig. 378–2). In the case of primary exposure, local itching and erythematous papules develop and last 1 week. More intense pruritus, vesiculation, and edema of 2 to 3 weeks' duration may occur after repeated exposure to infective larvae. Hookworm larvae migrating through the lungs rarely cause pulmonary symptoms.

Diagnosis

Hookworm infection is diagnosed by identification of the characteristic round eggs containing convoluted larvae. Direct smears of freshly passed stool using the Kato or other techniques are satisfactory for the diagnosis of moderately to heavily infected cases (>400 eggs/g of feces).

Treatment

Rx

Albendazole is the treatment of choice (Table 378–1).

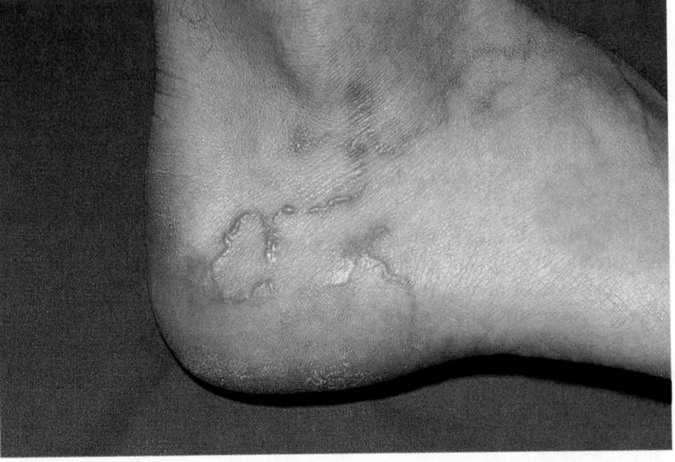

FIGURE 378–2 • Cutaneous larva migrans. Red, serpiginous lesions on the side of the foot. In the United States, the dog or cat hookworm (*Ancylostoma caninum* or *Ancylostoma braziliense*) is a common cause.

Prevention

The ideal method for preventing hookworm infection is improvement of hygienic conditions. Use of footwear, especially by children, is the only practical means of avoiding infection.

ASCARIASIS

Definition

A. lumbricoides are roundworms that are 2 to 3 cm long and that reside in the lumen of the jejunum and in the midileum. Infection occurs by the oral route when soil containing embryonated eggs is ingested. Larvae are released from eggs in the small intestine, penetrate the gut, and migrate to the liver and then lungs through the blood or lymphatic circulation. After maturation in the lungs over a 4-week period, the parasites ascend the respiratory tract and are swallowed. Adult worms reach sexual maturity (i.e., female worms release eggs that are detectable in feces) approximately 60 days after infection.

Epidemiology

Ascariasis affects approximately one fourth of the world's population and probably is the most prevalent helminthiasis of humans. Infection is common in Africa, Asia, and Latin America, especially in areas of high population density and poor sanitary conditions. The use of human feces as fertilizer, defecation in soil, and hand-to-mouth contact with contaminated soil are major factors that contribute to the spread of *Ascaris*. The ability of *Ascaris* eggs to remain viable in harsh environmental conditions (i.e., embryonated eggs remain infectious after exposure to freezing temperatures and desiccation for several weeks) also facilitates transmission.

Clinical Manifestations

Disease caused by *A. lumbricoides* is infrequent and generally correlates with the intensity of infection. Most infected individuals are asymptomatic.

Symptomatic cases can be divided into two categories on the basis of the phase of infection and site of pathology, that is, pulmonary or gastrointestinal tract. Pulmonary disease is caused by the migration of larvae in the small vessels of the lung and their subsequent rupture into alveoli. Tissue damage is thought to result from the host immune response, which includes production of immunoglobulin E (IgE) and eosinophilia. Transient pulmonary infiltrates, fever, cough, dyspnea, and eosinophilia lasting 1 to several weeks are the major clinical manifestations. This complex of symptoms and signs is frequently seasonal and coincidental with environmental changes that favor development of infective-stage larvae in eggs (e.g., spring rains that follow cold and dry periods). Intesti-

TABLE 378–1 TREATMENT FOR INTESTINAL NEMATODES

Nematode	Treatment
Hookworms	Albendazole, 400 mg one time. Do not give to pregnant women; iron supplementation (if warranted by anemia and complicating illnesses). Alternatives: Mebendazole, 100 mg orally bid for 3 days., or pyrantel pamoate, 11 mg/kg for 3 days; maximum daily dose not to exceed 1 g
Ascaris	Albendazole, 400 mg one time, or mebendazole, 100 mg orally bid for 3 days. Children with heavy infections, biliary or pancreatic tract obstruction: piperazine, 50–75 mg/kg for 2 days
Enterobius	Pyrantel pamoate, 11 mg/kg once, with a repeated dose 2 wk later; maximum single dose, 1 g. Several treatments may be required (every 3–4 months) if exposure continues (e.g., institutional setting). Alternatives include mebendazole, 100 mg, or albendazole 400 mg once, and repeat in 2 wk.
Trichuris	Mebendazole or albendazole, at same dosages as for ascariasis
Trichostrongylus	Pyrantel pamoate, 11 mg/kg once; maximum dose of 1 g
Anisakis	Surgical or endoscopic removal of worm from gastrointestinal tract
Capillaria	Mebendazole, 200 mg bid for 20 days. Alternative: albendazole, 400 mg once daily for 10 days. Supportive care: replace fluid and electrolytes, high-protein diet
Gnathostoma	For subcutaneous lesions: surgical removal. For central nervous system infection: albendazole, 400 mg bid for 21 days, or ivermectin, 200 µg/kg qd for 2 days

nal signs and symptoms result from obstruction caused by the presence of an exceptionally large number of parasites in the small intestine or migration of adult worms to unusual sites, such as the biliary tree or pancreatic duct. Intestinal obstruction almost always occurs in children younger than 6 years. The onset is sudden and characterized by colicky abdominal pain and vomiting. Heavily infected children are also susceptible to biliary disease or pancreatitis secondary to *Ascaris* lodging in the ducts draining these organs. A malabsorption syndrome characterized by steatorrhea and low vitamin A levels has been reported in Latin American children with ascariasis.

Diagnosis

Intestinal infection is diagnosed by the presence of the typical oval, thick-shelled *Ascaris* eggs in thick smears of fecal specimens. The existence of adult worms in pancreatic or biliary ducts should be suspected in children who have high egg outputs in conjunction with jaundice or pancreatitis. Pulmonary ascariasis cannot be diagnosed on the basis of identification of ova in feces because adult worms have not yet matured and reached the intestinal tract. Biopsy of the lung is unlikely to demonstrate larvae and is not recommended.

Treatment

Treatment for uncomplicated intestinal ascariasis is listed in Table 378–1. Treatment of obstruction of the pancreatic or biliary duct related to ascariasis is with piperazine citrate, which causes neuromuscular paralysis of the worms. No specific treatment is recommended for pulmonary ascariasis because the condition is self-limited. Mass chemotherapy successfully reduces worm loads but requires frequent treatment.

Prevention

The major means of preventing *Ascaris* infection is improvement of hygienic and socioeconomic conditions.

ENTEROBIASIS

Epidemiology

E. vermicularis or pinworm infection is cosmopolitan in its distribution. It is common in overcrowded settings and spreads rapidly in conditions in which person-to-person contact is frequent, such as in institutions for children.

Pathobiology

Infection occurs by the fecal-oral route. Embryonated eggs carried on the fingernails, bed clothing, or bedding are ingested and hatch in the upper small intestine. Larvae develop in the large bowel into adult worms that are 2 to 5 mm long. Female worms migrate nightly out of the rectum and deposit large numbers of ova (11,000 per worm) in the perianal and perineal areas. Larvae in the deposited eggs become infective within several hours of exposure to ambient oxygen. Infectivity is usually maintained for 1 to 2 days.

Clinical Manifestations

Most pinworm infections are asymptomatic or associated with perianal pruritus and consequent sleep deprivation. *E. vermicularis* is a rare cause of appendicitis and, when the adult worms follow an aberrant path of migration, vulvovaginitis, salpingitis, urethritis, or peritonitis.

Diagnosis

The diagnosis of pinworm infection is easily made by identifying ova on a piece of cellophane tape applied to the perirectal area in the morning. *E. vermicularis* eggs are oval and slightly flattened on one side. It is unusual to find eggs in feces or adult worms in the perianal area. Repeated examinations may be necessary.

Treatment

Treatment (see Table 378–1) is pyrantel pamoate or albendazole given to affected individuals and to close associates, such as family members. Although personal cleanliness is recommended as a means of limiting transmission, there is no clear-cut demonstration that it prevents infection.

TRICHURIASIS

T. trichiura or whipworm infection is similar to pinworm infection in that it is limited to the gastrointestinal tract and does not have a tissue migratory phase. Eggs containing infective larvae mature in warm, moist soil over a 2-week period. Ingested eggs hatch in the small bowel and subsequently develop in epithelial cells of the cecum and ascending colon into adult worms that are 40 mm in length. The body of the parasite protrudes into the colonic lumen. Its anterior portion has a whiplike shape.

Epidemiology

As is the case with most intestinal nematode infections, trichuriasis is most common in overcrowded areas with poor sanitation. The estimated prevalence worldwide is 800 million, with approximately 2 million cases in the southern United States. Children are more frequently infected than adults and more likely to have higher worm burdens.

Clinical Manifestations

Adults with trichuriasis are usually asymptomatic. In children with heavy infections (>10,000 eggs/g of feces), a syndrome of dysentery, growth retardation, and rectal prolapse has been described. The pathologic manifestations include infiltrates of eosinophils and neutrophils accompanied by epithelial denudation. Complicating diseases such as shigellosis and amebiasis may contribute to this condition in children.

Diagnosis

Whipworm infection is diagnosed by identification of football-shaped eggs in direct smears of fecal specimens.

Treatment

Mebendazole or albendazole at the same dosage indicated for ascariasis is satisfactory treatment, as listed in Table 378–1.

OTHER ANIMAL NEMATODIASES

Definition

Humans may serve as paratenic hosts for several nematodes that ordinarily parasitize the intestine of other mammals. These helminths are incapable of completing their life cycle in humans and display aberrant migration patterns in both intestinal and nonintestinal tissues.

Trichostrongylus

Several species of the genus *Trichostrongylus* infect humans and domestic ruminants. The infection is found widely in the Middle East, Far East, and Australia. Ova are passed in the stool of ruminants and hatch in the soil. Humans are incidentally infected when larvae are ingested with leafy vegetables. The adult worms live in the intestines and suck small amounts of blood; heavy infections result in anemia. Diagnosis is made by identifying ova, which resemble those of hookworm, in the stool. Treatment is explained in Table 378–1.

Anisakis

Anisakis is an intestinal nematode of marine mammals. Several species of saltwater fish are intermediate hosts. Human infection occurs when raw fish is eaten. The larvae of *Anisakis* and *Phocanema decipiens* have been implicated. Most cases have been reported in Japan or western Europe, particularly in Scandinavia. The larvae invade the wall of the small intestine or stomach, causing pain and, rarely, intestinal obstruction or perforation. Intestinal anisakiasis often resembles an acute abdomen, leading to laparotomy. Albendazole treatment is detailed in Table 378–1. The treatment of choice is surgical or endoscopic removal of worms. Infection is prevented by cooking or freezing fish before eating.

Capillaria philippinensis

Capillaria philippinensis infection has been reported primarily from the Philippines and Thailand, although the infection has been observed occasionally in Taiwan, Indonesia, Iran, and Egypt. This nematode is thought to parasitize birds, with fish and crustaceans serving as intermediate hosts. Humans are infected by eating the raw intermediate hosts. The ingested larvae mature and live in the crypts of the small intestine, where they reproduce. The result is often a heavy infection; up to 40,000 adult worms have been recovered at one autopsy. The clinical syndrome includes severe malabsorption and protein-losing enteropathy. The diagnosis is made by finding eggs or larvae in the stool; an intradermal test is also available. The treatment of choice is mebendazole or albendazole (see Table 378–1).

Gnathostoma spinigerum

Gnathostoma spinigerum is an intestinal nematode of dogs and cats; fish are intermediate hosts. The infection is endemic in rodents in the Far East and Thailand. Human infection has also been reported in South America. Infective larvae are ingested by humans in raw or undercooked fish. The larvae do not complete their life cycle in humans but migrate through the body. The most frequent site is subcutaneous tissue, where larvae are found in eosinophilic granulomas. A few weeks after infection, pruritic or painful subcutaneous nodules and swellings appear. These may be migratory and develop into abscesses. In central nervous system (CNS) gnathostomiasis, hemorrhagic tracts may be found in the brain. Fever, vomiting, and abdominal pain occur a few days after larvae are ingested. Paralysis of the extremities, encephalitis, and subarachnoid hemorrhage have been reported. Eye involvement with uveitis and orbital cellulitis represents a third variety.

Peripheral eosinophilia is usual in cutaneous gnathostomiasis; the diagnosis may be established by biopsy. In CNS infection, blood eosinophilia is an inconstant feature, but eosinophils are present in the cerebrospinal fluid (CSF), as in the case of angiostrongyliasis. Treatments are explained in Table 378–1. The infection may be prevented by thorough cooking of fish.

Other Parasites

Several nematodes that ordinarily parasitize the intestine of monkeys occasionally infect humans. *Oesophagostomum* has been reported from Africa, Asia, and Brazil; it is responsible for the formation of granulomas in the intestinal wall. *Ternidens deminutus* is sometimes found in the human colon in Africa and Asia; a heavy infection may cause anemia. *Physaloptera mordens,* also reported from Africa, may attach itself to the esophagus, stomach, or small intestine of humans. The definitive host of *Lagochilascaris minor* is unknown. About 30 human cases have been reported from Central America and South America, usually with worms invading the soft tissues of the neck, throat, and sinuses.

TOXOCARIASIS

Definition

Visceral larva migrans (VLM) and ocular larva migrans (OLM) are caused by ingestion and subsequent development and migration of embryonated eggs of the canine roundworm *Toxocara canis.* Roundworms of cats *(Toxocara cati)* and raccoons *(Baylisascaris procyonis)* also rarely cause VLM.

Epidemiology

Toxocariasis is endemic in temperate and tropical areas of the world. Most symptomatic cases occur in young children. This age group is most likely to be infected by virtue of frequent and intimate handling of dogs (especially newborn puppies that may be hyperinfected), playing in areas where dogs and cats defecate (e.g., public sandboxes), and the habit of geophagia. The potential for exposure to embryonated eggs is high in that *T. canis* infection is common in dogs (a 20% infection rate in dogs in the United States).

Pathobiology

In its normal canine host, *T. canis* organisms follow a route of migration similar to that described for *Ascaris.* Ingested larvae penetrate the small intestine, migrate to the lungs, are reswallowed, and develop into adult worms in the small intestine; the adult worms lodge there and release eggs that are passed in the feces. When embryonated *T. canis* eggs are ingested by humans, larvae also migrate throughout the body (i.e., lung, liver, brain, muscles, and occasionally eyes) but fail to complete development to the adult stage. Tissue necrosis caused by penetrating larvae and associated host inflammatory reactions, such as eosinophil-rich granulomas, are the underlying cause of disease.

Clinical Manifestations

Most children who ingest *T. canis* eggs are asymptomatic. VLM is the most common clinically defined entity attributable to *T. canis.* It occurs most frequently in children younger than 5 years (there are no published series of adults with VLM) and is characterized by fever with temperature less than 39° C; pulmonary symptoms, including wheezing and cough; and, less frequently, pain in the right upper quadrant. These symptoms have a gradual onset and resolve over 4 to 8 weeks. Physical signs include wheezing and hepatomegaly in about one fourth of cases. Larvae less commonly migrate to the brain and heart and cause focal neurologic defects and heart failure.

OLM has an incidence approximately one tenth that of VLM and affects children older than 8 to 10 years. Visual disturbances related to VLM are not distinguishable from those related to other causes of focal intraretinal granulomas or space-occupying lesions, such as tuberculosis and retinoblastoma. *T. canis* larvae may migrate intraretinally and produce transient and recurrent impairment of vision.

Diagnosis

VLM is diagnosed on the basis of suspicion of ingestion of *T. canis* eggs in a child with the symptoms previously described. Eosinophilia, elevated erythrocyte sedimentation rate, and generalized hypergammaglobulinemia are also consistent with the diagnosis. Biopsy to document the presence of larvae is insensitive and not recommended. An enzyme-linked immunosorbent assay (ELISA) for measuring anti-*Toxocara* antibodies is helpful if elevated immunoglobulin M (IgM) antibodies and a rise in titer between acute and convalescent phases are documented.

Differential Diagnosis

OLM represents a diagnostic dilemma in that it must be distinguished from intraretinal neoplasms and infections. Expert ophthalmologic consultation is necessary. Computed tomography and fluorescein angiography are helpful in diagnosis. Elevated anti-*Toxocara* antibody titers in aqueous fluid relative to serum values are consistent with OLM. It is unclear whether anthelmintics are useful for the treatment of OLM.

Treatment

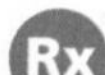

Most cases of VLM are not life-threatening and are self-limited. Treatment is therefore not required. In persons with severe pulmonary, cardiac, or neurologic involvement and high-grade eosinophilia (>10,000/mm^3 of blood), albendazole (400 mg given twice daily for 5 days) and corticosteroids may be used to reduce symptoms and shorten the course of the illness. No controlled studies, however, demonstrate the efficacy of chemotherapy.

VLM and OLM may be prevented by periodic deworming of dogs, especially puppies, and limiting their defecation in public places.

CUTANEOUS LARVA MIGRANS

Pathobiology

Animal hookworms, most frequently the dog parasite *A. braziliense* and less commonly *U. stenocephala* and *Bunostomum phlebotomum*, are the major causative agents of cutaneous larva migrans, or creeping eruption. *A. duodenale*, *N. americanus*, and *S. stercoralis* may produce a similar syndrome during the phase of infection that involves penetration of the skin.

The disease occurs when skin comes into direct and prolonged contact with hookworm larvae contained in the feces of dogs, cats, or humans. Moist areas visited by animals, such as vegetation near beaches and exposed soil covered by porches, are common sites in which humans may be infected. Cutaneous larva migrans in the United States is most prevalent in southern coastal regions.

Clinical Manifestations

Clinical manifestations result from penetration and migration of larvae in the epidermal-dermal junction of the skin. Within several hours of contact with exposed skin, the patient notices pruritus and raised erythematous serpiginous lesions. The lesions migrate approximately 1 cm each day and evolve into bullae. Multiple lesions may appear if large areas of the body have been exposed, as in sunbathing.

Treatment

Creeping eruption may be treated with 400 mg of albendazole per day for 3 days. If untreated, cutaneous larva migrans is self-limited; signs and symptoms resolve in several weeks to 2 months.

ANGIOSTRONGYLIASIS

Epidemiology

A. cantonensis is a cause of eosinophilic meningitis in Asia and the South Pacific. Small numbers of cases have also been reported in Cuba and Africa. *Angiostrongylus costaricensis* is a rare cause of gastrointestinal bleeding. The nematode is limited in its distribution to Central America and South America.

Etiology

Humans are infected with these rodent (primarily rat) nematodes after ingesting poorly cooked or raw intermediate mollusk hosts, such as snails, slugs, and prawns. Fresh vegetables may also be contaminated with infective larvae and serve as a vehicle of infection.

Clinical Manifestations

A. costaricensis larvae penetrate the mucosa of the terminal ileum, appendix, and ascending colon. The larvae subsequently develop into adult worms in the local lymphatics and mesenteric arterioles. Eggs released by the female worms elicit multiple eosinophil-rich granulomatous reactions that cause edematous, thickened bowel and necrosis from mesenteric blood vessel obstruction. Clinical presentations typically include right-sided abdominal pain, vomiting, and fever. Abnormal laboratory findings include leukocytosis with eosinophilia. Parasite larvae and eggs are not present in stools. A palpable mass derived from granulomatous lesions may be present and cause intestinal obstruction. Less frequently, gastrointestinal bleeding is the principal manifestation.

Diagnosis

In the case of *A. cantonensis* infection, ingested infective larvae penetrate the gut wall and migrate to small vessels of the meninges and, less commonly, the spinal cord and eye. An intense local inflammatory reaction ensues within 1 week. Fever, meningismus, and headache develop in association with eosinophilic pleocytosis of the CSF. Strabismus, paresthesias, and vomiting have been observed in a minority of cases. Diagnosis is based on a history of ingesting potentially contaminated foodstuffs and the presence of eosinophils in CSF. Larvae are usually not found in CSF. Other infectious causes of eosinophilic meningitis include *T. spiralis*, *Taenia solium*, *T. canis*, *G. spinigerum*, and *Paragonimus westermani*.

Treatment

Symptomatic *A. cantonensis* infection resolves over a 2-week period. The value of anthelmintic therapy has not been established. Analgesics and corticosteroids have been suggested to relieve symptoms.

Treatment for *A. costaricensis* is surgical. There is no demonstrated benefit of specific anthelmintic chemotherapy of human infection, although one report suggests that mebendazole and corticosteroids shorten the course of infection.

TRICHINELLOSIS

Definition

Infection by *T. spiralis* occurs when infective larvae are eaten in undercooked pork or other meats. Most infected individuals are asymptomatic. Clinical manifestations in heavily infected persons include diarrhea, myalgias, fever, and, less commonly, myocarditis and neurologic disease. Trichinellosis occurs in all areas of the world, including the Arctic and temperate regions. The incidence in the United States has decreased markedly over the past several decades.

Epidemiology

T. spiralis infection is enzootic in omnivorous and carnivorous animal populations, including rats, bears, and aquatic mammals of the Arctic. The nematode is introduced into domestic animals such as pigs and horses by feeding them garbage containing carcasses of these animals, most commonly rats. Human infection usually occurs in two settings: first, when undercooked or smoked pork products or beef contaminated with nematodes is eaten, and second, when flesh of poorly cooked wild game, such as bear or boar meat, is ingested. An important source of infection in Alaskan and Canadian Arctic native populations is uncooked walrus meat.

The annual incidence of human trichinosis in the United States has decreased dramatically over the past 60 years. This decline is primarily due to fewer cases related to ingestion of commercial pork products. Recent cases in the United States occur in point-source outbreaks associated with eating game or noncommercial pork products.

Pathobiology

Etiology

Infection is initiated by ingesting infective larvae encysted in striated muscle. Excystment occurs in the acid-pepsin environment of the stomach, and parasites develop into sexually mature adult worms in the upper to middle small intestine of the human host. Completion of the enteric phase of the parasite life cycle takes about 1 week, with adult worms remaining viable and productive of larval offspring for an additional 3 to 5 weeks. The systemic phase commences 1 week after infection, when larvae released by female worms migrate through blood vessels and lymphatics and invade multiple organ systems. Mature, third-stage larvae develop in host-derived nurse cells in striated skeletal and cardiac muscle, where they become encysted and remain viable for years.

As is the case with most helminthiases, the severity of symptoms is related to the total parasite load. Because adult worms are incapable of reproducing themselves, the number of infective larvae ingested is the most important determinant of worm load (i.e., number of larvae that invade muscle and other tissues).

Clinical Manifestations

Tissue-invasive *T. spiralis* larvae elicit an eosinophilic granulomatous reaction that may result in significant end-organ tissue damage and dysfunction. Skeletal muscle is the most frequent site involved. Myocardial damage, pulmonary infiltration, and focal neurologic damage caused by CNS invasion by larvae are seen in only the most heavily infected persons. The systemic phase of infection usually occurs 2 to 3 weeks after ingestion of infective larvae and may last for 2 months. Clinical manifestations typically include myalgias (especially of the gastrocnemius and masseter), periorbital edema, and fever. Myocardial damage may manifest as heart failure or dysrhythmias.

The enteric phase of infection may cause gastrointestinal signs and symptoms, such as diarrhea and abdominal cramps. These typically occur within 1 week of eating contaminated meat and last less than 2 weeks. Reports from the Canadian Arctic suggest that the *T. spiralis* larvae that infect walrus meat may cause diarrhea of 1 to 3 months' duration.

Diagnosis

A diagnosis of trichinellosis should be considered in individuals with generalized myalgias and eosinophilia (>600 eosinophils/mm^3). Serologic testing for *T. spiralis* antibodies is available at the Centers for Disease Control and Prevention. Elevation of IgM antibodies or a more than four-fold rise in titer between acute and convalescent phases of infection is helpful in making the diagnosis. The levels of creatine phosphate kinase and of serum immunoglobulins and the erythrocyte sedimentation rate are also increased for several weeks after infection. Muscle biopsy (e.g., gastrocnemius) may demonstrate larvae, although their absence does not exclude the diagnosis.

Treatment

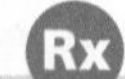

If patients present at a time when adult parasites are in the intestine (i.e., during the initial 1 to 2 weeks after infection, when gastrointestinal symptoms are prominent), albendazole is recommended at a dosage of 400 mg given twice daily for 8 to 14 days. It is not clear whether larvae in muscle are killed by this drug, and treatment is primarily symptomatic with antipyretics and analgesics. Although there are too few recent cases to establish a possible beneficial effect of corticosteroids, they may be useful to diminish the severity of inflammation when signs of myocarditis, neurologic disease (e.g., seizures, focal weakness), or pulmonary insufficiency develop.

Prevention

T. spiralis infection is prevented by killing larvae in meat products. This is achieved by heating until no trace of pink flesh remains. Freezing, smoking, or exposure to microwaves does not reliably kill the helminth.

STRONGYLOIDIASIS

Definition

S. stercoralis infection is endemic in warm climates worldwide, including the southern United States. In immunologically normal individuals, infection is usually asymptomatic or causes gastrointestinal dysfunction, manifested as abdominal pain, bloating, or bleeding. Persons who have deficient cell-mediated immunity can develop an autoinfective and hyperinfective life cycle of the nematode that markedly increases the total worm load. Life-threatening acute pulmonary disease and organ dysfunction related to dissemination of larvae to aberrant sites such as the brain, pancreas, and kidneys may result in immunocompromised hosts.

Epidemiology

S. stercoralis infection is endemic in Africa, Asia, Latin America, and areas of eastern and southern Europe. Prevalence rates based on stools examined for rhabditiform larvae vary from more than 40% in areas of sub-Saharan Africa to 1 to 7% in rural eastern Europe. In the United States, the infection is endemic in rural Appalachia and other parts of the South. Prevalences range from 0.4 to 3% in the United States. Refugees from Asia have a higher prevalence of infection than indigenous Americans. Surveys of homosexual men indicate a frequency of infection of 3.9%. It is likely that most studies of prevalence underestimate infection because they are based on examination of a single stool specimen, which is less sensitive than multiple examinations performed over days or weeks.

Strongyloidiasis is especially common in overcrowded situations in which sanitation and personal hygiene are poor, such as in institutions for retarded children and prisoner of war camps. An unusually high frequency of *S. stercoralis* infection has also been reported in persons with human T-cell lymphotropic virus type 1 (HTLV-1) infection.

Pathobiology

Etiology

S. stercoralis infection occurs when skin comes in contact with free-living filariform larvae in the soil. After penetrating the skin, the parasite embolizes to the small vessels of the lungs through the venous circulation. Rhabditiform larvae then break into the alveolar spaces, ascend the respiratory tree, and are swallowed. Further development to adult worms occurs in the duodenum and upper jejunum, where egg-laying parasites live in the mucosa and submucosa. Rhabditiform larvae are released from eggs and are passed from the body in stools. Infective filariform larvae develop in the soil by direct transformation from rhabditiform larvae or indirectly from free-living intermediate forms.

Several unusual features of the life cycle of *S. stercoralis* are crucial to understanding how this parasitic nematode causes life-threatening disease. First, unlike most human helminthic parasites, adult worms reproduce parthenogenetically in the gastrointestinal tract. The total worm burden in the host may therefore be greatly increased in the absence of repeated exposure to infective larvae in the environment. Second, rhabditiform larvae may develop into infective filariform larvae in the gastrointestinal tract and after passage in feces. Occurrence of the former process in immunocompromised hosts allows autoinfection, whereby larvae pass directly through the bowel (i.e., internal autoinfection) or perianal skin (i.e., external autoinfection) to reinitiate migration and development in the lungs. When this event is frequent, a hyperinfection syndrome ensues. Disseminated strongyloidiasis refers to a situation of hyperinfection in which the organisms also migrate to and cause pathology in organs not usually traversed by larvae, such as the CNS.

Pathogenesis

Adult worms and larvae penetrating the upper small bowel cause enteritis characterized histopathologically by eosinophil and mononuclear cell infiltration of the lamina propria. Edema and mucosal atrophy are present on gross examination. Ulcerative lesions with hemorrhages are present in the most severe cases. Filariform larvae in the lungs elicit an inflammatory response in the alveoli consisting of mononuclear cells and eosinophils. In hyperinfection syndrome, these may coalesce and result in alveolar hemorrhage.

Autoinfection leading to exceptionally high worm loads (i.e., hyperinfection) and disseminated strongyloidiasis occur in persons with deficient cell-mediated immunity. Groups at risk include persons who are chronically taking corticosteroids, renal transplant recipients, patients with Hodgkin's disease and other lymphomas, and leukemic patients. Because *S. stercoralis* may persist and the person may remain asymptomatic for decades after exposure, it is important to keep in mind that a change in immune status associated with these conditions may convert a previously asymptomatic infection to hyperinfection. In contrast, there is no correlation between an increased risk of disseminated strongyloidiasis and advancing acquired immunodeficiency syndrome (AIDS) marked by decreasing $CD4^+$ T-cell counts.

Clinical Manifestations

More than 50% of immunocompetent infected persons are asymptomatic. The frequency of clinical manifestations among infected immunocompromised subjects is unknown.

Signs and symptoms of *S. stercoralis* infection are attributable to the presence of adult worms in the upper gastrointestinal tract and larval invasion and to attendant host pathologic responses in the lung, skin, and aberrant sites of migration, such as the brain, eyes, pancreas, and kidney. Immunocompetent individuals rarely develop signs or symptoms attributable to larval migration outside the gut.

Gastrointestinal disease usually manifests as abdominal bloating, vague epigastric pain, and diarrhea with nausea. Symptoms are exacerbated by eating. Hematochezia and melena occur in less than 20% of subjects with intestinal strongyloidiasis. Major causes of morbidity related to *S. stercoralis* infection of the intestine are paralytic ileus, small bowel obstruction, and a malabsorption syndrome.

Pulmonary signs and symptoms in immunocompromised persons with hyperinfection syndrome are similar to those seen in the adult respiratory distress syndrome (i.e., acute onset of dyspnea, productive cough, and hemoptysis). These are accompanied by fever, tachypnea, hypoxemia, and respiratory alkalosis. *Strongyloides* larvae may also invade the CNS, pancreas, and eye and cause signs and symptoms attributable to tissue destruction in these sites.

Dermatologic manifestations include self-limited creeping eruption and, more commonly, larva currens, which results from migration of filariform larvae produced by a process of external autoinfection as described previously. The larvae elicit serpiginous erythematous papules and occasionally cause urticaria around the buttocks, upper thigh, and lower abdomen. Larva currens has been identified in former prisoners of war in the South Pacific.

Diagnosis

The unequivocal diagnosis of *S. stercoralis* infection depends on identifying larvae in host tissues or gastrointestinal and pulmonary secretions. The existence of filariform larvae in stools implies active autoinfection.

Intestinal strongyloidiasis is most easily diagnosed by identification of parasites in direct smears of freshly passed stools. Rhabditiform larvae are 225 to 380 mm long. Repeated examinations and concentration of stools increase the sensitivity of this method from approximately 25 to 80%. Examination of fluid obtained by duodenal aspiration or passage of a swallowed string into the upper small bowel may also be used if stool examination results are negative. Serologic tests are sensitive but not generally available. The differential diagnosis of intestinal *S. stercoralis* infection includes sprue, peptic ulcer, regional enteritis, and ulcerative colitis.

Hyperinfection syndrome and disseminated strongyloidiasis are diagnosed by identification of filariform larvae (500 to 600 mm long) in gastrointestinal secretions, as described previously, or in pulmonary tissues, secretions, or washings, such as those obtained by bronchoalveolar lavage or in sputum. Larvae have also been recovered from CSF, peritoneal washings, kidneys, urine, skin, and brains of immunocompromised persons.

Accompanying laboratory abnormalities frequently include eosinophilia. However, eosinophilia may not develop in immunocompromised hosts. Lack of eosinophilia is therefore not helpful in excluding strongyloidiasis in the differential diagnosis. The differential diagnosis of hyperinfection and disseminated strongyloidiasis includes overwhelming bacterial or fungal sepsis.

Complications

Disseminated strongyloidiasis is frequently accompanied by fungal or bacterial sepsis. Gram-negative enterococcal and polymicrobial septicemia has been observed. These infections probably result from translocation of gut organisms by migrating larvae.

Treatment

Rx

Uncomplicated intestinal strongyloidiasis should be treated with ivermectin (200 μg/kg body weight given daily for 1 to 2 days). Parasitologic cure rates are higher than 90%. Therapy may need to be extended for several more days in immunocompromised individuals, who should be closely monitored. Symptomatic improvement and failure to detect larvae in gastrointestinal secretions or other sites are indicative of cure. Corticosteroids and other immunosuppressive agents should be discontinued when possible.

Prevention

Infection is preventable by avoiding skin contact with contaminated soil. Immunocompromised patients in endemic areas should be advised to avoid walking barefoot. Persons residing in endemic areas who are to become immunosuppressed (e.g., for renal transplantation) should have their stools examined three times for the presence of larvae, and they should be treated if the examination result is positive. Because infected individuals may be incorrectly categorized as uninfected by this test, it is suggested by some authorities that prophylactic thiabendazole (50 mg/kg body weight given twice daily for 2 days, maximum of 3 g/day) or ivermectin be given in the month preceding iatrogenic immunosuppression. Positive serology for *S. stercoralis* is also an indication for treatment before immunosuppression.

SUGGESTED READINGS

Bethony J, Brooker S, Albonico M, et al: Soil-transmitted helminth infections: Ascaris, trichuriasis, and hookworm. Lancet 2006;367:1521–1532. *Comprehensive review.*

Hotez PJ, Brooker S, Bethony JM, et al: Hookworm infection. N Engl J Med 2004;351:799–807. *An excellent review of the biology and clinical consequences of human hookworm disease.*

Keiser PB, Nutman TB: *Strongyloides stercoralis* in the immunocompromised population. Clin Microbiol Rev 2004;17:208–217. *A good overview of the risk factors for hyperinfection in persons who are immunocompromised.*

Kuzucu A: Parasitic diseases of the respiratory tract. Curr Opin Pulm Med 2006;12:212–221. *Clinical review.*

Loukas A, Bethony J, Brooker S, et al: Hookworm vaccines: Past, present, and future. Lancet Infect Dis 2006;6:733–741. *Review of recent advances in the quest for a hookworm vaccine.*

Pozio E, Darwin Murrell K: Systematics and epidemiology of trichinella. Adv Parasitol 2006;63:367–439. *Review of the epidemiology of this infection.*

Slom TJ, Cortese MM, Gerber SI, et al: An outbreak of eosinophilic meningitis caused by *Angiostrongylus cantonensis* in travelers returning from the Caribbean. N Engl J Med 2002;346:668–675. *A complete description of the clinical, laboratory, and radiologic features of this condition in a large outbreak among travelers.*

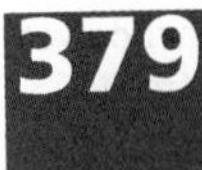

379 FILARIASIS

David O. Freedman

Definition

The filariases are a group of arthropod-borne parasitic diseases of humans caused by threadlike nematodes that in their mature adult stage reside in the lymphatics or in connective tissue (Table 379–1). Eight filarial species infect humans: *Wuchereria bancrofti, Brugia malayi, Brugia timori, Onchocerca volvulus, Loa loa, Mansonella streptocerca, Mansonella perstans,* and *Mansonella ozzardi.* Three species, *W. bancrofti, B. malayi,* and *O. volvulus,* which infect approximately 150 million individuals, are responsible for most human filarial disease in the world. Loiasis, however, is a relatively common affliction of returned travelers and expatriates.

Infection of the human host begins with the bite of an infected arthropod vector (see Table 379–1). Infective larvae are deposited into the skin or blood of a new host, where at least 3 to 12 months is required for the development of a mature adult female capable of producing larvae called *microfilariae.* To complete the life cycle, microfilariae, which circulate in blood or migrate through the skin, are ingested by another arthropod vector to develop into new infective larvae ready to be passed to the next human host in a blood meal. Generally, infection is established only with repeated and prolonged exposure to infective larvae. After successful infection, no multiplication of the adult worms occurs in the human host. Because adult worms live for 5 to 15 years, such infections are chronic diseases. Microfilariae live for approximately 5 to 15 months. The long asymptomatic incubation period significantly lessens the chance that a relevant travel history will be elicited in an individual who has the nonspecific symptoms that occur with many of the filarial infections.

Disease expression varies. In some filarial species, the adult parasite itself may provoke chronic inflammatory reactions in tissues, whereas in infection caused by other filariases, reaction to microfilariae migrating through tissues may incite the abnormality observed. Newly exposed individuals characteristically have acute symptoms that are exaggerated in comparison to those of chronically infected natives of the endemic area.

Definitive diagnosis of any of the filarial infections usually depends on the parasitologic demonstration of 170- to 300-μm-long and 5- to 9-μm-wide microfilariae either in blood or in skin snips (depending on the species; see Table 379–1). The presence or absence of a sheath, the arrangement of nuclei in the tail, and the tissue of origin are usually sufficient to differentiate the species. Geographic distribution of the different species may overlap. Diagnostic blood sampling must be timed during the day to account for the periodicity of every filarial parasite that is epidemiologically possible in the particular patient. Available serologic methods use crude heterologous antigen preparations. A positive result is not species specific, and individuals resident in endemic areas have antibodies regardless of whether they are currently infected. A positive result may be helpful in individuals originally from nonendemic areas who were presumably seronegative initially and are now infected with filarial parasites.

Diethylcarbamazine and ivermectin are the backbone of antifilarial treatment, but they are not active against all the different life cycle stages of a given filarial species. Diethylcarbamazine has substantial adulticidal effects against *L. loa* and the lymphatic filariases. Curative efforts with repeated courses of adulticidal therapy are more important in nonendemic individuals who will not be subsequently re-exposed to the parasite. Diethylcarbamazine is microfilaricidal to all species of human filaria except *M. ozzardi* and *M. perstans.* Ivermectin is not an adulticide and is microfilaricidal to *O. volvulus, W. bancrofti, Brugia* sp, *L. loa, M. ozzardi,* and *M. streptocerca.* Suppression of microfilaria production by adult female parasites that remain viable may vary from weeks to months. Treatment regimens differ according to whether the ultimate aim is treatment and cure of an individual patient or widespread, single-dose, community-based interruption of transmission by suppression of blood-borne or skin-dwelling microfilariae available to vectors. Albendazole, used as part of multidrug regimens in control programs, has antifilarial activity, but lack of rigorous controlled data precludes its use in first-line therapy for individual patients.

LYMPHATIC FILARIASIS

Etiology

W. bancrofti, B. malayi, and *B. timori* adults are threadlike worms that are convoluted in lymph nodes but have been shown by ultrasound to be extended into afferent lymph vessels. The females, which are about twice the size (80 to 100 mm long × 0.2 to 0.3 mm wide) of males, produce microfilariae that circulate in peripheral blood until ingestion by mosquito intermediate hosts. After a 1- to 3-week incubation, mosquitoes take a second blood meal, and infective larvae penetrate the skin at the puncture wound. An additional 4 to 12 months elapses until development into mature adults in the lymphatics of the new host.

Epidemiology

An estimated 120 million people are affected by lymphatic filariasis—90% with bancroftian and 10% with brugian filariasis. Humans are the only definitive host for *W. bancrofti,* which has no animal reservoir. *W. bancrofti* is found in 76 countries throughout the tropics and subtropics,

TABLE 379–1 COMMON FILARIAL PARASITES OF HUMANS

				Microfilariae		
Species	**Distribution**	**Vector**	**Primary Pathology**	**Primary Location**	**Periodicity**	**Presence of Sheath**
Wuchereria bancrofti	Tropics worldwide	Mosquitoes	Lymphatic, pulmonary	Blood, hydrocele fluid	Nocturnal, subperiodic	+
Brugia malayi	Southeast Asia, West Pacific	Mosquitoes	Lymphatic, pulmonary	Blood	Nocturnal, subperiodic	+
Brugia timori	Indonesia	Mosquitoes	Lymphatic	Blood	Nocturnal	+
Onchocerca volvulus	Africa, Central and South America	Black fly	Skin, eye, lymphatic	Skin, eye	None or minimal	–
Loa loa	Africa	Deer fly	Allergic	Blood	Diurnal	+
Mansonella perstans	Africa, South America	Midge	? Allergic	Blood	None	–
Mansonella streptocerca	Africa	Midge	Skin	Skin	None	–
Mansonella ozzardi	Central and South America	Midge	Vague	Blood	None	–

including areas of South America, the Caribbean, Africa, Asia, and the South Pacific. Two forms of the parasite are distinguished by the periodicity of their circulating microfilariae. Nocturnally periodic forms of the parasite, found in most endemic areas, have microfilariae detectable in blood primarily at night, with a peak between 10:00 PM and 2:00 AM. Subperiodic bancroftian filariasis is found only in the Pacific islands, with microfilariae circulating at all hours but with peak levels in the late afternoon. The natural vectors are *Culex quinquefasciatus* in urban settings and usually anopheline or aedean mosquitoes in rural areas.

B. malayi is restricted to an area of Asia from India in the west to Korea in the northeast. Foci also exist in Indonesia, Vietnam, Malaysia, China, and the Philippines. Two forms of *B. malayi* are distinguished. The nocturnally periodic form, which has no animal reservoir, is transmitted by *Mansonia* and *Anopheles* species in India, Sulawesi, Vietnam, and China. The nocturnally subperiodic form is transmitted by *Mansonia* species and coexists with periodic forms in Malaysia and Indonesia. Subperiodic *B. malayi* can produce a natural infection in cats. *B. timori*, transmitted by anophelines, has been reported from only two Indonesian islands.

Pathobiology

Microfilariae in blood are not associated with any disorder. The mature adult lymphatic-dwelling parasite induces a parasite-specific local inflammatory reaction, with cell-mediated, cytokine, and humoral components leading to hypertrophy of the vessel walls. The worm itself does not seem to cause blockage of the vessel. Endothelial and connective tissue proliferation leads to vessel dilation and intraluminal polyposis, which diminish normal lymphatic function. The resulting lymphedema is reversible in its early stages. Worm death leads to necrosis and a granulomatous reaction with infiltration of plasma cells, eosinophils, and giant cells. Over time, fibrosis and obstruction of lymph flow within the lumen result in irreversible elephantiasis of the affected part. Although some recanalization and collateralization of lymph vessels take place, lymphatic function remains compromised.

At an uncertain point during clinical evolution of the lymphatic insufficiency, extrinsic bacteria colonizing breaks in skin integrity begin to cause repeated limb infections in previously damaged vessels and become superimposed on other pathologic processes.

Separately, endosymbiotic *Wolbachia* bacteria live within *W. bancrofti* and *B. malayi* adult worms and are obligatory for these worms' development, viability, and fertility. *Wolbachia* major surface protein triggers the innate immune system through Toll-like receptor 2 (TLR2)- and TLR4-mediated mechanisms. *Wolbachia* bacteria are released from naturally dying adult worms, as well as those killed by standard antiparasitic drug regimens. Until recently, entirely asymptomatic individuals with microfilaremia but no overt clinical manifestations of filarial infection had been thought to have infection but not disease. Imaging of the lymphatic system with ultrasound and radionuclide lymphoscintigraphy and biopsy of affected tissue have demonstrated that lymphatic structural and functional abnormalities are often far advanced even before overt lymphatic insufficiency is clinically manifested.

Clinical Manifestations

The common clinical outcomes of lymphatic filariasis are asymptomatic microfilaremia, acute episodic adenolymphangitis (also called *filarial fever*), and chronic lymphatic obstruction. Clinically asymptomatic microfilaremia is the most common outcome of lymphatic filariasis. These individuals, however, almost uniformly have underlying lymphatic damage with impaired lymphatic function. Microscopic hematuria and low-grade proteinuria are common but of uncertain clinical significance.

Acute attacks of retrograde adenolymphangitis, accompanied by fever, chills, and malaise, each lasting 3 to 15 days, can occur up to 10 times per year and are often initial manifestations of progressive filarial disease. Patients usually give a clear history of pain, erythema, and tenderness in the affected lymph node region for hours or a day before onset of the lymphangitis. Some individuals may have only one or a few attacks in a lifetime. Adenolymphangitis most often affects the groin and, in male patients, the lymphatics of the genitalia and leads to funiculitis, orchitis, and epididymitis, but essentially any lymph node group and any body part may be involved. Patients with filarial fevers may be microfilaremic but often are not.

After months to years of acute episodes ranging from very insidious to severe, transient and then chronic obstructive disease develops as a result of lymphatic insufficiency. Pitting edema progresses to brawny edema, and thickening of subcutaneous tissue and hyperkeratosis develop. Fissuring of the skin develops along with nodular and papillomatous hyperplasia. Bacterial superinfection of limbs with such loss of skin surface integrity is manifested as typical cellulitis with a warm erythematous and edematous extremity. In many areas, the most common chronic manifestation is hydrocele, and scrotal lymphedema is seen in more advanced cases. Many patients give no history of earlier acute attacks, thus emphasizing the need for disrobing of all male patients to carry out a genital examination. Female patients occasionally have lymphedema of the vulva. If the retroperitoneal lymphatics are obstructed, rupture of the renal lymphatics leads to the development of intermittent chyluria. In endemic areas, the prevalence of chronic manifestations increases with age. Patients with chronic obstructive disease may be microfilaremic but most often are not. Attacks of acute adenolymphangitis often continue even in those with advanced disease.

Newly exposed individuals (e.g., long-term visitors, military personnel, migrants) characteristically have acute inflammatory symptoms with more rapid progression to chronic or irreversible abnormality than in those born in the endemic area. Prolonged, severe episodes of adenolymphangitis, often with genital involvement, may lead to the relatively rapid development of lymphedema and elephantiasis within 6 to 12 months of arrival. Disease abates quickly with removal of the patient from the endemic area. These individuals are uniformly amicrofilaremic.

Brugian filariasis differs in several respects from bancroftian filariasis. In *B. malayi* infection, only the lower part of the leg is affected, whereas in *W. bancrofti* infection, the thigh and lower part of the leg are involved. In brugian filariasis, infected superficial nodes, usually inguinal, may suppurate and form sterile abscesses that heal with a characteristic scar. In general, brugian filariasis is more clinically dramatic. An insidious onset of chronic lymphedema, as may be seen in bancroftian filariasis, is uncommon. Urogenital disease and chyluria do not occur.

Diagnosis

Definitive diagnosis often depends on parasitologic demonstration of the 250- to 320-μm-long microfilariae in blood. Diagnostic sampling must take into account the periodicity of the microfilariae in the area of exposure. A Giemsa-stained thick blood smear, performed as for the diagnosis of malaria, can detect heavily infected individuals but is relatively insensitive. Parasites may be concentrated by passage through a polycarbonate membrane filter (3-μm pore size). The filter itself is then stained and examined. Microfilariae of *W. bancrofti* have occasionally been found in urine but are not usually present in chyluric patients. Only an experienced pathologist can identify the sections of adult worms that are found incidentally in specimens of diverse human body tissues. Lymph node biopsy is not indicated in suspected filariasis unless neoplasia is also a diagnostic concern.

Serologic measurement of antifilarial antibodies is often not useful because existing assays cannot distinguish among the eight human filarial parasites. The assays cannot differentiate actively infected patients from those previously infected, and those merely exposed but not infected may also have positive findings. Cross-reactivity occurs with other helminth infections. A 10-minute rapid card test assay sensitive enough to detect circulating *W. bancrofti*–specific antigen liberated by adult worms (and present in blood both day and night) has dramatically advanced the serologic approach to diagnosis of filariasis. The card test is commercially available (*www.binax.com*) and is considered by most experts to be the "gold standard," but the test has not been approved by the U.S. Food and Drug Administration (FDA).

Ultrasound can be used to visualize rapidly moving ("dancing") adult worms or the dilated scrotal lymphatics of infected men. Such findings are pathognomonic for filarial parasites, and newer techniques are almost as sensitive as antigen detection techniques. Abnormalities detected by lymphoscintigraphy are not specific for filarial disease.

Bacterial infection, thrombophlebitis, or trauma may be mistaken for acute filarial adenolymphangitis. Filarial lymphangitis is retrograde, a characteristic that helps differentiate it from bacterial lymphangitis. In cases of orchitis and epididymitis, sexually transmitted diseases must be considered. Chronic lymphedema may be caused by malignancy, postoperative changes, congenital malformations, and renal or cardiac failure. Physical examination cannot distinguish a filarial from a nonfilarial cause of lymphedema or elephantiasis. A foreign body reaction to silica dust introduced into traumatized legs accounts for elephantiasis in some parts of the world. Patients with filarial lymphedema are often amicrofilaremic, and diagnosis therefore depends on the clinical history, epidemiologic features, and physical examination results and may be supported by a positive serologic or antigen assay result or, in men, by compatible scrotal ultrasonographic findings.

Treatment

Individual patients with current active infection by a lymphatic filariasial parasite, whether symptomatic or asymptomatic, should be treated with diethylcarbamazine (6 mg/kg/day in three divided doses for 2 to 3 weeks). FDA-approved diethylcarbamazine is available only through the Centers for Disease Control and Prevention (CDC) drug service (404-639-3670). Side effects are caused by dying parasites, not direct drug toxicity, and are proportional to the number of circulating microfilariae. Side effects include fever, chills, headache, dizziness, nausea, vomiting, and arthralgias, all usually occurring in the first 24 to 36 hours and then subsiding even with continued therapy. For highly parasitemic persons, the physician can initiate treatment with single doses of 50 to 100 mg of diethylcarbamazine on the first 2 days or premedicate the patients with steroids. Some patients may experience adenolymphangitis because of dying adult worms. In individual patients who will not be returning to endemic areas, attempts at adulticidal therapy with prolonged or repeated courses of diethylcarbamazine should be undertaken. The adult worm burden is reduced in most patients, but all parasites are eliminated in less than a quarter. If the patient remains microfilaremic, at least two repeat courses at several month intervals should be considered. Patients with lymphedema or elephantiasis should receive low-dose diethylcarbamazine daily for at least a year in an attempt to determine whether there is any reversible component of the chronic disease. Limb elevation, massage, use of elastic stockings, and prevention of superficial bacterial and fungal infection through meticulous hygiene are important in the care of a lymphedematous extremity. Suspected bacterial superinfection should be treated with antibiotics. In individuals with live adult worms visible by ultrasound in the scrotal lymphatics, serial studies may be performed to monitor the adulticidal effects of therapy.

Doxycycline, 200 mg/day for 8 weeks, has been shown to suppress *W. bancrofti* microfilaria production for up to 14 months and reduce but not eliminate adult worms. Without direct comparisons to standard diethylcarbamazine regimens, doxycycline must be regarded as experimental for this indication at present.

Single doses of diethylcarbamazine, ivermectin, or albendazole are microfilaricidal and may be used in community control programs in endemic areas in which the aim is to break transmission by suppression of microfilariae available to vectors. However, single-dose combination therapies are more effective in long-term suppression of microfilariae. Combinations containing diethylcarbamazine as one component are the most effective, and evidence for an additional benefit of adding albendazole to one of the other single drugs is lacking at this time.

Prognosis

Although the psychosocial morbidity associated with this deforming disease is profound, there is little mortality associated with lymphatic filariasis. It is likely that some untreated asymptomatic microfilaremic individuals become symptomatic, but factors determining such clinical changes are unknown. The determinants of which patients with chronic manifestations have a component that is reversible with therapy are not defined. Disease should not progress in those removed from an endemic area and adequately treated.

Prevention

Diethylcarbamazine has some value as a prophylactic agent in humans at a dose of 10 mg/kg on 2 consecutive days each month. Yearly mass treatment with a single dose of diethylcarbamazine significantly reduces the prevalence of infection within a community. Diethylcarbamazine-supplemented table salt can reduce the number of blood-borne microfilariae in the community to levels so low that transmission is interrupted. Vector control in endemic areas has proved difficult, but bed net programs may have some efficacy.

TROPICAL EOSINOPHILIA

Tropical pulmonary eosinophilia is a syndrome that develops in a small percentage of individuals infected with lymphatic filarial parasites. The characteristic patient is a male (4:1 male-to-female ratio) in his teens or 20s who is a resident of India, Pakistan, Sri Lanka, Brazil, or Southeast Asia. Characteristic clinical findings include paroxysmal coughing and wheezing that occur almost exclusively at night, weight loss, low-grade fever, adenopathy, and extreme blood eosinophilia. Chest radiographs generally show diffusely increased bronchovascular markings or mottled opacities in the middle and lower lung fields. Restrictive and obstructive abnormalities are found through pulmonary function tests. The total serum IgE level and antifilarial antibody levels are extremely elevated.

Tropical pulmonary eosinophilia is thought to occur as a result of unusually rapid immune-mediated clearance of blood microfilariae with trapping in the lung. The pulmonary symptoms result from allergic (IgE-mediated) and inflammatory reactions to the cleared parasites (*W. bancrofti* or *B. malayi*). Several reports have described microfilariae or their degenerating remnants in lung biopsy specimens, and eosinophils are present in bronchial lavage fluid. Untreated disease can progress to interstitial fibrosis.

The differential diagnosis of tropical pulmonary eosinophilia includes asthma, Löffler's syndrome (which can be caused by the migrating larval forms of other helminths), allergic bronchopulmonary aspergillosis, Churg-Strauss syndrome or other systemic vasculitides, chronic eosinophilic pneumonia, and idiopathic hypereosinophilic syndrome. The diagnosis of tropical pulmonary eosinophilia is usually confirmed by the coexistence of nocturnal wheezing, very high antifilarial titers, and rapid initial response to diethylcarbamazine therapy in a patient with the right geographic exposure. Diethylcarbamazine at a dose of 6 mg/kg/day for 14 to 21 days is the treatment of choice. Ivermectin is not useful for tropical pulmonary eosinophilia. Symptoms typically respond within a week, but relapse may occur even after an interval of years in 25% and necessitate repeat treatment.

ONCHOCERCIASIS (RIVER BLINDNESS)

Etiology

Transmission of *O. volvulus* occurs through the bites of black flies (*Simulium* species) that ingest microfilariae from the skin of an infected person. After development in the vector, infective larvae are transmitted to a new human host. Over a period of several months, the larvae develop into adult worms that are coiled within fibrotic subcutaneous nodules. Nine to 18 months after infection, each mature female worm begins to produce up to 2000 microfilariae per day, which migrate primarily through the skin and ocular tissues.

Adult female worms are 23 to 70 cm long, and the males are 3 to 6 cm long. Microfilariae are unsheathed, 200 to 300 μm long, and 6 to 9 μm wide. The average lifespan of an adult worm is 8 to 10 years, and that of microfilariae is 13 to 14 months. Two distinct strains or biotypes of *O. volvulus* are present in western Africa. The blinding or savanna strain is associated with the development of ocular disorders, whereas the nonblinding or forest strain is not generally associated with ocular disease.

Epidemiology

Onchocerciasis is endemic in 35 countries, 27 in equatorial Africa in a broad belt extending from the Atlantic coast to the Red Sea and more focally in 6 Latin American countries (i.e., Guatemala, Mexico, Venezuela,

Brazil, Colombia, and Ecuador) and in the Arabian peninsula (i.e., Yemen and Saudi Arabia). Current estimates are that approximately 18 million people are infected, 270,000 of whom are blind and another 500,000 of whom have severe visual disability. More than 99% of cases occur in sub-Saharan Africa, with almost half of them in Nigeria and Zaire. Because the black flies depend on well-oxygenated, fast-flowing waterways for egg laying and reproduction, the vectors and the disease are concentrated around streams and rivers, often in the most fertile farming areas.

O. volvulus–induced blindness is associated with a life expectancy that is decreased by at least 10 years over that of nonblinded individuals in the same area. However, more than the blinding disease, which affects only a small proportion of those infected, the pervasiveness of the chronic skin lesions and the intense pruritus caused by onchodermatitis make it a leading cause of morbidity in infected areas.

Pathobiology

Onchocerciasis predominantly affects the skin, the eyes, and the lymph nodes. The inflammatory reaction is elicited by microfilariae and not the adult worms, whose encapsulation seems to protect them from the immune response. Tissue damage results primarily from the host response to the secretion of toxic products by granulocytes, particularly granular proteins from eosinophils that adhere to microfilariae. Sclerosing keratitis, the major cause of blindness, is caused by a parasite antigen–specific, lymphocytic inflammatory reaction to dying intraocular microfilariae that appears to be dependent on T_H2 cytokines. As with *W. bancrofti*, endosymbiotic *Wolbachia* bacteria live within *O. volvulus* adult worms and are obligatory for the development, viability, and fertility of these worms. *Wolbachia* major surface protein triggers the innate immune system through TLR2- and TLR4-mediated mechanisms. With time, neovascularization and scarring of the cornea lead to loss of transparency and to blindness. Ongoing low-grade inflammation in the skin eventually leads to loss of elastic fibers and atrophy. Chronic inflammatory changes and fibrosis are seen in lymph nodes. Release of *Wolbachia* bacteria from naturally dying microfilaria in the skin, as well as those killed by standard antiparasitic drug regimens, accounts for the so-called Mazzotti reaction seen after treatment with diethylcarbamazine or ivermectin.

Clinical Manifestations

Dermatitis

The pruritus of onchocerciasis is often intractable and unresponsive to antipruritic medication. In heavily infected individuals in endemic areas, scratching and excoriation occur to the point of bleeding and even suicide. Episodes of localized rash, erythema, and angioedema may be superimposed on the ongoing dermatologic manifestations at any stage of disease. The five categories used to classify onchodermatitis are not mutually exclusive in a given patient, and the clinical findings are not necessarily specific for onchodermatitis. In type 1, acute papular onchodermatitis, the small, pruritic papules may be scattered on the limbs, shoulders, and trunk. Lesions may progress to become vesicular or pustular. In type 2, chronic papular onchodermatitis, the often flat-topped papules are larger but more variable in size and height than in the acute papular eruption. Lesions are less pruritic than in the acute eruption. In type 3, lichenified dermatitis (i.e., sowdah), an intensely pruritic eruption is limited to one limb, usually the leg, and consists of hyperpigmented papules and plaques with accompanying edema of the entire limb. In type 4, atrophy–premature atrophy, one or more of the structural elements of the skin degenerate, pruritus is uncommon, and fine wrinkles appear on the skin after pushing along the surface with one finger. Loss of elasticity can be demonstrated by slow return to the original position of skin pinched between two fingers. In type 5, depigmentation, areas of complete depigmentation occur over the anterior aspect of the shin along with islands of normally pigmented skin, also called "leopard skin." In short-term residents of endemic areas, an evanescent acute papular dermatitis is almost always the sole manifestation of infection.

Eye

Inflammation caused by the microfilariae of *O. volvulus* as they migrate through the eye is initially manifested as punctate keratitis or snowflake corneal opacities. Free microfilariae may be visible by slit lamp examination in the anterior chamber or aqueous humor but are rarely found in infected short-term visitors, who are typically very lightly infected. Long-standing infection with the savanna strain of *O. volvulus* leads to sclerosing keratitis characterized by a fibrovascular pannus. Iridocyclitis with flare and cells in the anterior chamber leads to the development of synechiae, raised intraocular pressure, and secondary glaucoma. Chorioretinitis and chorioretinal atrophy are the common manifestations of posterior ocular disease. Optic neuritis and optic atrophy occur in savannah regions. Infected short-term visitors do not have ocular involvement.

Subcutaneous Nodules

Asymptomatic, 0.5- to 3.0-cm subcutaneous onchocercomas, occurring most often over bony prominences, are freely movable encapsulated nodules that contain coiled masses of adult worms. In Latin America, the nodules are often located on the head and upper part of the body, whereas in Africa, the nodules occur most often over the hips and lower limbs. More than 80% of nodules are not palpable and, in lightly infected expatriates, are rarely detectable.

Lymphadenopathy

Lymphadenopathy is frequently found in the inguinal and femoral areas. When it occurs in the inguinofemoral nodes in a sling of stretched-out atrophic abdominal skin, the so-called hanging groin results. The lymph nodes are nontender and fibrotic.

Diagnosis

Definitive diagnosis depends on the demonstration of motile microfilariae in superficial, bloodless skin snips. For this type of skin biopsy, a thin piece of skin that has been tented up with a needle or a corneoscleral biopsy instrument is sliced with a razor blade to obtain 1 to 2 mg of skin bloodlessly. Six snips, one from over each scapula, iliac crest, and lateral aspect of each calf, are incubated with saline solution in microplate wells and examined microscopically. Deep punch biopsy of the skin is not necessary, and multiple skin snips have a higher yield than one random traumatic deep biopsy. When available, polymerase chain reaction amplification of parasite DNA directly from skin snips is far more sensitive than direct visualization. Blood contamination of a skin snip may cause one of the blood-borne microfilaria to escape into the specimen. If the patient has been in an area endemic for *M. streptocerca*, it is necessary to fix the skin and stain the microfilariae for identification. In well-equipped clinical settings, biopsy or ultrasound demonstration of adult parasites in any nodules that are present can be diagnostic. Elevated titers of antifilarial antibodies may support the diagnosis of onchocerciasis but should not be used alone. The total eosinophil count is not helpful diagnostically because it is often, but inconstantly elevated in onchocerciasis.

Scabies, insect bites, hypersensitivity reactions, miliaria rubra, and atopic or contact dermatitis enter the differential diagnosis of acute pruritic disease. In expatriates, Calabar swellings (see the discussion of loiasis), clinically similar episodes of localized rash and mild angioedema, can mimic onchodermatitis. Tuberculoid leprosy, streptocerciasis, and eczema should be considered if chronic skin changes are present. Dermatomycoses, previous trauma, and yaws can also cause hypopigmented skin lesions. The posterior eye lesions are not at all specific for onchocerciasis.

Treatment

No available nontoxic agent is able to kill the long-lived adult worms of *O. volvulus*. Repeated microfilaricidal therapy with ivermectin (150 μg/kg) in a single dose every 6 to 12 months is effective in ameliorating symptoms. For unclear reasons, pruritus in lightly infected expatriates may be refractory to therapy every 6 months, and many clinicians find it necessary to treat more aggressively for the first 2 years or so. The appropriate duration of therapy in those without further exposure is unknown, but it should probably be offered for at least 10 years. In *L. loa*–coinfected individuals with high levels of circulating microfilaremia, ivermectin therapy may precipitate a toxic encephalopathy. In areas endemic for loiasis, high microfilaremia should be ruled out before administration of ivermectin for onchocerciasis. Because of frequent unacceptable reactions to dying microfilariae ranging from urticaria and angioedema to hypotension and death, diethylcarbamazine should never be used for microfilaricidal treatment of onchocerciasis. Suramin (available from the CDC drug service) is adulticidal, but because of toxicity and even potentially life-threatening effects, it should be used only in extreme situations. Surgical removal of palpable nodules to reduce the microfilarial load and the ensuing disorder has been successful in some areas. Nodulectomy is appropriate for cosmetic reasons but cannot be expected to cure infection because most nodules are not palpable.

Doxycycline, 100 mg/day for 6 weeks, has been shown to suppress production of *O. volvulus* microfilariae for up to 18 months. Without direct comparisons to standard ivermectin regimens, doxycycline must be regarded as experimental for this indication at present.

Prognosis

Ivermectin is effective in reversing existing early skin and ocular abnormalities but must be given repeatedly because adult parasites again begin producing microfilariae with time. The atrophic skin changes, sclerosing keratitis, and established lesions in the posterior segment of the eye are not helped by therapy.

Prevention

There are no effective vaccines or chemoprophylactic drugs. For expatriates or others with sufficient resources, personal mosquito protection with repellents is probably of benefit. Building a sustainable infrastructure for mass community-based distribution of the microfilaricide ivermectin has now become the primary global control strategy. Annual mass treatment of an affected community with ivermectin, which is available free through a remarkable donation program by Merck, reduces the microfilariae available to vectors from the skin of infected individuals but is not thought to be an effective eradication strategy. There is no nonhuman reservoir of *O. volvulus*.

LOIASIS

Etiology and Epidemiology

L. loa, the African eye worm, is restricted to the rain forest area of central and western Africa. Its prevalence and endemicity are imprecisely defined, but loiasis appears to be most prevalent in Gabon, Cameroon, Congo, Nigeria, and the Central African Republic. Adult parasites (females are 50 to 70 mm long; males are 25 to 35 mm long) live a constantly migratory existence in subcutaneous tissue. Blood-borne microfilariae have a diurnal periodicity peaking between noon and 4:00 PM. Tabanid flies of *Chrysops* species are the vectors. In temporary residents, a shorter period of exposure appears to be necessary to acquire infection than with other filarial parasites.

Pathobiology

The pathogenesis of the angioedematous reaction that occurs in response to the adult worm is poorly understood. The extremely elevated serum IgE level and eosinophilia seen in newly infected individuals prone to Calabar swellings indicate a hypersensitivity reaction to adult worms or worm products.

Clinical Manifestations

More so than with other filarial infections, the clinical manifestations are much more exaggerated in short-term residents or visitors to endemic areas than in natives. Nonendemic persons, who are usually amicrofilaremic, have severe allergic symptoms with frequent and incapacitating Calabar swellings, pruritus, and urticaria. Calabar swellings are localized areas of evanescent erythema and angioedema (up to 5 to 10 cm in diameter) that occur primarily on the extremities and last 1 to 3 days. The subcutaneous adult organisms, which are large enough to be visible, only rarely migrate across the conjunctiva. Among endemic individuals, infection is most often asymptomatic with microfilaremia and has a much lower incidence of Calabar swellings and allergic manifestations. Eye worm occurs in up to 50% of these individuals. In chronically infected individuals, nephropathy and cardiomyopathy develop only rarely.

Diagnosis

Definitive diagnosis depends on demonstration of characteristic sheathed microfilariae on an afternoon blood film. Nonendemic individuals are usually amicrofilaremic, and the diagnosis often cannot be made parasitologically and must be based on the characteristic history, clinical findings, blood eosinophilia, and elevated antifilarial antibody titers. *O. volvulus*, *M. perstans*, *M. ozzardi*, and *M. streptocerca* all cause overlapping syndromes and must, if epidemiologically possible, be ruled out by a complete search for microfilariae in blood and skin. Occasionally, an adult *L. loa* is excised while crawling across the conjunctiva or under the skin. Definitive diagnosis sometimes occurs after initiation of diethylcarbamazine therapy and subcutaneous biopsy of a swelling developing at the site of a dying adult worm.

Treatment and Prognosis

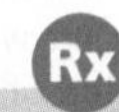

Diethylcarbamazine (6 to 10 mg/kg/day for 21 days) has both microfilaricidal and adulticidal effects. Decisions about repeat treatment should be based on clinical resolution, and multiple courses of diethylcarbamazine may be required before the signs and symptoms completely resolve. One course of therapy cures about half of those infected, and a second course cures half of the remaining infected individuals. Eosinophilia and antifilarial titers resolve slowly, even with effective therapy, and therefore should not be closely monitored as a test of cure. However, an antifilarial titer or eosinophilia that is increasing or unchanged after 6 months should prompt suspicion of failure of treatment given up until that time.

In patients with any microfilaremia, diethylcarbamazine therapy should be initiated with low doses of drug (50 mg/day) on the first few days, and pretreatment with corticosteroids should be considered. With microfilaremia levels greater than a few hundred microfilariae per milliliter of blood, diethylcarbamazine-induced inflammatory reactions to dying microfilariae may progress to encephalopathy and death. If available, apheresis to remove circulating microfilariae can be performed before initiating diethylcarbamazine therapy in these individuals. If this latter option is not available for highly microfilaremic individuals, limited data support the use of albendazole (200 mg twice daily for 21 days) because it appears to be moderately adulticidal without effects on microfilariae. Ivermectin is microfilaricidal but has no adulticidal effect and may cause toxic encephalopathy in highly microfilaremic individuals. If epidemiologically appropriate, onchocerciasis must be carefully ruled out before the initiation of diethylcarbamazine therapy for loiasis to prevent toxicity from dying *O. volvulus* microfilariae.

Prevention

Diethylcarbamazine is effective in preventing loiasis when taken in prophylactic doses of 300 mg/wk.

DRACUNCULIASIS

Dracunculiasis, or guinea worm disease, is caused by the helminth *Dracunculus medinensis* and is close to eradication. A global effort reduced its incidence from 3.5 million cases in 20 countries in 1986 to 16,000 cases in 2004, 91% of which occurred in Sudan and Ghana. The infection has been eradicated from the Indian subcontinent and remains in only 11 countries of sub-Saharan Africa.

Transmission to humans occurs through drinking water contaminated with tiny crustaceans called *copepods* that carry larval forms of the parasite. A year or so later, adult female worms up to 1 m long emerge through the skin, usually on the lower part of the leg or the foot. Transmission is perpetuated when the female releases thousands of larvae into the water if the human host immerses that part of the body in a source of drinking water. Emergence of the worm is accompanied by a painful blister that ruptures and ulcerates. Fever and allergic symptoms, including wheezing and urticaria, often precede rupture of the blister. Affected persons may be incapacitated for weeks or months, often coinciding with major planting or harvesting seasons. Secondary bacterial infection of the ulcer with abscess formation is common.

Emerging worms can be extracted by winding a few centimeters on a stick each day. Chemotherapy is ineffective. Worms may be removed surgically. Prevention is achieved through the provision of safe drinking water.

OTHER FILARIASES

Perstans Filariasis

M. perstans infection occurs commonly throughout central Africa and northeast South America, but exact numbers are unknown. The blood-borne microfilariae circulate without periodicity, and adults reside in serous body cavities (i.e., pleural, peritoneal, and pericardial) and in mesenteric, perirenal, and retroperitoneal tissue. Most individuals are asymptomatic or at most mildly symptomatic, but a distribution that overlaps with several other human filarids has hampered definition of distinct clinical features. Reported manifestations include transient angioedematous swellings, pruritus, fever, headache, arthralgias, abdominal pain, and neurologic syndromes. Pericarditis and hepatitis have been reported. Eosinophilia and elevated antifilarial antibody titers are often present. No reliable therapy exists. Diethylcarbamazine and ivermectin are clearly ineffective. Some success with albendazole (two 400-mg doses per day) or mebendazole (two 100-mg doses per day) for at least 1 month has been reported. Doxycycline trials are under way.

Streptocerciasis

M. streptocerca, transmitted by midges, was thought to be restricted to the tropical forest zone of Africa from Ghana to Zaire, but it has recently been described as far east as Uganda. The adult worms are subcutaneous, and the microfilariae, which have characteristic hooked tails, are found in the skin, most often on the upper part of the body. Ocular involvement does not occur. Infection is usually asymptomatic, but pruritus and acute or chronic papular dermatitis similar to onchodermatitis can affect the trunk and upper extremities in up to 24% of those infected. Inguinal adenopathy is common. In areas of epidemiologic overlap, skin snips must be stained to differentiate *M. streptocerca* from *O. volvulus.* Adult worms and microfilariae are killed by diethylcarbamazine (6 mg/kg/day for 2 weeks). Ivermectin in a single dose of 150 μg/kg is microfilaricidal.

Mansonella ozzardi

M. ozzardi is found only in Central and South America and certain islands of the Caribbean. The blood-borne microfilariae circulate without periodicity, and the location of adults is unclear. Adult worms have been recovered only twice, both times from the peritoneal cavity. Although it is generally considered nonpathogenic, articular pain, headache, fever, pulmonary symptoms, adenopathy, hepatomegaly, and pruritic skin eruptions are reported. Ivermectin in a single dose of 150 μg/kg appears to suppress microfilaremia reliably for at least several months but is probably not adulticidal. Diethylcarbamazine is ineffective.

Zoonotic Filarial Infections

Uncommonly, several animal filariae, including *Dirofilaria immitis* and *Dirofilaria repens* in dogs and *Dirofilaria tenuis* in raccoons, can infect humans. Their distribution is worldwide, and the organisms are found in nontropical and tropical climates. The parasites die in the larval stages before reaching maturity and cause few symptoms. Localization is to the lungs with *D. immitis* infection (appearing as coin lesions on chest radiographs) or to subcutaneous tissue and lymph nodes with the other *Dirofilaria* species. Subcutaneous lesions may be migratory. Zoonotic *Brugia* infection localizes to lymph nodes. Eosinophilia and positive antifilarial antibody titers are unusual. Surgical removal of lesions is diagnostic and curative, whereas chemotherapy is uniformly ineffective.

SUGGESTED READINGS

Adinarayanan S, Critchley J, Das PK, et al: Diethylcarbamazine (DEC)-medicated salt for community-based control of lymphatic filariasis. Cochrane Database Syst Rev 2007;CD003758. *Meta-analysis showing some efficacy of DEC-medicated salt in the prevention of filariasis.*

Enk CD: Onchocerciasis—river blindness. Clin Dermatol 2006;24:176–180. *Comprehensive review with a focus on the dermatologic manifestions of the infection.*

Ottesen EA: Lymphatic filariasis: Treatment, control and elimination. Adv Parasitol 2006;61:395–441. *Clinical review.*

Taylor MJ, Makunde WH, McGarry HF, et al: Macrofilaricidal activity after doxycycline treatment of *Wuchereria bancrofti:* A double-blind, randomised placebo-controlled trial. Lancet 2005;365:2116–2121. *Potential new or adjunctive therapy for lymphatic filariasis.*

Tisch DJ, Michael E, Kazura JW: Mass chemotherapy options to control lymphatic filariasis: A systematic review. Lancet Infect Dis 2005;5:514–523. *Definitive comparative analysis of chemotherapy trials.*

380 ARTHROPODS AND LEECHES

David Schlossberg

ARTHROPODS

The Pathogens

Arthropods are bilaterally symmetrical invertebrates with an exoskeleton, segmented bodies, and jointed appendages. In the phylum Arthropoda, six classes are important sources of disease in humans: Arachnida, Pentastomida, Chilopoda, Diplopoda, Crustacea, and Insecta. Table 380–1 lists these classes, and their members are discussed in this chapter.

Arthropods cause disease in humans directly and indirectly. They bite, sting, envenom, and evoke hypersensitivity reactions; they also serve as vectors for infectious pathogens. Arthropods are the link between humans and age-old scourges such as plague, typhus, and malaria.

Infections spread by arthropod vectors are listed in Table 380–2. They are each described in greater detail elsewhere in this text and are not reviewed further here.

TABLE 380–1 MEDICALLY IMPORTANT ARTHROPODS

Arachnida (four pairs of legs)
Acari—mites, ticks
Araneida—spiders
Scorpionida
Pentastomida—tongue worms
Chilopoda—centipedes
Diplopoda—millipedes
Crustacea
Copepoda—*Cyclops, Diaptomus*
Decapoda—shrimp, lobster, crayfish, crab
Insecta (three pairs of legs)
Anoplura—lice
Coleoptera—beetles
Diptera—flies (mosquitoes, black flies, midges, horse flies, deer flies, greenheads, tsetse flies, stable flies, sand flies, houseflies, bluebottle flies, cockroaches; myiasis)
Hemiptera—bed bugs, cone-nose bugs
Hymenoptera—ants, bees, wasps
Lepidoptera—moths, caterpillars
Siphonaptera—fleas

TABLE 380–2 ARTHROPOD VECTORS OF INFECTION

Mites	Rickettsialpox, scrub typhus
Ticks	Colorado tick fever, viral encephalitides (e.g., Powassan encephalitis, louping-ill), viral hemorrhagic fevers (e.g., Crimean-Congo hemorrhagic fever, Omsk hemorrhagic fever), tick-borne rickettsioses (e.g., Rocky Mountain spotted fever, Mediterranean tick fever), ehrlichiosis, anaplasmosis, relapsing fever, Lyme disease, babesiosis, tularemia
Crustaceans	Dracunculosis, nematode and cestode infestation, paragonimiasis
Lice	Typhus, trench fever, relapsing fever
Mosquitoes	Malaria, filariasis, viral encephalitides (e.g., West Nile encephalitis, Eastern equine encephalitis), dengue, yellow fever
Deer flies	Loiasis, tularemia
Black flies	Onchocerciasis
Tsetse flies	Trypanosomiasis
Sand flies	Leishmaniasis, bartonellosis, sand fly fever
Cone-nose bugs	Chagas' disease
Fleas	Plague, murine typhus, ? *Bartonella henselae, Rickettsia felis, Dipylidium caninum, Hymenolepis diminuta*

Scabies

Definition

Mites are small arachnids, about the size of a grain of sand. They have a single apparent body region with a fused cephalothorax and abdomen. The best-known mite, *Sarcoptes scabiei*, is the cause of scabies. It has a worldwide distribution and is associated with war, poverty, malnutrition, and sexual promiscuity. Although it causes dramatic skin manifestations, the scabies mite is not a vector for other infectious diseases.

Scabies is spread by skin-to-skin contact, such as shaking hands, sharing a bed, and having sexual relations. It is also spread by fomites because the mite is able to survive for 2 to 3 days away from human skin and may infect clothing, towels, and bed linen. Activated by warmth, the mite burrows under the skin to the bottom of the stratum corneum in 2.5 minutes. The female moves at a rate of 2 to 3 mm/day and lays eggs as she tunnels. The male (seldom seen because it is smaller than the female and dies a day or two after copulation) makes side chambers or branches in the female's burrows. Burrows contain mites, fecal pellets, and eggs. In 2 to 3 days a larva is born, and it eventually molts through nymphal stages to an adult. This cycles takes 10 to 17 days. During the female's lifespan of 4 to 5 weeks, she lays a total of 40 to 50 eggs.

Pathobiology

Scabies may take several forms. Nodular scabies forms red-brown papules and nodules in the groin, axillae, and genitalia. Histopathologically, these lesions are characterized by multinucleated cells that resemble the Reed-Sternberg cells of Hodgkin's disease. Bullous scabies is seen in infants and children and mimics bullous impetigo and pemphigus. In adults, vesicular scabetic lesions mimic dermatitis herpetiformis, especially when in a sacral and gluteal location. The mites that cause scabies in animals (i.e., mange) are transmissible to humans after direct contact with horses, dogs, and other infested species. These mites are unable to propagate in humans, although they may cause papules or vesicles. *Norwegian* or *crusted scabies* is seen predominantly in immunosuppressed or elderly patients; additional risk factors include diabetes mellitus, renal failure, and topical corticosteroids. Norwegian scabies occurs as a local or generalized dermatitis with scaling and crusting and may mimic psoriasis. When the extremities are involved, there may be heavy involvement of the nails. Itching is often minimal. In this disease, thousands of mites are present rather than the 3 to 50 organisms seen in typical scabies; thus, it is extremely contagious. The diagnosis is relatively easy to make because there are so many mites, and scrapings should demonstrate their presence. This form of scabies may be complicated by bacteremia.

Clinical Manifestations

Typical lesions are small papules over the female mite, with wavy or linear burrows indicating her path. Typical locations of lesions are the interdigital webs, wrist folds, elbows, axillae, feet, thighs, nipples in women, genitalia, buttocks, and belt line. Crusted, excoriated, pruritic papules on the penis or buttocks are almost pathognomonic for scabies. Infants may have involvement of the head, neck, palms, and soles, areas typically spared in adults, although geriatric and immunosuppressed adults (e.g., patients with acquired immunodeficiency syndrome [AIDS]) may also have head and neck involvement.

These lesions cause severe itching, especially at night. A generalized rash may occur separate from the burrows. Other secondary local phenomena include urticaria, eczematous plaques, excoriation, and impetigo. Superimposed streptococcal infection occasionally results in post-streptococcal glomerulonephritis.

Many of the clinical phenomena result from sensitization. The incubation period for the initial infection is 2 weeks to 2 months because time is required for sensitization. With subsequent infection, however, itching may begin in 1 to 4 days. During the prolonged incubation period patients may be entirely asymptomatic even though they can transmit the disease. A clue to the presence of scabies is the appearance of typical lesions and pruritus in multiple family members.

In elderly and immunosuppressed patients, the skin reaction may be muted, with pruritus but minimal inflammation. Outbreaks in nursing homes and early disease in AIDS patients may go undetected. Scabies may also be asymptomatic (i.e., *scabies incognito*) in patients receiving topical or systemic corticosteroids.

Diagnosis

The diagnosis is made by skin scrapings of burrows or papules. Burrows may be enhanced by applying washable ink or tetracycline (which fluoresces under Wood's light) to an area of suspected involvement. When the area is washed off, remaining ink or tetracycline may indicate the presence of burrows. For microscopic diagnosis, mineral oil is applied to a scalpel blade and allowed to flow onto a burrow or papule, which is then scraped gently (until pinpoint bleeding occurs). The oil and tissue mixture is then microscopically examined for mites, eggs, or fecal pellets.

Treatment

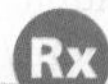

The preferred treatment of scabies is 5% permethrin (Elimite). This cream is applied from the neck to the feet and washed off 8 to 14 hours later. One application is usually adequate. In infants, the scalp, temple, and forehead are included. Crotamiton (Eurax) is also effective. It is applied from the neck down and repeated in 24 hours. The patient bathes and washes the crotamiton off 48 hours later. In infants, it is applied to the entire body. Lindane (Kwell) had been the mainstay of treatment for years, but it is limited in application as a result of toxicity; excessive absorption of lindane may result in central nervous system toxicity. It should not be used in individuals who have Norwegian scabies, premature infants, young children, pregnant or lactating mothers, or patients with a history of seizure disorder. In treating Norwegian scabies, the patient should take a bath first, apply permethrin, and repeat after 12 hours. This process should be repeated in a week, and an additional scraping should be done afterward in case further therapy is necessary.

Ivermectin—alone or in combination with other topical preparations—appears to be effective in the treatment of scabies, but ivermectin is not approved for this indication in the United States, and safety in pregnancy and in pediatric patients weighing less than 15 kg has not been established. Administered as a single oral dose

Rx

of 200 μg/kg, ivermectin has been especially helpful in treating Norwegian scabies because topical agents may have difficulty penetrating the crusts. Ivermectin has also been used in institutional outbreaks of scabies, in which it provides single-dose convenience for the treatment or prophylaxis of large numbers of patients. Some authorities recommend a second dose in patients with severe infection or after therapeutic failure. Resistance to ivermectin has emerged after intensive use in patients with multiple recurrences.

Nodular scabies may be treated by intralesional steroids. Antiscabietic medication is not effective in nodular scabies because there are no mites at this stage of the disease. Fortunately, its natural history is resolution with time.

In all of the therapies discussed, it is important to follow the manufacturer's instructions. Patients should trim their nails and scrub under their nails with a toothbrush, which is then discarded. Close contacts and family members who have had skin-to-skin contact should also be treated without waiting for lesions to appear. It is not necessary to clean furniture or carpets, but bed covers, pillow cases, sheets, outer clothes, and underwear, if used in the previous 48 hours, should be put in a hot water cycle or dry-cleaned.

After one course of treatment, scabies is no longer contagious. In the hospital, patients should be managed by contact isolation for 24 hours after the start of therapy. Clothes and linens should be placed in plastic laundry bags and handled only by personnel wearing gloves. Particular care should be taken for patients with Norwegian scabies because it is highly contagious; these patients should be isolated.

After therapy for scabies, pruritus may persist for 1 to 2 weeks. Most of the time pruritus does not indicate treatment failure, and symptomatic therapy with antipruritics is indicated. Treatment of scabies is summarized in Table 380–3.

TABLE 380–3 TREATMENT OF LICE AND SCABIES*

	Treatment	Alternatives
LICE		
Head lice Crab lice	1% Permethrin (Nix); clean clothing, headwear, and bedding	5% permethrin (Elimite) Pyrethrins (RID) Malathion (Ovide) Lindane (Kwell) Ivermectin†
Body lice	Clean clothing	
Eyelashes	Petrolatum	Trimethoprim-sulfamethoxazole Yellow oxide of mercury
Contacts	Treat sexual partners of patients with crab lice	
SCABIES		
Typical	5% Permethrin (Elimite) Clean clothes and bedding	Crotamiton (Eurax) Lindane (Kwell) Ivermectin†
Norwegian	5% Permethrin (Elimite) Clean clothes and bedding	Crotamiton (Eurax) Lindane (Kwell) Ivermectin†
Nodular	Intralesional steroids	
Contacts	Treat as for scabies	

*Manufacturers' instructions should be followed carefully with these products.
†Ivermectin is not approved for this indication in the United States, and safety in pregnancy and in pediatric patients weighing less than 15 kg has not been established.

Other Mites

Mites other than those that cause scabies generally do not cause permanent infestation. Most of them can bite and produce pruritic or allergic reactions. However, because their involvement with humans is transitory, treatment is symptomatic and involves elimination of the mite from a pet or the local environment. Topical therapy with corticosteroids and oral antihistamines are useful.

The follicle mite *(Demodex)* is an elongated, wormlike mite that occurs on the face and lives in hair follicles or sebaceous glands. It is frequently found in the absence of disease, although individual cases of rosacea, blepharitis, and perioral dermatitis have been attributed to *Demodex* infestation, and it has been described in patients infected with human immunodeficiency virus (HIV), in whom it may be a dermatologic manifestation of immune reconstitution disease. A variety of experimental treatments have been used with varied and anecdotal success, including topical crotamiton, sulfur and 5% permethrin, and both topical and oral metronidazole and ivermectin. Dust mites do not bite, but exposure to them may result in rhinitis, asthma, and childhood eczema. Infestation with these organisms requires treating the house by cleaning carpets, mattresses, and blankets and minimizing household humidity. Fowl mites infest humans in association with birds such as pigeons, and they are capable of biting and may cause a local dermatitis. Some of them are occasionally important vectors. For example, the fowl mite *Ornithonyssus sylviarum* can transmit the western equine encephalitis virus, and the viruses of St. Louis encephalitis and western equine encephalitis have been isolated from the chicken mite *Dermanyssus gallinae.*

A variety of food mites (e.g., *Pyemotes ventricosus*) are associated with cheese, cereal, sugar, flour, grain, dried vegetable products, eggs, and other foodstuffs. These mites penetrate the superficial epithelium and cause a papulovesicular or urticarial eruption. Occasionally, exposure to them results in fever, diarrhea, and anorexia. More commonly, it causes a chronic dermatitis; it has been held responsible for "grocer's itch," "copra itch," "dried fruit dermatitis," and "vanillism" (in those who work with vanilla pods). When inhaled, some of the food mites cause pulmonary infiltrates and peripheral eosinophilia, called *acariasis.*

The best known of the nonscabies mites is the harvest mite, chigger, or "red bug." These are *Trombicula* species and are the bane of picnickers and campers. They are bright orange to red and attach where clothing fits snugly, especially at the ankles, groin, and waist. They do not burrow but feed at a sweat pore or the base of a hair follicle for several days. It is the larval stage (not the adult) that attacks humans. Chigger larvae are tiny, about 0.2 mm long, in contrast to the 1-mm adults. The initial reaction to their bite is itching within 3 to 6 hours. Some patients experience a papular, urticarial, or vesicular rash, occasionally with fever and adenopathy. Treatment is a warm soapy bath or shower plus antipruritic lotions; topical corticosteroids or anesthetic ointments are also used. These mites are the vector for *Rickettsia tsutsugamushi* (scrub typhus) in central and eastern Asia.

An important mite associated with rats is *Ornithonyssus bacoti,* a vector of murine or endemic typhus *(Rickettsia typhi).* Another medically important vector is *Liponyssoides sanguineus,* the mouse mite, which transmits rickettsialpox *(Rickettsia akari)* to humans. This mite is capable of biting and is seen on rats and other rodents, as well as mice. Cheyletiellid mites are parasites of dogs, cats, rabbits, and other small mammals and are the cause of "walking dandruff" in these animals. They do not burrow but live on the keratin layer of the epidermis and produce a mangelike dermatitis in the animal. Humans, often pet owners, experience transient pruritus and a rash, typically papulovesicles on the flexor side of the arms, breasts, or abdomen. Cure in humans follows treatment of the pet.

The straw itch mite is also capable of biting; it is acquired by handling grain or sleeping on straw mattresses. The clover mite, associated with ivy, grass, clover, and fruit trees, may infest humans but does not bite.

Ticks

Like mites, ticks have a single, disc-shaped body region with a fused cephalothorax and abdomen. They are larger than mites, about the size of a pea. However, after feeding, engorged ticks may appear much larger. Conversely, the nymphs of some species may be extremely small, resembling a poppy seed (Fig. 380–1). Ticks are divided into soft and hard

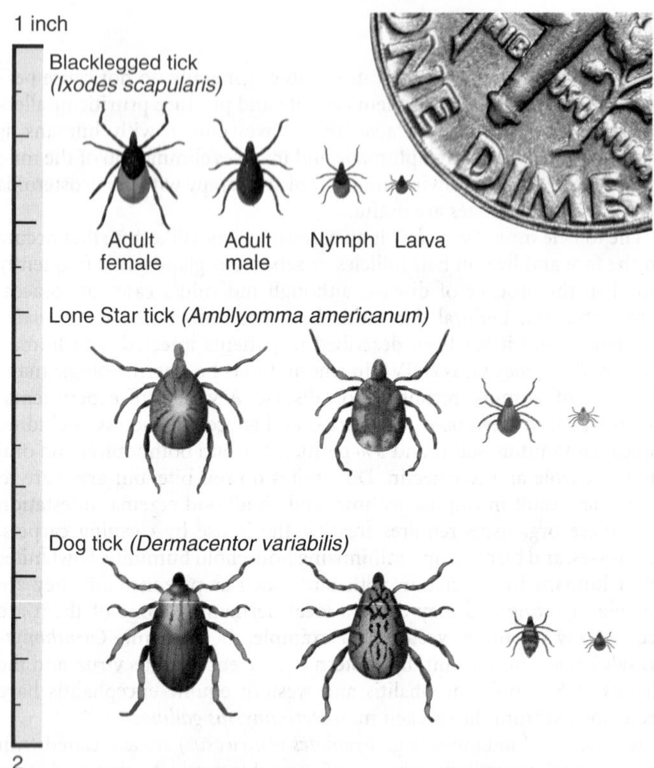

FIGURE 380–1 • Comparison of adult, nymph, and larval forms of three important tick species. A, The blacklegged tick or deer tick, *Ixodes scapularis* (formerly *Ixodes dammini*), is the main vector for Lyme disease in central and eastern United States. **B,** The Lone Star tick, *Amblyomma americanum,* transmits tularemia and human monocytic ehrlichiosis. **C,** The dog tick, *Dermacentor variabilis,* is the principal vector for Rocky Mountain spotted fever in the eastern United States (the related wood tick, *Dermacentor andersoni,* is the main vector for Rocky Mountain spotted fever in the western United States). (Courtesy of the Centers for Disease Control and Prevention.)

varieties based on a dorsal plate, or scutum. Most infections transmitted to humans are from hard ticks.

Ticks cause disease in a variety of ways. They transmit microorganisms that cause infection, they cause toxic and hypersensitivity reactions to their salivary secretions, and they directly inject toxin into a human host.

Most tick bites occur in the spring and summer. The bites are not usually painful or even symptomatic. Local swelling and erythema may result, and occasionally blistering or ecchymosis follows, sometimes complicated by necrosis and ulceration. In some cases a chronic granulomatous reaction may develop and persist for years.

Ticks do not fly, jump, or swim. They quest for host animals by waiting on low-lying vegetation and waving their legs or moving around on the plant and respond to nearby vibrations or carbon dioxide. After they contact their host, they move around to find a suitable location, often for 1 to 2 hours, before attaching to feed.

Ticks need time to transmit disease. For example, to transmit Rocky Mountain spotted fever, the tick has to feed for at least 8 to 14 hours before rickettsiae are released from its salivary glands. For Lyme disease, the tick needs at least 24 hours of feeding and possibly 72 hours to transmit disease efficiently. A tick removed while it is still wandering in search of a location for feeding or before it has had an adequate chance to feed is not likely to have spread disease to its human host.

Tick paralysis is not an infection, but an intoxication. Worldwide, 50 species of ticks cause paralysis in humans or animals. In North America there are six, including the species that also transmit Lyme disease, tularemia, Rocky Mountain spotted fever, ehrlichiosis, anaplasmosis, Colorado tick fever, and babesiosis; some ticks harbor more than one infectious agent, so it is possible to acquire multiple infections or both infection and tick paralysis simultaneously. The paralysis begins 5 to 7 days after attachment of the tick. It occurs most frequently in small girls. The child becomes irritable and lethargic; leg weakness develops and may progress to complete paralysis. The weakness can ascend and cause bulbar paralysis. Cranial nerve involvement includes the face and extraocular muscles. Eventually, respiratory paralysis supervenes, and death may occur. The patient remains afebrile. Characteristic features of this disease are its symmetry, the flaccid nature of the paralysis, normal pupils, intact sensory examination findings, clear sensorium, preservation of sphincter tone, lack of fever, and normal cerebrospinal fluid. Unusual manifestations can be extremely misleading and have included unilateral Bell's palsy, ataxia, chorea, and localized weakness of one arm or leg. These localized findings are attributed to the nearby location of the tick. For example, one-sided facial weakness has resulted from a paralytic tick in the ipsilateral ear. The differential diagnosis for tick paralysis is extensive, and tick paralysis has been misdiagnosed as Guillain-Barré syndrome, botulism, poliomyelitis, spinal cord compression, myasthenia gravis, and transverse myelitis. It is important to consider tick paralysis in a susceptible host; without removal the process may be fatal, but after the tick is removed, most patients improve within a few hours.

Tick removal has acquired an elaborate folklore. The safest and most efficient method is to grab the tick at the skin surface with tweezers or blunt forceps. The tick is then pulled steadily and gently out of the skin (see Fig. 348–2). None of the mouthparts should be left in the skin. The tick itself should be incinerated and the site disinfected. The best ways to prevent tick attachment are to keep pant legs tucked in boots or socks and use an effective repellent.

Spiders

Spider bites cause secondary infection, allergic reactions, and envenomation. Approximately 50 species bite humans, but a limited number cause severe disease in the United States: the widow *(Latrodectus),* the brown recluse *(Loxosceles),* the hobo spider *(Tegenaria),* the wolf spider *(Lycosa),* the fishing spider *(Dolomedes),* the green lynx spider *(Peucetia),* the jumping spider *(Phidippus),* and the yellow sac spider *(Cheiracanthium),* a greenish gray garden dweller that is the most common domestic spider in many areas of the United States. All these spiders except the widow may cause necrotic arachnidism. Bites from other spiders may be painful but are not dangerous. It is important for a bite victim to save the spider for identification.

The brown recluse, or *Loxosceles reclusa,* is the best known cause of necrotic arachnidism in the United States. These spiders have a 2- to 4-cm leg span. There is a violin-shaped marking from the eyes to the abdomen, with the base pointing forward. The brown recluse is not aggressive but hides in clothing and in the bathroom, attic, and closets. It bites only when threatened. Bites are painless until 3 to 8 hours afterward, and then the lesion ranges from a local urticarial reaction to full-thickness skin necrosis. Redness, swelling, and tenderness develop; sloughing, ulceration, and scabbing may follow. Some lesions show central blistering with ecchymosis surrounded by blanched skin, which in turn is surrounded by erythema. This is called the *red, white, and blue sign.* The lesion tends to extend downward gravitationally, "to flow downhill." Systemic reactions include fever, arthralgias, maculopapular rash, nausea, and vomiting. Treatment is controversial. Beyond the basic first aid measures of elevation, local wound care, ice packs, and tetanus immunization, a variety of specific interventions have been advocated but are of unproven benefit. Such interventions include antimicrobials, dapsone, antivenin, hyperbaric oxygen, corticosteroids, aspirin, heparin, antihistamines, dextran, vasodilators, nitroglycerin, and even stun guns. If used at all, surgical excision should be postponed until later in the course, when the venom is less likely to impair wound healing. Eventually, many patients require extensive plastic surgical repair.

The differential diagnosis for necrotic arachnidism is extensive, and many arachnologists contend that necrotic spider bites are widely overdiagnosed in the United States, particularly out of the native *Loxosceles* range of the south central and southwestern United States. Prominent mimics of necrotic arachnidism are listed in Table 380–4. The widow spider, found throughout North America, is also known as the hourglass, shoe-button, or po-ko-moo spider. It does not cause necrotic arachnidism but injects a neurotoxin (α-latrotoxin) into its victims. This toxin results in acetylcholine depletion at neuromuscular junctions. The bite causes pain at the bite site, which then spreads to local and regional muscle groups as a dull ache and sometimes numbness, followed by sweating, nausea, tremor, myalgias, muscle spasm, a boardlike abdomen, chest pain, paralysis, bradycardia, seizures, and rarely, death. Fortunately, less than 1% of bites are fatal.

TABLE 380–4 MIMICS OF NECROTIC SPIDER BITES
Other arthropod stings and bites
Pyogenic infection
Erythema chronicum migrans
Anthrax
Tularemia
Rickettsial eschar, e.g., *R. conorii*
Cutaneous leishmaniasis
Sporotrichosis, other mycoses
Herpes simplex
Vasculitis
Pyoderma gangrenosum
Neoplastic disease
Sweet's syndrome

The female spider (males do not bite humans) has a leg span of 3 to 4 cm. There is a red-orange hourglass on the ventral side of the abdomen; however, some species have red markings on the dorsal side, and in some, the hourglass is incomplete, appearing more like hatch marks. The wound should be cleaned and ice packs applied. Systemic therapy is undertaken with intravenous calcium gluconate, muscle relaxants, and tetanus toxoid. Antivenin is given if the envenomation is severe.

Tarantulas are large hairy spiders native to the southwestern United States, often inexplicably kept as pets. The tarantula bite is painful but without significant envenomation in humans, presumably because the spider is large enough to subdue its usual prey without much need for venom. The tarantula can also throw its hairs and provoke an urticarial response on the skin and keratitis if a hair lands in the eye.

Scorpions

In the United States, the only dangerous species of scorpions is *Centruroides exilicauda,* found in Arizona and New Mexico. Otherwise, scorpion bites in the United States are not serious unless the victim has a severe allergic reaction to them.

Scorpions inject a neurotoxic venom when they sting. The sting produces local swelling, pain, and numbness. Systemic signs may be neurologic (e.g., coma, tremor, paralysis of respiratory muscles, seizures), cardiac (e.g., hypertension, arrhythmias, pulmonary edema), and pancreatic. Scorpion bite is a common cause of pancreatitis in Brazil. Death may ensue within hours.

Therapy for bites includes ice packs and antihistamines. Some advocate applying a tourniquet and removing the venom from the wound by suction. Antivenin use is controversial. It has been suggested that patients receive nonopiate analgesics because opiates may have a synergistic effect with the venom of some scorpions.

Tongue Worm (Pentastomiasis)

Pentastomiasis is human infection by two genera of pentastomids, *Armillifer* and *Linguatula.* These wormlike arthropods are found principally in Asia and Africa and reside in the respiratory tract of birds, reptiles, dogs, and other mammals. Animals such as sheep or goats may also serve as intermediate hosts of the parasite, and when humans eat uncooked viscera or lymph nodes of these animals, gastric juices liberate the nymphs encapsulated in the viscera, and they ascend the esophagus and anchor themselves in the upper respiratory tract. This produces severe inflammation with violent coughing and occasionally causes asphyxiation. This syndrome is known as *halzoun* or *marrara syndrome,* referring to suffocation. Other symptoms include hemoptysis, sneezing, lacrimation, aural pruritus, coryza, facial edema, and vomiting.

Visceral infection is acquired by ingesting eggs in water contaminated with the sputum of animals harboring the pentastome in their upper respiratory tract. These eggs then hatch and develop into larvae that spread hematogenously through the body. This infection is usually asymptomatic and is discovered incidentally by the pathologist or radiologist as comma-shaped pleural or peritoneal calcifications. However, fatal infections do occur rarely.

Contact with Centipedes and Millipedes

Chilopods (i.e., centipedes) and diplopods (i.e., millipedes) are elongated, multisegmented arthropods. The centipede, or "hundred legger," has one pair of legs per segment and is a carnivore. Its bite produces a painful wound, and the larger species seen in the tropics and subtropics are also capable of secreting venom through their claws while holding their victim. The site of this envenomation may become ulcerated and necrotic, and patients may experience nausea, vomiting, and headache. Secondary infection is common. The wounds should be washed and cool compresses applied; antimicrobials should be given for secondary infection, and some patients have required administration of corticosteroids and local injection of anesthetic for the extreme pain.

The millipede, or "thousand legger," has two pairs of legs per body segment. This arthropod is a vegetarian and does not bite or sting. However, some tropical species emit a toxic fluid from glands on each segment when they are threatened. This fluid may cause local skin discoloration and burning, with the formation of blisters. If the eyes are contaminated, conjunctivitis or keratitis results and rarely causes blindness. Some species are able to squirt these secretions as far as 80 cm. Treatment includes washing the involved area of skin, and some advocate the application of solvents such as ether or alcohol to help remove the toxic fluid. If the eyes are involved, they should be irrigated copiously with water.

Crustaceans as a Source of Infection

Crustaceans may function as intermediate hosts of parasites that infect humans. Copepods are tiny aquatic arthropods that may be intermediate hosts of the guinea worm *Dracunculus medinensis,* the nematode *Gnathostoma spinigerum,* and the cestodes *Spirometra mansonoides* and *Diphyllobothrium latum.* The decapods include shrimp, lobster, crab, prawn, and crayfish. Land crabs and freshwater prawns may be host to the rat lungworm *Angiostrongylus* species; the lung fluke *Paragonimus westermani* is an occasional parasite of freshwater crabs and crayfish.

Lice Infestation

Lice are small (2 to 4 mm), dorsoventrally flattened, wingless insects that have mouthparts modified for piercing and sucking blood. They are parasites exclusively of humans and are seen in three varieties: *Pediculus humanus* var *capitis* (i.e., head louse), *Pediculus humanus* var *humanus* (i.e., body louse), and *Phthirus pubis* (i.e., crab louse).

Head Lice

Epidemiology

The head louse ("motorized dandruff") is usually transmitted by direct contact but can be spread by fomites such as combs, hats, brushes, headgear, earphones, bedding, upholstered furniture, and rugs. It is seen under circumstances of crowding and poor hygiene and is particularly common in schoolchildren, the elderly, and the senile. The organisms live for approximately 1 month on the scalp but are able to live only a few days (as long as a week) if removed from the warmth and blood meals available on the scalp.

Diagnosis

Infestation of scalp hairs can produce severe itching (although many cases are asymptomatic) and occasionally secondary pyogenic infection and cervical lymphadenopathy. Head lice favor hair in the back of the head. Lice may be visible crawling on hair shafts, and they may move quite rapidly, approximately 23 cm/min. However, they are few in number (usually <10), and it is much easier to identify the nits, the gray-white, glistening, oval eggs, 0.6 to 0.8 mm in diameter, that the lice attach to the base of scalp hairs. These nits are cemented securely to the hair shafts and are difficult to remove. They fluoresce under ultraviolet light (e.g., Wood's light), thus facilitating diagnosis, especially when large numbers of patients are screened.

Treatment

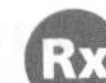

Patients should be treated with 1% permethrin (Nix), which has some ovicidal activity. It is available over the counter. The patient should shampoo, rinse, and dry the hair and then apply it to the hair and scalp. After 10 minutes it is rinsed off. Repetition in 1 week is necessary only if lice are seen again. As a result of growing resistance, there may be treatment failures with 1% permethrin, in which case 5% permethrin (Elimite) may be used. Other alternatives include pyrethrins with piperonyl butoxide (RID), Lindane (Kwell) (see precautions for lindane under the section on treatment of scabies), malathion (Ovide), or a single oral dose of ivermectin (200 µg/kg). Malathion is considered the treatment of choice by some if permethrin and pyrethrin therapy fails; however, malathion is flammable, so hair dryers and curling irons should be avoided during therapy. Furthermore, malathion is malodorous and requires a prolonged application time, although the recent literature suggests efficacy with 20-minute applications. Moreover, malathion's safety is not established for children younger than 2 years. Ivermectin is not approved for this indication in the United States, and safety in pregnancy and in pediatric patients weighing less than 15 kg has not been established. Because ivermectin has no ovicidal activity, a second dose after 10 days may be necessary to kill nymphs that subsequently hatch from nits. The manufacturers' instructions should be followed carefully with all of these products. When the patient is treated, all infested family members should be treated simultaneously, although prophylactic therapy is discouraged. Combing the nits reduces the number of viable ova and decreases the chance of relapse and treatment failure. Clothing that had contact with the patient's head should be washed and dried in a dryer or dry-cleaned.

Body Lice

Epidemiology

Body lice ("cooties") look like head lice but are slightly larger and have different clinical behavior. Body lice are seen in cold climates (because of heavy clothing) and under conditions of crowding and poor sanitation. They are most common in jails and crowded tenements and among military personnel. Unlike head lice, body lice are uncommon in affluent members of our society.

Clinical Manifestations

Lice and eggs are found in the seams of clothing, and very few lice are seen on the body of patients. The lice favor clothing fibers, especially wool, and live in the clothing, visiting the body only to feed. Clinically, the major manifestation is itching. Small red spots are produced, especially on the back and under the arm. Ultimately, excoriations, urticaria, pigmentary changes, and secondary infection may occur. "Vagabonds' disease" refers to the hyperpigmentation and thickening of the skin seen in chronic, untreated infestation. Body lice are also a vector for serious diseases of humanity, including typhus *(Rickettsia prowazekii)*, trench fever *(Bartonella quintana)*, and relapsing fever *(Borrelia recurrentis)*.

Treatment

Treatment of body lice requires only improved hygiene and cleaned clothing in mild cases. Heat kills both ova and lice in clothing. In severe cases and in epidemics, topical pediculicidal agents may be used.

Crab Lice

Pathobiology

Crab lice are transmitted predominantly by sexual contact, clothes, or infected hairs. During coitus, adult lice and nits are transmitted on broken hairs. Less frequently, they are transmitted by toilet seats or bedding. Though typically found on pubic hair, crab lice occasionally infect other short hairs of the body, including eyebrows, eyelashes, the edge of the scalp, moustache, and axilla.

Clinical Manifestations

Symptoms may not begin for 30 days after infection. On close inspection nits are visible, and the louse may be seen clinging to one or two hairs. Also evident in these infestations are dried serous fluid, blood, and louse feces. The combination of louse saliva and blood produces a blue-gray macule known as *macula cerulea.* The crab louse dies after 24 to 48 hours off the host.

Treatment

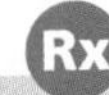

Treatment is similar to that for pediculosis capitis. It is important to clean bedding and clothing, which should be washed in hot water. Treatment failure often results from not treating other involved areas of the body. Infestation of the eyelid can be treated with petrolatum occlusions, yellow oxide of mercury ointment, or mechanical removal of nits. Oral trimethoprim-sulfamethoxazole has also been used to treat eyelid infestation; the mode of action may be eradication of the bacteria required by the lice for production of B vitamins and nit glue. Sexual partners and intimate contacts should be treated. A third of patients with pubic lice have other sexually transmitted diseases, including HIV infection, and should be screened for them. Children with pubic lice infestation in facial hair or eyes should be evaluated for the possibility of sexual abuse.

Symptomatic treatment of pruritus in all types of lice infestation consists of antihistamines, and in some cases topical corticosteroids may be applied to affected areas for additional symptomatic relief. Treatment of lice infestation is summarized in Table 380–3.

Beetle-Related Skin Injuries

Of the approximately 250,000 species of beetles, some are injurious to humans. The most common beetle injury is not from a bite or sting but from the formation of blisters. The best known blister beetle is *Lytta vesicatoria,* the Spanish fly. This beetle fills its breathing tube with air and closes its breathing pores to elevate body pressure. This maneuver forces the toxin cantharidin out through its leg joints. On human skin, cantharidin forms blisters within hours. Some of the blistering may evolve to ulceration and secondary infection. Clues to this cause of blisters are the presence of multiple blisters in the same stage of development and the lack of an accompanying rash. Sometimes the blisters form a line, reflecting the path of the beetle as it crossed the skin. When ingested, cantharidin causes nausea and abdominal pain. Cantharidin has been prepared commercially and used as a diuretic, aphrodisiac, and rubefacient. Other beetles, such as the carpet beetle, cause papulovesicular dermatitis.

Treatment of these beetle-related skin injuries is soap and water and wet compresses. Occasionally, topical or systemic corticosteroids are used.

Flies

The order Diptera contains the true flies, which transmit more disease than any other arthropod order. Prominent among the flies is the mosquito, a slender delicate insect that is a vector for disease throughout the world. *Anopheles* mosquitoes transmit malaria and filariasis; *Aedes* mosquitoes transmit viral encephalitis, dengue, yellow fever, and filariasis; and *Culex* mosquitoes transmit filariasis and viral encephalitis, including West Nile encephalitis, established in the United States in 1999. In addition to functioning as vectors, mosquito bites are irritating. The female mosquito lacerates human skin with her jaws and inserts a blood tube. Her salivary secretions contain an anticoagulant and cause local inflammation, pruritus, and urticaria. Mosquitoes prefer blacks to whites, young to old, warmth, strong scents, bright colors, and carbon dioxide, which is an effective attractant when humans and animals are grouped. The feeding habits of different mosquito species may differ. For example, *Aedes* mosquitoes are daytime feeders and usually inhabit urban areas, whereas *Anopheles* mosquitoes bite at dusk and are rural. *Culex* mosquitoes also bite at dusk or early evening. Although *Culex* mosquitoes are the main vector for West Nile virus in the United States, West Nile virus is also spread by *Aedes* and *Anopheles* species, both of which are established in the United States. Mosquito bites may be prevented by netting, protective clothing, and repellents. The most effective mosquito repellents are those that contain DEET (*N,N*-diethylmetatoluamide), with the longest duration of efficacy (up to 12 hours) in products containing concentrations of 50%. Other repellents, containing citronella, eucalyptus oil, alanine analogues, and soybean oil, are effective but for shorter durations than DEET. A product recently released in the United States contains picaridin, which has shown protection for up to 8 hours with a 20% solution in Europe and, unlike DEET, is odorless and does not damage clothing fabrics and plastics. However, the product currently available in the United States is only a 7% solution, for which no published data are available.

Black flies (i.e., buffalo gnats) are bloodsucking flies that are small (2 to 3 mm) and humpbacked. This fly injects an anesthetic compound into the wound so that the initial bite is not painful. Subsequently, the bitten area becomes pruritic, red, and swollen. Black flies transmit onchocerciasis in the tropics. Biting midges (i.e., punkies, gnats, no seeums, flying teeth) are tiny (1 to 1.5 mm). They cause immediate pain and erythema and eventually cause papulovesicles, with a nodular reaction that may last for months. These flies are small enough to pass through screens. Tabanid flies are large and colorful and include the horse flies, deer flies, and greenheads. They cause painful bites that often bleed because of the relatively large size of the fly and its bladelike mouthparts. Only the *Chrysops* (i.e., deer fly) is a vector of human disease in this group; it transmits loiasis in Africa and tularemia in the United States.

The Muscidae include *Glossina* species (e.g., tsetse flies), the vector of trypanosomiasis, and *Stomoxys* species (e.g., stable flies, storm flies, stinging flies, dog flies). The *Stomoxys* fly is slightly larger than the common housefly, and its resemblance has misled some patients into thinking that they were bitten by a housefly (which does not bite). The phlebotomid sand flies cause a painful bite and also transmit leishmania, *Bartonella bacilliformis,* and sandfly fever, a nonfatal viral disease. The bites of all of these flies are treated symptomatically by cleaning with soap and water, treating secondary infection with antimicrobials, and applying soothing topical ointments or corticosteroids. Nonbiting flies such as houseflies, flesh flies, and blowflies (i.e., bluebottle flies) can transmit disease, particularly that caused by gastrointestinal pathogens, by acting as mechanical vectors. They are also occasional causes of myiasis. Eye gnats do not bite but may transmit bacterial conjunctivitis and yaws.

Other than biting and acting as vectors of disease, flies may affect humans by causing *myiasis,* or infestation of the skin or a body orifice with fly larvae. A well-known example is the botfly found in the American tropics, which glues its eggs to a bloodsucking fly such as the mosquito; when the mosquito bites humans, the larvae leave the mosquito, hatch, and penetrate the skin of their new host. A similar form of myiasis is caused by the tumbu or mango fly in Africa, which lays its eggs on the ground or on soiled clothing. On direct contact with humans, the larvae penetrate the skin. The screwworm lays its eggs at the edge of wounds and may infect the nose, eyes, ears, and other body orifices. This larva often travels through tissues. Sarcophagid flies deposit their living larvae on the hosts. Some larvae migrate in tortuous channels and produce a type of larva migrans (i.e., hypoderma). Other flies that feed on decaying tissue occasionally cause myiasis in humans; the larvae enter living tissue after feeding on necrotic wounds. Usually confined to the skin or superficial wounds, myiasis can involve the genitourinary tract and the intestine. The larvae are usually passed spontaneously, although urethral involvement sometimes requires cystoscopy. Areas of cutaneous myiasis are frequently misdiagnosed as pyogenic infection, and this diagnosis should be kept in mind for a "boil" that is refractory to medical therapy if a patient has visited an endemic area.

Treatment of the cutaneous form requires mechanical removal by squeezing with tweezers or by excision. Covering the embedded larvae with strips of raw bacon fat or occlusive substances such as petrolatum encourages them to wriggle upward, where they are grasped more easily.

Exposure to Cockroaches

Cockroaches are important pests. They are able to consume any human or animal food, dead plant or animal material, leather, glue, fabrics, grease, hair, wallpaper, and bookbinding. They may function as mechanical vectors of pathogens and are sometimes intermediate hosts of helminths. Cockroaches can bite, but these bites are not particularly painful. Their glandular secretions can cause asthma when ingested, and cockroaches may be an important cause of asthma in children, in which group sensitization to cockroach allergens is commonly demonstrable.

Hemiptera: Bugs

Hemiptera are the true bugs and consist of bed bugs, cone-nose bugs, and wheel bugs. Bed bugs are 5-mm-long, flat, oval insects that resemble large ticks or small cockroaches. The most common species in temperate climates is *Cimex.* Bed bugs are not an important vector of disease, but their bites cause inflammation and occasionally produce hemorrhagic bullae. They are nocturnal feeders, have a distinct odor, and are capable of hiding successfully in the seams of mattresses, in couches, behind loose wallpaper, and under baseboards.

Cone-nose bugs are members of the reduviid family. They are 1 to 3 cm long and can fly. The best known of these bugs are the assassin bug (so named because it kills other insects) and the "kissing" bug (because it often bites around the lips and face). The kissing bug may transmit Chagas' disease, caused by *Trypanosoma cruzi.* Although some species of reduviid bugs produce painful bites that occasionally ulcerate and resemble necrotic arachnidism, the vectors of Chagas' disease produce painless bites. The bug defecates after eating, and it is the human host who scratches the trypanosomes into the skin. Although some species of cone-nose bugs are found throughout the United States, those that transmit Chagas' disease are found in Mexico, Central and South America, and only rarely in the southwestern United States.

The bites of all these bugs are treated symptomatically with topical antipruritic ointments and corticosteroids when needed, antihistamines for allergic reactions, and antimicrobials for secondary infections.

Hymenoptera Stings

The Hymenoptera include bees, wasps, and ants. These insects have an ovipositor designed to deposit eggs; however, the ovipositor has been modified to a stinging apparatus that injects venom, which causes severe local inflammation and sometimes elicits hypersensitivity. The familiar honeybee is yellow and black striped and has an ovipositor that is barbed; after the honeybee stings, the stinger and venom sacs are left in its victim, and the bee dies. During stinging, the honeybee releases pheromones that attract other bees to attack. "Killer bees" are Africanized honeybees imported to South America to improve honey production. However, multiple swarms escaped from experimental colonies and spread northward to Central America and the southern United States. The sting of the killer bee is not more toxic or allergenic than that of the domesticated honeybee, but the killer bee is more aggressive. Killer bees attack with less provocation; they sense intruders tens of meters from the colony and pursue them up to hundreds of yards away while exhibiting massive stinging behavior. Up to 50% of the bees in a killer bee colony are guard bees that respond to such threats. The bumble bee is not as aggressive as the honeybee but otherwise exhibits similar behavior and attacks perceived predators, particularly those that are darkly colored, moving, perspiring, or emitting carbon dioxide. Wasps include yellow jackets, hornets, and paper wasps. Yellow jackets are usually 1.5 to 2 cm long and are attracted to bright colors, perfumes, and human foods, especially those with high sugar content. They have familiar black bands and produce a large, honeycombed nest with a paper envelope. Hornets are larger than yellow jackets, 2.5 to 3.5 cm, and are brown, orange, and red. Paper wasps are the same size as yellow jackets but may be black, brown, red, or yellow. Their nest is a single open comb of gray paper, usually attached to a building or tree.

Of the 15 species of ants capable of stinging humans, 8 are found in the United States. The imported fire ants are the most troublesome. Found in the southeastern states, they bite and sting. They attach to the skin with their jaws and then pivot around their head to sting multiple times. The harvester ant, found in the western and southeastern states, stings its victim, and like the honeybee, its stinger may be torn off after envenomation. Velvet ants (i.e., wooly ants, cow killers, or mutillid wasps) look like ants but are wingless female wasps. They are red, orange, or yellow and achieve a size of 0.75 to 2.5 cm. Found in the western and southeastern states, they are capable of a painful sting.

The Hymenoptera produce local and systemic reactions. The local reaction is an area of inflammation that involves the immediate area of the sting, appears within 2 to 3 minutes, and abates within hours. Fire ant stings often develop into pustules, and lymphangitis may complicate harvester ant bites. Patients who have extensive local reactions have a slightly increased risk for future anaphylaxis. Local reactions themselves are not life-threatening except for instances of multiple stings (50 to 100 or more), which may be fatal as a result of toxicity rather than hypersensitivity. The effects of multiple stings suggest excessive histamine release, and antihistamines may therefore be appropriate in this setting. Otherwise, local reactions are treated with ice, elevation, local analgesics, corticosteroid creams, and lotions such as calamine. If a stinging apparatus remains in the skin, it should be removed. Systemic anaphylactic reactions are treated with epinephrine, corticosteroids, and antihistamines. Patients with severe Hymenoptera allergies should carry a preloaded epinephrine syringe, available in kit form, and should consider venom immunotherapy (Chapter 382).

Contact with Lepidoptera

Lepidoptera insects cause dermatologic and systemic disease through the hairs of caterpillars and moths. The caterpillars of several moth and butterfly families secrete venom from a gland at the base of specialized hairs or from cells lining the lower part of sharp spines. These hairs and spines can be irritating and allergenic when touched. An immediate burning sensation develops, followed by swelling, numbness, urticaria, extreme pain referred to regional lymph nodes, and rarely, headache, nausea, paralysis, and seizures. In the United States, the most bothersome varieties of caterpillar are the puss, IO, brown-tail, saddleback, and gypsy moth. The puss caterpillar is a particular problem in the southern United States. Puss caterpillars do not look like caterpillars, but like a teardrop-shaped tuft of yellow cotton. Some caterpillars, such as gypsy moth larvae, do not sting, but contact with their hair causes dermatitis, which has occurred in outbreak form in the northeastern United States. Some moths have scales or hairs that become airborne and cause urticaria, skin irritation, upper respiratory symptoms, and conjunctivitis. When occurring in great numbers, such airborne spread has caused epidemics on land or aboard ship. Treatment of caterpillar stings includes repeated stripping of the sting site with cellophane or adhesive tape to remove spines, local application of ice, antihistamines, calamine lotion, and corticosteroids. Zinc oxide and lime water have also proved helpful. Some advocate the use of meperidine, codeine, or intravenous calcium gluconate for pain in view of the poor analgesic effect of aspirin for these lesions. Systemic symptoms are treated with epinephrine, antihistamines, and corticosteroids.

Fleas

Fleas are small, brown, wingless insects that are flattened laterally. Human and animal (e.g., cat, dog, bird, rat) species may bite humans. Animal fleas can live for months without a host. If humans are available and a natural host is not accessible, fleas will bite. Their ability to jump several inches increases humans' vulnerability. Flea bites produce a punctate, hemorrhagic area initially, followed by a maculopapular, pruritic dermatitis. Typically, the papules are linear or clustered. The dermatitis may be more severe in previously sensitized patients. Most fleas feed on humans only transiently, but the chigoe flea (i.e., jigger, nigua, chica, pico, pique, or suthi), *Tunga penetrans*, burrows into the dermis, lays her eggs, and remains embedded in the skin. The chigoe is found in tropical America, Africa, the Near East, and India; lesions are most commonly seen between the toes and under the toenails. If it is found within the first 48 hours, a sterile needle can remove the flea. Later, surgical removal is usually necessary.

The term *sand flea* is used loosely by the lay public to indicate chigoes, cat fleas, dog fleas, human fleas, and tiny crustaceans found in seaweed along coastal beaches.

Other than the minor discomfort of bites or the focal persistence of the chigoe, fleas are vectors. The rat flea *Xenopsylla cheopis* is the most efficient vector of plague *(Yersinia pestis)* and murine typhus *(Rickettsia typhi)*. In the southwestern United States, a natural reservoir of plague exists among wild rodents, especially ground squirrels; domestic pets may then carry these infected fleas to their owner's home. Recent observations have associated *Bartonella henselae,* which causes cat-scratch disease, bacillary angiomatosis, and peliosis hepatis, with exposure to flea-infested cats. A newly described rickettsial agent, *Rickettsia felis,* is maintained in cat fleas by transovarian passage and uses the opossum as a reservoir host. It has caused a murine typhus–like illness in humans. Fleas may also act as mechanical vectors for numerous bacterial and viral infections by contaminated wind-borne feces that reach humans' mucous membranes. Several flea species act as intermediate hosts of the dog tapeworm *Dipylidium caninum* and the rat tapeworm *Hymenolepis diminuta* and infect humans when fleas are accidentally ingested.

DELUSORY PARASITOSIS

The psychiatric disorder delusory parasitosis can torture both the patient and physician. Typically, patients are elderly white women who have seen many physicians and then come to the examining physician with a container or small bag containing the suspected "bugs." Often, they claim that these bugs are in their vagina or rectum and emerge at night. Some patients have skin lesions from excoriation. After excluding true parasitosis and somatic disease, physicians should refer such patients for psychiatric evaluation. Some patients have responded to therapy with psychoactive agents such as pimozide or haloperidol.

Leeches and Other Annelids

Leeches are members of the phylum Annelida, class Hirudinea. They are segmented worms found in fresh and salt water and on land. Aquatic leeches are found in temperate and tropical climates. They attach to their swimming or wading hosts to acquire a blood meal. The bite of saltwater leeches is painful, whereas attachment of the freshwater variety may be asymptomatic. Smaller leeches may invade the upper respiratory or gastrointestinal tract, eye, nose, vagina, urethra, and anus. Thus, clinical manifestations in endemic areas include bleeding from the vagina or rectum, hoarseness, airway obstruction, hemoptysis, unilateral epistaxis, and severe anemia from unsuspected chronic infection of the airway or gastrointestinal tract. Bites of leeches often continue to bleed freely after the leech has stopped feeding because the leech injects hirudin, an anticoagulant that inhibits thrombin. Other allergens that the leech introduces may elicit anaphylaxis or a local hypersensitivity response, including bullae, urticaria, or necrotic ulceration.

In the Far East, land leeches attach themselves to travelers in tropical forests; they often crawl between the boot and sock and feed by penetrating the material of the sock. Treatment is removal, often facilitated by local anesthetic, salt solutions, alcohol, vinegar, or a lighted match. No mouthparts should be left behind. The wound is then cleaned and disinfected; residual bleeding can be stemmed with a styptic pencil. Leeches have been used in plastic surgery for tissue flaps and other tissues compromised by venous congestion. They have also been applied to sites of cutaneous ischemia in patients with purpura fulminans. Medicinal leech therapy has caused infection in as many as 20% of patients, although infection is not common after leech bites in the wild. These infections are usually due to *Aeromonas,* although leeches have also been shown to carry *Serratia,* other gram-negative enteric bacilli, and various rickettsial species. Most of the infections involve a surgical wound, with occasional bacteremia, and may be delayed by several days. In one patient, meningitis developed with leech therapy for a skin flap after cranial surgery.

Other marine annelids related to the leech can bite or envenom. The bloodworm, used as fish bait in North America, causes a painful bite that takes days to resolve. The bristle worm, found in Asia and the Gulf of Mexico and California, has chitinous spines filled with venom. A sting from one of these spines causes pain, rash, swelling, and occasionally skin necrosis. It is important to remove the spines in addition to applying topical soothing creams and ice.

SUGGESTED READINGS

Chosidow O: Clinical practice. Scabies. N Engl J Med 2006;354:1718–1727. *A case-based review.*

Golden DB, Kagey-Sobotka A, Norman PS, et al: Outcomes of allergy to insect stings in children, with and without venom immunotherapy. N Engl J Med

2004;351:668–674. *Immunotherapy was associated with a decreased risk of systemic reactions even 20 years after treatment is stopped.*

Ko CJ, Elston DM: Pediculosis. J Am Acad Dermatol 2004;50:1–12. *A review of head lice.*

Swanson LS, Vetter RS: Bites of brown recluse spiders and suspected necrotic arachnidism. N Engl J Med 2005;352:700–707. *Updates current knowledge of the brown recluse and related spiders, with emphasis on differential diagnosis and the overdiagnosis of necrotic arachnidism.*

381 VENOMOUS SNAKE BITES

G. Ralph Corey, James O. Armitage, and Steven A. Seifert

Five hundred of the approximately 2900 species of snakes are venomous, and more than 200 species have caused fatal envenomation in humans. Throughout the world, some estimate deaths at up to 100,000 annually, and hundreds of thousands of others suffer serious morbidity.

Epidemiology

The incidence of venomous snake bites varies enormously throughout the world. Snake-free areas consist primarily of islands, and Europe continues to be the continent with the lowest incidence of venomous snake bites. In the United States, it is estimated that up to 8000 venomous bites by native species occur each year, mostly by pit vipers (rattlesnakes, copperheads, cottonmouths), with fewer than 100 by coral snakes, the only native elapid. Fortunately, the number of fatalities, primarily caused by rattlesnakes, is below 10 per year. Children are at highest risk for complications. In addition, there are approximately 50 venomous snake bites a year in the United States by non-native (exotic) species, mostly in private collections, but also in zoos and academic institutions. In the past 10 years, human evenomation by more than 90 different non-native species has occurred. The majority are by viperids, with about 40% by elapids, mostly cobras. The case-fatality rate of exotic envenomation is two to three times higher than that of native species. Unprovoked attacks by venomous snakes are extremely unusual because humans are not seen as prey. Most bites occur on extremities when snakes are threatened by being trod on, by someone reaching where they did not look, or by intentional handling of venomous snakes. Prevention of snake bite is better than therapy.

Etiology

Venomous snakes belong to one of five families: Viperidae with its two subfamilies—Viperinae, or Old World vipers, and Crotalinae, or pit vipers, including rattlesnakes, copperheads, and water moccasins; Elapidae, including cobras, mambas, kraits, and coral snakes; Hydrophiidae (e.g., sea snakes); Atractaspididae (e.g., asps); and Colubridae, including boomslangs. Although all five categories contain venomous species, the two families responsible for more than 90% of venomous bites are Viperidae and Elapidae. In North America, pit vipers, named for the heat-sensitive organ between the eyes and nostrils that is used for hunting warm-blooded prey, are responsible for the majority of venomous snake bites.

In Europe, the only snake of importance is the adder, a viperid snake. Bites are uncommon and rarely fatal. Australia, on the other hand, is home to several very dangerous Elapidae: taipan, death adder, tiger snake, and eastern brown snake. As a result, there are many serious bites per year despite the low-density population. Fatalities are infrequent because of excellent treatment.

In Central and South America, pit vipers are the primary subfamily responsible for human envenomation; rattlesnakes (Crotalinae, *Sistrurus*) and the *Bothrops* species (*B. jararaca*, fer-de-lance) are responsible for the high morbidity and mortality. The largest venomous snake in the Americas is the bushmaster *(Lachesis muta muta)*. Africa is home to a large number of venomous species. Elapids (cobras and mambas) and the Old World vipers (e.g., saw-scaled viper, puff adder) are among the most prevalent and dangerous of all the world's snakes. In addition, because the health care system is less well developed, the mortality rate is high. The largest number of fatalities from snake envenomation occurs in Asia. In India and its eastern neighbors, elapids and viperids are prominent. Cobras, kraits, pit vipers, and saw-scaled and Russell's vipers inflict most of the injuries.

Pathogenesis

Snake venoms are complex poisons and often consist of dozens of components that immobilize and digest prey. Venom effects may be neurotoxic, cardiotoxic, hemotoxic, or myotoxic, and the presence or absence of particular components may be variable even within a single species.

Local swelling and bruising after a bite are caused by increased vascular permeability as a result of endothelial cell damage and are mediated by hydrolases, proteases, phospholipase A_2, polypeptide toxins, metalloproteinases, and the release of endogenous autacoids such as bradykinin and histamine. Snakes from the Viperidae and Elapidae families are primarily responsible for these effects.

Hemostatic abnormalities are frequent and varied. Procoagulants activate factors V, IX, and X, protein C (Russell's viper), and prothrombin (vipers) and cleave fibrinopeptide A from fibrinogen. Fibrinolytic activators result in a disseminated intravascular coagulation (DIC)-like picture without elevation of D-dimer (rattlesnakes). Snake venom hemorrhagins damage endothelium and increase the potential for serious bleeding, especially after viper bites. Intravascular hemolysis can occur after bites by *Bothrops* (e.g., fer-de-lance) and other species and results in severe anemia and acute renal failure.

Paralysis is the primary function of many types of venom of the Elapidae, Viperidae, and Hydrophiidae families. Presynaptic neurotoxins (e.g., β-bungarotoxins, crotoxin, and taipoxin) prevent acetylcholine release, and postsynaptic toxins (e.g., α-bungarotoxins and cobrotoxin) bind to acetylcholine receptors on the motor end plate.

Rhabdomyolysis occurs most commonly from the presynaptic neurotoxins of sea snakes, but myotoxins have also been found in Australasian elapids, Russell's viper, and selected rattlesnakes. Acute renal failure, hyperkalemia, and death often result. Other mechanisms of renal failure after envenomation include a direct renal toxin, hemoglobinuria after massive intravascular hemolysis, hypotension, and DIC.

Toxins that do not immobilize prey through neurotoxins may immobilize by causing hypotension. Some snakes (primarily vipers) produce an acute hypotensive syndrome just minutes after envenomation through the release of vasodilating autacoids. *Bothrops* species inhibit the breakdown of bradykinin and angiotensinogen (angiotensin-converting enzyme inhibitors). Vasodilation, diffuse vascular permeability, myocardial depression, and atrioventricular block all play roles in the hypotension caused by crotalines and elapids.

Clinical Manifestations

Pit Viper Envenomation

Swelling and pain are the first and most important findings of early envenomation. These symptoms often occur within 10 minutes and are followed by progressive proximal swelling and ecchymoses in the bitten extremity, although onset of the latter may be delayed for hours. Local swelling may be massive and compartment syndrome may occur, either from extrinsic tissue pressure or from intracompartmental venom injury. Necrosis may develop, typically over a period of several days, with the potential for tissue loss. Secondary infection may occur but is rare. The development of systemic symptoms such as nausea, diaphoresis, paresthesias, metallic taste, and dizziness may indicate more severe envenomation. Hypotension and bleeding manifestations (e.g., distant petechiae, gingival, gastrointestinal, hematuria, central nervous system) may also occur early and pose the greatest risk for death. During the first 24 hours, the white blood cell count is often increased, and various coagulation abnormalities, alone or in combination, may be seen, including thrombocytopenia, elevated fibrin split products with or without hypofibrinogenemia, and prolongations of the prothrombin time/international normalized ratio or activated partial thromboplastin time. Spontaneous bleeding is more likely with combined and severe coagulation system abnormalities. In patients with persistent hypotension, coma, acidosis, and oliguric renal failure presage death.

Progression of local injury may recur in the first 24 hours, particularly in patients treated with a Fab antivenin. Coagulation system disorders may persist despite antivenin and may also recur. After treatment with a Fab antivenin, recurrence of coagulation abnormalities typically takes place several days after treatment and may persist or recur for up to 3 weeks.

Coral Snake Envenomation

Unlike the pit vipers, local symptoms after coral snake bites are confined to paresthesias around the bite. Systemic symptoms are often delayed for 1 to 6 hours. With severe envenomation, perioral paresthesias, nausea, vomiting, hypersalivation, and euphoria give way to cranial nerve paralysis (e.g., ptosis, diplopia, dysphagia) and respiratory failure. Respiratory failure may develop within minutes of the onset of neurologic signs.

0	No envenomation: fang marks and minimal pain.
I	Minimal envenomation: fang marks, pain, 1 to 5 inches of edema, and erythema during the first 12 hours; no systemic symptoms.
II	Moderate envenomation: fang marks, pain, 6 to 12 inches of edema, and erythema in the first 12 hours; systemic symptoms may be present, along with rapid progression of signs from grade I; may be bloody ooze at bite site.
III	Severe envenomation: Fang marks, pain, edema greater than 12 inches in first 12 hours; systemic symptoms, including coagulation defects after pit viper bites; signs of grades I and II appear in rapid progression, with immediate systemic signs and symptoms.
IV	Very severe envenomation: local reaction develops rapidly; edema may involve ipsilateral trunk; ecchymoses, necrosis, and blebs and blisters develop; at tightly restrictive fascial planes, tension may become great enough to obstruct venous or even arterial flow.

FIGURE 381–1 • Grade I to IV scoring method for severity of snake bites.

Treatment

Rx

Expert assistance in managing a snake bite of any kind can be obtained by contacting the regional poison center at 1-800-222-1222.

On arrival at an emergency care facility, primary attention should be given to assessing and establishing the airway, breathing, and circulation. Supportive care is an important component of treatment and might include management of type I hypersensitivity reactions to snake venom or antivenin (e.g., epinephrine, H_1- and H_2-blockers), intravenous fluids, tetanus toxoid, airway protection, mechanical ventilation, pressors, pain medications, and later, débridement of necrotic tissue and physical therapy. Surgical treatment of tissue edema or compartment syndrome and antibiotics are rarely necessary.

Pit Viper Envenomation

Prehospital

Appropriate care consists of immobilization of a bitten extremity, consideration of the need to slow systemic absorption by dependent positioning, and most importantly, rapid transit to a hospital emergency department. Any treatment that increases or prolongs the local concentration of venom is likely to result in increased local injury and should be used only when life-threatening systemic effects (e.g., profound hypotension, anaphylaxis, severe bleeding) are seen. The application of a lymphatic constriction band (15 to 25 mm Hg) or a pressure immobilization bandage requires training and proper equipment and should be very rarely required. Popular prehospital treatments such as arterial or venous tourniquets, incision, suction, heat, cold, and electric shock are not helpful, can delay definitive treatment, and add additional trauma.

Hospital

The chance of a North American crotaline bite resulting in envenomation is around 80%. The onset of symptoms of pit viper envenomation is usually quickly obvious but may be delayed for many hours. Potentially "dry" bites should be observed for at least 10 to 12 hours.

The ultimate severity of envenomation becomes apparent only over time, and "mild" envenomation may progress to "severe," depending on the venom load, venom components, and host factors. A snake bite severity score (Fig. 381–1) can be used to assess the current degree of envenomation severity and to monitor response to treatment.

Definitive therapy for systemic symptoms of snake bite, including hypotension and coagulation abnormalities, is antivenin. Administration of blood product components is usually futile in the absence of adequate venom neutralization. With neutralization, the body replenishes platelets, fibrinogen, and clotting factors on its own. Blood products should be reserved for life-threatening bleeding and given in conjunction with additional antivenin.

In the past, because of the risks associated with antivenin therapy, treatment was restricted to patients with moderate envenomation

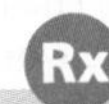

or greater. With the advent of a much safer ovine Fab antivenin, treatment has been advocated for any degree of envenomation, with the anticipated benefit that tissue injury and long-term morbidity may be minimized. However, the cost of antivenin therapy is significant, and whether there is a demonstrable benefit in mild cases is not known. Regardless, because of the inability to determine the venom load and ultimate classification of severity, if there are signs of progressive worsening of envenomation over time, definitive management is with antivenin.

The current crotaline snake antivenin in the United States, CroFab, was approved in October 2000. It consists of Fab antibodies to specific crotaline venoms that were raised in sheep. It is indicated and efficacious for all North American crotaline snakes. Because antivenin contains foreign proteins, hypersensitivity reactions are possible, including fatal anaphylaxis. To date with Fab antivenin, predominantly mild type I (immediate) hypersensitivity reactions have been reported in less than 7% of patients. Cutaneous sensitivity testing before administration is not recommended and, regardless, does not adequately predict the likelihood of a type I reaction in other settings. Type I hypersensitivity reactions are managed by stopping or slowing the rate of infusion and using standard therapies. It is usually possible to restart the infusion at a slower rate after treatment and to give the complete dose, although a risk-benefit reassessment should be made regarding the ongoing need for antivenin. Means of treating anaphylaxis should always be immediately available.

The initial dose of Fab antivenin is four to six vials regardless of patient weight because the object is to neutralize a specific quantity of injected venom. Additional doses may be repeated as needed to obtain initial control of the signs and symptoms of envenomation. Initial control includes reversal of systemic symptoms, cessation of progression of proximal swelling, and cessation of worsening or improvement in coagulation components. Repeated dosing of Fab antivenin after initial control (two vials every 6 hours for three doses) is recommended to prevent recurrence of local effects (Fig. 381–2).

Management of increased tissue pressure and possible compartment syndrome is controversial. Dermotomy may be considered in areas without true compartments (e.g., fingers) if the degree of swelling compromises circulation, although additional antivenin and elevation may reduce the swelling to such a degree that this procedure is not necessary. In practice, dermotomy is rarely required. If there is very tense tissue or compartment edema, intra-compartmental pressures should be measured directly. In general, additional antivenin is recommended for increased pressure (>30 mm Hg). Elevation is controversial because in other mechanisms of compartment

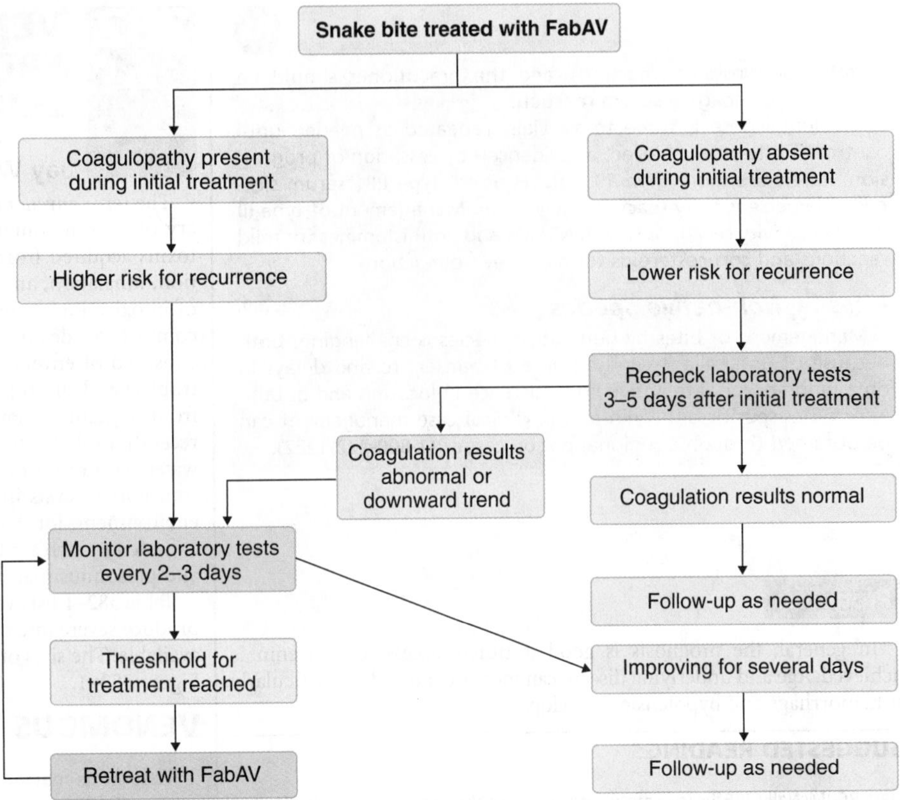

FIGURE 381–2 • Monitoring for coagulopathy in patients treated with Crotalidae polyvalent immune Fab (ovine) (FabAV).

syndrome it has been shown to result in decreased tissue perfusion. However, the mechanism of elevated compartment pressure in snake bite may be secondary to extrinsic tissue edema. In this case, elevation may result in proximal redistribution of tissue fluid with a reduction in extrinsic pressure on the compartment and thus a reduction in intracompartmental pressure. If there is either direct intracompartmental injection of venom or lymphatic drainage of venom into the compartment, a true compartment syndrome may occur, and elevation may be harmful, as with other mechanisms of this syndrome. Regardless, it has been shown in a porcine model of intracompartmental venom injection that fasciotomy does not improve tissue outcomes. Judicious elevation seems reasonable to add to additional antivenin in an effort to reduce compartment pressures before fasciotomy is contemplated. In the United States, reported fasciotomy rates vary from 4% to far less than 1% of cases.

Patients with early, severe coagulopathic abnormalities are at risk for recurrence of severe abnormalities of the same kind, with about 70% of those with early coagulation defects returning with late recurrences. The specific type of early coagulation abnormality and its severity generally predict the type and severity of recurrence. Optimal management of severe recurrence is undetermined, but patients with severe abnormalities in multiple coagulation systems (e.g., platelets and fibrinogen) or with comorbid conditions (e.g., advanced age, hypertension, bleeding diathesis, risk-taking behavior) are at increased risk for significant bleeding and are candidates for repeat dosing of Fab antivenin. Two vials should be given intravenously and the patient monitored and possibly treated daily until a clear improving trend is observed (see Fig. 381–2).

Post–acute Phase

In an effort to improve functional outcome, physical therapy should begin as soon as the acute phase of local injury has subsided, usually in 36 to 48 hours. Type III hypersensitivity reactions ("serum sickness," occurring 5 to 21 days after treatment), usually mild with Fab antivenin, occur in up to 25% of cases. Management of type III hypersensitivity reactions is with nonsteroidal anti-inflammatory drugs (NSAIDs) and antihistamines for mild reactions and corticosteroids for more severe reactions.

Coral Snake Envenomation

Prehospital

Appropriate care consists of immobilization of a bitten extremity and efforts to slow systemic absorption with the use of a pressure immobilization bandage. Because proper application of this technique requires training and it is frequently misapplied by untrained providers, a lymphatic constriction band (blood pressure cuff inflated to 15 to 25 mm Hg) may be safer, though possibly less effective. Most important is rapid transit to a hospital emergency department. Because local effects are minimal and neurologic toxicity may progress rapidly, there is little risk in the use of a properly applied pressure immobilization bandage or lymphatic constriction band. Popular prehospital treatments such as tourniquets, incision, suction, heat, cold, and electric shock are not helpful, can delay definitive treatment, and add additional trauma.

Hospital

The chance of a bite from an eastern coral snake resulting in envenomation is around 75%. The onset of neurologic symptoms may be quickly evident but may also be delayed for many hours. Because of minimal local effects and potentially delayed neurotoxicity, evenomation and the seriousness of such bites can easily be underestimated. The snake bite severity score is not valid for these snake bites. Potentially "dry" bites should be closely observed for at least 24 hours.

In the United States, a monovalent, equine IgG antivenin (Wyeth antivenin) is available for bites by the eastern coral snake *(Micrurus fulvius)* and also the Texas coral snake *(Micrurus fulvius tenere)*. It should be given at the first signs of envenomation. Skin testing is suggested by the manufacturer, although such testing should not delay administration in the event of life-threatening effects. Skin testing is also not adequately predictive of the risk for type I (imme-

diate) hypersensitivity reactions, and the practitioner should be prepared to manage a severe reaction.

The initial dose is three to six vials, repeated as needed until control of effects is achieved, as evidenced by cessation of progression. Rarely are more than 10 vials required. Type III ("serum sickness") hypersensitivity reactions may occur. Management of type III hypersensitivity reactions is with NSAIDs and antihistamines for mild reactions and corticosteroids for more severe reactions.

Bites by Non-native Species

Management of bites by non-native species is challenging, both because of unfamiliarity and because of barriers to and delays in obtaining appropriate antivenin. Assistance in locating and obtaining species-specific antivenin and in clinical case management can be obtained through a regional poison center (1-800-222-1222).

Prognosis

In general, the prognosis is good if timely access to antivenin is achieved. Age and underlying disease can increase morbidity, particularly if hemorrhage and hypotension develop.

SUGGESTED READINGS

Dart RC, McNally J: Efficacy, safety, and use of snake antivenoms in the United States. Ann Emerg Med 2001;37:181–188. *Overview of the various antivenins.*

Gold BS, Dart RC, Barish RA: Bites of venomous snakes. N Engl J Med 2002;347:347–356. *A comprehensive review of snakes, venoms, and treatments.*

Kularatne SA, Kumarasiri PV, Pushpakumara SK, et al: Routine antibiotic therapy in the management of the local inflammatory swelling in venomous snakebites: Results of a placebo-controlled study. Ceylon Med J 2005;50:151–155. *There was no benefit.*

382 VENOMS AND POISONS FROM MARINE ORGANISMS

Jay W. Fox

The term *envenomation* implies penetration by an organism for delivery of venom containing one or more toxins. In contrast, poisons are toxins acquired from the environment by mechanisms such as absorption, inhalation, and ingestion. In the marine environment, both forms of intoxication occur with effects ranging from mild irritation and discomfort to death. Previously, most clinically relevant intoxications consisted of envenomation from marine organisms found primarily in tropical and subtropical waters. However, severe outbreaks of poisoning from ingesting marine organisms containing toxins have occurred recently, probably because of increased microorganism growth in coastal waters as a result of a combination of eutrophication, aquaculture, and transport of cysts in the ballast of ships. Encroachment on the marine environment for recreation, living space, and food sources may be expected to increase the frequency of adverse encounters with venomous and poisonous marine organisms.

Table 382–1 lists venomous and poisonous marine organisms that can produce severe intoxication or death and indicates whether antivenom is available. The sites of action of some marine neurotoxins are depicted in Figure 382–1.

VENOMOUS MARINE ORGANISMS

Venomous marine organisms deliver their venom by biting and stinging (see Table 382–1). Envenomation involves penetration of the skin and may be complicated by bacterial infections, especially in situations involving deep puncture wounds and bites.

Sea Snakes

Sea snakes are members of the family Hydrophiidae and are generally found in tropical and subtropical waters. They are very common in the

TABLE 382–1 SIGNIFICANT VENOMOUS AND POISONOUS MARINE ORGANISMS

Organism	Type of Envenomation (Poisoning)	Primary Toxins	Antivenom Available
Sea snakes (Hydrophiidae)	Bite	Postsynaptic neurotoxin	Yes
Blue-ringed octopus (Octopodidae)	Bite	Postsynaptic neurotoxin (tetrodotoxin)	No
Cone shell (Conidae)	Bite	Presynaptic and postsynaptic neurotoxins	No
Box jellyfish *(Chironex fleckeri, Chiropsolmus quadrigatus)*	Sting	Hemolysins, proteinases, cardiotoxin, necrotoxins	Yes
Portuguese man-of-war *(Physalia physalis)*	Sting	Hemolysins, proteinases, cardiotoxin, necrotoxins	No; may be needed
Sea nettles *(Chrysaora quinquecirrha, Cyanea capillata)*	Sting	Hemolysins, proteinases, cardiotoxin, necrotoxins	No; generally no need
Sea anemone *(Anemonia sulcata)*	Sting	Neurotoxins	No; generally no need
Scorpionfish (Scorpaenidae)	Sting puncture	Hemolysins, necrotoxins?	Yes
Lionfish (Scorpaenidae)	Sting puncture	Hemolysins, necrotoxins?	No
Stonefish (Scorpaenidae)	Sting puncture	Hemolysins, necrotoxins?	Yes
Weeverfish (Trachinidae)	Sting puncture	Hemolysins, necrotoxins?	No
Stingrays (Rajiformes)	Sting puncture	?	No
Dinoflagellates		Ciguatera poisoning, ciguatoxins, maitotoxin (neurotoxins)	
Gambierdiscus toxicus	Poisonous (found in fish)		
Ptychodiscus brevis	Poisonous (found in shellfish)	Neurotoxic shellfish poisoning, neurotoxins	
Gonyaulax species	Poisonous (found in shellfish)	Paralytic shellfish poisoning	
Pyrodinium species	Poisonous (found in shellfish)	Saxitoxin, neosaxitoxin, and gonyautoxin	
Jania species	Poisonous (found in shellfish)	Okadaic acid (phosphatase inhibitors)	
Pufferfish (Tetraodontiformes)	Poisonous	Tetrodotoxin (neurotoxin)	No
Porcupinefish (Tetraodontiformes)	Poisonous	Tetrodotoxin (neurotoxin)	
Sunfish (*Mola* species)	Poisonous	Tetrodotoxin	

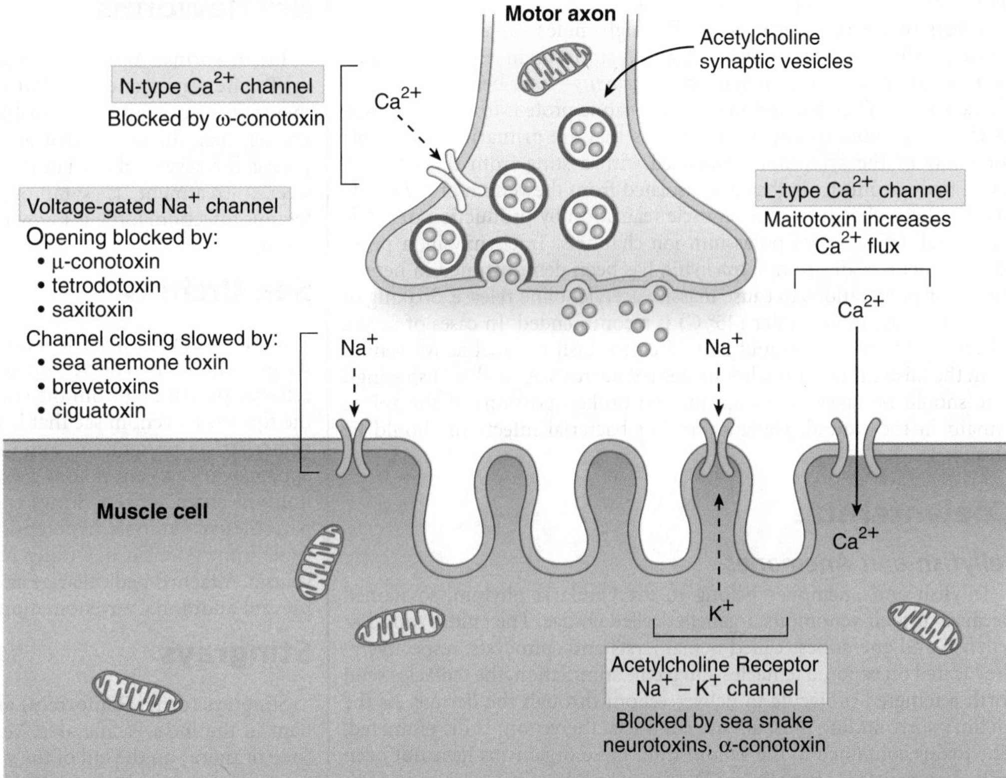

FIGURE 382–1 • Schematic representation of a motor axon synapse and the sites of action of various marine neurotoxins.

coastal waters of Thailand, Indonesia, the Persian Gulf, Australia, and India. One species of sea snake, *Pelaramis platurus,* the yellow-bellied sea snake, is found in the Pacific coastal waters of Central America. Sea snakes are very capable swimmers but do not come ashore and are relatively immobile on land. They inject their venom with two small maxillary fangs (2 to 4 mm long) containing ducts connected to venom glands located posterior and ventral to the maxillary bone. The relatively short length of the fangs prevents effective envenomation through most protective clothing such as dive suits. If the subject reacts to envenomation by forceful retraction, the fangs are often dislodged from the maxillary bone of the snake and may remain in the site—a condition that imposes an additional risk for infection.

Because of the nature of the venom and the size of the fangs, the sea snake bite itself is not generally painful. One or two small prick marks are present at the envenomation site, as occasionally are additional marks from the other teeth in the snake's mouth. The primary toxin in sea snake venom is a postsynaptic peptide neurotoxin that functions by blocking the acetylcholine receptor at neuromuscular junctions (see Fig. 382–1). The symptoms of sea snake envenomation are mainly neurologic and typically appear within 30 minutes to 2 hours after the bite. Ptosis, dysphagia, and nonrigid paralysis occur. In severe cases, respiratory failure may develop, and respiratory support may be necessary.

Mollusks

Blue-Ringed and Spotted Octopus

The blue-ringed and spotted octopuses (*Hapalochlaena maculosa* and *Hapalochlaena lunulata*), found in Australian waters, inject their venom by a relatively painless bite and produce two small puncture wounds. Hemorrhage at the site may occur. The major toxic component in the venom is tetrodotoxin, a postsynaptic neurotoxin that causes perioral and intraoral paresthesias, dysphagia, nausea, ataxia, aphonia, flaccid muscular paralysis, and respiratory distress or failure. Fatal envenomation has occurred.

Cone Shells

Cone shell venom is injected into victims through a hollow, harpoon-like tooth. The venom is primarily neurotoxic and causes paresthesias, hypotension, and respiratory impairment or failure. Seven superfamilies of neurotoxins have been identified in cone shell venom: A (families: α, ρ, αA, κA), M (families: μ, ψ), O (families: ω, κ, δ, μO, χ), P (family: spastics), S (family: σ), I (family: excitatory, κI), and T (families: τ, χ). All of the conotoxins are short polypeptides that demonstrate a variety of neurotoxic actions via targeting specific subtypes of ion channels, neurotransmitter receptors, or transporters (see Fig. 382–1). The bite is very painful and may be followed by systemic symptoms such as dysphagia, aphonia, pruritus, blurred vision, syncope, muscular paralysis, and respiratory and cardiac failure. In cases of severe envenomation, preparation for cardiovascular and respiratory support should be made. Rare cases of coagulopathy have been reported, and fatal envenomation has occurred.

Weeverfish, Scorpionfish, Stonefish, and Lionfish

Weeverfish belong to the Trachinidae family, whereas scorpionfish, stonefish, and lionfish all belong to the family Scorpaenidae. Members of the Scorpaenidae family are mostly found in tropical and subtropical waters. Weeverfish occur in European and African waters. All of these fish sting by using dorsal spines. The anal spines of Scorpaenidae fish and the opercular spines of Trachinidae fish can also deliver venom. The spines are encased in an integumentary sheath that is torn when the spine punctures the victim's skin. Venom glands are located at the base of the spine.

Few details are known regarding the biochemistry and pharmacology of the toxins in weeverfish venom. The sting of the weeverfish is extremely painful and may produce systemic effects such as aphonia, fever, chills, dyspnea, cyanosis, nausea, syncope, hypotension, and arrhythmias. The wound is edematous, erythematous, and ecchymotic. Bacterial infection is typical, and gangrene has developed in severe cases of infection. The venom may be somewhat heat labile, and soaking in tolerably hot water may relieve some pain and attenuate the effects of the venom. Death from a weeverfish sting is rare.

Scorpionfish *(Scorpanena)* are primarily found in tropical and subtropical waters and the Mediterranean. The stings of these fish have been described to be very similar to those of the weeverfish. Lionfish *(Pterois)* dwell in tropical waters; their stings are generally the most severe of all of the fish stings and occasionally cause death from hypotension. Because the venom is heat labile, soaking in hot water is recommended.

The stonefish *(Synanceja)* group is found throughout the Indo-Pacific area, China, Australia, and the Indian Ocean and is considered to be the most venomous. Symptoms are similar to those from the stings of members of the other groups. Similar high-molecular-weight toxins—verrucotoxin from *Synanceja verrucosa,* stonustoxin from *Synanceja horrida,* and cytolysin from *Synanceja trachynis*—have been isolated and characterized. They are multimeric, heat-labile protein toxins composed of α- and β-subunits and are the toxins that are primarily responsible for many of the symptoms associated with a sting from these fish. A lethal toxin, stonustoxin, has been isolated from the venom of *S. horrida* and has been shown to cause muscle relaxation by production of nitric oxide and activation of potassium ion channels. Trachynilysin, a pore-forming neurotoxin from *S. trachynis,* has been demonstrated in neuromuscular preparations to cause massive acetylcholine release. Soaking of the wound site in hot water (45° C) is recommended. In cases of severe blistering, the blisters should be excised to flush residual active venom from the blister fluid to ameliorate dermal necrosis. As with all fish stings, care should be taken to ensure that no broken portions of the spines remain in the wound; vigilance against bacterial infections should be observed.

Coelenterates

Jellyfish and Anemones

Jellyfish and anemones belong to the Cnidaria phylum, so named because of their venomous organelles called cnidae. The cnidae found in jellyfish and anemones (called nematocysts and spirocysts, respectively) are located on exposed tentacles. On tactile stimulation, the tentacles send forth a tethered projectile to deliver venom through the dermis. As the victim's surrounding musculature contracts, the venom is disseminated. The toxins contained in the venom from these organisms have not been fully documented. Hemolysins, DNAases, and histamine releasers have been identified in some venoms. Several peptide toxins have been characterized from the sea anemone *Anemonia sulcata;* they act similarly to α-scorpion toxins by inactivating the sodium channel.

Stings by jellyfish and anemones typically produce immediate pain at the site of envenomation, followed by erythematous and urticarial lesions. Anaphylaxis is not common in most situations unless previous sensitization has occurred. Depending on the severity of the sting, wheals and whiplike patterns at the sites of envenomation may appear within a few minutes or be delayed by several hours, followed in some cases by dermal necrosis. Recurrence of eruptions days after the envenomation has been reported. Systemic reactions may include muscle spasms and cramps, vomiting, nausea, diarrhea, diaphoresis, and in rare cases, cardiorespiratory failure.

Verapamil can suppress cardiac arrhythmia but does not ameliorate respiratory depression. Unfired nematocysts on tentacles adhering to the skin may be neutralized by vinegar or baking soda, depending on the species of jellyfish. Vinegar seems to be most useful for Portuguese man-of-war *(Physalia physalis)* and Australian blue bottle *(Physalia utriculus)* stings, whereas baking soda appears more efficacious for sea nettle *(Chrysaora quinquecirrha)* stings.

The box jellyfish *(Chironex fleckeri)* found in Australian waters is perhaps the most venomous jellyfish; it produces very severe stings that may cause death from hypotension, muscular and respiratory paralysis, and ultimately, cardiac arrest. Treatment of box jellyfish stings may require respiratory support and administration of an antivenin.

Sponges

Some sponges colonized by coelenterates produce toxins that can cause a pruritic, allergenic dermatitis or an irritant dermatitis. These toxins are delivered by the sharp spicules present in the sponges, which when handled penetrate the dermis. The toxins can cause the typical sponge diver's disease characterized by local burning and itching, which in severe cases may be accompanied by soft tissue edema and purulent vesiculation. Serious illness is rare.

Corals

Fire coral *(Millepora alcicornis)* is found in shallow tropical waters. Stings are a common consequence of brushing or rubbing against the coral. Envenomation produces a burning or stinging sensation, followed by severe pruritus. Edematous wheals may occur but generally dissipate over the course of several days. The site of envenomation should be soaked in dilute acetic acid or isopropanol to relieve pain.

Bristleworms

Bristleworms *(Annelida)* are segmented invertebrates found in tropical Pacific waters and the Gulf of Mexico. The bristles present on segments of the organism are capable of penetrating the skin and producing severely painful envenomation with pruritus and burning that may persist for several days. Local paresthesia is likely and may linger for weeks. Treatment is symptomatic, with consideration of possible tetanus infection. Little is known regarding the chemistry of bristleworm venom.

Sea Urchins

Of the echinoderms, sea urchins and sea stars are responsible for most stings in humans. The venom is delivered by the long spines and pedicellariae protruding from the sea urchin body. The spines are covered at the tips with a venom sac that is broken when it penetrates the skin. The pedicellariae, present on some species of sea urchins, are pincer-like appendages carrying venom glands. The toxins of sea urchin venom are not well characterized. Stings can produce pain, hemorrhage, aphonia, paresthesias, paralysis, hypotension, nausea, syncope, and respiratory distress. Immersion in hot water helps inactivate heat-labile toxins in the venom. Attached pedicellariae and embedded spines must be removed to prevent additional envenomation.

Stingrays

Stingrays (order Rajiformes) are found in most seas but are predominant in the Indo-Pacific area. Venom is delivered by stings from spines (one or more) on the tail of the stingray. Stingray spines are retroserrated on the margins and are covered by an integumentary sheath. Venomous glandular tissue is located at the base of the spines. On puncture of the skin, the sheath is torn by the serrated spine and venom flows along the two ventrolateral grooves of the spine into the surrounding tissue. One of the toxins identified in the venom is serotonin. The spines are often deeply embedded in the tissue and difficult to extract because of the retroserration. Care must be taken to remove all spine and sheath fragments. A sting produces severe pain and edema, which in extreme cases is accompanied by hemorrhage, syncope, vomiting, hypotension, and cardiac arrhythmia. In rare cases, death can occur, especially if the pericardial, peritoneal, or pleural cavities are penetrated. Soaking the wound in hot water inactivates some of the heat-labile toxins in the venom.

POISONOUS MARINE ORGANISMS

Marine poisoning nearly always results from consumption of fish or shellfish harboring various toxins. The causes of three types of marine poisoning are fish or shellfish containing toxins produced by dinoflagellates (i.e., ciguatera, neurotoxic shellfish, paralytic shellfish, and diarrhetic shellfish poisoning), fish that produce their own toxin (i.e., Tetraodontiformes fish), and fish containing significant levels of bacteria that have metabolized histidine to histamine, thereby resulting in pseudoallergic reactions.

Ciguatera Poisoning

Ciguatera toxins have been identified in more than 400 species of fish. During blooms of the dinoflagellate *Gambierdiscus toxicus,* toxins produced by these organisms concentrate in the fish to levels that are toxic to humans when ingested. The primary toxins responsible for ciguatera poisoning are ciguatoxins, which are cyclic polyethers that act as excitatory agents by binding to sodium channels. Maitotoxin, from the same dinoflagellate, is a water-soluble polyether and acts by enhancing calcium entry through L-type calcium channels. Symptoms of ciguatera poisoning generally appear within 2 to 12 hours after the ingestion of contaminated fish. Gastrointestinal symptoms, including diarrhea, abdominal pain, nausea, and vomiting, appear first, followed by neurologic and cardiovascular symptoms. Neurologic symptoms include aphonia, dental dysesthesias, fatigue, tremor, ataxia, pruritus, extremity and perioral dysesthesia, vertigo, headache, myalgia, arthralgia, temperature reversal, and hyporeflexia. Cardiovascular symptoms, such as bradycardia and hypotension, occur least often. There is no specific treatment of ciguatera poisoning; supportive, symptom-based therapy is indicated. Death from ciguatera poisoning has occurred but is rare.

Neurotoxic Shellfish Poisoning

Neurotoxic shellfish poisoning is caused by eating shellfish that contain brevetoxins produced by the dinoflagellate *Ptychodiscus brevis.* Brevetoxins are cyclic polyethers that function similarly to ciguatoxins. Gastrointestinal and neurologic symptoms of intoxication appear within 3 hours after toxic shellfish is eaten and are similar to those of ciguatera poisoning. Treatment is supportive. No deaths have been reported after neurotoxic shellfish poisoning.

Paralytic Shellfish Poisoning

Paralytic shellfish poisoning is significantly more severe than neurotoxic shellfish poisoning and predominantly involves neurologic symptoms with less pronounced gastrointestinal symptoms such as nausea, vomiting, and diarrhea. The toxins responsible for paralytic shellfish poisoning are from the dinoflagellate genera *Gonyaulax, Pyrodinium,* and *Jania* and are harbored in a variety of shellfish. The primary paralytic shellfish poisoning toxins—saxitoxin, neosaxitoxin, and gonyautoxin—are heterocyclic compounds that block nerve and muscle action potentials by binding to sodium channels. The site of binding overlaps with tetrodotoxin and results in paralysis. Symptoms appear soon after the consumption of contaminated shellfish (minutes to hours), beginning with circumoral and extremity paresthesias. Additional neurologic symptoms such as ataxia, arthralgia, dysphagia, dysmetria, diaphoresis, and tachycardia soon follow the initial paresthesias. Respiratory depression or failure can occur and may result in death, usually within 12 hours of the onset of symptoms. As with other shellfish poisoning, therapy is supportive, with close attention paid to potential respiratory distress or failure.

Diarrhetic Shellfish Poisoning

Diarrhetic shellfish poisoning is also caused by eating shellfish that are contaminated by dinoflagellate toxins. The two primary toxins associated with diarrhetic shellfish poisoning are okadaic acid and pectenotoxin. Okadaic acid is a polyether derivative of a 38-carbon fatty acid. It functions as an inhibitor of protein phosphatase 1 and 2A and causes smooth and cardiac muscle contraction. Symptoms of diarrhetic shellfish poisoning begin with abdominal cramps and nausea and progress to diarrhea. Additional, delayed symptoms occurring approximately 35 hours after ingestion may appear and include vomiting, vertigo, diarrhea, cramps, and headache. Treatment is supportive.

Tetraodontiformes (Pufferfish, Porcupinefish, and Sunfish) Poisoning

Pufferfish (i.e., blowfish, balloonfish, and toadfish), porcupinefish, and sunfish (*Mola* species) have a very potent toxin, tetrodotoxin, in their livers, gonads, intestines, and skin. The flesh of the fish (fugu) is a delicacy in Japan and is prepared by specially trained chefs to avoid serving significant amounts of toxins. Tetrodotoxin is a heterocyclic compound that binds at voltage-sensitive sodium channels (at an overlapping site with saxitoxin) to block sodium passage, thereby preventing nerve and muscle action potentials and resulting in paralysis. Symptoms occur rapidly (several minutes to several hours), beginning with circumoral paresthesias and progressing to widespread paresthesias. After the initial paresthesias, additional symptoms soon follow, including ataxia, weakness, aphonia, diaphoresis, excess salivation, dyspnea, dysphagia, weakness, and respiratory distress or failure. Gastrointestinal symptoms include nausea, vomiting, and diarrhea. Coagulopathies have been associated with tetrodotoxin intoxication. Respiratory intervention is crucial in light of the potential for complete flaccid paralysis. Without respiratory assistance, death is not unusual in cases of severe intoxication.

Scombroid Fish Poisoning

Scombroid poisoning is a pseudoallergic fish poisoning caused by the consumption of certain types of fish that have been improperly stored, including scombroid fish (e.g., tuna, mackerel, wahoo, bonito, albacore, skipjack) and nonscombroid fish (e.g., mahi-mahi, amberjack, sardines, and herring). The poisoning results from high levels of histamine and saurine present in the fish because of bacterial catabolism of histidine. The appearance of symptoms from intoxication is rapid (within minutes to hours), beginning with flushing of the skin, oral paresthesias, pruritus, urticaria, nausea, vomiting, diarrhea, vertigo, headache, bronchospasm, dysphagia, tachycardia, and hypotension. Therapy should follow a course for allergic reaction and anaphylaxis. The symptoms usually resolve in several hours.

SUGGESTED READINGS

Bedry R, Gabinski C, Paty MC: Diagnosis of scombroid poisoning by measurement of plasma histamine. N Engl J Med 2000;342:520–521. *Elevated levels of histamine in the appropriate clinical scenario is suggestive of scombroid poisoning.*

Chegini S, Metcalfe DD: Contemporary issues in food allergy: Seafood toxin–induced disease in the differential diagnosis of allergic reactions. Allergy Asthma Proc 2005;26:183–190. *A practical clinical overview.*

Hamilton B, Hurbungs M, Vernoux JP, et al: Isolation and characterisation of Indian Ocean ciguatoxin. Toxicon 2002;40:685–693. *Identification of a new, distinct ciguatoxin.*

Khoo HE: Bioactive proteins from stonefish venom. Clin Exp Pharmacol Physiol 2002;29:802–806. *Review of one of the most common venomous fish.*

Klsbister G, Kiernan MC: Neurotoxic marine poison. Lancet Neurol 2005;4:219–228. *Overview of marine poisoning from ingestion of marine animals.*

Salam AM, Albinali HA, Gehani AA, et al: Acute myocardial infarction in a professional diver after jellyfish sting. Mayo Clin Proc 2003;78:1557–1560. *An unusual complication.*

Terlau H, Olivera BM: Conus venoms: A rich source of novel ion channel–targeted peptides. Physiol Rev 2004;84:41–68. *A thorough review of conus toxins.*

383 ANTIVIRAL THERAPY (NON-HIV)

John H. Beigel and Frederick G. Hayden

Although some viral infections are self-limited, others can cause significant morbidity and mortality. Effective therapy is available for many of these infections. Emerging viral diseases such as coronaviruses and avian influenza, concern over viral agents of bioterrorism, and treatment of chronic viral diseases such as hepatitis B and C have led to a reinvigorated search for new antiviral agents. This chapter reviews currently available antiviral agents for the treatment of infections caused by viruses other than human immunodeficiency virus (HIV). Not all agents discussed are presently licensed in all countries.

MECHANISM OF ACTION

Currently available agents can be classified into those that directly inhibit viral replication at the cellular level (antivirals), those that modify the host response to infection (immunomodulators), and those that directly inactivate viral infectivity (antibodies, virucides, or microbicides). Antiviral agents can be further classified into two general mechanisms. First—and most numerous—are nucleic acid analogues that inhibit viral DNA or RNA synthesis by competing with endogenous nucleic acids for incorporation into the viral genome by viral DNA polymerase or RNA transcriptases. The second mechanism is inhibition of the functions of other essential viral enzymes or proteins, including those responsible for attachment or release from cells. For example, the principal antivirals for influenza viruses inhibit viral proteins responsible for either uncoating (M2 protein) or release and spread (neuraminidase).

Antiviral strategies that are not covered in this chapter include local destructive measures that destroy both host tissues and virus simultaneously, such as cryotherapy, laser, or podophyllin treatment of warts. Though effective, such measures are useful only for discrete or localized mucocutaneous infections. A number of topical virucidal agents have been and continue to be developed, and these agents may find utility in preventing transmission of certain viral infections.

ANTIVIRALS FOR HERPESVIRUS INFECTIONS

Acyclovir/Valacyclovir

Acyclovir, which is an acyclic analogue of the nucleoside guanosine, is converted to its active form via initial monophosphorylation by a virus-specific thymidine kinase (TK). Although normal human cells possess TK, the affinity of acyclovir for virus-specific TK is approximately 200 times greater than for human TK. The monophosphate then undergoes two additional host cell enzyme-mediated phosphorylations to acyclovir triphosphate, which selectively inhibits viral DNA polymerase, competitively and through chain termination. The higher concentrations of the activated form in infected cells and its affinity for viral polymerases result in low toxicity to normal host cells.

Valacyclovir is the L-valyl ester prodrug of acyclovir. Addition of the L-valyl ester fosters greater oral absorption, after which valacyclovir is converted to acyclovir; the prodrug provides three to five times greater bioavailability than oral acyclovir does.

Clinical Uses

Acyclovir and valacyclovir are used principally to treat infections caused by herpes simplex virus (HSV; Chapter 397) and varicella-zoster virus (VZV; Chapter 398) (Tables 383–1 through 383–4). Depending on country, acyclovir is available in a topical ointment and cream, oral capsules, and intravenous and ophthalmic formulations. Valacyclovir is available only as an oral capsule.

Oral acyclovir or valacyclovir decreases the duration of symptoms by approximately 50% and reduces the duration of viral shedding by about 90% in initial episodes of genital herpes. Two or 3 days of therapy appears to be sufficient for recurrent genital herpes. Chronic suppression is highly effective in reducing clinical and viral recurrences, and valacyclovir reduces the risk of transmitting genital HSV between heterosexual partners by 48%. [1] For herpes labialis (cold sores), 1 day of therapy with

TABLE 383–1 ANTIVIRALS FOR HERPESVIRUS INFECTIONS

Viral Infection	Drug	Route	Usual Adult Dosage
HERPES SIMPLEX VIRUS			
Genital herpes			
First episode	Acyclovir	PO	400 mg tid or 200 mg 5 times/day for 7–10 days
	Famciclovir	PO	250 mg tid for 7–10 days
	Valacyclovir	PO	1 g bid for 7–10 days
Recurrent	Acyclovir	PO	800 mg tid for 2 days or 400 mg tid or 200 mg 5 times/day for 5 days
	Famciclovir	PO	1000 mg bid for 2 doses
	Valacyclovir	PO	500 mg bid for 3 days or 1 g/day for 5 days
Suppression	Acyclovir	PO	400 mg bid or 200 mg tid
	Famciclovir	PO	250 mg bid
	Valacyclovir	PO	500 mg/day or 1 g/day (>10 episodes/yr)
Orolabial herpes	Penciclovir 1%	Topical	Apply cream every 2 hr while awake for 4 days
	Acyclovir 5%	Topical	Apply cream 5 times/day for 4 days
	Docosanol 10%	Topical	Apply cream 5 times/day until healing
	Valacyclovir	PO	2 g q12h × 2 doses
	Acyclovir	PO	400 mg 5 times/day for 5 days
	Famciclovir	PO	1500 mg single dose
Mucocutaneous disease	Acyclovir	IV	5 mg/kg/8 hr for 7–14 days
	Acyclovir	PO	400 mg 5 times/day for 7–14 days
	Valacyclovir	PO	500 mg or 1 g bid for 7–10 days
	Penciclovir	IV	5 mg/kg/8–12 hr for 7 days
Encephalitis	Acyclovir	IV	10–15 mg/kg/8 hr in 1-hr infusion for 14–21 days
Neonatal	Acyclovir	IV	10–20 mg/kg/8 hr for 14–21 days
Keratoconjunctivitis	Trifluridine	Topical	1 drop of 1% solution q2h up to 9 drops/day
	Vidarabine	Topical	½-inch ribbon of 3% ointment 5 times daily
CYTOMEGALOVIRUS			
Retinitis	Ganciclovir	IV	5 mg/kg/12 hr for 14–21 days (maintenance therapy is 5 mg/kg/day)
	Valganciclovir	PO	900 mg bid for 21 days (maintenance therapy is 900 mg/day)
	Cidofovir	IV	5 mg/kg once weekly × 2, then every other wk (maintenance therapy is 5 mg/kg q2wk)
	Foscarnet	IV	60 mg/kg/8 hr or 90 mg/kg q12h for 14–21 days (maintenance therapy is 90–120 mg/kg q2wk)
	Fomivirsen	Intravitreal	330 µg q2wk × 2, then q4wk (maintenance therapy is 330 µg q month)
VARICELLA-ZOSTER VIRUS			
Varicella in normal children	Acyclovir	PO	20 mg/kg (up to 800 mg) qid for 5 days
Varicella in immunocompromised hosts	Acyclovir	IV	10 mg/kg/8 hr or 500 mg/m²/8 hr for 7–10 days
Herpes zoster in immunocompromised hosts	Acyclovir	IV	10 mg/kg/8 hr for 7–10 days
Herpes zoster in normal hosts	Acyclovir	PO	800 mg 5 times daily for 7–10 days
	Valacyclovir	PO	1 g tid for 7 days
	Famciclovir	PO	500 mg tid for 7 days

TABLE 383–2 MECHANISMS OF EXCRETION AND THRESHOLDS FOR DOSE ADJUSTMENT

	Major Route of Elimination	Threshold for Adjustment in Renal Insufficiency/Failure	Adjustment for Hepatic Failure	Adjustment for Obesity
Acyclovir IV	Renal	CrCl < 50 mL/min/1.72 m²	No adjustment	Dose by ideal body weight
Acyclovir PO	Renal	CrCl < 25 mL/min/1.72 m²	No adjustment	Dose by ideal body weight
Valacyclovir	Renal	CrCl < 50 mL/min/1.72 m²	No adjustment	Unknown
Famciclovir	Renal	CrCl < 60 mL/min/1.72 m²	No adjustment	Unknown
Foscarnet	Renal	CrCl < 1.4 mL/min/kg	No adjustment	Unknown
Ganciclovir IV	Renal	CrCl < 70 mL/min/1.72 m²	No adjustment	Unknown
Valganciclovir	Renal	CrCl < 60 mL/min/1.72 m²	No adjustment	Unknown
Cidofovir	Renal	CrCl < 55 mL/min/1.72 m²	No adjustment	Unknown

TABLE 383–3 DRUG-DRUG INTERACTIONS

	Coadministered Drug	Risks/Toxicities	Possible Mechanism
Acyclovir	Fosphenytoin	Decreased phenytoin plasma concentration	Decreased phenytoin absorption
	Meperidine	Increased risk for CNS stimulation and excitation	Increased meperidine metabolites
	Mycophenolate	Increased plasma concentration of acyclovir	Competition for renal secretion
	Valproic acid	Decreased valproic acid plasma concentration	Decreased valproic acid absorption
	Varicella vaccine	Decreased varicella vaccine effectiveness	Inhibition of VZV
	Zidovudine	Increased lethargy and fatigue	Unknown
Valacyclovir	Mycophenolate	Increased risk for neutropenia	Unknown
Ganciclovir	Didanosine	Increased didanosine toxicity (neuropathy, diarrhea, pancreatitis)	Increased didanosine bioavailability
	Imipenem	Increased risk for CNS toxicity (seizures)	Unknown
	Mycophenolate	Increase in plasma concentration of ganciclovir	Competition for renal secretion
	Probenecid	Increase in plasma concentration of ganciclovir	Competition for renal secretion
	Tacrolimus	Increased risk for nephrotoxicity	Additive nephrotoxicity
	Zidovudine	Increased risk for hematologic toxicity (anemia, neutropenia)	Unknown
Valganciclovir	Probenecid	Increase in plasma concentration of ganciclovir	Competition for renal secretion
	Zidovudine	Increased risk for hematologic toxicity (anemia, neutropenia)	Unknown
Cidofovir	Aminoglycosides	Nephrotoxicity	Additive nephrotoxicity
	Foscarnet	Nephrotoxicity	Additive nephrotoxicity
	Pentamidine	Nephrotoxicity	Additive nephrotoxicity
Foscarnet*	Drugs that prolong QRS	Torsades de pointes	Additive toxicity/prolongation of QRS
	Renal toxic drugs	Nephrotoxicity	Additive nephrotoxicity
Idoxuridine	Boric acid	Eye irritation	Formation of precipitate

*Many classes of drugs have added toxicity when administered with foscarnet. Consult with a pharmacologist if uncertain about possible interactions.

TABLE 383–4 SIGNIFICANT ADVERSE EFFECTS (U.S. FDA BLACK BOX WARNING)

Drug	Black Box Synopsis
Cidofovir	Renal impairment, including renal failure Prehydrate and use probenecid Neutropenia May be carcinogenic and teratogenic and may cause hypospermia or aspermia
Foscarnet	Nephrotoxicity. Prehydrate Seizures related to minerals and electrolyte disturbances
Ganciclovir	Neutropenia, anemia, thrombocytopenia May be carcinogenic and teratogenic and may cause hypospermia or aspermia
Valganciclovir	Neutropenia, anemia, thrombocytopenia May be carcinogenic and teratogenic and may cause hypospermia or aspermia

oral valacyclovir improves time to healing and reduces pain, [2] whereas acyclovir ointment has no consistent clinical benefit.

Parenteral acyclovir is indicated for the initial treatment of mucosal or cutaneous HSV infection in immunocompromised patients, neonatal HSV infections, and disseminated or organ-invasive infections in immunocompetent patients. A subsequent switch to oral valacyclovir is possible in some circumstances. High-dose parenteral acyclovir is the therapy of choice for treating HSV encephalitis.

Acyclovir is also effective treatment of VZV infections, although higher doses are needed than for mucosal HSV infections (see Table 383–1). In adults treated within 24 hours of the development of a varicella rash, acyclovir decreases the severity of disease and number of lesions, but oral valacyclovir may be more effective than oral acyclovir. Intravenous acyclovir is warranted for initial treatment of varicella and zoster in immunocompromised hosts. Both acyclovir and valacyclovir chemoprophylaxis reduce the incidence of recurrent HSV in recipients of stem cell and solid organ transplants, but valacyclovir is superior for prevention of cytomegalovirus (CMV) disease.

Toxicity

Acyclovir and valacyclovir have excellent safety profiles and are generally well tolerated. Common side effects include nausea, vomiting, and headaches. Major adverse effects include renal dysfunction and central nervous system (CNS) toxicity. Dehydration and preexisting renal dysfunction predispose to the development of renal impairment. Neurologic side effects include tremor, myoclonus, confusion, lethargy, agitation, and hallucination. Renal dysfunction predisposes to the development of neurotoxicity. Neutropenia and other signs of bone marrow toxicity have also been reported rarely.

Antiviral Resistance

Despite widespread use of acyclovir, the development of HSV resistance in immunocompetent subjects is uncommon (prevalence <1%). However, antiviral resistance is higher in immunocompromised subjects, including those with HIV infection (prevalence of 5%) or bone marrow transplants (prevalence of up to 30%). Drug-resistant, refractory VZV infections can occur in highly immunocompromised patients. Intravenous foscarnet or cidofovir may be effective for infections caused by acyclovir-resistant viruses.

Penciclovir/Famciclovir

Penciclovir is an acyclic guanine analogue that unlike acyclovir, is not an obligate chain terminator and may be incorporated into DNA. Penciclovir demonstrates in vitro activity against VZV, HSV, and Epstein-Barr virus (EBV) comparable to that of acyclovir. The bioavailability of penciclovir after oral administration is less than 2%. In contrast, famciclovir is an oral prodrug that is deacetylated and oxidized in the liver to form penciclovir; penciclovir's bioavailability averages 77% after administration of famciclovir.

Clinical Uses

Penciclovir and famciclovir are used to treat HSV and VZV infections. Penciclovir is available as a topical cream and in some countries as an intravenous formulation. Famciclovir is available as a capsule.

Frequent applications of topical penciclovir reduce herpes labialis pain and lesions by about 1 day. [3] Famciclovir is approved for the treatment of recurrent HSV labialis and genital infections and herpes zoster, for which it is as effective as valacyclovir. However, it is also as effective orally as acyclovir when used to treat initial genital HSV infection. Intravenous penciclovir is useful for mucocutaneous infections in immunocompromised hosts.

Toxicity

Penciclovir is well tolerated as a topical cream, with the majority of adverse reactions being local irritation or mild erythema. Adverse effects of oral famciclovir include headache, dizziness, nausea, and diarrhea.

Antiviral Resistance

Penciclovir resistance in HSV has been very uncommon in immunocompetent subjects but, like acyclovir, more frequent in immunocompromised hosts (2.1%). Most acyclovir-resistant HSV isolates are cross-resistant to penciclovir.

Ganciclovir/Valganciclovir

Ganciclovir is an acyclic deoxyguanosine analogue with antiviral activity against multiple herpesviruses, including HSV, VZV, CMV, EBV, and human herpesvirus 8; it is much more active than acyclovir against CMV and EBV.

Oral ganciclovir's bioavailability is less than 10%. After administration of oral valganciclovir, which is an L-valyl prodrug of ganciclovir, bioavailability of ganciclovir averages 60%.

Clinical Uses

Ganciclovir is available as an oral capsule, a parenteral injection, and an ocular implant, whereas valganciclovir is available only as a tablet. Ganciclovir and valganciclovir are effective for treating CMV retinitis, [4] for which they are comparably active. In the absence of immune reconstitution, long-term suppression therapy is necessary.

They are also used for life-threatening CMV diseases (Chapter 399) in patients with acquired immunodeficiency syndrome (AIDS) and other immunocompromising conditions and for prevention of CMV disease in transplant patients. [5] For immunocompromised patients with organ-invasive CMV infections, ganciclovir provides clinical response rates of 70 to 90%, although response rates are lower for CMV pneumonitis after stem cell transplantation or CMV encephalitis in patients with AIDS. Long-term prophylaxis with ganciclovir or valganciclovir reduces the incidence of CMV disease after solid organ and stem cell transplantation, but this therapy has substantial side effects, including bone marrow suppression. These drugs can also be used as preemptive therapy for patients who have CMV viremia or antigenemia. Intravenous ganciclovir is the recommended agent for treating herpesvirus B infections, particularly those involving the CNS.

Toxicity

The most common adverse effect with ganciclovir and valganciclovir is bone marrow suppression, particularly neutropenia and thrombocytopenia, which occur in up to 50% of patients given intravenous ganciclovir. Fever, edema, phlebitis, headache, neuropathy, disorientation, nausea, anorexia, rash, and myalgias have also been reported with ganciclovir therapy. Intravitreal ganciclovir implants may cause vitreous hemorrhage and retinal detachment.

Antiviral Resistance

Ganciclovir resistance secondary to mutations in CMV kinase and sometimes DNA polymerase is related to the length of ganciclovir exposure and the degree of immunosuppression. Resistance may be associated with progressive disease during continued ganciclovir use; foscarnet or cidofovir are alternative treatments.

Cidofovir

Cidofovir, which is an acyclic phosphonate derivative of cytosine, is phosphorylated to its active diphosphate form by host cellular enzymes. Cidofovir diphosphate competitively inhibits viral DNA polymerase and viral DNA synthesis. Despite a short serum half-life, the antiviral effects are protracted because of prolonged intracellular concentrations of the phosphorylated metabolite.

Clinical Uses

Cidofovir is commercially available as an intravenous infusion. Investigational uses have included topical gel and intravitreal and intralesional injection.

Intravenous cidofovir is indicated for the treatment of CMV retinitis in AIDS patients who are failing ganciclovir or foscarnet therapy. Limited data suggest that intravenous cidofovir may be effective in other CMV infections (pneumonitis, gastroenteritis), acyclovir- or foscarnet-resistant HSV infections, certain forms of human papillomavirus disease, invasive adenoviral infections in transplant recipients, and possibly BK virus infection in renal transplant patients. In addition, in vivo and animal data suggest efficacy of cidofovir against smallpox, vaccinia, and monkeypox infections, although clinical trials are lacking.

Toxicity

Dose-related nephrotoxicity, characterized by increased serum creatinine, proteinuria, and tubular dysfunction, is the main side effect of intravenous cidofovir. Adequate hydration and concomitant oral probenecid reduce the risk. Other common side effects include diarrhea, asthenia, nausea, vomiting, neutropenia, fever, and rash. Iritis, intraocular pressure changes, loss of visual acuity, and uveitis have been reported with intravenous cidofovir. Intravitreal cidofovir is effective but locally toxic.

Antiviral Resistance

Sustained exposure to cidofovir does not easily induce resistance, although resistance has infrequently been described in HSV and CMV.

Foscarnet

Foscarnet is a pyrophosphate analogue that acts as a noncompetitive inhibitor of many viral RNA and DNA polymerases. Because foscarnet directly inhibits viral polymerases without metabolism, TK-deficient acyclovir-resistant HSV and VZV are susceptible to this agent.

Clinical Uses

Foscarnet is as effective for treatment of CMV retinitis in patients with AIDS as ganciclovir is, and combination therapy with ganciclovir may be superior to monotherapy with either agent for recalcitrant retinitis. [6] For extraretinal CMV disease, foscarnet has demonstrated efficacy similar to that of ganciclovir. The choice of agent may be dictated by the side effect profile. Foscarnet is also effective for the treatment of acyclovir-resistant HSV and VZV infections.

Toxicity

Nephrotoxicity with azotemia and proteinuria is dose limiting and occurs in more than a third of patients. A slow infusion rate and saline hydration reduce the risk. Other common side effects include anemia (30 to 50% of patients), granulocytopenia, diarrhea, nausea, vomiting, fever, seizures, paresthesias, headache, and genital ulcers. Marked electrolyte disturbances may develop, including hypophosphatemia, hypocalcemia, hypokalemia, and hypomagnesemia. Foscarnet can prolong the QT interval and be associated with cardiac arrhythmias, including ventricular tachycardia, ventricular fibrillation, and torsades de pointes.

Antiviral Resistance

The development of CMV resistance to foscarnet as a result of mutations in viral DNA polymerase is uncommon, except after prolonged administration. In AIDS patients with retinitis, foscarnet resistance is detectable in 13% of patients at 6 months and in 37% at 12 months.

Fomivirsen

Fomivirsen, which is an antisense oligonucleotide that inhibits CMV replication, is currently available as an intravitreal injection that is effective for both newly diagnosed and CMV retinitis failing usual therapies, 7 although direct comparisons with other agents are lacking. Intravitreal administration of fomivirsen may cause increased intraocular pressure, iritis, vitreitis, and cataracts in 10 to 20% of patients.

Brivudine

Brivudine, also known as bromovinyldeoxyuridine, is a thymidine analogue that is currently licensed for the treatment of herpes zoster in several European Union countries, but not the United States. Its efficacy is comparable to that of acyclovir, with similar time to crusting and cessation of pain. Common side effects include nausea, vomiting, abdominal discomfort, and anorexia.

Docosanol

Docosanol, which is a 22-carbon saturated fatty alcohol that inhibits intracellular penetration of lipid-enveloped viruses, is approved as a cream for the treatment of herpes labialis. Frequent topical applications have shown some reductions in time to cessation of pain and healing, but direct comparison to other agents is lacking. Local reaction, rash, and pruritus are common side effects.

Idoxuridine and Trifluorothymidine

Idoxuridine and trifluorothymidine are thymidine analogues that are phosphorylated by both viral and cellular TKs to active triphosphate derivatives that inhibit both viral and cellular DNA synthesis. The result is antiviral activity but also host cytotoxicity, which prevents safe systemic use. However, the tolerability of these compounds is adequate for topical use. Both idoxuridine and trifluorothymidine are available as ophthalmic formulations and are licensed for the treatment of herpetic keratitis. In direct comparison, trifluridine appears to be the more efficacious of these compounds. In addition, idoxuridine in dimethyl sulfoxide has been used topically in some countries for treating mucosal herpes infections. The most frequent adverse effects with trifluridine are transient burning or stinging on instillation and palpebral edema. Irritation and punctate corneal defects have been reported with idoxuridine.

Vidarabine

Vidarabine, an adenosine analogue, is now available only as an ophthalmic ointment indicated for acute keratoconjunctivitis and recurrent epithelial keratitis secondary to HSV. Its clinical activity appears to be superior to that of idoxuridine. Toxicities of the ointment include conjunctival injection, burning, and irritation.

ANTIVIRALS FOR INFLUENZA VIRUS INFECTIONS

Adamantanes (Amantadine, Rimantadine)

Amantadine and rimantadine are symmetrical tricyclic amines with activity against many influenza A viruses. By inhibiting the ion channel function of the M2 protein of influenza A, they interfere with uncoating of the virus and release of the viral genome.

Clinical Uses

Amantadine and rimantadine (Tables 383–5 through 383–7) decrease the length and severity of uncomplicated influenza A virus infection by susceptible strains if initiated within the first 2 days after the onset of symptoms, but it is uncertain whether they reduce the risk for complications. Both drugs are formulated for oral administration: capsules for amantadine and tablets for rimantadine, as well as pediatric syrups. In recent years marked increases in antiviral resistance in community isolates have limited the utility of these drugs.

Both rimantadine and amantadine are effective when used for prophylaxis against influenza A illness (overall 66% average for rimantadine and 74% for amantadine). In persons who take the drug for prophylaxis, subclinical infections may still develop and elicit immune responses that will protect them when exposed to antigenically related viruses.

Amantadine is also used in the treatment of parkinsonism, for drug-induced extrapyramidal reactions, and in the management of multiple sclerosis symptoms.

Toxicity

Amantadine causes CNS side effects in 10 to 30% of healthy young adults who take the standard adult dose of 200 mg/day; the frequency is

TABLE 383–5 ANTIVIRALS FOR INFLUENZA VIRUS INFECTIONS

Virus	Drug	Route	Usual Adult Treatment Dosage
Influenza A and B virus	Oseltamivir	PO	75 mg bid for 5 days
	Zanamivir	Inhalation	10 mg bid by inhaler for 5 days
Influenza A virus	Amantadine	PO	100 mg bid for 5 days
	Rimantadine	PO	100 mg bid for 5 days

TABLE 383–6 MECHANISMS OF EXCRETION AND THRESHOLDS FOR DOSE ADJUSTMENTS

	Major Route of Elimination	Threshold for Adjustment in Renal Insufficiency/Failure	Adjustment for Hepatic Failure	Special Adjustment for the Elderly
Amantadine	Renal	CrCl < 50 mL/min/1.72 m²	No adjustment	>65 yr: 100 mg daily
Rimantadine	Hepatic and renal	CrCl < 10 mL/min/1.72 m²	100 mg daily	100 mg daily
Oseltamivir	Renal	CrCl < 30 mL/min/1.72 m²	Unknown	
Zanamivir	Renal	No adjustment	Unknown	

TABLE 383–7 DRUG-DRUG INTERACTIONS

	Coadministered Drug	Risks/Toxicities	Possible Mechanism
Amantadine	Anticholinergics	Dry mouth, constipation, decreased urination, sedation, blurred vision	Additive anticholinergic effect
	Benztropine	CNS toxicity (confusion, hallucinations)	Unknown
	Bupropion	Nausea, vomiting, excitation, restlessness, postural hypotension	Unknown
	Triamterene	Incoordination, agitation, visual hallucinations	Decreased amantadine clearance
	Trimethoprim	CNS toxicity (insomnia, confusion)	Decreased amantadine clearance

TABLE 383–8 ANTIVIRALS FOR HEPATITIS VIRUS INFECTIONS

Viral Infection	Drug	Route	Usual Adult Dosage
Chronic hepatitis C (genotypes 1 and 4)	PEG-interferon alfa-2a	SC	180 μg weekly for 48 wk
	PEG-interferon alfa-2b	SC	1.5 μg/kg weekly for 48 wk
	Plus ribavirin	PO	800–1200 mg/day, depending on weight
Chronic hepatitis B	Interferon alfa-2b	SC/IM	5 MU/day or 10 MU 3 times weekly for 16–24 wk
	PEG-interferon alfa-2a	SC	180 μg weekly for 48 weeks
	Entecavir—naive	PO	0.5 mg daily. Optimal duration of therapy is unknown
	Lamivudine resistant	PO	1 mg daily. Optimal duration of therapy is unknown
	Lamivudine	PO	100 mg/day
	Adefovir	PO	10 mg/day
	Telbivudine	PO	600 mg/day

significantly lower with rimantadine. Neuropsychiatric side effects include anxiety, nervousness, insomnia, and particularly in the elderly or those with renal insufficiency, hallucinations, confusion, disorientation, and psychosis or coma. Amantadine or less often rimantadine is associated with an increased risk for seizures. Both drugs cause gastrointestinal side effects. Orthostatic hypotension occurs in 1 to 5%. Anticholinergic side effects, including dry mouth, occur in amantadine recipients.

Antiviral Resistance

Single point mutations in M2 confer high-level resistance to these drugs and make them ineffective. Such resistant variants emerge commonly during treatment and are transmissible. In 2005–2006, the frequency of resistance in influenza A (H3N2) viruses was as high as 92% in the United States. Resistance is also present in some H, N, and many H5N1 viruses.

Neuraminidase Inhibitors (Oseltamivir, Zanamivir)

Zanamivir and oseltamivir are sialic acid analogues that inhibit influenza virus neuraminidases by competitively interacting with the active enzyme site of influenza A and B viruses, including adamantine-resistant strains. Influenza neuraminidase cleaves terminal sialic acid residues and destroys the receptors recognized by viral hemagglutinin. These drugs inhibit this action, which is essential for release of virus from infected cells, prevention of viral aggregates, and spread within the respiratory tract.

Oseltamivir is administered orally as the phosphate prodrug, which is rapidly absorbed and hydrolyzed to the active form oseltamivir carboxylate. The oral bioavailability of zanamivir is poor, and it is currently licensed to be delivered as an orally inhaled powder.

Clinical Uses

Oseltamivir and zanamivir are effective for the treatment and prophylaxis of acute influenza A and B infections. Early treatment in adults decreases the duration and severity of illness, [8] well reduces lower respiratory tract complications, antibiotic use, and with oseltamivir, hospitalizations. Zanamivir is also effective in alleviating symptoms and decreasing the risk for lower respiratory complications. Both zanamivir and oseltamivir are highly effective for the prevention of influenza. [9]

Toxicity

The most common side effects with oseltamivir are nausea and vomiting. It may also be associated with headache, rash, and possibly abnormal transaminases. Zanamivir is generally well tolerated, but bronchospasm (sometimes severe) has been reported primarily in patients with underlying airway disease.

Antiviral Resistance

Oseltamivir resistance as a result of neuraminidase mutations has been detected during treatment of seasonal influenza, more often in children than adults and recently in H5N1-infected patients. In the immunocompromised host, and possibly in individuals with H5N1, the development of resistance is associated with treatment failure. Zanamivir retains activity against several oseltamivir-resistant variants.

ANTIVIRALS FOR HEPATITIS VIRUS INFECTIONS

Adefovir

Adefovir, which is an acyclic analogue of adenosine monophosphate, is administered orally as a prodrug, adefovir dipivoxil, which is rapidly converted enzymatically to adefovir in intestinal epithelium.

Clinical Uses

In chronic hepatitis B (Chapter 152), prolonged administration (Tables 383–8 through 383–11) is effective in improving liver histology, decreasing hepatitis B virus (HBV) DNA levels, and normalizing biochemical (alanine aminotransferase) markers in patients with hepatitis B e antigen (HBeAg)-positive [10] and HBeAg-negative chronic hepatitis B. [11] In addition, it has been shown to be effective against chronic HBV resistant to lamivudine, as well as in HIV-coinfected patients.

Toxicity

The major adverse effect is nephrotoxicity, manifested by increased serum creatinine and sometimes hypophosphatemia, both of which are usually reversible with discontinuation of the drug. Common side effects include asthenia, headache, nausea, vomiting, and diarrhea. In addition, severe exacerbation of hepatitis has occasionally been observed after cessation of therapy.

Section XXIII Infectious Diseases

TABLE 383–9 MECHANISMS OF EXCRETION AND THRESHOLDS FOR DOSE ADJUSTMENT

	Major Route of Elimination	Threshold for Adjustment in Renal Insufficiency/Failure	Adjustment for Hepatic Failure	Special Adjustment for Elderly
Adefovir	Renal	CrCl < 50 mL/min/1.72 m^2	No adjustment	
Entecavir	Renal	CrCl < 50 mL/min/1.72 m^2	No adjustment	
Lamivudine	Renal	CrCl < 50 mL/min/1.72 m^2	No adjustment	
Tenofovir	Renal	CrCl < 50 mL/min/1.72 m^2	No adjustment	
Ribavirin	Renal	CrCl < 50 mL/min/1.72 m^2	No adjustment	
PEG-interferon alfa-2a	Renal	CrCl < 50 mL/min/1.72 m^2	Progressive rise in alanine transaminase	>60 yr: consider reduction
Telbivudine	Renal	CrCl < 50 mL/min	No adjustment	

TABLE 383–10 DRUG-DRUG INTERACTIONS

	Coadministered Drug	Risks/Toxicities	Possible Mechanism
Lamivudine	Ribavirin	Lactic acidosis	Unknown
	Sulfamethoxazole	Increased risk for lamivudine adverse effects	Competition for renal secretion
	Trimethoprim	Increased risk for lamivudine adverse effects	Competition for renal secretion
	Zalcitabine	Increased zalcitabine and lamivudine exposure	Inhibition of phosphorylation
Tenofovir	Atazanavir	Decreased atazanavir concentration and/or increased tenofovir levels	Unknown
	Didanosine	Increased didanosine plasma concentration and risk for toxicity	Increased didanosine bioavailability
	Lopinavir	Increased tenofovir bioavailability	Unknown
	Ritonavir	Increased tenofovir bioavailability	Unknown
Ribavirin	Nucleoside analogues	Lactic acidosis	Unknown
	Interferon alfa-2b	Worsening mental depression, anger, and hostility	Unknown
Interferon alfa-2	Angiotensin-converting enzyme inhibitors	Hematologic abnormalities (granulocytopenia, thrombocytopenia)	Unknown
	Colchicine	Decreased interferon alfa-2a effectiveness	Unknown
	Theophylline	Theophylline toxicity (nausea, vomiting, palpitations, seizures)	Unknown
	Ribavirin	Worsening mental depression, anger, and hostility	Unknown

TABLE 383–11 SIGNIFICANT ADVERSE EFFECTS (U.S. FDA BLACK BOX WARNING)

Drug	Black Box Synopsis
Adefovir	Severe acute exacerbations of hepatitis B may occur with cessation of therapy Nephrotoxicity may occur in patients at risk for or undergoing renal dysfunction Lactic acidosis and severe hepatomegaly with steatosis
Entecavir	Lactic acidosis and severe hepatomegaly with steatosis; severe acute exacerbations of hepatitis B may occur with cessation of therapy
Lamivudine	Severe acute exacerbations of hepatitis B may occur with cessation of therapy Lactic acidosis and severe hepatomegaly with steatosis
Ribavirin	Monotherapy for hepatitis C is not effective Hemolytic anemia Teratogenic and/or embryocidal
Interferon alfa	May cause or aggravate neurophychiatric, autoimmune, ischemic, and infectious disorders
Telbivudine	Severe acute exacerbation of hepatitis B may occur with cessation of therapy Lactic acidosis and severe hepatomegaly with steatosis

Antiviral Resistance

Adefovir resistance secondary to point mutations in HBV polymerase develops in about 6% of patients after 3 years of adefovir therapy. Lamivudine generally retains activity against adefovir-resistant variants.

Entecavir

Entecavir, which is a deoxyguanosine nucleoside analogue with specific antiviral activity for hepadnaviruses, is more potent than lamivudine and also retains some activity against lamivudine-resistant HBV variants. It is well absorbed after oral administration, and its prolonged half-life (128 to 149 hours) allows for once-daily dosing.

Clinical Uses

Entecavir is approved for the treatment of chronic hepatitis B in adults with evidence of active viral replication and either persistent elevations in serum aminotransferases or histologically active disease. When compared with lamivudine, entecavir is more efficacious in reducing HBV DNA levels and normalizing serum aminotransferases, as well as in improving histologic abnormalities. 12 Higher doses are indicated for lamivudine-resistant infections.

Toxicity

Adverse effects reported during entecavir therapy include headache, fatigue, dizziness, nausea, abdominal pain, rhinitis, fever, diarrhea, cough, and myalgia.

Antiviral Resistance

Entecavir resistance, caused by specific mutations in HBV polymerase, appears to be uncommon, with no evidence after more than 1 year of drug exposure.

Lamivudine

Lamivudine is a deoxycytidine L-nucleoside analogue active against retroviruses and hepadnaviruses. The triphosphate inhibits HBV polymerase, and its incorporation into viral DNA results in termination of the DNA chain.

Clinical Uses

Prolonged lamivudine administration to patients with chronic hepatitis B suppresses viral replication, improves liver histology, reduces progression of fibrosis, and decreases the risk for late complications, but monotherapy with lamivudine appears to be inferior to monotherapy with interferon for sustained control of HBV replication. Combination therapy with lamivudine and interferon has shown inconsistent benefit when compared with either drug alone.

Toxicity

Adverse effects of lamivudine include diarrhea, headache, and elevated liver enzymes. Severe post-treatment exacerbations of hepatitis B, including fatalities, have occurred with discontinuation of lamivudine, more commonly in patients coinfected with HBV and HIV.

Antiviral Resistance

Lamivudine resistance, caused by mutations in HBV polymerase, is common during prolonged treatment of hepatitis B and emerges in about 20% of treated patients annually. Resistance is associated with increases in viral replication and aminotransferases.

Tenofovir

Tenofovir is a nucleotide analogue of adenosine monophosphate. The commercially available agent, tenofovir disoproxil fumarate, is an ester prodrug of tenofovir and gives an effective tenofovir bioavailability of 25%.

Clinical Uses

Tenofovir is not currently approved by the FDA for HBV infection but has shown benefits in HBV/HIV-coinfected patients failing interferon alfa and lamivudine. In such patients, the addition of tenofovir to lamivudine lowers HBV DNA levels, improves aminotransferase levels, and helps maintain suppressed HIV loads. 13 In individuals not infected with HIV, tenofovir is more effective than adefovir in suppressing HBV DNA at week 48.

Toxicity

Tenofovir is generally well tolerated, with the most common side effects being nausea, diarrhea, vomiting, and anorexia. Lactic acidosis with hepatic steatosis has been reported, primarily when used in combination with other nucleoside analogues. Acute exacerbations of hepatitis B have been reported after discontinuation of tenofovir in patients who are coinfected with HIV and HBV.

Antiviral Resistance

Mutations in HBV polymerase that confer reduced susceptibility to tenofovir occur during prolonged use (>12 months), although the clinical significance of these mutations remains to be defined.

Telbivudine

Telbivudine is a synthetic thymidine nucleoside analogue with activity against HBV, including some lamivudine-resistant variants. The triphosphate form competitively inhibits the HBV DNA polymerase (reverse transcriptase). Telbivudine is used for the treatment of chronic HBV. In comparative trials against lamivudine, telbivudine demonstrated greater biologic response at week 52 (60% vs 40% of subjects HBV DNA negative by PCR). Common side effects include headache, nausea, and vomiting. Severe acute exacerbations of hepatitis B have been reported in patients who have discontinued anti-HBV therapy. Myopathy, manifested by muscle aches and/or weakness with increased CPK, has rarely been reported.

Ribavirin

Ribavirin is a purine nucleoside with antiviral activity against some DNA viruses and many RNA viruses, including influenza A and B, parainfluenza, measles, respiratory syncytial virus (RSV), retroviruses, arenaviruses such as Lassa virus, and some hantaviruses.

Clinical Uses

Monotherapy with ribavirin for chronic hepatitis C (Chapter 152) has been shown to decrease serum alanine aminotransferase but not hepatitis C virus RNA levels. However, combination therapy with ribavirin and various interferons, most recently pegylated interferons, is superior to interferon monotherapy, improves viral clearance and liver histologic responses, and reduces complications, including mortality. Ribavirin plus pegylated interferon has become the standard treatment of chronic hepatitis C.

Aerosol administration of ribavirin has been used to treat RSV bronchiolitis and pneumonia in children and to treat influenza A and B infections. Limited benefit has been seen with oral ribavirin in uncomplicated influenza. Aerosol ribavirin combined with intravenous immunoglobulin, particularly with the anti-RSV monoclonal antibody palivizumab, appears to reduce the mortality of RSV infection in bone marrow transplant and other highly immunocompromised patients.

Systemic ribavirin reduces the mortality associated with Lassa fever and Asian (Korean) hemorrhagic fever with renal syndrome, 14 though not mortality in patients with hantavirus-associated cardiopulmonary syndrome. It appears to have activity in Congo-Crimean hemorrhagic fever and in Nipah virus infections. Ribavirin is often recommended as treatment of hemorrhagic fevers of unknown etiology (Chapter 404) or secondary to arenaviruses or bunyaviruses in the event that these viruses are used as biologic weapons.

Toxicity

Aerosol delivery may cause bronchospasm. Systemic ribavirin is frequently associated with hemolytic anemia (in up to 61% in some series) and sometimes with electrolyte abnormalities, including hypocalcemia and hypomagnesemia. Arrhythmias, pruritus, rash, nausea, and myalgia have been reported, as have neurologic side effects, including insomnia and irritability. Ribavirin is gonadotoxic and teratogenic in multiple species.

Interferons

Interferons are glycoprotein cytokines with a complex array of antiviral, immunomodulating, and antineoplastic properties. Interferons are currently classified as α, β, or γ, with the natural sources of these classes, in general, being leukocytes, fibroblasts, and lymphocytes, respectively. Each type of interferon can now be produced through recombinant DNA technology. Although the full mechanism of interferon's action is not defined, interferons generally induce synthesis of new cellular RNA and proteins that mediate antiviral effects through multiple different mechanisms.

Interferons generally require administration daily or several times per week. However, the combination of interferon with polyethylene glycol to form pegylated interferon significantly prolongs absorption, decreases elimination, and provides higher, more sustained plasma levels that enable administration once weekly.

Clinical Uses

In chronic active hepatitis B (Chapter 152), treatment with interferon alfa leads to loss of HBV DNA and biochemical and histologic improvement in about 25 to 40% of patients. Administration of PEG-interferon alfa-2a or alfa-2b for 48 weeks converts about 30% of patients to seronegative status after 6 months of treatment. 15 Combination therapy with interferon and lamivudine is not clearly superior to interferon alone.

In contrast to hepatitis B, combination therapy is the mainstay of treatment of hepatitis C (Chapter 152). Subcutaneous administration of PEG-interferon alfa-2a plus daily ribavirin for 48 weeks results in a sustained virologic response in about 55% of treated patients, as compared with less than a 30% response with interferon monotherapy. Patients with hepatitis C genotype 1 have lower levels of response than do patients with genotype 2 or 3 (46 vs. 76%); patients with genotypes 2 and 3 may need only 24 weeks of combination therapy. 16

Toxicity

Common side effects of interferon administration include influenza-like symptoms (fever, chills, headache, and malaise), but these symptoms usually become less severe with repeated treatments; tolerance develops in most patients within several weeks. Major toxicities have included bone marrow suppression, primarily granulocytopenia and thrombocytopenia, which are generally reversible when therapy is discontinued. Neuropsychiatric disturbance may be manifested by depression, anxiety, somnolence, confusion, and behavioral disturbance. Other side effects include profound fatigue and anorexia, weight loss, hypo or hyperthyroidism, alopecia, and cardiotoxicity with arrhythmias and reversible cardiomyopathy.

OTHER ANTIVIRALS

Imiquimod

Imiquimod and the related compound resiquimod are topical immune response modifiers that lack direct antiviral effects. Instead, these agents induce activation of immune cells (monocytes, macrophages, natural killer cells) to produce antiviral cytokines, particularly interferon-α and tumor necrosis factor-α.

Topical imiquimod cream is approved for the treatment of anogenital warts (Chapters 396 and 465). In immunocompetent patients, imiquimod leads to complete clearance of warts in 37% to 52% of patients. It may also be beneficial in patients with refractory cutaneous leishmaniasis (Chapter 369) and for molluscum contagiosum (Chapters 396 and 465). It is administered as a topical cream three times weekly for a maximum of 16 weeks and is washed off 6 to 10 hours after application.

Side effects are primarily local and include erythema, irritation, tenderness, and less often, erosion. The side effects usually resolve with cessation of the drug.

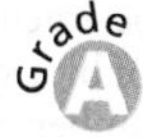

1. Corey L, Wald A, Patel R, et al: Once-daily valacyclovir to reduce the risk of transmission of genital herpes. N Engl J Med 2004;350:11–20.
2. Spruance SL, Jones TM, Blatter MM, et al: High-dose, short-duration, early valacyclovir therapy for episodic treatment of cold sores: Results of two randomized, placebo-controlled, multicenter studies. Antimicrob Agents Chemother 2003;47:1072–1080.
3. Boon R, Goodman JJ, Martinez J, et al: Penciclovir cream for the treatment of sunlight-induced herpes simplex labialis: A randomized, double-blind, placebo-controlled trial. Penciclovir Cream Herpes Labialis Study Group. Clin Ther 2000;22:76–90.
4. Martin DF, Sierra-Madero J, Walmsley S, et al: A controlled trial of valganciclovir as induction therapy for cytomegalovirus retinitis. N Engl J Med 2002;346:1119–1126.
5. Paya C, Humar A, Domiquez E, et al: Efficacy and safety of valganciclovir vs. oral ganciclovir for prevention of cytomegalovirus disease in solid organ transplant recipients. Am J Transplant 2004;4:611–620.
6. Combination foscarnet and ganciclovir therapy vs monotherapy for the treatment of relapsed cytomegalovirus retinitis in patients with AIDS. The Cytomegalovirus Retreatment Trial. The Studies of Ocular Complications of AIDS Research Group in Collaboration with the AIDS Clinical Trials Group. Arch Ophthalmol 1996;114:23–33.
7. Vitravene Study Group: Randomized dose-comparison studies of intravitreous fomivirsen for treatment of cytomegalovirus retinitis that has reactivated or is persistently active despite other therapies in patients with AIDS. Am J Ophthalmol 2002;133:475–483.
8. Nicholson KG, Aoki FY, Osterhaus AD, et al: Efficacy and safety of oseltamivir in treatment of acute influenza: A randomised controlled trial. Neuraminidase Inhibitor Flu Treatment Investigator Group. Lancet 2000;355:1845–1850.
9. Hayden FG, Atmar RL, Schilling M, et al: Use of the selective oral neuraminidase inhibitor oseltamivir to prevent influenza. N Engl J Med 1999;341:1336–1343.
10. Marcellin P, Chang TT, Lim SG, et al: Adefovir dipivoxil for the treatment of hepatitis B e antigen–positive chronic hepatitis B. N Engl J Med 2003;348:808–816.
11. Hadziyannis SJ, Tassopoulos NC, Heathcote EJ, et al: Adefovir dipivoxil for the treatment of hepatitis B e antigen–negative chronic hepatitis B. N Engl J Med 2003;348:800–807.
12. Lai CL, Rosmawati M, Lao J, et al: Entecavir is superior to lamivudine in reducing hepatitis B virus DNA in patients with chronic hepatitis B infection. Gastroenterology 2002;123:1831–1838.
13. Dore GJ, Cooper DA, Pozniak AL, et al: Efficacy of tenofovir disoproxil fumarate in antiretroviral therapy–naive and–experienced patients coinfected with HIV-1 and hepatitis B virus. J Infect Dis 2004;189:1185–1192.
14. Huggins JW, Hsiang CM, Cosgriff TM, et al: Prospective, double-blind, concurrent, placebo-controlled clinical trial of intravenous ribavirin therapy of hemorrhagic fever with renal syndrome. J Infect Dis 1991;164:1119–1127.
15. Janssen HL, von Zonneveld M, Senturk H, et al: Pegylated interferon alfa-2b alone or in combination with lamivudine for HBeAg-positive chronic hepatitis B: A randomised trial. Lancet 2005;365:123–129.
16. Hadziyannis SJ, Sette H Jr, Morgan TR, et al: Peginterferon-alpha2a and ribavirin combination therapy in chronic hepatitis C: A randomized study of treatment duration and ribavirin dose. Ann Intern Med 2004;140:346–355.

SUGGESTED READINGS

Darling JM, Fried MW: Optimizing treatment regimens in hepatitis C. Clin Liver Dis 2006;10:835–850. *Comprehensive clinical review.*

Jefferson T, Demicheli V, Rivetti D, et al: Antivirals for influenza in healthy adults: Systematic review. Lancet 2006;367:303–313. *Meta-analysis of all medications available for the treatment of influenza.*

384 THE COMMON COLD

J. Owen Hendley

Definition

The common cold, also known as upper respiratory infection, is an acute, self-limited illness caused by a virus. Nasal symptoms, including rhinorrhea and nasal obstruction, are invariably present (Chapters 272 and 452); sore or scratchy throat or cough, or both (Chapter 83), may also be present. There are no normal viral flora of the respiratory tract in humans (two possible exceptions are human herpesvirus type 6 in saliva and adenovirus, which can be recovered from adenoid tissue of otherwise healthy children by cocultivation with susceptible cells). In sharp contrast, luxuriant normal bacterial flora occur in the upper respiratory tract and mouth. Because viruses are not part of the normal flora, the viruses that cause colds must be passed from another human to produce the cold.

The Pathogens

Colds are common because viruses with few serotypes reinfect many times and viruses that infect an individual only once have multiple serotypes (Table 384–1). Rhinoviruses (rhino = "nose") cause at least 50% of colds in adults; coronaviruses (corona = "crown"; Chapter 389) and respiratory syncytial virus (RSV; Chapter 385) are each responsible for about 10%, and each of the other virus groups cause less than 5% of colds. With the use of molecular techniques, additional viruses that are

TABLE 384–1 IMMUNITY TO COMMON COLD VIRUSES

Virus	Number of Serotypes
SOLID IMMUNITY NOT PRODUCED BY INFECTION (REPEATED INFECTION WITH THE SAME SEROTYPE USUAL)	
Respiratory syncytial virus	1
Parainfluenza virus	4
Coronavirus	4
IMMUNITY PRODUCED BY INFECTION (REINFECTION WITH THE SAME SEROTYPE UNCOMMON)	
Rhinovirus	>100
Adenovirus	>33
Influenza	3 (type A subtypes change)
Echovirus	31
Coxsackievirus	
Group A	23
Group B	6

From Hendley JO: Immunology of viral colds. *In* Veldman JE, McCabe BF, Huizing EH, Mygind N (eds): Immunobiology, Autoimmunity, Transplantation in Otorhinolaryngology. Amsterdam, Kugler, 1985, pp 257–260.

Section XXIII Infectious Diseases

occasionally associated with wintertime colds have been detected, including metapneumovirus, which behaves like RSV, three new coronaviruses, and Bocavirus. Adults are susceptible to RSV and parainfluenza virus, but the illness in adults is usually a cold rather than the more severe involvement seen in infants. Some of the viruses that cause colds are characteristically associated with other syndromes. For example, influenza viruses (Chapter 387) cause febrile respiratory disease with lower tract involvement, adenoviruses (Chapter 388) are associated with pharyngoconjunctival fever or acute undifferentiated febrile illness, echoviruses and other enteroviruses (Chapter 402) are an important cause of aseptic meningitis, and coxsackievirus A (Chapter 402) causes herpangina.

Epidemiology

Colds are the most frequent disease of humans and the single most common cause of absenteeism from school and work. The frequency of colds varies with age. Even before the widespread proliferation of daycare centers, colds were particularly common in children younger than 6 years. In one study, infants younger than 1 year had an average of 6.7 colds per year, 1- to 5-year olds had 7.4 to 8.3 colds per year, and teenagers averaged about 4.5 colds per year. Mothers reported 4.5 colds and fathers 3.5 colds per year. The number of colds in adults may increase for several years because of exposure to young children, who commonly introduce new viruses to their families. In one study, for example, coworkers in an insurance company office with simultaneous rhinovirus colds were usually infected with different serotypes of virus, but each worker's serotype was found in family contacts.

In temperate climates, colds are epidemic in the winter months (Fig. 384–1). The epidemic starts with a sharp rise in frequency in September after children have returned to school; the incidence then remains at an almost constant level until spring. This epidemic curve is produced by successive waves of different viruses moving through the community. Although rhinovirus infections occur year-round, the epidemic is initiated by a sharp rise in rhinovirus infections in early fall. Parainfluenza viruses (Chapter 386) peak in October and November, followed by RSV and coronaviruses in winter months. Influenza viruses appear later in winter; then rhinovirus has a resurgence in spring. Summer colds are usually caused by rhinovirus or one of the enteroviruses. The wave of each virus moving through is not sharp, and two or three viruses may have overlapping peaks. Adenovirus and parainfluenza virus type 3 contribute to the burden of illness throughout the epidemic.

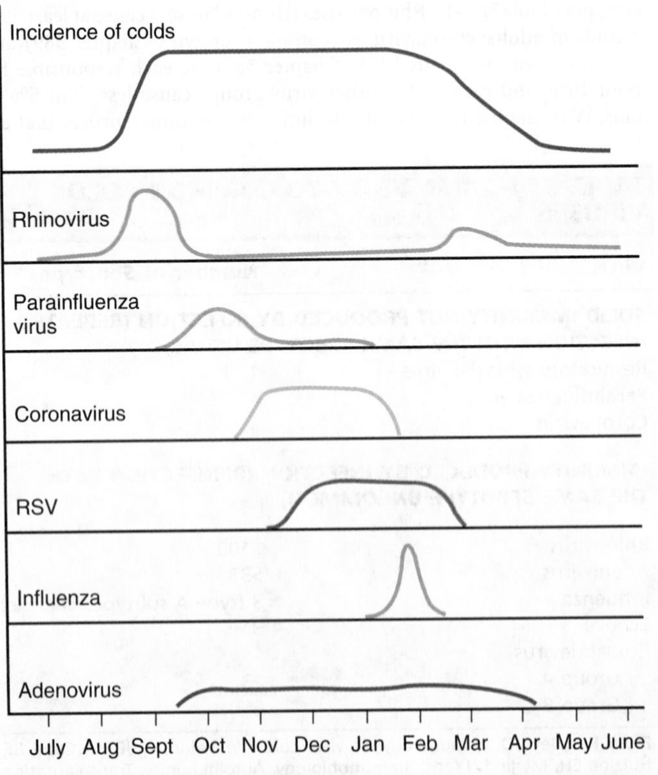

FIGURE 384–1 • Schematic diagram of the incidence of colds and frequency of the causative viruses. RSV = respiratory syncytial virus.

Determinants of the yearly epidemic of colds include human behavior, with more virus transmitted by higher indoor contact in colder months. Another determinant might be attributes of the viruses. Enveloped viruses, including RSV, parainfluenza virus, influenza virus, and coronavirus, may survive on environmental surfaces outside the host for longer periods in winter when the relative humidity of indoor (but not outdoor) air is low.

Transmission of viruses causing colds can occur by one or more of three mechanisms: (1) small-particle (<5 μm in diameter) aerosol in which virus may be suspended in air for an hour and infect by inhalation; (2) large-particle (>10 μm in diameter) airborne droplets that travel less than 1 m and infect by landing on a mucosal surface, such as conjunctiva or nasal mucosa; and (3) transfer of virus in the secretions of a person with a cold, by way of hand contact or contaminated environmental surfaces, to the fingers of uninfected persons, who then inoculate the virus onto their own conjunctival or nasal mucosa. Oral inoculation of rhinovirus or RSV does not result in infection, presumably because the stratified squamous epithelium of the mouth and oropharynx is not susceptible. The transmission route under natural conditions in the home has not been definitely established for any of the viruses. However, the importance of spread of colds in the home favors direct contact or large-droplet spread, or both, as the most likely cause. Influenza virus, however, can also be transmitted by small-particle aerosol.

Pathobiology

The histologic appearance of the nasal mucosa in biopsy specimens taken during a common cold cannot be distinguished from that of biopsy specimens taken 2 weeks after illness except for an increased number of polymorphonuclear leukocytes (PMNs) during illness. Infiltration of PMNs in the nose increases coincidently when symptoms appear in experimentally induced rhinovirus colds. Kinins (primarily bradykinin) also appear in the nasal secretions of infected volunteers at the time when they become ill, and their presence parallels cold symptoms. Viral infection of individual epithelial cells in the mucosa of the nose and nasopharynx can lead to elaboration of interleukin-8 (IL-8), which is a chemoattractant for PMNs, and to increased levels of IL-1β and IL-6. The possibility that cold symptoms might be ablated by blocking host response mediators without having to kill the virus holds promise for future research.

Clinical Manifestations

The clinical manifestations of colds are predominately subjective. In adults, rhinorrhea, nasal obstruction, and a scratchy or sore throat are usually noted. The rhinorrhea is usually clear early in illness and may become white or yellow-green. Malaise and nonproductive cough are common; sneezing is sometimes noted. Other common symptoms include sinus fullness and a "nasal" quality to the voice. Hoarseness is sometimes present.

Objective physical findings in an adult with a cold are usually minimal. The nasal mucosa may be red, but not to a degree that differs from normal. Mild erythema of the pharynx and redness around the external nares may be noted. Fever (temperature >38° C) is uncommon in an adult with a cold; the presence of fever suggests influenza or a bacterial complication of the cold. The symptoms of the cold generally abate in 5 to 7 days. Colds in infants and children, however, may be associated with more objective signs, such as moderate enlargement of the anterior cervical lymph nodes. Fever during the first 2 to 3 days of a cold is not unusual in young children, even when the child's parent or older sibling does not have an elevated temperature during a cold caused by the same virus. The usual duration of cold symptoms in children is 10 to 14 days.

Diagnosis

Self-diagnosis of a cold is usually accurate. Laboratory tests, including a white blood cell count and differential, are not helpful. Sloughed ciliated cells may be present, and PMNs would be expected in nasal secretions during viral colds. The differential diagnosis of a cold includes an intranasal foreign body in a child and allergic or vasomotor rhinitis

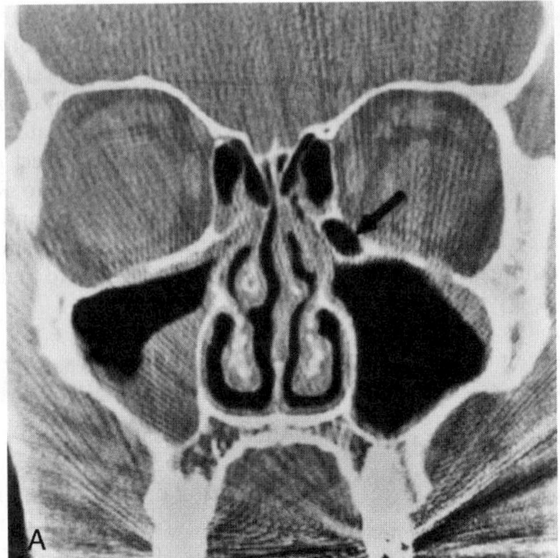

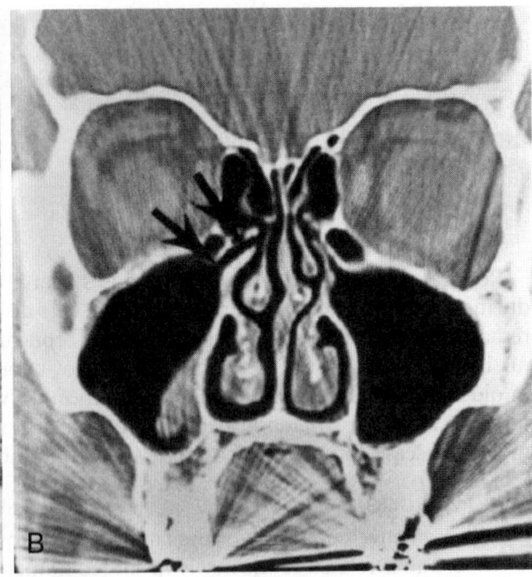

FIGURE 384–2 • Imaging of a cold. A sinus computed tomographic scan was performed in an adult during a symptomatic cold **(A)** and 2 weeks later **(B)**. The arrow in the left panel denotes an infraorbital air cell (Haller cell). Bilateral abnormalities were observed in the ethmoid and maxillary sinuses during the cold, with an air-fluid interface in the right maxillary sinus. Two weeks later, all abnormalities had cleared except for a residual density in the right maxillary sinus. The infundibulum (two arrows) draining the maxillary antrum was now open. (Courtesy of Dr. Jack M. Gwaltney, Jr., Department of Internal Medicine, University of Virginia School of Medicine, Charlottesville, VA.)

(Chapter 272) in adults and children. Examination of the nose should exclude a foreign body; the chronicity of symptoms with allergic or vasomotor rhinitis should differentiate these conditions from an acute cold.

Etiologic (virologic) diagnosis of a cold can be attempted by inoculation of a sample of nasal secretions into tissue cell cultures, but such testing is rarely needed or useful. Assays using polymerase chain reaction for detection of respiratory viruses can facilitate diagnosis when indicated, primarily during potential outbreaks that may affect immunocompromised hosts. Rapid tests for RSV antigen in nasal secretions are not reliable in adults. Detection of nucleoprotein of both A and B influenza may be useful to screen for these viruses.

Clinical differentiation between primary viral and secondary bacterial infection of the respiratory tract is a challenge because respiratory viruses may involve the middle ear or paranasal sinuses in the absence of bacterial infection. Tympanocentesis or maxillary sinus puncture provides definitive information of viral versus bacterial infection, but these tests are too invasive for routine use. Coronal computed tomography of the paranasal sinuses may show abnormalities in one or more sinuses (Fig. 384–2) in up to 87% of young adults during uncomplicated colds without bacterial infection. These abnormalities clear or markedly improve without antibiotic therapy in about 80% of cases.

Prevention

Vaccines to prevent common colds are unlikely to be useful given the multiplicity of immunotypes of some of the viruses and the lack of solid immunity to reinfection with other viruses. Prophylaxis with topical interferon applied intranasally for 5 days after one family member appears with a cold is moderately effective in preventing other family members from acquiring a cold, particularly colds caused by rhinovirus, but the practicality of this preventive approach is limited.

Probably the only practical, albeit imperfect means of preventing cold is to prevent virus from reaching the nasal or conjunctival mucosa by way of one's own hands. If transmission occurs by inhalation of airborne small particles or by adherence of large droplets to a mucosal surface, infection is inevitable for those who enjoy contact with other humans. However, if transmission occurs by self-inoculation with virus on contaminated fingertips, the simple measure of ridding the fingers of viable virus before touching one's eye or nose might be helpful. The virus can be removed physically by rinsing the hands. Applying a virucide to the hands might be another approach.

Treatment

Rx

Given the self-limited nature of colds, any treatment should be completely safe. Antibiotics have no place in therapy for uncomplicated colds because they neither hasten nor delay recovery from the cold, nor do they reduce the frequency of bacterial complications.

Rx

Because the subjective symptoms of a cold disappear in 7 days without intervention, a variety of actually ineffective treatments, such as vitamin C and zinc gluconate lozenges, have been reported to be effective as a result of inadequate "blinding" of placebo recipients. Herbal remedies are widely used, but evidence does not indicate any benefit. [1] No antiviral agents are currently available for treating colds, except those caused by influenza virus (Chapter 387).

Individual symptoms may be treated. Malaise may be relieved by analgesics (e.g., aspirin, acetaminophen, ibuprofen). Nasal congestion may be relieved by taking decongestants by mouth (pseudoephedrine, 60 mg three times a day) or by topical application (oxymetazoline 0.05%, two sprays into each nostril twice daily). Oral first-generation antihistamines (e.g., brompheniramine, chlorpheniramine, clemastine) may provide modest relief of sneezing and rhinorrhea in colds.

Prognosis

Secondary bacterial infection may complicate viral colds. Purulent rhinitis may respond to antibiotics, but their side effects appear to counterbalance any benefits. [2] Suppurative otitis media (Chapter 452), which occurs in some 5% of colds in preschool-aged children, may be heralded by a secondary fever with associated ear pain. Bacterial sinusitis (Chapters 272 and 452) is estimated to occur in 0.5% of colds, primarily in adults. Sinusitis is suggested by the presence of fever or facial pain, or both. Bacterial pneumonia is a rare complication. An important complication of viral colds in adults and children with underlying reactive airways disease or asthma (Chapter 87) is wheezing, which occurs in 30 to 50% of episodes of viral colds in prospective studies of patients with asthma. Colds in these patients produce a large burden of illness because up to 50% of asthma exacerbations in children and up to 20% of exacerbations in adults are associated with an identified virus.

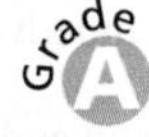

1. Turner RB, Bauer R, Woelkart K, et al: An evaluation of *Echinacea angustifolia* in experimental rhinovirus infections. N Engl J Med 2005;353:341–348.
2. Arroll B, Kenealy T: Are antibiotics effective for acute purulent rhinitis? Systematic review and meta-analysis of placebo controlled randomised trials. BMJ 2006;333:279.

SUGGESTED READINGS

Musher DM: How contagious are common respiratory tract infections? N Engl J Med 2003;348:1256–1266. *Reviews all the relevant viruses.*

Pratter MR: Cough and the common cold: ACCP evidence-based clinical practice guidelines. Chest 2006;129:72S–74S. *The common cold is probably the most usual cause of cough.*

Taverner D, Latte J: Nasal decongestants for the common cold. Cochrane Database Syst Rev 2007;1:CD001953. *Evidence of modest efficacy in reducing congestive symptoms.*

385 RESPIRATORY SYNCYTIAL VIRUS

Edward E. Walsh

Definition

Respiratory syncytial virus (RSV) causes yearly outbreaks of illness during the fall, winter, and early spring. Since its discovery in 1957, RSV remains the single most important cause of bronchiolitis and pneumonia in young infants and is a common cause of upper respiratory illness in older children and young adults. In addition, RSV causes serious respiratory infection in elderly people, adults with underlying cardiopulmonary disease, and those who are severely immunocompromised.

The Pathogen

RSV is an enveloped virus of the family Paramyxoviridae, genus *Pneumovirus,* and is related to the newly identified human metapneumovirus. The single-stranded negative-polarity RNA encodes 11 proteins, 8 of which are found in purified virions. Three transmembrane glycoproteins (G, attachment protein; F, fusion protein; SH protein) protrude from a lipid bilayer encompassing the nucleocapsid proteins (N, P, M2, polymerase) complexed with the genome. The matrix protein (M) is associated with the viral envelope. Two nonstructural proteins (NS1 and NS2) block the antiviral activity of interferon-α. Neutralizing antibodies are directed at F and G glycoproteins, whereas F, N, and M2 are primary targets for cytotoxic T cells. Two major virus groups (A and B), each with four to five subgroups, are distinguishable by antigenically divergent G proteins.

Epidemiology

As with influenza, worldwide RSV outbreaks occur annually. In the United States, epidemics generally begin in the southern states in late fall, move steadily north, and peak in February and March in colder climates. RSV causes approximately 100,000 hospitalizations and accounts for 60% of bronchiolitis and 25% of pneumonia cases in infants in the United States. Mortality is relatively low in U.S. infants, with an estimated 250 deaths annually; however, deaths are more common in underdeveloped countries. In the first year of life, nearly 70% of infants become infected, with the remainder being infected the following year. Family studies suggest that schoolchildren introduce RSV into the home and it is subsequently spread to parents and younger siblings, with infection rates of 43 and 62%, respectively. Like rhinovirus (Chapter 384), RSV is transmitted principally by direct contact with large-particle fomites from respiratory secretions, in contrast to the primary mode of spread of influenza virus, aerosolization.

Approximately 1 to 3% of primary infections result in hospitalization, but lower socioeconomic status, underlying prematurity, congenital cardiac abnormalities, bronchopulmonary dysplasia, and immunosuppression significantly increase the risk for serious disease. Recent genetic analysis has found that severe disease is associated with specific polymorphisms in the promoter regions of cytokine genes. Hospitalization is most frequent between the ages of 1 and 6 months, with a median age of 2 months. Maternally derived antibody appears to protect briefly in the first month of life, when serious lower respiratory symptoms are infrequent. Reinfection occurs frequently throughout life, although illness is less severe and hospitalization infrequent except for those with underlying cardiac or pulmonary conditions.

Though often not considered in adults, RSV infection is common and, in certain populations, may be severe. In a British study, RSV accounted for 17% of medically attended respiratory illnesses in those older than 45 years. RSV has been identified as a relatively common cause of community-acquired pneumonia in adults and ranked third behind pneumococcus and influenza in one large study. Elderly persons appear to be at highest risk, and outbreaks in nursing homes are common. In addition, RSV infection has been associated with 10% of hospitalizations for acute pulmonary symptoms in the winter among community-dwelling elderly persons, a rate similar to that for influenza. Infection rate and severity correlate inversely with levels of mucosal and serum antibody, respectively. RSV infection in severely immunocompromised adults, such as bone marrow transplant recipients and those with acute leukemia undergoing cytotoxic chemotherapy, is associated with 60% mortality rates when pneumonia develops.

Both RSV groups usually cocirculate during outbreaks, although group A strains generally dominate. Within groups, the prevailing genotypes shift annually and may reflect immune pressure in the susceptible population. Partial immunity to RSV develops over time, as indicated by resistance to both infection and illness. Experimental studies suggest that immunopathologic mechanisms, principally mediated by innate immune function, helper T cells and their cytokines, and leukotrienes, account for disease manifestations.

Clinical Manifestations

After an incubation period of 2 to 8 days, previously uninfected infants experience upper respiratory symptoms. Conjunctival injection, mucopurulent nasal discharge, cough, and low-grade fever (38° C) are typical and indistinguishable from those in other respiratory infections. Otitis media occurs commonly, generally in association with bacteria. After several days, lower respiratory tract symptoms develop in 25 to 50% of infants. Cough, wheezing, increased respiratory rate, use of accessory muscles, intercostal retractions, and cyanosis are seen as the disease progresses. Expiratory wheezes, rhonchi, and fine rales are the most common findings on lung examination. Sudden apnea may develop in the youngest infants. Mortality is rare in otherwise healthy infants but can reach 37% in infants with cardiac disorders. Hyperinflation and diffuse interstitial pneumonitis are the most frequent radiographic findings. Infiltrates are usually diffuse, but consolidation is seen in up to a fourth of patients.

High-titer virus shedding lasts 7 to 10 days, although immunocompromised infants may excrete virus for a month or longer. Interestingly, clinical symptoms may not correlate with prolonged shedding. Coinfection with other respiratory viruses is not uncommon but is not clinically discernible. Should bacterial superinfection develop, with *Streptococcus pneumoniae* and *Haemophilus influenzae* being the most frequent organisms isolated, treatment with antibiotics is indicated. Severe bronchiolitis has been linked to childhood asthma, although the precise contributions of RSV infection and allergic predisposition are unknown.

Illness in young adults typically lasts for 1 week and consists of nasal discharge, pharyngitis, and low-grade fever. The impact is not trivial because many have lower respiratory symptoms, especially wheezing, and miss work while seeking medical attention. Virus is shed at low titer for approximately 3 to 5 days. Elderly persons with RSV infection may experience cough, dyspnea, variable but generally low-grade fever, wheezing, and in some cases, respiratory failure. Large studies show that RSV is more often associated with wheezing than influenza is, whereas the reverse is true for high fever. In frail elderly persons, those with underlying chronic obstructive pulmonary disease or congestive heart failure, and those who are severely immunocompromised, severe disease with attack rates of 5 to 10% annually can develop. Nasal congestion followed by cough and wheezing is a clue to the presence of RSV. Attack rates in nosocomial outbreaks in nursing homes average 10 to 15%. Rales and wheezes are evident in a third of patients, and radiographically confirmed pneumonia is noted in approximately 10%. Among those hospitalized, bacterial superinfection occurs in about 8%, a rate similar to that seen during influenza virus infection.

RSV infection has been documented in up to 10% of bone marrow transplant recipients and those with acute leukemia during the winter months. The illness begins with upper respiratory symptoms but frequently spreads to the lower respiratory tract. If RSV infection occurs before marrow engraftment, pneumonia develops in half with an attendant mortality of 60 to 90%. Notably, this figure is somewhat higher than the mortality with influenza virus pneumonia in this population. Chest radiographs demonstrate diffuse interstitial and alveolar infiltrates. A useful clinical clue to the presence of RSV is the almost universal presence of radiographically proven sinusitis. The presence of upper respiratory tract symptoms distinguishes this illness from cytomegalovirus pneumonia.

Diagnosis

In the pediatric setting, a presumptive diagnosis is suggested by typical symptoms occurring during the epidemic season. In adults, the diagnosis is often never considered. Because the clinical picture of RSV is indistinguishable from that of other infectious agents of respiratory disease, especially in adults, laboratory confirmation is required if antiviral therapy is contemplated. In infants the sensitivity of viral culture is about 75%. Rapid diagnostic tests rely on detecting viral antigen or RNA in respiratory secretions. Immunofluorescence (IF) has a sensitivity of about 80%, whereas commercial enzyme immunoassay (EIA) is less sensitive and less specific than IF. Reverse transcription–polymerase chain reaction (RT-PCR) is considerably more sensitive than culture. In adults, diagnostic tests are significantly less sensitive: less than 50% for virus culture and 10% for IF and EIA. RT-PCR is very sensitive in adults and detects infection in three quarters of culture-negative seropositive cases. In immunocompromised adults, RSV antigen is found in only 15% of nasal secretions but in 90% of bronchoalveolar lavage specimens.

Treatment

Rx

Therapy for hospitalized infants includes hydration, oxygen, bronchodilators, and specific antiviral medication. Severely ill infants are commonly dehydrated and require intravenous fluid. Supplemental oxygen should be given to all infants with hypoxia. The effectiveness of nebulized bronchodilators such as salbutamol is variable, but a subset of infants respond. Glucocorticosteroids have not been shown to have benefit. Specific antiviral therapy is currently limited to inhaled ribavirin (1-β-D-ribafuranosyl-1,2,4-triazole-3-carboxamide), a nucleoside analogue with activity against several RNA viruses. Ribavirin is administered by aerosol, typically for 4 hours three times a day for 3 to 5 days, although longer therapy has been used. High-dose, short-duration (2 hours three times daily) treatment is considered equivalent. Some placebo-controlled clinical trials have demonstrated more rapid resolution of respiratory symptoms and hypoxia. The majority of infants do not require therapy, but ribavirin treatment may be indicated for infants at high risk for serious disease and those who are severely ill. There are no placebo-controlled studies of the effect of ribavirin in adults with severe RSV disease, although anecdotal data suggest benefit in immunocompromised adults with RSV pneumonia, especially if therapy is begun before respiratory failure develops. Finally, intramuscular humanized RSV monoclonal antibody has demonstrated benefit when administered prophylactically to high-risk infants with underlying cardiopulmonary disease or prematurity. Studies using monoclonal antibody, in combination with inhaled ribavirin, suggest benefit in the treatment of RSV pneumonia in immunosuppressed adults.

Prevention

Adherence to standard infection control principles (e.g., gloves, gowns, and frequent handwashing) can substantially reduce nosocomial spread. Health care personnel and visitors with symptoms suggestive of RSV infection should be medically evaluated before having contact with bone marrow transplant and other immunosuppressed persons at high risk for severe disease. A vaccine for prevention of RSV is not available, although both inactivated purified subunit and live attenuated vaccines are in clinical trials.

SUGGESTED READINGS

Falsey AR, Hennessey PA, Formica MA, et al: Respiratory syncytial virus infection in elderly and high-risk adults. N Engl J Med 2005;352:1749–1759. *Comprehensive report of the epidemiology and clinical impact of RSV infection in elderly and high-risk adults with cardiopulmonary disease, with a direct comparison to influenza virus infection.*

Falsey AR, Walsh EE: Respiratory syncytial virus infection in adults. Clin Microbiol Rev 2000;13:371–384. *A detailed review of RSV infection in adults, including the epidemiology, clinical disease, immunology, therapy, and prospects for vaccines.*

Hall CB: Respiratory syncytial virus and parainfluenza virus. N Engl J Med 2001;344:1917–1928. *A comprehensive review.*

Thompson WW, Shay DK, Weintranb E, et al: Mortality associated with respiratory syncytial virus in the United States. JAMA 2003;289:179–186. *A recent epidemiologic study of influenza and RSV.*

Ventre K, Randolph AG: Ribavirin for respiratory syncytial virus infection of the lower respiratory tract in infants and young children. Cochrane Database Syst Rev 2007;1:CD000181. *Ribavirin may decrease the duration of mechanical ventilation and length of hospital stay.*

386 PARAINFLUENZA VIRAL DISEASE

Edward E. Walsh

Definition

Parainfluenza viruses are important causes of a wide spectrum of respiratory illness in infants and young children, producing syndromes ranging from the common cold and otitis media to severe croup, bronchiolitis, and pneumonia. In older children and adults, illness is usually limited to the upper respiratory tract, although immunocompromised individuals may develop fatal respiratory failure.

The Pathogen

The parainfluenza viruses are enveloped single-stranded nonsegmented RNA viruses and belong to the family Paramyxoviridae, which also includes measles, mumps, and respiratory syncytial viruses (RSVs). The genome encodes six structural proteins, of which the hemagglutinin-neuraminidase (HN) and fusion (F) proteins are exposed on the bilayered lipid envelope that surrounds a helical nucleocapsid-RNA complex. The two surface proteins, which mediate attachment and penetration of the virus into susceptible mammalian cells, have retained antigenic stability for more than 30 years. There are four serotypes of human parainfluenza viruses, types 1 through 4, with two subgroups (A and B) of type 4 virus. Molecular analysis indicates significant genetic variability within major groups.

Epidemiology

The parainfluenza viruses are ubiquitous and have a worldwide geographic distribution. Spread principally by large-particle fomites and close person-to-person contact, each of the four serotypes displays somewhat different epidemiologic features.

Over the years, parainfluenza virus activity has displayed both endemic and epidemic patterns. Primary infection with parainfluenza viruses begins soon after birth, with each serotype favoring different age groups and distinct clinical syndromes. Significant overlap exists in this regard, precluding specific diagnosis based on clinical and epidemiologic grounds. Among the parainfluenza viruses, type 3 infects infants first, with more than 50% showing serologic evidence of infection in the first year of life. Parainfluenza virus type 3 is second only to RSV (Chapter 385) as a cause of bronchiolitis and pneumonia in this youngest age group and causes approximately 18,000 hospitalizations annually in the United States. Parainfluenza virus type 1exhibits a unique epidemiology with biennial outbreaks in the fall of odd-numbered years. Type 2 infections occur later in childhood, between ages 2 and 6. The peak incidence of infection with parainfluenza virus 1, manifested principally as croup, occurs between ages 1 and 2. The lower infection rate with parainfluenza type 1 and 2 viruses in very young infants suggests that maternally derived antibody is protective, in contrast to parainfluenza virus type 3 infection, in which maternal antibody has only limited benefit. Parainfluenza virus causes 18,000 to 35,000 croup hospitalizations in children younger than 5 years each year. After primary infection, a relatively brief period of immunity against homotypic reinfection develops; however, the fact that reinfections are common later in childhood highlights the lack of durable immunity.

Clinical Manifestations

Illness associated with primary parainfluenza virus infection varies by age and virus serotype, although substantial overlap occurs. Underlying medical conditions, such as cardiopulmonary or immune disorders, also influence the severity of disease. In general, parainfluenza virus types 1 and 2 are associated with croup whereas parainfluenza virus type 3 causes bronchiolitis and pneumonia. Other causes of croup include influenza A and RSV.

Infection typically starts with upper respiratory signs and symptoms, notably coryza, rhinorrhea, pharyngitis without cervical adenopathy, and low-grade fever. In 15%, signs of lower respiratory tract disease develop. If croup evolves, the child manifests a raspy, barking cough with notable inspiratory stridor, dyspnea, and respiratory distress. The latter symptoms, which may be spasmodic, are due to subglottic inflammation and edema. Typically, in mild to moderate illness symptoms last 3 to 5 days but may be quite unpredictable and result in sudden respiratory failure. In hospitalized infants, hypoxia is universal, and hypercarbia is present in half. In severe stridor, differentiation from epiglottitis caused by *Haemophilus influenzae* type b (Chapter 323) may be suggested by lateral neck radiography, which can show subglottic edema and narrowing, in contrast to epiglottic swelling. Although also a cause of croup, parainfluenza virus type 3 more commonly causes disease indistinguishable from RSV: tracheobronchitis, bronchiolitis, and pneumonia. Cough, rales, and wheezing associated with hypoxia and air trapping on radiography are common.

Reinfection with the parainfluenza viruses is less severe and typically causes cold symptoms in normal children and adults. However, as with RSV, some adults may develop severe disease requiring hospitalization and even ventilatory support. Fever, cough, dyspnea, and wheezing in association with nasal congestion are common. Radiographic changes, primarily lobar or interstitial infiltrates, are seen in 59% of hospitalized adults with this infection. Nursing home outbreaks with a high incidence of pneumonia have been reported, and parainfluenza viruses have been implicated in severe pneumonia in immunocompromised children and adults. In a report of more than 1000 bone marrow transplant recipients, 61 parainfluenza virus infections were documented. Many were nosocomial; 44% of the patients developed pneumonia and 27% died, with most having had preceding upper respiratory symptoms. The latter finding is clinically useful in distinguishing parainfluenza virus pneumonia from cytomegalovirus pneumonia in this group. In another study of 3577 bone marrow transplant recipients, nearly 8% developed parainfluenza infections; 90% were parainfluenza virus type 1, and the majority were community acquired. Approximately 25% developed lower respiratory disease, which carried 40% mortality. Unrelated donor status and steroids were statistically associated with infection and development of pneumonia, respectively. Coinfection, especially with *Aspergillus,* occurred in half of those with pneumonia. As with RSV infection, the most severe illnesses and 90% of the deaths related to parainfluenza virus pneumonia occur in the first 100 days after transplantation, when lymphopenia is most pronounced. Fever, cough, shortness of breath, and sputum production are the most common symptoms, and bilateral pulmonary infiltrates are the most common radiographic finding.

Diagnosis

Although the clinician may suspect parainfluenza virus on clinical and epidemiologic grounds, specific diagnosis requires isolating the virus or detecting viral antigen or RNA in respiratory secretions. Monkey kidney or human embryonic kidney cell cultures are optimal for virus recovery, generally in 5 to 10 days, with the exception of type 4 virus, which requires up to 3 weeks in culture. Indirect immunofluorescence tests are also available for rapid antigen detection and, although specific, are less sensitive than culture. Diagnosis of parainfluenza infection in adults may be more difficult than in children, but virus can usually be recovered from the nasal or pharyngeal secretions of bone marrow transplant recipients with pneumonia and also generally from bronchoalveolar specimens in this group. Reverse transcription–polymerase chain reaction is a highly sensitive and specific test.

Treatment

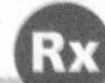

Specific antiviral treatment for parainfluenza virus is currently unavailable. Aerosolized ribavirin, approved for use in RSV infection, has in vitro activity against the parainfluenza viruses. No conclusions can be drawn from uncontrolled studies of ribavirin therapy of immunocompromised children and adults with severe parainfluenza virus pneumonia when administered at a dose of 20 mg/mL for 12 to 20 hours per day for 7 to 14 days with or without concomitant intravenous immune globulin.

Treatment of croup in children, under usual circumstances, includes mist and supplemental oxygen. Aerosolized bronchodilators (racemic epinephrine) have definite but only transient benefit, and corticosteroid use is controversial. Antibiotics are indicated only when bacterial superinfection is documented, an uncommon occurrence except for the immunocompromised host with pneumonia. Immunization to prevent parainfluenza virus infection with live attenuated vaccines is under study.

SUGGESTED READINGS

Chiu CY, Rouskin S, Koshy A, et al: Microarray detection of human parainfluenzavirus 4 infection associated with respiratory failure in an immunocompetent adult. Clin Infect Dis 2006;43:e71–e76. *Case report demonstrating the utility of a pan-viral DNA microarray for viral pathogen screening.*

Fry AM, Curns AT, Harbour K, et al: Seasonal trends of human parainfluenza viral infections: United States, 1990–2004. Clin Infect Dis 2006;43:1016–1022. *Describes distinct seasonal patterns for different serotypes.*

Hall CB: Respiratory syncytial virus and parainfluenza viruses. N Engl J Med 2001;344:1917–1928. *This review article describes the epidemiology and diseases associated with parainfluenza viruses.*

Nichols WG, Corey L, Gooley T, et al: Parainfluenza virus infections after hematopoietic stem cell transplantation: Risk factors, response to antiviral therapy, and effect on transplant outcome. Blood 2001;98:573–578. *A comprehensive review of the risk factors, outcome, and effect of therapy of parainfluenza virus infections in severely immunocompromised patients.*

387 INFLUENZA

Frederick G. Hayden

Definition

Influenza is an acute febrile respiratory illness that occurs in annual outbreaks of varying severity and unpredictably in worldwide epidemics (pandemics). The causative virus infects the respiratory tract, is highly contagious, and typically produces prominent systemic symptoms early in the illness. Influenza virus infection can produce various clinical syndromes in adults, including common colds, pharyngitis, tracheobronchitis, and pneumonia. Conversely, infections with other respiratory viruses, such as respiratory syncytial virus (RSV) (Chapter 385) or adenovirus (Chapter 388), may produce influenza-like illness. Influenza A viruses have caused three pandemics and one pandemic-like event in the 20th century (Table 387–1). The pandemic in 1918 to 1919 caused at least 500,000 deaths in the United States and over 40 million worldwide. Influenza epidemics are associated with enormous morbidity, economic loss, and often substantial mortality. Recent epidemics have caused on average more than 36,000 respiratory- and circulatory-related deaths and over 200,000 hospitalizations in the United States alone.

The Pathogen

Influenza viruses belong to the family Orthomyxoviridae and are divided into three types (A, B, and C) distinguished by their internal and external proteins (Table 387–2). The virion (Fig. 387–1) is a medium-sized, enveloped pleomorphic particle covered with two types of surface glycoprotein spikes, the trimeric hemagglutinin (H or HA) and the

TABLE 387–1 ANTIGENIC SUBTYPES OF INFLUENZA A VIRUS ASSOCIATED WITH PANDEMIC AND PANDEMIC-LIKE INFLUENZA

Year	Interval (yr)	Subtype Designation	Extent of Antigenic Change in Indicated Surface Protein*	Severity of Pandemic (Mortality)
1889	?42–59	H3N?	H+++N?	Severe
1918	18	H1N1†	H+++N+++	Very severe
1957	39	H2N2	H+++N+++	Severe
1968	11	H3N2	H+++N–	Moderate‡
1977	9	H1N1	H+++N+++	Negligible§

*Compared with antecedent or cocirculating virus.
†Formerly designated H0N1 (swine virus prototype) or Hsw1N1.
‡The population had some immunity to N2 neuraminidase.
§The older population was immune because of previous infection with earlier circulating, antigenically identical virus; it primarily affected those born after 1957.
+ = Minor change; ++ = moderate change; +++ = major change; – = no change.

TABLE 387–2 INFLUENZA VIRUS PROTEINS

Designation	Location (Approximate No. per Virion)	Function	Other
Hemagglutinin (HA)	Surface (500)	Cell attachment and penetration; fusion activity	Type-, subtype-, and strain-specific antigens; key antigen in inactivated vaccine
Neuraminidase (NA)	Surface (100)	Virus release and spread; enzymatic activity	Type-, subtype-, and strain-specific antigens; activity linked to risk for pneumonia; site of action of zanamivir, oseltamivir carboxylate
Membrane or M1 matrix	Internal (3000)	Major structural envelope protein; virus assembly	Type-specific antigen
M2	Surface (20–60)	Virus uncoating and assembly; ion channel	Influenza A only; site of action of amantadine/ rimantadine
Nucleoprotein (NP)	Internal (1000)	Associated with RNA and polymerase proteins	Type-specific antigen
Polymerase proteins (PB1, PB2, PA)	Internal (30–60)	RNA replication and transcription	Determinant of replication efficiency; probable site of action of ribavirin
NS1	Nonstructural (infected cells)	Regulation of virus replication	Interferon antagonist
NEP	Internal (130–200)	Nuclear export factor	Formerly NS2
PB1-F2	Nonstructural (infected cells)	Proapoptotic factor	Expressed from 1+ reading frame of PB1 of certain viruses

Adapted from Lamb RA, King RM: Orthomyxoviridae. *In* Fields BN, Knipe DM, Howley PM (eds): Fields Virology, 4th ed. Philadelphia, Lippincott Williams & Wilkins, 2001, p 1487.

tetrameric neuraminidase (N or NA). The envelope is composed of a lipid bilayer overlying the matrix (M1) protein that surrounds the segmented viral genome. The genome consists of eight segments of single-stranded RNA; influenza C viruses have seven segments and only a single surface glycoprotein. Whereas influenza B and C viruses are principally human pathogens, influenza A viruses primarily infect aquatic birds and sometimes other animal hosts, including other avians, swine, horses, marine mammals, cats, and dogs. Influenza A viruses are further classified into subtypes on the basis of their HA and NA glycoproteins. Sixteen HA and 9 NA subtypes are recognized in nature, but only 3 HAs (H1, H2, and H3) and 2 NAs (N1 and N2) have been documented thus far in epidemic and pandemic human influenza A viruses. Each strain is identified by type, subtype, site, sample number, and year of isolation.

Epidemiology

Antigenic Variation

Influenza viruses are unique among the respiratory viruses with regard to their extent of antigenic variation, epidemic behavior, and frequent association with excess mortality during community outbreaks. The changing antigenicity of the surface glycoproteins largely accounts for the continuing epidemics of influenza in humans. Antibody to HA neutralizes viral infectivity and is thus the major determinant of immunity. Anti-NA antibody limits viral replication and probably reduces the severity of infection. Variation involves either relatively minor (antigenic drift) or major (antigenic shift) changes in antigenicity. Significant antigenic variation is much less frequent with influenza B than with influenza A and may not occur with influenza C.

Antigenic drift refers to small changes that occur frequently (every year or every few years) within an influenza A or B virus. For example, the original H3N2 variant, A/Aichi/68, has undergone successive drifts resulting in epidemic strains that include the recent circulation of A/Wisconsin/67/2005–like viruses. Antigenic drift results from point mutations in the RNA segment coding for HA that cause amino acid substitutions in at least one of five antigenic sites on HA. Immunologic selection favors the new variant over the old for transmission because of the less frequent presence of antibody to the new virus in the population.

Antigenic shift results from the appearance of an influenza A virus with HA or with HA and NA glycoproteins new to humans or the possible reappearance of virus after decades of absence. Because of the lack of population immunity to the new strain, one that is transmissible from person to person can cause pandemic disease (see Table 387–1). Infection by one subtype does not provide cross-protection against another. The origin of new pandemic strains and the basis for their apparent recirculation remain incompletely defined. Avian influenza viruses have served as the reservoir of new genes for human pandemic viruses. Reassortment of gene segments may occur when two influenza viruses simultaneously infect a single cell, and reassortment events in which human viruses acquired avian genes led to both the 1957 and 1968 pandemic viruses. Because swine can support replication of both human and avian viruses, they have been postulated to serve as a mixing vessel for the generation of new strains or the host in which avian viruses can adapt to mammals. Frequent reassortment among human influenza A viruses occurs and has resulted in recent circulation of H1N2 viruses. In contrast, the 1918 pandemic virus was not such a reassortant virus but appears to be an avian virus that underwent mutational adaptation in a mammalian host, perhaps human or swine, before causing the pandemic.

Zoonotic infections occur from swine, poultry, or rarely other animals. Although avian influenza viruses do not generally cause infections directly in humans, bird-to-human transmission of avian subtype H5, H9, and H7 viruses has been documented. Initially recognized by a cluster of human cases in Hong Kong in 1997, an unprecedented epizootic of avian H5N1 infections has spread since 2003 to affect many areas of Asia, the Middle East, Europe, and Africa and has caused sporadic human illnesses with high mortality in more than 275 persons.

Epidemic or Interpandemic Influenza

An *epidemic* is an outbreak of influenza confined to one geographic location. In a given community, epidemics of influenza A virus infection

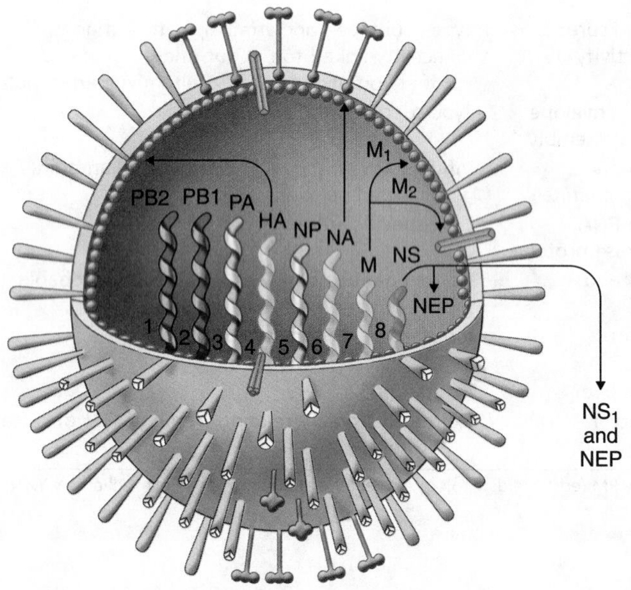

FIGURE 387–1 • Diagram of influenza virus structure. Eight segments of viral RNA are contained within the envelope and matrix (M1) shell. Each codes for one or two proteins that form the virus or regulate its intracellular replication. The presumed functions of each are listed in Table 387–2. (Courtesy of Dr. Robert G. Webster.)

often have a characteristic pattern. They usually begin rather abruptly, reach a sharp peak in 2 or 3 weeks, and last 6 to 10 weeks. Increased numbers of schoolchildren with febrile respiratory illness are often the first indication of influenza in a community. This outbreak is soon followed by illness in adults and 1 to 2 weeks later by increased hospital admission of patients with influenza-related complications. Hospitalization rates in high-risk persons increase two- to five-fold during major epidemics (Table 387–3). School and employment absenteeism increases, as frequently does mortality from pneumonia and influenza, especially in older persons during A/H3N2 epidemics. Epidemics occur almost exclusively during the winter months in temperate areas, but influenza activity may occur year-round in the tropics or display other patterns. Outbreaks sometimes occur in tour groups (land or ship) and in facilities during summer months, particularly after the appearance of a drift variant. Regional differences in the time and magnitude of occurrence of influenza outbreaks are common. During epidemics, overall attack rates typically range from 5 to 20% in adults. Attack rates of 40 to 50% are not uncommon in closed populations, including those in hospitals and nursing homes, and in certain highly susceptible age groups. Two different strains within a single subtype, two different influenza A subtypes (H1N1 and H3N2), or both influenza A and B viruses may cocirculate. In addition, simultaneous outbreaks of influenza A and RSV have occurred. Strains circulating at the end of one season's epidemic are sometimes responsible for the next season's outbreak (the so-called herald wave phenomenon). Furthermore, other than the association of influenza outbreaks with colder seasons, factors that allow an epidemic to develop or those responsible for its cessation when susceptible individuals still remain are unknown.

Pneumonia- and influenza-related deaths fluctuate annually, with peaks in the winter months. When such deaths exceed the expected threshold, it is due to influenza A or occasionally to influenza B virus or RSV activity. Although mortality is greatest during pandemics, substantial total mortality occurs with epidemics. During seasonal influenza, more than 85% of pneumonia- and influenza-related deaths occur in persons 65 years and older. Other cardiopulmonary and chronic diseases also result in increased mortality after influenza epidemics, so the overall influenza-associated mortality is about two- to four-fold higher than pneumonia- and influenza-related deaths.

Pandemic Influenza

Pandemics of influenza A result from the emergence of a new virus capable of sustained person-to-person transmission and to which the population contains no or limited immunity. The virus spreads worldwide and infects persons of all ages. The pandemics of 1957 and 1968 began in mainland China, and Southeast Asia has been postulated to be the epicenter for such strains. The interval between pandemics is variable (10 to 40 years) and unpredictable. The most severe pandemics have resulted when there were major antigenic alterations in both major surface antigens. Virulence is a multigenic characteristic that varies among strains and is not necessarily linked to transmissibility. The unique virulence of the 1918 H1N1 virus in causing severe viral pneumonia appears to be related in part to its HA, whereas the virulence of recent H1N1 viruses appears to be less than that of H3N2 viruses. After one or more waves of pandemic influenza, the level of immunity in the

TABLE 387–3 AGE-SPECIFIC RATES FOR ILLNESS AND MORTALITY DURING URBAN INFLUENZA EPIDEMICS

Age (yr)	Physician Visits per 100	ARD Hospitalizations per 10,000	Pneumonia- and Influenza-Related Mortality per 100,000
<5	28	43	3
5–14	14	5	1
15–44	10	8	1
45–54	9	13	10
55–64	10	21	10
≥65–	—	73	104

ARD = acute respiratory disease; P + I = pneumonia and influenza; — = not stated.
Adapted from Glezen WP: Anatomy of an urban influenza epidemic. *In* Hannoun C, Kendal AP, Klenk HD, et al (eds): Options for the Control of Influenza II. Amsterdam, Elsevier, 1993, p 12.

population increases, although excess mortality in younger adults may continue for some years. Repeated epidemics caused by strains showing antigenic drift within the subtype occur in subsequent years.

Pathobiology

Influenza virus infection is transmitted from person to person by virus-containing respiratory secretions. Large- and small-particle aerosols over short distances (1–2 meters) both appear to contribute, but transmission by other routes, including fomites, may be possible. Infection by avian viruses also can occur after direct contact with infected birds or their excreta, possibly, ingestion of contaminated food, and sometimes inoculation into the conjunctiva. Virtually all cells lining the respiratory tract can support viral replication, although receptors for avian viruses appear to be concentrated on cells in the distal bronchioles and alveoli. Once the virus initiates infection of the respiratory tract epithelium, successive cycles of viral replication infect large numbers of cells and result in destruction of ciliated epithelium through direct cytopathic effects or apoptosis. The incubation period, which averages 2 days and varies from 1 to 4 days, may be somewhat longer in infections caused by avian viruses. The quantity of virus in respiratory tract specimens correlates with the severity of illness and levels of host pro-inflammatory cytokine-chemokine responses, findings that support the importance of ongoing viral replication in producing illness. Elevated levels of pro-inflammatory cytokines such as interferon-α, interleukin-6, and tumor necrosis factor-α occur in blood and respiratory secretions and probably contribute to systemic symptoms and fever. The duration of viral replication depends on age and immune status. Shedding generally lasts for 3 to 5 days in adults, often into the second week in children, and may persist for weeks to months in immunocompromised hosts. Prolonged viral replication and excessive cytokine-chemokine responses have been found in H5N1 infections. Viremia or extrapulmonary dissemination is rarely associated with typical human influenza, but both occur in some patients with avian H5N1 infections, in whom gastrointestinal replication may also occur.

Nasal and bronchial biopsy specimens from persons with uncomplicated influenza reveal desquamation of the ciliated columnar epithelium. Individual cells show shrinkage, pyknotic nuclei, and loss of cilia. In addition, the lungs in fatal influenza may show necrotizing bronchitis, alveolar edema and hemorrhage, hyaline membrane formation, diffuse alveolar damage, and later, fibrosis and squamous metaplasia. Secondary bacterial infections develop as a result of altered bacterial flora, damage to bronchial epithelium with depressed mucociliary clearance, decreased polymorphonuclear and alveolar macrophage functions, accumulation of alveolar fluid, and possibly viral NA–mediated exposure of cellular receptors for bacteria.

Neutralizing, hemagglutination-inhibiting (HAI), anti-NA, complement-fixing, enzyme-linked immunosorbent assay, and immunofluorescent antibodies begin to develop in the sera of persons with primary influenza virus infection during the second week after infection and reach a peak by 4 weeks. Secretory antibodies develop in the upper respiratory tract and consist predominantly of IgA antibodies. Cell-mediated immune responses develop by 1 week after infection. Adaptive immunity to influenza appears to be largely subtype specific and durable for a particular strains. Protection against illness caused by human viruses is generally associated with serum HAI titers of 1:40 or greater, serum-neutralizing antibody titers of 1:8 or greater, or nasal-neutralizing antibody titers of 1:4 or greater.

Clinical Manifestations

Influenza Syndrome

An abrupt onset of feverishness, chilliness, rigors, headache, myalgia, and malaise is characteristic of influenza but occurs in less than two thirds of cases. Systemic symptoms predominate initially, and prostration occurs in more severe cases. Usually, myalgia and headaches are the most troublesome early symptoms, and their severity is related to the level of fever. Arthralgia is common. Sometimes ocular symptoms, including photophobia, tearing, burning, and pain on moving the eyes, are helpful diagnostically. Conjunctivitis is characteristic in avian H7 virus infections. Respiratory symptoms, particularly dry cough and nasal discharge, are also generally present at the onset but are overshadowed by the systemic symptoms. Nasal obstruction, hoarseness, and sore throat are likewise common. As systemic illness diminishes, respiratory complaints and findings become more apparent. Cough is the most frequent and troublesome symptom and may be accompanied by substernal discomfort or burning. Cough, lassitude, and malaise may persist for several weeks before full recovery.

Fever is the most important initial physical finding. The temperature usually rises rapidly to a peak of 38 to 40° C within 12 hours of onset, concurrently with systemic symptoms. Fever is usually continuous but may be intermittent, especially if antipyretics are administered. Typically, the duration of fever in adults is 3 days, but it may last from 1 to 5 or more days. Uncommonly, the fever takes a biphasic course. Early in the course of illness, the patient appears toxic, the face is flushed, and the skin is hot and moist. The eyes are watery and reddened. Clear nasal discharge is common. The mucosa of the nose and throat is hyperemic, but exudate is not observed. Small, tender cervical lymph nodes are often present. Transient scattered rhonchi or localized areas of rales are found in less than 20% of cases.

The pattern of illness just described occurs with any strain of influenza A or B virus. Illness is more frequent and severe in smokers, and attack rates are higher in children than in adults. Maximum temperatures are higher in children, cervical adenopathy may be more frequent, and gastrointestinal symptoms of nausea, emesis, or abdominal pain are more common. Women experience increased complications of influenza during the second and third trimesters of pregnancy. Symptoms may be protracted for some persons infected with human immunodeficiency virus (HIV), and they are also at higher risk for complications. Older adults, especially the infirm elderly, develop fever, muscle aches, sore throat, and headache less often but have higher rates of altered mental status and pulmonary complications. In sporadic illness attributable to H5N1 virus, upper respiratory complaints are less frequent, diarrhea is more common, and progressive viral pneumonia with high mortality is much more likely. Influenza C virus generally causes sporadic upper respiratory tract illness or febrile bronchitis.

Respiratory Complications

Three pneumonic syndromes have been described: primary influenza viral pneumonia, secondary bacterial pneumonia, and mixed viral and bacterial pneumonia. Influenza A and B virus infections may be associated with other respiratory tract complications, including exacerbations of chronic bronchitis, asthma, or cystic fibrosis; croup and bronchiolitis in young children; and otitis media, sinusitis, and rarely, parotitis or bacterial tracheitis. Apparently uncomplicated influenza causes tracheobronchitis frequently and is often accompanied by abnormal tracheobronchial clearance, airway hyperactivity, and dysfunction of small airways lasting weeks. A syndrome mimicking pulmonary embolism with transiently altered perfusion scans has also been described.

Primary influenza viral pneumonia is uncommon during epidemics but has accounted for up to 20% of pneumonias during pandemics and has been the principal manifestation of patients with H5N1 illness. It occurs predominantly in persons with underlying pulmonary and cardiac disorders, pregnancy, or immunodeficiency states, although up to 40% of reported cases and almost all patients with H5N1 have no recognized underlying disease. After a typical onset of influenza, there is rapid progression of fever, cough, dyspnea, and cyanosis. Bilateral pulmonary infiltrates, often consistent with adult respiratory distress syndrome, and hypoxia may evolve rapidly. Gram staining of sputum may show abundant polymorphonuclear leukocytes but scant bacterial flora. Sputum may be bloody. Viral cultures of sputum or tracheal aspirates usually yield high titers of influenza virus. Antibiotics are not helpful, and the value of antiviral or immunomodulator therapies is unproven.

Bacterial superinfection is often clinically distinguishable from primary viral pneumonia. Patients are most often elderly or have chronic medical conditions. After a typical influenza illness, a period of improvement lasting from 1 to 4 days may ensue. Recrudescence of fever is typically associated with increased cough, sputum production, often pleuritic chest pain, and a localized area of consolidation apparent on physical and chest radiographic examination. Gram staining and culture of sputum most often reveal *Streptococcus pneumoniae* (Chapter 311), *Staphylococcus aureus* (Chapter 310), including community-acquired methicillin-resistant *S. aureus*, or *Haemophilus influenzae* (Chapter 323). Such patients usually respond to specific antibiotic therapy, although staphylococcal infections may be particularly virulent and cause destructive pulmonary lesions. Invasive aspergillosis (Chapter 360) occurs rarely after influenza.

In addition, during an outbreak of influenza, many less distinct syndromes are observed; patients may have viral tracheobronchitis, milder forms of localized viral pneumonia, or mixed viral and bacterial infection. Many respond to antibiotics. Immunocompromised hosts, including transplant recipients and acute leukemia patients undergoing chemotherapy, may have high rates of pneumonia and mortality after influenza.

Nonpulmonic Complications

Reye's syndrome, which is a well-recognized hepatic and central nervous system (CNS) complication of influenza A and B virus infections in children and rarely in adults, is associated with salicylate use. Toxic shock syndrome (Chapter 312) caused by respiratory tract infection with toxin-bearing *S. aureus* occurs, and outbreaks of meningococcal infection have been associated with both influenza A and B virus infections. Myositis with tender leg muscles and elevated serum creatine kinase levels may develop uncommonly, more often in children. Rhabdomyolysis can be severe, and virus has been recovered from skeletal muscle. Disseminated intravascular coagulation (DIC; Chapter 181) develops rarely, as does renal failure related to DIC or myoglobinuria. Lymphopenia and thrombocytopenia are common in H5N1 disease; hemophagocytic syndrome may complicate it and rarely human influenza. Myocarditis or pericarditis occur uncommonly. Aseptic meningitis, myelitis, encephalopathy associated with acute illness, especially in children, and postinfluenzal encephalitis have been reported.

Diagnosis

In an individual case, influenza often cannot be distinguished from infection with a number of other viruses (and occasionally streptococcal pharyngitis; Chapters 312 and 455) that produce headache, muscle aches, fever, sore throat, or cough (or various combinations thereof). On the other hand, when public health authorities report an epidemic of influenza A and B virus infection in a given community and a patient is seen with typical illness, it is highly likely that these symptoms are caused by an influenza virus infection. In such circumstances, the presence of fever and cough has a positive predictive value of about 80% for laboratory-proven influenza in adults. Influenza virus is readily isolated from nasal, sputum, or tracheal secretion specimens in the first 2 or 3 days of illness. Throat samples have lower yield than nasal samples in infections by human viruses but appear to be superior to nasal samples for detection of H5N1 infections. Usually, infectious virus is recovered in cell culture within 48 to 72 hours. Immunofluorescence testing of respiratory cells or inoculated cell cultures (shell vials) can reduce time to detection. Commercially available enzyme immunoassays or NA detection–based assays can document influenza virus infection rapidly but may have limited sensitivity (50 to 70%) in adults; some do not distinguish between influenza A and B. The limited specificity of some assays makes their predictive value low, especially outside the influenza season. Detection of viral RNA by reverse transcription–polymerase chain reaction appears to be highly sensitive and specific; this is the rapid test of choice for suspected H5N1 illness. Serologic methods are less useful clinically because they require convalescent serum obtained 14 to 21 days after the onset of infection.

Prevention

The mainstay of prevention is influenza virus vaccine (Chapter 16). Inactivated vaccines given by intramuscular injection provide 70 to 90% protection in young and middle-aged adults against influenza illness when the vaccine matches the epidemic strain. Immunogenicity and hence protection rates are often lower in elderly persons, particularly infirm nursing home residents, and in immunosuppressed patients, including those with advanced HIV infection, transplant recipients, and chemotherapy patients. In institutionalized elderly people, immunization is 50 to 60% effective in preventing hospitalization and pneumonia and reduces influenza-related mortality by 70 to 80%. In ambulatory high-risk patients, immunization reduces hospitalizations from pneumonia, influenza, and cardiovascular disease, as well as all-cause mortality during the influenza season. Immunization also appears to be cost-effective in working adults, depending on the size of the epidemic. Immunization of school-aged children appears to reduce respiratory illness in household contacts and, in one Japanese study, excess deaths in the elderly. Immunization of health care providers reduces the risk of transmission to patients. An intranasal, live attenuated vaccine that is highly protective against influenza in children and to a lesser extent in adults is currently approved in the United States for persons aged 5 to 49 years.

The antigenic composition of vaccines is reviewed annually so that these trivalent vaccines contain the most recently circulating strains, usually two subtypes of influenza A and an influenza B virus. Both vaccines are grown in eggs, and episodic production problems have led to shortages of the inactivated vaccine. With inactivated vaccine, fever and systemic symptoms occur at rates comparable to those of adults given placebo but are more common in young children. Among adults, 25% or more may have mild local reactions at the site of injection. Persons with malignant disease should receive vaccine between courses of chemotherapy. Intranasal vaccine causes coryza and sore throat in adults. Studies of investigational H5 vaccines indicate that two doses of high–HA antigen content or coadministration with an adjuvant appear to be necessary for adequate immunogenicity.

The priority groups for seasonal vaccine continue to expand and include those at increased risk for influenza complications and their immediate contacts (Table 387–4), although vaccine can be safely administered to anyone trying to avoid influenza. Vaccine should be given each year in the fall, preferably October or November, before the influenza season. The vaccine is contraindicated in persons with chicken egg anaphylactic hypersensitivity. Inactivated vaccine does not cause exacerbation of asthma but may rarely be associated with Guillain-Barré syndrome in older adults.

Rimantadine and amantadine are 70 to 90% effective in preventing influenza A illness caused by susceptible strains. However, the recent global circulation of resistant H3N2 and H1N1 strains has made use of these agents unreliable. Transmission of resistant virus from drug-treated close contacts (households, nursing homes) may cause failure of prophylaxis and has been associated with failure to terminate nursing home outbreaks. Inhaled zanamivir and oral oseltamivir are highly effective for chemoprophylaxis of both influenza A and B virus infections (Table 387–5). Unimmunized persons can be given prophylaxis when an outbreak develops and be given inactivated vaccine simultaneously with cessation of prophylaxis after 14 days. Alternatively, if vaccine is not available or is a poor match or if the patient is highly immunosuppressed, administration may be continued for the duration of the outbreak. When given to patients and staff alike, these drugs may be helpful in managing nosocomial outbreaks. Patients hospitalized with human influenza should be managed with standard and droplet precautions; those hospitalized with sporadic illness caused by presumed H5N1 or other novel strains warrant airborne, droplet, and contact precautions, including eye protection.

Treatment Rx

Oral rimantadine or amantadine therapy shortens the duration of fever and systemic and respiratory symptoms in uncomplicated influenza A caused by susceptible strains by 1 to 2 days and speeds functional recovery (see Table 387–5). [1,2] The possible effectiveness of these drugs in preventing or treating the pulmonary complications of influenza is unknown. Rimantadine carries a lower risk for CNS side effects than amantadine does, but both may cause gastrointestinal upset. These agents are ineffective for influenza B infections. Antiviral resistance because of point mutations in the M2 gene emerges in 30% or more of treated persons, who sometimes transmit drug-resistant virus to close contacts. Circulating H3N2 and increasingly H1N1 viruses often show high-level resistance to this antiviral class, as do many human isolates of avian A/H5N1 virus, so these drugs are not recommended for routine use at present.

The NA inhibitors inhaled zanamivir and oral oseltamivir are active against both influenza A and B viruses. [2] Therapy within 2 days of the onset of illness reduces symptoms, time to functional recovery, and risk for lower respiratory complications, including bronchitis and pneumonia. Early oseltamivir therapy also decreases the risk for hospitalization. Zanamivir may be infrequently associated with bronchospasm, sometimes severe, and oseltamivir is associated with nausea or emesis.

TABLE 387–4 RECOMMENDED TARGET GROUPS FOR INFLUENZA IMMUNIZATION

GROUPS AT INCREASED RISK FOR COMPLICATIONS (RECOMMENDED)
Persons 50 years and older
Residents of nursing homes and other chronic care facilities
Patients with a chronic pulmonary (including asthma) or cardiac disorder
Patients with chronic metabolic disease (including diabetes), renal dysfunction, hemoglobinopathies, immunosuppression (including HIV infection), or conditions (including cognitive, neuromuscular) that compromise respiratory function or increase aspiration risk
Children and teens receiving long-term aspirin
Women who will be pregnant during the influenza season
Children 6 months to 5 years old
GROUPS IN CONTACT WITH HIGH-RISK PERSONS (RECOMMENDED)
Physicians, nurses, and other health care providers
Employees of nursing homes and chronic care and assisted-living facilities
Providers of home care to high-risk persons
Household contacts (parents, siblings, caregivers) and out-of-home caregivers of high-risk persons, including children 0–5 years old
OTHER GROUPS (ENCOURAGED)
Providers of essential community services (e.g., police, fire)
Travelers (including to the tropics, large organized groups, or to the Southern Hemisphere in its winter)
Students, dormitory residents
Anyone wishing to their reduce risk for influenza

HIV = human immunodeficiency virus.
Adapted from Centers for Disease Control and Prevention: Prevention and control of influenza: Recommendations of the Advisory Committee on Immunization Practices. MMWR Morb Mortal Wkly Rep 2006;55:2.

TABLE 387–5 ANTIVIRAL DOSE RECOMMENDATIONS IN ADULTS

Drug	Route	Treatment	Prophylaxis	Dose Reductions	Comment
Amantadine	Oral	100 mg bid	100 mg bid	Age >64 yr, Cl_{cr} <50–80 mL/min	Consider further dose reductions in elderly <70 kg
Rimantadine	Oral	100 mg bid	100 mg bid	Age >64 yr, Cl_{cr} <10 mL/min or severe hepatic dysfunction	Once-daily dosing (200 mg) is an alternative
Oseltamivir	Oral	75 mg bid	75 mg once daily	Cl_{cr} <30 mL/min	
Zanamivir	Inhaled	10 mg bid	10 mg once daily		Training in use of the inhaler device is important

The standard duration of treatment is 5 days; a longer duration might be considered for infections in immunosuppressed hosts or those caused by novel viruses. The duration of prophylaxis depends on the epidemiologic setting; durations of 2 weeks after immunization or 7 to 10 days for postexposure prophylaxis are appropriate. Antiviral prophylaxis may interfere with response to intranasal, live-attenuated but not to intramuscular, inactivated vaccine.
Cl_{cr} = creatine clearance.

Other symptomatic measures include antipyretics and cough suppressants. Aspirin should not be used, especially in children younger than 16 years, because of its association with Reye's syndrome.

Influenza viral pneumonia, including H5N1 disease, often requires intensive respiratory monitoring and ventilator support. Oral amantadine or rimantadine, intravenous ribavirin, aerosolized ribavirin, nebulized zanamivir, and oral oseltamivir have been used with uncertain benefit. [2] Intensive care unit complications, including ventilator-associated pneumonia, are common. Secondary bacterial pneumonia should be treated with appropriate antibiotics. When studies of sputum do not clearly indicate an infecting bacterium, antibiotics that are effective against the probable pathogens, including *S. aureus*, should be used.

Prognosis

The mortality rate from seasonal influenza is very low. Most patients make a full recovery, and 90% of influenza-related deaths occur in persons older than 65 years or at high risk because of comorbid conditions. In patients whose viral pneumonia progresses to respiratory failure, the mortality rate is about 50%. For the new H5N1 subtype, the mortality of confirmed cases has been about 60%.

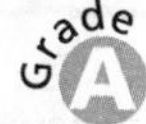

1. Jefferson T, Demicheli V, Di Pietrationi C, Rivetti D: Amantadine and rimantadine for influenza A in adults. Cochrane Database Syst Rev 2006;2:CD001169.
2. WHO Rapid Advice Guidelines on pharmacological management of humans infected with avian influenza A(H5N1) virus. Available at http://www.who.int/csr/disease/avian_influenza/guidelines/pharmamanagement/en/index.html.

SUGGESTED READINGS

Belshe RB, Edwards KM, Vesikari T, et al: Live attenuated versus inactivated influenza vaccine in infants and young children. N Engl J Med 2007;356:685–696. *Live attenuated vaccine had greater efficacy but was associated with a higher rate of all-cause hospitalization.*

Centers for Disease Control and Prevention: Prevention and control of influenza: Recommendations of the Advisory Committee on Immunization Practices. MMWR Recomm Rep 2006;55(RR-10):1–42. *Review of influenza epidemiology and recommendations for influenza immunization and antiviral use; updated on an annual basis.*

Centers for Disease Control and Prevention Influenza Website. Available at http://www.cdc.gov/cnidod/diseases/flu/weekly.htm. *Information on influenza surveillance, prevention, detection and control measures, as well as weekly updates on current activity levels in the United States.*

Jefferson T, Demicheli V, Rivetti D, et al: Antivirals for influenza in healthy adults: Systematic review. Lancet 2006;367:303–313. *Because of their low effectiveness, neuraminidase inhibitors should be used only in a serious epidemic or pandemic alongside other public health measures.*

World Health Organization Website. Available at http://www.wpro.who.int/health_topics/influenza/. *A frequently updated source.*

388 ADENOVIRUS DIESEASES

John J. Treanor

Definition

The adenoviruses are found in a variety of animal species, including humans, simians, horses, pigs, goats, and dogs. Specific disease syndromes or hosts are often associated with specific adenovirus serotypes (Table 388–1).

The Pathogen

The virus is nonenveloped and has a double-stranded DNA genome. The human adenoviruses are grouped into six subgenera (A to F) on the basis of differences in genome content, pattern of hemagglutination, and ability to cause tumors in experimental animals. In addition, at least 51 distinct serotypes are defined on the basis of neutralization tests. The majority of adenoviruses use the same cellular receptor as the coxsackieviruses (Chapter 402), called the coxsackievirus-adenovirus receptor (CAR).

Epidemiology

The adenoviruses can infect and cause disease in a variety of human epithelial tissues, including those of the eye, respiratory tract, gastrointestinal tract, and urinary bladder. Virus may be shed from either the gastrointestinal or respiratory tract for months after acute infection.

Many outbreaks of epidemic keratoconjunctivitis have been attributed to contamination of ophthalmologic equipment, such as tonometers. Sterilization of such equipment between patients, good handwashing, segregation of patients, and other infection control procedures are critical in terminating nosocomial outbreaks.

Most infections in immunologically competent individuals are subclinical.

Pathobiology

Adenoviruses appear to use multiple mechanisms to circumvent the host's immune response, including inhibition of the antiviral effects of interferons, downregulation of the expression of human leukocyte antigen molecules on the surface of infected cells, and inhibition of apoptotic cell death. They are capable of establishing persistent infection in some tissues.

Clinical Manifestations

NORMAL HOSTS

Eye Disease

Pharyngoconjunctival Fever

The syndrome of pharyngoconjunctival fever is seen predominantly in children and is characterized by bilateral conjunctivitis accompanied by mild pharyngitis without exudate. Fever, myalgias, and malaise may also be present. The eyes are itchy but not painful, with a boggy, hyperemic conjunctiva and watery discharge. Occasionally, the syndrome may be complicated by punctate keratitis.

Pharyngoconjunctival fever is highly contagious (see Table 388–1) and can be spread by contact with the eyes and mouth for 8 to 10 days after the onset of symptoms. The incubation period is 5 to 8 days. The illness is self-limited, with a duration of a few days to as long as 3 weeks. There is no specific therapy.

Epidemic Keratoconjunctivitis

In contrast to pharyngoconjunctival fever, epidemic keratoconjunctivitis occurs as unilateral disease in the majority of cases and is not generally accompanied by sore throat, fever, or systemic symptoms. The patient may complain of a mild foreign body sensation with watery tearing but is not in significant discomfort. Physical findings include a swollen eyelid, conjunctival hyperemia with edema and chemosis, and tender preauricular adenopathy. Keratitis eventually develops in about 80% of patients and is usually noted on about the eighth day of illness with the onset of pain, photophobia, lacrimation, and blepharospasm. Visual acuity may be temporarily reduced during the height of illness. Subepithelial corneal infiltrates can be detected in about a third of patients and may take weeks or months to resolve. Some cases of adenoviral conjunctivitis may result in prominent subconjunctival hemorrhage and resemble enteroviral acute hemorrhagic conjunctivitis.

TABLE 388–1 ADENOVIRUS SEROTYPES AND ASSOCIATED SYNDROMES

Host and Disease Category	Epidemiologic Features	Associated Adenovirus Serotypes
IMMUNOCOMPETENT HOSTS		
Pharyngoconjunctival fever	Epidemics in schools, families, and military personnel; associated with swimming pools	3, 7
Epidemic keratoconjunctivitis	Sporadic epidemics in schools, families, and industrial sites; may cause nosocomial outbreaks; more common in fall and winter	8, 19, 37
Endemic upper respiratory disease	Seen predominantly in children, families, and daycare settings	1, 2, 5
Acute lower respiratory tract disease	Most common in military recruits, but other healthy adults can also be affected	3, 4, 7, 14, 21
Acute hemorrhagic cystitis	Male preponderance	7, 11, 21, 35
Gastroenteritis	Predominantly in children <2 yr old	40, 41
IMMUNOCOMPROMISED HOSTS		
Transplantation		7, 11, 31, 34, 35
Acquired immunodeficiency syndrome		Multiple, 35, 42–47

Respiratory Disease

Upper Respiratory Tract Illness

Acute pharyngitis is the most common respiratory syndrome attributed to the adenoviruses (Chapter 388). Adenoviruses can cause an exudative tonsillitis similar to that caused by group A streptococci (Chapter 312). In children, common associated syndromes include otitis media, coryza, and undifferentiated fever. Overall, adenoviruses are associated with about 7% of acute febrile illnesses in children, with the peak incidence occurring between 6 months and 2 years of age. High secondary attack rates are seen in families or in the daycare setting.

Lower Respiratory Tract Illness

Adenoviruses have been etiologically implicated in approximately 10% of childhood pneumonias. Clinical features are nondescript, and chest radiographs are similar to those in other forms of viral pneumonia, with the exception that hilar adenopathy is more common in children with adenoviral pneumonia than with other forms of viral pneumonia. Mixed bacterial-viral pneumonia is often present and may be suggested by elevations in band forms in peripheral blood.

Adenoviruses can also be responsible for acute, febrile lower respiratory tract disease in healthy adults, seen most commonly in military recruits. The exceptional susceptibility of military recruits may be related to the special conditions of fatigue and crowding found in military training. Formerly well controlled by vaccination, adenoviruses types 4 and 7 have reemerged as an important cause of acute respiratory illness in recruits after the production of adenovirus vaccine was discontinued in the 1990s. The disease is manifested as an atypical pneumonia syndrome and clinically resembles *Mycoplasma* pneumonia (Chapter 338). Prodromal symptoms of upper respiratory tract infection are reported by most patients, and pharyngitis is often found on initial evaluation. Bacterial superinfection may occur, particularly with *Neisseria meningitidis.* Although the illness is typically mild, more severe disseminated infections and deaths have been reported. Radiographic patterns can include focal infiltrates that resemble acute bacterial pneumonia, as well as large pleural effusions.

Acute, severe lower respiratory tract disease has also been reported in healthy adults in civilian populations in a variety of settings. Nosocomial outbreaks of adenoviral respiratory disease in healthy adults and children in long-term care facilities, psychiatric hospitals, and hospitals have been reported.

Because adenoviruses are relatively rare causes of pneumonia in otherwise healthy civilian adults but are frequently shed asymptomatically, isolation of adenovirus from stool or respiratory secretions in normal adults with pulmonary infiltrates should be interpreted with caution.

Urinary Disease: Hemorrhagic Cystitis

Acute hemorrhagic cystitis may be caused by adenoviruses. The patient complains of gross hematuria and dysuria. The findings may be confused with glomerulonephritis, but laboratory tests of renal function remain normal, and fever and hypertension do not occur. Acute hemorrhagic cystitis is generally self-limited.

Gastrointestinal Disease: Gastroenteritis

Although multiple adenovirus serotypes may be shed in stool, only types 40 and 41, referred to as the enteric adenoviruses, have been convincingly associated with acute gastroenteritis (Chapter 305). These adenovirus types belong to subgroup F and differ from other adenoviruses in being acid stable and highly restricted in their ability to replicate in conventional cell culture.

Gastroenteritis caused by enteric adenovirus is a disease predominantly of children younger than 2 years. Clinical features include watery diarrhea and vomiting similar to what is seen with group A rotavirus infection (Chapter 403). In contrast to gastroenteritis associated with the rotaviruses and astroviruses, adenoviral gastroenteritis shows no significant seasonal variability. The frequency of illness is about 5 to 10% of that caused by rotavirus in the same age group. Adenoviruses are rarely causes of acute gastroenteritis in adults.

Other Syndromes Associated with Adenoviruses in Immunocompetent Hosts

Adenoviruses are often isolated in cases of pertussis-like syndrome, but there is no evidence that adenoviruses by themselves are important causes of whooping cough (Chapter 334). A toxic shock–like manifestation (Chapter 312) of disseminated adenovirus infection in a normal host has been reported. Adenoviruses have occasionally been isolated from cerebrospinal fluid in immunocompetent individuals with meningitis or meningoencephalitis and have been reported to be associated with an acute flaccid paralysis resembling polio (Chapter 402) in children. These viruses have also been implicated in sudden infant death syndrome. Adenoviruses may be detected in mesenteric lymph nodes at the time of surgery for intussusception (Chapter 146), and it is postulated that viral infection causes an acute mesenteric lymphadenitis that leads to the development of this condition. Adenoviruses have also been isolated from myocardial biopsy specimens in adults with acute myocarditis (Chapter 59), thus suggesting a role for adenoviruses in the pathogenesis.

DISEASE IN IMMUNOCOMPROMISED HOSTS

Transplantation

In contrast to infection in normal hosts, infection in immunocompromised subjects tends to be disseminated, with virus isolated from multiple body sites, including the lung, liver, gastrointestinal tract, and urine. The spectrum of serotypes includes those found in immunocompetent individuals and a markedly increased frequency of higher-numbered serotypes rarely found in immunologically normal subjects (see Table 388–1). The source of infection may be reactivation of latent virus, but nosocomial infection has also been documented.

In bone marrow transplant recipients (Chapter 184), adenoviruses may cause a hemorrhagic cystitis that can be confused with that related to cyclophosphamide. Differentiation between these two possibilities is generally achieved by virus culture and by the timing of cystitis in relationship to drug administration. Pneumonia, hepatic necrosis, gastroenteritis, and encephalitis may develop in individuals with cystitis. The case-fatality rate of disseminated infection can be as high as 60%. Resolution is associated with recovery of adenovirus-specific T cells.

Disseminated disease after liver transplantation (Chapter 158) frequently leads to loss of the transplanted liver but does not preclude successful transplantation of a new liver if one is available. Adenovirus infection has been associated with rejection of heart transplants. Adenovirus disease in renal transplant recipients (Chapter 133) is generally less severe; hemorrhagic cystitis is the most common problem, whereas pneumonia is rare.

Acquired Immunodeficiency Syndrome

Adenoviruses are also frequently isolated from the stool and urine of individuals with acquired immunodeficiency syndrome, particularly patients with relatively low $CD4^+$ lymphocyte counts. The most remarkable aspect of this situation is the isolation of a wide variety of serotypes in these patients (see Table 388–1), including new, higher-numbered serotypes isolated for the first time in such subjects. In addition, antigenically intermediate types have been isolated that possibly reflect recombination events made possible by prolonged virus replication in these hosts.

Because adenoviruses are often isolated from immunocompromised patients in conjunction with multiple other opportunistic pathogens, it is difficult to ascribe specific clinical syndromes to them. Described associations include pneumonia, meningoencephalitis, hepatitis, gastroenteritis, and colitis. Adenovirus in the large bowel has associated with chronic diarrhea.

Diagnosis

Adenovirus can be cultured efficiently from conjunctival swabs, respiratory secretions, urine, or stool in as little as 2 days by applying centrifugation culture systems coupled with detection by immunofluorescence. Other widely used methods of directly detecting viral antigen or nucleic acid in clinical specimens include enzyme immunoassays, immunofluorescence tests, and polymerase chain reaction techniques. Virus can be detected in the blood of immunocompromised individuals with disseminated disease and in healthy children with primary infections.

Prevention

Live adenovirus vaccines administered orally in enteric-coated capsules provide effective protection against serotypes 4 and 7 but are no longer in production. There is an active program to reintroduce these vaccines in the military. Adenovirus vaccines have not been used in civilian populations, partially because of the plethora of additional serotypes causing severe disease in these populations.

Treatment

Rx

Conjunctivitis

Therapy is generally supportive. Corticosteroids should be avoided in mild cases of conjunctivitis (Chapter 449) because symptoms generally recur when these agents are discontinued. In more severe cases of keratitis, mild topical corticosteroids may be used with cycloplegics as needed for iritis. Topical antibiotics may be administered to prevent bacterial superinfection. Topical cidofovir may decrease the frequency of severe corneal opacities but is associated with significant local toxicity.

Systemic Infections

No antiviral therapy has been proved to be effective in any systemic adenoviral syndrome. Cidofovir is highly active in cell culture and has been used to treat disseminated disease in immunosuppressed individuals; however, no controlled trials are available to evaluate its efficacy. In a case report, intravesicular application of cidofovir was effective in the treatment of hemorrhagic cystitis in an immunosuppressed child.

SUGGESTED READINGS

Goncalves MA, de Vries AA: Adenovirus: From foe to friend. Rev Med Virol 2006;16:167–186. *Review of the diseases that it causes and its potential use as a vector for gene therapy.*

Heemskerk B, Lankester AC, van Vreeswijk T, et al: Immune reconstitution and clearance of human adenovirus viremia in pediatric stem-cell recipients. J Infect Dis 2005;191:520–530. *Lymphocyte reconstitution appears to play a crucial role in clearance of human adenovirus viremia and survival of the host.*

Ison MG: Adenovirus infections in transplant recipients. Clin Infect Dis 2006;43:331–339. *A clinical review.*

Leen AM, Rooney CM: Adenovirus as an emerging pathogen in immunocompromised patients. Br J Haematol 2005;128:135–144. *Review of strategies to prevent and treat adenovirus infections in immunocompromised subjects.*

389 CORONAVIRUSES

Larry J. Anderson

Definition

Human coronaviruses were, until 2003, recognized as a frequent cause of common cold symptoms, occasionally a cause of lower respiratory tract disease, but rarely if ever a cause of serious disease. In 2003, a novel coronavirus was isolated from patients with outbreak-related severe acute respiratory syndrome (SARS). This virus, SARS coronavirus, was introduced into humans from an animal host and is the etiologic agent of the SARS outbreak. The virus that caused most of the cases during the 2003 outbreak appeared to have changed after its introduction from animals to humans to a virus adapted to human infection and to human-to-human transmission. The SARS outbreak demonstrated that coronaviruses can be serious human pathogens and led to an upsurge in clinical, epidemiologic, and laboratory studies of coronaviruses. Subsequent to discovery of the SARS coronavirus, two other novel human coronaviruses that are associated with respiratory disease have been discovered.

The Pathogens

Coronaviruses are members of the family *Coronaviridae,* which includes two genera, coronaviruses and toroviruses. Coronaviruses are single-stranded, positive-sense RNA viruses with a genome of approximately 30 kD, the largest genome among RNA viruses. These viruses were named coronaviruses because by electron microscopy they have club-shaped surface projections that give them a crownlike appearance. The genome encodes for four or five structural proteins (a spike protein [S], a small envelop protein [E], a membrane protein [M], a nucleocapsid protein [N], and sometimes a hemagglutinin-esterase protein [HE]) and multiple other proteins that participate in virus replication and assembly but are not incorporated into the virus. Coronaviruses have also been isolated from a variety of animals and birds and, in their respective species, cause a wide range of respiratory, gastrointestinal, neurologic, and systemic illnesses. The coronaviruses have been divided into three antigenic groups, with human and animal viruses comprising groups I and II and avian viruses group III. The first two human coronaviruses, 229E and OC43, are members of groups I and II, respectively. SARS coronavirus will probably be designated as a very distant member of group II, and the two most recent human coronavirus isolates, NL63 and HK1, are members of groups I and II, respectively. There is antigenic and genetic variability among human coronavirus isolates within the same antigenic group, but it is not known whether these differences contribute to differences in disease or protective immunity.

Epidemiology

The non-SARS coronaviruses are common pathogens of humans and appear to be transmitted through close contact that probably includes contamination of hands from person-to-person contact or fomites, followed by autoinoculation to the mucosal surfaces of the mouth, nose, or eyes and inhalation of infectious large droplets and possibly aerosols. Symptoms occur 2 to 4 days after infection and are usually those of the common cold. Coronavirus infections are detected early in life, and repeat infections can occur throughout life. One group noted that about 50% of children had antibodies against OC43 by 3 years of age and about 70% of adults had anti-OC43 antibodies. Studies looking for 229E- and OC43-like infections suggest that groups I and II human coronaviruses are associated with about 15% of cases of the common cold. In temperate climates, OC43 and 229E are generally detected between December and May. The extent of coronavirus infections varies from year to year, with peak activity occurring every 2 to 4 years. OC43 and 229E have also been implicated in nosocomial respiratory infections.

The epidemiology of infection with two newly identified human non-SARS coronaviruses, NL63 from antigenic group I and HK1 from antigenic group II, is yet to be determined. Initial studies suggest that NL63 may be associated with 2 to 5% of pediatric hospitalizations for acute respiratory illness.

Most documented infections with SARS coronavirus in humans have occurred in persons ill with a SARS-like illness during the 2002–2003 global outbreak. Some persons working in wild animal markets in China had serologic evidence of a SARS coronavirus–like infection acquired before the 2003 outbreak but reported no SARS-like disease. A few persons infected during the 2003 outbreak had a mild illness or were asymptomatic. It is likely that wild animal markets in Guangdong Province, China, played a key role in amplifying and introducing the virus into humans. The animal source of the outbreak virus, however, has not been determined. Studies in bats suggested they might possibly be the animal source of SARS coronavirus. Of the wild animal studied to date, only horseshoe bats from Hong Kong and several provinces in China have been found to have high rates of infection in nature. The SARS coronavirus–like viruses detected in the horseshoe bat, however, are too different from SARS coronavirus to be the progenitor of the outbreak virus. Although animals were the original source of human infections, global spread of SARS coronavirus occurred through human-to-human transmission and involved droplet, person-to-person, and fomite transmission and, in some instances, probably small-particle aerosol transmission. Most transmission occurred within households, hospitals, or other health care facilities, and little transmission occurred in the community. The fact that transmission appeared to occur only after the onset of illness and usually after the patient's illness had become serious and required hospitalization explains the importance of transmission in health care settings and the relative unimportance of transmission in the community.

Pathobiology

The human coronaviruses characterized to date, including SARS coronavirus, infect humans through the respiratory tract. The site of virus replication is determined, at least in part, by which cells express the respective receptors. The receptors for antigenic group I human coronaviruses 229E and the recently described NL63 are aminopeptidase N and angiotensin-converting enzyme 2 (ACE2), respectively. The receptors for the two group II human coronaviruses characterized to date, OC43 and the recently described HK1, have not yet been determined, but OC43 may use several cell surface molecules as receptors, including 9-*O*-acetylated neuraminic acid. The primary receptor for SARS coronavirus is ACE2, but the virus also binds to two C-type lectins expressed on dendritic cells, DC-SIGN and L-SIGN. Aminopeptidase N is expressed in various cells, including respiratory, gastrointestinal, kidney epithelial, and myeloid cells, but 229E is known to infect only respiratory epithelial cells. ACE2 is found in various tissues, including the lung, gastrointestinal tract, heart, and kidneys. The SARS coronavirus has consistently been detected in pneumocytes in the lung and enterocytes in the gastrointestinal tract and occasionally in other cells, including distal tubular cells in the kidney and macrophages in various tissues. Autopsy studies suggest that infection in the lung leads initially to diffuse alveolar damage and later to a repair process that includes fibrosis in the alveolar walls. It is not known whether NL63, which also uses ACE2 as its receptor, infects sites other than the respiratory tract.

It is likely that the illness associated with SARS and non-SARS coronavirus infections results from both the cytopathic effect of the virus and the host immune and inflammatory response to the viral infection. How this interplay contributes to disease, however, is not understood. The biphasic course of SARS in some patients, the onset of severe disease in the second week of illness, and the decrease in the number of lymphocytes suggest a role for the host response and virus-induced immune suppression in the disease process. The widespread use of steroids and ribavirin, both of which affect host immune responses, makes it difficult to evaluate relationships between measures of the immune response, such as serum cytokine levels, and disease.

Clinical Manifestations

Coronavirus infections are important causes of respiratory tract diseases. They have also been suggested but not proved to cause gastrointestinal and neurologic disease. Several groups have reported coronavirus-like particles in stool specimens from patients with gastroenteritis, but such particles have not been confirmed to be coronaviruses. Other groups have suggested but not documented an association between coronavirus and multiple sclerosis, a suggestion based on detection of RNA in brain tissue or T-cell cross-reactions between 229E and myelin basic protein.

SARS coronavirus and non-SARS coronaviruses cause very different respiratory illnesses. The best studied non-SARS coronaviruses known to infect humans are 229E and OC43. These two viruses are most often associated with a common cold–like illness. Adult volunteers inoculated intranasally with 229E had both respiratory symptoms, such as rhinorrhea, nasal congestion, sore throat, and cough, and systemic symptoms that included fever, headache, and malaise. Symptoms develop 2 to 4 days after inoculation, but about 30% of the volunteers who excreted virus had no associated illness. Symptoms usually persist for about 1 week but sometimes for as long as 3 weeks. Previous infection does not induce high levels of protective immunity. Humans can be reinfected with respiratory coronaviruses throughout life, and human volunteers could be symptomatically reinfected with the same strain of coronavirus 1 year after the first infection. As with other infections, the severity of disease varies among individual patients during the same outbreak and among groups of patients during different outbreaks in the same community. Lower respiratory tract disease has been reported for infection with both 229E- and OC43-like viruses in children and adults but is most often found in patients with compromised cardiac, pulmonary, or immune systems.

Initial reports suggested that infection with the two newly described non-SARS human coronaviruses NL63 and HK1 is associated with respiratory illness that is clinically similar to that associated with 229E and OC43 infection.

In contrast to the mild illness associated with 229E and OC43, SARS coronavirus infection nearly always resulted in a serious illness that required hospitalization, often in an intensive care unit, and had a high fatality rate. Radiologic evidence of pneumonia was seen in nearly all SARS coronavirus–infected persons, acute respiratory distress syndrome (ARDS) developed in up to 20% or more and required admission to an intensive care unit and mechanical ventilation, and nearly 10% of outbreak-associated patients died. The death rate was especially high, approaching 50%, in elderly patients and those with underlying illnesses. The initial clinical manifestation of SARS was often different from that seen with other viral respiratory infections. SARS coronavirus–infected patients often had systemic symptoms of fever, malaise, and myalgias from 2 to 10 days (rarely longer than 10 days) after exposure. Several days after the onset of systemic symptoms, lower respiratory tract symptoms of nonproductive cough and shortness of breath were noted. Unlike patients with most other respiratory virus infections, the majority of patients never experience upper respiratory tract symptoms such as rhinorrhea, sore throat, or nasal congestion (Table 389–1). As with other infections, the expected signs and symptoms with SARS coronavirus infection may be obscured or not present in elderly patients or those with underlying chronic illnesses. During the course of their illness, most SARS coronavirus–infected patients had elevated liver enzyme levels and lymphopenia, including a substantial drop in numbers of both $CD4^+$ and $CD8^+$ T cells. Some patients were reported to have a biphasic illness (i.e., initial improvement in symptoms followed by worsening of their condition). Patients whose illness failed to resolve often had progressive respiratory failure that led to death within weeks but sometimes months after the onset of illness. SARS coronavirus–infected patients with severe complications, for example, those who required intensive supportive care, also suffered complications associated with intensive supportive care, such as secondary bacterial infections. A more severe illness with infection has been associated with older age, the presence of underlying chronic illness, higher liver enzyme values, lower lymphocyte levels and platelet counts, and higher titers of virus or viral RNA. Asymptomatic or mild illness did occur but was uncommon. In studies of exposed health care workers and patients evaluated for SARS, less than 1% of those tested who did not have a SARS-like illness had definitive serologic evidence of SARS coronavirus infection (i.e., a positive neutralization test). Children had less severe illness than adults did and were more likely to be infected without having a SARS-like illness.

Although most survivors of SARS coronavirus infection appeared to achieve full recovery, as many as 25% had abnormal pulmonary findings such as ground-glass opacities on chest radiograph or abnormal pulmonary function test results (e.g., decreased diffusing capacity) 6 or more months after their illness.

Diagnosis

The etiologic diagnosis of most non-SARS coronavirus respiratory infections can be considered in patients with any respiratory tract symptoms, although such infections are most commonly associated with symptoms of the common cold. The role of non-SARS coronavirus infections in more serious lower respiratory tract infections in both otherwise healthy patients and those with chronic underlying conditions has been considered to be minor; this fact plus the lack of antiviral therapy has provided little impetus to develop good diagnostic tests. The emergence of SARS coronavirus has been associated with markedly improved diag-

TABLE 389–1 PERCENTAGE OF SARS CORONAVIRUS–INFECTED PATIENTS WITH SELECTED CLINICAL AND LABORATORY FEATURES OF SARS CORONAVIRUS INFECTION

	SARS Coronavirus—Infected Patients with Symptoms or Laboratory Findings (%)	
Clinical or Laboratory Finding	**At Hospital Admission**	**Sometime During the Illness**
Fever	90–100%	≈100%
Upper respiratory tract symptoms	10–25%	Not available
Cough or shortness of breath	40–75%	Up to 100%
Diarrhea	20–30%	40–70%
Elevated liver function test results	35–90%	70–100%
Pneumonia on chest radiograph	65–90%	90–100%
Lymphopenia*	50–90%	70–95%

*Both $CD4^+$ and $CD8^+$ lymphocyte counts are decreased.
SARS = severe acute respiratory syndrome.

nostic tests, and these tests make it possible to redefine our understanding of the clinical and epidemiologic features of coronavirus disease and situations in which a virus-specific diagnosis is important to patient management.

The diagnosis of SARS coronavirus infection, on the other hand, is critically important for patient management and the public health response to reemergence of SARS. Since the 2003 outbreak was controlled in June 2003, only 17 cases of SARS have been confirmed and none occurred after June 2004. Thirteen of these 17 cases resulted from laboratory exposure, including 7 secondary cases associated with 1 patient. The other four cases occurred in southern China and resulted from exposure in the community, presumably to SARS coronavirus–infected animals from wild animal markets. Three features of SARS cases provide the foundation for a strategy for considering SARS coronavirus infection in an ill patient. First, SARS has occurred only in persons who have been exposed to a patient with SARS, a location where SARS coronavirus transmission was occurring, a laboratory working on SARS coronavirus, or the location where SARS initially emerged (e.g., southern China). Second, most patients with SARS have radiographic evidence of pneumonitis by the time that they seek medical care, and nearly 100% have radiographic abnormalities by day 10 of their illness. Finally, SARS nearly always developed within 10 days of exposure. When no SARS transmission is known to be occurring, the trigger for considering the diagnosis should include radiograph-confirmed pneumonia in a person with some indication of exposure to SARS coronavirus within 10 days of the onset of illness. The following suggest a possible SARS exposure: (1) travel to mainland China, Hong Kong, or Taiwan or exposure to an ill traveler from these locations in the 10 days before onset of the illness; (2) working in a setting at risk for SARS, such as a health care worker with direct patient contact or a worker in a laboratory working with SARS coronavirus; or (3) being part of a cluster of cases of pneumonia of unknown etiology. Once SARS is being considered, a combination of the likelihood that an exposure actually occurred plus clinical signs and symptoms along with radiographic and laboratory test results should guide the clinician to include or exclude SARS. For example, exposure to a pneumonia case in China or a wild animal market in China would increase suspicion for SARS. It is possible that exposure to bats in China could also be an additional risk factor for acquiring SARS. Although horseshoe bats in China have been found to have a high infection rate with SARS coronavirus–like viruses, these viruses are distinct from those that infected humans and it is not known whether these viruses or other bat SARS coronavirus–like viruses will infect or cause disease in humans. SARS provides a reminder to clinicians of the importance of determining travel and work exposure in evaluating a patient's illness.

The tools to detect coronavirus infection have markedly improved with the development of polymerase chain reaction (PCR) tests for viral RNA. Because the human coronaviruses have been difficult to isolate in tissue culture (requiring specialized cell lines) and antigen detection enzyme-linked immunosorbent assay or immunofluorescent antibody assays have not been readily available, laboratory testing has been limited to a few research laboratories. PCR assays, including very sensitive real-time PCR, have been developed and can be designed to detect both known and previously unidentified coronaviruses. A variety of serologic assays can also be used to detect infection. Most of these assays detect IgG antibodies and require a rise in antibody titer between acute and convalescent phase serum specimens and thus are not usually helpful in managing the care of individual patients.

Laboratory confirmation of SARS coronavirus infection early in the illness proved to be problematic, even with very sensitive real-time PCR assays. Unlike most respiratory viral infections, the highest titer of virus, or viral RNA, was found in clinical specimens from the second week of illness. During the first week of illness, the best way to detect infection is by a sensitive PCR assay or a sensitive enzyme immunoassay (EIA) for N protein antigen applied to respiratory and serum specimens. Although sensitive PCR has been considered the best way to detect the SARS virus, several groups have reported that EIA for N protein applied to serum specimens can be a sensitive means of detecting virus during the first week of infection. During the second week of illness, respiratory and stool specimens are most likely to be positive for viral RNA. Because most populations are negative for SARS coronavirus antibodies, detection of serum SARS coronavirus antibodies was considered diagnostic of infection during the outbreak. Antibodies were sometimes detected early in the second week of illness but at times were not detected until 4 weeks into the illness. SARS coronavirus antibodies proved to be the most reliable indicator of infection. Because antibodies persist in serum, a specimen can be collected late without compromising the ability to detect antibodies. The results of serologic assays are not confounded by problems with specimen contamination, which is an important concern with the other most commonly used diagnostic assay, PCR. Finally, with rare exceptions, populations had no preexisting antibodies to SARS coronavirus during the 2003 outbreak, and thus a single positive antibody test from an ill person could be considered diagnostic of an acute SARS coronavirus infection. However, because few individuals have antibodies induced by other coronaviruses that cross-react with SARS coronavirus, when the likelihood of infection is low, a positive SARS coronavirus finding may need to be confirmed with additional tests (e.g., a neutralization assay). Tissue culture isolation, in situ or immunohistologic studies of tissue specimens, electron microscopy to detect virus-like particles, and immunofluorescent or EIA assays for viral antigens have also been used to detect infection. Because diagnosis of reemergence of SARS coronavirus will have substantial public health, social, and economic impact, a diagnosis of SARS should be confirmed by another laboratory experienced in SARS coronavirus diagnostics.

Treatment

There is no virus-specific treatment of non-SARS coronavirus infections, but the illnesses are mild and usually resolve in a few days to a week. Patients require symptomatic therapy or, uncommonly, management of complications of infection. Treatment of SARS coronavirus infection is more complex. As with non-SARS coronavirus, no antiviral drug has been proved to be effective, although several were used during the outbreak and a number have shown promise in in vitro studies. In addition, various strategies to manage ARDS associated with infection were attempted, including high doses of steroids. With the high death rate, fast pace of the outbreak, and no other information to guide treatment, clinicians turned to anecdotal reports, and early in the outbreak a combination of ribavirin, steroids, and various mechanical ventilation and oxygenation regimens became the standard of care for treating SARS patients. Later in the outbreak, with some in vitro data available to guide treatment, interferon alfa, SARS convalescent phase immune globulin, and lopinavir plus ritonavir were used to treat patients. Although many people were treated during the outbreak, there are few reports that include control groups sufficient to evaluate the efficacy of the various treatments, and we cannot be certain which, if any, therapies were beneficial. If SARS reemerges, in vitro and animal model studies of antiviral drugs and data from studies of ARDS from other causes can be used to guide treatment; ideally, patients will be treated in clinical studies so that the safety and efficacy of the treatment can be determined.

Prevention

There is no vaccine or other virus-specific therapy to prevent coronavirus infections. However, handwashing and other infection control measures are known to decrease the spread of other infections and will probably also decrease the spread of coronaviruses in the home, health care facilities, and other settings. Because health care facilities may contribute to the spread of many respiratory viruses, including SARS coronavirus, the Healthcare Infection Control Practices Advisory Committee and the Centers for Disease Control and Prevention developed "Respiratory Hygiene and Cough Etiquette Strategies for Healthcare Facilities." These strategies focus on reinforcing the need for patients with respiratory illnesses to cover their nose and mouth when coughing or sneezing, to use tissues to contain respiratory secretions, and to wash their hands after contact with respiratory secretions and for staff to use good infection control practices. Such reminders in the health care setting may promote such practices in other settings as well.

The 2003 SARS outbreak presented a serious challenge to global health, and the global public health, health care, political, and scientific communities responded quickly and—to the surprise and relief of many—effectively. Within 4 months of the initiation of rapid global spread in February 2003, the outbreak was contained and human-to-human transmission stopped. This was achieved without a vaccine or antiviral therapy but with careful and thorough implementation of the classic public health tools of case finding and management coupled with contact tracing and management. When implemented quickly and correctly, thorough case finding followed by prompt patient isolation with strict attention to infection control measures will prevent further spread. Similarly, rapid and thorough contact tracing will identify those most likely to become new patients so they can be monitored and placed in isolation at the first signs of illness, thereby stopping any further spread. The low risk of SARS transmission early in the illness and the very low rate of asymptomatic infection were key factors to the success of these preventive measures.

Because the reemergence of SARS could lead to global spread, the local, national, and global public health and health care communities need to be alerted quickly and updated regularly about new cases and the status of transmission. The World Health Organization very effectively monitored and updated the world on SARS transmission during the 2003 outbreak.

The cases of laboratory-acquired SARS coronavirus infection and the subsequent transmission of disease to others after one such case reinforce the importance of strict attention to safe laboratory practices. Such practices include handling the virus in the appropriate type of facility and under the appropriate standardized operating procedures, staff training, and medical surveillance programs for staff members.

Since SARS coronavirus was discovered, a number of candidate vaccines have been developed and evaluated for their ability to induce neutralizing antibodies and protect animals from challenge with SARS coronavirus. Two candidate vaccines have also been tested in a small number of humans for immunogenicity and safety. Although a number of vaccines show promise in in vitro and in animal model studies, none is likely to be ready for human use in the near future.

SUGGESTED READINGS

Chen WJ, Yang JY, Lin JH, et al: Nasopharyngeal shedding of severe acute respiratory syndrome–associated coronavirus is associated with genetic polymorphisms. Clin Infect Dis 2006;42:1561–1569. *Host polymorphisms in alleles IL-18 and IL-1A were associated with increased viral shedding.*

Cowling BJ, Muller MP, Wong IO, et al: Clinical prognostic rules for severe acute respiratory syndrome in low- and high-resource settings. Arch Intern Med 2006;166:1505–1511. *Predictors of poor outcome included thrombocytopenia and elevated serum LDH.*

Groneberg DA, Poutanen SM, Low DE, et al: Treatment and vaccines for severe acute respiratory syndrome. Lancet Infect Dis 2005;5:147–155. *A very good summary of the information that is presently available on antiviral drugs and vaccines for SARS.*

Lew TW, Kwek TK, Tai D, et al: Acute respiratory distress syndrome in critically ill patients with severe acute respiratory syndrome. JAMA 2003;290:374–380. *A report of clinical, epidemiologic, and laboratory features of SARS-infected patients in whom ARDS developed.*

Peiris JS, Guan Y, Yuen KY: Severe acute respiratory syndrome. Nat Med 2004;10:S88–S97. *Review of the SARS outbreak and laboratory and clinical features of SARS coronavirus infection.*

www.cdc.gov/ncidod/sars/index.htm. *This website contains background information on SARS and provides comprehensive guidance for the health care and public health communities on approaches to diagnosing and containing SARS and controlling a SARS outbreak.*

www.who.int/cxr/sars/en. *This website contains information on SARS and the global SARS outbreak and global strategies to diagnose and contain SARS and to control a SARS outbreak.*

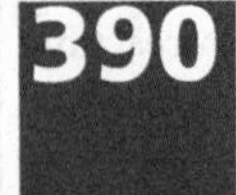

390 MEASLES (RUBEOLA VIRUS INFECTION)

Philip A. Brunell

Definition

Measles, which is an acute, highly contagious disease caused by rubeola virus, is characterized by fever, coryza, cough, conjunctivitis, and both an enanthem and an exanthem.

The Pathogen

The measles virus is an enveloped, negative-stranded RNA paramyxovirus (genus Morbillivirus) 120 to 250 mm in diameter, similar to other members of the Paramyxovirus family but lacking neuraminidase. Its single antigenic serotype has been remarkably stable throughout the world for many years, but sequencing has revealed geographic strain differences. The virus contains six major polypeptides that are responsible for a number of structural and functional properties, including hemagglutination (of primate erythrocytes), hemolysis, cell fusion, and others.

Epidemiology

Before the advent of measles vaccine, almost every child contracted measles, most before entering school. With the introduction of routine immunization against measles in the United States in 1963, the incidence of the disease has decreased to fewer than 100 cases per annum during the past several years, and indigenous transmission has been virtually absent. The largest recent measles outbreak in the United States occurred in 1998 to 1991, when more than 55,000 cases were reported and 123 people died of measles-related illnesses—almost half younger than 5 years. Ninety percent of fatal cases had not been vaccinated.

In recent years, outbreaks of measles in the United States have been small (<50 cases) and have involved either groups who refused vaccination or high-school and college students who were unvaccinated or received only one dose of measles vaccine. In March 2000, the Centers for Disease Control and Prevention concluded that measles is no longer endemic in the United States. Rather, cases are imported, with limited domestic spread. Cases have been reported in parents of adoptees from China. Because of an aggressive measles vaccination program by the Pan American Health Organization, the incidence of measles is now very low in Latin America and the Caribbean, and elimination of measles from the Americas appears to be an achievable goal. Unfortunately, measles is still very common in developing countries, especially among children, and it is estimated to cause about 400,000 deaths annually worldwide.

Measles is one of the most highly contagious infections, with almost all unprotected household contacts becoming infected. Demonstration of virus in nasopharyngeal secretions during the prodromal, preeruptive phase and in the first days of rash is in accord with epidemiologic evidence of contagiousness. Close physical proximity or direct person-to-person respiratory droplet contact is the usual requisite for infection, although airborne transmission has been documented.

An unmodified attack of measles is followed by lifelong immunity. Passively transferred maternal antibody protects young infants during the early months of life.

Pathobiology

Uncomplicated viral disease is associated with pathologic changes in tonsillar, nasopharyngeal, and appendiceal tissue during the prodrome. These changes consist of round cell infiltration and the presence of multinucleated giant cells. Giant cells are also observed in tissue cultures infected with measles virus. The skin and mucous membranes contain perivascular round cell infiltrates, along with congestion and edema. Koplik's spots are inflammatory lesions of the submucous glands with similar microscopic features.

Measles virus replicates in lymphoid tissue (e.g., spleen, thymus, lymph nodes) and can be isolated from monocytes and other mononuclear cells during acute infection. Cell-mediated immunity is impaired during measles; an example is transient suppression of the tuberculin reaction (also observed with measles vaccines). Improvement in eczema and allergic asthma and induction of remission in nephrosis have been noted. In severe disease, the magnitude of depression of the total lymphocyte count correlates with a lessened chance of recovery.

Infection of brain cells results in an incomplete viral replicative cycle with production of defective virions. Studies of patients with acute measles encephalomyelitis and those with late-onset, subacute sclerosing panencephalitis show high titers of antibodies in serum and cerebrospinal fluid to all the measles virus proteins except M.

Clinical Manifestations

After an incubation period that averages 11 days, measles is clinically manifested by symptoms of fever, malaise, myalgia, and headache. Within hours, the ocular symptoms of photophobia and conjunctival injection occur. The palpebral and, to a lesser extent, the bulbar conjunctivae are involved. There is usually no exudate. Sneezing, coughing, and nasal discharge occur almost simultaneously. Less commonly, hoarseness and aphonia may reflect laryngeal involvement. In this prodromal stage of 1 to 4 days' duration, the appearance of a rash may be heralded by tiny white (Koplik's) spots on the buccal mucosa. They are characteristically lateral to the molar teeth and typically mounted on a bluish red areola of injected mucosa, superimposed on a diffuse red background (Fig. 390–1). These spots, which generally appear a day or so before the rash and disappear within 2 days after its appearance, constitute a pathognomonic, diagnostic sign. The enanthem may also involve other mucous membranes such as the palpebral conjunctiva and vaginal lining.

The rash of measles follows the prodromal symptoms by 2 to 4 days, occasionally by as much as 7 days. It first appears behind the ears or on the face and neck as a blotchy erythema, spreads downward to cover the trunk, and finally involves the extremities (Fig. 390–2). The hands and feet may escape involvement. Initially, the eruption consists of discrete red macules that blanch with pressure. Subsequently, these lesions become papular, tend to coalesce, and may develop a red, nonblanching component. In adults, the rash is generally more extensive, with a greater tendency to become confluent and slightly more raised and redder than in children, particularly on the face. The rash fades in the order of its appearance; its disappearance about 5 days after onset may be attended by a fine, powdery desquamation that spares the hands and feet. In adults, malaise may continue for 1 to 2 weeks.

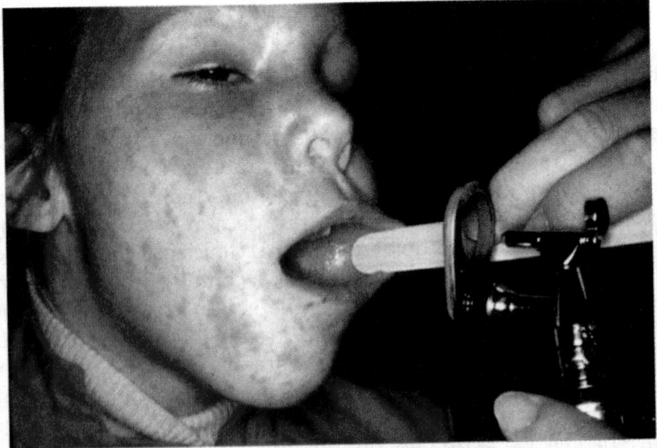

FIGURE 390–1 • Typical Koplik's spots.

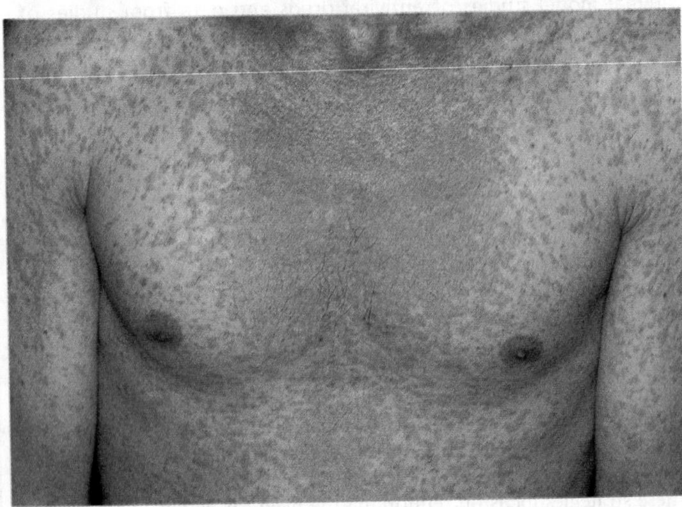

FIGURE 390–2 • Measles causes a classic maculopapular or morbilliform eruption.

The fever of measles may persist for about 6 days and frequently reaches temperatures of 40 or 41° C. Throughout the febrile period, productive cough and auscultatory evidence of bronchitis may be evident. These manifestations may persist after defervescence, and cough is often the last symptom to disappear.

Generalized lymphadenopathy accompanies the acute febrile illness and may persist for several weeks thereafter. Nausea and, less commonly, emesis appear to affect adults more often than children and are usually accompanied by slightly elevated serum aminotransferase levels.

Complications

The persistence or recurrence of fever and the development of leukocytosis are presumptive evidence of the common bacterial sequelae of otitis media or pneumonia. Laryngitis of sufficient severity to embarrass respiration has been observed. Keratoconjunctivitis is part of the acute phase. Electroencephalographic abnormalities have been described in about half the children with measles. Severe measles has been reported in pregnant women along with hepatitis and pneumonia; the latter is sometimes fatal. Premature labor has resulted in prematurity and stillbirths.

A rare (0.1%) but serious consequence of measles is a demyelinating encephalomyelitis (Chapter 439) that may appear 1 to 14 days after the onset of rash. This complication is associated with recurrence of fever, headache, vomiting, and stiff neck. Stupor and convulsions usually follow. Death ensues in about 10% of patients; more than half the survivors suffer permanent residuals of varying severity.

Other late sequelae of measles are thrombocytopenic purpura and exacerbation or activation of preexisting pulmonary tuberculosis. Subacute sclerosing panencephalitis is a late complication (Chapter 439).

In patients who are immunocompromised (e.g., those with acquired immunodeficiency syndrome [AIDS]), measles virus may induce an interstitial pneumonia characterized by giant cells and intracellular inclusion bodies that is often fatal. This reaction has also been reported in a human immunodeficiency virus (HIV)-positive measles vaccine recipient.

Diagnosis

The diagnosis of measles should be suspected during an outbreak or in a patient with a history of exposure or foreign travel to developed or developing countries. Before the appearance of rash, diagnosis may be difficult unless Koplik's spots are present. Finding an uncomfortable patient in a darkened room who has conjunctivitis, coryza, and cough should make the physician suspect measles. The rash in adults may be more violaceous, confluent, slightly raised, and more extensive than in children. A history of having received a single dose of measles vaccine does not preclude the diagnosis because two doses are recommended (Chapter 16).

Measles virus can be identified by isolation or reverse transcriptase polymerase chain reaction. Increased levels of a specific antibody may be detected as early as the first or second day of rash. Acute and convalescent sera are usually required. Demonstration of measles IgM is available in some laboratories. A presumptive diagnosis may be made if giant cells are detected in stained smears of nasal exudate in the preeruptive period.

Leukopenia is observed on the first day of rash, mainly because of a decrease in lymphocytes; subsequently, granulocytopenia ensues. Simultaneous with the onset of rash, measles-specific antibodies are detectable in serum. Roentgenographic evidence of pulmonary involvement is frequently seen in uncomplicated disease in the absence of leukocytosis and obvious bacterial infection.

Differential Diagnosis

The differential diagnosis (Table 390–1) includes consideration of rubella (Chapter 391), scarlet fever (Chapter 312), infectious mononucleosis (Chapter 400), secondary syphilis (Chapter 340), drug eruptions (Chapter 275), toxic shock syndrome (Chapter 312), and Kawasaki's disease (Chapters 291 and 465). Of value in excluding these possibilities are the milder course, postauricular nodes, and pinker rash of rubella; the sore throat, eventual desquamation, strawberry tongue, and leukocytosis of scarlet fever; and serologic test results for infectious mononucleosis. Fever, enanthem, and catarrh are uncommon with the cutaneous manifestations of drug hypersensitivity. Erythema infectiosum (Chapters 394 and 465) is usually an afebrile illness with rash on the cheeks, arms, and legs; there is little or no prodrome or accompanying respiratory tract involvement. Kawasaki's disease is rare in adults.

Prevention

Postexposure Prophylaxis

Attenuation of the natural disease by antibody prophylaxis may result in an illness of lessened severity, comparable to the milder infection seen in infants with illness modified by maternally acquired antibody. Fever alone may be observed, but some degree of exanthem is usually apparent. Koplik's spots may not appear. In general, the course is truncated and relatively uncomplicated. Lasting immunity is uncertain, and later routine immunization of these individuals is probably indicated.

Vaccination

A live attenuated vaccine has been the sole product licensed and used in the United States since 1967 (Chapter 16). This live virus vaccine produces immunity by infection. A second dose is now routinely recommended. In children older than 1 year, the rate of seroconversion after vaccination in recent years is 98 to 99%. Measles vaccine is generally given in combination with mumps and rubella (MMR) vaccine. Failure of measles immunization was much more common before 1980; the reasons are unclear but may include poor recall or faulty documentation of immunization, age at immunization, use of immune globulin with the vaccine, receipt of killed rather than live vaccine, and the type of live vaccine.

Vaccine recommendations depend on the measles experience in the community. The first dose of MMR is recommended at the age of 12 months. During epidemics, it may be given as monovalent measles vaccine to infants as young as 6 months, in which case it should be repeated in combination with mumps, rubella, and varicella (MMRV) (ProQuad) after the first birthday. A second routine dose of MMRV at school entry is recommended. All entering college students and beginning health care workers born after 1956 should show evidence of measles immunity: positive serologic test, physician-documented measles, or receipt of two doses of measles vaccine or, preferably MMRV. MMRV is licensed through age 12. Older persons should receive MMR. The immune status of persons contemplating foreign travel should be reviewed. A large number of military personnel have been reimmunized without significant side effects. Measles vaccine may be given at the same time as other live or killed vaccines.

Pregnancy, immunodeficiency, leukemia, other systemic malignant diseases, active tuberculosis, and administration of resistance-depressing drugs such as corticosteroids and antimetabolites are contraindications to live virus vaccination. Measles immunization of HIV-infected children is recommended, with the caveat to avoid severely immunocompromised individuals.

TABLE 390–1 A GUIDE TO THE DIFFERENTIAL DIAGNOSIS OF MEASLES

	Conjunctivitis	Rhinitis	Sore Throat	Enanthem	Leukocytosis	Tests Available
Measles	++	++	0	+	0	+
Rubella	0	0	0	0	0	+
Exanthem subitum	0	0	0	0	0	+
Enterovirus infection	0	0	±	0	0	+
Adenovirus infection	+	+	+	0	0	+
Scarlet fever	0	0	++	±	+	+
Infectious mononucleosis	0	0	++	±	±	+
Drug rash	0	0	0	0	0	0

0 = Not usually present or no test available; ± = variable in occurrence; + = present: test available (virus or bacterial culture, serology); ++ = present and severe.

The Measles Initiative is committed to reduce deaths by 90% in 2010 compared with those in 2000.

Recipients of killed vaccine who later receive live vaccine may have severe local and systemic reactions to reimmunization. Atypical measles has also been reported in some patients who received killed vaccine or live vaccine alone. Subsequent investigations showed that such patients failed to develop antibodies to the fusion (F) protein of the virus. Lack of antibodies to the cell fusion factor is believed to have permitted unrestricted replication of the virus. This fact, together with the anamnestic antibody response, is believed to have resulted in the clinical manifestations. High fever, pneumonia with pleural effusion, obtundation, and an exanthem that is hemorrhagic and most marked on the extremities may develop. In some instances, vesicular, macular, or maculopapular phases have been observed. The rash is sometimes accompanied by edema of the hands and feet. These patients have extraordinarily high titers of measles-specific antibodies and may also have elevated liver enzymes, disseminated intravascular coagulation, and marked myalgia. Nodular pulmonary changes have persisted in some patients. Some cases of pneumonia occurred in the absence of rash. Incorrect diagnoses on initial evaluation have included Rocky Mountain spotted fever (Chapter 348) and meningococcemia (Chapter 321) as a result of similarities in rash and toxicity. Because inactivated vaccines were available only from 1963 through 1967 in the United States, the past recipients are now adults.

Treatment

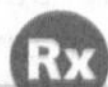

There is no specific antiviral therapy with demonstrated efficacy against measles, although ribavirin has been used in some cases. All children in developing countries in whom measles is diagnosed should receive two doses of vitamin A supplements given 24 hours apart to help prevent eye damage and blindness. Moreover, vitamin A supplementation has been shown to reduce the number of deaths from measles by 50%.

In the absence of complications, bedrest is the essence of treatment of this self-limited disease. Codeine sulfate may be useful to ameliorate headache and myalgia and for cough. Analgesics and antipyretics may be useful. Fluids should be encouraged. Bright light is not an ocular hazard, but photophobia may require darkening the patient's room.

The course of uncomplicated measles is not influenced by antimicrobial drugs, and their use during the acute illness has resulted in no decrease in the 10 to 15% rate of secondary bacterial complications such as otitis, sinusitis, and pneumonia. If careful observation of the patient is possible, rational therapy is based on promptly recognizing and defining the cause of complications, followed by starting the appropriate antimicrobial drug in proper dosage.

Prognosis

Uncomplicated measles is rarely fatal, and complete recovery is the rule. Fatalities are almost always the result of pneumonia in adults or children younger than 1 year. Heart failure is a common cause of death in patients older than 50 years. The prognosis is particularly poor for patients with AIDS and other immunocompromised patients.

The use of antimicrobial drugs after the usual secondary invaders appear reduces the case-fatality rate of measles sharply. Encephalitis occurs as frequently in mild as in severe measles (about 1 case per 1000). Subacute sclerosing panencephalitis develops about 7 years after measles and has essentially disappeared with widespread vaccine use.

SUGGESTED READINGS

Bedford H, Sengupta N, Elliman D, et al: Measles: Prevention. Clin Evid 2005;43:373–387. *A detailed review.*

Bojinova VS, Dinora PS, Belopitova LD, et al: Clinical and epidemiologic characteristics of subacute sclerosing panencephalitis in Bulgaria during the past 25 years (1978–2002). Eur J Pediatr Neurol 2004:8:89–94. *Emphasizes the impact of measles vaccination; the mean onset was 7 years after infection.*

Moss WJ, Griffin DE: Global measles elimination. Mat Rev Microbiol 2006;4: 900–908. *Review of the pathophysiology of this infection and the likelihood of worldwide elimination of the disease.*

Otten M, Kezaala R, Fall A, et al: Public health impact of accelerated measles control in the WHO African Region 2000–2003. Lancet 2005;366:832–839. *Strategies including vaccination have reduced measles by 91%.*

391 RUBELLA (GERMAN MEASLES)

Philip A. Brunell

Definition

Rubella is an acute, usually benign infectious disease characterized by a 3-day rash, generalized lymphadenopathy, fever, and minimal or no prodromal symptoms. Since 1941, it has been known that rubella causes congenital malformations when infection occurs during the early months of pregnancy.

The Pathogen

Rubella is a small, spherical, enveloped virus containing single-stranded RNA of positive polarity. Structural proteins include two enveloped glycoproteins and a nucleocapsid protein. The virus is classified as a togavirus, genus Rubivirus. It multiplies slowly in a variety of primary cell culture systems and in some continuous cell lines in most systems without detectable cytopathic effect.

Epidemiology

Before rubella vaccines were available, the disease was worldwide in distribution, produced major epidemics at 6- to 9-year intervals, and was recognized mainly in school-aged children. Rubella also produced outbreaks in settings such as military recruit bases and college campuses, where large numbers of susceptible young adults gathered in relatively crowded conditions. Since licensure of the vaccine in the United States in 1969, there has been strikingly altered epidemiology. No major epidemic has occurred since 1964–1965. In other nations where rubella vaccine has not been widely used, the epidemiology has remained unchanged. Because the disease may be quite nonspecific clinically, with nearly a third of adults experiencing infection without rash, epidemiologic reporting tends to underestimate its prevalence. Since 1966, congenital rubella has been a reportable disease.

It is probable that rubella is spread by the respiratory route and by close and sustained personal contact. The incubation period in experimentally infected individuals was found to be 12 to 23 days, with most cases occurring 14 to 15 days after exposure. Although virus was isolated as early as 7 days before and as late as 21 days after the onset of rash, infectivity is probably greatest throughout the period of prodromal symptoms and for as long as 7 days after appearance of the rash. Individuals with subclinical infection can also pass the virus; 20 to 50% of infections are asymptomatic. Infants with congenitally acquired infection may excrete virus in respiratory secretions and urine for months after birth and are contagious during this time. In hospital environments, especially in nurseries, newborns with congenital rubella had been a source of nosocomial infection of personnel involved in their care.

In most people, immunity is lifelong after initial infection. Authenticated second attacks are exceedingly rare and require serologic documentation because of the nonspecific nature of the clinical syndrome. Subclinical reinfection demonstrated by an increase in IgG serum antibody has been documented. Such reinfections are very rarely, if ever associated with viremia and thus pose little threat to pregnant women. IgM response has been used to distinguish primary infection from reinfection. The immunity that follows artificial immunization with live virus vaccine is apparently of equal duration, even though the antibody titers induced may be somewhat lower.

Pathobiology

Death from postnatal rubella is usually due to encephalitis. Accordingly, most autopsies describe only the brain findings. Since 1962 it has been possible to investigate the pathogenesis and to correlate clinical findings with virologic events. After initial invasion of the upper respiratory tract, virus spreads to local lymphoid tissue, where it multiplies and initiates a viremia of approximately 7 days' duration. Respiratory tract shedding of virus and the viremia rises to peak levels until the onset of rash, at which time the viremia becomes undetectable, whereas respiratory secretions contain diminishing quantities of virus over the succeeding 5 to 15 days. Specific serum antibodies can be demonstrated with the onset of rash, and circulating immune complexes are detectable soon thereafter.

Congenital Rubella

Necropsies of fetal and neonatal victims of intrauterine infection have shown a variety of embryonal defects related to developmental arrest involving all three germ layers.

The virus establishes chronic persistent infection in many tissues, with resultant intrauterine growth retardation. Delayed and disordered organogenesis produces embryopathic structural defects of the eye, brain, heart, and large arteries; continued viral infection during the fetal and postnatal period causes organ and tissue damage (e.g., hepatitis, nephritis, myocarditis, pneumonia, osteitis, meningitis, cochlear degeneration, and pancreatitis with the development of diabetes).

Clinical Manifestations

Postnatally Acquired Rubella

Twelve to 23 days after exposure, the onset of rubella is manifested by the appearance of a rash (Fig. 391–1) with mild accompanying constitutional symptoms of malaise and occasionally mild sore throat. Enlargement of the postauricular and suboccipital nodes generally appears about a week before the rash. Moderate fever may accompany or precede the rash. Generalized peripheral lymphadenopathy and, more rarely, splenomegaly may occur.

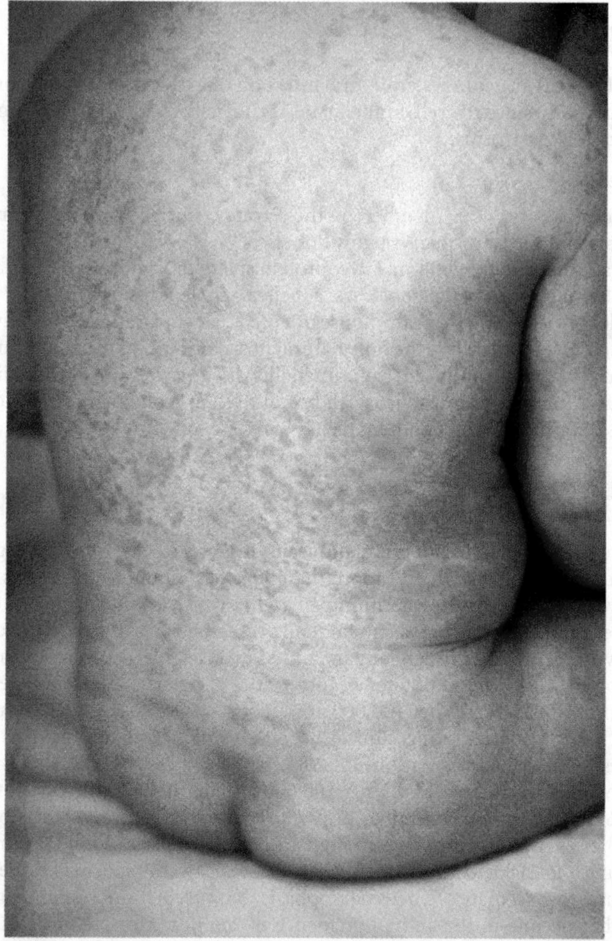

FIGURE 391–1 • Rash of rubella on the skin of a child's back. The distribution is similar to that of measles, but the lesions are less intensely red. (From Centers for Disease Control and Prevention Image Bank, Figure #712. Available at http://phil.cdc.gov/phil/home.asp. Accessed 11/3/06.)

The exanthem of rubella is usually apparent within 24 hours of the first symptoms as a faint macular erythema that first involves the face and neck. Characterized by its brevity and evanescence, it spreads rapidly to the trunk and extremities, sometimes leaving one site even as it appears at the next. The pink macules that constitute the rash blanch with pressure and rarely stain the skin. Rubella virus has been isolated from skin lesions, as well as from uninvolved sites. The truncal rash may coalesce, but the lesions on the extremities remain discrete. The eruption generally vanishes by the third day. Rubella may occur without rash. In the absence of an epidemic and serologic or virologic confirmation, clinical diagnosis of rubella is not reliable.

Complications

Recovery is almost always prompt and uneventful. In contrast to measles, secondary bacterial infections are not encountered with rubella. Transient polyarthralgia and polyarthritis are more common in adolescents and adults with rubella, particularly females. They appear 3 or more days after the onset of rash and usually last 5 to 10 days, but they may last as long as a month. The knees and joints of the hands and wrists are most often involved. Surveys during urban epidemics have revealed rates of 5 to 15% in males and 10 to 35% in females.

Thrombocytopenia, when sought by serial platelet counts, is common but rarely of clinical consequence. Hemorrhagic complications occur at an overall incidence of approximately 1 in 3000 and are more frequent in children. A meningoencephalitis of short duration may occur 1 to 6 days after appearance of the rash. Its incidence is estimated at 1 in 5000 cases, and it is fatal in approximately 20% of those afflicted. Rubella encephalopathy is not associated with demyelinization, in contrast to other viral encephalitides. Survivors may have electroencephalographic abnormalities, but intellectual function seems to be preserved.

Congenital Rubella

Congenital transplacental infection of the fetus occurs as a consequence of maternal infection, usually in the first 4 months of pregnancy. Virus is demonstrable in placental and fetal tissues obtained by therapeutic abortion at that time. If pregnancy is not interrupted, fetal infection persists, and on delivery of the infant, virus is recoverable from the throat, urine, conjunctivae, bone marrow, and cerebrospinal fluid of living infants and from most organs at autopsy. From 20 to 80% of infants born to mothers infected in the first trimester of pregnancy have stigmata of infection readily recognizable in the first year of life, including cardiac lesions (most commonly patent ductus arteriosus and peripheral pulmonic stenosis) and eye defects (e.g., cataracts, glaucoma, retinitis, microphthalmos). Most infants in whom virus is detectable do not have evidence of disease at birth or may simply have intrauterine growth retardation. In others, more severe disease occurs. Most prominent of these manifestations is hemorrhagic skin lesions related to extramedullary erythropoiesis, which disappears soon after birth. Hepatosplenomegaly with active hepatitis may persist for months. Other involvement includes interstitial pneumonia, meningoencephalitis, hearing loss of varying extent, and lesions of the long bones. A progressive panencephalitis simulating subacute sclerosing panencephalitis has been observed in the second decade after congenital infection. Long-term sequelae in infants with congenital rubella include psychomotor retardation, hearing loss, retinopathy, and diabetes.

A striking finding has been persistence of virus in the pharynx, urine, and cerebrospinal fluid for as long as 1 year after birth in 7% of infants. Infective virus was found in a congenital cataract after 3 years. This evidence of continuing viral synthesis occurs coincidentally with circulating antibody. The character of the antibody changes during the first months from maternal IgG to IgM, thus indicating a primary response of the infant to the persisting viral antigen. Studies of older infants and children with stigmata of congenital rubella show them to be free of demonstrable virus and to possess the IgG that characteristically persists after other viral infections.

Diagnosis

Rubella may be diagnosed clinically with assurance only during an epidemic. Distinction from measles may be made on the basis of a fainter rash, a milder course, and minimal or absent systemic complaints. Sore throat is a more prominent complaint in scarlet fever, the course of infectious mononucleosis is often more protracted, and splenomegaly is more frequent than in rubella. Specific diagnosis of rubella is made by isolating the virus in any of several cell culture systems or by demonstrating a rise in antibody by latex agglutination, hemagglutination inhibition, enzyme-linked immunosorbent assay, or complement fixation. Reverse transcriptase polymerase chain reaction is also available in some laboratories.

Treatment

Rx

There is no specific antiviral therapy. Few patients suffer discomfort severe enough to warrant symptomatic medication, but headache and myalgia or arthritis may be controlled by analgesics.

Prevention

Passive Immunization

Administration of gamma globulin to a pregnant woman may only mask her symptoms of infection and not protect the fetus from viral invasion. Thus, it should be considered for susceptible pregnant women exposed to rubella only when termination of pregnancy is not an option.

Active Immunization

Rubella may be prevented in children and adults by parenteral attenuated live virus vaccines produced in cell culture. Seroconversion rates after immunization are at least 98% with the current RA 27/3 vaccine. The vaccine is given in combination with the measles and mumps vaccinations (MMR-II live vaccine) as a 0.5 mL subcutaneous injection at 12 to 15 months of age and again at 4 to 6 years of age. It is now available in combination with mumps, measles, and varicella vaccines (MMRV) (ProQuad). However, use of this vaccine is approved only through 12 years of age. Two doses are now recommended. Joint symptoms are less common than with the older HPV 77-DE strain and occur in about 3% of children and up to 26% of adult females. Arthritis occurs 13 to 19 days after immunization and lasts 2 to 11 days. The fingers are most often affected, with the wrists and knees less commonly involved. Arthralgias generally begin 10 to 25 days after vaccination and last 1 to 9 days. Joint symptoms are less common in men than in women. In children, vaccination is attended by little or no reaction. Population-based studies have not established a relationship between rubella immunization and chronic arthropathy.

It was initially recommended in the United States that immunization be carried out principally in childhood. There is now a more aggressive attempt to immunize the remaining susceptible women and adolescent girls. Current policy recommends vaccinating all such persons who have no history of previous rubella immunization. Postpartum immunization of those found to be seronegative during pregnancy is encouraged. Although vaccine virus has occasionally been transmitted to the newborn by breast milk, it has proved to be of little consequence. Only nonpregnant individuals should be immunized, and contraception, when appropriate, should be carried out for at least 1 month after vaccination. Inadvertent administration of vaccine to pregnant women has occasionally resulted in attenuated vaccine virus infection of the fetus. However, in more than 500 such cases studied, no infant has been observed with congenital malformations as a result. The frequency of fetal infection with the RA 27/3 vaccine currently used is less than with the previous rubella vaccine. Use of vaccine in the United States prevented a large epidemic of rubella expected in the early 1970s and has reduced the reported annual occurrence from more than 50,000 cases, with epidemic peaks of 200,000 to 500,000. Since 2001, there have been no more than 25 rubella cases per annum and a total of 4 congenital rubella cases. Endogenous transmission has been interrupted, and most cases can be identified as foreign strains. A goal has been set to eliminate rubella and congenital rubella syndrome in the Western Hemisphere by 2010.

Prognosis

Complete recovery from postnatally acquired rubella is almost invariable. The rare deaths attributable to rubella follow the infrequent complication of meningoencephalitis. Infection in pregnancy constitutes a grave hazard to the fetus but not to the mother.

SUGGESTED READINGS

Achievements in public health: Elimination of rubella and congenital rubella syndrome—United States, 1969–2004 MMWR Morb Mortal Wkly Rep 2005;54(11):279–282. *A history of the elimination of rubella in the United States and plans for elimination in the Western Hemisphere.*

Dyer JA: Childhood viral exanthems. Pediatr Am 2007;36:21–29. *A clinical review.*

Madsen KM, Hviid A, Vestergaard M, et al: A population-based study of measles, mumps and rubella vaccination and autism. N Engl J Med 2002;347: 1477–1482. *Epidemiologic evidence against an association between vaccination and autism.*

Reef S: Rubella mass campaigns. Curr Top Microbiol Immunol 2006;304:221–229. *Review of the effects of mass rubella vaccination.*

392 MUMPS

John W. Gnann, Jr.

Definition

Mumps is an acute systemic viral infection that occurs most commonly in children, is usually self-limited, and is clinically characterized by nonsuppurative parotitis.

The Pathogen

Mumps virus is a member of the Paramyxoviridae family. Mumps virions are pleomorphic, roughly spherical enveloped particles with an average diameter of 200 nm. Glycoprotein spikes project from the surface of the envelope, which encloses a helical nucleocapsid composed of nucleoproteins and linear, nonsegmented, single-stranded, negative-sense RNA. Humans are the only natural hosts for mumps virus, although infection can be induced experimentally in a variety of mammalian species. In vitro, mumps virus can be cultured in many mammalian cell lines and in embryonated hens' eggs.

Epidemiology

In unvaccinated urban populations, mumps is a disease of school-aged children (5 to 9 years), and more than 90% have mumps antibodies by 15 years of age. Before the mumps vaccine was released in the United States in 1967, mumps was an endemic disease with a seasonal peak of activity occurring between January and May. The largest number of cases reported in the United States occurred in 1941, when the incidence of mumps was 250 cases per 100,000 population. In 1968, when the mumps vaccine was first entering clinical use, the incidence of mumps was 76 cases per 100,000 population. In 1985, only 2982 cases of mumps were reported, an incidence of 1.1 per 100,000 population, which represents a 98% decline from the number of cases reported in 1967. Epidemiologic studies of mumps epidemics in high schools, colleges, and military units during the 1980s demonstrated that outbreaks were principally due to failure to vaccinate. Renewed emphasis on vaccination resulted in a further decline in the annual incidence of mumps. More recent studies have attributed smaller mumps outbreaks in the 1990s to primary vaccine failure and possibly to waning vaccine-induced immunity. In 2003, the Centers for Disease Control and Prevention reported only 231 cases of mumps in the United States, the lowest annual total ever recorded.

Pathobiology

Mumps is highly contagious and can be transmitted experimentally by inoculation of virus onto the nasal or buccal mucosa, thus suggesting that most natural infections result from droplet spread of upper respiratory secretions. The average incubation period for mumps is 18 days. Primary viral replication takes place in epithelial cells of the upper respiratory tract, followed by spread of virus to regional lymph nodes and subsequent viremia and systemic dissemination. Because virus can be isolated from saliva for 5 to 7 days before and up to 9 days after the onset of clinical symptoms, an infected individual is potentially able to transmit mumps for a period of about 2 weeks. An estimated 30% of mumps infections in children are subclinical or associated only with nonspecific upper respiratory infection symptoms. Transient IgM antibody responses are detected early in the course of mumps infection, followed by the appearance of IgG antibody and cytotoxic T lymphocytes. Mumps-specific IgG can be detected during the first week of acute infection, peaks at 3 to 4 weeks, and persists for decades. Lifelong immunity follows natural infection. Patients who report more than one episode of mumps probably had parotitis of another cause.

Clinical Manifestations

Parotitis

Mumps usually begins with a short prodromal phase of low-grade fever, malaise, headache, and anorexia. Young children may complain of ear pain initially. The characteristic parotid tenderness and enlargement, in which the earlobe is lifted forward and obscures the angle of the mandible, then develops (Fig. 392–1). The parotid glands are involved most commonly, although other salivary glands may occasionally be enlarged. Parotitis may initially be unilateral, with swelling of the contralateral parotid gland occurring 2 to 3 days later; bilateral parotitis with symptomatic salivary gland involvement eventually develops in 70% of patients. Painful parotid gland enlargement progresses over a period of about 3 days, followed by defervescence and resolution of the parotid pain and swelling within about 7 days. Long-term sequelae of mumps parotitis are uncommon.

Aseptic Meningitis

Symptomatic meningitis occurs in 15% of cases and is the second most common manifestation of mumps. About 50% of patients with mumps parotitis have cerebrospinal fluid (CSF) pleocytosis, but many have no clinical evidence of meningitis. Signs and symptoms of meningeal inflammation (headache, neck stiffness, vomiting, and lethargy) plus high fever usually develop 4 to 5 days after the onset of parotitis, although the meningitis may occasionally precede the parotitis. Indeed, 40 to 50% of all cases of documented mumps meningitis occur in patients who never exhibit clinical parotitis. For unexplained reasons, symptomatic central nervous system (CNS) involvement with mumps is two to three times more common in males than in females. Examination of CSF usually reveals normal opening pressure and a mononuclear cell pleocytosis with an average cell count of 450/mm^3. A polymorphonuclear leukocyte predominance may be seen in some patients early during the course of mumps meningitis. CSF protein is generally normal or mildly elevated (<100 mg/dL). Hypoglycorrhachia, which is not usually seen in viral meningitis, may be present in 10 to 30% of patients with mumps meningitis. Mumps virus can be recovered from CSF. Whereas the symptoms of mumps meningitis typically resolve within 7 to 10 days, the CSF abnormalities may persist for up to 5 weeks. Mumps meningitis is generally benign, and significant neurologic complications are rare.

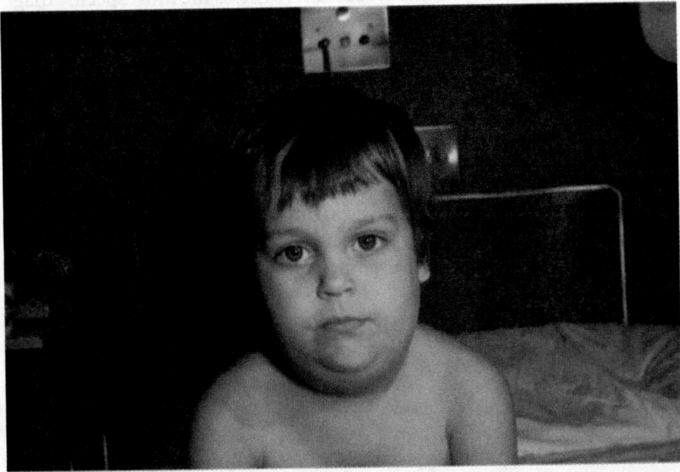

FIGURE 392–1 • Mumps. This child's face is displaying diffuse lymphedema of the neck caused by mumps virus infection of the parotid salivary glands. (From CDC Public Health Image Library #4491.)

Encephalitis

The spectrum of mumps-induced CNS disease ranges from mild "aseptic" meningitis (which is common) to severe encephalitis (which is rare). Some cases of encephalitis develop concurrently with the parotitis and are thought to result from direct extension of viral infection from the choroid plexus ependyma into parenchymal neurons. Other cases of mumps encephalitis occur 1 to 2 weeks after the onset of parotitis and may represent a demyelinating postinfectious encephalitis. Clinical findings in mumps encephalitis include obtundation (and less commonly delirium), generalized seizures, and high fever. Other neurologic findings can include focal seizures, aphasia, paresis, and involuntary movements. Recovery from mumps encephalitis is generally complete, although complications such as aqueductal stenosis with hydrocephalus, seizure disorders, and psychomotor retardation have been reported. The overall mortality from mumps encephalitis is 0.5 to 2.3%.

Orchitis

Epididymo-orchitis is rare in boys with mumps but occurs in 15 to 35% of postpubertal males with mumps. Orchitis is most often unilateral (bilateral involvement occurs in 17 to 38% of cases) and results from replication of mumps virus in the seminiferous tubules with resulting lymphocytic infiltration and edema. Orchitis typically develops within 1 week of the onset of parotitis, although orchitis (like mumps meningitis) can develop before or even in the absence of parotitis. Mumps orchitis is characterized by marked testicular swelling and severe pain accompanied by fever, nausea, and headache. The pain and swelling resolve within 5 to 7 days, but residual testicular tenderness can persist for weeks. Testicular atrophy may follow orchitis in 35 to 50% of cases; however, sterility is an uncommon complication even in men with bilateral orchitis.

Other Manifestations

Mumps can cause inflammation of other glandular tissues, including pancreatitis and thyroiditis. Oophoritis and mastitis have been reported in postpubertal women with mumps. Transient renal function abnormalities are common in mumps, and virus can be isolated readily from urine; significant renal damage is rare, however. Other infrequent manifestations of mumps include sensorineural deafness (either transient or permanent), arthritis, myocarditis, and thrombocytopenia. Maternal mumps infection during the first trimester of pregnancy results in an increased frequency of spontaneous abortions, but no clear association between congenital malformations and maternal mumps has been demonstrated.

Diagnosis

The diagnosis of mumps is usually based on clinical findings in a child with fever and parotitis, particularly if the individual is known to be susceptible and has been exposed to mumps during the preceding 2 to 3 weeks. An atypical clinical manifestation (e.g., meningitis or orchitis without parotitis) requires laboratory confirmation. Culturing for mumps virus is definitive but not universally available. Testing of acute and convalescent sera should demonstrate a diagnostic four-fold rise in mumps IgG antibody titer. Alternatively, finding mumps IgM antibody provides good evidence of recent infection. About 30% of patients have an elevated serum amylase level that may be due to parotitis or pancreatitis.

The differential diagnosis of a mumpslike syndrome includes infections caused by other viruses such as Epstein-Barr virus (Chapter 400), adenovirus (Chapter 388), influenza A virus (Chapter 387), parainfluenza virus (Chapter 386), coxsackievirus (Chapter 402), or lymphocytic choriomeningitis virus. Bacteria such as *Staphylococcus aureus* can cause suppurative parotitis. Parotid gland enlargement can also be associated with Sjögren's syndrome, sarcoidosis, amyloidosis, thiazide ingestion, iodine sensitivity, tumor, or salivary duct obstruction. Careful examination should distinguish parotitis from lymphadenopathy.

Treatment

Rx

Management of a patient with mumps consists of conservative measures to provide symptomatic relief and adequate hydration and nutrition. Treatment of orchitis includes bedrest, scrotal support, analgesics, and ice packs. Patients with significant CNS involvement require hospitalization for observation and supportive care. There is currently no established role for antiviral drugs, corticosteroids, or passive immunotherapy in the treatment of mumps.

Prevention

The cornerstone of mumps prevention is active immunization with the live attenuated mumps vaccine. In the United States, mumps vaccine is administered in combination with the measles and rubella vaccines (MMR) to children at 12 to 15 months of age and produces protective antibody levels in more than 95% of recipients. A second dose of MMR is recommended for children at 4 to 6 years of age. The mumps vaccine is also indicated for susceptible adults.

The Jeryl-Lynn strain of attenuated mumps virus used in the United States since 1967 is a very well tolerated vaccine, although rare instances of fever, parotitis, and possibly aseptic meningitis have been reported after immunization. In recent years, an increased frequency of cases of vaccine-related mumps meningitis has been recognized in other countries. These cases occurred after the administration of an MMR vaccine that contained the Urabe AM9 or Leningrad 3 strains of mumps virus. This problem has not been recognized in the United States, where the Jeryl-Lynn mumps vaccine continues to be used.

Questions regarding prevention often arise when an individual with no history of mumps (typically an adult male) is exposed to a patient with active mumps. The immune status of the exposed individual can be determined by serologic testing, although such testing may involve some delay. Detection of complement-fixing antibodies against V (hemagglutinin-neuraminidase) and S (nucleocapsid) antigens was previously the routine method for determining immune status but has been replaced by more sensitive and specific enzyme-linked immunosorbent assays. The mumps skin test is not a reliable indicator of immune status. The vast majority of adults born in the United States before 1957 were naturally infected and are therefore immune. Mumps vaccine can be safely administered to an individual of unknown immune status, although vaccine given to a susceptible individual after exposure to mumps may not provide protection.

Highly controversial reports have been published that suggest an etiologic association between the administration of MMR vaccine and the development of autism. Parental concerns generated by the adverse publicity have resulted in lower rates of immunization in some countries with consequent increases in infection rates. However, subsequent large-scale epidemiologic studies conducted in the United States and Europe have failed to demonstrate any link between the MMR vaccine and childhood autistic disorders.

For infection control purposes, patients with mumps require both standard precautions and droplet precautions. In the outpatient setting, a patient with suspected mumps should wear a mask and be isolated from other potentially susceptible persons. When a patient with mumps is hospitalized, a private room is required, caregivers should wear masks, and the patient should wear a mask when being transported.

SUGGESTED READINGS

Gupta RK, Best J, MacMahon E: Mumps and the UK epidemic 2005. BMJ 2005;330:1132–1135. *Description of the mumps outbreak in the UK and review of the diagnosis and treatment of the disease.*

Kancherla VS, Hanson IC: Mumps resurgence in the United States. J Allergy Clin Immunol 2006;118:938–941. *Description of the outbreak as well as a review about the virus and the possible mechanisms of vaccine failure.*

393 CYTOMEGALOVIRUS, EPSTEIN-BARR VIRUS, AND SLOW VIRUS INFECTIONS OF THE CENTRAL NERVOUS SYSTEM

Joseph R. Berger and Avindra Nath

CYTOMEGALOVIRUS

Human cytomegalovirus (CMV) is a ubiquitous herpesvirus that is acquired throughout life (Chapter 399). In children, CMV is an important and relatively common cause of congenital neurologic deficits. In the United States, 60 to 80% of adults have serologic evidence of infection. Primary infection is usually asymptomatic in young, healthy adults but may be associated with a transient mononucleosis-like syndrome. CMV results in major neurologic disability in the setting of immunosuppression, particularly in persons with acquired immunodeficiency syndrome (AIDS). In addition to retinitis, CMV may involve the brain, spinal cord, and peripheral nerves.

Cytomegalovirus Encephalitis

CMV encephalitis has several manifestations in patients with AIDS. The most typical is subacute, diffuse encephalopathy evolving over a period of weeks and characterized by headache, impaired cognition and sensorium, apathy, and social withdrawal. Neurologic examination reveals abnormal mentation and variable motor features, including hyperreflexia, ataxia, and weakness. CMV ventriculitis is characteristically present and is often associated with cranial neuropathy, nystagmus, and progressive ventricular enlargement. Other features may suggest brain stem encephalitis, including internuclear ophthalmoplegia, cranial nerve palsy, gaze paresis, ataxia, and quadriparesis. Rarely, CMV infection may be manifested as a cerebral mass lesion. Other findings in these patients include cerebral infarction resulting from CMV vasculitis, acute subarachnoid hemorrhage, and intracerebral hemorrhage. Virtually all patients with CMV encephalitis have systemic CMV infection. CMV myelitis, polyradiculitis, and multifocal neuritis may also occur with CMV encephalitis. Distinctive retinal lesions can often be seen ophthalmoscopically (Chapter 399).

Cerebral imaging studies are of limited sensitivity and low specificity in patients with CMV encephalitis. Ependymal or meningeal enhancement may be visualized, as well as areas of focal infarction or necrosis. Progressive ventricular enlargement should suggest CMV ventriculitis. Cerebrospinal fluid (CSF) findings are variable. Most patients have elevated protein levels. Glucose levels may be normal or decreased. Leukocytes may be absent, but CSF pleocytosis is usual. A marked pleocytosis with a polymorphonuclear leukocyte preponderance may occur in patients with CMV ventriculoencephalitis. CMV can rarely be cultured from CSF. CSF polymerase chain reaction (PCR) is the most specific diagnostic method, but the diagnosis is often difficult and relies on a high index of clinical suspicion.

Necrotizing Myelitis

Necrotizing myelitis secondary to CMV in human immunodeficiency virus (HIV)–infected patients is most commonly associated with polyradiculitis. Some cases of necrotizing myelitis in the absence of a typical polyradiculitis syndrome have been described, with patients displaying acute or progressive paraplegia and disturbances in urinary and rectal sphincter function. Reflexes are preserved or enhanced in the legs unless concurrent neuropathy is present. A sensory level may be demonstrable.

Polyradiculomyelitis

Neuromuscular pathology from CMV has been found in approximately a fourth of patients dying of AIDS. It is predominantly localized to the perineurial and epineurial regions. CMV polyradiculomyelitis in HIV-infected patients is manifested subacutely over a period of days to a few weeks. Initial symptoms of paresthesias or dysesthetic pain localized to the perineal and lower extremity regions are followed by rapidly progressive paraparesis with hypotonia and diminished or absent lower extremity reflexes. Urinary retention is characteristic, and rectal sphincter incontinence is common. Variable sensory findings are typically overshadowed by weakness. Babinski's signs and diminished sensation below a discrete level across the trunk are signs of an associated myelitis. With time, symptoms progress by ascending to involve the upper limbs and sometimes the cranial nerves. CSF examination generally reveals polymorphonuclear pleocytosis and prominent elevation of protein levels. Hypoglycorrhachia is frequently present. Findings on spinal magnetic resonance imaging (MRI) may be normal or reveal enhancement of the conus medullaris, cauda equina, meninges, and nerve roots. Electrophysiologic studies reveal axonal neuropathy with evidence of acute denervation. Variable slowing of nerve conduction may occur.

The appearance of acute cauda equina syndrome in a patient with AIDS is suggestive of CMV infection when a polymorphonuclear pleocytosis is present in CSF; however, the syndrome is not pathognomonic. Other conditions that may produce a cauda equina syndrome in AIDS patients include lymphomatous meningitis, syphilis, toxoplasmosis, other herpesviruses, and cryptococcal or bacterial meningitis. Progressive multifocal motor and sensory neuropathy that evolves over a period of weeks to months has also been seen in patients with CMV infection. Paresthesia and dysesthesia are quickly followed by prominent motor weakness involving both the upper and lower limbs asymmetrically. Neurogenic atrophy may be prominent. Nerve biopsy reveals necrotizing neuritis with mononuclear and polymorphonuclear infiltrates and cytomegalocytes localized around endoneurial capillaries in the nerve trunks and roots. Some patients may have necrotizing arteritis. PCR for CMV in CSF may be useful in establishing the diagnosis.

CMV neurologic complications should be treated with ganciclovir or foscarnet; however, evidence of their efficacy in these conditions is limited chiefly to case reports and small series. Cidofovir is a second-line agent. CMV strains resistant to both agents have emerged, and CMV encephalitis has developed in the presence of maintenance ganciclovir therapy for CMV retinitis. Combination (foscarnet and ganciclovir) or alternative therapies should be considered in patients already undergoing suppressive monotherapy or in those with persistent CSF pleocytosis. Maintenance therapy is required unless the patient experiences immune reconstitution, such as after highly active antiretroviral therapy (HAART) in an AIDS patient or discontinuation of immunosuppressive regimens in a transplant or cancer patient.

Prognosis

The prognosis for long-term survival, especially with AIDS, is very poor.

EPSTEIN-BARR VIRUS

Epstein-Barr virus (EBV), the cause of infectious mononucleosis (Chapter 400), is distributed worldwide. Its acquisition depends on population density and socioeconomic status. Individuals in areas of high population density and lower social strata acquire the virus in early childhood. However, seroepidemiologic studies indicate that virtually all persons are infected by EBV by 30 years of age.

Neurologic manifestations occur in 1 to 5% of patients with primary EBV infection and may be the only prominent clinical finding. The most common neurologic disorder associated with infectious mononucleosis is meningoencephalitis. This complication is rare in early childhood and is most often observed in persons between the ages of 15 and 25 years. Its onset may be gradual over a span of several days or be explosive. Fever, headache, mild stiff neck, confusion, lethargy, seizures, and hyperreflexia are the most typical features. Occasionally, focal neurologic features, including hemiparesis, focal seizures, and cerebellar and brain stem findings may be detected. The prognosis for patients with EBV meningoencephalitis is excellent, with complete resolution anticipated in 1 to 2 weeks.

SLOW VIRUS INFECTIONS OF THE CENTRAL NERVOUS SYSTEM

Human Immunodeficiency Virus and Human T-Lymphotrophic Virus Type 1

These viruses and their neurologic sequelae are considered in Chapters 401 and 417, respectively.

Subacute Sclerosing Panencephalitis and Progressive Rubella Panencephalitis

Subacute sclerosing panencephalitis (SSPE) is caused by the measles virus (Chapter 390). It usually affects children, but its onset can extend into young adulthood. Patients generally have a history of measles within the first 2 years of life, and it is speculated that such early host exposure allows the emergence of persistent defective virus replication. As a result of effective vaccination strategies against measles virus, its incidence has markedly decreased.

SSPE usually begins with cognitive and behavioral changes. It progresses to include motor dysfunction with prominent myoclonus, choreoathetosis, dystonia, and rigidity. Its course progresses over a period of 1 to 3 years to rigid quadriparesis and a vegetative state. The condition is more common in rural settings and affects males more often than females.

The electroencephalogram reveals periodic complexes with synchronous bursts of two or three high-amplitude slow waves per second, with recurrence at regular intervals of 5 to 8 seconds and a 1:1 relationship with myoclonic jerks. Computed tomography (CT) of the brain shows generalized atrophy. CSF protein, glucose, and cell levels are usually normal; CSF is characterized by a high immunoglobulin concentration, oligoclonal bands, and intrathecal synthesis of antibody to measles virus antigens. Serum measles antibody titers are also high. These findings are usually sufficiently characteristic for diagnosis; rarely, brain biopsy is needed for definitive diagnosis in atypical cases. Gray matter is most prominently involved. The pathologic features of SSPE include gliosis, loss of myelin, and perivascular infiltrates of lymphocytes and plasma cells in white and gray matter. Neuronal cell loss is seen in later stages of the illness. Intranuclear Cowdry type A inclusions containing viral nucleocapsids are identified in neurons and glia. Measles RNA can be detected in the brain by PCR.

Measles virus may also cause subacute encephalitis in an immunocompromised host. The prominence of cognitive and motor dysfunction in these patients resembles that of SSPE, but in the clinical setting its subacute onset and more rapid evolution and the presence of generalized seizures rather than myoclonus are distinctive. Brain abnormalities include abundant intranuclear inclusions, but inflammation is minimal, and neither serum nor CSF antibody titers against measles virus are high. For this reason, brain biopsy is generally needed for diagnosis.

Progressive rubella panencephalitis is a rare disorder resembling SSPE but caused by rubella virus (Chapter 391). It occurs as a complication of congenital rubella syndrome or, more typically, after childhood rubella. A hiatus of years separates early infection from the onset of neurologic deterioration, which is characterized by behavioral changes, cognitive impairment, cerebellar ataxia, spasticity, and sometimes seizures. Myoclonus is a less prominent feature than it is in SSPE. Electroencephalography shows generalized slowing. The course of illness is similar to that of SSPE—progression to coma, brain stem involvement, and death in 2 to 5 years. Serology or isolation of the virus from brain or peripheral blood lymphocytes confirms the cause.

With the advent of widespread measles and rubella immunization, these disorders have been nearly eliminated in the United States, although recently patients with atypical manifestations of SSPE have been recognized. There is no established, unequivocally effective treatment of SSPE or progressive rubella panencephalitis, but arrest of the disease has been reported in some patients with SSPE after long-term treatment with intrathecal interferon alfa.

Progressive Multifocal Leukoencephalopathy

Definition

This demyelinating disease is associated with infection of oligodendrocytes by JC virus (JCV), a papovavirus widely distributed in humans. JCV exhibits a neurotropism exclusive to glial cells. Progressive multifocal leukoencephalopathy (PML) was the first demyelinating disease to be unequivocally associated with a viral infection.

Epidemiology

Serologic studies indicate that by 5 years of age, approximately 10% of children have antibody to JCV and, by the age of 10 years, 40 to 60% have the antibody. Despite the wide dissemination of JCV infection, PML is rarely observed in the absence of underlying cellular immunosuppression. It is also rarely observed in childhood. Until the AIDS epidemic, PML was most commonly observed in patients with lymphoproliferative disorders. In a 1984 review, lymphoproliferative disorders were associated with 62.2% of PML cases, 6.5% of myeloproliferative diseases, 2.2% of carcinomatous diseases, 10.9% of a variety of acquired immunodeficiency states, and 5.6% of cases with no underlying disease. Since the inception of the AIDS epidemic in 1981, AIDS has been the disorder associated with PML in most cases. Before the introduction of HAART, PML would ultimately develop in 5% of AIDS patients, thus accounting for the explosive increased incidence of the disorder during the first 2 decades of the AIDS pandemic. Recently, PML has been reported to occur in association with the administration of natalizumab, an $\alpha 4\beta 1$ integrin inhibitor used in the treatment of multiple sclerosis and Crohn's disease.

Pathobiology

The cardinal feature of PML is demyelination, which is typically multifocal but occasionally unifocal (Fig. 393–1). These lesions may occur in any location in the white matter but have a predilection for the parieto-occipital regions. The lesions range in size from 1 mm to several centimeters; larger lesions may reflect the coalescence of multiple smaller lesions. The other histopathologic hallmark of PML is the presence of hyperchromatic, enlarged oligodendroglial nuclei and enlarged bizarre astrocytes with lobulated hyperchromatic nuclei. Electron microscopic examination reveals the JC virions, which are 28 to 45 nm in diameter and appear singly or in dense crystalline arrays in oligodendroglial cells and, less frequently, in reactive astrocytes.

Clinical Manifestations

The clinical hallmark of PML is the presence of focal neurologic symptoms and signs associated with radiographic evidence of white matter

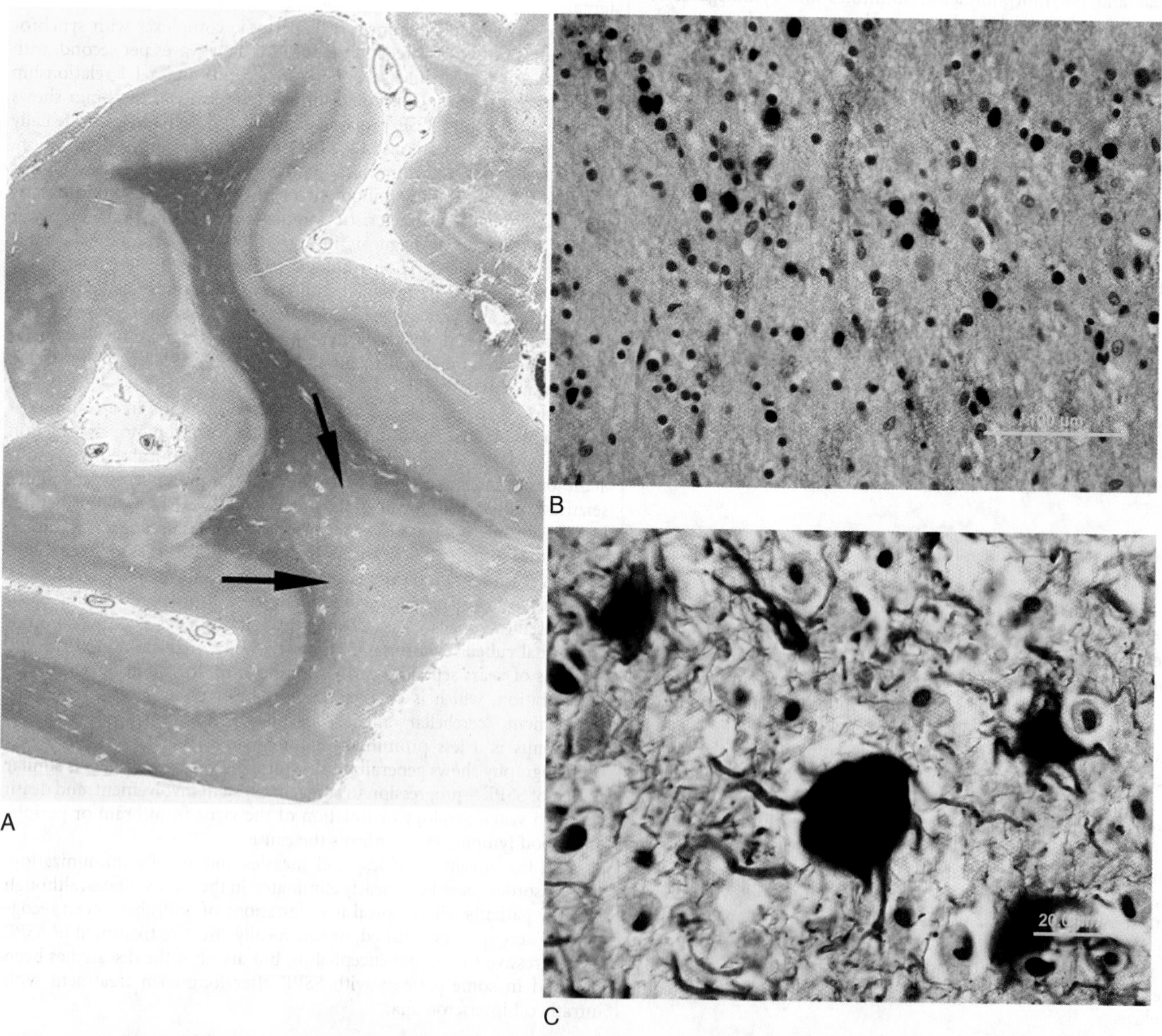

FIGURE 393–1 • Pathology of progressive multifocal leukoencephalopathy. A, An area of demyelination is seen in the white matter that fails to stain with Luxol fast blue dye. **B,** Immunohistochemical staining with antibody to papovavirus shows brown-staining nuclei in oligodendrocytes, indicative of JC virus infection. **C,** Immunohistochemical staining for glial fibrillary acidic protein shows large bizarre astrocytes. (Courtesy of Dr. Carlos Pardo, Johns Hopkins University, Baltimore.)

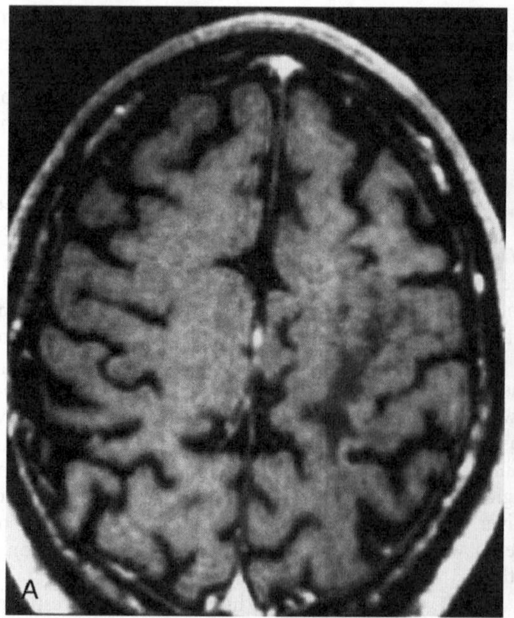

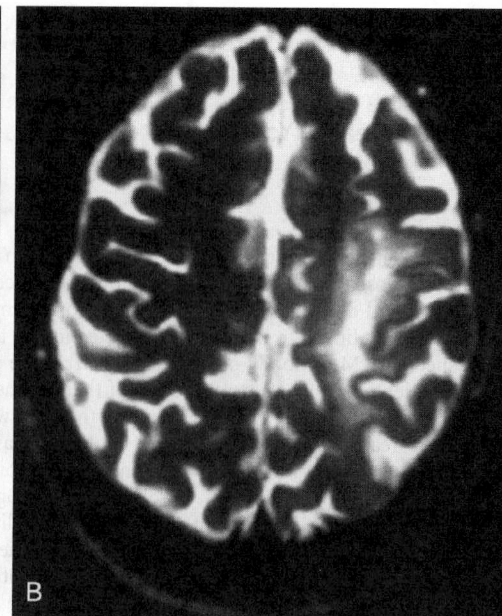

FIGURE 393–2 • Cranial magnetic resonance images of progressive multifocal leukoencephalopathy. A, A T1-weighted image shows a hypointense signal abnormality of the left frontal lobe white matter. **B,** On T2-weighted imaging, the lesion is hyperintense.

disease in the absence of a mass effect. The most common initial symptoms include weakness, speech abnormalities, and cognitive disturbances, each seen in approximately 40% of patients. Though rare in non-AIDS patients, headache may occur in as many as a third of patients with AIDS. Gait disturbances, sensory loss, and visual impairment all occur in approximately 20 to 30%. Seizures and brain stem symptoms are less common. Signs noted on physical examination parallel the reported symptoms, with weakness, typically a hemiparesis, detected in more than half of patients at initial evaluation. Gait abnormalities, cognitive problems, and language disorders (i.e., dysarthria and dysphasia) are observed in about a fourth of patients at initial contact. Limb and trunk ataxia reflecting cerebellar involvement is detected in as many as 10% but may occasionally result from severe impairment in position sense (i.e., sensory ataxia). Neuro-ophthalmic symptoms occur in 50% of patients with PML and are the initial manifestation in 30 to 45%. The most common visual deficit is homonymous hemianopia or quadrantanopia secondary to lesions of the optic radiations. Cortical blindness is present in as many as 5 to 8% of patients at the time of diagnosis. Other neuro-ophthalmic manifestations include optic agnosia, alexia without agraphia, and ocular motor abnormalities. Sensory disturbances occur with PML but are distinctly less common than impairment of strength or visual function.

Diagnosis

The diagnosis of PML may be strongly suggested by the clinical manifestations and the radiographic imaging results. When the former are coupled with a positive JCV PCR finding in CSF, the diagnosis of PML is virtually certain. Brain biopsy with demonstration of the characteristic histopathologic triad of PML coupled with immunohistochemical or electron microscopic evidence of JCV remains the "gold standard" for diagnosis.

CT of the brain reveals hypodense lesions of the affected white matter that generally have a "scalloped" appearance because of involvement of the subcortical arcuate fibers lying directly beneath the cortex. Cranial MRI shows a hyperintense lesion on T2-weighted images in the affected regions (Fig. 393–2) and usually shows a hypointense lesion on T1-weighted images. Contrast enhancement is seen in approximately 5 to 10% of pathologically confirmed cases of PML with either brain imaging technique. The enhancement observed is typically faint and at the periphery of lesions. In patients without AIDS, the lesions of PML have a predilection for the parieto-occipital lobes, but in AIDS patients, the lesions are more often found in the frontal lobes. Involvement of the basal ganglia, external capsule, and posterior fossa structures (i.e., cerebellum and brain stem) is also seen.

The results of routine analysis of CSF are not diagnostic, but CSF protein may be elevated. CSF PCR for JCV is of great value in diagnosis; though not always positive, it is highly specific.

Treatment

Rx

There is no effective therapy for PML. Although cytosine arabinoside prevents JCV replication in vitro, a randomized, double-blind trial in which it was administered intrathecally or intravenously in patients with AIDS-associated PML demonstrated no benefit. This lack of efficacy may have been a reflection of inadequate concentrations of the drug at the sites of infection. The improved understanding of the mechanism of viral entry into the cell via 5-HT2a receptors and clathrin-dependent endocytosis has led to an interest in using agents that block these pathways. However, their efficacy remains to be established. Spontaneous recovery in untreated patients makes it difficult to assess the results of experimental treatments in small or uncontrolled treatment trials.

Prognosis

Previously, PML was regarded as a fatal illness with mean survival times averaging 6 months. After the introduction of HAART, 50% of patients with AIDS-associated PML have demonstrated survival exceeding 12 months, often with partial or nearly complete clinical and radiographic recovery. Factors associated with a more benign course include the presence of PML as the heralding manifestation of AIDS, high or climbing $CD4^+$ T-lymphocyte counts, contrast enhancement of the lesions on radiographic studies, and any clinical or radiographic evidence of recovery. JCV-specific T lymphocytes appear to be critical for controlling the infection.

SUGGESTED READINGS

Koralnik IJ: Progressive multifocal leukoencephalopathy revisited: Has the disease outgrown its name? Ann Neurol 2006;60:162–173. *A review of JC virus and this clinical syndrome.*

Maschke M, Kastrup O, Diener HC: CNS manifestations of cytomegalovirus infections: Diagnosis and treatment. CNS Drugs 2002;16:303–315. *An overview, with emphasis on CMV in immunocompromised patients.*

Prashanth LK, Taly AB, Ravi V, et al: Adult onset subacute sclerosing panencephalitis: Clinical profile of 39 patients from a tertiary care centre. J Neurol Neurosurg Psychiatry 2005;77:630–633. *A large case series from India.*

Salehi HR, Delgado E, Wolf SM, et al: Subacute sclerosing panencephalitis with atypical features. Pediatr Neurol 2005;33:280–282. *A typical presentation of three U.S. cases.*

Yousry TA, Major EO, Ryschkewitsch C, et al: Evaluation of patients treated with natalizumab for progressive multifocal leukoencephalopathy. N Engl J Med 2006;354:924–933. *Risk of PML was estimated at 1 in 1000 patients over 17.9 months.*

394 B19 PARVOVIRUS

Neal S. Young

Definition

B19 parvovirus was discovered by Yvonne Cossart in the mid-1970s by electron microscopic observation of an anomalous precipitin reaction of a normal blood donor's sera (occupying position 19 in plate B). Human disease was first linked to B19 parvovirus infection by the observation of virus-specific IgM antibody or the virus itself in the sera of sickle cell disease patients suffering a complication of their disease called transient aplastic crisis. The common illness caused by the virus was identified later during outbreaks of fifth disease, a highly contagious rash illness of childhood long suspected of having a viral etiology. The ability of parvovirus to persist and be manifested as an isolated hematologic syndrome was demonstrated by the presence of the virus in fetal liver at autopsy of hydropic newborns and in immunosuppressed patients with chronic pure red cell aplasia at the National Institutes of Health.

The Pathogen

The parvoviruses form small icosahedral capsids of about 25 nm. They have a limited genome of single-stranded DNA. The approximately 5600 nucleotides of B19 parvovirus show remarkably little sequence variation among isolates; two variants, V9 and A6, are of uncertain clinical significance.

The Parvoviridae family contains many pathogenic animal viruses: feline panleukopenia virus, the cause of a fatal agranulocytosis in cats; canine parvovirus, which probably arose from the cat virus as a host range variant in the 1970s to produce a global pandemic and can cause fatal myocarditis in puppies; Aleutian mink virus infection, a model of immune complex pathology; and porcine parvovirus, responsible for fetal wastage in pig litters. Besides B19, other parvoviruses that have recently been isolated from human tissues are not clearly identified as pathogens.

Epidemiology

B19 infection is global; infectivity rates, inferred from the presence of antiparvovirus IgG antibody in sera, are similar in the United States, Europe, and Asia, and only isolated populations, Amazonian tribesman, and residents of remote islands off the coast of Africa have escaped exposure. B19 parvovirus infection is common in childhood, and half of 15-year-old adolescents have specific antiparvovirus B19 antibodies. Infection continues throughout adult life, and the great majority of the elderly are seropositive. In temperate climates, most infections occur in the spring, with small epidemics every few years being typical. Transmission is respiratory by droplet spread, and secondary infection rates among household contacts are very high. Nosocomial infection can occur, and B19 parvovirus has been transmitted in blood products, especially pooled components such as factor VIII and IX concentrates. Producers of plasma derivatives now voluntarily screen by quantitative measurement of B19 DNA to reduce the risk for iatrogenic transmission. The lack of a lipid envelope and the stable DNA genome make parvoviruses notoriously resistant to heat inactivation and solvent detergents.

Pathobiology

The biology of the Parvoviridae makes them especially dependent on helper function from host cells or other viruses. The autonomous parvoviruses propagate in actively dividing cells; the family Parvoviridae includes disease-causing animal parvoviruses. Adeno-associated viruses grow in tissue cultures infected with adenoviruses and herpesviruses and are popular vectors for gene transduction and therapy. B19 is the type member of the Erythrovirus genus, which includes very similar simian viruses, all of which are best propagated in erythroid progenitor cells, which are responsible for red blood cell production in the bone marrow. Active replication of virus can be detected by the presence of double-stranded intermediate forms by simple DNA hybridization methods. The transcription map of the erythroviruses differs markedly from that of other Parvoviridae. Only three genes produce proteins of known function. Many antigenic determinants recognized by the host immune system are located in helical loops that form the surface of each capsomere. Most of the capsid is composed of a major structural protein, called VP2, but about 5% of the capsid is a minor structural protein, VP1, which differs from VP2 only by an additional 226 amino acids at the amino terminus; this VP1-unique region is located external to the capsid surface and contains linear epitopes recognized by neutralizing antibodies.

The only known natural host cell of B19 parvovirus is the human erythroid progenitor. The tropism of the virus for an erythroid cell host mainly results from its cellular receptor, globoside, a neutral glycolipid also known as erythrocyte P antigen. Rare individuals with the p phenotype, who congenitally lack globoside on their erythrocytes, are genetically insusceptible to B19 parvovirus infection; they show no serologic evidence of previous infection, and their marrow erythroid progenitors proliferate normally in the presence of high concentrations of virus. Parvovirus kills erythroid progenitors by expression of its nonstructural protein, and it is possible that some cells, such as megakaryocytes, may be lysed by restricted expression of viral proteins in the absence of viral propagation.

The humoral immune response is dominant in B19 parvovirus infection. Natural antibody production correlates with disappearance of the virus from blood, and the presence of IgG appears to confer lasting protection against second infection. Parvovirus infection can persist if immunoglobulin production is defective such that antibody fails to neutralize the virus; reactivity of antibodies to the unique amino-terminal region of VP1 is especially important.

Clinical Manifestations

Fifth Disease

Most B19 parvovirus infections are asymptomatic. The most common manifestation of infection is erythema infectiosum, or fifth disease, a rash illness of childhood characterized by a "slapped cheek" appearance (Fig. 394–1). In volunteers inoculated intranasally with B19, nonspecific "flulike" complaints occurred early along with parvoviremia; the cutaneous eruption a week later corresponded to the appearance of antiviral

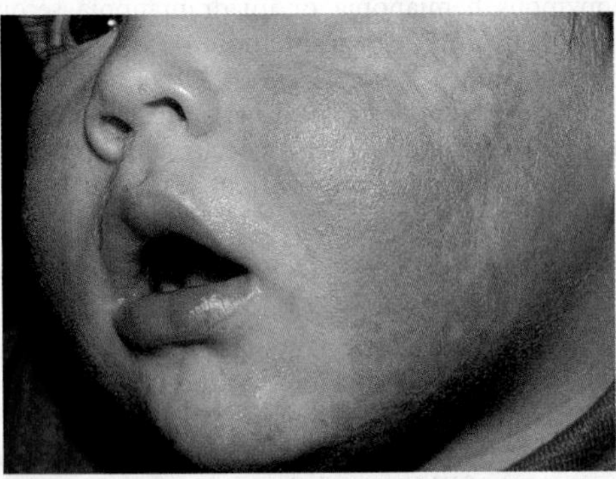

A

B

FIGURE 394–1 • Erythema infectiosum. In this infection by parvovirus B19, a child will develop prominent erythema of the cheeks, "slapped cheeks" **(A)**, followed by a lacelike erythema on the extremities **(B)** and buttocks. It is also known as fifth disease.

Section XXIII Infectious Diseases

antibodies. These more specific symptoms of B19 parvovirus infection are secondary to immune complex formation and deposition. Serologic testing generally shows seroconversion, IgM antibody, or the new presence of IgG antibody to parvovirus. The rash of fifth disease may be evanescent, and recurrences can be provoked by sunlight, heat, emotion, or exercise. Fifth disease can be confused with rubella. In adults, the rash is less characteristic and may be difficult to visualize in dark-skinned individuals.

B19 Arthropathy

In contrast to the mild course of B19 infection in children with fifth disease, acute parvovirus infection in adults, particularly middle-aged women, may cause significant arthropathy. Not only arthralgia but also a true inflammatory arthritis occurs in about 50% of older patients, and approximately 15% of new arthritis cases may be the sequelae of B19 parvovirus infection. Symmetrical joint involvement of the hands and occasionally the ankles, knees, and wrists can mimic rheumatoid arthritis, and a test for rheumatoid factor may be positive. B19 arthropathy usually resolves within a few weeks; even with persistent symptoms, joint destruction does not occur. Parvovirus is not the cause of rheumatoid arthritis, but case reports suggest that B19 infection may mimic, precipitate, or exacerbate a variety of rheumatologic diseases, including juvenile rheumatoid arthritis, systemic lupus erythematosus, and fibromyalgia.

Transient Aplastic Crisis

In persons with underlying hemolysis or a high demand for production of circulating erythrocytes, acute B19 parvovirus infection causes transient aplastic crisis, an abrupt cessation of red blood cell production that exacerbates or, in previously compensated states, provokes severe anemia. Erythropoiesis is temporarily suppressed in all B19 parvovirus infections, but hemoglobin levels ordinarily remain stable because of the long lifespan of erythrocytes. The anemic crises associated with low or absent reticulocytes in hereditary spherocytosis and sickle cell disease are virtually always secondary to B19 parvovirus infection. Parvoviremia is present in patients with transient aplastic crisis, and red cell production resumes once antibodies to the virus are produced and the infection is cleared. Transient aplastic crisis is generally a unique event in the patient's life, thus suggesting induction of long-lasting protective immunity. Though self-limited, aplastic crisis can lead to severe, occasionally fatal anemia that precipitates congestive heart failure and cerebrovascular accidents, and transfusion is frequently required. Early on, transient aplastic crisis was associated with a pathognomonic bone marrow morphology, absence of maturing erythroid precursors and the presence of "giant pronormoblasts" (Fig. 394–2)—these cells are now recognized as the cytopathic effect of parvovirus infection.

White blood cell and platelet counts may fall modestly during transient aplastic crisis, especially in patients with functioning spleens. Occasional cases of agranulocytosis may be due to B19; thrombocytopenia and pancytopenia have been reported, and B19 can precipitate a benign viral-associated hemophagocytic syndrome.

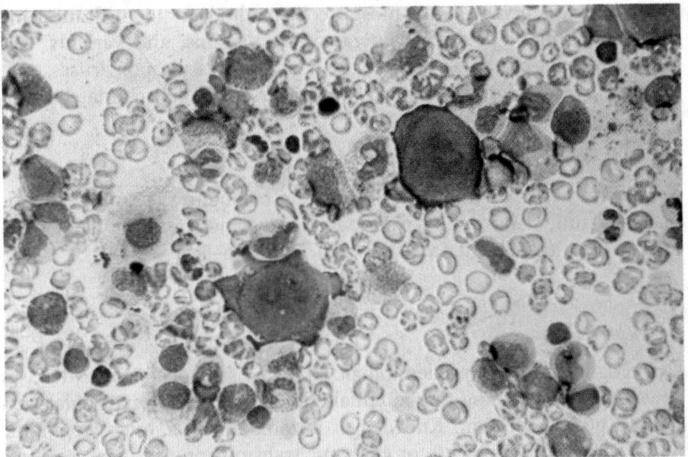

FIGURE 394–2 • Bone marrow aspirate of a patient with chronic pure red cell aplasia secondary to persistent B19 parvovirus infection. Mature erythroid precursors are absent, and giant pronormoblasts are typical of B19 infection.

Persistent Infection

B19 parvovirus persists in the absence of an appropriate host antibody response. In the absence of specific immunity, there are none of the clinical features of fifth disease but instead a purely hematologic syndrome of pure red cell aplasia; the anemia is severe and requires transfusion, and reticulocytes are absent from blood, as are erythroid precursors from marrow. Giant pronormoblasts in a suggestive clinical setting may lead to the diagnosis. Antibody to parvovirus is absent from blood, but the virus can readily be detected in the circulation, often at extremely high levels (>10^{12} genome copies/mL). Failure to produce neutralizing antibodies to B19 parvovirus occurs in patients with congenital immunodeficiency (Nezelof's syndrome), in those with iatrogenic immunodeficiency (chemotherapy or immunosuppressive drugs), or as a result of acquired immunodeficiency secondary to HIV-1. Pure red cell aplasia secondary to parvovirus may be the first manifestation of acquired immunodeficiency syndrome (AIDS).

Hydrops Fetalis

B19 parvovirus infection of the pregnant mother followed by transplacental transmission to the fetus can lead to an adverse outcome, either miscarriage or hydrops fetalis. Parvovirus infects the fetal liver, the site of erythrocyte production during early development. The swollen appearance in hydrops is the result of severe anemia, as well as perhaps myocarditis, contributing to congestive heart failure. Prospective studies have led to an estimated 30% risk of transplacental infection and 9% risk of fetal loss in women who are exposed to B19 during pregnancy. Infection during the second trimester poses the greatest risk for birth of a hydropic infant; B19 parvovirus probably accounts for 10 to 20% of all cases of nonimmune hydrops fetalis. The risk of spontaneous abortion resulting from first trimester infections has been more difficult to quantitate. The risk for infection increases in epidemic years and correlates with the level of contact of the pregnant woman with children. Although most B19 infections during pregnancy probably do not lead to either loss of the fetus or congenital anomalies, B19 infection is a relatively frequent cause of fetal death. Congenital malformations have not been consistently associated with intrauterine parvovirus infection. However, severe anemia at birth with a bone marrow histology consistent with either constitutional pure red cell aplasia (Diamond-Blackfan anemia) or congenital dyserythropoietic anemia has occurred in infants salvaged by in utero blood transfusions or exchange transfusion at birth.

Other Syndromes

Elevated levels of hepatic transaminases can accompany fifth disease, and parvovirus infection has been associated with severe, but self-limited hepatitis in a few children. The presence of B19 genetic sequences in cardiac tissue has led to a diagnosis of parvovirus myocarditis. Serologic and DNA evidence of B19 infection implicated parvovirus in some patients with necrotizing vasculitis, Kawasaki's disease, Henoch-Schönlein purpura, and giant cell arteritis. Glove-and-sock syndrome, an exanthem localized to the hands and feet and consisting of edema, erythema, paresthesia, and pruritus, has been linked to B19. Chronic fatigue syndrome may follow parvovirus infection. Meningitis, encephalitis, and a variety of neurologic complications may occur with fifth disease and parvovirus infection.

False-positive results arise when the diagnosis of infection rests on detection of amplified B19 genome by polymerase chain reaction, and furthermore, B19 parvovirus can persist at low levels in normal individuals for many months after infection.

Diagnosis

Because of the difficulty propagating B19 parvovirus in standard tissue culture, laboratory diagnosis relies on serologic and DNA tests (Table 394–1). Virus-specific antibodies are measured in standardized commercial solid-phase enzyme-labeled immunoassays, generally involving the use of capsid proteins generated in the baculovirus system. "Capture" formats are preferred to detect serum IgM, which is first bound to a solid phase coated with anti–μ-chain antibodies, followed by the addition of viral antigen and an antiviral monoclonal antibody. IgM antibodies are diagnostically positive in almost all cases of fifth disease at initial evaluation and appear within a few days of the onset of transient aplastic crisis, and IgM may persist for months after acute infection. IgG is usually

TABLE 394–1 DIAGNOSIS OF PARVOVIRUS B19

Disease	IgM	IgG	B19 Dot Blot*	B19 PCR
Fifth disease	+++	++	−	+
Polyarthropathy syndrome	++	+	−	+
Transient aplastic crisis	+/−	+/−	++	++
Persistent anemia	+/−	+/−	++	++
Hydrops/congenital infection	+/−	+	+/−	++
Previous infection	−	++	−	+/−

*Sensitivity about 10^6 genome copies per milliliter.
PCR = polymerase chain reaction.

assayed in conventional indirect assays. IgG circulates later than IgM, generally at the end of the first week of illness. Although titers of IgG are generally highest in the year after an acute infection, substantial interindividual variation and the presence of IgG in a large proportion of the population make measurement of IgG less helpful than other tests for diagnosis of parvovirus. DNA assays are required for persistent B19 infection, in which antibody production is absent or minimal. Parvovirus can also be found in the serum of patients with early transient aplastic crisis. Direct hybridization methods are reliable, and they detect clinically relevant viral titers of greater than 10^6 international units (orders of magnitude below levels present in both acute and persistent infection). Gene amplification methods are more sensitive but less reliable because of false-positive results. Virus can be detected in amniotic fluid, and both virus and IgM antibody to B19 are found in umbilical cord blood; mother's sera will show seroconversion during pregnancy, but maternal IgM may be negative at the onset of hydrops fetalis.

Prevention

Effective vaccines exist for animal parvoviruses, and human B19 infection can also probably be prevented. A recombinant immunogen in development for the human virus lacks DNA and is therefore noninfectious; the empty capsids have been engineered to overexpress the highly immunogenic minor structural protein VP1, and a single 2.5-μg dose of empty capsids elicited excellent neutralizing antibody responses in normal volunteers. Vaccination could prevent transient aplastic crisis in patients with sickle cell disease and other hemolytic anemias, pure red cell aplasia in some immunodeficient individuals, and hydrops if seronegative mothers were inoculated early in pregnancy.

Treatment

Rx

Most parvovirus infections in normal children and adults do not require specific therapy. Isolation of infected individuals is impractical, with the exception of hospitalized cases. Pure red cell aplasia and the underlying persistent B19 parvovirus infection can be dramatically terminated by discontinuation of immunosuppressive therapy or institution of effective antiretroviral drugs in patients with AIDS. Commercial immunoglobulins are a good source of antibodies to parvovirus, and persistent B19 infection responds to a 5- or 10-day course of IgG at 0.4 g/kg with a prompt decline in serum viral DNA, as measured by hybridization methods, accompanied by reticulocytosis and increased hemoglobin levels. This regimen has been curative in congenital immunodeficiency, but in AIDS, parvovirus often persists at lower levels and relapses of anemia may require repeated IgG administration. Immunoglobulin therapy can precipitate fifth disease rash and arthralgia. Hydrops fetalis may resolve spontaneously, but intrauterine blood transfusions have been used with apparent success. Chronic arthropathy has been treated symptomatically with anti-inflammatory drugs, and there is not a clear role for the administration of immunoglobulin. Equally important as recognizing parvovirus infection is avoiding misinterpretation of laboratory studies, such as positive IgG serology or borderline IgM and DNA tests, and misguided maneuvers that delay alternative appropriate treatments.

SUGGESTED READINGS

Broliden K, Tolfvenstam T, Norbeck O: Clinical aspects of parvovirus B19 infection. J Intern Med 2006;260:285–304. *A comprehensive review focusing on the clinical aspects of parvovirus B19.*

Chorba TL, Coccia P, Holman RC, et al: Role of parvovirus B19 in aplastic crisis and erythema infectiosum (fifth disease). J Infect Dis 1986;154:383–393. *The best epidemiologic study of parvovirus B19 in the community.*

Eid AJ, Brown RA, Patel R, et al: Parvovirus B19 infection after transplantation: A review of 98 cases. Clin Infect Dis 2006;43:40–48. *A review of the epidemiology and clinical spectrum of post-transplant parvovirus infection.*

Ergaz Z, Ornoy A: Parvovirus B19 in pregnancy. Reprod Toxicol 2006;21:421–435. *An excellent review of parvovirus B19 infection during pregnancy.*

Moore TL: Parvovirus-associated arthritis. Curr Opin Rheumatol 2000;12:289–294. *Reviews rheumatic complications of parvovirus B19 infection.*

Servey JT, Reamy BV, Hodge J: Clinical presentations of parvovirus B19 infection. Am Fam Physician 2007;75:373–376. *An excellent review.*

Young NS, Brown KE: Parvovirus B19. N Engl J Med 2004;350:586–597. *A recent and complete review of parvovirus B19 disease.*

395 SMALLPOX, MONKEYPOX, AND OTHER POXVIRUS INFECTIONS

Inger K. Damon

Definition

Human illness caused by a poxvirus is characterized by a cutaneous manifestation; illness may be localized or systemic, depending on the particular poxvirus and the route of introduction. DNA-based assays, including DNA sequencing, are the most precise methods for identification and differentiation of poxvirus genera, species, strains, and variants. The guanosine plus cytosine content of orthopoxviruses, yatapoxviruses, molluscum contagiosum virus, and parapoxviruses is approximately 33%, 32%, 60%, and 63%, respectively.

The Pathogens

All poxviruses described in this chapter belong to the family Poxviridae, subfamily Chordopoxvirinae. The genus and species of the viruses discussed in this chapter are shown in Table 395–1.

Epidemiology

Recognition of the epidemiologic characteristics of poxvirus diseases is valuable in assessing the potential etiologic agent of a particular suspected poxvirus lesion. Knowledge of zoonotic reservoirs, geographic localizations, and capacity for epidemic transmission is critical for clinical assessment and control measures. All human poxvirus infections are zoonotic in nature, with the exception of molluscum contagiosum and

TABLE 395–1 TAXONOMY OF POXVIRUSES KNOWN TO INFECT HUMANS

Genus	Species
Orthopoxvirus	Variola virus, vaccinia virus, cowpox virus, monkeypox virus
Parapoxvirus	Orf virus, milker's node virus, bovine papular stomatitis virus, sealpox virus
Yatapoxvirus	Tanapox virus (Yaba-like disease virus), Yaba monkey tumor virus
Molluscipoxvirus	Molluscum contagiosum virus

variola, which are solely human pathogens. Parapoxvirus and Molluscipoxvirus infections are endemic worldwide; Orthopoxvirus and Yatapoxvirus infections are geographically restricted, probably by the distribution of competent reservoir hosts. With the exception of variola virus (the causative agent of smallpox, a disease declared eradicated in 1980), none of these diseases are required to be reported to public health systems; furthermore, diagnostics are not widely available, so it is difficult to estimate disease incidence and prevalence with any certainty. In addition to variola virus, monkeypox and camelpox viruses are considered to be select agents by the U.S. government; they must be reported and appropriately handled if discovered, and if samples are maintained in the United States.

Orthopoxvirus

The epidemiology of smallpox, caused by the orthopoxvirus variola, is understood through detailed studies conducted during the end of the eradication campaign. Interhuman transmission of variola virus generally occurred through the inhalation of large airborne respiratory droplets of infectious variola virus. Transmission usually required prolonged face-to-face or other close contact, although airborne transmission over longer distances had been reported. Transmission via fomites or contact with infectious material from the rash also occurred. Aggregate data, collected during the smallpox eradication campaign, suggest a secondary attack rate of 58.4% in unvaccinated close or household contacts and a secondary attack rate of 3.8% in previously vaccinated close or household contacts. Case-fatality rates for variola major varied with the type of disease manifested, but aggregate rates of 10 to 30% in various outbreaks have been recorded. Severity of disease correlated with rash burden and was also more severe in children and pregnant women. Variola alastrim minor, a variant of variola with a case-fatality rate of less than 1%, has similar human-to-human disease transmission characteristics.

Monkeypox has a more complex epidemiology; the virus is zoonotic and two genetically discrete virus clades have been described, with apparent distinct clinical and epidemiologic parameters. Human infections in western and central Africa were first identified in 1970. Investigations in the Congo Basin country Zaire, now the Democratic Republic of Congo, demonstrated that human-to-human transmission of monkeypox was less prevalent than that of smallpox. The secondary attack rate in unvaccinated contacts of monkeypox cases was calculated to be 9.3% versus 37 to 88% for smallpox. Previous smallpox vaccination (3 to 19 years previously) appeared to be 85% protective in preventing disease acquisition in contacts and also ameliorated disease severity. Overall, the majority of cases identified acquired disease from presumed animal exposure; only 28% of cases were ascribed to person-to-person transmission. A case-fatality rate of approximately 10% was observed in unvaccinated persons, and the majority of fatalities and severest disease manifestations were observed in children younger than 5 years. Serosurveys suggested that subclinical infection may have occurred in up to 28% of close contacts of monkeypox patients in some communities, which may have contributed to the rarity of sustained generations of human-to-human transmission in household and other close contact situations.

Among primary cases, recent close contact—via hunting, skinning, killing, cooking, or playing with carcasses—was identified with *Cercopithicus, Colobus,* and *Cercocebus* (primate); *Cricetomys* (terrestrial rodent); and *Funisciurus* and *Heliosciurus* (squirrel species). Ecologic studies (using samples of animals collected in areas of western and central Africa surrounding human cases) demonstrated orthopoxvirus and sometimes monkeypox-specific seroprevalence in various members of these species, but not in *Cricetomys* species. Virus was found in only one euthanized, moribund squirrel species, *Funisciurus anerythrus.* The prevailing hypothesis was that squirrel species were the probable reservoir of disease. Near the end of the 1980s, disease surveillance waned after modeling studies based on the epidemiologic observations of secondary attack rates from human-to-human exposure suggested that a limited number of transmission events were feasible even with the low population immunity provided by waning vaccinia immunization rates in the populations of central Africa. The virus had not therefore adapted to survive solely through human infection and would not have the same human-to-human transmission dynamics of smallpox. This work also led to the recommendation not to continue routine smallpox vaccination.

Reemergence of disease was noted in 1996 in the Democratic Republic of Congo; a salient observation from a series of investigations was that more cases were derived from secondary human-to-human contact (88%) than seen in the 1981 to 1986 investigations (28%). This fact was attributed, in part, to a larger population of humans fully susceptible to disease because of cessation of routine smallpox vaccination in 1980 after eradication of smallpox. Another observation was that disease epidemiology showed more cases in the older child/young adult population. Disease mortality was observed to be lower (1%) than seen in 1981 to 1986. This may have been due to a smaller demographic of very young children (0 to 4 years old) being infected. Whereas previous ecologic serosurveys of animal populations had implicated tree squirrels, these investigations were the first to show orthopoxvirus seroprevalence in terrestrial rodents *(Cricetomys emini)* and in one domestic pig *(Sus scrofa).*

Monkeypox virus was introduced to the United States in 2003 via a consignment of animals from the west African country of Ghana. The virus was identified as belonging to a distinct clade of monkeypox that included previous west African monkeypox isolates, as well as isolates derived from earlier outbreaks in primate colonies. Detailed comparison of the clinical and epidemiologic characteristics of the U.S. cases (imported from western Africa) with Democratic Republic of Congo cases from 1981 to 1986 demonstrated significant differences in human disease manifestation: pronounced rash and more severe illness were seen in the Congo Basin cases. After controlling for age and vaccination status, disease severity remained more extreme in the Congo Basin than in the United States. Monkeypox-related mortality and human-to-human transmission were seen only in the Congo Basin. These data are suggestive of at least two populations of monkeypox virus being maintained in Africa.

Cowpox virus is found in Europe and Asia and is maintained in rodents; in Britain, the reservoirs are bank voles and wood mice. Human infection is a zoonosis. The domestic cat is the most common source of human infection, which probably explains the occurrence of cases in children; 26% of 54 cases occurred in children younger than 12 years. Most feline and human cases occur between July and October, with only occasional cases between January and June. No case of bovine cowpox has been detected since 1976.

Cowpox virus has a wide host range, and an interesting finding has been the occurrence of cowpox in a variety of captive exotic species in European zoos. Susceptible animals have included cheetahs, lions, anteaters, rhinoceros, elephants, and okapi, and infection has occasionally been transmitted to animal handlers.

Vaccinia is the live virus used in preparations of the smallpox vaccines used to eradicate smallpox. The origin of vaccinia is unknown, and no natural host for the virus is known. A number of vaccinia "variants" have been described. Buffalopox has been described in India, and human infection results from contact with infected animals. It is not known whether buffaloes are a reservoir or whether other wildlife is involved, as with cowpox. Similarly, there have been increasing reports of vaccinia viruses infecting cattle handlers in Brazil. Cantagalo virus has been classified as a vaccinia variant, but other similar but nonidentical vaccinia-like viruses have also been reported in the region.

Parapoxvirus

Human infection is an occupational hazard of farm workers, abattoir workers, veterinary surgeons, and students. It is most common in the lambing and calving seasons and among sheep workers.

Factors responsible for ongoing transmission have been attributed both to the environmental stability of orf virus in scab material (although infectivity wanes over time) and to the manifestation of chronic infections in some animals. There is no known latent state for this or any other poxvirus. Transmission of virus to humans and to animals is via direct contact with lesions or by fomites.

Molluscipoxvirus

Molluscum contagiosum virus occurs worldwide, and increasing reports of the disease have paralleled the number of reported cases of acquired immunodeficiency syndrome (AIDS). Traditional modes of transmission are associated with mild skin trauma such as abrasions, direct contact with a lesion, and in some cases fomites (e.g., shared towels). However, there is increasing evidence that the disease is sexually transmitted and that genital lesions are more common than lesions elsewhere on the body. The disease is a significant concern for individuals whose children are in daycare or school situations, where potential transmission to other children may exist. Secondary spread of lesions may occur by autoinoculation (excoriation of primary lesions and spread to areas of normal skin), as well as by shaving. No known animal reservoir exists.

Yatapoxvirus

Tanapox virus is restricted to Africa, principally to Kenya and the Democratic Republic of Congo, and probably has a simian reservoir. Cases of direct primate-to-human transmission via a break in skin have been described in animal handlers, although such cases appear to be extremely rare. Several factors have led to speculation that an insect or arthropod intermediary may be involved in the transmission of tanapox virus to humans. Furthermore, the seasonal variation of human tanapox infections follows the variations in local arthropod populations. No human-to-human transmission has been reported. Yaba monkey tumor virus causes localized infections after contact with infected primate lesions. Little is known about the epidemiology of this virus.

Pathobiology

Much of what is described about the pathogenesis of smallpox, the prototype of systemic human poxvirus disease, comes from experimental studies of variola infection of nonhuman primates or the closely related orthopoxviruses monkeypox, ectromelia, and rabbitpox systemic infections of susceptible hosts. These studies, in addition to clinical diagnostic investigations of human smallpox patients or autopsy data from deceased smallpox patients, comprise our understanding of the pathogenesis of human smallpox.

The majority of infections were initiated by inhalation of respiratory droplets and implantation of virus on the oropharyngeal and respiratory mucosa. No primary localized site of infection was evident if the route of exposure was by inhalation. Disease could also be introduced through suspensions of virus obtained from scabs of patients that were introduced percutaneously and constituted the practice of variolation. In these cases (when skillfully administered), illness was usually less virulent, a localized primary infectious lesion was present, and the asymptomatic incubation period was truncated.

In the model of pathogenesis that has been developed, after entry, virus moves to local lymph nodes and then disseminates to the reticuloendothelial system to replicate further. At this time the individual is asymptomatic. In 10 to 14 days, secondary viremia occurs and heralds the prodrome of symptomatic illness. During this time virus seeds the oropharynx and epidermis. The absence of a keratinized structure in the mucosa of the oropharynx leads to ulceration and release of virus in saliva; virus replicates in the epidermis to cause the characteristic macular, papular, and vesicular eruptions of smallpox.

Recent studies of intravenous variola infection of cynomolgus monkeys provide a model of illness that resembles some aspects of types of clinical smallpox with higher case-fatality rates and thus may yield additional information about the pathophysiologic processes that lead to fatal outcomes. In this model, high doses of variola are administered, and a few days after infection, virus is recoverable in the oropharynx, centrifugally distributed vesicular lesions are evident, and death ensues 3 to 10 days after infection. High levels of type I interferons, interleukin-6, and interferon-γ; D-dimers and thrombocytopenia suggestive of disseminated intravascular coagulation; and nitric oxide are measurable in plasma. Apoptosis with loss of T cells in lymphoid organs was also observed. These findings are consistent with those seen in sepsis. Of note, tumor necrosis factor-α (TNF-α) levels were minimal in the infected animals. In evaluation of host transcriptional responses in this variola infection model with the use of RNA extracted from peripheral blood mononuclear cells isolated at times during infection, there is a notable decrease in the expression of genes regulated by nuclear factor NF-κB and TNF-α. This is in contrast to what had been seen in bacterial infection of human mononuclear cells; the function of the TNF receptor homologue of variola (see later) may in part be responsible for these findings.

In humans, it is the rash that has been extensively studied during the pathogenesis of smallpox. The viral lesion primarily develops in the epidermis, although early changes of capillary dilation, endothelial cell swelling, and perivascular cuffing with lymphocytes, macrophages, plasma cells, and eosinophils are seen in the papillary layer of the dermis before development of the rash lesion. Subsequently, within the epidermis, the cells of the malpighian layer swell and vacuolate to undergo ballooning degeneration. B-type inclusions could be seen in the cytoplasm. The cytoplasm continues to enlarge, loss of nuclear material is noted, and coalescence of vacuoles via cell rupture creates reticulating degeneration of the middle and upper layers of the stratum spinosum. In the next stages, the vesicle is formed. Cells of the lower stratum spinosum and basal layer exhibit nuclear condensation, and nuclei fragment. The cavity of the vesicle (later the pustule) thus develops adjacent to the dermis, which permits the "deep-seated" feel of the smallpox pustular lesions. The cavity retains some cellular remnants that create a multiloculated appearance, also adding to the firmness of the lesion. When polymorphonuclear cells move into the cavity, pustulation occurs. High titers of virus are found within the lesions. In mucosal surfaces, the absence of a horny layer allows the necrosis caused by proliferation of virus within the epithelium to create ulcers and leads to liberation of large quantities of virus into the oropharynx. Evaluation of other organs in human smallpox has been done only in select autopsy cases. Mild pathologic changes are seen in the lungs.

Clinical Manifestations

Orthopoxvirus

Smallpox

Naturally acquired variola virus infection causing a systemic illness is characterized by fever and a distinctive rash. The World Health Organization (WHO) differentiated eight types of smallpox; their classification was largely based on the clinical categorization of disease seen in India (Table 395–2). The classic description of smallpox is based on ordinary forms of illness that were the most common clinical manifestations. After

TABLE 395–2 WORLD HEALTH ORGANIZATION SMALLPOX TYPES

WHO Smallpox Type	Clinical Definition
Variola sine eruptione	Fever, no rash
Modified	Like ordinary, with an accelerated course
Ordinary discrete	Fever, rash, areas of normal skin between pustules, even on the face
Ordinary semiconfluent	Fever, rash, pustules confluent on the face, discrete elsewhere
Ordinary confluent	Fever, rash, pustules confluent on the face and forearms
Flat	Fever, erythema, and edema of the skin; vesicles soft, flat, and bullous
Hemorrhagic, early	Fever (persistent), hemorrhages and petechiae, purpuric rash at illness onset
Hemorrhagic, late	Fever (persistent), rash, hemorrhage into the base of vesicles late in illness

an asymptomatic incubation period of 10 to 14 days (range, 7 to 17), fever quickly rose to about 103° F (38 to 40° C), and sometimes dermal petechiae appeared. Associated constitutional symptoms included backache, headache, vomiting, and prostration. Within a day or two after incubation, a systemic rash appeared that was characteristically centrifugally distributed (i.e., lesions present in greater numbers on the oral mucosa, face, and extremities than on the trunk). The fever typically abated as the rash developed. Lesions commonly appeared on the palms and soles. The rash lesions were initially macular and then advanced to the papular stage, at which point they enlarged and progressed to a vesicle by day 4 to 5 and a pustule by day 7. When lesions became pustular, the fever typically returned. Lesions became encrusted and scabbed by day 14 and then sloughed off. Skin lesions in the vesicular and pustular stages were deep seated and in the same stage of development in any one area of the body (Fig. 395–1). The ordinary disease type was subgrouped into three categories based on the extent of rash on the face and the body: confluent, semiconfluent, and discrete. In *ordinary confluent disease,* no area of skin was visible between vesiculopustular rash lesions on the trunk or the face. In *ordinary semiconfluent* and *discrete disease,* patches of normal skin were visible between rash lesions on the trunk and face, respectively. Less severe manifestations (modified smallpox or variola sine eruptione) occurred in both unvaccinated and, more commonly, vaccinated individuals. The mortality rate correlated with the rash burden.

Four main clinical types of variola can be subgrouped according to the WHO classification schema: (1) *ordinary smallpox* (≈90% of cases) produced viremia, fever, prostration, and rash, and mortality rates were generally proportional to the extent of rash and ranged as described earlier; (2) *(vaccine) modified smallpox* (5% of cases) produced a mild prodrome with few skin lesions in previously vaccinated people and had a mortality rate well under 10%; (3) *flat smallpox* (≈5% of hospitalized cases) produced slowly developing lesions that were difficult to ascertain because at the vesicular stage they appeared flush with the (edematous) skin and was almost always fatal; and (4) *hemorrhagic smallpox* (<1% of cases) induced bleeding into the skin and the mucous membranes and was invariably fatal. A discrete type of the ordinary form, with a typical febrile prodrome and rash, resulted from alastrim variola minor infection. Individuals with this form of disease were not nearly as moribund or "toxemic" as individuals with variola major infection.

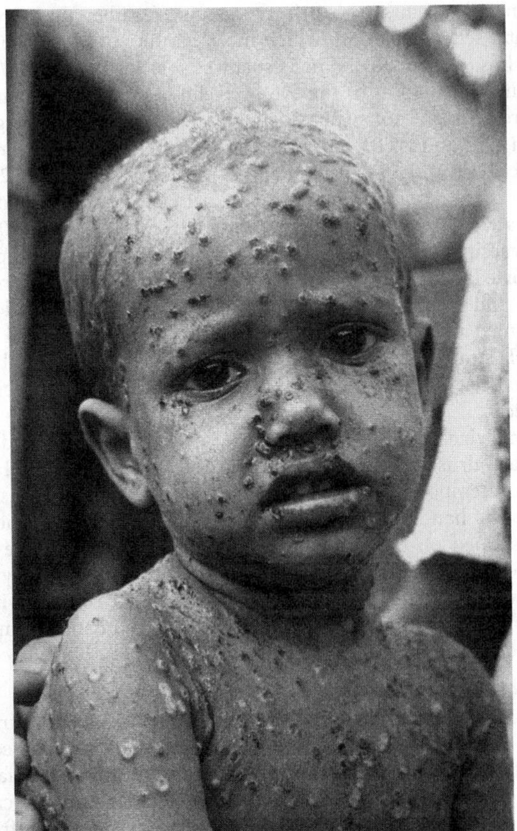

FIGURE 395–1 • Pustular lesions of smallpox and beginning of scarring on the face and upper part of the torso. (From the Public Health Information Library. Available at *http://phil.cdc.gov/phil/home.asp*—image 7055. Photo by Stan Foster.)

The most severe forms of smallpox, the flat and hemorrhagic varieties, did not appear to be dependent on the strain of variola circulating in an outbreak; hemorrhagic disease did not necessarily develop in contacts of hemorrhagic disease cases. Defects in the host immune response are believed to be responsible for these forms of disease. Previous vaccination was not necessarily protective against the hemorrhagic forms of disease but was suggested to be protective against flat forms of disease. Pregnant women were also prone to development of the hemorrhagic forms of disease; an increase in cortisone levels present during pregnancy was suggested to be one of the host factors responsible. Administration of cortisone to nonhuman primates challenged with variola led to severe disease manifestations with hemorrhagic features and worse outcomes. In studies of viremia during illness, as detected by growth of virus on chorioallantoic membrane, only in hemorrhagic forms of disease was viremia routinely detected during illness; evaluation of the host's sera demonstrated minimal antibody response to virus.

In flat smallpox, illness was heralded by the abrupt onset of fever to 38.3 to 38.9° C and appearance of the rash after 3 to 4 days. The oral enanthem was often confluent, and sloughing of rectal mucosal membranes was also reported. At the papulovesicular stage of disease, lesions appeared as small indentations (day 6) with hemorrhages in the bases and were surrounded by an erythematous ring. By day 7 or 8, the lesions appeared flat. Bullous lesions that would slough were reported. Fever persisted throughout the disease course, and respiratory complications were often observed by day 7 or 8 of illness. Thrombocytopenia, neutropenia, and lymphocytosis were reported. In hemorrhagic forms of smallpox, the timing of appearance of hemorrhagic manifestations led to the nomenclature of early and late forms. In addition, pathology studies support different pathogenic manifestations. These manifestations of smallpox were more prevalent in adults than in children. In early hemorrhagic disease, illness began with fever and typical prodromal symptoms; the fever never abated. Early after fever onset, petechiae and purpuric rashes became apparent; subconjunctival hemorrhages, hematuria, and vaginal bleeding were also seen. Patients usually died by day 6 of illness, well before any classic vesiculopustular rash was evident. In late hemorrhagic disease, after the onset of fever, typical maculopapular lesions developed, but the fever did not abate. The lesion evolved slowly, and areas of hemorrhage were evident at the base of the lesions. In some cases the lesions remained flat, whereas in others the lesions vesiculated. Bleeding occurred in the mucous membranes, thrombocytopenia was profound, and death occurred between days 8 and 10 of illness.

Monkeypox

In humans, clinical disease is believed to result from either respiratory, percutaneous, or permucosal exposure. Classic descriptions from the active surveillance program in Zaire (now the Democratic Republic of Congo) have historically provided most of our understanding of human monkeypox. After an incubation period of 7 to 17 days (mean, 12 days), a prodrome of fever, headache, backache, and fatigue begins. The cutaneous eruption evolves similar to that of smallpox. Lesions evolve in the same stage in any one part of the body from macules, papules, vesicles, to pustules, and then they crust and scar (Fig. 395–2). This is apparently more common in unvaccinated individuals; in previously vaccinated individuals, a pleomorphic manifestation of rash lesions was observed. After resolution of the rash, hypopigmentation is followed by hyperpigmentation of the scarred lesions. Pronounced lymphadenopathy clinically distinguishes monkeypox from smallpox; lymphadenopathy in the facial area (cervical, postauricular, submandibular, and inguinal) can be quite pronounced.

Vaccinia

Multiple-puncture vaccinia virus infection via a bifurcated needle is the current smallpox vaccination regimen used for laboratory personnel working with orthopoxviruses, public health care personnel, and military in the United States. Most commonly, the infection progresses through a standard course of events from vesicle to pustule. However, of all vaccines used today, the smallpox vaccine, which is composed of live, replicative vaccinia virus, has one of the highest rates of adverse events. Major complications include progressive vaccinia, eczema vaccinatum, generalized vaccinia, postvaccinial encephalitis, accidental infection, and carditis.

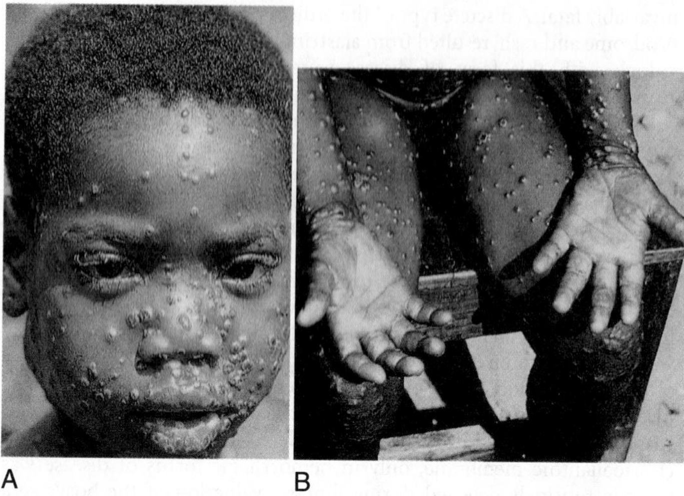

FIGURE 395–2 • Rash of monkeypox of the (A) head and (B) extremities in a 7-year-old girl in central Zaire. (From Peters W, Pasvol G: Tropical Medicine and Parasitology, 5th ed. New York, Mosby, 2002, p 238.)

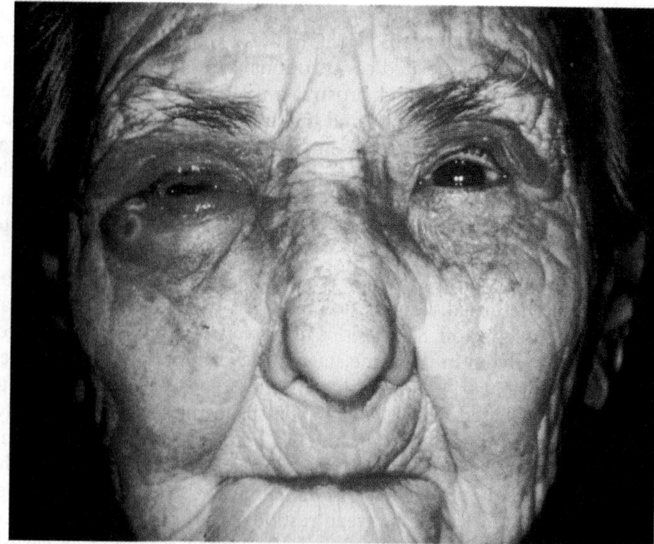

FIGURE 395–3 • Vaccinia autoinoculation of an eye. (From the Public Health Information Library. Available at *http://phil.cdc.gov/phil/home.asp*—image 3322.)

Progressive vaccinia, previously called vaccinia necrosum or vaccinia gangrenosum, is a rare and often fatal vaccine complication in persons with severe deficiencies in cellular immunity. In 1 year (1968) in the United States there were 5 cases among 6 million primary vaccinees and 6 cases among 8.6 million revaccinated persons; 4 of these 11 patients died. Progressive vaccinia is characterized by progressive, frequently painless growth and spread of the vaccine virus beyond the inoculation site, often leading to necrosis and sometimes metastases to other body sites. The possibility of progressive vaccinia should be considered if the vaccination site lesion continues to progress and expand without apparent healing more than 15 days after vaccination. Initially, limited or no inflammation is present at the inoculation site, and histopathologic examination shows an absence of inflammatory cells.

Eczema vaccinatum can occur in people with a history of atopic dermatitis (eczema), irrespective of disease severity or activity. This complication is the clinical consequence of local spread or dissemination from the primary vaccination site in such persons or the result of the skin of an individual with atopic dermatitis contacting the unscabbed vaccination site of another person. A localized or generalized papular, vesicular, or pustular rash anywhere on the body or localized to previous eczematous lesions is the clinical manifestation of eczema vaccinatum. Systemic illness with fever, malaise, and lymphadenopathy may occur. In the national U.S. surveillance of smallpox vaccination that was performed in 1968, there were 66 cases (no deaths) of eczema vaccinatum among 14.5 million vaccinees (4.6 cases/million) and 60 cases (1 death) among their several million contacts. In one study, early administration of vaccinia immune globulin (VIG) reduced mortality from 30 to 40% to 7%.

Generalized vaccinia is a nonspecific term that is used to describe a vesicular rash that develops after vaccination. Excluding dissemination associated with eczema vaccinatum and progressive vaccinia, it has been extremely rare to document virus in these lesions. True generalized vaccinia is believed to represent the end product of viremic spread of virus, and no predisposing factors have been identified. Generalized vaccinia is estimated to occur in about 242 of every million primary vaccinations.

Postvaccination encephalomyelitis (PVEM) is a rare, but serious complication that usually occurs only in primary vaccinees. The frequency of its occurrence differed widely from country to country and with the strain of vaccinia virus used in the vaccine. The incidence of PVEM was lower with the NYCBOH vaccinia virus strain (the U.S. vaccine strain) than with the strain used in other countries. No predisposing factors for PVEM are known, although host factors are believed to be important; the pathophysiology of PVEM is not well understood. Patients have variably displayed clinical and diagnostic features suggestive of a postimmunization demyelinating encephalomyelitis or direct viral invasion of the nervous system. This postvaccination reaction typically occurs 11 to 15 days after vaccination. Symptoms of PVEM include fever, headache, vomiting, confusion, delirium, disorientation, restlessness, drowsiness or lethargy, seizures, and coma. Cerebrospinal fluid can demonstrate elevated pressure but generally has a normal cell count and chemistry profile. A rare postvaccination encephalopathy (PVE) can also develop in infants younger than 2 years, similar to PVEM. The acute onset of PVE occurs earlier in the postvaccination period (6 to 10 days after vaccination), has the same symptoms as PVEM, and may also include hemiplegia and aphasia. The diagnosis of PVE or PVEM is one of exclusion in that no specific tests are available to confirm the diagnosis of this complication and many other infectious and toxic causes can result in similar clinical symptoms. Because this complication is not known to be the result of viral proliferation, the role of modern antiviral medications is unclear.

Accidental infection occurs when virus from the vaccination site is transferred to another site or to another person via intimate skin contact. This generally occurs with primary vaccinees rather than revaccinees. Accidental self-inoculation, which most commonly occurs on the face, mouth, lips, or genitalia, is not usually serious and requires no specific treatment. Inoculation of the eye or eyelid is more serious and can be sight threatening if not evaluated and treated appropriately (Fig. 395–3). Between 1963 and 1968, ocular vaccinia was observed in 348 persons; 259 were vaccinees and 66 were contacts of vaccinees. Of these, 22 had evidence of corneal involvement and 11 experienced permanent defects.

Cardiac adverse events are rare; none were reported before 2003 in any person vaccinated with the NYCBOH strain. Myocarditis and pericarditis, reported after vaccination with a different vaccine strain used in Europe and Australia and in the U.S. military population, were documented in 18 of 230,734 primary vaccinees immunized with the NYCBOH strain in 2002 and 2003. Arrhythmias and myocardial ischemia have also been described recently, but the association with vaccination is not as clear.

Vaccinia viruses in the Indian subcontinent (buffalopox) and in Brazil (Cantagalo virus and the related strains Aracatuba virus, Belo Horizante virus, Passatempo virus, and others) have been reported to cause human infection in handlers of buffaloes or cattle. Up to 10 lesions have been described on the hands or arms of human handlers; fever, lymphadenopathy, backache, and fatigue are also associated symptoms. Transmission is believed to occur by unprotected contact with active lesions present on animal teats and udders. Interhuman transmission of buffalopox to family members has been reported to occur via contact.

Cowpox

Cowpox also causes localized lesions in humans. Most information is available from a detailed analysis of 54 human cases investigated during 1969 to 1993. Lesions are generally restricted to the hands and face; most patients (72%) have only one lesion. Multiple lesions may be caused by multiple primary inoculations, by autoinoculation, and very infrequently by lymphatic or viremic spread. Occasionally, a very severe infection and death may occur, typically in immunosuppressed individuals.

The cowpox lesion passes through macular, papular, vesicular, and pustular stages before forming a hard black crust. The lesion is generally very painful, and erythema and edema are common at the late vesicular and pustular stages. Patients usually have lymphadenitis, fever, and general malaise, often referred to as "flulike" symptoms. These features are generally severe in children, and absence from school or work is common; 16 of 54 patients (30%) were hospitalized. Most patients take 6 to 8 weeks to recover, but in some cases up to 12 weeks may be required. Scarring is usually permanent.

Parapoxvirus

Lesions, such as from the orf virus, start as erythematous papules and progress to a "target' stage. This stage, seen 1 to 2 weeks after infection, has a red center surrounded by a white halo and an outer inflamed halo. Lesions progress to a nodular and then a papillomatous stage, which often has a "weeping" surface. In some patients, lesions may enlarge and persist for some weeks before resolving and may cause some concern. Resolution is via a crusting stage, which may last some weeks. Occasionally, very large granulomatous lesions occur and may require surgical removal.

Most patients have only one lesion, but multiple primary lesions may develop. Systemic reaction is relatively uncommon and the lesion is often not particularly painful. Lymphadenopathy is present in some patients, and lymphangitis is observed but is relatively uncommon. Erythema multiforme was reported in a third of patients reported in one case series.

Molluscum Contagiosum Virus

Molluscum infection occurs as a result of *molluscum contagiosum virus* coming in contact with nonintact skin. The characteristic lesion begins as a small papule and, when mature, is a discrete, 2- to 5-mm-diameter, smooth, dome-shaped, pearly or flesh-colored nodule that is often umbilicated. A cheesy, off-white or yellowish material is easily expressed from lesions. There are usually 1 to 20 lesions, but hundreds may occasionally be present. Because of multiple simultaneous infections or mechanical spread, the lesions may become confluent along the line of a scratch, and satellite lesions are sometimes seen.

In children, molluscum lesions occur mainly on the trunk and proximal ends of the extremities, and in adults, they tend to occur on the trunk, pubic area, and thighs; however, in all cases, infection can be transmitted to other parts by autoinoculation. In males infected with human immunodeficiency virus (HIV), molluscum lesions appear to occur along the beard line, and in persons with infections involving the face, there have been reports of ocular involvement. Individual lesions last for about 2 months, but the disease usually lasts 6 to 9 months. More severe and prolonged infection tends to occur in individuals with impaired cell-mediated immunity, including persons with HIV infection.

Yatapoxvirus

Tanapox infection begins with a short febrile (38 to 39° C) illness lasting 2 to 4 days that is sometimes accompanied by headache, backache, or prostration. The eruption of a lesion is frequently heralded by pruritus at the site of the outbreak. The lesion appears as a hyperpigmented macule, often with central elevation, and the macule then evolves to a papule with palpable induration. Fever and systemic symptoms wane as the lesion erupts. The papule then becomes more "pocklike" but contains no fluid; umbilication or the formation of a pseudocrust has been reported at this stage. Typically, the papule evolves into a firm, deep-seated, elevated nodule. At the end of the first week, the lesion is surrounded by erythema and indurated skin. Regional lymphangitis is common at this stage. During the next stage, lesions either ulcerate or become larger nodules (up to 2 cm in diameter). In an African series, the maximum lesion size was usually reached within 2 weeks, and then the local inflammatory response started to wane and the lesion began to granulate. Resolution of lesions occurred within 6 weeks.

Most cases (78% in one series) involve a solitary nodule; however, as many as 10 lesions have been described on one individual. Most lesions (72%) occur on the lower extremities, and the fewest occur on the face and areas normally covered by clothing. Infection appears to confer lifelong immunity.

Diagnosis

Before its eradication, smallpox as a clinical entity was relatively easy to recognize, but other exanthematous illnesses were mistaken for this disease. For example, the rash of severe chickenpox, caused by varicella-zoster virus, was often misdiagnosed as that of smallpox. However, chickenpox produces a centripetally distributed rash and rarely appears on the palms and soles. In addition, in the case of chickenpox, prodromal fever and systemic manifestations are mild, the lesions are superficial in nature, and lesions in different developmental stages may be present in the same area of the body. Other diseases and conditions that could be confused with vesicular-stage smallpox include monkeypox, generalized vaccinia, disseminated herpes zoster, disseminated herpes simplex virus infection, drug reactions (eruptions), erythema multiforme, enteroviral infections, scabies, insect bites, impetigo, and molluscum contagiosum. Diseases confused with hemorrhagic smallpox included acute leukemia, meningococcemia, and idiopathic thrombocytopenic purpura. The Centers for Disease Control and Prevention, in collaboration with numerous professional organizations, has developed a worksheet for evaluating patients for smallpox (available at *http://www.bt.cdc.gov/agent/smallpox/diagnosis/evalposter.asp*) and an algorithm for assessing the vesiculopustular stage of rash (available at *http://www.bt.cdc.gov/agent/smallpox/diagnosis/rashtestingprotocol.asp*).

Orthopoxvirus

Negative-stain electron microscopic evaluation of virion particles derived from clinical rash specimens or viral tissue culture has been a mainstay of orthopoxvirus diagnosis. The technique's primary utility is rapid discrimination of the large brick-shaped particles typical of orthopoxviruses from the viral forms characteristic of herpesviruses. Although a skilled negative-stain electron microscopist can differentiate orthopoxviruses from parapoxviruses (see later), it is not be feasible to differentiate the structure of orthopoxviruses from that of other genera of the poxvirus family of viruses.

Serologic tests are largely genus specific, detect IgG, and mostly cannot differentiate between species. Recent reports, however, have identified possible monkeypox-specific serologic tests, as well as orthopoxvirus IgM diagnostics. The latter appear helpful in differentiating recent orthopoxvirus infection from remote vaccination.

Nucleic acid–based tests are widely used to diagnose orthopoxvirus infections. A number of techniques using standard methods of band visualization on agarose gels, as well as real-time polymerase chain reaction (PCR) assays, have been reported. Viral tissue culture is used to demonstrate the presence of live, infectious material. The virus grows well in a number of tissue culture systems used in clinical microbiology laboratories; cytopathic effect is easily visualized in monkey kidney–derived cell lines.

If a diagnosis of smallpox is being contemplated, at this time variola virus should be grown only in laboratories with biosafety level 4 (BSL-4) containment and sanctioned by the WHO to use variola virus. Within the United States, current recommendations are for vaccinia (smallpox) vaccinated personnel to work with infectious orthopoxviruses in BSL-2 containment. Most laboratories that use monkeypox virus also use BSL-3 work practices.

Parapoxvirus

The differential diagnosis of parapoxvirus lesions can include ecthyma gangrenosum (a *Pseudomonas aeruginosa* infection in immunocompromised hosts), vaccinia or cowpox infection, cutaneous anthrax, erysipeloid, tularemia, or tumor. Clinical diagnosis of uncomplicated cases in patients with a known animal contact has been confused with anthrax. Farm workers recognize the infection and tend not to seek medical attention for routine cases. Consequently, a disproportionately large number of reported cases have no known contact with infected animals. Of approximately 500 cases surveyed during 1978 to 1995, some 45% had no such contact. Clinical diagnosis of such cases, particularly if severe or prolonged, may cause difficulty. In particular, large weeping granulomatous or papillomatous lesions may be misdiagnosed as malignancies, in one case resulting in unnecessary amputation.

With negative-stain electron microscopy, virions with the characteristic morphology of parapoxviruses are usually seen easily in lesion extracts, thereby providing a rapid, certain diagnosis of the genus. The virus can be grown in cell culture, but this is not routinely attempted in laboratories that do not maintain primary ovine or bovine cultures.

A number of methods derived from limited or complete genomic analysis have been used for nucleic acid detection (PCR) and laboratory diagnosis of infection. Species-specific and species-generic protein-based diagnostics have also been developed for parapoxviruses.

Molluscum Contagiosum Virus

The clinical appearance of molluscum lesions in normal cases is generally sufficiently characteristic to permit a clinical diagnosis. Brick-shaped virions can usually be seen in large numbers if the cheesy material expressed from the lesion is examined by negative-stain transmission electron microscopy. The virus has not been cultured in standard tissue culture systems. The characteristic histopathology of these lesions is diagnostic, but PCR methods have also been described for use in identifying molluscum contagiosum.

Yatapoxvirus

The limited geographic distribution of tanapox virus and the patient's travel history should be considered in the diagnosis of tanapox infection. Unique clinical features that allow differentiation of tanapox from other orthopoxvirus infections are the nodular nature of the rash lesion, the paucity of lesions, the benign disease course, and the protracted resolution of the rash. The solid nodular/ulcerated lesions are larger and develop more slowly than those of monkeypox, but they are smaller and develop more rapidly than those of tropical ulcers.

Tanapox virus can be detected by electron microscopy (the virions generally appear enveloped), but this finding would not exclude the possibility of infection with other morphologically similar brick-shaped poxviruses; nucleic acid testing on lesion extracts could be used for that purpose. Tanapox virus grows in a number of cell lines (e.g., owl monkey kidney, Vero, MRC-5, BSC-1), but not on chorioallantoic membrane.

Treatment and Prevention

Orthopoxvirus

Vaccination with smallpox vaccine has been the mainstay for prevention of orthopoxvirus infection and was the primary tool used in the eradication of smallpox. Currently, stockpiles of vaccine have been generated for use in the event that smallpox should reoccur. In the United States, however, recommendations for smallpox vaccine use are currently limited to laboratory personnel working with live, infectious orthopoxvirus, certain public health personnel, and certain members of the military.

An active area of research involves the development and evaluation of therapeutics for orthopoxvirus infections. Currently, no antiviral drugs have been licensed for the treatment of orthopoxvirus or other poxvirus illnesses. VIG is best used for the treatment of certain complications of vaccinia (smallpox) vaccine administration, but it may have utility in the treatment of certain other orthopoxvirus infections. No clear benefit has been shown for the use of this product alone in treating smallpox.

The most studied antiviral compounds are inhibitors of DNA polymerase. Some nucleoside analogue compounds with activity against herpesviruses do not have activity against poxviruses, most importantly, acyclovir and its derivatives. Other compounds with antiherpesvirus activity do show in vitro and in vivo activity against poxviruses, specifically, 5-iodo-2′-deoxyuridine, adenine arabinoside, and trifluorothymidine. Because of their systemic toxicity, these compounds have been used topically for the treatment of orthopoxvirus (and herpes) ocular infections. Many phosphonate nucleoside analogues, such as cidofovir, have antiorthopoxvirus activity. In vitro, cidofovir has been shown to be active against the orthopoxviruses cowpox, vaccinia, monkeypox, and variola. In in vivo studies, cidofovir has successfully protected challenged animals when given prophylactically or early in the evolution of disease, often before the onset of overt illness symptomatology. Cidofovir has known renal toxicity and is administered with hydration and probenecid. It has a long intracellular half-life but is not orally bioavailable; the alkoxyalkylester analogue of cidofovir, 1-*O*-hexadecyloxypropyl cidofovir (HDP-CDV), is orally bioavailable, and a preliminary report of the protective effect of HDP-CDV in aerosolized cowpox–challenged mice has appeared. Recent studies have shown promise for a compound with a viral target involved in virion maturation. The drug ST-246 has been shown to be effective in the treatment of animal models of systemic orthopoxvirus infection.

Other antivirals tested against orthopoxviruses have predicted cellular targets. Ribavirin, an inosine monophosphate dehydrogenase inhibitor, has in vitro activity against a number of orthopoxviruses and has shown antiorthopoxvirus activity in animal models of vaccinia-induced keratitis and mouse tail pock lesions. There are case reports of the use of ribavirin and VIG in the treatment of progressive vaccinia. Initial therapy with ribavirin alone was ineffective in stemming new lesions; however, with the addition of VIG, the development of new lesions was halted.

Parapoxvirus

Most workers at risk get infected at some stage, and reinfection is not uncommon. Individuals should take care not to spread infection by autoinoculation or to contacts, including animals. The vaccine used to control orf in sheep is fully virulent and has caused human infection. Work is under way to create live, attenuated viruses that can be used as vaccines. Treatment options are limited; anecdotal reports have described the use of topical cidofovir, and other options may be topical formulations of interferon-modulating compounds such as imiquimod.

Molluscum Contagiosum Virus

Molluscum contagiosum infection is benign and recovery is usually spontaneous, but treatment may be sought for cosmetic reasons, particularly for facial or multiple lesions. Various treatments have been tried, including cryotherapy, mechanical curettage, and chemical treatments such as podophyllin/podofilox, cantharidin, iodine, and tretinoin. Irritation has been a side effect of many of the chemical treatments. Topical application of a 3% cidofovir antiviral cream or suspension has been reported to be beneficial, as has the use of potentially immune-modulating cimetidine or topical imiquimod therapy. The absence of well-controlled trials makes it difficult to assess the efficacy of various therapeutic regimens. Covering of lesions and the use of proper hand hygiene after contact with lesions should prevent transmission in most situations. For individuals with AIDS and molluscum, the use of highly active antiretroviral therapy, with improvement in $CD4^+$ cell counts, appears to be efficacious.

Prognosis

Monkeypox and smallpox both cause human illness, with mortality reported to range from 10% to 40%; variola minor variants, however, had mortality rates of less than 1%. Yatapoxvirus infections are self-limited, and the illness resolves in the course of a few weeks. Parapoxvirus infections are manifested chiefly by localized symptoms, and in nonimmunocompromised hosts the lesions resolve over the course of a month. Molluscum contagiosum infection is benign and recovery is usually spontaneous, but treatment may be sought for cosmetic reasons, particularly for facial or multiple lesions; the duration of infection can be quite prolonged (months).

SUGGESTED READINGS

Bernard SM, Anderson SA: Qualitative assessment of risk for monkeypox associated with domestic trade in certain animal species, United States. Emerg Infect Dis 2006;12:1827–1833. *A qualitative assessment of the risk for monkeypox.*

Cono J, Casey CG, Bell DM; Centers for Disease Control and Prevention: Smallpox vaccination and adverse reactions. Guidance for clinicians. MMWR Recomm Rep 2003;52(RR-4):1–28. *A thorough review of vaccinia (smallpox) vaccine complications and their treatment.*

Dohil MA, Lin P, Lee J, et al: The epidemiology of molluscum contagiosum in children. J Am Acad Dermatol 2006;54:47–54. *A clinical overview.*

Likos AM, Sammons SA, Olson VA, et al: A tale of two clades: Monkeypox viruses. J Gen Virol 2005;86:2661–2672. *A general review.*

Malone JD: Pre-event smallpox vaccination for healthcare workers revisited—the need for a carefully screened multidisciplinary cadre. Int J Infect Dis 2007;11:93–97. *A review of pre-event smallpox vaccination for health care workers.*

Moore ZS, Seward JF, Lane JM: Smallpox. Lancet 2006;367:425–435. *A comprehensive review.*

Parrino J, Graham BS: Smallpox vaccines: Past, present, and future. J Allergy Clin Immunol 2006;118:1320–1326. *A review of the smallpox vaccine.*

Scaramozzino N, Ferrier-Rembert A, Favier AL, et al: Real-time PCR to identify variola virus or other human pathogenic orthopox viruses. Clin Chem 2007;53:606–613. *Real-time PCR provides a rapid method for the early detection and differentiation of smallpox and other human pathogenic orthopoxvirus infections.*

Sivapalasingam S, Kennedy JS, Borkowsky W, et al: Immunological memory after exposure to variola virus, monkeypox virus, and vaccinia virus. J Infect Dis 2007;195:1151–1159. *A review of immunologic memory after exposure to variola virus, monkeypox virus, and vaccinia virus.*

396 PAPILLOMAVIRUS

John M. Douglas, Jr.

Definition

Human papillomaviruses (HPVs) are a group of small DNA viruses that cause a variety of benign and malignant lesions of the skin and mucous membranes. The most commonly recognized HPV-associated diseases include warts (Chapter 466) at anogenital sites (condyloma acuminatum), other skin surfaces (common warts or verruca vulgaris), and the plantar surface of the foot (verruca plantaris).

In addition, HPV infection causes cervical squamous intraepithelial lesions, also known as cervical intraepithelial neoplasia (CIN), and is considered to be the etiologic agent of cancer of the cervix (Chapter 209) and possibly other anatomic sites as well.

The Pathogen

Papillomaviruses are nonenveloped, measure 55 nm in diameter, and have a double-stranded circular DNA genome of approximately 7900 base pairs enclosed by an icosahedral capsid. Their genomes comprise three functional regions: early genes (E), which are expressed soon after infection and control replication, transcription, and cellular proliferation; late genes (L), which are expressed in later stages of infection and encode the structural capsid proteins; and a noncoding upstream regulatory region. Papillomaviruses complete their life cycle only in terminally differentiated epithelial cells and thus are difficult to grow in cell culture. Papillomavirus taxonomy is based on a genotyping system involving the use of DNA sequence relatedness of the gene encoding L1, the major capsid protein, with different types defined as having less than 90% homology. Currently, more than 100 types of HPV have been well characterized, approximately 40 of which infect genital skin and mucosa. Of the genital types, approximately 15 are considered to be "high risk" because they are associated with high-grade squamous intraepithelial lesions and cervical and other genital tract cancers, whereas others are considered "low risk" because they are largely associated with genital warts and low-grade squamous intraepithelial lesions (Table 396–1).

Epidemiology

HPV infections are primarily transmitted by direct contact of skin or mucous membranes with an infected lesion. Genital HPV infection is typically contracted through sexual intercourse, although nonpenetrative genital contact, oral-genital contact, and manual-genital contact are also possible routes of transmission. In addition, genital HPV infection can be transmitted to the mouth and upper respiratory tract perinatally from infected mothers to newborns. For nongenital HPV infection, personal skin-to-skin contact also plays a primary role, although for plantar warts, fomite transmission from moist surfaces is likely to be an important source of infection. Both genital and nongenital infection can be transmitted to new sites by autoinoculation.

Overall, in the United States it is estimated that more than 6 million new infections of genital HPV occur annually in sexually active adolescents and adults and that the lifetime risk for infection is 50 to 80%, thus making genital HPV one of the most common sexually transmitted infections. The majority of infections are caused by high-risk types, with HPV 16 having the highest incidence. Acquisition of infection begins shortly after sexual debut, and there is an estimated 40% incidence of at least one type within 2 years of initiation of sex. Risk factors for infection include variables related to probable exposure (e.g., younger age, increased

TABLE 396–1 CLINICAL MANIFESTATIONS OF HUMAN PAPILLOMAVIRUS INFECTION AND ASSOCIATED TYPES

Clinical Manifestation	Associated HPV Types
Skin lesions	
Plantar warts	1, 2, 4
Common warts	1, 2, 4, 26, 27, 29, 41, 57, 65, 77
Flat warts	3, 10, 27, 28, 38, 41, 49, 75, 76
Butchers' warts	7
Epidermodysplasia verruciformis warts	2, 3, 5, 8–10, 12, 14, 15, 17, 19, 20–25, 36, 37, 46, 47, 50
Epidermodysplasia verruciformis–associated squamous cell cancers	5, 8, 14, 17, 20, 47
Nongenital mucosal lesions	
Mouth (focal epithelial hyperplasia)	13, 32
Recurrent respiratory papillomatosis	6, 11
Squamous cell cancers (oropharyngeal)	16, 18
Genital mucosal lesions	
Genital warts	6, 11, 30, 42–45, 51, 54, 55, 70
Squamous intraepithelial lesions	Low-risk types (both LSIL and HSIL): 6, 11, 40, 42–44, 54, 61, 70, 72, 81 High-risk types (HSIL): 16, 18, 31, 33, 35, 39, 45, 51, 52, 56, 58, 59, 68, 73, 82
Cancers (cervical, penile, anal, vulvar, vaginal)	16, 18, 31, 33, 35, 39, 45, 51, 52, 56, 58, 59, 68, 73, 82

HSIL = high-grade squamous intraepithelial lesion; LSIL = low-grade squamous intraepithelial lesion.
Modified from Douglas JM, Moreland A: Genital human papillomavirus infections. *In* Morse SA, Ballard RC, Holmes KK, et al (eds): Atlas of Sexually Transmitted Diseases and AIDS, 3rd ed. Edinburgh, Mosby; 2003, pp 261–278.

number of partners), susceptibility (e.g., lack of circumcision for men), and absence of prevention factors (e.g., lack of consistent condom use or immunization). Most infections are asymptomatic and clear without treatment, with only 10% estimated to persist longer than 2 years. Only such "persistent" HPV infections are associated with the development of high-grade squamous intraepithelial lesions and cancer. The prevalence of genital HPV infection is estimated to range from 15 to 25% in U.S. women. The prevalence of anogenital warts is estimated to be approximately 1% in the sexually active adult population. Cervical cancer has declined in developed countries since the initiation of cytologic screening programs, although an estimated 9700 cases and 3700 deaths still occur in the United States annually. However, the disease is a major problem in the developing world, where screening is limited, and it is the second most common cancer in women worldwide, with an estimated 470,000 cases annually.

Nongenital HPV infection is most typically recognized by common and plantar warts, especially in children and adolescents, where prevalence rates of 3 to 20% have been reported. All types and manifestations of HPV infection are more common in persons with impaired cell-mediated immunity, such as those infected with human immunodeficiency virus (HIV) or receiving immunosuppressive therapy.

Pathobiology

HPV infections cause disease by producing aberrant cell growth. In the case of cutaneous and low-risk genital types, lesions such as warts result from HPV-induced benign proliferation of epidermal layers. For high-risk genital types, precancerous and cancerous lesions result from replacement of the epithelium by undifferentiated cells as a result of HPV-induced interference with normal cellular growth.

Infection begins in the lowest and least well differentiated layer of the epithelium, the basal cells, where exposure is thought to be facilitated by microtrauma. Transcription and protein expression are highly coordinated with the level of cellular differentiation. In the basal layer, the viral genome becomes established in the nucleus as an episome that replicates in tandem with cellular replication, thus maintaining a stable copy number of viral genomes. As basal cells migrate up and differentiate in the superficial layers of the epithelium, full vegetative viral DNA replication and expression of structural proteins occur, with assembly of infectious virions in the most superficial layer of the epithelium, where they are released with the sloughing of dead cells during normal cellular turnover.

Based on a variety of epidemiologic and laboratory studies, persistent infection with HPV is firmly established as the cause of squamous cell carcinoma and adenocarcinoma of the cervix (Chapter 209) and is highly associated with other anogenital squamous cell cancers (Chapter 148). There are also associations with squamous cell cancer of the oropharynx (Chapter 200) and skin (Chapter 214). HPV DNA can be detected in more than 99% of cases of cervical cancer, with 70% of cancers being associated with the two most common high-risk types, HPV 16 and 18. The pathogenesis of HPV-induced cancer involves viral integration into the host genome with resulting disruption of the E2 transcription regulatory gene and increased expression of E6 and E7 proteins. These proteins have oncogenic activity and affect cell growth by binding with tumor suppressor proteins, E6 with p53 and E7 with the retinoblastoma tumor suppressor protein, thereby disrupting apoptosis and cell cycle regulation. Although persistent infection with high-risk types is "necessary" for the development of cervical cancer, it is not "sufficient" because cancer does not develop in the vast majority of infected women. There is evidence to support a variety of possible cofactors, including cigarette smoking, prolonged hormonal contraceptive use, multiparity, micronutrient deficiency, and other infections, including *Chlamydia trachomatis* and herpes simplex virus type 2. In addition, specific HLA alleles have been associated with both increased (e.g., DQB1*03, DRB1*1501, and DQB1*0602) and decreased (DRB1*13, DQB1*0603) risk for disease, whereas polymorphisms of the p53 gene and the tumor necrosis factor-α promoter region have been associated with increased susceptibility to disease.

The immune response after initial infection is less robust than for most viral infections, with measurable antibody developing in only an estimated 60% of infected individuals, often as long as 6 to 12 months after infection. The limited immune response is probably due to the superficial location of infection in the epithelium and the fact that the capsid proteins are not expressed except in the most well differentiated cells, which are the least accessible to antigen-presenting cells of the immune system. The dynamics of the immune response are quite different after the administration of L1-containing vaccines, with almost 100% seroconversion within several months and antibody levels approximately 10-fold higher than those after natural infection. The high efficacy of these vaccines, which are believed to produce primarily humoral immunity, support the importance of the antibody response in protection from infection. In contrast, once infection occurs, cellular immunity appears to be critical for clearance of infection, based on the experience of persons with impaired cell-mediated immunity, in whom persistent HPV infection and high-grade squamous intraepithelial lesions are common.

The histopathologic changes of warts include epithelial papillomatosis and acanthosis, with hyperkeratosis, parakeratosis, and hyperplasia of the parabasal cells. A characteristic feature is the presence in the upper epidermis of koilocytes, or large atypical keratinocytes with irregular, hyperchromatic nuclei surrounded by a perinuclear halo. Squamous intraepithelial lesions are characterized by hyperkeratosis, parakeratosis, and epidermal hyperplasia, with increased mitotic figures in the upper half of the epidermis; koilocytosis is common and often detected cytologically, but less prominent than in warts. Several classification systems have been used to classify these lesions and their probable risk for progression based on the proportion of the epithelium replaced by undifferentiated cells. The CIN system grades lesions as CIN 1 (with undifferentiated cells occupying the lower third), CIN 2 (with undifferentiated cells in the lower third to two thirds), and CIN 3/carcinoma-in-situ (CIS) (with undifferentiated cells across the full thickness of the epithelium). The newest classification, the Bethesda system, was originally developed for use with cytology but has increasingly been used for histologic classification; it includes only two categories, low-risk squamous intraepithelial lesions (CIN 1) and high-risk squamous intraepithelial lesions (CIN2 and CIN 3/CIS).

Clinical Manifestations

The clinical manifestations of HPV infection vary by anatomic site and viral type (see Table 396–1). Common warts are exophytic, hyperkeratotic papules that typically occur on the hands but can appear on any skin surface, including the genital skin. Plantar warts are caused by similar types of HPV; they are hyperkeratotic and endophytic and often very painful. In contrast, flat warts (verruca plana) are small flat-topped papules that occur more commonly on the face, hands, and legs and are caused by a relatively different group of nongenital HPV types. Epidermodysplasia verruciformis is an uncommon autosomal recessive disease that is usually manifested in childhood as diffuse warts that respond poorly to treatment. This syndrome, which is thought to be due to a selective defect in cell-mediated immunity because other opportunistic infections do not occur, is associated with two types of lesions: flat warts caused by the same HPV types as in normal hosts and scaly tinea versicolor–type lesions caused by a large number of unusual types. The latter are associated with the development of squamous cell cancer in sun-exposed areas. Similar skin lesions and, rarely, associated skin cancers can develop in other patients with acquired defects in cell-mediated immunity. Other uncommon lesions caused by unique HPV types include butchers' warts, which are verrucous lesions found on the hands of meat handlers, and focal epithelial hyperplasia, which consists of flat mucosal lesions of the oropharynx.

The majority of genital HPV infections do not produce recognized lesions and remain subclinical, detected only by HPV DNA testing. Anogenital warts are papillomatous growths that occur throughout the anogenital skin and mucosa, generally at sites of genital friction. Perianal warts, which are more common in persons with a history of anal intercourse, are often associated with intra-anal warts but can occur without such contact, presumably through autoinoculation. The warts can range from flat or papular lesions to the classic pedunculated, cauliflower-shaped condyloma acuminatum. They are typically caused by low-risk types (>90% are due to HPV 6 or 11), although warts caused by high-risk or multiple types can occur in immunocompromised patients. Warts are typically asymptomatic, noticed either by the patient as a "bump" or inadvertently during a genital examination, although they can cause itching, burning, pain, or rarely, bleeding or mechanical obstruction of the birth canal in pregnant women. Warts caused by genital types can also rarely occur in the mouth and upper respiratory tract, the latter producing a serious condition known as recurrent respiratory papillomatosis, which can cause hoarseness and even airway compromise.

Squamous intraepithelial lesions are most commonly found on the cervix as a result of cytologic screening, with confirmation by colposcopy and biopsy. Like warts, they also occur at other anogenital sites and, as for cervical lesions, are categorized either as low-risk/high-risk squamous intraepithelial lesions or as various stages of intraepithelial neoplasia (e.g., vulva—VIN; vagina—VaIN; anus—AIN; penis—PIN). At all sites, low-risk squamous intraepithelial lesions can be caused by either low- or high-risk types, whereas high-risk squamous intraepithelial lesions are always due to high-risk types. Most squamous intraepithelial lesions are not visible on mucosal surfaces without magnification, although they can appear as flat hyperpigmented papules known as bowenoid papulosis on the external genitalia.

Although the natural history of HPV infection is not fully characterized, the large majority of infections and premalignant lesions are self-limited in most immunocompetent patients. Whether infections no longer detectable have been cleared by the immune system or remain latent in the basal layer of the epithelium with the potential for reactivation is not clear, but the higher prevalence of detectable infection in advanced than in early HIV infection supports the possibility of long-term infection. Many, if not most clinical lesions resolve spontaneously, presumably as a result of the development of cell-mediated immunity. Spontaneous regression is estimated to occur in 25% of genital warts and more than 50% of common warts in children.

Estimates of the likelihood of regression versus the risk of progression to invasive cancer are 60% and 1% for CIN 1, 40% and 5% for CIN 2, and 32% and 12% for CIN 3. Traditionally, the various stages of precursor lesions have been viewed as a biologic continuum, with CIN 1 progressing through higher grades to invasive cancer. However, emerging data indicate that low-risk squamous intraepithelial lesions and high-risk squamous intraepithelial lesions may be distinct processes, with low-risk squamous intraepithelial lesions (CIN 1) being a manifestation of what is usually a transient productive infection characterized by the production of capsid protein (and probably infectious virions) and only minor cellular abnormalities and high-risk squamous intraepithelial lesions (CIN 2/3) representing proliferation of immature cells as a result of the activity of oncogenic proteins of high-risk types. In this model (Fig. 396–1), initial infection frequently leads to a usually transient low-risk squamous intraepithelial lesion and less frequently to persistent infection. Persistent infection can, in turn, lead directly to high-risk squamous intraepithelial lesions within several years of initial infection and can progress to invasive cancer over a period of several decades. The natural history of squamous intraepithelial lesions at other anogenital sites is less well defined, but they may be associated with higher rates of regression. Immunodeficient patients, such as those with HIV infection, have a lower rate of spontaneous regression of squamous intraepithelial lesions and may have a higher rate of progression to cancer.

Diagnosis

Both cutaneous (Fig. 396–2) and genital (Fig. 396–3) warts generally present an easily recognized clinical picture and can be diagnosed by history and physical examination without laboratory testing. The application of 3 to 5% acetic acid causes whitening of HPV lesions on genital mucosa ("acetowhitening") and may be useful with magnification in women; however, because its sensitivity and specificity have not been defined, it is not recommended for routine use.

The differential diagnosis of cutaneous warts includes seborrheic and solar keratoses, nevi, irritated acrochordons, clavi, and squamous cell carcinoma (Chapter 466); lichen planus (Chapter 464) can mimic flat warts and calluses of the foot or plantar warts. Genital warts must also be distinguished from the condyloma latum lesions of secondary syphilis (Chapter 340) and molluscum contagiosum (Chapters 395 and 466). Biopsy for histopathologic examination may be helpful for lesions that are atypical or not responsive to therapy, those suggestive of high-risk squamous intraepithelial lesions or cancer (e.g., pigmented, indurated, fixed, bleeding, or ulcerated), or lesions in immunocompromised patients.

The principal approach to the diagnosis of cervical squamous intraepithelial lesions is cytologic screening, with assessment of abnormal results by colposcopy and biopsy for histopathology. The one currently available virologic test for HPV is a DNA detection assay that can identify any of 13 high-risk types (16, 18, 31, 33, 35, 39, 45, 51, 52, 56, 58, 59, 68); results are reported as positive for any type or negative, but type-specific results are not available. This test is approved as an adjunct to cytology to enhance the sensitivity of screening in women older than 30 years and also for triage of women whose Papanicolaou tests show atypical

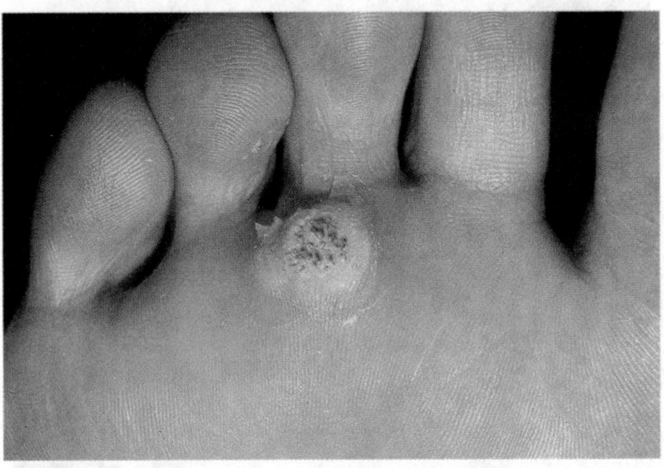

FIGURE 396–2 • Plantar wart. A hyperkeratotic, verrucous papule or plaque beneath a pressure point on the sole of the foot is charateristic. Human papillomavirus (HPV) types 1 (myrmecia), 2 (mosaic), and 4 are most common. Because plantar warts are driven into the skin by the pressure of walking or standing, they are usually the most treatment resistant.

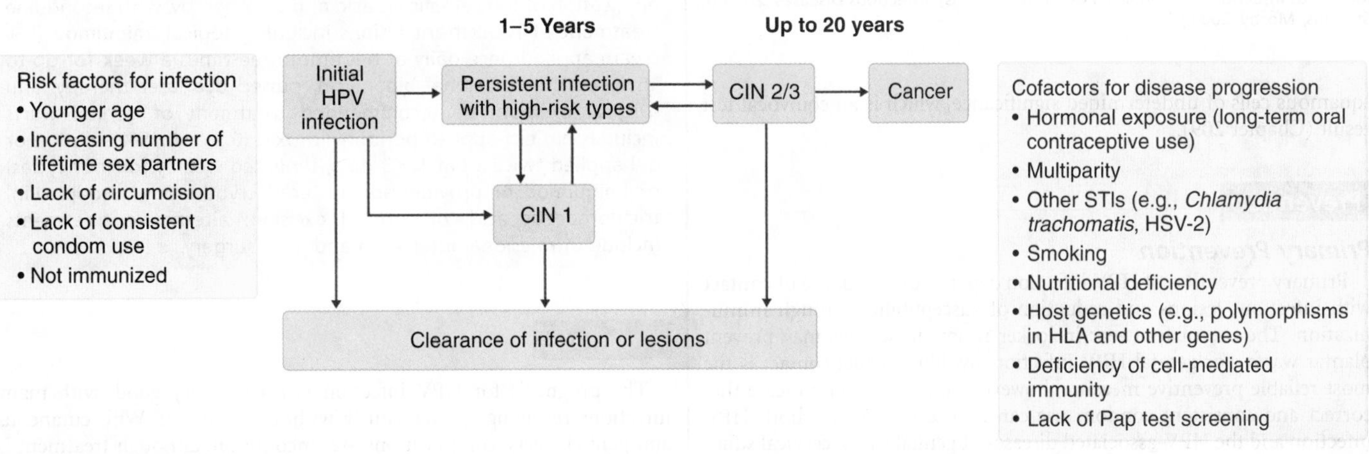

FIGURE 396–1 • Natural history of genital human papillomavirus (HPV) infection and cervical cancer. CIN = cervical intraepithelial neoplasia; HSV = herpes simplex virus; STIs = sexually transmitted infections.

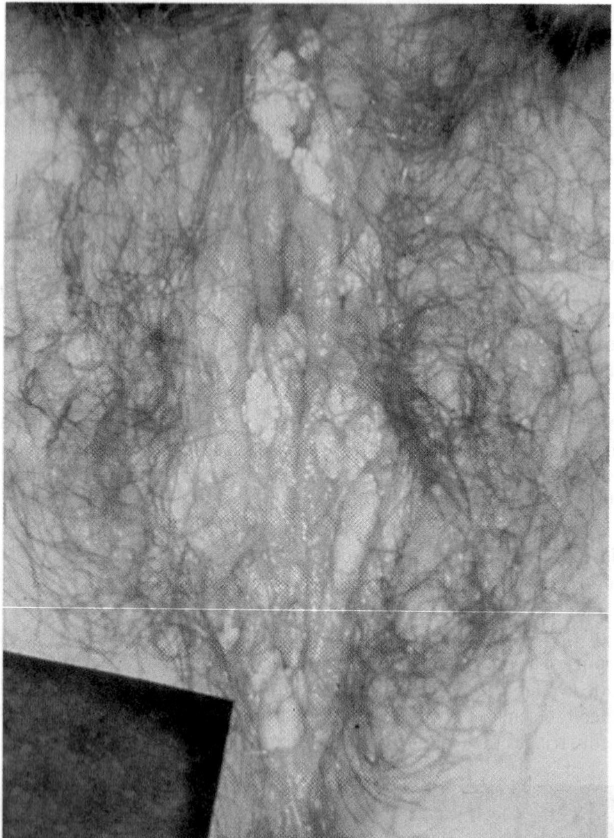

A

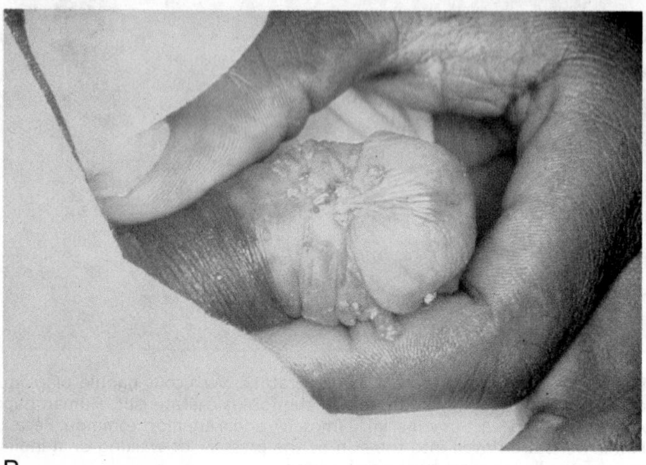

B

FIGURE 396–3 • Genital human papillomavirus (HPV) infection. A, Vulvovaginal HPV infection. **B,** Penile HPV infection. (From Vermund SH, MP Bhatta: Papillomavirus infections. *In* Cohen J, Powderly WG [eds]: Infectious Diseases, 2nd ed. St Louis, Mosby, 2004.)

squamous cells of undetermined significance, which is an equivocal test result (Chapter 209).

Prevention

Primary Prevention

Primary prevention of HPV infection depends on avoidance of contact with infectious lesions and reduction of susceptibility through immunization. The use of footwear in locker rooms in schools may prevent plantar warts. For genital HPV infection, avoiding sexual contact is the most reliable preventive measure; however, emerging data indicate that correct and consistent condom use can reduce the risk for both HPV infection and the HPV-associated diseases of genital warts, cervical squamous intraepithelial lesions, and cervical cancer. A newly licensed quadrivalent vaccine (types 6, 11, 16, 18) given in three doses over a period of 6 months is highly effective in susceptible persons for the prevention of CIN 1 and CIN 2/3, as well as genital warts and VaIN and VIN, caused by any of the four types. [1] This vaccine has recently been recommended for the routine immunization of 11- to 12-year-old girls, as well as females 13 to 26 years of age; girls 9 to 10 years of age may also be vaccinated at the discretion of the provider. The vaccine has no therapeutic benefit against existing infection or lesions and is most effective if given before initiation of sexual activity. Because it provides protection against only two of the high-risk types associated with cancer, immunized females will continue to need Pap test screening. In males, the vaccine is also immunogenic but is not yet recommended, pending completion of clinical trials.

Secondary Prevention

Pap test screening plus treatment of cervical squamous intraepithelial lesions is one of the most successful of all cancer prevention strategies. Current guidelines in the United States vary slightly among recommending organizations, but all agree that screening should begin within 3 years of initiation of sexual activity or by age 21 and continue at 1- to 3-year intervals. Women older than 30 who have had three negative Pap tests or a negative Pap test accompanied by a negative HPV test can be screened at 3-year intervals. Assessment by colposcopy and biopsy is recommended for most abnormal results, although women with atypical squamous cells of undetermined significance can be managed safely without colposcopy if an HIV test is negative.

Treatment depends on histologic staging and the results of colposcopy and is recommended for all CIN 2/3 lesions, with options including a loop electrosurgical excision procedure, cryosurgery, or laser surgery. Because CIN 1 usually regresses spontaneously, conservative management with close follow-up is an alternative to surgical therapy. The value of cytologic screening for anal intraepithelial lesions in HIV-positive homosexual men, among whom anal cancer is increased, is controversial but not currently recommended because of limited data on the natural history of these precursor lesions, the reliability of screening methods, and the safety and effectiveness of treatment.

Treatment

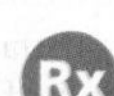

Management of HPV is directed toward diagnosis and treatment of the lesions themselves because there are no virus-specific therapies. Many lesions resolve spontaneously, so the goal of treatment is amelioration or prevention of symptoms or, in the case of high-grade squamous intraepithelial lesions, prevention of progression to cancer. Treatment generally involves destruction of lesions by physical techniques (e.g., surgical excision, cryotherapy, electrocautery, laser) or topically applied or injected cytotoxic agents (e.g., salicylic acid, bleomycin, podofilox, podophyllin resin, trichloroacetic acid) or immunomodulating agents (e.g., imiquimod, interferon). Because treatment does not eradicate infection in surrounding tissues, recurrent lesions are common.

Treatment of warts depends on their location and size, the patient's preferences, and the provider's experience. Recommended first-line treatment of common, flat, and plantar warts includes the application of topical salicylic acid and cryotherapy, with second-line treatment of recalcitrant lesions including topical imiquimod (5% cream applied once daily at bedtime three times a week for up to 16 weeks), intralesional bleomycin, pulsed dye laser therapy, and surgical excision. [2] Recommended treatment of genital warts includes patient-applied podophyllotoxin (0.5 or 0.15% solution or gel applied twice a day for 3 days, repeated weekly for four cycles) or imiquimod or provider-administered cryotherapy, podophyllin, trichloroacetic acid, or surgical excision; alternative treatments include intralesional interferon and laser surgery. [2]

Prognosis

The prognosis for HPV infection is usually very good, with many infections resolving spontaneously without treatment. With cutaneous and genital warts, complications are uncommon, although treatment is often prolonged because of recurrent lesions. Recurrent respiratory papillomatosis can be a severely disabling condition with the potential for airway compromise and multiple invasive procedures. Although cervical cancer can be a fatal condition, the prognosis for cervical squamous intraepithelial lesions is excellent if they are detected and treated adequately.

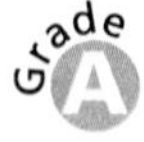

1. Centers for Disease Control and Prevention: Quadrivalent human papillomavirus vaccine. Recommendations of the Advisory Committee on Immunization Practices. MMWR Rep 2007;56:1–24.
2. Gibbs S, Harvey I, Sterling JC, Stark R: Local treatments for cutaneous warts. Cochrane Database Syst Rev 2004;4:CD001781.

SUGGESTED READINGS

Baseman JG, Koutsky LA: The epidemiology of human papillomavirus infection. J Clin Virol 2005;32S:S16-S24. *Comprehensive review.*

Center for Disease Control and Prevention; Workowski KA, Berman SM: Sexually transmitted disease treatment guidelines, 2006. MMWR Recomm Rep 2006;55(RR-11):1–94. *A careful review.*

Gravitt PE, Jamshidi R: Diagnosis and management of oncogenic cervical human papillomavirus infection. Infect Dis Clin North Am 2005;19:439–458. *Review of cervical cancer screening and role of HPV testing.*

Lacey CJN: Therapy for genital human papillomavirus–related disease. J Clin Virol 2005;32S:S82–S90. *Thorough review of the rationale and options for treatment of genital warts and squamous intraepithelial lesions.*

Snijders JF, Steenbergen RDM, Heideman DAM, et al: HPV-mediated carcinogenesis: Concepts and clinical implications. J Pathol 2006;208:152–164. *Review of the molecular basis for HPV-induced cervical carcinogenesis.*

Winer R, Hughes JP, Feng Q, et al: Condom use and the risk of genital human papillomavirus infection in young women. N Engl J Med 2006;354:2645–2654. *Condom use can reduce the risk for infection substantially.*

397 HERPES SIMPLEX VIRUS INFECTIONS

Richard J. Whitley

Definition

The Pathogen

Herpes simplex virus (HSV), a member of the family Herpesviridae, has been implicated in human infections since descriptions of cutaneous-spreading lesions in ancient Greek times. Scholars of Greek civilization define the word *herpes* to mean "to creep or crawl," in reference to the spreading nature of the observed skin lesions. More recently, infection has been defined by the spectrum of illnesses caused by HSV. In 1968, well-defined antigenic and biologic differences were demonstrated between HSV type 1 (HSV-1) and HSV type 2 (HSV-2). Of all the herpesviruses, HSV-1 and HSV-2 are most closely related, with approximately 60% genomic homology. HSV-1 was more frequently associated with nongenital infection and HSV-2 with genital disease. These two viruses can be distinguished most reliably by DNA restriction enzyme analysis; however, differences in antigen expression and biologic properties also serve as methods for differentiation.

Inclusion in the family Herpesviridae is based on the structure of the virion (Fig. 397–1). HSV contains double-stranded DNA at its central core, has a molecular weight of approximately 100 million, and encodes at least 80 polypeptides. The DNA core is surrounded by a capsid that consists of 162 capsomers arranged in icosapentahedral symmetry. The capsid is 100 to 110 nm in diameter. Tightly adherent to the capsid is the tegument, which consists of amorphous material. Loosely surrounding the capsid and tegument is a lipid bilayer envelope derived from host cell membranes. The envelope consists of polyamines, lipids, and glycoproteins. These glycoproteins confer distinctive properties to the virus and provide unique antigens to which the host is capable of responding. Notably, glycoprotein G (gG) provides antigenic specificity to HSV and therefore results in an antibody response that allows for distinction between HSV-1 (gG-1) and HSV-2 (gG-2).

Epidemiology

HSV infections occur worldwide and have been reported in both developed and underdeveloped countries. Animal vectors for human HSV

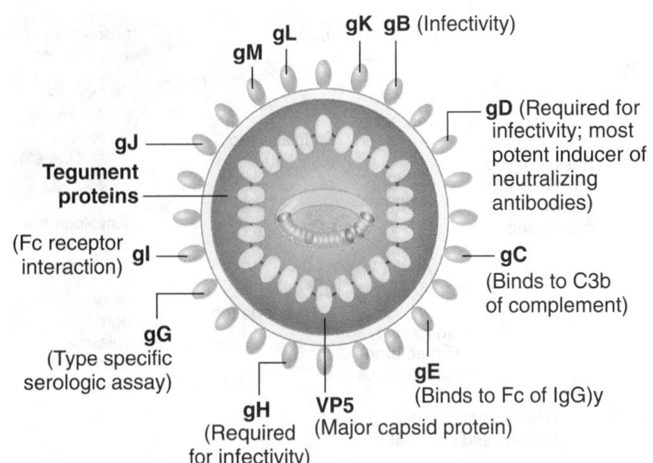

FIGURE 397–1 • Schematic diagram of the herpes simplex virion.

infections have not been described, and there is no seasonal variation in the incidence of HSV infections. HSV is transmitted from infected to susceptible individuals during close personal contact, and the virus must come in contact with mucosal surfaces or abraded skin for infection to be initiated. Because approximately a third of the world's population has recurrent HSV infections and because infection is rarely fatal, a large reservoir of HSV exists in the community.

Seroprevalence studies have demonstrated that acquisition of HSV-1 infection is related to socioeconomic factors. Antibodies, which indicate past infection, are found early in life among individuals of lower socioeconomic groups, presumably a consequence of crowded living conditions that provide a greater opportunity for direct contact with infected individuals. Antibodies develop in as many as 75 to 90% of individuals from lower socioeconomic populations by the end of the first decade of life. In contrast, only 30 to 40% of persons in the middle and upper socioeconomic groups are seropositive by the middle of the second decade of life.

Because infections with HSV-2 are usually acquired through sexual contact, antibodies to this virus are rarely found until the onset of sexual activity. There is a progressive increase in infection rates with HSV-2 in all populations beginning in adolescence. Overall, about one in five Americans has genital HSV-2 infection. As with HSV-1 infections, the rate of acquisition of HSV-2 infection appears to be related to socioeconomic factors. The number of sexual contacts is also an important risk factor for the acquisition of HSV-2. Genital herpes infection has been found to be a risk factor for another sexually transmitted virus: human immunodeficiency virus (HIV) (Chapter 409).

Localized, recurrent HSV-2 infection is the most common form of HSV infection during gestation. Transmission of infection to the fetus is most frequently related to shedding of the virus at the time of delivery. The incidence of cervical shedding in pregnant women with asymptomatic HSV infection is approximately 1%. Most infants in whom neonatal disease develops are born to women who are completely asymptomatic for genital HSV infection at the time of delivery and who have neither a past history of genital herpes nor a sexual partner reporting a genital vesicular rash. These women account for 60 to 80% of all women whose children acquire neonatal HSV infection.

Pathobiology

Replication of HSV is a multistep process (Fig. 397–2). After the onset of infection, DNA is uncoated and transported to the nucleus of the host cell. This step is followed by transcription of immediate-early genes, which encode for the regulatory proteins, and is followed by the expression of proteins encoded by early and then late genes. These proteins include enzymes necessary for viral replication and structural proteins.

Assembly of the viral core and capsid takes place within the nucleus. Envelopment at the nuclear membrane and transport out of the nucleus occur through the endoplasmic reticulum and the Golgi apparatus. Glycosylation of the viral membrane occurs in the Golgi apparatus. Mature

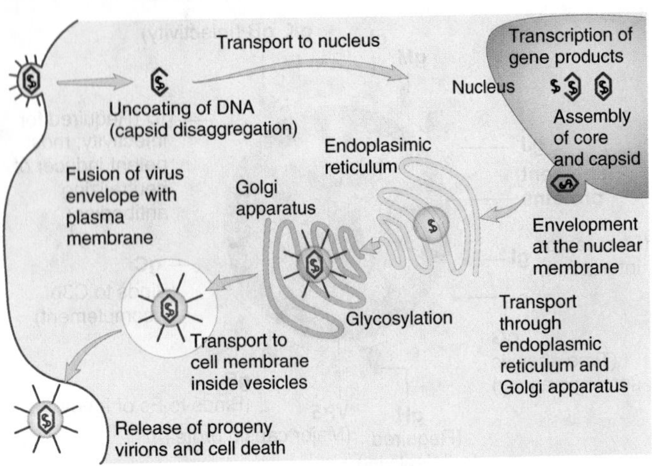

FIGURE 397–2 • Schematic diagram of replication of herpes simplex virus.

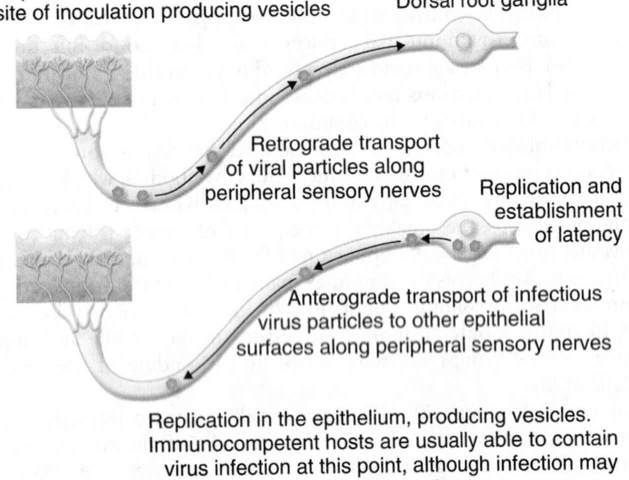

FIGURE 397–3 • Schematic diagram of primary herpes simplex virus infection.

virions are transported to the outer membrane of the host cell inside vesicles. Release of progeny virus is accompanied by cell death. Replication for all herpesviruses is considered inefficient, with a high ratio of noninfectious to infectious viral particles.

A critical factor for transmission of HSV, regardless of virus type, is intimate contact between a person who is shedding virus and a susceptible host. With inoculation onto skin or mucous membranes, HSV replicates in epithelial cells; the incubation period is 4 to 6 days (Fig. 397–3). As replication continues, cell lysis and local inflammation ensue and result in the characteristic vesicles on an erythematous base. Regional lymphatics and lymph nodes become involved as a result of draining of infected secretions from the area of viral replication. Viremia and visceral dissemination may develop, depending on the immunologic competence of the host. In all hosts, the virus generally ascends peripheral sensory nerves to reach the dorsal root ganglia. Replication of HSV within neural tissue is followed by spread of the virus to other mucosal and skin surfaces by means of peripheral sensory nerves. HSV replicates further in epithelial cells and reproduces the lesions of the initial infection until infection is contained through host immunity.

The histopathologic changes induced by HSV replication are similar in both primary and recurrent infection. Changes induced by viral infection include ballooning of infected cells and the appearance of condensed chromatin within the nuclei of cells, followed by subsequent degeneration of cellular nuclei. Cells lose intact plasma membranes and form multinucleated giant cells. They may also demonstrate intranuclear inclusions known as Cowdry type A bodies, which are suggestive but not

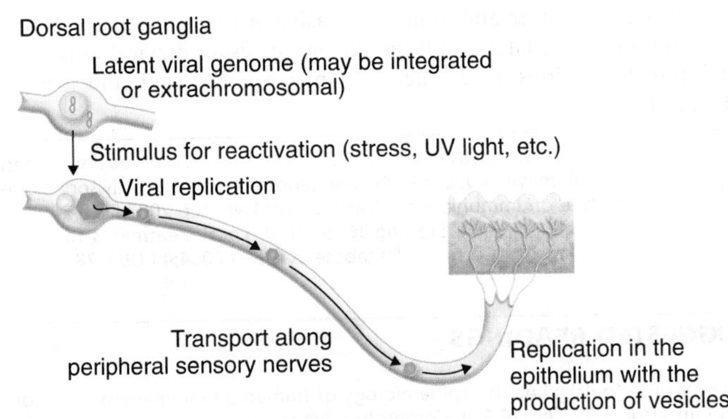

FIGURE 397–4 • Schematic diagram of herpes simplex virus latency and reactivation. UV = ultraviolet.

diagnostic of HSV infection. With cell lysis, clear vesicular fluid containing large quantities of virus forms between the epidermis and dermal layer. The dermis reveals an intense inflammatory response, more so with primary infection than with recurrent disease. As healing progresses, the clear vesicular fluid becomes pustular with the recruitment of inflammatory cells. The pustule then forms a scab; scarring is uncommon.

Vascular changes in the area of infection include perivascular cuffing and hemorrhagic necrosis. These changes are particularly prominent when organs other than skin are involved, as is the case with herpes simplex encephalitis or disseminated neonatal HSV infection. Local lymphatics can show evidence of infection with intrusion of inflammatory cells because of draining of infected secretions from the area of viral replication. As host defenses are mounted, an influx of mononuclear cells can be detected in infected tissue.

A unique characteristic of all herpesviruses is their ability to establish latent infection, persist in an apparently inactive state for varying amounts of time, and then be reactivated (Fig. 397–4). The latent viral genome may be either extrachromosomal or integrated into host cell DNA, depending on the virus.

Latency is established when HSV reaches the dorsal root ganglia after retrograde transmission through sensory nerve pathways. Latent virus may be reactivated and enter a replicative cycle at any point in time. Reactivation of latent virus is a well-recognized biologic phenomenon but not one that is understood from a molecular standpoint. Stimuli associated with the reactivation of latent HSV have included stress, menstruation, and exposure to ultraviolet light. Precisely how these factors interact at the level of the ganglia remains to be defined. Reactivation may be clinically asymptomatic, or it may produce life-threatening disease.

Clinical Manifestations

Gingivostomatitis

Gingivostomatitis (usually caused by HSV-1) occurs most frequently in children younger than 5 years. Illness is characterized by fever, sore throat, pharyngeal edema, and erythema, followed by the development of vesicular or ulcerative lesions on the oral and pharyngeal mucosa. Recurrent HSV-1 infections of the oropharynx are most frequently manifested as herpes simplex labialis (cold sores) and usually appear on the vermilion border of the lip (Fig. 397–5). Recurrences are triggered by fever, stress, and exposure to ultraviolet light, as well as other factors. Intraoral lesions as a manifestation of recurrent disease are uncommon.

Genital Herpes

Genital herpes is most frequently caused by HSV-2. However, an increasing percentage is being caused by HSV-1. Primary infection in women usually involves the vulva, vagina, and cervix. In men, initial infection is most often associated with lesions on the glans penis, prepuce, or penile shaft. In individuals of either gender, primary disease is associated with fever, malaise, anorexia, and bilateral inguinal adenopathy. Women frequently have dysuria and urinary retention as a result of urethral involvement. Aseptic meningitis develops in as many as 10% of individuals with primary infection. Sacral radiculomyelitis may occur in both

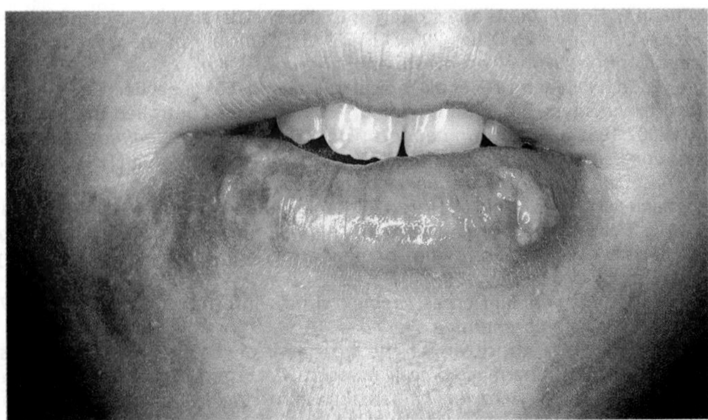

FIGURE 397–5 • Herpetic whitlow, classic grouped blisters.

men and women and results in neuralgias, urinary retention, or obstipation. Complete healing of primary infection may take several weeks. The first episode of genital infection is less severe in individuals who have previously had HSV-1 infections at other sites. Antibodies to HSV-1 appear to ameliorate the expression of HSV-2 clinical disease, although this effect is controversial.

Recurrent genital infections in either men or women can be particularly distressing. The frequency of recurrence varies significantly from one individual to another. Of note, viral DNA can be detected by polymerase chain reaction (PCR) in genital secretions three- to four-fold more frequently than symptomatic recurrences. A third of infected individuals have virtually no or few clinical recurrences, a third have approximately three recurrences per year, and another third have more than three per year. Several seroepidemiologic studies have found that between 25 and 65% of individuals in the United States have antibodies to HSV-2 and that seroprevalence is correlated with the number of sexual partners.

Herpetic Keratitis

Herpes simplex keratitis is usually caused by HSV-1 and is accompanied by conjunctivitis in many cases. It is considered the most common infectious cause of blindness in the United States. The characteristic lesions of HSV keratoconjunctivitis are dendritic ulcers best detected by fluorescein staining. Deep stromal involvement has also been reported and may result in visual impairment.

Other Cutaneous Manifestations

HSV infections can occur at any skin site. Common among health care workers are lesions on abraded skin or the fingers, known as *herpetic whitlow*. Similarly, in wrestlers, disseminated cutaneous lesions known as *herpes gladiatorum* may develop as a result of physical contact.

Diagnosis

Definitive diagnosis of HSV infection requires isolation of virus. Swabs of clinical specimens or other body fluids can be inoculated into susceptible cell lines and observed for the development of characteristic cytopathic effects. This technique is useful for the diagnosis of HSV-1 and HSV-2 infection because of their short replicative cycles.

In the absence of diagnostic virology facilities, cytologic examination of cells scraped from a clinical lesion may be useful in making a presumptive diagnosis of HSV infection. Material obtained from scraping the base of a lesion should be smeared on a glass slide and promptly fixed in cold ethanol. The slide can be stained according to the methods of Papanicolaou, Giemsa, or Wright. The presence of intranuclear inclusions and multinucleated giant cells is indicative, but not diagnostic of HSV infection. This method has a sensitivity of only 60 to 70% and should not be the sole diagnostic method used.

DNA amplification by PCR is gaining greater acceptance for routine diagnostic purposes. DNA amplification has become the diagnostic method of choice in assessing cerebrospinal fluid (CSF) specimens for evidence of HSV infection of the central nervous system. Furthermore, PCR has significantly improved sensitivity for confirming HSV as the etiology of lip and genital herpes infection.

In addition to new tests for viral DNA, type-specific serologic assays are commercially available. These tests are based on differences in HSV-1 and HSV-2 gG.

Treatment

Rx

Infections caused by HSV-1 and HSV-2 are amenable to therapy with antiviral drugs (Chapter 383). At present, intravenous acyclovir administration is the treatment of choice for mucocutaneous HSV infections in immunocompromised hosts, herpes simplex encephalitis, and neonatal HSV infections. [1] Intravenous acyclovir is also recommended for clinically severe initial genital herpes in immunocompetent hosts, including patients with complications such as urinary retention or aseptic meningitis, and they should receive 5 mg/kg of intravenous acyclovir every 8 hours for 5 to 7 days. Caution must be exercised when acyclovir is used intravenously because it may crystallize in the renal tubules when given too rapidly or to dehydrated patients.

Valacyclovir and famciclovir have improved pharmacokinetics over acyclovir. Thus, they should preferentially be used for the treatment of non–life-threatening HSV infection.

Immunocompromised individuals with non–life-threatening mucocutaneous HSV infections may be given oral acyclovir, valacyclovir, or famciclovir. Any of the three drugs is also useful in treating initial genital herpes. Recurrent episodes, however, are not as responsive to acyclovir.

HSV has been used for experimental gene therapy. By removing the $\gamma_1$34.5 gene, both neurovirulence and the propensity to establish latency are ablated. These engineered viruses are being experimentally tested in patients with glioblastoma multiforme and colorectal metastases to liver.

Prevention

At present, there are no licensed vaccines directed against HSV. Experimental vaccines for HSV-1 and HSV-2 remain under investigation. Acyclovir, valacyclovir, and famciclovir are being given to recipients of solid organ and bone marrow transplants in the immediate post-transplant period in an effort to prevent reactivation of latent disease. Valacyclovir has been proved to decrease person-to-person transmission of HSV-2.

NEONATAL HERPES SIMPLEX VIRUS INFECTION

Neonatal HSV infection is estimated to occur in approximately 1 in 3500 deliveries in the United States each year. Approximately 70% of cases are caused by HSV-2 and usually result from contact of the fetus with infected maternal genital secretions at the time of delivery. Manifestations of neonatal HSV infection can be divided into three categories: (1) skin, eye, and mouth disease; (2) encephalitis; and (3) disseminated infection. As the name implies, skin, eye, and mouth disease consists of cutaneous lesions and does not involve other organ systems. Involvement of the central nervous system may occur with encephalitis or disseminated infection and generally results in diffuse encephalitis. CSF assay characteristically reveals elevated protein levels and mononuclear pleocytosis. Disseminated infection involves multiple organ systems and can cause disseminated intravascular coagulation, hemorrhagic pneumonitis, encephalitis, and cutaneous lesions. Diagnosis is difficult in the absence of skin lesions, which occurs in as many as 36% of cases. The mortality rate for each disease classification varies from zero for skin, eye, and mouth disease to 5% for encephalitis and 25% for neonates with disseminated infection, even with appropriate antiviral treatment. In addition to the high mortality associated with these infections, morbidity is significant in that children with encephalitis or disseminated disease develop normally in only 40% of cases, even with appropriate antiviral therapy.

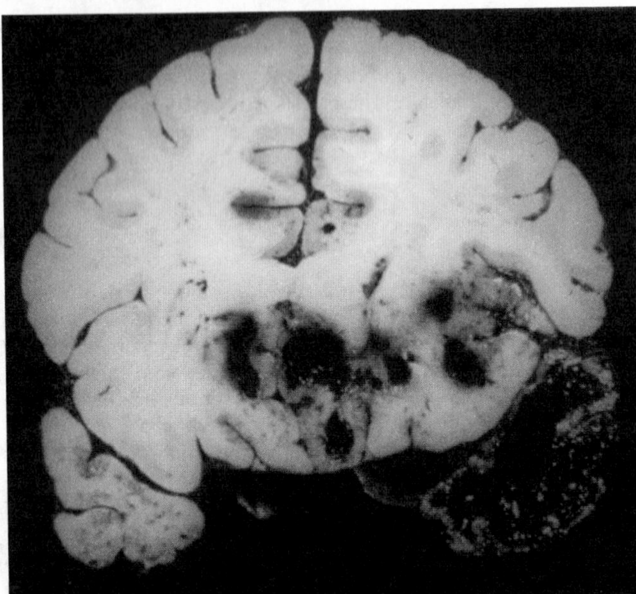

FIGURE 397–6 • Hemorrhagic necrosis in herpes simplex encephalitis.

HERPES SIMPLEX ENCEPHALITIS

Herpes simplex encephalitis is characterized by hemorrhagic necrosis of the temporal lobe (Chapter 439). Disease begins unilaterally and spreads to the contralateral temporal lobe (Fig. 397–6). It is the most common cause of focal, sporadic encephalitis in the United States today and occurs in approximately 1 in 150,000 individuals. Most cases are caused by HSV-1. The actual pathogenesis of herpes simplex encephalitis requires further clarification, although it has been speculated that primary or recurrent virus can reach the temporal lobe by ascending neural pathways, such as the trigeminal tracts or the olfactory nerves.

Clinical manifestations of herpes simplex encephalitis include headache, fever, altered consciousness, and abnormalities in speech and behavior, findings characteristic of temporal lobe involvement. Focal seizures also may occur. CSF findings in these patients are variable but usually consist of a pleocytosis with both polymorphonuclear leukocytes and monocytes present. The protein concentration is characteristically elevated, and the glucose level is usually normal. Diagnosis can be achieved by PCR evaluation of CSF in experienced laboratories. Mortality and morbidity are high, even with appropriate antiviral therapy. At present, the mortality rate is approximately 30% 1 year after treatment. In addition, approximately 50% of survivors have moderate or severe neurologic impairment.

HERPES SIMPLEX VIRUS INFECTIONS IN IMMUNOCOMPROMISED HOSTS

HSV infections in immunocompromised hosts, including patients with acquired immunodeficiency syndrome, are usually due to reactivation of latent infection and are clinically more severe, may be progressive, and require a longer time to heal. Manifestations of HSV infections in this patient population include pneumonitis, esophagitis, hepatitis, colitis, and disseminated cutaneous disease. Individuals suffering from HIV infection may have extensive perineal or orofacial ulcerations. HSV infections are also noted to be of increased severity in individuals with extensive burns.

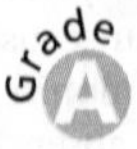

1. Watts DH, Brown ZA, Money D, et al: A double-blind, randomized, placebo-controlled trial of acyclovir in late pregnancy for the reduction of herpes simplex virus shedding and cesarean delivery. Am J Obstet Gynecol 2003;188:836–843.

SUGGESTED READINGS

Corey L, Wald A, Patel R, et al: Once daily valacyclovir to reduce the risk of transmission of genital herpes. N Engl J Med 2004;350:11–20. *Valacyclovir reduces the risk of transmission of genital herpes.*

Engelberg R, Carrell D, Krantz E, et al: Natural history of genital herpes simplex virus type 1 infection. Sex Transm Dis 2003;30:174–177. *Genital HSV-1 recurs infrequently, and the rate decreases further over time.*

Kleymann G: Novel agents and strategies to treat herpes simplex virus infections. Expert Opin Investig Drugs 2003;12:165–183. *Summary of the current therapeutic options, as well as investigational drugs.*

Mark KE, Corey L, Meng TC, et al: Topical resiquimod 0.01% gel decreases herpes simplex virus type 2 genital shedding: A randomized, controlled trial. J Infect Dis 2007;195:1324–1331. *In patients with HSV-2, topical resiquimod, an investigational immune response modifier and Toll-like receptor (TLR) 7 and 8 agonist, can reduce the frequency of mucosal activation.*

Weidmann M, Meyer-Konig U, Hufert FT: Rapid detection of herpes simplex virus and varicella-zoster virus infections by real-time PCR. J Clin Microbiol 2003;41:1565–1568. *Sensitivities of new assays are above 95% with nearly 100% specificity.*

Whitley RJ, Roizman B: Herpes simplex viruses infections. Lancet 2001;357:1513–1518. *A comprehensive overview.*

Vinh DC, Aoki FY: Famciclovir for the treatment of recurrent genital herpes: A clinical and pharmacological perspective. Expert Opin Pharmacother 2006;7:2271–2286. *A review of famciclovir for the treatment of recurrent genital herpes.*

Xu F, Sternberg MR, Kottiri BJ, et al: Trends in herpes simplex virus type 1 and type 2 seroprevalence in the United States. JAMA 2006;296:964–973. *The seroprevalence of HSV-2 and HSV-1 have declined.*

Yeung-Yue KA, Brentjens MH, Lee PC, et al: Herpes simplex viruses 1 and 2. Dermatol Clin 2002;20:249–266. *Overview of the pathogenesis and transmission of HSV infections, type-specific diagnostic tests, and new treatments such as cidofovir gel and resiquimod.*

398 VARICELLA (CHICKENPOX, SHINGLES)

Philip A. Brunell

Definition

Varicella, or chickenpox, is an acute communicable disease characterized by a generalized vesicular rash. Because it is highly contagious, most individuals contract it in childhood. Herpes zoster, caused by reactivation of varicella-zoster virus (VZV), is a dermatomal cutaneous eruption.

The Pathogen

Varicella is caused by VZV, a member of the alpha Herpesviridae subfamily. VZV has the characteristic structure of a herpesvirus with an envelope, a tegument, a capsid, and a core of double-stranded DNA. The DNA is organized with terminal and internal repeats flanking unique short and long segments containing about 125,000 base pairs coding for approximately 70 genes. There are at least six glycoproteins. Its thymidine kinase has been a target for antiviral agents. There is some diversity in the restriction enzyme patterns among isolates but there is only a single serotype. Although the human is the only known natural host, a closely related virus has been identified in a simian species.

Epidemiology

Varicella is a highly contagious disease. After continuing household exposure, as would occur in a family, almost all susceptible persons are infected. The subclinical attack rate is believed to be no more than 4%. The results of nonhousehold exposure are less predictable. Chickenpox may be most contagious the day before the onset of rash. The period of contagiousness lasts no more than 5 days after the appearance of the first lesion. Children may return to school at this time or earlier if the lesions are crusted. The incubation period is usually about 14 days. Ninety-nine percent of the cases occur 10 to 20 days after exposure. The disease is known to be spread by direct contact. Airborne spread has also been demonstrated, most notably in hospitals.

Spread of varicella in health care facilities is well documented. It has occurred from room to room by airborne spread as well as between patients and staff. Adults with herpes zoster who are hospitalized are less likely to cause secondary cases of chickenpox than are children. The reason is that hospitalized children are more likely to be susceptible to chickenpox than hospitalized adults. Isolation is recommended for hospitalized patients with varicella and for children or immunocompromised adults with herpes zoster. Adults with localized herpes zoster require less stringent isolation procedures.

Most cases of chickenpox occur in childhood. Before the widespread use of varicella vaccine, most children contracted chickenpox prior to school entry, often in out-of-home care; fewer than 2% of the cases occurred after the second decade. Now that an increasing proportion of children are vaccinated, the age of peak incidence has shifted to school age.

Less than 10% of hospital workers with a negative history of chickenpox are actually seronegative. Almost all individuals with a positive history are seropositive. A single attack of chickenpox usually confers lifetime immunity.

Disease transmission may be more efficient in temperate than in tropical climates. The reason for this is uncertain. In the United States, varicella occurs most commonly during the late winter and spring months, the peak being in about March. Since the advent of universal immunization, cases are more evenly distributed throughout the year.

Varicella is more common than other childhood diseases during the early months of life. After the first 2 weeks of life, the disease is generally mild. Maternal antibody transferred across the placenta may not be as effective in protecting infants against this disease as antibodies against other viruses. However, nursery outbreaks have been rare. Children who have varicella during the early months of life or who are exposed in utero have a greater risk for herpes zoster in childhood.

Pathobiology

Replication of virus is believed to occur initially in the epithelial cells of the mucosa of the upper respiratory tract. Because VZV produces a disseminated rash, blood stream distribution is assumed and virus can be isolated from white blood cells from 5 days before to 2 days after the appearance of rash. In uncomplicated chickenpox, rises in serum aminotransferase levels have been demonstrated. This observation suggests that there is also visceral involvement in the normal course of this disease.

After clinical recovery, the virus persists in the absence of clinical symptoms in a latent phase. During this time, DNA and some species of messenger RNA can be demonstrated in neurons in dorsal root ganglia. The segmental distribution of herpes zoster, which usually occurs decades after the initial VZV infection, is consistent with a dorsal root ganglion site for the latent virus. The vesicular lesions of varicella contain a predominance of polymorphonuclear leukocytes even during the early phase of vesicle formation. Multinuclear giant cells are occasionally found in the base of the lesions, often containing eosinophilic intranuclear (Cowdry type A) inclusions. Large amounts of virus can be demonstrated in vesicular fluid by electron microscopy, and virus can be isolated in DNA by PCR.

Postmortem descriptions of patients with varicella have usually involved immunocompromised subjects. In these cases, inflammatory changes are usually found in multiple organs, including the lung, liver, spleen, and skin, together with anoxic changes in the brain. Similar involvement is found in the newborn. Focal areas of necrosis and intranuclear eosinophilic inclusions are common. Changes in otherwise healthy individuals usually include myocardial and pulmonary lesions. On microscopic examination, the brain has demonstrated edema with some lymphocyte cuffing around the cerebral vessels.

Clinical Manifestations

Varicella is characterized by a generalized eruption that is centripetal in distribution; erythematous macules, papules, vesicles, and scabbed lesions may be present at the same time. The vesicles are superficial, with varying amounts of erythema at their bases. Adults tend to have considerably more erythema than children. During the early phase of the eruption, lesions are found on the face, scalp, and trunk. Often, lesions can be detected in the scalp before their appearance on the skin by running the fingers through the hair. Later, new lesions appear on the extremities. By this time, the earlier lesions have dried and crusted. Excoriations are common, attesting to the pruritic nature of the lesions. Mucous membranes of the conjunctiva and oropharynx are more frequently involved in adults than in children. New lesions continue to appear over a 3- or 4-day period, after which the rate of their appearance decelerates markedly.

In persons who have received vaccine previously, fewer than 50 lesions, many of which are abortive, are seen. Others have more extensive lesions resembling unmodified varicella. There is a striking variation in the extent of systemic symptoms associated with varicella. Most children have a mild illness with few systemic complaints and an average maximal temperature of about 38.3° C. It is more common for adults to have considerable malaise, muscle ache, arthralgia, and headache. These may precede the first skin lesions by 24 to 48 hours.

In immunocompromised subjects, the disease is often severe. Approximately 30% of children with leukemia or lymphoma who contract varicella and receive no prophylaxis or treatment develop progressive varicella. Vesicles continue to erupt into the second week of illness, accompanied by high fever. Lesions tend to be deep seated rather than superficial. Toward the end of the first week and the beginning of the second week, the lesions are more common on the extremities than on the trunk. Indeed, the distribution and appearance may resemble those with smallpox. Visceral involvement occurs in about 30% of these patients. The lung, liver, pancreas, and brain may be involved. Death occurs in about 9% of immunocompromised patients with unmodified varicella. Death is usually due to pulmonary involvement. Patients with human immunodeficiency virus (HIV) infections may have recurrent attacks of varicella in the absence of exposure or a persistent eruption that may continue for months, the latter usually in severely immunocompromised patients.

Varicella in pregnant women is believed to be more serious than in nongravid females; fatalities have been reported. The rate of fetal wastage is not increased. About 1% of infants born to mothers who have had varicella early in pregnancy, however, have been found at birth to have varicella embryopathy. Risk appears to be greatest during midpregnancy. The infants are born with cerebral damage and a variety of ocular findings, and characteristically they have a scarred, atrophic limb. The children are generally small for gestational age and may have other abnormalities as well. When mothers develop chickenpox within a few days of delivery, varicella of the newborn may occur. If maternal onset of varicella is between 5 and 10 days prior to birth, it is associated with a higher risk of serious disease and even death of the newborn.

Complications

Bacterial infections of the skin are the most common complication of chickenpox in childhood. The frequency of invasive streptococcal superinfection has increased. The rate of complications is much higher in adults than in children. Prior to the vaccine, although fewer than 2% of the reported cases occur after the second decade, almost 35% of the deaths occur in this group. A disproportionate rate of hospitalization is also found in adults. The major complications of varicella in adults are encephalitis and pneumonia.

Approximately 1 in 400 adults with chickenpox are hospitalized for pneumonia. In a prospective study, however, it was found that only 6% of young adults with chickenpox had respiratory symptoms, whereas 16% had roentgenographic evidence of pulmonary involvement.

Infection produces a diffuse interstitial type of pneumonia with hypoxia resulting from poor diffusion of gases. Diffuse calcification of the lung parenchyma may be found years after recovery.

Encephalitis in childhood is most commonly manifested by a cerebellitis, which usually occurs at the end of the first week or during the second week after the onset of rash. This complication is almost always self-limited. In contrast, an acute form of encephalitis usually occurring soon after the onset of rash often has a fulminating course; it is characterized by severe brain swelling. When Reye's syndrome was prevalent, as many as 20% of cases were preceded by chickenpox. A variety of other neurologic complications, including optic neuritis, transverse myelitis, and Guillain-Barré syndrome, may be associated with chickenpox. Hemorrhagic complications of chickenpox include thrombocytopenic purpura and purpura fulminans. Nephritis, myocarditis, hepatitis, and arthritis have also been described.

Diagnosis

In unimmunized persons, there is usually little difficulty in recognizing typical forms of chickenpox, particularly if there has been a history of exposure. The diagnosis may be more difficult in immunocompromised hosts because they may have features of progressive varicella with visceral involvement. The umbilicated lesions in a peripheral distribution late in the course in these patients may be mistaken for smallpox. In the latter infection, all the lesions appear simultaneously rather than in crops.

Modified cases of chickenpox may occur after passive or active immunization. These cases may require laboratory confirmation. The most common sources of confusion are insect bites, generalized herpes in the immunocompromised host, rickettsialpox, or "hand, foot, and mouth disease" caused by an enterovirus. The differentiation of disseminated herpes zoster from chickenpox may be difficult. The former usually has dermatomal involvement initially. Generalization usually does not occur until 3 to 5 days after onset of the zosteriform rash. In severely immunocompromised patients (e.g., bone marrow recipients), generalization may occur earlier and the clinical differentiation may be difficult. Fluorescence microscopy is a rapid and accurate method of confirming the diagnosis from vesicular scrapings. Virus can usually be isolated during the first 3 or 4 days after the onset of lesions. The virus is quite labile; it must be stored at –70° C if cultures cannot be inoculated immediately. Ideally, vesicular fluid should be collected in unheparinized capillary tubes and transferred directly into human embryonic lung fibroblasts at the bedside. Specimens from throat, urine, or stool are of little value for isolation of virus. Polymerase chain reaction can be used to demonstrate the presence of virus in vesicular fluid and throat swabs. This technique is particularly useful when viable virus cannot be obtained. It can also be used to distinguish vaccine from wild strains of virus.

Serologic confirmation of the diagnosis can be made using a variety of techniques. The enzyme-linked immunosorbent assay (ELISA) and the latex agglutination assay are the most generally available. The laboratory director should be consulted regarding appropriate time of collection of specimens as well as interpretation of data.

The immune status of contacts can be determined most reliably with the latex agglutination test. Because complement-fixing antibody is lost rapidly after infection, it cannot be used for determining susceptibility. Fluorescence antibody testing using fixed cells sometimes yields false-positive results. Commercial ELISAs have been unpredictable. A number of laboratories have developed tests for VZV immunoglobulin M (IgM). It was hoped that these might differentiate varicella from herpes zoster in cases in which this was unclear. Unfortunately, these tests have not been very useful because VZV IgM is present in the sera of many patients with acute herpes zoster.

Treatment

Rx

Major therapeutic objectives are the prevention of superinfection and relief of pruritus. The latter can be accomplished frequently by application of calamine lotion. Occasionally this does not suffice, and a systemic antipruritic agent such as trimeprazine may be necessary. It is advisable to trim and file nails to reduce the damage from scratching. Bacterial superinfection can best be prevented by encouraging daily bathing with an antibacterial soap. Following this with a colloidal starch bath may also be useful for relieving pruritus.

Relief of systemic symptoms may require additional medication such as acetaminophen, although this may increase pruritus. Salicylates are contraindicated because there is an association between their use and development of Reye's syndrome in children. Special care should be taken to be certain that over-the-counter medications containing salicylates are avoided. Necrotizing fasciitis caused by group A *Streptococcus* has been associated with the use of ibuprofen. The increased frequency has been shown in some studies to be due to the selection of more severe disease for treatment with this drug.

Some patients, particularly those who are immunocompromised, may require antiviral therapy. Intravenous acyclovir has been shown to be effective in immunocompromised children with varicella. A dose of 500 mg/m^2 repeated every 8 hours has been used. VZV is generally less sensitive to acyclovir than herpes simplex. For this reason, larger doses are required. Studies of the use of oral acyclovir in the treatment of varicella have demonstrated some efficacy. Newer drugs (e.g., valacyclovir and famciclovir) have been effective in treating zoster with less frequent dosing. Although oral therapy may be useful in adolescents and adults, immunocompromised patients who are sick enough to require antiviral therapy probably should be treated with parenteral rather than oral medication.

For patients who are not immunocompromised, either valacyclovir or famciclovir given as soon as possible after the onset and within

Rx

72 hours is the recommended treatments of zoster. Valacyclovir (Valtrex) 1000 mg is given three times daily for 7 days. Famciclovir (Famvir) 500 or 750 mg is given three times daily for 7 days. These have the advantage over acyclovir of requiring less frequent dosing. They reduce the time to healing and decrease immediate pain. Steroids are controversial and may have some significant side effects in older persons.

Patients receiving high doses of corticosteroids or other immunosuppressive drugs who have been exposed to chickenpox are at high risk for developing progressive varicella. Corticosteroids appear to be most deleterious when given during the incubation period. They have been used in the treatment of pneumonia after the eruption has occurred without any obvious deleterious effects.

Prevention

Live attenuated varicella vaccine is recommended for all children aged 1 through 12 years and for certain adults. There has been waning immunity and a tendency for more severe disease with increasing interval since immunization with a single dose. Therefore, two doses are given at least 4 weeks apart. A combined measles-mumps-rubella–varicella vaccine (MMRV) may be used through the 12th year of life. All those born after 1980 who do not have evidence of immunity should be immunized. Most adults, including those with a negative history, are immune to varicella. Assuring the immunity of child care providers, other institution-based workers, those traveling abroad, military personnel, and postpartum women is important. Immunity of health care workers should be ensured. Immunization during pregnancy should be avoided, but if it occurs it should be reported by calling 1-800-986-8999, the Merck Patient Service Center. Varicella immunity should be screened for during pregnancy and those judged to be susceptible should be immunized post partum. The vaccine is quite safe and effective. Breakthrough cases are generally mild but are contagious. Some vaccinees have developed a rash after immunization and may spread vaccine virus to contacts. Caution is advised when immunizing those who may come in contact with pregnant women or immunocompromised individuals. Except for relatively immunocompetent HIV-infected individuals, the latter should not be immunized.

An enhanced varicella vaccine containing at least a log more of vaccine virus has been found to reduce the frequency and severity of zoster and postherpetic neuralgia in those older than 60 years. This vaccine, Zostavax, is recommended for persons older than 60 years of age. 1

Patients in whom varicella develops should be isolated in a negative-pressure room if possible. Those who are susceptible and cannot be discharged should be isolated from the 10th to the 20th day after exposure. Screening for susceptibility with the latex agglutination test may be useful in grouping patients. This test is not as reliable for predicting protection of vaccinees. Increased immunization of health care workers and increased use of the vaccine in the general population should decrease the risk of health care–associated transmission related to exposure to varicella. However, cases occurring in health care workers exposed to zoster continue to be a problem.

Passive immunization is indicated for postexposure prophylaxis of some people. The only product currently available for use in the United States is not licensed by the Food and Drug Administration but is available as an investigational new drug (IND) (contact FFF Enterprises 24-hour telephone, 1-800-843-7477). Patients without evidence of immunity to varicella (i.e., without a history of disease or age-appropriate vaccination) who are at high risk for severe disease and complications, who have been exposed to varicella (e.g., through household contact), and from whom informed consent has been obtained are eligible to receive the IND application product under an expanded access protocol. The groups of patients recommended to receive VariZIG include the following: (1) immunocompromised patients (e.g., patients with bone marrow transplants); (2) neonates whose mothers have signs and symptoms of varicella around the time of delivery (i.e., 5 days before to 2 days after); (3) premature infants born at more than 28 weeks of gestation who are exposed during the neonatal period and whose mothers do not have evidence of immunity; (4) premature infants born at less than 28 weeks of gestation or who weigh less than 1000 g at birth and were exposed during the neonatal period, regardless of maternal history of varicella disease or vaccination; and (5) pregnant women.

A history of varicella is usually reliable in both adults and children. Children who have a negative history are usually susceptible. Serologic testing of adults with the latex agglutination test who have a negative history is useful if it does not delay passive immunization, which should be given as soon as possible after exposure and has not been shown to be effective if delayed more than 96 hours.

Varicella vaccine is recommended for postexposure prophylaxis of other persons without evidence of varicella immunity who have no contraindications to vaccination. The vaccine should be administered preferably within 96 hours and possibly up to 120 hours after exposure. If illness occurs, with or without postexposure vaccination, antiviral treatment (e.g., acyclovir) can be considered for adolescents and adults. Some experts also recommend administration of acyclovir orally from the seventh day after exposure for 7 days.

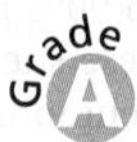

1. Oxman MN, Levin MJ, Johnson GR, et al: A vaccine to prevent herpes zoster and postherpetic neuralgia in older adults. N Engl J Med 2005;352:2271–2284.

SUGGESTED READINGS

Centers for Disease Control and Prevention (CDC): A new product (VariZIG) for postexposure prophylaxis of varicella available under an investigational new drug application expanded access protocol. MMWR Morb Mortal Wkly Rep 2006;55:209–210.

Chaves SC, Gargiullo P, Zhang JX, et al: Loss of vaccine-induced immunity to varicella over time. N Engl J Med 2007;356:1121–1129. *Because vaccine-induced immunity wanes over time, a second dose of varicella vaccine could improve protection from both primary vaccine failure and waning vaccine-induced immunity.*

Dworkin RH, Johnson RW, Breuer J, et al: Recommendations for the management of herpes zoster. Clin Infect Dis 2007;44(Suppl. 1):S1–26. *A review of the evidence-based recommendations for the management of patients with herpes zoster.*

Frangides CY, Pneumatikos I: Varicella-zoster virus pneumonia in adults: Report of 14 cases and review of the literature. Eur J Intern Med 2004;15:364–370. *A report on the current management and outcome of varicella pneumonia in adults.*

Heininger U, Seward J: Varicella. Lancet 2006;368:1365–1376. *A comprehensive overview.*

Jumaan AO, Yu O, Jackson LA, et al: Incidence of herpes zoster, before and after varicella-vaccination-associated decreases in the incidence of varicella, 1992–2002. J Infect Dis 2005;191:2002–2007. *The widespread use of varicella vaccine is not associated with an increased risk of zoster.*

Kimberlin DW, Whitley RJ: Varicella-zoster vaccine for the prevention of herpes zoster. N Engl J Med 2007;356:1338–1343. *A review of varicella zoster virus and the indications for the vaccine.*

van Wijck AJ, Opstelten W, Moons KG, et al: The PINE study of epidural steroids and local anaesthetics to prevent postherpetic neuralgia: A randomised controlled trial. Lancet 2006;367:219–224. *A single epidural injection in the acute phase modestly reduced zoster-associated pain for 1 month.*

399 CYTOMEGALOVIRUS

W. Lawrence Drew

Definition

Cytomegalovirus (CMV) is a member of the herpesvirus family and shares, with the other members, the ability to establish a long-lived latent infection. Most of the clinical disease caused by this virus results from reactivation of latent virus in immune-impaired patients, although primary infection in such patients and in antibody-negative fetuses can also be devastating.

The Pathogen

CMV has a linear, double-stranded DNA genome with about 250,000 base pairs that encode about 160 proteins. Microscopically, the hallmark of CMV infection is a large (cytomegalic), 25- to 35-μm cell containing a large central, basophilic intranuclear inclusion (Fig. 399–1), referred to as an "owl's eye."

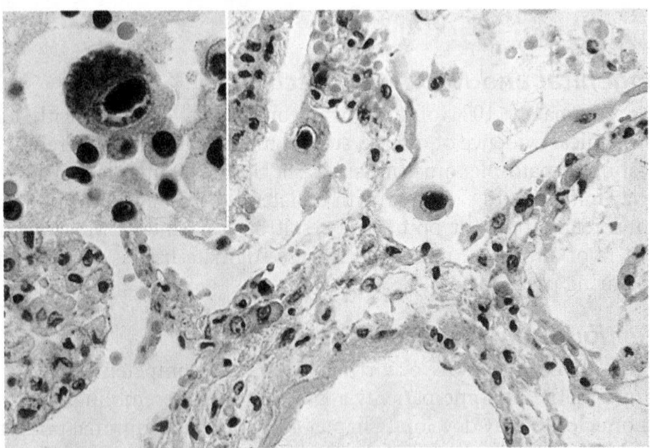

FIGURE 399–1 • Cytomegalovirus (CMV) pneumonia. A lung biopsy specimen was stained with hematoxylin and eosin and magnified 250-fold. The insert shows a CMV "owl's eye" inclusion.

Epidemiology

Multiple mechanisms account for the spread of this virus, including vertical (in utero, during vaginal delivery, and by breast milk) and horizontal contact (saliva, genital, urine). These routes of transmission lead, collectively, to a 15 to 20% seroprevalence by 15 years of age in developed countries, with a higher seroprevalence in lower socioeconomic settings. From that age on, there is a steady upward trend of 1 to 2% per year that is due in part to sexual transmission. As a result, approximately 50% of the general population of the United States is antibody positive by 35 years of age, and a 1% per year rate of increase occurs thereafter. In underdeveloped countries, up to 90% of persons may be seropositive by 2 years old. Presumably, crowded living conditions permit spread of the virus via bodily fluids. Two additional mechanisms of transmission include blood transfusion and organ transplantation. A final important epidemiologic fact is that reinfection with a different strain of CMV may occur in a CMV-seropositive person, especially those who are immunocompromised, pregnant, or sexually promiscuous.

Pathobiology

In fully immunocompetent individuals, CMV rarely causes clinically evident end-organ disease. When immune mechanisms are deficient, especially those mediated by $CD4^+$ and $CD8^+$ lymphocytes, latent virus replicates and causes both direct and indirect effects. Examples of direct virally mediated diseases are necrotizing CMV retinitis and esophagitis. In contrast, CMV pneumonitis is frequently manifested as subtle histologic alterations accompanied by limited viral replication, thus suggesting that immune-mediated injury may be the primary pathologic mechanism. Such injury may result from the upregulation and release of cytokines, including tumor necrosis factor-α, interferon-γ, and interleukin-2. Immune-mediated tissue injury may also be effected by $CD8^+$ cytotoxic T lymphocytes directed against CMV-infected target cells. The clinical manifestations of CMV infection reflect the range of cell types that CMV is capable of infecting, including meningoencephalitis, retinitis, enteritis, vasculitis, pneumonitis, myocarditis, lymphadenitis, hepatitis, adrenalitis, and pancreatitis.

The immune response to CMV infection involves both the humoral and cell-mediated arms, but the $CD8^+$ cytotoxic T-cell response appears to be the most important. The CMV envelope glycoproteins that participate in viral entry are gB, gH/gL, and gcII. Humoral immunity directed at gB has been detected in convalescent phase sera and has been shown to block viral entry, cell-to-cell transmission, and syncytium formation in CMV-infected cells.

Fundamental to the pathogenesis of CMV is latency, or persistence of the viral genome in host cells without evidence of productive viral replication. It is thought that monocytes and bone marrow progenitor cells are sites of human CMV latency. Reactivation from the latent state has classically been associated with immunosuppression. Exposure to a rich milieu of cytokines and growth factors results in the activation of signal transduction pathways, generation of increased levels of intracellular transcription factors, and production of viable virus.

Clinical Manifestations

Congenital and Neonatal Infection

Approximately 10% of newborns congenitally infected with CMV show clinical evidence of disease, such as microcephaly, intracerebral calcification, hepatosplenomegaly, and rash. Up to 700 infants may be born in the United States each year with unilateral or bilateral hearing loss or mental retardation (or both) as a result of congenital CMV infection. Mothers of almost all infants with these stigmata had a primary infection during pregnancy.

Infection in Immunocompetent Persons

Most CMV infections occurring in immunocompetent persons are asymptomatic. In some patients a clinical illness resembling infectious mononucleosis may develop (Chapter 400), but with minimal pharyngitis and lymphadenopathy. Atypical lymphocytosis develops in these patients, similar to Epstein-Barr virus infection, but they have a negative heterophile antibody test.

Infection in Transplant Recipients

When a CMV-seronegative recipient receives a solid organ from a CMV-seropositive donor, the resulting illnesses include the "CMV syndrome," characterized by fever, neutropenia, atypical lymphocytes, and often hepatosplenomegaly. CMV disease may also develop in the transplanted organ. For example, CMV hepatitis in liver transplant recipients is associated with fever, hyperbilirubinemia, and elevated liver enzymes; liver failure may ensue and necessitate retransplantation.

CMV pneumonia may occur after solid organ transplantation but is most common after stem cell transplantation. Fever, nonproductive cough, and dyspnea can progress rapidly. The diagnosis is suggested by interstitial to nodular infiltrates rather than alveolar densities on chest radiographs. In contrast to solid organ transplantation, CMV disease following stem cell transplantation usually results from reactivation of latent CMV in a seropositive recipient.

CMV may cause disease throughout the gastrointestinal tract. Colitis, which is the most common syndrome in transplant recipients, is manifested as diarrhea, weight loss, and fever. It is characterized by diffuse submucosal hemorrhages and ulcerations. CMV retinitis rarely occurs in transplant recipients

Infection in Patients with Acquired Immunodeficiency Syndrome

In the era before highly active antiretroviral therapy, CMV retinitis occurred in approximately a third of patients with acquired immunodeficiency syndrome (AIDS), most often in those with CD4 counts less than 50/mm^3. It usually begins unilaterally with visual blurring, floaters, decreased acuity, and loss of visual fields and progresses to blindness if untreated. Retinal examination reveals apparent hemorrhages and exudates (Fig. 399–2). CMV colitis is similar to that seen in transplant recipients, but esophagitis is also common and characterized by distal ulceration, which may be single but extensive. CMV neurologic disease occurs in multiple forms, including encephalitis and a polyradiculopathy/myelitis syndrome.

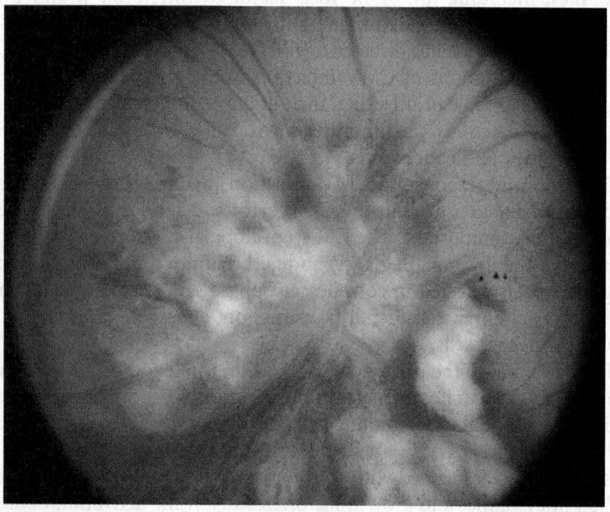

FIGURE 399–2 • Cytomegalovirus retinitis as seen by direct ophthalmoscopic examination.

Diagnosis

Culture

Historically, culture has been regarded as the "gold standard" for detecting CMV infection, but false-negative culture results do occur. Furthermore, CMV grows only in diploid fibroblast cell cultures and may require at least 4 to 6 weeks for detection. More rapid culture results may be achieved by centrifuging specimens in a shell vial seeded with diploid fibroblast cells and examining them after 1 to 2 days of incubation by indirect immunofluorescence. Interpretation of cultures positive for CMV may be difficult, particularly in immunosuppressed patients. For example, CMV may be present in saliva or urine in up to 60 to 90% of transplant recipients or patients with AIDS. Recovery from these sites, however, does not prove that CMV is the cause of a patient's pneumonia or fever. Identification of CMV in blood has greater diagnostic accuracy. Cytologic and histologic abnormalities are not sensitive measures of CMV infection, but they are specific and more indicative of CMV disease than culture of virus from the tissue.

CMV Antigen/Nucleic Acid Detection

Monoclonal antibodies can be used to detect CMV antigens directly in peripheral blood leukocytes (antigenemia) (Fig. 399–3). In addition to enhanced sensitivity, antigenemia offers the possibility of a quantitative assay. Assays of viral DNA by polymerase chain reaction or hybrid capture are also more sensitive than culture and at least comparable to antigenemia assays. These quantitative assays may be particularly useful for early detection of CMV disease and for monitoring therapy. Viral RNA assay may also be a useful indicator of viral replication.

Serology

Seroconversion is an excellent marker for primary CMV infection, but rises in IgG titers, even four-fold or greater, are not diagnostic of newly acquired infection. CMV-specific IgM antibody develops during primary infection but may reappear during reactivation of latent CMV. The presence of IgG antibody is a sensitive marker of past infection and is used to screen transplant recipients and donors, as well as certain blood product recipients and donors.

Prevention

Live attenuated CMV vaccines induce antibody formation, as well as cell-mediated immunity. However, the length of immunity, protection from future infection, and possible oncogenic properties of the vaccine are not known. Nonviable vaccines are being evaluated in clinical trials.

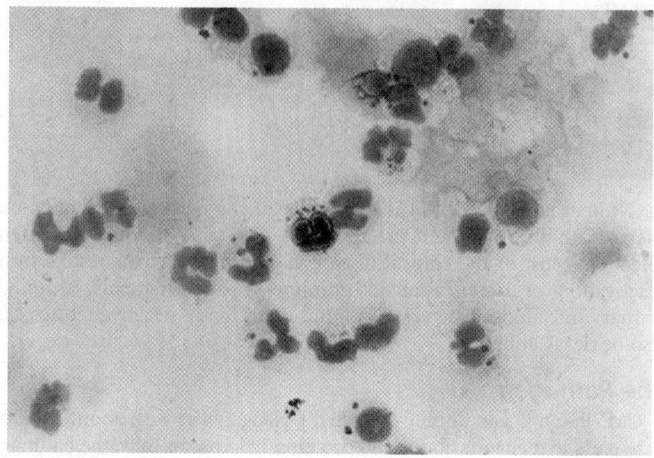

FIGURE 399–3 • Peripheral blood leukocytes stained with monoclonal antibody to cytomegalovirus pp65 antigen by the immunoperoxidase technique (magnification × 500).

Because CMV is transmitted by exchange of secretions or excretions, infection can be diminished by reducing exposure to body fluids. For example, both vaginal and anal intercourse are bidirectional risks for transmission.

The risk of acquiring CMV disease can be reduced in seronegative, immunosuppressed patients through the use of blood products or organ grafts from CMV-seronegative donors. Preemptive treatment is beneficial to prevent CMV disease in recipients of solid organ transplants. [1] Prophylactic administration of high-titer CMV antibody to transplant recipients reduces the risk for CMV disease, even though subclinical infections are not prevented. Acyclovir is of some benefit in preventing CMV disease in transplant recipients, but valganciclovir and ganciclovir are more protective. Universal prophylaxis is used less frequently for stem cell transplant recipients; instead, these patients may be monitored weekly (from day 10 to day 100 after transplantation) for CMV DNA or antigenemia, and antiviral therapy is introduced preemptively if positivity occurs. Thus, active infection is not prevented, but end-organ disease is avoided.

Treatment

Rx

Ganciclovir (dihydroxypropoxymethylguanosine [DHPG], Cytovene) is given intravenously, 5 mg/kg two times daily during initial induction (2 to 3 weeks), and maintenance therapy consists of 5 mg/kg once daily (Chapter 383). The oral form of ganciclovir is given at a dose of 3 g/day for maintenance treatment, but it has been largely replaced by valganciclovir, which achieves levels comparable to intravenous ganciclovir when given orally in a 900-mg dose. Administration of ganciclovir is indicated for the treatment of acute CMV disease, but granulocyte colony–stimulating factor may be needed to offset neutropenia. Initial response in retinitis (improvement or stabilization of vision or ophthalmoscopic appearance) occurs in approximately 75% of patients treated with ganciclovir alone. CMV retinitis can also be treated locally by implanting a sustained-release device. Ganciclovir together with CMV hyperimmune globulin may reduce the mortality of CMV pneumonia after stem cell transplantation from approximately 85% to 40%. CMV colitis may improve with ganciclovir therapy. Ganciclovir resistance may occur as a result of mutations in the phosphorylating gene or in the DNA polymerase gene.

Foscarnet, or phosphonoformic acid, blocks the pyrophosphate-binding site of viral DNA polymerase, thereby preventing cleavage of pyrophosphate from deoxyadenosine triphosphate. Resistance to foscarnet can develop because of mutations in DNA polymerase. The recommended initial therapy with foscarnet is 60 mg/kg intravenously every 8 hours or 90 mg/kg every 12 hours. The maintenance dosage ranges from 90 to 120 mg/kg daily. Adverse effects include renal impairment, anemia, hypocalcemia (especially ionized calcium), hypomagnesemia, and hypophosphatemia. Because of toxicity and the absence of an oral formulation, foscarnet is usually a second choice for treating CMV but may sometimes be used in combination with ganciclovir for serious infections such as retinitis.

Cidofovir, or 3-hydroxy-2-phosphonomethoxypropyl cytosine (HPMPC), appears to the cell as a nucleotide and does not require phosphorylation by viral-encoded enzyme. It is therefore active against the majority of ganciclovir-resistant CMV strains that have resistance mutations only in *UL97,* the phosphorylating gene. When polymerase, *UL54,* mutations occur in ganciclovir-treated patients, cross-resistance to cidofovir is frequent. These resistance mutations also occur in patients treated with cidofovir de novo. The drug has an extremely long half-life that permits intravenous administration as infrequently as every 2 weeks during maintenance treatment.

Cidofovir is nephrotoxic, especially to the proximal renal tubule, but this side effect can be diminished by prehydration and concomitant probenecid therapy. Cidofovir is as effective as the combination of oral ganciclovir plus a ganciclovir vitreal implant, [2] but its toxicities make it a second- or third-line agent for CMV.

Prognosis

In immunocompetent patients, the mononucleosis-like CMV syndrome resolves spontaneously. Infections in immunocompromised patients are much more serious and often result in failure of a transplanted solid organ. For CMV pneumonia, death is common even with antiviral therapy, especially after stem cell transplantation. In AIDS patients, CMV infection generally resolves when CD4 counts exceed 100/mm^3 but is a grave prognostic sign if counts do not recover to this level.

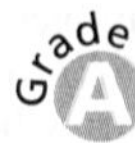

1. Strippoli GF, Hodson EM, Jones CJ, et al: Pre-emptive treatment for cytomegalovirus viremia to prevent cytomegalovirus disease in solid organ transplant recipients Cochrane Database Syst Rev 2006;1:CD005133.
2. The Studies of Ocular Complications of AIDS Research Group in Collaboration with the AIDS Clinical Trials Group: The ganciclovir implant plus oral ganciclovir versus parenteral cidofovir for the treatment of cytomegalovirus retinitis in patients with acquired immunodeficiency syndrome: The ganciclovir cidofovir cytomegalovirus retinitis trial. Am J Ophthalmol 2001;131:457–467.

SUGGESTED READINGS

Drew WL: Is combination antiviral therapy for CMV superior to monotherapy? J Clin Virol 2006;35:485–488. *The two approaches seem to be similar.*

Hodson E, Jones C, Strippoli G, et al: Immunoglobulins, vaccines or interferon for preventing cytomegalovirus disease in solid organ transplant recipients. Cochrane Database Syst Rev 2007;(2):CD005129. *A review of the use of IgG, anti CMV vaccines, or interferon for preventing symptomatic CMV disease in solid organ transplant recipients.*

Steininger C, Puchhammer-Stockl E, Popow-Kraupp T: Cytomegalovirus disease in the era of highly active antiretroviral therapy (HAART). J Clin Virol 2006;37:1–9. *A practical overview.*

400 EPSTEIN-BARR VIRUS INFECTION

Robert T. Schooley

Definition

Epstein-Barr virus (EBV), a member of the gamma human herpesvirus family, is the etiologic agent of infectious mononucleosis. In addition, the etiologic role of EBV in the pathogenesis of a number of neoplastic syndromes is increasingly becoming apparent.

Epidemiology

Ubiquitous in the human population, EBV is found in 90 to 95% of adults throughout the world. As in the case of other herpesviruses, infection with EBV is lifelong. The virus resides in B lymphocytes and is intermittently shed asymptomatically in oropharyngeal secretions, which accounts for the bulk of its transmission in the human population. The virus is not highly contagious; it is usually acquired during early childhood through sharing of saliva-bearing fomites or during adolescence through kissing, although it can be acquired at any decade of life. Thus, for example, EBV-seronegative platonic roommates of patients with acute infectious mononucleosis in college dormitory settings are not at higher risk for acquiring the virus than others in the college population. Although clusters of cases of infectious mononucleosis have been reported, these reports were generally made before the modern era of specific virologic diagnosis and now are not believed to be plausible. In addition to oropharyngeal spread, the virus can be transmitted by blood transfusion or through organ donation.

Most childhood EBV infections are clinically silent, but infection of adolescents and adults results in the clinical syndrome of infectious mononucleosis between 25 and 70% of the time, depending on the setting. The incidence of infectious mononucleosis is highest in the 15- to 24-year-old age group. Incidence rates in men and women are equal, but the peak incidence is 2 years earlier in women than in men. Incidence rates are lower in lower socioeconomic populations, in whom the likelihood of acquisition is greater in childhood than in adolescence.

Pathobiology

EBV enters B lymphocytes through the CD21 molecule (also known as the C3d receptor) on the surface of B cells or nasopharyngeal epithelial cells. Major histocompatibility complex class II molecules serve as secondary receptors on B cells. Once inside the cell, the virus expresses a series of nuclear proteins (termed Epstein-Barr nuclear antigens [EBNAs]), which in turn activate EBV-encoded latent membrane proteins and other gene products responsible for regulation of B-cell growth. This sequence of events leads to the transformation or immortalization of the B cell that is the phenotypic hallmark of B-cell infection. EBV-transformed B cells proliferate vigorously both in vivo and in vitro and maintain EBV within progeny cell nuclei in an episomal state. During acute EBV infection, up to 20% of peripheral blood B cells express EBNA.

The host response to acute EBV infection consists of a vigorous and coordinated cellular and humoral immune response. The humoral immune response includes IgM and IgG antibodies directed at the viral capsid (VCA) and to EBNA, as well as antibodies to antigens on the surface of sheep red blood cells. Sheep red blood cell–directed antibodies, termed *heterophile antibodies,* are useful diagnostically and are present in up to 90% of cases, although they are not always demonstrable at initial evaluation. These antibodies are probably an epiphenomenon in terms of host defense and are not cross-reactive with any known viral antigens.

The cellular immune response includes both natural killer and EBV-specific $CD4^+$ and $CD8^+$ T lymphocytes. The expansion of the $CD8^+$ subset of T lymphocytes during acute EBV infection includes a subset of large, activated cells demonstrable on standard peripheral blood smears as "atypical" lymphocytes. This vigorous cellular immune response is associated with an outpouring of cytokines, including tumor necrosis factor, interleukin-1, and interleukin-6, which are probably responsible for many of the symptoms and signs of infectious mononucleosis. Over a period of 4 to 6 weeks after initial evaluation in most patients, immune response mechanisms gain control of the EBV-driven B-cell proliferation and the virus enters into a lifelong period of symbiosis with the host. The virus is asymptomatically shed approximately 15% of the time in the oropharyngeal fluids of healthy human immunodeficiency virus type 1 (HIV-1)-seronegative adolescents and adults. The shedding rate increases significantly in patients with defects in cellular immunity, such as those that occur with HIV-1 infection or immunosuppression associated with organ allografts.

Clinical Manifestations

Most cases of acute EBV infection are clinically silent. The syndrome of infectious mononucleosis consists of the clinical triad of fever, sore throat, and lymphadenopathy, in association with an atypical lymphocytosis and the transient appearance of heterophile antibodies. Epidemiologic studies indicate that the incubation period between exposure and the onset of symptoms is generally 30 to 50 days. The onset of symptoms may be abrupt, or it may be heralded by a several-day nonspecific prodrome of malaise and low-grade fever. Although the classic syndrome includes fever, sore throat, and adenopathy, the findings may be dominated by only one or any combination of these symptoms. Other common clinical manifestations include headache, malaise, and anorexia. On physical examination, patients are usually febrile. Pharyngeal erythema, tonsillar enlargement, and cervical adenopathy are generally present. Mild periorbital edema may also be observed. Abdominal findings may include splenomegaly or hepatomegaly, or both. Although most patients will have mild splenomegaly at some point in their illness, splenic enlargement is usually maximal in the second or third week of illness and might not be detectable at the initial clinical manifestation of the illness. Adenopathy may be observed in noncervical regions, but it is usually much less prominent than in cervical regions. Approximately 5% of patients will exhibit a rash that may be macular, scarlatiniform, or urticarial in nature. If patients with acute EBV infection are given ampicillin or its derivatives, a pruritic maculopapular eruption will develop in 90 to 100% of them. Patients with an ampicillin-induced rash during acute EBV infection generally tolerate the drug and other penicillin products when administered after the infection has resolved.

Diagnosis

Because clinical manifestations of acute EBV infection vary from patient to patient and other organisms may cause similar clinical syndromes, laboratory tools are required to confirm an etiologic diagnosis. Heterophile antibodies to sheep red blood cells are classically used to diagnosis EBV-induced infectious mononucleosis. Though ultimately demonstrable in approximately 90% of symptomatic acute EBV infections, these antibodies are present in only about two thirds of patients at initial encounter. If antibodies are negative at the outset and clinical suspicion is high, repeat testing in the second or third week of the illness is warranted. Although EBV-specific antibodies remain the "gold standard" for the diagnosis of acute EBV infection, if heterophile antibodies are demonstrated in a straightforward case of infectious mononucleosis, it is not generally necessary to order EBV-specific serologic studies. IgM antibodies to the EBV capsid antigen (VCA) are the most useful serologic study in the diagnosis of acute EBV infection. Relatively high titers of IgG antibodies to VCA persist for life after initial infection and are not useful in making the diagnosis of acute EBV infection. Antibodies to EBNA are slower to arise than those to capsid antigens, and acute infection may be diagnosed by demonstration of seroconversion to this antigen. EBV-specific antibodies may be demonstrated by immunofluorescence or by enzyme-linked immunosorbent assay. If the diagnosis is based on the emergence of antibodies to EBNA, both tests should be performed in the same laboratory.

A number of other pathogens may be accompanied by clinical syndromes that can be mistaken for acute EBV infection. Cytomegalovirus is the organism most frequently associated with a clinical syndrome that is mistaken for EBV infection. Patients with cytomegalovirus infection are less likely to have an acute onset of illness, and pharyngitis is less frequently a prominent manifestation of the illness. *Toxoplasma gondii* infection can also be manifested as a nonspecific febrile illness that can be confused with infectious mononucleosis. Streptococcal pharyngitis and primary herpes stomatitis may occasionally cause symptoms that are mistaken for acute EBV infection. None of these syndromes are associated with heterophile antibodies or with other serologic evidence of acute EBV infection. The differential diagnosis is generally made by serologic studies directed at these organisms or by culture. Nonetheless, physicians should be cognizant that organisms such as group A β-hemolytic streptococci are also common in the human population and may be demonstrated in people whose symptoms are nonetheless due to acute EBV infection.

Prevention and Treatment

Rx

Because the virus is usually transmitted by asymptomatic oral shedders and is so common in the human population, epidemiologic interventions to prevent spread are not practical. No vaccine has been developed yet. The clinical course is generally self-limited and does not usually require specific therapeutic intervention beyond the use of aspirin or acetaminophen for antipyresis and mild pain relief, except in the presence of specific complications such as when lymphadenopathy threatens the airway or in certain cases of autoimmune hemolytic anemia or thrombocytopenia. Short courses of corticosteroids have been used to hasten symptomatic recovery in cases in which the symptoms are severe or refractory. Corticosteroids should not, however, be used routinely and should consist of no more than a 10- to 14-day tapering course that begins at a dose equivalent of 0.5 mg/kg of prednisone. Although EBV replication can be inhibited in vitro or in vivo by acyclovir and related antiviral agents, the symptoms of infectious mononucleosis are primarily driven by the immune response to the virus and follow the time of maximal viral replication. Antiviral agents have not been demonstrated to significantly accelerate resolution of symptoms or prevent complications of the disease.

Prognosis

Most patients recover uneventfully from the acute symptoms and signs of infectious mononucleosis over a 2- to 3-week period, although many patients may have a variable period of malaise and fatigue that can last for another 3 to 4 weeks. Some patients may take longer to make a full recovery and experience fatigue and difficulty concentrating for up to 6 months after diagnosis. Symptoms often wax and wane and can be extremely troublesome. Reassurance is usually the best approach to these patients. There is less evidence that corticosteroids are of benefit in this setting. Recovery may be less straightforward in patients with certain specific complications of acute EBV infection (outlined in the next section). Death from infectious mononucleosis is rare. When it does occur, it is most frequently associated with neurologic complications of the illness, splenic rupture, or the X-linked lymphoproliferative syndrome (discussed later).

Complications

Although most patients recover spontaneously from acute EBV infection, a number of complications may arise. In some patients, these complications dominate the clinical findings, and seroconversion may be the only evidence of acute EBV infection. The most serious complication of acute EBV infection arises in individuals with the X-linked lymphoproliferative syndrome. This syndrome occurs in males with mutations in the signaling lymphocyte activation molecule (SLAM)-associated protein that regulates T and natural killer cells. These otherwise healthy individuals have severe clinical symptoms, a large lymphocytosis consisting of T and B cells, and severe hepatitis. If patients survive the acute infection, the syndrome may evolve into progressive agammaglobulinemia or lymphoma in the following months.

A number of less severe, organ system–specific complications are seen substantially more frequently than the aforementioned X-linked lymphoproliferative syndrome. Patients should be specifically warned about splenic rupture, a complication attributable to splenomegaly and associated stretching of the splenic capsule that occurs most frequently in the second or third week of the illness, when other symptoms of the disease are abating. It is generally accompanied by trauma of some sort but can occasionally occur without an obvious antecedent event. Patients should be counseled against activities that might result in abdominal trauma for 6 to 8 weeks after the onset of symptoms. Left upper quadrant pain, especially pain radiating to the subscapular region, should raise this diagnostic consideration. As with other complications of acute EBV infection, splenic rupture may occur occasionally in patients without other prominent clinical manifestations of acute EBV infection. Other hematologic complications include autoimmune hemolytic anemia, thrombocytopenia, and neutropenia. These complications usually arise from a combination of self-reactive antibodies and hypersplenism and are generally self-limited and resolve with resolution of the illness. Corticosteroids may be of benefit in more severe cases of autoimmune hemolytic anemia or thrombocytopenia.

Neurologic complications are also reported during acute EBV infection. EBV DNA has been detected in brain tissue from rare patients with clinical manifestations compatible with herpes simplex encephalitis. Although these patients have a much better prognosis than those with herpes simplex encephalitis, they should receive parenteral acyclovir. Other neurologic complications include aseptic meningitis, cerebellitis, mononeuritis multiplex, Bell's palsy, Guillain-Barré syndrome, and transverse myelitis. These complications may be clinically dramatic but are usually self-limited and associated with full recovery in 85% of patients without specific antiviral therapy.

Mild hepatomegaly is not uncommon in acute infectious mononucleosis, and biochemical evidence of hepatitis is to be expected in virtually every case of acute infection. More severe hepatic complications are uncommon, although they have been reported. Renal, cardiac, pulmonary, and skeletal muscle complications are rare.

Other Clinical Manifestations of EBV Infection

In addition to infectious mononucleosis, EBV is also associated with neoplasia and lymphoproliferative disorders, which are seen most frequently in patients with defects in cellular immunity but are not restricted to such patients.

Post-transplant Lymphoproliferative Disease

EBV-driven B-cell proliferation that is insufficiently regulated in the presence of prolonged periods of severe T-cell immunodeficiency may result in a polyclonal proliferation of B cells that is initially similar to that seen in acute infectious mononucleosis. Though most frequently occurring in the setting of organ transplantation, especially when patients are immunosuppressed with agents directed specifically at T lymphocytes, such as anti-CD3 antibodies or cyclosporine, this syndrome can be seen in other conditions with similar levels and durations of immunodeficiency such as HIV-1 infection. Patients with this disorder often initially have fever, adenopathy, and splenomegaly. Intestinal B-cell proliferation is also common. If the immunodeficiency persists, the natural history of these disorders is that they often proceed from a polyclonal stage, which can be reversed with restoration of immunity, to a monoclonal or oligoclonal stage that is progressive despite restoration of cellular immunodeficiency. These tumors are less frequently seen in the current era in which allograft-associated immunosuppression is better targeted and less intense. The diagnosis is not generally difficult to make in the appropriate clinical setting and can be made histopathologically. There is some evidence that post-transplant lymphoproliferative disorder (PTLD) may be less frequent in patients who have received acyclovir or ganciclovir after transplantation, but these agents are less useful once the syndrome develops. Successful management depends on the extent to which the immunosuppressive condition can be reversed. Surgery or radiation therapy, or both, have also been used. Recently, there have been reports of successful therapy for PTLD with anti-CD20 antibodies.

Burkitt's Lymphoma

EBV was initially described in the setting of African Burkitt's lymphoma. The tumor is composed of small, noncleaved B cells and, unless aggressively treated, is rapidly fatal. This aggressive B-cell lymphoma with a predilection for the head and neck is endemic in equatorial Africa and is geographically linked to *Plasmodium falciparum* malaria. EBV DNA is readily demonstrable in tumor biopsy specimens, and high titers of antibodies to EBV structural antigens are found in plasma. Sporadic cases of abdominal B-cell lymphomas with a histologic appearance compatible with Burkitt's lymphoma are also observed but are associated with EBV only about 25% of the time. The tumor is likewise seen in patients with HIV-1 infection, but it is not as clearly associated with advanced immunodeficiency as other complications of HIV-1 infection are. Although an etiologic role for EBV in Burkitt's lymphoma is widely accepted, the molecular basis by which EBV causes the neoplasm has not yet been fully delineated. Despite the high-grade clinical behavior of the tumor, it should be vigorously treated because it is often quite responsive to combination chemotherapy with or without radiation therapy.

Hodgkin's Lymphoma

EBV is also associated with a subset of Hodgkin's lymphomas. The association between the tumor and EBV is best established in tumors of the lymphocyte-depleted or mixed-cellularity histologic subtypes. EBV DNA and proteins are detected in the Reed-Sternberg cells that are characteristic of Hodgkin's lymphoma. Therapy for EBV-associated Hodgkin's lymphoma is directed at the tumor. The specific approach used is based on the histology and extent of disease and is not determined in a given patient by its relationship to EBV.

Central Nervous System Lymphoma

EBV is also associated with central nervous system (CNS) lymphoma. This tumor was most frequently observed in the post-transplant setting before the HIV epidemic but is now the most frequent CNS neoplasm in HIV-1–infected individuals. The major differential diagnostic challenge is with *T. gondii* infection. Although a tissue-based diagnosis is definitive, noninvasive neurodiagnostic approaches coupled with the demonstration of EBV DNA in CSF by polymerase chain reaction can strongly support the diagnosis of lymphoma over that of *T. gondii* infection. Treatment involves radiation therapy but it is generally unsatisfactory.

Nasopharyngeal Carcinoma

EBV has also been associated with certain cases of nasopharyngeal carcinoma. This tumor is rare in Western countries, but it is much more frequent in southern China and in the Inuit population of Alaska. EBV-associated cases are more often less histologically differentiated than sporadic forms of nasopharyngeal carcinoma. EBV DNA is demonstrable in tumor tissue, and high titers of IgA and IgG antibodies to the EBV capsid antigens are found in plasma. The prognosis for this tumor is poor, although it is often treated with radiation therapy.

Oral Hairy Leukoplakia

This clinical manifestation of EBV infection is characterized by a corrugated or "hairy" plaquelike lesion that extends around the lateral aspects of the tongue. Oral hairy leukoplakia (OHL) is most often observed in individuals with chronic forms of cellular immunodeficiency, especially those with HIV-1 infection and CD4 cell counts less than 200/mm^3. It is most often clinically confused with mucocutaneous candidiasis but can be differentiated because its distribution is restricted to the lateral surface of the tongue and, unlike thrush, does not involve the buccal mucosa, palate, or pharynx and is not readily removed by superficial scraping. Biopsies demonstrate a characteristic histopathologic pattern, as well as the presence of EBV antigens and DNA within squamous epithelial cells. Although the lesions may be cosmetically troublesome, they are not generally painful. In the case of HIV-1–associated OHL, the lesions resolve with successful antiretroviral chemotherapy. If the immunosuppression cannot be reversed, OHL usually responds to valacyclovir, valganciclovir, or foscarnet.

Chronic Active EBV Infection

Infrequent patients with no apparent defect in cellular immunity have been described in which chronic EBV infection has been associated with persistent or intermittent hepatitis or interstitial pulmonary disease (or both). These rare patients with bona fide organ system disease should not be confused with those who have chronic fatigue syndrome. This nonspecific clinical syndrome, seen most frequently in young and middle-aged women, is characterized by malaise and difficulty concentrating and lacks objective physical findings. Although an etiologic or contributing role for EBV had been posited in the past, there is no convincing evidence that the virus plays a role in this condition.

SUGGESTED READINGS

Andreone P, Gramenzi A, Lorenzini S, et al: Posttransplantation lymphoproliferative disorders. Arch Intern Med 2003;163:1997–2004. *A well-organized review of the clinical manifestations and management of post-transplantation EBV-associated lymphoproliferative disorders.*

Candy B, Hotopf M: Steroids for symptom control in infectious mononucleosis. Cochrane Database Syst Rev 2006;3:CD004402. *There is insufficient evidence to recommend steroid treatment for symptom control in infectious mononucleosis.*

Choquet S, Leblond V, Herbrecht R, et al: Efficacy and safety of rituximab in B-cell post-transplantation lymphoproliferative disorders: Results of a prospective multicenter phase 2 study. Blood 2006;107:3053–3057. *Very well written description of the use of rituximab for the treatment of post-transplant lymphoproliferative disorders.*

Higgins CD, Swerdlow AJ, Macsween KF, et al: A study of risk factors for acquisition of Epstein-Barr virus and its subtypes. J Infect Dis 2007;195:474–482. *There is substantial evidence to support that EBV may be sexually transmitted.*

Latour S, Veillette A: Molecular and immunological basis of X-linked lymphoproliferative disease. Immunol Rev 2003;192:212–224. *A comprehensive review of the molecular basis of the EBV-associated X-linked lymphoproliferative syndrome.*

401 RETROVIRUSES OTHER THAN HUMAN IMMUNODEFICIENCY VIRUS

William A. Blattner

Definition

There are now three members of the human T-lymphotropic virus (HTLV) family: HTLV-1, discovered in 1979; HTLV-2, discovered in 1982; and HTLV-3, discovered in 2005 and about which little is known. HTLV-1 has been causally linked to adult T-cell leukemia/lymphoma (ATL) and to several chronic degenerative conditions, most notably HTLV-1–associated myelopathy/tropical spastic paraparesis (HAM/TSP), whereas disease associated with HTLV-2 is rare, and no disease associations have been established with HTLV-3.

The Pathogens

Within the taxa of RNA reverse-transcribing viruses, the HTLV viruses, along with bovine leukemia virus, are classified in the subfamily Retroviridae within the genus Deltaretrovirus (formerly termed oncovirus). The oncogenic properties of these viruses and their molecular structure distinguish them from the human immunodeficiency retroviruses HIV-1 and HIV-2 (Chapter 409), which are members of the genus Lentivirus. Both deltaretroviruses and lentiviruses are capable of prolonged asymptomatic infection. In vitro, however, HIV-1 and HIV-2 have cytopathic effects on human T cells, whereas HTLV-1 and HTLV-2 are capable of transforming T cells into immortalized cell lines. The HTLVs are diploid single-stranded RNA viruses that replicate through cDNA, a proviral intermediate, via reverse transcriptase, a viral enzyme.

Epidemiology

Geographically, HTLV-1 is widely disseminated worldwide and is estimated to infect 10 to 25 million persons, with the aggressive T-cell malignancy ATL developing in 1 to 5% and chronic inflammatory diseases, mainly HAM/TSP, developing in another 1 to 5% in their lifetime. Similar to HIV, molecular epidemiology suggests that the three major subtypes of HTLV identified in humans arose from separate interspecies transmission from simians to humans. Related to such interspecies transmission, there are three major lineages of HTLV-1: Melanesian (Papua New Guinea, Melanesia, and Australian aborigines), central African, and cosmopolitan groups. Within the cosmopolitan group are four subtypes: (A) transcontinental, (B) Japanese, (C) West African, and (D) North African. The virus from Melanesia differs molecularly from the Japanese and African strains by 5 to 10%, the result of independent evolution of the virus in these populations separated for tens of thousands of years. The stability of HTLV-1 in comparison to HIV-1 reflects the observation that HTLV favors viral expansion through proliferation of proviral DNA–harboring cells rather than infection of new cells by cell-free virions.

HTLV-1 is not universally present in all human populations but rather clusters geographically in southern Japan; Melanesia; Australia, in aboriginal peoples; West Africa and, via the slave trade from Africa, the Caribbean and the United States in African Americans; southern India; and the Mashad region of Iran. In the United States, HTLV-1 infection is often found in persons who migrate from these regions. HTLV-2 is found in Native American people throughout North, Central, and South America and in West Africa. Most HTLV-2 infections in the United States and Europe occur in injection drug users, in whom the virus is spread by needle sharing and other injection practices. Based on limited information, HTLV-3 occurs in West Africa.

Routes of Transmission

HTLV, like HIV-1, is transmitted sexually, perinatally, and by transfusion or injection drug use (Table 401–1).

Sexual Transmission

Sexual transmission of HTLV-1 from male to female and from female to male, as well as from male to male, has been documented. HTLV-1 transmission is cell associated and appears to be at least an order of magnitude less infectious than HIV-1. Coincidental infection with other sexually transmitted diseases, particularly those associated with ulcerative and inflammatory genital lesions, amplifies the risk of transmission. For HTLV-1, elevated viral load is linked to heightened transmission. In regions endemic for the virus, there is a characteristic age-dependent rise in HTLV-1 seroprevalence. This increase first becomes evident in the adolescent years; it is steeper in women than in men and continues in women after 40 years of age, whereas rates in men plateau around the age of 40. This pattern reflects more efficient male-to-female transmission. For HTLV-2, the rates for both genders are equal, thus suggesting that there may be differences in the kinetics of transmission between the two viruses.

TABLE 401–1 TRANSMISSION OF HTLV-1 AND HTLV-2

Mode of Transmission	HTLV-1	HTLV-2
MOTHER TO INFANT		
Transplacental	Yes	Not known
Breast milk	Yes	Probable
SEXUAL		
Male to female	Yes	Yes
Female to male	Yes	Yes
Male to male	Yes	Not known
PARENTERAL		
Blood transfusion	Yes	Yes
Intravenous drug use	Yes	Yes
COFACTORS		
Ulcerative genital lesions	Yes	Not known
Cellular transfusion products	Yes	Yes
Sharing of "works"*	Yes	Yes
ELEVATED VIRUS LOAD		
Mother to infant	Yes	Not known
Heterosexual	Yes	Not known

*Intravenous paraphernalia, such as needles.
HTLV-1/2 = human T-lymphotropic virus type I/II.

Perinatal Transmission

For HTLV-1, transmission through breast-feeding is more efficient than in utero or perinatal transmission. On average, 20% of infants breast-fed by HTLV-1–positive mothers seroconvert to HTLV-1, whereas only 1 to 2% of bottle-fed infants of HTLV-1–positive mothers become infected. In contrast, in utero and perinatal transmission accounts for virtually all HIV-1 transmission in the West, and breast-feeding accounts for an additional 15 to 20% of infant HIV infection in Africa. This difference may reflect the fact that maternal antibody to HTLV-1 transmitted across the placenta appears to neutralize perinatal HTLV-1 but not the highly mutable HIV-1. HTLV-2 is detectable in breast milk and, similar to HTLV-1, accounts for many childhood infections.

Transfusion and Injection Drug Use

Parenteral transmission, either through transfusion or injection drug use, is a major source of HTLV infection. Among blood donors in the United States, more than half of HTLV infections are due to HTLV-2. Among injection drug users, the vast majority of infections are due to HTLV-2; it is projected that HTLV-2 is more efficiently transmitted by this route than HTLV-1 is.

Both HTLV-1 and HTLV-2 are transmitted in association with cellular components, unlike HIV-1, which is transmitted by cells, plasma, or plasma products. Approximately 50% of the recipients of HTLV-1/HTLV-2–positive blood seroconvert as compared with more than 95% for HIV-1.

The only documented illness linked to HTLV-1 or HTLV-2 transfusion-associated transmission is the HTLV-associated demyelinating neurologic syndrome HAM/TSP. Leukemia has not been associated with transfusion of HTLV-positive blood. Among U.S. blood donors who are confirmed to be HTLV positive (slightly less than half are HTLV-1 positive and the others are HTLV-2 positive), the major risk factors are intravenous drug use, birthplace in an area in the Caribbean or Japan endemic for the virus, or sexual contact with a person with this profile.

Coinfection with HTLV-1 and HIV-1 appears to increase the progression to acquired immunodeficiency syndrome (AIDS) through unexplained mechanisms, possibly related to the cell-proliferative effects of HTLV-1 on HIV-1–infected T cells. Such a relationship has not been shown for HTLV-2. Other modes of transmission involving "casual contact" are not a source of infection. Health care and laboratory workers who experience a needlestick or skin or mucous membrane exposure in the absence of protective barriers have little or no risk for infection but should be monitored.

Pathobiology

Virology

The HTLV viruses, which are single-stranded RNA viruses that contain a diploid genome, replicate through a DNA intermediary that integrates into the genome of the target T cell as a provirus, thereby resulting in lifelong infection. HTLV-1 is approximately 100 nm in diameter and has a thin, electron-dense outer envelope and an electron-dense, roughly spherical core. The total provirus genome contains 9032 nucleotides with two identical sequences termed long terminal repeats (LTRs) at the 5′ and 3′ ends of the genome, which contain regulatory elements that control virus expression and virion production. The retroviral structural genes (*gag* and *pol*) code for large overlapping polyproteins that are later processed into functional peptide products by virally encoded protease and cellular proteases. The encoding genes of the virus are *gag* (group-specific antigen), *pol* (polymerase/integrase/protease), and *env* (envelope), and it has a series of regulatory genes, *tax* and *rex,* and several smaller gene products that regulate infection and virus expression. Tax protein plays a central role in enhancing the transcription of viral and cellular gene products that promote viral replication and transformation of human T lymphocytes. Through binding to the LTR, Tax promotes transcriptional activation of the viral genome and, by binding to key regulatory proteins of the cell, promotes cell activation and disease pathogenesis. Through binding to regulatory enhancers of the cell and through abrogation of key suppressor genes, Tax not only promotes cellular growth but also appears to have an impact on pathogenesis of the disease (see later). Rex stabilizes viral mRNA, essential for export of full-length Gag/Pol and single-spliced Env mRNA from the nucleus to the cytoplasm.

Viral Life Cycle

The life cycle of the HTLVs involves attachment, membrane fusion, and reverse transcription from an RNA template to a circular DNA provirus that is transported to the cell nucleus and integrated into the host genome. Both cell-free and cell-to-cell transmission of HTLV-1 has been documented, but once infected, viral expansion is primarily achieved through proliferation of proviral DNA–harboring cells rather than through repeated cycles of cell-to-cell infection. Glut-1, the major vertebrate glucose transporter, is the cellular receptor for HTLV-1 attachment to the cell. Given the ubiquity of this receptor, the cellular trophism of HTLV-1 for $CD4^+$ cells and HTLV-2 for $CD8^+$ cells appears to involve postinfection transcriptional mechanisms; in contrast, HIV targets $CD4^+$ cells through direct binding with a cell-specific receptor. After uptake and uncoating, viral RNA is transcribed by *reverse transcriptase,* an RNA-dependent DNA polymerase complexed to the RNA in the core of the virus particle, into double-stranded DNA. This double-stranded viral DNA is integrated into the host cell nucleus by the virally encoded integrase, which results in lifelong cell infection. The viral LTR elements are essential for integration and regulation of viral genome expression.

Pathogenesis of Adult T-Cell Leukemia

HTLV-1 is integrally involved in the pathogenesis of ATL through a multistage process that includes clonal integration of virus (sometimes including partial viral sequences that always include *tax*) into active cellular gene sequences. The clonal pattern of integration indicates that ATL is derived from a single transformed tumor cell that evolved from a virus infection *before* transformation rather than afterward as a passenger virus. Tax interacts with numerous cellular proteins to reprogram cellular processes to alter transcription, cell cycle regulation, DNA repair, and apoptosis, thereby allowing cells with potential carcinogenic mutations to survive and escape cell death.

In some healthy carriers, T-cell polyclonal and oligoclonal proliferations develop that can later progress to malignancy or may disappear spontaneously. Morphologically distinct "flower cells," which represent T cells with deeply lobulated nuclei resembling ATL leukemic cells, are seen on peripheral blood smears of healthy carriers but do not always presage risk for subsequent disease.

Pathogenesis of Myelopathy/Spastic Paraparesis

Viral overproduction, as measured by high viral loads, appears to result from defective host immune responses characterized by very high levels of cytotoxic T cells. Local pathologic changes in neuronal tissue may result from immune-mediated damage caused by misdirected responses to molecular mimics of viral proteins.

ADULT T-CELL LEUKEMIA/LYMPHOMA

Clinical Manifestations

The most common malignancy caused by HTLV-1 is ATL, a type of T/natural killer cell lymphoma in the new World Health Organization classification (Table 401–2). The subtypes of ATL (acute, chronic, smoldering, and lymphoma [Fig. 401–1]) have different clinical features and prognoses. These tumors represent high-grade lymphomas (Chapter 196), usually of large, medium, or pleiotropic morphology (or combined morphology) and advanced clinical stage, and they are associated with a poor prognosis.

The acute form of ATL is characterized by an aggressive, mature T-cell lymphoma whose clinical course is often associated with a high white blood cell count, hypercalcemia, and cutaneous involvement. Other cases resemble T-prolymphocytic leukemia and are termed *chronic ATL.* Smoldering ATL may clinically resemble mycosis fungoides/Sézary syndrome, with cutaneous involvement manifested as erythema or as infiltrative plaques or tumors. Sometimes a long prodrome of signs (e.g., cutaneous rashes) and symptoms (e.g., fevers) is noted before transformation to an acute, rapidly fatal form of disease occurs.

The cumulative lifetime incidence of ATL in persons infected with HTLV-1 is approximately 2.5%, so about 2500 to 5000 cases per year occur in the approximately 10 to 25 million infected persons worldwide. Studies of mothers of children with ATL emphasize that early life exposure is associated with the greatest risk for subsequent disease. In the United States, which has a low prevalence of infection, it is estimated that approximately 30 cases occur per year. In areas endemic for HTLV-1 such as southern Japan and the Caribbean Islands, ATL accounts for half or more of adult lymphoid malignancies. In one series of pediatric cases of ATL, four of the eight patients shared a homozygous deletion in the p16 gene locus, and deletion of exons 7 and 8 of p53 were detected in another child, thus suggesting that a genetic predisposition interacts with viral infection to accelerate disease progression.

Diagnosis

The diagnosis should be considered in an adult with mature T-cell lymphoma and hypercalcemia or cutaneous involvement (or both), particularly if the individual is from a known risk group or endemic region.

TABLE 401–2 HTLV-ASSOCIATED DISEASES

Diagnosis	Nature of Syndrome	Strength of Association
HTLV-1–ASSOCIATED DISEASES		
Adult T-cell leukemia/ lymphoma	Aggressive lymphoproliferative malignancy of mature T lymphocytes	Strong
HTLV-associated myelopathy/ tropical spastic paraparesis	Chronic progressive demyelinating syndrome of the long motor tracts of the spinal cord	Strong
Polymyositis	Degenerative inflammatory syndrome of skeletal muscles	Probable
Sporadic inclusion body myositis	Recently described HTLV-associated inflammatory muscle disease	Possible
Infective dermatitis	Chronic generalized eczema of skin in children; potential for preleukemia and immunodeficiency	Strong
Uveitis	Inflammatory infiltration of the uvea of the eye	Strong
HTLV-associated arthritis	Large-joint polyarthropathy; rheumatoid factor positive with HTLV-1–positive cells infiltrating the synovia	Possible
Immunodeficiency	Subclinical (e.g., decreased PPD response and clinical tuberculosis in western Africa) or clinical (e.g., poor response to therapy for symptomatic strongyloidiasis)	Possible
Miscellaneous clinical conditions	Case reports or case series of Sjögren's syndrome, interstitial pneumonitis, small cell lung cancer with monoclonal HTLV-1 integration, and invasive cervical cancer	Uncertain
HTLV-2–ASSOCIATED DISEASES		
HTLV-associated myelopathy	Increased numbers of cases among blood donors	Definite but rare

*HTLV-1/2 = human T-lymphotropic virus type 1/2; PPD = purified protein derivative.

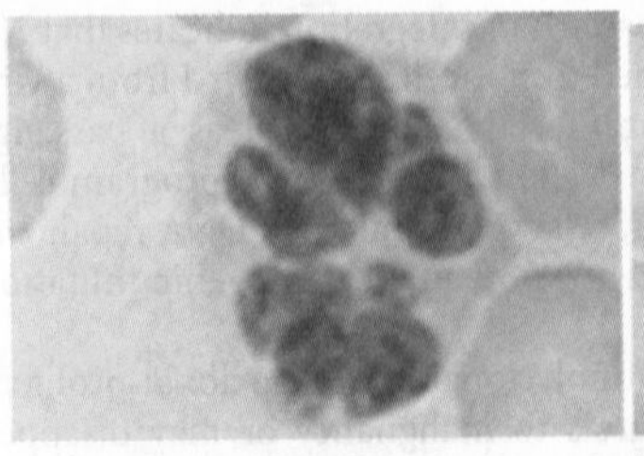

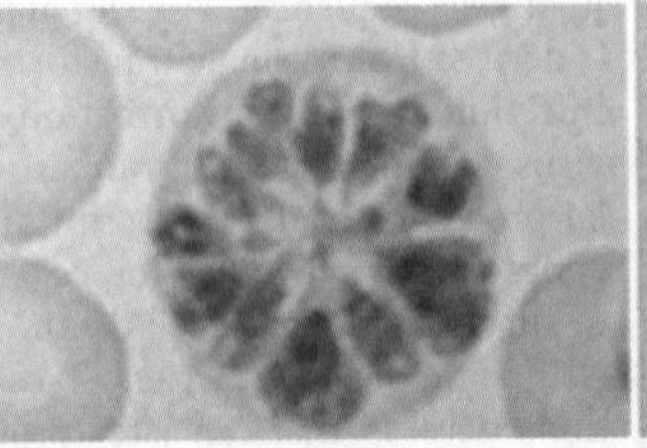

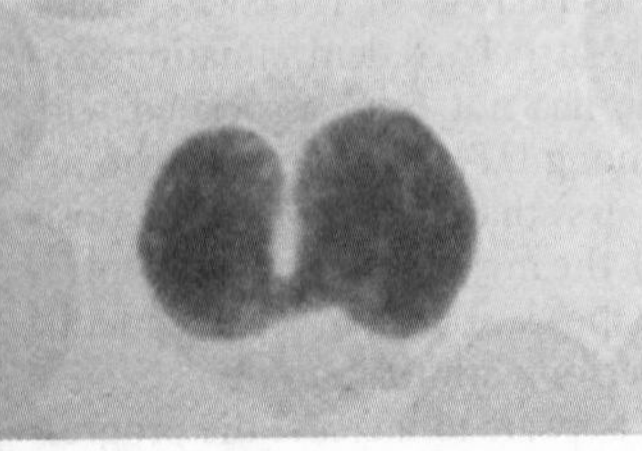

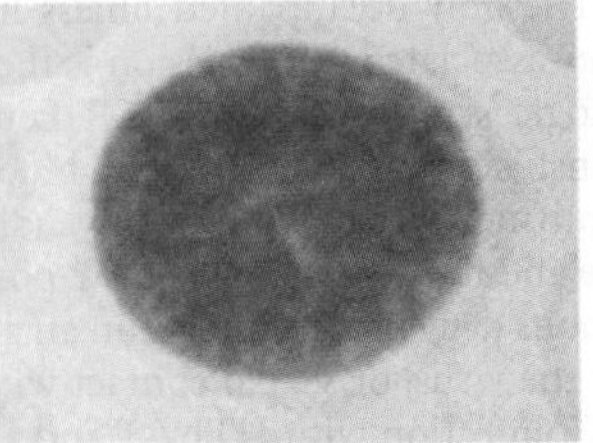

FIGURE 401–1 • Photomicrographs demonstrating the morphologic features of leukemic cells observed in different subtypes of adult T-cell leukemia/lymphoma (ATL). A and B, Polylobulated morphology of the acute type, with the highly characteristic "flower cell" shown in **B. C,** Typical cleaved cell seen in chronic-type ATL. **D,** Typical morphology of smoldering ATL. (Courtesy of K. Yamaguchi and K. Takatsuki.)

The diagnosis is established by testing serum for HTLV-1 antibodies. HTLV-1 and HTLV-2 are routinely detected through blood bank screening assays and confirmed by Western blotting. Polymerase chain reaction (PCR) is another technique that is useful in research settings for detecting and distinguishing the type of virus and quantifying cell-associated virus as a marker of disease. A particularly distinctive morphology includes the so-called flower cells, which represent a sine qua non of HTLV-1–associated leukemia (see Fig. 401–1). Cells with this morphology are also seen in apparently healthy carriers and may presage the risk for future ATL. Occasional cases with characteristic clinical features are antibody negative but provirus positive as detected by PCR in blood cells or in biopsy specimens.

Treatment

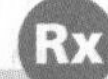

Many hematologists recommend watchful waiting for patients with smoldering or chronic ATL, but conventional chemotherapy, including prednisone with or without cyclophosphamide, is sometimes used. More aggressive therapy is associated with high rates of infection.

The acute and lymphoma types of ATL are aggressive high-grade lymphomas, but some respond to multidrug regimens, such as vincristine, cyclophosphamide, prednisolone, and doxorubicin (VEPA), sometimes with methotrexate (VEPA-M), or to even more complex 9- and 10-drug regimens Although initial response rates are higher than 50% and complete remissions are achieved in 20% of cases, these responses can be short lived, with relapses occurring in weeks to months, often involving the central nervous system (CNS). Recent reports suggest a therapeutic role for allogeneic hematopoietic stem cell transplantation, with a reported 3-year overall survival rate of 45% and a relapse-free survival rate of 34%. Some patients may respond to a combination of zidovudine and interferon.

Prognosis

Smoldering ATL has a relatively good prognosis, with a 5-year survival rate of 70% (Fig. 401–2). The chronic subtype has a 5-year survival rate of 20%, which although dismal, is better than the 5-year survival rate of 5% observed in the acute and lymphoma types. Most patients with the latter types of ATL die within 6 months of diagnosis. Significant prognostic factors include poor performance status at diagnosis, age older than 40 years, extensive disease, hypercalcemia, and high serum lactate dehydrogenase levels. Death usually results from rapid growth of tumor cells, hypercalcemia, bacterial sepsis, and opportunistic and other infectious complications.

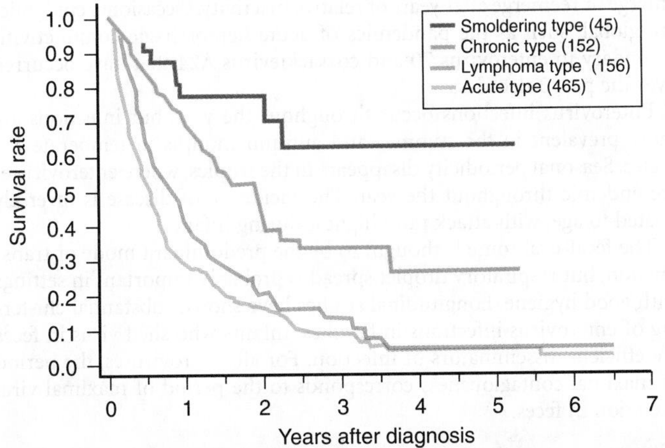

FIGURE 401–2 • Survival by adult T-cell leukemia/lymphoma (ATL) subtype after polychemotherapy in Japan. Poorest survival is observed in patients with acute and lymphoma-type ATL. (From Tsukasaki K, Ikeda S, Murata K, et al: Characteristics of chemotherapy-induced clinical remission in long survivors with aggressive adult T-cell leukemia/lymphoma. Leuk Res 1993;17:157.)

HTLV-ASSOCIATED MYELOPATHY/ TROPICAL SPASTIC PARAPARESIS

Clinical Manifestations

HTLV-1 is linked to a neurologic syndrome known as HAM/TSP that results from demyelination of the long motor neurons of the spinal cord; it is associated with a variety of symptoms, including stiff gait, spasticity, lower extremity weakness, back pain, urinary incontinence and impotence, and (rarely) ataxia. Symptoms often begin with a stiff gait and progress (usually slowly) to increasing spasticity and weakness, with incontinence and impotence developing later. In some cases, isolated lesions of the CNS are detected on a nuclear magnetic resonance scan. In contrast to classic multiple sclerosis, HAM/TSP is characterized by a generally slow, progressive course, absence of waxing and waning symptoms, and demyelination of long motor neurons rather than the CNS. However, some cases are acutely progressive, especially in those associated with transfusion of HTLV-1–positive blood.

The lifetime incidence is approximately half the rate for ATL, with approximately 1 to 2% of carriers affected. HAM/TSP is approximately two times more likely to develop in females. The majority of adult cases occur in the 30- to 50-year-old age group, but cases have occurred in children as young as 3 years of age. These patterns suggest that the latency period for HAM/TSP is shorter than that for ATL and that both early-life and adult exposure causes disease.

Diagnosis

The diagnosis is suspected in patients with unexplained CNS disease and loss of pyramidal tract functions and is confirmed by testing sera for HTLV-1 antibodies. Oligoclonal immunoglobulin bands in the cerebrospinal fluid of patients with HAM/TSP react to HTLV-1 antigens.

Treatment

Corticosteroids reduce symptoms in approximately 40% of cases, especially in early disease or patients with rapid progression. Cyclophosphamide also benefits some patients. Pentoxifylline, a phosphodiesterase inhibitor that decreases tumor necrosis factor-α and interferon-γ levels and upregulates interleukin-4 (IL-4) and IL-10, improves motor disability, especially spasticity, thus suggesting that correction of the imbalanced T_H1 cytokine response may be of benefit in ameliorating the clinical symptoms. A small study of interferon alfa therapy showed sustained improvement in motor performance during and for up to 6 months after completion of such therapy. Treatment with danazol, an androgenic steroid, has resulted in improvement in urinary and fecal incontinence but not in the underlying neurologic deficit.

Prognosis

The prognosis of HAM/TSP has historically been poor, with inexorable progressive neurologic deterioration. However, recent therapeutic advances hold hope for improved outcomes.

OTHER HTLV-ASSOCIATED CONDITIONS

HAM/TSP is the prototype for a series of immune-mediated syndromes characterized by a high viral load, immune activation, and an indirect pathogenic mechanism produced by virally induced perturbations in immune function. Examples include skeletal muscle polymyositis, sporadic inclusion body myositis, uveitis (30 to 40% of cases in areas endemic for HTLV), large-joint arthropathy, and Sjögren's syndrome. Carriers of HTLV-1 also have elevated rates of invasive cervical cancer, tuberculosis, parasitic infestations (e.g., strongyloidiasis), scabies, and refractory generalized eczema.

More than a dozen HAM/TSP cases associated with HTLV-2 have been reported. In some instances the clinical pattern has features of the ataxic form, but most demonstrate the more typical spastic paraparesis. Preliminary data suggest that this syndrome is infrequent in comparison to its occurrence in HTLV-1 carriers. One prospective study of HTLV-2–positive drug users showed an excess of asthma-related deaths and an increased frequency of skin and soft tissue infections.

Prevention

Patients identified as HTLV positive based on blood bank screening must be told that complications related to HTLV-1 infection are rare and that HTLV-2 is hardly ever responsible for clinical disease. Second, it should be emphasized that these viruses are not easily transmitted. Third, the patient should be clearly counseled concerning the distinction between HTLV and HIV because the greatest fear that patients may experience is that they have the "AIDS virus." Other guidelines for prevention include the following:

1. Blood for donation should be screened before transfusion, and positive donors should be deferred from donating.
2. HTLV-1/HTLV-2–positive mothers should be discouraged from breast-feeding to prevent mother-to-infant transmission (except in particular settings, such as in the tropics, where diarrheal disease in non–breast-fed infants presents a high risk for morbidity and mortality).
3. Condoms should be used by discordant couples, but given the relatively low frequency of sexual transmission per sexual encounter, couples who desire a pregnancy could time unprotected sexual intercourse to coincide with periods of maximal fertility. Such decisions, however, require careful discussion between the physician and patient.

Postexposure prophylaxis with zidovudine is not recommended because the efficacy of such prophylaxis for HTLV infection has not been established. Vaccines containing whole virus and recombinant HTLV-1 envelope antigens have successfully prevented HTLV-1 infection in monkeys and in a rabbit model. However, a vaccine for humans is unlikely to be a high priority because of the relatively low incidence of clinical disease.

SUGGESTED READINGS

Araujo AO, Silva MT: The HTLV-1 neurological complex. Lancet Neurol 2006;5:1068–1076. *Clinical review.*

Fukushima T, Miyazaki Y, Honda S, et al: Allogeneic hematopoietic stem cell transplantation provides sustained long-term survival for patients with adult T-cell leukemia/lymphoma. Leukemia 2005;19:829–834. *The estimated 3-year survival rate of 45% and disease-free survival rate of 34% were far better than for historical controls.*

Heneine W, Wolfe ND, Carr JK, et al: Emergence of unique primate T-lymphotropic viruses among central African bushmeat hunters. Proc Natl Acad Sci U S A 2005;102:7994–7999. *Emphasizes the zoonotic spread of HTLV.*

Matsuoka M, Jeang KT: Human T-cell leukaemia virus type 1 (HTLV-1) infectivity and cellular transformation. Nat Rev Cancer 2007;7:270–280. *Review of the pathophysiology of HTLV-1 associated cellular transformation.*

Nose H, Saito M, Usuku K, et al: Clinical symptoms and the odds of human T cell lymphotropic virus type 1-associated myelopathy/tropical paraparesis (HAM/STP) in healthy virus carriers. J Neurovirol 2006;12:171–177. *Brisk reflexes and flower cell–like lymphocytes were the major predicators.*

402 ENTEROVIRUS INFECTIONS

John F. Modlin

Definition

The human enteroviruses are ubiquitous, positive-stranded RNA viruses that are directly or indirectly transmitted from person to person. Polioviruses (Chapter 440), the prototypical enteroviruses, are the cause of paralytic poliomyelitis, a disease that has been eradicated in the United States and other developed countries and is targeted for global eradication. The nonpolio enteroviruses continue to be responsible for a wide spectrum of diseases, most commonly in infants and young children but also in adults.

TABLE 402–1 CLASSIFICATION OF HUMAN ENTEROVIRUSES

Species	Serotypes
Polioviruses	1–3
Group A coxsackieviruses	1–24
Group B coxsackieviruses	1–6
Echoviruses	1–34
Enteroviruses	68–72

The Pathogens

The enteroviruses belong to the family Picornaviridae, a large family of morphologically identical, approximately 30-nm, nonenveloped viruses with a capsid formed from four polypeptides that encloses a linear, single-stranded RNA genome about 7.4 kilobases in length. The enterovirus genome is divided into three regions: a highly conserved 5′ noncoding region of approximately 743 nucleotides that interacts with cellular ribosomes to initiate translation, a continuous-coding region of about 6625 nucleotides, and a 3′ poly-A end region of variable length. Host cell susceptibility to enterovirus infection is defined by the presence of specific membrane receptor proteins.

The enteroviruses are traditionally divided into five subgenera: polioviruses, group A coxsackieviruses, group B coxsackieviruses, echoviruses, and "newer" enteroviruses, based on differences in host range and pathogenic potential (Table 402–1). Each subgenus contains a number of unique serotypes that are distinguished from one another on the basis of neutralization by specific antisera. A total of more than 90 serotypes have now been identified. A new classification scheme divides all nonpolio enteroviruses into four groups designated A through D based on homology within the RNA region coding for the VP1 capsid protein, which contains the major epitopes associated with neutralization.

Epidemiology

Only poliovirus infections are nationally reportable. However, the prevalence of nonpolio enterovirus infections is known to rise progressively until 15 years of age, when 90% of the adult population has type-specific neutralizing antibodies, depending on the serotype tested and the socioeconomic class of the population surveyed. The 10 most common serotypes of nonpolio enterovirus isolates account for about 85% of all enterovirus isolates (Table 402–2). In urban areas of the United States, usually one to three serotypes predominate each season, but some serotypes are isolated from year to year, whereas other serotypes may emerge or reemerge after years of relative inactivity. Occasional epidemics are global, such as the pandemics of acute hemorrhagic conjunctivitis secondary to enterovirus 70 and coxsackievirus A24 that have occurred over the past 3 decades.

Enterovirus infections occur throughout the year, but infections are more prevalent in the summer and autumn months in temperate climates. Seasonal periodicity disappears in the tropics, where enteroviruses are endemic throughout the year. The incidence of disease is inversely related to age, with attack rates highest during infancy.

The fecal-oral route is thought to be the predominant mode of transmission, but respiratory droplet spread is probably important in settings with good hygiene. Longitudinal studies have shown substantial clustering of enterovirus infections in families. Infants who shed virus in feces are efficient disseminators of infection. For all enteroviruses, the period of maximal contagiousness corresponds to the period of maximal viral excretion in feces.

Pathobiology

After initial replication in the oropharynx, enteroviruses, unlike other picornaviruses, survive transit through the acidic environment of the

TABLE 402–2 MOST COMMON ENTEROVIRUS SEROTYPES SUBMITTED BY STATE AND LOCAL PUBLIC HEALTH LABORATORIES TO THE CDC, 2000–2001

Enterovirus Serotype	Percentage
Echovirus 18	22.0
Echovirus 13	20.8
Coxsackievirus B5	11.9
Coxsackievirus B2	6.3
Echovirus 6	6.1
Echovirus 11	4.5
Coxsackievirus A9	4.0
Echovirus 9	3.3
Coxsackievirus B4	3.2
Echovirus 4	3.1
Coxsackievirus B3	2.4
Coxsackievirus B1	2.0
Echovirus 30	1.8
Echovirus 25	1.2
Enterovirus 71	1.1
Total	93.5

From Centers for Disease Control and Prevention (CDC): Enterovirus surveillance—United States, 2000–2001. MMWR Morb Mort Wkly Rep 2002; 51(46):1047–1049.

stomach and reach the lower intestinal tract, where they replicate more extensively in submucosal lymphatic tissues and give rise to a transient viremia, which then targets reticuloendothelial tissue such as the liver, spleen, bone marrow, and deep lymph nodes. At this point, virus replication is usually controlled by host defense mechanisms, and the patient experiences no illness or only brief, nonlocalized symptoms. However, in a minority of infected persons, further replication of virus results in sustained viremia and dissemination to the central nervous system (CNS), heart, and other target organs, with replication of virus in these locations. Both virus-induced cell lysis and the host's inflammatory response are thought to contribute to clinical disease. The maximal duration of viral excretion is 3 to 4 weeks from the pharynx and 5 to 6 weeks in feces.

Immunity to enterovirus infections is serotype specific. Neutralizing IgG antibody is detected in serum by 7 to 10 days after infection and plays an important role in recovery from enterovirus infection, as evidenced by the development of persistent infection in persons with B-cell immunodeficiency and by protection against subsequent infection with virus of the same serotype. IgA antibody appears in nasal and alimentary secretions 2 to 4 weeks after infection and persists for at least 15 years. Secretory IgA antibody is also present in the colostrum and milk of immune women. Maternal antibodies passively acquired either transplacentally or via milk prevent or modify enterovirus infections in early infancy.

Macrophage function is also critical for viral clearance. By comparison, inhibition of T-lymphocyte function has little effect on virus replication in vivo, and persons with abnormal cell-mediated immunity are not predisposed to serious or prolonged enterovirus infections unless they have accompanying B-cell dysfunction. Even though T lymphocytes do not contribute to the inhibition of enterovirus replication, there is evidence that induction of natural killer cell activity and T-lymphocyte immune responses contribute to necrosis of enterovirus-infected cells in vivo and to development of the host's inflammatory response. Inflammation may persist long after viral replication has ceased, and ongoing cardiac damage may be mediated by virus-induced antibodies against cardiac antigens or by cytotoxic T-lymphocyte-mediated myocyte lysis.

Clinical Manifestations

The incubation period for enterovirus infections is typically 3 to 5 days. Infected persons may excrete virus in throat secretions or feces for several days before the onset of symptoms and continue to excrete virus in feces for several weeks thereafter. However, the period of maximum communicability is believed to be early in illness, when viral shedding is greatest.

At least 50 to 80% of nonpolio enterovirus infections are asymptomatic. Most symptomatic infections result in brief, undifferentiated febrile illnesses that are often accompanied by symptoms of upper respiratory tract infection or one of many types of rash, but a wide range of clinical syndromes are observed (Table 402–3). Disease syndromes considered characteristic of enteroviruses, such as aseptic meningitis or pericarditis, are less common manifestations of infection. Some syndromes (e.g., viral meningitis) are caused by many enterovirus serotypes, some are predominately caused by certain enterovirus subgroups (e.g., pleurodynia and myocarditis by group B coxsackieviruses), and other diseases are mostly associated with individual enterovirus serotypes.

Age, gender, physical activity, and immune status of the host are also important determinants of the severity of disease. Pregnancy may enhance the severity of enterovirus infections. Enterovirus illnesses may be more frequent and more severe in persons who exercise vigorously before the onset of symptoms.

Diagnosis

Laboratory diagnosis of enterovirus infection may be accomplished by cell culture, polymerase chain reaction (PCR), or serologic methods. Cell culture is being supplanted by more rapid and sensitive PCR-based assays.

A presumptive diagnosis of enterovirus infection can usually be reported by the laboratory within 3 to 5 days after identification of a characteristic cytopathic effect in any of three or four appropriately chosen cell lines, which usually include primary monkey kidney cells and human embryonic cells. Group B coxsackieviruses and echoviruses are recovered readily, but only a few serotypes of group A coxsackieviruses (e.g., A9, A16) and the "newer" enteroviruses grow readily in routinely used cell lines. Isolates may be confirmed as enteroviruses with the use of a monoclonal antibody to a broadly reactive VP1 epitope. The opportunity to recover virus in cell culture is optimized by sampling of multiple sites.

Reverse transcriptase–PCR is a rapid, sensitive, and specific method of detecting enterovirus RNA in clinical specimens. With cerebrospinal fluid (CSF) specimens from patients with aseptic meningitis, PCR detects enterovirus RNA in 66 to 86% of cases, as compared with viral isolation rates of approximately 30%. Experience with non-CSF specimens is more limited, but PCR has detected enterovirus RNA from throat swabs, serum, urine, and stool. The sensitivity with urine specimens is somewhat lower than with other specimens. PCR has detected enterovirus RNA in only a minority of endomyocardial biopsy specimens from patients with acute myopericarditis. Further characterization of enteroviruses may include sequencing portions of the capsid-coding regions of the viral RNA to assign the nonpolio enterovirus isolates to one of four classes and predict the serotype.

The microneutralization test is the most specific method for determination of antibodies to enteroviruses. Because microneutralization is serotype specific, it has limited usefulness in the routine diagnosis of nonpolio enterovirus infections as a result of the low feasibility of testing with multiple live viral antigens and because methods based on neutralization are relatively insensitive, poorly standardized, and labor-intensive. Type-specific immunoassays are more versatile methods that are now offered in commercial laboratories to assay antibodies against the more common enterovirus serotypes. Serum IgM antibody to group B coxsackieviruses can often be detected early in the course of illness, but positive test results are not serotype specific and may occur during infections with enteroviruses of other classes.

Prevention

The success of vaccination against poliomyelitis suggests that a similar approach would prevent nonpolio enterovirus infections as well. However, vaccines have not been developed against the other human enteroviruses. Preexposure administration of immune globulin, which is known to reduce the risk for paralytic poliomyelitis, may also prevent

TABLE 402–3 CLINICAL MANIFESTATIONS OF NONPOLIO ENTEROVIRUS INFECTIONS*

Clinical Syndrome	Group A Coxsackieviruses†	Group B Coxsackieviruses	Echoviruses‡	Enteroviruses
Asymptomatic infection	All serotypes	All serotypes	All serotypes	All serotypes
Undifferentiated febrile illness ("summer grippe") with or without respiratory symptoms	All serotypes	All serotypes	All serotypes	68, 70, 71
Aseptic meningitis (often associated with an exanthem)	1, 2, 3, 4, 5, 6, 7, 8, 9, 10, 11, 14, 16, 17, 18, 22, 24	1, 2, 3, 4, 5, 6	1, 2, 3, 4, 5, 6, 7, 8, 9, 10, 11, 12, 14, 16, 17, 18, 19, 20, 21, [22], [23], 25, 30, 31, 33	70, 71
Encephalitis	2, 4, 5, 6, 7, 9, 10, 16	1, 2, 3, 4, 5	2, 3, 4, 6, 7, 9, 11, 14, 17, 18, 19, [22], 25, 30, 33	70, 71
Paralytic disease (poliomyelitis-like)	4, 5, 6, 7, 9, 10, 11, 14, 16, 21, 24	1, 2, 3, 4, 5, 6	1, 2, 4, 6, 7, 9, 11, 14, 16, 17, 18, 19, 30	70, 71
Myopericarditis	1, 2, 4, 5, 7, 8, 9, 14, 16	1, 2, 3, 4, 5, 6	1, 2, 3, 4, 6, 7, 8, 9, 11, 14, 16, 17, 19, [22], 25, 30	
Pleurodynia	1, 2, 4, 6, 9, 10, 16	1, 2, 3, 4, 5, 6	1, 2, 3, 6, 7, 8, 9, 11, 12, 14, 16, 19, [23], 25, 30	
Herpangina	1, 2, 3, 4, 5, 6, 7, 8, 9, 10, 16, 22	1, 2, 3, 4, 5	6, 9, 11, 16, 17, [22], 25	71
Hand-foot-and-mouth disease	4, 5, 7, 9, 10, 16	2, 5	7	71
Exanthems	2, 4, 5, 6, 7, 9, 10, 16	1, 2, 3, 4, 5	2, 4, 5, 6, 9, 11, 16, 18, 25	71
Common cold	2, 10, 21, 24	1, 2, 3, 4, 5	2, 4, 8, 9, 11, 20, 25	
Lower respiratory tract infections (bronchiolitis, pneumonia)	7, 9, 16	1, 2, 3, 4, 5	4, 8, 9, 11, 12, 14, 19, 20, 21, 25, 30	68, 71
Acute hemorrhagic conjunctivitis§	24			70
Generalized disease of the newborn	3, 9, 16	1, 2, 3, 4, 5	3, 4, 6, 7, 9, 11, 12, 14, 17, 18, 19, 20, 21, [22], 30	

*A great many enterovirus serotypes have been implicated in most of these syndromes, at least in sporadic cases. The serotypes listed are those that have been clearly and/or frequently implicated. Serotypes with a strong association are underlined, and those with the strongest association are double underlined.
†Because isolation of many of the group A coxsackieviruses requires suckling mouse inoculation, they are likely to be underreported as causes of illness.
‡Echovirus types [22] and [23] were found to differ substantially in nucleotide and amino acid sequence from other enteroviruses and to have three rather than four capsid proteins. Consequently, they have been reclassified as parechoviruses 1 and 2, the first members of a new genus, Parechovirus, within the Picornavirus family. The epidemiologic and clinical features of these two parechoviruses are similar to those of the echoviruses.
§Conjunctivitis without hemorrhage is frequently seen in association with other manifestations in patients infected with many group A and group B coxsackieviruses and echoviruses, especially coxsackieviruses A9, A16, and B1 to B5 and echoviruses 2, 7, 9, 11, 16, and 30.

nonpolio enterovirus disease, but this strategy is rarely applicable to clinical practice.

In the setting of a community epidemic or a patient hospitalized with enterovirus illness, simple hygienic measures such as handwashing and careful disposal or autoclaving of potentially infected feces and secretions should be practiced. Gown and mask procedures or isolation of the patient is unwarranted. Pregnant women, especially those near term, should be advised to avoid contact with patients suspected of having enterovirus illness.

Treatment

Rx

The majority of enterovirus infections are self-limited and do not require antiviral therapy. Exceptions may include acute myocarditis and life-threatening infections in B cell–deficient patients. Therapeutic options for these more serious infections are very limited. Serum immune globulin and intravenous immune globulin have been given to individual, persistently infected B cell–deficient patients with mixed results and have been used in nonrandomized trials in children with myocarditis with uncertain effect.

Effective antiviral drugs for enterovirus infections are neither licensed nor currently available. The most promising experimental agents bind to a pocket in the viral capsid and alter virus attachment and uncoating. An example is pleconaril, which inhibits the replication of most enterovirus serotypes at concentrations of less than 0.1 μg/mL in vitro and has a favorable pharmacologic and safety profile. Placebo-controlled trials of pleconaril in patients with enterovirus meningitis demonstrate significant reductions in the duration and severity of headache and a shorter period of viral shedding when the drug is administered within 24 hours of symptom onset.

SPECIFIC CLINICAL SYNDROMES

Central Nervous System Infections

Viral Meningitis

The group B coxsackieviruses and echoviruses together cause the majority of cases of acute viral meningitis (Chapter 437); the most common serotypes include group B coxsackievirus serotypes 2 through 5 and echovirus serotypes 4, 6, 9, 11, 13, 16, 30, and 33. Widespread outbreaks of viral meningitis caused by single echovirus serotypes occur roughly every 5 to 12 years.

Clinical Manifestations and Diagnosis

The typical patient has a brief prodrome of fever, pharyngitis, chills, and a prominent headache. Meningismus, when present, varies from mild to severe, and Kernig's and Brudzinski's signs are present in about a third of patients. The total CSF cell count usually falls within the range of 10 to 500 cells/mm^3 but may occasionally exceed 1000/mm^3. Cell counts less than 10/mm^3 occur in a small minority of cases. Early in the clinical course there is often an increased proportion of neutrophils in CSF, but the differential invariably shifts to a predominance of lymphocytes within 1 to 2 days. In general, the CSF glucose concentration is normal and the CSF protein concentration is normal or slightly elevated. Enteroviruses can be detected in CSF and other specimens by PCR genomic amplification or by cell culture. For confirmed or suspected enterovirus meningitis cases, PCR sensitivity ranges from 66 to more than 90%. The overall sensitivity of virus isolation from the CSF of patients with aseptic meningitis is 30 to 35%, but concomitant culture of serum, upper respiratory secretions, urine, and stool will enhance the likelihood of virus recovery.

Treatment and Prognosis

Hospital admission is not necessary for all cases, but it may be advisable when disturbances in consciousness, muscle weakness, or a petechial rash suggest the possibility of a more serious illness. When bacterial meningitis cannot be excluded because of previous antibiotic treatment, administration of appropriate antibiotics is advisable after performing a Gram stain and bacterial culture. In most cases, treatment consists only of relief of symptoms. Analgesics are usually given to older children and adults to alleviate headache. Pleconaril, an orally administered enterovirus capsid–stabilizing drug, may reduce the duration of headache and other symptoms but is not licensed by the Food and Drug Administration.

Serious complications are rare, although adults may experience a more prolonged period of fever and headache than infants and children do. Some adult patients may take weeks to return to normal activity.

Encephalitis

Encephalitis (Chapter 439), which is an unusual manifestation of coxsackievirus and echovirus infection, may or may not include symptoms of meningitis. The enteroviruses account for less than 5% of all cases of encephalitis and for 11 to 22% of all cases that are proved to be viral. Children and young adults are most frequently affected.

Clinical Manifestations and Diagnosis

Clinical findings range from lethargy, drowsiness, and personality change to seizures, paresis, and coma. Abnormalities detected by brain imaging or electroencephalography reflect the extent and severity of brain involvement. In a minority of cases, a specific cause has been proved by isolation of virus from brain tissue or CSF; in others, the cause of encephalitis has been inferred by isolating virus from a mucosal site or by serology.

Prognosis

Most patients who contract coxsackievirus and echovirus encephalitis after the neonatal period recover fully, although permanent neurologic sequelae and rare deaths do occur.

Limb Paralysis and Other Neurologic Complications of Coxsackievirus and Echovirus Infections

Sporadic cases of flaccid motor paralysis have been associated with several coxsackievirus and echovirus serotypes, including enterovirus 71. Paralytic disease caused by the nonpolio enteroviruses is characteristically less severe than poliovirus-associated paralysis. Muscle weakness is more common than flaccid paralysis, and the paresis is not usually permanent.

Transverse myelitis (coxsackievirus B4 and echovirus 5) and Guillain-Barré syndrome (coxsackievirus serotypes A2, A5, and A9 and echovirus serotypes 6 and 22) have been reported in a small number of patients.

Enterovirus 71 Infections

Enterovirus 71 can cause encephalitis and aseptic meningitis. Enterovirus 71 is unique among the nonpolio enteroviruses as a cause of epidemic paralysis in which localized outbreaks have involved small numbers of patients over a period of several years and regional epidemics have involved hundreds to thousands of persons within a single season. Brain stem encephalitis associated with high mortality as a result of pulmonary edema and rapid cardiovascular collapse has also developed in some infants and young children.

Acute Hemorrhagic Conjunctivitis

Acute hemorrhagic conjunctivitis is a highly contagious, self-limited ocular infection characterized by pain, swelling of the eyelids, and subconjunctival hemorrhage. Large-scale epidemics caused by enterovirus 70 and coxsackievirus A24 occur predominantly in crowded coastal areas of tropical countries during the hot, rainy season. Infection is transmitted from fingers or fomites directly to the eye, and contagion is favored by crowding and unsanitary living conditions. Antibody prevalence rates are highest in children younger than 10 years, but attack rates for clinical disease are greatest in young adults, thus suggesting that many infections in children are mild or unapparent.

Clinical Manifestations and Diagnosis

Eye disease occurs suddenly and peaks within 24 hours. The main symptoms are a burning, foreign body sensation, ocular pain, photophobia, swelling of the eyelids, and watery discharge. The most distinctive sign is subconjunctival hemorrhage, which is present in 70 to 90% of patients with enterovirus 70 but much less frequent in cases caused by coxsackievirus A24. Small follicles appear on the tarsal conjunctiva within 3 to 5 days in 90% of patients, and a fine punctate, erosive epithelial keratitis can be demonstrated by slit lamp examination after staining with fluorescein. The preauricular lymph nodes are often enlarged and tender by the second day of illness.

Prevention and Treatment

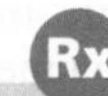

Treatment is symptomatic. Contagion can be prevented by careful handwashing, use of separate towels, and sterilization of ophthalmologic instruments.

Prognosis

Recovery is usually noticeable by the second or third day. The keratitis may persist for several weeks but almost never leads to permanent scarring. More than 200 cases of acute motor paralysis indistinguishable from poliomyelitis have been reported in association with enterovirus 70.

Exanthems

Coxsackieviruses and echoviruses cause a wide variety of exanthems (Chapter 465), which are sometimes associated with enanthems, but only hand-foot-and-mouth disease is sufficiently distinctive to permit a reliable etiologic diagnosis on clinical grounds alone. Otherwise, enteroviral exanthems occur in the setting of acute febrile illnesses that mimic other infective exanthems such as measles (Chapter 390), rubella (Chapter 391), and purpura fulminans (Chapter 465).

Enterovirus exanthems themselves cause little morbidity. Fine maculopapular, rubelliform rashes occurring during the summer months are common manifestations of echovirus infection. The rash, which characteristically appears simultaneously with fever, begins on the face and then spreads to the neck, chest, and extremities. It is characterized by innumerable nonpruritic, faint pink macules 1 to 3 mm in diameter. Multiple cases may occur sequentially in the same household.

Petechial and purpuric rashes have been described with echovirus 9 and coxsackievirus A9 infections. These rashes may easily be confused with meningococcal disease, especially if aseptic meningitis occurs simultaneously.

Hand-Foot-and-Mouth Disease

Coxsackievirus A16 is the most common cause of the distinctive vesicular eruption known as hand-foot-and-mouth disease (Fig. 402–1), although other enteroviruses, including enterovirus 71, can also cause the syndrome. Children younger than 10 years are often the source of spread of the disease to other family members. Patients complain of a sore throat or sore mouth and may have difficulty eating. The illness begins with fever, which may persist for 1 to 2 days, and is characterized by vesicles on the buccal mucosa and tongue. Several of these lesions may coalesce to form bullae, which frequently ulcerate by the time that they are seen by a physician. In about 75% of patients, peripherally distributed, tender cutaneous lesions occur on the hands and feet, where either the extensor surfaces or the palms and soles may be involved, and sometimes on the buttocks or genitalia. Skin biopsy demonstrates subepidermal lesions with a mixed lymphocytic and polymorphonuclear perivascular inflammatory response in the overlying epidermis. The disease itself requires only symptomatic management and is almost invariably self-limited, although disease caused by enterovirus 71 can be accompanied by severe CNS disease and deaths.

Herpangina

Herpangina, which is a vesicular enanthem of the tonsillar fauces and soft palate, is accompanied by fever, sore throat, and pain on swallowing. Group A coxsackieviruses are the most common viruses recovered from patients with herpangina. Illness begins suddenly with fever, headache, vomiting, and myalgia. Sore throat and pain on swallowing are prominent symptoms and precede appearance of the enanthem by several hours to a day. The enanthem begins as punctate macules, which evolve over a 24-hour period to 2- to 4-mm erythematous papules that vesiculate and then ulcerate centrally. The lesions, which usually number two to six but rarely a dozen, are moderately painful. The fever subsides in 2 to 4 days, but the ulcers may persist for up to a week. Patients with herpangina do not appear very ill and require only symptomatic treatment for sore throat.

Acute Respiratory Disease

Enteroviruses commonly cause undifferentiated febrile illnesses with sore throat and occasionally cough or coryza, especially during the summer and fall. These upper respiratory tract illnesses are generally indistinguishable from disease caused by other agents such as rhinoviruses (Chapter 384) and *Mycoplasma pneumoniae* (Chapter 97), unless accompanied by aseptic meningitis, hand-foot-and-mouth disease, or other clinical features suggesting enterovirus infection. Severe lower respiratory tract enterovirus infections are very uncommon. The best characterized enterovirus respiratory pathogens are coxsackieviruses A21 and A24, which produce illness resembling the common cold, except for a higher incidence of fever. Outbreaks of coxsackievirus A21 illness have been reported in military populations.

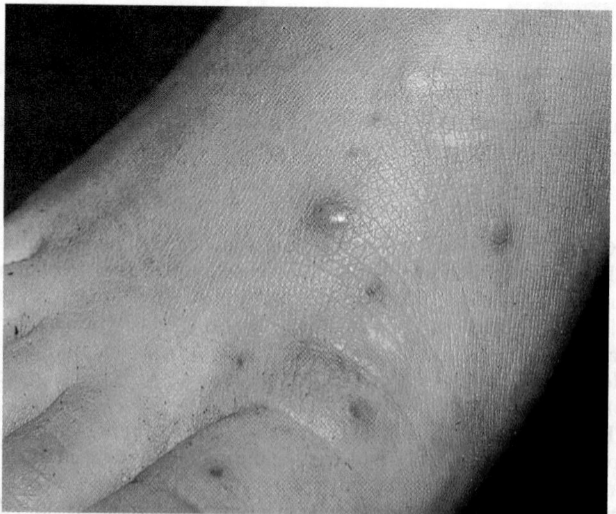

FIGURE 402–1 • Hand-foot-and-mouth disease. Silver-gray vesicles on the dorsal foot.

Myositis

Pleurodynia

Pleurodynia (Chapter 100), which is an acute infection of skeletal muscle, is most commonly caused by group B coxsackieviruses. It results in sharp, spasmodic pain in the chest (Chapter 48) or upper part of the abdomen. Pleurodynia occurs in adolescents and adults more often than in young children, and multiple family members may be attacked almost simultaneously or in rapid sequence.

Clinical Manifestations and Diagnosis

Patients experience an abrupt onset of fever and spasmodic chest wall or abdominal wall pain. The most common location is the vicinity of the costal margin, on one or both sides or occasionally the subxiphoid region, but any thoracic, paraspinal, or abdominal muscle groups may be involved. Periumbilical pain and pain in the lower abdominal quadrants also occur, especially in children. A few patients experience pain in neither the chest nor the abdomen but instead in the neck or limbs; in these cases, the diagnosis can be made only by association with other more typical cases in the family. The hallmark of pleurodynia is the spasmodic and paroxysmal character of the pain. The same pain can be elicited by pressure on affected muscles, and palpable, often visible muscle swelling may be a subtle finding. Auscultation of the chest or abdomen reveals no abnormalities. Not surprisingly, pleurodynia is readily confused with many other illnesses, including pneumonia (Chapter 97), pulmonary infarction (Chapter 99), myocardial ischemia (Chapter 70), and the preeruptive phase of herpes zoster (Chapter 398). Abdominal pain in epidemic pleurodynia may resemble a variety of causes of acute abdomen.

Treatment and Prognosis

Rx

Analgesics are useful in relieving pain. Most patients are ill for 4 to 6 days, but approximately 25% of patients experience multiple recurrences, often after they have been free of pain for a day or more and have felt well enough to return to work or school. Late relapses may occur in some patients who have been free of symptoms for a month or longer. Debility out of all proportion to the apparent severity of the illness is occasionally observed for several months during convalescence, but all patients eventually recover completely.

Myositis in Other Skeletal Muscles

Several different enterovirus serotypes have been associated with generalized polymyositis (Chapter 290) and focal myositis of the thighs or other large muscle groups. Clinical myositis is manifested by fever, chills, weakness, hypotonia, tenderness, and edema of the involved muscles. Myoglobinemia, myoglobinuria, and an elevated creatine kinase level are often found. Most reported patients have recovered rapidly. A dermatomyositis-like illness (Chapter 290) occurs in B cell–deficient immunocompromised patients with persistent enterovirus infections.

Myopericarditis

The enteroviruses account for at least half of acute myopericarditis cases (Chapter 59 and 77). Although disease is most commonly due to group B coxsackieviruses, other enteroviruses are also cardiotropic. Virus replication in cardiac myocytes results in scattered myocyte necrosis and infiltration of neutrophils, lymphocytes, plasma cells, and macrophages.

A chronic inflammatory response persists for weeks to months after replicating virus is no longer present in the heart, and this lingering response may be due to virus-induced, cytotoxic T-lymphocyte destruction of myocytes or an autoimmune process. Healing is accompanied by a variable degree of interstitial fibrosis and evidence of myocyte loss.

Clinical Manifestations and Diagnosis

Enteroviral myopericarditis occurs at all ages but has a special predilection for physically active adolescents and young adults. An upper respiratory tract illness often precedes the onset of cardiac manifestations by 7 to 14 days. The most common symptoms are dyspnea, chest pain, fever, and malaise. A transient pericardial friction rub may be observed with pericardial inflammation. Enlargement of the cardiac silhouette on the chest radiograph, a gallop rhythm, and other signs of heart failure are noted in about 20% of patients with myocardial involvement. Electrocardiographic abnormalities, which are invariably present, include ST segment elevations and nonspecific ST segment and T wave abnormalities (Chapter 77). More severe myocardial disease may lead to the development of Q waves, ventricular tachyarrhythmias, and heart block. Echocardiography may confirm the presence of acute ventricular dilation or a diminished cardiac ejection fraction. Serum levels of cardiac biomarkers are frequently elevated.

Acute myocardial infarction (Chapter 72) associated with chest pain, arrhythmias, and heart failure may be difficult to distinguish from myopericarditis. Although coxsackieviruses have been isolated on numerous occasions from pericardial fluid or by open myocardial biopsy, such specimens are rarely available. The diagnosis often rests on circumstantial evidence provided by recovery of the agent from the oropharynx or feces or on serologic evidence of recent infection by a group B coxsackievirus.

Treatment and Prognosis

Rx

Treatment consists of bedrest, pain relief, and management of arrhythmias and heart failure (Chapter 58). Randomized trials of immunosuppressive therapy, including prednisone, have failed to show any consistent treatment effect. Persistent electrocardiographic abnormalities, cardiomegaly, and chronic heart failure are indications of permanent myocardial injury that occur in about a third of adult patients overall with acute myopericarditis; these abnormalities may ultimately lead to a diagnosis of dilated cardiomyopathy. Chronic constrictive pericarditis has occurred after intervals of 5 weeks to 1 year.

Chronic Meningoencephalitis in Agammaglobulinemic and Other Immunocompromised Patients

Enteroviruses are responsible for persistent, sometimes fatal CNS infections in patients with hereditary or acquired defects in B-lymphocyte function, including children with X-linked agammaglobulinemia and adults with common variable immunodeficiency (Chapter 271). In some recipients of hematopoietic stem cell transplants (Chapter 184), enteroviral infections disseminate and contribute to fatal outcomes.

Clinical Manifestations and Diagnosis

Most cases have been caused by echoviruses. Symptoms include headache, mild nuchal rigidity, lethargy, weakness, ataxia, and seizures. Physical examination may reveal papilledema, motor weakness, or tremors. These clinical manifestations may fluctuate in severity or steadily progress. Persistent skeletal muscle involvement causes a dermatomyositis-like syndrome in more than 50% of these patients, and some patients also have chronic hepatitis.

CSF exhibits lymphocytic pleocytosis and a higher protein concentration than usually seen in cases of acute enteroviral aseptic meningitis. An enterovirus can be repeatedly recovered from CSF over a period of months to years, but in some cases virus is isolated intermittently from CSF or detected only by PCR.

Treatment and Prognosis

Routine use of intravenous immune globulin in patients with B-cell immunodeficiency is effective in preventing chronic enterovirus infections, but this therapy appears to be less useful for the treatment of patients who have previously been infected. For many patients, possibly most, the disease ends fatally without specific therapy.

Other Enterovirus Infections

Acute hepatitis is described in association with group B coxsackievirus and echovirus infections; in general, these cases are mild and self-limited. Data indicate that 2 to 20% of patients with acute pancreatitis (Chapter 147) have concurrent enteroviral infection. Orchitis has been observed in adolescent boys during infection with coxsackievirus A9, group B coxsackieviruses 2, 4, and 5, and echovirus 6.

SUGGESTED READINGS

Barnard DL: Current status of anti-picornavirus therapies. Curr Pharm Des 2006;12:1379–1390. *Review of current options, some of which are in routine use.*

Cuba IPV Study Collaborative Group: Randomized, placebo-controlled trial of inactivated poliovirus vaccine in Cuba. N Engl J Med 2007;356:1536–1544. *With the exception for seroconversion against type 2, vaccination with two or three doses of IPV resulted in a rate of seroconversion of at least 90%.*

Palacios G, Oberste MS: Enteroviruses as agents of emerging infectious diseases. J Neurovirol 2005;11:424–433. *A comprehensive review.*

403 ROTAVIRUSES, NOROVIRUSES, AND OTHER GASTROINTESTINAL VIRUSES

Albert Z. Kapikian

Definition

Viral gastroenteritis (i.e., acute infectious nonbacterial gastroenteritis, epidemic diarrhea, winter vomiting disease, or sporadic infantile gastroenteritis) is a common acute infectious disease that affects all age groups; it is characterized by vomiting or watery diarrhea, or both, and may be accompanied by fever, nausea, anorexia, and malaise. It ranges from a mild, self-limited illness of short duration to life-threatening dehydration, especially in infants and young children.

The impact of diarrheal illnesses globally is staggering. These illnesses are the third most common cause of death in children younger than 5 years, accounting for almost 2 million deaths annually, or 18% of all deaths in this age group; the greatest toll, by far, occurs in developing countries.

The Pathogens

Noroviruses

In 1972, Kapikian and colleagues, using immune electron microscopy (IEM), discovered the first virus-like particles that could be implicated as an important cause of acute gastroenteritis in a stool specimen derived from a gastroenteritis outbreak in Norwalk, Ohio. The 27-nm human

TABLE 403–1 VIRUSES ASSOCIATED WITH ACUTE GASTROENTERITIS IN HUMANS

Virus	Size (nm)	Epidemiology	Important As a Cause of Hospitalization
Rotavirus			
Group A	70	Single most important cause (viral or bacterial) of endemic severe diarrheal illness in infants and young children worldwide (in cooler months in temperate climates)	Yes
Group B	70	Outbreaks of diarrheal illness predominantly in China in adults (mostly) and children	No
Group C	70	Sporadic cases and occasional outbreaks of diarrheal illness in children	
Enteric adenovirus	70–80	Endemic diarrheal illness in infants and young children	No
Norovirus	27–32	Most important cause of outbreaks of nonbacterial gastroenteritis in older children and adults in families, communities, and institutions; frequently associated with ingestion of food Also implicated in diarrheal illnesses of infants and young children with the use of recently developed sensitive assays	No (but in infants and young children it has emerged as second in importance to, but considerably below the rotaviruses)
Sapovirus	28–40	Sporadic cases and occasional outbreaks of diarrheal illness in infants and young children primarily and in the elderly	No
Astrovirus	28	Sporadic cases and occasional outbreaks of diarrheal illness in infants, young children, and the elderly	No

Adapted from Kapikian AZ: Viral gastroenteritis. JAMA 1993;269:627–630.

Norwalk virus is the prototype strain of a group of fastidious, nonenveloped, approximately 27- to 32-nm particles that are now called noroviruses (Table 403–1). The human noroviruses share a similar size and shape but lack a distinctive structural appearance by electron microscopy (EM). They have a positive-sense, single-stranded RNA genome, a buoyant density of 1.33 to 1.41 g/cm^3 in cesium chloride, and a single, primary, virion-associated protein with a molecular mass of approximately 60,000 daltons. They have not been grown in cell culture.

The noroviruses include at least four serotypes by IEM: the Norwalk, Hawaii, Snow Mountain, and Taunton viruses. Other viruses such as the Montgomery County, Southampton, Lorsdale, Desert Shield, Toronto, and Otofuke agents have not been characterized serotypically. Though lacking the distinctive cuplike surface indentations of the "classic" caliciviruses (Latin *calix*, cup), the Norwalk and related viruses are now classified in a separate genus named Norovirus in the family Caliciviridae. Other noncultivatable human enteric viruses that are associated with gastroenteritis in infants and young children or with outbreaks in the elderly have the classic calicivirus morphology. These classic caliciviruses belong to a separate genus named Sapovirus (derived from Sapporo virus) in the family Caliciviridae; they have been associated primarily with pediatric gastroenteritis, and their role in causing severe diarrhea requiring hospitalization appears to be relatively minor.

Rotavirus

In 1973, Bishop and associates, also using EM, discovered rotavirus particles in duodenal biopsy specimens from infants and young children hospitalized with acute gastroenteritis. Rotaviruses have emerged as the major known cause of severe diarrhea of infants and young children worldwide.

Rotaviruses, which are classified in the genus Rotavirus, family Reoviridae, are etiologic agents of diarrhea in humans and in numerous animal and a few avian species. They are 70 nm in diameter, are nonenveloped, and possess a distinctive double-layered capsid that surrounds a third layer, the core, which contains the genome consisting of 11 segments of double-stranded RNA. The virions have a density of 1.36 g/cm^3 in cesium chloride. Rotaviruses possess three important antigenic specificities—group, subgroup, and serotype—that are mediated by different proteins: group and subgroup by VP6 (encoded by RNA segment 6) and serotype by VP7, a glycoprotein that is one of the two major neutralization antigens located on the outer capsid (encoded by RNA segment 7, 8, or 9). The other outer capsid protein, VP4, which is encoded by RNA segment 4 and protrudes from the smooth outer surface as a series of 60 short spikes about 12 nm long, also induces neutralizing antibodies. VP4 is the hemagglutinin in certain strains. Antibodies to both VP4 and VP7 are associated with protection against rotavirus illness. Most animal and human rotaviruses share the common group antigen and are classified as group A rotaviruses, and they are further divided into subgroups. There are 11 human rotavirus serotypes as defined by VP7 neutralization (also designated "G" [for glycoprotein] serotypes), 5 of which (numbers 1, 2, 3, 4, and 9) are of the greatest epidemiologic importance worldwide. Based on neutralization of VP4 (also designated "P" [for protease sensitive]), a binary serotyping system has been developed. Sequence analysis and nucleic acid hybridization of VP4 have also been used to characterize the VP4 genotype of various strains. Thus, there are 12 human rotavirus serotypes or genotypes as defined by VP4. The human rotaviruses have been grown efficiently in cell culture.

Several human and animal rotavirus strains have been discovered that do not share the common group antigen and are classified as non–group A rotaviruses (groups B to G). Group B rotavirus has been responsible for widespread outbreaks of severe gastroenteritis in adults in China, and a relatively small number of group C rotaviruses have been recovered from individuals with gastroenteritis in various countries. In this chapter, however, the term *rotavirus* is used to describe only rotaviruses belonging to group A, unless specified otherwise.

Other Agents

Other viral agents associated with gastroenteritis include enteric adenoviruses (Chapter 388) belonging to types 40 and 41 (70 to 80 nm in diameter), astroviruses (28 to 30 nm), small round viruses (20 to 30 nm) other than the noroviruses, putative coronavirus-like particles (100 to 150 nm), the pleomorphic fringed toroviruses (100 to 140 nm), 35-nm "picobirnaviruses," and an antigen representing certain pestiviruses. The importance of these agents in causing severe infantile diarrhea requiring hospitalization and in epidemic viral gastroenteritis appears to be relatively minor, although the enteric adenoviruses and astroviruses have been firmly established as etiologic agents of acute gastroenteritis. About a third of severe episodes of gastroenteritis in developed countries have yet to be associated with an etiologic agent.

Epidemiology

Norovirus

The noroviruses are the major etiologic agents of acute nonbacterial gastroenteritis, which typically occurs as a sharp outbreak affecting adults, school-aged children, and family contacts. The location or source of contamination responsible for these outbreaks includes settings such as schools, camps, recreational areas, nursing homes, hospitals, swimming facilities, cruise ships, and restaurants or events with catered meals. Noroviruses were detected in 217 (93%) of 233 nonbacterial gastroenteritis outbreaks that were evaluated in the United States by the Centers for Disease Control and Prevention (CDC) between July 1997 and June 2000. In another CDC study, noroviruses were the leading cause of both the total number of cases of gastroenteritis annually in the United States and the number of cases that were food-borne; they accounted for an estimated 23 million total cases, 40% of which were food-borne. In addition, noroviruses are estimated to cause 50,000 hospitalizations and 310 deaths in the United States annually. Studies of acute gastroenteritis in general practices in the Netherlands indicated that bacterial and viral agents were detected with nearly equal frequency (with norovirus and rotavirus each at 5%), whereas in a population-based cohort study of gastroenteritis, viral agents were detected more frequently than bacterial agents, with noroviruses being the leading pathogens (11%). In the United States, antibody to the Norwalk virus is acquired gradually in childhood and somewhat more rapidly in the adult years such that by the age of 50 years, at least 50% of individuals have serum antibody. In developing countries, infants and young children acquire Norwalk virus antibody at an earlier age. With sensitive assays, noroviruses are detected frequently in infants and young children, and they are now a distant second in importance after rotaviruses (Fig. 403–1).

Noroviruses are most likely transmitted by the fecal-oral route; however, Norwalk virus has also been detected in vomitus. Although sporadic cases attributed to person-to-person transmission may occur, the explosive nature of outbreaks associated with noroviruses often suggests a common source of infection, such as water or food. Common-source outbreaks have been attributed to contamination of community and noncommunity public water systems, stored water on cruise ships, and recreational swimming water, as well as the ingestion of various foods such as tainted oysters, lettuce, potato salad, coleslaw, and cake frosting.

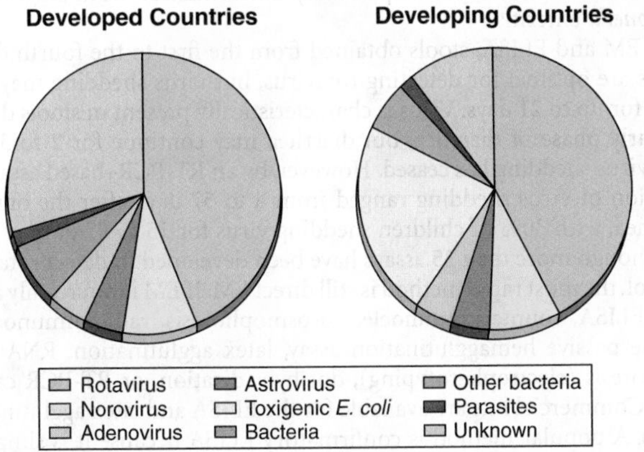

FIGURE 403–1 • Estimates of the roles of etiologic agents in severe diarrheal illnesses requiring hospitalization of infants and young children in developed and developing countries. (Adapted from Kapikian AZ: Viral gastroenteritis. JAMA 1993;269:627–630.)

Norovirus infections have been detected in individuals with travelers' diarrhea, but this agent is not considered to be an important cause of this disease. Secondary person-to-person transmission to contacts is relatively common.

The incubation period in Norwalk virus challenge studies ranges from 10 to 51 hours, with means ranging from 24 to 37 hours, and illnesses characteristically last approximately 24 to 48 hours. Norovirus outbreaks occur throughout the year without a peak season.

Rotavirus

Rotaviruses are the major known etiologic agents of severe diarrhea in infants and young children in most areas of the world. They are usually associated with sporadic or endemic gastroenteritis, which differs from the epidemic viral gastroenteritis associated with noroviruses in the following characteristics: (1) rotavirus does not usually occur in sharp outbreaks; (2) rotavirus is consistently the most important cause of severe diarrheal illness in infants and young children; (3) rotavirus does not normally cause illness in adults; and (4) the attack rate in family contacts of index cases is low, although subclinical infections occur frequently in contacts. In contrast to norovirus infections, most infants and young children (approximately 90%) in developed and developing countries experience a rotavirus infection (as determined from antibody prevalence) by about 3 years of age.

In developed countries, rotaviruses are associated with approximately 35 to 52% of acute diarrheal illnesses requiring hospitalization of infants and young children. It is estimated that rotaviruses are responsible for approximately 2.7 million episodes of diarrheal illness, 600,000 outpatient visits, 55,000 to 70,000 hospitalizations (including nosocomial), and 20 to 60 deaths annually in the United States in infants and children younger than 5 years (Fig. 403–2).

A similar pattern is also usually observed in developing countries, where rotaviruses are the single most frequently detected pathogens in children younger than 2 years who have severe gastroenteritis; bacterial agents play an important, but lesser role in such areas. It is estimated that worldwide more than 600,000 infants and children younger than 5 years die of rotavirus diarrhea each year (i.e., more than 1400 deaths each day), with the greatest toll and risk, by far, in developing countries.

In temperate climates, rotavirus gastroenteritis has a characteristic seasonal occurrence, with a peak prevalence in the winter months. In tropical countries it occurs throughout the year, with less pronounced peaks. Rotavirus diarrhea occurs most frequently in children between approximately 6 months and 24 months of age. The low frequency of clinical illness in neonates with rotavirus infection is an unusual paradox that has not been explained, although the protective role of maternal antibodies is considered to be of prime importance.

Rotavirus gastroenteritis occurs infrequently in adults, but subclinical infections are common. It has been observed in individuals with travelers' diarrhea but is not thought to be an important cause of this illness.

Rotaviruses are transmitted by the fecal-oral route, although respiratory transmission also remains a possibility because there is such rapid acquisition of serum antibody during the first 2 years of life, regardless of hygienic conditions. Nosocomial rotavirus infections occur frequently. The incubation period of rotavirus illness is approximately 2 to 4 days.

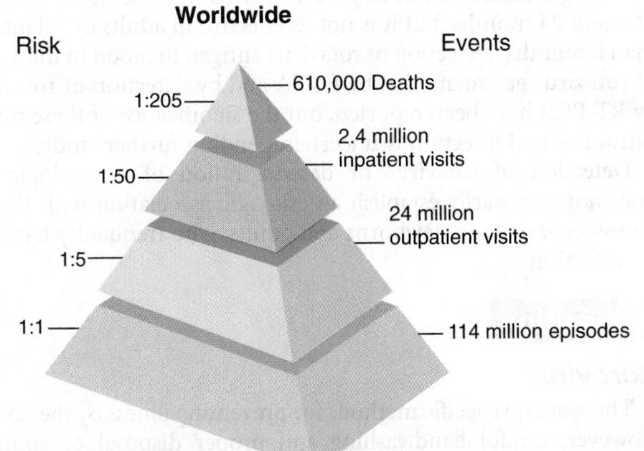

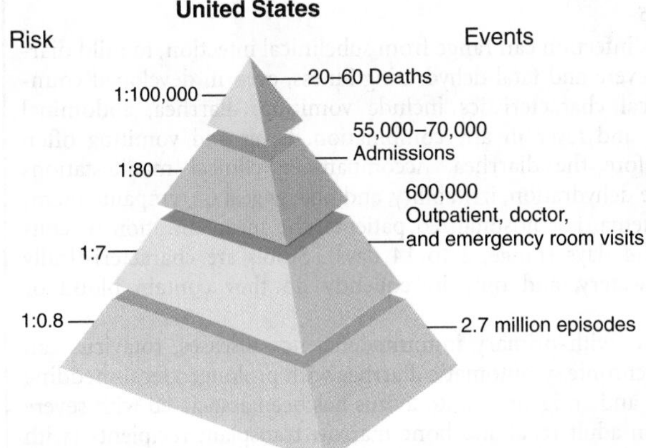

FIGURE 403–2 • Annual burden of rotavirus disease worldwide and in the United States in infants and children younger than 5 years. (Adapted from Glass RI, Parashar UD, Bresee JS, et al: Rotavirus vaccines: Current prospects and future challenges. Lancet 2006;368:323–332).

Pathobiology

Norovirus

Histopathologic lesions after Norwalk or Hawaii virus infection are characterized by reversible involvement of the upper jejunum. The jejunal mucosa remains intact, with marked broadening and blunting of the villi and shortening of the microvilli, along with mononuclear cell infiltration and cytoplasmic vacuolization. Functional alterations may include transient malabsorption of fat, D-xylose, and lactose, as well as a significant decrease in levels of small intestinal brush border enzymes (i.e., alkaline phosphatase and trehalase). Adenylate cyclase activity in the jejunum is not elevated. Delay in gastric emptying may be responsible for the nausea and vomiting associated with these agents. Although immunity to Norwalk virus has been observed in approximately 50% of adults, it appears to correlate inversely with the level of serum or local jejunal antibody. Innate genetic resistance seems to be an important protective factor for Norwalk virus but not for Snow Mountain virus.

Rotavirus

The major histopathologic lesions are characterized by reversible involvement of the proximal portion of the small intestine. The mucosa remains intact, with shortening of the villi, mononuclear cell infiltration of the lamina propria, distended cisternae of the endoplasmic reticulum, mitochondrial swelling, and sparse, irregular microvilli. Functional alterations may include impaired D-xylose absorption and depressed levels of disaccharidases (i.e., maltase, sucrase, and lactase). The nonstructural protein NSP4, with enterotoxin activity (encoded by gene 10), has been shown to induce diarrhea in a mouse model by its effect on calcium regulation. Its role in humans awaits further study.

Although significant levels of serum antibodies correlate with resistance to illness, the role of local intestinal immunity has not been evaluated as extensively. Animal studies indicate that antibody in the small intestine is the major determinant of resistance to illness. A high rate of subclinical infection in neonates is well documented and may be related to passively acquired maternal antibody, host factors, or naturally attenuated rotaviruses that are able to persist in newborn nurseries. The absolute mechanisms of resistance to rotavirus illness remain controversial.

Clinical Manifestations

Norovirus

Clinical characteristics include nausea, vomiting, diarrhea, anorexia, and abdominal discomfort in any combination. Accompanying clinical manifestations may also include myalgias, low-grade fever, headache, and chills. In children, vomiting occurs more often than diarrhea, whereas the opposite pattern is observed in adults. The onset of illness may be abrupt and marked by vomiting or diarrhea, or both. The illness is usually mild and characteristically lasts about 24 to 48 hours. However, severe gastroenteritis has been observed in various age groups and has contributed to the death of elderly, debilitated individuals.

The stools are characteristically loose and watery; blood, mucus, and leukocytes are not typically present. A transient decrease in the T-cell, B-cell, and null cell lymphocyte subpopulations has been observed.

Rotavirus

Rotavirus infection can range from subclinical infection, to mild diarrhea, to a severe and fatal dehydrating illness, even in developed countries. Clinical characteristics include vomiting, diarrhea, abdominal discomfort, and fever in any combination. Fever and vomiting often develop before the diarrhea. Accompanying clinical manifestations may include dehydration, irritability, and pharyngeal or tympanic membrane erythema. For hospitalized patients, the mean duration of confinement is 4 days (range, 2 to 14 days). Stools are characteristically loose and watery, and only infrequently do they contain blood or leukocytes.

In patients with primary immunodeficiency diseases, rotavirus can also induce chronic symptomatic diarrhea with prolonged fecal shedding of the virus and antigenemia. Rotavirus has been associated with severe symptoms in adult renal and bone marrow transplant recipients (with deaths in the latter group) and in children with severe combined immunodeficiency. Rotavirus infections are also associated with necrotizing enterocolitis and hemorrhagic gastroenteritis in neonates, but they do not appear to have an important role in acute diarrhea in human immunodeficiency virus–positive adults. Outbreaks of rotavirus gastroenteritis among elderly individuals in nursing homes can cause fatalities. Ultrasound examination of infants with wild-type rotavirus infection demonstrates thickening of the distal ileum and lymphadenopathy, both of which might predispose to intussusception.

Diagnosis

Norovirus

The diagnosis relies on detection of virus in stool or a serologic response to a virus-specific antigen. Tests include IEM and enzyme-linked immunosorbent assay (ELISA). A polymerase chain reaction (PCR) procedure is available for research use. By IEM, shedding of Norwalk virus is maximal at or shortly after the onset of illness and minimal at 72 hours after onset. However, by RT-PCR, the peak of virus shedding is 25 to 72 hours after challenge, and virus is detectable for at least 7 days. The characteristic absence of fecal leukocytes in Norwalk infection may be helpful for differentiation from *Shigella* (Chapter 330) and *Salmonella* (Chapter 329) enteritis.

A tentative diagnosis of norovirus infection can be made during an outbreak if (1) bacterial or parasitic pathogens are not detected, (2) vomiting is present in at least 50% of cases, (3) the incubation period is 24 to 48 hours, and (4) the mean or median duration of illness is 12 to 60 hours. These criteria are highly specific (99%) and moderately sensitive (68%) in discriminating between etiologically confirmed outbreaks caused by noroviruses or bacteria.

Rotavirus

Diagnosis requires detection of the virus or demonstration of a significant serologic response to rotavirus in paired acute and convalescent sera. The epidemiologic pattern related to the age of the patient, the temporal occurrence of illness, and the signs and symptoms of illness, however, may suggest the diagnosis. The usual absence of fecal leukocytes in rotavirus diarrhea may help in early differentiation from *Shigella* and *Salmonella* enteritis.

By EM and ELISA, stools obtained from the first to the fourth day of illness are optimal for detecting rotavirus, but virus shedding may continue for up to 21 days. Virus is characteristically present in stools during the early phase of diarrhea, but diarrhea may continue for 2 to 3 days after virus shedding has ceased. However, by an RT-PCR–based assay, the duration of virus shedding ranged from 4 to 57 days after the onset of diarrhea, with 30% of children shedding virus for 25 to 57 days.

Although more than 25 assays have been developed to detect rotavirus in stool, the most rapid method is still direct EM. If EM is not readily available, ELISA, counterimmunoelectro-osmophoresis, radioimmunoassay, reverse passive hemagglutination assay, latex agglutination, RNA electrophoresis (electropherotyping), dot hybridization, or RT-PCR can be used. Commercial kits are available for the ELISA and latex agglutination assays. A popular method is confirmatory ELISA because it is simple to perform, is sensitive, does not require specialized equipment, and has a negative serum antibody control for detecting nonspecific reactions. Serotyping by ELISA or genotyping by RT-PCR remains a research tool.

There are many assays for detecting a serologic response, but most remain research tools. Complement fixation is an efficient assay for detecting a serologic response to rotavirus in patients between the ages of 6 and 24 months, but it is not as effective in adults or infants younger than 6 months. Detection of rotavirus antigen in blood in the acute phase of rotavirus gastroenteritis by ELISA and by detection of rotavirus RNA by RT-PCR have been reported, but the significance of these findings for extraintestinal infection is uncertain pending further study.

Detection of rotavirus or demonstration of a serologic response does not necessarily establish an etiologic association with the patient's illness, especially in newborns and adults, who frequently have subclinical infection.

Prevention

Norovirus

There are no specific methods for preventing illness by the noroviruses. However, careful handwashing and proper disposal of contaminated material should minimize transmission. Hygienic preparation of food and measures to decrease contamination of drinking water or swimming facilities should limit the frequency of Norwalk virus outbreaks. Active immunization against these viruses is not yet feasible.

Rotavirus

In August 1998, a quadrivalent rotavirus vaccine (RotaShield) was licensed by the U.S. Food and Drug Administration (FDA) for the immunization of infants at 2, 4, and 6 months of age. However, in July 1999, after more than 1 million doses of vaccine had been given, the CDC recommended suspending further vaccination because postlicensure surveillance suggested that the vaccine was linked with cases of intussusception. The manufacturer (Wyeth Laboratories) subsequently withdrew the vaccine from the market. The population-attributable risk for intussusception with the vaccine was estimated to be approximately 1 in 10,000 infants from CDC case-control and cohort studies.

Since that time, two new live, oral rotavirus vaccines have been developed and have undergone unusually large clinical trials because of the RotaShield experience. One is a pentavalent human-bovine rotavirus reassortant vaccine (RotaTeq) with G1-4 and P1A specificity. It was shown to be safe, immunogenic, and highly effective for preventing severe rotavirus diarrhea [1] and was licensed in the United States in early 2006 and recommended by the Advisory Committee on Immunization Practices for routine use in infants at 2, 4, and 6 months of age. The other, a monovalent human rotavirus vaccine (Rotarix) with G1:P1A specificity, was also safe and highly effective when given at 2 and 4 months of age [2]; this vaccine was first licensed in Mexico and the Dominican Republic in 2004, in Brazil in 2005, and in the European Union countries in early 2006. Neither vaccine was linked with intussusception in placebo-controlled studies in 60,000 to 70,000 infants. However, postmarketing studies will be monitored for safety. In this regard, very recently (Feb 13, 2007), the FDA released an "FDA Public Health Notification" entitled "Information on RotaTeq and Intussusception," which describes postmarketing reports of 28 cases of intussusception in infants in the United States following RotaTeq administration, with approximately half of the cases occurring 1 to 21 days after vaccination. The number of cases did not exceed the expected number of naturally occurring background cases. However, in order to "assess whether RotaTeq may be associated with an increased risk of intussusception and, if so, to what degree," the FDA encouraged reporting of any cases that might be associated with vaccination. The FDA also updated the RotaTeq label and Patient Product Information "to include postmarketing reports of intussusception" and also noted that "The dosage and administration schedule remains unchanged in the label."

A monovalent lamb rotavirus (G10P[12]) vaccine was licensed in 2001 in China, but postlicensure efficacy evaluations have not been completed.

Breast milk is considered to confer some degree of protection against clinically significant rotavirus diarrhea during infancy. Prophylactic oral administration of human serum globulin containing rotavirus antibody to low-birthweight neonates provides significant protection against rotavirus diarrhea. Passive oral immunization of infants and young children with bovine colostrum that contains antibodies to human rotavirus is also effective in preventing rotavirus illness.

Treatment

Rx

Because the noroviruses characteristically cause mild, self-limited gastroenteritis, replacement of fluid and electrolyte loss with an oral rehydration solution (ORS; see later) is usually sufficient. By comparison, rotavirus gastroenteritis may lead to severe dehydration in infants and young children, so early replacement of fluids and electrolytes is essential; intravenous fluids can be used effectively, but oral rehydration therapy is also safe and effective. [1] The recommended World Health Organization ORS is composed of the following: sodium, 90 mmol/L; chloride, 80 mmol/L; potassium, 20 mmol/L; trisodium citrate dihydrate, 10 mmol/L; and glucose, 111 mmol/L, for an overall osmolarity of 311 mOsm/L. Sodium bicarbonate, 30 mmol/L, may be substituted for the trisodium citrate dihydrate. However, an oral glucose-electrolyte solution containing 75 mmol/L sodium, 65 mmol/L chloride, 20 mmol/L potassium, 10 mmol/L citrate, and 75 mmol/L glucose, for an overall osmolarity of 245 mOsm/L, is even more effective for avoiding unscheduled intravenous therapy. [3] After the initial calculated fluid deficit is corrected by administration of ORS, ongoing diarrheal or vomiting fluid losses should be replaced with ORS, volume for volume, until the diarrhea or vomiting stops. The infant's usual diet should be

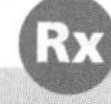

resumed when the rehydration therapy is completed. If oral rehydration fails to correct the fluid and electrolyte loss, if the patient has severe persistent vomiting and is unable to drink, or if the patient is severely dehydrated or in a state of shock or near shock or has depressed consciousness (see later), intravenous therapy must be given immediately. In patients with severe dehydration, intravenous therapy should be used until the patient is able to drink fluids, as needed. Beverages containing high concentrations of simple sugars, such as commercial carbonated drinks, should be avoided during a diarrheal illness. Rice-based ORS is effective in rehydrating infants and young children hospitalized with mild to moderate dehydration caused by diarrhea associated with various pathogens, including rotavirus.

Patients with vomiting can generally be treated with ORS if it is administered in frequent, small amounts (e.g., 5 mL/min). Oral rehydration therapy should not be given to infants and young children with depressed consciousness because of the possibility of fluid aspiration.

In a limited study, chronic rotavirus illness in immunodeficient children has been treated effectively by oral intake of pooled human milk that contained rotavirus antibody. Oral administration of preparations containing rotavirus antibody has produced conflicting results regarding their efficacy for the treatment of normal children during episodes of rotavirus gastroenteritis.

Oral administration of bismuth subsalicylate can significantly reduce the severity and duration of abdominal cramps and decrease the median duration of gastrointestinal symptoms from 20 to 14 hours. However, bismuth subsalicylate is not recommended for acute diarrhea in infants and young children because of concern about its toxic effects. Loperamide, anticholinergic agents, adsorbents, or lactobacillus-containing compounds are also not recommended for acute diarrhea in infants or young children. Randomized placebo-controlled studies suggest that oral racecadotril (an enkephalinase inhibitor that is not available in the Unites States) or nitazoxanide (an antiprotozoal agent), 7.5 mg/kg orally for 3 days [4] may significantly reduce the duration of severe rotaviral diarrheal illness in hospitalized pediatric patients. However, these findings remain to be confirmed in various settings.

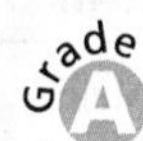

1. Vesikari T, Matson DO, Dennehy P, et al: Safety and efficacy of a pentavalent human-bovine (WC3) reassortant rotavirus vaccine. N Engl J Med 2006;354:23–33.
2. Ruiz-Palacios GM, Perez-Schael I, Velazquez FR, et al: Safety and efficacy of an attenuated vaccine against severe rotavirus gastroenteritis. N Engl J Med 2006;354:11–22.
3. Choice Study Group: Multicenter, randomized, double-blind clinical trial to evaluate the efficacy and safety of a reduced osmolarity oral rehydration salts solution in children with acute watery diarrhea. Pediatrics 2001;107:613–618.
4. Rossignol JF, Abu-Zekry M, Hussein A: Effect of nitazoxanide for treatment of severe rotavirus diarrhoea: Randomised double-blind placebo-controlled trial. Lancet 2006;368:124–129.

SUGGESTED READINGS

Atmar RL, Estes MK: The epidemiologic and clinical importance of norovirus infection. Gastroenterol Clin North Am 2006;35:275–290. *An excellent review of the clinical manifestations and pathogenesis of norovirus infection, as well as the diagnostic and therapeutic approaches to this disease.*

Blanton LH, Adams SM, Beard RS, et al: Molecular and epidemiologic trends of caliciviruses associated with outbreaks of acute gastroenteritis in the United States, 2000–2004. J Infect Dis 2006;193:413–421. *A comprehensive survey of the role of caliciviruses in outbreaks of acute gastroenteritis in the United States.*

Glass RI, Parashar UD, Bresee JS, et al: Rotavirus vaccines: Current prospects and future challenges. Lancet 2006;368:323–332. *A comprehensive perspective on the past, present, and future of rotavirus vaccines.*

Parashar UD, Alexander JP, Glass RI: Prevention of rotavirus infection among infants and children: Recommendations of the Advisory Committee on Immunization Practices (ACIP). MMWR Recomm Rep 2006;55(RR-12):1–13. *Consensus guidelines.*

Parashar UD, Gibson CJ, Bresee JS, et al: Rotavirus and severe childhood diarrhea. Emerg Infect Dis 2006;12:304–306. *Estimates on the importance of rotavirus disease.*

VIRAL HEMORRHAGIC FEVERS

Michael Bell

Definition

Viral hemorrhagic fever is a nonspecific syndrome that can be caused by several different viruses (Table 404–1) from the families Flaviviridae, Bunyaviridae, Arenaviridae, and Filoviridae. All contain RNA, and most are zoonotic (Chapter 349). However, they differ in their modes of transmission, animal reservoirs, and ability to be transmitted directly from human to human. Both arthropod-borne and rodent-associated viruses cause viral hemorrhagic fevers. The rodent-associated viruses do not require an arthropod vector but are transmitted directly to vertebrates by infectious excreta or secretions of the rodent. The reservoir and natural mode of transmission for the African hemorrhagic fever viruses Marburg and Ebola are not known, but amplification of transmission of both routinely occurs in health care settings. Primary infections caused by these viruses are geographically restricted by the natural range and habitats of their respective vector or reservoir species. Because of the increasing prevalence of international travel, however, infected individuals may be encountered anywhere on the planet.

Clinical Manifestations

The syndrome begins as an acute febrile illness that may be accompanied by a range of symptoms and signs, including headache, pharyngitis, myalgia, nausea, vomiting, and conjunctival injection. Mild to moderate bleeding diatheses and capillary fragility can occur, and severe cases can progress rapidly to sepsis syndrome (Chapter 109), multiorgan failure, and death. Shock has been attributed to both antigen-antibody complexes and direct viral cytopathic effects that alter capillary permeability. Several viruses cause disease-specific pathologic changes, including hepatocellular damage with yellow fever, meningoencephalitis with tick-borne flavivirus infections, and renal tubular necrosis with hantaviruses causing hemorrhagic fever with renal syndrome.

Prevention

Control of epidemic and endemic disease requires interruption of the specific transmission cycle. Interventions may include vaccination of reservoir mammals, arthropod vector control, peridomestic rodent control, public education to avoid vectors, and infection control to prevent the spread of infections that are transmitted from human to human or during medical procedures. Vaccines are available or are under development for yellow fever, dengue, Junin, and Ebola hemorrhagic fever viruses. For most of these infections, the role of specific antiviral therapy is limited.

VECTOR-BORNE HEMORRHAGIC FEVERS

Yellow Fever

The Pathogen

Yellow fever virus is in the genus Flavivirus of the family Flaviviridae. They are enveloped, spherical viruses approximately 40 nm in diameter with single-stranded, negative-sense RNA genomes. They replicate in arthropod and vertebrate cells and can be grown in arthropod and vertebrate tissue cultures, suckling mice, and several primate species. Mosquitoes become infective 9 to 30 days after feeding on a viremic vertebrate, with this incubation period being shorter at higher temperatures.

Epidemiology

Worldwide, there are an estimated 200,000 cases of yellow fever each year and as many as 30,000 deaths. The disease is endemic in Africa and South America, with the latter experiencing mostly sporadic infections in forestry and agricultural workers exposed to forested environments.

TABLE 404–1 CLINICAL PARAMETERS OF VIRAL HEMORRHAGIC FEVERS*

Disease	Viral Agent	Incubation Period (Days)	Clinical Syndromes: Hemorrhage	Hepatitis	Encephalitis	Nephropathy	ARDS	Case-Fatality Rate (%)
Yellow fever	Yellow fever	3–6	Major	Major	Absent	Moderate	Absent	2–20
Dengue hemorrhagic fever	Dengue 1-4	5–8	Moderate	Moderate	Absent	Absent	Absent	2–10
Rift Valley fever	Rift Valley fever	3–6	Major	Major	Moderate	Absent	Absent	0.2–10
Crimean-Congo hemorrhagic fever	Crimean-Congo hemorrhagic fever	2–9	Major	Major	Minor	Absent	Absent	30–50
Kyasanur Forest disease	Kyasanur Forest disease	3–8	Minor	Minor	Moderate	Absent	Absent	5–10
Omsk hemorrhagic fever	Omsk hemorrhagic fever	3–8	Minor	Minor	Moderate	Absent	Absent	0.4–2.5
Hemorrhagic fever with renal syndrome	Hantaan, Puumala, Dobrava, Seoul	2–42	Moderate	Rare	Minor	Major	Absent	2–5
Hantavirus pulmonary syndrome	Sin Nombre	12–16	Minor	Minor	Absent	Minor	Major	40–50
Venezuelan hemorrhagic fever	Guanarito	7–14	Moderate	Rare	Rare	Minor	Absent	33
Brazilian hemorrhagic fever	Sabiá	8–12	Major	Minor	Minor	Minor	Absent	33
Argentine hemorrhagic fever	Junin	10–14	Minor	Rare	Moderate	Minor	Absent	10–20
Bolivian hemorrhagic fever	Machupo	7–14	Moderate	Rare	Moderate	Minor	Absent	15–30
Lassa fever	Lassa	3–16	Minor	Major	Minor	Minor	Absent	15
African hemorrhagic fever	Marburg	3–9	Major	Major	Minor	Absent	Absent	20–30
	Ebola	3–18	Major	Major	Minor	Absent	Absent	53–88

*This table appeared as Table 375–1 in Cecil Textbook of Medicine, 22nd edition and was compiled by Dr. Robert Shope.
ARDS = adult respiratory distress syndrome.

Natural infection is maintained among primates and mosquitoes in tropical South America as far north as Panama and in sub-Saharan Africa, particularly in the moist savannah zones of western and central Africa during the rainy season. Yellow fever is not found in Asia, although *Aedes aegypti* mosquitos capable of transmitting the virus are present. To prevent introduction of the virus into the mosquito population, India and other Asian nations require proof of vaccination for travelers arriving from regions in which yellow fever is endemic.

Two patterns of yellow fever transmission are recognized: urban and sylvan. The two are clinically indistinguishable.

Urban yellow fever occurs in towns, cities, and semirural areas, where it is transmitted by *A. aegypti* mosquitoes. Mosquitoes acquire yellow fever virus from an infected human during the first few days of fever and, after an extrinsic incubation period ranging from 4 to 18 days, can transmit the infection to other humans for the life of the mosquito. *A. aegypti* breeds near human habitations where there is stagnant water, such as in discarded tires, jars, cisterns, or drains. Yellow fever was endemic in large urban centers such as Havana, Rio de Janeiro, and Guayaquil and was a common cause of death before enactment of mosquito control measures and subsequent elimination of the disease in the early 1900s. The last recorded urban yellow fever case in the Americas occurred in Trinidad in 1954. In Africa, *A. aegypti* remains prevalent in cities, and yellow fever outbreaks still occur there. Although *A. aegypti* accounts for the majority of yellow fever transmission, some African transmission is also maintained by other *Aedes* species, including *Aedes bromeliae, Aedes africanus* (which breeds in tree holes), *Aedes luteocephalus,* and *Aedes furcifer-taylori,* the latter found in savannah and forest-savannah transition zones of western Africa.

Sylvan yellow fever is an incidental infection of humans. The virus is maintained between primates and forest canopy mosquitoes. Humans are infected when they come in contact with infective mosquitoes in the forest or when an infected primate brings the virus to the forest periphery where transmission to humans can be established by anthropophagous mosquitoes.

Although young males are more likely to come in contact with forest environments and are thus more likely to be infected with sylvan yellow fever, individuals of all ages and either sex are susceptible to the virus. Vaccination and natural infection both result in long-term immunity. Epidemics occur when virus-bearing mosquitoes are introduced to non-immune populations, such as age groups not covered by previous immunization or those born since a previous outbreak.

Pathobiology

Yellow fever principally affects the liver, kidneys, heart, and lymphoid tissues. Gross pathologic findings include icteric skin and petechial hemorrhages, which may be widespread; an icteric, fatty liver of normal size; a soft, flabby heart; and swollen, pink-gray kidneys. Small effusions may be present in the peritoneal and pleural spaces.

Characteristic histologic features in fatal cases include diffuse fatty degeneration and coagulative necrosis of hepatocytes in the midzone of the hepatic lobule, with relative sparing of the central zone. Coagulated contents of hepatocytes stain with eosin and produce reddish pink Councilman's bodies, visible under low-power microscopy. Renal lesions include fatty changes with tubular necrosis, and nephritis or nephritic syndrome may be seen, along with accumulation of proteinaceous material in the proximal tubules. Fatty infiltration of the myocardium may involve not only muscle fibers but also the sinoatrial node and bundle of His. Perivascular cerebral hemorrhages and cerebral edema may be seen.

Viral replication occurs in hepatocytes and myocytes and is presumed to mediate damage to these cells. Hepatocellular damage accounts for jaundice and loss of synthetic capacity, thereby resulting in a prolonged prothrombin time. Some fatal cases have coagulopathies, including thrombocytopenia; increased prothrombin, partial thromboplastin, and thrombin times; diminished factor VIII and fibrinogen levels; and elevated fibrin split products.

Clinical Manifestations

Most cases of yellow fever are abrupt, brief, and self-limited. Inapparent infections are common, and symptomatic illness is usually relatively mild.

The incubation period is generally 3 to 6 days, whereupon a sudden onset of fever (40° C or higher) and headache develops in symptomatic cases. Mild illness resolves spontaneously after 48 hours or less. More severe illness is accompanied by prostration, myalgia, nausea, and vomiting. Bradycardia relative to fever (Faget's sign) and mild proteinuria are present.

Hemorrhagic fever, which is the most severe manifestation of yellow fever, is characterized by severe headache, myalgias, nausea, jaundice, and dehydration. Minor gingival bleeding and epistaxis may occur. There may be several days of quiescence, usually around the fourth day of illness, at which time clinical deterioration with hepatorenal failure ensues. Significant gastrointestinal bleeding, including black vomitus, emesis of fresh blood, and melena, may occur, and genitourinary bleeding may be seen. Albuminuria may lead to oliguria or anuria. Meningoencephalitis has been documented. Heart failure with myocardial depression develops, and ST segment changes can be seen on the electrocardiogram; in rare cases, late cardiac sequelae may occur. Secondary infectious complications include suppurative parotitis subsequent to dehydration and bacterial pneumonia. Recovery is complete if the patient survives. In fatal cases, death usually occurs on about the seventh or eighth day of illness.

Early in the infection there may be leukopenia with relative neutropenia, thrombocytopenia, and prolongation of the clotting and prothrombin times. The serum bilirubin level is typically elevated and ranges from 10 to 20 mg/dL or higher in severe cases. Aminotransferase elevations peak between days 5 and 10 of severe illness. Hypoglycemia is seen in cases with severe liver involvement. The prothrombin and partial thromboplastin times are increased; platelets and clotting factors II, V, VII, IX, and X are decreased. Albuminuria is initially minimal but rises to levels of 3 to 5 g/L or higher on day 4 or 5 of illness. Biliuria and casts are seen. Cerebrospinal fluid (CSF) may show elevated protein and opening pressure; cell counts are normal.

Diagnosis

The diagnosis may be made by detecting viral antigen, currently either by identification of RNA with reverse transcription–polymerase chain reaction (RT-PCR) or by detection of antigen in blood during viremia with an antigen capture enzyme-linked immunosorbent assay (ELISA). However, isolation of virus is the "gold standard" of diagnosis in locations where appropriate laboratory capacity is available. Virus may be isolated from blood during the first 3 days of illness, and later it can be isolated from liver and other postmortem specimens. Postmortem diagnosis can be made by histopathologic examination of the liver with immunohistochemical stains against specific antigens.

Serologic diagnosis is made by using antibody capture ELISA to detect IgM. A four-fold or greater change in specific antibody titer between acute and convalescent sera is diagnostic. Complement fixation, hemagglutination inhibition, and ELISA tests are preferred in field settings because they are quicker, but neutralization tests can also be used. Other flaviviruses (dengue, West Nile, and St. Louis encephalitis) may have cross-reactive serology with yellow fever virus.

Differential Diagnosis

Mild cases of yellow fever are characterized by a nonspecific syndrome indistinguishable from many other acute febrile illnesses. In severe forms, fulminant viral hepatitis (Chapter 151), severe malaria (Chapter 366), leptospirosis (Chapter 344), relapsing fever (Chapter 343), and other viral hemorrhagic fevers must be considered.

Prevention

Vaccination

Vaccination with the 17D yellow fever vaccine protects against all strains of the virus despite minor antigenic differences among strains from different regions. This vaccine is administered only at designated yellow fever vaccination centers, the locations of which can be provided by local health departments or the U.S. Centers for Disease Control and Prevention (CDC) Travelers' Health Yellow Fever website. Although yellow fever is a rare cause of illness in travelers, most countries have regulations and requirements for yellow fever vaccination that must be met before entering the country after being in an area with endemic yellow fever. Individuals for whom vaccine is contraindicated should obtain a waiver letter before travel or delay travel to an area with active yellow fever transmission.

Yellow fever vaccine (Chapter 16), which is a live virus vaccine that has been used for several decades, is approved for adults and children older than 9 months. Administration of immune globulin does not interfere with the antibody response to yellow fever vaccine. A single dose confers immunity lasting 10 years or more. If a person is at continued risk for yellow fever infection, a booster dose is needed every 10 years. Yellow fever vaccine generally has few side effects; mild headache, muscle pain, or other minor symptoms develop in less than 5% of recipients 5 to 10 days after vaccination. Contraindications to vaccination include age younger than 6 months because of a risk of viral encephalitis; pregnancy because of a theoretical risk of vertical infection; individuals with egg allergy; or immunosuppression as a result of symptomatic human immunodeficiency virus infection, malignancy, or immunosuppressive therapy, among other conditions. Individuals should be evaluated on a case-by-case basis to determine whether the risk of contracting yellow fever outweighs a contraindication to vaccination.

Vector Control

Individuals living in areas infested with *A. aegypti* should eliminate potential breeding sites, primarily artificial containers that hold water. Items that collect rainwater or are used to store water (e.g., plastic containers, 55-gallon drums, buckets, or used automobile tires) should be covered or properly discarded. Pet and animal watering containers and vases with fresh flowers should be emptied and scoured at least once a week to eliminate the mosquito eggs and larvae and thus reduce the number of mosquitoes. Air-conditioned buildings or the use of screens on windows and doors can reduce the risk of being bitten by mosquitoes indoors, and appropriate use of repellents containing 20 to 30% DEET (diethyltoluamide) on exposed skin decreases the risk of being bitten when outdoors.

Treatment

Treatment of yellow fever is supportive and includes analgesia and antiemetics. Aspirin and other medications that may exacerbate a potential coagulopathy should be avoided. Electrolyte balance should be maintained, and careful parenteral fluid and blood transfusion may be used with attention to fluid status. Experience with hemodialysis is limited, and the usefulness of heparin for disseminated intravascular coagulation (DIC) (Chapter 181) in this setting is unclear. Secondary infections should be treated promptly.

Secondary Prevention

Patients should be protected from mosquitoes, either by window screens or by a bed net, to prevent secondary transmission by mosquitoes to other patients or health care personnel. Standard precautions for infection control should be used when caring for patients.

Prognosis

Most cases are asymptomatic or mild. However, 10 to 20% may have fulminant disease, with a case-fatality rate greater than 50%, mostly in settings with limited capacity for supportive care.

Dengue Hemorrhagic Fever

The Pathogen

Dengue virus, which is in the genus Flavivirus of the family Flaviviridae, is an enveloped, spherical virus with a single-stranded, negative-sense RNA genome. It replicates in arthropod and vertebrate cells. Dengue virus is the etiologic agent of dengue fever (Chapter 405). Mosquitoes become infective 8 to 11 days after feeding on a viremic vertebrate and remain infective for life.

Epidemiology

The basic epidemiology of dengue hemorrhagic fever is the same as described for dengue fever, with transmission from person to person by *Aedes* mosquitoes (most often *A. aegypti*) in the domestic environment. Less than 7% of dengue virus infections result in dengue hemorrhagic fever. An estimated 250,000 cases of dengue hemorrhagic fever occur annually worldwide, with more than 12,000 attributed deaths.

Dengue viruses are distributed throughout tropical and subtropical zones of Southeast Asia (all four serotypes), the Pacific Islands (type 2), western Africa (types 1 and 2), eastern Africa (type 2), the Caribbean (types 1 and 4), and the Americas (types 2 and 3). Dengue hemorrhagic fever has been reported in all these areas except Africa.

In hyperendemic regions such as Southeast Asia, dengue hemorrhagic fever is seen primarily in children between 4 and 12 years of age. Elsewhere, all ages may be affected. Since World War II, epidemics of dengue hemorrhagic fever have been seen with increasing frequency in areas where dengue virus is present, most commonly Southeast Asia, the Pacific Islands, and most recently, the Caribbean and South America.

Pathobiology

Although dengue hemorrhagic fever can occur with primary dengue infection, the majority of cases have been associated with infection of hosts already sensitized by a previous dengue infection of different serotype. With secondary infection, an anamnestic antibody response results in rapid formation of antigen-antibody complexes. These complexes have been shown to enhance infectivity of the dengue virus in monocytes through facilitation of cell entry.

Dengue virus infects macrophages, lymphocytes, and endothelial cells. In dengue hemorrhagic fever, the lymphoreticular system shows loss of lymphocytes in T-cell-dependent zones. An Arthus-like reaction with monocytic and lymphocytic perivascular infiltration without necrosis may be seen in skin. Monocyte infection is also believed to mediate rapid activation of complement via the classical pathway and perhaps by the alternative pathway as well, ultimately resulting in increased vascular permeability and a cascade of coagulation defects, including thrombocytopenia and clotting abnormalities. The process develops quickly and, if not managed effectively, can lead to shock and death in just a few hours.

Grossly, on postmortem examination, focal hemorrhages, vascular congestion, and edema are evident in multiple organs. Pleural and peritoneal effusions are present.

Clinical Manifestations

Dengue hemorrhagic fever is characterized by thrombocytopenia and loss of intravascular volume because of capillary leakage; hemorrhage, despite the name, is not a major aspect of the disease. Patients may progress to shock and, without effective supportive treatment, multiorgan failure and death.

Initial symptoms are those of dengue fever, with a sudden onset of high, continuous fever, headache, myalgias, pharyngitis, facial flushing, anorexia, nausea, and right upper quadrant and epigastric abdominal tenderness. High fever may persist for as long as a week. Application of a tourniquet to an extremity (tourniquet test) demonstrates easy bruising. Fine petechiae can be seen on the face, soft palate, and extremities as a result of the underlying thrombocytopenia and capillary abnormality. Gingival bleeding and epistaxis occur in some cases. Progression to dengue hemorrhagic fever may be heralded by severe abdominal pain, persistent vomiting, hypothermia, or altered mental status (e.g., irritability or depressed level of consciousness). Patients experience hypotension and tachycardia on about the third to seventh day of illness. Pleural and peritoneal effusions are common, and hemoconcentration is reflected by an approximately 20% increase in the patient's hematocrit. White blood cell counts may be normal or slightly high, with lymphocytosis and atypical lymphocytes. Elevated transaminases and blood urea nitrogen are seen.

Diagnosis

Laboratory diagnosis is the same as for dengue fever (Chapter 405). Rapid diagnosis, which is possible with RT-PCR techniques, is important in facilitating prompt supportive care.

Confirmatory testing may involve either isolation of virus or detection of specific antibodies. Isolation of virus is performed on serum specimens collected during the first 5 days of fever. Serologic diagnosis requires paired sera obtained during initial illness and after the sixth day of fever. Antidengue antibodies are nonspecific and may cross-react with other flaviviruses, including West Nile and St. Louis encephalitis viruses. Commercial kits vary in sensitivity and specificity, so critical results should be confirmed by a reference laboratory. Paired sera may be sent to the state health department for testing or be forwarded for testing at the CDC.

Prevention

Prevention and control of dengue hemorrhagic fever are as described for dengue fever (Chapter 405).

Treatment

Rx

Treatment is supportive and focuses on maintenance of intravascular volume, preservation of electrolyte and acid-base balance, and correction of coagulation abnormalities. Resuscitation should be initiated promptly at the first signs of shock, with fluid administration managed carefully to avoid fluid overload. Medications that inhibit coagulation or increase the potential for gastritis and hemorrhage (e.g., salicylates, nonsteroidal anti-inflammatory drugs, steroids) should be avoided. Heparin may be used for DIC (Chapter 181) cautiously in refractory cases. Standard precautions for infection control should be used when caring for patients.

Prognosis

Uncorrected, shock may progress to metabolic acidosis and severe bleeding (usually epistaxis or from upper gastrointestinal, genitourinary, or gingival sites). Patients generally recover or die within a day of the onset of shock. The case-fatality rate of dengue hemorrhagic fever is as high as 50% without treatment; with appropriate supportive care, estimates range from 2 to 10%. If patients survive, there are usually no sequelae after dengue hemorrhagic fever.

Tick-Borne Flavivirus Diseases: Kyasanur Forest Disease and Omsk Hemorrhagic Fever

The Pathogen

Both Kyasanur Forest disease and Omsk hemorrhagic fever are caused by flaviviruses that are enveloped and contain single-stranded RNA genomes. They are antigenically related to each other but do not provide cross-immunity. Both are transmitted transovarially and trans-stadially in ticks. Other closely related viruses include those responsible for central European tick-borne encephalitis, Russian spring-summer encephalitis, and Powassan encephalitis.

Epidemiology

Kyasanur Forest disease was originally described in what is now Karnataka, India, in the Kyasanur forest. Omsk hemorrhagic fever originated in the oblasts of Omsk and Novosibirsk in the former Soviet Union. Both Kyasanur Forest disease and Omsk hemorrhagic fever are transmitted to humans by ixodid ticks and are maintained in rodent and other vertebrate hosts. Cattle grazing at the forest fringe, though not infected, are thought to serve as amplifying hosts that greatly increase the number of infectious ticks to which humans are exposed. In addition to tick-borne transmission, Omsk hemorrhagic fever has been transmitted by direct contact with infectious muskrat carcasses. Infections in laboratory workers have been common, though generally mild.

Pathobiology

Fatal cases may demonstrate scattered hemorrhagic and necrotic areas in the lungs, liver, gastrointestinal tract, and kidneys. Reticuloendothelial proliferation is seen in Kyasanur Forest disease, with marked erythrophagocytosis in the spleen.

Clinical Manifestations

Incubation periods range from 3 to 8 days. Kyasanur Forest disease is an acute, usually self-limited illness characterized by fever, headache, myalgias, conjunctivitis, soft palate vesicles, cough, bradycardia, nausea, vomiting, and diarrhea. Lymphadenopathy and hepatomegaly are seen, but jaundice is uncommon. Hemorrhagic signs are limited to minor upper gastrointestinal and genitourinary bleeding, epistaxis, and hemoptysis. Most infections resolve by day 10, but approximately 20% of patients have a biphasic illness with recrudescence after 1 to 2 weeks that may last a week and be accompanied by meningoencephalitis.

Leukopenia, thrombocytopenia, and albuminuria are seen. CSF in the presence of meningoencephalitis may show elevated protein levels but is otherwise normal.

Omsk hemorrhagic fever is clinically very similar to Kyasanur Forest disease, though with a greater frequency of sequelae that include hair loss, deafness, and neuropsychiatric abnormalities.

Diagnosis

The diagnosis may be made by isolation of the virus or detection of RNA by PCR from blood collected during the first 10 days of illness or by serologic assessment of acute and convalescent sera.

Prevention

Measures to prevent tick attachment, including repellents and protective clothing, should be used by individuals entering affected areas. Environmental spraying of forest tracts with acaricides can reduce tick populations. A chick embryo–derived Kyasanur Forest disease vaccine is in use in endemic regions. A mouse brain–derived Omsk hemorrhagic fever vaccine has been used for those at risk of occupational exposure.

Treatment

Treatment is supportive, as described for dengue and yellow fever. Standard precautions for infection control should be followed when caring for patients.

Prognosis

For Kyasanur Forest disease, the case-fatality rate is approximately 5%. Convalescence is long, but sequelae are not reported. The case-fatality rate with Omsk hemorrhagic fever is less than 3%.

Crimean-Congo Hemorrhagic Fever

The Pathogen

Crimean-Congo hemorrhagic fever is caused by a virus of the Nairovirus genus, family Bunyaviridae. The virus has a single-stranded RNA genome, is enveloped and spherical, and replicates in suckling mice and several cell culture systems.

Epidemiology

Crimean-Congo hemorrhagic fever is a tick-borne infection whose distribution includes parts of the former Soviet Union, the Balkan nations, Iraq, Iran, the Indian subcontinent, Afghanistan, northwestern China, the Middle East, and most of sub-Saharan Africa, including South Africa. The disease was first characterized in the Crimea in 1944 as Crimean hemorrhagic fever. It was recognized in 1969 as the cause of illness in the Congo, thus the current name.

The virus is harbored and transmitted in nature, principally by ixodid ticks of the genus *Hyalomma* but also by ticks of the genera *Rhipicephalus, Boophilus,* and *Amblyomma.* The virus is transmitted transovarially and trans-stadially among ticks, with amplification in vertebrates, including hares, hedgehogs, sheep, and cattle. In Africa, antibodies against Crimean-Congo hemorrhagic fever have been found in giraffes, rhinoceros, elands, buffalos, kudus, zebras, and dogs.

Transmission to humans occurs through contact with infected animal blood or ticks. Crimean-Congo hemorrhagic fever can be transmitted from one infected human to another by contact with infectious blood or body fluids. Outbreaks have been reported in military personnel, campers, and persons tending sheep and cattle. Health care personnel have been infected through contact with infectious human blood and tissue. Health care–associated spread as a result of improper sterilization of medical equipment, reuse of injection needles, and contamination of medical supplies has been documented.

Pathobiology

After initial inoculation, the virus is spread by blood and the lymphatic circulation and achieves high levels in multiple organs, including the liver. Diffuse foci of necrosis and hemorrhage are seen, with Councilman's bodies in hepatocytes. DIC occurs within the first 3 days of illness.

Clinical Manifestations

After an incubation period of 2 to 9 days, patients have a sudden onset of fever with symptoms that include headache, myalgia, pharyngitis, conjunctivitis, nausea, vomiting, diarrhea, and abdominal pain. Petechiae may be seen on the soft palate, and jaundice and hepatomegaly may be present. In severe cases, mood alterations and confusion may be noted. As the illness progresses, large ecchymoses, severe epistaxis, and persistent bleeding at injection sites can be seen, usually beginning on about the fourth day of illness and lasting approximately 2 weeks. Aminotransferase and serum bilirubin levels are often elevated in late illness. Evidence of DIC is seen (abnormal prothrombin, activated partial thromboplastin, and thrombin times and increased fibrin degradation products).

Multiple organ system failure may lead to death, usually during the second week of illness. Other potentially lethal complications include severe blood loss, cerebral hemorrhage, and pulmonary edema.

Diagnosis

Laboratory diagnosis can be made by a positive serologic test result, evidence of viral antigen in tissue by immunohistochemical staining and microscopic examination, or identification of viral RNA sequences in blood or tissue in a patient with a clinical history compatible with Crimean-Congo hemorrhagic fever. Virus or nucleic acid is easily detected during the first 8 days of illness. Antibodies are detectable by immunofluorescence and ELISA in surviving patients. Specific IgM and IgG are present by days 7 to 9 of illness.

Prevention

Measures to prevent tick attachment, including repellents and protective clothing, should be used by individuals in high-risk settings, such as livestock enclosures in affected areas. Treatment of livestock to reduce the tick burden may reduce transmission to humans. Handling of blood and tissue of sick sheep and cattle should be minimized and undertaken with appropriate safety and hygiene precautions.

Treatment

Rx

Treatment is supportive, including monitoring and correction of volume status and electrolyte imbalances, support of the coagulation system, careful sedation, and pain control. Careful fluid management is necessary to avoid fluid overload. Standard precautions for infection control should be used, including appropriate management of sharp items such as injection needles, appropriate protection against contact with blood and body fluids, and the use of barriers to prevent splashes onto mucous membranes when procedures are performed.

Prognosis

Although improvement is usually seen on approximately day 10, patients may remain weak and listless for more than a month. Patients who recover do not demonstrate sequelae. The case-fatality rate has ranged from 15% to as high as 70% in some outbreaks.

RODENT-BORNE HEMORRHAGIC FEVERS

Hemorrhagic Fever with Renal Syndrome

The Pathogen

Hemorrhagic fever with renal syndrome encompasses a group of clinically similar illnesses caused by hantaviruses from the family Bunyaviridae. Hantaviruses have a single-stranded RNA genome and are enveloped. Hemorrhagic fever with renal syndrome includes Korean hemorrhagic fever, epidemic hemorrhagic fever, and nephropathia epidemica. The viruses that cause hemorrhagic fever with renal syndrome include Hantaan, Dobrava-Belgrade, Seoul, and Puumala.

Epidemiology

Hantaan virus is widely distributed in eastern Asia, particularly in China, Russia, and Korea. Puumala virus is found in Scandinavia, western Europe, and Russia. Dobrava virus is found primarily in the Balkans, and Seoul virus is found worldwide. In the Americas, viruses in the same family cause a different disease known as hantavirus pulmonary syndrome.

Hantaviruses are carried and transmitted by rodents. The striped field mouse *Apodemus agrarius* is a carrier in Korea and other parts of Asia; the bank vole *Clethrionomys glareolus* carries the virus in Finland and west of the Ural Mountains; and *Rattus rattus* and *Rattus norvegicus* serve as reservoirs in urban areas of Japan, Korea, North America, and Europe. Human exposure occurs through contact with the urine, droppings, or saliva of infected rodents or after exposure to dust from their nests. Humans may also become infected by the introduction of infectious material through broken skin or onto mucous membranes of the eyes, nose, or mouth. Occupational exposure may occur (e.g., among laboratory personnel and field biologists) through rodent bites from infected animals, and health care–associated transmission has been reported.

Pathobiology

Human cells infected with hantaviruses do not demonstrate the cytopathic effects of viral replication. The associated syndrome of illness appears to be immune mediated, consistent with the presence of specific antibodies and T cells at the onset of symptoms. Virus is present in blood only during the initial stage of infection and is usually absent at the time that severe symptoms begin. On postmortem examination, viral antigens are found prominently in the endothelial cell layers of the lungs and kidneys. Vascular endothelium is affected, with markedly increased capillary permeability. Retroperitoneal edema is seen, and petechial hemorrhages are widespread. Larger visceral and cerebral hemorrhages can occur (e.g., myocardium, pituitary). Acute tubulointerstitial nephritis is seen, with inflammatory cell infiltration in some cases.

Clinical Manifestations

After an incubation period of 1 to 2 weeks and in some cases as long as 8 weeks, there is the sudden onset of a febrile phase, with symptoms including intense headaches, myalgia, nausea, abdominal pain, and blurred vision. Conjunctivitis or rash may be present. Late features of illness usually appear after approximately 5 days and consist of a hypotensive phase that may lead to shock, manifestations of vascular leakage, and acute renal failure with fluid overload. Laboratory findings include a rising hematocrit, leukocytosis, thrombocytopenia, and heavy proteinuria with decreased renal function. The hypotensive phase lasts approximately 4 days and is followed by an oliguric phase, during which extravascular fluid is resorbed. Hypertension and pulmonary edema may be seen. The diuretic phase with return of renal function may, in contrast, be accompanied by marked electrolyte and fluid imbalance, which if not appropriately managed can lead to death.

In general, only 20% of patients manifest severe illness, but the severity of illness also varies with the etiologic agent. Hantaan and Dobrava virus infections cause more severe illness, whereas Seoul and Puumala are usually milder.

Diagnosis

In the presence of a consistent clinical history, the diagnosis of hemorrhagic fever with renal syndrome may be confirmed by serologic tests (e.g., immunofluorescence, ELISA, and neutralization tests), which become positive at the end of the first week of illness. Hantavirus antigen in tissue can be detected by immunohistochemical staining and histologic examination. Rapid tests to identify viral RNA in blood or tissue may be positive early in the course of illness. Specific antibody titers peak at 2 weeks after the onset of illness and last for many years.

Prevention

Rodent control is essential for preventing infections. Rodent populations near human communities should be addressed, with particular attention to exclusion of rodents from homes. Contact with rodent urine, droppings, saliva, and nesting materials should be avoided.

Treatment

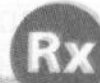

Treatment is supportive, with careful management of fluid and electrolyte balance and volume status. Dialysis may be necessary in cases of severe fluid overload or hyperkalemia with renal failure. Intravenous ribavirin (Chapter 412), preferably given within the first 5 days of illness, has been shown to shorten illness and decrease the risk for death. Standard precautions for infection control should be used when caring for patients.

Prognosis

Recovery may take weeks or months. The case-fatality rate depends on the virus and ranges from 5 to 15% with Hantaan virus to less than 1% for Puumala virus infection.

Hantavirus Pulmonary Syndrome

Definition

Hantaviruses that cause hantavirus pulmonary syndrome belong to a genus in the bunyavirus family of viruses. The viruses are enveloped, with RNA genomes. Sin Nombre virus (SNV) was first isolated from rodents collected during investigation of the hantavirus pulmonary syndrome outbreak in the Four Corners region. Black Creek Canal virus and Monongahela virus have been isolated in association with subsequent clusters of hantavirus pulmonary syndrome in Florida and West Virginia.

Epidemiology

Viruses causing hantavirus pulmonary syndrome are carried by New World rats and mice (family Muridae, subfamily Sigmodontinae). Although the viruses do not cause illness in their rodent hosts, infected rodents shed virus in saliva, urine, and feces for months or for life. Several hantaviruses, each carried by a specific rodent host, can cause hantavirus pulmonary syndrome. Widely distributed throughout the Americas, these rodents are generally associated with rural environments; species that enter houses and outbuildings, such as the deer mouse (*Peromyscus maniculatus*) and white-footed mouse (*Peromyscus leucopus*), are most likely to be encountered by humans. The deer mouse is the reservoir for SNV, the main cause of hantavirus pulmonary syndrome in the United States. On average, about 10% of deer mice may be infected with SNV. Other viruses causing hantavirus pulmonary syndrome include New York virus, carried by the white-footed mouse; Black Creek Canal virus, carried by the cotton rat; and Bayou virus, carried by the rice rat. However, in addition to being more likely to be found in peridomestic settings, both the deer mouse and white-footed mouse typically have higher population densities than other rodents do, a feature that has been associated with an increased likelihood of human infection. Hantavirus pulmonary syndrome is more common in South America than in North America; numerous South American hantaviruses and associated rodent species have been identified thus far, although most have not been linked to human illness.

Human infection occurs through exposure to infectious rodent saliva or excreta, including inhalation of infectious material in dust and aerosols created by activities such as sweeping. Direct inoculation into broken skin, such as by rodent bites, and mucous membrane exposure have led to human infections. Disturbing or entering rodent-infested buildings, especially structures that are seasonally closed, has been strongly associated with the acquisition of hantavirus pulmonary syndrome. Occupational risk has been related to work activities of grain farmers, field biologists, and agricultural, mill, construction, utility, and feedlot workers, although in many cases peridomestic exposure has occurred as well.

Pathobiology

The pathology of hantavirus pulmonary syndrome is characterized primarily by pulmonary lesions with involvement of the spleen, liver, and lymph nodes. Viral antigens are found in the capillary endothelia of affected tissues, which demonstrate varying degrees of capillary dilation and edema. Interstitial pneumonitis is seen with edema and monocytic infiltration. In addition to prominent impairment of vascular endothelium and alterations in permeability, myocardial depression also contributes to the multifaceted shock syndrome that typifies severe disease.

Clinical Manifestations

Hantavirus pulmonary syndrome is a febrile illness characterized by a biphasic pattern with acute respiratory compromise, capillary leakage, and myocardial depression without significant hemorrhagic features. The illness begins with a 3- to 5-day prodrome of fever, chills, myalgia, headache, and gastrointestinal symptoms. Hantavirus pulmonary syndrome is seldom correctly diagnosed at this nonspecific stage.

The second, or cardiopulmonary, phase usually begins on the seventh day of illness with the onset of cough, tachypnea, hypoxia, pulmonary edema, and hypotension with low cardiac output. The syndrome progresses rapidly, and hospitalization and mechanical ventilation are commonly required within 24 hours of onset of the second phase. In fatal cases, myocardial depression develops and progresses to sinus bradycardia, ventricular tachycardia, or fibrillation.

Only about 30% of patients with hantavirus pulmonary syndrome have radiographic evidence of pulmonary edema on initial evaluation. Within 48 hours, essentially all have interstitial edema, and two thirds have extensive bibasilar or perihilar air space disease.

Clinical laboratory findings include an elevated hematocrit, elevated neutrophil count with a left shift, thrombocytopenia, and circulating immunoblasts. DIC develops only very rarely, in sharp contrast to hemorrhagic fever with renal syndrome.

Diagnosis

Because onset of the cardiopulmonary phase of hantavirus pulmonary syndrome occurs after the viremia has subsided, viral isolation from human specimens has not been useful for diagnosis. Serologic evidence of hantavirus pulmonary syndrome includes the presence of hantavirus-specific IgM or a four-fold rise in titer of hantavirus-specific IgG detected by ELISA, hantavirus-specific RNA sequences detected by PCR in clinical specimens, and hantavirus antigen detected by immunohistochemistry.

Laboratory testing is generally performed or confirmed at a reference laboratory. Immunohistochemical testing of formalin-fixed tissues with specific monoclonal and polyclonal antibodies can be used to detect hantavirus antigens and diagnose hantavirus pulmonary syndrome on postmortem specimens. To select which patients to test, a screening case definition can be used for assessment of patients who do not have a predisposing medical condition (e.g., chronic pulmonary disease, malignancy, trauma, burn, and surgery) that would account for adult respiratory distress syndrome (ARDS): (1) a febrile illness with bilateral diffuse interstitial edema that may radiographically resemble ARDS, along with respiratory compromise requiring supplemental oxygen, developing within 72 hours of hospitalization and occurring in a previously healthy person or (2) an unexplained respiratory illness resulting in death, with an autopsy examination demonstrating noncardiogenic pulmonary edema without an identifiable cause.

Prevention

Rodent control is essential for preventing hantavirus infections. Rodent populations near human communities should be addressed, with particular attention to exclusion of rodents from homes. Contact with rodent urine, droppings, saliva, and nesting materials should be avoided.

Treatment

Rx

Treatment of hantavirus pulmonary syndrome is supportive, with administration of antipyretics, analgesics, and appropriate antimicrobial therapy. Intravenous ribavirin is not effective treatment of hantavirus pulmonary syndrome despite its effectiveness in the treatment of hemorrhagic fever with renal syndrome. If hantavirus pulmonary syndrome is strongly suspected, patients should be immediately transferred to an intensive care unit for hemodynamic and laboratory monitoring and resuscitation. Cardiac function should be closely monitored, with inotropic and vasopressor support provided as needed. Hydration should be provided with care because of the potential for capillary leakage. Supplemental oxygen and equipment and materials for intubation and mechanical ventilation should be readily available for sudden onset of respiratory failure. Standard precautions for infection control should be used when caring for patients.

Arenaviral Hemorrhagic Fevers (Argentine, Bolivian, Venezuelan, and Brazilian Hemorrhagic Fevers; Lassa Fever)

Definition

Arenaviruses are a family of enveloped, pleomorphic RNA viruses associated with rodent-transmitted diseases in humans. Each virus is usually associated with a particular rodent host species in which it is maintained. Viewed in cross section, a pattern of ribosomes gives these viruses a characteristic grainy appearance for which the Latin *arenosus* ("sandy") is applied. The arenaviruses are divided into two groups: the New World or Tacaribe complex and the Old World or LCM/Lassa complex. New World viruses include Junin virus, which causes Argentine hemorrhagic fever; Machupo virus, which causes Bolivian hemorrhagic fever; Guanarito virus, which causes Venezuelan hemorrhagic fever; and Sabia, which causes Brazilian hemorrhagic fever. Of the Old World viruses, Lassa virus causes Lassa fever in West Africa, and related serotypes are found throughout sub-Saharan Africa.

Epidemiology

Each of the arenaviruses is associated with one or more closely related rodent species that are the natural reservoir for that virus. The Tacaribe complex viruses are associated with New World rats and mice (family Muridae, subfamily Sigmodontinae), including *Calomys musculinus, Calomys laucha,* and *Akodon arenicola,* which carry Junin virus; *Calomys callosus,* which carries Machupo virus; and *Zygodontomys brevicauda,* which carries Guanarito virus. The LCM/Lassa complex viruses are associated with Old World rats and mice (family Muridae, subfamily Murinae). Lassa virus is carried by *Mastomys natalensis.* Tacaribe virus, an exception thus far, was not isolated from a rodent but from a bat.

Arenaviruses generally cause chronic infections without evident illness in their rodent hosts. Some Old World arenaviruses are vertically transmitted in rodents during pregnancy and are thus maintained in the rodent population. New World arenaviruses are believed to spread among adult rodents by salivary inoculation (e.g., by biting). Rodents shed the viruses in their urine or droppings, thereby contaminating the immediate environment.

Humans become infected incidentally when they have contact with infectious rodent excreta or material soiled by infected rodents. Human exposure reflects the overlap of human activities with specific rodent habitats. Thus, agricultural workers are at risk of exposure to rodent species that nest in field settings (e.g., Junin virus infection during corn harvesting in northern Argentina), whereas peridomestic rodents are likely to be encountered in woodsheds, attics, cabins, and similar structures related to human dwellings (e.g., domestic and peridomestic transmission of Machupo virus in Bolivia and Lassa virus in Liberia, Sierra Leone, and parts of Nigeria).

Human exposure can occur when handling rodent nest material during cleaning, by ingestion of food contaminated by rodents, or by exposure to infectious material through abraded or broken skin. Activities such as sweeping to remove a rodent nest can generate infectious dust that contains dried rodent urine or saliva. Inhalation of such dust may result in infection.

Lassa and Machupo viruses have been associated with secondary transmission from human to human and with health care–associated transmission. Both are generally due to contact with infectious blood or body fluids from an infected individual, either directly or from intermediate contaminated objects, such as medical equipment. Laboratory personnel have been infected with Sabia while working with infectious material.

Pathobiology

These infections are characterized by severe systemic illness with multiorgan involvement. Neither microscopic nor gross findings on postmortem examination tend to be sufficient to explain the observed severity of illness or death. Focal necrotic lesions may develop in the liver, kidneys, and adrenal cortex. Evidence of altered vascular permeability may be seen; petechial hemorrhages, ecchymoses, and mucosal hemorrhages are diffusely present. Thrombocytopenia and hemorrhage are most common among the South American hemorrhagic fevers and less so in Lassa fever; vasculitis and DIC are uncommon. Viremia tends to be of relatively high titer and may last as long as 3 weeks.

Clinical Manifestations

Incubation periods range from 1 to 2 weeks for the South American hemorrhagic fevers and from 3 to 16 days for Lassa fever. All these infections are characterized by a gradual onset of fever, chills, and malaise. Symptoms may include headache, retro-orbital pain, myalgia, anorexia, nausea, and vomiting. Fever is nonremitting. Pharyngitis is not a prominent feature of the South American hemorrhagic fevers, whereas exudative pharyngitis and mouth ulcers are commonly seen with Lassa fever. In addition, patients may have conjunctivitis, facial edema, lymphadenopathy, upper body rash, or petechiae. Jaundice and liver enlargement are not characteristic. Laboratory findings include leukopenia, thrombocytopenia, and albuminuria with casts.

Hypotension with relative bradycardia becomes prominent during the second week of illness. Bleeding is not massive and usually takes the form of epistaxis, gingival bleeding, or upper gastrointestinal and genitourinary tract bleeding. Though common in South American hemorrhagic fevers, bleeding is seen in less than 20% of patients with Lassa fever. Transient hair loss may occur. Neurologic signs are common in South American hemorrhagic fever; nearly 50% of patients have cerebellar signs with tremor of the tongue and hands, and as many as 25% progress to encephalopathy and seizures. CSF remains normal in these patients. Neurologic signs are less common during acute illness with Lassa fever; however, unilateral or bilateral eighth cranial nerve damage occurs in about 29% of patients and can result in permanent hearing loss. Acute illness resolves after 7 to 15 days and is followed by prolonged convalescence over a period of several weeks, during which patients may experience diaphoresis and lightheadedness. Death occurs as a result of hypovolemic shock, usually in the second week of illness.

Diagnosis

Laboratory confirmation of the clinical diagnosis may be made by isolation of virus from cell culture of blood, CSF, or throat washings taken during the viremic phase of illness and from postmortem tissues in fatal cases. Isolation of virus requires laboratory facilities with appropriate biosafety capacity. Detection of viral antigen, IgG, and IgM may be accomplished by ELISA or immunofluorescence testing, or both. Immunohistochemical staining of postmortem tissue specimens can identify viral antigen. RT-PCR for detection of viral RNA may offer rapid diagnostic information but has thus far been predominantly a research tool.

Prevention

Rodent control measures are an important aspect of control of arenaviral infections associated with peridomestic rodent hosts. Trapping in and around human habitations with effective exclusion of rodents, removal of rodent food sources, and closed rodent-proof storage of human food supplies is required. Rodent nests and carcasses should be handled carefully, with gloves if possible and attention to hand hygiene and environmental cleaning afterward. Sweeping and activities that raise dust should be avoided. Mopping or wet cleaning is presumed to be safer. A live attenuated vaccine for Junin virus has proved efficacious in Argentina.

Treatment

Treatment is supportive, with careful attention to fluid balance and electrolyte management. Overly aggressive volume administration may precipitate pulmonary edema, especially in later stages of infection. Specific immune plasma against Junin virus has been used to treat Argentine hemorrhagic fever with some success. Ribavirin administered intravenously at 60 mg/kg/day for 4 days, followed by oral administration of 30 mg/kg/day for an additional 6 days, appears to be beneficial. Standard precautions for infection control with the addition of contact isolation should be used when caring for patients.

Prognosis

Case-fatality rates range from 25 to 30% for South American hemorrhagic fevers. In hospitalized patients with Lassa fever, the case-fatality rate is 15 to 20%; however, the overall mortality is approximately 1% among all patients with Lassa fever. Mortality is increased in women in the third trimester of pregnancy; 95% of affected pregnancies end in fetal death.

HEMORRHAGIC FEVERS TRANSMITTED FROM HUMAN TO HUMAN

Filoviral Hemorrhagic Fevers (Marburg and Ebola)

Definition

Filoviruses are enveloped, filamentous RNA viruses of the order Mononegavirales, family Filoviridae. They are composed of two groups, Marburg and Ebola, with Marburg virus being the single representative of the former. Ebola viruses include four species: Zaire, Sudan, Cote d'Ivoire, and Reston. Although various potential reservoirs, including bats, have been postulated, the true natural host species for these viruses remains unknown.

Marburg virus is named for the German city where along with Yugoslavia, laboratory personnel died in 1967 after exposure to African green monkeys from Uganda. Ebola virus is named for the river in the former Zaire where a hemorrhagic fever initially identified in 1976 involved human-to-human transmission, as well as spread by contaminated injection equipment.

Epidemiology

Ebola Reston was identified as the cause of severe illness in cynomolgus monkeys imported to the United States from the Philippines. Laboratory personnel working with the monkeys were serologically confirmed to have become infected, but they did not experience symptomatic illness.

In contrast, all of the other aforementioned filoviruses cause severe hemorrhagic fever with a high case-fatality rate and efficient transmission among humans. Ebola and Marburg viruses have caused outbreaks throughout sub-Saharan Africa, with infection originating in the Sudan, Uganda, Kenya, Zimbabwe, the Democratic Republic of Congo, Gabon, and Cote d'Ivoire.

In a series of filoviral outbreaks, a consistent pattern of insertion and amplification has been observed wherein an individual acquires infection from an unidentified source, becomes ill, and transmits the infection to close contacts, usually family members who provide care during the illness, persons who provide burial services that involve contact with infectious body fluids, or persons who have direct contact with blood, emesis, or other body fluids from the infected individual. Initial spread within a family or residential group is followed by health care–associated transmission after an infectious individual seeks care or is taken to a hospital. These diseases are efficiently spread to cleaners, students, nurses, and physicians who in the course of providing care have unprotected contact with infectious material. Health care amplification of the outbreak is exacerbated by limited health care resources and hygienic infrastructure and generally leads to international efforts to support infection control and outbreak response.

Transmission from human to human is associated with direct contact, percutaneous inoculation, or splashing of infectious blood or body fluids onto mucous membranes. Illness has not been observed in individuals without such contact or exposure despite living with infected patients in poorly ventilated dwellings. Health care–associated transmission by reuse of injection equipment can occur.

Pathobiology

Filoviral infection affects all organs, with necrosis seen in the spleen, lymph nodes, testes, ovaries, kidneys, and liver. Tissue damage mirrors sites of viral replication, as indicated by evidence of viral antigen on immunohistochemical and in situ hybridization studies. Monocytes, in particular, Kupffer cells, and endothelial cells are directly affected, with capillary endothelium manifesting increased permeability. Lymphoid depletion and necrosis may be extensive.

Clinical Manifestations

After an incubation period ranging from 2 to 21 days (Ebola hemorrhagic fever) or 3 to 9 days (Marburg hemorrhagic fever), infected patients have an abrupt onset of fever with initial symptoms that include headache, pharyngitis, myalgia, and weakness. Incubation periods may be shorter in patients infected by direct percutaneous inoculation of infectious material.

The initial findings are nonspecific and, in endemic areas, difficult to distinguish from more common infections such as malaria (Chapter 366), typhoid fever (Chapter 329), rickettsial infections (Chapter 348), and other viral infections such as measles (Chapter 390). Subsequently, patients may have abdominal and chest pain, diarrhea, vomiting, rash, conjunctivitis, hiccups, and hemorrhagic symptoms, including epistaxis, gingival bleeding, hematemesis, melena, genitourinary bleeding, and persistent oozing from injection sites. By the third or fourth day of illness, delirium, agitation, and lethargy are common. Patients who survive may experience prolonged fatigue, anorexia, hair loss, or neuropsychiatric symptoms.

Early leukopenia and thrombocytopenia may be followed by lymphocytosis with atypical lymphocytes. Aminotransferase levels, amylase level, and the prothrombin time may be increased, and DIC (Chapter 181) may be seen. Albuminuria and electrocardiographic changes may be present.

Diagnosis

Diagnostic laboratory confirmation of filoviral hemorrhagic fever can be made by antigen capture ELISA, IgM ELISA, PCR, and isolation of virus. Patients who die may not have a detectable antibody response; however, antigen can be detected by PCR of blood or gingival brushings, virus can be isolated from postmortem tissue and blood specimens, and immunohistochemistry can identify antigen in these specimens. Electron microscopy can demonstrate characteristic filoviral morphology.

Prevention

Primary Prevention

Given an unknown reservoir, primary prevention measures are limited. Public education on avoidance of known high-risk practices, such as traditional funeral practices and consumption of primate flesh, has been attempted, although penetration and acceptance are limited by cultural, traditional, and economic imperatives. Protection of health care facilities and personnel in areas likely to be affected is paramount. Routine use of basic infection control, hygiene, and disinfection practices must be implemented to ensure that health care–associated exposure to infectious blood or body fluids will not occur.

Secondary Prevention

Standard precautions for infection control should be used when caring for patients, with the addition of contact and droplet precautions, including eye protection to prevent splashes of blood or body fluids reaching the conjunctivae. Handling of soiled items and infectious waste must protect not only health care personnel but also community members. A dedicated site for waste disposal with appropriate security may be necessary if routine autoclaving and disinfection are not available. Environmental disinfection with an appropriate hospital disinfectant should be prioritized to ensure that secondary transmission from contaminated surfaces does not occur. Use of sharp implements should be minimized.

Treatment

Rx

Treatment is supportive with judicious fluid and electrolyte management. Pulmonary edema may occur rapidly with intravenous hydration. Analgesia and sedation may be helpful in agitated patients. Procedures and medications that potentiate bleeding should be avoided. Although hemodialysis for renal failure and fluid overload may be considered, the patient's increased bleeding risk and exposure of health care personnel to infectious blood should be taken into consideration. Heparin therapy for DIC may be useful, but its efficacy is not established in filoviral disease.

Prognosis

Death usually occurs around the ninth day of illness secondary to hypovolemic shock and multiple organ failure. The case-fatality rate is lower for Ebola Sudan (50 to 60%) than for Zaire (78 to 90%). Although Marburg hemorrhagic fever has had a relatively low (22%) case-fatality rate in patients cared for in a well-resourced hospital setting, recent experience in Angola and the Democratic Republic of Congo has demonstrated a higher rate (80 to 90%), more consistent with Ebola hemorrhagic fever.

SUGGESTED READINGS

Barnett ED: Yellow fever: Epidemiology and prevention. Clin Infect Dis 2007;44:850–856. *Comprehensive review of the epidemiology of yellow fever.*

Bausch DG, Nichol ST, Muyembe-Tamfum JJ, et al: Marburg hemorrhagic fever associated with multiple genetic lineages of virus. N Engl J Med 2006;355:866–869. *A detailed series of 154 cases.*

Ergonul O: Crimean-Congo haemorrhagic fever. Lancet Infect Dis 2006;6:203–214. *Comprehensive review.*

Marty AM, Jahrling PB, Geisbert TW: Viral hemorrhagic fevers. Clin Lab Med 2006;26:345–386. *A detailed review.*

Mertz GJ, Hjelle B, Crowley, M, et al: Diagnosis and treatment of New World hantavirus infections. Curr Opin Infect Dis 2007;101:169–175. *A practical overview.*

Pattnaik P: Kyasanur forest disease: An epidemiological review in India. Rev Med Virol 2006;16:151–165. *Comprehensive review.*

Tuboi SH, Costa ZG, da Costa Vasconcelos PF, et al: Clinical and epidemiological characteristics of yellow fever in Brazil: Analysis of reported cases 1998–2002. Trans R Soc Trop Med Hyg 2007;101:169–175. *The case fatality rate was 44% in 251 hospitalized patients.*

Wilder-Smith A, Schwartz E: Current concepts: Dengue in travelers. N Engl J Med 2005;353:924–932. *Practical review.*

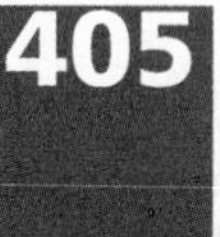

405 ARTHROPOD-BORNE VIRUSES CAUSING FEVER AND RASH SYNDROMES

Stanley J. Naides

COLORADO TICK FEVER

Definition

Colorado tick fever is an acute, often self-limited, typically biphasic febrile illness that is common in the Rocky Mountain areas, the Sierra Nevada and Wasatch ranges, and the Black Hills mountain areas. The virus is transmitted through the bite of the hard-shelled tick *Dermacentor andersoni* (Rocky Mountain wood tick), and the disease's range corresponds to the vector's range. Other coltiviruses, such as the Salmon River, Eyach, Banna, Beijing, and Gansu viruses, have also been implicated in human disease.

The Pathogen

The causative agent, Colorado tick fever virus, is a member of the Coltivirus genus, family Reoviridae. Coltiviruses have a genome consisting of 12 double-stranded RNA segments. Colorado tick fever virus is the prototype member.

Epidemiology

D. andersoni is found at elevations of 4000 to 10,000 ft. Seasonal temperatures tend to influence the range, with the vector being found at higher elevations in warmer seasons and at lower elevations in colder seasons. Human exposures usually occur during outdoor recreational activities in these areas. Occasional exposure occurs in nonendemic areas from ticks exported out of the endemic region in clothes, hiking equipment, or baggage. Infections generally take place between March and September, when the adult tick is most plentiful. Ticks are most abundant in south-facing dry and rocky slope habitats that favor small rodent hosts (e.g., chipmunks, ground squirrels, marmosets), with underbrush cover, burrows, and humidity for the ticks. Colorado tick fever virus is found in nymphal and adult ticks that overwinter on the rodent host, in which viremia persists for weeks to months. As many as 14% of *D. andersoni* ticks in the endemic area carry Colorado tick fever virus. Humans are an incidental host. Fewer than 50 cases were reported annually in Colorado beginning in 1992. The actual number of cases is probably significantly larger and includes subclinical, mild, and unreported cases.

The geographic range of Colorado tick fever may be larger than the well-recognized endemic mountain areas. Serologically confirmed cases in California have been attributed to the Colorado tick fever–related virus S1-14-03, which is transmitted by *Dermacentor variabilis* (American dog tick). Salmon River virus causes a Colorado tick fever–like illness in rafters on the Salmon River in Idaho. Another similar virus, Eyach virus, has been implicated in neurologic illness in France and Germany and has been isolated from the deer ticks *Ixodes ricinus* and *Ixodes ventalloi*.

Pathobiology

Colorado tick fever virus replicates in bone marrow CD34+ stem cells and leads to mild to moderate leukopenia and thrombocytopenia. The virus also replicates in committed erythrocyte precursors and may be detected in circulating erythrocytes up to 4 weeks after infection.

Clinical Manifestations

Patients report a tick bite or exposure in 90% of cases, but there is no notable local reaction to the tick bite. After a mean incubation of 3 to 4 days (range, 0 to 14 days), sudden-onset fever develops in association with malaise, chills, myalgia, weakness, headache, photophobia, retro-orbital pain, and cutaneous hyperesthesia. Conjunctival and oropharyngeal injection, palatal enanthem, lymphadenopathy, and splenomegaly may be present. The absence of prominent respiratory and gastrointestinal symptoms helps exclude other febrile illnesses. A petechial or maculopapular exanthem, found in 15% of patients, may be confused with the rash of Rocky Mountain spotted fever (Chapter 348). The illness has a "saddleback" fever pattern consisting of resolution of the initial fever within 1 week and recrudescence after a 2- to 3-day hiatus. A third fever episode may occur.

Leukopenia develops 5 to 6 days after onset of the illness. Mild thrombocytopenia and anemia may occur.

Myocarditis, pneumonitis, hepatitis, orchitis, and epididymitis may complicate adult infection, and aseptic meningitis or encephalitis may occur in up to 10% of childhood infections.

Diagnosis

Clinical diagnosis is confirmed by demonstration of the Colorado tick fever viral genome or specific acute phase IgM antibody. The viral genome may be detected up to 6 weeks after infection by nucleic acid–based methods such as reverse transcriptase polymerase chain reaction (RT-PCR) on blood or stored blood clots. Virions in circulating erythrocytes may be detected by immunofluorescent antibody labeling. Anti–Colorado tick fever virus IgM antibody is detected by antibody capture enzyme-linked immunosorbent assay (ELISA) or complement fixation. Neutralization assays using Vero or BHK-21 cells have been helpful.

Differentiating Colorado tick fever from Rocky Mountain spotted fever (Chapter 348) may be difficult before the appearance of the typical rash of the latter. However, Rocky Mountain spotted fever does not have a saddleback fever pattern and is 20 times less common than Colorado tick fever in the western endemic area.

Treatment

Rx

Treatment is supportive. Aspirin is contraindicated to avoid complicating thrombocytopenia.

Prognosis

Extreme weakness and malaise may persist for weeks to months after final resolution of the fever. Older patients have a prolonged recovery. Seventy percent of patients older than 30 years may still have fatigue 3 weeks after the fever, whereas children and adolescents may recover completely within a week. Rare instances of maternal-fetal transmission have been reported. Full recovery eventually occurs, except when the disease course is complicated by neurologic insult. Patients should refrain from donating blood for 6 months.

DENGUE

Definition

Dengue is an acute febrile illness characterized by severe muscle and joint pain, rash, malaise, and lymphadenopathy. The severity of the musculoskeletal complaints gave rise to the sobriquet *break bone fever.* Dengue occurs in the tropical and subtropical climes of the Caribbean, Central and South America, Asia, and Africa. The mosquito range extends into the southeastern United States, where dengue reemerged in the 1980s. After World War II, a global pandemic has been associated with erosion of mosquito control programs, human populations that have spread into rural settings, accelerated population movement as a result of travel by airplane, and large areas that have experienced deterioration in public health infrastructure. Tens of millions of individuals are infected annually.

The Pathogen

Dengue is a member of the Flaviviridae family, which consists of single-stranded RNA viruses with a lipid envelope approximately 50 nm in diameter. There are four serotypes of dengue: DEN-1, DEN-2, DEN-3, and DEN-4. There is no cross-protection among the serotypes, so individuals can experience dengue after infection with another serotype. Infection with a second serotype places the individual at risk for the development of hemorrhagic fever (Chapter 404).

Epidemiology

Dengue is transmitted to humans by the bite of female *Aedes aegypti* and *Aedes albopictus* mosquitoes. *A. albopictus* has become the dominant pest mosquito in many urban centers. Members of the two mosquito species acquire dengue virus by biting humans, typically during the day. Zoonotic life cycles involving nonhuman primates (i.e., chimpanzees, gibbons, and macaques) and canopy-dwelling forest *Aedes* species have been demonstrated in western Africa and Malaysia. The mosquitoes nest in stagnant water around human dwellings; they are not typically encountered in the forest. In the human host, dengue virus may reach a titer of greater than 10^8 median infectious doses (MID_{50})/mL. The mosquito becomes infected when taking its meal from a viremic host. The virus continues replication in the midgut epithelium and salivary glands of female mosquitoes, which remain infectious for life. Within 8 to 12 days of the initial infection, the mosquito's salivary glands become infected and virus is shed with saliva during the next blood meal. A given mosquito may infect multiple individuals, especially in view of its skittishness during feeding: slight movement of the host interrupts its meal, after which it returns to the original or another host.

The incubation period is typically 4 to 7 days but may range from 3 to 14 days. During outbreaks in the southeastern United States and Puerto Rico, the risk for infection may be as high as 79% in naive hosts, and clinical disease may develop in up to 20%. Immunity against the infecting serotype is probably lifelong, but individuals remain susceptible to the remaining serotypes. Peak transmission occurs after increased rainfall, when rainwater collected in household containers allows expansion of mosquito populations. Epidemics tend to occur in 3- to 5-year cycles, but interepidemic cases occur regularly. Dengue is a particular risk to visitors to the tropics.

Pathobiology

Dengue hemorrhagic fever (Chapter 404) and dengue shock syndrome are forms of dengue reinfection characterized by capillary leakage and hemorrhage. Previous infection with an alternative serotype allows antibody to the previously encountered serotype to combine with the newly infecting serotype. Although the first exposed serotype antibody is not neutralizing, it does allow enhanced antibody-mediated macrophage uptake, thereby leading to a macrophage activation state. Macrophage excretion of vasoactive inflammatory mediators results in vascular leak; severe vascular leak causes shock. Endothelial cell swelling and perivascular edema may occur. Rarely, dengue shock syndrome may occur in primary infection. Variation in a strain's ability to generate enhancing antibody, as well as differences in virulence, may account for differences in clinical behavior.

Clinical Manifestations

Dengue infection is often subclinical. When symptomatic, dengue may be manifested as classic dengue, dengue hemorrhagic fever, or dengue shock syndrome. Patients may also have mild illness characterized by nonspecific fever, anorexia, and headache.

Classic dengue, which typically occurs in nonindigenous older children and adults, is characterized by sudden-onset fever, severe frontal headache, retro-orbital pain, myalgias, and in many cases, nausea, vomiting, rash, lymphadenopathy, and arthralgias. Patients may experience generalized weakness, altered taste, rigors, and cutaneous hyperesthesia.

Physical examination demonstrates fever, relative bradycardia, scleral injection, ocular pressure tenderness, and pharyngeal injection. A transient macular rash appears on days 1 or 2 of illness. On days 2 and 3 of illness, fever and other symptoms may improve. The fever is typically, but not consistently biphasic. After a hiatus of typically 2 days, fever and other symptoms recrudesce, though less severely. Generalized, nontender lymphadenopathy of the posterior cervical, epitrochlear, and inguinal regions may develop. Rash also recurs, appearing as 2- to 5-mm speckles of pallor surrounded by erythema and occasionally accompanied by burning dysesthesias of the palms and soles. The rash may desquamate.

In severe cases, dengue shock syndrome is accompanied by hypotension, narrowed pulse pressure, and shock.

Diagnosis

An adequate travel history and knowledge of community disease occurrence can lead to consideration of dengue in the differential diagnosis. Viremia is of adequate intensity in infections with DEN-1, DEN-2, and DEN-3 to allow viral isolation. Viremia in DEN-4 infections is often less intense and more difficult to detect through inoculation of mosquito cells in vitro. Detection of IgM antibody confirms recent infection, but cross-reactivity with other flaviviruses prevents serotype-specific diagnosis. Neutralization testing is more specific with hemagglutination inhibition, and complement fixation testing for IgG in paired sera is helpful.

Leukopenia develops by the second day of fever, reaches 2000 to 4000 cells/mL by day 4 or 5, and is associated with granulocytopenia. In dengue hemorrhagic fever, thrombocytopenia of less than 100,000 cells/mL and a prolonged prothrombin time are characteristic. Mild to moderate proteinuria and a few casts may be detected. Aspartate transaminase levels may be increased.

Treatment and Prognosis

Rx

Treatment is supportive. Initial resuscitation with lactated Ringer's solution is indicated in children with moderately severe dengue shock syndrome, and 6% hydroxyethyl starch is preferred for children with severe shock. 1 Classic dengue resolves abruptly in 5 to 7 days, but fatigue and depression may linger for weeks; survival is uniform. The prognosis for dengue hemorrhagic fever (Chapter 404) and dengue shock syndrome depends on early diagnosis and introduction of supportive measures.

WEST NILE FEVER VIRUS

Definition

West Nile fever is an acute febrile illness associated with malaise, rash, headache, myalgia, and lymphadenopathy.

Infection involves a bird-mosquito-human cycle. Viremia develops in all varieties of birds. Bats, cats, chipmunks, domestic rabbits, horses, skunks, and squirrels may be infected.

The Pathogen

West Nile fever virus is a flavivirus transmitted by a variety of mosquito species. The mosquito vector varies: *Culex univittatus, Culex pipiens,* and *Culex molestus* in the Middle East and Africa; *Mansonia metalliicus* in Uganda; and *Culex tritaeniorhynchus* in Asia. *C. pipiens, Culex quinquefasciatus, Culex nigripalpus,* and *Culex tarsalis* are probably vectors in North America, although at least 25 other mosquito species carry the virus.

Epidemiology

Virus transmission involves mosquitoes and wild birds, with mammals, including humans, as incidental end-stage hosts. In endemic areas, more than 60% of young adults have antibodies, thus suggesting a high prevalence of inapparent or undifferentiated febrile illness in children. There is no gender predominance.

Between 0.5 and 1% of infected individuals experience a more severe illness. Incubation is typically 3 to 14 days but may be as short as 1 day.

West Nile virus emerged in the United States in New York in the summer of 1999 and by September 2006 had spread through 36 states and the District of Columbia. In the American outbreak, birds of the Corvidae family (e.g., crows, jackdaws, ravens) were often affected, and recognition of increased death in crow populations continues to serve as a sentinel for the presence of West Nile virus. *C. pipiens* is the major vector in the United States. In addition to mosquito transmission, the virus has been transmitted by a transplanted organ, via blood transfusion, transplacentally, and in the laboratory.

Pathobiology

West Nile virus grows in a variety of cells in vitro and produces cytopathic effects in *A. albopictus* cells. Individuals in whom encephalitis develops show evidence of diffuse brain inflammation and neuronal degeneration.

Clinical Manifestations

Most cases remain asymptomatic, but aseptic meningitis or encephalitis (Chapter 406) may occur in the elderly and, less commonly, the very young. Most symptomatic cases are mild, with fever, malaise, headache, nausea, anorexia, generalized lymphadenopathy, and myalgia. Like Colorado tick fever and dengue, West Nile fever may be biphasic. Nonpruritic, maculopapular, or roseolar rash occurs on the chest, back, and arms in half the patients, beginning during or with resolution of the fever. Rash persists for up to 1 week and then resolves with desquamation. Patients may experience vomiting, diarrhea, abdominal pain, and pharyngitis. Anterior myelitis or hepatitis may also occur. Disease is usually milder in children than in adults.

Diagnosis

West Nile virus may be isolated from up to 77% of patients with West Nile fever on the first day of illness, but viral isolation is less common in patients with encephalitis (Chapter 406). Low-titer viremia may persist for the first 5 days of illness. Tests for virus-specific antibody using ELISA or immunofluorescence are available. RT-PCR may detect viral RNA in human samples and in avian and insect specimens.

Treatment

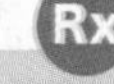

Treatment is supportive. The clinical value of antiviral agents is unknown.

Prognosis

Illness generally persists 3 to 6 days before rapid recovery. The prognosis is excellent, but mortality rates of 10% or higher occur in patients with encephalitis (Chapter 406).

PHLEBOTOMUS FEVER

Definition

Phlebotomus fever (i.e., sandfly fever, pappataci, and 3-day fever) is an acute, mild, self-limited febrile illness transmitted through the bite of *Phlebotomus* flies.

The Pathogen

Phlebotomus fever viruses are members of the genus Phlebovirus, family Bunyaviridae. The latter consists of a group of single-stranded

RNA viruses that are 80 to 120 nm in diameter, possess a lipid envelope, and have three segments in the genome. A related virus, the Toscana virus hosted by *Phlebotomus perniciosus,* causes a similar illness in central Italy, Cyprus, Spain, and Portugal.

Epidemiology

The virus's distribution parallels the distribution of *Phlebotomus* flies found throughout the Mediterranean basin, Middle East, and western India and Pakistan. In Central America, *Lutzomyia* fly species may transmit the virus. These tiny sandflies pass through mosquito netting to feed in the early evenings. Virus is maintained by transovarial and transstadial transmission. During outbreaks, humans may serve as a reservoir. Human infection is more common in rural areas during the summer months. The incubation period is 2 to 6 days. Sandflies spread by hopping, thus limiting their travel range. Use of insect sprays locally is effective in decreasing risk.

Clinical Manifestations

Sandfly fever virus causes an acute febrile illness associated with malaise, headache, photophobia, ocular pain, altered taste, myalgias, and arthralgias. Myalgias may be localized to specific regions (e.g., the chest) and simulate regional syndromes such as pleurodynia. A macular or urticarial rash may appear. Examination may show relative bradycardia after the first day, conjunctival injection, mild papilledema, or small palatal vesicles. Fever lasts 2 to 4 days and then subsides. Weakness and malaise may persist during convalescence. About 15% of patients experience recrudescence in 2 to 12 weeks. Aseptic meningitis may occur with mild cerebrospinal fluid pleocytosis. Peripheral leukopenia and lymphopenia may be present early in the illness. However, leukopenia may be delayed in some patients until the third day of illness, and a rebound relative lymphocytosis may be encountered.

Diagnosis

The diagnosis of phlebotomus fever is confirmed by isolation of virus after intracerebral inoculation of suckling mice, detection of the viral genome by RT-PCR, or detection of specific IgM antibody by ELISA.

Treatment and Prognosis

Rx

Treatment is supportive, and recovery is complete. Ribavirin (Chapter 383) has been proposed as a therapeutic option.

RIFT VALLEY FEVER

Rift Valley fever, which is an acute-onset, febrile illness, is often associated with epizootic waves of spontaneous abortion in livestock.

Definition

The Rift Valley fever virus is a member of the family Bunyaviridae, genus Phlebovirus, but unlike other members of the genus, it is transmitted by *Aedes* mosquitoes.

Epidemiology

Rift Valley fever occurs throughout most of Africa, with the majority of epizootic outbreaks occurring in eastern and southern Africa. Rift Valley fever was first documented in Saudi Arabia and Yemen in 2000. The principal initial vectors are probably the *Aedes* species associated with flooding. Shallow pools along rivers and streams play an important role as mosquito breeding sites. Feeding on nearby livestock allows a local epizootic outbreak and amplification of the virus in local mosquito populations, including *C. pipiens* in Egypt and *Culex theileri* in eastern Africa.

Hemorrhagic fever in humans is typically seen 1 to 2 weeks after a wave of abortion in livestock. Initial human cases usually occur in those who have close contact with livestock. The virus is highly transmissible through aerosolization. Although the risk for severe human infection is less than 1%, the extensive exposure associated with outbreaks can lead to significant morbidity and mortality. For example, in the 1977–1978 Egyptian outbreak associated with movement of camels from Sudan, an estimated 200,000 people were infected, with 600 deaths. Zinga virus, isolated in central Africa and Madagascar and shown to be responsible for mild human illness, is a strain of Rift Valley fever virus.

Pathobiology

Rift Valley fever virus grows well in a variety of cell cultures and has cytopathic effects. After infection by a mosquito bite, virus is transported through the lymphatics to regional lymph nodes, where replication allows amplification of the input inoculum and development of viremia with systemic spread. Virus replication in liver, spleen, lymph node, adrenal, lung, and kidney tissues is highly cytopathic. In severe cases, hepatic necrosis and, rarely, focal brain necrosis may occur. Encephalitis is not associated with viremia, thus suggesting that this sequela is immune mediated rather than a direct viral effect. Inflammatory cell infiltration is associated with focal necrosis in the brain. Spontaneous abortion is common in livestock, but fetal loss in humans is not clearly correlated with viral infection.

Clinical Manifestations

Most human infection is mild, with abrupt-onset fever, chills, and malaise. However, about 0.5% of infections cause a severe hemorrhagic fever associated with hepatic necrosis and disseminated intravascular coagulopathy. Recovery is complicated by retinal vasculitis or encephalitis, which occurs in less than 0.5% of patients 1 to 4 weeks after recovery and is associated with recurrent fever. In severe cases, focal brain necrosis and encephalitis may lead to hallucinations, stupor, coma, and death.

Diagnosis

Intense viremia allows detection of virus through inoculation of suckling mouse brain or a variety of cells in culture. Specific IgM and IgG are detectable by ELISA applied to acute and convalescent (after 1 to 2 weeks) paired sera.

Treatment and Prognosis

Treatment is supportive. Ribavirin (Chapter 383) has been proposed as a therapeutic option. The prognosis is good in the absence of retinitis or encephalitis. In endemic areas, vaccination of livestock is the most effective preventive measure.

CHIKUNGUNYA FEVER

Definition

Chikungunya fever is a febrile arthritis that occurs in sporadic cases and in epidemics.

The Pathogen

Chikungunya is a member of the family Togaviridae, genus Alphavirus. Chikungunya virus is transmitted by mosquitoes, principally *Aedes* species, but also *Mansonia africana* and other genera. Known animal reservoirs are monkeys, baboons, and in Senegal, *Scotophilus* bat species. During outbreaks, humans are the major reservoir.

Chikungunya is an enveloped, single-stranded RNA virus 60 to 70 nm in diameter.

Epidemiology

Chikungunya, which is endemic in sub-Sahara Africa, India, the Philippines, and Southeast Asia, also recently appeared in the French island La Reunion and spread to Seychelles, Mauritius, and Mayotte Islands before arising in India, China, Malaysia, and European countries. Outbreaks typically occur after heavy rains. In urban settings, outbreaks are explosive. In a 1964 epidemic in Bangkok, Thailand, an estimated 40,000 persons in an urban area of 2 million were infected. In endemic areas, seroprevalence rates may be as high as 90%, thus suggesting that time required for loss of herd immunity is the reason for prolonged absence of cases in a region after an outbreak. Globalization may contribute to increasing propensity for spread. An outbreak in Malaysia from 1998 to 1999 was attributed to migrant workers from endemic areas. After inoculation, the incubation period is typically 2 to 3 days but ranges from 1 to 12 days.

Pathobiology

Intense viremia develops within 48 hours of the mosquito bite and wanes 2 to 3 days later. Onset of hemagglutination inhibition and neutralizing antibodies clears the viremia. Superficial capillaries in rash-involved skin demonstrate erythrocyte extravasation and perivascular cuffing. The virus adsorbs to human platelets and causes them to aggregate. Synovitis probably results from direct chikungunya viral infection of synovium.

Clinical Manifestations

Chikungunya fever is characterized by an explosive onset of fever and severe arthralgia. Constitutional symptoms, fever to 40° C, rigors, headache, photophobia, retro-orbital pain, conjunctival injection, pharyngitis, anorexia, nausea, vomiting, abdominal pain, tense lymphadenopathy, and myalgias are common. A maculopapular rash located on the torso, extremities, and occasionally the face, palms, and soles occurs in most patients 1 to 10 days after onset of the illness. The appearance of rash is often associated temporally with initial defervescence; rash may recur with fever and may be pruritic. Isolated petechiae and mucosal bleeding may occur, but significant hemorrhage is rare. Desquamation may occur when the rash resolves. The initial acute illness may last 2 to 3 days (range, 1 to 7 days). Fever may recrudesce after a 1- to 2-day hiatus. Polyarthralgia is migratory and predominantly affects the small joints of the hands, wrists, feet, and ankles, with less prominent involvement of the large joints. Previously injured joints may be more severely affected. Stiffness and swelling may occur, but large effusions are uncommon. Synovial fluid shows decreased viscosity with poor mucin clot and 2000 to 5000 white blood cells per milliliter.

Diagnosis

Chikungunya fever must be differentiated from dengue and o'nyong-nyong fever. Chikungunya virus may be isolated from blood during the initial 2 to 4 days of illness. In some patients, viral antigen may be detected in acute sera by hemagglutination assay as a result of the intensity of the viremia. Specific IgM antibody may be detected for 6 months or longer. Hemagglutination inhibition and neutralization antibodies develop as the viremia is cleared. Complement fixation antibodies are positive by the third week and slowly decrease over the subsequent year. RT-PCR offers more rapid diagnosis than viral culture or antibody testing does.

Treatment and Prognosis

Rx

Treatment is supportive. Nonsteroidal anti-inflammatory agents are useful. During the acute arthritis, range-of-motion exercises lessen stiffness. In most cases, mild joint symptoms may last months. Destructive arthropathy is rare and may be associated with low-titer rheumatoid factor, thus suggesting an unrelated, underlying inflammatory arthritis. Approximately 10% of patients have joint symptoms 1 year after infection. Symptoms in children tend to be milder; arthralgia and arthritis are milder and briefer in duration.

O'NYONG-NYONG FEVER

Definition

O'nyong-nyong means "joint breaker" in the Acholi dialect of northwestern Uganda, where o'nyong-nyong fever first appeared in February 1959.

The Pathogen

O'nyong-nyong fever is clinically similar to chikungunya fever, and the viruses share antigenic similarity. O'nyong-nyong virus is also a member of the family Togaviridae, genus Alphavirus.

Epidemiology

Within 2 years of its appearance in 1959, the o'nyong-nyong fever virus spread through Uganda and the surrounding region and affected 2 million people. Serologically determined attack rates ranged from 50 to 60%, with case rates of 9 to 78%. Disease spread at a rate of 2 to 3 km daily. After the epidemic, the virus was not detected again until it was isolated from *Anopheles funestus* mosquitoes in Kenya in 1978. *Anopheles gambiae* also serves as a vector. Serologic surveys suggested that o'nyong-nyong virus is endogenous, but cases were not detected again until 1996–1997, during an outbreak in south central Uganda. An outbreak in western Côte d'Ivoire occurred in 2003. The nonhuman vertebrate reservoir for o'nyong-nyong virus is not known. The incubation period lasts at least 8 days.

Igbo-ora (meaning "the disease that breaks your wings") virus is a variant of o'nyong-nyong, with 98.5% homology between the two at the genomic level. Igbo-ora is serologically similar to chikungunya and o'nyong-nyong viruses. In 1984, an epidemic of fever, rash, arthralgia, and myalgia occurred in four villages in the Ivory Coast. The virus was isolated from *A. funestus* and *A. gambiae* mosquitoes and from affected individuals.

Pathobiology

Little is known about the pathobiology of o'nyong-nyong fever.

Clinical Manifestations

Illness begins with a sudden onset of polyarthralgia and polyarthritis. Between 4 and 7 days later, rash begins with improvement in joint symptoms. The rash is uniform in nature, begins on the face, and then spreads to the torso and extremities and occasionally to the palms. The rash lasts 4 to 7 days before fading. Fever is not prominent, but postcervical lymphadenopathy may be marked. Arthralgia is incapacitating in most patients for up to a week, but residual joint pain may persist for months.

Diagnosis

O'nyong-nyong fever is difficult to differentiate from chikungunya fever and may also be mistaken for measles. Specific hemagglutination inhibition and complement fixation tests are available. Mouse antisera raised against chikungunya virus react equally well with o'nyong-nyong virus, but o'nyong-nyong antisera do not react well with chikungunya virus. O'nyong-nyong–specific RT-PCR is available in reference laboratories.

Treatment and Prognosis

Rx

Treatment is symptomatic. Although residual joint pain often persists, there does not appear to be any long-term sequelae.

MAYARO FEVER

Definition

Mayaro fever is an acute febrile illness characterized by fever, rash, arthralgia, and arthritis. Mayaro virus was first recognized in Trinidad in 1954. It has caused recorded outbreaks in Bolivia and Brazil and is endemic in the rain forest region where Bolivia, Brazil, and Peru share borders. Mayaro virus has a monkey reservoir and is transmitted to humans by *Haemagogus* mosquitoes dwelling in the tropical rain forest canopy.

The Pathogen

Mayaro virus is a member of the family Togaviridae, genus Alphavirus.

Epidemiology

Mayaro virus was responsible for an outbreak in Belterra, Brazil, in 1988. Eight hundred of 4000 exposed latex gatherers became infected, with a clinical attack rate of 80%. Cases of imported Mayaro virus infection have been documented in the United States after travel from the endemic Brazil-Bolivia-Peru interborder region. Mayaro virus has been isolated from a bird in Louisiana, thus raising the specter of emergence of Mayaro virus in North America.

Pathobiology

Viremia occurs during the first 1 to 2 days of illness.

Clinical Manifestations

Illness is characterized by a sudden onset of fever, headache, dizziness, chills, and arthralgia in the small joints of the hands and feet. About 20% of patients have joint swelling. Unilateral inguinal lymphadenopathy is occasionally seen. Leukopenia is common. Fever resolves after 2 to 5 days, but a maculopapular rash then develops on the trunk and extremities of about two thirds of patients and lasts about 3 days.

Diagnosis

Mayaro virus may be isolated from blood by growth in Vero or C6/36 cells. RT-PCR with ELISA is available. A specific IgM is also available as an antibody capture ELISA.

Treatment and Prognosis

Rx

Recovery is complete, although some patients have persistent arthralgia 2 months later.

ROSS RIVER FEVER VIRUS (EPIDEMIC FEBRILE POLYARTHRITIS)

Ross River fever virus causes an acute-onset, febrile illness characterized by rash and arthralgia. Ross River virus is a member of the family Togaviridae, genus Alphavirus.

Epidemiology

Epidemics of fever and rash have been observed in Australia since 1928. Isolation of Ross River virus from mosquitoes, its serologic association with epidemic polyarthritis, and isolation of the virus from epidemic polyarthritis patients in Australia confirmed Ross River virus as the etiologic agent of epidemic polyarthritis. Seroprevalence has been observed in endogenous populations in Papua New Guinea, western New Guinea, the Bismarck Archipelago, Rossel Island, and the Solomon Islands. An outbreak in the Fiji Islands affected more than 40,000 individuals in 1979 to 1980. A similar epidemic occurred in the Cook Islands early in 1980. Antibodies to Ross River virus are not found in individuals west of Weber's line, a hypothetical line separating the Australian geographic zone from the Asiatic zone. Endemic cases and epidemics occur in tropical and temperate regions in Australia. Queensland and New South Wales have a particularly high annual incidence associated with higher rainfall. High rainfall usually precedes epidemic periods, with cases subsequently occurring from spring through fall. Seroprevalence may reach just 6 to 15% in temperate coastal zones but is 27 to 39% in the plains of the Murray Valley river system. In Queensland, annual rates of disease range from 31.5 to 288.3 per 100,000 person years.

Aedes vigilax is the major vector on the eastern coast of Australia and *Aedes camptorhynchus* in the salt marshes of southern Australia. *Culex annulirostris* is a freshwater breeding vector. Other Australian *Aedes* species and *Mansonia uniformis* may also serve as vectors. In outbreaks in the Pacific islands, *Aedes polynesiensis, A. aegypti, A. vigilax,* and *C. annulirostris* may have contributed to transmission. Domestic animals, rodents, and marsupials may serve as intermediate hosts.

Most infected individuals become symptomatic. Although male and female infection rates are similar, there is a predominance of women among cases. Children have a case–attack rate ratio lower than that of adults. The incubation period is 7 to 11 days.

Barmah Forest virus, another alphavirus found in Australia in 1986, may be manifested in a fashion similar to epidemic febrile polyarthritis. The number of cases reported annually has been increasing since its initial discovery.

Pathobiology

Ross River viral antigen may be detected in monocytes and macrophages early in infection, but intact virus is not identifiable by electron microscopy or cell culture. Dermal vessels show mild perivascular mononuclear cell infiltrates, mostly T lymphocytic, in erythematous and purpuric areas. Vessels in purpuric areas also show erythrocyte extravasation. Antigen can be demonstrated in epithelial cells in erythematous or purpuric skin and in the perivascular zone in erythematous skin. However, viral antigens have not been found in normal skin. Synovium undergoes lining cell hypertrophy and sublining vascular proliferation and mononuclear cell infiltration. Viral RNA can be identified by RT-PCR. Synovial fluid cell counts range from 1500 to 13,800 cells/mL and consist of monocytes, vacuolated macrophages, and a few neutrophils. Animal models of infection indicate that Ross River virus targets bone, joint, and skeletal muscle and elicits an inflammatory response mediated by the innate immune system.

Clinical Manifestations

Arthralgia typically occurs abruptly, followed in 1 to 2 days by a macular, papular, or maculopapular rash that may be pruritic. Most patients have severe, incapacitating arthralgia in an asymmetrical and migratory distribution. Commonly affected joints are the metacarpophalangeal joints, finger interphalangeal joints, wrists, knees, and ankles. The shoulder, elbow, toe, spine, hip, and temporomandibular joints may also be affected. Arthralgias are worse in the morning and after periods of inactivity. A third of patients have synovitis. Polyarticular swelling and tenosynovitis are common. Up to a third of patients have paresthesias or palm or sole pain. Classic carpal tunnel syndrome may occur.

In some individuals, rash may precede or follow the joint symptoms by 11 or 15 days, respectively. Occasionally, vesicles, papules, or petechiae are seen. The trunk and extremities are typically involved, but the palms, soles, and face may also be involved. Rash resolves by fading to a brownish discoloration or by desquamation. Fever tends to be mild to moderate and lasts 1 to 3 days. Headache, nausea, and myalgia are common. Mild photophobia, respiratory symptoms, and lymphadenopathy may occur.

Diagnosis

In the Australian epidemics before 1979, patients were antibody positive at the time of initial evaluation. However, in the Pacific island epidemics of 1979 to 1980, patients remained viremic and serologically negative for up to a week after the onset of symptoms. Virus in serum is stable for up to a month at 0 to −10° C. Current testing in Australia is performed with an indirect ELISA. The presence of specific IgM or evidence of seroconversion to IgG positivity supports a recent infection.

Treatment and Prognosis

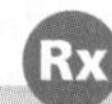

Treatment is supportive. Nonsteroidal anti-inflammatory drugs provide relief of joint pain. Half of all patients return to activities of daily living within 4 weeks despite residual polyarthralgia. Joint symptoms may recur, but episodes gradually resolve. In some patients, joint symptoms may persist for up to 3 years. Mild exercise tends to improve the joint symptoms.

SINDBIS

Sindbis virus causes a sudden-onset, febrile illness associated with arthralgia and rash. It is known as Ockelbo disease in Sweden, Pogosta disease in Finland, and Karelian fever in the Karelian Isthmus of Russia. *Aedes, Culex*, and *Culiseta* mosquitoes transmit the virus to humans, with birds serving as intermediate hosts. Sindbis virus is the prototype alphavirus used for molecular virology studies of its genus.

Epidemiology

The virus was first isolated from *Culex* mosquitoes in the Egyptian village of Sindbis in 1952. Outbreaks frequently occur in the forested areas of Sweden, Finland, and the Karelian Isthmus, but sporadic cases and small outbreaks have occurred in Uganda, South Africa, Zimbabwe, central Africa, and Australia. Individuals involved in outdoor activities or occupations are at greatest risk.

Pathobiology

Skin lesions show perivascular hemorrhage, lymphocytic infiltrates, edema, and areas of necrosis. Virus has been isolated from skin lesions. Antiviral IgM may persist for years, thus raising the possibility that Sindbis virus arthritis is associated with viral persistence and a direct viral effect on the synovium.

Clinical Manifestations

Arthralgia and rash are the initial symptoms, although one may precede the other by a few days. Arthralgia and arthritis involve the small joints of the hands and feet, wrists, elbows, ankles, and knees. Occasionally, arthralgia involves the spine. Tendinitis is common, often involving the Achilles and hand extensor tendons. Fever, if present, tends to be mild to moderate. Constitutional symptoms, headache, fatigue, malaise, nausea, vomiting, pharyngitis, and paresthesias may be present but are not usually severe. Macular rash typically begins on the torso and then involves the arms, legs, palms, soles, and occasionally the head. Macules evolve to papules that have a tendency to vesiculate. Vesiculation is prominent on pressure points, including the palms and soles. As the eruption fades, a brownish discoloration is left. Vesicles on the palms and soles may become hemorrhagic. Rash may recur during convalescence.

Diagnosis

Specific IgM detected by enzyme immunoassay supports a diagnosis of Sindbis virus infection. IgM titers may wane over a period of 3 to 4 years.

Treatment and Prognosis

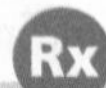

Treatment is supportive. Nonerosive chronic arthropathy is common in Sweden and Finland, with up to half of all patients having joint symptoms 2.5 years after infection. In a few cases, symptoms may persist for up to 6 years.

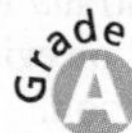

1. Wills BA, Nguyen MD, Dong TH, et al: Comparison of three fluid solutions for resuscitation in dengue shock syndrome. N Engl J Med 2005;353:877–889.

SUGGESTED READINGS

Attoui H, Mohd Jaafar F, de Micco P, et al: Coltiviruses and seadornaviruses in North America, Europe, and Asia. Emerg Infect Dis 2005;11:1673–1679. *A review of viruses in the Colorado tick fever group.*

Centers for Disease Control and Prevention (CDC): Chikungunya fever diagnosed among international travelers—United States, 2005–2006. MMWR Morb Mortal Wkly Rep 2006;55(38):1040–1042. *Detailed review of 4 of the 12 cases.*

Ferguson DD, Gershman K, LeBailly A, et al: Characteristics of the rash associated with West Nile virus fever. Clin Infect Dis 2005;41:1204–1207. *Overview of 15 cases with an emphasis on maculopapular rash on days 5 to 12 of illness.*

Kurkela S, Manni T, Vaheri A, et al: Causative agent of Pogosta disease isolated from blood and skin lesions. Emerg Infect Dis 2004;10:889–894. *A thorough review of this prototype virus.*

Ligon BL: Reemergence of an unusual disease: The chikungunya epidemic. Semin Pediatr Infect Dis 2006;17:99–104. *A timely report on reemergent chikungunya fever.*

Petersen LR, Marfin AA: West Nile virus: A primer for the clinician. Ann Intern Med 2002;137:173–179. *A concise, lucid review of this virus emerging in the United States.*

Wilder-Smith A, Schwartz E: Dengue in travelers. N Engl J Med 2005;353:924–932. *A clinical review with helpful pictures.*

406 ARTHROPOD-BORNE VIRUSES AFFECTING THE CENTRAL NERVOUS SYSTEM

Thomas P. Bleck

Arthropod-borne viruses (also termed "arboviruses") that affect the central nervous system (CNS) share a number of clinical and epidemiologic similarities, have an RNA genome, but do not form a formal virologic taxonomic group. These viruses generally have avian or small mammalian reservoirs and are transmitted to humans and other large mammals incidentally when an infected mosquito or other arthropod obtains a blood meal.

Epidemiology

Most human disease is subclinical; a few patients have a brief febrile illness resembling influenza, and a small percentage, usually at the extremes of age, suffer meningitis or encephalitis. The diseases (Table 406–1) reflect the quotidian and seasonal characteristics of their insect vectors, but the clinician must remember to elicit a travel history to match the epidemiology to the patient. Other viruses of the same genera cause hemorrhagic fever (Chapter 404), and other less frequently encountered arboviruses are also capable of producing encephalitis.

Many of these agents cause notifiable disease in the United States: St. Louis, West Nile (Fig. 406–1), Powassan, eastern equine, western equine, and the California serogroup encephalitis viruses. Case definitions and additional information are available at *http://www.cdc.gov/epo/dphsi/casedef/encephalitis_arboviral_current.htm*.

The diseases described here are zoonoses (Chapter 349; i.e., illnesses caused by viruses transmitted from animals to humans). They are more prevalent in the tropics and subtropics and are usually localized because of ecologic restrictions on their transmission.

Pathobiology

Two pathologic processes are common to the arboviral encephalitides: neuronal and glial damage mediated by intracellular viral infection and migration of immunologically active cells into the perivascular space and brain parenchyma. Endothelial cell swelling and proliferation, destruction of myelin sheaths in deep white matter areas, and vasculitis are present in some arboviral encephalitides.

After a bite by an infected arthropod, viral replication occurs in local tissues and regional lymph nodes. Viremia, which seeds extraneural

TABLE 406–1 ARTHROPOD-BORNE VIRUSES ASSOCIATED WITH HUMAN ENCEPHALITIS

Virus	Insect Vector	Common Vertebrate Hosts	Geographic Distribution
TOGAVIRIDAE			
Alphaviruses	Mosquitoes		
Eastern equine encephalitis	*Culiseta* sp, *Aedes* sp, *Coquillettidia* sp		Eastern United States and Gulf Coast, Caribbean region, South America
Western equine encephalitis	*Culiseta* sp, *Culex* sp		Western United States, Canada
Venezuelan equine encephalitis	*Aedes* sp, *Culex* sp, *Psorophora* sp, and *Mansonia* sp		South America, Central America, Florida and southwestern United States
FLAVIVIRIDAE			
Japanese serocluster	Mosquitoes		
Japanese encephalitis (JE)	*Culex* and *Aedes* sp		East and Southeast Asia, India, Australia
West Nile encephalitis	*Aedes* sp, *Culex* sp, and others		Africa, Middle East, North America
St. Louis encephalitis	*Culex* sp		Western Hemisphere
Murray Valley encephalitis	*Culex* sp		Australia
Tick-Borne Encephalitis Complex			
Central European encephalitis	*Ixodes* sp	Goats, sheep	Europe, Russia
Russian spring-summer encephalitis	*Ixodes* sp		Europe, northern and central Asia
Kyasanur Forest disease	*Haemaphysalis spinigera*	Rodents, insectivores	India
Omsk hemorrhagic fever	*Dermacentor reticulatus*	Rodents	Central Asia
Powassan	*Ixodes* sp	Squirrels, groundhogs	North America, Russia
Louping ill	*Ixodes ricinus*	Small mammals, sheep, birds	British Isles
Langat	*Ixodes* sp	Rodents	Malaysia, Thailand, parts of former Soviet Union
BUNYAVIRIDAE			
California encephalitis	*Aedes melanimon, Aedes dorsalis*	Rodents, rabbits	California
La Crosse encephalitis	*Aedes triseriatus*	Chipmunks, squirrels	Eastern and midwestern United States

tissues, occurs and persists, depending on the extent of replication in extraneural sites, the rate of viral clearance by the reticuloendothelial system, and the appearance of humoral antibodies. The sites of extraneural infection vary among the viruses. Many alphaviruses and flaviviruses involve striated muscle and endothelium, whereas Venezuelan encephalitis virus is associated with myeloid and lymphoid tissue invasion. During viremia, the neural parenchyma may be invaded, but the mode of penetration of virus across the blood-brain barrier is not completely understood. Possible mechanisms include passive movement of virus across vascular membranes and viral replication in the cerebral capillary endothelium. Factors increasing vascular permeability promote nervous system invasion. In experimental animal infection, flaviviruses enter the CNS via the olfactory epithelium.

The immature brain is more susceptible to damage by western equine encephalitis, Venezuelan equine, and California serogroup encephalitis viruses (Table 406–2). St. Louis encephalitis and West Nile virus principally affect the elderly, whereas Japanese encephalitis and eastern equine encephalitis have a bimodal incidence and strike both children and elderly persons. In endemic areas, immunity accumulated with increasing age may reduce the incidence of disease in older persons for some viruses; however, the reasons for the increased severity of illness with other viruses remain unknown.

Clinical Manifestations

Clinical symptoms and signs vary among the viral causes (see later), although all share common signs and symptoms of encephalitis (Chapter 439).

Diagnosis

Diagnosis depends on a careful history encompassing exposure to vertebrate animals and arthropod vectors, age, season, and travel, including the geographic site of exposure. Laboratory confirmation of infection is essential. The virus may be isolated from acute phase serum or whole blood in laboratory animals or in tissue culture. Neutralization, complement fixation (CF), hemagglutination inhibition (HI), fluorescent antibody, and enzyme-linked immunosorbent assay (ELISA) of acute and 3-week convalescent sera can also produce the correct diagnosis. Antigen detection and IgM capture ELISA often permit diagnosis on initial evaluation and within a week of the onset of illness in most cases. Sensitive nucleic amplification assays using reverse transcriptase polymerase chain reaction (RT-PCR) are under development for a number of the arboviruses and may lead to earlier diagnosis.

Differential Diagnosis

The most important initial consideration is to differentiate arboviral encephalitides from other acute CNS infections, including infections other than encephalitis (Chapters 437 and 438) and treatable causes of encephalitis (Chapter 439). The early prodrome resembles influenza (Chapter 387). Bacterial meningitis (Chapter 437; especially early or partially treated), infective bacterial endocarditis (Chapter 76), brain abscess (Chapter 438), subdural empyema (Chapter 438), and cerebral thrombophlebitis may mimic viral encephalitis, and the cerebrospinal fluid (CSF) profile is sometimes similar. Other infections that occasionally cause meningoencephalitis resembling arthropod-borne viral encephalitis include tuberculosis (Chapter 345), cryptococcosis (Chapter 357),

Cumulative Human Disease Cases by County—2006

Alabama, 2006

County	Cases
Jefferson County	2
Mobile County	3
Cumulative Total Entire State:	5

Arkansas, 2006

County	Cases
Bradley County	1
Cleburne County	1
Drew County	1
Hempstead County	1
Jefferson County	5
Lafayette County	2
Lawrence County	1
Lonoke County	1
Nevada County	1
Pulaski County	5
Saline County	1
Sebastian County	2
Washington County	1
Yell County	1
Cumulative Total Entire State:	23

Arizona

County	Cases
Apache County	1
Cochise County	2
Coconino County	1
Gila County	1
Maricopa County	25
Mohave County	1
Pima County	11
Pinal County	2
Santa Cruz County	1
Cumulative Total Entire State:	45

California

County	Cases
Alameda County	1
Butte County	30
Colusa County	2
Contra Costa County	8
El Dorado County	1
Fresno County	8
Glenn County	12
Imperial County	1
Kern County	45
Kings County	1
Lake County	1
Los Angeles County	10
Marin County	1
Merced County	2
Modoc County	2
Mono County	1
Napa County	1
Nevada County	1
Orange County	5
Placer County	7
Riverside County	3
Sacramento County	11
San Bernardino County	1
San Diego County	1
San Joaquin County	8
San Luis Obispo County	1
Santa Clara County	5
Shasta County	2
Solano County	6
Stanislaus County	10
Sutter County	11
Tehama County	3
Tulare County	4
Ventura County	3
Yolo County	25
Yuba County	3
Cumulative Total Entire State:	237

Colorado

County	Cases
Adams County	7
Bent County	3
Boulder County	57
Broomfield County	4
Crowley County	2
Delta County	33
Denver County	3
Eagle County	1
El Paso County	2
Elbert County	1
Garfield County	1
Jefferson County	6
La Plata County	2
Larimer County	32
Logan County	4
Mesa County	36
Montrose County	10
Morgan County	1
Otero County	3
Phillips County	1
Prowers County	4
Pueblo County	5
Weld County	55
Cumulative Total Entire State:	273

Connecticut

County	Cases
Fairfield County	2
Hartford County	1
New Haven County	5
Cumulative Total Entire State:	8

Florida

County	Cases
Escambia County	2
Palm Beach County	1
Cumulative Total Entire State:	3

Georgia

County	Cases
Cobb County	1
Dekalb County	1
Dougherty County	3
Fulton County	2
Cumulative Total Entire State:	7

Idaho

County	Cases
Ada County	177
Adams County	6
Bannock County	3
Bingham County	26
Blaine County	10
Boise County	2
Bonneville County	22
Butte County	1
Camas County	2
Canyon County	148
Cassia County	2
Clearwater County	1
Custer County	3
Elmore County	53
Fremont County	3
Gem County	12
Idaho, continued	
Gooding County	36
Idaho County	2
Jefferson County	9
Jerome County	9
Kootenai County	9
Lemhi County	1
Lincoln County	5
Madison County	3
Minidoka County	17
Owyhee County	20
Payette County	18
Twin Falls County	31
Valley County	2
Washington County	17
Cumulative Total Entire State:	642

Illinois

County	Cases
Adams County	1
Bond County	1
Brown County	1
Clay County	1
Cook County	77
Crawford County	2
Dekalb County	1
Dupage County	32
Effingham County	2
Franklin County	1
Jefferson County	2
Jo Daviess County	1
Kane County	2
Kendall County	2
Lake County	10
Macoupin County	1
Madison County	1
McHenry County	3
McLean County	3
Monroe County	1
Morgan County	1
Moultrie County	1
Ogle County	1
Richland County	1
Rock Island County	1
Saint Clair County	2
Sangamon County	3
Stephenson County	1
Will County	18
Woodford County	2
Cumulative Total Entire State:	176

Indiana

County	Cases
Allen County	1
Blackford County	1
Clinton County	1
Elkhart County	3
Jackson County	1
La Porte County	1
Lake County	10
Marion County	1
Noble County	1
Porter County	5
Saint Joseph County	1
Vanderburgh County	1
Wabash County	1
Cumulative Total Entire State:	28

Iowa

County	Cases
Adair County	1
Carroll County	1
Cass County	1
Cerro Gordo County	1
Dickinson County	1
Emmet County	3
Hardin County	1
Henry County	1
Jackson County	1
Kossuth County	1
Lee County	1
Marion County	1
O'Brien County	1
Plymouth County	3
Pottawattamie County	1
Ringgold County	1
Shelby County	1
Sioux County	1
Wapello County	1
Washington County	1
Woodbury County	3
Cumulative Total Entire State:	27

Kansas

County	Cases
Barton County	1
Chase County	1
Cheyenne County	1
Douglas County	1
Finney County	1
Gray County	1
Harvey County	3
Johnson County	3
Kiowa County	1
Neosho County	1
Pawnee County	2
Pratt County	1
Reno County	2
Rooks County	1
Rush County	2
Sedgwick County	1
Cumulative Total Entire State:	23

Louisiana

Parish	Cases
Ascension Parish	16
Assumption Parish	1
Avoyelles Parish	1
Bossier Parish	2
Caddo Parish	3
Calcasieu Parish	5
De Soto Parish	1
East Baton Rouge Parish	5
Jefferson Parish	7
Lafayette Parish	1
Lafourche Parish	2
Livingston Parish	2
Orleans Parish	10
Ouachita Parish	5
Rapides Parish	5
Saint Bernard Parish	1
Saint Tammany Parish	26
Tangipahoa Parish	11
Union Parish	1
Vermilion Parish	1
Vernon Parish	1
Washington Parish	5
Webster Parish	2
West Baton Rouge Parish	1
Cumulative Total Entire State:	115

Maine

County	Cases
Cumberland County	2
Waldo County	1
York County	3
Cumulative Total Entire State:	6

Maryland

County	Cases
Baltimore City	2
Baltimore County	1
Cumulative Total Entire State:	3

Massachusetts

County	Cases
Barnstable County	9
Bristol County	19
Essex County	7
Hampden County	4
Middlesex County	5
Norfolk County	4
Plymouth County	6
Suffolk County	1
Worcester County	2
Cumulative Total Entire State:	57

FIGURE 406–1 • Cases of human West Nile Virus in the United States in 2006. (Data accessed September 19, 2006 from http://diseasemaps.usgs.gov/wnv_us_human.html.)

Cumulative Human Disease Cases by County—2006

Michigan

County	Cases
Alcona County	2
Alger County	1
Allegan County	7
Alpena County	1
Antrim County	1
Barry County	2
Bay County	9
Benzie County	1
Berrien County	10
Cass County	1
Charlevoix County	1
Chippewa County	5
Clinton County	6
Crawford County	3
Delta County	1
Gladwin County	1
Grand Traverse County	2
Gratiot County	1
Hillsdale County	1
Houghton County	3
Huron County	1
Ingham County	15
Ionia County	4
Iosco County	1
Iron County	1
Kalamazoo County	4
Kalkaska County	2
Kent County	5
Lake County	5
Leelanau County	1
Lenawee County	9
Luce County	1
Manistee County	1
Marquette County	2
Mason County	2
Mecosta County	1
Midland County	4
Missaukee County	1
Montcalm County	1
Montmorency County	1
Muskegon County	15
Newaygo County	3
Oceana County	4
Ogemaw County	1
Ontonagon County	1
Oscoda County	1
Otsego County	4
Ottawa County	7
Roscommon County	2
Saginaw County	71
Saint Joseph County	3
Shiawassee County	1
Tuscola County	5
Van Buren County	4
Washtenaw County	12
Wayne County	9
Wexford County	9
Cumulative Total Entire State:	273

Minnesota

County	Cases
Anoka County	34
Carver County	1
Chisago County	1
Dakota County	29
Goodhue County	1
Hennepin County	120
Isanti County	1
Pine County	1
Ramsey County	47
Rice County	1
Scott County	6
Wabasha County	1
Washington County	21
Cumulative Total Entire State:	264

Mississippi

County	Cases
Adams County	1
Bolivar County	2
Desoto County	1
Hancock County	1
Hinds County	5
Humphreys County	1
Kemper County	1
Lamar County	1
Lauderdale County	1
Lawrence County	1
Leake County	4
Lincoln County	1
Madison County	7
Marion County	2
Pearl River County	1
Pike County	4
Rankin County	4
Smith County	1
Sunflower County	1
Tallahatchie County	2
Warren County	2
Washington County	4
Winston County	1
Yazoo County	1
Cumulative Total Entire State:	50

Missouri

County	Cases
Adair County	1
Barry County	2
Boone County	4
Buchanan County	4
Callaway County	1
Cape Girardeau County	1
Cole County	7
Dent County	1
Douglas County	1
Franklin County	2
Gasconade County	3
Henry County	1
Howell County	4
Iron County	1
Jasper County	2
Jefferson County	8
Johnson County	1
Laclede County	3
Lewis County	1
Marion County	1
Newton County	2
Perry County	1
Pike County	1
Polk County	1
Pulaski County	1
Ralls County	6
Reynolds County	1
Saint Charles County	6
Saint Francois County	1
Saint Louis City	3
Taney County	2
Texas County	2
Washington County	3
Webster County	3
Wright County	2
Cumulative Total Entire State:	84

Montana

County	Cases
Yellowstone County	1
Cumulative Total Entire State:	1

Nebraska

County	Cases
Adams County	2
Burt County	2
Butler County	2
Chase County	1
Cheyenne County	1
Clay County	1

Nebraska *(continued)*

County	Cases
Custer County	1
Dodge County	3
Douglas County	15
Fillmore County	2
Gage County	2
Hall County	3
Hamilton County	1
Kearney County	1
Lancaster County	13
Lincoln County	4
Madison County	3
Nemaha County	1
Otoe County	1
Phelps County	2
Polk County	3
Richardson County	1
Saline County	2
Sarpy County	7
Saunders County	2
Scotts Bluff County	2
Seward County	2
Stanton County	1
Valley County	3
Wayne County	2
York County	5
Cumulative Total Entire State:	91

Nevada

County	Cases
Carson City	5
Churchill County	9
Douglas County	7
Elko County	13
Eureka County	1
Lyon County	3
Washoe County	5
Cumulative Total Entire State:	43

New Hampshire

County	Cases
Hillsborough County	12
Merrimack County	1
Rockingham County	5
Cumulative Total Entire State:	18

New Jersey

County	Cases
Atlantic County	1
Bergen County	2
Camden County	2
Essex County	2
Gloucester County	1
Hunterdon County	1
Mercer County	3
Monmouth County	6
Morris County	3
Ocean County	15
Passaic County	1
Somerset County	1
Union County	1
Warren County	1
Cumulative Total Entire State:	40

New Mexico

County	Cases
Chaves County	1
Colfax County	1
Cumulative Total Entire State:	2

New York

County	Cases
Albany County	6
Bronx County	2
Chautauqua County	2
Columbia County	1
Cortland County	4
Erie County	5
Herkimer County	1
Jefferson County	1
Kings County	3
Lewis County	5

New York *(continued)*

County	Cases
Livingston County	3
Monroe County	8
Nassau County	5
Niagara County	12
Onondaga County	19
Ontario County	3
Orleans County	4
Oswego County	1
Putnam County	1
Queens County	13
Richmond County	50
Saratoga County	1
Schuyler County	1
Seneca County	7
Suffolk County	62
Tompkins County	7
Wayne County	2
Yates County	1
Cumulative Total Entire State:	235

New Mexico

County	Cases
Chaves County	1
Colfax County	1
Cumulative Total Entire State:	2

North Dakota

County	Cases
Barnes County	1
Bowman County	1
Burleigh County	1
Cass County	5
Foster County	1
Ramsey County	1
Cumulative Total Entire State:	10

Ohio

County	Cases
Allen County	2
Ashland County	2
Ashtabula County	1
Butler County	1
Clark County	2
Cuyahoga County	1
Defiance County	2
Franklin County	1
Fulton County	2
Geauga County	5
Hamilton County	1
Hancock County	1
Knox County	1
Lake County	15
Licking County	1
Lorain County	4
Lucas County	4
Mahoning County	2
Marion County	2
Medina County	3
Mercer County	1
Ottawa County	3
Paulding County	1
Portage County	3
Richland County	2
Sandusky County	2
Stark County	4
Summit County	3
Tuscarawas County	1
Union County	1
Williams County	1
Wood County	4
Wyandot County	2
Cumulative Total Entire State:	81

Oklahoma

County	Cases
Tulsa County	4
Cumulative Total Entire State:	41

FIGURE 406–1, cont'd

Cumulative Human Disease Cases by County—2006

Oregon	
Baker County	1
Malheur County	2
Cumulative Total Entire State:	3

Pennsylvania	
Beaver County	1
Berks County	1
Blair County	1
Bucks County	2
Butler County	2
Cambria County	1
Centre County	1
Crawford County	3
Cumberland County	1
Erie County	14
Franklin County	2
Jefferson County	1
Lackawanna County	1
Lebanon County	1
Lehigh County	3
Lycoming County	1
Mercer County	3
Montgomery County	1
Northampton County	1
Pike County	1
Somerset County	1
Venango County	1
Washington County	1
Westmoreland County	3
Cumulative Total Entire State:	48

South Carolina	
Charleston County	11
Cumulative Total Entire State:	11

South Dakota	
South Dakota, 2006	
Brookings County	1
Brown County	1
Butte County	2
Clay County	3
Kingsbury County	1
Minnehaha County	1
Roberts County	4
Shannon County	1
Todd County	1
Turner County	3
Cumulative Total Entire State:	18

Texas	
Bowie County	3
Brazos County	6
Camp County	1
Denton County	1
Ellis County	1
Franklin County	1
Harris County	100
Jefferson County	2
McLennan County	1
Smith County	1
Wharton County	1
Cumulative Total Entire State:	118

Utah	
Carbon County	1
Davis County	3
Emery County	1
Grand County	1
Salt Lake County	48
Uintah County	2
Utah County	12
Weber County	7
Cumulative Total Entire State:	75

Vermont	
Addison County	1
Chittenden County	7
Cumulative Total Entire State:	8

Virginia	
Arlington County	1
Augusta County	1
Cumulative Total Entire State:	2

West Virginia	
Greenbrier County	1
Lincoln County	1
Cumulative Total Entire State:	2

Wisconsin	
Adams County	2
Ashland County	2
Barron County	2
Brown County	2
Calumet County	2
Chippewa County	2
Clark County	2
Columbia County	2
Dane County	7
Dodge County	2
Door County	2
Douglas County	2
Dunn County	1
Eau Claire County	4
Fond du Lac County	5
Forest County	3
Grant County	3
Green County	1
Iron County	3
Jackson County	2
Jefferson County	2
Juneau County	1
Kenosha County	3
Kewaunee County	1
La Crosse County	2
Langlade County	2
Lincoln County	2
Manitowoc County	2
Marathon County	3
Marinette County	3
Marquette County	2
Milwaukee County	2
Monroe County	3
Oneida County	3
Outagamie County	2
Ozaukee County	3
Pepin County	2
Polk County	1
Portage County	2
Price County	2
Racine County	2
Rock County	3
Saint Croix County	3
Sauk County	2
Sawyer County	2
Sheboygan County	4
Taylor County	1
Vilas County	3
Walworth County	2
Washburn County	2
Washington County	5
Waukesha County	2
Waupaca County	1
Waushara County	2
Winnebago County	3
Wood County	2
Cumulative Total Entire State:	133

Wyoming	
Campbell County	3
Fremont County	2
Goshen County	2
Natrona County	1
Sweetwater County	2
Cumulative Total Entire State:	10

FIGURE 406–1, cont'd

histoplasmosis (Chapter 353), coccidioidomycosis (Chapter 354), Rocky Mountain spotted fever (Chapter 348), leptospirosis (Chapter 344), falciparum malaria (Chapter 366), trichinosis (Chapter 378), *Naegleria* meningitis (Chapter 437), typhoid fever (Chapter 329), Lyme disease (Chapter 342), and *Mycoplasma* pneumonia (Chapter 338).

Acute meningoencephalitis may result from infections with other viruses, including herpesviruses (Chapter 397), human immunodeficiency virus (Chapter 407), mumps virus (Chapter 392), enteroviruses (Chapter 402), lymphocytic choriomeningitis virus (Chapter 437), rabies (Chapter 441), influenza (Chapter 387), and the exanthematous viral infections of childhood (Chapters 390 and 391). The exposure history, the presence of similar disease in the community, and summer-fall occurrence are principal clues to an arboviral etiology. Enteroviruses (Chapter 402) also cause summer-fall outbreaks, but the predominant syndrome is aseptic meningitis, and the occurrence of rash or pleurodynia is a helpful clue. Herpes simplex encephalitis (Chapter 439) presents an important diagnostic challenge because effective therapy is available and should be started quickly. The presence of localizing neurologic signs, localizing findings on computed tomography (CT) or magnetic resonance imaging (MRI), or detection of herpes simplex DNA in CSF by PCR help distinguish herpes simplex encephalitis from the arboviral encephalitides.

Noninfectious diseases of the CNS such as stroke (Chapter 431) may rarely be confused with viral encephalitis. Subarachnoid hemorrhage (Chapter 432) produces meningismus, fever, headache, and neurologic signs that mimic an infectious etiology. Metabolic encephalopathies occasionally have features suggesting infectious encephalitis. Neoplastic or granulomatous diseases involving the CNS and a variety of diseases of uncertain etiology (Behçet's disease [Chapter 447], Reye's syndrome, acute multiple sclerosis [Chapter 436], and systemic lupus erythematosus [Chapter 287]) must be considered in the differential diagnosis as well.

Prevention

Control can be achieved by interrupting the cycle, including vaccination of reservoir animals, vector control, and education on vector avoidance. Practical measures include wearing long-sleeved clothing, using

TABLE 406–2 FEATURES OF ARBOVIRAL ENCEPHALITIDES IMPORTANT IN THE UNITED STATES

	Eastern Equine Encephalitis	Western Equine Encephalitis	Venezuelan Equine Encephalitis	West Nile Encephalitis	St. Louis Encephalitis	California Serogroup Encephalitis
Annual U.S. cases of symptomatic disease	10	0–2 cases, mostly infants and children	Rare, mostly children	Up to 3000, mostly >40 yr	0–2000, mostly >50 yr	10–50, mostly children
Time of year	Late summer, early fall	Early and mid-summer	Summer	Summer, fall	Mid to late summer	July–September
Case-fatality rate	50–70%, highest in children <15 yr and adults >55 yr	3–5% in children	35% in children, <10% in older persons	14–19%, 30% in adults >70 yr	9% overall; 0% <20 yr, 30% >65 yr	<1%
Residual damage	30–50%, especially in children	33% in infants	Frequent in children	50%, more frequent in elderly	Frequent in elderly	Probably rare
Cerebrospinal fluid findings	500–2000 cells, predominantly neutrophils	<500 cells, predominantly lymphocytes	<500 cells, predominantly lymphocytes	<500 cells, predominantly lymphocytes	<500 cells, predominantly lymphocytes	<500 cells, predominantly lymphocytes

insect repellents, limiting outdoor activities during peak mosquito season, and eliminating standing pools of water. Vaccines are currently available for Japanese encephalitis.

Treatment

Treatment is symptomatic and may include bedrest, antipyretics, and analgesics. In some situations, early empirical treatment of herpes simplex encephalitis (Chapter 397) may be appropriate while the diagnostic evaluation to document arboviral encephalitis proceeds.

EASTERN EQUINE ENCEPHALITIS

Epidemiology

Human disease is relatively rare, with fewer than 10 cases occurring each year in the Gulf Coast and Atlantic states, usually in association with an equine epizootic involving 100 to 300 animals. Outbreaks generally occur during the late summer and early fall. The occurrence of equine cases or outbreaks of fatal encephalitis in penned exotic birds precedes the appearance of human cases by several weeks or more. Epizootics of eastern equine encephalitis have been reported in the Caribbean (Hispaniola) and South America.

In temperate areas, eastern equine encephalitis virus circulates between wild birds and *Culiseta melanura* mosquitoes in a freshwater swamp habitat. Equine epizootics and associated human cases result from extension of the transmission cycle to involve *Aedes* and *Coquillettidia* mosquitoes, which feed on horses and humans.

Pathobiology

The brain is grossly edematous and congested, and the inflammatory response is predominantly polymorphonuclear. The areas most affected are the basal ganglia, thalamus, hippocampus, and frontal and occipital cortices. Focal vasculitis, endothelial cell swelling, intravenous and arteriolar thrombus formation, demyelination, necrosis, neuronolysis, and neuronophagia are prominent.

Clinical Manifestations

Onset is abrupt, with high fever, vomiting, and somnolence. Stupor, coma, myoclonus, and generalized convulsions appear within 24 hours to as long as 10 days later. Autonomic disturbances (sialorrhea) may be prominent, and respiratory difficulty and cyanosis are frequent. In children, facial, periorbital, or generalized edema may be present.

A striking peripheral leukocytosis with immature neutrophils occurs frequently in patients with eastern equine encephalitis. CSF examination reveals 500 to 2000 white blood cells/mL (predominantly neutrophils). As the total cell count falls, neutrophils may persist as a significant fraction. Red blood cells may be present, protein is elevated, and the glucose level is normal.

Diagnosis

Brain CT and MRI are frequently abnormal and reveal lesions in the basal ganglia, thalami, and brain stem. The virus can rarely be isolated from blood or CSF. Serologic diagnosis by demonstrating a rise in antibody titer in appropriately timed paired sera is the most practical and available test. Because of the rapid course of the clinical disease, sera should be obtained at 2- to 3-day intervals during the acute phase of illness.

Prevention

An experimental formalin-inactivated chick embryo cell culture vaccine is used to protect laboratory and field workers. Reduction of mosquito populations by appropriate use of insecticides may be effective in threatened or established outbreaks.

Treatment

Treatment is supportive. Control of fever, intracranial pressure, seizures, fluid and electrolyte disturbances, and the airway is critical. Although attempts at immunologic therapy have been reported, no controlled data are available.

Prognosis

The case-fatality rate is 50 to 70%. Mortality, like incidence, is highest in children younger than 15 years and in persons older than 55 years, with no gender predilection. Death usually occurs during the first week; in surviving patients, recovery begins during the second week and may progress rapidly. Good functional recovery is associated with a long prodromal course and absence of coma. Residual damage, found in 30 to 50% of patients, is often severe, especially in children, and is characterized by mental retardation, spastic paralysis, and radiographic evidence of brain atrophy.

WESTERN EQUINE ENCEPHALITIS

Epidemiology

Few cases of western equine encephalitis have been reported in the past decade; the most recent epidemic occurred in Colorado in 1987. Epidemics occur in early or mid summer and may follow heavy snow melt or flooding, conditions favorable for breeding of mosquitoes. Cases of encephalitis in equines often precede the appearance of human disease. The illness principally affects residents of rural communities, and the incidence is higher in males than in females.

The ratio of inapparent to apparent infection is also age dependent and ranges from about 1:1 in infants younger than 1 year, 58:1 in children 1 to 4 years old, to more than 1000:1 in persons older than 14 years. Western equine encephalitis virus also occurs in South America. Equine epizootics in Argentina have been associated with human cases.

Western equine encephalitis virus circulates between wild birds and *Culex tarsalis* mosquitoes. *C. tarsalis* is responsible for infection of humans and equines, which have low or undetectable viremia and do not perpetuate the chain of transmission. In temperate areas, transmission ceases during the winter months.

Pathobiology

Pathologic examination of the brains of infants reveals massive parenchymal destruction; children dying months or years after the acute insult often have large cystic lesions in many areas of the brain. In older children and adults, acute western equine encephalitis is characterized by focal necrosis and perivascular cuffing, predominantly in the basal ganglia and thalami but also in deep cerebral white matter.

Clinical Manifestations

The disease usually begins with an influenza-like illness consisting of fever, headache, malaise, and myalgia lasting 1 to 4 days. Somnolence, lethargy, photophobia, vomiting, and neck stiffness may follow; neurologic involvement may rapidly progress to stupor, coma, and seizures. Pareses, cranial nerve deficits, tremors, and abnormal reflexes may be present. In fatal cases, patients die 1 to 2 days after coma develops. Congenital infections have been documented and result in severe and progressive neurologic deterioration.

Leukocytosis and a shift to the left are common. The CSF contains less than 500 white blood cells/mL (at first polymorphonuclear, then mononuclear) and an elevated protein concentration (usually 90 to 110 mg/dL).

Diagnosis

Viral isolation from blood or CSF is almost never successful. Diagnosis is achieved by demonstrating a rise in HI, fluorescent antibody, CF, ELISA, or neutralizing antibody titers in appropriately timed (10 to 14 days apart) paired sera. Demonstration of IgM antibodies in serum or CSF by ELISA provides a presumptive diagnosis.

Prevention

An experimental formalin-inactivated vaccine grown in chick embryo cell culture has been used to protect laboratory workers but is not indicated for others. In threatened or ongoing epidemics, residents should be advised to use protective clothing, insect repellents, and window screens and to restrict outdoor activity in the early morning, late afternoon, and evening (times of greatest mosquito activity). Public health measures include spraying insecticides aimed at the adult *C. tarsalis* vector.

Treatment

There is no specific therapy for western equine encephalitis. Supportive therapy is similar to that discussed earlier for eastern equine encephalitis.

Prognosis

Western equine encephalitis is most severe in infants and young children. The case-fatality rate is between 3 and 5%. Survivors generally experience sudden and rapid recovery. However, about a third of surviving infants suffer mental retardation, cerebellar damage, choreoathetosis, and spastic paralysis. Children with protracted illnesses in whom convulsions develop during the acute stage are more likely to suffer long-term neurologic sequelae. Adults may have a prolonged convalescent syndrome, but objective residua are rare.

VENEZUELAN EQUINE ENCEPHALITIS

Six antigenic subtypes of Venezuelan equine encephalitis (I to VI) with several antigenic variants of subtypes I and III are recognized serologically. Subtypes IAB and IC are responsible for epidemics involving humans and equines. In Florida, subtype II is enzootic and produces sporadic human disease. Methods of transmitting Venezuelan equine encephalitis virus as a biologic warfare agent were developed in the 1960s; an epidemic of Venezuelan equine encephalitis, especially if humans and horses become ill simultaneously, could represent an attack rather than naturally occurring illness.

Epidemiology

Before 1973, large equine epizootics occurred at 5- to 10-year intervals in Venezuela, Colombia, Ecuador, and Peru and involved many thousands of animals with mortality rates as high as 40%. Associated human morbidity was also great (up to 32,000 clinical cases). The disease was quiescent for several years but has reemerged in the past decade. The last major outbreak occurred in Venezuela and Colombia in 1995, with more than 85,000 human cases. Laboratory infections are common in unvaccinated persons working with the virus or infected animals.

A large variety of mosquito vectors, including species of the genera *Aedes, Psorophora,* and *Mansonia,* transmit subtypes IAB and IC during epizootic epidemics. Equines are the principal viremic hosts. Virus may be present in the pharyngeal excretions of human patients; contact or aerosol person-to-person spread, though possible, is not epidemiologically important.

The other members of the Venezuelan equine encephalitis viral complex, including subtype II in Florida, have enzootic transmission cycles involving *Culex* mosquitoes and small forest rodents and marsupials. Human disease is sporadic and relatively uncommon.

Pathobiology

Pathologic changes in the CNS include edema, congestion, meningeal and perivascular inflammation, intracerebral hemorrhage, neuronal degeneration, and vasculitis. In addition, hepatocellular degeneration and necrosis, widespread lymphoid depletion and follicular necrosis, and interstitial pneumonitis are frequent. Congenitally infected fetuses demonstrate massive and widespread necrosis of brain tissue, hemorrhage, and resorption of brain material resulting in hydranencephaly.

Clinical Manifestations

The predominant syndrome is a self-limited influenza-like illness; encephalitis develops in only about 4% of infected persons, principally children younger than 15 years. Subclinical infections are rare.

After an incubation period of 2 to 5 days, there is a sudden onset of fever, chills, malaise, and headache, followed by myalgias, nausea, vomiting, and occasionally diarrhea. Physical examination reveals fever, tachycardia, conjunctival injection, and in some cases, nonexudative pharyngitis. The acute illness generally subsides in 4 to 6 days, and convalescent symptoms may last up to 3 weeks. A biphasic course has sometimes been noted; acute symptoms can reappear after a brief remission, within a week after initial onset.

When it occurs, severe encephalitis is characterized by meningeal signs, seizures, tremor, stupor, coma, spastic paralysis, abnormal reflexes, cranial nerve palsies, and central respiratory failure. Residual neurologic damage occurs in severe cases. Infections of pregnant women acquired during the first and second trimester may result in fetal encephalitis and death.

The peripheral leukocyte count is often low, with a decrease in both lymphocytes and neutrophils, or normal with relative lymphopenia. In patients with CNS signs, the CSF contains up to 500 cells/mL, predominantly lymphocytes. Serum lactate dehydrogenase and aspartate aminotransferase concentrations may be elevated.

Diagnosis

In contrast to the other arboviral encephalitides, Venezuelan equine encephalitis virus can be isolated from blood or from throat swabs or washings during the first 3 or 4 days of illness. Serodiagnosis is usually more practical and is achieved by testing appropriately timed paired sera by HI, CF, ELISA, neutralization, or IgM immunoassay.

Prevention

An experimental live, attenuated vaccine made from subtype IAB is used for adult laboratory personnel. It provides solid immunity to subtype IAB and its closest relative (IC), but incomplete protection against other heterologous Venezuelan equine encephalitis viruses. Epidemics and epizootics can be prevented by effective vaccination of equines. Spraying insecticides to reduce adult (infective) mosquito populations is the only means of immediate control in the face of an ongoing epidemic. Individual protection against mosquitoes is advised.

Treatment

Rx

No specific therapy is available, and treatment of encephalitis cases is supportive.

Prognosis

The case-fatality rate in children 5 years or younger with encephalitis is approximately 35%, but in older persons it is less than 10%.

JAPANESE ENCEPHALITIS

Epidemiology

Japanese encephalitis virus causes epizootics of clinical encephalitis in equines. The disease occurs throughout Asia, including Japan, the Korean peninsula, Taiwan, the People's Republic of China, Okinawa, Vietnam, the Philippines, Burma, Malaysia, Bangladesh, east and south India, Sri Lanka, Thailand, and Indonesia. More than 30,000 clinical cases occur annually. Japanese encephalitis is a summertime disease in temperate areas but occurs sporadically year-round in the tropics. Epidemics are most frequent at the northern fringe of the tropical zone. It is a predominantly rural disease, and the incidence in males is often higher than in females. In hyperendemic areas, more than 70% of adult populations surveyed have antibodies, and children younger than 15 years are principally affected by the disease. In areas without a high prevalence of background immunity (e.g., northern India), however, all age groups are affected. In Japan, where schoolchildren have been protected by vaccination campaigns targeted at this age group, encephalitis has become prominent in the elderly. The ratio of clinically inapparent to apparent infection is higher than 500:1 in children and decreases with age; in Korea, the ratio in American servicemen was estimated at 25:1.

Pathobiology

Neuropathologic changes and the distribution of lesions are similar to those described for St. Louis encephalitis (see later).

Clinical Manifestations

Manifestations of Japanese encephalitis include abrupt fever, headache, and gastrointestinal symptoms. Meningeal irritation develops within 24 hours and is followed on the second or third day by the appearance of irritability, impaired consciousness, seizures (especially in children), muscular rigidity, parkinsonian findings, ataxia, coarse tremor, involuntary movements, cranial nerve deficits, paresis, hyperactive deep tendon reflexes, and pathologic reflexes. Weight loss and dehydration are often striking findings. In mild cases, fever subsides after the first week, and neurologic signs resolve by the end of the second week after onset. In severe cases, hyperpyrexia, progressive neurologic dysfunction, and coma result in death, usually between the 7th and 10th days. About 25% of patients undergo a prolonged recovery, with permanent sequelae often remaining. The occurrence of such sequelae correlates with severity of the acute stage of illness, and young children are most susceptible. Cardiorespiratory complications are frequent during the acute stage in these patients. A poor prognosis is associated with protracted high fever, frequent or prolonged seizures, high protein content in CSF, the Babinski sign, and early respiratory depression. Fetal death from transplacental Japanese encephalitis infection has been reported.

Diagnosis

Moderate peripheral leukocytosis and neutrophilia occur early in the disease. Pleocytosis (predominantly lymphocytic), protein elevation, and normal glucose in CSF are usual findings.

MRI in Japanese encephalitis reveals edema in the basal ganglia, thalami, and focal area of the cerebral cortex; evidence of hemorrhage in these areas may likewise be present. Enhancement may also be noted in the meninges, brain stem, and spinal cord.

Virus is rarely isolated from blood. Virus is also rarely recovered from the CSF of patients who live but may be recovered from the CSF of a third of patients who die. HI and neutralizing antibodies appear during the first week, and CF antibodies appear during the second week. Cross-reactions with other flaviviruses make serodiagnosis difficult. Specific IgM antibodies in serum or CSF are detectable by immunoassays in more than three fourths of patients at the time of hospital admission.

Prevention

The inactivated, partially purified mouse brain vaccines produced in Japan are safe and effective in preschool- and school-aged children. A vaccine produced in Japan is available to U.S. citizens traveling to high-risk areas. However, generalized urticaria and angioedema may occur in 0.3% of recipients, and anecdotal cases of encephalomyelitis have been reported; as a result, the precise indications for vaccination of travelers are unclear. Because three doses of the inactivated vaccine are used and approximately 1 month is required to confer protection, vaccination is not a practical measure in the event of an ongoing epidemic. Reduction of vector mosquito populations by applying insecticides may help abort outbreaks. Immunization of swine is an ancillary control strategy.

Treatment

Rx

Treatment is supportive (see Eastern Equine Encephalitis). A randomized trial of interferon-alfa showed no benefit.

Prognosis

The case-fatality rate is probably about 25%. Sequelae such as mental impairment, emotional lability, choreoathetosis, tremor, parkinsonism, autonomic disturbances, paralysis, and psychiatric disturbances have been reported in up to 75% of patients.

WEST NILE FEVER AND ENCEPHALITIS

Before 1996, the predominant clinical manifestation of West Nile virus was a brief influenza-like illness, sometimes with a rash (Chapter 405) but infrequently with neurologic manifestations. Epidemics since then in Romania, Israel, and North America have added meningitis, meningoencephalitis, and myelitis to the list of disorders attributable to the virus. Sequence analysis of various isolates of the virus indicate two lineages. The first includes viruses from North America, Europe, Israel, western Africa, India, Russia, and Australia, and the second includes viruses from sub-Saharan Africa and Madagascar.

Epidemiology

See Chapter 405.

Clinical Manifestations

The majority of infected persons are asymptomatic. Fever develops in about 20%, and CNS manifestations are seen in less than 1%, although this percentage is higher in the elderly (Chapter 405). In those in whom clinical manifestations develop, an incubation period of 1 to 6 days is followed by the abrupt onset of symptoms, usually without a prodrome. The temperature rises quickly to 38.3 to 40° C, with rigors in a third of patients. Symptoms include drowsiness, severe frontal headache, ocular pain, myalgia, and pain in the abdomen and back. A small number of patients have dryness of the throat, anorexia, and nausea. Cough is common. Examination shows facial flushing, conjunctival injection, and coating of the tongue. Generalized lymphadenopathy had been a prominent feature in past epidemics but is no longer commonly reported. The spleen and liver are occasionally slightly enlarged. The temperature curve may be biphasic. A pale roseolar maculopapular rash, predominantly on the trunk and upper part of the arms, may appear from the second to fifth day but is now less common as well; it may be evanescent (several hours) or persist until defervescence, and it does not desquamate. Vesicular lesions occur rarely. The illness lasts 3 to 5 days in 80% of patients.

In the past decade the incidence of CNS disease has increased in several epidemics, apparently because of a true increase in the invasiveness and neurovirulence of the virus. The virus causes a syndrome resembling poliomyelitis (Chapter 440), with prominent lower motor neuron dysfunction (acute flaccid paralysis with asymmetrical weakness and decreased deep tendon reflexes but preserved sensory function), which may be seen independently or with signs of meningoencephalitis. In some patients, prolonged, possibly permanent ventilatory failure requiring mechanical ventilation develops. A parkinsonian syndrome has also been noted, but it generally remits after months. Some patients may have seizures, cranial nerve involvement, ataxia, tremors, or myoclonus. Acute inflammatory polyneuropathy (e.g., Guillain-Barré syndrome; Chapter 436) has also been reported. Other rare complications include myocarditis, pancreatitis, and hepatitis. Convalescence is often prolonged, lasting several weeks with prominent symptoms of fatigue. Lymph node enlargement requires several months to regress. Laboratory findings often include leukocytosis, whereas 10 to 15% of patients have leukopenia.

Diagnosis

CSF examination may reveal a lymphocytic pleocytosis (<1800 cells/mL) with some increase in protein but a normal glucose concentration. Although West Nile virus may be isolated from the blood of three fourths of patients with West Nile fever on the first day of illness (Chapter 405), patients with West Nile encephalitis appear less likely to be viremic, and isolation of virus from CSF is infrequent. Viral RNA is detected in CSF by RT-PCR in about 50% of cases. IgM antibody capture immunoassay, which is the test of choice, is more sensitive than RT-PCR. IgM antibodies may remain detectable for up to 500 days after infection, so their presence should suggest acute infection only in the presence of compatible clinical manifestations. In some situations, cross-reactions with other flaviviruses, particularly St. Louis encephalitis virus, may complicate the interpretation of IgM immunoassays.

Treatment

Rx

Treatment is symptomatic and similar to that suggested for eastern equine encephalitis. Patients may require prolonged mechanical ventilation for either the polio-like syndrome or Guillain-Barré syndrome. The Guillain-Barré syndrome seen in West Nile patients does not appear to respond to plasma exchange. A large trial of intravenous immunoglobulin is under way. Ribavirin has activity against West Nile virus, but its clinical utility is unknown.

Prognosis

The overall case-fatality rate is 4 to 14%, but it is higher in the elderly. Risk factors for death include more severe weakness or coma, immunocompromise, and failure to produce virus-specific IgM. The prognosis for neurologic recovery is guarded, with about half the patients still reporting difficulties 1 year after the illness.

ST. LOUIS ENCEPHALITIS

Etiology

St. Louis encephalitis virus, a member of the family Flaviviridae, shares close antigenic relationships with Japanese encephalitis, Murray Valley encephalitis, and West Nile viruses and is related to yellow fever (Chapter 404) and dengue viruses (Chapters 405 and 406). Strains associated with *Culex pipiens*–borne epidemics in the eastern United States are distinct from endemic strains transmitted by *C. tarsalis* in the western states.

Epidemiology

The virus is present in all parts of the Western Hemisphere, but epidemics occur only in North America and some Caribbean islands. During epidemic years, the virus has been responsible for up to 80% of all reported cases of encephalitis of known etiology in the United States. Epidemics of up to 2000 cases have taken place, mainly in urban-suburban localities of the Ohio-Mississippi River basin and in eastern and central Texas and Florida. Small outbreaks have also occurred in the western United States. Epidemics generally take place between July and September but may arise later in the year in warm areas such as Florida. Previous exposure and immunity to dengue may provide a degree of cross-protection against clinical St. Louis encephalitis. The inapparent-to-apparent infection ratio is 800:1 in children up to 9 years of age, 400:1 in persons aged 10 to 49 years, and 85:1 in persons older than 60 years.

In most of the eastern United States, St. Louis encephalitis virus circulates between wild birds and *C. pipiens* mosquitoes, which breed in polluted water. In Florida and in parts of the Caribbean, *Culex nigripalpus* is the principal vector. The cycle in the western United States also involves wild birds, but the vector is *C. tarsalis*, also that of western equine encephalitis. Because of the similar ecology of St. Louis encephalitis and western equine encephalitis viruses in the west, mixed outbreaks occur, mostly in rural, agricultural areas.

Above-average summer temperatures and conditions such as deficient rainfall, which create stagnant pools suitable for *C. pipiens* breeding, are associated with epidemics in the eastern United States. St. Louis encephalitis in the western states is favored by warm spring temperatures, heavy snow melt, and flooding.

Pathobiology

Pathologic changes in fatal cases are limited to microscopic findings. Leptomeningitis is characterized by lymphocytic inflammation. Parenchymal changes consist of lymphocytic perivascular cuffing, cellular nodule formation, and neuronal degeneration.

Clinical Manifestations

Three clinical syndromes are recognized: febrile headache, aseptic meningitis, and encephalitis. After an incubation period of 4 to 21 days, a variable period of nonspecific symptoms, including fever (38 to 41° C), headache, malaise, drowsiness, myalgia, and sore throat, may be followed by an acute or subacute onset of meningeal or encephalitic signs, or both. Nausea, vomiting, and photophobia are common.

Neurologic abnormalities occur in up to 25% of patients. Extrapyramidal abnormalities and altered consciousness are the most significant findings. Other findings include meningismus, cranial nerve deficits (particularly the facial nerve), abnormal reflexes, tremors, myoclonic twitching, nystagmus, and ataxia. Motor abnormalities are infrequent, and sensory changes are extremely uncommon. Seizures occur in 10% of patients and are a poor prognostic sign, as is a persistent high temperature of 40 to 41° C. Signs of markedly increased intracranial pressure are unusual. A Guillain-Barré–like syndrome (Chapter 436) has occasionally been associated with St. Louis encephalitis, both as an acute manifestation and during the convalescent period.

In uncomplicated cases of St. Louis encephalitis, a moderate peripheral neutrophilic leukocytosis and shift to the left are noted. CSF pressure is elevated, protein is mildly elevated, and glucose is normal; a pleocytosis of up to 500 cells/mL is present, with an early neutrophilia predominance changing to lymphocytes within days. Serum creatine kinase, aspartate aminotransferase, and aldolase levels are frequently elevated. The electroencephalogram typically shows polymorphic delta activity, most prominently in the frontal and temporal regions; electrographic seizures are common. CT scans are normal, but MRI may show edema involving deep structures such as the substantia nigra. Hypo-osmolality, presumably as a result of the syndrome of inappropriate antidiuretic hormone secretion (Chapter 243), is noted in a third of patients.

Genitourinary tract symptoms (urgency, frequency, incontinence, and retention), microscopic hematuria, pyuria, proteinuria, and elevated blood urea nitrogen are frequent. St. Louis encephalitis viral antigen in cells of the urinary sediment has been detected by fluorescent techniques and virus-like particles in urine by immuno-electron microscopy.

Diagnosis

St. Louis encephalitis virus is rarely isolated from blood or CSF obtained during the acute phase of illness. Serologic diagnosis is achieved by demonstrating changing antibody titers; the HI, fluorescent, ELISA, and neutralizing tests demonstrate antibody within the first week after onset, and titers rise during the ensuing 2 weeks. CF antibodies appear 10 to 20 days after onset. Rapid, early diagnosis is possible by detection of IgM antibodies by ELISA in serum and CSF. Serologic cross-reactions may occur in persons with previous exposure to dengue, West Nile, and other related flaviviruses. RT-PCR provides a more specific diagnosis, but its sensitivity is uncertain.

Prevention

No vaccine is available for St. Louis encephalitis. Surveillance of viral activity in vectors and avian hosts is used to define the risk for human infection and initiate vector control efforts. In an established outbreak, avoiding mosquito bites and spraying to reduce infected adult mosquitoes are the only effective means of control.

Treatment

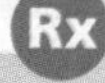

Treatment is supportive.

Prognosis

A convalescent syndrome characterized by weakness, fatigue, nervousness, tremulousness, sleeplessness, irritability, depression, difficulty concentrating, and headaches occurs in 30 to 50% of older persons and clears in 80% of them within 3 years. The overall case-fatality rate is approximately 9%. Mortality is negligible in persons younger than 20 years but rises steeply after 55 years to approximately 30% in patients older than 65 years. Approximately 50% of the deaths occur during the first week and 80% occur within 2 weeks after onset.

MURRAY VALLEY ENCEPHALITIS AND ROCIO ENCEPHALITIS

Murray Valley encephalitis and Rocio encephalitis, which are similar to Japanese encephalitis in their pathogenesis and clinical features, are caused by closely related flaviviruses. Murray Valley encephalitis has occurred in small epidemics in the Murray and Darling River valleys of Victoria and New South Wales, Australia. The virus is endemic in northern Australia and New Guinea, where it is maintained in a bird-mosquito cycle. Rocio encephalitis has caused epidemics of 1000 or more cases in São Paulo State, Brazil.

TICK-BORNE ENCEPHALITIS

Pathogens

A complex of six antigenically related tick-borne flaviviruses cause encephalitis: Powassan, tick-borne encephalitis, louping ill, Kyasanur Forest disease, Omsk hemorrhagic fever, and Langat viruses. The predominant syndrome is hemorrhagic fever (Chapter 404), but meningoencephalitis may be a component of the disease spectrum. Two subtypes of tick-borne encephalitis virus (Central European encephalitis and Russian spring-summer encephalitis) are distinguished by serologic tests, are ecologically distinct, and differ in virulence for humans. Powassan and louping ill viruses are rare causes of encephalitis in North America and the British Isles, respectively. These viruses are easily distinguished serologically from mosquito-borne flaviviruses but induce cross-reactions within the complex.

Epidemiology

Tick-borne encephalitis occurs in Europe (including eastern Europe and Ukraine), southern Scandinavia, and far eastern Russia during the summer months, which corresponds to peak tick vector populations. Several hundred to more than 2000 cases are reported annually, with morbidity rates of up to 20 per 100,000 inhabitants. Adults older than 20 years are mainly affected, and persons frequenting wooded areas that are heavily tick infested are at highest risk. In Europe the disease is relatively mild (case-fatality rate of 1 to 2%), but in the Far East it is severe (20 to 25%).

In Europe the vector of tick-borne encephalitis is *Ixodes ricinus* and, in the Far East, *Ixodes persulcatus.* The tick vector also serves as a reservoir for the virus. Larval ticks parasitize small rodents, which serve as amplifying viremic hosts during the spring and summer. Large vertebrates (goats, sheep, cattle) are hosts for nymphal and adult ticks. Outbreaks have occurred in families or groups of individuals ingesting unpasteurized milk or cheese from goats or sheep.

Clinical Manifestations

Inapparent infections are common. Symptomatic tick-borne encephalitis in Europe typically (but not invariably) has a biphasic course beginning 7 to 14 days after exposure with an influenza-like illness that lasts 1 week, followed by a period of clinical remission for several days and then an abrupt onset of aseptic meningitis or meningoencephalitis. The meningoencephalitis is usually benign, although severe paralytic illness, myelitis, myeloradiculitis, and bulbar forms may occur.

In the Far East, tick-borne encephalitis begins suddenly with fever, headache, and gastrointestinal symptoms, followed rapidly by the appearance of depressed sensorium, coma, convulsions, and paralysis. Bulbar paralysis and cervical myelitis are frequent findings. In fatal cases, death occurs in the first week after onset. Aseptic meningitis and milder forms of encephalitis also occur. Chronic forms of tick-borne encephalitis have been described, with active clinical and pathologic abnormalities present a year or more after onset.

Diagnosis

Brain MRI in patients with tick-borne encephalitis shows evidence of edema in the basal ganglia, thalami, and brain stem in about 20% of cases.

MRI of the spinal cord may show anterior horn cell lesions corresponding to lower motor neuron weakness on examination.

Isolation of virus from blood is also possible during the early phase of illness. Serologic diagnosis is achieved by the HI, CF, neutralization, or ELISA techniques.

Prevention

In eastern Europe and the former Soviet Union, vaccines are used in high-risk groups (forestry and agricultural workers, military personnel). In Austria, immunization of the general population has resulted in a marked decline in incidence. Avoiding tick exposure by wearing protective clothing and using repellents may be recommended in areas of high tick-borne encephalitis activity.

Treatment

Rx

Treatment is supportive (see Eastern Equine Encephalitis).

Prognosis

In European tick-borne encephalitis, convalescence is often prolonged, and residual paralysis may follow in severe cases. In the Far East, survivors frequently have residual paralysis, especially lower motor neuron paralysis of the upper extremities or shoulder girdle as a result of spinal cord involvement.

Louping Ill Encephalitis

Louping ill causes encephalitis in sheep (rarely in cattle, horses, and swine) in Scotland, northern England, and Ireland. Sporadic human cases have been recognized. Louping ill virus is maintained in nature by *I. ricinus* ticks and a variety of hosts, including small mammals, ground-dwelling birds (grouse), and probably sheep. The clinical features of louping ill resemble the European form of tick-borne encephalitis.

Powassan Virus Encephalitis

Powassan virus encephalitis has been documented in a small number of cases in the northeastern United States and eastern Canada. The virus is not associated with animal disease. The transmission cycle of Powassan virus involves *Ixodes cookei, Ixodes marxi,* and possibly other tick species, along with mammals, particularly rodents and carnivores. Powassan encephalitis is characterized by fever and nonspecific symptoms, followed by encephalitic signs, which are frequently severe. Peripheral blood and CSF changes are similar to those described for other forms of flaviviral encephalitis. The case-fatality rate is about 50%, and residual paralysis may persist in survivors.

Section XXIII Infectious Diseases

CALIFORNIA SEROGROUP ENCEPHALITIS

At least four members of the California serogroup of the Bunyaviridae family (Bunyavirus genus)—La Crosse, California encephalitis, Jamestown Canyon, and snowshoe hare virus—cause encephalitis. California encephalitis virus occurs in the western United States (California, New Mexico, Utah, Texas) and has been implicated in only three human cases. In contrast, La Crosse virus, distributed more widely in the eastern half of the United States and southern Canada, is a major human pathogen. Jamestown Canyon and snowshoe hare viruses have also been implicated in sporadic cases of human encephalitis in the north central United States and Canada. California serogroup viruses have been implicated in human disease in China and the former Soviet Union.

Epidemiology

California serogroup encephalitis occurs as an endemic rather than an epidemic disease, with individual or small clusters of cases scattered across affected areas. Seventy to 115 cases are reported each year, generally between July and September, with a peak incidence in August. The virus primarily affects persons younger than 15 years living in rural and suburban areas characterized by deciduous hardwood forests. It is most prevalent in the north central states, where it is responsible for as many as 20% of cases of acute CNS infection in children. Focal "hot spots" (communities, even backyards) of recurrent summertime viral activity are recognized. The inapparent-to-apparent infection ratio has been estimated variably at between 26:1 and 157:1.

The vector of La Crosse virus is *Aedes triseriatus,* which breeds both in forest tree holes and in artificial containers, notably discarded tires. This vector also serves as a reservoir for La Crosse virus. Wild rodents (squirrels, chipmunks) contribute to the cycle of transmission as viremic hosts. Humans acquire the disease by being bitten by an infected mosquito.

Aedes communis, Aedes stimulans, A. triseriatus, and possibly anopheline mosquitoes are involved in transmitting Jamestown Canyon virus, and deer are the principal vertebrate hosts.

Pathobiology

Histopathologic features in the CNS are qualitatively similar to those of other viral encephalitides. However, absence of inflammatory lesions in the cerebellum, medulla, and spinal cord may be a distinguishing feature of La Crosse infection.

Clinical Manifestations

The clinical spectrum of California serogroup virus infection includes nonspecific febrile illness, aseptic meningitis, and meningoencephalitis. The disease begins with fever, headache, sore throat, and gastrointestinal symptoms. In mild cases, CNS signs appear on the third day after onset and subside within 7 to 8 days. In the more severe form, neurologic signs appear within 24 to 48 hours of onset, usually in the form of generalized seizures, elevated intracranial pressure, and altered consciousness, and persist longer. Encephalitis may be quite severe in the acute stage, but the disease is almost always self-limited; death is extremely rare.

The peripheral white blood cell count is elevated, with a predominance of polymorphonuclear cells and a shift to the left. CSF contains up to 500 lymphocytes/mL, normal or mildly elevated protein, and a normal glucose concentration. The electroencephalogram reveals generalized slowing in the delta and theta range; focal delta wave activity related to cortical destruction and focal seizures are also common findings.

Diagnosis

In contrast to the other arboviral encephalitides, brain MRI in patients with California serogroup encephalitides may show lesions involving the temporal lobe in a pattern similar to that of herpes simplex encephalitis. The virus cannot be recovered from blood or CSF obtained during the acute phase. Diagnosis is best achieved by counterimmunoelectrophoresis, HI, CF, fluorescent, ELISA, and neutralization tests for antibody in paired acute and convalescent sera. The most practical, sensitive, and reliable methods are the HI test with La Crosse viral antigen and IgM antibody capture ELISA. Viral RNA can be detected in CSF or brain tissue by RT-PCR, although the sensitivity of the test remains to be determined.

Prevention

There is no vaccine for California encephalitis, although research involving DNA-based vaccines appears promising. Vector control methods are of uncertain usefulness in this disease. In defined "hot spots" of recurrent viral activity, breeding sites for *A. triseriatus* should be eliminated, particularly by draining or eliminating standing water (e.g., discarded tires or birdbaths) and filling holes in trees. Parents should protect children by limiting exposure and using mosquito repellents.

Treatment

Treatment is supportive.

Prognosis

The case-fatality rate is less than 1%. The risk for permanent neuropsychiatric sequelae is unclear, but hemiparesis and persistent seizure disorders have been reported.

SUGGESTED READINGS

Campbell GL, Marfin AA, Lanciotti RS, Gubler DJ: West Nile virus. Lancet Infect Dis 2002;2:519–529. *An excellent summary of current understanding of the virus and the disease.*

Carson PJ, Konewko P, Wold KS, et al: Long-term clinical and neuropsychological outcomes of West Nile virus infection. Clin Infect Dis 2006;43:723–730. *Multiple somatic complaints and defects in motor skills are common long-term sequelae.*

Kumar R, Tripathi P, Singh S, et al: Clinical features in children hospitalized during the 2005 epidemic of Japanese encephalitis in Uttar Pradesh, India. Clin Infect Dis 2006;43:123–131. *Thrombocytopenia and abnormal serum transaminase levels were prominent features.*

Mackenzie JS, Gubler DJ, Petersen LR: Emerging flaviviruses: The spread and resurgence of Japanese encephalitis, West Nile and dengue viruses. Nat Med 2004;10:S98–S109. *A comprehensive review.*

Romero JR, Newland JG: Diagnosis of viral encephalitides: Zoonotic-associated viruses. Pediatr Infect Dis J 2006;25:741–742. *A concise guide to diagnostic studies.*

Shlim DR, Solomon T: Japanese encephalitis vaccine for travelers: Exploring the limits of risk. Clin Infect Dis 2002;35:183–188. *A useful discussion of the variables for making a decision about the vaccine.*

Solomon T, Dung NM, Willis B, et al: Interferon alfa-2a in Japanese encephalitis: A double-blind placebo-controlled trial. Lancet 2003;361:821–826. *Interferon has been used frequently in JE; this study shows it is no more useful than placebo.*

Sejvar JJ: The evolving epidemiology of viral encephalitis. Curr Opin Neurol 2006;19:350–357. *An excellent recent review.*

Wurtz R, Paleologos N: LaCrosse encephalitis presenting like herpes simplex encephalitis in an immunocompromised adult. Clin Infect Dis 2000;31:1113–1114. *Medial temporal lobe focal encephalitis is not always due to herpes simplex virus.*

Section XXIV

Human Immunodeficiency Virus and the Acquired Immunodeficiency Syndrome

407 HUMAN IMMUNODEFICIENCY VIRUS INFECTION AND ACQUIRED IMMUNODEFICIENCY SYNDROME: A GLOBAL OVERVIEW

Peter Piot

In the quarter century since acquired immunodeficiency syndrome (AIDS) was first recognized, the global AIDS epidemic has arguably become not only the most serious health threat of the early 21st century but also one of the greatest impediments to social and economic progress in heavily affected countries.

With 4.3 million new human immunodeficiency virus (HIV) infections occurring in 2006, the global epidemic shows no sign of slowing, particularly in low- and middle-income countries, where about 95% of infected persons live. The cumulative impact of the epidemic is already devastating, most so in high-prevalence sub-Saharan countries, including crippling stresses on health and other essential services, major declines in life expectancy, and deepening poverty.

Although there has been a quantum increase in financial resources and political commitment to address AIDS since the beginning of this decade, much faster progress on these and several other fronts is needed if the world is to achieve the Millennium Development Goal of halting and beginning to reverse the epidemic by 2015.

A DYNAMIC EPIDEMIC

As of the end of 2006, an estimated 39.5 million (range, 34.9 to 47.1 million) people were living with HIV infection. In 2005 alone, an estimated 4.1 million people became infected with HIV, and 2.9 million AIDS deaths occurred.

The epidemic is now truly globalized, with major epidemic foci in every continent. Though interrelated, each of these epidemics has a different dynamic and course, often changing over time. Regional epidemiologic trends are extensively discussed in Chapter 410.

Globally, HIV infection is a sexually transmitted infection, with sexual transmission being responsible for roughly 80% of the world's HIV infections. Unprotected heterosexual intercourse accounts for the large majority of cases of HIV infection in developing countries. Unprotected sexual intercourse between men is responsible for between 4 and 6% of the global total of people living with HIV, including the largest share of infections in most industrialized countries and in Latin America.

Mother-to-child transmission of HIV during pregnancy, delivery, or breast-feeding is the second leading mode of spread of HIV and causes roughly 600,000 new infections annually.

Transmission through injection drug use continues to play a major role in HIV epidemics in several regions of the world, particularly eastern Europe and Asia. Worldwide, there are approximately 13 million injection drug users, and in some regions more than 50% of them are infected with HIV.

The epidemic is becoming increasingly entrenched in women and young people worldwide. Approximately half of all adults living with HIV are female; in sub-Saharan Africa, almost 60% are, with females accounting for 76% of young people (15 to 24 years of age) living with HIV. It is estimated that young people (15- to 24-year-olds) account for 35% of the annual total of new HIV infections. This trend is especially alarming because today's youth generation is the largest in history.

Despite the epidemic's continued expansion, there is strong evidence, including evidence from some of the poorest countries of the world, that the spread of HIV can be reversed or prevented on a large scale. In addition to the well-known successes of Brazil, Senegal, Thailand, and Uganda in stabilizing or lowering HIV infection rates, a small but growing number of countries, in every region but eastern Europe and central Asia, have reduced HIV prevalence through sound prevention efforts. Declines in national HIV prevalence across all ages have recently been documented in the Bahamas, Barbados, Kenya, Rwanda, and Zimbabwe, as well as in urban areas of Burkina Faso, Côte d'Ivoire, and Haiti. Additionally, among 11 sub-Saharan African countries that provided data, 3 reported declines of 25% or more in HIV prevalence among young people (15 to 24 years old) nationally, and another 3 reported such declines in capital cities between 2001 and 2005. HIV prevalence among young adults has also been declining in four southern states in India. In Cambodia and Thailand, steady ongoing declines in HIV prevalence are continuing. Although the exact mix of reasons for the fall in HIV prevalence in these countries varies, in every one there is strong evidence of changes in sexual behavior: people have increased their use of condoms, are delaying the first time that they have sexual intercourse, and are having fewer sexual partners.

THE EXCEPTIONAL IMPACT OF AIDS

AIDS is now the world's leading cause of death in both women and men aged 15 to 59 years, with one in every six deaths in this age group being due to AIDS, about twice as many as caused by ischemic heart disease or tuberculosis. By primarily affecting the young adults on whom societies depend—for their economic future and for the transmission of values and skills to children—AIDS undermines the very foundations of society.

Life expectancy in the African countries worst affected by AIDS is likely to be up to 30 years lower by 2010 than it would have been without AIDS, unless there is a vast and sustained increase in access to antiretroviral treatment. Put in context, this fall in life expectancy is almost twice that caused anywhere in Europe by the combined impacts of the First World War and the 1918–1919 influenza epidemic.

AIDS deepens poverty and magnifies ongoing demographic and economic crises. Studies of AIDS-affected households in southern Africa document sharp drops (between 66 and 80%) in monthly income because of the need to cope with AIDS-related illness. In Cambodia, where infection levels are significantly lower than in sub-Saharan Africa, it is projected that AIDS will slow the rate of reduction in poverty by 60% between 2003 and 2015. In the Russian Federation, AIDS is magnifying the ongoing demographic crisis.

AIDS diminishes the agricultural labor force and depletes family income normally used to purchase food, thereby aggravating food shortages. The southern African food crisis in 2002–2003 and 2005 resulted not just from drought but also from weakening of agriculture because of AIDS. By 2020, the agriculture work force in Botswana, Namibia, and Zimbabwe is projected to be over 20% smaller—and over 10% smaller in another eight African countries—than it would have been in the absence of AIDS.

By killing adults in their prime reproductive period, AIDS is creating an unprecedented crisis of orphans and vulnerable children, with as yet poorly understood intergenerational effects. In the 10 sub-Saharan countries where 15% or more of all children have lost one or both parents, AIDS was the primary cause of orphaning in 6 countries and increased orphaning levels by 25 to 40% in the remaining countries.

The losses so far are only a fraction of the impact to come, given the rapid spread of HIV together with the long lag between infection and the onset of severe illness. In heavily affected countries, the longer-term result could be the unraveling of economic and social development, in large part because vital knowledge will not be transferred between generations. In 2000, the United Nations Security Council declared AIDS a threat to global security.

THE NEED FOR AN EXCEPTIONAL RESPONSE WORLDWIDE

AIDS is now firmly on the global political agenda. The sixth Millennium Development Goal, agreed to by all world leaders at the United Nations in 2000, provides that the world will halt and begin to reverse HIV/AIDS by 2015. Inclusion of AIDS in the foremost global goals for the early 21st century not only recognizes the independent significance of the epidemic itself but also acknowledges the impact of AIDS on the world's prospects for reducing poverty, preventing childhood deaths, and providing education for all.

In 2001 at a special session of the United Nations General Assembly, member states unanimously adopted a Declaration of Commitment on HIV/AIDS in which a blueprint for action was established. The declaration recognizes that sound national AIDS responses engage both health and non–health-related sectors and work to prevent new infections, provide life-preserving care and treatment to those who are living with HIV infection, and mitigate the epidemic's impact on children, affected families, vulnerable populations, and society at large. In addition, countries committed to mobilizing vastly increased resources—including the establishment of a Global Fund—and to grounding national responses in respect for human rights and recognition of the role of gender inequality.

Between 2001 and 2005, financing for the AIDS response of low- and middle-income countries increased from roughly $1.6 to $8.3 billion, with about 31% coming from developing countries themselves in 2005.

The increase in financing and significant reductions in the price of antiretroviral drugs in developing countries have led to a sea change in terms of global access to antiretroviral therapy. Between December 2003 and June 2006, the number of people in low- and middle-income countries receiving antiretroviral therapy increased from 400,000 to 1.6 million, with countries in sub-Saharan Africa experiencing a 10-fold rise in antiretroviral use (from 100,000 to 1 million). Even with such remarkable progress, only 24% of those needing therapy had access.

HIV prevention coverage has also risen. Between 2001 and 2005, the number of people receiving HIV counseling and testing quadrupled in more than 70 countries surveyed, from roughly 4 million people in 2001 to 16.5 million in 2005. Significant increases were also reported in the number of secondary school students receiving AIDS education and the number of pregnant women who were offered services to prevent mother-to-child transmission.

Nevertheless, by 2005, prevention programs were reaching only a minority of those at highest risk—9% of men who have sex with men and less than 20% of injection drug users—and globally less than 8% of pregnant women had access to interventions to prevent mother-to-child transmission of HIV.

As financial resources for the response have increased, global attention has increasingly focused on scaling up national AIDS programs by making the best use of available financing. In 2003–2004, a strong global consensus developed in favor of key principles for rapid implementation of national AIDS programs. Known as the 'Three Ones," these principles provide for a single, agreed-upon AIDS action framework that provides the basis for coordinating the work of all partners, one national AIDS coordinating authority with a broad-based multisectoral mandate, and one agreed country-level monitoring and evaluation system.

At the June 2006 High Level Meeting on AIDS, United Nations member states reaffirmed the 2001 Declaration of Commitment on HIV/AIDS and committed themselves further to scaling up comprehensive HIV prevention, treatment, care, and support programs toward universal access by 2010. In the Political Declaration on HIV/AIDS, member states recognized the need to fund all credible national AIDS plans and to mobilize $20 to $23 billion annually by 2010 for the AIDS response in low- and middle-income countries.

Placing the world on track toward universal access to HIV prevention and treatment will require not only faster progress on mobilizing financial resources but also real political and public commitment for making certain that the lessons of effective practice are rapidly translated into broad-based programs in every country.

Building on that emergency effort of massively scaling up HIV programs, a full-scale and comprehensive response needs to be sustained over at least another generation because the epidemic is still evolving and is likely to persist for an as yet unclear period. Only a sustained response at increasingly high levels can move us from the piecemeal progress of recent years to real success.

SUGGESTED READINGS

Beyrer C: HIV epidemiology update and transmission factors: Risks and risk contexts—16th International AIDS Conference epidemiology plenary. Clin Infect Dis 2007;44:981–987. *An epidemiologic update.*

Centers for Disease Control (CDC): Revised recommendations for HIV testing of adults, adolescents, and pregnant women in health-care settings. MMWR 2006;55[No. RR-14]. *HIV testing recommendations.*

Centers for Disease Control (CDC): The global HIV/AIDS pandemic, 2006. MMWR Morb Mortal Wkly Rep 2006;55:841–844. *A global overview.*

Frieden TR, Das-Douglas M, Kellerman SE, et al: Applying public health principles to the HIV epidemic. N Engl J Med 2005;353:2397–2402. *More effective epidemic control using proven strategies would save between 4 and 5.4 billion dollars per year.*

Goldie SJ, Yazdanpanah Y, Losina E, et al: Cost-effectiveness of HIV treatment in resource-poor settings—the case of Côte d'Ivoire. N Engl J Med 2006; 355:1141–1153. *Use of antiretrovirals and trimethoprim-sulfamethoxazole prophylaxis is a cost-effective strategy.*

Piot P: AIDS: From crisis management to sustained strategic response. Lancet 2006;368:526–530. *A public health update.*

Sawires S, Dworkin S, Fiamma A, et al: Male circumcision and HIV/AIDS: Challenges and opportunites. Lancet 2007;369:708–713. *Circumcision reduces the infection rate in men by about 50%.*

Simon V, Ho DD, Karim, QA: HIV/AIDS epidemiology, pathogenesis, prevention, and treatment. Lancet 2006;368:489–504. *A clinical update.*

UNAIDS/WHO 2006 Global Report. Available at http://www.unaids.org/en/HIV_data/2006GlobalReport/default.asp. *Report of the global burden.*

WHO/UNAIDS: Progress on scaling up access to HIV treatment in low and middle-income countries, June 2006. Available at http://www.who.int/hiv/toronto2006/FS_Treatment_en.pdf. *A progress report.*

408 IMMUNOPATHOGENESIS OF HUMAN IMMUNODEFICIENCY VIRUS INFECTION

Paul E. Sax and Bruce D. Walker

CLINICAL CONSEQUENCES OF HIV INFECTION

The clinical consequences of human immunodeficiency virus (HIV) infection are due to the ability of this retrovirus to infect crucial cells of the immune system. This infection occurs because the primary target for the virus is lymphocytes expressing the cell surface marker CD4, which serves as a receptor that binds the envelope protein of the virus. These lymphocytes, also called *help-inducer lymphocytes,* orchestrate myriad immune functions. HIV infection can be considered a disease of the immune system characterized by the progressive loss of $CD4^+$ lymphocytes. Immunodeficiency results not only from a lack of effective immunity against HIV itself but also because the virus damages CD4 cell subsets that are crucial for containing other pathogens, thus explaining the problems encountered with so-called opportunistic pathogens that are not seen in persons with intact immunity.

Although the immune system ultimately fails to control HIV infection, emerging data indicate that at least partially effective virus-specific immune responses are generated. These responses contribute to the long, asymptomatic phase that typically follows infection by keeping the virus partially contained, but in most infected persons the immune system ultimately fails and disease progression ensues. There are notable exceptions, however. With the HIV epidemic now in its third decade, a small group of individuals have been identified who seem to be able to control HIV infection for 20 or more years, without the need for antiviral drug therapy. These persons, probably representing much less than 1% of those infected, suggest that persistent immune control can be achieved. Understanding of the immunology related to HIV provides insight not only into the clinical sequelae of infection but also into the prospects for development of effective therapeutic and prophylactic vaccines against HIV.

Immunopathogenesis of Acute HIV Infection

The acute phase of HIV infection is associated with nonspecific symptoms common to many viral infections, including fever, sore throat, malaise, swollen lymph nodes, and often a transient maculopapular rash. The symptoms are probably a result not only of virus replication but also the immune response that is being generated.

In the early days after infection, virus replication increases dramatically, with plasma viral loads reaching an excess of 10 million virus particles per milliliter of plasma in most persons. This replication occurs mainly in CD4-bearing lymphocytes in gut-associated lymphoid tissue (GALT) and particularly in those bearing the CCR5 coreceptor required for virus entry. This early and massive infection results in a profound reduction in CD4 cell number in GALT, accompanied by a much more modest decline in the peripheral blood CD4 cell count. Estimates are that more than 50% of memory CD4 cells are infected and lost in this early phase of infection.

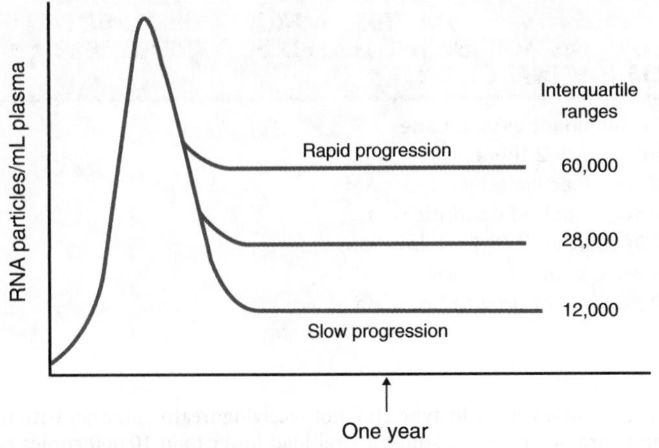

FIGURE 408–1 • Steady-state viral load after acute HIV-1 infection. Plasma viremia reaches a mean peak of greater than 10 million viral particles per milliliter of plasma during acute HIV infection and then drops precipitously coincident with the appearance of virus-specific immune responses. The differences in steady-state viral load relate to, among other things, differences in immune selection pressure, viral attenuation, HLA type of the infected person, and differences in viral coreceptors needed for viral entry.

Countering this early viral replication is the generation of an adaptive immune response that consists of humoral (antibody-mediated) and cellular (cell-mediated) immunity.

The initial peak in viremia is brought to an average steady-state level of about 30,000 copies within 6 months of infection (Fig. 408–1), most likely as a result of the generation of partially effective antiviral immune responses. Among these responses is the generation of virus-specific $CD4^+$ helper T cells, which orchestrate a coordinated humoral and cellular immune response. Because CD4 is a receptor for the virus and HIV has the unique ability to infect activated CD4 cells preferentially, these cells that are attempting to respond to the virus are infected and probably partially deleted in the early phase of infection when the viral load is so high. This leaves most infected persons with an impaired ability to fight HIV infection.

Lymphocytes bearing the CD8 cell surface marker, called *cytotoxic T lymphocytes,* are generated and their appearance correlates with the initial dramatic decrease in plasma viral load. Functioning of these cells is impaired in the absence of an adequate virus-specific $CD4^+$ helper T-cell response, however, thus explaining the lack of effective long-term control of infection. The difficulty with immune control is exacerbated by the continued evolution of the virus within an infected person. Infidelity of the viral reverse transcriptase allows the generation of multiple closely related, yet distinct viruses within a given person. In the same way that partial antiviral drug pressure allows the generation of drug resistance mutations, partial antiviral immune pressure permits the gradual development of mutations within key sites targeted by the immune responses that have been generated.

In contrast to the rapid generation of cellular immune responses, the antibody response to HIV is slower to develop. The standard enzyme-linked immunosorbent assay for HIV antibody may be negative during the early phase of acute infection. Antibodies can generally be detected within a few weeks of infection; many of these antibodies are directed against virion debris, and a smaller number can neutralize infectious virus. However, as these antibodies are generated, viral mutations in the envelope protein ensue and allow the virus to escape immune detection. New waves of neutralizing antibodies are generated, but the virus continues to outpace this response by the development of additional mutations in the highly variable envelope protein. The ability of the virus to escape neutralizing antibodies is one of the major problems with HIV infection and represents a major hurdle for vaccine development. Those antibodies that do develop are usually only weakly neutralizing, in part because of the heavy sugar coating on the envelope of the virus that keeps crucial neutralization sites masked from the immune system. Figure 408–2 provides an overview of immune responses to HIV.

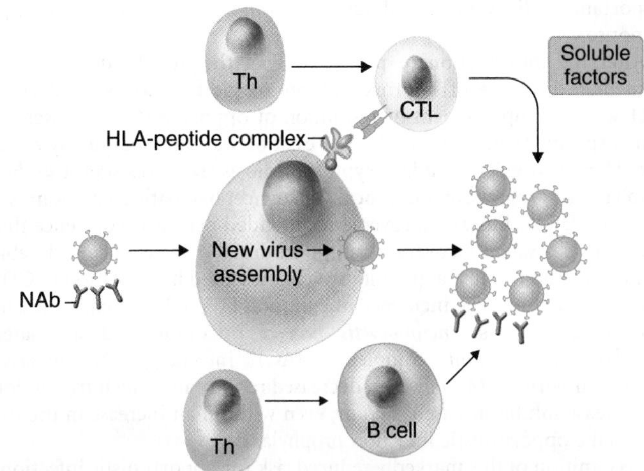

FIGURE 408–2 • Immune responses to HIV. Virus-infected cells produce progeny virions within approximately 2 days. After viral entry, virion proteins are presented at the cell surface in the groove of an HLA class I molecule. This complex is recognized by cytotoxic T lymphocytes (CTLs), which can directly lyse infected cells and secrete soluble factors that inhibit viruses that may have been released already. B cells produce neutralizing antibodies that directly neutralize free virions. B-cell function and CTL function are critically dependent on signals received from $CD4^+$ helper T cells.

CLINICAL IMPLICATIONS OF HIV-RELATED IMMUNOLOGY

Absolute CD4 Cell Count: Measurement and Interpretation

The most important clinical application of HIV-related immunology is measurement and interpretation of the absolute CD4 cell count. This value is derived from multiplying the number of lymphocytes on a complete blood count by the percentage of $CD4^+$ lymphocytes, the latter determined by flow cytometry. CD4 cells are composed of many different specificities—not only those that are specific for HIV but also those that are specific for other pathogens, including opportunistic pathogens. The CD4 cell count does not provide any indication of the specific function of the CD4 cells, only a cumulative number of cells present. It is currently recommended that patients have this test performed at the time of HIV diagnosis and then again approximately every 3 to 4 months, usually in conjunction with an HIV RNA (viral load) test. Less expensive and more rapid techniques of measuring the absolute CD4 cell count are under development; they are likely to be of great utility in resource-poor settings where flow cytometry is unavailable.

The risk for HIV-related complications correlates strongly with the absolute count and the CD4 percentage, although presently only the absolute count is formally incorporated into guidelines for initiation of antiretroviral therapy (ART) or prevention of opportunistic infections. This relationship is due to the fact that as more CD4 cell decline occurs, the individual subsets that orchestrate effective immunity against a variety of pathogens drop below a crucial threshold. From an epidemiologic perspective, patients with CD4 cell counts less than 200 cells/mm^3 or a CD4 percentage less than 14% meet the Centers for Disease Control and Prevention case definition for acquired immunodeficiency syndrome (AIDS), even in the absence of an HIV-related opportunistic infection. Some clinicians make a further distinction of 50 cells/mm^3 as another important threshold (often called *advanced HIV disease*) because these patients are at particularly high risk for opportunistic infections and HIV-related death.

CD4 Cell Counts, Immune Responses, and Antiretroviral Therapy

For treatment-naïve patients, potent ART with at least three active agents has a rapid, predictable effect on lowering HIV RNA levels, with a corresponding (albeit slower) increase in the CD4 cell count. Recovery of the CD4 cell count in response to ART has been shown to be the most important predictor of clinical outcome, even more so than the virologic response.

After the introduction of potent ART in the mid-1990s, the most immediate evidence of improved immunologic function secondary to ART was the improvement or resolution of opportunistic processes for which specific therapy either did not exist or was only marginally effective. These processes included cryptosporidiosis, azole-resistant *Candida* esophagitis, progressive multifocal leukoencephalopathy, and Kaposi's sarcoma. These clinical improvements provided persuasive evidence that the immune system recovery resulting from ART was of a considerable qualitative and not just a quantitative (as measured by the absolute CD4 cell count) nature. The incidence of common HIV-related opportunistic infections, such as *Pneumocystis jiroveci* pneumonia, disseminated *Mycobacterium avium* complex (MAC) infection, and invasive cytomegalovirus (CMV) disease, decreased rapidly after the introduction of protease inhibitor–based therapy, even without an increase in the use of specific opportunistic infection prophylaxis.

Recognition of this markedly reduced risk for opportunistic infections with ART-associated increases in CD4 cell counts led to clinical studies of withdrawing specific prophylaxis for patients who have experienced ART-induced increases in CD4 numbers above certain thresholds. These studies thus far have uniformly shown that this strategy is safe, and as a result, recent guidelines for prevention of opportunistic infections have incorporated stopping strategies for the prophylaxis of most conditions (see Chapter 412 for discussion of prophylaxis therapy). Because antibody responses to vaccinations are improved with higher CD4 cell counts, these guidelines now recommend deferring certain vaccinations (e.g., pneumococcal vaccine) until the CD4 count has risen to greater than 200 cells/mm^3.

Discordant CD4/HIV RNA Responses

ART-induced increases in the CD4 cell count are much more variable from patient to patient than reduction in HIV RNA is. Although most patients experience at least a 100-cell/mm^3 increase after 12 months of therapy, some have an even more robust response, whereas others have hardly any increase at all. Factors found in some studies to be associated with poor CD4 responses include older age, high baseline HIV RNA levels and low CD4 cell counts, hepatitis C coinfection, and receipt of a non–protease inhibitor–containing regimen. Some genetic factors are involved as well, including the patient's chemokine receptor CCR5 and multidrug resistance (MDR1) transporter genotype. These genetic tests are not currently available to clinicians on a routine basis, however.

Because some patients do not experience a sustained significant increase in CD4 cell counts, there has been long-standing interest in using immune-based therapy to boost this response. Several studies have shown that patients with HIV who are given interleukin-2 plus ART in a variety of different dosing strategies have a significantly greater CD4 response than do patients receiving ART alone. Further studies of interleukin-2 are ongoing to establish whether this increase in CD4 cells translates into clinical benefit because the therapy has a high rate of subjective adverse effects (mostly flulike symptoms) and is costly. Another randomized study demonstrated that growth hormone can augment both absolute and naïve CD4 cell responses, as well as increase thymic size. Again, the clinical benefits of this approach are unknown.

A different form of discordant HIV RNA and CD4 response is seen when there is a continued increase or stability in the CD4 cell count despite a rebounding HIV RNA level. This situation has been observed most commonly in patients treated with a regimen that includes a protease inhibitor and two nucleoside reverse transcriptase inhibitors and accounts in part for the ongoing excellent prognosis of HIV patients receiving this therapy despite the high rates of virologic breakthrough seen in clinical practice. Several possible explanations for this HIV RNA–CD4 "disconnect" phenomenon have been proposed. They are not mutually exclusive and include (1) emergence of antiviral-resistant HIV strains with impaired virulence ("fitness") as compared with wild-type virus, (2) reduced CD4 cell turnover as compared with untreated controls, and (3) the prolonged time that the HIV RNA level remains below the pretreatment baseline, even after clear emergence of drug resistance. The duration of this immunologic benefit from ART despite virologic rebound varies among patients, but in one study it persisted for a mean of 72 weeks. In another study, the rate of CD4 decline was substantially slower in patients treated with ART who had multidrug-resistant virus than in those with wild-type HIV not receiving treatment, even with the same viral load. In this study, a viral load lower than 10,000 copies per milliliter or a reduction of viremia to 2 log below the pretreatment set point was associated with a CD4 gain, regardless of whether the viral load was undetectable.

TABLE 408–1 SELECTED IMMUNOTHERAPEUTIC APPROACHES BEING TESTED FOR TREATMENT OF HIV INFECTION

Recombinant virus vaccines
Interleukin-2 therapy
Whole inactivated viral vaccines
Antigen-pulsed dendritic cells
CD4$^+$ and/or CD8$^+$ T-cell infusions
Passive antibody infusions
Recombinant growth hormone

Immune Reconstitution Syndromes

Improvements in immune function after starting ART can sometimes lead to dramatic worsening of preexisting opportunistic infections, either infections that have been diagnosed previously (e.g., CMV retinitis) or infections that were clinically unapparent (most commonly disseminated MAC) (Chapter 412). These *immune reconstitution inflammatory syndromes* probably result from eliciting a previously weak or absent host inflammatory response that becomes much stronger as a result of ART. In a typical case, a patient with a severely depleted CD4 cell count (usually <50 cells/mm^3) starts a potent ART regimen and has a prompt decline in HIV RNA and an increase in the CD4 cell count. Several weeks to months later, the patient may have fevers, night sweats, and on computed tomography, dramatic focal lymphadenitis—any or all of the mesenteric, thoracic, inguinal, cervical, and axillary sites may be involved. On biopsy, pathology reveals acid-fast organisms and granulomatous inflammation. In the United States, this would most commonly be MAC disease, but an identical manifestation has been reported with tuberculosis. With CMV retinitis, a patient with indolent retinal disease may suddenly contract a brisk vitritis, a response that was distinctly unusual in the pre-ART era. Analogous immune reconstitution syndromes have been described for several common HIV-related opportunistic infections, including *P. jiroveci* pneumonia, cryptococcosis, toxoplasmosis, and progressive multifocal leukoencephalopathy.

Optimal management of these syndromes is still being defined. Targeted treatment of the underlying opportunistic infection and continuation of ART are desirable, and the latter is especially important because most patients in whom immune reconstitution inflammatory syndromes develop are severely immunocompromised. If symptoms are particularly prolonged or severe, palliative corticosteroids may be required, though only when the risk of further immunosuppression is warranted based on the severity of the syndrome.

Prospects for Immune Augmentation as Treatment of HIV Infection

The apparent ability of the immune system to contain HIV replication at least partially has led to great interest in immune augmentation as a treatment of chronic HIV infection, but results thus far have been largely disappointing. Early treatment of acute HIV infection can lead to augmentation in the CD4$^+$ T-cell response to HIV and to transient control of viremia when therapy is stopped, but the durability of control has been disappointing—again probably because of the ability of the virus to mutate key epitopes targeted by the immune system. Many approaches are being undertaken to augment immunity in HIV-infected persons (Table 408–1). Prominent among these is therapeutic immunization, in which persons already infected are immunized to boost immune responses. The hypothesis that increasing or broadening the HIV-specific CD4$^+$ and CD8$^+$ T-cell responses would allow better immune control has yet to be proved in humans, but encouraging data have been generated in animal models of AIDS virus infection, and numerous studies of this approach are likely to be seen in the next few years.

SUGGESTED READINGS

Brenchley JM, Price DA, Schacker TW, et al: Microbial translocation is a cause of systemic immune activation in chronic HIV infection. Nat Med 2006;12:1365–1371. *Circulating lipopolysaccharide, presumably from translocated intestinal flora, is increased in patients with HIV.*

Miller MF, Haley C, Koziel MJ, Rowley CF: Impact of hepatitis C virus on immune restoration in HIV-infected patients who start highly active antiretroviral therapy: A meta-analysis. Clin Infect Dis 2005;41:713–720. *This systematic review of eight trials involving more than 6000 patients found that HIV⁺ patients coinfected with HCV have a less robust CD4 response to potent antiretroviral therapy.*

Robertson J, Meier M, Wall J, et al: Immune reconstitution syndrome in HIV: Validating a case definition and identifying clinical predictors in persons initiating antiretroviral therapy. Clin Infect Dis 2006;42:1639–1646. *Patients with more advanced illness are at increased risk of developing immune reconstitution syndrome.*

Scriba TJ, Zhang HT, Brown HL, et al: HIV-1–specific CD4⁺ T lymphocyte turnover and activation increase upon viral rebound. J Clin Invest 2005;115:443–450. *There was no decline in HIV-1–specific CD4 cells when ART was discontinued and HIV viremia rose.*

Simon V, Ho DD, Karim QA: HIV/AIDS epidemiology, pathogenesis, prevention, and treatment. Lancet 2006;368:489–504. *A clinical update.*

409 BIOLOGY OF HUMAN IMMUNODEFICIENCY VIRUSES

George M. Shaw

DISCOVERY OF HUMAN IMMUNODEFICIENCY VIRUSES

Identification of human immunodeficiency virus type 1 (HIV-1) as the causative agent of acquired immunodeficiency syndrome (AIDS) just 3 years after the clinical syndrome was initially described represents a remarkable scientific achievement that had its roots in earlier discoveries of animal and human retroviruses (Chapter 401). The selective loss of $CD4^+$ helper T lymphocytes in patients with the disease implicated an agent with T-lymphocyte tropism. As expected for an etiologic agent, HIV-1 was shown to be uniformly present in subjects with AIDS and to reproduce the hallmark of disease in tissue culture, destruction of T lymphocytes.

HUMAN IMMUNODEFICIENCY VIRUS TYPE 1

General Biologic Properties

Soon after its discovery, HIV-1 was shown to be biologically, structurally, and genetically distinct from human T-lymphotropic virus type 1 (HTLV-1) and type 2 (HTLV-2) and more like members of the lentivirus subfamily of retroviruses (Chapter 401). Unlike the leukemia viruses, which lead to immortalization of lymphocytes in vitro and in vivo, HIV-1 exhibits pronounced cytopathic properties for lymphocytes and causes syncytia formation and cell death. Morphologically, HIV-1 differs from HTLV-1 and other type C oncogenic retroviruses in exhibiting a dense, cylindrical core surrounded by a lipid envelope typical of lentiviruses (Fig. 409–1).

The structural organization of HIV-1 is shown diagrammatically in Figure 409–2. Like all retroviruses, HIV-1 is a single-stranded, plus-sense RNA virus. The RNA-dependent DNA polymerase, or reverse transcriptase, is packaged within the virion core and is responsible for replicating the single-stranded RNA genome through a double-stranded DNA intermediate, which serves as the precursor molecule for proviral integration within the host cell genome. The major structural core proteins of HIV-1 are the p24 capsid protein and the p18 matrix protein. Surrounding the viral core protein structures is a bilayered lipid envelope that is derived from the outer limiting membrane of the host cell as the virus buds from the cell surface during replication. Studding this outer viral membrane are the envelope glycoproteins gp120 and gp41, which are encoded by virus-specific genes and are responsible for cell attachment and entry.

The life cycle of HIV-1 is shown diagrammatically in Figure 409–3. Features of this life cycle distinguish retroviruses from all other viruses.

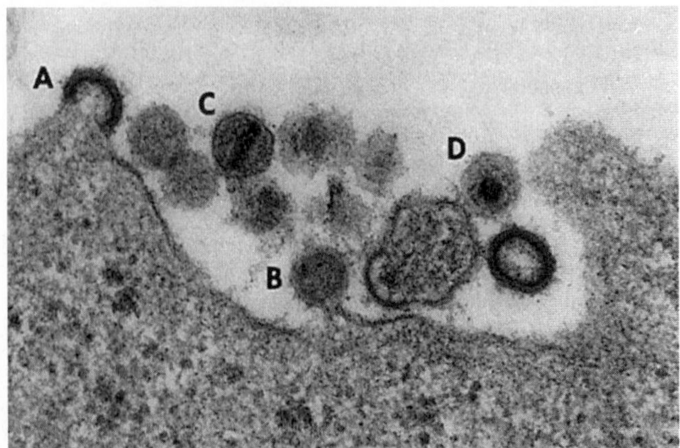

FIGURE 409-1 • Transmission electron micrograph of HIV-1. Virions are shown at all stages of morphogenesis: early (A) and late (B) budding forms and cell-free mature virions (C and D) with condensed central cores. Virion diameter is approximately 110 nm.

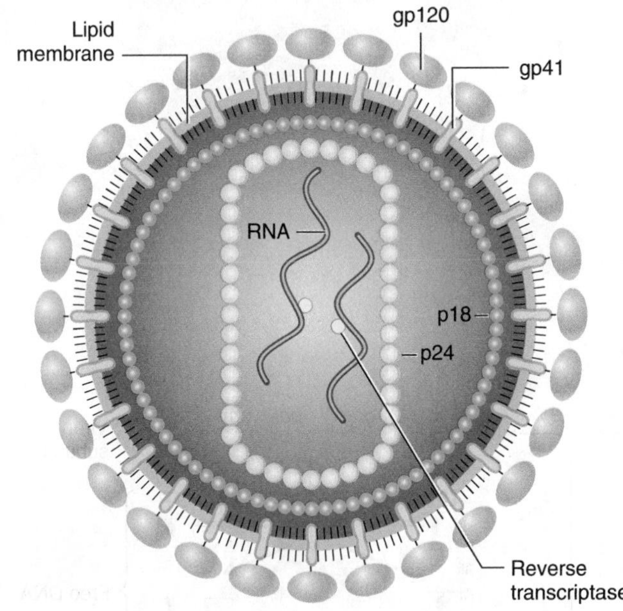

FIGURE 409-2 • Structure of HIV-1. (Adapted from RC Gallo: The AIDS virus. Sci Am 1987(Jan);256(1):46–56. Copyright © 1987 by Scientific American, Inc., and George V. Klein.)

The cell-free virion first attaches to the target cell through a specific interaction between the viral envelope and the host cell membrane. The specificity of this interaction between virus and cell results from a high-affinity interaction between the viral gp120 envelope glycoprotein and the target cell–associated CD4 molecule and leads to a conformational change in gp120 and subsequent interaction with a member of the cellular chemokine receptor family (CCR5 or CXCR4). These highly specific interactions among gp120, CD4, and CCR5/CXCR4 culminate in fusion of the viral and cellular membranes and internalization of the nucleoprotein-viral complex. Reverse transcription catalyzed by viral reverse transcriptase generates a double-stranded DNA copy of the viral RNA within the nucleoprotein complex, and this copy migrates to the nucleus, where covalent integration of viral DNA into host chromosomes leads to formation of the provirus. Subsequent expression of viral DNA is controlled by a combination of viral and host cellular proteins that interact with viral DNA and RNA regulatory elements. Transcribed viral mRNA is translated into viral proteins, and new virions are assembled at the cell surface, where genomic-length viral RNA, reverse transcriptase, structural and regulatory proteins, and envelope glycoproteins are assembled. Because the HIV-1 provirus is covalently integrated within the host cell chromosome, it represents a stable component of the host genome. Relevant to subsequent discussions of viral pathogenesis, the integrated provirus may remain transcriptionally latent or may exhibit high levels of gene expression with explosive production of progeny virus.

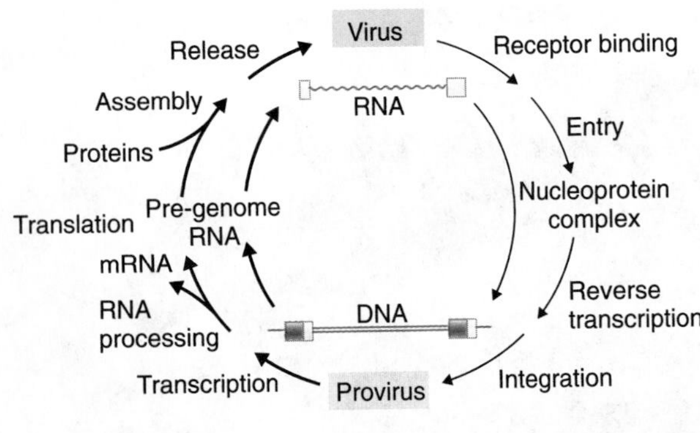

A

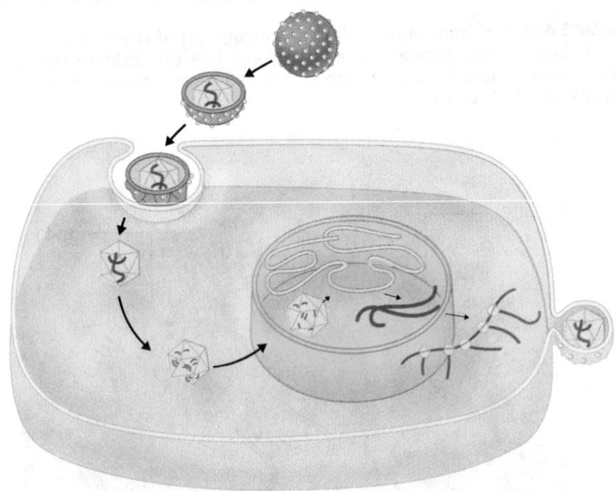

B

Cap β gag pol env An Viron subunit
R U5 U3 R
LTR LTR
Free DNA
Virus particle
gag pol env Provirus
SD SA
Cap An Genome + mRNA
Psi
Cap env An
Splice
+
Viral proteins
P CHO

C

FIGURE 409–3 • Different representations of the HIV-1 life cycle. A, Thick arrows denote amplification of viral products that may occur in the latter half of the replication cycle. **B,** A pictorial overview of the virus life cycle outlined in A. **C,** Major transformations of retroviral genetic information during the life cycle. A_n = poly(A) tract; Cap = 5′-methyl-G nucleotide; CHO = glycosylation site; LTR = long terminal repeat; P = phosphorylation site; Psi = viral packaging signal sequence; S_A = splice acceptor site; S_D = splice donor site. (From Varmus H, Brown P: Retroviruses. *In* Berg DE, Howe MM [eds]: Mobile DNA. Washington, DC, American Society for Microbiology, 1989, p 53.)

Molecular Structure and Function of HIV-1

The genomic organization of HIV-1 is shown diagrammatically in Figure 409–4. The HIV-1 genome, like other retroviral genomes, is diploid and consists of two identical viral RNA molecules assembled in a hydrogen-bonded 70S complex. These genomic subunits are plus strands of viral RNA in that they have the same chemical polarity as the mRNA from which viral products are translated. Like eukaryotic mRNA, the genomic viral RNA contains a 5′-methyl-G nucleotide, a poly(A) tract of 100 to 200 nucleotides at its 3′ end, and a number of methylated(A) residues. Host cell–derived tRNA incorporated within the virion is base-paired over a stretch of 18 nucleotides to the primer-binding site of the genomic viral RNA near its 5′ terminus and serves to prime the synthesis of minus-strand DNA during the initial stages of viral replication after infection.

The HIV-1 genome is bounded by long terminal repeat (LTR) elements and contains genes encoding the structural and enzymatic proteins (gag, pol, and env) found in all other replication-competent retroviruses. In addition to these genes, HIV-1 contains genes encoding other viral functions unique to this family of viruses that are responsible for their biologic behavior. The LTR sequences of HIV-1 direct and regulate expression of the viral genome (Fig. 409–5).

The *gag* gene encodes a precursor protein (p55) of 55 kD that is cleaved into four smaller products with the linear order NH_2-p18-p24-p9-p7-COOH. These proteins constitute the core protein structure of the virus and subserve nucleic acid and lipid membrane binding functions. The gag proteins of HIV-1, like those of other retroviruses, are synthesized as a polyprotein precursor that is subsequently cleaved during the viral maturation process. This facilitates assembly of the different components of the virus core structure into a three-dimensional configuration that when cleaved by a specific virus-derived protease, acquires the specialized functions characteristic of the mature virion. The polymerase gene products are translated from the same genomic RNA message as the gag proteins but in a different, overlapping reading frame as a result of ribosomal frame shifting. The *pol* gene encodes three proteins that are cleaved from a larger precursor polypeptide. These genes include NH_2–protease (p13)–reverse transcriptase (p66/p51)–integrase (p31)–COOH. The HIV-1 protease plays a critical role in virus biology in that it acts specifically to cleave gag and pol precursor polypeptides into functionally active proteins. The reverse transcriptase of HIV-1 is a magnesium-requiring, RNA-dependent DNA polymerase responsible for replicating the RNA viral genome. The integrase protein is required for proviral integration into the host cell genome.

The envelope gene (*env*) encodes a glycosylated polypeptide precursor (gp160) that is cleaved to form the exterior envelope glycoprotein (gp120) and the transmembrane glycoprotein (gp41), the latter of which anchors the envelope complex to the virus surface. In recent years, much has been learned about the structure and function of the HIV-1 envelope. The gp120/gp41 heterodimer exists as a trimeric spike complex on the virion surface and must serve two separate, but essential functions: mediation of virus binding and entry into cells and avoidance of neutralization by virus-specific antibodies. The former task is accomplished by sequential gp120 binding to cell-associated CD4 followed by a chemokine receptor, which triggers a gp41-mediated fusion event. The latter function results from a combination of carbohydrate cloaking of the exposed viral env surface, mutation of exposed env epitopes, and masking of conserved env receptor surfaces by conformational or energetic barriers to antibody binding.

Within the HIV-1 genome, additional genes serve important viral functions and distinguish HIV-1 from oncogenic retroviruses. They include the *vif*, *vpr*, and *vpu* genes located between *pol* and *env*; the *nef* gene located 3′ to *env* and extending into the U3 region of the viral LTR; and the *tat* and *rev* genes, both of which exist as bipartite coding exons in the central and 3′ end of the virus. The *tat* gene encodes a 14-kD protein that upregulates HIV-1 expression at transcriptional and post-transcriptional levels and is thus essential for HIV-1 replication. The target sequence for *tat*-mediated upregulation of HIV-1 expression is the *trans*-acting responsive region (TAR) of the LTR, which interacts with cellular factors to bind and activate TAR (see Fig. 409–5). The *rev* gene encodes a 20-kD protein that is required for transport of unspliced and singly spliced viral mRNA from the nucleus to cytoplasm. In the absence

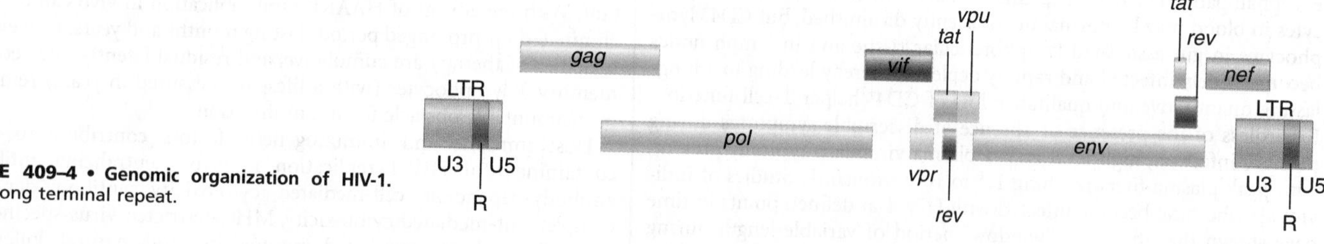

FIGURE 409–4 • Genomic organization of HIV-1. LTR = long terminal repeat.

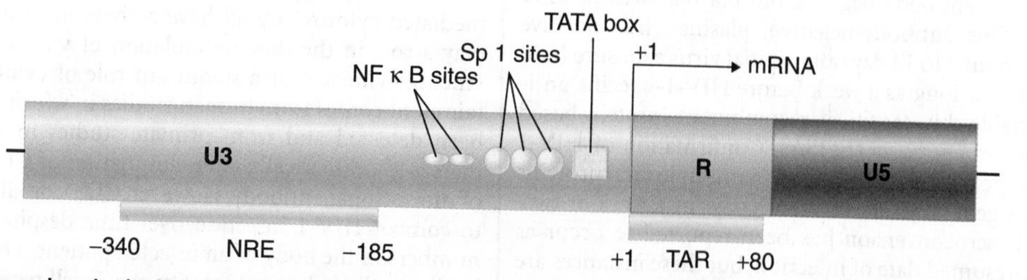

FIGURE 409–5 • Regulatory regions in the long terminal repeat (LTR) of HIV-1. Deletion mutant studies of the LTR have identified at least five regions for gene expression, including the TATA box and promotor, where RNA polymerase binds and transcription is initiated (+1); a negative regulatory element (NRE) located between nucleotides −340 and −185, deletion of which increases the level of gene expression directed by the viral LTR; enhancer elements (NFκB and Sp-1) located between nucleotides −137 and −17; and a *trans*-acting responsive region (TAR) located between nucleotides +1 and +80, which represents the putative binding region for regulatory factors responsible for tat-mediated transcriptional activation.

of *rev,* gag and env mRNA transcripts become multiply spliced and gag and env proteins are not made. The *vif* gene encodes a protein product of 23 kD that suppresses the antiretroviral cellular enzyme apoB mRNA–editing enzyme–catalytic polypeptide–like 3G (APOBEC3G), thereby enabling the production of infectious virions. The *vpr* gene encodes a protein of 15 kD that induces G_2/M cell cycle arrest, thereby enhancing virus production. The *vpu* gene encodes a 16-kD protein that is involved in virus assembly and release. The *nef* gene encodes a 27-kD protein that facilitates viral pathogenesis by downregulating cell surface–bound CD4, altering T-cell activation, and interfering with major histocompatibility complex (MHC) antigen presentation.

In summary, HIV-1 encodes the usual structural and enzymatic proteins typical of other replication-competent retroviruses, including gag, pol, and env, but it also encodes a group of at least six regulatory or auxiliary proteins (vif, vpr, vpu, tat, rev, and nef) whose activities are critically important in regulating the life cycle and pathogenesis of the virus.

Cell Tropism

The hallmark of AIDS is selective depletion of $CD4^+$ helper-inducer T lymphocytes. This defect is believed to result largely from the selective tropism of HIV-1 for this population of cells based on the high affinity of the viral gp120 envelope protein for the CD4 molecule (k_d = 4×10^{-9} M). CD4 normally serves as a ligand for MHC type II interactions, but in HIV-1 infection, it is used as the primary receptor molecule for HIV-1 targeting. This has been shown conclusively by studies demonstrating (1) direct complexing of gp120 and CD4 during viral infection, (2) inhibition of viral attachment and infection by anti-CD4 monoclonal antibodies that prevent gp120 binding, and (3) the ability of recombinant CD4 to confer susceptibility to HIV-1 infection to transfected human cells that normally do not express CD4.

CD4 expression alone is not sufficient to mediate HIV-1 entry. Coreceptors essential for virus entry include members of the chemokine receptor family, which are G protein–coupled receptors for pro-inflammatory chemokines. They include CCR5, which normally responds to the chemokines RANTES, MIP-1α, and MIP-1β, and CXCR4, which normally binds SDF-1. CCR5 and CXCR4 are differentially expressed on normal human cells that serve as targets of HIV-1 infection and are importantly involved in the cellular and tissue tropism of HIV-1 and in virus transmission and pathogenesis.

A variety of cell types other than helper-inducer T lymphocytes are known to express CD4 on their surface and are capable of replicating HIV-1. Such cells include blood monocytes, tissue macrophages, Langerhans cells in skin, and microglial and multinucleated giant cells in the central nervous system (CNS). These cells generally express smaller amounts of CD4 on their cell surface, but in each case they express one or more coreceptor molecules. Infection of such cells is believed to play an important role in the pathogenesis of AIDS. Other cell types, including neurons, glial cells, gastrointestinal epithelial cells, and kidney epithelium, can support HIV-1 infection, but the pathophysiologic significance of such findings in regard to viral pathogenesis in vivo is uncertain.

Viral Pathogenesis

Retroviral diseases are typically characterized by restricted viral gene expression, latency, and lifelong persistence of virus in the face of substantial host immune responses. From cohort studies of individuals infected with HIV-1 before the era of highly active antiretroviral therapy (HAART), it was estimated that AIDS develops in 26 to 36% of infected individuals within 7 years of infection and that lesser signs of immune dysfunction develop in an additional 40%. This protracted clinical course suggested that expression of the HIV-1 genome in vivo was to some degree downregulated as compared with in vitro infection of lymphocytes by HIV-1, which is characterized by explosive lytic viral infection.

Figure 409–6 depicts the natural history of HIV-1 infection of humans in relation to clinical symptoms, immune function, and viral replication. Initial infection with HIV-1 frequently causes an acute viral syndrome with protean manifestations but typically characterized by fever, lymphadenopathy, pharyngitis, and rash. Other symptoms and signs that may occur with acute HIV-1 infection include myalgias, arthralgias, leukopenia, thrombocytopenia, nausea, diarrhea, headache, and

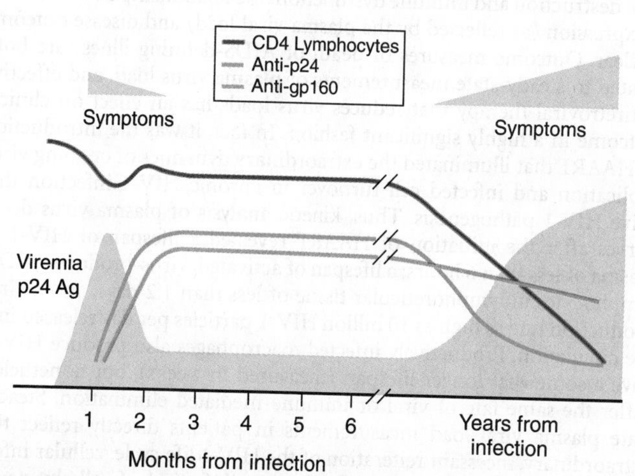

FIGURE 409–6 • Natural history model for HIV-1 infection. Viremia denotes cell-free virus in plasma, p24 Ag denotes circulating viral p24 antigen in plasma, and anti-p24 and anti-gp160 correspond to antibodies to viral core and envelope proteins.

encephalopathy. During this primary phase of infection, $CD4^+$ lymphocytes in blood may be normal or transiently diminished, but $CD4^+$ lymphocytes in gut-associated lymphoreticular tissue and in lymph nodes become widely infected and rapidly depleted, thereby leading to a long-lasting quantitative and qualitative loss of $CD4^+$ helper T-cell function. Regardless of the presence or absence of discernible symptoms during primary infection, high-level HIV-1 plasma viremia is typically present, with peak plasma titers reaching 10^6 to 10^7 virions/mL. Studies of individuals who have become infected with HIV-1 at defined points in time have shown that there is a "window" period of variable length during which the patient is HIV-1 antibody negative but plasma virus positive and highly infectious. This antibody-negative, plasma virus–positive period generally begins about 7 to 14 days after initial virus exposure (and infection) and persists for as long as a week before HIV-1–specific antibodies are first detectable by sensitive recombinant protein-based enzyme-linked immunosorbent assay (ELISA). Confirmation of HIV-1 infection based on the appearance of antibodies to multiple viral proteins on Western immunoblot generally follows within days or a week or two. In some cases, antibody seroconversion has been reported to occur as long as months after a presumed date of infection, but these instances are believed to be rare. Although HIV-1 replication is downregulated by host defense mechanisms and resolution of the acute pro-inflammatory infectious state, virus replication is not abrogated. Even during the clinically quiescent stages of infection, substantial viral replication ensues and leads to progressive $CD4^+$ cell destruction. This serves as the rationale for clinical studies examining the risk-benefit ratio of antiviral therapy initiated at the earliest stages of infection, a question that has still not been answered.

The precise biologic mechanisms responsible for the cytopathic effects and immunosuppressive properties of HIV-1 in vivo are unknown. Molecularly cloned HIV-1 proviral DNA, transfected into human cells, has been shown in cell culture experiments to contain all the necessary information to generate infectious and cytopathic virus. Expression of HIV-1 proteins in activated lymphocytes leads to cell cycle arrest in G_2 and cell death within approximately 2 days. HIV-1 alone exerts direct cytopathic activity against $CD4^+$ lymphocytes in vitro and in vivo. Expression of only the HIV-1 envelope on lymphocytes is sufficient to induce fusion of cells with normal uninfected $CD4^+$ bystander cells, thus suggesting that syncytium formation mediated by gp120-CD4 interaction may contribute to cell loss in vivo. Other mechanisms of $CD4^+$ cell loss may also be operative. Cell-free HIV-1 gp120 envelope protein adsorbs to $CD4^+$ cells and may serve as an antigen for mediating antibody-dependent cell-mediated cytotoxicity and, when processed by antigen-presenting cells, be a target for direct T-cell cytotoxicity. In the CNS of infected individuals, in which the predominant cell types infected with HIV-1 are cells of the monocyte-macrophage lineage, additional mechanisms of cellular and organ dysfunction are involved. These mechanisms are believed to include the elaboration of cytotoxic factors from infected cells and interference with neurotropic factors leading to the clinically recognized AIDS dementia complex.

Despite uncertainties regarding precise mechanisms of $CD4^+$ lymphocyte destruction and immune dysfunction, the relationship between HIV-1 expression (as reflected by the plasma viral load) and disease outcome is clear. Outcome measures of death or AIDS-defining illness are both related to steady-state measurements of plasma virus load, and effective antiretroviral therapy that reduces virus loads has an effect on clinical outcome in a highly significant fashion. In fact, it was the introduction of HAART that illuminated the extraordinary dynamics of ongoing virus replication and infected cell turnover in chronic HIV-1 infection that drive HIV-1 pathogenesis. Thus, kinetic analysis of plasma virus decay curves after the initiation of HAART revealed a lifespan of HIV-1 in plasma of less than 6 hours; a lifespan of activated, virus-producing $CD4^+$ lymphocytes in lymphoreticular tissue of less than 1.2 days; and a virus production rate as high as 10 billion HIV-1 particles per day released into the circulation. Productively infected macrophages also produce HIV-1, have a somewhat longer lifespan (measured in weeks), but nonetheless suffer the same fate of viral or immune-mediated elimination. Steady-state plasma viral load measurements in patients directly reflect this extraordinary, incessant reiteration of the HIV-1 life cycle: cellular infection, virus production, cell death, de novo infection of cells by newly released virus, and so on. It is not surprising that clinical outcome as measured by time to diagnosis of AIDS or time to death from AIDS is significantly related to the steady-state plasma viral load, although other factors, including activated T-cell levels, are also prognostically important. With the advent of HAART, viral replication in vivo can be all but eliminated for prolonged periods lasting months and years. However, the toxicities of therapy are cumulative, and residual latently infected $CD4^+$ memory T lymphocytes (with a lifespan measured in years) remain an insurmountable obstacle to cure of infection.

Host immune and immunogenetic factors contribute to partial containment of HIV-1 replication in vivo. Neutralizing antibodies, antibody-dependent cell-mediated cytotoxicity, antibody-dependent complement-mediated cytotoxicity, MHC-restricted virus-specific cytotoxic T-lymphocyte-mediated cytotoxicity, and natural killer cell–mediated cytotoxicity all have activity against HIV-1 in vitro and may play a role in the downmodulation of viral replication. The most convincing evidence for a significant role of cytotoxic T cells in virus containment comes from human studies in which virus escape mutants have been detected and from primate studies in which plasma virus loads increased dramatically after elimination of $CD8^+$ cells by administration of monoclonal antibody. However, $CD8^+$, or killer, T cells lose their ability to combat HIV-1 infection over time despite their persistence in large numbers in the body of an infected patient. This "T-cell exhaustion" may be due to the enhanced activity of a T-cell receptor protein, programmed death 1 (PD-1), whose ligand (PD-L1) is located on antigen-presenting cells. This interaction diminishes the capacity of these T cells to be activated, most likely reflecting a normal pathway for dampening immune responses to prevent the consequences of uncontrolled cytotoxicity. Blocking the interaction between T-cell receptor PD-1 and its ligand PD-L1 may help reinvigorate T cells that have become exhausted because of chronic infection. This approach is currently being studied as therapy for HIV-1 infection.

Genetic variability is a hallmark of HIV-1. The variability of the HIV-1 genome is characteristic of retroviruses because reverse transcription of viral RNA into proviral DNA and transcription of proviral DNA into genomic viral RNA are not subject to cellular proofreading mechanisms. The rate of nucleotide misincorporation by the viral reverse transcriptase is on the order of 10^{-4} per nucleotide per replication cycle. Because the HIV-1 genome is 10^4 nucleotides long, this high rate of nucleotide misincorporation means that virus strains that infect patients or that are isolated from patients must be described as a "quasi-species" composed of populations of viruses with highly related, but distinct viral genomes. Such variation in the HIV-1 genome leads to viral resistance to reverse transcriptase, protease, and entry inhibitors and to escape from the cellular and humoral arms of the adaptive immune system. Genetic variability can also lead to other biologic changes in the virus over time, including altered cellular tropism. Patients in whom predominant virus strains develop that use the CXCR4 coreceptor, for example, generally have an accelerated decline in $CD4^+$ cell counts and a less favorable clinical prognosis. On a global population level, the variability in HIV-1 can be recognized in the phylogenetic relationships among circulating virus strains. HIV-1 viruses globally are composed of three distinct groups: M, N, and O. Group M is responsible for more than 99% of infections worldwide. Groups N and O are largely restricted to west-central Africa. It is believed that HIV-1 groups M, N, and O represent separate introductions of virus into the human population from African primates sometime early in the 20th century. Group M viruses can be further subdivided by phylogeny into subtypes A through K. Although these phylogenetic distinctions allow molecular epidemiologic tracking of HIV-1 at a population level, there is little evidence to suggest that the various virus groups and subtypes differ in any clinically meaningful manner. All are pathogenic in humans.

HUMAN IMMUNODEFICIENCY VIRUS TYPE 2

After discovery of HIV-1 as the cause of epidemic AIDS in the United States, Europe, and Asia, patients in western Africa with AIDS-like symptoms were identified whose sera reacted more strongly with a simian immunodeficiency virus (SIV_{MAC}) isolated from captive rhesus macaques in U.S. primate centers than with HIV-1. Identification of patients with serologic reactivity for SIV_{MAC} raised the possibility that certain African human and simian populations could be infected with immunodeficiency viruses related to, but distinct from HIV-1. An extensive survey of African primate species for such viruses led initially to the identification of distinct SIV viruses in African green monkeys (SIV_{AGM}), mandrills

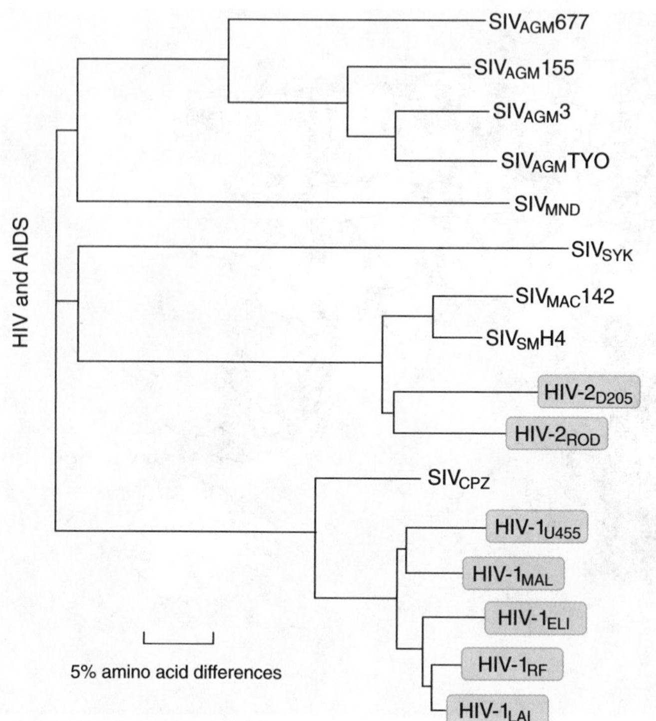

FIGURE 409–7 • Phylogenetic relationships among primate lentiviruses inferred from pol protein sequences. Independent isolates of simian immunodeficiency viruses (SIVs) obtained from the African green monkey (AGM), mandrill (MND), Sykes (SYK), rhesus macaque (MAC), sooty mangabey (SM), and chimpanzee (CPZ) are depicted along with representative isolates of HIV-1 and HIV-2 (boxed). The horizontal branch lengths are drawn to scale and can be used to determine the percent difference in pol protein sequences between the different virus strains. There are five major and roughly equidistant phylogenetic lineages of viruses: SIV$_{AGM}$, SIV$_{MND}$, SIV$_{SYK}$, SIV$_{MAC}$/SIV$_{SM}$/HIV-2, and SIV$_{CPZ}$/HIV-1. HIV-1 and HIV-2 appear as members of larger viral lineages composed of simian- and human-derived viruses. Such relationships are indicative of cross-species transmission. (Adapted from Hahn BH: Viral genes and their products. *In* Broder S, Merigan TC, Bolognesi D [eds]: Textbook of AIDS Medicine. Baltimore, Williams & Wilkins, 1994, p 21.)

(SIV$_{MND}$), sooty mangabeys (SIV$_{SM}$), and chimpanzees (SIV$_{CPZ}$) (Fig. 409–7). At least 31 naturally infected primate species in Africa are now recognized to harbor lentiviruses.

West African patients with AIDS-like symptoms and healthy individuals at risk for AIDS were identified who were infected with a virus closely related to SIV$_{SM}$. This virus was isolated, molecularly cloned, and shown through sequence analysis to represent a second major class of human immunodeficiency viruses called HIV-2. Though originally limited geographically to western Africa, HIV-2 has now been identified in patients in Europe, the United States, South America, and India. HIV-2 is approximately 40 to 50% similar to HIV-1 in overall nucleotide sequence homology. There are two major differences in the genomic organization of HIV-1 and HIV-2. The *vpu* gene of HIV-1 is not present in HIV-2, and HIV-2 contains an additional gene, *vpx*, in its central region that is not present in HIV-1. Vpx is an 18-kD protein involved in nuclear transport of the HIV-2 preintegration complex in nondividing cells. Antigenically, HIV-2 and HIV-1 are distinct, with greatest cross-reactivity in structural proteins and least in envelope proteins. Licensed ELISA tests to detect HIV-1 infection include HIV-2 antigens as well.

Like HIV-1, HIV-2 selectively infects CD4$^+$ cells. Although HIV-2 can cause profound immunodeficiency and an AIDS syndrome indistinguishable from that caused by HIV-1, evidence suggests that HIV-2 is less virulent than HIV-1 and causes disease in a smaller fraction of individuals and over a more protracted period.

The discovery of two distinct types of human immunodeficiency viruses (HIV-1 and HIV-2) having closely related counterparts in African primates (SIV$_{CPZ}$ in chimpanzees and SIV$_{SM}$ in sooty mangabeys, respectively), along with epidemiologic findings revealing Africa as the geographic source of all human and simian immunodeficiency viruses, suggested a cross-species (zoonotic) origin for HIV-1 and HIV-2. This conclusion has been confirmed by molecular epidemiologic studies that have unequivocally identified the chimpanzee subspecies *Pan troglodytes troglodytes* in west-central Africa as the source of the HIV-1 pandemic and the sooty mangabey (*Cercocebus atys*) in western Africa as the source of HIV-2.

SUGGESTED READINGS

Heeney JL, Dalgleish AG, Weiss RA: Origins of HIV and the evolution of resistance to AIDS. Science 2006;313:462–466. *A comprehensive review.*

Keele BF, Van Heuverswyn F, Li Y, et al: Chimpanzee reservoirs of pandemic and nonpandemic HIV-1. Science 2006;313:523–526. *Discovery of ancestral HIV-1 lineages in wild-living chimpanzees from southern Cameroon.*

Lederman MM, Penn-Nicholson A, Cho M, et al: Biology of CCR5 and its role in HIV infection and treatment. JAMA 2006;296:815–826. *A review including possible therapeutic avenues involving this receptor.*

Persaud D, Zhou Y, Siliciano JM, Siliciano RF: Latency in human immunodeficiency virus type 1 infection: No easy answers. J Virol 2003;77:1659–1665. *Comprehensive review of HIV-1 latency and implications for therapy.*

Quinn TC, Wawer MJ, Sewankambo N, et al: Viral load and heterosexual transmission of human immunodeficiency virus type 1. Rakai Project Study Group. N Engl J Med 2000;342:921–929. *An important study that established the relationship between HIV viral load in the infected partner and the risk for HIV transmission.*

Simon V, Ho DD, Karim QA: HIV/AIDS epidemiology, pathogenesis, prevention, and treatment. Lancet 2006;368:489–504. *A clinical update.*

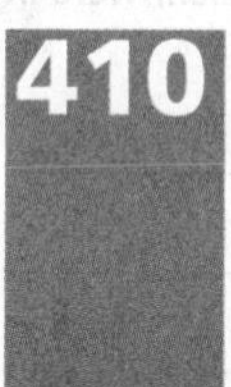

EPIDEMIOLOGY OF HUMAN IMMUNODEFICIENCY VIRUS INFECTION AND ACQUIRED IMMUNODEFICIENCY SYNDROME

Thomas C. Quinn

HISTORICAL PERSPECTIVE

Twenty-five years after initial recognition of acquired immunodeficiency syndrome (AIDS) in the United States, the disease has become epidemic in every country of the world. Initially reported as a disease primarily affecting homosexual men, AIDS was rapidly identified in many other risk groups, and it became evident that it was caused by an infectious agent transmitted through sexual activities, parentally through blood transfusions and injection drug use, and perinatally from mother to infant. Early investigations in the 1980s demonstrated that the etiologic agent of AIDS was human immunodeficiency virus (HIV), which existed in two types, HIV-1 and HIV-2. After the development of diagnostic assays for HIV antibody, it became possible to track and monitor the escalating spread of HIV throughout the world, definitively define the modes and probabilities of transmission, and study the natural history of HIV infection. Within years of its recognition, HIV disseminated rapidly throughout the world, caused a massive epidemic, and became one of the leading causes of death worldwide. Prevention efforts and treatment with antiretroviral drugs have tempered the spread and decreased the fatality rate in some countries, but in developing countries where the social, demographic, cultural, and economic impact of the AIDS epidemic has been the greatest, these gains have been too limited and too slow to reverse the escalating trend of the epidemic.

GLOBAL STATISTICS

By August 2006, approximately 65 million people had become infected with HIV since the beginning of the epidemic in 1981. Of these individuals, more than 27 million people had already died of AIDS, and it became ranked as one of the leading causes of death throughout the world. According to estimates by the Joint United Nations Program on HIV/AIDS (UNAIDS), 38.6 million people were living with HIV by August 2006 (Fig. 410–1). In 2005 alone, 4.1 million people became newly

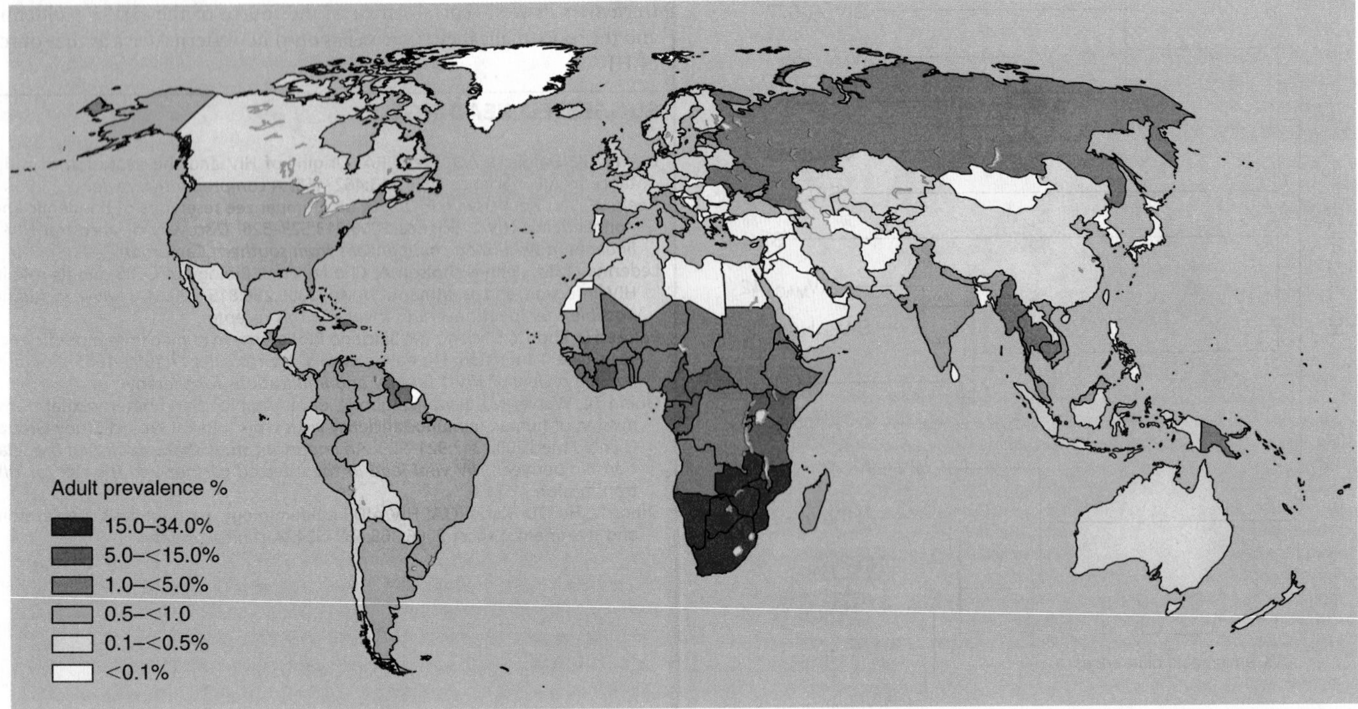

FIGURE 410–1 • A total of 38.6 million people (33.4 to 46.0 million) were living with HIV infection or AIDS in 2005 as estimated by UNAIDS. The adult prevalence of HIV infection is shown by country. (Data from UNAIDS.)

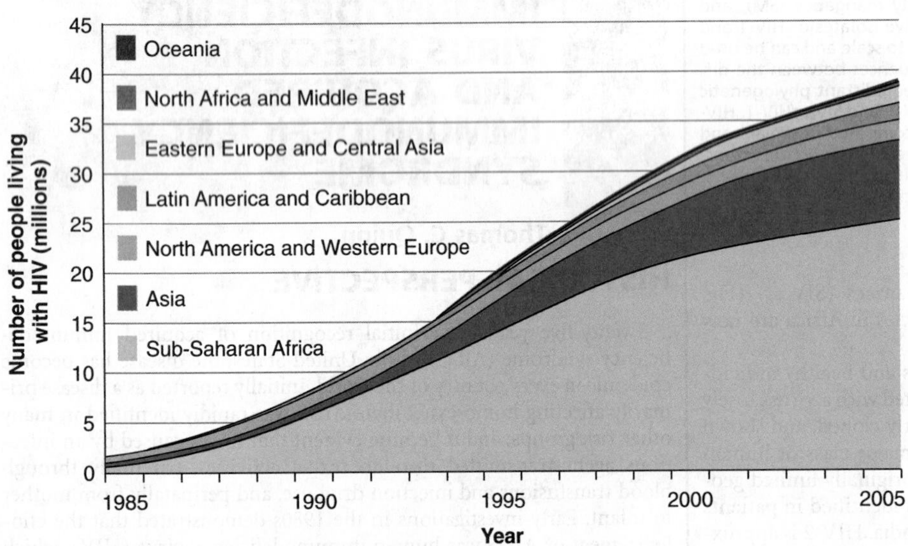

FIGURE 410–2 • Estimated number of adults and children living with HIV by region, 1986 to 2005. (Data from UNAIDS.)

infected, half of whom were young individuals between the ages of 15 and 24 years. Nearly 90% of all new infections occurred in developing countries; 50% occurred in women; and the major mode of transmission was heterosexual transmission, although infections continue to spread at high rates among men who have sex with men (MSM). Injecting drug use remains the second leading mode of transmission responsible for the rapid spread of HIV throughout Asia, eastern Europe, and other developed countries of the world. Perinatal transmission also continues to occur in developing countries, where access to antiretroviral drugs to prevent mother-to-infant transmission is limited or nonexistent. In 2005, 700,000 children became newly infected, and 18 million children have been orphaned by the premature deaths of their parents from AIDS. In 2005, 3.1 million people died of AIDS, including 570,000 children.

From these epidemiologic trends (Fig. 410–2), it is projected that within the next 8 years an additional 45 million people could become infected with HIV in 126 low- and middle-income countries, which have the most concentrated or generalized epidemics, unless the world succeeds in mounting a drastically expanded global prevention and treatment effort. It is anticipated that more than 40% of these new infections will occur in Asia, the Pacific, and eastern Europe, although it is apparent that the epidemic will continue to devastate nearly all countries of the African continent. During the next decade, without full access to treatment and care in many countries, millions of individuals will join the ranks of the more than 35 million people who have already died.

DEMOGRAPHIC, SOCIAL, AND ECONOMIC IMPACT OF HIV AND AIDS

AIDS is the leading cause of death in sub-Saharan Africa and the fourth largest killer worldwide. The average life expectancy in sub-Saharan Africa is now 47 years; it would have been 62 years without AIDS (Fig. 410–3). Life expectancy at birth in Botswana has dropped to a level not seen in that country since the 1950s. Even in Haiti, life expectancy is nearly 6 years less than it would have been in the absence of AIDS. In Asia, Cambodia has experienced a reduction in life expectancy of 4 years. Current HIV prevalence levels merely hint at the greater lifetime probability of being infected with AIDS. In Lesotho, it is estimated that a person who is 15 years old has a 74% chance of being infected with HIV by his or her 50th birthday.

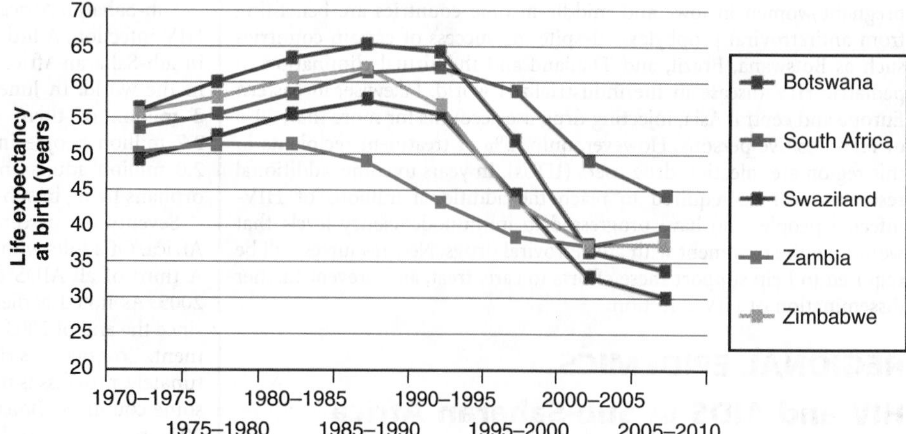

FIGURE 410–3 • Impact of AIDS on life expectancy in five African countries between 1970 and projected to 2010. (From the United Nations Population Division, 2004. World Population Prospects: The 2004 Revision Database.)

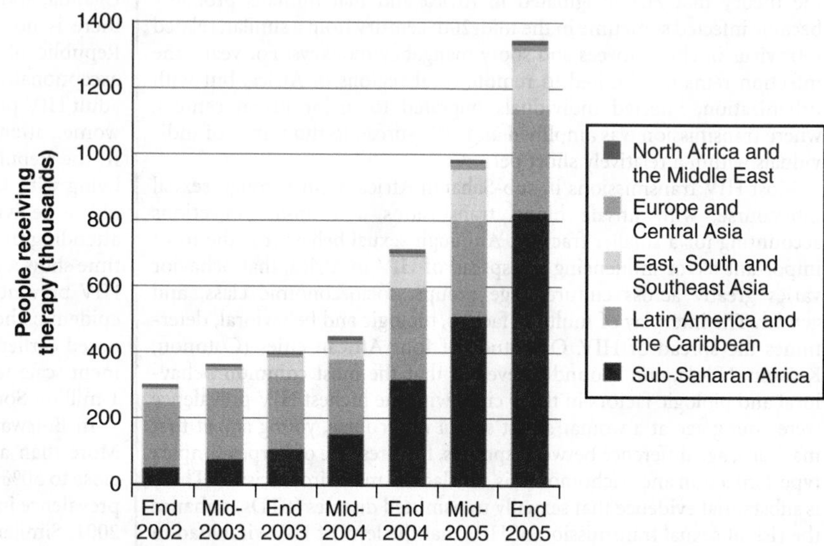

FIGURE 410–4 • Estimated number of people receiving antiretroviral therapy in low- and middle-income countries from 2002 through 2005. (Data from World Health Organization and UNAIDS.)

According to one report, AIDS is expected to cause a decline in life expectancy in 51 countries over the next 20 years. Seven nations in sub-Saharan Africa now have life expectancies less than 40 years, and this number will increase by 11 countries over the next 7 years. The declining life expectancies will soon reach levels that have not existed since the 19th century. In Zimbabwe and South Africa, the infant mortality rate is higher than it was in 1990. Five African nations will experience more deaths than births by 2010, with a resultant decrease in population. Life expectancy will drop to just 27 years in Botswana and Mozambique in the next 8 years, and Swaziland will have an estimated life expectancy of 33. In Zimbabwe, Zambia, and Namibia, the expected lifespan will be 34 years. In contrast, the overall life expectancy in an African without AIDS would be 70 years by 2010.

THE GLOBAL RESPONSE

At a 2001 special session of the United Nations General Assembly on AIDS, 189 nations agreed that AIDS was a national and international security issue of the highest priority. The representatives of these countries—and later the G8 leaders—signed a historic declaration of commitment on HIV/AIDS that promised innovative responses, coordinated efforts, and accountability for progress against the epidemic. The declaration set a comprehensive list of time-bound targets to support the millennium development goal of halting and beginning to reverse the epidemic by 2015. Shortly thereafter, the Global Fund for AIDS, Tuberculosis, and Malaria raised funds from private donations and industrialized countries to help support access to care and treatment within developing countries. This initiative was complemented by President Bush's Emergency Plan for AIDS Relief, which committed $15 billion over a 5-year period to provide treatment for 2 million HIV-infected individuals and care for 7 million, as well as provide additional resources for enhancing prevention efforts to prevent further transmission. As of June 2006, more than 1.6 million persons were accessing antiretroviral therapy (ART) against HIV in low- and middle-income countries (Fig. 410–4). This represented more than a four-fold increase since December 2003, when global efforts to expand access to ART began to increase significantly. Overall, ART coverage in these countries increased from 7% in 2003 to 24% in June 2006. Of the 38.6 million people infected with HIV worldwide, approximately 6.8 million in low- and middle-income countries are now estimated to require ART. Over the past year the number of people receiving treatment in these countries increased by about 300,000 every 6 months.

Scale-up in sub-Saharan Africa has been most dramatic, increasing from 100,000 people receiving treatment in 2003 to more than 1 million in June 2006—a 10-fold increase. Sixty-three percent of all people now receiving treatment in low- and middle-income countries are living in sub-Saharan Africa, as compared with 25% in late 2003. Data from countries in sub-Saharan Africa, Asia, Latin America, and the Caribbean now indicate that 20 countries with at least 1000 people needing ART are providing treatment to at least 50% of people who need it. Coverage by region ranges from 5% in North America and the Middle East and 13% in eastern Europe and central Asia to 75% in Latin America and the Caribbean. Sub-Saharan Africa now has the second highest percentage after Latin America in coverage, although this region still accounts for 70% of unmet treatment need in low- and middle-income countries. Unfortunately, not all have equal access to therapy, even within countries with middle to high prevalence. For example, an estimated 800,000 children younger than 15 years now require ART, but only 60,000 to 100,000 are receiving treatment. Children account for approximately 14% of AIDS death. Nearly 90% of children infected with HIV are African. The median proportion of HIV-infected children receiving treatment is just 8% in sub-Saharan Africa. Similarly, less than 10% of HIV-infected pregnant women in low- and middle-income countries are benefiting from antiretroviral prophylaxis despite the success of certain countries such as Botswana, Brazil, and Thailand and the virtual elimination of pediatric HIV disease in the industrialized world. Likewise, in eastern Europe and central Asia, injecting drug use accounts for more than 70% of HIV-positive persons. However, only 25% of treatment recipients in this region are injection drug users (IDUs). In years to come, additional resources will be required to reach the additional millions of HIV-infected people who have progressed to immunodeficiency levels that would require treatment with antiretroviral drugs. New resources will be required to help support these efforts to care, treat, and prevent further dissemination of HIV infection.

REGIONAL EPIDEMICS

HIV and AIDS in Sub-Saharan Africa

Sub-Saharan Africa represents the epicenter of the global HIV/AIDS pandemic (Table 410–1). Studies in the late 1990s and early 2000 support the theory that HIV originated in Africa and that humans probably became infected sometime in the mid-20th century from a similar, related retrovirus in chimpanzees and sooty mangabey monkeys. For years, the infection remained limited to remote rural regions of Africa, but with urbanization, infected individuals migrated to major urban centers, where transmission was amplified and HIV spread to thousands of individuals within a relatively short period.

Most HIV transmissions in sub-Saharan Africa occur through sexual intercourse, with unsafe blood transfusions and unsafe injections accounting for a smaller fraction. Although sexual behavior is the most important factor influencing the spread of HIV in Africa, that behavior varies greatly across cultures, age groups, socioeconomic class, and gender. The interplay of multiple factors, biologic and behavioral, determines the spread of HIV. One study of four African cities (Cotonou, Kisumu, Ndola, and Yaounde) revealed that the most common behavioral and biologic factors in those cities with the highest HIV prevalence were young age at a woman's first sexual intercourse, young age at first marriage, age difference between spouses, the presence of herpes simplex type 2 infection and trichomoniasis, and lack of male circumcision. There is substantial evidence that sexually transmitted diseases (STDs) enhance the risk of sexual transmission of HIV, that the level of HIV viral load in an individual enhances the probability of infectiousness, and that male circumcision is associated with a reduced risk of transmission. Although the complex interplay of factors makes it difficult to estimate the probable growth of the epidemic within the region, evidence from the past 25 years demonstrates that HIV can spread rapidly and widely from very low seroprevalence levels.

Sub-Saharan Africa remains the worst affected region in the world for HIV infection. A little more than a tenth of the world's population lives in sub-Saharan Africa, but it is home to 64% of all people living with HIV in the world. In June 2006, 24.5 million people were living with HIV, 2 million of them children younger than 15 years. Approximately 2.7 million people in the region became newly infected in 2005, and 2.0 million adults and children died of AIDS. There were 12 million orphans living in sub-Saharan Africa in 2005.

Seventy-five percent of all women living with HIV are in sub-Saharan Africa. Of adults with HIV in Africa, 59% are women and 41% are men. A third of all AIDS deaths globally occurred in sub-Saharan Africa in 2005. As noted earlier, access to ART has increased more than 10-fold since the end of 2003, and more than a million people now receive treatment. Coverage has risen from 2 to 23% between 2003 and 2006. Unfortunately, progress is uneven, with coverage reaching or exceeding 50% in some countries (Botswana, Namibia, and Uganda) but remaining below 20% in most others. Southern Africa accounts for a quarter of all people receiving ART in sub-Saharan Africa.

Although some countries in sub-Saharan Africa such as Kenya, Uganda, and Zimbabwe have shown recent declines in HIV prevalence, there is no evidence of any decline in southern Africa, including the Republic of South Africa, Botswana, Namibia, and Swaziland, where exceptionally high infection levels continue. In Swaziland, the national adult HIV prevalence is estimated at 33.4%. HIV prevalence in pregnant women attending antenatal clinics rose from 4% in 1992 to 43% in 2004. In the Republic of South Africa, an estimated 5.5 million people were living with HIV in 2005. An estimated 18.8% of adults (15 to 49 years old) were living with HIV in 2005. Almost one in three pregnant women attending public antenatal clinics were living with HIV, and trends over time show a gradual increase in HIV prevalence. Although South Africa's HIV prevention efforts have not made a significant impact against the epidemic, there has been considerable progress on the treatment front as noted earlier. South Africa accounts for a large percentage of the treatment scale-up in sub-Saharan Africa, but as of 2006, nearly 80% of the 1 million South Africans in need of ART were still without treatment.

In Botswana, the national adult HIV prevalence was 24.1% in 2005. More than a third of pregnant women attending antenatal clinics and close to 50% of women 30 to 34 years of age were infected with HIV. The prevalence in pregnant women has generally remained at 34 to 37% since 2001. Similarly, Lesotho has a national adult HIV prevalence of 23.2%, with 27% documented in women attending antenatal clinics. A third of pregnant women 25 to 34 years of age were infected. In Namibia, the prevalence of HIV infection is 19.6% among all adults, with an HIV prevalence of 42% in antenatal clinics in selected areas. In neighboring Mozambique, Malawi, and Zambia, HIV prevalence has been documented between 16 and 17%. There is wide geographic variation,

TABLE 410–1 REGIONAL HIV AND AIDS STATISTICS AND FEATURES AT THE END OF 2002

Region	Adults and Children Living with HIV/AIDS	Adults and Children Newly Infected with HIV	Adult Prevalence Rate*	Main Modes of Transmission for Adults Living with HIV/AIDS
Sub-Saharan Africa	25,000,000	3,200,000	7.2%	Hetero
North Africa and Middle East	440,000	67,000	0.2%	Hetero, IDU
South and Southeast Asia	7,600,000	990,000	0.7%	Hetero, IDU
East Asia and Pacific	680,000	140,000	0.1%	IDU, hetero, MSM
Oceania	78,000	8,200	0.5%	MSM, Hetero
Latin America	1,600,000	200,000	0.6%	MSM, IDU, hetero
Caribbean	330,000	30,000	1.6%	Hetero, MSM
Eastern Europe and central Asia	1,500,000	270,000	0.9%	IDU, Hetero, MSM
Western Europe	720,000	22,000	0.3%	MSM, IDU, Hetero
North America	1,300,000	43,000	0.9%	MSM, IDU, hetero
Total	38,600,000	4,900,000	1.1%	

*The proportion of adults (15 to 49 years of age) living with HIV infection or AIDS in 2005 using 2005 population numbers.
Hetero = heterosexual transmission; IDU = transmission through injecting drug use; MSM = sexual transmission among men who have sex with men.

however, with HIV infection levels in pregnant women ranging from less than 10% in some places to as high as 30% in others.

In the countries of eastern Africa, HIV prevalence has either decreased or remained stable in the past several years. In Uganda, which saw a steep decline in HIV prevalence during the mid and late 1990s, adult HIV prevalence was estimated at 6.7% in 2005. However, recent trends in 2006 suggest that HIV prevalence may be increasing in selected areas, in part because of a decrease in mortality with access to ART but potentially because of increasing incident rates as a result of decreasing condom use and an increased percentage of multiple partners. In neighboring Kenya, Eritrea, Tanzania, Burundi, and Rwanda, the HIV epidemic has been stable in recent years, with prevalence rates ranging from 2% in Eritrea to 7% in Kenya, Tanzania, Burundi, and Rwanda. In Ethiopia, HIV prevalence has stabilized in urban areas but appears to be increasing in more distant rural areas, where access to treatment and care is more limited.

Western Africa is less severely affected than other parts of sub-Saharan Africa, with national adult HIV prevalence rates of 2% in several countries. The highest rate in the region is in Côte d'Ivoire: 7.1%. Nigeria has the third largest number of people living with HIV in the continent, 2.9 million, but it is also the most populous country in Africa, with more than 110 million people. Infection levels vary radically across the country from 2.6% in the southwest to 6.1% in the north central zones. HIV continues to spread rapidly among female sex workers and their clients, as well as in the general population. In some urban populations, more than 10% of adults are infected and the annual incidence is as high as 3%. Within the years to come, more resources will be required to reach the additional millions of HIV-infected people who have progressed to immunodeficiency levels that would require treatment with antiretroviral drugs. New resources will be required to help support these efforts to care, treat, and prevent further dissemination of HIV infection.

Over the past decade, AIDS has become the leading cause of death and years of productive life lost throughout the continent. Excess deaths attributable to HIV are highest in the 25- to 34-year-old group, usually a group with low mortality. Nearly 90% of deaths in this age group are in excess of background rates and were attributable to HIV. Because AIDS deaths are concentrated in childhood and young adult age groups, their effects are substantial, with life expectancy reduced by more than 20 years in several countries. Demographic projections have estimated that population growth will decline more rapidly than expected and that the size of the African population in 2005 will be smaller than it would have been without AIDS. HIV or AIDS cases will put an increasing strain on health care systems, which are already overburdened, and on individual households that are trying to manage with limited economic resources. Care and support for children orphaned by AIDS will become a growing concern throughout the region.

HIV and AIDS in Asia and the Pacific

After sub-Saharan Africa, Asia and the Pacific have the second largest number of HIV-infected individuals in the world, estimated at 8.3 million people. In 2005, 1 million adults and children became newly infected, in part because of the explosive growth of the HIV epidemic in China, India, and several other countries in Southeast Asia. With the exception of Cambodia, Myanmar, and Thailand, national HIV prevalence levels remain comparatively low in most countries of Asia and the Pacific, to some extent because of their large population base. For example, in China, Indonesia, and India, where large numbers of people are infected, national HIV prevalence rates in these highly populous countries do not provide the full impact of the epidemic. India's national adult HIV prevalence rate of 1% offers little indication of the serious situation facing the country. An estimated 5.2 million people were living with HIV at the end of 2005—the second highest figure in the world after South Africa. HIV prevalence in women attending antenatal clinics was higher than 1% in Andhra Pradesh, Karnataka, Maharashtra, Manipur, Nagaland, and Tamil Nadu.

Throughout the region, injecting drug use remains one of the most prominent modes of transmission of HIV. More than 50% of IDUs have already acquired HIV in Malaysia, Myanmar, Nepal, Thailand, Indonesia, Manipur, and southern China. Very high rates of needle sharing have been documented among users in Bangladesh and Vietnam, along with evidence that a considerable proportion of sex workers in Vietnam also inject drugs.

China, with a fifth of the world's population, has also witnessed a dramatic escalation of the HIV epidemic in the past decade. A total of 650,000 Chinese individuals are estimated to be living with HIV. The HIV epidemic is particularly severe among IDUs, who account for almost half (44%) of all HIV infections. HIV prevalence exceeds 50% in IDUs in Xinjiang, Yunnan, and Sichuan provinces. To compound the tragedy of the epidemic in China, reports from Henan province in central China demonstrate that tens of thousands and possibly more rural villagers became infected by selling their blood to collecting centers that did not follow basic blood donation safety procedures. It has been estimated that 150,000 people have been infected through these practices. There are new signs of heterosexually transmitted HIV epidemics in at least three provinces–Guangdong, Guangxi, and Yunnan—where HIV prevalence rates have been documented at 11 to 15% among sentinel sex workers in 2000. Several other factors highlight the swift escalation of HIV infection in China. STDs quadrupled between 1997 and 2002, thus suggesting that unprotected sex with nonmonogamous partners is increasing in China. There is massive population mobility. Approximately 100 million Chinese are temporarily or permanently away from their registered addresses, and increasing socioeconomic disparities add to the likelihood of HIV spread.

Indonesia, the world's fourth most populous country, is another example of how quickly the AIDS epidemic can emerge. After more than 10 years of negligible HIV prevalence, the infection rate among IDUs, sex workers, and blood donors in some regions is rapidly increasing. In one drug treatment center in Jakarta, HIV prevalence rose from 15.4% in 2000 to more than 40% by 2002. Papua New Guinea has also reported the highest HIV infection rates among the Pacific Island countries and territories. Studies in the capital of Port Moresby showed high HIV prevalence levels in female sex workers (17%) and attendees of STD clinics (7%) in 1999. Even though the Philippines have maintained a low HIV prevalence, higher rates of STDs among Filipino sex workers, their clients, and MSM indicate low levels of condom use and the potential for rapid spread of HIV.

In some countries of Southeast Asia where HIV rose rapidly in the 1990s, strong prevention programs have limited the spread, most notably in Thailand, Cambodia, and Myanmar. Furthermore, the increased access to ART has coincided with a drastic drop in AIDS-related deaths. Despite these advances, AIDS is still a leading cause of death in Thailand, and 1.4% of the country's 63.6 million people are infected with HIV. Although STDs and heterosexual transmission have declined as a result of the government's prevention programs, HIV continues to spread rapidly among IDUs and MSM.

HIV and AIDS in Eastern Europe and Central Asia

The HIV epidemic has increased faster in eastern Europe and central Asia between 2000 and 2006 than in any other area of the world. In 2005, there were an estimated 1.5 million people living with HIV, a 20-fold increase in less than a decade. In recent years, the Russian Federation has experienced an exceptionally steep rise in reported HIV infections, 90% of which have been attributed to injecting drug use. It is estimated that nearly 1% of the young people in eastern Europe and central Asia are injecting drugs, which places these individuals and their sex partners at high risk for being infected with HIV. In one study in Moscow, secondary school students acknowledged that 4% injected drugs. In countries such as Azerbaijan, Georgia, Tajikistan, and Uzbekistan, HIV has experienced explosive growth. Similar explosive high rates of HIV are being documented among IDUs and heterosexuals at risk for STDs in other countries of the Commonwealth of Independent States, in the Baltic states, and in Romania.

In Estonia, Latvia, and Lithuania, major HIV outbreaks are also occurring in selected populations such as prison inmates. In one prison in Lithuania, 15% of inmates were HIV positive, thus confirming the role of prisons in the spread of HIV in many countries of the region. The concentration of large numbers of young people in overcrowded prisons or juvenile justice facilities, often marked by an abundance of drugs but a scarcity of HIV information, clean needles, or condoms, provides fertile ground for the rapid spread of HIV among inmates and, on their eventual release, into the wider population.

Initially driven by injecting drug use among young people, heterosexual transmission of HIV has become a prominent mode of spread in

Belarus and Ukraine. With an estimated adult HIV prevalence rate of 1.4%, Ukraine is one of the most severely affected countries in the region. Three fourths of HIV infections in Ukraine are related to injecting drug use, but the proportion of sexually transmitted infection is increasing. Although many of these infections may occur in sex partners of IDUs, the trend may also indicate spread into the wider population of these countries. Studies in Donesk, Moscow, and St. Petersburg revealed HIV prevalence rates of 13 to 17% among sex workers. In the Russian Federation in the Ukraine, up to 30% of female IDUs are also involved in commercial sex work. In Odessa, 67% of sex workers who inject drugs were HIV positive. The public health efforts to stem the tide of the epidemic in these countries are limited and, in some cases, nonexistent. In contrast, HIV prevalence remains low in Poland, the Czech Republic, Hungary, and Slovenia, where well-designed national HIV/AIDS programs are in operation. If effective interventions are not implemented in the more severely affected countries, it is likely that the situation will become dramatically worse over the next 5 years.

HIV and AIDS in Latin America and the Caribbean

An estimated 1.9 million adults and children are living with HIV in Latin America and the Caribbean. Twelve countries in this region have an estimated HIV prevalence of 1% or greater among pregnant women. In several Caribbean countries, adult HIV prevalence rates are surpassed only by the rates experienced in sub-Saharan Africa, which makes this region the second most affected in the world. Haiti remains the worst affected, with an estimated national prevalence higher than 3.8%, along with the Bahamas, where the prevalence is 3.5%.

AIDS is the leading cause of death in some countries of the Caribbean basin. In Haiti, the Bahamas, and Guyana, the number of deaths in 15- to 34-year-olds is 2.5 times higher than it would have been in the absence of AIDS. The estimated 100,000 AIDS deaths in 2005 have further increased the ranks of children orphaned by epidemics in this region. About 330,000 of the orphans are living in Latin America (130,000 of them in Brazil) and 250,000 in the Caribbean (200,000 in Haiti alone).

Homosexual and heterosexual transmission continues to be the major modes of transmission throughout the region, although there is evidence that spread of HIV is increasing through sharing of infected drug equipment. Population mobility, spurred by high rates of unemployment and poverty, is emerging as a significant factor in the epidemic's growth in this region. Central America's geographic position also makes it an important transit zone for people moving between the rest of the region and North American countries. Appropriately, protecting vulnerable populations on the move, including adolescent girls and young women, is now the focus of a regional prevention program in Central America. In Mexico, adult HIV prevalence in the wider population is still well under 1%, but prevalence rates are higher in specific population groups—6% in IDUs and 15% in MSM. There is significant overlap between IDUs and MSM, especially in Brazil and the southern Latin American countries, where injecting drug use is a growing social phenomenon. Injecting drug use is also a major route of HIV transmission in Argentina, Chile, and Uruguay.

Despite many constraints, the region has made progress in provision of treatment and care. In Brazil, an estimated 170,000 of 209,000 infected people were receiving state-sponsored treatment by the end of 2005, including 30,000 IDUs. By reducing HIV-related morbidity through treatment, Brazil's treatment and care program is estimated to have avoided 234,000 hospitalizations in a 4-year period, thereby demonstrating a cost-effective approach to care. Argentina, Costa Rica, Uruguay, and Cuba now guarantee free and universal access to drugs through the public sector, and sharp reductions have recently been secured in Honduras and Panama. Unfortunately, access to antiretrovirals remains unequal across the region, largely because of discrepancies in drug prices in different countries. Unless overcome, economic difficulties within some countries will continue to plague the region, thus facilitating further economic decline and the spread of HIV.

HIV and AIDS in Western Europe

More than 720,000 HIV-infected individuals reside in western Europe, with trends similar to those witnessed in the United States, Australia, and New Zealand. The introduction of combination ART in 1996 to 1998 has dramatically reduced HIV-related mortality, although this trend has leveled off in the past 6 years. Longer survival of people living with HIV has led to a steady increase in the number of people living with the virus in high-income countries.

The HIV epidemic in western Europe is a result of a multitude of epidemics that differ in their timing, scale, and effects on populations. A larger proportion of new HIV diagnoses in western European countries occur through heterosexual intercourse. More than half of the new HIV infections in the United Kingdom resulted through heterosexual sex, as compared with 33% in 1998. In Ireland, a similar trend is visible, with numbers of heterosexually transmitted HIV infection increasing fourfold between 1998 and 2001. Unsafe sex between men remains an important factor of spread in most European countries, particularly in the United Kingdom, Germany, Netherlands, and Spain. Injecting drug use remains a major mode of transmission in Spain, France, and Portugal, but like other countries in Europe, about a fourth of all HIV infections are now heterosexually transmitted. Most data from high-income countries demonstrate that the epidemic has shifted into the poor and marginalized sections of society. Underscoring the need for renewed prevention efforts, especially among young people, are findings of increases in high-risk behavior, less frequent condom use, and higher rates of STDs in several countries. In the United Kingdom, for example, rates of gonorrhea, syphilis, and chlamydial infections have more than doubled since 1995, and increases have been found in other western European countries as well.

HIV and AIDS in the United States

By 2005, more people than ever were living in the United States with HIV—1.2 million (see Table 410–1). Nationally, the adult HIV prevalence was estimated at 0.6%. This increase reflects mixed results in the U.S. effort to combat its epidemic. More people with HIV are living longer because of ART, but on the other hand, the early gains made on prevention have not been sustained (Fig. 410–5). The number of new recorded HIV cases in 33 states with confidential name-based reporting has varied only slightly since the late 1990s. Half of all HIV infections in men, women, and children diagnosed in 2005 were in MSM.

Another aspect of the U.S. epidemic is that more women are being infected with HIV through unprotected heterosexual exposure and injecting drug use. Overall, nearly 20% of new HIV infections are attributable to injecting drug use. The main risk factor for women who acquire HIV during sex is the risk behavior of their male partners, such as injecting drug use, commercial sex, or sex with other men. As in Latin America, women living in impoverished and marginal circumstances appear to be at disproportional risk for HIV infection. In North Carolina, HIV-positive women were considerably more likely to be unemployed, requiring public assistance, and exchanging sex for money and gifts.

As the U.S. epidemic evolves, it is becoming more an epidemic of African Americans and other minorities. African Americans make up 12% of the U.S. population but account for 50% of new HIV diagnoses. Hispanics represent 14% of the population but account for 18% of new HIV diagnoses. Among African Americans and Hispanics, most men infected with HIV were exposed during sex with other men (49% and 59%, respectively), whereas most women with HIV become infected heterosexually (78% and 73%, respectively). African American women are over 10 times more likely to be infected with HIV than white women are. AIDS continues to be the leading cause of death in African American women aged 25 to 34 years and ranks in the top three causes of death for African American men aged 25 to 54 years. African Americans are about half as likely to receive ART as other population groups, and twice as many African Americans as whites die of AIDS. In the United States, the challenge of slowing the rate of new HIV infections overlaps with the need to provide diagnosis, treatment, and care services more equitably.

With an epidemic that is nearly into its third decade, complacency has increased, and prevention efforts have dwindled as a result of declining mortality. Multiple studies illustrate that prevention efforts are not reaching the large number of at-risk individuals who engage in unsafe sex. Rates of sexually transmitted infections among MSM have been documented in the United States, Australia, Great Britain, Canada, and other developed countries. Rates of gonorrhea, syphilis, and chlamydia have more than doubled in the past 5 years among MSM in selected U.S. and European cities. Renewed efforts to enhance prevention efforts, particularly in HIV care clinics, are being echoed throughout all these countries.

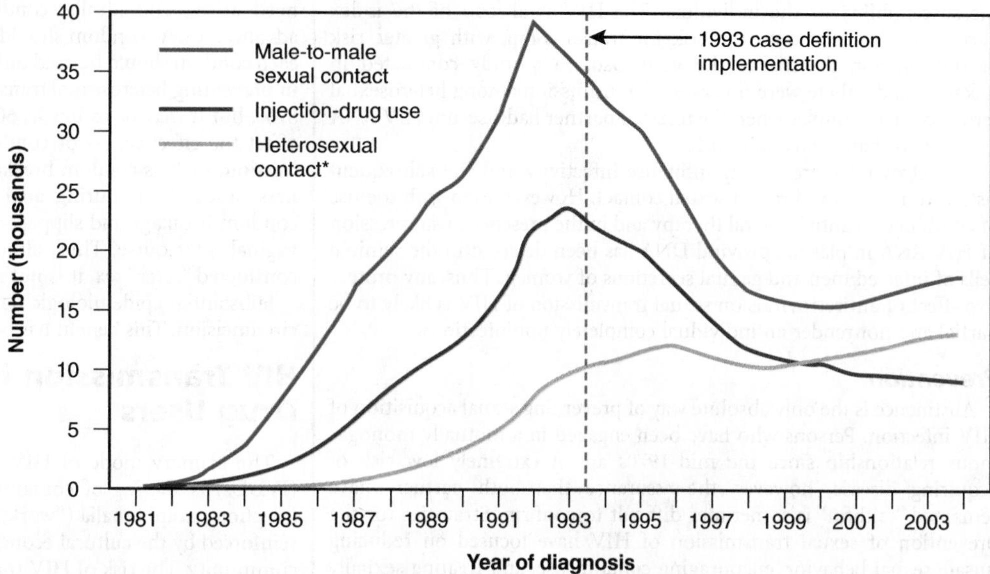

FIGURE 410–5 • Number of AIDS cases by major transmission category in the year of diagnosis for the United States, 1981 to 2004. (Data from Centers for Disease Control and Prevention, Morbidity and Mortality Weekly Report.)

SUGGESTED READINGS

Beyrer C: HIV epidemiology update and transmission factors: Risks and risk contexts—16th International AIDS Conference epidemiology plenary. Clin Infect Dis 2007;44:981–987. *An epidemiologic review.*

Centers for Disease Control and Prevention (CDC): HIV prevalence, unrecognized infection, and HIV testing among men who have sex with men—five U.S. cities, April 2004–June 2005. MMWR Morb Mortal Wkly 2005;54(24):597–601. *Provides disturbing data regarding the continuing epidemic of HIV among men who have sex with men, with evidence of a resurgence in unsafe sex practices and rising HIV incidence.*

Centers for Disease Control and Prevention: Epidemiology of HIV/AIDS—United States, 1981–2005. MMWR Morb Mortal Wkly Rep 2006;55(21):589–592. *Reviews the epidemiology and spread of HIV within the United States over a 25-year period, starting with the initial recognition of AIDS in men who have sex with men but escalating to be a leading cause of mortality in minority populations.*

Centers for Disease Control and Prevention (CDC): Racial/ethnic disparities in diagnoses of HIV/AIDS—33 states, 2001–2005. MMWR 2007;56:189–193. *Fifty-one percent of new diagnoses of HIV in this period were in African Americans.*

Schwartlander B, Grubb I, Perriens J: The 10-year struggle to provide antiretroviral treatment to people with HIV in the developing world. Lancet 2006;368:541–546. *Provides insight into the global response to provide antiretroviral therapy to all HIV-infected people living in developing countries, illustrating the challenges, the successes, and the failures.*

UNAIDS: AIDS epidemic update: December 2005. UNAIDS/05.19E. Geneva, World Health Organization, 2006. *Provides the latest statistics and epidemiologic trends for the AIDS epidemic through December 2005.*

UNAIDS: Report on the global AIDS epidemic. Joint United Nations Programme on HIV/AIDS, 06.20E, May 2006. *Provides an in-depth review of the global epidemic from 1981 through June 2006. It not only covers the statistics of the epidemics but also provides an excellent review of the impact of the epidemic on people and societies, as well as the global response.*

411 PREVENTION OF HUMAN IMMUNODEFICIENCY VIRUS INFECTION

Carlos del Rio

Prevention of human immunodeficiency virus (HIV) infection requires a thorough understanding of the epidemiology of HIV infection and knowledge of the science of human behavior. Only then can science-based prevention strategies be designed and implemented. HIV has been identified in virtually every body fluid and tissue, including blood, semen, vaginal secretions, saliva, tears, breast milk, cerebrospinal fluid, amniotic fluid, urine, and fluid obtained from bronchoalveolar lavage. In most instances, the virus resides in lymphocytes present within body fluids; therefore, any fluid that contains lymphocytes could theoretically be implicated in spread of the virus. Nonetheless, no cases of HIV transmission have been documented through any body fluids except blood and fluids grossly contaminated with blood, semen, vaginal secretions, and breast milk. HIV has also been transmitted through transplanted organs, including kidney, liver, heart, pancreas, and bone.

A number of preventive interventions have been evaluated and proved to reduce HIV-associated risk behavior across a variety of populations. In general, these programs are theory driven and emphasize the development of cognitive, social, and technical skills associated with safer sex and drug use practices. In addition, many of these interventions are clearly cost-effective and, if implemented, would dramatically change the course of the epidemic. For example, a review of studies on preventive interventions for HIV/acquired immunodeficiency syndrome (AIDS) in Africa has shown that targeted condom distribution, blood screening, administration of nevirapine to prevent mother-to-child transmission, and treatment of sexually transmitted infections are all cost-effective. The advent of antiretroviral therapy has resulted in new challenges in the field of HIV prevention, and concern about reports of an upsurge in sexually transmitted infections among people known to be infected with HIV has resulted in new guidelines for the incorporation of HIV prevention into the medical care of HIV-infected persons.

MODES OF HIV TRANSMISSION AND PREVENTION

Sexual Transmission

HIV infection is a sexually transmitted disease (STD). Like other STDs, HIV spreads bidirectionally and appears to be more efficiently transmitted from male to female. The per-act risk for acquisition of HIV has been estimated to be 5 per 10,000 for insertive unprotected penile-vaginal intercourse to 50 per 10,000 for receptive unprotected anal intercourse. Sexual contact is the predominant mode of HIV transmission throughout the world. However, the geographic distribution of cases attributable to homosexual or heterosexual transmission varies markedly. In the United States, most sexually transmitted cases reported have occurred through male homosexual activity, and heterosexual transmission accounts for a smaller, albeit growing proportion of cases. In contrast, heterosexual transmission is the leading mode of transmission worldwide and is the primary mode of disease acquisition in Africa. Sexual transmission of HIV is relatively inefficient, but behavioral and biologic factors influence the likelihood of HIV transmission in a given sexual encounter. In particular, the coexistence of an STD (most notably the presence of genital ulcerative disease) greatly increases the infectiousness as well as the susceptibility of the individual. The HIV viral load of the index partner is also related to the risk for transmission, with greater risk of transmission the higher the viral load. In a study conducted in Rakai, Uganda, there were no cases of transmission among heterosexual serodiscordant couples when the infected partner had a serum HIV RNA level of less than 1500 copies/mL.

Antiretroviral therapy may influence infectivity and the subsequent risk of transmission through sexual contact. However, even with the use of combination antiretroviral therapy and in the presence of suppression of HIV RNA in plasma, proviral DNA has been detected in the seminal cells of infected men and genital secretions of women. Thus, any protective effect of antiretrovirals on sexual transmission of HIV is likely to be partial and not render an individual completely noninfectious.

Prevention

Abstinence is the only absolute way of preventing sexual acquisition of HIV infection. Persons who have been engaged in a mutually monogamous relationship since the mid-1970s are at extremely low risk of acquiring disease; however, the assurance that both partners have remained "faithful" is sometimes difficult to confirm. Strategies for the prevention of sexual transmission of HIV have focused on reducing unsafe sexual behavior, encouraging condom use, and treating sexually transmitted infections. Gender-tailored, culturally congruent behavioral interventions can reduce transmission to uninfected females. 1

In situations in which a decision to engage in sexual activity has been made and the HIV status of the partner is positive, unknown, or in doubt, safe sexual practices ("safe sex") should be implemented (Table 411–1). Mutual masturbation is considered "safe," assuming that it is nontraumatic and not followed by the ingestion of body fluids such as semen or vaginal secretions. Transmission of HIV has never been documented to occur through saliva; however, no group of patients has ever been studied who engage in deep "French" kissing as their sole means of sexual activity. Because HIV exists in saliva, albeit in very low titer, deep French kissing cannot be considered absolutely safe, even though the likelihood of HIV transmission is extremely low. Condom use is the most effective means of preventing HIV infection among individuals who engage in oral, vaginal, or anal intercourse. Consistent use of latex condoms has been shown to be effective in the prevention of HIV transmission at both an individual and population level. Multiple epidemiologic studies of heterosexual couples in which one partner is HIV positive and the other is HIV negative indicate that correct and consistent use of condoms can significantly reduce transmission of HIV and other STDs.

To be effective, however, the condom should be made of latex and must be used properly. Natural skin condoms should not be used because they do not prevent HIV transmission. Nonoxynol 9, a spermicide with some antiviral activity, enhances the protective effects of condoms and should be used in conjunction with condoms as a spermicidal jelly or impregnated into the latex condom itself. Petroleum-based lubricants enhance the likelihood of rupture of latex condoms and should be avoided. If needed, water-based lubricants such as K-Y jelly should be used.

Both partners should be knowledgeable about the correct use of condoms. Discussions regarding condom use should occur before the need arises, and ideally, condom placement should be practiced in advance. A new condom should be used for each act of intercourse, and each condom should be used only one time. The effectiveness of condoms in preventing heterosexual transmission of HIV has been estimated to be 87%, but it may be as low as 60% or as high as 96%. Many factors can affect the effectiveness of condoms in reducing the risk of HIV transmission, such as condom breakage, leakage, and slippage. The effectiveness of condoms during anal intercourse is probably lower because condom breakage and slippage may be considerably higher than during vaginal intercourse. Thus, although condom use during intercourse is considered "safer" sex, it is not absolutely safe.

Substantial epidemiologic data support a protective benefit for male circumcision. This benefit has been confirmed in a randomized trial. 2

TABLE 411–1 SAFE AND UNSAFE SEXUAL PRACTICES IN ORDER OF 'SURENESS' OF SAFETY

SAFE
Abstinence
Monogamous relationship with a confirmed seronegative partner
Manual sex (manual masturbation)
Kissing
Intercourse with a latex condom (used in combination with nonoxynol 9)
UNSAFE
Intercourse with a "natural skin" condom
Intercourse with a latex condom lubricated with petroleum-based lubricants
Unprotected oral-genital sex
Unprotected vaginal intercourse
Unprotected anal intercourse

HIV Transmission in Intravenous Drug Users

The primary mode of HIV transmission in intravenous drug users (IVDUs) is sharing of contaminated needles and syringes. Sharing of injection paraphernalia ("works") is commonplace among IVDUs and is reinforced by the cultural economic and legal environment in the IVDU community. The risk of HIV transmission is highest among IVDUs who share needles and use drugs that are injected more often, such as cocaine. HIV is frequently transmitted from IVDUs to their sexual partners through heterosexual and homosexual activity, and ultimately, the virus may be transmitted to their children through perinatal exposure. Many cases of heterosexual transmission, including transmission from prostitutes, are associated with intravenous drug use.

Prevention

The primary mode of preventing HIV transmission in IVDUs is to stop the use of intravenous drugs in the first place. Education programs that are culturally sensitive and geared to young audiences have the best chance of preventing drug use. Access to treatment centers is the best approach for individuals already using intravenous drugs. However, approximately 80% of active drug users in the United States are not in substance abuse treatment because of either choice or the unavailability of treatment centers. For IVDUs who do not wish to seek treatment or who are unable to gain access to treatment, the most effective way to prevent HIV infection is to avoid sharing needles and works. Where works are in short supply, needles and syringes should be cleaned after each use, preferably with readily accessible virucidal cleansers such as chlorine bleach (diluted 1:10). Some communities have adopted programs that provide free needles and syringes for IVDUs, and there is strong evidence that these programs, when implemented properly, are effective in reducing HIV transmission and do not result in increased drug use among participants. Voluntary HIV testing and outreach programs that rigorously maintain confidentiality can be effective in reducing transmission to sexual partners of IVDUs. To be effective, antibody testing should be combined with intensive pretest and post-test counseling.

The efficacy of many community programs is limited, however, by cultural barriers, including lack of trust, fear of prosecution, misconceptions regarding the prevalence of HIV infection within the local drug-using population, and the use of ineffective language in delivering anti-HIV messages by program staff. When combined with the relative paucity of intravenous drug treatment resources, HIV education among IVDUs that ultimately results in behavioral changes remains a challenging HIV prevention goal.

Transmission of HIV through Blood Products and Other Tissues

HIV has been transmitted through the transfusion of single-donor blood and blood products, including whole blood, fresh-frozen plasma, packed red blood cells, cryoprecipitate, clotting factors, and platelets. Before May 1985, when the Red Cross began testing the blood supply for evidence of HIV antibodies, 0.04% of 1,200,000 donations in the United States were estimated to be HIV positive and an estimated 29,000 blood or blood product recipients were exposed to HIV. Because many died of underlying conditions for which the transfusion was required, only an estimated 10,000 to 12,000 individuals who received blood products from HIV-infected donors survived long enough for AIDS to develop. Confidential donor exclusion, as well as the institution of HIV antibody screening in 1985, followed by additional testing for antibodies to HIV-2 and p24 antigen in 1996 and nucleic acid testing in 2002, has reduced the risk of HIV infection through the transfusion of blood or blood products to approximately 1 in 2,135,000.

HIV transmission by liver, heart, kidney, pancreas, bone, and possibly skin transplantation has been reported. In contrast, relatively avascular tissues such as corneas and processed tissues have not been associated with transmission.

Prevention

Aggressive efforts by the American Red Cross have greatly reduced the risk of HIV transmission through transfusion in the United States. Voluntary self-deferral of donors at risk for HIV acquisition in the community was initiated in 1983. The effectiveness of self-deferral is limited, however, by social pressures. Some high-risk individuals may view blood donation as a means of being tested for HIV and provide erroneous screening information to receive free, confidential evaluation of their HIV status. Other at-risk individuals may be coerced to participate in blood donation drives at work. Potentially infected donors may feel uncomfortable excusing themselves from donation and provide false information on screening to avoid possible disclosure of a high-risk lifestyle to their coworkers. Self-deferral programs are most effective when free, voluntary testing centers are readily available elsewhere in the community and when blood drives encourage potential donors to come to donation centers by themselves and not in groups.

The institution of HIV antibody testing of donated blood and blood products in 1985 has had the most dramatic effect on lowering the incidence of transfusion-related transmission. When combined with voluntary self-deferral and nucleic acid testing, the blood supply has become relatively free of HIV. Heat inactivation processes for cryoprecipitate and clotting factor concentrates have virtually eliminated transmission of HIV through use of these products. Other products, such as immune globulin preparations and hepatitis B vaccines, are produced by methods that inactivate HIV and have never been associated with transmission of HIV.

Organ and tissue donors should be evaluated and serologically screened in a manner similar to blood donors. In addition, donations of semen and bone from a living donor may be quarantined until subsequent testing has definitively ruled out the possibility of delayed seroconversion in the donor.

Transmission of HIV to Health Care Workers

Transmission of HIV in the health care delivery setting has been the subject of intense investigation throughout the course of the epidemic. The percentage of health care workers with AIDS who have "no identified risk" for HIV infection has remained low (<10%) and has not increased over time despite the dramatic increase in the number of AIDS cases and concomitant exposure of health care workers to patients with HIV disease. More importantly, detailed studies examining the risk of specific exposures, such as needlestick injuries and mucous membrane exposure, have demonstrated very low risk of disease acquisition in the workplace. More than 3628 health care workers have been prospectively examined in carefully designed surveillance studies at 10 high-incidence medical centers. The overall risk of seroconversion after a percutaneous needlestick from a known HIV-positive source is 0.3% per exposure. Percutaneous injury, usually inflicted by a hollow-bore needle, is the most common mechanism of occupational HIV transmission. In a retrospective study conducted by the Centers for Disease Control and Prevention (CDC) it was found that the risk of transmission of HIV to health care workers was increased when the device causing the injury was visibly contaminated with blood, when the device had been used for insertion into a vein or artery, when the device caused a deep injury, or when the source patient died within 2 months after the exposure. Although mucous membrane exposure to HIV-positive blood has resulted in seroconversion in at least five health care workers, the risk of transmission is estimated to be 0.09%. No transmission has occurred after exposure to body fluids other than blood or fluids heavily contaminated with blood. Although the potential for HIV transmission to health care providers clearly exists, the risk of infection is inherently low and can be further minimized by following routine precautions to prevent transmission.

Prevention

In August 1987, the CDC published guidelines designed to minimize health care worker exposure to blood and body fluids that may be infected with blood-borne pathogens such as HIV. The guidelines, updated in June 2001 (available at *http://www.aidsinfo.nih.gov/guidelines/*), remain the principal mode of HIV prevention among health care workers today. These so-called universal precautions are based on the premise that any patient may be infected with blood-borne infectious agents and it may be difficult, if not impossible, to differentiate those with infection from their uninfected counterparts. All specimens containing blood or blood-tinged fluids obtained from *any* patient should be considered hazardous and handled as such (Table 411–2).

TABLE 411–2 SUMMARY OF UNIVERSAL PRECAUTIONS
Specimens, including blood, blood products, and body fluids, obtained from all patients should be considered hazardous and potentially infected with transmissible agents.
Handwashing should be performed before and after patient contact, after removing gloves, and immediately if hands are grossly contaminated with blood.
Gloves should be worn when hands are likely to come in contact with blood or body fluids.
Gowns, protective eyewear, and masks should be worn when splashing, splattering, or aerosolization of blood or body fluids is likely to occur.
Sharp objects ("sharps") should be handled with great care and disposed of in impervious receptacles.
Needles should never be manipulated, bent, broken, or recapped.
Blood spills should be handled by initial absorption of the spill with disposable towels, cleaning the area with soap and water, followed by disinfecting area with a 1:10 solution of household bleach.
Contaminated reusable equipment should be decontaminated by heat sterilization or, when heat is impractical, with a mycobactericidal cleanser.
Pocket masks or mechanical ventilation devices should be available in areas where cardiopulmonary resuscitation procedures are likely.
Health care workers with open lesions or weeping dermatitis should avoid direct patient contact and should not handle contaminated equipment.
Private rooms are not required for routine care; select circumstances, however, such as the presence of a concomitant transmissible opportunistic disease, may warrant respiratory, enteric, or contact isolation.

Handwashing is the cornerstone of universal precautions, as it is with all infection control practices. Gloves should be worn when spillage of blood or body fluids is likely. Gloves should *never* be washed and should be changed after soiling or after gross contamination, with handwashing immediately after the gloves are removed. Handwashing may be performed with soap and water or with the use of commercially available alcohol-based cleansing gels. Gowns, protective eyewear, and masks are not usually needed except in circumstances in which splattering or splashing of blood-containing fluids is likely to occur. Masks should always be worn in situations in which eyewear is required. Reusable equipment should be cleaned of visible organic material, placed in an impervious bag, and returned to central supply for decontamination. Although heat is the single best decontamination method, chemical agents that possess mycobactericidal activity are effective against hepatitis B virus and HIV and are acceptable alternatives when heat inactivation is impractical. Blood spills should be cleaned with appropriate caution. After putting on gloves and using other appropriate barrier precautions, excess blood should be removed with absorbent materials (e.g., paper towels) and the area then cleaned with soap and water and disinfected with a 1:10 solution of sodium hypochlorite (i.e., household bleach) and water. Health care workers with denuded skin, open lesions, or active dermatitis should avoid direct patient contact and should not process contaminated equipment or materials. Private rooms are not generally required for patients known to be HIV infected unless a concomitant opportunistic disease is present that requires respiratory, enteric, or contact isolation. Food service should be provided as usual on reusable dishware.

Because *all* blood and body fluids should be handled as being potentially hazardous and *all* patients presumed to be infected, it makes little sense to identify infected patients or their specimens with "blood and body fluid" labels. The use of such labels on known infected patients implies that unlabeled specimens or specimens from patients of unknown status are less hazardous and may be handled with less care. Studies have shown that more than half of specimens containing antibodies to hepatitis B surface antigen or HIV went to the laboratory unlabeled.

Handling of sharp instruments ("sharps") represents the greatest risk of HIV transmission to health care workers. Although injuries from sharps cannot be entirely eliminated, the number of exposures can be reduced substantially by adhering to guidelines put forth in universal precautions. Before a sharp instrument is used, thought should be given to where the instrument will be disposed after use. Impervious containers should be readily available in all patient care areas and identified by the health care worker *before* the use of sharps. These containers should be checked frequently and should not be allowed to overfill. Used needles should never be manipulated, bent, broken, or recapped. Recapping of needles is the single most common activity that results in needlestick injuries. Technologic developments that do not rely on health care worker compliance such as self-sheathing needles have also been important in decreasing the risk of needlestick injury.

Despite their logical basis and relative ease of implementation, universal precautions have not been used routinely by many health care providers. Studies have shown that more than 50% of health care workers engage in inadequate infection control practices, even in high-impact AIDS centers, and up to 40% of needlestick exposures were judged to be preventable. Although lack of adequate education may partly explain these findings, implementation of infection control practices has generally been poor historically. Between 200 and 400 health care workers die each year as a result of hepatitis B acquired on the job. The use of universal precautions helps minimize the transmission of many transmissible diseases in addition to HIV.

Even in the best of circumstances, accidental mucous membrane and percutaneous exposure to blood from HIV-infected patients does occur. Each institution and health care facility should adopt procedures for managing such exposure based on guidelines published by the CDC (see Suggested Readings). The essential elements of management after needlestick or mucous membrane exposure include defining the type of exposure, appropriately evaluating the donor (patient) and recipient (health care worker) at the time of exposure, and providing follow-up of the health care worker for at least 1 year after exposure.

Proposed definitions of the types of exposure are summarized in Table 411–3. Health care workers with any kind of parenteral exposure should be counseled and evaluated for possible acquisition of HIV and should receive routine prophylaxis against hepatitis B virus. The source patient (donor) should be evaluated for HIV infection; if the donor's HIV status is unknown, the donor should be informed about the incident and encouraged to allow voluntary, confidential screening of blood for HIV and hepatitis B antibody. If a patient refuses or cannot give consent, that patient should be considered to be infected. In cases in which exposure to HIV is documented or presumed to have occurred, the health care worker should be evaluated serologically for the presence of HIV as soon as possible after the exposure (baseline) and again at 6 weeks, 12 weeks, 24 weeks, and 1 year after the exposure to determine whether HIV transmission has occurred. The health care worker should report any acute illnesses that occur during the follow-up period, especially during the first 6 to 12 weeks after exposure. Exposed workers should follow the recommended guidelines for preventing HIV transmission, including using safe sexual practices; refraining from blood, semen, and organ donation; and avoiding breast-feeding. If the source patient is seronegative for HIV and has no clinical manifestations of HIV disease, no further follow-up of the exposed health care workers is necessary, although some workers prefer follow-up for their own peace of mind. Serologic testing should be made available to all health care workers who are concerned about potential on-the-job exposure.

For occupational exposure to HIV among health care workers, the CDC recommended in 1990 the use of zidovudine for postexposure prophylaxis. This recommendation was further supported by a case-control study in which it was shown that the risk of HIV seroconversion after occupational exposure was decreased by approximately 81% with the use of zidovudine. Subsequent recommendations have incorporated the newer antiretroviral drugs, as well as risk stratification for the type of exposure, in the management of occupational exposure to HIV. The current CDC recommendations are different, depending on the type of exposure and the clinical status of the source patient. For less severe exposures (e.g., a solid needle or a superficial injury), two nucleosides are recommended (e.g., zidovudine and lamivudine). For more severe exposures (e.g., large-bore hollow needle, deep puncture, visible blood in the device, or a needle used in a patient's artery or vein), a regimen that includes

TABLE 411–3 CDC RECOMMENDATIONS FOR POSTEXPOSURE PROPHYLAXIS (PEP) FOR PERCUTANEOUS AND MUCOUS MEMBRANE EXPOSURE TO HIV

Exposure Type	HIV Positive, Class 1*	HIV Positive, Class 2†	HIV Status or Source Unknown	HIV Negative
Percutaneous exposure: less severe (e.g., solid needlestick)	Recommend basic 2-drug PEP‡	Recommend expanded ≥3-drug PEP	No PEP, but should consider 2-drug PEP if source has HIV risk factors	No PEP
Percutaneous exposure: more severe (e.g., large-bore hollow needlestick)	Recommend expanded 3-drug PEP‡	Recommend expanded ≥3-drug PEP	No PEP, but should consider 2-drug PEP if source has HIV risk factors	No PEP
Mucous membrane exposure: small volume (e.g., few droplets)§	Consider basic 2-drug PEP¶	Recommend basic 2-drug PEP	Generally no PEP warranted	No PEP
Mucous membrane exposure: large volume (e.g., major blood splash or prolonged contact)	Recommend basic 2-drug PEP	Recommend expanded ≥3-drug PEP	Generally no PEP warranted, but should consider 2-drug PEP if source has HIV risk factors	No PEP

*Asymptomatic patient with HIV infection, low viral load (<1500 copies/mL). If drug resistance is suspected, obtain expert consultation regarding the choice of antiretroviral regimen. PEP should not be delayed while awaiting consultation.
†Symptomatic patient with HIV, high viral load (>1500 copies/mL), AIDS, or acute seroconversion syndrome.
‡Basic PEP refers to dual nucleoside therapy (e.g., zidovudine plus lamivudine); expanded PEP includes dual nucleosides combined with a potent protease inhibitor (such as lopinavir-ritonavir). PEP should be discontinued if the source patient is later determined to be HIV negative.
§Body fluids considered to be potentially infectious include blood, blood products, cerebrospinal fluid, amniotic fluid, menstrual discharge, inflammatory exudates, pleural fluid, peritoneal fluid, pericardial fluid, and any fluid visibly contaminated with blood. All other fluids are considered noninfectious.
¶Consider PEP indicates that PEP is optional and should be individualized for each situation based on the nature of the exposure and the opinion of the exposed health care worker and the treating clinician.
Adapted from Henderson D, Gerberding J: Occupational and nonoccupational exposure management. *In* Dolin R, Masur H, Saag M (eds): AIDS Therapy, 2nd ed. New York, Churchill-Livingstone, 2003, pp 327–346; and Panlilo AL, Cardo DM, Grohskopf LA, et al: Updated U.S. Public Health Service guidelines for the management of occupational exposures to HIV and recommendations for postexposure prophylaxis. MMRW Recomm Rep 2005;54(RR-9):1–17.

three antiretrovirals is recommended (e.g., zidovudine, lamivudine. and lopinavir/ritonavir). Postexposure prophylaxis should be initiated as soon as possible, preferably within hours of exposure, and administered for 4 weeks.

The U.S. Public Health Service has established a National Clinicians' Post-Exposure Prophylaxis Hotline (PEPline) to provide expert consultation about the management of health care workers with potential HIV exposure. The PEPline can be accessed at 1-888-448-4911 or through the Internet at *http://www.ucsf.edu/hivcntr/Hotlines/PEPline.*

Transmission from Infected Health Care Workers to Their Patients

Transmission of HIV from a health care worker to patients has been documented in two instances: in a dental practice in Florida and from an orthopedic surgeon in France. The Florida cluster of cases was reported in July 1990. Six patients are believed to have acquired infection from the dentist based on the absence of other risk factors in the patients and the high degree of homology between the virus isolated from the dentist and those isolated from the patients. Although each patient underwent an invasive procedure in the dental office, the precise mode of transmission remains unknown. Aside from these two instances, investigation of 22,759 patients of 53 other HIV-infected health care workers has not identified other episodes of transmission of HIV from health care worker to patient.

Two patients undergoing nuclear medicine procedures have been reported to have been infected through inadvertent intravenous injection of blood or other material from HIV-infected patients. In addition, transmission of HIV through percutaneous or mucocutaneous exposure to blood or other body substances has occurred in homes in which health care has been provided. Transmission of HIV from patient to patient through improper sterilization or reuse of contaminated needles and syringes has been reported in Romania and the former Soviet Union. Routine use of universal precautions should minimize the risk of transmission from HIV-infected patients to health care providers and vice versa.

PREVENTION INTERVENTIONS FOR HIV-POSITIVE INDIVIDUALS

Increases in high-risk sex practices and STDs among HIV-infected individuals have prompted considerable concern over increased risk of transmission of HIV infection and have led to initiatives to increase STD screening and risk reduction measures in the HIV-infected population. The available evidence indicates that risk reduction counseling is effective, and improved attention to risk reduction counseling in the HIV medical care setting is needed. The CDC 2006 STD treatment guidelines (see Suggested Readings) recommend that all patients with newly diagnosed HIV infection undergo screening for gonorrhea, chlamydial infection, hepatitis B and C virus infection, and syphilis. Screening for curable STDs (gonorrhea, chlamydial infection, and syphilis) should be performed at least annually in sexually active patients. The CDC, Health Resources and Services Administration, National Institutes of Health, and Infectious Diseases Society of America have also published joint recommendations for incorporating HIV prevention into the HIV medical care setting. These guidelines reflect four basic priorities: (1) screening for risky behavior and STDs, (2) providing general and tailored risk reduction messages to patients, (3) when indicated, referring patients for additional risk reduction services and other services that may affect risk reduction (e.g., substance abuse treatment), and (4) ensuring that patients are provided with partner counseling and referral services.

VACCINE DEVELOPMENT

Education and behavior modification are the only means of HIV prevention currently available. During the past few years, significant effort has been directed toward the development of an effective vaccine against HIV. Although substantial progress has been achieved, several obstacles remain. Despite enormous advances in understanding the immunopathogenesis of HIV infection, the precise mechanism of protective immunity remains unknown. Without such knowledge, it is difficult to develop vaccines that ensure targeting the appropriate arm of the immune system that confers long-term protective immunity. Another obstacle is the lack of correlation of data from animal models to the potential protective effects of vaccines in humans. Although vaccine research has been continuing for many years, it was only recently that results of the first phase III efficacy trial with a candidate vaccine were reported. Unfortunately, this study showed lack of efficacy of an envelope gp120 vaccine. Over the next few years, more than 30 clinical trials of candidate HIV vaccines will be taking place in different parts of the world, yet the prospects for an effective vaccine that will be simple enough to allow its implementation in developing countries where the impact of AIDS is most severe are not promising. Thus, even when an effective vaccine is developed, education will remain the cornerstone of HIV prevention.

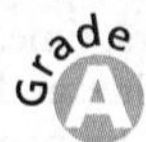

1. DiClemente RJ, Wingood GM, Harrington KF, et al: Efficacy of an HIV prevention intervention for African American adolescent girls: A randomized controlled trial. JAMA 2004;292:202–209.
2. Gray RH, Kigozi G, Serwadda D, et al: Male circumcision for HIV prevention in men in Rakai, Uganda: A randomised trial. Lancet 2007;369:657–666.

SUGGESTED READINGS

Balzarini J, Van Damme L: Microbicide drug candidates to prevent HIV infection. Lancet 2007;369:787–797. *Given the current lack of availability of antiretroviral drugs in developing countries, low-cost microbicides to prevent sexually transmitted HIV infections should be given high priority.*

Centers for Disease Control and Prevention: Updated U.S. Public Health Service guidelines for the management of occupational exposures to HIV and recommendations for postexposure prophylaxis. MMWR Recomm Rep 2005;54(RR-9):1–17. *A comprehensive summary of guidelines for the management of health care worker exposure to HIV. A "must" for employee health and infection control counselors. Extensive reference list.*

Chou R, Huffman LH, Fu R, et al: Screening for HIV: A review of the evidence for the U.S. Preventive Services Task Force. Ann Intern Med 2005;143:55–73. *Benefits of HIV screening appear to outweigh harm, with the highest yield coming from screening higher-prevalence populations.*

Gray RH, Wawer MJ, Brookmeyer R, et al: Probability of HIV-1 transmission per coital act in monogamous, heterosexual, HIV-1–discordant couples in Rakai, Uganda. Lancet 2001;357:1149–1153. *A carefully performed study demonstrating the likelihood of transmission to be 0.01 to 0.2% per coital act, depending on the plasma viral load.*

Koblin BA, Chesney MA, Husnik MJ, et al: for the EXPLORE Study Team: High-risk behaviors among men who have sex with men in 6 US cities: Baseline data from the EXPLORE Study. Am J Public Health 2003;93:926–932. *About half the men reported unprotected receptive and insertive anal sex in the previous 6 months, with alcohol and drug use being associated with this risky behavior.*

Pradier C, Bentz L, Spire B, et al: Efficacy of an educational and counseling intervention on adherence to highly active antiretroviral therapy: French prospective controlled study. HIV Clin Trials 2003;4:121–131. *This simple program improved adherence to HAART.*

412 TREATMENT OF HUMAN IMMUNODEFICIENCY VIRUS INFECTION AND ACQUIRED IMMUNODEFICIENCY SYNDROME

Henry Masur, Letha Healey, and Colleen Hadigan

HISTORY

When the first cases of acquired immunodeficiency syndrome (AIDS) were recognized in the United States in the late 1970s, strategies for patient management focused on prompt diagnosis and treatment of opportunistic infections. Clinicians recognized that this strategy resulted in short survival. The median time to death after the first AIDS-defining opportunistic process was about 9 months, and most patients died within 2 years of this initial opportunistic process. By the mid-1980s, there was growing enthusiasm for chemoprophylaxis against the most common opportunistic infections, although at that time trimethoprim-sulfamethoxazole (TMP-SMX) was the only agent marketed that seemed to be useful. TMP-SMX prophylaxis was found to be protective against *Pneumocystis jiroveci* pneumonia (PCP) and against toxoplasmosis and certain bacterial infections. TMP-SMX chemoprophylaxis was highly effective in preventing opportunistic complications and prolonging survival. Chemoprophylaxis against *Mycobacterium avium* complex and improved survival became feasible when rifabutin and then clarithromycin and azithromycin were developed. Chemoprophylaxis against *Mycobacterium tuberculosis* was also shown to prolong survival in high-prevalence areas.

With the licensing of zidovudine in 1987, treatment of the underlying retroviral cause of immunosuppression became possible for the first time. Monotherapy with nucleosides (zidovudine, didanosine, zalcitabine, and stavudine) in that era slowed the immunologic decline caused by human immunodeficiency virus (HIV), reduced the number of HIV-related opportunistic infections, and prolonged survival. The combination of anti-infective chemoprophylaxis and nucleoside antiretroviral therapy (ART) represented a multifaceted approach to improving the quality and duration of survival. The antiviral and immunologic-enhancing effects of the early nucleoside agents were modest in potency, however, and lacked durability. Within 6 to 18 months, nucleoside-resistant virus developed in many patients. As patients' viral loads returned to their pre–nucleoside therapy levels, CD4$^+$ T-lymphocyte counts began to decline, and patients again became susceptible to opportunistic processes.

The development of more potent ART agents in the mid-1990s, and the recognition that combination therapy was more effective than monotherapy, led to regimens that provided more potent and durable virologic and immunologic effects and better clinical benefit. These regimens have been a major advance in the management of patients infected with HIV who have access to medical care and who are capable and willing to take these drugs. Given their toxicity and their inconvenience, taking these drugs has been no small challenge for patients in every social and economic stratum. For many patients who can tolerate and adhere to these regimens, the quality and duration of survival have improved dramatically. The development of combination regimens formulated into once-daily single-tablet formulations has been a major development in terms of facilitating administration.

Current strategies focus on determining how to develop a regimen for an individual patient that has durable efficacy and safety (i.e., how to maximize the likelihood that the patient will have prolonged survival free of disease-related or drug-related complications). These strategies depend on early recognition of HIV infection (i.e., before the occurrence of severe immunosuppression or devastating clinical events) and access to a full range of adequate medical services. Such strategies require determination of which drug regimens are proven to be durably safe and effective. These approaches also require individualization of regimens to maximize the likelihood of long-term patient adherence and minimize the likelihood that drug toxicity or drug interactions will adversely affect the quality or duration of the patient's survival.

TREATMENT

Treatment of HIV and AIDS can be organized into three major areas: (1) ART, (2) prophylaxis for opportunistic infections, and (3) treatment of HIV-related complications. These treatments need to be used with the goal of preventing HIV-related complications with as little disruption as possible in the patient's lifestyle and treating complications when they occur expeditiously, before they become debilitating or life-threatening.

Antiretroviral Therapy

ART should be initiated before sufficient immunologic decline develops in HIV-infected patients to place them at substantially increased risk for HIV-related complications. Although this general approach is a logical principle for therapy, it is difficult to put into practice. Many patients do not recognize the utility of being screened for HIV infection if they engage in high-risk behavior. Many continue to come to medical attention for the first time when acute PCP or cryptococcal meningitis develops and their CD4$^+$ T-lymphocyte counts are already low (e.g., <200 cells/mL). Public health strategies that emphasize widespread testing are a logical approach to reducing transmission in the United States, as well as in other nations.

For patients who do come to medical attention when their CD4$^+$ T-lymphocyte counts are still relatively high, clinicians must realize that although the CD4$^+$ T-lymphocyte count is a reliable indicator of susceptibility to opportunistic infections, susceptibility is a continuum and the CD4$^+$ T-lymphocyte thresholds at which susceptibility to specific opportunistic infections begins are only approximations. Waiting to start ART until the CD4$^+$ T-lymphocyte count is 200 cells/mL does not guarantee that PCP will be prevented because 5 to 10% of cases of PCP occur at CD4$^+$ T-lymphocyte counts greater than 200 cells/mL and some cases occur at counts of 400 to 500 cells/mL. Other opportunistic processes, such as pneumococcal pneumonia, tuberculosis, Kaposi's sarcoma, and lymphoma, can occur with enhanced incidence at any CD4$^+$ T-lymphocyte count. At every CD4$^+$ T-lymphocyte count, HIV-infected patients have some increased risk for opportunistic infection. The issue for the health care provider and the patient to address is the point at which susceptibility to infection increases sufficiently to warrant the toxicity, inconvenience, drug interactions, and cost of ART.

Susceptibility can be assessed by factors other than the CD4$^+$ T-lymphocyte count alone. Plasma HIV viral load and a history of any HIV-related complication are factors that should be part of the equation to determine susceptibility to immunologic progression and clinical complications. Other laboratory parameters, such as the cytotoxic T-lymphocyte count, in vitro assays of lymphocyte function, and cytomegalovirus (CMV) plasma viral load, predict susceptibility to opportunistic infections, but it is less clear how to use these assays to make clinical decisions.

ART is not likely to be effective unless the patient is committed and able to adhere to the ART regimen and the clinician is skilled at managing the regimen. Studies have shown that the likelihood of achieving a durable virologic response (i.e., plasma viral load below the limit of detection of the assay system used) depends on adherence. There is a direct relationship between missing doses of the ART regimen and the development of HIV drug resistance. If a patient is not fully invested in taking the drugs regularly or is unable to adhere because of psychiatric, social, economic, or medical issues, initiation of ART may not be indicated. Active drug and alcohol abuse, mental illness, including depression, concomitant medical problems, poor clinician-patient relationship, history of drug toxicity, and fear of drug toxicity are strong predictors of poor adherence. Directly observed therapy can be a successful strategy for improving adherence, but this approach is not practical in most settings. The success of directly observed therapy programs, however, emphasizes the importance of regimen adherence to a durable virologic and immunologic response.

Successful management of HIV therapy also requires an experienced clinician. In the 1980s there was considerable emphasis on "mainstreaming" HIV-infected patients (i.e., encouraging general internists, family practitioners, and a variety of other primary care providers to care for patients with HIV infection). Since that era, management has become dramatically more complex. Studies show that clinicians with experience are more likely to follow current standards and guidelines than clinicians with less experience are. When feasible, patients should be managed by clinicians who have considerable experience and the capacity to keep abreast of the rapidly evolving field.

Principles of Antiretroviral Therapy

Most experts recommend that a major goal of ART should be complete inhibition of HIV replication. Inhibition of viral replication should prevent HIV-related immunologic decline and promote immune reconstitution. Proviral HIV integrates into host cells in a latent form, however. The absence of detectable plasma viral RNA does not indicate that no virus is present: virus may be present in plasma at levels below the detection capability of the laboratory assay; virus may be present in body compartments other than blood, such as lymphoid tissue or the central nervous system (CNS); and provirus may be present in a variety of cells that can act as reservoirs for HIV, such as memory T cells. Long-term inability to detect plasma HIV RNA does not ensure eradication of the virus. This concept is supported by the observation that if ART is discontinued in treated patients who have had no detectable virus for several years, plasma HIV RNA levels virtually always return to pretherapy levels within a few weeks of stopping therapy.

HIV has an extremely high mutation rate. Resistance to therapeutic agents can emerge rapidly, especially when viral loads are high. Resistance to reverse transcriptase inhibitors is associated with amino acid substitutions in the reverse transcriptase enzyme. Resistance to protease inhibitors is associated with amino acid substitutions in the protease enzyme. Chemically important resistance can occasionally occur in untreated patients as a result of spontaneous mutations. For some drugs, a single mutation can produce clinically important resistance. For other drugs, significant resistance occurs only if several mutations take place. Most clinically important resistance, however, occurs as a result of selective pressure from ART. This resistance can be assessed by genotypic and phenotypic assays. It can emerge rapidly; for example, with nevirapine monotherapy, resistance can emerge within the first few days of treatment. Resistance can even emerge after a single dose of nevirapine because of the long half-life of this compound, which essentially exposes the patient to many days of monotherapy. Early experience with zidovudine showed that zidovudine resistance emerged during the initial 6 to 12 months of therapy. Current concepts of therapy emphasize the use of combination regimens that include at least one potent agent so that viral replication is minimized and mutation rates conferring resistance occur infrequently.

Initiating Antiretroviral Therapy

Patients with acute HIV infection (i.e., those in the process of seroconverting) and patients who have seroconverted in the previous 6 months should be considered for early therapy. About 40 to 90% of acutely infected patients experience symptomatic illnesses, and if the patient or health care provider considers the possibility that the symptoms might have been related to high-risk behavior, HIV infection can potentially be identified by serologic and virologic assays. In theory, this therapy should reduce the viral load in lymphoid tissue during the period before an effective host immune response is initiated and subsequently lead to lower viral loads and higher CD4$^+$ T-lymphocyte counts. The long-term clinical benefit of treating acute or early HIV infection has not been shown conclusively, however, and the potential benefits of treating acute HIV infection must be weighed against the disadvantages of toxicity, cost, and inconvenience. Many clinicians would offer at least 2 to 6 months of this therapy in an effort to reduce viral replication in lymphoid tissue and produce a lower plasma HIV viral load. It is often difficult to stop such therapy when both the patient and the clinician witness the rapid fall in plasma viral load and the rebound in CD4$^+$ T-lymphocyte cell count.

Chronically infected patients with CD4$^+$ T-lymphocyte counts less than 200 cells/mL have been shown by clinical end point studies to benefit from ART in terms of longer disease-free survival. For patients with CD4$^+$ T-lymphocyte counts less than 200 cells/mL and for those with symptomatic HIV-related disease (i.e., patients who have an opportunistic infection, neoplasm, or some other disease entity related to HIV infection) and CD4$^+$ T-lymphocyte counts greater than 200 cells/mL, there is relatively uniform consensus that ART is indicated.

In patients with CD4$^+$ T-lymphocyte counts greater than 200 cells/mL, there have been no clinical end point studies to show conclusively when therapy should be initiated. Observational studies provide some important clues, however. Figure 412–1 shows the relationship between CD4$^+$ T-lymphocyte count and plasma HIV viral load during a 3-year follow-up of untreated patients in the Multicenter AIDS Cohort Study. This figure indicates that the CD4$^+$ T-lymphocyte count and plasma HIV viral load influence the 3-year risk for progression to AIDS. These data by themselves do not prove which patients would respond to therapy or which patients would respond best. These data do indicate, however, that for some patients (e.g., those with CD4$^+$ T-lymphocyte counts >350 cells/mL or plasma viral loads <3000 copies/mL), the risk for progression is so low that therapy could logically be withheld until the risk was substantially higher, such as when the CD4$^+$ T-lymphocyte count had fallen substantially (e.g., <200 cells/mL) or the plasma HIV viral load had risen substantially (e.g., >55,000 copies/mL).

Observational data from ART-treated patients provide important information related to the decision when to initiate therapy. An analysis of data from 13 European and North American studies assessed the risk for progression in drug-naive patients who started ART and had plasma HIV viral loads less than 100,000 copies/mL. The 3-year probability of death or AIDS-defining disease was 15.8% for patients who initiated therapy when the CD4$^+$ T-lymphocyte count was 0 to 49 cells/mL, 12.5% if the count was 50 to 99 cells/mL, 9.3% if the count was 100 to 199 cells/mL, 4.7% if the count was 200 to 349 cells/mL, and 3.4% if the count was 350 cells/mL or higher. These data support the proposition that therapy should be initiated before the CD4$^+$ T-cell count decreases to less than 200 cells/mL. The data do not, however, show an escalating benefit of initiating therapy at CD4$^+$ T-lymphocyte counts that are incrementally higher than 200 cells/mL. There is no consensus regarding the exact CD4$^+$ T-cell count at which ART should be initiated, as long as ART is started before the count decreases to less than 200 cells/mL. Many experts would initiate therapy when the CD4$^+$ T-lymphocyte count falls below 350 cells/mL. Few experts would start ART at counts greater than 350 cells/mL unless there were extenuating circumstances, such as a rapidly falling CD4$^+$ T-lymphocyte count, a high viral load, or a clinical event such as an AIDS-defining illness or another opportunistic infection.

Data from the same European/North American analysis also showed that there is a dramatic increase in risk for disease progression in patients with a viral load greater than 100,000 copies/mL, regardless of the CD4$^+$ T-lymphocyte count. Many experts would recommend that ART be initiated at viral loads greater than 55,000 copies/mL, especially in patients with CD4$^+$ T-lymphocyte counts less than 350 cells/mL. The guidelines of the U.S. Public Health Service/Infectious Diseases Society of America for HIV-infected adults and adolescents regarding when to initiate ART are shown in Table 412–1.

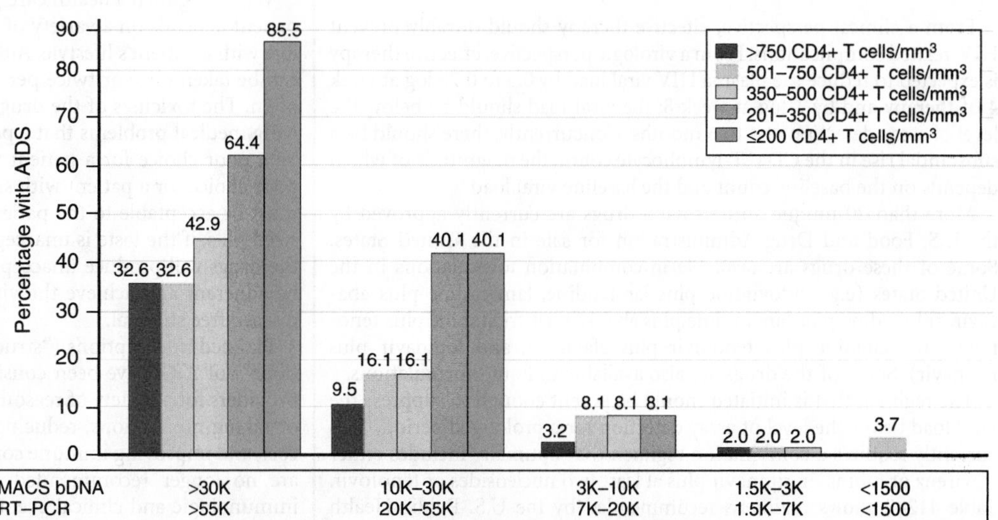

FIGURE 412–1 • Likelihood of AIDS developing within 3 years. MACS = Multicenter AIDS Cohort Study; RT-PCR = reverse transcriptase polymerase chain reaction.

TABLE 412–1 INDICATIONS FOR INITIATING ANTIRETROVIRAL THERAPY FOR CHRONICALLY HIV-1–INFECTED PATIENTS

Clinical Category	CD4⁺ Cell Count	Plasma HIV RNA	Recommendation
AIDS-defining illness or severe symptoms (AI)	Any value	Any value	Treat
Asymptomatic (AI)	$CD4^+$ T cells <200/mL	Any value	Treat
Asymptomatic (BII)	$CD4^+$ T cells >200/mL but ≤350/mL	Any value	Treatment should be offered after full discussion of the pros and cons with each patient
Asymptomatic (CII)	$CD4^+$ T cells >350/mL	≥100,000	Most clinicians recommend deferring therapy, but some clinicians will treat
Asymptomatic (DII)	$CD4^+$ T cells >350/mL	<100,000	Defer therapy

Modified from Guidelines for the Use of Antiretroviral Agents in HIV-1–Infected Adults and Adolescents, October 10, 2006. Available at http://www.aidsinfo.nih.gov.

TABLE 412–2 ANTIRETROVIRAL REGIMENS RECOMMENDED FOR TREATMENT OF HIV-1 INFECTION IN ANTIRETROVIRAL-NAIVE PATIENTS

	Column A (NNRTI or PI options—in alphabetical order)				Column B (Dual-NRTI options—in alphabetical order)
Preferred components	*NNRTI* efavirenz[1] (AII)	*or*	*PI* Atazanavir + ritonavir (AIII) Fosamprenavir + ritonavir (2×/day) (AII) Lopinavir/ritonavir[2] (2×/day) (AII) (co-formulated)	+	Tenofovir/emtricitabine[3] (co-formulated) (AII); *or* Zidovudine/lamivudine[3] (co-formulated) (AII)
Alternative to preferred components	*NNRTI* nevirapine[4] (BII)	*or*	*PI* Atazanavir[5] (BII) Fosamprenavir (BII) Fosamprenavir + ritonavir (1×/day) (BII) Lopinavir/ritonavir (1×/day) (BII) (co-formulated)		Abacavir/lamivudine[3] (co-formulated) (BII) Didanosine + (emtricitabine or lamivudine) (BII)

[1]Efavirenz is not recommended for use in the first trimester of pregnancy or in sexually active women with childbearing potential who are not using effective contraception.
[2]The pivotal study that led to the recommendation of lopinavir/ritonavir as a preferred PI component was based on twice-daily dosing. A smaller study has shown similar efficacy with once-daily dosing but also showed a higher incidence of moderate to severe diarrhea with the once-daily regimen (16% vs. 5%).
[3]Emtricitabine may be used in place of lamivudine and vice versa.
[4]Nevirapine should not be initiated in women with $CD4^+$ T cell count >250 cells/mm^3 or in men with $CD4^+$ T cell count >400 cells/mm^3 because of increased risk of symptomatic hepatic events in these patients.
[5]Atazanavir must be boosted with ritonavir if used in combination with tenofovir.
NRTI = nucleoside reverse transcriptase inhibitor; NNRTI = non-nucleoside reverse transcriptase inhibitor; PI = protease inhibitor.
Modified from Guidelines for the Use of Antiretroviral Agents in HIV-1–Infected Adults and Adolescents, October 10, 2006. Available at http://www.aidsinfo.nih.gov.

What Antiretroviral Regimen Should Be Initiated?

Criteria for Assessing Efficacy of a Regimen

From a clinical perspective, effective therapy should durably prevent HIV-related complications. From a virologic perspective, effective therapy is expected to reduce the plasma HIV viral load by 0.5 to 0.75 log at week 4 of therapy and by 1 log at week 8; the viral load should be below the level of assay detection at 4 to 6 months. Concurrently, there should be a substantial rise in the $CD4^+$ T-lymphocyte count, the magnitude of which depends on the baseline count and the baseline viral load.

More than 20 unique antiretroviral drugs are currently approved by the U.S. Food and Drug Administration for sale in the United States. Some of these drugs are available in combination formulations in the United States (e.g., zidovudine plus lamivudine, lamivudine plus abacavir, zidovudine plus lamivudine plus abacavir, emtricitabine plus tenofovir, emtricitabine plus tenofovir plus efavirenz, and lopinavir plus ritonavir). Some of the drugs are also available in liquid formulations.

The regimen that is initiated should be potent enough to suppress the viral load below the level of assay detection for a prolonged period. This currently requires a combination regimen that optimally includes either efavirenz or lopinavir-ritonavir plus at least two nucleosides or tenofovir. Table 412–2 shows regimens recommended by the U.S. Public Health Service/Infectious Diseases Society of America guidelines at the time that this chapter was written. Currently, regimens consisting of efavirenz, nevirapine, or lopinavir-ritonavir plus lamivudine and either zidovudine or tenofovir are popular. Three-drug regimens appear to be as good as four-drug regimens for initial treatment.

Which regimen a health care provider should choose for an individual patient depends on a variety of factors. The regimen should be compatible with a patient's lifestyle. Adherence is more likely with regimens that can be taken once or twice per day than with those that are taken more often. The toxicities of the drugs must be compatible with other underlying medical problems that a patient has. For example, nelfinavir might be a poor choice for a patient with diarrhea, and ritonavir might be a poor choice for a patient with significant underlying liver disease. Drugs must be acceptable to the patient; if the patient cannot swallow certain sized pills, if the taste is unacceptable, or if the patient is convinced that the drugs will produce unacceptable toxicity, the patient is not likely to be adherent and achieve the virologic results that would produce long disease-free survival.

Planned interruptions ("structured" or "strategic treatment interruptions") of ART have been considered by some patients and health care providers for a variety of reasons, including reducing the lifestyle burden of taking medications, reducing medication-related toxicity, decreasing cost, and improving immune control of HIV infection. These approaches are no longer recommended in most situations because of adverse immunologic and clinical events after interruption of treatment. When ART is stopped, the HIV viral load in virtually all patients returns to pretherapy values within several weeks, which may result in irreversible loss of $CD4^+$ T lymphocytes.

Immune-based therapies have been used in an attempt to augment immunity against HIV-associated infections and tumors. Interleukin-2, given subcutaneously 5 days every 2 months for several cycles, has been shown to increase $CD4^+$ T-lymphocyte counts in a substantial fraction of patients. It is not yet clear whether these increases in $CD4^+$ T-lymphocyte count correlate with improved prognosis. Immune-based therapies offer a different approach to ART that could theoretically be used in addition to or instead of ART.

Changing a Failing Regimen

The initial ART regimen may need to be changed because of toxicity, drug availability, cost, patient preference, or lack of efficacy. The initial decision to start therapy and considerations to change a regimen are important because of the limited number of antiretroviral agents that could be used in subsequent regimens. A long-term strategy needs to be developed for each patient, with a focus on what approach might be available if the current one fails. If adherence is poor, a period of no ART might be a better choice than a new regimen so that viruses resistant to all available drugs do not develop. Similarly, if a patient's viral load were detectable but less than 5000 copies/mL and the $CD4^+$ T-lymphocyte count were stable and greater than 200 to 350 cells/mL, it might be reasonable to consider maintaining the current regimen rather than switching to a more complex regimen that would expose the patient to other previously untried classes of drugs, although many experts would be reluctant to allow even that degree of viral replication to persist.

Lack of efficacy can be defined in a variety of ways: (1) failure to meet the virologic milestones noted earlier; (2) repeated detection of virus after initial suppression to levels below assay detection that are not attributable to vaccination, intercurrent infection, or test methodology; (3) $CD4^+$ T-lymphocyte counts that either fail to increase or decline; and (4) clinical deterioration. In terms of their implications for therapy, each of these aspects of failure must be interpreted in context. A patient with a high initial viral load (e.g., >1 million copies/mL) whose viral loads are declining might be recommended to remain on a regimen if the viral load was still declining at 6 months or was stable at a low level. Similarly, a patient who started a regimen when the $CD4^+$ T-lymphocyte count was low and in whom an opportunistic infection developed at a time when the HIV viral load was below the level of assay detection might be unlikely to benefit from a different ART regimen. Decisions about changing therapies must also consider what treatment options are feasible in view of previous drug exposure, viral resistance, drug tolerability, and drug availability.

There are many reasons for treatment to fail. Poor patient adherence is probably the most common cause, and clinicians may find it especially difficult to identify this factor. Altered drug pharmacokinetics resulting from abnormal absorption or metabolism of the drug may also be a factor. Drug interactions with licensed drugs or "alternative" medicines may be relevant. The patient may have acquired a drug-resistant virus when initially infected, or the patient's virus may have become resistant during therapy. These causes of regimen failure must be investigated carefully to maximize the likelihood that the next regimen will succeed.

Changes in therapy mandated by lack of regimen efficacy should be guided by the results of resistance testing. The relative merits of genotypic and phenotypic assays have not been well delineated, however, and there are no well-validated algorithms on how to interpret these tests. Careful consideration should be given to past history regarding the efficacy and tolerability of specific drugs and the results of resistance. Enfuvirtide, a fusion inhibitor, can provide significant benefit to patients who have done poorly despite multiple antiviral drugs when it is used as part of a combination regimen. Other new drugs, especially those with novel mechanisms of action, show similar promise.

Potential Complications of Antiretroviral Regimens

As with any medication, each antiretroviral agent is associated with toxicities. Some are class specific, such as mitochondrial toxicities with nucleoside analogues or rash or CNS dysfunction with non-nucleoside reverse transcriptase inhibitors. Others are drug specific, such as stone formation and interstitial nephritis with indinavir, diarrhea with nelfinavir, or a unique hypersensitivity reaction with abacavir. The occurrence of these toxicities is not usually predictable; however, a specific HLA genotype (HLA-B*5701) has been associated with abacavir hypersensitivity responses, thus for the first time showing that the likelihood of a particular toxicity may be predicted.

Certain toxicities deserve special mention. Chronic compensated hyperlactemia occurs during treatment with nucleoside and nucleotide reverse transcriptase inhibitors (NRTIs). In a few cases (about 1.3 cases per 1000 person years of NRTI exposure), decompensated lactic acidosis accompanied by hepatic steatosis and hepatomegaly can occur and is associated with high mortality. Risk factors for this potentially fatal syndrome include female gender, obesity, prolonged use of nucleosides, late-stage pregnancy or the postpartum period, and the use of didanosine and stavudine combination therapy during pregnancy. The lactic acidosis syndrome is manifested as nonspecific gastrointestinal symptoms, including nausea, abdominal pain, vomiting, diarrhea, weakness, myalgias, paresthesias, and hepatomegaly. Hepatic enzymes may be normal or only slightly elevated. Elevated lactate levels may be associated with an anion gap, elevated creatine phosphokinase and lactate dehydrogenase, and an enlarged fatty liver on computed tomography. Therapy consists of discontinuing all nucleoside analogue drugs. Bicarbonate infusions and hemodialysis may be helpful. It is not clear how safe it is to rechallenge the patient with any nucleoside drug.

Mitochondrial dysfunction in association with NRTIs may be accompanied by several complications, including peripheral neuropathy, cardiomyopathy, myopathy, pancreatitis, and lipoatrophy. Although antiretroviral drug toxicity can contribute to these conditions, it is possible that HIV itself or opportunistic infections, or both, may also play an etiologic role.

HIV infection and ARTs have been associated with body fat abnormalities or lipodystrophy. Loss of peripheral fat or lipoatrophy, most notable in the face and extremities, as well as abnormal accumulation of abdominal and dorsocervical fat, may be seen, each alone or in combination. Although there is no uniform definition of lipodystrophy and prevalence reports vary, lipodystrophy is estimated to affect a third or more patients treated with ART regimens. As previously noted, recent research has linked lipoatrophy most closely to NRTIs in association with mitochondrial toxicity. Although causality has not been established, lipid accumulation may be a consequence of protease inhibitors, more so than NRTIs. It remains unknown whether fat distribution abnormalities represent various manifestations of a single pathologic process, but increasingly they seem to represent distinct entities or toxicities of ART. When fat maldistribution occurs, it can be disfiguring and distressing. There is growing evidence that switching ART to regimens with less mitochondrial toxicity (e.g., switching from stavudine-, didanosine-, or zidovudine-containing regimens) can result in improvements in lipoatrophy over a period of many months or years.

Before the advent of ART, HIV infection was associated with reduced high-density lipoprotein cholesterol and elevated triglycerides. ART, in particular most protease inhibitors, is associated with elevated total serum cholesterol and fasting triglycerides. Evidence is mounting that these atherogenic lipid profiles are important factors contributing to the accelerated atherosclerosis manifested as increased risk for cardiovascular and cerebrovascular disease independent of other recognized risk factors such as age, tobacco use, and family history. Most clinicians monitor and treat these lipid abnormalities as they would manage abnormalities in a non–HIV-infected patient. When implementing lipid management programs, however, careful consideration must be given to drug interactions, especially interactions between protease inhibitors and β-hydroxy-β-methylglutaryl-coenzyme A reductase inhibitors (statins). Replacing a protease inhibitor with either abacavir or a non-NRTI may be effective in reducing the lipid elevations.

Elevations in lipids alone do not appear to account for all the excess risk for cardiovascular disease observed in HIV-infected patients receiving ART. Other factors, possibly related to drug toxicity, are probably implicated. For example, insulin resistance and diabetes are increasingly identified in HIV-infected patients, in particular in patients treated with ART. As with hyperlipidemia, the use of certain protease inhibitors is linked to impaired insulin sensitivity and potential risk for diabetes; however, other ART agents and abnormalities in fat distribution may also contribute to these observations. The combination of insulin resistance, hyperlipidemia, and abnormal fat distribution represents many of the components of metabolic syndrome, a condition known to be associated with increased risk for diabetes and cardiovascular disease. Therefore, accelerated atherosclerosis may be due in part to this combination of factors, as well as traditional risk factors as indicated earlier.

Hepatotoxicity is an important complication of ART. Serum transaminase elevations have been reported with all licensed protease inhibitors and non-NRTIs and have been associated with nucleoside agents as well. In some patients, the transaminase elevations are mild and unassociated with symptoms. In other cases, symptomatic hepatitis or associated hepatic steatosis with or without lactic acidosis requires cessation of the drug. Among the non-NRTIs, nevirapine has the greatest potential for causing symptomatic hepatitis. Manifestations often include fever, rash, and eosinophilia and usually occur within 12 weeks of initiating therapy. Protease inhibitor–associated liver enzyme abnormalities can occur at any juncture during therapy. Ritonavir-containing regimens are particularly likely to be associated with hepatic toxicity. Hepatitis C, hepatitis B, alcohol, elevated baseline liver function test results, and other hepatotoxic drugs are risk factors for the development of protease inhibitor–associated liver toxicity.

Decreased bone mineral density and avascular necrosis are complications of HIV infection that appear to be associated with HIV and ART. However, pathologic fractures have not yet been reported often as a complication of the decreased bone density. Avascular necrosis of the hips and other joints appears to be a separate and distinct syndrome, possibly associated with previous steroid use. There are few data to guide the development of preventive or therapeutic strategies for these bone disorders.

Prophylaxis of Opportunistic Infection

Prevention of Opportunistic Infections

Early during the AIDS epidemic, it became clear that a strategy of treating opportunistic infections as they occurred had many disadvantages. Patients experienced discomfort, expense, and inconvenience; damage to organs such as the lungs, brain, or eye was often not completely reversible; the opportunistic infection frequently accelerated progression of the HIV disease; and many of the opportunistic infections were associated with substantial mortality. Chemoprophylaxis was an attractive strategy because the most common life-threatening opportunistic infection associated with HIV, PCP, was being successfully prevented in oncology patients and a similar strategy seemed feasible in patients with HIV infection. Because the period of susceptibility to opportunistic infections in patients with HIV infection could be measured by $CD4^+$ T-lymphocyte counts, a strategy of chemoprophylaxis seemed particularly attractive for patients whose immunity could not be restored with ART or immunomodulating therapies.

Chemoprophylaxis regimens are available for most treatable HIV-associated opportunistic infections. Tables 412–3 and 412–4 summarize regimens that are recommended for primary and secondary chemoprophylaxis. [2,3] Table 412–5 summarizes the $CD4^+$ T-lymphocyte counts at which chemoprophylaxis should be implemented. Chemoprophylaxis for various pathogens should be started when the $CD4^+$ T-lymphocyte count declines to specific levels (depending on the pathogen) to prevent an initial episode of disease (primary prophylaxis). This prophylaxis can be stopped if immunity is augmented by ART but must be restarted if immunity again declines to designated thresholds. Similarly, if an opportunistic infection develops, suppressive therapy (secondary prophylaxis) is indicated for life for most opportunistic infections unless immunity is restored by ART.

The regimens recommended in Tables 412–3 and 412–4 have been shown to prevent primary and subsequent occurrence of disease. The use of these regimens improves patient survival in several instances (PCP, *M. avium* complex disease, and *M. tuberculosis*) and decreases patient morbidity. Several caveats about the use of chemoprophylaxis are worth noting, however. First, some opportunistic infections occur at $CD4^+$ T-lymphocyte counts above the recommended thresholds for starting chemoprophylaxis. Of PCP cases, 5 to 10% occur at $CD4^+$ T-lymphocyte counts greater than 200 cells/mL. In some instances, clinical information, such as the development of oral candidiasis or substantial weight loss, may provide clues that the patient is clinically more immunosuppressed than the laboratory parameters would predict. A high viral load (e.g., >100,000 copies/mL) may also suggest that earlier institution of chemoprophylaxis is warranted. Second, patients may be unable to tolerate certain chemoprophylactic agents. TMP-SMX is often associated with intractable pruritus or rash and cannot be used by many patients with HIV infection. Third, no chemoprophylactic regimen is completely effective. Some regimens fail because of poor adherence, but some fail because of poor host immune response or pathogen resistance. Prescribing a chemoprophylactic regimen does not guarantee that the targeted disease will never develop. Finally, a decision to use a chemoprophylactic agent depends on the balance between its benefit in terms of efficacy and its disadvantages in terms of toxicity, inconvenience, drug interactions, ecologic effects (e.g., effects on producing resistance in targeted and bystander organisms), and cost. Some effective drugs, such as fluconazole for *Candida* and *Cryptococcus* and oral ganciclovir or valganciclovir for CMV, have not been recommended because their disadvantages were judged to outweigh the benefits.

TABLE 412–3 PROPHYLAXIS TO PREVENT FIRST EPISODES OF OPPORTUNISTIC DISEASE IN ADULTS AND ADOLESCENTS INFECTED WITH HIV

		Preventive Regimens	
Pathogen	**Indication**	**First Choice**	**Alternatives**
STRONGLY RECOMMENDED AS STANDARD OF CARE			
Pneumocystis jiroveci	$CD4^+$ count <200/mL or oropharyngeal candidiasis	Trimethoprim-sulfamethoxazole (TMP-SMX), 1 double-strength tablet PO qd, or TMP-SMX, 1 single-strength tablet PO qd	Dapsone, 50 mg PO bid or 100 mg PO qd; dapsone, 50 mg PO qd, plus pyrimethamine, 50 mg PO weekly, plus leucovorin, 25 mg PO weekly; dapsone, 200 mg PO, plus pyrimethamine, 75 mg PO, plus leucovorin, 25 mg PO, weekly; aerosolized pentamidine, 300 mg every month via Respirgard II nebulizer; atovaquone, 1500 mg PO qd; TMP-SMX, 1 double-strength tablet PO 3 times a week
Mycobacterium tuberculosis			
Isoniazid sensitive	Tuberculin skin test reaction (5 mm), previous positive tuberculin skin test result without treatment, or contact with a case of active tuberculosis regardless of tuberculin skin test result	Isoniazid, 300 mg PO, plus pyridoxine, 50 mg PO, qd × 9 mo; or isoniazid, 900 mg PO, plus pyridoxine, 100 mg PO, twice a week × 9 mo	Rifampin, 600 mg PO qd × 4 mo, or rifabutin, 300 mg PO qd × 4 mo; Pyrazinamide, 15–20 mg PO qd × 2 mo, plus either rifampin, 600 mg PO qd × 2 mo, or rifabutin, 300 mg PO qd × 2 mo*

TABLE 412–3 PROPHYLAXIS TO PREVENT FIRST EPISODES OF OPPORTUNISTIC DISEASE IN ADULTS AND ADOLESCENTS INFECTED WITH HIV—cont'd

		Preventive Regimens	
Pathogen	**Indication**	**First Choice**	**Alternatives**
Isoniazid resistant	Same as above; high probability of exposure to isoniazid-resistant tuberculosis	Rifampin, 600 mg PO, or rifabutin, 300 mg PO, qd × 4 mo	Rifampin, 600 mg PO, or rifabutin, 300 mg PO, qd × 2 mo*
Multidrug (isoniazid and rifampin) resistant	Same as above; high probability of exposure to multidrug-resistant tuberculosis	Choice of drugs requires consultation with public health authorities. Depends on susceptibility of isolate from source patient	—
Toxoplasma gondii	IgG antibody to *Toxoplasma* and $CD4^+$ count <100/mL	TMP-SMX, 1 double-strength tablet PO qd	TMP-SMX, 1 single-strength tablet PO qd; dapsone, 50 mg PO qd, plus pyrimethamine, 50 mg PO weekly, plus leucovorin, 25 mg PO weekly; dapsone, 200 mg PO, plus pyrimethamine, 75 mg PO, plus leucovorin, 25 mg PO, weekly; atovaquone, 1500 mg PO qd, with or without pyrimethamine, 25 mg PO qd, plus leucovorin, 10 mg PO qd
Mycobacterium avium complex	$CD4^+$ count <50/mL	Azithromycin, 1200 mg PO weekly, or clarithromycin, 500 mg PO bid	Rifabutin, 300 mg PO qd; azithromycin, 1200 mg PO weekly, plus rifabutin, 300 mg PO qd
Varicella-zoster virus (VZV)	Significant exposure to chickenpox or shingles for patients who have no history of either condition or, if available, negative antibody to VZV	Varicella-zoster immune globulin (VZIG) is no longer available, but VARIZIG is currently available, administered ≤96 hr after exposure, ideally within 48 hr	
GENERALLY RECOMMENDED			
Streptococcus pneumoniae	$CD4^+$ count >200/mL	23-Valent polysaccharide vaccine, 0.5 mL IM	None
Hepatitis B virus	All susceptible (anti-HBs–negative) patients	Hepatitis B vaccine, 3 doses	None
Influenza virus	All patients (annually, before influenza season)	Inactivated trivalent influenza virus vaccine: one annual dose (0.5 mL) IM	Oseltamivir, 75 mg PO qd, or zanamivir, 10 mg per inhalation device qd (influenza A or B)
Hepatitis A virus (HAV)	All susceptible (anti-HAV–negative) patients at increased risk for HAV infection (e.g., illicit drug users, men who have sex with men, hemophiliacs) or with chronic liver disease, including chronic hepatitis B or C	HAV vaccine: 2 doses	None
EVIDENCE FOR EFFICACY BUT NOT ROUTINELY INDICATED			
Cryptococcus neoformans	$CD4^+$ count <50/mL	Fluconazole, 100–200 mg PO qd	Itraconazole capsule, 200 mg PO qd
Histoplasma capsulatum	$CD4^+$ count <100/mL, endemic geographic area	Itraconazole capsule, 200 mg PO qd	None

*Should generally not be offered unless no reasonable alternatives are available.
Modified from Guidelines for the Use of Antiretroviral Agents in HIV-1–Infected Adults and Adolescents, 2005. Available at http://www.aids.info.nih.gov.

TMP-SMX is the agent of choice for prevention of PCP. It should be started when the $CD4^+$ T-lymphocyte count decreases to 200 cells/mL, when oral candidiasis develops (regardless of the $CD4^+$ T-cell count), or when the patient has had a previous episode of PCP. Prophylaxis should be continued as long as the $CD4^+$ T-lymphocyte count remains less than 200 cells/mL. Several regimens of TMP-SMX are effective: one double-strength tablet per day, one single-strength tablet per day, and one double-strength tablet three times weekly are all recommended. The daily regimens seem to be more effective than the three-times-per-week regimen. TMP-SMX can be associated with a variety of toxicities, including rash, fever, pruritus, nausea, vomiting, nephritis, hyperkalemia, and aseptic meningitis. For reasons that have not been well delineated, rash occurs at an unusually high frequency in HIV-infected patients who take TMP-SMX. Lower-dose regimens (e.g., a single-strength rather than a double-strength tablet or three times weekly rather than daily) seem to be better tolerated. Gradual dose escalation may also improve the

TABLE 412–4 PROPHYLAXIS TO PREVENT RECURRENCE OF OPPORTUNISTIC DISEASE (AFTER CHEMOTHERAPY FOR ACUTE DISEASE) IN ADULTS AND ADOLESCENTS INFECTED WITH HIV

		Preventive Regimens	
Pathogen	**Indication**	**First Choice**	**Alternatives**
RECOMMENDED AS STANDARD OF CARE			
Pneumocystis jiroveci	Previous *P. jiroveci* pneumonia	Trimethoprim-sulfamethoxazole (TMP-SMX), 1 double-strength tablet PO qd TMP-SMX, 1 single-strength tablet PO qd	Dapsone, 50 mg PO bid or 100 mg PO qd; dapsone, 50 mg PO qd, plus pyrimethamine, 50 mg PO weekly, plus leucovorin, 25 mg PO weekly; dapsone, 200 mg PO, plus pyrimethamine, 75 mg PO, plus leucovorin, 25 mg PO, weekly; aerosolized pentamidine, 300 mg every month via Respirgard II nebulizer; atovaquone, 1500 mg PO qd; TMP-SMX, 1 double-strength tablet PO 3 times a week
Toxoplasma gondii	Previous toxoplasmic encephalitis	Sulfadiazine, 500–1000 mg PO qid, plus pyrimethamine, 25–50 mg PO qd, plus leucovorin, 10–25 mg PO qd	Clindamycin, 300–450 mg PO q6–8h, plus pyrimethamine, 25–50 mg PO qd, plus leucovorin, 10–25 mg PO qd; atovaquone, 750 mg PO q6–12h, with or without pyrimethamine, 25 mg PO qd, plus leucovorin, 10 mg PO qd
Mycobacterium avium complex	Documented disseminated disease	Clarithromycin, 500 mg PO bid, plus ethambutol, 15 mg/kg PO qd; with or without rifabutin, 300 mg PO qd	Azithromycin, 500 mg PO qd, plus ethambutol, 15 mg/kg PO qd; with or without rifabutin, 300 mg PO qd
Cytomegalovirus	Previous end-organ disease	Oral valganciclovir, 900 mg PO qd	Ganciclovir, 5–6 mg/kg IV 5–7 days/wk or 1000 mg PO tid; or foscarnet, 90–120 mg/kg IV qd; or (for retinitis) ganciclovir sustained-release implant, q6–9mo, plus valganciclovir, 900 mg PO qd Cidofovir, 5 mg/kg IV every other week, with probenecid, 2 g PO 3 hr before the dose, followed by 1 g PO 2 hr after the dose and 1 g PO 8 hr after the dose (total of 4 g) Fomivirsen, 1 vial (330 μg) injected into the vitreous, then repeated every 2–4 wk
Cryptococcus neoformans	Documented disease	Fluconazole, 200 mg PO qd	Amphotericin B, 0.6–1.0 mg/kg IV 1–3 times a week; itraconazole, 200-mg capsule PO qd
Histoplasma capsulatum	Documented disease	Itraconazole capsule, 200 mg PO qd	Amphotericin B, 1.0 mg/kg IV weekly
Coccidioides immitis	Documented disease	Fluconazole, 400 mg PO qd	Amphotericin B, 1.0 mg/kg IV weekly; itraconazole, 200-mg capsule PO bid
Salmonella (non-typhi)	Bacteremia	Ciprofloxacin, 500 mg PO bid for several months	Antibiotic chemoprophylaxis with another active agent
RECOMMENDED ONLY IF SUBSEQUENT EPISODES ARE FREQUENT OR SEVERE			
Herpes simplex virus	Frequent/severe recurrences	Acyclovir, 200 mg PO tid or 400 mg PO bid	Valacyclovir, 500 mg PO bid; famciclovir, 500 mg PO bid

Modified from Guidelines for the Use of Antiretroviral Agents in HIV-1–Infected Adults and Adolescents, 2006. Available at http://www.aids.info.nih.gov.

tolerability of TMP-SMX prophylaxis. Evidence of enzyme mutations in *Pneumocystis,* which probably confer sulfonamide resistance, raises the ominous possibility that this useful prophylactic and therapeutic agent may lose the impressive efficacy that it has enjoyed to date.

Alternatives to TMP-SMX include dapsone, dapsone-pyrimethamine, sulfadiazine-pyrimethamine, atovaquone, and aerosolized pentamidine. These regimens are not as effective as TMP-SMX in preventing PCP. In addition, TMP-SMX provides protection against toxoplasmosis, bacterial pneumonia, and enteric infections. None of the alternative regimens provides protection against all these pathogens, and all have associated toxicities.

Clarithromycin or azithromycin is the chemoprophylactic agent of choice for *M. avium* complex in HIV-infected patients with $CD4^+$ T-lymphocyte counts less than 50 cells/mL. Each of these agents is more effective than placebo, and each is preferred over rifabutin because the latter is less effective and associated with multiple complex drug interactions. Clarithromycin and azithromycin provide additional protection against bacterial pneumonia. These drugs are relatively well tolerated; however, the weekly regimen of azithromycin can be associated with considerable nausea. Azithromycin causes fewer drug interactions than clarithromycin does and is preferred by some clinicians when multiple other drugs metabolized by the cytochrome P-450 system are being used.

Prophylaxis for *M. tuberculosis* is an important aspect of the management of HIV-infected patients, especially in communities in which tuberculosis is common. Purified protein derivative (PPD) screening for all patients with newly diagnosed HIV and regular screening thereafter are important for identifying subclinically infected patients because HIV-infected individuals have such a high likelihood for reactivation of latent tuberculosis. Latently infected patients (defined as a PPD reaction ≥5 mm for this patient population) or patients recently exposed to active tuberculosis should be treated with one of the recommended regimens with careful attention to the toxicities and interactions of the regimen chosen.

Immunization of patients with pneumococcal vaccine also seems to be important for preventing upper and lower respiratory disease. Immunization with pneumococcal vaccine is probably more effective when the $CD4^+$ T-lymphocyte count is greater than 200 cells/mL than when it is less than 2000 cells/mL. If patients received initial immunization when their $CD4^+$ T-lymphocyte count was less than 200 cells/mL, it is logical to reimmunize them if their counts subsequently rise. Immunization of patients with hepatitis A and hepatitis B vaccines is also logical, especially

TABLE 412–5 CRITERIA FOR STARTING, DISCONTINUING, AND RESTARTING PROPHYLAXIS FOR OPPORTUNISTIC INFECTIONS IN ADULTS WITH HIV INFECTION*

Opportunistic Illness	Criteria for Initiating Primary Prophylaxis	Criteria for Discontinuing Primary Prophylaxis	Criteria for Restarting Primary Prophylaxis	Criteria for Initiating Secondary Prophylaxis	Criteria for Discontinuing Secondary Prophylaxis	Criteria for Restarting Secondary Prophylaxis
Pneumocystis jiroveci pneumonia	$CD4^+$ <200 cells/mL or oropharyngeal candidiasis	$CD4^+$ >200 cells/mL for 3 mo	$CD4^+$ <200 cells/mL	Previous *P. jiroveci* pneumonia	$CD4^+$ >200 cells/mL for 3 mo	$CD4^+$ < 200 cells/mL
Toxoplasmosis	IgG antibody to *Toxoplasma* and $CD4^+$ <100 cells/mL	$CD4^+$ >200 cells/mL for 3 mo	$CD4^+$ <100–200 cells/mL	Previous toxoplasmic encephalitis	$CD4^+$ >200 cells/mL sustained (e.g., >6 mo), completed initial therapy, and asymptomatic for *Toxoplasma*	$CD4^+$ <200 cells/mL
Disseminated *Mycobacterium avium* complex (MAC)	$CD4^+$ <50 cells/mL	$CD4^+$ >100 cells/mL for 3 mo	$CD4^+$ <50–100 cells/mL	Documented disseminated disease	$CD4^+$ >100 cells/mL sustained (e.g., >6 mo), completed 12 mo of MAC therapy, and asymptomatic for MAC	$CD4^+$ <100 cells/mL
Cryptococcosis	None	Not applicable	Not applicable	Documented disease	$CD4^+$ >100–200 cells/mL sustained (e.g., >6 mo), completed initial therapy, and asymptomatic for cryptococcosis	$CD4^+$ <100–200 cells/mL
Histoplasmosis	None	Not applicable	Not applicable	Documented disease	Therapy for 1 year $CD4^+$ >150 cells/mL *Histoplasma* antigen <4 ng/mL	$CD4^+$ <150 cells/mL
Coccidioidomycosis	None	Not applicable	Not applicable	Documented disease	No criteria recommended for stopping	Not applicable
Cytomegalovirus retinitis	None	Not applicable	Not applicable	Documented end-organ disease	$CD4^+$ >100–150 cells/mL sustained (e.g., >6 mo) and no evidence of active disease with regular ophthalmic examination	$CD4^+$ <100–150 cells/mL

Modified from Guidelines for the Use of Antiretroviral Agents in HIV-1–Infected Adults and Adolescents, 2005. Available at http://www.aids.info.nih.gov.

if patients are at high risk of acquiring such infections and they have concomitant hepatitis C.

Primary chemoprophylaxis for fungal or herpesvirus diseases is not currently recommended. Primary prophylaxis may be effective, but the benefits are currently thought to be outweighed in the United States and western Europe by the effects of prophylaxis on pathogen resistance and by the toxicity and cost of drugs that target diseases that are usually readily treatable.

Treatment of Acute Opportunistic Infections

Minimizing the effect of acute opportunistic infections on the lifestyle and survival of patients depends on prompt recognition of such diseases and expeditious institution of appropriate therapy. Patients and health care providers need to be familiar with the signs and symptoms of HIV-associated opportunistic infections and neoplasms so that diseases can be treated early, before manifestations are severe.

The manifestations of HIV-related opportunistic infections often differ from manifestations in other patient populations. PCP, for instance, is usually much less acute in patients with HIV infection than in those receiving high-dose corticosteroids or antineoplastic chemotherapy. CMV disease is associated with retinitis or colitis most often in patients with HIV disease and only rarely with pneumonitis; in contrast, organ transplant recipients almost always manifest pneumonitis, and retinitis rarely develops. *M. avium* complex is common in patients with HIV infection but rare in patients with most other causes of immunosuppression. Similarly, therapy for various opportunistic infections may also differ. Certain drugs may not be tolerated as well by HIV-infected patients as by other immunosuppressed patients; the unusually high incidence of rash associated with TMP-SMX is a good example of this phenomenon. Drug regimens need to be continued for longer periods: unless the immune competence can be augmented substantially by ART, the likelihood of recurrence for most HIV-associated infections is so high that lifelong suppressive or maintenance therapy (e.g., secondary prophylaxis) must be maintained. Drug-drug interactions are often important considerations, especially if patients are receiving ART; rifampin, rifabutin, and fluconazole are examples of drugs that may have clinically important drug interactions with antiretroviral agents that could require dose modifications of either the antiretroviral agent or the drug used to treat the opportunistic infection. HIV-infected patients frequently have multiple concurrent opportunistic infections. Patients are often being treated or receiving prophylaxis for multiple infections simultaneously, thereby leading to potential additive toxicities or drug interactions. Finally, HIV-infected patients are administered multiple courses of antimicrobial agents, often for prolonged periods. These patients have the potential for the development of drug-resistant pathogens themselves, and they are exposed to drug-resistant pathogens in clinics, hospitals, and other group settings. They are at high risk for disease caused by drug-resistant pathogens, such as *M. tuberculosis, P. jiroveci, Streptococcus pneumoniae,* and *Candida.* All these issues support the concept that optimal management should emphasize identification of the specific organism causing a specific syndrome because the range of possible etiologic agents is broad and the adverse consequences of unnecessary drugs are magnified in patients with HIV as compared with many other populations.

The manifestations and treatment of specific opportunistic and nonopportunistic pathogens are discussed in Chapters 300 to 408. Additional chapters detail pulmonary disease (Chapter 414), skin disorders (Chapter 415), hematologic problems (Chapter 416), gastrointestinal disease (Chapter 413), and neurologic disorders (Chapter 417). Several additional syndromes deserve particular mention.

Fever is a common finding in patients with HIV infection. As noted earlier, patients with HIV infection are susceptible to a wide range of processes that can cause fever, including opportunistic and nonopportunistic infections, neoplasms, and drug toxicities. The $CD4^+$ T-lymphocyte cell count is a valuable indicator of the likelihood for opportunistic pathogens. At high $CD4^+$ T cell counts (e.g., >300 cells/mL), the evaluation should probably be similar to that for non–HIV-infected healthy individuals, although patients do have enhanced predisposition to certain processes, notably pneumococcal disease, tuberculosis, and specific neoplasms such as lymphoma and Kaposi's sarcoma.

Fever and Wasting

Early in the HIV epidemic, patients often sought care for fever of several weeks' or months' duration, associated with considerable weight loss. This is less common in the era of effective ART, but it still occurs in the United States and western Europe and is especially common in emerging countries. Many of the opportunistic infections associated with HIV infection can cause this syndrome. In some patients, chronic cough, chronic diarrhea, abnormal liver function test results, and other focal findings can lead to a directed evaluation. Some patients have no focal or localizing findings. In such patients, methodical evaluation is required with specific attention to the possibility of pulmonary or disseminated tuberculosis, disseminated *M. avium* complex or fungal disease, lymphoma, and endocrine abnormalities such as adrenal insufficiency. Diagnostic evaluations that merit special consideration include mycobacterial blood cultures and serum cryptococcal and *Histoplasma* antigen testing. Extensive imaging procedures should be considering before initiating empirical therapy.

Retinitis

Ocular manifestations are one of the most common complications of HIV infection. When patients have visual complaints, it is important to determine the anatomic location of the lesion (e.g., cornea, choroid, retina, cranial nerve, or occipital lobe) to establish the appropriate diagnostic and therapeutic approach.

CMV retinitis is the most common vision-threatening lesion. Patients almost universally have positive serum anti-CMV IgG levels and $CD4^+$ T-lymphocyte cell counts less than 50 cells/mL. CMV causes irreversible necrosis of the retina, although treatment can restore some vision as edema of the retina subsides. Untreated, CMV retinitis causes progressive loss of vision in both eyes.

The diagnosis of CMV retinitis can be made during routine retinal examination (dilated indirect ophthalmoscopy) performed by an experienced ophthalmologist. Examination with a direct ophthalmoscope evaluates just 10% of the total retinal area; disease can be excluded only by a full funduscopic evaluation. Polymerase chain reaction (PCR) of the aqueous or vitreous can be used to document CMV, as can retinal biopsy, but such procedures are almost never used given the characteristic clinical findings. In patients with CMV retinitis, CMV disease may also be present or eventually develop in other anatomic locations, such as the colon or CNS.

The goal of therapy for CMV retinitis is to arrest progression of the disease, prevent further spread of infection, and preserve visual function. Therapy with one of the recommended modalities (e.g., oral valganciclovir, intravenous ganciclovir or foscarnet, or an ocular implant plus oral valganciclovir) is usually effective; maintenance therapy is necessary lifelong unless ART leads to substantial immunologic reconstitution. If such reconstitution occurs, immune reconstitution syndromes can cause substantial ocular pathology.

Other pathogens can also cause retinitis. Varicella-zoster virus (VZV) can cause acute retinal necrosis ($CD4^+$ T-lymphocyte count >50 cells/mL) or progressive outer retinal necrosis ($CD4^+$ T-lymphocyte count <50 cells/mL). The former often responds to acyclovir; the latter usually does not. Toxoplasmosis can likewise cause retinitis. Experienced ophthalmologists can generally distinguish *Toxoplasma* retinochoroiditis from CMV or VZV disease or from pathology caused by herpes simplex virus, mycobacteria, or fungi. However, such diagnoses can be difficult to establish based solely on funduscopic examination.

Central Nervous System Mass Lesions

In the era before ART, focal brain lesions developed in 10% of patients, and the majority of such patients came to attention when their $CD4^+$ T-lymphocyte counts were less than 100 cells/mL. Initial signs and symptoms range from focal deficits (hemiparesis, aphasia, diplopia, seizures) to generalized weakness or altered mental status. Neuroimaging is important to confirm the clinical diagnosis of a mass lesion and to distinguish among general diagnostic categories (e.g., bacterial brain abscess, tumor, opportunistic infection, or progressive multifocal leukoencephalopathy [PML]). Neuroimaging does not, however, provide a microbiologic diagnosis. Positron emission tomography with radiolabeled glucose to measure tissue metabolism or single-photon emission computed tomography to measure metabolically linked cerebral blood flow appears to be useful for distinguishing tumors (e.g., lymphoma) from infections (e.g., toxoplasmosis).

The majority of focal contrast-enhancing brain lesions in HIV-infected patients are caused by cerebral toxoplasmosis (25 to 50%) or primary CNS lymphoma (20 to 30%). On magnetic resonance imaging or computed tomography, these lesions are often associated with surrounding edema. Although primary CNS lymphoma typically involves solitary brain lesions and cerebral toxoplasmosis is more commonly associated with multiple lesions, these diagnoses cannot be distinguished solely by neuroradiographic parameters.

Toxoplasmosis almost always occurs as a result of reactivation of previously acquired disease in patients with CD4⁺ T-lymphocyte counts less than 50 cells/mL. Almost all patients have positive IgG serum antibodies against *Toxoplasma* if serology is performed by a reference laboratory. The diagnosis of toxoplasmosis is usually established by either response to empirical therapy or brain biopsy. Cerebrospinal fluid (CSF) examination is rarely helpful in establishing toxoplasmosis as the diagnosis.

The majority of patients with cerebral toxoplasmosis (65 to 90%) respond rapidly to standard two-drug anti-*Toxoplasma* therapy with pyrimethamine (200 mg orally once, followed by 75 mg daily) plus either sulfadiazine (1 to 1.5 g orally every 6 hours) or clindamycin (600 mg orally/intravenously every 6 hours). Clinical improvement is generally seen within several days, and neuroradiographic improvement occurs within 2 to 3 weeks. Failure to reach these milestones should raise suspicion of other diagnoses, such as lymphoma. Patients who respond should be treated for a minimum of 6 weeks after resolution/stabilization of the clinical and radiologic abnormalities. Lifelong suppressive therapy is necessary to prevent recurrences (80% recurred in the pre-ART era without secondary prophylaxis), unless the patient responds immunologically to ART.

Primary CNS lymphoma and generalized lymphoma both occur in patients who are usually naive to ART and commonly have less than 100 cells/mL. Both diseases progress rapidly, with high morbidity and mortality. HIV-associated primary CNS lymphoma occurs most often in patients with $CD4^+$ T-lymphocyte counts of 100 cells/mL or lower. Epstein-Barr viral DNA can be detected by PCR in the CSF of almost all patients.

Most authorities recommend treatment of primary CNS lymphoma with combination chemotherapy; lesions are highly responsive to irradiation, but radiation is associated with considerable morbidity and a dismal prognosis.

PML involves white matter lesions and is generally clinically distinct from the manifestations of toxoplasmosis or lymphoma. Patients usually have subacute limb weakness, sensory loss, gait difficulties, cognitive impairment, or any combination of these findings.

Magnetic resonance imaging shows predominantly white matter lesions with no contrast enhancement or mass effect. JC viral DNA can be demonstrated by PCR examination of CSF.

The prognosis for PML is dismal: most patients die within 4 months unless they have a robust immunologic response to ART. No specific therapy has been shown to be effective for PML.

Diarrhea

Chronic diarrhea is a common problem for patients with HIV infection and $CD4^+$ T-lymphocyte counts below 100 to 200 cells/mL. See Chapter 413 for detailed information.

Parasitic and Fungal Infections Acquired Outside the United States

In patients who live in emerging countries or those who have traveled to such areas, latent infections may reactivate once they return to the United States or emigrate there. Leishmaniasis, Chagas' disease, and malaria are examples of parasitic diseases that can be more frequent and more severe in patients with HIV infection than in those without HIV infection. Leishmania, for example, can reactivate years after residence in an endemic area such as the Mediterranean basin or Brazil and be associated with fever, cytopenia, and hepatosplenomegaly. Therapy with liposomal amphotericin B or pentavalent antimony is effective, although treatment may have to be lifelong unless immunity is reconstituted with highly active ART. Similarly, *Trypanosoma cruzi* can be manifested as a focal cerebral mass lesion or lesions years after residence in an endemic area; therapy with benznidazole or nifurtimox has been used successfully.

Immune Reconstitution Syndromes

When patients with HIV infection initiate ART, their augmented immune response may produce clinical syndromes that seem to represent immunologic or inflammatory reactions rather than disease progression from proliferating organisms. Within days, weeks, or months after ART is started and sometimes before the $CD4^+$ T-lymphocyte count has risen, patients may manifest such a syndrome. These syndromes may involve pathogens not previously recognized; patients who initiate ART when their $CD4^+$ T-lymphocyte count is less than 50 cells/mL may have lymphadenopathy secondary to previously unrecognized *M. avium* complex or pulmonary disease from cryptococcosis. These syndromes may also involve sites that were recognized to be involved by opportunistic infections but that seemed to be well controlled; patients who initiate ART many months after apparently successful treatment of CMV retinitis or cryptococcal meningitis may experience deterioration in vision or severe headache. Immune reconstitution syndromes are most often associated with *M. tuberculosis, Cryptococcus neoformans,* and *M. avium* complex; the frequency depends on their prevalence in a given geographic area.

Some of these syndromes do not seem to be associated with active infection (e.g., immune reconstitution uveitis after CMV retinitis). Others, such as mycobacterial lymphadenitis, are associated with organisms that can be identified by histology and culture. Data regarding managing these syndromes are largely anecdotal. It is not clear when specific or pathogen-directed therapy is indicated or how long this therapy should be continued. It is also not clear what role topical or systemic anti-inflammatory agents should play. Most clinicians would continue ART unless immune reconstitution manifestations were life-threatening or intolerable; nonsteroidal anti-inflammatory agents and corticosteroids can be used, although there are no helpful guidelines about when to use these agents other than to use good clinical judgment.

The potential for immune reconstitution syndrome should be a consideration when deciding whether to start ART soon after the onset of an opportunistic infection. Initiation of ART may be the only promising intervention for certain infections that have limited specific options, such as cryptosporidiosis or PML. However, for PCP, tuberculosis, or pulmonary histoplasmosis, for example, for which specific therapy is quite effective, initiation of ART may cause more organ dysfunction if an immune reconstitution response occurs.

Treatment of HIV/AIDS-Associated Complications

Treatment of HIV-Associated Neoplasms

Therapy for HIV-associated lymphoma, Kaposi's sarcoma, human papillomavirus–associated neoplasms, and other malignant processes such as primary effusion cell lymphoma and multicentric Castleman's disease is detailed in Chapter 416. Early in the HIV epidemic there was little optimism that these neoplastic processes could be treated successfully. More recent studies, however, suggest that even for HIV-associated lymphoma, rates of remission and long-term survival are improving. When treating HIV-associated neoplasms, particular attention to antiretroviral regimens, drug toxicities, drug interactions, and chemoprophylaxis for HIV-associated opportunistic infections is required if the prognosis is to be optimized.

Treatment of Pregnant HIV-Infected Patients

Women with HIV infection who are pregnant should be offered therapy based on the same virologic, immunologic, and clinical parameters as nonpregnant women. [4] The goal of therapy is to provide maximal virologic suppression to optimize the health of the mother and minimize transmission of virus to the fetus. The choice of drugs and the timing of initiating therapy may, however, be influenced by the pregnancy.

Most antiretroviral drugs are safe in pregnant women, to the extent they have been studied. Many of the toxicities caused by antiretroviral agents may contribute to parallel complications of pregnancy, however (e.g., the hyperglycemia associated with protease inhibitors may exacerbate pregnancy-associated diabetes). There are specific concerns regarding the use of nucleosides during pregnancy, especially stavudine and didanosine, in view of their association with hepatic steatosis and lactic acidosis in several pregnant women. There is also particular concern about the association of efavirenz with fetal abnormalities in monkeys. Finally, combination ART may be associated with an increased risk for preterm delivery. Antiretroviral regimens must be chosen carefully and monitored.

Transmission of HIV from mother to fetus has been observed at all maternal plasma HIV RNA levels. There does seem to be a correlation, however, between the HIV plasma RNA copy number and the risk of transmission. Clinical trials have shown that ART can greatly reduce the likelihood that virus will be transmitted to the fetus or infant. Zidovudine monotherapy and nevirapine monotherapy have been most carefully studied, and both seem to be safe for the mother and fetus and are effective in substantially reducing the rate of maternal-fetal transmission.

However, monotherapy is no longer indicated in settings in which combination ART is feasible. Moreover, it has become apparent that single-dose nevirapine monotherapy can produce HIV resistance because of the long half-life of nevirapine. It is logical to use combination ART regimens for treating the mother to lower her viral load effectively and produce durable viral suppression.

Current guidelines indicate that combination ART, usually including zidovudine, should be recommended for infected women who meet the standard criteria for treatment or who have HIV RNA levels greater than 1000 copies/mL, regardless of immunologic or clinical status. Women who are in the first trimester of pregnancy may prefer delaying therapy until after 10 to 12 weeks of gestation if they are concerned about the teratogenicity of drugs administered during the early part of their pregnancy. Women who are not receiving zidovudine or nevirapine but who have HIV plasma RNA levels less than 1000 copies/mL seem to have a low risk of transmitting HIV to their offspring. There are no clear guidelines about how best to manage pregnant women whose virus is resistant to zidovudine and nevirapine.

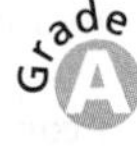

1. U.S. Public Health Service/Infectious Diseases Society of America: Guidelines for using antiretroviral agents among HIV-infected adults and adolescents. Recommendations of the Panel on Clinical Practices for the Treatment of HIV. Available at AIDSINFO.nih/gov/guidelines.
2. U.S.I Public Health Service/Infectious Diseases Society of America: Guidelines for prevention of opportunistic infections in persons with HIV infection. Available at AIDSINFO.nih/gov/guidelines.
3. National Institutes of Health/Centers for Disease Control and Prevention/Infectious Diseases Society of America: Guidelines for treatment of opportunistic infections in persons with HIV infection. Available at AIDSINFO.nih/gov/guidelines
4. U.S. Public Health Service Task Force: Recommendations for use of antiretroviral drugs in pregnant HIV-1–infected women for maternal health and interventions to reduce perinatal HIV-1 transmission in the United States. Available at AIDSINFO.nih/gov/guidelines.

SUGGESTED READINGS

Braitstein P, Brinkhof MW, Dabis F, et al: Mortality of HIV-1-infected patients in the first year of antiretroviral therapy: Comparison between low-income and high-income countries. Lancet 2006;367:817–824. *Patients in resource-poor settings have increased mortality rates in the first months on therapy.*

Hammer SM, Saag MS, Schechter M, et al: Treatment for adult HIV infection: 2006 recommendations of the International AIDS Society—USA panel. JAMA 2006;296:827–843. *Expert guidelines for the use of antiretroviral therapy.*

Goldie SJ, Yazdanpanah Y, Losina E, et al: Cost-effectiveness of HIV treatment in resource-poor settings—the case of Côte d'Ivoire. N Engl J Med 2006;355:1141–1153. *A cost and clinical analysis of treatment strategies.*

Lockman S, Shapiro RL, Smeaton LM, et al: Response to antiretroviral therapy after a single, peripartum dose of nevirapine. N Engl J Med 2007;356:135–147. *Women who received a single dose of nevirapine to prevent perinatal transmission of HIV-1 had higher rates of virologic failure with subsequent nevirapine-based antiretroviral therapy that did women without previous exposure to nevirapine.*

May MT, Sterne JA, Costagliola D, et al: HIV treatment response and prognosis in Europe and North America in the first decade of highly active antiretroviral therapy: A collaborative analysis. Lancet 2006;368:451–458. *Review of this remarkable success story.*

413 GASTROINTESTINAL MANIFESTATIONS OF HUMAN IMMUNODEFICIENCY VIRUS AND ACQUIRED IMMUNODEFICIENCY SYNDROME

John G. Bartlett

The gastrointestinal tract is an especially common site for clinical expression of human immunodeficiency virus (HIV) infection and is an important factor in both morbidity from opportunistic infections in late-stage disease and gastrointestinal complications from antiretroviral agents or other drugs. Nearly all opportunistic infections occur when the $CD4^+$ T-cell count is less than 200/mL, and almost all seem to respond well to immune reconstitution with antiretroviral therapy.

ORAL LESIONS

Oral candidiasis ("thrush") is encountered at some time in 80 to 90% of all patients with advanced stages of HIV infection. The usual finding is white patches that show yeast forms and pseudohyphae on potassium hydroxide preparation. Thrush is often asymptomatic, or it may cause mouth pain, dysphagia, and taste change. The diagnosis is usually made by visual appearance. Treatment consists of topical agents (e.g., nystatin, clotrimazole troches) or oral therapy with azoles. Because relapse rates are high, continuous therapy with topical agents or azoles is often necessary.

Oral hairy leukoplakia (Chapter 415) is characterized by white patches consisting of white fibrillar projections that are usually located on the tongue and are often confused with thrush. Oral hairy leukoplakia is generally asymptomatic, but some patients complain of pain or voice changes; symptomatic patients usually respond to treatment with acyclovir. Herpes simplex virus (HSV) (Chapter 397) often causes painful oral lesions characterized by typical vesicles on an erythematous base that break down to form ulcers. Herpetic oral lesions are common in the general population, but they tend to be more severe and prolonged in patients with advanced HIV infection. The usual treatment is acyclovir, famciclovir, or valacyclovir given orally; severe cases may require intravenous acyclovir or, for acyclovir-resistant strains, foscarnet given parenterally. The major source of confusion is aphthous ulcers of unknown origin, which seem to respond best to thalidomide or to corticosteroids given topically or systemically.

Patients with Kaposi's sarcoma (Chapter 416) may have involvement of the oral cavity, most frequently with typical purplish raised lesions on the palate, although any site in the oral cavity may be involved. Most are asymptomatic; symptomatic lesions generally respond to irradiation, laser treatments, or vinblastine injections.

Periodontal disease, with gingivitis or periodontitis, is relatively common. Treatment consists of topical chlorhexidine (Peridex) or systemically administered metronidazole.

ESOPHAGITIS

Dysphagia or odynophagia in a patient with advanced HIV infection and thrush usually indicates *Candida* esophagitis, and most patients are treated empirically with fluconazole. Alternative causes of esophagitis include esophageal ulcers, most commonly caused by cytomegalovirus (CMV), or aphthous ulceration, infrequently caused by HSV (Table 413–1). Endoscopy is recommended for patients with atypical symptoms and those who fail to respond to fluconazole. Some cases are caused by fluconazole-resistant *Candida* species and require intravenous amphotericin B or caspofungin. HSV may be treated with acyclovir, CMV responds to ganciclovir or valganciclovir, and aphthous ulcers are optimally treated with systemic corticosteroids or thalidomide.

GASTRIC LESIONS

Patients with acquired immunodeficiency syndrome (AIDS) often have gastric achlorhydria; less common are Kaposi's sarcoma and opportunistic infections. Gastric intolerance to medications is common, especially with zidovudine, didanosine, all protease inhibitors, macrolides, trimethoprim-sulfamethoxazole, and pentamidine. Symptoms include nausea, vomiting, anorexia, and epigastric pain and generally resolve promptly when use of the implicated drug is discontinued.

SMALL BOWEL AND COLON LESIONS

Acute or chronic diarrhea is a frequent complication and may be caused by medications, opportunistic infections, or common sources occurring in the general population such as viral gastroenteritis or irritable bowel syndrome. The antiretroviral agents that most commonly cause diarrhea are nelfinavir, didanosine, and saquinavir. Treatment with antibacterial agents may be complicated by *Clostridium difficile*–associated diarrhea or colitis, which is now the most frequent enteric pathogen in AIDS patients (Chapter 319).

TABLE 413–1 ESOPHAGEAL COMPLICATIONS OF HIV INFECTION

Agent	Frequency* (%)	CD4⁺ Count	Clinical Features	Diagnosis	Treatment
Candida	50–70	<200/mL	Odynophagia, thrush, diffuse pain, usually afebrile	Usually treated empirically; endoscopy shows plaques	Fluconazole
Cytomegalovirus (CMV)	10–20	<50/mL	Odynophagia, focal pain, usually febrile	Biopsy of ulcer to show CMV inclusions	Ganciclovir or valganciclovir
Herpes simplex virus (HSV)	2–5	<200/mL	Odynophagia, oral HSV lesions common, usually afebrile	Biopsy of ulcer to show HSV inclusions	Acyclovir
Idiopathic	10–20	<300/mL	Odynophagia, focal pain, usually afebrile	Negative biopsy of ulcer	Prednisone or thalidomide

*Approximate frequency in HIV-infected patients with odynophagia.

TABLE 413–2 AGENTS OF ACUTE AND CHRONIC DIARRHEA

Agent	Frequency* (%)	CD4⁺ Count	Clinical Features	Diagnosis	Treatment
ACUTE DIARRHEA					
Salmonella	5–15	Any	Watery diarrhea, fever	Stool and blood culture	Fluoroquinolone
Clostridium difficile	10–15	Any	Cramps, watery diarrhea, fever	Stool toxin assay	Metronidazole or vancomycin
Enteric viruses	15–30	Any	Watery diarrhea, usually afebrile	None	Symptomatic
Idiopathic	25–40	Any	Variable	Negative culture, O&P examination, *C. difficile* toxin	Symptomatic
CHRONIC DIARRHEA					
Cryptosporidium	10–30	<100/mL	Watery diarrhea, fever variable, may have devastating fluid losses	Stool O&P with AFB	HAART
Microsporidia	15–30	<100/mL	Watery diarrhea, afebrile	Stool trichrome stain	Albendazole (*Encephalitozoon intestinalis* only) HAART
Isospora belli	1–3	<100/mL	Watery diarrhea	Stool O&P with AFB	TMP-SMX
Mycobacterium avium	10–20	<50/mL	Watery diarrhea, fever, wasting	Blood culture	Clarithromycin and ethambutol
Cytomegalovirus	15–40	<50/mL	Watery or bloody diarrhea, fever, fecal WBCs	Colon biopsy	Ganciclovir or valganciclovir
Idiopathic	20–30	Any	Watery diarrhea	Negative culture, O&P, *C. difficile* toxin, endoscopy	Symptomatic

*Frequency in HIV-infected patients with acute or chronic diarrhea; with chronic diarrhea, frequency of a CD4⁺ count less than 200/mL.
AFB = acid-fast bacillus; HAART = highly active antiretroviral therapy; O&P = ova and parasites; TMP-SMX = trimethoprim-sulfamethoxazole; WBCs = white blood cells.

Diagnosis

The differential diagnosis must include consideration of medication effects, CD4⁺ count, distinction between acute versus chronic diarrhea, and clinical features of inflammatory (colonic) versus secretory (small bowel) diarrhea. The duration that separates acute and chronic diarrhea is 3 weeks. Characteristic features of inflammatory diarrhea are colitis, clinical symptoms of cramps and fever with small-volume "fraction" stools, and stool examinations showing leukocytes or blood, or both. Secretory diarrhea is usually caused by small bowel pathology; the diarrhea is watery and large volume, and stool studies are negative for fecal leukocytes and blood. The CD4⁺ count that generally defines vulnerability to opportunistic enteric pathogens is 200/mL, although the common forms (i.e., CMV colitis, microsporidiosis, chronic cryptosporidiosis, and disseminated *Mycobacterium avium*) are usually seen only with CD4⁺ counts less than 50/mL.

The most common infectious causes of acute diarrhea in HIV-infected patients are *C. difficile*, salmonellosis, and enteric viruses (Table 413–2). When the CD4⁺ count is greater than 200/mL, the differential diagnosis includes the same pathogens seen in immunocompetent patients. HIV-infected patients do not appear to be uniquely susceptible to *C. difficile*, but this complication is relatively common because they often take antibiotics. The only enteric pathogen responsible for acute diarrhea to which HIV-infected patients are uniquely susceptible is *Salmonella*. The diagnostic evaluation is the same as that for immunocompetent patients and is based on the severity of symptoms, the epidemiology, and the probability of inflammatory diarrhea because these enteric pathogens (i.e., *Salmonella, Shigella, Campylobacter jejuni, C. difficile,* and *Escherichia coli* O157) are more likely to be serious and treatable. Treatment is the same as for persons without HIV infection, except that salmonellosis is usually treated with antibiotics and for a longer period. With CD4⁺ counts less than 200/mL, especially if less than 50/mL, acute diarrhea may represent the early stages of enteric infection caused by pathogens more commonly associated with chronic diarrhea.

Opportunistic pathogens that cause chronic diarrhea are much more closely associated with the $CD4^+$ count. With counts greater than 200/mL, the usual causes are medications, idiopathic or functional bowel disease, inflammatory bowel disease, and occasionally, chronic parasitic infections such as cryptosporidiosis, giardiasis, or amebiasis. With $CD4^+$ counts less than 200/mL, the "big four" enteric pathogens are *Cryptosporidium parvum,* microsporidia (*Enterocytozoon bieneusi* and *Encephalitozoon intestinalis*), *M. avium,* and CMV; less common is *Isospora belli.*

The diagnostic evaluation is dictated by the symptoms and $CD4^+$ count. Standard screening tests for HIV-infected patients who have diarrhea that is severe, chronic, and not associated with medication include a stool culture for enteric pathogens, ova and parasite examination twice with acid-fast stain (to detect *Cryptosporidium, Isospora,* and *Cyclospora*), stool stain and microscopy for microsporidia (≈1000 magnification with trichrome stain), *C. difficile* toxin assay (especially with recent antibiotic use), and stool analysis for fecal leukocytes and red blood cells. Endoscopy is generally reserved for patients with severe or persistent symptoms and a negative evaluation with noninvasive studies. Endoscopy is often necessary to establish the diagnosis of CMV colitis or enteritis.

Treatment

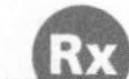

Treatment of chronic infectious diarrhea in an HIV-infected patient is determined by the severity of symptoms and pathogen. In nearly all cases, the most important facet of care is immune reconstitution with antiretroviral agents. With chronic cryptosporidiosis and most cases of CMV colitis and microsporidiosis, this is the only intervention that is likely to be effective. Nonspecific interventions that are commonly used and are effective include antiperistaltic agents such as loperamide and diet modification, including small, frequent, bland feedings without caffeine, fat, milk, or milk products. Antimicrobial recommendations are summarized in Table 413–2: cryptosporidiosis is commonly treated with paromomycin, but evidence of benefit by this or other antimicrobials is sparse. *E. intestinalis* responds to albendazole, but *E. bieneusi* causes 80% of microsporidia cases and cannot be treated with antimicrobials. CMV is usually treated with intravenous ganciclovir or oral valganciclovir, but response is modest and recurrence rates are high. *M. avium* generally responds to standard treatment, but therapy must be lifelong unless immune reconstitution takes place.

ADVERSE REACTIONS TO ANTIRETROVIRAL AGENTS

Gastrointestinal complications of antiretroviral agents are common and important because they often interfere with adherence to antiretroviral drugs, which is critical for virologic control and response, and because they may represent potentially life-threatening complications. Gastrointestinal intolerance with nausea, vomiting, and abdominal pain may occur with all antiretrovirals but is especially common with zidovudine, didanosine, ritonavir, amprenavir, and indinavir. All are dose related, and tolerance to protease inhibitors may be worsened with the use of ritonavir boosting. Diarrhea is also common, but secretory diarrhea is especially frequent with nelfinavir; this can usually be controlled with loperamide or calcium. Life-threatening complications attributed to antiretroviral agents include pancreatitis (didanosine and stavudine), lactic acidosis (zidovudine, didanosine, stavudine), and hepatotoxicity (nevirapine). Pancreatitis occurs in 1 to 9% of didanosine recipients, is more common in patients with other risk factors for pancreatitis, and is associated with the typical symptoms of severe abdominal pain with elevated amylase and lipase. Lactic acidosis results from mitochondrial toxicity caused by nucleoside analogues, primarily stavudine, zidovudine, and didanosine (although any nucleoside may be the cause). The usual manifestation is prolonged nucleoside exposure, gastrointestinal symptoms, including weight loss, and an elevated blood lactate level, generally greater than 5 mmol/mL. Treatment of pancreatitis and lactic acidosis is largely supportive, recovery is often prolonged, and the inducing agent should be avoided.

TUMORS

Tumors of the gastrointestinal tract associated with HIV infection include Kaposi's sarcoma, non-Hodgkin's lymphoma, cloacogenic carcinoma of the rectum, and squamous cell carcinoma of the rectum and anus (see Chapter 416). The most common of these tumors is Kaposi's sarcoma, which has been found in gut tissue at autopsy in 40 to 50% of persons with typical cutaneous lesions. Endoscopy characteristically shows raised red nodules, but histologic confirmation is difficult because of the depth of the pathologic changes. Most are asymptomatic; less common manifestations include diarrhea, subacute intestinal obstruction, protein-losing enteropathy, and rectal ulcer. The lymphomas associated with HIV infection are generally high-grade B-cell lymphomas that are extranodal in origin. The gastrointestinal tract is affected in up to 20% of patients, and any site may be involved from the oral cavity to the rectum.

AIDS ENTEROPATHY

Endoscopy in patients with advanced AIDS often shows morphologic changes in the small bowel in the absence of evidence of a superimposed opportunistic infection. Characteristic features are villous blunting, a reduced villus-crypt ratio, and an inappropriately low number of mitotic figures. In the absence of an enteric pathogen, the findings are sometimes referred to as *AIDS enteropathy.* Studies of gastrointestinal function in the presence of AIDS enteropathy typically show malabsorption with abnormal D-xylose and ^{14}C-glycerol-tripalmitin absorption tests. The cause of these changes is unknown, but the major considerations include direct invasion by HIV, an opportunistic infection that has not been detected, or a consequence of immune suppression.

MALNUTRITION AND WASTING

The average patient with late-stage AIDS loses 15 to 20% of baseline weight. Protein-calorie malnutrition is a common and important sequela that may accelerate progressive immunosuppression. Factors contributing to malnutrition include a hypermetabolic state associated with chronic infection (especially with fever), oral lesions causing pain, esophageal lesions resulting in dysphagia, reduced taste sensation, depression, HIV-associated subcortical dementia, gastrointestinal side effects of medications, hypogonadism, and AIDS enteropathy. Many patients lose weight with sequential opportunistic infections that is not regained during asymptomatic intervals. Therapy for wasting depends on the severity, cause, patient gender, and response. Immune reconstitution with antiretroviral therapy has been associated with remarkable weight gain. Prevention of opportunistic infections is an important factor in stabilizing weight. A number of pharmacologic agents are in common use, with variable responses in terms of the amount and quality of weight gained (fat versus muscle). The most commonly used agents for wasting are appetite stimulants (e.g., megestrol acetate, dronabinol), testosterone, or synthetic anabolic steroids (e.g., oxandrolone, nandrolone).

HEPATOBILIARY DISEASE

The prevalence of markers for hepatitis B (i.e., hepatitis B surface antigen [HBsAg], antibody to HBsAg, or antibody to hepatitis B core antigen) is 35 to 80% in AIDS patients, which is a reflection of their prevalence among homosexual men, intravenous drug abusers, and hemophiliacs. HBsAg is found in 5 to 10% of patients. Hepatitis C virus (HCV) infection is found in up to 90% of injection drug users and patients with hemophilia. It is clear that the course of HCV infection is accelerated by HIV coinfection, but evidence for the reverse is less impressive.

The preferred treatment of chronic HCV infection is pegylated interferon plus ribavirin, but indications are confounded by drug interactions and toxicity when used with antiretroviral agents, the uncertain natural history of HCV infection, and high rates of intolerance to HCV drugs. Patients coinfected with hepatitis B virus (HBV; HBsAg positive) are challenging because some drugs given for HIV are also active against HBV, including lamivudine, tenofovir, and emtricitabine. Hepatitis flares may result from several interventions, including immune reconstitution, development of HBV resistance to lamivudine, and discontinuing drugs that are active against HBV. Hepatotoxic drugs commonly taken by HIV-infected patients include all antiretroviral agents, as well as azoles, sulfonamides, isoniazid, and rifampin. With nucleosides (zidovudine, stavudine, didanosine), lactic acidosis with steatosis may develop; the manifestation is typical of lactic acidosis (e.g., nausea, vomiting, abdominal pain, weight loss) combined with elevated transaminase levels and characteristic features on liver scans. With non-nucleoside reverse transcriptase inhibitors, there is a particular problem with nevirapine because it may cause a serious life-threatening syndrome characterized by fever, gastrointestinal symptoms, and hepatic necrosis. This reaction is most common in the first 6 to 12 weeks of treatment and in treatment-naive patients with baseline $CD4^+$ counts of greater than 250/mL for women and greater than 400/mL for men. It is best to avoid nevirapine in this setting; if nevirapine is necessary, frequent monitoring is required. All protease inhibitors may cause hepatotoxicity; rates are highest with ritonavir. This is usually a dose-related toxicity, and therapy should be changed when transaminase levels exceed five times the upper limits of normal.

Cholestasis from papillary stenosis and sclerosing cholangitis are most often caused by *Cryptosporidium,* Microsporida, or CMV or are idiopathic. The usual manifestation is right upper quadrant pain and laboratory evidence of cholestasis in patients with late-stage AIDS. Diagnosis and treatment are usually established with endoscopic retrograde cholangiopancreatography. Treatment directed against an identified pathogen is generally unsuccessful.

SUGGESTED READINGS

Abubakar I, Aliyu SH, Arumugam C, et al: Prevention and treatment of cryptosporidiosis in immunocompromised patients. Cochrane Database Syst Rev 2007;CD004932. *Meta-analysis confirming that there is no evidence for an effective treatment of this disease in immunocompromised individuals.*

Dworkin MS, Williamson JM, for the Adult/Adolescent Spectrum of HIV Disease Project: AIDS wasting syndrome: Trends, influence on opportunistic infections, and survival. J Acquir Immune Defic Syndr 2003;33:267–273. *The incidence is declining.*

Falco V, Rodriguez D, Ribera E, et al: Severe nucleoside-associated lactic acidosis in human immunodeficiency virus–infected patients. Clin Infect Dis 2002;34:838–846. *A review of 60 reported cases showing that the most common manifestation is GI symptoms with weight loss, the most commonly implicated nucleotide reverse transcriptase inhibitor is stavudine, and the mortality rate is directly related to the lactic acid level.*

Gan I, May G, Raboud J, et al: Pancreatitis in HIV infection: Predictors of severity. Am J Gastroenterol 2003;98:1278–1283. *Outcomes are similar to those in non–HIV-infected patients.*

Koziel MJ, Peters MG, et al: Viral hepatitis in HIV infection. N Engl J Med 2007;356:1445–1554. *Clinical review.*

Lewthwaite P, Gill GV, Hart CA, et al: Gastrointestinal parasites in the immunocompromised. Curr Opin Infect Dis 2005;18:427–425. *Comprehensive clinical review.*

Pienaar ED, Young T, Homes H: Interventions for the prevention and management of oropharyngeal candidiasis associated with HIV infection in adults and children. Cochrane Database Syst Rev 2006;CD003940. *Meta-analysis of the efficacy of several antifungal medications in the treatment and prevention of oral thrush in the setting of HIV.*

Thom K, Forrest G: Gastrointestinal infections in immunocompromised hosts. Curr Opin Gastroenterol 2006;22:18–23. *Clinical review.*

Vazquez JA, Skiest DJ, Nieto L, et al: A multicenter randomized trial evaluating posaconazole versus fluconazole for the treatment of oropharyngeal candidiasis in subjects with HIV/AIDS. Clin Infect Dis 2006;42:1179–1186. *Randomized trial showing equivalent efficacy of the two medications in initial treatment response but perhaps improved long-term outcomes in patients who received posaconazole.*

414 PULMONARY MANIFESTATIONS OF HUMAN IMMUNODEFICIENCY VIRUS INFECTION AND ACQUIRED IMMUNODEFICIENCY SYNDROME

Laurence Huang

Definition

Respiratory symptoms are common in persons with human immunodeficiency virus (HIV) infection, and HIV-infected persons are subject to a wide spectrum of pulmonary diseases, both HIV-associated (Table 414–1) and non–HIV-associated. The spectrum of HIV-associated pulmonary diseases encompasses opportunistic infections, neoplasms, and other pulmonary disorders. Table 414–1 lists the most frequent pulmonary diseases seen in HIV-infected persons in the United States. In other parts of the world, these frequencies may be strikingly different. Although each pulmonary disease has characteristic clinical and radiographic findings, they can vary and often overlap.

Diagnosis

Initial Diagnostic Approach

The frequency of HIV-associated opportunistic infections and the need for prompt treatment of these infections often focus the initial diagnostic approach and management on identifying and treating possible infectious causes. However, HIV-infected persons may have HIV-associated neoplasms or other disorders. In addition, risk factors for HIV infection such as injection drug use may also contribute to pulmonary disease (e.g., endocarditis with septic pulmonary emboli). Finally, HIV-infected persons may have preexisting pulmonary disease (e.g., asthma), or pulmonary disease unrelated to their HIV infection (e.g., pulmonary embolism) may develop and be the cause of their symptoms. Therefore, in the proper clinical context, clinicians must also consider noninfectious HIV-associated pulmonary diseases and non–HIV-associated disorders before embarking on an exhaustive search for HIV-associated opportunistic infections.

Clinical Setting

The clinical setting in which the patient is encountered and evaluated has an impact on the relative frequency of pulmonary diseases seen (Table 414–2). This point has been established by several different studies. The Pulmonary Complications of HIV Infection Study, an observational cohort study that monitored more than 1150 HIV-infected subjects for 5 years at six sites across the United States, found that patients seen at an outpatient clinic with respiratory illness more often had upper respiratory tract infections and acute bronchitis than pneumonia secondary to bacteria or *Pneumocystis jirovecii* (formerly *Pneumocystis carinii*). However, neither of the former conditions typically necessitates hospitalization, whereas a significant number of patients with the latter diseases require hospitalization. The most common pulmonary diseases in hospitalized HIV-infected patients are bacterial pneumonia, followed by *Pneumocystis* pneumonia, both of which are significantly more frequent than the next most common diagnoses: tuberculosis, pulmonary Kaposi's sarcoma (KS), and *Cryptococcus neoformans* pneumonia. The Pulmonary Complications of HIV Infection Study found that the most common pulmonary disease in patients requiring critical care was *Pneumocystis* pneumonia, followed by bacterial pneumonia.

The geographic location of the clinic or hospital may also influence the frequency of different diagnoses. In specific populations or particular geographic regions, mycobacterial and endemic fungal pneumonias become important considerations. In endemic areas, diseases caused by *Histoplasma capsulatum* or *Coccidioides immitis* are among the most frequent infections seen.

TABLE 414–1 HIV-ASSOCIATED PULMONARY DISEASES

Opportunistic Infections			
BACTERIAL	**MYCOBACTERIAL**	**FUNGAL**	**VIRAL/PARASITIC**
Streptococcus pneumoniae	*Mycobacterium tuberculosis*	*Pneumocystis jirovecii**	Cytomegalovirus
Haemophilus species	*Mycobacterium kansasii*	*Cryptococcus neoformans*	*Toxoplasma gondii*
Pseudomonas aeruginosa	*Mycobacterium avium* complex	*Histoplasma capsulatum*	
Staphylococcus aureus		*Coccidioides immitis*	
Klebsiella pneumoniae		*Aspergillus* species (esp. *fumigatus*)	

Neoplasms and Selected Noninfectious Diseases		
NEOPLASM	**LYMPHOPROLIFERATIVE DISORDERS**	**MISCELLANEOUS DISORDERS**
Kaposi's sarcoma	Nonspecific interstitial pneumonitis	Pulmonary hypertension
Non-Hodgkin's lymphoma	Lymphocytic interstitial pneumonitis	Chronic obstructive pulmonary disease
		Sarcoidosis
		Immune reconstitution syndromes

*The form of *Pneumocystis* that infects humans is *Pneumocystis jirovecii* (formerly *Pneumocystis carinii*).

Laboratory Findings

CD4⁺ Lymphocyte Count

The $CD4^+$ cell count remains an excellent indicator of an HIV-infected patient's risk for development of a specific opportunistic infection or particular neoplasm, and it is an essential component of the diagnostic approach. Many of the HIV-associated pulmonary diseases become primarily manifested once a patient's $CD4^+$ cell count has declined to less than a characteristic range, and these diseases only occasionally occur in a patient whose $CD4^+$ cell count is greater than that range (Table 414–3). The exceptions are diseases that can develop in persons without underlying immunodeficiency, such as bacterial pneumonia, tuberculosis, and non-Hodgkin's lymphoma. These diseases can occur with any $CD4^+$ cell count in HIV-infected patients. However, their incidence increases as the $CD4^+$ cell count declines. One study found that the risk for bacterial pneumonia in HIV-infected subjects with a $CD4^+$ cell count less than 200 cells/μL was more than $5^1/_2$ times greater than that for subjects whose $CD4^+$ count was higher than 500 cells/μL. In addition, as the $CD4^+$ cell count declines, the incidence of bacterial pneumonia accompanied by bacteremia (especially *Streptococcus pneumoniae*) and the incidence of *Mycobacterium tuberculosis* infection accompanied by extrapulmonary or disseminated disease increase, features that have important implications for diagnosis.

At $CD4^+$ cell counts lower than 200 cells/μL, *Pneumocystis* and *C. neoformans* pneumonias both become significant diagnoses to consider. A review from the Clinical Center of the National Institutes of Health found that 46 of 49 patients (94%) in whom *Pneumocystis* pneumonia was diagnosed had a $CD4^+$ cell count less than 200 cells/μL. The Multicenter AIDS Cohort Study demonstrated that HIV-infected subjects with a $CD4^+$ cell count less than 200 cells/μL at study entry had nearly a five-fold greater risk for *Pneumocystis* pneumonia than did subjects who had a $CD4^+$ cell count greater than 200 cells/μL at entry. Finally, the Pulmonary Complications of HIV Infection Study reported that 95% of 145 cases of *Pneumocystis* pneumonia occurred in subjects whose $CD4^+$ cell count was lower than 200 cells/μL (median $CD4^+$ cell count, 29 cells/μL).

At $CD4^+$ cell counts less than 100 cells/μL, pneumonias secondary to *Pseudomonas aeruginosa* and *Toxoplasma gondii* and lung involvement by KS are increasingly diagnosed. One study of 64 HIV-infected patients with pulmonary toxoplasmosis diagnosed by bronchoalveolar lavage (BAL) reported a mean $CD4^+$ cell count of 40 cells/μL; 82% had a $CD4^+$ count of less than 50 cells/μL, and only 4% had a count greater than 200 cells/μL. A series of 168 consecutive HIV-infected patients with pulmonary KS diagnosed by bronchoscopy reported a median $CD4^+$ cell count of 19 cells/μL; 68% had a $CD4^+$ count less than 50 cells/μL, and only 4% had a count greater than 200 cells/μL.

Finally, at $CD4^+$ cell counts less than 50 cells/μL, diseases caused by nontuberculous mycobacteria (*Mycobacterium avium* complex), endemic (*H. capsulatum, C. immitis*) and nonendemic (*Aspergillus* species) fungi, and cytomegalovirus increasingly become important diagnoses to consider. These diseases are usually accompanied by extrapulmonary or disseminated disease, which can dominate the clinical findings. In many of these cases, the patient may have minimal or no respiratory complaints and the chest radiograph is often normal. One review noted respiratory complaints in 53% of HIV-infected patients with disseminated histoplasmosis and a normal chest radiograph in 43%.

History

Patient Background

A number of important diagnostic clues are contained in a patient's personal and medical background that may help suggest specific diagnoses (see Table 414–2).

Health Habits and Mode of HIV Transmission

A patient's health-related habits and mode of acquiring HIV influence the relative frequency of various HIV-related and non–HIV-related pulmonary diseases. HIV-associated KS is seen almost exclusively in men who report having sexual relations with other men. Bacterial pneumonia and tuberculosis are more common in HIV-infected patients who are injection drug users than in HIV-infected patients without a history of injection drug use. Furthermore, injection or other illicit drug use can cause a variety of non–HIV-related pulmonary diseases such as endocarditis-associated septic pulmonary emboli, pulmonary talcosis–interstitial lung disease, aspiration pneumonia secondary to respiratory depression, and drug-induced pulmonary edema.

HIV-infected patients who smoke tobacco are at increased risk for a variety of smoking-related respiratory illnesses and diseases. Both bacterial bronchitis and bacterial pneumonia are more common in HIV-infected cigarette smokers than in HIV-infected nonsmokers or former smokers. This is especially the case in persons with a $CD4^+$ cell count lower than 200 cells/μL. In addition, HIV-infected patients who report a long history of cigarette use may have manifestations of chronic obstructive pulmonary disease or respiratory bronchiolitis–interstitial lung disease as the cause of their symptoms. Although it is currently debated whether HIV infection itself is associated with an increased risk for lung carcinoma, most cases of lung cancer reported in HIV-infected patients have developed in persons with a history of cigarette smoking.

Travel and Residence

Travel to or residence in a geographic region that is endemic for fungi such as *C. immitis, H. capsulatum,* or *Penicillium marneffei* is a strong determinant of the risk for exposure, infection, and ultimately disease. HIV-infected patients without such a history are unlikely to have been exposed and infected and therefore are unlikely to contract these diseases. However, clinicians caring for patients in nonendemic areas would be wise to query their patients for details on their residence and travel history if the findings are suggestive of an endemic fungal infection.

Tuberculosis is more common in certain geographic areas and in certain populations. HIV-infected patients who were born in or have

TABLE 414–2 DIAGNOSTIC APPROACH TO PULMONARY DISEASE IN HIV-INFECTED PERSONS: CLUES

CLINICAL SETTING

Ambulatory care/outpatient clinic: URI > acute bronchitis > bacterial pneumonia > *Pneumocystis* pneumonia
Hospital: bacterial pneumonia > *Pneumocystis* pneumonia > tuberculosis > pulmonary Kaposi's sarcoma
Intensive care unit: *Pneumocystis* pneumonia > bacterial pneumonia

CD4⁺ CELL COUNT (see Table 414–3)
PATIENT BACKGROUND

HIV transmission category: MSM—increased incidence of Kaposi's sarcoma; IDU—increased incidence of bacterial pneumonia, tuberculosis
Habits: cigarettes—increased incidence of bacterial bronchitis, bacterial pneumonia, COPD, RB-ILD, bronchogenic carcinoma
Travel and residence: assess risk for endemic fungal diseases, tuberculosis

MEDICAL BACKGROUND AND USE OF PROPHYLAXIS

Previous disease: increased incidence of recurrence of bacterial pneumonia, *Pneumocystis* pneumonia, fungal pneumonias
Prophylaxis/maintenance: decreased incidence of disease—*Pneumocystis* pneumonia, fungal pneumonias, tuberculosis (if PPD$^+$)

SYMPTOMS AND SIGNS

Respiratory symptoms: especially cough (productive or nonproductive) and symptom duration
Symptoms suggesting extrapulmonary or disseminated disease
Physical examination of the chest: focal or nonfocal findings
Signs suggesting extrapulmonary or disseminated disease

LABORATORY TESTS

White blood cell count: elevated or if normal, elevated relative to baseline—bacterial pneumonia
Serum lactate dehydrogenase: elevated—nonspecific but classically seen in *Pneumocystis* pneumonia
Arterial blood gas: nonspecific but useful for prognosis, management decisions (e.g., admit and whether corticosteroids are indicated for *Pneumocystis* pneumonia)

CHEST RADIOGRAPH (see Table 414–4)

COPD = chronic obstructive pulmonary disease; IDU = injection drug users; MSM = men who have sex with men; PPD = purified protein derivative (in HIV-infected person, PPD is considered positive if ≥5-mm induration); RB-ILD = respiratory bronchiolitis–interstitial lung disease; URI = upper respiratory tract infection.

TABLE 414–3 CD4⁺ CELL COUNT RANGES FOR HIV-ASSOCIATED PULMONARY DISEASES

ANY CD4⁺ CELL COUNT

Bacterial pneumonia (most often *Streptococcus pneumoniae, Haemophilus* species)
Mycobacterium tuberculosis pneumonia
Non-Hodgkin's lymphoma
Nonspecific interstitial pneumonitis
Pulmonary hypertension
Chronic obstructive lung disease

CD4⁺ CELL COUNT <200 CELLS/μL

Pneumocystis pneumonia
Cryptococcus neoformans pneumonia

CD4⁺ CELL COUNT <100 CELLS/μL

Bacterial pneumonia caused by *Pseudomonas aeruginosa*
Toxoplasma gondii pneumonia
Pulmonary Kaposi's sarcoma

CD4⁺ CELL COUNT <50 CELLS/μL

Mycobacterium avium complex—usually associated with disseminated disease
Histoplasma capsulatum—usually associated with disseminated disease
Coccidioides immitis—usually associated with disseminated disease
Aspergillus species (most often *A. fumigatus*) pneumonia
Cytomegalovirus pneumonia—usually associated with disseminated disease

traveled to a country with a high prevalence of tuberculosis and patients who are homeless or previously incarcerated are at higher risk for exposure to *M. tuberculosis.* Patients who have a positive purified protein derivative tuberculin skin test (defined as ≥5-mm induration in HIV-infected persons), especially if recent converters, are at increased risk for the development of tuberculosis.

Medical Background and Use of Prophylaxis

Many HIV-related opportunistic infections recur, and the current manifestation may be due to recurrence or relapse of a previous pulmonary disease (see Table 414–2). Bacterial infections are often recurrent, and patients with recurrent episodes of bacterial pneumonia are subject to the development of airway damage or bronchiectasis, which in turn predisposes them to further bacterial infections. Patients with previous *Pneumocystis* pneumonia are at high risk for recurrence, especially if their CD4⁺ cell count remains less than 200 cells/μL. If the CD4⁺ count rises to greater than 200 cells/μL with antiretroviral therapy, prophylaxis against *Pneumocystis* can be safely discontinued in the majority of patients. Similarly, patients with previous cryptococcosis, coccidioidomycosis, or histoplasmosis are at high risk for relapse. Patients with a positive purified protein derivative reaction and no evidence of active tuberculosis should receive therapy for latent tuberculosis infection; failure to do so places the patient at high risk for tuberculosis. In HIV-infected patients, adherence to the prescribed regimen lessens the probability of disease, whereas failure to adhere to the regimen frequently results in recurrent or relapsed disease, or both.

Diagnostic Evaluation (See Table 414–2)

Symptoms

Respiratory symptoms are a frequent complaint in HIV-infected persons, and symptoms increase in frequency as the CD4⁺ cell count declines. In general, respiratory symptoms are nonspecific. All of the HIV-associated pulmonary diseases may be accompanied by cough, dyspnea, or pleuritic chest pain, or any combination of these symptoms. However, each pulmonary disease has a characteristic manifestation, and particular aspects of these symptoms may be useful in suggesting a specific diagnosis. For example, in patients who complain of a cough, it is important to determine whether the cough is productive of purulent sputum or nonproductive. The two most common HIV-associated pulmonary diseases encountered in many hospital settings are bacterial pneumonia and *Pneumocystis* pneumonia; most patients with bacterial pneumonia have a cough productive of purulent sputum, whereas most patients with *Pneumocystis* pneumonia have a nonproductive cough. In one study, subjects with a productive cough were 2½ times more likely to have bacterial pneumonia than were subjects without such complaints. Similarly, subjects with a nonproductive cough were more than two times more likely to have *Pneumocystis* pneumonia than were subjects without such complaints. The duration of symptoms may also be useful. Bacterial pneumonias caused by *S. pneumoniae* and *Haemophilus* species characteristically have an acute onset and a symptom duration of 3 to 5 days. In contrast, *Pneumocystis* pneumonia usually has a subacute onset and a typical symptom duration of 2 to 4 weeks. Thus, in an HIV-infected patient with a CD4⁺ cell count lower than 200 cells/μL (and hence at risk for both pneumonias), the presence of cough productive of purulent sputum with a symptom duration of a few days favors the diagnosis of bacterial pneumonia. In contrast, the absence of purulent sputum with a symptom duration of a few weeks strongly favors the diagnosis of *Pneumocystis* pneumonia. Patients with mixed clinical findings may well have dual infections (*Pneumocystis* and bacterial pneumonias).

Constitutional symptoms such as fever, night sweats, and weight loss may suggest the presence of a systemic or disseminated disease. Fever and weight loss may be the sole complaints associated with disseminated mycobacterial or fungal disease, or they may be "B" symptoms associated with non-Hodgkin's lymphoma.

Extrapulmonary symptoms, when present, are often useful in suggesting a specific diagnosis. Although HIV-infected patients can have multiple concurrent illnesses, many of the HIV-associated pulmonary diseases have important extrapulmonary manifestations that account for their nonpulmonary findings. For example, the presence of respiratory symptoms and headache in a patient with a $CD4^+$ cell count less than 200 cells/μL should suggest the possibility of *C. neoformans* pneumonia and meningitis. In fact, although the lungs are the portal of entry for *Cryptococcus,* many patients have asymptomatic or minimally symptomatic pulmonary disease and the diagnosis is suggested only by the presence of extrapulmonary symptoms. In one series, 84% of 106 patients with *C. neoformans* infection had meningitis; cough or dyspnea was present in less than a third of these patients (31%).

Signs

HIV-infected patients with pneumonia may be febrile, tachycardic, and tachypneic. The presence of systemic hypotension often suggests a fulminant disease process (e.g., bacterial septicemia). Pulse oximetry frequently reveals a decrease in oxygen saturation and provides an estimate of the severity of the disease. The presence of exercise-induced oxygen desaturation is reported to be a sensitive indicator of *Pneumocystis* pneumonia.

Examination of the lungs may suggest a cause of the respiratory symptoms. Patients with bacterial pneumonia often have focal lung findings suggestive of consolidation or pleural effusion, or both. In contrast, patients with *Pneumocystis* pneumonia most often have a normal lung examination and only a minority have inspiratory crackles (usually bilateral). Abnormal findings on lung examination may be the result of a nonpulmonary disease. For example, rales in association with an S_3 cardiac gallop and elevated jugular venous pressure suggest a cardiac etiology.

The remainder of the physical examination may also suggest a cause of the respiratory symptoms. Altered mental status in an HIV-infected patient with pulmonary disease whose $CD4^+$ cell count is lower than 200 cells/μL suggests *C. neoformans* with neurologic involvement. A patient with focal neurologic findings and pulmonary disease may have concurrent *T. gondii* encephalitis and pneumonitis. The presence of mucocutaneous KS lesions may point to pulmonary KS. However, the absence of KS lesions on the skin and mucous membranes does not preclude the possibility of significant visceral disease, including the lung. One series found that 15% of 168 patients with pulmonary KS diagnosed by bronchoscopic visualization had no evidence of concurrent or preexisting mucocutaneous Kaposi's sarcoma. An abdominal examination revealing hepatosplenomegaly suggests either disseminated mycobacterial or fungal disease or non-Hodgkin's lymphoma.

Laboratory Tests

Laboratory tests may provide important clues to the diagnosis of pulmonary disease (see Table 414–2). In general, however, HIV-infected patients typically have a host of laboratory abnormalities that are nonspecific or due to conditions unrelated to the pulmonary disease. Laboratory tests that may be useful include a complete blood count with a white blood cell (WBC) count and differential, serum lactate dehydrogenase (LDH), and arterial blood gas (ABG) analysis. These tests also serve as prognostic markers and as baseline values for subsequent measurements. Serial measurements are useful in any patient who fails to exhibit a clinical response or who worsens despite appropriate therapy.

White Blood Cell Count

The WBC count is frequently elevated and a left shift is present as well in persons with bacterial pneumonia. This elevation may be relative to the baseline value in a patient whose baseline WBC count is less than the normal laboratory range. HIV-infected patients with neutropenia are at higher risk for bacterial and certain fungal infections, such as those caused by *Aspergillus* species.

Serum Lactate Dehydrogenase

Serum LDH is often elevated in patients with *Pneumocystis* pneumonia. However, it may be elevated in other pulmonary (including bacterial pneumonia and tuberculosis) and nonpulmonary conditions. Despite its diagnostic limitations, the degree of LDH elevation has been shown to correlate with prognosis and response to therapy. Patients with *Pneumocystis* pneumonia and an initial markedly elevated or increasing serum LDH level despite treatment of *Pneumocystis* pneumonia have a poor prognosis.

Arterial Blood Gases

As in any population, ABGs are frequently abnormal in HIV-infected patients with significant pulmonary disease. The findings of hypoxemia, an increased alveolar-arterial oxygen difference, and hypocapnia with respiratory alkalosis are nonspecific. However, ABG analysis is useful for prognosis, as well as clinical decisions regarding whether to admit the patient and whether adjunctive corticosteroids are indicated in patients with *Pneumocystis* pneumonia.

Imaging

Chest Radiograph

The chest radiograph is the cornerstone for evaluation of pulmonary diseases in HIV-infected patients. Because each of these diseases has a characteristic radiographic appearance, the radiograph can narrow the diagnostic possibilities and suggest a diagnostic approach (Table 414–4).

Bacterial pneumonia is currently the most common pulmonary disease seen in HIV-infected persons at many institutions in the United States. The most frequently identified pathogens are *S. pneumoniae, Haemophilus* species, and *P. aeruginosa.* Classically, chest radiographs of HIV-infected patients with bacterial pneumonia demonstrate focal, segmental, or lobar consolidation, similar to that observed in non–HIV-infected persons (Fig. 414–1). However, this finding may be more frequent in pneumonias caused by *S. pneumoniae* and to a lesser extent *Haemophilus* species than in community-acquired *P. aeruginosa.* One study reported that a classic lobar alveolar pattern was seen in 67% and a diffuse alveolar pattern in 10% of 21 HIV-infected patients with *S. pneumoniae* pneumonia. Another study found similar proportions in 34 HIV-infected patients with *H. influenzae* pneumonia; in this study, focal or diffuse lobar infiltrates were noted in 74%. However, a different series of 12 HIV-infected patients with *H. influenzae* pneumonia reported that the findings may be clinically and radiographically indistinguishable from those of *Pneumocystis* pneumonia. The patients complained of nonproductive cough and dyspnea with a median symptom duration of 4 weeks. On chest radiograph all had bilateral interstitial or mixed interstitial-alveolar infiltrates, similar to *Pneumocystis* pneumonia. In contrast, a study of 16 HIV-infected patients with *P. aeruginosa* pneumonia found that the pneumonia was community acquired in 15 (94%). Chest radiographs revealed cavitary infiltrates on admission in 50%, and an additional 19% had pulmonary infiltrates that subsequently cavitated. The frequency of cavitary infiltrates in *P. aeruginosa* pneumonia was also noted in a study of 58 HIV-infected patients with *P. aeruginosa* infection, 25 of whom had pneumonia. Of these 25 patients, 24% had cavitary pneumonia. Thus, the presence of cavitary pneumonia may be more suggestive of *Pseudomonas* than either *Streptococcus* or *Haemophilus.*

Tuberculosis can have a variety of chest radiographic findings, including upper lung zone infiltrates, often with cavitation (Fig. 414–2), middle or lower lung zone consolidation (or both) mimicking bacterial pneumonia (Fig. 414–3), miliary or nodular disease, and pleural effusions or intrathoracic adenopathy (or both). The frequency with which each of these specific findings is seen is influenced by the patient's $CD4^+$ cell count. HIV-infected patients with a $CD4^+$ cell count well above 200 cells/μL are more likely to have a radiograph that has upper lung zone infiltrates and cavitation than are patients with a $CD4^+$ count lower than 200 cells/μL. In this latter group, patients are as likely or more likely to have a radiograph demonstrating mid or lower lung zone involvement (or both) or diffuse involvement and are more likely to have associated intrathoracic adenopathy. One study of radiographic findings in HIV-infected patients with tuberculosis found that the proportion of patients with cavitary infiltrates declined significantly as the $CD4^+$ cell count decreased from 400 cells/μL or more to less than 200 cells/μL, whereas the proportion with noncavitary infiltrates and with intrathoracic

TABLE 414–4 CHARACTERISTIC CHEST RADIOGRAPH FINDINGS FOR SELECTED PULMONARY DISEASES*

Pulmonary Disease	Author (Year), Patients	Distribution	Pattern	Associated Findings
Bacteria[†]	Selwyn (1998), 99	Focal (71%) Diffuse (29%)	Lobar (54%) Interstitial (17%) Nodular (10%)	Cavitation (1%) Pleural effusion (7%) Adenopathy (2%)
Mycobacterium tuberculosis, CD4⁺ count ≥400 cells/μL	Abouya (1995), 30	Miliary (0%)	Cavitary (63%) Noncavitary (33%)	Pleural effusion (3%) Adenopathy (0%)
M. tuberculosis, CD4⁺ count of 200–399 cells/μL	Abouya (1995), 36	Miliary (6%)	Cavitary (44%) Noncavitary (44%)	Pleural effusion (11%) Adenopathy (14%)
M. tuberculosis, CD4⁺ count <200 cells/μL	Abouya (1995), 45	Miliary (9%)	Cavitary (29%) Noncavitary (58%)	Pleural effusion (11%) Adenopathy (20%)
Pneumocystis jirovecii	DeLorenzo (1987), 104	Bilateral (95%) Diffuse (48%)	Interstitial or mixed (88%) Alveolar (12%)	Cysts (7%) Honeycomb lesions (4%)
Cryptococcus neoformans	Batungwanayo (1994), 37	Diffuse (76%)	Interstitial or mixed (76%) Alveolar (19%) Nodular/nodules (5%)	Cavitation (11%) Adenopathy (11%) Pleural effusion (5%)
Cytomegalovirus	Salomon (1997), 18	Normal (33%)	Reticular-granular (33%) Alveolar (22%) Nodular (11%)	Cavitation (11%) Cyst (6%) Pleural effusion (33%) Adenopathy (11%)
Cytomegalovirus	Rodriguez-Barradas (1996), 17	Bilateral (71%) Unilateral (29%)	Interstitial (82%) Alveolar (18%)	Pleural effusion (12%)
Toxoplasma gondii	Rabaud (1996), 43	Normal (23%) Bilateral (58%)	Interstitial (53%) Nodular (16%)	Pleural effusion (7%) Pneumothorax (2%)
Kaposi's sarcoma	Gruden (1995), 76	Normal (3%) Bilateral (96%) Diffuse or mid–lower lung zones (92%)	Bronchial wall thickening ± coalescence (95%) Nodules (78%)	Kerley's B lines (71%) Pleural effusion (53%) Adenopathy (16%)
Non-Hodgkin's lymphoma	Eisner (1996), 38	Normal (3%)	Nodules (40%) or mass (24%) Lobar (40%) Reticular (24%)	Cavitation (3%) Pleural effusion (44%) Adenopathy (21%)

*Chest radiograph findings can vary significantly, depending on a number of factors, including the severity of disease and the use of prophylaxis.
[†]The characteristic chest radiograph manifestation is influenced by the specific bacteria (see text).

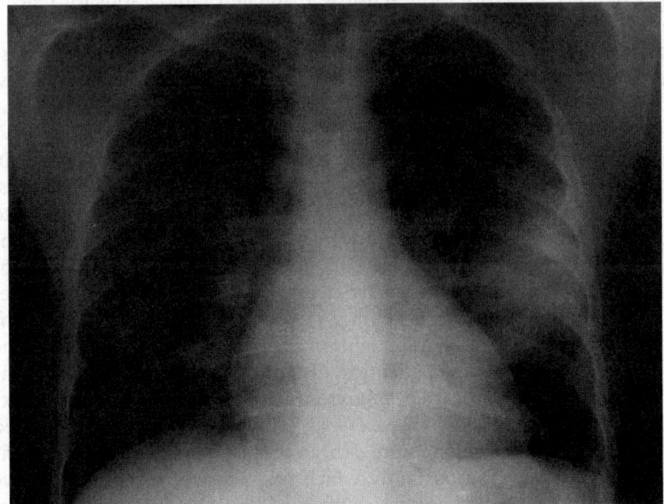

FIGURE 414–1 • Chest radiograph of an HIV-infected person, CD4⁺ cell count greater than 200 cells/μL, revealing left lingular consolidation. Sputum and blood cultures were positive for *Streptococcus pneumoniae.* (Courtesy of Laurence Huang, MD, and Chin Tang Huang, MD.)

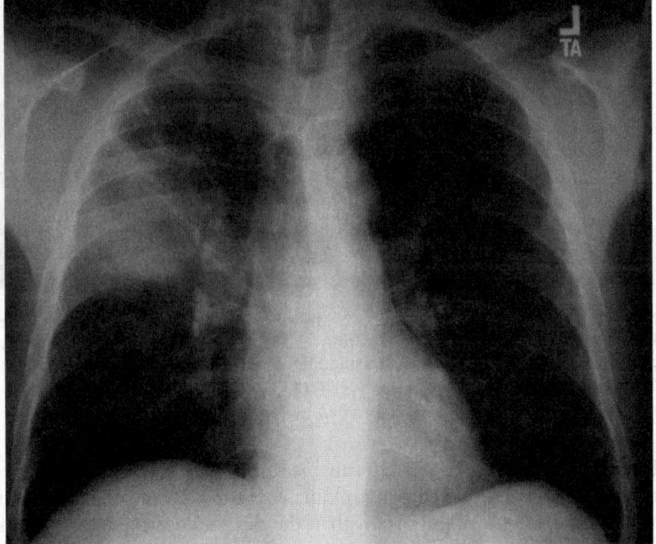

FIGURE 414–2 • Chest radiograph of an HIV-infected person, CD4⁺ cell count greater than 200 cells/μL, demonstrating a right upper lobe infiltrate with areas of cavitation. Sputum acid-fast bacillus stain was positive, and multiple sputum cultures grew *Mycobacterium tuberculosis.*

adenopathy increased significantly as the CD4⁺ count declined. Thus, the radiographic key to diagnosis of tuberculosis is knowledge of the patient's CD4⁺ cell count and patterns common at that CD4⁺ count.

Classically, *Pneumocystis* pneumonia is characterized by bilateral interstitial-reticular or granular opacities (Fig. 414–4). Often, the opacities are symmetrical, and they are diffuse when the disease is severe. One large study revealed that 87.5% of HIV-infected patients with *Pneumocystis* pneumonia had either an interstitial pattern (75%) or a mixed interstitial-alveolar pattern (12.5%) whereas the remaining patients had an alveolar pattern. In addition, 7% had thin-walled cysts (pneumatoceles) (Fig. 414–5) and 4% had honeycomb lesions. Infiltrates were bilateral in 95% and involved the entire lung in 48%. Importantly, this study predates the widespread use of *Pneumocystis* prophylaxis. Several reports have described the radiographic findings in patients receiving aerosolized pentamidine prophylaxis; these radiographs characteristically reveal an upper lung zone predominance mimicking mycobacterial disease.

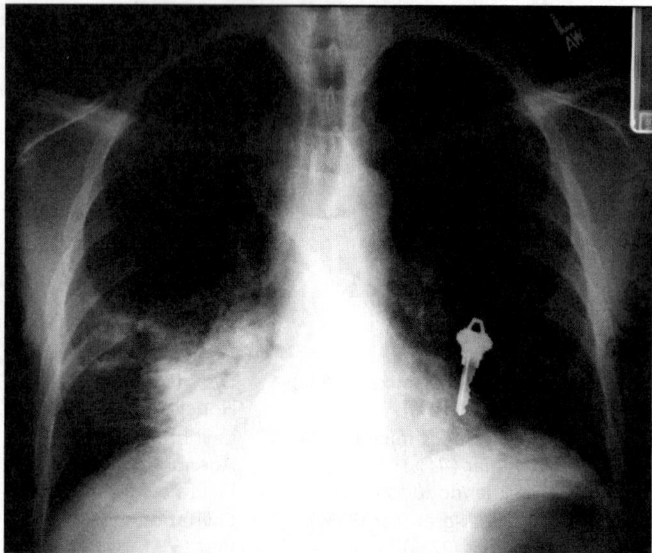

FIGURE 414–3 • Chest radiograph of an HIV-infected person, CD4⁺ cell count less than 200 cells/μL, revealing right lower lung zone consolidation with air bronchograms. Sputum culture grew *Mycobacterium tuberculosis* that was resistant to rifampin treatment alone. In this case, the key to the diagnosis of tuberculosis was knowledge of the patient's CD4⁺ cell count and an understanding that tuberculosis can be manifested in this manner in such an individual.

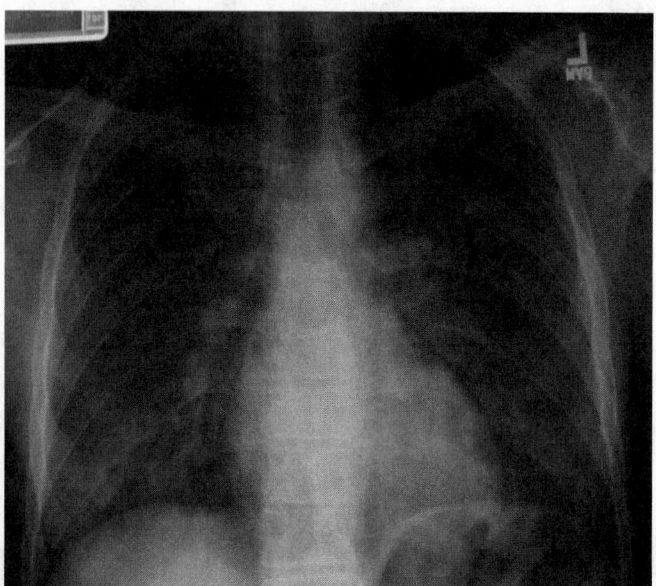

FIGURE 414–4 • Chest radiograph of an HIV-infected person, CD4⁺ cell count less than 200 cells/μL, demonstrating the characteristic bilateral, reticular-granular opacities of *Pneumocystis* pneumonia. Bronchoscopy with examination of bronchoalveolar lavage fluid revealed *Pneumocystis jirovecii.*

However, upper lung zone predominance can also be seen in patients who never received aerosolized pentamidine, and the pattern present (reticular, granular) is more important than the distribution in suggesting the diagnosis of *Pneumocystis* pneumonia.

Similar to tuberculosis, *C. neoformans* pneumonia can have a variety of chest radiographic findings. Although bilateral interstitial-reticular infiltrates are the most common radiographic manifestation (mimicking *Pneumocystis* pneumonia), pulmonary involvement by *Cryptococcus* can also result in an alveolar or nodular pattern, thin-walled cysts or cavities, nodules, masses (Fig. 414–6A and B), intrathoracic adenopathy, and pleural effusions.

Pulmonary KS is characteristically accompanied by bilateral opacities in a central or perihilar distribution (Fig. 414–7). One study of 76 HIV-infected patients with pulmonary KS diagnosed by bronchoscopy (in which BAL was negative for infectious organisms) found that 95% of chest radiographs demonstrated peribronchial cuffing and tram track

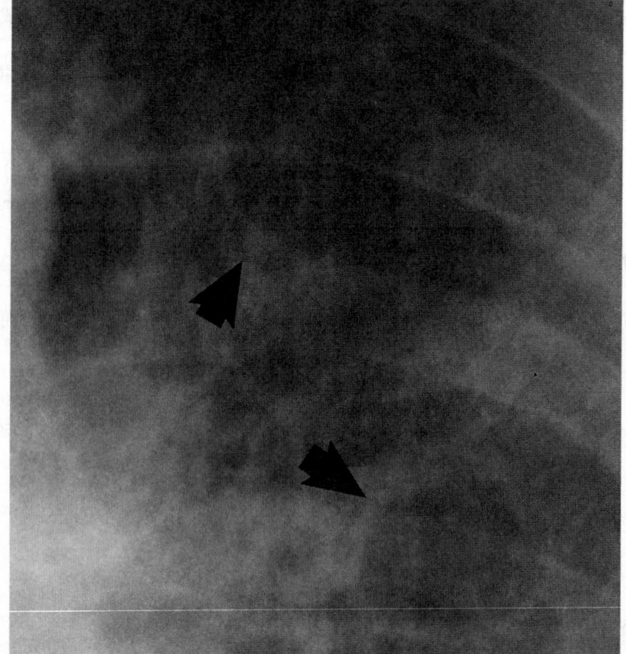

FIGURE 414–5 • Close-up of the left lung from a chest radiograph of an HIV-infected person, CD4⁺ cell count less than 200 cells/μL. Two thin-walled cysts (arrows) are present as a result of *Pneumocystis* pneumonia.

opacities with (45%) or without (50%) more extensive perihilar coalescent opacities. Small nodules (50%) or nodular opacities (28%) were seen in 78%, Kerley's B lines in 71%, and pleural effusions in 53% of the radiographs. No patient had either Kerley's B lines or pleural effusions without concurrent parenchymal findings. Sixteen percent of these patients had hilar or mediastinal lymph node enlargement, a finding that is often better appreciated on chest computed tomography (CT).

Chest Computed Tomography

Chest CT scans are more sensitive than chest radiographs for detecting the presence and defining the characteristics and extent of pulmonary disease. However, a CT scan is unnecessary in most evaluations because the clinical and chest radiographic findings often suggest a single or a few diagnoses to consider primarily. There are a number of specific clinical scenarios in which chest CT scans may be of particular use in HIV-infected patients. High-resolution CT (HRCT) is extremely useful in cases of clinically suspected *Pneumocystis* pneumonia in which the chest radiograph is normal or unchanged, a phenomenon that occurs in up to 39% of reported series. When *Pneumocystis* pneumonia is suspected clinically, dismissing the possibility of the disease based on a normal or unchanged radiograph could have catastrophic consequences. Nevertheless, the majority of patients with symptoms suggestive of *Pneumocystis* pneumonia whose radiograph is normal or unchanged do not have the disease. Subjecting these patients to diagnostic procedures such as bronchoscopy or to empirical *Pneumocystis* treatment with its associated toxicities is also ill advised. In these cases, a sensitive follow-up test is needed to select which patients require either diagnostic procedures or empirical therapy and, as importantly, which patients require neither invasive procedures nor *Pneumocystis* treatment. Chest HRCT is one such test because patients with *Pneumocystis* pneumonia and a normal chest radiograph have patchy areas of ground-glass opacity on HRCT (Fig. 414–8). Although the presence of ground-glass opacity is nonspecific and it may be seen in a number of pulmonary disorders, its absence strongly argues against the presence of *Pneumocystis* pneumonia.

Chest CT can also be useful in suggesting a diagnosis in cases in which the chest radiograph reveals multiple pulmonary nodules. Finding a predominance of nodules less than 1 cm in diameter in a centrilobular distribution strongly suggests the presence of an opportunistic infection, whereas a predominance of nodules greater than 1 cm in diameter is suggestive of neoplasm. When the nodules are mostly less than 1 cm in diameter, the presence of intrathoracic adenopathy, especially if low attenuation (another use for CT), indicates that mycobacterial (or fungal) disease is probable. When the nodules are mostly greater than 1 cm in

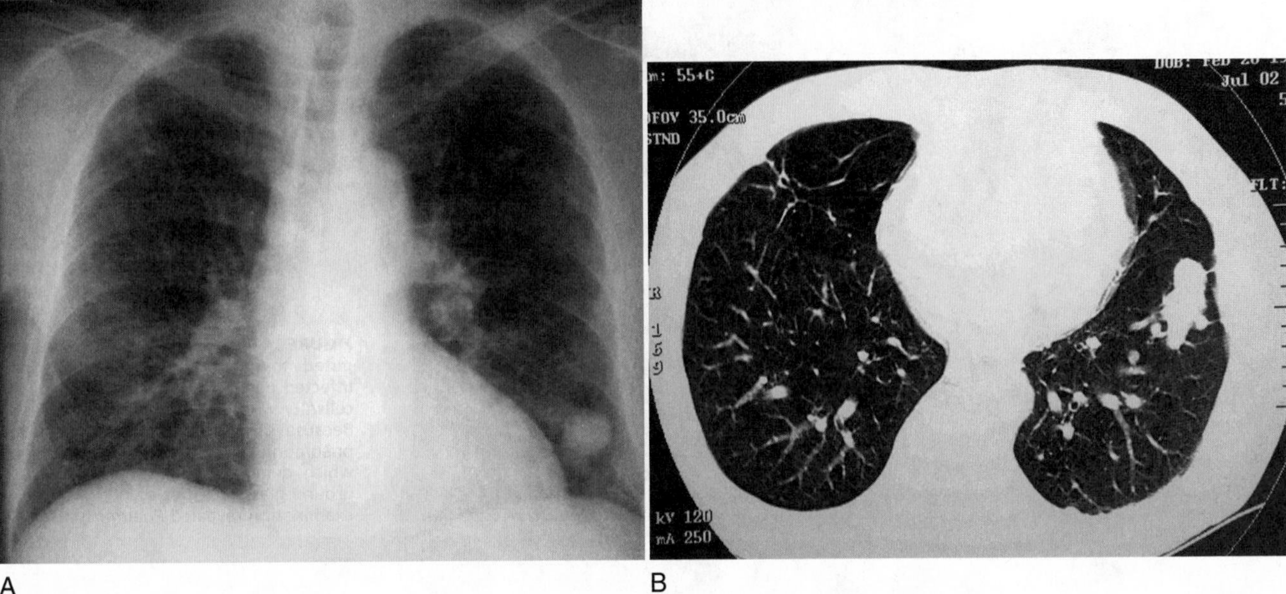

FIGURES 414–6 • A and B, Chest radiograph and chest computed tomography (CT) scan of an HIV-infected person, CD4⁺ cell count less than 200 cells/μL. A multilobulated noncalcified mass measuring 4.6 × 2.4 cm is present in the left lower lobe with multiple adjacent satellite nodules. Culture from CT-guided transthoracic needle aspiration revealed *Cryptococcus neoformans.*

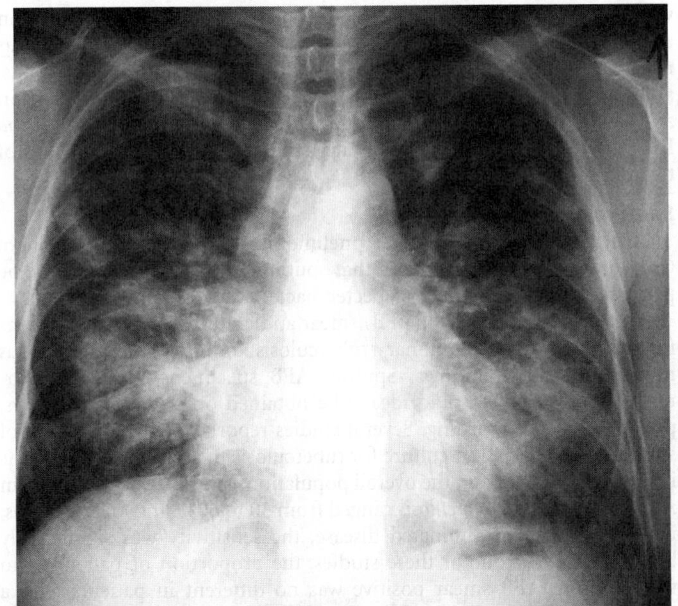

FIGURE 414–7 • Chest radiograph of an HIV-infected person, CD4⁺ cell count less than 100 cells/μL, with the characteristic bilateral, middle, and lower lung zone, predominantly central distribution of abnormalities of pulmonary Kaposi's sarcoma. The patient had no evidence of mucocutaneous Kaposi's sarcoma, and the diagnosis of pulmonary disease was made by bronchoscopy with visualization of characteristic erythematous-violaceous Kaposi's sarcoma lesions throughout the visible airway (see Fig. 414–12).

diameter, the finding of associated peribronchovascular thickening inevitably results in a diagnosis of pulmonary KS.

HIV-infected patients may initially be suspected of having disseminated mycobacterial or fungal disease. In these patients, the chest radiograph may reveal little or no parenchymal lung involvement. However, chest CT may reveal intrathoracic adenopathy, which if low attenuation, strongly suggests these infections. Finally, chest CT scans are useful in guiding diagnostic procedures such as bronchoscopy, transthoracic needle aspiration (see Fig. 414–6B), and surgical procedures.

Pulmonary Function Tests

Pulmonary function testing can be useful in the evaluation of respiratory complaints in HIV-infected patients (Fig. 414–9). In patients complaining of dry cough or dyspnea (or both) whose chest radiograph is normal, spirometry may diagnose airflow obstruction that is often responsive to bronchodilators. Pulmonary function testing frequently reveals a restrictive ventilatory defect with decreased lung volumes and increased airflow in patients with *Pneumocystis* pneumonia. In addition, the diffusing capacity for carbon monoxide (DLCO) is a sensitive, but nonspecific indicator of *Pneumocystis* pneumonia, and a normal DLCO makes the diagnosis of *Pneumocystis* pneumonia extremely unlikely. One study demonstrated that the combination of a chest radiograph followed by DLCO if the radiograph was normal or unchanged identified more than 97% of 80 cases of *Pneumocystis* pneumonia. Importantly, the sensitivity of a DLCO value less than or equal to 75% of predicted after a normal or unchanged radiograph was 90% (its specificity was 53%).

Selected Diagnostic Tests

The approach to the evaluation of HIV-infected patients with suspected pulmonary disease begins with consideration of the spectrum of pulmonary diseases outlined in Table 414–1. After a careful history and physical examination supplemented by selected laboratory tests and a chest radiograph, the goal is to arrive at a probable diagnosis (or at most a few diagnoses) for which specific diagnostic tests can be ordered and appropriate treatment can be initiated (Figs. 414–10 and 414–11). The next section provides a discussion of selected diagnostic tests (Table 414–5).

Blood Cultures

Blood cultures can be obtained for bacterial, fungal, and mycobacterial assays. Because *S. pneumoniae* is the most frequent cause of bacterial pneumonia and because pneumococcal pneumonia is often accompanied by bacteremia in HIV-infected patients (especially when the CD4⁺ cell count is less than 200 cells/μL), blood cultures should always be performed in patients with suspected bacterial pneumonia. When positive, blood cultures are specific for the diagnosis, and in an era of increasing antibiotic resistance, the utility of drug susceptibility testing cannot be overemphasized. Tuberculosis and many of the fungal pneumonias may be manifested as extrapulmonary or disseminated disease with minimal or absent respiratory complaints and normal chest radiographs. For this reason, mycobacterial and fungal blood cultures should usually be obtained in cases of suspected tuberculous or fungal infection, especially if the CD4⁺ cell count is below 200 cells/μL.

Serology

Serum cryptococcal antigen (sCRAG) is an extremely sensitive test for the presence of cryptococcemia and cryptococcal meningitis, and a negative sCRAG test virtually rules out the diagnosis of cryptococcal meningitis. However, sCRAG may be negative in HIV-infected patients who have isolated cryptococcal pneumonia. In one study of HIV-infected

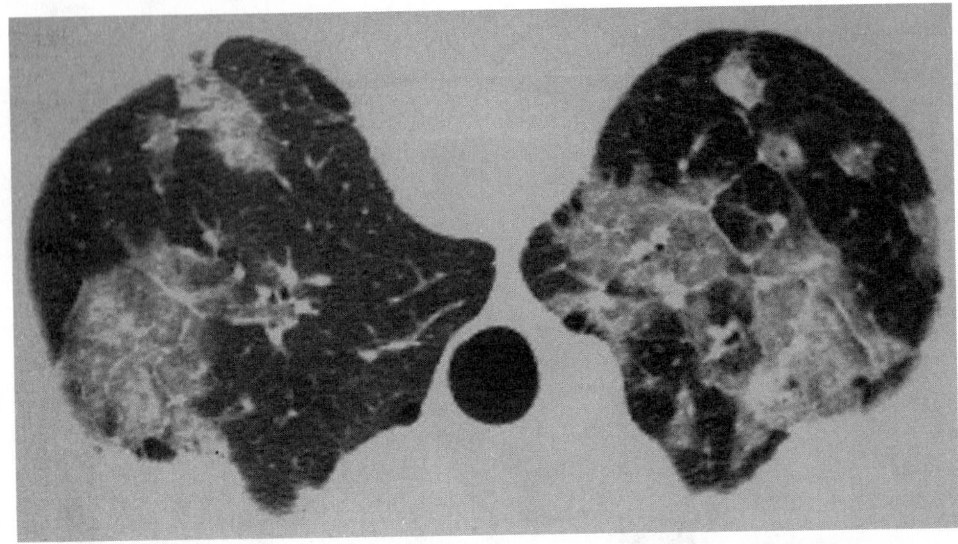

FIGURE 414–8 • Chest high-resolution computed tomography (HRCT) scan of an HIV-infected person, CD4+ cell count less than 200 cells/μL, whose chest radiograph was normal. Because of clinical suspicion of *Pneumocystis* pneumonia (PCP), the patient underwent HRCT, which demonstrates the characteristic patchy ground-glass opacities of PCP. Induced sputum examination revealed *Pneumocystis jirovecii*.

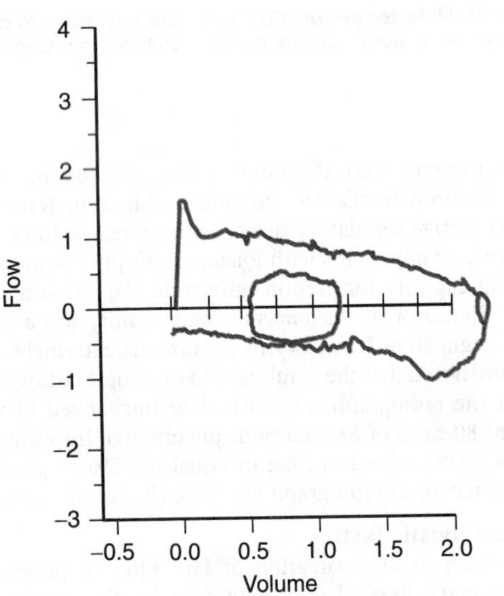

FIGURE 414–9 • Flow-volume loop of an HIV-infected person, CD4+ cell count less than 50 cells/μL. Evidence of a fixed large airway (in this case, tracheal) obstruction is apparent.

patients with cryptococcal pneumonia, sCRAG was positive in only 8 of 26 patients (31%) in whom it was determined. However, sCRAG is extremely specific for cryptococcal infection; false-positive tests are rare but may result from infection with *Trichosporon beigelii.* Therefore, sCRAG should be determined in all patients with suspected cryptococcal disease; patients positive for sCRAG should undergo an evaluation to determine the extent of disease (i.e., lumbar puncture for possible meningitis), whereas those negative for sCRAG but with respiratory complaints or chest radiograph findings should undergo further pulmonary evaluation (i.e., bronchoscopy with BAL). There appears to be little to no utility in measuring serial sCRAG titers in patients with cryptococcal disease.

Similar to sCRAG, *H. capsulatum* polysaccharide antigen (HPA) is a sensitive test for the presence of disseminated histoplasmosis. However, the HPA test may be negative in patients with mild or localized disease. The antigen, which can be measured in blood and other fluids (including BAL) but is most commonly assayed from urine, should be determined in patients with suspected histoplasmosis. In the proper clinical context, a positive result indicates *H. capsulatum* infection. However, patients with a positive HPA test should have appropriate material (i.e., blood) sent for fungal culture because fungal pathogens such as *P. marneffei, Blastomyces dermatitidis,* and *Paracoccidioides braziliensis* may cause a false-positive result. One final important benefit of serial HPA testing is its use in diagnosing relapsed disease; a 2-unit increase is associated with relapsed disease.

Most cases of *T. gondii* encephalitis result from reactivation of latent infection. In studies of central nervous system toxoplasmosis, up to 97% of HIV-infected patients were positive for *Toxoplasma* IgG, with a smaller percentage being positive for *Toxoplasma* IgM. In a study of 64 patients with pulmonary toxoplasmosis, *Toxoplasma* IgG was positive in 92% in whom previous serology results were available, and an additional 5% in this study seroconverted (IgA, IgM, and IgG all detected after previous negative results) at the time that toxoplasmosis was diagnosed. Thus, although positive *Toxoplasma* IgG merely indicates previous infection and cannot be taken as proof of acute toxoplasmosis, negative *Toxoplasma* IgG, especially if accompanied by negative IgM, makes the diagnosis of toxoplasmosis unlikely.

Sputum

Most patients with bacterial pneumonia have a productive cough. Current guidelines recommend that sputum Gram stain and culture be performed in patients with suspected bacterial pneumonia.

Sputum acid-fast bacilli (AFB) smear and culture are the foundations for the diagnosis of pulmonary tuberculosis and other nontuberculous mycobacterial pneumonias. Sputum AFB specimens—either spontaneous or induced—should ideally be obtained on 3 consecutive days, preferably in the morning. Several studies report that the sensitivity of sputum AFB smear and culture for tuberculosis in HIV-infected patients is similar to that seen in the overall population. The sensitivity of sputum AFB smear for *M. tuberculosis* ranged from 50 to 60% in two large series; in persons with disseminated disease, the sensitivity was significantly higher (90%). In one of these studies, the proportion of patients who were sputum AFB smear positive was no different in patients with a normal chest radiograph and those with an abnormal radiograph. Thus, all patients with suspected tuberculosis, even if respiratory complaints and chest radiograph findings are absent, should have three sputum specimens sent for AFB smear and culture. Patients with a positive AFB smear must be presumed to have tuberculosis, and appropriate measures must be instituted while awaiting either culture or nucleic acid amplification test results. Patients with three negative sputum AFB smear results may still have tuberculosis detected on culture or determined by clinical and radiographic response but are at reasonably low likelihood for transmission, so respiratory isolation (if hospitalized) can be discontinued. Whereas a single positive sputum AFB culture result for *M. tuberculosis* is diagnostic of tuberculosis, the same cannot be said for a sputum specimen positive for a nontuberculous mycobacteria (i.e., *Mycobacterium kansasii, M. avium* complex). In these patients, a positive sputum culture result can be due to colonization, and determination of when these mycobacteria are causing pulmonary disease relies on a constellation of clinical, radiographic, and microbiologic criteria.

Most patients with *Pneumocystis* pneumonia have a dry, nonproductive cough, and sputum must be induced. Sputum induction should be performed in a properly engineered room to minimize transmission of infectious microorganisms. Sputum induction is a sensitive diagnostic test for *Pneumocystis* pneumonia, with a reported sensitivity ranging

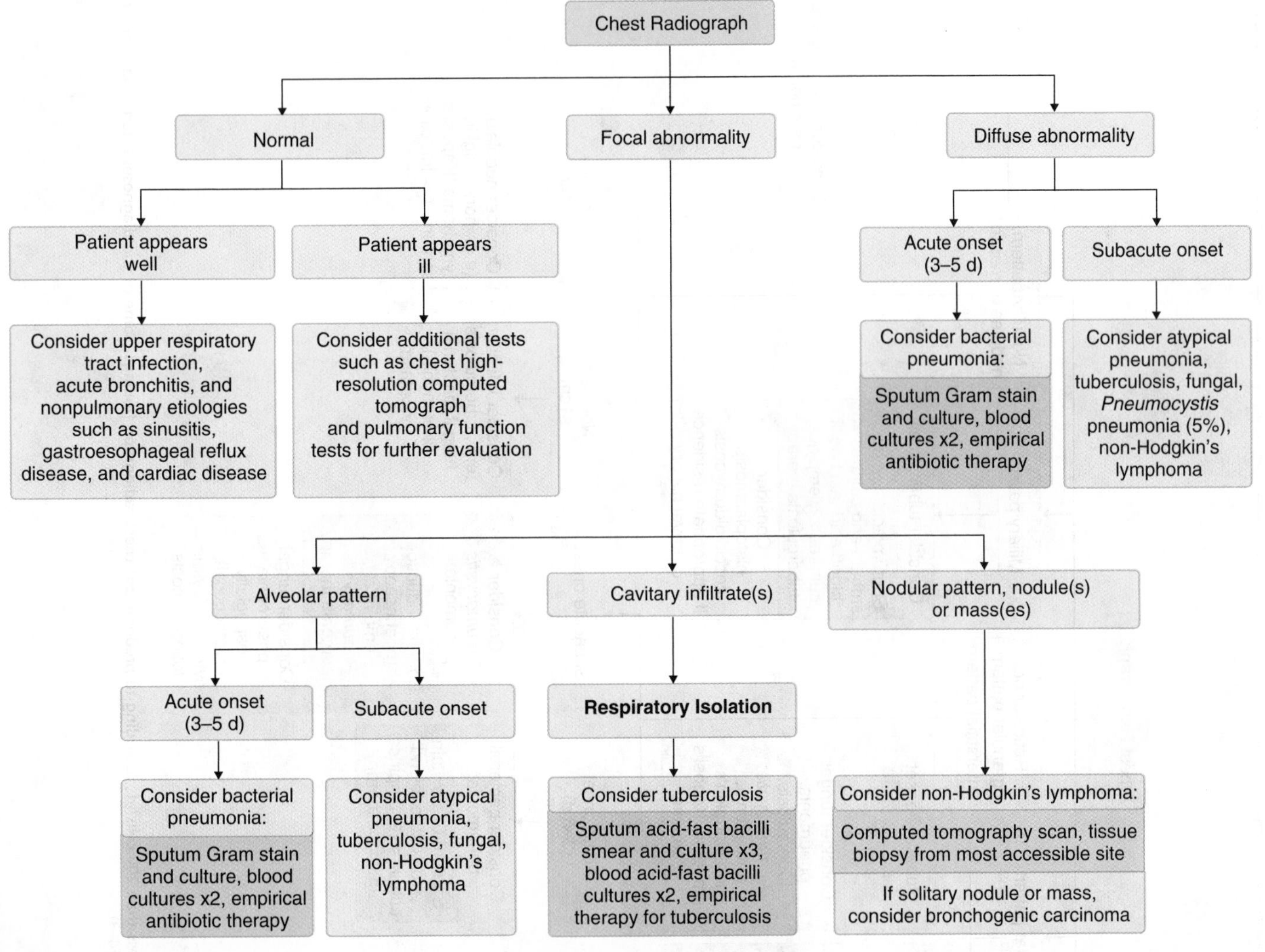

FIGURE 414–10 • Diagnostic approach to an HIV-infected patient, CD4⁺ greater than 200 cells/μL, according to predominant chest radiograph findings.

from 55% in early studies to 95% with fluorescent antibody testing. At institutions where sputum induction is performed, the need for bronchoscopy is decreased. In one study of 992 HIV-associated diagnoses of *Pneumocystis* pneumonia over a 4-year period, sputum induction accounted for 800 of the 992 (81%) diagnoses; the remainder were diagnosed by bronchoscopy. In addition, induced sputum diagnosed cases of certain bacterial, mycobacterial, fungal, and parasitic pneumonias and suggested the presence of bacterial bronchitis/bronchopneumonia. Recent studies have examined the utility of polymerase chain reaction (PCR)-based assays applied to noninvasive respiratory specimens (i.e., oropharyngeal washing or oral gargle) and have reported encouraging results. These PCR-based assays appear to be sensitive diagnostic tests, but they are less specific than standard microscopy in that patients without clinical *Pneumocystis* pneumonia have been demonstrated to have positive assay results. Nevertheless, these assays are typically available only in a research setting. Thus, sputum induction should be the initial diagnostic test for patients with suspected *Pneumocystis* pneumonia at institutions where it is available.

Although experience is limited when compared with that for tuberculosis and *Pneumocystis* pneumonia, sputum examination or culture, or both, can occasionally diagnose fungal pneumonias, including *C. neoformans, H. capsulatum,* and *C. immitis,* but not invasive *Aspergillus* disease, nontuberculous mycobacterial pneumonia (e.g., *M. kansasii*), and *T. gondii* and other parasitic pneumonias (e.g., *Strongyloides stercoralis*).

Bronchoscopy

Bronchoscopy is a mainstay in the diagnosis of HIV-associated pulmonary disease. It should be considered for any patient with pulmonary disease whose severity warrants prompt and accurate diagnosis, for patients with suspected pulmonary KS, for patients in whom the diagnosis is unclear despite less invasive diagnostic tests (e.g., sputum), and for patients who are failing empirical therapy for a presumed pathogen.

Bronchoscopy with BAL is the "gold standard" diagnostic test for *Pneumocystis* pneumonia, and it is the initial test of choice at institutions where either sputum induction is unavailable or its sensitivity is low. Numerous studies report that the sensitivity of BAL alone for *Pneumocystis* pneumonia is 95 to 98% or greater. Bronchoscopy with BAL can be performed in patients with suspected *Pneumocystis* pneumonia whose induced sputum examination is negative. In a study of 992 cases of *Pneumocystis* pneumonia diagnosed over a 4-year period, only 2 of the 992 episodes (0.2%) were diagnosed *solely* by transbronchial biopsy (TBBX). This is not to imply that TBBX is an insensitive test for *Pneumocystis* pneumonia but to demonstrate that most cases of *Pneumocystis* pneumonia can be diagnosed by other, less invasive (sputum induction) or less risky (BAL) procedures. However, there are institutional differences in the sensitivity of BAL, and both BAL and TBBX are warranted at institutions where the yield of these two procedures is complementary.

Bronchoscopy is an important modality for diagnosing cryptococcal pneumonia, especially if the disease is limited to the lungs. One study reported that BAL fluid culture was positive in 27 of 33 HIV-infected patients (82%) with cryptococcal pneumonia in whom it was performed. These results are similar to another study in which 23 of 27 HIV-infected patients (85%) with pulmonary cryptococcosis had a positive BAL fluid culture. In this study, two of the patients with a negative BAL fluid culture had a positive BAL CRAG and the remaining two had pleural cryptococcosis that was diagnosed by pleural fluid culture, as well as pleural fluid CRAG.

Bronchoscopy with a thorough visual inspection of the airways is the procedure of choice for the diagnosis of pulmonary KS. In these patients, neither transbronchial nor endobronchial biopsy adds to the yield when

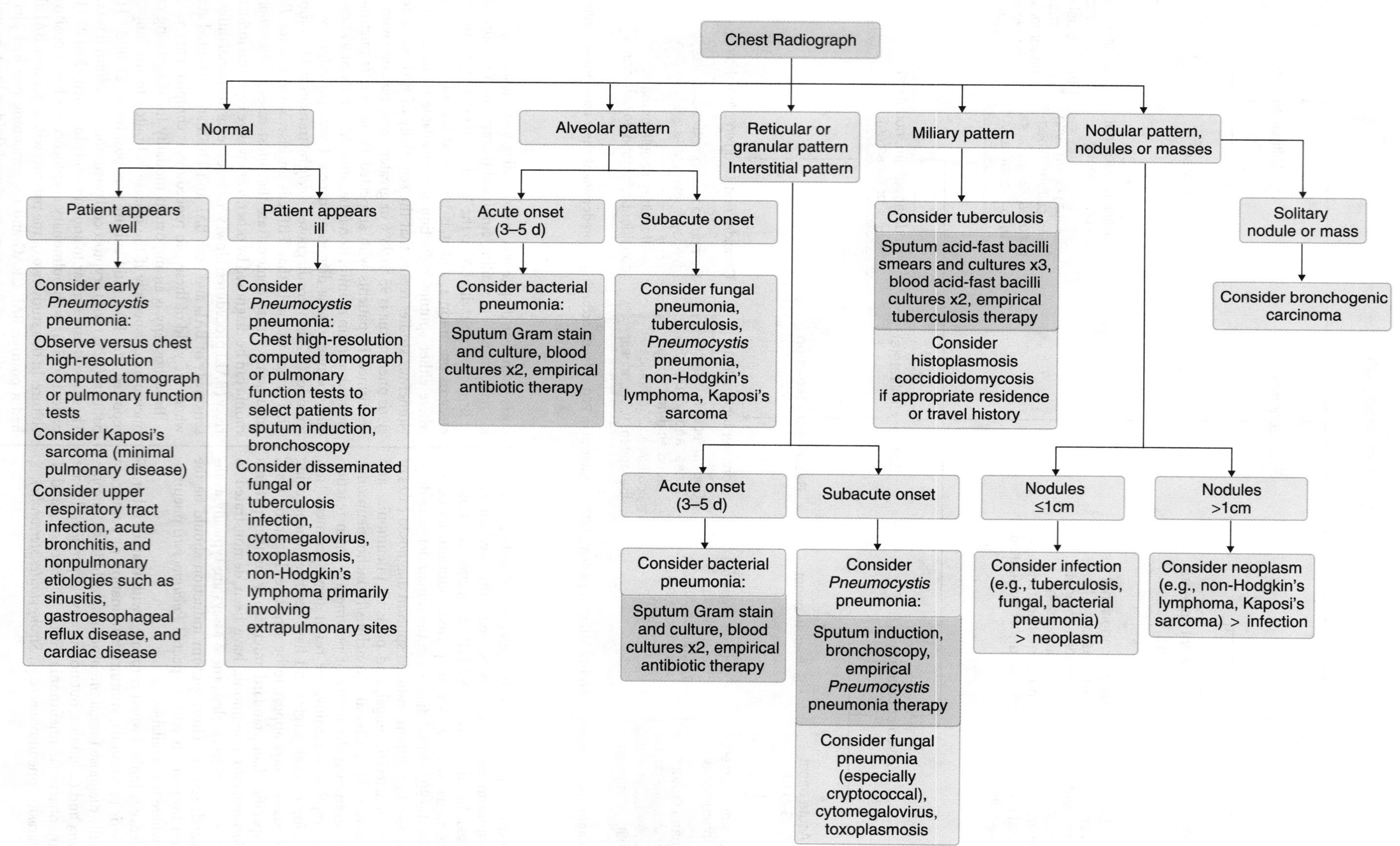

FIGURE 414–11 • Diagnostic approach to an HIV-infected patient, CD4+ cell count less than 200 cells/μL, according to predominant chest radiograph findings. Some of the diagnoses listed usually occur when the CD4+ cell count is below 100 cells/μL or even below 50 cells/μL (see Table 414–3).

TABLE 414–5 **DIAGNOSTIC TESTS FOR SELECTED PULMONARY DISEASES***

Pulmonary Disease	Serology or Blood Cultures	Sputum	BAL and/or TBBX	Pleural Fluid	Important Other Sites†	Suggestive Tests
Bacteria	**Blood cultures (esp. *Streptococcus pneumoniae*)**	**Gram stain and culture**	Rarely, quantitative cultures	**Consider (esp. if concern for empyema)**		WBC count increase (may be relative to the patient's baseline)
Mycobacterium tuberculosis	**Blood cultures**	**AFB smear and culture × 3**	Occasionally, BAL and TBBX	**Consider (with biopsy)**	Lymph node Liver Spleen Bone marrow	
Pneumocystis jirovecii	? SAM‡	**Induced sputum examination**	**BAL ± TBBX** (depends on respective sensitivities at the institution)	Rarely		HRCT—GGO; PFTs—decreased DLCO; O_2 saturation—decreased with exercise
Cryptococcus neoformans	**Serum CRAG§ Blood cultures**	Occasionally	**BAL**	Rarely	Cerebrospinal fluid Skin	
Cytomegalovirus	? PCR	No	**TBBX**	No	Retina GI tract	
Toxoplasma gondii	***T. gondii* IgG, IgM**	Occasionally	**BAL**	Rarely	Central nervous system	Head CT/MRI with multiple lesions
Kaposi's sarcoma	? HHV-8	No	**Visualization of lesions ± TBBX**	No	Mucocutaneous Lymph node GI tract	Gallium negative
Non-Hodgkin's lymphoma	No	No	**TBBX, Wang needle biopsy**	**Cytology**	Extranodal disease	

*Tests in **BOLD** are the usual diagnostic tests of choice. Other tests should be considered if the tests of choice are nondiagnostic.
†Many of the pulmonary diseases have important extrapulmonary sites of involvement that may dominate the clinical findings. In such cases, pulmonary disease (if classic findings) may be presumed in selected patients if the diagnosis is established from another site.
§Serum CRAG may be negative in isolated cryptococcal pneumonia.
‡S-Adenosylmethionine (SAM) levels have been reported to be significantly lower in HIV-infected patients with PCP than in HIV-infected patients without PCP and healthy control subjects.
AFB = acid-fast bacilli; BAL = bronchoalveolar lavage; CRAG = cryptococcal antigen; CT = computed tomography; DLCO = diffusing capacity for carbon monoxide; GGO = ground-glass opacities; GI = gastrointestinal; HHV-8 = human herpes virus 8 (Kaposi's sarcoma herpes virus, KS-HV); HRCT = chest high-resolution computed tomography; MRI = magnetic resonance imaging; PFTs = pulmonary function tests; TBBX = transbronchial biopsies; WBC = white blood cell.

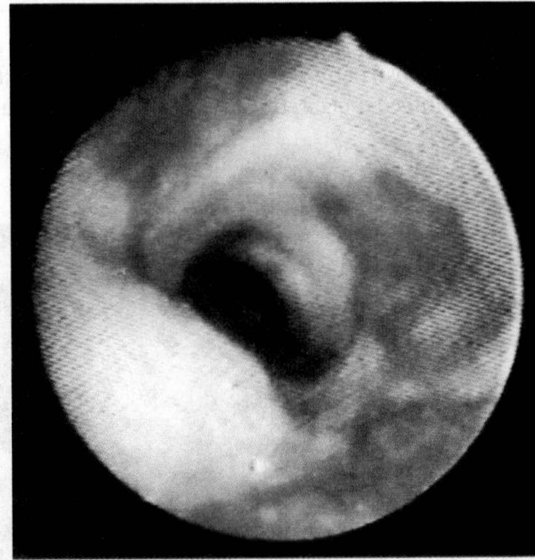

FIGURE 414–12 • Characteristic Kaposi's sarcoma lesions located in the trachea in an HIV-infected person, CD4+ cell count less than 100 cells/μL. Concurrent bronchoalveolar lavage also revealed *Pneumocystis* pneumonia.

the characteristic KS lesions are seen (Fig. 414–12). However, the absence of visible KS lesions does not preclude their presence in more distal airways, nor does it preclude the possibility of parenchymal Kaposi's sarcoma involvement. In these select patients, TBBX can occasionally establish the diagnosis.

Bronchoscopy with BAL may diagnose *M. tuberculosis* (although the diagnostic yield improves with the addition of TBBX), *H. capsulatum*, *C. immitis*, and *T. gondii* pneumonia. Bronchoscopy with TBBX (or other biopsy specimen) is required to establish a definitive diagnosis of *Aspergillus* and cytomegalovirus pneumonia. Similarly, biopsy is an important tool in the diagnosis of non-Hodgkin's lymphoma pulmonary disease.

Other Procedures

Diagnostic thoracentesis should be considered for any HIV-infected patient with evidence of pleural effusion in whom other tests are nondiagnostic or there is a concern for empyema. In most situations, pleural fluid culture or cytology in the case of non-Hodgkin's lymphoma can establish the diagnosis. However, in patients with pleural effusion and suspected tuberculosis, the diagnostic yield is improved with the addition of pleural biopsy.

CT-guided transthoracic needle aspiration is an important and useful diagnostic procedure for selected patients. HIV-infected patients with focal parenchymal lesions, most often peripheral lung nodules or masses that may be beyond the reach of a bronchoscope, are ideal candidates for CT-guided aspiration. In one study of 32 HIV-infected patients undergoing this procedure, a diagnosis was established in 27. Mediastinoscopy should be considered for patients with a mediastinal mass or adenopathy, or both. Video-assisted thoracoscopic surgery can be an important procedure in selected patients.

Occasionally, despite all these efforts, HIV-infected patients with pulmonary disease may elude definitive diagnosis. In such patients, consideration should be given to open lung biopsy, although results have been mixed. Even though open lung biopsy often provides important new information, patients who undergo this procedure are frequently already so ill that this new information fails to translate into improved survival.

Complications

Noninfectious Complications

The focus of the evaluation and management of respiratory symptoms in an HIV-infected patient is frequently placed on opportunistic infections and their prompt diagnosis and treatment. However, several noninfectious complications associated with HIV infection warrant discussion.

Kaposi's Sarcoma

The overwhelming majority of HIV-infected patients with KS are men who have sexual relations with other men (Chapter 416). Clinically symptomatic pulmonary KS occurs at the lower range of CD4$^+$ cell counts, but tracheobronchial lesions may be seen in patients with higher CD4$^+$ counts who are undergoing bronchoscopy for other reasons. Most patients with pulmonary KS have mucocutaneous disease.

Pulmonary KS is characterized by nonproductive cough, dyspnea, and occasionally fever. Chest pain and hemoptysis are less frequently noted. Symptoms are usually present for weeks or months but may also progress rapidly in a manner indistinguishable from opportunistic infection. Pulmonary KS is characteristically accompanied by bilateral middle to lower lung zone opacities in a central or perihilar distribution. Typical chest radiograph findings include linear densities (bronchial wall thickening), nodules or nodular opacities of varying size, Kerley's B lines, pleural effusions, and intrathoracic adenopathy. Chest CT scans often demonstrate the characteristic peribronchovascular distribution with associated nodules.

The diagnosis of pulmonary KS is usually established by bronchoscopy. The finding of characteristic endobronchial, reddish purple, flat or slightly raised lesions is sufficient to diagnose pulmonary disease in the proper clinical context (see Fig. 414–12). Most patients with chest radiograph findings suggestive of pulmonary KS have endobronchial KS lesions seen below the level of the carina. However, the absence of lesions in the observable airway does not preclude more distal airway disease or parenchymal, pleural, or nodal involvement. When there is strong clinical suspicion for pulmonary KS but no endobronchial lesions are seen, TBBX should be considered to establish the diagnosis. A significant proportion of patients with pulmonary KS have concurrent opportunistic infection, and patients undergoing evaluation for pulmonary KS should be concomitantly evaluated for opportunistic infection.

Non-Hodgkin's Lymphoma

Most HIV-infected patients with non-Hodgkin's lymphoma have widely disseminated disease and extranodal involvement (Chapter 416). Frequent extranodal sites include the liver, spleen, bone marrow, meninges, and gastrointestinal tract, whereas intrathoracic involvement is seen in a smaller proportion. Occasionally, the lung is the only site involved. Patients with non-Hodgkin's lymphoma can have a wide range of CD4$^+$ cell counts. In one study, the median CD4$^+$ cell count was 100 cells/μL, and 75% of patients had a CD4$^+$ cell count lower than 50 cells/μL.

When the lungs are involved, the most common symptoms are cough and dyspnea, with pleuritic chest pain and hemoptysis occurring less frequently. Classic B symptoms such as fever, sweats, and weight loss are also common features. The most frequent parenchymal lung findings on chest radiograph are multiple nodular opacities or masses, lobar infiltrates, and diffuse interstitial infiltrates. Occasionally, a solitary nodule or mass is seen. Pleural effusions are the most common radiographic abnormality; they are seen in 40 to 70% of cases and may occur in the absence of parenchymal disease. Hilar and mediastinal adenopathy is found in up to 60% of patients.

The diagnosis of non-Hodgkin's lymphoma requires demonstration of malignant lymphocytes on cytology or biopsy specimens. Persons with isolated intrathoracic involvement should undergo bronchoscopy with biopsy or CT-guided transthoracic needle aspiration. Other options include mediastinoscopy, thoracoscopy, and open lung biopsy. For patients with effusions, pleural fluid cytology or biopsy, or both, are often diagnostic.

Nonspecific Interstitial Pneumonitis

Nonspecific interstitial pneumonitis (NSIP) has been reported with various frequencies in HIV-infected patients. Because it is a histologic diagnosis, its incidence depends partly on the frequency that biopsy is performed during the diagnostic evaluation. Symptoms of NSIP include dyspnea, nonproductive cough, and fever. These clinical features are indistinguishable from *Pneumocystis* pneumonia. However, NSIP may occur at CD4$^+$ cell counts higher than 200 cells/μL, whereas *Pneumocystis* pneumonia rarely does. Chest radiographic findings in NSIP are nonspecific and usually indistinguishable from *Pneumocystis* pneumonia, and as with *Pneumocystis* pneumonia, patients with NSIP can have a normal radiograph. One study of NSIP found that 44% of 36 patients had a normal radiograph. The most common radiographic abnormality seen was a diffuse interstitial pattern. Other abnormalities include pleural effusions, alveolar infiltrates, and nodules. Pulmonary function tests often reveal a mildly decreased diffusing capacity. The diagnosis of NSIP requires histologic confirmation and exclusion of other causes.

Lymphocytic Interstitial Pneumonitis

The most striking feature of HIV-associated lymphocytic interstitial pneumonitis (LIP) is the effect of age on its incidence. LIP has been a frequent acquired immunodeficiency syndrome–defining diagnosis in children but is rare in adults. Symptoms of LIP include slowly progressive dyspnea, nonproductive cough, and fever indistinguishable from opportunistic infection. The chest radiograph is nonspecific in patients with LIP and characteristically shows bilateral reticulonodular "interstitial" infiltrates with a lower lung zone predominance. Hilar or mediastinal adenopathy is occasionally seen and can potentially be used to distinguish LIP from *Pneumocystis* pneumonia. Pulmonary function tests often reveal a restrictive ventilatory defect and decreased diffusing capacity. Chest CT scans demonstrate small (2 to 4 mm) nodules, frequently in a peribronchovascular distribution, or diffuse areas of ground-glass opacity (Fig. 414–13). The diagnosis of LIP requires histologic confirmation by biopsy.

Pulmonary Arterial Hypertension

Numerous reports of pulmonary arterial hypertension in HIV-infected patients are scattered throughout the literature. The characteristic clinical manifestation is progressive dyspnea, with nonproductive cough, chest pain, and syncope or near-syncope seen in a minority. Chest radiograph findings include cardiomegaly and prominence of the pulmonary arteries. Most often, a chest radiograph or an electrocardiogram with evidence of right ventricular hypertrophy first suggests the diagnosis of pulmonary hypertension. Patients in whom pulmonary hypertension is diagnosed should undergo a thorough evaluation for secondary causes, including underlying cardiac (i.e., left ventricular failure, valvar disease) and pulmonary diseases (i.e., chronic obstructive pulmonary disease, recurrent pulmonary emboli).

Chronic Obstructive Pulmonary Disease

HIV-infected patients are subject to the entire spectrum of pulmonary disease, including the obstructive lung diseases. Reports and studies have suggested that HIV-infected cigarette smokers may be at greater risk for

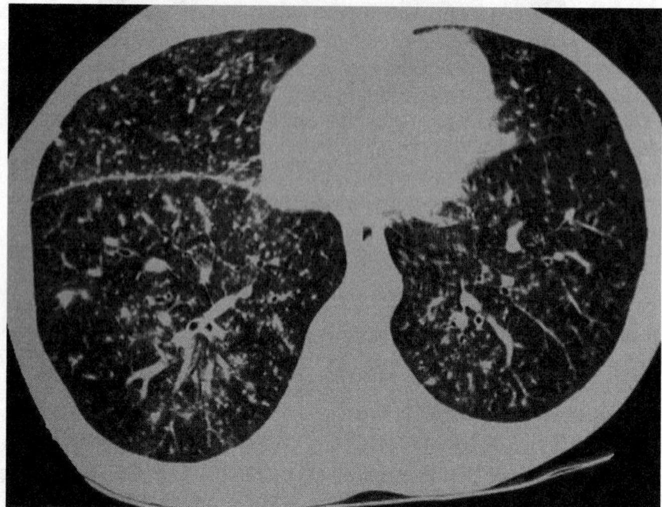

FIGURE 414–13 • Chest high-resolution computed tomography scan of an HIV-infected person, CD4$^+$ cell count less than 200 cells/μL. Lymphocytic interstitial pneumonitis was diagnosed by transbronchial biopsy.

the development of emphysema than HIV-infected nonsmokers or non-immunocompromised cigarette smokers. In addition to cigarette smoking, repeated opportunistic pulmonary infections may eventually result in the development of chronic bronchitis and bronchiectasis. The clinical and radiographic findings, diagnosis, and management of obstructive lung disease in HIV-infected patients are identical to that in immunocompetent patients, including the use of inhaled corticosteroids, when indicated.

Sarcoidosis

Several cases of sarcoidosis in HIV-infected patients have been reported. In these cases the clinical and radiographic manifestations, diagnosis, and clinical course with corticosteroid therapy were similar to cases of sarcoidosis in non–HIV-infected persons.

Immune Reconstitution Syndromes

The initiation of combinations of potent antiretroviral therapy and the subsequent improvement in immune function have also resulted in several syndromes that have important clinical implications (Chapter 412). Interestingly, in some of the examples provided, the use of antiretroviral therapy transiently exacerbates the disease, whereas in others, its use is seemingly solely responsible for the reported improvements. Finally, in some cases, the use of antiretroviral therapy has been associated with the development of pulmonary disease that is host mediated.

The transient worsening of clinical symptoms and signs and chest radiograph findings of tuberculosis after the initiation of appropriate antituberculous therapy has been well recognized. These paradoxical reactions are thought to represent an enhanced antituberculous immune response, and they usually resolve with continued therapy alone. HIV-infected patients in whom tuberculosis develops and who receive concurrent antiretroviral and antituberculous therapy appear to have an increased incidence of paradoxical worsening. One study found that 36% of HIV-infected tuberculosis patients receiving these dual therapies exhibited a paradoxical reaction versus 7% of HIV-infected tuberculosis patients who received tuberculosis therapy alone and 2% of tuberculosis patients without concomitant HIV infection. Another study noted transient worsening on serial chest radiographs in 45% of HIV-infected tuberculosis patients receiving dual HIV and tuberculosis therapy. The radiographic findings consisted of new or worsening parenchymal disease in 32%, new or worsening intrathoracic lymphadenopathy in 23%, and new or worsening pleural effusion in 19%. The diagnosis of paradoxical reaction must be one of exclusion. HIV-infected tuberculosis patients with suspected paradoxical reactions must also be thoroughly evaluated for progressive tuberculosis resulting from drug resistance or patient nonadherence and for the presence of a concurrent, superimposed opportunistic infection.

Similar to tuberculosis, paradoxical reactions in HIV-infected patients have been reported in patients receiving concurrent therapy for HIV and opportunistic infection, including important pulmonary pathogens such as *Pneumocystis* and *Cryptococcus.*

In contrast to the paradoxical reactions observed in the setting of opportunistic infection, the use of antiretroviral therapy, often in the absence of specific chemotherapy, has resulted in clinical regression and, occasionally, complete resolution of KS lesions (including pulmonary KS).

Whether the addition of antiretroviral therapy to standard treatment of opportunistic infection is beneficial—or potentially harmful if paradoxical reactions develop—in patients with opportunistic infections is a largely unanswered question. A few retrospective studies have suggested that the use of potent antiretroviral therapy in critically ill HIV-infected patients may be associated with improved survival. Given the still significant mortality associated with respiratory failure from opportunistic infections, this question is particularly important with regard to HIV-associated pneumonia.

Improved immune function may also play a role in the development of host-mediated pulmonary disease. There are several reports of sarcoidosis or a sarcoidosis-like disease that developed after the initiation of antiretroviral therapy. In addition, hypersensitivity pneumonitis to avian antigen that developed only after the patient's immune function improved with antiretroviral therapy has been described. Diseases in which the host's immune response plays an essential role in pathogenesis can be expected to become more prevalent as more HIV-infected patients receive potent antiretroviral therapy.

SUGGESTED READINGS

Grant AD, Charalambous S, Fielding KL, et al: Effect of routine isoniazid preventive therapy on tuberculosis incidence among HIV-infected men in South Africa: A novel randomized incremental recruitment study. JAMA 2005;293:2719–2725. *Enrollment in a clinic offering primary isoniazid preventive therapy to HIV-infected adults reduced tuberculosis incidence by 38% overall, although the incidence remained high (9.0 per 100 person-years).*

Grubb JR, Moorman AC, Baker RK, et al: The changing spectrum of pulmonary disease in patients with HIV infection on antiretroviral therapy. AIDS 2006;20:1095–1107. *An update addressing the influence of antiretroviral treatment.*

Huang L, Quartin A, Jones D, et al: Intensive care of patients with HIV infection. N Engl J Med 2006;355:173–181. *The optimal approach to patients with HIV infection in the ICU requires awareness of their complex management issues.*

Kanmogne GD: Noninfectious pulmonary complications of HIV/AIDS. Curr Opin Pulm Med 2005;11:208–212. *A helpful review.*

Lawn SD, Bekker LG, Miller RF: Immune reconstitution disease associated with mycobacterial infections in HIV-infected individuals receiving antiretrovirals. Lancet Infect Dis 2005;5(6):361–373. *Excellent review of immune reconstitution to mycobacterial infections in HIV-infected persons.*

Thomas CF Jr, Limper AH: *Pneumocystis* pneumonia. N Engl J Med 2004; 350:2487–2498. *A scholarly review.*

415 SKIN MANIFESTATIONS IN PATIENTS WITH HUMAN IMMUNODEFICIENCY VIRUS INFECTION

Toby Maurer

From the beginning of the epidemic, skin disease has often been the initial feature of infection with human immunodeficiency virus (HIV). Cutaneous manifestations are often predictive of the stage of immunosuppression and long-term prognosis. Morbidity from skin diseases, particularly from opportunistic infections, has decreased with the advent of antiretroviral treatment (ART), although there are still significant dermatologic problems for patients in the post-ART era. Cutaneous manifestations seen in patients with HIV may be categorized as infectious, neoplastic, inflammatory, or related to ART.

INFECTIOUS MANIFESTATIONS

HIV Seroconversion Exanthem

Frequently observed in acute HIV infection is an infectious mononucleosis–like illness that precedes seroconversion by 2 to 6 weeks. The rash is characterized by erythematous macules and papules ranging from 2 mm to a few centimeters, particularly on the upper part of the trunk and face with relative sparing of the peripheries. It is commonly accompanied by aphthous or penile ulceration, or both. There is evidence that very early after infection, HIV goes to dendritic cells in skin and causes an inflammatory response, which may explain the rash. At this stage the viral load may be very high and is suggestive of acute HIV seroconversion, although the HIV antibody test is likely to remain negative.

Viruses

Herpes Zoster

Herpes zoster is often observed even at relatively normal CD4$^+$ counts and may therefore be the first feature of HIV infection. In any patient younger than 50 years with zoster, risk factors for HIV should be explored and consideration given to HIV testing (Chapter 398). Zoster infection may be multidermatomal or disseminated and, if it involves the eye, treatment with intravenous acyclovir should be considered. Antiviral treatment should be started at any time during the disease course (not only within the first 48 hours as with zoster not associated with HIV). Less severe disease normally responds to standard treatment. There have been a few reports of a verrucous chronic form of zoster occurring in more severely immunosuppressed patients; this form of zoster is usually associated with acyclovir resistance.

Herpes Simplex Virus

Infection with herpes simplex virus (HSV) should always be considered in patients with HIV who have mucocutaneous ulcerations (Fig. 415–1), particularly in the anogenital area. Patients with CD4$^+$ counts below 200 may require higher doses of acyclovir to treat the infection. (See Table 415–1 for conditions occurring at CD4$^+$ counts less than 200 in patients not receiving ART.) Patients who fail to respond may have HSV with acyclovir resistance, and alternative agents such as foscarnet or cidofovir may be required. The presence of HSV clinically or subclinically increases the likelihood of HIV transmission. There also appears to be synergy between HSV and HIV, which may mean faster progression of HIV disease.

Human Papillomavirus

Human papillomavirus infection (Chapter 396) is very common in all stages of HIV infection. Common, flat, genital, and plantar warts are all seen with increased frequency. Patients with significant immunosuppression may have particularly extensive warts that are recalcitrant to standard treatment. Most patients commencing on ART often notice considerable improvement or resolution of the warts. However, some patients receiving ART will not clear their warts despite improvement in the CD4$^+$ count, suppressed viral load, and resolution of all other opportunistic infections. The reasons for this observation remain obscure. Treatment modalities include cryotherapy, surgery, laser, topical salicylic acid preparations, podophyllin, intralesional bleomycin, and contact sensitization immunotherapy. Imiquimod has proved to be a useful modality for genital warts but appears to be less effective in the HIV setting.

Molluscum Contagiosum

Molluscum contagiosum is a poxvirus that causes a self-limited papular umbilicated eruption commonly seen in children. It is rarer to see in adults and, when on the face, persistent, or severe, raises the possibility of HIV coinfection. It tends to occur when the CD4$^+$ count falls below 200. First-line treatment is ART because molluscum contagiosum is invariably cleared with rising CD4$^+$ counts. Ablative treatments such as cryotherapy or curettage will treat individual lesions more expeditiously but can leave scarring; however, without ART the lesions are likely to recur.

TABLE 415–1 CONDITIONS COMMON IN PATIENTS WITH CD4$^+$ COUNTS LESS THAN 200 AND NOT RECEIVING ANTIRETROVIRAL THERAPY

Photodermatitis
Psoriasis, difficult to control or more than 50% of the body
Pruritic papular eruption of HIV
Prurigo nodularis
Oral hairy leukoplakia
Molluscum contagiosum
Eosinophilic folliculitis

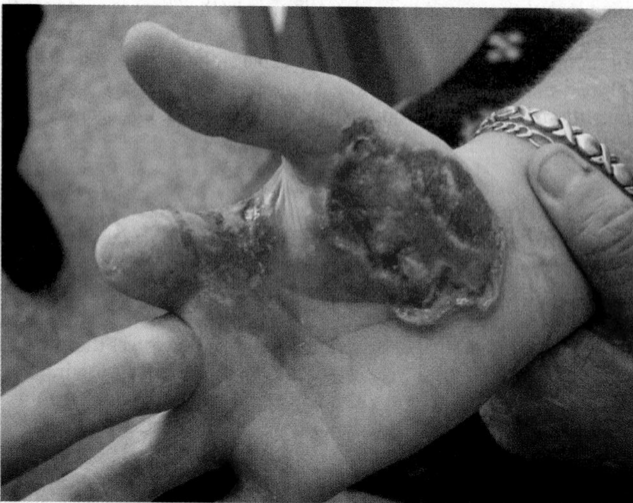

FIGURE 415–1 • Chronic herpes simplex infection.

Epstein-Barr Virus (Oral Hairy Leukoplakia)

Oral hairy leukoplakia (OHL) is characterized by nonpainful white plaques with a feathered edge, particularly on the lateral border of the tongue. It is associated with Epstein-Barr virus and is very rare in immunocompetent hosts. OHL can occur at any CD4$^+$ count and may therefore be the initial feature of HIV infection. (See Table 415–2 for diseases not affected by the CD4$^+$ count.) The appearance of OHL was a poor prognostic indicator before ART. There is no specific treatment of OHL, although it tends to resolve when patients are taking ART. Superinfection with *Candida* sp should be considered if the lesions are painful.

Bacteria

Staphylococcus aureus

Infections with *Staphylococcus aureus* are commonly seen in HIV disease. Staphylococcal folliculitis (Fig. 415–2) tends to be more severe or refractory to treatment than in patients who are HIV negative. Other cutaneous manifestations of staphylococcal infection include cellulitis, ecthyma (necrotic plaques), or rarely, botryomycosis. Treatment of folliculitis includes antiseptic washes such as chlorhexidine solution, eradication of nasal carriage with mupirocin ointment, and occasionally,

TABLE 415–2 CONDITIONS THAT CAN PRESENT AT ANY CD4$^+$ COUNT

Eczema
Xerosis
Tinea/onychomycosis
Kaposi's sarcoma
Warts
Syphilis

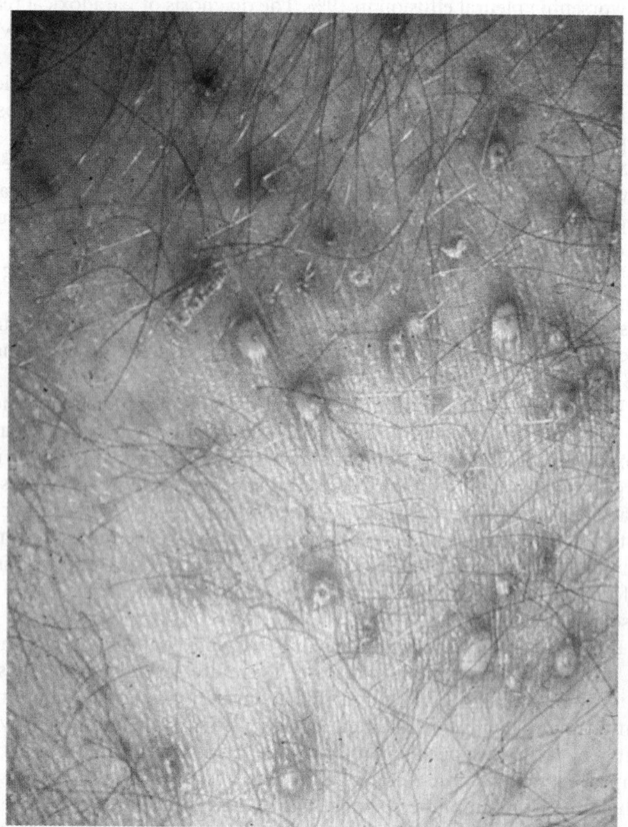

FIGURE 415–2 • Staphylococcal folliculitis.

systemic antibiotics. More severe infections may require intravenous antibiotics. There has been concern that patients with HIV are at increased risk for the development of infections with methicillin-resistant *S. aureus* (MRSA). Rifampicin is often used to clear MRSA, but caution should be used in patients receiving ART because rifampicin is a potent inducer of cytochrome P-450 and will therefore interfere with protease inhibitors.

Bartonella

Bacillary angiomatosis is caused by *Bartonella* species (most commonly *Bartonella henselae* and *Bartonella quintana*). Occult infection with *Bartonella* should be considered in any HIV-infected patient with fever of unknown origin. The cutaneous lesions appear as purple papules, nodules, or ulcers in HIV-positive individuals. Clinically, they may resemble lesions of Kaposi's sarcoma (KS) and may also be confused with pyogenic granuloma or cutaneous lymphoma. These lesions should always be biopsied and tissue sent for culture. Bacillary angiomatosis responds to antibiotics such as macrolides, which will be needed for at least a 2-month course of treatment. Bacillary angiomatosis can be associated with visceral disease; in particular, the liver and spleen may be affected.

Syphilis

Syphilis (Chapter 340) is frequently seen in patients with HIV infection. Its cutaneous manifestations are protean, and therefore syphilis should be considered in any patient infected with HIV who has a new cutaneous eruption. An example of a secondary syphilis exanthem is shown in Figure 415–3. Primary, secondary, and tertiary forms of syphilis may be manifested clinically as they are in HIV-negative individuals, although atypical findings are not uncommon. Serology is not as reliable in HIV infection, and skin biopsy may be useful in establishing the diagnosis. First-line treatment is with penicillin, but a longer duration of therapy will be required in patients coinfected with HIV. Follow-up titers of syphilis serology should be documented to ensure adequate treatment and central nervous system clearance.

Fungi

Candida

Oral candidiasis is commonly seen in patients with immunodeficiency, including HIV infection. It is characterized by white, cheesy plaques and papules loosely adherent to the tongue and oropharynx. Topical therapies include clotrimazole troches and nystatin oral suspension. First-line oral treatment is with fluconazole, although there is emerging resistance in *Candida* species, including *Candida albicans,* the most common species associated with thrush. Second-line treatment is with oral itraconazole, although it is unclear whether pulsed therapy is preferable.

Dermatophytes

The prevalence of dermatophyte infection is not more frequent in HIV-infected patients than in control groups. However, increased severity and variability in manifestations of dermatophyte infection are seen in HIV coinfection. Tinea corporis and tinea cruris can occur at all stages of immunosuppression and may be successfully treated with topical antidermatophytic preparations such as ketoconazole or terbinafine. Treatment of onychomycosis is systemic therapy with oral antifungals, although onychomycosis recurrence rates have not been studied.

Other Fungi

Cryptococcus neoformans is a yeast that tends to cause clinical problems when patients are profoundly immunosuppressed (CD4$^+$ count <100). It commonly affects the central nervous system and causes meningitis, but it can affect the skin and give rise to papules indistinguishable from molluscum contagiosum. *Histoplasma capsulatum* and *Penicillium marneffei* may morphologically resemble molluscum.

Infestations

Scabies

Scabies is caused by infestation with the mite *Sarcoptes scabiei* and is commonly seen in HIV infection. It can be manifested as the classic rash of scabies with burrows affecting the finger and toe webs and widespread excoriated papules with a predilection for the axillae, nipples, and genitalia. It can also appear as crusted scabies with hyperkeratotic plaques that tend not to be pruritic. Combination treatment with a topical agent such as permethrin or benzoyl benzoate and systemic treatment with ivermectin tablets is recommended for crusted scabies. Topical agents may be sufficient for classic scabies. Lindane lotion is often used to treat scabies, but there have been reports of lindane-resistant scabies and neurologic side effects attributed to this treatment.

TUMORS

Kaposi's Sarcoma

KS is the most common HIV-associated malignancy, but since the introduction of ART, there has been a significant decrease in its incidence. It is characterized by dusky, purple nodules and plaques with a predilection for the extremities and the oral mucosa (Fig. 415–4). Poor prognostic factors include lymphedema and internal organ involvement. It is caused by human herpes virus 8, also known as Kaposi's sarcoma–associated virus. The virus may be transmitted vertically, sexually, or casually, and its presence is necessary for the development of KS. First-line treatment consists of ART, with the addition of chemotherapy for aggressive or unresponsive KS.

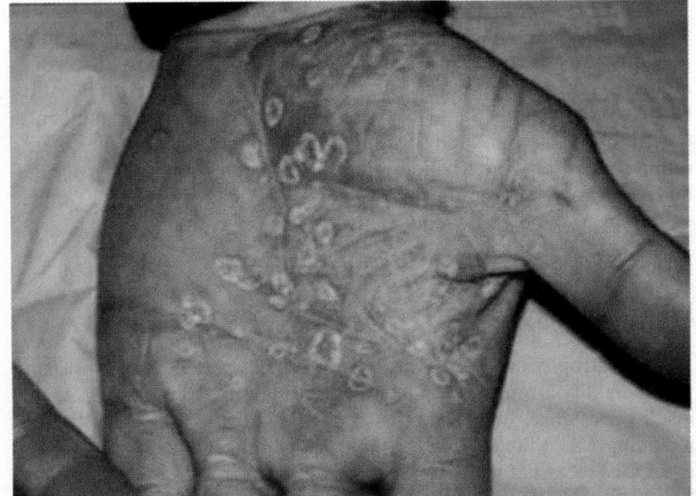

FIGURE 415–3 • Secondary syphilis.

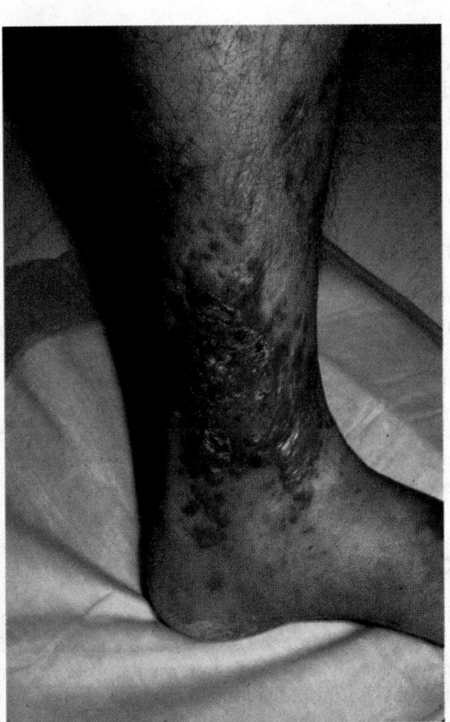

FIGURE 415–4 • Kaposi's sarcoma.

Section XXIV HIV and AIDS

Malignant Melanoma

Malignant melanoma may have an increased incidence in HIV-positive patients. There is some evidence that malignant melanoma behaves more aggressively in HIV-infected patients, and therefore more extensive primary surgical treatment and closer follow-up of patients should be considered, as well as maximizing immune function with appropriate ART.

Nonmelanoma Skin Cancer

There appears to be a three-fold increased risk for the development of nonmelanoma skin cancer in patients with HIV disease. The clinical manifestations of squamous cell carcinoma (SCC) and basal cell carcinoma (BCC) do not appear to be any different than in the uninfected population. However, in the context of HIV infection, SCC behaves more aggressively and is associated with reduced survival. Management of SCC is surgical excision, whereas curettage and electrodesiccation may be appropriate for BCC lesions on the extremities or trunk. Surgical excision should be the treatment of choice for BCC on the face.

INFLAMMATORY MANIFESTATIONS

Seborrheic Dermatitis

Seborrheic dermatitis is a common dermatosis in the general population, but it has a strikingly increased prevalence in HIV-infected patients, and the frequency increases with more severe immunosuppression. It appears as orange-red scaly patches affecting the scalp, eyebrows, nose, and cheeks. Seborrheic dermatitis can also affect the central portion of the chest and genitalia. It responds well to a combination of topical antifungals such as econazole or ketoconazole and low-potency corticosteroids. The condition also tends to improve when patients are taking ART.

Atopic Dermatitis

Atopic dermatitis is common in HIV-infected patients. As with other dermatoses, it improves with ART, but in patients with a $CD4^+$ nadir greater than 200, it tends to be more persistent. Treatment is with topical steroids and emollients as in the HIV-uninfected population. Topical pimecrolimus and tacrolimus are licensed for the treatment of atopic dermatitis, but their safety has not been demonstrated in HIV infection.

Psoriasis

HIV infection can be associated with severe psoriasis as the $CD4^+$ count drops. This observation is paradoxical because psoriasis is thought to be a T-cell-mediated disease but may be explained by immune dysregulation. Topical treatments, systemic retinoids, and ultraviolet phototherapy are all reasonable treatment options. Immunosuppressive agents such as methotrexate and cyclosporine should be avoided if possible. ART invariably reduces the severity of psoriasis.

Papular Pruritic Eruption of HIV

Papular pruritic eruption is commonly seen in Africa in association with HIV. It should be considered in the differential diagnosis of any widespread itchy dermatosis, but it does appear to be a separate entity. Papular pruritic eruption has a rather nondescript appearance of red excoriated papules on the trunk and limbs. Other itchy skin diseases such as eczema or eosinophilic folliculitis should be considered in the differential diagnosis. Recent evidence has suggested that exaggerated arthropod bite reactions may be the predominant cause. Potent topical corticosteroids and, anecdotally, ART have been of benefit.

Eosinophilic Folliculitis

Eosinophilic folliculitis is characterized by edematous papules and pustules on the face and upper part of the trunk (Fig. 415–5). These lesions are intensely itchy, and skin biopsy is helpful in ruling out other causes of folliculitis. Eosinophilic folliculitis tends to be seen when $CD4^+$ counts are less than 200 and may improve with ART. Treatments such as itraconazole, retinoids, and phototherapy are all effective.

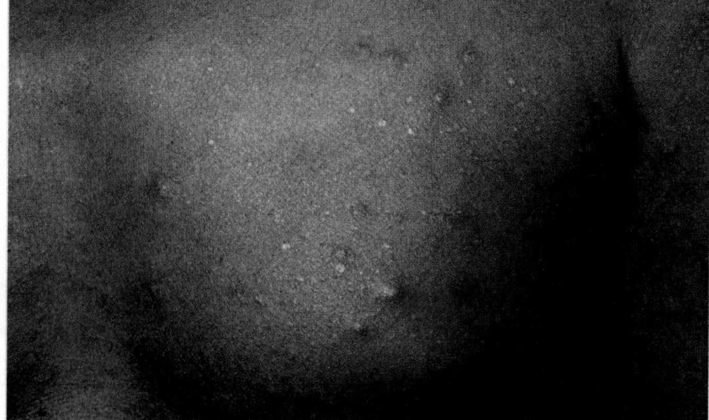

FIGURE 415–5 • Eosinophilic folliculitis.

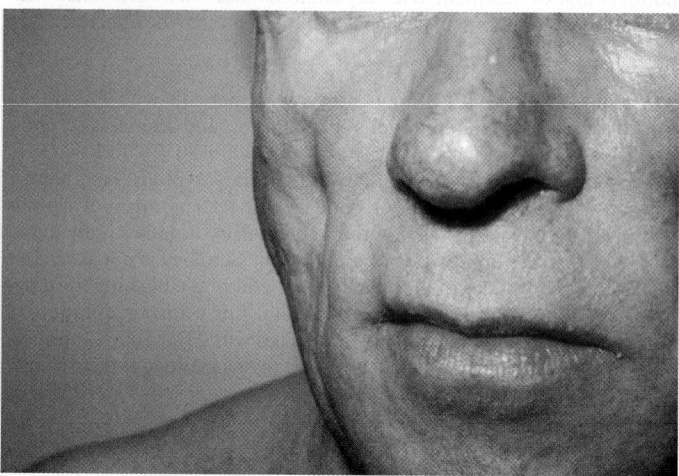

FIGURE 415–6 • HIV-associated facial lipoatrophy.

TABLE 415–3 MOST COMMON SKIN DISEASES SINCE THE ADVENT OF ANTIRETROVIRALS
Acne
Staphylococcal infections of the soft tissue and skin
Erythema nodosum
Eosinophilic folliculitis
Lipodystrophy

Prurigo Nodularis

In patients with prurigo nodularis, symmetrically distributed papules and nodules develop on the limbs and trunk with sparing of the mid-portion of the back (because of inaccessibility for scratching). It is commonly seen in HIV infection and is sometimes associated with hepatitis C virus coinfection. Standard treatment options include emollients, potent topical steroids, and sedating antihistamines such as chlorpheniramine or hydroxyzine. Thalidomide is often effective in recalcitrant cases but requires careful monitoring for peripheral neuropathy, and women of childbearing potential require effective contraception.

METABOLIC MANIFESTATIONS

HIV Lipodystrophy Syndrome

Lipodystrophy syndrome was first described in 1998 and consists of peripheral lipoatrophy, central lipohypertrophy, lipid abnormalities, and insulin resistance. It is likely that it is caused by a number of factors, including ART (Table 415–3), although it is unlikely that a single agent is responsible. Cutaneous facial lipoatrophy tends to be the most problematic dermatologic aspect, with significant associated psychological morbidity (Fig. 415–6). Currently, no treatments are effective for lipodystrophy syndrome, although surgical correction with dermal fillers may improve the cosmetic appearance.

SUGGESTED READINGS

Di Lorenzo G, Konstantinopoulos PA, Pantanowitz L, et al: Management of AIDS-related Kaposi's sarcoma. Lancet Oncol 2007;8:167–176. *Review of recent advances in the treatment of Kaposi's sarcoma.*

Hawkins T: Appearance-related side effects of HIV-1 treatment. AIDS Patient Care STDS 2006;20:6–18. *Review of the many dermatologic side effects of HIV treatment and their impact on treatment adherence.*

Lehloenya R, Meintjes G: Dermatologic manifestation of the immune reconstitution inflammatory syndrome. Dermatol Clin 2006;24:549–570. *Comprehensive review of the dermatologic manifestations of the IRIS syndrome.*

Mocroft A, Kirk O, Clumeck N, et al: The changing pattern of Kaposi sarcoma in patients with HIV, 1994–2003: The EuroSIDA Study. Cancer 2004;100: 2644–2654. *Demonstrates the changing clinical spectrum.*

Nagot N, Ouedraogo A, Foulongne V, et al: Reduction of HIV-1 RNA levels with therapy to suppress herpes simplex virus. N Engl J Med 2007;22:790–799. *Treatment of HSV significantly reduces genital and plasma HIV RNA levels.*

Nguyen P, Vin-Christian K, Ming ME, et al: Aggressive squamous cell carcinomas in persons infected with the human immunodeficiency virus. Arch Dermatol 2002;138:758–763. *Emphasizes the different natural histories in HIV-infected patients.*

Strick LB, Wald A, Celum C: Management of herpes simplex virus type 2 infection in HIV type 1–infected persons. Clin Infect Dis 2006;43:347–356. *Comprehensive clinical review.*

Zancanaro PC, McGirt LY, Mamelak AJ, et al: Cutaneous manifestations of HIV in the era of highly active antiretroviral therapy: An institutional urban clinic experience. J Am Acad Dermatol 2006;54:581–588. *Large case series describing the common dermatologic conditions in patients with various levels of immunosuppression.*

Zetola NM, Klausner JD: Syphilis and HIV infection: An update. Clin Infect Dis 2007;44:1222–1228. *Comprehensive clinical review.*

416 HEMATOLOGY AND ONCOLOGY IN PATIENTS WITH HUMAN IMMUNODEFICIENCY VIRUS INFECTION

Paul A. Volberding

Hematologic disorders and unusual cancers were important and early warnings of the human immunodeficiency virus (HIV) epidemic and remain significant clinical problems despite progress in antiretroviral (ARV) drug development. The remarkable and specific reduction in peripheral CD4$^+$ lymphocytes almost immediately connected early cases to an underlying immune deficiency. This was further underscored by the increased incidence of a cancer, Kaposi's sarcoma (KS), previously seen in immunosuppressed renal transplant recipients. Acquired immunodeficiency syndrome (AIDS)-associated cancers were also important in the early epidemic and attracted oncologists who adapted cancer care models to AIDS. These systems, comprehensive and multidisciplinary with community-based palliative components, were ideal when no therapy could reverse the underlying fatal HIV infection.

Hematologic disorders can be caused by HIV infection itself as a consequence of its immune deficiency or can be side effects of drugs used to treat HIV or to manage associated conditions. Both HIV-related malignancies and hematologic disorders have changed with the advent of effective ARV therapy. Study of these clinical problems affords insight into the consequences of immune deficiency and its reversal and highlights the benefits and limitations of ARV therapy.

HEMATOLOGIC DISORDERS IN HIV INFECTION

Disorders in all major blood cell lines were recognized early in the HIV epidemic. The underlying biology of HIV-associated hematologic disease is complex, often involving multiple lineages and mechanisms of pathogenesis. HIV itself infects cells involved in hematopoiesis and can cause cytopenia. HIV infection also causes both immune activation and immune deficiency. The former, analogous to inflammation, can cause anemia of chronic disease, whereas the dysregulation of lymphocyte subsets can disrupt the balance of cytokines and other factors needed for normal myelopoiesis. The combination of immune activation and dysregulation can also contribute to hypergammaglobulinemia and reticuloendothelial activation and result in accelerated cellular destruction. The effect of ARV therapy on HIV-associated hematologic disease is similarly complex. ARV drugs have well-described direct hematologic toxicities, whereas their ability to reverse established immune deficiency and to control HIV infection within marrow reduces the incidence and severity of many HIV-associated hematologic disorders.

Red Blood Cell Dysfunction and Anemia

The prevalence of anemia in HIV infection varies by threshold definition and patient demographics. Before the advent of effective ARV therapy, estimates ranged as high as 75%. Prevalence was increased in women, African Americans, and those with advanced disease stage.

Epidemiology

Anemia in HIV-infected patients can be caused by many factors (Table 416–1). Those unrelated to HIV infection, such as hemoglobinopathies, should always be considered in the differential diagnosis.

HIV-associated anemia is usually caused by decreased red blood cell (RBC) production. RBC loss from bleeding or intravascular hemolysis can occur but is less common. Decreased RBC production is seen with chronic inflammation, nutritional deficiencies, erythropoietic defects, and marrow suppression as a result of infection or drug therapy.

Anemia of chronic disease follows ineffective iron utilization in the setting of inflammation. Iron studies typically show reductions in serum

TABLE 416–1 CAUSES OF ANEMIA IN HIV-INFECTED PATIENTS

CAUSED PREDOMINANTLY BY DECREASED RED BLOOD CELL PRODUCTION

- Anemia of chronic disease
- Hypogonadism and decreased erythropoietic effect
- Infections and cancers in marrow
  - *Mycobacterium avium intracellulare*
  - *Mycobacterium tuberculosis*
  - Parvovirus
  - *Bartonella henselae*
  - *Bartonella quintana*
  - Other non-Hodgkin's lymphomas
- Nutritional deficiency
  - Iron deficiency
- Drug effects
  - Zidovudine
  - Trimethoprim-sulfamethoxazole
  - Ganciclovir
  - Amphotericin
  - Cytotoxic chemotherapeutics
  - Others

CAUSED PREDOMINANTLY BY ACCELERATED RED BLOOD CELL LOSS

- Hypersplenism
  - HIV
  - Portal hypertension from hepatitis C, hepatitis B with cirrhosis
- Hemolysis
  - Microangiopathy—thrombotic thrombocytopenic purpura
  - Others
  - Intravascular hemolysis secondary to oxidative stress in glucose-6-phosphate dehydrogenase deficiency
    - Dapsone
    - Others

iron and transferrin concentration. RBCs are typically normochromic and normocytic. In HIV-infected patients, this anemia presumably reflects the chronic infection of lymphocytes and ongoing immune activation and cytokine dysregulation. Direct HIV infection of precursor hematopoietic cells may also be involved. The frequency and severity of this anemia are often reduced with the use of effective ARV therapy.

Inadequate Erythropoietic Production

Relative or absolute hypogonadism is common in HIV infection and probably contributes to reduced erythropoietic effect. This anemia may respond to testosterone replacement. Total testosterone and free serum levels should be evaluated in HIV-infected men with anemia. The role, if any, of testosterone deficiency in HIV-infected women with anemia is uncertain.

Infections and Malignancies within Marrow

Bone marrow can be infected by a variety of opportunistic pathogens, especially *Mycobacterium avium-intracellulare* and *Mycobacterium tuberculosis.* The causative relationship of such infections to anemia is complicated by the advanced HIV disease stage of many of these patients, which may itself cause marrow failure. Chronic parvovirus B19 infection in an HIV-infected patient can cause anemia with RBC aplasia on bone marrow examination. This uncommon cause of HIV-related anemia is rarely seen with effective ARV therapy. It responds to replacement of IgG that contains parvovirus B19 antibodies. Bacillary angiomatosis, seen with *Bartonella henselae* or *Bartonella quintana* infection, can also result in anemia. This condition can cause skin lesions resembling those of KS and responds to antibiotic therapy. HIV-associated cancers, particularly non-Hodgkin's lymphoma (NHL), can involve bone marrow. Extensive involvement may result in anemia and other types of cytopenia but is uncommon.

Nutritional Deficiencies

Advanced-stage HIV disease, particularly before the use of effective ARV therapy, leads to severe wasting and complex nutritional deficiencies. Although common deficiencies of vitamins such as folate and B_{12} should be considered, they are less common than iron deficiency as a cause of anemia in HIV infection.

Iron Deficiency

Iron deficiency is an uncommon but not rare cause of anemia in HIV-infected persons. It is most often seen in women and injection drug users. Women may, of course, have iron deficiency separate from their HIV infection, and this cause of anemia should always be considered. KS rarely causes sufficient gastrointestinal blood loss to lead to iron deficiency.

Drug Toxicity

Anemia is most common with the ARV drug zidovudine (ZDV). ZDV and the other thymidine analogue reverse transcriptase inhibitor stavudine (d4T) both cause macrocytosis, whereas ZDV causes a relative RBC aplasia, presumably by interference with normal thymidine utilization. The macrocytosis seen with ZDV and d4T is quite predictable and has been used to assess drug adherence. Within the first several months of ZDV use, mean corpuscular volume increases to the range of 100 to 110 fmol/L. The other ARV drugs are not commonly associated with anemia.

A variety of drugs used to treat HIV-associated conditions can cause bone marrow suppression with resulting anemia, neutropenia, or thrombocytopenia. Such drugs include trimethoprim-sulfamethoxazole, ganciclovir, amphotericin, and many cytotoxic chemotherapeutic agents.

Red Blood Cell Antibodies

HIV infection is associated with polyclonal gammopathy as a result of dysregulation and altered balance of the $CD4^+$ and $CD8^+$ cell populations of T lymphocytes and corresponding B-cell function. RBC antibodies are not uncommon in HIV infection and cause a positive direct Coombs antiglobulin test. This is not usually associated with hemolysis and requires no specific therapy.

Clinical Manifestations

Anemia from accelerated RBC loss in HIV infection is uncommon. Frank bleeding is rare in HIV-infected patients, except in those with concomitant conditions such as portal hypertension from coincident cirrhosis associated with hepatitis B virus (HBV) or hepatitis C virus (HCV) infection. Hypersplenism, most often also seen with portal hypertension, may lead to anemia and other types of cytopenia. Finally, hemolytic anemia (as well as methemoglobinemia) can occur with microangiopathic disease or as a consequence of oxidative stress from some drugs, particularly dapsone, when used in patients with underlying glucose-6-phosphate dehydrogenase deficiency.

Anemia in HIV infection causes fatigue and decreased exercise tolerance with resultant decreased quality of life. Anemia also predicts accelerated disease progression and shortened survival. This association is seen even after adjusting for baseline $CD4^+$ cell counts and plasma HIV load.

Clinical evaluation of anemia in HIV infection is similar to that in other disease settings (Chapter 162) and should explore both HIV-related and HIV-unrelated causes. Reversible causes are especially important to identify. Peripheral cell counts, including reticulocytes, are obtained, as well as careful review of the peripheral smear. Iron studies can help differentiate between anemia of chronic disease and iron deficiency. Underlying malignancies and opportunistic infections must be considered, as should exposure to drugs with potential bone marrow suppression, especially ZDV. Bone marrow biopsy is rarely indicated specifically for anemia.

Treatment

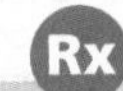

Potent ARV therapy has changed the frequency and severity of anemia in HIV infection, although it has not eliminated this problem. Even with ZDV, severe anemia is uncommon because the drug is currently used in a multiagent regimen where immune recovery reduces this adverse effect. It should be noted, however, that rapid and severe ZDV-related anemia is common in Africa, perhaps as a result of coinfection with malaria or other pathogens.

Anemia in HIV is managed according to its etiology. Reversible causes such as iron deficiency or unnecessary exposure to a toxic drug should be addressed, as should bone marrow infections or malignancies. ARV therapy should be started if other indications exist. Whether anemia should be considered an independent reason for ARV therapy is not known. Replacement therapy with testosterone in the case of hypogonadism may be considered. RBC transfusion is indicated for the acute onset of severe anemia, especially in a patient with underlying cardiovascular disease. Transfusion carries its own set of risks and should be performed only when other options are limited.

The use of replacement erythropoietin in HIV-infected patients is approved in the United States solely for ZDV-associated anemia. It has been studied in the broader population of HIV-associated anemia of chronic disease and does raise hemoglobin levels as in other patient groups. Such use has improved baseline quality-of-life measures. Whether erythropoietin replacement in this setting is cost-effective has not been proved, not is there any proven effect on disease progression or survival, although improved outcome has been reported in some studies in those who recovered from anemia.

White Blood Cell Dysfunction

Apart from lymphocytes, the primary pathogenic target of HIV infection, the white blood cell population, is relatively spared in HIV disease in comparison to other cell lines. Neutrophils are affected to some degree, whereas eosinophils and monocytes usually remain normal in number.

Neutrophils

Considering the devastating effect of HIV infection on lymphocytes, neutrophils are relatively spared. Neutrophil morphology is unaffected, absent drug toxicity or nutritional defects. Although neutropenia is not uncommon, it is rarely severe. Neutropenia in HIV infection is most commonly a manifestation of drug toxicity. Drugs used to treat or prevent opportunistic infections (such as trimethoprim-sulfamethoxazole) or malignancies are common offenders. Neutrophil function is similarly well preserved in HIV infection, especially in earlier-stage disease. Although mucocutaneous candidal infections are very common in HIV disease, dissemination is extremely rare, even with advanced $CD4^+$

depletion. Presumably, preserved neutrophil function prevents these and related infections. Still, bacterial infections are common in HIV-infected persons and may be managed appropriately.

Lymphocytes

The total lymphocyte count may be decreased in advanced HIV disease but is not a reliable surrogate for actual CD4$^+$ cell enumeration. This is unfortunate because the cost of CD4$^+$ counts remains an important barrier for effective ARV therapy in many international settings, although new devices for easy testing in the field may overcome this hurdle. Lymphocyte subset analysis, possible even early in the HIV epidemic, highlights the striking CD4$^+$ depletion of HIV infection, although the mechanism for this loss remains, surprisingly, an active research question.

CD8$^+$ lymphocytes are less directly involved by HIV infection. CD8$^+$ cell number is relatively preserved until the most advanced disease stage. This cell population is, however, of research interest and may be important in overall HIV disease pathogenesis.

Platelet Dysfunction and Thrombocytopenia

HIV infection is associated with thrombocytopenia. Immune thrombocytopenia (ITP), though never common, was more often seen in the early years of the epidemic—in up to 8.7% with advanced AIDS. Its severity varied, but as with non–HIV-associated autoimmune or idiopathic thrombocytopenic purpura, bleeding was uncommon.

Epidemiology

The cause of platelet suppression is not fully clear. Increased splenic clearance of platelets with hypersplenism is a factor, but whether platelets are coated with nonspecific antibodies from immune activation and polyclonal gammopathy or with specific platelet antibodies, as some often suggest, remains uncertain. Although HIV may infect megakaryocytes, accelerated platelet loss appears to be more important than decreased production. Further anecdotal evidence supporting accelerative clearance is the observation that platelet counts tended to normalize in late HIV disease, presumably because of decreased reticuloendothelial function and hence less platelet clearance.

Treatment

Rx

Therapy for HIV-associated ITP (HIV-ITP) resembles that for ITP without HIV infection. Splenectomy is successful in many cases. Splenectomy also results in an increase in peripheral CD4$^+$ cell counts. Corticosteroids are likewise effective in HIV-ITP, although many fear the use of immunosuppressants in the setting of an acquired immunodeficiency disease. Other treatments with some reported success in HIV-ITP include interferon alfa, danazol, intravenous IgG/RhoGAM, and plasmapheresis. ZDV was also shown to raise platelet counts, even as monotherapy before the use of multidrug regimens. Whether ZDV has any independent nonviral effect is unclear.

The advent of effective ARV regimens has reduced the incidence of severe HIV-ITP. HIV-ITP should prompt the initiation of ARV therapy should other indications exist. It should otherwise be managed essentially as it is in non–HIV-infected persons, with corticosteroids in a tapering dose as the initial management strategy.

Thrombotic Thrombocytopenic Purpura

Thrombotic thrombocytopenic purpura (TTP), often involving some combination of microangiopathy, renal disease, and neurologic disorders, has been reported to be increased in HIV infection. Most of these series, however, are very small, with an uncertain relationship to HIV. Management and outcome in these reports resemble those for TTP in patients without HIV infection. Response to plasmapheresis and immunoglobulin replacement is typically rapid. The effect of effective ARV therapy on this condition—either on its incidence or on its disease course—is unknown.

Thrombosis

Reports of increased deep vein thrombosis in HIV infection are relatively rare, which is perhaps surprising in the setting of a chronic viral infection. Reports may reflect the overlap between two relatively common diseases. Deep vein thrombosis in an HIV-infected person should be evaluated and managed as for noninfected patients.

Bone Marrow in HIV Infection

Numerous reports early in the HIV epidemic identified alterations in bone marrow morphology and suggested ways in which bone marrow biopsy might affect patient management. These conclusions may require adjustment in the era of effective ARV therapy. In the absence of opportunistic infections or malignancies, the marrow is not strikingly abnormal. Relative RBC aplasia may be seen in anemic patients, and plasma cell number is often increased, but not usually to a striking degree. The marrow findings may resemble mild cases of myelodysplasia. Marrow has been considered a site to diagnose opportunistic infections but has little added utility over peripheral blood culture. Marrow can be affected by HIV-related malignancies and is commonly biopsied to stage HIV-related lymphoma. Bone marrow biopsy is not required in the evaluation of KS.

HIV ONCOLOGY

After 25 years of investigation, HIV is still not directly implicated in oncogenesis. Most HIV-associated cancers seem to result from HIV-induced activation of other viral coinfections, especially human herpesvirus 8 (HHV8), from defects in "immune surveillance," or from immune activation.

HIV-related cancers have been profoundly affected by the common use of effective ARV therapy. The incidence of some has declined sharply, and even advanced-stage KS has regressed after initiation of ARV therapy. Some cancers are less affected, whereas others—perhaps those less directly linked in a causative manner to HIV—have been marginally changed, if at all.

Kaposi's Sarcoma

Reports of KS in previously healthy young men heralded the onset of the AIDS epidemic. The striking novelty of this cancer in this population, along with simultaneous reports of previously rare infections, allowed almost immediate recognition of underlying immune impairment.

Before the HIV epidemic KS was an uncommon, relatively indolent tumor that primarily affected the skin of the distal end of the lower extremity in elderly men. It was more common in men of Jewish descent and those residing in southern Europe. This "classic" KS rarely required systemic therapy. KS also followed early kidney transplantation. Less common in modern transplantation with lower doses of more targeted immunosuppressants, post-transplant KS was believed to result from a combination of immune suppression and intense antigenic stimulation. KS was also seen before the HIV epidemic in east central Africa, especially Uganda, where it was and remains extremely common. As a result, KS was speculated to arise from immune deficiency, along with intriguing suggestions of genetic, environmental, or hormonal factors explaining the predominance of affected men in all settings.

In the setting of HIV, especially before the use of effective ARV therapy, KS affected a very specific subpopulation in the Western World. Women and children were almost always spared, and men with KS typically reported sexual contact with other men as their probable source of HIV infection. These and other observations fueled early speculation that an agent, sexually transmitted between men, might be involved in the pathogenesis of KS. These predictions have proved true with the identification of a new human herpesvirus, HHV8, as a causative or contributing agent of KS and other malignancies.

In the early HIV epidemic, KS was a common initial manifestation of AIDS and was included as an AIDS-defining condition. In the population of men who have sex with other men (MSM), it was present in nearly 50% of new AIDS cases before the use of effective ARV therapy. In contrast, KS was seen in only 2% of new AIDS cases in women, and most of them reported sexual contact with MSM. KS rarely developed in HIV-infected children in the United States.

Epidemiology

The viral etiology of KS, later shown to be due to HHV8 infection, was suggested by its distinctive epidemiology. HHV8, a gamma herpes virus, was discovered after viral gene sequences characteristic of this viral family were found in KS lesions, but not in adjacent normal tissue. HHV8 infects B lymphocytes, macrophages, and endothelial cells. Lytic and latent forms are seen in KS lesions. The precise mechanism of oncogenesis remains unclear but is dramatically accelerated in the setting of HIV coinfection.

HHV8 is a common infection. In one multicenter study its prevalence in all U.S. blood donors was estimated at 3.5%. In HHV8-endemic areas of sub-Saharan Africa, children are infected by puberty, probably from salivary transmission. In San Francisco, HHV8 prevalence was already high in MSM before the HIV epidemic. In the United States, the higher prevalence in MSM suggests sexual transmission.

Chronic HHV8 infection, as opposed to seropositivity, is required for the development of KS. HHV8 plasma titers correlate with KS incidence and disease progression rates. Together, these observations suggest a rationale for HHV8 therapy to prevent or treat KS. The incidence of KS was reduced in several clinical trials of antiherpes therapy in HIV-infected adults. These studies, however, were very small and not powered to detect this effect, and gamma herpes viruses, including HHV8, are relatively resistant to antiviral control. Whether such approaches offer promise for prevention or treatment of KS requires much further research.

Clinical Manifestations

KS results from proliferation of endothelial cells. At least in later stages it is a true malignancy showing monoclonality and growth independence. Histologically, KS is characterized by both a proliferation of spindle-shaped cells and poorly formed vascular channels, often with extensive RBC extravasation.

KS lesions typically involve the visible skin surface, although internal lesions may be seen in essentially any organ. Cutaneous lesions are generally violaceous, occasionally with surrounding ecchymosis. They are nodular and range in size from several millimeters to 2 cm in diameter, although multiple lesions can coalesce into large tumor plaques. Lesions are nonpruritic and painless except in advanced stages. KS lesions can appear simultaneously in widely separated regions rather than as a primary site with metastatic spread. Lesions may appear in clusters, may be symmetrical, and may be somewhat linear and appear to follow skin creases. KS lesions may appear on scars or other sites of previous trauma. Lesions are also common in the oral cavity, where they correlate with gastrointestinal involvement.

KS in the gastrointestinal tract is common, and bulky disease can cause obstruction. Frank hemorrhage is uncommon. Pulmonary involvement with KS is typically evidenced by reticulonodular, patchy infiltrates on chest radiograph. Pleural effusions, if seen, are often hemorrhagic with no evident malignant cells on cytology. Advanced KS disease can cause intractable lymphedema, especially common in the lower extremities and head and neck.

Treatment and Prognosis

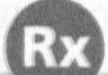

KS lesions are usually quite distinct in appearance, but biopsy confirmation is essential. HHV8 is invariably present. Bacillary angiomatosis may resemble KS morphologically but is distinguished histologically.

ARV therapy is currently regarded as the treatment of choice for HIV-associated KS because it is remarkably active. The incidence of KS has fallen precipitously (5- to 10-fold) with wide use of ARV therapy. Moreover, established KS often responds rapidly after initiation of ARV therapy. In one series, 90% of patients responded, with complete and durable resolution in 18 of 20 cases. ARV therapy may decrease HHV8 viremia. Several preliminary reports suggest an especially active KS response with HIV protease inhibitors. This possibility is being explored in ongoing clinical trials. An immune response inflammatory syndrome has also been reported in KS after initiation of ARV therapy.

Before the use of effective ARV therapy, KS was treated with a variety of cytotoxic agents. Vinblastine, administered either systemically or intralesionally, was later replaced by paclitaxel, anthracyclines, or etoposide. Monotherapy is generally preferred over more aggressive drug combinations. Biologic agents, including interferon alfa, retinoids, and tumor necrosis factor inhibitors, are also active against KS. Radiation therapy may be useful for systematic control of bulky KS plaques causing pain or lymphatic obstruction. Despite the vascular proliferation of KS lesions histologically, experimental angiogenesis inhibitors have not yet proved active in treating KS.

Non-Hodgkin's Lymphoma

NHL is the second malignancy whose incidence is clearly increased in HIV infection. NHL in HIV occurs in two distinct forms, of peripheral or central nervous system (CNS) origin.

Epidemiology

Peripheral NHL

HIV-associated peripheral NHL (HIV-NHL) is a B-cell tumor. The malignancy is often of moderate- to high-grade classification. The most common histologic variants are intermediate-grade large cell and high-grade immunoblastic lymphomas. HIV-NHL is often advanced at initial evaluation. Extranodal sites are common in HIV-NHL, but rare otherwise. NHL arising in the bile duct, in the appendix, or as a solitary parenchymal pulmonary nodule has been reported. Intravascular NHL has also been seen, occasionally in vessels within the CNS.

The epidemiology of peripheral HIV-NHL is much less interesting than that of KS. Both sexes are equally affected, as are HIV-infected children and adolescents. The $CD4^+$ cell count at diagnosis is typically only moderately suppressed in HIV-NHL.

The cause of peripheral HIV-NHL is unknown. Epstein-Barr virus (EBV) is not consistently found, and the tumor is HHV8 negative.

Central Nervous System HIV-NHL

High-grade B-cell NHL can arise within the CNS in HIV-infected patients. This occurs at a much higher rate and is considered diagnostic of AIDS. This distinction, however, is seldom required because CNS NHL is almost always seen in HIV-infected persons with strikingly advanced stages of immune deficiency. The median $CD4^+$ cell count in one report, for example, was 12 cells/mL. Given the close relationship between immune deficiency and risk for CNS NHL, it is not surprising that the common use of effective ARV therapy has led to a striking reduction in the incidence of this malignancy.

Clinical Manifestations

Apart from frequent occurrence in extranodal sites, peripheral HIV-NHL closely resembles the disease in HIV-uninfected individuals. It can be an aggressive tumor with rapid enlargement, pain, and erythema. Nodes are usually asymmetrically affected and have a firm, rubbery consistency on palpitation. Any unusual mass or asymmetrical lymphadenopathy should prompt diagnostic procedures in an HIV-infected patient. "B" symptoms may be present but are neither sensitive nor specific for HIV-NHL.

Peripheral HIV-NHL is typically an aggressive malignancy—unsurprising given the high-grade histology, advanced stage at diagnosis, and underlying immune deficiency. Apart from the inherent risk for opportunistic infections in these cases, the disease course is not specifically affected by HIV infection. Progression can occur at local or distant sites, and CNS involvement (distinct from primary CNS HIV-NHL) is commonly seen.

CNS NHL is typically associated with signs and symptoms of a space-occupying mass. Although the specific manifestation depends on the precise location, as well as the size and rate of tumor growth, sensory and motor deficits are common, as are seizures. Headache, fever, and personality changes are less common than in the frequent differential diagnostic considerations of CNS toxoplasmosis or cryptococcal meningitis.

Treatment and Prognosis

Peripheral HIV-NHL is diagnosed and staged similar to when HIV is not present (Chapter 196). Bone marrow biopsy, thoracic and abdominal imaging, and cerebrospinal fluid (CSF) examination are routine. Conventional histologic examination and immunoassays are used to evaluate specimens, and cell surface markers are determined by flow analysis.

HIV-NHL generally requires systemic combination chemotherapy. It is seldom so localized that it benefits from local radiation therapy and does not, itself, respond to ARV therapy as seen with KS. Various regimens have been commonly used. CHOP (cyclophosphamide, hydroxydaunomycin, Oncovin [vincristine], and prednisone) is usually considered a first-line regimen in standard doses. The addition of rituximab does not significantly increase response rates or survival and is associated with an increased risk for bacterial infection. A more aggressive regimen based on prolonged chemotherapy infusion has also been used with success. This regimen includes etoposide, vincristine, doxorubicin, cyclophosphamide, and prednisone.

Because of the high risk for CNS relapse, prophylactic treatment with methotrexate or cytosine arabinoside is recommended.

The use of ARV therapy in patients with HIV-NHL improves survival. Most practitioners would fully treat the NHL before initiating ARV therapy because drug interactions between the drug regimens are common. If, however, ARV therapy has already been initiated in a patient with newly diagnosed HIV-NHL, most would continue it during NHL chemotherapy. In one series, HIV-NHL patients treated with ARV therapy had a median duration of survival of 30 months as compared with only 6.1 months in the group not receiving ARV therapy.

The common use of ARV therapy has decreased the incidence of HIV-NHL by more than two-fold. This is less of a reduction than with KS, however, and HIV-NHL has thus become the most common HIV-related malignancy, even though its absolute prevalence is reduced from the era before effective ARV therapy was available.

CNS NHL is diagnosed by brain imaging and tissue biopsy. Although a solitary mass is common, several may be seen, especially if magnetic resonance imaging is used, which is more sensitive than computed tomography. Positron emission tomography is also useful. The most common site is deep in the white matter, and periventricular sites are disproportionately involved. CNS toxoplasmosis is more typically multicentric, but imaging alone cannot reliably differentiate most cases. CNS NHL is much more suspect if the patient has no serum *Toxoplasma* antibodies, although many patients with CNS NHL are also *Toxoplasma* antibody positive. Essentially all CNS NHL cases in the HIV setting are EBV positive. Finding EBV on CSF polymerase chain reaction (PCR) in a patient with advanced-stage HIV and CNS imaging typical of CNS NHL has been considered adequate by some to establish this diagnosis, but many still demand tissue confirmation, usually obtained by stereotactic brain biopsy. CSF cytology is relatively insensitive, with 80% of cases showing no malignant cells. Flow analysis of malignant cells is characteristic for NHL; essentially all are $CD20^+$.

The aggressive nature of CNS NHL, the relative isolation of the body compartment affected from systemic chemotherapy, and the severe underlying immune deficiency combine to limit survival. Before the common use of ARV therapy, the median duration of survival was measured in weeks. The use of effective ARV therapy has improved this expectation and allows the implementation of more aggressive systemic therapy for CNS NHL, but it remains a serious disease. In one series, the median survival without radiation or ARV therapy was 29 days, whereas six of seven ARV-treated patients were alive 667 days after diagnosis.

Given the severe underlying immune deficiency and the high mortality rate from opportunistic infections in early series, beginning effective ARV therapy as soon as possible is indicated. Mass lesions can be palliated with combined chemotherapy and brain irradiation, although neurologic impairment is common in longer-term survivors. The use of ARV therapy may allow high-dose systemic chemotherapy alone, particularly high-dose methotrexate with leucovorin rescue. Radiation therapy can be used to control recurrent disease, unfortunately still an expected part of this tumor's disease course.

Primary Effusion Lymphoma

Primary effusion lymphoma (PEL) is an interesting HIV-related malignancy, often grouped with peripheral NHL but distinct in many respects. PEL was first reported in HIV-infected patients. These lymphomas arise as a malignant, exudative effusion in essentially any body cavity and thus have also been called body cavity lymphomas. These cancers are quite rare. Even rarer are solid tumor variants, with only several reported cases. Some of these malignancies are plasmablastic tumors related to multicentric Castleman's disease (MCD).

PEL typically occurs in advanced HIV disease. Like KS, PEL is closely associated with HHV8 infection. HHV8 infects B lymphocytes, but the precise mechanism of malignant transformation has not yet been established.

Clinical Manifestations

PEL has been reported in many body cavities. Pleural and pericardial disease is the most frequent, but peritoneal and synovial sites are also seen. Fever and other "B" symptoms are present in many patients. The diagnosis must be considered with any localized effusion in an HIV-infected patient, and the diagnosis of PEL should prompt HIV testing in a patient not known to be so infected.

The effusion is exudative with a lymphocyte predominance. HHV8 DNA PCR is positive in essentially all cases.

Treatment and Prognosis

Even though response to chemotherapy is expected, complete resolution is rare. PEL is treated with systemic chemotherapy. Although no large series or controlled trials are reported, standard doses of CHOP regimens are often used. ARV therapy is also typically initiated, analogous to the situation in CNS NHL, but PEL does not, itself, respond to ARV treatment. Effective ARV therapy has decreased the incidence of PEL and prolongs survival, but it remains an aggressive malignancy with a short median duration of survival. Median survival in one series was 6.2 months.

Multicentric Castleman's Disease

MCD is a lymphoproliferative disorder associated with overexpression of interleukin-6. MCD in the HIV-infected population is associated with HHV8 infection. Though "benign," the proliferation is often extensive, with diffuse nodal enlargement, splenomegaly, and "B" symptoms seen in the majority of cases. MCD has high potential for malignant transformation, with KS, HIV-NHL, and PEL all seen in high frequency.

Clinical Manifestations

MCD is commonly accompanied by diffuse lymphadenopathy, hepatic and splenic enlargement, and a variety of systemic signs and symptoms. In some series, pulmonary manifestations were common and anemia was also frequent. Lymph node biopsy is essential for diagnosis. Histologic patterns vary, but B cells predominate. EBV studies are not consistently positive, whereas HHV8 DNA is typically detected.

Treatment and Prognosis

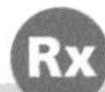

MCD carries a high risk for the simultaneous or subsequent development of an HIV-related malignancy. Depending in part of the predominant histologic pattern of MCD at biopsy, progression may be toward HIV-NHL or PEL/KS. MCD itself responds to low-dose chemotherapy, such as vinblastine, which may prolong survival. The effect of ARV therapy on MCD has been incompletely examined but should be initiated.

Human Papillomavirus–Associated Anal-Cervical Disease

Human papillomavirus (HPV) infection is sexually transmitted and, unsurprisingly, is often seen in combination with HIV, also a sexually transmitted infection. Numerous studies have documented this epidemiologic linkage. Connecting HPV to those cancers with which it is associated, however, is more controversial in terms of an HIV relationship. Both cervical and anal cellular atypia are common in patients dually infected with HIV and HPV. Some reports suggest a higher frequency of higher-grade or premalignant atypia in such populations, although HIV did not increase the risk for high-grade atypia. Similarly, both cervical and anal cancers have been diagnosed in HIV-infected persons. It is less established, however, whether these cancers are actually seen more frequently as a result of HIV infection. HPV infection is common in the MSM population (with or without HIV infection), and anal cancer is clearly more common in the MSM community. However, studies are as yet inconsistent in establishing a higher risk for anal cancer in persons with HIV infection than in MSM not infected with HIV. Cervical cancer is also seen in HIV-infected women but, again, not at a clearly higher frequency than in non–HIV-infected women. More effective ARV therapy has not led to a declining incidence of these cancers as opposed to those more directly associated with HIV infection or to a decrease in the frequency of premalignant atypia.

Nonetheless, an association between HPV infection, HIV infection, and cervical and anal cancer is expected to exist and may become more evident as survival is prolonged with effective ARV therapy. Moreover, regardless of any cause-and-effect relationship, it is clear that proliferative changes with a potential for malignant transformation occur frequently in HIV-infected persons. These observations have led to increasingly strong recommendations for regular physical and cytologic examination of cervical and anal tissue in HIV-infected patients. Standard Papanicolaou (PAP) testing has been adapted for anal examination and is increasingly routine. Abnormal PAP cytology should prompt further diagnostic and therapeutic approaches, although proof of improved outcome with specific algorithms remains under investigation. The role and prophylactic effect of the recently approved HPV vaccine have not yet been evaluated.

Hepatitis C, Hepatitis B, and Hepatocellular Cancer

HIV infection accelerates the disease course of both hepatitis B and hepatitis C. Both are associated with an increased risk for hepatocellular cancer (HCC). In the case of HCV infection, this risk requires underlying cirrhosis. HCC in an HBV-infected patient can arise without cirrhosis. It is not clear that screening for HCC should be affected by HIV infection because of the relative insensitivity and nonspecific nature of all techniques. Perhaps more importantly, this association should increase interest in developing effective antivirals for HBV and HCV infection. If effective, such antivirals would presumably prove useful in decreasing the risk for malignancy, particularly since each infection is potentially curable.

Cancers in HIV-Infected Persons Not Proved To Be Linked Causally

A wide variety of cancers have been diagnosed in HIV-infected persons. This may, of course, represent the coincidence of common diseases. Such cancers may, in fact, increase as a larger number of people survive HIV infection for prolonged periods as a result of effective ARV therapy. Some causal relationship may exist, though difficult to prove, and the natural history of cancers may be altered by HIV infection.

Hodgkin's lymphoma has been most closely linked to HIV infection. Several epidemiologic studies have shown an increased incidence in HIV-infected persons. Other reports suggest an altered histology with less favorable subtypes, including mixed cellularity and lymphocyte depletion seen at a higher frequency with an associated impact on outcome. Not all reports show a causative relationship, however, and the management of individual patients is probably not specifically changed in the setting of HIV infection.

Other cancers, including lung cancer and myeloma, have been reported to be potentially linked to HIV infection. Again, given the prolonged survival now possible in HIV-infected persons, further studies will be of particular interest.

Future Directions

HIV-related hematologic and malignant diseases were vital indicators of the AIDS epidemic. They remain significant clinical problems, although their severity and frequency have altered, in some cases dramatically, after the common use of effective ARV therapy. Research will continue to investigate the causative relationship between HIV infection and these problems. This research may also be able to elucidate the relationship between the inflammation, immune activation, and immune deficiency expected to underlie these disorders. Because many HIV-related cancers require the participation of a second virus, this work will also provide strong motivation for the development of vaccines and antivirals directed at these viruses. Such research, if positive, could well benefit an even broader population.

SUGGESTED READINGS

Bower M, Palmieri C, Dhillon T: AIDS-related malignancies: Changing epidemiology and the impact of highlly active antiretroviral therapy. Curr Opin Infect Dis 2006;19:14–19. *Review of the postive impact of HAART on the incidence of AIDS-related cancers.*

Cattelan AM, Calabro ML, De Rossi A, et al: Long-term clinical outcome of AIDS-related Kaposi's sarcoma during highly active antiretroviral therapy. Int J Oncol 2005;27:779–785. *A good review of the positive impact of potent antiretroviral therapy on Kaposi's sarcoma.*

Cheung MC, Pantanowitz L, Dezube BJ: AIDS-related malignancies: Emerging challenges in the era of highly active antiretroviral therapy. Oncologist 2005;10:412–426. *Summarizes newer treatment approaches and the effect of antiretroviral therapy.*

Chin-Hong PV, Vittinghoff E, Cranston RD, et al: Age-related prevalence of anal cancer precursors in homosexual men: The EXPLORE study. J Natl Cancer Inst 2005;97:896–905.

Di Lorenzo G, Konstantinopoulos PA, Pantanowitz L, et al: Management of AIDS-related Kaposi's sarcoma. Lancet Oncol 2007;8:167–176. *Review of recent advances in the treatment of Kaposi's sarcoma.*

Evans SR, Krown SE, Testa MA, et al: Phase II evaluation of low-dose oral etoposide for the treatment of relapsed or progressive AIDS-related Kaposi's sarcoma: An AIDS Clinical Trials Group clinical study. J Clin Oncol 2002;20:3236–3241. *Of 36 patients, 25 stabilized or improved.*

Lim ST, Tupule A, Espina BM, Levine AM: Weekly docetaxel is safe and effective in the treatment of advanced-stage acquired immunodeficiency syndrome–related Kaposi sarcoma. Cancer 2005;103:417–421. *Only 5 of 12 patients had even a partial response.*

Marti-Carvajal A, Cordona A, Rodriquez M: Interventions for treating AIDS-associated Hodgkins lymphoma in treatment-naïve adults. Cochrane Database Syst Rev 2007;CD006149. *Meta-analysis of the treatments available for this disease highlighting the need for additional investigation.*

Marti-Carvajal AJ, Sola I: Treatment for anemia in people with AIDS. Cochrane Database Syst Rev 2007;CD004776. *Meta-analysis of the treatments for anemia in the setting of AIDS showing some potential benefit of rHuEPO.*

Moscicki AB, Ellenberg JH, Crowley-Nowick P, et al: Risk of high-grade squamous intraepithelial lesion in HIV-infected adolescents. J Infect Dis 2004; 190:1413–1421. *Emphasizes the relationship between HIV and risk for cervical cancer.*

Novitzky N, Thomson J, Abrahams L, et al: Thrombotic thrombocytopenic purpura in patients with retroviral infection is highly responsive to plasma infusion therapy. Br J Haematol 2005;128:373–379. *An informative clinical series.*

Pantanowitz L, Schlecht HP, Dezube BJ: The growing problem of non–AIDS-defining malignancies in HIV. Curr Opin Oncol 2006;18:469–478. *Review of the current epidemiology of cancers in HIV-infected patients.*

Ratner L, Lee J, Tang S, et al: Chemotherapy for human immunodeficiency virus–associated non-Hodgkin's lymphoma in combination with highly active

antiretroviral therapy. J Clin Oncol 2001;19:2171–2178. *Modified or full-dose CHOP is safe and effective.*
Semba RD, Shah N, Strathdee SA, Vlahov D: High prevalence of iron deficiency and anemia among female injection drug users with and without HIV infection. J Acquir Immune Defic Syndr 2002;29:142–144.
Stebbing J, Sanitt A, Nelson M, et al: A prognostic iindex for AIDS-associated Kaposi's sarcoma in the era of highly active antiretroviral therapy. Lancet 2006;367:1495–1502. *Four prognostic factors were identified to obtain an accurate prognostic index.*
Volberding PA, Baker KR, Levine AM: Human immunodeficiency virus hematology. Hematology Am Soc Hematol Educ Program 2003:294–313. *This three-part review includes an overview of antiretroviral therapy, HIV-associated lymphomas, and hematologic manifestations of HIV.*
Waterston A, Bower M: Fifty years of multicentric Castleman's disease. Acta Oncol 2004;43:698–704. *Reviews the clinical picture and management of multicentric Castleman's disease; focuses on the association with HIV infection.*

417 NEUROLOGIC COMPLICATIONS OF HUMAN IMMUNODEFICIENCY VIRUS INFECTION

Joseph R. Berger and Avindra Nath

The neurologic complications of human immunodeficiency virus (HIV) infection can affect any portion of the neuraxis. They can be broadly divided into two large groups: those that are the consequence of HIV per se and those that are secondary in nature and occur chiefly as a result of the associated immunosuppression (Table 417–1). With respect to the former group, some of these disorders, such as acute HIV meningitis, are relatively rare, whereas others, such as HIV dementia and HIV-associated peripheral neuropathy, are very common. HIV meningitis generally occurs at the time of seroconversion, but other disorders such as HIV dementia, HIV myelopathy, and HIV peripheral neuropathy are typically not observed until advanced stages of immunosuppression.

The most common neurologic complications occurring as a secondary consequence of the virus are opportunistic infections. The most frequent of such infections are central nervous system (CNS) toxoplasmosis (Chapter 370), cryptococcosis (Chapter 357), tuberculosis (Chapter 345), cytomegalovirus (Chapter 399), and JC virus, which results in progressive multifocal leukoencephalopathy (PML). However, many noninfectious complications occur as well. Primary malignancies of the brain also appear to be associated with HIV infection. The incidence of primary CNS lymphoma is remarkably high. Unlike non–AIDS-associated primary CNS lymphoma, in which Epstein-Barr virus (EBV) can be recovered from only 50% of tumors, all AIDS-related primary CNS lymphomas have been associated with EBV infection. A wide variety of toxic and metabolic complications have been observed in HIV-infected patients, including Wernicke's encephalopathy and vitamin B_{12} deficiency. Drugs, particularly antiretroviral agents, have also been associated with neurologic complications. Certain nucleoside analogues (e.g., the "d" drugs ddI, ddC, and d4T; see Table 417–5) are frequently associated with peripheral neuropathy, and it has been proposed that zidovudine causes a mitochondrial myopathy. Finally, a wide variety of cerebrovascular disorders have been associated with HIV infection. Thrombotic ischemic stroke in this population has been attributed to an as yet undefined procoagulant tendency. Certain infections seen with increased frequency in patients infected with HIV, such as syphilis, tuberculosis, and cryptococcosis, may be associated with stroke. Additionally, CNS vasculitis has occasionally been observed with HIV infection, either from HIV or from an associated infection.

TABLE 417–1 CLASSIFICATION OF THE NEUROLOGIC COMPLICATIONS OF HIV INFECTION

Direct	Indirect
Acute meningitis	Opportunistic infections
Chronic meningitis	Neoplasms
Encephalopathy	Toxic/metabolic
Myelopathy	Drug effects
Peripheral neuropathy	Cerebrovascular disease
Myositis/myopathy	

Few HIV-infected individuals will escape experiencing one or more of these complications during their lifetime. They are responsible for a significant amount of morbidity and mortality. Not infrequently, more than one neurologic condition coexists in the same patient, which is often a source of confusion because one of the illnesses may be appropriately diagnosed and treated yet the patient continues to deteriorate. Furthermore, one must also consider that any neurologic abnormalities observed are the consequence of more pedestrian disorders, such as radiculopathy secondary to disc herniation, and are unrelated to the HIV infection. In patients not responding to appropriate therapy for a proven disorder, careful clinical reevaluation is essential.

HIV DEMENTIA

Definition

In 1983, 2 years after the initial description of acquired immunodeficiency syndrome (AIDS), an encephalitis accompanying the illness was described in 18 of 50 persons with AIDS-related neurologic disease. HIV dementia has subsequently been referred to by a number of names, including subacute encephalitis, multinucleated giant cell encephalitis, AIDS dementia complex, and HIV-associated cognitive/motor disorder.

A spectrum of increasing cognitive impairment has been described in association with HIV infection. Individuals with a clear abnormality in one cognitive ability are described as having a *neuropsychological deficit.* When abnormalities exist in two or more cognitive spheres, the term *neuropsychological impairment* has been proposed. Individuals with a *minor cognitive/motor disorder* have cognitive impairments with mild functional deficits, and those with marked functional impairment are referred to as having *HIV dementia.* By definition, HIV dementia requires that there be no delirium and no other etiology to explain the deficit.

Epidemiology

In the pre-antiretroviral era, HIV dementia was observed more commonly. Early studies suggested that it was evident in more than 50% of preterminal patients. The MultiCenter AIDS Cohort found an incidence of 4% coincident with the diagnosis of AIDS, and dementia developed in 7% within 1 year of the development of AIDS and in 14% within 2 years. Other studies have found slightly higher rates. After the introduction of combination antiretroviral therapy (ART) in 1996, the incidence rate of HIV dementia appeared to decline substantially; however, the prevalence of the disorder appeared to increase. The latter finding may be the result of prolonged survival of affected patients. Recent studies suggest that the incidence of HIV dementia may be climbing toward pre-ART levels. HIV dementia has been regarded as a disorder that occurs in the setting of advanced immunosuppression. Indeed, in the pre-ART era, the average CD4 count in an affected person was below 200 cells/mm^3. However, in the recent past, the average CD4 count has exceeded 500 cells/mm^3. Greater susceptibility at the extremes of age has been suggested, but it remains chiefly a disorder of young adult males in the United States and western Europe, the group that is most often infected with HIV. Congenitally infected children may exhibit delayed development. Genetic factors such as *APOE4* and polymorphisms in chemokine monocyte chemotactic protein-1 and tumor necrosis factor receptor have been identified as risk factors for the development of HIV dementia. Drug abuse and anemia may also predispose patients to the development of HIV dementia.

Pathobiology

HIV enters the brain early after the initial infection. In all likelihood, the virus enters the brain in infected mononuclear cells, although it is possible that it also enters as cell-free virus. HIV can be demonstrated in the brain as early as 2 weeks after infection. The viral infection largely remains confined to invading macrophages in the brain, microglial cells and multinucleated giant cells, usually in perivascular areas. HIV can also infect astrocytes, where it can remain latent for extended periods. Infection of other cell types is a rare event. Viral replication within these cells results in the elaboration of more virus in CNS tissues. The brain may thus be an important reservoir for HIV. Certain proteins of the virus, Tat and gp120, have been demonstrated to have a significant pernicious effect on neuronal function and viability either through direct toxic effects on neurons or by stimulation of glial cells, which in turn produce neurotoxic metabolites—cytokines and chemokines. Similarly, the perivascular, HIV-infected inflammatory cells produce a wide variety of chemokines and cytokines that have also been demonstrated to have similar deleterious effects. Therefore, there appear to be parallel paths, direct viral neurotoxicity and toxicity from inflammatory byproducts, that lead to the development of HIV dementia.

On gross examination, the brain typically exhibits cortical atrophy, sulcal widening, ventricular dilation, and frequently, meningeal fibrosis. Histopathologic examination shows multinucleated giant cells, microglial nodules, white matter pallor, astrogliosis, and perivascular inflammation (Fig. 417–1). The multinucleated giant cell, which is a syncytium of macrophages, has been regarded as the hallmark of infection, but it may be absent in the setting of HIV dementia. Concomitant vacuolar myelopathy is seen in as many as 40% of patients.

Clinical Manifestations

Most commonly, patients describe impaired memory, poor concentration, and difficulty reading. They often find it difficult to recall a passage recently read. Other frequent symptoms include gait problems, depression, and tremors, and patients may appear apathetic and slow or become socially withdrawn. Headaches, fatigue, and sexual dysfunction are frequent. The most commonly observed physical findings are psychomotor slowing with bradyphrenia and impaired rapid repetitive and alternating movements, hyperreflexia, increased tone, facial masking, frontal release signs (snout, glabellar, involuntary grasp), and abnormal ocular motility. The dementia has the features of a subcortical dementia not inconsistent with the relatively marked disease burden observed in dopaminergic basal ganglia. Screening tools for HIV dementia have been proposed (Table 417–2) and a battery of specific neuropsychological tests used (Table 417–3). Staging of the disease along a continuum has been widely adopted (Table 417–4).

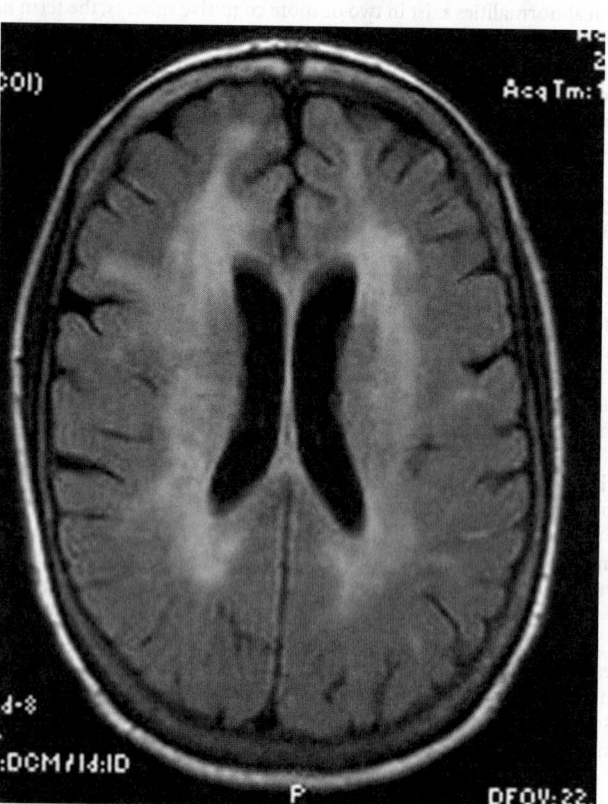

FIGURE 417–1 • Magnetic resonance image of the brain in HIV dementia. The FLAIR image shows confluent areas of signal hyperintensity adjacent to ventricles.

Diagnosis

Computed tomography of the head typically shows brain atrophy, but findings may be normal. Central atrophy is generally more pronounced than cortical atrophy. In children, calcification of the basal ganglia is often observed. Similar findings are seen on magnetic resonance imaging (MRI). Basal ganglia hyperintensity is seen rarely on T2-weighted images and may resolve during the course of ART. White matter hyperintensities are also commonly detected on T2-weighted images and fluid-attenuated inversion recovery (FLAIR) sequences (Fig. 417–2). These lesions may be discrete and focal or large and confluent. They are generally symmetrically distributed and may be confused with lesions of PML. Unlike PML lesions, they are typically not hypointense on T1-weighted sequences.

Treatment

Rx

Whether ART needs to cross the blood-brain barrier remains controversial, but prudence dictates that highly CNS penetrant ARTs would best be used. Table 417–5 provides a list of ARTs with their respective cerebrospinal fluid–plasma ratios, which may provide a proxy for CNS penetration. A variety of other therapies have been proposed for the treatment of HIV dementia that chiefly address the proposed inflammatory pathway of the pathogenesis of the disorder. To date, none have been established to be effective. The flow chart in Figure 471–3 provides an algorithm for the management of HIV dementia.

Prognosis

In the pre-ART era, the life expectancy of patients with HIV dementia was less than 6 months. The institution of effective ART has considerably increased the life expectancy of affected patients, and partial recovery of neurocognitive deficits may be seen.

HIV MYELOPATHY

A broad spectrum of myelopathies occur with HIV infection (Table 417–6). HIV causes a distinct myelopathy referred to as HIV vacuolar myelopathy. Evident in 20 to 55% of autopsies, this myelopathy is underrecognized clinically. It is characterized by an insidious onset of leg weakness and gait abnormality that usually occurs during the course of advanced HIV infection. Sensory complaints include vague leg discomfort and distal paresthesias. Bowel and bladder dysfunction is seen frequently. Physical examination reveals spastic paraparesis with lower extremity hyperreflexia, a spastic-ataxic gait, and impaired sensation with vibratory and position perception disproportionately affected. The sensory loss may be asymmetrical, but the presence of a discrete sensory level should suggest an alternative cause of the myelopathy. MRI of the spinal cord is usually normal but may show cord atrophy or hyperintense signal abnormalities within the cord on T2-weighted images. The value of spinal MRI lies in excluding other diagnostic possibilities, particularly structural abnormalities of the cord. Somatosensory evoked potentials generally demonstrate delayed conduction. Although findings on gross examination of the cord and dura are usually normal, histopathologic examination typically reveals loss of myelin with spongy degeneration, axonal preservation, microglial nodules, and multinucleated giant cells involving the lateral and posterior columns of the spinal cord. The pathogenesis of this disorder remains obscure. The clinical and pathologic features are suggestive of vitamin B_{12} deficiency, but no consistent

TABLE 417–2 HIV DEMENTIA SCREENING TEST

Maximum Score	Score	
		MEMORY REGISTRATION Give 4 words to recall (dog, hat, green, peach), 1 second to say each. Then ask the patient all 4 after you have said them
4	( )	**ATTENTION** Anti-saccadic eye movements: 20 commands __________errors of 20 trails ≤3 errors = 4; 4 errors = 3; 5 errors = 2; 6 errors = 1; >6 errors = 0
6	( )	**PSYCHOMOTOR SPEED** Ask patient to write the alphabet in uppercase letters horizontally across the page (use the back of this form) and record the time: __________sec ≤21 sec = 6; 21.1–24 sec = 5; 24.1–27 sec = 4; 27.1–30 sec = 3; 30.1–33 sec = 2; 33.1–36 sec = 1; >36 sec = 0
4	( )	**MEMORY RECALL** Ask for 4 words from Registration above. Give 1 point for each correct. For words not recalled, prompt with a "semantic" clue, as follows: animal (dog); piece of clothing (hat), color (green), fruit (peach). Give ½ point for each correct after prompting.
2	( )	**CONSTRUCTION** Copy the cube below; record the time: __________sec <25 sec = 2; 25–35 sec = 1; 35 sec = 0

TOTAL SCORE: __________/16

From Power C, Selnes OA, Grim JA, McArthur JC: HIV dementia scale: A rapid screening test. J Acquir Immune Defic Syndr Hum Retrovirol 1995;8:273–278.

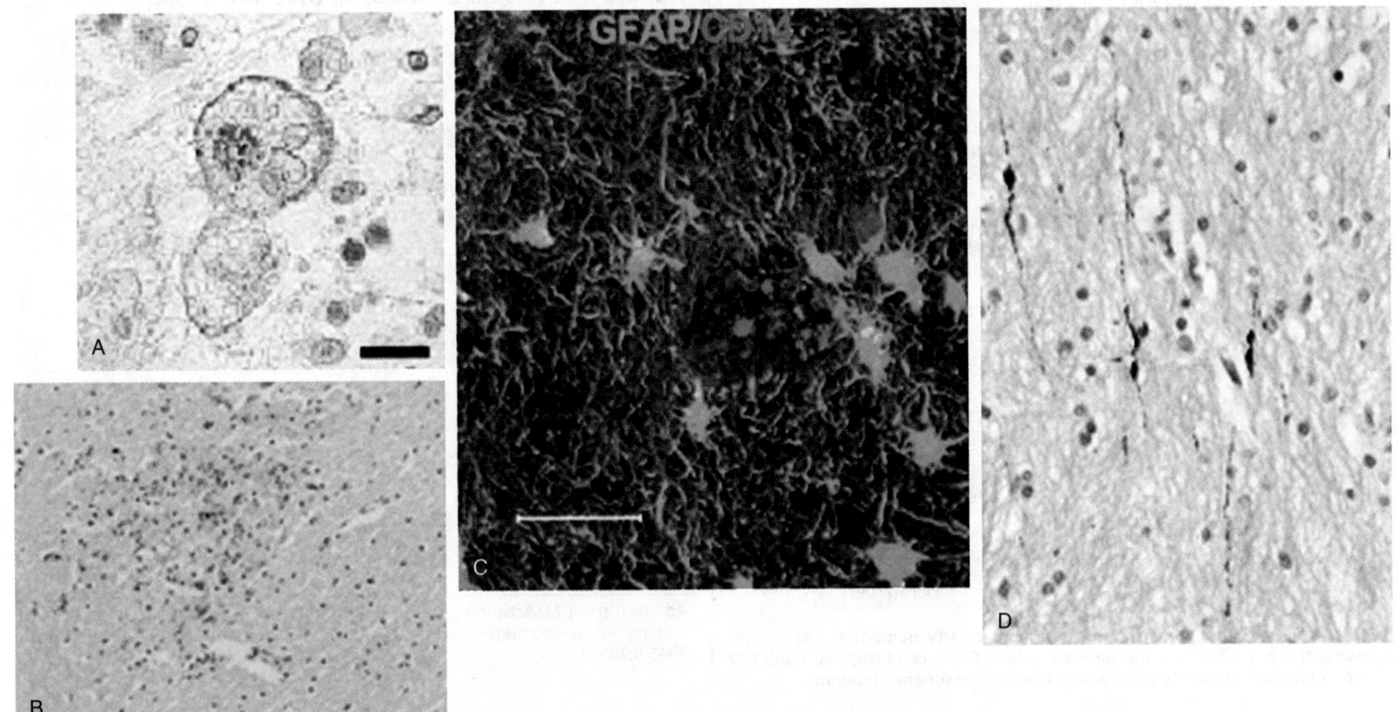

FIGURE 417–2 • Histopathology of HIV dementia. A, Multinucleated giant cell immunostaining for HIV antigen. **B,** A microglia nodule shows a collection of inflammatory cells. The HIV-infected cells are immunostained for HIV antigen and are brown. **C,** A confocal photomicrograph shows astrocytosis. The astrocytes are stained blue with antibody to glial acidic fibrillary protein (GFAP). The macrophages are immunostained with antibody to CD14 (red). (Courtesy of Carlos Pardo, Johns Hopkins University, Baltimore.) **D,** In neurons immunostained with antibody to amyloid precursor protein, beading of the neuritis suggests interruption of axonal flow. (Courtesy of Chris Zink, Johns Hopkins University, Baltimore.)

TABLE 417–3 NEUROPSYCHOLOGICAL BATTERY PROPOSED FOR EVALUATING HIV DEMENTIA

Fine motor control
- Grooved pegboard
- Finger tapping

Rapid sequential problem solving
- Trail making A & B
- Digit symbol

Visuospatial problem solving
- Block design

Spontaneity
- Verbal fluency

Visual memory
- Visual reproduction

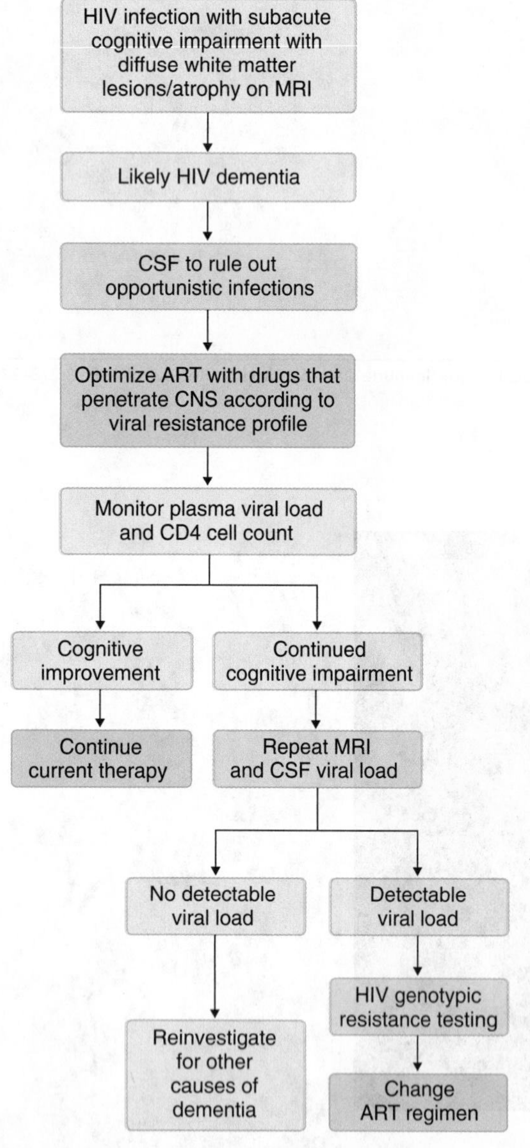

FIGURE 417–3 • Flow chart for the treatment of HIV dementia. ART = antiretroviral therapy; CNS = central nervous system; CSF = cerebrospinal fluid; HIV = human immunodeficiency virus; MRI = magnetic resonance imaging.

TABLE 417–4 MEMORIAL SLOAN KETTERING SCALE FOR HIV DEMENTIA

Stage 0 (normal)	Normal mental and motor function
Stage 0.5 (equivocal or subclinical)	Absent, minimal, or equivocal symptoms without impairment of work or capacity to perform activities of daily living
Stage 1 (mild)	Able to perform all but the more demanding aspects of work or activities of daily living
Stage 2 (moderate)	Able to perform all the basic activities of daily self-care but cannot work or maintain the more demanding aspects of daily life
Stage 3 (severe)	Major intellectual incapacity or motor disability with slowing
Stage 4 (end stage)	Nearly vegetative

From Price RW, Brew BJ: The AIDS dementia complex. J Infect Dis 1988;158: 1079–1083.

TABLE 417–5 CEREBROSPINAL FLUID–PLASMA RATIOS FOR ANTIRETROVIRAL THERAPIES

	Cerebrospinal Fluid–Plasma Ratio
NUCLEOSIDE REVERSE TRANSCRIPTASE INHIBITORS	
Zidovudine (AZT)	0.3–1.35
Stavudine (d4T)	0.16–0.97
Abacavir (ABC)	0.3–0.42
Didanosine (ddI)	0.16–0.19
Lamivudine (3TC)	0.11
Zalcitabine (ddC)	0.09–0.37
Emtricitabine	0.04
NUCLEOTIDE REVERSE TRANSCRIPTASE INHIBITORS	
Tenofovir	<0.05
FUSION INHIBITORS	
Enfuvirtide	NA
NON-NUCLEOSIDE REVERSE TRANSCRIPTASE INHIBITORS	
Nevirapine (NVP)	0.28–0.45
Delavirdine	0.02
Efavirenz	0.01
PROTEASE INHIBITORS	
Indinavir	0.02–0.76
Saquinavir	<0.05
Nelfinavir	<0.05
Ritonavir	<0.05
Amprenavir	<0.05
Lopinavir	<0.05
Atazanavir	0.0021–0.0226
Fosamprenavir	<0.05

Adapted from McArthur JC, Haughey N, Gartner S, et al: Human immunodeficiency virus–associated dementia: An evolving disease. J Neurovirol 2003;9:205–221.

TABLE 417–6 SPECTRUM OF MYELOPATHIES IN HIV INFECTION

HIV ASSOCIATED
Vacuolar myelopathy
Acute myelitis
Relapsing remitting encephalomyelitis
Spinal myoclonus
VIRAL
Cytomegalovirus
HTLV-1 and HTLV-II
Varicella-zoster virus
Measles virus
Progressive multifocal leukoencephalopathy
BACTERIAL
Mycobacterium tuberculosis
Treponema pallidum
Pseudomonas cepacia
FUNGAL
Cryptococcus immitis
Aspergillus sp
Nocardia
PARASITIC
Toxoplasma gondii
Schistosoma
MALIGNANCY
Primary CNS lymphoma
Metastatic CNS lymphoma
Other tumors (e.g. glioma)
VASCULAR
Necrotizing vasculitis
Disseminated intravascular coagulation
TOXIC/METABOLIC
Vitamin B_{12} deficiency
Protease inhibitor epidural lipomatosis

CNS = central nervous system; HTLV = human T-lymphotropic virus.

abnormalities are found in serum vitamin B_{12} levels or its metabolites, and replacement therapy with cyanocobalamin or *S*-methyl-L-methionine has not proved to be beneficial. The most effective management appears to be ART coupled with physical therapy.

HIV PERIPHERAL NEUROPATHY

Although a large number of peripheral neuropathies have been described in association with HIV infection, the one most commonly observed is a distal symmetrical sensorimotor peripheral neuropathy that ultimately affects at least a third of all HIV-infected persons. This neuropathy is seen more often in advanced disease. The patient typically complains of "burning feet." Distal paresthesias and numbness are reported and the pain may be debilitating. Distal vibratory, pinprick, and temperature sensory perception are diminished, and a positive Romberg test is often present. Ankle jerks are depressed or absent, and mild weakness of the toes with associated atrophy of the intrinsic muscles of the foot is frequently noted. Nerve conduction studies show reduced sensory nerve action potentials and conduction velocities. Nerve conduction amplitudes are reduced disproportionately to the reduction in conduction velocity. Electromyography may demonstrate features consistent with either acute or chronic denervation. Skin biopsy shows a reduction in cutaneous nerve fibers.

A clinically indistinguishable neuropathy may be seen with some of the antiretroviral agents, particularly with ddI, ddC, and d4T. The neuropathy associated with these agents appears to be dose dependent. Other drugs used in treating AIDS or its complications, such as hydroxyurea, isoniazid, vincristine, and thalidomide, may also result in a similar peripheral neuropathy. Discontinuing the use of these drugs should result in improvement in the neuropathic features; however, a phenomenon referred to as "coasting," in which continued worsening of the neuropathy occurs after discontinuation of the offending agent, may be observed over a period of several months.

Shortly after seroconversion, a demyelinating peripheral neuropathy identical to Guillain-Barré syndrome or chronic inflammatory polyradiculoneuropathy may be observed if it progresses over a duration of 3 or more weeks. An autoimmune process is the probable pathogenesis, and these neuropathies respond to therapy routinely used in the treatment of these conditions. In rare instances, mononeuritis multiplex may be seen with HIV infection.

HIV MYOPATHY

Several forms of muscle disease occur with HIV infection and, as with other neurologic disorders, may be due to HIV or be secondary to other processes. Among the latter are myopathies associated with drugs such as zidovudine and cholesterol-lowering agents, opportunistic infections, neoplastic infiltrates, and vasculopathies. HIV myopathy mirrors the clinical and laboratory findings of classic polymyositis. It is characterized by a progressive symmetrical weakness of the limb girdle and neck flexor muscles. Fatigue, myalgias, and wasting are observed in up to 50% of affected persons. Muscle enzymes, creatine phosphokinase and aldolase, are elevated and the electromyogram shows short, brief, polyphasic unit action potentials. Muscle biopsy reveals myofibrillar necrosis, phagocytosis, variation in fiber size, and regeneration and degeneration typically with endomysial inflammatory infiltrates. This myopathy is rare, with an incidence less than 1%, and has been observed in any stage of HIV infection. All patients with weakness who are taking a nucleoside reverse transcriptase inhibitor (NRTI) should have blood lactate levels measured because of an association between a newly described neuromuscular weakness syndrome and lactic acidosis in patients taking NRTIs. The contribution of zidovudine to the genesis of HIV-associated myopathy remains controversial. As in non-HIV polymyositis, corticosteroid therapy is beneficial and can be administered with tolerable side effects.

SUGGESTED READINGS

Ances BM, Ellis RJ: Dementia and neurocognitive disorders due to HIV-1 iinfection. Semin Neurol 2007;27:86–92. *Comprehensive clinical review.*

Cornblath DR, Hoke A: Recent advances in HIV neuropathy. Curr Opin Neurol 2006;19:446–450. *Comprehensive clinical review.*

Ellis R, Langford D, Masliah E: HIV and antiretroviral therapy in the brain: Neuronal injury and repair. Nat Rev Neurosci 2007;8:33–44. *Review of the current understanding of HIV infection of the CNS and the implications for therapy.*

McArthur JC, Brew B, Nath A: Neurological complications of HIV infection. Lancet Neurol 2005;4:543–555. *A comprehensive review.*

Section XXV

Neurology

418 APPROACH TO THE PATIENT WITH NEUROLOGIC DISEASE

Robert C. Griggs, Ralph F. Józefowicz, and Michael J. Aminoff

Clinical Manifestations

The symptoms of nervous system diseases are a part of everyday experience for most normal people. Slips of the tongue, headaches, backache and other pains, dizziness, lightheadedness, numbness, muscle twitches, jerks, cramps, and tremors all occur in totally healthy persons. Mood swings with feelings of elation and depression, paranoia, and displays of temper are equally a part of the behavior of completely normal people. The rapid increase in information about neurologic diseases coupled with the intense interest of people in all walks of life in medical matters has focused public attention on both common and rare neurologic conditions.

Most older people are concerned that they or their spouse have or are developing Alzheimer's disease or stroke, or both. The almost ubiquitous tremor of the elderly prompts concern about Parkinson's disease. Many younger patients are concerned about multiple sclerosis or brain tumor, and few normal people lack one or more symptoms suggesting the diagnosis of a serious neurologic disease. For most of these and other common diagnoses, the results of imaging and other tests are typically normal when symptoms first appear, and such tests should not be performed to reassure the patient or physician. Moreover, the widespread availability of neurodiagnostic imaging and electrophysiologic, biochemical, and genetic testing has led to the detection of "abnormalities" in many young and most elderly persons. In evaluating a patient's symptoms, it is imperative that a clinical diagnosis be reached without reference to a neurodiagnostic laboratory finding. Patients with disorders such as headache, anxiety, or depression do not usually have abnormal laboratory results. Abnormalities noted on various neurodiagnostic studies are often incidental findings whose treatment may be justified and necessary, but they do not improve the patient's symptoms. Abnormalities detected incidentally that are not accompanied by signs or symptoms may, as for disorders such as hypertension, require aggressive evaluation and treatment, but in general, the adage that it is difficult to improve an asymptomatic patient should be kept in mind. Thus, in elderly patients, few imaging or electrophysiologic studies are interpreted as "normal," but in the absence of specific complaints consistent with the findings, treatment and even further evaluation should reflect an estimate of the specificity and sensitivity of the test, as well as the likelihood that the patient will require and benefit from treatment. It is a good rule of thumb that one should never perform (or refer to the result of) a neurodiagnostic procedure without a specific diagnosis or at least a differential diagnosis in mind.

It is important to allow patients to describe any symptoms in their own words. Direct questions are often necessary to fully characterize the problem, but suggested terms or descriptors for symptoms are frequently grasped by a patient unfamiliar with medical terminology and then parroted to subsequent interviewers. The patient's terms should always be used when recording symptoms. Terms such as *lameness, weakness, numbness, heaviness, cramps,* and *tiredness* may each mean pain, weakness, or alteration of sensation to some patients.

Diagnosis

History

In neurologic diagnosis, the history usually indicates the nature of the disease or the diagnosis, whereas the neurologic examination localizes it and quantitates its severity. For many diseases, the history is almost the only avenue to explore. Examples of such disorders include headaches, seizures, developmental disorders, memory disorders, and behavioral diseases. In arriving at a diagnosis, the following points are useful. Consider the entire medical history of the patient. Early life events or long-standing processes such as head or spine trauma, unilateral hearing or visual loss, poor prowess in sports, poor performance in school, spinal curvature, or bone anomalies are easily overlooked but may point to the underlying disease process.

Consider the tempo and duration of the symptoms. Have the symptoms been progressive without remission, or have there been plateaus or periods of return to normal? Cerebral mass lesions (tumor, subdural) tend to have a progressive but fluctuating course; seizures and migraine, an episodic course; and strokes, an abrupt, ictal onset with worsening for 3 to 5 days, followed by partial or complete recovery.

Can one disease account for all of the symptoms and signs? The clinician should formulate a diagnostic opinion in anatomic terms: Is the history suggestive of a single (e.g., stroke or tumor) focus or multiple sites of nervous system involvement (e.g., multiple sclerosis)? Or is the process a disease of a *system:* vitamin B_{12} deficiency, myopathy, or polyneuropathy?

The neurologic history is the most important component of neurologic diagnosis. A careful history frequently determines the cause and allows one to begin localizing the lesions, which aids in establishing whether the disease is diffuse or focal. Symptoms of acute onset suggest a vascular cause or seizure, symptoms that are subacute in onset suggest a mass lesion such as a tumor or abscess, symptoms that have a waxing and waning course with exacerbations and remissions suggest a demyelinating cause, and symptoms that are chronic and progressive suggest a degenerative disorder.

The history is often the only way of diagnosing neurologic illnesses that typically have normal or nonfocal findings on neurologic examination. These illnesses include many seizure disorders, narcolepsy, migraine and most other headache syndromes, the various causes of dizziness, and most types of dementia. The neurologic history may often provide the first clues that a symptom is psychological in origin. The following are points to consider when obtaining a neurologic history:

- *Carefully identify the chief complaint or problem.* Not only is the chief complaint important in providing the first clue to the physician about the differential diagnosis, but it is also the reason why the patient is seeking medical advice and treatment. If the chief complaint is not properly identified and addressed, the proper diagnosis may be missed and an inappropriate diagnostic work-up may be undertaken. Establishing a diagnosis that does not incorporate the chief complaint frequently focuses attention on a coincidental process irrelevant to the patient's concerns.
- *Listen carefully to the patient for as long as necessary.* A good rule of thumb is to listen initially for at least 5 minutes without interrupting the patient. The patient often volunteers the most important information at the start of the history. During this time, the examiner can also assess mental status, including speech, language, fund of knowledge, and affect, and observe the patient for facial asymmetry, abnormalities in ocular movements, and an increase or a paucity of spontaneous movements as seen with movement disorders.
- *Steer the patient away from discussions of previous diagnostic test results and the opinions of previous caregivers.* Abnormal results of laboratory studies may be incidental to the patient's primary problem or may simply represent a normal variant.
- *Take a careful medical history, medication history, psychiatric history, family history, and social and occupational history.* Many neurologic illnesses are complications of underlying medical disorders or are due to adverse effects of drugs. For example, parkinsonism is a frequent complication of the use of metoclopramide and most neuroleptic agents. A large number of neurologic disorders are hereditary, and a positive family history may establish the diagnosis in many instances. Occupation plays a major role in various neurologic disorders, such as carpal tunnel syndrome (in machine operators and people who use computer keyboards) and peripheral neuropathy (caused by exposure to lead or other toxins).
- *Interview surrogate historians.* Because patients with dementia or altered mental status are generally unable to provide exact details of the history, a family member may need to provide the key details required to make an accurate diagnosis. This situation is especially common with patients who have dementia and certain right hemispheric lesions with various agnosias (lack of awareness of disease) that may interfere with their ability to provide a cogent history. Surrogate historians also provide missing historical details for patients with episodic loss of consciousness, such as syncope and epilepsy.
- *Summarize the history for the patient.* Summarizing the history is an effective way to ensure that all details were covered sufficiently to make

a tentative diagnosis. Summarizing also allows the physician to fill in historical gaps that may not have been apparent when the history was initially taken. In addition, the patient or surrogate may correct any historical misinformation at this time.

- *End by asking what the patient thinks is wrong.* This question allows the physician to evaluate the patient's concerns about and insight into the condition. Some patients have a specific diagnosis in mind that spurs them to seek medical attention. Multiple sclerosis, amyotrophic lateral sclerosis, Alzheimer's disease, and brain tumors are diseases that patients often suspect may be the cause of their neurologic symptoms.

Diagnostic Challenges

Two common situations provide special challenges to the diagnostic skills of the physician.

Physical Abuse As a Cause of Neurologic Symptoms

Traumatic injury inflicted by family members or others is usually difficult to detect by the medical history and examination. Physically battered babies, abused children, battered women, and traumatized seniors are often unable or unwilling to complain of this cause or contribution to symptoms. The only method to prevent overlooking this frequent cause of common problems is systematic consideration of the possibility in every patient and awareness of the (often subtle) signs that suggest physical trauma: ecchymoses or fractures (often attributed to a logical cause), denial of expected symptoms, failure to keep appointments, and unexplained intensification of neurologic symptoms (headache, dizziness, ringing in the ears, blackouts).

Alcoholism and Drug Abuse

See Chapters 31 and 32. A host of neurologic disorders can be the result of intentional ingestion of toxins (Chapter 111). Patients do not give an accurate account of their use of these agents. Consequently, physical signs and laboratory screening test results that give evidence of drug-related hepatic and other metabolic abnormalities may point to a major underlying problem.

ACUTE NEUROLOGIC DISORDERS REQUIRING IMMEDIATE DIAGNOSIS AND TREATMENT

Most neurologic diagnoses are arrived at by a careful, thorough history and an appropriately complete examination. However, the tempo of illness and the availability of life-saving treatment that is effective only if administered within minutes of first evaluating a patient dictate rapid action in several specific circumstances. Coma (Chapter 428), repetitive seizures (Chapter 426), acute stroke (Chapters 431 and 432), suspected meningitis and encephalitis (Chapters 437 and 439), head and spine trauma (Chapter 422), and acute spinal cord compression are diagnosed by clinical and laboratory assessment, and urgent treatment must be instituted as soon as ventilation and cardiac status are stabilized.

NEUROLOGIC EXAMINATION

The neurologic examination is always tailored to the clinical setting of the patient. A complete neurologic examination of a child is much different from that of an elderly adult, and the examination of a patient with specific complaints focuses on findings pertinent to that patient. Thus, more detailed testing of cognition is indicated in patients with behavioral or memory disturbance, and more detailed testing of sensation should be performed in patients with complaints of pain, numbness, or weakness.

However, many tests of neurologic function are routinely indicated in all patients because they provide a baseline for future examination and are frequently helpful in detecting unsuspected neurologic disease in apparently normal persons or in patients whose symptoms initially suggest disease outside the nervous system. It is particularly important to perform all routine tests in patients with abnormalities in one sphere of neurologic dysfunction; otherwise, erroneous localization of a lesion or disease process is likely. It is essential for a physician to have extensive experience in the routine assessment of normal persons in order to recognize and quantitate deviations from normal.

The General Examination

Specific neurologic symptoms or signs should prompt attention to the assessment of general findings. Head circumference should be measured in patients with central nervous system (CNS) or spinal cord disease (normally 55 ± 5 cm in adults). Head enlargement is occasionally a normal, often hereditary variant but should suggest a long-standing anomaly of the brain or spinal cord. The skin should be inspected for cafe au lait maculae, adenoma sebaceum, vascular malformations, lipomas, neurofibromas, and other lesions (Chapter 444). Neck range of motion, straight leg raising, and spinal curvature (scoliosis) should be assessed. Carotid auscultation for bruits is indicated in all older adults; carotid palpation is seldom informative. In patients with bladder, bowel, or leg symptoms, a rectal sphincter examination for tone and ability to contract voluntarily is usually indicated. Limitation of joint range of motion or painless swelling of joints is often a sign of an unsuspected neurologic lesion.

Neurologic Examination

The various aspects of the detailed neurologic examination are considered in specific symptom and disease sections noted later. The five major divisions of the examination should be assessed in all patients. During a careful medical history, mental status is often adequately assessed: level of consciousness, orientation, memory, language function, affect, and judgment. If any of these functions are abnormal, more detailed testing is needed. Cranial nerve function that should be tested in all patients includes visual acuity (with and without correction); optic fundi; visual fields; pupils (size and reactivity to direct and consensual light); ocular motility; jaw, facial, palatal, neck, and tongue movement; and hearing.

Examination of the motor system (Chapter 447) is essential in all patients because incipient weakness is generally overlooked by the patient. Muscle tone (flaccid, spastic, or rigid), muscle size (atrophy or hypertrophy), and muscle strength can be assessed rapidly. Muscle strength testing should always assess specific functional activities, including the ability to walk on heel and toe, sit up from a supine position, rise from a deep knee bend or deep chair, lift the arms over the head, and make a tight fist. Gait, stance, and coordination are assessed. The patient should be observed for tremor and other abnormal movements and the muscles inspected for fasciculations.

Sensory testing (Chapter 446) need not be detailed unless there are sensory symptoms. However, vibration perception in the toes and the normality of perception of pain, temperature, and light touch in the hands and feet should be assessed.

Muscle stretch reflexes and plantar responses should always be assessed by evaluating right/left symmetry and disparity between proximal or distal reflexes or arm versus leg reflexes. Biceps, triceps, brachioradialis, quadriceps, and ankle reflexes should be quantitated from 1 to 4 (4 = clonus; 3 = spread; 2 = brisk; 1 = hypoactive).

The Comatose Patient

The rapid examination required for a patient with an altered state of consciousness is much different from that of an alert, aware individual (Chapter 428). Many aspects of the neurologic examination cannot be tested: cognitive function, subtleties of sensory perception, specific motor functions, coordination, gait, and stance. Moreover, the muscle stretch reflexes are likely to fluctuate from one moment to the next, and minor asymmetries are much less important than in an awake patient. Instead, attention should focus on examination of (1) the level of consciousness, (2) respiratory pattern, (3) eyelid position and eye movements, (4) pupils, (5) corneal reflexes, (6) optic fundi, and (7) motor responses. Particular elements of the general examination must also be assessed quickly: evidence of cranial and spine trauma, tenderness of the skull to percussion, nuchal rigidity (but not in patients with head or neck trauma), and evidence of physical abuse.

COMMON COMPLAINTS OF POSSIBLE NEUROLOGIC ORIGIN

Weakness

It is axiomatic that patients typically have motor signs before motor symptoms and, conversely, sensory symptoms before sensory signs. Thus, patients with even severe weakness may not report symptoms of weakness. Somewhat paradoxically, patients who complain of "weakness" often do not have confirmatory findings on examination that document the presence of weakness.

TABLE 418–1 DISORDERS COMMONLY ACCOMPANIED BY "WEAKNESS"

Disorders of the motor unit
Upper motor neuron lesions—spasticity
Basal ganglia disorders—rigidity
General medical conditions
Heart failure
Respiratory insufficiency
Renal, hepatic, and other metabolic disease
Alcoholism and other toxin-related disease
Psychiatric and behavioral disorders
Depression
Malingering

Weakness, when actually a symptom of neurologic disease, is frequently caused by diseases of the motor unit (Chapters 435, 447, and 448) and is usually reported by a patient in terms of loss of specific functions, for example, difficulty with tasks such as climbing stairs, rising from a chair, sitting up, lifting objects onto a high shelf, or opening jars. Symptoms may also reflect the consequences of weakness such as frequent falls or tripping. Such symptoms can be remarkably quantitative. A patient with leg muscle weakness who is falling even as infrequently as once a month almost invariably has severe weakness of the knee extensor muscles and can be shown on examination to have a knee extension lag: an inability to lift the leg fully against gravity and to lock the knee.

The symptom of "weakness" without findings of weakness on examination is not generally the result of neuromuscular disease but can be a sign of neurologic disease outside the motor unit or, more commonly, a symptom of disease outside the nervous system altogether (Table 418–1).

Fatigue

The complaints of "fatigue," "tiredness," and "lack of energy" are even less likely than the symptom of "weakness" to reflect definable neurologic disease. With the exception of neuromuscular junction disorders such as myasthenia gravis, fatigue is rarely a complaint of diseases of the motor unit. Fatigue can be a sign of upper motor neuron disease (corticospinal pathways) and is a common complaint of established multiple sclerosis and other multifocal CNS disease. Similarly, any process that produces bilateral corticospinal tract or extrapyramidal disease can cause fatigue. Examples include motor neuron disease (Chapter 435), spinal cord disease in the cervical cord region (Chapter 423), and Parkinson's disease (Chapter 433). In addition, disorders that impair sleep (Chapter 429) may include fatigue as a complaint.

"Fatigue," like "weakness," is much more often than not a sign of disease outside the central and peripheral nervous system. Depression and other psychiatric and behavioral disorders (Chapter 420), as well as the medical illnesses associated with a complaint of weakness, are all frequent causes of fatigue.

Chronic fatigue syndrome, as well as many cases of fibromyalgia (Chapter 295), has fatigue as a dominant, disabling symptom. These disorders are defined in part by the absence of consistent neurologic findings and lack of demonstrable pathology in the nervous system.

Spontaneous Movements

Muscle tremors, jerks, twitches, cramps, and spasms (Chapter 434) are all frequent symptoms. The cause of spontaneous movements can reside at any level of the nervous system. In general, movements that occur in an entire limb or in more than one muscle group concurrently are caused by CNS disease. Movements confined to a single muscle are likely to be a reflection of disease of the motor unit (including the motor neurons of the brain stem and spinal cord). When spontaneous movements of a muscle are associated with severe pain, patients often use the term *cramp.* Cramp is a medically defined disorder that reflects the intense contraction of a large group of motor units. Leg cramps are occasionally a sign of an underlying disease of the anterior horn cell, nerve roots, or peripheral nerve; however, cramps are frequent in normal persons and particularly common in older patients, and they are usually benign. When severe, cramps can produce such intense muscle contraction that muscle injury is produced and muscle enzyme (e.g., creatine kinase) levels are elevated in blood.

The rare muscle diseases in which an enzyme deficiency interferes with substrate utilization as fuel for exercise (e.g., McArdle's disease) are often associated with severe, exercise-provoked muscle *contractures.* These contractures are electrically silent on electromyography (EMG), in contrast to the intense motor unit activity seen with cramps. Contractures must not be confused with the limitation of joint range of motion resulting from long-standing joint disease or long-standing weakness—also termed contractures.

The intense muscle contractions of *tetany* are frequently painful. Although tetany is usually a reflection of hypocalcemia (Chapter 266), it can occasionally be seen without demonstrable electrolyte disturbance. Tetany results from hyperexcitability of peripheral nerves. Similarly, in the syndrome of *tetanus* produced by a clostridial toxin (Chapter 320), intensely painful, life-threatening muscle contractions arise from hyperexcitable peripheral nerves. A number of toxic disorders such as strychnine poisoning and black widow spider envenomation produce similar neurogenic spasms.

Muscle Pain

Acute muscle pain in the absence of abnormal muscle contractions is an extremely common symptom. When such pain occurs after strenuous exercise or in the context of an acute viral illness (e.g., influenza), it probably reflects muscle injury. In such patients, the serum creatine kinase level is often raised. It is uncommon for this frequent and essentially normal sign of muscle injury to be associated with weakness or demonstrable ongoing muscle pathology. *Chronic* muscle pain is a common symptom but is seldom related to a definable disease of muscle.

Episodic and Intermittent Weakness

The complaint of attacks of severe weakness or paralysis occurring in a patient with baseline normal strength is an uncommon symptom. It is typical of the periodic paralyses and may also be seen with episodic ataxias and myotonic disorders (Chapter 447). All of these disorders are ion channelopathies. These channelopathies (e.g., the calcium channelopathy hypokalemic periodic paralysis) are rare but treatable disorders (Chapter 447). Episodic weakness is also seen in patients with neuromuscular junction disorders such as myasthenia gravis and the myasthenic syndrome (Chapter 448). Occasionally, patients with narcolepsy complain of intermittent paralysis as a reflection of *sleep paralysis* (Chapter 429).

Loss of Balance

Unsteadiness of gait is a common symptom. When associated with complaints of dizziness or vertigo (Chapter 454), disease of the labyrinth, the vestibular nerve, the brain stem, or the cerebellum is a probable cause. When unsteadiness and loss of balance are unassociated with dizziness, particularly if the unsteadiness appears to be out of proportion to other symptoms of the patient, a widespread disorder of sensation or motor function is likely.

Abnormal Gait and Posture

The ability to stand and to walk in a well-coordinated, effortless fashion requires the integrity of the entire nervous system. Relatively subtle deficits localized to one part of the central or peripheral nervous system produce characteristic abnormalities (Table 418–2).

Sensory Symptoms

Sensory symptoms can be negative or positive. Negative symptoms represent a loss of sensation, such as a feeling of numbness. Positive symptoms, by contrast, consist of sensory phenomena that occur without normal stimulation of receptors and include paresthesias and dysesthesias. *Paresthesias* may include a feeling of tingling, crawling, itching, compression, tightness, cold, or heat and are sometimes associated with a feeling of heaviness. The term *dysesthesias* is used correctly to refer to abnormal sensations, often tingling, painful, or uncomfortable, that occur after innocuous stimuli, whereas *allodynia* refers to painful perception from a stimulus that is not normally painful. For some patients, it may be difficult to distinguish paresthesias and dysesthesias from pain. *Hypesthesia* and *hypalgesia* denote a loss or impairment of touch or pain

TABLE 418–2 CHARACTERISTIC GAIT DISORDERS

Specific Disorder	Location of Lesion	Characteristics
Spastic gait	Bilateral corticospinal pathways within the thoracic or cervical cord or in the brain	Legs stiff, feet turning inward, "scissoring"
Hemiparetic gait	Unilateral central nervous system, cervical cord, or brain	Affected leg circumducted, foot extended, arm flexed
Sensory ataxia	Posterior columns of the spinal cord or peripheral nerve	Wide-based, high steps; Romberg's sign present
Cerebellar ataxia	Brain stem or cerebellum	Wide-based steps; Romberg's sign absent
Parkinsonian gait	Basal ganglia	Shuffling, small steps
Dystonic gait	Basal ganglia; also corticospinal pathways	Abnormal posture of the arms, head, neck
Gait disorder of the elderly	Multifactorial: bihemispheric disease, spinal cord disease, impaired proprioception, muscle weakness	Stooped posture, wide-based steps; often retropulsion
Steppage gait	Distal muscle weakness	High steps ("steppage")
Waddling gait	Proximal muscle weakness	Both legs circumducted to allow locking of the knees
Antalgic gait	Non-neurologic; reflects disease of joints, bones, or soft tissue	Minimizes pain in the hip, spine, leg
Hysterical gait	Psychiatric or behavioral disorder	Reeling side to side, associated astasia-abasia, bizarre arm and trunk movements

sensibility, respectively. By comparison, *hyperesthesia* and *hyperalgesia* indicate a lowered threshold to tactile or painful stimuli, respectively, such that there is increased sensitivity to such stimuli.

With the use of a wisp of cotton, a pin, and a tuning fork, the trunk and extremities are examined for regions of abnormal or absent sensation. Certain instruments are available for quantifying sensory function, such as the computer-assisted sensory examination, which is based on the detection of touch, pressure, vibratory, and thermal sensation thresholds.

Alterations in pain and tactile sensibility can generally be detected by clinical examination. It is important to localize the distribution of any such sensory loss in order to distinguish between nerve, root, and central dysfunction. Similarly, abnormalities in proprioception can be detected by clinical examination when patients are unable to detect the direction in which a joint is moved. In severe cases there may be pseudoathetoid movements of the outstretched hands, sensory ataxia, and sometimes postural and action tremors.

Disorders of peripheral nerves commonly lead to sensory disturbances that depend on the population of affected nerve fibers (Chapter 446). Some neuropathies are predominantly large-fiber neuropathies. Appreciation of movement and position is impaired, and paresthesias are common. Examination reveals that vibration, position, and movement sensations are impaired, and movement becomes clumsy and ataxic. Pain and temperature appreciation is relatively preserved. The tendon reflexes are lost early. In other neuropathies it is the small fibers especially that are affected; spontaneous pain is common and may be burning, lancinating, or aching in quality. Pain and temperature appreciation is disproportionately affected in these neuropathies, and autonomic dysfunction may be present. Examples of small-fiber neuropathies include certain hereditary disorders, Tangier disease, and diabetes. Most sensory neuropathies are characterized by a distal distribution of sensory loss, whereas sensory neuronopathies are characterized by sensory loss that may also involve the trunk and face and tends to be particularly severe. Sensory changes in a radiculopathy conform to a root territory; in cauda equina syndromes, sensory deficits involve multiple roots and may lead to saddle anesthesia and loss of the normal sensation associated with the passage of urine or feces.

Lesions of the *posterolateral columns* of the cord, such as occur in multiple sclerosis (Chapter 436), vitamin B_{12} deficiency (Chapter 443), and cervical spondylosis (Chapter 423), often lead to a feeling of compression in the affected region and to a Lhermitte sign (paresthesias radiating down the back and legs on neck flexion). Examination reveals ipsilateral impairment of vibration and joint position senses, with preservation of pain and temperature appreciation. Conversely, lesions of the *anterolateral region* of the cord (as by cordotomy) or *central* lesions interrupting fibers crossing to join the spinothalamic pathways (as in syringomyelia; Chapter 444) lead to impairment in pain and temperature appreciation with relative preservation of vibration, joint position sense, and light touch. Motor deficits may also be present and help localize the lesion. Upper motor neuron dysfunction (Chapter 435) from cervical lesions leads to quadriplegia, whereas more caudal lesions lead to paraplegia; lesions below the level of the first lumbar vertebra may simply compress the cauda equina and result in lower motor neuron deficits from a polyradiculopathy, as well as impairment of sphincter and sexual function.

NEUROLOGIC DIAGNOSTIC PROCEDURES

Lumbar Puncture

Sampling of cerebrospinal fluid (CSF) via lumbar puncture is crucial for accurate diagnosis of meningeal infections and carcinomatosis (Fig. 418–1). CSF analysis is also helpful in evaluating patients with central or peripheral nervous system demyelinating disorders and with intracranial hemorrhage, particularly when imaging studies are inconclusive.

The CSF formula often provides an important clue to the pathologic process involved (Table 418–3). An elevated white blood cell (WBC) count is seen with infections and other inflammatory diseases, as well as with carcinomatosis. The WBC differential cell count may point to a specific class of pathogen: polymorphonuclear leukocytes suggest a bacterial process, whereas mononuclear cells suggest a viral, fungal, or immunologic cause. The CSF glucose concentration is typically reduced in bacterial and fungal infections, as well as with certain viral infections (e.g., mumps virus) and with sarcoidosis. The CSF protein concentration is elevated in a variety of disorders, including most infections and demyelinating neuropathies.

Specialized tests that can be performed on CSF include oligoclonal banding, a pathologic pattern of banding on CSF electrophoresis that is seen in up to 90% of patients with multiple sclerosis. The bands, which

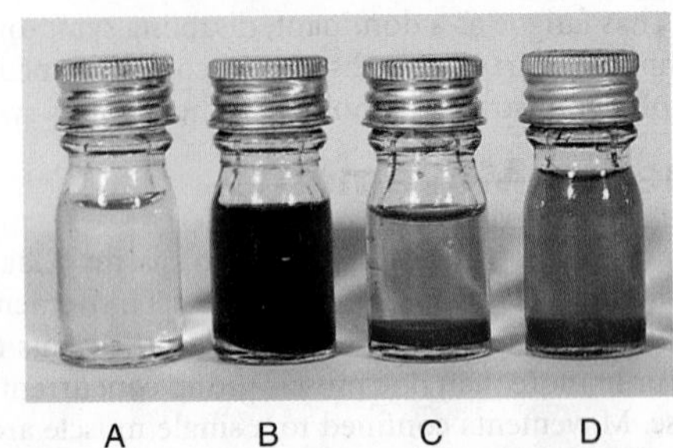

FIGURE 418–1 • Cerebrospinal fluid (CSF) examination. A, Normal crystal-clear CSF. **B,** Blood in the CSF, which could result from a traumatic (bloody) tap or from subarachnoid hemorrhage. In a traumatic tap, subsequent tubes of CSF are usually less bloody. **C,** Centrifuged CSF in a traumatic tap. The supernatant is nearly clear. **D,** CSF from a patient with subarachnoid hemorrhage. There is blood at the bottom of the tube and the supernatant is yellow (xanthochromic) as a result of breakdown of blood cells in the CSF before the lumbar puncture. (From Forbes CD, Jackson WD: Color Atlas and Text of Clinical Medicine, 3rd ed. London, Mosby, 2003, with permission.)

TABLE 418–3 CHARACTERISTIC CEREBROSPINAL FLUID FORMULAS

	Turbidity and Color	Opening Pressure	WBC (Cells/mm³)	Differential Cells	RBC Count	Protein	Glucose
Normal	Clear, colorless	70–180 mm H_2O	0–5	Mononuclear	0	<60 mg/dL	>2/3 serum
Bacterial meningitis	Cloudy, straw colored	↑	↑↑	PMNs	0	↑↑	↓
Viral meningitis	Clear or cloudy, colorless	↑	↑	Lymphocytes	0	↑	Normal
Fungal and tuberculous meningitis	Cloudy, straw colored	↑	↑	Lymphocytes	0	↑↑	↓↓
Viral encephalitis	Clear or cloudy, straw colored	Normal to ↑	↑	Lymphocytes	0 (Herpes ↑)	Normal to ↑	Normal
Subarachnoid hemorrhage	Cloudy, pink	↑	↑	PMNs and lymphocytes	↑↑	↑	Normal (early); ↓ (late)
Guillain-Barré syndrome	Clear, yellow	Normal to ↑	0–5	Mononuclear	0	↑	Normal

PMN = polymorphonuclear leukocyte; RBC = red blood cell; WBC = white blood cell.

represent monoclonal immunoglobulins that are locally synthesized in the CNS, are not specific for multiple sclerosis and may be seen with other inflammatory and noninflammatory conditions, including systemic lupus erythematosus, human immunodeficiency virus infection, and stroke.

CSF polymerase chain reaction is a rapid, sensitive, and specific test for the diagnosis of herpes simplex encephalitis (Chapter 439), for which it has replaced brain biopsy as the diagnostic procedure of choice. The CSF VDRL (Venereal Disease Research Laboratory) assay is a specific, though insensitive test for neurosyphilis (Chapter 341).

A lumbar puncture should not be performed in patients who have an obstructive, noncommunicating hydrocephalus or a focal CNS mass lesion causing raised intracranial pressure because reducing CSF pressure acutely in these settings via lumbar puncture may result in cerebral or cerebellar herniation. Lumbar puncture may be safely performed in patients with a *communicating* hydrocephalus, such as with idiopathic intracranial hypertension (pseudotumor cerebri), and it may even be an effective treatment in selected patients with this condition.

Electroencephalography

Electroencephalography is the recording and measurement of scalp electrical potentials to evaluate baseline brain functioning and paroxysmal brain electrical activity suggestive of a seizure disorder.

Electroencephalography is performed by securing 20 electrodes to the scalp at predetermined locations based on an international system that uses standardized percentages of the head circumference, the "10-20 system." Each electrode is labeled with a letter and a number, the letter identifying the skull region (Fp = frontopolar; F = frontal; P = parietal; C = central; T = temporal; O = occipital) and the number identifying the specific location, with odd numbers representing left-sided electrodes and even numbers right-sided electrodes. These electrodes are then connected in various combinations of pairs to generate voltage potential differences, and the potentials are recorded on a chart recorder.

To delineate the spatial distribution of the changing electrical field for an electroencephalogram (EEG), an orderly arrangement of electrode pairs is used, and each specific arrangement is known as a *montage.* Montages are generally of two types: *referential,* in which each electrode is connected to a single reference electrode such as the ear, and *bipolar,* in which electrodes are connected sequentially to one another to form a chain. A standard EEG generally records about 30 minutes of brain activity, both in the awake state and in the first two stages of sleep. Various activating procedures are used during the recording of an EEG, including hyperventilation and photic stimulation. These activating procedures may precipitate seizure discharges in some patients with seizure disorders, thereby increasing the sensitivity of the test.

The amplitudes of scalp electrical potentials are quite low, averaging 30 to 100 μV. They represent a summation of excitatory postsynaptic potentials and inhibitory postsynaptic potentials that are largely generated by the pyramidal cells in layer 4 of the cerebral cortex. Action potentials are of too brief a duration to have an effect on the EEG.

The EEG is analyzed with respect to symmetry between each hemisphere, wave frequency and amplitude, and the presence of spikes (20 to 70 msec) and sharp waves (70 to 200 msec), which may indicate a seizure focus. Electroencephalographic frequencies are divided into four categories as follows:

Delta: <4 Hz
Theta: 4–7 Hz
Alpha: 8–13 Hz
Beta: >13 Hz

The normal waking EEG (Fig. 418–2A) in a patient with eyes closed contains rhythms of alpha frequency in the occipital leads and beta frequency in the frontal leads. Normal sleep causes a generalized slowing of electroencephalographic frequencies and an increase in amplitude in each stage of sleep such that stage 4 sleep consists of greater than 50% large-amplitude delta rhythms. EEG abnormalities are of two types: abnormalities in background rhythm and abnormalities of a paroxysmal nature (Table 418–4).

The major usefulness of electroencephalography is for diagnosis and categorization of a seizure disorder (see Fig. 418–2B). EEGs are neither highly sensitive nor completely specific for diagnosing seizures. Because seizures are paroxysmal events, it is not unusual for an EEG to be normal—or only minimally abnormal—in a patient with epilepsy if it is recorded during an interictal phase (the period between seizures). Only about 50% of patients with seizures show epileptiform activity on the first EEG. Repeating the EEG with provocative maneuvers, such as sleep deprivation, hyperventilation, and photic stimulation, may increase this percentage to 90%. Conversely, about 1% of adults and 3.5% of children who are neurologically normal and who never had a seizure have epileptiform activity on an EEG.

The EEG may provide clues to the diagnosis of certain neurologic conditions, including viral encephalitis, prion disorders, and some forms of coma. In each of these situations, the EEG can have specific patterns that suggest a specific neurologic diagnosis. In herpes simplex encephalitis, periodic lateralizing epileptiform discharges emanating from the temporal lobes are frequently present. Triphasic slow waves are common in hepatic encephalopathy (Fig. 418–2C) but are a nonspecific finding. Creutzfeldt-Jakob disease is characterized by the presence of bilateral synchronous repetitive sharp waves. The EEG is also helpful in evaluating comatose patients, in confirming brain death when an apnea test cannot be performed because of cardiac instability, and for staging sleep in polysomnography.

In the past, the EEG was often used for localizing neurologic lesions such as stroke, brain tumor, or abscess. With the advent of neuroimaging, EEG is almost never used for these purposes.

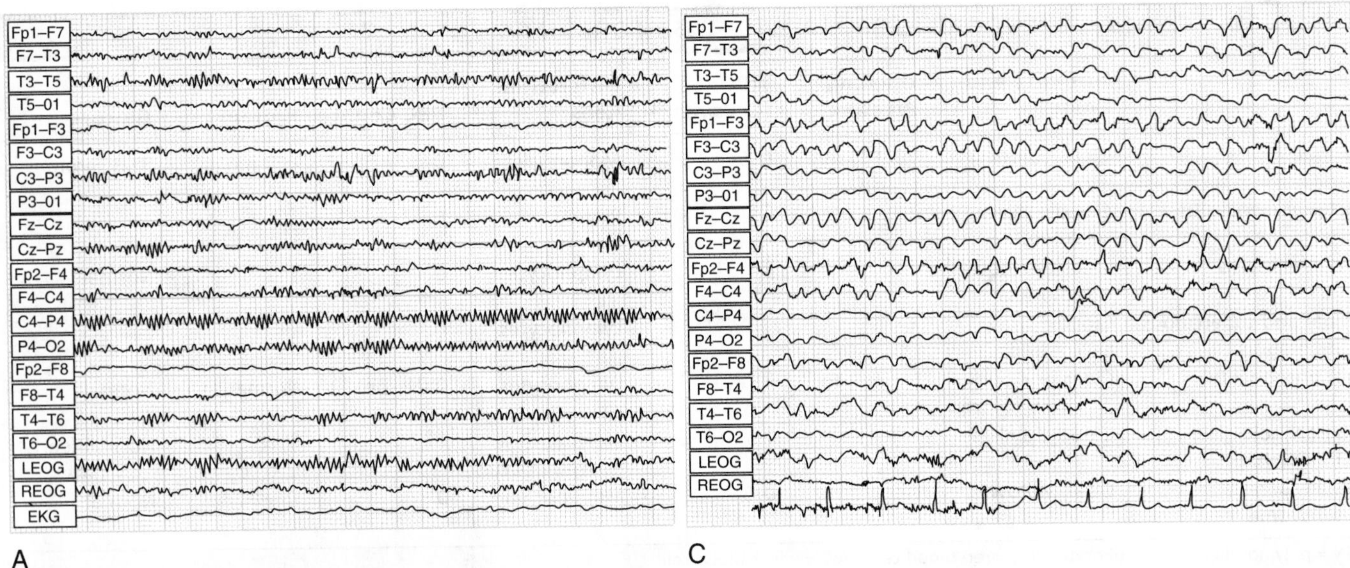

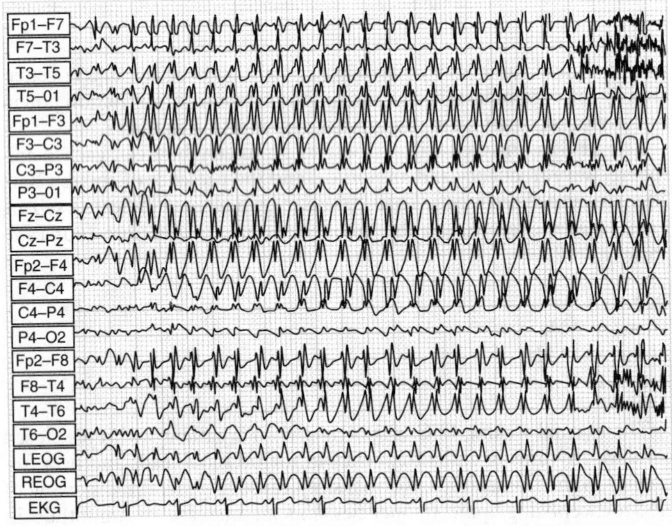

FIGURE 418–2 • Normal and abnormal electroencephalograms (EEGs). A, The EEG of a normal awake adult. **B,** A 3-Hz spike and wave activity, a pattern seen in absence epilepsy. In each record, channels 1 through 8 and 11 through 18 represent left- and right-sided bipolar electrode placements, respectively. Channels 9 and 10 represent midline bipolar electrode placements, and channels 19 and 20 represent the left and right electro-oculograms (eye movements). Each major horizontal division represents 1 second. **C,** Triphasic slow waves, a pattern seen in hepatic or other metabolic encephalopathies.

TABLE 418–4 ELECTROENCEPHALOGRAPHIC ABNORMALITIES

Electroencephalographic Abnormality	Clinical Correlate
BACKGROUND RHYTHM ABNORMALITIES	
Generalized slowing	Most metabolic encephalopathies
Triphasic waves	Hepatic, renal, and other metabolic encephalopathies
Focal slowing	Large mass lesions (tumor, large stroke)
Electrocerebral inactivity with lack of response to all stimuli	Brain death
PAROXYSMAL ABNORMALITIES	
3-Hz spike and wave, augmented by hyperventilation	Absence epilepsy
3- to 4-Hz spike and wave in light sleep or with photic stimulation	Primary generalized epilepsy
Central to midtemporal spikes	Benign rolandic epilepsy, other partial epilepsies
Anterior temporal spikes or sharp waves	Simple or complex partial seizures of mesial temporal origin
Hypsarrhythmia (high-voltage chaotic slowing with multifocal spikes)	Infantile spasms (West's syndrome)
Burst suppression	Severe anoxic brain injury, barbiturate coma

Nerve Conduction Study

A nerve conduction study (NCS) is the recording and measurement of the compound nerve and muscle action potentials elicited in response to an electrical stimulus.

To perform a motor NCS, a surface (active) recording electrode is placed over the belly of a distal muscle that is innervated by the nerve in question. A reference electrode is placed distally over the tendon. The nerve is then supramaximally stimulated at a predetermined distance proximal to the active electrode, and the resultant compound motor action potential (CMAP) is recorded. The terminal latency, amplitude, and duration of the evoked potential are measured directly, and the conduction velocity is calculated from the latencies of the evoked potentials with stimulation at two different points: the distance between the two

TABLE 418–5 NERVE CONDUCTION STUDY ABNORMALITIES

Abnormality	Clinical Correlate
Reduced CMAP amplitude	Axonal neuropathy
Prolonged terminal latency	Demyelinating neuropathy Distal compressive neuropathy
Conduction block	Severe focal compressive neuropathy Severe demyelinating neuropathy
Slowed conduction velocity	Demyelinating neuropathy

CMAP = compound muscle action potential.

points (conduction distance) is divided by the difference between the corresponding latencies (conduction time) to derive a calculated velocity (conduction velocity = distance ÷ time).

To perform a sensory NCS, the active recording electrode is placed over the portion of the skin innervated by the nerve in question, and a sensory nerve action potential is recorded after electrical stimulation of the nerve, similar to that noted for a motor NCS. NCS abnormalities include reduced amplitudes, prolonged terminal latencies, conduction block, and slowed conduction velocities (Table 418–5).

An NCS is helpful in documenting the existence of a neuropathy, quantifying its severity, and noting its distribution (i.e., whether it is distal, proximal, or diffuse). In addition, an NCS can provide information on the modality involved (i.e., motor versus sensory) and can suggest whether the lesion is axonal or demyelinating. An NCS is also helpful in diagnosing compressive mononeuropathies, such as carpal tunnel syndrome, ulnar palsy, peroneal nerve palsy, and tarsal tunnel syndrome.

F Wave and H Reflex

The F wave and H reflex are ways of looking at the conduction characteristics for proximal portions of nerves, including the nerve roots. The F wave is a late CMAP evoked intermittently from a muscle by a *supramaximal* electrical stimulus to the nerve, and it is due to antidromic activation (backfiring) of alpha motor neurons. F waves can be elicited from practically all distal motor nerves. The H reflex is a late CMAP that is evoked regularly from a muscle by a *submaximal* stimulus to a nerve, and it is due to stimulation of Ia afferent fibers (a spinal reflex). The H reflex can be routinely obtained from calf muscles only with stimulation of the tibial nerve in the popliteal fossa.

F waves are helpful in diagnosing Guillain-Barré syndrome, in which demyelination is often confined to the proximal portions of nerves early in the course of the disease. The H reflex is often absent in patients with acute S1 radiculopathy.

Repetitive Stimulation Study

A repetitive stimulation study (RSS) is a method of measuring electrical conduction properties at the neuromuscular junction. To perform an RSS, a surface recording electrode is placed over a muscle belly, and the nerve innervating that muscle is electrically stimulated with a supramaximal stimulus at a certain frequency. A series of electrical potentials are then recorded whose amplitude is roughly proportional to the number of muscle fibers that are being activated.

An RSS is helpful in diagnosing neuromuscular junction disorders, such as myasthenia gravis and myasthenic syndrome (Lambert-Eaton syndrome). In myasthenia gravis, the amplitudes of evoked potentials become progressively smaller with repetitive stimulation in clinically involved muscles. Clinically uninvolved muscles often do not demonstrate this decrement. In myasthenic syndrome, an *increment* is seen in the amplitudes of evoked potentials with rapid repetitive electrical stimulation.

Electromyography

EMG is the recording and study of insertional, spontaneous, and voluntary electrical activity of muscle. It allows physiologic evaluation of the motor unit, including the anterior horn cell, peripheral nerve, and muscle.

TABLE 418–6 ELECTROMYOGRAPHIC ABNORMALITIES

Abnormality	Clinical Correlate
INSERTIONAL ACTIVITY	
Prolonged	Acute denervation Active (usually inflammatory) myopathy
SPONTANEOUS ACTIVITY	
Fibrillations and positive waves	Acute denervation Active (usually inflammatory) myopathy
Fasciculations	Chronic neuropathies Motor neuron disease (rare fasciculations may be normal)
Myotonic discharges	Myotonic disorders Acid maltase deficiency
VOLUNTARY ACTIVITY	
Neuropathic potentials: large-amplitude, long-duration, polyphasic potentials	Chronic neuropathies and anterior horn cell diseases
Myopathic potentials: small-amplitude, short-duration, polyphasic potentials	Chronic myopathies Neuromuscular junction disorders
RECRUITMENT	
Reduced	Chronic neuropathic disorders
Rapid	Chronic myopathies

EMG is performed by inserting a needle electrode into the muscle in question and evaluating the motor unit action potentials both visually (on the oscilloscope screen) and aurally (over the loudspeaker). Muscles are typically studied at rest and during voluntary contraction. During EMG, the electrical activity of muscle is studied in four settings (Table 418–6): (1) *insertional activity* (occurring within the first second of needle insertion), (2) *spontaneous activity* (electrical activity at rest), (3) *voluntary activity* (electrical activity with muscle contraction), and (4) *recruitment pattern* (change in electrical activity with maximal contraction).

EMG is helpful when evaluating patients with weakness in that it can help determine whether the weakness is due to anterior horn cell disease, nerve root disease, peripheral neuropathy, or an intrinsic disease of muscle itself (myopathy). EMG can differentiate acute denervation from chronic denervation and may thus give an indication about the time course of the lesion causing the neuropathy. In addition, based on which muscles have an abnormal EMG pattern, it is possible to determine whether the neuropathy is due to a lesion of a nerve root (radiculopathy), the brachial or lumbosacral plexus (plexopathy), an individual peripheral nerve (mononeuropathy), or multiple peripheral nerves (polyneuropathy).

EMG is also helpful in differentiating active (inflammatory) myopathies from chronic myopathies. Active myopathies include dermatomyositis, polymyositis, inclusion body myositis, and some forms of muscular dystrophy, such as Duchenne's dystrophy. Chronic myopathies include the other muscular dystrophies, the congenital myopathies, and some metabolic myopathies. Myotonic dystrophy and myotonia congenita produce characteristic myotonic discharges.

It may take several weeks for a muscle to develop EMG signs of acute denervation after nerve transection. For this reason, EMG performed in the acute setting after nerve injury should be interpreted with caution, and it may need to be repeated at a later date.

Evoked Potentials

Evoked potentials are ways of measuring conduction velocities for sensory pathways in the CNS by means of computerized averaging techniques. Three types of evoked potentials are routinely performed: visual, brain stem auditory, and somatosensory.

Pattern Reversal Visual Evoked Responses

The pattern reversal visual evoked response (PVER) assesses the function of central visual pathways, in particular the optic nerves. To perform this test, EEG electrodes are placed over the occipital regions of the scalp and the patient is asked to look at the center of a black-and-white checkerboard screen with one eye patched. The color of the checks alternates about twice per second, a process known as pattern reversal. The scalp potentials elicited by approximately 100 such pattern reversals are then recorded and signal-averaged by a computer. This signal averaging cancels the random EEG activity and differentially amplifies the evoked potential. A single waveform (P 100) is recorded for each eye, and its latency is measured. Normal latency for the P 100 waveform is approximately 100 msec. A prolonged P 100 latency in one eye, in the absence of ocular pathology, implies slowed conduction velocity in the optic nerve and suggests demyelination of that nerve. PVER testing is helpful when multiple sclerosis is suspected clinically and it is necessary to document the presence of a second demyelinating lesion in the CNS that may not be clinically evident (Fig. 418–3).

Brain Stem Auditory Evoked Responses

The brain stem auditory evoked response (BAER) assesses function in the central auditory pathways in the brain stem. EEG electrodes are placed over the vertex and mastoid process, and a series of clicks at a frequency of 5 Hz are delivered to each ear separately for 3 minutes. The scalp potentials elicited by the clicks are then recorded and signal-averaged by a computer. This signal averaging cancels the random EEG activity and differentially amplifies the evoked potential. A series of five waves are recorded for each ear, and each wave corresponds to a different point in the central auditory pathway (Table 418–7). The wave latencies for the right and left ears are compared, and a delay in any of the latencies suggests a lesion at that point in the central brain stem auditory pathway. BAER testing is helpful in diagnosing acoustic schwannoma and other tumors in the cerebellopontine angle.

Somatosensory Evoked Responses

The somatosensory evoked response (SER) assesses conduction in the central somatosensory pathways in the posterior columns of the spinal cord, brain stem, thalamus, and primary sensory cortex in the parietal lobes. To perform SER testing, recording electrodes are placed over Erb's point and the cervical spine (for medial or ulnar nerve stimulation), over the popliteal fossa and lumbar spine (for peroneal or tibial nerve stimulation), and over the scalp. A series of 1000 to 2000 electrical shocks at a frequency of 5 Hz are delivered to the median or ulnar nerve (for an upper extremity SER) or to the peroneal or tibial nerves (for a lower extremity SER). The scalp potentials elicited by the electrical shocks are then recorded and signal-averaged by a computer. This signal averaging cancels the random EEG activity and differentially amplifies the evoked potential. A series of waves are recorded for each nerve stimulated, with each wave corresponding to a different point in the somatosensory pathways in the spinal cord, brain stem, and cerebral cortex. The wave latencies for the right and left limbs are compared, and a delay in any of the latencies suggests a lesion at that point in the somatosensory pathways.

SER testing, like PVER, is helpful when multiple sclerosis is suspected clinically and it is necessary to document the presence of a second demyelinating lesion in the CNS that may not be clinically evident. SER testing is also useful for monitoring spinal cord function intraoperatively in patients undergoing spinal surgery.

Electronystagmography

Electronystagmography accurately records eye movements and nystagmus after certain provocative maneuvers. To perform this test, disc electrodes are placed over the bridge of the nose and lateral to each outer canthus, and the electrical leads from these discs are connected to an oscilloscope. Because the cornea is electropositive and the retina is electronegative, these electrodes accurately record lateral eye movements. The patient is first observed for spontaneous nystagmus with the eyes open and closed and then for nystagmus evoked with lateral gaze, for nystagmus induced by hot and cold air instilled in the outer ears (caloric induced), and for positional nystagmus. The latter is performed by rotating the patient in a specialized chair. Spontaneous nystagmus suggests a vestibular pathologic lesion, as does an imbalance in the nystagmus evoked by these maneuvers in the right and left ears.

TABLE 418–7 BRAIN STEM EVOKED RESPONSE WAVE GENERATORS

Wave	Location
I	Auditory nerve
II	Cochlear nucleus
III	Superior olivary nucleus
IV	Lateral lemniscus
V	Inferior colliculus

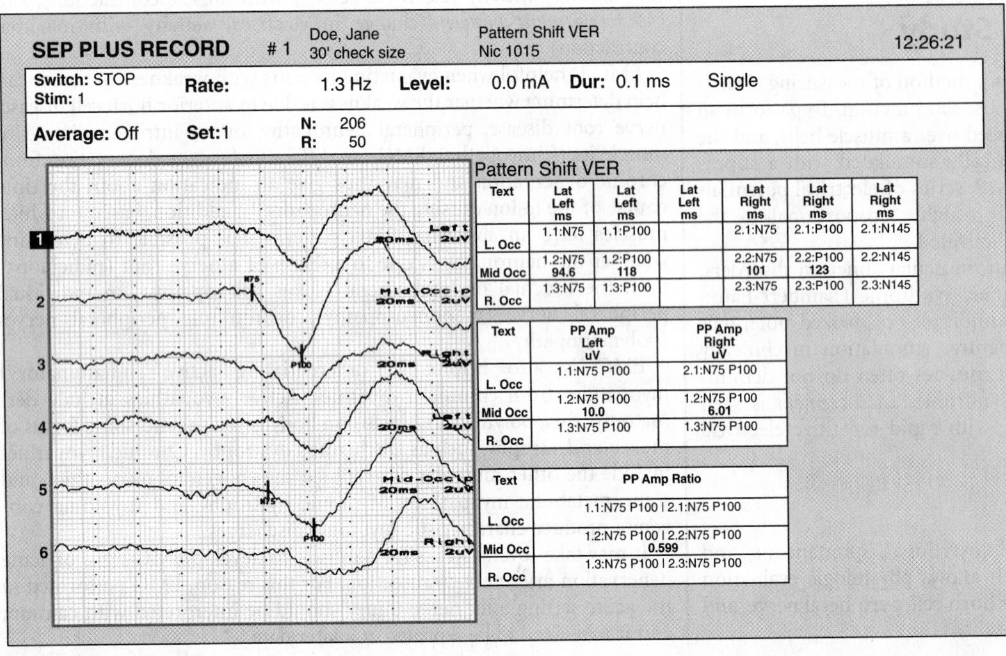

FIGURE 418–3 • Abnormal pattern reversal visual evoked response in a patient with multiple sclerosis. The prolonged P 100 wave latency with left eye stimulation suggests a conduction defect in the left optic nerve. The top three channels represent right eye stimulation and the bottom three channels represent left eye stimulation. Each horizontal division represents 20 msec.

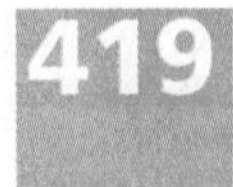

RADIOLOGIC IMAGING PROCEDURES

David Hackney

ROLE OF IMAGING IN CLINICAL EVALUATION

The primary imaging technique to diagnose diseases of the brain and spine is magnetic resonance (MR); x-ray computed tomography (CT) is typically reserved for instances in which bone detail is needed or emergent situations in which its speed and absence of contraindications have made it the dominant modality. Diagnostic imaging often is used to confirm a suspected clinical diagnosis and to exclude conditions that may mimic the expected diagnosis. It is always wise to have a specific diagnosis or differential diagnosis in mind before viewing neuroimages. Given that diagnostic imaging continues to undergo rapid changes in technology, the answer changes frequently to the question, What is the best way to evaluate this disease?

Computed Tomographic Scanning

Basis of CT Imaging

Normal intracranial structures have a narrow range of electron density, and there is essentially no contrast on plain radiographic images of the brain. With CT, the slightly higher density of gray matter is seen compared with the lower density of white matter. The cerebrospinal fluid has a markedly lower density than the brain, whereas blood in arteries and veins has a higher density. Calcified structures such as the calvaria, choroid plexus, and arterial plaques are much higher density. Administration of intravenous contrast agents only slightly increases the density of the normal brain and also provides information on the integrity of the blood-brain barrier.

Advantages of CT

Rapid Image Acquisition

Typical high-quality images of the brain require 10 to 20 seconds for the entire study to be obtained. It takes far more time to position the patient in the machine than it does to do the scan. This speed is important in acutely ill patients, in patients who are uncooperative, or in situations that require imaging of large portions of the body.

Compatibility

MR imaging is limited by the requirement that the patient and any necessary monitors and implants be placed inside a powerful magnetic field and subjected to radio frequency pulses. Many patients, such as those who have pacemakers, cannot be imaged with MR. CT is free of such limitations.

Simplicity of Interpretation

Although modern equipment can produce a huge number of images, including arteriograms, venograms, and perfusion information, all contrast on CT images is due to differences in electron density. Therefore, the appearance of the images is determined by a single parameter, and the images are relatively easy to interpret.

Disadvantages of CT

CT provides only one piece of information, the spatial distribution of electron density. If the disease of interest does not change electron density, it will be invisible on CT. Because many processes can raise or lower electron density, the image intensity on CT has limited specificity.

MR Imaging

Basis of MR Imaging

Unlike CT, the signal intensity of MR does not have a single simple interpretation. Signal intensity is determined by proton density (a reflection of "water concentration") as well as by a number of MR parameters including the longitudinal relaxation rate (T1), the transverse relaxation (T2), the diffusion coefficient, the magnetization transfer ratio, the homogeneity of magnetic susceptibility, and complex functions of the motion of tissues. Because of the large number of parameters that determine signal intensity on MR, the images reflect many physiologic processes with far more specificity than does CT.

Advantages of MR

Combinations of imaging options can detect and measure blood flow, determine the age of hemorrhage, display sequential physiologic changes after stroke, and detect developmental and neoplastic lesions. An abnormality identified on CT is often better characterized by MR. MR does not require ionizing radiation.

Contrast Imaging

Both CT and MR can display regions of breakdown of the blood-brain barrier. The standard contrast agents administered intravenously do not cross the normal vessels of the brain. However, a variety of processes will lead to leakiness of these vessels and resulting "contrast enhancement." Although CT and MR contrast agents differ in the mechanisms by which they produce increases in density (CT) or changes in T1 (MR), both approaches provide nearly identical information about the integrity of the blood-brain barrier. Because of its higher contrast-to-noise ratios, MR is more sensitive for detecting contrast enhancement than is CT.

Radiation Doses

As the radiation doses increase with modern multirow detector technology, thinner sections, and more indications for CT imaging, this advantage of MR becomes more important. However, if CT is appropriately monitored, the doses will rarely be high enough to cause medical concern except in children and young adults.

Anatomic and Physiologic Specificity

Because many brain structures have identical electron densities but differ on many MR parameters, MR can resolve anatomic structures that are invisible on CT. Similarly, MR can display many physiologic changes that do not alter electron density.

Disadvantages of MR

Resolution and Localization

MR can achieve exquisite spatial resolution, but at the expense of prolonged imaging times and the inconvenience of highly specialized hardware with limited general applicability. In routine applications, MR images are acquired at resolutions similar to or lower than those of CT. The major advantage of MR over CT for brain and spine imaging is the high contrast between differing tissues and pathologic processes, not spatial resolution. Spatial localization is comparable for MR and CT, but MR is not as good near air-filled structures, such as the paranasal sinuses or mastoid bones, or near metallic implants. When highly accurate spatial information is required to plan treatment (e.g., stereotactic radiosurgery), MR images are often supplemented with CT.

Rapidity of Image Acquisition

Although some MR images are acquired in a fraction of a second, MR approaches may take several minutes. For example, imaging of the brain in a patient with a stroke may take 15 seconds with CT, whereas MR in the same patient could take 30 minutes.

Compatibility

The powerful magnetic fields of MR instruments pose hazards to patients and staff. Patients on monitors or ventilators must be converted to nonmagnetic, MR-compatible equivalents before they can enter the magnet room. Medical implants may be inactivated or damaged by a powerful magnetic field, and some common devices may malfunction (e.g., some pacemakers will react to the MR pulse sequences by driving the pacing at unacceptable rates). Finally, the design of MR magnets, with long, relatively narrow bores, makes it difficult to monitor critically ill patients. Some large patients do not fit into the magnet, and some patients find the restricted vision and movement intolerable.

Simplicity of Interpretation

Because of the large number of factors that determine image signal intensity, the large number of artifacts, and the nearly infinite choices in how to acquire the images, interpretation of an MR image is often complex and difficult compared with a CT scan.

APPROACH TO COMMON CLINICAL SYNDROMES

On the basis of the relative advantages and disadvantages of MR, CT, and other neuroimaging modalities, different clinical entities can and should be assessed differently (Table 419–1).

TABLE 419–1 STRENGTHS AND WEAKNESSES OF SELECTED IMAGING MODALITIES

Modality	Strengths	Weaknesses
Computed tomography (CT)	Fast; best test for acute intraparenchymal or subarachnoid hemorrhage and calcification; easy to monitor patients; excellent for bones	Less sensitive to parenchymal lesions than MR; potential for significant reaction to contrast material; radiation exposure
Conventional angiography	Best imaging modality for aneurysms, vascular malformations, and vasculitis	Invasive and often lengthy; risk of stroke and other complications
Conventional myelography	Good images of nerve roots and small osteophytic lesions; accurate for bony stenosis; useful in patients with contraindications to MR	Invasive, with risk of complications from lumbar puncture and instillation of contrast material; does not image intramedullary lesions well
CT myelography	Excellent for imaging nerve roots and detecting root compression from degenerative processes	Invasive, with risk of complications from lumbar puncture and instillation of contrast material
Magnetic resonance imaging (MRI)	Noninvasive; no radiation; multiplanar; extremely sensitive, safe contrast agent	Less sensitive than CT for detection of subarachnoid hemorrhage and calcification; less sensitive for bony skull fractures; contraindicated in patients with implanted metallic devices or foreign bodies; the patient must be able to cooperate and tolerate confined space; time-consuming relative to CT
Magnetic resonance angiography (MRA)	Noninvasive; good for screening for extracranial and intracranial vascular disease; may be performed with or without contrast agent	Need cooperative patient; technically demanding; may overestimate the degree of vascular stenosis (noncontrast MRA); cannot image distal vessels optimally without contrast agent; may miss small lesions (e.g., aneurysms)
Positron emission tomography (PET)	Limited role in helping to distinguish radiation necrosis from tumor; helpful in the diagnosis of Alzheimer's disease and epilepsy	Requires a cyclotron to generate radioisotopes with a short half-life; lower resolution and less available than MRI or CT
Single-photon emission computed tomography (SPECT)	Useful in epilepsy; sensitive for diffuse pathologic processes; easier to use than PET	Lower resolution than PET, MRI, or CT
Proton magnetic resonance spectroscopy	Localization of seizure focus; may help diagnose and classify dementias, such as Alzheimer's disease; may distinguish brain tumors from other mass lesions; may distinguish radiation necrosis from recurrent tumor	Specificity not yet determined; not routinely available; lower resolution; time-consuming
Ultrasonography	Fast; easy to use; can be performed at the bedside to assess vessel patency	Does not assess the vertebral arteries; less sensitive and specific than MRA; cannot visualize vessels in the upper neck and cranial base
Transcranial Doppler (TCD)	Fast; easy to use; assesses vascular velocities quantitatively; can assess cerebral vasospasm and occluded vessels.	Does not provide images of vessels

Stroke

For the initial evaluation of patients who present clinically with stroke (Chapters 431 and 432), the first and most valuable imaging test is CT. Although MR often provides important complementary information, CT quickly detects hemorrhage, identifies its location, and estimates its age. CT will also identify previous cerebral infarctions.

Ischemic Stroke

In acute ischemic cerebral infarction without bleeding (Fig. 419–1), the CT scan is typically normal for the first 1 to 3 hours. However, the changes start to appear within the next 3 to 9 hours, relatively earlier in larger infarctions and in embolic infarctions. The initial sign is faint loss of the normal contrast between gray matter and white matter, often first recognized in the insular cortex, and the cortex gradually begins to swell. By 12 hours, early signs of infarction are routinely evident. By 24 hours, the loss of distinction between gray and white matter is readily evident, and there is usually localized swelling of the involved region. As the margins of the infarcted tissue become better defined, the difference in density between normal and affected tissue becomes greater. Brain swelling, which reflects edema in the infarcted tissue, often continues to worsen during 48 to 72 hours. As swelling subsides in the ensuing weeks, it is eventually replaced by atrophy. The density of the involved tissues continues to decrease, and normal contrast between gray and white matter is lost permanently. Smaller infarctions and strokes caused by emboli may progress through these stages more rapidly than large ones.

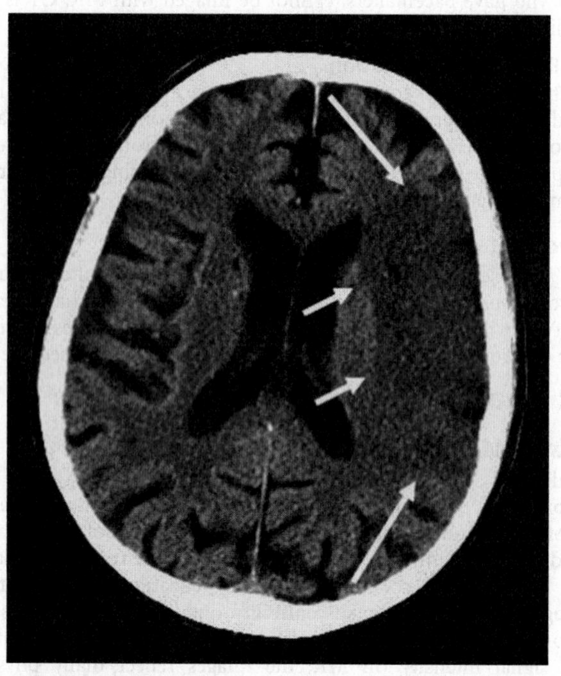

FIGURE 419–1 • Acute cerebral infarction.

The localization of ischemic lesions can provide insight about the cause of stroke. Characteristic anatomic distributions, for example, along the border between brain supplied by the anterior cerebral artery and brain supplied by the middle cerebral artery, suggest low flow in proximal vessels, a condition that results in "watershed" or "border zone" infarctions. Because these small vessels are distributed over a wide area, emboli do not produce this pattern of infarction; rather, this pattern implies a proximal stenosis or occlusion, so the diagnostic evaluation should focus on the carotid or vertebral arteries.

Subarachnoid Hemorrhage

Ruptured intracranial aneurysms are the most common cause of subarachnoid hemorrhage (Chapter 432). Although MR imaging may be as sensitive as CT for detecting subarachnoid hemorrhage, it is less specific, and the speed of CT scanning and its wide availability have made it the preferred initial imaging modality. With CT, the pattern of hemorrhage often suggests whether an aneurysm is the likely cause as well as the location of the aneurysm or other bleeding lesion. On CT, the blood fills the cerebrospinal fluid–containing cisterns most densely near the source of hemorrhage, a finding that can be difficult to see on MR. If subarachnoid hemorrhage has occurred, further evaluation of the patient often includes a noninvasive imaging method to confirm the cause and source of bleeding and to provide preliminary anatomic information. Either CT angiography or MR arteriography can display the three-dimensional anatomy of aneurysms with sufficient detail for therapy to be planned, but surgical treatment generally requires a pre-procedure catheter arteriogram (Chapter 432).

Intraparenchymal Hemorrhage

Intraparenchymal hemorrhages (Fig. 419–2) arise from hemorrhagic infarction, arteriovenous malformations, amyloid angiopathy, hypertensive hemorrhage, underlying neoplasm, and aneurysmal bleeding (Chapter 432). CT permits rapid diagnosis and provides information on location and possible pressure on nearby structures. The location of the hematoma, its proximity to major arterial branch points, and any associated subarachnoid hemorrhage or other findings can be helpful in suggesting the cause. Arteriovenous malformations often have visible, enlarged veins. Amyloid is typically lobar with a predilection for the parietal and occipital lobes. Hypertensive bleeding typically occurs in the basal ganglia, thalamus, pons, and cerebellum. Hematomas with underlying neoplasms often present with prominent edema shortly after the hemorrhage, whereas edema does not develop until 1 to 3 days later in other causes of hemorrhage.

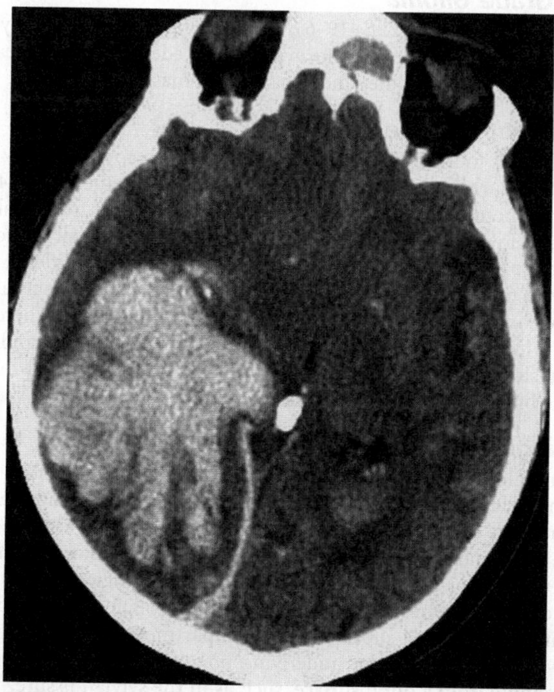

FIGURE 419–2 • Intraparenchymal hematoma.

Trauma

CT is the first-line method for evaluation of the brain after trauma (Chapter 422) because it is compatible with the many support and monitoring devices that accompany severely traumatized patients and it is rapid, requiring suspension of active treatment for only a few seconds during testing. Most of the important findings will be visible on CT without a need for the administration of intravenous contrast material.

Subdural Hematoma

Subdural hematomas (Fig. 419–3) usually have a classic concavo-convex shape and arise from bleeding of bridging veins that cross the subdural space on their way from the brain to the dural venous sinuses. Because, unlike epidural hematomas, they are contained externally by the dura, they do not cross the midline or the dural margins but rather are confined to the infratentorial or supratentorial space. Subdural hematomas become clinically important when they are large enough to cause mass effect. The severity of a mass effect from a subdural hematoma is judged by local effacement of sulci, compression of the adjacent lateral ventricles, midline shift, and evidence of herniation. However, subdural hematomas can continue to enlarge after the initial injury, so even a small subdural hematoma requires observation and usually follow-up imaging. MR imaging is better than CT for delineating the anatomy of a subdural hematoma and for estimating the age of the lesion. In general, however, the MR examination will have been performed for reasons other than a history of head trauma.

Epidural Hematoma

Epidural hematomas (Fig. 419–4) classically arise from bleeding of meningeal arteries or less commonly from tears of the dural venous sinuses. Because of high flow from their arterial or venous source, they can expand rapidly and dramatically. They are often associated with calvarial fractures. Epidural hematoma is distinguished from subdural hematoma by the characteristic biconvex configuration of the epidural hematoma, the ability of an epidural hematoma to cross divisions of the dura (such as the falx or tentorium), and the usual presence of underlying fractures.

Both subdural hematomas and epidural hematomas are typically hyperdense on CT images at initial presentation and decrease in density over time. Initially, the settling of red blood cells within the hematoma creates a high-density sediment of loosely packed cells, with lower density serum above. The cells then lyse, and the debris is resorbed. Over time, the density on CT decreases to approach that of the cerebrospinal fluid, and the collections usually decrease in size. Chronic subdural hematoma may change configuration and assume a biconvex shape, similar to an

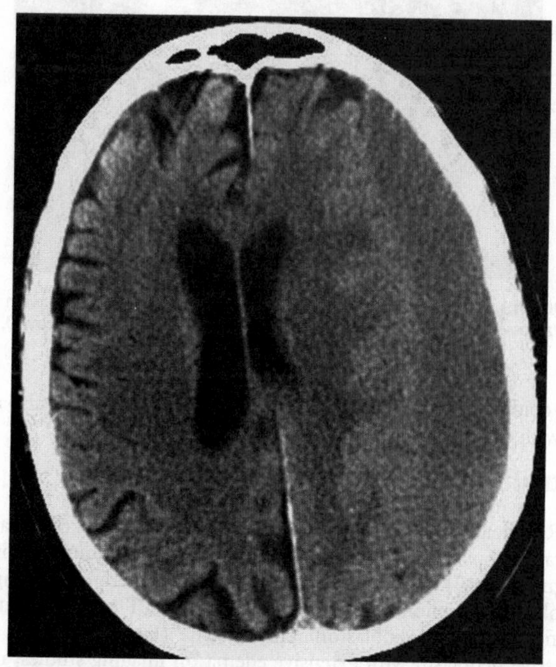

FIGURE 419–3 • Subdural hematoma.

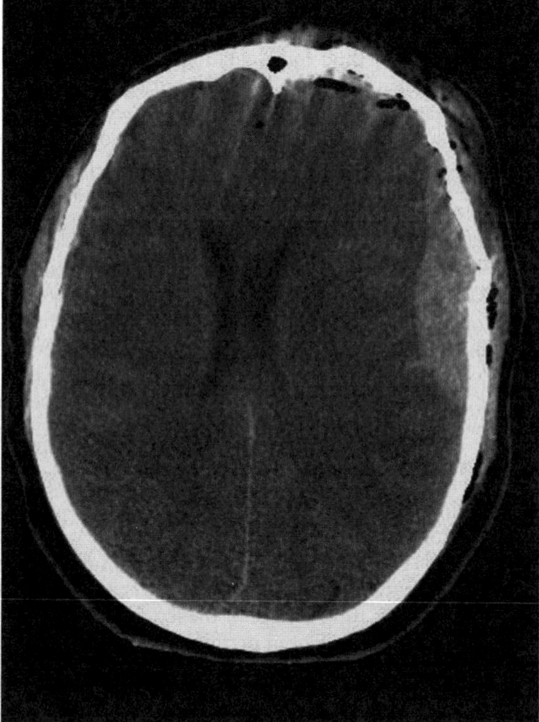

FIGURE 419–4 • Epidural hematoma.

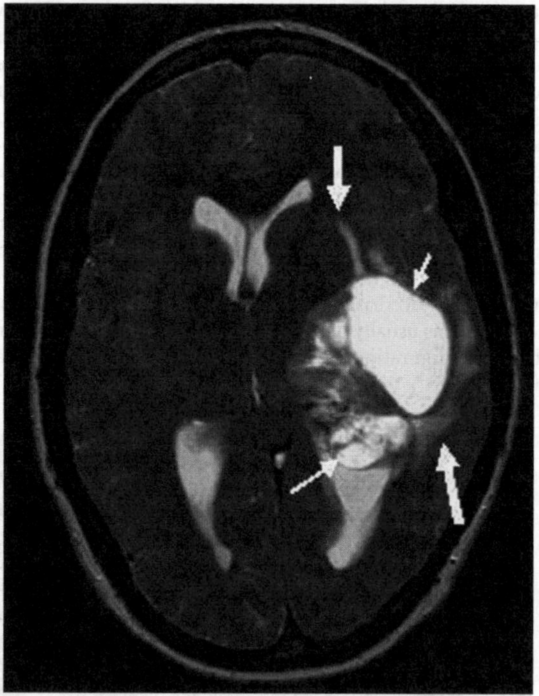

FIGURE 419–5 • T2-weighted MR image of a malignant glioma with edema (large arrows) and necrosis (uniform high signal regions, small arrows).

acute epidural hematoma, but with a low density. Trauma is also associated with contusion and diffuse axonal injury (Chapter 422).

Neoplasms

MR is the preferred modality for the detection and characterization of all brain neoplasms (Chapter 199). However, many tumors are initially recognized on CT scans. For certain tumors, such as craniopharyngiomas and oligodendrogliomas, calcifications seen on CT can contribute to a specific diagnosis. Glioblastoma multiforme (Fig. 419–5) is a highly aggressive neoplasm with extensive edema on imaging studies; neovascularity results in loss of the blood-brain barrier and consequent enhancement after the administration of contrast material. These tumors are often necrotic with central nonenhancing regions that are low density on CT and appear fluid filled on MR. If there is evidence of necrosis, the enhancement tends to be inhomogeneous and ringlike. There is extensive abnormal high signal on T2-weighted and FLAIR images in the adjacent white matter. These regions contain both edema and infiltrating tumor. Unlike simple edema, the combination of infiltrating tumor with edema can extend across the corpus callosum.

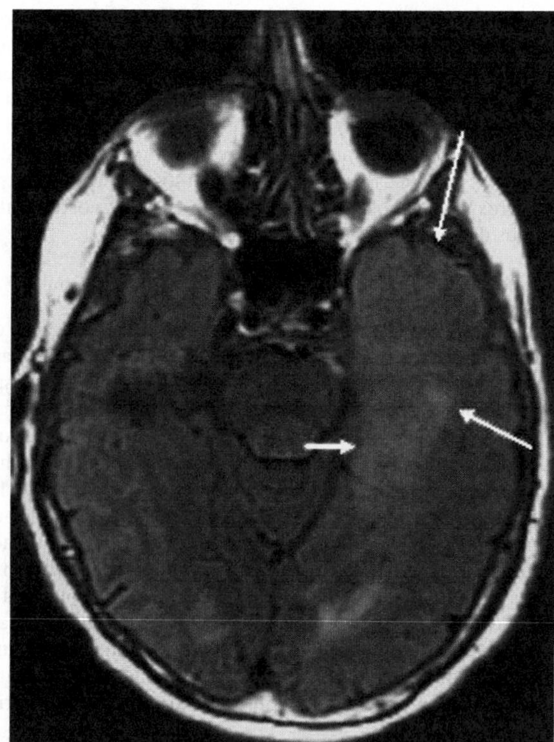

FIGURE 419–6 • Low-grade glioma. Axial MR image emphasizing T2 contrast (FLAIR technique) shows a diffuse infiltrating glioma, with only mild local mass effect, as well as loss of contrast between gray and white matter and loss of sulci due to swelling.

Low-Grade Glioma

Low-grade gliomas (Fig. 419–6), which are far less aggressive, typically show no enhancement and no evidence of edema. They appear well defined on imaging studies and produce less mass effect.

Metastatic Disease

Metastases to the brain present on imaging with approximately spherical shape, surrounding edema, and contrast enhancement (Fig. 419–7). They can become necrotic and difficult to distinguish from malignant gliomas. However, they do not infiltrate the brain, so they do not have the diffuse growth pattern of grade 3 or grade 4 gliomas. Edema associated with metastases does not cross the corpus callosum. Metastases can display contrast enhancement and are frequently multiple. Therefore, a solitary lesion with central necrosis and extensive edema could be a metastasis or a glioblastoma. A lesion with infiltration diffusely throughout the brain will not be a metastasis.

Meningioma

Meningiomas (Chapter 199), which are common tumors of the meninges, are usually histologically benign, but atypical and malignant variants can display aggressive behavior. Meningiomas usually have a broad attachment to dural surfaces along the inner margin of the calvaria, the falx, or the tentorium (Fig. 419–8). Meningiomas may invade these dural structures, crossing the midline through the falx, spanning the infratentorial and supratentorial compartments through the tentorium, or growing into the underlying bone. Meningiomas rarely may arise remote from a dural surface, such as in the sylvian fissure.

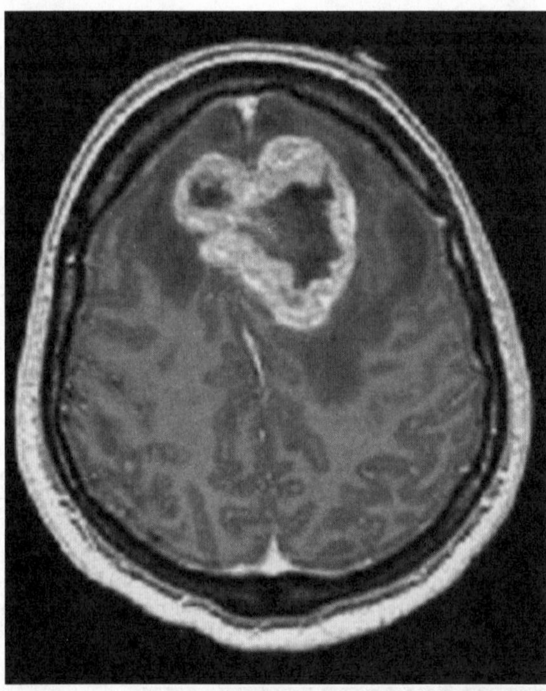

FIGURE 419–7 • Metastatic disease. T1-weighted MR image after administration of contrast agent. Melanoma metastasis with extensive necrosis and thick-walled enhancement.

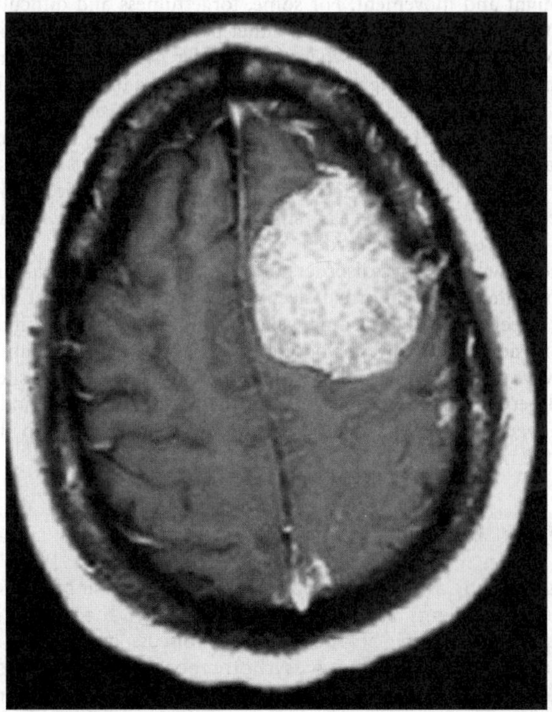

FIGURE 419–8 • Meningioma. T1-weighted contrast MR image.

Acoustic Neuroma

Acoustic neuromas (Chapter 199) usually can be diagnosed reliably with contrast-enhanced MR (Fig. 419–9). They arise at the meatus of the internal auditory canal and widen this structure. These tumors can grow deeply into the canal and into the cerebellopontine angle cistern. They enhance after administration of contrast material.

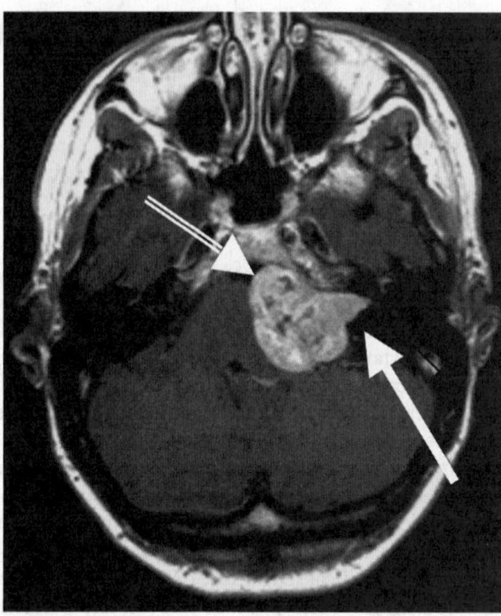

FIGURE 419–9 • Acoustic neuroma. T1-weighted axial MR image after administration of contrast agent. A large acoustic neuroma widens the left internal auditory canal (solid arrow) and compresses the brain stem (hollow arrow).

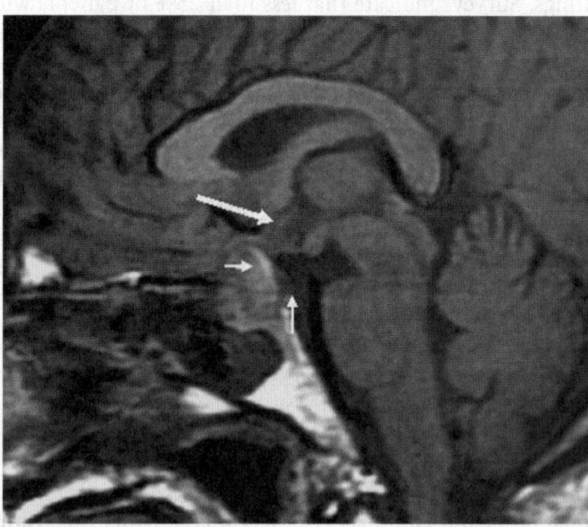

FIGURE 419–10 • Pituitary adenoma. Sagittal T1-weighted MR image before administration of contrast agent demonstrates a large mass in the sella turcica (small arrows), extending into the suprasellar cistern (large arrow). This tumor arises from the pituitary gland, so no normal pituitary is visible.

Pituitary Adenoma

Pituitary adenomas (Chapter 242) are best evaluated with MR imaging, by which the mass itself, enlargement of the sella, extension into the cavernous sinuses, and involvement of the optic chiasm are clearly seen (Fig. 419–10). Sagittal and coronal studies usually display a region of decreased signal on precontrast T1-weighted images and delayed enhancement after administration of contrast material.

SUGGESTED READINGS

Henson JW, Gaviani P, Gonzalez RG: MRI in treatment of adult gliomas. Lancet Oncol 2005;6:167–175. *A summary of MR imaging in adult gliomas, with principles applicable to other brain tumors.*

Macapinlac HA: Positron emission tomography of the brain. Neuroimaging Clin N Am 2006;16:591–603. *Outlines the current clinical use for PET imaging in the brain.*

Mukherjee P: Diffusion tensor imaging and fiber tractography in acute stroke. Neuroimaging Clin N Am 2005;15:655–665. *An advanced application of MR imaging for stroke.*

420 PSYCHIATRIC DISORDERS IN MEDICAL PRACTICE

Randolph B. Schiffer

BEHAVIORAL AND BEHAVIORALLY RELATED DISORDERS

As age-specific mortality decreases because of medical progress in treatment and prevention of infectious, nutritional, cardiovascular, and malignant disorders, the behavioral and behaviorally related disorders assume greater importance. According to the World Health Organization, 5 of the 10 leading causes of disability worldwide are psychiatric conditions: unipolar depression, substance abuse, bipolar disorder, schizophrenia, and obsessive-compulsive disorders.

Psychiatric morbidity is common among patients in ambulatory general medical settings, both in developed and in underdeveloped countries. General medical physicians can expect one in four of the patients whom they see to have active, diagnosable psychiatric disease. The most common diagnoses in medical settings are depression, generalized anxiety disorder, somatoform disorders, substance abuse, and personality disorders. These disorders are associated with substantial psychosocial morbidity and they are all treatable. Initial recognition and treatment of these disorders must occur in general medical settings because of shortages of psychiatrists and limitations in access to psychiatric expertise in managed care settings. Surveys indicate that less than 25% of patients with these mental illnesses are recognized and treated by primary care providers.

Psychiatric disorders are accompanied by a series of variable signs and symptoms, or syndromes, and diagnosis is still based on these clinical features despite increasing knowledge about the neurobiologic bases of these conditions. As yet, there are no reliable laboratory tests for diagnosis. All psychiatric diseases have a spectrum of severity, and available therapies probably work best during their milder phases. This chapter outlines the clinical features and therapeutics for the psychiatric syndromes that occur most frequently in general medical settings.

SYNDROMES

Depression and Risk of Suicide

Depression

Several depressive-spectrum disorders are included in the current edition of the American Psychiatric Association's *Diagnostic and Statistical Manual of Mental Disorders* (DSM-IV). Dysthymia is a syndrome of milder symptoms, but other patients have major depressive symptoms and can be suicidal.

When the pattern of recurrence is one of depressive syndromes only, the disorder is called a *unipolar depressive disorder.* When manic-like episodes are included (see later), the disorder is called a *bipolar disorder.*

Epidemiology

Lifetime prevalence rates for major depressive disorders are 15 to 20% in the United States. The exact prevalence is not known because of variable methods of ascertainment and diagnosis. Point prevalence rates for major depression in urban U.S. populations range from 2 to 4% for men and 4 to 6% for women.

Pathobiology

Several lines of evidence suggest that a genetic contribution exists for major depression. Occurrences of major depressive episodes clearly cluster in families. In general, increased rates of bipolar and unipolar disorders are present in first-degree relatives of patients with a bipolar disorder, and increased rates of unipolar depressive disorder are present in first-degree relatives of patients with unipolar disorders. These relatives have lifetime risks ranging from 10 to 20% for major depressive disorders, with perhaps a higher risk for depressive-spectrum disorders. This degree of increased risk is about three to five times that of the normal population. Twin and adoption studies are consistent with a genetic contribution to major depressive disorders, but studies suggest that other factors are also important. These life experience risk factors interact with the genetic constitution of each individual to determine the actual risk for depression. More recent techniques of molecular genetics, such as genomic mismatch scanning, repeat expansion detection, and mitochondrial DNA analysis, are beginning to contribute to our understanding of the genetics of affective disturbances, but as yet no discrete susceptibility genes for depression have been identified.

Neurochemical hypotheses for depression postulate that decreased availability of norepinephrine or serotonin at transmitter-specific synapses in the brain is associated with depression and that increased levels of these substances are associated with mania. Studies have generally supported the hypothesis that catecholamine and indolamine metabolism is important in mood states, although the relationships are complex. Almost all drugs with antidepressant properties affect catecholamine and indolamine availability at the synapse in the central nervous system.

Evidence also suggests that neuroendocrine function is altered in many people with major depressive disorders. Overactivity of the hypothalamic-pituitary-adrenocortical axis has been the most prominent of these neuroendocrine disturbances. This overactivity is reflected in higher levels of circulating cortisol in depressed patients than in controls, in addition to higher levels of cerebrospinal fluid (CSF) cortisol, increased excretion of urinary free cortisol, and cortisol resistance to dexamethasone suppression.

Clinical Manifestations and Diagnosis

The symptoms of depression are variable for each individual and are sometimes difficult to recognize. Behavior and cognition can be affected, as can mood and affect. Some people experience depression as a slowing of thought and movement. For some, forgetfulness and difficulty concentrating are prominent features. Other patients manifest agitation and even psychotic experiences when the disorder is severe. This variability in clinical features among patients can be used as a basis for classifying a major depressive episode into subtypes—agitated, psychotic, and others.

The core clinical features of the depressive disorders are included in the diagnostic criteria for a major depressive episode and for dysthymia (Table 420–1). These disorders tend to recur, and chronic, milder syndromes of depression, such as dysthymia, can evolve in time to the more severe major depressive disorder.

Patients with affective disorders often have a disturbance in circadian rhythm reflected as abnormal sleep patterns. Complaints of difficulty falling asleep and early morning wakening are reliable clinical indicators of depression. Electroencephalographic studies show a relative absence of slow-wave sleep (stages 3 and 4) in depressed individuals and a shortened period between the onset of sleep and the first dreaming period (rapid eye movement [REM] latency). These disturbances in sleep improve when the mood disturbance improves.

Treatment

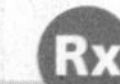

Diagnosis of a depressive disorder is the beginning of therapy. Depressed patients are usually relieved when their suffering is recognized and they are permitted to discuss it. The treatment plan must be individualized. A psychotherapeutic strategy (discussed later) should be considered for each patient before a drug is selected. Emerging clinical trials indicate that the combination of antidepressant medication and psychotherapy (see later) is superior to either alone in the treatment of depression. [1] These treatments should generally be initiated in primary care settings, followed by psychiatric consultation for nonresponders. Treatments should be continued for 6 to 12 months, with the goal of resolution of the depressive syndrome rather than just improvement.

Medical Therapy

Antidepressant drugs available in the United States (Table 420–2) vary in their structure and function. Second-generation medications (selective serotonin re-uptake inhibitors [SSRIs], bupropion, duloxetine, mirtazapine, and venlafaxine) are generally equivalent to each other therapeutically [2] and have fewer side effects than tricyclic antidepressants do.

TABLE 420–1 DIAGNOSTIC CRITERIA FOR DEPRESSIVE DISORDERS

MAJOR DEPRESSIVE EPISODE

1. At least five of the following symptoms have been present during the same 2-week period and represent a change from previous functioning; at least one of the symptoms is either depressed mood or loss of interest or pleasure
   A. Depressed mood most of the day, nearly every day
   B. Markedly diminished interest or pleasure in all, or almost all, activities most of the day, nearly every day
   C. Significant weight loss or weight gain when not dieting or decrease or increase in appetite nearly every day
   D. Insomnia or hypersomnia nearly every day
   E. Psychomotor agitation or retardation nearly every day; observable by others
   F. Fatigue or loss of energy nearly every day
   G. Feelings of worthlessness or excessive or inappropriate guilt (which may be delusional) nearly every day
   H. Diminished ability to think or concentrate, or indecisiveness, nearly every day
   I. Recurrent thoughts of death, recurrent suicidal ideation without a specific plan, or a suicide attempt or a specific plan for committing suicide
2. It cannot be established that an organic factor initiated and maintained the disturbance
3. The disturbance is not a normal reaction to the death of a loved one
4. At no time during the disturbance have there been delusions or hallucinations for as long as 2 weeks in the absence of prominent mood symptoms (i.e., before the mood symptoms developed or after they have remitted)
5. Not superimposed on schizophrenia, schizophreniform disorder, delusional disorder, or psychotic disorder; no other specific diagnosis

DYSTHYMIA

1. Depressed mood for most of the day for at least 2 years
2. The presence, while depressed, of two or more of the following:
   A. Poor appetite
   B. Insomnia or hypersomnia
   C. Low energy or fatigue
   D. Low self-esteem
   E. Poor concentration or difficulty making decisions
   F. Feelings of hopelessness
3. During the 2-year period, the person has never been without the symptoms for longer than 2 months at a time
4. No major depressive episode has been present during the first 2 years of the disturbance
5. There has not been an intermixed manic episode
6. The disturbance does not occur during the course of a psychotic disorder
7. The symptoms are not caused by the physiologic effects of a substance
8. The symptoms cause significant distress or functional impairment

Rx

Selective Serotonin Re-uptake Inhibitors

SSRIs are the initial therapy for depressive illness. They block the re-uptake of serotonin at presynaptic membranes, with relatively little effect on noradrenergic, cholinergic, histaminergic, or other neurochemical systems. As a result, they are associated with fewer side effects than the tricyclic antidepressants are. Additional advantages of SSRIs over the older tricyclic antidepressants include once-daily dosing and the ability to initiate treatment at the target dose for most patients. For sertraline, the dose is 50 mg once daily for almost all patients. The dosage can be increased to 100 mg/day after 3 weeks if there is no evidence of improvement. For nonresponders, the dose can be increased to 150 or 200 mg/day. Paroxetine can be started at 20 mg once daily and increased at similar intervals to 50 mg. Escitalopram may be taken on a once-daily schedule, beginning at 10 mg/day and increased after 4 to 6 weeks to 20 mg. Although plasma levels of these drugs and their metabolites are available in some laboratories, large clinical trials suggest that measurement of plasma levels is not a useful guide to clinical response.

Concerns about SSRIs include their adverse effects on sexual function and not as well established efficacy late in life. The greatest concern, however, is the occasional association of these drugs with impulsive self-destructive or violent behavior; this concern has resulted in a Food and Drug Administration warning.

Atypical Antidepressants

Amoxapine is an antidepressant with some dopamine-blocking properties. It is associated with extrapyramidal side effects. This drug has a theoretical advantage in depressed patients with psychotic features.

Rx

Trazodone and nefazodone inhibit the re-uptake of serotonin (5-HT) at the synapse and exhibit antagonism for a serotonin receptor subtype (5-HT_2). The absence of prominent anticholinergic side effects is a specific advantage for nefazodone. Trazodone has some sedating properties, which makes it useful in agitated patients with disturbed sleep, particularly elderly persons.

Venlafaxine is a phenylethylamine antidepressant that inhibits the re-uptake of serotonin and norepinephrine. It is selective for these two neurochemical systems and shows little in vitro binding to cholinergic, histaminergic, or dopaminergic receptors.

Bupropion is a novel monocyclic compound that inhibits the re-uptake of dopamine but has little effect on other adrenergic systems. *Mirtazapine*, a tetracyclic piperazinoazepine that is an analogue of mianserin, is an antidepressant that has been available in Europe. It is a presynaptic α_2-blocker that increases the release of norepinephrine and serotonin. It also blocks 5-HT_2 and 5-HT_3 receptors and histamine H_1 receptors. Common side effects include weight gain, dizziness, dry mouth, and constipation. It is a reasonable alternative for patients who do not respond to SSRIs.

Duloxetine combines SSRI-like pharmacologic properties with inhibition of norepinephrine re-uptake. This agent is also approved for the treatment of pain syndromes associated with peripheral neuropathy.

Tricyclic Antidepressants

The tricyclic antidepressants are thought to affect depressed mood by inhibiting synaptic re-uptake of norepinephrine and serotonin. Some of these agents, such as desipramine and nortriptyline, have a relatively greater effect on norepinephrine re-uptake

TABLE 420–2 DRUGS FOR DEPRESSION (BY STRUCTURAL GROUP)

Drug	Trade Name	Initial Dose Range	Target Dose Range	Side Effects	Comments
TRICYCLIC ANTIDEPRESSANTS					
Imipramine	Tofranil	10–75 mg	100–300 mg	Dry mouth, constipation, postural hypotension, tachyarrhythmia	
Desipramine	Norpramin	10–75 mg	100–200 mg		
Amitriptyline	Elavil	10–50 mg	100–300 mg		
Trimipramine	Surmontil	25–75 mg	200–300 mg		
Nortriptyline	Pamelor	10–50 mg	75–150 mg		
Protriptyline	Vivactil	10–30 mg	20–50 mg		
Doxepin	Sinequan	25–75 mg	75–300 mg		
TETRACYCLIC					
Maprotiline	Ludiomil	25–75 mg	100–300 mg		
SELECTIVE SEROTONIN RE-UPTAKE INHIBITORS					
Fluoxetine	Prozac	10–20 mg/day	10–80 mg/day	Nervousness, insomnia, tremor, agitation, headache, weight loss	
Sertraline	Zoloft	50 mg/day	50–200 mg/day		
Paroxetine	Paxil	20 mg/day	20–50 mg/day		
Fluvoxamine	Luvox	50 mg/day	50–300 mg/day		
Escitalopram	Lexapro	10 mg/day	10–20 mg/day		
MONOAMINE OXIDASE INHIBITORS					
Phenelzine	Nardil	15–45 mg	45–75 mg	Hypertensive crises; sedation, tremor	Patients taking these drugs must be on a tyramine-free diet
Tranylcypromine	Parnate	10–20 mg	20–30 mg		
ATYPICAL OR NONTRICYCLIC ANTIDEPRESSANTS					
Amoxapine	Asendin	25–75 mg	100–300 mg		
Trazodone	Desyrel	25–75 mg/day in divided doses	300 mg/day in divided doses	Priapism	Helpful as second drug for sleep disturbance
Nefazodone	Serzone	100 mg bid	200–400 mg	Headache and drowsiness sometimes associated	As effective as imipramine
Venlafaxine	Effexor	25 mg tid	200–275 mg/day, tid dosing	Hypertension	Serotonin/norepinephrine re-uptake inhibitor; may be effective in treatment of resistant depression
Mirtazapine	Remeron	15 mg/day	30–45 mg/day	Somnolence, weight gain	Increase at 1- to 2-wk intervals
Bupropion	Wellbutrin	100 mg bid	300 mg/day, tid dosing	Affects dopamine and norepinephrine re-uptake	May be especially helpful for atypical depression
Duloxetine	Cymbalta	20 mg/day	30 mg bid	Nausea, weight loss	Additionally useful in pain syndromes

Rx

systems. Others, such as amitriptyline, have a broader effect on serotonin systems. As a group, however, the tricyclic antidepressants have the disadvantage that they affect neurochemical systems that are not thought to be essential for antidepressant efficacy, including the histaminergic, adrenergic, and acetylcholinergic systems. Tricyclic antidepressants have a wide range of side effects such as postural hypotension, cardiac tachyarrhythmias, urinary retention, and constipation. These drugs are considered second-line agents for the treatment of depression, to be used in patients in whom treatment with SSRIs fails or in patients who have special complicating medical conditions, such as spastic bladder or parkinsonism. In these latter situations, the side effects of the tricyclic agents may be beneficial.

Monoamine Oxidase Inhibitors

The monoamine oxidase inhibitors used in psychiatric practice are irreversible inhibitors of both forms (A and B) of brain monoamine oxidase. These drugs are rarely used now because of their potentially dangerous interactions with dietary tyramine and other agents that have sympathomimetic or serotoninergic properties.

Prognosis

Depressive disorders should generally be considered to be chronic and recurring. Up to 70% of patients who have one major depression episode will have another. When antidepressant medications are discontinued, clinical surveillance should be continued according to the individual circumstances of each patient.

Risk of Suicide

Suicide is a uniquely human behavior for which we have only a limited psychobiologic understanding. Completed suicides are common in the United States and account for some 30,000 deaths each year. A much greater number of people attempt suicide, with variable degrees of intentionality. The most powerful associated features for completed suicide are current depression, alcohol abuse, and chronic medical illness. Suicide rates are highest for men older than 69 years, and rates are higher in whites and Native Americans than in other racial groups.

Most people who commit suicide have seen a physician within the previous month. Analysis of these physician visits suggests that clinical clues were probably conveyed but not adequately appreciated by the treating clinicians, in part because of the difficulty of recognizing depression in ambulatory general medical settings. When there is any suspicion

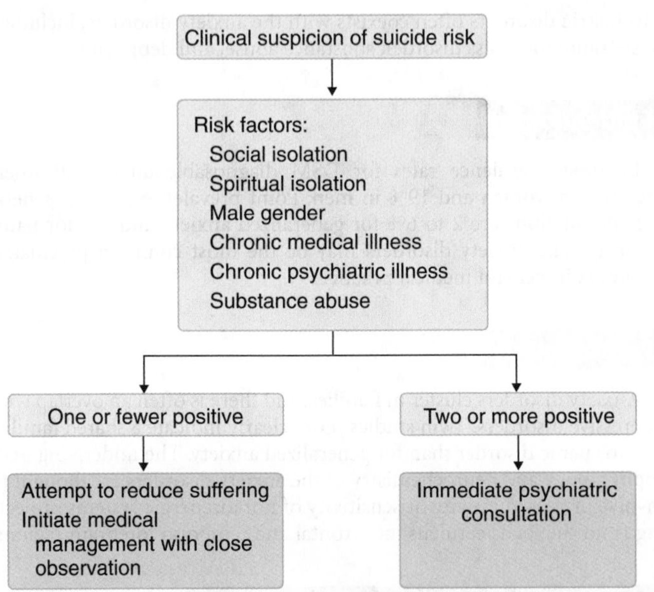

FIGURE 420–1 • Approach to a depressed patient at potential risk for suicide.

about potential suicide, it is important to ask patients directly. When depressive symptoms are more severe or when they include features of agitation or delusional ideas, the risk for suicide is greater (Fig. 420–1). Older age, male gender, and intercurrent alcohol abuse are also risk factors. Social isolation is a powerful risk factor, as is chronic painful medical illness. Consultation with a psychiatrist is essential for high-risk patients.

Bipolar Disorders

Definition

Bipolar disorders (previously called *manic-depressive disorders*) are characterized by swings in mood from depressive episodes to manic episodes. Normal behavior is usually seen between episodes. Psychotic features may accompany the manic phases of these disorders. There is little difficulty in recognizing the illness over a longitudinal course. If patients are examined only briefly at a particular moment in time, however, manic excitement can be confused with schizophrenic psychosis. The severe depressive phase of bipolar illness can also be misconstrued as a catatonic state. During the acute phases, bipolar disorders should be managed by psychiatrists.

Epidemiology

The lifetime risk for the development of bipolar illness ranges from 0.6 to 0.9%. The annual new-case incidence is 9 to 15 per 100,000 in men and 7.4 to 32 per 100,000 in women. The average age at onset of bipolar disorder is about 30 years, but about 20% of patients have an onset before 20 years of age. In women, onset of the condition has a bimodal distribution, with one peak falling between 20 and 30 years and the other far earlier, but the age at onset of bipolar illness overlaps enough that the differential diagnosis of a psychotic illness in a young person is difficult and may change as the clinical picture evolves over time.

Pathobiology

There is familial risk for bipolar illness, with 72% concordance in monozygotic twins and 19% concordance in same-sex dizygotic twins. The genetic loci associated with risk for bipolar disorder are not yet known and may vary with the phenotypic subtypes of the syndrome. The underlying neuropathophysiology of bipolar illness may differ somewhat from that of the major depressive disorders and may overlap with other psychiatric disorders, including the schizophrenias.

TABLE 420–3 MAJOR DIAGNOSTIC CRITERIA FOR A MANIC EPISODE

A distinct period of abnormally and persistently elevated, expansive, or irritable mood lasting at least 1 week (or any duration if hospitalization is necessary)

During the period of mood disturbance, at least three of the following symptoms have persisted (four if the mood is only irritable) and have been present to a significant degree:

1. Inflated self-esteem or grandiosity
2. Decreased need for sleep (e.g., feels rested after only 3 hours of sleep)
3. More talkative than usual or feels pressure to keep talking
4. Flight of ideas or subjective experiences that thoughts are racing
5. Distractibility (i.e., attention too easily drawn to unimportant or irrelevant external stimuli)
6. Increase in goal-directed activity (socially, at work or school, or sexually) or psychomotor agitation
7. Excessive involvement in pleasurable activities that have a high potential for painful consequences (e.g., engaging in unrestrained buying sprees, sexual indiscretions, or foolish business investments)

The mood disturbance is sufficiently severe to cause marked impairment in occupational functioning or in usual social activities or relationships with others to necessitate hospitalization to prevent harm to self or others

The symptoms are not due to the direct effects of a substance (e.g., drugs of abuse, medication) or a general medical condition (e.g., hyperthyroidism)

Clinical Manifestations and Diagnosis

The manic phase of bipolar disorder is characterized by an expansive, euphoric mood in which the patient is subject to grandiose plans and ideas (Table 420–3). Despite this expansiveness and grandiosity, patients who are frustrated or confronted often become irritable and sometimes aggressive. The patient can be psychotic in the manic phase, with delusions and hallucinations consistent with grandiosity; persecutory delusions (i.e., feelings of being controlled) may also be present. At times, it is difficult to distinguish an excited schizophrenic patient from a manic patient until either a depressive episode occurs or the course deteriorates into a schizophrenic process. In all instances, it is crucial to exclude metabolic and other medical disorders, particularly in older patients.

Almost half of patients with bipolar disorder have at least two or three episodes of illness, and a third experience seven or more episodes after the pattern has started. Each episode of illness, whether manic or depressive, can last 4 to 13 months; some become chronic, and some cease much sooner. Shorter durations are usually related to the effectiveness of treatment. Although some patients rapidly alternate between extremes over a period of 2 to 4 days, most episodes have a longer duration, and a manic phase frequently follows a depressive phase.

Treatment

Treatment of bipolar disorder has to approach two phases of the disease: the acute relapse, which may be mania, depression, or both, and long-term prevention of relapse. Treatment of an acute relapse is usually undertaken in the hospital, especially for patients who have manic features or severe depressive symptoms. Psychotropic drugs are the mainstay of this phase of treatment, and a combination of lithium and an antipsychotic drug such as olanzapine is most commonly used. [3] Antiepileptic drugs such as valproate or carbamazepine can be substituted for lithium in the treatment of acute manic and mixed phases of bipolar disorder.

Treatment to prevent relapse has historically relied on lithium or an antiepileptic drug. Olanzapine is associated with a substantial risk for adverse effects on various cardiovascular risk factors, including glucose tolerance, cholesterol levels, and blood pressure (Chapter 460). Integration of a psychotherapy, either cognitive or supportive (see later), with medications is optimal for preventing relapses.

Before lithium therapy is begun, a complete blood cell count, urinalysis, electrolytes, creatinine level, blood urea nitrogen level, thyroid function studies, and a baseline electrocardiogram should be obtained. Chronic medical illnesses, especially renal insufficiency, can be contraindications to lithium therapy. Lithium carbonate is available in 300-mg tablets or capsules, and a 300-mg slow-release tablet is available. The starting dose of lithium carbonate for acute mania is generally 300 mg three or four times per day. Lithium has a half-life of 24 to 36 hours, and it takes at least 4 days to achieve a steady state. Its specific therapeutic effectiveness is not evident until at least 4 to 10 days after the institution of therapy. The serum level of lithium should be monitored and the dose adjusted accordingly. The dosage should be adjusted upward by a full or half tablet after the serum level is checked during this time. Adequate levels for acute illness are 0.8 to 1.4 mEq/L. For maintenance therapy, blood levels of about 0.4 mEq/L are desirable. The dose and blood level should be titrated, however, against clinical effectiveness for each patient. Doses are usually given twice daily because absorption from the gastrointestinal tract is rapid and serum drug levels peak within 1 to 2 hours. Elevation of serum lithium levels to more than 2 mEq/L is toxic and a medical emergency requiring immediate hospitalization and possibly hemodialysis (Chapter 133). Side effects of the long-term use of lithium include the development of mild leukocytosis, hypothyroidism, diabetes insipidus, and renal tubular damage. Many patients have a tremor that can be embarrassing and occasionally interferes with activities.

Olanzapine is administered once daily, starting at 10 mg and increasing in 5-mg steps to 20 mg/day, if necessary. Monitoring for drug-induced change in weight, total cholesterol, triglycerides, and serum glucose should be performed at initiation of treatment and at 3-month intervals thereafter. Management of these cardiovascular risk factors should be carried out as for the population at large if in the judgment of the treating clinician the olanzapine is of substantial benefit for the patient. Valproate is initiated at 750 mg/day in divided doses, with increases every 3 to 4 days until a serum trough concentration greater than 50 µg/mL is achieved. Most patients require 1000 to 2500 mg/kg/day in divided doses two or three times per day.

Prognosis

Relapse episodes of bipolar disorder produce major disruptions in psychological, social, and vocational function. Divorce and job loss are common. Long-term, residual symptoms are more common. Most bipolar patients will face one or more relapses during the course of what must be considered a lifelong disease. Their long-term functional outcome depends on the frequency and severity of the affective episodes, response to treatment, and the care and quality with which that treatment is applied. Mortality with bipolar illness averages 2 to 2.5 times the age-expected rate; 8 to 10% of patients commit suicide.

Anxiety Disorders

Definition

The anxiety disorders, which occur across the entire lifespan, are accompanied by an array of neuropsychiatric symptoms, including nervousness, fearfulness, sleeplessness, dyspnea, chest pain, gastrointestinal distress, and others. These disorders generally occur in two patterns: (1) chronic, generalized anxiety and (2) episodic, panic-like anxiety. Episodic anxiety is often context dependent, such as the performance anxiety of a musician before an audience. When panic attacks occur, however, they are qualitatively different from generalized anxiety. The patient typically experiences a sudden onset of intense fear, arousal, and somatic symptoms without provocation. Panic attacks are often confused with systemic medical illnesses such as angina pectoris or epilepsy. A spectrum of related psychiatric disorders often coexists with the anxiety disorders, including post-traumatic stress disorder, substance abuse, and depression.

Epidemiology

Lifetime prevalence rates for DSM diagnosable anxiety disorders are 30% in women and 19% in men. Point prevalence rates in general U.S. populations are 2 to 6% for generalized anxiety and 1% for panic disorder. The anxiety disorders may be the most common psychiatric disorders in general medical practice.

Pathobiology

Anxiety disorders cluster in families, and there is often an overlap with depressive disorders. Twin studies more clearly indicate a shared familial risk for panic disorder than for generalized anxiety. The underlying neurophysiology and neurochemistry of the anxiety disorders are thought to involve increased activity or sensitivity of noradrenergic systems projecting from the locus ceruleus into frontal and temporal forebrain regions.

Clinical Manifestations and Diagnosis

Diagnostic criteria for generalized anxiety disorder (DSM-IV) emphasize the presence of unrealistic or excessive worry and apprehension about two or more life circumstances for a period of 6 months or longer, during which time the person has been bothered more days than not by these concerns. At least six symptoms from Table 420–4 must be present during these periods.

Panic attacks are characterized by the sudden onset of intense apprehension, fear, or a sense of impending doom. These attacks are often spontaneous and may overlap with the more generalized anxiety disorder described earlier (Table 420–5).

Treatment

In acute anxiety or panic disorder, the short-term efficacy of pharmacologic agents as measured by panic-free rates is high, with success rates of 50 to 70%. Four classes of medications have been shown to be effective in reducing recurrent panic attacks: SSRIs, tri-

TABLE 420–4 DIAGNOSTIC SYMPTOMS FOR ANXIETY AND PANIC

MOTOR TENSION

Trembling, twitching, or feeling shaky
Muscle tension, aches, or soreness
Restlessness
Easy fatigability

AUTONOMIC HYPERACTIVITY

Shortness of breath or smothering sensations
Palpitations or accelerated heart rate (tachycardia)
Sweating or cold, sweaty hands
Dry mouth
Dizziness or lightheadedness
Nausea, diarrhea, or other abdominal distress
Flashes (hot flashes) or chills
Frequent urination
Trouble swallowing or "lump in throat"

VIGILANCE AND SCANNING

Feeling keyed up or on edge
Exaggerated startle response
Difficulty concentrating or "mind going blank" because of anxiety
Trouble falling or staying asleep
Irritability

TABLE 420–5 DIAGNOSTIC CRITERIA FOR PANIC DISORDERS

One or more panic attacks (discrete periods of intense fear or discomfort) have occurred that (1) were unexpected (i.e., did not occur immediately before or on exposure to a situation that almost always caused anxiety) and (2) were not triggered by situations in which the person was the focus of others' attention

Either four attacks have occurred within a 4-week period or one or more attacks have been followed by a period of at least 1 month of persistent fear of having another attack

At least four of the following symptoms developed during at least one of the attacks:
- Shortness of breath (dyspnea) or smothering sensations
- Dizziness, unsteady feelings, or faintness
- Palpitations or accelerated heart rate (tachycardia)
- Trembling
- Sweating
- Choking
- Nausea or abdominal distress
- Depersonalization or derealization
- Numbness or tingling sensations (paresthesia)
- Flashes (hot flashes) or chills
- Chest pain or discomfort
- Fear of dying
- Fear of "going crazy" or of doing something uncontrolled

During at least some of these attacks at least four of the symptoms developed suddenly and increased in intensity within 10 minutes of the beginning of the first symptom noticed in the attack

Rx

cyclic antidepressants, benzodiazepines, and monoamine oxidase inhibitors. Drugs from all four classes have roughly comparable efficacy. Treatment is generally initiated with either SSRIs or benzodiazepines. All the available SSRIs in the United States have support from clinical trials to justify their use in the treatment of panic disorder. The doses of SSRIs for panic disorder should be at the high end of the ranges presented in Table 420–2. Alprazolam has been studied more extensively than other benzodiazepines for the treatment of panic disorder. Typically, its dosing is initiated at 0.5 mg twice daily and increased to 6 to 8 mg/day if clinically necessary to control symptoms. Many patients require ongoing pharmacotherapy, and others have symptoms despite treatment.

For generalized or chronic anxiety, the antidepressants are much less efficacious. The short-term relief afforded by almost any benzodiazepine is dramatic in generalized anxiety, but habituation and addiction are common, so caution should be exercised. If the generalized anxiety symptoms have any situational quality, other therapeutic measures should be considered before benzodiazepines are prescribed. Variations of cognitive behavioral psychotherapy should be tried, including reassurance, education, relaxation exercises, hypnosis, and other psychotherapies. Environmental alterations may be considered at home or at work, depending on the individual's specific anxiety symptoms. When a psychopharmacologic intervention is prescribed, it should be given for a defined period of 1 to 4 weeks while the situation is reassessed by the physician. Antihistamines such as diphenhydramine, 25 mg three times a day, can be tried in some patients. Buspirone is a nonbenzodiazepine antianxiety agent that sometimes provides relief at doses of 5 mg twice a day initially. The benzodiazepines presented in Table 420–6 are effective in many

TABLE 420–6 DRUGS FOR ANXIETY AND PANIC

Drug	Trade Name	Initial Dose	Target Dose Range	Side Effects	Comments
SEDATIVE HYPNOTICS					
Chloral hydrate	Noctec	500 mg	500–1000 mg	Sedation; overdose risk	Seldom appropriate
Meprobamate	Miltown	200 mg tid	1200–1600 mg		
ANTIHISTAMINES					
Diphenhydramine	Benadryl	25 mg PO qhs	50 mg	Dry mouth, mental confusion	Most useful at bedtime for associated sleep
Hydroxyzine	Atarax	50 mg PO qhs	100 mg	Dry mouth, mental confusion	Most useful at bedtime for associated sleep
BENZODIAZEPINES					
Lorazepam	Ativan	0.5 mg PO	2–10 mg, tid dosing		Also effective for generalized anxiety
Diazepam	Valium	5 mg PO	5–10 mg bid	Addictive	Abuse potential in many
Triazolam	Halcion	0.125 mg	0.25–0.5 mg hs		
Chlordiazepoxide	Librium	5 mg bid	10–30 mg		
Temazepam	Restoril	7.5 mg hs	15–30 mg		
Alprazolam	Xanax	0.25 mg bid	2–8 mg/day	Ataxia, drowsiness	
Clorazepate	Tranxene	7.5 mg hs	15–60 mg/day		
Flurazepam	Dalmane	15 mg hs	30–60 mg	Ataxia, drowsiness	Abuse potential
Oxazepam	Serax	10 mg bid	60–120 mg/day		
Clonazepam	Klonopin	0.25 mg/day	1–3 mg/day	Sedation, ataxia	Long duration of action permits once-daily dosing
Buspirone	BuSpar	5 mg bid	20–30 mg/day	Nervousness, headache	No dependence with prolonged use
Zolpidem	Ambien	10 mg hs	10 mg hs	Habituation, drowsiness	Most useful on an as-needed basis
β-BLOCKERS					
Propranolol	Inderal	20 mg bid	Individualize, 40–120 mg/day	Bradycardia, mental confusion	Does not block the fear component of anxiety or panic

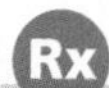

patients. Lorazepam is often the first used because it is relatively short acting (half-life of 10 to 15 hours) and easier to titrate in elderly or medically ill patients. Because its half-life is shorter than that of drugs such as diazepam, lorazepam must be taken at least twice and often three times per day. A dosage of 0.5 mg twice daily is the initial regimen for most patients. The dose should be increased by 0.5 mg/day at 3-day intervals until the target symptoms resolve or sedative side effects supervene. Elderly patients should always be watched carefully for an ataxic gait. For all patients, opportunities to taper or reduce the drug dose should be sought.

Somatoform Disorders

Definition

The somatoform disorders (Table 420–7) are a heterogeneous group of psychiatric disorders that share the common feature of mimicking medical or neurologic disease; their categorization may undergo revision in the future. The mimicry may involve an exaggeration of the severity or disability of an actual medical illness, or it may consist entirely of simulating a medical illness that is not present. In the lexicon of general medicine, some of these disorders are called "functional," some are called "pain syndromes," and some are called "conversion" or "Munchausen" syndromes. These disorders are quite common in general medical settings, where they account for as many as 25% of cases seen in primary and secondary care settings.

Epidemiology

Good epidemiologic data about the somatoform disorders are lacking. Cross-sectional studies of patients attending general neurology practices indicate prevalence rates of 15 to 20% in these populations. Disorder-specific and population-based studies are not available for these disorders.

Pathobiology

There are as yet no credible neurobiologic explanations for the somatoform disorders. Freud and colleagues believed that the symptoms were produced by a process of primary gain in which the expressed somatoform disorder provided a partial solution to an intrapsychic problem or conflict. The primary gain is not usually readily discernible because the patient is almost always unaware of it.

The *secondary gain* associated with a conversion illness refers to the clearly visible financial gain or relief from responsibility conferred by the sick role. These gains may be seen in many guises, such as disability pensions, relief from work, enhanced attention from family and physicians, and litigation payouts.

Clinical Manifestations and Diagnosis

Conversion Disorder

The essential feature of a conversion disorder is the mimicry of a discrete general medical or neurologic syndrome by a psychiatric process. Conversions typically do not conform to known anatomic systems but instead follow the individual's unconscious conceptualization of neurologic function. Conversion disorders may be episodic, as in conversion seizures, or chronic and persistent, as in the case of sensory loss or weakness. To make a valid diagnosis of conversion disorder, two features should be established: failure of the disorder to respect known neuroanatomy and neurophysiology and some positive association with unintentional psychological motivation.

Factitious Disorder

In a factitious disorder, the motivation for production of the symptom or sign must be more deliberate than in a conversion disorder but still not fully conscious. The individual may self-administer a drug or other material to create physical signs. Generally, these patients are aware of the behavior that constitutes the factitious syndrome, but they are not aware of why they are doing it.

Munchausen's syndrome, which is perhaps the best known of the factitious disorders, is defined as a repetitious pattern of medical attention–seeking behavior in which the individual has dramatic but untruthful complaints. The somatic complaints typically involve organ systems, such as abdominal pain, and tend to generate painful or invasive medical interventions.

Malingering

Malingering refers to the deliberate production of false or grossly exaggerated physical or psychological symptoms to achieve some obvious reinforcement. The secondary gain for malingering syndromes is usually obvious, such as an insurance settlement or relief from arduous duty or responsibility.

Hypochondriasis

In hypochondriasis, patients have an abnormal and emotionally heightened relationship with their medical symptoms. The symptoms

TABLE 420–7 SOMATOFORM DISORDERS

Disorder	Features
Somatization disorder	Chronic, multisystem disorder characterized by complaints of pain, gastrointestinal and sexual dysfunction, and pseudoneurologic symptoms. Onset is usually early in life, and psychosocial and vocational achievements are limited
Conversion disorder	Syndrome of symptoms or deficits mimicking neurologic or medical illness in which psychological factors are judged to be of etiologic importance
Pain disorder	Clinical syndrome characterized predominantly by pain in which psychological factors are judged to be of etiologic importance
Hypochondriasis	Chronic preoccupation with the idea of having a serious disease. The preoccupation is usually poorly amenable to reassurance
Body dysmorphic disorder	Preoccupation with an imagined or exaggerated defect in physical appearance
OTHER SOMATOFORM-LIKE DISORDERS	
Factitious disorder	Intentional production or feigning of physical or psychological signs when external reinforcers (e.g., avoidance of responsibility, financial gain) are not clearly present
Malingering	Intentional production or feigning of physical or psychological signs when external reinforcers (e.g., avoidance of responsibility, financial gain) are present
Dissociative disorders	Disruptions of consciousness, memory, identity, or perception judged to be due to psychological factors

may be related to an actual neuromedical disorder, or they may occur within the spectrum of normal physiology. A hypochondriacal individual fears the symptoms but is preoccupied with them at the same time. Social or vocational impairment occurs and is poorly responsive to reassurance from physicians.

Pain Disorder

In somatoform pain disorder, chronic and persistent pain has no neuromedical explanation nor objective manifestations. Pain clinics generally classify these disorders as "complex regional pain syndrome" (Chapter 28), but the results of physical treatments are often disappointing. Analgesic addiction is all too often the final, common psychiatric pathway for these patients.

Treatment

Rx

The long-term goal of treatment of somatoform disorders is to enable the patient to convert from a medical to a psychiatric patient. Cognitive behavioral therapy can improve hypochrondriachal manifestations and improve functioning. [4] This process requires patience and flexibility on the part of the physician. General medical interventions may be invoked initially, including biologic tests, medical rehabilitation, and pharmacotherapy. These interventions may make sense if an underlying medical disease is present or the patient adamantly views the illness as a physical one. The danger of biologic interventions is that they may strengthen the patient's conviction that the illness is physical.

If a pharmacologically accessible psychiatric symptom complex such as anxiety or depression accompanies the somatoform disorder, it may be helpful to initiate psychopharmacologic treatment. For the pain syndromes that represent masked addictions (Chapter 32), opportunities should be sought to promote the patient's entry into a drug treatment program.

Character Disorders

Definition

Behavior includes more than cognition and emotion; action and style are additional dimensions that are essential to success and satisfaction in life. Sustained dysfunctional patterns of coping with the world that involve dysfunctional patterns of action and style are called *character disorders* or *personality disorders.*

Pathobiology

All individuals have an enduring set of behavioral traits with which they faces life's challenges. These predispositions for the most part do not depend on context, and they are not easily changed from one time to another. These traits manifest themselves in style and action, especially in relationships with others. An individual is typically unaware of these qualities because they are formed in childhood as enduring aspects of personality. Qualities of character include honesty, timeliness, reliability, aggressiveness, and submissiveness.

Clinical Manifestations and Diagnosis

Some individuals have clusters of maladaptive traits that cause recurrent psychosocial difficulties (Table 420–8). In DSM-IV, these disorders are classified as Axis II disorders as opposed to the Axis I classification of the more overt major psychiatric disorders. The personality disorders have a spectrum of severity with poorly specified boundaries and thresholds. It makes clinical sense to think of "personality styles" when the maladaptive traits are less severe. The personality disorders also differ from the Axis I disorders in that they are mostly manifested in interpersonal relationships. It is difficult to imagine the diagnosis of a passive-aggressive personality style in a setting that did not include other people. Often the best clue to the diagnosis of character pathology is the pattern of behavior that the patient shows in relating to the physician. Personality disorders are difficult to recognize. Patients are not consciously aware of the data that validate their diagnoses, and they are typically sensitive when dysfunctional patterns of behavior are clarified. Physicians often do not "see" the personality disorders unless such patients provoke their physicians to feel angry or rejected.

TABLE 420–8 CHARACTER DISORDERS

Personality Type	Characteristic Behavior Patterns
Paranoid	Distrust and suspiciousness
Schizoid	Detachment from social relationships, with a restricted range of emotional expression
Schizotypal	Eccentricities in behavior and cognitive distortions; acute discomfort in close relationships
Antisocial	Disregard for rights of others; a defect in the experience of compunction or remorse for harming others
Borderline	Instability in interpersonal relationships, self-image, and affective regulation
Histrionic	Emotional overreactivity, theatrical behavior, and seductiveness
Narcissistic	Persisting grandiosity, need for admiration, and lack of empathy for others
Avoidant	Social inhibition, feelings of inadequacy, and hypersensitivity to negative evaluation
Dependent	Submission and clinging behavior
Obsessive-compulsive	Rigid, detail-oriented behavior, often associated with compulsions to perform tasks repetitively and unnecessarily

Treatment

Psychopharmacology is of limited value for the interpersonal dimensions of these disorders. The goal of management is to help patients increase their awareness of the dysfunctional interpersonal traits so that they become more self-conscious about how others are affected by their behavior. Although longer-term psychotherapies must be performed by psychiatric clinicians, general medical physicians can often provide the initial clarifying interventions. Variants of the psychotherapy type described as "interpersonal" (see later) are the most effective approach to patients who show character disorder behavior patterns in practice settings.

Schizophrenic Disorders

Definition

Schizophrenia is the "heart of madness" and is still the archetypal psychotic mental disorder. *Psychosis* is defined as a psychiatric disorder that disrupts reality testing or thought processes. Schizophrenia most often starts in late adolescence.

Epidemiology

The prevalence of schizophrenia in the general population is about 1%, with an incidence of about 0.5 per 1000 person years. The prevalence rate is eight times as great in the lower as in the higher socioeconomic groups. Because the parents of schizophrenics have a social class distribution similar to that of the general population, the lower position of the patients seems to be a result of the illness rather than the cause of it.

Of schizophrenics, 70% become ill between the ages of 15 and 35. The illness affects men and women in equal proportion over the entire lifespan. The age of peak onset risk is 15 to 24 years in men and 25 to 34 years in women. There are slight ethnic differences, with a higher incidence in Scandinavian countries and in nonwhites.

Pathobiology

Schizophrenia is a neuropsychiatric disorder with both structural and functional deficits in a variety of neural circuits interconnecting the prefrontal cortex, striatum, thalamus, and brain stem. It is not yet known to what extent these neurobiologic substrates are determined by genetics and to what extent they are determined by early developmental experiences. The evidence for genetic facilitation in schizophrenia is strong, but as in other psychiatric disorders, no single gene seems to be involved, and concordance in monozygotic twins is only 50 to 60%. The onset of clinical symptoms is often precipitated by adverse psychosocial events in early adult life. The emotional structures and patterns in families are also thought to be important in generating or maintaining some of the schizophrenic symptoms.

Clinical Manifestations and Diagnosis

The characteristic symptoms of schizophrenia fall into two broad categories described as positive and negative symptoms. Positive features include behavior such as delusions and hallucinations. Negative features include symptoms such as restricted affect, anhedonia, and apathy. When a thought process disturbance is the predominant clinical feature, the schizophrenic disorder is described as disorganized. The course of schizophrenia is usually marked by a decline in psychosocial functioning, with a tendency for the patient to become downwardly mobile in social strata. For most patients it becomes a chronic illness characterized by relapses.

Schizophrenia is defined as a long-term mental illness because psychotic features are required to persist for 6 months (Table 420–9). Psychosocial deterioration from a previous level of functioning is also required as part of the definition of schizophrenia. When a psychotic mental illness has persisted for less than 6 months, it is inadvisable to use the diagnosis of schizophrenia. Schizophrenia also tends to be characterized by acute relapses of psychotic features over time. With the first episode of any psychotic illness, an affective disorder or a systemic medical illness should be considered; psychotic episodes secondary to toxic drug reactions, sleep deprivation, and medical causes invariably persist for less than 6 months.

Subtypes of schizophrenia are defined by the predominant symptoms at the time of the most recent clinical evaluation. Subtypes include the paranoid type, the disorganized type, the catatonic type, and an undifferentiated type. Catatonic symptoms involve either markedly retarded motor behavior (often to the point of no voluntary movement; patients retain any posture into which they are passively placed) or markedly agitated motor behavior. In the paranoid forms of schizophrenia, the paranoid delusions are often the only major symptoms and tend to remain stable over time. The term *schizophrenia, residual type* is used when positive symptoms of psychosis have abated but the patient continues to have poor psychosocial function.

Treatment and Prognosis

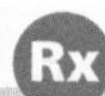

During a 25- to 30-year period, about a third of patients with schizophrenia show some recovery or remission, but the remaining patients have major residual symptoms or require long-term hospitalization. Management requires the establishment of a long-term psychotherapeutic relationship with the patient or the patient's family system, which can facilitate monitoring of the clinical course, recognition of early signs of decompensation, and enhanced compliance with psychopharmacologic treatments. Psychotherapy for schizophrenia is supportive (see later), educational, and rehabilitative in an attempt to prevent or minimize the chronic psychosocial deterioration that can occur in the course of the disease. Protected vocational and living situations are often important constituents of long-term treatment plans.

Long-term antipsychotic medication is essential to reduce relapses (Table 420–10). The initial pharmacologic therapy for psychosis should begin with the administration of one of the newer, "atypical" antipsychotic drugs. This group of drugs includes olanzapine, risperidone, quetiapine, ziprasidone, aripiprazole, and clozapine. Cloza-

TABLE 420–9 SCHIZOPHRENIA AND OTHER PSYCHOTIC DISORDERS

CHARACTERISTIC SYMPTOMS

At least two of the following, each present for a major portion of time during a 1-month period (or less if successfully treated)*:
- Delusions
- Hallucinations
- Disorganized speech (e.g., frequent derailment, "jumping from one topic to another," or incoherence)
- Grossly disorganized or catatonic behavior
- Negative symptoms (i.e., affective flattening, alogia, or avolition)

SOCIAL/OCCUPATIONAL DYSFUNCTION

For a significant portion of the time since the onset of the disturbance, one or more major areas of functioning (e.g., work, interpersonal relationships, or self-care) are markedly below the level achieved before the onset (or when the onset is in childhood or adolescence, failure to realize the expected level of interpersonal, academic, or occupational achievement)

DURATION

Continuous signs of the disturbance persist for at least 6 months. This 6-month period must include at least 1 month of characteristic symptoms as described above (i.e., active-phase symptoms) and may include periods of prodromal or residual symptoms. During these prodromal or residual periods, signs of the disturbance may be manifested by only negative symptoms or two or more of the characteristic symptoms present in an attenuated form (e.g., odd beliefs, unusual perceptual experiences)

SCHIZOAFFECTIVE AND MOOD DISORDER EXCLUSION

Schizoaffective disorder and mood disorder with psychotic features have been ruled out because (1) no major depressive or manic episodes have occurred concurrently with the active-phase symptoms or (2) if mood episodes have occurred during active-phase symptoms, their total duration has been brief in relation to the duration of the active and residual periods

SUBSTANCE/GENERAL MEDICAL CONDITION EXCLUSION

The disturbance is not due to the direct effects of a substance (e.g., drugs of abuse, medication) or a general medical condition

*Note: Only one characteristic symptom is required if delusions are bizarre or hallucinations consist of a voice keeping up a running commentary on the person's behavior or thoughts or involve two or more voices conversing with each other.

TABLE 420–10 DRUGS FOR PSYCHOSIS

Class	Generic Name	Trade Name	Acute Dose per 24 hr	Maintenance Dose	Side Effects
Phenothiazine/Aliphatic	Chlorpromazine	Thorazine	25–1000 mg PO 25–400 mg IM	25–400 mg PO	EPMD, hyperprolactinemia
Phenothiazine/ Piperazine	Perphenazine	Trilafon	8–64 mg PO 15–30 mg IM	12–24 mg PO	EPMD
	Fluphenazine	Prolixin	2.5–40 mg PO 5–20 mg IM	12.5–50 mg IM decanoate weekly	
	Trifluoperazine	Stelazine	1–5 mg PO		
Phenothiazine/ Piperidine	Thioridazine	Mellaril	25–800 mg PO	25–30 mg PO	EPMD, risk for retinal degeneration
	Mesoridazine	Serentil	50–400 mg PO	200–400 mg PO	
Butyrophenone	Haloperidol	Haldol	2–25 mg PO 6–30 mg IM	1–15 mg PO 25–200 mg IM	EPMD; can cause dysphoria at low to moderate doses decanoate monthly
Thioxanthene	Chlorprothixene	Taractan	30–100 mg PO	100–300 mg	
	Thiothixene	Navane	2–5 mg PO	5–10 mg PO	Intramuscular form available
Dibenzoxazepine	Loxapine	Loxitane	50–250 mg PO	60–100 mg	
Dihydroindole	Molindone	Moban	50–225 mg PO	20–200 mg	Less likely to reduce the seizure threshold
Benzisoxazole	Risperidone	Risperdal	2–4 mg PO	2–20 mg	Low incidence of extrapyramidal effects
Dibenzodiazepine	Olanzapine	Zyprexa	5–15 mg PO	5–10 mg PO	Fewer extrapyramidal effects; fatal agranulocytosis; sedating
	Clozapine	Clozaril	200–400 mg	200–600 mg	
Diphenylbutylpiperidine	Pimozide	Orap	10–30 mg	10–30 mg	
Phenylindole	Quetiapine	Seroquel	25 mg bid	300–400 mg/day	Low incidence of extrapyramidal effects
	Ziprasidone	Geodon	40–80 mg bid	40–80 mg bid	
Piperazinil/ dihydrocarbostyril	Aripiprazole	Abilify	10 mg/day	20–30 mg/day	Hyperglycemia

EPMD = extrapyramidal movement disorders.

pine cannot be considered first-line therapy because of its hematopoietic and hepatic side effects (Chapter 460). These agents are termed *atypical* because of their side effect spectrum, which differs significantly from that of the older, traditional antipsychotic agents such as haloperidol and chlorpromazine. As a group, the newer drugs cause less acute motor system side effects than the older drugs do and may have a lower long-term risk for tardive dyskinesias.

The relative effectiveness of these second-generation (atypical) antipsychotic drugs may not fully justify their widespread use. For example, a large randomized trial found that the efficacy of the first-generation antipsychotic drug perphenazine was equal to that of a series of second-generation drugs, including olanzapine, quetiapine, risperidone, and ziprasidone. [5] Of note was that 74% of patients in this study were unable to take their medication for the full 18-month target duration because of side effects.

As a group, the newer antipsychotic agents exacerbate cardiovascular disease risk factors such as hypertension, glucose tolerance, and hyperlipidemia. These adverse effects are significant for many patients and require continuous monitoring, usually on an every-3-month schedule (Chapter 460). The decision whether to manage such cardiovascular risk factors as in the general population while continuing the drug or to substitute an antipsychotic agent from another class must be based on the clinician's judgment of the substantive value of an individual drug for an individual patient.

Typical initial regimens include risperidone, 2 mg twice daily, with an increase to a total dose of 6 to 10 mg/day after 1 week if tolerated. Antipsychotic efficacy is usually seen in this target dose range for risperidone, with a 4- to 6-week delay for some effects. An alternative is olanzapine, which can be administered once daily. A starting dose for olanzapine is 5 mg daily, with 5-mg increases at weekly intervals to the 15- to 20-mg range if symptoms do not improve and side effects are tolerable. The aggressiveness of the dosing regimen is dictated to some extent by the quality and severity of the psychotic symptoms. The antipsychotic benefit from these drugs may be immediate, occur gradually over a period of weeks, or be delayed for 4 to 6 weeks. Additional psychotropic agents are sometimes added during the early days of treatment. A benzodiazepine (e.g., alprazolam, 0.25 mg three times daily) may be added when agitation and sleep disturbance are severe. The most frequent limiting factor in the dosing of antipsychotic drugs is the appearance of extrapyramidal side effects, including dystonia, akathisia (restlessness), and parkinsonism.

An additional risk with the use of antipsychotic drugs is the development of tardive dyskinesia. Tardive dyskinesia (Chapter 434) is a syndrome of involuntary movements, usually choreoathetoid, that can affect the mouth, lips, tongue, extremities, or trunk. Though generally associated with use of neuroleptics for 6 months or more, tardive dyskinesia can occur with shorter administration. Patients receiving neuroleptics should be evaluated periodically for these abnormal movements. Rates of tardive dyskinesia with the atypical antipsychotic medications are considerably lower than with the traditional ones but are not zero. The cause of tardive dyskinesia is not known, but it is believed to represent the development of dopaminergic hypersensitivity in extrapyramidal motor systems.

Drugs for Psychosis

Drugs that affect dopaminergic function by blocking mesolimbic dopamine receptors have the demonstrated ability to improve a variety of psychotic symptoms. The older antipsychotic drugs show broad-spectrum dopamine receptor–blocking properties; they affect all receptor subtypes, as well as nigrostriatal neurons (substantia nigra pars compacta, A9) and limbic dopaminergic neurons (ventral tegmental area, A10). Consequently, these drugs have many motor system side effects. The newer antipsychotic agents have variable effects on dopamine receptor subtypes and other neurochemical systems such as serotonin.

Risperidone

Concomitant blockade of D_2 receptors in the basal ganglia has been presumed to underlie the production of extrapyramidal syndromes by traditional antipsychotic drugs. More recently, psychopharmacologic research has turned to agents that simultaneously block D_2 and serotonin (5-HT_2) receptors. These agents have fewer extrapyramidal side effects and may be more broadly effective for the negative symptoms of schizophrenia than the traditional antipsychotic drugs are. In vitro evidence indicates that risperidone has 20-fold higher affinity for 5-HT_{2A} receptors than for D_2 receptors.

Clozapine

Clozapine was developed in Austria and Germany in the 1960s. Because of its tricyclic-like structure, it was hoped that it might be an antidepressant. Instead, it turned out to be an antipsychotic drug with no extrapyramidal side effects. Clozapine is a dibenzodiazepine with atypical properties and side effects. It possesses strong anticholinergic properties in addition to serotonin-blocking properties. It produces proportionally greater suppression of mesolimbic as opposed to striatal dopamine systems. Clozapine blocks D_2 receptors, as do other antipsychotic drugs, but it also produces a relatively greater blockade of D_1 systems, which may account for its altered pattern of efficacy and the absence of tardive dyskinesia as a side effect.

Clozapine can cause fatal agranulocytosis. An overview of available reports indicates that agranulocytosis occurs in 0.05 to 2% of patients given clozapine, a rate higher than that found in patients given other antipsychotic drugs. The agranulocytosis does not seem to be dose related. In most cases there is a several-week prodrome with a declining peripheral white blood cell count, but this prodrome is not always seen. Discontinuation of the medication does not consistently prevent progression to agranulocytosis. Most cases occur within 3 months after initiating treatment. Weekly monitoring of hematologic function is indicated for all patients receiving clozapine.

Olanzapine

Olanzapine blocks 5-HT_2 receptors in addition to a spectrum of dopamine receptor subtypes, including D_1, D_2, and D_4. It also has some anticholinergic and α_1-blocking properties. This spectrum of pharmacologic properties generates fewer extrapyramidal side effects than most older antipsychotic drugs do.

Quetiapine

Quetiapine has actions and uses similar to clozapine. It is associated with a lower incidence of agranulocytosis. Because of reports of cataracts with prolonged use, semiannual slit lamp examinations are recommended for patients taking quetiapine.

Ziprasidone

Ziprasidone is a newly approved antipsychotic drug that favorably affects positive and negative symptoms in schizophrenia. It has low rates of extrapyramidal side effects but can cause akathisia. It has been associated with a prolonged QT interval on the electrocardiogram.

Aripiprazole

Aripiprazole is the newest of the atypical antipsychotic drugs available in the United States. It is a mixed agonist/antagonist across several subtypes of dopamine and serotonin receptors.

PSYCHOPHARMACOLOGY AND PSYCHOTHERAPY

General Approach to Psychopharmacology

Some general clinical guidelines should be followed in the use of all psychotropic drugs. The physician should select in advance the symptoms that are targets for therapy, such as agitation, sleep disturbance, or depression. In addition, the clinician should establish clinical guideposts to judge the efficacy of the therapy. If the targeted symptoms fail to improve after some defined period, the therapy should be stopped or changed, or consultation should be sought.

Dosing and Timing

The two most common errors made by nonpsychiatrists who use psychopharmacologic agents are inadequate dosing and not waiting long enough to observe the expected effect. For all agents, the first approach to a suboptimal response should be to increase the dose of the selected drug either to a predetermined total daily target or to a maximal tolerated dose. Second, the physician must wait for a predetermined time, usually 4 to 6 weeks for antidepressant and antipsychotic drugs, to allow evidence of clinical efficacy to emerge.

Clinical Familiarity

Effective use of these drugs, as with other pharmacologic agents, requires practical expertise that comes only from experience. Clinicians should not attempt to become familiar with all psychopharmacologic drugs equally but should develop experience-based familiarity with one or two agents from each category.

General Approach to Psychotherapy

Of the total scope of ambulatory psychiatric morbidity, 90% is treated by primary care and other nonpsychiatric physicians. Restriction of these general medical therapies to psychopharmacology is too narrow in view of increasingly persuasive evidence of the efficacy of psychotherapies for neurotic psychiatric illness. At present, however, there is no generally accepted model by which to bring psychotherapeutic skills into the general medical setting. It has been argued persuasively for decades that nonpsychiatric physicians perform various forms of psychotherapy on a regular basis through the relationships that they already have with their patients. These practitioners can work to improve their psychotherapeutic effectiveness.

Theory of the Therapeutic Relationship

The patient comes to the physician because of an experienced need. There is almost always a perceived need for help that may be more or less developed and conceptualized, depending on the individual patient. It is from this fundamental need for assistance that the possibility of a therapeutic relationship arises. Nonpsychiatric physicians may underestimate the emotional depth and potential psychotherapeutic power of this therapeutic relationship. This relationship already exists in nascent form with many of their patients and is an underused therapeutic tool.

Psychotherapeutic Strategies

The fundamental skills of psychotherapy are largely generic and independent of technical expertise. These skills include empathy, sensitivity to emotional cues, the capacity to listen actively, and the ability to intervene with corrective information at acceptable time points as patients talk. When psychopharmacologic agents are prescribed, clinicians should generally craft some complementary psychotherapy in parallel. Several general approaches can be used.

Cognitive Behavioral Therapy

Behavioral therapy is a psychotherapy based on the general principle that interventions should be focused on behavior, thoughts, and emotions that are present at a given time. Such a hypothesis underlies most of our educational endeavors and is readily understandable to most physicians. Key elements of this psychotherapeutic technique are clarification, education, and emotional support. This strategy is commendable as a first-line therapeutic strategy for most mild psychiatric problems. This approach is similar to the approach that physicians use for other clinical problems.

Psychodynamic Therapy

Psychodynamic psychotherapy refers to more time-limited versions of psychotherapy that derive from psychoanalytic theory. One of the basic tenets of such therapies is that we do not fully understand ourselves, our motivations, our feelings, the ways in which we affect others, and the ways in which we are affected by important experiences earlier in life. The healing process of the dynamic or insight-oriented therapies is to increase this self-understanding. Freud allowed his patients to think and speak freely during his sessions with them while he listened intently for clues about meanings and motivations that were not quite consciously understood by the patients. He described resistances that patients showed to keep painful feelings and conflicts from emerging into conscious life, and he wrote about transference, or the application to the physician of emotional attachment behavior that derives from other areas of the patient's life experience. One of the major advantages of this perspective is that it permits the clinician to take full account of the strengths of individuals as they have expressed themselves across their entire life course. The technical skills most important in this technique include active listening, empathic connections with the patient, and the ability to make interpretive connections to previous life events.

Interpersonal Therapy

The interpersonal approach to psychotherapy is directed explicitly at the group system in which a patient lives or works, as opposed to the patient as an individual. It is a relationship-oriented psychotherapy. An approach to the family is a variation of interpersonal therapy and is performed whenever the physician brings family members into the examination room. Couples therapy is also a form of interpersonal psychotherapy and is the most common type of family therapy performed by nonpsychiatric clinicians. In these therapies, the physician addresses some difficulty in the interpersonal system. The relationship patterns of the system must be considered, and the positive strengths must be identified. The problem must be amenable to definition within such a relationship system. The simplest metaphor to use for interpersonal therapy in medical settings is the system-wide impact of the medical illness being experienced by the identified patient.

Guideline

A rough guideline to set a work plan for a medical psychotherapy might consider the following technical points:

Diagnosis: Define the problem in psychosocial terms in a way that makes sense to the patient and family.

Work plan: Set an initial number of talking visits and specify the frequency and duration of each visit.

Strategy: Consider the overview strategies outlined here, and consider which strategies might be best applicable to the situation at hand.

Consultation: Be prepared to request a psychiatric consultation.

Grade A

1. March J, Silva S, Petrycki S, et al: Treatment for Adolescents with Depression Study (TADS) Team: Fluoxetine, cognitive-behavioral therapy, and their combination for adolescents with depression: Treatment for Adolescents with Depression Study (TADS) randomized controlled trial. JAMA 2004;292:807–820.
2. Hansen RA, Gartlehner G, Lohr KN, et al: Efficacy and safety of second-generation antidepressants in the treatment of major depressive disorder. Ann Intern Med 2005;143:415–426.
3. Tohen M, Greil W, Calabrese JR, et al: Olanzapine versus lithium in the maintenance treatment of bipolar disorder: A 12-month, randomized, double-blind, controlled clinical trial. Am J Psychiatry 2005;162:1281–1290.
4. Barsky AJ, Ahern DK: Cognitive behavior therapy for hypochondriasis: A randomized controlled trial. JAMA 2004;291:1464–1470.
5. Lieberman JA, Stroup TS, McEvoy JP, et al: Effectiveness of antipsychotic drugs in patients with chronic schizophrenia. N Engl J Med 2005;353:1209–1223.

SUGGESTED READINGS

Benazzi F: Bipolar disorder—focus on bipolar II disorder and mixed depression. Lancet 2007;369:935–945. *A comprehensive review of bipolar II disorder and mixed depression.*

Katon WJ: Panic disorder. N Engl J Med 2006;354:2360–2367. *A case-based review.*

Kroenke K, Spitzer RL, Williams JB, et al: Anxiety disorders in primary care: Prevalence, impairment, comorbidity, and detection. Ann Intern Med 2007;146:317–325. *An overview of the current prevalence, impairment, and comorbidity of anxiety disorders in a primary care setting and a description of a method to enhance detection.*

Mann JJ: The medical management of depression. N Engl J Med 2005;353:1819–1834. *Overview of treatment options.*

Mayou R, Kirmayer LJ, Simon G, et al: Somatoform disorders: Time for a new approach in DSM-V. Am J Psychiatry 2005;162:847–855. *Diagnosis and treatment review.*

Schneier FR: Social anxiety disorder. N Engl J Med 2006;355:1029–1036. *Also known as social phobia, it is one of the most common psychiatric disorders.*

Vieweg WVR, Julius DA, Fernandez A, et al: Post-traumatic stress disorder: Clinical features, pathophysiology, and treatment. Am J Med 2006;119:383–390. *A detailed review.*

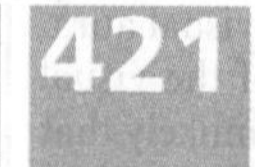

421 HEADACHES AND OTHER HEAD PAIN

F. Michael Cutrer and Michael A. Moskowitz

Definition

Headache is a very common complaint encountered by practitioners in almost every specialty of medicine and surgery. More than 90% of the population experience headache of one type or another at least once during life. The very common occurrence of headache sometimes leads to an underestimation of its potential importance as a symptom. Although headaches may be associated with minor trauma or febrile illness, they may also result from potentially life-threatening central nervous system (CNS) disease. Fortunately, most patients with recurrent or chronic headaches suffer from a primary headache disorder for which no ominous underlying source can be found. Though reassuring, this lack of identifiable cause does not diminish the patient's suffering or economic loss.

Pathobiology

A headache signifies activation of the primary afferent fibers that innervate cephalic blood vessels, chiefly meningeal or cerebral blood vessels. Most nociceptive fibers innervating these structures arise from pseudounipolar neurons located within the trigeminal ganglia (first division), although some may be located within the upper cervical ganglia. Stimuli activating these fibers are quite variable and can range from direct mechanical traction by a tumor to chemical irritation caused by CNS infection or subarachnoid blood. In patients with so-called *secondary headache disorders,* headaches result from an identifiable structural or inflammatory source. In these patients, treatment of the primary abnormality often results in resolution of the headache. However, most patients with chronic headaches have *primary headache disorders,* such as migraine or tension headache, for which the results of physical examination and laboratory studies are generally normal. With the absence of an identifiable cause, the mode of trigeminal activation in migraine has been hotly debated. Traditional theories have been dominated by two points of view.

The *vasogenic theory* is that intracranial vasoconstriction is responsible for symptoms of the migraine aura and that the headache results from rebound dilation and distention of cranial vessels and activation of perivascular nociceptive axons. This theory is based on the observations that (1) extracranial vessels distend and pulsate during a migraine attack in many patients, thus implying that cranial vessels might be of primary importance; (2) stimulation of intracranial vessels in awake patients results in an ipsilateral headache; and (3) substances that cause vasoconstriction, such as ergot alkaloids, abort headache, whereas vasodilators, such as nitrates, can provoke an attack.

The alternative hypothesis, the *neurogenic theory,* identifies the brain as the generator of migraine and proposes that the susceptibility of any individual to migraine attacks reflects thresholds intrinsic to the brain; the vascular changes occurring during migraine are the result rather than the cause of the attack. Supporters of the neurogenic hypothesis point to the observation that migraine attacks are often accompanied by a range of focal (in the aura) and vegetative (in the prodrome) neurologic symptoms that cannot be explained simply by vasoconstriction within a single neurovascular distribution.

It is likely that elements of both theories explain some of the pathophysiology of migraine and other primary headache disorders. Imaging (i.e., magnetic resonance imaging [MRI] and positron emission tomography [PET]) and genetic studies confirm that migraine and related headaches are disorders of neurovascular regulation.

Brain-Initiated Events

Clinical and experimental observations suggest that the brain, though usually insensate, can activate or sensitize (directly or indirectly) trigeminal nerve fibers within the meninges. One example in which headache is initiated by events within the brain occurs in migraine with visual aura. Imaging studies during migraine attacks implicate a cortical spreading depression–like phenomenon as the mechanism in migraine visual aura. The decreased levels of deoxyhemoglobin in affected areas of the visual cortex during the opening seconds of the visual aura make it unlikely that ischemia is the cause of the visual scintillations. In this form of migraine, endogenous neurophysiologic (cortical spreading depression–like) events in the neocortex may promote the release of nociceptive substances (e.g., potassium, protons, arachidonate metabolites) from the neocortex into the interstitial space. Within the Virchow-Robin spaces, the released substances accumulate to levels sufficient to activate or sensitize the trigeminovascular fibers that surround the pial vessels supplying the draining neocortex. Under steady-state conditions, the brain vigorously maintains equilibrium of its extracellular environment, and ions or transmitters normally released from cellular compartments are rapidly taken up in glia and neurons at rates that maintain constant levels of these ions, transmitters, and neuromodulators. Blood vessels provide a backup clearance mechanism that is not invoked in normal conditions. However, before the onset of headache, mechanisms associated with spreading oligemia may enhance release of the various substances, block uptake and inactivation—thereby increasing extracellular levels—and overwhelm the normal clearance mechanisms. The substances released may discharge or sensitize small unmyelinated nociceptive fibers and provide the trigger for headache or sensitize perivascular afferents to blood-borne or other as yet unidentified factors. The headache latency (20 to 40 minutes) observed in migraine may reflect the time needed for extracellular levels to exceed a threshold for axonal depolarization and for sensitization to occur within peripheral and central neurons. In this formulation, the brain becomes a master switch, a transducer. Triggering events, such as those associated with emotional stress, fatigue, bright lights, and too little (or too much) sleep, modulate activity within regions of the brain that are physically contiguous to the meningeal vessels innervated by the trigeminal nerve. In susceptible individuals, these events may provide a sufficient trigger for subsequent neurophysiologic events that lead to chemical activation of meningeal fibers. The photophobia, nausea, and vomiting associated with migraine are probably related to the consequences of meningeal irritation because similar symptoms also occur during meningeal infection or when blood enters the subarachnoid space. This pathogenetic framework for migraine is consistent with the currently understood principles of neurobiology and the physiology of pain. However, some of the details will require revision as data emerge from additional experimental studies in humans and animals.

Central Nervous System Dysfunction

Several observations and recent studies are consistent with the notion that CNS dysfunction may underlie migraine and cluster headache. For example, unilateral headaches tend to occur on the side corresponding to the dysfunctional hemisphere. In addition, studies of cluster headache and migraine without aura have shown changes in blood flow in the hypothalamus and the rostral brain stem, respectively. Furthermore, MRI has shown an increased deposition of nonheme iron in patients with migraine. Another MRI study showed an increase in subclinical white matter lesions within the cerebellum of patients with migraine headache; subjects with frequent migraines with aura had more cerebellar lesions. In each case, the pain develops from trigeminal activation in sensitized axons as a consequence of actual or threatened tissue injury.

PRIMARY HEADACHE DISORDERS

Migraine

Epidemiology

Migraine is the second most common primary headache disorder and has a prevalence of about 12%. It affects women disproportionately (approximately 18.2% of women vs. 6.5% of men in the United States) and commonly afflicts the population during the most productive years of life (peak prevalence, 25 to 45 years old).

Pathobiology

Genetics

A higher than expected prevalence of migraine has been observed in the relatives of migraine patients. In one large family study drawn from the general population, the risk for migraine in relatives of patients with migraines was three times higher than the risk in controls. Data from large twin registries have consistently revealed higher concordance rates for migraine in monozygotic twins than in dizygotic pairs. One study of more than 2500 monozygotic and 5000 dizygotic twin pairs estimated that 40 to 50% of the susceptibility to migraine is genetically based. Although migraine is widely thought to reflect an autosomal dominant condition, segregational analysis has failed to identify any single mendelian pattern of transmission. During the past few years, several novel migraine susceptibility genes have been identified in families by linkage analysis. These novel polymorphisms map to loci on chromosomes 19 (19p13), 6 (6p12.2-21.1), X (Xq24-28), and 4 (4q24) for the more common types of migraine, whereas loci for uncommon subtypes have been proposed on chromosomes 19 (19p13), 1 (1q21-23;1q31), and most recently 2 (2q24) as discussed later.

Familial Hemiplegic Migraine

Perhaps the most compelling genetic evidence to date comes from the identification of specific genetic loci for familial hemiplegic migraine. Familial hemiplegic migraine is an autosomal dominant disorder characterized by transient hemiplegia during the aura phase of a migraine attack. This rare migraine subtype has been linked to point mutations in the gene *CACNL1A4* located on chromosome 19p13 in 50% of affected families. Other genetic mutations in groups of families with familial hemiplegic migraine have been linked to chromosomes 1q31 (*ATP1A2* gene encoding an N^+/K^+ pump) and 2q24 (*SCN1A* gene coding for a voltage-gated sodium channel), thus implying genetic heterogeneity. Except for cerebellar atrophy in cases of disease that can be mapped to 19p13, no obvious clinical distinctions can be identified between affected families with and without this abnormal gene. The defective gene on chromosome 19 codes for the α_1-subunit of a brain-specific P/Q calcium channel that is coupled to the release of neurotransmitters and is expressed throughout the human brain. The mutant channel has been shown to cause increased calcium influx in response to depolarizations that are insufficient to open unmutated channels. It is unclear how sustained neurologic deficits and migraine result from a defect in an ion channel that operates (i.e., opens and shuts) in milliseconds.

Clinical Manifestations and Diagnosis

Migraine falls into two categories: *migraine without an aura* (previously called common migraine), which occurs in about 85% of patients, and *migraine with an aura* (previously called classic migraine), which occurs in about 15 to 20% of patients. Migraine patients with and without an aura may report prodromal symptoms that begin 24 to 48 hours before a headache attack. These symptoms can include hyperactivity, mild euphoria, lethargy, depression, craving for certain foods, fluid retention, and frequent yawning. Prodromal symptoms should not be confused with the migraine aura that consists of transient episodes of focal neurologic dysfunction appearing 1 to 2 hours before the onset of a migraine headache and resolving within 60 minutes. The aura symptoms may be of different types, and more than a single symptom type may be present within a given aura. Typical aura symptoms include homonymous (rarely monocular) visual disturbance, classically an expanding scotoma with a scintillating margin; unilateral paresthesias or numbness (or both), often affecting the hands and feet or the perioral region of the face; unilateral weakness; and dysphasia or other language disturbances. Sometimes aura symptoms localize to the brain stem and may include vertigo, dysarthria, tinnitus, fluctuating hearing loss, diplopia, bilateral weakness, ataxia, bilateral paresthesias, and a decreased level of consciousness. *Basilar migraine* is the diagnosis in patients in whom brain stem symptoms predominate. In many patients, basilar attacks are intermingled with more typical migraine attacks. Dizziness is frequently reported as a feature of an otherwise typical attack of migraine without an aura. Bilateral paresthesias can also occur with anxiety and hyperventilation.

The headache phase of a migraine attack (with or without aura) consists of 4 to 72 hours of unilateral throbbing head pain that is of moderate to severe intensity, worsened by routine physical exertion, and associated with nausea, photophobia, and phonophobia. *Complicated migraine* or *migraine with a prolonged aura* refers to migraine attacks associated with aura symptoms that persist for more than 1 hour but less than 1 week with normal neuroimaging studies. If symptoms persist for more than 1 week or result in neuroimaging abnormalities, migrainous infarction is likely. In general, migrainous infarction develops in the context of stereotypical aura symptoms.

Status Migrainosus

Migraine attacks that persist for longer than 72 hours despite treatment are classified as *status migrainosus.* During *status migrainosus,* headache-free periods of less than 4 hours (sleep not included) may occur. Status migrainosus is usually associated with prolonged use of analgesics and may require inpatient treatment with detoxification.

Treatment

Rx

Migraine therapy includes nonpharmacologic and pharmacologic interventions. Nonpharmacologic treatment consists of behavior modification techniques such as avoidance of triggering factors (e.g., ingestion of particular foods or food additives, strong smells, glaring light) and establishment of regular meals and consistent sleeping patterns. Other techniques to minimize the effects of environmental stress, such as biofeedback, relaxation training, rational motive therapy, self-hypnosis, and meditation, are sometimes helpful.

Medical Therapy

Pharmacologic treatment of migraine includes abortive therapy to shorten the attack or decrease the severity of the headache. In patients with infrequent and uncomplicated attacks, abortive medications are often sufficient. If migraines cause disability more than 3 days per month, daily prophylactic treatment may be taken to decrease the frequency and, less often, the severity of attacks. If taken at the time of attacks, prophylactic agents are usually ineffective, and agents used for treatment during an attack provide little protection against subsequent attacks. The use of analgesic medications for more than 3 days per week (including over-the-counter formulations) may increase the frequency and severity of headaches. In some cases, intermittent migraine progresses to a syndrome of daily severe headaches despite the use of escalating prophylactic medication or analgesics. Only nonsteroidal anti-inflammatory drugs (NSAIDs), ergotamine, and valproic acid are useful during an attack and for prevention.

Patients should be provided with a variety of treatments that may be taken in a manner appropriate to the severity of their symptoms.

Mild Attacks

Mild attacks may be treated with simple analgesics such as acetaminophen (suggested dose, 650 to 1000 mg) or NSAIDs (aspirin, 900 to 1000 mg; ibuprofen, 1000 to 1200 mg; naproxen, 500 to 825 mg; and ketoprofen, 75 to 150 mg). Mild to moderate attacks during pregnancy may be treated with acetaminophen if nonpharmacologic treatments are ineffective. *Moderate headaches* may respond to the combination of acetaminophen, isometheptene mucate (a mild vasoconstrictor, 65 mg), and dichloralphenazone (a mild sedative, 100 mg). Infrequent headaches of moderate to severe intensity may be treated with butalbital, a barbiturate, combined with caffeine, aspirin, or acetaminophen. Oral opiates have little place in the treatment of chronic, recurrent, primary headaches and should be avoided until alternatives, including NSAIDs and serotonin agonists such as dihydroergotamine or sumatriptan, have been considered. However, opiates (e.g., acetaminophen, 325 mg, with codeine, 30 mg) may be the only viable option during pregnancy or in patients with severe vascular disease; if so, they should be used with caution, and the risks associated with opiate use, including rebound headaches and dependency, should be discussed with patients before treatment is initiated.

A number of abortive agents with vasoconstrictive properties are available, but patients with uncontrolled hypertension or a history of coronary artery disease or angina should not be given any of these drugs.

Rx

Moderate to Severe Attacks

Moderate to severe attacks may be treated outside the hospital with dihydroergotamine (1 to 2 mg intranasally); with oral, intranasal, or subcutaneous formulations of serotonin $5\text{-HT}_{B/D}$ receptor agonists (e.g., sumatriptan, 25 to 100 mg orally, 20 mg intranasally, or 6 mg subcutaneously); or with second-generation sumatriptan-like drugs (e.g., naratriptan, 2.5 mg; zolmitriptan, 5 mg; rizatriptan, 10 mg; eletriptan, 40 mg; frovatriptan, 2.5 mg; or almotriptan, 12.5 mg). The second-generation drugs are similar to sumatriptan in overall efficacy and mechanism, but they may have a faster onset of action and fewer coronary vasoconstrictive properties. Ergotamine (2 mg sublingually or 1 to 2 mg orally), which is the longest established antimigraine agent, is typically given early in the migraine attack and can be effective if the associated nausea and peripheral vasoconstriction can be tolerated.

Very Severe Attacks

Very severe attacks sometimes require the administration of intravenous or intramuscular agents in the emergency department. Dihydroergotamine, an injectable hydrogenated ergot, has less potent peripheral arterial vasoconstrictive effects than ergotamine does and is usually effective even when given well into an attack. Dihydroergotamine may be administered subcutaneously (1 mg) or intravenously (0.5 to 1 mg). Given intravenously, dihydroergotamine causes less nausea than ergotamine does, but an antiemetic is still required before intravenous use. Meperidine (100 mg), an opioid analgesic, is frequently administered intramuscularly, especially in combination with an antiemetic (e.g., promethazine, 25 mg), to treat severe migraine attacks. With alternatives available, the use of parenteral opioids should be limited to patients with infrequent, severe attacks for whom other treatments are contraindicated.

Intravenous Neuroleptics

For patients who are nonresponsive or have contraindications to vasoactive abortive agents, intravenous neuroleptics may be given to treat severe or prolonged migraine attacks. Intravenous chlorpromazine, 10 mg, [1] may be used in this setting and repeated in 1 hour if no response is seen. The hypotension that sometimes accompanies the use of intravenous chlorpromazine may be avoided by administering 500 mL of normal saline intravenously before chlorpromazine (10 mg). Alternatively, intravenous prochlorperazine (10 mg over a 5-minute period) can be given without prior saline infusion and repeated after 30 minutes.

Prevention

In general, preventive treatment is recommended if headaches limit work or normal daily activity 3 or more days per month, if the symptoms accompanying headache are severe or prolonged, and if previous migraine was associated with a complication (e.g., cerebral infarction). Preventive treatment is largely empirical, and the drugs currently used were discovered serendipitously while being developed for the treatment of other disorders. The response rate in controlled clinical trials of prophylactic treatment is rarely more than 50% better than placebo. [2] Increased appetite and weight gain are common side effects of most prophylactic agents. Treatment should be initiated at low doses and gradually titrated to headache improvement or the onset of side effects. Groups 1 to 5 of the following list are generally considered first-line agents and tend to be associated with fewer or less potentially serious side effects. The prophylactic agents fall into eight groups:

1. β-Adrenergic blockers: propranolol (40 to 240 mg), atenolol (50 to 150 mg), nadolol (20 to 80 mg), timolol (20 to 60 mg), metoprolol (50 to 300 mg)
2. NSAIDs: aspirin (1000 to 1300 mg), naproxen (480 to 1100 mg), ketoprofen (150 to 300 mg)
3. Tricyclic antidepressants: amitriptyline (10 to 120 mg), nortriptyline (10 to 75 mg)

4. Calcium-channel antagonists: verapamil (120 to 480 mg), flunarizine (5 to 10 mg)
5. Anticonvulsants: divalproex sodium (750 to 1000 mg), gabapentin (900 to 1800 mg), topiramate (100 to 400 mg), lamotrigine (50 to 300 mg)
6. Serotoninergic drugs: methysergide (4 to 8 mg), cyproheptadine (8 to 20 mg)
7. Monoamine oxidase inhibitor: phenelzine (30 to 60 mg)
8. Angiotensin II receptor blocker: candesartan (16 mg)

Only a single prophylactic agent, lamotrigine, has been shown to have a specific effect in patients with migraine aura. [3] Unfortunately, comparative data on prophylactic treatments are sparse. A comorbid condition is sometimes an indication or contraindication to a specific type of drug.

Cluster Headache

Epidemiology

Cluster headache, which is much less common than tension-type headache or migraine, affects 0.4 to 2.4 persons per 1000 in the general population. Unlike patients with migraine headaches, those with cluster headaches usually seek medical consultation because of the intense pain that accompanies their attacks. As a result, physicians encounter cluster headache more frequently than would be predicted from its actual prevalence. The condition is more common in men than in women (male-to-female ratio of 6:1) and usually begins in the third through the sixth decades of life. Although cluster headaches may cease during pregnancy, attacks seldom correlate with menses.

Pathobiology

The cause of cluster headaches is not defined. Like other vascular headaches, they are presumed to develop from events that ultimately activate the trigeminovascular system. In the complete form of the disease, patients with cluster headache manifest pain referred to the first and second trigeminal divisions, sympathetic dysfunction (i.e., Horner's syndrome), sympathetic activation (i.e., sweating of the forehead and face), and parasympathetic activation (i.e., lacrimation and nasal congestion). This constellation of symptoms and signs is best explained by the presence of a single lesion at the point at which fibers from the ophthalmic and maxillary trigeminal division converge with projections from the superior cervical and sphenopalatine ganglia. This plexus is located within the cavernous sinus, and narrowing of the cavernous carotid artery has been observed in selected cases of cluster headache. PET-based functional imaging studies of blood flow during acute cluster attacks show areas of increased flow in the inferior portion of the hypothalamus on the same side as the headache. This finding is consistent with the clinical cyclicity exhibited by cluster headaches reported by many patients.

There is an increased concordance of cluster headache in monozygotic twins. Moreover, studies of relatives of patients with cluster headache have found a frequency 13 times higher than expected by chance.

Clinical Manifestations

Cluster headaches consist of recurrent episodes of unilateral, orbital, supraorbital, or temporal head pain usually accompanied by ipsilateral autonomic signs, including conjunctival injection, lacrimation, rhinorrhea, nasal congestion, ptosis, miosis, eyelid edema, and facial sweating. The attacks last 15 minutes to 3 hours and occur as infrequently as every other day to as frequently as eight attacks per day. The syndrome derives its name from the characteristic clusters or periods of frequent headaches that last weeks to months and are separated by periods of months or years of headache-free remission. Chronic symptoms without remission may develop in about 10% of patients. During a cluster period, the headache attacks often assume a temporal cyclicity, with occurrence at almost the same time every day. Exposure to small amounts of nitrates or alcohol may trigger an acute attack during a cluster period.

Treatment

During cluster headaches, oxygen inhalation (100%) delivered at a rate of 8 L/min for 15 minutes through a loose-fitting facemask is a safe and effective treatment of acute attacks, particularly in patients younger than 50 years who have episodic cluster headaches. Patients who respond to oxygen usually do so within 10 minutes. Inhalation of oxygen does not cause nausea and is not contraindicated in patients with coronary artery disease or peripheral vascular disease. Ergotamine tartrate, the classic treatment of cluster headache, is effective and well tolerated by many patients. Because of more rapid absorption, sublingual administration (1 mg) is generally preferred to oral administration (1 mg). Intranasal dihydroergotamine (1 mg) reduces the severity of cluster headaches, but not their duration. Subcutaneous administration of sumatriptan (6 mg), which is usually successful in alleviating acute cluster headaches, reduces pain and conjunctival injection within 15 minutes in most patients. Vasoconstrictive medications such as ergotamines and sumatriptan should be used with caution for cluster headache in patients who are at increased risk for coronary artery disease.

For many years ergotamine tartrate was the only prophylactic agent used for cluster headache. It is effective and well tolerated in doses of 2 to 4 mg/day given orally or by suppository. The ergot derivative methysergide (4 to 8 mg/day) is effective in about 70% of episodic cases. Retroperitoneal, pleural, or pericardial fibrosis is a severe potential side effect of long-term use. Because patients with cluster headache generally require treatment for less than 2 to 3 months, methysergide, if available, can be used with more safety than in migraine. Lithium carbonate, which was effective in chronic cluster headache in more than 20 open-label clinical trials, may also be beneficial in the episodic form of the disease. Because of the narrow range between toxic and therapeutic doses, it is important to monitor the serum lithium level 12 hours after the last dose. Average daily doses of lithium carbonate (600 to 900 mg) should be titrated according to the serum lithium level; the usual therapeutic range is 0.3 to 0.8 mmol/L, but low lithium levels may still be therapeutic. NSAIDs and thiazide diuretics may increase serum lithium levels. Verapamil (240 to 480 mg/day) is often effective as a prophylactic agent against cluster headache; it has relatively few side effects when compared with other prophylactic agents, and a double-blind trial found it to be as effective as lithium. Prophylactic medication dosages are usually tapered and then discontinued within 3 to 6 weeks after recurrent cluster headaches cease.

Corticosteroids are often used to treat the episodic and the chronic forms of cluster headache, even though evidence for their effectiveness is largely limited to open trials. Prednisone is frequently used in dosages of 60 to 80 mg/day for 1 week, followed by a taper in dosage over a period of 2 to 4 weeks.

Tension-Type Headache

Epidemiology

Tension-type headache is the most common of the primary headache disorders, with a lifetime prevalence between 30 and 78%. Tension-type headaches are more common in women than in men and most often begin in the second decade of life. In both sexes, the prevalence decreases with increasing age, and socioeconomic factors do not contribute to risk. Although no studies have been conducted in twins, genetic factors are not as prominent in the condition as in migraine or other headache syndromes.

Pathobiology

Tension-type headache is not well understood and defies a single or simple pathophysiologic explanation. In one model, headache pain is viewed as the sum of nociceptive input onto brain stem neurons from vascular structures, myofascial and muscular sources, and descending supraspinal modulation. The relative importance of these three factors varies among patients and among attacks in the same patient.

Clinical Manifestations

Tension-type headache occurs in episodic and chronic forms, which differ in their response to treatment and possibly in their pathophysiology. Pericranial muscle spasm or tenderness may or may not be present in either form. Episodic tension-type headache consists of recurrent attacks of tight, pressing (bandlike), bilateral, mild to moderate head pain that last from minutes to days. Tension-type headaches do not worsen with routine physical exertion and are not associated with nausea, although photophobia or phonophobia may be present. In the chronic form, characteristic tension-type headaches occur at least 15 days per month.

Treatment

Rx

Episodic tension-type headaches usually respond to simple analgesics such as acetaminophen (650 to 1000 mg) or to NSAIDs such as aspirin (900 to 1000 mg), ketoprofen (12.5 to 75 mg), ibuprofen (200 to 800 mg), and naproxen (250 to 500 mg). More severe, episodic tension-type headaches may respond to higher doses of NSAIDs or to combination remedies that contain isometheptene mucate or butalbital. Frequent use of analgesics can increase the number of headaches, so caution is advised whenever analgesic use regularly exceeds 3 days per week. Chronic tension-type headaches occasionally require prophylactic treatment. Tricyclic antidepressants decrease the frequency and severity of attacks; amitriptyline is the drug of choice, but its use may be limited by sedation, dry mouth, or other anticholinergic side effects. To avoid these side effects, therapy should be started at low doses (10 mg) given at bedtime and increased slowly until satisfactory improvement is achieved or intolerable side effects appear. Nortriptyline (50 to 100 mg each evening), doxepin (25 to 75 mg/day), maprotiline (10 to 25 mg/day), and fluoxetine (10 to 20 mg/day) are other antidepressants that are sometimes effective in chronic tension-type headache.

Chronic Daily Headache

Definition

The term *chronic daily headache* may be applied to any headaches occurring more than 15 days per month for at least 1 month. By this definition, the term includes several clinically distinct syndromes, including cluster headache, hemicrania continua, chronic paroxysmal hemicrania, and chronic tension-type headache.

Epidemiology

The typical patient with chronic daily headache is a woman in her 30s or 40s with a history of episodic migraine or tension-type headache beginning in the teens or 20s. Over a period of months to years, the patient's headaches gradually increase in severity and frequency to the point where consecutive headache-free days are rare.

Clinical Manifestations

Chronic daily headache is often used more narrowly to include headaches that occur on a daily or almost daily basis (>15 days/mo), have features of migraine and tension-type headache, and are frequently but not always associated with overuse of analgesic medications. Patients meeting these criteria account for a major proportion of those seen in headache specialty clinics and are often the most difficult headache patients to treat.

Diagnosis

The headaches are often of two types. More frequent headaches are of mild to moderate intensity and have a pressure-like or mildly throbbing quality and mild photophobia or phonophobia, but no associated nausea or vomiting. The duration of these milder headaches is variable and ranges from several hours to constant (although waxing and waning). Superimposed are severe attacks that occur as frequently as three times per week and as infrequently as once or twice per month. The more severe attacks are usually, but not always throbbing and may be associated with nausea, photophobia, phonophobia, and sometimes vomiting. Severe attacks may be preceded by a migrainous aura. The patient often exhibits features of depression or anxiety. Frequently, the patient is taking one or more daily analgesics, sometimes in an effort to preempt a headache. Chronic daily headaches are called *transformed migraine* when the migrainous component is prominent. When headaches begin without an antecedent migraine or tension-type headache but with many features of tension-type headache, they are often labeled new daily persistent headaches. Chronic daily headache is often accompanied by other paroxysmal symptoms that are frequently as distressing as the head pain. These symptoms may include dizziness (i.e., vertiginous and nonspecific forms), tinnitus, extreme phonophobia, fluctuating fatigue or mood alteration, and feelings of depersonalization. It is unclear whether these symptoms are fragments of underlying migraine or a mood disorder; they often resolve with improvement in the headaches.

Treatment

Rx

Overuse of medications is the most common exacerbating factor in chronic daily headache, and withdrawal of the overused medication usually improves the condition. The medications most often overused include butalbital combinations, ergotamines, oral analgesics containing caffeine in combination with acetaminophen or NSAIDs, and opiate combinations. However, chronic daily headache may develop in the absence of medication, and it does not always improve after analgesic withdrawal.

Less Common Primary Headache Syndromes

Paroxysmal Hemicrania

This uncommon syndrome has many features of cluster headache, including severe intensity, unilateral orbital or temporal location, and autonomic signs (e.g., conjunctival injection, tearing, rhinorrhea) ipsilateral to the pain, and it occurs in two forms. In the episodic form, the patient experiences bouts of several headaches per day for days or weeks at a time. These bouts are then separated by period of remission, during which no headaches occur. In the chronic form, there are no remissions and the headaches occur several times per day for months at a time. The attacks of paroxysmal hemicrania are shorter in duration (5 to 20 minutes) than cluster headache and have a higher frequency (generally more than five per day). The syndrome is more predominant in females and is generally responsive to indomethacin (150 mg/day or less).

Hemicrania Continua

Hemicrania continua is an unusual headache syndrome in which constant unilateral head pain of moderate to severe intensity underlies unprovoked brief episodes of sharp jabbing pain in a similar location.

Benign Cough Headache

Benign cough headache consists of severe bilateral head pain of sudden onset that follows coughing or other Valsalva maneuvers. It is a benign disorder that responds to indomethacin (25 to 50 mg) in about 90% of cases. However, the diagnosis of benign cough headache requires the exclusion of structural lesions with MRI because cough headache may sometimes result from posterior fossa tumors or a Chiari malformation, which may require surgical treatment. In rare instances, purely cough headaches that occur in association with a Chiari malformation may improve with suboccipital decompression. However, headaches with migrainous features often worsen significantly after suboccipital decompression.

Exertional or Orgasmic Headache

In some individuals, exertion or various types of exercise may trigger bilateral throbbing or pressure-like headaches that persist for several minutes up to 48 hours. Headaches may also develop during sexual activity, including coitus and, less frequently, during masturbation. These headaches usually begin with bilateral nonthrobbing pain that escalates as sexual excitement increases and reaches a crescendo at orgasm. Exertional and orgasmic headaches may occur in the absence of intracranial disorders; however, in rare cases, coital headache may be associated with unruptured cerebral aneurysms. The possibility of an aneurysm should be excluded. Exertional headache can sometimes be prevented by taking ergotamine (1 to 2 mg) or indomethacin (25 to 50 mg) before the planned exertion.

Hypnic Headaches

Hypnic headaches constitute a rare primary headache syndrome of the elderly (mean age of onset, 60 years or older). Hypnic headaches, which persist for 15 to 60 minutes and typically awaken patients from sleep about the same time each night, are in some ways similar to cluster headaches. However, unlike cluster headache, hypnic headaches are more diffuse, are often bilateral and throbbing, and are not associated with the autonomic symptoms of cluster headache. The differential diagnosis includes temporal arteritis and mass lesions. After exclusion of organic disease with an imaging study and erythrocyte sedimentation rate (ESR), treatment with low-dose lithium (300 mg every night) or caffeine may induce remission. If headaches return, careful upward titration of the dosage may be necessary. Lithium should be used with caution in older patients, especially in the presence of dehydration, renal disease, and diuretic or NSAID therapy.

SECONDARY HEADACHE DISORDERS

Headache may be the initial complaint in a host of CNS and systemic abnormalities (Table 421–1). Many of the disorders are given detailed consideration in other chapters. However, a few of the most prominent abnormalities that may result in chronic headache are discussed briefly.

Giant Cell Arteritis

Epidemiology and Clinical Manifestations

Giant cell arteritis (Chapter 292) is an inflammatory vasculitis involving branches of the temporal arteries. It most often affects individuals older than 60 years and can result in rapid and permanent loss of vision from granulomatous occlusion of the posterior ciliary or central retinal arteries. Features suggestive of temporal arteritis include orbital or frontotemporal head pain, described as dull and constant with superimposed jabbing sensations; aggravation of pain by cold temperatures; pain in the jaw or tongue pain on chewing (jaw claudication); accompanying constitutional or musculoskeletal symptoms such as weight loss, anemia, and polymyalgia rheumatica; elevated liver function test values; and decreased visual acuity, visual field cuts, pale or swollen optic disc, retinal splinter hemorrhages (i.e., anterior ischemic neuropathy) or a pale retina, and cherry-red spot (i.e., central retinal artery infarction).

Diagnosis

The ESR, which should be measured in all suspected patients, is elevated in 95% of cases. Definitive diagnosis is made by biopsy of the temporal artery, which can be performed within 48 hours after the initiation of treatment with steroids. When the diagnosis is suspected, prompt treatment with corticosteroids is necessary to avoid visual loss, which often becomes bilateral (75% of cases) after unilateral loss.

Treatment Rx

In patients with an elevated ESR, intravenous methylprednisolone (50 to 100 mg every 12 hours for 48 hours) should be followed by oral prednisone (80 to 100 mg/day for 14 to 21 days), with gradual taper over a period of 12 to 24 months. The tapering rate should be guided by serial ESR measurements.

Substance-Induced Headaches

Headaches may occur with acute exposure or as a result of withdrawal from many types of substances (Table 421–2).

TABLE 421–1 SECONDARY HEADACHE DISORDERS

HEADACHES ASSOCIATED WITH CRANIAL VASCULAR ABNORMALITIES

Subarachnoid hemorrhage
Intracerebral, epidural, and subdural hematoma
Unruptured vascular malformation
- Arteriovenous malformation
- Saccular aneurysm

Carotid or vertebral artery dissection
Carotidynia
Cerebral intra-arterial occlusion
Venous thrombosis
Arterial hypertension

HEADACHES ASSOCIATED WITH NONVASCULAR INTRACRANIAL DISORDERS

Intracranial neoplasms
Carcinomatous meningitis
High- and low-pressure headaches
Inflammatory disorders
- Temporal (giant cell) arteritis
- Tolosa-Hunt syndrome
- Intracranial sarcoidosis
- Wegener's granulomatosis

Intracranial infection
- Acute meningitis
- Meningoencephalitis
- Brain abscess

HEADACHES ASSOCIATED WITH SYSTEMIC ABNORMALITIES

Systemic infection: viral, bacterial, treponemal, etc.
Substance-induced headaches, exposure, and withdrawal
Metabolic disturbance
- Hypoxia, altitude sickness, sleep apnea
- Hypercapnia
- Hypoglycemia
- Dialysis

HEAD AND FACIAL PAIN ASSOCIATED WITH DISORDERS OF CRANIAL NERVES

Trigeminal neuropathy
Neuralgias
- Trigeminal neuralgia
- Glossopharyngeal neuralgia
- Occipital neuralgia

Herpes zoster

HEAD AND FACIAL PAIN ASSOCIATED WITH DISORDERS OF OTHER CRANIAL STRUCTURES

Glaucoma
Sinusitis
Temporomandibular joint disease
Dental pain
Neck abnormalities

Headaches Associated with Increased Intracranial Pressure

Headache may occur when an alteration in intracranial pressure (Chapter 199) causes compression or traction on pain-sensitive vascular, meningeal, or neural structures in the apex or base of the brain. Most commonly, these headaches are bilateral and frontotemporal, although their location is variable. Causes of elevated intracranial pressure include a mass lesion (Chapter 199), blockage of cerebrospinal fluid (CSF) circulation, hemorrhage, hypertensive encephalopathy (Chapter 66),

TABLE 421–2 SUBSTANCES INDUCING HEADACHE

AFTER ACUTE EXPOSURE
Alcohol
Amphotericin B
Azithromycin
Carbon monoxide
Cimetidine
Cocaine or crack
Danazol
Diclofenac
Dipyridamole
Estrogen or birth control pills
Fluconazole
Indomethacin
Monosodium glutamate
Nifedipine
Nitrates or nitrites
Ondansetron
Phenylethylamine
Ranitidine
Reserpine
Timolol ophthalmic drops
Tyramine
Verapamil
AFTER WITHDRAWAL FOLLOWING CHRONIC USE
Alcohol
Barbiturates
Caffeine
Ergotamine
Opiate analgesics

venous sinus thrombosis (Chapter 431), hyperadrenalism or hypoadrenalism (Chapter 246), altitude sickness (Chapter 94), tetracycline, and vitamin A intoxication (Chapter 237). In most instances, the source of the headache and raised pressure are identifiable. Treatment of the underlying condition generally improves the headache.

Intracranial Tumor

One of the most common concerns of patients seeking evaluation of chronic headaches is that their headache represents a space-occupying lesion such as a tumor (Chapter 199) or large vascular abnormality. Fortunately, most chronic headaches do not arise from a tumor or other structural lesion. Headaches in patients with brain tumors are usually dull and bifrontal, although they tend to be worse on the side of the tumor. The headaches are more often qualitatively similar to tension-type headaches than to migraines and tend to be intermittent and of moderate intensity; they are accompanied by nausea in about half the cases and are generally resistant to common analgesics. Classic brain tumor headache (i.e., progressive and beginning in the morning) is not typical. Factors that should increase suspicion of an intracranial tumor include papilledema, new neurologic deficits, initial attack of prolonged headache occurring after the age of 45 years, previous malignancy, cognitive abnormality, and altered mental status.

Idiopathic Intracranial Hypertension

Idiopathic intracranial hypertension (pseudotumor cerebri [Chapter 199]) is a syndrome composed of headache, papilledema, and transient visual symptoms that occur in the absence of CSF abnormalities, except for elevated intracranial pressure. The syndrome is not associated with hydrocephalus or another identifiable cause. In adults, females have an 8 to 10 times higher incidence than males do. The prototypical patient is an overweight woman of childbearing age. The diagnosis is made by lumbar puncture (CSF pressure higher than 250 mm Hg; normal CSF composition) after excluding a mass lesion by neuroimaging. Visual field testing often reveals an enlarged blind spot. Spontaneous recovery may eventually occur, but treatment to reduce intracranial pressure is generally indicated to prevent visual loss. Simple measures such as weight reduction should be attempted whenever appropriate. Drug therapies are usually attempted next and include medications such as acetazolamide and furosemide, which are aimed primarily at reducing CSF production. Furosemide, a potent loop diuretic, must be given with potassium supplementation and may cause hypotension. If drug treatment is ineffective, repeated lumbar puncture may sometimes be useful, although frequent lumbar puncture is not without a risk of complications, including post–lumbar puncture headache, spinal epidermoid tumor, or infection. If other treatments fail, surgical options include optic nerve fenestration and ventricular-peritoneal shunting of CSF (Chapter 199).

Headache Associated with Decreased Intracranial Pressure

Decreased intracranial pressure (<50 to 90 mm H_2O), which is usually caused by a decrease in CSF volume, is commonly associated with dull, throbbing, sometimes severe headaches that are probably caused by reduced brain buoyancy and subsequent traction on pain-sensitive meningeal and vascular structures (Chapter 199). Low-pressure headaches often become more intense on standing or sitting upright and may be relieved by lying down. The headaches may be accompanied by dizziness, visual symptoms, photophobia, nausea, vomiting, and diaphoresis. Although low-pressure headaches may begin spontaneously, they most commonly follow lumbar puncture. Other possible causes include intracranial surgery, ventricular shunting, trauma, and various systemic medical conditions such as severe dehydration, postdialysis status, diabetic coma, uremia, or hyperpnea. If the headache is prolonged, the possibility of a persistent CSF leak may be investigated by radioisotope cisternography or computed tomographic myelography. Post–lumbar puncture headaches can be caused by excessive leakage of CSF through a dural tear caused by the lumbar puncture needle. Headaches follow 10 to 30% of lumbar punctures and occur twice as frequently in women as in men. The headache may begin minutes to several days after the lumbar puncture and can persist for up to 2 weeks.

Treatment strategies include oral fluid or salt intake, intravenous fluids, CO_2 inhalation, methylxanthines such as theophylline (200 mg three times daily), caffeine (500 mg intravenously), or an intrathecal autologous blood patch (Chapter 199).

Head and Facial Pain Associated with Disorders of Cranial Nerves

Trigeminal neuralgia, also known as *tic douloureux,* usually occurs in older patients. The sharp, often electric shock–like pain of trigeminal neuralgia occurs in a rapid series of jabs (lasting seconds to minutes) in one or more divisions of the trigeminal nerve. The volleys of jabbing may be provoked by stimulation of areas on the face quite discrete from the site of pain and are usually followed by brief refractory periods. When trigeminal neuralgia occurs in persons younger than 40 years, a specific cause can frequently be found, such as demyelination (e.g., multiple sclerosis, especially when bilateral) and compression by vascular abnormalities or tumors (e.g., myeloma, metastatic carcinoma, cholesteatoma, chordoma, acoustic neuromas, trigeminal neuromas). In the elderly, trigeminal neuralgia has a prevalence of 155 per million and a female-to-male ratio of 3:2. Among older individuals with trigeminal neuralgia, microvascular compression of the trigeminal nerve root is often present. Because of the association with structural lesions (i.e., demyelinative or neoplastic), the initial evaluation should include MRI to detail the cerebellopontine angle and the entry foramen (e.g., V_1 superior orbital fissure, V_2 foramen rotundum, V_3 foramen ovale). In the absence of a structural cause, treatment usually consists of drugs such as carbamazepine (400 to 1200 mg), valproate (500 to 1500 mg), phenytoin (200 to 500 mg), baclofen (40 to 80 mg), or clonazepam (2 to 6 mg). Therapy with any of these agents must be initiated slowly. Patients who fail to respond to medication should be considered for microvascular decompression surgery.

Glossopharyngeal neuralgia is characterized by paroxysmal pain within the distribution of the vagus and glossopharyngeal nerves. The pain is paroxysmal, unilateral, and sudden in onset, and it has a jabbing or briefly persistent (square wave) quality. The pain is most often felt in or around the ear, tongue, jaw, or larynx, and it can be triggered by swallowing, talking, chewing, clearing the throat, yawning, or tasting spicy food or cold liquids. Although pain is usually followed by a brief refractory period, attacks can occur more than 20 times per day and may awaken sufferers from sleep. The intermittent pain may be superimposed on a dull, constant pain in the same area. Rarely, the pain of glossopharyngeal neuralgia is followed by bradycardia, syncope, or asystole, presumably resulting from the intense glossopharyngeal outflow and vagal efferent discharge. The usual cause of glossopharyngeal neuralgia appears to be microvascular compression, although abscess and tumor are sometimes associated. Medical treatment is similar to that for trigeminal neuralgia and includes the slow introduction of carbamazepine (400 to 1200 mg), gabapentin (900 to 1800 mg), or baclofen (40 to 80 mg). Cases refractory to adequate medical treatment often respond to microvascular decompression.

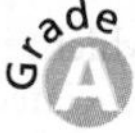

1. Bigal ME, Bordini CA, Speciali JG: Intravenous chlorpromazine in the emergency department treatment of migraines: A randomized controlled trial. J Emerg Med 2002;23:141–148.
2. Ramadan NM: Migraine headache prophylaxis: Current options and advances on the horizon. Curr Neurol Neurosci Rep 2006;6: 95–99.
3. Lampl C, Katsarava Z, Diener HC, et al: Lamotrigine reduces migraine aura and migraine attacks in patients with migraine with aura. J Neurol Neurosurg Psychiatry 2005;76:1730–1732.

SUGGESTED READINGS

Cady RK, Dodick DW, Levine HL, et al: Sinus headache: A neurology, otolaryngology, allergy, and primary care consensus on diagnosis and treatment. Mayo Clin Proc 2005;80:908–916. *A clinical review.*

Detsky ME, McDonald DR, Baerlocher MO, et al: Does this patient with headache have a migraine or need neuroimaging? JAMA 2006;296:1274–1283. *An excellent review that focuses on the diagnosis of a migraine headache and when to refer a patient to neuroimaging.*

Dodick DW: Clinical practice. Chronic daily headache. N Engl J Med 2006;354:158–165. *An excellent review of the diagnosis and management of chronic daily headache.*

May A: Cluster headache: Pathogenesis, diagnosis, and management. Lancet 2005;366:843–855. *A comprehensive review.*

Silberstein SD: Migraine. Lancet 2004;363:381–391. *Overview of diagnosis and management, with an emphasis on triptans.*

Stovner LJ, Hagen K, Jensen R, et al: The global burden of headache: A documentation of headache prevalence and disability worldwide. Cephalalgia 2007;3:193–210. *Globally, the percentages of the adult population with an active headache disorder are 11% for migraine, 42% for tension-type headache, and 3% for chronic daily headache.*

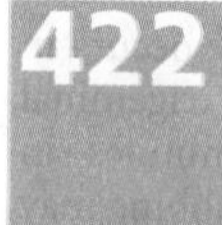

422 TRAUMATIC BRAIN INJURY AND SPINAL CORD INJURY

Geoffrey S. F. Ling

Traumatic brain injury and traumatic spinal cord injury are all too common preventable diseases. Traumatic brain injury is the leading cause of traumatic death and disability (Chapter 113). Approximately 1.4 million cases per year result directly in about 52,000 deaths in the United States annually—almost a third of all injury-related deaths. The majority of traumatic brain injuries are due to falls (Chapters 23 and 427), motor vehicle accidents, and assaults (Chapter 15). An additional approximately 11,000 cases of severe spinal cord injury occur each year in the United States, primarily the result of motor vehicle accidents, falls, sports-related injuries, and work-related accidents (Chapters 15 and 113). The majority of patients with traumatic brain and spinal cord injuries are young adult males.

Over the past 20 years, the marked improvement in overall mortality associated with traumatic brain and spinal cord injuries can largely be ascribed to improved care in intensive care units, early aggressive neurosurgical intervention, and prevention of long-term conditions such as deep vein thrombosis and decubitus ulcers. The almost 5.5 million survivors of traumatic brain and spinal cord injuries in the United States often require extended rehabilitation. Because the majority of these patients are young and otherwise in good physical health at the time of injury, many need chronic care for decades. It is important to note that even minor injury can lead to major disability; approximately 75% of patients who are classified as having mild to moderate traumatic brain injury continue to have residual symptoms months later, and many of these patients are unable to return to gainful employment.

Pathobiology

Traumatic injury to the central nervous system has two phases. The first is neuronal injury and occurs as a direct result of the initiating traumatic event. The second or late phase, which is caused by multiple neuropathologic processes, can continue for days to weeks after the initial insult.

Primary Injury Phase

The primary injury phase is immediate, and its damage, which can cause death almost instantaneously, is often complete by the time that medical care can be instituted. In closed compartment injury to the head or spine, the direct impact of neuronal tissue against the bony vault and shearing of neurovascular structures result in wounding. Because the neuronal structures reside in a fluid-filled compartment, these structures often lag behind the bony structure as it moves during sudden stopping of the body in motion. Thus, the structures will strike both anteriorly and posteriorly against the inner bony table, and a coup-contrecoup lesion will result. If a rotational component is present, the structures will torque, twist, and shear, thereby causing diffuse axonal injury. Motor vehicle accidents are particularly injurious because of the sudden deceleration. In penetrating lesions, the moving projectile will tear neural, vascular, and support structures as it traverses through the brain or spinal cord. If the projectile is moving at high velocity, such as a bullet, the vacuum created by its wake will give rise to tissue cavitation. The temporary cavity, which will ultimately collapse, may be many-fold larger than that of the projectile itself; the transient expansion of surrounding tissue will be sufficient to cause substantial irreversible damage.

Secondary Injury Phase

The delayed secondary phase of injury, which begins quickly after the primary phase and can continue for a prolonged period, involves both neurons and glia. Most neurologic injury is thought to be related to this secondary injury, when "neuron suicide" is caused by processes such as hypoxia, ischemia, inflammation, and the effects of free radicals, excitatory amino acids, and certain ions (e.g., calcium).

The injured brain is more susceptible to hypoxic-ischemic states. The most commonly affected areas are the hippocampus and "watershed" areas. It has been hypothesized that delayed neurologic compromise can be attributed to delayed ischemia.

Diffuse microvascular damage is due to early loss of cerebral vascular autoregulation and loss of integrity of the blood-brain barrier, with resulting endothelial changes such as the formation of intraluminal microvilli. Although the clinical significance of this injury is uncertain, it may play a role in the development of cerebral edema.

Diffuse axonal injury, which consists of shearing of axons in cerebral white matter, causes neurologic deficits such as nonfocal encephalopathy. The consequences of this type of injury can be delayed for up to 12 hours after the initial trauma.

Clinical Manifestations

Traumatic Brain Injury

The signs and symptoms of traumatic brain injury vary with its severity. Patients suffering from mild traumatic brain injury often experience headache, difficulty concentrating, anxiety, and disrupted sleep; findings on clinical examination are normal, but detailed neuropsychological testing may reveal mild cognitive abnormalities. With moderate traumatic brain injury, patients may have an abnormal sensorium, motor and sensory involvement, and impaired language; the results of neurologic examination will be abnormal. In very severe traumatic brain injury, patients are comatose; at best, they may exhibit some eye opening and decorticate or decerebrate posturing to stimulation.

Focal injuries cause neurologic deficits related to the site of impact. The orbitofrontal and anterior temporal lobes are most commonly affected. Extreme vigilance is needed to recognize the development of delayed hematomas and edema, which can be manifested days later.

In traumatic brain injury there may be a transient increase in systemic arterial pressure. Apnea or cerebral dysfunction may develop. Depending on the degree of injury, spontaneous resolution may be delayed, and laceration of the microvasculature will exacerbate this injury.

Traumatic Spinal Cord Injury

Spinal Cord Syndromes

There are three main spinal cord syndromes: Brown-Séquard, central cord, and anterior cord syndrome. In Brown-Séquard syndrome, the deficits are referable to a lesion of a lateral half of the cord; findings consist of loss of ipsilateral motor, touch, proprioception, and vibration sensation, as well as contralateral pain and temperature sensation. Central cord, or "man in a barrel," syndrome is manifested as bilateral loss of motor function involving the upper extremities but sparing the lower extremities. Proximal weakness is greater than distal weakness. Pain and temperature sensation is generally reduced, whereas proprioception and vibration are usually spared. Anterior cord syndrome is manifested by deficits referable to bilateral anterior and lateral spinal cord columns or funiculi. There is loss of touch, pain, and temperature sensation and motor function below the level of the lesion, but the posterior column functions of proprioception and vibratory sensation remain intact.

Spinal Shock

After acute traumatic spinal cord injury, patients may suffer from "spinal shock," or temporary loss of spinal reflexes below the level of injury. Clinically, there is loss of deep tendon reflexes, the bulbocavernosus reflex, and the anal wink. In high cervical injuries, the lower reflexes (bulbocavernosus and anal wink) may be preserved. Some patients demonstrate the "Schiff-Sherrington" phenomenon, in which reflexes are affected above the level of injury. There may also be loss of autonomic reflexes leading to neurogenic shock, ileus, and urinary retention.

Diagnosis

Traumatic Brain Injury

The Glasgow Coma Scale score (Table 422–1) should be calculated promptly, and a detailed neurologic examination should be performed to determine the extent of injury and the severity of impairment. Important clinical signs of occult injury may be revealed on a general physical examination. For example, a scalp laceration should be palpated for evidence of an underlying skull fracture. Periorbital ecchymosis ("raccoon eyes") and postauricular ecchymosis ("Battle's sign") are concerning for a basal skull fracture. A clear or blood-tinged watery discharge from the nose or ear may be a cerebrospinal fluid leak.

Intracranial bleeding caused by traumatic brain injury includes subdural hematoma, epidural hematoma, intraparenchymal hemorrhage, contusion, and traumatic subarachnoid hemorrhage (Chapter 432). The most common is subdural hematoma, which is the basis of approximately 50% of admissions for head injury. Epidural hematoma accounts for about 3%. An associated skull fracture, especially at the temporoparietal junction, increases the incidence of epidural hematoma, usually by disruption of the middle meningeal artery.

Imaging

A computed tomography (CT) scan without contrast should be obtained as soon as possible after the initial clinical assessment. The need for neuroimaging is best determined by using the Glasgow Coma Scale score and a validated clinical prediction instrument such as the Canadian CT Head Rule (Table 422–2). In any patient suspected of having suffered

TABLE 422–1 GLASGOW COMA SCALE SCORE

Best Eye Response	Best Verbal Response	Best Motor Response
1 = No eye opening	1 = No verbal response	1 = No motor response
2 = Eye opening to pain	2 = Incomprehensible sounds	2 = Extension to pain
3 = Eye opening to verbal command	3 = Inappropriate words	3 = Flexion to pain
4 = Eyes open spontaneously	4 = Confused	4 = Withdrawal from pain
	5 = Orientated	5 = Localizing pain
		6 = Obeys commands

To calculate the score, sum the numbers from each of the three columns.

TABLE 422–2 DECISION RULES FOR DETERMINING INDICATIONS FOR CT SCAN IN PATIENTS WITH MINOR HEAD INJURY

			Reported Validity (%)*	
Study	**Patient Population**	**Indications for CT Scan**	**Sensitivity**	**Specificity**
Canadian CT Head Rule†	GCS score of 15, loss of consciousness, no neurologic deficit, age >3 yr	High-risk patients: GCS score <15 at 2 hr after injury, suspected skull fracture, any sign of basal skull fracture, vomiting (≥2 times), age ≥65 y‡ Medium-risk patients: retrograde amnesia >30 min, dangerous mechanism (pedestrian vs. motor vehicle, ejection from motor vehicle, fall from height >1 m or 5 stairs)§	100	24.5
New Orleans Criteria¶	GCS score of 13–15, loss of consciousness, no neurologic deficit, no seizure, no anticoagulation, age >16 yr	Headache, vomiting, seizure, intoxication, short-term memory deficit, age ≥60 yr, or injury above the clavicles	98.4	49.6

*Validity for identifying patients with traumatic CT findings.
†Stiell IG, Wells GA, VAndemheen K, et al: The Canadian CT Head Rule for patients with minor head injury. Lancet 2001;357:1391–1396.
‡High-risk patients in whom a CT scan is mandatory.
§Medium-risk patients in whom a CT scan if recommended but close clinical observation is an alternative.
¶Haydel MJ, Preston CA, Mills TJ, et al: Indications for computed tomography in patients with minor head injury. N Engl J Med 2000;343:100–105.
CT = computed tomography; GCS = Glasgow Coma Scale.

TABLE 422–3 AMERICAN ACADEMY OF NEUROLOGY: DIAGNOSIS AND MANAGEMENT OF CONCUSSION

Grade 1 (Mild)*	Grade 2 (Moderate)†	Grade 3 (Severe)‡
Remove from duty/work/play	Remove from duty for the rest of the day	Take to the emergency department
Examine immediately and at 5-minute intervals	Examine frequently for signs of CNS deterioration Physician's neurologic examination as soon as possible (within 24 hours)	Neurologic evaluation, including appropriate neuroimaging
May return to duty/work if clear within 15 minutes	Return to duty after 1 full asymptomatic week (after being cleared by the physician)	Consider hospital admission

Grade of Concussion	Return to Play/Work
Grade 1 (first)	15 minutes
Grade 1 (second)	1 week
Grade 2 (first)	1 week
Grade 2 (second)	2 weeks
Grade 3 (first) (brief loss of consciousness)	1 week
Grade 3 (first) (long loss of consciousness)	2 weeks
Grade 3 (second)	1 month
Grade 3 (third)	Consult a neurologist

*Mild: transient confusion, no loss of consciousness, symptoms associated with concussion (such as amnesia) or mental status changes lasting less than 15 minutes.
†Moderate: transient confusion, no loss of consciousness, symptoms lasting longer than 15 minutes.
‡Severe: any loss of consciousness.

a head injury, the severity of the concussion should be assessed (Table 422–3). A subdural hematoma (see Fig. 419–3) is blood that accumulates above the brain but below the dura; on CT imaging it appears as a crescentic or concave opacity overlying the brain. An epidural hematoma (see Fig. 419–4) is blood that accumulates below the skull but above the dura; it appears as a convex or lenticular opacity on CT imaging. Skull fractures are best diagnosed with the use of CT bone windows.

Traumatic Spinal Cord Injury

A detailed neurologic examination is needed to identify the level of the injury and the severity of any deficits, as well as document the degree of neurologic dysfunction at the earliest time possible. The level of the injury is the lowest spinal cord segment with intact motor and sensory function. Normal neurologic findings in patients with a clear sensorium obviate the need for imaging studies. However, any complaints of pain over the spine, numbness, tingling, or weakness should raise suspicion of spinal cord injury. In particular, a complaint of "burning hands" suggests traumatic spinal cord injury.

The time of injury should be recorded as accurately as possible. The prognosis for neurologic improvement is better if the lesion is incomplete as opposed to complete. During the acute period, serial examinations must be performed frequently.

If spinal cord injury is suspected, the patient should be appropriately immobilized, such as with a rigid collar and back board. In patients who are able to cooperate with a neurologic examination, are not intoxicated, and do not have painful distracting injuries (such as a femoral fracture, which would interfere with the leg motor and sensory examination), normal neurologic findings effectively rule out cervical spine disease.

Imaging

In patients in whom a cervical injury cannot be excluded, the radiologic evaluation should begin with plain radiographs of the bony spine, with further neuroimaging of any abnormalities that are found. Bony vertebrae should be examined with CT and the spinal cord with magnetic resonance imaging (MRI). Intervertebral and paravertebral soft tissue are best studied with MRI. A chest radiograph is usually indicated to provide images of the lower cervical and thoracic vertebrae; the presence of a pleural effusion in the setting of a possible thoracic spine injury suggests a hemothorax.

Ligamentous Injury versus Spinal Cord Injury

If plain radiographs of the cervical spine are normal but the patient still complains of neck pain, a ligamentous injury should be considered. Ligamentous injury can be evaluated by flexion-extension radiographs of the cervical spine. If pain prevents an adequate study, patients should be kept in a rigid cervical collar for 3 to 5 days until the pain and muscle spasm resolve. If studies at that time are normal, the patient will no longer require the collar. Conversely, abnormal results warrant surgical evaluation to determine whether further immobilization or surgical correction is necessary.

Treatment

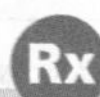

The immediate goals of therapy are to arrest ongoing injury, preserve and if possible restore neurologic function, and avoid secondary medical complications. To achieve this goal, an organized team approach is essential. Despite major research efforts, current clinical treatment is largely confined to supportive measures: maintaining perfusion pressure, minimizing intracompartment hypertension (e.g., increased intracranial pressure [ICP]), and indirectly treating edema.

Traumatic Brain Injury

Initial Management

It is crucial that prehospital providers optimize perfusion and oxygenation because the duration and severity of hypoxia and hypotension in this critical early period have dramatic consequences on clinical outcome. Treatment begins with immediate attention to airway and cardiopulmonary function, early identification of the potential for traumatic brain injury, and minimization of secondary insults such as hypoxia and ischemia.

Patients with mild or moderate traumatic brain injury often have returned to normal or are rapidly recovering by the time that they reach an emergency department. The critical element is the duration of amnesia or loss of consciousness (see Table 422–3). Longer periods of abnormal sensorium are associated with higher grades of concussion, and higher grades of concussion necessitate longer periods of convalescence.

Severe Traumatic Brain Injury

Patients with Glasgow Coma Scale scores of 8 or less are considered to have severe traumatic brain injury. With this level of impaired consciousness, even with an intact gag reflex, patients are unable to protect their airway adequately. Intubation should be performed with either an endotracheal or a nasotracheal tube, depending on clinical circumstances. The patient should be in a rigid neck collar with the head elevated 30 degrees. The neck collar is used not only to protect the cervical spine until appropriate imaging can be performed but also to keep the head midline to avoid compromising venous drainage.

Rx

If intracranial hypertension is suspected, patients should be given mannitol intravenously at a dose of 0.5 to 1.0 g/kg. Intravenous steroids are of no benefit acutely and increase mortality at 2 weeks after the injury. 1 Hyperventilation may be also tried but has a potential to exacerbate ischemia; if used, the goal should be hyperventilation to a PCO_2 of 34 to 36 mm Hg. Another therapeutic option is administration of a 30-mL intravenous dose of 23% hypertonic saline through a central venous catheter to lower elevated ICP acutely. Continuous infusion of 3% hypertonic saline through a central venous catheter may be started at a rate of 75 to 100 mL/hr with the goal of a serum sodium level of 150 to 155 mM/L to maintain ICP below 20 mm Hg. Induced hypothermia for traumatic brain injury remains controversial because of conflicting results from clinical trials.

In addition to ICP control, cerebral perfusion must be maintained. The goal is to maintain cerebral perfusion pressure, which is the difference between mean arterial pressure and ICP, higher than 60 mm Hg. Volume resuscitation is the first therapeutic intervention, with the aim of achieving euvolemia or only slight hypervolemia to a central venous pressure (CVP) goal of 4 to 6 mm Hg. Furthermore, to treat elevated ICP, an osmolar gradient between the systemic vasculature and the brain is needed. Thus, intravenous hyperosmolar solutions may be used, including normal saline, hypertonic saline (e.g., 3% sodium solutions), or colloids such as albumin solutions. The initial goal is 310 mOsm or a serum sodium level of 150 to 155 mM/L. If a cerebral perfusion pressure greater than 60 mm Hg cannot be achieved with intravenous fluids alone, vasoactive pharmacologic agents such as norepinephrine (beginning at 2 μg/min by continuous intravenous infusion) and phenylephrine (100 μg/min) may be required. Invasive hemodynamic monitoring with an arterial pressure line and CVP catheter may be needed.

Types of Injury

Certain lesions require prompt surgical intervention, whereas others do not. Penetrating wounds, intracerebral hemorrhage with a mass effect (including subdural and epidural blood), and bone injury (such as a displaced fracture and vertebral subluxation) require emergency surgical evaluation for intervention. However, focal, hypoxic-anoxic, diffuse axonal, and diffuse microvascular injuries do not warrant surgical intervention; treatment remains primarily with the critical care clinician. Skull fractures and intracranial hemorrhages require neurosurgical evaluation. In general, if a fracture is displaced more than the thickness of the skull, it needs to be elevated.

If a surgical lesion is not identified, the patient should be admitted to an intensive care unit. If the patient is still at a Glasgow Coma Scale score of 8 or less, an ICP-monitoring device should be used. An intraventricular catheter provides the most reliable data. It is also a treatment option because it allows drainage of cerebrospinal fluid. However, a subdural bolt and fiberoptic catheter are less invasive alternatives.

Pharmacologic Coma and Surgical Decompression

If ICP remains poorly controlled after the aforementioned efforts, pharmacologic coma or surgical decompression is considered. The postulated effect of pharmacologic coma on ICP is through reduction of cerebral metabolism. If the decision to use pharmacologic coma is made, pentobarbital can be administered at a loading dose of 5 mg/kg intravenously, followed by an infusion of 1 to 3 mg/kg/hr. Another option is propofol (loading dose of 2 mg/kg intravenously, followed by an infusion of up to 5 mg/kg/hr). Continuous electroencephalographic monitoring is helpful because the target response is burst suppression. Barbiturates and propofol are myocardial depressants, so aggressive cardiovascular management is often necessary to achieve the desired cerebral perfusion pressure. Recalcitrant elevated ICP despite these interventions is an ominous sign; serious consideration should be given to frontal or temporal lobe decompression and hemicraniectomy.

Complications

If the patient is agitated, an evaluation should be made to determine whether the patient is in pain or poorly tolerating mechanical ventilation. If pain is a concern, a narcotic analgesic such as fentanyl (50 to 100 μg intravenously) or morphine (1 to 2 mg intravenously) should be administered. Because these agents are easily reversed by naloxone, periodic reassessment of neurologic status can be performed. If agitation alone is the issue, haloperidol (0.5 to 2 mg intravenously), a nonsedating agent that still maintains the ability to perform a neurologic examination, should be considered.

The PO_2 level should be maintained at approximately 100 mm Hg. Phenytoin (loading dose of 1000 g intravenously followed by a maintenance dose of 300 mg/day intravenously) reduces seizures during the first week after traumatic brain injury, but its later usefulness is less clear. Fever greatly increases cerebral metabolism; antipyretic interventions such as acetaminophen and cooling blankets should be used as needed. Gastric stress ulcers may be prevented with H_2 antagonists such as ranitidine (50 mg intravenously three times daily) or proton pump inhibitors such as omeprazole (20 mg/day orally). Low-dose heparin (5000 units subcutaneously twice daily) or a low-molecular-weight heparin such as enoxaparin (40 mg/day subcutaneously) and pneumatic stockings should be instituted to avoid deep vein thrombosis. A nasogastric or orogastric tube should be placed for nutrition. Feeding should be initiated as soon as practical, usually on the second day after injury. Because cerebral edema is a concern, hyperosmotic feeding should be instituted. If ileus is present, total parenteral nutrition (TPN; Chapter 236) should be given.

After the first 6 to 12 hours, effort should be made to reduce hyperventilation. Otherwise, the metabolic compensation to chronic hyperventilation negates the ameliorative effects of the respiratory alkalosis.

Regular neurologic examinations and monitoring of ICP and cerebral perfusion pressure are useful to guide ongoing therapy. Generally, the peak period of cerebral edema is from 48 to 96 hours after traumatic brain injury. Thereafter, cerebral edema spontaneously resolves, often associated with clinical improvement.

Recovery

Recovering patients may experience "postconcussive syndrome," which is primarily manifested as headache. Other symptoms may include difficulty concentrating, changes in appetite, sleep abnormalities, and irritability. In general, postconcussive syndrome lasts a few weeks after injury, but it can persist beyond a year or more. Therapies are based on the patient's symptoms. For headache, nonsteroidal anti-inflammatory agents (such as ibuprofen at an oral dose of 400 to 600 mg), migraine drugs (such as sumatriptan at an oral dose of 25 to 50 mg), and biofeedback may be considered. For cognitive dysfunction, neuropsychological testing may be helpful in determining appropriate intervention.

Traumatic Spinal Cord Injury

Initial Management

Emergency management of traumatic injury to the spinal cord begins with the basics of airway, breathing, and circulation. A secure airway is essential. For patients suffering from high cervical lesions, spontaneous ventilation will be lost. Cervical lesions below C5 may also be associated with impaired ventilatory capability. If there is any concern that the airway or ventilatory effort is compromised, emergency intubation is required. In a patient in whom the cervical spine has not been imaged, the preferred method is nasotracheal intubation under fiberoptic guidance. Other approaches are nasotracheal (blind) or orotracheal intubation, provided that in-line traction is applied.

Other immediate concerns are bleeding and circulation. Hypotension may be due to either neurogenic shock or hypovolemia. For neurogenic shock, vasopressive pharmacologic agents such as phenylephrine (beginning as a continuous intravenous infusion at 100 μg/min with titration to clinical effect) may be needed. If tachycardia is present, hypovolemia is more likely, so fluid resuscitation would be more appropriate.

Targeted Therapy

If closed compartment spinal cord injury is identified, immediate pharmacologic therapy with methylprednisolone should be

Rx

instituted. The initial dose is a 30-mg/kg intravenous bolus followed by a continuous infusion of 5.4 mg/kg/hr for 1 day if treatment is started within 3 hours of injury. When treatment is begun between 3 and 8 hours after injury, the infusion should be continued for 48 hours. 2 The utility of methylprednisolone in penetrating traumatic spinal cord injury has not been demonstrated, and it should not be used.

At this time, the decision for surgical intervention should be based on the stability of the anterior, middle, and posterior vertebral columns. The anterior column consists of the anterior half of the vertebral body and the vertebral disc. The middle column is the posterior half of the body and the disc. The posterior column is composed of the arch, facets, and ligaments. In general, if two of the three columns are damaged, surgical stabilization is needed. If immediate surgery is not indicated, the patient should be admitted to the intensive care unit for further management.

Acute and Subacute Management

Patients with severe spinal cord injuries require close cardiovascular and ventilatory care, supportive care for bladder and bowel function, approaches to avoid pressure ulcers (Chapter 23), and general measures similar to those used for patients with traumatic brain injury.

Neurogenic Shock and Dysautonomia

After traumatic spinal cord injury, patients are at risk for neurogenic shock and dysautonomia. Lesions of the cervical and thoracic spine disrupt the descending sympathetic pathways to the intermediolateral cell column of the thoracolumbar spinal cord, thereby leading to peripheral vasodilation and hypotension. If the lesion is at T3 or above, sympathetic tone to the heart is compromised. In this setting, hypotension is accompanied by bradycardia, thus producing the neurogenic shock triad of bradycardia, hypotension, and peripheral vasodilation.

Initial therapy for dysautonomia should be fluid administration to restore an adequate circulating volume with a target CVP of 4 to 6 mm Hg. A hematocrit of 30 is optimal for perfusion of the central nervous system, so blood can be used if the patient is anemic. If blood is not required, either colloid (e.g., albumin solutions) or crystalloid (e.g., normal saline) may be used. If there is a suspicion of cardiac or pulmonary disease, a pulmonary artery catheter may be needed briefly to assess fluid status and the relationship between pulmonary pressure and CVP.

Once adequate circulating volume has been achieved, hypotension should be managed with vasopressive agents such as phenylephrine (see earlier), norepinephrine (see earlier) or dopamine (beginning at 1 μg/kg/min by continuous intravenous infusion) (Chapter 107), with the goal of a mean arterial pressure of 85 mm Hg or greater. Symptomatic bradycardia can be treated with atropine (1 mg intravenously).

Ventilatory Compromise

An injury at C5 or higher results in diaphragmatic denervation and requires complete ventilatory assistance. Proper management requires endotracheal or nasotracheal intubation and mechanical ventilation, with an appropriate tidal volume (6 to 10 mL/kg), an FIO_2 to achieve a PO_2 between 80 and 100 mm Hg, and a rate to give a PCO_2 of 40 mm Hg. Positive end-expiratory pressure should also be given to minimize atelectasis (Chapter 106). If the patient does not show signs of ventilatory recovery within 2 weeks of intubation, a tracheostomy should be considered.

Lesions below C5 may also be associated with inadequate spontaneous ventilation. Midcervical lesions may be associated with intact, but compromised diaphragm function. If suspected, a "sniff" test under fluoroscopy can be performed to determine whether both hemidiaphragms are functioning properly. If not, intubation/tracheostomy with volume-controlled ventilation may be needed. If intact, pressure support ventilation may be sufficient (Chapter 106) to achieve an appropriate tidal volume.

Cervical lesions at C6 and below spare the phrenic nerves but may disrupt innervation of the intercostal muscles. The primary finding is decreased cough and an inability to increase ventilation when needed, thereby leading to atelectasis and pneumonia; assisted elimination of tracheal secretions is essential.

Thromboembolic Disease

Thromboembolic disease (Chapters 81 and 99) is a leading cause of morbidity and mortality after traumatic spinal cord injury. Prolonged immobility of the lower extremities leads to deep venous thrombosis in up to 70% of spinal cord–injured patients. Patients should receive prophylaxis with intermittent compression devices (e.g., pneumatic stockings). Anticoagulation therapy with warfarin to a therapeutic goal of an international normalized ratio of 2 to 3 should begin after the first 72 hours. An inferior vena cava filter may be placed if anticoagulation therapy is contraindicated.

Visceral Function

The abdominal wall musculature is innervated by T7 to T12. The stomach, small bowel, liver, pancreas, and proximal two thirds of the colon receive innervation from T5 to L2. Spinal cord injury at these levels or above may impair visceral function. For ileus, a nasogastric tube should be placed to decompress the stomach. Parental nutrition should be started as soon as possible. Enteral feeding should be delayed until gastrointestinal motility returns, usually within 2 to 3 weeks.

Stress-induced peptic ulcer disease occurs in nearly a third of patients without prophylaxis. H_2-receptor antagonists such as ranitidine (50 mg intravenously three times daily) or a proton pump inhibitor such as omeprazole (20 mg/day orally) reduce the incidence of ulcers.

Bladder tone may be lost because of spinal shock. A Foley catheter should be placed for a minimum of 5 to 7 days to drain the bladder and evaluate volume and renal status. After spinal shock has resolved, autonomic dysreflexia may occur as a result of bladder distention. Clinical signs such as sweating, skin flushing, and hypertension may be present. Clinical examination with palpation and percussion will reveal a distended bladder, which can be treated by bladder training or intermittent catheterization.

Nutrition

Until enteral feeding can begin, parenteral nutrition should be used. Ideally, TPN should be started. However, if TPN is not possible, peripheral parenteral nutrition should be used until TPN (Chapter 236) can begin. Energy expenditures of 19 kcal/kg/day for high cervical injuries to 35.8 kcal/kg/day for injuries at T10 and below have been reported. A caloric level of 80% of the Harris-Benedict prediction should be used for quadriplegic patients. The full Harris-Benedict predicted amount should be used in patients with thoracic spine injuries and below.

Other Therapy

Patients with traumatic spinal cord injury have a propensity for the development of decubitus ulcers and pressure sores (Chapter 23). Mechanical kinetic beds, regular log rolling (every 2 hours), and padded orthotics are all useful in minimizing this complication. Orthotics, physical therapy, and occupational therapy (for cervical cord injury) are also important to minimize contractures and begin the rehabilitation process.

Prognosis

Traumatic Brain Injury

The most useful prognostic indicator after traumatic brain injury is the neurologic examination at initial evaluation. For patients with severe traumatic brain injury, the initial Glasgow Coma Scale score is the most reliable prognostic indicator. The lower the initial Glasgow Coma Scale score, the less likely a patient will have meaningful neurologic or functional recovery. After traumatic brain injury, 40% of patients with a score of 8 have a good recovery versus only 7% when the score is 3. Furthermore, only 27% of patients with a score of 3 survive versus 88% of patients with a score of 8. Patients in whom the Glasgow Coma Scale

TABLE 422–4 AMERICAN SPINAL INJURY ASSOCIATION IMPAIRMENT SCALE

Grade	Injury Type	Definition	Likelihood of Recovery*
A	Complete	No motor or sensory function below the lesion	15.5% (cervical) and 7% (thoracic)
B	Incomplete	Sensory but no motor function	47%
C	Incomplete	Some motor strength (<3)	84%
D	Incomplete	Motor strength >3	84%
E	None	Sensory and motor function normal	100%

Data from Coleman WP, Geisler FH: Injury severity as primary predictor of outcome in acute spinal cord injury: Retrospective results from a large multicenter clinical trial. Spine J 2004;4:373–378.

score remains the same or worsens over a period of 6 hours do worse clinically than those whose score improves. Further prognostic stratification at 24 hours can be based on pupillary responses, motor responses, and age (see Fig. 428–1).

A subsequent head injury before full recovery from even a mild traumatic brain injury may occasionally result in "second impact syndrome," which can worsen the clinical outcome. When seen (mostly in children and adolescents), coma develops rapidly after the second injury, often within minutes. There is decreased autoregulation, diffuse cerebral edema, and intracranial hypertension. Second impact syndrome is associated with high mortality.

Traumatic Spinal Cord Injury

For traumatic spinal cord injury, the completeness of the injury is the most useful predictor (Table 422–4). A grade "A" or complete motor and sensory deficit below the lesion has a poor prognosis. If such a lesion persists for 24 hours, there is little likelihood of meaningful recovery. On the other hand, even severe partial injuries have a higher probability of recovery.

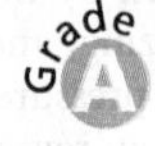

1. CRASH Trial Collaborators: Final results of MRC CRASH, a randomized placebo-controlled trial of intravenous corticosteroid in adults with head injury—outcomes at six months. Lancet 2005;365: 1957–1959.
2. Bracken MB, Shepard MJ, Holford TR, et al: Administration of methylprednisolone for 24 or 48 hours or tirilazad mesylate for 48 hours in the treatment of acute spinal cord injury. Results of the Third National Acute Spinal Cord Injury Randomized Controlled Trial. National Acute Spinal Cord Injury Study. JAMA 1997;277: 1597–15604.

SUGGESTED READINGS

Gunnarsson T, Fehlings MG: Acute neurosurgical management of traumatic brain injury and spinal cord injury. Curr Opin Neurol 2003;16:717–723. *Provides the standard approach.*

Hadley MN, Walters BC, Grabb PA, et al: Guidelines for the management of acute cervical spine and spinal cord injuries. Clin Neurosurg 2002;49:407–498. *Consensus-based guidelines.*

Haydel MJ: Clinical decision instruments for CT scanning in minor head injury. JAMA 2005;294:1551–1553. *One million persons per year in the United States have a head injury that requires emergency evaluation, but only 1% need neurosurgical treatment.*

Patel HC, Bouamra O, Woodford M, et al: Trends in head injury outcome from 1989 to 2003 and the effect of neurosurgical care: An observational study. Lancet 2005;366:1538–1544. *Treatment only in non-neurosurgical centers was associated with a 26% increase in mortality and a 2.15-fold increase in the odds of death versus treatment in a neurosurgical center.*

Ropper A, Gorson K: Concussion. N Engl J Med 2007;356:166–172. *A clinical review.*

Smits M, Dippel DW, Steyerberg EW, et al: Predicting intracranial traumatic findings on computed tomography in patients with minor head injury: The CHIP prediction rule. Ann Intern Med 2007;146:397–405. *The CHIP prediction rule may be useful for the selective use of CT in patients with minor head injury with or without loss of consciousness.*

Stiell IG, Clement CM, Rowe BH, et al: Comparison of the Canadian CT Head Rule and the New Orleans Criteria in patients with minor head injury. JAMA 2005;294:1511–1518. *With a Glasgow Coma Score of 13 to 15, the Canadian CT Head Rule found all patients who might benefit from CT-guided therapy.*

Vincent JL, Berre J: Primer on medical management of severe brain injury. Crit Care Med 2005;33:1392–1399. *A comprehensive overview.*

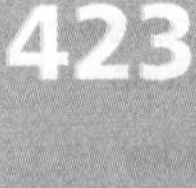

423 MECHANICAL AND OTHER LESIONS OF THE SPINE, NERVE ROOTS, AND SPINAL CORD

Michael J. Aminoff

Definition

The individual vertebrae are separated by intervertebral discs that cushion the spine during various physical activities. Each disc consists of a thick outer fibrous portion called the *annulus fibrosus,* within which is a soft, gelatinous, inner central portion called the *nucleus pulposus,* a remnant of the notochord. Posterior to the vertebral bodies, the vertebral arches (composed of paired pedicles anteriorly and laminae posteriorly) and transverse processes enclose the spinal cord in the spinal canal, and the posterior spinous process projects posteriorly (Fig. 423–1). Paraspinal muscles help support the spine.

Pathobiology

The intervertebral discs are not pain sensitive, but pain may arise from the ligaments connecting the vertebrae, facet joints, vertebral periosteum, outer layer of the annulus fibrosus, and spinal nerve roots. The paraspinal muscles are also pain sensitive and are probably the most common source of neck or back pain.

The spinal canal contains the spinal cord and the spinal and autonomic roots. Its size varies at different levels and between individuals. It tends to be more spacious in the cervical and lumbar regions than in the thoracic region. A congenitally narrow spinal canal (i.e., spinal stenosis) predisposes to neurologic dysfunction as a consequence of minor degenerative changes or disc protrusion. Such stenosis is common in the cervical and lumbar regions. In adults, the cord ends as the conus medullaris at about the level of the first lumbar vertebra; below this level, the spinal canal is occupied by the descending nerve roots that constitute the cauda equina. The cervical cord segments are at approximately the same level as the cervical vertebral bodies, the thoracic cord segments are generally one or two levels higher than the corresponding vertebral segments, and much of the lumbar and sacral cord is found between T10 and L1. The nerve roots in the cauda equina have to descend in the subarachnoid space before exiting at their various foramina. The absence of a C8 vertebral body but presence of a C8 spinal segment means that roots above C8 exit above the corresponding vertebral body whereas the remaining nerve roots exit below their respective vertebral bodies.

Thirty-one paired spinal nerves emerge from the spinal cord: 8 in the cervical, 12 in the thoracic, 5 in the lumbar, 5 in the sacral, and 1 in the coccygeal region. Each spinal nerve has anterior and posterior roots that connect it with the cord. The fibers in the posterior roots originate primarily in the dorsal root ganglia, which are situated distally along the posterior roots, shortly before they unite with the anterior roots and usually within the entrance of the bony intervertebral foramen. The axons in the anterior roots arise mainly from cells in the anterior and lateral gray columns of the spinal cord.

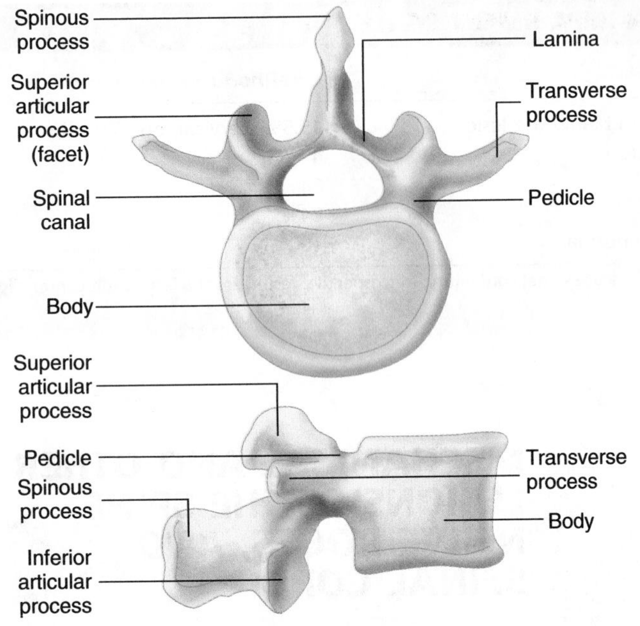

FIGURE 423–1 • Normal vertebral anatomy.

Shortly after passing through the intervertebral foramina, the spinal nerves divide into anterior and posterior rami. The posterior rami supply the skin over the back of the neck and trunk and the paraspinal musculature. The anterior rami innervate the anterolateral aspect of the trunk and limbs. The anterior rami contribute to the limb plexus, where the fibers are reorganized to form the various peripheral nerves to the extremities: the brachial plexus to the arms and the lumbar and sacral plexus to the legs.

The pattern of any motor or sensory deficits is helpful in localizing a lesion involving the cord or nerve roots (Fig. 423–2). A *myotome* designates a group of muscles that have common innervation from the same segment of the spinal cord and therefore from the same nerve root. Most muscles belong to more than one myotome because they are typically innervated by two or more adjacent cord segments and nerve roots. The designation *dermatome* refers to the cutaneous territory innervated by a single nerve root. Adjacent dermatomes overlap considerably.

NECK AND BACK PAIN

Epidemiology

Neck or back pain is one of the most common reasons for medical consultation, but it is usually short lived and responds to symptomatic measures. Most patients with acute neck or back pain, with or without radicular symptoms, have musculoskeletal or degenerative disorders that do not require specific treatment and are often self-limited. However, the possibility of more serious abnormalities that require specific treatment should always be excluded. Among young patients (<40 years) with low back pain, almost 90% have had more than one attack of pain, and most attacks have lasted for less than 2 weeks. Approximately 85% of patients with low back pain cannot be given a definitive diagnosis. Similarly, approximately a third of adults in the general population report neck pain within the previous year, the prevalence increasing with advancing age; almost 14% report chronic neck pain (i.e., pain exceeding 6 months' duration).

Clinical Manifestations

Local pain and tenderness may occur as a result of irritation of nerve endings at the site of pathology, such as in the vertebral periosteum. Similarly, degeneration or protrusion of intravertebral discs causes pain by compression of nerve endings in the annulus fibrosus or posterior longitudinal ligaments. Pain of muscle or ligamentous origin or related to a herniated disc is usually alleviated by recumbency. In contrast, the pain of vertebral metastases is often aggravated by recumbency and may be relieved by sitting up.

Referred Pain

Referred pain arises from deep structures and is felt at a distant site within the same spinal segment. It often has a deep aching quality and is sometimes accompanied by tenderness at the site of referral. Pain may be referred to the spine from pelvic or abdominal viscera and is usually not affected by the position of the spine. Pain may also be referred from the spine to other regions. For example, disease of the upper lumbar spine may lead to pain in the groin or anterior aspect of the thighs, and disease of the lower lumbar spine may cause pain in the buttocks and back of the thighs.

Musculoskeletal Pain

Musculoskeletal pain typically follows unaccustomed exercise but occasionally occurs spontaneously, often on awakening in the morning. It may be related to spasm of the paraspinal muscles as a result of injury or structural abnormality of the spine. Chronic neck pain is a well-recognized complication of whiplash (acute flexion-extension) injuries. Trigger points may be present and define certain myofascial pain syndromes. The pain is exacerbated by activity or movement and relieved by rest. Range of motion may be restricted by pain or muscle spasm. Localized tenderness is common. In the absence of a history of injury and any significant neurologic findings, detailed investigation is usually unrewarding. Patients can be managed conservatively. There is no agreement about the optimal duration of immobilization or bedrest. Physical therapy is often recommended for the treatment of acute low back pain, but the extent of any benefit is unclear. There is little evidence that traction, ultrasound, diathermy, or manipulation is helpful. Nonsteroidal analgesics are usually sufficient to relieve pain, but in severe cases narcotics may be required; in patients with chronic pain, tricyclic antidepressant drugs are often helpful. Muscle relaxants may relieve painful muscle spasm.

Radicular Pain

Radicular pain may occur from compression, angulation, or stretching of nerve roots as produced by disc protrusion, degenerative spinal disease, or metastatic deposits. Less commonly, radicular pain occurs in certain medical disorders such as diabetes mellitus. The pain has a dermatomal distribution but may also be felt in muscles supplied by the affected root. It is usually sharp in character. Coughing, sneezing, and straining typically exacerbate the pain by increasing intraspinal pressure, as do maneuvers that stretch the nerve roots. Examination may reveal sensory changes in the dermatomal distribution of the affected root, weakness and atrophy in a myotomal distribution, and depression of tendon reflexes subserved by the affected root, but examination is often normal. In patients with weakness, not all muscles within the myotome are necessarily affected. *Cauda equina syndromes* are typically associated with bilateral radicular pain; saddle anesthesia and sphincter dysfunction are common, and examination reveals bilateral root dysfunction.

Spinal Cord Disease

Spinal cord disease, especially compression of the long tracts, may lead to an unpleasant sensation in the extremities that is also enhanced by increased intraspinal pressure or movements that stretch the cord (e.g., neck flexion, straight leg raising). Neck or back pain may also be conspicuous. The associated signs vary with the extent of the lesion and speed of its development. Acute cord compression, as from epidural hemorrhage, is associated with pain and the rapid onset of a paraparesis or quadriparesis that may not be reversed by decompressive surgery. In contrast, a gradually evolving compressive lesion may be painless and leads to a slowly progressive deficit that often recovers after decompression. Laterally situated lesions lead to a Brown-Séquard syndrome, posterior lesions to bilateral posterior column dysfunction with impaired position and vibration appreciation, anterior lesions to weakness, and intramedullary lesions to a dissociated sensory loss with impairment of pain and temperature appreciation and preservation of posterior column sensation.

Diagnosis

History

Patients often first notice the onset of neck or back pain when awakening in the morning, commonly after unaccustomed activity. The

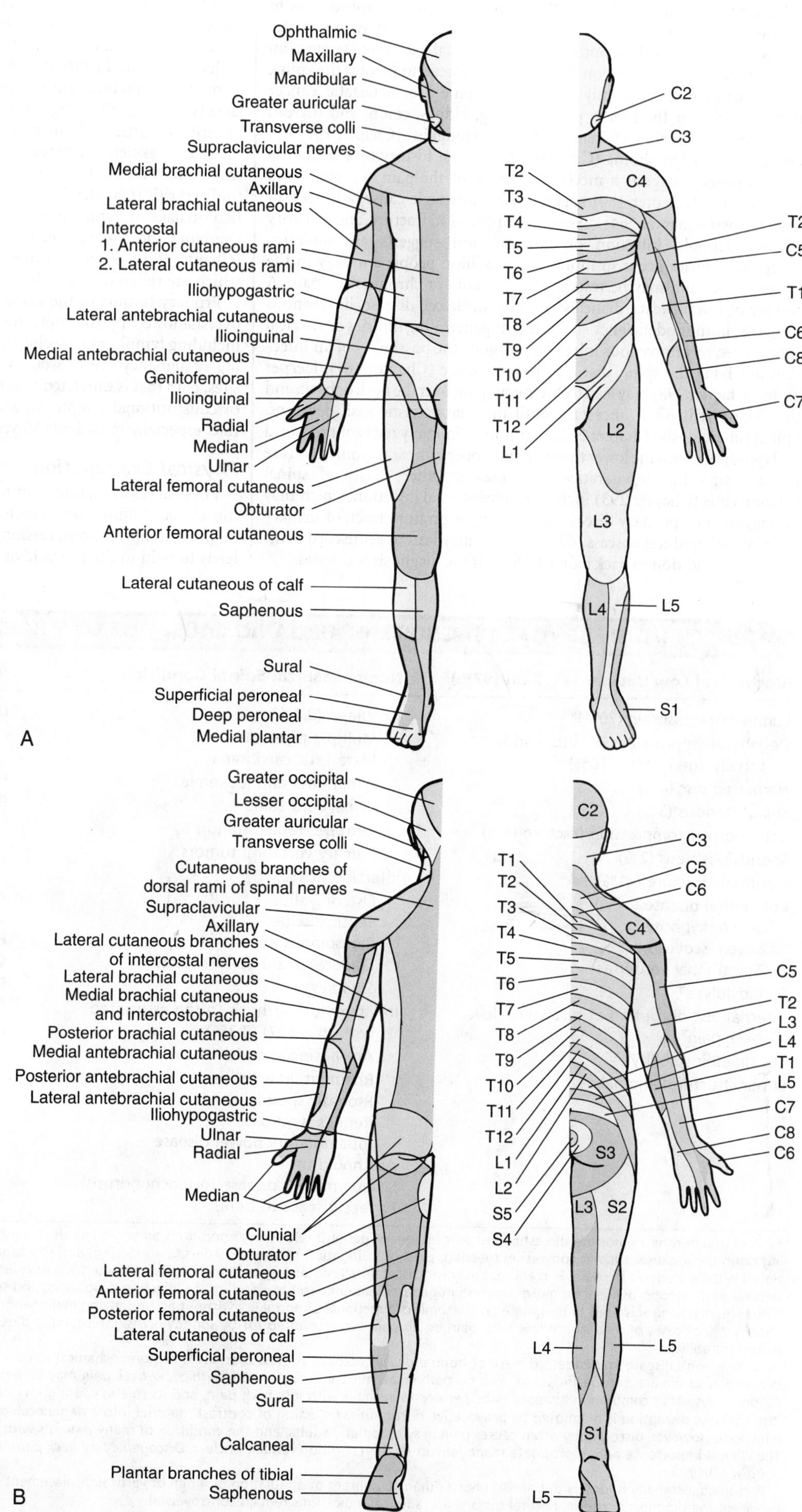

FIGURE 423–2 • Cutaneous innervation. The segmental (dermatomal) distribution is shown on the left side of the body, and the peripheral nerve distribution is shown on the right side of the body. **A,** Anterior view. **B,** Posterior view.

character and distribution of the pain are helpful in determining the probable underlying cause (Table 423–1) and hence further approaches to its investigation. A history of cancer raises the possibility of metastatic disease, whereas local symptoms, such as rectal bleeding, suggest an undiagnosed neoplastic lesion that may have spread to involve the spine. Malignancies that frequently involve the spine are metastatic cancer (Chapter 199) of the breast, prostate, lung, kidney, colon, and thyroid gland; multiple myeloma (Chapter 215); and Hodgkin's (Chapter 197) and non-Hodgkin's lymphoma (Chapter 196). A past history of a structural spinal disorder suggests a mechanical cause of the pain, a history of a coagulopathy (Chapter 180) suggests a hemorrhagic cause, a history of osteoporosis (Chapter 264) suggests a compression fracture, and a history of subarachnoid infection or inflammation suggests arachnoiditis. Whiplash injuries occur in more than 1 million people annually in the United States and may be responsible for acute or chronic neck pain. A history of fever, sweats, diabetes mellitus, sickle cell disease, intravenous drug use, immunodeficiency states, recent penetrating injuries or surgical procedures, or intravenous injections suggests the possibility of an infection involving the spine, disc, or epidural space (Chapter 181). Herpes zoster (Chapter 398) may lead to cutaneous pain over the neck or back, and the diagnosis is often uncertain until the characteristic rash develops. Spinal tuberculosis (Chapter 345) is common in many parts of the world and typically affects the lower thoracic and upper lumbar region, which are unusual sites for degenerative disc disease. Other causes of spinal osteomyelitis (Chapter 293) include staphylococcal infection, which may be suggested by primary disease of the skin, respiratory tract, or urinary tract. Spinal epidural abscess (Chapter 438) may lead to acute cord compression in addition to back pain and fever if the diagnosis is delayed.

Forced flexion or extension movements of the neck from trauma may lead to significant injury or compression fractures. Compression fractures of the vertebrae occur especially in patients with osteoporosis (Chapter 264) and therefore most commonly in patients who are elderly or have a family history of osteoporosis, chronic corticosteroid use, or immobility. Fractures are also especially likely in patients with osteomalacia (Chapter 265) or Paget's disease (Chapter 268) and may lead to complications, particularly in patients with ankylosing spondylitis, diffuse idiopathic skeletal hyperostosis, and spinal stenosis. Minor cervical trauma may lead to pain and significant deficits in patients with rheumatoid arthritis (Chapter 285). Injury may also lead to epidural or subdural hemorrhage or hematomyelia, which is typically heralded by severe pain overlying the site of bleeding (Chapter 422). Ankylosing spondylitis (Chapter 286) generally causes early morning stiffness and back pain, which are relieved by activity.

Primary tumors of the spine and spinal cord are uncommon and are overshadowed by the more frequent occurrence of secondary tumors, including lymphoma, myeloma, and cancer. Among the features suggesting malignancy are constant unremitting pain in atypical or multiple sites, pain that is unrelated to activity or posture, the presence of systemic or constitutional symptoms, and an elevated erythrocyte sedimentation rate, especially in patients 55 years or older.

Physical Examination

Physical examination commonly reveals spasm of the paraspinal muscles and limitation of spinal movement. Local tenderness may also be present. Spinal compression should be suspected when neck flexion leads to pain in the thoracic or lumbar region or when Lhermitte's sign

TABLE 423–1 DIFFERENTIAL DIAGNOSIS OF ORGANIC CAUSES OF LOW BACK PAIN*

Mechanical Low Back or Leg Pain (97%)†	Nonmechanical Spinal Conditions (~1%)‡	Visceral Disease (2%)
Lumbar strain, sprain (70%)§	Neoplasia (0.7%)	Disease of pelvic organs
Degenerative processes of discs and facets, usually age related (10%)	Multiple myeloma	Prostatitis
Herniated disc (4%)	Metastatic carcinoma	Endometriosis
Spinal stenosis (3%)	Lymphoma and leukemia	Chronic pelvic inflammatory disease
Osteoporotic compression fracture (4%)	Spinal cord tumors	Renal disease
Spondylolisthesis (2%)	Retroperitoneal tumors	Nephrolithiasis
Traumatic fracture (<1%)	Primary vertebral tumors	Pyelonephritis
Congenital disease (<1%)	Infection (0.1%)	Perinephric abscess
Severe kyphosis	Osteomyelitis	Aortic aneurysm
Severe scoliosis	Septic discitis	Gastrointestinal disease
Transitional vertebrae	Paraspinous abscess	Pancreatitis
Spondylolysis‖	Epidural or subdural abscess	Cholecystitis
Internal disc disruption or discogenic low back pain¶	*Shingles*	Penetrating ulcer
Presumed instability**	Inflammatory arthritis (often associated with HLA-B27) (0.3%)	Cardiac or pericardial disease
Other structural anomalies	Ankylosing spondylitis	Pulmonary or pleural disease
	Rheumatoid arthritis	
	Psoriatic spondylitis	
	Reiter's syndrome	
	Inflammatory bowel disease	
	Arachnoiditis	
	Scheuermann's disease (osteochondrosis)	
	Paget's disease of bone	

*Values in parentheses indicate the estimated percentages of patients with these conditions among all adult patients with low back pain in primary care, excluding nonorganic causes such as conversion reaction, psychosis, litigation-related disorders, malingering, and substance abuse. Diagnoses in italics are often associated with neurogenic leg pain. Percentages may vary substantially according to demographic characteristics or referral patterns in a practice. For example, spinal stenosis and osteoporosis will be more common in geriatric patients, spinal infections in injection drug users, and so forth.
†The term *mechanical* is used to designate an anatomic or functional abnormality without an underlying malignant, neoplastic, or inflammatory disease. Approximately 2% of cases of mechanical low back pain or leg pain are accounted for by spondylolysis, internal disc disruption, or discogenic low back pain and presumed instability.
‡Scheuermann's disease and Paget's disease of bone probably account for less than 0.1% of nonmechanical spinal conditions.
§*Strain* and *sprain* are nonspecific terms with no pathoanatomic confirmation. *Idiopathic low back pain* may be a preferable term.
‖Spondylolysis is as common in asymptomatic persons as in those with low back pain, and its role in causing low back pain remains ambiguous.
¶Internal disc disruption is diagnosed by provocative discography (injection of contrast material into a degenerated disc, with assessment of pain at the time of injection). However, discography often causes pain in symptomatic adults, and the condition of many patients with positive discograms improves spontaneously. The clinical importance and appropriate management of this condition remain unclear. *Discogenic low back pain* is used more or less synonymously with *internal disc disruption*.
**Presumed instability is loosely defined as greater than 10 degrees of angulation or 4 mm of vertical displacement on lateral flexion and extension radiographs. However, the diagnostic criteria, natural history, and surgical indications remain controversial.
From Deyo RA, Weinstein JN: Low back pain. N Engl J Med 2001;344:363–370.

is positive. Focal tenderness over a spinous process suggests vertebral involvement by tumor or infection. In patients with low back pain, the examination should include maneuvers that stretch different nerve roots. Hip flexion with the knee extended stretches the L5 and S1 roots and may reproduce pain in the back, buttocks, and posterior of the thighs, whereas hip extension with the leg straight and the patient prone (i.e., reverse straight leg raising sign) stretches the upper lumbar roots and may cause pain in the anterior thigh or medial calf region. Neurologic examination is important, and the presence of any deficits mandates further evaluation. The distribution of any abnormalities suggests the probable site of pathology.

General physical examination is also important in patients with back pain and should include rectal and pelvic examinations. When pain is referred to the back and is related to visceral disease, abdominal palpation may reproduce it.

Differential Diagnosis

Most cases of low back pain are caused by mechanical conditions, including lumbar muscle strain or sprain, degenerative processes of discs and facets, herniated discs, spinal stenosis, and osteoporotic compression fractures (see Table 423–1). Nonmechanical spinal conditions and systemic diseases are important but unusual causes of low back pain.

Imaging and Other Tests

In general, imaging procedures are not required for patients with uncomplicated neck or back pain of less than 1 month's duration (Fig. 423–3). However, even in patients older than 50 years or with symptoms suggestive of systemic disease, plain radiography and basic blood tests can virtually exclude an underlying systemic disease. Imaging studies of the neck or back are required when clinical examination reveals a likely cause, such as a fracture, or when pain does not respond to conservative measures over a period of several weeks. Imaging studies, especially computed tomography (CT) and magnetic resonance imaging (MRI), are important in patients at particular risk for a neoplastic or infectious cause of the pain and are also helpful in confirming spinal osteomyelitis or tuberculosis and in guiding bone biopsy. The presence of a focal or progressive neurologic deficit or pain in uncommon sites (e.g., lower thoracic region) also requires investigation, usually by MRI. However, many asymptomatic middle-aged or elderly subjects have MRI abnormalities of the spine, and the clinical relevance of any structural abnormalities may therefore be uncertain (Table 423–2). Electrophysiologic studies, particularly electromyography and nerve conduction studies, are sometimes helpful in showing the functional significance of anatomic abnormalities and additionally are important as a means of diagnosing a radiculopathy.

Children with low back pain usually require further investigation. Acute pain may be related to developing scoliosis, disc disease, or spondylolisthesis. Discitis may also be responsible.

Treatment

Rx

If a cervical fracture is suspected after trauma, the neck is immobilized and radiographs taken (Chapter 422). Acute hemorrhage may require evacuation, and infection requires antimicrobial

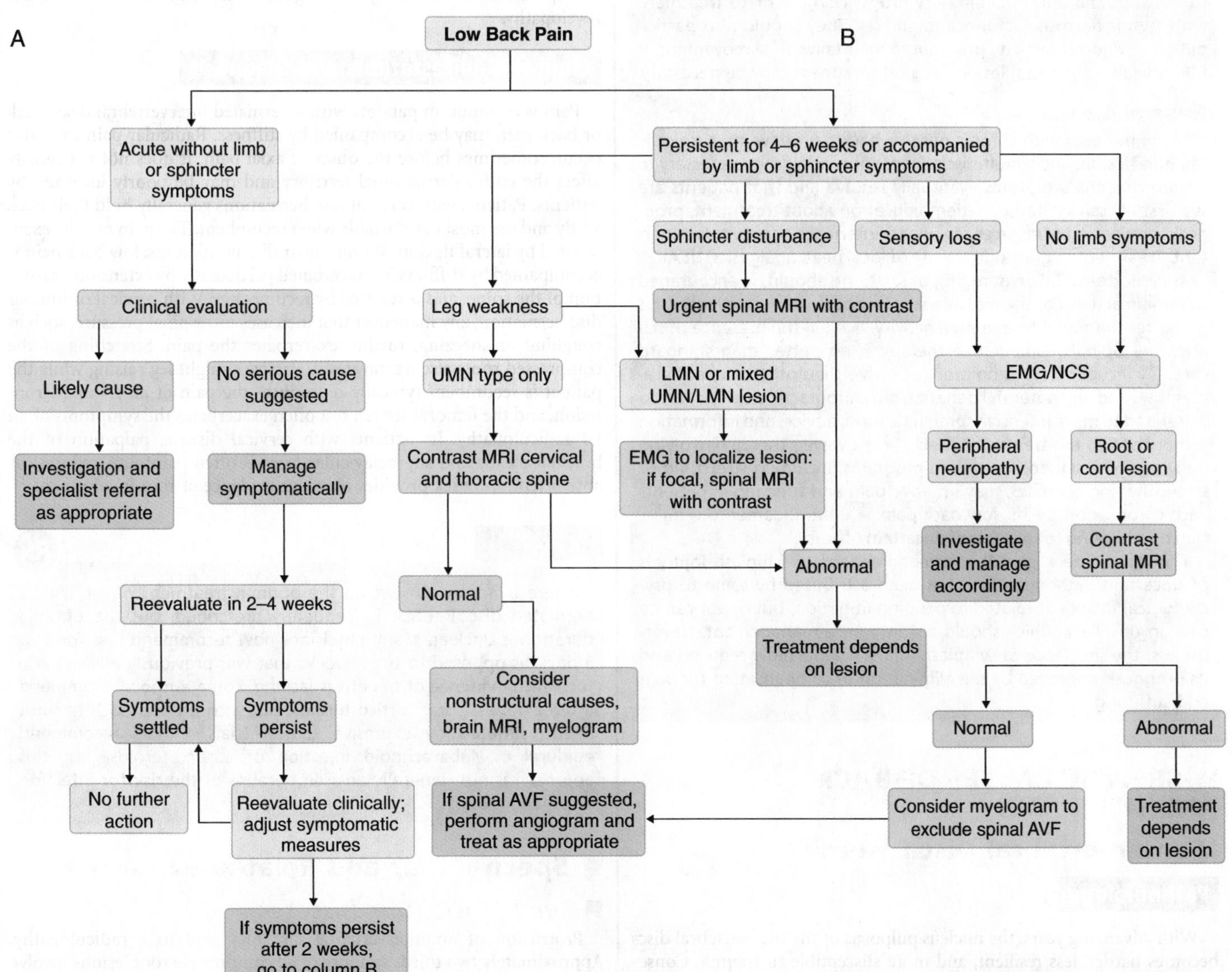

FIGURE 423–3 • Management of patients with low back pain. AVF = arteriovenous fistula; EMG/NCS = electromyography and nerve conduction studies; LMN = lower motor neuron; MRI = magnetic resonance imaging; UMN = upper motor neuron.

TABLE 423–2 REPRESENTATIVE RESULTS OF MAGNETIC RESONANCE IMAGING STUDIES IN ASYMPTOMATIC ADULTS

		Anatomic Findings				
Study	**Subjects**	**Herniated Disc**	**Bulging Disc**	**Degenerative Disc**	**Stenosis**	**Annular Tear**
Boden et al.	Volunteers <60 yr old	22	54	46	1	NR
	Volunteers ≥60 yr old	36	79	93	21	NR
Jensen et al.	Volunteers (mean age, 42 yr)	28	52	NR	7	14
Weishaupt et al.	Volunteers (mean age, 35 yr)	40	24	72	NR	33
Stadnik et al.	Patients referred for head or neck imaging (median age, 42 yr)	33	81	72	NR	56

NR = not reported.
From Deyo RA, Weinstein JN: Low back pain. N Engl J Med 2001;344:363–370.

therapy and, in some instances, drainage. Even in the absence of confirmatory evidence, a trial of antituberculous therapy may be necessary in those at high risk for spinal tuberculosis, such as the elderly, the immunocompromised, and those who have come from high-risk areas such as the Indian subcontinent.

Patients with ankylosing spondylosis (Chapter 286) may respond to nonsteroidal anti-inflammatory drugs (NSAIDs) or to treatment with tumor necrosis factor-α antagonists. They should also participate in a vigorous activity program to maintain spinal movement. If MRI reveals a structural lesion, surgical treatment may be necessary.

General Measures

Many patients with chronic neck or back pain have no surgically remedial lesion, and a multidisciplinary approach is then necessary to ensure that the symptoms eventually resolve and that patients are successfully rehabilitated. Patient education about treatment, prognosis, prevention of recurrences, and maintenance of activity is important. Treatment may include the use of local heat, analgesics, NSAIDs, or tricyclic drugs (taken at night), but patients should be encouraged to remain active. For the treatment of low back pain, strict bedrest is no better than symptom-limited activity, even in the presence of sciatica. [1] Spinal manipulative therapy is no better than standard care, [2] acupuncture is no more effective than other active therapies, [3] and any potential benefit from chiropractic care appears to be related to more intensive communication, advice, and information rather than to the treatment itself. [4] However, therapy involving individually designed, supervised programs, including stretching or strengthening exercises, may improve pain and function in patients with chronic nonspecific low back pain. [5] Intraligamentous injection of sclerosing solutions is of uncertain efficacy.

The chronic neck pain that sometimes follows whiplash injury is of uncertain pathogenesis. It has been attributed by some to psychological factors or related to pending litigation, but doubt can be cast on this view, which should not influence management. Nevertheless, the incidence of whiplash injury is reportedly reduced and its prognosis improved by the elimination of compensation for pain and suffering.

SPECIFIC CAUSES OF BACK AND NECK PAIN

Intervertebral Disc Disease

Pathobiology

With advancing years, the nucleus pulposus of the intervertebral discs becomes harder, less resilient, and more susceptible to trauma. Consequently, tears tend to develop in the annulus, through which a portion of the nucleus pulposus may herniate. Herniation is generally in a lateral direction and may lead to compression of the nerve roots as they enter the intervertebral foramina, but it sometimes occurs centrally and results in compression of the spinal cord or cauda equina. In some instances, the protruded disc material loses its continuity with the nucleus pulposus and becomes a free fragment within the spinal canal.

Disc herniations occur most commonly in the lumbosacral or cervical region. Early recognition of thoracic disc herniations is important, however, because there is only limited space in the thoracic portion of the spinal canal and delay in diagnosis may lead to an irreversible myelopathy.

Clinical Manifestations and Diagnosis

Pain is common in patients with a herniated intervertebral disc. Neck or back pain may be accompanied by stiffness. Radicular pain may also occur, sometimes before the onset of axial pain. It does not necessarily affect the entire dermatomal territory and may be poorly localized by patients. Patients with cervical disc herniations generally hold their neck stiffly and are most comfortable when recumbent. The pain may be exacerbated by lateral flexion. With lumbar disc herniations, low back pain is accompanied by stiffness, is exacerbated particularly by extension or rotation of the spine, and is relieved by recumbency. With cervical or lumbar disc herniation, any maneuver that increases intraspinal pressure, such as coughing or sneezing, further exacerbates the pain. Stretching of the compressed roots also aggravates it. Passive straight leg raising while the patient is recumbent typically reproduces the pain of an L5 or S1 root lesion, and the femoral stretch test often exacerbates the symptoms of an L4 radiculopathy. In patients with cervical disease, palpation of the brachial plexus and supraclavicular fossa is often painful. A reduced or absent tendon reflex provides objective evidence of root involvement.

Treatment

There is no agreement on the optimal treatment of an acutely herniated disc. Bedrest is frequently prescribed, but the optimal duration is unclear. Many physicians now recommend rest for 2 or 3 days, as opposed to the 2 weeks that was previously advised and for which evidence of benefit is lacking. Some authors recommend a brief dose of oral corticosteroids, but such an approach has not been validated by extensive clinical trials. Others recommend epidural or subarachnoid injection of corticosteroids, but this approach is not generally advised because of the risk for infection or inflammation.

Specific Disc and Related Syndromes

Lumbosacral Disc Disease

Protrusion of an intervertebral disc may lead to a radiculopathy. Approximately two thirds or more of all compressive root lesions involve the lumbosacral roots. The L5 and S1 roots are involved most commonly. Multiple lumbosacral radiculopathies may occur with protrusion of a

TABLE 423–3 DIAGNOSIS OF LOWER LUMBAR AND SACRAL RADICULOPATHY

	Pain	Weakness (Selected Muscles)	Sensory Loss	Reflex Loss
L4	Across the thigh and medial aspect of the leg to the medial malleolus	Quadriceps Thigh adductors Tibialis anterior	Medial part of the leg	Knee
L5	Posterior aspect of the thigh and lateral aspect of the calf, dorsum of the foot	Extensor digitorum brevis and longus Peronei	Dorsum of the foot	
S1	Buttock and posterior aspect of the thigh, calf and lateral border of the foot	Extensor digitorum brevis Peronei Gastrocnemius Soleus	Sole or lateral border of the foot	Ankle
S2–4	Posterior aspect of the thigh, buttocks, genitalia	Gastrocnemius Soleus Abductor hallucis Abductor digiti quinti pedis Sphincter muscles	Buttocks, anal region, genitalia	Bulbocavernosus Anal

single intervertebral disc that compresses the roots as they descend in the cauda equina. Lumbosacral polyradiculopathies may also result from spinal stenosis and, in rare instances, from lateral disc protrusion, but bilateral involvement is then often asymmetrical.

Clinical Manifestations and Diagnosis

An L5 or S1 radiculopathy is generally associated with low back pain and sciatica. An L5 root lesion leads to a footdrop and an S1 lesion to weakness of plantar flexion and eversion. S2 radiculopathies are often bilateral, probably because the sacral fibers are more medially situated in the cauda equina and therefore subject to midline compression. With involvement of sacral fibers, disturbances in bladder and bowel function are important complications (Table 423–3).

Treatment

Rx

In patients with severe sciatica, early surgery provides more rapid symptomatic relief than does the strategy of conservative therapy until surgery is needed, but both yield similar 1-year outcomes. [6] In another a randomized trial of patients between the ages of 25 and 65 years with at least 2 years of chronic low back pain and evidence of disc degeneration at L4–5 or L5–S1, lumbar fusion was better than continued medical therapy; posterolateral fusion, posterolateral fusion combined with internal fixation, and posterolateral fusion combined with internal fixation and interbody fusion provided similar benefits. [7] A successful response to surgical treatment is common when symptoms correlate with objective physical signs and with an associated structural abnormality that is visualized by imaging. A central disc prolapse may lead to bilateral sciatica and to early sphincter involvement; early investigation is therefore warranted when either of these features is present.

Lumbar Spinal Stenosis

Lumbar spinal stenosis is an important cause of disability in middle-aged or elderly patients. Superimposed minor disc disease then leads to symptoms that may be disabling. The disorder can be congenital or acquired. The congenital disorder is caused by a reduction in the normal dimensions of the spinal canal and occurs in achondroplastic dwarfs. Acquired lumbar stenosis is usually caused by degenerative disease of the spine and is typically associated with hyperplasia, fibrosis, and cartilaginous changes in the annulus, posterior longitudinal ligament, and ligamentum flavum. Spondylolisthesis (i.e., anterior or posterior displacement of one vertebral body on the next) or spondylolysis, a defect in the pars interarticularis, may contribute to spinal stenosis, as may other anatomic abnormalities. Acquired stenosis may also be related to injury, bony overgrowth such as occurs in Paget's disease, ankylosing spondylitis, rheumatoid arthritis, and diffuse idiopathic skeletal hyperostosis.

Clinical Manifestations and Diagnosis

Patients have pain that is brought on by activity and released by rest or leaning forward. The pain involves the lower part of the back and one or both legs, typically in a radicular distribution, and may be accompanied by numbness or weakness. Examination often reveals no abnormality, except perhaps for a depressed knee or ankle reflex. If examination is performed after activity, a radicular motor or sensory deficit is sometimes found. The results of straight leg raising may be normal. MRI is the most sensitive technique for detecting the disorder.

Treatment

Conservative treatment with NSAIDs and exercise to reduce lumbar lordosis is sometimes beneficial. The choice among NSAIDs (Chapter 28) is arbitrary and depends on the preference of individual physicians because no evidence suggests that one preparation is superior to another. In many cases, however, surgical intervention is the only means of relieving intolerable symptoms.

Cauda Equina Syndrome

An acute cauda equina syndrome occurs after spinal trauma or central lumbosacral disc protrusion. Patients may have bilateral sciatica and saddle anesthesia; disturbances in bladder or bowel function are common and are characterized by frequency, retention, or incontinence. The normal sensation associated with the passage of urine or feces may be lost, and impotence is common. Examination reveals bilateral root dysfunction and, frequently, perianal anesthesia and a lax anal sphincter. Investigations involve urgent imaging to define any surgically remedial lesion. Compressive lesions require urgent decompression—hematomas should be evacuated, and disc protrusions should be treated by laminectomy and excision.

Cervical Disc Disease

Definition

The cervical nerve roots occupy about 30% of the space in the intervertebral foramina that they traverse, accompanied by radicular vessels. The first cervical root exits between the occiput and the C1 vertebra and the subsequent cervical roots exit above their correspondingly numbered vertebra, except for the C8 root, which exits between the C7 and T1 vertebrae (because there is no C8 vertebra).

Pathobiology

Roots may be compressed by a protruded intervertebral disc or by pathology involving the facet joint or joints of Luschka. Disc herniation is the most common cause and occurs especially at the C5–6 and C6–7

TABLE 423–4 DIAGNOSIS OF CERVICAL RADICULOPATHY

	Pain	Weakness (Selected Muscles)	Sensory Loss	Reflex Loss
C5	Neck, shoulder, and interscapular region; lateral aspect of the arm	Deltoid Spinati Rhomboids	Lateral border of the shoulder and upper part of the arm	Biceps (brachioradialis)
C6	Shoulder; lateral aspect of the forearm, and the first two digits	Biceps Brachioradialis Extensor carpi radialis	Lateral aspect of the forearm and the first two digits	Brachioradialis (biceps)
C7	Interscapular region, posterior of the arm, midforearm	Triceps Extensor carpi and digitorum Flexor carpi radialis	Midforearm and middle digit	Triceps
C8	Medial aspect of the forearm and hand	Extensor carpi and digitorum Flexor digitorum (sublimis and profundus) Flexor carpi ulnaris	Medial aspect of the forearm and hand and the fourth and fifth digits	Finger flexors (triceps)
T1	Medial aspect of the arm to the elbow	Intrinsic hand muscles	Medial aspect of the arm to the elbow	

levels, affecting the C6 and C7 roots, respectively. The mechanism by which these various disorders cause radicular pain is unknown.

Clinical Manifestations and Diagnosis

The pain, which is often attributed to compression, angulation, or stretch of the nerve roots, generally subsides with time, even though the anatomic abnormality persists and the root therefore remains distorted. Most patients complain of neck or arm pain. Associated paresthesias are often poorly localized. Weakness is sometimes conspicuous. Table 429–4 summarizes the clinical features of the most common cervical radiculopathies.

Although there is considerable variation in the clinical findings between different patients, single-root involvement can generally be diagnosed by clinical means. Weakness in a myotomal distribution is assessed by evaluating different muscles supplied by the same nerve root but by different peripheral nerves in order to exclude more distal pathology. Motor and sensory function in the lower extremities and gait are evaluated to detect evidence of cord compression.

The Spurling test helps localize symptoms to the cervical spine. The extended neck is rotated and flexed to the side of symptoms, and careful pressure is then applied to the top of the head in a downward direction. Exacerbation of pain or numbness in the extremity supports a diagnosis of cervical root disease, but the lack of such a response does not exclude a radiculopathy. The maneuver should be discontinued if symptoms are reproduced or exacerbated in this way.

Plain radiographs of the cervical spine may be abnormal, but such abnormalities are commonly encountered in asymptomatic subjects. Electromyography is therefore often important in showing the functional relevance of any anatomic abnormalities detected by imaging studies. MRI is the most useful imaging approach because it provides good delineation of soft tissues.

Treatment Rx

Treatment is individualized. Many patients improve without surgical treatment and can therefore be managed conservatively with a soft collar, NSAIDs, or in some instances, traction. The value of other physical measures (e.g., heat, massage, and ultrasound) is unclear; a brief course of oral steroids is sometimes prescribed but is of uncertain benefit. Surgical decompression (discectomy) is necessary in patients with severe pain that is unresponsive to 10 to 12 weeks of conservative measures and in those with a progressive neurologic disturbance.

Cervical Spondylosis

Epidemiology and Pathobiology

Cervical spondylosis is a common cause of dysfunction in patients older than 55 years. Typically, there is bulging or herniation of intervertebral discs, along with osteophytes and ligamentous hypertrophy that is sometimes accompanied by subluxation. The underlying primary pathology is usually degenerative disease of the intervertebral discs. This is followed by reactive hyperostosis with osteophyte formation related to the disc and adjacent vertebral bodies, as well as the facet joints and joints of Luschka. Other associated pathologic findings include thickening of the ligamentum flavum, disc herniation, and a congenitally narrow spinal canal. Ischemia of the cord or roots from compression or distortion of small blood vessels may contribute to the neurologic deficit.

Clinical Manifestations and Diagnosis

Cervical spondylosis can be categorized by the anatomic location of the pathology. The lateral syndrome is characterized primarily by radicular pain and focal neurologic deficits that reflect root dysfunction; gait is usually unaffected. In contrast, the medial syndrome is associated with signs of cord involvement and especially with pyramidal tract findings in the legs and a gait disturbance. Many patients have root and cord involvement (i.e., combined syndrome). Pain in the neck may be accompanied by a root deficit in one arm, a clumsy hand, spastic paraparesis, and gait disturbance. A common manifestation is spastic paraparesis. Sudden quadriplegia or paraplegia after trivial injuries or a fall in an elderly person is often caused by spondylotic myelopathy. In all of these syndromes, neck movement may exacerbate the symptoms. Patients with cervical dystonia frequently have severe degenerative disease of the spine and are at greater risk for the development of spondylotic myelopathy.

Examination often reveals a lower motor neuron deficit in one or both upper limbs and a pyramidal tract deficit in the legs. Sensory changes are also present in a distribution that depends on the site of involvement.

Differential Diagnosis

When sensory findings are inconspicuous, the differential diagnosis of spondylotic myelopathy includes amyotrophic lateral sclerosis. The difficulty in diagnosis is compounded by the common occurrence of degenerative changes in the cervical spine in asymptomatic elderly persons and their coexistence in those with other neurologic disorders. Other causes of spastic paraparesis occurring in middle-aged or elderly persons must be excluded. Involvement of the hands in patients with spondylotic myelopathy may be of the lower motor neuron type in those with involvement of the C8–T1 segments or the upper motor neuron type in those with more rostral pathology. Extreme lateral herniation of a cervical disc may occasionally lead to compression of the vertebral artery and therefore to ischemia in the posterior circulation.

Imaging

Plain radiographs show disc space narrowing, osteophyte formation, and variable spondylolisthesis. Plain radiographs of the cervical spine in flexion and extension and surface coil MRI are particularly helpful in diagnosing spinal canal stenosis (i.e., anteroposterior canal diameter of less than 11 mm), herniated discs, and intradural pathology. MRI also indicates whether the most prominent compression is anterior or posterior in patients with cervical spondylosis, thereby helping to guide treatment.

Treatment

Rx

Surgical decompression is generally advised in patients with progressive neurologic dysfunction or a fixed deficit of less than 12 months' duration. The value of surgery, however, is uncertain. Surgery may involve an anterior or posterior approach. The efficacy of various surgical approaches is difficult to determine because the natural history of the disorder is unclear, methods of assessing outcome are not standardized, and postoperative complications are often not stated. The most optimistic figures suggest that between 15 and 30% of patients do not benefit from surgery, and several older studies indicate that up to 25% of patients worsen after laminectomy. A summary of the literature suggests that between 25 and 75% of patients improve after surgery and between 5 and 50% worsen after it. Given the uncertainties of the natural history, it is not clear whether benefit is related to surgery or occurs despite it. Regardless of the difficulty in determining its precise value, surgery is so widely accepted as a therapeutic option that it is difficult to withhold it in patients who are deteriorating despite conservative measures.

Measurement of cervical mobility is helpful in selecting patients who are more likely to deteriorate because patients with spinal hypermobility are more prone to deteriorate without surgery. Patients without major deficits or whose disorder is nonprogressive should be treated conservatively and monitored over time. Those with a greater level of disability when first seen are usually referred for surgical treatment, which is also indicated to arrest a progressive course.

Surgical treatment includes posterolateral or anterolateral approaches, as well as laminectomy, foraminotomy, and neurolysis, which may be combined with osteophyte excision.

Posterior Approach

The posterior approach allows good visualization of affected nerve roots, facilitates removal of any constricting material, and permits enlargement of the intervertebral foramen. In patients with diffuse spinal stenosis, laminectomy is the preferred approach, but it does not reduce any dynamic forces affecting the cord and may increase cervical mobility, which is associated with an increased risk for neurologic complications. In a few patients, increased radicular or cord deficits develop after surgery via the posterior approach.

Anterior Approach

The anterior approach permits easier decompression of roots and cord and removal of disc material. In patients with cervical spondylotic myelopathy, herniated discs and osteophytic spurs are indications for surgery by this approach. Fusion is favored by some surgeons, but the need for it is uncertain. Cord or root damage after surgery via the anterior approach occurs in a few instances, and other complications have also been described, including esophageal perforation, damage to various nerves (e.g., brachial plexus, superior laryngeal nerve, hypoglossal nerve, and sympathetic nerves), epidural hemorrhage, and damage to major blood vessels.

DISORDERS OF THE SPINAL CORD

Inflammatory Disorders Involving the Spinal Cord

Compression of the spinal cord or nerve roots may occur as a result of inflammatory diseases such as spinal osteomyelitis or tuberculosis, acute or chronic meningitis, sarcoidosis, and the connective tissue diseases. When the inflammatory process involves the subarachnoid space, root involvement is often multifocal and difficult to explain on the basis of a lesion at one site or level.

Spinal Arachnoiditis

Spinal arachnoiditis may follow the introduction of blood or foreign substances into the intrathecal space, but in some instances, it arises without obvious precipitating cause. It has sometimes followed epidural steroid therapy or related procedures. Spinal arachnoiditis is characterized by neck or back pain, often accompanied by radicular pain at the level of involvement. Cord involvement occurs less commonly but in severe cases may lead to paraplegia. The diagnosis is established by imaging studies, which sometimes reveal evidence of associated cord cavitation. Spinal fluid typically shows an increased protein concentration; in some instances there may be mild pleocytosis and a reduced glucose concentration. No specific treatment is available for spinal arachnoiditis other than lysis of adhesions and opening of subarachnoid cysts, unless an infective organism can be identified.

Acute Disseminated Encephalomyelitis

Acute disseminated encephalomyelitis (Chapter 439) is an acute monophasic neurologic illness that develops a few days after viral infection (e.g., measles or herpes zoster) and certain bacterial infections (e.g., *Mycoplasma pneumoniae*). Patients have symptoms of encephalitis or myelitis. The myelitis is manifested by flaccid paralysis of one or more limbs, most commonly the legs, variable sensory loss that may produce a sensory level, and loss of sphincter function. The tendon reflexes are often depressed initially, but the plantar responses are extensor. Cerebrospinal fluid typically shows a lymphocytic pleocytosis and an increased protein concentration. In severe cases, spinal cord necrosis occurs and may be associated with a fatal outcome (i.e., acute necrotizing hemorrhagic leukoencephalomyelitis). In patients who succumb, pathologic examination reveals perivenular mononuclear cell infiltration with demyelination; cord lesions are typically subpial in location.

Multiple Sclerosis

Multiple sclerosis (Chapter 436) is a disorder characterized by involvement of different regions of the central white matter at different times by an inflammatory process. The disorder commonly begins in young adult life and may follow a chronic, progressive, or relapsing and remitting course. Clinical onset usually consists of the acute development of a focal neurologic deficit that progressively worsens over several days and then shows partial or complete remission over a period of several weeks or longer. After a variable interval of a few days to many years, another attack occurs. With succeeding attacks, remission is often incomplete, and patients are left with a neurologic deficit that becomes increasingly severe as further attacks occur. In most patients, signs of progressive myelopathy become increasingly conspicuous with advancing disease. Eventually, the spinal cord may become atrophic. Further details of the clinical course, cause, diagnosis, and treatment of the disease are provided in Chapter 436.

Neuromyelitis Optica

Neuromyelitis optica (Devic's disease) refers to acute myelopathy accompanied by retrobulbar or optic neuritis. It appears to be a distinct entity as opposed to a form of multiple sclerosis or acute disseminated encephalomyelitis (Chapter 439).

Progressive Necrotizing Myelopathy

Progressive necrotizing myelopathy may occur at any age but is seen especially in young adults, usually after an infectious illness, or in patients with a known malignancy, usually small cell cancer of the lung or lymphomas such as Hodgkin's disease. Typically, patients complain of pain in the back or legs, sometimes accompanied by paresthesias. The legs then become weak and eventually paralyzed. The tendon reflexes are often lost initially, but after a variable interval, spasticity and hyperreflexia develop. Sensory deficits may be conspicuous, and sphincter disturbances are usual. The disorder follows a progressive course that eventually leads to respiratory disturbances and bulbar signs. A somewhat similar disorder has been described in patients with spinal vascular malformations under the eponym of Foix-Alajouanine syndrome. There is no specific treatment. Pathologic examination shows necrotic areas in the cord, especially in the thoracic region; in long-standing cases the cord is atrophic.

Transverse Myelitis

The designation *transverse myelitis* (Chapter 436) is used for an intrinsic lesion that interrupts most of the large tracts across the greater part of the horizontal extent of the cord at the level of the lesion. The term implies an inflammatory process, but in most instances this has not been clearly established. Transverse myelitis may occur as a feature of multiple sclerosis or Devic's disease, but it is generally an isolated event occurring after viral infections and in other contexts in which the cause is less clear or unknown. Patients typically have back pain, leg weakness, sensory disturbances below the level of the lesion, and sphincter dysfunction, especially urinary retention. Its onset is usually acute or subacute, from a few hours to several days, but the disorder sometimes evolves over a period of several weeks. Weakness is typically associated initially with flaccidity and hyporeflexia, but spasticity and hyperreflexia subsequently develop. A sensory level may be present over the trunk, and a band of hyperesthesia sometimes occurs just above this level. High-dosage corticosteroid treatment has been advocated for acute transverse myelitis. Although no controlled clinical trials have been conducted, methylprednisolone (500 mg every 12 hours for 3 days) followed by a tapering schedule of prednisone is often used. The prognosis is variable. About a third of patients show no recovery whatsoever; such an outcome is especially likely when the onset is abrupt, the deficit is severe, or pain is conspicuous at the onset. Nevertheless, some patients with severe transverse myelitis may make a good recovery, and there is no means of accurately predicting the outcome at an early stage.

Acute transverse myelitis sometimes occurs in heroin addicts and usually involves the thoracic cord, although it has occasionally affected other regions. Its cause is uncertain, but the speed of onset suggests a vascular origin. An acute myelitis may rarely occur in various connective tissue diseases, especially systemic lupus erythematosus. Other causes of an acute cord lesion must always be excluded, including iatrogenic myelopathies (e.g., after irradiation or intrathecal administration of methotrexate), vitamin B_{12} deficiency, and the myelopathies discussed earlier.

Vascular Disorders Involving the Spinal Cord

The spinal cord is supplied by the anterior and paired posterior spinal arteries, which are fed by segmental vessels at different levels. The posterior spinal arteries receive numerous feeders along their length. The anterior spinal artery, in contrast, is supplied by only a limited number, but usually by three or more vessels in the cervical and upper thoracic region, one in the midthoracic region between T4 and T8, and caudally by a single large vessel, the artery of Adamkiewicz, which generally arises from a segmental artery between about T9 and L2, most commonly on the left side. The anterior and posterior spinal arteries give off branches that form a fine network around the spinal cord, from which radially oriented branches supply much of the white matter and the posterior horns of the gray matter. The central or sulcocommissural arteries are the main branches of the anterior spinal artery. They originate in various numbers at each segmental level, in the anterior longitudinal fissure, and supply one or other lateral half of the cord. Through these vessels, blood is supplied to the gray matter and the innermost portions of the white matter.

Venous drainage of the cord is similarly organized into interconnecting anterior and posterior systems. An anteromedian group of intrinsic veins empties through the central veins into the anterior median spinal vein in the anterior longitudinal fissure. This venous system in particular drains the capillaries of the gray and white commissures, the medial columns of the anterior horns, and the anterior funiculi. The rest of the cord drains through radially oriented veins that connect with the posterolateral venous system running longitudinally on the surface of the cord. The veins on the surface of the cord drain via the medullary veins through the intervertebral foramina and converge there with the radicular veins draining the nerve roots and with communications from the anterior and posterior epidural and paravertebral plexuses.

Ischemic Myelopathy

Ischemia may contribute to the neurologic deficit that occurs in patients with space-occupying lesions and those with post-traumatic or postirradiation myelopathy. Wasting of the intrinsic muscles of the hands may result from compression of the anterior spinal artery in patients with lesions of the foramen magnum.

Disease of the abdominal aorta (Chapter 78) may cause an ischemic myelopathy. Aortic occlusion, dissecting or nondissecting aortic aneurysms, inflammatory aortitis, and emboli involving the aorta may all lead to cord dysfunction, as may surgery involving the aorta, especially in the region of origin of the artery of Adamkiewicz. Imaging studies such as aortography and mediastinal angiography can also lead to ischemic myelopathy. Aortic coarctation of the adult type may cause cord ischemia below the narrowed segment, and neurogenic intermittent claudication may occur because of the diversion of blood from the cord by retrograde flow in the anterior spinal artery to bypass the narrowed region. In classic coarctation, a cervicothoracic myelopathy may result from cord compression by enlarged collateral vessels or from a steal phenomenon, and rupture of aneurysmally distended vessels may lead to subarachnoid hemorrhage. Management involves surgical treatment of the coarctation.

Severe hypotension of any cause has been associated with ischemic myelopathy. The cord is involved particularly in the watershed regions where the anterior spinal artery is most remote from segmental feeding vessels. Some physicians regard the midthoracic region as being especially vulnerable to such ischemia.

When acute ischemia leads to transverse myelopathy, patients have the sudden onset of a flaccid areflexic paraplegia or quadriplegia, analgesia and anesthesia below the level of the lesion, and retention of urine and feces. Back pain is sometimes conspicuous at the level of the lesion. Curiously, occlusion of the spinal arteries by atherosclerotic or inflammatory processes, by emboli from the heart, or by fragments of nucleus pulposus is rare. Rapid exposure to high altitude or decompression of divers may lead to nitrogen emboli. Pathologic involvement of the posterior spinal arteries is so uncommon that many physicians doubt that it can be recognized clinically. The syndrome attributed to it consists of ipsilaterally impaired vibration and postural sense below the level of the lesion, along with segmental anesthesia and areflexia. An ipsilateral pyramidal tract deficit, mild and usually transient, also occurs if the lateral funiculus is affected. Anterior spinal artery occlusion, in contrast, is well described and leads to sudden, severe back pain, sometimes associated with radicular pain; this pain is followed by the rapid onset of flaccid paraplegia or quadriplegia, together with urinary and fecal retention. With recovery from spinal shock, an upper motor neuron syndrome develops below the level of the lesion, and neurogenic atrophy occurs in muscles supplied by the infarcted segments. A dissociated sensory loss is characteristic, with impairment of temperature and pain appreciation but relative sparing of light touch and joint position sense. The prognosis for recovery is poor, especially if improvement fails to occur within the first 36 to 48 hours.

Venous infarction of the cord occurs most commonly in association with an arteriovenous malformation but is occasionally related to sepsis, malignant disease, or vertebral disorders. Sudden back pain heralds the onset of weakness and sensory loss in the legs, with accompanying retention of urine and feces. The deficit may progress over the next few days to that of an acute transverse myelopathy, and a fatal outcome is common.

Embolism of nucleus pulposus material has been reported, particularly in women, who experience acute neck or back pain, followed within a few minutes by rapidly progressive limb weakness and sensory loss to all modalities. The cervical region is affected most commonly. Infectious complications may lead to death. Diagnosis in life is usually difficult, but autopsy reveals characteristic emboli in the spinal vessels. The manner in which the fibrocartilage of the nucleus pulposus enters into the circulatory system is unclear.

Neurogenic Intermittent Claudication

The development of pain or a neurologic deficit after exercise or with certain postures that extend the lumbar spine, with relief by rest or change in posture (i.e., leaning forward), has been designated *neurogenic intermittent claudication.* It may involve the spinal cord or the cauda equina. In contrast to the intermittent claudication of peripheral vascular disease, symptoms typically begin in part of a lower limb and then spread, often in a radicular distribution. Moreover, peripheral vascular disease is typically associated with reduced or absent peripheral pulses, a proximal arterial bruit, and cutaneous evidence of impaired circulation.

Examination may reveal no abnormalities unless performed while the patient is symptomatic, during which motor, sensory, or reflex changes may be found. Imaging studies confirm the presence of spinal stenosis or a structural abnormality involving the cord or cauda equina. The most common cause of intermittent claudication of the cord is probably a spinal vascular malformation.

Hemorrhage

Hematomyelia (i.e., hemorrhage into the spinal cord) or spinal subarachnoid hemorrhage may occur as a result of trauma, spinal vascular malformations, intradural spinal neoplasms, coarctation of the aorta, or ruptured spinal aneurysms. It may be associated with connective tissue diseases, blood dyscrasias, or anticoagulant therapy. In some instances, no cause can be identified.

Spinal Subarachnoid Hemorrhage

Spinal subarachnoid hemorrhage is heralded by the onset of sudden severe pain that begins at the site of bleeding but spreads rapidly to the rest of the back and, with cervical lesions, to the head. Dysfunction of the cord or nerve roots may result from compression by blood or a blood clot and lead to weakness, sensory disturbances, and impaired sphincter function. Signs of meningeal irritation are present. A spinal bruit or cutaneous vascular malformation suggests a spinal origin of the hemorrhage. CT can confirm the presence of blood in the subarachnoid space, and MRI may reveal a spinal vascular malformation. When MRI is unrevealing, myelography is performed with a large volume of contrast medium and the patient examined in the prone and supine positions. The prognosis reflects the cause and severity of the hemorrhage. Decompressive surgery may be necessary. An underlying spinal vascular malformation requires angiographic definition, followed by occlusion of feeding vessels by embolization or surgery. Neoplastic lesions may necessitate surgical treatment, and blood dyscrasias, anticoagulant-induced hemorrhage, or connective tissue diseases require appropriate medical management.

Intramedullary Hemorrhage

Intramedullary hemorrhage also leads to a neurologic deficit, but pain may be less conspicuous, especially if the hemorrhage remains confined within the spinal cord. Further evaluation is conducted as for spinal subarachnoid hemorrhage.

Spinal Subdural Hemorrhage

Spinal subdural hemorrhage may occur spontaneously or after trauma or lumbar puncture, especially in patients with blood dyscrasias or those receiving anticoagulant drugs. Sudden severe back pain is followed by a compressive myelopathy or cauda equina syndrome. CT or MRI is helpful in identifying the underlying lesion. Complete recovery may follow early evacuation of the hematoma, whereas an irreversible neurologic deficit can result from delaying surgery. The risk for spinal subdural hemorrhage is reduced in patients with predisposing hematologic disorders by correcting the underlying abnormality via transfusion before lumbar puncture. In patients with thrombocytopenia, platelet transfusion should be considered before lumbar puncture when the platelet count is less than 20,000/mm^3 or is dropping rapidly.

Spinal Epidural Hemorrhage

Spinal epidural hemorrhage results most commonly from trauma but also occurs in patients with epidural vascular malformations or tumors or hemorrhagic disorders. It sometimes occurs spontaneously or after a spinal tap or epidural anesthesia, especially in patients receiving anticoagulant drugs. Sudden severe back pain, sometimes accompanied by radicular pain, is usually the initial feature and is enhanced by activities that increase pressure in the vertebral venous plexus. A cord or cauda equina syndrome then develops after a variable interval. Clinical distinction of epidural from subdural hemorrhage may be impossible. MRI is helpful in detecting the hemorrhage, defining its anatomic site, and distinguishing it from other epidural lesions. Urgent evacuation is necessary to prevent irreversible neurologic damage.

Spinal Vascular Malformations

Pathobiology

A variety of vascular malformations occur in relation to the spinal cord and meninges. Arteriovenous fistulas, the most common and clinically important, consist of an abnormal communication between the arterial and venous systems without intervening capillaries. Telangiectases and cavernous malformations are uncommon and usually asymptomatic, although hemorrhage occasionally leads to a focal neurologic deficit.

Most spinal arteriovenous fistulas are located in the thoracolumbar region, are extramedullary, are supplied by vessels that do not supply the cord, and are so situated that the arteriovenous shunt is dural in location. In contrast, 20 to 30% of fistulas are located in the cervical or upper thoracic segments, and they are often intramedullary, are supplied by vessels contributing to the anterior spinal circulation, have multiple feeding vessels, and consist of an arteriovenous shunt that is usually of large volume.

Diagnosis

Spinal arteriovenous fistulas may be accompanied by subarachnoid hemorrhage or, more commonly, by myeloradiculopathy. Spinal subarachnoid hemorrhage occurs in about 10% of all spinal arteriovenous fistulas and has an overall mortality rate of approximately 15%; approximately half of survivors of the first hemorrhage will have another unless the underlying malformation is treated. The myeloradiculopathy typically has a gradual onset and progression but sometimes follows a relapsing and remitting course. Initial symptoms consist most commonly of pain or sensory disturbances, but by the time of diagnosis, many patients are found to have a more severe neurologic deficit characterized by weakness, sensory deficits, pain, and impaired sphincter function. Symptoms of neurogenic claudication of the cord or cauda equina are common. With thoracolumbar malformations, examination typically reveals a mixed upper and lower motor neuron deficit in the legs and a sensory disturbance. With cervical lesions, a mixed motor deficit in the arms is associated with an upper motor neuron deficit in the legs and sensory changes below the level of the lesion. The presence of a spinal bruit is helpful in suggesting the diagnosis, but its absence does not exclude it. The myeloradiculopathy may progress with rapidity and cause severe disability unless the underlying malformation is treated. It is probably related to cord ischemia; venous hypertension causes a reduction in the arteriovenous pressure gradient across the spinal cord and therefore a reduction in intramedullary blood flow. An acute onset or exacerbation of symptoms, however, may be related to intramedullary hemorrhage or to intravascular thrombosis. Radicular symptoms are presumably related to ischemia or compression of nerve roots.

Imaging

MRI permits easy visualization of the spinal cord, but it sometimes fails to detect a vascular malformation, in which case myelography should be undertaken when the diagnosis is suspected. The characteristic finding consists of serpiginous defects in the column of contrast material as a result of vascular impressions. The examination should be performed with a large volume of contrast medium and with the patient screened in the prone and supine positions. Spinal angiography is important in defining the anatomic features of the arteriovenous fistula and the normal blood supply to the spinal cord, but it is not indicated when myelography fails to suggest the diagnosis.

Treatment

Depending on the angiographic findings, surgical excision, embolic occlusion of feeding vessels, or both can be undertaken. Motor deficits are more likely to improve than other symptoms, and sphincter disturbances improve in only abut a third of cases; symptoms in the lower thoracic region tend to improve more than those from more rostral lesions. Treatment may not be possible for arteriovenous fistulas that are anterior to or within the spinal cord and are fed by the anterior spinal artery or one of its feeding vessels. However, interventional radiologic procedures involving embolization of some of the feeding vessels may still be possible in such circumstances.

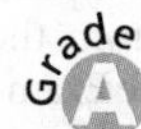

1. Hagen KB, Jamtvedt G, Hilde G, et al: The updated Cochrane review of bed rest for low back pain and sciatica. Spine 2005; 30:542–546.
2. Assendelft WJ, Morton SC, Yu EI, et al: Spinal manipulative therapy for low back pain. Cochrane Database Syst Rev 2004;1:CD000447.

3. Manheimer E, White A, Berman B, et al: Meta-analysis: Acupuncture for low back pain. Ann Intern Med 2005;142:651–663.
4. Hertzman-Miller RP, Morgenstern H, Hurwitz EL, et al: Comparing the satisfaction of low back pain patients randomized to receive medical or chiropractic care: Results from the UCLA low-back pain study. Am J Public Health 2002;92:1628–1633.
5. Hayden JA, van Tulder MW, Tomlinson G: Systematic review: Strategies for using exercise therapy to improve outcomes in chronic low back pain. Ann Intern Med 2005;142:776–785.
6. Peul WC, van Houwelingen HC, van den Hout WB, et al: Surgery versus prolonged conservative treatment for sciatica. N Engl J Med 2007;356:2245–2256.
7. Fritzell P, Hagg O, Wessberg P, et al: Swedish Lumbar Spine Study Group: Lumbar fusion versus nonsurgical treatment for chronic low back pain: A multicenter randomized controlled trial from the Swedish Lumbar Spine Study Group. Spine 2001;26:2521–2532.

SUGGESTED READINGS

Balague F, Mannion AF, Pellise F: Clinical update: Low back pain. Lancet 2007;369:726–728. *A comprehensive review.*

Carette S, Fehlings MG: Cervical radiculopathy. N Engl J Med 2005;353:392–399. *A case-based review.*

Carragee EJ: Persistent low back pain. N Engl J Med 2005;352:1891–1898. *A practical overview.*

Cenzato M, Versari P, Righi C, et al: Spinal dural arteriovenous fistulae: Analysis of outcome in relation to pretreatment indicators. Neurosurgery 2004; 55:815–822. *Comparison of outcome in relation to pretreatment status after surgical or endovascular treatment.*

Deyo RA, Nachemson A, Mirza SK: Spinal-fusion surgery—the case for restraint. N Engl J Med 2004;350:722–726. *Caution about adding spinal fusion to simple laminectomy or discectomy.*

Jarvic JG, Deyo RA: Diagnostic evaluation of low back pain with emphasis on imaging. Ann Intern Med 2002;137:586–597. *Review of the yield of various diagnostic tests.*

Novy J, Carruzzo A, Maeder P, et al: Spinal cord ischemia: Clinical and imaging patterns, pathogenesis, and outcomes in 27 patients. Arch Neurol 2006; 63:1113–1120. *A review of spinal cord ischemia.*

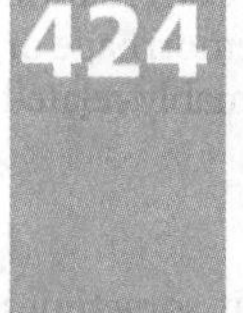

424 REGIONAL CEREBRAL DYSFUNCTION: HIGHER MENTAL FUNCTIONS

David S. Knopman

Definition

Higher mental function is at the core of what defines competent, independent individuals. Impairment of higher mental function can be broadly classified into four categories. Mental retardation is a form of cognitive impairment that is present from infancy. Acquired forms of cognitive impairment are delirium, dementia, and focal cognitive disorders. Delirium (Chapter 26) is defined by its acute or subacute onset and coexistent alterations in alertness. Dementia (Chapter 425) represents acquired cognitive impairment that is usually gradual in onset and not associated with alterations in alertness. Focal cognitive disorders involve only one aspect of cognition: memory, language, visuospatial cognition, or executive cognitive functioning, each of which is supported by a different cerebral region.

For the majority of patients in a non-neurology practice, a global description such as "normal mental function" or "cognitively impaired" will suffice. "Cognitive impairment" then becomes a diagnosis that subsumes all forms of altered higher mental function regardless of which domains are affected or how severely they are affected.

Clinical Manifestations and Diagnosis

An informal conversation with a patient lacks sensitivity for detecting cognitive impairment. If cognitive impairment is suspected from the patient's history, formal assessments such as the Mini-Mental State Examination (see Table 25–4) should be performed. Bedside evaluations of orientation, memory, language, reasoning, and visuospatial functions derive an overall view of cognitive function but do not automatically translate into diagnoses because alertness, cooperation, education, native language, sensorimotor function, and mood must be taken into account. Although scores on bedside mental status examinations correlate strongly with severity and prognosis, they provide only rough guides to cognitive ability and cannot localize a cognitive deficit anatomically in the brain. If cognitive dysfunction is discovered in the course of the bedside examination, further exploration of individual cognitive domains must be undertaken.

MEMORY FUNCTION AND AMNESIC DISORDERS

Definition

Human memory operates over a wide time range, from seconds to decades and with quantities of information ranging from a single word to a lifetime's experience. Each neural system that achieves this monumental dynamic range has its own brain localization (Table 424–1).

Declarative memory describes the type of learning and retrieval of facts and information that occur with conscious attention and intent; examples include remembering conversations, events, and intentions. Declarative memory includes semantic and episodic components. Semantic memory refers to the brain's storehouse of knowledge, words, and facts. Episodic memory refers to learning and recall of specific events. Retention of information for more than a few seconds, in the face of exposure to additional facts, details, or events, requires declarative episodic memory to store and organize information suitable for later recall. It is this declarative, episodic memory system that is assessed as "memory" in the clinical setting. Anterograde amnesia is the clinical manifestation of disturbances in declarative episodic memory. "Anterograde" refers to the failure to learn and hence recall new information on an ongoing basis. Most disorders of memory also exhibit retrograde amnesia, a disturbance of the ability to retrieve information from the past.

Immediate recall of information with zero delay and zero intervening information is a very short-term declarative memory function. Immediate memory is capable of storing an image of an auditory message in exact form, but only a small amount and for a short period. The fidelity of immediate memory recall accuracy drops off dramatically over seconds, particularly if intervening sensory stimuli attract attention. A comparable system exists in the visual modality in that the memory acts like a photograph that fades rapidly. From a clinical perspective, immediate memory is separate from declarative episodic memory. Immediate recall is generally used as a marker of attention and alertness and not memory per se. Loss of immediate recall is not usually indicative of memory loss.

Pathobiology

The hippocampal formations are the anatomic structures of importance for the declarative episodic memory system. The hippocampal formations are imaged well with magnetic resonance imaging (MRI) (Fig. 424–1). The principal input to the hippocampus comes through the entorhinal cortex from multimodal association areas in the frontal, parietal, and temporal neocortex. A second important input is a cholinergic pathway that originates in the septum of the medial-orbital frontal lobe. There are two principal output circuits of the hippocampal formations. One is via the subiculum back to multimodal association areas. The other hippocampal efferent pathway projects via the fornix to the mammillary bodies. The projection from the mammillary bodies passes through the medial thalamus to the ventral anterior nucleus of the thalamus, then to the posterior cingulate, and then back to the entorhinal cortex. The hippocampal circuit is believed to facilitate the formation of memory in association neocortices. The hippocampus does not store a particular learned fact, but rather it enables the appropriate region in a multimodal association cortical region to do so.

Lesions in one hippocampal formation will not generally have as devastating an impact on episodic memory as bilateral lesions will. However, in older people who may have subclinical bilateral hippocampal pathology, a unilateral lesion, particularly in the dominant hemisphere, may produce a dense anterograde amnesia. Lesions in the columns of the fornix, mammillary bodies, and medial thalamus have also been linked to anterograde amnesia.

TABLE 424–1 DESCRIPTION OF MEMORY SYSTEMS

Type of Memory Function	Regional Localization	Learning Efficiency	Time Span until Effective Retrieval	Capacity	Clinical Testing Techniques	Examples in Daily Life
Declarative episodic memory	Hippocampus, medial thalamus	Single exposure	Decades	Very large, with rehearsal and elaboration	Recall of 3–4 words after 5 minutes	Recall of recent events and conversations
Declarative semantic memory	Temporal-parietal association cortices	Capable of single exposure; enhanced with repetition	Decades	Very large, perhaps limitless	Confrontation naming, general knowledge	Vocabulary, knowledge of life events from remote past
Attention span, "immediate memory"	Primary auditory or visual cortex	Single exposure only	Seconds	Very small: 7 ± 2 digits (auditory)	Digit span	Dialing a telephone number after hearing it or reading it in a phone book
Working memory	Lateral frontal cortex	Single exposure only	Seconds	Small	Digits backward	Supporting many mental activities, such as mental arithmetic, abstract reasoning
Procedural memory	Basal ganglia, probably association neocortices	Requires extensive training	Decades	Moderate	Experimental laboratory methods only	Retention of motor skills, e.g., riding a bicycle or typing

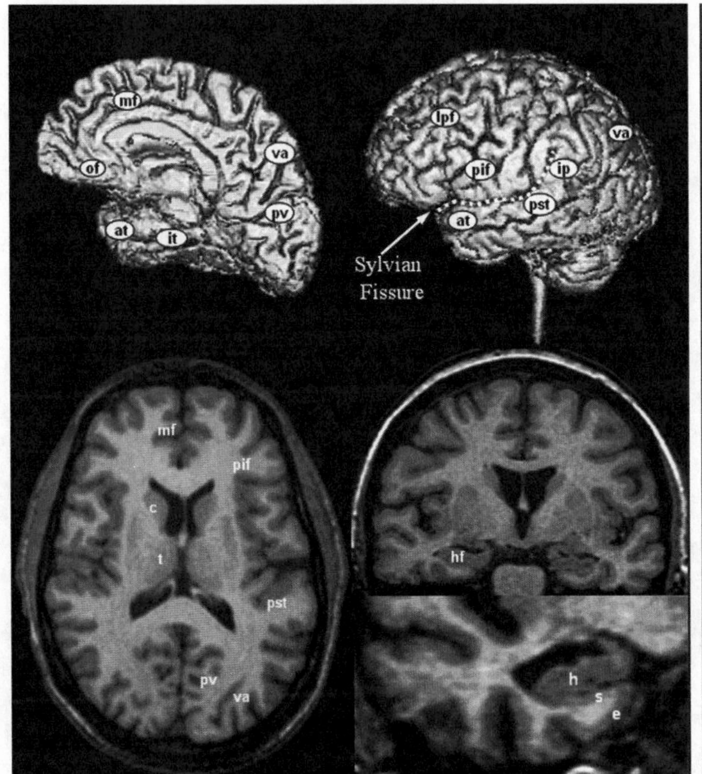

FIGURE 424–1 • Magnetic resonance images of normal brain. Upper left, Midsagittal view; **upper right,** left lateral view; **lower left,** axial view through the head of the caudate and body of the thalamus; **lower right,** coronal view through the mammillary bodies, with a magnified view of the medial temporal lobe. at = anterior temporal; c = caudate nucleus; e = entorhinal cortex; h = hippocampus; hf = hippocampal formation; ip = inferior parietal cortex; it = inferior temporal; lpf = lateral prefrontal cortex; mf = medial frontal cortex; of = orbital frontal cortex; pif = posterior inferior frontal cortex (Broca's area); pst = posterior superior temporal; pv = primary visual cortex (area 17); s = subiculum; t = temporal; va = visual association cortex (areas 18, 19). (Courtesy of Maria Shiung and Clifford Jack, MD.)

Clinical Manifestations

Patients with anterograde amnesia have poor or no recollection of events, conversations, or observations. Family members report that patients repeat themselves in conversation or re-ask the same questions over the course of a few minutes to hours. Patients will generally forget important events and conversations, even when they were fully engaged in them. They will lose track of the date and the time of day. They will forget appointments, even with reminders. Generally, patients with anterograde amnesia will fail to encode most events and happenings around them. The consequences of such memory failure are usually more evident to family and acquaintances of patients with the disorder than they are to the patients themselves. Anosognosia (lack of awareness) for the deficit of anterograde amnesia is very common, though not universal. Patients who most vehemently complain of memory loss are often suffering from depression rather than focal cognitive dysfunction.

Because some degree of forgetting is ubiquitous in human experience, it is challenging to distinguish between "everyday" forgetting and forgetting that is pathologic. All adults occasionally misplace important items, overlook an appointment, or forget some part of a conversation. In cognitively normal individuals, distraction, preoccupation, inattention, exhaustion, sleep deprivation, or other major life stressors inevitably produce some instances of excess forgetting. Pathologic forgetting as a result of a brain disorder produces a much greater degree of forgetting than occurs in the course of normal daily life, but there is no formulaic description of the boundary at which normal forgetting ends and pathologic forgetting begins.

Diagnosis

The diagnosis of anterograde amnesia begins with the complaint of memory impairment from the patient or from someone close to the patient. Testing of memory can be performed at the bedside in alert patients. The patient is asked to learn three or four words and recall them after 1 or 2 minutes. A patient with severe anterograde amnesia will recall none or at most one of the words, whereas individuals with normal memory can recall all of the words or all but one.

In patients with questionable memory difficulties, assessment by an experienced neuropsychologist is often a necessary part of the evaluation. Standardized tests of memory have greater precision and reliability and involve the use of lengthier material to be remembered and a longer delay between learning and recall.

Determining the Cause

Alzheimer's disease is the most common disorder in which anterograde amnesia occurs (Chapter 425). In Alzheimer's disease, anterograde amnesia is usually the dominant cognitive symptom, particularly early in the illness. Hippocampal atrophy is common (see Fig. 425–3). Anterograde amnesia also occurs in other dementing illnesses, such as vascular dementia and dementia with Lewy bodies.

Strokes can damage regions involved in episodic memory. Occlusion of the medial temporal branch of the posterior cerebral artery causes infarction of the hippocampus. Infarction in the territory of penetrating branches of the tip of the basilar artery causes bilateral medial thalamic infarcts.

Anterograde amnesia may be a major residual deficit after herpes simplex encephalitis (Chapter 397). Herpes simplex encephalitis has a predilection to damage structures at the base of the cerebral hemispheres; frequently, the temporal lobes are severely damaged. Korsakoff's syndrome, the residual of the encephalopathy of thiamine deficiency (Chapter 443), is characterized by profound anterograde amnesia. Hemorrhagic necrosis of the mammillary bodies occurs in Korsakoff's syndrome. Survivors of closed head injuries (Chapter 422) may have anterograde amnesia because the medial temporal lobes are vulnerable to trauma as a result of their close proximity to the temporal bone. Survivors of an episode of anoxic-ischemic encephalopathy may also have dense anterograde amnesia. The pyramidal neurons of the CA1 region of the hippocampus are particularly vulnerable to hypoxic injury.

The syndrome of transient global amnesia involves anterograde amnesia, but the duration of the amnesia is a matter of 6 to 12 hours rather than the weeks or months in post-traumatic amnesia or the permanent deficits in Alzheimer's disease or Korsakoff's syndrome. Transient global amnesia generally affects middle-aged or elderly individuals. Its cause is not known, although it is not usually due to typical cerebrovascular disease or epilepsy. Electroencephalography is typically not specifically abnormal, but diffusion-weighed MRI often shows distinctive abnormalities of the hippocampus a day or more after the onset of transient global amnesia.

THE APHASIAS

Definition

Aphasia is a disorder of language at the conceptual level. Aphasics may have difficulty with producing language, comprehending language, or both.

Pathobiology

In more than 99% of right-handed individuals, language is localized to the left hemisphere. In left-handed individuals, language is also predominantly localized to the left hemisphere, although varying degrees of bilateral or rarely right hemispheric dominance may be seen. The hemisphere involved in language is referred to as the dominant hemisphere. Anatomic differences in the temporal and parietal lobes of the dominant hemisphere versus the other hemisphere also reflect the specialization for language.

In clinical practice, lesions in the dominant hemisphere's auditory association areas cause receptive language dysfunction. The critical regions are located in the superior temporal lobes adjacent to the primary auditory cortex and in the adjacent supramarginal and angular gyri of the inferior parietal lobule, an area known as Wernicke's area. Lesions in the dominant hemisphere's lateral inferior posterior frontal lobes, often referred to as Broca's area, result in expressive language deficits. Loss of access to one's vocabulary for either understanding spoken language or expressing oneself results from lesions in any portion of the region of the dominant hemisphere around the sylvian fissure, including the lateral posterior inferior frontal lobe, the inferior parietal lobule, and the superior and middle temporal gyri. Coronal and axial MRI scans give a detailed view of the critical language regions (see Fig. 424–1).

Clinical Manifestations

The language comprehension difficulties in aphasia must be distinguished from hearing disorders (Chapter 454), and the motor speech dysfunction in aphasia must be distinguished from dysarthria. Errors of articulation in aphasia reflect altered conceptual selection of what is to be said. In aphasia, mispronunciation of a sound within one word may be followed by perfect pronunciation of the same sound in a different word. In dysarthria, by comparison, the errors in articulation or phonation are consistent.

Aphasia has three principal components: impaired verbal comprehension, disordered verbal expression, and impaired naming. Disorders of reading, writing, and sentence repetition are additional elements of the aphasia syndrome. Disordered verbal comprehension may range from profound to mild. When profound, patients are unable to grasp the meaning of single words. In milder forms of disordered comprehension, patients may be able to follow one-step, but not two- or three-step commands. Usually, the comprehension difficulty involves both spoken and written language, but each can be affected separately. Anomia, which is an inability to produce names of people or objects, is common in almost all aphasic syndromes.

In expressive aphasic syndromes, written material and spoken speech are most often affected in parallel. In the expressive aphasias, speech is labored, and it lacks the normal melody and variation in intonation that characterize normal speaking. Melody and intonation are referred to as the prosody of speech. Speech is often grammatically impoverished. The number of words per utterance is greatly reduced, thus giving the speech a choppy, staccato character. These features are referred to as speech apraxia. Nonfluency is a related term that describes the reduced number of words and the terseness of verbal output. In some aphasic syndromes, speech is often degraded by anomia and paraphasic errors (word or syllable substitutions), even when fluency, melody, and intonation are preserved.

Specific Aphasic Syndromes

Specific, common aphasic syndromes exhibit various combinations of receptive and expressive difficulty (Table 424–2).

Wernicke's Aphasia

In Wernicke's aphasia, verbal comprehension of both written and verbal language is severely impaired. Patients with Wernicke's aphasia have difficulty understanding the meaning of individual words and may not be able to follow any command of greater than one step. Their speech is fluent but marred by paraphasia and anomia. Wernicke's aphasics tend to lack awareness of the extent of their communicative difficulties and are often unaware that the words they are uttering are fundamentally incorrect. The location that typically causes Wernicke's aphasia is the dominant posterior superior temporal lobe or inferior supramarginal gyrus (see Fig. 424–1).

Broca's Aphasia

Broca's aphasia is a syndrome in which expressive language is prominently affected. Patients with Broca's aphasia have nonfluent, labored speech. The lesion location that typically causes Broca's aphasia is the dominant posterior inferior frontal lobe (see Fig. 424–1). Patients with Broca's aphasia have largely preserved comprehension and, as a result, are acutely aware of their difficulties and become frustrated with them. Depression is common in Broca's aphasics.

Global Aphasia

Global aphasia occurs when both expressive and receptive problems are present. Global aphasia often appears acutely after a major dominant hemisphere infarction, hemorrhage, or traumatic brain injury.

Anomia

Anomia is at the milder end of the spectrum of language disorders. Some anomic aphasics also have difficulty with sentence repetition, even in the presence of relatively preserved comprehension and verbal expressive abilities. There is some controversy whether this latter syndrome, called conduction aphasia, represents a disconnection between the

TABLE 424–2 MAJOR APHASIC SYNDROMES

Aphasia Syndrome	Regional Localization	Spontaneous Speech Abnormalities	Auditory Comprehension	Confrontation Naming	Sentence Repetition
Broca's aphasia	Lateral inferior frontal	Nonfluent, labored, agrammatic	Preserved	Poor	Poor
Wernicke's aphasia	Posterior superior temporal–parietal supramarginal gyrus	Fluent, many paraphasic errors, very little information content	Very impaired	Poor	Poor
Global aphasia	Major portions of the frontoparietal operculum and superior temporal lobe	Nonfluent or virtually absent	Very impaired	Poor	Poor
Anomic aphasia	Small lesion somewhere in the perisylvian region	Fluent, may contain some paraphasias	Normal or mildly impaired	Poor to moderately impaired	Preserved or impaired

perisylvian centers for comprehension and expression or whether it represents a lesion in the cortical auditory areas involved in immediate auditory memory.

Ideomotor Apraxia

Ideomotor apraxia is a disorder at the interface between comprehension and execution of facial or limb motor actions. Patients with ideomotor apraxia have no paresis of the face or limb musculature and are able to carry out simple tasks, but they are unable to execute more complex tasks or commands. For example, in a woman who is able to name a comb and use her right hand to point to parts of her body, ideomotor apraxia can be demonstrated if she is unable to indicate through her actions how she would use the comb.

Diagnosis

The diagnosis of aphasia is made by listening to the patient speak and by examining comprehension, naming ability, reading, and writing in a standardized fashion. Often, the diagnosis of aphasia is made during attempts to obtain a history from the patient. It is helpful to prompt patients to speak about a neutral topic, such as what they had for their last meal or what they did the previous day. Listening to their spontaneous speech allows the examiner to characterize its fluency, grammatical form, articulation, melody, and intonation, as well as difficulty finding words, the presence of paraphasias, and the overall information content.

Comprehension should be examined formally by asking the patient to perform tasks that range from one to at least three steps. Naming can be tested by asking the patient to name a series of common objects, such as the parts of the hand and arm (e.g., thumb, palm, knuckles, wrist, elbow). In general, the more commonly a word is used in the language, the easier it will be to name, whereas infrequent words are harder for aphasics. Reading and writing should also be tested.

Portions of the dominant perisylvian cerebral cortex may be damaged by infarction (Chapters 431 and 432), hemorrhage, and other space-occupying brain lesions such as neoplasm (Chapter 199) or abscesses (Chapter 438). Aphasia secondary to stroke has an abrupt onset, usually with some subsequent improvement. Recovery from aphasia after a stroke may occur as ischemic zones around an infarction eventually regain function. Regions remote from the infarction may also be synaptically depressed acutely after a stroke ("diaschisis") but eventually regain function. Finally, regions in the nondominant hemisphere may become more active over the course of recovery. Aphasia that has a gradual and slowly progressive onset occurs in the degenerative dementia syndromes of progressive aphasia and semantic dementia (Chapter 425).

Treatment 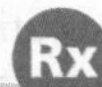

Speech therapy may be helpful for patients in the first few months after a brain injury that causes aphasia.

CORTICAL DISORDERS OF VISUAL FUNCTION AND HEMISPATIAL NEGLECT

Definitions

Cortical disorders of vision and spatial cognition are due to lesions in the occipitoinferotemporal or occipitoposteroparietal lobes. The principal disorders of cortical visual functioning are alexia (impaired reading), object agnosia (impaired recognition of visual forms), and prosopagnosia (impaired face recognition). The principal disorders of spatial cognition are simultanagnosia (impaired integration of complex visual scenes), dressing apraxia, and visual hemispatial neglect (lack of awareness of the personal or extrapersonal hemispace). A diagnosis of a cortical visual disorder requires integrity of primary visual function from the cornea to the lateral geniculate nuclei.

Pathobiology

Higher visual function is localized to a network centered in the occipital lobe and includes the inferior temporal and posterior parietal lobes (see Fig. 424–1). From area 17, processing of visual information passes to the visual association areas 18 and 19. From there it proceeds in several directions. Disorders of higher visual function can be related to a ventral or to a dorsal pathway. The ventral pathway from the visual centers to the medial temporal lobe links visual information to meaning ("What is the object?"). The dorsal visual processing pathway that links the visual centers to the parietal lobes is concerned with locating objects in space and determining spatial relationships among objects in order to grasp a complete visual scene ("Where is the object?"). Cortical control of the extraocular muscles in the parietal lobes is an integral part of the process whereby the eyes are directed to various elements of a visual scene so that the individual elements are synthesized into a coherent ensemble.

Alexia occurs as a result of lesions in the ventral pathway of the dominant hemisphere. Object agnosia may also occur with lesions, usually bilateral, in the ventral pathway. Simultanagnosia, dressing apraxia, and hemispatial neglect are syndromes caused by lesions in the dorsal pathway. Simultanagnosia usually requires bilateral posterior parietal lesions. Dressing apraxia and hemispatial neglect arise from unilateral lesions, most often in the nondominant hemisphere. Cortical blindness is a consequence of bilateral occipitoparietal pathology.

Clinical Manifestations

Alexia may occur as an isolated deficit, or it may occur in the context of other evidence of aphasia. Patients may be able to recognize individual letters but are unable to recognize a string of letters as a word. In pure alexia, auditory comprehension of words and sentences is preserved. Patients with object agnosia may be unable to identify objects visually, but they will be able to recognize the object based on its characteristic sound or how it feels to touch. In simultanagnosia, patients may be able to identify small objects easily if they happen to appear within the narrow viewing area at the center of their visual field. At the same time, such patients will fail to grasp the bigger visual picture. They may appear to be functionally blind. This clinical picture is referred to as Balint's syndrome.

Patients with cortical disorders usually have difficulty with visuoconstructional tasks such as copying figures or drawing simple objects such as a flower, a house, or a clock. Dressing apraxia represents a deficit of practical significance in which patients are unable to comprehend the orientation of articles such as a shirt or a blouse and to manipulate them.

The most severe form of a cortical disorder of visuospatial processing is that of cortical blindness. In this condition, in which the anterior visual pathways can be reasonably believed to be intact, patients appear functionally blind. On occasion, they also exhibit anosognosia for the blindness and claim that they can see. This latter condition is referred to as Anton's syndrome.

Hemispatial neglect occurs in the setting of acute strokes involving the nondominant perisylvian region. Even when there is no hemianopia as measured by single visual stimuli, presentation of double simultaneous stimuli to the patient reveals unawareness in the nondominant field. Hemispatial neglect can be demonstrated at the bedside with a task such as drawing a clock. A patient with hemispatial neglect will fail to place the numbers on the nondominant side (i.e., the left side in a right-handed person). Patients with hemispatial neglect may sometimes deny that their paretic limb belongs to them.

Diagnosis

Information about visual functioning can be obtained by the history. The patient or the patient's informant may report that the patient cannot read, cannot read a clock, or cannot find objects when asked to get something off a table or out of a cupboard. There is often a history of motor vehicle accidents in which the patient failed to see another vehicle, the curb, or the side of a garage. Patients may report difficulty recognizing people's faces, even though they are able to recognize them by their voices or by other cues.

Bedside tests that screen for visuospatial deficits include either copying a simple geometric design or drawing an object. Intersecting pentagons and a cube are objects used clinically. Clock drawing is a brief, but informative exercise. Reading of words or commands and naming of objects can be done at the bedside as well. Face recognition is more difficult to assess at the bedside. Formal testing of visuospatial function in the neuropsychology laboratory involves the use of specially designed instruments to characterize visual processing.

The etiology of lesions that cause deficits in cortical vision and spatial cognition ranges from focal cerebrovascular disease, neoplasms, infectious processes, and brain trauma to neurodegenerative disorders. When a stroke causes a disorder of cortical visuospatial processing or hemispatial neglect, the time course is usually that of an abrupt onset. Space-occupying brain lesions such as neoplasms or brain abscesses that cause cortical visual disorders do so on a subacute basis. Disordered visuospatial function may also appear insidiously when caused by the degenerative disorder posterior cortical atrophy.

EXECUTIVE COGNITIVE DYSFUNCTION AND CONTROL OF PERSONAL BEHAVIOR

Definitions

Integrative abilities that are broadly referred to as executive cognitive function include mental agility, abstract reasoning, and problem solving. Executive cognitive function represents processes that support mental flexibility, adaptability, focus, and tenacity. Control of personal actions and regulation of interpersonal relationships are also closely related to executive cognitive dysfunction. The term "comportment" denotes how a person behaves, particularly toward other people.

Pathobiology

The anatomic basis of executive cognitive function and comportment is a network of brain regions anchored by the prefrontal and anterior temporal lobe neocortex (see Fig. 424–1). These regions receive input from multiple cortical and subcortical regions. The caudate nucleus is a site for a major frontal lobe efferent pathway. The medial thalamus is a major afferent source to the frontal lobes. The anterior temporal lobes are also part of the same integrative circuitry as the prefrontal regions. Lesions in the lateral prefrontal regions are associated with slowing of cognitive processing, difficulty with set shifting (switching from one idea or task to another), difficulty initiating tasks, and loss of mental flexibility. The frontal and anterior temporal lobes are involved in the modulation of personal behavior and interpersonal relationships. Patients with lesions in the medial prefrontal lobes are often apathetic and lack initiative. Patients with lesions in the orbital frontal or right anterior temporal lobe may exhibit disinhibition, impulsivity, and a striking loss of ability to interpret or predict the feelings of others.

Traumatic brain injury (Chapter 422) is a common cause of frontal lobe and anterior temporal damage. The orbital frontal, frontal polar, and anterior temporal regions are particularly vulnerable to contusions because of their proximity to the skull. Patients with traumatic brain injuries may also suffer diffuse white matter damage as a result of shear injuries. Disconnection of the frontal and anterior temporal lobes from other parts of the brain can produce executive cognitive dysfunction and altered control of personal behavior.

Clinical Manifestations

Executive cognitive functioning and control and regulation of behavior are usually affected concurrently. Patients with executive dysfunction are deficient in goal-oriented behavior; they lose the ability to predict the consequences of their actions or words. Patients with executive dysfunction also exhibit poor mental agility and inflexibility in their thinking and control of their actions. They are easily distracted and exhibit a tendency to perseverate, in which the answer to a prior question is repeated in response to subsequent questions. They are disinhibited; as a consequence, when asked to recall a specific event, they may glibly answer with a fabrication, a phenomenon referred to as confabulation.

Patients with lateral prefrontal pathology exhibit poor performance on tests of abstract reasoning and mental agility. In a test such as verbal similarities, they tend to be very concrete and narrowly focused. They become easily distracted and are slow in performing tasks that require sustained attention. Because of their mental rigidity and difficulty in set shifting, they do poorly on tests that require the ability to vary their response strategies, such as verbal fluency tests.

Patients with medial frontal lesions are often profoundly apathetic and lack initiative and motivation. They may be laconic and completely unable to express emotion, whether it be anger, sadness, or elation. They tend to be indifferent to their surroundings, a state referred to as "abulia." The majority of patients with substantial prefrontal or anterior temporal lobe pathology lack insight into the extent of their inappropriate behavior.

In contrast, other patients with altered comportment exhibit different manifestations of dysregulation of personal actions and interpersonal behavior. These alterations may include difficulty controlling impulsivity, poor social graces manifested as rude behavior or caustic comments, a disregard for the feelings of others (loss of empathy), and a general failure to understand what constitutes acceptable behavior in a particular social context. If the underlying disease is progressive, gross alterations in table manners and loss of interest in maintaining personal hygiene may appear. Inappropriate sexual behavior may occur. Patients with prominent disease of the frontal lobes may also exhibit hyperorality, which is a compulsion to put nonfood objects into their mouths. Hyperorality can be life-threatening, depending on the substance ingested.

Diagnosis

The clinical history is essential for documenting the characteristic changes in personality, behavior, and interpersonal relationships. The history must almost always be obtained from an informant who knows the patient well because the patient may assert that there are no problems.

Mental status examination is an integral part of the diagnosis of an executive cognitive disorder. Simply interacting with the patient may be quite revealing. The patient may exhibit abulia, disinhibition, socially inappropriate behavior, or easy distractibility. Tests of executive cognitive function that are suitable for bedside use include verbal similarities and differences, the digits backward test, reciting the months of the year backward, or spelling a word backward. Verbal fluency, which is a very useful test of mental flexibility and set shifting, is tested by asking patients to produce as many words as they can that begin with a particular letter of the alphabet in 60 seconds. Often, a patient with a frontal lesion will quickly produce two or three words and then stop.

Bedside testing of executive cognitive dysfunction provides only a superficial view of the cognitive domain. Assessment in the neuropsychology laboratory gives a more refined estimate of the degree of executive dysfunction.

Space-occupying lesions of the frontal lobes such as neoplasms or brain abscesses can lead to the cognitive and behavioral syndromes of frontal lobe dysfunction. With these diseases, executive cognitive dysfunction and alteration of control of personal behavior develop over a period of weeks.

Neurodegenerative diseases such as frontotemporal lobar degeneration (Chapter 425) are associated with dysfunction and brain loss in the prefrontal (see Fig. 425–4) and anterior temporal lobes. These disorders may produce the entire spectrum of executive cognitive dysfunction and altered control of personal behavior over a period of a year or longer.

Some diseases that do not directly damage the frontal or anterior temporal neocortex may cause executive cognitive dysfunction and alteration of control of personal behavior because of the interconnectedness of the frontal and anterior temporal lobes with other cortical and subcortical regions. Multiple sclerosis (Chapter 436), a disorder of white matter pathways, may cause abnormalities in cognition and behavior of the frontal type. Similarly, Huntington's disease (Chapter 434) and progressive supranuclear palsy, which affect the caudate nuclei, may also resemble a frontal cognitive and behavioral syndrome, with executive cognitive dysfunction and alterations in comportment.

Treatment

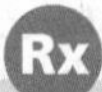

Cognitive-behavioral therapies offer modest, but definite benefit for patients with aphasia and for patients with mild attention deficits and mild memory deficits caused by brain injury. 1

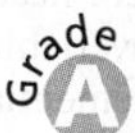

1. Cicerone KD, Dahlberg C, Malec JF, et al: Evidence-based cognitive rehabilitation: Updated review of the literature from 1998 through 2002. Arch Phys Med Rehabil 2005;86:1681–1692.

SUGGESTED READINGS

Knibb JA, Xuereb JH, Patterson K, et al: Clinical and pathological characterization of progressive aphasia. Ann Neurol 2006;59:156–165. *A comprehensive review.*

Miyashita Y: Cognitive memory: Cellular and network machineries and their top-down control. Science 2004;306:435–440. *A review of cognitive and basic science aspects of memory.*

Quinette P, Guillery-Girard B, Dayan J, et al: What does transient global amnesia really mean? Review of the literature and thorough study of 142 cases. Brain 2006;129(Pt 7):1640–1658. *A comprehensive review of transient global amnesia.*

Tekin S, Cummings JL: Frontal-subcortical neuronal circuits and clinical neuropsychiatry. An update. J Psychosom Res 2002;53:647–654. *A review of the neuroanatomic basis and behavioral functions of the frontal lobe system.*

425 ALZHEIMER'S DISEASE AND OTHER DEMENTIAS

David S. Knopman

DEMENTIA

Definition

Dementia, which is a disorder of cognition, interferes with daily functioning and results in loss of independence (Table 425–1). The majority of dementias are of gradual onset, are progressive in course, and occur in persons with previously normal cognition. However, none of these features are necessary aspects of the definition of dementia. Some dementias, such as those caused by an acute neurologic illness secondary to stroke, encephalitis, or head trauma, may begin abruptly and then remain static for long periods. Conversely, a small subset of dementias, such as Creutzfeldt-Jakob disease (Chapter 442), have a rapid onset and a course that can run for less than a year. Dementia may also occur in persons with developmental disabilities and long-standing cognitive deficits.

TABLE 425–1 DEFINITION OF DEMENTIA

Based on evidence from the history and mental status examination, a disorder characterized by the presence of at least two of the following:
- Impairment in learning and retaining new or recently acquired information (impairment in episodic declarative memory)
- Impairment in handling complex tasks and reasoning abilities (impairment in executive cognitive functions)
- Impaired visuospatial ability and geographic orientation
- Impaired language functions

The cognitive disturbance significantly interferes with work, usual social activities, or relationships with others

The cognitive disturbance and the consequences for daily functioning represent a significant decline from a previous level of functioning

The cognitive disturbance does not occur exclusively during the course of delirium (which includes reversibility as a criterion)

The disturbance is not better accounted for by a major psychiatric diagnosis

Epidemiology

The prevalence and incidence of dementia increase with advancing age. Dementia is very uncommon before 50 years of age. In individuals older than 65, the prevalence of dementia of all types is about 7%. In the age range 65 to 69 years, the prevalence of dementia is only 1 to 2%, but it increases to 20 to 25% in the 85- to 89-year-old age range and continues to rise steadily thereafter. The incidence of new cases of dementia is about 1 per 100 per year at the age of 70 years and rises to about 2 to 3 new cases per 100 per year by about age 80. Incidence rates continue to rise into the ninth and tenth decades of life. With the dramatic increase in longevity in North America, the societal burden of dementia has risen substantially.

In absolute numbers, far more women than men have dementia because women live longer. However, men and women have an equal age-adjusted risk for the development of dementia. There are no racial or ethnic differences in the risk for dementia.

Pathobiology

Dementia is the culmination of dysfunction in the cerebral hemispheres, especially the association cortices, hippocampal formations, their supporting subcortical nuclear structures such as the caudate nuclei and thalamus, and their white matter interconnections (see Fig. 424–1). Specific diseases that cause dementia do so by affecting particular parts of the cerebral cortex, subcortical nuclei, or the underlying white matter pathways linking different cortical regions.

Clinical Manifestations

Any of the major domains of cognition—declarative episodic memory, executive cognitive functioning, visuospatial function, or language—may be affected in dementia (Chapter 424). Because Alzheimer's disease is the most common dementia, anterograde amnesia is typically present first and most intensely in the majority of dementia patients. In other dementing illnesses, deficits in the other cognitive domains may be dominant. A pervasive and nearly invariant aspect of dementia is a loss of insight (anosognosia) into the extent of one's cognitive and functional losses.

Neuropsychiatric symptoms are also common in dementia. Apathy and loss of initiative are almost always present. Depression and anxiety are frequent, as are irritability, paranoia, delusional thinking, and hallucinations. Daily functioning of patients with dementia is compromised.

In early dementia, difficulty in managing finances, medications, independent travel, preparation of meals, and keeping appointments is likely to be present. In more advanced disease, difficulty in basic activities of daily living such as bathing, dressing, toileting, and feeding oneself becomes evident. Dementias secondary to cerebrovascular or Lewy body disease are often associated with specific abnormalities in strength, coordination, gait, or balance. Alzheimer's disease, the most common dementia, typically has no associated motor abnormalities.

Diagnosis

Clinical Examination

Dementia is strictly a clinical diagnosis based on evidence of cognitive dysfunction in both the history and the mental status examination. The key elements of the history flow from the definition of dementia: What is the evidence for impairment in one or more domain of cognition? What is the evidence that daily functioning is affected? The mental status examination is necessary to establish that alertness is preserved (i.e., the patient does not have delirium; Chapter 26) and to determine what specific areas of cognition exhibit directly observable impairment. For diagnosing the syndrome of dementia, no laboratory test supersedes the clinical history and the mental status examination. Laboratory testing is critical, however, for determining the cause of the dementia.

Bedside testing of mental status is based on the principles of cognitive neurology (Chapters 26 and 424). For distinguishing moderate or severe dementia from normal cognitive states, a bedside mental status examination such as the Mini-Mental State Examination (Table 25–4) is accurate. However, for mild dementia, bedside mental status examinations lack sensitivity (i.e., they fail to diagnose some cases of mild dementia). For patients with suspected mild dementia, neuropsychometric testing is a useful adjunct to the bedside examination. The neurologic examination is also important for evaluating signs of specific causes of dementia, including signs of cerebrovascular disease (e.g., hemiparesis; Chapter 430) and signs of extrapyramidal disease (e.g., rigidity, bradykinesia, resting tremor; Chapter 433).

Differential Diagnosis

Dementia must be distinguished from other disorders of cognition (Fig. 425–1). Delirium (Chapter 26) also affects cognition directly; key features distinguishing it from dementia include impaired arousal and attention. Delirium is almost always of sudden onset, whereas the majority of cases of dementia are of gradual onset.

Primary psychiatric diseases (Chapter 420) such as major depression, bipolar disorder, and schizophrenia may also impair cognition. In dementia, however, the impairment in cognition is typically equivalent or more pervasive than the changes in mood and behavior.

The principal diseases that cause dementia are three neurodegenerative diseases—Alzheimer's disease, Lewy body disease, and frontotemporal lobar degeneration—and cerebrovascular disease (Fig. 425–2). The neurodegenerative diseases that cause dementia are typically slow and insidious in onset and inexorably progressive. Dementia secondary to cerebrovascular disease may be of either sudden or gradual onset.

Many much less common secondary causes account for less than 2% of all dementias. Drug intoxication (Chapter 32), metabolic disorders (Chapter 428), central nervous system infections (Chapters 437 and 439), and brain structural lesions (Chapter 199) are typically subacute in onset; if diagnosed and treated early, the cognitive deficits improve or resolve completely. A number of medications such as sedatives, pain medications, corticosteroids, digoxin, and others cause mental confusion, particularly but not always at toxic levels (Chapter 111). Metabolic disorders that may also cause subacute confusion and produce a cognitive disorder include hypothyroidism or hyperthyroidism (Chapter 244), vitamin B_{12} deficiency (Chapter 170), chronic liver disease (Chapter 157), chronic renal failure (Chapter 131), and hypocalcemia or hypercalcemia (Chapter 266). Chronic viral infections of the brain, especially human immunodeficiency virus, frequently cause dementia (Chapter 417). Chronic meningitides in the differential diagnosis of dementia include cryptococcal meningitis (Chapter 358), tuberculous meningitis (Chapter 346), and tertiary syphilis (Chapter 340). Finally, structural lesions of the brain, including primary and metastatic tumors (Chapter 199), chronic subdural hematomas (Chapter 422), and normal-pressure hydrocephalus (Chapter 199), can cause a syndrome resembling dementia that consists of a subacute or slowly progressive decline in cognition with few or no other neurologic symptoms or signs.

Prognosis

Except for the secondary causes of dementia and the rare dementing illnesses caused by single episodes of brain injury such as severe head trauma or anoxic encephalopathy, dementia is a condition that invariably leads to worsening of cognition and function. Almost all dementia patients progress from mild stages to severe dementia over the course of several years, if they do not die prematurely. The rate of cognitive decline is quite variable among individuals and, of course, also varies with the

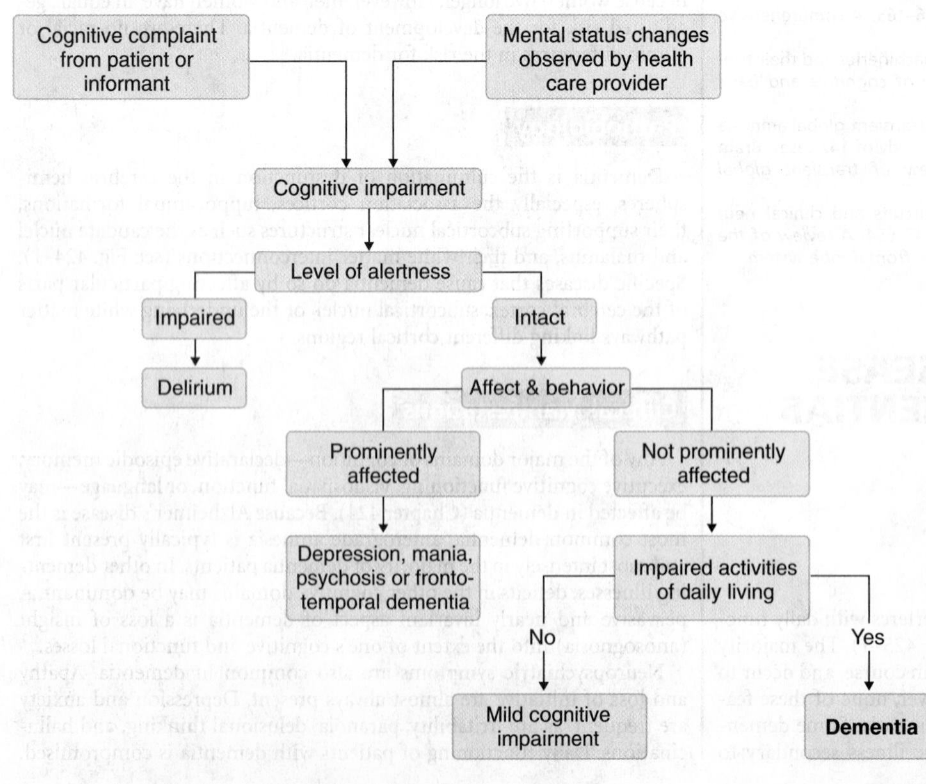

FIGURE 425–1 • Flow diagram for establishing the diagnosis of dementia.

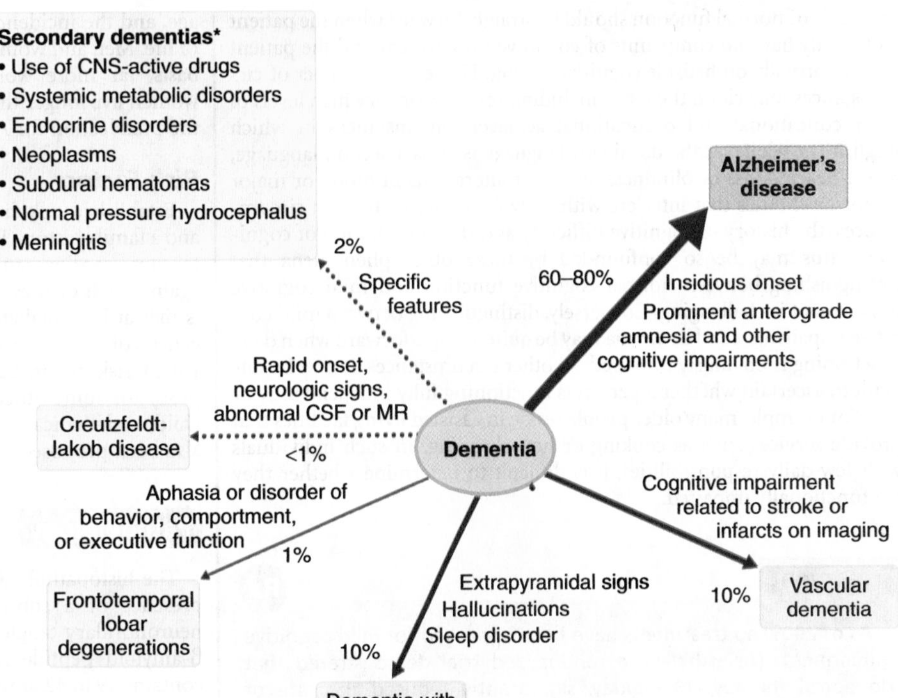

FIGURE 425–2 • Flow diagram for the differential diagnosis of dementia. The percent contributions of various diagnoses are approximate. *The list of secondary causes of dementia is not exhaustive. CSF = cerebrospinal fluid; MR = magnetic resonance imaging.

specific disease. In general, dementia can be said to decrease life expectancy by half when compared with the life expectancy of nondemented individuals.

End-of-Life Care

The terminal stage and end-of-life care issues (Chapter 3) associated with the common dementias are usually quite similar. Dementia itself does not directly cause death, but it is strongly linked to reduced survival. Patients with dementia typically die of the same illnesses that affect debilitated individuals, such as sepsis, pneumonia, pulmonary embolism, or heart disease.

Most patients with dementia experience their terminal illnesses in hospitals or extended care facilities. Given the inexorably progressive nature of most dementing illnesses and their likelihood of producing severe and completely disabling cognitive and functional impairment, it is widely accepted that patients with end-stage dementia should receive conservative care. Feeding tubes and ventilatory support should not generally be considered.

MILD COGNITIVE IMPAIRMENT

Definition

Mild cognitive impairment represents the transition between the state of normal cognition and dementia. Patients with mild cognitive impairment have abnormalities in a specific aspect of cognition to such an extent that it is clearly different from normal performance but does not interfere with daily functioning to any appreciable degree. More than one domain of cognition may be affected. The amnesic form of mild cognitive impairment, in which declarative episodic memory is impaired, is the most common. Alterations in attention, concentration, and mental agility may also be seen (Table 425–2). The term "cognitively impaired, not demented" includes patients whose mild cognitive impairment may progress to dementia but also encompasses anyone who is neither cognitively normal nor demented, such as individuals with stable, lifelong cognitive impairment.

Epidemiology

The prevalence and incidence of mild cognitive impairment are not yet fully characterized, in part because variations in the definition greatly alter estimates of prevalence. However, limited data indicate that mild cognitive impairment is nearly as prevalent as dementia itself.

TABLE 425–2 DIAGNOSTIC CRITERIA FOR AMNESIC MILD COGNITIVE IMPAIRMENT

The presence of a new memory complaint, preferably corroborated by an informant
Objective evidence of an impairment in episodic declarative memory (for age)
Normal general cognitive functions
No substantial interference with work, usual social activities, or other activities of daily living
No dementia

Pathobiology

Mild cognitive impairment is a risk state for the subsequent development of dementia. Alzheimer's disease, followed by cerebrovascular disease and Lewy body disease, is the most common underlying cause.

Clinical Manifestations

Patients with mild cognitive impairment may have more insight into their emerging cognitive difficulties than do patients with dementia. Hence, some patients with mild cognitive impairment may themselves seek medical consultation because of concern about their memory or their thinking. They or their family members may report a milder extent of many of the symptoms of dementia. Patients with mild cognitive impairment forget recent events and conversations or have trouble with mental flexibility, multitasking, problem solving, or completing mentally challenging activities at the speed that they once did. Mental status testing will sometimes corroborate the complaints, but neuropsychometric testing may be needed to document impairment. Other patients with mild cognitive impairment may have virtually no insight into their memory loss but the impairment is diagnosed after family members force the patient to undergo an evaluation.

Diagnosis

The principal alternative diagnoses when mild cognitive impairment is suspected are that the person is cognitively intact or has dementia. The diagnosis of normal function should be straightforward when the patient and family have no complaints of cognitive impairment and the patient scores normally on bedside cognitive testing. However, a number of circumstances may cloud the issue, including very low or very high levels of prior educational and occupational achievement, instances in which English (or whatever the dominant language is) was a second language, severe hearing loss or blindness, or major alterations in mood or major motor disabilities that interfere with daily functioning. In such circumstances, the history of cognitive difficulty and the examination of cognitive status may be so confounded by these other phenomena that distinguishing between normal cognitive function and mild cognitive impairment is challenging. Conversely, distinguishing between mild cognitive impairment and dementia may be quite straightforward when daily functioning is obviously impaired. In other circumstances, it may be difficult to ascertain whether a person is functioning fully independently or not. For example, many older people reside in assisted living facilities that provide services such as cooking or housekeeping. In such individuals with few daily responsibilities, it is difficult to determine whether they are functionally impaired.

Treatment

Rx

As of 2005, no treatments have been approved for mild cognitive impairment. Nevertheless, a randomized trial demonstrated that donepezil therapy, 10 mg/day, significantly reduced the rate of development of dementia secondary to Alzheimer's disease at 1 year but not at 3 years. 1

Prognosis

Mild cognitive impairment should be viewed as a risk state for the subsequent development of dementia. Using the definition of amnesic mild cognitive impairment in Table 425–2, the rate of evolution from mild cognitive impairment to dementia is 15% per year.

ALZHEIMER'S DISEASE

Definition

Alzheimer's disease is defined as a dementing illness in which anterograde amnesia is a dominant symptom (Table 425–3). The clinical diagnosis implies that the causative pathology is of the Alzheimer type, whereas the pathologic diagnosis rests on the findings of characteristic histopathology.

Epidemiology

Between 60 and 80% of all dementing illness is due to Alzheimer's disease. Among all individuals older than 65 years, the prevalence of Alzheimer's disease is estimated to be about 5%. As with dementia in general, the prevalence doubles in every 5-year interval after 65 years of age, and the incidence continues to rise into the 10th and 11th decades of life. Men and women may be equally affected, although on an absolute basis, far more women have prevalent Alzheimer's disease because women live longer than men. There are no ethnic or racial differences in the predilection for Alzheimer's disease.

TABLE 425–3 DIAGNOSTIC CRITERIA FOR THE ANTEROGRADE AMNESIC SYNDROME OF ALZHEIMER'S DISEASE

Dementia (as defined in Table 425–1) with:
- Major impairment in learning and retaining new information and at least one other domain of cognitive impairment:
  - Impairment in handling complex tasks and reasoning abilities (impairment in executive cognitive functions)
  - Impaired visuospatial ability and geographic orientation
  - Impaired language functions

The cognitive disturbance is of insidious onset and is progressive, based on evidence from the history or serial cognitive examinations

The cognitive disturbance is not better accounted for by a systemic disease or another brain disease

Risk Factors

Established risk factors for Alzheimer's disease include advancing age and a family history. Putative risk factors include diabetes mellitus, hypertension, cardiovascular disease, and head trauma; evidence for and against each of these four conditions is inconclusive, but the consensus is that at least diabetes and hypertension may play a role in the pathogenesis of Alzheimer's disease. Low educational achievement is also a consistent risk factor, but most experts believe that educational level is a proxy for some other factor, such as socioeconomic status or the early childhood medical and psychosocial environment. Protective factors have also been proposed, but their status is much debated.

Pathobiology

The histopathologic diagnosis of Alzheimer's disease is based on the presence of a substantial cerebral burden of neuritic plaques and neurofibrillary tangles. Neuritic plaques consist of a core of aggregated β-amyloid peptide surrounded by degenerating neurons. β-Amyloid contains 39 to 42 amino acids and is proteolytically derived from a larger protein, the amyloid precursor protein. In a low-powered microscopic section of frontal, temporal, or parietal cortex, at least six neuritic plaques should be visible to make the diagnosis of Alzheimer's disease.

Pathophysiology

The progression of changes of β-amyloidosis follows a roughly predictable pattern in Alzheimer's disease. The presence of increasing numbers of β-amyloid peptide–containing deposits in neuritic plaques in the neocortex is associated with increasing severity of dementia. For many years it was assumed that the plaques themselves were toxic. Instead, it is the soluble aggregates of β-amyloid in oligomeric (consisting of a small number of monomers) forms that may be the key pathogenic molecules.

Neurofibrillary tangles accumulate in the entorhinal cortex and hippocampus to a slight degree with advancing age, but the presence of neurofibrillary tangles in the temporal lobe neocortex or other neocortical association areas establishes the diagnosis of Alzheimer's disease. Neurofibrillary tangles are intracellular aggregates of the microtubule-associated protein tau. It is believed that neurofibrillary tangles represent a nonspecific response to a toxin, which is β-amyloid in the case of Alzheimer's disease. The precise nature of the link between β-amyloidosis and neurofibrillary tangle formation remains elusive, although increasingly sophisticated manipulations of transgenic models of Alzheimer's disease suggest that β-amyloid oligomers trigger a conformational change in the tau protein. The altered tau protein self-aggregates and forms neurofibrillary tangles.

The location of neurofibrillary tangles corresponds much more faithfully to the clinical evolution of specific symptoms and the severity of Alzheimer's disease than do the anatomic location and abundance of neuritic plaques. In Alzheimer's disease, the most intense burden of neurofibrillary tangles is in the entorhinal cortex and hippocampi, precisely the regions that are involved in declarative episodic memory. Hippocampal atrophy is characteristic, and reductions in hippocampal volume may be observed on magnetic resonance imaging (MRI) (Fig. 425–3). The appearance of neurofibrillary tangles in neocortical association areas in the temporal, parietal, and frontal lobes follows after involvement of the hippocampal and limbic areas. Reflecting the spread to association neocortex, language functions, visuospatial functions, and executive cognitive functions typically become impaired some time after declarative episodic memory dysfunction occurs.

The most consistent neurotransmitter deficit in Alzheimer's disease is in cholinergic neurotransmission. The cells of origin of hippocampal and neocortical cholinergic projections are located in the septum, diagonal band, and nucleus basalis. Neurofibrillary tangles accumulate in the neurons in these regions as Alzheimer's disease develops, but there is also neurochemical evidence that these neurons are stressed much earlier in the disease.

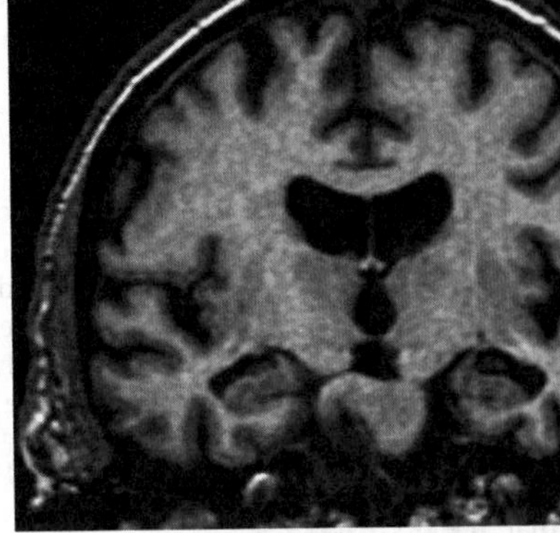
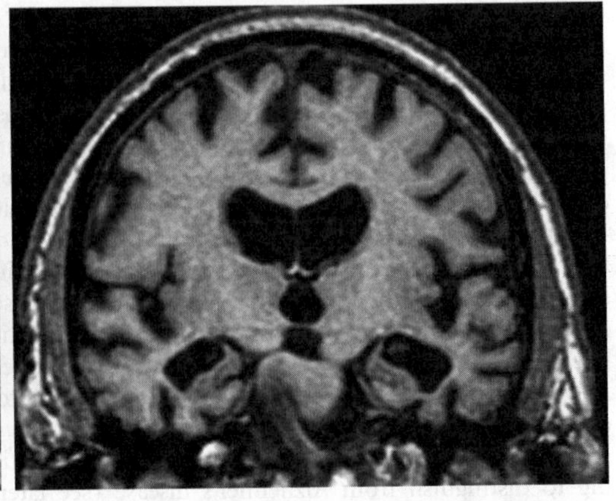

FIGURE 425–3 • Serial coronal images from a magnetic resonance image of a patient with Alzheimer's disease. The scan on the left was performed when the patient was clinically normal. The scan on the right was performed 11 years later when the patient was demented. Hippocampal atrophy has increased dramatically from the first to the subsequent scan. (Courtesy of Maria Shiung and Clifford Jack.)

Genetics

The overwhelming majority of Alzheimer's disease is due to sporadic (not genetic) disease. However, in a very small number of instances, Alzheimer's disease occurs as an autosomal dominant disease. The three known genes involved in autosomal dominant Alzheimer's disease all are directly involved in the production of β-amyloid peptide. The first is the amyloid precursor protein (APP) gene, located on chromosome 21q21.3. Eighteen known mutations in this gene lead to excess production of β-amyloid and are reliably associated with a very early onset (20 to 50 years of age) of Alzheimer's disease. Another line of evidence implicating the APP gene to Alzheimer's disease is the invariable appearance of the pathology of Alzheimer's disease in individuals with Down syndrome (trisomy 21; Chapter 39), who have an extra copy of the APP gene as a result of the trisomy.

The other two genes associated with autosomal dominant Alzheimer's disease are the presenilin 1 and 2 genes, located on chromosomes 14q24.3 and 1q31.42. A large number of presenilin 1 mutations account for the majority of autosomal dominant Alzheimer's disease. Both genes code for a similar protein known as presenilin. Presenilin is involved in degradation of the APP molecule at the gamma cleavage site. It is believed that the Alzheimer's disease–causing mutations in presenilin 1 and 2 lead to a "toxic gain of function" that produces excess β-amyloid peptide. The presenilin mutations are also associated with early-onset (40 to 60 years of age) Alzheimer's disease.

Studies of the familial aggregation of Alzheimer's disease have shown that later-onset disease also displays genetic risks, but only one gene has been definitively linked to later-onset Alzheimer's disease. That gene, located on chromosome 19q13.2, encodes apolipoprotein E (apo E), a protein involved in lipid transport. In humans, three allelic variants of apo E are determined by differences in the amino acids cysteine and arginine at positions 112 and 158 of the 299–amino acid protein. One of the allelic variants, with arginine at both positions, designated the ε4 variant, is strongly associated with a 14-fold increased risk for Alzheimer's disease in homozygotes and a 3-fold increase in heterozygotes. In many series, almost 50% of Alzheimer's disease patients but only about 25% of nondemented controls have at least one copy of the apo E ε4 allele. The presence of an apo E ε4 allele does not always cause Alzheimer's disease in that the disease never develops in some carriers of the genotype. The mechanism by which the apo E ε4 allele predisposes to Alzheimer's disease is not established, but the tertiary structure of the apo E protein with arginine at positions 112 and 158 may lead to impaired binding to β-amyloid, which in turn reduces the clearance of β-amyloid from cells.

Clinical Manifestations

The early course of Alzheimer's disease is dominated by difficulties with anterograde amnesia. Some of the usual complaints include forgetting recent events and conversations, misplacing items, problems with keeping track of the date, getting lost in familiar surroundings, and problems with remembering to complete tasks. The frequency and severity of the memory lapses progress from occasional difficulty to more pervasive and consistent failure.

In mild Alzheimer's disease, declarative episodic memory function may be lost. Familiarity and access to previous knowledge may allow patients to function in their usual daily routines as long as nothing out of the ordinary is required of them. They may still retain the ability to prepare simple meals and to take walks in their neighborhood without getting lost. However, even in mild Alzheimer's disease, medication-taking errors and difficulty managing money or balancing a checkbook are likely to occur. Traveling to unfamiliar places often accentuates confusion. Changes in personality commonly accompany the cognitive losses. Apathy, loss of initiative, and loss of interest in previous hobbies and pastimes are ubiquitous in early Alzheimer's disease.

As the disease progresses, the ability to perform necessary daily tasks becomes more and more difficult to the point that the patient will need assistance preparing meals, paying bills, taking transportation, and keeping house. As the disease moves into the severe stages, assistance and supervision in basic activities such as bathing, dressing, toileting, and eating become necessary.

In the terminal stages of the disease, all communicative abilities may be lost. Mobility may still be preserved until late in the disease. Alzheimer's disease patients commonly die of illnesses that strike other debilitated elderly individuals, such as sepsis, pneumonia, and congestive heart failure.

The duration of the course of clinical Alzheimer's disease is long but quite variable. The time from mild dementia to death may be as short as 2 to 3 years or may be well over a decade. For patients in whom mild dementia is diagnosed, about 10% per year reach the stage of severe dementia.

Rarely, Alzheimer's disease is associated with prominent symptoms in cognitive domains other than memory. The most common of the atypical syndromes is one in which profound visuospatial deficits occur without the typical severe anterograde amnesia. This syndrome is referred to as posterior cortical atrophy.

Diagnosis

The diagnosis of Alzheimer's disease, like that of dementia itself, is largely a clinical one based on the history and examination. The key elements in the history are a gradual onset and insidious progression of cognitive impairment, especially anterograde amnesia. The mental status examination should demonstrate impairment in short-term memory and other cognitive deficits. Alzheimer's disease should be thought of as a diagnosis of inclusion: if the history and examination are compatible with Alzheimer's disease and if certain exclusions can be verified, the diagnosis can be made with confidence.

No laboratory tests can confirm the diagnosis of Alzheimer's disease with sufficient sensitivity and specificity. For example, the presence of the apo E ε4 allele increases diagnostic accuracy only marginally after considering the history and physical examination. Findings on MRI, such as a decreased hippocampal volume, are useful when atrophy is present, but hippocampal atrophy is neither sensitive nor specific enough to be useful in diagnosis. Positron emission tomography with fluorodeoxyglucose or with newer amyloid-binding agents has yet to deliver the necessary precision or predictive abilities to warrant use in routine practice.

Differential Diagnosis

A number of other conditions that bear similarity to Alzheimer's disease must be excluded on clinical or laboratory grounds (see Fig.

425–2). One is dementia with Lewy bodies, which is suggested by the presence of parkinsonism, prominent visual hallucinations, and a specific sleep disorder. At autopsy, Lewy body pathology and Alzheimer's disease pathology often coexist, thus suggesting that the diagnoses overlap. Frontotemporal lobar degeneration is suggested by prominent behavioral and personality changes or by prominent language difficulties early in the course. Hippocampal sclerosis has unique neuropathologic findings but is virtually impossible to distinguish from Alzheimer's disease by clinical features. Other neurodegenerative conditions in the differential diagnosis of Alzheimer's disease include Huntington's disease (Chapter 434), progressive supranuclear palsy, corticobasal degeneration, amyotrophic lateral sclerosis (Chapter 435), and Wilson's disease (Chapter 230); however, these diseases invariably have prominent motor manifestations early in their course.

Dementia caused by cerebrovascular disease is particularly challenging to distinguish from Alzheimer's disease (see later). The fact that Alzheimer's disease and cerebrovascular disease often coexist requires clinicians to consider both simultaneously.

Prevention and Treatment

There are no established preventive therapies. Although a healthy diet, physical exercise, and stimulating cognitive leisure activities are sensible, they have not been shown to protect against Alzheimer's disease. Treatment of diabetes (Chapters 247 and 248) and hypertension (Chapter 66) is beneficial for other reasons, but it is not clear that such treatment alters the course of Alzheimer's disease.

Once Alzheimer's disease becomes symptomatic, support for family caregivers is a critical intervention that cannot be overemphasized. Support groups through the Alzheimer's Association (available at *www.alz.org*) can benefit families coping with the disease.

Important safety issues include supervision of medications, supervision of finances, and close scrutiny of motor vehicle operation. Operation of other potentially dangerous tools, firearms, appliances, and equipment should also be carefully monitored or avoided. Patients with Alzheimer's disease often wander and can become lost long distances from home. Patient identification can prevent tragic occurrences *(www.alz.org/Media/newsreleases/2003/033003wandering.asp).*

Evidence-Based Treatments

Two classes of drugs are approved for the treatment of Alzheimer's disease: cholinesterase inhibitors and memantine, a glutamate receptor antagonist. The rationale for the use of cholinomimetic drugs (donepezil, 5 or 10 mg/day, galantamine, 16 or 24 mg/day, or rivastigmine, 6 to 12 mg/day) is the reduced levels of cholinergic markers in the neocortex of patients dying of Alzheimer's disease. All three agents have been shown to delay progression of symptoms at 6 to 12 months in patients with mild to moderate Alzheimer's disease, but not at 3 years. [1-5] Furthermore, there is no compelling evidence that they alter its biologic progression. Individual patients often do not show any clear benefits of treatment.

Memantine, which is a low- to moderate-affinity, uncompetitive *N*-methyl-D-aspartate receptor antagonist that acts on glutamate neurotransmission, also delays the progression of functional decline [6] at a dose of 10 mg twice per day. It is not clear why modulation of glutamate neurotransmission is beneficial in Alzheimer's disease, and studies of memantine in patients with mild to moderate Alzheimer's disease have not yet been published.

One study of patients with moderately severe Alzheimer's disease showed that vitamin E was effective in delaying progression, but recent studies showed no benefit in subjects with mild cognitive impairment. [1] By comparison, donepezil appears to be beneficial for severe [7] as well as mild disease.

Prognosis

Alzheimer's disease is inevitably progressive, and severe cognitive impairment and complete dependence on others develop in virtually all patients, unless they die prematurely. Alzheimer's disease also contributes to premature death; the mortality rate in patients with Alzheimer's disease is about 10% per year.

Future Directions

Intensive research on the pathogenesis of Alzheimer's disease is elucidating information on production and degradation of the β-amyloid molecule and mechanisms of induction of tau aggregation. Research is also focusing on the development of biomarkers, CSF markers, and imaging techniques for the early diagnosis of Alzheimer's disease. A number of therapeutic agents are also being studied.

VASCULAR DEMENTIA

Definition

Vascular dementia is a dementing illness in which the underlying cause is cerebral infarction. For a cognitive disorder to be attributed to cerebrovascular disease from a neuropathologic perspective, there must be sufficient cerebral infarction in locations known to be responsible for the cognitive deficits in the absence of other neurodegenerative neuropathologic changes (Table 425–4). When cerebrovascular disease produces cognitive impairment that is not severe enough to meet the criteria for dementia, it is referred to as vascular cognitive impairment.

Epidemiology

In clinical studies, as many as 20% of dementia patients have cerebrovascular disease. Like Alzheimer's disease, it is less common in patients younger than 65 years and increases steadily thereafter. In neuropathologic studies, about 25% of all cases of dementia have some vascular component. Roughly half that number are relatively pure vascular dementia; the remainder consists of vascular disease mixed with Alzheimer's disease pathology. Men and women are equally affected.

Risk Factors

Risk factors for vascular dementia include cardiovascular disease, diabetes, and hypertension. There are no known protective factors other than treatment of these risk factors. Populations with high rates of generalized vascular disease should have higher rates of vascular dementia, but competing mortality from cardiovascular disease may obscure part of the relationship. In the first year after a stroke, the risk for development of dementia is about nine-fold higher than the rate in persons without a stroke; the risk remains about two-fold higher in subsequent years.

Pathobiology

The majority of vascular disease causing cognitive impairment is due to atherosclerosis. One mechanism is through large infarctions, such as those secondary to occlusive disease in major cerebral vessels, including

TABLE 425–4 DIAGNOSTIC CRITERIA FOR THE SYNDROME OF DEMENTIA CAUSED BY CEREBROVASCULAR DISEASE (VASCULAR DEMENTIA)

Dementia as defined in Table 425–1

Clinically important cerebrovascular disease is demonstrable by *either* of the following:

- Onset of the cognitive disturbance *or* dramatic worsening of an existing disturbance that occurred within 3 months of a stroke, where stroke is defined as a focal neurologic deficit of acute onset in which the symptoms and signs persist for more than 24 hours
- Neuroimaging evidence of bilateral brain infarctions rostral to but including the thalamus

the carotid arteries and the anterior, middle, and posterior cerebral arteries (Chapter 430). A second mechanism of infarction is at the arteriolar level, with lacunar infarctions in the thalamus, basal ganglia, and subcortical white matter. Both these processes can be detected by brain MRI. Infarcts in the hippocampal formations, medial thalamus, caudate nuclei, and parietal association areas are highly likely to produce cognitive impairment, but not necessarily dementia. Microinfarcts, which are small zones of infarction that are not visible to the naked eye but can be observed with light microscopy, may also contribute to the dementia. The simultaneous presence of Alzheimer's disease pathology is common in vascular dementia.

There are other uncommon causes of vascular dementia. Cerebral autosomal dominant arteriopathy with subcortical infarcts and leukoencephalopathy (CADASIL) is a very rare inherited disease that usually becomes clinically evident between the ages of 30 and 50 years and causes severe white matter disease, headaches, and dementia. The cause of CADASIL is mutations in the *notch3* gene on chromosome 19q12. Cerebral amyloid angiopathy, a β-amyloidosis in which the β-amyloid peptide accumulates in the media of small to medium-sized arteries in the leptomeninges and superficial cortex, causes cerebral hemorrhages that if occurring in sufficient number and in critical locations, may lead to dementia. Cerebral amyloid angiopathy is also seen in Alzheimer's disease, but its hemorrhagic manifestations may occur in individuals with little evidence of Alzheimer's disease clinically and modest evidence pathologically. Cerebral vasculitis (Chapter 291) is a very rare cause of dementia.

Clinical Manifestations

The spectrum of cognitive changes in patients with cerebrovascular disease is broad. The more common cognitive syndromes in cerebrovascular disease include mild cognitive impairment, a dementia with prominent anterograde amnesia, and a dementia with prominent changes in personality and executive function. Some patients with vascular cognitive impairment without dementia may have deficits in only one domain (Chapter 424). A number of aphasia syndromes occur as a result of cerebral infarction or hemorrhage in the perisylvian regions of the dominant hemisphere. Infarction or hemorrhage in the occipitotemporal or occipitoparietal regions may produce one of the disorders of visual cognition, such as alexia or visual agnosia. Infarcts in the caudate nuclei, particularly if they are bilateral, may produce a cognitive syndrome that includes both amnesia and disordered executive function, thus mimicking dementia. Large infarcts in the right parietal lobe can also produce dementia. Infarcts in the medial thalami or in the hippocampal formations can produce isolated amnesia.

The evolution of symptoms in vascular dementia does not follow a stereotypical pattern. In some, the dementia syndrome may remain static. In others, new strokes may lead to substantial declines in cognition and function. Some patients with vascular dementia may experience a gradually declining illness. Patients with vascular cognitive impairment without dementia or vascular dementia may also have other neurologic signs typical of patients with cerebrovascular disease, such as hemiparesis, hemianopia, hemisensory changes, or cranial nerve abnormalities.

Diagnosis

The diagnosis of vascular dementia is based on the neurologic history and examination. Brain imaging, preferably with MRI, is essential for establishing the presence of infarcts. The cardinal diagnostic features of vascular dementia are that (1) the cognitive disorder should have begun within 3 months of a clinical stroke event and (2) there should be multiple, bilateral infarcts in the cerebral hemispheres visible on brain imaging studies. The presence of a temporal link between the onset or worsening of cognitive impairment and a stroke is important in demonstrating that cerebrovascular disease is etiologically relevant to the cognitive impairment. Brain imaging of infarcts in the cerebral cortex, basal ganglia, thalamus, and cerebral white matter has obvious value for establishing the presence of cerebrovascular disease. In contrast to actual infarcts on imaging, the presence of white matter hyperintensities without infarcts on brain MRI is much less specific.

The accuracy of the clinical diagnosis of vascular dementia is generally lower than that of Alzheimer's disease. The combination of (1) a temporal relationship between dementia and a stroke and (2) imaging evidence of bilateral infarcts is diagnostically specific for vascular dementia but is insensitive. Broader diagnostic criteria (see Table 425–4) are more sensitive but less specific. The usual alternative diagnosis is Alzheimer's disease, and there is typically no way to be certain whether and how much Alzheimer's disease pathology is simultaneously present.

Prevention and Treatment

Some cases of vascular dementia should be preventable. With early, lifelong aggressive treatment of diabetes (Chapters 247 and 248), hypertension (Chapter 66), and hyperlipidemia (Chapter 217), the number of cerebral infarcts should be reduced, with a corresponding reduction in the number of cases of vascular dementia. Evidence for this link comes from large-scale studies in which the treatment of hypertension reduced the frequency of strokes and incident dementia. Once vascular dementia develops, cholinesterase inhibitors have shown some benefit in patients, [8] but the major goal is to prevent future strokes.

Prognosis

Patients with vascular dementia can often be expected to have severe cardiovascular disease and a greater likelihood of future strokes and cardiac ischemic events. Survival of patients with vascular dementia is poorer than that of patients with Alzheimer's disease.

DEMENTIA WITH LEWY BODIES

Definition

Dementia with Lewy bodies is a multifaceted dementing disorder in which the underlying pathology includes Lewy bodies in limbic and cortical structures (Table 425–5). Some clinicians make a distinction between patients in whom parkinsonism preceded the cognitive disorder and those in whom the cognitive disorder occurred either simultaneously with or before the movement disorder. This distinction may be somewhat useful in clinical practice, but there are very few clinical or neuropathologic differences based on different sequences of signs and symptoms. The diagnosis of dementia with Lewy bodies is similar in principle to diagnosing both dementia and Parkinson's disease (Chapter 433) in the same individual, but dementia with Lewy bodies is a term with broader connotations because of the presence of other features (hallucinations, fluctuations, and sleep disorder) that may be more apparent than the movement disorder.

Epidemiology

Dementia with Lewy bodies is about a quarter as common as Alzheimer's disease. Lewy body pathology becomes more common with advancing age, and the prevalence of dementia with Lewy bodies increases with advancing age as well. As with the other dementias, there

TABLE 425–5 DIAGNOSTIC CRITERIA FOR THE DEMENTIA SYNDROME ASSOCIATED WITH LEWY BODY PATHOLOGY

Dementia as defined in Table 425–1
The cognitive disturbance is of insidious onset and is progressive, based on evidence from the history or serial cognitive examinations
The presence of at least two of the following:
Parkinsonism (rigidity, resting tremor, bradykinesia, postural instability, parkinsonian gait disorder)
Prominent, fully formed visual hallucinations
Substantial fluctuations in alertness or cognition
Rapid eye movement sleep behavior disorder (see Chapter 429)
The disturbance is not better accounted for by a systemic disease or another brain disease

are no known ethnic or racial differences, but dementia with Lewy bodies may be more common in men. There are no known risk factors for dementia with Lewy bodies. Dementia develops in up to 30% of patients with Parkinson's disease, and advancing age is the major risk factor.

Pathobiology

The pathology of dementia with Lewy bodies is a mixture of Lewy body pathology and Alzheimer's pathology. Generally, the more intense the Lewy body pathology, the less abundant the Alzheimer pathology. Lewy bodies, which are intraneuronal inclusions that contain α-synuclein, are found in the nucleus basalis, pars compacta of the substantia nigra, locus ceruleus, other brain stem structures, amygdala, cingulate gyrus, and neocortex. The earliest locations of Lewy bodies are the brain stem, where they affect nuclei involved in sleep and arousal, the substantia nigra, the locus ceruleus, and cranial nerve nuclei IX and X. Typically, the nucleus basalis, transentorhinal cortex, cingulate gyrus, and neocortex become involved later.

In Lewy body pathology, the α-synuclein protein becomes misfolded and aggregates intraneuronally. Mutations in the α-synuclein gene have been seen in a few families with autosomal dominant Parkinson's disease, but the vast majority of cases of dementia with Lewy bodies are sporadic.

Clinical Manifestations

The clinical manifestations of dementia with Lewy bodies include four major abnormalities: the cognitive disorder, the neuropsychiatric disorder, the motor disorder, and the disorder of arousal. The cognitive disorder may differ from Alzheimer's disease, although there is considerable overlap. In a typical patient with dementia with Lewy bodies, visuospatial deficits, impaired concentration, and impaired attention dominate the picture. In some patients, the deficits in executive functions may be similar to what is seen in frontotemporal lobar degeneration. Anterograde amnesia is usually present but milder than in Alzheimer's disease. Language deficits are not prominent. The neuropsychiatric manifestations of dementia with Lewy bodies, including prominent apathy, loss of initiative, and depression, may be more disabling than the cognitive symptoms. The motor manifestations include bradykinesia, gait disturbances, postural disturbances, and rigidity. Rest tremor is less common in dementia with Lewy bodies in patients in whom the cognitive disorder appears before the parkinsonism. Visual hallucinations, fluctuations in alertness, and REM sleep disorders are part of a broader disorder of arousal and regulation of sleep and wakefulness. Visual hallucinations are often very graphic, detailed, and bizarre, perhaps because the sleep phenomenon of dreaming intrudes into wakefulness. Patients with dementia with Lewy bodies have large fluctuations in their alertness and arousal from day to day.

REM sleep behavior disorder (Chapter 429) is a parasomnia in which patients exhibit dream enactment behavior, often with violent, threatening overtones. Patients typically relate that they feel as though they are being chased by something or someone. Their behavior, while they are asleep, consists of excessive talking, calling out or shouting, and thrashing about, often to the point of striking a bed partner or falling out of bed. The REM sleep behavior disorder may precede the development of Parkinson's disease and dementia with Lewy bodies by years.

Diagnosis

The diagnosis of dementia with Lewy bodies is based on clinical information that corroborates the presence of abnormalities in cognition, motor function, neuropsychiatric behavior, and arousal. Formal neuropsychological testing is often helpful in evaluating memory, executive function, and visuospatial function in a detailed manner. Neuroimaging has only a limited role in the diagnosis of dementia with Lewy bodies.

Differential Diagnosis

Other disorders that must be considered in patients with dementia and a movement disorder include progressive supranuclear palsy, which can resemble dementia with Lewy bodies in terms of both the dementia and the motor disorder. In progressive supranuclear palsy, patients are much less likely to have disorders of arousal and typically have other distinctive signs and symptoms, including the characteristic supranuclear gaze palsy and other brain stem findings. The corticobasal degenerations, which are members of the family of frontotemporal lobar dementias (see later), may also produce a movement disorder and dementia. Huntington's disease (Chapter 434) is associated with dementia and a movement disorder, but the movement disorder of Huntington's disease includes prominent chorea and athetosis, neither of which is present in dementia with Lewy bodies.

Normal-pressure hydrocephalus (Chapter 199) is a rare disorder typically characterized by the triad of a gait disorder, dementia, and urinary incontinence. Normal-pressure hydrocephalus can be suspected when computed tomography or MRI shows ventricular enlargement that is out of proportion to the amount of sulcal widening. Predicting a favorable response to ventriculoperitoneal shunting in suspected normal-pressure hydrocephalus has proved to be very difficult. Imaging studies that measure CSF flow through the aqueduct of Sylvius or that measure flow of radiolabeled CSF with radionuclide cisternography have not been useful. Clinical response to the removal of a high volume (e.g., 30 mL) of CSF through lumbar puncture is sometimes used to select patients for surgery, although its positive and negative predictive value is unclear. Normal-pressure hydrocephalus is very rare relative to dementia with Lewy bodies and Alzheimer's disease.

Treatment

Rx

Management of patients with dementia with Lewy bodies is challenging because of the simultaneous appearance of a cognitive disorder, a neuropsychiatric disorder, a motor disorder, and a sleep disorder. Treatment of the motor disorder is accomplished with antiparkinsonian drugs such as levodopa or dopaminergic agonists (see Chapter 433). Treatment with these agents should be instituted for dementia with Lewy bodies if there are prominent gait or balance problems that threaten safety and interfere with independence. These medications may worsen hallucinations and exacerbate confusional states, but this concern should not preclude a treatment trial if the motor symptoms pose safety risks or interfere with independence. Cholinesterase inhibitors, which do not exacerbate parkinsonian symptoms, have a beneficial effect on neuropsychiatric symptoms but not clearly on the cognitive disorder. [9]

Hallucinations and agitation impair quality of life for the patient and family and often require treatment. Some antipsychotic agents that might otherwise control these symptoms dramatically exacerbate the parkinsonism in dementia with Lewy bodies. Atypical antipsychotics are usually recommended, but there is insufficient experience from controlled clinical trials. Many movement disorder specialists prefer to use quetiapine in doses of 25 to 200 mg/day or clozapine at 6.25 to 50 mg/day [10] because these agents appear to have the lowest rate of extrapyramidal side effects. However, it is not possible to make any strong statements about the relative efficacy of atypical antipsychotics in treating the hallucinations in dementia with Lewy bodies, especially in view of the possibility that atypical antipsychotic agents may be associated with higher than expected mortality.

The REM sleep behavior disorder (Chapter 429) can be disabling, but there are no controlled clinical trials to inform treatment. Some sleep disorder specialists typically use either melatonin, 3 to 12 mg, or clonazepam, 0.5 to 2 mg, at bedtime.

Treatment of depressive symptoms may substantially improve a patient's functioning. Use of one of the newer generation of antidepressants, such as sertraline in a dose of 25 to 100 mg/day or citalopram in a dose of 10 to 20 mg/day, may be beneficial and does not necessarily interfere with management of the other symptoms (see Chapter 420).

Prognosis

As opposed to patients with Alzheimer's disease, some studies show that patients with dementia with Lewy bodies have a more rapidly progressive course and poorer survival. As a result of the combination of manifestations, patients with dementia with Lewy bodies may become disabled sooner in their course.

TABLE 425–6 DIAGNOSTIC CRITERIA FOR FRONTOTEMPORAL DEMENTIA

Based on evidence from the history and mental status examination, a disorder characterized by the early *and* predominant presence of *either* of the following:
- Decline in regulation of personal or social interpersonal conduct (as characterized by loss of empathy for the feelings of others; socially inappropriate behavior that is rude, caustic, irresponsible, or sexually explicit; mental rigidity; inflexibility in interpersonal relationships or emotional blunting; disregard for personal hygiene and grooming; deviations in previous dietary preferences or habits)
- Impairment in mental agility, reasoning, or handling of complex tasks out of proportion to impairment in the domains of declarative episodic memory or visuospatial abilities

The cognitive or behavioral disturbances are of gradual onset and are progressive, based on evidence from the history or serial cognitive examinations

The cognitive disturbance significantly interferes with work, usual social activities, or relationships with others

The cognitive disturbance and the changes in daily functioning represent a significant decline from a previous level of functioning

Not occurring exclusively during the course of delirium

The disturbance is not better accounted for by a major psychiatric diagnosis, a systemic disease, or another brain disease

Future Directions

Because the REM sleep behavior disorder often precedes the development of dementia with Lewy bodies, early diagnosis offers an opportunity for early intervention. Progress in understanding the production and degradation of α-synuclein may lead to more specific therapies.

FRONTOTEMPORAL LOBAR DEGENERATION

Definition

The frontotemporal lobar degenerations are a group of neurodegenerative disorders with distinctive clinical manifestations and a predilection for the prefrontal and anterior temporal neocortices. The most common clinical syndrome is a disorder of behavior and personal relationships (comportment) with a loss of executive functions (Table 425–6). This syndrome is often called simply frontotemporal dementia. Other syndromes in the clinical spectrum of frontotemporal lobar degeneration involve different aspects of language or motor dysfunction of the limbs.

Epidemiology

Unlike Alzheimer's disease, the frontotemporal lobar degenerations have a peak age at onset in the 50- to 70-year-old range, and the incidence declines after age 70. In patients with dementia who are younger than 70 years, frontotemporal lobar degeneration makes up 10 to 20% of cases. However, across the entire age spectrum, the frontotemporal lobar degenerations are much less common than Alzheimer's disease, dementia with Lewy bodies, or vascular dementia. Both men and women are affected equally. There are no known risk factors for the frontotemporal lobar degenerations except a family history.

Pathobiology

The clinical syndrome in frontotemporal lobar degeneration is determined by the lobar location of the pathology. Right prefrontal or anterior temporal pathology and brain atrophy produce behavioral syndromes like frontotemporal dementia. Left frontal involvement tends to produce progressive nonfluent aphasia. Predominant left temporal lobe involvement may give rise to progressive anomic aphasia syndrome or semantic dementia.

On histopathologic grounds, the frontotemporal lobar degenerations can be divided into those that have inclusions containing the microtubule-associated protein tau versus those that do not. Among the tau-positive varieties are Pick's disease, in which intracellular tau-positive inclusions known as Pick bodies are seen. Several other pathologic tau-positive subtypes occur, including progressive supranuclear palsy, corticobasal degeneration, and a disorder associated with mutations in the tau gene. At least 30 mutations in the tau gene on chromosome 17q21 are associated with autosomal dominant frontotemporal lobar degeneration syndromes. The most common is a mutation of proline to leucine at codon 301, located in exon 10. Each of the mutations has a slightly different clinical and neuropathologic phenotype. The tau gene undergoes alternative splicing that results in six isoforms of the tau protein. Pathologic mutations appear to disrupt splicing of alterative isoforms of tau protein, which in turn adversely affects the binding of tau to microtubules in neurons. Reduced binding of tau to microtubules is deleterious to microtubule function and neuronal integrity.

The tau-negative frontotemporal lobar degenerations are almost equally common. Immunostaining has shown distinctive ubiquitin-containing inclusions that contain the TDP-43 protein. Mutations in the progranulin gene, also on chromosome 17q21, have been linked to this form of frontotemporal lobar degeneration.

Clinical Manifestations

The clinical manifestations of the syndrome of frontotemporal dementia begin insidiously. Apathy, loss of initiative, and flattening of affect are common early symptoms. As the disease progresses, the entire spectrum of behavioral changes associated with disease of the frontal and anterior temporal lobes appears. On cognitive assessments, patients may have preserved memory functions, but they typically have difficulty with tests of executive cognitive function. When frontotemporal dementia progresses to moderate or severe stages, the behavioral changes remain prominent, but the disease becomes harder to distinguish from other dementias such as Alzheimer's disease.

In some patients with frontotemporal lobar degeneration, signs and symptoms of motor neuron disease develop, such as weakness, atrophy, and fasciculation in the limbs or the bulbar musculature (Chapter 435). In other patients with frontotemporal lobar degeneration, asymmetric limb apraxia develops that is part of the corticobasal syndrome. Features of progressive supranuclear palsy may also appear in patients who are found to have frontotemporal dementia syndrome.

Frontotemporal lobar degeneration can be manifested as a progressive nonfluent aphasia in which patients experience a feeling of hesitancy in selecting words in their speech, a problem that may be difficult for others to appreciate at first. Anomia is an early sign. Gradually, the patient's speech becomes more hesitant and labored. Eventually, a nonfluent, apractic, agrammatic speech develops. In other cognitive domains, progressive nonfluent aphasics, as well as progressive anomic aphasics, often have no deficits. As the diseases progress, however, a pervasive cognitive disorder develops in some patients. Other progressive nonfluent aphasics may eventually become virtually mute, even though they may appear to have preserved memory and visuospatial functions.

Semantic dementia is a disorder that involves dissolution of the meaning of words or objects. A patient with semantic dementia becomes unable to access knowledge about words (alexia), objects (object agnosia), and people's faces (prosopagnosia). The most striking demonstration of the deficit in semantic dementia is when a patient can produce the name of an object, a watch for example, but then when asked what a watch is for, they cannot do so. Often, patients with semantic dementia have preservation of the ability to learn a list of words, even if their knowledge of the meaning of the words is diminished.

Diagnosis

Frontotemporal lobar degeneration must first be suspected on clinical grounds, based on the appearance of one of the distinctive clinical syndromes such as frontotemporal dementia (see Table 425–6) or one of the aphasic subtypes. Neuropsychological testing can also aid in the diagnosis by detecting abnormalities in executive function and verifying that

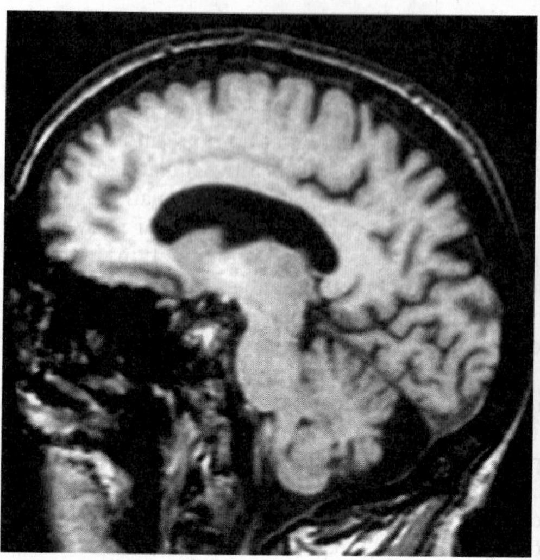

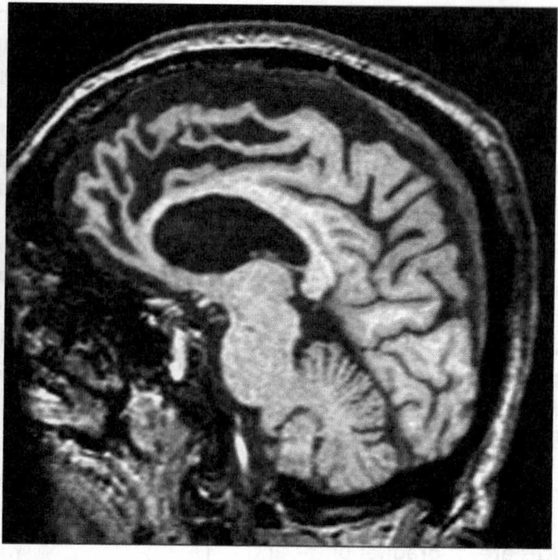

FIGURE 425–4 • Parasagittal image from a magnetic resonance image of a patient with frontotemporal dementia (left). Atrophy of the frontal lobes is dramatic when compared with the brain of a normal individual (right). (Courtesy of Maria Shiung and Clifford Jack.)

memory function is preserved, as it often is. For all of the frontotemporal lobar degeneration syndromes, MRI showing focal atrophy of the frontal (Fig. 425–4) or temporal lobes is highly likely to be diagnostic. Imaging with fluorodeoxyglucose-enhanced positron emission tomography can also be useful when the clinical diagnosis is uncertain and MRI is nondiagnostic.

Treatment

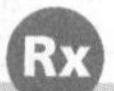

There is no symptomatic therapy specifically for frontotemporal lobar degeneration. In patients with agitation, paranoia, delusions, or obsessive behavior, atypical antipsychotics (e.g., quetiapine, 25 to 200 mg/day) are used, but no controlled clinical trials are available. There are no preventive treatments of frontotemporal lobar degeneration.

Prognosis

Specific frontotemporal lobar degeneration syndromes have dramatic differences in their clinical course and outcome. In patients with motor neuron signs and symptoms, the prognosis is usually poor, with survival of only about 2 years from the time of diagnosis. Patients with semantic dementia and progressive nonfluent aphasia have much more protracted and gradual trajectories; survival for more than 10 years is not uncommon. Frontotemporal dementia itself can also exhibit a more protracted course.

Future Directions

Drugs that delay or prevent the pathologic consequences of tau protein dysfunction could be of great value for many patients with frontotemporal lobar degeneration.

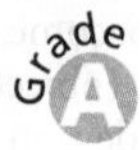

1. Petersen RC, Thomas RG, Grundman M, et al: Vitamin E and donepezil for the treatment of mild cognitive impairment. N Engl J Med 2005;352:2379–2388.
2. Raskind MA, Peskind ER, Wessel T, et al: Galantamine in AD: A 6-month randomized, placebo-controlled trial with a 6-month extension. Neurology 2000;54:2261–2268.
3. Rogers SL, Farlow MR, Doody RS, et al: A 24-week, double-blind, placebo-controlled trial of donepezil in patients with Alzheimer's disease. Neurology 1998;50:136–145.
4. Rosler M, Anand R, Cicin-Sain A, et al: Efficacy and safety of rivastigmine in patients with Alzheimer's disease: International randomised controlled trial. BMJ 1999;318:633–640.
5. AD2000 Collaborative Group: Long-term donepezil treatment in 565 patients with Alzheimer's disease (AD2000): Randomised double-blind trial. Lancet 2004;363:2105–2115.
6. Reisberg B, Doody R, Stoffler A, et al: Memantine in moderate-to-severe Alzheimer's disease. N Engl J Med 2003;348:1333–1341.
7. Winblad B, Kilander L, Eriksson S, et al: Donepezil in patients with severe Alzheimer's disease: Double-blind, parallel-group, placebo-controlled study. Lancet 2006;367:1057–1065.
8. Erkinjuntti T, Kurz A, Gauthier S, et al: Efficacy of galantamine in probable vascular dementia and Alzheimer's disease combined with cerebrovascular disease: A randomised trial. Lancet 2002; 359:1283–1290.
9. McKeith IG, Del Ser T, Spano P, et al: Efficacy of rivastigmine in dementia with Lewy bodies: A randomised, double-blind, placebo-controlled international study. Lancet 2000;356:2031–36.
10. The Parkinson Study Group: Low-dose clozapine for the treatment of drug-induced psychosis in Parkinson's disease. N Engl J Med 1999;340:757–763.

SUGGESTED READINGS

Blennow K, de Leon MJ, Zetterberg H: Alzheimer's disease. Lancet 2006; 368:387–403. *Clinical review.*

Farlow MR, Cummings JL: Effective pharmacologic management of Alzheimer's disease. Am J Med 2007;120:388–397. *A practical review.*

Gauthier S, Reisberg B, Zaudig M, et al: Mild cognitive impairment. Lancet 2006;367:1262–1270. *A comprehensive review.*

Kertesz A, McMonagle P, Blair M, et al: The evolution and pathology of frontotemporal dementia. Brain 2005;128:1996–2005. *A description of a large series of cases of frontotemporal dementia and progressive aphasia with autopsy confirmation.*

Knopman DS: Dementia and cerebrovascular disease. Mayo Clin Proc 2006;81:223–230. *Review of what is known and not known about vascular dementia.*

McKeith IG, Dickson DW, Lowe J, et al: Diagnosis and management of dementia with Lewy bodies: Third report of the DLB Consortium. Neurology 2005;65:1863–1872. *Description of clinical and pathologic criteria for the diagnosis of dementia with Lewy bodies.*

426 SEIZURES AND EPILEPSY

Susan S. Spencer

Definition

The term *epilepsy* includes disorders or syndromes with widely variable pathophysiologic findings, clinical manifestations, treatments, and prognoses. Individuals with epilepsy are identified by the tendency for and occurrence of recurrent seizures. A seizure is a paroxysmal, hypersynchronous, excessive neuronal discharge of variable extent. However, the word *seizure* is not synonymous with the word *epilepsy.* Any brain can generate a single or even multiple seizures under appropriate provocative circumstances. It is the tendency to have recurrent seizures, not necessarily with provocation, that makes the diagnosis of epilepsy. More than one seizure must occur before the diagnosis of epilepsy is made.

The clinical appearance and electroencephalographic (EEG) correlates of recurrent seizures allow classification of the seizure as either partial onset or generalized onset. An individual with epilepsy may have one or multiple specific types of seizures. Knowledge of demographic variables, the circumstances in which the seizures occur, and the results of diagnostic examinations are combined with the type of seizures to allow identification and classification of an epileptic syndrome (see Table 426–3). The diagnosis of a specific epileptic syndrome carries real meaning with respect to pathophysiology, duration of treatment, and prognosis.

The word *epilepsy* has many implications for the individual and for society. Frequently, it carries considerable stigma and leads to psychosocial, educational, and vocational obstacles and impairments. Nonetheless, substantial if not complete control of seizures is now possible with medical treatment in most patients, and remission often occurs. Even in patients with a poor response to medical treatment, surgical or other interventions may control the seizures.

Epidemiology

Epilepsy, which is the most common chronic neurologic condition, affects individuals of all ages, with a peak incidence in childhood and in the elderly. In the United States, the incidence of all types of epilepsy is 35 to 52 per 100,000, varying by age: 60 to 70 per 100,000 per year in young children (<5 years), 45 per 100,000 in adolescents, as low as 30 per 100,000 in the early adult years, but rising through the sixth and seventh decades back to 60 to 70 per 100,000 and reaching as high as 150 to 200 per 100,000 in individuals older than 75 years. The incidence in males is higher at every age. Estimates of the prevalence of epilepsy range from 4.7 to 6.9 per thousand, but its prevalence is much higher in less developed countries for all age groups.

Specific Causes

The cause of epilepsy remains undetermined in more than 50% of patients. The etiology varies with the age group and with the region of the country or the world. In childhood, most epilepsies are idiopathic, whereas in adults, most are secondary to identifiable causes. The most common cause of epilepsy worldwide in developed countries is stroke/vascular disease (10 to 17%), followed closely by head trauma, developmental/congenital disorders, infection, neoplasm, and degenerative disorders, especially Alzheimer's disease. The spectrum is dependent on age, with trauma/congenital/infectious causes most frequent in children and vascular disease/neoplasm accounting for greater than 25% of cases in patients older than 60 years.

Comorbid diseases are common in patients with epilepsy. The most frequent are mental retardation (cognitive disorders and learning disabilities) and psychiatric disorders, but motor deficits are also common. The presence and severity of mental retardation are related to the risk for epilepsy: 7 to 18% in children with mild mental retardation (IQ of 50 to 70) and greater than 37% in children with severe mental retardation (IQ <50). Cognitive deficits are common in adults with epilepsy of many causes, including stroke, dementia, and neoplasm.

Isolated symptomatic seizures that occur without a diagnosis of epilepsy are related to specific causes that overlap but differ from the causes of recurrent epileptic seizures and syndromes (Table 426–1). In young children, infection is the leading cause of acute symptomatic seizures, with trauma the second most common.

TABLE 426–1 SOME COMMON CAUSES OF ACUTE SECONDARY "SYMPTOMATIC" SEIZURES

Metabolic
Hypernatremia, hyponatremia, hypocalcemia, hypoxia, hypoglycemia, hyperglycemia (nonketotic hyperosmolar), renal failure
Drug induced
Theophylline, meperidine, tricyclic antidepressants, phenothiazines, lidocaine, quinolones, penicillins, selective serotonin re-uptake inhibitors, isoniazid, antihistamines, cyclosporine, interferons, cocaine, lithium, amphetamines, alcohol (withdrawal), benzodiazepines (withdrawal), barbiturates (withdrawal)
Infections
Sepsis, encephalitis (viral), abscess (intracerebral, subdural, epidural), meningitis (bacterial)
Endocrine
Hyperthyroidism, hypothyroidism, peripartum
Other systemic conditions
Sickle cell crisis, hypertensive encephalopathy, systemic lupus erythematosus, polyarteritis, eclampsia, high fever (any cause)
Central nervous system neoplasms
Central nervous system trauma
Vascular
Arrhythmia, stroke, intracerebral hemorrhage, hypotension

Pathobiology

Partial seizures involve a localized region or collection of cells in a specific area that display bursting behavior: the epileptic neuronal aggregate. Prolonged depolarization caused by a shift in calcium conductance results in firing of multiple sodium-dependent action potentials. The spontaneous or stimulation-induced bursting behavior produces a paroxysmal depolarization shift, which is the intracellular correlate of an interictal spike, the characteristic of EEG recordings in patients with epilepsy (see Fig. 426–3).

When a seizure occurs, the bursting cells in the epileptic neuronal aggregate recruit neighboring neurons by the accumulation of extracellular potassium, accumulation of calcium presynaptically, and activation of *N*-methyl-D-aspartate receptors. The seizure is characterized by continuous high-frequency firing of neurons, with spread of excitatory activity into neighboring neurons representing propagation of the partial seizure. Propagation occurs locally and also through longer anatomic pathways and circuits. Eventually, this firing is interrupted by repolarization. Hyperpolarization characterizes the postictal state.

The occurrence of seizures depends on the interaction of inhibitory and excitatory influences, including ion channel behavior, variations in protein expression, and variable membrane receptor properties. Seizures can be precipitated by alterations in metabolic status, sleep, lighting, sensory stimulation, drugs, toxins, ion status, or synaptic activity, even in individuals without local accumulations of bursting neurons—in which case they are termed acute secondary or "symptomatic" seizures, which does not constitute epilepsy.

The ways in which neurons develop the tendency to cause seizures—epileptogenesis—are not well understood but may include neuronal loss and reorganization and alterations in receptor responses, basic membrane function, or ion channel regulation. Developmental, genetically determined features clearly play a role.

In the generalized epilepsies, in which onset of the seizure is manifested by diffuse clinical and EEG changes that involve many or all areas of the brain, an alteration in the normal oscillatory rhythms that characterize the circuits of pyramidal neocortical neurons and neurons of the nucleus reticularis of the thalamus may be the cause. The nucleus reticularis of the thalamus controls the activity of T-type calcium currents in thalamic relay neurons through cells utilizing γ-aminobutyric acid as a neurotransmitter (GABAergic input). The thalamic relay neurons project to and regulate the excitability of cortical pyramidal neurons. Influences on this system, such as blockade of T-type calcium currents, prevent absence seizures. In generalized tonic-clonic seizures, the substantia nigra appears to play a role by acting through GABAergic inhibitory neurotransmission.

Genetics

Most of the common epileptic syndromes have complex inheritance patterns that have eluded definition. Many of the epilepsies with mendelian inheritance are rare disorders related to alterations in ion channels: benign neonatal convulsions associated with mutations in the potassium channel genes *KCNQ2* and *KQCNQ3;* generalized epilepsy with febrile seizures associated with mutations in the voltage-gated sodium channel genes *SCN1A, SCN2A, SCN3A,* and *SCN1B* and with mutations in the GABA receptor gene *(GABRG2);* severe myoclonic epilepsy of infancy associated with mutations in the sodium channel gene *SCN1A;* juvenile myoclonic epilepsy associated with mutations in the GABA receptor gene *GABRG1;* and autosomal dominant nocturnal frontal lobe epilepsy associated with mutations in the neuronal nicotinic acetylcholine receptor genes *CHRNA4* and *CHRNB2.* Other genetic epileptic syndromes for which specific mendelian genetics are now known include a variety of progressive disorders characterized by childhood seizures, developmental decline, and demonstrable structural abnormities. Such syndromes include progressive myoclonic epilepsy of Unverricht-Lundborg associated with *EPM1,* which encodes cystatin B, and progressive myoclonic epilepsy of Lafora associated with *EPM2;* neuronal ceroid lipofuscinoses associated with *CLN1, CLN2, CLN3, CLN5,* and *CLN8;* and a list of developmental disorders of neuronal migration resulting in various forms and locations of aberrant cortical cellular collections. Among these disorders are lissencephaly (associated with *LIS1,* which encodes a subunit of platelet-activating factor acetylhydrolase, a microtubule-associated protein), subcortical band heterotopia (associated with doublecortin *DCX,* or *XLIS*), and periventricular nodular heterotopia (associated with the filamin 1 gene *FLN1,* which encodes an actin-binding protein).

There is growing appreciation of both the genotypic variability associated with a single phenotype and the phenotypic variability associated with alterations in single identified genes. Nevertheless, the rapidly evolving understanding of the genetic determinants may lead to more rational classification and treatment.

Clinical Manifestations

The earliest manifestation of a partial seizure can be subjective and recognized by patients as an "aura." The most common aura is experiential: a feeling of déjà vu or jamais vu. Other auras include feelings of impending doom, fear, euphoria, or an odd sensation in the stomach, often rising toward the head. Such auras are typical in seizures beginning in the temporal lobe, but similar auras may occur with seizures originating from other lobes and are therefore not of localizing value. Rarely, the aura may be pleasant. Autonomic symptoms that may herald the onset of a seizure or be part of the clinical manifestations of a partial seizure include pallor, diaphoresis, olfactory or gustatory sensations, urge to defecate, dizziness, vertigo, nausea, and salivation.

Complex sensory phenomena may accompany or precipitate seizures and must be distinguished from psychiatric disorders. Auditory hallucinations are much more likely to be psychiatric than seizure related, although seizures that originate in the Heschl gyrus area include buzzing or ringing in the ears. Seizures can be precipitated by hearing music (so-called musicogenic epilepsy), presumably secondary to activation of portions of the auditory cortex as a form of reflex epilepsy; in these situations, an actual auditory stimulus, not a hallucinatory phenomenon, is present. Similarly, visual hallucinations can be complex in temporal lobe seizures but are unformed in simple partial seizures from the occipital cortex. Transient pain is rarely associated with seizures.

Vocalization is a common accompaniment of seizure activity. Frequently, the vocalization is not intelligible language but rather consists of repetitive phrases that become incorporated into the seizure activity; the vocalization may have originally been part of a reaction to the oncoming seizure. Thus, patients may repetitively state "help me, help me" or "oh God, oh God" at the onset of a seizure but have no recall of the event. Intelligible and intact language output during seizures excludes dominant hemisphere involvement in the seizure. Vertigo and dizziness are common at the onset of a seizure and are usually associated with involvement of the lateral temporal or occipital cortex.

Diagnosis

History

The diagnosis of epilepsy is based on historical information. However, because epilepsy may involve a change of consciousness, diagnosis can be problematic. In localization-related seizures, the patient has intact consciousness at the start of the seizure and can report what transpires up to the point when consciousness is altered. With generalized seizures, patients lose consciousness immediately and can report only the postictal state. Thus, for grand mal seizures, patients may report only awakening and noting of muscle aching, incontinence, a bloody pillow, or disarray in their surroundings. Nocturnal seizures may not come to light until individuals share a bed with someone. Simple partial seizures that are subjective in nature may be disregarded or underreported by patients who fear the consequences of reporting them and not come to medical attention until a more severe seizure is recognized by others. Dating the onset of symptoms is dependent on asking the appropriate question. Moreover, seizures may have been misdiagnosed as hypoglycemia, panic attacks, or migraine and not be reported at all.

Because patients have limited or no recall, the history from others is crucial. Observers contribute valuable information about the patient's activity, responses, and appearance (changes in color, diaphoresis, respirations, vocalization, and muscle tone), which are essential to characterize the type of seizure and to distinguish seizures from syncope (Chapter 427) and other paroxysmal disorders affecting the nervous system. The setting in which the events occur (time of day, activity, ambient temperature, position, and sleeping or waking state) is important. Seizures, especially frontal lobe seizures, can occur predominantly or even exclusively during sleep. Seizures can occur in any position. The seizure threshold is lowered by fasting, lack of sleep, stress, fever, hyperventilation, strobe lights, withdrawal of certain drugs (e.g., alcohol, benzodiazepines, barbiturates), and use of illegal and legal toxic substances (see Table 426–1).

The history should also define any familial paroxysmal disorders. The possibility that events called "seizures" represent ischemic or other processes demands that historical features thought to relate to cardiovascular disease, movement disorders, and a family history of syncope be obtained. The psychiatric history not only influences the diagnosis but may also modify the manifestation of the seizure disorder and the history provided by the patient. In mood disorders (particularly anxiety), treatment may interact to obscure the diagnosis of seizures; for example, benzodiazepines suppress seizure activity, even though they are not the usual choice for chronic use. Conversely, depression (Chapter 420) is treated with many drugs that lower the seizure threshold (e.g., tricyclic antidepressants, selective serotonin re-uptake inhibitors).

Physical Examination

Seizures resulting from injury or from congenital, traumatic, neoplastic, immunologic, infectious, metabolic, or toxic causes may be associated with other findings that point to specific causes. Atrial fibrillation, arrhythmia, or heart failure suggests cardiovascular or ischemic causes of seizures. Neurologic deficits in the distribution of a specific cerebral vessel suggest an ischemic cause. Seizures characterized by abnormal motor activity can be confused with movement disorders, and some movement disorders (Chapter 434) produce repetitive motor activity that is incorrectly attributed to seizures. The vocalization of Tourette's syndrome (Chapter 434) can be mistaken for vocalization in frontal lobe epilepsy, and vice versa. Paroxysmal dystonias and ataxias (Chapter 434) may be misdiagnosed as epilepsy with motor features.

Types of Epileptic Seizures

The current classification of epileptic seizures into diagnostic entities relies on clinical features and their accompanying EEG patterns. Seizures are divided into two main categories, partial and generalized, defined on the basis of involvement, at least at their start, of a localized region of the brain (partial) or the whole brain (as far as can be determined). In generalized seizures, consciousness is lost immediately. In partial seizures, consciousness may or may not be lost; by definition, partial seizures are simple, without alteration of consciousness, or complex, with altered consciousness. The specific types of seizures determine the epileptic syndrome and dictate the choice of drugs for treatment (see later).

Partial Seizures

Partial seizures have their origin in the gray matter of a localized area of the brain, although the size of this localized region remains unspecified. To observe any change on a simultaneous EEG recording, a cortical area of at least 6 cm^2 must participate in the electrical discharge, but demonstration of such EEG phenomena is not essential for diagnosis. Partial seizures from small or deep brain foci often show no change on surface EEG recordings. The manifestations of partial seizures are as diverse as the functions of the brain. The sequence of symptoms and signs gives information on the cerebral localization of dysfunction (Table 426–2).

In partial seizures, the neuronal discharge representing the partial seizure may remain confined to the region where it began (as an "aura" or more objective simple partial event), or it may spread to involve additional brain areas. Thus, a simple partial seizure of occipital lobe origin might begin with flashing lights in the contralateral visual field and then progress to involve additional occipital lobe regions ipsilaterally or contralaterally or propagate (along known anatomic pathways) to ipsilateral

TABLE 426–2 CHARACTERISTICS OF PARTIAL SEIZURES FROM DIFFERENT LOBES AND REGIONS

TEMPORAL LOBE SEIZURES

Medial temporal
- Aura (70–90%): epigastric sensation, déjà vu, emotions, indescribable feelings
- Arrest of activity (30–50%)
- Simple automatisms at onset; complex later, usually ipsilateral to the region where the seizure began
- Later, contralateral tonic motor activity secondary to spread of seizure activity—usually to the arm
- Confusion
- Consciousness may be preserved
- Lengthy (1–3 minutes)

Lateral temporal (neocortical)
- Early, auditory hallucinations, vertigo
- Contralateral motor/sensory abnormalities
- Later, complex visual/auditory hallucinations
- Receptive aphasia
- Spread to medial areas results in signs/symptoms of medial temporal lobe syndrome (see above)

FRONTAL LOBE SEIZURES

Rolandic
- Contralateral upper extremity clonic activity
- Postictal paralysis common

Supplementary motor
- Mainly tonic, contralateral arm extension
- Fencing posture (contralateral head turning and arm extension)
- Speech arrest or vocalization
- Preservation of consciousness
- Brief (10–20 seconds)
- No postictal findings

Frontopolar
- Contralateral tonic, often with secondary generalization
- Ipsilateral head and eye deviation
- Later, contralateral turning, axial clonic jerks

Dorsolateral frontal
- Prominent contralateral motor, tonic or clonic
- Contralateral head/eye deviation
- Speech arrest

Orbital frontal
- Mainly complex partial
- Autonomic disturbance
- Loud vocalization
- Bilateral motor and gestural automatisms, ambulation
- Olfactory hallucinations

Cingulate
- Complex motor/gestural automatisms (bilateral)
- Autonomic signs
- Urinary incontinence
- Asymmetrical tonic activity
- No loss of consciousness

PARIETAL LOBE SEIZURES

Sensory symptoms, usually contralateral face, hand, and arm, with positive or negative phenomena
- Positive phenomena: tingling, need to move, feeling of movement, tongue crawling, formed visual hallucinations, nausea, pain, metamorphopsia
- Negative phenomena: loss of awareness of body part (asomatognosia), numbness

Then, complex partial ± secondary generalization
- Dominant hemisphere: language disturbance
- Nondominant hemisphere: metamorphopsia, asomatognosia
- Paracentral: generalized sensory phenomena, secondary generalization
- Inferior: vertigo, disorientation

OCCIPITAL LOBE SEIZURES

Simple partial onset with elementary visual sensations (in the contralateral field, center, or moving across the field), decreased vision (white or black), sensation of eye movement, forced blinking, oculoclonic activity, ocular flutter

Contralateral head and eye deviation

Then, complex partial ± secondary generalization; the spread pattern determines subsequent characteristics
- Infrasylvian spread causes medial temporal syndrome
- Lateral suprasylvian spread causes motor/sensory signs
- Medial suprasylvian spread causes supplementary motor syndrome
- The same patient may have variable suprasylvian and infrasylvian spread in individual seizures

or contralateral temporal or frontal lobe regions (inferior or suprasylvian propagation). If consciousness is altered, it is termed a *complex partial seizure.*

A special instance of propagation in the frontal lobe occurs in seizures with onset in the rolandic area. The initial circumscribed contralateral clonic activity propagates in the primary motor strip. This seizure activity "marches" from hand to arm to leg area ipsilaterally, a process referred to as a jacksonian march. After the clonic motor activity ends, patients are often weak; a postictal or Todd paralysis may last hours or even a day or two, with gradual resolution.

Simple partial seizures originating from any region can become complex partial seizures, and unilateral simple or complex partial seizures can progress to involve bilateral brain areas, thereby resulting in secondary generalized seizures. Such secondary generalized seizures usually take the form of generalized tonic-clonic events rather than another type of generalized seizure in the international classification.

The evolution of the clinical seizure reflects the evolution of the EEG changes, which in turn reflects the pathophysiology of the process, with a simultaneous rhythmic, localized discharge (often in the 4- to 7-Hz range) becoming higher in amplitude and lower in frequency as the seizure continues (Fig. 426–1). The EEG characteristics do not, however, influence the ultimate consequence, the specific seizure diagnosis, localization of the seizure, diagnosis of a specific syndrome, or selection of appropriate therapy.

Some seizures that begin in the association cortex have bizarre or extremely brief clinical manifestations, without postictal deficits. This sequence may occur in frontal lobe seizures, which may not be immediately appreciated as bona fide seizures. The stereotyped nature of the clinical events, with identification of EEG changes if present, may be the only way to make an appropriate diagnosis. The diagnosis can be even more challenging if the seizure spreads to different cortical regions during different seizure episodes, thereby producing variable constellations of clinical findings.

Partial seizures can also occur as a series of single events without intervening normal behavior, termed "complex or simple partial status epilepticus." Simple partial status epilepticus appears as typical, repetitive, simple partial seizures, whereas complex partial status epilepticus is characterized by persistent confused behavior, quite different from what is observed in individual complex partial events, even though it is a result of repeated complex partial seizure events. EEG findings may be normal in a simple partial seizure, and they may remain normal during simple partial status epilepticus, but the diagnosis is usually evident from the clinical features. In complex partial status epilepticus, EEG recordings show continuous abnormalities that are not of the same nature as seen in single seizures in that individual. The most common are a slow background with superimposed rhythmic high-amplitude sharp waves or repetitive rhythmic seizure discharges. Complex partial status epilepticus is most frequent with frontal lobe seizures but can occur in temporal lobe seizures as well. The factors that precipitate complex partial status epilepticus are not well defined, nor are the implications for treatment or prognosis.

"Nonconvulsive status epilepticus" is a cause of confusion or impaired mental status in patients with various neurologic diagnoses (i.e., trauma, stroke) in the acute intensive care unit setting. Clinical suspicion should prompt an EEG study, which is essential for diagnosis.

TABLE 426–3 INTERNATIONAL CLASSIFICATION OF EPILEPTIC SYNDROMES (CONDENSED)

PRIMARY/IDIOPATHIC
Localization related
Benign epilepsy with centrotemporal spikes
Autosomal dominant nocturnal frontal lobe epilepsy
Generalized
Juvenile myoclonic epilepsy
Juvenile absence epilepsy
Severe myoclonic epilepsy of infancy
Progressive myoclonic epilepsies
Generalized epilepsy with febrile seizures plus
SECONDARY/SYMPTOMATIC
Localization related
Mesial temporal lobe epilepsy
Neoplasm (primary, metastatic)
Infection (abscess, encephalitis, meningitis, syphilis, cysticercosis, Lyme disease, tuberculosis, fungal disease, herpes)
Vascular (stroke, transient ischemic attack, migraine, hemorrhage)
Developmental (migrational)
Perinatal
Traumatic
Degenerative (e.g., Alzheimer's disease)
Immunologic (e.g., multiple sclerosis)
Generalized
West's syndrome
Lennox-Gastaut syndrome
Tuberous sclerosis
Sturge-Weber syndrome

Generalized Seizures

The international classification of epileptic seizures recognizes six distinct types of generalized seizures: tonic-clonic, absence, tonic, atonic, clonic, and myoclonic. All can involve both hemispheres at their onset, but one type of generalized seizure (tonic-clonic) may evolve by "secondary generalization" of a partial seizure. The subcortical structures that presumably contribute to these seizures are not entirely defined. The distinctive EEG patterns observed with generalized seizures differ from the lateralized EEG patterns of partial seizures and can be produced by stimulation of subcortical structures, particularly certain thalamic nuclei.

Generalized Tonic-Clonic Seizures

A generalized tonic-clonic seizure is also termed a *grand mal seizure* or *convulsion.* It is the most dramatic and common of the generalized seizures and arguably the most dramatic event in clinical medicine. Tonic-clonic seizures disrupt any situation in which they occur and frighten even the most informed or experienced bystanders. They may begin with a "cry" as a result of abrupt air movement across the glottis from sudden tonic muscle contraction. The patient becomes diffusely stiff, usually with limb and body extension and often with arching of the back. Breathing is suspended, cyanosis occurs, and urinary incontinence is common. EEG recordings show generalized high-amplitude rapid spiking, although interpretation is impeded by the intense muscle artifact. After 15 to 60 seconds, the tonic activity gives way to clonic, rhythmic jerking of all four extremities, and the EEG spiking is also interrupted. The rhythmic contractions gradually become slower in frequency until the event stops; the patient is apneic, comatose, and diaphoretic and within 60 seconds begins stridorous breathing with foaming and gasping. Patients who have generalized tonic-clonic seizures in public often prompt bystander resuscitation efforts, although such patients begin spontaneous respiration within 1 minute or so. Postictal stupor lasts a variable length of time. The patient generally sleeps for 2 to 8 hours and then complains of severe headache, sore muscles, a bitten tongue, and inability to concentrate for a day or more. After generalized tonic-clonic seizures, some individuals have severe memory loss that gradually improves, sometimes over a period of weeks. When the generalized tonic-clonic convulsion ends, the EEG findings mirror the patient's clinical appearance. At first it is nearly flat and then shows very slow recovery through different stages of less marked slowing of background rhythms, with normal rhythms resuming within 24 to 48 hours. Generalized tonic-clonic seizures can occur secondarily from a partial-onset seizure as the sole type of seizure or with other generalized seizures in certain inherited, generalized epileptic syndromes. Generalized tonic-clonic seizures are also what is seen in response to many metabolic, toxic,

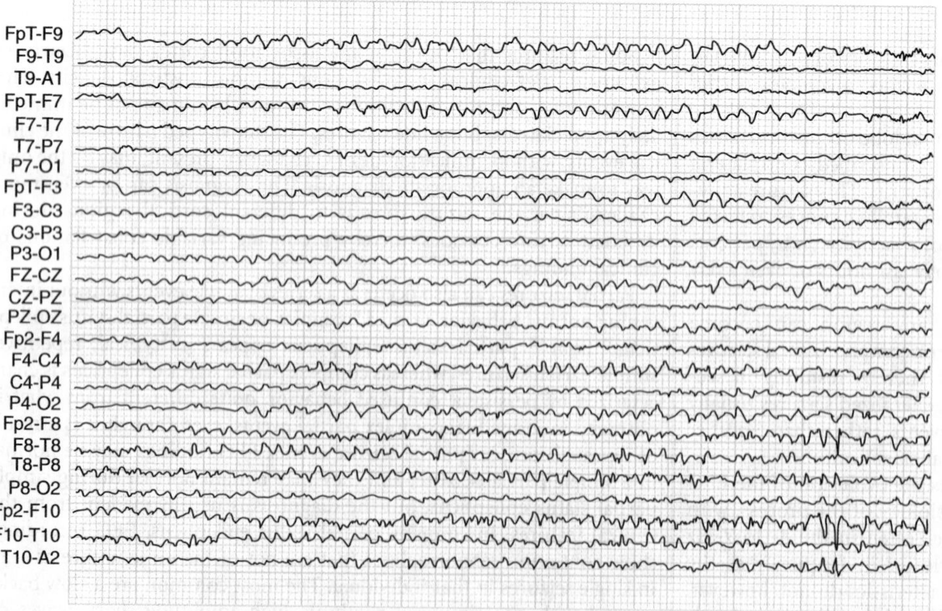

FIGURE 426–1 • Partial seizure. An electroencephalogram shows the first 10 seconds of a complex partial seizure discharge, with 5-Hz rhythmic theta activity in channels recorded in the right temporal scalp (Fp2–F8, F8–T8, T8–P8, Fp2–F10, F10–T10).

traumatic, or ischemic insults (see Table 426–1)—termed *acute symptomatic seizures*—but these do not qualify for the diagnosis of epilepsy.

Absence Seizures

An absence seizure, which is the second most common type of generalized seizure and is synonymous with the term "petit mal," describes a momentary lapse of awareness. The patient has no perception of any aspect of the event and may or may not realize that some time was lost, although individuals often lose their place in reading or their train of thought. Simultaneous with the "absence," the EEG recording shows a high-amplitude, 3-Hz spike and wave discharge, rarely lasting longer than 2 to 10 seconds, that occurs in both hemispheres but is predominantly frontal (Fig. 426–2). The discharge and the event involve both hemispheres at once; there are no focal or localized EEG discharges or lateralized behavioral manifestations. Because consciousness is immediately lost at the onset, there is no aura. There are also no residual postictal symptoms. Because these seizures begin in childhood, school teachers are often the first to notice them. The "absence" may be accompanied by brief eye blinking or myoclonic movement, particularly if the event (as judged by EEG recordings) extends beyond 10 seconds. These seizures can occur many times a day but are not associated with progressive neurologic disease. They can also occur in a more continuous form, with resultant confusion, another cause of "nonconvulsive status epilepticus."

ATYPICAL ABSENCE SEIZURES. Some patients with extensive bilateral brain disease have a variation of this generalized seizure type designated "atypical absence." The event is similar in terms of the brief loss of contact, but the spike and wave discharge observed on a simultaneous EEG recording is slightly slower in frequency and longer in duration; there is also more motor, autonomic, or automatic activity. "Atypical absence" seizures are usually part of symptomatic generalized epileptic syndromes (see later).

Myoclonic Seizures

Myoclonic seizures are brief episodes of sudden motor contraction, often flexion of the upper extremities, that appear as muscle jerks. These movements can be focal, with one arm involved, or bilateral and massive, with involvement of both upper extremities and the trunk. There is no acknowledged loss of consciousness, but the episodes are so momentary that consciousness is difficult to evaluate. Myoclonic seizures often appear in the setting of other generalized types of seizures in degenerative or inherited syndromes with bilateral cerebral involvement, and they may also be associated with abnormal cerebral function. Myoclonic seizures most commonly occur in the morning, just after awakening, and they can crescendo in frequency to culminate in a generalized tonic-clonic seizure. Generalized EEG discharges accompany myoclonic seizures but may be difficult to distinguish from muscle artifact.

Atonic and Tonic Seizures

Atonic forms of generalized seizures are also associated with generalized EEG abnormalities. These brief motor events are characterized by a sudden increase or decrease in muscle tone, often causing falls and injuries. Such seizures frequently occur in children with diffuse central nervous system (CNS) disease and multiple types of seizures.

Diagnostic Studies

The electroencephalogram (Chapter 419) is the most important diagnostic study in epilepsy. Most patients with epilepsy do not have a seizure recorded on a routine 30- to 40-minute EEG study, but interictal abnormalities on a routine EEG study can be highly suggestive of an epileptic disorder. Spikes or sharp waves in a restricted distribution associated with a localization-related seizure (Fig. 426–3) or in a generalized distribution associated with generalized epilepsy (see Fig. 426–2) rarely occur in the normal population. Spikes may not be present on a single interictal EEG recording, but interictal spikes are seen in more than 80% of individuals with localization-related epilepsy if three or more interictal EEG studies are performed. The generalized spikes or spike and wave complexes or polyspikes associated with generalized seizures are more frequent and therefore easier to see on routine EEG recordings, especially if hyperventilation and photic stimulation are used. The highest likelihood of detecting abnormal interictal activity on an EEG recording is in the 24-hour period after a seizure. Focal slowing and asymmetry may also be demonstrated, but such findings are not necessarily associated with epilepsy; however, they do establish a localized region of brain dysfunction or injury. By comparison, diffusely increased or decreased background activity can occur with a variety of medications and does not help in the diagnosis of epilepsy.

Brain magnetic resonance imaging (MRI), which can demonstrate the structural correlate of most diagnoses associated with secondary "symptomatic" seizures, should always be performed in patients with new-onset seizures. Functional imaging techniques, including single-photon emission computed tomography (SPECT) for determination of blood flow and positron emission tomography (PET) for analysis of metabolism, are useful, especially in individuals with uncontrolled seizures. Regions of the brain that generate frequent seizure activity also demonstrate interictal hypoperfusion and hypometabolism, findings that can help establish a diagnosis of intractable epilepsy and localize a region for surgical treatment.

Metabolic and toxic screening (Chapter 111) can point to other systemic disorders or causes of seizures. Endocrine disorders are not usually a cause of epilepsy but will worsen its clinical picture.

Lumbar puncture is not helpful unless there is a possibility of hemorrhage, infection, or immunologic disease as the underlying cause. These

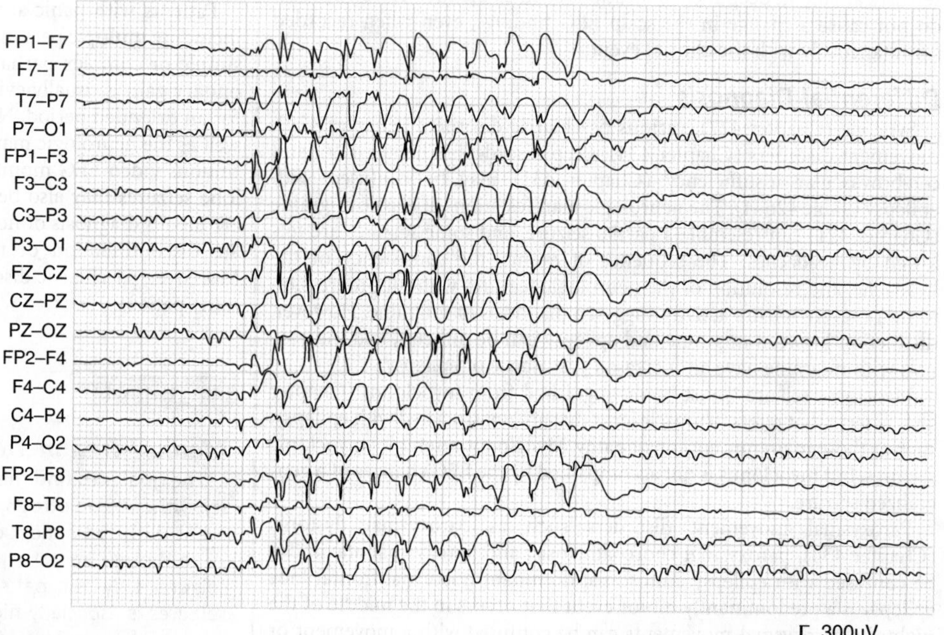

FIGURE 426–2 • Absence seizure. The 3-Hz spike and wave pattern of absence epilepsy emerges from a normal electroencephalographic (EEG) background and abruptly stops with resumption of normal activity. Shorter bursts of this type or single spike and wave forms are interictal; when they are longer, clinical absence seizures accompany the EEG findings. The discharge is strictly regular, bilateral, and most prominent in frontal leads (Fp1–F7, Fp1–F3, F2–C2, Fp2–F4, Fp2–F8).

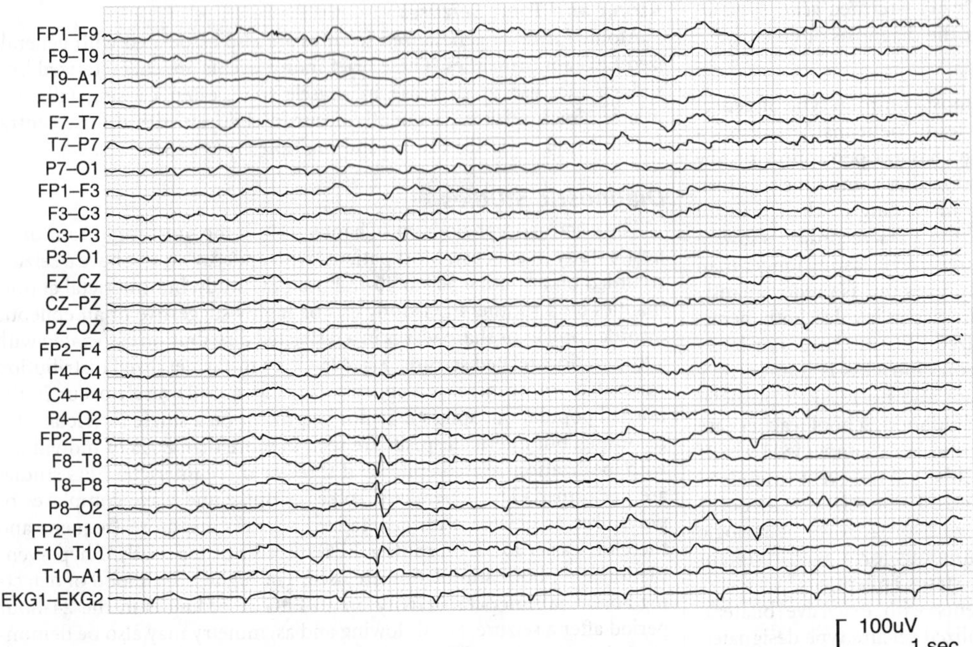

FIGURE 426–3 • Interictal EEG in localization-related epilepsy. The interictal spike discharge is demonstrated, with phase reversal across channels F8–T8, T8–P8, F10–T10, and T10–A2 that localizes the spike to T8, T10 (right anterior inferior temporal lobe). Spikes are highly correlated with the presence of partial epilepsy.

entities typically have systemic manifestations that suggest a need for lumbar puncture.

With the history, EEG recordings, and MRI, a definitive diagnosis of epilepsy and its cause can be made in up to 50% of patients. In other patients, the information is insufficient or inconsistent, but the physiologic and CNS abnormalities surrounding the actual event allow it to be placed provisionally into a specific diagnostic category nearly 80% of the time. Intensive 24-hour EEG and videotape monitoring in an inpatient epilepsy unit, while withdrawing the patient from medications and using provocative maneuvers such as sleep deprivation, can increase diagnostic sensitivity.

The serum prolactin level is elevated two-fold or more within 5 minutes after generalized tonic-clonic and some complex partial seizures; it rises to a maximum at 15 minutes and declines to baseline by 1 hour. This level can be a useful adjunct to diagnosis. An EEG recording during a spontaneous event can distinguish syncope and cerebral ischemia, which are manifested as diffuse rhythmic slowing, from epileptic events, which are characterized by rhythmic sharp, slow, spike or spike-wave discharges. However, some seizures, especially simple partial seizures and seizures arising in deep medial locations such as the medial frontal lobe, do not cause a change in the scalp EEG findings, even when recorded simultaneously with the clinical event.

Differential Diagnosis

Syncope (Chapter 427), various psychiatric disorders (Chapter 420), movement disorders (Chapter 434), sleep disorders (Chapter 429), and cerebrovascular insufficiency (Chapter 431) may be confused with epilepsy (Table 426–4). The neurologic manifestations of classic migraine (Chapter 421) can resemble a partial seizure, and some seizures are followed by headaches. The sequence of events, the consistency of the headache, and resolution of the neurologic features without progression to more severe seizure activity suggest a diagnosis of migraine. However, distinction between migraine and epilepsy can be difficult, and individuals with migraine have an increased prevalence of epilepsy.

Myoclonic seizures must be distinguished from myoclonus (Chapter 434), a term that refers to muscle jerks that are unassociated with epilepsy, such as those in uremic encephalopathy. Myoclonus resembles myoclonic seizures, but myoclonus is not accompanied by the EEG changes of a generalized seizure.

Paroxysmal movement disorders such as paroxysmal dystonia (Chapter 434), paroxysmal choreoathetosis, and paroxysmal ataxia can be confused with epilepsy. Autosomal dominant nocturnal frontal lobe epilepsy is a predominantly motor event that occurs in the middle of the night; its paroxysmal movements can be confused with a movement or sleep disorder. Video EEG monitoring may be necessary for diagnosis.

TABLE 426–4 PAROXYSMAL DISORDERS IN THE DIFFERENTIAL DIAGNOSIS OF EPILEPTIC SEIZURES

Vascular/perfusion disorders
Migraine, syncope, transient global amnesia, transient ischemic attack, arrhythmia/hypoperfusion
Movement disorders
Tics, paroxysmal dystonia, paroxysmal choreoathetosis, paroxysmal ataxia
Sleep disorders
Night terrors, sleep walking, sleep myoclonus
Psychiatric disorders
Panic disorder, dissociative disorder, psychogenic (nonepileptic) seizures, multiple personality disorder
Other
Breath-holding spells, paroxysmal vertigo

Patients with panic attacks and dissociative disorders (Chapter 420), including multiple personality disorder, can experience events that mimic simple or complex partial seizures. With such nonepileptic events, secondary gain is usually evident, and similar behavior may have occurred for an extended period. Nevertheless, the peculiarities of such attacks, as well as the neurologic manifestations of some patients, may require continuous video EEG monitoring for diagnosis, especially because frontal lobe seizures may also be associated with similar peculiar behavior. An erroneous diagnosis of nonepileptic seizures poses a risk for inappropriate discontinuation of medication, with resulting status epilepticus. Moreover, psychiatric disorders and epileptic seizures may coexist in the same patient.

Treatment

Medical Treatment

The goal is to find the drug or drugs that suppress all seizure activity without side effects. Even for a single seizure, prophylactic treatment with antiepileptic drugs delays the time to the next seizure, [1] although most experts recommend treatment after a single seizure only for patients in whom the likelihood of recurrent seizures is especially high. The presence of abnormal EEG changes, abnormal neurologic findings, a lesion on MRI, or a history of

Rx

significant brain injury increases the risk for recurrent seizures sufficiently to consider treatment after only one seizure. If a seizure occurs in the setting of an acute correctable metabolic or other provocation, long-term treatment is not indicated.

After two unprovoked seizures, the risk for recurrence is 70%. Initiation of treatment is typically indicated except in specific benign and self-limited syndromes, such as febrile seizures and benign epilepsy with centrotemporal spikes.

Specific drugs are effective for specific types of seizures, and some drugs can worsen other types of seizures (Table 426–5). Knowledge of individual drugs as they relate to age, sex, comorbid conditions, drug interactions, sedation, tolerance, mood, and withdrawal is critical in the drug selection process.

Drugs that cause enzyme induction (e.g., carbamazepine, phenytoin, phenobarbital, oxcarbazepine, topiramate) or inhibition (e.g., valproic acid) can be difficult to manage when additional medications are used for independent conditions, such as oral contraceptives. For these settings and in the elderly, gabapentin and levetiracetam are particularly useful because they have no appreciable drug interactions. The newer drugs are more expensive, whereas phenobarbital costs only pennies per dose and is preferable in many undeveloped countries and for individuals with limited resources.

As early as the 1980s, a randomized comparison study of carbamazepine, phenytoin, primidone, and phenobarbital for newly diagnosed partial seizures, with or without secondary generalization, found that all four drugs had similar efficacies but that the side effects of primidone and phenobarbital made carbamazepine and phenytoin preferable. [2] In a more recent meta-analysis of randomized clinical trials of antiepileptic drugs as monotherapy in newly diagnosed epilepsy, none of the newer antiepileptic drugs showed more efficacy than the traditional drugs, although tolerability was better in some situations. However, methodologic concerns may limit the applicability of these data to general treatment considerations. In trials comparing carbamazepine with lamotrigine monotherapy, for example, efficacy was equivalent, but more

Rx

carbamazepine-treated patients withdrew from the trial because of side effects. [3] In other randomized trials, valproate was as good as [4] or better than [5] topiramate and carbamazepine. The overall data indicate that there is not indisputable advantage of any single agent in terms of efficacy of monotherapy in patients with newly diagnosed epilepsy, so side effects, toxicity profiles (Table 426–6), and the type of seizure are of major importance in guiding therapy. For example, carbamazepine, oxcarbazepine, phenytoin, topiramate, lamotrigine, gabapentin, levetiracetam, and zonisamide could all be considered for initial treatment of partial epilepsy, with lamotrigine representing a potentially cost-effective alternative to carbamazepine. [6] Final selection would depend on age, gender, weight, psychiatric status, employment, concomitant medications, and pregnancy concerns relevant to the individual. Similarly, treatment of absence seizures would be equally appropriate with valproic acid, lamotrigine, and ethosuximide, so the accompanying seizure types, gender, age, and other aspects of the clinical setting would guide drug selection.

Treatment with the initial drug controls seizures completely in more than 50% of patients with newly diagnosed epilepsy. After failure of the first monotherapy, only 14 to 20% of patients with partial seizures will be successfully controlled with any alternative single drug. In combination therapy, drugs with differing mechanisms of action are used, but side effects are additive, and selection of combinations is not straightforward. Sometimes combining drugs with similar mechanisms is facilitative. Unfortunately, after failing monotherapy trials, less than 10% of patients have complete control of seizures with dual therapy.

Medical intractability occurs more often in patients with frequent seizures, multiple types of seizures, abnormal neurologic findings, a brain lesion, onset in the first year of life, or abnormal EEG findings consisting of either spike and slow wave activity or multifocal abnormalities. However, the most valuable predictor of medical intractability in epilepsy is the etiology. Patients with seizures secondary to mesial temporal sclerosis associated with mesial temporal

TABLE 426–5 ANTIEPILEPTIC DRUG SELECTION BY SEIZURE TYPE

	First or Alternative Monotherapy (Alphabetical Order)	Useful Combinations (Any A + Any B)		Other Useful Alternatives (Monotherapy or Polytherapy)
		A	B	
Partial seizures (complex or simple) with or without secondarily generalized seizures	Carbamazepine (CBZ) Gabapentin (GBP) Lamotrigine (LTG) Levetiracetam (LEV) Oxcarbazepine (OXC) Phenytoin (PHT) Topiramate (TPM) Valproate (VPA) Zonisamide (ZNS)	CBZ LTG OXC PHT	GBP LEV TPM VPA ZNS	Acetazolamide (ACZ) Chlorazepate (CLZ) Clonazepam (CLN) Phenobarbital (PB) Primidone (PRM) Felbamate (FBM)
Tonic clonic seizures, tonic seizures, atonic seizures	Carbamazepine Lamotrigine Levetiracetam Oxcarbazepine Phenytoin Topiramate Valproate Zonisamide	CBZ LTG OXC PHT	LEV TPM VPA ZNS	Acetazolamide Chlorazepate Clonazepam Felbamate (FBM) Phenobarbital Primidone
Absence seizures	Ethosuximide (ETH) Lamotrigine Valproate Topirimate	LTG VPA	ACZ CLN ETH TPM	Acetazolamide Clonazepam Phenobarbital Primidone
Myoclonic seizures	Clonazepam Valproate Zonisamide Levetiracetam	VPA	CLZ ZNS LEV	Phenobarbital

TABLE 426–6 CHARACTERISTICS OF MAJOR ANTIEPILEPTIC DRUGS

Name	Total mg/day (Usual Schedule)	Therapeutic Range (μg/mL)	Prominent Side Effects	Other Effects	Other Issues
Carbamazepine	400–1600 (bid)	4–12	Diplopia, fatigue, hyponatremia	Mood stabilizer	Enzyme inducer
Gabapentin	600–6000 (tid, qid)	2–12	Fatigue	Treatment of pain	No drug interactions
Lamotrigine	100–600 (bid)	4–18	Insomnia, headache, tremor, anxiety	Mood stabilizer	Risk for Stevens-Johnson syndrome; slow start-up
Levetiracetam	500–3000 (bid)	3–63	Mood change, irritability, lethargy		No drug interactions
Oxcarbazepine	300–2400 (tid)	6–40	Diplopia, hyponatremia, sedation	Mood stabilizer	
Phenobarbital	60–240 (hs)	15–40	Fatigue, depression, sedation	Joint pain	Enzyme inducer
Phenytoin	200–600 (bid)	10–20	Fatigue, hirsutism, gingival hypertrophy	Treatment of some pain	Enzyme inducer
Topiramate	50–600 (bid)	2–12	Anorexia, weight loss, kidney stones, speech disturbance, distal paresthesias	Headache prophylaxis, mood stabilizer	Enzyme inducer
Valproate	500–6000 (tid)	50–100	Weight gain, hair loss, tremor	Headache prophylaxis, mood stabilizer	Enzyme inhibitor, parkinsonian effects in elderly
Zonisamide	100–600 (hs)	10–40	Anorexia, kidney stones, dizziness, distal paresthesias	Mood stabilizer	

Rx

lobe epilepsy or developmental (migrational) substrates are most difficult to manage medically; only 40 to 50% of such patients are controlled as compared with a seizure-free rate of 65 to 80% in patients with newly diagnosed epilepsy of vascular or neoplastic cause.

Antiepileptic drugs and concomitant use of other drugs may alter serum levels. Antiepileptic drug levels (see Table 426–6) can establish the optimal therapeutic ranges for the individual, thereby allowing assessment of treatment failures as being caused by noncompliance, drug interactions, or incorrect prescribing. Phenytoin, carbamazepine, oxcarbazepine, topiramate, and phenobarbital induce hepatic enzymes, which may necessitate increasing the dose of other drugs. Similarly, enzyme inhibitors such as valproic acid or macrolide antibiotics can cause toxic levels of antiepileptic drugs. Carbamazepine induces the enzymes that metabolize it, so the initial dose needs to be increased later. Valproic acid inhibits clearance of lamotrigine, thereby allowing use of approximately half the dose of lamotrigine that would otherwise be needed to achieve the same serum level.

Treatment of Refractory Epilepsy

When seizures fail to respond to antiepileptic drug treatment, potential causes to be considered include incorrect diagnosis, incorrect drug selection, lack of compliance, factors that lower the seizure threshold, factors that reduce medication effects because of enhanced metabolism or reduced absorption, and factors that directly activate the CNS (Table 426–7). However, an estimated 15% or more of patients with partial-onset seizures are unresponsive to medical treatment, and resection of a cerebral region identified to be the origin of intractable partial seizures offers the possibility of cure. Removal of an epileptogenic region requires accurate identification of the region, as well as documentation of a lack of functional consequences after its removal. Video EEG monitoring with seizure recording from scalp electrodes, MRI protocols with special attention to areas commonly associated with refractory seizures (e.g., the medial temporal and frontal lobes), and functional neuroimaging, including PET (metabolism) and SPECT (perfusion), are routinely used. Neuropsychological evaluation, both for localizing

TABLE 426–7 CONSIDERATIONS IN REFRACTORY EPILEPSY

- Incorrect diagnosis
  - Nonepileptic disorder (see Table 426–4)
  - Seizure type
- Incorrect drug selection
- Lack of compliance
- Other drugs causing reduced levels of antiepileptic drugs
- Other medications that exacerbate seizures
  - Interferons
  - Lithium
  - Phenothiazines
  - Antidepressants
  - Isoniazid
  - Theophylline
  - Antihistamines
- Illicit drug use
  - Cocaine
  - Amphetamines
- Drug withdrawal
  - Alcohol
  - Barbiturates
  - Benzodiazepines
- Comorbid conditions exacerbating epilepsy
  - Diabetes mellitus
  - Sleep disorder
  - Psychosis
  - Pregnancy
- Other central nervous system–activating factors
  - Heat (hot tubs, saunas, fever, exercise)
  - Sleep loss
  - Fasting
  - Stress
  - Hyperventilation

Rx

areas of dysfunction and for establishing the level of functional activity in tissue being considered for possible resection, is an essential component of the evaluation. Good performance on measures of verbal memory, generally believed to rely on the dominant medial temporal lobe, may be used as an indicator of excessive risk of memory loss from contemplated resection of dominant medial temporal lobe structures when seizures localize to that region. Sometimes, EEG localization of the area of seizure onset requires implantation of intracranial or subdural electrodes or grids, which are also used for electrical stimulation to map cortical function in the nearby regions of the brain.

Surgical Interventions

In a randomized trial, resective surgery for intractable medial temporal lobe epilepsy achieved a 58% seizure-free rate at 1 year versus 8% in the control group. 7 Although 20% of patients relapse with long-term follow-up, reintroduction of antiepileptic drugs can control the seizures in some patients.

When intractable epilepsy is associated with multifocal seizures, when the onset of seizures occurs in functionally critical brain regions, or when localization is not possible, resection cannot be attempted. Alternative surgical interventions, including corpus callosum section or multiple subpial transection, may be of benefit. These usually palliative procedures functionally disconnect epileptogenic tissue from other brain regions, thereby preventing propagation of seizures and resulting in smaller, partial events. Callosotomy severs the major interhemispheric commissure and stops generalized seizures in most patients, but at the cost of considerable morbidity. Multiple subpial transection involves vertical cuts in the cortex to a depth of about 4 mm, placed 4 to 5 mm apart, in the identified region or regions of seizure generation to sever the horizontal connections that allow the seizure to propagate while maintaining the vertical, functional columns.

Electrical Stimulation

Electrical stimulation is now used to treat medically refractory epilepsy when surgery is not indicated. Programmed, intermittent stimulation of the vagus nerve in the neck with implanted leads attached to a battery placed subcutaneously in the upper part of the chest can reduce the frequency of seizures in approximately a third of patients by about 30%. Electrodes implanted to stimulate cortical epileptogenic locations are under study.

Management Issues in Women with Epilepsy

Hormonal cycling, pregnancy, and the long-term effects of certain antiepileptic drugs influence the management of epilepsy in women. Estrogen lowers the seizure threshold, whereas progesterone raises it, and changes in hormone levels during the menstrual cycle may aggravate seizures perimenstrually, less often at midcycle. In many women these changes do not cause difficulty with control of the seizure, but some women have seizures more frequently or even only with their menses (i.e., catamenial epilepsy). Although levels of antiepileptic drugs may fluctuate with the menstrual cycle, altering drug doses at mid or end cycle is generally difficult. Catamenial epilepsy is sometimes improved by the administration of an oral contraceptive pill; Depo-Provera may also reduce perimenstrual seizures. Enzyme-inducing antiepileptic drugs, particularly phenytoin, carbamazepine, phenobarbital, primidone, and topiramate, reduce estrogen levels by enhancing its metabolism, so oral contraceptives with higher doses of estrogen may be necessary, or alternative methods of contraception may be preferable.

Pregnancy itself has no consistent effect on the frequency of seizures, and the response varies not only among women but also among pregnancies in individual women. Generalized tonic-clonic seizures during pregnancy may pose a risk to the developing fetus. Whether complex partial seizures have similar negative effects on fetal development is not known. Simple partial seizures do not pose any risk unless they progress to a complex partial or generalized tonic-clonic event.

Although most of the antiepileptic drugs double the risk (to 4 to 6%) of major malformations in the developing fetus, it is usually important to maintain an effective antiepileptic drug level for each patient during pregnancy. Valproic acid is the most teratogenic of the commonly used antiepileptic drugs, with a substantial risk for spina bifida; it should be avoided in pregnancy and possibly in all women of childbearing age. Carbamazepine is also associated with an increased risk for spina bifida, but less so. The teratogenic effects of newer antiepileptic drugs are still unclear. With use of a single drug at the lowest possible dose, more than 90% of women with epilepsy have normal pregnancies and deliver normal babies without complications.

Most antiepileptic drugs reach breast milk only in low concentrations, so breast-feeding is possible. Occasionally, however, somnolence from absorption of even small amounts of antiepileptic drugs by the nursing infant may interrupt successful feeding.

Women of childbearing age and particularly women with epilepsy should routinely take 1 to 3 mg of folate per day. Long-term bone loss in women taking antiepileptic drugs, especially those that induce cytochrome P-450, is treated prophylactically with supplemental calcium and vitamin D.

Epileptic Syndromes

The syndromic diagnosis of epilepsy (see Table 426–3) uses the classification of the type or types of seizures, as well as information about the setting in which seizures occur, the patient's neurologic and cognitive status, age at onset, family history, and results of diagnostic studies, including imaging. Selection of specific drug treatment depends on the types of seizures present (see Table 426–5). The need for lifelong treatment, the risk of genetic transmission, the likelihood of concurrent neurologic diseases, the risk of comorbid conditions, and the long-term prognosis are critical factors that can be addressed only with knowledge of the specific epileptic syndrome.

The first issues in syndromic diagnosis are whether the epilepsy is related to a localized brain region or is generalized and whether it has an identified cause (symptomatic of or secondary to a detectable brain lesion) or not (idiopathic). Sometimes epilepsy is presumed to be symptomatic but no clear cause can be identified; these cases are called cryptogenic. Thus, the syndromic classification of epilepsies first divides syndromes into localization related versus generalized (see Table 426–3) and into symptomatic versus idiopathic. Other variables are then used to define the specific syndromes within these groups. Although most generalized epilepsies are idiopathic (and genetic) and most localization-related epilepsies are symptomatic with an identifiable brain lesion or cause, idiopathic epilepsy syndromes can be associated predominantly or exclusively with partial onset seizures (localizations related), and symptomatic epilepsy syndromes can be associated predominantly or exclusively with generalized seizures.

Generalized Epileptic Syndromes

Benign neonatal convulsions, which occur in previously healthy newborns on about day 5, may be partial or generalized tonic seizures. Mutations in two potassium channel genes *(KCNQ2, KCNQ3)* have been associated with this syndrome. Potassium channel regulation may be age dependent and therefore account for the age-related appearance of the seizures. The EEG recording is abnormal and shows rhythmic slow wave activity or spiking with seizures. The seizures are refractory to treatment, are recurrent over a brief interval, and disappear within a month. About 90% of such infants subsequently have normal development, whereas 10% have subsequent seizures in this idiopathic, generalized epileptic syndrome.

In generalized epilepsy with febrile seizures plus, febrile seizures occur in combination with a variety of other nonfebrile types of seizures, including myoclonic, absence, atonic, tonic-clonic, and partial seizures. Mutations in at least four different ion channel genes, including voltage-gated sodium channels *(SCN1A, SCN2A, SCN3A)* and GABA receptors *(GABRG2)*, have been identified.

In the syndrome of severe myoclonic epilepsy of infancy, which is also associated with various *SCN1A* mutations, myoclonic seizures

Rx

are associated with other types of seizures, including absence, atonic, and partial seizures. The seizures are difficult to treat and are associated with developmental and cognitive decline after 1 to 2 years of normal development.

Childhood absence epilepsy begins in early to mid childhood, usually with autosomal dominant inheritance, and is characterized by absence seizures, rarely with other types of generalized seizures. It is self-limited in about 40% of cases. It occurs in the setting of otherwise normal brain structure and function. The seizures are accompanied by a characteristic 3-Hz spike and wave EEG discharge, which appears in short bursts between seizures and in continuous runs during seizures (see Fig. 426–2). Earlier onset may be associated with a tendency to remit, whereas onset after 12 years of age is more likely to be accompanied by generalized tonic-clonic seizures and persist into adulthood.

Juvenile myoclonic epilepsy usually starts in the second decade with generalized tonic-clonic and myoclonic seizures. Mutations in GABA receptors, including *GABRG1,* can be found. Seizures typically occur in the morning, immediately after awakening. A proportion of these patients have had absence seizures as well. The EEG recording may be similar to the 3-Hz spike-wave of absence epilepsy, but the spike-wave pattern can be faster. The seizures are especially linked to sleep deprivation and tend to appear in college students. Lifetime treatment is generally needed.

West's syndrome is a catastrophic, usually secondary generalized epileptic syndrome that appears before the age of 12 months and ceases by the age of 5 years, often to be replaced by other symptomatic generalized epilepsy syndromes such as Lennox-Gastaut (see later). Tuberous sclerosis (Chapter 444) and hypoxia are among the common causes, but West's syndrome can also be idiopathic. The syndrome comprises a triad of so-called infantile spasms (synonymous terms include myoclonic spasms, jackknife convulsions, salaam seizures), developmental arrest, and an EEG pattern called hypsarrhythmia (a markedly abnormal EEG pattern with high-amplitude slowing and superimposed multifocal spikes, polyspikes, and spike and slow wave complexes). Associated abnormalities often include developmental delay, porencephaly, atrophic lesions, calcifications, and agenesis of the corpus callosum.

Lennox-Gastaut syndrome, a secondary or cryptogenic generalized epilepsy found in children with mental retardation, is characterized by the occurrence of multiple generalized types of seizures, including atypical absence, generalized tonic-clonic, tonic, atonic, and partial seizures. The EEG pattern is a spike-wave variation but slower than the 3 Hz associated with absence seizures, more characteristically between 2 and 2.5 Hz. It often appears after West's syndrome has resolved.

Febrile seizures are acute secondary seizures that are not considered epilepsy because seizures occur only when provoked by fever. The seizures begin after 6 months of age and generally do not continue beyond the age of 6 years. Usually, the febrile seizure diathesis is left untreated because the prognosis is benign. When seizures occur in the setting of a neurologic abnormality or are prolonged or complicated, the risk for later epilepsy is increased.

Localization-Related Epileptic Syndromes

Benign rolandic epilepsy, which is also called benign epilepsy with central temporal spikes, is an age-related partial seizure disorder with onset between 3 and 13 years of age; it is characterized by almost exclusively nocturnal partial motor or sensory seizures with facial or oral onset and with frequent secondary generalization. The family history is positive for epilepsy diagnoses in nearly 50% of cases. The EEG recording shows spiking in the central/temporal region. In some cases, the disorder may not require treatment because it usually remits spontaneously (97%) and is not associated with any known brain abnormality.

Autosomal dominant nocturnal frontal lobe epilepsy is characterized by clusters of brief seizures that occur during sleep and are manifested by turning prone, vocalization, and violent thrashing lasting 10 seconds, followed by immediate return to sleep. The syndrome is caused by mutations in genes for neuronal nicotinic acetylcholine receptors *(CHRNA4, CHRNB2);* the inheritance pattern appears to be autosomal dominant with variable penetrance. Seizures begin in childhood and persist, but they are not associated with other clinical manifestations or evidence of structural or functional brain abnormalities.

Lobar epilepsies are epileptic syndromes that begin in the temporal, parietal, occipital, and frontal lobes. Each of these lobes has subdivisions and regions, which can result in different clinical manifestations and EEG findings. Causes include neoplastic, traumatic, developmental, infectious, and ischemic diseases. Clinical characteristics are consistent with seizures originating in each specific cortical location (see Table 426–2).

Mesial Temporal Lobe Epilepsy

Mesial temporal lobe epilepsy is the most common partial (lobar) epilepsy in adults. It is characterized by recurrent simple and complex partial seizures that originate in mesial temporal/limbic structures, as documented by EEG seizure recordings obtained from implanted electrodes placed in the medial temporal regions. Various components of the mesial temporal limbic network (including the hippocampus, entorhinal cortex, amygdala, neocortical areas of the frontal and temporal lobes, and dorsal medial thalamus) are probably involved in the pathogenesis of these seizures. Mesial temporal sclerosis, also called hippocampal sclerosis, is characterized by neuronal loss and gliosis, mostly in the CA1 and CA3 regions of the hippocampus, with mossy fiber reorganization seen as sprouting of neuropeptide Y and dynorphin interneurons into the inner third of the dentate molecular layer. Whether the neuronal loss is secondary or primary and whether neuronal reorganization has a critical role in the epileptogenic process are not known.

The seizures of mesial temporal lobe epilepsy begin at 5 to 15 years of age. Seizures have mostly complex partial manifestations with altered consciousness, typically beginning with an aura of a rising epigastric sensation or a feeling of déjà vu, followed by oral and alimentary automatisms and later by contralateral arm dystonia and ipsilateral arm automatisms. The seizures are lengthy (lasting minutes), rarely generalize, and typically occur three to five times a month. Auras without following seizures are common. Up to 70% of patients have a risk factor, such as lengthy and complicated seizures before the age of 4 years, frequently associated with fever or with encephalitis, meningitis, or trauma. However, the characteristic seizures generally begin some years later. Most cases are sporadic, but there are familial forms of mesial temporal lobe epilepsy. Hippocampal atrophy and increased hippocampal T2 signal are best seen on coronal MRI, and widespread hypometabolism is seen in the temporal lobe on PET. Material-specific (verbal or visual) memory impairment corresponds to primary involvement of the dominant or nondominant hippocampus. EEG recordings show temporal lobe spikes interictally (see Fig. 426–3), as well as rhythmic 4- to 7-Hz discharges over the appropriate temporal lobe during seizures (see Fig. 426–1).

Less than 40% of patients with newly diagnosed mesial temporal lobe epilepsy will be controlled with medications, although familial cases are more easily managed medically. Up to 80% of patients with medically refractory seizures become seizure free, usually without medications, after resection of the responsible anterior temporal lobe and hippocampal structures.

Status Epilepticus

Status epilepticus is a medical emergency in which seizures occur continuously or repeatedly without intervening resumption of consciousness. Although the standard diagnostic criteria require a duration of 30 minutes, even 5 minutes of generalized tonic-clonic seizures cause hypoxia, lactic acidosis, muscle breakdown, and CNS toxicity as a result of excessive excitatory neurotransmitters, and longer durations cause progressively more severe long-term morbidity and mortality. Immediate intervention with parenteral agents to stop the seizures is mandatory. Prompt attention to defining the cause of the status epilepticus must also be given. Stabilization of airway and vascular status and initiation of assessment of the diagnostic possibilities are immediately followed by the use of intravenous benzodiazepines (e.g., lorazepam, 0.1 mg/kg given at

Rx

2 mg/min). Diazepam (10 mg intravenously) is an alternative. If seizures continue for 10 to 15 minutes, intravenous phenytoin at 20 mg/kg (or fosphenytoin in a similar phenytoin-equivalent dose) should be administered. If seizures do not respond within an additional 15 minutes, barbiturates (phenobarbital, 20 mg/kg intravenously) or a continuous drip of midazolam (0.1 to 2 mg/kg/hr), pentobarbital (0.5 to 3 mg/kg/hr), or propofol (2 to 4 mg/kg/hr) can be used. In refractory cases, the next step is general anesthesia for 24 hours.

Prognosis

After a single, first seizure, only 25% of patients have a recurrent seizure. Risk factors for recurrence include the presence of a brain lesion or injury or abnormal EEG findings. The risk for future recurrence rises to 70% after a second seizure.

The prognosis with treatment for individuals with two or more unprovoked seizures is excellent. The majority of patients without risk factors who have been seizure free for 5 years can be successfully withdrawn from medications. Remission is less likely for adults with more frequent seizures, a greater number of seizures before diagnosis, multiple types of seizures, or abnormal EEG or neurologic findings. Most remissions occur early, and response to treatment can also be predicted early: only 60% of patients who do not achieve control of seizures with medical treatment in the first year will ever remit, and only 10% of patients uncontrolled after 4 years can anticipate successful response to any medical regimen.

In population-based studies, idiopathic epilepsy has little effect on mortality rates, but secondary "symptomatic" epilepsy increases mortality rates two- to six-fold. Most of the increase in mortality among patients with epilepsy has been related to the underlying cause, but seizure-related causes of death include status epilepticus, injury, and SUDEP (sudden unexplained death in epilepsy). The pathophysiology of SUDEP, which occurs more often in individuals with frequent seizures and generalized tonic-clonic seizures, is unknown, although pulmonary edema is usually found on autopsy and hypoventilation is considered a likely mechanism. There is speculation that ion channel defects may cause both the epilepsy and cardiac abnormalities that predispose to SUDEP. The decreased mortality after successful control of seizures is related, in part, to a reduced risk for SUDEP.

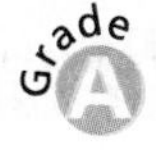

1. Marson A, Jacoby A, Johnson A, et al: Immediate versus deferred antiepileptic drug treatment for early epilepsy and single seizures: A randomised controlled trial. Lancet 2005;365:2007–2013.
2. Mattson RH, Cramer JA, Collins JF, et al: Comparison of carbamazepine, phenobarbital, phenytoin, and primidone in partial and secondarily generalized tonic-clonic seizures. N Engl J Med 1985;313:145–151.
3. Brodie MJ, Richens A, Yuen AWC: Double-blind comparison of lamotrigine and carbamazepine in newly diagnosed epilepsy. Lancet 1995;345:476–479.
4. Privitera MD, Brodie MJ, Mattson RH, et al: Topiramate, carbamazepine and valproate monotherapy: Double-blind comparison in newly diagnosed epilepsy. Acta Neurol Scand 2003;107:165–175.
5. Marson AG, Al-Kharusi AM, Alwaidh M, et al: The SANAD study of effectiveness of valproate, lamotrigine, or topiramate for generalised and unclassifiable epilepsy: An unblinded randomised controlled trial. Lancet 2007;369:1016–1026.
6. Marson AG, Al-Kharusi AM, Alwaidh M, et al: The SANAD study of effectiveness of carbamazepine, gabapentin, lamotrigine, oxcarbazepine, or topiramate for treatment of partial epilepsy: An unblinded randomised controlled trial. Lancet 2007;369:1000–1015.
7. Wiebe S, Blume W, Girvin J, et al: A randomized controlled trial of surgery for temporal lobe epilepsy. N Engl J Med 2001; 345:311–366.

SUGGESTED READINGS

Bleck TP: Refractory status epilepticus. Curr Opin Crit Care 2005;11:117–120. *An overview of treatment of status, with a useful approach to refractory cases.*

Glauser T, Ben-Menachem E, Bourgeois B, et al: ILAE treatment guidelines: Evidence-based analysis of antiepileptic drug efficacy and effectiveness as initial monotherapy for epileptic seizures and syndromes. Epilepsia 2006;47: 1094–1120. *Comprehensive review of the literature.*

Gutierrez-Delicado E, Serratosa J: Genetics of the epilepsies. Curr Opin Neurol 2004;17:147–153. *A current summary of newly identified genetic epilepsy syndromes.*

Hirtz D, Berg AT, Bettis D, et al: Practice parameter: Treatment of the child with a first unprovoked seizure. Report of the QSS of the AAN and the Practice Committee of the CNS. Neurology 2003;60:166–175. *Insight into the outcome of childhood epilepsy, with guidance on treatment.*

LaRoche SM, Helmers SL: The new antiepileptic drugs: Scientific review. JAMA 2004;291:605–614.; LaRoche SM, Helmers SL: The new antiepileptic drugs: Clinical applications. JAMA 2004;291:615–620. *Review of newer agents and their therapeutic roles.*

427 SYNCOPE

Roger P. Simon

Definition

Syncope is the phenomenon of loss of consciousness associated with loss of postural tone (Chapters 48 and 62). The episode is caused by global impairment of blood flow to the brain; occasionally, hypoperfusion may be confined to the cerebral hemispheres or the brain stem, and involvement of either structure produces unconsciousness. Syncope must be differentiated from seizures (Chapter 426), which may be manifested similarly but have different pathophysiology and therapy.

History

Because most spells of episodic loss of consciousness occur outside medical observation, the history is the most critical part of the evaluation. If multiple spells have occurred, their similarity should be established so that small pieces of history from one spell or another may be combined into a pathophysiologic profile. Each syncopal episode should be reviewed in detail with attention paid to the three key elements: events and symptoms preceding the spell, what happened during the spell of unconsciousness, and the time course of regaining orientation after consciousness is regained. The first of these elements can be obtained from the patient, but the second and frequently the third cannot. Accordingly, information from a witness is essential to the evaluation and should be obtained by phone calls, interviews, or revisits scheduled to include persons who have witnessed one or more spells.

Before the Spell

What position was the patient in when each spell began? Seizures or cardiac arrhythmias can occur in any body position, but vasovagal syncope rarely and orthostatic hypotension never begin with the patient recumbent. In patients with recurrent syncope, if even a single episode began in the recumbent posture, vasovagal and orthostatic causes are virtually excluded.

What prodromal symptoms were appreciated before loss of consciousness? Symptoms of cerebral hypoperfusion should be sought, including lightheadedness, dizziness (but uncommonly vertigo), bilateral tinnitus, nausea, diffuse weakness, and finally, dimming of vision from retinal hypoperfusion. This prodrome establishes the pathophysiology of the syncopal spell as that of cerebral hypoperfusion; such hypoperfusion may be of cardiac, orthostatic, or reflex cause. Loss of consciousness so rapid that a prodrome is absent may occur with seizures and with some cardiac arrhythmias such as asystole, which causes loss of consciousness within 4 to 8 seconds in the upright position but requires 12 to 15 seconds in the recumbent position. Palpitations (Chapter 62) during the prodrome suggest a tachyarrhythmia (Chapters 63 and 64) but may also occur with vasovagal events.

What was the activity of the patient immediately before the onset of symptoms? Identification of extreme exertion (cardiac), an emotional or painful stimulus (vasovagal), a rapid change in posture (orthostatic), and straining at urination (situational) can help in identifying the cause.

During the Event

What events do witnesses describe as occurring during the episode of unconsciousness? Although body stiffening and limb jerking are well-known motor phenomena occurring during the loss of consciousness associated with generalized seizures, very similar motor movements can result from cerebral hypoperfusion. These motor movements occur especially if cerebral blood flow is not rapidly restored by termination of an arrhythmia or by falling to a recumbent posture in the setting of reflex or vasovagal syncope. Such muscle jerking is often multifocal and can be synchronous or asynchronous. In contrast to epileptic seizures, which generally produce tonic-clonic activity for at least 1 to 2 minutes (Chapter 426), muscle jerking in syncope rarely persists longer than 30 seconds. If an arrhythmia continues or the patient is physically maintained upright (e.g., fainting in a phone booth or while sitting on a toilet), tonic stiffening of the body takes place (i.e., opisthotonos) and is followed by jerking movements of the limbs. Occasionally, motor movements identical to a tonic-clonic seizure occur, and a mistaken diagnosis of epilepsy can be made. Urinary incontinence during the spell is frequently used to support or refute a diagnosis of epilepsy; however, fainting with a full bladder can result in incontinence, whereas seizures with an empty bladder will not. Tongue biting favors seizures.

After the Event

Over what time frame were consciousness and orientation regained? This aspect of the history is the most useful in dealing with the differential diagnosis of seizures as the cause of a syncopal-like spell. Recovery of orientation and consciousness after vasovagal or reflex-mediated syncope occurs simultaneously. Recovery of orientation after syncope of cardiac origin is proportional to the duration of the unconsciousness but is usually rapid (0 to 10 seconds); with periods of malignant arrhythmia producing unconsciousness of 2 minutes, confusion on waking lasts less than 30 seconds. After seizures, however, the period of confusion, often with agitation, continues for 2 to 20 minutes after recovery of consciousness.

Pathobiology

Neurocardiogenic Syncope

The term *neurocardiogenic syncope* (Table 427–1) is used to describe spells of transient cerebral hypoperfusion in the absence of a demonstrable cardiac cause. The mechanism of the peripheral vasodilation and hypotension may be vagotonic, situational, or of unclear origin. A common phenomenon is activation of cardiopulmonary baroreceptors and mechanoreceptors resulting in inappropriate peripheral pooling of blood, inappropriate bradycardia, and in some, a combination of both. The prodrome (i.e., lightheadedness, tinnitus, and visual dimming) and the pattern of recovery (i.e., simultaneous recovery of consciousness and orientation) are reasonably consistent regardless of the precise cause.

Vasovagal Syncope

Vasovagal spells, or simple faints, are the most common cause of syncope. These episodes occur in all age groups, are equally common in men and women, and may be more frequent in some families. Precipitating factors include pain (especially medical instrumentation), trauma, fatigue, blood loss, or prolonged motionless standing. Vagally mediated hypotension and bradycardia combine to produce cerebral hypoperfusion with a resultant prodrome of lightheadedness, nausea, tinnitus, diaphoresis, salivation, pallor, and dimming of vision. Tachycardia may be the initial manifestation. The spells typically begin in the standing or sitting position, but medical instrumentation (e.g., phlebotomy or insertion of an intrauterine device) can induce episodes when the patient is horizontal. The patient loses consciousness and postural tone and then falls with flaccid or stiff limbs; the eyes are usually open, often with an upward gaze. The patient is pale and diaphoretic and has dilated pupils. Tonic posturing or a few symmetrical or asymmetrical myoclonic jerks may occur, especially if the patient is maintained in a semi-upright position. These jerking movements are not epileptic; concomitant electroencephalographic (EEG) recordings show generalized slow waves. Consciousness is recovered rapidly when the patient becomes horizontal. Postictal confusion is absent. Symptoms of nervousness, dizziness, nausea, and urge to defecate may persist, and syncope can recur on standing.

Situational Syncope

Vagally mediated neurocardiogenic syncope can be induced by micturition, defecation, or swallowing or can occur during episodes of glossopharyngeal neuralgia. Syncope during micturition occurs before, during, or after micturition in the upright position. Vagally mediated bradycardia is causative. Micturition syncope is most frequent after arising from the recumbency of sleep to urinate. Though much less common, a similar syndrome can occur with defecation. Brain stem reflexes triggering vagally induced bradyarrhythmias, with resultant syncope, can occur as a result of swallowing, with or without the association of severe pain in the tonsillar pillar, which may radiate to the ear (i.e., glossopharyngeal neuralgia). The pain can be prevented by carbamazepine (400 to 1000 mg/day orally) (Chapter 426). In refractory cases, 300 mg of phenytoin (Dilantin) each day can be added.

A nonvagally mediated situational syncope occurs with coughing (i.e., cough syncope). In predisposed patients, the coughing increases intrathoracic venous pressure, which is transmitted to the intracranial veins; the resultant transient increase in intracranial pressure is adequate to impair blood flow. Spells can occur in any position. A prodrome is absent, and impaired consciousness lasts only a few seconds.

Carotid Sinus Syncope

Carotid sinus syncope results when vagal stimulation from the carotid sinus produces hypotension or bradycardia. The syndrome is uncommon, has a male preponderance, and affects mainly patients older than 60 years. Use of propranolol, digitalis, or methyldopa may predispose to carotid sinus syncope. Carotid sinus massage may be diagnostic and can be performed in an outpatient setting, although only in the absence of carotid bruits or a history of ventricular tachycardia, recent stroke, or myocardial infarction. Induction of asystole for 3 seconds or longer,

TABLE 427–1 CAUSES OF SYNCOPE AND THEIR PREVALENCE IN VARIOUS SERIES

NEUROCARDIOGENIC CAUSES

Vasovagal (8–41% of patients)
Situational (1–8% of patients)
- Micturition
- Defecation
- Swallow
- Cough

Carotid sinus syncope (0.4% of patients)
Neuralgias
Psychiatric disorders
Medications, exercise

ORTHOSTATIC HYPOTENSION (4–10% OF PATIENTS)
DECREASED CARDIAC OUTPUT

Obstruction to flow (1–8% of patients)
- Obstruction to left ventricular outflow or inflow: aortic stenosis, hypertrophic obstructive cardiomyopathy, mitral stenosis, myxoma
- Obstruction to right ventricular outflow or inflow: pulmonic stenosis, pulmonary embolism, pulmonary hypertension, myxoma

Other heart disease
- Pump failure, myocardial infarction, coronary artery disease, coronary spasm, tamponade, aortic dissection

Arrhythmias (4–38% of patients)
- Bradyarrhythmias: sinus node disease, second- and third-degree atrioventricular block, pacemaker malfunction, drug-induced bradyarrhythmias
- Tachyarrhythmias: ventricular tachycardia, torsades de pointes (e.g., associated with congenital long QT syndrome or acquired QT prolongation), supraventricular tachycardia

NEUROLOGIC AND PSYCHIATRIC DISEASES (3–32% OF PATIENTS)

Migraine
Transient ischemic attacks

UNKNOWN (13–41% OF PATIENTS)

Adapted from Kapoor W: Approach to the patient with syncope. *In* Braunwald E, Goldman L (eds): Primary Cardiology, 2nd ed. Philadelphia, Saunders, 2003.

hypotension, or both constitute a positive test result. False-positive results are common, however, especially in the setting of contralateral carotid occlusion, because the ipsilateral massage transiently occludes the ipsilateral carotid and thereby prevents bilateral carotid blood flow. Symptomatic bradycardia can be treated by pacemaker implantation.

Psychiatric Syncope

Neuropsychiatric syncope is a diagnosis of exclusion but is suggested by young age, frequent spells, multiple symptoms (e.g., dizziness, vertigo, lightheadedness, numbness), and duplication of the patient's symptoms by hyperventilation with the mouth open for 2 to 3 minutes. Whereas syncope and seizures occur with the eyes open, often with gaze deviation, psychogenic events frequently begin with eye closing.

Orthostatic Hypotension

Postural hypotension can result in syncope that may be recurrent. The history confirms that the patient is in the upright posture during the spells, that the prodromal symptoms are those of cerebral hypoperfusion, and that the symptoms are relieved with recumbency. The diagnosis is supported by detecting a decrease of 30 mm Hg or greater in systolic pressure or a 10-mm Hg or greater decrease in diastolic pressure between testing in the recumbent versus the upright posture. The many causes include drugs, polyneuropathies, and neurodegenerative disorders (Chapters 433, 445, and 446).

Cardiogenic Syncope

Syncope that occurs during exercise or is associated with palpitations suggests a cardiac cause. A family history may be found in certain cases of prolonged QT interval syndrome. Cardiogenic syncope (Chapter 62) occurs in the setting of organic heart disease producing obstruction to inflow (e.g., myxoma, constrictive pericarditis) or outflow (e.g., aortic or pulmonic stenosis, hypertrophic cardiomyopathy) or as a result of bradyarrhythmia or tachyarrhythmia (Chapters 63 and 64). Premonitory symptoms may be caused by cerebral hypoperfusion (i.e., faintness, tinnitus, and dimming of vision), but these symptoms may be absent with bradyarrhythmias because of the rapid fall in cardiac output and precipitous decline in cerebral blood flow resulting in abrupt loss of consciousness, particularly in the upright posture. Evaluation for arrhythmias should begin with a rhythm strip, which provides a 5% yield, followed by Holter monitoring for 24 hours; symptoms occur during monitoring in approximately 20% of patients. With recurrent events, long-term ambulatory loop electrocardiography (ECG) is useful in recording the rhythm during a spell and thus confirming or excluding an arrhythmic cause. This technique identifies another 25 to 50% of patients studied. Electrophysiologic testing (Chapter 65) is often used in an attempt to induce arrhythmias in patients who have organic heart disease or a conduction block on ECG (especially in the elderly at risk for syncope-induced trauma); the yield is approximately 50%.

Cerebrovascular Syncope

Loss of consciousness can be a component of a basilar artery transient ischemic attack (Chapter 431), but unconsciousness alone is virtually never the initial symptom. Other brain stem symptoms always precede or accompany syncope. Vertigo is most frequent, but diplopia or visual field disturbances, hemifacial or perioral numbness, and dysarthria or ataxia are also common. Recovery of consciousness may require 30 to 60 minutes. These patients, who are at risk for basilar artery stroke, should be treated with aspirin, undergo formal noninvasive evaluation of their cerebral arteries, and be considered for other treatments appropriate for their symptoms and anatomy (Chapter 431).

Subclavian artery stenosis may result in retrograde blood flow from the vertebral artery to one arm, with resultant brain stem hypoperfusion (i.e., subclavian steal syndrome). An asymmetry in upper extremity blood pressure averaging 45 mm Hg is nearly always present. Brain stem symptoms similar to those in basilar transient ischemic attacks occur and can include loss of consciousness; a subsequent stroke resulting from subclavian steal is rare. Syncope may also occur in up to 10% of patients with basilar artery migraine (Chapter 421). It can have a postural (orthostatic) manifestation or be associated with other basilar artery symptoms.

Syncope in the Elderly

The elderly often have multiple factors contributing to syncope, including situational, reflex, cardiac, cerebrovascular, and neurologic (Chapter 23). Orthostatic syncope is particularly likely to occur 15 to 75 minutes after a meal or following a rapid change in posture, even in the absence of neurologic or gastrointestinal disease. The postprandial reduction in systolic pressure in a normal elderly person is approximately 14 mm Hg, as compared with 24 mm Hg in those with a history of syncope. Medications with hypotensive side effects (antihypertensive agents, sedatives, antidepressants, antianginal medications, and antiparkinsonian medications, particularly fluoxetine, haloperidol, and L-dopa), even if administered at standard doses, commonly induce symptomatic hypotension in the elderly. Protracted episodes of unresponsiveness lasting up to 4 hours occasionally occur in the elderly, especially while in the hospital. Investigations are not revealing. A disorder of the sleep cycle may be responsible.

Diagnosis

The history and physical examination guide the approach to further diagnostic testing (Tables 427–2 and 427–3 and Fig. 427–1). In patients without evidence of structural heart disease or cerebrovascular disease, typical symptoms may be reproduced during head-up tilt-table testing (Chapter 62), such as tilting the table to 70 degrees for up to 45 minutes; sensitivity may be increased by the addition of an isoproterenol infusion to mimic catecholamine release. Of patients identified in this manner, a third have a vasodepressor response and two thirds have a cardioinhibitory response.

Patients with a history of exercise-induced syncope, ischemic heart disease detected by history or electrocardiographic abnormalities, or auscultatory evidence of organic heart disease should be studied initially by echocardiography and then by exercise stress testing. A history suggestive of bradyarrhythmia (i.e., rapid loss of consciousness) or tachyarrhythmia (i.e., palpitations preceding the syncope) should be investigated with 24-hour Holter monitoring or long-term loop monitoring (Chapter 62). In patients with recurrent, difficult-to-diagnose syncope, an implantable loop recorder is better than the combination of tilt testing, an external loop recorder, and electrophysiologic testing. [1]

Routine EEG testing is not helpful; even in epileptic patients a single EEG study may be normal. Epilepsy is a clinical diagnosis. Particularly suggestive is prolonged postictal confusion. Structural brain diseases are rarely a cause of episodic loss of consciousness, and routine brain imaging studies are not indicated. Carotid Doppler (Chapter 431) studies may show various degrees of stenosis, especially in older patients. However, unconsciousness requires bihemispheric dysfunction; thus, unilateral carotid stenosis alone does not cause syncope. Transcranial Doppler studies or magnetic resonance angiography of the basilar artery is indicated only if brain stem ischemic symptoms are present in addition to loss of consciousness; false-positive tests are common, especially with increasing age.

Treatment

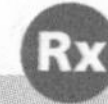

Treatment should be directed at the cause of syncope, such as valve replacement for aortic stenosis (Chapter 75); medications for obstructive, hypertrophic cardiomyopathy (Chapter 59); medications, cardioversion, a pacemaker, or an implantable cardioverter-defibrillator for arrhythmias (Chapters 62, 63, and 64); and fluid repletion for orthostatic hypotension.

Patients with neurocardiogenic syncope should be counseled on how to prevent episodes by avoiding situations that provoke their symptoms and to increase their intake of fluid and salt. Patients should also be taught how to tense their arms and legs and grip their hands during prodromal symptoms to increase peripheral resistance and systemic blood pressure. [1]

If neurocardiogenic syncope recurs despite education and lifestyle changes, fludrocortisone (0.1 mg/day, starting dose) may be used to expand intravascular volume. Midodrine, an α_1-receptor agonist and vasoconstrictor (2.5 mg three times daily) and paroxetine, a selective serotonin re-uptake inhibitor (20 mg/day), have each been effective in randomized trials of neurocardiogenic syncope. [3] Randomized trials have shown mixed results with β-blockers (e.g., atenolol, metoprolol, and propranolol). A double-blind randomized trial of pacing therapy failed to show a reduction in recurrence in patients with vasovagal syncope. [4]

TABLE 427–2 CLINICAL FEATURES SUGGESTING SPECIFIC CAUSES

Symptom or Finding	Diagnostic Consideration
After sudden unexpected pain, fear, unpleasant sight, sound, or smell	Vasovagal
Prolonged motionless standing	Vasovagal
Well-trained athlete after exertion (without heart disease)	Vasovagal
During or immediately after micturition, cough, swallowing, or defecation	Situational syncope
Syncope with throat or facial pain (glossopharyngeal or trigeminal neuralgia)	Neurocardiogenic syncope with neuralgia
With head rotation, pressure on the carotid sinus (as in tumors, shaving, tight collars)	Carotid sinus syncope
Immediately on standing	Orthostatic hypotension
Medication that may lead to long QT syndrome, orthostasis, or bradycardia	Drug induced
Associated with headaches	Migraine, seizures
Associated with vertigo, dysarthria, diplopia	Transient ischemic attack, subclavian steal, basilar migraine
With arm exercise	Subclavian steal
Confusion after a spell or loss of consciousness for more than 5 minutes	Seizure
Differences in blood pressure or pulse in the two arms	Subclavian steal or aortic dissection
Syncope and murmur with changing position (from sitting to lying, bending, turning over in bed)	Atrial myxoma or thrombus
Syncope with exertion	Aortic stenosis, pulmonary hypertension, mitral stenosis, obstructive hypertrophic cardiomyopathy, coronary artery disease
Family history of sudden death	Long QT syndrome, Brugada's syndrome
Brief loss of consciousness, no prodrome, with heart disease	Arrhythmias
Frequent syncope, somatic complaints, no heart disease	Psychiatric illness

From Kapoor WN: Syncope. N Engl J Med 2000;343:1856–1862.

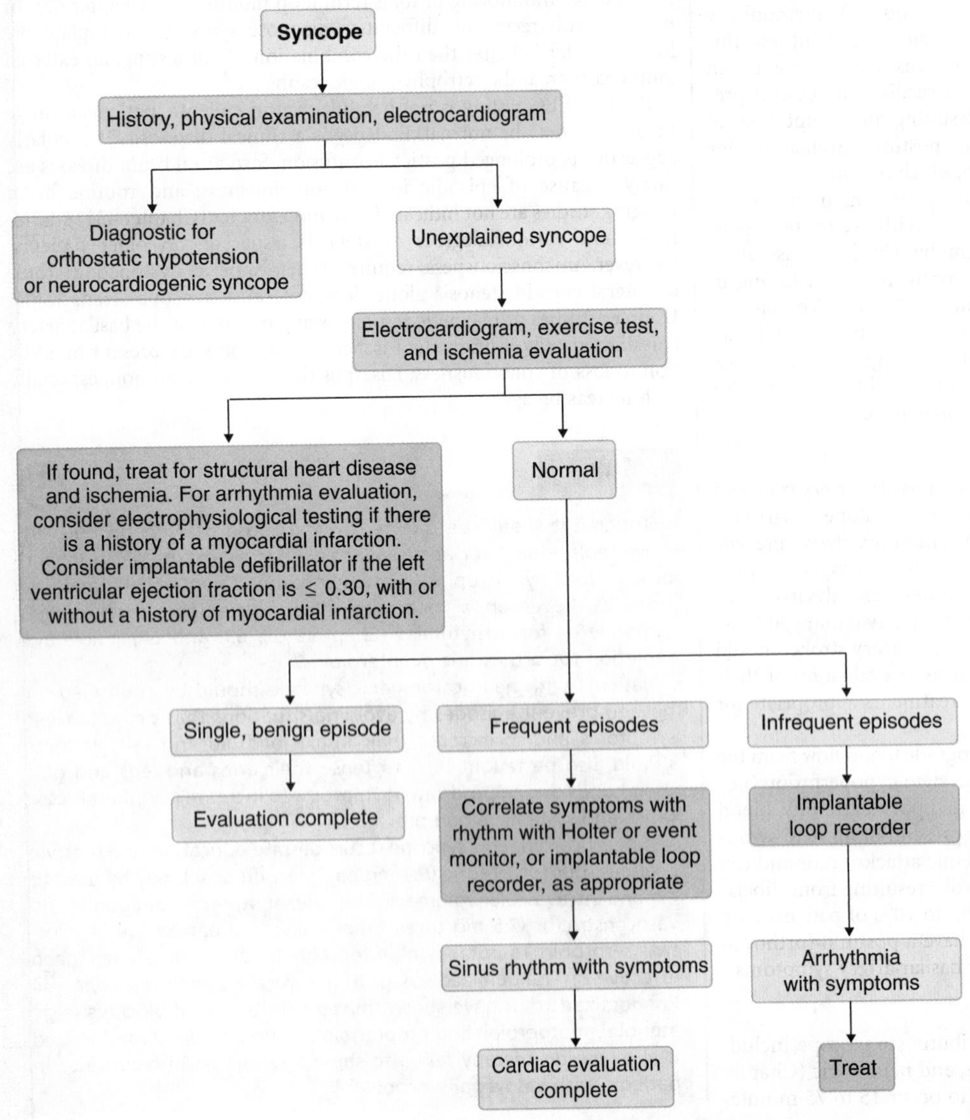

FIGURE 427–1 • Diagnostic approach to a patient with syncope. CT = computed tomography; ECG = electrocardiogram; EEG = electroencephalogram; EPS = electrophysiologic study; NSR = normal sinus rhythm. (Adapted from Linzer M, Yang EH, Ester NA, et al: Diagnosing syncope. Part 1. Value of history, physical examination, and electrocardiography. The Clinical Efficacy Assessment Project of the American College of Physicians. Ann Intern Med 1997;126:989–996; and Linzer M, Yang EH, Ester NA, et al: Diagnosing syncope. Part 2. Unexplained syncope. The Clinical Efficacy Assessment Project of the American College of Physicians. Ann Intern Med 1997;127:76–86. From Braunwald E, Goldman L [eds]: Primary Cardiology, 2nd ed. Philadelphia, Saunders, 2003.)

TABLE 427–3 DIAGNOSTIC CRITERIA FOR NEUROCARDIOGENIC SYNCOPE

Criteria	Points
Any one of bifascicular block, asystole, supraventricular tachycardia, diabetes	−5
Blue color noted by bystander	−4
Age at first syncope >35 years	−3
Remembers something about the spell	−2
Presyncope or syncope with prolonged sitting or standing	1
Sweating or warm feeling before a spell	2
Presyncope or syncope with pain or a medical procedure	3

Classify as neurocardiogenic syncope if points are ≥−2.
Reproduced from Sheldon R, Rose S, Connolly S, et al: Diagnostic criteria for vasovagal syncope based on a quantitative history. Eur Heart J 2006;27:344–350.

Prognosis

The occurrence of syncope predicts a substantial risk for recurrence of syncope. Patients with cardiac causes have higher mortality rates than do those with noncardiac causes or those without a definable cause. However, syncope does not itself increase the risk for death; mortality is associated with the underlying cardiac disease regardless of whether syncope has been a symptom.

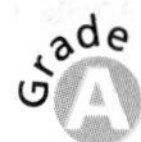

1. Krahn AD, Klein GJ, Yee R, et al: Randomized assessment of syncope trial: Conventional diagnostic testing versus a prolonged monitoring strategy. Circulation 2001;104:46–54.
2. van Dijk N, Quartieri F, Blanc JJ, et al: Effectiveness of physical counterpressure maneuvers in preventing vasovagal syncope: The Physical Counterpressure Manoeuvres Trial (PC-Trial). J Am Coll Cardiol 2006;48:1652–1657.
3. Di Girolamo E, Di Iorio C, Sabatini P, et al: Effects of paroxetine hydrochloride, a selective serotonin reuptake inhibitor, on refractory vasovagal syncope: A randomized, double-blind, placebo-controlled study. J Am Coll Cardiol 1999;33:1227–1230.
4. Connolly SJ, Sheldon R, Thorpe KE, et al: Pacemaker therapy for prevention of syncope in patients with recurrent severe vasovagal syncope: Second Vasovagal Pacemaker Study (VPS II): A randomized trial. JAMA 2003;289:2224–2229.

SUGGESTED READINGS

Grubb BP: Neurocardiogenic syncope. N Engl J Med 2005;352:1004–1010. *A useful, current overview.*

Strickberger SA, Benson DW, Biaggioni I, et al: AHA/ACCF scientific statement on the evaluation of syncope. Circulation 2006;113:316–327. *Comprehensive review.*

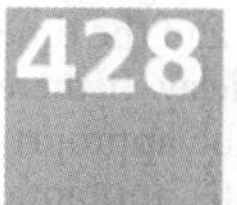

428 COMA AND DISORDERS OF AROUSAL

Roger P. Simon

COMA

Definition

Consciousness requires an intact and functioning brain stem reticular activating system and its cortical projections. The reticular formation begins in the midpons and ascends through the dorsal midbrain to synapse in the thalamus for its thalamocortical connections. Knowledge of this anatomic substrate provides the short list of regions to be investigated while searching for a structural cause of coma; a brain stem lesion or bihemispheric dysfunction must satisfy these anatomic requirements or it is not the cause of the patient's unconsciousness. In addition to structural lesions, the diffuse effects of meningeal inflammation (Chapter 437), metabolic encephalopathy, or seizure (Chapter 426) also satisfy the anatomic requirements and complete the differential diagnosis of a patient in coma.

Pathobiology

Meningeal Irritation

Meningeal irritation caused by infection (Chapter 437) or blood (Chapter 432) in the subarachnoid space is among the most important early considerations in the evaluation of coma because it is treatable and, especially with purulent meningitis, may not be diagnosed by brain imaging (Table 428–1). The mechanism by which inflammatory processes in the subarachnoid space result in unconsciousness is incompletely understood. Potential mechanisms include a combination of the release of humoral factors such as interleukin-1, tumor necrosis factor, and arachidonic acid metabolites (promoting blood-brain barrier permeability); progression of inflammation with the production of reactive oxygen species and nitric oxide; vasogenic cerebral edema; altered cerebral blood flow; and perhaps an increase in neurotoxic excitatory amino acid neurotransmitters. Later, vasculitis and thrombosis of meningeal veins may result in diffuse cortical and white matter necrosis.

Hemispheric Mass Lesions

Hemispheric mass lesions result in coma by expanding across the midline laterally to compromise both cerebral hemispheres or by impinging on the brain stem to compress the rostral reticular formation. These processes have been referred to as *lateral* or *uncal herniation* (i.e., lateral movement of the brain) and *transtentorial herniation* (i.e., vertical movement of hemispheric contents across the cerebellar tentorium, which separates the hemispheric compartment from the brain stem and posterior fossa). Although horizontal or vertical movement of the brain in isolation may produce coma, a combination of these processes is the most common cause. At the bedside, clinical signs of an expanding hemispheric mass evolve in a level-by-level, rostral-to-caudal manner (Fig. 428–1). Hemispheric lesions of adequate size to produce coma are readily seen on brain imaging.

Brain Stem Mass Lesions

Brain stem mass lesions produce coma by directly compromising the reticular formation. Because the pathways for lateral eye movements (i.e., pontine gaze center, medial longitudinal fasciculus, and oculomotor [third cranial nerve] nucleus) traverse the reticular activating system, impairment of reflex eye movements is often the critical element in clinical diagnosis. A comatose patient without impairment of reflex lateral eye movements does not have a mass lesion compromising brain stem structures in the posterior fossa. This aspect of the examination is therefore critical for rapid diagnosis because computed tomography (CT) is not able to detect some lesions in this region. Posterior fossa lesions may also compromise cortical function by upward herniation across the cerebellar tentorium or by blocking flow of cerebrospinal fluid from the lateral ventricles, thereby resulting in the dangerous state of noncommunicating hydrocephalus.

Metabolic Abnormalities

Metabolic abnormalities characterize syndromes caused by the presence of *exogenous toxins* (drugs) or *endogenous toxins* (organ system failure) and result in diffuse dysfunction of the nervous system without lateralized signs such as hemiparesis or unilateral pupillary dilation. A diagnosis of "metabolic encephalopathy" indicates that the examiner has found no focal anatomic features by examination or neuroimaging studies to explain coma but does not state that a specific metabolic cause has been established. Such global impairment of brain function is particularly typical of endogenous toxins (i.e., organ system failure). Drugs (i.e., exogenous toxins; Chapter 111) have a predilection for affecting the reticular formation in the brain stem and producing paralysis of reflex eye movement on examination.

TABLE 428–1 CAUSES OF COMA WITH NORMAL COMPUTED TOMOGRAPHIC SCAN RESULTS

MENINGEAL CAUSES
Subarachnoid hemorrhage (uncommon)
Bacterial meningitis
Encephalitis
Subdural empyema
EXOGENOUS TOXINS
Sedative drugs or barbiturates
Anesthetics or γ-hydroxybutyrate*
Alcohol
Stimulants
Phencyclidine†
Cocaine or amphetamine‡
Psychotropic drugs
Cyclic antidepressants
Phenothiazines
Lithium
Anticonvulsants
Opioids
Clonidine§
Penicillins
Salicylates
Anticholinergics
Carbon monoxide/cyanide/methemoglobinemia
ENDOGENOUS TOXINS, DEFICIENCIES, OR DERANGEMENTS
Hypoxia or ischemia
Hypoglycemia
Hypercalcemia
Osmolar
Hyperglycemia
Hyponatremia
Hypernatremia
Organ system failure
Hepatic encephalopathy
Uremic encephalopathy
Pulmonary insufficiency (CO_2 narcosis)
Seizures
Prolonged postictal state
Spike-wave stupor
Hypothermia or hyperthermia
Multifocal disorders manifested as metabolic coma
Disseminated intravascular coagulopathy
Sepsis
Pancreatitis
Vasculitis
Thrombotic thrombocytopenic purpura
Fat emboli
Hypertensive encephalopathy
Diffuse micrometastases
Brain stem ischemia
Basilar artery stroke
Brain stem or cerebellar hemorrhage
Conversion or malingering

*General anesthetic similar to γ-aminobutyric acid; recreational drug and bodybuilding aid characterized by rapid onset and rapid recovery, often with myoclonic jerking and confusion; deep coma (2 to 3 hours; Glasgow Coma Scale score = 3) with maintenance of vital signs.
†Coma associated with cholinergic signs: lacrimation, salivation, bronchorrhea, and hyperthermia.
‡Coma after seizures or status epilepticus (i.e., a prolonged postictal state).
§An antihypertensive agent active through the opiate receptor system; overdose common when used to treat narcotic withdrawal.

Seizures

Generalized seizures (Chapter 426) produce diffuse, abnormal electrical discharges throughout the reticular formation and cortex, thus satisfying the anatomic criteria for coma. In the late stages of status epilepticus, motor movements may be subtle even though seizure activity is continuing throughout the brain. After seizures stop, the abnormal electrical activity is followed by an inhibitory state, which may be prolonged. This so-called postictal state produces coma; if the inciting seizures are not witnessed, prior seizures can be a cause of unexplained coma.

Clinical Manifestations

Coma is a sleeplike state from which the patient cannot be aroused. It is sleeplike in that the eyes are closed and remain closed in the face of vigorous stimulation. A poorly responsive state in which the eyes are open, an agitated confused state, or delirium does not constitute coma but may represent early stages of the same disease processes causing coma and should be investigated in the same manner.

Diagnosis

History

The history, if obtainable, may be particularly helpful. A premonitory headache supports a diagnosis of meningitis, encephalitis, or intracerebral or subarachnoid hemorrhage. A preceding period of confusion or delirium points to a diffuse process such as meningitis or the effects of endogenous or exogenous toxins. A sudden apoplectic onset of coma is particularly suggestive of ischemic or hemorrhagic stroke affecting the brain stem or subarachnoid hemorrhage or intracerebral hemorrhage with intraventricular rupture. Lateralized symptoms of hemiparesis or aphasia before coma occur with hemispheric masses.

Physical Examination

The physical examination is critical, accomplished quickly, and diagnostic. Three issues must be addressed. Does the patient have meningitis? Are there signs of a mass lesion? Is this a diffuse syndrome of exogenous or endogenous metabolic cause?

Identify Meningitis

Though not invariably present and having varying sensitivity with regard to cause (i.e., very common with acute pyogenic meningitis [Chapter 437] and subarachnoid hemorrhage [Chapter 432], less common with indolent, fungal meningitis), the presence of signs of meningeal irritation on examination is the central clue to the diagnosis. Missing these signs results in time-consuming additional tests such as brain imaging and risks the loss of a narrow therapeutic window of opportunity. Passive neck flexion should be carried out in all comatose patients unless head and neck trauma is likely to have occurred. When the neck is passively flexed in an attempt to bring the chin within a few fingerbreadths of the chest, patients with irritated meninges reflexively flex one or both knees. This sign, Brudzinski's reflex, is usually asymmetrical and not dramatic, but any evidence of knee flexion during passive neck flexion requires that the spinal fluid be examined.

In the absence of lateralized signs (e.g., hemiparesis) indicating a superimposed mass lesion, a spinal puncture should be performed immediately. Although rare cases of herniation have been reported after lumbar puncture in children with bacterial meningitis, the urgency of diagnosis and treatment at the point of coma is paramount, and the time required for brain imaging may cause a fatal therapeutic delay. If there are lateralized, focal signs suggesting a mass lesion, it may be appropriate to obtain blood for culture and immediately initiate antibiotic therapy, perform either a CT scan or magnetic resonance imaging [MRI], and then perform a lumbar puncture if there is no evidence of a mass lesion. Cerebrospinal fluid cell count, glucose level, and protein content are unchanged, and Gram stain and culture often produce positive findings despite a short period of antibiotic treatment. The presence of bacterial antigens in cerebrospinal fluid or blood can also be determined.

Separate Structural from Metabolic Causes of Coma

Structural and metabolic causes of coma can be distinguished by neurologic examination. Because the evaluation and potential treatment modalities for structural versus metabolic coma are widely divergent and

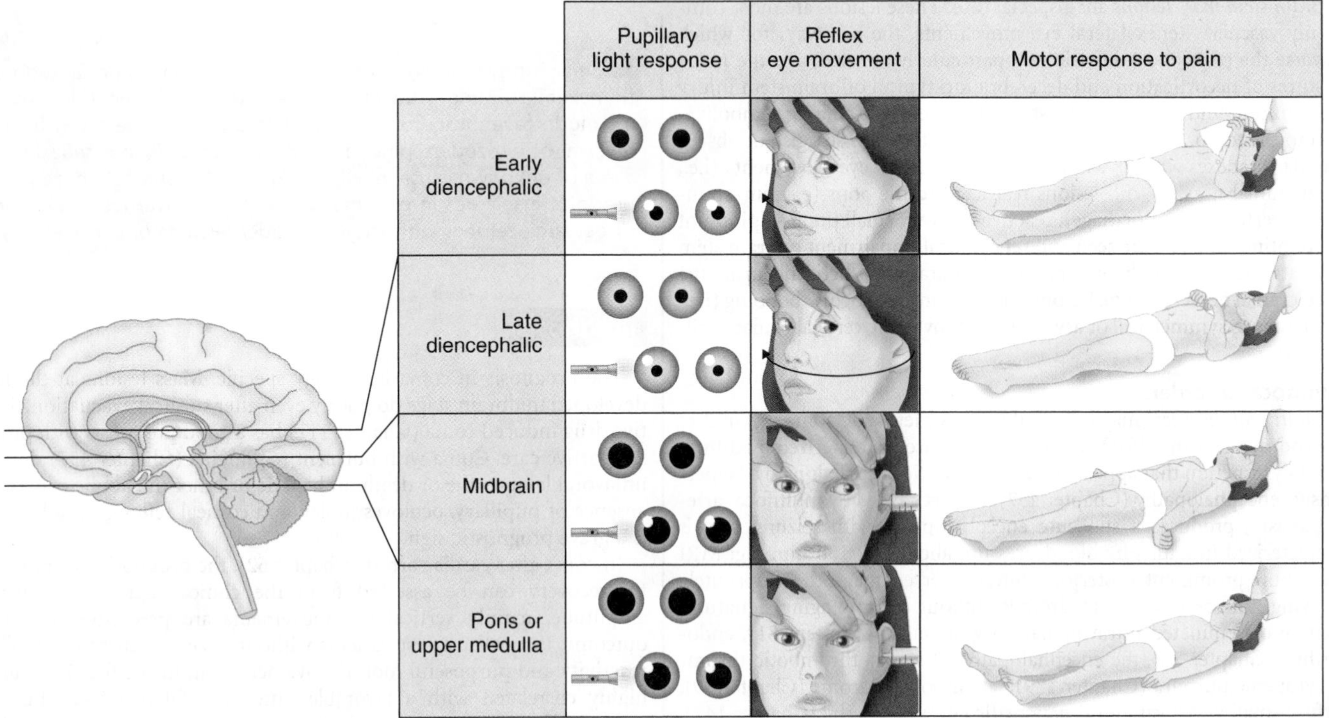

FIGURE 428–1 • Evolution of neurologic signs in coma from a hemispheric mass lesion as the brain becomes functionally impaired in a rostral caudal manner. Early and late diencephalic levels are levels of dysfunction just above (early) and just below (late) the thalamus. (From Aminoff MJ, Greenberg DA, Simon RP: Clinical Neurology, 3rd ed. Norwalk, CT, Appleton & Lange, 1996.)

the disease processes in both are often rapidly progressive, initiating the evaluation in a medical or surgical direction may be life-saving. This task is accomplished by focusing on three features of the neurologic examination: the motor response to a painful stimulus, pupillary function, and reflex eye movements.

Functioning of the motor system provides the clearest indication of a mass lesion. Elicitation of a motor response requires the application of a painful stimulus to which the patient will react. The arms should be placed in a semiflexed posture and a painful stimulus applied to the head or trunk. Strong pressure on the supraorbital ridge or pinching of skin on the anterior aspect of the chest or inner part of the arm is useful; nail bed pressure makes the interpretation of upper limb movement difficult.

The neurologic signs from an expanding hemispheric mass lesion evolve in stages (see Fig. 428–1), and asymmetry of such signs strongly supports a mass lesion as the cause. However, these motor movements, especially early in coma, are most frequently fragments of abnormal, asymmetrical flexion and extension in the arms rather than complete decorticate and decerebrate postures. A small amount of asymmetrical flexion or extension of an arm in response to a painful stimulus carries the same implications as the full-blown postures. Hemispheric masses at their early stage (early diencephalic, i.e., compromising the brain above the thalamus) produce appropriate movement of one upper extremity toward the painful stimulus. Any asymmetrical impairment in contralateral arm movement reflects a hemiparesis. Such lateralized motor movement in a comatose patient establishes the working diagnosis of a hemispheric mass. As the mass expands to involve the thalamus (i.e., late diencephalic), the response to pain is reflex arm flexion associated with extension and internal rotation of the legs (i.e., decorticate posturing); asymmetry of the response in the upper extremities is seen. With further rostral-caudal compromise at the midbrain level, the reflex posturing changes in the arms such that both arms and legs respond by extension (i.e., decerebrate posturing); at the midbrain level, the asymmetry in motor function tends to be lost. With further compromise at the level of the pons, the most frequent finding is no response to painful stimulation, although spinal-mediated movements of leg flexion may occur.

Metabolic lesions do not compromise the brain in a progressive, level-by-level, rostral-to-caudal manner as hemispheric masses do and rarely produce the asymmetrical motor signs typical of masses. Reflex posturing may be seen (e.g., hepatic encephalopathy), but it lacks the asymmetry of decortication from a hemispheric mass and is not associated with the loss of pupillary reactivity at the stage of decerebration.

Pupillary Reactivity

Functioning of the pupils reflects the structural integrity of the midbrain. If the pupils constrict to a bright light, the midbrain is intact, whereas if they do not, the midbrain has been compromised. In cases of mass lesions, the loss of pupillary reactivity from a hemispheric mass is asymmetrical, with the pupil homolateral to the mass losing reactivity before its contralateral fellow. A midbrain pupil may be large and unreactive if sympathetic pathways in the brain stem have not been compromised but is more commonly found at midposition (5 mm) because of parasympathetic (third cranial nerve) and sympathetic (brain stem) injury.

In metabolic coma, one feature is central to the examination: pupillary reactivity. Such reactivity is seen both early in coma, when an appropriate motor response to pain may be retained, and late in coma, when no motor responses can be elicited. The reaction is lost only when coma is so deep that the patient requires ventilatory and blood pressure support.

Reflex Eye Movements

The presence of inducible lateral eye movements reflects the integrity of the pons (i.e., vestibular nucleus, pontine gaze center, and sixth cranial nerve moving the eye laterally). The medial longitudinal fasciculus traverses the dorsal pons to connect with the third cranial nerve (i.e., moving the eye medially). This system may first be compromised at the midbrain level, with loss of medial eye movement in the eye homolateral to a mass, but it becomes clearly impaired by pontine dysfunction when no eye movements are inducible. These *reflex eye movements* (see Fig. 428–1) are brought about by passive head rotation to stimulate the semicircular canal input to the vestibular system (i.e., doll's-eyes maneuver) or by inhibition of the function of one semicircular canal by infusion of ice water against the tympanic membrane (i.e., caloric testing).

In *metabolic coma,* reflex eye movements may be lost or retained. Lack of inducible eye movement with the doll's-eyes maneuver in the setting of preserved pupillary reactivity is virtually diagnostic of coma induced by drug toxicity. Caloric testing is not useful in drug-induced coma because it may produce any of the following: delayed downward ocular deviation, ipsilateral adduction with incomplete contralateral abduction, ipsilateral abduction with contralateral adduction, or no response. With metabolic coma of non–drug-induced origin, such as organ system failure or electrolytic or osmolar disorders, full reflex eye movements are preserved.

Brain stem mass lesions are a special case. These lesions are most commonly vascular. Reflex lateral eye movements, the pathways for which traverse the pons and midbrain, are particularly affected, and the reflex postures of decortication and decerebration typical of brain stem injury are common findings. Lesions restricted to the midbrain (e.g., embolization to the top of the basilar artery) are manifested as sluggish or absent pupillary reflexes with or without impaired medial eye movements (i.e., third cranial nerve). With lesions restricted to the pons (e.g., intrapontine hypertensive hemorrhage), reactive but very small pupils—pinpoint or "pontine" pupils—are seen and reflect focal impairment of brain stem sympathetic fibers with preservation of parasympathetic fibers in the third cranial nerve. Pontine lesions may also produce ocular bobbing (i.e., spontaneous symmetrical or asymmetrical rhythmic vertical ocular oscillations).

Multifocal Disorders

Multifocal disorders may be manifested as metabolic coma. A number of syndromes of multifocal vascular disease are characterized by diffuse brain dysfunction that appears to be a metabolic encephalopathy. Hypertensive encephalopathy (Chapter 432), in part caused by multifocal arterial spasm, produces a subacute encephalopathy with seizures and is characterized in adults by blood pressure above 250/150 mm Hg; MRI may show prominent posterior white matter edema. Other subacutely evolving, diffuse vascular syndromes without neuroimaging signatures include disseminated intravascular coagulopathy (Chapter 181), endocarditis (Chapter 76), the encephalopathy of sepsis, thrombotic thrombocytopenic purpura (Chapter 179), fat emboli syndrome (Chapter 99), diffuse small vessel vasculitis, pancreatic encephalopathy (Chapter 147), and venous thrombosis, particularly affecting the superior sagittal sinus.

Consider Seizures

The diagnosis of a seizure is usually obvious from the history or observation. The return to an agitated confusional state and then consciousness over a period of a few minutes solves any diagnostic problem (Chapter 426). However, a prolonged alteration in consciousness after an unwitnessed seizure may produce diagnostic confusion. Such prolonged postictal states follow seizures that affect an acutely or chronically impaired brain, such as in patients with dementia, mental retardation, encephalitis, multifocal vascular disease (e.g., hypertensive encephalopathy), acute metabolic impairment of brain function (e.g., hyponatremia, hypernatremia, hypoglycemia, or hyperglycemia), or drug toxicity. In a postictal state, the examination can detect reactive pupils and inducible eye movements (in the absence of overtreatment with anticonvulsants) and may detect up-going toes; if the onset of the seizure was in a focal motor area of the cortex, there may be a prolonged hemiparesis (i.e., Todd's paresis). Nonconvulsive seizures, particularly spike-wave stupor, may occur in a patient without a history of epilepsy. The diagnosis is made by electroencephalography.

Treatment

Rx

General Measures

Emergency management of a patient with a decreased level of consciousness includes ensuring airway adequacy and support of ventilation and circulation. Blood should be drawn for determination of serum glucose and electrolyte levels, hepatic and renal function, prothrombin and partial thromboplastin times, complete blood cell count, and drug screen. Intravenous administration of 25 g of dextrose (typically 50 mL of 50% dextrose) should be routine to treat possible hypoglycemic coma. The glucose level is poorly correlated with the level of consciousness in patients with hypoglycemia, with coma, stupor, and confusion reported with blood glucose concentrations of 2 to 28, 8 to 59, and 9 to 60 mg/dL, respectively. Because administration of dextrose alone can precipitate or worsen Wernicke's encephalopathy in thiamine-deficient patients, 100 mg of thiamine should be given intravenously.

Specific Measures

Specific treatments are aimed at the cause of the coma. Mild therapeutic hypothermia improves short-term neurologic recovery and survival in patients who are comatose after a cardiac arrest.  Possible opiate overdose should be treated with naloxone (0.4 to 1.2 mg intravenously). The specific benzodiazepine antagonist flumazenil (0.2 mg intravenously, repeated once and followed by 0.1 mg intravenously to a total of 1 to 3 mg) can be given for the reversal of benzodiazepine-induced coma or conscious sedation. In coma of unknown cause, however, administration of flumazenil can precipitate seizures in patients with polydrug overdoses consisting of benzodiazepines with tricyclic antidepressants or cocaine.

Rx

Prognosis

The prognosis in coma is etiology specific. Mass lesions at the fully developed midbrain stage do poorly even after surgical evacuation. Sedative drug induced coma (Chapter 111) has a good prognosis with proper supportive care. Coma with purulent meningitis (Chapter 437) doubles unfavorable outcome or death. In hepatic or other metabolic comas, the absence of pupillary, oculovestibular, and corneal reflexes on admission is a grave prognostic sign.

In coma after cardiac arrest (Chapter 62), the prognosis for meaningful recovery can be assessed from the clinical signs. Brisk, small-amplitude, mainly vertical eye movements are predictive of a fatal outcome. In cardiac arrest patients without seizures, return of pupillary reactivity and purposeful motor movements within the first 72 hours is highly correlated with a favorable outcome (Table 428–2). Bilateral absence of somatosensory evoked responses in the first week predicts death or a persistent vegetative state.

After traumatic head injury (Chapter 422), young patients (<20 years) are more than three times as likely to survive as those older than 60 years. On examination at 24 hours, an absent motor response to pain combined with an absent pupillary response is a strong predictor of mortality, whereas localization of a painful stimulus with preserved pupillary reactivity is a highly favorable finding, especially in the young (Fig. 428–2). Unexpected late recoveries do occur.

COMA-LIKE STATES

Coma-like states include the locked-in syndrome and psychogenic unresponsiveness, as well as the persistent vegetative state, minimally conscious state, and brain death.

TABLE 428–2 PROBABILITY (%) OF RECOVERING INDEPENDENT FUNCTION FROM COMA AFTER CARDIAC ARREST

	Days after Cardiac Arrest			
Sign	**0**	**1**	**3**	**7**
From Levy et al. (*N* = 210)				
No verbal response	13	8	5	6
No eye opening	11	6	4	0
Unreactive pupils	0	0	0	0
No spontaneous eye movements	6	5	2	0
No caloric response	5	6	6	0
Extensor posturing	18	0	0	0
Flexor posturing	14	3	0	0
No motor response	4	3	0	0
From Edgren et al. (*N* = 131)				
No eye opening to pain	31	8	0	0
Absent or reflex motor response	25	9	0	0
Unreactive pupils	17	7	0	0

Data from Levy DE, Caronna J, Singer BH, et al: Predicting outcome from hypoxic-ischemic coma. JAMA 1985;253:1420–1426. Copyright © 1985, American Medical Association. Data from Edgren E, Hedstrand U, Kelsey S, et al: Assessment of neurological prognosis in comatose survivors of cardiac arrest. BRCT I Study Group. Lancet 1994;343:1055–1059. Copyright © by The Lancet Ltd., 1994.

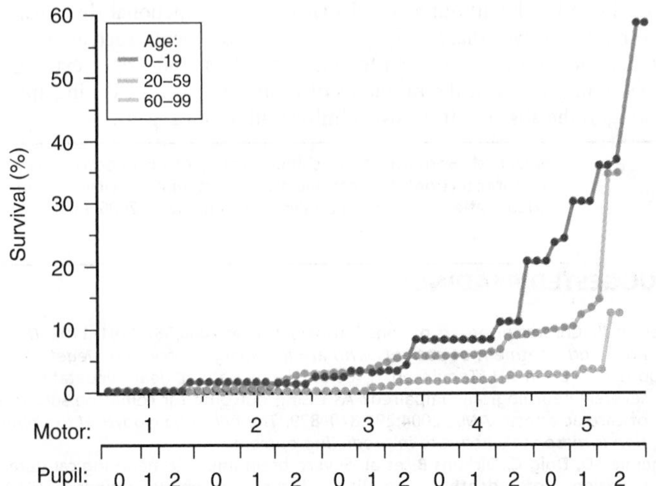

FIGURE 428–2 • Survival after traumatic coma based on age and clinical examination results at 24 hours. Motor: no response (1), reflex extension (2), reflex flexion (3), complex flexion (4), localization of pain (5). Pupils: no reactivity (0), unilateral reactivity (1), bilateral reactivity (2). (From Mamelak AN, Pitts LH, Damron S: Predicting survival from head injury 24 hours after injury: A practical method with therapeutic implications. J Trauma 1996;41:91–99.)

Locked-in Syndrome

Patients with locked-in syndrome are those in whom a lesion, usually hemorrhage or an infarct, transects the brain stem at a point below the reticular formation (therefore sparing consciousness) but above the ventilatory nuclei of the medulla (therefore precluding death). Such patients are awake, with eye opening and sleep-wake cycles, but the descending pathways through the brain stem necessary for volitional vocalization or limb movement have been transected. Voluntary eye movement, especially vertical, is preserved, and patients open and close their eyes or produce appropriate numbers of blinking movements in answer to questions. The electroencephalogram is usually normal because of normal cortical function. The mortality rate is high (40 to 70%), and most patients who recover are left with major deficits. Recovery to independence can occur, however, over a period of weeks to 3 to 4 months. Early recovery of lateral eye movements has been suggested as a particularly positive prognostic feature. Magnetic stimulation of the motor cortex to produce motor evoked potentials may be an additional positive prognostic feature. Survival in the locked-in state has lasted as long as 18 years.

Psychogenic Unresponsiveness

Psychogenic unresponsiveness is a diagnosis of exclusion. The neurologic examination shows reactive pupils and no reflex posturing to pain. Eye movements during the doll's-eyes maneuver demonstrate volitional override rather than the smooth, uninhibited, reflex lateral eye movements of coma. Ice water caloric testing arouses the patient because of the discomfort produced or induces cortically mediated nystagmus rather than the tonic deviation typical of coma. The slow, conjugate, roving eye movements of metabolic coma cannot be imitated and therefore exclude psychogenic unresponsiveness. The slow, often asymmetrical and incomplete eye closure that follows passive eyelid opening of a comatose patient cannot be feigned. These signs therefore exclude psychogenic coma. Conscious patients usually exhibit some voluntary muscle tone in the eyelids during passive eye opening. The electroencephalographic finding in patients with psychogenic unresponsiveness is normal wakefulness with reactive posterior rhythms on eye opening and eye closing.

Persistent Vegetative State

Whereas coma represents a state lacking wakefulness and awareness, patients in a vegetative state have awakened from coma but have not regained awareness. Wakefulness is manifested by eye opening and sleep-wake cycles.

Pathobiology

The neuroanatomic characteristics of the vegetative state dictate that the reticular activating system of the brain stem be intact to produce wakefulness but that the connections to the cortical mantle be interrupted, thereby precluding awareness. These anatomic requirements for a vegetative state are satisfied most commonly by diffuse axonal injury, laminar necrosis of the cortical mantle, or thalamic necrosis. Such pathologic alterations occur as the sequelae of a number of acute or chronic conditions affecting the brain.

Common causes include trauma (Chapter 422) with resultant diffuse axonal injury, hypoxia-ischemia secondary to cerebral hypoperfusion from cardiac arrest (Chapter 62) with ensuing death of the selectively vulnerable neurons in the cortical mantle (i.e., laminar necrosis), bihemispheric infarctions (Chapter 431), cortical injury after purulent meningitis (Chapter 437) or encephalitis (Chapter 439), exposure to nervous system toxins (particularly carbon monoxide; (Chapter 111), and prolonged hypoglycemia (Chapter 249). The sequelae of cerebral hypoperfusion may in particular affect the hemispheric watershed areas and the thalamus. A vegetative state usually evolves from coma but can develop as the end stage of neurodegenerative diseases in adults or children or accompany severe developmental abnormalities of the brain such as anencephaly.

Clinical Manifestations

Clinically, patients in a persistent vegetative state have signs associated with an intact reticular formation: they open their eyes and have sleep-wake cycles, although the cycles are irregular in timing. Their brain stem reflexes are intact: pupils react, and eye movements occur spontaneously and with the doll's-eyes maneuver. More complex brain stem reflexes are also seen, such as yawning, chewing, swallowing, and uncommonly, making guttural vocalizations. The brain stem reflexes of arousal and startle are preserved as well, so eye opening occurs with loud sounds and blinking may occur with bright lights. Tearing may be seen. Spontaneous roving eye movements, which are particularly characteristic, involve very slow movements of constant velocity, are uninterrupted by saccadic jerks, and cannot be volitionally mimicked. These eye movements can be particularly distressing to family members because the patient appears to be looking about the room and, at some point, the roving eyes are pointed at the observer, who may perceive the patient to be "looking at" or following him or her throughout the room. The lack of quick directed saccadic eye movements in the presence of continual fixed-velocity roving eye movements differentiates a willed response from reflex eye movements. The brain stem origin of the eye movements is further documented by their being readily redirected by the oculocephalic (doll's-eyes) reflex. The limbs may move, but motor responses are only primitively purposeful, such as grasping an object that contacts the hand. Pain usually produces decorticate or decerebrate postures or fragments of these movements.

Diagnosis

CT and MRI depict the sequelae of the causative injury but are not diagnostic of a persistent vegetative state. Magnetic resonance spectroscopy shows a decrease in the neuronal marker *N*-acetylaspartate. Positron emission tomography shows decreased cerebral blood flow and use of glucose, but such results are rarely diagnostic.

A vegetative state is diagnosed after 1 month in a patient without detectable awareness of the environment. A vegetative state is called persistent after 3 months if the brain injury was medical and after 12 months if it was traumatic. The determination that *persistent* equals *permanent* cannot be stated absolutely; prediction of which patients will become persistently vegetative early in the vegetative state is particularly difficult in cases of trauma. Lesions of the corpus callosum and dorsolateral brain stem seen on MRI between 6 and 8 weeks after trauma correlate with persistence of the vegetative state at 1 year.

Prognosis

Rare patients show late improvement, but none regain normal function. Partial recovery to the level of communication and comprehension has been reported in 3% of patients after 5 years, but improvement to independence in activities of daily living is even more uncommon. Although lack of awareness defines the vegetative state, patients may recover slightly beyond this criterion. Such minimally responsive patients present difficult ethical considerations for care.

Brain Death

Irreversible cessation of cardiopulmonary function precludes function of the brain. The opposite is true as well. Death of the organism can therefore be determined on the basis of death of the brain. Although some details may be dictated by local law, the standard criteria for the diagnosis of brain death in the United States are those established by the President's Commission report in 1981. This standard permits a diagnosis of brain death on documentation of irreversible cessation of all brain function, including those of the brain stem; the presence of seizures is not compatible with the diagnosis.

Diagnosis

The absence of hemispheric function is documented by unreceptivity and unresponsiveness, usually assessed in the setting of painful stimulation; the patient does not rouse, groan, grimace, or withdraw limbs. Purely spinal reflexes may be maintained: deep tendon reflexes, plantar flexion reflex, plantar withdrawal, and tonic neck reflexes. Decorticate or decerebrate posturing is not compatible with the diagnosis. Absence of brain stem function is assessed by region. Lack of midbrain function is documented by the absence of a pupillary light reflex (most easily assessed by viewing the bright light of an ophthalmoscope through its magnifying lens when focused on the iris). Unreactive pupils may be at midposition (as they will be in death) or dilated, as they often are in the setting of a dopamine infusion. Lack of pontine function is documented by the absence of a response to corneal stimulation and the absence of inducible eye movements: no eye movement toward the side of irrigation of the tympanic membrane with 50 mL of ice water. The oculocephalic response (doll's eyes) is always absent in the setting of absent oculovestibular testing. Cessation of medullary function is documented by the apnea test: no ventilatory movements in the setting of maximum CO_2 stimulation. The test is performed by disconnecting the ventilator from the endotracheal tube. Oxygen can be supplied by diffusion from a cannula placed through the endotracheal tube (6 L/min). In the absence of ventilation, P_{CO_2} passively rises 2 to 3 mm Hg/min. Because a P_{CO_2} of 60 mm Hg produces the maximum ventilatory stimulus required for the confirmation of apnea, a period of about 10 minutes is required for the P_{CO_2} to reach that level from a normal baseline. A Pa_{CO_2} greater than 60 mm Hg adequately stimulates the ventilatory drive within 60 seconds in a functioning brain.

Documentation of irreversibility requires that the cause of the coma be known and that it be adequate to explain the clinical findings of brain death. Irreversibility based on clinical criteria cannot be determined in the setting of sedative drugs or hypothermia (<32.2° C) or in the presence of shock or neuromuscular blockade.

Confirmatory tests may be useful. An isoelectric electroencephalogram is frequently used. However, deep coma from sedative drugs or hypothermia below 20° C can produce electroencephalographic flattening. Patients clinically brain dead may have residual electroencephalographic activity (i.e., alpha coma-like activity, low-voltage fast waves, or sleeplike slowing with spindle activity), which may persist for a number of days after a brain death diagnosis. The absence of cerebral blood flow is the most definitive confirmatory test and is most unequivocally demonstrated by angiography. Transcranial Doppler techniques and nuclear imaging with technetium are used in some centers.

Sequential testing is necessary for a clinical diagnosis of brain death. The period of observation required is at least 6 hours in all cases and at least 24 hours in the setting of anoxic-ischemic brain injury.

Prognosis

With the confirmation of brain death, asystole usually occurs within days (mean, 4 days), even if ventilatory support is continued. Recovery after appropriate documentation of brain death has never been reported. Removal of the ventilator results in terminal rhythms, most often complete heart block without a ventricular response, junctional rhythms, or ventricular tachycardia. Purely spinal motor movements, such as arching of the back, neck turning, stiffening of the legs, and upper extremity flexion, may occur in the moments of terminal apnea (or during apnea testing in the absence of passive administration of oxygen).

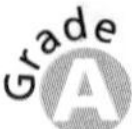

1. Holzer M, Bernard SA, Hachimi-Idrissi S, et al: Hypothermia for neuroprotection after cardiac arrest: Systematic review and individual patient data meta-analysis. Crit Care Med 2005;33:414–418.

SUGGESTED READINGS

Bernat JL: Chronic disorders of consciousness. Lancet 2006;367:1181–1192. *Diagnosis and treatment of patients who are minimally conscious or vegetative.*

Booth CM, Boon RH, Tomlinson G, et al: Is this patient dead, vegetative, or severely neurologically impaired? Assessing outcome for comatose survivors of cardiac arrest. JAMA 2004;291:870–879. *The neurologic physical examination is reasonably accurate in predicting outcome.*

Shemie SD, Doig C, Dickens B, et al: Severe brain injury to neurological determination of death: Canadian forum recommendations. CMAJ 2006;174:S1–S13. *Consensus recommendations.*

Stevens RD, Bhardwaj A: Approach to the comatose patient. Crit Care Med 2006;34:31–41. *Comprehensive review.*

Wood KE, Becker BN, McCartney JG, et al: Care of the potential organ donor. N Engl J Med 2004;351:2730–2739. *Attention to brain death issues in the setting of organ donation.*

429 DISORDERS OF SLEEP

Mark W. Mahowald

Definition

Wake/sleep complaints are second only to complaints of pain as the reason that patients seek medical attention. Undiagnosed and untreated wake/sleep complaints extract an enormous toll at the personal level in terms of misery and at the societal level in socioeconomic consequences. Knowledge of sleep and its disorders has rapidly expanded over the past half century, particularly with the discovery that sleep is far more than the passive absence of wakefulness. Sleep is an active brain process that includes two divergent states: non–rapid eye movement (NREM) and rapid eye movement (REM) sleep. A complex array of neurotransmitters, neuropeptides, and circulating humoral sleep-promoting factors interact with multiple areas of the central nervous system to determine wakefulness, REM sleep, and NREM sleep.

Pathobiology

Wakefulness is controlled by the reticular activating system of the rostral brain stem, which projects to the thalamus and cortex. Inhibition of these projections, which is modulated by neurons in the pons and midbrain, results in sleep. REM sleep, during which most dreaming occurs, is generated within the tegmentum of the pons with modulation from the norepinephrine- and serotonin-containing neurons of the locus ceruleus and the dorsal raphe nucleus. Electrical events generated in the pontine reticular formation (i.e., ponto-geniculo-occipital [PGO] waves) are propagated through the oculomotor and visual system during REM sleep simultaneously with rapid eye movements. PGO waves are suppressed by norepinephrine, and serotonin neuronal systems suppress PGO waves and REM; cholinergic neurons are stimulatory. PGO input can induce an action potential in neurons below their usual threshold. Such PGO-facilitated activity in the visual system may play a role in the random imagery of dreaming.

Hypocretins (orexins) are sleep modulatory neuropeptides made in the lateral hypothalamus with projections to the locus ceruleus and dorsal raphe, as well as to the thalamus, where they modulate the release of excitatory (glutamate) and inhibitory (γ-aminobutyric acid) neurotransmitters. Disruption of this system induces narcolepsy in animals, and hypocretin neurotransmission is deficient in most narcoleptic patients.

TABLE 429–1 STAGES OF SLEEP

Sleep Stage	EEG	Eye Movements	EMG Activity	Imagery
Wakefulness	Alpha and beta activity (low voltage fast)	Random, rapid	Active, spontaneous	Vivid, external
Non-REM sleep (NREM)				
Stage I (drowsiness)	Theta activity	Slow, rolling	Attenuated, episodic	Dulled
Stage II (light sleep)	Sleep spindles, K complexes	Slow or absent	Attenuated	Nonvivid
Stage III and IV (slow wave sleep)	Delta activity	Absent	Attenuated	
REM sleep	Low amplitude, irregular	Abrupt, rapid eye movements	Absent	Vivid, bizarre

EEG = electroencephalogram; EMG = electromyogram; REM = rapid eye movement.

Stage of Sleep

Sleep stages in humans are defined electroencephalographically and behaviorally (Table 429–1). Sleep includes NREM and REM sleep. NREM sleep can be divided into four stages. In *stage I NREM* sleep, patients are drowsy and may maintain some environmental awareness. The electroencephalogram (EEG) loses its alpha rhythm (8 to 13 Hz) and develops theta (3 to 7 Hz) activity; vertex potentials (i.e., negative deflections recorded from the midline) occur, especially in response to sensory stimuli. Slow lateral eye movements occur, and spontaneous motor activity, as monitored by electromyography (EMG), is diminished. Stage I represents about 5% of normal sleep.

Stage II NREM sleep is characterized by sleep spindles (12 to 14 Hz), vertex sharp waves, and K complexes (i.e., biphasic, high-voltage slow waves often followed by sleep spindles). Slow lateral eye movements may persist. EMG activity is further reduced. Stage II NREM sleep represents 50 to 60% of sleep and increases with age.

Stages III and IV NREM sleep are characterized by slow or delta waves (<4 Hz) and are therefore called delta sleep or deep sleep. If 20 to 50% of the EEG is delta activity, the patient is in stage III sleep; if delta activity is 50% or more, the sleep event is called stage IV. Deep sleep constitutes 10 to 20% of sleep time (less with advancing age). EMG activity is diminished. Eye movements are not seen, and ventilation is regular.

In REM sleep, the EEG resembles that of waking, with low-voltage, mixed frequencies. Abrupt rapid eye movements and irregular ventilation and heart rate are present. Penile tumescence occurs, and muscle tone is depressed because of suppression of activity in all somatic muscles except the diaphragm. REM sleep occupies 20 to 25% of sleep time. Dreaming occurs during all stages of NREM sleep and during REM sleep.

There is some evidence that procedural (i.e., motor learning such as typing) and declarative (i.e., episodic learning such as recalling places or events) memory consolidation occurs during REM sleep. REM sleep time increases after task training. After episodic learning, memory consolidation is accomplished during slow wave sleep by rapid reactivation of the hippocampal neurons previously activated by the place or event to be remembered. Alternatively, it has been hypothesized that dream sleep functions as a random stimulator of the cortex to remove weak memories and thus permit only stronger memories to be retained.

Clinical Manifestations

Most sleep complaints fall into four categories: hypersomnia (excessive daytime sleepiness), insomnia (trouble falling or staying asleep), circadian rhythm (biologic clock) disorders, and parasomnias (complex behavior arising during the sleep period).

Hypersomnia is typically manifested as the tendency to fall asleep in inappropriate or undesirable settings such as at work, while talking with others, or while driving. Sleepiness from any cause can result in impaired sustained attention, with adverse, occasionally disastrous socioeconomic consequences in the classroom, in the workplace, or on the highways. The most common cause of hypersomnia is volitional sleep deprivation for social or economic reasons. Volitional sleep deprivation can usually be diagnosed by the history or sleep diary. Nonvolitional sleep deprivation–related sleepiness is almost always due to an underlying sleep disorder, most commonly either obstructive sleep apnea or narcolepsy (Table 429–2).

TABLE 429–2 CAUSES OF HYPERSOMNIA (EXCESSIVE DAYTIME SLEEPINESS*)

Sleep deprivation
Obstructive sleep apnea (see Chapter 101)
Narcolepsy
Circadian rhythm disorders
Shift work sleep disorder
Jet lag
Advanced and delayed sleep phase syndrome
Restless legs syndrome (may be associated with extreme daytime sleepiness but is always manifested as insomnia)
Drug use
Syndromes associated with subjective sleepiness but usually without true, verifiable sleepiness by objective testing
Depression
Chronic pain
Insomnia

*Excessive daytime sleepiness is usually confirmed by objective testing.

Diagnosis

Subjective

Sleep Diaries and Sleepiness Scales

Sleep diaries kept for a period of 2 or 3 weeks may reveal valuable information about a patient's subjective perception of wakefulness and sleep. One useful scale is the Epworth Sleepiness Scale (Table 429–3), which is frequently used as a screening tool for identifying excessive daytime sleepiness and generally correlates with other measures of sleep propensity. A score higher than 11 suggests a high probability of a sleep problem. This scale may be limited by its lack of sensitivity in that there may be a striking discrepancy between self-perceived sleepiness and the physiologic sleepiness that can be documented by formal sleep studies.

Objective

Polysomnography

Polysomnography (Chapter 101) determines states of sleep and wakefulness by recording eye movements, submental EMG, and the EEG. If sleep-disordered breathing is suspected, additional monitoring such as oral/nasal airflow, chest/abdominal movement, hemoglobin oxygen saturation, and transcutaneous or end-tidal CO_2 is used.

Multiple Sleep Latency Test

The multiple sleep latency test, which assesses the tendency to fall asleep during normal waking hours, consists of five 20-minute nap opportunities at 2-hour intervals. An all-night polysomnograph is generally performed the night before to determine the quality and quantity of the preceding night's sleep. Normal, fully rested adults do not usually fall asleep in less than 10 minutes and uncommonly display REM sleep during daytime naps. Patients with narcolepsy typically fall asleep in 5 minutes or less and often display REM sleep on at least two of the daytime naps. This test is not generally performed in the setting of obstructive

TABLE 429–3 EPWORTH SLEEPINESS SCALE

How likely are you to doze off or fall asleep in the following situations, in contrast to just feeling tired? This refers to your usual way of life in recent time. Even if you have not done some of these things recently, try to work out how they would have affected you. Use the following scale to choose the most appropriate number for each situation.

0 = would never doze
1 = slight chance of dozing
2 = moderate chance of dozing
3 = high chance of dozing

Situation	Chance of Dozing
Sitting and reading	________
Watching TV	________
Sitting and inactive in a public place (theater or meeting)	________
As a passenger in a car for an hour without a break	________
Lying down to rest in the afternoon when circumstances permit	________
Sitting and talking to someone	________
Sitting quietly after lunch (without alcohol)	________
In a car, while stopped for a few minutes in the traffic	________
TOTAL	________

From Johns MW: A new method for measuring daytime sleepiness: The Epworth Sleepiness Scale. Sleep 1991;14:540–545.

sleep apnea because an explanation for the hypersomnia should have been identified by the preceding all-night polysomnograph.

Actigraphy

Analysis of sleep diaries may be insufficient to verify a tentative diagnosis in patients with reported insomnia or suspected wake/sleep cycle abnormalities. In such cases, definitive objective data may be obtained by actigraphy, in which a small, wrist-mounted device records activity plotted against time—usually over a period of 1 to 3 weeks. There is direct correlation between the rest/activity recorded by the actigraph and the wake/sleep pattern as determined by polysomnography.

SPECIFIC SLEEP DISORDERS

Obstructive Sleep Apnea

Obstructive sleep apnea (Chapter 101), which is the most common medical disorder causing hypersomnia, affects more than 2% of adult women and 4% of adult men. It is seen primarily in overweight people who are loud snorers, but it may also occur in children and thin individuals.

Obstructive sleep apnea is characterized by collapse of the upper airway during sleep. This upper airway collapse may be associated with a fall in the blood oxygen level and results in repetitive arousal (up to 100 per hour of sleep) to reestablish upper airway airflow. These brief arousals are not perceived by the individual but result in excessive daytime sleepiness. Obstructive sleep apnea is described in detail in Chapter 101.

Narcolepsy

Epidemiology and Pathobiology

Narcolepsy affects 1 in 2000 individuals. It has a clear genetic component, with more than 90% of affected individuals carrying the HLA-DR2/DQ1 (under current nomenclature, HLA-DR15 and HLA-DQ6) gene, which is found in less than 30% of the general population. Despite a genetic component, the risk in a first-degree relative is only 1 to 2%, but this risk represents a 10- to 40-fold increase over the general population. Thus, the genetic component is neither necessary nor sufficient to cause narcolepsy.

Hypocretin-1 is an excitatory neuropeptide found in a very circumscribed group of neurons confined to the hypothalamic region. Patients with narcolepsy have lost hypocretin cells, possibly by an immune-mediated phenomenon.

Clinical Manifestations

Narcolepsy is characterized by the tendency to fall asleep inappropriately during the daytime, particularly during sedentary or nonstimulating activities, despite having obtained an adequate amount of sleep the preceding night. Other symptoms of narcolepsy include (1) cataplexy (sudden brief spells of muscle weakness), often triggered by emotionally laden events; (2) hypnagogic (occurring at sleep onset) or hypnopompic (occurring at sleep offset) hallucinations; (3) sleep paralysis (awakening to find the entire body paralyzed—with the exception of being able to breathe and move the eyes); (4) automatic behavior; and (5) disrupted nighttime sleep.

Patients with narcolepsy do not sleep more per 24 hours than non-narcoleptics do; instead, they are unable to maintain the normal boundaries of wakefulness, NREM sleep, and REM sleep. The automatic behavior (driving past the desired freeway exit, putting clothing into the refrigerator) represents an admixture of wakefulness and NREM sleep, with enough wakefulness to perform complex behavior but not enough for conscious awareness of the behavior. Sleep paralysis and cataplexy represent the simultaneous occurrence of REM sleep–related muscle paralysis and wakefulness. If the paralysis intrudes into wakefulness, the result is cataplexy; if it persists into wakefulness from a period of REM sleep, sleep paralysis results. The waking hallucinations represent the release of sleep-related dreaming into wakefulness, and the disrupted nighttime sleep is a manifestation of the "state boundary dyscontrol" aspect of narcolepsy. Sleep paralysis and hypnagogic/hypnopompic hallucinations, but not cataplexy, are often experienced by people who do not have narcolepsy—particularly in the setting of sleep deprivation.

Diagnosis

Sleep laboratory evaluation of patients with narcolepsy includes polysomnography and the multiple sleep latency test. Results of the all-night polysomnograph will usually be unremarkable. The multiple sleep latency test will demonstrate objective hypersomnolence, and REM sleep may be present during the daytime naps.

Levels of hypocretin-1 are undectable in the cerebrospinal fluid (CSF) of most patients with narcolepsy who experience cataplexy and are HLA-DQB1*0602 positive. Absent CSF hypocretin-1 levels are not found in any conditions that could be confused clinically with narcolepsy, thus suggesting that CSF hypocretin determinations could be of value in the diagnosis of narcolepsy in difficult cases.

Treatment

Rx

Stimulant medications such as methylphenidate, methamphetamine, dextroamphetamine, and modafinil 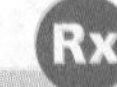 are generally effective and well tolerated. The response to medication is variable, and clinical judgment is needed to titrate to an effective dose. Dependency, tolerance, or abuse of stimulant medication is uncommon in patients with narcolepsy, and there is no indication for "drug holidays." Cataplexy is often controlled by tricyclic antidepressants, selective serotonin re-uptake inhibitors, or venlafaxine. γ-Hydroxybutyrate has been used in difficult cases.

Insomnia

Insomnia (Table 429–4) is defined not simply by total sleep time but rather by difficulty with initiation, maintenance, quality, and duration of sleep sufficient to impair functioning in the awake state.

Epidemiology

Insomnia, the most prevalent sleep complaint, affects up to 10 to 20% of the adult population and is second only to the complaint of pain as a reason to seek medical attention.

TABLE 429–4 CLASSIFICATION OF ADULT INSOMNIA

PRIMARY INSOMNIA
Idiopathic insomnia—Insomnia arising in infancy or childhood with a persistent, unremitting course
Psychophysiologic insomnia—Insomnia caused by a maladaptive conditioned response in which the patient learns to associate the bed environment with heightened arousal rather than sleep; its onset is often associated with an event causing acute insomnia, with the sleep disturbance persisting despite resolution of the precipitating factor
Paradoxical insomnia (sleep-state misperception)—Insomnia characterized by a marked mismatch between the patient's description of sleep duration and objective polysomnographic findings
SECONDARY INSOMNIA
Adjustment insomnia—Insomnia associated with active psychosocial stressors
Inadequate sleep hygiene—Insomnia associated with lifestyle habits that impair sleep
Insomnia caused by a psychiatric disorder—Insomnia secondary to an active psychiatric disorder, such as anxiety or depression
Insomnia caused by a medical condition—Insomnia secondary to a condition such as restless legs syndrome, chronic pain, nocturnal cough or dyspnea, or hot flashes
Insomnia caused by a drug or substance—Insomnia secondary to consumption or discontinuation of medication, drugs of abuse, alcohol, or caffeine

Reproduced with permission from The New England Journal of Medicine. Silber M: Clinical practice. Chronic insomnia. N Engl J Med 2005;353:803–810.

Pathobiology

There is growing evidence that some insomniacs may be in a constant state of hyperarousal because many are actually less sleepy during the day than normal subjects are as measured by objective daytime nap studies, and some also have increased 24-hour metabolic activity.

Many people with insomnia have identifiable psychiatric or psychological problems, and untreated insomnia is a risk factor for the future development of psychiatric problems such as depression (Chapter 420) or substance abuse (Chapter 32). Importantly, the relationship between insomnia and psychiatric conditions is bidirectional: depression may cause insomnia, and insomnia may cause depression.

Clinical Manifestations

Patients with insomnia complain of an inability to sleep long enough or well enough to awaken feeling rested or restored despite having an adequate amount of time to devote to sleep. Sleep deprivation as a result of inadequate time to devote to sleep is not insomnia. Many patients complain of nonrestorative sleep. Daytime consequences include feeling tired or fatigued or having trouble concentrating. True excessive daytime sleepiness (inappropriate or uncontrollable sleep episodes during the day) is extremely rare in insomniacs.

Diagnosis

Insomnia is a clinical diagnosis. Sleep diaries and actigraphy may be very helpful in difficult cases. Formal sleep studies are rarely indicated unless there is reason to suspect a coexisting sleep disorder such as obstructive sleep apnea.

Treatment

Rx

Behavioral therapy for insomnia (Table 429–5) can be quite effective [1-4] but may be very time consuming. Over-the-counter sleep aids are of little benefit.

TABLE 429–5 COGNITIVE BEHAVIORAL THERAPY FOR INSOMNIA

STIMULUS-CONTROL THERAPY
Go to bed only when sleepy
Use the bedroom only for sleeping and sex
Go to another room when unable to sleep in 15 to 20 minutes, read or engage in other quiet activities, and return to bed only when sleepy; repeat if necessary
Have a regular wake time regardless of the duration of sleep
Avoid daytime napping
SLEEP-RESTRICTION THERAPY
Reduce time in bed to the estimated total sleep time (minimum, 5 hr)
Increase time in bed by 15 minutes every week when the estimated sleep efficiency (ratio of time asleep to time in bed) is at least 90%
RELAXATION THERAPY
Physical component: progressive muscle relaxation, biofeedback
Mental component: imagery training, meditation, hypnosis
COGNITIVE THERAPY
Education to alter faulty beliefs and attitudes about sleep, such as that a minimum of 8 hours of sleep a night is required for health
SLEEP-HYGIENE EDUCATION
Correct extrinsic factors affecting sleep, such as environmental disruption (pets or snoring bed partner); bedroom temperature; fixation on the bedside clock; use of alcohol, nicotine, or caffeine; lack of exercise or exercise too close to bedtime

Reproduced with permission from The New England Journal of Medicine. Silber M: Clinical practice. Chronic insomnia. N Engl J Med 2005;353:803–810.

Although medications used to treat depression are often prescribed to treat insomnia, there is very little evidence that they are effective in the treatment of insomnia not associated with depression. Nevertheless, if patients with insomnia are physiologically hyperaroused, a case may be made for chronic administration of sedative-hypnotic agents. Three classes of medications are approved for the treatment of insomnia: the benzodiazepines (e.g., temazepam, 15 to 30 mg at bedtime; triazolam, 1.25 to 2.5 mg at bedtime; or estazolam, 1 to 2 mg at bedtime), the newer, nonbenzodiazepines (e.g., zolpidem, 5 to 10 mg at bedtime; zolpidem controlled release, 6.25 to 12.5 mg at bedtime; zaleplon, 5 to 10 mg at bedtime; or eszopiclone, 1 to 3 mg at bedtime), and a melatonin agonist (ramelteon, 8 mg at bedtime). Combined behavioral and pharmacologic treatments are often effective. Benzodiazepines may be safely and effectively administered for longer than 3 weeks. Tolerance, abuse, and dependency can be associated with chronic benzodiazepine administration in patients with well-documented sleep disorders, but the incidence of these complications is relatively low. Melatonin is normally secreted by the pineal gland (Chapter 241) in synchronization with the light/dark cycle. Its effect on sleep is variable, and its efficacy in treating insomnia has been disappointing.

Restless Legs Syndrome

Restless legs syndrome, which is one of the most common causes of severe insomnia, is a neurologic sensory/movement disorder that affects 5 to 15% of the general population. It is described in detail in Chapter 434.

Disorders of Circadian Rhythm

Definition

Most living creatures follow a relentless and pervasive daily rhythm of activity and rest that is ultimately linked to the geophysical light/dark cycle. Plants, animals, and even unicellular organisms show daily variations in metabolic activity, locomotion, feeding, and many other functions. The importance of the light/dark cycle on the human biologic clock is underscored by the fact that only a third of totally blind humans will be entrained to the environment, a third will have a 24-hour cycle that is out of phase with the environment, and the remaining third have a free-running pattern that is longer than 24 hours.

Epidemiology

In the absence of blindness, the etiology of primary circadian dysrhythmias is unknown. There is good evidence that genetic factors contribute in some cases.

Pathobiology

The function of the biologic clock is to promote wakefulness. Normally, maximal wakefulness occurs during daylight hours. For reasons that are not understood, the biologic clocks of people with circadian dysrhythmias are inexorably out of synchronization with the environment, thus making it difficult or impossible to adjust to demands of the environment.

Exposure to bright light has a potent effect on the biologic clock, and exposure at strategic times of the wake/sleep cycle results in a change in the underlying rhythm. For example, evening light exposure may delay the clock, whereas morning light exposure may advance it.

Clinical Manifestations and Diagnosis

The primary symptom of disorders of circadian rhythm is an inability to sleep during the desired sleep time. Once asleep, there is no abnormality of sleep per se, only an abnormality of the timing of sleep. The result is often a complaint of insomnia if sleep is attempted during the "wake" cycle of the clock or a complaint of sleepiness if wakefulness is attempted during the clock's sleep period. Wake/sleep schedule disorders fall into two categories: (1) primary malfunction of the biologic clock per se and (2) secondary malfunction as a result of environmental effects on the underlying clock. The primary disorders may be difficult to diagnose because they typically masquerade as other sleep, medical, or psychiatric disorders, such as hypersomnia, insomnia, substance (sedative-hypnotic or stimulant) abuse, or psychiatric conditions.

The diagnosis is made by the history. Most people, if asked what their wake/sleep pattern would be if they had 3 weeks of vacation without any constraints on their wake/sleep activities (meals, work, school, family activities), can provide an accurate estimate of their inherent wake/sleep pattern. Sleep diaries and actigraphy may be helpful in difficult cases. The secondary disorders (such as jet lag and shift work) are usually immediately apparent on simple questioning of the patient.

Treatment

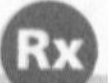

The mainstays of treatment of the primary circadian dysrhythmias are chronotherapy and phototherapy.

Chronotherapy

In chronotherapy, the desirable total sleep time is determined by sleep logs during a "free-running" period. The patient then delays or advances the onset of sleep by a few hours every day and sleeps only the predetermined number of hours until the onset of sleep is at the desired time, at which point the patient attempts to maintain that time. This method requires several days of free time and can be difficult if sleeping quarters cannot be kept dark and quiet during the several day sleeps required.

Phototherapy

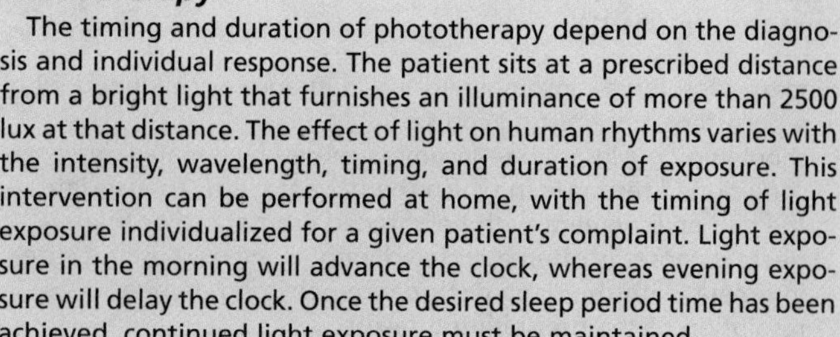

The timing and duration of phototherapy depend on the diagnosis and individual response. The patient sits at a prescribed distance from a bright light that furnishes an illuminance of more than 2500 lux at that distance. The effect of light on human rhythms varies with the intensity, wavelength, timing, and duration of exposure. This intervention can be performed at home, with the timing of light exposure individualized for a given patient's complaint. Light exposure in the morning will advance the clock, whereas evening exposure will delay the clock. Once the desired sleep period time has been achieved, continued light exposure must be maintained.

Jet Lag, Shift Work, and Persistent Primary Circadian Dysrhythmias

The best way to manage jet lag is to assume the wake/sleep pattern of the destination site immediately. Sedative/hypnotic medication may reduce sleep-onset insomnia associated with jet lag. Jet lag usually resolves at a rate of 1 day per time zone change.

Management of shift work may be difficult; options include stimulant medications and exposure to bright light at night or sedative/hypnotic medication and protection of the sleep environment during the day (or both). The biologic clocks of night shift workers virtually never completely adjust to the night shift because the drive home in the morning resets the clock every day and workers tend to sleep at conventional times during nights off.

Treatment with medications is justified in patients who have persistent symptoms despite chronotherapy and phototherapy. For example, modafinil, 100 to 200 mg during the night shift, is effective for the excessive sleepiness and loss of attention of shift work sleep disorder. [5] In addition, administration of 3 mg of melatonin 4 to 5 hours before the desired onset of sleep may be of benefit.

Delayed Sleep Syndrome

In delayed sleep phase syndrome, the patient falls asleep late and rises late. There is a striking inability to fall asleep at an earlier, more desirable time. This syndrome may be manifested as either sleep-onset insomnia or daytime hypersomnia, particularly in the morning. Delayed sleep phase syndrome is the most common of the primary circadian dysrhythmias and may, in part, be the consequence of societal increases in opportunities for nighttime activity. Combinations of chronotherapy, phototherapy, and medications may be effective in "resetting" the clock, as for circadian dysrhythmias. Unfortunately, the treatment regimen must be maintained, or the clock will again become delayed.

Advanced Sleep Phase Syndrome

Individuals suffering from advanced sleep phase syndrome fall asleep early and awaken earlier than desired. They are unable to remain awake until the desired time, falling asleep in the early evening and awakening in the very early hours of the morning. This syndrome may be manifested as hypersomnia, particularly in the evening, or sleep maintenance insomnia. Patients complain of interruption of evening activities by their sleepiness. They may avoid evening social activities for fear of the intrusive sleepiness. The undesirable early morning awakenings in this condition may lead to a misdiagnosis of depression. Bright light exposure in the evening may delay the clock to a more acceptable pattern.

Other Abnormalities of Circadian Rhythm

Other, less common circadian dysrhythmias include a "non–24-hour wake/sleep pattern" in which the wake/sleep period is longer than 24 hours and sleep begins at a later time each cycle, as well as an "irregular wake/sleep pattern" characterized by a completely chaotic and unpredictable wake/sleep pattern.

Parasomnias

Parasomnias are defined as unpleasant or undesirable behavioral or experiential phenomena occurring predominately or exclusively during sleep. Initially attributed to psychiatric disease, it is now clear that parasomnias are the manifestation of a wide variety of completely different conditions, most of which are diagnosable and treatable. The common parasomnias are examples of "dissociated sleep states," which represent the simultaneous admixture of wakefulness with either NREM sleep (disorders of arousal such as sleepwalking or sleep terrors) or REM sleep (REM sleep behavior disorder). The parasomnias, like narcolepsy, support the concept that wake and sleep are not mutually exclusive states and that sleep is not necessarily a global brain phenomenon.

Isolated, often bizarre sleep-related events may be experienced by perfectly normal individuals, and most do not warrant further extensive or expensive evaluation. However, serious attention should be paid to complaints of sleep-related behavior that is potentially violent or injurious. In these cases, formal sleep studies using a full EEG montage with continuous audiovisual monitoring is indicated to establish a correct diagnosis and treatment plan.

Disorders of Arousal

Disorders of arousal tend to arise from NREM sleep and usually occur in the first third of the sleep cycle and rarely during naps. They are common in childhood and usually decrease in frequency with increasing age.

Disorders of arousal may be triggered by febrile illness, alcohol, prior sleep deprivation, physical activity, emotional stress, or medications. They are not caused by significant underlying psychiatric problems.

Clinical manifestations vary across a broad spectrum ranging from confusional arousal to somnambulism (sleepwalking) to sleep terrors. Some patients perform more specialized behavior, such as sleep-related eating and sleep-related sexual activity, without conscious awareness.

Treatment

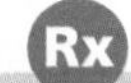

Most disorders of arousal, such as simple sleepwalking or sleep terrors, require no treatment other than reassurance of their benign nature. If the behavior is bothersome or potentially injurious, medical management with benzodiazepines (e.g., clonazepam, 0.5 to 1.0 mg ½ hour before bedtime), tricyclic antidepressant medications (e.g., imipramine, 25 to 50 mg ½ hour before bedtime), or behavioral treatment in the form of self-taught relaxation exercises is often effective.

Rapid Eye Movement Sleep Behavior Disorder

The most common and best-studied REM sleep parasomnia is the REM sleep behavior disorder.

Epidemiology and Pathobiology

REM sleep behavior disorder predominately affects males (about 90%) and usually begins after the age of 50 years. Acute REM sleep behavior disorder is often due to undesirable side effects of prescribed medications, most commonly antidepressant medications, particularly the selective serotonin re-uptake inhibitors. Chronic REM sleep behavior disorder, which may be preceded by a lengthy prodrome of REM sleep behavior disorder, can be idiopathic or associated with neurodegenerative disorders, particularly the synucleinopathies (Parkinson's disease, multiple system atrophy, or dementia with Lewy bodies), in which it may be the first symptom and precede other manifestations of the underlying process by more than 10 years (Chapter 433). There is also a higher incidence of REM sleep behavior disorder in patients with narcolepsy, in whom this tendency may be aggravated by the tricyclic antidepressants or selective serotonin re-uptake inhibitors prescribed to treat cataplexy.

Clinical Manifestations

In these patients, somatic muscle atonia—one of the defining features of REM sleep—is absent, thereby permitting the acting out of dream mentation, often with violent or injurious results. The initial complaint is that of vigorous sleep behavior usually accompanying vivid dreams. Such behavior may result in repeated injury, including ecchymoses, lacerations, and fractures.

Diagnosis

The diagnosis may be suspected by the clinical history, but formal sleep studies are indicated. Patients with REM sleep behavior disorder will demonstrate increased EMG activity during REM sleep, thus confirming the clinical suspicion.

Treatment

The benzodiazepine clonazepam (0.5 to 2.0 mg ½ hour before bedtime) is a highly effective treatment of REM sleep behavior disorder, with a sustained response rate of nearly 90%, although its mechanism of action is unknown.

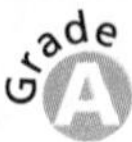

1. U.S. Modafinil in Narcolepsy Multicenter Study Group: Randomized trial of modafinil as a treatment for the excessive daytime somnolence of narcolepsy. Neurology 2000;54:1166–1175.
2. Edinger JD, Wohlgemuth WK, Radtke RA, et al: Cognitive behavioral therapy for treatment of chronic primary insomnia. A randomized controlled trial. JAMA 2001;285:1856–1864.
3. Morin CM, Colecchi C, Stone J, et al: Behavioral and pharmacological therapies for late-life insomnia. A randomized controlled trial. JAMA 1999;281:991–999.
4. Jacobs GD, Pace-Schott EF, Stickgold R, et al: Cognitive behavior therapy and pharmacotherapy for insomnia. A randomized controlled trial and direct comparison. Arch Intern Med 2004;164:1888–1896.
5. Czeisler CA, Walsh JK, Roth T, et al. for the U.S. Modafinil in Shift Work Sleep Disorder Study Group: Modafinil for excessive sleepiness associated with shift-work sleep disorder. N Engl J Med 2005;353:476–486.

SUGGESTED READINGS

Collup NA: Obstructive sleep apnea syndromes. Semin Respir Crit Care Med 2005;26:13–24. *A comprehensive review.*

Dauvilliers Y, Arnulf I, Mignot E: Narcolepsy and cataplexy. Lancet 2007;369:499–511. *A detailed review of these syndromes.*

Eckert DJ, Jordan AS, Merchia P, et al: Central sleep apnea: Pathophysiology and treatment. Chest 2007;131:595–607. *Comprehensive review.*

Howard ME, Desai AV, Grunstein RR, et al: Sleepiness, sleep-disordered breathing, and accident risk factors in commercial vehicle drivers. Am J Respir Crit Care Med 2004;170:1014–1021. *Nearly 25% of drivers reported excessive daytime sleepiness, more than 50% had sleep-disordered breathing, and the risk for accidents was increased in the sleepiest drivers.*

Kamel NS, Gammack JK: Insomnia in the elderly: Cause, approach, and treatment. Am J Med 2006;119:463–469. *A comprehensive review.*

Lu BS, Zee PC: Circadian rhythm sleep disorders. Chest 2006;130:1915–1923. *Clinical review.*

Mahowald MW, Cramer Bornemann M, Schenck CH: Parasomnias. Semin Neurol 2004;24:283–292. *A detailed review.*

Silber MH: Clinical practice. Chronic insomnia. N Engl J Med 2005;353:803–810. *A thorough review.*

Trenkwalder C, Paulus W, Walters AS: The restless legs syndrome. Lancet Neurol 2005;4:465–475. *A comprehensive review.*

430 APPROACH TO CEREBROVASCULAR DISEASES

Justin A. Zivin

Definition

Stroke is the generally preferred term for a group of diseases that are of abrupt onset and cause neurologic damage (Fig. 430–1). Approximately 85% of strokes are caused by a sudden onset of inadequacy of blood flow to some or all of the brain (Chapter 431). The remaining strokes are divided between hemorrhage (Chapter 432) into brain tissue (parenchymatous hemorrhage) and hemorrhage into the spaces surrounding the brain, most frequently the subarachnoid space. A commonly used synonym for stroke was *cerebrovascular accident,* but

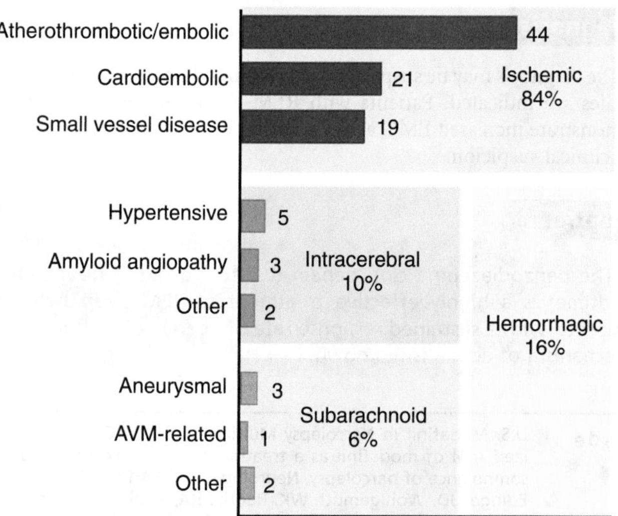

FIGURE 430–1 • Classification of cerebrovascular disease. AVM = arteriovenous malformation.

this term has lost favor because strokes are not really accidents. Well-established prophylactic and acute therapies are now available, and diagnostic tools have improved markedly. Management of strokes has become much more rational and successful.

Epidemiology

Stroke is the second leading cause of mortality worldwide and the third most common cause of death in the industrialized world (after heart disease and all types of cancer combined). It is the most common cause of adult disability in the United States. In China and Japan, stroke is the most frequent cause of death.

In the United States, the annual incidence and death rate for stroke declined steadily for most of the 20th century. In more recent years, the rate of decline has slowed, however, and the incidence of stroke may be increasing. About 750,000 new strokes reach medical attention per year in the United States, and strokes cause about 150,000 deaths annually. At any given time there are about 3 million stroke survivors in the United States. Incidence rates in western European countries are slightly higher than in the United States, and several eastern European countries, China, and Japan have much higher rates based at least partly on smoking and on environmental and dietary factors.

The rate of stroke approximately doubles with each decade after the age of 55. Blacks and Hispanics have about twice the risk of whites, and men have about a 40% higher incidence of stroke than women do. Hypertension increases the risk by four-fold, smoking nearly doubles the risk, and diabetes increases the risk two- to six-fold. Carotid stenosis and atrial fibrillation are perhaps the strongest risk factors. Other factors that increase risk include obesity, hypercholesterolemia, physical inactivity, alcohol abuse, hyperhomocysteinemia, drug abuse, and use of oral contraceptive agents.

Pathobiology

Cerebrovascular Anatomy

Strokes are usually caused by abnormalities in the cerebral circulation. Anatomic variations are frequent, however, and the territory receiving its blood supply from a given artery is not entirely predictable; as a result, stroke syndromes may not correlate well with the location of the vascular injury. Appropriate imaging studies are needed to provide detailed information about each individual patient. In many situations, noninvasive imaging is adequate. For vascular anomalies such as stenosis, malformations, and aneurysms, angiography is crucial for diagnosis because an understanding of the anatomy is necessary to develop treatment plans.

Four major arteries supply the brain: the bilaterally paired internal carotid and vertebral arteries (Fig. 430–2). The left common carotid artery arises directly from the aortic arch, but the right originates from branches of the aorta. The right common carotid artery is a branch of the innominate artery, and the left and right vertebral arteries originate from the subclavian arteries.

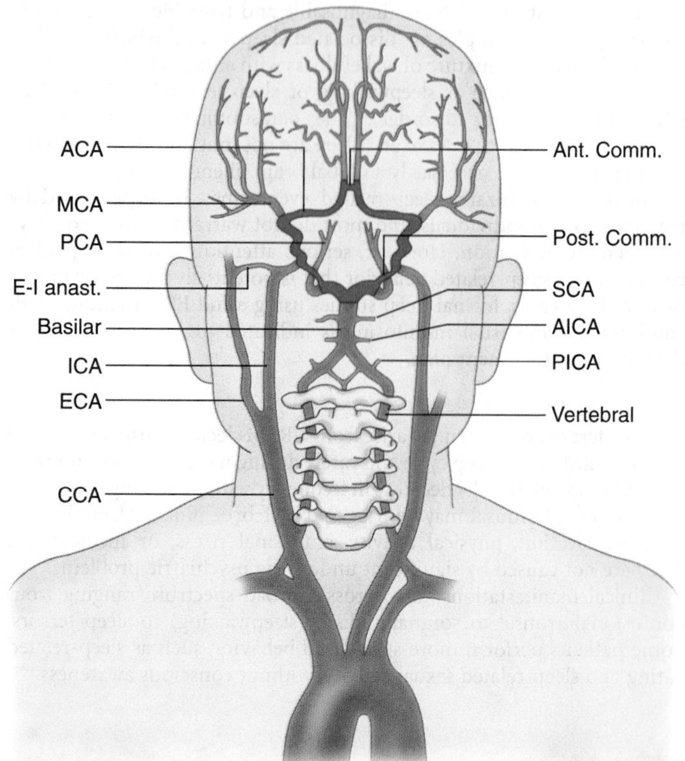

FIGURE 430–2 • Extracranial and intracranial arterial supply to the brain. Vessels forming the circle of Willis are highlighted. ACA = anterior cerebral artery; AICA = anterior inferior cerebellar artery; Ant. Comm. = anterior communicating artery; CCA = common carotid artery; ECA = external carotid artery; E-I anast. = extracranial-intracranial anastomosis; ICA = internal carotid artery; MCA = middle cerebral artery; PCA = posterior cerebral artery; PICA = posterior inferior cerebellar artery; Post. Comm. = posterior communicating artery; SCA = superior cerebellar artery. (Modified from Lord R: Surgery of Occlusive Cerebrovascular Disease. St Louis, Mosby, 1986.)

Internal Carotid Arteries

In most individuals, each common carotid artery bifurcates into an internal and external carotid artery just below the angle of the jaw and approximately at the level of the thyroid cartilage. The internal carotid artery (ICA) enters the skull through the foramen lacerum and travels a short distance within the petrous portion of the temporal bone. It then enters the cavernous sinus before penetrating the dura and ascends above the clinoid processes to divide into the anterior cerebral artery (ACA) and middle cerebral artery (MCA). The portion of the ICA that lies between the cavernous sinus and the supraclinoid process forms an S shape and is sometimes termed the *carotid siphon.* The ICA gives off its first important branches at the supraclinoid level: the ophthalmic, posterior communicating, and anterior choroidal arteries, usually in that order. In some cases, the ophthalmic artery arises from the ICA within the cavernous sinus.

External Carotid Arteries

Branches of the external carotid artery sometimes form anastomoses that provide collateral circulation to the ICA. These branches include the facial artery and the superficial temporal artery. Both vessels may anastomose with the supratrochlear branches of the ophthalmic artery. In instances of ICA occlusion below the level of the ophthalmic branch, the facial and superficial temporal arteries sometimes supply blood through the ophthalmic branch to the distal ICA.

Vertebral-Basilar Arteries

Anatomic variation is considerably more common in the vertebral artery system than in the ICA. The paired vertebral arteries usually arise from the subclavian arteries, but their origins may be more proximal on the aortic arch, or they may form a common branch of the thyrocervical trunk. The vertebral arteries generally enter the foramina of the sixth cervical vertebra or, much less commonly, the fourth, fifth, or seventh vertebral foramina. The vertebral arteries ascend through the transverse foramina and exit at C1, where they turn nearly 90 degrees posteriorly to pass behind the atlantoaxial joint before penetrating the dura and entering the cranial cavity through the foramen magnum. The portion of the vertebral artery that loops behind the atlantoaxial joint is prone to mechanical deformation, and excessive rotation of the head may cause arterial narrowing and reduction of blood flow to the ipsilateral vertebral artery.

Intracranially, the vertebral arteries are lateral to the medulla oblongata and then course ventrally and medially, where they unite rostrally at the medullopontine junction to form the basilar artery. The basilar artery ultimately bifurcates at the pontomesencephalic junction to form the posterior cerebral arteries (PCAs).

In a few individuals, the right or left vertebral arteries terminate before reaching the basilar artery, which consequently is supplied, proximally, by a single vertebral artery. The vertebral arteries usually have medial branches that turn caudally and unite to form the anterior spinal artery, as well as lateral branches supplying the dorsolateral medulla and posterior cerebellum, called the *posterior inferior cerebellar arteries.*

Circle of Willis

The circle of Willis, which is at the base of the brain, is formed by the union of the right and left ACAs via the anterior communicating artery, the MCAs, and the PCAs via the posterior communicating arteries. Anomalies of the circle of Willis occur frequently; in large autopsy series of normal individuals, more than half show an incomplete circle of Willis. The most common sites for these abnormalities, which are usually manifested as hypoplasia or absence, are the posterior communicating arteries and the ACAs.

Anterior Cerebral Arteries

The ACAs travel medially above the optic chiasm and pass rostrally toward the interhemispheric fissure, where they arch caudally to lie just dorsal to the corpus callosum. In a small fraction of normal individuals, the A1 segment of the ACA (the portion between the origin at the MCA and the first major branch, the anterior communicating artery) is hypoplastic or absent, which leaves its distal portion to be supplied by the opposite ACA via the anterior communicating artery. Branches of the ACA normally supply the frontal poles, the superior surfaces of the cerebral hemispheres where their distal branches anastomose with those of the MCA, and all of the medial surfaces of both cerebral hemispheres with the exception of the calcarine cortex (Figs. 430–3 and 430–4). Cortical areas served by the ACA include the motor and sensory cortex of the legs and feet, the supplementary motor cortex, and the paracentral lobule.

The A1 and A2 segments (the portions between the anterior communicating artery and the genu of the corpus callosum) give off many small branches that penetrate the anterior perforated substance of the brain. These small penetrating branches include all of the anterior and some of the medial lenticulostriate arteries. Usually, there is a dominant medial striate vessel called the *recurrent artery of Heubner,* which commonly arises from the A1 segment of the ACA. This artery penetrates the perforated substance of the brain and, along with the other small perforators, supplies the anterior and inferior portions of the anterior limb of the internal capsule, the anterior and inferior head of the caudate nucleus, the anterior globus pallidus and putamen, the anterior hypothalamus, the olfactory bulbs and tracts, and the uncinate fasciculus.

Anterior Choroidal Artery

The anterior choroidal artery arises from the supraclinoid portion of the ICA in most people. It travels caudally and medially over the optic tract, to which it provides a few small branches, and enters the brain via the choroidal fissure. Many important brain structures receive blood flow from the anterior choroidal artery, including portions of the anterior hippocampus, uncus, amygdala, globus pallidus, tail of the caudate nucleus, lateral thalamus, geniculate body, and a large portion of the most inferior, posterior limb of the internal capsule.

Middle Cerebral Artery

The MCA provides flow to most of the lateral surface of the cerebral hemispheres and is the vessel most frequently involved in ischemic stroke. As the main MCA trunk passes laterally toward the sylvian fissure, it gives rise to some of the medial and all of the lateral lenticulostriate arteries. These arteries supply the putamen, the head and body of the caudate nucleus, the lateral globus pallidus, the anterior limb of the internal capsule, and the superior portion of the posterior limb of the internal capsule. The MCA extends into the sylvian fissure, where it branches into several smaller arteries grouped into a superior division, which feeds the cortical surface above the fissure, and an inferior division, which supplies the cortical surface of the temporal lobe. The territory of the MCA includes the major motor and sensory areas of the cortex, the areas for contraversive eye and head movement, the optic radiations, the auditory sensory cortex, and in the dominant hemisphere, the motor and sensory areas for language.

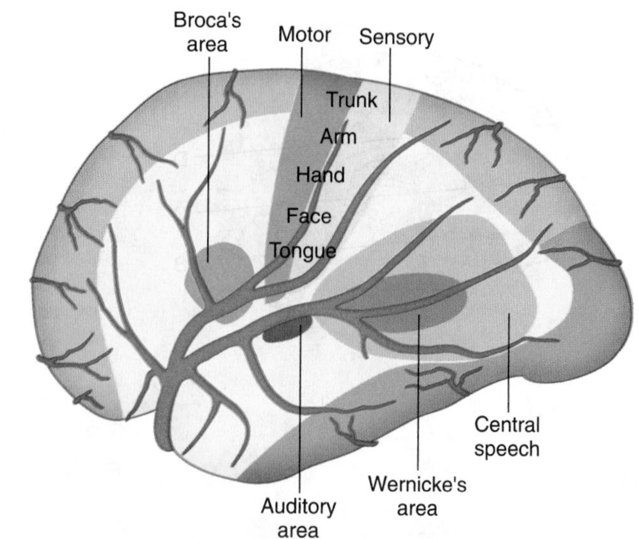

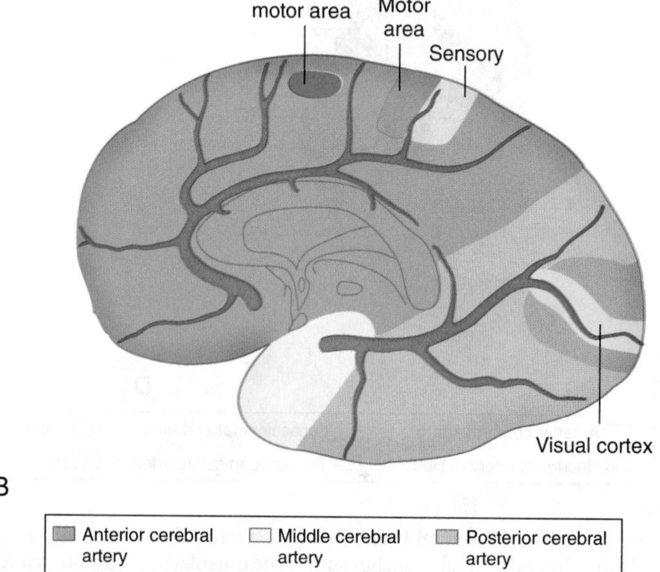

FIGURE 430–3 • Surface cerebral arterial anatomy. Lateral **(A)** and medial **(B)** views of the cerebral hemisphere show the surface distributions of the anterior, middle, and posterior cerebral arteries.

Posterior Cerebral Arteries

Blood flow to both PCAs derives in most people from the basilar artery and infrequently from the ICA. Sometimes the ICA is the origin of one PCA and the other PCA originates from the basilar artery. The PCAs pass dorsal to the third cranial nerves and across the cerebral peduncles, then ascend upward along the medial edge of the tentorium, where they branch into anterior and posterior divisions. The anterior division supplies the inferior surface of the temporal lobe, where its terminal branches form an anastomosis with branches of the MCA. The posterior division supplies the occipital lobe, where its terminal branches anastomose with the ACA and the MCA. In its most proximal course along the base of the brain, the PCA gives off several groups of penetrating arteries commonly called the *thalamogeniculate,* the *thalamoperforating,* and the *posterior choroidal* arteries. The red nucleus, the substantia nigra, medial portions of the cerebral peduncles, the nuclei of the thalamus, the hippocampus, and the posterior hypothalamus receive blood from these penetrating branches.

Brain Stem Blood Supply

The ventral medial portion of the brain stem receives its blood supply from short paramedian vessels, the ventrolateral region receives its blood

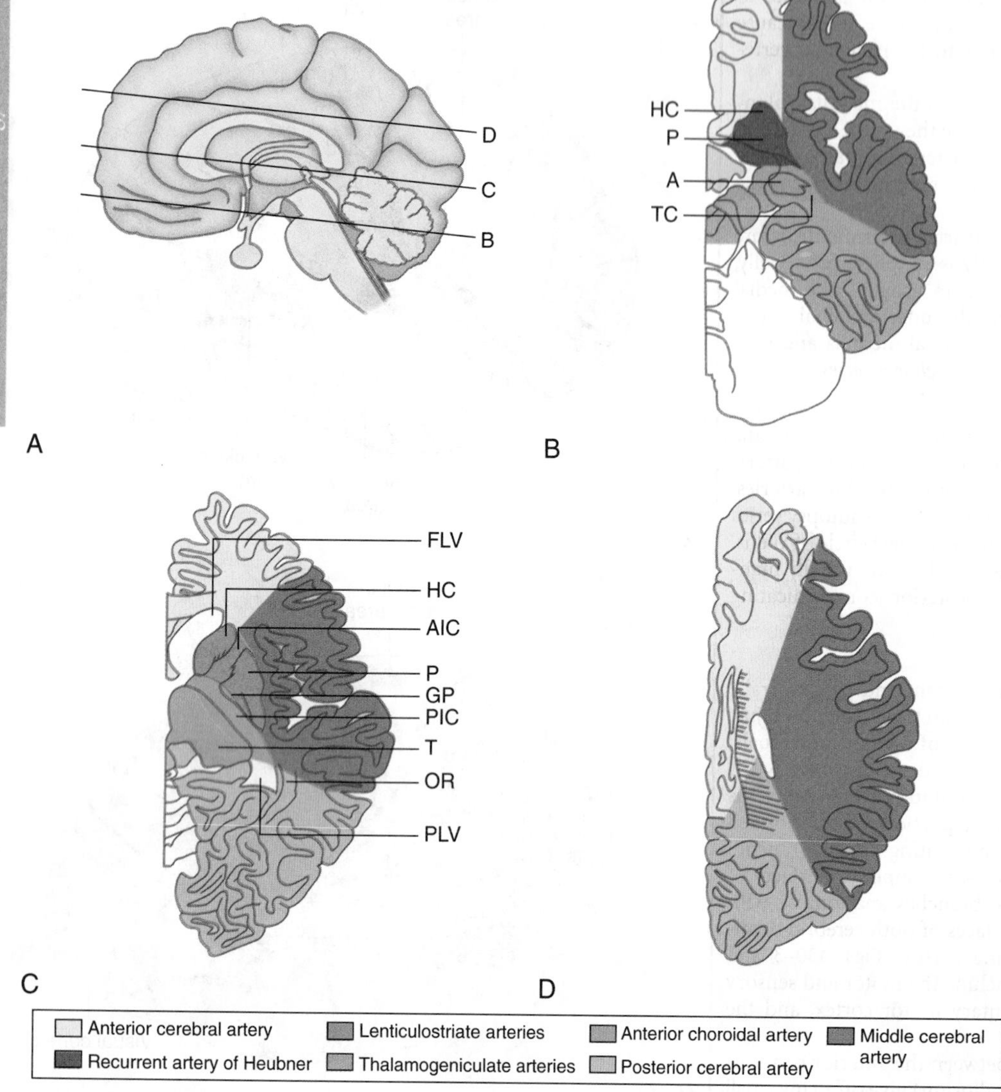

FIGURE 430–4 • Arterial supply of the deep brain structures. A, Sagittal view of the brain showing the computed tomography (CT) planes through which views **B, C,** and **D** were taken. **B,** CT plane through the head of the caudate nucleus (HC), putamen (P), amygdala (A), tail of the caudate nucleus (TC), hypothalamus, temporal lobe, midbrain, and cerebellum. **C,** CT plane through the frontal horn of the lateral ventricle (FLV), head of the caudate nucleus (HC), anterior and posterior limbs of the internal capsule (AIC, PIC), putamen (P), globus pallidus (GP), thalamus (T), optic radiations (OR), and posterior horn of the lateral ventricle (PLV). **D,** CT plane through the centrum semiovale. (Modified from De Armond S, Fusco MM, Dewey MM: Structure of the Human Brain, a Photographic Atlas, 3rd ed. New York, Oxford University Press, 1989, with permission.)

from short circumferential branches of the vertebral or basilar arteries, and long circumferential branches supply the dorsolateral brain stem and cerebellum (Fig. 430–5). These vessels include the posterior inferior cerebellar arteries, which arise from the vertebral arteries, and the anterior inferior and superior cerebellar arteries, which arise from the basilar artery.

The pyramids, the inferior olives and medial lemnisci, the medial longitudinal fasciculi, and the emerging fibers of the hypoglossal nerve derive blood from the vertebral arteries. Longer branches from the vertebral arteries and posterior ICAs supply the spinothalamic tracts, the vestibular nuclei, the sensory nuclei of the fifth cranial nerve, the descending fibers of the sympathetic nervous system, the restiform body, and the emerging fibers of the vagus and glossopharyngeal nerves. The most cephalad and dorsal segment of the medulla includes the vestibular and cochlear nuclei, which along with the posterior portion of the cerebellum, receive flow from the posterior inferior cerebellar artery.

The basilar artery gives rise to perforating branches as it spans the ventral midline pons and midbrain. These short perpendicular branches distribute blood to the paramedian structures, including the corticospinal tracts, the pontine reticular nuclei, the medial lemnisci, the medial longitudinal fasciculi, and the pontine reticular nuclei. The anterior ICA feeds blood to the lateral pons, including the emerging seventh and eighth cranial nerves, the trigeminal nerve root, the vestibular and cochlear nuclei, and the spinothalamic tracts. It also branches to the most dorsal and lateral of these structures on its dorsal course toward the cerebellum.

At the midbrain level, the basilar artery lies in the midline in the interpeduncular fossa. Short branches pass laterally and dorsally on both sides to supply the cerebral peduncles, the emerging fibers of the third nerve, medial portions of the red nuclei, the medial longitudinal fasciculus, the oculomotor nuclei, and the midbrain reticulum. The superior cerebellar arteries contribute to the dorsal midbrain supply, including that of the colliculi and the superior portion of the cerebellum on each side.

Venous Drainage

The veins in the brain, in contrast to those in many other parts of the body, often do not accompany the arteries. Cortical veins drain into the superior sagittal sinus, which runs between the cerebral hemispheres. Deeper structures drain into the inferior sagittal sinus and great cerebral vein (of Galen), which join at the straight sinus (Fig. 430–6). The straight sinus runs along the attachment of the falx cerebri and tentorium to join with the superior sagittal sinus at the torcular Herophili, from which the two transverse sinuses arise. Each transverse sinus passes laterally toward the petrosal bone to become the sigmoid sinus, which exits the skull into the internal jugular vein. Each cavernous sinus communicates with its contralateral twin and surrounds the ipsilateral carotid artery. Both drain into the petrosal sinuses, which drain into the sigmoid sinus.

Normal Physiology

Cerebral Metabolism and Blood Flow

Although the brain is normally about 2% of body weight in humans, it is supplied with approximately 14% of the resting cardiac output. The energy demands to support normal brain activity in conscious humans are equal, on a per-weight basis, to the demands of the most metabolically active tissues, such as the heart and kidney. Aerobic glucose metabolism in a normal, conscious human brain consumes an average of 140 μmol of oxygen and 24 μmol of glucose per 100 g of brain each minute. Normal brain activities, such as thinking or sleeping, do not alter the total blood flow, glucose use, or oxygen uptake in the brain, but they do change the patterns of blood supply and energy use in specific brain areas.

The brain extracts approximately 10% of available blood glucose in a single pass, yet only 80% of this glucose is used to generate energy. About

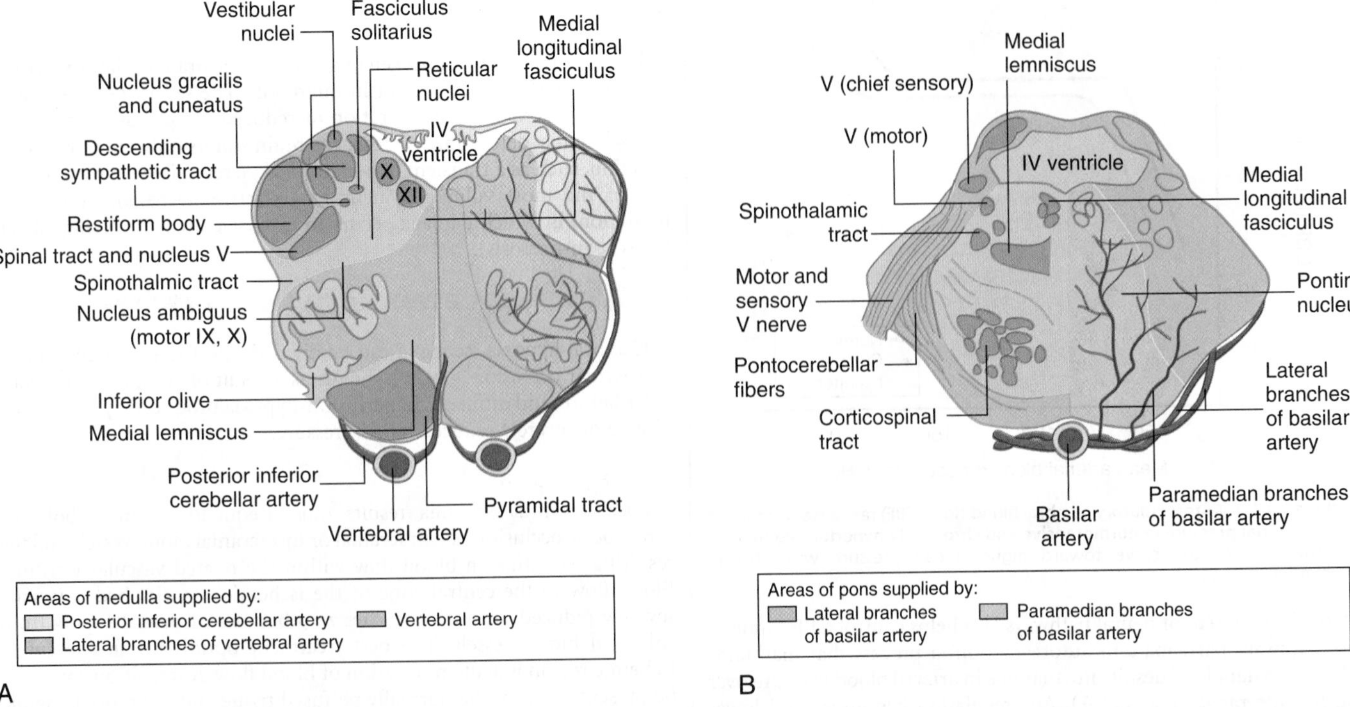

FIGURE 430–5 • Brain stem blood supply. A, Cross section of the medulla oblongata at the level of the hypoglossal nuclei (XII). Short branches of the vertebral and anterior spinal arteries supply the medulla. Longer circumferential branches, including the posterior inferior cerebellar artery, supply the lateral portions of the medulla. **B,** Cross section of the midpons region. The medial portion receives blood supply from short, perforating basilar artery branches. More laterally, the blood supply comes from lateral basilar artery branches.

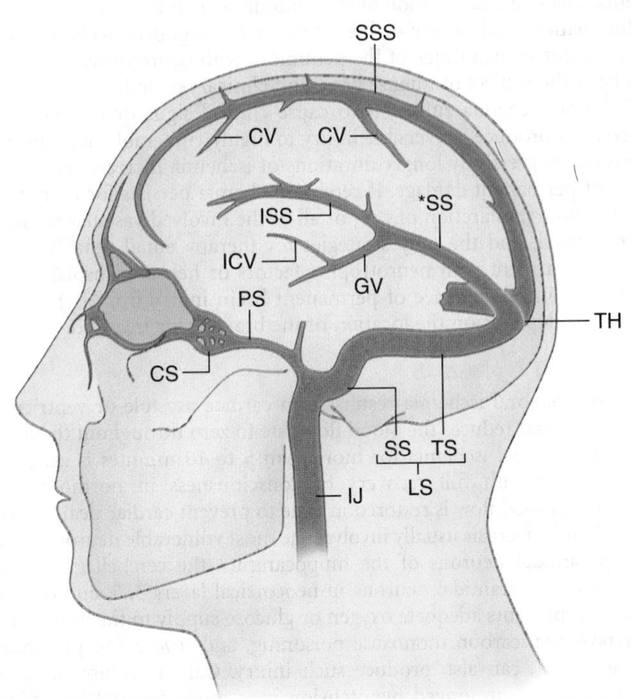

FIGURE 430–6 • Venous drainage of intracranial structures. CS = cavernous sinus; CV = cortical veins; GV = great vein of Galen; ICV = internal cerebral vein; IJ = internal jugular vein; ISS = inferior sagittal sinus; LS = lateral sinus; PS = petrosal sinus; SS = sigmoid sinus; *SS = straight sinus; SSS = superior sagittal sinus; TH = torcular Herophili; TS = transverse sinus. (From Gates P, Barnett HJ, Mohr JP, et al [eds]: Stroke: Pathophysiology, Diagnosis and Management. New York, Churchill Livingstone, 1986.)

10 to 15% of glucose is metabolized to lactate, which may be lost to the circulation; the remainder is used for the synthesis of neurotransmitters, fats, and to a small degree, proteins. Each mole of glucose metabolized by the brain through glycolysis and the mitochondrial respiratory chain yields approximately 30 mol of adenosine triphosphate (ATP) instead of the theoretical maximum of 38 mol.

In contrast to most other tissues, the brain stores little glucose, glycogen, or high-energy phosphates (ATP, phosphocreatine) but instead relies on continuous, well-regulated blood flow to satisfy its needs for energy. Cerebral blood flow (CBF) averages 50 mL/100 g of brain per minute in a normal, conscious human. In the absence of this flow, the brain has sufficient high-energy stores to support its metabolic needs for only a few minutes. The vascular reserves of oxygen and glucose are small, as illustrated by the fact that all changes in synaptic activity, whether related to thinking, talking, or directing muscular activity, are tightly coupled, temporally and anatomically, to an almost instantaneous increase in local CBF. The mechanisms responsible for this coupling of blood flow to metabolic activity have not been fully elucidated, but the relationship is well established, under normal conditions, and provides a basis for the use of imaging methods to assess regional brain activity. Regional CBF can be precisely quantified with positron emission tomography. Other less invasive techniques such as magnetic resonance imaging and single-photon emission computed tomography provide qualitative measurements of local CBF (Chapter 419). The brain's functional activities result in a frequently and rapidly changing pattern of regional metabolic and blood flow values that reflect moment-to-moment changes in activity. On a larger scale, the low stores and high metabolic rate of the brain are responsible for the rapid loss of consciousness and subsequent irreversible damage that accompanies loss of the critical energy sources of the brain, glucose and oxygen.

The coupling of CBF to regional synaptic and metabolic activity is only one of several mechanisms known to regulate normal CBF. Another is alteration of carbon dioxide. Hypercapnia dilates and hypocapnia constricts cerebral resistance vessels so that CBF shows a linear relationship to $Paco_2$ within the normal range. This physiologic response to $Paco_2$ can be exploited clinically to treat cerebral herniation. Increases in intracranial pressure (ICP) in the absence of adequate intracranial volume may force the hemispheres through the tentorium or the cerebellum through the foramen magnum. Mechanical hyperventilation to a $Paco_2$ of 20 to 25 mm Hg reduces CBF by approximately 40 to 45% and normal adult cerebral blood volume from 50 to approximately 35 mL. Though seemingly small, this reduction sometimes suffices to retard the progression of herniation and is the fastest way to reduce ICP. The response is short-lived, however, and brain and blood HCO_3^- and H^+ ions controlling blood vessel tone re-equilibrate within 30 to 60 minutes. More definitive therapy must be initiated quickly.

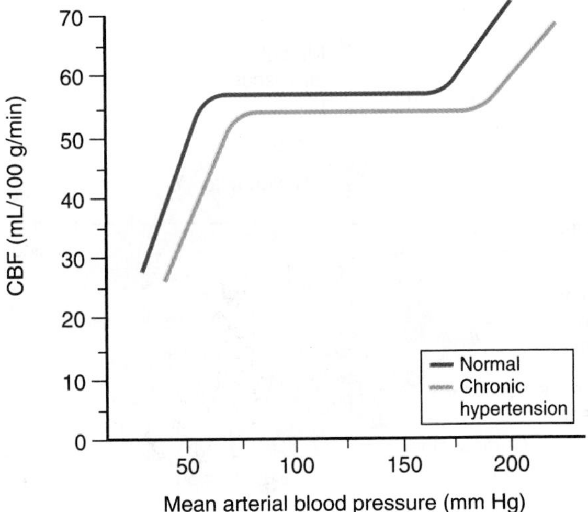

FIGURE 430–7 • Autoregulatory cerebral blood flow (CBF) response to changes in mean arterial pressure in normotensive and chronically hypertensive people. Note the shift of the curve toward higher mean pressure with chronic hypertension.

A complex system of neural pathways also helps control CBF. Some of these pathways participate in autoregulation, a process that maintains CBF at a constant level despite fluctuations in arterial blood pressure over a fairly wide range (Fig. 430–7). Autoregulation has upper and lower limits; at a mean arterial pressure greater than about 150 mm Hg, blood flow increases and capillary pressure rises, whereas at a mean arterial pressure less than 50 mm Hg, CBF falls. In patients with chronic hypertension, the upper and lower autoregulatory limits are shifted toward higher systemic pressure. Consequently, a rapid therapeutic reduction in blood pressure to levels that would be normal in most people carries the risk of further lowering CBF in hypertensive patients who have ongoing cerebral ischemia. Long-term treatment with antihypertensive agents readjusts the autoregulatory curve toward more normal values. Conversely, excessive reduction of blood pressure in previously normal patients to a mean arterial pressure of less than approximately 50 mm Hg inevitably leads to loss of autoregulation, possible expansion of an ischemic zone, or production of global cerebral ischemia. These injuries are seen in patients who are treated too aggressively with antihypertensive agents in the immediate aftermath of a stroke and in patients who are anesthetized during surgical procedures.

Blood-Brain Barrier

The brain's extracellular ionic and molecular environment is tightly regulated. Small changes in extracellular concentrations of Na^+, K^+, and Ca^{2+} ions or neurotransmitters, including glutamate, acetylcholine, and norepinephrine, alter neuronal function. Intracellular communication within the brain, perhaps its most important basic function, depends on a carefully controlled extracellular space. The blood-brain barrier (BBB), which has evolved to protect this milieu, is composed of unique endothelial cells that lack the usual transendothelial channels and closely abut one another in tight junctions. This anatomy protects the brain against the fluctuating composition of blood and reduces the entry of potentially toxic compounds. A negative consequence is that the BBB prevents the entry of polar molecules into the brain, thus limiting the utility of many drugs, small molecules, and proteins, which cannot gain entry into the brain by the oral or intravenous routes.

The entry of nutrients and egress of metabolic waste across the BBB can occur by simple diffusion, facilitated transport, or active transport. Lipid-soluble compounds can diffuse rapidly across endothelial cell membranes, whereas some polar compounds can be transported by special carrier molecules that are driven either by concentration gradients (facilitated transport) or through the expenditure of energy (active transport). Gas molecules, such as oxygen and carbon dioxide, freely diffuse across plasma membranes and rapidly equilibrate between blood and brain. Glucose, a highly polar molecule, enters the brain on a special glucose transporter. The rate of brain glucose transport is normally two to three times faster than the metabolism of glucose, but because glucose uptake depends so highly on its blood concentration, a reduction in blood glucose level to a third of normal, caused by either ischemia or hypoglycemia, may compromise normal brain energy metabolism.

CEREBRAL ISCHEMIA

Inadequate delivery of oxygen or glucose to the brain initiates a cascade of events that ultimately result in infarction. The severity of the insult, defined by the degree and duration of reduced blood flow, hypoxia, or hypoglycemia, determines whether the brain suffers only temporary dysfunction, such as a transient ischemic attack; irreversible injury to only a few of the most vulnerable neurons (selective necrosis); or cerebral infarction, in which damage occurs to extensive areas involving all cell types (pan-necrosis).

Types of Cerebral Hypoxia-Ischemia

Cerebral hypoxia-ischemia can be divided into focal ischemia caused by vascular occlusion, global ischemia as a result of complete cardiovascular failure, and diffuse hypoperfusion-hypoxia produced by respiratory disease or severely reduced blood pressure.

Focal Ischemia

Focal cerebral ischemia results most frequently from embolic or thrombotic occlusion of extracranial or intracranial blood vessels and the resulting reduction in blood flow within the related vascular territory. Blood flow to the central zone of the ischemic vascular bed is usually severely reduced but rarely reaches zero because of partial supply from collateral blood vessels. The best treatment option for this intensely ischemic region is acute restoration of blood flow. A transition zone may be present between the normally perfused tissue and the more ischemic central core. This rim of moderately deprived tissue has been called the *ischemic penumbra*. It is thought that brain cells in the penumbra remain viable for a longer time than do cells in the ischemic core. This marginally viable tissue may die if inadequate blood flow persists but may be salvaged by restoring flow or, possibly, by neuroprotective therapeutic agents. The size and duration of the penumbra are unknown in any individual patient and poorly defined by current diagnostic techniques. In more recent years, salvage of the penumbra with neuroprotective agents has been the subject of intense basic and clinical research.

Cerebral ischemia sufficient to cause clinical signs or symptoms, if severe, can produce irreversible injury to highly vulnerable neurons in 5 minutes. Progressively longer durations of ischemia increase the probability of permanent damage. If cerebral ischemia persists for more than about 6 hours, infarction of part or all of the involved vascular territory is completed, and the only strategies for therapy entail rehabilitation, such as treatment with neurotrophic factors or neural transplantation. Whether clinical evidence of permanent brain injury from ischemia is detectable depends on the location of the brain tissue involved.

Global Ischemia

Global cerebral ischemia results from cardiac asystole or ventricular fibrillation that reduces the blood flow rate to zero throughout the brain and body. Global ischemia for more than 5 to 10 minutes is generally incompatible with full recovery of consciousness in normothermic humans. If blood flow is restored in time to prevent cardiac death, selective ischemic necrosis usually involves the most vulnerable neurons in the CA1 pyramidal neurons of the hippocampus, the cerebellar Purkinje cells, and the pyramidal neurons in neocortical layers 3, 5, and 6. Anything that prevents adequate oxygen or glucose supply to the brain, such as hypoxemia, carbon monoxide poisoning, and severe and prolonged hypoglycemia, can also produce such injury. Cardiac resuscitation or other causes of prolonged hypotension may cause cerebral infarction, particularly in border zones that lie between the terminal branches of major arterial supplies, often termed *watershed zones*.

Diffuse Hypoxia

Diffuse cerebral hypoxia initially causes cerebral dysfunction but not irreversible brain injury. Individuals with cerebral hypoxia from high altitude, pulmonary disease, or severe anemia can exhibit confusion, cognitive impairment, and lethargy. The onset of coma heralds permanent brain damage. With acute changes in Pao_2 from normal to less than 40 mm Hg or a decrease in the hemoglobin concentration to less than 7 g/dL, compensatory increases in CBF become inadequate, and clinical signs and symptoms of cerebral hypoxia develop. A slower onset of reduced oxygenation, such as caused by moving to high elevations or the gradual development of anemia, permits compensation by a variety of mechanisms; if hypoxia increases, however, the compensation ultimately fails.

Neuropathology of Cerebral Ischemia

Four general classes of histopathologic damage can occur. Cerebral infarction caused by focal vascular occlusion is characterized by destruction of all cellular elements: neurons, glia, and endothelial cells (pannecrosis). Cerebral infarcts are initially grossly pale (anemic) or hemorrhagic (showing gross petechial bleeding). Later, necrotic tissue is removed and replaced by a glial scar or a cavity. Transient arrest of the cerebral circulation (global ischemia) can cause selective *ischemic necrosis* of highly vulnerable neurons. Using conventional stains, histologic change begins to outline the margins between living and dying neurons and glia within a few hours, although the full extent of damage may not be evident for several days. The neurologic functionality of the cells is irreversibly lost within the first 6 hours. Newer imaging techniques can reveal abnormal cell function much more rapidly than conventional histology can.

Cerebral *autolysis* is observed most frequently in brain-dead patients who are maintained on mechanical ventilators for more than a few days; it reflects enzymatic autodigestion of brain tissue. *Demyelination* of the central hemispheric white matter is usually a consequence of carbon monoxide poisoning or other prolonged periods of moderately severe hypoxemia or cerebral hypoperfusion. Development of these lesions may take several days, and the onset of neurologic dysfunction may be delayed. Patients may have a lucid interval after such an injury and subsequently manifest neurologic symptoms. Within these lesions, nerve cell axons are demyelinated, and oligodendroglial cells die.

Ischemic Cascade

In severe ischemia, energy-rich compounds become depleted within minutes. As energy-dependent membrane pumps fail, neuronal and glial cell membranes depolarize and allow the influx of Ca^{2+} ions. Elevated intracellular Ca^{2+} and other second messengers activate lipases and proteases, which release membrane-bound free fatty acids that denature proteins. Depolarization of presynaptic terminals releases abnormally high concentrations of excitatory neurotransmitters, such as glutamate, which may elevate metabolic demand at a time when energy supplies are inadequate and thus exacerbate the injury. If blood flow is restored within 5 minutes and there are no other complicating factors such as hyperglycemia, these events are completely reversible. As the duration of ischemia increases, selectively vulnerable neurons die first; if ischemia persists for hours or longer, cerebral infarction develops. Prompt restoration of blood flow permits full functional recovery and maintenance of tissue integrity. Tissues with partial depletion of ATP and impaired calcium homeostasis may benefit from pharmacologic therapies that reduce calcium movement through voltage- and neurotransmitter-dependent ion channels. Many other neuroprotective strategies have also been shown to be effective in animal models, including prevention of the detrimental actions of excitatory neurotransmitters, inhibition of many biochemical pathways leading to cell death, and therapies that may delay the denaturation of proteins. Thus far, however, none of these therapies has proved useful in clinical trials in stroke patients.

Leukocytes

More recently, the role of leukocytes in ischemic damage has been recognized. Two proposed mechanisms of injury are (1) microvascular occlusion from direct mechanical obstruction and damage to the endothelium and (2) infiltration into central nervous system tissue and cellular cytotoxic injury. The white blood cell–mediated damage may be irreversible even if blood flow is restored.

White blood cells require considerable deformation to pass through capillaries. When activated by chemotactic substances during ischemia, their cytoplasmic stiffness increases, and they adhere to capillary endothelium. Under conditions of reduced perfusion pressure, white blood cells may obstruct the microcirculation. This leukocyte capillary plugging may be the major cause of the *no-reflow phenomenon,* which is defined as incomplete restoration of normal blood flow after a period of ischemia. Areas of parenchyma that might be viable when blood flow returns are inadequately reperfused. This phenomenon was a laboratory curiosity until the advent of thrombolytic therapy; it may now be a cause of apparent stroke in evolution or the development of increased neurologic deficits after apparently successful thrombolysis.

Leukocytes may potentiate injury by toxic damage to vascular endothelium and by transendothelial migration to the parenchyma. Release of leukocyte granule contents, which include reactive oxygen metabolites and membrane phospholipases, can injure the endothelium and is usually responsible for removing necrotic tissue after irreversible damage. The resultant effects include increased endothelial permeability, interstitial edema, expansion and injury of individual cells (endothelial, glial, and neuronal), vasoconstriction, and generation of substances that induce further leukocyte adhesion.

Anoxic Encephalopathy

In industrialized countries, out-of-hospital cardiac arrest (Chapter 62) occurs in 0.04 to 0.13% of the total population per year. Only a minority of these patients will survive the arrest and be discharged with a good neurologic outcome, in part because of the risk for anoxic encephalopathy. If brain stem function is preserved but the cerebral hemispheres are destroyed, the patient enters a persistent vegetative state (Chapter 428).

CEREBRAL HEMORRHAGE

Bleeding into the subarachnoid space from a ruptured aneurysm or other vascular malformation produces a chemical (sterile) meningitis and can induce vasospasm, particularly in the vessels constituting the circle of Willis. If the vasospasm is sufficiently severe, it can result in cerebral infarction and death.

Intraparenchymal hemorrhage may be relatively benign. Bleeding into a region of previous infarction, called *hemorrhagic transformation,* causes no additional functional loss. Primary parenchymatous hemorrhage damages tissue in several ways, however. If a large vessel ruptures, the amount of bleeding into the brain can be severe. The portion of the vascular distribution distal to the site of rupture is no longer supplied with blood, and infarction results. At the site of rupture, bleeding into the brain may cause traumatic injury to the exposed tissue, and blood or its breakdown products in the parenchyma damage brain tissues. In addition, the extravascular blood in the brain parenchyma increases total brain volume, and the edema that forms rapidly in and around the site of bleeding increases the intracranial contents. Because cranial capacity is fixed, ICP increases rapidly, and cerebral herniation may occur.

The biochemical pathology caused by exposure of brain tissue to blood has not been established. Hypertension is closely associated with intracerebral hemorrhage. Research suggests that the matrix metalloproteinases in vessel walls are activated, thereby leading to degradation of vascular tissue with subsequent bleeding.

Cerebral Edema

A pathologic increase in the water content of brain tissue (edema) eventually develops in all types of ischemic and hemorrhagic stroke. Brain swelling and raised ICP relate proportionally to the volume of accumulated water; in some instances, edema can cause neurologic deterioration and death by herniation syndromes.

The intracranial space contains the brain, which weighs approximately 1400 g, about 75 mL of blood, and approximately 75 mL of cerebrospinal fluid (CSF). An increase in the volume of any of these contents must be accompanied by a decrease in another component because the intracranial cavity is of relatively fixed size and surrounded by bone. Normally the brain's tissue volume is constant, whereas intracranial blood and CSF vary reciprocally to maintain normal ICP. A variety of mechanisms can compensate for increased intracranial contents to a limited extent, including displacement of CSF into other cranial compartments, reduction of venous blood volume, reduction of normal cerebral interstitial fluid, and chronic cerebral atrophy. If there is a rapid increase in extravascular blood, reduced venous outflow, blockage or resorption of CSF, or cerebral edema, ICP markedly increases.

Brain edema is categorized on the basis of pathophysiologic and anatomic criteria as intracellular or interstitial. Intracellular edema, also called *cytotoxic edema,* develops as energy-dependent membrane ion pumps fail; as a result, Na^+ and other osmoles enter the cell and draw water in from the interstitial and vascular compartments. This process can begin within a few hours after the onset of ischemia. Cell swelling occurs predominantly in astrocytes, but neurons, oligodendroglial cells, and endothelial cells are also involved.

Interstitial edema, also called *vasogenic edema,* occurs later than the intracellular form. Damage to endothelial cells of the BBB allows macromolecules, such as plasma proteins, to enter the cerebral interstitial space accompanied by osmotically bound water. Interstitial edema after cerebral infarction progressively worsens for about 3 days after a stroke. Fluid accumulation within the vicinity of damaged endothelial cells and the zone of infarction can raise the local water content of brain by 10%. The osmolality of ischemic brain increases from 310 to approximately 350 mOsm. The intracellular accumulation of water increases from a normal value of approximately 79 to 81% of brain weight.

If cerebral circulation is reestablished before permanent brain injury develops, the intracellular edema resolves without permanent sequelae. A large increase in the brain's volume can, however, lead to transtentorial herniation of the cerebral hemispheres or to cerebellar herniation. These syndromes can result in irreversible global ischemia of the hemispheres or crushing of the brain stem, loss of cerebral control of the circulation, and death from respiratory arrest. The edema-induced increase in ICP usually reaches a maximum about 3 days after the onset of a stroke. If a patient has a large stroke and survives after the third day, the patient is unlikely to die as a result of that stroke.

SUGGESTED READINGS

Candelise L, Gattinoni M, Bersano A, et al: Stroke-unit care for acute stroke patients: An observational follow-up study. Lancet 2007;369:299–305. *Patients with acute stroke may benefit from hospitalization on a specialty stroke unit.*

Goldstein LB, Simel DL: Is this patient having a stroke? JAMA 2005; 293:2391–2402. *A case-based review.*

Savitz SI, Caplan LR: Vertebrobasilar disease. N Engl J Med 2005;352:2618–2626. *A comprehensive overview.*

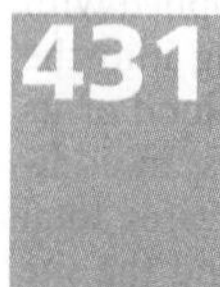

431 ISCHEMIC CEREBROVASCULAR DISEASE

Justin A. Zivin

Definition

Ischemic stroke is caused by insufficient blood flow to part or all of the brain. Focal stroke is conventionally defined as a neurologic deficit lasting more than 24 hours that is caused by reduced blood flow in an artery supplying part of the brain; the reduced blood flow ultimately results in infarction. Strokes are distinguished from transient ischemic attacks (TIAs) in that TIAs have historically been defined, arbitrarily, as ischemia-induced neurologic deficits persisting for less than 24 hours. Current thinking is that nearly all TIAs resolve more rapidly and a deficit that persists for more than 1 or 2 hours is likely to be associated with permanent brain damage, often demonstrable by computed tomography (CT) or magnetic resonance imaging (MRI), despite complete clinical recovery. The important distinction between a TIA and a stroke is whether the ischemia has caused brain infarction or selective ischemic necrosis, a difference that may not be possible to distinguish within the first few hours after the onset of symptoms but commonly becomes apparent retrospectively. During the early phases, when acute therapy is potentially beneficial, it is impossible to predict whether a patient will recover because the treatment is effective only if given before it is known whether the symptoms will resolve spontaneously.

Ischemic strokes are differentiated from hemorrhagic strokes (Chapter 432) by the lack of extravasated blood in the brain parenchyma. There are two main classifications of ischemic stroke. *Thrombosis* and *embolism,* which are caused by arterial occlusion with either a thrombus that forms locally at the site of an atherosclerotic plaque or an embolic clot, are responsible for 65% of all strokes. Emboli are produced when a piece of a larger clot breaks off from a mural thrombus in the heart or a more proximal artery and lodges downstream at a point where the diameter of the vessel has decreased in size so that the clot can no longer pass through the arterial lumen. It is often impossible to distinguish a thrombus from an embolus by imaging methods or histopathologic material, so the two processes are classified together. *Small vessel strokes,* commonly called *lacunes,* are caused by occlusion of small arterioles and account for about 20% of strokes. The histologic lesion in blood vessels in these strokes is classically called lipohyalinosis, which does not help in identifying the cause of these strokes. Some of these strokes are caused by local vascular abnormalities, but others are almost certainly caused by small emboli. The other 15% or so of strokes are caused by hemorrhage (Chapter 432).

Epidemiology

Hypertension is the most important risk factor for ischemic and hemorrhagic stroke (Chapter 66). The incidence of stroke increases directly in relation to the degree of elevation of systolic and diastolic arterial blood pressure above threshold values. More important, there has been conclusive evidence for more than 30 years that control of hypertension prevents strokes. Meta-analyses of randomized controlled trials confirm an approximate 30 to 40% reduction in stroke risk with lowering of blood pressure.

Approximately 7 to 10% of men and 5 to 7% of women older than 65 years have asymptomatic carotid stenosis of greater than 50%. Epidemiologic studies suggest that the rate of unheralded stroke ipsilateral to a stenosis is about 1 to 2% annually.

Nonvalvar atrial fibrillation (Chapter 63) carries a 3 to 5% annual risk for stroke, with the risk becoming even higher in the presence of advanced age, previous TIA or stroke, hypertension, impaired left ventricular function, and diabetes mellitus.

In epidemiologic studies, the risk for stroke in smokers is almost double that in nonsmokers, but the risk becomes essentially identical to that of nonsmokers by 2 to 5 years after quitting. The relative risk for stroke is two to six times greater for patients with insulin-dependent diabetes (Chapter 247). Patients with sickle cell disease (Chapter 167) have a markedly increased risk for stroke. Hyperlipidemia also increases the risk for stroke, and reduction of low-density lipoprotein cholesterol levels with statins reduces this risk. Some evidence suggests that abdominal obesity in men and obesity and weight gain in women are independent risk factors for stroke. Weight reduction in overweight people is recommended, but weight loss has not been proved to reduce the risk for stroke.

Epidemiologic studies have found that consumption of fruits and vegetables is associated with a lower risk for stroke, but no randomized trials have proved the value of changing dietary habits. Heavy alcohol consumption may be a risk factor for ischemic and hemorrhagic stroke.

Postmenopausal hormone replacement therapy has been shown to increase the risk for stroke. The absolute risk for stroke remains low, however, in otherwise healthy, low-risk patients. Meta-analysis suggests an increase in the relative risk for stroke in women taking oral contraceptives, but the absolute risk for stroke is small. Women who smoke, are hypertensive or diabetic, have migraine headaches, or have previously suffered thromboembolic events may be at increased risk for stroke when taking oral contraceptives.

Pathobiology

The precise signs and symptoms of ischemic stroke depend primarily on the region deprived of blood flow. The tempo with which deficits develop has important clinical implications.

Pattern of Development of Strokes

Shortly after the onset of vascular occlusion, it is common for symptoms and signs to fluctuate and either to improve or to deteriorate, often rapidly. Some patients may be in denial and anticipate that their symptoms will resolve, thereby resulting in delay in seeking medical care until sufficient time has elapsed that acute therapy is useless.

If the symptoms resolve completely in 1 or 2 hours, the patient has had a TIA. The basis for this resolution is unclear. Possibilities include dissolution of an embolus with subsequent restoration of normal regional blood flow, decrease in vasospasm, and improvement in perfusion secondary to increased collateral flow.

Ischemic episodes that ultimately develop into infarction often fluctuate for several hours after onset. Early in the course it is impossible to predict what will happen. Recovery may stop suddenly, and deficits may plateau or increase. Persistence of any neurologic deficit beyond 2 hours, even if the patient subsequently recovers fully, is nearly always accompanied by some degree of tissue destruction.

Hours to days after the abnormality becomes stable, increased neurologic deficits may develop, a deterioration termed *stroke in evolution.* Probable reasons include reperfusion injury, clot extension, or a new stroke in the same vascular distribution. Compromised cardiac output and systemic hypotension resulting from myocardial ischemia, cardiac arrhythmias, or heart failure may also contribute in some cases. Patients may appear to have stroke in evolution because of systemic disorders, such as electrolyte imbalances or glucose abnormalities that initially appear to be exacerbations of a stroke but are really comorbid problems that do not cause extension of the infarct. Cerebral edema may increase neurologic deterioration in large strokes by causing herniation syndromes. Secondary bleeding into an infarct can occur; ordinarily, this process does not increase neurologic deficits unless the blood extends into an area outside the initial boundaries of the infarction or causes a mass effect and increased intracranial pressure. The term *stroke in evolution* describes a clinical picture rather than a specific pathologic process.

Complete versus Incomplete Strokes

A stroke is called *complete* if the total area of the brain supplied by an occluded vessel is damaged. If so, prophylactic therapies to prevent further extension are of no benefit. If there is some cellular damage (loss of neurons) but not cystic pan-necrosis, the stroke is called *incomplete.* If a stroke is incomplete, additional tissue in the vascular distribution is at risk, and prophylaxis should be considered. Distinguishing between complete and incomplete strokes based on clinical findings can be impossible, particularly during the early phases of a stroke. At present, no diagnostic method can reliably identify threatened tissue. Distinction between a complete and an incomplete stroke, as a practical matter, is often based on whether a patient has all the manifestations of one of the common stroke syndromes or just some of them.

Common Causes and Pathogenesis Of Stroke

Atherosclerosis

Atherosclerosis (Chapter 69) is the most common disorder that leads to stroke. Atherosclerotic plaques are thought to cause stroke in three ways: (1) mural thrombosis forms at the site of an atherosclerotic lesion, and the clot obstructs the artery at that location; (2) ulceration or rupture of a plaque leads to formation of a clot and distal embolization; and (3) hemorrhage into a plaque obstructs the artery. The clinical manifestations of a stroke depend on the rate of occlusion. If occlusion occurs slowly, there may be time for collateral blood supply to develop, and a stroke is avoided. If the occlusion is abrupt, a stroke ensues, and the degree of damage depends on the extent of collateral supply that is available to the territory of the brain supplied by the occluded vessel. If collateral supply is marginal, just enough blood may pass through the stenotic region to maintain minimally adequate blood flow. In these circumstances, neurologic function may become critically dependent on changes in blood pressure, and small decreases can cause a stroke or recurrent TIAs.

More frequently, a platelet-fibrin thrombus forms on the roughened surface of an atherosclerotic plaque. The thrombus can break off and float distally in the blood stream, eventually becoming lodged in a distal, smaller branch; this process is termed *artery-to-artery embolization.* These embolic occlusions are more likely to be symptomatic because the more distal end vessels have no collateral supply. The amount of territory that is deprived of blood is smaller, however, and symptoms are usually less severe than with occlusion of the main stem of a vessel. The most common locations for an intravascular thrombus to form are the base of the aorta, the bifurcation of the common carotid artery, or the point at which the vertebral arteries originate from the subclavian arteries.

Emboli of Cardiac Origin

Emboli originating from the heart may lodge in any part of the body; however, because about 20% of the normal cardiac output goes to the brain, it is a common site of cardioembolism. Thrombus formation and release of emboli from the heart are promoted by arrhythmias and by structural abnormalities of the valves and chambers. The frequency of the various types of stroke produced by cardioembolism can only be estimated. Although some strokes are clearly embolic in origin and others are unquestionably thrombotic, it is generally impossible to distinguish them pathologically. There is no diagnostic test to prove that a thrombus or embolus is of cardiac origin.

Mural Thrombi

Myocardial infarction may produce a region of dyskinetic myocardium that predisposes to the formation of mural thrombi (Chapter 72). Anterior wall myocardial infarction is associated with the highest frequency of thromboembolic strokes. Cardiomyopathies (Chapter 59), such as those caused by alcohol abuse or viral infections, also produce dyskinesia that promotes mural thrombi and can result in cerebral embolization, as can any cause of severe heart failure (Chapter 58). In some instances, a cardiac mural thrombus may release numerous pieces that produce a shower of emboli and cause several simultaneous strokes at various locations in the brain.

Valvular Heart Disease

Rheumatic heart disease (Chapter 313), which is now rare in industrialized countries, is associated with systemic emboli, especially in patients who have mitral stenosis (Chapter 75). Acute or subacute infectious endocarditis (Chapter 76) produces vegetations on heart valves, and these vegetations can embolize to the cerebral circulation. Endocarditis caused by staphylococci, fungi, or yeast is often extensive enough to occlude large intracranial arteries. Infective endocarditis is associated with other forms of cerebrovascular disease, including intracerebral hemorrhage, subarachnoid hemorrhage, and mycotic aneurysm (Chapter 432). Strokes can occur during the acute phases of the disease, and the combination of fever, a new murmur, and petechiae should prompt collection of blood for culture and consideration of empirical treatment with antibiotics. Anticoagulants may increase the risk for intracerebral hemorrhage in patients with bacterial endocarditis.

Nonbacterial endocarditis (Chapter 59), which is usually associated with various types of cancer, can also give rise to vegetations that produce cerebral embolization and cause focal strokes or diffuse encephalopathy, sometimes in the form of disseminated intravascular coagulopathy. Systemic lupus erythematosus (Chapter 287) is associated with atypical verrucous (Libman-Sacks) endocarditis in which friable vegetations form on the leaflets of any of the heart valves and can rarely produce cerebral embolization.

In patients with prosthetic heart valves, the incidence of stroke is 1 to 5% per year despite oral anticoagulation (Chapter 75). Mechanical valves have a higher risk than biologic valves do. Many studies have suggested that anticoagulants reduce but do not completely eliminate cerebral embolization in these patients.

Arrhythmias

Atrial fibrillation, independent of the presence or absence of valvar disease, is a proven cause of embolic stroke and increases the relative risk, when compared with age-matched controls, to about 5% per year (Chapter 63). Approximately 15% of all ischemic strokes are associated with nonvalvar atrial fibrillation. Most patients with atrial fibrillation never have a stroke, however. The strokes are often large and disabling, but minor strokes, silent strokes, and TIAs can occur. Most ischemic strokes in patients with atrial fibrillation are due to embolism from left atrial mural thrombi. The risk for atrial fibrillation–associated strokes is increased in patients who have chronic hypertension. The risk for embolic stroke is highest shortly after the development of atrial fibrillation, but embolism can also accompany cardioversion to normal sinus rhythm regardless of whether the conversion is spontaneous, induced by medication or electrical.

Paradoxical Emboli

Embolic occlusion of intracranial vessels can be of venous origin. The embolic material gains access to the arterial circulation through various cardiac defects, such as a patent foramen ovale, atrial septal defect (Chapter 68), or arteriovenous malformation. When venous emboli enter the heart, a right-to-left shunt allows the emboli to enter the arterial circulation. A patent foramen ovale has been detected in 40% of patients with acute ischemic stroke of uncertain origin, and it is often assumed that paradoxical embolization is the cause of the stroke. Patients with an atrial septal aneurysm and a patent foramen ovale are at highest risk.

Clinical Manifestations

The clinical manifestations are summarized in Table 431–1.

Internal Carotid Artery

The common carotid artery bifurcation, at the origin of the internal carotid artery (ICA), is the most frequent site of atherosclerotic lesions

TABLE 431-1 CLINICAL MANIFESTATIONS OF ISCHEMIC STROKE

Occluded Blood Vessel	Clinical Manifestations
ICA	Ipsilateral blindness (variable) MCA syndrome (see below)
MCA	Contralateral hemiparesis, sensory loss (arm, face worst) Expressive aphasia (dominant) or anosognosia and spatial disorientation (nondominant) Contralateral inferior quadrantanopsia
ACA	Contralateral hemiparesis, sensory loss (worst in leg)
PCA	Contralateral homonymous hemianopia or superior quadrantanopia Memory impairment
Basilar apex	Bilateral blindness Amnesia
Basilar artery	Contralateral hemiparesis, sensory loss Ipsilateral bulbar or cerebellar signs
Vertebral artery or PICA	Ipsilateral loss of facial sensation, ataxia, contralateral hemiparesis, sensory loss
Superior cerebellar artery	Gait ataxia, nausea, dizziness, headache progressing to ipsilateral hemiataxia, dysarthria, gaze paresis, contralateral hemiparesis, somnolence

ACA = anterior cerebral artery; ICA = internal carotid artery; MCA = middle cerebral artery; PCA = posterior cerebral artery; PICA = posterior inferior cerebellar artery.

of the cerebral vasculature. Occlusion of the ICA is often clinically silent if the circle of Willis is complete. It is often impossible to distinguish ICA occlusion from similar damage to the middle cerebral artery (MCA) on clinical examination (see later). Because the ophthalmic artery originates from the ICA, however, TIAs of the ICA may be manifested as transient monocular blindness (also called *amaurosis fugax*). Severe stenosis of the ICA, particularly if bilateral, can cause hypoperfusion of the cerebral hemispheres and symptoms in border zones between the MCA and other major vascular territories (watershed areas), especially if superimposed on generalized hypoperfusion secondary to severe hypotension.

Anterior Cerebral Artery

Isolated occlusion of the anterior cerebral artery (ACA), which is relatively rare in comparison to strokes in other major branches of the circle of Willis, accounts for about 2% of all cerebral infarcts. The principal symptoms associated with occlusion of an ACA distal to the anterior communicating artery are upper motor neuron weakness and cortical sensory deficits (neglect) in the contralateral leg. Other manifestations of ACA occlusion can include urinary incontinence, generalized depression of psychomotor activity (abulia), and transcortical motor aphasia manifested as loss of verbal fluency with preserved ability to repeat. Bilateral occlusion may occur because the origins of the two ACAs are separated by only a short stretch of anterior communicating artery, and there are frequent anomalies in which both ACAs originate from a common source. Bilateral damage usually causes a patient to be mute, with severe mood disturbances and long-lasting incontinence from bilateral damage to the frontal lobes.

Middle Cerebral Artery

Strokes in the distribution of the MCA are the most common type of focal stroke, and such strokes cause approximately two thirds of all infarcts. Occlusion of the stem of the MCA often results in massive, devastating infarction of much of the hemisphere. Edema during the first 3 to 4 days may lead to severely increased intracranial pressure and herniation. The classic picture of occlusion of the MCA stem is contralateral weakness and sensory loss in the face and arm (with relative sparing of the leg) and homonymous hemianopia on the side of the weakness; initially, there may be depressed consciousness and deviation of gaze toward the side of the lesion. There is little chance of substantial recovery. In right-handed people, occlusion of the left MCA produces global aphasia in which the patient can neither understand the speech of others nor produce meaningful speech. In the nondominant hemisphere, unilateral neglect, anosognosia (unawareness of the deficit), and spatial disorientation occur.

Occlusion of branches of the MCA produces partial syndromes. An embolus to the MCA frequently lodges in one of its two main divisions. Occlusion of the superior division can cause dense sensorimotor deficits in the contralateral face and arm without initial impairment of alertness. Later, some neurologic function may recover, and the aphasia may decrease. Strokes of the inferior division in the dominant hemisphere characteristically produce receptive aphasia of the Wernicke type (severe loss of speech comprehension with preserved spoken and written language). Damage to either hemisphere can result in contralateral loss of integrated sensation, such as perception of shapes (stereognosis). Occlusion of more distal branches causes less clinical damage.

Posterior Cerebral Artery

In about three quarters of people, both posterior cerebral arteries (PCAs) arise from the basilar artery; in most others, one PCA arises from the basilar artery and the other arises from the ICA. In a few individuals, both PCAs originate from the ICAs. As a consequence, the syndromes associated with occlusion of the PCA are highly variable. Strokes of the perforating branches most frequently cause complete contralateral hemianesthesia with loss of all sensation and complete hemianopia on that side. Macular (central) vision may be spared because of collateral blood supply from the MCA. Difficulty reading (dyslexia) and performing calculations (dyscalculia) may occur. Recovery is often good, but the initial numbness may be replaced by paresthesias or excruciating pain; this Dejerine-Roussy syndrome is caused by damage to the thalamus. Involvement of the subthalamic nucleus may produce hemiballismus, with wild flinging movements of the limbs on one side of the body. Distal branch occlusions of the PCA cause partial syndromes; occlusion of the terminal branch can produce a variety of incomplete visual field deficits, although the loss is characteristically congruous (superimposable) in both visual fields.

Vertebral and Basilar Arteries

Characteristic of occlusion of the blood supply to the brain stem are "crossed syndromes" (i.e., contralateral loss of strength and selected contralateral and ipsilateral sensory symptoms below the level of the lesion, in addition to ipsilateral motor and sensory deficits localized to the level of the lesion). Weber's syndrome is caused by a mesencephalic lesion that produces an ipsilateral third cranial nerve palsy resulting from damage to the oculomotor nerve, as well as contralateral weakness.

The vertebral arteries are the principal blood supply for the medulla. The posterior inferior cerebellar artery is usually a branch of the vertebral artery. The consequences of occlusion of the posterior inferior cerebellar artery are variable, but lateral medullary infarction (Wallenberg's syndrome) is classically produced. In about 80% of cases, occlusion of the vertebral artery causes lateral medullary syndrome, which consists of severe vertigo, nausea, vomiting, nystagmus, ipsilateral ataxia (of the cerebellar type), and ipsilateral Horner's syndrome (ptosis, myosis, and decreased sweating). The syndrome also includes ipsilateral loss of facial pain and temperature sensation and contralateral loss of these sensory modalities in the trunk and limb. Partial syndromes are the rule; a complete lateral medullary syndrome is rare, so it is often misdiagnosed.

The basilar artery supplies most of the brain stem, and occlusion of this artery produces a variety of syndromes. Obstruction of the basilar artery trunk is often fatal because the main motor and sensory pathways between the cerebral hemispheres and the remainder of the body are compact and travel through the brain stem. The findings in occlusion of the basilar artery consist of a combination of bilateral sensory and motor long-tract signs, cerebellar dysfunction, and cranial nerve abnormalities: paralysis or weakness of all extremities and the bulbar muscles, impaired vision with various visual field defects, bilateral cerebellar ataxia, and a variety of sensory disturbances ranging from normal to total anesthesia. Coma may occur, or the locked-in syndrome may develop in which consciousness is preserved but the victims are unable to move anything voluntarily except their eyes or eyelids. It is possible to communicate with these patients and demonstrate normal mental status by codes involving eye movements.

Occlusion of the various branches of the basilar artery produces a large variety of syndromes. Because the pathways are so closely spaced in the brain stem, even small brain infarctions can cause substantial motor and sensory deficits. The characteristic findings are crossed syndromes with motor and sensory dissociation, unless the findings are bilateral. Distinguishing mild vertebrobasilar ischemia from the common causes of dizziness is occasionally difficult (Chapter 427), but ischemia is rarely a cause of isolated vertigo in the absence of other brain stem signs or symptoms.

Diagnosis

The history gives initial clues about the site and severity of a stroke, and the physical examination helps refine a hypothesis on the location of the lesion. Based on this information, definitive laboratory testing can proceed efficiently.

History

As the name implies, stroke ordinarily starts at a clearly identifiable time. The most important aspect of the history, which must be elicited from a patient or accompanying observers if a stroke is suspected, is the time of onset of symptoms. If abnormalities began within the preceding 3 hours, the patient should be managed as an acute emergency, and thrombolytic therapy may be indicated. Patients may be confused, anxious, or aphasic, and they may not remember the duration of symptoms. It may be necessary to try to associate the onset of symptoms with events that the patient or accompanying persons can identify accurately. Did the patient wake up with symptoms? In this case the symptoms must be assumed, in terms of considering acute treatment, to have started at the time that the patient was last known to be in a premorbid state—usually at the time of going to sleep. Was the patient watching television, and if so, what program was it? Consultation with the program guide in the newspaper can be used to assign a time of onset. Was an ambulance called, and if so, what time was the patient first examined by paramedics? This information is usually available in the ambulance records.

TIAs may not be distinguishable from a stroke during the early phases, but TIAs usually resolve within the first hour or two. Rapid progression of deficits or the presence of headache occurs more often in patients with intracerebral hemorrhage (Chapter 432). Although intracerebral hemorrhage is responsible for only about 15% of strokes, hemorrhages generally produce more severe symptoms that cannot be denied. By comparison, patients with minor strokes or predominantly sensory symptoms are often in a state of denial and do not seek medical care until long after vessel occlusion. Because ischemic strokes are nearly always painless, they do not awaken patients from sleep and are frequently discovered at the time of normal awakening in the morning. There is some diurnal variation in the onset of stroke, with a peak in the late morning.

Physical Examination

The neurologic examination (Chapter 418) is a cost-effective method for initiating a diagnostic evaluation, and it often helps localize the site of the lesion. The cardiovascular examination (Chapter 48) should focus on measurement of arterial blood pressure, including measurement in both arms to evaluate the possibility of aortic dissection (Chapter 78) or vascular abnormalities that result in reduced blood flow to the brain when the arms are exercised (subclavian steal). The greatest risk factor for stroke is preexisting hypertension. In many patients, transient hypertension develops in the immediate aftermath of a stroke, however, so it is important to determine whether a patient has had sustained hypertension (Chapter 66). Extremely elevated blood pressure at initial evaluation can lead to heart failure, which may have to be managed urgently. If hypertension is a transient manifestation of acute stroke, aggressive reduction may cause hypotension and enlarge the infarct. The pulse may reveal arrhythmias, such as atrial fibrillation, that can result in cerebral embolism. Cardiac murmurs may suggest valvular lesions (Chapter 75) that can cause cerebral embolism. Bruits of the carotid arteries can be produced by atherosclerotic disease of the arteries, and such disease is associated with embolic and thrombotic strokes. Evidence of peripheral vascular disease (Chapter 79) may be a reflection of generalized atherosclerosis.

Ophthalmoscopic visualization of retinal cholesterol or platelet-fibrin emboli suggests more proximal atherosclerotic disease. Examination of the retinal vessels may also reveal signs of chronic hypertension or diabetes (arteriovenous crossing defects or retinal hemorrhages; Chapter 449).

The neurologic examination usually suggests the location and size of the stroke. If the patient's mental status is depressed, bilateral cerebral lesions or a brain stem lesion is suggested. Multiple smaller strokes may lead to dementia. Speech is commonly affected, with various aphasic patterns suggesting the site of the lesion. Testing of strength, sensation, and deep tendon reflexes provides information about the patterns of the deficits and suggests the site of the vascular lesion. Plantar stimulation (Babinski's sign), which is a classic finding in patients with damage to the long tracts, indicates upper motor neuron damage caused by stroke. However, during the early phases of a large stroke, reflexes may be depressed rather than hyperactive.

Laboratory Examination

Hematologic Tests

A complete hemogram, including a platelet count, is essential to evaluate for polycythemia (Chapter 172), thrombocytosis, bacterial endocarditis (Chapter 76), and severe anemia. An erythrocyte sedimentation rate is also a useful screening test because it may be elevated in patients with hypercoagulable states (Chapter 182) and is markedly elevated in patients with giant cell arteritis (Chapter 292). A blood glucose level must be checked because hyperglycemia and hypoglycemia can produce focal and global neurologic deficits, sometimes mimicking stroke. Diabetes (Chapter 247) increases the risk for stroke, and stroke may be the initial symptom of diabetes. A prothrombin time and partial thromboplastin time should be obtained in patients who may have received anticoagulants before the onset of stroke to determine whether they have been taking their medications or the anticoagulation is excessive.

Although moderate hyperlipidemia is not a proven risk factor, extremely high lipid levels are strongly associated with stroke. Antiphospholipid antibodies are elevated in some patients with immune-related diseases. Measurement of protein C, protein S, antithrombin III, blood viscosity, and platelet function (Chapter 182) and tests for homocysteinuria, collagen vascular diseases (Chapter 277), amyloidosis (Chapter 296), and syphilis (Chapter 340) should be performed in selected cases.

Cardiovascular Testing

Patients with acute myocardial infarction or a new or chronic atrial arrhythmia may have suffered an embolic stroke. A standard electrocardiogram and rhythm strip should be obtained at initial evaluation to determine whether acute myocardial ischemia or arrhythmia is present. Echocardiography is indicated urgently only in patients with a history of cardiac disease and an abnormal electrocardiogram; if no cause for the stroke is identified, however, particularly if the patient is relatively young, echocardiography is generally indicated.

Noninvasive Brain Imaging

Brain imaging (Chapter 419), which is essential to verify causes of focal neurologic dysfunction, can generally distinguish ischemic stroke from other diseases. The most important disorders to differentiate from acute ischemic stroke are intracerebral hemorrhage (Chapter 432), subarachnoid hemorrhage (Chapter 432), and brain tumors (Chapter 199).

CT is the standard initial imaging study (Fig. 431–1). Non–contrast-enhanced imaging usually detects intracerebral hemorrhage. Signals indicating tissue hypodensity, particularly in the region of the brain appropriate to the neurologic deficits, and loss of the distinction between gray and white matter are often observed 3 to 24 hours after the onset of stroke. These findings cannot predict the size of the infarction, however, and noncontrast CT findings may be normal for 3 to 24 hours after an ischemic stroke. The hypodensity typically becomes progressively more apparent over the first 3 to 24 hours and is usually readily detectable by 24 hours in patients with large infarcts. Small ischemic strokes in the brain stem can produce major neurologic dysfunction and may not be detected by CT. Contrast enhancement of CT scans seldom improves detection of acute stroke, but it may distinguish ischemic lesions from some types of neoplasms.

CT is currently the only imaging method useful for deciding whether to administer thrombolytic therapy. Detection of hemorrhage in areas of infarction is important because it precludes thrombolytic therapy. Small hemorrhages may be detected by CT scanning during the first few hours but may not have clinical importance. Hemorrhages become more

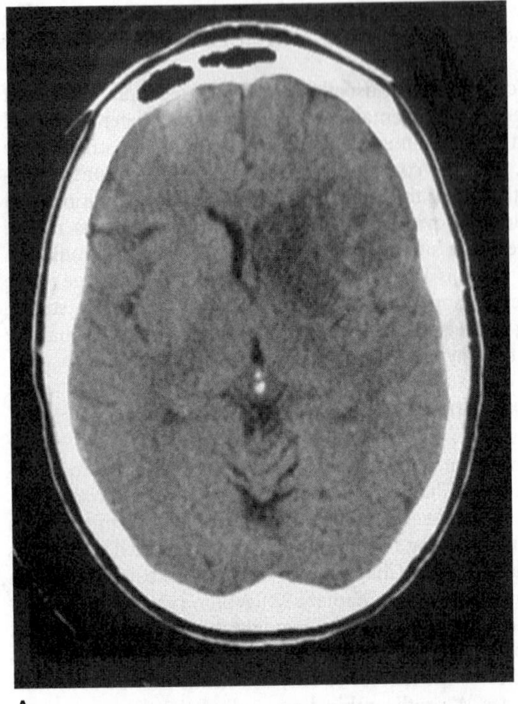

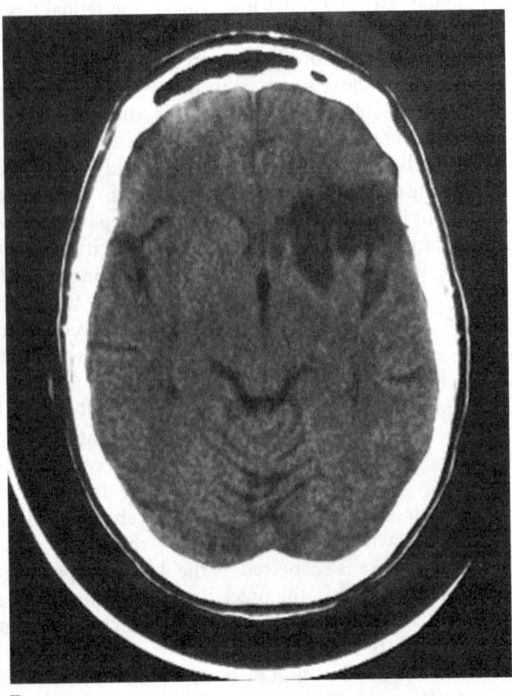

FIGURE 431–1 • Computed tomographic imaging. A, A computed tomography (CT) scan of a patient with a left hemisphere infarction 6 to 24 hours after the onset of symptoms shows a hypodense area in the basal ganglia region and compression of the frontal horn of the lateral ventricle. **B,** A CT scan shows the chronic infarction 1 year later; atrophy and loss of tissue volume are visible. (Courtesy of Gregory W. Albers, Stanford University, Stanford, CA.)

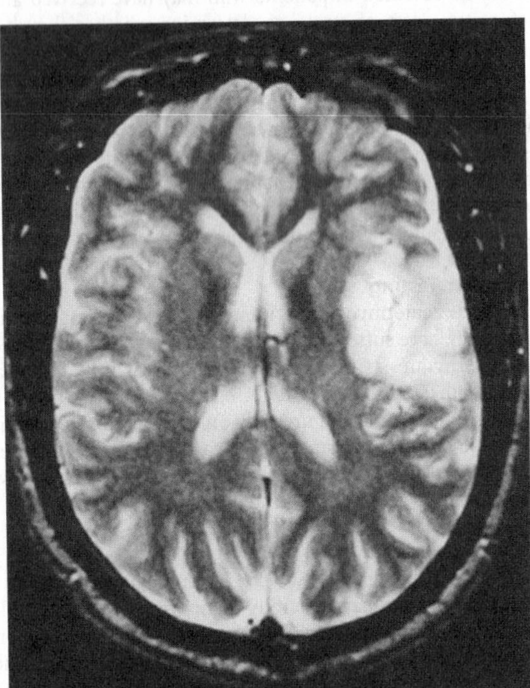

FIGURE 431–2 • Magnetic resonance imaging showing early ischemic changes obtained 6 hours after the onset of right-sided weakness in a patient with an occluded left internal carotid artery. (Courtesy of Gregory W. Albers, Stanford University, Stanford, CA.)

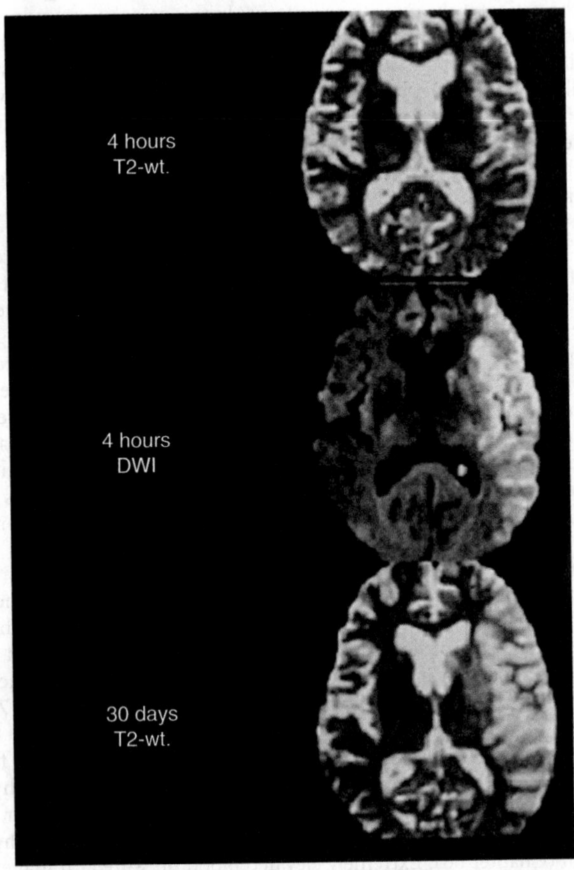

FIGURE 431–3 • Magnetic resonance imaging (MRI) showing possible advantages of diffusion-weighted imaging (DWI) relative to conventional MRI at early times after vascular occlusion. Top, Conventional T2-weighted MRI 4 hours after symptom onset that appears normal. **Middle,** At the same time, a DWI scan shows abnormalities in the left hemisphere. **Bottom,** Repeat T2-weighted MRI 1 month later showed an infarction in the same location as the initial DWI scan. (Courtesy of Gregory W. Albers, Stanford University, Stanford, CA.)

evident with time and appear on repeat scans hours to weeks after infarction. Whether this apparent increase in the detection of hemorrhage is due to a progressive increase in the size of the initial hemorrhage or to alterations in the extravasated blood is not known.

MRI is more sensitive than CT for detecting early ischemia (Fig. 431–2). MRI sequences can identify tissue or blood flow abnormalities within minutes after the onset of ischemia (Fig. 431–3). These early indicators of tissue injury are qualitative and have not been shown to predict the ultimate volume of the lesion or whether the tissue damage is irreversible. MRI cannot be used in patients who have ferromagnetic materials within their bodies, is often impossible to use in critically ill patients, and renders the patient inaccessible for several minutes. No MRI sequences successfully distinguish ischemia from hemorrhage, especially during the early phases of injury, when decisions regarding whether thrombolysis should be administered are needed. CT remains the imaging procedure of choice for acute patient management.

Lumbar Puncture

Lumbar puncture is no longer performed routinely in the evaluation of a patient with stroke because CT detects intracerebral hemorrhage more reliably (Chapter 419). CT can also usually identify blood in the subarachnoid space, although lumbar puncture is more sensitive for this purpose and can give some indication about when the bleeding occurred (Chapter 432). After subarachnoid hemorrhage, erythrocytes hemolyze. As hemoglobin is metabolized, cerebrospinal fluid becomes xanthochromic. Lumbar puncture is required to determine whether a patient has neurosyphilis (Chapter 340), although screening blood testing should be conducted first. Lumbar puncture is also occasionally indicated if there is concern that a patient may have bacterial meningitis (Chapter 437).

Noninvasive Cerebrovascular Examination

Ultrasonography provides an estimate of luminal diameter and the direction and speed of blood flow. B-mode ultrasonography, which produces real-time images of the carotid vessels, and range-gated pulsed Doppler, which is guided visually by the B-mode image, can detect increased blood velocity through a stenotic lumen. The combination of the location of the Doppler frequency signal and the B-mode image provides a noninvasive method for analyzing the condition of the extracranial circulation. Limitations of the technique include (1) access to only the portion of the carotid circulation that lies between the clavicles and the mandible (in approximately 10% of patients, the carotid bifurcation lies above the angle of the jaw, thus making ultrasonography difficult or impossible); (2) absorption of sound waves by calcium within a mural plaque, a process that may "shadow" and obscure a plaque on a distal vessel wall; and (3) echolucency of acute thrombi, which can be indistinguishable from flowing blood. The direction and velocity of blood flow in the intracranial blood vessels originating from the circle of Willis can be examined with low-frequency pulsed transcranial Doppler. Although these methods are useful screening techniques with essentially no risk to the patient, the "gold standard" for defining the status of the cerebral vasculature remains cerebral angiography. Moreover, ultrasound technique is critically dependent on the training and skill of the technician; there is considerable variation among different laboratories, and the clinician must confirm new or suspicious findings with repeat examinations or other tests.

CT and MR angiography can visualize the larger cerebral vessels and detect abnormalities such as stenosis, aneurysms, or arteriovenous malformations. These methods lack sensitivity for small lesions, however, and the degree of stenosis tends to be exaggerated.

Cerebral Angiography

Cerebral angiography is reserved for patients who are suspected to have a surgically correctable lesion. Arterial vessels are displayed initially, and delayed images can outline the venous system. Patients commonly receive anticoagulants during the procedure. The images give high-quality resolution of the vessels but do not provide quantitative information about blood flow. This method is the only one that has been proved to be useful for selecting patients who can benefit from carotid endarterectomy.

Angiography, particularly in patients with abnormal vasculature, can itself cause stroke and result in permanent neurologic deficits or death. The rate of injury varies in different surveys but is about 0.5% in good facilities. Angiography requires exposure to ionizing radiation, may be associated with adverse reactions to the contrast material, and involves a fluid load that poses a risk to patients with severe cardiac disease.

Other Techniques

Single-photon emission computed tomography provides only qualitative blood flow rates. Positron emission tomography quantitatively measures blood flow or brain metabolism. CT and MRI methods for measurement of cerebral blood flow and metabolism are in development. None of these techniques have yet been shown to be useful for the management of stroke patients (Chapter 419).

Differential Diagnosis

The characteristic feature of ischemic stroke is the abrupt, painless onset of a neurologic deficit. Blood supply is lost in the distribution of a terminal vessel, and loss of function begins within seconds. The brain does not have pain receptors in its parenchyma, so the symptoms are painless unless the dura mater, which does have pain fibers, is stretched or irritated. One type of stroke that can evolve slowly is subdural hematoma (Chapter 432), which may be distinguishable from ischemic stroke because a hematoma produces deficits more slowly. Focal symptoms and signs of tumors (Chapter 199) of various types typically evolve over a period of weeks or longer, except in uncommon cases in which a tumor erodes a vessel and causes bleeding or crushes it and causes infarction. TIAs cannot initially be distinguished from strokes, but they generally resolve within the first 1 or 2 hours.

Other neurologic disorders can be manifested as an abrupt onset of neurologic abnormalities. Migraine (Chapter 421) with or without aura may simulate stroke or TIA because of its associated hemiparesis or other focal deficits. Migraine is primarily an exquisitely painful, throbbing, unilateral headache that sometimes has an aura (symptoms preceding the headache) of scintillating scotomas (flashing lights). Complicated migraine (migraine accompanied by focal deficits) can rarely evolve into a true ischemic stroke, probably because of the decreased blood flow that often accompanies migraine.

Seizures (Chapter 426) can be confused with TIAs. Many seizures produce tonic (sustained) or clonic (rapid) motor activity or positive sensory phenomena. Strokes and TIAs produce weakness and sensory loss without involuntary motor activity. Seizures can sometimes be associated with these negative symptoms, particularly in the postictal state after (unobserved) seizures. The patient generally returns to the premorbid state after a seizure, however. Serial observations usually permit the differentiation of stroke from seizure, but early differentiation may be difficult and require laboratory testing, particularly an electroencephalogram. In a few patients with stroke, especially with emboli, a seizure occurs at the onset of the stroke.

Hyperglycemia and hypoglycemia can cause focal neurologic deficits. Most patients have a history of diabetes, and the glucose abnormality is substantial at the time of focal neurologic deficits.

Hemorrhagic stroke (Chapter 432) cannot generally be definitively distinguished from ischemic stroke on the basis of the history or clinical examination. Primary hemorrhages are often severe at onset and may result in headache and rapidly evolving deficits. Ischemic strokes are normally painless and characterized by a fixed deficit or a stuttering onset followed by rapid waxing and waning fluctuations. Headaches can occur in conjunction with many ischemic strokes, however, and the only way to distinguish infarct from hemorrhage definitively is with a CT scan.

Brief global cerebral anoxia causes syncope without any permanent sequelae. Prolonged diffuse ischemia, by contrast, can have devastating consequences. The most common causes are cardiac asystole or other forms of overwhelming cardiopulmonary failure. Aortic dissection (Chapter 78), global hypoxia, or carbon monoxide poisoning (Chapter 94) can cause a similar picture. Clinically, these disorders result in unconsciousness. If ischemia persists for more than 4 to 5 minutes, patients often remain in a coma, sometimes evolving into the vegetative state, in which brain stem functions are preserved but the patient has no higher cortical function (Chapter 428). If patients do not regain consciousness within 2 or 3 days, the prognosis for return of independent function is poor. Prompt and aggressive effort to restore cardiovascular circulation is most important. Clinical trials have shown that induced hypothermia within minutes to hours improves outcome in adults who remain comatose after initial resuscitation from out-of-hospital ventricular fibrillation cardiac arrest. [1]

In young patients, hypoxia caused by near-drowning in cold water may result in resistance to prolonged hypoxic ischemic damage. Therapeutic hypothermia has not yet been proved useful in adults with stroke.

Treatment

Acute Stroke

Thrombolytic therapy is the only safe and effective method for acute management of ischemic stroke of typical cause (i.e., atherosclerotic and embolic stroke). Multiple randomized, placebo-controlled trials have been conducted to evaluate intravenous tissue plasminogen activator (t-PA), streptokinase, and intra-arterial recombinant prourokinase. Meta-analyses provide support for the efficacy and safety of this approach if patients are treated within 3 hours after the onset of symptoms. [2] Obstacles to thrombolytic treatment include the need to redesign and implement acute stroke care systems, delay of patients in reaching medical facilities, and insufficient expertise in the use of thrombolysis by many physicians.

Rx

The recommended therapy with intravenous t-PA requires adherence to relatively stringent eligibility criteria (Table 431–2 and Fig. 431–4). Therapy must be started within 3 hours after the onset of stroke. Before initiating therapy, a non–contrast-enhanced CT scan should be obtained to exclude patients with intracranial hemorrhage. Blood pressure limits are a maximum of 185 mm Hg systolic or 110 mm Hg diastolic. If blood pressure exceeds these limits, it should be lowered with an antihypertensive drug such as labetalol before initiating t-PA. In addition, patients who have had major surgery or serious trauma within the preceding 2 weeks or evidence of gastrointestinal bleeding should not be treated. The recommended dose of intravenous t-PA is 0.9 mg/kg to a maximum of 90 mg, administered as a 10% initial bolus with the remainder given over a 60-minute period.

Treatment should begin as soon as possible, and even patients with mild strokes or rapidly resolving deficits probably merit treatment. Patients with severe strokes, as evidenced by major clinical deficits or early signs of a large infarct by CT scan, do not fare well regardless of whether they are treated. Treatment 3 to 6 hours after the onset of ischemic stroke is not currently recommended, although one study of intra-arterial prourokinase given 3 to 6 hours after the onset of an ischemic stroke showed benefit from such therapy. Streptokinase is not of benefit. Intra-arterial t-PA has been used in patients who are not candidates for intravenous t-PA, but there are no controlled studies of this form of treatment.

Acute anticoagulation with various forms of heparin or warfarin is of no benefit in patients with ischemic stroke. Patients with stroke in evolution, in which deficits increase over the first day after the onset of the stroke, commonly receive anticoagulants, but there is no strong evidence that such therapy is effective. Vital signs and neurologic status should be monitored. After the acute stroke has stabilized and begun to improve, hypertension must be treated. Blood pressure is often transiently elevated in the initial hours after a stroke and should not be rapidly lowered except as a prelude to t-PA therapy (see earlier).

If a patient has suffered an acute myocardial infarction, the preferred therapy is primary angioplasty (Chapter 73). It is uncertain what dose of t-PA should be administered if a patient simultaneously has a stroke and myocardial infarction. If a patient is a candidate for coronary artery bypass graft surgery and is found to have surgically correctable carotid stenosis, the more urgent procedure should generally be performed first.

There is an increased risk for pulmonary embolism and deep vein thrombosis in patients with ischemic stroke, particularly those with neurologic deficits that produce immobility. In these patients, prophylactic low-dose subcutaneous heparin or low-molecular-weight heparin (Chapter 35) is recommended unless there are other contraindications to anticoagulation.

TABLE 431–2 TISSUE PLASMINOGEN ACTIVATOR THERAPY FOR ACUTE ISCHEMIC STROKE

Clinical manifestation—focal neurologic deficits

Patient selection
- Therapy must be started within 3 hr of the onset of acute ischemic stroke symptoms
- A baseline CT scan must be obtained before initiation of therapy

Contraindications
- Evidence of intracranial hemorrhage on pretreatment evaluation
- Suspicion of subarachnoid hemorrhage
- Recent intracranial surgery, serious head trauma, or previous stroke
- History of intracranial hemorrhage
- Uncontrolled hypertension at the time of treatment—>185 mm Hg systolic or >110 diastolic—that cannot be reduced with acute antihypertensive therapy
- Seizure at stroke onset
- Active internal bleeding
- Intracranial neoplasm, AVM, or aneurysm
- Known bleeding diathesis, including but not limited to
  - Oral anticoagulation with a prothrombin time >15 sec
  - Heparin administration within the preceding 48 hr and an elevated activated partial thromboplastin time at initial evaluation
  - Platelet count <100,000/mm^3

Warnings
- Patients with a severe neurologic deficit (NIH Stroke Scale >22) at initial evaluation have an increased risk for ICH
- Patients with major early infarct signs on CT (edema or mass effect) are probably >3 hr since vessel occlusion

Dosing information for acute ischemic stroke
- 0.9 mg/kg to a maximum dose of ≤90 mg
- 10% of the total dose administered as an IV bolus over a 1-min period
- 90% of the remainder infused continuously over a 60-min period

Follow-up
- Monitor vital signs and neurologic status
- Maintain blood pressure at ≤185/≤110 mm Hg
- No anticoagulant or antiplatelet therapy for 24 hr

Modified from package insert for Activase, Genentech, Inc., South San Francisco, CA.
AVM = arteriovenous malformation; CT = computed tomography; ICH = intracranial hemorrhage; NIH = National Institutes of Health.

UNUSUAL CAUSES OF STROKE

Atrial Myxoma

Atrial myxomas (Chapter 59) are the most common type of primary cardiac tumor and are found in about 0.05% of autopsies of young adults with ischemic strokes or TIAs. Nonspecific constitutional symptoms are frequent, and less than half of myxomas produce emboli. When these tumors do produce emboli, the danger period usually lasts days to weeks. Metastasis can rarely cause cerebral aneurysms. Other primary and metastatic cardiac tumors can embolize neoplastic tissue or thrombus.

Vasculitis

Vasculitis (Chapters 287, 291, and 292) can produce focal or multifocal cerebral ischemia by means of inflammation and necrosis of extracranial or intracranial blood vessels. Segmental inflammation of cerebral blood vessels is associated with cerebral ischemia acutely at the site of involvement.

Vasculitis of the central nervous system (CNS) is often manifested as cognitive disturbances, headache, and seizures. Because the vascular damage is commonly diffuse, these nonfocal neurologic abnormalities occur more frequently with vasculitis than with focal ischemic disorders. The diagnosis is often difficult to make because the signs and symptoms are frequently nonspecific. The angiographic appearance of a "beadlike" segmental narrowing of cerebral blood vessels, when present, is virtually diagnostic, but cerebral angiograms are often normal in histologically proven cases. Definitive diagnosis requires the demonstration of characteristic inflammatory histopathology in leptomeningeal or cortical biopsy specimens. Because of the segmental and highly focal nature of the inflammatory process, the histopathology may go undetected at biopsy despite a positive angiogram.

Primary CNS vasculitis, Behçet's disease (Chapter 297), Takayasu's arteritis (Chapters 78 and 291), and temporal arteritis (Chapter 292) are notable for their infrequent involvement of the peripheral nervous system. By contrast, hypersensitivity and systemic necrotizing vasculitides frequently produce polyneuropathies. Primary CNS arteritis (Chapter 291), giant cell arteritis (Chapter 292), and vasculitis associated with certain CNS infections may be manifested initially or solely as neurologic abnormalities.

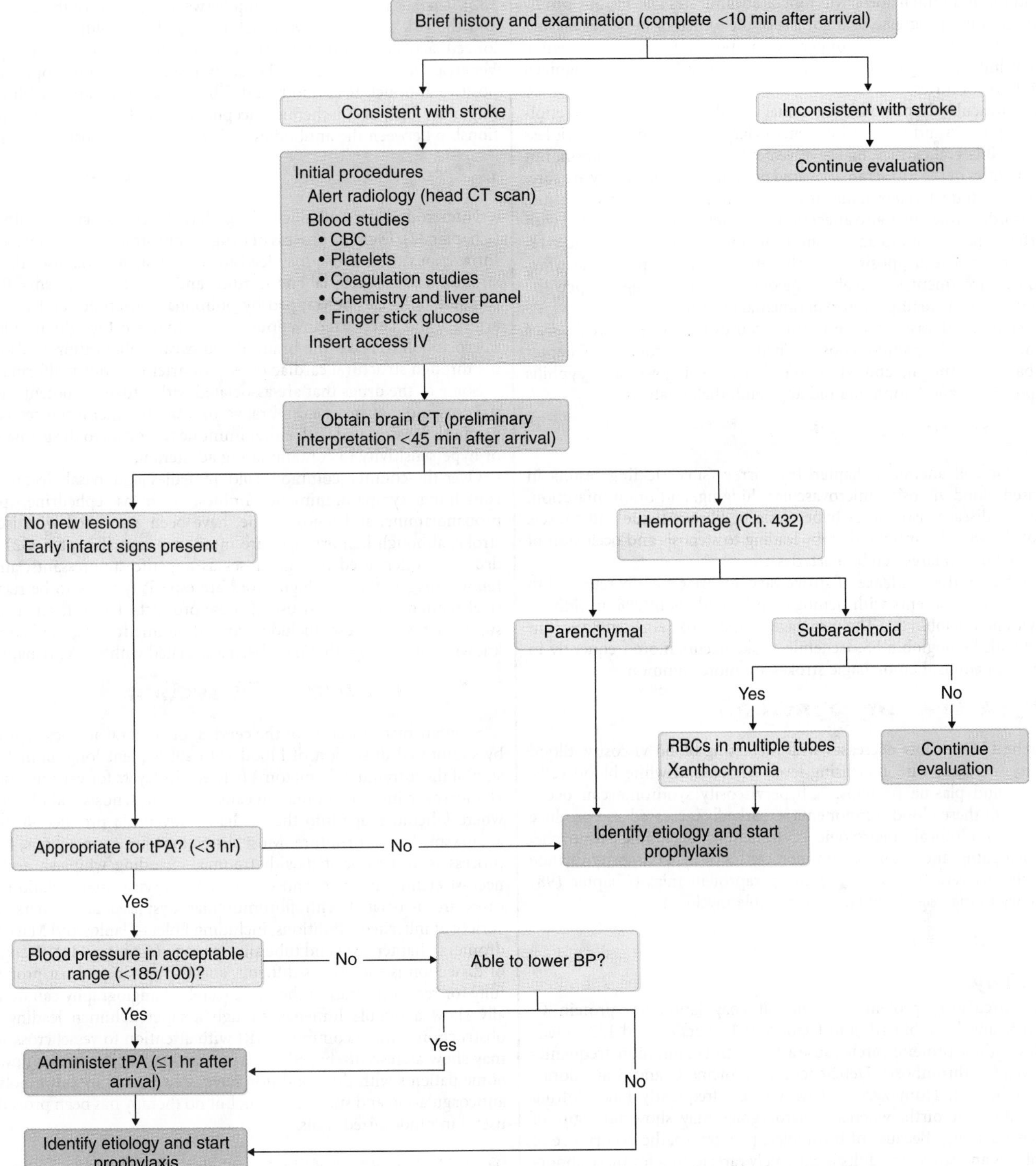

FIGURE 431–4 • Algorithm for the emergency evaluation of a patient with suspected stroke. BP = blood pressure; CBC = complete blood count; CT = computed tomography; RBCs = red blood cells; tPA = tissue plasminogen activator.

Primary arteritis of the CNS causes headache and other encephalopathy-like symptoms in young or middle-aged individuals. The course is usually insidiously progressive but may wax and wane for periods of several months. A few of these patients initially have a strokelike episode.

Giant cell arteritis (Chapter 292) can affect any medium or large artery in the body. When it is present in the cerebral vasculature, it is called *temporal arteritis* and is characterized by panarteritis, including intimal proliferation, destruction of the internal elastic lamina, and thickening of the media. Luminal obstruction is caused by edema, thickening of the intima, and thrombosis. A prominent inflammatory infiltrate consisting of mononuclear cells, giant cells, and eosinophils with granuloma formation is present with active disease. Giant cell arteritis is the most common angiitis causing ischemic stroke. Temporal arteritis predominantly affects patients older than 55 years. Symptoms include fever, malaise, weight loss, and headache. In many patients, constitutional symptoms consistent with polymyalgia rheumatica may coexist, including jaw, neck, and facial pain and morning stiffness. Pain over the temporal arteries and an erythrocyte sedimentation rate greater than 50 mm/hr are frequently, but not always present. Biopsy of the superficial temporal artery provides a definitive diagnosis; because of the segmental nature of the vasculitis, however, serial sections must be examined or the characteristic histology may be missed. The diagnosis is important to establish because early initiation of corticosteroid therapy (e.g., prednisone, 60 mg/day) may decrease the risk for acute ischemic blindness or stroke (Chapter 292). This treatment can be started shortly before performing the biopsy.

Takayasu's arteritis, also called *pulseless disease* (Chapters 78 and 291), is a chronic, idiopathic inflammatory disorder, primarily of young women. It affects mainly the aortic arch, the large brachiocephalic arteries, and the abdominal aorta. Mononuclear infiltrates and fibrous proliferation produce progressive narrowing of the lumen of these vessels and thus reduced flow into the upper extremities and cerebral ischemia. Though initially diagnosed in Japanese families, it has been recognized in Western countries.

Fibromuscular dysplasia is a segmental vasculopathy of unknown etiology (Chapters 78 and 126). Its frequency in large angiographic series is less than 1%. Bilateral extracranial involvement of the ICA is common, but abnormalities of the intracranial carotid or vertebrobasilar artery are rare. Dysplasia of the arterial wall may involve the intima, media, or adventitia. This disorder, which may also affect the renal arteries and is associated with hypertension, can lead to aneurysm formation and cervicocephalic arterial dissection. The diagnosis is made by cerebral angiography. Little information on treatment is available; angioplasty and stenting to open the narrowed lumen are unproven experimental procedures.

Other types of vasculitis are unusual causes of stroke. Such diseases include Wegener's granulomatosis (Chapter 291); sarcoidosis (Chapter 95); bacterial, fungal, and viral infections; meningovascular syphilis (Chapter 341); and lymphomatoid angioendotheliomatosis.

Hemoglobinopathies

In sickle cell anemia (Chapter 167), irreversible sickling results in increased blood viscosity, microvascular sludging, and brain infarction. Sickle cell disease also causes hyperplasia of fibrous tissue and muscle cells of the vascular intima, thereby leading to stenosis and occlusion of some medium to large cerebral arteries.

Estimates of the incidence of stroke vary but are generally reported to be 8 to 17% in patients with hemoglobin SS and about 2% in individuals with hemoglobin SA. The mean age at first stroke is about 8 years in people with hemoglobin SS. Ischemic stroke occurs more frequently in children. In adults, hemorrhagic strokes are more common.

Hyperviscosity Syndrome

Cerebral blood flow decreases with increasing blood viscosity. Blood viscosity increases with increasing levels of red and white blood cells, platelets, and plasma proteins. A hyperviscosity syndrome can occur when any of these blood components is markedly increased and produce focal or multifocal neurologic dysfunction, including headache, encephalopathy, and seizures. Common causes of hyperviscosity include polycythemia vera (Chapter 172) and paraproteinemias (Chapter 198) secondary to macroglobulinemia or multiple myeloma.

Coagulation Disorders

Hereditary

Four circulating proteins that inhibit coagulation are protein C, protein S, antithrombin III, and factor V (Chapters 81 and 182). Deficiencies of these proteins rarely cause arterial strokes but more frequently cause venous thrombosis. Deficiencies of proteins C and S are dominantly inherited. Homozygotes have serious, frequently fatal clotting abnormalities at birth, whereas heterozygotes may show no signs of hypercoagulability. Because of incomplete penetrance, the occurrence of thrombosis and stroke in adults is extremely rare; testing for these abnormalities should be undertaken only in unusual cases. Antithrombin III is vitamin K independent and synthesized in the liver. Deficiency should be suspected in young patients with a history of recurrent deep vein thrombosis or pulmonary embolism, especially if there is a similar family history. Inheritance is autosomal dominant with incomplete penetrance. Arterial stroke is rare.

Acquired

Cancer and pregnancy, including the postpartum period, are associated with hypercoagulable states that predispose to arterial and venous thrombosis (Chapters 81, 182, and 189). Although a variety of clotting abnormalities may be present, no tests have been devised to detect patients at risk for stroke. No treatments have been proved to be useful for strokes associated with these conditions.

Antiphospholipid Antibodies

The antiphospholipid antibody syndrome is associated with cerebral arterial and venous infarction, particularly in young adults (Chapter 182). There is no clear relationship between the levels of these antibodies and the risk for stroke. Other laboratory abnormalities include a prolonged activated partial thromboplastin time, biologic false-positive Venereal Disease Research Laboratory results, thrombocytopenia, and a positive antinuclear antibody test. There is an association with atypical migraine, TIA, and ischemic encephalopathy. The reason for the relationship between the antibodies and cerebral thrombosis is unknown.

Drug-Related Causes of Stroke

Numerous legal and illicit drugs have been associated with stroke (Chapter 32). Even the process of drug administration may cause a stroke. Intravenous drug abuse may lead to septicemia and diseases that cause strokes, such as bacterial endocarditis and mycotic aneurysms. Particles of adulterants can be trapped by pulmonary arterioles and cause local arteritis and later arteriovenous shunts that are thought to allow the microemboli to reach the brain. Paradoxical embolization is also possible through structural cardiac defects or arteriovenous malformations.

Some of the drugs that are associated with stroke are potent vasoconstrictors and may initiate cerebral vasospasm. In other instances, cerebral vasculitis is associated with either immune responses to the primary drug or hypersensitivity to contaminating adulterants.

Over-the-counter common cold remedies and nasal decongestants containing sympathomimetic amines, such as ephedrine, phenylpropanolamine, and fenoxazoline, have been associated with ischemic stroke, although hemorrhages are more common (Chapter 432). These drugs are often used in high doses as appetite suppressants, and case reports suggest that the high doses are especially likely to be related to stroke, often after the first use of these products. Herbs taken as dietary supplements may also include sympathomimetics (e.g., ephedra, also known as *ma huang*) that have been associated with stroke (Chapter 36).

Cervical Artery Dissection

Spontaneous dissection of the cervical or cerebral arteries is produced by subintimal dissection of blood with subsequent longitudinal extension of the intramural hematoma between its layers for various distances. Hemorrhage into the intima can cause luminal stenosis and obstruction, whereas hemorrhage into the media or adventitia produces a pseudoaneurysm that can rupture. Most dissections are spontaneous, but this process is also associated with trauma, including whiplash and other neck-stretching injuries, and chiropractic cervical manipulation. Some cases are associated with fibromuscular dysplasia and others with a variety of inherited conditions, including Ehlers-Danlos and Marfan syndromes (Chapter 281) and tuberous sclerosis (Chapter 444). Recognition of dissection is sometimes difficult, and the physician must probe carefully for recent injuries to the neck. Cerebral angiography can occasionally show a double lumen, although a tapered lumen leading to an obstruction is more common. MRI with attention to vessel cross section may show a crescent-shaped hyperintense mass adjacent to a flow void. Some patients with this condition have been treated by thrombolysis or anticoagulation and surgical repair, but no therapy has been proved to be useful in randomized trials.

Homocystinuria

Homocystinuria (Chapter 223) is associated with a variety of disorders, including dislocated ocular lenses, bone deformities, mental retardation, and accelerated atherosclerosis of large and medium-sized arteries. Strokes commonly occur before 20 years of age. Detection of homocystine in urine is the diagnostic test of choice. Individuals with modest increases in serum homocystine levels may also have an increased risk for stroke. Treatment with a diet low in methionine and supplements of cysteine and pyridoxine (vitamin B_6) can decrease the plasma level of methionine. Folate administration may also be helpful because it is necessary for methylation of homocystine. Vitamin therapy has not been proved to reduce the risk for stroke in patients with homocystinuria, however.

Fat Embolism

Fat embolism (Chapter 99) is mostly a complication of long bone trauma (Chapter 113), intramedullary manipulation during orthopedic procedures, contusions of soft tissues, and severe trauma to large fat deposits. Strokes typically occur several days after the trauma. Clinical features of cerebral embolization depend on the sites within the brain that are affected. Diffuse embolization can produce encephalopathy or seizures, but more discrete lesions can cause focal neurologic deficits. The condition is probably underdiagnosed clinically and at autopsy. Peripheral features that suggest the diagnosis include petechiae and fat emboli visible on ophthalmoscopic examination. Laboratory abnormalities include hypoxemia, anemia, lipuria, and disorders of blood coagulation. The chest radiograph commonly shows bilateral fluffy infiltrates.

Air Embolism

Air embolism can occur with a variety of surgical procedures, particularly cardiac surgery, and as a complication of neurosurgical procedures performed with the patient in the sitting position. Trauma can produce pneumothorax, and air may enter the pulmonary vein and subsequently lodge in the brain. Extended underwater dives and too rapid an ascent can cause the air in the blood to come out of solution and form bubbles that can be pumped into the cerebral circulation (caisson disease). Arterial gas embolism can cause disturbances in cortical function, including seizures and focal deficits. Segmental areas of pallor may be observed on the tongue, marbling of the skin may be seen, and air emboli can be detected on funduscopic examination. When caused by rapid decompression, barotrauma is treated in a decompression chamber.

Moyamoya

Moyamoya disease is a chronic, noninflammatory occlusive vasculopathy of unknown etiology. It is a rare condition that is most common among the Japanese. It has a bimodal age distribution, with peaks in the first and fourth decades. Diagnostic criteria include stenosis or occlusion involving the bifurcation of the ICA and proximal portions of the ACA and MCA, the presence of unusual netlike ("puff of smoke") collateral arteries arising from the circle of Willis, and bilateral occurrence. In adults, the clinical manifestation is usually hemorrhages. Moyamoya is diagnosed by cerebral angiography. No treatment has been proved to be effective.

Cerebral Venous Sinus Thrombosis

Thrombosis of a cerebral venous sinus may be manifested as headache, focal neurologic deficits, seizures, altered mental status, and papilledema. With obstruction of the superior sagittal sinus, veins draining into the sinus from the superior and medial surfaces of both cerebral convexities are commonly obstructed; in its early stages, the condition can result in bilateral weakness and sensory changes in the legs. The presence of bilateral leg weakness should alert the clinician to the possibility of sinus thrombosis. Seizures occur more often with venous than with arterial occlusion. The most dangerous form of venous disease arises when the superior sagittal sinus is occluded, but obstruction of a transverse sinus or one of the major veins over the cerebral convexity can also produce major damage. These venous occlusions occur most commonly in association with coagulopathies, often in the puerperal period, or in patients with disseminated cancer. The transverse sinus can be occluded as a consequence of inner ear infections, a condition called *otitic hydrocephalus*.

The differential diagnosis of venous obstruction can include an arterial stroke, but the findings more often suggest a diffuse process, such as herpes simplex encephalitis or meningitis. The diagnosis depends on the recognition of impaired venous flow, which can be suspected on routine CT or MRI and confirmed by CT or MR angiography; conventional angiography is rarely needed. Unfractionated dose-adjusted heparin (see Table 81–4) and perhaps low-molecular-weight heparin may be safe and effective for cerebral venous sinus thrombosis during the acute phase, even in the presence of hemorrhagic infarction caused by the sinus thrombosis. Oral warfarin anticoagulation is generally continued for 3 to 6 months with the usual target international normalized ratio of 2.0 to 3.0.

Rare Genetic Causes

More than 50 genetic disorders have strokes as at least one of their features, but the prevalence of these abnormalities is low, so strokes produced by monogenetic anomalies are relatively rare. Cerebral autosomal dominant arteriopathy with small subcortical infarcts and leukoencephalopathy (CADASIL) is characterized by recurrent strokes resulting in multiple deep infarcts and dementia, without the usual risk factors for stroke. It has an autosomal dominant pattern of inheritance. The mean age at onset is approximately 40 years, and dementia ensues within 10 to 15 years. Migraine with aura often precedes the strokes by several years. The responsible gene on chromosome 19 results in mutations of the Notch3 receptor protein. As is true of all these genetic causes of stroke, treatment is symptomatic. Antenatal diagnosis is possible in these disorders.

Fabry's disease (angiokeratoma corporis diffusum) (Chapter 223) is an X-linked disease that causes a reduction in α-galactosidase A enzyme activity. Patients have diseases of the skin, eyes, and kidneys, as well as frequent neurologic complications that result from either vascular occlusion or, infrequently, intracerebral hemorrhage related to the accumulation of glycolipids in small and medium-sized arteries. The gene encoding this enzyme is located at Xq22. Enzyme replacement therapy is of benefit (Chapter 223).

Neurofibromatosis (Chapter 444) is associated with strokes as a result of occlusion of the internal carotid arteries or the proximal part of the anterior cerebral circulation. Histologically, arterial lesions consist of hyperplasia of the intimal layer with fragmentation and reduplication of the elastic layer. Cerebral aneurysms can also occur. The diagnosis of type I neurofibromatosis is usually based on clinical findings. *DNA-based testing* of the NF1 gene is available clinically but is infrequently needed for diagnosis.

Marfan syndrome (Chapter 281), which is an autosomal dominant disorder of the fibrillin gene on chromosome 15, affects the skeletal, ocular, cardiovascular, and central nervous systems. Expression is highly variable, and only one system may be involved. Involvement of large arteries, such as the aorta and carotid arteries, is common and may cause death. The most life-threatening problem is dissection of these arteries. Pathologically, the disease results from defective fibrillin, which is an important component of connective tissue.

Prevention and Treatment of Stroke and Transient Ischemic Attack

Rx

Primary Prevention

Risk factors for stroke fall into two general categories, nonmodifiable and modifiable (Table 431–3). Within the modifiable group are risk factors that are well documented and others that are not. Blood pressure control (Chapter 66) is the most important primary prevention strategy. It is especially important in patients with diabetes, in whom tight control of hypertension with angiotensin-converting enzyme inhibitors substantially reduces the incidence of stroke. Statins are recommended in patients who meet the criteria for treating hyperlipidemia (Chapter 217). Smoking cessation (Chapter 30) is routinely recommended, but there are no prospective randomized trials to prove that cessation of smoking reduces the risk for stroke. Anticoagulation markedly reduces the risk for stroke in patients with atrial fibrillation (Chapter 63), and blood transfusion is the usual treatment to prevent strokes in patients with sickle cell disease (Chapter 167).

Prophylactic Carotid Interventions

In asymptomatic patients, ipsilateral carotid endarterectomy benefited patients who had a 60% or greater reduction in diameter of the artery without ulceration, provided that the perioperative complication rate was less than 3%, a rate that requires a skilled surgeon.  Clinical trials of carotid artery angioplasty and stent placement are under way, but these procedures cannot be routinely recommended yet in asymptomatic patients.

Secondary Prevention in Patients with Previous Stroke or Transient Ischemic Attack

All the risk factor reductions that are recommended for primary prevention are also recommended in patients who have suffered a previous stroke or TIA and have no contraindication. In addition, specific medical and surgical therapies should be considered.

TABLE 431–3 WELL-DOCUMENTED MODIFIABLE RISK FACTORS FOR STROKE

Factor	Prevalence (%)	Relative Risk	Risk Reduction with Treatment
Hypertension (by age group)			38%
50 yr	20	4	
60 yr	30	3	
70 yr	40	2	
80 yr	55	1.4	
90 yr	60	1	
Smoking	25	1.8	50% within 1 yr, baseline after 5 yr
Diabetes	20	1.8–6.	Reduction of stroke risk in hypertensive diabetics with blood pressure control. No demonstrated benefit in stroke reduction with tight glycemic control
Asymptomatic carotid stenosis	2–8	2	50%
Hyperlipidemia			
Adults <35 yr	8-9	1.8	20–30% with statins in patients with known coronary disease
Men >55 yr	25	2.6	
Women >65 yr	40		
Atrial fibrillation (nonvalvular)			
50–59 yr	0.5	4	68% warfarin
60–69 yr	1.8	2.6	21% aspirin
70–79 yr	4.8	3.3	
80–89 yr	8.8	4.5	

Modified from Goldstein LB, Adams R, Becker K, et al: Primary prevention of ischemic stroke. Stroke 2001;32:280–299.

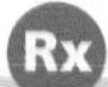

Medications

Aspirin and other antiplatelet agents reduce the odds of nonfatal stroke by 31% when used in patients with known vascular disease (Chapter 35). All patients who have sustained a stroke and have no contraindication should receive an antiplatelet agent to reduce the risk for recurrent stroke. The optimal dose of aspirin has not yet been established, and doses of 50 to 1300 mg/day have been used. Clopidogrel, 75 mg/day, instead of or in addition to aspirin appears to be no better than aspirin alone [4] but is substantially more expensive. Warfarin anticoagulation is not superior to antiplatelet agents in preventing recurrent strokes, except in patients with atrial fibrillation or another cardiac source of emboli. The addition of dipyridamole to aspirin can benefit high-risk patients with prior cerebral ischemia. [5] The risks for cerebral hemorrhage with warfarin exceed the potential benefit for prevention of ischemic stroke. [6] In patients with previous cerebrovascular disease or high-risk conditions, aggressive cholesterol reduction with 40 mg of simvastatin or 80 mg of atorvastatin reduces the rate of stroke by 25% or more. [7]

Surgery

Carotid endarterectomy reduces the cumulative risk for any ipsilateral stroke at 2 years from 26 to 9% in patients with a 70 to 99% symptomatic (i.e., previous TIA or nondisabling stroke) internal carotid stenosis and from 22 to 16% at 5 years in patients with a 50 to 70% symptomatic stenosis. [8] Patients with less than a 50% symptomatic stenosis do better with medical management alone.

Devices

Carotid artery stents can restore patency to stenotic arteries with an efficacy and safety comparable to that of open endarterectomy in experienced centers. Intra-arterial clots can also be extracted under radiologic guidance with a corkscrew-like device inserted into the common or internal carotid artery for occlusion of the anterior circulation or into the subclavian artery for occlusion of the posterior circulation and then advanced to remove clot located in medium or large intracranial vessels (ICA, MCA, vertebral artery, basilar artery, PCA, or ACA). Using proximal balloon occlusion to arrest flow, the corkscrew device can grab and hold the clot as it is extracted from the patient's artery. Currently, however, outcomes appear to be better with endarterectomy than with stenting, suggesting that stenting should be reserved for selected situations.

Prognosis and Rehabilitation

Patients who receive care in specialized, acute stroke units are less likely to die, more likely to go home, and more likely to be independent 3 months later. In most clinical trials, about 15% of patients with ischemic stroke die within the first 3 months. Immediate causes of death include herniation because of brain swelling or neurologic dysfunction directly related to the stroke. Deaths that occur days after stroke and are not directly related to neurologic dysfunction are commonly produced by pulmonary embolism or pneumonia. Most large population studies report that about 20% of patients who survive a stroke require long-term institutionalization and that 33 to 50% of the others are left with substantial disability. Stroke is the most common cause of adult disability in the United States. Most functional recovery takes place during the first month, but some continued slow improvement is possible for 1 year. The most common long-term cause of death in patients with stroke is myocardial infarction.

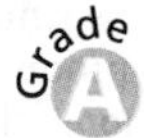

1. Hypothermia after Cardiac Arrest Study Group: Mild therapeutic hypothermia to improve the neurologic outcome after cardiac arrest. N Engl J Med 2002;346:549–556.
2. The ATLANTIC, ECASS, and NINDS rt-PA Study Group Investigators: Association of outcome with early stroke treatment: Pooled analysis of ATLANTIC, ECASS, and NINDS rt-PA stroke trials. Lancet 2004;363:768–774
3. MRC Asymptomatic Carotid Surgery Trial (ACST) Collaborative Group: Prevention of disabling and fatal strokes by successful carotid endarterectomy in patients without recent neurological symptoms: Randomised controlled trial. Lancet 2004;363: 1491–1502.
4. Bhatt DL, Fox KA, Hacke W, et al: Clopidogrel and aspirin versus aspirin alone for the prevention of atherothrombotic events. N Engl J Med 2006;354:1706–1717.
5. The ESPRIT Study Group: Aspirin plus dipyridamole versus aspirin alone after cerebral ischaemia of arterial origin (ESPRIT): Randomised controlled trial. Lancet 2006;367:1665–1673.
6. Chimowitz MI, Lynn MJ, Howlett-Smith H, et al: Comparison of warfarin and aspirin for symptomatic intracranial arterial stenosis. N Engl J Med 2005;352:1305–1316.
7. The Stroke Prevention by Aggressive Reduction in Cholesterol Levels (SPARCL) investigators: High-dose atorvastatin after stroke or transient ischemic attack. N Engl J Med 2006;355:549–559.
8. Barnett HJM, Taylor DW, Eliasziw M, et al: The North American Symptomatic Carotid Endarterectomy Trial Collaborators: Benefit of carotid endarterectomy in patients with symptomatic moderate or severe stenosis. N Engl J Med 1998;339:1415–1425.
9. Mas J, Chatellier G, Beyssen B, et al: Endarterectomy versus stenting in patients with symptomatic severe carotid stenosis. N Engl J Med 2006;355:1660–1671.

SUGGESTED READINGS

American College of Cardiology Foundation, American Society of Interventional and Therapeutic Neuroradiology, Society for Cardiovascular Angiography and Interventions, et al: ACCF/SCAI/SVMB/SIR/ASITN 2007 clinical expert consensus document on carotid stenting: A report of the American College of Cardiology Foundation Task Force on Clinical Expert Consensus Documents (ACCF/SCAI/SVMB/SIR/ASITN Clinical Expert Consensus Document Committee on Carotid Stenting). J Am Coll Cardiol 2007;49:126–170. *Comprehensive review and recommendations on carotid stenting.*

Goldstein LB, Adams R, Alberts MJ, et al: AHA/ASA Guideline—primary prevention of ischemic stroke. Circulation 2006;113:e873–e923 Web Site Feature. *A consensus overview.*

Goldstein LB, Simel DL:. Is this patient having a stroke? JAMA 2005; 293:2391–2402. *A case-based review.*

Johnston SC, Rothwell PM, Nguyen-Huynh MN, et al: Validation and refinement of scores to predict very early stroke risk after transient ischaemic attack. Lancet 2007;369:283–292. *Validation of the prognostic scores used to assess patients who suffer transient ischemic attacks.*

Khaja AM, Grotta JC: Established treatments for acute ishaemic stroke. Lancet 2007;369:319–330. *Comprehensive review.*

Kizer JR, Devereux RB: Patent foramen ovale in young adults with unexplained stroke. N Engl J Med 2005; 353:2361–2372. *Considers patent foramen ovale and other sources of emboli that can cause stroke.*

Sacco RL, Adams R, Albers G, et al: Guidelines for prevention of stroke in patients with ischemic stroke or transient ischemic attack. Stroke 2006;37:577–617. *Evidence-based review.*

Savitz SI, Caplan LR: Vertebrobasilar disease. N Engl J Med 2005;352:2618–2626. *A comprehensive overview.*

Stam J: Thrombosis of the cerebral veins and sinuses. N Engl J Med 2005;352: 1791–1798. *A scholarly review.*

Wahlgren N, Ahmed N, Dávalos A, et al: Thrombolysis with alteplase for acute ischaemic stroke in the Safe Implementation of Thrombolysis in Stroke-Monitoring Study (SITS-MOST): An observational study. Lancet 2007;369: 275–282. *Confirms that intravenous alteplase is safe and effective in routine clinical use when used within 3 hours of stroke onset.*

432 HEMORRHAGIC CEREBROVASCULAR DISEASE

Justin A. Zivin

Approximately 15% of all strokes are due to intracranial hemorrhage. Hemorrhagic stroke can be diffuse (i.e., bleeding into the subarachnoid or intraventricular spaces) or focal (i.e., intraparenchymal hemorrhage). About two thirds of intracranial bleeding are predominantly subarachnoid hemorrhages, whereas about a third are intracerebral hemorrhages. Subarachnoid hemorrhage is usually caused by rupture of vessels on or near the surface of the brain or ventricles (e.g., aneurysms, vascular malformations), with bleeding mainly into the cerebrospinal fluid (CSF) spaces. Intracerebral hemorrhage is most frequently caused by the rupture of arteries that are within the brain substance (e.g., hypertensive hemorrhage, vascular malformations) but do not extend to the CSF spaces. Both types of hemorrhagic stroke have high mortality rates, depending on subtype and location. Prevention is the mainstay of management because there are no sufficiently efficacious therapies for hemorrhage-induced cerebral injury.

SUBARACHNOID HEMORRHAGE

Epidemiology

In the United States, about 30,000 new cases of subarachnoid hemorrhage occur each year and predominantly involve young adults. Both genders are equally affected, and the rate may be twice as high in African Americans as in whites. Rupture of aneurysms is by far the most common cause of nontraumatic subarachnoid hemorrhage. Advances in diagnostic imaging have improved the detection of intracranial aneurysms, but most cases are not discovered until after rupture.

Risk factors include cigarette smoking, binge drinking, illicit drugs, phenylpropanolamine, and other sympathomimetic agents. Although hypertension is well established as a risk factor for ischemic stroke, the relationship of nonmalignant hypertension to subarachnoid hemorrhage is less well documented; the decline in hypertension in the general population has not been accompanied by a decrease in the incidence rate of subarachnoid hemorrhage.

Pathobiology

The principal causes of subarachnoid hemorrhage are aneurysms and arteriovenous malformations (AVMs), but trauma can also cause subarachnoid bleeding (Chapter 422). Rare causes of subarachnoid hemorrhage include vasculitis, central nervous system neoplasms (Chapter 199), and hematologic disorders such as hemophilia, disseminated intravascular coagulopathy, and thrombocytopenic purpura.

Clinical Manifestations

The classic symptom of a subarachnoid hemorrhage is a very rapidly developing, severe headache, typically called the "worst headache of my life," that is sometimes accompanied by a stiff neck. Aneurysms may generate prodromal signs and symptoms as they gradually expand or cause sentinel (warning) leaks that produce focal or generalized head pain. Such sentinel headaches are frequently severe, and they may be accompanied by nausea or vomiting and may cause meningeal irritation.

Arterial blood pressure is often elevated, and body temperature usually increases, particularly during the first few days after bleeding as subarachnoid blood products produce chemical meningitis. Transient alterations in mental status occur in nearly half the patients, particularly if intracranial pressure exceeds cerebral mean arterial pressure. Patients can remain in coma for several days, depending on the location of the aneurysm and the amount of bleeding.

Acute subarachnoid hemorrhage causes meningeal irritation; nuchal rigidity and photophobia can require several hours to develop. Ophthalmoscopic observation reveals well-circumscribed, bright red, preretinal hemorrhages, known as subhyaloid hemorrhages and thought to be a result of increased intracranial pressure, raised retinal venous pressure, and dissection of blood along the optic nerve sheath. Focal neurologic dysfunction is not usually a prominent feature unless an aneurysm compresses surrounding brain structures, a jet of blood dissects directly into a clinically eloquent brain region, or vasospasm subsequently develops.

Diagnosis

Laboratory Findings

A complete blood cell count, including platelets, should be obtained, and clotting times should be determined to assess whether the patient has an infection or clotting abnormalities. Blood should also be sent for electrolyte analysis to serve as a baseline for detecting later complications.

Imaging

The patient should then be sent immediately for emergency computed tomography (CT). A scan performed within 24 hours of onset generally reveals an area of high signal attenuation consistent with hemorrhage; if blood is present in the subarachnoid space, it is seen within the basal cisterns in more than 90% of patients. By 48 hours after onset, the sensitivity of CT declines to about 75%. Conventional magnetic resonance imaging (MRI) sequences (T1- or T2-weighted scans) are less sensitive than CT scans.

The location of subarachnoid hemorrhage by CT suggests the source of bleeding. High signal attenuation in the basal cisterns, sylvian fissure, or intrahemispheric fissure often indicates rupture of a saccular aneurysm, whereas higher concentrations of blood over the convexities or within the superficial parenchyma of the brain are more consistent with rupture of an AVM or a mycotic aneurysm. A large amount of blood in the subarachnoid space increases the likelihood of subsequent vasospasm. A contrast-enhanced CT scan may aid in the identification of an AVM and some large aneurysms.

An electrocardiogram should be performed to detect peaked or inverted T waves and increased U waves. These abnormalities and subsequent arrhythmias have been attributed to multifocal myocardial necrosis caused by elevated levels of circulating catecholamines.

If the CT findings are normal but the index of suspicion remains high for subarachnoid hemorrhage, a lumbar puncture is usually diagnostic. A traumatic lumbar puncture (i.e., penetration of the needle into a small blood vessel of the venous plexus on the anterior wall of the spinal canal) produces a declining number of red blood cells in subsequent tubes, whereas subarachnoid hemorrhage produces a relatively constant number of red blood cells in each tube. In the presence of bloody fluid, one of the CSF samples should be centrifuged immediately and the supernate examined for the presence of hematin or xanthochromia by visual inspection. Red blood cells in CSF begin to lyse within a few hours, and the centrifuged supernate then appears pink. Later (about 10 hours), as the hemoglobin is converted to bilirubin, the fluid becomes slightly yellow. Opening CSF pressure is generally elevated and may remain so for many days. CSF samples obtained within the first day may show a white blood cell count consistent with the normal circulating white cell–to–red cell ratio (about 1:1000). Chemical meningitis is produced by the presence of blood or breakdown products within the subarachnoid space, and CSF samples contain increased numbers of polymorphonuclear and mononuclear cells relative to red blood cells. The CSF glucose concentration is usually normal shortly after the onset of bleeding, but as chemical meningitis develops, the glucose level may decline, rarely to less than 40 mg/dL. After a subarachnoid hemorrhage, the protein content of CSF is generally elevated, consistent with contamination by blood (the usual ratio is 1 mg/dL of protein for every 1000 red blood cells).

Cerebral angiography remains the definitive study to identify the source of subarachnoid hemorrhage. When the diagnosis of aneurysmal subarachnoid hemorrhage seems highly probable, the timing and need for a cerebral angiogram should be determined by surgical considerations. If doubt exists, angiography should be performed with minimal delay. Because many patients have multiple cerebral aneurysms, the carotid and vertebral artery systems should be examined angiographically. The initial cerebral angiogram fails to detect the source of bleeding in about 20% of patients; such patients are thought to have a fairly good prognosis, with only a 1 to 2% annual risk for recurrent hemorrhage. Failure to detect the bleeding source can be due to obliteration of the aneurysm because of clot or may be due to the small size of the ruptured aneurysm. A superficial venous angioma, a spinal cord aneurysm, or a spinal AVM also will not be seen on a cerebral angiogram. The presence of back pain or neurologic signs localized to the spinal cord at onset should prompt a search for a spinal source of hemorrhage. If the initial angiogram is negative and no other clues to the bleeding site can be found, repeat cerebral angiography is usually performed within a few weeks; MRI or CT with and without contrast may also be helpful.

Treatment Rx

Treatment of Complications

If a patient does not die immediately after a subarachnoid hemorrhage, a number of neurologic complications can occur. Some result from blood in the subarachnoid space, and other concerns include rebleeding from the same aneurysm, cerebral vasospasm and its ischemic consequences, hydrocephalus caused by blockage of CSF outflow pathways, and seizures. Non-neurologic complications include cardiac and electrolyte abnormalities.

Rebleeding

If an aneurysm is not repaired promptly, it can rupture again. A new headache or neurologic worsening suggests repeat rupture, which can be diagnosed only if a repeat CT scan or lumbar puncture shows the presence of new blood in the subarachnoid space. Approximately 30% of patients with aneurysmal subarachnoid hemorrhage rebleed during the first month, and the incidence is highest during the first 2 weeks after the initial episode. Patients with unrepaired aneurysms who survive their initial bleeding for more than 1 month have a 2 to 3% annual risk of rebleeding.

Vasospasm

A common cause of death and disability in patients with aneurysmal subarachnoid hemorrhage is cerebral vasospasm. The vessels at the base of the brain become narrowed, thereby reducing blood flow; if the vasospasm is severe, it can produce infarction of the brain distal to the site of the spasm. The vessels that go into spasm are often different from the artery that was responsible for the initial bleeding. Vasospasm has been reported in up to 75% of patients after subarachnoid hemorrhage, and delayed neurologic deficits develop in as many as 30% of patients with vasospasm. The onset of vasospasm is typically between days 3 and 14 after bleeding, but this complication can develop as late as 3 weeks after subarachnoid hemorrhage. The arteries of the circle of Willis and their major branches are the usual initial site of spasm, with more distal arteries becoming involved later. The amount and location of blood detected within the basal cisterns on CT correlate with the incidence and location of vasospasm. The pathogenesis of cerebral vasospasm is unknown.

Cerebral angiography, which is the best established method to diagnose vasospasm, shows narrowing of the dye column. However, other methods such as transcranial Doppler ultrasonography or magnetic resonance angiography are increasingly being used. Transcranial Doppler has high specificity, but its sensitivity is not as good as that of angiography.

Hydrocephalus

Acute hydrocephalus occurs in up to two thirds of patients within 3 days after subarachnoid hemorrhage. Hydrocephalus is caused by obstruction of CSF outflow pathways at the level of the fourth ventricle and the pacchionian granulations lining the venous sinuses. Increasing age, a history of hypertension, intraventricular hemorrhage, focal neurologic findings, a decreased level of consciousness, and hyponatremia are associated with risk for the development of hydrocephalus. Chronic ventricular enlargement occurs in as many as 60% of patients within 1 month after subarachnoid hemorrhage and is often asymptomatic. Several forms of treatment have been advocated for the management of hydrocephalus, including repeated lumbar puncture and shunt placement, but their value has not been proved.

Seizures

Seizures may occur shortly after subarachnoid hemorrhage in 15 to 90% of patients. Seizures are thought to be caused by cortical damage from bleeding into the neocortex or from ischemic necrosis related to vasospasm. The development of persistent epilepsy is unusual. Prophylactic anticonvulsant therapy has not been useful.

Non-neurologic Complications

Cardiac complications occur as a consequence of subarachnoid hemorrhage. In the acute phases of subarachnoid hemorrhage, electrocardiographic patterns can mimic acute myocardial infarction (Chapter 72). A pattern of deep inverted T waves across the pericardium is classic. Appropriate biomarker assays and repeat electrocardiograms are needed to document true myocardial damage.

Hyponatremia (Chapter 117) is the most common electrolyte abnormality after subarachnoid hemorrhage. Sodium loss, which is typically mild, may occur in up to 25% of patients. The natriuresis has been attributed to inappropriate levels of antidiuretic hormone (Chapter 243), but this hypothesis has not been proved. Hyponatremia can itself result in a decreased level of consciousness and seizures, but it is often impossible to distinguish the effects of hyponatremia from the other possible causes of these neurologic abnormalities.

SPECIFIC CAUSES AND THEIR TREATMENT AND PROGNOSIS

Saccular Aneurysms

Definition and Epidemiology

Saccular or "berry" aneurysms, which account for 80 to 90% of all intracranial aneurysms, are thin-walled outpouchings that protrude from the arteries of the circle of Willis or its major branches; 85% are located at branching points (Fig. 432–1). Because of the local weakness and degeneration of the media, the intima bulges outward and is covered only by the adventitia. A saccular aneurysm may be an incidental finding on a scan or be detected at autopsy in patients who die of other diseases; in symptomatic cases, however, the sack gradually enlarges and ultimately ruptures.

Saccular aneurysms are rarely detected in children, and the incidence of subarachnoid hemorrhage increases with age; therefore, it seems clear

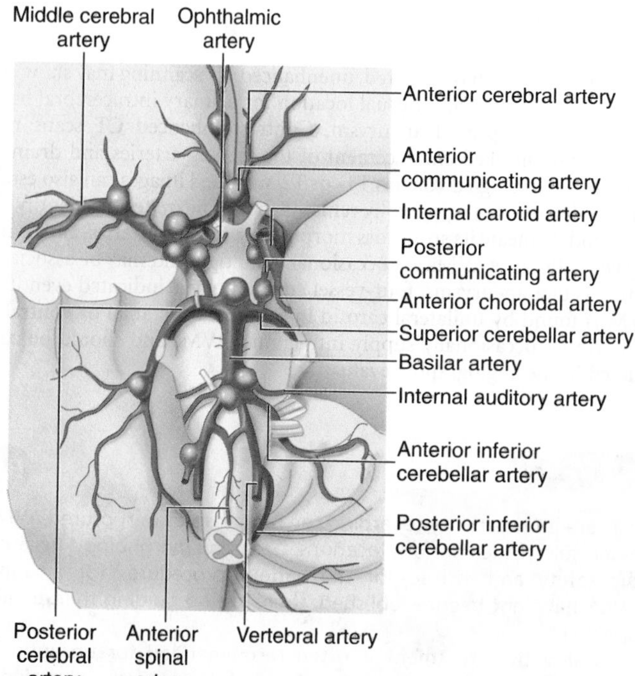

FIGURE 432–1 • Saccular aneurysms. Saccular or berry aneurysms typically develop at the bifurcations of arteries on the undersurface of the brain.

that congenital wall defects develop into aneurysms only after some time. Congenital defects in the muscle and elastic tissue of the arterial media are observed at autopsy in up to 80% of normal vessels of the circle of Willis. It is postulated that these defects gradually degenerate over time as they are exposed to pulsatile arterial blood pressure. Multiple aneurysms are found in about 15% of people with at least one aneurysm. Because the incidence of aneurysmal subarachnoid hemorrhage is approximately 1 in 10,000, it is evident that most saccular aneurysms do not rupture.

Pathobiology

Approximately 10 to 20% of patients with known aneurysms have a family history. Diseases that are associated with intracranial saccular aneurysms include polycystic kidney disease (Chapter 128), Marfan and Ehlers-Danlos syndromes (Chapter 281), fibromuscular dysplasia (Chapter 78), pseudoxanthoma elasticum (Chapter 281), systemic lupus erythematosus (Chapter 287), and sickle cell anemia (Chapter 167). Screening of other family members is often recommended when two or more members of a family have aneurysms.

Treatment

Rx

Primary Prevention of Bleeding

Because the natural history of aneurysms may be highly variable and the risk-benefit ratio for the various invasive techniques is unknown, expectant waiting may sometimes be the best option. However, an aneurysm may rupture without warning, and the uncertainty is unacceptable to some patients and physicians. Medical therapies may delay the time of rupture but cannot repair the lesion.

Treatment of Aneurysms That Have Bled

Medical Treatment

Medical management of a ruptured aneurysm aims to reduce the risk of rebleeding and cerebral vasospasm and prevent other medical complications before and after surgical intervention. The only form of medical therapy that has been useful in treating subarachnoid hemorrhage patients is the voltage-regulated calcium-channel antagonist nimodipine. Although it does not reduce the frequency of vasospasm, nimodipine (60 mg orally every 4 hours for 21 days) lowers the incidence of cerebral infarction by about a third.

Rx

General support consisting of bedrest, analgesics for headache, and gentle sedation as needed is provided to quiet the patient. Stool softeners can minimize straining. Hypertension should be treated appropriately but not aggressively (Chapter 66) because elevated blood pressure may represent a normal compensatory mechanism, particularly in a chronically hypertensive patient, and excessive reduction may cause extension of the infarct. There is no conclusive evidence that modification of blood pressure in patients with acute subarachnoid hemorrhage is of benefit. Antifibrinolytic drugs, including tranexamic acid and ε-aminocaproic acid, may reduce rebleeding, but any such benefit is outweighed by an increased incidence of infarction.

Interventional Therapies

The objectives of interventional procedures are to exclude the aneurysm from the circulation or relieve pressure on adjacent brain tissue caused by expansion of the sack. The optimal timing of these therapies is uncertain, but many surgeons recommend treatment as soon as possible after the subarachnoid hemorrhage.

An electrical current applied to a detachable coil threaded into an aneurysm via percutaneous angiography causes the surrounding blood to clot. The coil is detached and left in place, and the catheter is then removed. This approach is more effective than surgical clipping for achieving disability-free survival in patients who have had ruptured aneurysms. 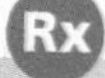 With very large aneurysms, for which use of a coil is not possible, wrapping the sack with various types of material to prevent it from rupturing or growing is sometimes performed. Indirect procedures include various methods of occluding the feeding artery; if there is sufficient collateral supply, the risk of infarction may be less than that of spontaneous rupture of the aneurysm with subsequent extensive subarachnoid hemorrhage.

Prognosis

Mortality and morbidity rates differ among studies. About 12% of subarachnoid hemorrhage victims die before reaching medical attention. By 30 days, approximately 50% die, but 30-day survivors generally survive for at least a year. An equally high mortality rate accompanies each episode of rebleeding. Approximately 25% of survivors have persistent neurologic deficits.

Fusiform Aneurysms

Fusiform aneurysms are so named because they are elongated dilations (i.e., ectasia) of large arteries associated with atherosclerosis. These aneurysms typically develop in the basilar artery but also may affect the internal, middle, and anterior cerebral arteries of individuals with widespread arteriosclerosis and hypertension. These aneurysms may progressively dilate and become tortuous, thereby producing neurologic dysfunction, most frequently by compressing surrounding structures. Thrombi may form in them and embolize distally to cause ischemic strokes. Typically, ectatic aneurysms of the basilar artery compress cranial nerves and cause facial pain (V), hemifacial spasm (VII), and hearing loss with vertigo (VIII). Fusiform aneurysms may mimic pituitary and suprasellar mass lesions or cerebellopontine angle tumors. Fusiform aneurysms rarely rupture; if they do, they are difficult to treat surgically because their shape and stiff walls generally preclude easy surgical clipping, and total occlusion is usually required.

Mycotic Aneurysms

Infected emboli, usually originating on an infected heart valve (Chapter 76), may lodge in a distal branch of a cerebral artery and cause small areas of infarction or microabscesses. In arteries that do not rupture immediately, focal arteritis and mycotic aneurysms, also known as septic aneurysms, may develop. Mycotic aneurysms are frequently multiple and can be found distally in the cerebral arteries. Rates of rupture of these aneurysms may be as high as 10%. Such lesions may be detected by noninvasive imaging studies, but the definitive test is contrast-enhanced angiography, for which the indications are controversial. Aside from treatment of the underlying infection, other treatments are not established.

Vascular Malformations

Epidemiology

About 1% of all strokes and 10% of intracerebral hemorrhages are caused by vascular malformations. The prevalence of AVMs is approximately 0.5%, and the annual incidence of hemorrhage is between 1 and 3 cases per 100,000 people. Familial cases occur but are rare.

Pathobiology

Conventional classifications of cerebrovascular malformations are based on the histologic appearance of the vessels and the intervening neural parenchyma. The most frequent type of vascular malformation is an AVM, which has a core of dysplastic vessels (i.e., nidus), feeding arteries, and draining veins. In the nidus, arteries connect directly to veins without intervening capillaries to produce a low-resistance, high-flow shunt that ultimately dilates feeding arteries and thickens the walls of the draining veins. The classic arteriographic appearance includes an early draining vein. Ordinarily, there is no intervening neural tissue in the nidus. The nidus is the usual site of hemorrhage in an AVM.

The next most common lesions are cavernous malformations (i.e., cavernous angiomas or hemangiomas), which are composed of small-caliber sinusoidal vascular channels that are commonly thrombosed. The low flow rate through these vessels makes them difficult to detect by angiography, and they are unlikely to hemorrhage; these malformations also do not contain neural tissue. Cavernous AVMs are often associated with venous malformations, which are composed of small veins separated by normal parenchyma. Smaller venous channels drain into a dilated venous trunk that ultimately drains into a large vein and sinus in the brain. The classic angiographic appearance is a caput medusa in the late venous phase. These anomalies are readily detected by CT, but they rarely hemorrhage.

A cerebral varix is a single dilated vein that seldom causes clinical symptoms. Telangiectasis, also called capillary malformation, is a cluster of enlarged capillaries surrounded by normal parenchyma. These lesions are too small to be detected by conventional imaging methods and are usually noted as petechiae that are found incidentally at autopsy; these benign lesions rarely hemorrhage.

Clinical Manifestations

Although increasing numbers of probably asymptomatic vascular malformations are being diagnosed by brain imaging as part of the evaluation of nonspecific headaches, about 50% of AVMs are manifested as intracranial hemorrhage, a lower proportion initially present as seizures, and the remainder cause progressive neurologic disability as the first symptom. Hemorrhage, which is the most feared complication of an AVM, has an associated mortality rate of 10 to 15%. The mortality and morbidity rates associated with AVMs are somewhat less than for aneurysms. The initial hemorrhage tends to occur during the second through fourth decades, and hypertension before the hemorrhage is uncommon. The risk for acute rebleeding averages approximately 6 to 7%. In the next 5 years the rate is about 2% per year, and it is 1 to 2% per year thereafter. If this rebleeding rate is maintained for life, a young individual who has a hemorrhagic AVM faces a 50 to 60% chance of an incapacitating or fatal subsequent hemorrhage during a normal lifespan.

AVMs can bleed into the subarachnoid space, the brain parenchyma, or the ventricular system. Focal neurologic abnormalities depend on the severity of the bleeding and the location of brain parenchyma that has been affected. The frequency of cerebral vasospasm after hemorrhage from an AVM is less than that for aneurysmal bleeding.

Approximately 30% of patients who have an AVM are initially evaluated for seizures, which often have a focal onset. Focal neurologic deficits independent of seizures can develop, possibly caused by vascular thrombosis and perhaps by shunting of blood through arteriovenous fistulas away from normal brain tissue.

Diagnosis

If a hemorrhage has occurred, unenhanced CT scanning may show evidence of bleeding in an unusual location for primary intracerebral hemorrhage or a ruptured aneurysm. Contrast-enhanced CT scans may demonstrate marked enhancement of the feeding arteries and draining veins. MRI with signal void on T1- or T2-weighted images can also establish the diagnosis. Angiography remains the definitive test to identify the AVM and delineate its size, gross morphology, feeding arteries, and draining veins. Because AVMs are occasionally multiple and may be associated with saccular aneurysms, four-vessel angiography is indicated even if an AVM is found by unilateral carotid injection. Extracranial or contralateral arteries occasionally supply intracranial AVMs and should be considered in the angiographic evaluation.

Treatment

Rx

There is uncertainty regarding the prognosis of unruptured AVMs as a result of their various locations, sizes, and morphology. Because the safety and efficacy of the various procedures for treating AVMs have not been established, there are no guiding therapeutic principles.

Conservative treatment is often recommended for unruptured AVMs manifested as seizures or headache, especially in patients older than 55 to 60 years. This approach emphasizes control of hypertension, avoidance of anticoagulants, and use of anticonvulsants to control seizures.

If an AVM has ruptured and the patient has recovered from the initial hemorrhage, the two goals of interventional therapy are to remove the AVM completely and avoid deterioration of neurologic dysfunction. Removal can be curative, but it is important to eliminate residual abnormal vessels, which may produce hemorrhages, especially if reduction of outflow increases perfusion pressure within the remaining anomalous vasculature. However, it is particularly dangerous to perform these procedures in critical neurologic areas, such as in or near the speech centers.

Therapeutic options include surgical resection of the AVM, embolization of the feeding arteries, and radiation-induced thrombosis. In some cases, combinations of these treatments are used. Selective embolization of the lesion via the transfemoral angiographic approach is commonly the initial procedure, with the goal of reducing blood flow through the AVM. Embolization may be performed in stages to reduce the size of the lesion sequentially, but endovascular treatment seldom obliterates an AVM. A risk of embolization is that embolic material may escape from the AVM and occlude normal vessels.

Stereotactic radiosurgery can eliminate an AVM but is satisfactory only for small lesions. The therapeutic effect of this technique is delayed because the abnormal vessels shrink gradually after the procedure.

Direct surgical intervention involves the use of microsurgical techniques. If the AVM is large, the procedures are often performed in stages to reduce blood flow in an adjacent region and make subsequent surgery easier. Surgery is considered successful if the postoperative angiogram shows no residual AVM. However, long-term occlusion rates are unknown, and recanalization with recurrent hemorrhage is possible.

PRIMARY INTRACEREBRAL HEMORRHAGE

Definition

Primary nontraumatic intracerebral hemorrhage (i.e., hemorrhage that does not result from ischemic injury) occurs predominantly as a consequence of chronic, poorly controlled hypertension (Chapter 66). Less frequently, a ruptured vascular malformation or amyloid angiopathy is responsible. Intracerebral hemorrhage can also be caused by a bleeding diathesis and certain drugs of abuse (Table 432–1).

TABLE 432–1 CAUSES, MEANS OF DIAGNOSIS, AND CHARACTERISTICS OF INTRACEREBRAL HEMORRHAGES

Causes	Primary Means of Diagnosis	Characteristics
Hypertension	Clinical history	Rupture of small arterioles related to degenerative changes induced by uncontrolled hypertension
Amyloid angiopathy	Clinical history	Rupture of small and medium-sized arteries with deposition of β-amyloid protein; manifested as lobar hemorrhages in people older than 70 years
Arteriovenous malformation	MRI or angiogram	Rupture of abnormal small vessels connecting arteries and veins
Intracranial aneurysm	MRI or angiogram	Rupture of a saccular dilation from a medium-sized artery; usually associated with subarachnoid hemorrhage
Cavernous angioma	MRI or angiogram	Rupture of abnormal capillary-like vessels with intermingled connective tissue
Venous angioma	MRI or angiogram	Rupture of an abnormal dilation of venules
Venous sinus thrombosis	MRI or angiogram	Result of hemorrhagic venous infarction
Intracranial neoplasm	MRI or angiogram	Result of necrosis and bleeding within hypervascular neoplasms
Coagulopathy	Clinical history	Most commonly associated with the use of anticoagulants or thrombolytics
Vasculitis	Serologic and cerebrospinal fluid markers, brain biopsy	Rupture of small or medium-sized arteries with inflammation and degeneration
Cocaine or alcohol abuse	Clinical history	Underlying vascular abnormalities may be present
Hemorrhagic transformation	CT	Hemorrhage in the region of cerebral infarction as a result of ischemic damage to the blood-brain barrier

Modified from Qureshi AI, Tuhrim S, Broderick JP, et al: Spontaneous intracerebral hemorrhage. N Engl J Med 2001;344:1450–1460.

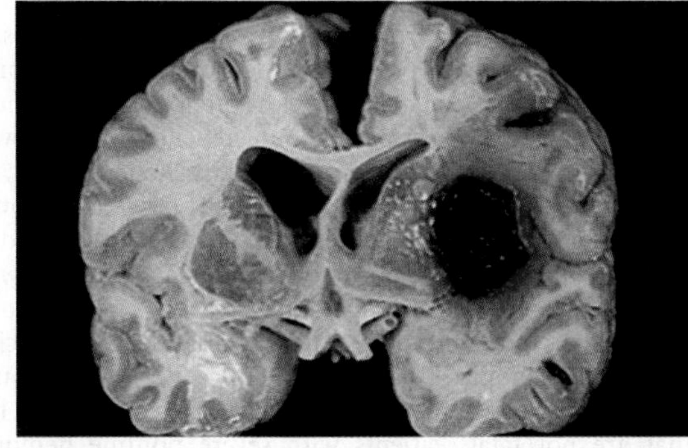

FIGURE 432–2 • Pathology specimen showing a large basal ganglia parenchymal hemorrhage in the left hemisphere. (Courtesy of Gregory W. Albers, Stanford University, Stanford, CA.)

Epidemiology

In the United States, primary intracerebral hemorrhage is responsible for 10 to 15% of strokes and about 80% of all intracranial hemorrhages. The average annual incidence in the United States is approximately 0,000. Intracerebral hemorrhage has the highest mortality rate of all subtypes of stroke, and almost 60% of affected patients die within the first year. The risk for primary intracerebral hemorrhage in blacks is about 40% higher than in whites. Worldwide, the incidence of intracerebral hemorrhage ranges from 10 to 40 per 1 million people, with the rate in Japan being at the top end of this range. Age-adjusted rates for men are about 50% higher than those for women. As with ischemic stroke, the incidence appears to be declining in the industrialized world, concurrent with the decline in hypertension.

Pathobiology

Primary intracerebral hemorrhage typically consists of a large, confluent area of blood that clots (Fig. 432–2). Most bleeding occurs at or near bifurcations of arteries with prominent degeneration of the media and smooth muscle. Several weeks later, the blood is slowly removed by phagocytosis, and after several months, only a small, collapsed cavity lined by hemosiderin-containing macrophages may remain. Rupture into the ventricles with bleeding into the subarachnoid space commonly occurs with large hemorrhages. Edematous parenchyma rapidly develops around the clot. Although hemorrhage may destroy brain tissue locally, histologic examination suggests that displacement of normal brain tissue and dissection of blood along fiber tracts account for much of the pathology. Viable and salvageable neural tissue may exist in the vicinity of the hematoma.

The most important risk factor for intracerebral hemorrhage is hypertension, particularly in people who are younger than 55 years, smokers, and poorly compliant with antihypertensive medications. Excessive chronic alcohol consumption also increases the risk for intracerebral hemorrhage. A less well established risk factor is a low serum cholesterol concentration (<160 mg/dL).

Hypertension is associated with hemorrhage in various locations throughout the brain, especially in the external capsule–putamen, internal capsule–thalamus, central pons, and cerebellum (Fig. 432–3). A smaller number of hemorrhages occur in the subcortical white matter, especially in the frontal, temporal, and occipital lobes.

Evidence, especially from serial CT scans, shows that hematomas expand for many hours after the onset of bleeding in many patients. Bleeding may cease when the lesion grows to a size sufficient to produce increased tissue pressure with consequent tamponade.

Amyloid (congophilic) angiopathy is a pathologic diagnosis that is more frequently made in people older than 55 years. This condition, which is unrelated to generalized amyloidosis and is occasionally hereditary, commonly produces multiple, small hemorrhages. It often appears in the brains of patients with Alzheimer's disease (Chapter 425) and has been associated with nonhypertensive hemorrhage in unusual lobar locations in the cerebral hemispheres. Amyloid deposits, chemically similar to those in Alzheimer's plaques, are seen in the media and adventitia of small and medium-sized arteries.

Anticoagulation, thrombolysis, and various hematologic abnormalities (Chapters 179 to 181) are associated with intracerebral hemorrhages. Warfarin anticoagulation to conventional intensities (i.e., international normalized ratio of 2.0 to 3.0) has been associated with a risk for intracranial hemorrhage of approximately 1% per year in many stroke-prone patients (Chapter 35). This rate is about 7 to 10 times greater than the risk in similar patients who have not undergone anticoagulation. On average, when such hemorrhages occur, the fatality rate is about 60%. Predictors are advanced age, previous ischemic stroke, hypertension, and the intensity of anticoagulation.

The most feared complication of thrombolytic therapy for acute myocardial infarction (Chapter 72) or ischemic stroke (Chapter 431) is intracerebral hemorrhage. When tissue plasminogen activator (t-PA) is administered within 3 hours after the onset of stroke symptoms, the intracerebral hemorrhage rate is 6.5% as compared with 0.5% in placebo patients; 50% of the patients who sustain these hemorrhages die. However, the overall benefit of t-PA therapy in appropriate patients persists because the increased risk for hemorrhage is more than counterbalanced by the improvement in ischemic strokes (Chapter 431).

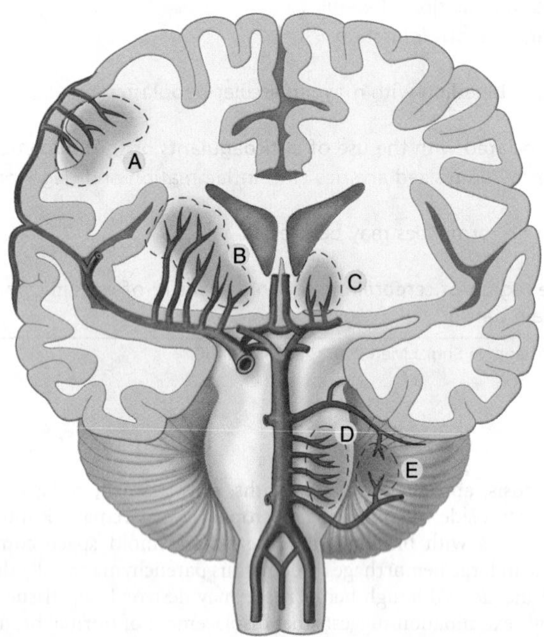

FIGURE 432–3 • Typical sites and sources of intracerebral hemorrhage. Intracerebral hemorrhages most commonly involve the cerebral lobes and originate from penetrating cortical branches of the anterior, middle, or posterior cerebral arteries (A); the basal ganglia and originate from ascending lenticulostriate branches of the middle cerebral artery (B); the thalamus and originate from ascending thalamogeniculate branches of the posterior cerebral artery (C); the pons and originate from paramedian branches of the basilar artery (D); and the cerebellum and originate from penetrating branches of the posterior inferior, anterior inferior, or superior cerebellar arteries (E). (From Qureshi AI, Tuhrim S, Broderick JP, et al: Spontaneous intracerebral hemorrhage. N Engl J Med 2001;344:1450–1460.)

Cerebral hemorrhages also occur in patients with leukemia (Chapter 194), polycythemia vera (Chapter 172), thrombocytopenia (Chapter 179), hemophilia (Chapter 180) and other clotting abnormalities, infectious and noninfectious vasculitis, intracranial neoplasms, and venous thrombosis. In addition, intracerebral hemorrhage can occur in patients who abuse various sympathomimetic agents and cocaine (Chapter 32).

Clinical Manifestations

The neurologic abnormalities caused by intracerebral hemorrhage do not differ from those caused by ischemic strokes (Chapter 431) because destruction of neural tissue is the basis of the neurologic dysfunction caused by both entities. The signs and symptoms are related to the location of the lesion. Because the site of intracerebral hemorrhage often differs from that of ischemic strokes, characteristic patterns of neurologic loss may be more frequently associated with intracerebral hemorrhage than with ischemic strokes (Table 432–2). Hemorrhages may grow as the bleeding continues, whereas ischemic lesions usually do not change in size after vascular occlusion; as a result, hemorrhages characteristically cause progressively increasing loss of neurologic function until a plateau is reached, whereas ischemic strokes may fluctuate or remain static after the early phases of the stroke. Subsequent deterioration in the level of consciousness after an intracerebral hemorrhage occurs in about a fourth of patients who are initially alert.

Intracranial hemorrhages in each of the four typical locations produce characteristic findings. Patients with massive *putaminal hemorrhages* become lethargic or comatose within minutes to hours after onset and concurrently experience contralateral weakness (including the face) with contralateral hemianopia and gaze paresis (i.e., eyes deviated toward the side of the hemorrhage). *Cerebellar hemorrhages* initially spare the brain stem, and consciousness is generally preserved in the early stages. Occipital headache may be the first symptom. The usual findings are unsteady gait, ataxia, nausea, and vomiting, which is often severe and repetitive. A variety of eye movement abnormalities may be present. Weakness is not prominent at onset, but with progression and brain stem compression, focal or bilateral weakness and coma develop, often rapidly. Further deterioration can result from herniation of cerebellar tissue downward through the foramen magnum or upward across the tentorium; hydrocephalus may be caused by obstruction of CSF flow. With continued bleeding or tissue swelling, severe brain stem damage ensues and causes rapid demise of the patient. Less frequent are *thalamic hemorrhages,* which cause patients to lose consciousness relatively rapidly; those who survive often experience contralateral hemiparesis, sensory deficits, and homonymous hemianopia. *Pontine hemorrhage* was once thought to produce coma invariably, but modern imaging detects smaller hemorrhages that are not fatal. Patients with severe pontine hemorrhages become comatose, usually with very small but detectable reactive pupils. Oculovestibular responses are often lost early, vomiting can occur at

TABLE 432–2 CLINICAL FEATURES OF COMMON HYPERTENSIVE HEMORRHAGES

	Site of Hemorrhage			
Clinical Features	**Putaminal**	**Thalamic**	**Pontine**	**Cerebellar**
Unconsciousness	Later	Later	Early	Late
Hemiparesis	Yes	Yes	Quadriparesis	Late
Sensory change	Yes	Yes	Yes	Late
Hemianopia	Yes	Yes	No	No
Pupils				
Size	Normal	Small	Small	Normal
Reaction	Yes	Yes or no	Yes or no	Yes
Gaze paresis				
Size	Contralateral, sometimes ipsilateral	Contralateral	Ipsilateral	Ipsilateral
Response to calorics	Yes	Yes	No	Yes or no
Downward eye deviation	Yes	No	No	
Ocular bobbing	No	No	Sometimes	Sometimes
Gait loss	No	No	Yes	Yes
Vomiting	Occasional	Occasional	Often	Severe

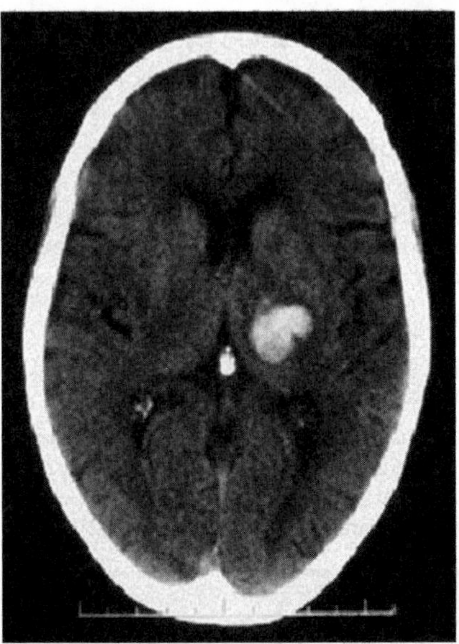

FIGURE 432–4 • Intracerebral hemorrhage. A computed tomographic scan shows a parenchymal hemorrhage involving the left thalamus and posterior internal capsule. (Courtesy of Gregory W. Albers, Stanford University, Stanford, CA.)

onset, and these patients generally have quadriplegia and bilateral extensor posturing. Patients may be "locked-in" (Chapter 428).

Lobar hemorrhages, which are more characteristic of amyloid angiopathy than hypertension, usually originate at the junctions between gray and white matter in the cerebral hemispheres. Such hemorrhages account for about a third of intracerebral hemorrhages and are approximately as common as putaminal hemorrhages. The clinical manifestation depends on the location of the hemorrhage. Most patients are elderly because amyloid angiopathy and hypertension are relatively frequent in this age group. Nonspecific symptoms, including headache, nausea, and vomiting, probably occur with about the same frequency but with less intensity than in deep, hypertensive hemorrhages. Coma and seizures are uncommon, possibly because most of these hemorrhages are comparatively small and located in subcortical white matter.

Diagnosis

Intracerebral hemorrhage often cannot be distinguished from other types of strokes based on clinical findings alone. The test of choice for making the diagnosis is a non–contrast-enhanced CT scan (Fig. 432–4) that shows areas of hemorrhage as zones of increased density, which may or may not have associated regions of decreased density indicating infarction. Primary parenchymal hemorrhages typically display homogeneous areas of increased density and a mass effect (i.e., shift of normal tissue from its usual location), whereas hemorrhagic infarctions are characterized by areas of increased density (i.e., blood) interspersed with areas of decreased density (i.e., infarction).

MRI findings depend on the precise imaging sequence and the age of the hemorrhage. The sensitivity and specificity of MRI for the diagnosis of hemorrhage, particularly in the presence of infarction, are unknown. MRI is able to detect small lesions, particularly in the posterior fossa, better than CT can, but how much of the lesion is hemorrhage or hypoperfusion is uncertain. Cerebral angiography is not needed for the acute evaluation of hemorrhages, but it is commonly used later to identify a suspected aneurysm or AVM that may be considered for intervention.

Treatment

General Measures

The usual medical management of acute parenchymal hemorrhage has been supportive, with initial care directed at maintenance of the airway, oxygenation, nutrition, and prevention and treatment of secondary complications. Optimal blood pressure treatment is uncertain, although the general guidelines for excessive hypertension and reduction of cerebral perfusion apply as for ischemic strokes (Chapter 431). There is no accepted protocol for the management of increased intracranial pressure; osmotherapy, hyperventilation, and neuromuscular paralysis rarely are beneficial. Fluid management should maintain euvolemia; fluid restriction or volume expansion is not of proven value. Seizures are particularly harmful in critically ill patients and are treated despite lack of data from randomized trials. Maintenance of normal body temperature is theoretically desirable because fever may accelerate tissue destruction.

Medical Therapy

Intravenous administration of recombinant factor VIIa within 4 hours after onset reduces the volume of hemorrhage and surrounding cerebral edema, as measured by CT, and improves neurologic outcomes at 90 days despite an increase in ischemic stroke and myocardial infarction. [2] Larger trials of this promising therapy are in progress. Small clinical trials of corticosteroids, glycerol, and hemodilution have not demonstrated benefit, and corticosteroids may increase the risk for infectious complications.

Surgical Therapy

The goal of surgical treatment of intracerebral hemorrhage is to remove as much blood clot as possible as quickly as possible. Ideally, surgery should remove the underlying cause, such as an AVM, and prevent hydrocephalus. Early surgical intervention to evacuate intracerebral hematomas within 24 hours is no better than medical therapy. [3] However, patients who have cerebellar hemorrhages and are deteriorating because of brain stem compression and hydrocephalus caused by ventricular obstruction are still recommended by some for removal of the clot or amputation of part of the cerebellum, although no proof exists to support this approach.

Prognosis

In recent series, the 30-day case-fatality rate averaged 30 to 50%. Most early deaths result from the direct neurologic consequences of the hemorrhage; the severity of bleeding (e.g., size, extension into ventricles) and level of neurologic function are the best predictors of poor outcomes. Supratentorial hemorrhages smaller than 30 mL rarely lead to death unless they are located in the thalamus. The long-term prognosis for various degrees of recovery is similar or better than that of cerebral infarctions of comparable severity. The risk for recurrent intracerebral hemorrhage has not been well studied, but the risk for at least one rebleeding episode may be as high as 25% over the next several years. The risk for intracerebral hemorrhage can be reduced by appropriate treatment. Control of mild to moderate hypertension decreases the risk for hemorrhagic stroke by a third to half (Chapter 66).

HYPERTENSIVE ENCEPHALOPATHY

Definition

Hypertensive encephalopathy is usually defined as malignant hypertension associated with central nervous system abnormalities (Chapter 66). Malignant hypertension is commonly defined as sustained, elevated arterial blood pressure, with diastolic levels of 130 mm Hg or greater and systolic pressure in excess of 200 mg Hg. Abnormal funduscopic findings include papilledema, retinal linear hemorrhages, or extravascular cotton-wool exudates. Hypertensive encephalopathy is classically characterized by rapidly evolving severe hypertension associated with headache, nausea, vomiting, visual disturbances, seizures, confusion, stupor, and ultimately, coma. Focal neurologic signs are common.

Pathobiology

The pathogenesis of hypertensive encephalopathy remains unclear. Pathologic findings include purpura in the brain, retinal hemorrhages, papilledema, and fibrinoid arteriolar lesions of the glomeruli. Diffuse fibrinoid necrosis and thrombotic occlusion of arterioles cause microinfarctions and petechial hemorrhages, and these changes lead to distal ischemia. Ring hemorrhage around a thrombosed precapillary is the characteristic microscopic lesion of hypertensive encephalopathy. Multiple, compacted petechiae can resemble a hematoma.

Clinical Manifestations and Diagnosis

Hypertensive encephalopathy is associated with hypertension of any cause and can occur in patients of any age. Severe headache is the most frequent manifestation. Nausea, vomiting, impaired vision, and dizziness are common. Confusion, stupor, and coma with generalized seizures may develop. Retinal changes characteristic of severe hypertension are common and often include hemorrhages or papilledema, but arteriolar narrowing may be the only abnormality. Because there are no pathognomonic findings in this disorder, it is a diagnosis of exclusion.

Uremic encephalopathy also occurs in patients with renal failure (Chapter 131). Uremia can cause altered mental status and seizures, and differentiation from hypertensive encephalopathy may be difficult. However, uremia is usually accompanied by metabolic acidosis or water intoxication, which may differentiate it from hypertensive encephalopathy, and correction of the uremia by dialysis may help clarify the picture.

Other complications of hypertension to be considered in the differential diagnosis of hypertensive encephalopathy include hemorrhagic and ischemic strokes. Focal neurologic signs predominate in these other conditions, whereas mental status changes are characteristic of hypertensive encephalopathy. Increased intracranial pressure from obstructive hydrocephalus (Chapter 199), brain tumor (Chapter 199), or subdural hematoma (Chapter 422) can elevate blood pressure and slow the pulse, but encephalopathy and markedly elevated blood pressure are absent.

Treatment

Rx

Therapy should be initiated immediately, but the rate of decrease in blood pressure should be controlled to avoid hypotension (Chapter 66). Seizures can usually be stopped with intravenous diazepam (10 mg); in eclamptic patients (Chapter 259), fosphenytoin (15 to 20 mg phenytoin equivalent per kilogram intravenously) or magnesium sulfate (4 g intramuscularly every 4 hours as needed) are often used, particularly because they may not depress the respiratory drive of the fetus as much as some other drugs do. Prompt delivery of the fetus may be quite helpful.

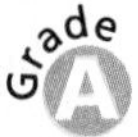

1. Molyneux AJ, Kerr RSC, Yu L-M, et al: International subarachnoid aneurysm trial (ISAT) of neurosurgical clipping versus endovascular coiling in 2143 patients with ruptured intracranial aneurysms: A randomised comparison of effects on survival, dependency, seizures, rebleeding, subgroups, and aneurysm occlusion. Lancet 2005;366;809–817.
2. Mayer SA, Brun NC, Begtrup K, et al: Recombinant activated factor VII for acute intracerebral hemorrhage. N Engl J Med 2005; 352:777–785.
3. Mendelow AD, Gregson BA, Fernandes HM, et al: Early surgery versus initial conservative treatment in patients with spontaneous supratentorial intracerebral haematomas in the International Surgical Trial in Intracerebral Haemorrhage (STITCH): A randomised trial. Lancet 2005;365:387–397.

SUGGESTED READINGS

Brisman JL, Song JK, Newell DW: Cerebral aneurysms. N Engl J Med 2006;355:928–939. *Comprehensive review.*

Gould DB, Phalan FC, van Mil SE, et al: Role of COL4A1 in small-vessel disease and hemorrhagic stroke. N Engl J Med 2006;354:1489–1496. *Mutation of this gene is associated with small vessel intracerebral bleeding.*

Johnston SC, Higashida RT, Barrow DL, et al: Recommendations for the endovascular treatment of intracranial aneurysms: A statement for healthcare professionals from the Committee on Cerebrovascular Imaging of the American Heart Association Council on Cardiovascular Radiology. Stroke 2002; 33:2536–2544.

Stapt C, Mohr JP, Choi JH, et al: Invasive treatment of unruptured brain arteriovenous malformations is experimental therapy. Curr Opin Neurol 2006;19:63–68. *A scholarly review explaining the need for an ongoing randomized trial.*

Van Gijn J, Kerr RS, Rinkel GJ: Subarachnoid haemorrhage. Lancet 2007;369:306–318. *Comprehensive review.*

433 PARKINSONISM

Anthony Lang

Parkinsonism is a clinical syndrome that consists of four cardinal signs: tremor, rigidity, akinesia, and postural disturbances (TRAP). Parkinson's disease is a common cause of the TRAP syndrome, but there are numerous other causes (Table 433–1).

PARKINSON'S DISEASE

Epidemiology

Parkinson's disease, which is the second most common neurodegenerative disorder after Alzheimer's disease, occurs in approximately 1 in 1000 in the general population and in 1% of persons older than 65 years. Men are affected slightly more often than women (3:2).

TABLE 433–1 DIFFERENTIAL DIAGNOSIS OF PARKINSONISM

PARKINSON'S DISEASE
Sporadic
Genetic
Autosomal dominant (e.g., α-synuclein gene mutations, duplications, triplications; *LRRK2* mutations)
Autosomal recessive (e.g., *parkin, DJ-1, PINK-1*)
SECONDARY PARKINSONISM
Neurodegenerative diseases (sporadic or genetic)
Progressive supranuclear palsy*
Multiple-system atrophy*
Corticobasal degeneration*
Dementia with Lewy bodies*
Alzheimer's disease*
ALS-parkinsonism-dementia complex of Guam
Huntington's disease
Neuroacanthocytosis
Spinocerebellar ataxias (e.g., SCA-3, SCA-2)
Wilson's disease
Pantothenate kinase–associated neurodegeneration (Hallervorden-Spatz syndrome)
Neuroferritinopathy
Calcification of the basal ganglia (Fahr's disease)
Dopa-responsive dystonia
Drugs*
Neuroleptics, metoclopramide, prochlorperazine, tetrabenazine, reserpine, cinnarizine, flunarizine, α-methyldopa, lithium
Toxic
MPTP, manganese, carbon monoxide, mercury
Infectious
Encephalitis lethargica
Other encephalitis, including HIV
Subacute sclerosing panencephalitis
Creutzfeldt-Jakob disease
Vascular*
Atherosclerosis
Amyloid angiopathy
Neoplastic
Brain tumor
Other mass lesions
Normal-pressure hydrocephalus*
Head trauma
Multiple sclerosis

*See Table 433–4 for additional details.
ALS = amyotrophic lateral sclerosis; HIV = human immunodeficiency virus; MPTP = 1-methyl-4-phenyl-1,2,3,6-tetrahydropyridine.
Adapted from Cloutier M, Lang AE: Movement disorders: An overview. *In* Factor SA, Lang AE, Weiner WJ (eds): Drug Induced Movement Disorders. Malden, MA, Blackwell, 2005, pp 3–19.

Pathobiology

The cause of Parkinson's disease is believed to be a variable combination of poorly understood genetic and environmental factors. Both autosomal dominant and recessive genes can cause classic Parkinson's disease. The protein α-synuclein, which is the chief constituent of the hallmark cytoplasmic inclusion, the Lewy body (Chapter 425), is critical in the pathogenesis of Parkinson's disease. Abnormal aggregation of the protein, either from mutations in the α-synuclein gene or as a result of excessive production of the normal protein because of gene duplications or triplications, is associated with varying disease phenotypes. Other defined genetic abnormalities may be associated with classic later-onset Parkinson's disease, including *LRRK2,* which is currently the most common cause of autosomal dominantly inherited Parkinson's disease, or with early-onset parkinsonism, typically found in the autosomal recessive forms associated with *parkin,* DJ-1, and *PINK1.* Other genes in which mutations may increase the risk for development of Parkinson's disease include the glucocerebrosidase gene *(GBA)* in Ashkenazi Jews.

Although monogenetic forms of Parkinson's disease are uncommon, knowing that parkin is an E-3 ubiquitin protein ligase has implicated the ubiquitin proteasome system in the pathogenesis of Parkinson's disease. Proteasome inhibitors, which may be present in the environment, are being studied for their potential to cause parkinsonism in animals. Such findings support the "environmental hypothesis" of sporadic Parkinson's disease, similar to the discovery that the selective neurotoxin 1-methyl-4-phenyl-1,2,3,6-tetrahydropyridine (MPTP) is oxidized to the active toxin MPP^+, which is a selective inhibitor of complex I of the mitochondrial electron transport chain. This knowledge, combined with recognition of the importance of dopamine (see later), has implicated oxidative stress in the pathogenesis of Parkinson's disease. Other proposed pathogenetic factors include excitotoxicity and inflammation.

Pathology

Many of the features of Parkinson's disease are due to loss of dopamine in the neostriatum (especially the putamen) secondary to loss of the pigmented dopaminergic neurons in the substantia nigra pars compacta (SNc) of the midbrain. Approximately 60% of these dopaminergic neurons will have degenerated before clinical features of the disease develop.

In addition to the prominent degenerative changes in the SNc (cell loss, gliosis, abnormal deposition of aggregated α-synuclein as Lewy bodies and Lewy neurites), pathologic changes are also evident in other brain stem nuclei, in cortical regions, and in peripheral autonomic neurons. Indeed, it has been suggested that Parkinson's disease may begin in the lower brain stem and the olfactory system, where it causes early loss of the sense of smell, and only later involves the substantia nigra. Independent of the order of involvement, it is likely that the widespread extranigral neurodegenerative changes account for the many symptoms that do not respond to dopamine replacement and that become increasingly problematic as the disease progresses.

Clinical Manifestations

Typically, the symptoms begin in one limb. This asymmetry often persists into later stages of the disease.

Motor Symptoms

The classic "resting tremor" of Parkinson's disease has characteristic clinical features. The tremor has a frequency of 4 to 6 cycles per second, typically with a "pill rolling" character when it involves the hand. It is generally present with the limb in complete repose and typically subsides when the limb moves and takes up a new position, although the tremor may reemerge ("reemergent tremor") within a short time after maintaining the new position. Because resting tremor diminishes or subsides with action, it may not be disabling but can be embarrassing and may be associated with aching or fatigue of the affected limb. Resting tremor is usually accentuated by stress (e.g., by asking the patient to perform mental calculations). It is also characteristically present in the upper limbs while walking. A higher-frequency (e.g., 7 to 10 Hz) postural and kinetic tremor is also common in patients with various causes of parkinsonism.

Rigidity

Rigidity is a form of increased muscle tone appreciated best on slow passive movements. It may be characterized as "cogwheel" when a tremor is superimposed or as "lead pipe" when it is not. Rigidity is "activated" or accentuated on examination by asking the patient to move the limb opposite the one being tested. Patients may complain of stiffness, but rigidity is not usually disabling.

Akinesia

Akinesia or bradykinesia comprises a variety of disturbances of movement, including slowness, reduced amplitude, fatiguing, and interruptions in ongoing movement. This disabling aspect of parkinsonism interferes with all voluntary activities and accounts for many of the well-known features of parkinsonism: lack of facial expression with reduced blinking (hypomimia or masked facies—the "reptilian stare"), soft monotonous speech (hypophonia), impaired swallowing resulting in drooling (sialorrhea), small handwriting (micrographia), reduced arm swing while walking, shortened stride and shuffling gait, difficulty arising from a low chair, and problems turning over in bed. Arrests in ongoing movement ("motor block") can interfere with a variety of activities, but these are best appreciated as freezing of gait. Bradykinesia is evident on inspection and elicited by testing rapid repetitive and alternating movements: finger tapping, opening and the closing the fist, pronating and supinating the wrist, and toe and heel tapping.

Postural Disturbances

Postural disturbances include a flexed posture in the limbs and trunk (stooped, simian posture), as well as postural instability resulting in imbalance and falls. Patients may complain of being unable to stop themselves from going forward (propulsion) or backward (retropulsion). Clinical assessment of postural instability includes the "pull test," in which the examiner abruptly pulls the patient off balance while being ready to catch the patient in the event of a fall.

Other Symptoms

In addition to the motor features of parkinsonism, a variety of non-motor features are extremely common and include pain and other sensory disturbances; dysautonomic complaints, such as urinary urgency and frequency; orthostatic faintness; constipation; male erectile dysfunction; sleep abnormalities, including rapid eye movement behavioral disorder (Chapter 429); anxiety; fatigue; depression; and cognitive disturbances, including dementia. As the disease progresses, more resistant features develop, including "axial" motor disturbances (speech and swallowing abnormalities, freezing, and postural instability), as well as neurobehavioral and cognitive dysfunction.

Complications

In addition to the manifestations of the disease itself, complications of drug therapy include motor and non–motor-related fluctuations and psychiatric or behavioral disturbances. Thus, in the later stages of the disease, the clinical picture often fluctuates from hour to hour and even from minute to minute; accordingly, patients exhibit the classic features of parkinsonism, which may improve considerably in response to medication, symptoms that persist despite the peak benefit of medication, and symptoms that occur as a complication of dopaminergic medication (Table 433–2).

Diagnosis

Testing for monogenetic forms of Parkinson's disease (e.g., parkin) is becoming available, but guidelines for its use have not yet been developed. Given the classic clinical manifestations, the diagnostic evaluation focuses largely on ways to exclude other causes of parkinsonism (Table 433–3). Young-onset patients should have Wilson's disease excluded by determination of 24-hour urine copper and serum ceruloplasmin and by slit lamp examination (Chapter 230). Findings on magnetic resonance imaging are generally normal in Parkinson's disease, but it is indicated to exclude other diagnoses (Table 433–4). Positron emission tomography, which can assess the presynaptic and postsynaptic sides of the nigrostriatal dopamine system, is useful for research, but the most common ligand, $[^{18}F]$ fluorodopa, does not reliably distinguish Parkinson's disease from many other neurodegerative diseases that mimic it. The same

TABLE 433–2 PROBLEMS IN LATE-STAGE PARKINSON'S DISEASE

Problem	Symptoms
LATER TREATMENT-RESISTANT SYMPTOMS	
Motor	Dysarthria Dysphagia Freezing of gait (on-period freezing) Postural instability with falls
Non–motor*	Dysautonomia, weight loss Sensory symptoms, including pain (some may be responsive to levodopa) Changes in mood or behavior (depression, anxiety), sleep disturbances (excessive daytime sleepiness often caused by or aggravated by dopaminergic medication) Fatigue Cognitive dysfunction and dementia
RELATED TO TREATMENT AND DISEASE	
Motor fluctuations	Wearing off of drug effect (predictable end-of-dose deterioration, morning akinesia), increased latency to benefit ("delayed-on"), dose failures ("no-on") On-off phenomenon, more rapid and unpredictable fluctuations Concomitant fluctuations of non–motor-related symptoms that may be as disabling as motor symptoms (or more so)
Dyskinesias (abnormal involuntary movements)	Peak-dose dyskinesias: chorea, athetosis, and less often, more prolonged dystonia, typically worse on the initially affected side Diphasic dyskinesia ("beginning-of-dose" and "end-of-dose" dyskinesias): mixtures of choreoathetosis, ballism, dystonia, alternating movements (especially in legs) Off-period dystonia: most often involving the legs and feet (including morning foot dystonia)
Psychiatric disturbances	Vivid dreams and nightmares Rapid eye movement sleep behavior disorder (may develop before parkinsonism)* Visual hallucinations with clear sensorium Hallucinations with confusion Mania, hypersexuality, problem gambling, dopaminergic drug addiction Paranoid psychosis

*These symptoms sometimes occur earlier in the course of the illness.
Adapted from Lang AE, Lozano AM: Parkinson's disease—second of two parts. N Engl J Med 1998;339:1130–1143.

TABLE 433–3 CLINICAL CLUES TO AN ALTERNATIVE (NON-PARKINSON'S DISEASE) CAUSE OF PARKINSONIAN SIGNS AND SYMPTOMS

Extraocular movements—e.g., nystagmus, limitation of vertical gaze, especially with slowing of downward saccadic eye movements
Early and prominent dysarthria/dysphagia
Prominent or early abnormal neck postures: flexion or extension
Ataxia—limb, gait (impaired tandem gait)
Lower body distribution with relative sparing of upper limb function
Early postural instability/falls/freezing
Dysautonomia (early/prominent), prominent hypotensive response to dopaminergic medication
Pyramidal tract signs—very brisk reflexes, clonus, extensor plantar responses
Peripheral nerve dysfunction—loss of reflexes, distal sensory loss, weakness
Apraxia/cortical sensory changes
Early severe dementia
Poor response to levodopa

limitations apply to evaluation of the dopamine transporter by single-photon emission computed tomography. The finding of increased echogenicity in the SNc of the midbrain on transcranial ultrasound may be more specific in diagnosing Parkinson's disease, but the data are not conclusive.

Treatment

Rx

Treatment of Parkinson's disease is directed at slowing the progression ("neuroprotective" or "disease-modifying" treatments); improving symptoms, typically by restoring dopaminergic tone medically or by correcting basal ganglia neurophysiology surgically ("symptomatic"); or attempting to restore or regenerate the damaged neurons ("neurorestorative" or "neuroregenerative" therapy).

Medical Treatment

To date, no medical treatment (Table 443–5) has been proved to modify the progressive course of Parkinson's disease. The selective monoamine oxidase B (MAO-B) inhibitor selegiline may exert a mild neuroprotective effect, and there may also be a disease-modifying effect of the newer MAO-B inhibitor rasagiline [1] and coenzyme Q10.

Early treatment in a patient with little or no disability may entail only education, psychological support, encouragement to remain active and become involved in an exercise program, and ongoing follow-up. When symptoms begin to interfere with function, mildly effective drugs such as an MAO-B inhibitor, amantadine, and anticholinergics (the latter predominantly for tremor in younger patients) may provide adequate benefit (see Table 443–5). When symptoms are more pronounced or inadequately controlled with these approaches, dopaminergic therapy should be introduced. In patients younger than 65 years who are cognitively intact and lack other major medical problems, initial therapy with a dopamine agonist may delay the development of motor complications. [2] However, these drugs result in more excessive sleepiness, leg edema, "impulse control disorders" (such as pathologic gambling,

Text continued on p. 2733.

TABLE 433–4 DISEASES THAT MUST BE DISTINGUISHED FROM PARKINSON'S DISEASE

Diagnosis	Important Distinguishing Clinical Features	Response to Levodopa/Comments (Including Imaging)
Multiple-system atrophy (MSA) (includes striatonigral degeneration, sporadic olivopontocerebellar atrophy, and Shy-Drager syndrome) MSA-P = a predominant parkinsonian manifestation MSA-C = a predominant cerebellar manifestation (mixed features are common)	Early dysautonomia (including orthostatic hypotension and sexual impotence) and bladder dysfunction (with autonomic and nonautonomic components) Cerebellar dysfunction Pyramidal tract signs Stimulus-sensitive myoclonus of the hands and face Extreme forward neck flexion (anterocollis) Mottled, cold hands Inspiratory stridor Prominent dysarthria	Good response initially evident in 20% and sustained partial response in ≈15% Dyskinesias or motor fluctuations possible; cranial dystonia may be prominent Patient is wheelchair bound despite response to levodopa (early loss of postural reflexes, with or without ataxia) MRI (including diffusion-weighted imaging and gradient echo sequences) often shows diagnostic changes in the stratum in MSA-P and "hot-crossed bun sign" in the pons in MSA-C
Progressive supranuclear palsy	Supranuclear vertical ophthalmoplegia Other oculomotor and eyelid disturbances Axial rigidity greater than limb rigidity Early falls, speech and swallowing disturbances Nuchal extension Cognitive or behavioral changes Possibly a higher incidence of hypertension than in Parkinson's disease and other neurodegenerative causes of parkinsonism	Good response rarely evident; benefit only to classic parkinsonian features such as limb rigidity, bradykinesia, and rare examples of tremor at rest MRI often demonstrates profound midbrain atrophy (midline sagittal view)
Corticobasal (cortical-basal ganglionic) degeneration	Apraxia, cortical sensory loss, alien-limb phenomenon Pronounced asymmetrical rigidity Limb dystonia Stimulus-sensitive myoclonus Aphasia Cognitive dysfunction (frontotemporal dementia)	Usually negligible MRI may show a pronounced asymmetrical cortical atrophy
Vascular parkinsonism	"Lower-half " parkinsonism with gait disturbances predominating, often with minimal or much milder upper body involvement Additional neurologic deficits (e.g., pyramidal tract signs, pseudobulbar palsy)	Usually poor Imaging demonstrates multiple infarcts involving the basal ganglia and subcortical white matter
Dementia with Lewy bodies	Early dementia (cognitive profile somewhat different from that of Alzheimer's disease) Spontaneous hallucinations, fluctuating cognitive status, falls Pronounced sensitivity to the extrapyramidal side effects of neuroleptic drugs Parkinsonism may be similar to typical Parkinson's disease, although rigidity may be more prominent than bradykinesia or tremor	Motor features may respond well; psychiatric side effects of dopaminergic drugs are typically dose limiting
Alzheimer's disease	Early dementia (memory loss, apraxia, aphasia) Tremor uncommon Spontaneous hallucinations less common than in dementia with Lewy bodies	Poor
Normal-pressure hydrocephalus	"Lower-half" parkinsonism ("gait apraxia") Urinary complaints (frequency, urgency, incontinence) Cognitive disturbances	Generally poor Imaging demonstrates ventriculomegaly out of proportion to cortical atrophy
Drug-induced parkinsonism	All the classic features of parkinsonism (tremor may be less common than in Parkinson's disease) Usually symmetrical signs and symptoms Other drug-induced movement disorders (e.g., tardive dyskinesia with neuroleptics)	Usually poor because of ongoing dopamine receptor blockade; may aggravate movements of tardive dyskinesia

For evidence-based recommendations on investigation of parkinsonism, see Suchowersky O, Reich S, Perlmutter JS, et al: Practice parameter: Diagnosis and prognosis of new onset Parkinson disease (an evidence-based review): Report of the Quality Standards Subcommittee of the American Academy of Neurology. Neurology 2006;66:968–975.
Adapted from Lang AE, Lozano AM: Parkinson's disease—first of two parts. N Engl J Med 1998;339:1044–1053.

TABLE 433–5 DRUGS FOR PARKINSON'S DISEASE

Class	Drug	Usual Starting Dose	Usual Final Dosage	Important Adverse Effects	Comments	Indications
Anticholinergic	Many (e.g., benztropine, trihexyphenidyl)	Benztropine or trihexyphenidyl, 1–2 mg 2–3 times per day	Varied	Peripheral effects, e.g., dry mouth, blurred vision, constipation, difficulties with urination Central effects, e.g., confusion, memory problems, hallucinations	Relatively contraindicated in the elderly and contraindicated in patients with cognitive disturbances	Early treatment of tremor
Miscellaneous	Amantadine	100 mg once per day	100 mg 2 or 3 times per day	Confusion, visual hallucinations; livedo reticularis, swelling of the ankles; dose reduction or drug withdrawal necessary in the presence of renal failure	Previously considered a dopaminergic drug, now thought to act primarily through NMDA antagonist effects	Early treatment; later for dyskinesias
Dopamine precursor	Levodopa given with peripheral dopa decarboxylase inhibitor (carbidopa [in 4:1 and 10:1 ratios] or benserazide [4:1]*)	5.0–12.5 mg (4:1 preparation) 3 times per day (with meals to reduce nausea and vomiting)	Varied; begin with 3-times-daily schedule (controlled-release levodopa-carbidopa may be given twice daily at first); late in the disease patients may require multiple doses per day (sometimes >2 g/day). Initially give with meals to reduce GI upset; later avoid meals to improve absorption and reliability of response	Peripheral and central dopaminergic side effects Peripheral: nausea, vomiting, and orthostatic hypotension Central: motor fluctuations, dyskinesias, psychiatric disturbances	Peripheral side effects often controlled by additional carbidopa or the peripheral dopamine receptor blocker domperidone* Controlled-release formulations often less bioavailable with less reliable absorption (more "dose failures" later on)	Formulations: Immediate release—for early and later treatment Controlled-release (with carbidopa [4 : 1] or benserazide [4 : 1]*)—for predictable motor fluctuations (wearing off) and nighttime akinesia Stalevo (with carbidopa and entacapone)—for wearing off Parcopa (orally disintegrating tablets for faster absorption)—for patients with problematic long latency to benefit of individual doses Duodopa* (used with a pump for duodenal infusions)—for problematic motor fluctuations
Dopamine agonists Ergot derived	Bromocriptine	1.25 mg 3 times per day with meals	30–40 mg/day	Peripheral and central dopaminergic side effects; pedal edema, excessive daytime sleepiness Pleuropulmonary reaction, retroperitoneal fibrosis, erythromelalgia	Peripheral side effects often well controlled with domperidone* Rare pulmonary, retroperitoneal, and skin effects possibly caused by ergot derivation (drug withdrawal usually required)	Early and adjunctive therapy

	Pergolide	0.05 mg once per day ×2 days, increasing slowly thereafter	3–5 mg/day	As for bromocriptine; cardiac valvopathy	As for bromocriptine	Not the first agonist because it causes restrictive cardiac valve disease
	Cabergoline*	0.5–1 mg once per day	2–6 mg/day	As for pergolide	As for pergolide Long half-life allows once-daily dosage	As for pergolide, although advantage of a long half-life may outweigh this concern
	Lisuride*	0.1–0.2 mg 1–3 times per day	2–5 mg/day	As for bromocriptine	As for bromocriptine	Uncertain whether cardiac valve abnormalities occur Parenteral formulations allow chronic infusion (pump) therapy
Non–ergot derived	Ropinirole	0.25 mg 3 times per day	Up to 24 mg/day in 3 divided doses	Similar peripheral and central dopaminergic side effects to those of ergot-derived dopamine agonists, with the probable exceptions of pleuropulmonary reaction, retroperitoneal fibrosis, erythromelalgia, and cardiac valvulopathy	Effective as first-line and adjunctive therapy; dopamine D_3 agonist effects may contribute to efficacy	De novo therapy shown to be associated with less motor complications than with levodopa Implications of less progressive loss of dopamine terminal function on imaging uncertain
	Pramipexole	0.125 mg 3 times per day	Up to 4.5 mg/day in 3 divided doses	As for ropinirole	As for ropinirole, possibly greater "D_3-preferring" effects—may account for antidepressant effect	As for ropinirole
	Rotigotine*	4.5 mg/day (10 cm^2)	Transdermal patch (4.5–27.0 mg/day; 10–60 cm^2)	As for ropinirole Additional adverse effects related to skin patch application (dermatitis)	May be effective for both first-line and adjunctive therapy	Utility and patient acceptance still being explored
	Apomorphine	3–5 mg SC injection	Parenteral agent given as needed or as continuous infusion	Peripheral and central dopaminergic side effects Local skin reactions, including nodule formation	Concomitant antiemetic (e.g., domperidone,* trimethobenzamide) needed	Late-stage problematic motor fluctuations Long-term use of infusions may reduce dyskinesias, as well as motor fluctuations
Monoamine oxidase B inhibitors	Selegiline	5 mg once per day	5 mg 2 times per day	Dopaminergic effects of other drugs possibly accentuated, insomnia, confusion	Last dose given at midday to avoid insomnia	Early mild disease Predictable motor fluctuations (wearing off)
	Zydis selegiline	1.25 mg once per day	1.25 or 2.5 mg/day (wafer formulation)	As for selegiline	As for selegiline Absorbed from the buccal mucosa, thereby avoiding first-pass hepatic metabolism and methamphetamine metabolite of selegiline	As for selegiline
	Rasagiline	1 mg once per day	1–2 mg once per day	As for selegiline		Preliminary evidence suggests possible disease-modifying effects As for selegiline

Continued

TABLE 433-5 DRUGS FOR PARKINSON'S DISEASE—cont'd

Class	Drug	Usual Starting Dose	Usual Final Dosage	Important Adverse Effects	Comments	Indications
Catechol *O*-methyltransferase inhibitors	Tolcapone	100 mg 3 times per day	100 or 200 mg 3 times per day (at 6-hr intervals)	Effects of levodopa accentuated Diarrhea in approximately 5% of patients Hepatotoxicity	Dose of levodopa may have to be reduced by as much as 25%; diarrhea (sometimes explosive) typically forces discontinuation Ongoing monitoring of liver function tests required (second-line COMT inhibitor)	Motor fluctuations, especially wearing off (probably more effective than entacapone)
	Entacapone	200 mg with each dose of levodopa	200 mg 4–10 times per day (given with doses of levodopa)	Effects of levodopa accentuated	As for tolcapone; diarrhea possibly less frequent Liver function monitoring unnecessary	As for tolcapone Available in a combination tablet with levodopa/carbidopa (Stalevo)
Atypical neuroleptics	Clozapine	12.5 mg hs	Wide range (6.25–150 mg/day), usually <75 mg/day	Agranulocytosis, sedation, hypotension, sialorrhea	Very low risk of worsening parkinsonism; agranulocytosis rare (<1%) and reversible if discovered early (requires regular monitoring of complete blood count)	Drug-induced psychosis Other "off-label" indications include drug-resistant tremor and possibly levodopa-induced dyskinesias
	Quetiapine	12.5–25 mg hs	25–150 mg/day	Sedation May worsen parkinsonism	Probably less ineffective than clozapine	Drug-induced psychosis
Acetylcholinesterase inhibitors	Donepezil	5 mg once per day	5–10 mg/day	Peripheral cholinergic side effects: nausea, vomiting, diarrhea Increased tremor, worsening of other Parkinson features		Dementia Possibly effective for psychotic symptoms
	Rivastigmine	1.5 mg twice per day	3–12 mg/day	As for donepezil		As for donepezil

*Unavailable in the United States.
COMT = catecholamine *O*-methyltransferase; GI = gastrointestinal; NMDA = *N*-methyl-D-aspartate.
For evidence-based treatment recommendations, see Suchowersky O, Gronseth G, Perlmutter J, et al: Practice parameter: Neuroprotective strategies and alternative therapies for Parkinson disease (an evidence-based review): Report of the Quality Standards Subcommittee of the American Academy of Neurology. Neurology 2006;66:976–982; Pahwa R, Factor SA, Lyons KE, et al: Practice parameter: Treatment of Parkinson disease with motor fluctuations and dyskinesia (an evidence-based review): Report of the Quality Standards Subcommittee of the American Academy of Neurology. Neurology 2006;66:983–995; and Miyasaki JM, Shannon K, Voon V, et al: Practice parameter: Evaluation and treatment of depression, psychosis, and dementia in Parkinson disease (an evidence-based review): Report of the Quality Standards Subcommittee of the American Academy of Neurology. Neurology 2006;66:996–1002.

Rx

hypersexuality, binge eating, and shopping), and hallucinations than levodopa does. If a full dose of a dopamine agonist does not provide adequate clinical benefit or has intolerable side effects, levodopa should be initiated. In older patients, in those with cognitive dysfunction (more prone to hallucinations with dopamine agonists), and in circumstances that require more rapid improvement of pronounced disability, levodopa should be the initial drug used.

Alleviating Symptoms

Levodopa is the most effective treatment of Parkinson's disease, but it is associated with a variety of side effects (see Table 433–2). For the first year or more the benefit of levodopa lasts throughout the day with little symptomatic variability. However, in time the duration of benefit declines, with worsening of symptoms first thing in the morning (morning akinesia) and for a variable time before scheduled daytime doses (wearing-off/end-of-dose akinesia). Within 2 to 5 years of initiating treatment, up to 50% of patients may also experience involuntary movements (chorea, athetosis, dystonia), most often at the peak action of the medication. These complications, which are generally more prominent and occur earlier in patients with onset of disease at a younger age, reflect the short half-life of levodopa combined with the underlying progressive loss of presynaptic dopamine neurons and result in nonphysiologic "pulsatile" stimulation of striatal dopamine receptors, which then induces "neuroplastic" changes in postsynaptic striatal neurons. Initially, these complications rarely cause major disability.

Although initiating therapy with a dopamine agonist rather than levodopa may be associated with a delay in the onset of these motor problems, the clinical benefit is generally less than with levodopa, and all patients eventually require the addition of levodopa to control symptoms. No data support delaying levodopa, and some data suggest that levodopa could have a neuroprotective effect. [3] Even as Parkinson's disease progresses, most of the classic features continue to respond even after 20 years of treatment. It is not clear that delaying motor complications in the first 5 years of treatment by the initial use of a dopamine agonist improves long-term outcome or quality of life.

There is no advantage to starting a controlled-release rather than an immediate-release preparation of levodopa. Whether prolonging the duration of action of levodopa by blocking its metabolism (e.g., by a catecholamine *O*-methyltransferase [COMT] inhibitor) and thus resulting in less pulsatile stimulation of postsynaptic dopamine receptors from the outset will result in a delay in motor complications is unknown. Motor fluctuations that develop during levodopa therapy are managed by a number of approaches (see Table 433–5), including increasing the frequency of the dose, using a controlled-release preparation, prolonging the action by blocking metabolism (MAO-B or COMT inhibition), or adding a dopamine agonist. For example, adding rasagiline or entacapone to levodopa provides significant incremental benefits. [4]

Medical management of Parkinson's disease often includes a variety of other agents, for example, drugs directed at treatment of orthostatic hypotension (Chapter 427), depression (Chapter 420), anxiety (Chapter 420), urinary frequency and urgency (Chapters 24 and 124), and male erectile dysfunction (Chapter 253). Management of late-stage Parkinson's disease requires skill with polypharmacy and an understanding of the complicated benefit-risk ratios of the many drugs needed.

Surgical Treatment

Surgical therapy, which involves deep brain stimulation of the subthalamic nucleus, improves the symptoms of Parkinson's disease [5] and permits lower doses of antiparkinson medications, whereas deep brain stimulation of the internal segment of the globus pallidus may provide a less consistent and durable response. Thalamic deep brain stimulation is of limited utility because it is effective only for tremor. The best predictor of a good response to deep brain stimulation of the subthalamic nucleus is the patient's ongoing clinical response to levodopa. Apart from tremor, which may be resistant to the highest tolerable dose of levodopa, symptoms that are resistant to the peak effect of levodopa (e.g., dysarthria, postural instability with falls) also fail to respond to deep brain stimulation. The typical good candidate for deep brain stimulation of the subthalamic nucleus is an otherwise healthy, relatively young, cognitively intact, and psychiatrically stable patient who still responds well to levodopa but is suffering from disabling motor fluctuations and dyskinesias. Double-blind randomized trials of transplantation of fetal substantia nigra into the stratum have not only failed to show significant efficacy but have also been associated with the side effect of transplant-induced off-medication dyskinesias. [6] A double-blind randomized trial of bilateral intraputamenal infusion of glial-derived neurotrophic factor failed to confirm the benefits found in unblinded studies.

Prognosis

Parkinson's disease progresses inexorably over a period of many years; the speed and course of progression vary considerably from patient to patient. Some patients maintain an excellent response to treatment and seem to change very little over prolonged follow-up, but most patients note increasing disability, with the development of many symptoms that are poorly responsive to medications. Factors such as poor postural stability, falls, dysarthria, dysphagia, dysautonomia, excessive daytime sleepiness, and dementia contribute to the disability and increased mortality.

Future Directions

Gene therapies directed at either modifying neurotransmitter function or inducing neuroregeneration and other cell-based therapies are under development. Future treatments must also address the widespread, multisystemic nature of the disease, especially symptoms that are unrelated to nigrostriatal dopamine deficiency and that fail to respond to current therapies.

OTHER CAUSES OF PARKINSONISM

The numerous causes of parkinsonism (see Table 433–1) are sometimes termed "akinetic-rigid syndrome," "Parkinson's syndrome," "atypical parkinsonism," or even "Parkinson-plus syndrome" to emphasize that these patients commonly demonstrate additional clinical features indicative of the more widespread and particularly more severe pathologic involvement of areas beyond the dopaminergic SNc. These other parkinsonism conditions are generally associated with "postsynaptic" changes that result in a poor or unsustained response to levodopa, and this unresponsiveness serves as one of the most important of several clues that the parkinsonism features are caused by conditions other than Parkinson's disease (see Table 433–4) (i.e., "parkinsonism minus" a levodopa response; see Table 433–3).

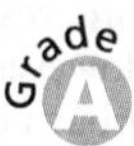

1. Siderowf A, Parkinson Study Group: A controlled, randomized, delayed-start study of rasagiline in early Parkinson disease. Arch Neurol 2004;61:561–566.
2. Holloway RG, Shoulson I, Kieburtz K, et al: Pramipexole vs levodopa as initial treatment for Parkinson disease—a 4-year randomized controlled trial. Arch Neurol 2004;61:1044–1053.
3. Fahn S, Shoulson I, Kieburtz K, et al: Levodopa and the progression of Parkinson's disease. N Engl J Med 2004;351:2498–2508.
4. Rascol O, Brooks DJ, Melamed E, et al: Rasagiline as an adjunct to levodopa in patients with Parkinson's disease and motor fluctuations. Lancet 2005;365:947–954.
5. Deuschl G, Schade-Brittinger C, Krack P, et al: A randomized trial of deep-brain stimulation for Parkinson's disease. N Engl J Med 2006;355:896–908.
6. Olanow CW, Goetz CG, Kordower JH, et al: A double-blind controlled trial of bilateral fetal nigral transplantation in Parkinson's disease. Ann Neurol 2003;54:403–414.

SUGGESTED READINGS

Goetz CG, Poewe W, Rascol O, et al: Evidence-based medical review update: Pharmacological and surgical treatments of Parkinson's disease: 2001 to 2004. Mov Disord 2005;20:523–539. *An update of evidence-based treatments published in* Movement Disorders *in 2002 (vol 17, Suppl. 4).*

Hely MA, Morris JGL, Reid WGJ, et al: Sydney multicenter study of Parkinson's disease: Non-L-dopa–responsive problems dominate at 15 years. Mov Disord 2005:20:190–199. *Shows the increased mortality and progressive disability, especially that attributable to non-dopaminergic aspects of the disease.*

Krack P, Batir A, Van Blercom N, et al: Five-year follow-up of bilateral stimulation of the subthalamic nucleus in advanced Parkinson's disease. N Engl J Med 2003;349:1925–1934. *Showed persistent marked benefit in off-medication symptoms but gradual worsening of on-medication features, particularly axial symptoms and bradykinesia.*

Miyasaki JM, Shannon K, Voon V et al: Practice parameter: Evaluation and treatment of depression, psychosis, and dementia in Parkinson disease (an evidence-based review): Report of the Quality Standards Subcommittee of the American Academy of Neurology. Neurology 2006;66:996–1002. *Evidence-based review of these neuropsychiatric features of Parkinson's disease.*

Nutt JG, Wooten GF: Diagnosis and initial management of Parkinson's disease. N Engl J Med 2005;353:1021–1027. *A practical review.*

Schüpbach WM, Maltête D, Houeto JL, et al: Neurosurgery at an earlier stage of Parkinson disease: A randomized controlled trial. Neurology 2007;68:267–271. *Small trial suggesting that subthalamic nucleus stimulation should be considered early in the course of disease.*

Suchowersky O, Gronseth G, Perlmutter J, et al: Practice parameter: Neuroprotective strategies and alternative therapies for Parkinson disease (an evidence-based review): Report of the Quality Standards Subcommittee of the American Academy of Neurology. Neurology 2006;66:976–982. *A comprehensive evidence-based review.*

Suchowersky O, Reich S, Perlmutter JS, et al: Practice parameter: Diagnosis and prognosis of new onset Parkinson disease (an evidence-based review): Report of the Quality Standards Subcommittee of the American Academy of Neurology. Neurology 2006;66:968–975. *A comprehensive evidence-based review.*

434 OTHER MOVEMENT DISORDERS

Anthony Lang

Definition

Movement disorders are first divided into hypokinetic and hyperkinetic categories. *Hypokinetic disorders,* which are characterized by akinesia, bradykinesia, and rigidity, are parkinsonian syndromes and are discussed elsewhere (Chapter 433). The common *hyperkinetic movement* disorders (Table 434–1) are defined by their specific clinical phenomena.

Clinical Manifestations and Diagnostic Approach

The traditional approach to a neurologic symptom is first to address localization within the nervous system (i.e., "Where is the lesion?") followed by an evaluation of the origin ("What is the lesion?"). The neurologic examination is critical in determining the localization of the lesion, and generally the history, including the nature of onset and the progression of the symptoms, determines the most likely diagnosis. However, when a movement disorder is the predominant problem, the approach is somewhat different. The pathophysiology of most movement disorders is complex and often poorly understood. Many of these disorders are the result of dysfunction of different circuits in the brain, and it is often impossible to ascertain a specific anatomic localization. Instead, an accurate appreciation of the clinical phenomena is the first important step in evaluating these patients. The clinician must observe and examine the patient to define the type of movement disorder that best describes the clinical picture. This accurate characterization then allows the generation of a differential diagnosis for the specific movement disorder. The age and nature of onset, the distribution, the progression of symptoms, a family history of similar or related symptoms, and the presence of systemic signs then help to determine the most likely explanation for that movement disorder.

TABLE 434–1 HYPERKINETIC MOVEMENT DISORDERS
Tremor
Chorea
Ballism
Dystonia
Athetosis
Tics
Myoclonus
Startle
Stereotypies
Miscellaneous

TREMOR

Tremor, which is a rhythmic, sinusoidal movement of a body part, is caused by regular, either synchronous or alternating, contractions of reciprocally innervated muscles. Tremors are classified based on whether they occur at rest (weight fully supported against gravity) or in action. Resting tremors are typically seen in Parkinson's disease and other parkinsonism syndromes (see Table 433–1). Action tremors are further divided into postural, kinetic, or intention tremors. A *postural tremor* is seen with the maintenance of a posture against gravity (e.g., when the arms are outstretched in front of the body). A *kinetic tremor* is seen with a voluntary movement of the limb (e.g., a tremor in an upper limb when performing the finger-to-nose test). An *intention tremor* increases in amplitude on approaching a target.

Clinical Manifestations

Most action tremors (Table 434–2) combine postural and kinetic components. All tremors worsen with stress, including performing an affected activity in public. Initially, a tremor may be evident only when one attempts fine, dextrous tasks such as threading a needle, soldering, or using a screwdriver. More severe tremors interfere with activities such as handwriting, fastening buttons, shaving, eating soup with a spoon, or drinking from a cup. Patients often adapt or use compensatory measures, such as switching an activity to a less affected hand (e.g., shaving with the nondominant hand), using two hands to drink, drinking only from an incompletely filled glass or cup, or completely avoiding more challenging feeding activities in public. Severe action/intention tremors can cause handwriting to become completely illegible and can result in dependence on others for care.

Head tremors, which may be side to side, up and down, or mixed, are rarely disabling but are often a source of embarrassment. Tremor of the larynx, which causes the voice to quaver, is best appreciated by asking the patient to sustain a note. Action tremor of the lower limbs is assessed by having the patient hold the foot up to a target (e.g., the examiner's hand) and then perform a heel-knee-shin test.

Most upper limb action tremors affect many activities to a similar extent. Less commonly, tremors can affect a single task in isolation *(task-specific tremors),* the most common being a primary writing tremor. *Orthostatic tremor* is apparent in the legs and in antigravity muscles only when the patient is standing in one spot and subsides during walking or leaning against a wall; these patients commonly complain of a tremendous sense of insecurity while standing and a fear of falling. Electrophysiologic assessment demonstrates a very characteristic high-frequency tremor (14 to 16 Hz).

Enhanced Physiologic Tremor

A 7- to 12-Hz tremor is found in everyone on electrophysiologic recording. This physiologic tremor is enhanced and may become symptomatic in a variety of circumstances including fatigue, anxiety, and excitement. This same tremor may be accentuated by drugs and systemic processes.

Essential Tremor

Essential tremor affects up to 5% of the general population after the age of 60 years. Essential tremor is often inherited in an autosomal dominant fashion, with the phenotype showing genetic heterogeneity from at least three different genes as well as environmental influences. The age of onset may be as early as the first or second decade of life, but the tremor may be

TABLE 434–2 DIFFERENTIAL DIAGNOSIS OF TREMOR AND RHYTHMIC MOVEMENT DISORDERS

ENHANCED PHYSIOLOGIC TREMOR

Metabolic disorders
- Hyperthyroidism
- Hyperparathyroidism
- Hypoglycemia
- Pheochromocytoma

Drugs
- Caffeine
- Theophylline
- Amphetamines
- Lithium
- Valproic acid
- Antidepressants
- Amiodarone
- β-Agonists
- Others

Withdrawal of drugs
- Benzodiazepines
- Alcohol
- Others

Fever, sepsis

Anxiety, stress, fatigue

PRIMARY OR IDIOPATHIC TREMOR

Essential tremor
Task-specific tremor
Orthostatic tremor
Idiopathic palatal tremor

TREMOR ASSOCIATED WITH CENTRAL NERVOUS SYSTEM DISEASES

Tremor with parkinsonian syndromes
- Idiopathic Parkinson's disease
- Multiple system atrophy
- Progressive supranuclear palsy
- Corticobasal degeneration
- Neuroleptic-induced parkinsonism

Wilson's disease
Multiple sclerosis
Fragile X premutation–tremor/ataxia syndrome
Stroke
Arteriovenous malformation
Tumor
Head trauma
Midbrain tremor (Holmes' tremor)

TREMOR ASSOCIATED WITH PERIPHERAL NEUROPATHIES

PSYCHOGENIC TREMOR

OTHER RHYTHMICAL MOVEMENT DISORDERS

Rhythmic movements in dystonia ("dystonic tremor")
Rhythmic myoclonus (including "myoclonic tremor")
Asterixis
Clonus
Epilepsia partialis continua
Hereditary chin quivering
Spasmus nutans
Head bobbing with hydrocephalus
Nystagmus

Adapted from Cloutier M, Lang AE: Movement disorders: an overview. *In* Factor SA, Lang AE, Weiner WJ (eds): Drug Induced Movement Disorders. Malden, MA, Blackwell, 2005, pp 3–19.

delayed until the mid-60s. Patients first become aware of a mild postural and action tremor in the hands, which is indistinguishable from an enhanced physiologic tremor and may result in little functional impairment for many years until it gradually interferes with activities. Older patients with large-amplitude, lower-frequency tremors can have a resting component that is often misdiagnosed as Parkinson's disease (see Table 433–1). At least 50% of patients note improvement or complete amelioration of tremor following the ingestion of a small amount of ethanol.

Treatment

Rx

Treatment of essential tremor does not influence the course of the illness and therefore is justified only when the tremor interferes with function. First-line drug treatment includes trials of a noncardioselective β-adrenergic blocker (e.g., propranolol, ≤320 mg/day) or primidone (starting in a low dose of 25 to 62.5 mg at night and increasing to 500 to 750 mg/day). 1 Other drugs that have been shown to be effective in double-blind crossover trials include gabapentin (1200 to 1800 mg/day), topiramate (≤400 mg/day), and alprazolam (0.125 to 3 mg/day), 1 but many patients remain resistant to all drugs. If disability is substantial, thalamic deep brain stimulation or thalamotomy can be of major benefit, but a few patients suffer permanent neurologic sequelae owing to intracranial hemorrhage or other postoperative complications.

CHOREA

Chorea (Table 434–3) consists of irregular, random, brief, flowing movements that often flit from one body part to another in an unpredictable and purposeless sequence. Patients may incorporate choreiform movements into a voluntary movement to mask them. The severity varies from the appearance of being slightly fidgety or restless, to striking, continuous movements involving the whole body. Many patients with chorea seem unaware of their movements, whereas others can be very troubled and disabled.

Huntington's Disease

Definition and Epidemiology

Huntington's disease is a fully penetrant autosomal dominant neurodegenerative disorder caused by an expanded trinucleotide (CAG) repeat in the gene for the protein *huntingtin*. The prevalence is approximately 10 per 100,000.

Pathobiology

Huntington's disease is characterized neuropathologically by neuronal loss accompanied by intraneuronal inclusions and gliosis, especially in the caudate nucleus, the putamen (the striatum), and the cerebral cortex. Understanding how these changes result from the expanded polyglutamine tract in the mutated huntingtin protein is the goal of current research.

Clinical Manifestations

Symptoms typically begin between the ages of 30 and 55 years, but 5 to 10% of patients have an onset before the age of 20 years (juvenile HD), and a few patients begin to have symptoms quite late in life. Symptoms include a combination of a movement disorder, psychiatric disturbances, and cognitive dysfunction. Early on, the movement disorder is predominantly chorea, but parkinsonism and dystonia develop later. Some patients, especially those with juvenile onset, have a more rapidly progressive akinetic-rigid/dystonic form (the Wesphal variant). Psychiatric manifestations, which are universal but widely variable, include personality changes, impulsiveness, aggressive behavior, depression, and paranoid psychosis. These psychiatric symptoms may precede the motor manifestations, and psychotropic drug therapy may be incorrectly blamed for the subsequent development of the movement disorder. Cognitive changes result in progressive "subcortical dementia" with disturbed attention, concentration, judgment, and problem-solving that differs from the typical "cortical dementia" of Alzheimer's disease. Oculomotor dysfunction, most often manifested by difficulties with refixating the gaze and a resulting tendency to use head thrusts, is another common feature.

Diagnosis

The diagnosis is confirmed by genetic testing. Normal alleles of the *IT15* gene have fewer than 30 CAG repeats, whereas 40 or more repeats invariably result in clinical illness. An earlier age of onset correlates with larger numbers of CAG repeats.

TABLE 434–3 DIFFERENTIAL DIAGNOSIS OF CHOREA

GENETIC DISORDERS

Benign hereditary chorea
Huntington's disease
Huntington-like conditions
Neuroacanthocytosis
Dentatorubropallidoluysian atrophy
Wilson's disease
Hallervorden-Spatz disease
Spinocerebellar ataxias
Ataxia-telangiectasia
Tuberous sclerosis

INFECTIONS/PARAINFECTIOUS CAUSES

Sydenham's chorea
Acquired immunodeficiency syndrome (including complications)
Encephalitis and postencephalitic disorders
Creutzfeldt-Jakob disease

DRUGS

Levodopa, dopaminergic agonists, amphetamines, anticholinergics, anticonvulsants, neuroleptics, antidepressants, oral contraceptives, antihistaminics

ENDOCRINOLOGIC/METABOLIC CONDITIONS

Hyperthyroidism
Hypoparathyroidism
Chorea gravidarum
Acquired hepatolenticular degeneration

IMMUNOLOGIC DISORDERS

Systemic lupus erythematosus
Antiphospholipid syndrome
Henoch-Schönlein purpura

VASCULAR DISORDERS

Stroke
Hemorrhage
Arteriovenous malformation
Polycythemia rubra vera

OTHER CONDITIONS

Cerebral palsy
Kernicterus
Head trauma
Cardiopulmonary bypass with hypothermia
Neoplastic and paraneoplastic syndromes

Adapted from Cloutier M, Lang AE: Movement disorders: an overview. *In* Factor SA, Lang AE, Weiner WJ (eds): Drug Induced Movement Disorders. Malden, MA, Blackwell, 2005, pp 3–19.

Treatment and Prognosis

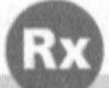

Current care for patients with Huntington's disease involves a multidisciplinary team of clinical geneticists, neurologists, psychiatrists, psychologists, social workers, occupational and physical therapists, speech therapists, nutritionists, and nurses. Genetic counseling for patients and family members is critical. Chorea may be extremely responsive to drugs that reduce central dopamine activity, including standard dopamine receptor blocking neuroleptic drugs, such as haloperidol (3 to 30 mg/day), pimozide (0.5 to 10 mg/day), or fluphenazine (0.5 to 20 mg/day), or dopamine depleting agents such as tetrabenazine (50 to 200 mg/day) or reserpine (0.75 to 5 mg/day).

TABLE 434–4 DIFFERENTIAL DIAGNOSIS OF BALLISM

Focal lesions in basal ganglia
- Vascular: stroke (including infarction and hemorrhage), cavernous angioma, postsurgical complications
- Neoplastic: metastases; primary central nervous system tumors
- Infections: cryptococcosis; toxoplasmosis; tuberculoma
- Inflammatory: multiple sclerosis
- Iatrogenic: subthalamotomy; thalamotomy

Immunologic: systemic lupus erythematosus; scleroderma; Behçet's disease
Nonketotic hyperglycemia
Hypoglycemia
Sydenham's chorea
Head injury
Drugs
- Anticonvulsants
- Oral contraceptives
- Levodopa

Adapted from Cloutier M, Lang AE: Movement disorders: an overview. *In* Factor SA, Lang AE, Weiner WJ (eds): Drug Induced Movement Disorders. Malden, MA, Blackwell, 2005, pp 3–19.

These agents should be reserved for patients with disabling chorea because they may be associated with increased parkinsonism, postural instability, depression, sedation, and other adverse effects. Unfortunately, physical function may not improve significantly even when the chorea is controlled. Psychiatric symptoms (e.g., anxiety, psychosis, depression) can be managed effectively with the same strategies as in other psychiatric disease (Chapter 420). The disease progresses to institutionalization and death over the course of approximately 15 years.

Other Choreas

Most of the non-neurodegenerative causes of chorea (see Table 434–3) can be excluded by a careful history (including a detailed drug history) and a focused set of investigations including, in appropriate circumstances, wet preparation of peripheral blood for acanthocytes, immunologic studies (including anticardiolipin antibodies), endocrine assessment (hyperthyroidism, pregnancy), and neuroimaging. *Sydenham's chorea,* which is a late component of rheumatic fever (Chapters 312 and 314), is presumably the result of immunologic cross-reactivity between the causative group A β-hemolytic streptococcus and the basal ganglia. This disorder is infrequently seen in North America but is more common in developing countries. Sydenham's chorea usually affects children and young adults, and it is more common in girls before puberty. Adults with a past history of Sydenham's chorea in childhood may develop chorea during pregnancy or in response to taking oral contraceptive agents or estrogen preparations.

Ballism

Ballism, which is considered an extreme form of chorea, involves large amplitude, random, often violent flinging movements of the proximal limbs (Table 434–4). It is most often a consequence of an acute cerebral insult, such as a stroke, and it usually involves one side of the body, particularly the arm, hence the term *hemiballism.* When a causative lesion can be demonstrated, it typically involves the region of the subthalamic nucleus or the striatum. When the condition is caused by a stroke, movements usually subside spontaneously over days to weeks, although they may persist indefinitely in some patients. Treatment often requires the use of medication that antagonizes the effects of dopamine in the brain, including dopamine receptor blockers (neuroleptics such as haloperidol, 3 to 30 mg/day) or dopamine depleter (e.g., tetrabenazine, 50 to

200 mg/day). Functional neurosurgery (e.g., pallidotomy, deep brain stimulation) can be considered in patients with refractory, persistent cases.

DYSTONIA

Definition and Pathobiology

In *dystonia,* sustained muscle contractions result in twisting and repetitive movements and abnormal postures. Dystonia can be classified according to its origin (Table 434–5). *Primary dystonia* includes syndromes in which the only phenotypic expressions are dystonia and tremor. These diseases can be hereditary or sporadic. *Dystonia-plus* is characterized by a combination of dystonia with other neurologic signs resulting from a known or presumed genetic defect without an underlying progressive neurodegenerative process; *dopa-responsive dystonia* and *myoclonus-dystonia* are examples of such diseases. *Secondary dystonias* are the result of acquired injury to the central nervous system. *Heredodegenerative dystonias* include a large number of genetic as well as idiopathic neurodegenerative diseases.

Clinical Manifestations

Common forms of dystonia include eyelid enclosure (blepharospasm), jaw opening or closing (oromandibular dystonia), pulling or turning of the neck in any one or combination of directions (cervical dystonia: rotatory torticollis, laterocollis, retrocollis, anterocollis), hyperadduction and less often excessive abduction of the vocal cords (laryngeal dystonia or spasmodic dysphonia), abnormal posturing and tightness of the hand while writing or using the hand for other tasks (writer's cramp, manual dystonia), abnormal posturing of the trunk or pelvis (axial dystonia), or abnormal posturing of the lower limb, including plantar flexion and inversion of the foot. The movements are often slow and sustained, although they may also be rapid *(dystonic spasms).* Slower, sinuous writhing dystonic movements, particularly present in the distal limbs, are referred to as *athetosis.* Dystonia is often made worse by activity *(action dystonia),* and a unique aspect of dystonia is that only selected acts may be affected, with complete sparing of all other activities in the same limb *(task-specific dystonia).* In some patients, dystonia remains isolated and action specific over many years, whereas in others it progresses to involve adjacent muscles *(overflow dystonia)* and may eventually be present at rest, in which case joint contractures may result. Another common feature of dystonia is its transient improvement with the use of a sensory trick *(geste antagoniste),* such as lightly touching the chin to relieve severe cervical dystonia or the lid to relieve disabling blepharospasm. Patients with dystonia, independent of cause, often have additional postural and action tremors, phenotypically similar to essential tremor. Some patients also demonstrate more irregular, coarse, lower-frequency rhythmic movements called *dystonic tremor.*

TABLE 434–5 CLASSIFICATION AND CAUSES OF DYSTONIA

PRIMARY DYSTONIAS (PRIMARY TORSION DYSTONIA)

Familial (several genetic causes and types)
Sporadic, usually adult-onset, focal, or segmental

DYSTONIA-PLUS

Dystonia with parkinsonism
- Dopa-responsive dystonia
- Dopamine-agonist responsive dystonia (e.g., aromatic acid decarboxylase deficiency)

Myoclonus-dystonia

SECONDARY DYSTONIAS

Perinatal cerebral injury
- Athetoid cerebral palsy
- Delayed-onset dystonia
- Pachygyria
- Kernicterus

Encephalitis
- Reye's syndrome
- Subacute sclerosing leukoencephalopathy
- Wasp sting
- Creutzfeldt-Jakob disease
- Human immunodeficiency syndrome

Head trauma
Thalamotomy
Brain stem lesion
Primary antiphospholipid syndrome
Stroke
Arteriovenous malformation
Hypoxia
Brain tumor
Multiple sclerosis
Central pontine myelinolysis
Cervical cord injury
Peripheral injury
Drugs
Toxins
Hypoparathyroidism
Psychogenic conditions

HEREDODEGENERATIVE DYSTONIAS

X-linked
- Lubag
- Deafness-dystonia-optic atrophy syndrome (Mohr-Tranebjaerg)
- Pelizaeus-Merzbacher disease
- Lesch-Nyhan syndrome

Autosomal dominant
- Rapid-onset dystonia-parkinsonism
- Juvenile parkinsonism (e.g., from mutations in the parkin gene)
- Huntington's disease
- Machado-Joseph disease (SCA3) and other SCAs
- Dentatorubropallidoluysian atrophy

Autosomal recessive
- Wilson's disease
- Niemann-Pick disease type C
- GM1 gangliosidosis
- GM2 gangliosidosis
- Metachromatic leukodystrophy
- Homocystinuria
- Glutaric acidemia
- Triose-phosphate isomerase deficiency
- Hartnup's disease
- Ataxia-telangiectasia
- Hallervorden-Spatz disease
- Juvenile neuronal ceroid lipofuscinosis
- Neuroacanthocytosis
- Intranuclear hyaline inclusion disease
- Hereditary spastic paraplegia with dystonia

Probably autosomal recessive
- Familial basal ganglia calcifications
- Progressive pallidal degeneration
- Rett's syndrome

Mitochondrial
- Leigh's disease
- Leber's disease
- Other mitochondrial cytopathies

Sporadic, with parkinsonism
- Parkinson's disease
- Progressive supranuclear palsy
- Multiple system atrophy
- Corticobasal degeneration

Adapted from Cloutier M, Lang AE: Movement disorders: an overview. *In* Factor SA, Lang AE, Weiner WJ (eds): Drug Induced Movement Disorders. Malden, MA, Blackwell, 2005, pp 3–19.

Dystonia is often classified according to the site of involvement: focal, only one body part (e.g., blepharospasm, cervical dystonia, writer's cramp); segmental, two or more contiguous body parts; multifocal, two or more noncontiguous body parts; generalized, legs and other body areas; and hemidystonia, unilateral (generally a causative focal brain lesion is found most often involving the putamen).

Diagnosis and Prognosis

For diagnostic and prognostic purposes, dystonia also may be distinguished by age of onset as childhood-onset, adolescent-onset, or adult-onset dystonia. The younger the age of onset, the more likely it will be that a cause can be defined. Conversely, isolated dystonia beginning in adult life is most often an "idiopathic" disorder; further investigations are typically unrewarding and are usually not indicated. Likewise, independent of the cause, dystonia beginning in childhood commonly progresses to segmental or generalized involvement, whereas adult-onset dystonia usually remains focal or segmental.

Specific Dystonias

Primary (Idiopathic) Dystonias

Primary dystonia accounts for up to 90% of patients with a pure dystonic syndrome. To date, no consistent neuropathologic changes have been found in the small numbers of brains affected by primary dystonia that have been studied.

When symptoms begin in *childhood,* a definable genetic cause is often identified, the most common being DYT1 resulting from the autosomal dominant inheritance of a GAG deletion in the *torsin A* gene *(Oppenheim's dystonia).* This disorder is more common in persons of Ashkenazi Jewish descent. The dystonia often begins in the first decade of life and can progress to severe disability, although the spectrum of disease, even within the same family, can be quite varied, and penetrance is relatively low (~40%). Genetic testing is available but is recommended only when the age of onset in the patient or another affected family member is less than 26 years. Increasing numbers of other genetic forms of primary dystonia are being defined, but genetic testing is not yet available for most of them.

Adult-Onset Idiopathic Dystonia

Adult-onset idiopathic dystonia is the most common type of dystonia seen in general neurologic practice. The dystonia typically begins in the face, neck, or arm and may remain focal and nonprogressive or spread only to contiguous muscles after many years. The cause of this disorder is not known, although a positive family history may be noted if multiple family members can be examined.

Dystonia-Plus

Dopa-responsive dystonia, which usually results in dystonia beginning in the first decade of life, most often in the lower limbs, sometimes can be mistaken for hereditary spastic paraplegia (Chapter 435) or cerebral palsy. Most patients with dopa-responsive dystonia have a mutation in the *GCH1* gene, which results in reduced production of dopamine. Approximately 75% of patients have notable worsening of dystonia as the day progresses *(diurnal variation).* Exercise often aggravates the dystonia. Patients commonly demonstrate some degree of bradykinesia (especially in the legs) and postural instability. Rare adult-onset disease may result in a pure parkinsonian phenotype. Dopa-responsive dystonia should be considered in all children with dystonia. Symptoms are exquisitely sensitive to low doses of levodopa (typically as little as 50 mg/day of levodopa), and this treatment allows patients to live a normal life without the usual complications seen in Parkinson's disease (Chapter 433).

Myoclonus Dystonia

Myoclonus dystonia, which usually begins within the first decade of life, combines dystonia with separate multifocal myoclonic jerks. Myoclonus dystonia is genetically heterogeneous; the most common definable cause is a mutation in the ε-sarcoglycan gene. The dystonia in these patients most often involves the neck or upper limbs, is mild, and is often overlooked. The disorder can also include psychopathology, such as obsessive-compulsive behavior. A characteristic feature of this disorder is the marked ameliorative effect of ethanol on both the myoclonus and the dystonia, a feature that sometimes results in alcohol abuse.

Other Dystonias

Dystonia may be a symptom of many diseases. The nature and extent of the investigations undertaken depend on such factors as age of onset, clues provided on the history, and additional neurologic or systemic features on examination. *Wilson's disease* (Chapter 230) is an important consideration in the diagnosis of dystonia beginning in children and young adults.

Treatment

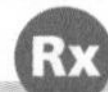

Ideally, treatment is directed at the underlying cause (e.g., dopa-responsive dystonia, Wilson's disease). Unfortunately, cause-specific treatment usually is not possible, so a variety of symptomatic treatments may be tried, often unsuccessfully, in an attempt to reduce disability.

Focal injections of botulinum toxin are now usually the first choice for treatment of focal and segmental dystonias. [2] This approach can improve the condition of patients with cranial (blepharospasm, oromandibular dystonia) and cervical dystonia. Patients with task-specific limb dystonias (e.g., writer's cramp) often benefit less because weakness of the treated muscles, which is the most common side effect of this therapy, can impair other important upper limb functions.

Young patients in particular can tolerate and benefit from high doses of drugs such as trihexyphenidyl (6 to 40 mg/day, but sometimes as much as 100 mg/day). Muscle relaxants, including benzodiazepines (diazepam, 10 to 100 mg/day) and baclofen (40 to 120 mg/day), may provide some benefit. Dopamine depleting (e.g., tetrabenazine, 50 to 200 mg/day) and blocking (e.g., haloperidol, 3 to 30 mg/day) agents are occasionally helpful (more often effective in tardive dystonia than in other types). Neurosurgical treatments, particularly deep brain stimulation of the internal segment of the globus pallidus, [3] can be considered in medically refractory, disabling dystonia, especially in patients with idiopathic dystonia (e.g., DYT1, adult-onset cervical dystonia).

TICS

Epidemiology and Pathobiology

Tics are repetitive, stereotyped movements (motor tics) or vocalizations (vocal tics). Transient tics are extremely common in childhood, and simple tics may begin in childhood and persist throughout adult life. Most tics (Table 434–6) are primary or idiopathic and have no identifiable cause. Secondary tics are caused by a defined underlying brain disease or environmental factor.

Clinical Manifestations

Tics vary in terms of complexity, from abrupt, brief, meaningless movements or sounds (*simple motor tics* such as eye blinking, nose wrinkling, or head jerking; *simple vocal/phonic tics* such as sniffing, throat clearing, or grunting) to more sustained, more deliberate, almost meaningful gestures or utterances (*complex motor tics* such as touching, hand shaking, and jumping; *complex vocal tics* such as echolalia [repeating others], palilalia [repeating oneself] and coprolalia [uttering profanities]). The frequency of the tics in an individual patient varies markedly over minutes, hours, days, weeks, and years.

Diagnosis

Various characteristics help to differentiate tics from other abnormal movements. Tics are often described by patients as being "semivoluntary" in response to an inner, irresistible urge. Premonitory sensory symptoms occasionally precede the tic, generally in the same general anatomic area as the tic itself. Relief is often associated with the production of the tic. Tics can be partially or completely voluntarily suppressed for variable periods, but often at the expense of mounting inner tension and psychologic discomfort. Performing the tic or sometimes even substituting

TABLE 434–6 ETIOLOGIC CLASSIFICATION OF TICS

PRIMARY OR IDIOPATHIC TICS
Transient motor or phonic tics
Chronic motor or phonic tics
Adult-onset tics
Tourette's syndrome
SECONDARY TICS
Genetic disorders
Neuroacanthocytosis
Huntington's disease
Hallervorden-Spatz disease
Idiopathic dystonia*
Tuberous sclerosis*
Chromosomal disorders
Infections
Sydenham's chorea
PANDAS†
Encephalitis and postencephalitic disorders
Creutzfeldt-Jakob disease
Neurosyphilis
Drugs
Methylphenidate, amphetamines, cocaine, levodopa, carbamazepine, phenytoin, phenobarbital, lamotrigine, neuroleptics
Developmental disorders
Mental retardation
Pervasive developmental disorders/autism
Other causes
Head trauma
Stroke
Carbon monoxide poisoning
Cardiopulmonary bypass with hypothermia
RELATED DISORDERS
Mannerisms, stereotypies
Compulsions
Self-injurious behavior

*Tics have been described with these conditions but may simply be coincidental.
†Pediatric autoimmune neuropsychiatric disorders associated with streptococcal infections. The existence of this disorder remains somewhat controversial.
Adapted from Cloutier M, Lang AE: Movement disorders: an overview. *In* Factor SA, Lang AE, Weiner WJ (eds): Drug Induced Movement Disorders. Malden, MA, Blackwell, 2005, pp 3–19.

another more acceptable behavior for the socially inappropriate tic alleviates the tension. Many patients report that some tics occur in response to a typical urge, whereas the same or different tics may be unexpected and totally involuntary.

Tourette's Syndrome

Epidemiology and Pathobiology

The exact relationship between childhood tics and Gilles de la Tourette's syndrome remains uncertain. Tourette's syndrome is a common disorder, with prevalence estimates varying from 10 to 700 per 100,000. There is a male preponderance of 3:1 for the classic syndrome, but female patients manifest obsessive-compulsive features more often than tics. The cause of Tourette's syndrome is unknown, but epidemiologic studies support an autosomal dominant, sex-influenced trait.

Clinical Manifestations and Diagnosis

The criteria for this disorder include the presence of multiple motor and at least one vocal tic beginning before the age of 21 years (typically between ages 2 and 10 years), lasting for more than 1 year, waxing and waning symptoms over time (new tics replacing old ones; previous tics sometimes recurring years after they had originally resolved), and the absence of other explanatory medical conditions. Involuntary swearing (coprolalia), a highly publicized feature of the syndrome, is present in fewer than 10% of patients and is usually manifested by aborted forms such as "fu" and "shi." Patients commonly exhibit a variety of comorbid disorders including obsessive-compulsive disorder, attention-deficit disorder (with or without hyperactivity), impulse control problems, and other behavioral disturbances.

Treatment

Most patients who fulfill diagnostic criteria for Tourette's syndrome have mild symptoms that do not require treatment; education, reassurance, and follow-up are often sufficient. When tics (isolated or as part of Tourette's syndrome) interfere with social and physical function, low-dose clonazepam (0.5 to 4 mg/day) may be effective. Clonidine (0.05 to 0.5 mg/day) is variably effective in controlling tics and may be useful for impulse control and symptoms of attention-deficit/hyperactivity disorder (ADHD); alternatively, guanfacine (0.5 to 4 mg/day) can be used. The most effective treatments for disabling tics are the dopamine receptor blockers such as risperidone (0.5 to 16 mg/day), haloperidol (0.5 to 20 mg/day), pimozide (0.5 to 10 mg/day), and fluphenazine (0.5 to 20 mg/day), but caution is required in view of the potential for important side effects, including tardive dyskinesia, with long-term use. An alternative without this complication is the dopamine depletor tetrabenazine (50–200 mg/day dopamine). Dopamine agonists such as pergolide (0.15 to 1 mg/day) may also reduce tic severity. Injected botulinum toxin may be effective for simple motor tics of the face and neck and may also reduce the urge to perform the tic. Comorbid ADHD can be treated safely with stimulant therapy (e.g., methylphenidate, 2.5 to 60 mg/day) without a significant risk of increasing the severity of tics. [4] Obsessive-compulsive symptoms may respond well to selective serotonin re-uptake inhibitors (e.g., clomipramine, 25 to 250 mg/day; paroxetine, 10 to 60 mg/day; or citalopram, 10 to 40 mg/day). Behavioral disorders, which remain a major therapeutic challenge, may require a variety of psychotherapeutic or behavioral modification approaches. Promising preliminary reports of deep brain stimulation require confirmation in controlled clinical trials.

Prognosis

The natural history of Tourette's syndrome is to stabilize and often improve in adolescence. Approximately 50% of patients have a complete or partial remission at this time.

MYOCLONUS

Definition

Myoclonus (or myoclonic jerks) consists of sudden, brief, shocklike, involuntary movements that result from both active muscle contraction (positive myoclonic jerks) and brief inhibition of ongoing muscle activity (negative myoclonic jerks). The most common form of negative myoclonic jerk is *asterixis.*

Pathobiology

Myoclonus generally arises in the central nervous system, although rare peripheral causes are described, and it is distinct from abnormal muscle activity associated with peripheral nervous system diseases, such as fasciculations or myokymia. Myoclonus can be classified according to origin (Table 434–7), including physiologic, essential, epileptic, and symptomatic forms. Physiologic myoclonus, such as hypnic (sleep) jerks and hiccups, occurs in normal healthy subjects. Patients with essential myoclonus, which may be sporadic or inherited, often have additional postural tremor or dystonia, and this disorder is probably the same as what is now referred to as *myoclonus-dystonia* (see Dystonias, earlier). Epileptic myoclonus arises in the context of seizures (Chapter 426), including many inherited generalized epileptic syndromes and the progressive myoclonic epilepsies. Symptomatic myoclonus occurs in association with a large number of encephalopathic states.

TABLE 434–7 CLASSIFICATION AND CAUSES OF MYOCLONUS

PHYSIOLOGIC MYOCLONUS	Parkinson's disease
Sleep myoclonus	Multiple system atrophy
Anxiety-induced myoclonus	Huntington's disease
Exercise-induced myoclonus	Dentatorubropallidoluysian atrophy
Hiccups	Mitochondrial cytopathies
Benign infantile myoclonus during feeding	Dementias
ESSENTIAL MYOCLONUS	Alzheimer's disease
Essential myoclonus*	Creutzfeldt-Jakob disease
Hereditary	Dementia with Lewy bodies
Sporadic	Viral encephalopathies
Myoclonus-dystonia*	Subacute sclerosing panencephalitis
EPILEPTIC MYOCLONUS	Encephalitis lethargica
Fragments of epilepsy	Herpes simplex encephalitis
Isolated epileptic myoclonic jerks	Arbovirus encephalitis
Photosensitive myoclonus	Human immunodeficiency virus infection
Myoclonic absences	Postinfectious encephalitis
Epilepsia partialis continua	Metabolic disorders
Idiopathic stimulus-sensitive myoclonus	Hepatic failure
Childhood myoclonic epilepsies	Renal failure
Infantile spasms	Dialysis dysequilibrium syndrome
Lennox-Gastaut syndrome	Hyponatremia
Cryptogenic myoclonus epilepsy	Hypoglycemia
Juvenile myoclonic epilepsy of Janz	Nonketotic hyperglycemia
Benign familial myoclonic epilepsy	Infantile myoclonic encephalopathy
Baltic myoclonus (Unverricht-Lundborg)	Multiple carboxylase deficiency
SYMPTOMATIC MYOCLONUS	Biotin deficiency
Storage disease	Toxins
Lafora body disease	Bismuth
Lipidoses	Heavy-metal poisoning
Neuronal ceroid lipofuscinosis	Methylbromide, dichlorodiphenyltrichloroethane (DDT)
Sialidosis	Drugs (multiple)
Spinocerebellar degeneration	Physical encephalopathies
Friedreich's ataxia	Posthypoxic myoclonus (Lance-Adams)
Ataxia-telangiectasia	Post-traumatic status
Other spinocerebellar degenerations	Heat stroke
Basal ganglia degenerations	Electric shock
Wilson's disease	Decompression injury
Idiopathic torsion dystonia	Focal central nervous system damage
Hallervorden-Spatz disease	Stroke
Progressive supranuclear palsy	Post-thalamotomy status
Corticobasal degeneration	Tumor
	Trauma
	Spinal cord lesions
	Paraneoplastic syndromes
	Psychogenic myoclonus

*Probably represents the same entity.
Adapted from Cloutier M, Lang AE: Movement disorders: an overview. *In* Factor SA, Lang AE, Weiner WJ (eds): Drug Induced Movement Disorders. Malden, MA, Blackwell, 2005, pp 3–19.

Clinical Manifestations and Diagnosis

Myoclonic jerks are very short, typically lasting less then 150 milliseconds. Myoclonus can be spontaneous, action induced, and/or reflex (induced by various sensory stimuli). Spontaneous myoclonus occurs at rest, without any provocation. Action myoclonus occurs during purposeful movement and is often very disabling owing to its interference with volitional activity. Reflex myoclonus can be triggered by visual, auditory, or somesthetic stimuli. The distribution of myoclonus may be focal, segmental, multifocal, or generalized. When myoclonus involves more than one body area, the movements may be synchronous or asynchronous. Myoclonus can be intermittent or repetitive, and it sometimes is rhythmic (e.g., usually originating in the brain stem or spinal cord). *Palatal myoclonus*, recently redesignated as *palatal tremor*, is a rhythmic movement disorder originating in the brain stem and involving the soft palate as well as the eyes, facial muscles, neck, and limbs; it is commonly the result of a focal lesion (e.g., stroke, demyelination) in the connections between the dentate nucleus of the cerebellum and the inferior olives of the medulla.

Diagnosis

Myoclonus can be classified according to the anatomic site of origin, usually with the assistance of detailed electrophysiologic assessments. These sites may be cortical, subcortical (e.g., thalamus; lower brain stem [reticular myoclonus]), or spinal (two types: spinal segmental and propriospinal).

Treatment

Rx

Management of myoclonus, when possible, should be directed specifically at the underlying cause. Drug treatment includes a variety of anticonvulsant medications, most notably clonazepam (1.5 to 15 mg/day), valproic acid (10 to 15 mg/kg/day), carbamazepine (600 to 1200 mg/day), and levetiracetam (1000 to 4000 mg/day). Postanoxic action myoclonus (the Lance-Adams syndrome) in some patients who survive severe cerebral anoxia may also respond to 5-hydroxytryptophan (400 to 2800 mg/day) given with carbidopa (75 to 300 mg/day).

HYPEREXPLEXIA

A disorder related to myoclonus, known as *hyperexplexia,* manifests as excessive response to startle. It may be inherited (startle disease, most often caused by a mutation in the α_1-subunit of the glycine receptor gene). Some patients demonstrate only generalized body jerking or an exaggerated startle response that habituates poorly after repeated stimuli. Others also experience disabling stiffness in response to sudden unexpected stimuli such as loud sound. The disorder responds well to clonazepam (1.5 to 15 mg/day) therapy.

OTHER MOVEMENT DISORDERS

Drug-Induced Movement Disorders

All the movements listed in Table 434–1 can be induced by medications. Neuroleptic drugs, which block postsynaptic dopamine receptors, particularly the D2 subtype, can result in a variety of movement disorder syndromes, including acute dystonic reactions, akathisia, drug-induced parkinsonism (including "the rabbit syndrome" with perinasal/perioral rest tremor), the neuroleptic malignant syndrome, and a variety of later-onset, often persistent, movements referred to as *tardive dyskinesia.*

Acute Dystonic Reactions

Acute dystonic reactions are most often seen in young patients who are receiving potent antipsychotic agents (e.g., young male patients receiving high doses of haloperidol for acute psychosis), but they also occur in patients receiving dopamine receptor blockers, including metoclopramide as antiemetic therapy. Symptoms range from overt dystonic postures of the face and neck, to involuntary prolonged deviation of the eyes (oculogyric crises), to simple slurring of speech and difficulty coordinating the tongue. Symptoms often vary from moment to moment and can increase with anxiety and improve with relaxation or reassurance. Acute dystonic reactions are self-limited and respond rapidly to a parenteral injection of an anticholinergic drug such as benztropine (2 mg intravenously followed by 2 mg three times daily orally for a variable duration depending on neuroleptic use) or an antihistaminic such as diphenhydramine (50 mg intravenously followed by oral benztropine).

Akathisia

Akathisia refers to a sense of restlessness and a need to move. Typically, the patient performs a variety of purposeful or semipurposeful, often complex, movements in response to an uncomfortable subjective restlessness, including pacing when standing, marching in place, rocking, shifting weight, moving legs when sitting, picking at clothing or hair, rubbing body parts with hands, and other similar movements. Akathisia is most often a side effect of medications, especially neuroleptic drugs and selective serotonin re-uptake inhibitors (Chapter 420). Symptoms occur in a dose-related fashion and usually resolve on drug withdrawal. Akathisia is a common reason for psychiatric patients to comply poorly with their medications; management includes adjustment of the dose or type of antipsychotic agent and trials of β-blockers (e.g., propranolol, 80 mg/day) or antiparkinson agents, such as anticholinergics (e.g., benztropine (6 mg/day) or amantadine (200 to 300 mg/day). Rare patients experience a very disabling and persistent form referred to as *tardive akathisia.* Akathisia is also sometimes seen in patients with Parkinson's disease.

Neuroleptic Malignant Syndrome

The *neuroleptic malignant syndrome* (Chapters 458 and 460) is an uncommon but severe, sometimes fatal, complication of neuroleptic therapy. Patients usually manifest a combination of features including fever, marked rigidity, changes in level of arousal, and autonomic instability. Laboratory abnormalities include a marked increase in the serum creatine kinase level and the blood leukocyte count. Management involves early recognition, withdrawal of the causative agent, systemic supportive therapy, a dopamine agonist (most experience has been with the older agent bromocriptine (≤60 mg/day), and, when necessary, dantrolene sodium (50 to 600 mg/day orally or ≤10 mg/kg/day intravenously) to reduce muscle contraction.

Tardive Dyskinesia

Epidemiology and Pathobiology

The term *tardive dyskinesia* encompasses a wide variety of abnormal movements caused by chronic neuroleptic therapy. The cumulative 5-year incidence rate in patients taking classic neuroleptics is approximately 25%, and the incidence may continue to increase almost linearly beyond that point. The propensity to develop tardive dyskinesia on newer "atypical" neuroleptics appears to be much lower.

Clinical Manifestations

Tardive dyskinesia generally begins after a minimum of 6 weeks of treatment. One of the most common forms involves the lower facial muscles and has been given a variety of names including "orobuccolinguomasticatory dyskinesia." The movements generally comprise repetitive chewing and smacking movements with the tongue, either protruding between the lips ("fly-catching" movements) or pushing into the cheek ("bonbon sign"). Although the movements are somewhat choreic, they are not as random as true chorea. The more stereotypic, repetitive nature of the movements, involving not only face but also the limbs (e.g., piano playing movements of the fingers, rocking or thrusting of the pelvis), has encouraged the more recent term "tardive stereotypies." Many patients with classic orofacial tardive dyskinesia seem unaware of the presence of the movements and are not disabled by them, but others are embarrassed or otherwise impaired.

Tardive akathisia and tardive dystonia are less common but particularly disabling subtypes of tardive dyskinesia. Rarer forms include tardive tics (tourettism), tardive tremor, tardive myoclonus and even tardive oral or genital pain.

Treatment and Prognosis

Treatment is often unsatisfactory. The dopamine depletor tetrabenazine (50 to 200 mg/day) is often very effective. Prevention is the most important consideration. The physician must regularly re-assess the need for ongoing neuroleptic therapy, consider switching to an atypical agent when possible, and routinely evaluate the patient for the presence of early subtle clinical features, such as mild pursing of the lips or rolling movements of the tongue in the mouth. Unfortunately, tardive dyskinesia may persist for many years despite withdrawal of neuroleptic treatment in up to 50% of patients.

Restless Legs Syndrome

Epidemiology

Restless legs syndrome (Chapter 429) is now recognized as an extremely common disorder affecting between 3 and 29% of the general population. Women are affected more frequently than men. Although the incidence increases with age, it can also affect children, in whom it may be confused with "growing pains" or ADHD.

Pathobiology

Restless legs syndrome is most often "primary" or idiopathic, in which case it is frequently inherited in an autosomal dominant fashion. Restless legs syndrome also may be secondary to other causes, including peripheral neuropathy, uremia, pregnancy, and iron deficiency, and it may occur more commonly than by chance in some neurodegenerative disorders such as Parkinson's disease. The pathophysiology of restless legs syndrome is uncertain, but central iron dysregulation may somehow alter central dopamine. Serum ferritin levels are often low, even in the presence of normal values of hemoglobin, hematocrit, iron, and iron binding capacity.

Clinical Manifestations and Diagnosis

In restless legs syndrome, as in akathisia, movements occur because of the subjective need to move. However, unlike in akathisia, the patient typically complains of a variety of sensory disturbances in the legs, including pins and needles, creeping or crawling sensations, aching, itching, stabbing, heaviness, tension, burning, or coldness. Occasionally, similar symptoms are appreciated in the upper limbs. These symptoms are usually experienced during periods of prolonged inactivity, especially with recumbency in the evening, and are often associated with insomnia (Chapter 429). The discomfort appears particularly during the transition from wake to sleep in the evening and often follows a circadian pattern, peaking between midnight and 4 AM. Symptoms are typically relieved only by movement or stimulation of the legs; although these maneuvers are effective while they are being performed, the discomfort usually returns as soon as the individual becomes inactive or returns to bed to try to sleep. Patients often have significant problems with immobility during long automobile drives or plane flights.

In approximately 80% of patients, this condition is associated with another movement disorder, periodic leg movements in sleep, sometimes inappropriately termed nocturnal myoclonus. These periodic, slow, sustained (1 to 2 seconds) movements range from synchronous or asynchronous dorsiflexion of the toes and feet to triple flexion of one or both legs. In 15% of patients, more rapid myoclonic movements or slower, prolonged dystonic-like movements of the feet and legs are present while patients are awake. In the absence of evidence of a secondary cause of restless legs syndrome, the only useful routine test is a serum ferritin level.

Treatment

Rx

Dopamine agonists (e.g., pramipexole, 0.125 to 1.5 mg at bedtime) or ropinirole (1 to 4 mg at bedtime) [5] are the treatments of choice in moderate to severe restless legs syndrome and can be very effective. Levodopa preparations (100 to 300 mg of levodopa at bedtime; consider controlled-release preparation) are also effective but are more often associated with disabling rebound symptoms early in the morning or during the day *(augmentation)*. Patients with milder symptoms may respond to gabapentin (300 to 2400 mg/day). Opiate agonists (e.g., oxycodone, 5 mg at bedtime; codeine, 30 mg at bedtime; propoxyphene, 65 mg or N-100 mg at bedtime) and less often benzodiazepines (e.g., clonazepam, 0.5 to 2 mg at bedtime) may also be effective. Tolerance or loss of original benefit may occur with all these treatments. Iron replacement is indicated in patients with reduced serum ferritin levels (325 mg ferrous sulfate two to three times per day for 3 to 4 months until ferritin levels exceed 50 μg/L and iron saturations surpass 20%).

Painful Legs and Moving Toes

Another uncommon but well-defined movement disorder of the lower limbs has been termed *painful legs and moving toes.* Patients typically complain of a deep pulling or searing pain in the lower limbs, associated with continuous involuntary wriggling or writhing of the toes. Occasionally, the ankle and less commonly more proximal muscles of the legs are involved. Rarely, a similar problem is seen in the upper limbs as well. Various treatments have been tried without much benefit to the pain, which is typically the major concern of the patient.

Other Abnormal Movements

Numerous abnormal movements are caused by dysfunction of the peripheral nerves (e.g., fasciculations, myokymia); these movements are usually easily separated from the movement disorders described earlier. *Hemifacial spasm* is a common disorder in which irregular clonic and tonic movements involve the muscles innervated by the facial nerve, usually owing to compression of the seventh nerve as it exits the brain stem, most often by a normal small artery or vein and less often by a mass lesion or inflammatory process. Eyelid twitching is usually the first symptom, followed at variable intervals by lower facial muscle involvement. A magnetic resonance image with careful assessment of the posterior fossa is necessary to exclude secondary causes. Treatment usually involves injections of botulinum toxin into selected facial muscles, although surgical decompression can be curative.

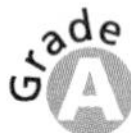

1. Zesiewicz TA, Elble R, Louis ED, et al: Practice parameter: Therapies for essential tremor—Report of the quality standards subcommittee of the American Academy of Neurology. Neurology 2005;64:2008–2020.
2. Jankovic J, Esquenazi A, Fehlings D, et al: Evidence-based review of patient-reported outcomes with botulinum toxin type A. Clin Neuropharmacol 2004;27:234–244.
3. Kupsch A, Benecke R, Müller J, et al: Pallidal deep-brain stimulation in primary generalized or segmental dystonia. N Engl J Med 2006;355:1978–1990.
4. Kurlan R, Goetz CG, McDermott MP, et al: Treatment of ADHD in children with tics: A randomized controlled trial. Neurology 2002;58:527–536.
5. Bogan RK, Fry JM, Schmidt MH, et al: Ropinirole in the treatment of patients with restless legs syndrome: A US-based randomized, double-blind, placebo-controlled clinical trial. Mayo Clin Proc 2006;81:17–27.

SUGGESTED READINGS

Correll CU, Leucht S, Kane JM: Lower risk for tardive dyskinesia associated with second-generation antipsychotics: A systematic review of 1-year studies. Am J Psychiatry 2004;161:414–425. *A systematic review showing the reduced risk of tardive dyskinesia with the newer "atypical" neuroleptics.*

Hening W: Current guidelines and standards of practice for restless legs syndrome. Am J Med 2007;120:S22–S27. *A practical overview.*

Leckman JF: Tourette's syndrome. Lancet 2002; 360:1577–1586. *A useful review.*

Pahwa R, Lyons KE: Essential tremor: Differential diagnosis and current therapy. Am J Med 2003;115:134–142. *A useful review.*

Postuma RB, Lang AE: Hemiballism: Revisiting a classic disorder. Lancet Neurol 2003;2:661–668. *A detailed review.*

Tarsy D, Simon DK: Dystonia. N Engl J Med 2006;355:818–829. *Comprehensive review.*

Trenkwalder C, Paulus W, Walters AS: The restless legs syndrome. Lancet Neurol 2005;4:465–475. *A detailed review.*

Walker FO: Huntington's disease. Lancet 2007;369:218–228. *Comprehensive review.*

435 AMYOTROPHIC LATERAL SCLEROSIS AND OTHER MOTOR NEURON DISEASES

Eva L. Feldman

Definition

Motor neuron diseases are a heterogeneous group of disorders that selectively affect upper or lower motor neurons, or both (Table 435–1). Upper motor neurons are large cerebral and bulbar motor neurons whose dysfunction leads to decreased strength, spasticity, and hyperreflexia. Lower motor neurons are located in the ventral spinal cord; lesions result in decreased strength, tone, and reflexes accompanied by fasciculations and atrophy. Pure upper motor neuron disorders are most commonly acquired, whereas pure lower motor neuron disorders are frequently inherited. The most common acquired motor neuron disease, amyotrophic lateral sclerosis (ALS), usually includes dysfunction of both

TABLE 435–1 MAJOR MOTOR NEURON DISEASES

HEREDITARY
Autosomal dominant
Familial ALS
Autosomal recessive
Spinal muscular atrophy
Type I: acute, infantile (Werdnig-Hoffmann disease)
Type II: late infantile
Type III: juvenile and adult types (Kugelberg-Welander disease)
X-Linked
Bulbospinal muscular atrophy (Kennedy's syndrome)
ACQUIRED
Acute
Anterior poliomyelitis
Chronic
Sporadic ALS
Postpoliomyelitis syndrome, motor neuron loss associated with spinocerebellar degeneration, multisystem atrophy, Creutzfeldt-Jakob disease
ALS-like syndromes
Motor neuron disease with gammopathy or paraproteinemia, heavy metal intoxication, hexosaminidase A deficiency, paraneoplastic motor neuronopathy
Primary lateral sclerosis

ALS = amyotrophic lateral sclerosis.

upper and lower motor neurons. Recent advances in the molecular genetics of hereditary motor neuron diseases have improved their classification and have led to advances in defining potential underlying causes of acquired motor neuron disorders.

AMYOTROPHIC LATERAL SCLEROSIS

Definition and Epidemiology

Sporadic ALS accounts for approximately 80% of all cases of acquired motor neuron disease, whereas the remaining 20% of patients have either only lower motor neuron signs or a familial form of ALS (FALS). The 80% of patients who have sporadic ALS present with spasticity, hyperreflexia, and Babinski's sign (upper motor neuron signs) in the setting of progressive muscle wasting and weakness (lower motor neuron signs). ALS has an estimated annual incidence of 2 per 100,000 with a worldwide prevalence of 4 to 6 per 100,000.

Pathobiology

Autosomal dominant familial ALS is an adult-onset disease that is clinically and pathologically indistinguishable from sporadic ALS. The protein cytosolic copper-zinc superoxide dismutase (SOD1) is mutated in several families affected by familial ALS, and more than 90 mutations in SOD1 (mostly missense) occur in patients with familial ALS. However, SOD1 mutations account for only approximately 20% of cases of familial ALS. Another gene implicated in familial ALS is alsin (also known as *ALS2*), which is a guanine-nucleotide-exchange factor that is essential for normal cytoskeletal dynamics. A mutant gene product of *ALS2* is present in a slowly progressive, early-onset form of familial ALS. Linkage to chromosomes 16, 18, and 20 has also been reported in separate families with familial ALS, thereby implicating additional undiscovered genes.

The importance of the work on familial ALS lies in the finding that affected patients are clinically identical to patients with sporadic ALS, a feature suggesting a common mechanism of disease. Sporadic ALS may represent an acquired age-associated change in SOD1 function with resultant oxidative injury to the nervous system. Other potential causes of sporadic ALS include altered protein trafficking, glutamate excitotoxicity or neurotoxicity, abnormal accumulations of neurofilaments, and altered neurotropism.

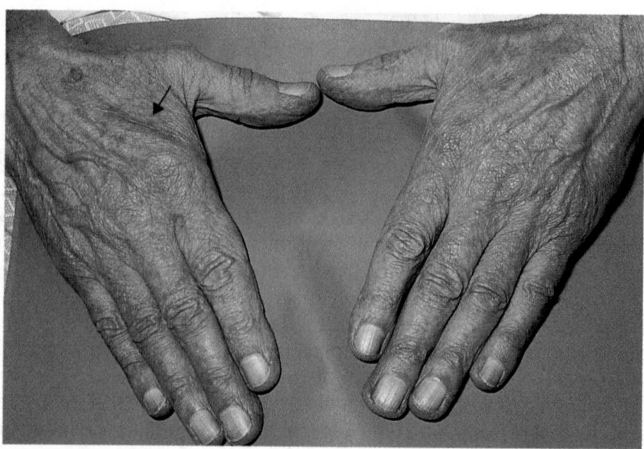

FIGURE 435–1 • Motor neuron disease. This patient has progressive muscular atrophy and presented with fasciculation and wasting of the muscles between the thumb and index finger on the dorsal (arrow) and palmar surfaces. Wasting in the right hand was followed by the development of similar wasting in the left hand and subsequently by progressive wasting and fasciculations elsewhere.

Pathology

At autopsy, patients with ALS have brain stem and spinal cord atrophy with loss of motor neurons and associated extensive gliosis. In the cortex, large pyramidal cell loss leads to degeneration of the corticospinal tracts and gliosis of the lateral spinal cord columns. As with other denervating disorders, patients have loss of ventral nerve roots, with histologic evidence of denervation and reinnervation in affected muscle groups.

Clinical Manifestations

ALS is a disorder of upper and lower motor neurons. This combination results in a complex clinical syndrome. Painless, progressive weakness is the usual presenting sign and symptom of ALS. Usually focal in onset, weakness then spreads to contiguous muscle groups. Weakness is accompanied by muscle atrophy (Fig. 435–1). Head "ptosis" resulting from weakness of neck extensor muscles with head droop is often present. Individuals frequently experience muscle cramps. Spasticity is common, and patients may complain of spontaneous clonus. With more long-standing disease, foot and hand deformities are seen as a result of tendon imbalance and secondary joint contractures.

ALS can manifest initially with bulbar dysfunction, although more commonly bulbar signs and symptoms are seen in the presence of extremity and truncal weakness. Individuals experience dysarthria, or impaired speech, which may be flaccid or spastic or of a mixed flaccid-spastic quality. Dysphagia with choking is common and places patients at a high risk of aspiration. The absence of spontaneous swallowing results in sialorrhea, or drooling.

Weakness of respiratory muscles is common and is the presenting symptom in rare cases in ALS. Early in ALS, individuals complain of dyspnea with exertion and frequently sigh at rest. With disease progression, dyspnea at rest, inability to sleep in a supine position (orthopnea), sleep apnea, and morning headaches are present. Constitutional symptoms reflect loss of muscle mass and difficulties with swallowing and breathing. Individuals experience weight loss and frequently complain of fatigue.

Several aspects of neurologic function are usually spared in ALS, including mentation, extraocular movements, bowel and bladder function, and sensation. However, approximately 1 to 2% of patients with ALS have dementia and ophthalmoplegia, usually reflecting ocular apraxia. Although bladder function is usually reported as normal, detailed study of bladder function reveals that nearly one third of patients with ALS experience urgency and obstructive micturition.

Debate continues about whether a disorder termed *primary lateral sclerosis* is a subtype of upper motor neuron ALS or is a separate entity. In this rare condition, individuals present with slowly progressive spastic paraparesis or quadriparesis, with no evidence of lower motor neuron involvement, either by clinical examination or diagnostic testing. Individuals with these presenting signs and symptoms should undergo the same diagnostic procedures and require similar treatment strategies as patients with sporadic ALS. Some patients with primary lateral sclerosis have an autosomal recessive form of hereditary spastic paraplegia.

Diagnosis

The El Escorial World Federation of Neurology criteria provide a set of guidelines for the diagnosis of ALS. In these criteria, the body is divided into four regions: (1) bulbar (jaw, face, palate, larynx, and tongue), (2) cervical (neck, arm, hand, and diaphragm), (3) thoracic (back and abdomen), and (4) lumbosacral (back, abdomen, leg, and foot). The diagnosis of definite ALS is made when upper and lower motor neuron signs are present in the bulbar region and two other spinal regions or in three spinal regions. Individuals with upper and lower motor neuron signs in two spinal regions alone are classified as having probable ALS; possible ALS is diagnosed when dysfunction is present in only one region or when an individual presents with only upper motor neuron signs in two regions or lower motor neuron signs are rostral to upper motor neuron signs.

When the clinical findings suggest a diagnosis of ALS, nerve conduction studies with repetitive stimulation and electromyography (EMG) confirm lower motor neuron degeneration and exclude disorders of the neuromuscular junction, such as myasthenia gravis (Chapter 448), and of peripheral nerve and muscle. Neuroimaging of the brain and spinal cord is often needed to confirm the expected normal anatomy present in ALS and to exclude structural pathologic processes. Routine clinical laboratory tests are necessary to exclude ALS-related syndromes. These tests include complete blood cell count and routine chemical analyses, thyroid studies, serum protein electrophoresis, serum immunoelectrophoresis with immunofixation, and measurements of serum VDRL (Venereal Disease Research Laboratory) parameters, creatine kinase, erythrocyte sedimentation rate, antinuclear antibody, rheumatoid factor, and, when clinically indicated, hexosaminidase A, parathyroid hormone, and paraneoplastic antibodies. Additional tests may be warranted on the basis of the patient's clinical presentation. The EMG, neuroimaging, and clinical laboratory tests exclude the most common ALS-related disorders (Table 435–2): polyradiculopathy with myelopathy, postpolio syndrome, multifocal motor neuropathy, motor neuron disease with paraproteinemia, heavy metal intoxication, hexosaminidase A deficiency, paraneoplastic motor neuronopathy, and syringomyelia and syringobulbia.

Treatment and Prognosis

Rx

For direct disease treatment, the only drug currently available is riluzole (2-amino-6-trifluoromethoxy benzothiazole). Riluzole blocks release of glutamic acid and may slow the progression of disease by disrupting glutamate-mediated neurotoxicity. 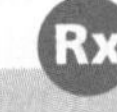 Administered at 50 mg twice a day, riluzole is generally well tolerated, although some patients experience nausea and general asthenia. Over the past decade, double-blind, placebo controlled trials of antiepileptic agents, antibiotics, antioxidants, protease inhibitors, platelet inhibitors, and growth factors have shown no benefit for the treatment of ALS.

Combining the results of several clinical epidemiology studies, the mean duration between the onset of symptoms and death in sporadic ALS ranges from 27 to 43 months, and the median duration is from 23 to 52 months. The average 5-year survival is 25%. The mean disease duration of primary lateral sclerosis is much longer, with an average of 224 months between symptoms and death. The relentless progression and poor prognosis of ALS require that patients receive attentive, supportive care.

A multidisciplinary approach is essential and is best coordinated by a dedicated ALS nurse or other health care professional. Symptomatic treatment is frequently required for sialorrhea, pseudobulbar symptoms, cramps, and spasticity. A social worker should help the patient cope with a sense of general fear, anxiety, and depression. A physical therapist should provide the patient with exercises for stretching and flexibility and should recommend needed bracing and adaptive walking devices. An occupational therapist should arrange adaptive devices to improve functional independence. As swallowing function decreases and speech becomes more difficult, a speech pathologist is helpful to oversee barium swallow tests and to obtain augmentative communication devices. For patients who undergo percutaneous endoscopic gastrostomy, a dietitian assists in selection of proper feedings. Pulmonary specialists are often helpful in determining when noninvasive ventilation techniques, such as bilevel positive airway pressure, will be helpful for pulmonary symptoms and in assisting in the long-term care of patients who choose to become ventilator dependent.

SPINAL MUSCULAR ATROPHIES

Definition

The spinal muscular atrophies (SMAs) are hereditary, progressive motor neuron disorders that can begin in utero, during infancy, in childhood, or in adulthood. SMA types 1 to 3 and bulbospinal muscular atrophy (BSMA), also known as Kennedy's syndrome, are more readily diagnosed than other SMAs because their genetic characteristics are defined. Other disorders include distal hereditary motor neuropathy types I and II, upper limb–predominant hereditary motor neuropathy (type V), proximal SMA, and scapuloperoneal syndromes resulting from SMAs (see Table 435–1).

TABLE 435–2 DIFFERENTIAL DIAGNOSIS OF AMYOTROPHIC LATERAL SCLEROSIS CLASSIFIED BY ANATOMY OF THE NERVOUS SYSTEM

Anatomic Site	Possible Disorder
Muscle	Idiopathic inflammatory myopathy (especially IBM), distal myopathy, nemaline myopathy, isolated neck extensor myopathy, metabolic myopathy, oculopharyngeal dystrophy
Neuromuscular junction	MG, Lambert-Eaton myasthenic syndrome
Roots, plexus, nerve	Radiculopathy, diabetic polyradiculoneuropathy, infectious polyradiculopathy, plexopathies, mononeuropathies, motor neuropathies
Anterior horn cells	Spinal muscular atrophy, BSMA, monomelic amyotrophy, paraneoplastic motor neuropathy, progressive postpolio muscular atrophy, hexosaminidase deficiency
Spinal cord	Spondylotic myelopathy, syringomyelia, MS, adrenomyeloneuropathy, vitamin B_{12} deficiency, familial spastic paraparesis, HTLV-1 myelopathy
Central nervous system	Parkinson's disease, Creutzfeldt-Jakob disease, multisystem atrophy, Huntington's disease, brain stem stroke, brain stem glioma, foramen magnum tumors
Systemic disorders	Hyperthyroidism, hyperparathyroidism

BSMA = bulbospinal muscular atrophy, HTLV-1 = human T-lymphotropic virus type 1, IBM = inclusion body myositis, MG = myasthenia gravis, MS = multiple sclerosis.

Epidemiology

The estimated carrier frequency of a survival motor neuron mutation is 1 in 50. SMA 1 (Werdnig-Hoffmann disease) has a cumulative incidence of disease of 1 in 8000 births.

Pathobiology

SMAs 1 to 3 represent the first class of neurologic disorders in which a developmental defect in neuronal apoptosis is the most likely cause. Linkage to chromosome 5q13 led to the identification of the survival motor neuron *(SMN)* genes, two copies of which exist on 5q13. The form of SMA with the earliest onset and most severe disease, SMA 1 (Werdnig-Hoffmann disease), is caused by homozygous deletions in exons 7 and 8 of the telomeric gene copy (SMNt). Mutations that convert SMNt to the centromeric copy result in a milder disease phenotype, SMA 2 (late infantile) and SMA 3 (Kugelberg-Welander disease). The *SMN* gene is highly expressed in spinal neurons and is involved in RNA splicing. Deletions of exons 5 and 6 or complete absence of another gene on 5q13, the neuronal apoptosis inhibitor *(NAIP)*, occur in 45 to 65% of patients with SMA 1 and in 20 to 40% of individuals with SMA 2 and 3. *NAIP* mutations may modify the severity of SMA.

Pathology

At autopsy, patients with SMA have atrophic spinal cords with loss of α-motor neurons and evidence of motor neuron degeneration and gliosis. Ventral roots are atrophic, and muscle groups supplied by these motor neurons and roots are atrophied and show microscopic evidence of denervation and reinnervation.

Clinical Manifestations

The onset of SMA 1 (Werdnig-Hoffmann disease), by definition, occurs either in utero or within the first 3 months of life. Infants present with severe diffuse weakness, hypotonia, reduced or absent reflexes, and tongue fasciculations. The usual cause of death is respiratory failure; 50% of infants die by age 7 months and 95% by 17 months.

Individuals with SMA 2 (late infantile form) and SMA 3 (Kugelberg-Welander disease) are less severely affected than those with SMA 1. SMA 2 is considered an intermediate phenotype. The onset occurs in children younger than 18 to 24 months. These children may never stand or walk, develop early scoliosis and respiratory insufficiency, and have a shortened lifespan. SMA 3 is the mildest phenotype, with onset frequently in later childhood or even in the teen years. These individuals have proximal, symmetrical weakness but stand and walk independently. With time, slow and mild loss of function usually takes place. Death occurs in adulthood, and whether SMA 3 shortens an individual's lifespan remains uncertain.

Diagnosis

The diagnosis of SMAs 1 to 3 is made by genetic testing in a patient with appropriate clinical signs and symptoms. Ninety-five percent of affected individuals have SMN deletions. Currently, carrier testing can be performed only by linkage analysis. Prenatal diagnosis is available. EMG and muscle biopsy, which are often performed before the diagnosis has been considered, reveal evidence of denervation but are unnecessary if a molecular diagnosis is established. Cerebrospinal fluid analysis is normal, and serum creatine kinase levels are elevated only in SMA 3.

It is important to distinguish SMA 1 from infantile botulism (Chapter 320), which can have a similar initial clinical picture. EMG with high-frequency repetitive nerve stimulation shows a decrement in botulism but not in SMA. Examination of the stool for botulinum can confirm the diagnosis of infantile botulism. SMA 2 and SMA 3 can be distinguished from chronic inflammatory demyelinating polyneuropathy by the presence of normal cerebrospinal fluid protein and normal nerve conduction studies in SMA. SMA 3 and the hereditary motor sensory neuropathies (Charcot-Marie-Tooth disease; Chapter 446) can be clinically similar. In addition to genetic testing, key diagnostic differences lie in normal nerve conduction studies in individuals with SMA 3 compared with abnormal studies in individuals with hereditary motor sensory neuropathies.

Treatment and Prognosis

No treatment is currently available, although trials with ciliary neurotrophic factor, brain-derived neurotrophic factor, gabapentin, and riluzole are under way. In SMA 2 and SMA 3, children benefit from passive and active physical therapy, lightweight braces, and, if necessary, surgery to correct scoliosis.

BULBOSPINAL MUSCULAR ATROPHY

Definition and Etiology

BSMA was first described by Kennedy and colleagues; consequently, it is also called Kennedy's syndrome. It is an X-linked recessive disorder. Incidence and prevalence have not been defined, but it is commonly held that BSMA is the most common form of adult-onset SMA.

Pathobiology

BSMA is a trinucleotide-repeat disorder with a CAG expansion encoding for a polyglutamine tract in the first exon of the androgen receptor gene on chromosome Xq11-12. Nuclear inclusions, aggregates, and aberrant proteolytic processing of the mutant androgen receptor are observed in bulbar and spinal motor neurons, which may lead to the pathologic features. It is not known why this mutation causes motor neuron disease instead of the testicular feminization caused by other androgen receptor mutations.

Pathology

At autopsy, patients with BSMA have findings similar to those of SMA 3. Mild brain stem and spinal cord atrophy with loss of α-motor neurons are seen, as are evidence of motor neuron degeneration and gliosis. Muscle biopsy reveals denervation and reinnervation in affected muscle groups.

Clinical Manifestations

The mean onset of BSMA is 30 years, with a range of 15 to 60 years. Gynecomastia occurs in 50% of affected individuals. Patients present with facial, tongue, and proximal weakness. Dysphagia, dysarthria, and masseter muscle weakness are common. Weakness is symmetrical and slowly progressive over decades; patients generally become dependent on canes or walkers in the fifth or sixth decades of life. Fasciculations are present largely in the face, and tendon reflexes are reduced or absent. Individuals frequently experience a mild postural tremor and a mild loss of vibratory sensation. No upper motor neuron signs are present.

Diagnosis

The diagnosis of BSMA is made when a patient with appropriate clinical signs and symptoms has positive genetic test results. Individuals affected at a younger age and more severely have more CAG expansion and longer polyglutamine tracts. The absence of upper motor neuron signs distinguishes BSMA from ALS. EMG and a muscle biopsy, which are often performed because creatine kinase levels are frequently elevated (up to 10-fold), reveal evidence of chronic denervation, which differentiates BSMA from muscular dystrophy and other myopathies.

Treatment and Prognosis

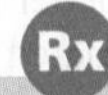

No specific treatment is available. Lifespan is usually unaffected, and therapy consists of supportive care, such as ambulatory aids.

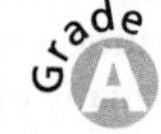

1. Bensimon G, Lacomblez L, Meininger V, et al: ALS/Riluzole Study Group: A controlled trial of riluzole in amyotrophic lateral sclerosis. N Engl J Med 1994;330:585–591.

SUGGESTED READINGS

Andersen PM, Borasio GD, Dengler R, et al: EFNS task force on management of amyotrophic lateral sclerosis: Guidelines for diagnosing and clinical care of patients and relatives. Eur J Neurol 2005;12:921–938. *A consensus overview.*

Boillee S, Yamanaka K, Lobsiger CS, et al: Onset and progression in inherited ALS determined by motor neurons and microglia. Science 2006;312:1389–1392. *A pathophysiologic description.*

Pasinelli P, Brown RH: Molecular biology of amyotrophic lateral sclerosis: Insights from genetics. Nat Rev Neurosci 2006;7:710–723. *Review of the postulated pathophysiology of ALS.*

Pestronk A: Neuromuscular Disease Center. St. Louis, MO, Washington University School of Medicine, Neuromuscular Disease Center, 2006. URL: http://www.neuro.wustl.edu/neuromuscular/. *Comprehensive collection of motor neuron disorders with key links to salient information on genetics, recent basic research, and therapy. This website is user friendly, is updated continuously, and is invaluable for the clinician.*

436 MULTIPLE SCLEROSIS AND DEMYELINATING CONDITIONS OF THE CENTRAL NERVOUS SYSTEM

Peter A. Calabresi

The disorders of myelin encompass a wide range of diseases in which either myelin is not formed in a normal fashion (dysmyelinating disease) or normally formed myelin is destroyed or not maintained appropriately (demyelinating disease) (Table 436–1). Dysmyelinating diseases are uncommon and include an array of leukodystrophies that have a genetic basis. Demyelinating diseases are much more common and include multiple sclerosis (MS), which represents more than 95% of all types of disorders of central nervous system (CNS) myelin.

Some disorders of myelin actually have a distinct pathogenesis in which the disruption of myelin is secondary. Further, in many of the diseases of myelin, the axon degenerates as a result of loss of trophic support from loss of myelin or because of increased susceptibility to injury in the absence of myelin. This observation has led to the recent hypothesis that axonal loss is the underlying substrate for permanent disability in MS, adrenoleukodystrophy, and perhaps other diseases of myelin.

MULTIPLE SCLEROSIS

Definition

MS is a disease characterized by multifocal areas of demyelination in the brain and spinal cord, with associated inflammatory cell infiltrates, reactive gliosis, and axonal degeneration. It typically presents in young adults with episodic neurologic dysfunction. Although the exact origin of MS remains enigmatic, evidence suggests that it is an immune mediated attack on myelin, with secondary disruption of axons leading to progressive disability over time in the majority of afflicted patients.

Epidemiology

The annual incidence of MS varies by location and ranges between 1.5 and 11/100,000 people. MS is second only to trauma as the most common cause of neurologic disability in young adults. More recent studies suggest that the incidence rate has increased, in part because of better recognition of more cases at an earlier stage. The prevalence is estimated at 350,000 to 400,000 in the United States and more than 1,000,000 worldwide, but these numbers may be underestimates owing to incomplete recognition of the disease even in developed countries.

MS occurs two- to 2.5-fold more frequently in women than in men, a sex predilection that is common in autoimmune diseases. The disease most often presents in the third to fourth decades of life, but with an incidence age range from postpubertal teenagers to persons in their 50s. Rare cases occur in infants or in patients in their 60s, but extreme caution is warranted in these situations to exclude alternative processes. In many of the late-onset cases, symptoms were present in younger years and were attributed to other causes.

TABLE 436–1 DISEASES OF MYELIN

IDIOPATHIC
Recurrent or chronic progressive demyelination (multiple sclerosis and its variants)
Monophasic demyelination (may be the first clinical episode of multiple sclerosis)
Optic neuritis
Acute transverse myelitis
Acute disseminated encephalomyelitis; acute hemorrhagic leukoencephalopathy
VIRAL INFECTIONS
Progressive multifocal leukoencephalopathy
Subacute sclerosing panencephalitis (Chapter 439)
NUTRITIONAL AND METABOLIC DISORDERS (Chapter 443)
Combined systems disease (vitamin B_{12} deficiency)
Demyelination of the corpus callosum (Marchiafava-Bignami disease)
Central pontine myelinolysis
ANOXIC-ISCHEMIC SEQUELAE (Chapter 428)
Delayed postanoxic cerebral demyelination
Progressive subcortical ischemic encephalopathy
LEUKODYSTROPHIES PRIMARILY AFFECTING CENTRAL NERVOUS SYSTEM MYELIN
Adrenoleukodystrophy (Schilder's disease)
Pelizaeus-Merzbacher disease (sudanophilic leukodystrophies)
Spongy degeneration
Vanishing white matter disease
Others (Alexander's disease, Canavan's disease)
Leukodystrophies of the central and peripheral nervous system
Metachromatic leukodystrophy
Globoid cell leukodystrophy (Krabbe's disease)

MS is most common in people of Northern European descent, and whites acquire multiple sclerosis at nearly twice the rate of African Americans in the United States. In many areas of the world, MS is more prevalent in temperate latitudes (approaching 1 in 500 in some locations) and becomes less common toward the equator (1 in 20,000 or rare case reports only in some locations), perhaps explained, in part, by migration patterns of people with the same gene pools. However, the absence of complete genetic penetrance in monozygotic twin studies suggests an environmental component to the disease. Indeed, an outbreak of MS was documented on the Faeroe Islands following World War II, and numerous other clusters have been reported, although an environmental trigger has not been identified.

Pathobiology and Genetics

Monozygotic twins with MS show a concordance rate of between 15 and 50%, compared with only 3 to 5% concordance in dizygotic twins, consistent with a strong but incomplete role for genes in causing MS. The lifetime risk of MS is increased to 2 to 4% in individuals with a first-degree relative with MS compared with the general population risk of 0.1%. In addition, between 10 and 20% of patients with MS have a first-degree relative with another autoimmune disease, commonly rheumatoid arthritis, systemic lupus erythematosus, or autoimmune thyroid disease. Hashimoto's disease and Crohn's disease also may be more common in patients with MS. Genetic modeling of the disease strongly argues against a single MS gene and suggests that many different genes predispose to MS and account for its many phenotypes. Linkage and association studies have identified the human leukocyte antigen (HLA) or major histocompatibility complex (MHC) region on chromosome 6 as one genetic determinant for MS. The MHC class II region, involved in presentation of antigen to CD4+ T cells, is the most strongly associated locus. The HLA-DR2 allele and, more specifically, the molecular haplotype HLA-DRB*1501 allele have repeatedly been implicated. Other loci of interest on other chromosomes, including chromosome 1, continue to be investigated, but the associations appear less strong.

Pathology

Pathologically, most cases are characterized by multifocal areas of demyelination and gross gliotic scar in the brain and spinal cord. Classic locations of these lesions, called *plaques,* are the optic nerves, periventricular white matter, deep white matter, juxtacortical white matter, corpus callosum, cerebellar peduncles, and dorsolateral spinal cord. However, there may be a bias toward recognition of lesions in white matter because of the relative ease of detecting demyelination and inflammation in white versus gray matter. Indeed, more recent pathologic studies have confirmed demyelination, neuritic damage, and atrophy in the cortex and deep gray matter. At the microscopic level, one usually sees multiple areas of perivenular inflammatory cell infiltrates with extravasation into the surrounding tissue parenchyma. In the acute active plaque, the CD4 helper T cell is prominent in the perivenular areas. Increasingly large numbers of CD8 cytotoxic T cells have been documented in brain tissue, especially in the parenchyma. Most parenchymal inflammatory cells are CD68 positive macrophages and microglia. In addition to the influx of circulating immune cells, prominent astroglial activation and even oligodendrocyte precursor cell proliferation occur in response to injury. Over time, the inflammation becomes less prominent in the center of the plaque, but a chronic active rim of inflammation with microglial activation exists at a well-demarcated border between abnormal and normal unharmed myelin. This characteristic of MS is seldom seen in other disorders of myelin. Although oligodendrocytes may survive, proliferate, and result in partial remyelination (shadow plaques) in some early cases, this process is hardly ever complete in MS. Over time, remyelination is less successful, and oligodendrocyte progenitor cells appear unable to differentiate into mature myelinating oligodendrocytes.

The number of damaged axons correlates with the extent of inflammation. Further, axonal damage and even neuronal apoptosis is seen in the cortex. Atrophy of both the brain and spinal cord, which occurs more rapidly in MS than in normal aging, reflects loss of both myelin and axons.

No consistent microbial cause has been discerned from careful examination of MS tissues for known infectious pathogens. Differential expression of the human herpes virus type 6, which is acquired by most people in childhood, has been noted in oligodendrocytes of patients with MS, but whether this virus is a cofactor in demyelination or just a bystander remains unclear. Evidence suggests the possibility that the earliest event in MS may be an insult to the oligodendrocytes, with subsequent activation of resident immune cells and secondary recruitment of other immune cells only at later stages.

Some pathologists believe that four distinct subtypes of MS can be discerned, in which the pathologic characteristics are consistent in every lesion, thereby allowing classification of patients with differing pathologic categories rather than just describing evolution of lesions over time. Type I lesions are characterized by typical perivenular inflammatory infiltrates consisting mainly of T cells, with early preservation of oligodendrocytes. Type II lesions are similar to type I but have an additional humoral component with immunoglobulin G (IgG) deposition and complement activation. Type III lesions are distinguished by not being based around venules and by prominent loss of myelin-associated glycoprotein, with evidence for oligodendrocyte apoptosis. Type IV lesions have inflammatory infiltrates more similar to types I and II but also have oligodendrocyte loss as in type III. These varying pathologic features may begin to explain clinical subtypes of the disease.

Pathogenesis

It remains possible that the autoimmune hypothesis is wrong and that the inflammation observed in MS is secondary to an as yet uncharacterized primary degenerative process. Proponents of this theory cite evidence from pathologic features of hyperacute cases, in which the oligodendrocytes appear to die before any systemic immune response occurs, as well as recent data revealing neuronal and axonal death or demyelination in the absence of inflammation.

Macrophages and microglia, which comprise the majority of cells within the parenchymal infiltrate in chronic MS plaques, are potent antigen-presenting cells and express HLA and costimulatory molecules. Activated macrophages and microglial also have effector functions including release of cytokines that are partly (interleukin-6 [IL-6], tumor necrosis factor-α) or completely distinct from the T cells (IL-1β, IL-12, and IL-23). In high concentrations, these cytokines may damage oligodendrocytes and neurons, and activate T cells.

Clinical Manifestations

Presenting Symptoms

MS, which can present in many ways across a broad age range, may initially masquerade as a variety of different illnesses (see Table 436–1; Table 436–2). In a classic presentation, a young white person, more often a woman, will have the acute to subacute onset of impaired vision or sensation. Fatigue, depression, bladder urgency, weakness, impaired balance, and impaired coordination are also common symptoms. The often remarkably mild nature of the first symptoms often dissuades the patient

TABLE 436–2 CONDITIONS THAT CAN BE MISTAKEN FOR MULTIPLE SCLEROSIS AND OTHER DISEASES OF MYELIN

VASCULAR DISEASE
Small vessel cerebrovascular disease
Vasculitides
Arteriovenous malformation
CADASIL
Antiphospholipid antibody syndrome
STRUCTURAL LESIONS
Craniocervical junction posterior fossa or spinal tumors
Cervical spondylosis or disc herniation
Chiari malformation or syrinx
DEGENERATIVE DISEASES
Hereditary myelopathy
Spinocerebellar degeneration
INFECTIONS
HTLV-1 infection
HIV myelopathy or HIV-related cerebritis
Neuroborreliosis (e.g., Lyme disease)
JC virus/progressive multifocal leukoencephalopathy
Neurosyphilis
OTHER INFLAMMATORY CONDITIONS
Systemic lupus erythematosus
Sjögren's syndrome
Sarcoidosis
MONOFOCAL OR MONOPHASIC DEMYELINATING SYNDROMES
Transverse myelitis
Optic neuritis
Neuromyelitis optica/Devic's disease
Acute disseminated encephalomyelitis
OTHER CONDITIONS
Hashimoto's thyroiditis with or without encephalopathy
Nonspecific MRI abnormalities related to migraine, aging, or trauma

HIV = human immunodeficiency virus; HTLV = human T-cell lymphotropic virus; MRI = magnetic resonance imaging, CADASIL = cerebral autosomal dominant arteriopathy with subcortical infarcts and leukoencephalopathy.

from seeking medical attention or is insufficiently impressive to stimulate the physician to order diagnostic tests. Furthermore, patients may initially have few objective neurologic findings, especially between attacks.

Paresthesias of a limb that are circumferential and do not follow a dermatome suggest a spinal cord lesion; these symptoms often manifest distally and then ascend to involve more proximal parts of the limb, spread to the contralateral limb, or progress from a leg to an arm. Similarly, bandlike sensations around a limb or the torso also suggest a myelopathic process.

Incomplete transverse myelitis is a focal (partial) spinal cord syndrome that is usually inflammatory and does not follow vascular territories. It is a common presentation of MS.

Lhermitte's symptom, an electrical sensation moving down the spine into the limbs on flexion of the neck, is characteristic of cervical myelitis from any cause, including MS. Frank loss of sensation is less common as an early symptom or sign but is seen in more advanced cases. Burning, electrical, or deep aching sensations are also common in MS.

Sensory Abnormalities

On examination, the most common sensory findings are loss of vibration perception, most prominent in the feet, and incomplete spinal cord levels to pin prick or vibration, which are often more notable in a graded fashion rather than at a distinct level. Such sensory levels may be asymmetrical and differ by sensory modality because of isolated demyelination in the dorsal columns as compared with the spinothalamic tracts. Patchy or seemingly nonanatomic focal areas of impaired sensation can occur, and some patients describe bizarre sensations such as water dripping or bugs crawling on an area of the body.

Visual Effects

Optic neuritis (Chapter 450) is a classic presenting syndrome, typically with visual symptoms in one eye. In optic neuritis, patients often complain of pain over the lateral eyebrow and worsening on lateral eye movement. The visual impairment may be described as looking through frosted glass or a veil. The scotoma or area of greatest loss can often be mapped in a centrocecal distribution (central focal point to the blind spot laterally), which in mild cases may be evident only as desaturation to red color using the head of a pin. More severe cases may result in total loss of light perception. In most acute cases of optic neuritis, the inflammation is retrobulbar (behind the disc), so no immediate changes are visible on the optic disc, thereby leading to the aphorism "the patient sees nothing and the doctor sees nothing." However, there should be a relative afferent papillary defect (Marcus-Gunn pupil; Chapter 450) with paradoxical dilation of the affected eye to direct light on swinging a flashlight from the unaffected eye in which consensual constriction was induced. In cases of bilateral optic neuritis (new or old), this abnormality may not be seen. Patients usually spontaneously recover substantial vision after weeks to months. Later, the optic disc may become pale, especially in the temporal region, a finding reflecting damage to the axons following inflammation and demyelination, even with recovery of normal visual acuity. Patients often have more subtle chronic visual impairment for colors and low contrast visual acuity and contrast sensitivity.

Visual impairment from impaired tracking of eye movements owing to brain stem or cerebellar disease most commonly occurs in the setting of an acute lesion affecting the medial longitudinal fasciculus, which is the neurologic pathway that yokes the eyes together on lateral saccades. Patients may experience frank diplopia or just blurred vision, especially when they look off to one side rapidly, such as when looking over one's shoulder while driving. The neurologic sign of this problem is called *internuclear ophthalmoplegia* (Chapter 450) and manifests as slowed or absent adduction of one eye with abducting nystagmus of the other eye. It may occur bilaterally or may exist in milder forms, such that the adduction lag is imperceptible to the human observer. Blurred vision from cerebellar damage with nystagmus is very common in MS and is often worse on extreme lateral or vertical gaze. *Oscillopsia,* the sensation that the environment is moving when it actually is not, is another symptom of impaired cerebellar coordination of the eyes. Saccadic eye movement or loss of smooth pursuit is also common in MS and also can be seen in numerous neurologic conditions or with aging.

Motor Symptoms

The most common motor symptoms of MS are weakness and impaired coordination in a leg, with ascending involvement from distal to proximal and commonly spreading to the contralateral leg or ipsilateral arm. The lesion causing these symptoms is more commonly in the cervical spinal cord rather than the thoracic spinal cord, even when the first sign is partial footdrop. It is likely that axons that must conduct impulses over the longest distance (entire length of the spinal cord) from a site of inflammatory demyelination will become symptomatic before axons delivering signals to closer synapses (adjacent anterior horn cells in the cervical cord). Clinically, the weakness may be severe and may result in an obvious paralysis or be so subtle as to be undetectable. Heat-induced fatigue and weakness, as manifested by focal symptoms (slapping of a foot or dragging a leg) occurring after 15 to 20 minutes of exercise and resolving with rest, are characteristic of early demyelinating disease. The early absence of associated hyperreflexia and plantar extensor responses (Babinski's sign) may make it difficult to document corticospinal tract involvement. Later, in more established MS, classic corticospinal tract signs are often evident and manifest clinically as spastic gait (either hemiparetic or paraparetic), muscle cramps, and clonus (sustained reflex loop), sometimes occurring with positional changes and mistaken for signs of a cerebellar tremor.

Ataxia may occur as a result of impaired delivery of sensory information up the spinal cord or from demyelination of cerebellar pathways in the brain stem or cerebellum. Often, the two are mixed and may be confounded further by visual loss and impaired ability to compensate by fixing on the environment; this combination commonly causes dizziness in crowds, in which fixation may be further obscured. Appendicular dysmetria resulting in tremor on reaching for an object is a common cause of impaired coordination and dexterity. Lower extremity and truncal ataxia may result in a wide-based (drunk) gait. Other movement disorders such as postural tremor and titubation (head tremor) are much less common in MS. *Myokymia* (wormlike muscle movements) under the skin, especially around the face, however, is fairly common. Pseudoathetosis and parkinsonism can be seen in severe cases.

Organ Dysfunction

Bladder symptoms are extremely common, but often are not volunteered, so specific questions must be asked. A careful bladder history may reveal isolated or mixed patterns of urinary frequency, urgency, incontinence, and/or retention. Careful delineation of a spastic bladder (detrusor muscle spasm) causing incontinence from an atonic bladder or spasm of the external sphincter (the latter two are causes of retention) leading to overflow incontinence is critical to designing an appropriate therapeutic strategy (Chapter 24). Urinary tract infections (Chapter 307), which are commonly the result of bladder dysfunction, may aggravate the underlying symptoms of MS.

Bowel dysfunction commonly manifests as constipation (Chapter 138), which may be primary (related to spinal cord involvement) or secondary (related to self-induced dehydration to manage urinary frequency or to side effects of anticholinergic drugs). Bowel incontinence secondary to an incompetent anal sphincter is less common and most often occurs as an isolated episode of fecal urgency, sometimes related to dietary change or diarrheal illness.

Sexual dysfunction is also common and underdiscussed in MS. In men, erectile dysfunction is frequent. In women and men, loss of libido and inability to achieve orgasm can occur as a result of medication, loss of sensation, heat-induced worsening of symptoms, physical barriers to intercourse (impaired mucosal moisture, spasticity, and pain), depression, or disorders of body image.

Systemic Symptoms

Fatigue, which is common in MS, may be linked to depression but often occurs independently and can be the most disabling symptom of the disease. A sleep history is important to exclude daytime fatigue resulting from disrupted sleep secondary to pain, cramps, bladder frequency, sleep apnea, periodic limb movements, depression, or disrupted sleep-wake cycles. Daytime fatigue even after a good night of sleep may occur in midafternoon and may be described as being "unplugged" or completely drained. Many patients obtain benefit from a short daytime nap.

Sensitivity to heat, which is a classic symptom of MS, occurs only in some patients. Even minor elevations of the body temperature can dramatically worsen symptoms. Symptoms usually (but not always) improve on cooling. Cooling devices can prevent this phenomenon, but there is no persistent benefit of cooling below normal body temperature. Some patients complain of worsened symptoms in cold weather, likely related to increased dysfunction of already stiff muscles and increased pain.

Pregnancy

Many women with MS successfully have multiple children, and the activity of MS lessens during the course of pregnancy, especially by the third trimester, when the frequency of exacerbations is reduced by approximately two thirds. Relapses are more frequent in the first 6 postpartum months, but no evidence indicates that pregnancy changes the natural history of the disease. Breast-feeding does not alter the course of MS, but it is contraindicated for patients who resume disease-modifying drugs following delivery.

Types of Multiple Sclerosis

The three major clinical types of MS are relapsing remitting, secondary progressive, and primary progressive. Approximately 85 to 90% of patients present with relapsing remitting MS, characterized by acute or subacute episodes of new or worsening old neurologic symptoms that increase in severity, plateau, and then partly or completely remit. Patients may have no detectable residual deficit, or they may accumulate significant permanent disability from an attack. Most patients with relapsing remitting MS convert to secondary progressive MS after 20 to 40 years. This stage of the disease is defined by at least 6 months of progressive worsening without evidence of a relapse. Some patients with secondary progressive MS also have interposed relapses distinct from their periods of progressive worsening, although these episodes become less frequent with time. Primary progressive MS, which is characterized by progressive deterioration from the onset for at least 1 year without a history of distinct relapses, occurs in approximately 10 to 15% of patients. It is more common in middle-aged men and typically has more involvement of the spinal cord and fewer inflammatory brain lesions.

Several other uncommon types of MS also are described. Progressive relapsing MS refers to a fairly uncommon variant of MS (6%), in which a relapse ensues after an initially primary progressive course. Acute progressive MS (Marburg's disease) causes acute or subacute progressive neurologic deterioration leading to severe disability within days to a month in a patient with no prior history of MS. This rare form of the disease may progress to a quadriplegic, obtunded state with death as a result of intercurrent infection, aspiration, or respiratory failure from brain stem involvement.

Diagnosis

The diagnosis of MS rests on demonstrating evidence of at least two inflammatory demyelinating lesions referable to different locations within the CNS, occurring at different times (usually ≥1 month apart), and for which no better explanation exists. Diagnostic criteria allow for the diagnosis to be made on clinical grounds alone as long as appropriate exclusionary testing is performed (Table 436–3). Clinical evidence of a lesion requires objective findings on examination, not just a symptom. Further, repeated episodes of neurologic dysfunction that could be explained based on one lesion (e.g., a cervicomedullary junction lesion causing brain stem, cerebellar, and corticospinal tract dysfunction) is not enough evidence to diagnose MS.

Laboratory Findings

Magnetic Resonance Imaging

No definitive diagnostic laboratory test exists for MS, but magnetic resonance imaging (MRI) of the brain is extremely useful and should be performed in all patients in whom MS is a diagnostic consideration. More than 95% of patients with clinically definite MS have an abnormal brain MRI, and the presence of high-signal, bright lesions is so characteristic of MS that a normal brain MRI should suggest an alternative diagnosis. Brain MRI is also useful in predicting future MS at the time of a clinically isolated demyelinating syndrome. Specific MRI findings (Table 436–4) allow for confirmation of disease disseminated in space (different parts of the brain or spine) as well as fulfilling evidence for dissemination in time (a new inflammatory T2 lesion occurring 3 months after a clinically isolated demyelinating syndrome in a location different from the original presenting lesion, without a better explanation). MS plaques typically appear as high-signal (white) areas on fluid attenuation inversion recovery (FLAIR) T2-weighted images, which allow for the best discrimination of these lesions by suppressing high-signal from cerebrospinal fluid (CSF) in the ventricles (Fig. 436–1). Lesions generally range in size from 2 mm to 2 cm; larger plaques occasionally resemble a tumor. Features of an MRI lesion suggesting MS include an elliptical shape, discrete borders, lack of mass effect, and gadolinium enhancement. Typical locations include the periventricular area (perpendicular to and or abutting the walls of the ventricles) (Fig. 436–2), the corpus callosum, the cerebellar peduncles, the brain stem, the juxtacortical area, and the dorsolateral spinal cord (Fig. 436–3). Cortical and deep gray matter lesions also occur but are less clearly seen on conventional MRI. Gadolinium enhancement, which suggests permeability of the blood-brain barrier, is correlated with new or active inflammation in lesions (Fig. 436–4). Lesions that enhance on a T1-weighted sequence usually have a concomitant lesion in the same location on a T2-weighted image. However, T2-weighted lesions may form without evident enhancement. Gadolinium enhancement typically persists for 2 to 8 weeks and thus may be missed on intermittent scans. Persistent areas of low signal on T1-weighted images before contrast (black holes) correlate with pathologic evidence of axonal loss and atrophy (Fig. 436–5).

TABLE 436–3 2005 REVISIONS TO THE MCDONALD DIAGNOSTIC CRITERIA FOR MULTIPLE SCLEROSIS

Clinical Presentation	Additional Data Needed for Diagnosis of Multiple Sclerosis
Two or more attacks; objective clinical evidence of two or more lesions	None*
Two or more attacks; objective clinical evidence of one lesion	Dissemination in space, demonstrated by: (1) MRI† or (2) Two or more MRI-detected lesions consistent with MS plus positive CSF or (3) Await further clinical attack implicating a different site
One attack; objective clinical evidence of two or more lesions	Dissemination in time, demonstrated by: (1) MRI‡ or (2) Second clinical attack
One attack; Objective clinical evidence of one lesion (monosymptomatic presentation; clinically isolated syndrome)	(1) Dissemination in space, demonstrated by: (a) MRI† or (b) Two or more MRI-detected lesions consistent with MS plus positive CSF and (2) Dissemination in time, demonstrated by: (a) MRI or (b) Second clinical attack

*Must rule out other causes (e.g., Table 436–2)
CSF = cerebrospinal fluid; MRI = magnetic resonance imaging; MS = multiple sclerosis.
Adapted with permission from Polman CH, Reingold SC, Edan G, et al: Diagnostic criteria for multiple sclerosis: 2005 revisions to the "McDonald Criteria." Ann Neurol 2005;58:840–846.

Table 436–4 MAGNETIC RESONANCE IMAGING CRITERIA IN MULTIPLE SCLEROSIS (INTERNATIONAL PANEL RECOMMENDATIONS: 2005)

DISSEMINATION IN TIME
Detection of gadolinium enhancement at least 3 months after the onset of the initial clinical event, if not at the site corresponding to the initial event
OR
Detection of a new T2 lesion if it appears at any time compared with a reference scan done at least 30 days after the onset of the initial clinical event*
DISSEMINATION IN SPACE (THREE OF THE FOLLOWING)†
At least one gadolinium-enhancing lesion or nine T2 hyperintense lesions if there is no gadolinium enhancing lesion
At least one infratentorial lesion
At least one juxtacortical lesion
At least three periventricular lesions
DIAGNOSIS OF PRIMARY PROGRESSIVE MULTIPLE SCLEROSIS
One year of disease progression (retrospectively or prospectively determined) plus two of the following:
a. Positive brain magnetic resonance imaging (nine T2 lesions or four or more T2 lesions with positive visual-evoked potentials)
b. Positive spinal cord magnetic resonance imaging (two focal T2 lesions)
c. Positive cerebrospinal fluid (isoelectric focusing evidence of oligoclonal immunoglobulin G bands or increased immunoglobulin G index, or both).

*Caution: Determination that a T2 lesion is indeed new can be challenging. A new T2 lesion must be of sufficient size and location to reflect one that could not have been missed previously for technical reasons of slice orientation, thickness or spacing, tissue contract, patient motion, or other artifacts. This judgment requires standardized scanning procedures, with emphasis on careful repositioning, as well as input from qualified evaluators experienced in multiple sclerosis imaging.

†A spinal cord lesion is equivalent to an infratentorial brain lesion; an enhancing spinal cord lesion is considered to be equivalent to an enhancing brain lesion, and individual spinal cord lesions can contribute together with individual brain lesions to reach the required number of T2 lesions.

From Polman Ch, Reingold SC, Edan G, et al: Diagnostic criteria for multiple sclerosis: 2005 revisions to the "McDonald Criteria." Ann Neurol 2005;58:840–846, with permission.

Cerebrospinal Fluid

Examination of the CSF is useful in many cases but is not mandatory in patients with a typical clinical presentation and MRI evidence of disseminated disease. CSF evaluation includes cell counts, total protein, glucose, oligoclonal bands with a paired serum sample, and an IgG index. The presence of myelin basic protein is not specific for MS because it can be elevated secondary to any disruption of CNS tissue. Oligoclonal bands in the CSF or an elevated IgG index provides evidence for intrathecal production of immunoglobulins, and oligoclonal bands are common in MS but can occur with infection or other immune-mediated processes; the test lacks both specificity for MS and has a sensitivity of only approximately 85 to 90% of patients with clinically definite MS. In clinically isolated demyelinating syndromes (see later), the sensitivity is even lower (~50%).

CSF evaluation is generally recommended if an alternative diagnosis is considered, especially if one suspects an infectious process (e.g., fever, sweats, unusual travel history, tick bite, or rash). CSF analysis may also be useful if clinical or MRI criteria are incomplete to provide confirmation of the diagnosis.

Evoked Potential Tests

Evoked potentials (Chapter 418) may also be useful in some situations to document objective evidence of slowed conduction owing to demyelination in locations different from those recognized clinically. However, visual evoked potentials, brain stem auditory evoked potentials, and somatosensory evoked potentials are less sensitive and less specific for MS than is high-resolution MRI.

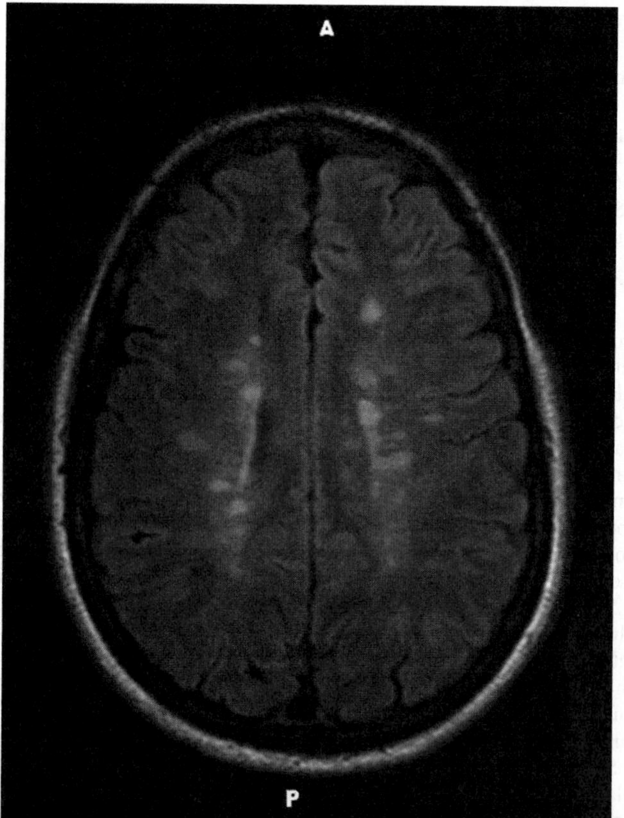

FIGURE 436–1 • Axial fluid attenuation inversion recovery image of the brain from a patient with multiple sclerosis revealing classic multiple periventricular and deep white matter high signal lesions.

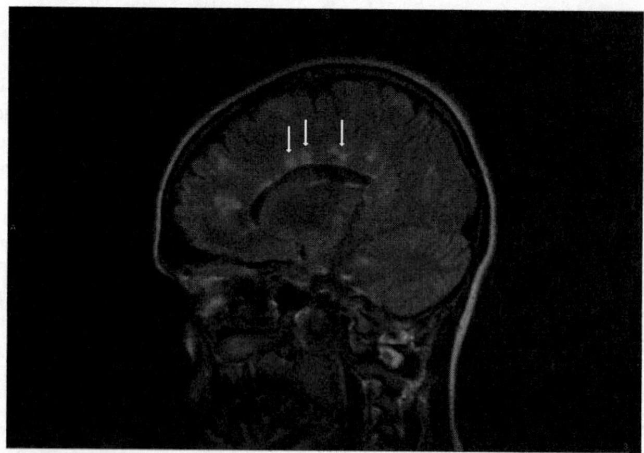

FIGURE 436–2 • Sagittal fluid attenuation inversion recovery image of the brain from a patient with multiple sclerosis revealing classic periventricular lesions radiating outward from the ventricles (arrows).

Differential Diagnosis

The diagnosis of MS may be so clear that it is recognized by the patient and is readily confirmed by the primary physician or so obscure that even experienced specialists disagree. Many processes (see Table 436–2) can mimic the clinical, radiologic, and CSF findings associated with MS, and there is no "gold standard" diagnostic test that is 100% sensitive and specific for the disease.

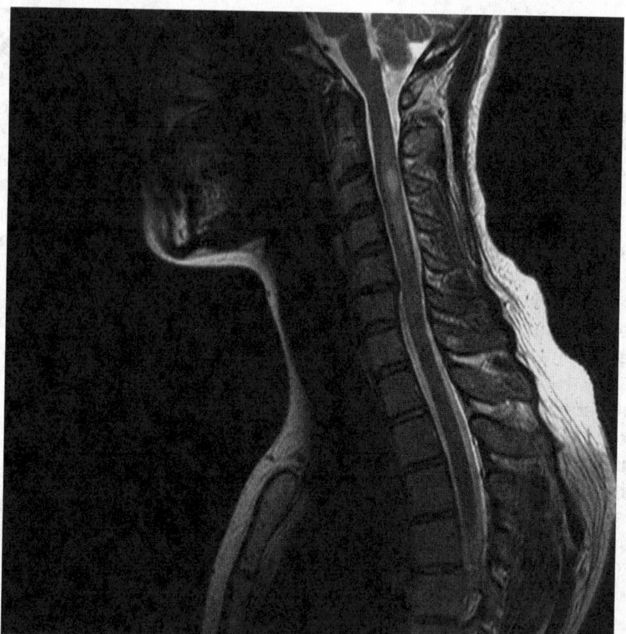

FIGURE 436–3 • Sagittal T2-weighted image of the brain and cervical spine from a patient with multiple sclerosis. The image shows a high-signal plaque from C3-C5 in the spinal cord.

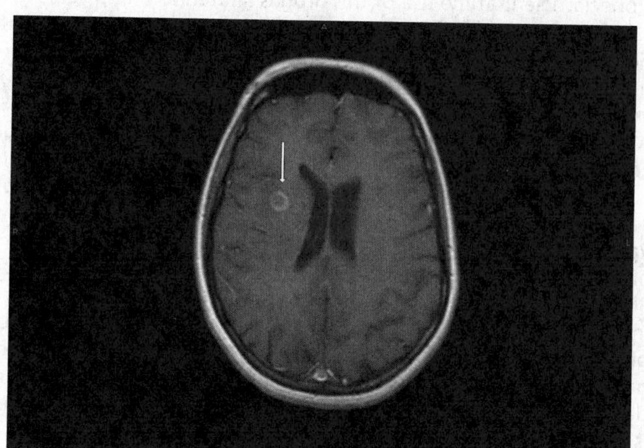

FIGURE 436–4 • Axial T1-weighted image after gadolinium contrast showing an actively inflamed ring-enhancing lesion in a patient with MS.

Processes that mimic MS include structural lesions, especially of the base of the brain and of the spinal cord, where one lesion can cause symptoms referable to many different tracts and at different perceived locations in the body. Chiari malformations with or without syrinx (Chapter 444), disc herniation (Chapter 423), cervical spondylosis, and low-grade tumors (Chapter 199) can produce symptoms of MS both in newly presenting patients and in patients who truly have MS but who also have a second process.

Various infectious diseases can mimic MS. Examples include human T-cell lymphotropic virus types I and II (virally associated myelopathy/tropical spastic paraparesis; Chapter 402), human immunodeficiency virus (neuropathy, myelopathy, cognitive impairment, CNS white matter changes; Chapter 407), neuroborreliosis (Lyme disease; Chapter 342), neurosyphilis, and herpes viruses (Epstein-Barr virus (Chapter 400), cytomegalovirus (Chapter 399), herpes simplex virus (Chapter 397), varicella-zoster virus myelitis (Chapter 398), and JC virus (progressive multifocal leukoencephalopathy; Chapter 399).

Other inflammatory diseases that usually involve other parts of the body can concomitantly affect the CNS or rarely present in the CNS. Examples include sarcoidosis (Chapter 95), systemic lupus erythematosus (Chapter 287), Sjögren's syndrome (Chapter 289), and vasculitides (Chapter 291). Ischemic vascular disease secondary from any cause also

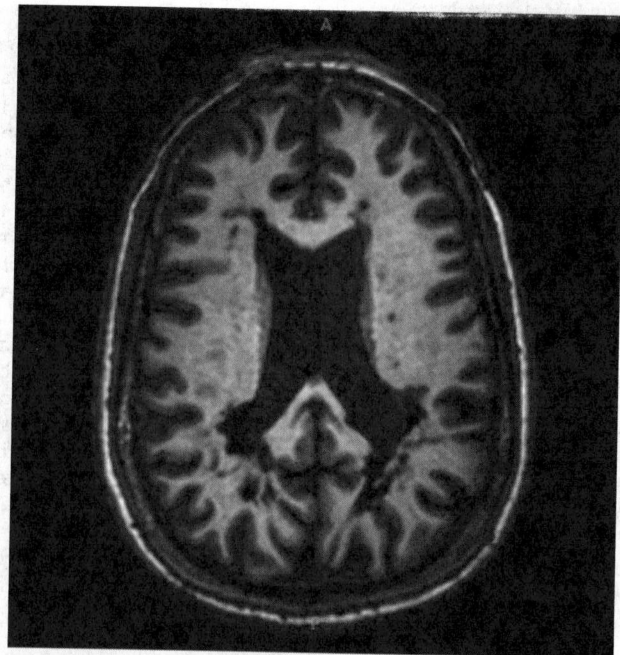

FIGURE 436–5 • Axial T1-weighted images showing numerous areas of T1 low signal ("black holes"), ventricular enlargement, and diffuse atrophy.

can resemble MS. Metabolic or nutritional disorders that can mimic MS include vitamin B_{12} deficiency and methylmalonic acidemia (in some cases distinct from cyanocobalamin deficiency). Central pontine myelinolysis (Chapter 443) secondary to overly rapid correction of sodium is rarely mistaken for MS. Thyroid disease (Chapter 244) may mimic the fatigue of MS and may cause dysesthesias and disorders of the optic nerve and muscles.

Monophasic demyelinating syndromes with or without multiple other lesions often, but not always, progress to become MS (see later). Spinocerebellar atrophy and hereditary myelopathy cause slowly progressive disease but do not cause sensory and visual abnormalities.

Treatment

The treatment of MS can be divided into drugs designed to relieve symptoms, drugs designed to modify the course of the disease, and nondrug measures. In addition, numerous drugs can target specific aspects of MS: depression, fatigue, muscle spasticity, pain, insomnia, bladder, bowel, and sexual dysfunction. Before considering a symptomatic therapy, the patient should be educated about the purpose of the drug and its side effect profile. On learning that these drugs have no long-term impact on disease activity, patients may elect not to use them for relief of symptoms alone. Symptomatic therapies are best started at low doses and frequently require titration to obtain the optimal balance between efficacy and side effects.

Treatment of Specific Symptoms

Depression and emotional lability are common symptoms of MS. In addition to appropriate supportive care and counseling, antidepressant therapy with one of the "activating" serotonergic or noradrenergic drugs (fluoxetine, sertraline, citalopram, escitalopram, venlafaxine, or bupropion) can be of benefit (see Table 420–2). If anxiety and panic symptoms predominate, a less activating drug such as paroxetine may be preferable. Patients with concomitant pain or insomnia may benefit more from a sedating tricyclic (amitriptyline or nortriptyline) given at bedtime.

Spasticity can be managed by physical therapy, stretching, and institution of either baclofen (5 to 160 mg in divided doses) or tizanidine (2 to 32 mg in divided doses). Either drug should be started as a single agent at a low dose, generally three to four times a day,

Rx

but a larger dose at bedtime is often the best tolerated and may target nocturnal symptoms. Decreasing muscle tone can result in weakness. Baclofen should never be discontinued abruptly because of the potential for a severe withdrawal reaction.

Bladder urgency resulting from detrusor muscle spasm can be managed effectively with anticholinergics such as oxybutynin (5 to 20 mg in divided doses) or tolterodine (1 to 4 mg), but these agents can cause temporary urinary retention. Bladder ultrasonography permits accurate bedside assessment of postvoid residual volume to determine whether a patient is retaining excessive amounts of urine. Urinary retention may be improved by removing drugs known to induce it. Primary urinary retention is difficult to treat with drugs, but external sphincter spasm can be treated with α_{1a}-adrenergic receptor blockers such as tamsulosin (0.4 to 0.8 mg) and doxazosin (1 to 8 mg). Bethanechol (10 to 150 mg in divided doses) may be tried for an atonic bladder, but intermittent catheterization is often required. Alternative causes of bladder symptoms such as urinary tract infections, prostatic enlargement, or anatomic changes following pregnancy should be considered and managed separately.

Painful dysesthesias and paroxysmal dystonic spasms may be managed effectively with antiepileptic drugs (gabapentin, 300 to 5400 mg/day in divided doses; pregabalin, 75 to 600 mg/day in divided doses; or carbamazepine, 100 to 2400 mg/day in divided doses) or tricyclic antidepressants (amitriptyline, 10 to 150 mg; or nortriptyline, 10 to 50 mg). Patients with trigeminal neuralgia (Chapter 421) may respond to these drugs or to baclofen, misoprostol, botulinum toxin, or decompression surgery.

Sexual dysfunction in MS is often multifactorial. Patients with erectile dysfunction usually respond well to the phosphodiesterase inhibitors, which enhance penile vasodilation (Chapter 253). Education regarding the use of lubrication, alternative sensory stimulation, and the adverse effect of heat can improve sexual function.

Systemic Treatments

Corticosteroids (e.g., intravenous methylprednisolone, 1 g/day for 3 to 5 days) shorten the duration and severity of symptoms from an acute exacerbation but have no effect on long-term disability. Oral corticosteroids used in equivalent dosage are probably equally efficacious and safe. Intravenous immunoglobulin and plasma exchange have been reported occasionally to benefit steroid refractory patients, but randomized placebo-controlled trials have failed to show consistent benefits, perhaps because only patients with type II disease (humoral component) are likely to respond.

Six disease-modifying agents have been approved by the U.S. Food and Drug Administration: interferon-β (IFN-β)1b (Betaseron), IFN-β1a (Avonex), IFN-β1a (Rebif), glatiramer acetate (Copaxone), natalizumab (Tysabri), and mitoxantrone (Novantrone). The first five agents were approved for relapsing remitting MS, and mitoxantrone is indicated for worsening forms of MS and for secondary progressive MS.

The three IFN-β drugs [1-3] and glatiramer acetate [4] reduce the relapse rate by approximately one third. IFN-β1b (8 million IU, subcutaneously every other day) and IFN-β1a (30 μg intramuscularly weekly [Avonex] or 22 to 44 μg subcutaneously three times a week [Rebif]). The more frequently dosed interferons appear to have more rapid onset of action, perhaps based on their dosing regimen, as compared with weekly IFN-β1a (30 μg weekly IM). However, weekly IFN-β1a Aronex is less immunogenic and results in only a 3% incidence of neutralizing antibodies, which reduce efficacy, as compared with 20 to 30% for the other IFN-β preparations. The major side effects of IFN-β are a flulike reaction (low-grade fever, chills, and myalgias 6 to 24 hours after the injection), local reactions at the injection site (pain, erythema, and rarely necrosis), and elevated aminotransferase levels (rarely severe hepatitis). These side effects can be managed by initiating the drug slowly and by prophylaxis with acetaminophen and nonsteroidal anti-inflammatory agents, and they improve in the majority of patients after 3 to 6 months.

Glatiramer acetate is a copolymer of four amino acids designed to mimic myelin basic protein; given as 20 mg/day subcutaneously, it also reduces relapses by about one third and is well tolerated by most patients. [4] Major side effects are local reactions at the injection site, swelling, hives, and a rare, self-limited (15 to 20 minutes) systemic reaction consisting of chest pain, palpitations, and anxiety. No monitoring of blood tests is required for this medication. The effect of glatiramer acetate on MRI T2-weighted and gadolinium-enhancing lesions is less dramatic than for the IFNs (30% reduction) perhaps because its primary effect is not at the blood-brain barrier.

Natalizumab is a monoclonal antibody directed against the α4-integrin chain of the leukocyte adhesion molecule VLA-4. In a large phase III trial, this drug, at a dose of 300 mg intravenously every 4 weeks, was shown to reduce relapses by 68% compared with placebo and reduced gadolinium enhancing lesions by 92%. [5] However, two cases of JC virus infection of the brain causing progressive multifocal leukoencephalopathy occurred in patients taking this drug in combination with IFN-β1a and resulted in the temporary suspension of its marketing. The risk appears to be 1 per 1000 patients at 18 months

Mitoxantrone, which is an anthracenedione antineoplastic agent with potent immunosuppressive activity, has been approved to slow progression of neurologic disability and to reduce the relapse rate in patients with relapsing remitting MS and secondary progressive MS. [6] The recommended dose is a 5- to 12-mg/m² intravenous infusion every 3 months. In a phase III, randomized, placebo-controlled, multicenter trial of 188 patients, the number of treated relapses was reduced by 67%. Side effects of mitoxantrone include nausea and alopecia. The lifetime use of this drug is limited to 2 to 3 years (or a cumulative dose of 120 to 140 mg/m²) because of its cardiotoxicity. Heart failure or asymptomatic decreases in left ventricular ejection fraction can occur even after one to four doses, so careful monitoring is mandatory. The risk of leukemia is increased, but less than 1%. A complete blood count, including platelets, should be done before each course of mitoxantrone therapy, and women of childbearing age should have a pregnancy test and should know the results before each dose, regardless of whether or not they are using birth control. Patients should be made aware that mitoxantrone may impart a blue-green color to the urine for 24 hours after administration. It also may cause bluish discoloration of the sclera. Other forms of immunosuppression including methotrexate, azathioprine, mycophenolate mofetil, anti-CD52 (CAMPATH), cladribine, and cyclophosphamide also appear to have some efficacy in MS, although no definitive clinical trials have been done with these agents, and none is as yet approved for MS by the Food and Drug Administration.

Nondrug Approaches to Well-Being

Nonmedical treatment of MS is a critical part of managing the disease. Patients derive benefit from a health care team approach consisting of an experienced MS physician, nurse, social worker, therapist, and counselor, with appropriate referral to other subspecialties as needed. Alternative and complementary therapies (Chapter 36) are commonly used by patients with MS, and the risks and benefits of these approaches must be discussed with the patient.

Prognosis

The average lifespan of patients with MS is about 8 years less than normal, a finding reflecting a bimodal distribution in which many patients live a normal lifespan and a few die at a significantly younger age owing to aggressive disease, severe disability, infection, or suicide. Most patients presenting with relapsing remitting MS convert to secondary progressive MS after 20 to 40 years. Only one third of patients will require use of a wheelchair, but 50% may need assistive devices, and nearly two thirds will have disability that prevents them from working. African Americans and men of all races tend to have a more aggressive course and are more likely to become disabled. Institution of immunomodulating therapy early on in the course of the disease may slow progression of disability, but no long-term follow-up data are available to quantify the extent of this benefit.

OTHER DISEASES OF MYELIN

Monofocal and Monophasic Demyelinating Processes

Optic Neuritis and Transverse Myelitis

Optic neuritis (Chapter 450) and transverse myelitis are inflammatory processes that can occur as entities distinct from MS or as part of MS (see earlier). In addition, optic neuritis and transverse myelitis can occur together in the syndrome called *neuromyelitis optica* (Devic's disease).

Optic Neuritis

Optic neuritis (Chapter 450) is an inflammatory disease that usually involves the retrobulbar portion of the optic nerve and sometimes parts of the optic chiasm. Although optic neuritis is most often associated with MS (50 to 75%), it also can be seen as an isolated idiopathic disorder (25 to 50%), as part of neuromyelitis optica, or associated with other inflammatory and infectious diseases such as systemic lupus erythematosus, Sjögren's syndrome, sarcoidosis, Lyme disease, syphilis, and human immunodeficiency virus infection. The pathobiologic features are thought to be similar to those of MS and are characterized by idiopathic inflammatory demyelination followed by secondary axonal injury.

Clinical Manifestations and Diagnosis

The clinical presentation, which typically is monocular visual loss with pain that worsens with lateral eye movement, is similar regardless of whether it presents as part of MS (see the earlier discussion of the visual effects of MS) or not. When it involves the optic nerve head, it is called *papillitis* and, in bilateral cases, can be impossible to differentiate from papilledema. Optic neuritis can also be mimicked by anterior segment, choroidal, or retinal diseases. Optic neuritis is distinguished from optic neuropathy, which is a chronic, generally noninflammatory condition of the optic nerve caused by tobacco or nutritional amblyopia, ischemia, Leber's disease, or other rare hereditary diseases (Chapter 450).

Treatment

Rx

Among patients with optic neuritis, the 10-year risk of developing MS is 38%; patients who have one or more typical lesions on a baseline brain MRI have a 56% risk, whereas those with no lesions have a 22% risk. Treatment with intravenous methylprednisolone as in MS may shorten the duration and severity of the attack, but no definitive evidence indicates that it changes the long-term outcome. Oral prednisone alone, without prior treatment with intravenous methylprednisolone, may increase the risk for recurrent optic neuritis and should be avoided. Data support the use of IFN-β drugs in patients whose optic neuritis is at high risk for conversion to MS (two or more typical brain MRI lesions).

Transverse Myelitis

Transverse myelitis is a rare (~1/100,000) monophasic inflammatory process of the spinal cord that is usually distinct from MS in that it involves either the entire cross section or is longitudinally extensive along three vertebral body segments rostrocaudally. Transverse myelitis may be idiopathic or associated with inflammatory diseases (systemic lupus erythematosus, Sjögren's syndrome, vasculitis, or MS), infectious diseases, or vascular diseases (antiphospholipid antibody syndrome or dural venous fistula).

Clinical Manifestations and Diagnosis

In its fulminant form, transverse myelitis causes complete loss of motor and sensory function below the affected level of the spinal cord and causes concomitant bowel, bladder, and sexual dysfunction. Autonomic involvement can be seen in cervical and high thoracic spine cases. Transverse myelitis may also manifest in an incomplete or partial form, which is more commonly associated with MS.

Treatment and Prognosis

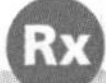

Treatment is usually with methylprednisolone (1000 mg intravenously for 3 to 5 days), followed by specific treatment of any identifiable underlying disease process. The prognosis is worse than in MS in that significant recovery is seen in fewer than 50% of patients, and many patients remain completely paralyzed after the initial attack. Plasma exchange or cyclophosphamide may be considered in steriod refractory cases.

Neuromyelitis Optica

Neuromyelitis optica is now recognized as a distinct entity from MS in that there usually are no cerebral lesions visible on MRI, the optic neuritis is often bilateral and temporally associated with a fulminant transverse myelitis, and a specific IgG directed against aquaporin 4 strongly predicts this process. Neuromyelitis optica may be similar to what is called *opticospinal MS* in Japan. There is no proven effective treatment, but patients are usually given anti-inflammatory and immunosuppressive medications. The prognosis is generally poor; most patients sustain disabling visual loss and weakness.

Acute Disseminated Encephalomyelitis

Acute disseminated encephalomyelitis and its hyperacute form, acute necrotizing hemorrhagic encephalopathy, are thought to be forms of monophasic immune-mediated inflammatory demyelination. They differ from MS in that they are typically monophasic, whereas MS is by definition multiphasic or chronically progressive. However, no reliable clinical or pathologic criteria are available to differentiate the two processes, which may represent a continuum. Patients may present with fever, headache, meningeal signs, and altered consciousness, which are exceedingly rare in MS. There is no known effective treatment. Large numbers of patients, especially children, make remarkable recoveries, but the necrotizing form can be severely disabling or fatal.

Leukodystrophies

The leukodystrophies represent a variety of diseases formerly characterized by their common clinical and pathologic characteristics of white matter and, presumably, myelin. Many of these diseases now have a defined biochemical and genetic basis, and some (e.g., Alexander's disease) are no longer considered dysmyelinating diseases.

Adrenoleukodystrophy and Adrenomyeloneuropathy

Adrenoleukodystrophy and adrenomyeloneuropathy, which are caused by impaired ability of the peroxisomes to metabolize very long-chain fatty acids, represent different phenotypes resulting from the same X-linked, incompletely recessive genetic defect. Impaired oxidation of very long-chain fatty acids results from deficient function of the enzyme lignoceroyl–coenzyme A ligase. The defective gene maps to Xq28 and codes for a peroxisomal membrane protein (ALDP), which is a member of a large family of proteins referred to as the adenosine triphosphate binding cassette (ABC) transporters, specifically *ABCD1*.

Childhood cerebral adrenoleukodystrophy, which is the most common form of the disorder, comprises 45% of all cases; it is seen only in male patients, with an onset at ages 4 to 11 years. Adolescent (5%) and adult (3%) cerebral forms progress at a similar or slower rate compared with the childhood form.

Clinical Manifestations

Adrenomyeloneuropathy begins in young men as slowly progressive paraparesis with hypogonadism, impotence, sphincter disturbances, variable adrenal insufficiency, and axonal neuropathy affecting mainly the lower extremities. A rare acute inflammatory form with rapid progression and dementia may occur. A similar, but usually milder, disorder can be seen in up to 20% of women who are heterozygous for the disease.

Diagnosis

Diagnosis is established in male patients by finding elevated very long-chain fatty acids in the plasma. DNA-based diagnosis in carriers is reliable and is recommended in women because of false-negative results using the plasma assay.

Treatment

Rx

Treatment is unsatisfactory. A 4:1 mixture of glyceryl trioleate and glyceryl trierucate (i.e., "Lorenzo's oil") normalizes plasma very long-chain fatty acids within 4 weeks and has few side effects. Although clinical trials suggested that treatment in presymptomatic patients delayed or prevented the onset of disease, this treatment is ineffective after symptoms have begun, and the disease progresses relentlessly.

Pelizaeus-Merzbacher Disease

Pelizaeus-Merzbacher disease is an extremely rare, chronic, familial leukodystrophy usually caused by a genetic defect in the myelin proteolipid (PLP; lipophilin) protein gene. In classic Pelizaeus-Merzbacher disease, age at onset varies between 3 months and 9 years, the age at death varies between 6 years and 25 years, and the longest duration of the disease is approximately 24 years. The disease manifests as a slowly progressive myelopathy, often with cerebellar and cognitive involvement. The diagnosis is established by genetic testing for mutations in the *PLP* gene. No specific treatment exists for Pelizaeus-Merzbacher disease.

Metachromatic Leukodystrophy

Metachromatic leukodystrophy usually results from a recessively inherited defect in the lysosomal enzyme arylsulfatase A. Absence of arylsulfatase A results in the accumulation of sulfatide in both central and peripheral myelin and myelin-forming cells; instability of the myelin membranes results in the breakdown of myelin. Metachromatic leukodystrophy is generally divided into four subtypes: congenital, late infantile (most common), juvenile, and adult. It appears in all ethnic groups and has an overall frequency of 1 in 40,000.

The clinical manifestation are variable and may include progressive spastic paraparesis, extrapyramidal signs, seizures, and peripheral neuropathy. Brain MRI usually shows large confluent symmetrical high-signal areas in the cerebral white matter, brain stem, and cerebellum, but a more patchy appearance resembling MS is occasionally seen in adult cases. At present, no satisfactory treatment exists. Some evidence suggests that bone marrow transplantation delays the onset in presymptomatic patients and may slow progression of the disease.

Globoid Cell Leukodystrophy

Globoid cell leukodystrophy is characterized biochemically by accumulation of galactocerebroside in cerebral white matter as a result of deficient galactocerebroside β-galactosidase activity. The disease is transmitted as an autosomal recessive trait and affects infants in the first 2 to 3 months of life, initially manifesting with behavioral changes and failure to achieve developmental milestones. Rare late-onset cases present with progressive motor impairment and, less frequently, visual failure. Neuropathologic examination reveals marked loss of myelin throughout the brain, with the presence of round or oval macrophages and large, irregular, multinucleated cells, termed *globoid cells,* that are filled with galactocerebroside. Accumulation of galactosylsphingosine (psychosine) is thought to cause destruction of oligodendrocytes and marked reduction of myelin formation.

Canavan's Disease

Canavan's disease is a fatal, progressive leukodystrophy with an autosomal recessive inheritance, caused by mutations in the gene for aspartoacylase, an enzyme that hydrolyzes *N*-acetylaspartate into L-aspartate and acetate. Aspartoacylase deficiency results in elevated levels of its substrate molecule, N-acetylaspartate, brain edema, and dysmyelination. Clinically, the disease manifests with retardation, seizures, and diffuse, symmetrical white matter degeneration in the subcortical areas, with involvement of the globus pallidum on MRI. No treatment is available.

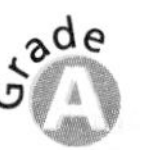

1. The IFN-β Multiple Sclerosis Study Group: Interferon beta-1b is effective in relapsing-remitting multiple sclerosis. I. Clinical results of a multicenter, randomized, double-blind, placebo-controlled trial. Neurology 1993;43:656–661.
2. Jacobs LD, Cookfair DL, Rudick RA, et al: Intramuscular interferon beta-1a for disease progression in relapsing multiple sclerosis: The Multiple Sclerosis Collaborative Research Group (MSCRG). Ann Neurol 1996;39:285-294, 1998;51:285–294.
3. PRISMS Study Group (Prevention of Relapses and Disability by Interferon beta-1a Subcutaneously in Multiple Sclerosis): Randomised double-blind placebo-controlled study of interferon beta-1a in relapsing/remitting multiple sclerosis. Lancet 1998;352:1498–1504.
4. Johnson KP, Brooks BR, Cohen JA, et al: Copolymer 1 reduces relapse rate and improves disability in relapsing-remitting multiple sclerosis: Results of a phase III multicenter, double-blind placebo-controlled trial. Neurology 1995;45:1268–1276.
5. Polman C, O'Connor PW, Havrdovra E, et al: A randomized, placebo-controlled trial of natalizumab for relapsing multiple sclerosis. N Engl J Med 2006;354:899–910.
6. Hartung H-P, Gonsette R, Konig N, et al: Mitoxantrone in progressive multiple sclerosis: A placebo-controlled, double-blind, randomized, multicentre trial. Lancet 2002;360:2018–2025.

SUGGESTED READINGS

Balcer LJ: Clinical practice: Optic neuritis. N Engl J Med 2006;354:1273–1280. *A practical review.*

Frohman EM, Racke MK, Raine CS: Multiple sclerosis—the plaque and its pathogenesis. N Engl J Med 2006;354:942–955. *A scholarly review.*

Kappos L, Antel J, Giancarlo C, et al: Oral fingolimod (FTY720) for relapsing multiple sclerosis. N Engl J Med 2006;355:1124–1140. *Proof-of-principle randomized trial found reductions in gadolinium-enhanced lesions after six months.*

Keegan M, Konig F, McClelland R, et al: Relation between humoral pathological changes in multiple sclerosis and response to therapeutic plasma exchange. Lancet 2005;366:579–582. *Patients with MS with type II disease are more likely to respond favorably to plasma exchange than are patients with type I or III.*

Kuhle J, Pohl C, Mehling M, et al: Lack of association between antimyelin antibodies and progression to multiple sclerosis. N Engl J Med 2007;356:371–378. *Serum antibodies against MOG and MBP are not associated with an increased risk of progression to multiple sclerosis.*

Lennon VA, Wingerchuk DM, Kryzer TJ, et al: A serum autoantibody marker of neuromyelitis optica: Distinction from multiple sclerosis. Lancet 2004;364:2106–2112. *NMO-IgG is a specific marker autoantibody of neuromyelitis optica.*

Lublin FD: Clinical features and diagnosis of multiple sclerosis. Neurol Clin 2005;23:1–15. *A clinical review.*

Moser HW, Raymond GV, Dubey P: Adrenoleukodystrophy: New approaches to a neurodegenerative disease. JAMA 2005;294:3131–3134. *A comprehensive review.*

437 MENINGITIS: BACTERIAL, VIRAL, AND OTHER

Morton N. Swartz

BACTERIAL MENINGITIS

Definition

Meningitis is an inflammation of the arachnoid, the pia mater, and the intervening cerebrospinal fluid (CSF). The inflammatory process extends throughout the subarachnoid space about the brain and spinal cord and regularly involves the ventricles. Pyogenic meningitis is usually an acute infection with bacteria that evoke a polymorphonuclear response in the CSF. One of its major forms, that caused by meningococci, is considered in Chapter 321. Tuberculous meningitis (Chapter 345) is a less acute form of bacterial meningitis, characterized initially by modest polymorphonuclear pleocytosis that rapidly progresses to one with a lymphocytic predominance. Fungal meningitides are considered with the endemic and opportunistic mycoses (Chapters 352 to 361).

Epidemiology

In the 1990s, the number of cases of community-acquired bacterial meningitis declined by 55%, primarily owing to the introduction of routine immunization of infants with the *Haemophilus influenzae* type b polysaccharide-protein conjugate vaccines. This practice resulted in a 94% decrease in the number of cases of *H. influenzae* meningitis.

The relative frequencies with which the different bacterial species cause community-acquired meningitis depend on age (Fig. 437–1). In individuals older than 18 years *Streptococcus pneumoniae* (62%) is the most common cause. *Listeria monocytogenes* accounts for 8% of cases of bacterial meningitis overall but has peak frequencies (~20%) in the neonatal period and in those 60 years of age and older. Group B *Streptococcus* is increasing in frequency in adults, commonly in persons older than 50 years and with comorbid conditions. Meningococcal meningitis is the only common type that occurs in outbreaks; its relative frequency among the meningitides depends on whether statistics have been gathered in a hyperendemic area or during epidemic or interepidemic periods. Simultaneous mixed bacterial meningitis is rare, occurring in the setting of neurosurgical procedures, penetrating head injury, erosion of the skull or vertebrae by adjacent neoplasm, or intraventricular rupture of a cerebral abscess; the isolation of anaerobes should strongly suggest the latter two of these situations. Meningitis involving anaerobes may also occur very rarely as a result of an intestinal-meningeal fistula following surgery and radiation therapy for colorectal cancer. In approximately 10% of patients with pyogenic meningitis, the bacterial cause cannot be defined.

Over the past several decades, gram-negative bacillary meningitis has doubled in frequency in adults, a change reflecting more frequent and extensive neurosurgical procedures as well as other nosocomial factors. *L. monocytogenes* has increased 8- to 10-fold as a cause of bacterial meningitis in large urban general hospitals. *Listeria* infections appear to be food-borne (dairy products, processed meats, uncooked vegetables) and especially involve the following groups: organ transplant recipients; patients in hemodialysis units; other patients receiving corticosteroids, anti–tumor necrosis factor-α neutralizing agents (e.g., infliximab and etanercept) and cytotoxic drugs; patients with liver disease; pregnant women; and neonates. Meningitis caused by coagulase-negative staphylococci now represents approximately 3% of cases in large urban hospitals. It occurs as a complication of neurosurgical procedures and may present a particular therapeutic problem because of the methicillin resistance of many of the involved strains. Rarely, bacterial meningitis complicates invasive neurodiagnostic (e.g., myelographic) and therapeutic procedures (spinal puncture and rhizotomy). Whereas in the past those infections were usually caused by *Pseudomonas aeruginosa*, other gram-negative bacilli, and *Staphylococcus aureus*, currently, viridans streptococci are the agents most often associated with meningitis complicating diagnostic myelography and percutaneous trigeminal rhizotomy.

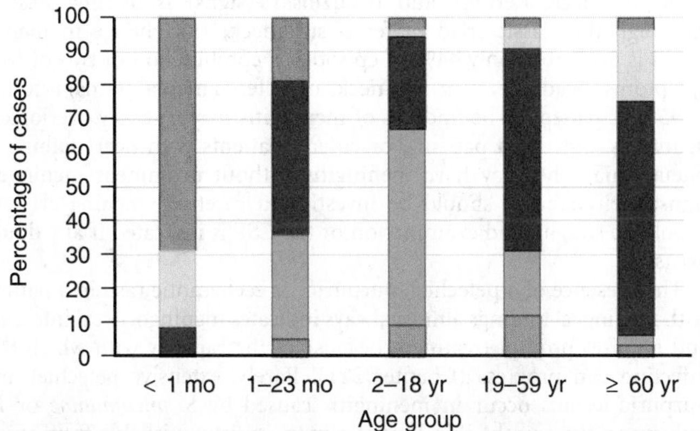

FIGURE 437–1 • Pathogenic agents of bacterial meningitis in adults by age group. Red = group B *Streptococcus;* yellow = *Listeria monocytogenes;* blue = *Streptococcus pneumoniae;* green = *Neisseria meningitidis;* brown = *Haemophilus influenzae.* (From Schuchat A, Robinson K, Wenger JD, et al: Bacterial meningitis in the United States in 1995. N Engl J Med 1997;337:970–976. Copyright 1997, Massachusetts Medical Society. All rights reserved.)

In large urban tertiary care general hospitals, approximately 40% of cases of bacterial meningitis in adults are of nosocomial origin. In this category, the leading causes are gram-negative bacilli (primarily *Escherichia coli* and *Klebsiella*), which account for approximately 40% of nosocomial episodes, as well as various streptococci, *S. aureus,* and coagulase-negative staphylococci, each responsible for approximately 10% of nosocomial cases.

The clinical setting in which meningitis develops may provide a clue to the specific bacterial cause. Meningococcal disease, including meningitis, may occur sporadically and in cyclic outbreaks. In the past, military recruits were particularly susceptible, but now meningococcal vaccine (polysaccharides of groups A, C, Y, and W135) is protective. Other high-risk groups include those living in close quarters such as crowded classrooms or jails; meningococcal vaccine is also advised for freshmen in college dormitories (Chapter 16). Meningococcal infections also occur worldwide in endemic form. In industrialized countries, serogroups C and B (the latter particularly of one clonal complex) have accounted for the majority of infections. In developing countries, serogroups A and, to a lesser extent, C are dominant. In sub-Saharan Africa, the so-called meningitis belt, recurrent yearly waves of serogroup A meningococcal infections occur.

Predisposing factors for the development of pneumococcal meningitis include acute otitis media (Chapters 311 and 452), with or without mastoiditis, which is present in approximately 20% of adult patients. Pneumonia is present in approximately 15% of patients with pneumococcal meningitis, a much higher frequency than in meningitis caused by *H. influenzae* or *Neisseria meningitidis.* Acute pneumococcal sinusitis is occasionally the initial focus from which infection spreads to the meninges. A significant head injury (recent or remote) precedes approximately 10% of episodes of pneumococcal meningitis, and CSF rhinorrhea (usually caused by a defect or fracture in the cribriform plate) is present in approximately 5% of patients. Cochlear implants, particularly those that include a positioner, have been implicated in cases of childhood bacterial meningitis, particularly episodes resulting from *S. pneumoniae.* Occasionally, patients with central nervous system (CNS) shunts develop meningitis caused by *S. pneumoniae.* Meningitis occurring in young children with sickle cell anemia is most likely to be caused by *S. pneumoniae.* Alcoholism (Chapter 31) is an underlying problem in 10 to 25% of adults with pneumococcal meningitis in urban hospitals. The estimated annual incidence of bacterial meningitis (primarily pneumococcal) among patients infected with human immunodeficiency virus (HIV) is 150-fold higher than in the general population.

S. aureus meningitis is seen most commonly as a complication of a neurosurgical procedure, after penetrating skull trauma, or occasionally secondary to staphylococcal bacteremia and endocarditis. Meningitis caused by *gram-negative bacilli* takes one of three forms: neonatal meningitis, meningitis after trauma or neurosurgery, or spontaneous meningitis in adults (e.g., bacteremic *Klebsiella* meningitis in a patient with diabetes mellitus). The most common causes of gram-negative bacillary meningitis in the adult are *E. coli* (~30%) and *Klebsiella-Enterobacter* (~40%). The most frequent causes of bacterial meningitis in patients with neoplastic disease are gram-negative bacilli (particularly *P. aeruginosa* and *E. coli*), *L. monocytogenes, S. pneumoniae,* and *S. aureus.* Meningitis caused by group A streptococci is uncommon but occasionally occurs after acute otitis media, more often in children than adults. *H. influenzae* type b meningitis in an adult should raise the question of the presence of an underlying anatomic or immunologic defect.

Pathobiology

Pathology

The purulent exudate is distributed widely in the subarachnoid space and is most abundant in the basal cisterns and about the cerebellum initially, but it also extends into the sulci over the cerebrum. Although no direct invasion of cerebral tissue by the infecting organism or the inflammatory exudate occurs, the subjacent brain becomes congested and edematous. The effectiveness of the pial barrier accounts for the finding that cerebral abscess does not complicate bacterial meningitis. Indeed, when these two processes coexist, the sequence usually has been that of an initial abscess subsequently leaking its contents into the ventricular system and thus producing meningitis.

Structures adjacent to the meninges may show a variety of pathologic changes secondary to bacterial meningitis. *Cortical thrombophlebitis* results from venous stasis and adjacent meningeal inflammation. Infarction of cerebral tissue may follow. *Involvement of cortical and pial arteries* with peripheral aneurysm formation and vascular occlusion or narrowing (related to spasm and/or arteritis) of the supraclinoid portion of the internal carotid artery at the base of the brain occurs in approximately 15% of patients with meningitis. Anterior and middle cerebral arteries may have markedly increased intracerebral blood flow velocities (an index of stenosis or arterial spasm) on transcranial Doppler ultrasonography, corresponding to focal cerebral signs. In fulminating cases (particularly meningococcal meningitis), *cerebral edema* may be marked even though the pleocytosis is only moderate. Rarely, such patients develop temporal lobe and cerebellar herniation, resulting in compression of the midbrain and medulla. *Damage to cranial nerves* occurs in areas where dense exudate accumulates; the third and sixth cranial nerves are also vulnerable to damage by increased intracranial pressure. *Ventriculitis,* which probably occurs in most cases of bacterial meningitis, rarely progresses to *ventricular empyema. Hydrocephalus* can develop during meningitis from obstruction of CSF flow within the ventricular system (obstructive hydrocephalus) or extraventricularly (communicating hydrocephalus). *Subdural effusions* are sterile transudates that develop over the cerebral cortex and can be demonstrated readily by computed tomography (CT) as low-density areas about the cerebrum; rarely such effusions become infected and produce subdural empyema.

Pathogenesis

Bacteria may reach the meninges by several routes: (1) systemic bacteremia, (2) direct ingress from the upper respiratory tract or skin through an anatomic defect (e.g., skull fracture, eroding sequestrum, meningocele), (3) passage intracranially through venules in the nasopharynx, (4) spread from a contiguous focus of infection (infection of the paranasal sinuses, leakage of a brain abscess), or (5) nosocomial meningitis after CSF drainage procedures. Bacteremic spread to the meninges is probably the most frequent path of infection. However, not all bacteremic organisms have the same likelihood of causing meningitis. Bacteremia with *H. influenzae* and *N. meningitidis* is usually initiated by pharyngeal adhesion and colonization by an infecting strain. Adhesion of such strains, as well as of *S. pneumoniae,* to mucosal surfaces is abetted by their capacity to produce immunoglobulin A proteases (cleaving this antibody in the hinge region) and thus inactivating this local antibody defense. *N. meningitidis* adhesion to nasopharyngeal cells is effected by fimbriae or pili and promoted by prior damage to ciliated cells such as from smoking or viral infections. Meningococci invade the nasopharyngeal mucosal cells by means of endocytosis and are transported to the abluminal side in membrane-bound vacuoles. *H. influenzae,* in contrast, invades intercellularly by causing separation of apical tight junctions between columnar epithelial cells. When these meningeal pathogens gain access to the blood stream, their intravascular survival is aided by the presence of polysaccharide capsules that inhibit phagocytosis and confer resistance to complement-mediated bactericidal activity.

After entry into the blood stream, specific bacterial adhesion to elements of the blood-brain barrier is likely, as indicated by the preferential binding of fimbriated strains of *E. coli* to the endothelial cell surface of cerebral capillaries and the epithelial cell surface of the choroid plexus and ventricles. Once established in any part of the meninges, infection quickly extends throughout the subarachnoid space. Bacterial replication proceeds relatively unhindered because low CSF levels of complement early in meningeal inflammation result in minimal or no opsonic or bactericidal activity and because surface phagocytosis of unopsonized organisms is meager in such a fluid environment. Secondary bacteremia may follow meningeal infection and may itself contribute to continuing further inoculation of the CSF.

Pathophysiology

Bacterial components (e.g., pneumococcal cell walls or lipoteichoic acid, *H. influenzae* lipopolysaccharide) are major elicitors of meningeal inflammation by causing release into the subarachnoid space of various proinflammatory cytokines such as interleukin-1 and tumor necrosis factor from endothelial and meningeal cells, macrophages, and microglia. Cytokines appear to enhance the passage of leukocytes by inducing several families of adhesion molecules that interact with corresponding receptors on leukocytes. Cytokines can also increase the binding affinity of a leukocyte selectin, leukocyte-adhesion molecule, for its endothelial cell receptor, and may thereby contribute further to neutrophil trafficking into the subarachnoid space.

Once within the subarachnoid space, neutrophils are further activated to release products such as prostaglandins, matrix metalloproteinases, and toxic oxygen metabolites that increase local vascular permeability and may cause direct neurotoxicity. Endothelial intercellular tight junctions and subendothelial basal lamina (matrix metalloproteinases may have a role) are disrupted, increased pinocytotic vesicles appear in endothelial cells, and albumin escapes across postcapillary venules into the subarachnoid space.

The foregoing inflammatory changes can contribute to development of increased intracranial pressure and alterations in cerebral blood flow. Cerebral edema is commonly caused by increased permeability of the blood-brain barrier (vasogenic) and may result from cellular swelling in the brain as a result of toxic molecules released by bacteria and neutrophils (cytotoxic), and sometimes increased CSF pressure may result primarily from obstruction of CSF outflow related to inflammation at the level of the arachnoidal villi (interstitial). Cerebral blood flow, which depends on mean arterial pressure, appears to be increased in the very early stages of meningitis, but subsequently it decreases, substantially in some patients, in whom it may be responsible for ensuing neurologic injury. Localized regions of marked hypoperfusion, attributable to focal vascular inflammation or thrombosis, can occur in patients with normal blood flow. Impairment of cerebral blood flow autoregulation, as measured by transcranial Doppler ultrasonography of the middle cerebral artery, occurs in the early phase of acute bacterial meningitis and causes cerebral blood flow to correspond directly with mean arterial blood pressure with attendant hyperperfusion or hypoperfusion of the brain. On recovery, the ability of the cerebral vasculature to maintain a constant level of perfusion despite variations in mean arterial pressure is restored.

Clinical Manifestations

History

Acute-onset fever, generalized headache, vomiting, and stiff neck are common to many types of meningitis (Table 437–1). Most of patients with community-acquired pyogenic meningitis have had an antecedent or accompanying upper respiratory tract infection or nonspecific febrile illness, acute otitis (or mastoiditis), or pneumonia. Myalgias (particularly in meningococcal disease), backache, and generalized weakness are common symptoms. The illness usually progresses rapidly, with development of confusion, obtundation, and loss of consciousness. Occasionally, the onset may be less acute, with meningeal signs present for several days to a week.

General Physical Findings

Evidence of meningeal irritation (drowsiness and decreased mentation, stiff neck, Kernig's and Brudzinski's signs) is usually present. Although the classic triad of fever, stiff neck, and change in mental status is present in only 44% of episodes, a combination of two of four symptoms (headache, fever, stiff neck, and altered mental status) is found in 95% of patients. The findings of meningitis may be easily overlooked in infants, obtunded patients, or elderly patients with heart failure or pneumonia, who may have meningitis without prominent meningeal signs; their lethargy should be investigated carefully, meningeal signs should be sought, and examination of the CSF is indicated if any doubt exists.

The presence of a petechial, purpuric, or ecchymotic rash in a patient with meningeal findings almost always indicates meningococcal infection and requires prompt treatment because of the rapidity with which this infection can progress (Chapter 321). Rarely, extensive petechial and purpuric lesions occur in meningitis caused by *S. pneumoniae* or *H. influenzae.* Very rarely, skin lesions almost indistinguishable from those of meningococcal bacteremia occur in patients who have acute *S. aureus* endocarditis and who also have meningeal signs and pleocytosis (secondary either to staphylococcal meningitis or to embolic cerebral infarction). Usually one or two of the lesions in such a patient are those of

TABLE 437–1 CHARACTERISTICS OF THE STUDY POPULATION*

Characteristic	Episodes of Meningitis (N = 696)
Duration of symptoms <24 hr	48%
Predisposing conditions	
Otitis or sinusitis	25%
Pneumonia	12%
Immunocompromise†	16%
Symptoms on presentation	
Headache	87%
Nausea	74%
Neck stiffness	83%
Triad of fever, neck stiffness, and change in mental status	44%
Focal neurologic deficits	33%
Aphasia	23%
Hemiparesis	7%
Indexes of CSF inflammation	
Opening pressure (mm H_2O)‡	370 ± 130
White cell count§	
Mean (cells/mm^3)	7753 ± 14,736
<100/mm^3	7%
100–999/mm^3	14%
>999/mm^3	78%
Protein (g/L)	4.9 ± 4.5
CSF/blood glucose ratio	0.2 ± 0.2
Positive blood culture‖	66%
Blood tests	
ESR (mm/hr)¶	46 ± 37
C-reactive protein (g/L)**	225 ± 132
Thrombocyte count (platelets/mm^3)††	198,000 ± 100,000

*The study included 671 patients who had a total of 696 episodes of community-acquired meningitis. Plus–minus values are means ± SD.
†Immunocompromise was defined by the use of immunosuppressive drugs, a history of splenectomy, or the presence of diabetes mellitus or alcoholism, as well as patients infected with the human immunodeficiency virus.
‡The CSF pressure was measured in 216 patients.
§The CSF leukocyte count was determined in 659 patients; CSF specimens from 14 patients had too many leukocytes for an exact count to be performed.
‖Blood culture was performed in 611 patients.
¶The ESR was determined in 549 patients.
**C-reactive protein levels were determined in 394 patients.
††The thrombocyte count was determined in 653 patients.
CSF = cerebrospinal fluid; ESR = erythrocyte sedimentation rate.
Data from 696 cases reported in van de Beek D, de Gans J, Spanjaard L, et al: Clinical features and prognostic factors in adults with bacterial meningitis. N Engl J Med 2004;351:1849–1859.

purulent purpura; aspiration of material reveals staphylococci on Gram staining. In the summer, viral aseptic meningitis may produce meningeal signs, macular and petechial skin lesions, and pleocytosis of several hundred cells, sometimes with neutrophils predominating initially.

Neurologic Findings and Complications

Cranial nerve abnormalities, involving principally the third, fourth, sixth, or seventh nerve, occur in 5 to 10% of adults with community-acquired meningitis and usually disappear shortly after recovery. Persistent sensorineural hearing loss occurs in 10% of children with bacterial meningitis, and another 16% have a transient conductive hearing loss. The most likely sites of involvement in persistent sensorineural deafness appear to be the inner ear (infection or toxic products possibly spreading from the subarachnoid space along the cochlear aqueduct) and the acoustic nerve. In children, permanent hearing impairment is more common after meningitis caused by *S. pneumoniae* than by *H. influenzae* or *N. meningitidis.*

Seizures (focal or generalized; Chapter 426) occur in 20 to 30% of patients and may result from readily reversible causes (high fever or hypoglycemia in infants; penicillin neurotoxicity when large doses are administered intravenously in the presence of renal failure) or, more commonly, from focal cerebral injury related to arterial hypoperfusion and infarction, cortical venous thrombosis, or focal edema and cerebritis. Seizures can occur during the first few days or can appear with associated focal neurologic deficits caused by vascular inflammation some days after the onset of the meningitis. In adults with seizures accompanying meningitis, *S. pneumoniae* is more commonly the cause, but alcohol withdrawal is a confounding factor.

Brain swelling and increased CSF pressure are associated with seizures, sixth- and third-nerve dysfunction, abnormal reflexes, reduced consciousness or coma, dilated and poorly reactive pupils, decerebrate posturing, hypertension, bradycardia, and irregular respirations. In approximately one fourth of fatal cases of community-acquired meningitis in adults, cerebral edema accompanied by temporal lobe herniation is observed at autopsy.

Papilledema is rare (1%) in bacterial meningitis even with high CSF pressures, probably because the patient is seen early in the process before changes have occurred in the nerve head. The presence of this sign should indicate the possibility of another associated or independent suppurative intracranial process (subdural empyema, brain abscess). Marked central hyperpnea sometimes occurs in patients with severe bacterial meningitis; CSF acidosis (principally caused by increased lactic acid levels) provides much of the respiratory stimulus.

Focal cerebral signs (principally hemiparesis, dysphasia, visual field defects, and gaze preference) occur in approximately one third of adults with community-acquired bacterial meningitis. These signs may develop during early meningitis secondary to occlusive vascular processes or some days later. In addition, cerebral blood flow velocity may be decreased in the presence of increased intracranial pressure and may lead to temporary or lasting neurologic dysfunction. It is important to distinguish these vascular effects from postictal changes (Todd's paralysis), which usually persist for no more than several hours.

Diagnosis

The diagnosis of bacterial meningitis is not difficult in a febrile patient with meningeal symptoms and signs developing in the setting of a predisposing illness. The diagnosis may be less obvious in an elderly, obtunded patient with pneumonia or a confused alcoholic patient in impending delirium tremens.

When the diagnosis of bacterial meningitis is entertained, blood cultures should be obtained, CSF examined and cultured, and antimicrobial therapy instituted promptly. If a mass lesion (cerebral abscess, subdural empyema) is suspected from the history, clinical setting, or physical findings (papilledema, focal cerebral signs), CT should be performed. *Bacterial meningitis is a medical emergency requiring immediate diagnosis and rapid institution of antimicrobial therapy.* Delay in performing a diagnostic lumbar puncture to obtain a CT scan should be avoided except in patients with findings suggestive of a parameningeal collection or other intracranial mass lesions. In such patients, it is critical to initiate antimicrobial therapy aimed at meningitis of unknown origin or brain abscess before CT is performed. Patients with community-acquired meningitis rarely have significant CT abnormalities in the absence of focal neurologic findings.

Laboratory Findings

Cerebrospinal Fluid Examination

Initial CSF pressure is usually moderately elevated (200 to 300 mm H_2O in the adult). Striking elevations (≥450 mm H_2O) occur in occasional patients with acute brain swelling complicating meningitis in the absence of an associated mass lesion.

Gram-Stained Smear

By the time of hospitalization, most patients with pyogenic meningitis have large numbers (≥10^5/mL) of bacteria in the CSF. Careful examination of the Gram-stained smear of the spun sediment of CSF reveals the etiologic agent in 60 to 80% of cases. In most instances when gram-positive diplococci (or short-chaining cocci) are observed on a stained CSF smear, they are pneumococci. In certain clinical settings, it is important to distinguish pneumococci from the relatively penicillin-resistant *Enterococcus,* an occasional cause of nosocomial meningitis that requires an aminoglycoside in addition to penicillin in treatment by latex particle agglutination. Rarely, three species may morphologically mimic *Neisseria* in the CSF or may suggest a mixed infection with short gram-negative rods and meningococci: *Acinetobacter baumannii, Moraxella* sp, and *Pasteurella multocida.* Culture of the CSF reveals the etiologic agent in 80 to 90% of patients with bacterial meningitis.

Special Testing Procedures

Broad-range 16S ribosomal DNA polymerase chain reaction (PCR) has been used in CSF for diagnosis of bacterial meningitis in patients for whom antimicrobial therapy is begun before lumbar puncture or when cultures are negative and a bacterial origin is still suspected. The use of this technique in routine diagnostic laboratories has been limited by its time-consuming and technically demanding nature. Specific real-time PCR for the diagnosis of pneumococcal and meningococcal meningitis currently is available only in the research setting. The sensitivity and specificity of rapid antigen testing by latex agglutination are highest (>90%) for *H. influenzae,* lower for *S. pneumoniae,* and considerably lower for *N. meningitidis.* Gram-stained smears almost invariably show the causative microorganism when the latex agglutination test result is truly positive. Latex agglutination testing may be most useful when the CSF cell count is abnormal, the Gram stain is negative, and blood and CSF cultures are unrevealing at 48 hours (at which time a stored sample of the initial CSF specimen can be tested). Occasionally, when only rare organisms of ambiguous morphology or Gram-staining properties are seen, latex agglutination may be helpful in providing a more specific diagnosis.

Cell Count

The normal CSF white blood cell count is less than 5 cells/mm^3 (all mononuclear). The cell count in untreated meningitis usually ranges between 100 and 10,000/mm^3, with polymorphonuclear leukocytes predominating initially (>80%) and lymphocytes appearing subsequently. The cell count in *L. monocytogenes* meningitis tends to be lower (median, 585/mm^3) than in other types of community-acquired pyogenic meningitis. Extremely high cell counts (>50,000/mm^3) may occur rarely in primary bacterial meningitis but also should raise the possibility of intraventricular rupture of a cerebral abscess. Cell counts as low as 10 to 20/mm^3 may be observed early in bacterial meningitis, particularly that caused by *N. meningitidis* and *H. influenzae.* Occasionally, in granulocytopenic patients or in elderly persons with overwhelming pneumococcal meningitis, the CSF may contain very few leukocytes and yet may appear grossly turbid because of the presence of a myriad of organisms. Meningitis caused by several bacterial species *(Mycobacterium tuberculosis, Borrelia burgdorferi, Treponema pallidum, Leptospira* sp, *Francisella tularensis, Brucella* sp) characteristically produces lymphocytic pleocytosis. With *L. monocytogenes* meningitis in the adult, there is usually a polymorphonuclear response, but lymphocytes may predominate in rare instances.

Glucose

The CSF glucose is reduced to values of 40 mg/dL or less (or <50% of the simultaneous blood level) in 50% of patients with bacterial meningitis; this finding can be valuable in distinguishing bacterial meningitis from most viral meningitides or parameningeal infections. However, a normal CSF glucose value does not exclude the diagnosis of bacterial meningitis. The simultaneous blood glucose level should be determined because patients with diabetes mellitus (or those who are receiving intravenous glucose infusions) have an elevated CSF glucose level that can be appreciated only on comparison with the simultaneous blood level; however, it may take 90 to 120 minutes for equilibration to occur after major shifts in the level of glucose in the circulation. The hypoglycorrhachia characteristic of pyogenic meningitis appears to result from interference with normal carrier-facilitated diffusion of glucose and increased utilization of glucose by host cells.

Protein

The level of protein in the CSF is usually elevated to more than 100 mg/dL, and higher values are more commonly observed in pneumococcal meningitis. Extreme elevations, 1000 mg/dL or more, may indicate subarachnoid block secondary to the meningitis.

Other Abnormalities

Elevated levels of lactic acid occur in pyogenic meningitis, but other conditions (cerebral ischemia, metabolism of CSF neutrophils, hypoxia) may also increase CSF lactate concentrations. Although lactic dehydrogenase levels are higher in patients with bacterial meningitis than in patients with viral infections of the CNS, these alterations are not helpful in determining the specific etiologic agent.

Blood and Respiratory Tract Cultures

Bacteremia is demonstrable in approximately 80% of patients with *H. influenzae* meningitis, 50% of patients with pneumococcal meningitis, and 30 to 40% of patients with meningococcal meningitis. Cultures of the upper respiratory tract are not helpful in establishing an etiologic diagnosis.

Determining serum creatinine and electrolytes is important in view of the gravity of the illness, the occurrence of specific abnormalities secondary to the meningitis (syndrome of inappropriate secretion of antidiuretic hormone), and problems with therapy in the presence of renal dysfunction (seizures and hyperkalemia with high-dose penicillin therapy). In patients with extensive petechial and purpuric skin lesions, evaluation for coagulopathy is indicated. Elevated serum procalcitonin levels have been used to distinguish bacterial meningitis from that of viral origin, but CSF examination (Gram stain, white blood cell count, glucose, culture) usually provides more direct and specific information.

Radiologic Studies

In view of the frequency with which pyogenic meningitis is associated with primary foci of infection in the chest, nasal sinuses, or mastoid, radiographs of these areas should be taken when clinically indicated at the appropriate time after antimicrobial therapy is begun. Initial head CT is not indicated in most patients with bacterial meningitis. For example, among patients who undergo head CT before lumbar puncture for suspected meningitis, only approximately 5% have a mass effect on CT. Baseline clinical features associated with abnormal CT findings include age older than 60 years, history of CNS disease, seizure within the prior week, abnormal level of consciousness, abnormal visual fields, limb drift, and aphasia. In patients without any of these clinical findings, only approximately 1% have a mass effect on CT that would raise concerns regarding lumbar puncture.

Specific changes that may be observed on CT during meningitis include cerebral edema and enlargement of the subarachnoid spaces, contrast enhancement of the leptomeninges and the ependyma, or patchy areas of diminished density owing to associated cerebritis and necrosis. In patients who have meningitis and whose clinical status deteriorates or fails to improve, the CT scan may help demonstrate suspected complications: sterile subdural collections or empyema; ventricular enlargement secondary to communicating or obstructive hydrocephalus; prominent persisting basilar meningitis; extensive areas of cerebral infarction resulting from occlusion of major cerebral arteries, veins, or venous sinuses; or marked ventricular wall enhancement, suggesting ventriculitis or ventricular empyema. Rarely, cerebral hemorrhage identifiable on CT may complicate acute bacterial meningitis in adults. In approximately 10% of adults with bacterial meningitis, cranial CT findings (mastoid or sinus wall defect, eroding retrobulbar mass, pneumocephalus) are indicative of disruption of the dural barrier.

Rarely, paraparesis or tetraparesis resulting from myelitis may complicate bacterial meningitis. In this situation, T2-weighted magnetic resonance imaging (MRI) can be helpful to exclude spinal cord compression by an extramedullary mass.

Differential Diagnosis

Headache, fever, stiff neck, confusion, vomiting, and pleocytosis are features of meningeal inflammation and are common to many types of meningitis (e.g., bacterial, fungal, viral, chemical) and also to some parameningeal processes. The CSF findings are most helpful in distinguishing among these processes (Chapters 438 and 439). Although a lymphocyte-predominant pleocytosis without hypoglycorrhachia is characteristic of viral (usually enteroviral or herpes simplex virus type 2 [HSV-2]) meningitis or meningoencephalitis (HSV-1), the initial CSF finding may be a polymorphonuclear response (of ≤60%) that quickly becomes mononuclear. HSV-1 encephalitis is suggested by neurologic findings (dysphasia, hemiparesis, olfactory hallucinations, and other temporal lobe signs, seizures), MRI abnormalities in the orbitofrontal and medial temporal lobes, and distinctive electroencephalographic changes in the temporal lobe or lobes. The rash, fever, and headache of Rocky

Mountain spotted fever (Chapter 348) may suggest meningococcal infection, but the geographic and seasonal predilections of the former can provide clues. Approximately 10% of patients hospitalized with Rocky Mountain spotted fever have CSF cell counts higher than 100/mm^3 (>70% polymorphonuclear), and thus the condition may initially be confused with bacterial meningitis. Acute subarachnoid hemorrhage (Chapter 432) may be confused with bacterial meningitis because of headache, stiff neck, and vomiting. However, subarachnoid hemorrhage usually has a more abrupt onset without prodromal fever and with evidence of subarachnoid blood on CT scanning or CSF examination.

In the patient who has meningitis but whose CSF does not reveal the etiologic agent on a Gram-stained smear, particularly when the CSF glucose is normal and the polymorphonuclear pleocytosis is atypical, certain treatable processes that can mimic bacterial meningitis should be considered in the differential diagnosis:

1. *Parameningeal infections.* The presence of infections (chronic ear or nasal accessory sinus infections, lung abscess) predisposing to brain abscess, epidural (cerebral or spinal) abscess, subdural empyema, or pyogenic venous sinus phlebitis should be sought (Chapter 438). Neurologic findings may appear in the course of primary bacterial meningitis, but their presence should alert the physician to the need for close scrutiny for the presence of a space-occupying infectious process in the CNS. Neurologic symptoms or findings antedating the onset of meningeal symptoms should suggest the possibility of a parameningeal infection. The isolation of an anaerobic organism should suggest the possibility of intraventricular leakage of a cerebral abscess.
2. *Bacterial endocarditis.* Bacterial meningitis may occur during bacterial endocarditis (Chapter 76) caused by pyogenic organisms such as *S. aureus* and enterococci. In subacute bacterial endocarditis, sterile embolic infarctions of the brain may produce meningeal signs and pleocytosis containing several hundred cells, including polymorphonuclear leukocytes. A history of dental manipulation, fever, and anorexia antedating the meningitis should be sought; careful examination for heart murmurs and peripheral stigmata of endocarditis is indicated.
3. *"Chemical" meningitis.* The clinical and CSF findings (polymorphonuclear pleocytosis and even reduced glucose level) of bacterial meningitis may be produced by chemically induced inflammation. Acute meningitis after diagnostic lumbar puncture or spinal anesthesia may result from bacterial or chemical contamination of equipment or anesthetic agent. Chemical meningitis, characterized by polymorphonuclear pleocytosis, hypoglycorrhachia, and a latent period of 3 to 24 hours, occurs after 1% of metrizamide myelograms. Endogenous chemical meningitis resulting from material from an epidermoid tumor or a craniopharyngioma leaking into the subarachnoid space can produce polymorphonuclear pleocytosis and hypoglycorrhachia; birefringent material may be seen on polarizing microscopy of the CSF sediment.

Complications

Non-neurologic Complications

Shock. When shock occurs in pyogenic meningitis, it is usually a manifestation of accompanying intense bacteremia, as in fulminant meningococcemia, rather than of the meningitis itself. Management is guided by the principles of septic shock therapy (Chapter 109), with appropriate modifications for heart failure (Chapter 58).

Coagulation Disorders. Coagulopathies (Chapter 180) are frequently associated with the intense bacteremias (usually meningococcal, occasionally pneumococcal) and hypotension that can accompany meningitis. The changes may be mild, such as thrombocytopenia (with or without prolongation of prothrombin and partial thromboplastin times), or more marked, with clinical evidence of disseminated intravascular coagulation (Chapter 181).

Septic Complications

Endocarditis. Patients with pneumococcal meningitis, particularly those with concomitant bacteremia and pneumonia, can develop acute endocarditis (Chapter 76), most commonly on the aortic valve. In such patients, febrile relapse and a new cardiac murmur may appear shortly after completion of antimicrobial therapy for meningitis.

Pyogenic Arthritis. Septic arthritis may result from the bacteremia associated with meningitis caused by *S. pneumoniae, N. meningitidis,* or *H. influenzae.*

Prolonged Fever

With appropriate antimicrobial treatment of community-acquired bacterial meningitis, patients become afebrile within 2 to 5 days. Sometimes fever persists or recurs after an afebrile period. In the patient with persisting headache, obtundation, and cerebral findings, inadequate drug therapy or neurologic sequelae (cortical venous thrombophlebitis, ventriculitis, subdural collections) are important considerations. Reevaluation of the CSF, particularly Gram-stained smear and culture, is essential under these circumstances. Drug fever (Chapters 302 and 303) may be responsible in the patient who continues to show clinical improvement in all other respects. Metastatic infection (septic arthritis, purulent pericarditis, thoracic empyema, endocarditis) may be the cause of continuing or recurrent fever. A syndrome, likely immunologic, consisting of fever, arthritis, and pericarditis 3 to 6 days after initiation of effective antimicrobial therapy of meningococcal meningitis occurs in approximately 10% of patients (Chapter 312).

Recurrent Meningitis

Repeated episodes of bacterial meningitis generally indicate a host defect, either in local anatomy or in antibacterial and immunologic defenses (e.g., recurrent *N. meningitidis* infections in patients with congenital or acquired deficiencies of complement, particularly late-acting components). Approximately 10% of episodes of pneumococcal meningitis in adults are recurrent meningitis, but only 0.5% of patients with community-acquired meningitis caused by other microorganisms have recurrent attacks. *S. pneumoniae* is the cause of one third of episodes of community-acquired recurrent meningitis; various streptococci, *H. influenzae,* and *N. meningitidis* are the causes of another one third of episodes. In contrast, in nosocomial recurrent meningitis, gram-negative bacilli and *S. aureus* are the causes of approximately 60% of episodes. A history of head trauma is much more frequent in patients with recurrent meningitis. Organisms may enter the subarachnoid space directly, through a defect in the cribriform plate (the most common site), in association with the empty sella syndrome, by means of a basilar skull fracture, through an erosive sequestrum of the mastoid, through congenital dermal defects along the craniospinal axis (usually evident before adult life), or as a consequence of penetrating cranial trauma or neurosurgical procedures. The anatomic defect may produce a frank CSF leak (rhinorrhea or, less commonly, otorrhea) or may entrap a vascular cuff of meninges that may subsequently serve as a direct route for organisms to reach the meninges. CSF rhinorrhea may be intermittent, and meningitis may occur months or years after head injury.

Any patient with bacterial meningitis, particularly if meningitis is recurrent, should be evaluated carefully for any congenital or post-traumatic defects. The presence of CSF rhinorrhea should be sought at admission and subsequently (rhinorrhea may clear during active meningitis only to recur when inflammation has resolved). Clinical clues suggesting the presence of a CSF fistula through the cribriform plate, pericranial air sinuses, or temporal bone include (1) salty taste in the throat, (2) positionally dependent rhinorrhea (rhinorrhea only in the lateral recumbent or prone position suggests an otic or sphenoid origin), (3) anosmia (cribriform plate leak), and (4) hearing loss or full feeling in the ear, often with a finding of fluid or bubbles behind the tympanic membrane (leakage into the middle ear). Quantitative determination of glucose and chloride content of nasal secretions and detection by protein electrophoresis of a transferrin band unique to CSF can definitively establish the presence of CSF rhinorrhea.

Recurrent pneumococcal meningitis may occur without apparent predisposing circumstances, and cryptic CSF leaks should be sought actively in such patients by CT scanning of the frontal and mastoid regions and by radioisotope techniques. Radioiodine-labeled albumin is introduced intrathecally, and pledgets of cotton placed in the nares are subsequently examined for the radionuclide. Intrathecal introduction of fluorescein as a visual tracer (under ultraviolet light) can be employed similarly to detect active leaks. Surgical closure of CSF fistulas should be performed to prevent further episodes of meningitis. Extracranial approaches through the ethmoidal sinuses can repair cribriform plate or sphenoidal sinus dural defects and can avoid the higher morbidity associated with craniotomy.

In most patients with CSF otorrhea and rhinorrhea after an acute head injury, the leak ceases in 1 or 2 weeks. *Persistent rhinorrhea for more than 4 to 6 weeks is an indication for surgical repair.* Prolonged administration of penicillin does not prevent pneumococcal meningitis and may encourage infection with more drug-resistant species.

Treatment

Rx

Antimicrobial Agents

Antimicrobial therapy should be begun promptly in this life-threatening emergency. Subsequent management should be undertaken with close monitoring, often in an intensive care unit. Treatment should be aimed at the most likely causes based on clinical clues, such as the age of the patient, the presence of a petechial or purpuric rash, a recent neurosurgical procedure, and CSF rhinorrhea. If the infecting organism is observed on examination of the Gram-stained smear of the CSF sediment, specific therapy is initiated. If the etiologic agent is not seen on the smear from a patient with suspected bacterial meningitis or if lumbar puncture is delayed because a head CT is needed, empirical antimicrobial therapy should be initiated (Table 437–2).

With the exception of rifampin and chloramphenicol, the commonly used antimicrobial agents do not readily penetrate the normal blood-brain barrier, but the passage of penicillin and other antimicrobial agents is enhanced in the presence of meningeal inflammation. Antimicrobial drugs should be administered intravenously throughout the treatment period; the dose should not be reduced as the patient improves because normalization of the blood-brain barrier during recovery reduces the achievable CSF drug levels. Bactericidal drugs (penicillin, ampicillin, third-generation cephalosporins) are preferred whenever possible, and CSF levels of antibiotics at least 10 to 20 times the minimal bactericidal concentration appear to be needed for optimal therapy. Several antimicrobial drugs (first- or second-generation cephalosporins, clindamycin) do not provide effective levels in the CSF and should not be used.

Empirical Treatment

Initial treatment of presumed bacterial meningitis when the etiologic agent cannot be identified on a Gram-stained smear of CSF is based on available clinical clues. In older children and adults, therapy with vancomycin and a third-generation cephalosporin (cefotaxime or ceftriaxone) is recommended (see Table 437–2). In adults more than 50 years of age and in high-risk groups, ampicillin is added to vancomycin in addition to a third-generation cephalosporin because of the role of *L. monocytogenes* (susceptible to ampicillin but not to third-generation cephalosporins), because of penicillin-resistant pneumococci, and because of the increased frequency of aerobic gram-negative bacilli in nosocomial meningitis and meningitis in immunocompromised patients. In the penicillin-allergic individual, trimethoprim-sulfamethoxazole is a suitable alternative in *Listeria* meningitis. In special settings, such as nosocomial meningitis associated with neurosurgical procedures or penetrating head trauma, more resistant species such as methicillin-resistant *S. aureus*, coagulase-negative staphylococci, and *P. aeruginosa* may be responsible; in these situations, vancomycin in addition to cefepime is indicated as initial therapy.

Meningitis of Specific Bacterial Cause

Pneumococcal Meningitis. The treatment of choice for pneumococcal meningitis in the adult historically has been penicillin, with van-

TABLE 437–2 INITIAL EMPIRICAL THERAPY FOR COMMUNITY-ACQUIRED AND NOSOCOMIAL PURULENT MENINGITIS BASED ON AGE AND CLINICAL SETTING

Predispositions	Likely Pathogens	Preferred Antimicrobials	Alternative Antimicrobials
Age			
<1 mo	Group B streptococcus, *Escherichia coli, Listeria monocytogenes, Klebsiella* sp	Ampicillin plus cefotaxime	Ampicillin plus aminoglycoside
1–23 mo	*Streptococcus pneumoniae, Neisseria meningitidis,* group B streptococci, *Haemophilus influenzae, Escherichia coli*	Vancomycin* plus ceftriaxone or cefotaxime	Meropenem (? plus vancomycin*)
2–50 yr	*Neisseria meningitidis, Streptococcus pneumoniae*	Vancomycin* plus ceftriaxone or cefotaxime	Meropenem (? plus vancomycin*)
>50 yr	*Streptococcus pneumoniae, Neisseria meningitidis, Listeria monocytogenes*	Vancomycin* plus ceftriaxone or cefotaxime plus ampicillin	Vancomycin* plus ceftriaxone or cefotaxime plus trimethoprim-sulfamethoxazole
Impaired immunity	*Listeria monocytogenes,* gram-negative bacilli, *Streptococcus pneumoniae*	Ampicillin plus ceftazidime plus vancomycin*	Trimethoprim-sulfamethoxazole plus meropenem
Cerebrospinal fluid leak or basilar skull fracture	*Streptococcus pneumoniae,* various streptococci, *Haemophilus influenzae*	Vancomycin* plus cefotaxime or ceftriaxone	Vancomycin* plus meropenem
After neurosurgery or penetrating trauma	*Staphylococcus aureus,* coagulase-negative staphylococci, aerobic gram-negative bacilli (including *Pseudomonas aeruginosa*)	Vancomycin* plus cefepime	Vancomycin* plus ceftazidime, or vancomycin* plus meropenem
Cerebrospinal fluid shunts (external or internal)	Coagulase-negative staphylocci, *Staphylococcus aureus,* aerobic gram-negative bacilli (including *Pseudomonas aeruginosa*), *Propionibacterium acnes*	Vancomycin* plus cefepime	Vancomycin* plus ceftazidime, or vancomycin* plus meropenem

*If dexamethasone is also administered, consideration should be given to addition of rifampin.
Modified from Tunkel AR, Hartman BJ, Kaplan SL, et al: IDSA practice guidelines for the management of bacterial meningitis. Clin Infect Dis 2004;39:1267–1284.

comycin (or chloramphenicol) as a reasonable alternative for patients allergic to penicillin (see later). However, penicillin-resistant pneumococcal strains are found worldwide, including 25% of clinical isolates in the United States. Thus, antimicrobial susceptibilities should be determined for all pneumococcal isolates from CSF, blood, or sterile body fluids (Table 437–3). Approximately 9% of pneumococcal isolates from cases of meningitis in the United States are resistant to third-generation cephalosporins, with a minimal inhibitory concentration greater than or equal to 2 μg/mL. If the minimal inhibitory concentration for cefotaxime or ceftriaxone (≤1.0 μg/mL) indicates a susceptible isolate, cefotaxime or ceftriaxone would be the drug of choice. If the isolate is highly penicillin resistant or is resistant to 1.0 μg/mL ceftriaxone or cefotaxime, alternative therapy (vancomycin with or without rifampin intravenously) is indicated. Because of the increasingly wide distribution of highly resistant strains, initial therapy (pending susceptibility testing) with cefotaxime (or ceftriaxone) in addition to vancomycin intravenously is recommended. When initial adjunctive therapy with dexamethasone is used (see later) along with vancomycin, it should be borne in mind that vancomycin levels in the CSF may be reduced by the concomitant corticosteroid use.

TABLE 437–3 ANTIMICROBIAL THERAPY OF COMMUNITY-ACQUIRED BACTERIAL MENINGITIS OF KNOWN CAUSE IN ADULTS OR CHILDREN

Organism	Preferred Therapy Antimicrobial	Alternative Therapy Antimicrobial
STREPTOCOCCUS PNEUMONIAE		
Penicillin MIC <0.1 μg/mL	Penicillin G or ampicillin	Cefotaxime or ceftriaxone or vancomycin or chloramphenicol
Penicillin MIC 0.1–1 μg/mL	Ceftriaxone or cefotaxime	Vancomycin or meropenem or cefepime
Penicillin MIC ≥2.0 μg/mL	Vancomyin* (plus cefotaxime or ceftriaxone)	Moxifloxacin or gatifloxacin
Cefotaxime or ceftriaxone MIC ≥1.0 μg/mL	Vancomycin* (plus cefotaxime or ceftriaxone)	Moxifloxacin or gatifloxacin
NEISSERIA MENINGITIDIS		
Penicillin MIC <0.1 μg/mL	Penicillin G or ampicillin	Ceftriaxone or cefotaxime or chloramphenicol
Penicillin MIC 0.1–1.0 μg/mL	Ceftriaxone or cefotaxime	Chloramphenicol, meropenem or gatifloxacin or moxifloxacin
HAEMOPHILUS INFLUENZAE		
β-Lactamase negative	Ampicillin	Ceftriaxone or cefotaxime or cefepime or chloramphenicol
β-Lactamase positive	Ceftriaxone or cefotaxime	Cefepime or chloramphenicol; or gatifloxacin or moxifloxacin
LISTERIA MONOCYTOGENES		
	Ampicillin† or penicillin G†	Trimethoprim-sulfamethoxazole or meropenem
STREPTOCOCCUS AGALACTIAE		
(group B streptococci)	Ampicillin† or penicillin G†	Cefotaxime or ceftriaxone

*Addition of rifampin should be considered. Consider intrathecal (or intraventricular vancomycin [5–20 mg/day]) if not responding to intravenous therapy.
†Addition of intravenous gentamicin should be considered.
MIC = minimal inhibitory concentration.
Tunkel AR, Hartman BJ, Kaplan SL, et al: IDSA practice guidelines for the management of bacterial meningitis. Clin Infect Dis 2004;39:1267–1284.

Although resistance to chloramphenicol is unusual among pneumococcal isolates from the United States, chloramphenicol has poor bactericidal activity against penicillin-resistant isolates from children with meningitis in South Africa. The relative chloramphenicol resistance of such strains may not be discerned on usual laboratory testing but it is revealed when the minimum bactericidal concentration is determined. For this reason, vancomycin is preferred to chloramphenicol for initial treatment of pneumococcal meningitis in the highly penicillin-allergic patient.

The β-lactam antibiotic meropenem is as effective as cefotaxime for meningitis caused by *S. pneumoniae, N. meningitidis,* and *H. influenzae* in adults and in children. Cefepime also is similar to ceftriaxone and cefotaxime for infection with *S. pneumoniae, N. meningitidis,* and *H. influenzae,* and it has greater activity than these antibiotics against *Enterobacter* sp and *P. aeruginosa.*

Meningococcal Meningitis. Penicillin G and ampicillin intravenously, in the doses used to treat meningitis caused by penicillin-susceptible pneumococci, successfully treat *N. meningitidis* meningitis resulting from susceptible strains. Meningococci resistant to penicillin have been isolated occasionally in Spain (≤50% of strains), South Africa, and Canada but rarely in the United States. Most of these isolates have been only intermediately resistant to penicillin (minimal inhibitory concentration, 0.1 to 1.0 μg/mL), although rare strains have had high-level resistance related to β-lactamase production and require third-generation cephalosporins such as ceftriaxone, which is as effective as the potentially more toxic chloramphenicol. 1 Nevertheless, "meningitis doses" of penicillin or ampicillin may provide CSF levels that are sufficient for infections with some strains of intermediately penicillin-resistant *N. meningitidis.*

***Haemophilus Influenzae* Meningitis.** At present, 25 to 35% of isolates of *H. influenzae* type b in the United States are β-lactamase producers and are ampicillin resistant; cefotaxime or ceftriaxone is the initial therapy of choice (see Table 437–3), with cefepime as an alternative. Chloramphenicol combined with ampicillin is another acceptable alternative; if the isolate proves susceptible to ampicillin, the chloramphenicol may be discontinued. Although more than 50% of isolates are chloramphenicol resistant in some areas of Spain, fewer than 1% of isolates have been resistant in the United States.

Staphylococcal Meningitis. For the treatment of adult meningitis caused by methicillin-susceptible *S. aureus* or in the penicillin-allergic patient, vancomycin is the alternative of choice (Tables 437–4 and 437-5). Because penetration of vancomycin into the CSF is limited, adjunctive intrathecal (or intraventricular) therapy with vancomycin (without preservative) is occasionally used when CSF cultures have remained positive after 48 hours of intravenous therapy alone and CSF levels can be monitored. For adult meningitis caused by methicillin-resistant *S. aureus,* intravenous vancomycin (with adjunctive intrathecal vancomycin as needed) is the treatment of choice. In severe or refractory cases, the addition of rifampin is warranted.

Gram-Negative Bacillary Meningitis. Cefotaxime or ceftriaxone (see Tables 437–4 and 437-5) is used to treat meningitis known to be caused by susceptible gram-negative bacilli (e.g., *E. coli, Klebsiella, Proteus*). It should not be used to treat meningitis caused by less susceptible species such as *P. aeruginosa* and *Acinetobacter.* Initial treatment (on the basis only of findings on a Gram-stained smear of CSF)

TABLE 437–4 THERAPY FOR NOSOCOMIAL MENINGITIS OF KNOWN BACTERIAL CAUSE IN ADULTS

Organism	Therapy of Choice	Alternative Therapy
STAPHYLOCOCCUS		
AUREUS		
Methicillin susceptible	Nafcillin or oxacillin; in difficult cases may add rifampin	Vancomycin, or meropenem
Methicillin resistant	Vancomycin; in difficult cases may add rifampin	Linezolid or trimethoprim-sulfamethoxazole
COAGULASE-NEGATIVE	Vancomycin; may consider addition of rifampin	Linezolid
***ENTEROCOCCUS* SP**		
Ampicillin susceptible	Ampicillin plus gentamicin	Vancomycin plus gentamicin
Ampicillin resistant	Vancomycin plus gentamicin	Linezolid
Ampicillin and vancomycin resistant	Linezolid	
ESCHERICHIA COLI* AND OTHER ENTEROBACTERIACEAE	Cefotaxime or ceftazidime	Meropenem or aztreonam, or ampicillin or trimethoprim-sulfamethoxazole
PSEUDOMONAS AERUGINOSA*	Cefepime or ceftazidime	Meropenem or aztreonam or ciprofloxacin

*Selection of specific antimicrobial drug should be based on in vitro susceptibility results, with consideration given to the addition of aminoglycoside (e.g., tobramycin, gentamicin or amikacin).

TABLE 437–5 DOSES OF ANTIMICROBIAL DRUGS IN TREATMENT OF BACTERIAL MENINGITIS*

Antimicrobial Drug	Adults (24-hr Dose)	Infants and Children (24-hr Dose)
β-LACTAMS		
Penicillin G	24 million U, q4h aliquots	300,000 U/kg, q4h aliquots
Ampicillin	12 g, q4h aliquots	300 mg/kg, q4h aliquots
Nafcillin	10–12 g, q4h aliquots	200 mg/kg, q4h aliquots
Oxacillin	10–12 g, q4h aliquots	200 mg/kg, q4h aliquots
Aztreonam (a monobactam)	6–8 g, q6–8h aliquots	
Meropenem (a carbapenem†)	6 g, q8h aliquots	120 mg/kg, q8h aliquots
CEPHALOSPORINS		
Cefotaxime	12 g, q4h aliquots	200–300 mg/kg, q6h aliquots
Ceftriaxone††	4 g, q12h aliquots	80–100 mg/kg, q12h aliquots
Ceftazidime	6 g, q8h aliquots	150 mg/kg, q8h aliquots
Cefepime	6 g, q6–8h aliquots	150 mg/kg, q8h aliquots
AMINOGLYCOSIDES		
Gentamicin§	5 mg/kg, q8h aliquots	7.5 mg/kg, q8h aliquots
Tobramycin§	5 mg/kg, q8h aliquots	7.5 mg/kg, q8h aliquots
Amikacin§	15 mg/kg, q8h aliquots	20–25 mg/kg, q8h aliquots
FLUOROQUINOLONES		
Ciprofloxacin	800–1,200 mg, q8–12h aliquots	—
Gatifloxacin‖	400 mg, q24h dosing	—
Moxifloxacin‖	400 mg, q24 h dosing	—
OTHERS		
Chloramphenicol	4–6 g, q6h aliquots	75–100 mg/kg, q6h aliquots
Vancomycin¶	2–3 g, q 6–8h aliquots	50–60 mg/kg, q6h aliquots
Rifampin	600 mg, q 24h dosing	10–20 mg/kg, q12–24h aliquots
Trimethoprim-sulfamethoxazole**	20 mg/kg, q6h aliquots	20 mg/kg, q6h aliquots
Linezolid	1200 mg, q12h aliquots	30 mg/kg, q8h aliquots

*Dosages are intravenous and for patients with normal renal and hepatic function.
†Use may be associated with seizures, but much less so than with imipenem.
††4 g maximum daily dose.
§Peak and trough serum levels should be monitored.
‖No data are available on the optimal dosage required for bacterial meningitis.
¶Monitoring of trough serum levels is advisable; they should be maintained at concentrations of 15–20 μg/mL. If the patient is not responding well, one may need to monitor cerebrospinal fluid levels, and if low, temporarily increase daily dose accordingly or add adjuvant intrathecal vancomycin (5–20 mg), as in treatment of methicillin-resistant *Staphylococcus aureus* meningitis.
**Dosage based on the trimethoprim component of the combination.

Rx

of adults with gram-negative bacillary meningitis is listed in Table 437–4. After identifying the specific pathogen and determining its drug susceptibilities, alterations in antimicrobial therapy may be indicated. If the organism is *P. aeruginosa*, ceftazidime or cefepime should be used (see Table 437–4 and 437-5).

Zoonotic Meningitis. Uncommonly, systemic or bacteremic zoonotic infections are complicated by bacterial meningitis. *F. tularensis* (Chapter 332) meningitis, a rare complication of tularemia, develops approximately a week after onset of infection. Illness is acquired from direct (or airborne) contact with wild rabbits or squirrels, with domestic animals, or through tick bites. Tularemia occurs throughout the United States, particularly in the Southeast and Midwest. The CSF formula usually consists of lymphocytic pleocytosis (several hundred to 2000 cells/mm^3), hypoglycorrhachia, and increased protein concentration. Treatment of adults consists of chloramphenicol (4 g/day intravenously, in 6-hourly aliquots) in addition to either gentamicin (3 to 5 mg/kg/day intravenously, in 8-hourly aliquots) or streptomycin (15 mg/kg intramuscularly, every 12 hours for 3 days followed by 7.5 mg/kg every 12 hours for the remainder of treatment). The duration of therapy is 14 days or longer.

Brucella meningitis (Chapter 331) is a subacute or chronic process, often accompanied by other manifestations of neurobrucellosis (encephalitis, polyradiculitis, myelitis). Infection is transmitted to humans in endemic areas (Central and South America, Mediterranean littoral, Arabian peninsula) from ingestion of unpasteurized milk or cheese or direct contact with domestic animals. Neurobrucellosis occurs in 2 to 5% of patients with brucellosis. CSF findings consist of lymphocytic pleocytosis (<500 cells/mm^3), hypoglycorrhachia, and an elevated protein level, findings that could mistakenly suggest tuberculous meningitis. Diagnosis is based on the demonstration of antibody in serum and CSF or by isolation of *Brucella* from blood; the microorganism is isolated from CSF only in a minority of cases. Treatment of adults involves the three-drug combination of doxycycline (200 mg/day), rifampin (600 mg/day), and trimethoprim-sulfamethoxazole (20 mg/kg/day, based on trimethoprim component, in 6-hourly aliquots) intravenously for several months, depending on the clinical and CSF responses.

Streptococcus suis is an uncommon cause of meningitis seen in pig breeders, butchers, and abattoir workers in Europe, Canada, and China. *S. suis* meningitis, which is an acute illness with brisk neutrophilic pleocytosis, is often initially mistaken for pneumococcal meningitis on the basis of Gram stain of the CSF. Treatment of adults consists of penicillin (12 to 24 million U/day, in 4-hourly aliquots) or ampicillin (12 g/day, in 4-hourly aliquots) intravenously for 10 to 14 days.

Bacillus anthracis (Chapter 317) is a rare cause of meningitis, most often developing as a complication of inhalation anthrax following exposure to aerosols of anthrax spores in the setting of large-scale processing of wool and hides or a bioterrorism attack (Chapter 19). Anthrax meningitis is an acute process characterized by a hemorrhagic or serohemorrhagic CSF with a neutrophilic predominance (several thousand cells/mm^3), hypoglycorrhachia, an elevated protein level, and prominent large Gram-positive bacilli on stained smear. Treatment of adults initially includes ciprofloxacin (400 mg at 12-hour intervals) in addition to penicillin (24 million U/day, in 4-hourly aliquots) and chloramphenicol (4 g/day, in 6-hourly aliquots) intravenously. Whether all drugs are continued (or treatment is narrowed to one or two antimicrobials) and the duration of treatment depend on whether the meningitis is of suspected bioterrorist origin (Chapter 19) or from cutaneous anthrax resulting from animal (or animal product) exposure (Chapter 317). Consultation with infectious disease and public health authorities should be sought.

Duration of Therapy

The frequency of CSF examinations depends on the clinical course, but a repeated examination should be done in 24 to 48 hours if there has not been satisfactory improvement or if the causative microorganism is a more resistant gram-negative bacillus or a highly penicillin-resistant (or cephalosporin-resistant) *S. pneumoniae,* especially in patients who are receiving adjunctive dexamethasone therapy. Routine "end-of-treatment" CSF examination is unnecessary in most patients with the common types of community-acquired bacterial meningitis. Meningococci are rapidly eliminated from the circulation and CSF with appropriate antimicrobial therapy, which should be continued for 4 to 7 days after the patient becomes afebrile. If the patient has responded well, a follow-up lumbar puncture is not necessary. *H. influenzae* meningitis should be treated for 7 to 10 days. Follow-up CSF examination may be omitted in patients who have responded with rapid clinical resolution of the meningitis. In pneumococcal meningitis, antimicrobial treatment should be continued for 10 to 14 days, and follow-up examination of the CSF should be performed, particularly when the patient has coexistent mastoiditis. More prolonged therapy is indicated with concomitant parameningeal infection. Meningitis caused by *L. monocytogenes* should be treated for 21 days. Treatment of gram-negative bacillary meningitis with parenteral antimicrobials is prolonged, usually for a minimum of 3 weeks (particularly in patients with a recent neurosurgical procedure) to prevent relapse. Repeated examinations of the CSF are necessary both during and at the conclusion of treatment to determine whether bacteriologic cure has been achieved. When treating meningitis resulting from vancomycin-resistant *Enterococcus faecium* with linezolid, an antibiotic that is bacteriostatic, approximately 4 weeks of therapy is indicated.

Other Aspects of Treatment

Adjunctive Corticosteroids

In children, the routine use of dexamethasone administered intravenously (either 0.15 mg/kg every 6 hours for 4 days or 0.4 mg/kg every 12 hours for 2 days) either at the time of or 10 to 20 minutes before initiating antimicrobial therapy (third-generation cephalosporin) has no effect on mortality but reduces the incidence of neurologic sequelae (primarily bilateral sensorineural hearing loss). However, the benefits are seen predominantly in *H. influenzae* type b meningitis, the incidence of which has been sharply reduced by the use of protein-conjugate vaccines. In a randomized double-blind study in adults with community-acquired bacterial meningitis, adjunctive dexamethasone therapy (10 mg every 6 hours intravenously for 4 days) significantly reduced the proportion of patients with an unfavorable neurologic outcome from 25 to 15% or a fatal outcome from 15 to 7%. 2 Adverse events were not increased in those receiving dexamethasone. Notably, the risk of gastrointestinal bleeding was not increased in the dexamethasone-treated group. Dexamethasone's beneficial effect was most evident in the subgroup of patients with pneumococcal meningitis, in whom unfavorable outcomes were reduced from 52 to 26% and deaths from 34 to 14%. In this trial, adjuvant dexamethasone was not beneficial in patients with meningococcal meningitis, but the number of patients in this subgroup was small. Based on these data, adjunctive dexamethasone (0.15 mg/kg every 6 hours for 2 to 4 days, with the initial dose 10 to 20 minutes before or simultaneously with the initial dose of antimicrobial therapy) is recommended in adults with suspected or demonstrated pneumococcal meningitis. Continuation of dexamethasone requires demonstration of gram-positive diplococci on the CSF Gram stain or positive blood or CSF cultures for *S. pneumoniae.* When vancomycin is used in treatment of meningitis resulting from highly cephalosporin-resistant *S. pneumoniae,* as is recommended in the United States, the addition of rifampin should be considered because dexamethasone may reduce the CSF concentration of vancomycin (see Table 437–3).

Elevated Cerebrospinal Fluid Pressure (Brain Swelling)

Occasional patients with acute bacterial meningitis experience marked brain swelling (CSF pressure >450 mm H_2O), which may lead to temporal lobe or cerebellar herniation after lumbar puncture. To decrease the possibility of this complication when the pressure is noted to be this high, only a small amount of CSF should be removed for analysis (the amount present in the manometer), and a 20% solution of mannitol (0.25 to 0.5 g/kg) should be infused intravenously over 20 to 30 minutes while monitoring (if possible) the decline of CSF pressure to a lower level before the spinal needle is removed.

Rx

Continued control of increased intracranial pressure, if needed thereafter, may be effected with additional mannitol; dexamethasone (10 mg intravenously, followed by 0.15 mg/kg every 6 hours) should be used in patients with brain swelling regardless of the suspected bacteriologic cause of meningitis.

In the stuporous patient or one with respiratory insufficiency and markedly increased intracranial pressure, use of a ventilator to reduce the arterial carbon dioxide pressure to between 25 and 32 mm Hg is reasonable, and the patient's head should be elevated to 30 to 45 degrees. Intubation should be performed with minimal stimulation to avoid an appreciable further rise in pressure; pharmacologic aids to intubation, such as succinyl choline and opioids, with possible use of adjunctive intravenous lidocaine, are recommended. Subsequently, transient increases in intracranial pressure associated with hyperactive airway reflexes can be mitigated by intratracheal instillation of lidocaine before vigorous suctioning. With continued marked and fluctuating elevations of intracranial pressure, use of a continuous intracranial monitoring device may be warranted.

Hypotension

Initial hypovolemia or hypotension, if present, should be treated with fluid to prevent significantly decreased cerebral blood flow. Over the next 24 to 48 hours, inappropriate secretion of antidiuretic hormone may contribute to further brain swelling; in such cases, fluid should be restricted to 1200 to 1500 mL daily in adults if possible, although a study in children suggests that routine fluid restriction does not improve outcome and that the resulting decrease in extracellular water may increase the likelihood of hypovolemia and an adverse outcome.

Supportive Care

Patients with acute bacterial meningitis should receive constant nursing attention in an intensive care unit to ensure prompt recognition of seizures and to prevent aspiration. If seizures occur, they should be treated in adults acutely with diazepam (administered slowly intravenously in a dose of 5 to 10 mg) or lorazepam (4 to 8 mg). Maintenance anticonvulsant therapy can be continued thereafter with intravenous phenytoin (Chapter 426) until the medication can be administered orally. Sedation should be avoided because of the danger of respiratory depression and aspiration.

Surgery

Surgical treatment of an accompanying pyogenic focus such as mastoiditis should be undertaken when recovery from the meningitis is as complete as possible but under continuing antibiotic administration. Rarely, the mastoid infection (e.g., Bezold's abscess) is so hyperacute that early drainage may be required after 48 hours or so of antibiotic therapy when the acute meningeal process has subsided somewhat.

Prognosis

Prompt treatment of bacterial meningitis usually results in rapid recovery of neurologic function. Persistent or late-onset obtundation and coma without focal findings suggest brain swelling, subdural effusion, hydrocephalus, loculated ventriculitis, cortical thrombophlebitis, or sagittal sinus thrombosis. The last three conditions are commonly associated with fever and continuing pleocytosis.

The mortality rate for community-acquired bacterial meningitis in adults varies with the etiologic agent and the clinical circumstances. With current antimicrobial therapy, the mortality rate for *H. influenzae* meningitis is less than 5% and that for meningococcal meningitis is approximately 10%. The highest mortality is with pneumococcal and *L. monocytogenes* meningitis, for which the rates are approximately 20% and 20 to 30%, respectively.

The mortality rate for gram-negative bacillary meningitis, commonly nosocomial in origin, has been 20 to 30% in adults, but it appears to be decreasing. The mortality rate for recurrent community-acquired meningitis in adults (~5%) is strikingly lower than the 20% rate for nonrecurrent episodes. Poor prognostic factors include advanced age, the presence of other foci of infection, underlying diseases (leukemia, alcoholism), obtundation, seizures within the first 24 hours, and delay in instituting appropriate therapy.

Residual neurologic damage remains in 10 to 20% of patients who recover from bacterial meningitis. Approximately 25% of adults considered clinically well recovered (expected to function independently and to resume activities of daily life including work) from pneumococcal meningitis show neuropsychological abnormalities, mainly loss of cognitive speed, when they are examined 6 to 24 months after hospital discharge. Developmental delay and speech defects are each observed in approximately 5% of children. In infants surviving neonatal meningitis, significant sequelae are much more frequent (15 to 50%).

Prevention

Vaccination

Effective vaccines are now available for many subtypes of *H. influenzae* type b [3] (Chapter 323) and many meningococcal [4] (Chapter 321) infections that cause meningitis. Adherence to recommended vaccination (Chapter 16) substantially reduces meningitis from each of those organisms.

Chemoprophylaxis

Prompt prophylaxis of close contacts (individuals who frequently slept and ate in the same household with the patient, girlfriend, or boyfriend) is warranted because up to one third of secondary cases of meningococcal disease develop within 2 to 5 days of illness in the initial case. Only hospital personnel who were in close contact with a patient (mouth-to-mouth resuscitation, initial examination before institution of respiratory precautions) are at special risk. Commonly, rifampin orally is used for prophylaxis: for adults (other than pregnant women), 600 mg twice daily for 2 days; for children, 10 mg/kg twice daily for 2 days. Alternatively, for adults ciprofloxacin (500 mg), ofloxacin (400 mg), or azithromycin (500 mg), each given orally as a single dose, may be employed. Another choice is ceftriaxone intramuscularly as a single dose for adults (250 mg) or children (125 mg).

Widespread use of *H. influenzae* b polysaccharide protein-conjugate vaccine in developed countries has largely eliminated need for chemoprophylaxis of close childhood contacts of cases of *H. influenzae* meningitis or invasive infection. However, prophylaxis would be indicated for unimmunized close household contacts of an index case (e.g., recent immigrants) younger than 6 years. If two or more cases of invasive *H. influenzae* b disease occur among children at a daycare center, prophylaxis of other unimmunized attendees is warranted. Rifampin (20 mg/kg orally) once daily for 4 days is recommended for such children.

Future Directions

Use of a pneumococcal protein polysaccharide conjugate-vaccine containing the seven most common pneumococcal types (PCV-7) in children has reduced the incidence of invasive infections in this age group, and a reduction of nasopharyngeal carriage of *S. pneumoniae,* including antibiotic-resistant serotypes contained in the vaccine, has been observed. Development of a PCV containing principal pneumococcal polysaccharide types for adults could possibly provide protection as well for this population against invasive pneumococcal infections, including meningitis. The quadrivalent (groups A,C,Y,W-135) conjugate meningococcal vaccine (MCV-4), recently recommended for 11 and 12 year olds should lead to a reduction in meningococcal infections, including meningitis, in adolescents and adults.

VIRAL MENINGITIS

Definition

The nonspecific term *aseptic meningitis* describes an inflammatory process involving the meninges, usually accompanied by mononuclear pleocytosis, without evidence of pyogenic bacterial infection on Gram stain or culture. The definition encompasses various processes that produce similar clinical pictures and inflammatory responses: *viral meningitis, atypical and nonpyogenic bacterial and fungal meningitis, chemically induced meningitis, drug-induced meningitis, neoplastic meningitis, meningeal inflammation caused by adjacent pyogenic infections,* and *meningitis associated with autoimmune hypersensitivity diseases.* Aseptic meningitis, which is usually an acute or subacute process, can be further divided into types by duration of illness *(chronic versus chronic-intermittent)* and by distinctive cellular responses in the CSF (e.g., *eosinophilic meningitis*).

Many of the viruses causing meningitis may also cause infection of the brain parenchyma (encephalitis; Chapter 439) or spinal cord. Sometimes, parenchymatous involvement and meningeal involvement occur simultaneously in the same patient and are referred to as meningoencephalitis and meningomyelitis, respectively.

Epidemiology

Most cases of community-acquired aseptic meningitis are the result of viruses, principally enteroviruses, which account for more than 60% of viral meningitides and for 90% of those for which an etiologic agent is identified (Table 437–6). Enteroviruses are members of the picorna (small RNA) virus family, which consists of approximately 60 serotypes: 28 echoviruses, 23 group A and 6 group B coxsackie viruses, 4 numbered enteroviruses (68 to 71), and 3 polioviruses. The most common serotypes implicated in viral meningitis from year to year have been echoviruses 4, 6, 9, 11, 16, and 30 (most recently 13 and 33) and coxsackie B serotypes 2 to 5. Currently, poliovirus infections (Chapter 402) are limited to parts of Asia and Africa, although rare cases occur secondary to attenuated vaccine strains.

TABLE 437–6 AGENTS OF VIRAL MENINGITIS

COMMON
NONARTHROPOD VIRUSES
Picornavirus (RNA)
Enterovirus
Echovirus
Coxsackie A
Coxsackie B
Enterovirus 70, 71
Poliovirus
Herpes simplex type 2 (HSV-2) (DNA)
ARTHROPOD-BORNE VIRUSES (ARBOVIRUSES)
Togavirus (Alphavirus, RNA)
Eastern equine encephalitis (EEE)
Western equine encephalitis (WEE)
Venezuelan equine encephalitis (VEE)
Flavivirus (RNA)
St. Louis encephalitis (SLE)
West Nile virus (WNV)
Bunyavirus (RNA)
California encephalitis
UNCOMMON
Arenavirus (RNA)
Lymphocytic choriomeningitis (LCM)
Paramyxovirus RNA)
Mumps
Retrovirus (RNA)
Human Immunodeficiency virus (HIV-1)
RARE
Herpes virus (DNA)
Herpes simplex type 1 (HSV-1)
Epstein-Barr virus (EBV)
Cytomegalovirus (CMV)
Varicella-Zoster virus (VZV)
Human herpes virus type 6 (HHV-6)
Adenovirus (DNA)
Coltivirus (RNA)
Colorado tick fever
Bunyavirus (RNA)
Toscana virus (a Phlebovirus)

Many viruses that produce the clinical picture of aseptic meningitis, such as arthropod-borne viruses, HSV-1, enterovirus 71, lymphocytic choriomeningitis, mumps, HIV-1, cytomegalovirus, and Epstein-Barr virus, can also produce the clinical picture of meningoencephalitis and encephalitis (Chapter 439). Some viruses also involve the spinal cord, including anterior horn cells (poliovirus) or dorsal root ganglia (HSV-2).

Enterovirus

An estimated 10 to 15 million clinical enteroviral infections (Chapter 402) occur annually in the United States, and these include an estimated 50,000 to 75,000 cases of enteroviral meningitis. In temperate climates, enteroviral meningitis peaks during the summer and fall, especially in children. Serotypes tend to cycle with varying periodicity, and outbreaks are related to lack of prior exposure to a particular serotype. Serotype-specific protective antibodies develop following infection, so subsequent episodes of enteroviral meningitis are uncommon and are caused by a different serotype.

Humans are the only known reservoir of enteroviruses. Enteroviral infection is spread predominantly by the fecal-oral route and occasionally by the respiratory route.

Herpes Simplex Virus

Herpes simplex (Chapter 397) accounts for 1 to 3% of all episodes of aseptic meningitis and occurs most commonly in sexually active adults or adolescents. Among individuals with primary genital herpes (HSV-2) infection, up to 36% of women and 13% of men have symptoms of aseptic meningitis. Recurrences of genital herpes are common and are sometimes accompanied by aseptic meningitis. More than 80% of cases of benign recurrent aseptic meningitis are caused by HSV-2. In contrast, HSV-1 CNS infection almost always presents as encephalitis rather than aseptic meningitis.

Arboviruses

Although the most common form of CNS infection caused by arboviruses (Chapters 406 and 407) is encephalitis, aseptic meningitis also may occur. These vector-borne viruses are introduced subcutaneously by a mosquito (e.g., West Nile Virus), tick (e.g., Colorado tick fever), or sandfly (e.g., Toscana virus). Birds, which are vectors of mosquito-borne arboviruses, may not obviously be sick, although West Nile virus may cause prominent die-offs of corvide species, especially crows and blue jays, that provide clues of an outbreak affecting humans.

The geographic spread in the United States of the alphavirus infections (Eastern equine encephalitis, Western equine encephalitis, Venezuela equine encephalitis) is determined by the range of their individual mosquito vectors. Eastern equine encephalitis occurs sporadically or as focal outbreaks in the summer in the Eastern and Gulf coasts, most frequently in children and elderly persons. Western equine encephalitis occurs predominantly in the Western states, and Venezuela equine encephalitis is found in Florida. Saint Louis encephalitis infections were originally recognized in the Midwest, but sporadic cases and outbreaks have occurred more recently in most parts of the United States; it is the most common arbovirus causing aseptic meningitis in the United States. West Nile virus infections first appeared in the United States in 1999 and now account for approximately 3000 cases of meningitis and another 3000 cases of encephalitis annually.

Mumps

Mumps (Chapter 392) was the leading identifiable cause of viral meningitis before widespread immunization in the 1960s. Episodes occurred most frequently in the winter and spring. Mumps is now an uncommon form of viral meningitis in the United States.

Lymphocytic Choriomeningitis

Lymphocytic choriomeningitis virus is transmitted to humans by rodents through direct contact, through ingestion of animal-contaminated food, or via aerosol or an animal bite. Cases tend to occur in early winter when mice seek shelter in homes. Outbreaks have occurred following exposure to pet or laboratory hamsters. Currently, lymphocytic choriomeningitis is infrequently a cause of aseptic meningitis.

Pathobiology

The two basic routes for virus to gain access to the CNS are hematogenous (enteroviral infection) or neuronal (HSV infection). Enteroviruses pass through the stomach, where they resist the acid pH, and proceed to the lower gastrointestinal tract. Some virus also undergoes replication in the nasopharynx and spreads to regional lymphatics. After presumably binding to specific enterocyte receptors, the virus breaches the epithelial lining and undergoes primary replication in a permissive cell. From there, the virus progresses to Peyer's patches, where further replication occurs. A minor enterovirus viremia then seeds the CNS, heart, liver, and reticuloendothelial system. Following extensive replication at the latter sites, a major viremia ensues, often accompanying the onset of clinical illness. The mechanism by which the enterovirus enters the CNS is presumed to involve crossing the blood-CSF barrier's tight endothelial junctions and then entering the CSF, likely at the choroid plexus.

In contrast, HSV infections may reach the CNS via the neuronal route: in HSV-1 encephalitis, from oral sites via the trigeminal and olfactory nerve; in HSV-2 (and the rare HSV-1) aseptic meningitis, by spread from a primary genital lesion and ascent along sacral nerve roots to the meninges. After subsidence of the primary infection, HSV-1 may remain dormant in the trigeminal or olfactory root ganglia only to reactivate at a later date, enter the temporal lobe, and produce encephalitis. Similarly, HSV-2 may remain latent in sacral root ganglia until subsequent reactivation causes later episodes of aseptic meningitis.

Clinical Manifestations

Enteroviral Meningitis

The clinical features of enteroviral meningitis (Chapter 402) in older children and adults often begin abruptly with headache (85 to 100%), fever (80 to 100%), and stiff neck (50 to 80%). In some patients, the course is biphasic, with the initial prodromal phase characterized by low-grade fever and nonspecific symptoms (malaise, sore throat, diarrhea), followed by a second phase at which time the meninges are seeded, with development of higher fever, nausea, vomiting, myalgias, photophobia, and stiff neck. Other enteroviral syndromes, particularly pleurodynia or pericarditis resulting from coxsackieviruses, may coexist. Rash may be a manifestation of infections caused by echoviruses, particularly echovirus type 9, coxsackieviruses A9 and A16, and enterovirus 71; the latter three cause hand-foot-and-mouth disease, which may occur alone or accompany aseptic meningitis. Echovirus 9 epidemics often produce syndromes of exanthem, enanthem (small, grayish-white lesions resembling Koplik's spots on the buccal mucosa), and aseptic meningitis, either alone or in combination; a maculopetechial rash in the presence of a meningitic syndrome must be differentiated from meningococcal meningitis.

Neurologic abnormalities affecting the cerebrum are rarely observed, because such cases would be defined as encephalitis or meningoencephalitis rather than enteroviral meningitis. In agammaglobulinemic individuals who acquired enteroviral CNS infection, meningitis may progress to a chronic meningoencephalitis with multiple neurologic features, including headache, seizures, ataxia, weakness, hearing loss, obtundation, and coma.

The clinical course of enteroviral meningitis is benign, even in the minority of patients in whom the onset is acute, even fulminant. Symptoms subside within a week in children but may continue for several weeks in adults.

Herpes Simplex Virus Type 2 Meningitis

Aseptic meningitis is a common complication of primary genital HSV-2 infection (Chapter 397); up to 36% of women and 13% of men have headache (developing over 2 to 3 days), stiff neck, and photophobia. Clinical features of meningitis occur 3 to 12 days after appearance of genital lesions and usually last for 4 to 7 days. Neurologic complications occur in up to 37% of patients, and include dysesthesias or paresthesias in the perineum or sacral area, urinary retention, and constipation; evidence of transverse myelitis with motor weakness in the lower extremities, hyporeflexia, paraparesis occasionally ensues. Recurrent episodes of HSV-2 meningitis may occur at intervals of months or years in 20% of patients. In recurrent HSV-2 meningitis, fever may occur but is not as prominent as in bacterial or acute enteroviral meningitis. Recurrent vesicular lesions, paresthesias, or dysesthesias in areas of prior genital herpes may or may not precede individual recurrences of meningitis. Between recurrences, CSF findings and clinical manifestations return to normal. In patients who have had neurologic complications with a first episode of HSV-2 meningitis, the findings subside within 6 months.

Mumps Meningitis

Symptomatic CNS disease, principally meningitis or meningoencephalitis, occurs in 1 to 10% of patients with mumps parotitis (Chapter 392), but pleocytosis occurs in more than 50% of patients with mumps, most of whom lack CNS symptoms. When meningitis occurs in mumps, it usually follows parotitis by 4 to 10 days, but it may precede parotitis by up to 1 week. The typical features of viral meningitis (headache, fever, vomiting) are each present in 50 to 100% of patients. Stiff neck (40 to 90%) is common, and abdominal pain (perhaps complicating pancreatitis or oophoritis) or orchitis (in ≤20% of men with mumps) may be present. Other complications of mumps may involve the nervous system (eighth nerve damage, transient facial nerve paralysis and, rarely, fifth nerve palsy) but are usually independent of mumps meningitis or meningoencephalitis. The incubation period of mumps is 18 to 21 days. When mumps meningitis occurs in the absence of clinical parotitis, it is difficult to distinguish it from other forms of viral meningitis.

When meningitis complicates mumps, fever, which had been low grade, rises to 103° F or higher and persists at this level for 3 or 4 days. Most cases are uncomplicated, with approximately a 10-day duration of illness and complete recovery. However, symptomatic mumps meningitis may persist for more than 14 days in some patients.

Lymphocytic Choriomeningitis Virus Meningitis

Lymphocytic choriomeningitis infections are uncommon, and clinical illness occurs after an incubation period of 1 to 3 weeks. Illness begins with a grippelike syndrome of fever, rigors, malaise, myalgias, anorexia, and photophobia. Sore throat and arthralgias or arthritis of the digits are noted by some patients. Orchitis or parotitis occurs rarely. This grippelike illness lasts 1 to 3 weeks in humans, but 15% of patients have a biphasic illness with transient improvement and then recrudescence, 1 to 2 days later, of fever, photophobia, and more prominent headache. Meningeal signs are observed during the second phase. The duration of lymphocytic choriomeningitis meningitis, like that of mumps meningitis, tends to be longer than the 7 to 10 days for enteroviral meningitis.

Human Immunodeficiency Virus Meningitis

Initial infection with HIV-1 (Chapter 406) is symptomatic in 40 to 90% of patients but frequently is overlooked. The interval between exposure and onset of symptoms is 2 to 4 weeks. This acute illness resembles mononucleosis, with fever, malaise, lymphadenopathy, arthralgias, myalgias, anorexia, nausea, headache, and morbilliform rash. A few patients with this initial syndrome have manifestations of aseptic meningitis (headache, photophobia, nausea, vomiting, and stiff neck). Occasionally, encephalopathy or cranial nerve palsies (seventh, eighth, and fifth) develop. Symptoms of the initial HIV-1 aseptic meningitis syndrome last several weeks and then subside. Occasionally, manifestations similar to those of the initial infection may appear later in the course of untreated infection.

Diagnosis

Cerebrospinal Fluid Examination

CSF findings in all types of viral meningitis are similar and consist of a predominantly lymphocytic pleocytosis, usually 50 to 1000 but occasionally up to several thousand/mm^3, a normal glucose concentration, and a mildly elevated protein level, usually less than 150 mg/dL. During the first 24 to 48 hours of enteroviral meningitis, a predominance of neutrophils (55 to ≤90%) is observed in approximately 50% of patients; subsequently, the principal cells in the CSF change to lymphocytes. Occasionally, no pleocytosis is noted in patients proven by culture or PCR to have early enteroviral meningitis. Rarely, hypoglycorrhachia occurs in meningitis resulting from mumps or lymphocytic choriomeningitis or in infants with enterovirus.

Polymerase Chain Reaction versus Culture or Antibody Detection

The recent development of reverse-transcription PCR for enteroviruses can reduce detection time to as little as 5 hours, thereby shortening hospital stays and minimizing the unnecessary use of antimicrobial agents. Sensitivity in CSF is 85 to 100%, with a specificity of 90 to 100%. The test is available in research settings, large hospitals, and commercial laboratories. By comparison, viral culture of enterovirus from CSF has a sensitivity of only 65 to 75% and takes 4 to 8 days.

HSV-2 can be cultured from CSF in approximately 75% of patients with aseptic meningitis during an initial episode of genital HSV-2 infection, but it is rarely isolated from CSF during meningitis associated with recurrent genital herpes. PCR for HSV-2 DNA is usually positive in CSF of patients with initial episodes of meningitis and is positive in approximately 80% of patients with benign recurrent lymphocyte meningitis.

Diagnosis can be made retrospectively by demonstrating seroconversion in antibody to gG-2 antigen in HSV-2 meningitis. A fourfold rise in titer to mumps or lymphocytic choriomeningitis virus between acute and convalescent sera also is diagnostic. Serodiagnosis is not practical for sporadic enteroviral meningitis because of the specificity of antibodies to individual serotypes.

Differential Diagnosis

The most important process to distinguish from viral meningitis is bacterial meningitis. A predominance of CSF neutrophils, hypoglycorrhachia, and bacteria on Gram-stained smear or culture indicate bacterial meningitis. An early neutrophilic predominance in CSF combined with a maculopetechial rash in enteroviral meningitis may mimic meningococcemia with meningitis. Occasional bacteria and fungi cause meningitis with a predominantly lymphocytic pleocytosis similar to that of most viral meningitides (Table 437–7). Epidemiologic considerations and clinical findings aid in distinguishing leptospiral, Lyme borrelial, and syphilitic meningitis, whereas hypoglycorrhachia suggests tuberculous and cryptococcal meningitis.

Prevention and Treatment

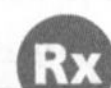

Introduction of live-attenuated mumps vaccine in the United States reduced mumps from the leading cause of aseptic meningitis and meningoencephalitis to the point at which it occurs only rarely. Chronic enteroviral meningitis and meningoencephalitis in agammaglobulinemic patients have been controlled by parenteral (even intrathecal) administration of immune globulin.

TABLE 437–7 NONVIRAL INFECTIOUS CAUSES OF ASEPTIC MENINGITIS

Uncommon	Rare
BACTERIAL	**BACTERIAL**
Leptospira interrogans serovars	*Mycoplasma pneumoniae*
Borrelia burgdorferi	*Ehrlichia chaffeensis*
Treponema pallidum	*Listeria monocytogenes*
Mycobacterium tuberculosis	*Borrelia recurrentis* and *Borrelia hermsii*
Brucella sp	*Chlamydia psittaci*
Parameningeal infections	Staphylococcal enterotoxin or TSST-1
Subacute bacterial endocarditis	*Rickettsia rickettsii* and *Rickettsia prowazekii*
Partially treated bacterial (pyogenic) meningitis	
FUNGAL	**FUNGAL**
Cryptococcus neoformans	*Blastomyces dermatitidis*
Coccidioides immitis	*Sporothrix schenckii*
Histoplasma capsulatum	*Candida* sp
	PROTOZOAN
	Trypanosoma brucei sp
	Toxoplasma gondii
	Acanthamoeba sp

Rx

No approved antiviral chemotherapy is available for enteroviral meningitis. Pleconaril, a drug that prevents viral attachment to host cells, can produce clinical improvement in agammaglobulinemic patients with chronic enteroviral meningoencephalitis.

Intravenous acyclovir (5 to 10 mg/kg every 8 hours) is used to treat hospitalized, symptomatic patients with HSV-2 meningitis, particularly when the disease is associated with primary genital herpes, although it has not been shown in clinical trials to alter the course of illness. In patients with frequent recurrences of HSV meningitis, it is reasonable to attempt prophylaxis with oral antivirals: valacyclovir (500 mg once daily), famciclovir (250 mg twice daily), or acyclovir (400 mg twice daily).

Prognosis

The course and outcome in enteroviral meningitis are almost always benign, although approximately 1% of patients have subsequent abnormalities, probably reflecting a meningoencephalitic process. Most viral meningitides are self-limited, but some cause chronic or recurrent illness. Persistent meningitis or meningoencephalitis, sometimes fatal, can occur in individuals with hereditary (usually X-linked agammaglobulinemia or common variable immunodeficiency) deficiencies in B-lymphocyte function. HIV-1 may produce a prolonged meningeal inflammation. HSV-2 infection is the most common viral cause of recurrent episodes of aseptic meningitis.

OTHER MENINGITIDES

Nonviral Infectious Causes of Aseptic Meningitis

Categories of aseptic meningitis other than viral meningitides include nonviral infectious processes (see Table 437–7), noninfectious processes (Table 437–8), chronic meningitides (Table 437–9), recurrent meningitis

TABLE 437–8 NONINFECTIOUS CAUSES OF ASEPTIC MENINGITIS

DRUG HYPERSENSITIVITY

SYSTEMIC DISEASE

Systemic lupus erythematosus
Familial Mediterranean fever
Behcet's syndrome
Wegener's granulomatosis
Cogan's syndrome
Sarcoidosis
Still's disease
Kawasaki's disease
Lead poisoning

NEOPLASTIC DISEASE

Metastatic carcinomatous meningitis
Central nervous system tumors (meningeal gliomatosis, dysgerminomas, ependymomas)
Tumors that leak inflammatory materials into cerebrospinal fluid (squamous cells in epidermoid tumors of the posterior fossa, cholesteatomas)

INFLAMMATORY PROCESSES INVOLVING CENTRAL NERVOUS SYSTEM STRUCTURES PRIMARILY

Chemical meningitis following myelography (water-soluble nonionic contrast)
Continuous spinal and epidural anaesthesia, post-neurosurgery inflammation
Granulomatous cerebral vasculitis
Vogt-Koyanagi-Harada syndrome

TABLE 437–9 INFECTIOUS CAUSES OF CHRONIC (PERSISTENT) LYMPHOCYTIC MENINGITIS

Causative Conditions	Other CSF Findings
BACTERIAL	
Mycobacterium tuberculosis	Usually <500 white blood cells/mm^3; low glucose; high protein
Borrelia burgdorferi (Lyme disease)	Normal glucose, elevated protein
Treponema pallidum (secondary syphilitic meningitis; tertiary meningovascular syphilis)	Elevated protein; Venereal Disease Research Laboratory positive in CSF and serum
Brucella sp (uncommon)	Often low glucose; elevated protein
Tropheryma whippelii (rare)	Periodic acid–Schiff–positive cells on meningeal biopsy
Partially treated bacterial meningitis	Mixture of PMNs and lymphocytes; bacteria on Gram stain and culture
Parameningeal infections	Lymphocytes or mixed lymphocytic-PMN response; normal glucose
FUNGAL	
Cryptococcus neoformans	Low glucose; elevated protein; budding yeast on India ink or fungal wet mount; antigen detectable
Coccidioides immitis	Often low glucose; may have 10–20% eosinophils; elevated protein; presence of complement-fixing antibody
Histoplasma capsulatum	Low glucose; complement-fixing antibodies in CSF; antigen detectable in urine, CSF, serum
Blastomyces dermatitidis	Low glucose
Candida sp	Low glucose; may have PMN or lymphocyte predominance; fungal stain may be positive
Aspergillus sp	Lymphocytes or PMNs predominate
Sporothrix schenckii (sporotrichosis)	Low glucose; protein, 200–800 mg/dL
PROTOZOAL	
Toxoplasma gondii	Usually picture is that of an encephalitis; often in patients with AIDS; pleocytosis is mild (<60 cells/mm^3) and protein mildly elevated
Trypanosoma gambiense or *Trypanosoma rhodesiense*	Meningoencephalitis is stage II of disease; elevated protein and immunoglobulin M; trypanosomes on Giemsa-stained smear
VIRAL	
Mumps	Rarely, low glucose
Lymphocytic choriomeningitis	Rarely, low glucose
Echovirus (in patients with congenital agammaglobulinemia)	Occasionally, low glucose
HIV-1	Cell counts lower (10–20/mm^3) than in acute self-limited meningitis at clinical onset of HIV infection; or may develop during course of AIDS

AIDS = acquired immunodeficiency syndrome; CSF = cerebrospinal fluid; HIV = human immunodeficiency virus; PMN = polymorphonuclear leukocyte.

TABLE 437–10 CAUSES OF CHRONIC (RECURRENT) MENINGITIS

INFECTIONS
Herpes simplex type 2
LEAKAGE OF CONTENTS FROM CENTRAL NERVOUS SYSTEM TUMORS (CHEMICAL MENINGITIS)
Epidermoid tumors
Craniopharyngiomas
Cholesteatomas
DRUG HYPERSENSITIVITY WITH REPEATED USE OF AGENT
INFLAMMATORY PROCESSES
Behçet's syndrome
Systemic lupus erythematosus
Mollaret's meningitis
Vogt-Koyanagi-Harada syndrome

(Table 437–10), and eosinophilic meningitis (Table 437–11). Nonviral infectious causes are uncommon or rare compared with viral or acute suppurative meningitis. Some of the bacterial causes (e.g., *Leptospira* serovars, *B. burgdorferi, Brucella* sp, *T. pallidum*) produce lymphocytic pleocytosis; others (partially treated bacterial meningitis, subacute bacterial endocarditis with embolic cerebral infarcts) produce mixed neutrophilic-mononuclear pleocytosis; and *M. tuberculosis,* while producing a lymphocytic response with developing hypoglycorrhachia, may show a predominantly neutrophilic response in a minority of patients early in the disease. Although patients with *L. monocytogenes* infection usually have neutrophilic pleocytosis, this infection may suggest aseptic meningitis because of its sometimes indolent onset and, occasionally, an early predominantly lymphocytic response in young children. Fungal (e.g., *Cryptococcus neoformans, Coccidioides immitis, Histoplasma capsulatum*) meningitides are associated with a predominantly mononuclear response, sometimes with a small percentage of eosinophils, particularly in coccidioidal meningitis (Chapter 354). Patients with Rocky Mountain spotted fever (Chapter 348), an acute disease with a maculopetechial rash, may exhibit confusion. When examined, the CSF in approximately 20% of such patients shows pleocytosis of 10 to 100 or more cells/mm^3, with either a neutrophilic or lymphocytic predominance. The clinical picture may suggest either enteroviral or meningococcal disease.

Epidemiologic factors are important in raising suspicion of nonviral aseptic meningitis. Leptospirosis (Chapter 344) may be suggested by a history of recent direct or indirect exposure to animals (e.g., dogs, rodents, dairy cattle) and their urine. Neurobrucellosis (Chapter 331) is suggested by the recent ingestion of unpasteurized cheese from the Mediterranean littoral, Middle East, or Mexico or by work as a veterinarian or in an abattoir. Specific endemic mycoses may be a consideration with residence in southwestern United States (coccidioidomycosis; Chapter 354) and the Mississippi river valley (histoplasmosis; Chapter 353). The setting of immunosuppression by drugs or illness such as

TABLE 437–11 CAUSES OF EOSINOPHILIC MENINGITIS*

Causative Conditions	Source
PARASITIC DISEASE	
Angiostrongylus cantonensis	Ingestion of raw shellfish; Pacific
Taenia solium (cysticercosis)	Fecal-oral transmission of *Taenia solium* eggs
Gnathostoma spinigerum	Ingestion of raw fish; Japan, Southeast Asia
Baylisascaris procyonis	Accidental ingestion of *Baylisascaris procyonis* eggs from raccoon feces
Trichinella spiralis (trichinosis)	Ingestion of poorly cooked pork
Schistosoma sp	Exposure of skin to fresh water; Africa, Middle East
Echinococcus granulosus	Contact with infected dogs passing eggs in feces
Toxoplasma gondii	Ingestion of meat containing cysts or food contaminated with oocysts from cat feces
Toxocara canis (visceral larva migrans)	Ingestion of infective eggs from dog feces
FUNGAL INFECTIONS	
Coccidioides immitis	Southwestern United States
NEOPLASTIC DISEASE	
Lymphoma, leukemia, metastatic carcinoma	
Hypereosinophilic syndrome (myeloproliferative disorder)	
INFLAMMATORY PROCESSES	
Sarcoid	
Drug hypersensitivity	
Presence of foreign body in the central nervous system	

*Percentage of eosinophils varies from as little as 6% to the majority of cells.

acquired immunodeficiency syndrome would raise the possibility of *C. neoformans* (Chapter 357) or *L. monocytogenes* (Chapter 316). Sexual promiscuity and the macular rash of secondary syphilis could suggest *T. pallidum* (Chapter 340) as the cause in a patient with lymphocytic meningitis.

Noninfectious Causes of Aseptic Meningitis

Noninfectious causes fall into four principal categories (see Table 437–8): drug hypersensitivity; systemic processes such as systemic lupus erythematosus and other collagen-vascular diseases; neoplastic disease, primary or metastatic, infiltrating the leptomeninges; and inflammatory processes primarily involving the CNS. Although a mononuclear cell predominance is found in the CSF in most noninfectious aseptic meningitides, there are several important exceptions. Drug hypersensitivity meningitis usually causes a neutrophilic response, although occasionally mononuclear cells or eosinophils predominate. In systemic lupus erythematosus (Chapter 287), the pleocytosis may be predominantly lymphocytic or neutrophilic (sometimes several thousand/mm^3) with a normal CSF glucose level. Hypoglycorrhachia is a feature of few noninfectious aseptic meningitides and suggests malignant disease or sarcoidosis. Various drugs, most commonly the nonsteroidal anti-inflammatory drugs, also have been implicated in aseptic meningitis.

Chronic (Persistent) Lymphocytic Meningitis

Chronic meningitis is defined by the clinical syndrome of headache, stiff neck, altered mental status, nausea, and vomiting, with or without cranial nerve palsies (e.g., III, IV, VI, VII, VIII) and evidence of myelopathy or radiculopathy, and an inflammatory response in the CSF for 4 weeks or longer. Obstruction of CSF flow may produce hydrocephalus and papilledema.

Infectious Causes

Among the more common bacterial causes of this syndrome, *M. tuberculosis* (Chapter 345) is most important to identify because, if untreated, it is almost always fatal within 4 to 8 weeks (see Table 437–9). Similarly, parameningeal infections (Chapter 438) must be recognized and treated promptly because surgery is often necessary to provide a specific bacteriologic diagnosis and prevent neurologic residua. Tuberculosis should be suspected in patients with a prior history of a tuberculous illness, a history of recent exposure, HIV infection or another immunosuppressed state, fever and night sweats, sixth cranial nerve palsies, stroke related to arteritis, or lesions on the chest radiograph. The purified protein derivative skin test may be negative in patients with recently acquired or overwhelming disease. Acid-fast smear and culture of concentrated CSF can provide the diagnosis, and PCR can be very helpful. When clinical and CSF findings suggest the diagnosis, treatment should be initiated while one awaits culture results.

Parameningeal infections (Chapter 438) should be suspected when chronic meningitis with focal neurologic signs develops in the setting of chronic otitis media or sinusitis, pleuropulmonary infection, or right-to-left cardiopulmonary shunting. Contrast-enhanced CT or MRI scans of the head are important to delineate brain abscess, sinus infection, and epidural or subdural infections.

Meningitis may accompany skin, mucous membrane, and lymph node features of secondary syphilis (Chapter 340), or it may occur alone. Individual cranial nerves (II to VII) may be involved; visual abnormalities, hearing loss, and facial palsy are most frequent. Fluorescent treponema antibody–absorbed or microhemagglutination–*T. pallidum* serologic studies are helpful in distinguishing the process from biologic false-positive Venereal Disease Research Laboratory (or rapid plasma reagent) results in serum.

Lyme disease meningitis (Chapter 342) should be suspected based on epidemiologic grounds (geographic location, season, tick exposure) and associated clinical features (erythema chronicum migrans rash, Bell's palsy, radiculopathy). Diagnosis involves enzyme-linked immunosorbent assay with Western blot confirmation.

Noninfectious Causes

Noninfectious causes of meningitis include malignant disease, chemical meningitis, and primary inflammatory conditions (Table 437–12). Malignant disease may be diagnosed by cytologic examination of large volumes of CSF. Contrast-enhanced MRI may disclose thickening of the meninges and nerve roots, but meningeal biopsy may be required for diagnosis. Chemical meningitis from prior subarachnoid injection may persist, with xanthochromia in the CSF; meningeal inflammation may be identified on contrast-enhanced CT or MRI scans.

Meningeal or CNS sarcoid (Chapter 95) may be isolated or occur with other organ involvement, such as pulmonary granulomas, lymphadenopathy, or myopathy. Neurologic findings can include diabetes insipidus and cranial nerve palsies. Wegener's granulomatosis (Chapter 291) may produce meningeal inflammation and cranial nerve palsies, often in association with air sinus disease. The diagnosis is suggested by lesions on the chest radiograph, microscopic hematuria, skin lesions, peripheral neuropathy, and serum antineutrophil cytoplasmic antibodies. Systemic lupus erythematosus (Chapter 287) aseptic meningitis may be accompanied by other neurologic manifestations (seizures, encephalopathy, stroke and transverse myelopathy), systemic manifestations (rash, arthritis), and antinuclear and anti-DNA antibodies.

Chronic (Intermittent) Meningitis

In chronic intermittent meningitis, all clinical and CSF abnormalities resolve completely between episodes without antimicrobial therapy (see

TABLE 437–12 NONINFECTIOUS CAUSES OF CHRONIC (PERSISTENT) LYMPHOCYTIC MENINGITIS

Causative Conditions	Other CSF Findings
NEOPLASMS	
Metastatic: lung, breast, stomach, pancreas B-cell lymphoma, melanoma, leukemia Central nervous system: Meningeal gliomatosis, meningeal sarcoma, cerebral dysgerminoma; epidermoid tumors/cysts	Low glucose; elevated protein, cytologic examination; polarizing microscopy; clonal B-lymphocyte markers
CHEMICAL INFLAMMATION	
Endogenous: epidermoid tumor, craniopharyngioma	Low glucose; elevated protein
Exogenous: recent injection into subarachnoid space	Low glucose; elevated protein
PRIMARY INFLAMMATORY PROCESSES	
Central nervous system sarcoid	Often low glucose; elevated protein; elevated angiotensin converting enzyme levels in CSF (and serum)
Wegener's granulomatosis	Elevated protein
Behcet's syndrome	Elevated protein
Isolated granulomatous angiitis of central nervous system	Elevated protein
Systemic lupus erythematosus	Elevated protein
?Chronic idiopathic benign meningitis	Elevated protein

CSF = cerebrospinal fluid.

Table 437–10). Uncommonly, a patient may have several episodes resulting from different viral agents. The major causes of recurrent aseptic meningitis are infections (almost always viral and resulting from HSV-2), endogenous chemical meningitis, drug hypersensitivity with meningitis following each use, and inflammatory and autoimmune diseases.

In HSV-2 recurrent meningitis, lymphocytes predominate, with the cell numbers approximately 40% higher in the initial episode than in recurrences. Leakage of material from intracranial epidermoid cysts produces 1000 to 5000 cells/mm^3 (~80% polymorphonuclear leukocytes) initially, with subsequent mononuclear cell predominance. Occasionally, polarizing microscopy may demonstrate keratin and cholesterol crystals in CSF of patients with endogenous chemical meningitis. In Behcet's syndrome (Chapter 291), the CSF formula may consist predominantly of mononuclear cells or polymorphonuclear leukocytes. Mollaret's meningitis, a syndrome of benign recurrent meningitis usually caused by HSV-2, initially is associated with neutrophils and monocytes in the CSF without hypoglycorrhachia, but subsequently transitions to a predominantly lymphocytic pleocytosis. Vogt-Koyanagi-Harada syndrome, a rare uveomeningoencephalitis, consists of recurrent meningitis/meningoencephalitis and anterior or posterior uveitis, followed by vitiligo, poliosis, alopecia, and dysacousia; the CSF cellular response is mononuclear, and an autoimmune origin, directed against a melanocyte antigen, has been suggested.

Chronic Meningitis with Predominantly Neutrophilic Pleocytosis

Chronic persistent neutrophilic meningitis (Table 437–13) is defined by the following combination: (1) clinical features consistent with meningitis; (2) initial CSF formula of >50% neutrophils, hypoglycorrhachia, and elevated protein concentration; (3) antimicrobial therapy that would be appropriate for usual causes of bacterial meningitis; (4) negative smears and cultures for bacteria on the initial CSF specimen; and (5) repeat CSF examination 7 days or more after initial analysis showing 50% or greater neutrophils, hypoglycorrhachia, and elevated protein concentration.

Among the bacterial causes (see Table 437–13) are organisms (*Actinomyces israelii* and *Arachnia propionica* [Chapter 350]) that can be isolated by culture only under anaerobic conditions. Coexisting pulmonary lesions may suggest *Nocardia* (Chapter 351) or *M. tuberculosis* (Chapter 345) as the cause, although the initial polymorphonuclear pleocytosis present in some cases uncommonly persists much beyond a week before changing to a lymphocytic predominance. *Brucella* (Chapter 331) and endemic invasive mycotic infections would be suggested by epidemiologic considerations. Other fungal causes may be diagnosed, particularly in immunocompromised patients, by antigen testing by enzyme-linked immunosorbent assay (*Aspergillus* sp galactomannan; Chapter 360), or meningeal biopsy may be required.

Occasionally, exogenous chemical meningitis secondary to intrathecal injection of antimicrobials, chemotherapeutic agents, or contrast media may produce persisting pleocytosis and hypoglycorrhachia resulting from sclerosing arachnoiditis well after the inciting medication has been withdrawn. Systemic lupus erythematosus (Chapter 287) can produce a variety of meningitides, including acute lymphocytic or neutrophilic aseptic meningitis, as well as chronic persistent lymphocytic or neutrophilic CSF responses.

Eosinophilic Meningitis

The presence of 5% or greater eosinophils in CSF is uncommon and suggests parasitic disease, certain fungal infections such as coccidioidal or candidal meningitis, neoplastic diseases, or a few inflammatory processes (see Table 437–11). In most cases, eosinophils are mixed with lymphocytes, which predominate; the highest percentage of eosinophils (≤70%) is seen with meningitis caused by migrating larvae of the raccoon ascarid, *Baylisascaris procyonis* (Chapter 378), and the rat lung worm, *Angiostrongylus cantonensis* (Chapter 378). In fungal meningitides, particularly those resulting from *C. immitis* (Chapter 354), the CSF response is primarily mononuclear with 6 to 20% eosinophils; hypoglycorrhachia may be a feature of *C. immitis* and *Candida* meningitis (Chapter 359) and of neoplastic processes and sarcoid.

Most patients with eosinophilic meningitis, except those with cases resulting from trichinosis (Chapter 378) or drug hypersensitivity, present with prolonged symptoms suggesting chronic meningitis. Most patients with cases of parasitic or neoplastic origin have evidence of cerebral involvement as well.

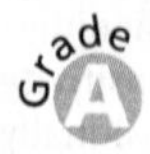

1. Nathan N, Borel T, Djibo A, et al: Ceftriaxone as effective as long-acting chloramphenicol in short-course treatment of meningococcal meningitis during epidemics: A randomised non-inferiority study. Lancet 2005;366:308–313.
2. De Gans J, Van de Beek D: Dexamethasone in adults with bacterial meningitis. N Engl J Med 2002;347:1549–1556.
3. Obonyo CO, Lau J: Efficacy of *Haemophilus influenzae* type b vaccination of children: A meta-analysis. Eur J Clin Microbiol Infect Dis 2006;25:90–97.
4. Prevention and control of meningococcal disease: Recommendations of the Advisory Committee on Immunization Practices (ACIP). MMWR Recomm Rep 2000;49:1–10.

TABLE 437–13 CAUSES OF CHRONIC (PERSISTENT) MENINGITIS WITH NEUTROPHIL PREDOMINANCE

Uncommon	Other CSF Findings
BACTERIAL	
Nocardia asteroides	Low glucose; markedly elevated protein; culture positive
Actinomyces israelii	Low glucose; elevated protein, anaerobic culture positive
Arachnia propionica	Low glucose; elevated protein; anaerobic culture positive
FUNGAL	
Candida sp	Low glucose; elevated protein; culture positive
Aspergillus sp	Low glucose; elevated protein; enzyme immunoassay or enzyme-linked immunosorbent assay for *Aspergillus galactomannan*
Zygomycetes	Low glucose; elevated protein
Dematiaceous fungi	Low glucose; protein may be markedly elevated
NONINFECTIOUS	
Systemic lupus erythematosus	Low glucose; elevated protein
Chemical meningitis	Low glucose; protein may be markedly elevated
Very Rare	
BACTERIAL	
Brucella sp	Low glucose; elevated protein
Mycobacterium tuberculosis	Low glucose; elevated protein; polymerase chain reaction positive for *Mycobacterium tuberculosis* DNA
FUNGAL	
Pseudoallescheria boydii	Low glucose; protein may be markedly elevated
Coccidioides immitis	Low glucose; protein elevated; presence of complement-fixing antibody
Blastomyces dermatitidis	Low glucose; protein elevated; antigen detection possible in CSF and urine
Histoplasma capsulatum	Low glucose; protein mildly elevated; complement-fixing antibodies in CSF; antigen detectable in CSF, urine, serum

CSF = cerebrospinal fluid.

SUGGESTED READINGS

Hoogman M, van de Beek D, Weisfeldt M, et al: Cognitive outcome in adults after bacterial meningitis. J Neurol Neurosurg Psychiatry 2007 Mar 12; Epub ahead of print. *Cognitive impairment of variable severity was present in one-third of adults affer pneumococcal or meningococcal meningitis.*

Straus SE, Thorpe KE, Holroyd-Leduc J: How do I perform a lumbar puncture and analyze the results to diagnose bacterial meningitis? JAMA 2006;296:2012–2022. *A review of the indications, risks, and results of this diagnostic procedure.*

Tunkel AR, Hartman BJ, Kaplan SL, et al: IDSA practice guidelines for the management of bacterial meningitis. Clin Infect Dis 2004;39:1267–1284. *The most authoritative, thorough, and well-referenced presentation of current recommendations for diagnosis and treatment of bacterial meningitis.*

van de Beek D, de Gans J, Spanjaard L, et al: Clinical features and prognostic factors in adults with bacterial meningitis. N Engl J Med 2004;351:1849–1859. *Only 44% presented with the triad of fever, stiff neck, and altered mental status, but 95% had at least two of the following four characteristics: fever, headache, stiff neck, or altered mental status.*

van de Beek D, de Gans J, Tunkel AR, et al: Community-acquired bacterial meningitis in adults. N Engl J Med 2006;354:44–53. *A practical review.*

Weisfelt M, van de Beek D, Spanjaard L, et al: Clinical features, complications, and outcome in adults with pneumococcal meningitis: a prospective case series. Lancet Neurol 2006;5:123–129. *Predictors of adverse outcome were the Glasgow coma scale score, cranial nerve palsies, a CSF WBC count less than 1000/mm³, and a high CSF protein concentration; in-hospital mortality was 30%.*

438 BRAIN ABSCESS AND PARAMENINGEAL INFECTIONS

Avindra Nath

Brain abscess affects the brain's parenchyma directly, whereas parameningeal infections produce suppuration in potential spaces covering the brain and spinal cord (epidural abscess and subdural empyema) or produce occlusion of the contiguous venous sinuses and cerebral veins (cerebral venous sinus thrombosis).

BRAIN ABSCESS

Epidemiology

The frequency of various causes of brain abscess (Table 438–1) in the population has been difficult to ascertain because of wide variations among case series, in part as a result of referral patterns. In addition, case series of children with brain abscesses contain a sizable contingent of cases related to cyanotic congenital heart disease or otogenic infection. Cryptogenic abscesses seem to be accounting for a greater percentage of cases in more recent series, perhaps related to the presence of a patent foramen ovale. Males predominate in virtually all series of brain abscess. Terminally ill patients in whom medical care may be withdrawn may be found to have abscesses at autopsy, but these abscesses are typically of little clinical importance.

Pathobiology

Brain abscesses are collections of purulent material (neutrophils and necrotic tissue) caused by infection with a variety of bacterial, fungal, and parasitic organisms. The infection begins with perivascular infiltrates

TABLE 438–1 CONDITIONS THAT PREDISPOSE TO THE DEVELOPMENT OF BRAIN ABSCESS

- Otogenic
  - Otitis media
  - Mastoiditis
- Dental
- Cardiac
  - Cyanotic heart disease
  - Tetralogy of Fallot
  - Patent foramen ovale
  - Infective endocarditis
- Pulmonary
  - Pulmonary arteriovenous fistula
  - Lung infection
    - Lung abscess
    - Bronchiectasis
- Esophageal strictures
- Cerebral infarcts and tumors
- Penetrating and nonpenetrating head injury
- Postoperative neurosurgical procedure (trauma and non–trauma related)
- Dermal sinus tracts
- Sepsis
- Immunosuppression
- Unknown mechanism

and infiltration of neutrophils into the brain parenchyma (cerebritis). With time, the developing abscess is characterized by a purulent exudate that includes necrotic brain tissue, as well as viable and necrotic neutrophils. Granulation tissue develops at the interface between necrotic and viable tissue, and eventually, the abscess is walled off by a fibrous capsule. Formation of the capsule depends on the virulence of the organism and the immune status of the individual. More virulent organisms are associated with larger lesions, more necrosis, earlier ependymitis, and more frequent areas of inflammatory escape outside the collagen capsule. Immunocompromised patients, such as human immunodeficiency virus (HIV)-infected patients with *Toxoplasma* abscesses, are unable to mount an immune response to form a capsule and hence respond well to antibiotic therapy alone.

Clinical Manifestations

The clinical picture reflects a triad of the infectious nature of the lesion, focal brain involvement, and an increasing intracranial mass effect (Table 438–2). One or two elements may be absent in a given case, particularly early in the course. Among infectious symptoms, fever is present at onset or early in the course in only about 60% of cases. Neck stiffness is an infrequent complaint, and meningeal signs are elicited in about 30% of cases.

Focal neurologic deficits depend on the site of the lesion, which in turn will be determined by the causal or predisposing condition. In some patients, seizures precede the diagnosis. The early deficits in patients with temporal lobe lesions, which are typically caused by spread of an otogenic abscess, are contralateral homonymous superior quadrantic visual field defects and, if in the dominant hemisphere, aphasia. Motor deficits eventually occur in 40 to 50% of supratentorial abscesses. Cerebellar abscesses, which are often caused by aural-mastoid infections, are characterized by ipsilateral limb ataxia; there may also be abnormal head positioning, forward and away from the side of the lesion, and nystagmus that is slow and coarse on looking to the side of the abscess and rapid on looking away. Patients with multiple brain abscesses may have multifocal signs or encephalopathy. Patients with *Toxoplasma* (Chapter 370) brain abscesses often have movement disorders because these abscess frequently localize to the basal ganglia. In fact, nearly all patients with HIV infection in whom hemiballism or hemichorea is present have *Toxoplasma* brain abscesses.

Headache is an important initial symptom in 80 to 90% of patients with bacterial abscess but is less frequent (≈20%) in patients with fungal abscesses. Symptoms of increased intracranial pressure, such as nausea, depressed level of consciousness, and papilledema, occur less often. The development of headache in a patient with a known chronic anaerobic infection, such as aural-mastoid, paranasal sinus, or pulmonary suppuration, suggests the possibility of brain abscess. Similarly, the development of headache in a child with cyanotic congenital heart disease is often related to a brain abscess.

Diagnosis

Examination of the cranium, ears, paranasal sinuses, oral cavity, heart, and lungs may provide important clues to the etiology, as may overt signs of other sites of infection. Cultures of blood and sputum may identify the organism and its antimicrobial sensitivity. In patients with signs of raised intracranial pressure, lumbar puncture may be contraindicated.

TABLE 438–2 BRAIN ABSCESS: INITIAL FEATURES IN 123 CASES

Feature	%
Headache	55%
Disturbed consciousness	48%
Fever	58%
Nuchal rigidity	29%
Nausea, vomiting	32%
Seizures	19%
Visual disturbance	15%
Dysarthria	20%
Hemiparesis	48%
Sepsis	17%

Magnetic resonance imaging (MRI) allows detection of early changes, such as brain edema, and is preferable to computed tomography (CT). In the early cerebritis stage, T2-weighted MRI shows abnormally high signal intensity corresponding to low signal intensity on the T1-weighted images. The fluid-attenuated inversion recovery (FLAIR) sequence provides superior visualization of brain edema. On T1-weighted images, the area of cerebritis that is seen initially as a low–signal intensity, ill-defined area later progresses to a central cavity with slightly higher signal intensity than cerebrospinal fluid (CSF), surrounded by edema that is slightly hypointense in comparison to brain parenchyma. Later stages of infection show central necrosis and formation of a rim of slightly high signal intensity on T1-weighted images (Fig. 438–1). Gadolinium administration shows a ring-enhancing lesion. Diffusion-weighted imaging helps differentiate abscesses from brain tumors; an abscess cavity demonstrates high signal with decreased apparent diffusion coefficient values, whereas necrotic tumor cavities demonstrate the opposite.

Surgical aspiration or excision of the lesion may be necessary to establish a microbial diagnosis. Gram stain and culture from abscess fluid, with proper handling, have high yield, with or without previous antibiotic therapy. If immediate surgery is planned, antibiotics can be deferred until culture material has been acquired. Multiplex polymerase chain reaction testing is now being developed for rapid identification of bacterial organisms and detection of antibiotic resistance genes.

Treatment

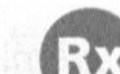

Brain abscess requires urgent intervention. Because of the risk for cerebral herniation with large lesions, treatment of cerebral edema (intravenous dexamethasone, 16 to 24 mg/day in four divided doses) may be needed even while initiating surgical intervention. Corticosteroids often decrease edema within 8 hours but may retard the formation of a capsule around the brain abscess, may suppress the immune system, and may decrease penetration of antibiotics; hence, they should be used for short periods, usually only until surgical decompression by needle drainage or surgical removal is possible. A trial of nonsurgical treatment may be considered in patients with (1) small lesion size; (2) an already identified pathogen; (3) no

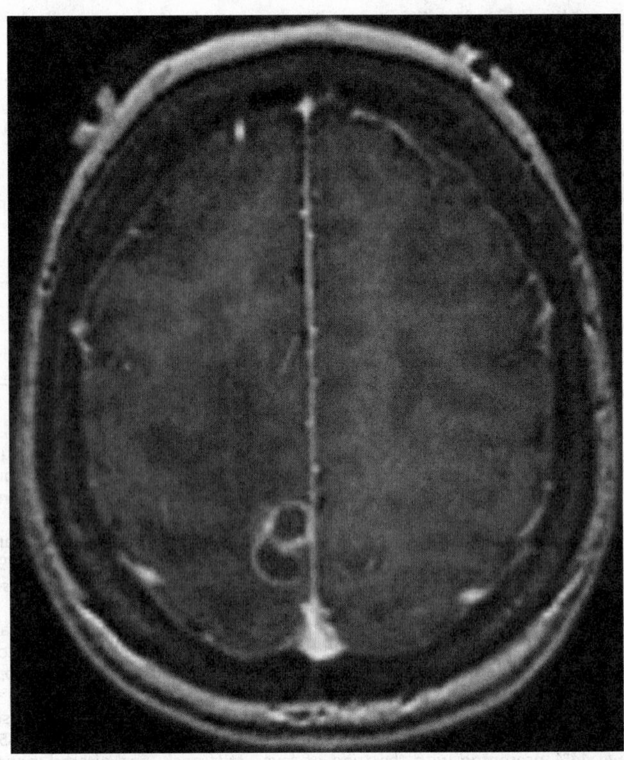

FIGURE 438–1 • Brain abscess. Magnetic resonance imaging with gadolinium shows a mutiloculated ring-enhancing lesion caused by *Nocardia* infection.

TABLE 438–3 COMMON PATHOGENS AND EMPIRICAL THERAPY FOR BRAIN ABSCESS

Predisposing Condition	Common Pathogens	Antimicrobial Agents
Dental abscess	Streptococci, *Bacteroides fragilis*	Penicillin + metronidazole
Chronic otitis	*Bacteroides fragilis, Pseudomonas, Proteus, Klebsiella*	Cefotaxime or ceftriaxone + metronidazole; ceftazidime or cefepime for *Pseudomonas*
Sinusitis	Streptococci, *Haemophilus, Staphylococcus*	Cefotaxime, ceftriaxone, or nafcillin + metronidazole
Penetrating trauma or post surgical	*Staphylococcus, Pseudomonas, Enterobacter,* streptococci	Nafcillin or vancomycin + ceftriaxone or cefotaxime + metronidazole
Bacterial endocarditis or drug use	Mixed flora, streptococci, *Staphylococcus*	Nafcillin or vancomycin + ceftriaxone or cefotaxime + metronidazole
Congenital heart disease	Streptococci	Cefotaxime or ceftriaxone
Pulmonary infection	*Nocardia, Bacteroides fragilis,* streptococci, mixed flora	Penicillin + metronidazole + trimethoprim-sulfamethoxazole
HIV infection	*Toxoplasma gondii*	Pyrimethamine + sulfadiazine + folinic acid

Rx

symptoms or signs of increased intracranial pressure requiring neurosurgical intervention; (4) a deep or inaccessible lesion; (5) multiple abscesses; (6) a contraindication to surgery (e.g., a bleeding diathesis); (7) a short duration of symptoms, which suggests that the lesion is in the cerebritis stage; and (8) availability of monitoring with MRI. Patients with acquired immunodeficiency syndrome and suspected cerebral toxoplasmosis (Chapter 370) should receive antimicrobial therapy initially.

Successful antibiotic management of brain abscess is based on knowledge of proved or suspected pathogens, as well as familiarity with a drug's spectrum of activity and penetration into the central nervous system. When surgery cannot be performed, empirical antibiotic therapy must be initiated even if the organism cannot be isolated from the abscess (Table 438–3).

Prognosis

In general, brain abscesses have a high mortality rate of about 15%, even in the modern era with neuroimaging techniques. In post-transplant patients and those with deep hemispheric or brain stem abscesses, mortality rates may exceed 80%. Other factors associated with a poor prognosis include extremes of age, multiple abscesses, and diagnostic delay in the absence of systemic signs of infection. Impaired level of consciousness is a poor prognostic sign even with early hospitalization and rapid diagnosis. Anaerobic and gram-negative organisms and culture-negative cases also have a poor prognosis.

SPINAL EPIDURAL ABSCESS

Definition

Infection within the epidural space around the spinal cord is an uncommon, but readily treatable potential cause of paralysis and death. The epidural space surrounds the dural sac and is limited by the posterior longitudinal ligament anteriorly, the ligamenta flava and the periosteum of the laminae posteriorly, and the pedicles of the spinal column and the intervertebral foramina containing their neural elements laterally. The space communicates with the paravertebral space through the intervertebral foramina. Superiorly, the space is closed at the foramen magnum. Caudally, the space is closed by the sacrococcygeal ligament. The epidural space contains loose areolar connective tissue, semiliquid fat, lymphatics, arteries, an extensive plexus of veins, and the spinal nerve roots.

Epidemiology

Spinal epidural abscesses can result from hematogenous spread of infection; risk factors include intravenous drug use, organ transplantation, chronic steroid use, malignancy, and diabetes. Local infection after acupuncture for back pain or epidural analgesia can also cause epidural abscesses. Cutaneous sites of infection are the most common remote sources, especially in intravenous drug users. Abdominal, respiratory tract, and urinary sources are also common. Osteomyelitis may be a cause of either direct extension or hematogenous spread, particularly when associated with sepsis. Contiguous spread may occur from epidurally placed catheters, psoas abscesses, decubitus ulceration, perinephric and retropharyngeal abscesses, or surgical sites. Minor back trauma has been implicated in causing a paraspinal hematoma, which may subsequently be seeded hematogenously. *Staphylococcus aureus* is the most common organism isolated from spinal epidural abscesses.

Pathobiology

Because the dura mater about the cord is adherent to the vertebral column anteriorly, more epidural abscesses lie posteriorly, and because no anatomic barriers separate the spinal segments in the posterior epidural space, such abscesses usually extend over several vertebral segments. Spinal cord dysfunction probably reflects toxic processes secondary to inflammation, as well as venous thrombosis, thrombophlebitis, ischemia secondary to compression of the spinal arteries, and edema.

Clinical Manifestations

The presence of a risk factor (>80% of patients) in the setting of neurologic deficits or back or radicular pain should suggest a spinal epidural abscess. The clinical manifestations can be divided into four stages (Table 438–4). Back pain (71%), fever (66%), tenderness of the spine with focal percussion (17%), spinal irritation (20%), and headache (3%) are common. Radicular pain can be mistaken for sciatica, a visceral abdominal process, chest wall pain, or cervical disc disease. Clinical signs are often substantially greater than would be predicted from the anatomic extent of pus or granulation tissue. If the condition goes unrecognized at this stage, the symptoms can evolve, over a period of hours to days, to paralysis below the spinal level of infection.

Diagnosis

The differential diagnosis includes compressive and inflammatory processes involving the spinal cord: transverse myelitis (Chapter 436), herniation of an intervertebral disc (Chapter 423), epidural hemorrhage (Chapter 423), or metastatic tumor (Chapter 199), none of which are associated with evidence of systemic infection. Blood leukocytosis may not be present, but the sedimentation rate is often elevated. Other infectious processes that may produce back or neck pain or tenderness must be excluded: bacterial meningitis (Chapter 437), perinephric abscess, disc space infection (Chapter 423), and bacterial endocarditis (Chapter 76).

TABLE 438–4 INITIAL CHARACTERISTICS OF 915 SPINAL EPIDURAL ABSCESSES

STAGE 1	
Back pain	71%
Fever	66%
STAGE 2	
Radicular pain	20%
STAGE 3	
Muscle weakness	26%
Sphincter incontinence	24%
Sensory deficits	13%
STAGE 4	
Paralysis	31%
Quadriplegia	3%

From Reihsaus E, Waldbaur H, Seeling W: Spinal epidural abscess: A meta-analysis of 915 patients. Neurosurg Rev 2000;23:175–204.

Lumbar puncture should be avoided in patients suspected of having a spinal epidural abscess for fear of spreading the infection to the subarachnoid space and causing meningitis. Gadolinium-enhanced MRI (Fig. 438–2) is the method of choice for diagnosis, but MRI findings in patients undergoing epidural analgesia can resemble those of epidural spinal abscess, even when no infection is present.

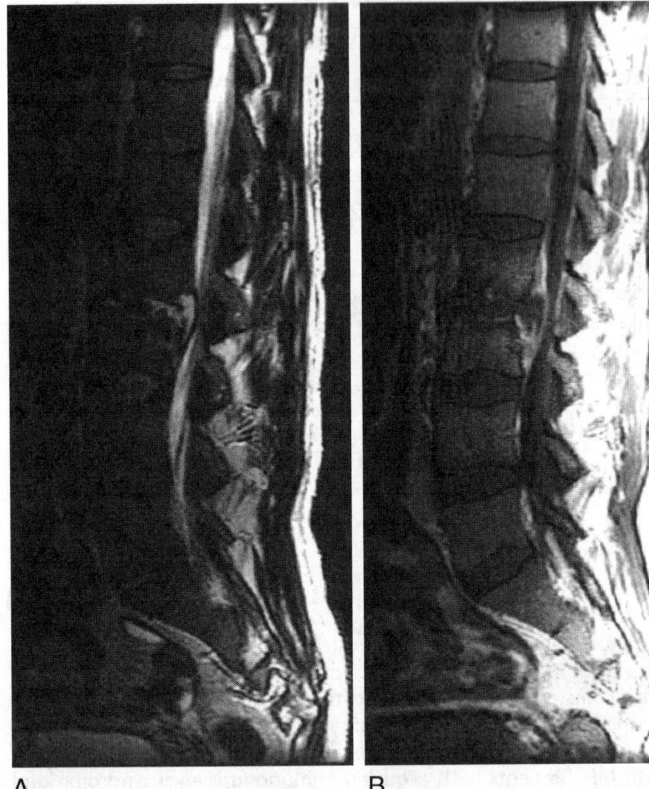

FIGURE 438–2 • Epidural abscess. A and B, Magnetic resonance images of the lumbosacral spine shows a lesion in the epidural space compressing the thecal sac. (Courtesy of Drs. Martin Pomper and Dima Hammoud, Johns Hopkins University.)

Treatment

Rx

Patients with a progressing neurologic deficit should undergo urgent surgical drainage; CT-guided aspiration may be useful, and antibiotics plus percutaneously guided needle aspiration appears to be at least as good as antibiotics plus surgery. Unless culture results and sensitivities dictate otherwise, empirical therapy should cover *S. aureus* (nafcillin, 2 g every 6 hours; vancomycin, 1 g every 12 hours for methicillin-resistant strains). Additional gram-negative coverage with a third-generation cephalosporin (e.g., cefotaxime, 2 g every 6 hours, or ceftriaxone, 2 g every 12 hours) or a quinolone (e.g., ciprofloxacin, 400 mg every 12 hours) should be considered for severe disease. Rifampin (300 mg every 12 hours) may be added because of its ability to penetrate the abscess cavity. Intravenous therapy should be continued for 3 to 4 weeks, except in the presence of osteomyelitis (6 to 8 weeks).

Prognosis

The mortality associated with spinal epidural abscess is about 15%. Most patients achieve complete recovery.

SUBDURAL EMPYEMA

Subdural empyema is an infection in the space between the dura and the arachnoid. It usually results from infected paranasal sinuses and rarely from infected mastoid sinuses by extension of thrombophlebitis from the sinuses into the subdural space. The infection is most commonly unilateral because bilateral spread is prevented by the falx. The empyema may evolve to cause cortical vein thrombosis, cerebral abscesses, or purulent meningitis.

Clinical Features and Diagnosis

The most common symptoms are headache, fever, a neurologic deficit, and a stiff neck. However, subdural empyema may progress and cause signs of raised intracranial pressure, such as vomiting, altered level of consciousness, seizures, and papilledema. A high degree of suspicion is needed to establish the diagnosis early in the course of the illness. In patients with complicated sinusitis, the symptoms of subdural empyema may be attributed to the sinusitis.

MRI with gadolinium enhancement and diffusion-weighted images is particularly useful in visualizing the subdural infection as a crescent-shaped mass with an enhancing rim over the cerebral convexities and below the inner table of the skull. CSF evaluation is useful only if there is accompanying meningitis. In a patient with signs of raised intracranial pressure, lumbar puncture should be avoided because of the risk for herniation.

Treatment

Surgical drainage of the empyema is mandatory. Intravenous antibiotic therapy is also necessary and is based on the organisms isolated at the time of craniotomy.

Prognosis

Mortality rates in most series are about 25%, with severe neurologic sequelae remaining in 20% of survivors. Accompanying venous sinus thrombosis or brain abscess carries a poor prognosis.

VENOUS SINUS THROMBOSIS SECONDARY TO INFECTION

The venous sinus system itself lacks valves, thereby permitting retrograde propagation of clots or infections that emanate from structures located in the central portion of the face or the middle ear.

Septic Cavernous Sinus Thrombosis

Definition

The cavernous sinuses are the most caudal dural venous chambers at the base of the skull. The paired structures lie on either side of the pituitary fossa, immediately above the midline sphenoid sinus. The cavernous sinus encloses the "cavernous portion" of the internal carotid artery, as well as the third, fourth, and sixth cranial nerves en route to the apex of the orbit.

Epidemiology and Pathobiology

The infection usually spreads from the paranasal sinuses, dental abscesses, or other infections affecting the orbit or middle third of the face. *S. aureus* is the most common organism. Streptococci, pneumococci, and gram-negative bacilli are less common; anaerobic infection has also been reported. Many cases of idiopathic intracranial hypertension (Chapter 199) are due to thrombosis in the lateral sinuses.

Clinical Manifestations

Cavernous sinus thrombosis may be manifested as an acute, fulminant disease or have an indolent, subacute manifestation. Fever and other systemic symptoms from sepsis may be present. Clinical symptoms and signs are related to anatomic structures within the cavernous sinuses or drained by them: unilateral periorbital edema, headache, photophobia, proptosis, ophthalmoplegia, pupillary dilation, decreased corneal reflex, and periorbital sensory loss. Obstruction of venous drainage from the retina can result in papilledema, retinal hemorrhages, and visual loss. The infection can spread rapidly (24 to 48 hours) via the intercavernous sinuses to the contralateral cavernous sinus. Thrombus can extend to other dural venous sinuses, adjacent vascular structures, or the brain parenchyma.

Diagnosis

The diagnosis is made on clinical grounds and confirmed by radiographic studies. Radiologic evaluation includes sinus imaging, particularly the sphenoid and ethmoid sinuses. MRI using flow parameters and an MR venogram is very sensitive and may reveal deformity of the cavernous portion of the internal carotid artery, a heterogeneous signal from the abnormal cavernous sinus, and an obvious hyperintense signal of thrombosed vascular sinuses. MRI with intravenous gadolinium can demonstrate venous thrombosis by illustrating a lack of the normal "flow void" within vascular structures. Cranial CT scans are less helpful but may show a subtle increase in the size and enhancement of the thrombosed sinus. MR angiography may demonstrate extrinsic narrowing of the intracavernous portion of the internal carotid artery.

Treatment and Prognosis

Rx

Blood cultures are often negative, so delays in diagnosis are common. Even when the diagnosis is established, empirical antimicrobial treatment may not provide full coverage.

Treatment consists of prompt drainage of infected paranasal sinuses or other identifiable source of infection, as well as specific antistaphylococcal agents (Chapter 310). Heparin anticoagulation without a loading dose is sometimes initiated to reduce morbidity from associated brain ischemia, but experience in septic venous thrombosis is limited as compared with the more frequent use of anticoagulation in nonseptic venous thromboses. Despite modern therapy, mortality rates remain as high as 44%.

Lateral Sinus Thrombosis

Septic thrombosis of the lateral sinus results from acute or chronic infections of the middle ear.

Clinical Manifestations and Diagnosis

Symptoms consist of ear pain and fever followed by headache, nausea, vomiting, loss of hearing, and vertigo, usually evolving over a period of several weeks. Symptoms or signs suggestive of otitis media (Chapter 452), including mastoid swelling, may be seen. Sixth cranial nerve palsies can occur, but other focal neurologic signs are rare. In some patients with nonseptic lateral sinus thrombosis, headache may be the only symptom. Papilledema occurs in 50% of cases, and elevated CSF pressure is present in most, especially with occlusion of the right lateral sinus, which is the major venous conduit from the superior sagittal sinus (Fig. 438–3).

CSF is usually normal, although a parameningeal inflammatory profile (mild pleocytosis, slight elevation in protein level, and a normal glucose level) may be seen. The diagnosis is confirmed by MR venography.

Treatment

Treatment includes intravenous antibiotics to cover staphylococci, anaerobes, and gram-negative bacilli such as *Proteus* and *Escherichia coli* (nafcillin, 2 g every 6 hours, or vancomycin, 1 g every 12 hours; plus cefotaxime, 2 g every 6 hours, or ceftriaxone, 2 g every 12 hours; plus metronidazole, 7.5 mg/kg every 6 hours, or clindamycin, 300 mg every 6 hours; plus ciprofloxacin, 400 mg every 12 hours). Surgical drainage (mastoidectomy or tympanoplasty) may be required to eradicate the nidus of infection and to determine the antibiotic susceptibility of the organism. If the sinus contains pus, it must be opened so that the septic thrombus can be removed. Unless vision is compromised, increased intracranial pressure seldom requires specific treatment such as drainage or placement of a shunt.

Prognosis

Broad intravenous antibiotic coverage and eradication of the perisinus infection, which may require surgical drainage, early in the course of the illness lead to a good prognosis. Neurologic sequelae may include a sixth nerve palsy, ataxia, and hearing loss.

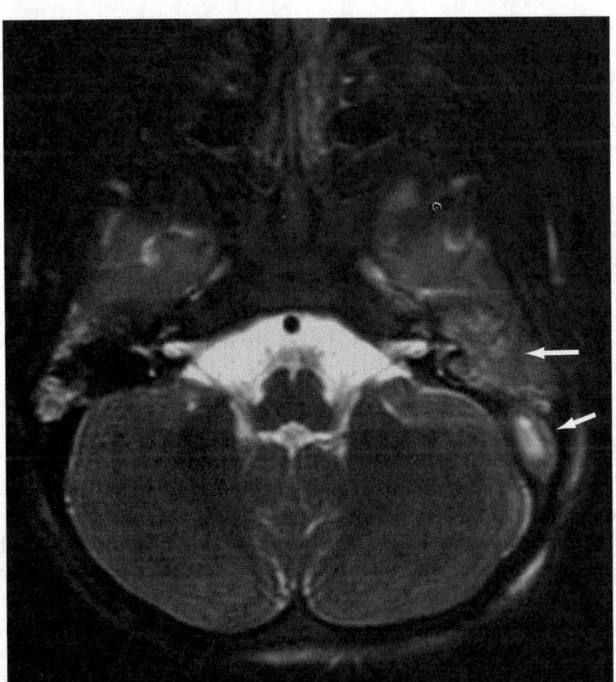

FIGURE 438–3 • **Lateral sinus thrombosis.** Magnetic resonance imaging shows a thrombus in the lateral sinus (thin arrow) with accompanying mastoiditis (thick arrow). (Courtesy of Drs. Martin Pomper and Dima Hammoud, Johns Hopkins University.)

Septic Sagittal Sinus Thrombosis

Although superior sagittal sinus thrombosis is the most common form of venous sinus thrombosis and is frequently associated with the use of oral contraceptives, septic sagittal sinus thrombosis is an uncommon condition that occurs as a consequence of purulent meningitis, infections of the ethmoid or maxillary sinuses spreading via venous channels, compound infected skull fractures, or rarely, neurosurgical wound infections.

Clinical Manifestations and Diagnosis

Symptoms are primarily related to the elevated intracranial pressure and can evolve rapidly to stupor and coma. Seizures and hemiparesis may result from cortical infarction. Early recognition and treatment are necessary because septic sagittal sinus thrombosis carries a high mortality rate. The rate of progression, severity of symptoms, and prognosis are all related to the location of thrombosis. Obstruction of the anterior third of the sinus produces less intense symptoms and evolves more slowly.

CSF abnormalities are frequent, including enough red blood cells that the CSF can sometimes be mistaken for a subarachnoid hemorrhage; the opening pressure is increased in proportion to the extent of sagittal sinus involvement. A septic sagittal sinus is best visualized during the venous phase of cerebral angiography or MR venography. The diagnosis can also be made by MRI, which demonstrates an abnormal increase in signal intensity (absent flow void) within the affected venous sinus. Contrast-enhanced CT scanning may reveal a contrast void lying at the junction of the transverse and sagittal sinuses (the region of the torcular); this so-called delta sign is an intraluminal clot surrounded by contrast material.

Treatment

Rx

Intravenous antibiotics should be directed at organisms recovered from the meningeal process or the meningeal site. *S. aureus* (Chapter 310), β-hemolytic streptococci (Chapter 312), pneumococci (Chapter 311), and gram-negative aerobes such as *Klebsiella* sp (Chapter 328) are the most common organisms. Associated paranasal sinusitis should be drained surgically.

Prognosis

If the thrombosis progresses to involve the middle and posterior thirds of the sinus, deterioration progresses rapidly, and the prognosis is poor with a mortality rate of nearly 30%.

NEUROLOGIC COMPLICATIONS OF INFECTIOUS ENDOCARDITIS

Neurologic complications develop in nearly a third of patients with infective endocarditis (Chapter 76), and neurologic manifestations are the initial symptom in 20% of patients with infective endocarditis. In nearly 30% of patients, the neurologic complications occur within 2 weeks after the initiation of treatment. Stroke is the most common manifestation; the majority of strokes are due to cerebral emboli, and others are due to intracerebral hemorrhage. Infective endocarditis should always be considered in a patient with a fever and stroke.

Pathobiology

Cerebral embolization occurs as a result of dislodgement or disruption of the cardiac vegetations that frequently cause occlusion of cerebral blood vessels. Emboli occurring before the initiation or completion of treatment with antibiotics may contain microorganisms capable of causing metastatic infections such as abscesses, arteritis, meningitis, or mycotic aneurysms. Most cerebral emboli involve small or moderate-sized blood vessels, and multiple cerebral emboli are common. Intracranial hemorrhage is usually due to rupture of a mycotic aneurysm (Chapter 432), septic erosion of the arterial wall without the formation of an aneurysm, or hemorrhagic transformation of a large cerebral infarct. About 20% of patients with mycotic aneurysms have multiple aneurysms; involvement of the middle cerebral artery and its branches occurs in more than 75% of patients, unlike congenital aneurysms, which occur predominantly in the circle of Willis. Mycotic aneurysms develop as a result of either septic embolization into the vasa vasorum or direct penetration through the wall of the artery. Streptococci and staphylococci account for nearly 90% of all mycotic aneurysms.

Clinical Manifestations

Patients usually have focal neurologic deficits attributable to the region of the infarct or seizures. Patients with multiple microemboli are often found to have an altered or fluctuating level of consciousness not adequately explained by other abnormalities.

Most patients with mycotic aneurysms have a sudden, often fatal subarachnoid or intracerebral hemorrhage without warning signs. Warning signs, if present, include severe localized headache, ischemic events, seizures, and cranial nerve abnormalities. In some patients, mycotic aneurysms may be asymptomatic and resolve with antibiotic therapy.

Diagnosis

MRI is the modality of choice for the diagnosis of cerebral infarcts, a CT scan is the best test for hemorrhage, and an MR angiogram is preferred for diagnosing an aneurysm. CSF evaluation is useful if accompanying meningitis or a slow leak from an aneurysm is suspected but not visualized with these imaging tests.

Treatment

Rx

Treatment of patients with infective endocarditis and cerebral emboli requires prevention of embolization with appropriate antibiotic therapy and sometimes cardiac surgery (Chapter 76). Anticoagulation is contraindicated in patients with cerebral infarcts and septic emboli because of the high risk of complications from intracerebral bleeding.

Patients with unruptured aneurysms smaller than 7 mm in diameter, proximal aneurysms, multiple aneurysms, ruptured aneurysms without an intracerebral hematoma, and aneurysms for which excision is likely to cause a neurologic deficit can be monitored conservatively with serial MRI and MR angiography. All other aneurysms require surgical excision of the aneurysm and the adjacent septic vessel wall. Patients who cannot undergo surgery may be candidates for endovascular embolization of the aneurysmal vessel.

Prognosis

Mortality rates in patients with infective endocarditis and cerebral emboli range from 30 to 80%. Mortality is high if there is hemorrhagic transformation of the infarct. Mortality in patients with ruptured mycotic aneurysms is 80%, and even patients with unruptured aneurysms have a mortality rate of 30%.

SUGGESTED READINGS

Cumurciuc R, Crassard I, Sarov M, et al: Headache as the only neurological sign of cerebral venous thrombosis: A series of 17 cases. J Neurol Neurosurg Psychiatry 2005;76:1084–1087. *Seventeen of 123 consecutive cases had new ipsilateral or bilateral headaches, normal head CT, and normal CSF; MR and/or MR venography was required for diagnosis.*

Darouiche RO: Spinal epidural abcess. N Engl J Med 2006;355:2012–2020. *A comprehensive review.*

Khouzam RN, El-Dokla AM, Menkes DL: Undiagnosed patent foramen ovale presenting as a cryptogenic brain abscess: Case report and review of the literature. Heart Lung 2006;35:108–111. *PFOs are an increasingly common finding in patients without other known predisposing causes.*

McClelland S, Hall WA: Postoperative central nervous system infection: Incidence and associated factors in 2111 neurosurgical procedures. Clin Infect Dis 2007;45:55–59. *The incidence was 0.3% for bacterial meningitis and 0.2% for brain abscess, with 50% caused by* S. aureus.

Prasad KN, Mishra AM, Gupta D, et al: Analysis of microbial etiology and mortality in patients with brain abscess. J Infect 2006;53:221–227. *Organisms were found by culture in 75% of cases and by Gram stain in an additional 6%.*

Stam J, De Bruijn SF, DeVeber G: Anticoagulation for cerebral sinus thrombosis. Cochrane Database Syst Rev 2002;(4):CD002005. *Anticoagulation appears to be safe and was associated with a non-statistically significant reduction in death.*

Stam J: Thrombosis of the cerebral veins and sinuses. N Engl J Med 2005;352:1791–1798. *A comprehensive review.*

439 ACUTE VIRAL ENCEPHALITIS

Avindra Nath and Joseph R. Berger

Definitions

The term *viral meningitis* refers to infection of the leptomeninges, *viral encephalitis* refers to infection of the brain parenchyma, and *viral meningoencephalitis* is sometimes used when both the meninges and brain parenchyma appear to be infected, although viral encephalitis is almost always accompanied by meningeal inflammation. When the spinal cord and brain are involved, the term *viral encephalomyelitis* may be used. The nonspecific term *aseptic meningitis* refers to an inflammatory process of the meninges accompanied by a predominantly mononuclear cell pleocytosis and not caused by pyogenic bacterial infection. Although viral infections are the most common cause of aseptic meningitis, infections by other types of organisms, chemical irritation of the meninges, carcinomatous meningitis, and reactions to certain medications can cause a similar clinical picture and cerebrospinal fluid (CSF) profile. In this chapter, acute central nervous system (CNS) infections caused by a variety of viruses are considered together because of their largely indistinguishable clinical features. Viral infections causing more distinct neurologic symptoms and signs are described separately in subsequent sections.

Epidemiology

Viral encephalitis is a relatively common disorder. In one study in Rochester, Minnesota, for example, the incidence of viral encephalitis was greater than 7 per 100,000 person years. In general, a specific cause is identified in only about 10 to 15% of cases of meningoencephalitis in the United States.

Implicated Viruses

Many viruses can cause acute encephalitis or meningitis (Table 439–1), whereas others may result in subacute or chronic encephalitis (Table 439–2). Enteroviruses (Chapter 402), which are the most common cause of aseptic meningitis, are small, nonenveloped RNA viruses of the picornavirus family with numerous serotypes. More than 50 have been associated with meningitis or encephalitis. Japanese encephalitis virus is the most common cause of encephalitis worldwide in humans. It has a high morbidity and mortality rate. Although an effective vaccine has been available since 1960, only small populations in Asia have been vaccinated.

Arboviruses include agents of several families, including Bunyaviridae, Togaviridae, and Flaviviridae, that are transmitted by mosquitoes or ticks (Chapter 405). More than 15 different arboviruses have been associated with encephalitis in various areas of the world. In the United States, the most important are California encephalitis (most cases involve the La Crosse subtype), eastern and western equine encephalitis, St. Louis encephalitis, and Colorado tick fever. Less common in the United States are Venezuelan equine encephalitis and Powassan encephalitis. West Nile encephalitis (Chapter 405) was first observed in the United States in 1999 and has rapidly spread across the continent.

Herpes simplex virus type 1 (HSV-1; Chapter 397) is the most common identified cause of encephalitis in the Western world. It causes severe encephalitis, usually with characteristic focal features reflecting its predilection for the mesial temporal and orbital frontal lobes. By comparison, HSV-2 causes aseptic meningitis in association with genital herpes and has been implicated as a cause of recurrent viral meningitis called Mollaret's meningitis. Lymphocytic choriomeningitis virus, an arenavirus, is a sporadic cause of meningitis and occasionally encephalitis. Human immunodeficiency virus (HIV) may cause aseptic meningitis and, rarely, acute meningoencephalitis (Chapter 417), usually at the time of seroconversion. These neurologic complications of HIV are to be distinguished from HIV dementia. Adenoviruses (Chapter 388) are respiratory viruses that only rarely cause meningitis or severe childhood encephalitis. Cytomegalovirus (Chapter 399) and varicella-zoster virus (Chapter 398) cause encephalitis, but only in immune-compromised individuals.

The acute neurologic disease associated with measles (Chapter 390), vaccinia (Chapter 395), or rubella infections (Chapter 391) is usually a sequela of infection termed *postinfectious encephalomyelitis.* Postinfectious encephalomyelitis occasionally follows influenza and parainfluenza virus infections.

Epidemiologic Patterns

Each virus causing CNS infection has its own epidemiologic pattern (see Table 439–1). Because of the predominance of enteroviruses and arboviruses, the overall incidence of viral meningitis and encephalitis peaks in the late summer. Enteroviruses (Chapter 402), which are transmitted by the fecal-hand-oral route, often involve young children, with rapid spread in families or social groups.

The geographic and seasonal incidence of arbovirus infection (Chapter 406) relates to the life cycle of arthropod vectors and animal reservoirs, as well as their contact with humans. Eastern equine encephalitis virus is limited largely to the Atlantic and Gulf coasts, whereas western equine encephalitis virus is confined to the western two thirds of the country, with the highest incidence west of the Mississippi River Valley. The latter virus causes many more human infections than the eastern virus does, but encephalitis develops in only 1 in 100 infected persons. St. Louis encephalitis virus causes disease in both rural and urban areas over a large part of the United States. In rural areas, the virus has the same pattern as western equine encephalitis virus, but in urban areas, more explosive outbreaks can occur. In recent years, the La Crosse subtype of the California encephalitis virus has been related every year to cases spread widely over the United States, particularly in the East and Midwest and mostly in children. Colorado tick fever occurs in the Rocky Mountain area; meningitis develops in about 18% of infected patients, but encephalitis is rare. Venezuelan encephalitis has spread to Florida and the southwestern states and produces an influenza-like illness in most of those infected; however, acute encephalitis develops in about 3%. Powassan virus is a rare cause of encephalitis in Canada and along the northern border of the United States.

West Nile encephalitis was introduced into the United States in 1999; the first cases were reported in New York, but by 2003, it had caused disease in nearly 10,000 persons in 46 states. Contaminated blood transfusions can cause the disease, and currently all blood donations in the United States are tested for West Nile virus RNA by nucleic acid amplification tests.

Tick-borne encephalitis virus is endemic in many parts of Europe and northern Asia, and in these regions it causes more than 10,000 cases of severe CNS disease in humans each year. The virus is primarily transmitted to humans when infected ticks take a blood meal, but infections from the consumption of unpasteurized milk, primarily from goats, occur in certain regions.

Lymphocytic Choriomeningitis

Lymphocytic choriomeningitis virus is the major zoonotic (a human infection that is naturally transmitted from any vertebrate animal) virus causing meningitis and encephalitis. Humans acquire the infection by contact with dust or food contaminated by the excreta of the common house mouse. Human disease is more common in winter, when the natural host tends to move indoors. Lymphocytic choriomeningitis virus has also been found in hamsters, and human infections have been traced to both laboratory and pet hamsters.

Mumps

Mumps virus (Chapter 392) spreads by the respiratory route, with infection occurring throughout the year but with the incidence increasing during spring. Although mumps virus infects both sexes equally, meningoencephalitis develops in males three times more frequently than in females. Japanese encephalitis is geographically the most widely distributed of all the arthropod-borne viruses.

TABLE 439–1 VIRUSES ASSOCIATED WITH ACUTE CENTRAL NERVOUS SYSTEM INFECTION

	Season	Mortality (%)	Morbidity (%)
NON–ARTHROPOD-BORNE VIRUSES			
RNA VIRUSES			
Picornaviruses (enteroviruses)	All year (tropics); summer and fall (temperate regions)		
Polioviruses			
Coxsackieviruses, group A			
Coxsackieviruses, group B			
Echoviruses		0	Rare
Enteroviruses 70, 71		Rare	Rare
Togaviruses			
Rubella	Spring	Rare	Rare
Arenavirus			
Lymphocytic choriomeningitis	Winter	Rare	Rare
Rhabdovirus			
Rabies	All year		>95
Orthomyxoviruses	Winter and spring		
Influenza			
Parainfluenza			
Paramyxoviruses	Winter and spring		
Measles			
Mumps			
Nipah		35	15
Retroviruses	All year		
Human immunodeficiency virus, type 1		100	
DNA VIRUSES			
Herpesviruses	All year		
Herpes simplex, type 1		15	60
Adenoviruses		Rare	Rare
ARTHROPOD-BORNE VIRUSES			
RNA VIRUSES			
Togaviruses			
Eastern equine encephalitis	Summer	50	30
Western equine encephalitis	Summer	5	30
Venezuelan equine encephalitis	Summer	10	<5
Flaviviruses			
Mosquito-borne encephalitis viruses			
Japanese encephalitis (Asia)	Summer	30	30
St. Louis encephalitis	Summer and fall	<10	10
Murray Valley encephalitis (Australia, New Guinea)		20	40
West Nile virus	Summer and fall		
Tick-borne encephalitis viruses	Summer	50	5
Russian spring-summer encephalitis	Spring and summer		
Louping ill (British Isles)			
Powassan virus (Canada, Northern United States)	Spring and summer	<5	Rare
Kyasanur Forest virus (India)	Summer	Rare	Rare
Bunyaviruses			
California encephalitis	Spring and summer		
La Crosse virus		Rare	Rare
Snowshoe hare virus (Canada)			
Jamestown Canyon virus			
Orbivirus			
Colorado tick fever	Spring and summer	Rare	Rare

Pathobiology

Events leading up to development of the acute viral encephalitides can be divided into three stages. The first involves exposure of an external body surface to the virus, usually with local replication of the "inoculum." In the case of enteroviruses, the infecting virus is contained in body fluids or excreta from infected persons and transferred by direct contact or within contaminated environmental materials. On ingestion, the virus replicates within Peyer's patches of the lamina propria of the lower intestinal tract. The arboviruses, by contrast, are introduced by an arthropod bite. The next stage involves systemic viremia and amplification of virus in visceral organs; a secondary viremia may lead to invasion and replication within the nervous system or meninges. With the exception of rabies virus and the neurotropic herpesviruses, viruses that cause acute encephalitis or meningitis typically reach the nervous system hematogenously, thereby explaining the widespread distribution of cerebral dysfunction associated with most of the encephalitides.

The third stage is viral replication within the nervous system. Infection of neurons, glial cells, and even the vascular endothelium leads to cellular dysfunction and sometimes cell death. Inflammatory responses follow. Clinical symptoms and signs depend on the distribution of infection and on both the direct effect of the virus and secondary

TABLE 439–2 VIRUSES ASSOCIATED WITH SUBACUTE OR CHRONIC NERVOUS SYSTEM INFECTION

	Neurologic Syndrome
RNA VIRUSES	
Togavirus	
Rubella	Progressive rubella panencephalitis
Paramyxovirus	
Measles	Subacute sclerosing panencephalitis
Retroviruses	
Human immunodeficiency virus type 1	HIV dementia
Human T-cell lymphotropic virus type 1	HTLV-I–associated myelopathy
DNA VIRUSES	
Herpesviruses	
Herpes simplex type 2	Mollaret's meningitis
Human herpes virus type 6	(?) Subacute encephalitis
Varicella-zoster	Herpes zoster, subacute encephalitis
Epstein-Barr	Subacute encephalitis
Cytomegalovirus	Ventriculitis and encephalitis
Papovaviruses	
JC virus	Progressive multifocal leukoencephalopathy

inflammatory reactions in the tissue. The relative contribution of each to brain dysfunction depends on the particular infecting virus. The remarkable degree of recovery in many patients suggests that some viruses may not result in permanent neuronal injury or death and that secondary inflammatory and immune responses contribute significantly to the clinical manifestations.

Clinical Manifestations

Most acute viral encephalitides produce similar symptoms, with variations depending on the particular virus. Neurologic symptoms are often preceded or accompanied by fever, malaise, or myalgia; gastrointestinal disturbance; respiratory symptoms; or rash. These manifestations are followed by headache, photophobia, stiff neck, and other signs of meningeal irritation, usually with an intensity milder than that of bacterial meningitis.

When encephalitis is present, evidence of diffuse or, less commonly, focal brain dysfunction accompanies or overshadows signs of meningeal irritation. Patients characteristically exhibit altered attention and consciousness ranging from confusion to lethargy or coma. Motor function may be abnormal, with weakness, altered tone, or incoordination reflecting dysfunction of the cortex basal ganglia or cerebellum. Severe cases may be accompanied by difficult-to-control generalized or focal seizures. Some patients exhibit myoclonus or tremor. Hypothalamic involvement may lead to hyperthermia or hypothermia, autonomic dysfunction with vasomotor instability, or diabetes insipidus. Abnormalities in ocular motility, swallowing, or other cranial nerve functions are uncommon. Spinal cord infection is usually inconspicuous but can result in flaccid weakness, with acute loss of reflexes in the most severe cases. Spinal cord involvement, in particular, involvement of anterior horn cells, is most common with polio virus (Chapter 440). Focal symptoms other than seizures are generally minor and overshadowed by generalized brain dysfunction; nevertheless, some patients may have hemiparesis, visual disturbance, or sensory loss. Focal involvement of limbic structures is particularly characteristic of rabies encephalitis (Chapter 441). Some patients with West Nile encephalitis may have a combination of encephalitis and Guillain-Barré syndrome. Tick-borne encephalitis involves predominantly the neurons in the spinal cord, brain stem, and cerebellum; involvement of the brain stem accounts for the high morbidity rate. An acute hemorrhagic encephalitis is most often caused by HSV-1 infection but may rarely be caused by flaviviruses such as Japanese B encephalitis, West Nile, and tick-borne encephalitis.

The time course of acute viral encephalitis varies. The onset may occur within a matter of hours or evolve more slowly over a few days. Usually, the maximum deficit appears within 1 to 4 days.

Diagnosis

Laboratory Findings

When viral encephalitis is suspected, examination of CSF is essential. If major focal signs are present, however, a computed tomography (CT) scan should be performed first to exclude a mass lesion. The presence of 10 to 1000 mononuclear cells per cubic millimeter (pleocytosis) is characteristic. On occasion, early examination may show acellular fluid or predominance of polymorphonuclear leukocytes, but the typical mononuclear pleocytosis soon evolves; repeat lumbar puncture may be warranted in the appropriate clinical setting. CSF pressure may be elevated, whereas the glucose level is characteristically normal or only modestly reduced. The protein content is usually elevated (50 to 100 mg/dL). Though not part of routine examination, elevated immunoglobulin levels and oligoclonal bands may be observed. An increased protein content and pleocytosis may persist for weeks or months after convalescence; oligoclonal bands can be detected for an even longer period.

Systemic laboratory findings vary, depending on the etiologic agent. Generally, the white blood cell count is not elevated, but either elevations or depressions can be seen, usually with a lymphocytic predominance. Involvement of the salivary glands or pancreas in mumps (Chapter 392) may elevate the serum amylase level.

Neurodiagnostic tests generally reveal nonspecific abnormalities, with the notable exception being herpes simplex encephalitis, which shows areas of hyperintensity in the mesiotemporal and frontal lobes and edema on T2-weighted and fluid-attenuated inversion recovery (FLAIR) magnetic resonance imaging (MRI). CT and MRI findings are usually normal early in the course of the nonherpetic viral encephalitides, but diffuse cerebral edema and multifocal areas of parenchymal injury with contrast enhancement may appear in more severe cases. The greatest value of these neuroimaging procedures lies in excluding alternative diagnoses.

Virology

With few exceptions, the neurologic and laboratory findings accompanying the acute viral meningoencephalitides are insufficiently distinct to allow an etiologic diagnosis, and it may even be difficult to distinguish these disorders from a number of nonviral diseases. The epidemiologic setting (e.g., time of year, exposure to insects, the local community) and accompanying systemic manifestations may be helpful in presumptive diagnoses. Thus, involvement of the nervous system by mumps virus is usually suspected from associated clinical parotitis or pancreatitis, although the neurologic disease can be the sole or initial clinical manifestation; conversely, a certain history of previous mumps eliminates this diagnostic possibility.

Several enterovirus infections (Chapter 402) produce a rash, which usually accompanies the onset of fever and persists for 4 to 10 days. In infections by coxsackieviruses A5, 9, and 16 and echoviruses 4, 6, 9, 16, and 30, the rash is typically maculopapular and nonpruritic and may be confined to the face and trunk or may involve the extremities, including the palms and soles. Echovirus 9 infections can cause a petechial rash resembling meningococcemia. Herpangina, characterized by gray vesicular lesions on the tonsillar fossae, soft palate, and uvula, can accompany group A coxsackievirus infection (Chapter 402). In coxsackievirus A16 and, rarely, other group A serotype infections, a vesicular rash may involve the hands, feet, and oropharynx. The encephalitis related to Epstein-Barr virus (Chapter 400) occurs in the setting of acute mononucleosis. The principally postinfectious encephalitides related to measles (Chapter 390) and varicella (Chapter 398) follow overt systemic diseases with characteristic rashes.

Because no specific treatment exists for acute viral meningitis and encephalitis (except those caused by herpes) in immune-competent patients and because the signs and symptoms are often nonspecific, exclusion of other diagnoses becomes important. The following disorders are potentially confusing diagnostically: partially treated bacterial meningitis (Chapter 437); rickettsial infections (Chapter 348); Lyme disease (Chapter 342); meningitis caused by a variety of nonpyogenic organisms, including *Mycobacterium tuberculosis* (Chapter 345) and *Cryptococcus neoformans* (Chapter 357) and other fungi; parameningeal bacterial infections (Chapter 438); brain abscess (Chapter 438); subacute bacterial endocarditis (Chapter 76); and the cerebral vasculitides (Chapter 291). Among noninfectious causes, trimethoprim-sulfamethoxazole, nonsteroidal analgesics, OKT3 antibody given for immunosuppression, intravenous immunoglobulin, and certain other drugs may occasionally cause aseptic meningitis. Without a CSF examination, the differential diagnosis becomes even broader and encompasses additional toxic and vascular diseases. Most alternative diagnoses can be suspected or eliminated by the history, the CSF profile, or brain imaging.

Despite the absence of effective treatment, a specific virologic diagnosis is useful both for prognosis in the individual patient and for epidemiologic implications for the populations at risk. Diagnosis usually relies on serology, although direct detection of the organism in CSF, blood, or stool may sometimes be achieved. Selection of tests and their interpretation depend on the particular organism. Almost all acute viral syndromes occur in the setting of a first encounter with the agent, which then results in lasting immunity. In these cases, seroconversion documented by a four-fold or greater rise in antibody titer between acute and convalescent sera is a principal means of diagnosis, although virus-specific IgM antibodies provide a rapid and accurate method of early diagnosis. A notable exception is herpes simplex encephalitis, in which antibody titers must be more cautiously interpreted (see Chapter 397). Attempts at direct viral isolation are of limited value in clinical management and must be tailored to the suspected agent. Arboviruses and enteroviruses can be isolated from blood but are seldom recoverable at the time of clinically evident meningitis or encephalitis. During acute disease, coxsackieviruses and echoviruses are most readily isolated from stool or CSF and, in some cases, from throat washings. Lymphocytic choriomeningitis virus can be isolated from blood or CSF. Mumps virus may be isolated from saliva, throat washings, or CSF. HSV-2 may be cultured from CSF or identified in genital lesions. Polymerase chain reaction screening of CSF undoubtedly improves specific diagnoses, but it is still not widely available.

Prevention

Effective vaccines for polio, measles, mumps, and rubella have dramatically reduced the frequency of these infections in countries with effective vaccination strategies (Chapter 16). Similarly, vaccination against Japanese encephalitis has been effective in controlling the infection in Asia. A vaccine against varicella (Chapter 398) has similarly encouraging early results. Rabies (Chapter 441) is the only infection for which the vaccine may be given after exposure to the virus.

Treatment

Rx

Effective antiviral therapy is available against HSV-1 (acyclovir, 10 mg/kg intravenously every 8 hours for 2 weeks), cytomegalovirus, and varicella-zoster virus, the latter two of which cause encephalitis in immune-compromised patients only. These antiviral drugs target virus-specific enzymes such as thymidine kinase. In immunosuppressed patients, long-term therapy may be necessary. Several antiretroviral drugs are also available that provide only temporary control of the virus because drug-resistant strains of HIV frequently emerge. Treatment of acute viral encephalitis and meningitis (except herpes) is directed at relief of symptoms, supportive care, and prevention and management of complications.

Strict isolation is not essential, although careful handwashing precautions and handling of stool should be instituted when enteroviral infection is suspected. Persons with measles, chickenpox, rubella, or mumps virus infections should observe the usual precautions of isolation from susceptible individuals. Isolation should also be considered for severely immunosuppressed patients, patients with an exanthematous encephalitis, and those with a potentially contagious viral hemorrhagic fever. Arboviruses are not characteristically spread from person to person because they require an intermediate insect vector.

The headache and fever of meningitis can usually be managed with judicious doses (650 to 1000 mg orally every 4 hours as needed, maximum of 4 g/day) of acetaminophen. Severe hyperthermia (>40° C) may require vigorous therapy with a cooling blanket or ice packs; however, mild temperature elevations may serve as a natural defense mechanism and are best left untreated. Patients with severe encephalitis often become comatose, but vigorous support and avoidance of complications are essential because some may achieve remarkable recovery. Meticulous care in an intensive care unit setting with respiratory and nutritional support is indicated.

Although seizures sometimes complicate encephalitis, prophylactic anticonvulsants are not routinely recommended. If seizures develop, they can usually be managed with phenytoin, valproate, or phenobarbital because these drugs can be given parentally and blood levels can be monitored (see Chapter 426). If status epilepticus ensues, appropriately vigorous therapy should be instituted to prevent secondary brain injury and hypoxia. Similarly, secondary bacterial infections should be sought and promptly treated. Steroids should probably be generally avoided in the treatment of encephalitis because of their inhibitory effects on host immune responses.

Prognosis

Full recovery from viral meningitis usually occurs within 1 to 2 weeks of onset, although some patients describe persistence of fatigue, lightheadedness, and asthenia for months. The prognosis of encephalitis depends on its cause (see Table 439–1). Arbovirus encephalitides have variable mortality rates. Eastern equine encephalitis has the highest mortality rate of all arboviruses, whereas California virus has the lowest. Mortality rates for most viral encephalitides are greater in children younger than 4 years and in the elderly. Nonfatal encephalitis caused by eastern equine, western equine, West Nile, and St. Louis viruses has a relatively high rate of neurologic sequelae. Encephalitis associated with mumps or lymphocytic choriomeningitis virus rarely leads to death, and sequelae are infrequent. The most common complication after mumps meningoencephalitis is sensorineural deafness. Hydrocephalus from aqueductal stenosis has been reported as a late sequela of mumps meningitis and encephalitis in children.

SUGGESTED READINGS

Steiner I, Budka H, Chaudhuri A, et al: Viral encephalitis: A review of diagnostic methods and guidelines for management. Eur J Neurol 2005;12:331–343. *Evidence-based recommendations regarding diagnosis and treatment.*

Tyler KL, Pape J, Goody RJ, et al: CSF findings in 250 patients with serologically confirmed West Nile virus meningitis and encephalitis. Neurology 2006;66:361–365. *CSF findings are correlated with clinical manifestation and outcome.*

440 POLIOMYELITIS

Avindra Nath and Joseph R. Berger

Definition

Poliomyelitis (acute anterior poliomyelitis, infantile paralysis) is an acute illness caused by the three strains of poliovirus. The disease selectively destroys the motor neurons of the spinal cord and brain stem, thereby resulting in flaccid asymmetrical weakness. Through the mid-20th century, poliomyelitis was one of the most feared of all human infectious diseases; however, it is now almost entirely preventable by vaccination.

Etiology

The antigenically different strains of poliovirus (types 1, 2, and 3) are classified in the genus Enterovirus within the family Picornaviridae. They are small (approximately 27 nm), roughly spherical particles with icosahedral symmetry that contain a single-stranded RNA core surrounded by a protein capsid. The majority of disease is caused by the type 1 strain. Lacking a lipid envelope, the polioviruses are resistant to lipid solvents and are stable at low pH.

Epidemiology

Since the World Health Assembly resolved in May 1988 to eradicate poliomyelitis, the estimated number of polio cases globally has declined more than 99%, and nearly 55% of the world's population is considered polio free. About 80% of the world's cases occur in India, although some African countries, particularly those engaged in ongoing warfare, continue to have low immunization rates with high rates of disease. In the United States, the number of cases of paralytic poliomyelitis has fallen to just a few cases yearly because of the widespread use of an effective vaccine (Chapter 16). Polio is more frequent during the summer in temperate zones but has a more even distribution throughout the year in tropical areas. Poliovirus is acquired by the oral route and subsequently replicates in the oropharynx and lower gastrointestinal tract. It may be secreted for a week or two in saliva and for more prolonged periods in feces, which provide the major avenue of host-to-host transmission. Spread of polioviruses is greatly influenced by standards of hygiene, and the greatest risk occurs within families or other crowded circumstances.

Paralysis is an unusual complication of poliovirus infection. During an epidemic, only 1 to 2% of infections result in neurologic symptoms and signs; another 4 to 8% of infected persons suffer nonspecific (minor) illness. Although polio occurs most commonly in preschool children, other factors increase the incidence of paralytic disease, including advanced age, recent strenuous exercise, tonsillectomy, pregnancy, and impairment of B-lymphocyte (antibody) defenses. Immunity to each of the three types of poliovirus is lifelong, but infection with one strain does not protect against subsequent infection by another. In the United States, the incidence of poliomyelitis from live attenuated strains, though extremely rare, parallels that of wild-type virus occurring in nonimmunized subjects.

Pathobiology

Polioviruses selectively infect specific neuronal populations and induce highly stereotyped pathologic processes; in this manner they contrast with most of the viruses that cause acute encephalitis or meningitis. The unique susceptibility of anterior horn cells (motor neurons) may be due to the presence of a higher density of viral receptors or spread of the virus along motor nerve fibers.

The poliovirus invades the nervous system only after prior systemic replication. An initial alimentary phase with local replication in the intestinal mucosa and spread to the local lymphatics is followed by viremia, which seeds the nervous system. The virus may replicate in skeletal muscle and be transported via peripheral nerves to the spinal cord; this mechanism of spread may contribute to the myalgia that precedes the onset of weakness. Convalescent poliomyelitis is characterized by loss of motor neurons and denervation atrophy of their associated skeletal muscles.

Clinical Manifestations

Acute poliomyelitis is separated into two distinct phases: "minor illness" and "major illness." The minor illness coincides with viremia and consists of fever, headache, and sore throat, which resolve within 1 to 2 days. In some patients this phase is followed by the major illness, which is characterized by an abrupt onset of fever, headache, vomiting, and meningismus. Cerebrospinal fluid (CSF) pleocytosis is present at this stage. The symptoms of aseptic meningitis resolve within 5 to 10 days. Asymmetrical muscle weakness, which is the hallmark of the illness, is typically preceded by intense myalgia. The proximal muscles are more commonly involved, and legs are involved more often than arms. In mild cases, paralysis affects only parts of muscles rather than selective peripheral nerve or nerve root distributions. Sensory changes are lacking. The paralysis may render one limb useless yet entirely spare the contralateral arm or leg. Acute urinary retention develops in about 50% of patients. The trunk musculature is least commonly affected. The affected muscles are flaccid, and deep tendon reflexes may be absent. Atrophy develops rapidly, usually beginning within a week in paralyzed muscles and progressing over the ensuing weeks. The motor deficit rarely progresses for more than 3 to 5 days.

In 10 to 15% of cases and especially in young adults, the lower brain stem motor nuclei are affected. Involvement of the ninth and tenth cranial nerve nuclei leads to paralysis of the pharyngeal and laryngeal musculature (bulbar poliomyelitis). Parts of the facial muscles may be involved, either unilaterally or bilaterally. Less often, the tongue and muscles of mastication are paralyzed. External oculomotor weakness occurs rarely, and the pupils are invariably spared. Direct involvement of the brain stem reticular formation can disrupt breathing and swallowing and produce serious disturbances in cardiovascular control, including hypertension, hypotension, and cardiac arrhythmias.

Diagnosis

In poliomyelitis, CSF shows increased protein content and pleocytosis with a normal glucose concentration. The virus is more commonly isolated from the nasopharynx or stool than from CSF. Molecular diagnosis with polymerase chain reaction is now the technique of choice for identifying the poliovirus serotype and for differentiating between wild and vaccine strain poliomyelitis.

Differential Diagnosis

Because of its rarity in the United States, poliomyelitis may present diagnostic difficulties. Its early phases must be differentiated from other acute meningitides; when paralysis ensues, a major differential diagnosis is postinfectious polyneuropathy or Guillain-Barré syndrome (Chapter 446). Illnesses virtually identical to poliomyelitis have been reported rarely with other enteroviruses, the flaviviruses, (such as Japanese B and West Nile virus infection), tick-borne encephalitis, and human immunodeficiency virus infection. Furthermore, motor neuron disease has been reported with some herpes virus infections (Chapter 397) such as cytomegalovirus, Epstein-Barr virus, and varicella-zoster virus. Other infectious illnesses that must be considered in the differential diagnosis are rabies, Lyme disease, *Mycoplasma, Borrelia,* diphtheria, and botulism. Careful neurologic examination can distinguish other entities that might be confused with poliomyelitis because they affect different areas of the neuraxis (peripheral nerve, spinal cord, neuromuscular junction, or muscle).

Treatment

Rx

No specific treatment is available, but supportive care is important in reducing pain during the acute attack and in maintaining vital functions to ensure survival. Bedrest and treatment of pain are recommended during the myalgic phase. Important measures include preventing contractures, maintaining airway and cardiovascular stability, and preventing bed sores and excessive mobilization of calcium. Acute respiratory failure requiring intubation and intermittent positive pressure ventilation may develop rapidly. If prolonged ventilation is needed or coexisting bulbar weakness is present, tracheostomy may be necessary to protect the airway.

Prognosis

Death in patients with poliomyelitis is usually the result of bulbar involvement and is attributable to respiratory and cardiovascular impairment. Mortality has been considerably reduced with modern management of respiratory insufficiency. Patients who survive an episode of acute paralytic poliomyelitis usually recover considerable motor function. Generally, motor improvement begins within the first weeks after onset, and 60% of eventual recovery is achieved by 3 months.

The Postpolio Syndrome

In a number of patients with previous poliomyelitis, further motor deterioration develops later in life. In some, this worsening relates simply to musculoskeletal decompensation or other factors but does not involve new weakness. However, other persons suffer a true loss of strength, termed *postpolio syndrome.* This disorder is characterized by an insidiously progressive weakness typically beginning 30 or more years after an attack of poliomyelitis. Most commonly, it adds to the weakness of already affected muscles; less often, weakness develops in muscles previously thought to be normal. This weakness is often accompanied by fasciculations, and additional atrophy may develop. Muscle biopsy shows type grouping consistent with chronic denervation-reinnervation. Overall, the prognosis is good, with slow progression of further weakness, which only rarely leads to a severe increase in disability or death. The most likely pathogenesis consists of senescence of the surviving expanded motor units. In all cases it is imperative to exclude coincidental unrelated disease.

Prevention

Poliomyelitis can be prevented by live attenuated or killed polio vaccines, which are now given routinely. The practice of immunization has relaxed as the threat of development of paralytic poliomyelitis has become less conspicuous. The World Health Organization plan to eradicate polio has had a substantial impact; however, polio is still endemic in some countries and vaccine-associated polio also occurs.

SUGGESTED READINGS

Alexander LN, Seward FJ, Santibanez TA, et al: Vaccine policy changes and epidemiology of poliomyelitis in the United States. JAMA 2004;292:1696–1701. *The change to inactivated polio virus vaccine has eliminated vaccine-induced polio.*

Howard RS: Poliomyelitis and the postpolio syndrome. BMJ 2005;330:1314–1319. *Useful review.*

Sejvar JJ: West Nile virus and "poliomyelitis." Neurology 2004;63:206–207. *In the United States, West Nile virus is now a much more frequent cause of acute anterior horn cell disease than poliomyelitis is.*

Trojan DA, Cashman NR: Postpoliomyelitis syndrome. Muscle Nerve 2005;31:6–19. *This uncommon syndrome is of concern to the thousands of patients who had poliomyelitis before its prevention.*

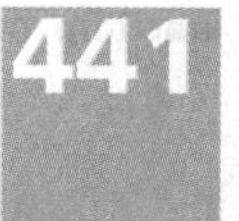

441 RABIES

Avindra Nath and Joseph R. Berger

Definition

Rabies is a viral infection with nearly worldwide distribution. It affects principally wild and domestic animals, but it also results in a devastating, almost invariably fatal encephalitis in humans.

Rabies virus is a bullet-shaped, enveloped, single-stranded RNA virus classified in the Rhabdoviridae family (*rhabdos,* Greek for *rod*) and Lyssavirus genus (*lyssa,* Greek for *frenzy*). It has particular neurotropic properties, and unlike many of the other viruses causing acute encephalitis, it appears to require central nervous system (CNS) infection as an essential part of its life cycle.

Epidemiology

The epidemiology of rabies varies in different parts of the world, with two patterns being recognized. In *sylvatic rabies,* infection is maintained in wildlife reservoirs. In the United States (Fig. 441–1), rabies is endemic in the striped skunk in the Midwestern states and California, in the raccoon in the southeastern and mid-Atlantic states, in the red fox in northern New York and adjacent regions of Canada, and in the gray fox in parts of the southwestern states. Domestic dogs, which are at risk of acquiring rabies from exposure to these animals, may in turn bite humans. Bat rabies has a wide geographic range, and reports of human rabies have been associated with contact with bats without an actual bat bite. In western Europe, human rabies is rare and more often results from direct contact with wildlife than from contact with domestic dogs or cats. This pattern contrasts with that in much of Asia, Africa, and Latin America, where *urban rabies* is maintained as an epizootic infection in the domestic dog, and human disease is far more common. Viral strains differ among various animal hosts. Human-to-human transmission can also occur.

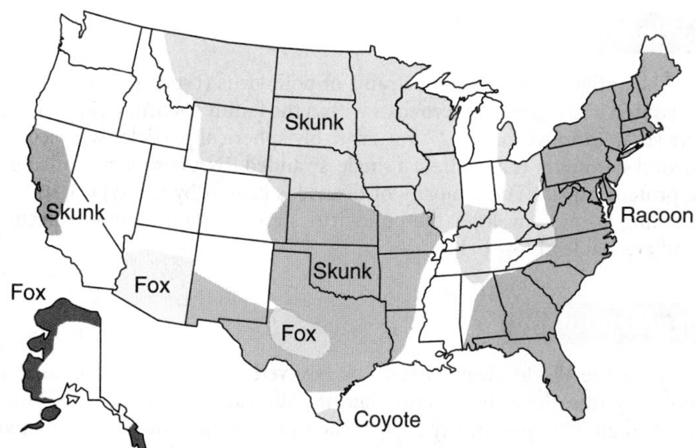

FIGURE 441–1 • Distribution of rabies in the United States. (Available from http://www.cdc.gov/ncidod/dvrd/rabies/Epidemiology/Epidemiology.htm.)

Pathobiology

Pathogenesis

Viral transmission to animals and humans characteristically results from the bite of a rabid animal, although cases have been transmitted by aerosol in the laboratory or in a bat cave and by transplantation of infected corneal tissue and solid organs. After the virus breaches the protective epithelium, it reaches the CNS through peripheral nerves and exploits retrograde axoplasmic transport by using the neuronal microtubulin network. The interval between the bite and the onset of disease ranges from days to more than a year, but in most cases it is 1 to 2 months. This delay may be related to amplification of the virus in peripheral tissues, particularly skeletal muscle, before it gains access to the CNS through motor and sensory nerves. The incubation period is shorter, 20 to 30 days, in post-transplant patients. Viral entry is mediated via the nicotinic acetylcholine receptor at the neuromuscular junction. The p75 neurotropic receptor can also mediate viral entry into neurons. It is this delay that provides the opportunity for the virus to be eliminated by host immune mechanisms and by prophylactic postexposure immunization after a rabid animal bite. After virus enters peripheral and CNS pathways, immune defenses are unable to suppress further replication and spread of infection.

The CNS is involved in subsequent transmission of the virus by infected animals in two essential ways: (1) infection of certain brain regions, in particular, the limbic system, causes characteristic behavioral changes in the rabid animal that lead to increased biting activity, and (2) antegrade or centrifugal transport of the virus from the brain to highly innervated areas (e.g., the salivary glands, cornea, skin) leads to shedding of the virus. In concert, these two aspects of infection ensure transmission and survival of the virus in the wild. They also have practical diagnostic implications for human disease. The characteristic altered behavior in humans often results in a distinct clinical picture that distinguishes rabies from other viral encephalitides. Antegrade virus transport also affords a means of diagnosing rabies by isolation from saliva or immunohistochemical staining of various tissues, including corneal impressions, buccal mucosa, or skin, where the virus can be found in cutaneous nerves innervating hair follicles. Humoral immune responses and neutralizing antibodies generated by rabies vaccine are important in tempering the virus; however, animal studies suggest that cell-mediated immune responses are also critical.

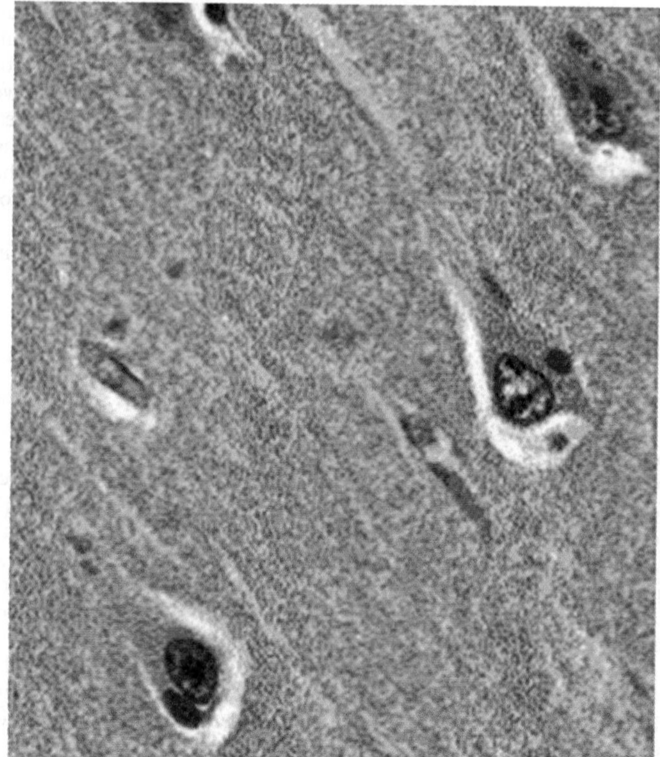

FIGURE 441–2 • Histopathology of rabies encephalitis. The pathognomonic eosinophilic Negri bodies are present in pyramidal neurons. (Courtesy of Drs. S.K. Shankar and A. Mahadervan, National Institute of Mental Health and Neurosciences, Bangalore, India.)

Pathology

Negri bodies, which are eosinophilic neuronal intracytoplasmic inclusion bodies composed of viral nucleoprotein, are pathognomonic of rabies virus infection but are observed in only 75 to 80% of cases (Fig. 441–2). At autopsy, infection is usually widespread in the brain, but the brain stem, spinal cord, hippocampus, basal ganglia, cortex, and other structures are also prominently involved. The relationship of viral infection of neurons and the attendant inflammatory reaction to the clinical manifestations remains incompletely understood. Rabies infection of neurons may alter their membrane properties or synaptic transmission.

Clinical Manifestations

Clinical rabies usually begins with a prodrome of nonspecific malaise, fever, and headache. More specific local symptoms at the site of the original bite include itching, paresthesia, or other sensations that begin in the area of the healed wound and then spread to a wider region as a result of ganglioneuritis. No accompanying sensory loss occurs.

Within a few days, the full-blown illness takes one of two forms: encephalitic *(furious)* or paralytic *(dumb)* rabies, perhaps depending on the source and strain of the infecting virus. In its initial phase, encephalitic rabies is often distinguished from other viral infections by irritability and muscle hyperactivity. Periods of lucidity may alternate with confusion and intense anxiety precipitated by internal or external stimuli. Hydrophobia, with intense reflexive contraction of the diaphragm and accessory respiratory and other muscles, is induced by attempts to drink or even by the mere sight of water. Similarly, blowing or fanning air on the chest may induce intense laryngeal, pharyngeal, or other muscle spasms (i.e., aerophobia). High fever persists throughout the illness. Patients may also have spontaneous inspiratory spasms and autonomic dysfunction (i.e., hypersalivation, nonreactive pupils, and piloerection). Seizures are rare.

Paralytic rabies is less common and is often misdiagnosed. Patients demonstrate weakness, usually beginning in the bitten extremity and spreading to involve all four limbs and the facial muscles early in the course. Consciousness and sensory function are spared. Areflexia often suggests Guillain-Barré syndrome (Chapter 446). As the disease progresses, it may converge with the encephalitic form and be accompanied by irritative phenomena. Both forms evolve into lethargy and coma with prominent respiratory and cardiovascular dysfunction. Patients may have arrhythmias and irregular breathing patterns such as cluster or periodic respirations. Patients die of respiratory failure or cardiovascular collapse within a mean interval of 4 to 7 days from onset. Intensive supportive care may rarely extend survival. Rare patients with partial vaccine-induced immunity have survived with intensive care.

Diagnosis

Rabies is usually suspected on the basis of a history of an animal bite or other exposure. However, in as many as a third of cases, no such history is obtained. Reverse transcriptase–polymerase chain reaction can detect rabies virus RNA in CNS tissue, saliva, cerebrospinal fluid (CSF), tears, skin biopsy samples, and urine within 3 days of the onset of clinical features. Definitive antemortem diagnosis can also be established by immunohistochemical identification of rabies virus antigen in hair follicle nerve endings of biopsied skin, usually obtained from the nape of the neck, buccal mucosa, or corneal impressions. Isolation of virus from saliva or the presence of antirabies antibodies in blood in the absence of vaccination or in CSF may also establish the diagnosis.

Magnetic resonance imaging is nondiagnostic and may show hyperintense lesions in areas of the cortex, periventricular region, basal ganglia, and elsewhere on T2-weighted fluid-attenuated inversion recovery (FLAIR) images. Enhancement with gadolinium usually occurs only in late stages of the illness. Findings on computed tomography of the brain are typically normal. CSF examination generally reveals normal or slightly raised pressure, a normal cell count, mildly increased protein (<100 mg/mL), and normal glucose; a lymphocytic pleocytosis is occasionally observed. Postmortem diagnosis is usually made by immunohistochemical examination of the brain.

The differential diagnosis depends on the clinical manifestation and the epidemiologic setting. Paralytic rabies is most often confused with Guillain-Barré syndrome (Chapter 446) or poliomyelitis (Chapter 440), whereas the encephalitic form must be differentiated from other viral and infectious encephalitides (Chapter 439), tetanus (Chapter 319), and toxic encephalopathies. In geographic regions where vaccine is prepared with neural tissue (still the practice in many regions of the world with the highest rates of rabies), allergic encephalomyelitis remains a principal differential diagnosis.

Treatment

Rx

Death usually occurs within 1 week of the onset of symptoms, and the disease has been regarded as invariably fatal. However, one reported survivor was treated with ribavirin at a loading dose of 33 mg/kg followed by a maintenance dose of 16 mg/kg every 6 hours. After a cumulative total of 276 mg/kg of ribavirin had been administered, ribavirin was reduced to 8 mg/kg for nine doses. The patient also received amantadine (200 mg/day for 3 weeks) and was managed in a coma that was induced with ketamine and midazolam.

Prevention

Prevention relies on public health measures to reduce animal reservoirs and on postexposure immune prophylaxis to abort viral penetration of the CNS after a rabid bite or other contact. Although clinical rabies is a rare disease in the United States and western Europe, the need to consider active prophylaxis is a common clinical issue. Postexposure prophylaxis is uniformly successful if the protocol is followed rigorously (see later), but even slight deviations from the protocol can result in treatment failure and lead to the development of rabies. The physician first determines the type of possible exposure. An open wound or disrupted mucous membrane exposed to saliva may warrant postexposure prophylaxis, whereas contact of saliva with intact skin may not. Although evidence-based practice guidelines have not been developed, bite wounds warrant an organized, standardized approach to care to help prevent complications. The first step in management is to administer prompt local wound care by thoroughly washing the wound with soap and water and then applying iodine or 70% ethanol. Besides rabies, tetanus prophylaxis and antibiotic prophylaxis may also be needed. The epidemiologic setting, which is important in determining the likelihood that the biting animal may be rabid, often requires consultation with local health authorities to ascertain which animals carry rabies in the geographic region.

In the absence of previous vaccination, both passive (i.e., rabies immune globulin of human origin) and active (i.e., diploid cell vaccines) immunizations are administered. Rabies immunoglobulin (20 IU/kg) should be injected in and around the wound, and the remaining volume should be given intramuscularly at a site distant from the vaccine site. Safe, tissue culture–derived vaccines with a low incidence of major adverse reactions are now available. Five doses of rabies vaccine (1 mL each) should be given in the deltoid muscle on days 0, 3, 7, 14, and 28 in individuals not previously immunized against rabies virus.

SUGGESTED READINGS

http://www.cdc.gov/mmwr. *Website hosted by the Centers for Disease Control and Prevention, which periodically updates current practice recommendations for immunization for rabies and other infectious diseases.*

Jackson AC: Rabies: New insights into pathogenesis and treatment. Curr Opin Neurol 2006;19:267–270. *A comprehensive review.*

Morgan M, Palmer J: Dog bites. BMJ 2007;334:413–417. *A review of this topic, including rabies.*

Rupprecht CE, Gibbons RV: Prophylaxis against rabies. N Engl J Med 2004;351:2626–2635. *A careful review.*

Srinivasan A, Burton EC, Kuehnert MJ, et al: Transmission of rabies virus from an organ donor to four transplant recipients. N Engl J Med 2005;352:1103–1111. *This report highlights the challenges of preventing and detecting transmission of unusual pathogens through transplantation.*

Willoughby RE, Tieves KS, Hoffman GM, et al: Survival after treatment of rabies with induction of coma. N Engl J Med 2005;352:1508–2514. *A well-documented case report.*

442 PRION DISEASES

Martin Zeidler

Definition

Prion diseases are a group of relentlessly progressive and fatal human and animal neurodegenerative conditions associated with the deposition of abnormal prion protein (PrP) in the brain. The most common human form is Creutzfeldt-Jakob disease (CJD), a syndrome that can be manifested as a genetic, infectious (including "variant"), or sporadic disorder. All forms of prion disease are experimentally transmissible to animals.

Epidemiology

The annual incidence of CJD is approximately one per million. The majority of cases arise sporadically (i.e., appear to occur randomly). Sporadic CJD has a mean age at onset of 65 years (range, 14 to 92) and no clear sex or racial bias. About 10 to 15% of human prion disease is inherited (autosomal dominant) as familial CJD or the extremely rare disorders fatal familial insomnia and Gerstmann-Sträussler-Scheinker disease. Infectious (variant) CJD has been reported in several settings. More than 260 cases of iatrogenic variant CJD have been documented to be due to medical treatment with pituitary-derived hormones, dura mater grafts, or contaminated neurosurgical instruments.

Kuru

Kuru is a prion disease confined to the people originating from a number of adjacent valleys in the mountainous interior of Papua New Guinea. It was first described in 1955 and was subsequently shown to have arisen from infection by brain tissue as a result of the practice of ritualistic cannibalism. Since the cessation of this practice toward the end of the 1950s, the disease has become rare.

Bovine Spongiform Encephalopathy

Bovine spongiform encephalopathy (BSE or mad cow disease), a prion disease of cattle, was first recognized in the mid-1980s in the United Kingdom. An epidemic ensued and reached a peak in 1989. More than one million infected cattle were thought to have been used for human food in the United Kingdom, and the first cases of the human form of BSE (termed variant CJD) were identified in 1995. Human cases have subsequently been reported in more than 160 people in the United Kingdom, more than 15 in France, and rare individuals in Canada, Hong Kong, Italy, Japan, the Netherlands, Saudi Arabia, Spain, Portugal, and the United States. Probable cases of human-to-human transmission of variant CJD via blood transfusion have been identified.

Chronic wasting disease is a prion disease of deer that is prevalent in the United States. Transmission to humans has not been documented.

Pathobiology

The term "prion" derives from *pro*teinaceous *in*fectious particle (the "o" and "i" being switched for convenience). PrP is a normal protease-sensitive membrane protein. In the disease state, PrP is converted into a malrotated form that is protease resistant and forms amyloid. Once formed, this abnormal PrP promotes the conversion of more normal PrP to the malrotated form. It is hypothesized that mutations associated with familial prion disease lead to the production of unstable PrP, which has a tendency to twist into the abnormal form. In sporadic CJD, the malrotated PrP is thought to occur as a rare spontaneous event. In the infective form of disease, the inoculated malrotated PrP initiates the chain reaction of converting normal host PrP to the malrotated form. How the deposition of abnormal PrP leads to the characteristic neuropathologic features of prion disease (cortical spongiform change, proliferation of astrocytes, and neuronal loss) is unclear.

Clinical Manifestations

The classic diagnostic triad of sporadic CJD is rapidly progressive dementia, myoclonus, and a characteristic periodic electroencephalogram (EEG). Patients usually demonstrate (in order of decreasing frequency) cognitive decline, ataxia, or visual disturbance, either alone or in combination. Less common initial features include behavioral disturbance or rapid evolution resembling a stroke. Dementia is invariably present during the course of the illness. Myoclonus (electric shock–type movements), though a rare initial feature, is observed at some stage in 80% of cases. Visual abnormalities include nonspecific blurring, visual field defects, perceptual abnormalities, and occasionally, hallucinations. Seizures virtually never occur at presentation and are observed later in the clinical course in only 10% of patients. As the disease progresses, multifocal central nervous system (CNS) failure occurs with increasing global cognitive dysfunction, urinary incontinence, ataxia, and dependency; the patient eventually becomes bed bound, rigid, mute, and unresponsive.

Physical signs correspond with the global CNS involvement and may include a combination of cerebellar, pyramidal, and extrapyramidal signs. Primitive reflexes, paratonic rigidity (involuntary, but apparently active resistance to passive limb movement), cortical blindness, and akinetic mutism are also common, whereas lower motor neuron signs are rarely observed. Myoclonus, which is probably the most important clinical sign, usually shows some asymmetry; is typically arrhythmic, asynchronous, and sensitive to stimuli; and is noted most frequently in the limbs but also commonly affects the body and face. Stimulus-sensitive myoclonus or a startle reaction can occur in response to a sudden noise, visual threat, touch, or muscle stretch; however, myoclonus can usually also be noted at rest.

Although dementia and myoclonus are common to all human prion disease, there are differences in the phenotypes of the various subtypes. Variant CJD is typically first manifested as painful sensory disturbance or psychiatric symptoms, and the mean age at death is 29 years. Familial disease on average develops a decade earlier than sporadic CJD and has a highly variable phenotype, including a course clinically identical to sporadic disease and an illness with a prolonged prodrome of psychiatric disturbance that can extend for more than a decade. The clinical course of iatrogenic CJD relates to the mode of infection: peripherally acquired disease (e.g., after human growth hormone injections) tends to be characterized by progressive cerebellar ataxia, whereas central infection (e.g., contaminated neurosurgical instruments) leads to an illness more akin to typical sporadic CJD.

Diagnosis

Routine blood test results are usually normal. Cerebrospinal fluid (CSF) characteristically lacks a pleocytosis or fall in glucose, but an elevated protein level (only very rarely greater than 100 mg/dL) occurs in about 40% of cases. Detection of 14-3-3 protein, a marker of neuronal damage, in CSF has high specificity (94%) and sensitivity (84%) for the diagnosis of sporadic CJD when measured in patients with a reasonable likelihood of CJD.

Familial CJD can be diagnosed by analysis of the PrP gene. More than 20 different point or insert mutations have been identified. A methionine/valine (M/V) polymorphism at codon 129 of the PrP gene has been shown to influence susceptibility to sporadic CJD, as well as clinical phenotype and neuropathology. To date, all cases of variant CJD have been homozygous for methionine at codon 129. Differences in electrophoretic motility of PrP (designated types 1 and 2) occur in sporadic CJD. Combining electrophoresis with codon 129 status leads to six molecular strains: MM1, MM2, MV1, MV2, VV1, and VV2. The molecular strain has been reported to correlate with clinical subtype; for example, the rare VV1 cases are characterized by a long duration (average of 21 months), early age at onset (average of 45), and lack of a periodic EEG.

The EEG is usually abnormal and often shows nonspecific slowing. Characteristic periodic complexes, which are sharp waves occurring every 0.5 to 2 seconds, occur in approximately two thirds of cases, and this appearance is strongly supportive of a diagnosis of sporadic CJD, although it is rarely seen in variant CJD or other conditions such as Alzheimer's disease.

Brain magnetic resonance imaging (MRI) shows bilateral high signal in the striatum in about two thirds of patients with sporadic CJD but in only 7% of controls. About 80% of cases may have linear areas of cortical high signal on diffusion-weighted imaging. The characteristic MRI appearance of variant CJD is bilateral hyperintensity in the pulvinar of the thalamus, a finding observed in about 90% of patients.

Differential Diagnosis

Conditions that most often mimic CJD are Alzheimer's disease, vascular dementia, and dementia with Lewy bodies (Chapter 425). Treatable disorders that can cause a CJD-like illness include Hashimoto's encephalopathy (Chapter 244), drug-induced states (reported with bismuth, amitriptyline, mianserin, lithium, and baclofen), limbic encephalitis, cerebral vasculitis (Chapter 291), and Wilson's disease (Chapter 230).

Treatment

Rx

No medication has been shown to alter the course of genetic, sporadic, or variant CJD. Information on patient care and infection control issues has been published by the World Health Organization and is available at *http://whqlibdoc.who.int/hq/2000/WHO_CDS_CSR_APH_2000.3.pdf.*

Prognosis

The median survival of patients with sporadic CJD is 4.5 months (mean, 8 months), and only 4% survive longer than 2 years. The average duration of variant CJD is 14 months. The duration of illness in iatrogenic CJD relates to the route of infection: disease acquired by parenteral growth hormone injection is more prolonged than in centrally infected cases (e.g., via neurosurgical instruments). The survival of patients with familial prion disease relates to the associated mutation and ranges from months to many years.

OTHER RARE PRION DISEASES

Gerstmann-Sträussler is a rare disease of progressive cerebellar dysfunction associated with mutations in the PrP gene at codons 102, 117, or 198.

Fatal familial insomnia is associated with mutation of asparagine for aspartate at codon 178. Patients have intractable insomnia, often have sympathetic hyperactivity, and may demonstrate other characteristics of CJD.

Future Directions

Much is unknown about the nature and properties of the transmissible agent associated with prion disease. Furthering our understanding of these issues will, it is hoped, lead to presymptomatic screening, methods to identify and remove infectivity from biologic and food products, and development of a treatment to reverse or prevent the disease.

SUGGESTED READINGS

Bosque P: Molecular types of Creutzfeldt-Jakob disease: The strange diversity of prions. Neurology 2005;65:1520–1521. *Succinct consideration of this puzzling infectious agent.*

Collinge J, Whitfield J, McKintosh E, et al: Kuru in the 21st century—an acquired human prion disease with very long incubation periods. Lancet 2006;367:2068–2074. *Kuru provides the principal experience of epidemic human prion disease.*

Collins SJ, Lawson VA, Masters CL: Transmissible spongiform encephalopathies. Lancet 2004;363:51–61. *A useful review.*

Shiga Y, Miyazawa K, Sato S, et al: Diffusion-weighted MRI abnormalities as an early diagnostic marker for Creutzfeldt-Jakob disease. Neurology 2004;63:443–449. *Imaging can be useful for CJD.*

Westergard L, Christensen HM, Harris DA: The cellular prion protein (PrP[C]): Its physiological function and role in disease. Biochim Biophys Acta 2007;1772:629–644. *Review of the proposed functions for PrP(C), including protection against apoptotic and oxidative stress, uptake of copper, transmembrane signaling, formation and maintenance of synapses, and adhesion.*

443 NUTRITION- AND ALCOHOL-RELATED NEUROLOGIC DISORDERS

John C. M. Brust

Neurologic disease is associated with deficiency of certain nutrients. In developing countries, such deficiencies are usually the result of starvation or a restricted diet. In developed countries, the major causes are alcoholism (Chapter 31) and, less often, malabsorption syndromes (Chapter 143), chronic illness with cachexia, food faddism, psychiatric disease, infantile malnutrition, and rarely, genetic disorders. The most clearly defined nutritional disorders of the nervous system are associated with a deficiency of particular vitamins—organic compounds that are required for normal metabolic functions but are not synthesized in the body (Chapter 237). Vitamins are either water soluble or fat soluble, and deficiency of fat-soluble vitamins is a feature of malabsorption disorders (e.g., unavailability of bile acids, pancreatic insufficiency, sprue). With the exception of cobalamin, deficiency of water-soluble vitamins is generally secondary to inadequate intake. Such malnutrition seldom produces selective avitaminosis, and the resulting neurologic symptoms and signs therefore reflect multiple deficiencies.

NUTRITION-RELATED NEUROLOGIC DISORDERS

Excessive intake of certain fat-soluble vitamins can be toxic. Symptomatic hypervitaminosis is less often encountered with water-soluble vitamins, which are much more rapidly excreted.

Inadequate Intake of Water-Soluble Vitamins

Thiamine (Vitamin B_1)

Thiamine in the body is converted to thiamine pyrophosphate, which is a coenzyme in a number of steps in glucose metabolism. Although the adult daily requirement seldom exceeds 2 mg, limited body storage means that inadequate intake can produce symptomatic deficiency in only a few weeks or months. In developing countries, thiamine deficiency most often produces beriberi with high-output cardiac failure and sensorimotor polyneuropathy. Acute thiamine deficiency can cause fatal lactic acidosis. In North America and Europe, thiamine deficiency most often affects alcoholics and causes the Wernicke-Korsakoff syndrome (see later).

Niacin

Epidemiology and Pathobiology

Niacin, also called nicotinic acid, is converted in the body to nicotinamide adenine dinucleotide (NAD) or nicotinamide adenine dinucleotide phosphate (NADP), which are coenzymes in tissue respiration. Deficiency of niacin or its precursor tryptophan causes pellagra, which in developed countries is most often encountered in alcoholics, in whom additional nutritional deficiencies are likely to be present. A pathologic characteristic is widespread central nervous system (CNS) neuronal chromatolysis.

Clinical Manifestations and Diagnosis

Pellagra is characterized by a triad of dermatologic, gastrointestinal, and neurologic symptoms. An erythematous and later hyperpigmented rash appears on light-exposed areas. Glossitis and enteritis can be severe and give rise to nausea, vomiting, and watery or bloody diarrhea. Neurologic abnormalities include altered mentation (irritability, insomnia, and fatigue progressing to depression, impaired memory, dementia, psychosis, delirium, or coma), sensorimotor polyneuropathy, myelopathy, myoclonus, seizures, cerebellar ataxia, parkinsonism, retinitis, and optic atrophy. When niacin is used to treat hyperlipidemia, large doses are associated with flushing, vomiting, diarrhea, hepatic dysfunction, lactic acidosis, delirium, and retinal maculopathy.

Treatment and Prognosis

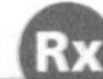

Treatment of pellagra is administration of niacin or nicotinamide plus other vitamins. Response is usually rapid, but mental abnormalities can be permanent.

Pyridoxine (Vitamin B_6)

Vitamin B_6 consists of pyridoxine, pyridoxol, and pyridoxamine, each of which is converted in the body to pyridoxal phosphate, a cofactor for several enzymes. More common than dietary deficiency of pyridoxine are conditions of pyridoxine dependency. Neonates and infants with recessively inherited glutamic acid decarboxylase deficiency have seizures that are refractory to conventional anticonvulsants but responsive to pyridoxine in doses several times the daily requirement.

Pathobiology

Pyridoxine is a cofactor for the trans-sulfuration of homocysteine to cystathionine. Pyridoxine deficiency will therefore aggravate hyperhomocysteinemia in patients with low levels of folic acid or cobalamin, thereby potentially further increasing the risk for cardiovascular disease.

Isoniazid inhibits an enzyme that converts pyridoxine to its active form, and hydralazine converts pyridoxine to an inactive hydrazone; peripheral neuropathy or even CNS symptoms can develop in patients receiving either of these drugs unless supplemental pyridoxine is given.

Clinical Manifestations and Diagnosis

Pyridoxine deficiency causes seizures and sensorimotor polyneuropathy and probably contributes to the neurologic manifestations of pellagra. Severe sensory polyneuropathy affects persons taking pyridoxine in megadoses (2 to 6 g/day for 2 to 40 months; doses in excess of 100 mg/day are never indicated and are unwise because the lower limit of toxicity has not been defined).

Treatment and Prognosis

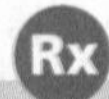

Treatment of deficiency consists of administration of pyridoxine plus other vitamins. Toxic polyneuropathy usually improves after pyridoxine withdrawal but often requires months to years.

Cobalamin (Vitamin B_{12})

Deficiency of cobalamin (Chapter 237) damages the entire neuraxis, with combinations of polyneuropathy, myelopathy ("combined systems disease," "subacute combined degeneration"), encephalopathy, and less often, optic neuropathy.

Epidemiology

Cobalamin deficiency is present in up to 15% of elderly people, who often have other reasons for cognitive and gait disturbance. The diagnosis is thus easy to overlook.

Pathobiology

Nitrous oxide oxidizes cobalamin, thereby inactivating the cobalamin-dependent enzyme methionine synthase. Chronic recreational use of nitrous oxide can produce the symptoms and signs of subacute combined degeneration in the presence of normal serum cobalamin levels (or precipitate such symptoms in subjects with low levels).

Patients with acquired immunodeficiency syndrome (AIDS) often have low serum cobalamin levels, which seem to predict more rapid progression of disease and increased neurologic abnormalities. Vacuolating myelopathy pathologically indistinguishable from combined systems disease is commonly found at autopsies of AIDS patients, including those with normal serum cobalamin levels (Chapter 417). A possible cause is human immunodeficiency virus–or cytokine-induced derangement of cobalamin-dependent transmethylation pathways.

Pathologic features include swelling and vacuolization of myelin sheaths in the CNS, initially affecting the dorsal columns of the spinal cord and then the corticospinal tracts; eventually, over a period of months or years, these changes become widespread and diffuse. Frontal lobe white matter may show patchy demyelination.

Clinical Manifestations

More than a third of patients with documented cobalamin deficiency have neurologic symptoms and signs, which often precede other symptoms. Some patients have earlier fatigue, glossitis, anorexia, vomiting, weight loss, generalized weakness, or syncope as a result of severe anemia. In the great majority of patients, the earliest neurologic symptoms are sensory and consist of paresthesias and numbness in the hands and feet and gait ataxia secondary to proprioceptive loss. The sensory loss is due to peripheral neuropathy, myelopathy, or both. With progression, leg weakness and impaired manual dexterity are noted. Hyperactive tendon reflexes and extensor plantar responses reflect corticospinal tract involvement; decreased tendon reflexes also occur as a result of peripheral neuropathy. Mental symptoms, which rarely occur without other neurologic abnormalities, include memory loss, personality change, dementia, and paranoid psychosis with hallucinations ("megaloblastic madness"). Less frequent symptoms include impotence, urinary incontinence, decreased visual acuity, and anosmia. Nerve conduction studies reveal sensorimotor polyneuropathy with both demyelinating and axonal features.

Diagnosis

More than a fourth of patients with cobalamin deficiency and neurologic symptoms have normal hematocrit levels, mean erythrocyte volumes, or both, and the neurologic abnormalities tend to be more severe in these patients than in those with anemia or macrocytosis. Furthermore, some patients with clinically significant cobalamin deficiency have low-normal serum cobalamin levels. The diagnosis in such instances can be confirmed by the presence of increased serum levels of methylmalonic acid and homocysteine (Chapter 170). Conversely, in subjects with falsely low serum cobalamin levels—a not uncommon occurrence—clinically significant cobalamin deficiency can be excluded by finding normal serum levels of these metabolites.

Treatment

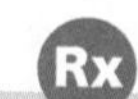

Treatment of cobalamin deficiency is administration of vitamin B_{12}, which can be given orally in high doses except in patients with malabsorption (Chapter 170). With treatment, improvement may take 3 months to begin and then may continue over a period of months or even years. Most patients either make a complete neurologic recovery or improve.

Folic Acid

By donating a methyl group to cobalamin, folic acid becomes available to participate in DNA synthesis; folate supplementation in patients with cobalamin deficiency probably accounts for some, but not all cases of neurologic impairment in the absence of anemia. Folate deficiency results in megaloblastic anemia.

Although low serum folate levels have been associated with depressive disorders and with cognitive decline in the elderly, folate deficiency has not been established as a cause of central or peripheral nervous system disease in adults (Chapters 170 and 237). In the United States, fortification of flour provides roughly 0.2 mg of folic acid daily, a dose that can prevent the occurrence of neural tube defects such as spina bifida and anencephaly. Additional supplementation of 0.4 mg daily is currently recommended for women who might become pregnant. Some studies suggest increasing benefit with up to 5 mg daily. Such doses would mandate monitoring of serum cobalamin levels or prophylactic addition of cobalamin supplementation.

Deficiency of either cobalamin or folate results in elevated blood levels of homocysteine, which is a risk factor for occlusive vascular disease. Although supplemental folic acid, cobalamin, and pyridoxine lower homocysteine levels, they have not been shown to reduce the incidence of recurrent stroke. [1]

Elderly persons with elevated homocysteine levels also have worse cognitive function and more cognitive decline. Supplementation of folate has improved cognitive outcome in some studies but not in others, so no definitive recommendations can be made at this time.

Other Water-Soluble Vitamins

Because other deficiencies are nearly always present, the role of riboflavin, pantothenic acid, or biotin deficiency in neurologic or other disease is difficult to determine. Anecdotal reports and animal experiments suggest a possible relationship to sensory polyneuropathy and myalgia. Ascorbic acid deficiency causes bleeding, which can affect either the central or the peripheral nervous system.

Excessive or Inadequate Intake of Fat-Soluble Vitamins

Vitamin A (Retinol)

Retinol is necessary for the integrity of epithelial tissue and the retina. Deficiency, associated with malnutrition, malabsorption, liver disease, myxedema, diabetes mellitus, or renal failure, causes visual loss secondary to both retinal and corneal damage.

Hypervitaminosis A, most often affecting adolescents taking excessive dosage for acne, causes increased intracranial pressure, which if prolonged, can result in visual loss.

Vitamin D (Calciferol, Cholecalciferol)

Synthesized in the skin, vitamin D is further metabolized in the liver and kidney to its active form 1,25-dihydroxycholecalciferol (Chapter 263). Deficiency is associated with malnutrition, lack of sunlight, malabsorption, liver disease, renal failure, and phenytoin or barbiturate administration; in addition, several hereditary disorders are characterized by vitamin D resistance. Hypovitaminosis D causes rickets in children and osteomalacia in adults. Severe bone disease can produce spinal cord or nerve root symptoms, and hypocalcemia causes tetany, altered mentation, and seizures. Myopathic weakness is described.

Hypervitaminosis D (Chapter 266), from excessive vitamin D intake, malignant or granulomatous disease, hyperparathyroidism, or other endocrinopathy, causes life-threatening hypercalcemia with bone, kidney, and neurologic disease; symptoms include weakness, lassitude, impaired memory, dementia, depression, paranoia, hallucinations, delirium, and coma. Treatment includes saline administration, furosemide diuresis, and sometimes corticosteroids.

Vitamin E (Tocopherols, Tocotrienols)

Vitamin E (Chapter 237) reduces peroxide production, and deficiency occurs in malabsorption disorders, including biliary atresia and cystic fibrosis. In the hereditary disorder abetalipoproteinemia (Bassen-Kornzweig syndrome), steatorrhea, acanthocytosis, decreased serum levels of cholesterol and triglycerides, retinitis pigmentosa, ophthalmoplegia, peripheral neuropathy, and spinocerebellar degeneration with ataxia, amyotrophy, and dorsal column and pyramidal signs are seen. Another hereditary disorder, isolated vitamin E deficiency, clinically resembles Friedreich's ataxia; a hereditary abnormality in vitamin E absorption is the cause.

Vitamin E's antioxidant properties have led to clinical trials in a variety of disorders. Its value in the prevention of cardiovascular disease and some types of cancer is controversial. The weight of evidence suggests that vitamin E is not beneficial in altering the rate of progression of Alzheimer's disease [2] (Chapter 425).

Although the recommended daily allowance of vitamin E is 30 IU, most supplements contain 200 to 800 IU. Reports of possible toxicity include hemorrhagic stroke in men who smoke and acceleration of disease in patients with retinitis pigmentosa.

Vitamin K (Phytonadione, Menaquinones)

Neurologic symptoms in patients with vitamin K deficiency are the result of bleeding. Intracranial hemorrhage may occur in the setting of trauma or hemorrhagic disease of the newborn.

ALCOHOL-RELATED DISORDERS

Alcohol intoxication and withdrawal are discussed in Chapter 31.

Wernicke-Korsakoff Syndrome

Wernicke's and Korsakoff's syndromes are clinically distinct, but they share the same pathology, and each is the result of thiamine deficiency. In alcoholics and others with low thiamine stores, administration of glucose can precipitate acute Wernicke's syndrome.

Pathobiology

The characteristic pathologic lesions of Wernicke's syndrome include loss of neuronal processes, gliosis, and sometimes endothelial proliferation and petechiae—these changes involve the medial thalamus and hypothalamus, midbrain periaqueductal gray matter, and floor of the fourth ventricle. In the cerebellum, neuronal loss affects Purkinje cells especially and is maximal in the vermis. In Korsakoff's syndrome, the lesions are predominantly in the diencephalon and the temporal lobes.

Clinical Manifestations

Wernicke's syndrome evolves over a period of days to weeks and has three features that may occur alone or together: (1) abnormal eye movements, which usually begin with nystagmus and lateral rectus or horizontal gaze paresis and progress to complete ophthalmoplegia, usually with pupillary sparing; (2) ataxia of gait and stance, often accompanied by lower limb intention tremor and dysmetria (the arms are not usually affected, and dysarthria is usually absent); and (3) altered mentation, the earliest signs of which are inattentiveness, mental slowing (abulia), and impaired memory. If patients are not treated, they become lethargic, and their condition progresses to coma and death.

Korsakoff's syndrome is manifested by memory loss, both antegrade and retrograde, out of proportion to the other features. Prominent manifestations include confabulation as well as disorientation to time and place.

Diagnosis

The diagnosis of thiamine deficiency is supported by decreased levels of erythrocyte transketolase, and the lesions of Wernicke's syndrome can sometimes be identified with magnetic resonance imaging (MRI). If the diagnosis is suspected, however, treatment must not be delayed.

Prevention, Treatment, and Prognosis

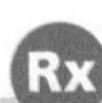

Patients receiving parenteral glucose as part of parenteral alimentation or in an acute setting for the diagnosis and treatment of unexplained seizures or coma should also be given parenteral thiamine (50 to 100 mg) and other water-soluble vitamins, as should persons with suspected Wernicke's syndrome. The therapeutic response is often dramatic. Eye movements sometimes begin to improve within a few hours and, except for residual nystagmus, may be normal within 1 or 2 weeks. Ataxia tends to improve less completely; more than half of patients are left with a broad-based, unsteady gait. Drowsiness, inattentiveness, and apathy tend to clear with treatment, but Korsakoff's syndrome often persists. Once established, the memory disorder is permanent in the majority of patients.

Peripheral Neuropathy

Eighty percent of patients with Wernicke-Korsakoff syndrome also have peripheral neuropathy (Chapter 446), and many alcoholics have peripheral neuropathy without other neurologic symptoms or signs (Chapter 31).

Clinical Manifestations

The earliest symptoms are usually sensory and consist of paresthesias or pain in the feet and later the hands. Absent ankle tendon reflexes and impaired distal vibratory and pain sensation generally precede proprioceptive loss or weakness, but progression to a severe sensorimotor disorder can occur, with proximal as well as distal weakness in addition to vagal symptoms (e.g., hoarseness, dysphagia) and autonomic signs (e.g., tachycardia, postural hypotension). Thiamine deficiency and direct ethanol toxicity each contribute to different features of peripheral neuropathy in alcoholics. Alcoholic neuropathy in the absence of nutritional deficiency is largely sensory, with burning pain, slow progression, and loss of small fiber axons on sural nerve biopsy. Thiamine deficiency neuropathy in nonalcoholics is motor dominant, with rapid progression and loss of large axonal fibers.

Treatment and Prognosis

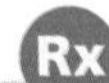

With replacement of thiamine and other vitamins, as well as abstinence from alcohol, symptoms usually improve.

Cerebellar Degeneration

Many alcoholics manifest cerebellar vermal degeneration without other clinical or histologic evidence of Wernicke-Korsakoff syndrome, thus raising the possibility that cerebellar degeneration, though more likely nutritional than toxic in origin, may be less related than Wernicke-Korsakoff syndrome to thiamine deficiency per se.

Clinical Manifestations and Diagnosis

The typical finding is a broad-based ataxic gait with little or no limb ataxia or dysarthria.

Treatment and Prognosis

With abstinence and vitamin replacement, patients usually improve, albeit often incompletely.

Optic Neuropathy

Optic neuropathy in alcoholics—formerly called "tobacco-alcohol amblyopia"—is also nutritional in origin, but the particular deficiencies are uncertain, and the possibility of additional direct toxicity from ethanol, or even the cyanide in tobacco smoke, remains controversial. Bilateral visual loss, usually with central or centrocecal scotomas, may evolve subacutely with swollen optic discs. Improvement follows treatment with multivitamins, but residual visual impairment and temporal disc pallor are often present.

Alcoholic Dementia

In experimental animals, ethanol is directly toxic to neurons, and evidence continues to mount that such toxicity in humans can cause dementia (Chapter 425) in the absence of nutritional disturbance. In nonalcoholics with thiamine deficiency and beriberi, full-blown Wernicke-Korsakoff syndrome infrequently develops, which raises the possibility that excessive ethanol plus nutritional deficiency can produce a pathologic condition that neither insult would cause alone. If ethanol neurotoxicity alone causes clinically significant cognitive disturbance in humans, it is important to identify a safe threshold dose. In fact, a number of population-based studies have shown that high doses of ethanol are associated with dementia but low to moderate doses decrease the risk for both vascular and Alzheimer-type dementia. A special protective effect of red wine, perhaps related to its antioxidant properties, has been suggested in some studies.

Clinical Manifestations and Diagnosis

Whereas Korsakoff's syndrome is predominantly an amnestic disorder affecting recent memory, alcoholics with dementia not evidently caused by nutritional deficiency are more likely to have cognitive dysfunction in additional domains (e.g., executive function, working memory, or abstracting), but the distinction is not clear-cut. Alcoholics often have enlarged cerebral ventricles and widened sulci on imaging. Brain shrinkage sometimes improves with abstinence from alcohol, but whether radiographic improvement is associated with improved mental function is uncertain.

Treatment and Prognosis

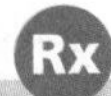

Treatment of alcoholic dementia consists of abstinence and nutritional supplementation. Progression of cognitive dysfunction after abstinence suggests an additional disorder such as Alzheimer's disease.

Myopathy

Patients with alcoholic myopathy are often malnourished, but direct toxicity is more important than nutritional deficiency. Other factors, most importantly hypokalemia, are often present and contribute to the muscle necrosis and myoglobinuria. The myopathy (Chapter 447) can be either chronic, with progressive proximal weakness, or acute, with rhabdomyolysis (Chapter 114), severe muscle weakness and pain, and myoglobinuria causing renal failure. Serum creatine kinase levels are elevated, and findings on electromyography are reflective of myopathy. Alcoholic cardiomyopathy (Chapter 59), a low-output state distinguishable from beriberi heart disease, often coexists. Symptoms sometimes begin or accelerate during a binge, and improvement follows abstinence.

Marchiafava-Bignami Disease

Marchiafava-Bignami disease, which occurs almost exclusively in alcoholics, is defined by characteristic demyelinating lesions of the corpus callosum. The cause of Marchiafava-Bignami disease, including the role—if any—of nutritional deficiency, is unknown. Early symptoms include depression, paranoia, psychosis, or dementia. Major motor seizures are common, and hemiparesis, aphasia, abnormal movements, and ataxia can progress to coma and death over a few months. Computed tomography (CT) and MRI can detect the lesions; in a few cases, clinical improvement has been accompanied by regression of the CT or MRI abnormalities.

Alcoholic Liver Disease

In the United States, most deaths from cirrhosis in people older than 45 years are caused by ethanol, and hepatic encephalopathy (Chapter 157) must always be considered in an alcoholic with altered mentation. A syndrome of altered mentation, myoclonus, and myelopathy sometimes follows portocaval shunting in alcoholic cirrhotics. Some alcoholics with repeated bouts of hepatic encephalopathy have a tendency for the development of "acquired chronic hepatocerebral degeneration," with dementia, dysarthria, ataxia, tremor, choreoathetosis, and asterixis.

Hypoglycemia

Hypoglycemia (Chapter 249) in alcoholics is the consequence of decreased intake, lack of liver glycogen stores, and in particular, failure of gluconeogenesis secondary to depletion of NAD (a cofactor for the ethanol-metabolizing enzyme alcohol dehydrogenase). Symptomatic hypoglycemia (e.g., seizures or coma) therefore often occurs in the midst of a binge and is easily mistaken for intoxication or withdrawal. The result can be permanent brain damage.

Alcoholic Ketoacidosis

Ethanol-induced impairment of fatty acid oxidation, coupled with vomiting and dehydration at the end of a binge, can lead to the accumulation of β-hydroxybutyric acid and lactic acid, obtundation, and Kussmaul respirations (Chapters 31 and 119). Blood glucose may be normal, low, or elevated. Other causes of acidosis with a large anion gap, including methanol or ethylene glycol poisoning, must be excluded.

Fetal Alcohol Syndrome

Ethanol is teratogenic. Intrauterine exposure to large doses results in characteristic facial anomalies, growth deficiency, and mental retardation, which can be severe and lifelong. Exposure to lesser amounts can cause subtle cognitive and behavioral abnormalities without other somatic features. Binge drinking is especially dangerous, but a safe level of intake has not been defined, and much of the damage seems to occur early in pregnancy, before a woman is aware that she is pregnant.

Central Pontine Myelinolysis

Caused by overvigorous correction of hyponatremia (Chapter 117), central pontine myelinolysis is not restricted to alcoholics, but they are especially vulnerable. The major clinical sign is quadriparesis, and corresponding lesions in the basis pontis can sometimes be seen by MRI. Prevention is more effective than treatment, which is simply supportive. In most patients who survive, clinical signs improve.

Other Risks and Abnormalities (Chapter 31)

Alcoholics are often immunocompromised. Altered mentation must always raise the possibility of CNS infection, especially bacterial or tuberculous meningitis. Independently of tobacco, ethanol increases the risk for carcinoma of the mouth, esophagus, larynx, liver, and breast.

Alcoholics often have coagulopathies, including thrombocytopenia (Chapter 179). Acute brain or spinal injury or chronic subdural hematoma must not be overlooked, especially in intoxicated subjects, who are at higher risk for injuries (Chapter 422).

As with coronary artery disease, low to moderate doses of ethanol decrease the risk for ischemic stroke, whereas higher amounts increase it. Ethanol in any amount increases the risk for hemorrhagic stroke in a dose-dependent fashion.

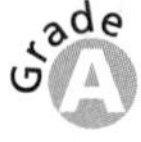

1. Toole JF, Malinow MR, Chambless LE, et al: Lowering homocysteine in patients with ischemic stroke to prevent recurrent stroke, myocardial infarction, and death: The vitamin Intervention for Stroke Prevention (VISP) randomized controlled trial. JAMA 2004;291:565–575.
2. Peterson RC, Thomas RG, Grundman M, et al: Vitamin E and donepezil for the treatment of mild cognitive impairment. N Engl J Med 2005;352:2379–2388.

SUGGESTED READINGS

Day E, Bentham P, Callaghan R, et al: Thiamine for Wernicke-Korsakoff syndrome in people at risk from alcohol abuse. Cochrane Database Syst Rev 2004;(1):CD004033. *There is insufficient evidence from RCTs to guide the dose, frequency, route, or duration of thiamine prophylaxis.*

Durga J, van Boxtel MP, Schouten EG, et al: Effect of 3-year folic acid supplementation on cognitive function in older adults in the FACIT trial: A randomised, double blind, controlled trial. Lancet 2007;369:208–216. *The 3-year change in memory, information processing speed, and sensorimotor speed were significanly better in the folic acid group.*

Klein M, Weksler N, Gurman EM: Fatal metabolic acidosis caused by thiamine deficiency. J Emerg Med 2004;26:301–303. *In these case reports, thiamine deficiency was initially overlooked as a cause of refractory lactic acidosis.*

Koike H, Iijima M, Sugiura M, et al: Alcoholic neuropathy is clinicopathologically distinct from thiamine deficiency neuropathy. Ann Neurol 2003;54:19–29. *A definitive study correlating clinical features with whole blood thiamine levels and sural nerve histopathology.*

Koike H, Sobue G: Alcoholic neuropathy. Curr Opin Neurol 2006;19:481–486. *A useful review.*

McMahon JA, Green TJ, Skeaff CM, et al: A controlled trial of homocysteine lowering and cognitive performance. N Engl J Med 2006;354:2764–2772. *Homocysteine lowering with B vitamins did not improve cognitive performance.*

Zhong C, Jin L, Fei G: MR imaging of nonalcoholic Wernicke encephalopathy: A follow-up study. AJNR Am J Neuroradiol 2005;26:2301–2305. *Distinctive abnormal MRI signals are useful for diagnosis and prognosis.*

444 CONGENITAL, DEVELOPMENTAL, AND NEUROCUTANEOUS DISORDERS

A. James Barkovich and Ruben I. Kuzniecky

MALFORMATIONS OF THE CEREBRAL CORTEX

The heterogeneous malformations of cerebral cortical development result from disturbed development of cells that normally participate in formation of the cerebral cortex. The known causes include intrauterine infection, intrauterine ischemia, and chromosomal mutations (i.e., germline, mosaic, and large deletions). When small areas of the brain are involved, epilepsy typically develops in the first or second decade, and patients have minor static neurologic dysfunction and normal intellect. Patients with larger areas of involved brain often have cognitive deficits and more severe neurologic dysfunction in addition to epilepsy. Malformations are best established by magnetic resonance imaging (MRI).

Balloon Cell Cortical Dysplasia

Focal cortical dysplasia is caused by abnormal neuronal and glial proliferation. The histology is characterized by cortical dyslamination, neuronomegaly, and dysplastic "balloon cells." Affected patients often have intractable partial epilepsy that correlates with the anatomic location of the lesion. Seizures may begin at any age but most frequently within the first 2 decades. If extensive regions of the brain are involved, patients may have neurologic impairment such as mental subnormality and hemiparesis. The diagnosis can be made with cranial MRI by detecting focal gyral thickening or blurring of the cortical–white matter junction on T1-weighted images and signal changes in subjacent white matter on T2-weighted or FLAIR (fluid-attenuated inversion recovery) images, but some lesions may be undetectable. Management includes medical control of seizures; however, surgical resection of the epileptogenic focus is often necessary for complete remission (Chapter 426).

Lissencephaly and Band Heterotopia Spectrum

The term *lissencephaly* (meaning smooth brain) describes a group of disorders caused by arrested migration of neurons to the cerebral cortex. Lissencephaly is diagnosed in childhood; most patients have severe developmental delay, microcephaly, intractable seizures, and premature death. Most affected children have mutations of chromosome 17p13.3 (*LIS1*) or Xq22 (*DCX*); patients with the former mutation have more severe cortical malformation of the posterior cerebrum, and some have the Miller-Dieker syndrome, whereas those with the latter have more severe malformation of the anterior cerebrum and are often born to mothers with band heterotopia (i.e., double cortex). MRI shows a smooth cortex with minimal sulcation. Band heterotopia is a less severe form of lissencephaly that is usually seen in women with mutation of *DCX*. The clinical manifestations of band heterotopia are variable; seizures and mild to severe developmental delay are most common. MRI studies are diagnostic for the condition and demonstrate a band of gray matter beneath a nearly normal cortex. The thickness of the band correlates with the ultimate neurologic outcome. Management consists of seizure control and genetic counseling.

Subependymal Nodular Heterotopia

Multiple bilateral gray matter nodules in the walls of the lateral ventricles characterize subependymal nodular heterotopia. It may be X-linked (*FIL1* at Xq28), with males much more severely affected. Clinical features include seizures starting at any age and various degrees of mental impairment (generally mild in females and severe in males). Diagnosis is by MRI, which demonstrates the typical gray matter nodules (Fig. 444–1). Treatment consists of antiepileptic agents (Chapter 426) and genetic counseling.

Polymicrogyria-Schizencephaly Complex

Polymicrogyria is caused by failure of cortical organization as a result of in utero injury or mutation of a gene such as *GPR56* (16q13). Schizencephaly is thought to represent a more extensive injury or mutation in which the entire cerebral mantle is affected. Clinical features include developmental delay, pyramidal signs, motor speech dysfunction, and epilepsy; in general, the clinical abnormalities are more severe with more extensive or bilateral lesions. The diagnosis is established by MRI, which can delineate a number of syndromes. Treatment is directed at control of seizures (Chapter 426).

MALFORMATIONS OF THE CRANIOVERTEBRAL JUNCTION AND SPINAL CORD

Developmental anomalies of the vertebral bodies (i.e., hemivertebrae, butterfly vertebrae, nonsegmentation of two or more adjacent vertebrae [Klippel-Feil anomaly], and transitional vertebrae) are frequently encountered on radiographs of patients with pain in the neck or back. Most of these anomalies are asymptomatic unless they lead to scoliosis or to accelerated degenerative changes of the spine, in which case they may cause pain or neurologic symptoms. Neurologic disability is likely if the anomalies are associated with underlying anomalies of the spinal cord, if they compress neural structures, or if they alter the flow of cerebrospinal fluid (CSF).

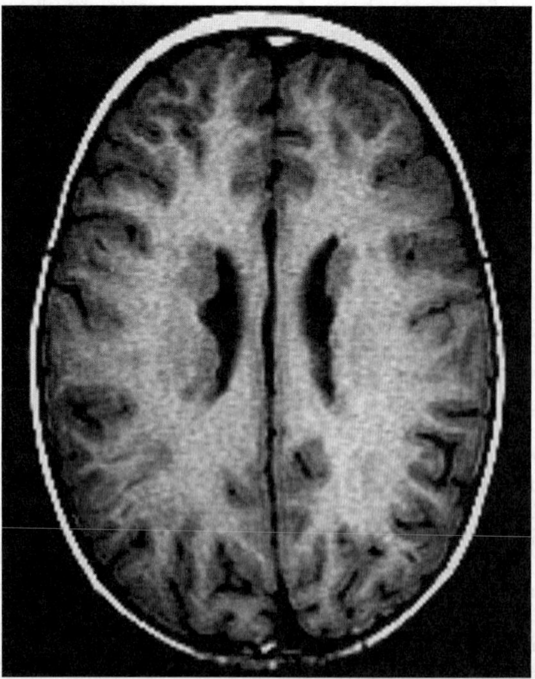

FIGURE 444–1 • Subependymal nodular heterotopia. A T1-weighted magnetic resonance imaging shows subependymal heterotopia in a young man with epilepsy.

Chiari Malformations

Chiari I

Chiari I malformations consist of inferior ectopia and compression of the cerebellar tonsils. This abnormality is often incidental and asymptomatic. When clinical manifestations develop, they result from compression of neural structures or CSF pathways and may include headaches accentuated by straining or coughing, lower cranial neuropathies, downbeat nystagmus, progressive ataxia, posterior column signs, or dissociated anesthesia of the trunk and extremities. Although the malformation is often congenital, symptoms typically begin in the third and fourth decades or even later. Symptoms attributable to the Chiari malformation may be difficult to separate from those of associated syringohydromyelia or syringobulbia (discussed later). Similar signs and symptoms may result from multiple sclerosis (Chapter 436) or from other causes of neural compression at the craniocervical junction, including bony anomalies, metabolic bone diseases that lead to invagination of the base of the skull, and tumors. Definitive diagnosis is made with MRI, which shows the compressed tonsils extending through the foramen magnum into the cervical subarachnoid space (Fig. 444–2). Treatment is surgical: decompression of the craniocervical junction.

Chiari II

Chiari II malformations (i.e., Arnold-Chiari malformations) are characterized by caudal elongation of the cerebellum and lower brain stem through the foramen magnum. Open spinal dysraphism (i.e., myelomeningocele) and hydrocephalus are almost always present. Symptoms are those of dysfunction of the brain stem, cerebellum, and spinal cord. Brain stem dysfunction may result from intrinsic malformation or compression of neural structures at the C1 level. Other brain anomalies are common, especially anomalies of the corpus callosum and gray matter heterotopia. Treatment is surgical repair of the myelomeningo-

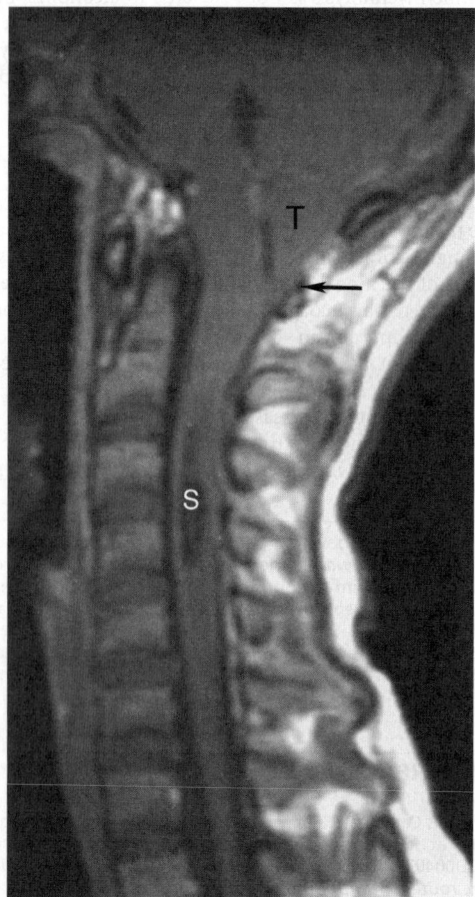

FIGURE 444–2 • Chiari I malformation. A sagittal magnetic resonance image shows low, pointed cerebellar tonsils (i.e., Chiari I malformation, T) that extend to the level of C1 (black arrow) and a dilated central canal of the spinal cord (i.e., syringohydromyelia, S).

cele, relief of hydrocephalus, and occasionally, cervical bone decompression. The prognosis depends on the level (i.e., better for sacral, worse for thoracic) and extent of the myelomeningocele and on the severity of associated brain anomalies.

Tethered Spinal Cord

In a tethered spinal cord, an anomalous filum terminale results in a lack of normal ascent of the conus medullaris to the L1 vertebral level or an ischemic or metabolic disturbance of the most caudal portions of the spinal cord. Associated spinal anomalies are common and may include diastematomyelia (i.e., split cord malformation), spinal lipomas, dermal sinuses, and fibrolipomas of the filum terminale. An increased incidence of cord tethering occurs in patients with anorectal malformations (i.e., anomalies of the genitourinary and lower gastrointestinal tract). Patients typically have urinary incontinence in conjunction with lower extremity weakness and spasticity. Males may manifest impotence. Symptoms can occur at any age but typically develop in childhood or adolescence during periods of rapid growth. Cutaneous anomalies such as focal hypertrichosis, hemangiomas, and nevi may be seen over the lumbar spine.

The differential diagnosis includes multiple sclerosis, tumors in the region of the conus medullaris, and lumbosacral hypogenesis. Definitive diagnosis is made with MRI, which shows diminished pulsations of the spinal cord, a low conus medullaris (i.e., below the bottom of the L2 vertebral body), or a thickened (i.e., more than 1 mm in diameter at the L5-S1 level) or fat-containing filum terminale.

Treatment consists of surgical release of the tethered cord. If surgery results in adequate untethering, symptoms typically do not progress and may improve.

Syringohydromyelia

Syringohydromyelia is a condition in which the central canal of the spinal cord (i.e., hydromyelia), the substance of the spinal cord (i.e., syringomyelia), or the brain stem (i.e., syringobulbia) is expanded by the presence of fluid under pressure. Occasionally, focal areas of mildly (2 to 3 mm) dilated central canal are discovered incidentally when MRI is performed for reasons unrelated to suspected spinal cord symptoms. The long-term prognosis for patients with such lesions, if no associated cause is found, is considered to be good. Most experts believe that syringes form as a result of alterations in the flow of CSF that cause variations in pressure in different parts of the subarachnoid space. The variations in pressure create hydrostatic forces that drive CSF into the spinal cord. Causes of these alterations in CSF pressure include bony narrowing of the foramen magnum (as in achondroplasia or basilar invagination, Chiari I and II malformations, and intramedullary and extramedullary tumors) and subarachnoid scarring (from trauma, hemorrhage, or infection). In patients with Chiari II malformations, hydrocephalus may result in syrinx formation. Rostral or caudal extension of the cyst may subsequently result from rapid changes in intraspinal pressure, such as those caused by coughing, straining, or sneezing.

Clinical Manifestations

Symptoms of syringohydromyelia most commonly begin in late adolescence or early adulthood and progress irregularly, with long periods of stability. Classically, patients have asymmetrical segmental weakness and atrophy of the hands and arms, loss of upper limb deep tendon reflexes, and dissociated sensory loss (with impaired perception of pain and temperature but preservation of light touch and proprioception) in the neck, arms, and upper part of the trunk. In the legs, muscle tone is increased, and the reflexes are hyperactive. Some patients experience deep pain in the neck and arms. However, the clinical manifestations depend on the cross-sectional and vertical extent of cordal involvement; symptoms may be unilateral or confined to the lower extremities. Extension into the medulla may cause nystagmus or lower cranial neuropathies. Moreover, symptoms from the syrinx may be difficult to differentiate from those of the associated craniocervical junction anomaly. Post-traumatic syringes are characterized by a latent period of up to 20 years or longer. Ascending and descending levels of weakness or sensory impairment typically develop in affected patients.

Diagnosis

The diagnosis is made by MRI (see Fig. 444–2), which defines the extent of the syrinx. In addition, MRI may show the associated craniocervical junction lesion, arachnoidal scarring, or tumor that is the cause. Electromyography reveals active and chronic denervation in the muscles of affected extremities. Nerve conduction studies are typically normal because the lesion is located central to the dorsal root ganglia. CSF is normal unless an inflammatory or neoplastic process is the cause.

Treatment

If possible, treatment is directed at the cause of the syrinx. In patients with Chiari II malformations, adequate shunting of the lateral ventricles may result in collapse of the syrinx. Syringohydromyelia in patients with spinal tumors is treated by resecting the tumor. Patients with altered CSF dynamics caused by narrowing of the craniocervical junction are treated by decompression of the bony foramen magnum, sometimes accompanied by dural grafts to increase the size of the subarachnoid space. Patients with arachnoidal scarring are typically treated by insertion of a syringopleural or syringoperitoneal shunt. Treatment of patients with benign extramedullary tumors and craniocervical junction lesions may arrest the process and provide long-term relief of symptoms. In patients with arachnoidal scarring, the relief is often only transient.

NEUROCUTANEOUS DISORDERS

The neurocutaneous syndromes are congenital disorders characterized by dysplastic and neoplastic lesions primarily involving the nervous system and skin. Of the more than 40 syndromes, the most important are neurofibromatosis, tuberous sclerosis, and the Sturge-Weber and von Hippel-Lindau syndromes.

Neurofibromatosis Type 1

Epidemiology

Neurofibromatosis encompasses a wide spectrum of syndromes with neurocutaneous lesions. Although at least eight variants have been described, only two are well-recognized, genetically distinct entities: NF1 and NF2. NF1 corresponds to the classic disorder described by von Recklinghausen and has a prevalence of 1 in 3000 births. Although it is an autosomal dominant disease, approximately 50% of cases are clinically sporadic, with a high mutation rate.

Pathobiology

Neurologically important lesions in neurofibromatosis include neurofibromas, plexiform neurofibromas, optic pathway gliomas, and astrocytomas of the brain and spinal cord. Hamartomas and meningiomas may also develop.

Molecular genetic studies have demonstrated that most mutations in *NF1* occur in the parental germline. The *NF1* gene is located on chromosome 17q and encompasses about 350 kilobases of genomic DNA that encode a protein designated as neurofibromin. Neurofibromin appears to be expressed in most tissues and has multiple functions, including acting as a tumor suppressor compound; a major myelin protein is also embedded in the *NF1* gene. Although pathogenic mutations in *NF1* are identified in approximately 75% of clinical cases, there does not appear to be any correlation between particular genotypes and phenotypes.

Clinical Manifestations

Clinical criteria for the diagnosis of NF1 include two or more of the following: (1) six or more cafe au lait macules larger than 5 mm in prepubertal patients and larger than 15 mm in postpubertal individuals, (2) two or more neurofibromas of any type (Fig. 444–3) or one plexiform neurofibroma, (3) axillary or inguinal freckling, (4) sphenoid bone dysplasia, (5) optic pathway glioma, (6) Lisch nodules (i.e., iris

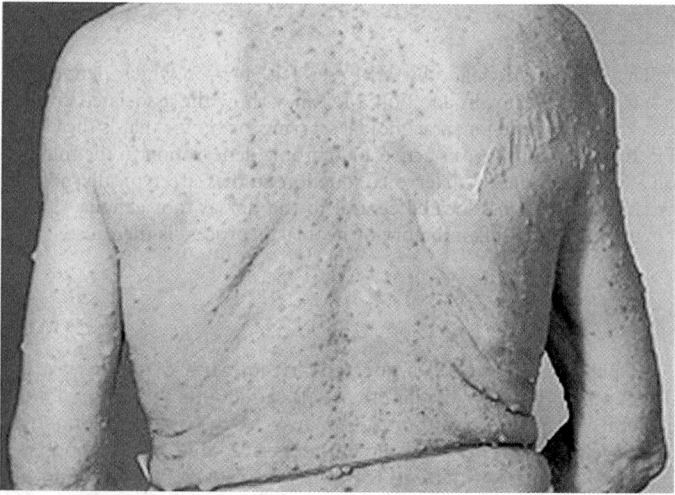

FIGURE 444–3 • Multiple neurofibromas covering the back of a patient with neurofibromatosis type 1.

hamartomas), and (7) a family history of NF1. Other manifestations may include learning difficulties, epilepsy, and mental retardation. Important complications may include scoliosis, gastrointestinal neurofibromas, pheochromocytomas (Chapter 246), and vascular dysplasia, including renal artery stenosis.

Diagnosis

The diagnosis is based on clinical criteria, sometimes supplemented by neuroimaging findings such as cerebellar, basal ganglia, and brain stem foci of dysmyelination, optic pathway gliomas, vascular dysplasia, and nerve sheath tumors.

Treatment

Rx

Most patients with NF1 do not require treatment. Subcutaneous neurofibromas may be painful or disfiguring and can be excised surgically. Intraspinal and intracranial tumors are approached surgically. Optic nerve gliomas may be treated with radiation, but treatment may not affect the outcome. Genetic counseling is important and must be provided to all patients and families in whom NF1 is present.

Neurofibromatosis Type 2

NF2, or central neurofibromatosis, is an autosomal dominant syndrome with high penetrance.

Epidemiology

The prevalence of this disorder, approximately 1 in 50,000 individuals, is much lower than that of NF1.

Pathobiology

The classic pathologic abnormality in NF2 is bilateral eighth cranial nerve schwannomas. However, multiple meningiomas and multiple other schwannomas are also common features of NF2. Spinal cord ependymomas, meningioangiomatosis, and cerebral microhamartomas can also occur.

The *NF2* gene is located on chromosome 22q. The gene product (merlin) is a cytoskeletal protein with unknown function.

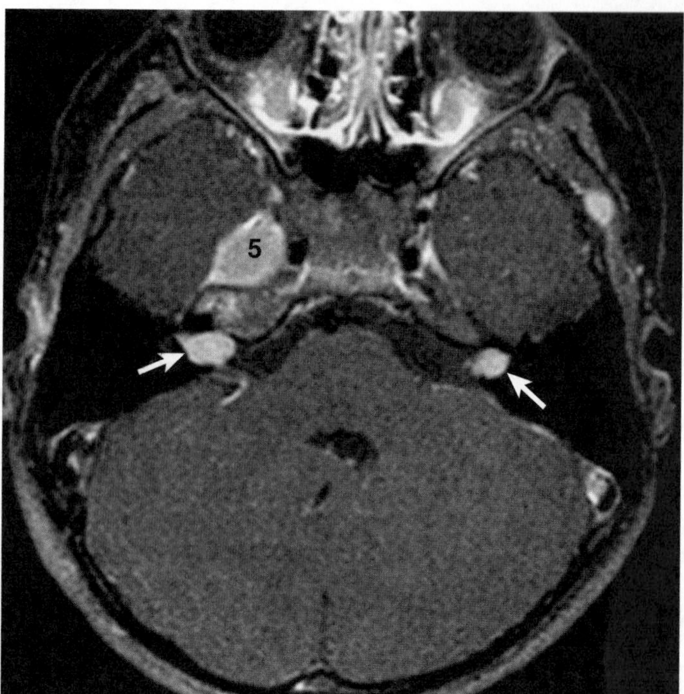

FIGURE 444–4 • Postcontrast axial T1-weighted image of a patient with neurofibromatosis type 2. Enhancing bilateral eighth nerve schwannomas (arrows) are present. Other schwannomas such as those of cranial nerve V (5) are common.

Clinical Manifestations

Although skin lesions may be present in up to 30% of patients with NF2, the diagnosis is based on the presence of the following criteria: (1) bilateral eighth cranial nerve schwannomas detected by MRI (Fig. 444–4) or (2) a first-degree relative with NF2 and (a) a unilateral eighth nerve schwannoma or (b) two tumors from among the following—meningioma, neurofibroma, other schwannoma, glioma, or juvenile subcapsular lenticular opacity.

The mean age at the onset of symptoms in patients with NF2 is approximately 22 years. Absence of the characteristic MRI findings in children (<12 years) does not exclude the disease. Cutaneous lesions such as cafe au lait macules and neurofibromas can be seen in up to 70%, and approximately 40% of patients have cataracts, often evident in childhood.

Treatment

Treatment is related to the complications of the illness. Surgical treatment may be indicated in patients with intramedullary spinal tumors. Surgical treatment of schwannomas and meningiomas may be indicated to preserve function or to relieve compression of adjacent structures. Family members should be screened regularly with hearing tests and contrast-enhanced MRI. Genetic counseling should be provided to affected families.

Tuberous Sclerosis

Epidemiology

In tuberous sclerosis complex (TSC), which may occur as a familial autosomal dominant syndrome or in sporadic form with a high rate of spontaneous mutations, hamartomatous lesions involve multiple organs at different stages in the course of the disease. The incidence of this disorder is 1 in 10,000 to 50,000.

Pathobiology

TSC affects tissues from different germ layers. Cutaneous and visceral lesions may occur, including adenoma sebaceum, cardiac rhabdomy-

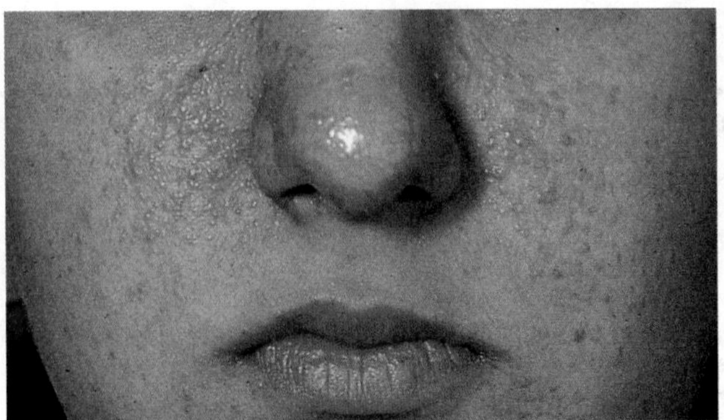

FIGURE 444–5 • Facial angiofibroma, typical of tuberous sclerosis. (From Forbes CD, Jackson WD: Color Atlas and Text of Clinical Medicine, 2nd ed. London, Mosby, 1996.)

omas, and renal angiomyolipomas. The central nervous system (CNS) lesions seen in this disorder include hamartomas of the cortex, hamartomas of the ventricular walls, and subependymal giant cell tumors, which typically develop in the vicinity of the foramina of Monro.

Molecular genetic studies have defined at least two loci for TSC. In *TSC1*, the abnormality is localized on chromosome 9q34, but the nature of the gene protein, called hamartin, remains unclear. No missense mutations occur in *TSC1*. In *TSC2*, the gene abnormalities are on chromosome 16p13. This gene encodes tuberin, a guanosine triphosphatase–activating protein. The specific function of this protein is unknown. In *TSC2*, all types of mutations have been reported; new mutations occur frequently. Few differences have yet been observed in the clinical phenotypes of patients with mutation of one gene or the other.

Clinical Manifestations

Criteria for diagnosis have been established and include primary criteria such as hypomelanotic skin macules (i.e., ash-leaf spots, sometimes visible at birth), shagreen patches, facial angiofibromas (Fig. 444–5), subungual fibromas, and imaging evidence of multiple calcified subependymal nodules, cortical tubers, or multiple retinal hamartomas. Retinal hamartomas can be seen ophthalmoscopically in about half of the patients. Diagnosis of this condition is usually clinical and confirmed by identification of calcified or uncalcified hamartomas on imaging studies.

Treatment

Rx

Treatment is directed at complications of the disease, particularly epilepsy. Neurosurgical intervention may sometimes be indicated for epilepsy and for symptomatic treatment of complications such as hydrocephalus resulting from midline giant cell tumors. Serial cardiac and renal ultrasound may be indicated in some patients because benign tumors of these organs may enlarge rapidly. The disorder is autosomal dominant, so genetic counseling is of paramount importance in familial cases.

Sturge-Weber Syndrome

Epidemiology

Sturge-Weber syndrome is a sporadic, noninherited abnormality, even though a few familial cases have been reported. The true incidence and prevalence of this disorder are poorly established, although reports have indicated that it occurs in fewer than 5 in 100,000 births.

The characteristic neurologic feature of this disorder is capillary angiomatosis of the pia mater. Associated cerebral cortical calcifications are generally seen in a pericapillary distribution and are progressive.

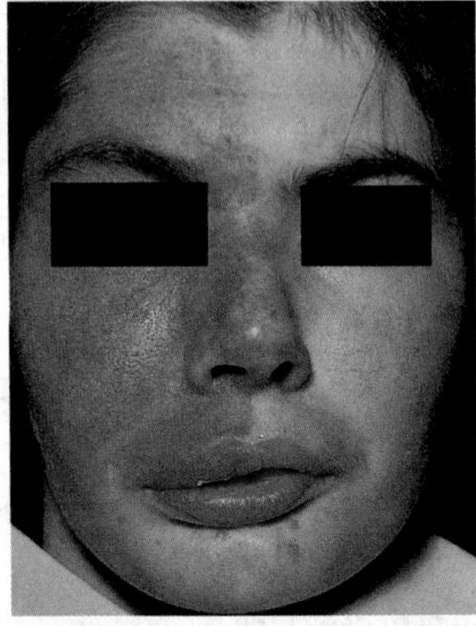

FIGURE 444–6 • Sturge-Weber syndrome. This patient has a classic diffuse capillary hemangioma in the distribution of the ophthalmic, nasociliary, and maxillary branches of the trigeminal nerve. The lesion extends backward over the anterior two thirds of the crown of the head. (From Forbes CD, Jackson WD: Color Atlas and Text of Clinical Medicine, 2nd ed. London, Mosby, 1996.)

Clinical Manifestations

The hallmark of this disorder includes the presence of facial vascular nevi (e.g., port-wine stain) (Fig. 444–6), epilepsy, cognitive deficits, and sometimes hemiparesis or hemiplegia, hemianopsia, or glaucoma. Most patients have epilepsy, the severity of which may correlate with the developmental status and the presence of hemiparesis. However, seizures never develop in some patients. A forme fruste of the syndrome has also been described without the usual skin lesion.

Diagnosis

The diagnosis is generally based on the presence of a facial nevus and imaging confirmation of intracranial pathology. MRI with contrast may be indicated in some patients, particularly those with the forme fruste of the disorder and those in whom surgery is being contemplated. Although the intracranial lesion is ipsilateral to the facial nevus in most cases, contralateral and bilateral lesions have been described.

Treatment

Treatment is usually aimed at the epilepsy (Chapter 426). Surgical excision of epileptogenic areas corresponding to the abnormality has been successful in some individuals. When the disorder is characterized by early, intractable epilepsy and infantile hemiplegia, hemispherectomy can improve the seizures and neurodevelopmental outcome.

von Hippel-Lindau Disease

Pathobiology

von Hippel-Lindau disease (i.e., CNS angiomatosis) is an autosomal dominant disorder caused by a defective tumor suppressor gene at chromosome 3p25-p26 and characterized by retinal angiomas (Chapter 449), brain (usually cerebellar) and spinal cord hemangioblastomas, renal cell carcinomas (Chapter 207), endolymphatic sac tumors, pheochromocytomas (Chapter 246), papillary cystadenomas of the epididymis, angiomas of the liver and kidney, and cysts of the pancreas, kidney, liver, and epididymis. Both sexes are affected equally. The diagnosis is established if the patient has more than one CNS hemangioblastoma, one hemangioblastoma with a visceral manifestation of the disease, or one manifestation of the disease and a known family history.

Clinical Manifestations

Symptoms typically begin during the third or fourth decade. Retinal inflammation with exudate, hemorrhage, and retinal detachment from the retinal angiomas typically antedates the cerebellar complaints, but this order is not constant. Moreover, the ocular findings are nonspecific, and the retinal detachment may mask the underlying lesion. Headache, vertigo, and vomiting result from cerebellar tumors. Other findings such as dysdiadochokinesia, dysmetria, and Romberg's sign are common. It is rare for patients to be seen initially with symptoms of spinal cord or visceral lesions. Rarely, patients may have hearing loss from tumors of the endolymphatic sac.

Treatment

Treatment is symptomatic. Retinal detachments and tumors are treated by laser therapy. Large brain tumors, renal cell carcinomas, pheochromocytomas, epididymal tumors, and endolymphatic sac tumors are treated surgically; smaller CNS tumors may be treated by gamma knife. A high index of suspicion and repeated imaging studies are necessary to detect the tumors before they metastasize or become unresectable.

SUGGESTED READINGS

Barkovich AJ, Kuzniecky RI, Jackson GD, et al: A developmental and genetic classification for malformations of cortical development. Neurology 2006;65:18731887. *Classification of these disorders based on their embryology, morphology, and genetics.*

Crino PB, Nathanson KL, Henske EP: The tuberous sclerosis complex. N Engl J Med 2006;355:1345–1356. *A comprehensive overview.*

Lonser RR, Glenn GM, Walther M, et al: von Hippel-Lindau disease. Lancet 2003;361:2059–2067. *A detailed review.*

Theos A, Korf BR: Pathophysiology of neurofibromatosis type 1. Ann Intern Med 2006;144:842–849. *A comprehensive review.*

445 AUTONOMIC DISORDERS AND THEIR MANAGEMENT

Clifford B. Saper

This chapter discusses disorders of the peripheral autonomic nervous system and disorders of central integration of autonomic control (Table 445–1). Central regulation of autonomic response is closely tied to neuroendocrine control, and both are often affected by central nervous system disorders. Aspects of neuroendocrine disease are discussed in Chapters 241, 242, and 243.

DISORDERS OF PERIPHERAL AUTONOMIC FUNCTION

The peripheral autonomic nervous system consists of three main divisions: (1) *parasympathetic,* or outflow from the cranial nerves and the low lumbar and sacral spinal cord; (2) *sympathetic,* or autonomic outflow from the thoracic and high lumbar segments of the spinal cord; and (3) *enteric* nervous system, or neurons that are intrinsic to the wall of the gut. Knowledge of the different types of neurotransmitters and receptors associated with the peripheral autonomic nervous system has made available a wide range of drugs to modify autonomic responses (Table 445–2).

TABLE 445–1 DISORDERS OF THE AUTONOMIC NERVOUS SYSTEM

PERIPHERAL AUTONOMIC DISORDERS

- Pandysautonomias
  - Acute pandysautonomia
  - Tetanus
  - Chronic autonomic neuropathy
  - Familial dysautonomia
  - Idiopathic autonomic insufficiency (Shy-Drager syndrome)
- Regional dysautonomia
  - Horner's syndrome
  - Paraspinal tumors
  - Somatosympathetic dysreflexia
  - Complex regional pain syndrome
- Disorders of specific autonomic functions
  - Pupillary disorders
    - Horner's syndrome
    - Oculomotor paresis
  - Cardiovascular disorders
  - Glossopharyngeal neuralgia
  - Carotid sinus hypersensitivity
  - Sweating disorders
    - Hyperhidrosis
    - Anhidrosis
  - Gastrointestinal disorders
    - Disorders of motility
    - Vomiting
  - Genitourinary disorders
    - Incontinence
    - Urinary retention
    - Spastic bladder
    - Impotence

DISORDERS OF CENTRAL AUTONOMIC INTEGRATION

- Emotional disorders
  - Panic disorder
  - Psychosomatic illness
  - Cardiac arrhythmias
- Thermoregulatory disorders
  - Poikilothermia
  - Paroxysmal hypothermia
  - Hyperthermia and fever
  - Neuroleptic malignant syndrome
- Feeding disorders
  - Hyperphagia and obesity
  - Hypophagia and inanition
- Disorders of fluid and electrolyte regulation
  - Hypernatremia, hyperosmolality, and absence of thirst
  - Hyperdipsia, hyponatremia, and water intoxication
  - Paroxysmal hyponatremia
- Central reproductive disorders
- Arousal disorders
  - Hypersomnolence
  - Insomnia

Pandysautonomias

Acute Pandysautonomia

Widespread failure of the autonomic nervous system may evolve acutely or subacutely as part of a parainfectious inflammatory polyneuropathy. In rare cases, autonomic neuropathy predominates and, when severe, may be life-threatening. Wide swings in blood pressure and heart rate occur but usually reverse themselves in a few minutes. In most patients the Trendelenburg position is sufficient to maintain cerebral perfusion during hypotensive periods. Various cardiac arrhythmias may occur, presumably from instability of autonomic innervation of the cardiac conducting system. The presence of ganglionic acetylcholine receptor antibodies may be diagnostic of an autoimmune origin. Any arrhythmias must be treated gingerly because the underlying conduction abnormalities are neurogenic in origin and may change rapidly. There is anecdotal evidence that intravenous immune globulin (2 g/kg in divided doses administered over a period of 2 to 5 days) can cause rapid improvement, as in other forms of Guillain-Barré syndrome.

Tetanus

A similar subacute pandysautonomia is also seen in severe cases of tetanus (Chapter 319). Tetanus toxin, elaborated by *Clostridium tetani* organisms in an infected wound, is transported by autonomic as well as motor axons back to the spinal cord, where it is taken up by and inactivates the terminals of inhibitory interneurons. Treatment of the motor manifestations of tetanus by paralyzing and sedating the patient does not control the autonomic storm. Up to 40% of patients who have tetanus

TABLE 445–2 SYSTEMIC EFFECTS OF SOME COMMONLY USED AUTONOMIC DRUGS

Receptor Type	Drug Type (Example)	Tissue	Effect
Muscarinic cholinergic	Antagonist (atropine)	Pupil	Mydriasis
		Salivary gland	Dry mouth
		Bronchi	Dilation
		Heart	Tachycardia
		Gut	Decreased motility and secretion
α-Adrenergic	Antagonist (phenoxybenzamine)	Blood vessels	Vasodilation
α_1-Adrenergic	Agonist (phenylephrine)	Blood vessels	Vasoconstriction
	Antagonist (prazosin)	Blood vessels	Vasodilation
β-Adrenergic	Agonist (isoproterenol)	Heart	Increased rate and contractility
β_1-Adrenergic	Antagonist (metoprolol)	Blood vessels	Decreased rate and contractility
β_2-Adrenergic	Agonist (terbutaline)	Bronchi	Dilation

TABLE 445–3 PERIPHERAL NEUROPATHIES THAT MAY HAVE AN AUTONOMIC COMPONENT

AUTONOMIC SYMPTOMS OFTEN PROMINENT

Guillain-Barré syndrome
Amyloid neuropathy
Diabetic neuropathy
Acute intermittent porphyria
Vacor (rat poison)

AUTONOMIC SYMPTOMS MAY OCCUR

Renal failure
Toxic neuropathies
- Vinca alkaloids
- Perhexiline maleate
- Thallium
- Arsenic
- Mercury
- Organic solvents
- Acrylamide

Vasculitis
- Systemic lupus erythematosus
- Rheumatoid arthritis
- Mixed connective tissue disease

Thiamine deficiency
Leprosy
Hereditary autonomic neuropathies
Fabry's disease

and require intensive care suffer cardiac arrest as a result of an arrhythmia; such patients are generally easily resuscitated with standard measures.

Chronic Autonomic Neuropathy

The axons of the peripheral autonomic nervous system are generally of small caliber and thinly myelinated or unmyelinated. Certain polyneuropathies have a predilection for small-diameter axons and result in autonomic changes. *Amyloid neuropathy* (Chapter 296) often includes a gastrointestinal motility disorder or orthostatic hypotension. Similarly, *diabetic neuropathy* (Chapter 247), although it is often dominated by sensory or motor complaints, may cause widespread autonomic failure. The neuropathy of *acute intermittent porphyria* (Chapter 229) or certain toxic agents such as *Vacor* (a rat poison) may have a prominent autonomic component. Acute poisoning with *organophosphate insecticides* (Chapter 111) that block acetylcholinesterase results in a hypercholinergic state, including miosis and cardiac slowing, that lasts for several days; the neuropathy that follows several weeks later does not usually have a strong autonomic component. Other peripheral neuropathies with an autonomic component are listed in Table 445–3. The hypercholinergic state from acute organophosphate poisoning may be treated with atropine, 10 μg/kg intravenously as necessary, to prevent cardiac slowing or gastrointestinal distress.

Degenerative Dysautonomia

Childhood familial dysautonomia of the Riley-Day type is most commonly recessively inherited in Ashkenazi Jewish children. Symptoms referable to the autonomic nervous system and relative indifference to pain are present from birth.

Pure Autonomic Failure in Adults

In middle age or late adult life, *pure autonomic failure* may develop as a chronic degenerative condition as a result of loss of neurons in the autonomic ganglia, as well as in the preganglionic cell groups in the medulla and spinal cord. Pure autonomic failure may have an autoimmune cause in patients with ganglionic acetylcholine receptor antibodies. However, in most cases, Lewy body–type degeneration (Chapter 425) is present in the brain stem, thus suggesting that this disorder is part of the spectrum of Parkinson's disease (Chapter 433). Similarly, 10 to 20% of patients with Parkinson's disease have some degree of autonomic failure, and these patients also have Lewy bodies and loss of pigmented neurons in sympathetic ganglia as well as in the brain.

Clinical Manifestations

The initial complaints often result from orthostatic hypotension, but signs or symptoms of sweating or pupillary, gastrointestinal, genitourinary, or other autonomic abnormalities are elicited by the history and physical examination.

Diagnosis

Pure autonomic failure is distinguished from non-neurologic causes of orthostatic hypotension by the lack of compensatory tachycardia, which indicates impairment of either the peripheral or central components of the baroreceptor reflex. Severe autonomic neuropathy affecting the glossopharyngeal or vagus nerves may also impair the baroreceptor response but is typically associated with other evidence of sensory or motor neuropathy. Other cardiovascular signs include loss of sinus arrhythmia and absence of normal overshoot in diastolic blood pressure during phase IV of the Valsalva maneuver. An abnormally accentuated blood pressure response to intravenous infusion of norepinephrine is consistent with widespread denervation supersensitivity, and tests of autonomic function can establish the diagnosis (Table 445–4).

Shy-Drager Syndrome

The combination of findings in pure autonomic failure must be distinguished from a superficially similar disorder, *Shy-Drager syndrome* (Chapter 433), which is characterized by degeneration of central autonomic control nuclei. Shy-Drager syndrome is part of a spectrum of *multiple systems atrophy* in which there is evidence of cerebellar and extrapyramidal involvement but no evidence of peripheral autonomic degeneration on formal testing (see Table 445–4). Loss of neurons is seen in the basal ganglia, substantia nigra, pons, cerebellum, inferior olives, and brain stem autonomic nuclei, but not in autonomic ganglia. No Lewy bodies are present, but glial fibrillary inclusions containing α-synuclein may be found. The movement disorder in patients with Parkinson's disease improves with L-dopa/carbidopa, but in multiple systems atrophy the response is poor. Carbidopa, however, can worsen blood pressure control in both conditions by blocking dopa decarboxylase in sympathetic ganglion cells.

Treatment

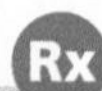

Orthostatic hypotension is generally the most disabling aspect of autonomic degeneration. Treatment with elastic stockings or even entire lower body compression suits can improve standing blood pressure by limiting blood pooling in the lower part of the body. Treatment with fludrocortisone, a mineralocorticoid (0.1 mg once to three times a day), expands intravascular blood volume and causes an elevation in blood pressure in all positions. Midodrine, the prodrug of a direct sympathetic agonist, can improve vasoconstrictor response. [1] A starting dose of 10 mg three times a day may increase blood pressure in all positions. In patients treated with either drug, the head of the bed should be elevated in recumbency to minimize hypertensive effects on the brain. L-Dihydroxyphenylserine, which is a synthetic precursor of norepinephrine, has shown encouraging results in clinical trials, [2] but it may require residual sympathetic neuronal function to be useful; it has not been approved by the Food and Drug Administration at the time of publication. Drinking 480 mL of water at room temperature can reduce the decrease in orthostatic blood pressure by up to 20 mm Hg 30 minutes later and be a useful adjunct to other therapies. [3]

Regional Dysautonomia

Horner's Syndrome

The segmental organization of the sympathetic nervous system can result in regional disturbances of function. The most common of these disturbances is *Horner's syndrome*, which is caused by injury to the cranial sympathetic innervation arising from the superior cervical ganglion.

Clinical Manifestations and Diagnosis

The most common cause of new-onset Horner's syndrome is atherosclerotic disease affecting the vasa nervorum originating in the carotid artery. However, Horner's syndrome may also be seen when an intrathoracic or cervical tumor involves the sympathetic chain. Miosis, ptosis, and anhidrosis may occur if the ascending sympathetic fibers are injured below the level at which they enter the skull with the internal carotid artery. Damage to sympathetic fibers along the course of the intracranial carotid artery produces only oculosympathetic paresis (Raeder's syndrome). This difference is only of marginal value clinically because Horner's syndrome produced by extracranial lesions is often incomplete. Lesions of the central descending sympathoexcitatory pathway, which runs through the lateral portions of the brain stem from the hypothalamus to the spinal cord, may produce a central Horner's syndrome characterized by miosis and ptosis, as well as loss of sweating over the entire ipsilateral half of the body. Postganglionic Horner's syndrome can be differentiated from preganglionic or central lesions by pharmacologic testing (see Table 445–4).

The diagnosis is usually obvious from the history and physical examination. To determine the underlying cause, evaluation of Horner's syndrome of recent onset should include radiographic or magnetic resonance examination of the pulmonary apices and paracervical area.

TABLE 445–4 TESTS OF AUTONOMIC FUNCTION

Test	Interpretation
PUPILLARY RESPONSES	
4% cocaine	Pupillodilation indicates release of normal catecholamine stores
1% hydroxyamphetamine	Pupillodilation indicates denervation supersensitivity
1% phenylephrine	Pupillodilation indicates denervation supersensitivity
0.1% epinephrine	Pupillodilation indicates denervation supersensitivity
0.1% pilocarpine	Pupilloconstriction indicates denervation supersensitivity
2.5% methacholine	Pupilloconstriction indicates denervation supersensitivity
SWEATING RESPONSES	
Thermal sweating	Regional absence of sweating indicates sympathetic cholinergic denervation
Galvanic skin response	Increased conductivity under mild stress indicates normal adrenergic innervation
1:1000 pilocarpine	Intradermal injection causes axon reflex sweating
1:10,000 acetylcholine	Intradermal injection causes direct activation of sweat glands
AXON REFLEX	
1:1000 histamine	Intradermal injection normally causes wheal and flare
CARDIOVASCULAR RESPONSES	
Orthostatic challenge	Pulse normally increases and diastolic blood pressure decreases <15 mm Hg
Carotid sinus massage	Normally causes decrease in blood pressure and heart rate
RR interval	Normally increases during inspiration (sinus arrhythmia)
Valsalva maneuver	Longest to shortest RR interval ratio normally ≥1.4
Cold pressor test	Immersing hand in ice water normally increases blood pressure and heart rate
Plasma catecholamines	Normally increase response to standing or stress
Norepinephrine infusion, 0.05 µg/kg/min	Diastolic blood pressure increase ≥20 mm Hg indicates supersensitivity
GENITOURINARY, RECTAL RESPONSES	
Cremasteric reflex	Stroking skin or thigh normally causes testicular retraction
Anal wink reflex	Scratching perianal skin normally causes anal sphincter contraction
Bulbocavernosus reflex	Squeezing glans penis or clitoris normally causes anal sphincter contraction

Treatment and Prognosis

Rx

No treatment is necessary except as indicated for the underlying disease. The prognosis depends on what is causing the Horner's syndrome, such as a tumor or an infarct, but the defect is generally permanent.

Spinal Epidural Tumors

Spinal epidural tumors (Chapter 199) that compress the spinal cord may cause loss of sweating over the dermatomes caudal to the tumor. This deficit can be appreciated by running the handle of a tuning fork down the skin in the paraspinal region. The smooth movement is interrupted by the dry skin below the level of the lesion. Occasionally, compression of a midthoracic spinal root, which carries visceral sensory fibers, by a disc or tumor may be manifested as abdominal pain.

The diagnosis is made by magnetic resonance imaging. If the primary tumor has been diagnosed, the epidural metastasis is usually treated with dexamethasone (100 mg intravenously, followed by 10 mg every 6 hours) and radiation therapy. However, if the epidural tumor is the first manifestation of the cancer, surgery may be needed for decompression and diagnosis.

Previous Spinal Cord Injury

In patients with preexisting spinal cord transection, a noxious stimulus below the level of the transection may produce either local sympathetic reflex responses (segmental sweating) or more generalized spinal reflex patterns (e.g., hypertension with bladder overfilling). Stimulation of pain fibers at any level results in both local (spinospinal) and generalized (spinobulbospinal) somatosympathetic reflex responses, including sweating, vasoconstriction, and pupillodilation. Paraplegic patients with sympathetic responses should be evaluated for evidence of occult disease that might cause pain in an intact individual.

Complex Regional Pain Syndrome

After injury to peripheral nerves, aberrant regeneration may result in severe pain, a condition known as *complex regional pain syndrome.* The role of sympathetic nerves in mediating the chronic pain (reflex sympathetic dystrophy) remains controversial. Normally innocuous sensory stimulation, such as covering the affected limb with a sheet or with clothing, may cause excruciating burning pain associated with variable autonomic changes. Atrophic changes in skin and bone may reflect abnormal sympathetic innervation or disuse. Although regional sympathetic block alleviates the pain in some patients, injection of placebo can have similar effects, and removal of the affected sympathetic ganglion rarely produces permanent relief.

Disorders of Specific Autonomic Functions

Pupils

Anisocoria, or asymmetry in pupillary size, may reflect a deficit of sympathetic innervation of the smaller pupil (causing miosis) or parasympathetic innervation of the larger pupil (causing mydriasis) (Chapter 450). Because both oculosympathetic and oculomotor (parasympathetic) innervation participate in lid elevation, ptosis, if present, generally indicates the abnormal eye. Anisocoria may be long-standing and of little clinical significance, but pupillary asymmetry of recent onset should be evaluated by a neurologist. Impairment of sympathetic innervation of the iris (pupillodilator) muscle is not always accompanied by ptosis or a sweating deficit (Horner's syndrome). The pupilloconstrictor fibers travel in the dorsomedial part of the oculomotor nerve, where they may be selectively impaired by temporal lobe herniation or by an aneurysm of the posterior communicating artery. Pharmacologic testing may aid in identification of the pupillary abnormality (see Table 445–4). A common factitious cause of a unilaterally dilated pupil is the instillation of atropinic eye drops; the situation is exposed when the pharmacologically dilated pupil does not respond even to strong solutions of pilocarpine. Another common cause of a large, poorly reactive pupil is *Adie's syndrome,* an idiopathic condition involving degeneration of the ciliary ganglion. The abnormal pupil usually shows sector paralysis, but dilates and responds to light after a period in complete darkness. Abnormalities of accommodation are more mild. The abnormal pupil responds briskly to 0.1% pilocarpine (see Table 445–4), and concomitant loss of tendon reflexes is seen in most cases.

Although Adie's syndrome is sometimes accompanied by other autonomic abnormalities, such as changes in sweating, these associated abnormalities are rarely symptomatic, and there is no specific treatment. The pupillary abnormalities and areflexia are permanent.

Cardiovascular

The baroreceptor reflex is an important protective response that induces bradycardia and peripheral vasodilation to counteract an acute increase in blood pressure—or the reverse response during hypotension. The afferent fibers for the response run in the glossopharyngeal (carotid sinus) and vagus (aortic depressor) nerves, whereas the efferent response includes both parasympathetic and sympathetic components. Injury to the glossopharyngeal or carotid sinus nerves in the neck (often by a tumor) can cause episodic attacks of hypotension and bradycardia, often manifested as syncope. In most cases, an associated pain or paresthesia is located in the cutaneous distribution of the glossopharyngeal nerve (in the external auditory meatus or the pharynx), known as *glossopharyngeal neuralgia* (Chapter 421). The situation is analogous to tic douloureux, which is characterized by intermittent volleys of firing in the affected nerve. Atropine or a transvenous pacemaker may prevent the bradycardia associated with the attacks, but loss of vasoconstrictor tone sometimes results in symptomatic hypotension despite these maneuvers. Anticonvulsants, including phenytoin (starting at 100 mg three times daily), carbamazepine (starting at 200 mg three times daily), or oxcarbazepine (starting at 300 mg twice daily), may prevent the attacks; doses are adjusted to the minimum necessary to prevent attacks for each patient. The final doses are often much lower than those required to treat epilepsy.

Carotid Sinus Syncope

Carotid sinus syncope (Chapter 427) occurs most commonly in elderly individuals with carotid atherosclerosis. Even mild pressure over the carotid bulb, such as a tight shirt collar, can produce a full-blown carotid sinus response resulting in syncope. The diagnosis is made by gently compressing the carotid artery below the angle of the jaw while the electrocardiogram is monitored. Facilities for cardiac resuscitation must be immediately available in case the compression results in sinus arrest. Vigorous massage should be avoided because it may dislodge an embolus and result in a transient or even permanent neurologic deficit. Treatment of carotid sinus hypersensitivity is the same as that for glossopharyngeal neuralgia (see the previous paragraph).

Neurocardiogenic Syncope

Neurocardiogenic (vasovagal) syncope (Chapters 61 and 427) typically occurs in young people during dehydration, during prolonged standing, or in response to a painful or emotional stimulus. It is believed to be due to venous pooling that results in decreased venous return to the heart, which in turn activates atrial mechanoreceptors that cause reflex slowing of the heart rate with a fall in vasomotor tone and hence blood pressure. Activation of other visceral mechanoreceptors (e.g., lung, bladder, gut) is also thought to trigger this response, as in patients with cough or micturition syncope. Postural orthostatic tachycardia syndrome is a related disorder in which the upright posture produces tachycardia instead of bradycardia. Tilt-table testing can be used in an attempt to provoke an attack, but both the sensitivity and specificity of the test are suboptimal. β-Blockers (e.g., atenolol, 25 to 50 mg/day) and midodrine (5 mg three times daily) have been used with variable success (Chapter 427).

Sweating

Human sweat glands are innervated by both noradrenergic sympathetic fibers (mediating emotional responses) and cholinergic sympathetic fibers (thermal sweating). Certain somatosympathetic reflexes can produce generalized or regional sweating in response to innocuous or noxious somatosensory stimuli.

Hyperhidrosis

Hyperhidrosis, or pathologically increased sweating, can be generalized or focal, most commonly involving the palms of the hands and the soles of the feet. Drugs that interrupt α-adrenergic transmission (phenoxybenzamine, 10 mg three times daily) or muscarinic transmission (propantheline, 15 mg three times daily) may be effective, particularly in combination. In extreme cases, regional sympathectomy has been performed, but this procedure sometimes results in a compensatory increase in sweating in adjacent regions.

Idiopathic Anhidrosis

Idiopathic anhidrosis may be segmental or generalized. This rare condition is sometimes associated with Adie's syndrome (Ross' syndrome), but in other cases no other signs of autonomic impairment are noted. In some patients the impairment is preganglionic and in others postganglionic, as judged by the axon reflex sweating response (see Table 445–4). In most patients studied the deficits were stable and did not progress to involve other autonomic functions.

Gastrointestinal

Disorders of intestinal motility may be due to damage to the parasympathetic innervation of the gut or to dysfunction of the enteric nervous system itself (Chapter 138). Specific abnormalities of esophageal contraction and colonic tone have been noted in patients suffering from depression and may predict response to antidepressant medication. A wide range of dysmotility syndromes, from difficulty swallowing to gastroparesis and severe constipation, are seen in patients with Parkinson's disease, perhaps because of involvement of the enteric neurons by the underlying degenerative disorder.

Vomiting is a neurally mediated gastrointestinal reflex that is coordinated by neurons in the medullary reticular formation. Chemical emetic agents such as certain narcotics or dopaminergic agonists act at the area postrema, a chemosensory zone on the fourth ventricular surface of the medulla, to elicit the vomiting reflex. Local dopaminergic and serotoninergic connections are thought to mediate the response, and antidopaminergic drugs such as prochlorperazine (5 to 10 mg orally every 6 hours) or blockers of the serotonin 5-HT_3 receptor (e.g., ondansetron, 8 mg orally every 8 hours) may act at the level of the area postrema to suppress vomiting; use of the two types of drugs together is even more efficacious. Intractable vomiting without any gastrointestinal abnormalities has been reported in certain patients with tumors involving the medullary cell groups controlling vomiting or their connections. Treatment of the tumor with steroids and radiation therapy generally results in improvement.

Genitourinary

The urinary bladder is composed of interlacing smooth muscle fibers of the detrusor covered by an internal mucous membrane and an outer serosa. The detrusor is innervated by local parasympathetic ganglion cells, which in turn are controlled by preganglionic neurons located in the intermediolateral column at the second through fourth sacral segments. Additional motor neurons located in the ventral horn at the same levels constitute Onuf's nucleus. Their axons run through the pelvic nerve to innervate the striated accessory muscles of micturition (including the external urethral sphincter) in the pelvic floor. Neurons of Onuf's nucleus are strikingly preserved in motor neuron disease but are lost along with autonomic preganglionic cells in Shy-Drager syndrome. The internal sphincter at the bladder neck is innervated via the hypogastric nerve by sympathetic prevertebral pelvic ganglia whose preganglionic innervation arises from the intermediolateral column at the T12–L1 level.

Bladder relaxation during filling and subsequent coordination of micturition are under control of Barrington's nucleus and the adjacent pontine reticular formation, near the locus ceruleus. Brain stem control of micturition is, in turn, under voluntary regulation by areas within the cerebral sensory and motor cortex. When bladder fullness is sensed and the environmental conditions are appropriate, micturition is initiated by Barrington's nucleus, under forebrain control. External sphincter pressure decreases and thereby results in reflex relaxation of the internal sphincter and contraction of the bladder.

Forebrain impairment results in loss of voluntary control of micturition but does not otherwise affect the complex sensory and motor program that results in normal voiding. Incontinence in such patients can be managed with adult diapers or external urinary collection devices without the risk of frequent urinary tract infections or damage to the upper urinary tract. Injury to the bulbospinal pathway from Barrington's nucleus to the sacral intermediolateral column, however, causes major disruption of coordinated bladder function. Immediately after spinal cord injury there is a period of spinal shock during which the bladder does not undergo reflex contraction as it fills. Such patients require urinary catheterization to prevent vesical and renal damage.

One to 2 weeks after injury, spinal reflex control of the bladder returns. Some patients can induce reflex bladder emptying by somatosensory stimulation, such as stroking the skin over the thigh. The bladder reflexively contracts at a lower volume but does not empty completely *(spastic bladder)*. In other patients, detrusor action is not coordinated with sphincter opening, and bladder contraction against a closed sphincter can cause ureteral reflux *(sphincter dyssynergia)*. Injury to sensory nerves supplying the bladder may also cause overfilling and incomplete emptying, thus indicating the importance of sensory feedback in bladder control. Patients with significant postvoid residual urine are at increased risk for urinary tract infections, but bladder overfilling with elevated pressures greater than 40 cm H_2O may ultimately be a greater problem. Elevations in pressure greater than 40 cm H_2O may require continuous or intermittent catheterization to prevent damage to the upper urinary tract.

Pharmacologic intervention aimed at augmenting or suppressing autonomic motor responses of the bladder or internal sphincter has only limited value (Chapter 24). Bethanechol, a cholinergic agonist (10 to 15 mg three times daily), is used to augment bladder contraction to improve emptying. It is most effective in combination with an α-adrenergic blocker, such as terazosin (1 to 10 mg daily), that simultaneously reduces pressure at the internal sphincter. Baclofen (10 mg three times daily) may be used to decrease spastic contraction of the external sphincter. Drugs that have atropinic properties, including a surprising variety of antiarrhythmic, antihistamine, neuroleptic, and antidepressant medications, may inhibit bladder contraction and result in overfilling and urinary retention (Table 445–5).

Erectile function (Chapter 253) in males is under parasympathetic control at the same sacral levels as the urinary system. Sensory afferent fibers travel via the pudendal nerve, whereas parasympathetic motor fibers run in the pelvic nerve. Sympathetic innervation via the hypogastric nerve contracts the seminal vesicles during ejaculation and closes the bladder neck to prevent retrograde emission. Although supraspinal influences are of great importance, reflex erection and ejaculation can occur in patients after spinal injury. Neurogenic impotence can result either from damage to the descending pathways relaying forebrain influence from the hypothalamus to the sacral preganglionic neurons or from injury to the sensory or parasympathetic motor innervation of the penis. A variety of drugs that block either parasympathetic or sympathetic function can interfere with erectile function (Table 445–6). Because erections normally occur several times nightly during periods of rapid eye movement sleep, it is possible to document organic disorders of erection by measuring penile tumescence overnight.

DISORDERS OF INTEGRATIVE CONTROL OF THE AUTONOMIC NERVOUS SYSTEM

Pathobiology

The autonomic nervous system is under three levels of central control. The *preganglionic* neurons located in the medulla and the spinal cord provide the final common pathway for central autonomic control. Each

TABLE 445–5 SOME COMMONLY PRESCRIBED DRUGS THAT MAY IMPAIR URINARY FUNCTION

Antiarrhythmics
Atropine
Disopyramide
Antihistamines
Diphenhydramine
Neuroleptics
Haloperidol
Chlorpromazine
Antidepressants
Amitriptyline
Imipramine
Antiparkinsonian agents
Amantadine
Dopa/carbidopa
Bromocriptine
Benztropine
Trihexyphenidyl
Antispasmodics
Baclofen

of these neurons integrates the input from many sources, including afferents from higher levels of the nervous system and local reflex responses. A series of *brain stem* and *spinal* cell groups coordinate *reflex control* of the autonomic nervous system. These nuclei receive cranial (parasympathetic) and spinal (sympathetic) afferent information and control a variety of important reflexes (e.g., swallowing, maintaining blood pressure, initiation of voiding). Both the preganglionic neurons and the brain stem reflex neurons are under the control of *forebrain integrative* cell groups that coordinate autonomic function with behavior and with endocrine control.

TABLE 445–6 SOME COMMONLY PRESCRIBED DRUGS THAT MAY IMPAIR ERECTILE FUNCTION

DRUGS CAUSING IMPOTENCE

Parasympatholytics
- Atropine
- Amitriptyline

Sympatholytics
- Methyldopa
- Guanethidine
- Clonidine
- Propranolol
- Prazosin

Vasodilators
- Hydralazine

Diuretics
- Hydrochlorothiazide

Antihistaminergic
- Cimetidine

DRUGS CAUSING PRIAPISM

Chlorpromazine
Thioridazine
Trazodone
Prazosin
Dopa/carbidopa

The hypothalamus is the most important area for integration of behavior with autonomic responses and with neuroendocrine control of the anterior and posterior pituitary glands (Fig. 445–1). Because the hypothalamus consists of tightly packed, interwoven pathways and cell groups, it is unusual for an injury to selectively involve a single functional system. Nevertheless, considerable progress has been made in determining the anatomic substrates for specific integrative functions, and disorders of these systems are occasionally encountered (Table 445–7). In addition, autonomic dysfunction is a frequent concomitant of emotional disorders.

Emotional Disorders

Portions of the insular and cingulate areas of the cerebral cortex and the amygdala are believed to regulate autonomic responses to emotional stress. In healthy individuals, stress can induce sympathetic responses such as pupillodilation, dry mouth, and increases in blood pressure. In patients with *panic disorder* (Chapter 420), such autonomic responses can become overwhelming and convince the patient that a serious organic problem exists. Positron emission tomography studies show increased metabolism in structures of the medial temporal lobe and the insular cortex during panic attacks. After eliminating the possibility of pheochro-

TABLE 445–7 REGIONAL HYPOTHALAMIC SYNDROMES

Region	Normally Regulates	Disorders
Preoptic	Blood volume, pressure, and electrolytes	Paroxysmal hyponatremia Essential hypernatremia
	Thermoregulation	Paroxysmal hypothermia
Tuberal	Gastrointestinal tract and feeding	Hyperphagia (ventromedial lesions) Hypophagia (lateral lesions)
	Reproduction	Hypogonadism
	Emotions	Rage responses
Posterior	Arousal	Hypersomnolence
	Descending autonomic and motor pathways	Poikilothermia

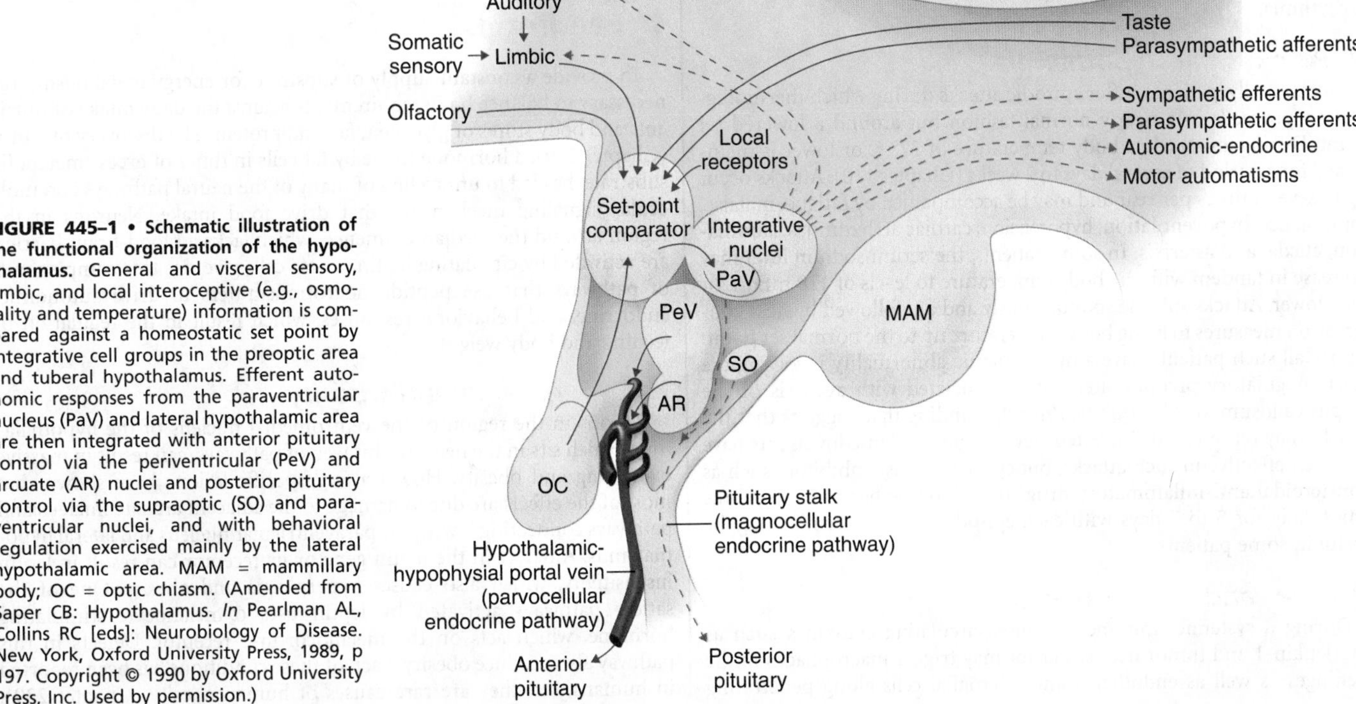

FIGURE 445–1 • Schematic illustration of the functional organization of the hypothalamus. General and visceral sensory, limbic, and local interoceptive (e.g., osmolality and temperature) information is compared against a homeostatic set point by integrative cell groups in the preoptic area and tuberal hypothalamus. Efferent autonomic responses from the paraventricular nucleus (PaV) and lateral hypothalamic area are then integrated with anterior pituitary control via the periventricular (PeV) and arcuate (AR) nuclei and posterior pituitary control via the supraoptic (SO) and paraventricular nuclei, and with behavioral regulation exercised mainly by the lateral hypothalamic area. MAM = mammillary body; OC = optic chiasm. (Amended from Saper CB: Hypothalamus. *In* Pearlman AL, Collins RC [eds]: Neurobiology of Disease. New York, Oxford University Press, 1989, p 197. Copyright © 1990 by Oxford University Press, Inc. Used by permission.)

mocytoma (Chapter 246), anxiolytic drugs (such as lorazepam, 1 to 2 mg three times daily) or antidepressant medications (such as citalopram, 20 mg/day) are usually helpful.

Some individuals under chronic emotional stress are subject to a variety of syndromes involving disruption of autonomic control of the internal organs. Although *psychosomatic illness* is often thought to be nonorganic and may respond to psychotherapeutic drugs, considerable evidence suggests that some organic disorders seen in anxious patients may also be caused by autonomic dysregulation. For example, individuals under stress may suffer erosive gastritis, gastric ulcers, and irritable bowel syndrome as a result of autonomic dysfunction. Perhaps the most serious problems are encountered in patients with preexisting cardiac abnormalities, who may have cardiac arrhythmias under stressful conditions. Retrospective studies of victims of sudden death caused by lethal ventricular arrhythmias indicate a much higher incidence of behavioral stress in the period preceding the attack. β-Adrenergic blockers, such as atenolol, 25 mg/day, may be useful in reducing the frequency of such arrhythmias.

Thermoregulatory Disorders

Thermoresponsive neurons in the medial preoptic area monitor brain temperature and regulate autonomic, endocrine, and somatomotor responses to match body temperature to a set point, which is normally 37° C in humans. Control of body temperature requires shifting blood flow between deep and superficial vascular beds and regulating conservation of body fluids (increased urination in the cold, increased sweating in the heat). Hence, thermoregulation is tightly linked to control of blood pressure, volume, and electrolyte composition, which are also regulated by neurons around the anteroventral tip of the third ventricle (see later).

Poikilothermia

Poikilothermia, defined as fluctuation in body temperature of more than 2° C with changes in ambient temperature, may result when lesions in the posterior hypothalamus or midbrain damage hypothalamic pathways for autonomic as well as behavioral thermoregulation. Relative poikilothermia can also result from metabolic disorders such as sedative drug ingestion (Chapter 32), hypoglycemia (Chapter 249), or hypothyroidism (Chapter 244), and a mild form is often seen in old age. Such patients are dangerously susceptible to lowered environmental temperature. Conversely, patients with relative poikilothermia or those taking anticholinergic drugs that prevent thermal sweating may experience dangerously elevated body temperatures during periods of hot weather. *Heat stroke* (Chapter 110), in which body temperature may exceed 42° C, is often fatal and requires prompt treatment by cooling the patient in an ice bath and expanding body fluids. Death is often a result of ventricular arrhythmia.

Paroxysmal Hypothermia

Occasionally, patients suffer episodic attacks during which thermoregulation proceeds in a nearly normal fashion but around a lowered set point. During an attack, a body temperature of 32° C or lower is maintained for a period of several days to 2 weeks (Chapter 110). Attacks occur up to several times per year and may be accompanied by fatigue, malaise, somnolence, hypoventilation, hypotension, cardiac arrhythmias, lacrimation, ataxia, and asterixis. In some patients, the serum sodium level may decrease in tandem with the body temperature to levels of 110 mEq/L or even lower. Attacks subside spontaneously and are followed by heat conservation measures to bring body temperature up to the normal set point. Nearly all such patients have a hypothalamic abnormality involving the thermoregulatory preoptic area (often associated with agenesis of the corpus callosum, or *Shapiro's syndrome*), a finding that suggests that the attacks may represent an "inverted" fever response. Anticonvulsants have not been effective in such attacks, but cyclooxygenase inhibitors such as nonsteroidal anti-inflammatory drugs (e.g., indomethacin, 25 mg three times daily for 5 to 7 days with each episode of hypothermia) may be useful in some patients.

Fever and Hyperthermia

During a systemic immune response, circulating cytokines such as interleukin-1 and tumor necrosis factor may trigger macrophages in the meninges as well as endothelial and microglial cells along penetrating venules at the borders of the brain to produce prostaglandins. These lipid mediators can cross the blood-brain barrier and act on neurons in the anteromedial preoptic area to reset the body's thermoregulatory set point upward. This process activates a coordinated set of autonomic, endocrine, and behavioral responses that increase thermogenesis and conserve heat. Drugs that inhibit the generation of prostaglandins are the mainstay of treatment of fever, but the wisdom of treating low-grade fever (<38.5° C) during an infectious illness has engendered considerable debate. An elevated body temperature may improve the function of certain immune cells while impairing the defenses of invading microorganisms.

Any physical injury to the brain that allows entry into the brain of macrophages or activates microglial cells to produce cytokines induces a febrile response as well. Hence, fever may be seen after head trauma, intracranial surgery, or cerebral hemorrhage or infarction. "Central neurogenic fever" is often proposed as a mechanism for fever of unknown origin, and a continuously elevated body temperature may be produced in animals by lesions that transect the anterior hypothalamus or the caudal pons. However, an inflammatory signal acting on the hypothalamus is generally responsible in cases in which body temperature fluctuates.

Malignant Hyperthermia

Malignant hyperthermia (Chapters 110, 114, 447, and 458), which is caused by an autosomal dominant disorder of skeletal muscle, can occur in patients who have been exposed to certain drugs. During induction of anesthesia, particularly with halothane and succinylcholine, certain patients sustain sudden massive muscle contractions accompanied by a rapid increase in body temperature to 42° C or greater. Circulatory and respiratory collapse and death can ensue unless immediate treatment with intravenous dantrolene (1 to 10 mg/kg) and supportive measures are instituted. This disorder is often associated with muscle central core disease and is due to a defect in regulation of the calcium release channel in muscle sarcoplasmic reticulum. The disorder is genetically heterogeneous, so preoperative pharmacologic testing of a muscle biopsy sample from suspected family members (with the caffeine-halothane contracture test) is still recommended.

Neuroleptic Malignant Syndrome

Muscular rigidity and elevated body temperature can occasionally be seen during treatment with neuroleptic drugs or after withdrawal of dopaminergic agonists. The pathogenesis of this *neuroleptic malignant syndrome* (Chapters 110, 433, and 434) is not understood, although it may reflect a febrile response in a patient with parkinsonian rigidity and drug-induced impairment of thermoregulation. Treatment with dopaminergic agonists such as bromocriptine, 5 to 15 mg three times daily, or in severe cases, dantrolene, 1 to 10 mg/kg, may provide faster resolution of the hyperthermia.

Feeding Disorders

To provide a constant supply of substrate for energy metabolism, it is necessary to balance body requirements against the daily intake of nutrients and body stores of glycogen, fat, and protein. The discovery of leptin (Chapter 239), a hormone made by fat cells in times of excess metabolic substrate, has led to unraveling of many of the neural pathways and molecular signaling mechanisms that drive food intake. Neurons in the region around the median eminence, which lacks a blood-brain barrier, are activated by circulating leptin. These cells give rise to a complex web of pathways that use peptide neurotransmitters to drive autonomic, endocrine, and behavioral responses, which result in the regulation of feeding and body weight.

Hyperphagia and Obesity

Lesions in the region of the ventromedial nucleus of the hypothalamus, which sits in the heart of this web of pathways, can result in massive overeating and obesity. However, cell-specific lesions have shown that most of the effects are due to damage to the adjacent arcuate nucleus and pathways connecting it with the paraventricular nucleus and lateral hypothalamus. A defect in the leptin gene or its receptor can result in leptin insensitivity, which also causes hyperphagia and obesity. One of the satiety pathways activated by leptin uses α-melanocyte–stimulating hormone, which acts on the melanocortin-4 receptor. Defects in this pathway also produce obesity. Each of these conditions has been reported in humans, but they are rare causes of human obesity (Chapter 239).

Conversely, ghrelin, a hormone produced by the stomach, causes hunger; reducing the ghrelin signal may be critical to maintaining weight loss.

Kleine-Levin Syndrome

Kleine-Levin syndrome is a poorly understood disorder in which patients, typically adolescent boys, have episodic attacks of somnolence in which they often sleep up to 20 hours per day. When awake, they appear dull and often confused and consume enormous quantities of food. Attacks may last up to 2 weeks and can recur several times per year. Pathologic verification of the site of the lesion in typical cases is lacking, but a similar syndrome may be seen acutely in encephalitis involving the hypothalamus.

Prader-Willi Syndrome

Prader-Willi syndrome (Chapter 39), a congenital disorder caused by a deletion in chromosome 15, is characterized by mental retardation, hypogonadism, and hyperphagia, often with massive obesity. Patients with Prader-Willi syndrome have elevated ghrelin levels, which may drive feeding behavior, but the causes of high ghrelin levels and other aspects of the syndrome remain unknown.

Hypophagia and Inanition

Large lesions in the region of the lateral hypothalamic area at the level of the ventromedial nucleus result in aphagia, which may recover to hypophagia and regulation around a new, lower body weight set point. Such lesions, which must be bilateral, are usually devastating, and selective impairment of eating on this basis has rarely been reported in adults. More often, patients with hypothalamic damage and inanition are somnolent and show a variety of endocrine abnormalities. No evidence of injury to the hypothalamus has been found in patients with anorexia nervosa (Chapter 238).

Central Disorders of Fluid and Electrolyte Regulation

The medial preoptic area around the anteroventral tip of the third ventricle plays a critical role in regulating blood pressure, volume, and electrolyte composition. Endocrine control (mineralocorticoids and especially vasopressin), autonomic regulation (control of blood flow in different vascular beds and innervation of sweat glands and the kidney, especially the juxtaglomerular apparatus controlling renin release), and behavioral response (drinking) all play important roles in this process. Disorders of the release of vasopressin by neurons whose cell bodies are located in the supraoptic and paraventricular nuclei are covered in Chapters 117 and 243. Coordinated central disorders of fluid regulation are rare.

Hypernatremia, Hyperosmolality, and Absence of Thirst

Neurogenic hypernatremia is a rare disorder marked by impairment of the normal responses to osmolar stimuli. Hence, there are deficits in the vasopressin response to increased sodium and osmolality, as well as absence or relative deficiency of thirst. The vasopressin response to hypovolemia may be maintained, and the preservation of habitual drinking of water (often related to meals) may be sufficient to maintain serum osmolality under normal conditions. During hot weather, when loss of water is increased through evaporation of sweat, patients often fail to increase their water consumption adequately and may suffer attacks of fatigue, fever, muscle cramps and tenderness, and even myoglobinuria (associated with hypokalemia). With very high serum sodium levels, patients may experience confusion or even become stuporous, and some may die (Chapter 117).

The hypothalamic injury giving rise to essential hypernatremia has been accurately localized in a few cases to the preoptic area in the region of the anteroventral third ventricle. Treatment consists of training the patient to drink adequate amounts of fluid, particularly during hot weather. Spironolactone (25 to 50 mg/day), chlorpropamide (250 mg/day), and thiazide diuretics (e.g., hydrochlorothiazide, 25 to 50 mg/day) have been used to reduce serum sodium and increase potassium.

Hyperdipsia, Hyponatremia, and Water Intoxication

Excessive water drinking in the absence of either hypovolemia or serum hyperosmolality is termed *primary hyperdipsia* and must be distinguished from the compensatory hyperdipsia of diabetes insipidus (Chapter 243), diabetes mellitus (Chapters 247 and 248), and polyuric renal failure (Chapter 131). In the absence of inappropriate vasopressin secretion, symptoms of water intoxication such as stupor, delirium, or convulsions are infrequent. Most severe hyperdipsia occurs in persons who have psychiatric disturbances. The only treatment is to restrict access to fluids until the psychiatric problem is controlled.

Paroxysmal Hyponatremia

Many patients with paroxysmal hypothermia (see earlier discussion) suffer simultaneous hyponatremia, which may be sufficiently severe (serum sodium <110 mEq/L) to cause symptoms of confusion or even convulsions. The serum sodium concentration is regulated around the reduced set point but may respond to fluid restriction.

Central Reproductive Disorders

Reproductive hormonal control, behavior, and the associated autonomic responses are controlled by neurons in the preoptic area close to those that regulate fluid and electrolyte control and by cells in the ventromedial hypothalamus close to neurons that regulate feeding. Although this contiguity may seem anomalous, reproductive capacity is closely tied to nutritional status (and leptin is a main regulator of both). In addition, sexual function and fetal maintenance rely on control of blood flow in specific vascular beds, which must be coordinated with control of body temperature and fluid balance. The change in body temperature that accompanies ovulation (Chapter 256) and the fluid shifts seen in the perimenstrual period in women are examples of this integration. Male erectile function (Chapter 253), which is dependent on sacral parasympathetic innervation of the penis, may be affected by diseases of the peripheral autonomic nervous system, as well as by psychogenic factors acting at the level of the forebrain.

Disorders of Arousal, Sleep, and Circadian Rhythms

The function of the autonomic nervous system is to augment the activity of various organ systems to deal with perturbations in internal homeostasis. Of all the body's organs, the single most important one to activate during an external threat is the brain. The ascending activating system, which runs from the rostral pons and caudal midbrain to the diencephalon, increases the responsiveness of the forebrain to external stimuli and may be considered a cerebral component of the autonomic system.

The hypothalamus plays a key role in inhibiting the arousal system during sleep and stabilizing the waking state during the day (Chapter 429). Loss of neurons in the ventrolateral preoptic nucleus can cause insomnia, whereas selective loss of the orexin (or hypocretin) neurons in the lateral hypothalamus causes excessive daytime sleepiness with attacks of loss of muscle tone *(cataplexy)* known as *narcolepsy.* Both wake and sleep systems are governed by a circadian system, under control of the suprachiasmatic nucleus, that organizes daily cycles of autonomic, endocrine, and behavioral functions. Work outside the normal circadian day, such as experienced by shift workers and physicians, can cause substantial impairment of alertness and cognitive function.

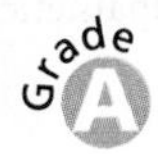

1. Low PA, Gilden JL, Freeman R, et al: Efficacy of midodrine vs. placebo in neurogenic orthostatic hypotension. A randomized, double-blind multicenter study. JAMA 1997;277:1046–1051.
2. Kaufmann H, Saadia D, Voustianiouk A, et al: Norepinephrine precursor therapy in neurogenic orthostatic hypotension. Circulation 2003;108:724–728.
3. Shannon JR, Diedrich A, Biaggioni I, et al: Water drinking as a treatment for orthostatic syndromes. Am J Med 2002;112:355–360.

SUGGESTED READINGS

Eisenach JH, Atkinson JL, Fealey RD: Hyperhidrosis: Evolving therapies for a well-established phenomenon. Mayo Clin Proc 2005;80:657–666. *A detailed overview.*

Goldstein DS, Robertson D, Esler M, et al: Dysautonomias: Clinical disorders of the autonomic nervous system. Ann Intern Med 2002;137:753–763. *A comprehensive overview.*

Grubb BP: Clinical practice: Neurocardiogenic syncope. N Engl J Med 2005;352:1004–1010. *A thorough review.*

Klein CM, Vernino S, Lennon VA, et al: The spectrum of autoimmune autonomic neuropathies. Ann Neurol 2003;53:752–758. *Redefines the pathophysiology and subgroups of peripheral autonomic failure based on the presence of ganglionic acetylcholine receptor antibodies.*

Saper CB, Scammell TE, Lu J: Hypothalamic regulation of sleep and circadian rhythms. Nature 2005;437:1257–1263. *An up-to-date review of the regulation of sleep and circadian rhythms of activity, body temperature, and hormones.*

Shibao C, Gamboa A, Diedrich A, et al: Management of hypertension in the setting of autonomic dysfunction. Curr Treat Options Cardiovasc Med 2006;8:105–109. *Overview of this difficult clinical problem, suggesting that nighttime transdermal nitroglycerin (0.1 to 0.2 mg/hr) or nifedipine (30 mg orally) is useful.*

Taylor RS, Van Buyten JP, Buchser E: Spinal cord stimulation for complex regional pain syndrome: A systematic review of the clinical and cost-effectiveness literature and assessment of prognostic factors. Eur J Pain 2006;10:91–101. *Reviews evidence suggesting benefits from this treatment.*

Vinik AI, Ziegler D: Diabetic cardiovascular autonomic neuropathy. Circulation 2007;115:387–397. *A comprehensive review.*

446 PERIPHERAL NEUROPATHIES

Michael E. Shy

APPROACH TO PERIPHERAL NEUROPATHIES

Definition and Pathobiology

Peripheral neuropathy is a general term for disorders affecting peripheral nerves. The peripheral nervous system consists of motor, sensory, and autonomic neurons that extend outside the central nervous system (CNS) and are ensheathed by Schwann cells or ganglionic satellite cells. The peripheral nervous system includes the dorsal and ventral spinal roots, spinal and cranial nerves, sensory and motor terminals, and part of the autonomic nervous system. Motor neurons extend from their cell body in the ventral horn of the spinal cord to the neuromuscular junctions at the muscle that they innervate. The cell bodies of primary sensory neurons lie outside the spinal cord in the dorsal root ganglia, where they extend peripherally to specialized sensory end organs, including nociceptors, thermoreceptors, and mechanoreceptors. Central projections from dorsal root ganglia enter the spinal cord through the dorsal roots. At each spinal segment, the ventral roots, which carry motor axons, and the dorsal roots, which carry sensory axons, join to form mixed sensorimotor nerves. In the cervical, brachial, and lumbosacral areas, the mixed spinal nerves form plexuses from which arise the major anatomically defined limb nerves. Each mixed nerve is composed of large numbers of myelinated and nonmyelinated nerve fibers of varying diameter. The large myelinated axons include motor neurons and large fiber sensory nerves that mediate position and vibration sense. Small, thinly myelinated and nonmyelinated axons primarily provide nociception and autonomic functions. Preganglionic sympathetic autonomic fibers begin in the intermediolateral column of the spinal cord and synapse in ganglia of the sympathetic trunk. Preganglionic parasympathetic fibers travel long distances from their cell bodies in the brain stem or sacral spinal cord to reach terminal ganglia near the organs that the parasympathetic fibers innervate.

Clinical Manifestations

Symptoms of peripheral neuropathy include weakness, sensory loss, abnormal balance, and autonomic dysfunction. Weakness in peripheral nerve disease is often distal and more severe in the legs than the arms. Deep and superficial muscles that are innervated by the peroneal nerve, such as the tibialis anterior and peroneus brevis and longus muscles, often cause more symptoms than do the plantar flexion muscles innervated by the tibial nerve, such as the gastrocnemius. As a result, tripping on a carpet or curb and spraining one's ankle are frequent symptoms of neuropathy. In the hands, symptoms typically involve fine movements, such as using buttons or zippers and inserting and turning keys in locks. Cramps, the painful knotting of a muscle, frequently occur with motor or sensorimotor neuropathies.

The sensory symptoms of neuropathy may involve small, thinly myelinated or nonmyelinated fibers subserving pain and temperature, as well as large myelinated fibers subserving position sense. Common symptoms of small fiber sensory neuropathy include feeling as though the feet are "walking on pebbles" or "ice cold" and difficulty determining whether bath water is hot or cold with the foot. Painful dysesthesias, such as feeling as though the feet are "on fire," "on hot coals," or "stuck with pins," are also associated with small fiber abnormalities. Similar symptoms occur less frequently in the hands because most neuropathies are dependent on the length of the nerves; as a general rule, sensory symptoms begin in the hands when sensory symptoms in the legs have progressed up to the knee. An exception is when the patient also has carpal tunnel syndrome, which is often manifested as pain and tingling in the hands and can awaken patients from sleep. Large fiber sensory loss usually impairs balance, which may be worse in a crowd or at night when vision cannot overcome the loss of proprioception. Loss of proprioception is also frequently length dependent, so a patient may improve balance by lightly touching a wall with the hand because nerves from the arm improve proprioceptive input to the brain.

Autonomic symptoms are frequent in neuropathies associated with diabetes or amyloidosis and include urinary retention or incontinence, abnormalities of sweating, constipation alternating with diarrhea, and light-headedness when standing. Impotence is frequent.

Diagnosis

Systematic Approach to Patients with Peripheral Neuropathy

Evaluation begins with the history and physical examination to demonstrate peripheral nerve disease and proceeds to neurophysiologic testing to characterize whether the process is demyelinating or axonal. Other specific tests are then ordered (Fig. 446–1).

Peripheral neuropathies usually affect both motor and sensory nerves, thereby causing both weakness and sensory loss. However, certain neuropathies are predominantly sensory, such as diabetes, or motor, such as multifocal motor neuropathy (Tables 446–1 and 446–2). Most neuropathies are symmetrical as well as length dependent. Pronounced asymmetries in symptoms suggest specific disorders, such as mononeuritis multiplex or hereditary neuropathy with liability to pressure palsies. It is also useful to know whether symptoms are acute (<1 month), subacute (<6 months), or chronic (>6 months). For example, Guillain-Barré syndrome develops over a period of days to weeks, whereas chronic inflammatory demyelinating polyneuropathy (CIDP) evolves over months and inherited neuropathies may develop over years.

Neurologic Examination

Wasting of muscle is a prominent feature of many sensorimotor or motor neuropathies, regardless of whether they are primary axonal or primary demyelinating disorders, because even demyelinating neuropathies are associated with secondary axonal degeneration. Atrophy frequently occurs in muscles of dorsiflexion, such as the tibialis anterior, and in intrinsic hand muscles, such as the first dorsal interosseus. Fasciculations, which appear as small twitches of the muscle, are sometimes present, particularly in axonal neuropathies.

Weakness is often most pronounced in foot dorsiflexion and eversion and in the intrinsic hand muscles. In the lower extremities, weakness usually progresses to the muscles of plantar flexion before more proximal muscles become involved. For most sensorimotor or motor neuropathies, symmetry is the rule.

Sensory loss is usually in a stocking-glove distribution in both large and small fiber neuropathy. Cold, erythematous, or bluish discolored feet suggest loss of small fiber function. Large fiber sensory loss, or "sensory ataxia," in the upper extremities can often be detected by an inability of the patient to locate the thumb accurately with the opposite index finger while the eyes are closed or by the presence of a characteristic irregular tremor (pseudoathetosis) of the fingers.

The sensory examination should include vibration, position, and light touch, as well as pain and temperature. It is important to determine the degree and extent of sensory loss, in addition to the pattern of deficits (symmetrical or asymmetrical; distal or generalized; focal, multifocal, or diffuse).

The complete absence of reflexes early in the course of a neuropathy suggests a demyelinating neuropathy (Chapter 436); for example, the

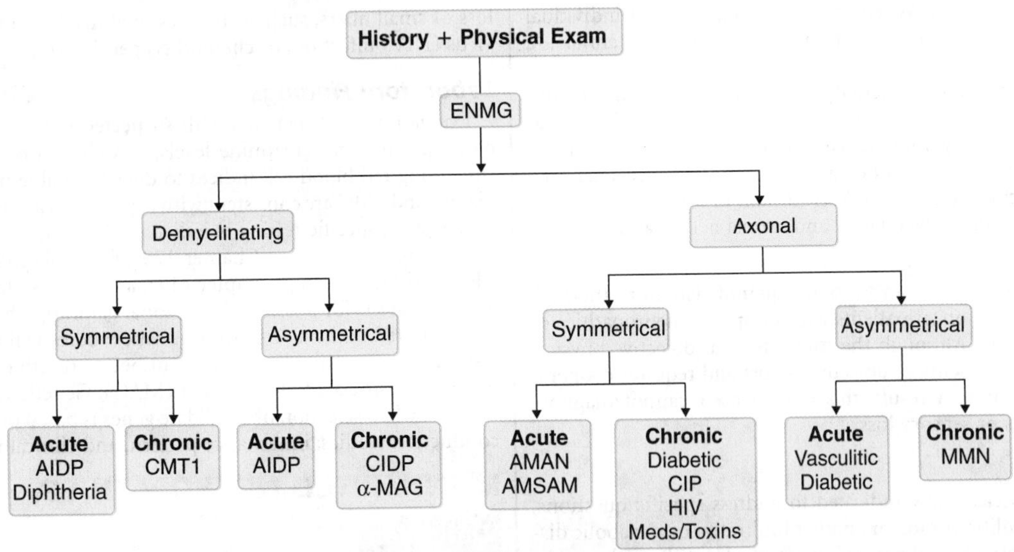

FIGURE 446–1 • A systematic approach to evaluate neuropathy. The diseases listed are examples of neuropathies associated with specific neurophysiologic and clinical findings. Diabetic distal, predominantly sensory neuropathies are manifested as chronic axonal neuropathies; acute asymmetrical neuropathies can also occur with diabetes. Most neuropathies caused by toxins or by side effects of medication are chronic, symmetrical axonal neuropathies. AIDP, AMAN, and AMSAN are subtypes of Guillain-Barré syndrome. These and other examples are discussed in more detail in the text. AIDP = acute inflammatory demyelinating polyradiculoneuropathy; AMAN = acute motor axonal neuropathy; AMSAN = acute motor and sensory axonal neuropathy; CIDP = chronic inflammatory polyradiculoneuropathy; CIP = chronic illness polyneuropathy; CMT1 = Charcot-Marie-Tooth disease type 1, a genetic disorder; HIV = human immunodeficiency virus–related neuropathy; α-MAG = anti–myelin-associated glycoprotein; MMN = multifocal motor neuropathy.

TABLE 446–1 PREDOMINANTLY SENSORY NEUROPATHIES

Classification	Subgroup	Type	Fibers
Genetic		HSAN	Large, small
Inflammatory/immune	Monoclonal gammopathy	Anti-MAG (early on)	Mainly large
	Vasculitis	Sjögren's syndrome	Large, small
	Paraneoplastic	Anti-Hu	Large
Metabolic	Diabetic	Distal symmetrical polyneuropathy	Large, small
Infectious	HIV	HIV neuropathy	Small
	Herpes zoster	Focal radiculoneuropathy	Small
	Leprosy	Tuberculoid	Small
Toxic/deficiency	Medications	Vincristine	Small
		Paclitaxel	Large
		Cisplatin	Large
		Thalidomide	Large
		NRTIs	Small
	Toxins	Thallium	Small
		Acrylamide	Large
		Pyridoxine (B_6)	Large, small
	Deficiency states	Vitamin B_1	Large, small
		Vitamin B_{12}	Large
		Vitamin E	Large
Idiopathic	Frequent		Large, small

HIV = human immunodeficiency virus; HSAN = hereditary sensory and autonomic neuropathy; MAG = myelin-associated glycoprotein; NRTIs = nucleoside reverse transcriptase inhibitors.

absence of reflexes in early childhood is often the first detectable abnormality in children with inherited demyelinating neuropathies. Alternatively, the absence of ankle reflexes but the presence of normal patellar or upper extremity reflexes is common in "dying back" (length dependent) axonal neuropathies, both acquired and inherited. Reflexes may be present in small fiber neuropathies.

On gait testing, subtle weakness in the feet can be detected by an inability of the patient to heel walk. Sensory ataxia can be appreciated by a wide-based gait or inability to tandem walk.

Neurologic Testing

Neurophysiology

Electromyography (EMG) and nerve conduction studies can determine whether a neuropathy is primarily demyelinating or axonal and can confirm whether the process is symmetrical or asymmetrical (Chapter 418).

Motor nerve conduction velocities measure conduction over the main body of nerves but not their proximal or distal portion. Distal motor latencies and F wave latencies measure velocities over the distal and proximal portions of the nerves. When slowing is roughly the same over the proximal, distal, and main portion of the nerve, the slowing is said to be uniform. When the slowing is multifocal or asymmetrical, either along the same nerve or between different nerves, the slowing is said to be nonuniform. Slowed conduction velocities (to less than 70% of normal) suggest that the neuropathy is primarily demyelinating.

The sensory nerve action potential is a summation of action potentials from individual large-diameter sensory axons. In axonal neuropathies, amplitudes of the compound muscle action potential or sensory nerve action potential are reduced. When there has been a loss of individual sensory axons, amplitudes of the sensory nerve action potential are reduced.

The presence of spontaneous activity such as fibrillations or positive sharp waves by EMG suggests that an acute or active process is damaging axons and denervating muscle. The presence of large, polyphasic motor units suggests partial reinnervation of muscle by regenerating axons (i.e., a more chronic process). Recruitment of motor units is also reduced in patients with demyelinating and axonal neuropathies.

Quantitative Sensory Testing

Quantitative sensory testing can assess and quantify vibratory, thermal, or painful sensory function in patients with peripheral neuropathies or other sensory disorders. Although the stimulus is an objective physical event, the response represents a subjective report and requires cooperation from the patient; as a result, this test by itself cannot diagnose sensory neuropathies or sensory loss.

Nerve Biopsy

Nerve biopsy is occasionally indicated to address specific questions, such as whether vasculitis, tumor, or another infiltrative or metabolic disorder is present. Biopsy of sural nerves is performed just above the ankle. After biopsy, patients lose sensation over the region on the lateral aspect of the foot that is innervated by the sural nerve, and transient painful dysesthesias may develop around the biopsy site. Teased sural nerve fiber analysis can demonstrate segmental demyelination or remyelination, and electron microscopy can demonstrate features of nerve regeneration and identify specific pathologic processes. Epidermal skin biopsies with quantification of the loss of small epidermal nerve fibers may aid in the diagnosis of sensory neuropathies, particularly in neuropathies that involve a loss of small fibers, such as diabetes mellitus, human immunodeficiency virus (HIV) infection, or chemotherapeutic drugs.

Laboratory Findings

Evaluation of all patients with suspected neuropathy should include blood glucose and creatinine levels, as well as a complete blood count (including red blood cell indices to detect possible macrocytosis). If the history and EMG are consistent with exposure to a toxin or a vitamin deficiency state, specific testing is indicated. Most, if not all patients should also have a vitamin B_{12} (Chapter 170), rapid plasmin reagent (Chapter 340), and HIV testing (Chapter 417), as well as serum immunofixation electrophoresis for possible monoclonal gammopathy (Chapter 198).

In selected patients, electrodiagnostic studies will suggest the need to test for specific antibodies, such as antibodies reacting to ganglioside GM_1 or myelin-associated glycoprotein (MAG). Genetic testing is most cost-effective when selection of candidate genes is based on the patient's nerve conduction studies, inheritance pattern, and clinical findings.

INHERITED NEUROPATHIES

Definition

Inherited neuropathies are frequently called Charcot-Marie-Tooth disease (CMT) based on the names of the three physicians who initially characterized the disorders in the late 19th century. They are also referred to as hereditary motor and sensory neuropathies, hereditary motor neuropathies, or hereditary sensory and autonomic neuropathies, depending on their clinical manifestation. Autosomal dominant forms are subdivided into demyelinating (CMT1) and dominantly inherited axonal (CMT2) forms based on electrophysiologic and neuropathologic criteria. X-linked (CMTX) and autosomal recessive (CMT4) forms are also seen. Each type of CMT is subdivided according to the specific genetic cause of the neuropathy. For example, the most common form of CMT1, termed CMT1A, is caused by a duplication of a fragment of chromosome 17 containing the peripheral myelin protein 22-kD *(PMP22)* gene (see later). Currently, mutations in more than 30 genes have been identified as causes of inherited neuropathies (available at *http://molgen-www.uia.ac.be/CMTMutations/*) (Table 446–3).

Epidemiology

The prevalence of CMT is about 1 in 2500, without ethnic predisposition. The 17p11.2 duplication causing CMT1A accounts for 60 to 70% of CMT1 patients, CMTX1 for approximately 10 to 20% of CMT cases, CMT1B for less than 5% of patients, and CMT2 for about 20% of cases. The prevalence of hereditary neuropathy with liability to pressure palsies is not known, but about 85% of patients with clinical evidence of this syndrome have a chromosome 17p11.2 deletion.

TABLE 446–2 PREDOMINANTLY MOTOR NEUROPATHIES

Classification	Subgroup	Type
Genetic		HMN
Inflammatory/immune	Guillain-Barré	AMAN
	Multifocal motor neuropathy	MMN
	Critical illness myopathy	CIM
Toxic/deficiency	Medications	Dapsone
	Toxins	Lead (adults)

AMAN = acute motor axonal neuropathy; HMN = hereditary motor neuropathy.

TABLE 446–3 INHERITED NEUROPATHIES

Disorder	Locus/Gene	Inheritance	Protein	Mutation (Frequency)	Testing Method	Type of Testing
HEREDITARY MOTOR AND SENSORY NEUROPATHIES						
CMT1A	17p11.2/*PMP22*	AD	Peripheral myelin protein 22	Duplication (98%)	Pulsed-field gel electrophoresis, FISH, Southern blot	Clinical
				Point mutation (2%)	Sequencing, mutation scanning, mutation analysis	
HNPP	17p11.2/*PMP22*	AD	Peripheral myelin protein 22	Deletion (80%)	Mutation analysis, FISH, long PCR-RFLP, Southern blot	Clinical
				Point mutation/small deletion (20%)	Sequencing	
CMT1B	1q22/*MPZ*	AD	Myelin protein zero	Point mutation	Sequencing, mutation scanning, mutation analysis	Clinical
CMT1C	16p13.1-p12.3/*LITAF*	AD	SIMPLE			Research

TABLE 446–3 INHERITED NEUROPATHIES—cont'd

Disorder	Locus/Gene	Inheritance	Protein	Mutation (Frequency)	Testing Method	Type of Testing
CMT1D	10q21.1-q22.1/*EGR2*	AD	Early growth response protein 2	Point mutation	Sequencing, mutation scanning, mutation analysis	Clinical
CMT2A	1p36.2/*MFN2*	AD	Mitofusin 2	Point mutation	Direct DNA, linkage analysis	Research
CMT2B	3q21/*RAB7*	AD	Ras-related protein Rab-7	Point mutation	Direct DNA, linkage analysis	Research
CMT2C	12q23-24/unknown	AD	Unknown		Direct DNA, linkage analysis	
CMT2D	7p15/*GARS*	AD	Glycyl-tRNA synthetase	Point mutation	Direct DNA, linkage analysis	Research
CMT2E	8p21/*NEFL*	AD	Neurofilament triplet L protein	Point mutation	Sequencing	Clinical
CMT2F	7q11-21/unknown	AD	Unknown		Linkage	Research
CMT4A	8q13-q21.1/*GDAP1*	AR	Ganglioside-induced differentiation protein-1	Point mutation	Sequencing	Clinical
CMT4B1	11q22/*MTMR2*	AR	Myotubularin-related protein 2	Point mutation		Research
CMT4B2	11p15/*CMT4B2*	AR	SET binding factor 2	Point mutation		Research
CMT4C	5q32/*KIAA1985*	AR	KIAA1985	Point mutation		Research
CMT4D	8q24.3/*NDRG1*	AR	NDRG1 protein	Point mutation		Research
CMT4E	10q21.1-q22.1/*EGR2*	AR	Early growth response protein 2	Point mutation	Mutation analysis, sequencing	Clinical
CMT4F	19q13.1-q13.2/*PRX*	AR	Periaxin	Point mutation	Mutation analysis, sequencing	Clinical
CMTX	Xq13.1/*GJB1*	X-linked	Gap junction β-1 protein (connexin 32)	Point mutations, deletions (rare)	Sequencing, mutation scanning, mutation analysis	Clinical
DISTAL HEREDITARY MOTOR NEUROPATHIES						
dHMN I	Unknown	AD	Unknown			Research
dHMN II	12q24.3/unknown	AD	Unknown			Research
dHMN III	1q21-23/unknown	AR	Unknown			Research
dHMN V	7p15/*GARS*	AD	Glycyl-tRNA synthetase	Point mutation		Research
dHMN VI	Unknown	AR	Unknown			Research
dHMN VII	2q14/unknown	AD	Unknown			Research
dHMN Jerash	9p21.1-p12/unknown	AR	Unknown			Research
ALS4	9q34/unknown	AD	SETX	Point mutation		Research
HMN Dynactin	2p13/*DCTN1*	AD	Dynactin	Point mutation		Research
HEREDITARY SENSORY AND AUTONOMIC NEUROPATHIES						
HSAN I	9q22.1-q22.3/*SPTLC1*	AD	Serine palmitoyltransferase light chain 1	Point mutations	Sequencing	Clinical
HSAN II	Unknown	AR	Unknown			Research
HSAN III (Riley Day)	9q31/*IKBKAP*	AR	IκB kinase complex–associated protein	2 mutations account for 99% of affected patients of Ashkenazi Jewish descent	Mutation analysis, quantitative PCR	Clinical
HSAN IV	1q21-q22/*NTRK1*	AR	Tyrosine kinase for nerve growth factor	Point mutation		Research

CMT = Charcot-Marie-Tooth disease; FISH = fluorescence in situ hybridization; HNPP = hereditary neuropathy with liability to pressure palsies; dHMN = distal hereditary motor neuropathy; HSAN = hereditary sensory and autonomic neuropathy; PCR = polymerase chain reaction; RFLP = restriction fragment length polymorphism.

Pathobiology

Pathology

Segmental demyelination, remyelination, and axonal loss are characteristic features of the various demyelinating forms of CMT1. In Dejerine-Sottas neuropathy, the demyelination is more severe. In CMT1, onion bulbs of concentric Schwann cell lamellae are usually present on nerve biopsies, with loss of both small- and-large diameter myelinated fibers and sometimes axons. Focal, sausage-like thickenings of the myelin sheath (tomacula) are characteristic of hereditary neuropathy with liability to pressure palsies but may also be found in other forms of CMT1, particularly CMT1B. In CMT1, disability typically correlates better with secondary axonal degeneration than with demyelination itself, thereby demonstrating the importance of Schwann cell–axonal interactions in demyelinating disease (Fig. 446–2).

Genetics

Mutations in *PMP22* and *MPZ* cause CMT1, and mutations in *GJB1* cause CMTX1. All three genes code for myelin proteins. Mutations in the neurofilament light *(NEFL)*, mitofusin 2 *(MFN2)*, and *dynactin* genes cause CMT2; all three genes have roles in the axonal cytoskeleton and axonal transport. LITAF/SIMPLE, the myotubulin-related proteins 2 and 13, and RAB7 are involved in intracellular trafficking. MFN2 and ganglioside-induced differentiation-associated protein-1 (GDAP1) are nuclearly encoded mitochondrial proteins.

Clinical Manifestations

Despite phenotypic variability, the typical clinical course of CMT1 and CMT2 patients includes normal development before weakness, and

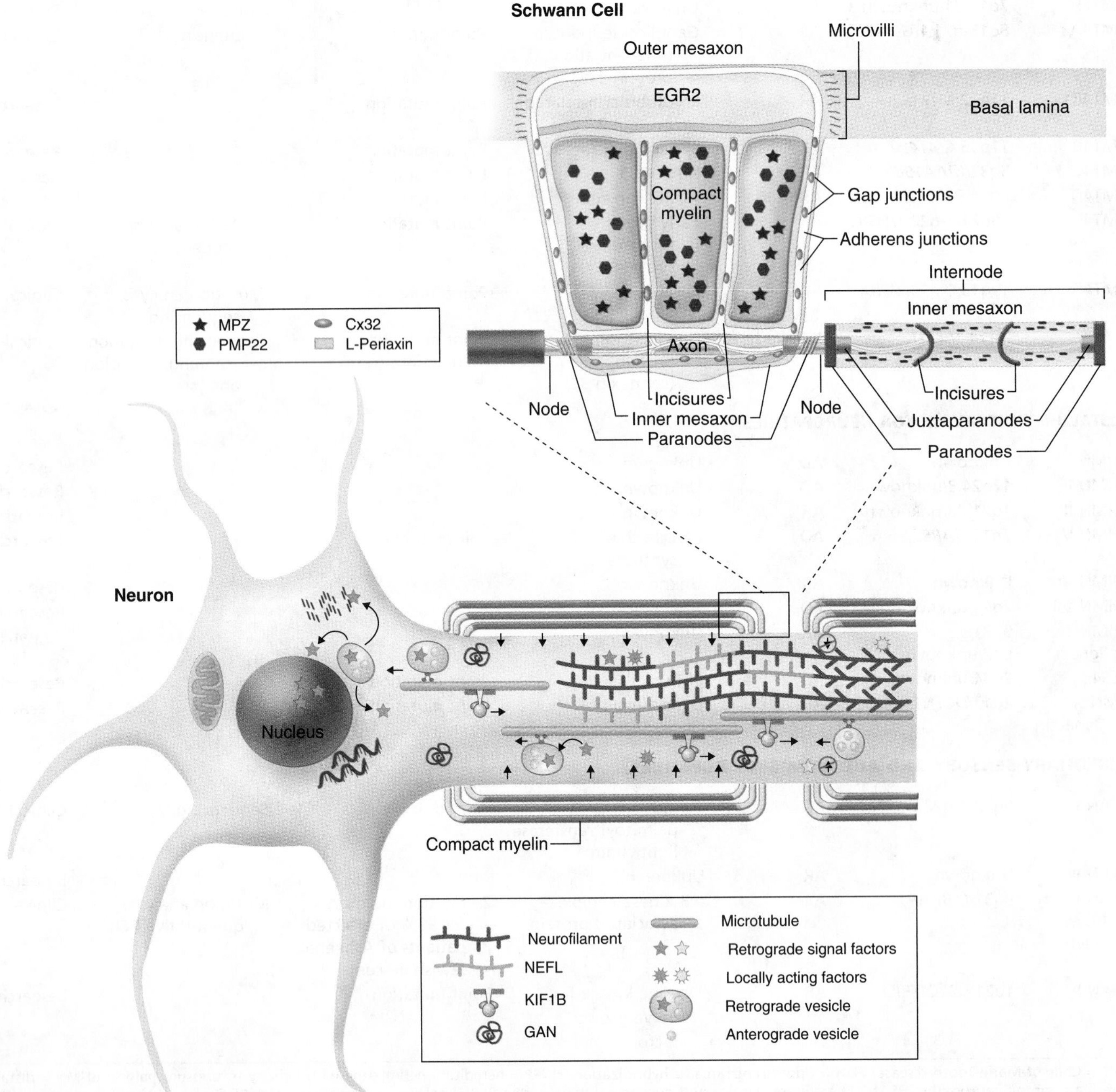

FIGURE 446–2 • Schematic view of an axon and its myelinating Schwann cell. Proteins mutated in inherited peripheral neuropathies are shown in color at their cellular location. In the upper part of the panel, the myelinating Schwann cell has been unraveled to show the nucleus and regions of both compact myelin and noncompact myelin. Cytoskeletal elements within the axon are also illustrated. (From Shy ME, Garbern JY, Kamholz J: Hereditary motor and sensory neuropathies: A biological perspective. Lancet Neurol 2002;1:110–118.)

sensory loss appearing gradually within the first 2 decades of life. Affected children are often slow runners and have difficulty with activities that require balance (e.g., skating, walking across a log). Ankle-foot orthoses are frequently required by the third decade. Fine movements of the hands for activities such as turning a key or using buttons and zippers may be impaired, but the hands are rarely as affected as the feet. Most patients remain ambulatory throughout life and have a normal lifespan.

A minority of CMT patients have a more severe phenotype with delayed motor milestones and onset in infancy, termed *Dejerine-Sottas neuropathy.* Especially severe cases are classified as congenital hypomyelination if myelination appears to be disrupted during embryologic development. Many patients have de novo autosomal dominant disorders, and the term Dejerine-Sottas neuropathy is currently used primarily to denote severe early-onset clinical phenotypes regardless of the inheritance pattern. Patients with hereditary motor neuropathies sometimes have mild sensory abnormalities, and patients with hereditary sensory and autonomic neuropathies usually have some weakness. The same mutations in the same gene *(GARS)* cause both CMT2D and hereditary motor neuropathy type V.

Diagnosis

Molecular testing, performed after the family history, neurologic examination, and neurophysiologic testing have suggested the probable candidate genes (GeneClinics—available at *www.geneclinics.org*), is the "gold standard" for the diagnosis of inherited neuropathies. Nerve conduction velocity testing can distinguish between demyelinating and axonal neuropathies. Most CMT1 patients, particularly those with CMT1A, have a uniformly slow nerve conduction velocity of about 20 m/sec. Asymmetrical slowing, which is characteristic of hereditary neuropathy with liability to pressure palsies, may be found in patients with missense mutations in *PMP22, MPZ, EGR2,* and *GJB1.* Although CMT2 is characterized by axonal loss and reduced compound muscle action potential or sensory nerve action potential amplitudes, virtually all forms of CMT1 have axonal loss as well as demyelination.

Differential Diagnosis

Inherited neuropathies must be distinguished from acquired neuropathies (see later). Additionally, genetic disorders of the CNS such as hereditary spastic paraplegia or leukodystrophies (Chapter 436) may mimic inherited neuropathies by causing length-dependent weakness, sensory loss, and foot deformities such as pes cavus; these patients will frequently have upper motor neuron signs, such as increased reflexes or Babinski's signs, and do not have neurophysiologic evidence of neuropathy.

Treatment

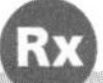

There is no specific therapy for the inherited neuropathies, but clinical and genetic counseling and symptomatic and rehabilitative treatment are important. A detailed family history and often examination of family members are required for prognosis and genetic counseling.

Ankle-foot orthoses to correct footdrop may return gait and balance to normal for years. Foot surgery is sometimes offered to correct inverted feet, pes cavus, and hammertoes. Surgery may improve walking, alleviate pain over pressure points, and prevent plantar ulcers. However, foot surgery is generally unnecessary and does not improve weakness and sensory loss.

Ascorbic acid, antagonists to progesterone, and subcutaneous injections of neurotrophin 3 have benefited animal models of CMT1A or small numbers of CMT1A patients. Clinical trials of these agents are needed.

INFLAMMATORY/IMMUNOLOGIC NEUROPATHIES

Guillain-Barré Syndrome

Definition

Guillain-Barré syndrome refers to acquired, inflammatory peripheral neuropathies that have (1) an acute onset, (2) elevated cerebrospinal fluid (CSF) protein levels with low CSF cell counts (cyto-albumologic dissociation), and (3) a monophasic illness with at least partial recovery. Guillain-Barré syndrome is subdivided into acute inflammatory demyelinating polyneuropathy, acute motor and sensory axonal neuropathy, acute motor axonal neuropathy, and the Miller-Fisher syndrome (Table 446–4).

TABLE 464–4 INFLAMMATORY AND IMMUNE-RELATED NEUROPATHIES

Disorder	Type	Clinical Traits	Pathobiology	Treatment*
Guillain-Barré syndrome	AIDP	Acute flaccid weakness, sensory loss	Demyelination, lymphocyte infiltration	Plasma exchange, IVIG
	AMAN/AMSAN	Acute flaccid weakness, no sensory loss in AMAN	Molecular mimicry, association with *Campylobacter jejuni*	? Plasma exchange or IVIG
	Fisher's syndrome	Acute ataxia, ophthalmoparesis and areflexia	Anti-GQ1b antibodies	? Plasma exchange or IVIG
CIDP		Slower onset of weakness, sensory loss	Inflammatory/immune-mediated demyelination	Corticosteroids, plasma exchange, IVIG
Monoclonal gammopathy	IgM	Sensory > motor	Particularly anti-MAG	Immune suppression (Chapter 198)
	IgG	Sensorimotor	Many probably chance associations, osteosclerotic myeloma, solitary plasmacytoma; POEMS may be immune mediated	Treatment of myeloma
Multifocal motor neuropathy		Pure motor	Focal demyelination, antibodies to GM_1 frequent	IVIG

*Typical regimens: IVIG, 0.4 g/kg/day × 5 days for a total of 2 g/kg; may be repeated monthly as needed. Corticosteroids: prednisone, 60 to 80 mg/day for up to 3 months, followed by gradual tapering, depending on the clinical response, with a goal to about 20 mg on an alternate-day regimen.

AIDP = acute idiopathic demyelinating polyneuropathy; AMAN = acute motor axonal neuropathy; AMSAN = acute motor and sensory axonal neuropathy; CIDP = chronic inflammatory polyradiculoneuropathy; IVIG = intravenous immune globulin; MAG = myelin-associated glycoprotein; POEMS = polyneuropathy, organomegaly, M protein, skin changes.

Epidemiology

Acute inflammatory demyelinating polyneuropathy, the demyelinating form, accounts for up to 97% of cases of Guillain-Barré syndrome in North America and Europe. It is a sporadic disorder with an incidence of 0.6 to 1.9 cases per 100,000 in North America and Europe. Men are more likely to be affected than women (2:1). In 60% of cases, acute inflammatory demyelinating polyneuropathy is preceded by a respiratory tract infection (e.g., cytomegalovirus, Epstein-Barr virus) or gastroenteritis *(Campylobacter jejuni)*. Acute motor axonal neuropathy and acute motor and sensory axonal neuropathy are rare in North American and Europe but more frequent in China, Japan, Mexico, Korea, and India.

Pathobiology

All forms of Guillain-Barré syndrome probably result from postinfectious molecular mimicry in which nerve antigens are attacked by the immune system because they resemble antigens presented by microbes, in particular, *C. jejuni*. For example, the HS/0:19 serotype of *C. jejuni* is common in northern Chinese patients with Guillain-Barré syndrome and has also been isolated from such patients in Ireland and the United States. Assays with antiganglioside antibodies, bacterial toxins, and lectins have characterized potential immunogenic regions of diarrhea-associated *C. jejuni* strains, but no definitive antigen or antibody has been identified as being responsible for Guillain-Barré syndrome.

Clinical Manifestations

Weakness, which is the most common initial symptom in both acute inflammatory demyelinating polyneuropathy and acute motor and sensory axonal neuropathy, can be mild, such as difficulty walking, or severe, such as total quadriplegia and respiratory failure. Bilateral weakness of facial muscles (facial diplegia) occurs in about 50% of cases. The most common manifestation is leg weakness that subsequently "ascends" into the arms. Although Guillain-Barré syndrome has been described as an "ascending paralysis," proximal weakness is common, and 5% of cases have isolated cranial nerve involvement that subsequently descends into the limbs. Sensory loss occurs in the majority of patients. The autonomic nervous system is involved in about 65% of patients.

Length-dependent weakness without sensory loss develops in patients with acute motor axonal neuropathy, including cranial nerve involvement in about 25%. Miller-Fisher syndrome consists of the triad of ophthalmoplegia, ataxia, and areflexia. Facial weakness, ptosis, and pupillary abnormalities may be present. Nerve conduction velocities in Miller-Fisher syndrome are generally normal, unlike the case with acute inflammatory demyelinating polyneuropathy.

Diagnosis

The diagnosis of acute inflammatory demyelinating polyneuropathy and acute motor and sensory axonal neuropathy is based on the history, physical examination, and CSF evaluation. Deep tendon reflexes are decreased or absent and the CSF is abnormal with cyto-albuminologic dissociation. The weakness is symmetrical. The presence of CNS abnormalities should cast doubt on the diagnosis. Acute inflammatory demyelinating polyneuropathy is distinguished from acute motor and sensory axonal neuropathy by nerve conduction studies. In both acute inflammatory demyelinating polyneuropathy and acute motor and sensory axonal neuropathy, the CSF should have fewer than five white blood cells (WBCs)/mL. If the CSF cell count is greater than 50 WBCs/mL, another diagnosis, such as HIV infection (Chapter 417) or Lyme disease (Chapter 342), should be considered. Elevated CSF protein may not be apparent in the first 7 to 10 days of the illness; in up to 10% of cases, CSF protein levels remain normal. Approximately 5% of patients with Guillain-Barré syndrome have Miller-Fisher syndrome, and more than 85% of these patients have polyclonal antibodies that react with the ganglioside GQ_{1b}.

Differential Diagnosis

The differential diagnosis varies in different parts of the world. Historically, poliomyelitis (Chapter 440) was the major cause of acute flaccid quadriparesis. In North America, polio has been eradicated, but other viral illnesses may induce polio-like syndromes: ECHO 70 (Chapter 402), coxsackievirus (Chapter 402), West Nile virus (Chapter 405), and rarely, rabies (Chapter 441). Because these diseases are not demyelinating disorders, they can be distinguished from acute inflammatory demyelinating polyneuropathy by their normal nerve conduction velocity. However, the results of electrodiagnostic studies are similar in both acute motor axonal neuropathy and the polio-like syndromes, thus making distinction between acute motor axonal neuropathy and these syndromes difficult.

Tick paralysis (Chapter 405), caused by a toxin within the tick, can mimic Guillain-Barré syndrome, particularly in children. Usually, removal of the tick is associated with improvement within hours, although progression can occur. Progression is particularly likely in Australia, where the toxin differs from that found in North America.

Botulism (Chapters 319 and 448) rapidly produces a flaccid paralysis. Patients have ophthalmoplegia, bulbar weakness, dry mouth, constipation, and orthostatic hypotension, but sensory symptoms do not develop. Other entities that can mimic Guillain-Barré syndrome are acute spinal cord compression (Chapter 423), acute transverse myelitis (Chapter 436), and vascular myelopathies, all of which are characterized by decreased reflexes before the development of upper motor neuron signs such as increased reflexes. Carcinomatous or lymphomatous meningitis can also cause a rapidly developing quadriparesis, but both are associated with elevated CSF WBC counts.

Treatment

Rx

Patients with Guillain-Barré syndrome require hospitalization because of the potential for respiratory compromise. Pulmonary function tests should be performed frequently; a vital capacity of less than 1 L or a negative inspiratory force of less than −70 suggests that ventilator support may be needed in an intensive care unit setting. Autonomic instability and difficulty swallowing also need to be monitored.

Nonspecific therapies directed at modulating the immune system are effective in Guillain-Barré syndrome. For example, plasma exchange, usually four exchanges of 1.5 L of plasma spread over a 10-day period, is considered the "gold standard" therapy. [1] Two plasma exchanges may be sufficient in mild cases, and six exchanges are not superior to four in severely affected patients. This therapy should ideally be administered within the first 2 weeks and not later than 4 weeks from clinical onset.

Intravenous immunoglobulin (IVIG) therapy, given as 2 g/kg divided over 2 to 5 days within the first 2 weeks, is as effective as plasma exchange. [1] Because plasma exchange and IVIG are equally effective, at least in the first 2 weeks, IVIG is often preferred for its convenience unless there are contraindications, such as low serum IgA levels, renal failure, or severe hypertension.

Ten percent of patients with Guillain-Barré syndrome relapse after initially responding to plasma exchange or IVIG; they usually respond to a second cycle of the previously effective treatment. The combined use of plasma exchange followed by IVIG does not improve the prognosis.

Corticosteroids in different forms (intravenous methylprednisolone, oral prednisolone or prednisone, intramuscular adrenocorticotropic hormone) are not of benefit. A recent trial of intravenous methylprednisolone (500 mg/day for 5 days) in association with IVIG versus IVIG alone showed a slight initial advantage for the combined treatment but no benefit in terms of long-term disability.

Prognosis

Fifty percent of patients progress to their nadir, or maximum disability, within 2 weeks, 75% within 3 weeks, and more than 90% within 4 weeks of the onset of symptoms. With modern supportive care, acute mortality is about 2%. After a brief period of stabilization, slow spontaneous recovery occurs over a period of weeks or months. Most patients undergo either complete recovery or are left with minor sequelae; about 20% have a persistent disability. The long-term prognosis depends at least in part on the extent of axonal loss. Patients with low compound muscle action potential amplitudes in the upper extremities are more likely to have a poor prognosis.

Patients with acute motor axonal neuropathy will recover after approximately 2 months, but the extent of recovery may be less than in Guillain-Barré syndrome. In general, the prognosis for recovering from Miller-Fisher syndrome is excellent.

Chronic Inflammatory Demyelinating Polyradiculoneuropathy

Definition

CIDP is a chronic acquired demyelinating sensorimotor neuropathy that may be monophasic, relapsing, or progressive. By definition, CIDP develops over at least a 2-month period versus acute inflammatory demyelinating polyneuropathy, which it otherwise resembles.

Epidemiology

CIDP occurs in all age groups with a mean age range of 30 to 50 years. Women are slightly more likely to be affected than men. Antecedent events are less common than in Guillain-Barré syndrome; they occur in around 30% of patients and include upper respiratory infections, gastrointestinal infections, vaccinations, surgery, and trauma.

Pathobiology

CIDP is considered an autoimmune disorder based on pathologic findings in nerve biopsy samples from patients and on animal models such as experimental allergic neuritis in which a similar disorder follows immunization with peripheral nervous system myelin components and Freund's adjuvant. Nerve biopsy shows macrophage-mediated segmental demyelination, occasional endoneurial lymphocytic T-cell infiltrates, and endoneurial edema. The major histocompatibility complex class I and II antigens are upregulated, and there are often deposits of immunoglobulins and complement split products on the outer Schwann cell membranes or myelin sheaths. CIDP can be passively transferred to animals by patient sera, but no clear autoantigen has been identified.

Clinical Manifestations

Weakness and sensory loss begin insidiously and progress over a period of months to years. Weakness is commonly proximal as well as distal. Patients can become bedridden. Loss of proprioception from damage to large-diameter sensory nerves may affect balance and result in an action tremor. Deep tendon reflexes are usually absent or markedly decreased. Facial weakness (15%), ptosis or ophthalmoparesis (5%), and papilledema occur occasionally. Variant forms include pure motor, pure sensory, and multifocal disease.

Diagnosis

Diagnosis is based on clinical symptoms and signs, electrodiagnostic studies, and CSF examination. Nonuniform, asymmetrical slowing on nerve conduction studies is characteristic. One portion of a nerve may have different conduction than another. For example, if damage is primarily in the spinal roots, proximal conduction velocities and F wave latencies may be most affected. Compound muscle action potentials are generally reduced because of the concomitant axonal degeneration that occurs with demyelinating neuropathies. However, temporal dispersion and conduction block may also reduce the amplitude of muscle action potential in any demyelinating neuropathy. Sensory nerve conduction is also slow in CIDP, but because sensory nerve action potentials are often not detectable, sensory conduction velocity may be unmeasurable.

CSF results resemble those of acute inflammatory demyelinating polyneuropathy: WBC counts are usually less than 10 cells/mm^3, and protein levels are higher than 60 mg/dL. CSF cell counts higher than 50/mm^3 suggest another diagnosis, such as HIV infection or hematologic malignancy. CSF protein levels may be normal early in the course of CIDP.

Differential Diagnosis

CIDP is distinguished from acute inflammatory demyelinating polyneuropathy by its time course. A similar manifestation can also occur in diabetes, lymphoma, monoclonal gammopathies (see later), and asymmetrical inherited neuropathies (see earlier).

Treatment

Rx

Corticosteroids are effective in more than two thirds of patients with CIDP. A standard approach is to use oral prednisone (1 mg/kg/day) for 6 to 8 weeks, followed by slow tapering over a 3- to 12-month period to a maintenance level of about 0.1 mg/kg/day. A response to prednisone may take months to occur, and occasional patients may worsen before they respond. As a result, plasma exchange [2] or IVIG [3, 4] is often used as initial treatment.

Because of the side effects of long-term corticosteroids or the lack of response to them, azathioprine, cyclosporine, cyclophosphamide, methotrexate, mycophenolate mofetil, rituximab, and interferon alfa or beta have been used with variable success in uncontrolled reports.

Neuropathy Associated with Monoclonal Gammopathy

Definition

Monoclonal gammopathy refers to the presence in the β-γ region of serum protein electrophoresis of an abnormal spike (variably termed a paraprotein, monoclonal protein, or M protein) consisting of immunoglobulins of the same isotype, all produced by a single clone of abnormally proliferating lymphocyte/plasma cells. In some cases the M protein is part of a malignant lymphoproliferative disease such as multiple myeloma, solitary plasmacytoma (IgG and IgA), Waldenström's macroglobulinemia (IgM) (Chapter 198), lymphoma (Chapter 196), chronic lymphocytic leukemia (IgM) (Chapter 195), primary amyloidosis (Chapter 296), or cryoglobulinemia (Chapter 198). In most instances, however, monoclonal gammopathy is not initially associated with any of theses disorders and is classified as a monoclonal gammopathy of uncertain significance (MGUS), although in patients with MGUS the gammopathy may evolve into a malignant form (Chapter 198).

Epidemiology

Monoclonal gammopathy occurs in up to 8% of patients with peripheral neuropathy of unknown etiology. However, MGUS is frequent, being found in 1% of the population older than 50 years and in 3% older than 70 years, and most subjects with MGUS do not have neuropathy. In some cases the co-occurrence of neuropathy and M protein may be a coincidence, but in other cases the M protein is clearly related to the neuropathy.

The prevalence of neuropathy is higher in patients with IgM versus IgG or IgA M proteins. The prevalence of symptomatic neuropathy associated with IgM monoclonal gammopathy in patients older than 50 years is approximately 20 per 100,000. In half of such patients, the M protein reacts with either the HNK1 carbohydrate moiety of MAG or with other glycoproteins (MPZ, PMP22) and glycolipids (sulfoglucuronylparagloboside [SGPG] and lactosaminylparagloboside [SGLPG]). IgM M proteins associated with neuropathy may also bind to other neural antigens.

In patients with IgG monoclonal gammopathy and neuropathy, the relationship is less clear than with IgM. Although about 10% of patients with multiple myeloma have neuropathy, in most cases the M protein does not react with a neural antigen, and patients do not improve with immunotherapy (see later). Conversely, approximately 50% of patients with the osteosclerotic form of myeloma have neuropathy, often associated with the non-neurologic manifestations of organomegaly, endocrine abnormalities, and brown, tannish discoloration of the skin). Collectively, the *M* protein, *p*olyneuropathy and other features are referred to by the acronym POEMS (Chapter 198). Similarly, about 50% of patients with light chain amyloidosis have neuropathy.

Pathobiology

In patients with IgM M proteins that immunoreact with MAG, nerve biopsies demonstrate segmental demyelination with deposits of M protein and complement. High titers (>1:10,000) of anti-MAG IgM antibodies are associated with neuropathy, and intraneural or systemic injection of anti-MAG IgM M proteins causes complement-mediated demyelination of nerves in animals.

Clinical Manifestations

Most patients with anti-MAG neuropathies are initially seen in their sixth to seventh decade of life with dysesthesias and paresthesias in their legs and unsteadiness while walking because of loss of proprioception. Physical examination shows a length-dependent large fiber sensory neuropathy. Weakness may develop later.

Diagnosis

Nerve conduction velocities are slow (around 25 m/sec) with pronounced delays in distal motor latencies, thus prompting the designation *distal acquired demyelinating symmetrical neuropathy* to distinguish the disorder from CIDP.

Treatment

Treatment of neuropathies associated with monoclonal gammopathy is similar to that for CIDP (see earlier). However, patients with anti-MAG–related neuropathies do not respond as well to treatment as do patients with CIDP. Anecdotal data support the benefit of rituximab in some patients.

Prognosis

Progression of the neuropathy of monoclonal gammopathy disables about 25% of patients after 10 years and 50% after 15 years. The course of patients with osteosclerotic myeloma and neuropathy depends on the response to treatment of the myeloma. In patients whose myeloma responds to treatment, more than 50% have improvement in neuropathy. In other patients with sensorimotor neuropathies associated with plasma cell dyscrasias, the course is variable and the M protein may not be related to their neuropathy.

Multifocal Motor Neuropathy and Lewis-Sumner Syndrome

Definition

Multifocal motor neuropathy is characterized by progressive, distal more than proximal, asymmetrical limb weakness, mostly affecting the upper limbs with minimal or no sensory impairment.

Epidemiology

The prevalence of multifocal motor neuropathy is estimated at 2 per 100,000. Men are more frequently affected than women (2.6:1). Initial symptoms develop in 80% between the ages of 20 and 50 years, with a mean age at onset of 40. Lewis-Sumner syndrome occurs less frequently than multifocal motor neuropathy.

Pathobiology

Multifocal motor neuropathy is considered to be an autoimmune neuropathy based on its clinical improvement with immunologically based therapies and because of a frequent association with antiglycolipid antibodies. Patients often have serum antibodies that react with ganglioside GM_1, and these titers decrease during effective treatment. GM_1 is highly represented in neural membranes at the nodes of Ranvier, compact myelin, and the motor end plate at the neuromuscular junction. A blocking effect on mouse distal motor nerve conduction has been induced in vitro by sera from multifocal motor neuropathy patients with and without high anti-GM_1 antibody titers. These data support the presence of serum factors responsible for conduction block in the sera of patients with multifocal motor neuropathy, although these factors are not invariably related to anti-GM_1 antibodies.

Clinical Manifestations

The usual pattern is progressive, distal, asymmetrical arm weakness, often in the distribution of a single nerve. In a minority of patients, weakness may start proximally or in the legs. The disease will frequently affect other nerves, occasionally with a crossed distribution (i.e., one arm and the contralateral leg). Asymmetry and predominance of arm weakness may become less evident as the disease progresses. Localized muscle atrophy may be mild or absent in the early stage of the disease but can become prominent later as a result of axonal degeneration.

Fasciculations, cramps, and myokymia occur in patients with multifocal motor neuropathy and those with amyotrophic lateral sclerosis (Chapter 435), thereby making distinction between the two disorders difficult. Marked asymmetry in the degree of clinical findings and electrophysiologic abnormalities between contiguous nerves is suggestive of multifocal motor neuropathy rather than amyotrophic lateral sclerosis. Cranial nerve involvement or respiratory failure as a result of unilateral or bilateral phrenic nerve palsy rarely occurs in multifocal motor neuropathy. The presence of sensory loss suggests Lewis-Sumner syndrome.

Diagnosis

The diagnosis is established by the presence of multifocal, persistent partial conduction blocks on motor but not sensory nerve conduction studies. Lewis-Sumner syndrome has sensory loss as well as weakness, with conduction block in both sensory and motor nerves.

Treatment

IVIG (2 g/kg) is the initial treatment of multifocal motor neuropathy, and almost 80% of patients respond within a week. However, improvement is typically brief (3 to 6 weeks), so repeated treatments are required indefinitely. Clinical improvement is often accompanied by a reduction or resolution of the motor conduction block in some, but not all nerves, but it does not consistently correlate with a reduction in antiganglioside antibody titers. Patients may eventually become refractory to IVIG, and another agent may be needed, such as rituximab or azathioprine. Plasma exchange and corticosteroids are generally ineffective and have been associated with worsening neuropathy in some patients.

PARANEOPLASTIC NEUROPATHIES

Definition

Paraneoplastic neuropathies (Chapter 189) are a "remote effect of cancer" not caused by metastatic invasion of neural tissue; radiation therapy or chemotherapy; metabolic, vascular, or hormonal disturbances; or opportunistic infections. It is hypothesized that they are the result of host immune responses to a tumor antigen or antigens that are also present in neural tissues.

Epidemiology

Paraneoplastic syndromes occur in less than 1% of patients with cancer, and peripheral neuropathy is only one of the paraneoplastic syndromes. Although more than 25% of patients with cancer have evident neuropathy on neurologic examination, the relationship to malignancy is unclear in most. Paraneoplastic neuropathy may develop before, during, or after the tumor is diagnosed. In certain tumors, neuropathies are distinctive and should prompt a thorough investigation for cancer. For example, small cell carcinoma of the lung (Chapter 201) is by far the most common underlying neoplasm, followed by carcinoma of the stomach, breast, colon, rectum, ovary, and prostate.

Pathobiology

Subacute sensory neuropathy, the most characteristic paraneoplastic neuropathy, results from an immune-mediated ganglionitis that destroys sensory neurons in the dorsal root ganglia. Mononuclear inflammatory infiltrates composed of $CD4^+$ and prominent $CD8^+$ T cells, along with plasma cells, are found in the stroma surrounding the dorsal root ganglion neurons. Other findings include atrophy of the dorsal roots; loss of sensory neurons, which appear to be replaced by a proliferation of satellite cells (Nageotte's nodule); axonal degeneration; and secondary degeneration of the dorsal column of the spinal cord. Inflammatory infiltrates can also be found in peripheral nerves or muscle. Sural nerve biopsies typically reveal only loss of myelinated nerve fibers and are not useful for diagnosis.

Clinical Manifestations

Subacute sensory neuropathy is characterized by subacute, progressive impairment of all sensory modalities and is associated with severe sensory ataxia and areflexia. Subacute sensory neuropathy may precede the diagnosis of tumor by months or even years.

At onset, patients may have shooting pain and burning sensations. Other symptoms include numbness, tingling, and a progressive sensory loss that may be asymmetrical. Symptoms usually progress rapidly to involve all four limbs, the trunk, and face. Findings may then stabilize, although by this time the patient is often totally disabled. Occasional patients have an indolent course.

Neurologic examination reveals loss of deep tendon reflexes and involvement of all modalities of sensation; large fiber modalities such as vibration and joint position sense are most severely affected. The loss of position sense may lead to severe sensory ataxia with pseudoathetoid movements of the hands and an inability to walk despite normal strength. Cranial nerve involvement may cause sensorineural deafness, loss of taste, and facial numbness. The frequent asymmetrical pattern of symptoms sometimes suggests a radiculopathy or plexopathy.

A paraneoplastic encephalomyelitis characterized by patchy, multifocal neuronal loss in regions of the cerebral hemispheres, the limbic system, the cerebellum, the brain stem, the spinal cord, and autonomic ganglia often develops in patients with subacute sensory neuropathy. Autonomic symptoms include impotence, dry mouth, and constipation.

Diagnosis

The diagnosis is based on recognizing the typical neuropathy in the setting of malignancy. The results of routine laboratory studies are generally normal. The diagnosis is supported by finding serum polyclonal IgG anti-Hu antibodies, also called antineuronal antibodies type 1, or by indirect immunofluorescence or immunohistochemistry and confirmed by Western blot analysis.

Nerve conduction studies typically demonstrate small-amplitude or absent sensory nerve action potentials. Motor conduction velocities and F wave studies are most often normal. Needle EMG usually demonstrates normal motor unit morphology and recruitment patterns with no signs of denervation, except in unusual cases in which there is also involvement of the spinal motor neurons. In rare cases, motor conduction abnormalities with axonal and demyelinating features occur in association with involvement of the dorsal root ganglia.

Subacute painful, asymmetrical neuropathy or neuronopathy in an elderly patient should prompt a search for carcinoma of the lung because small cell lung cancer accounts for more than 80% of the associated tumors. Subacute sensory neuropathy has also been reported in patients with adenocarcinoma of the lung, breast, ovary, stomach, colon, rectum, and prostate, as well as Hodgkin's and non-Hodgkin's lymphoma. In patients with no evidence of cancer, detection of anti-Hu antibodies should prompt a computed tomography study of the chest with special attention to the mediastinal lymph nodes. The use of whole body positron emission tomography with fluorodeoxyglucose has been advocated for early diagnosis in patients with anti-Hu antibodies or clinical suspicion of subacute sensory neuropathy because it may reveal neoplastic adenopathy months before computed tomography or magnetic resonance imaging can detect them.

Treatment

Subacute sensory neuropathy responds poorly to plasma exchange, IVIG, or various immunosuppressant medications, even when such treatment is started early in the course of the disease, possibly before the loss of sensory neurons. Even successful treatment of the tumor rarely induces remission of subacute sensory neuropathy, but the symptoms may stabilize.

Other Neuropathies Possibly Associated with Cancer

Sensorimotor Neuropathy

Sensorimotor neuropathy occurs in approximately 25% of patients with all type of tumors. The neuropathy can have an acute or subacute onset, with a progressive or relapsing/remitting course. Because no antineuronal antibody has been specifically associated with these neuropathies, their paraneoplastic nature is not established. Severe or relapsing neuropathies often precede the diagnosis of cancer, but the search for malignancy is generally limited to a chest radiograph, stool samples for blood, and routine blood tests. There are no specific treatments of these neuropathies, and their progression does not necessarily correlate with that of the malignancy.

Paraneoplastic Vasculitis of Nerves

A nonsystemic vasculitic neuropathy, which may also involve muscle, occurs with various types of tumor, including small cell lung cancer, lymphoma, and carcinoma of the kidney, stomach, and prostate. Neurologic symptoms may develop either before or after the tumor is diagnosed. The neuropathy is subacute and progressive and usually affects older men. Like many paraneoplastic disorders, these neuropathies often do not respond well to treatment, which is similar to that for the vasculitic neuropathies (see later).

VASCULITIC NEUROPATHIES

Definition

Vasculitic neuropathies (Table 446–5) are typically manifested as painful acute or semiacute axonal mononeuritis multiplex. There is acute motor and sensory loss in multiple nerve territories. The number of nerves involved may be extensive enough to make the distinction between a multifocal and diffuse neuropathy difficult. Occasionally, vasculitic neuropathy can be manifested as sensory neuropathy, trigeminal neuropathy, compressive neuropathy, or autonomic neuropathy. Neuropathy can occur in systemic vasculitis associated with other organ systems, as well as in nonsystemic vasculitis affecting just nerve and muscle.

Epidemiology

Systemic vasculitic neuropathy is more common than nonsystemic vasculitic neuropathy. Peak ages at onset of both are the fifth to eighth decades, but vasculitis can occur at any age. Neuropathy, particularly mononeuritis multiplex, is common in several forms of systemic vasculitis. Rheumatoid arthritis (Chapter 285) evolves into systemic rheumatoid vasculitis in 5 to 15% of patients, and vasculitic neuropathy will develop in about 50% of these patients. More than 50% of patients with Churg-Strauss syndrome (Chapter 291), 40 to 50% with Wegener's granulomatosis (Chapter 291), 35 to 75% with polyarteritis nodosa (Chapter 291), and a majority of patients with mixed cryoglobulinemia (Chapter 198) have neuropathy. Patients with Sjögren's syndrome (Chapter 289) are often initially found to have sensory neuropathies. Neuropathies are uncommon in systemic lupus erythematosus.

TABLE 446–5 SYSTEMIC VASCULITIS AND NEUROPATHY

Type	Serology Features	Associated Features	Usual Neuropathy Type	Neuropathy Prevalence
Rheumatoid arthritis	RF 80–90%	Arthralgias, arthritis frequent; multiple organs	Mononeuritis multiplex and sensorimotor neuropathy	50% of patients with vasculitis
Churg-Strauss	c-ANCA <30% p-ANCA <50%	Eosinophilia Asthma	Mononeuritis multiplex	20% of patients
Wegener's granulomatosis	c-ANCA 75–90% p-ANCA <20%	Pulmonary and renal	Mononeuritis multiplex	15% of patients
Polyarteritis nodosa	c- and p-ANCA rare	Multiple organs, 30% hepatitis B	Mononeuritis multiplex	60% of patients
Mixed cryoglobulinemia	No	Hepatitis C, purpura frequent	Mononeuritis multiplex	20–90% of patients
Sjögren's	α-Ro/SS-A 60%, α-La/SS-B 50%	Dry eyes, dry mouth; women 90%	Sensory	25% of patients
Systemic lupus erythematosus	ANA screen >90%	Multiorgan	Sensorimotor neuropathy	5–20% of patients

ANA = antinuclear antigen; p- and c-ANCA = perinuclear and cytoplasmic antineutrophil cytoplasmic antibodies; RF = rheumatoid factor; α-Ro/SS-A and α-La/SS-B = antibodies to the Ro/SS-A and La/SS-B antigens.

Pathobiology

In patients with mononeuritis multiplex, axonal degeneration develops as a result of nerve ischemia caused by the vasculitic process. Immune-mediated inflammation and necrosis of blood vessel walls occlude the vessel's lumen, thereby resulting in ischemic damage. Small arteries or arterioles (50 to 300 μm) are most commonly affected, particularly those that occur in watershed areas between the distribution of the major nutrient arteries of proximal nerves. True nerve infarcts are rare.

The immune-mediated inflammation is associated with antibody-antigen complexes that are deposited in the wall of the blood vessel. Antibodies also bind directly to endothelial cell antigens. In both circumstances, complement is activated, as evidenced by deposition of membrane attack complex. Chemotactic factors then recruit neutrophils, which release proteolytic enzymes and generate toxic oxygen free radicals.

The sensory neuropathy of Sjögren's syndrome probably results from the infiltration of dorsal root ganglia by cytotoxic T cells. Some patients with systemic vasculitis have symmetrical neuropathies rather than mononeuritis. The pathogenesis of such cases is not defined.

Clinical Manifestations

Patients typically have a relatively sudden onset of painful, focal or multifocal weakness or sensory loss. These symptoms reflect ischemia anywhere along the length of the nerve or nerves, generally in the lower extremities. Onset usually occurs rapidly (hours to days) as a result of the abrupt, ischemic etiology.

Diagnosis

Nerve biopsy of clinically affected sensory nerves (sural, superficial peroneal, or superficial radial) is often necessary and is justified because therapy may be aggressive and long-term. Superficial peroneal nerve biopsy may be combined with muscle biopsy from the same incision. Pathologic features diagnostic of vasculitis occur in 60% of patients, and less specific features such as multifocal loss of fibers occur in others. Findings diagnostic of vasculitis include destruction of the vessel and inflammation within the vessel wall. Fibrinoid necrosis, vessel wall scarring, recanalization, neovascularization, and hemosiderin are common, but not essential histopathologic features of vasculitis.

Although nerve biopsy is the "gold standard" for diagnosis, clinical, serologic, and electrophysiologic findings can suggest the diagnosis. For example, EMG and nerve conduction velocity studies can distinguish between mononeuritis multiplex and a symmetrical neuropathy. It is essential to confirm nerve conduction velocity abnormalities in a nerve before biopsy, which is always required before treatment. An acute or subacute onset of asymmetrical weakness or sensory loss in the distribution of individual nerves suggests mononeuritis multiplex, particularly in the setting of a known connective tissue disorder. Systemic symptoms, such as unexplained weight loss and purpura, or constitutional symptoms, such as fever, myalgias, arthralgias, pulmonary disease, abdominal complaints, rashes, or night sweats, suggest systemic vasculitis in a patient with mononeuritis multiplex.

The erythrocyte sedimentation rate is usually elevated in the systemic vasculitides but is normal in nonsystemic cases. Perinuclear and cytoplasmic antineutrophil cytoplasmic antibody (p-ANCA and c-ANCA) suggests Wegener's granulomatosis (Chapter 291) or Churg-Strauss syndrome (Chapter 291). Hepatitis C (Chapters 151 and 152) is usually associated with the presence of cryoglobulins. Serum complement levels, extractable nuclear antigen, angiotensin-converting enzyme levels, serum protein electrophoresis, and HIV serology are generally indicated. CSF analysis is not usually helpful in cases of vasculitic neuropathy but may be needed to exclude infectious (e.g., Lyme disease [Chapter 342]) or other inflammatory causes.

Differential Diagnosis

Acute or subacute mononeuritis multiplex may also result from diabetes, sarcoidosis, Lyme disease, and malignant infiltration of nerves. Multifocal motor neuropathy with conduction block and Lewis-Sumner syndrome can resemble vasculitic mononeuritis multiplex. Sensory neuropathies similar to those in Sjögren's syndrome may occur in patients with diabetes, paraneoplastic syndromes associated with anti-Hu antibodies, and pyridoxine deficiency.

Treatment

Systemic Vasculitis

Corticosteroid therapy is used for most vasculitic neuropathies (Chapter 291). Oral prednisone (1 mg/kg) is appropriate for relatively mild cases, but intravenous methylprednisolone (1000 mg/day for 3 to 5 days) may be indicated as initial treatment in severe cases. Daily dosing is commonly used for the first 2 months or longer if the disease remains active. Subsequently, the dose is gradually tapered, with a transition to alternate-day dosing and discontinuation depending on the clinical picture and associated systemic features.

Corticosteroid treatment may be adequate for Churg-Strauss syndrome, but additional medication is generally needed in other forms of systemic vasculitic neuropathy. In most cases of Wegener's granulomatosis and microscopic polyangiitis, combined therapy with glucocorticoids and oral cyclophosphamide (2 mg/kg/day) or weekly oral methotrexate is used. Azathioprine (2 to 3 mg/kg/day) is also used.

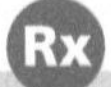

Nonsystemic Vasculitis

Because patients with nonsystemic vasculitic neuropathy may recover spontaneously or have a relatively benign course, low-dose or alternate-day oral prednisone (60 to 80 mg/day) is often adequate therapy. Azathioprine or weekly methotrexate can be used as a glucocorticoid-sparing agent. Doses such as 60 mg of prednisone on alternate days, 2 to 3 mg/kg/day of azathioprine, or 7.5 to 15 mg/wk of methotrexate, are reasonable starting doses that can ultimately be tapered if the treatments prove effective.

Prognosis

Most systemic and nonsystemic vasculitis responds to treatment, and patients make at least partial recovery with gradual return of function after a static period. The prognosis of patients with nonsystemic vasculitis is better than that of patients with systemic vasculitis, with fewer episodes of nerve damage; the disease may be monophasic or relapsing/remitting over a period of years, and most patients recover the ability to walk.

CRITICAL ILLNESS NEUROPATHY

Definition

Critical illness polyneuropathy is an acute or subacute axonal length–dependent neuropathy that occurs in critically ill patients, not as a direct consequence of their underlying illness. The neuropathy is monophasic and recovers, at least in part, if the patient survives the underlying illness.

Epidemiology

The incidence of critical illness polyneuropathy is uncertain because of variable diagnostic criteria. Moreover, it frequently accompanies critical illness myopathy (Chapter 447), which may be indistinguishable from it. Critical illness polyneuropathy frequently occurs in patients with systemic inflammatory response syndrome (Chapters 107 and 109), a generalized inflammatory host response to severe illness; up to 70% of patients with sepsis have a length-dependent axonal neuropathy.

Pathobiology

Nerve biopsies have identified perivascular lymphocytic infiltration, macrophages, and cytokines such as interleukin-1β, interferon-γ, and interleukin-12. Ischemia caused by a sepsis-induced abnormal distribution of capillary blood flow, nutritional deprivation, and hypoglycemia has also been implicated in critical illness polyneuropathy.

Clinical Manifestations

The typical finding is rapid development of profound limb weakness days to weeks after acquiring a severe illness that necessitated intensive care unit admission and ventilator support. Weakness is length dependent, beginning in the feet and hands, although proximal weakness is also frequent. Respiratory muscles are often involved, and inability to wean from the ventilator is a common problem. Elicitable deep tendon reflexes distinguish critical illness polyneuropathy from acute inflammatory demyelinating polyneuropathy. Sensory findings are typically absent, but sensory testing is difficult to perform in a severely disabled patient with underlying medical problems.

Diagnosis

Laboratory studies are rarely helpful. CSF protein is normal, unlike the case with acute inflammatory demyelinating polyneuropathy. A lack of cells also excludes infectious or inflammatory disorders. Creatine kinase levels are normal, unlike critical illness myopathy, in which such levels may be elevated.

Motor conduction velocities are normal with reduced or absent compound muscle action potential amplitudes. Critical illness polyneuropathy is a predominantly motor disorder, so sensory conduction velocities and sensory nerve action potential amplitudes are normal. Abnormal spontaneous activity from axonal damage may occur within 1 to 3 weeks of onset. The presence of neuropathic and myopathic abnormalities suggest that critical illness polyneuropathy and critical illness myopathy coexist.

Differential Diagnosis

Distinguishing between critical illness myopathy and critical illness polyneuropathy can be difficult. Glucocorticoids and neuromuscular blocking agents predispose to critical illness myopathy (Chapter 447), which occurs in up to 5% of critically ill patients and is also manifested as rapidly progressive weakness of the limbs and diaphragm. Muscle biopsy and special electrical techniques are often needed to diagnose critical illness myopathy. If patients with critical illness myopathy survive their critical illness, their long-term prognosis may be better than that of patients with critical illness polyneuropathy.

Acute inflammatory demyelinating polyneuropathy can mimic critical illness polyneuropathy but can be distinguished by slow nerve conduction velocity and abnormal CSF. Acute motor axonal neuropathy or acute motor and sensory axonal neuropathy may be more difficult to distinguish, particularly if sepsis or another underlying disorder induces an abnormal CSF; nevertheless, the presence of antiganglioside antibodies may help distinguish these disorders from critical illness polyneuropathy. Myasthenia gravis (Chapter 448), botulinum toxin (Chapter 319), acetylcholinesterase inhibitor poisoning (Chapter 111), and other toxins can cause a similar clinical picture.

Treatment

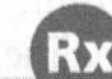

The main treatment is directed at the underlying disease or diseases, such as sepsis. Glucocorticoids and neuromuscular blocking agents should be avoided if possible because both have been associated with critical illness myopathy.

Prognosis

In-hospital mortality has been reported to be as high as 84% in patients with critical illness polyneuropathy as compared with 50% in similarly ill patients without it. Although most patients improve if they survive their underlying illness, up to 10% have persistent severe limb weakness and are ventilator dependent. Most patients have at least some evidence of weakness 2 years after discharge.

DIABETIC AND OTHER METABOLIC NEUROPATHIES

Definition

Diabetic peripheral neuropathies can be separated into two large groups; (1) symmetrical, predominantly sensory or autonomic neuropathies (or both) and (2) asymmetrical mononeuropathies or plexopathies (Table 446–6).

Epidemiology

Diabetes (Chapter 247) is the most common cause of neuropathy in the Western world. In the United States alone, more than 17 million people have diabetes. Diabetic neuropathy occurs in 8 to 70% of patients with diabetes, depending on the criteria used to diagnose neuropathy, and patients with retinopathy or overt albuminuria are over twice as likely to have neuropathy. Distal symmetrical polyneuropathies are the most common diabetic neuropathy, but distal autonomic neuropathy is also common. For example, impotence develops in 20 to 60% of diabetic men, but widespread autonomic dysfunction develops in less than 5% of diabetic patients.

TABLE 446–6 DIABETIC NEUROPATHIES

Type	Etiology	Frequency
SYMMETRICAL		
Distal sensory polyneuropathy	Possible metabolic, inflammatory, vascular	Frequent
Autonomic neuropathy	Possible metabolic, inflammatory, vascular	Frequent
ASYMMETRICAL		
Lumbosacral radiculoplexus neuropathy	Vascular	Less frequent
Truncal radiculopathy	Vascular	Less frequent
Cranial neuropathies	Vascular	Less frequent
Compressive neuropathies	Unknown	Frequent (especially carpal tunnel syndrome)

Pathobiology

Distal Symmetrical Polyneuropathy and Autonomic Neuropathy

The pathogenesis of distal symmetrical polyneuropathy and autonomic neuropathy involves both microvascular and metabolic abnormalities, with a causal link between increased blood glucose levels and the development and progression of diabetic neuropathy. The mechanisms by which hyperglycemia causes nerve dysfunction include activation of the polyol pathway, extensive glycation, altered diacylglycerol/protein kinase activity, and oxidative stress. Evidence from animal models suggests a role for neurotrophic factors, in particular, nerve growth factor, which selectively supports small fiber sensory and sympathetic neurons.

Acute Asymmetrical Neuropathies

The focal nature of these diabetic neuropathies is presumed to result from occlusion of endoneurial arterioles with resultant ischemic damage to the nerve. Changes suggestive of vasculitis are observed in epineurial and perineurial blood vessels in about 50% of cases, and perivascular lymphocytic infiltrates are common.

Clinical Manifestations

Distal Sensory Polyneuropathy and Autonomic Neuropathy

Distal symmetrical polyneuropathy is typically manifested as insidious symmetrical sensory loss of small (pain and temperature) and large (proprioception) fiber modalities. Paresthesias or painful dysesthesias (e.g., burning or tingling feet) are common, though not invariable. An unsteady gait may be the initial finding. Weakness is usually minimal, even in the distal foot muscles. Ankle reflexes are generally absent, although patellar reflexes may be present. Feet and distal calves are often cold and erythematous. Slow distal proximal progression of sensory symptoms and signs is the rule. By the time that symptoms reach the knees, abnormalities often begin in the hands.

When sensory changes reach the level of the knees, symptoms of autonomic neuropathy often begin: gastroparesis, which may alternate with diarrhea, orthostatic hypotension, anhidrosis, cardiac arrhythmias, and impotence. Autonomic abnormalities can be the most disabling component of diabetic neuropathy.

Acute Asymmetrical Neuropathies

Asymmetrical, acute neuropathies cause focal or multifocal symptoms, depending on the peripheral nerve or nerves affected. They are usually accompanied by acute pain in the afflicted region. The pain may be deep and aching or throbbing and lancinating. Most cases of acute focal or multifocal diabetic neuropathy eventually resolve, at least partially. Pain may resolve within a few months, whereas weakness may take a year or more to recover and may persist. Characteristic manifestations include the following:

1. *Diabetic lumbosacral radiculoplexus neuropathy:* Patients are frequently elderly with type 2 diabetes (Chapter 248). Asymmetrical pain in the upper part of the thigh is followed by progressive weakness and atrophy of the proximal leg muscles. Progression to the other leg occurs frequently. In about 50% of those affected, autonomic symptoms also develop, including orthostatic, gastrointestinal, and sexual dysfunction. Weakness may progress for up to 6 months. About 50% of patients require a wheelchair for ambulation, and many require opiates for pain. After the nadir, the patient will usually stabilize for several months, followed by progressive improvement. As many as 50% of patients do not regain full ambulation.
2. *Truncal radiculopathy:* An acute, focal onset of pain and sensory loss develop over a region of the trunk. In extreme cases, the abdominal wall muscles may become weak, resembling a hernia. As with diabetic lumbosacral radiculoplexus neuropathy, at least partial improvement will probably occur after a period of months, but the pain is difficult to control.
3. *Cranial neuropathies:* The classic manifestation is an acute oculomotor nerve palsy in which retro-orbital pain is followed by diplopia and ptosis. Pupillary fibers are often spared, thereby distinguishing the disorder from lesions that compress the oculomotor nerve and cause a dilated pupil. Similar findings may occur with the trochlear (fourth nerve) or abducens nerves. Bell's palsy is more frequent in diabetic patients and is less likely to involve taste than in patients without diabetes.
4. *Compressive mononeuropathies:* Compressive neuropathies, such as carpal tunnel syndrome, occur more frequently in diabetic patients for unclear reasons. It is not known whether the response of carpal tunnel syndrome to treatment is as effective as when these mononeuropathies occur independently of diabetes.

Diagnosis

Distal Sensory Polyneuropathy

The diagnosis of distal symmetrical polyneuropathy is based on identification of a predominantly sensory length–dependent neuropathy in the presence of either type 1 or type 2 diabetes. Neuropathy can develop independently of good control of blood sugar. Clinically similar neuropathies occur in patients with glucose abnormalities that are detectable only by oral glucose tolerance testing. Nerve conduction studies usually show low-amplitude or nondetectable sensory nerve action potential amplitudes; when detectable, sensory conduction may be slightly slow. Compound muscle action potential amplitudes are often reduced. Motor conduction studies are slightly slowed even if there is only minimal motor involvement clinically. Needle EMG in distal muscles typically demonstrates changes characteristic of chronic denervation. Occasional fibrillations and positive sharp waves may also be present.

Acute Asymmetrical Neuropathy

The focal neuropathies tend to occur in older patients with type 2 diabetes. The characteristic syndromes are diagnosed on the basis of their clinical manifestations and association with diabetes. EMG may demonstrate pronounced denervation in affected muscles. Concomitant evidence of distal symmetrical polyneuropathy is often present clinically and by electrophysiologic studies.

Treatment

Distal Symmetrical Polyneuropathy

An important treatment goal in distal symmetrical polyneuropathy is prevention of osteomyelitis and the resultant amputation of toes and feet. Because patients often do not sense injuries to their feet, diligence in foot care is important. Specific treatments to reverse or

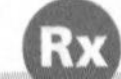

halt progression of the distal symmetrical polyneuropathy in diabetic patients are not yet available. Current therapy is based on control of hyperglycemia, management of symptoms, and foot care. Aggressive control of blood glucose (Chapter 247) remains the only treatment proven to delay the onset and slow progression of distal symmetrical polyneuropathy. There is, however, no HbA_{1c} threshold below which patients avoid risk for neuropathy. Combination therapy with gabapentin and morphine in low doses is effective treatment of pain when less aggressive treatments fail (Chapter 28). 5

Acute Asymmetrical Neuropathy

Although acute asymmetric neuropathy generally improves spontaneously, improvement may take months and remain incomplete. Intravenous corticosteroids, IVIG, or plasma exchange may improve the speed and extent of recovery, but these treatments are not of established benefit. Pain management is similar to that just described. Because the pain in patients with diabetic lumbosacral radiculoplexus neuropathy and truncal radiculopathy is focal, topical therapy may be effective.

INFECTIOUS NEUROPATHIES

Neuropathies Associated with HIV Infection

The peripheral nervous system may be involved in all phases of HIV infection (Chapter 417). The most common peripheral neuropathy is a distal, painful, sensory axonal polyneuropathy that is very similar to the toxic neuropathy caused by nucleoside reverse transcriptase inhibitors (NRTIs), including zidovudine, zalcitabine, didanosine, stavudine, and lamivudine. When an iatrogenic neuropathy is suspected, discontinuation of NRTIs may improve symptoms. Conversely, a neuropathy caused by HIV is likely to stabilize or improve with antiretroviral treatment.

Inflammatory neuropathies such as chronic or acute inflammatory demyelinating polyneuropathy can also occur in the early stages of HIV infection; the CSF cyto-albumin dissociation usually seen with these conditions may not be evident in these patients because of a mild CSF mononuclear pleocytosis. The response of these neuropathies to plasma exchange or IVIG is generally good. In later stages of HIV infection, cytomegalovirus (Chapter 399) may cause either an acute lumbosacral polyradiculopathy as a result of direct invasion of nerve roots or a mononeuritis multiplex through a vasculitic mechanism.

Neuropathies Associated with Herpes Zoster

Varicella-zoster virus (Chapter 398) usually remains latent in cranial or spinal ganglia after resolution of a systemic infection. Reactivation, which tends to occur in elderly persons or immunocompromised patients, causes a vesicular skin eruption accompanied by pruritus and dysesthesias. Herpes zoster normally undergoes spontaneous resolution but is frequently followed by a severe post-herpetic neuralgia, which is defined as pain persisting for more than 6 weeks after the rash appears. Early treatment with oral acyclovir (800 mg, five times daily for 7 days) may reduce both the duration of the acute phase and the chance of post-herpetic neuralgia developing, which is usually treated with symptomatic drugs for neuropathic pain (Chapter 28).

The use of concomitant corticosteroids to treat herpes zoster is controversial because of concern that suppressing cell-mediated immunity might exacerbate viral spread. There is little evidence supporting this concern, but the evidence is also not strong that combining corticosteroids with acyclovir leads to a better outcome than does treatment with acyclovir alone.

Neuropathy Associated with Lyme Disease

Borrelia burgdorferi causes a disease with three stages (Chapter 342). In the first stage, shortly after and in the same area of a tick bite, a nonpruritic rash (erythema migrans) appears and spontaneously disappears after a few weeks. The second stage is frequently associated with neurologic complications such as lymphocytic meningitis and focal and multifocal peripheral and cranial neuropathies; characteristic manifestations are unilateral or bilateral facial palsy and radiculitis. The third stage is associated with severe neurologic complications, including encephalopathy, encephalomyelitis, and a predominantly sensory axonal polyneuropathy. A lymphocytic pleocytosis in CSF and demonstration of *B. burgdorferi* infection in serum or CSF are the main laboratory findings. Treatment is discussed in Chapter 342.

Neuropathy Associated with Leprosy

Leprosy (Chapter 347) is the most common cause of peripheral neuropathy in developing countries, although it is infrequent in the Western world. Leprosy may be manifested in different forms, depending on the host's immune system. Patients with normal cell-mediated immunity are more likely to have a tuberculoid form characterized by hypopigmented skin lesions associated with decreased sensation. In patients with abnormal cell-mediated immunity, the more severe lepromatous form with large disfiguring lesions may develop. A mononeuritis multiplex pattern with prominent superficial sensory loss is the most typical clinical manifestation of leprosy.

If treated early, neuropathies in leprosy can improve significantly. World Health Organization recommendations call for combination therapy that includes dapsone (50 to 100 mg/day or 200 to 250 mg/wk), rifampicin (600 mg monthly), and clofazimine (100 mg/day) (Chapter 347).

Neuropathy Associated with Diphtheria

Although vaccination has made diphtheria (Chapter 315) rare in developed countries, it is still an important cause of subacute neuropathy in developing countries. Some strains of *Corynebacterium diphtheriae* produce a potent neurotoxin that causes palatal weakness, accommodation deficits, and extraocular palsies. This acute manifestation is followed by an ascending paralysis secondary to a demyelinating neuropathy that shares many clinical features with acute inflammatory demyelinating polyneuropathy.

The neuropathy caused by the neurotoxin usually resolves with resolution of the infection. The diphtheria organism can be eradicated by therapy with antibiotics such as erythromycin (2 g/day intravenously divided twice daily for adults) or penicillin (procaine penicillin G, 1.2 million U/day intramuscularly divided twice daily for 14 days). However, the neuropathy, as with other manifestations of the disease, generally requires treatment with diphtheria antitoxin, a hyperimmune antiserum produced in horses. Depending on the severity of the disease, antitoxin is administered intramuscularly or intravenously (80,000 to 120,000 units for extensive disease with a duration of 3 or more days) (Chapter 315).

TOXIC AND DEFICIENCY SYNDROMES

In Western countries, toxic neuropathies are frequently the side effects of medications rather than a result of environmental exposure. In most cases, iatrogenic neuropathy is manifested as a length-dependent or "dying-back" axonal neuropathy. Treatment requires a correct diagnosis (Table 446–7) and discontinuation of the drug, but improvement is often slow and may take several months.

Compressive Neuropathies

Peripheral nerves are vulnerable to chronic compression in many sites: median nerve compression at the wrist within the carpal tunnel *(carpal tunnel syndrome)*, median nerve compression in the upper part of the forearm, ulnar nerve compression in the hand *(cubital tunnel syndrome)*, ulnar nerve compression at the elbow or wrist, tibial nerve compression behind the medial malleolus *(tarsal tunnel syndrome)*, and peroneal nerve compression over the lateral fibular head.

TABLE 446–7 TOXIC AND DEFICIENCY NEUROPATHIES

Associated with antineoplastic agents: vincristine, paclitaxel (Taxol), cisplatin, suramin, thalidomide
Associated with antimicrobials: chloroquine, dapsone, isoniazid, metronidazole, nitrofurantoin
Associated with cardiac medications: amiodarone, perhexiline, hydralazine
Associated with other medications: colchicine, tacrolimus, gold salts, phenytoin, disulfiram (Antabuse), pyridoxine (vitamin B_6)
Associated with heavy metals: lead, arsenic, mercury, thallium
Associated with chemical compounds: acrylamide, carbon disulfide, ethylene glycol, hexacarbons, organophosphate esters, vacor
Deficiency neuropathies: vitamin B_1 deficiency, vitamin B_{12} deficiency, vitamin E deficiency

Carpal Tunnel Syndrome

Entrapment of the median nerve at the wrist reflects the limited space available for the median nerve because of the surrounding bone, joint, ligaments, tendons, and synovium. Repetitive motion of the fingers is an exacerbating element. Other precipitating factors include trauma, osteoarthritis, synovial cysts, myxedema (Chapter 244), and amyloid deposition (Chapter 296). Mild symptoms typically involve paresthesias of the first three digits, often occur overnight, and are relieved by shaking or elevating the hands. In more severe disease, objective sensory loss in the median nerve distribution, weakness of median-innervated muscles such as the abductor pollicis brevis, and prolongation of nerve conduction across the carpal tunnel (prolonged distal latency) are characteristic. The diagnosis is supported by identification of *Tinel's sign,* in which tapping the carpal tunnel elicits paresthesias in the median nerve distribution, and by paresthesias produced by sustained flexion of the wrist *(Phalen's sign).* Treatment begins with splinting of the wrist in slight dorsiflexion during sleep. Injection of corticosteroids into the carpal tunnel provides temporary benefit. [6] More severe carpal tunnel syndrome is treated surgically by release of the carpal ligament. [7]

Bell's Palsy

Unilateral facial paralysis of acute onset frequently occurs on an idiopathic basis (Bell's palsy). The diagnosis is one of exclusion. Facial nerve palsies also occur in the setting of *herpes zoster oticus* (Chapter 398), in which they are typically associated with otalgia and varicelliform lesions affecting the external ear, ear canal, or tympanic membrane. Facial paralysis of a lower motor neuron type can be caused by carcinomatous meningitis (Chapter 199), sarcoidosis (Chapter 95), Lyme disease (Chapter 342), and HIV infection (Chapter 417).

Primary tumors of the facial nerve can occur with apparently rapidly developing facial paralysis. Facial paralysis can also occur in primary *CNS disease* affecting the pontomedullary junction, such as stroke or multiple sclerosis (Chapter 436).

Clinical Manifestations and Diagnosis

Most cases of facial paralysis are idiopathic. Patients typically notice facial paralysis on inspection in the mirror in the morning. Facial paralysis may be heralded or accompanied by pain behind the ear. The severity of paralysis varies widely.

Treatment

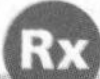

Bell's palsy can be associated with herpes simplex virus infection, and some advocate early treatment with acyclovir. Oral corticosteroids administered early in the course with rapid tapering may improve the prognosis, but this widely used therapy remains unproven. In severe cases, protection of the cornea from drying and injury is essential.

Prognosis

The prognosis is favorable in most cases, but about 10% of patients achieve little recovery. Aberrant regeneration of the facial nerve can cause synkinesias, such as "jaw winking" (when the eye is closed) or tearing accompanying salivation ("syndrome of crocodile tears").

Trigeminal Neuralgia (Tic Douloureux)

Trigeminal neuralgia and other painful cranial neuralgias are discussed in Chapter 421.

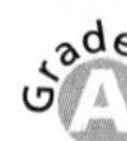

1. Plasma Exchange/Sandoglobulin Guillain-Barré Syndrome Trial Group: Randomised trial of plasma exchange, intravenous immunoglobulin, and combined treatments in Guillain-Barré syndrome. Lancet 1997;349:225–230.
2. Hahn AF, Bolton CF, Pillay N, et al: Plasma-exchange therapy in chronic inflammatory demyelinating polyneuropathy. A double-blind, sham-controlled, cross-over study. Brain 1996;119:1055–1066.
3. Mendell JR, Barohn RJ, Freimer ML, et al: Randomized controlled trial of IVIG in untreated chronic inflammatory demyelinating polyradiculoneuropathy. Neurology 2001;56:445–449.
4. Hughes R, Bensa S, Willison H, et al: Randomized controlled trial of intravenous immunoglobulin versus oral prednisolone in chronic inflammatory demyelinating polyradiculoneuropathy. Ann Neurol 2001;50:195–201.
5. Gilron I, Bailey JM, Tu D, et al: Morphine, gabapentin, or their combination for neuropathic pain. N Engl J Med 2005;352:1324–1334.
6. Dammers JW, Veering MM, Vermeulen M: Injection with methylprednisolone proximal to the carpal tunnel: Randomized double-blind trial. BMJ 1999;319:884–886.
7. Hui AC, Wong S, Leung CH, et al: A randomized controlled trial of surgery vs steroid injection for carpal tunnel syndrome. Neurology 2005;64:2006–2007.

SUGGESTED READINGS

Corbett CF: Practical management of patients with painful diabetic neuropathy. Diabetes Educ 2005;41:523–524, 526–528. *A rational approach to the treatment of painful diabetic neuropathies.*

England JD, Asbury AK: Peripheral neuropathy. Lancet 2004;363:2151–2161. *A guide to etiology, evaluation, and patient support groups.*

Freeman R: Autonomic peripheral neuropathy. Lancet 2005;365:1259–1270. *A comprehensive review.*

Hughes RA, Cornblath DR: Guillain-Barré syndrome. Lancet 2005;366:1653–1666. *Overview of pathogenesis, diagnosis, and treatment.*

Juurlink DN, Stukel TA, Kwong J, et al: Guillain-Barré syndrome after influenza vaccination in adults: A population-based study. Arch Intern Med 2006;166:2217–2221. *There was small but significantly increased risk of GBS after influenza vaccination, but the overall rates of GBS did not increase upon institution of a universal immunization program.*

Köller H, Kieseier BC, Jander S, et al: Chronic inflammatory demyelinating polyneuropathy. N Engl J Med 2005;352:1343–1356. *Chronic motor or sensory (or both) dysfunction in the absence of other underlying causes may respond to immunosuppressants.*

Lacomis D: Clinical utility of peripheral nerve biopsy. Curr Neurol Neurosci Rep 2005;5:41–47. *Indications for the prudent use and interpretation of sural nerve biopsies.*

Latronico N, Peli E, Botteri M: Critical illness myopathy and neuropathy. Curr Opin Crit Care 2005;11:126–132. *Overview of pathophysiologic mechanisms and methods for rapid diagnosis.*

Mutation database of inherited peripheral neuropathies (IPNDB). Available at http://www.molgen.ua.ac.be/CMTMutations/default.cfm. *An up-to-date listing of known mutations in genes causing inherited neuropathies.*

Nobile-Orazio E: Treatment of dysimmune neuropathies. J Neurol 2005;252:385–395. *A detailed review.*

Pagnoux C, Guillevin L: Peripheral neuropathy in systemic vasculitides. Curr Opin Rheumatol 2005;17:41–48. *A review of the disorders as well as potential pathogenic mechanisms of these neuropathies.*

Rudnicki SA, Dalmau J: Paraneoplastic syndromes of the peripheral nerves. Curr Opin Neurol 2005;18:598–603. *Thorough review of the immunologic associations.*

Shy ME: Therapeutic strategies for the inherited neuropathies. Neuromolecular Med 2006;8:255–278. *A review of the molecular basis and therapeutic approaches.*

Singleton JR, Smith AG, Russell J, et al: Polyneuropathy with impaired glucose tolerance: Implications for diagnosis and therapy. Curr Treat Options Neurol 2005;7:33–42. *Addresses the relationship between abnormal glucose tolerance tests and painful sensory neuropathies.*

Umapathi T, Chaudhry V: Toxic neuropathy. Curr Opin Neurol 2005;18:574–580. *Review of the causes of toxic neuropathy and potential therapeutic options.*

van Tulder M, Malmivaara A, Koes B: Repetitive strain injury. Lancet 2007;369:1815–1822. *A comprehensive review.*

447 MUSCLE DISEASES

Richard J. Barohn

APPROACH TO MUSCLE DISEASES

Definition

Diseases of skeletal muscle, termed myopathies, are disorders in which there is a primary structural or functional impairment of muscle. Myopathies therefore do not include diseases of the central nervous system (CNS), lower motor neurons (motor neuron disease), peripheral nerves, or neuromuscular junction that secondarily produce muscle weakness. Myopathies can be differentiated from other disorders of the motor unit by characteristic clinical and laboratory findings (Table 447–1). In addition, the disorders of muscles can be categorized and subdivided so that it is generally possible to recognize a particular myopathy on the basis of its distinctive features (Table 447–2).

Pathobiology

A single motor unit consists of four components: (1) a motor neuron, (2) its peripheral axon and terminal branches, (3) the neuromuscular junctions at each terminal nerve ending, and (4) all of the skeletal muscle fibers innervated by the axon. The number of muscle fibers innervated by a single motor unit varies from muscle to muscle. Muscles subserving finely coordinated movements, such as the ocular muscles, can have fewer than 10 muscle fibers in a motor unit. Powerful proximal limb muscles have large motor units with 1000 or 2000 fibers innervated by a single motor neuron. Individual fibers from different motor units intermingle randomly in the muscle. The muscle also contains connective tissue and blood vessels. Each of these tissues can be affected in myopathic disorders.

The muscle fibers consist of thick and thin filaments (myofibrils) arranged in repeating units, or sarcomeres, that are limited by Z discs. The thin filaments (actin, troponin, and tropomyosin) are anchored to the Z discs and interdigitate between the thick filaments (myosin) in the central region (A band) of the sarcomere. The myofibrils are associated with transverse (T) tubules, sarcoplasmic reticulum (SR), glycogen, and mitochondria. The head of each myosin molecule acts as a cross-bridge between myosin and actin. T tubules are inward projections of the muscle fiber surface membrane and serve to propagate the action potential into the muscle fiber. The SR contains calcium and partially surrounds the T tubules. Depolarization of T tubules triggers the opening of calcium channels and release of calcium from the SR into the myofilament space. Calcium then binds to troponin on the thin filaments, which acts on tropomyosin to allow repeated binding of the myosin cross-bridges to actin. The conformational change in the myosin-actin cross-bridge moves the thin filaments toward the center of the sarcomere, and the Z discs are pulled closer together to produce muscle fiber contraction. This contraction is an energy-dependent process that requires adenosine triphosphate (ATP), which is split by an ATPase on the cross-bridge.

The myofibrils and associated constituents are surrounded by the sarcolemmal membrane and basal lamina (Fig. 447–1). Many muscular dystrophies are caused by genetic defects in this region. The sarcolemmal components are known as the dystrophin-glycoprotein complex, a trans-sarcolemmal complex of proteins and glycoproteins that link the subsarcolemmal cytoskeleton to the extracellular matrix. The role of the dystrophin-glycoprotein complex is to provide structural support to the sarcolemma during muscle contraction and stretch. In addition, the dystrophin-glycoprotein complex may have a role in the regulation of intracellular calcium and in signal transduction.

Dystrophin is a rod-shaped molecule on the cytoplasmic side of the skeletal and cardiac sarcolemma. It consists of an amino-terminal domain that binds to the cytoskeletal thin actin filaments. The mid-rod domain and the carboxy-terminal domain are important in linking dystrophin to the other glycoproteins of the dystrophin-glycoprotein complex. These dystrophin-glycoprotein complex components are the dystroglycan complex (α, β), the sarcoglycan complex (α, β, γ, δ), and the syntrophin complex (α, β1, β2).

Closely adherent to the extracellular portion of the sarcolemma is the basal lamina, which is composed of collagen types I and IV, heparin sulfate proteoglycan, entactin, fibronectin, and laminin. Laminin is a heterotrimer composed of α, β, and γ chains held together by disulfide bonds. Merosin is the collective name for laminins that share a common α_2 chain. α-Dystroglycan binds to laminin and anchors the basal lamina to the sarcolemma. Another group of transmembrane proteins that are distinct from the dystrophin-glycoprotein complex are the integrins, which link the extracellular matrix to the sarcolemma. Integrins also bind merosin to skeletal muscle, and this interaction appears to be as important as the α-dystroglycan linkage in providing structural stability. In

TABLE 447–2 CLASSIFICATION OF MYOPATHIES

HEREDITARY

Muscular dystrophies
Congenital myopathies
Myotonias and channelopathies
Metabolic myopathies
Mitochondrial myopathies

ACQUIRED

Inflammatory myopathies
Endocrine myopathies
Myopathies associated with systemic illness
Drug-induced/toxic myopathies

TABLE 447–1 CLINICAL FINDINGS DIFFERENTIATING MUSCLE FROM NERVE DISEASE

Finding	Myopathy	Anterior Horn Cell Disease	Peripheral Neuropathy	Neuromuscular Junction Disease
Distribution	Usually proximal, symmetrical	Distal, asymmetrical, and bulbar	Distal, symmetrical	Extraocular, bulbar, proximal limb
Atrophy	Slight early, marked late	Marked early	Moderate	Absent
Fasciculations	Absent	Frequent	Sometimes present	Absent
Reflexes	Lost late	Variable, can be hyperreflexic	Lost early	Normal
Pain	Diffuse in myositis	Absent	Variable, distal when present	Absent
Cramps	Rare	Frequent	Occasional	Absent
Sensory loss	Absent	Absent	Usually present	Absent
Serum creatine kinase	Usually elevated	Occasionally slightly elevated	Normal	Normal

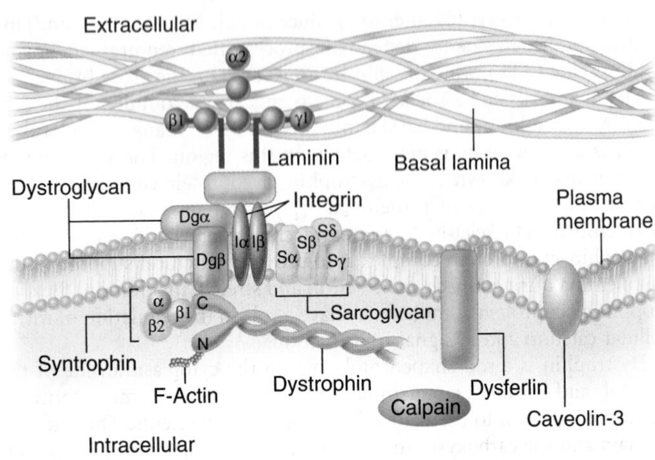

FIGURE 447–1 • The dystrophin-glycoprotein complex and related proteins.

addition, integrins are important in transducing signals from the extracellular matrix to the cell.

Clinical Manifestations

Symptoms of muscle disease can be divided into "negative" and "positive" complaints.

Negative Symptoms

The most common symptom of a patient with muscle disease is weakness. An inability to perform activities because of proximal muscle weakness is the most common symptom in a myopathic disorder (see later). However, occasional patients with myopathies can complain of poor handgrip (difficulty opening jar tops and turning door knobs) or tripping because of ankle weakness secondary to distal muscle weakness. Some myopathies involve "proximal" cranial muscles. Other crucial points in the history concern the age at onset of symptoms. Was the weakness (or other symptoms) first apparent at birth or was the onset in the first, second, third, or later decade? It is important to determine the tempo of the disease. Patients should be asked whether the weakness is present all the time or intermittently. Myopathies can be manifested as either fixed weakness (muscular dystrophies, inflammatory myopathies) or episodic periods of weakness with normal strength interictally (periodic paralysis secondary to channelopathies, metabolic myopathies secondary to certain disorders in the glycolytic pathway). Disorders of muscles can have acute (<4 weeks), subacute (4 to 8 weeks), or chronic (>8 weeks) periods over which the weakness evolves. The disorders with episodic weakness have acute weakness that can return to normal strength within hours or days. The tempo of the disorders with persistent weakness can vary from (1) acute or subacute in some inflammatory myopathies (dermatomyositis and polymyositis) to (2) chronic slow progression over a period of years (most muscular dystrophies) or to (3) fixed weakness with little change over decades (congenital myopathies). Finally, both constant and episodic myopathic disorders can cause symptoms that may be monophasic or polyphasic (relapsing).

Objective weakness is the most reliable symptom of a patient with a myopathy. Many patients who complain of generalized global "weakness" or fatigue are not weak and do not have a disorder of muscle, particularly if the findings on neurologic examination are normal. On the other hand, abnormal fatigability after exercise can result from certain metabolic and mitochondrial myopathies, and it is important to define the duration and intensity of exercise that provoke it.

Positive Symptoms

Myalgia

Muscle pain (myalgia) is a nonspecific complaint that accompanies some myopathies. Myalgias may be episodic (e.g., metabolic myopathies) or nearly constant (e.g., inflammatory muscle disorders). However, muscle pain is surprisingly uncommon in most muscle diseases, and limb pain is more likely to be due to bone or joint disorders. It is rare for a muscle disease to be responsible for diffuse aching pain and discomfort in muscle if the results of neurologic examination and laboratory studies are normal.

Muscle Cramps

A specific category of muscle pain is the involuntary muscle cramp. Cramps are usually localized to a particular muscle region and last from seconds to minutes. They are generally benign, occur in normal individuals, do not reflect an underlying disease process, and are seldom a feature of a primary myopathy. Cramps can occur with dehydration (Chapter 117), hyponatremia (Chapter 117), azotemia (Chapter 121), and myxedema and in disorders of the motor neuron (especially amyotrophic lateral sclerosis) or nerve.

Muscle Contractures

Muscle contractures are uncommon but can superficially resemble cramps. They usually last longer than cramps and are provoked by exercise in patients with glycolytic enzyme defects. They can be distinguished from cramps with needle electromyography (EMG). Contractures are electrically silent, whereas cramps are associated with rapidly firing motor unit discharges. Muscle contractures should not be confused with fixed tendon contractures.

Myotonias

Myotonia is impaired relaxation of muscle after forceful voluntary contraction. Patients may complain of muscle stiffness or persistent contraction in almost any muscle group, particularly those involving the hands and eyelids. They will note difficulty releasing their handgrip after a handshake, unscrewing a bottle top, or turning a doorknob. If they shut their eyes forcefully, they have difficulty opening their eyelids. With repeated exercise, the myotonia improves: the so-called warm-up phenomenon. Paramyotonia is the paradoxical phenomenon in which exercise makes the myotonia worse. Myotonia is due to repetitive depolarization of the muscle membrane. Exposure to cold worsens myotonia and paramyotonia.

Rhabdomyolysis

Patients who complain of exercise-induced weakness and myalgias should be asked whether their urine has ever turned dark or red during or after these episodes, which is indicative of myoglobinuria. Myoglobinuria follows excessive release of myoglobin from muscle during periods of rapid muscle destruction (Chapter 114).

Diagnosis

The most important aspect of evaluating a patient with a myopathy is the information obtained from the history (Chapter 418). After taking the history, the physician should formulate a reasonable preliminary diagnosis that places the patient into one of the categories in Table 447–2. The findings on physical examination (Chapter 418), in particular the pattern of weakness, help further define the diagnosis.

History

A detailed family history should be obtained to look for autosomal dominant, recessive X-linked, and vertical maternal (mitochondrial) patterns of transmission. Identifying a particular hereditary pattern is of help in diagnosis and genetic counseling.

Potential precipitating factors should be explored. Is the patient taking legal or illegal drugs or exposed to myotoxins? Does exercise provoke weakness, pain, or dark urine? Are episodes of weakness associated with or preceded by a fever, a feature of carnitine palmitoyltransferase (CPT) deficiency? Does the ingestion of a high-carbohydrate meal precede the weakness, suggestive of a periodic paralysis? Does cold exposure precipitate muscle stiffness, suggestive of myotonia?

Neurologic Examination

It is important to grade muscle power at the bedside. All muscle groups should be tested bilaterally. Knee extension and hip flexion should be tested in the seated position, knee flexion should be tested prone, and knee abduction should be tested in the lateral decubitus position. Assessment of muscle strength is usually based on the Medical Research Council of Great Britain (MRC) grading scale:

5—Normal power
4—Active movement against gravity and resistance
3—Active movement against gravity
2—Active movement only with gravity eliminated
1—Trace contraction
0—No contraction

It is important to watch the patient perform functional activities: walking (to look for a wide-based waddling gait with hyperlordosis, which is a sign of pelvic muscle weakness); rising from a chair, from a squat, or from a seated position on the floor (Gowers' sign); or climbing stairs (noting whether the patient needs to use the arms, another sign of proximal weakness in the lower extremities). An inability to walk on the heels or toes can indicate weakness in the distal leg muscles. Observe the patient talk and smile to determine whether facial weakness is present. Does the patient have the so-called horizontal smile, indicative of lower facial muscle weakness? Is the patient unable to close the eyes completely when asked to do so, indicative of upper facial muscle weakness? Are the upper eyelids lowered so that they touch the pupil, indicative of ptosis? Is the patient's speech nasal, indicative of palatal muscle involvement?

Finally, if the patient complains of muscle stiffness, myotonia should be sought by asking the patient to squeeze the examiner's finger and then observing whether the patient has an inability to relax the handgrip. Additionally, the muscles can be directly percussed with a reflex hammer. Observe for a slow persistent contraction and delayed relaxation. The muscles that can be most easily percussed to look for myotonia are the thenar and wrist/finger extensor muscle groups. Facial myotonia can also be observed after forceful voluntary eye closure. The patient will be unable to open the eyes easily after this maneuver.

The sensory examination should be normal in patients with muscle disease. Reflexes are usually present early in the disease process. Once the myopathy is advanced and the muscles are extremely weak, reflexes can become hypoactive or unobtainable. Evidence of damage to upper motor neurons (spasticity, extensor plantar responses, clonus) is present in myopathies only if there is coincidental CNS disease.

Pattern of Weakness

Once the muscles have been inspected and tested for power and functional activity has been observed, an attempt should be made to place the patient in one of the patterns of muscle weakness that can occur in myopathic disorders. The various patterns of muscle weakness can be divided into six broad groups:

1. The pattern (most common) of weakness that is exclusively or predominantly found in the proximal muscles of the legs and arms—the so-called limb-girdle distribution. The neck flexor and extensor muscles can also be affected. This pattern of weakness can be seen in many hereditary and acquired myopathies and is therefore the least specific in arriving at a particular diagnosis. It is not known why most myopathic disorders selectively involve the proximal muscles.
2. The pattern of distal weakness in the upper extremities (extensor muscle group) or lower extremities (anterior or posterior compartment muscle groups). Selective weakness and atrophy in distal extremity muscles are more often features of neuropathies (Chapter 446) and are uncommonly due to a primary muscle disease. When this pattern of weakness is determined to be due to a myopathic rather than a neuropathic disorder, a diagnosis of distal myopathy is appropriate. Examples include myotonic dystrophy, distal dystrophies (see later), titinopathy, zaspopathy, and inclusion body myositis.
3. The pattern of proximal upper extremity weakness of the periscapular muscles and distal lower extremity weakness of the anterior compartment—the scapuloperoneal pattern. The scapular muscle weakness is usually accompanied by scapular winging. When this pattern is associated with facial weakness, it is highly suggestive of facioscapulohumeral dystrophy. Other hereditary myopathies can be associated with a scapuloperoneal syndrome, for example, scapuloperoneal dystrophy, Emery-Dreifuss dystrophy, acid maltase deficiency, and some congenital myopathies.
4. The pattern of distal upper extremity weakness in the distal forearm muscles (wrist and finger flexors) and proximal lower extremity weakness involving the knee extensors (quadriceps). This pattern is essentially pathognomonic of inclusion body myositis. In addition, the weakness is often asymmetrical between the two sides, a pattern that is uncommon in most myopathies.
5. Predominant involvement of the ocular or pharyngeal muscles. The combination of ptosis, ophthalmoplegia without diplopia, and pharyngeal weakness should suggest the diagnosis of oculopharyngeal dystrophy, especially if the onset is in middle age or later. Ptosis and ophthalmoplegia without prominent pharyngeal involvement are hallmarks of many of the mitochondrial myopathies. Ptosis and facial weakness without ophthalmoplegia or pharyngeal weakness are common features of myotonic dystrophy. Therefore, the presence of ocular or pharyngeal muscle involvement can suggest a particular muscle disorder. Patients with ocular or pharyngeal involvement can also have the typical pattern of limb-girdle weakness.
6. Prominent neck extensor weakness. Some myopathic conditions have such a dramatic degree of weakness of the neck extensor muscles that the term *dropped head syndrome* is used. The neck flexors may or may not be weak. Neck extensor weakness can also occur with myopathies such as those with a limb-girdle pattern of weakness. Prominent neck extensor weakness is common in two other neuromuscular diseases: amyotrophic lateral sclerosis (Chapter 435) and myasthenia gravis (Chapter 448).

These six patterns of myopathy have limitations but are useful in narrowing the differential diagnosis. Patients with neuromuscular diseases other than myopathies can also have one of these weakness patterns.

Laboratory Studies

The results of the laboratory studies (blood tests, EMG, muscle biopsy, molecular studies) serve to confirm the preliminary diagnosis arrived at from the history and physical examination.

Serum Enzymes of Muscle Origin

Creatine kinase (CK) occurs in high concentration in the sarcoplasm of skeletal and cardiac muscle. The MM isoenzyme of CK predominates in skeletal muscle, MB occurs primarily in cardiac muscle, and BB is found mainly in brain. When skeletal muscle is injured, CK can leak into blood. Therefore, an elevated serum CK level is present in many muscle diseases. However, the absence of an elevated serum CK level does not exclude a myopathy, particularly in patients with severe muscle atrophy. In addition, elevation of the serum CK level does not necessarily imply that the muscle is the primary site of abnormality. The CK level is often elevated in normal individuals for days after strenuous voluntary exercise. Involuntary prolonged muscle contraction from a generalized motor seizure or tetany can elevate the CK level. The serum CK level is above the normal range in some African individuals, in individuals with large muscles, and after minor muscle trauma (e.g., EMG). Finally, other neuromuscular disorders such as motor neuron disease can produce up to a five-fold increase in the CK level. The serum CK level is normal in peripheral neuropathies and neuromuscular junction disorders.

The serum CK level is the most sensitive for muscle disease, and it is rarely necessary to measure other enzymes that can be released from injured skeletal muscle, such as aspartate aminotransferase (AST), alanine aminotransferase (ALT), or lactate dehydrogenase (LDH), all three of which are also elevated in hepatic disease. Because AST, ALT, and LDH are often measured in large screening chemical panels, their elevation should prompt measurement of CK to determine whether the source is muscle or liver. If a patient with an inflammatory myopathy is treated with a drug that may have hepatotoxicity as a side effect, it is not sufficient to measure ALT and AST levels; the liver-specific enzyme γ-glutamyltransferase should be monitored.

In general, CK isoenzymes are not helpful in the evaluation of myopathy. Elevated CK-MM levels are typical of muscle disease, but the CK-MB level is also elevated in myopathies and does not indicate that cardiac disease is present.

Electromyography and Muscle Biopsy

EMG is the electrophysiologic assessment of the neuromuscular system (Chapter 418). It consists of a nerve conduction study and needle EMG. A muscle specimen can be obtained through either an open or a closed (needle or punch) biopsy procedure. The biopsy should sample a muscle that is moderately weak. Biopsy specimens should generally not be taken from severely weak (MRC grade 2 or less) muscles. Muscles that have recently been studied by needle EMG often have artifacts from the procedure.

The muscle biopsy findings can establish whether there is evidence of either a neuropathic or a myopathic disorder. A neuropathy can produce denervation atrophy with small angular fibers, groups of atrophic fibers, and as a result of reinnervation, groups of fibers of the same histochemical type and target fibers. These features should not be present in a myopathy. Typical myopathic abnormalities include central nuclei, both small and large hypertrophic round fibers, split fibers, and degenerating and regenerating fibers. Inflammatory myopathies are characterized by mononuclear inflammatory cells in the endomysial and perimysial connective tissue between fibers and occasionally around blood vessels. Atrophy of fibers located on the periphery of a muscle fascicle, or perifascicular atrophy, is a common finding in a particular inflammatory myopathy, dermatomyositis. Any long-standing chronic myopathy can produce an increase in connective tissue and fat. Mitochondrial disorders are suggested by the identification of ragged red fibers on Gomori stain and various abnormal staining patterns on oxidative stains.

Electron microscopy (EM) evaluates the ultrastructural components of muscle fibers. In most myopathic disorders, EM is not usually required to make a pathologic diagnosis. However, EM is important in the study of certain disease states with abnormal light microscopic findings: congenital myopathies (e.g., nemaline rod, central core) and mitochondrial disorders.

Molecular Genetic Studies

The specific molecular genetic defect is known for an increasing number of myopathies. Molecular genetic testing is important for both diagnosis and carrier detection.

Other Tests

Electrolyte, endocrine, and immunologic tests are indicated to establish specific medical diagnoses. A decrease in the serum creatinine level is a useful indicator of decreased muscle mass.

Forearm exercise testing in patients with a suspected metabolic myopathy is often performed to determine whether there is a defect in the glycolytic enzyme pathway. After vigorous exercise, serum lactate and ammonia levels are measured. In disorders such as phosphorylase deficiency (McArdle's disease), the characteristic elevation in the serum lactate level after exercise is absent.

Urinalysis can detect the presence of myoglobinuria, which should be suspected if the urine is positive for blood but no red blood cells are seen.

Imaging studies include computed tomography, magnetic resonance imaging (MRI), and ultrasound. MRI can show specific regional myopathies and help with muscle biopsy when it is unclear from the neurologic examination and EMG which muscle should be selected for biopsy.

MUSCULAR DYSTROPHIES

Muscular dystrophies are inherited myopathies characterized by progressive muscle weakness and degeneration and by subsequent replacement with fibrous and fatty connective tissue. Historically, muscular dystrophies were categorized by their distribution of weakness, age at onset, and inheritance pattern. Advances in molecular understanding of the muscular dystrophies have defined the genetic mutation and abnormal gene product for many of these disorders (Table 447–3).

Dystrophinopathies

The dystrophinopathies include X-linked disorders resulting from mutations of the large dystrophin gene located at Xp21. Dystrophin is a large 427-kD subsarcolemmal cytoskeletal protein that along with other components of the dystrophin-glycoprotein complex, provides support to the muscle membrane during contraction. The large size of the gene (2.4 megabases) accounts for the high mutation rate. Large deletions, several kilobases to more than 1 million base pairs, can be demonstrated in approximately two thirds of patients; duplications occur in 5% of cases, and the remainder have small mutations that are not readily detectable. Mutations disrupting the translational reading frame of the gene result in near-total loss of dystrophin (Duchenne's muscular dystrophy), whereas in-frame mutations result in the translation of semi-functional dystrophin of abnormal size or amount (Becker's muscular dystrophy).

Duchenne's Muscular Dystrophy

Epidemiology and Pathobiology

The incidence of Duchenne's muscular dystrophy is 1 in 3500 male births, and the prevalence approaches 1 per 18,000 males. A third of cases result from a new mutation. Most patients with Duchenne's muscular dystrophy have a frameshift mutation and total deficiency of dystrophin. Deficiency of dystrophin weakens the sarcolemma and thus permits the influx of calcium-rich extracellular fluid, which then activates intracellular proteases and complement and leads to fiber necrosis.

Clinical Manifestations

Duchenne's dystrophy is manifested as early as 2 to 3 years of age with delays in motor milestones and difficulty running. The proximal muscles are the most severely affected early (limb-girdle pattern), and the course is relentlessly progressive.

Cardiac muscle is also affected. Although patients are generally asymptomatic, heart failure and arrhythmias can occur late in the disease.

The smooth muscle of the gastrointestinal tract is also involved, and intestinal pseudo-obstruction occurs. The average intelligence quotient of affected boys is 1 SD below the normal mean, thus suggesting CNS involvement.

Diagnosis

A dystrophin gene deletion (or less often a duplication) can be detected by analysis of DNA from leukocytes (by polymerase chain reaction) in a blood sample in approximately two thirds of patients. The DNA from a muscle sample can be similarly tested, but it is no more specific than leukocyte DNA analysis. If the patient falls into the third of patients in whom a deletion cannot be detected, muscle biopsy is required to demonstrate dystrophin deficiency by either Western blot or immunostaining. Muscle biopsy will also demonstrate typical features of a muscular dystrophy: variability in fiber size, fiber necrosis and regeneration, and replacement with connective tissue and fat.

Serum CK levels are markedly elevated at birth (20 to 100 times normal). They remain elevated but tend to decline over the course of the disease, after severe loss of muscle mass has occurred. EMG shows fibrillation potentials and myopathic motor units. EMG and muscle biopsy are not necessary in Duchenne's dystrophy if the diagnosis can be established by molecular studies of lymphocytes.

Up to 90% of patients can have an abnormal electrocardiogram (ECG) consisting of tall right precordial R waves and deep left precordial Q waves. Echocardiography shows either hypokinesis or dilation of ventricular walls.

Prognosis

Patients begin to fall frequently by 5 to 6 years of age, have difficulty climbing stairs by the age of 8, and are usually confined to a wheelchair by 12 years of age. Joint contractures commonly appear between 6 and 10 years. Initially, calf hypertrophy is often present, but after ambulation is lost, all muscles atrophy. Paraspinal muscle weakness leads to progressive kyphoscoliosis. The proximal tendon reflexes (biceps, quadriceps) disappear by the age of 10, although gastrocnemius reflexes are often preserved until late in the disease. Respiratory function gradually declines, and decreased vital capacity can be detected after the age of 10. Most patients die of respiratory complications in their 20s.

Becker's Muscular Dystrophy

Epidemiology and Pathobiology

Becker's dystrophy is a milder form of dystrophinopathy and varies in severity, depending on the genetic lesion. It is less common than Duchenne's, with an incidence of 5 per 100,000 and prevalence of 2.4 per 100,000. Most patients with Becker's dystrophy have a non–frame-shifting mutation, so a reduced amount of an abnormal dystrophin is produced and results in a milder syndrome than Duchenne's muscular dystrophy.

Clinical Manifestations

The pattern of weakness resembles that of Duchenne's muscular dystrophy, but it is less severe. The mean age at onset of symptoms is later, between 5 and 15 years. Calf hypertrophy is often prominent, and patients may complain of exercise-induced calf pain as an early symptom. Patients usually remain ambulatory after the age of 15, and the average age when a wheelchair is required is 30 years. Children with Duchenne's

TABLE 447–3 MUSCULAR DYSTROPHIES

Disease	Mode of Inheritance	Gene Mutation Location	Gene Defect/Protein
X-LINKED MD			
Duchenne's/Becker's	XR	Xp21	Dystrophin
Emery-Dreifuss	XR	Xq28	Emerin
LIMB-GIRDLE MD			
LGMD 1A	AD	5q22-34	Myotilin
LGMD 1B	AD	1q11-21	Lamin A/C
LGMD 1C	AD	3p25	Caveolin-3
LGMD 2A	AR	15q15	Calpain-3
LGMD 2B*	AR	2p12	Dysferlin
LGMD 2C	AR	13q12	γ-Sarcoglycan
LGMD 2D	AR	17q12	α-Sarcoglycan
LGMD 2E	AR	4q12	β-Sarcoglycan
LGMD 2F	AR	5q33	δ-Sarcoglycan
LGMD 2G	AR	17q11	Telethonin
LGMD 2H	AR	9q31	E3 ubiquitin ligase
LGMD 2I	AR	19q13.3	Fukutin-related protein 1
LGMD 2J	AR	2q31	Titin
CONGENITAL MD			
WITH CNS INVOLVEMENT			
Fukuyama's CMD	AR	9q31-33	Fukutin
Walker-Warburg CMD	AR	9q31-33	?Fukutin
Muscle-eye-brain CMD	AR	1p	Glycosyltransferase
WITHOUT CNS INVOLVEMENT			
Merosin-deficient, classic type	AR	6q2	Laminin-2 (merosin)
Merosin-positive, classic type	AR	?	Not known
Integrin-deficient CMD	AR	12q13	Integrin α7
Rigid-spine syndrome	AR	1p3	Selenoprotein NI
DISTAL MD			
Late adult-onset 1A (Welander)	AD	2p15	Unknown
Late adult-onset 1B	AD	2q31	Titin
Early adult-onset 1A (Nonaka)	AR	9p1-q1	GNE
Early adult-onset 1B (Miyoshi)[†]	AR	2q12-14	Dysferlin
Early adult-onset 1C (Laing)	AD	14	MPD1
OTHER MD			
Facioscapulohumeral	AD	4q35	Deleted chromatin
Oculopharyngeal	AD	14q11	Poly(A) binding protein 2
Myotonic dystrophy type 1	AD	19q13	RNA accumulation
Myotonic dystrophy type 2	AD	3q	RNA accumulation
Myofibrillar myopathy	AD	11q21-23	β-Crystallin
	AD		Zasp
	AD	2q35	Desmin
Bethlem myopathy	AD	21q22	Collagen VI

*Probably the same condition as Miyoshi distal MD.
[†]Probably the same condition as LGMD 2B.
AD = autosomal dominant; AR = autosomal recessive; CMD = congenital muscular dystrophy; CNS = central nervous system; GNE = UDP-*N*-acetylglucosamine 2-epimerase/*N*-acetylmannosamine kinase; LGMD = limb-girdle muscular dystrophy; MD = muscular dystrophy; XR = X-linked recessive.

muscular dystrophy cannot lift their head fully against gravity (MRC grade <3), whereas less severe, "outlier" children and those with Becker's dystrophy retain this ability. Cardiac abnormalities are similar to those described for Duchenne's muscular dystrophy.

Diagnosis

DNA analysis from blood leukocytes will show an Xp21 deletion in about 60% of cases. Results of immunostaining and Western immunoblot for dystrophin on muscle extracts reveal that the protein is not absent, as in Duchenne's muscular dystrophy, but is reduced in amount or abnormal in size. The serum CK level is moderately elevated, and needle EMG shows electrophysiologic signs of a myopathy, similar to the findings in Duchenne's muscular dystrophy.

Prognosis

Most patients with Becker's dystrophy experience slow progression. Death may occur from respiratory or cardiac complications after 40 years of age.

Other Dystrophinopathies

Other, milder dystrophinopathy phenotypes include exercise intolerance associated with myalgias, muscle cramps, or myoglobinuria;

minimal limb-girdle weakness or quadriceps myopathy; asymptomatic elevation of the serum CK level; cardiomyopathy with only mild muscle weakness; and fatal X-linked cardiomyopathy without muscle weakness. The different dystrophin phenotypes are determined by the site of the mutation in the dystrophin gene and the effect or lack of effect of the mutation on expression of the cardiac isoform of dystrophin.

Female Carriers and Prevention

The daughters of males with a dystrophinopathy are obligate carriers of the mutated dystrophin gene, as are the mothers of affected children who also have a family history of Duchenne's or Becker's muscular dystrophy. Mothers and sisters of index cases of isolated Duchenne's or Becker's dystrophy are at risk for being carriers. There is a 50% chance that males born to carrier females will inherit the disease, and 50% of the carrier's daughters will become carriers themselves. Female carriers are generally asymptomatic, but they may rarely demonstrate moderate limb-girdle weakness.

The CK level is elevated in about 50% of female carriers. A more accurate method of carrier detection is to look for an Xp21 deletion, which will be present if the affected males in the family are among the 60% who have a dystrophin gene deletion (or duplication). If a deletion is not present, linkage analysis of families can be performed. Prenatal genetic testing can be performed on amniotic fluid cells or chorionic villi.

Treatment

Rx

Controlled trials with prednisone, 0.75 mg/kg/day, in Duchenne's dystrophy have demonstrated moderate improvement in strength and delay in progression to a wheelchair or braces. 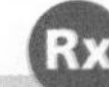 Short-term and medium-term creatine supplements can improve muscle strength. 2 Prednisone also delays respiratory compromise, but it cannot prevent deterioration and death. Side effects of therapy include weight gain, growth delay, and changes in behavior. Gene therapy for the dystrophinopathies and other muscular dystrophies with known genetic mutations is still in preclinical stages. Trials of myoblast transfer from the normal fathers of patients with Duchenne's dystrophy to their affected sons found no effect.

Emery-Dreifuss Dystrophy

Emery-Dreifuss dystrophy is an X-linked muscular dystrophy. The mutated gene in the Xq28 region codes for a protein product, emerin. Emerin is a 254–amino acid protein that localizes to the nuclear membranes of skeletal, cardiac, and smooth muscle fibers; its function is unknown.

Clinical Manifestations

The disease is characterized by the clinical triad of (1) early contractures of the elbows, ankles, and posterior cervical muscles; (2) slowly progressive muscle weakness, usually in a scapulohumeroperoneal distribution; and (3) cardiomyopathy with atrial conduction defects. The early elbow contractures are often an important phenotypic key to the diagnosis.

Diagnosis

The serum CK level is either normal or only moderately elevated. Muscle biopsy shows a range of myopathic changes but fewer dystrophic features than in Duchenne's or Becker's dystrophy. The ECG can demonstrate sinus bradycardia, prolongation of the PR interval, or more severe degrees of conduction block. Definitive diagnosis can be made by either leukocyte DNA analysis or immunostaining of muscle or skin tissue for emerin. The normal emerin perinuclear staining pattern in these tissues will be absent in Emery-Dreifuss dystrophy.

Prognosis

Although Emery-Dreifuss dystrophy usually begins in childhood, most patients remain ambulatory into their third or fourth decades. The cardiac conduction defects are potentially lethal and frequently require a pacemaker.

Bethlem Myopathy

Bethlem myopathy clinically resembles Emery-Dreifuss dystrophy because of a similar pattern of weakness and early contractures. However, Bethlem myopathy has no cardiac involvement, and the inheritance pattern is autosomal dominant. At least some cases of Bethlem myopathy are due to a mutation in the α_1 and α_2 subunits of collagen VI located on chromosome 21q.

Rigid-Spine Syndrome

The rigid-spine syndrome is a disorder in which muscle contractures involve the spine, as well as other joints. The genetic defect has been localized to chromosome 1p3, and the presumed gene product is selenoprotein. Because of the severe contractures, it must be distinguished from Emery-Dreifuss dystrophy and Bethlem myopathy. In most cases, the disease is sporadic and manifested in infancy as hypotonia, proximal weakness, and delayed motor milestones. The serum CK level is mildly elevated. Muscle biopsies demonstrate nonspecific myopathic features. Throughout the first decade, the child experiences progressive, severe scoliosis and limitations of spinal mobility, as well as elbow and knee contractures. The spinal deformities continue until about 7 to 13 years of age, at which time the disease appears to stabilize.

Limb-Girdle Muscular Dystrophies

Limb-girdle muscular dystrophies (LGMDs) include a large number of hereditary muscular dystrophies with a limb-girdle pattern of weakness. LGMDs are either autosomal recessive (the majority) or autosomal dominant and thus are clinically distinguished from the dystrophinopathies by an equal occurrence in both sexes. When LGMD occurs in early childhood, it resembles Duchenne's dystrophy and has been termed severe childhood recessive muscular dystrophy. Milder phenotypes can resemble Becker's dystrophy. The laboratory features (serum CK, EMG, muscle biopsy) are consistent with a muscular dystrophy. At least 10 subtypes of LGMD have been established on the basis of genetic mutations and the resulting protein defects. The less common autosomal dominant forms have been labeled type 1 (LGMD 1A, 1B, 1C, etc.), the autosomal recessive disorders are type 2 (LGMD 2A, 2B, etc.), and the list continues to grow.

Autosomal Recessive Limb-Girdle Muscular Dystrophies

A number of the autosomal recessive LGMDs are due to defects in one of the sarcoglycan components of the dystrophin-glycoprotein complex, termed sarcoglycanopathies (LGMD 2C, 2D, 2E, 2F).

The protein mutated in LGMD 2C, α-sarcoglycan, was previously known as adhalin—Arabic for "muscle." These disorders may account for as many as 20% of the muscular dystrophies that have a Duchenne or Becker phenotype. LGMD 2C and 2D usually begin in childhood; LGMD 2E and 2F have a more variable age at onset, even within families. These LGMDs are not associated with intellectual impairment or cardiac abnormalities, in contrast to the dystrophinopathies.

The sarcoglycans are important components of the dystrophin-glycoprotein complex, but the exact role of these proteins is unknown. A deficiency in one of the sarcoglycans results in destabilization of the entire sarcoglycan complex. The results of muscle biopsy show normal dystrophin; however, immunostaining for each of the sarcoglycans is absent or diminished, regardless of the primary sarcoglycan mutation.

Other autosomal recessive LGMDs have known protein mutations that are not part of the dystrophin-glycoprotein complex. LGMD 2A, with an age at onset of between 3 and 30 years (mean, 13), is due to a genetic mutation producing a deficiency in the muscle-specific proteolytic enzyme calpain-3. Calpains are nonlysosomal intracellular cysteine proteases. In patients with LGMD 2B, weakness develops between the ages of 13 and 35 and CK levels are elevated up to 200 times normal. The LGMD 2B mutation localizes to a region on 2p13 that codes for a protein recently named dysferlin. Dysferlin shares amino acid sequence homology with the *C. elegans* spermatogenesis factor FER-1. LGMD 2B is also of interest because affected individuals can have one of two distinct phenotypes: limb-girdle or a distal myopathy pattern (see the later discussion of distal muscular dystrophy). How a mutation in the same protein can result in such dissimilar clinical manifestations is unclear.

Autosomal Dominant Limb-Girdle Muscular Dystrophies

The autosomal dominant LGMDs all have their onset in childhood or early adult life. Linkage to chromosome locations is known for LGMD 1A and 1B; the molecular defect for LGMD 1C produces a protein deficiency of caveolin-3. Caveolins may act as scaffolding proteins on which caveolin-interacting lipids and proteins are organized. Caveolin-3 is not considered part of the dystrophin-glycoprotein complex, although it is localized to the sarcolemma by immunostaining.

Differential Diagnosis of Limb-Girdle Syndromes

All patients with limb-girdle syndromes need to be investigated by EMG and muscle biopsy. In those with a positive family history, the differential diagnosis includes inherited metabolic myopathies (e.g., acid maltase deficiency or a lipid storage myopathy), morphologically distinct congenital myopathies or their late-onset variants (e.g., nemaline, central core, and myotubular myopathies), or the anterior horn cell disease spinal muscular atrophy. In sporadic cases of a limb-girdle syndrome, the differential diagnosis includes the same diseases and also inflammatory myopathies (polymyositis, inclusion body myositis, or sarcoidosis confined to muscle), endocrine myopathies, sporadic Duchenne's dystrophy, Duchenne's or Becker's dystrophy manifested in female carriers, other dystrophinopathies, and sporadic Emery-Dreifuss dystrophy before the appearance of joint contractures or cardiomyopathy.

Congenital Muscular Dystrophies

The congenital muscular dystrophies are a group of autosomal recessive disorders in which the onset of hypotonia and proximal weakness occurs during the prenatal period; muscle biopsy shows dystrophic findings. Affected infants often have joint contractures of the elbows, hips, knees, and ankles (arthrogryposis). Congenital muscular dystrophies can be broadly divided into those without and those with clinical evidence of CNS involvement (severe mental retardation, seizures, and visual loss from cerebro-ocular dysplasia). However, many patients without severe brain disease clinically, the so-called classic type, usually demonstrate cerebral hypomyelination on MRI. The congenital muscular dystrophies with significant brain and eye involvement generally have progressive courses and result in death by 10 to 12 years of age. Classic-type congenital muscular dystrophies without clinical CNS involvement have a more benign outlook with a nonprogressive course; affected patients may eventually walk independently.

Fifty percent of classic-type congenital muscular dystrophy is associated with a deficiency of the basal lamina protein α_2-laminin, also known as merosin. Merosin is bound to the dystrophin-glycoprotein complex and anchors the basal lamina to the sarcolemma. Merosin-negative congenital muscular dystrophy can be diagnosed by immunostaining of muscle or skin. Other congenital muscular dystrophies without clinical CNS involvement are associated with a deficiency of integrin, a trans-sarcolemmal protein that is not part of the dystrophin-glycoprotein complex. Fukuyama-type congenital muscular dystrophy, occurring primarily in Japan, is associated with mutations in the gene encoding for a protein named fukutin. The same genetic defect probably accounts for the Walker-Warburg cerebro-ocular dysplasia syndrome. Fukutin is not associated with the sarcolemma and appears to be a secreted protein, but its function is unknown.

Facioscapulohumeral Dystrophy

Epidemiology and Pathobiology

Inheritance of facioscapulohumeral dystrophy is autosomal dominant with high penetrance and variable expression within families. Affected family members may be unaware of their mild deficits, thus making examination of relatives of suspected patients very important. The incidence of facioscapulohumeral dystrophy is 1 in 20,000. Facioscapulohumeral dystrophy has been linked to the telomeric region of chromosome 4q35. Although the gene has not been isolated, a deletion in this region is present in virtually all patients with facioscapulohumeral dystrophy.

Clinical Manifestations

The disease is initially manifested in childhood or adult life. It involves the facial muscles early and then descends to the scapular stabilizers (serratus anterior, rhomboid, trapezius, latissimus dorsi), the muscles of the upper part of the arm (biceps, triceps), and the anterior leg muscles. Early physical signs include failure to bury the eyelashes on forced eye closure, an expressionless face, winging of the scapulas when the arms are raised, and prominent indentation of the anterior axillary folds. The deltoids are relatively spared when compared with the other proximal arm muscles. Distal muscle weakness occurs first in the tibialis anterior and may result in footdrop and lead to a scapuloperoneal pattern of weakness. Later, wrist and finger extensor weakness may develop.

Diagnosis

The serum CK level is normal or mildly elevated. Muscle biopsy shows moderate myopathic changes, but a prominent mononuclear inflammatory infiltrate can be confused with polymyositis. However, these patients do not respond to immunosuppressive therapy. A variant is associated with sensorineural hearing loss and with retinal telangiectasia and painless blindness (Coats' disease).

Differential Diagnosis

Scapuloperoneal muscular dystrophy is an autosomal dominant disorder that can resemble facioscapulohumeral dystrophy, but without facial weakness. In these families there is no linkage to chromosome 4q35.

Prognosis

The rate of progression and the extent to which the pelvic girdle and forearm muscles are eventually affected vary considerably between and within families. In general, cases with early onset have a worse prognosis. Some patients experience a late exacerbation of weakness after years of little or slow progression. Approximately 20% of these patients will eventually require a wheelchair. Joint contractures are uncommon.

The Myotonic Dystrophies

Type 1 myotonic dystrophy (DM-1) is an autosomal dominant multisystemic disorder that affects skeletal, cardiac, and smooth muscle and other organs, including the eyes, endocrine system, and brain.

Epidemiology

DM-1 is the most common muscular dystrophy, with an incidence of 13.5 per 100,000 live births and a prevalence of 3 to 5 per 100,000. DM-1 can occur at any age, but the usual onset of symptoms is in the late second or third decade. However, some affected individuals may remain free of symptoms their entire life. The severity generally worsens from one generation to the next. A severe form with onset in infancy is known as congenital DM-1.

Pathobiology

The molecular defect in DM-1 is abnormal expansion of CTG repeats in a protein kinase gene on chromosome 19q13.2. Affected individuals have more than 50 CTG repeats, and the severity of the disease directly correlates with the size of the expanded triplet repeat. The protein kinase encoded by this gene has been termed myotonin. Studies of transgenic animals suggest that some, if not all manifestations of DM-1 result from the accumulation of abnormal RNA transcribed by the lengthy trinucleotide repeat on chromosome 19.

Clinical Manifestations

Typical patients exhibit facial weakness with temporalis muscle wasting, frontal balding, ptosis, and weakness of the neck flexor muscles (Fig. 447–2). Weakness of the extremities usually begins distally and progresses slowly to affect the limb-girdle muscles proximally. Weakness is a

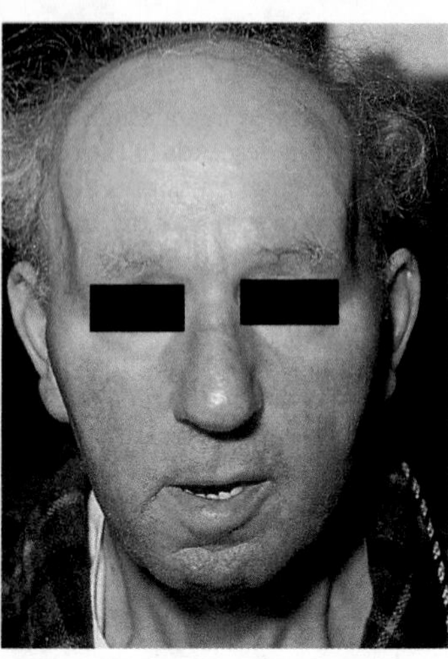

FIGURE 447–2 • Myotonic dystrophy in a 50-year-old man. His appearance is typical, with facial weakness, atrophy of the temporal muscles and sternomastoids, and frontal baldness, which gives a "monklike" appearance. (From Forbes CD, Jackson WF: Color Atlas and Text of Clinical Medicine, 3rd ed. London, Mosby, 2003.)

more common symptom than muscle stiffness or myotonia, although patients may complain of an inability to relax the fingers after a handgrip. Patients may be areflexic, but findings on sensory examination are normal.

Associated manifestations include posterior subscapular cataracts, testicular atrophy and impotence, intellectual impairment, and hypersomnia from both central and obstructive sleep apnea. Respiratory muscle weakness may be severe. Elevated serum glucose levels occur as a result of end-organ unresponsiveness to insulin, but frank diabetes mellitus rarely develops. Involvement of smooth muscle in the gastrointestinal tract can produce dysphagia, reduced gut motility, and chronic pseudo-obstruction. Cardiac conduction defects are common and can produce sudden death. Chronic hypoxia can lead to cor pulmonale. Affected females may have a high rate of fetal loss.

Diagnosis

The serum CK level is normal or mildly increased. Muscle biopsies show excessive number of central nuclei, type 1 atrophy, and other nonspecific myopathic changes. EMG shows myopathic motor units in addition to myotonic potentials.

The diagnosis can be established by documenting an increased number of CTG expansions on chromosome 19q13.2 in leukocytes from a blood sample. Marked expansion of the CTG repeat usually occurs in the children of mothers with DM-1, thus accounting for anticipation and the severe phenotype of congenital DM-1.

Differential Diagnosis

A second myotonic dystrophy locus (DM-2) on chromosome 3q involves mutations that expand a tetranucleotide repeat sequence. The clinical features of DM-2 are similar, but weakness is more often proximal than in DM-1. DM-2 is also referred to as proximal myotonic myopathy (PROMM). A similar abnormality in RNA transcription is probably responsible for DM-2. Proximal extremity weakness and myalgias are characteristic of DM-2. Patients with DM-2 may have less cardiac muscle or other organ involvement than those with DM-1.

Treatment Rx

In both DM-1 and DM-2, the myotonia is generally less symptomatic than weakness and may not require treatment. Phenytoin, usually 300 mg daily, is the safest drug for myotonia; quinine, tocainide, and mexiletine can exacerbate cardiac conduction abnormalities. Annual ECGs are recommended, and a pacemaker may be necessary. Positive pressure ventilation devices may assist DM-1 patients who have sleep apnea (Chapter 101). Sedatives and opiates should be used with caution because they can depress the ventilatory drive. Patients with myotonic dystrophy are at risk for pulmonary and cardiac complications during general anesthesia. Braces can assist patients with footdrop.

Prognosis

The prognosis is extremely variable. Patients with mild weakness and myotonia can have very little progression, whereas those with severe weakness, cardiac conduction defects, and progressive disease have a shortened life expectancy.

Distal Dystrophies

Although a number of myopathies can have prominent distal weakness as a feature, some genetically distinct entities are classified as distal muscular dystrophies. There are two late adult-onset autosomal dominant forms.

Welander's Distal Dystrophy

Welander's distal dystrophy occurs in Scandinavia and is manifested between the fourth and sixth decades as selective weakness and atrophy of the forearm extensor and intrinsic hand muscles and then involves the anterior leg and small foot muscles. Tibial muscular dystrophy has been observed in Finnish, French, and U.S. patients and initially involves the anterior tibial muscles and later the distal ends of the upper extremities. A mutation in titin is responsible. The protein defect for autosomal recessive Nonaka distal muscular dystrophy (also known as hereditary inclusion body myopathy) has been identified in uridine diphosphate-*N*-acetylglucosamine 2-epimerase/*N*-acetylmannosamine kinase (GNE). GNE is involved in the post-translational glycosylation of proteins to form glycoproteins. Disturbed glycosylation is therefore now recognized as a molecular genetic defect for the muscular dystrophies. Serum CK level can be elevated in all of these disorders. Examination of muscle biopsy specimens shows variable degrees of dystrophic changes. All these disorders have progressive courses and over time can involve the proximal muscles and lead to loss of ambulation.

Myofibrillar Myopathy

Myofibrillar myopathy (also known as desmin myopathy) is a heterogeneous group of muscular dystrophies that can be manifested as either distal or limb-girdle patterns of weakness. Myofibrillar myopathy is not a single disorder: some kindreds have a molecular defect in the αβ-crystallin chaperone protein on 11q21-23, others have a mutation in the desmin gene on 2q35, and still others have a mutation in Zasp (a Z disc–related protein). In most kindreds the disorder is inherited in an autosomal dominant fashion, but sporadic cases occur. Cardiomyopathy is common.

Oculopharyngeal Muscular Dystrophy

Oculopharyngeal muscular dystrophy is inherited as an autosomal dominant disorder. The molecular genetic defect is increased expansion of a triplet GCG repeat on chromosome 14q11 within the poly(A) binding protein 2 gene *(PABP2)*. The function of PABP2 and the means by which mutation of this protein leads to muscle disease are unknown. This disease is manifested in the fifth or sixth decade as progressive ptosis followed by dysphagia. Later, all external ocular and other extremity muscles may become affected. Diplopia does not develop. Extremity weakness usually occurs in a limb-girdle pattern, but some variants have distal involvement. The serum CK level is normal or slightly increased. Patients may benefit from surgical correction (cricopharyngeal myotomy) for achalasia or a gastric feeding tube. Progression of the disease is usually slow. Death can result from aspiration pneumonia or starvation if adequate nutrition is not addressed.

CONGENITAL MYOPATHIES

Congenital myopathies (Table 447–4) are distinguished from dystrophies in three respects: (1) characteristic morphologic alterations are

TABLE 447–4 MORPHOLOGICALLY DISTINCT CONGENITAL MYOPATHIES

Central core myopathy
Nemaline (rod) myopathy
Centronuclear (myotubular) myopathy
Severe X-linked recessive form
Milder autosomal recessive and dominant forms
Congenital fiber-type disproportion
Multicore/minicore myopathy
Fingerprint body myopathy
Sarcotubular myopathy
Reducing body myopathy
Trilaminar myopathy
Hyaline myopathy with focal lysis of myofibrils
Myofibrillar myopathy

demonstrated on biopsy, (2) they are manifested at birth as hypotonia and subsequent delayed motor development, and (3) most are relatively nonprogressive and more benign than the muscular dystrophies. However, there are exceptions to all three generalizations. Onset can occur later in childhood and even in early adulthood, and some congenital myopathies have a severe course and fatal outcome. Moreover, the molecular defect of some congenital myopathies can result in the phenotype of a muscular dystrophy.

Common clinical findings include reduced muscle bulk, slender body build and a long, narrow face with skeletal abnormalities (high-arched palate, pectus excavatum, kyphoscoliosis, dislocated hips, pes cavus), and absent or reduced muscle stretch reflexes. Most patients have limb-girdle weakness, although distal weakness occurs in some families. Serum CK is moderately elevated or normal, and EMG usually shows a myopathic pattern but may be normal. Inheritance patterns are variable.

Central Core Myopathy

Central core myopathy is autosomal dominant, but sporadic cases occur. The disorder is associated with a mutation on chromosome 19q13.1 in the ryanodine receptor gene. Some patients with malignant hyperthermia also have mutations in this gene, and thus the disorders may be allelic. The mechanism by which defects in the ryanodine receptor gene lead to these disorders is unknown.

Nemaline Myopathy

The histologic characteristic of nemaline myopathy, a congenital myopathy, is the presence of rods, or nemaline (Greek *nema* = "thread") bodies, within muscle fibers. Nemaline myopathy can occur as an autosomal recessive or dominant condition. In most autosomal recessive families the disorder has been linked to 2q; nebulin is the probable candidate gene. In some autosomal dominant families, however, nemaline myopathy has been linked to a mutation in the α-tropomyosin gene on chromosome 1q. Other cases are sporadic. Clinically, the myopathy can be manifested as a severe neonatal form with respiratory (diaphragm) involvement that is generally fatal within the first year of life or as a mild static or slowly progressive condition present from birth or early childhood.

Centronuclear (Myotubular) Myopathy

The histologic hallmark of centronuclear (myotubular) myopathy is the presence of large central nuclei within many muscle fibers. The molecular defect is a mutation in the myotubularin gene on Xp28. Myotubularin is a phosphatase important in muscle cell growth and differentiation. As with nemaline myopathy, there are severe neonatal varieties and static or slowly progressive forms with onset from birth to adulthood. Ptosis and ophthalmoparesis commonly occur in all forms of centronuclear myopathy and may distinguish these patients from those with other congenital myopathies. The severe infantile form is usually X-linked recessive and is associated with respiratory insufficiency; most patients die in infancy, but a few survive into childhood, usually with major disabilities.

TABLE 447–5 METABOLIC AND MITOCHONDRIAL MYOPATHIES

GLYCOGEN METABOLISM DEFICIENCIES
Type II: α-1,4-Glucosidase (acid maltase)
Type III: Debranching
Type IV: Branching
Type V: Phosphorylase (McArdle's disease)*
Type VII: Phosphofructokinase (Tarui's disease)*
Type VIII: Phosphorylase B kinase*
Type IX: Phosphoglycerate kinase*
Type X: Phosphoglycerate mutase*
Type XI: Lactate dehydrogenase*
LIPID METABOLISM DEFICIENCIES
Carnitine palmitoyltransferase*
Primary systemic/muscle carnitine deficiency
Secondary carnitine deficiency
β-Oxidation defects
Medications (valproic acid)
PURINE METABOLISM DEFICIENCIES
Myoadenylate deaminase deficiency*
MITOCHONDRIAL MYOPATHIES
Pyruvate dehydrogenase complex deficiencies (including Leigh's syndrome)
Progressive external ophthalmoplegia (PEO)
Autosomal dominant with multiple mitochondrial DNA deletions
Adenine nucleotide translocator 1 (ANT1)
TWINKLE
Polymerase gamma
Kearns-Sayre syndrome
Mitochondrial encephalopathy with lactic acidosis and strokelike episodes (MELAS)
Myoclonic epilepsy and ragged red fibers (MERRF)
Mitochondrial neurogastrointestinal encephalomyopathy (MNGIE)
Mitochondrial depletion syndrome
Leigh's syndrome and neuropathy, ataxia, and retinitis pigmentosa (NARP)
Succinate dehydrogenase deficiency *

*Deficiency can produce exercise intolerance and myoglobinuria.

Congenital Fiber-Type Disproportion

The distinguishing morphologic finding in congenital fiber-type disproportion is an increased number of small type 1 muscle fibers. The genetic defect is unknown. Most patients have an onset at birth with hypotonia, and the course of the disorder is nonprogressive and relatively benign.

METABOLIC MYOPATHIES

Metabolic myopathies include (1) glucose/glycogen metabolism disorders, (2) lipid metabolism disorders, and (3) mitochondrial disorders. A fourth group involving the utilization of adenine nucleotides is more controversial (Table 447–5).

Glucose/Glycogen Metabolism Disorders

Glucose and its storage form glycogen are essential for the short-term, predominantly anaerobic energy requirements of muscle. Disorders of glucose and glycogen metabolism (grouped under the term glycogenoses) have two distinct clinical patterns. One group of disorders has dynamic manifestations consisting of exercise intolerance, pain, cramps, and myoglobinuria (types V, VII, VIII, IX, X, XI). The second, static group is associated with fixed weakness without features of exercise intolerance or myoglobinuria (types II, III, IV). Occasionally, there is overlap between the two groups. Of the 11 distinct glycogenoses, only glucose 6-phosphate (type I) and liver phosphorylase (type VI) deficiencies do not affect muscle. The glycogenoses that affect muscle are usually transmitted as autosomal recessive traits, except for phosphoglycerate kinase, which is X linked.

Glycogenoses with Exercise Intolerance/Myoglobinuria

The common clinical features of the glycogenoses characterized by exercise intolerance/myoglobinuria (myophosphorylase [type V], phosphofructokinase [PFK, type VII], phosphorylase B kinase [PBK, type VIII], phosphoglycerate kinase [PGK, type IX], phosphoglycerate mutase [PGM, type X], and LDH [type XI] deficiencies) are exercise intolerance in childhood followed by exertion-induced muscle pain and myoglobinuria in the second or third decade. Many patients note a "second-wind" phenomenon after a period of brief rest so that they can continue the exercise at the previous level of activity. The muscle pain is caused by electrically silent contractures and is not associated with depletion of ATP; the mechanism is not understood. Strength examination, CK levels, and findings on EMG between attacks are usually normal early in the disease but may become abnormal with advancing age. After episodes of severe myoglobinuria with rhabdomyolysis, needle EMG can show myopathic units and fibrillations. After forearm exercise, the venous lactate level fails to rise in myophosphorylase, PFK, and PGK deficiencies and rises only partially in PBK, PGM, and LDH deficiencies. Muscle biopsy shows scattered necrotic and regenerating fibers, especially after an episode of rhabdomyolysis.

In PFK deficiency, hyperuricemia and gout occur in some cases, and there is mild hemolytic anemia caused by a partial erythrocyte enzyme defect. PGK mutations result either in severe hemolytic anemia and neurologic deficits but no myopathy or in a myopathy with only the features described earlier. LDH deficiency is associated with a rash because M-lactate dehydrogenase is the dominant form of the enzyme expressed in skin.

Histochemical stains are readily available for myophosphorylase and PFK, but definitive diagnosis requires biochemical analysis to document the enzyme deficiency or molecular testing to define specific mutations. Mutations have been identified for all the glycogenoses except PBK deficiency. Oral sucrose ingestion improves exercise tolerance in patients with myophosphorylase deficiency. [3] Otherwise, no specific treatment is available for these disorders, but aerobic exercise training and a high-protein diet have been proposed as sensible strategies.

Glycogenoses with Fixed Weakness and No Exercise Intolerance

α-Glucosidase Deficiencies

α-Glucosidase, also known as acid maltase, is a lysosomal enzyme that breaks down glycogen to glucose; when its level is deficient, glycogen accumulates within lysosomes, as well as freely in the cytoplasm of cells. Mutations have been identified in the α-glucosidase gene on chromosome 17q21.

Clinical Manifestations

There are three clinical variants. The infantile type (Pompe's disease) is manifested in early infancy as generalized and rapidly progressive weakness and heart, tongue, and liver enlargement. There is widespread glycogen excess in tissues, including lower motor neurons. Death results from cardiorespiratory failure before the age of 2 years.

The childhood (juvenile) type is manifested in infancy or early childhood as a myopathy. Weakness is more proximal than distal, and there may be calf enlargement simulating muscular dystrophy. Glycogen excess is less marked and confined to muscle. The heart, but not the liver may be involved. Death results from respiratory failure before the age of 20.

The adult type is manifested between the second and seventh decades of life either as slowly progressive limb muscle weakness that mimics limb-girdle dystrophy or in a scapuloperoneal pattern. These patients often experience insidious ventilatory muscle weakness leading to respiratory failure. The adult form does not affect the heart or liver.

Diagnosis

In all three types, the serum CK level is moderately increased. The EMG in affected muscles shows myopathic changes and excessive abnormal electrical irritability, including myotonic discharges, particularly in the paraspinous muscles. However, there is no clinical myotonia. Muscle biopsy demonstrates a vacuolar myopathy with high glycogen content and acid phosphatase reactivity in the vacuoles. The diagnosis is confirmed by demonstrating α-glucosidase deficiency in either muscle, skin fibroblasts, or lymphocytes.

Differential Diagnosis

Danon's disease has clinical and histologic features similar to those of the adult form of α-glucosidase deficiency, including glycogen accumulation. The defect is a mutation in lysosome-associated membrane protein (LAMP).

Treatment and Prognosis

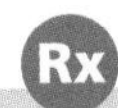

Enzyme replacement therapy with intravenous recombinant α-glucosidase (Myozyme) can be life-saving [4] and was recently approved by the Food and Drug Administration for the infantile, childhood, and adult forms of the disease. With the advent of effective therapy, the prognosis is likely to improve.

Debranching Enzyme Deficiency

Debranching enzyme deficiency is a rare disease that can affect the liver, heart, or skeletal muscle. The gene for the enzyme maps to chromosome 1p21. The disease is most commonly manifested in childhood as hepatomegaly with fasting hypoglycemia that spontaneously resolves by adulthood. Patients less frequently have a disabling myopathy that affects both proximal and distal muscles and can appear in childhood or (more commonly) in adult life. Affected patients can experience exercise intolerance. There may be a depressed lactate response on forearm testing, but myoglobinuria is rare. The CK level is elevated, and the EMG shows myopathic changes and abnormal electrical irritability.

Branching Enzyme Deficiency

Deficiency of the branching enzyme is manifested in infancy as progressive liver and cardiac dysfunction, which leads to death in the first years of life. Muscle weakness is variable; if weakness is present, the tongue is severely affected.

Disorders of Fatty Acid Metabolism

Lipids are essential for the aerobic energy needs of muscle during sustained exercise. Serum long-chain fatty acids, which are the primary lipid fuel for muscle metabolism, are transported into the mitochondria as carnitine esters and are metabolized via β-oxidation. CPT I converts cytoplasmic acyl coenzyme A (acyl-CoA) to acylcarnitine, which is then transported into mitochondria by carnitine acyltransferase in exchange for carnitine. CPT II on the inner mitochondrial membrane reconstitutes acyl-CoA. A deficiency of carnitine, CPT, or the enzymes of β-oxidation can lead to impaired muscle lipid metabolism.

As with glycogen pathway defects, the myopathic manifestations of fatty acid metabolism can consist of dynamic exercise intolerance with myoglobinuria or static weakness with a lipid storage myopathy. A lipid storage myopathy can be caused by primary carnitine deficiency or by another defect in fatty acid oxidation with secondary carnitine deficiency. In addition, some disorders of lipid metabolism can produce multiorgan metabolic crises with hepatic failure and altered mental status (Reye's syndrome). Most lipid disorders occur sporadically; they are believed to be autosomal recessive.

Carnitine Palmitoyltransferase Deficiency

CPT occurs in two forms: types I and II. Deficiency of CPT I may be manifested in infancy or childhood as hepatic dysfunction. It causes a Reye syndrome–like illness with hypoketotic hypoglycemia, encephalopathy, hyperammonemia, and liver dysfunction.

Deficiency of CPT II typically causes exertional myalgias and myoglobinuria. The disorder is autosomal recessive, and mutations in the CPT

II gene on chromosome 1p32 have been identified. These attacks are distinct from those associated with glycolytic defects in that they occur after prolonged exercise, fasting, febrile illness, or other provocations that may increase muscle dependence on free fatty acids. Unlike patients with McArdle's disease, those with CPT deficiency tolerate brief, intense exercise and have no second-wind phenomenon. Muscle strength and the CK level are normal at rest. Serum and muscle carnitine levels are typically normal. EMG is normal except for myopathic changes after episodes of rhabdomyolysis. Ammonia and lactate levels rise normally after forearm exercise. Findings on muscle biopsy are usually normal except for evidence of muscle myopathic injury after rhabdomyolysis. Diagnosis requires assay of CPT activity in muscle. Although there is no specific treatment, increasing intake of carbohydrates and the frequency of meals prevents episodes of rhabdomyolysis.

Carnitine Deficiency

Primary carnitine deficiencies may cause a generalized systemic illness or a disorder confined to muscle. In the systemic form, the impaired transport of carnitine into multiple tissues results from nonfunctional high-affinity carnitine receptors. Patients have a myopathy with cardiac involvement, as well as episodes of hepatic dysfunction with hypoketotic hypoglycemia and altered mental status. Abnormal lipid storage is seen on muscle biopsy. Carnitine levels are reduced in serum, muscle, and other tissues. There is no urinary excretion of organic acids to suggest a secondary metabolic illness. Patients with this condition improve with carnitine supplementation.

When the disease is limited to muscle, patients are usually seen in childhood with limb-girdle myopathy. Patients have diminished muscle uptake of carnitine and a fixed lipid storage myopathy but a normal serum carnitine level. Carnitine replacement has been of inconsistent benefit.

Secondary Carnitine Deficiency

Most carnitine deficiencies are secondary to enzyme defects in β-oxidation (e.g., acyl-CoA dehydrogenase deficiencies), mitochondrial dysfunction, renal disease, impaired metabolism of medications such as valproic acid, or other metabolic disorders. Defects in lipid metabolism lead to accumulation of acyl-CoA molecules, which are converted to acylcarnitines, forms that are more readily excreted in urine. This process leads to negative carnitine balance and, ultimately, to carnitine deficiency. Impaired metabolism of valproic acid may similarly lead to excretion of valproylcarnitine and secondary carnitine deficiency. Most of these illnesses occur in early childhood or infancy and lead to Reye syndrome–like episodes. Some surviving adults experience a lipid storage myopathy with the clinical phenotype of a limb-girdle syndrome. Muscle biopsy reveals lipid storage. The free carnitine level is diminished, but that of esterified carnitine may be increased, especially after oral supplementation of depleted carnitine stores. Abnormal urinary excretion of organic acids is a critical clue to differentiate these disorders from primary carnitine deficiency. Different metabolic blocks in fatty acid metabolism lead to the excretion of distinct urinary acylcarnitine species, which can be distinguished by mass spectroscopy. Carnitine supplementation produces variable results, but some patients have fewer or less severe attacks. Some cases of multiple flavin-dependent dehydrogenase deficiency respond to riboflavin.

Disorders of Purine Nucleotide Metabolism: Myoadenylate Deaminase Deficiency

Myoadenylate deaminase (MAD), which is an enzyme in the purine nucleotide cycle, provides a short-term supply of ATP in muscle by catalyzing the conversion of adenosine monophosphate to inosine monophosphate through the removal of ammonia. If MAD is absent, less ATP is formed. MAD deficiency has been found in patients with exertional muscle pain and occasionally myoglobinuria. Forearm exercise results in a normal rise in the lactate level but no increase in the ammonia level. Muscle biopsy shows absent staining for MAD. The gene for MAD is on chromosome 1p13-21 and is mutated in most patients with MAD deficiency. However, the frequency of this mutation in the "normal" population is high, and patients without symptoms may have biochemical evidence of MAD deficiency. Therefore, it is still unclear whether MAD deficiency results in a metabolic myopathy or whether the enzyme deficiency is coincidental.

Mitochondrial Myopathies

Mitochondrial myopathies produce slowly progressive weakness of the limb-girdle or external ocular and other cranial muscles and abnormal fatigability on sustained exertion; some affect multiple organs or systems, in addition to muscle. In many mitochondrial myopathies, a substantial proportion of the muscle fibers contain subsarcolemmal and intermyofibrillar accumulations of structurally and functionally abnormal mitochondria. These fibers appear "ragged red" with trichrome stain and may fail to react for cytochrome *c* oxidase. Other laboratory features frequently seen in mitochondrial myopathies are an elevated serum lactic acid level on exertion or at rest, as well as a modestly elevated CK level and myopathic findings on EMG. Cerebrospinal fluid protein is often elevated.

Mitochondrial DNA encodes for 22 transfer RNAs (tRNAs), 2 ribosomal RNAs (rRNAs), and 13 messenger RNAs (mRNAs). The 13 mRNAs are translated into polypeptide subunits of the respiratory chain complex. A mutation in a mitochondrial tRNA gene can impair proper translation of the 13 mitochondrial mRNAs. However, the 13 proteins encoded by the mitochondrial genome account for less than 5% of mitochondrial proteins; the majority are encoded by nuclear DNA and are translated in the cytoplasm and transported into mitochondria.

Mitochondrial diseases can arise from mutations in nuclear or mitochondrial DNA. During fertilization, essentially all of the mitochondria are contributed by the mother's ovum; thus, all mutations in mitochondrial DNA either are maternally transmitted or arise de novo in the maternal ovum or in early embryonic life. However, because the majority of mitochondrial proteins (95%) are encoded from nuclear genes, mitochondrial disorders can also have autosomal dominant and even X-linked hereditary patterns.

From a biochemical standpoint, mitochondrial disorders can be due to defects proximal to the respiratory chain (involving substrate transport and utilization) or within the respiratory chain. Viewed in this way, the derangements in lipid metabolism can be considered "mitochondrial" dysfunctions. Acetyl-CoA feeds into the mitochondria to enter the Krebs cycle and the respiratory chain. However, the lipid disorders generally do not have structural defects of mitochondria or a "mitochondrial myopathy" phenotype. Among the exceptions are substrate utilization abnormalities secondary to pyruvate dehydrogenase complex defects, which can produce X-linked Leigh's syndrome or subacute necrotizing encephalomyopathy. Although muscle biopsy may show ragged red fibers, the CNS abnormalities overshadow the neuromuscular abnormalities.

Most mitochondrial disorders are due to biochemical defects in the mitochondrial respiratory chain that can involve coenzyme Q and the five distinct enzyme complexes: complex I (reduced nicotinamide adenine dinucleotide–coenzyme Q oxidoreductase); complex II (succinate dehydrogenase); complex III (coenzyme Q–cytochrome *c* oxidoreductase); complex IV (cytochrome *c* oxidase); and complex V (ATPase synthetase). Defects in the electron transport complexes are associated with marked clinical, biochemical, and genetic heterogeneity because each complex is composed of multiple subunits, different subunits of a given complex are encoded by different genes, some subunits of a given complex are encoded by mitochondrial rather than nuclear DNA, and some subunits are tissue specific.

Specific Mitochondrial Disorders Affecting Muscle

Progressive External Ophthalmoplegia

Severe ptosis and progressive external ophthalmoplegia are clinical hallmarks of mitochondrial disease. Ptosis is often the initial symptom and is generally first noted in childhood. As the ophthalmoplegia progresses, it often becomes complete. Patients do not have diplopia. A limb-girdle weakness pattern may occur with varying degrees of severity. Muscle biopsy reveals characteristic ragged red fibers, and EM shows structurally abnormal mitochondria with "parking lot" paracrystalline inclusions.

Progressive external ophthalmoplegia secondary to mitochondrial disease is associated with single or multiple mitochondrial DNA deletions. Patients with single mitochondrial deletions have the Kearns-Sayre syndrome, which includes retinitis pigmentosa, heart block, hearing loss, short stature, ataxia, delayed secondary sexual characteristics, peripheral neuropathy, and impaired ventilatory drive. The syndrome develops before 20 years of age. Kearns-Sayre syndrome, which is due to single large mitochondrial deletions, occurs as a sporadic mutation only.

By comparison, progressive external ophthalmoplegia with multiple mitochondrial deletions is autosomal dominant; in some kinships the defects have been localized to both chromosomes 10q22-23 and 3ql4-21, and maternally inherited point mutations in mitochondrial tRNA have been reported. This disease, which has a later onset of symptoms than Kearns-Sayre syndrome does, is often accompanied by various degrees of encephalomyopathy and neuropathy.

Myoclonic Epilepsy and Ragged Red Fibers

Patients affected by myoclonic epilepsy with ragged red fibers have varying symptoms of myoclonus, generalized seizures, ataxia, dementia, sensorineural hearing loss, and optic atrophy, as well as limb-girdle weakness. Some patients also have a sensorimotor peripheral neuropathy, cardiomyopathy, and cutaneous lipomas. Ptosis and ophthalmoparesis are not usually present. Most patients have a point mutation in the mitochondrial DNA encoding for tRNA, and the disease is maternally inherited.

Mitochondrial Encephalomyopathy with Lactic Acidosis and Strokelike Episodes

Patients with mitochondrial encephalomyopathy with lactic acidosis and strokelike episodes (MELAS) have normal early development, experience migraine-like headaches and strokes before 40 years of age, and have lactic acidosis. Other features frequently include dementia, hearing loss, episodic vomiting, ataxia, and coma, as well as diabetes. Ptosis and ophthalmoparesis are uncommon. MELAS is inherited maternally and is caused by mitochondrial DNA mutations encoding for tRNA. Dichloroacetate seemed beneficial in anecdotal reports, but a placebo-controlled trial demonstrated that dichloroacetate causes peripheral neuropathy and is not of benefit.

Mitochondrial Neurogastrointestinal Encephalomyopathy

Mitochondrial neurogastrointestinal encephalomyopathy (MNGIE) is associated with sensorimotor polyneuropathy, ophthalmoplegia, leukoencephalopathy on MRI of the brain, and chronic intestinal pseudo-obstruction (POLIP syndrome). Patients have distal as well as proximal weakness and ptosis. There are multiple mitochondrial DNA deletions similar to those found in autosomal dominant progressive external ophthalmoplegia. MNGIE has been localized to chromosome 22q13 in some families.

Mitochondrial DNA Depletion Syndrome

Mitochondrial DNA depletion is an autosomal recessive syndrome that is manifested at birth or shortly afterward as generalized hypotonia and weakness. Other features can include cardiomyopathy, renal tubular defects, seizures, and liver failure. Infants experience respiratory failure, and many die within the first year of life. There is also a benign infantile form in which the hypotonic infants can survive and appear normal by 2 or 3 years of age.

Leigh's Syndrome

Leigh's syndrome usually occurs in infancy or early childhood and consists of altered mental status, generalized weakness or hypotonia, vomiting, ataxia, ptosis and ophthalmoplegia, seizures, and respiratory failure. The molecular genetic characteristics are heterogeneous. The disease is generally fatal.

Mitochondrial Myopathies Associated with Recurrent Myoglobinuria

Recurrent myoglobinuria provoked by exercise is uncommon in mitochondrial disorders. Between attacks, the patient is normal. This genetically heterogeneous group of disorders includes multiple mitochondrial DNA deletions (autosomal recessive inheritance), mitochondrial point mutations (maternal inheritance), and nuclear DNA mutations encoding for succinate dehydrogenase (complex II).

CHANNELOPATHIES (NONDYSTROPHIC MYOTONIAS AND PERIODIC PARALYSES)

The myotonias are grouped into dystrophic and nondystrophic disorders. The nondystrophic myotonias and the periodic paralyses are caused by mutations of various ion channels in muscle (Table 447–6). The term *channelopathies* is often used to describe this group of disorders.

Chloride Channelopathies

Myotonia congenita is due to point mutations in the muscle chloride channel gene on chromosome 7q35. Both the autosomal dominant form (Thomsen's disease) and the autosomal recessive form (Becker's myotonia) are benign and associated with muscle hypertrophy and with action, percussion, and electrical myotonia. Cold increases the myotonia, and sustained exercise improves it (warm-up phenomenon). There is no involvement of the heart or other organs. Patients with Thomsen's disease are not weak, but those who have Becker's myotonia congenita have fluctuations in strength and may experience limb-girdle weakness. Patients with myotonia congenita seldom complain of pain, a feature that distinguishes them from those who have proximal myotonic myopathy (PROMM or DM-2). The membrane defect consists of markedly reduced chloride conductance with resulting hyperexcitability and afterdepolarization that produces involuntary myotonic potentials. Many patients do not require treatment, but drugs such as quinine, procainamide, phenytoin, and mexiletine may be effective in reducing symptomatic myotonia.

Sodium Channelopathies

Several autosomal dominant disorders are due to point mutations in the voltage-dependent sodium channel *(SCN4A)* gene on chromosome 17q23-25. All have symptoms that begin in the first decade and continue throughout life, and there is considerable clinical overlap between the disorders. Patients with paramyotonia congenita (Eulenburg's disease) have paradoxical myotonia in that the myotonia increases with repetitive movements; for example, after several attempts, patients cannot open their eyelids. Muscle stiffness is worsened by cold temperature. The myotonia can be treated with sodium-channel blockers such as mexiletine.

Hyperkalemic periodic paralysis (Chapter 118) is characterized by attacks of weakness lasting 1 or 2 hours. Attacks are precipitated by fasting, by rest after exercise, or by ingestion of potassium-rich foods or compounds. During attacks, patients are areflexic with normal sensation, and there is no ocular or respiratory muscle weakness. The serum potassium level may or may not be increased during the attack, and therefore a more appropriate term may be potassium-sensitive periodic paralysis. Strength is generally normal between attacks, but some patients can have mild interictal limb-girdle weakness. Some families with potassium-sensitive periodic paralysis also have either myotonia or paramyotonia. Episodes of weakness are rarely serious enough to require acute therapy; oral carbohydrates or glucose may improve the weakness. Treatment options to prevent attacks include acetazolamide, dichlorphenamide, 5 thiazide diuretics, β-agonists, and preventive measures such as a low-potassium, high-carbohydrate diet and avoidance of fasting, strenuous activity, and cold (Chapter 118).

Sodium-channel myotonias are a group of potassium-sensitive disorders caused by molecular defects in the sodium channel but not characterized by periodic paralysis or paramyotonia phenotypes. These disorders include acetazolamide-responsive myotonia, myotonia fluctuans (myotonia that fluctuates on a daily basis), and myotonia permanens.

Calcium Channelopathies

Hypokalemic periodic paralysis (Chapter 118) is due to abnormal muscle membrane excitability arising either from mutations in the muscle calcium-channel α-subunit on chromosome 1q31-32 or, in a small proportion of cases, from a mutation in the skeletal muscle sodium channel. The α_1-subunit of the calcium channel contains the dihydropyridine receptor, which acts as a pore for conducting calcium ions in the T tubule. The mutation produces a reduction in the calcium current in the T tubule. During attacks, there is an influx of potassium into muscle cells, and the muscles become electrically inexcitable. Patients have increased sensitivity to the effects of insulin on potassium flux. However, the mechanism through which the shift in potassium from the extracellular to the intracellular space is associated with functional impairment of the calcium-channel dihydropyridine receptor is unknown.

Hypokalemic periodic paralysis is an autosomal dominant condition. It is the most frequent form of periodic paralysis, is more common in males, and has reduced penetrance in females. Attacks begin by adolescence and are aggravated by exercise, sleep, stress, alcohol, or meals rich in carbohydrates and sodium. The episodes last from 3 to 24 hours. A

TABLE 447–6 CHANNELOPATHIES AND RELATED DISORDERS

Disorder	Pattern of Clinical Features	Inheritance	Chromosome	Gene
Chloride channelopathies				
Myotonia congenita				
Thomsen's disease	Myotonia	Autosomal dominant	7q35	*CLC1*
Becker's disease	Myotonia and weakness	Autosomal recessive	7q35	*CLC1*
Sodium channelopathies				
Paramyotonia congenita	Paramyotonia	Autosomal dominant	17q13.1-13.3	*SCNA4A*
Hyperkalemic periodic paralysis	Periodic paralysis with myotonia and paramyotonia	Autosomal dominant	17q13.1-13.3	*CNA4A*
Hypokalemic periodic paralysis	Periodic paralysis	Autosomal dominant	17q13.1-13.3	*SCNA4A*
Potassium-aggravated myotonias				
Myotonia fluctuans	Myotonia	Autosomal dominant	17q13.1-13.3	*SCNA4A*
Myotonia permanens	Myotonia	Autosomal dominant	17q13.1-13.3	*SCNA4A*
Acetazolamide-responsive myotonia	Myotonia	Autosomal dominant	17q13.1-13.3	*SCNA4A*
Calcium channelopathies				
Hypokalemic periodic paralysis	Periodic paralysis	Autosomal dominant	1q31-32	Dihydropyridine receptor
Schwartz-Jampel syndrome (chondrodystrophic myotonia)	Myotonia, dysmorphic	Autosomal recessive	1q34.1-36.1	Perlecan
Rippling muscle disease	Muscle mounding/stiffness	Autosomal dominant	1q41	Caveolin-3
Andersen-Tawil syndrome	Periodic paralysis, cardiac arrhythmia, skeletal abnormalities	Autosomal dominant	17q23	*KCNJ2* (Kir 2.1)
Brody's disease	Delayed relaxation, no EMG myotonia	Autosomal recessive	16p12	Calcium ATPase
Malignant hyperthermia	Anesthetic-induced delayed relaxation	Autosomal dominant	19q13.1	Ryanodine receptor

ATPase = adenosine triphosphatase; EMG = electromyogram.

vague prodrome of stiffness or heaviness in the legs can occur, and if the patient performs mild exercise, a full-blown attack may be aborted. Rarely, the ocular, bulbar, and respiratory muscles can be involved in severe attacks. Early in the disease, patients have normal interictal examination findings except for eyelid myotonia (about 50%). Later, the frequency of attacks can diminish, but many patients have proximal weakness; in occasional patients, this weakness produces severe incapacity.

Preventive measures include a low-carbohydrate, low-sodium diet and drugs such as acetazolamide, dichlorphenamide, spironolactone, and triamterene (Chapter 118). Acute attacks are treated with oral potassium every 30 minutes until strength improves; the ECG must be monitored. In severe episodes, particularly in patients with gastrointestinal symptoms, parenteral potassium therapy may be necessary.

Other Forms of Periodic Paralysis, Channelopathies, and Muscle Stiffness

Andersen's syndrome is an autosomal dominant disorder with periodic paralysis (hypo-, hyper-, or normo-kalemic), distinctive facial features (hypertelorism, short stature, low-set ears), a prolonged QT interval, and life-threatening ventricular arrhythmias. The genetic defect has been localized to chromosome 17q23 and is caused by a defect in the inward rectifying potassium channel gene *KCNJ2* encoding Kir2.1.

Rippling muscle disease is an autosomal dominant disorder characterized by localized transient swelling or rippling of muscle induced by percussion or exercise. A pedigree has been localized to chromosome 1q41. Patients complain of tightness in the thighs or upper part of the arms.

Brody's disease is characterized by exercise-induced impaired relaxation and stiffness, but with no abnormalities indicated by muscle percussion or on EMG. The disorder is autosomal recessive and in some cases is caused by mutations in the SR calcium ATPase gene of type 2 muscle fibers located on chromosome 16p12.

Schwartz-Jampel syndrome is an autosomal recessive disorder of ATPase that occurs in early childhood and consists of chondrodystrophy, short stature, bone and joint deformities, hypertrichosis, blepharophimosis, and muscle stiffness. A mutation in perlecan is responsible for some cases. There is delayed muscle relaxation clinically resembling myotonia, but the EMG shows nonvariable (nonmyotonic) continuous high-frequency electrical activity.

Malignant hyperthermia (Chapters 110, 114, 445, and 458) is characterized by severe muscle rigidity, fever, and tachycardia precipitated by depolarizing muscle relaxants and inhaled anesthetic agents such as halothane. The symptoms usually occur during surgery but can first be noticed in the postoperative period. Patients may have previously undergone anesthesia without symptoms. During attacks, the CK level is markedly elevated and myoglobinuria develops. The disorder is caused by excessive calcium release by the SR calcium channel, the ryanodine receptor. Some patients have mutations in the ryanodine receptor gene on chromosome 19q13, which is the same gene mutated in central core disease. However, malignant hyperthermia appears to be genetically heterogeneous, and the defect in other families has been localized to different chromosomes. The symptoms are treated with dantrolene, and at-risk patients should not be given known provocative anesthetic agents. The occurrence of malignant hyperthermia in one member of a family should prompt consideration of whether other family members could also be at risk.

Neuromyotonia, or *Isaacs' syndrome*, is an autoimmune disorder with antibodies directed against voltage-gated potassium channels on peripheral nerves. Therefore, it is an acquired channelopathy, not a primary myopathy, that has a major secondary effect on muscle activity.

Inactivation of these channels makes the motor nerve hyperexcitable and produces continuous muscle fiber activity that persists even during sleep. Clinically, there is involuntary muscle activity with stiffness, twitches, fasciculations, and continuous small, undulating movements of the overlying skin (myokymia). Patients may also experience excessive sweating, a peripheral neuropathy, and stiffness. EMG documents the myokymic potentials and very high-frequency bursts (150 to 300 Hz) of spontaneous motor activity, termed *neuromyotonia.* Some cases are associated with neoplasms: thymoma (with or without myasthenia gravis), small cell lung carcinoma, and lymphoma. The CK level can be mildly elevated, cerebrospinal fluid shows elevated protein and oligoclonal bands, and voltage-gated potassium channel antibodies are present in serum. Treatment consists of immunosuppressive agents, symptomatic therapy with phenytoin or carbamazepine, or removal of the malignancy. An autosomal dominant form of neuromyotonia exists; it is associated with ataxia or a peripheral neuropathy.

Stiff-Person Syndrome

Stiff-person syndrome, an acquired autoimmune condition, is characterized by severe muscle stiffness of the proximal and especially the paraspinous muscles. The muscle spasms produce hyperlordosis, and all movements are slow and laborious. There is excess motor unit activity because of autoantibodies to glutamic acid decarboxylase, which is a major enzyme in the synthesis of γ-aminobutyric acid; the result is disinhibition in the CNS. The CK level is elevated, and EMG shows resting continuous motor unit activity that the patient cannot voluntarily suppress. Some patients also have antibodies to islet cells and thus are susceptible to the development of diabetes mellitus. Symptomatic treatment consists of diazepam; immunosuppressive treatment and intravenous immune globulin can markedly improve the condition.

Evaluation of Periodic Paralysis

In any patient with hypokalemia or hyperkalemia who is initially being evaluated for an attack of periodic paralysis, secondary causes need to be excluded (Table 447–7). In the primary forms of periodic paralysis, the serum potassium level decreases or increases but may be within the normal range during attacks; it is normal between attacks. By contrast, in secondary periodic paralysis caused by potassium wastage or retention, the serum potassium level is always markedly reduced or elevated during and even between attacks.

TABLE 447–7 SECONDARY CAUSES OF PERIODIC PARALYSIS

HYPOKALEMIC

Thyrotoxic
Primary hyperaldosteronism (Conn's syndrome)
Renal tubular acidosis (e.g., Fanconi's syndrome)
Juxtaglomerular apparatus hyperplasia (Barter's syndrome)
Gastrointestinal potassium wastage
Villous adenoma
Laxative abuse
Pancreatic non–insulin-secreting tumors with diarrhea
Nontropical sprue
Barium intoxication
Potassium-depleting diuretics
Amphotericin B
Licorice
Corticosteroids
Toluene toxicity
p-Aminosalicyclic acid
Carbenoxolone

HYPERKALEMIC

Addison's disease
Hypoaldosteronism
Excessive potassium supplementation
Potassium-sparing diuretics
Chronic renal failure

Thyrotoxic periodic paralysis resembles hypokalemic periodic paralysis. It is most common in Asian and Latin American young male adults. β-Adrenergic blocking agents reduce the frequency and severity of attacks, but the ultimate treatment is directed against the thyrotoxicosis (Chapter 244).

During an attack of periodic paralysis, potassium levels should be measured every 15 to 30 minutes to determine the direction of change when muscle strength is worsening or improving. An ECG is useful to demonstrate the changes of hypokalemia or hyperkalemia. The CK level is usually elevated during an attack but normal between attacks. Findings on routine EMG are normal between attacks, but the compound motor action potential may decline in amplitude after exercise (exercise test) and thus corroborate the presence (but not the cause) of periodic paralysis. Muscle biopsy between attacks may demonstrate vacuoles or tubular aggregates within fibers. Provocative testing for hypokalemic periodic paralysis consists of giving oral or intravenous glucose with or without insulin; for hyperkalemic periodic paralysis, testing consists of giving repeated doses of oral potassium under close supervision with cardiac monitoring and intravenous access.

INFLAMMATORY AND OTHER MYOPATHIES

Inflammatory Myopathies

Inflammatory myopathies (Chapter 290) include a heterogeneous group of acquired, nonhereditary disorders (Table 447–8) that are characterized by muscle weakness and evidence of inflammation on muscle biopsy. Most patients have elevated CK levels, myopathic findings on EMG, and a limb-girdle distribution of weakness. Occasionally, inflammatory myopathies have distal, focal, or other selective involvement of particular muscles. Most inflammatory myopathies are considered idiopathic; although the cause is unknown, an autoimmune origin is suspected. The three major categories of idiopathic inflammatory myopathy

TABLE 447–8 CLASSIFICATION OF INFLAMMATORY MYOPATHIES

IDIOPATHIC

Polymyositis
Dermatomyositis
Inclusion body myositis
Overlap syndromes with other connective tissue disease (scleroderma, systemic lupus erythematosus, mixed connective tissue disease, Sjögren's syndrome, rheumatoid arthritis, polyarteritis nodosa)
Sarcoidosis and other granulomatous myositis
Behçet's syndrome
Inflammatory myopathies and eosinophilia
  Eosinophilic polymyositis
  Diffuse fasciitis with eosinophilia
Focal myositis
Myositis ossificans

INFECTIOUS

Bacterial: *Staphylococcus aureus*, streptococci, *Escherichia coli, Yersinia* sp, *Legionella* sp, gas gangrene *(Clostridium welchii)*, leprous myositis, Lyme disease *(Borrelia burgdorferi)*
Viral: acute myositis after influenza or other viral infections (adenovirus, coxsackievirus, echovirus, parainfluenza virus, Epstein-Barr virus, arbovirus, cytomegalovirus), retrovirus-related myopathies (HIV, HTLV-1), hepatitis B and C
Parasitic: trichinosis *(Trichinella spiralis)*, toxoplasmosis *(Toxoplasma gondii)*, cysticercosis, sarcosporidiosis, trypanosomiasis *(Taenia solium)*
Fungal: *Candida, Cryptococcus*, sporotrichosis, actinomycosis, histoplasmosis

HIV = human immunodeficiency virus; HTLV-1 = human T-lymphotropic virus 1.

are dermatomyositis, polymyositis, and inclusion body myositis. These inflammatory myopathies are clinically, histologically, and pathogenically distinct (Table 447–9). Polymyositis and dermatomyositis are covered in detail in Chapter 290.

Clinical Manifestations and Diagnosis

Inclusion body myositis is characterized by an insidious onset of slowly progressive proximal and distal weakness. The slow evolution of the disease process contributes to the delay in diagnosis, which averages 6 years from the onset of symptoms. Inclusion body myositis typically begins after 50 years of age and is the most common inflammatory myopathy in the elderly. Men are more commonly affected than women. These patients have a distinctive pattern of muscle involvement consisting of early weakness and atrophy of the quadriceps (knee extensors), volar forearm muscles (wrist and finger flexors), and tibialis anterior (ankle dorsiflexors). Involvement of these muscle groups is frequently asymmetrical, in contrast to the symmetrical weakness in dermatomyositis and polymyositis. Patients have difficulty making a fist because of finger flexor weakness. Some degree of shoulder and hip girdle weakness is often present as well. Facial weakness occurs in a third of patients, and dysphagia occurs in nearly half. Although most patients have no sensory symptoms, evidence of a distal sensory peripheral neuropathy can be detected in nearly 30% of patients through clinical examination and electrophysiologic testing. Quadriceps muscle stretch reflexes are usually decreased when quadriceps atrophy is severe. Myalgias do not occur, but as the quadriceps muscles progressively weaken and genu recurvatum develops, patients frequently complain of knee pain. Patients do not have associated pulmonary, cardiac, or malignant disorders. No or only slight elevations in the CK level are seen, and the erythrocyte sedimentation rate is usually normal. Muscle biopsy is essential to establish the diagnosis of inclusion body myositis.

Treatment and Prognosis

Although immunotherapy can improve strength and function in patients with dermatomyositis and polymyositis, inclusion body myositis is usually refractory to immunosuppressive therapy, and intravenous gamma globulin is also ineffective. Life expectancy is normal, but patients frequently require a cane or wheelchair for long distances and some patients become severely incapacitated within 10 to 15 years of onset. Many patients with so-called steroid-resistant or refractory polymyositis in fact have inclusion body myositis.

Rx

Other Idiopathic Inflammatory Myopathies

Overlap Syndromes

The term *overlap syndromes* denotes a group of disorders in which an inflammatory myopathy occurs in association with another well-defined connective tissue disorder, including scleroderma (Chapter 288), systemic lupus erythematosus (Chapter 287), Sjögren's syndrome (Chapter 289), rheumatoid arthritis (Chapter 285), mixed connective tissue disease, and polyarteritis nodosa (Chapter 291). Clinical and histologic features of either dermatomyositis or polymyositis can develop in up to 10% of each of these disorders. The myositis associated with overlap syndromes may be more responsive to immunosuppressive treatment than polymyositis is.

Eosinophilic Polymyositis

Eosinophilic polymyositis usually occurs as part of the hypereosinophilic syndrome (Chapter 176). Peripheral eosinophilia in the absence of parasitic infection is associated with a multisystemic disorder of muscle, peripheral nerve, lung, heart, skin, and CNS. Response to immunosuppressive therapy is inconsistent, and the prognosis is generally poor.

Diffuse Fasciitis with Eosinophilia

In diffuse fasciitis with eosinophilia, also known as Shulman's syndrome, peripheral eosinophilia is associated with painful scleroderma-like skin changes, contractures, myalgia, arthralgia, and fever. However, unlike eosinophilic polymyositis, the heart, lungs, and other organs are not involved. Laboratory features include hypergammaglobulinemia, elevated erythrocyte sedimentation rate, and occasionally, an elevated CK level. Full-thickness biopsy from the skin to muscle is required to demonstrate the thickened fascia infiltrated by eosinophils and lymphocytes. The inflammation can invade adjacent underlying muscle. The

TABLE 447–9 IDIOPATHIC INFLAMMATORY MYOPATHIES: CLINICAL AND LABORATORY FEATURES

	Sex	Typical Age at Onset	Rash	Pattern of Weakness	CK Level	Muscle Biopsy	Response to IS Therapy	Common Associated Conditions
Dermatomyositis	F > M	Childhood and adult	Yes	Proximal > distal	Increased (up to 50× normal)	Perimysial and perivascular inflammation; $CD4^+$ T cells, B cells; MAC, Ig, C deposition on vessels	Yes	Myocarditis, interstitial lung disease, vasculitis, other connective tissue diseases, malignancy
Polymyositis	F > M	Adult	No	Proximal > distal	Increased (up to 50× normal)	Endomysial inflammation; $CD8^+$ T cells, Macros	Yes	Myocarditis, interstitial lung disease, other connective tissue diseases; ?malignancy
Inclusion body myositis	M > F	Elderly (>50 yr)	No	Proximal = distal; predilection for finger/wrist flexors, knee extensors	Increased (<10× normal)	Endomysial inflammation; $CD8^+$ T cells, Macros; rimmed vacuoles; amyloid deposits; EM: 15- to 18-nm tubulofilaments	No	Neuropathy

C = complement; CK = creatine kinase; F = female; Ig = immunoglobulin; IS = immunosuppressive; M = male; MAC = membrane attack complex; Macros = macrophages.

prognosis is good, and patients usually respond rapidly to corticosteroid treatment. Relapses are infrequent.

Granulomatous Myopathy with and without Sarcoidosis

Patients with sarcoidosis (Chapter 95) can have asymptomatic granulomas in muscle or an elevated CK level. Occasionally, these patients have nodular swellings of subcutaneous tissue and underlying muscle. These lesions have histopathologic features indicative of sarcoid. Patients can also experience focal muscle pain or a generalized limb-girdle weakness pattern reflecting muscle involvement by sarcoid granulomas. Patients with symptomatic weakness are generally treated with corticosteroids but respond poorly.

Giant cell or granulomatous myopathy can occur in the absence of sarcoidosis. Most affected patients also have myasthenia gravis or thymoma (Chapter 448). Myocarditis can be part of the disease process. These patients generally improve with corticosteroids.

Behçet's Syndrome

Behçet's syndrome (Chapter 297), a multisystem disorder, is usually associated with mucocutaneous and ocular manifestations but may rarely be associated with myositis and myocarditis. The myositis can be focal or generalized, and there is a predilection for the calves. The myositis often responds to immunosuppressive therapy.

Focal Myositis

Focal myositis is an uncommon disorder that can develop at any age. It is manifested as a solitary, painful, and rapidly expanding skeletal muscle mass and must be distinguished from sarcoidosis, Behçet's disease, polyarteritis nodosa, or muscle tumors (sarcoma or rhabdomyosarcoma). The leg is the most common site of involvement, but myositis can occur in any region. The serum CK level is usually normal. Biopsy of lesions shows mononuclear inflammatory cells in the endomysium with muscle fiber necrosis. The myositis generally resolves spontaneously or after immunosuppressive treatment with corticosteroids. In rare cases, focal myositis is the heralding sign of typical polymyositis.

Infectious Myositis

Viral

An acute viral myositis can occur in the setting of an upper respiratory tract infection caused by an influenza virus (Chapter 387). In addition to typical influenza-associated myalgias, these patients have proximal weakness, an elevated CK level, and myopathic motor units indicated on EMG. The disorder is self-limited, but when severe it is often associated with myoglobinuria and occasionally with renal failure. A similar syndrome can complicate infections with coxsackievirus, parainfluenza virus, mumps virus, measles virus, adenovirus, cytomegalovirus, hepatitis B virus, herpes simplex virus, Epstein-Barr virus, respiratory syncytial virus, and echovirus.

An inflammatory myopathy can occur in the setting of human immunodeficiency virus infection in either the early or later stages of acquired immunodeficiency syndrome (Chapter 413). The neurologic manifestation of type 1 human T-lymphotropic virus infection typically consists of spastic paraparesis, but myositis can also develop.

Bacterial

Pyomyositis refers to focal or multifocal abscesses associated with bacterial infection of muscle. Pyomyositis is more common in the tropics, in developing countries, and among intravenous drug users. It usually arises as an extension of an infection in adjacent tissues or from hematogenous spread. The most common organisms involved are *Staphylococcus aureus* (Chapter 310), *Streptococcus* sp (Chapter 312), *Escherichia coli* (Chapter 314), *Yersinia* sp (Chapter 333), and *Legionella* sp (Chapter 335). Treatment consists of antibiotics for the underlying infection and, in severe infections, incision and drainage of abscesses.

Fungal

Fungal infections of muscle can occur rarely, usually in immunocompromised individuals. Candidiasis (Chapter 359) is the most common fungal myositis. Diffuse muscle pain, weakness, and fever are associated with a papular erythematous rash.

Parasitic

Trichinosis (Chapter 378) is the most common parasitic disease that can produce a diffuse inflammatory myositis and be confused with idiopathic polymyositis. Ingested larvae from undercooked pork migrate to muscle, with the subsequent development of fever, myalgias, weakness, myocarditis, and CNS manifestations. There is a peripheral eosinophilia, the CK level is elevated, and antibodies against *Trichinella spiralis* can be demonstrated 3 to 4 weeks after infection. Therapy consists of thiabendazole; in severe cases, corticosteroids may be indicated. An inflammatory myopathy can also occur in the course of cysticercosis (*Taenia solium;* Chapter 375) and toxoplasmosis (*Toxoplasma gondii;* Chapter 370).

Myopathies Caused by Endocrine Systemic Disorders, Toxins, and Myoglobinuria

Fatigue can be a symptom of any endocrine disorder, but objective muscle weakness secondary to a myopathy is less common. The serum CK level is often normal except in hypothyroidism (Chapter 244). EMG shows normal findings or myopathic motor units, but generally without spontaneous electrical activity. The histologic alterations in muscle are often nonspecific. Muscle symptoms improve with successful treatment of the underlying endocrinopathy.

Adrenal/Glucocorticoid Disorders

Excess corticosteroids can result from endogenous Cushing's disease (Chapter 245) or can be due to exogenous glucocorticoid administration (Chapter 33). Iatrogenic corticosteroid myopathy (or atrophy) is the most common endocrine-related myopathy. However, muscle weakness is rarely the initial manifestation of Cushing's disease, and other factors contribute to the weakness in virtually all instances of corticosteroid myopathy. Women are more susceptible to corticosteroid atrophy than men are, and divided daily doses are more toxic than single or alternate-day doses. Muscle biopsy shows type 2 muscle fiber atrophy, and the serum CK level and findings on EMG are normal. Therapy consists of reducing the corticosteroid dosage to the lowest possible level. Exercise and adequate nutrition prevent and may improve weakness. Muscle strength returns to normal within 1 to 4 months after therapy is stopped.

Addison's Disease

Addison's disease (adrenal insufficiency; Chapter 245) is often associated with fatigue, but objective signs of myopathy are rare. Electrolyte disturbances can produce weakness and, when hyperkalemia occurs, simulate periodic paralysis (see earlier).

Thyroid Disorders

Patients with hyperthyroidism (Chapter 244) often have some degree of weakness, but it is rarely the initial manifestation of thyrotoxicosis. Weakness is predominantly proximal, especially in the shoulder region, and there may be atrophy. Weakness of extraocular muscles and proptosis occur in Graves' disease. Thyrotoxic periodic paralysis was described earlier. Hypothyroid myopathy (Chapter 244) is associated with proximal weakness and myalgias, muscle enlargement, slow relaxation of the reflexes, and a marked (up to 100-fold) increase in the serum CK level.

Parathyroid Disorders

Hyperparathyroidism (with hypercalcemia and hypophosphatemia; Chapter 266) can be associated with proximal weakness, atrophy, and pain, especially in the setting of osteomalacia. Patients may also experience hoarseness, dysphagia, and neck extensor weakness. Hypoparathyroidism (with hypocalcemia and hyperphosphatemia) is not usually associated with a myopathy; however, paresthesias and tetany with Chvostek's sign and Trousseau's phenomenon can occur in hypocalcemic patients (Chapter 266).

Pituitary Disorders

Acromegaly (Chapter 242) can be associated with mild proximal weakness, but not generally until late in the disease. Muscles can look enlarged despite being weak. Weakness as a result of nerve, root, or spinal cord compression is a more likely cause of the weakness. Panhypopituitarism results in weakness and fatigability, probably because of the combined influence of thyroid and adrenal deficiencies.

Diabetes Mellitus

Progressive, painless proximal weakness in a diabetic patient is seldom, if ever the result of diabetes-related myopathy. Asymmetrical, usually painful proximal leg weakness can occur from an ischemic radiculoplexopathy ("amyotrophy"). Rarely, acute muscle infarction can develop in the quadriceps or hamstring muscles.

Vitamin Deficiency

Vitamin E deficiency as a result of malabsorption can produce a myopathy along with gait ataxia and neuropathy (Chapters 237 and 443). Vitamin D deficiency (from decreased intake or impaired absorption or metabolism) may also lead to chronic muscle weakness.

Systemic Amyloid Myopathy

The most common neurologic complication in various types of amyloidosis (Chapter 296) is a predominantly sensory-autonomic neuropathy. Amyloid deposition in muscle is frequent, but the muscle involvement is usually subclinical. Occasionally, amyloidosis is manifested as or associated with an overt myopathy characterized by muscle enlargement, macroglossia, stiffness, exertional muscle pain, and proximal or diffuse weakness. EMG shows myopathic features in proximal muscles with or without distal neuropathic changes. The amyloid deposits, identified by their metachromasia and affinity for Congo red stain, appear between and around the mural elements of the small vessels and extend into the interstitial spaces, where they tightly surround individual muscle fibers.

Myositis Ossificans

The localized form of myositis ossificans appears as a tender swelling after trauma to a muscle. After a few months, the lesion becomes hard and ossified. Therapy consists of excision. The generalized form is an autosomal dominant disease with variable expression that begins in childhood, involves many muscles, and causes progressive rigidity of body parts. The initial lesions appear in fascia and dermis and are associated with inflammation, hemorrhage, and proliferation of connective tissue. Cartilage and bone formation occur at a later stage. Other congenital malformations (microdactyly of the great toe, exostoses, absence of the upper incisors or ear lobules, and hypogenitalism) are found in most patients. There is no effective therapy.

Toxic Myopathies

Many drugs have been associated with muscle damage, but it may occur more often with exposure to specific drugs (Table 447–10). Most drug-induced myopathies can produce proximal weakness, an elevated CK level, myopathic findings on EMG, and abnormalities on muscle biopsy. Symptoms generally improve after stopping the medication. Several drugs can produce an inflammatory myopathy on muscle biopsy, including penicillamine and cimetidine. Zidovudine causes a mitochondrial myopathy. A number of drugs can produce a necrotizing or vacuolar myopathy, including amiodarone, colchicine, chloroquine, and cyclosporine. Emetine (ipecac) produces proximal weakness and a myofibrillar myopathy. Isoretinoic acid, a vitamin A analogue used for acne, infrequently causes myalgias, elevation of the serum CK level, and reversible muscle damage.

Clofibrate, gemfibrozil, the statins, and niacin can all produce a rapidly progressive myopathy with elevated CK levels, weakness, pain, and myoglobinuria. An acute necrotizing myopathy associated with myoglobinuria occurs in chronic alcoholics after a bout of drinking (Chapter 31). Illicit drugs such as heroin, cocaine, amphetamines, and pentazocine can produce rhabdomyolysis through direct toxic effects, status epilepticus, or prolonged loss of consciousness, immobility, and secondary pressure.

Focal muscle injury can be caused by injection of certain drugs, particularly pentazocine and meperidine. Muscle necrosis is followed by fibrous connective tissue replacement and induration.

TABLE 447–10 TOXIC MYOPATHIES

INFLAMMATORY
Cimetidine
D-Penicillamine
Procainamide
L-Tryptophan
L-Dopa
NONINFLAMMATORY NECROTIZING OR VACUOLAR
Cholesterol-lowering agents
Chloroquine
Colchicine
Emetine
ε-Aminocaproic acid
Labetalol
Cyclosporine and tacrolimus
Isoretinoic acid (vitamin A analogue)
Vincristine
Alcohol
RHABDOMYOLYSIS AND MYOGLOBINURIA
Cholesterol-lowering drugs
Alcohol
Heroin
Amphetamine
Toluene
Cocaine
ε-Aminocaproic acid
Pentazocine
Phencyclidine
MALIGNANT HYPERTHERMIA
Halothane
Ethylene
Diethyl ether
Methoxyflurane
Ethyl chloride
Trichloroethylene
Gallamine
Succinylcholine
MITOCHONDRIAL
Zidovudine
MYOTONIA
2,4-D-Chlorophenoxyacetic acid
Anthracene-9-carboxycyclic acid
Cholesterol-lowering drugs
Chloroquine
Cyclosporine
MYOSIN LOSS
Nondepolarizing neuromuscular blocking agents
Intravenous glucocorticoids

Critical Illness Myopathy

Also known as acute quadriplegic myopathy, critical illness myopathy develops in a patient in the intensive care setting and is often discovered when a patient is unable to be weaned off a ventilator. The cause of the diffuse weakness is prolonged daily use of either (often both) high-dose intravenous glucocorticoids (usually methylprednisolone) or nondepolarizing neuromuscular blocking agents (e.g., vecuronium). Patients often have had sepsis and multiorgan failure. The serum CK level is moderately elevated, and EMG shows myopathic units and fibrillations. On nerve conduction studies, motor amplitudes are small, and occasionally a decremental response can be seen on repetitive stimulation. The diagnosis can be confirmed by muscle biopsy, which shows loss of myosin thick filaments on EM. Treatment is supportive after discontinuing the offending agents. Strength recovers over a period of weeks or months, and patients can usually be weaned off the ventilator. Critical illness myopathy must be distinguished from critical illness neuropathy (Chapter 446) and can occasionally coexist with it.

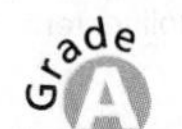

1. Griggs RC, Moxley RT, Mendell JR, et al: Duchenne dystrophy: Randomized controlled trial of prednisone (18 months) and azathioprine (12 months). Neurology 1993;43:520–527.

2. Kley R, Vorgerd M, Tarnopolsky M: Creatine for treating muscle disorders. Cochrane Database Syst Rev 2007;1:CD004760.
3. Vissing J, Haller RG: The effect of oral sucrose on exercise tolerance in patients with McArdle's disease. N Engl J Med 2003;349:2503–2509.
4. Klinge L, Straug V, Neudorf U, et al: Safety and efficacy of recombinant acid alpha-glucosidase (rhGAA) in patients with classical infantile Pompe disease: Results of a phase II clinical trial. Neuromuscul Disord 2005;15:24–31.
5. Tawil R, McDermott M, Brown R, et al: Randomized trials of dichlorphenamide in the periodic paralyses. Ann Neurol 2000;47:46–53.

SUGGESTED READINGS

Day JW, Ricker K, Jacobsen JF, et al: Myotonic dystrophy type 2. Molecular, diagnostic, and clinical spectrum. Neurology 2003;60:657–664. *Thorough review.*
Nizar C, Duygu S, Engel AG: Sporadic late onset nemaline myopathy. Neurology 2005;65:1158–1164. *Definitive review.*
Schapira AH: Mitochondrial disease. Lancet 2006;368:70–82. *A comprehensive review.*
Venance S, Cannon SC, Fialho D, et al: The primary periodic paralyses: Diagnosis, pathogenesis and treatment. Brain 2006;129:8–17. *Definitive review.*

448 DISORDERS OF NEUROMUSCULAR TRANSMISSION

Angela Vincent and John Newsom-Davis

Definition

Neuromuscular transmission depends on the release of acetylcholine from synaptic vesicles that are stored in the terminal boutons of the motor nerve axon (Fig. 448–1). Invasion of the motor nerve terminal by the action potential opens voltage-gated calcium channels, resulting in the Ca^{2+}-dependent release of the vesicular contents into the synaptic space. Acetylcholine binds to the acetylcholine-gated ion channels (acetylcholine receptors) on the postsynaptic membrane, leading to the opening of these channels and a local depolarization, the end plate potential. If the end plate potential exceeds the critical firing threshold, voltage-gated sodium channels open (sited at the bottom of the postsynaptic folds), generating the muscle action potential that propagates along the muscle fiber and activates muscle contraction. The action of acetylcholine is terminated by its dissociation from the acetylcholine receptors, which close spontaneously after 1 to 4 msec; hydrolysis of acetylcholine by acetylcholinesterase; and acetylcholine diffusion from the synaptic cleft. Meanwhile, in the motor nerve terminal, the voltage-gated calcium channels close spontaneously, and the resting membrane potential is restored through the transient opening of voltage-gated potassium channels.

The extent to which the amplitude of the end plate potential exceeds the threshold for activation of the voltage-gated sodium channels is called the safety factor. In healthy individuals, the amplitude decreases during repeated activity but does not fall below the threshold for activation of the action potential; thus, neuromuscular transmission is not compromised. However, if there is a reduction in the amplitude, failure of neuromuscular transmission at any individual neuromuscular junction may occur. Causes include defects in the release of acetylcholine, the postsynaptic response to acetylcholine, or the number or sensitivity of the voltage-gated sodium channels. Morphologic changes to the pre- or postsynaptic components or to the basal lamina between them may also influence the efficacy of transmission. Although myasthenia gravis and some neurotoxic envenomations (Chapter 381) are the most common disorders of neuromuscular transmission, a number of different conditions have been implicated (Table 448–1).

AUTOIMMUNE DISEASES

Myasthenia Gravis

Epidemiology

Myasthenia is the commonest disorder of neuromuscular transmission, with a prevalence of about 15 per 100,000 in Western countries. All races can be affected. It can occur at any age from about year 1 onward, showing a small peak in the third decade. It is being increasingly recognized in elderly persons, with the annual incidence rising above 5 per 100,000 in individuals older than 70 years, making it important in the differential diagnosis of limb or bulbar muscle weakness in older people.

Myasthenia gravis itself is heterogeneous and can be divided into different subtypes; the relative frequency of these different forms is not known, but relatively mild childhood forms are more frequent than older cases in some Asian countries. Neonatal myasthenia gravis, caused by the placental transfer of maternal antibodies to the acetylcholine receptor or to the muscle-specific kinase, affects up to one in eight babies born to mothers with myasthenia gravis. Autoimmune myasthenia gravis needs to be distinguished from congenital myasthenic syndromes, which are caused by gene mutations.

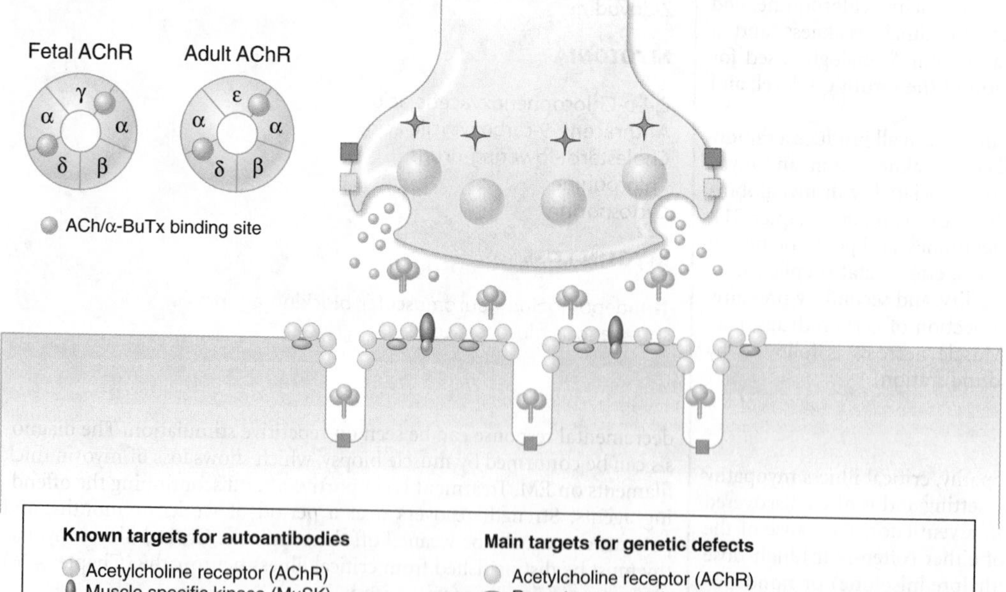

FIGURE 448–1 • Diagrammatic representation of the neuromuscular junction, indicating the ion channels, receptors, enzymes, and associated proteins that are the most frequent targets for autoimmune diseases (left) or mutations in genetic diseases (right). The acetylcholine receptor exists in fetal and adult isoforms as illustrated at top left. The replacement of the fetal form by the adult form takes place toward the end of gestation in humans. Voltage-gated sodium channels are located at the bottom of the postsynaptic folds.

TABLE 448–1 DISORDERS OF NEUROMUSCULAR TRANSMISSION

Disease	Target	Pathobiology
AUTOIMMUNE		
Myasthenia gravis	Acetylcholine receptors	Antibodies to the acetylcholine receptor in 85% of patients reduce the number of acetylcholine receptors and the amplitude of the end plate potential Antibodies to muscle-specific kinase in up to 10% of patients—mechanism not known
Transient neonatal myasthenia	Acetylcholine receptors, muscle-specific kinase	Maternal antibodies cause transient disease in neonates; not seen commonly if mother receiving treatment
Arthrogryposis	Fetal acetylcholine receptor	Maternal antibodies that inhibit fetal acetylcholine receptor function paralyze the baby in utero, leading to joint contractures; very rare cause of arthrogryposis
Lambert-Eaton myasthenic syndrome	Voltage-gated calcium channels	Antibodies to voltage-gated calcium channels in 90% of patients reduce the number of voltage-gated calcium channels, the release of acetylcholine, and the amplitude of the end plate potential
Acquired neuromyotonia	Voltage-gated potassium channels	Antibodies to voltage-gated potassium channels in 40% of patients probably lead to spontaneous and repetitive motor unit discharges
GENETIC		
Acetylcholine receptor deficiency	Acetylcholine receptor	Recessive mutations in acetylcholine receptor genes reduce the expression of the acetylcholine receptor
Acetylcholine receptor deficiency		Recessive mutations in rapsyn gene reduces anchoring of acetylcholine receptors on the postsynaptic membrane
Acetylcholine receptor kinetic abnormalities	Acetylcholine receptor	Dominant or recessive mutations in acetylcholine receptor genes cause kinetic defects—slow and fast channel syndromes
Choline acetyltransferase deficiency	Choline acetyltransferase	Recessive mutations in the gene for choline acetyltransferase, which synthesizes acetylcholine, reduce the release of acetylcholine
Acetylcholinesterase deficiency	Acetylcholinesterase	Recessive mutations in the collagen tail (Col Q) that anchors acetylcholinesterase at the neuromuscular junction cause absence of acetylcholinesterase
Arthrogryposis	Can occur with rapsyn and δ-subunit acetylcholine receptor mutations	Fetal akinesia
CMS with proximal muscle weakness (limb girdle type)	Dok-7	Recessive mutations in Dok-7 impair interactions with MuSK and lead to a "synaptopathy"
NEUROTOXIC		
Botulism	Presynaptic acetylcholine release	Botulinum toxin gains entry into the presynaptic motor nerve and cleaves proteins involved in the release of acetylcholine
Envenomation following bites from snakes, spiders, scorpions, and so on	Varied sites of action	Neurotoxins specific for voltage-gated calcium channels, voltage-gated potassium channels, acetylcholinesterase, acetylcholine receptors, voltage-gated sodium channels, and other targets are frequent in many animal venoms and either inhibit or enhance function
Drugs/insecticides	Varied sites of action	Muscle relaxants and other drugs Many antibiotics and quinine-related drugs can alter neuromuscular transmission at high doses Organophosphates and other insecticides block acetylcholinesterase

Pathobiology

Pathophysiology

Myasthenia gravis is the result of a defect in neuromuscular transmission. The postsynaptic response to acetylcholine, the end plate potential, is reduced so that the threshold for activation of the muscle action potential is not reached. At a severely affected end plate, this deficiency can occur at the initiation of contraction, but it is most common during repetitive activity when the end plate potential naturally declines. This phenomenon, occurring across many end plates within a muscle, is responsible for the decrement in the amplitude of the compound muscle action potential on repetitive nerve stimulation that is diagnostic of a disorder of neuromuscular transmission.

In myasthenia gravis, the reduced end plate potentials result from loss of functional acetylcholine receptors on the postsynaptic membrane and also from morphologic damage to the membrane. This damage leads to loss of acetylcholine receptor–containing membrane and to simplification of the postsynaptic folds, which contain the voltage-gated sodium channels. The result is a raised threshold for generation of the action potential, further compromising neuromuscular transmission. These changes are caused by antibodies to the acetylcholine receptors in most patients. The pathophysiology in patients without detectable antibodies to the acetylcholine receptor, including patients with muscle-specific kinase antibodies, is not well studied.

Like most synapses, the neuromuscular junction is highly regulated. If the nerve is cut, leading to loss of neuromuscular transmission, the muscle responds by upregulating the expression of acetylcholine receptors that revert to a fetal phenotype (see Fig. 448–1). Alternatively, if the activity of the postsynaptic muscle decreases, the motor nerve attempts to compensate. Consequently, in myasthenia gravis, there is some increase in the release of acetylcholine from the motor nerve and an increase in the synthesis of acetylcholine receptors in the muscle fiber.

Direct block of function preventing ACh binding and ion channel opening

A

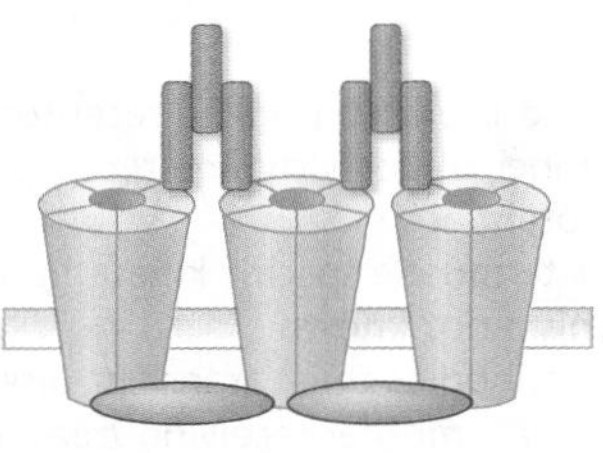

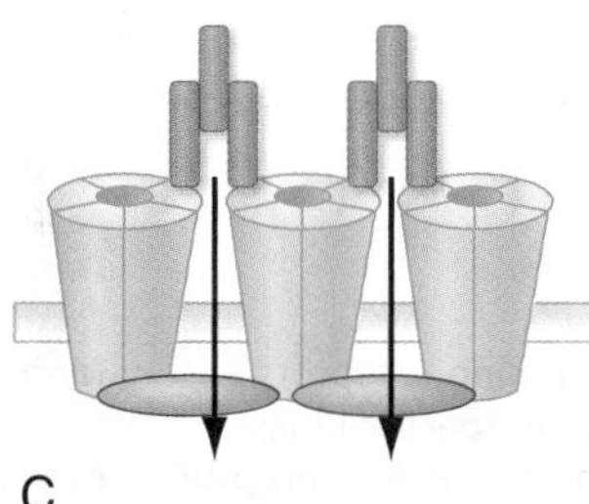

FIGURE 448–2 • Mechanisms of loss of the acetylcholine receptor (AChR) at the neuromuscular junction. Antibodies can act (a) by directly blocking ACh binding or ion channel function; (b) by cross-linking the AChRs in the membrane, thereby leading to increased internalization and degradation; or (c) by complement-dependent lysis of the AChR-containing postsynaptic membrane. In myasthenia gravis, complement-dependent lysis is likely to be the most important mechanism overall. Interestingly, there is no evidence of complement-dependent mechanisms in either the Lambert-Eaton myasthenic syndrome or acquired neuromyotonia, in which cross-linking of the respective ion channels with increased internalization is the main mechanism.

Pathogenesis

Myasthenia gravis is an antibody-mediated autoimmune disease. Evidence includes its association with other autoimmune diseases, most often thyroid disease, and, in younger patients, with an increased incidence of the human leukocyte antigen HLA-B8,DR3 haplotype that also is associated with several other autoimmune diseases. Placental transfer of autoantibodies from myasthenic mothers can cause transient symptoms of neonatal myasthenia. Conversely, removal of the antibodies by plasma exchange (plasmapheresis) produces a marked improvement in symptoms, starting within days and lasting a few weeks. Moreover, injection of patients' plasma into mice causes weakness with loss of acetylcholine receptors. In addition, experimental animals immunized against purified acetylcholine receptors develop clinical and pathologic changes of myasthenia gravis.

The antibodies act by three main mechanisms (Fig. 448–2). First, a few antibodies directly inhibit the binding of acetylcholine to the acetylcholine receptor and cause a pharmacologic-like blockade of function. Second, because of their divalence, antibodies can bind simultaneously to two adjacent acetylcholine receptors through the α-subunits that are present in duplicate in each receptor to form acetylcholine receptor–antibody complexes that are internalized and degraded by the muscle fiber, leading to loss of acetylcholine receptors. Third, most of the antibodies are immunoglobulin G1 (IgG1) subclass, a subclass that binds and activates complement. As a result, the membrane attack complex is activated, leading to destruction of the postsynaptic membrane and probably causing the morphologic damage that is frequently seen. All of these effects are strictly limited to the neuromuscular junction; the remainder of the muscle fiber is essentially normal.

The acetylcholine receptor antibodies are IgG, high affinity, and highly specific for the native human acetylcholine receptor. Although the antibodies are the effector mechanism for the loss of acetylcholine receptors, their characteristics indicate that specific antibody production requires helper T cells that can recognize acetylcholine receptor epitopes. The thymus gland, which is often abnormal in myasthenia, is at least one site where the immune response occurs. In early-onset myasthenia gravis (see later), the thymus is often "hyperplastic," with numerous T- and B-cell lymphocytic infiltrates in the medulla. These infiltrates are very similar to the germinal centers that are found in lymph nodes, and some of them can be shown to contain B cells that express surface immunoglobulin specific for acetylcholine receptors. Plasma cells are also present and synthesize acetylcholine receptor antibodies. In the thymic medulla, there are muscle-like "myoid" cells that have acetylcholine receptors on their surface in both normal and myasthenic individuals; these cells probably provide the antigenic stimulus responsible for the germinal center formation and acetylcholine receptor antibody production in myasthenia gravis. Numerous attempts to characterize the T-cell response in myasthenia have been only partly successful, perhaps because the number of such T cells in patients with an ongoing highly specific autoimmune disease is small.

In late-onset myasthenia gravis, the thymus is probably normal for age. In patients without acetylcholine receptor antibodies, the thymus gland is more likely to appear normal for age, particularly in patients with muscle-specific kinase antibodies (see later). However, in patients without either acetylcholine receptor or muscle-specific kinase antibodies, some lymphocytic infiltrates and germinal centers can be present.

Thymoma

Thymoma occurs in about 10% of myasthenic patients, reaching a peak in middle age. Thymomas are epithelial cell tumors and correspond mainly to the World Health Organization type B1 and B2. The epithelial cells attract large numbers of T lymphocytes, which may be sensitized to the acetylcholine receptor in the tumor and then exported to the periphery. Myasthenia gravis can also arise several years after thymoma removal.

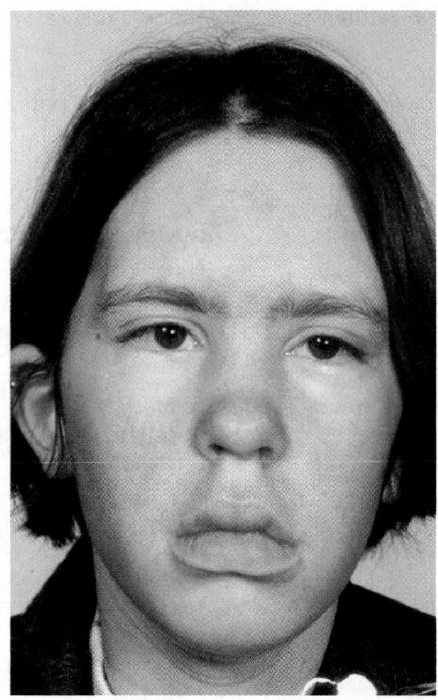

FIGURE 448–3 • Marked ocular and facial muscle weakness in a young female with myasthenia gravis.

Clinical Manifestations

Myasthenia gravis arises with fatigable muscle weakness, that is, painless weakness that increases with muscle use and improves after rest. In many patients, the weakness starts in the eye muscles, resulting in double vision or ptosis (drooping eyelids). In others, it may first affect bulbar muscles or limb muscles (Fig. 448–3). Virtually any skeletal muscle may be involved as the illness progresses. Typically, the weakness varies in distribution and severity from day to day or from week to week, and it is often worse in the evening. It may first appear following an infection. Established weakness can increase with anxiety, with infection, or with the menstrual period and tends to improve with rest.

Ocular muscle weakness is characterized by ptosis (often asymmetrical) and diplopia that initially can be transient and first noticed while driving, for example. Severity can range from mild unilateral ptosis or minimal diplopia to profound bilateral ptosis, which obscures vision, combined with almost complete ophthalmoplegia. Bulbar symptoms include weakness of mouth closure, difficulty in chewing, a "snarling" smile, nasal or slurred speech that can noticeably deteriorate as speech continues, impaired swallowing sometimes associated with nasal regurgitation of fluids, reduced tongue movements, and head droop related to neck weakness.

Limb muscle involvement is common, and proximal muscles are usually more involved than distal. Proximal weakness of the legs can lead to collapse when walking and can be misinterpreted as a functional (psychogenic) disorder. Weakness of elbow extension and of finger abduction may be prominent. By contrast, ankle dorsiflexion is rarely affected except in severe disease.

Respiratory muscle involvement is less common but can be life threatening, especially if associated with dysphagia. Selective involvement of the diaphragm can cause severe breathlessness in the supine posture. Wasting is uncommon but can affect the facial muscles and tongue, for example, in long-standing disease. Tendon reflexes are typically brisk. Bladder disturbances are rare, and sensory symptoms do not occur.

Subtypes of Myasthenia Gravis

Several subgroups can be distinguished on the basis of clinical and pathologic criteria, as set out subsequently, and can help to inform treatment protocols.

Ocular Myasthenia Gravis

Ocular myasthenia gravis describes symptoms that are confined to extraocular muscles. If they remain localized for at least 2 years, subsequent generalization of weakness is unlikely. Acetylcholine receptor antibody levels are generally low and are undetectable in about 50%. Thymoma is rare in this group. The neuromuscular junction of ocular muscles shows structural and physiologic differences from typical limb muscles. Ocular weakness is often the presenting symptom not only in myasthenia gravis but also in neurotoxin poisoning, for example, botulism. Thus physiologic factors or accessibility of the neuromuscular junctions of ocular muscles to circulating factors may make them particularly vulnerable to antibodies in myasthenia gravis.

Generalized Myasthenia Gravis with Acetylcholine Receptor Antibodies

Among patients with generalized disease and acetylcholine receptor antibodies, there are three clinical subgroups. Early-onset myasthenia gravis is more frequent in females and associates strongly with HLA-A1,B8,DR3. The thymus is often hyperplastic. Acetylcholine receptor antibody titers are usually high and decline to varying degrees after successful treatments, including thymectomy.

Late-onset myasthenia gravis is becoming increasingly common with the aging of the population and, when arising with bulbar weakness, may be mistaken for amyotrophic lateral sclerosis (Chapter 435) or brain stem cerebrovascular disease. Among older patients, males are more frequently affected, and the thymus is usually normal for age. Thymoma-associated myasthenia gravis is an important distinction because thymectomy or other specific tumor therapy is required. Most patients with thymomas and myasthenia gravis present between the ages of 30 and 60 years.

Generalized Myasthenia Gravis with Muscle-Specific Kinase Antibodies

About 15% of all myasthenic patients with generalized symptoms do not have detectable acetylcholine receptor antibodies. A variable proportion of these patients have antibodies to another neuromuscular junction protein, the muscle-specific kinase. Muscle-specific kinase antibodies are mainly IgG4 and are absent or very infrequent in patients with acetylcholine receptor antibody–positive myasthenia gravis, patients with persistent ocular myasthenia gravis, or patients with thymoma. Muscle-specific kinase antibodies are found relatively often in younger females, including children, with marked ocular, bulbar, neck, or respiratory muscle weakness but are seen less frequently in older patients. It is not yet clear how these antibodies cause the neuromuscular junction defect.

Generalized Myasthenia Gravis with neither Acetylcholine Receptor nor Muscle-Specific Kinase Antibodies

There remain some patients with generalized myasthenia gravis who have neither acetylcholine receptor nor muscle-specific kinase antibodies. These patients can develop severe disease but in general respond better to treatment than muscle-specific kinase antibody–positive patients. It is possible that they have acetylcholine receptor antibodies at levels not detected by current laboratory tests.

Diagnosis

Diagnosis is based on the clinical features, serologic testing for specific antibodies, clinical electrophysiology, and, if doubt still remains or specialized facilities are not available, the clinical response to anticholinesterase medication (Table 448–2). Mediastinal imaging is needed to exclude a thymoma in patients with acetylcholine receptor antibodies.

Acetylcholine receptor antibodies are present in about 85% of patients with generalized symptoms but only 50% of patients with purely ocular involvement. In the absence of acetylcholine receptor antibodies, the diagnosis can be more difficult, but detection of muscle-specific kinase antibodies can be helpful.

The electrophysiologic abnormality is an abnormally large decrement (>10%) in the amplitude of the compound muscle action potential upon stimulation with 3 Hz, with increased jitter or blocking on single-fiber electromyography (EMG). In patients with muscle-specific kinase antibodies, EMG abnormalities may be detectable only in facial muscles. These EMG changes are not specific for myasthenia gravis but can occur in any disorder that interferes with neuromuscular transmission.

Intravenous edrophonium (Tensilon), a short-acting cholinesterase inhibitor, transiently improves myasthenic weakness but requires an appropriate medical setting, including resuscitative facilities and the availability of atropine, because of the risk of adverse events and severe cholinergic reactions, including syncope. A test dose of 2 mg is given intravenously, followed 30 seconds later by 6 to 8 mg if no adverse event has occurred. The equivalent doses in children are a 20 μg/kg test dose followed by 60 to 80 μg/kg. Some patients improve sufficiently with the test dose that it is not necessary to give the full dose. An alternative pharmacologic test in adults is a single dose of subcutaneous or intramuscular neostigmine (1 to 2.5 mg) or of oral pyridostigmine (60 mg).

Differential Diagnosis

Congenital acetylcholine receptor deficiency syndromes (see later) should be considered in patients who have clinical and EMG evidence of myasthenia but are seronegative for acetylcholine receptor and muscle-specific kinase antibodies. Lambert-Eaton myasthenic syndrome almost always arises with difficulty in walking; ocular symptoms are rare, and specific laboratory tests are available (see later). The ocular muscle involvement that characterizes the Miller-Fisher syndrome is more rapid in onset than is usual in myasthenia gravis and is associated with GQ1b antibodies. Mitochondrial myopathy may show signs that are similar to those of myasthenia gravis (e.g., asymmetrical ptosis and limitation of eye movements), and there may be increased jitter on single-fiber EMG, but this condition and oculopharyngeal dystrophy can be distinguished from myasthenia gravis by the nonfluctuating weakness and by muscle biopsy. In neurasthenia and chronic fatigue syndrome (Chapter 298), the laboratory tests for myasthenia gravis are negative.

Treatment and Prognosis

Many patients respond to oral pyridostigmine 30 to 60 mg four or five times daily; in patients with mild disease, this dose may adequately control symptoms. Doses in excess of 90 mg are likely to cause gastrointestinal side effects, abdominal cramps and diarrhea, which can be controlled with oral propantheline bromide (Pro-Banthine) 15 mg or loperamide 2 mg.

Neonatal Myasthenia Gravis

Pyridostigmine 5 to 10 mg can be given every 4 hours to about an hour before a feeding. Close monitoring and respiratory support in a special unit may be required.

Ocular Myasthenia

Diplopia can sometimes be helped by the use of prisms. Ocular symptoms responding incompletely to pyridostigmine are often improved or completely corrected by low-dose prednisone therapy (e.g., 5 mg every other day) increasing by 5 mg at weekly intervals either until symptoms are completely controlled or until a ceiling dose (e.g., 1 mg/kg) is reached. When remission is established, the dose can be slowly reduced (e.g., by 5 mg at 2-weekly intervals) until symptoms recur and then adjusted upward to define the effective minimal dose. Full withdrawal of prednisone is usually followed by a symptomatic relapse. Most centers do not recommend thymectomy for nonthymomatous ocular myasthenia gravis. In patients who fail to respond adequately to prednisone or who are intolerant of the medication, the addition of azathioprine (2 to 2.5 mg/kg

TABLE 448–2 DIAGNOSTIC EVALUATION OF SYNDROMES CAUSING REDUCED NEUROMUSCULAR TRANSMISSION

Characteristic	Acetylcholine Receptor Myasthenia Gravis	Muscle-Specific Kinase Myasthenia Gravis	Seronegative Myasthenia Gravis	Neonatal Myasthenia Gravis	Lambert-Eaton Myasthenic Syndrome	Congenital Myasthenic Syndrome	Botulism	Mitochondrial Myopathy
Onset birth, recovery within 2 months	–	–	–	+	–	–	–	–
Onset birth plus arthrogryposis	–	–	–	+	–	Rapsyn or AChR δ-subunit mutations	–	–
Onset at <1 year and persistent	–	–	–	–	–	Any CMS. Rapsyn-AChR deficiency and SCS may arise later	+	±
Infantile apneas	–	–	–	±	–	AChR-ε, rapsyn, or ChAT mutation		
Acetylcholine receptor antibody positive	+	–	–	±	–	–	–	–
Muscle-specific kinase antibody positive	–	+	–	±	–	–	–	–
Voltage-gated calcium channels antibody positive	–	–	–	–	+	–	–	–
EMG decrement >10%	±	±	±	±	±	±	±	–
EMG jitter increased	+	+ especially face muscles	+	+	+	+	+	±
Post-tetanic potentiation	–	–	–	–	+	–	+	–
Acetylcholinesterase inhibitor response	+	Often weak	+	+	Often weak	Except SCS and ChAT deficiency	±	–
Thymoma	±	–	–	–	–	–	–	–

AChR = acetylcholine receptor; ChAT = choline acetyltransferase; CMS = congenital myasthenic sydrome; EMG = electromyogram; SCS = slow channel syndrome.

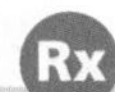

body weight) or ocular muscle surgery is an option. However, the diagnosis should be reviewed in patients who show no improvement with high-dose prednisone treatment.

Thymoma

Thymoma usually requires surgery, but removal of the tumor typically does not result in improvement in muscle weakness. If the tumor is found to be locally invasive, radiotherapy is indicated. If tumor spread is more extensive, chemotherapy is necessary.

Generalized Nonthymomatous Myasthenia Gravis

When generalized symptoms are inadequately controlled by pyridostigmine, thymectomy is often recommended empirically even for patients without a thymoma, especially patients younger than 45 years, despite the absence of trials and no clear consensus from observational data. However, many patients respond to alternate-day prednisone, started at a low dose (e.g., 10 mg qod) and increasing by 5 to 10 mg per dose to 1.0 to 1.5 mg/kg. Because starting prednisone can temporarily exacerbate the disease, patients are usually best managed in the hospital, especially if they have bulbar or respiratory muscle involvement. When remission is established, the dose can be reduced by 5 to 10 mg every 2 weeks (or more slowly) until symptoms recur, when it can then be adjusted upward, aiming to define the effective minimal dose. Prophylactic treatment for steroid-induced bone disease should be considered in all patients (Chapter 264).

Additional immunosuppressive medication is likely to be required in patients who can be controlled only by high-dose prednisone or who are intolerant of it. Azathioprine 2.5 mg/kg/day is often the medication of choice. In fact, a randomized double-blind trial comparing azathioprine plus prednisone with placebo plus prednisone showed that the combined treatment was better tolerated, allowed a substantially lower dose of prednisone to be used, and was associated with fewer relapses than prednisone alone. 1 Mycophenolate 1 g/kg twice daily, cyclosporin 3 to 5 mg/kg daily, and methotrexate 5 to 15 mg weekly are options for those intolerant of azathioprine, but results of long-term randomized studies using the latter therapies have not yet been reported. When remission has been achieved, doses can be reduced slowly and cautiously; full withdrawal is likely to be followed by relapse.

Plasmapheresis (plasma exchange) or immunoglobulin infusion 2 can lead to short-term improvement, typically lasting 4 to 6 weeks, and can be used to prepare patients for thymectomy, to cover the initiation of prednisone therapy, or to control an exacerbation of myasthenic weakness. These two treatments are equally efficacious. 3 An immunoglobulin infusion of 1 g/kg given on day 1 only is as effective as 1 g/kg given on day 1 and again on day 2. 4 Because of the short-lived benefits of these therapies, they must be accompanied by additional immunosuppressive therapy, as noted previously.

Prognosis

The increasing use of immunologic therapies, coupled with advances in critical care, has improved the prognosis in nonthymomatous myasthenia gravis. Many patients can expect substantial improvement or remission with a normal life expectancy. The prognosis is less good, however, in those with invasive thymoma.

The Lambert-Eaton Myasthenic Syndrome

Definition and Epidemiology

The Lambert-Eaton myasthenic syndrome is a rare disorder that can occur in paraneoplastic (Chapter 189) and nonparaneoplastic forms and affects all races. The incidence of the former is much higher, but its shorter survival results in a similar prevalence of the two types. The paraneoplastic form affects about 2% of patients with small cell lung cancer (Chapter 201) and can also occur with lymphoma (Chapter 196). The nonparaneoplastic form associates with HLA-A1, -B8, and -DR3, as in myasthenia gravis.

Pathobiology

Lambert-Eaton myasthenic syndrome is an antibody-mediated presynaptic disorder characterized by a reduced number of acetylcholine quanta (vesicles) released by each nerve impulse. End plate potentials recorded from intercostal muscle biopsies are consequently much reduced in amplitude. During repetitive nerve stimulation, the end plate potential amplitude increases, probably because of build up of calcium in the motor nerve terminal, leading to increased release of acetylcholine. Freeze-fracture electron microscopic studies of motor nerve terminals show that the "active zone" particles, which represent voltage-gated calcium channels, are reduced in number and disorganized. IgG can be identified bound to the presynaptic nerve terminal at the sites of acetylcholine release. Similar changes can be reproduced in mice injected with IgG from patients with the Lambert-Eaton myasthenic syndrome, indicating that the electrophysiologic and morphologic changes are due to antibodies. The mice have reduced end plate potential amplitudes and quantal contents, and IgG is bound to their motor nerve terminals. The IgG also interferes with transmitter release from postganglionic parasympathetic and sympathetic neurons in injected mice, providing an explanation for the autonomic dysfunction observed in many patients.

The antibodies in Lambert-Eaton myasthenic syndrome appear to act principally by cross-linking the voltage-gated calcium channels on the surface of the presynaptic motor nerve membrane, leading to their clustering and internalization. There is no evidence that the antibodies activate complement, and the motor nerve terminal is morphologically intact. Direct inhibition of voltage-gated calcium channel function by antibody is infrequent.

Clinical Manifestations

Almost all patients present with difficulty in walking, which exhibits a rolling characteristic. Weakness in ocular, bulbar, and respiratory muscles is less common than in myasthenia gravis. Weakness predominantly affects proximal muscles, which may show augmentation of strength during the first few seconds of a maximum contraction. Reflexes are absent or depressed but can increase following 10 seconds of maximum contraction of the muscle (post-tetanic potentiation). Autonomic symptoms (dry mouth, constipation, erectile dysfunction) are present in most patients. Occasionally, cerebellar ataxia may be present. Patients with nonparaneoplastic Lambert-Eaton myasthenic syndrome may have other autoimmune diseases, notably vitiligo.

Diagnosis

Diagnosis is based on the clinical features, on a positive serum voltage-gated calcium channel antibody test, and on the characteristic EMG findings (see Table 448–2). Antibodies specific for the α1A (P/Q) subtype of voltage-gated calcium channels are found in 90% of patients, both with and without small cell lung cancer. Patients may not respond convincingly to intravenous edrophonium. On EMG, the amplitude of the resting compound muscle action potential is reduced, but it increases by more than 100% following 10 seconds of voluntary contraction of the muscle or during high-frequency (40 Hz) nerve stimulation. Chest imaging is required in those at risk for tumor.

Differential Diagnosis

Botulinum poisoning (Chapter 319) causes blockade of presynaptic transmitter release at the neuromuscular junction as well as EMG changes similar to those in the Lambert-Eaton myasthenic syndrome. Botulinism is detected by finding the toxin in serum or the *Clostridium botulinum* bacteria in the wound or feces. Myopathies (Chapters 290 and 447) can mimic Lambert-Eaton myasthenic syndrome clinically, but autonomic changes do not occur, EMG findings are different, and muscle biopsy is abnormal.

Treatment and Prognosis

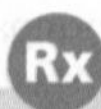

Plasma exchange leads to clinical improvement within a few days in acutely ill patients, and most patients respond to immunosuppressive drugs or intravenous immunoglobulin therapy. Intravenous immunoglobulin therapy (1 g/kg for 1 to 2 days) improves strength, with an associated decline in specific antibody. [5] Patients may also respond to plasmapheresis.

Specific tumor treatments (resection, local radiotherapy, chemotherapy) often lead to improvement of the neurologic disorder. Most patients respond to 3,4-diaminopyridine (10 to 20 mg four times daily; *this drug had not been approved by the U.S. Food and Drug Administration at the time of publication*), which increases transmitter release from motor nerve terminals; however, excessive doses can lead to seizures.

Long-term immunosuppressive treatment with prednisone, azathioprine, or cyclosporin may be required in those with severe weakness, using doses similar to those described previously for myasthenia gravis.

ACQUIRED NEUROMYOTONIA

Definition and Epidemiology

Neuromyotonia, or Isaacs' syndrome, is a rare disorder primarily characterized by myokymia (spontaneous undulating muscle contractions) that can be intermittent or continuous and may be present during sleep or general anesthesia. It results from the hyperexcitability of motor nerves. A milder variant, the cramp-fasciculation syndrome, is more common. Autoimmunity underlies many cases.

Pathobiology

Neuromyotonia may be associated with other autoimmune diseases or other autoantibodies, and cerebrospinal fluid analysis may show oligoclonal bands. In about 15% of patients, it is paraneoplastic, usually associated with thymoma and occasionally with lung cancer. Evidence for an antibody-mediated pathogenesis includes improvement following plasma exchange, passive transfer to mice by patients' plasma/IgG, and the effects of patients' IgG on cultures of dorsal root ganglia or neuroblastoma cell lines.

Antibodies to voltage-gated potassium channels can be detected in about 40% of patients by radioimmunoprecipitation. Occasionally, neuromyotonia appears to be triggered by infection.

Clinical Manifestations

Acquired neuromyotonia is rare, and the clinical presentation is heterogeneous. There is a combination of muscle stiffness, cramps, myokymia (visible undulation of the muscle), pseudomyotonia (e.g., failure to relax after fist clenching), and weakness. Increased sweating is common. Myokymia persists during sleep. Cramp-fasciculation syndrome shares some features with neuromyotonia. Some patients have sensory symptoms, including transient or continuous paresthesias, dysesthesia, and numbness, and a proportion have central nervous system features of an encephalopathy, including insomnia, hallucinations, delusions, and mood change. Rare cases have constipation and cardiac irregularities.

Diagnosis

EMG shows spontaneous motor unit discharges that occur as distinctive doublet, triplet, or multiplet bursts with high intraburst frequency (40 to 300 per second), longer continuous bursts, and postactivation contraction. The abnormal muscle activity may be generated at different sites throughout the length of the nerve, but in most cases it is principally distal. Antibodies to voltage-gated potassium channels are found in 40% of patients. The differential diagnosis includes neuromyotonia caused by acquired and inherited neuropathies and by voltage-gated potassium channel gene mutations (Kv1.1) that can associate with episodic ataxia.

Treatment and Prognosis

Neuromyotonia can be improved by anticonvulsant drugs, such as carbamazepine (up to 800 to 1000 mg daily), phenytoin (up to 300 mg daily), or lamotrigine (up to 100 mg daily), that downregulate sodium channel function, thereby reducing the hyperexcitability of nerves. Plasma exchange and intravenous immunoglobulins, using the same regimen as for myasthenia gravis, may be followed by short-term improvement. Immunosuppressive medications, again using the same drugs as for myasthenia gravis, are effective in some patients.

GENETIC MYASTHENIC SYNDROMES

Epidemiology

These conditions (see Table 448–1) are rare inherited disorders, mostly autosomal recessive except for the slow channel syndrome, that result from mutations in genes encoding key proteins at the neuromuscular junction. Their frequency in the population is unknown but could be as high as 3 per million.

Pathobiology

The genetic mutations can be presynaptic, synaptic, or postsynaptic. The most common site for mutations is the acetylcholine receptor ε-subunit gene, where the mutations can be single nucleotide substitutions or deletions and usually result in complete loss of function of the acetylcholine receptor ε-subunit. Because this subunit replaces the acetylcholine receptor γ-subunit around the time of birth, the babies are normal in development but show weakness during late pregnancy and in the neonatal period. Survival probably depends on the continued expression of the γ-subunit. Acetylcholine receptor deficiency can also result from defects in the gene for rapsyn, a cytoplasmic protein required for the clustering of the acetylcholine receptors at the neuromuscular junction. Single nucleotide changes in genes for any of the acetylcholine receptor subunits can affect acetylcholine-induced receptor channel openings, leading to kinetic defects. In the fast channel syndrome, the result is reduced function of acetylcholine receptor, whereas in the slow channel syndrome, the channel opens for prolonged periods, resulting in subsynaptic accumulation of ions and degenerative changes.

Mutations in the ColQ gene, which gives rise to the collagen tail that anchors acetylcholinesterase in the synaptic cleft, are uncommon. The resulting continuous exposure of the postsynaptic membrane to acetylcholine leads to degenerative changes and progressive muscle weakness. Mutations in choline acetyltransferase, the enzyme responsible for the synthesis of acetylcholine, do not necessarily lead to dysfunction at rest; during repetitive activity, however, the amount of acetylcholine in each packet decreases, with consequent failure of neuromuscular transmission. Mutations in Dok-7 cause a "synaptopathy" with small, simplified neuromuscular junctions.

Clinical Manifestations

There may be a history of fetal akinesia. Most cases present in infancy with hypotonia and with difficulties in feeding and breathing. Arthrogryposis multiplex congenita often associates with rapsyn mutations. Life-threatening episodic apneas can occur with mutations in choline acetyltransferase or rapsyn. However, some patients do not present until adolescence or young adulthood, including some with rapsyn mutations and the slow channel syndrome. The age at presentation can differ even within a family.

Diagnosis

The EMG findings in the acetylcholine receptor deficiencies and fast channel syndromes are similar to those in typical myasthenia gravis. In the slow channel syndrome and acetylcholinesterase deficiency syndrome there may be a double response to a single nerve stimulus (see Table 448–2). Most patients show a response to cholinesterase inhibitors (edrophonium or neostigmine), with the exception of the slow channel syndrome and acetylcholinesterase deficiency. DNA screening for congenital myasthenic syndromes is essential. Genetic analysis can confirm the diagnosis, although there remain many families in which the faulty gene has not been identified. A precise genetic diagnosis can help in treatment, prognosis, and counseling.

The principal differential diagnoses are spinal muscular atrophy, infant botulism, hereditary neuropathies, and congenital myopathies or muscular dystrophies. Onset in early childhood, adolescence, or adulthood, as can occasionally occur, may mean that the genetic nature of the disorder is not recognized or initially leads to the incorrect diagnosis of seronegative myasthenia gravis.

Treatment and Prognosis

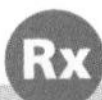

Many of the congenital myasthenic syndromes respond to acetylcholinesterase inhibitors as used for myasthenia gravis. However, no specific treatment is available for acetylcholinesterase deficiency (ColQ mutations). For the slow channel syndrome, some adult patients have responded to fluoxetine, but the use of fluoxetine in children or adolescents requires psychiatric supervision. Although these congenital disorders can be fatal during infancy, usually because of apneic episodes during infections, most tend to be nonprogressive and stable or even may improve during adolescence or adult life. The exceptions are the slow channel syndrome and acetylcholinesterase deficiency, which, owing to the excess acetylcholine receptor activations that they cause, can be associated with progressive degenerative changes at the neuromuscular junction.

Grade A

1. Palace J, Newsom-Davis J, Lecky B, et al: A randomized double-blind trial of prednisolone alone or with azathioprine in myasthenia gravis. Myasthenia Gravis Study Group. Neurology 1998;50:1778–1783.
2. Zinman L, Ng E, Bril V: IV immunoglobulin in patients with myasthenia gravis: A randomized controlled trial. Neurology 2007;68:837–841.
3. Gajdos P, Chevret S, Clair B, et al: Clinical trial of plasma exchange and high-dose intravenous immunoglobulin in myasthenia gravis. Myasthenia Gravis Clinical Study Group. Ann Neurol 1997;41:789–796.
4. Gajdos P, Tranchant C, Clair B, et al: Treatment of myasthenia gravis exacerbation with intravenous immunoglobulin: A randomized double-blind clinical trial. Arch Neurol 2005;62:1689–1693.
5. Bain PG, Motomura M, Newsom-Davis J, et al: Effects of intravenous immunoglobulin on muscle weakness and calcium-channel autoantibodies in the Lambert-Eaton myasthenic syndrome. Neurology 1996;47:678–683.

SUGGESTED READINGS

Engel AG, Sine SM: Current understanding of congenital myasthenic syndromes. Curr Opin Pharmacol 2005;5:308–321. *A review of the genetic forms of myasthenia.*

Maddison P, Newsom-Davis J: Treatment for Lambert-Eaton myasthenic syndrome. Cochrane Database Syst Rev CD003279, 2005. *A systematic review of therapy.*

Schneider-Gold C, Gajdos P, Toyka KV, et al: Corticosteroids for myasthenia gravis. Cochrane Database Syst Rev CD002828, 2005. *A systematic review of steroid therapy.*

Vermino S: Autoimmune and paraneoplastic channelopathies. Neurotherapeutics 2007;4:305–314. *A practical review.*

Vincent A, McConville J, Farrugia ME, et al: Seronegative myasthenia gravis. Semin Neurol 2004;24:125–133. *A review of the pathogenesis of myasthenia gravis without acetylcholine receptor antibodies.*

Section XXVI

Eye, Ear, Nose, and Throat Diseases

DISEASES OF THE VISUAL SYSTEM

Aaron Fay

GENERAL APPROACH TO VISUAL LOSS

Diminished vision often brings patients to medical attention. The cause may be primarily ophthalmic (e.g., cataract) or systemic (e.g., hypertensive retinal detachment). Frequently, patients do not recognize their visual loss until it is brought to their attention by the examining physician or by a paramedical professional.

Ocular physiology and neurophysiology provide essentially identical corrected visual potential in all individuals, unlike the broad range of hearing thresholds seen in a healthy population. Therefore, any deviation from that norm (so-called 20/20 vision) requires thorough investigation until a cause can be identified. Another important purpose of routine ophthalmic examination is the identification of asymptomatic local (e.g., choroidal melanoma) or systemic (e.g., diabetes mellitus) pathology in patients with normal acuity and no subjective complaints.

Evaluation of Ocular Function

Diagnosis

Although the most objective and common measure of vision is line letter *acuity,* vision also includes perception of color, motion, contrast, brightness, field, and depth. The latter qualities are less frequently evaluated during screening because there is greater variation between individuals and because objective, reproducible scales have not been standardized. Visual acuity, however, is limited by retinal anatomy and remains remarkably consistent among individuals. Normal acuity describes accurate resolution of a flat object that subtends an angle of 1 degree on the human retina. The "20/20" line on a visual acuity chart consists of letters that, when held 20 feet from the subject, subtend an angle of 5 degrees; each individual segment of those letters subtends an angle of 1 degree and must be resolved to identify the letter (Fig. 449–1). Letters half that size, held at half that distance, subtend the same angle (10/10 visual acuity). When a subject demonstrates an inability to resolve printed forms subtending 1 degree of arc, vision is substandard and leads to functional disability (Table 449–1). The cause may lie anywhere along the visual pathway from the tear film to the visual cortex of the occipital lobe (Fig. 449–2).

Whether chief complaint or incidental finding, poor visual acuity should prompt complete ophthalmic evaluation. Examination of *pupillary response* provides the most objective measure of ocular function. The swinging light test for *relative afferent pupillary defect* (RAPD, Marcus Gunn pupil) is performed by alternately illuminating the pupils while examining the direct (ipsilateral) and consensual (contralateral) responses. An optic nerve or, rarely, a central nervous system lesion interfering with afferent conduction produces a paradoxical dilation of the involved side on direct illumination. Pathologic processes of the anterior segment, including dense cataract, and of the posterior segment do not produce RAPD. Severe amblyopia may occasionally produce RAPD. *Confrontational visual fields* are performed independently in each eye to detect gross quadrantic defects. *Color vision* testing plates are used as a sensitive indicator of optic nerve function. Extraocular motility is assessed for nerve or muscle abnormalities.

Intraocular tension is determined most accurately by applanation tonometry, in which an applanation prism is used to depress the cornea. Increased intraocular tension may indicate glaucoma, whereas decreased intraocular tension may indicate retinal detachment or a ruptured globe. Corneal thickness and rigidity also influence these measurements. Correct binocular *alignment* (orthophoria) is determined by corneal light reflexes; cover tests using prisms provide greater detail. *Binocular function* may be assessed using polarized glasses and targets at distance and near.

Sudden visual loss is commonly due to circulatory conditions or trauma (Table 449–2). Prompt evaluation is critical, although the condition may be irreversible.

Clinical Evaluation

Anatomic Evaluation

Anatomic evaluation of the eye begins with external examination of the eye and lids and ocular adnexa. Exophthalmos or enophthalmos is recorded with an exophthalmometer relative to the lateral orbital rim. Eyelid position and lesions are noted. The orbital rim and regional lymph nodes are palpated. The globe is ballotted for resistance to retropulsion.

Slit lamp biomicroscopy proceeds in orderly fashion to evaluate lid contour, lesions, and lashes. The conjunctiva, sclera, and cornea are examined for injection, discharge, and inflammation. The anterior chamber is examined for proteinaceous exudate (flare) and inflammatory or red blood cells. The lens and anterior vitreous are examined.

Gonioscopy may be performed using various mirrored lenses to view the angle structures and evaluate angle closure, neovascularization, or tumors. Dilated fundus examination with an indirect ophthalmoscope provides a panoramic view of the fundus. Specific attention is paid to the optic nerve head, retinal vessels, and macular region. The peripheral retina is best seen with scleral depression.

Ancillary Studies

Numerous electrophysiologic and radiographic tests may be used to complement the ophthalmic physical examination. Automated perimetry utilizing static stimuli of variable intensity has replaced manual visual field testing in most offices. Computerized statistical analysis allows more accurate comparison between serial examinations. Automated perimetry has been the "gold standard" for long-term follow-up of glaucoma over the past decade. More recently, nerve fiber layer laser scanners have been used to detect early defects in the nerve (ganglion cell) fiber layer of the retina that precede measurable visual field loss. Corneal topography, pachymetry, and specular microscopy can be used to detect subclinical abnormalities and are required for refractive surgical evaluation. Electroretinography may help distinguish specific retinal diseases, and measurement of visual evoked potentials is used to assess visual cortex function.

Among the more common imaging studies is fluorescein angiography of the retina and choroid. Fluorescein solution is injected intravenously into the antecubital fossa while timed photographs are taken through light filters. Similar tests with different dyes can help define macular lesions. A-scan ultrasonography is used to determine the axial length of an eye, most commonly to determine the appropriate power of implanted intraocular lenses in patients undergoing cataract extraction. B-scan ultrasonography provides excellent intraocular imagery when the fundus cannot be viewed directly, such as in cases of intraocular hemorrhage, advanced cataracts, or miotic pupils. Ultrasound biomicroscopy can provide detailed images of the anterior segment. Computed tomography is preferred to evaluate orbital structures, whereas magnetic resonance imaging produces greater detail for optic nerve and central nervous system lesions.

Specific Conditions

Refractive Error

The most frequent cause for diminished visual acuity is refractive error: light rays entering the eye are not properly brought into focus on the retina. Patients with refractive errors are said to be ametropic. Eyes that focus light perfectly on the retina at rest are called emmetropic. In the absence of ophthalmic pathology, best-corrected visual acuity should equal emmetropic vision. In other words, all patients should be correctable to 20/20 vision unless other pathology is present.

Myopia

Myopia is a common condition in which the refracting power of the eye at rest is too great in relation to the axial length of the eye; the focused image of an object held at infinity (approximated at a distance of 20 feet) lies anterior to the retina (Fig. 449–3).

Physiologic Myopia

Physiologic myopia, which is more common than pathologic myopia, results from a mismatch between the refracting power of the optical elements of the eye and the axial length of the globe when neither of these components lies outside the normal range. The refracting power of a normal human eye is approximately 65 diopters (D), with the cornea and tear film contributing 45 D and the crystalline lens contributing 20 D.

TABLE 449–1 VISUAL ACUITIES REQUIRED FOR COMMON DAILY TASKS

20/20	Physiologic vision
20/30–20/100	Driver's license, varies by state
20/50	Newspaper print
20/70	Large-print *Reader's Digest*
20/100	Write a check
20/200	Legally blind
20/400	Paper currency

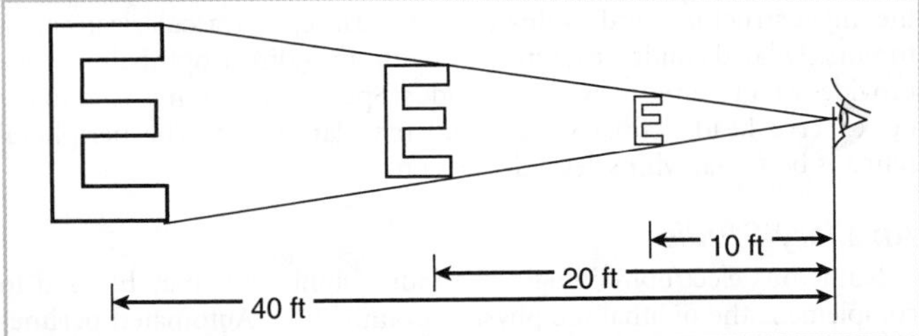

FIGURE 449–1 • Snellen visual acuity. The most common test for visual acuity describes the eye's ability to resolve linear images at a test distance of 20 feet, approximating infinity (parallel rays of light). A 20/20 E subtends 5 minutes of arc at a distance of 20 feet, with each segment of the E subtending 1 minute of arc. The larger letters (e.g., 20/30, 20/40) are determined by the distance at which they subtend an angle of 5 minutes. Thus, an E that subtends 5 minutes at 40 feet, if viewed clearly at 20 feet, indicates 20/40 visual acuity.

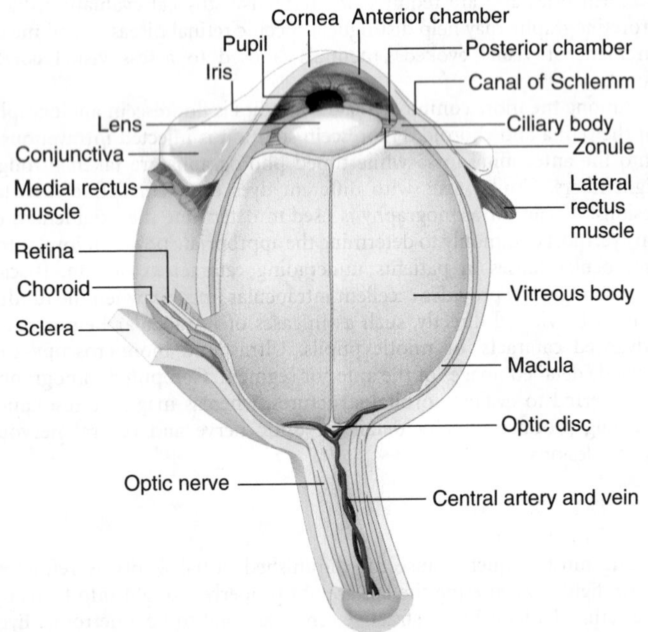

FIGURE 449–2 • Anatomy of the eye.

TABLE 449–2 DIFFERENTIAL DIAGNOSIS OF SUDDEN VISUAL LOSS

Unilateral	Bilateral
Amaurosis fugax (carotid artery stenosis)	Eclampsia
Central retinal artery occlusion	Vertebrobasilar infarct
Occipital lobe infarct	Trauma
Temporal arteritis	
Nonarteritic anterior ischemic optic neuropathy	
Hemorrhage	
Preretinal (high altitude, Valsalva)	
Vitreous	
Aqueous (hyphema)	
Trauma	

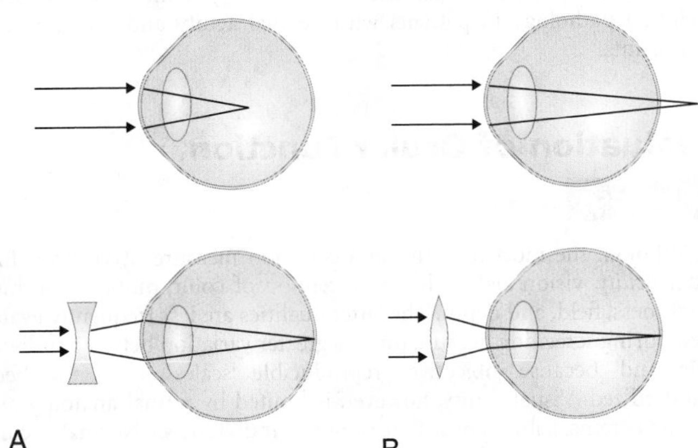

FIGURE 449–3 • Myopia/hyperopia. A, In the myopic eye, parallel rays of light are focused anterior to the retina. A divergent lens can be used to compensate for the mismatch between refracting power and axial length. **B,** The hyperopic eye requires the additional power of a convergent lens to bring images into focus on the retina.

The average axial length of the human eye is approximately 24 mm. Physiologic myopia usually ranges from about 0.5 to about 8.0 D, where the eye appears normal on physical and radiographic evaluation. Onset begins in the second decade and may progress through the third decade. Physiologic myopia is not thought to be heritable, but there appears to be an increased frequency of the disorder among higher socioeconomic groups and among those with greater academic training. Although the cause is not clear, several laboratory and epidemiologic studies indicate that prolonged accommodation as experienced through extensive reading may contribute to progression of physiologic myopia; well-lighted reading conditions may mitigate this effect.

Physiologic myopia is usually treated with spectacle or soft contact lens correction. Photorefractive keratectomy (PRK) uses laser energy to ablate the anterior surface of the central cornea, directly creating a new refractive surface. Laser in situ keratomileusis (LASIK) involves surgical elevation of an anterior corneal flap, stromal ablation, and replacement of the flap. Laser vision correction (PRK and LASIK) is now widely accepted as the standard for surgical correction of myopia and other refractive errors, with 95% of patients achieving visual acuity of 20/40 or better. Mild to moderate hyperopia can also be treated with LASIK. The most common complications include glare symptoms, dry eye, and undercorrection or overcorrection. Rare but serious complications include epithelial ingrowth, diffuse keratitis, and flap dislocation. Other refractive surgical techniques include intracorneal lenses, phakic intraocular lenses, clear lens extraction with intraocular lens implantation, thermal distortion of the cornea, and intracorneal rings to alter the central corneal curvature reversibly. These procedures are not widely performed because of the success of laser vision correction. Clear lens extraction and phakic intraocular lenses are gaining popularity because of the introduction of pseudoaccommodative lenses that may also mitigate presbyopia. Intraocular surgery always carries a risk of surgical complication, and even seemingly uneventful cases may be subject to vision-threatening endophthalmitis. Because physiologic myopia tends to progress into the third decade of life, a minimum of 12 months of stable refractive error should be demonstrated before an irreversible refractive procedure is performed.

Pathologic Myopia

Pathologic myopia is a heritable condition in which the eye is abnormally long; the refracting apparatus is usually normal. Refractive error in pathologic myopia is usually greater than about 8.0 D. *Peripapillary atrophy* is common: The internal scleral surface of the elongated globe is incompletely covered by retina and retinal pigmented epithelium, and a white or yellow crescent or ring of bare sclera may be seen around the optic nerve. The optic discs may be tilted, making estimation of optic nerve cupping difficult. An outpouching of the posterior globe (posterior staphyloma) with broad areas of retinal pigmented epithelium alteration may be seen. Patients with pathologic myopia are predisposed to retinal tears and holes, retinal detachment, subretinal bleeding, and choroidal neovascularization. Pathologic myopia may be associated with systemic disorders, including trisomy 21, Cornelia de Lange's syndrome, Stickler's syndrome, and Marfan syndrome. Dilated fundus examination should be performed at frequent intervals, and patients should be alerted to symptoms of retinal detachment (flashing lights, floaters). Pathologic myopia may be managed with spectacles or contact lenses. Refractive procedures are less successful in pathologic myopia because of high refractive errors and posterior segment anomalies. Surgical and laser procedures may be required to treat retinal and choroidal lesions.

Hyperopia

Hyperopia is an ametropic condition in which the refracting power of the eye is insufficient to bring the focused image of an object held at infinity onto the retina; the image lies posterior to the retinal plane. Hyperopia is the normal condition in infants and young children. Adolescent and adult hyperopia is not usually associated with anatomic abnormalities of the posterior segment. Many patients with hyperopia are able to overcome their refractive deficiency by accommodating even when viewing at distance. Accommodation is an active process in which parasympathetic stimulation of the circular ciliary muscle relaxes the lens zonules, allowing the lens to relax into a more spherical conformation with greater refracting power. The ability to accommodate diminishes with age. Emmetropes rely on accommodation to focus at near; they require near correction as they lose the ability to accommodate, usually entering the sixth decade (presbyopia). Hyperopes, however, may require near correction earlier in life because much of their accommodative power is used to offset the distance refractive error, and small decreases in accommodative ability may be symptomatic (hyperopic presbyopia).

In addition to blurred vision, hyperopia may incite headaches in young adults because increasing effort is required to focus at intermediate distances. Hyperopia is managed with periodic cycloplegic refraction and spectacle or contact lens correction. LASIK can be used to treat up to 5 D of hyperopia.

Astigmatism

Astigmatism is a condition in which the corneal surface is asymmetric: light is refracted differently along different axes. In regular astigmatism, the steepest corneal axis lies 90 degrees away from the flattest corneal axis, a configuration geometrically labeled an ellipsoid cap. Regular astigmatism can usually be corrected with cylindrical and spherical spectacle lenses or with rigid contact lenses. Some forms of astigmatism can also be corrected with laser ablation of the cornea. Irregular astigmatism may produce an array of corneal configurations, usually owing to corneal ectasias such as keratoconus or corneal scarring. Irregular astigmatism is not correctable with spectacles but may be correctable with rigid contact lenses.

OPHTHALMIC DISORDERS USUALLY NOT ASSOCIATED WITH SYSTEMIC DISEASE

Congenital Disorders

Oculogenesis is initiated between 22 and 25 days of gestation when the neural tube begins to close and the optic pits first appear; retinal vascularization is completed shortly after birth, as is uveal pigmentation. Because of this very long developmental process, many systemic congenital syndromes display protean ocular manifestations. The congenital disorders limited to the eye and discussed here may be treatable or may have catastrophic consequences if not detected early.

Amblyopia and Strabismus

Normal development of visual pathways depends on simultaneous and appropriate retinal stimulation in early childhood. *Amblyopia,* or incomplete visual development, is commonly categorized according to cause as strabismic, anisometropic, or deprivational. Amblyopia may be minimized or prevented by early diagnosis and intervention.

Strabismus

Misalignment of the eyes, or *strabismus,* causes disparate images to be cast simultaneously on the two retinas. Children are able to avoid diplopia by involuntarily suppressing one of the images. Left and right images are sometimes suppressed alternately, in which case excellent vision may develop in each eye, but binocular vision does not develop in either situation. More frequently, one eye is constantly suppressed, preventing normal visual development in that eye.

Esotropia

Esotropia, in which the eyes are deviated inward, is the most common strabismus of childhood. Congenital esotropia may not manifest until 3 or 4 months of age and is therefore often termed *infantile esotropia.* There is usually a large angle deviation; cross fixation, in which each inward-turned eye is used to view the contralateral visual field, is not uncommon. Infantile esotropia must be distinguished from pseudostrabismus, in which a broad nasal bridge and prominent epicanthal folds create an illusion of esotropia by obscuring the nasal sclera; in this condition, however, corneal light reflexes are symmetrical and (later) alternate cover testing will show no movement. Abduction should be demonstrated to differentiate congenital esotropia from congenital bilateral sixth cranial nerve palsies. Family history of strabismus confers an increased risk, but no inheritance pattern has been determined. Infantile esotropia is most frequently seen in otherwise normal children, but it occurs with increased frequency in several systemic conditions including cerebral palsy, prematurity, hydrocephalus, and trisomy 21. Cycloplegic refraction should be performed, and patching of one eye may be needed; however, surgery is almost always required to straighten the eyes. Binocular vision can rarely be produced.

Anisometropia

Anisometropia is a condition in which the refractive states of the two eyes differ. One eye may focus a clear image on the retina without accommodation while the contralateral image is blurred, leading to unilateral amblyopia. Children can be seen squinting the affected eye, especially in bright sunlight. Cycloplegic refraction, spectacle or contact lens correction, and occlusive or pharmacologic penalization, or both, of the favored eye may reverse visual loss if instituted before 9 years of age.

Deprivational amblyopia may be caused by any opacity along the visual axis. *Congenital blepharoptosis* resulting from dysgenesis of the levator palpebrae superioris may require early surgical intervention. *Eyelid hemangiomas* may produce ptosis by mechanical effects, and they can also cause amblyopia by inducing an astigmatism. These benign, red, elevated lesions appear within the first few weeks of life and generally involute by age 10. Indications for treatment with intralesional corticosteroid injection, surgical resection, or pulsed-dye laser ablation include pupillary occlusion and induced refractive error. Most *congenital cataracts* incompletely occlude the pupil and permit normal vision to develop. *Complete congenital lenticular opacification,* however, may cause amblyopia if not removed within the first few weeks of life.

Glaucoma

The clinical triad of epiphora, photophobia, and blepharospasm is characteristic of congenital glaucoma. It is thought to result from anomalous aqueous outflow and may be seen in isolation or with other ocular and systemic abnormalities. *Congenital open-angle glaucoma* produces a large eye (buphthalmos) and megalocornea. Examination under anesthesia is required to evaluate the optic nerve head and anterior chamber angle. Medical therapy may provide temporary benefit, but early surgical intervention is indicated. Congenital glaucoma is rare compared with adult-onset open-angle glaucoma.

The rudimentary stump of iris present in congenital *aniridia* produces glaucoma within the first decade by blocking aqueous outflow through the trabecular meshwork. Congenital aniridia is inherited in an autosomal dominant pattern; 13% of cases are sporadic. Patients with congenital sporadic aniridia are at risk for Wilms' tumor and the WAGR syndrome (Wilms' tumor, aniridia, genitourinary anomalies, and mental retardation). Congenital glaucoma may be seen with any of the anterior segment dysgeneses. Genetic investigation and counseling are advised.

Leukocoria

A white pupil, which may result from anterior or posterior segment pathology (Table 449–3), requires prompt and thorough ophthalmic investigation. *Leukocoria* is the most frequent presenting sign in patients with retinoblastoma, the most common intraocular malignancy of childhood. *Retinoblastoma* may be inherited or sporadic, bilateral or unilateral. Calcification is commonly demonstrated radiographically, and involved eyes are usually normal in size. Early, aggressive intervention

TABLE 449–3 DIFFERENTIAL DIAGNOSIS OF LEUKOCORIA

Retinoblastoma
Cataract
Persistent hyperplastic primary vitreous
Retinopathy of prematurity (retrolental fibroplasia)
Coats' disease (retinal telangiectasia)
Retinal detachment
Toxocariasis
Familial exudative vitreo-retinopathy (FEVR)

with irradiation or surgery, or both, may be sight saving and lifesaving. Any disorder that produces congenital leukocoria may be confused with retinoblastoma. The *retinal telangiectasia* of Coats' disease produces unilateral leukocoria through exudative retinal detachment; 85% of patients are boys, and the disease is not heritable. Calcification is distinctly uncommon. Treatment consists of vascular ablation and management of retinal detachment.

Persistent hyperplastic primary vitreous is associated with unilateral microphthalmos in otherwise normal infants. Leukocoria is produced by a retrolenticular vascularized membrane or by induced cataract. Calcification is rare. Although visual prognosis is poor, early vitrectomy or lensectomy may prevent amblyopia and glaucoma. *Familial exudative vitreoretinopathy* is an autosomal dominant, bilateral peripheral retinal disorder that produces retinal exudation and detachment. Incomplete vascularization of the temporal retina is seen in full-term, otherwise healthy infants. Severity may be asymmetric, and prognosis is variable.

Congenital cataracts are relatively common, occurring in 1 in 2000 live births. Cases may be found in association with other ocular or systemic disorders or may be isolated; one third of cases are inherited (usually autosomal dominant). Intrauterine chemical or radiation insult and TORCH (toxoplasmosis, other infections, rubella, cytomegalovirus, and herpes) infections have been implicated. Severity is variable and related to morphology and cause. Metabolic disorders such as galactosemia may produce total, bilateral lenticular opacity resulting in nystagmus and irreversible amblyopia; focal cataracts are less visually devastating. Traumatic cataracts may result from child abuse.

Genetic Disorders

Hereditary disorders primary to the eye are far too numerous to address. Many ophthalmic syndromes and diseases that are not commonly considered hereditary exhibit patterns of inheritance in a minority of cases. The following representations highlight some of the more common and more interesting entities that demonstrate familial patterns in a majority of cases.

Mitochondrial Transmission

Among the ophthalmic disorders inherited through mitochondrial DNA are *Leber's hereditary optic neuropathy* and *chronic progressive external ophthalmoplegia* (CPEO). Leber's hereditary optic neuropathy became the first human disease for which mitochondrial inheritance was definitively demonstrated. Symptoms are limited to subacute, bilateral, progressive loss of vision. Males are affected in 60 to 90% of cases. Onset occurs in the second and third decades. Vision is generally reduced to 20/200 or worse sequentially in the two eyes over a period of months. Clinical findings include optic disc hyperemia with telangiectatic, tortuous retinal vessels; optic nerve pallor (atrophy) is seen in the late stages. Treatment is limited to use of low vision aids.

CPEO frequently manifests as bilateral blepharoptosis in the first and second decades. The paralysis is called external because the extraocular muscles are primarily involved; the iris dilator, iris sphincter, and ciliary muscles are spared. Vision is usually spared, although funduscopic examination reveals deterioration of the retinal pigmented epithelium in the macular region. The condition may occur in isolation or with cardiac conduction abnormalities and arrhythmias: the Kearns-Sayre syndrome. Muscle biopsy specimens demonstrate ragged red fibers. Systemic corticosteroids are contraindicated because they have reportedly precipitated hyperosmolar nonketotic coma in patients with Kearns-Sayre syndrome.

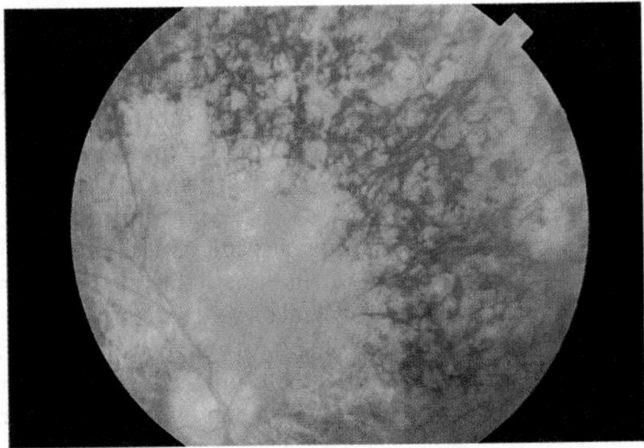

FIGURE 449–4 • Retinitis pigmentosa. Fundus photograph shows "bone spicule" pigmentation of the midperipheral fundus, waxy pallor of the optic disc, and attenuated retinal vessels, the most consistent finding in retinitis pigmentosa. (Courtesy John I. Loewenstein, MD.)

Autosomal Dominant Transmission

The corneal dystrophies are bilateral, inherited disorders that may produce pain and visual loss or may go entirely unnoticed. Autosomal dominant transmission is the rule. Corneal dystrophies are characterized by particular layer of corneal involvement, material deposition, age at onset, and treatment of symptoms.

Recurrent corneal erosions commonly result from *map-dot-fingerprint dystrophy*, the most common corneal dystrophy. This epithelial basement membrane disorder produces patterned irregularities for which it is named. Epithelial cells are stripped away with seemingly trivial trauma, such as with lid opening on wakening, producing severe pain out of proportion to clinical signs. Symptoms first appear in middle age. Methods of treatment range from hypertonic saline drops to mechanical anterior corneal puncture to excimer laser ablation.

Corneal stromal dystrophies rarely produce epithelial erosion but may cause decreased visual acuity. The focal, hyaline deposits of *granular dystrophy* produce modest visual disturbance and may recur in a corneal graft. *Lattice dystrophy* is characterized by amyloid deposition in the anterior stroma and may or may not be associated with systemic amyloidosis. Recurrence in a corneal graft is common. *Macular dystrophy* produces large, confluent areas of acid mucopolysaccharide in patients with a metabolic defect in the production or breakdown of keratan sulfate. Macular dystrophy is the only common corneal dystrophy that shows autosomal recessive transmission.

Thickened protuberances of Descemet's membrane, corneal edema, and painful subepithelial bullae are characteristic of *Fuchs' endothelial dystrophy*. Visual acuity is worse after sleep, when prolonged lid closure limits evaporation from the corneal surface. Transmission is autosomal dominant, but sporadic cases are seen. Temporizing treatment may include hypertonic solutions and bandage contact lenses. Fuchs' dystrophy is one of the most common indications for penetrating keratoplasty (corneal transplant).

Autosomal Recessive Transmission

Retinitis Pigmentosa

Retinitis pigmentosa (RP) is a group of photoreceptor dystrophies in which rod and cone photoreceptors degenerate. Nyctalopia (night blindness) and gradual, progressive loss of peripheral vision are typical features. Although the appearance of the fundus varies greatly, signs in advanced stages include attenuation of retinal vessels, waxy pallor of the optic disc, and "bone spicule" pigmentation of the peripheral fundus in a majority of cases (Fig. 449–4). Early in the disease, the fundus can appear normal.

Prevalence in the United States is approximately 1 in 3000. Approximately 20% of RP cases show autosomal recessive transmission, about 43% are autosomal dominant, about 8% are X-linked recessive, about 23% are isolated cases, and the inheritance pattern cannot be determined in about 6% of cases (e.g., patients who are adopted). Hundreds of genetic defects have been identified in dozens of responsible genes; many additional RP genes remain to be discovered. Perimetry may be useful to document progression, but an electroretinogram (ERG) is required for definitive diagnosis. The ERG typically demonstrates progressive loss of function of rod photoreceptors early in the disease; cones are affected to varying degrees.

The spotty pigmentation of the fundus so often associated with RP may be seen with a number of treatable disorders, including infectious and inflammatory chorioretinitis, vascular occlusions, drug toxicity, and retinal detachment. RP associated with congenital deafness is called Usher's syndrome.

Education of patients is critical in RP. The only therapy known to slow the course of the disease in the common forms of RP is oral supplements of vitamin A palmitate (15,000 units/day). Patients taking these supplements should be monitored for liver toxicity, although toxicity has been seen only in patients taking far higher doses. Vitamin E supplements may worsen the disease. In most cases, the disease is slowly progressive over decades. Central visual acuity may remain surprisingly good despite severe constriction of the visual field. Patients whose visual field is reduced to 20 degrees are considered legally blind in most states. Low vision aids are useful in many cases. Genetic counseling should be provided. Some authorities advise limiting light exposure with the use of tinted glasses, although this approach has not been proved to be of benefit.

Leber's Congenital Amaurosis

Leber's congenital amaurosis is considered by some authorities to be a variant of RP in which the degeneration of photoreceptors is so rapid that little to no vision is present in the first years of life. Infants are usually brought to medical attention within the first 6 months of life when nystagmus develops or delay of visual maturation is otherwise evident. Transmission is autosomal recessive. Affected patients do not respond to visual stimuli on examination, and pupils show variable reactivity. Fundus findings range from normal to heavily spiculed. Multiple, small, white choroidal foci may be seen. The ERG demonstrates generalized photoreceptor dysfunction. No treatment is available.

Gyrate Atrophy of the Choroid

Gyrate atrophy of the choroid is another autosomal recessive degeneration of the fundus. Progressive visual loss and night blindness begin in the first decade. Severely constricted visual fields are present in adults with the disease. The peripheral fundus appearance may be dramatic, showing geographic areas of retinal pigmented epithelial dropout and choroidal atrophy with hyperpigmented borders. The central retina may become involved later as these patches become confluent. The disease is associated with defects in ornithine aminotransferase, which result in elevated serum levels of ornithine. The ERG is abnormal early in the disease. Diagnosis is based on fundus findings and serum ornithine levels. Treatment requires dietary restriction of arginine. Differential diagnosis includes pathologic myopia, choroideremia, RP, and other causes of chorioretinal atrophy.

X-Linked Transmission

Choroideremia

Choroideremia may be confused with gyrate atrophy owing to its similar fundus appearance. It is an X-linked recessive condition that results in progressive atrophy of the choriocapillaris beginning in the first decade. Hyperpigmented areas are generally not seen. Night blindness is often the presenting symptom, whereas visual acuity gradually decreases to the 20/200 level by the fourth decade. Female carriers are asymptomatic but may show subtle fundus signs.

Dyschromatopsia

Nearly all forms of congenital *dyschromatopsia* demonstrate X-linked recessive transmission. Three distinct cone photoreceptor subtypes provide color perception in most humans. The pigment of each subtype demonstrates specific peak wavelength absorption. Patients lacking red cones are said to demonstrate protanopia, whereas those lacking green cones are labeled deuteranopes. Congenital tritanopia, or absence of blue cones, is extremely rare and shows autosomal dominant inheritance.

Most cases of color blindness represent a relative deficiency or abnormality of one of the cone populations rather than a total absence. Genetic defects in coding for cone pigments usually result in subtle shifts in peak wavelength absorption such that color matching responses in affected individuals are incongruous with those in normal subjects, but color differences are perceived nonetheless. Blue-yellow confusion is seen more frequently in acquired dyschromatopsia and may herald optic nerve disease.

Exogenous Infections

Exogenous ocular infections may involve any of the ocular or periocular tissues. Signs and symptoms reflect focality, chronicity, and the infectious pathogen. Treatment may range from modifications in hygiene to surgical débridement.

Blepharitis

Inflammation of the eyelids may produce itching and redness of one or both eyes. *Anterior blepharitis* primarily involves the eyelash follicles, which are located within the anterior lamella of the eyelid. *Staphylococcus aureus* is the most common infectious agent. If untreated, the condition becomes chronic and may lead to corneal and conjunctival inflammation (blepharoconjunctivitis). Patients are advised to clean the eyelids and eyelashes rigorously using a cotton-tipped applicator or washcloth daily. Ophthalmic antibiotic ointment (bacitracin or erythromycin) is more effective than eyedrops to treat the lid margin. *Seborrheic blepharitis* is an anterior blepharitis in which crusting and oily material may envelop individual cilia. Treatment focuses on eyelid hygiene.

Meibomitis

The inflammation of *meibomitis* is localized to the posterior lamella, where the meibomian gland orifices exit the tarsal plate. Slit lamp examination reveals inspissated glands from which white material may be expressed with manual pressure to the eyelid. Vision may be impaired, and the conjunctiva may be inflamed by hyperviscous secretions that enter the tear film. Treatment requires daily eyelid hygiene. Warm, dilute solutions of baby shampoo and a clean washcloth may be used to massage the eyelid margin. Some patients improve with oral doxycycline (50 to 100 mg by mouth twice daily for 3 months), and half of patients may have rosacea (Chapter 465). Chronic, refractory unilateral blepharitis can be caused by a sebaceous carcinoma.

Hordeolum

Acute, focal infection of a meibomian or Zeiss gland is called a *hordeolum.* Commonly termed a *stye,* a hordeolum may be painful and may produce blepharoptosis when it occurs in the upper lid. Hordeola are usually self-limited infections, but they may progress to preseptal cellulitis in which the surrounding lid tissue becomes erythematous, edematous, and warm (Fig. 449–5). Hordeola usually respond to warm compresses over a period of days, whereas preseptal cellulitis requires systemic antibiotics (see later).

Chalazion

Chalazion (Fig. 449–6) describes a chronically inspissated meibomian gland. Glandular secretions become fossilized within the tarsal plate, producing a firm, nonmobile subcutaneous nodule. Extravasation into adjacent soft tissue may produce chronic granulomatous inflammation with enlargement of the chalazion, internal or external erosion, spontaneous drainage, or focal cellulitis. Conservative treatment involves warm soaks with or without antibiotic ointment. Incision and curettage are usually reserved for large lesions or those persisting despite more than 1 month of conservative treatment. Recurrent, isolated chalazia may respond to local corticosteroid injection, although hypopigmentation and tissue necrosis are risks of this treatment. Multiple chronic chalazia may

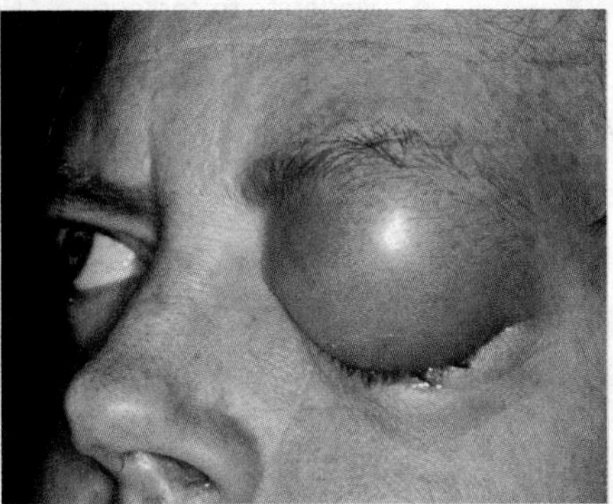

FIGURE 449–5 • Eyelid abscess. Preseptal cellulitis, commonly resulting from minor penetrating trauma, may evolve into an abscess. Treatment requires incision and drainage followed by systemic antibiotics.

Section XXVI Eye and ENT

respond to systemic antibiotics. Chalazia may increase in size during pregnancy. Chronic, nonresponsive chalazia, especially when accompanied by loss of eyelashes, must be evaluated to exclude *sebaceous cell carcinoma.*

Periocular cellulitis may involve deep orbital structures or may be confined to preseptal tissues. In either case, it may produce warm, erythematous eyelid edema and associated pain. Fever and leukocytosis are not uncommon. A history of an insect bite or other skin perforation is frequently elicited in cases of *preseptal cellulitis,* whereas ethmoidal sinusitis is the leading risk factor for *orbital cellulitis.* Treatment is critically dependent on proper diagnosis.

Cellulitis

Clinical signs of *preseptal cellulitis* are limited to external soft tissues as described. Decreased visual acuity, RAPD, limited ocular motility, and pronounced chemosis herald postseptal involvement. In the presence of orbital signs, computed tomographic scans of the orbit and sinuses should be obtained. If untreated, *orbital cellulitis* may extend intracranially.

Preseptal cellulitis is treated with oral antibiotics in an outpatient setting. First-generation cephalosporins are generally effective against *Streptococcus pneumoniae* and staphylococcal species. *Haemophilus influenzae,* found in pediatric patients, produces a characteristic violaceous discoloration. Infants and young children with preseptal cellulitis are admitted for intravenous therapy with antibiotics. Orbital cellulitis requires hospital admission with intravenous administration of antibiotics in all age groups. Lack of clinical improvement in 24 to 36 hours may suggest another process. *Orbital pseudotumor* in adults and *rhabdomyosarcoma* in children must be excluded.

Dacryocystitis

Acute dacryocystitis (Fig. 449–7) produces pain, redness, and swelling of the lacrimal sac. Patients may experience purulent discharge from the lacrimal puncta, and secondary conjunctivitis is common. Symptoms of *chronic dacryocystitis* may be limited to epiphora. Both are associated with nasolacrimal duct obstruction. Digital massage of the lateral nasal wall may cause mucopurulent reflux through the lacrimal punctum. Initial treatment with oral antibiotics may quell any acute inflammation, but definitive treatment requires dacryocystorhinostomy.

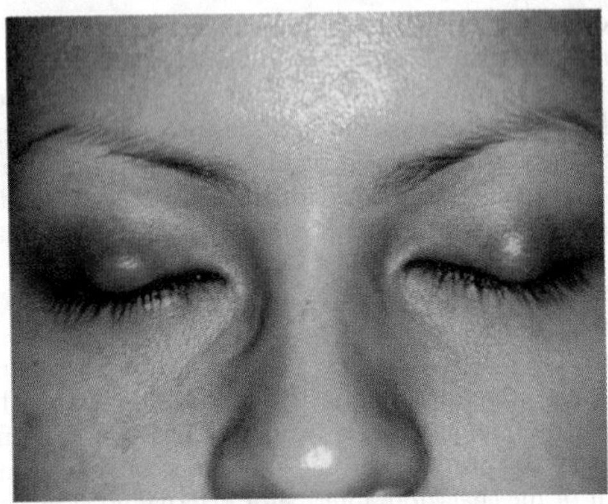

FIGURE 449–6 • Bilateral chalazion in the upper eyelids.

Conjunctivitis

Conjunctivitis is a frequent complaint in which patients experience redness, itching, and foreign body sensation, with discharge ranging from watery to hyperpurulent. It must be differentiated from a corneal abrasion (Fig. 449–8) and other causes of a red, painful eye (Table 449–4).

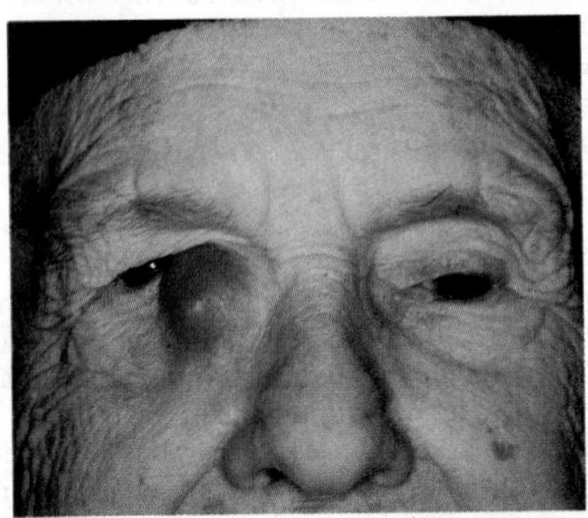

FIGURE 449–7 • Acute dacryocystitis. External photograph shows erythema and edema in the region of the lacrimal sac. Pressure applied to the lesion produces purulent reflux through the canaliculi. Conservative treatment requires oral antibiotics and warm compresses. Pointing lesions such as the one pictured require incision and drainage.

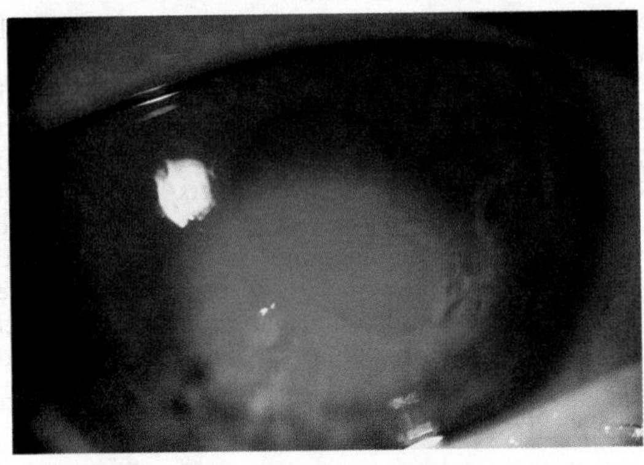

FIGURE 449–8 • Corneal abrasion. Corneal epithelial defects are best observed with topical fluorescent stain under blue illumination. Pain is often out of proportion to clinical findings. Prophylactic topical antibiotics are required until the epithelium has healed. (Courtesy Deborah P. Langston, MD.)

TABLE 449–4 DIFFERENTIAL DIAGNOSIS OF COMMON CAUSES OF INFLAMED EYE*

Feature	Acute Conjunctivitis	Acute Iritis†	Acute Glaucoma‡	Corneal Trauma or Infection
Incidence	Extremely common	Common	Uncommon	Common
Discharge	Moderate to copious	None	None	Watery or purulent
Vision	No effect on vision	Slightly blurred	Markedly blurred	Usually blurred
Pain	None	Moderate	Severe	Moderate to severe
Conjunctival injection	Diffuse: more toward fornices	Mainly circumcorneal	Mainly circumcorneal	Mainly circumcorneal
Cornea	Clear	Usually clear	Steamy	Change in clarity related to cause
Pupil size	Normal	Small	Moderately dilated and fixed	Normal or small
Pupillary light response	Normal	Poor	None	Normal
Intraocular pressure	Normal	Normal	Elevated	Normal
Smear	Causative organisms	No organisms	No organisms	Organisms found only in corneal ulcers related to infection

*Other less common causes of red eyes include endophthalmitis, foreign body, episcleritis, and scleritis.
†Acute anterior uveitis.
‡Angle-closure glaucoma.

The majority of cases are caused by viral infections that typically begin unilaterally and progress to involve both eyes. Viral conjunctivitis is caused most frequently by adenovirus species. Transmission is by direct contact with an infected individual. *Epidemic keratoconjunctivitis* caused by adenovirus subtypes 7, 11, and 18 may spread rapidly through a school, summer camp, or physician's office. Patients diagnosed with viral conjunctivitis should be isolated from other patients; examining rooms and waiting areas should be disinfected.

Viral Conjunctivitis

Viral conjunctivitis produces inferior palpebral conjunctival lymphoid follicles evident on slit lamp examination. There may be copious watery discharge, but mucopurulent discharge is uncharacteristic. Conjunctival hemorrhage suggests an alternative pathogen. Preauricular lymphadenopathy may be present, and a history of upper respiratory tract infection is common. Vision may be compromised by immune infiltration of the corneal stroma. The disease is self-limited, and treatment is aimed at patients' comfort. Cool compresses are often soothing. Patients are advised to wash their hands frequently. When viral conjunctivitis has been diagnosed, antibiotic solutions and ointments are not required, and topical corticosteroids are contraindicated in the acute stage. Although viral particles may be recovered from infected individual for up to 2 to 3 months, most patients are believed to be contagious for 1 to 2 weeks.

Bacterial Conjunctivitis

Bacterial conjunctivitis (Fig. 449–9) represents fewer than 5% of all cases of conjunctivitis. Infection with staphylococcal species appears as chronic mild mucoid discharge and crusting and may be associated with chronic blepharitis or dacryocystitis. Symptoms may improve with erythromycin or bacitracin ointment, but treatment should be targeted at underlying infectious sources. Acute bacterial conjunctivitis caused by *Haemophilus* or streptococcal species may be seen in epidemic or isolated form. Transmission may be through direct contact or through fomites. Moderate purulent discharge is seen. There may be mild edema of the conjunctiva (chemosis) and lids. Slit lamp examination of the inferior palpebral conjunctiva reveals a fine papillary response. The disease is usually self-limited but responds well to broad-spectrum antibiotic solutions, including gentamicin and the combination of polymyxin B with trimethoprim.

Hyperacute Purulent Conjunctivitis

Hyperacute purulent conjunctivitis caused by *Neisseria gonorrhoeae* is transmitted through sexual contact. Copious green pus is produced, and the lids are often extremely edematous. Preauricular lymphadenopathy is common. Immediate intervention is critical to prevent perforation of corneal ulcers caused by bacterial exotoxins. Gram stain and culture of the conjunctiva should be performed. Copious irrigation with saline solution is required to dilute the exotoxins. Systemic antibiotics are required. Third-generation cephalosporins may be given intramuscularly or intravenously. Adjunctive topical treatment with ciprofloxacin, gentamicin, or bacitracin may be useful.

Adult Inclusion Conjunctivitis

Adult inclusion conjunctivitis is produced through sexual transmission of *Chlamydia trachomatis.* This chronic conjunctivitis produces conjunctival follicles in association with preauricular lymphadenopathy and is refractory to many antibiotic regimens. If untreated, the disease may linger for many months. Systemic treatment with erythromycin or azithromycin is required. *Trachoma* is a chronic cicatricial conjunctivitis resulting from repeated infection with particular chlamydial subspecies (Chapter 339). Endemic in many developing countries, it is the world's leading cause of corneal blindness. The superior palpebral conjunctiva develops white, linear scars that can cause the eyelid to roll inward (cicatricial entropion). Trichiasis, inverting of the eyelashes, eventually leads to corneal vascularization and opacification. Medical treatment requires systemic erythromycin or tetracycline, whereas surgical epilation or eyelid reconstruction may be required for cicatricial changes.

Allergic Conjunctivitis

Allergic conjunctivitis is commonly associated with atopy, hay fever, and allergic rhinitis. Itching is usually the prominent symptom, although foreign body sensation is common as well. Watery discharge occurs. Supportive treatment includes cool compresses and topical vasoconstrictors or antihistamines such as naphazoline or levocabastine. Long-term treatment with mast cell stabilizers can be extremely effective in treating chronic symptoms.

Keratitis

Keratitis caused by herpes simplex virus usually represents secondary ocular infection (Fig. 449–10). Primary infection may go unnoticed or may be limited to a periocular vesicular dermatitis or blepharoconjunctivitis. Viral particles lie dormant within the trigeminal ganglion indefinitely or may reinfect the corneal epithelium or stroma. Herpes simplex *epithelial* keratitis produces a characteristic dendritic epithelial defect and is believed to represent active viral infection. Treatment is with topical trifluridine drops nine times daily or vidarabine ointment five times daily. Oral acyclovir can be given (400 mg orally three times daily for 1 to 3 weeks), and long-term acyclovir (400 mg twice daily for 6 months) decreases the risk of recurrent keratitis by 50%. Isolated stromal manifestations are believed to represent immunologic activity against the virus. Treatment with topical corticosteroids (typically, prednisolone acetate 1%, one drop four times a day to start and then tapered over 1 month depending on the response) reduces the risk of corneal opacification. However, steroids should not be used if active infection is suspected, and they should be accompanied by topical or systemic antiviral prophylaxis (e.g., trifluridine, one drop every 4 hours while awake or acyclovir 400 mg by mouth three times a day).

Bacterial Keratitis

Bacterial keratitis may appear as a minor peripheral corneal opacity or a large central suppurative ulcer. Symptoms include pain, redness, photophobia, and decreased vision. Fluorescein staining reveals an epithelial defect with underlying opacity. Gross or microscopic epithelial trauma is the primary risk factor. The risk of bacterial keratitis is five times greater in contact lens wearers and increases among those who sleep with lenses in place. Gram-positive cocci are the most common pathogens, but *Pseudomonas* is most common in patients who wear contact lenses. Identification of the pathogen requires Gram stain and culture of corneal scrapings. Empirical treatment with topical fourth-generation fluoroquinolones (e.g., moxifloxacin, gatifloxacin) is common outside academic

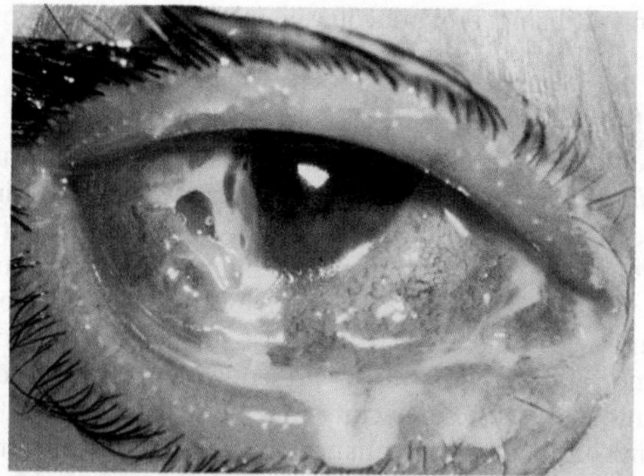

FIGURE 449–9 • Bacterial conjunctivitis. Purulent discharge and conjunctival hyperemia suggest bacterial conjunctivitis. Viral conjunctivitis produces watery discharge, foreign body sensation, preauricular lymphadenopathy, and conjunctival follicles seen on slit lamp examination. (Reproduced with permission from the American Academy of Ophthalmology.)

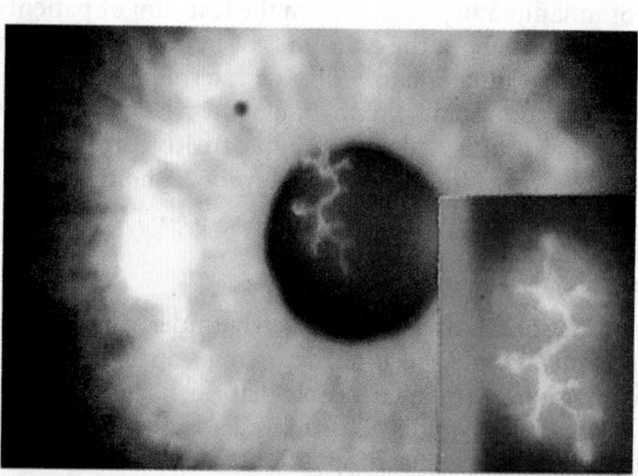

FIGURE 449–10 • Herpes simplex corneal epithelial keratitis in diffuse light and in light passed through a cobalt blue filter after fluorescein staining (inset). Note the dendritic staining pattern characteristic of herpes simplex.

centers for less severe cases, but these agents may need to be administered as frequently as every 15 minutes. More severe cases require hospital admission and topical application of fortified antibiotic solutions every 10 to 15 minutes. Systemic antibiotics are not routinely used. Perforation may be treated with bandage contact lens, cyanoacrylate (Crazy Glue), or penetrating keratoplasty. Fungal infection, suspected after injury with vegetable matter, often requires early surgical débridement.

Endophthalmitis

Endophthalmitis, or inflammation of the intraocular cavity, may be exogenous or endogenous, and it may be infectious or sterile. Exogenous infectious endophthalmitis follows surgical or nonsurgical penetrating trauma. Incidence is estimated at 0.1% after intraocular surgery and 5% after penetrating injury. The primary symptom is decreased vision. Vitritis and anterior uveitis are evident on examination. Corneal, conjunctival, retinal, and choroidal involvement is variable. Toxin-producing gram-positive species and gram-negative species produce rapid onset necrosis of the vitreous and other intraocular structures. *Propionibacterium acnes* and *Staphylococcus epidermidis* are indolent organisms causing more subtle presentations. Endophthalmitis is a rare but potentially catastrophic complication of cataract surgery. Visual acuity should continually improve in the weeks after surgery. *Any decrease in visual acuity or increase in pain during the postoperative period requires immediate examination.*

Endophthalmitis requires sampling of the aqueous and vitreous for Gram stain and culture. *P. acnes* and *S. epidermidis* may require injection of intravitreal antibiotics. More virulent infections require pars plana vitrectomy with intravitreal corticosteroids and intravenous antibiotics. Prognosis is variable and depends on the specific pathogen. Treatment of indolent infections may result in excellent postoperative vision, but aggressive pathogens can completely destroy intraocular tissues within several hours, eliminating all useful vision.

Idiopathic Inflammatory and Autoimmune Disorders

Ocular or periocular tissues may be the primary focus of isolated idiopathic or autoimmune inflammation. Pain is a common symptom. Vision is variably reduced. Treatment is aimed at reducing symptoms and limiting tissue destruction because the underlying cause is poorly understood.

Keratoconjunctivitis Sicca

Keratoconjunctivitis sicca, commonly called dry eye syndrome, results from deficiency of any of the tear film layers. Symptoms include gritty, foreign body sensations, burning, photophobia, and decreased visual acuity. The cornea and conjunctiva may stain with fluorescein, although rose Bengal and lisamine green are more sensitive stains. Idiopathic inflammation of the lacrimal and salivary glands resulting in keratoconjunctivitis sicca and xerostomia is called Sjögren's syndrome (Chapter 289) and is more common in women. Secondary complications include recurrent corneal erosion, keratitis, and corneal opacification. A number of medications can also cause dry eyes (Table 449–5).

Artificial tears, administered no more than four times a day, and lubricating ointments at night are a traditional initial treatment regimen, often in combination with temporary or permanent punctal occlusion, but the presence of inflammatory mediators in the tear film of patients with dry eye raises questions about the usefulness of punctual occlusion. Because dry eye is often an inflammatory disorder, steroid protocols are becoming more common; some ophthalmologists recommend loteprednol 0.5% eyedrops four times a day as an initial treatment. [1] Cyclosporine 0.05% eyedrops (one drop in each eye every 12 hours) have become a mainstream second- or third-line intervention over the past 2 years. [2]

Scleritis

Episcleritis is inflammation immediately underlying the conjunctiva. Pain, if present, is mild. Sectoral hyperemia, distinguished from conjunctivitis by radially oriented vessels that do not move with the conjunctiva, is dramatically reduced with instillation of phenylephrine 2.5% or 10%, but even a single drop of the 10% solution can produce acute arterial hypertension. Episcleritis is self-limited, although oral or topical nonsteroidal anti-inflammatory medications such as flurbiprofen or diclofenac may hasten resolution. In contradistinction to scleritis, episcleritis is not usually related to systemic rheumatoid disease.

TABLE 449–5 PARTIAL LIST OF SYSTEMIC MEDICATIONS CAUSING DRY EYE

Medication	Class
Ibuprofen	Nonsteroidal anti-inflammatory
Diphenhydramine	Antihistamine
Triprolidine	Antihistamine
Chlorpheniramine	Antihistamine
Atenolol	β-Blocker
Metoprolol	β-Blocker
Propranolol	β-Blocker
Clonidine	α-Agonist
Scopolamine	Anticholinergic
Amiodarone	Antiarrhythmic
Thiabendazole	Antinematode
Isotretinoin*	Retinoid

*Severe, long-term dry eye with onset up to several years after treatment. All others tend to abate with cessation.

Scleritis frequently manifests as severe pain and redness. Fifty percent of cases are associated with systemic disease. Vision may be reduced when the posterior sclera is involved. There may be diffuse or sectoral hyperemia that is nonmobile and does not blanch with instillation of phenylephrine. Scleral thinning may occur, but perforation is rare. Uveitis and keratitis may occur secondarily. Diagnostic evaluation includes ultrasonography or magnetic resonance imaging, or both, as well as laboratory tests to identify infectious or autoimmune connective tissue disease. Treatment may require topical or oral nonsteroidal anti-inflammatory medications or corticosteroids. Refractory cases may require cytotoxic drugs.

Mooren's Ulcer

Mooren's ulcer is a progressive, idiopathic peripheral corneal thinning thought to be an autoimmune phenomenon. The condition may be unilateral or bilateral, and pain is common. Perforation is rare except with trauma. Topical corticosteroids, mucolytics, and cytotoxic agents have been used. Bandage contact lenses and conjunctival recession or advancement have also been used with variable success.

Ocular Cicatricial Pemphigoid

Ocular cicatricial pemphigoid is a vesicular conjunctivitis named for its relentless destruction of the ocular surface. Involvement before age 60 is rare. Initial symptoms of foreign body sensation and burning reflect chronic conjunctivitis. Ruptured epithelial bullae destroy conjunctival goblet cells, leading to profound dry eye. The conjunctival fornices may be obliterated. Mild trauma or surgery may increase inflammation. Patients with ocular cicatricial pemphigoid demonstrate antibodies to the conjunctival basement membrane, and other mucous membranes may be affected. Dapsone is the first-line treatment, although it is contraindicated in patients with glucose-6-phosphate dehydrogenase deficiency. Cytotoxic medications or corticosteroids may be helpful. Surgical reconstruction utilizing oral mucous membrane autografts or amniotic membrane allografts can be effective in severe cases.

Orbital Pseudotumor

Nonspecific, idiopathic orbital inflammation has been called *orbital pseudotumor.* The inflammation may involve the lacrimal gland (dacryoadenitis), extraocular muscles (myositis), orbital fat, sclera, or optic nerve sheath (optic perineuritis). Inflammation primarily involving the orbital apex produces painful external ophthalmoplegia, the Tolosa-Hunt syndrome. Pain is the most frequent symptom in orbital pseudotumor, although many cases present with proptosis and limitation of ocular movements; visual acuity may be reduced. Orbital computed tomography or magnetic resonance imaging is generally required to exclude mass lesions; biopsy may be indicated in atypical cases. A dramatic response to systemic corticosteroids within 24 hours is common. A poor clinical response should suggest an alternative diagnosis. Corticosteroids must be tapered slowly over months to prevent recurrence.

Irradiation may be required if corticosteroids cannot be discontinued successfully, and steriod-sparing immunomodulators are under investigation (e.g., mycophenolate mofetil).

Iritis

Patients with *iritis* complain of pain, photophobia, and blurred vision. More than 50% of cases are unrelated to systemic disease. Perilimbal conjunctival injection may be present, and slit lamp examination demonstrates inflammatory cells and protein exudate (flare) in the anterior chamber. Initial episodes are usually treated symptomatically with prednisolone acetate 1% suspension four times a day and cycloplegic drugs (cyclopentolate 1 or 2% twice daily). Repeated episodes require systemic evaluation for autoimmune and infectious causes.

Central Serous Retinopathy

Central serous retinopathy occurs unilaterally as acutely decreased visual acuity and metamorphopsia in young to middle-aged adults. Patients are usually well educated and employed in stressful occupations. Visual acuity may range from 20/40 to 20/200. Fundus examination demonstrates a central, serous elevation of the neurosensory retina. Fluorescein angiography is useful in diagnosis. The disease is self-limited, although permanent visual deficits have been reported. Focal laser treatment reduces duration of symptoms but does not improve final outcome.

Neoplastic Diseases

Neoplasms primary to the eye and adnexa are vast. External lesions are often categorized as pigmented or nonpigmented. Intraocular metastases are about 10 times more common than primary intraocular tumors.

Hemangioma

The eyelid *hemangioma* is a pediatric lesion that manifests in the first several weeks of life. The so-called strawberry nevus enlarges over several months but generally begins to involute after 1 year of age. Potential complications include blepharoptosis, astigmatism, and amblyopia. The orbit may be involved. Large tumors may require intralesional or systemic corticosteroids during the proliferating phase. Pulsed-dye laser treatment increases the rate of involution of superficial cutaneous lesions. Interferon should be avoided because of the risk of irreversible spastic diplegia. Surgical excision is effective in many cases, although most ophthalmologists continue to recommend observation.

Rhabdomyosarcoma

Rhabdomyosarcoma is the most common primary orbital malignancy of children. Proptosis, ptosis, and lid ecchymosis are most common on presentation; visual loss is variable. History of incidental trauma may be misleading. Orbital computed tomography may be useful, but biopsy is required for definitive diagnosis. Systemic evaluation for metastases (including chest radiography, lumbar puncture, and bone marrow biopsy) should be initiated emergently. Survival rates exceeding 90% have been achieved with focal irradiation (4000 to 6000 cGy) and systemic chemotherapy (vincristine and actinomycin D).

Basal Cell Carcinoma

Basal cell carcinoma, the most common eyelid malignancy, occurs 40 to 50 times more often than either squamous or sebaceous malignancies. These lesions are typically pearly, umbilicated nodules, although morphology varies widely and includes deeply pigmented tumors. They are most commonly located on the lower eyelid. Excision with clear surgical margins is generally curative. Basal cell carcinoma rarely metastasizes, and local recurrence can be treated with excision. Caruncular lesions may extend into deep tissues and therefore warrant orbital imaging before surgery.

Squamous Cell Carcinoma

Although *squamous cell carcinoma* occurs much less frequently than basal cell carcinoma, it carries the risk of metastasis. Squamous cell carcinoma is found most frequently on the lower lid, where actinic exposure is greatest. Advanced cases may involve the orbit and sinuses and require systemic evaluation. Surgical excision is required.

Sebaceous Cell Carcinoma

Sebaceous cell carcinoma arises from the sebaceous glands of the eyelids. Chronic chalazia that destroy local lid architecture should raise the possibility of sebaceous cell carcinoma, as should chronic unilateral blepharitis. The tumor is aggressive, tends to demonstrate pagetoid (intraepithelial) spread through the conjunctiva, and requires excisional surgery. Metastasis is not uncommon. Sebaceous cell carcinoma associated with visceral malignancy is termed *Muir-Torre syndrome.*

Malignant Melanoma

Malignant melanoma (Chapter 214) of the conjunctiva may arise de novo, from nevi, or in areas of *primary acquired melanosis.* Unilateral conjunctival pigmentation in lightly pigmented persons may exhibit cellular atypia, in which case the individual is at risk for melanoma. Conjunctival melanoma may be pigmented or amelanotic. Tumor thickness greater than 0.8 mm portends a greater likelihood of metastasis. Early local excision with adjunctive cryotherapy is often curative. Intraocular malignant melanoma is the most common primary intraocular tumor. Malignant melanoma arises in the choroid or ciliary body and may extend through the sclera to involve the conjunctiva. Choroidal malignant melanoma may arise de novo or from a previously identified choroidal nevus. Tumor thickness greater than 3 mm, breadth greater than 10 mm, or rapid enlargement suggests malignant melanoma. The liver is the most common site of metastasis, and liver enzymes are the most sensitive screening tool. In cases without metastases, treatment is controversial and may involve focal irradiation, laser ablation, excision, or enucleation. Orbital invasion of any of these tumors requires exenteration (complete removal of all orbital contents.)

Retinoblastoma

Retinoblastoma, the most common intraocular malignancy of childhood, may be inherited as an autosomal dominant trait or may be sporadic. Genetic study of retinoblastoma, a prototypic genetic malignancy, gave rise to the Knudson two-hit hypothesis. Normal development relies on a tumor suppressor gene located on the long arm of chromosome 13. One normal allele is sufficient to suppress tumorigenesis. Familial retinoblastoma may result from autosomal dominant transmission of one defective allele, in which all the cells in the body are affected. Bilateral or multicentric disease is common in this situation, and the abnormal gene is passed on to future offspring. Sporadic retinoblastoma results from mutations during embryogenesis. Mutation early in embryogenesis affects all the cells in the body, in which case a de novo germline defect is created. Bilateral or multicentric disease is common in this situation as well. Late mutation in embryogenesis produces nontransmissible, unilateral, unifocal disease. In any of these settings, the second allele suffers somatic mutation in a developing retina cell. Patients most frequently present with leukocoria or strabismus, and 90% are diagnosed by age 3. Enucleation is recommended in unilateral cases, and extension of tumor cells along the transected optic nerve is the most significant prognostic factor. Radiation, laser ablation, cryotherapy, and chemotherapy may be used in bilateral cases to treat the second eye. Survivors are at risk for other malignancies, including osteogenic sarcoma.

Intraconal orbital tumors generally produce axial proptosis and decreased vision. Orbital venous malformation, erroneously termed *cavernous hemangioma* in the ophthalmic literature, is the most common orbital tumor. These lesions are benign, vascular endothelial malformations that may be intraconal or extraconal. Orbital images reveal a well-circumscribed tumor. Significant pain should suggest another diagnosis. Excision is indicated by compromised vision, optic neuropathy, globe displacement, or proptosis.

Primary Optic Nerve Tumors

Primary optic nerve tumors include *meningioma* and *glioma.* Optic nerve meningiomas are slow-growing tumors seen in middle-aged individuals; women are affected more often than men. Vision may be gradually reduced or may remain normal. Characteristic computed tomographic images reveal primary involvement of the neural sheath. Serial examinations and images are performed to detect posterior progression. Threat of chiasmal involvement is the primary indication for excision, although this is somewhat controversial. Optic nerve *glioma* may be seen in children with von Recklinghausen's disease (Chapter 444) or tuberous sclerosis (Chapter 444). Bilateral optic nerve glioma is pathognomonic for neurofibromatosis type 1. Isolated optic nerve glioma in adults is rare but more aggressive and often lethal.

Degenerative Conditions

Cataract

Cataract, or opacification of the crystalline lens, is the leading cause of blindness in the world and the leading cause of visual loss in Americans older than 40. Prevalence of cataract in the United States has been estimated as 50% for persons older than 75. The great majority of cases represent normal aging changes in which progressive yellowing of the lens nucleus (nuclear sclerosis) and hydration of the lens cortex are seen. Genetic predisposition to senile cataract has been hypothesized but not proved. Prolonged exposure to ultraviolet radiation has been shown to be cataractogenic. Surgical extraction is required to improve vision; there is no known medical treatment.

Nearly all patients older than 50 demonstrate some degree of degenerative lens changes when examined by slit lamp. Visual disability depends on the extent of lenticular changes as well as on the visual demands of the patient. Very rarely is cataract extraction medically indicated. Mature, swollen cataracts may induce phacomorphic glaucoma by narrowing the anterior chamber angle. Hypermature, liquefied cataracts may leak lens protein and thereby cause phacoantigenic uveitis. In the majority of cases, however, elective cataract extraction serves to restore lost vision. There is no urgency in most cases, and patients who are told they must have cataract surgery in the absence of disabling visual complaints should beware.

Congenital cataracts may be associated with metabolic disease, result from intrauterine TORCH infections, or be familial. Traumatic cataracts result from hydration after penetrating injury to the lens. Some cataracts may be characteristic in color or location, such as the sunflower cataract of Wilson's disease (Chapter 230) or the posterior subcapsular cataract often resulting from systemic corticosteroid use (Chapter 33).

Cataract extraction with intraocular lens implantation has become a very successful procedure in the developed world. Potential complications include cystoid macular edema, astigmatism, retinal detachment, and endophthalmitis. Current methods of surgery include small, self-sealing incisions performed under local (retrobulbar) or topical anesthesia. Prognosis for visual recovery is excellent barring any concomitant eye disease such as diabetic retinopathy, glaucoma, or macular degeneration.

Glaucoma

Glaucoma is best defined as atrophy of the retinal ganglion cell layer in the presence of elevated intraocular pressure. The classical clinical triad consists of elevated intraocular tension, atrophic cupping of the optic nerve head, and characteristic visual field loss. Normal tension glaucoma has been described. Elevated intraocular pressure has not been clearly defined as causative. Many experts view glaucoma as a vascular optic neuropathy, whereas others favor an endogenous toxic etiology. Early in the disease, findings are variable, and the diagnosis is difficult to make; many patients are categorized as "glaucoma suspects" on the basis of one or more risk factors and should be examined every 4 to 6 months. Risk factors include family history of glaucoma, increasing age, diabetes mellitus, obesity, and ocular trauma. Glaucoma is the leading cause of blindness among blacks.

Primary Open-Angle Glaucoma

Primary open-angle glaucoma, the most common glaucoma, occurs in 15% of individuals older than 80 years. The anterior chamber angle anatomy appears normal, but aqueous outflow is reduced. Progressive visual field loss begins in the periphery and occurs so insidiously that affected individuals may be unaware until late in the disease course. Intraocular tension measurement is an effective, if imperfect, screening method, and all adults should be screened. Medical treatment attempts to reduce aqueous production by the ciliary body or to increase outflow through the trabecular meshwork or uvea. Topical β-blockers, carbonic anhydrase inhibitors, miotics, and prostaglandin analogues may be additive in their effects. Refractory cases may require laser or cryoablative procedures. Filtering surgery is used to produce a subconjunctival outflow conduit in advanced cases.

Angle-Closure Glaucoma

Angle-closure glaucoma constitutes an ophthalmic emergency. Patients present with a red, painful eye. Nausea and vomiting are common. The pupil is usually fixed in a mid-dilated position, and the cornea appears cloudy because of pressure-driven edema. The iris is bowed forward by posterior accumulation of aqueous humor, thereby sealing off the anterior chamber angle. Risk factors include narrow anterior chamber angles, for which the contralateral eye may provide diagnostic clues. Emergent treatment (Table 449–6) requires topical administration of a β-adrenergic antagonist, an α-adrenergic agonist, and carbonic anhydrase inhibitors. Systemic pressure-lowering medications include carbonic anhydrase inhibitors, glycerol, isosorbide, and mannitol. Some ophthalmologists advocate anterior chamber paracentesis (aqueous tap). Definitive treatment requires peripheral iridotomy, usually performed with a laser after the initial crisis is resolved. The contralateral eye is treated prophylactically on an elective basis. Chronic angle closure may result from prolonged intraocular inflammation and secondary fibrosis of the anterior chamber angle.

Secondary glaucomas arise in the setting of mature cataract, intraocular inflammation, or gross anatomic distortion. Inflammatory debris may clog the trabecular meshwork in uveitis. Angle recession glaucoma may follow blunt trauma up to several years after the inciting event. Congenital glaucoma may be primary or may result from malformation such as aniridia causing mechanical dysfunction of the trabecular meshwork. Retinal ischemia from diabetic retinopathy or vascular occlusion may cause neovascularization of the anterior chamber angle, leading to neovascular glaucoma. Treatment requires panretinal laser photocoagulation.

Age-Related Macular Degeneration

Age-related macular degeneration (ARMD) is an idiopathic atrophy of the photoreceptors and retinal pigmented epithelium. Genetic variations in complement factor H have been associated with an increased risk of macular degeneration in several independent studies. Many of the pathologic changes may be seen without visual loss. In this case, the term *age-related maculopathy* is used. Because these findings do not necessarily portend an ominous progression, "macular degeneration" should be reserved for individuals with visual loss. Amsler grid home monitoring is advised to detect acute visual field loss and metamorphopsia, which is focal image distortion often caused by focal retinal elevation.

Nonexudative ("dry") macular degeneration manifests as painless, progressive loss of central vision (Fig. 449–11). Pigmentary mottling is seen in the macular area of the fundus, and drusen are evident. Drusen are lipofuscin deposits beneath the retinal pigmented epithelium basement membrane. Drusen may be discrete (hard), indistinct (soft), or confluent. Focal retinal pigmented epithelium detachment is common. There is no known treatment for nonexudative ARMD. Risk factors include smoking, hypertension, and hypercholesterolemia. Some believe that

TABLE 449–6 MEDICAL TREATMENT OF ACUTE ANGLE-CLOSURE GLAUCOMA

1. Systemic
   a. Acetazolamide, 500 mg orally in one dose
   b. Isosorbide, 50–100 g orally in one dose, *or* mannitol, 1–2 g/kg intravenously over 1 hour
2. Topical (administered at 5-minute intervals) β-blocker (e.g., timolol 0.5%) one drop, repeat every 15 minutes ×4
   Pilocarpine* 1–2%, one drop, repeat every 15 minutes ×4
3. Place patient in supine position
4. Refer to ophthalmologist
5. Definitive treatment requires peripheral iridotomy

*Not given to aphakic or pseudophakic patients.

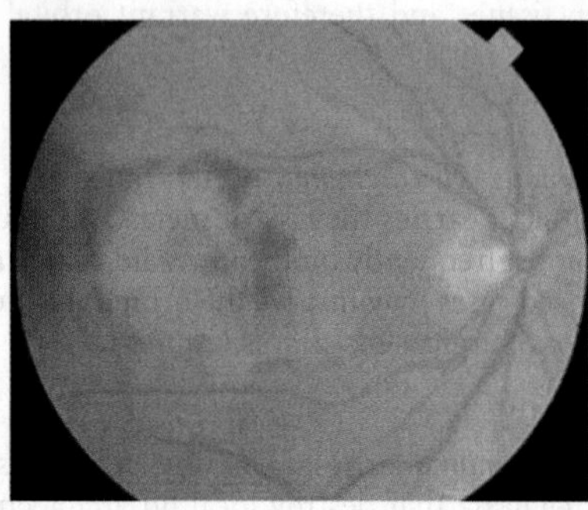

FIGURE 449–11 • **Wet, atrophic age-related macular degeneration.**

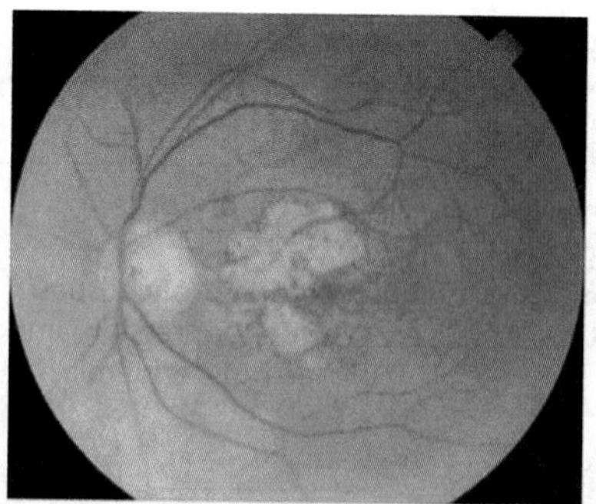

FIGURE 449–12 • Dry, atrophic age-related macular degeneration.

ultraviolet exposure is an additional risk factor. Low vision aids may be extremely useful. The Age-Related Eye Disease Study (AREDS) demonstrated the efficacy of vitamin supplementation in retarding progression of moderate ARMD to severe ARMD. Vitamins C and E, β-carotene, zinc, and copper were shown to be effective in large doses specified in the study protocol leading to AREDS-compliant formulations now marketed by several companies (Bausch and Lomb, Preservision or ICAPS, AREDS Formula). 3 β-Carotene (a vitamin A precursor) of this quantity is not recommended for cigarette smokers because of an increased risk of lung cancer.

Choroidal neovascularization is the main complication of "wet" ARMD (Fig. 449–12). Breaks in Bruch's membrane permit the choriocapillaris access to the subretinal space. Submacular hemorrhage is common in these cases. Intravitreal antiangiogenic medications such as ranibizumab have been effective in a broad range of cases and are now indicated for all angiographic subtypes of subretinal neovascularization. 4 Approximately 10% of proliferative lesions may be treated prophylactically with photocoagulation to decrease the likelihood of severe visual loss, and surgical excision of subretinal membranes may be indicated in even fewer cases. Photodynamic therapy, however, is applicable in 60 to 70% of cases of choroidal neovascularization that are not amenable to thermal photocoagulation because of their location or character. Photodynamic therapy involves the use of intravascular light sensitizers, such as verteporfin, that permit selective coagulation of choroidal vessels without damaging the overlying retina. This technique has been most effective in treating small areas of "classical" neovascularization as determined angiographically.

Retinal Detachment

Retinal detachment, or separation of the neurosensory retina from the retinal pigmented epithelium, may be classified as tractional, exudative, or rhegmatogenous. Tractional retinal detachments are most commonly associated with severe, proliferative diabetic retinopathy or follow nondiabetic vitreous hemorrhage. Tractional membranes form from organized hemorrhage and drag the retina as they contract. Exudative elevations are seen with malignant hypertension, posterior inflammation, or choroidal disease. Serous fluid accumulates in the subretinal space and produces a smooth, domed, dependent detachment. Rhegmatogenous retinal detachment results from a break in the retina secondary to intraocular involutional changes or trauma.

Rhegmatogenous detachments are by far the most common form of retinal detachment. Symptoms include acute decrease in acuity, photopsia (flashing lights), and floaters. There may be associated vitreous hemorrhage, and more than 90% of cases demonstrate red blood cells in the vitreous (Shafer's sign). Retinal breaks may occur from trauma, posterior vitreous detachment, or retinal atrophy. The vitreous gradually liquefies (syneresis) in middle-aged to elderly individuals and remains firmly adherent to the retina anteriorly. Vitreous traction can produce a tear that allows liquefied vitreous access to the subretinal space. Trauma can produce a similar scenario in younger individuals. Approximately 25% of rhegmatogenous retinal detachments are found in patients with lattice degeneration of the retina, which is present in 10% of adults. Focal vitreous liquefaction occurs over the lattice lesions, whereas the vitreous is firmly attached at the lesion's perimeter. Atrophic retinal holes can also lead to rhegmatogenous detachment.

Not all rhegmatogenous retinal detachments require immediate intervention. Acute, symptomatic cases must be repaired, although the timing of surgery depends on the threat or presence of macular involvement and the condition of the eye. Patients with vitreous hemorrhage should adhere to strict bed rest with the head elevated to optimize visualization of the fundus. Asymptomatic or chronic detachments may be observed in some cases. Surgical treatment requires identification and closure of the break or breaks, usually through scleral buckling procedures, with or without vitrectomy, and laser photocoagulation to induce a chorioretinal adhesion in the area of the break. Other procedures include retinopexy (intraocular gas injection) and cryotherapy. *Proliferative vitreoretinopathy* is a rare but potentially devastating complication of retinal breaks in which fibrovascular proliferation distorts the retina and intraocular surface.

Corneal and Conjunctival Degeneration

Actinic exposure of the conjunctiva and cornea may cause degenerative changes. *Pingueculae* are yellowish elevations of the interpalpebral conjunctiva in which the substantia propria demonstrates elastotic degeneration. Ultraviolet radiation is thought to induce fibroblasts to produce altered collagen. Lesions encroaching on the nasal or temporal cornea and demonstrating identical histopathologic findings are known as *pterygia.* Programmed degeneration of the cornea may be seen in *keratoconus.* The central cornea is thinned, resulting in a conical shape. Keratoconus has been associated with atopy and eye rubbing. Patients present with severe astigmatism, usually in the second decade, which may progress until age 30. Rigid contact lenses correct astigmatism in many cases; other patients require penetrating keratoplasty, which has been very effective in these cases. Calcium deposition at the level of the corneal epithelial basement membrane is seen clinically as *band keratopathy.* Usually seen in elderly persons or in degenerated eyes, band keratopathy may be amenable to chelation with disodium ethylenediaminetetraacetic acid.

Vascular Conditions

Infarction of the optic nerve head is called *anterior ischemic optic neuropathy.* Many cases are related to vasculitides, whereas others are nonarteritic (idiopathic). Patients present with acute, painless, unilateral loss of vision. Most patients are between 50 and 75 years old. Other risk factors include a small optic disc with very little cupping, hypertension, and diabetes mellitus. Disc edema may be sectoral. Visual field loss is usually altitudinal (superior or inferior hemianopsia), and sectoral atrophy ensues; 25% of patients suffer contralateral disease. Optic nerve sheath fenestration is ineffective in acute cases but may be useful in rare cases that progress over days.

Systemic Effects of Ocular Medications

Many ophthalmic solutions may produce systemic side effects even when administered in small doses (Table 449–7). Manual punctal occlusion after instillation of drops helps to increase ocular penetration and to limit systemic uptake through the nasal mucosa. Because many patients cannot follow this protocol, they can be alternatively instructed to close their eyes for 1 minute after instilling the drops. *β-Adrenergic antagonists* are among the most commonly prescribed ophthalmic solutions. Patients with asthma may experience bronchospasm or bradycardia; others may experience lethargy or impotence. The miotic drug *pilocarpine* is a direct-acting parasympathomimetic that may produce acute, severe headache, especially in younger patients. *Echothiophate* is an acetylcholinesterase inhibitor and may produce cholinergic symptoms, including diarrhea and hypersalivation. Concomitant administration of succinylcholine should be avoided. *Atropine* and other muscarinic antagonists may be used to paralyze the ciliary muscle and dilate the pupil. Systemic effects may include tachycardia and fever. Severe cases may be treated with physostigmine. The α-adrenergic medication *phenylephrine* may produce rapid hypertension when given as a 10% topical solution. *Carbonic anhydrase inhibitors* may be administered topically and do not seem to carry the risk of central nervous system effects and aplastic anemia seen with systemic administration.

OPHTHALMIC MANIFESTATIONS OF SYSTEMIC DISEASES

Congenital Disorders

Sturge-Weber Syndrome

Systemic nonhereditary congenital disorders with frequent ocular manifestations include *Sturge-Weber* syndrome (Chapter 444) and prematurity. Sturge-Weber syndrome (encephalofacial angiomatosis) is defined as facial nevus flammeus (port-wine stain) with cerebral lesions

TABLE 449–7 SIDE EFFECTS OF SOME COMMON EYE MEDICATIONS

Class	Indication	Generic Name	Trade Name	Systemic Side Effects
α_2-Agonists	Glaucoma	Apraclonidine Brimonidine	Iopidine Alphagan	Dry mouth, dry nose
β-Blockers	Glaucoma	Timolol	Timoptic, Betimol	Bradycardia, bronchospasm, hypotension, fatigue, depression, impotence, hypertriglyceridemia
		Betaxolol Carteolol Levobunolol Metipranolol	Betoptic Ocupress Betagan OptiPranolol	
Prostaglandin analogues	Glaucoma	Latanoprost, etc.	Xalatan Rescula Travatan	Trichomegaly, iridal hyperpigmentation
Topical NSAIDs	Moderate inflammation, cystoid macular edema	Acular		
Cycloplegics	Amblyopia treatment, iritis	Atropine Homatropine Cyclopentolate	Cyclogyl	Dry mouth, tachycardia, somnolence
Antihistamines	Seasonal allergies	Ketotifen Levocabastine Olopatadine	Zaditor Livostin Patanol	Headache
Mast cell stabilizers	Seasonal allergy, giant papillary conjunctivitis	Cromolyn Lodoxamide	Crolom, Opticrom Alomide	Headache
Vasoconstrictors	Hyperemia, allergy	Naphazoline	Vasocon-A Naphcon-A	Rebound hyperemia

NSAID = nonsteroidal anti-inflammatory drug.

or seizures. Diffuse involvement of the choroid, termed choroidal hemangioma in the ophthalmic literature, can be seen. The characteristic fundus is diffusely red, the so-called tomato catsup fundus. Children may remain asymptomatic, although retinal detachment is a common complication in adults. Glaucoma is a risk in patients with facial port-wine stains and may require surgical filtration.

Retinopathy of Prematurity

Premature and low-birth-weight infants who receive supplemental oxygen therapy are at risk to develop *retinopathy of prematurity,* an incomplete vascularization of the peripheral retina that may progress to retinal neovascularization, retinal detachment, and blindness in its most severe form. Previously called retrolental fibroplasia, it may produce leukocoria and be confused with retinoblastoma. Normal retinal vascularization begins at 16 weeks' gestation and is completed at 40 weeks' gestation. Although retinopathy of prematurity may rarely occur even in full-term infants, those at greatest risk weigh less than 1250 g at birth or have a gestational age younger than 28 weeks. The pathophysiology of retinopathy of prematurity has not been fully elucidated.

Initial examination of low-birth-weight infants should be performed before the child is discharged from the neonatal intensive care unit at approximately 4 weeks of age. Subsequent examinations to identify progression depend on the initial findings. The international classification of retinopathy of prematurity reflects the degree and location of fibrous proliferation and provides guidelines for intervention. Approximately 8% of infants who weigh less than 1250 g at birth require treatment. Of the infants who ultimately require treatment, more than 90% do so between 34 and 42 weeks after conception. Observation may be adequate in many cases in which spontaneous regression is seen. When treatment is required, laser or cryoablation of peripheral retinal tissue is usually adequate. More severe cases require pars plana vitrectomy and scleral buckling.

Genetic Disorders

The list of genetic abnormalities that exhibit ocular signs and symptoms is staggering.

Sickle cell disease (Chapter 167) is one of the more common causes of retinal vascular occlusive disease. Patients with SC disease are at greater risk for ocular complications than patients with SS disease. Like arterioles elsewhere in the body, peripheral retinal vessels may become occluded, producing focal infarction. Subsequent neovascularization may result in vitreous hemorrhage and retinal detachment. Neovascular fronds may undergo spontaneous regression or may require photocoagulation. Characteristic comma-shaped conjunctival vessels may be noted on slit lamp evaluation.

Trisomy 21 (Chapter 39) has been associated with strabismus, myopia, keratoconus, and cataract. Optometric and surgical interventions are based on the severity of systemic and ocular abnormalities. *Kearns-Sayre syndrome* (Chapter 59), a mitochondrial cytopathy demonstrating autosomal dominant inheritance, results in progressive external ophthalmoplegia. Diplopia is not common, and there is no known treatment. Either *ocular albinism* or *oculocutaneous albinism* may manifest as foveal hypoplasia, poor vision, and nystagmus. The former results from a decreased number of melanosomes and shows X-linked transmission. The latter results from decreased melanin granules within each melanosome and shows autosomal recessive transmission. Photophobia is common. Low vision aids may be of some help. *Marfan syndrome* (Chapter 281) is associated with many findings common to connective tissue disorders, including high myopia, lenticular subluxation, cataract, and colobomas. Lensectomy may be required. Inheritance is autosomal dominant.

Multisystem congenital hamartomatous diseases have been curiously called *phakomatoses* in the ophthalmic literature. *Von Hippel–Lindau disease* (Chapter 444), or *angiomatosis retinae,* is transmitted in autosomal dominant fashion. Early photocoagulation of retinal capillary hemangiomas may prevent exudation and retinal detachment. Cerebellar and visceral hemangiomas are common, and patients are at risk for renal cell carcinoma and pheochromocytoma. The ocular hamartomas of *von Recklinghausen's neurofibromatosis* (Chapter 444) include optic nerve glioma (astrocytic hamartoma), iris Lisch nodules, and plexiform neurofibromas of the eyelids. The optic nerve tumors are slowly progressive, producing painless loss of vision and proptosis. Approximately 50% of patients with neurofibromatosis develop optic nerve gliomas; bilateral tumors are pathognomonic for neurofibromatosis type 1. Lisch nodules are not seen in neurofibromatosis type 2. *Tuberous sclerosis* (Chapter 444) is less frequently associated with optic nerve gliomas, but retinal glial hamartomas are seen in combination with angiofibromas of the eyelids. Transmission is autosomal dominant.

Infections

Systemic infection may cause uveitis, endophthalmitis, retinitis, or choroiditis. Systemic severity often does not correlate with ocular activity. Ophthalmic manifestations may initiate diagnosis or may occur late in the disease.

Tuberculosis (Chapter 345) involves the uvea in approximately 1% of pulmonary cases. Iridocyclitis and diffuse choroiditis are the most common manifestations. Symptoms include painless progressive visual loss. Small yellow choroidal lesions may be seen, and retinal periphlebitis may occur secondarily. Intermediate- and second-strength purified protein derivative testing may be positive. Clinical response to a 3-week trial course of isoniazid strongly suggests tuberculosis.

Ocular complications of acquired *syphilis* (Chapter 340) occur in approximately 5% of patients with secondary syphilis, although symptoms may occur during any stage of the disease. Nearly any ocular structure may be involved. The more common presentations include anterior uveitis, neuroretinitis, and the syphilitic Argyll Robertson pupil in which miotic pupils react poorly to light but briskly to accommodation. Congenital syphilis produces "salt and pepper" pigmentation of the fundus.

Nerve fiber layer infarcts seen clinically as "cotton-wool" spots are the most common ocular manifestation of *acquired immunodeficiency syndrome* (AIDS) (Chapter 413). In combination with retinal hemorrhage, these lesions may mimic cytomegalovirus retinitis, another common finding in patients with AIDS. Additional ocular findings in AIDS include opportunistic infections of the retina, choroid, and optic nerve as well as cranial nerve palsies. Kaposi's sarcoma may occur in the lids, orbit, or conjunctiva.

Cytomegalovirus Retinitis

Cytomegalovirus retinitis may appear as subacute unilateral visual loss or vitreous floaters in immunocompromised patients. Large areas of hemorrhagic infarction are seen with minimal vitritis (Fig. 449–13). Intravenous ganciclovir (2.5 to 5.0 mg/kg every 8 to 12 hours intravenously for 2 to 3 weeks of induction) or foscarnet (e.g., 60 mg/kg intravenously every 8 hours for 2 weeks, with maintenance dose of 60 mg/kg daily for 5 to 7 days/week, adjusted on the basis of renal responses) and intravitreal ganciclovir (200 μg in 0.1 mL of water injected with a 30-gauge needle one to three times each week) are the mainstays of treatment. Even with aggressive treatment, recurrences are seen in up to 50% of cases. Herpes zoster and herpes simplex viruses may produce fulminating necrosis of the retina, *progressive outer retinal necrosis,* in patients with AIDS.

Toxoplasmosis

Until recently, ocular *toxoplasmosis* (Chapter 370) was thought to represent reactivation of congenital disease in nearly all cases; however, studies now suggest that many cases of toxoplasmosis retinitis are acquired after birth. Symptoms include reduced vision and floaters. The typical retinal fundus lesion comprises an active yellow satellite adjacent to an old chorioretinal scar with a dense overlying vitritis, the so-called headlight in the fog. Antibody titers, even in undiluted serum, are significant. Treatment requires combinations of systemic pyrimethamine, clindamycin, sulfonamides, prednisone, and folinic acid. These regimens are moderately efficacious and potentially toxic; treatment is therefore limited to severe intraocular inflammation that threatens the macular area. The toxoplasmosis fundus lesions seen in AIDS patients may differ morphologically from those seen in immunocompetent patients.

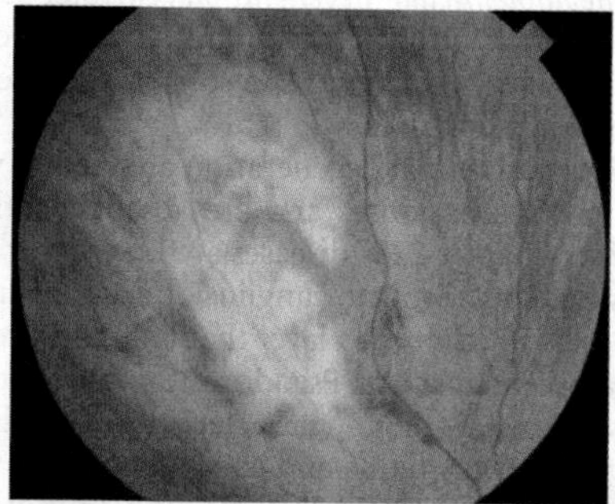

FIGURE 449–13 • Cytomegalovirus retinitis.

Idiopathic Inflammatory and Autoimmune Disorders

Autoimmune diseases may produce incidental ocular findings or may have their greatest effects in ocular tissues.

Dysthyroid Ophthalmopathy

Dysthyroid ophthalmopathy, commonly but erroneously called *Graves' ophthalmopathy* (Chapter 244), may be seen in hyperthyroid, euthyroid, or hypothyroid individuals. The orbital tissues and thyroid gland appear to be common targets of the same autoimmune process. Inflammation of the extraocular muscles and orbital fat causes proptosis, corneal exposure, and limited ocular motility (Fig. 449–14). Optic neuropathy may result from extreme proptosis with stretching of the nerve or from compression at the orbital apex. Lid retraction is common. Patients present with pain, decreased vision, diplopia, and vascular congestion. Active inflammation may be treated with systemic corticosteroids (e.g., initial dose of prednisone of 1 mg/kg/day for 1 week, tapered over 4 to 6 weeks). External beam irradiation, previously used as an alternative to prednisone, has been shown to be ineffective. Aggressive topical lubrication must be used. Emergent surgical decompression may be required when the optic nerve is threatened, but it may not reduce (and may exacerbate) inflammation. Surgical decompression of severe proptosis is usually deferred until inflammation is controlled and the clinical examination is stable for several months. Active inflammation generally subsides after 1 to 12 months. Secondary surgeries to correct chronic exposure, diplopia, and lid malposition may then be considered.

Sarcoidosis

Sarcoidosis (Chapter 95) is a common cause of intraocular inflammation among people of African descent, and chronic uveitis is seen in 25% of sarcoid patients. Sarcoid may also involve the optic nerve, cranial nerves, and lacrimal glands. Anterior uveitis is treated topically with prednisolone acetate in decreasing doses, depending on degree of inflammation, and with daily cycloplegics (cyclopentolate 2%, atropine 1%). Posterior uveitis, dacryoadenitis, and neurologic manifestations require systemic corticosteroids, but the doses have not been standardized.

Uveitis

Uveitis accompanies many autoimmune diseases, and there is often no correlation between ocular and systemic inflammatory activity. *Ankylosing spondylitis* (Chapter 286) is associated with acute, recurrent anterior uveitis in 25% of patients. Anterior uveitis or conjunctivitis is seen in nearly all patients with reactive arthritis (Chapter 286). Two to 12% of patients with *inflammatory bowel disease* (Chapter 144) develop anterior uveitis, which is also commonly found in patients with *psoriatic arthritis* but not with psoriasis alone (Chapters 286 and 464). Symptoms include decreased vision and photophobia. Treatment with topical corticosteroids (e.g., prednisolone acetate 1%, one drop in the affected eye or eyes every 1 to 6 hours while awake) is usually sufficient to control the ocular disease.

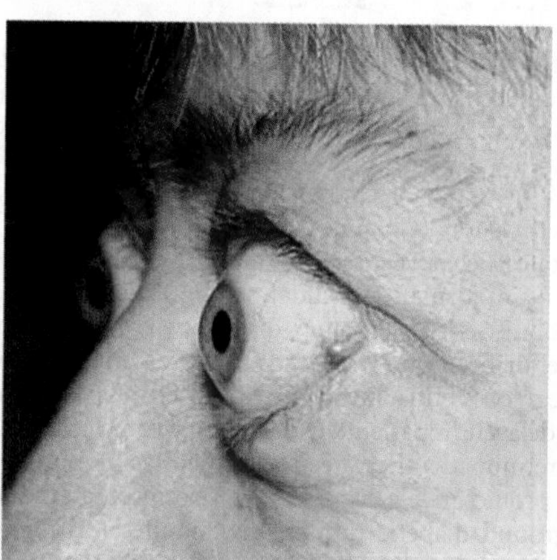

FIGURE 449–14 • Graves' ophthalmopathy with characteristic exophthalmos and eyelid retraction.

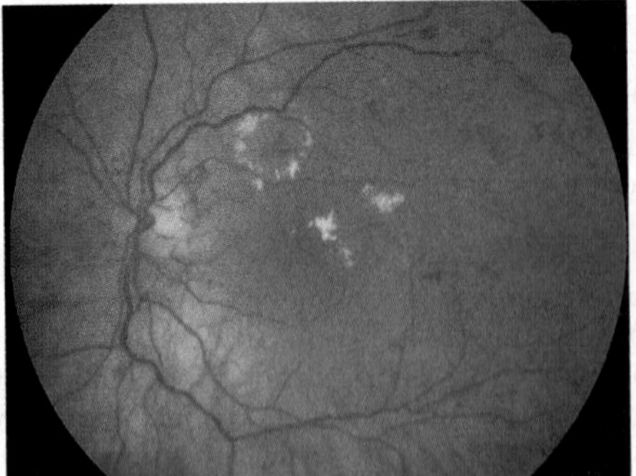

FIGURE 449–15 • Diabetic retinopathy. Fundus photograph of background (nonproliferative) diabetic retinopathy demonstrates scattered dot and blot intraretinal hemorrhages and retinal exudates. A circinate exudate is seen surrounding a microaneurysm.

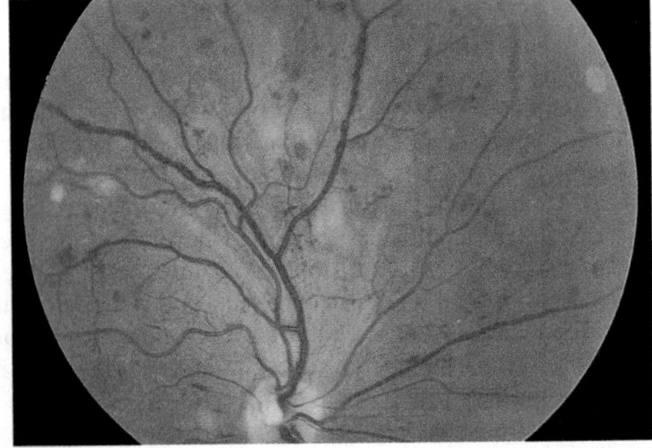

FIGURE 449–16 • Severe proliferative diabetic retinopathy with cotton-wool spots, intraretinal microvascular abnormalities, and venous bleeding. (From Yanoff M, Duker JS: Ophthalmology. London, CV Mosby, 1999, with permission.)

Juvenile Rheumatoid Arthritis

Chronic anterior uveitis may severely reduce vision in patients with *juvenile rheumatoid arthritis* (Chapter 285). The ocular disease is insidious and devastating; routine examinations are critical. Pauciarticular juvenile rheumatoid arthritis carries an 80 to 90% risk of uveitis, whereas uveitis is rarely seen in patients with systemic onset. Girls have a fourfold higher risk of uveitic involvement compared with boys. Patients are usually free of symptoms on diagnosis and must be carefully screened for eye involvement. Cataract is the rule, resulting from either inflammation or corticosteroid treatment. Early intervention with topical corticosteroids (e.g., prednisolone acetate 1%, one drop in the affected eye or eyes every 1 to 6 hours) may delay progression, and oral or intravenous corticosteroids may be required in advanced cases. Megadose pulsed intravenous corticosteroids (1 to 2 g intravenously in a single dose) may be equally efficacious while minimizing systemic side effects.

Uveomeningeal Syndrome

Vogt-Koyanagi-Harada syndrome (uveomeningeal syndrome), typically seen among more heavily pigmented peoples, may produce anterior or posterior uveitis. Decreased vision is the primary ocular symptom. Periocular vitiligo and whitening of the lashes (poliosis) may be seen. Chorioretinitis may lead to exudative retinal detachment. Early treatment with topical or systemic corticosteroids may delay or prevent severe visual loss.

Stevens-Johnson Syndrome

Stevens-Johnson syndrome, an idiosyncratic vesicular mucocutaneous eruption (Chapter 465), may be triggered by medications or infectious agents. Adolescents are most frequently affected. Conjunctival involvement may lead to cicatrization and obliteration of the fornices with secondary entropion, loss of mucus-producing goblet cells, and corneal opacification. Aggressive lubrication in the acute stage may mitigate these sequelae. Reconstructive grafting with mucous membranes and amniotic membranes may be helpful. Penetrating keratoplasty alone is rarely successful.

Metabolic Diseases

Systemic metabolic diseases demonstrate protean ocular findings. Select metabolic diseases may be evident only in the eye. In either case, ocular findings can assist in diagnosis and ongoing evaluation.

Diabetic Retinopathy

Diabetic retinopathy (Chapter 247) is a leading cause of blindness in the United States. Selective loss of pericytes in the retinal capillaries leads to microaneurysm formation, exudation, capillary obliteration, and neovascularization. Twenty years after diagnosis, virtually all patients with juvenile-onset diabetes and two thirds of those with adult-onset diabetes have some degree of retinal involvement. Onset and progression of retinal findings are delayed in patients with tight glycemic control. [5]

Diabetic retinopathy has been classified as nonproliferative (Fig. 449–15) or proliferative (Fig. 449–16). Nonproliferative disease, also called background diabetic retinopathy, manifests as microaneurysms, intraretinal hemorrhages, subretinal exudation, venous beading, and intraretinal vascular abnormalities. Macular edema, the most frequent cause of visual loss, is common in this stage. Macular edema meeting the criteria of the Early Treatment Diabetic Retinopathy Study [6] is treated with focal laser photocoagulation. This study concluded that focal laser photocoagulation reduced the incidence of moderate visual loss by 50% in patients who demonstrated clinically significant macular edema, defined as (1) retinal thickening within 500 μm of the fovea, (2) subretinal exudates within 500 μm of the fovea with adjacent retinal thickening, or (3) an area of retinal thickening of greater than one disc diameter, any part of which lies within one disc diameter of the fovea.

Retinal ischemia is thought to be the primary stimulus to proliferative diabetic retinopathy, in which extraretinal fibrovascular tissue grows along the posterior vitreous scaffold. Neovascularization at the optic disc or elsewhere may lead to vitreous hemorrhage and acute loss of vision. Fibrous organization produces tractional detachment of the retina. Proliferative disease meeting the criteria set forth in the Diabetic Retinopathy Study is treated with panretinal laser photocoagulation. This multicenter, randomized study [7] determined that panretinal laser photocoagulation reduced the incidence of severe visual loss from 16 to 6% in patients at high risk for vitreous hemorrhage. These patients were defined by (1) neovascularization of greater than one third of the optic nerve head, (2) neovascularization elsewhere associated with vitreous hemorrhage, (3) any degree of neovascularization of the disc associated with vitreous hemorrhage, or (4) any two of the following: retinal hemorrhages in four quadrants, venous beading in two quadrants, or intraretinal microvascular anomalies in one quadrant. Advanced cases may require pars plana vitrectomy with peeling of preretinal fibrovascular membranes.

Diabetics are at increased risk for painless, isolated cranial nerve palsies, most frequently involving cranial nerve III or VI and generally resolving in 6 to 8 weeks. Multiple cranial nerve palsies should prompt thorough and rapid investigation including magnetic resonance imaging of the brain with careful attention to the brain stem and cavernous sinus. In the setting of acute hyperglycemia, accumulation of lenticular sorbitol may lead to lenticular swelling. Secondary refractive errors may linger for 6 to 8 weeks after glycemic control is realized; spectacle correction may change dramatically over this period, and prescription should be delayed until the examination stabilizes.

Wilson's Hepatolenticular Degeneration

Accumulation of copper in the posterior cornea may aid in the diagnosis of *Wilson's hepatolenticular degeneration* (Chapter 230), although its appearance usually lags neurologic symptoms. This characteristic Kayser-Fleischer ring fades after treatment. The so-called sunflower cataract is seen less frequently in such cases.

Corneal clouding and retinal degeneration are seen to varying degrees in specific mucopolysaccharidoses and are absent in others. *Tay-Sachs* and *Niemann-Pick* (Chapter 223) diseases are known for the appearance of a foveal cherry-red spot owing to ganglioside accumulation within perifoveal ganglion cells, which form a layer that is absent over the fovea and thickest in the adjacent macula. Pseudoxanthoma elasticum (Chapter 281) is often associated with its characteristic angioid streaks of the retina. *Gyrate atrophy* of the retina and choroid occurs in the presence of increased serum ornithine caused by ornithine aminotransferase deficiency. Progressive geographic atrophy eventually involves the macula.

Corneal, conjunctival, and retinal crystalline deposits may be seen in *cystinosis*. Vision is usually unaffected, but corneal involvement may cause photophobia (pain on exposure to light). Conjunctivitis, iritis, and scleritis experienced during attacks of gout (Chapter 294) usually abate with systemic control.

Neoplastic Diseases

Metastatic ocular disease and systemic neoplastic proliferations involving the eye are far more common than primary ocular malignancy. Pediatric metastases tend to involve the orbit, whereas the vascular choroid is usually affected in adults. Choroidal metastases are seen most commonly with adenocarcinoma of the breast in women (Chapter 208); primary lung tumors (Chapter 201) are the leading cause in men. Together, breast and lung carcinomas account for 70% of ocular metastases. Left eye involvement surpasses right eye involvement by a ratio of 3:2 because of the direct connection between the aorta and the left common carotid artery. Decreased visual acuity is the leading symptom. In the case of breast carcinoma, nearly 70% of patients already carry the diagnosis when choroidal disease is detected. In contrast, choroidal metastases from lung disease may be the initial finding in 90% of cases. Disfiguring surgery such as enucleation or orbital exenteration should be limited to patients with severe pain.

Multiple Myeloma

Ocular findings in *multiple myeloma* (Chapter 198) include uveal protein-filled cysts and retinal hemorrhages second to hyperviscosity. Orbital involvement is rare, but periocular osteolytic lesions may be seen. Patients should undergo ophthalmic examination at the time of diagnosis. External beam radiation may be dramatically effective. Although B-cell *lymphoma* (Chapter 196) of the large cell variety is the most common lymphoma to involve the eye, it involves the eye with much less frequency than does leukemia. *Leukemic* ocular disease (Chapters 194 and 195) may masquerade as a chronic, unilateral "uveitis" or may cause white-centered retinal hemorrhages similar to the Roth spots (Fig. 449–17) seen in infectious endocarditis (Chapter 76). Focal irradiation maybe used to augment systemic treatment with either entity.

Orbital and conjunctival lymphomas are usually the small B-cell mucosa-associated lymphoid tissue (MALT) variety. Approximately 50% of cases ultimately include systemic disease, sometimes decades later. Systemic evaluation should include chest, abdominal, and pelvic magnetic resonance imaging as well as serum protein electrophoresis and possibly bone marrow biopsy. External beam radiation is used to treat isolated periocular disease, whereas systemic chemotherapy is required for systemic involvement.

Vascular Diseases

Because the retinal vasculature is uniquely accessible for direct visual inspection, nearly all systemic vascular diseases manifest ocular changes.

Hypertension

Chronic *hypertension* (Chapter 66) produces characteristic retinal vascular findings that can be used to identify and assess progression of the disease. Arterial narrowing, nicking at arteriovenous crossings, nerve fiber layer infarcts, and intraretinal hemorrhages characterize hypertensive retinopathy. Arteriolar sclerosis heightens the arterial light reflexes. Moderately sclerosed arterioles demonstrate "copper wiring," whereas severely sclerosed vessels show "silver wiring." Acute hypertension may produce optic nerve edema (Fig. 449–18) and serous retinal detachments that shift dramatically when the patient changes position. These detachments usually resolve without significant sequelae if blood pressure is brought under control.

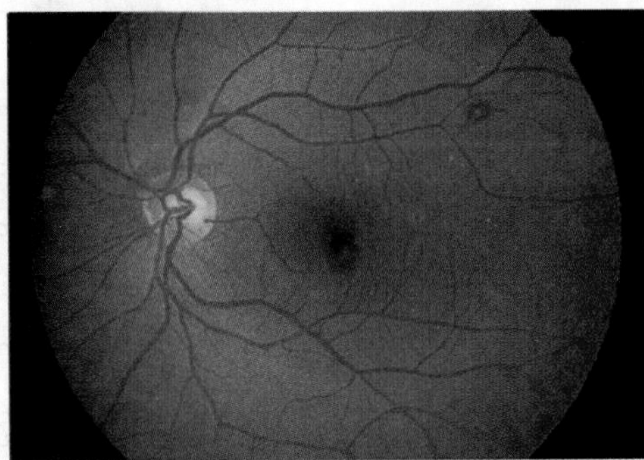

FIGURE 449–17 • Roth's spots. Multiple white-centered hemorrhages in a man with recurrent subacute bacterial endocarditis. White-centered hemorrhages are also seen with leukemia and diabetes. The small white scars are probably the residua of previous episodes.

Hypertension may be implicated in retinal vascular occlusions. *Branch retinal vein occlusion* may cause macular edema and decreased visual acuity or may be asymptomatic. Occlusion typically occurs at an arteriovenous crossing where a common adventitia binds the vessels together and causes compression of the venule wall by the sclerotic arteriole. Sectoral hemorrhages are seen. Regional photocoagulation may help to resolve macular edema but rarely improves functional outcome and is therefore not frequently advised. Neovascularization is a rare complication, and most eyes maintain a favorable prognosis. *Central retinal vein occlusion* (Fig. 449–19) is a more severe disease entity. Ischemic and nonischemic varieties are recognized and are most accurately differentiated by ERG. The characteristic fundus appearance includes dilated tortuous vessels in all quadrants as well as variable degrees of retinal hemorrhage. Nonischemic occlusion may result from hyperviscosity, whereas ischemic occlusion is thought to represent arteriolar impingement on the central retinal vein at the level of the lamina cribrosa. Neovascularization of the iris or retina, occurring in up to 52% of cases, usually occurs 3 months after the initial insult. Panretinal photocoagulation should be deferred until neovascularization is detected.

In contrast to venous occlusive disease, *central retinal artery occlusion* (Fig. 449–20) is not generally associated with systemic hypertension. Emboli result most commonly from carotid stenosis (Chapter 430), but endocarditis and cardiac thromboemboli are other potential sources. Unilateral sudden loss of vision is typical. Amaurosis fugax, or transient unilateral visual loss, may precede frank occlusion and warrants urgent carotid evaluation. Fundus examination reveals a characteristic cherry-red spot that reflects diffuse opacification of the infarcting macula contrasted to the hyperpigmented fovea. An RAPD is present. An acute reduction in intraocular pressure by means of ocular massage, anterior chamber paracentesis, or systemic carbonic anhydrase inhibitors may dislodge a proximal embolus, allow reperfusion of the fovea, and return some useful vision if performed within several hours of onset. *Branch retinal artery occlusion* may go unnoticed by the patient despite a permanent visual *scotoma* (focal visual field defect).

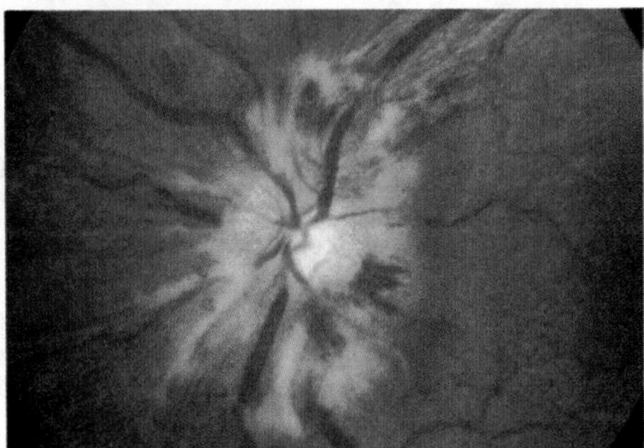

FIGURE 449–18 • Papilledema in a young person. Note disc swelling, hemorrhages, and exudates, with preservation of the physiologic cup.

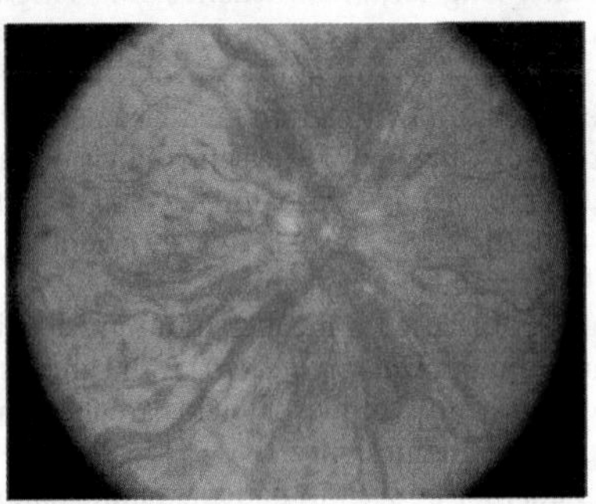

FIGURE 449–19 • Central retinal vein occlusion with diffuse intraretinal hemorrhages in all four quadrants.

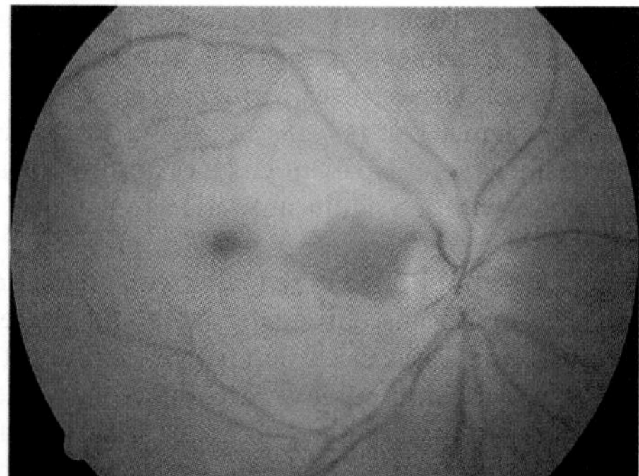

FIGURE 449–20 • Central retinal artery occlusion. Fundus photograph shows diffuse retinal edema. The heavily pigmented fovea with its uniquely thin inner retina produces a cherry-red spot against the dusky macula. In this case, a small area of retina adjacent to the optic disc is spared, owing to the presence of a cilioretinal artery.

Temporal Arteritis

Temporal arteritis (Chapter 292) is an important cause of visual loss among elderly persons. Symptoms include sudden, unilateral loss of vision. Headache, jaw claudication, scalp tenderness, weight loss, and malaise are common. Visual loss may result from arteritic optic neuropathy or associated central retinal artery occlusion. The erythrocyte sedimentation rate (ESR) is elevated. Systemic corticosteroids (prednisone, 1 to 2 mg/kg/day) should be initiated as soon as the diagnosis is suspected, and temporal artery biopsy should be performed within 7 days after beginning treatment. Corticosteroids are tapered slowly over months, and many patients require perpetual low-dose corticosteroid treatment as guided by following the ESR. If untreated, approximately 65% of patients lose vision in the contralateral eye.

Wegener's Granulomatosis

Orbital involvement in *Wegener's granulomatosis* (Chapter 291) usually indicates extension from nasal or sinus mucosa and may produce proptosis. Ocular vasculitis may cause inflammation in any of the ocular tissues. Retinal involvement in *polyarteritis nodosa* (Chapter 291) is usually limited to the small vessels, although central retinal artery occlusion can occur. Cranial nerve palsies are not uncommon. The occlusive vasculitis of *Behçet's disease* (Chapter 291) produces retinal vasculitis and iridocyclitis in patients aged 20 to 40 years. Hypopyon (layering of leukocytes within the anterior chamber) can be seen in one third of cases. Topical corticosteroids are used to treat anterior disease, whereas systemic corticosteroids and cytotoxic agents may be required for posterior disease.

Ocular Effects of Systemic Medications

Thousands of systemic medications have been implicated in reports of ocular side effects (Table 449–8). Therefore, patients taking systemic medications often require periodic surveillance to identify ocular toxicity. A few of the more common associations are described here.

Chloroquine and *hydroxychloroquine* may cause decreased color vision and visual field defects at high doses. Chloroquine toxicity is thought to occur after a cumulative dose of 300 g, whereas hydroxychloroquine may cause symptoms after long-term maintenance of 750 mg/day. The fundus develops a typical bull's-eye pattern, and corneal whorls may be seen. Symptoms are not reversible and tend to progress after drug cessation. Annual fundus examination with automated visual field test is indicated.

Pigmentary maculopathy may arise as blurred vision in patients taking *thioridazine* or *chlorpromazine.* Approximately 800 mg/day of the former or 1200 mg/day of the latter is believed sufficient to cause toxicity. Patients should be examined every 6 months.

Any of the commonly used antituberculous medications may cause optic neuropathy, although *ethambutol* carries the greatest risk. Pupillary response, color vision, acuity, and visual fields are the clinical parameters used to assess optic nerve function.

Cornea verticillata may be seen in patients taking *amiodarone* because of lysosomal accumulations within the epithelial basement membrane. *Fabry's disease* produces similar changes, as can other medications.

TABLE 449–8 SYSTEMIC MEDICATIONS WITH OCULAR EFFECTS

Agent	Effect
Chloroquine	Dyschromatopsia, visual field defects
Hydroxychloroquine	Dyschromatopsia, visual field defects
Thioridazine	Blurred vision
Chlorpromazine	Blurred vision
Digoxin	Yellow vision
Ethambutol	Optic neuritis
Amiodarone	Corneal whorls, pigmentary retinopathy
Corticosteroids	Glaucoma, cataract
Plaquenil	Pigmentary maculopathy
Tamoxifen	Retinopathy
Neuroleptics	Nystagmus
Compazine	Oculogyric crisis
Vitamin A	Pseudotumor cerebri
5-Fluorouracil	Canalicular stenosis (tearing)
Isotretinoin	Severe dry eye (long-term effect)

Corneal whorls are usually reversible when caused by drug toxicity, and they rarely interfere with vision.

Systemic *corticosteroids* are associated with the same ocular side effects as topical corticosteroids, including glaucoma and posterior subcapsular cataract.

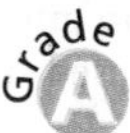

1. Pflugfelder SC, Maskin SL, Anderson B, et al: A randomized, double-masked, placebo-controlled, multicenter comparison of loteprednol etabonate ophthalmic suspension, 0.5%, and placebo for treatment of keratoconjunctivitis sicca in patients with delayed tear clearance. Am J Ophthalmol 2004;138:444–457.
2. Perry HD, Doshi-Carnevale S, Donnenfeld ED, et al: Efficacy of commercially available topical cyclosporine A 0.05% in the treatment of meibomian gland dysfunction. Cornea 2006;25:171–175.
3. Clemons TE, Rankin MW, McBee WL: Age-Related Eye Disease Study Research Group. Cognitive impairment in the age-related eye disease study: AREDS Report No. 16. Arch Ophthalmol 2006;124:537–543.
4. Rosenfeld PJ, Brown DM, Heier JS, et al: Ranibizumab for neovascular age-related macular degeneration. N Engl J Med 2006; 355:1419–1431.
5. Diabetes Control and Complications Trial Research Group: Progression of retinopathy with intensive versus conventional treatment in the Diabetes Control and Complications Trial. Ophthalmology 1995;102:647–661.
6. Early Treatment Diabetic Retinopathy Study Research Group: Early photocoagulation for diabetic retinopathy. ETDRS report #9. Ophthalmology 1991;98:766–785.
7. Photocoagulation treatment of proliferative diabetic retinopathy. Clinical application of Diabetic Retinopathy Study (DRS) findings, DRS Report Number 8. The Diabetic Retinopathy Study Research Group. Ophthalmology 1981;88:583–600.

SUGGESTED READINGS

Asbell PA, Dualan I, Mindel J, et al: Age-related cataract. Lancet 2005;365: 599–609. *A comprehensive review.*

de Jong P: Age-related macular degeneration. N Engl J Med 2006;355:1474–1485. *A clinical overview.*

Holmes JM, Clarke MP: Amblyopia. Lancet 2006;367:1343–1351. *A comprehensive review.*

Lynn WA, Lightman S: The eye in systemic infection. Lancet 2004;364:1439–1450. *A useful review.*

Sakimoto T, Rosenblatt MI, Azar DT: Laser eye surgery for refractive errors. Lancet 2006;367:1432–1447. *A comprehensive review.*

Vitale S, Cotch MF, Sperduto RD: Prevalence of visual impairment in the United States. JAMA 2006;295:2158–2163. *Visual impairment due to uncorrected refractive error is common in the U.S.*

Wirbelauer C: Management of the red eye for the primary care physician. Am J Med 2006;119:302–306. *A comprehensive review.*

Wong TY, Mitchell P: Hypertensive retinopathy. N Engl J Med 2004;351: 2310–2317. *Excellent review with clear color pictures.*

NEURO-OPHTHALMOLOGY

Robert W. Baloh

A mechanistic understanding of vision impairment along with disturbances in pupillary and oculomotor control lies close to the heart of diagnosing neurologic disorders.

VISION

One of the most difficult diagnostic problems is vision loss that cannot be explained by obvious abnormalities of the eye. To evaluate such a patient properly, the examining physician must be familiar with the anatomy and physiology of the afferent visual system. The afferent visual pathways cross the major ascending sensory and descending motor systems of the cerebral hemispheres and in their anterior portion are intimately related to the vascular and bony structures at the base of the brain. Not surprisingly, localization of lesions within the afferent visual pathways has great value in neurologic diagnosis.

Anatomy of the Visual Pathways

Light entering the eye falls on the retinal rods and cones, which transduce the stimulus into neural impulses to be transmitted to the brain. The distribution of visual function across the retina takes a pattern of concentric zones increasing in sensitivity toward the center, the fovea. The fovea consists of a "rod-free" central grouping of approximately 100,000 slender cones. The ganglion cells subserving these cones send their axons directly to the temporal aspect of the optic disc, where they form the papillomacular bundle. Axons originating from ganglion cells in the temporal retina curve above and below the papillomacular bundle and form dense arcuate bands.

The arteries supplying the optic nerve and retina derive from branches of the ophthalmic artery. The central retinal artery approaches the eye along each optic nerve and pierces the inferior aspect of the dural sheath about 1 cm behind the globe to enter the center of the nerve. The artery emerges in the fundus at the center of the nerve head, from which it nourishes the inner two thirds of the retina by superior and inferior branches. Anastomotic branches derived from the choroidal and posterior ciliary arteries, the ciliary system, supply the choroid, optic nerve head, and outer retinal layers, including the photoreceptors. In about 10% of the population, the macula is supplied by a retinociliary artery, a branch of the ciliary system. Venous drainage from the retina and nerve head flows primarily via the central retinal vein, whose course of exit from the eye parallels that of entry of the artery.

What each eye "sees" is termed its *visual field* (Fig. 450–1). The nasal side of the left retina and the temporal side of the right see the left side of the world, and the upper half of each retina sees the lower half of the world. Behind the eyes the optic nerves pass through the optic canal to form the optic chiasm. In the chiasm, nerves from the nasal half of each retina decussate and join the fibers from the temporal half of the contralateral retina. From the chiasm, the optic tracts pass around the cerebral peduncles to reach the lateral geniculate ganglia. The orientation of the visual field is rotated 90 degrees in the lateral geniculate such that images from the inferior visual field project to the medial half whereas images from the superior visual field project to the lateral half. The geniculocalcarine radiation initially fans out into superolateral and inferolateral projections, the latter passing around the lateral ventricle and for a short distance into the temporal lobe (Meyer's loop) before turning posteriorly to reach the striate cortex of the occipital lobe. In the occipital lobe, the striate cortex (area 17) lies along the superior and inferior bands of the calcarine fissure, with macular fibers projecting most posteriorly to the occipital pole and more peripheral retinal projections lying more anteriorly.

Localization of Lesions within Visual Pathways

Monocular vision loss is due to a lesion in one eye or optic nerve. Binocular visual loss, on the other hand, can result from disease located anywhere in the visual pathways from the corneas to the occipital poles. Lesions involving the optic chiasm produce nonhomonymous visual abnormalities (e.g., the bitemporal hemianopia illustrated by lesion 3 in Fig. 450–1). Optic tract abnormalities are comparatively rare but produce characteristic visual changes. The fibers serving identical points in the homonymous half fields do not fully commingle in the optic tract, so lesions damaging this structure produce incongruous homonymous hemianopia. Lesions of the geniculate nuclei, optic radiations, or visual cortex produce congruent hemianopic field defects that may go unrecognized unless the hemianopia intrudes on macular vision. Postgeniculate visual loss can be differentiated from pregeniculate visual loss by (1) a normal funduscopic appearance, (2) intact pupillary light reactions, and (3) appropriate lesions on brain imaging.

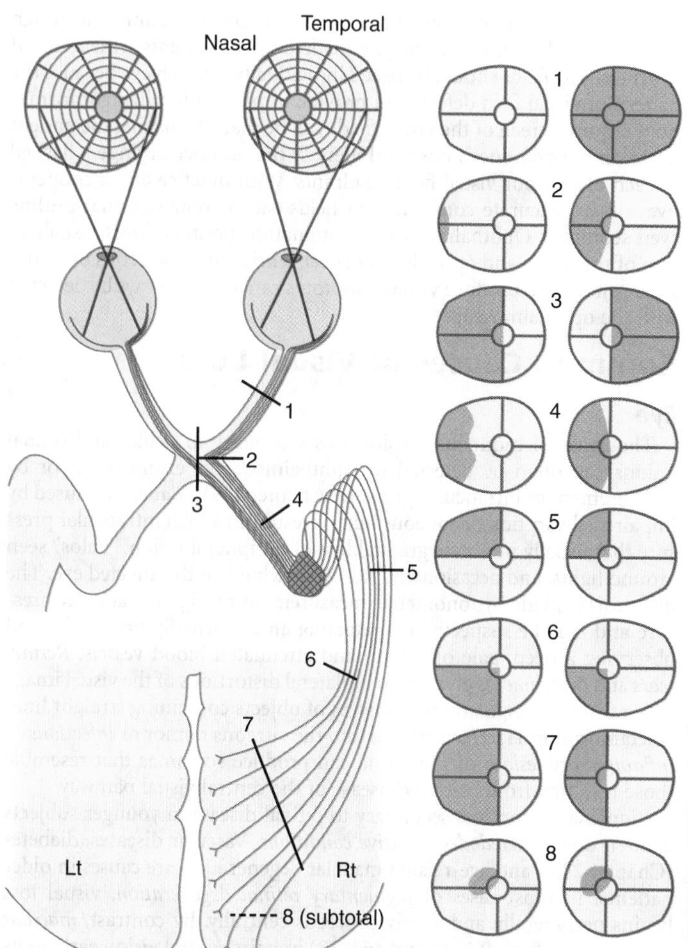

FIGURE 450–1 • Visual fields that accompany damage to the visual pathways. 1, Optic nerve: unilateral amaurosis. 2, Lateral optic chiasm: grossly incongruous, incomplete (contralateral) homonymous hemianopia. 3, Central optic chiasm: bitemporal hemianopia. 4, Optic tract: incongruous, incomplete homonymous hemianopia. 5, Temporal (Meyer's) loop of the optic radiation: congruous partial or complete (contralateral) homonymous superior quadrantanopia. 6, Parietal (superior) projection of the optic radiation: congruous partial or complete homonymous inferior quadrantanopia. 7, Complete parieto-occipital interruption of the optic radiation: complete congruous homonymous hemianopia with psychophysical shift of the foveal point, often sparing central vision and resulting in "macular sparing." 8, Incomplete damage to the visual cortex: congruous homonymous scotomas, usually encroaching at least acutely on central vision.

Examination of the Afferent Visual System

Visual function is most commonly assessed by "best-corrected visual acuity" (Chapter 449). If visual acuity is not normal, it must be determined whether acuity can be improved with lenses or at least with the use of a pinhole. The normal reference is recognition of letters at an idealized 20 feet, and acuity charts are designed with even larger letters that are normally recognized at proportionally greater distances. Thus, if one reads letters at 20 feet no better than those normally perceived at 40 feet, vision is recorded as 20/40. Small visual charts that are easily carried in the physician's case permit quick and fairly accurate bedside appraisal of acuity.

Visual fields can be tested at the bedside by confrontation, and rough estimates of their integrity can be made even in patients with reduced alertness. The fields should be tested individually for each eye because the pattern of visual field defects can provide important localizing information. A quick screen of the visual fields can be made by having the patient fixate on the examiner's nose and identify the number of fingers flashed in each of the four visual field quadrants. With practice and a cooperative subject, accurate confrontation fields can be obtained that outline even scotomas. Ophthalmoscopic examination permits direct visualization of the retina and optic disc. Corneal, lenticular, or vitreous opacities severe enough to produce visual symptoms can almost always be detected with the ophthalmoscope.

Common Causes of Visual Loss

Eye

The cause of monocular vision loss secondary to ocular and retinal lesions can often be detected by ophthalmoscopic examination or by measurement of intraocular pressure (Chapter 449). *Glaucoma* caused by impaired absorption of aqueous humor results in a high intraocular pressure that usually produces gradual loss of peripheral vision, "halos" seen around lights, and occasionally, pain and redness in the affected eye. The diagnosis is made by tonometric measurement of high intraocular pressure and may be suspected by palpating an abnormally firm globe and observing a deep, pale optic cup and attenuated blood vessels. *Retinal tears* and *detachments* give rise to unilateral distortions of the visual image seen as sudden angulations or curves of objects containing straight lines (metamorphopsia). *Hemorrhages* into the vitreous humor or *infections* or *inflammatory lesions* of the retina can produce scotomas that resemble those resulting from primary disease of the central visual pathway.

Binocular vision loss secondary to retinal disease in younger subjects is often due to *heredodegenerative conditions.* Vascular diseases, diabetes (Chapter 247), and age-related macular degeneration are causes in older patients. In most cases of *pigmentary retinal degeneration,* visual loss begins peripherally and slowly proceeds centrally. By contrast, *macular degeneration* (Figs. 465–11 and 465–12) impairs central vision early in its course. A common variant in the complement factor H (*CFH*) gene is associated with a markedly increased risk for the development of age-related macular degeneration.

Optic Nerve

Acute or subacute monocular vision loss as a result of optic nerve disease is most commonly produced by demyelinating disorders, vascular obstruction, neoplasm, or hereditary optic neuropathy. Demyelinating disease of the nerve head (*optic neuritis* or *papillitis*) produces disc edema along with loss of central vision in the affected eye only; subjectively unrecognized scotomas may sometimes be found in the other eye. Demyelination of the optic nerve behind the point where the retinal vein emerges (*retrobulbar neuritis*) initially leaves a normal-looking disc but a central or paracentral scotoma. With chronic demyelinating disorders, the optic disc becomes pale and atrophic. In more than 50% of patients initially seen with optic neuritis, typical symptoms and signs of multiple sclerosis eventually develop (Chapter 436). If associated periventricular white matter lesions are present on magnetic resonance imaging (MRI), treatment with high-dose steroids (intravenous methylprednisolone, 1 g/day for 3 days, followed by oral prednisone, 1 mg/kg/day for 11 days) and interferon beta reduces the short-term risk for development of multiple sclerosis. Intraocular arterial occlusion may produce either central visual loss or an altitudinal field defect (*ischemic optic neuropathy*). Common causes of transient monocular vision loss and their differential features are listed in Table 450–1. *Tumors* (Chapter 199) invading the optic nerve or space-occupying lesions compressing it anywhere between the orbit and chiasm cause gradually decreasing central vision or a sector defect of the peripheral visual field. With such chronic lesions, the affected optic nerve becomes visibly atrophic.

Acute binocular vision loss resulting from bilateral optic nerve disease is most often caused by demyelinating disease or by toxic or nutritional factors (Chapter 443). In younger persons and those lacking a clear history of toxic exposure, demyelinating lesions overwhelmingly predominate. Symptoms are of abrupt or subacute onset with visual blurring, which may progress rapidly to blindness within hours or days. There may be pain about the eyes, particularly with movement. *Leber's optic neuropathy,* caused by a mutation in mitochondrial DNA, typically begins painlessly and centrally in one eye, with the second eye affected weeks to months later.

Papilledema is disc edema secondary to increased intracranial pressure (Fig. 449–18). Vision is normal except under one of two circumstances: (1) acute transient episodes of amaurosis lasting a few seconds and attributable to acute increases in intracranial pressure (plateau waves) and (2) progressive loss of peripheral vision with long-standing, severe papilledema caused by compression of the optic nerve head. Table 450–2 gives the main differential points between papilledema and optic neuritis. Subacute or chronic binocular vision loss secondary to optic nerve disease can result from *toxic* and *nutritional* causes or from *inherited optic atrophy.* The latter sometimes accompanies spinocerebellar degeneration but may selectively affect the optic nerve. With either cause, visual loss is painless and primarily affects central vision; ophthalmoscopy shows optic atrophy.

TABLE 450–2 DIFFERENTIATION OF OPTIC NEURITIS FROM PAPILLEDEMA

	Optic Neuritis	Papilledema
Central-cecocentral vision loss	Present	Absent
Distribution	Usually unilateral	Usually bilateral
Ocular pain on movement	Present	Absent
Direct light reflex	±Reduced	Intact
CT and MRI of head	White matter plaques	Tumor, venous occlusion, etc.
Visual evoked responses	Abnormal	Normal
Lumbar puncture pressure	Normal	Elevated

CT = computed tomography; MRI = magnetic resonance imaging.

TABLE 450–1 COMMON CAUSES OF TRANSIENT MONOCULAR VISION LOSS

Category (Typical Duration)	Causes	Differential Features
Thromboembolism (1–5 min)	Atherosclerosis	Other atherosclerotic vascular disease, associated crossed hemiparesis, angiography (carotid atheroma)
	Cardiac	Valvar disease, mural thrombi, atrial fibrillation, recent myocardial infarction
	Blood dyscrasia	Blood tests positive for sickle cell anemia, macroglobulinemia, multiple myeloma, polycythemia, etc.
Vasospasm (5–30 min)	Migraine	Ipsilateral headache, other classic aura, family history
Vascular compression (few seconds)	Increased intracranial pressure	Precipitated by position change, Valsalva maneuver, or pressure waves
	Tumor	Associated slowly progressive monocular visual loss
Vasculitis (1–5 min)	Temporal arteritis	Associated headache, polymyalgia rheumatica, palpable temporal artery, elevated sedimentation rate

Chiasm and Optic Tract

Patients with lesions of the optic chiasm or optic tract are often unaware of visual impairment until the deficit encroaches on central vision in one or both eyes. Intrinsic or extrinsic neoplasms and parachiasmal arterial aneurysms are the most common lesions in this location. Gliomas that arise within the chiasm or optic tract are rare in adulthood. Extrinsic lesions compressing the chiasm or tract include *pituitary adenomas* (Chapter 242), *dysgerminomas, craniopharyngiomas, meningiomas* (Chapter 199), and large *aneurysms* of the carotid or basilar artery (Chapter 430). The diagnosis rests on finding the characteristic visual field abnormalities (bitemporal hemianopia for chiasm and incongruous homonymous hemianopia for optic tract lesions) and identifying the lesion with computed tomography or MRI. Pituitary apoplexy secondary to acute hemorrhage into the gland (Chapter 242) can result in sudden vision loss; prompt neurosurgical intervention under steroid coverage is required for most patients.

Visual Radiations and Occipital Cortex

Lesions involving the postgeniculate visual pathways most often result from *vascular damage, traumatic injuries, neoplasms,* or rarely, *inflammatory* or *degenerative disorders* involving the cerebral white matter. Their localization can be deduced by the resulting visual field defects. Vascular disease of the occipital lobes is the most common cause of homonymous visual field defects in the middle-aged and elderly population. *Anton's syndrome* refers to cerebral visual loss with denial of a visual defect. Affected patients not only deny the fact that they are blind but also confabulate details of their visual environment from memory. Anton's syndrome results from bilateral lesions involving the parieto-occipital lobes or in the setting of metabolic encephalopathy. The reversible *posterior leukoencephalopathy syndrome,* which is characterized by headache, seizures, and cortical visual loss, is associated with an abrupt increase in blood pressure and with immunosuppressive therapy after transplantation.

PUPILLARY CONTROL

The neuromechanisms that control pupil size and reactivity are complex, yet they can be evaluated by simple clinical procedures. The diameter of the pupil is determined by the antagonistic actions of the iris sphincter and dilator muscles, with the latter playing a minor role. If the sphincter muscle is severed or ruptured, it does not retract toward one quadrant but rather continues to function, except in the altered segment. Therefore, pupillary response can be evaluated even in the presence of significant damage to the iris.

Anatomy and Localization of Lesions within Pupillary Pathways

The size of the pupil is governed by tonic balance between sympathetic and parasympathetic innervation of the muscles of the iris. Sympathetic stimulation dilates the pupil, whereas parasympathetic stimulation constricts it. In the normal resting state, light entering the eye provides the major stimulus governing the size of the pupil (Fig. 450–2). Light activates the retinal rods and cones, with maximal sensitivity in the macular area. The optic nerve fibers follow the crossed and uncrossed visual pathways to the pregeniculate portion of the optic tracts, where the receptor fibers for light diverge to the pretectal nucleus located at the midbrain-diencephalic junction. Interneurons project from this nucleus to the Edinger-Westphal nuclei atop the midbrain third nerve nuclear complex of either side. From that point, paired parasympathetic efferents leave the midbrain in the third nerves, travel in the interpeduncular space across the petroclinoid ligament and edge of the tentorium, traverse the cavernous sinus, and then enter the orbit through the superior orbital fissure. In the orbit, the parasympathetic efferents synapse in the ciliary ganglion, from which ciliary nerves enter the eye to reach the pupillary muscles.

The principal sympathetic control of the pupil originates in the ventral lateral hypothalamus (first-order neuron), from which fibers descend ipsilaterally through the brain stem tegmentum and thence to the cervical cord, where they synapse with preganglionic neurons in the intermedial lateral column of the upper three thoracic segments. Preganglionic fibers (second-order neurons) emerge with the ventral roots of C8, T1, and T2 and ascend in the neck to synapse in the superior cervical ganglion adjacent to the base of the skull. Postganglionic (third-order

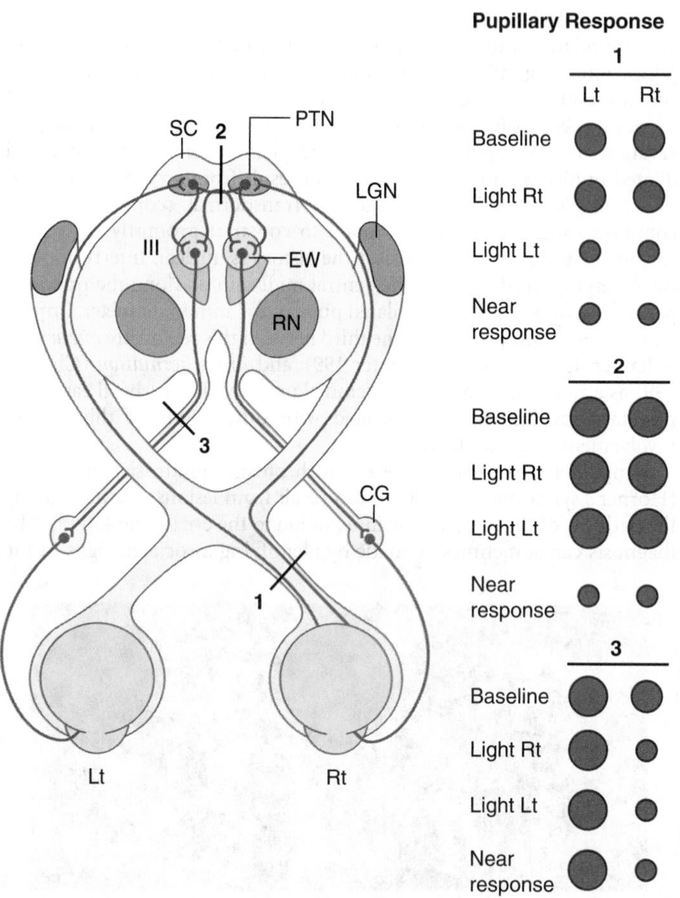

FIGURE 450–2 • Pupillary responses associated with lesions of the (1) optic nerve, (2) pretectum, and (3) oculomotor nerve. Baseline is obtained with fixation on a distant target and the near response with a target in front of the nose. CG = ciliary ganglion; EW = Edinger-Westphal nucleus; LGN = lateral geniculate nucleus; PTN = pretectal nucleus; RN = red nucleus; SC = superior colliculus.

neurons) pupillary fibers accompany the internal carotid artery through the skull and then leave it to follow the ophthalmic branch of the trigeminal nerve to reach the pupillodilator muscle of the eye.

Examination of the Pupil

The pupillary response to light should be examined in a dimly lighted room, where the pupils are naturally dilated. First, the size and symmetry of the pupils are assessed by shining a dim light onto the face from below so that both pupils are seen simultaneously in the indirect illumination. To test light reactivity, gaze is directed at a distant object (so that constriction secondary to convergence is minimal), and first one and then the other pupil is illuminated with a bright light source. If a pupil reacts poorly to direct light, it is observed as the opposite eye is illuminated (consensual response). Pupils that react poorly to light should be tested for reactivity to the near reflex by first having the patient gaze at a distant object and then quickly fixate on an object just in front of his or her nose. *Light-near dissociation* refers to a pupil that does *not* react to light but does accommodate by constricting to a near target.

Common Causes of Pupillary Abnormalities

With so-called benign pupillary dilation or *physiologic anisocoria,* there is a long-standing difference in the size of the two pupils with normal reflex reactions; the disparity remains constant during constriction and dilation. Lesions compressing or damaging the pretectal region interrupt the afferent light reflex bilaterally to produce dilated and light-fixed pupils (e.g., lesion 2, Fig. 450–2). Pupillary constriction to the near response is preserved until late stages. Tumors of the pineal gland (e.g., dysgerminomas) and *localized infarctions* are the most common lesions in this location. *Adie's tonic pupil* (Fig. 450–3) is a medium to large (3 to

6 mm) pupil that constricts little or not at all to light and very slowly to accommodation but constricts with the instillation of dilute (0.125%) pilocarpine (Fig. 450–4). The condition usually affects one eye (occasionally both), is more common in women 25 to 45 years of age, and carries no serious implications. It most likely results from postviral denervation of the pupillary muscles. Unexplained unilateral or bilateral dilated pupils as an isolated finding can result from *accidental or intentional instillation of mydriatic drugs.* Transdermal scopolamine is a common cause. Failure of the pupil to constrict promptly with pilocarpine (1%) gives the diagnosis if the history is unclear. Interruption of the emerging third nerve in the ventral midbrain or along the proximal part of its course produces a dilated pupil 6 to 7 mm in diameter. Important causes of compression of the third nerve in this region are *aneurysms* (Chapter 430), *neoplasia* (Chapter 199), and *brain herniation* (Chapter 199) as a result of increased intracranial pressure. In nearly all cases, the pupillary involvement is associated with other signs of third nerve involvement (see later text).

Sympathetic paralysis of the eye with ptosis, anhidrosis, and miosis (Horner's syndrome; Fig. 450–5) can result from lesions anywhere along the pathway of the sympathetic innervation to the eye (Table 450–3). The diagnosis can sometimes be made by identifying associated signs in the brain stem or neck or along the carotid artery. *Argyll Robertson pupils* are small (1 to 2 mm), unequal, irregular, and fixed to light; they constrict minimally to accommodation. Their principal cause is tertiary neurosyphilis (Chapter 340).

OCULOMOTOR CONTROL

Abnormal eye movements can result from disturbances at several levels. Disconjugate eye movements result from lesions in the individual ocular muscles, the myoneural junctions, the oculomotor nerves and their three paired nuclei in the brain stem, and the internuclear medial longitudinal fasciculus (MLF), which yokes the eyes in horizontal movements. Supranuclear lesions typically produce disorders of conjugate gaze (gaze palsies).

Anatomy and Localization of Lesions within the Oculomotor Pathways

Nuclear and Internuclear Pathways

The abducens (sixth) nerve supplies the lateral rectus muscle. Selective involvement of the abducens nerve anywhere along its pathway leads to

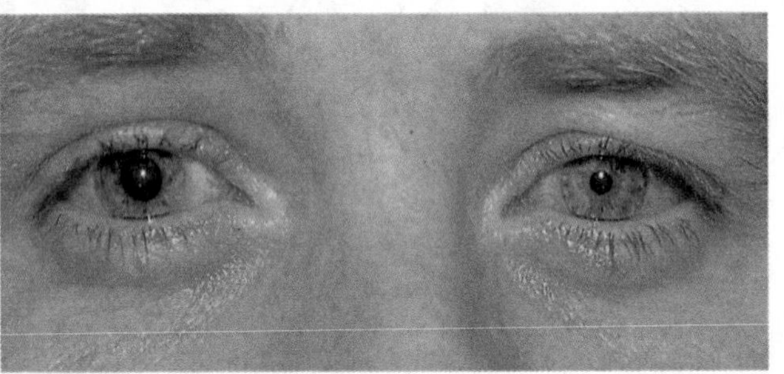

FIGURE 450–3 • Adie's tonic pupil in the right eye of a young woman. The affected pupil is "tonic"; that is, it responds slowly to light and accommodation but on rapid testing appears unresponsive. The site of the lesion is usually obscure, but the condition is benign. There may be associated areflexia. (From Forbes CD, Jackson WF: Color Atlas and Text of Clinical Medicine, 3rd ed. London, Mosby, 2003.)

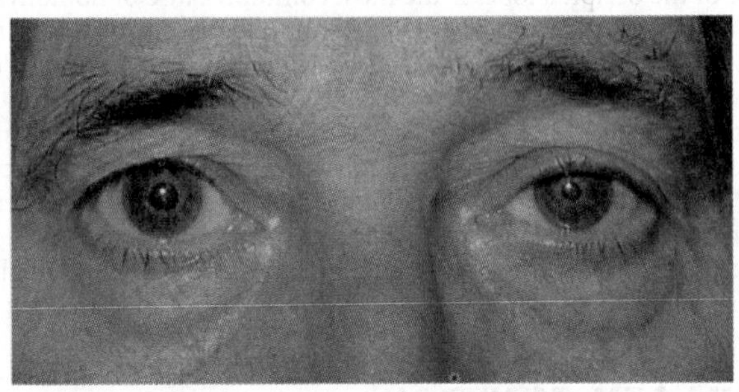

FIGURE 450–5 • Horner's syndrome. Note the characteristic ptosis of the left eye associated with constriction of the pupil (miosis). This patient had syringomyelia, but Horner's syndrome has many possible causes. (From Forbes CD, Jackson WF: Color Atlas and Text of Clinical Medicine, 3rd ed. London, Mosby, 2003.)

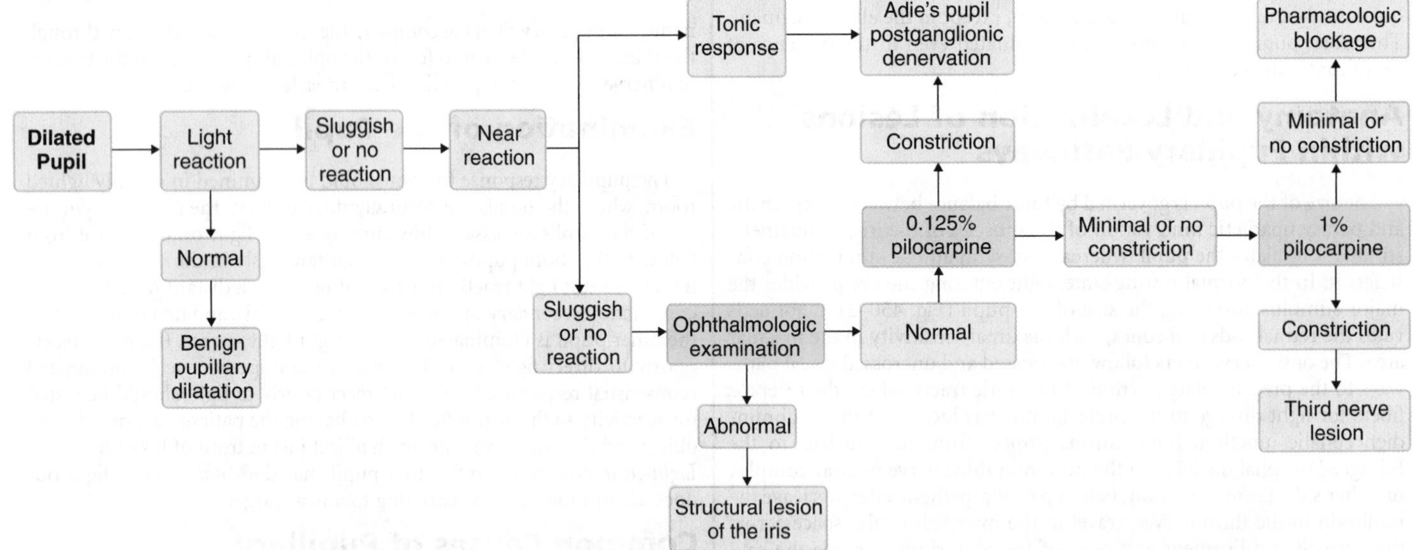

FIGURE 450–4 • Use of pilocarpine to help differentiate between different causes of a dilated pupil.

TABLE 450–3 HORNER'S SYNDROME RESULTS FROM LESIONS IN MULTIPLE LOCATIONS

Location of Lesion	Neuron Involved	Type of Lesion	Associated Symptoms and Signs
Lateral brain stem	1st order	Infarction, glioma	Vertigo, nystagmus, imbalance, numbness, weakness
Apex of lung	2nd order	Lung cancer, trauma	Often none
Neck	3rd order	Carotid dissection or inflammation	Pain, monocular visual loss, hemiparesis

isolated weakness of abduction of the affected eye. Destruction of the abducens nucleus in the brain stem results in a conjugate gaze paralysis (ipsilateral) because in addition to oculomotor neurons, the nucleus contains interneurons destined for the contralateral medial rectus nucleus. The trochlear (fourth) nerve supplies the contralateral superior oblique muscle, which turns in and depresses the eye. Patients with superior oblique weakness note an increase in diplopia with head tilt toward the side of weakness and often tilt their head in the opposite direction. At rest there is slight upward deviation of the involved eye, and downward movement is impaired when the affected eye is turned in. Patients typically complain of diplopia when reading or going down stairs. The third (oculomotor) cranial nerve supplies the remaining ocular muscles. Involvement of the third nerve nucleus in the midbrain always produces at least some bilateral oculomotor weakness; the superior rectus division of the nucleus supplies the contralateral superior rectus muscle (all other divisions supply ipsilateral muscles). Peripheral third nerve paralysis can result from lesions damaging the structure anywhere from its course within the ventral midbrain to where it enters the orbit via the superior orbital fissure. When complete, third nerve palsy produces a widely dilated pupil, severe ptosis, and an externally deviated eye held in position by unopposed contraction of the lateral rectus muscle. In such conditions, the continued trochlear action reveals itself by intorsion of the eye when the subject attempts to look down.

The MLF interconnects the abducens nucleus in the pons with the contralateral oculomotor nuclear complex in the midbrain. It terminates cephalad in the interstitial nucleus in the rostral midbrain and can be traced as far caudad as the thoracocervical region of the spinal cord (coordinating nuchal-ocular control). Lesions involving the MLF characteristically produce internuclear ophthalmoplegia (INO), in which the eyes are conjugate in the primary position but disconjugate on lateral gaze. With fully developed INO on lateral gaze away from the side of the lesion, the contralateral eye abducts and shows nystagmus, whereas the ipsilateral adducting eye does not move nasally because of failure of ascending impulses to reach the medial rectus division of the third nerve nucleus. Adduction for convergence is usually relatively maintained.

Supranuclear Pathways

Pathways descending from the frontal eye fields in the frontal lobe through the superior colliculi to the contralateral brain stem regulate rapid voluntary eye movements (*saccades*) (Table 450–4). Pathways descending from the parieto-occipital and frontal regions to the ipsilateral brain stem subserve slow visual tracking (smooth pursuit—foveal target; optokinetic—full-field target). For the vestibulo-ocular reflex, primary afferent neurons in the inner ear synapse with neurons in the vestibular nuclei, which in turn synapse with appropriate oculomotor neurons to produce compensatory eye movements. The *convergence* center is located in the rostral-dorsal midbrain near the vertical gaze center.

Examination of Eye Movements

Fixation and gaze holding are tested by having the patient look center, right, left, up, and down. Each position should be held steady and unwavering with the observer carefully documenting abnormal movements or ocular disconjugacies. Each supranuclear oculomotor control system is examined separately. *Saccades* are tested by having the patient alternately fixate on two targets such as the examiner's finger and nose; the speed and accuracy are noted. *Smooth pursuit* is tested by slowly moving a target back and forth and up and down and observing the patient's ability to produce smooth tracking movements. If the target velocity is low, normal subjects should be able to pursue without requiring catch-up saccades. The *vestibulo-ocular reflex* is evaluated with the head-thrust test (Chapter 454). *Convergence* is tested by having the patient follow a target moving from far to near. The degree of convergence depends to some extent on the cooperation of the patient. A clear sign that the patient is attempting to converge is simultaneous pupillary constriction.

Common Causes of Abnormal Oculomotor Control

Strabismus (Ocular Misalignment)

A comitant (same in all directions of gaze) strabismus present since childhood is usually a benign *congenital disorder.* Latent congenital strabismus can become manifested in adulthood in association with a systemic illness. An acquired skew deviation (vertical displacement of the ocular axes) indicates a lesion within the otolith-ocular pathways (generally the brain stem). Incomitant strabismus can result from restrictive disease of the orbit or from abnormal muscle or oculomotor nerve function. The presence of mechanical restriction is confirmed by the use of forced duction testing (Fig. 450–6). (After a topical anesthetic is applied to the eye, the ophthalmologist grasps the muscle insertion with large blunt-toothed forceps. Failure of the eye to deviate fully in the pulled direction implies restriction.) Common causes of *orbital restrictive disease* include dysthyroid ophthalmopathy (Chapter 244), orbital pseudotumor, trauma, and orbital mass lesions (Chapter 449). Variable strabismus that increases with fatigue suggests *myasthenia gravis* (Chapter 448). A Tensilon test can usually confirm the diagnosis (see Fig. 450–6). If both restrictive disease and myasthenia gravis (Chapter 448) have been excluded, most patients with incomitant strabismus have processes affecting the oculomotor nuclei, their fascicles, or the cranial nerves themselves. Common causes of an *isolated third nerve palsy* in an adult include aneurysm (Chapter 430), small-vessel occlusive disease (including diabetes mellitus (Chapter 247), trauma (Chapter 422), and neoplasm. Typically, third nerve lesions secondary to vascular disease spare the pupil. Vascular disease and trauma are by far the most common causes of *isolated trochlear nerve palsy.* The abducens nerve is particularly vulnerable to isolated traumatic involvement because of its long pathway outside the brain stem. Lesions that produce increased intracranial pressure (Chapter 199) can lead to abducens nerve dysfunction regardless of the location and produce a "false localizing sign." Other common causes of *isolated sixth nerve palsy* are vascular disease (Chapter 430), trauma (Chapter 422), and neoplasm. About a fourth of cases with cranial nerve palsy (third, fourth, or sixth nerves) remain undiagnosed.

Internuclear Ophthalmoplegia

INO (Fig. 450–7) may be unilateral or bilateral, partial or complete, depending on the location of the lesion and the degree of damage to the MLF. *Demyelinating* and small *vascular lesions* are the most common cause of unilateral INO unaccompanied by other ocular palsies or brain stem signs. Larger brain stem lesions that damage one or more oculomotor nuclei plus the MLF often produce combinations of disconjugate eye movements coupled with nuclear oculomotor palsies. Myasthenia gravis (Chapter 448) can produce an ophthalmoparesis resembling INO as a result of greater involvement of the medial rectus than the lateral rectus. Demyelinating diseases (Chapter 436) are the most common causes of bilateral INO involvement.

TABLE 450–4 SUPRANUCLEAR OCULOMOTOR CONTROL SYSTEMS

System	Description	Function	Key Anatomic Structures
Saccade	Fast conjugate voluntary movements	Move the fovea to a new target of interest	Frontal eye field, superior colliculus, pretectum—vertical, pontine—horizontal, cerebellar dentate nucleus
Smooth pursuit/ optokinetic	Slow conjugate tracking	Match eye velocity to target velocity	Occipital, parietal, pons, cerebellar flocculus
Vestibulo-ocular	Slow conjugate compensatory eye movements	Keep eyes stable when head moves	Pontomedullary region
Vergence	Slow disconjugate tracking	Focus on near and far targets	Pretectum, tectum

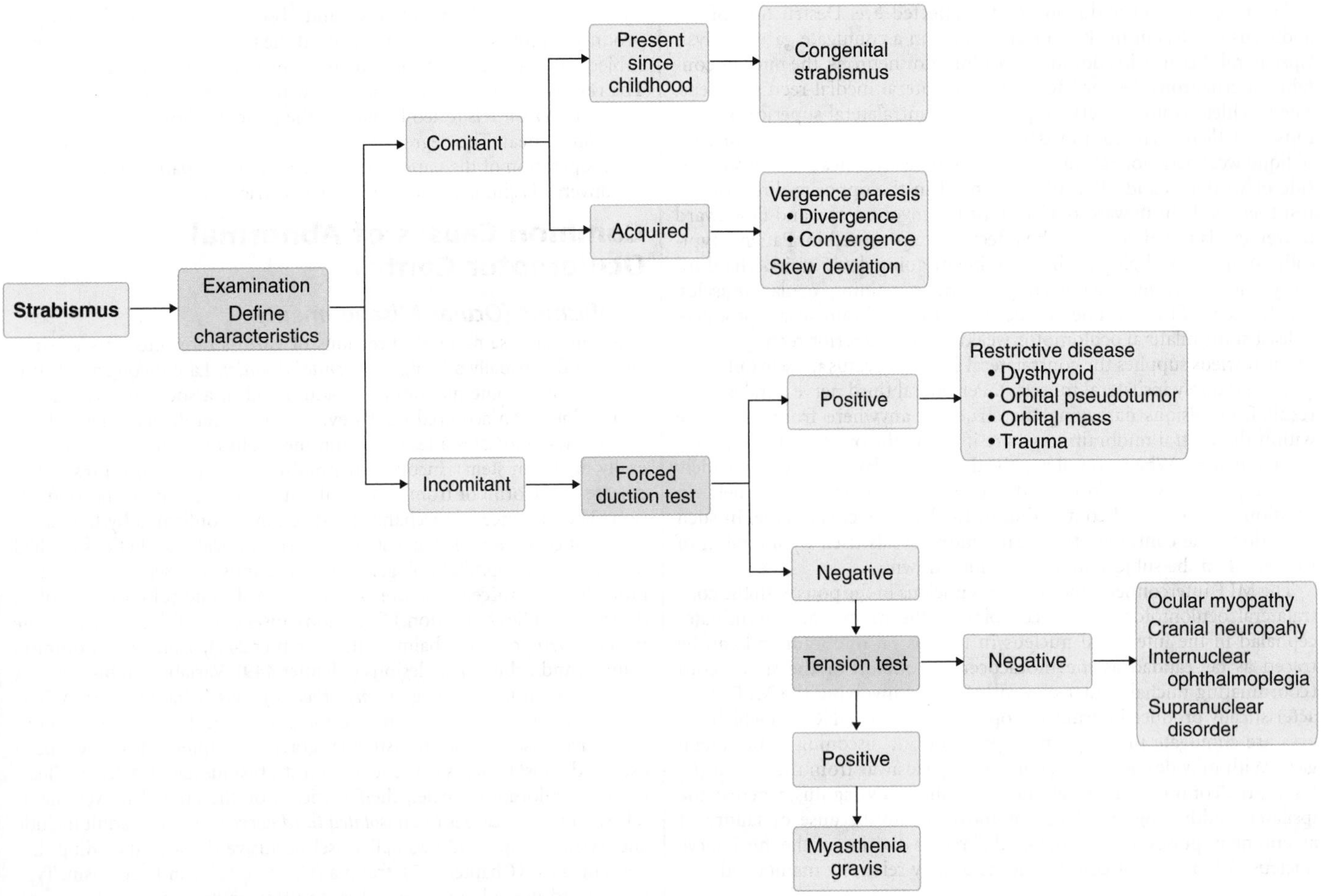

- Strabismus → Examination: Define characteristics
  - Comitant
    - Present since childhood → Congenital strabismus
    - Acquired → Vergence paresis
      - Divergence
      - Convergence

      Skew deviation
  - Incomitant → Forced duction test
    - Positive → Restrictive disease
      - Dysthyroid
      - Orbital pseudotumor
      - Orbital mass
      - Trauma
    - Negative → Tension test
      - Negative → Ocular myopathy; Cranial neuropahy; Internuclear ophthalmoplegia; Supranuclear disorder
      - Positive → Myasthenia gravis

FIGURE 450–6 • Diagnostic tests that help differentiate between common causes of strabismus.

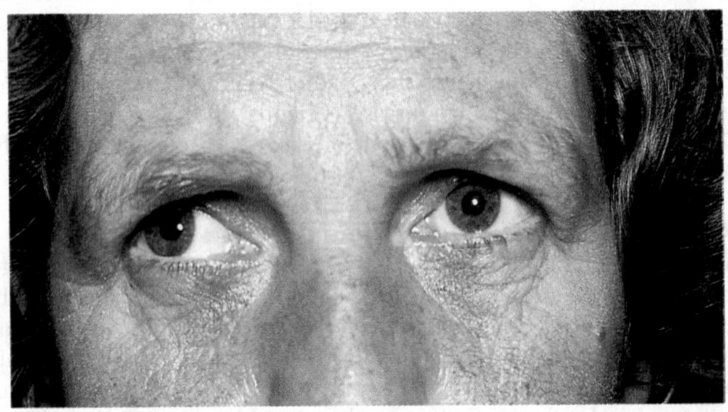

FIGURE 450–7 • Internuclear ophthalmoplegia may be an initial feature of brain stem involvement in multiple sclerosis. On lateral gaze to the right, adduction of the left eye is incomplete. On convergence, eye movement was normal. The lesion is in the left medial longitudinal bundle, between the nucleus in the pons and the third nerve nucleus on the opposite side. (From Forbes CD, Jackson WF: Color Atlas and Text of Clinical Medicine, 3rd ed. London, Mosby, 2003.)

Disorders of Conjugate Gaze

Acute lesions involving a frontal eye field (e.g., hemorrhage or infarction [Chapters 431 and 432]) result in a transient inability to direct the eyes contralaterally. Vertical eye movements are not affected by unilateral lesions. Bilateral damage to the frontal eye fields or their descending pathways may produce an inability to move the eyes voluntarily (horizontal or vertical) despite preserved reflex eye movements, a condition called *oculomotor apraxia.* Lesions involving the horizontal gaze center in the pons produce an ipsilateral paralysis of conjugate gaze and tonic deviation of the eyes to the contralateral side (Chapter 449). Lesions of the pretectum selectively impair vertical gaze, with the vertical upgaze center being slightly rostral and dorsal to the vertical downgaze center. Patients with the *dorsal midbrain syndrome* (Parinaud's syndrome) have a conjugate upgaze paresis. When they attempt to make upward saccades, convergence retraction nystagmus develops. As noted earlier, impaired convergence and light-near dissociation of the pupillary reflexes are also part of the syndrome. The most common causes of the dorsal midbrain syndrome include tumors of the pineal gland (Chapter 241) (dysgerminomas), hydrocephalus (Chapter 199), and localized infarction. With the so-called locked-in syndrome (secondary to basilar artery thrombosis [Chapter 431]), voluntary horizontal eye movements are absent; the patient's only remaining motor functions are vertical eye and lid movements.

Nystagmus

Spontaneous nystagmus can be congenital or acquired. *Congenital nystagmus* typically has a high frequency and variable waveform (usually pendular) and is highly fixation dependent. It generally remains horizontal in all positions of gaze. The lifelong history and lack of symptoms confirm the diagnosis. Spontaneous nystagmus resulting from a *peripheral vestibular* lesion (i.e., in the labyrinth or vestibular nerve) usually has combined horizontal and torsional components (Table 450–5). The nystagmus resolves within a few days of the acute lesion. Acquired persistent spontaneous nystagmus indicates a lesion in the brain stem or cerebellum, or both. The latter is often purely vertical, horizontal, or torsional. Spontaneous *downbeat nystagmus* is commonly seen with lesions of the cerebellum or cervicomedullary junction (e.g., Arnold-Chiari malformation [Chapter 444]).

Gaze-evoked nystagmus is always in the direction of gaze and is usually present with and without fixation. It is most commonly produced by the ingestion of *drugs* such as phenobarbital, phenytoin, alcohol, and diazepam (Chapter 111). It can also occur in patients with such varied conditions as myasthenia gravis (Chapter 448), multiple sclerosis (Chapter 436), and cerebellar atrophy. Asymmetrical horizontal gaze-evoked nystagmus is caused by a structural brain stem or cerebellar lesion (particularly at the cerebellopontine angle), with the lesion generally being on the side of the larger-amplitude nystagmus (Brun's nystagmus).

TABLE 450–5 KEY DISTINGUISHING FEATURES OF PERIPHERAL AND CENTRAL TYPES OF SPONTANEOUS AND POSITIONAL NYSTAGMUS

Type of Nystagmus	Peripheral (End Organ and Nerve)	Central (Brain Stem and Cerebellum)
Spontaneous	Unidirectional, fast phase away from the lesion, combined horizontal torsional, inhibited with fixation	Bidirectional or unidirectional; often pure horizontal, vertical, or torsional; *not* inhibited with fixation
Static positional	Fixed or changing direction, inhibited with fixation	Fixed or changing direction, *not* inhibited with fixation
Paroxysmal positional	Vertical-torsional, occasionally horizontal-torsional, vertigo prominent, fatigability, latency	Often pure vertical, vertigo less prominent, no latency, nonfatigable

Rebound nystagmus is a type of gaze-evoked nystagmus that either disappears or reverses direction as the eccentric gaze position is held. When the eyes are returned to the primary position, nystagmus occurs in the direction of the return saccade. Rebound nystagmus occurs in patients with cerebellar atrophy and focal structural lesions of the cerebellum; it is the only variety of nystagmus thought to be specific for cerebellar involvement. *Disconjugate gaze-evoked nystagmus* most commonly results from lesions of the MLF (see earlier discussion), but it can also occur with other lesions of the brain stem involving the oculomotor nuclei. Positional nystagmus is discussed in Chapter 454.

Other Ocular Oscillations

Ocular bobbing consists of a fast conjugate downward eye movement followed by a slow return to the primary position. The phenomenon accompanies severe displacement or destruction of the pons or, less often, metabolic central nervous system depression. *Ocular myoclonus* consists of continuous rhythmic pendular oscillations, most often vertical, at a rate of 1 to 3 beats per second; it often accompanies palatal myoclonus and has a similar pathogenesis. *Square-wave jerks* and *ocular flutter* consist of brief, intermittent, horizontal oscillations (back to back saccades) arising from the primary gaze position. These types of ocular oscillation are most commonly seen with cerebellar disease but can also accompany more diffuse central nervous system disorders. *Opsoclonus* consists of rapid, chaotic, conjugate, repetitive saccadic eye movements (dancing eyes). Opsoclonus accompanies the cerebellar dysfunction, with the most chaotic varieties associated with brain stem encephalitis or the remote effects of systemic neoplasm, especially neuroblastoma in children. *Ocular dysmetria* refers to overshooting and undershooting of saccadic eye movements, often followed by multiple attempts at refixation. It reflects cerebellar dysfunction.

SUGGESTED READINGS

Balcer LJ: Clinical practice. Optic neuritis. N Engl J Med 2006;354:1273–1280. *Reviews, diagnosis, and treatment of this common disorder.*

Chhabra VS, Newman NJ: The neuro-ophthalmology of pituitary tumors. Compr Ophthalmol Update 2006;7:225–240. *Review of the neuro-ophthalmologic manifestations of pituitary disease.*

Jacobs DA, Galetta SL: Neuro-ophthalmology for neuroradiologists. Am J Neuroradiol 2007;28:3–8. *Focuses on common neuro-ophthalmologic problems with localizing value on neuro-imaging.*

451 DISEASES OF THE MOUTH AND SALIVARY GLANDS

Troy E. Daniels

More than 200 primary lesions or diseases occur in the oral mucosa, gingiva, teeth, jaws, and minor or major salivary glands. In addition, secondary abnormalities of the oral mucosa or salivary glands can be caused by systemic diseases or drugs. The most common or important of these diseases may be observed during physical examination and are often part of a systemic process.

ORAL MUCOSAL DISEASES

Acute Ulcerations

Painful short-term ulcerations are usually caused by mechanical trauma, immunologic mechanisms, and bacterial or viral infections (Table 451–1). Soon after formation, oral mucosal ulcers become covered by a white to gray pseudomembrane, analogous to scabs on dry epidermis. Pseudomembrane-covered ulcers are distinguished from the white hyperkeratotic lesions by their clinical features of pain, a flat surface, and an erythematous periphery. Traumatic ulcers are characteristically located on the tongue or inside the cheeks or lips, are close to the chewing surfaces of the teeth, and have irregular borders.

Aphthous Ulcers

These idiopathic recurrent ulcers, which afflict about 20% of the population, are found on all areas of the oral mucosa except the hard palate, gingiva, and vermilion, which are keratinized (Fig. 451–1). They form well-defined circular lesions that may be single or multiple. There are three clinical forms: (1) minor, which are flat and less than 1 cm in diameter and last 5 to 10 days; (2) major, which have raised borders, are greater than 1 cm, and often last for weeks or months; and (3) herpetiform, which are usually clusters of very small ulcers that resemble recurrent herpetic lesions but are not preceded by vesicles and do not occur on keratinized mucosa. A viral pathogenesis has not been established for any of these forms. Lesions clinically identical to minor aphthous ulcers occur in Behçet's syndrome (Chapter 291). Aphthous ulcers are occasionally associated with anemias or gluten-sensitive enteropathy and may become more frequent and severe in association with human immunodeficiency virus (HIV) infection (Table 451–2).

Minor or herpetiform aphthous ulcers may not require treatment. Topical steroids, such as fluocinonide gel or ointment, can reduce the severity and duration of the lesions only if applied with prodromal symptoms or earliest signs. Major aphthae usually require treatment by topical or systemic corticosteroids and occasionally are biopsied to exclude neoplasia.

Viral Ulcers

Several types of virus (most commonly herpes simplex type 1; Chapter 397) cause multiple oral mucosal vesicles that last only a few hours or days and then become irregular shallow ulcers. In the initial infection by herpes simplex virus, usually in children, numerous vesicles may appear on any oral mucosal site (primary herpetic gingivostomatitis), accompanied by malaise, headache, fever, and cervical lymphadenopathy. Patients previously exposed to this virus may develop recurrent (secondary) lesions as clusters of small vesicles, most commonly on the lips (herpes labialis) and less commonly on the keratinized mucosa of the gingiva or hard palate (Fig. 451–2). Such lesions contain live virus and tend to recur at the same site but less frequently with increasing age.

Similar mucosal vesicles may also accompany the initial infection by the varicella-zoster virus in children with chickenpox (Chapter 398), and unilateral lesions may occur if herpes zoster (Chapter 398) affects branches of the trigeminal nerve. Uncommonly, oral mucosal ulcers may be caused by different types of coxsackievirus (Chapter 402), appearing on any oral site in hand-foot-and-mouth disease or on the soft palate or pharynx in herpangina. After infection by the measles (rubeola) virus, small ulcers (Koplik's spots) may form on the inside of the cheeks 1 to 2 days before development of the skin rash (Chapter 390).

TABLE 451–1 ORAL MUCOSAL ULCERS

Type/Disease	Clinical Features
INSIDIOUS ONSET, CHRONIC	
Multiple or bilateral	Shallow ulcers on mucosa, skin, or both
Pemphigus vulgaris	Begin as short-duration blisters
Mucous membrane pemphigoid	Begin as short-duration blisters
Lichen planus	Bilaterally symmetrical lesions (associated with hyperkeratosis and/or erythema)
Lupus erythematosus	Asymmetric lesions, with or without systemic lupus (associated with hyperkeratoses and/or erythema)
Drug reaction	Variable lesions; appropriate history of drug use (e.g., penicillamine, gold)
Epidermolysis bullosa	Begin as blisters; lifelong history
Solitary	Indurated or cratered ulcers
Squamous cell carcinoma	Most common on tongue, oropharynx, lip, mouth floor
Adenocarcinomas, various	Most commonly on palate, cheeks, mouth floor
Tuberculosis	Usually painful
Actinomycosis	Often associated with draining sinus
Deep mycoses (particularly histoplasmosis, coccidioidomycosis)	Associated with systemic infection
Midline granuloma	Associated with necrosis, may perforate palate
ACUTE ONSET, OFTEN SELF-LIMITING	
Clusters	Usually small and shallow ulcers; history of blisters
Primary herpes simplex	Any oral mucosal site, associated with fever, malaise
Recurrent herpes simplex	Only on gingiva, hard palate, or lip (keratinized mucosa)
Varicella-zoster	Unilateral lesions along neural distribution
Herpangina	Usually on oropharynx
Measles (rubeola)	Precede skin rash; associated with fever, malaise
Solitary or multiple (without clustering)	Variable, usually without history of blisters
Traumatic ulcers	Usually solitary; history of trauma
Recurrent aphthae	Circular, often multiple, only on nonkeratinized mucosa
Behçet's syndrome	Oral lesions similar to recurrent aphthae
Erythema multiforme	Multiple lesions, often involve lower labial mucosa; can be recurrent or chronic
Drug reaction	Appropriate history of drug use
Necrotizing sialometaplasia	Deep ulcers, usually on palate
Primary syphilis	Solitary, indurated, painless, any site
Gonorrhea	Painful, surrounded by erythema, any site

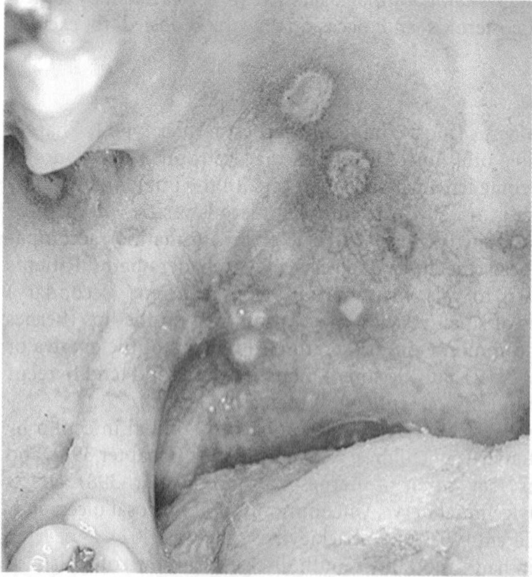

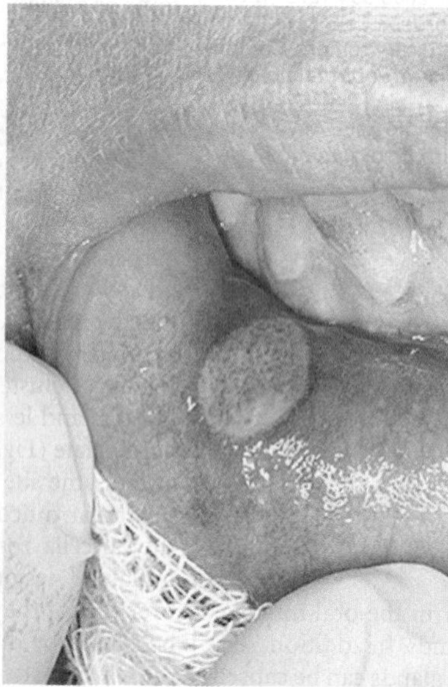

FIGURE 451–1 • Aphthous ulcers. Left, A cluster of minor aphthae on the soft palate and buccal mucosa, present about 1 week. **Right,** A major aphthous ulcer on the labial mucosa, present about 3 weeks.

Erythema Multiforme

In this potentially recurrent mucocutaneous disease, painful oral mucosal ulcerations develop rapidly in as many as half of patients. The lesions may be confined to the mouth, with no skin involvement. The affected patients, usually young adults with minimal or no systemic symptoms, have irregularly shaped ulcers that can be small and few or involve large areas of the mucosa; the most common site is the lower labial mucosa. These lesions can be distinguished from those of primary herpes by the absence of oral vesicles and systemic symptoms or by the presence of characteristic skin lesions (Chapter 465). A major variant of this disease is Stevens-Johnson syndrome, in which ocular, genital, and other lesions may accompany the oral lesions.

Venereal Infections

Primary syphilis may arise as a solitary, indurated, painless ulcer on the oral mucosa that resolves spontaneously in 4 to 6 weeks (Chapter 340). Uncommonly, *Neisseria gonorrhoeae* may cause oral ulcers, usually in the pharynx, which may be confused with oral ulcers of other causes.

TABLE 451–2 ORAL LESIONS ASSOCIATED WITH HUMAN IMMUNODEFICIENCY VIRUS INFECTION

Kaposi's sarcoma
Candidiasis:
Pseudomembranous lesions
Hyperplastic lesions
Erythematous lesions
Other opportunistic fungal infections (e.g., histoplasmosis or coccidioidomycosis)
Aphthous ulcers (increased frequency, duration, or size)
Virus-associated epithelial hyperplasias
Hairy leukoplakia
Oral wart
Focal epithelial hyperplasia (Heck's disease)
Condyloma acuminatum
Herpes zoster
Exaggerated forms of gingivitis and inflammatory periodontal disease
Decreased salivary gland function
Parotid gland enlargement (lymphoepithelial lesion)
Non-Hodgkin's lymphoma

Oral Squamous Cell Carcinoma

About 4% of all cancers occur in the mouth, commonly as squamous cell carcinomas of the mucosal epithelium (Chapter 200). Oral carcinoma occurs usually in the fifth decade or beyond, in men twice as frequently as in women, and is associated with long-term use of tobacco in more than 80% of cases (see Table 467–1).

Oral carcinoma usually arises as a chronic, indurated, cratered ulcer, but early lesions of squamous cell carcinoma may appear as white or red macules (Table 451–3; Fig. 451–3). About 15% of oral carcinomas arise within a preexisting white plaque (leukoplakia). The overall 5-year survival is approximately 50%, but early treatment of small, localized lesions can lead to survival rates as high as 90%.

TABLE 451–3 WHITE AND RED ORAL MUCOSAL LESIONS

WHITE LESIONS (PLAQUES)
Squamous cell carcinoma (early)
Frictional keratosis
Leukoplakia (idiopathic)
Smokeless tobacco–associated lesions
Nicotine stomatitis (palate)
Lichen planus (reticular and plaque types)
Pseudomembranous candidiasis (thrush)
Hyperplastic candidiasis (candidal leukoplakia)
Hairy leukoplakia (HIV-associated; usually on lateral tongue)
Geographic tongue
Mucous patch or condyloma latum of secondary syphilis
Pseudomembrane-covered ulcers (see Table 451–1)
RED LESIONS (MACULAR, MACULOPAPULAR)
Squamous cell carcinoma (early)
Erythroplakia (epithelial dysplasia)
Erythematous (atrophic) candidiasis
Median rhomboid glossitis
Mucocutaneous diseases (see Table 451–1)
Angular cheilitis
Telangiectasias and purpuras
Kaposi's sarcoma (blue to purple color)

HIV = human immunodeficiency virus.

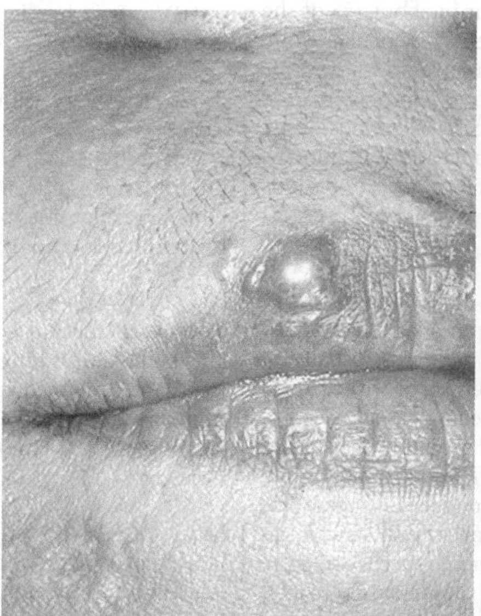

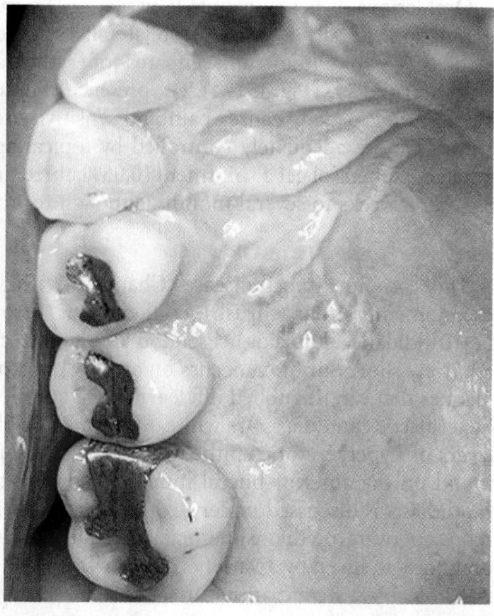

FIGURE 451–2 • Clusters of recurrent herpes simplex vesicles. Left, on the lip; **right,** on the hard palate, both present 2 to 3 days, in different patients.

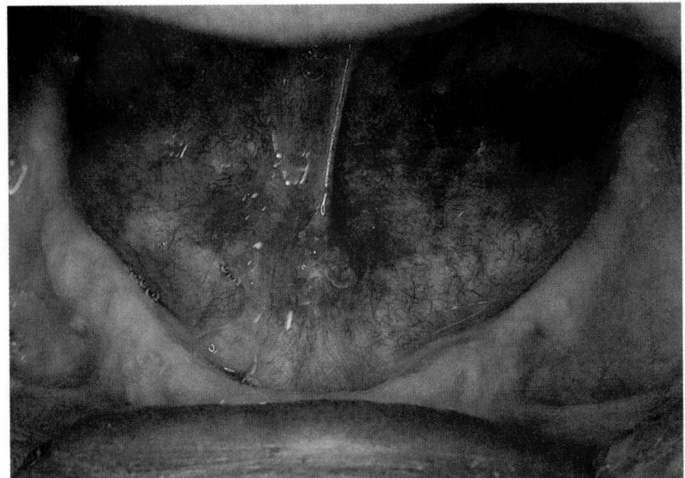

FIGURE 451–3 • Squamous cell carcinoma. Biopsy of this area of erythroplakia with slight induration in the anterior mouth floor exhibited squamous cell carcinoma.

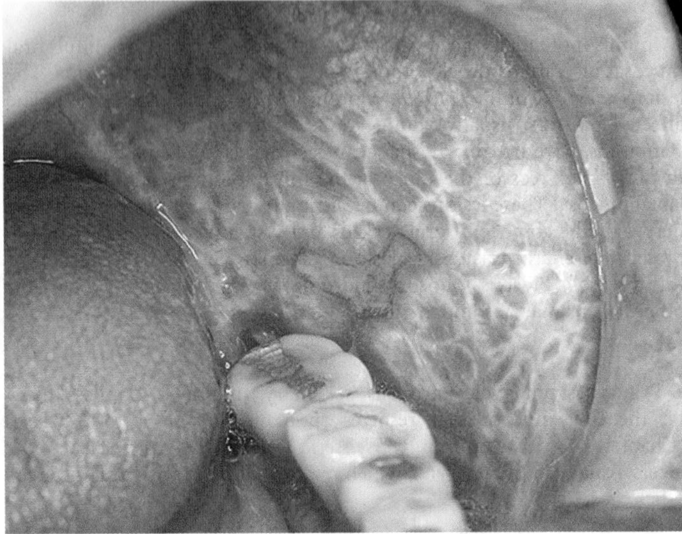

FIGURE 451–4 • Lichen planus. A similar-appearing lesion is also present on the right buccal mucosa.

Other Chronic Ulcerations

Several mucocutaneous diseases can cause chronic multifocal oral mucosal lesions composed of ill-defined areas of erythema and ulceration. They are among the most difficult oral lesions to diagnose and are discussed subsequently with the red lesions (see Table 451–3). Several microbial infections can lead to indurated, chronic oral mucosal ulcerations with moderate symptoms (see Table 451–1).

White Lesions

White plaques are commonly found in the mouth but, like ulcerations, have a wide variety of causes and outcomes (see Table 451–3). The term leukoplakia applies to a white plaque that does not rub off and whose appearance does not indicate another disease. Leukoplakia can occur in any area of the mouth and usually exhibits benign hyperkeratosis on biopsy (see Fig. 200–1). On long-term follow-up, 2 to 6% of these lesions undergo malignant transformation into squamous cell carcinoma. Areas of leukoplakia with a corrugated surface or mixed with areas of erythema are often found in the lower labial or buccal vestibule of patients who use smokeless tobacco.

Frictional keratoses are often found posterior to the lower molar teeth as irregular white plaques and on the buccal mucosa as white lines adjacent to the dental occlusion. Unlike leukoplakia, these lesions rarely become malignant.

Lichen Planus

Oral lesions of lichen planus (Chapter 464) occur in about 1% of the population, usually as multiple, bilaterally symmetrical reticular white plaques, with or without adjacent areas of erythema (atrophy or erosion) or irregular ulcers (Fig. 451–4). The presence of mucosal atrophy, erosion, or ulceration usually causes pain and sensitivity to certain foods. Most lesions can be adequately controlled by topical application of fluocinonide or clobetasol gel or ointment (0.05%, three times a day) for periods of several weeks to several months, although recurrence is common.

Oral Candidiasis

This common fungal disease (Chapter 359) has three clinical forms: pseudomembranous (thrush), erythematous (atrophic), and hyperplastic (candidal leukoplakia). Pseudomembranous candidiasis, usually of relatively short duration, occurs on any site and consists of white fungal plaques that can be rubbed off, leaving a red or bleeding base. Lesions of hyperplastic candidiasis are white, have fungal hyphae within the surface layers of hyperkeratotic epithelium, do not rub off, and are most often found on the anterior buccal mucosa or on the tongue. Erythematous candidiasis is discussed under Red Lesions. All forms of oral candidiasis represent overgrowth or superficial infection by *Candida* species from the oral flora, induced by a variety of causes including suppression of bacterial flora by systemic antibiotics, chronic salivary dysfunction, uncontrolled diabetes mellitus or anemia, and immunosuppression (especially in HIV-infected patients).

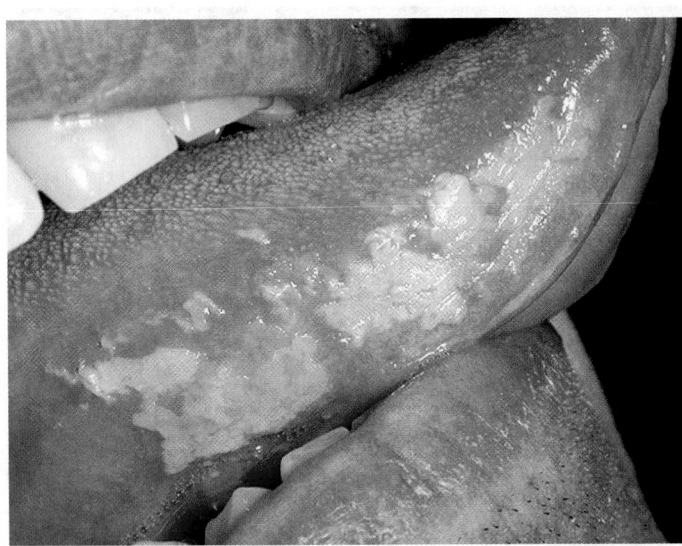

FIGURE 451–5 • Hairy leukoplakia. These white plaques were the first visible sign of human immunodeficiency virus infection.

Hairy Leukoplakia

This lesion is a white plaque occurring most frequently on the lateral surfaces of the tongue bilaterally in immunosuppressed persons, usually HIV infected (Fig. 451–5). *Candida* may be present in the surface layers, but the lesion is not eliminated by effective antifungal therapy, and it contains large quantities of Epstein-Barr virus. Its diagnosis by biopsy should be followed by an HIV antibody test.

Geographic Tongue

Also called *benign migratory glossitis,* this benign idiopathic condition affects the dorsal tongue of about 2% of the population. It is characterized by well-defined areas of atrophied filiform papillae bordered by arcs of normal or hyperplastic filiform papillae and by gradual changes in the location of these lesions over time (Fig. 451–6). Treatment is usually not necessary.

Secondary Syphilis

Secondary syphilis may manifest as a well-defined white plaque on the labial or palatal mucosa, called *condyloma latum* (or "split papule," because of their lobulated periphery).

Red Lesions

Solitary red macules or plaques ("erythroplakia") are less common in the mouth than white lesions but should be viewed with concern because they may exhibit microscopic dysplasia, carcinoma in situ, or carcinoma (see Table 451–3 and Fig. 451–1). One exception is a red macule occurring in the midline of the posterior dorsal tongue, classified as median rhomboid glossitis, which is an idiopathic but uniformly benign condition that is often associated with localized overgrowth of *Candida* species.

Erythematous (Atrophic) Oral Candidiasis

This chronic condition is characterized by erythema and atrophy of the filiform papillae on the dorsal tongue or by patchy, ill-defined erythema on the palate, tongue, or buccal mucosa (Fig. 451–7). It is usually accompanied by symptoms of oral mucosal burning and sensitivity to certain foods. It occurs most commonly in patients with chronic salivary hypofunction (e.g., Sjögren's syndrome or anticholinergic drug effects), but it also occurs in patients who wear removable dentures, in whom mucosal erythema is confined to the denture-bearing area.

Topical or systemic antifungal drugs are necessary to resolve these lesions. In patients who have clinically apparent salivary production, fluconazole (200 mg on the first day, then 100 mg every day for 2 to 4 weeks) is the drug of choice. However, systemic antifungal drugs may not be effective in patients who have severe salivary hypofunction and insufficient saliva to convey the drug from blood stream to the oral mucosa. In such patients, with remaining natural teeth, oral antifungal preparations (troches or pastilles), all of which contain cariogenic amounts of sucrose or glucose, *must not be used* to avoid enhancing dental caries. Instead, slow oral dissolution (15 to 20 minutes) of vaginal nystatin tablets (100,000 U, twice a day for 2 weeks to 2 months), which contain little or no caries-supporting carbohydrates, is safe and effective when patients take frequent sips of water to aid in dissolving the tablets. Effective topical or systemic treatment significantly improves oral symptoms. Treatment of denture-associated candidiasis requires concurrent treatment of the denture.

The treatment end point is reached when mucosal burning symptoms cease, the patient can again tolerate acidic or spicy foods, and filiform papillae on the dorsal tongue have returned to normal; this recovery takes from 2 to 12 weeks, depending on patients' salivary production and treatment compliance. Recurrence is common in patients with chronic salivary hypofunction or immunosuppression, which necessitates recurring or long-term treatment using a noncariogenic topical antifungal drug that provides a sufficient duration of oral mucosal contact (e.g., vaginal tablets).

Angular Cheilitis

Erythema or crusting of the labial angles is usually caused by *Candida* (see Fig. 451–7). It is usually associated with intraoral candidiasis, and in such cases topical treatment of the angular cheilitis with clotrimazole (1% cream) must be accompanied by intraoral or systemic antifungal treatment as described previously.

Mucocutaneous Diseases

The mucocutaneous diseases of pemphigus vulgaris, mucous membrane pemphigoid, atrophic or erosive lichen planus, and lupus erythematosus can cause similar-appearing oral lesions. Their diagnosis requires examination of a biopsy specimen by routine histopathology and direct immunofluorescence to identify characteristic deposits of various inflammatory proteins.

The first lesions of pemphigus vulgaris are usually oral mucosal vesicles that rapidly rupture, leaving painful erosions or ulcerations. These are followed by development of skin lesions. Rarely, the lesions remain confined to the mouth (Chapter 465).

Lesions of mucous membrane (cicatricial) pemphigoid are usually confined to the oral mucosa or conjunctivae and occur in patients older than 50 years. They begin as vesicles that quickly rupture, leaving ulcers that are chronic but only moderately symptomatic. Use of topical fluocinonide or clobetasol (0.05% gel or ointment, three times a day, 4 to 12 weeks) for several months, as described for lichen planus, is sometimes sufficient to treat the oral lesions, but some patients also need systemic treatment (Chapter 465).

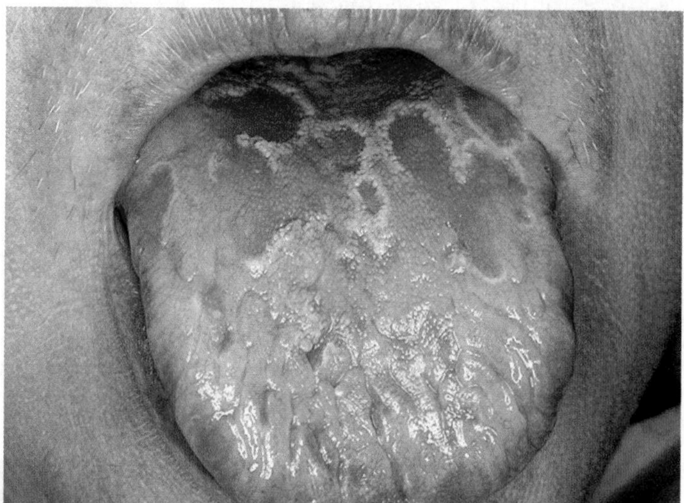

FIGURE 451–6 • Geographic tongue. The distribution of these changes on the dorsal tongue may change over time, but they are asymptomatic and diagnosed by their characteristic appearance.

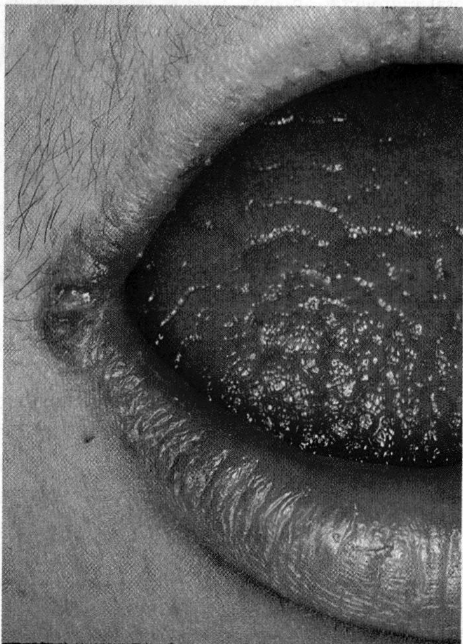

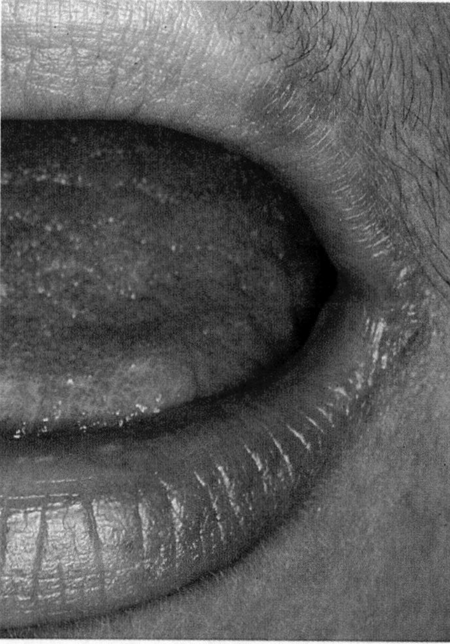

FIGURE 451–7 • Erythematous oral candidiasis. Left, Erythematous candidiasis in a 26-year-old woman with primary Sjögren's syndrome, exhibiting symptomatic angular cheilitis, atrophic mucositis, and lingual papillary atrophy. **Right,** Asymptomatic and normal-appearing mucosa after treatment with appropriate topical antifungal drugs (see text).

TABLE 451–4 PIGMENTATIONS OF THE ORAL MUCOSA (BROWN OR GRAY-BLACK IN COLOR)

INCREASED MELANIN PRODUCTION (FLAT LESIONS)
Oral melanotic macule
Ephelis (vermilion border)
Systemic diseases: Addison's disease, von Recklinghausen's disease of skin, Albright's syndrome, Peutz-Jeghers syndrome
PROLIFERATION OF MELANIN-PRODUCING CELLS (FLAT OR RAISED LESIONS)
Pigmented cellular nevi (benign and premalignant types)
Atypical melanocytic hyperplasia, melanoma in situ, radial growth phase of melanoma
Malignant melanoma
NONMELANIN PIGMENTATION
Amalgam tattoo
Focal deposition of systemically distributed metal (lead, bismuth, mercury, others) usually at sites of chronic inflammation
Systemically administered drugs (chloroquine, minocycline, ketoconazole, cyclophosphamide)

Oral mucosal lesions of lupus may occur in patients who have systemic lupus erythematosus (SLE), in patients who do not have SLE but later develop that disease, or in patients who do not develop SLE (Chapter 287). In this latter group, the lesions of mucosal lupus may be analogous to the skin lesions of chronic discoid lupus. Lesions of oral lupus are usually solitary or bilaterally asymmetric. They take the form of reticular hyperkeratotic figures associated with erythema, often resembling lichen planus. The lesions can be controlled by topical fluocinonide (0.05%, three times a day, 2 to 4 weeks), intralesional triamcinolone suspension (5 mg/mL), or possibly systemic treatment of SLE.

Lesions of Kaposi's sarcoma associated with HIV infection often appear first on the oral mucosa, especially the palate. They begin as macules with a blue or purple color, at which time they need to be distinguished from purpura. Later, they spread radially and expand vertically (Chapter 416).

Pigmentations

Brown or gray-black macules on the oral mucosa are relatively common and range from benign to highly malignant. They may be caused by localized increase in melanin production, proliferation of melanin-producing cells, or deposition of local or systemically distributed pigmented substances (Table 451–4). Mucosal pigmentation may occur after long-term administration of hydroxychloroquine, minocycline, ketoconazole, methyldopa, or cyclophosphamide. Malignant melanoma can occur at any oral mucosal site, but about 85% develop on the hard palatal mucosa or gingiva, or both. Diagnosis of any of these conditions is usually established by biopsy and knowledge of relevant underlying conditions.

ORAL SOFT TISSUE TUMORS

In addition to the malignant neoplasms described, a variety of oral benign soft tissue tumors are usually treated by excisional biopsy.

Connective Tissue Hyperplasias

The most common oral soft tissue tumors are small, pedunculated masses of hyperplastic fibrous connective tissue covered by normal-appearing mucosa (Table 451–5). Solitary lesions are usually found on the inside of the cheeks or lips. Similar lesions may be present at the border of an ill-fitting denture or may occur in clusters on the hard palate under an ill-fitting denture (palatal papillomatosis).

Generalized or multifocal enlargement of the gingiva (gingival hyperplasia) may be caused by chronic administration of phenytoin, cyclosporine, and many of the calcium-channel blocking drugs (e.g., diltiazem, verapamil, or nifedipine; Fig. 451–8). It can also be associated with a hereditary defect or be caused by an infiltration of atypical white blood cells in some types of leukemia (particularly acute monocytic leukemia; Chapter 194) or by uncontrolled diabetes mellitus (Chapter 247).

TABLE 451–5 ORAL SOFT TISSUE TUMORS

CONNECTIVE TISSUE HYPERPLASIA (NORMAL-APPEARING OVERLYING MUCOSA)
Irritation fibroma
Denture-associated hyperplasia
Palatal papillomatosis
Generalized gingival hyperplasia
Drug-induced (phenytoin, nifedipine, cyclosporine)
Hereditary
REACTIVE HYPERPLASIA (ERYTHEMATOUS OVERLYING MUCOSA)
Pyogenic granuloma/pregnancy tumor
Peripheral giant cell granuloma
Inflammatory gingival hyperplasia
Hyperplastic lingual tonsil
EPITHELIAL MASSES (USUALLY IRREGULAR WHITE SURFACE)
Papilloma/oral wart
Squamous cell carcinoma
Verrucous carcinoma
Focal epithelial hyperplasia (Heck's disease)
Condyloma acuminatum (venereal wart)
Keratoacanthoma (on lips)
SALIVARY DUCT OBSTRUCTION (MINOR SALIVARY GLANDS)
Mucocele/ranula (usually fluctuant)
Salivary stone (sialolith)
SUBEPITHELIAL NEOPLASMS
Primary connective tissue or salivary gland tumors
Metastatic lesions (especially in the mandible)
Lymphoma (especially in the palate or posterior mandible)
Focal or generalized leukemic infiltrates in the gingiva (especially with acute monocytic leukemia)

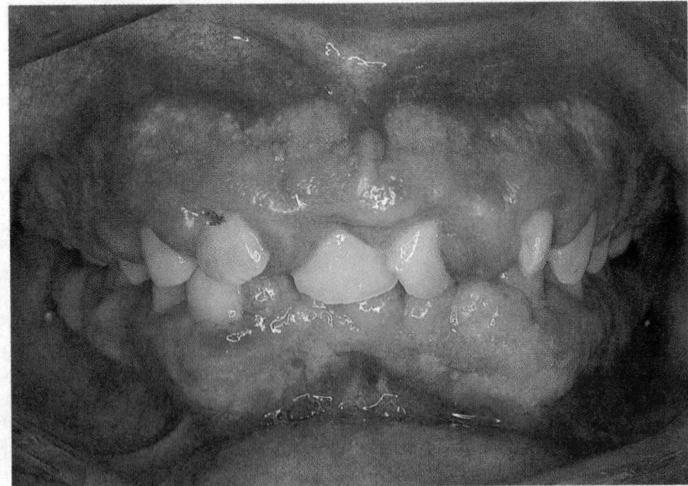

FIGURE 451–8 • Drug-induced gingival hyperplasia. Similar clinical lesions may occur with prolonged use of various drugs or as a hereditary condition (see text).

Reactive Hyperplasias

Small masses with surfaces that are ulcerated or only partially covered by normal-appearing mucosa usually represent reactive lesions in the form of pyogenic granulomas (whose frequency increases during pregnancy), peripheral giant cell granulomas, or lymphoid hyperplasia of the lingual or other tonsillar tissue. The granulomas are most often located on the gingiva. Rarely, such lesions may represent a metastatic neoplasm.

Epithelial Tumors

Small, white, wartlike epithelial masses are common and can occur in any area of the oral mucosa (Fig. 451–9). They are occasionally classified as epithelial neoplasms, but most do not continue to grow. Human papillomavirus types 2, 6, 11, 13, 32, and 57 have been identified in these wartlike lesions, which are usually classified generically as papillomas. A large wartlike lesion on the oral mucosa should raise the suspicion of verrucous carcinoma.

Mucus Retention Lesions (Mucoceles)

Mucoceles are small, chronic or recurring vesicles or bullae that occur commonly on the inside of the cheeks and lips, the posterior palate, and the mouth floor. They are caused by injury to one of the many submucosal minor salivary glands, resulting in extravasation of mucus, which causes granulomatous inflammation or blockage of the excretory duct, leading to cyst formation. Both types of lesions require conservative surgical excision because simple incision and drainage are usually followed by recurrence.

SALIVARY GLAND DISEASES

Primary Diseases of Salivary Glands

Patients with enlargement of a major or minor salivary gland usually present a diagnostic challenge (Table 451–6). More than 20 types of benign or malignant salivary gland neoplasms may appear as unilateral enlargement of a major gland that is firm and nontender to palpation or as a firm submucosal nodule on the palate or the labial or buccal mucosa. Uncommonly, unilateral major gland enlargement may be reactive—for example, lymphoepithelial lesion or chronic sialadenitis from duct obstruction or inadequately treated bacterial sialadenitis. Observation of any of these lesions should be followed by appropriate imaging and biopsy.

Unilateral major salivary gland enlargement that is markedly painful or tender to palpation and has a purulent exudate or nothing expressible from the duct suggests bacterial sialadenitis. Any exudate should be cultured, and initial treatment should be with an oral penicillinase-resistant antibiotic, such as cloxacillin or dicloxacillin, 500 mg, every 6 hours.

Bilateral Salivary Gland Enlargement and Decreased Salivary Secretion Associated with Systemic Diseases

The best-known cause of bilateral salivary gland enlargement is infection by the mumps virus (Chapter 392) in children. However, the prevalence of mumps decreased in the United States by more than 98% after the introduction of an effective vaccine in 1967, and now there are only a few hundred to a few thousand cases per year. Uncommonly, a less acute, mumpslike illness may occur in adults in association with cytomegalovirus (Chapter 399), influenza (Chapter 387), or Coxsackie A (Chapter 402) virus infection.

Sjögren's syndrome (Chapter 289) is characterized in about one third of patients by gradual development of firm, nontender or only slightly tender, bilateral enlargement of major salivary glands. The enlargement is chronic and may slowly wax and wane. In most patients, however, gradually progressive salivary hypofunction can impair speech and swallowing and be associated with a unique pattern of progressive dental caries and difficulty in wearing dentures. In severe cases, the oral mucosa is dry and sticky, saliva is not expressible from the major ducts, and about one

TABLE 451–6 CAUSES OF SALIVARY GLAND ENLARGEMENT

USUALLY UNILATERAL
Benign or malignant salivary gland neoplasms (more than 20 different histopathologic types)
Bacterial infection
Chronic sialadenitis (single gland)
USUALLY BILATERAL AND ASSOCIATED WITH SALIVARY HYPOFUNCTION
Viral infection (mumps, cytomegalovirus, influenza, Coxsackie A)
Sjögren's syndrome (benign lymphoepithelial lesion)
Chronic granulomatous diseases (sarcoidosis, tuberculosis, leprosy)
Recurrent parotitis of childhood
Human immunodeficiency virus infection/acquired immunodeficiency syndrome
BILATERALLY SYMMETRIC, SOFT, NONTENDER, PAROTID ONLY
Sialadenosis (asymptomatic parotid enlargement), idiopathic or associated with:
Diabetes mellitus
Hyperlipoproteinemia
Hepatic cirrhosis
Anorexia/bulimia
Chronic pancreatitis
Acromegaly
Gonadal hypofunction
Phenylbutazone use

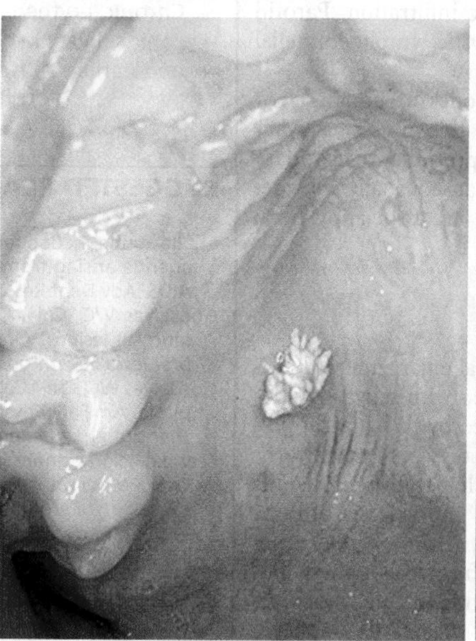
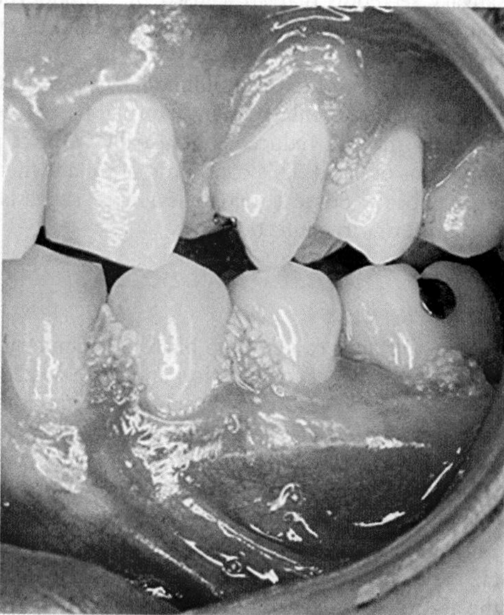

FIGURE 451–9 • Papillary epithelial tumors. Left, A solitary squamous papilloma. **Right,** multiple gingival papillomas, occurring in all quadrants, from condyloma acuminatum, associated with papilloma virus subtype 6 or 11.

TABLE 451–7 CAUSES OF DECREASED SALIVARY SECRETION

TEMPORARY

Effects of short-term drug use (e.g., antihistamines)
Virus infections (e.g., mumps)
Dehydration
Psychogenic conditions (e.g., anxiety)

CHRONIC

Effects of chronically administered drugs (particularly antidepressants, monoamine oxidase inhibitors, neuroleptics, parasympatholytics, some combinations of drugs for treating hypertension)
Chronic diseases:
- Sjögren's syndrome
- Sarcoidosis
- Human immunodeficiency virus or hepatitis C infection
- Depression
- Diabetes mellitus (uncontrolled)
- Amyloidosis (primary or secondary)
- Central nervous system diseases

Other effects of treatment
- Therapeutic radiation to the head and neck
- Graft-versus-host disease

Absent or malformed glands (rare)

third of patients have signs and symptoms of erythematous candidiasis (see earlier discussion) (see Fig. 451–7).

The salivary component of Sjögren's syndrome is diagnosed from a labial salivary gland biopsy specimen containing three to five minor glands and exhibiting focal lymphocytic sialadenitis in the absence of nonspecific chronic sialadenitis or abnormalities indicative of another disease, such as noncaseating granuloma. A patient's symptoms of oral dryness (xerostomia) are important but are subjective and can be caused by a wide variety of conditions (Table 451–7). Results from salivary function measurement or imaging are not diagnostically specific to Sjögren's syndrome.

Several chronic granulomatous diseases, such as sarcoidosis (Chapter 95), tuberculosis (Chapter 345), and leprosy (Chapter 347), can cause bilateral enlargement and decreased function of salivary glands. The clinical and serologic features of sarcoidosis may closely mimic those of Sjögren's syndrome, and the distinction is best made by minor salivary gland biopsy.

A few adult patients with HIV infection and most children who are infected in utero develop major salivary gland enlargement and reduced salivary secretion that are caused by lymphocytic infiltration. Parotid gland enlargement usually represents a solid or cystic lymphoepithelial lesion (see Table 451–2).

Recurrent parotitis of childhood includes episodes of unilateral or bilateral parotid enlargement. During flares of this illness, salivary secretion may be reduced, but usually without prominent secondary symptoms or signs. This condition, of unknown cause, usually subsides after puberty. Some serologic evidence suggests an association with Epstein-Barr virus infection.

Asymptomatic Parotid Enlargement (Sialadenosis)

Parotid glands can develop bilateral, symmetrical enlargement that is soft and nontender to palpation and not associated with salivary hypofunction (see Table 451–6). Diagnosis is established by this clinical presentation and the presence of one of the systemic diseases known to be associated with it: diabetes mellitus (Chapter 247), hyperlipoproteinemia (Chapter 225), hepatic cirrhosis (Chapter 157), anorexia or bulimia (Chapter 238), chronic pancreatitis (Chapter 147), acromegaly (Chapter 242), and gonadal hypofunction. It can also result from use of phenylbutazone or be a reaction to iodine-containing contrast media. Biopsy of the affected glands is not indicated for diagnosis.

Impaired Salivary Secretion without Gland Enlargement

The common symptom of dry mouth (xerostomia) is most often a side effect of chronically administered drugs. Many classes of drugs reduce unstimulated salivary secretion through anticholinergic or other mechanisms (see Table 451–7). Patients experience these symptoms soon after beginning to use the drug but produce enough saliva during a meal for normal chewing and swallowing. However, the symptoms and associated dental caries are dose dependent and gradually increase with prolonged use of the drug. The classes of drugs producing the most profound effects are most tricyclic antidepressants, most neuroleptics, monoamine oxidase inhibitors, and all anticholinergics. A combination of drugs for treatment of hypertension may cause symptoms of dry mouth but usually not to the extent of the drugs listed.

Several systemic diseases affect salivary secretion. As noted earlier, most patients with Sjögren's syndrome, some with sarcoidosis, and a few patients with HIV infection experience symptoms of dry mouth to various degrees, with or without salivary gland enlargement. In addition, patients who have primary or secondary amyloidosis with salivary gland deposition may develop impaired secretion. The symptom of xerostomia is more prevalent in individuals who also exhibit symptoms of depression but are not taking any drugs. Furthermore, studies done before the availability of antidepressant drugs showed that symptoms of depression were associated with decreased salivary secretion.

Irradiation of the head and neck region to treat a malignant tumor usually produces profound dry mouth during therapy. Secretory capacity recovers only slightly in the months following treatment for patients with solid tumors but recovers significantly for those with multifocal tumors (e.g., Hodgkin's disease).

Treatment

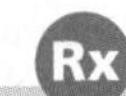

Significant chronic salivary hypofunction from any cause produces a risk for dental caries (decay) in approximate proportion to the secretory impairment, but caries can largely be prevented if appropriate measures are taken as soon as the hypofunction begins. Remaining teeth should be protected by a comprehensive dental caries prevention program, monitored by a dentist and including frequent application of appropriate topical fluorides, removal of dental plaque, counseling on control of cariogenic dietary carbohydrates, and placement of appropriate dental restorations as necessary.

Symptomatic treatment of mild to moderately severe salivary hypofunction can include sialagogues such as sugar-free hard candies or chewing gum, regular sips of water, and use of saliva substitutes at night. Symptoms of severe hypofunction can be improved by prescribing oral pilocarpine, 5 mg four times a day, or cevimeline, 30 mg three times a day, if not contraindicated.

Chronic erythematous oral candidiasis is a frequent sequela of chronic salivary hypofunction, and its treatment and retreatment, as noted earlier, substantially improve the patient's oral symptoms.

SUGGESTED READINGS

Challacombe S, Coogan M, Williams D, Greenspan J: Overview and research agenda arising from the 5th World Workshop on Oral Health and Disease in AIDS. Adv Dent Res 2006;19:5–9. *A comprehensive view of HIV-related lesions.*

Gonsalves WC, Chi AC, Neville BW: Common oral lesions: Part I. Superficial mucosal lesions. Am Fam Physician 2007;75:501–507. *An excellent review of oral lesions with good illustrations.*

Gonsalves WC, Chi AC, Neville BW: Common oral lesions: Part II. Masses and neoplasia. Am Fam Physician 2007;75:509–512. *An excellent review of oral lesions that present as masses.*

Mandel I, Surattanont F: Bilateral parotid swelling: A review. Oral Surg Oral Med Oral Pathol Oral Radiol Endod 2002;93:221–237. *Discussion of the various causes of bilateral parotid enlargement, which is almost always associated with an underlying systemic disease or process.*

Pihlstrom BL, Michalowicz BS, Johnson NW: Periodontal diseases. Lancet 2005;366:1809–1820. *A comprehensive overview.*

Scully C: Aphthous ulceration. N Engl J Med 2006;355:165–172. *Topical therapy such as lidocaine or protective bioadhesives might be helpful.*

452 APPROACH TO THE PATIENT WITH NOSE, SINUS, AND EAR DISORDERS

Andrew H. Murr

Patients with nose, sinus, and ear disorders may present with a variety of chief complaints. Nasal symptoms most commonly relate to rhinorrhea or congestion, both of which may be due to allergic, infectious, inflammatory, or structural causes. Sinus disorders, which commonly arise as a feeling of stuffiness or congestion but sometimes also manifest as pain or even headache (Chapter 421), have a similar set of causes. Common ear complaints include pain, loss of hearing (Chapter 454), and vestibular symptoms (Chapter 454), commonly described by the patient as dizziness but recognized by the physician as vertigo that is different from the lightheadedness that characterizes presyncope and syncope (Chapter 427). Epistaxis, which is bleeding from the nose, is usually easy to distinguish from hemoptysis from the bronchial tree (Chapter 83) or hematemesis from the gastrointestinal tract (Chapter 137).

Loss of hearing (Chapter 454) and vestibular symptoms (Chapter 454) are discussed elsewhere, as are smell, the related sensation of taste (Chapter 453), and the details of head and neck tumors (Chapter 200). This chapter focuses on the approach to patients with other common nose, sinus, and ear complaints.

NASAL AND SINUS COMPLAINTS

Rhinitis and Sinusitis

Definition

Rhinitis is generally defined as any inflammatory process in the nose, with the common result being a sensation of excess mucous or nasal congestion. The patient may have a sensation of fluid dripping from the nose, either coming from the nose anteriorly or coming from the nose posteriorly. Anterior nasal drainage may be perceived by the patient as being accompanied by an activity such as eating (gustatory rhinitis) and may be visible to an observer. Posterior nasal drainage is more nebulous and subjective, but it is very common and is referred to as postnasal drip.

In general, acute rhinitis and sinusitis describe inflammatory conditions of the nose and sinuses that last less than 4 weeks. Chronic rhinitis and sinusitis persist for more than 3 months despite treatment. Recurrent acute rhinitis and sinusitis are defined by exacerbations that occur four or more times per year and last 7 to 10 days per episode. Subacute rhinitis and sinusitis define symptoms that persist between 4 weeks and 12 weeks and resolve completely with treatment.

Epidemiology

The most common reason that a patient seeks the advice of a physician in the United States concerns problems relating to rhinitis and sinusitis. Over 20 million visits by patients per year are devoted to this complaint, and billions of dollars are spent on medications that are expected to improve the condition.

Pathobiology

Humans normally produce about 2 L of mucus per day from their nasal lining. The nose functions primarily as a humidification and filtration system, with a clean and refreshed nasal mucous blanket serving to trap particulate matter and organisms. The nasal and sinus lining consists of a ciliated respiratory epithelium; the cilia function in a highly organized and orderly fashion under normal circumstances to transport particulate matter trapped in the mucous blanket in a consistent fashion to allow the mucus to be swallowed, thereby avoiding deposition in the bronchi. The nose also serves as the organ of olfaction (Chapter 453) to allow patients to discern tastes and avoid spoiled foods that could cause illness.

The parasympathetic nervous system controls both vascular tone and mucus production in the nose. Inflammatory conditions, such as a common cold, can cause the nasal and sinus lining to swell, highlighting the nasal cycle governed by parasympathetic neural control. In a normal state, one side of the nose is relatively decongested and one side of the nose is relatively congested owing to vascular engorgement. This vascular dilatation allows humidification and warming of inspired air and can also affect the ability to discern odors in the process of olfaction. During rhinitis, the inflammation exaggerates the normal relative comparison between the decongested and congested sides of the nose and can be perceived as an uncomfortable nasal stuffiness that shifts from side to side over several hours.

Sinusitis differs from rhinitis because the term implies an infectious etiology rather than physiologic dysfunction. Nevertheless, many different mechanisms of inflammation besides infection may give rise to what is currently generally termed sinusitis.

Clinical Manifestations

When normal nasal mucosal function is lost, patients often complain of nasal crusting or obstruction, hypersecretion or postnasal drip, coughing, facial pressure, and fatigue. Nasal obstruction that shifts from side to side during the day is common in many types of rhinitis and may be considered an exaggeration of normal physiology.

Major symptoms of sinusitis (Table 452–1) include facial pressure, facial congestion or fullness, nasal obstruction, nasal discharge, and anosmia. Minor symptoms include headache, halitosis, fatigue, dental pain, cough, and ear pressure. Major signs include purulence in the nose noted on examination and, in acute sinusitis, fever. Pain is a frequent complaint with acute sinusitis but infrequent in chronic sinusitis. Patients with chronic sinusitis often note a dull facial pressure that seems to worsen with dependency. Patients with acute sinusitis may have discrete facial pain or dental pain but also have obvious purulent nasal discharge, often with a frank fever. It is important to note that facial pain is not a symptom of chronic sinusitis in the absence of other nasal signs and symptoms. Generally, sinusitis is thought to be present on the basis of at least two major factors, one major factor and two minor factors, or purulence on nasal examination.

Diagnosis (Fig. 452–1)

History

A thorough history should probe whether patients have tried over-the-counter or prescription medications, including antihistamines, decongestants, mucolytics, analgesics, mast cell stabilizers, and even steroids, and whether they have helped improve the condition. In addition, other prescription medications have side effects that affect nasal physiology, including birth control pills, antihypertensive medications that cause systemic vasodilation, aspirin, steroids, and antibiotics. Specific questions regarding allergies are important, including seasonality or environmental triggers, the presence or absence of pets, food sensitivities, recent changes in environment, and living conditions, with a focus on old or new carpets, mattresses, furnace filters, or freshly painted interior walls. A patient should be questioned about past allergy skin testing or other testing.

A recent history of other family members or coworkers being ill suggests an infectious process. An astute physician often suspects an

TABLE 452–1 MAJOR AND MINOR SINUSITIS FACTORS

Major Factors	Minor Factors
Facial pain or pressure (in conjunction with other nasal symptoms)	Headache
Facial fullness	Halitosis
Nasal obstruction	Fatigue
Nasal discharge or purulence	Dental pain
Fever (in acute rhinosinusitis)	Fever (in nonacute rhinosinusitis)
	Cough
	Ear pressure or fullness

Section XXVI Eye and ENT

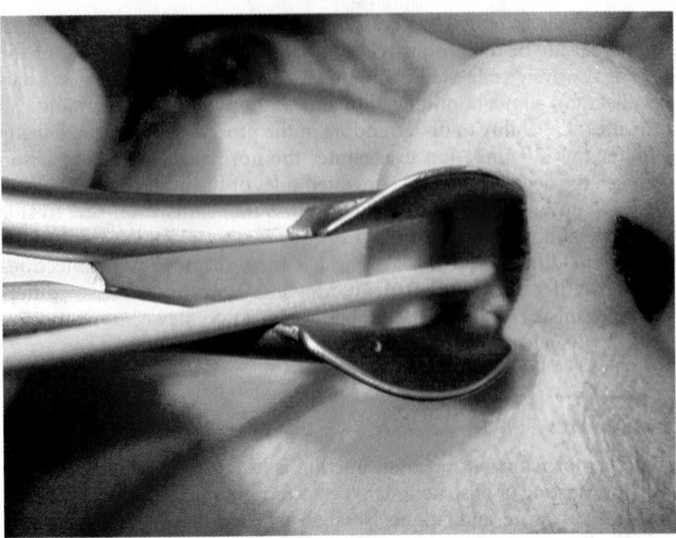

FIGURE 452–1 • The caudal aspect of the septum is often the site of origin of anterior epistaxis.

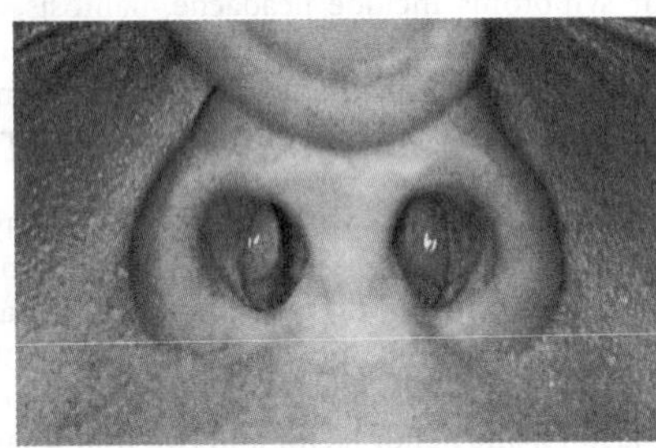

FIGURE 452–2 • Edematous inferior turbinates narrowing the nasal airway in a patient with hay fever. (From Dhillon RS, East CA [eds]: Ear, Nose and Throat and Head and Neck Surgery, 2nd ed. Edinburgh, Churchill Livingstone, 1994, p 34.)

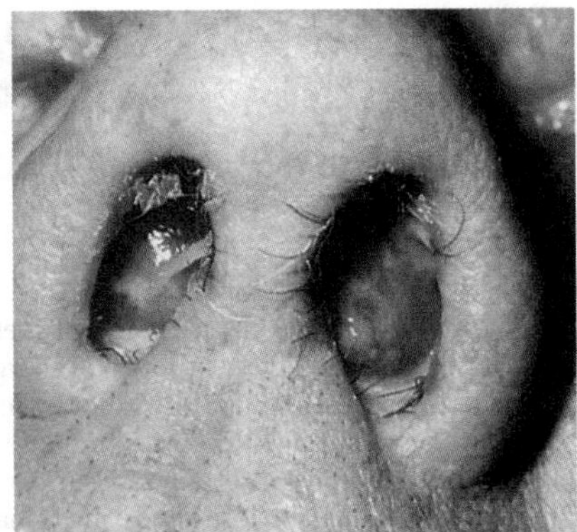

FIGURE 452–3 • Bilateral nasal polyps in the nasal vestibules. A polyp can easily be confused with a normal inferior turbinate. (From Dhillon RS, East CA [eds]: Ear, Nose and Throat and Head and Neck Surgery, 2nd ed. Edinburgh, Churchill Livingstone, 1994, p 36.)

infectious process by noting the similarity and time course of symptoms in other patients; this information can be related to patients so that they know what to expect in terms of time course and recovery. A careful past medical history should determine whether relevant conditions such as prior nasal surgery or trauma, granulomatous diseases, cystic fibrosis (Chapter 89), rheumatologic conditions, immune deficiencies (Chapter 271), or other problems may be contributing factors. Unilateral nasal congestion raises a concern for either an anatomic abnormality such as a septal deviation, perhaps related to prior trauma, a polyp or other neoplastic mass, or perhaps even a foreign body.

Physical Examination

The nose should be inspected with a nasal speculum to assess the nasal septal anatomy, the most caudal aspect of the inferior turbinates (Fig. 452–2), and the possibility of large nasal polyps (Fig. 452–3) or other masses. In allergic rhinitis, the physical examination may reveal pale and swollen inferior turbinates, whereas copious nasal secretion are more apparent in viral infections. By spraying the nose with a topical decongestant such as phenylephrine (Neo-Synephrine), the middle meatus, which is the air space between the middle turbinate and lateral nasal wall, can often be visualized to assess for nasal polyps or purulent discharge. Examination of the mouth, oropharynx, and posterior pharyngeal wall, with a tongue blade if necessary, can sometimes identify a stream of postnasal discharge or pus. Sinus palpation and transillumination, although part of the art of medicine, are not sufficiently reliable for diagnosis. The patient's ability to open the mouth without limitation helps exclude trismus, which can sometimes be caused by a deep neck infection.

A complete examination of the head and neck should look for signs of recent or old trauma such as ecchymosis under the eyelids, swelling of the soft tissue of the face, or a deviation of the nasal dorsum. The neck should be palpated for adenopathy (Chapter 174) or other masses.

A basic eye examination should assess pupillary function, extraocular movements, and possible nystagmus (Chapter 450). An ear examination should assess the tympanic membranes bilaterally. In patients with an abnormality of the membrane or concomitant complaints of hearing loss or disequilibrium (Chapter 454), pneumotoscopy using an air bulb attached to the otoscope can be used to insufflate the ear canal and assess for mobility of the tympanic membrane; decreased mobility suggests a middle ear effusion. Weber and Rinne testing using a tuning fork screens for conductive hearing loss, especially unilateral.

Endoscopic examination of the nose, almost always by a specialist, is the "gold standard" for evaluating rhinitis and sinusitis. A flexible or rigid fiberoptic scope can allow fine inspection of the septum, turbinates, middle meatus, and sphenoethmoid recess as well as direct inspection of the nasopharynx, orifice of the eustachian tube, and the fossa of Rosenmüller, which is just rostral to the eustachian tube in the nasopharynx and is often the site of origin of nasopharyngeal carcinoma (Chapter 200). Flexible endoscopy can further inspect the oropharynx, larynx, and most of the hypopharynx (Chapter 455).

Laboratory Findings

Cultures

Cultures of the nostril or lower nasal cavity are not useful and are not recommended. An endoscopically guided culture by a specialist may help guide treatment for acutely ill immunocompromised patients, cases of refractory chronic rhinosinusitis, or patients whose sinusitis is suspected of causing secondary meningitis, epidural or subdural abscess, brain abscess, orbital involvement, or cavernous sinus thrombosis.

Other Tests

A nasal smear can reveal eosinophils, which are consistent with allergic rhinitis (Chapter 272). Likewise, skin testing or radioallergosorbent testing can help pinpoint allergic triggers (Chapter 270). In patients with acute sinusitis, a white blood cell count with differential may be useful. In patients with chronic sinusitis, serum immunoglobulin levels can be helpful: highly elevated immunoglobulin E (IgE) levels can raise suspicions for allergic fungal sinusitis, whereas low levels of IgG and other subclasses suggest immunodeficiency (Chapter 271). If the patient has chronic nasal crusting as a primary complaint, screening serologies for sarcoid (Chapter 95), Wegener's granulomatosis (Chapter 291), T-cell lymphomas (Chapter 196), syphilis (Chapter 340), tuberculosis (Chapter 345), Sjögren's syndrome (Chapter 289), and other chronic inflammatory diseases can be considered. In a patient with a lifelong history of sinusitis since childhood, cystic fibrosis should also be considered (Chapter 89).

Imaging

Noncontrast computed tomographic (CT) scanning is indicated for patients with known or suspected rhinitis and sinusitis. CT scans are generally ordered to document the presence of disease or the effects of treatment to improve the disease. CT scan examination is also used to evaluate complications of sinusitis or to investigate sinusitis in immunocompromised patients. Finally, the CT scan is critical prior to any surgical treatment of the sinuses. Opacification or other findings on a CT scan (Fig. 452–4) can often differentiate among the various causes of sinusitis. Plain

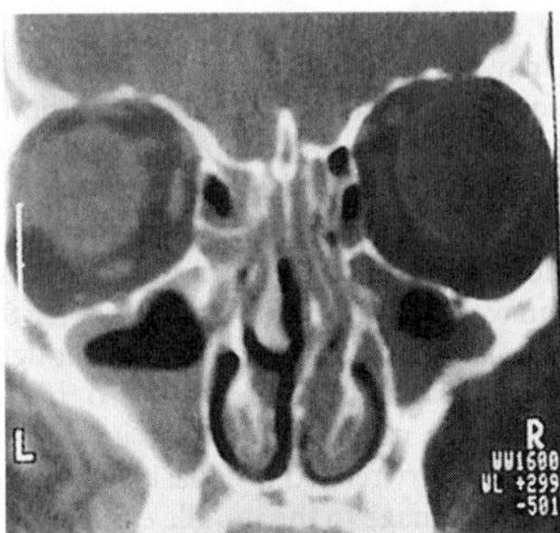

FIGURE 452–4 • Coronal computed tomography scan showing bilateral acute pansinusitis. There is a fluid level in the left maxillary sinus, which, if aspirated, can be sent for microbiology. (From Dhillon RS, East CA [eds]: Ear, Nose and Throat and Head and Neck Surgery, 2nd ed. Edinburgh, Churchill Livingstone, 1994, p 50.)

films have little utility and are not generally recommended. Magnetic resonance imaging (MRI) is occasionally helpful.

Differential Diagnosis

A rapid onset of symptoms present for a short time suggests a viral upper respiratory infection, especially if the patient also has typical systemic symptoms, such as arthralgias, myalgias, fever, chills, gastrointestinal symptoms, and cough in addition to nasal congestion, postnasal drip, and headache. By comparison, acute bacterial rhinosinusitis arises with facial pressure and purulent postnasal discharge. Often, viral disease can progress to a secondary bacterial infection, which can become chronic. The acute onset of inhalant allergy is often seasonal or can be traced to a particular precipitant (Chapter 272). Allergic rhinitis typically responds to an empirical trial of antihistamines, whereas viral or bacterial rhinitis does not.

Chronic sinusitis must be differentiated from rhinitis, which is not accompanied by the same degree of incessant inflammation. Types of rhinitis include gustatory rhinitis associated with eating, rhinitis of pregnancy, rhinitis associated with abuse of topical vasoconstrictors, rhinitis associated with illicit drug use (e.g., cocaine or methamphetamine), rhinitis of aging, vasomotor rhinitis presumably related to a hypersecretory state mediated by the parasympathetic nervous system, and perennial allergic rhinitis, whose hallmark is a lack of seasonality.

Chronic sinusitis may be caused by chronic viral infection, chronic bacterial infection, chronic fungal infection, and chronic allergy. It is often difficult to pinpoint a specific cause, but the common underlying factor is often inflammatory in nature. Whereas maxillary antral punctures were used for diagnosis and treatment in the pre-CT era, endoscopically guided culture techniques combined with CT imaging are now the standard of care, except in acute bacterial maxillary sinusitis, for which surgical decompression is desirable, or in some cases of refractory sinusitis in immunocompromised patients or in the intensive care unit, where direct culture can guide antibiotic therapy.

Nasal polyps may be caused by Samter's triad (asthma, aspirin sensitivity, and nasal polyposis related to upregulation of leukotrienes caused by prostaglandin blockade). Human papillomavirus (Chapter 396) may cause an inverted papilloma, which responds to surgical excision but can transform to frank malignancy. Polyps are also seen in patients with cystic fibrosis (Chapter 89) and allergic fungal sinusitis, which is manifested by an elevated IgE level, positive fungal cultures (usually for aspergillosis), Charcot-Leyden crystals on histopathology, characteristic densities on CT imaging, and nasal polyposis that is often, but not always, unilateral. Antral choanal polyps may extend into the nasal cavity or nasopharynx and cause obstruction.

CT imaging can reveal mucoceles, blocked individual sinuses that continue to secrete mucus and can slowly erode bone, expand to involve the eye and brain, or become acutely infected. A mycetoma, which is an isolated "fungus ball" of a sinus, has a characteristic hyperdensity within a sinus opacification. Unilateral nasal polyposis is suggestive of antral choanal polyps, malignancy, inverted papilloma, or allergic fungal sinusitis; early biopsy is recommended. Mucus retention cysts, often present in the maxillary sinus, are manifested by a spherical opacification; an estimated 10% of the population has a mucus retention cyst, which is often asymptomatic.

Treatment

Medical Therapy

Viral rhinitis is treated with supportive care, including fluid replacement and treatment of the febrile component of the syndrome with acetaminophen or nonsteroidal anti-inflammatory medications. Steam has a mild decongestant effect, and vitamin C and good nutrition may help hasten the resolution of symptoms. Oral decongestants (such as pseudoephedrine 120 mg every 12 hours for several days), mucolytics (such as guaifenesin 200 to 400 mg every 4 to 6 hours for several days), and ipratropium bromide (0.03 or 0.06%, two sprays on each side of the nose every 12 hours for several days) are of potential benefit.

Allergic rhinitis (Chapter 272) responds to various antihistamines, such as diphenhydramine hydrochloride (25 to 50 mg every 4 to 6 hours), loratadine (5 mg twice a day or 10 mg a day), cetirizine hydrochloride (10 mg a day), and fexofenadine hydrochloride (60 mg twice a day or 120 mg a day), and topical nasal steroids, including triamcinolone acetonide (two sprays [55 μg] to each side of the nose every day), mometasone furoate (two sprays [50 μg] to each naris every day), fluticasone propionate (two sprays [50 μg] to each naris every day), and budesonide (two sprays [32 μg] to each naris every day). Oral steroids such as prednisone and methylprednisolone in various doses are sometimes useful as well. Allergic desensitization is sometimes recommended when a discrete allergen elicits a strong reaction in a patient. Allergic desensitization may specifically be beneficial in some inflammatory disorders, such as allergic fungal sinusitis. [1] Nasal polyps frequently respond to oral steroids, either in a tapered burst dose or, in rare cases, in small amounts of titrated daily oral steroids such as prednisone or methylprednisolone.

Bacterial sinusitis should be treated with antibiotics directed toward *Haemophilus influenzae, Moraxella catarrhalis, Streptococcus pneumoniae,* and *Staphylococcus aureus.* Antibiotics such as amoxicillin 500 mg three times a day or erythromycin 500 mg twice a day for 2 to 3 weeks with a subsequent follow-up examination to document resolution are reasonable first-line coverage. β-Lactamase–stable antibiotics are used as a second-line treatment, as are antibiotics that have good anaerobic coverage: amoxicillin with clavulanic acid at 875 mg twice a day for β-lactamase stability or clindamycin at 300 mg three times a day for anaerobic coverage. The use of antifungals including itraconazole in an oral or aerosolized form and amphotericin B in an aerosolized form is controversial in the treatment of chronic sinusitis. [2]

Surgical Therapy

Surgery is recommended in patients with mucoceles, inverted papilloma, antral choanal polyps, juvenile nasopharyngeal angiofibroma, and malignancies. Surgery can correct septal deviations and anatomically related nasal obstruction. Surgery on the inferior turbinates may be beneficial in refractory rhinitis. Surgery for benign nasal polyposis can improve symptomatic control and reduce the need for oral steroids. Functional endoscopic surgery, which is designed to preserve mucociliary function and is performed with endoscopes through the nostril without large incisions, can be useful in recurrent acute sinusitis and in chronic rhinosinusitis.

Epistaxis

For a patient with epistaxis, it is first critical to determine the severity of the blood loss. Persistent bleeding may result from warfarin, antiplatelet agents, or any underlying platelet or (Chapter 179) clotting deficiency (Chapter 180). Physical examination should focus on inspection of the anterior septum, which is the most frequent point of origin for epistaxis. Often, dilated blood vessels on the caudal septum can be seen upon anterior rhinoscopy (Fig. 425–5). The combination of unilateral otitis media, epistaxis, nasal congestion, and a neck mass would be concerning for nasopharyngeal carcinoma. Rare tumors that can arise with bleeding include juvenile nasal angiofibromas in male patients.

Epistaxis can be treated by local pressure, packing (using nasal sponges, balloons, or petroleum jelly–impregnated 1/2 inch by 72 inch gauze), humidification, and hydration. Hospitalization and transfusion are rarely required. Offending medications should be reduced in dose or discontinued temporarily if possible. Occasionally, lasers are used or other types of cautery can address a specific bleeding area.

EAR PAIN

Definition

Ear pain (Table 452–2) is discomfort perceived by a patient in the area of the temporal bone. Although the discomfort can often be localized by the patient, at times the cause of the discomfort may in fact be distant from the site where the pain is felt. This referred pain can be due to problems in the oral cavity, oropharynx, hypopharynx, or larynx.

Pathobiology

The ear is well supplied with sensory nerves and is positioned on the side of the skull. The ear is divided into the outer ear or pinna and ear canal; the middle ear, which encompasses the tympanic membrane and ossicles; and the inner ear, which includes the cochlea and the vestibular canals, including the utricle and saccule. In general, otalgia is due to problems in the outer or middle ear. The trigeminal nerve innervates the anterior superior quadrant of the pinna, whereas the C2 and C3 cervical cutaneous nerves innervate the rest of the majority of the outer ear. However, there are contributions by ninth and tenth nerves in the ear canal and even a small patch of sensory innervation by the seventh nerve in the posterior superior ear canal. It is the overlap in distribution of the ninth and tenth cranial nerves that establishes the anatomic basis for referred otalgia in diseases of the oral cavity, oropharynx, and larynx. Therefore, ear pain may be due to inflammatory conditions of the skin of the outer ear, the ear canal, or the middle ear, or it may be due to disease processes unrelated to the ear itself.

Clinical Manifestations

Patients with ear pain often present with complaints referable directly to the ear itself. In cases of otitis externa, frankly obvious erythema and swelling of the ear canal may be present. Even minute physical manipulation of the ear may be excruciating. In chondritis of the pinna, which may be related to rheumatologic disorders, infection, or trauma, the entire pinna may be swollen and painful. Hearing loss accompanying otalgia may indicate middle ear disease, especially otitis media. Patients sometimes complain of pain in the ear after air travel or driving from a mountainous region. Quick changes in pressure, such as are encountered in scuba diving, may indicate barotrauma (Chapter 94), in which the eustachian tube is unable to compensate rapidly enough for the pressure changes that are encountered. Pain may also be a post-traumatic symptom from relatively minor percussion injury, more severe head trauma, or percussion injury related to a blast. Pain related to noise exposure may also indicate damage to the middle ear or even inner ear. Deep-seated boring pain over the temporal area accompanied by retro-orbital pain can be due to petrous apex disease, including petrous apicitis.

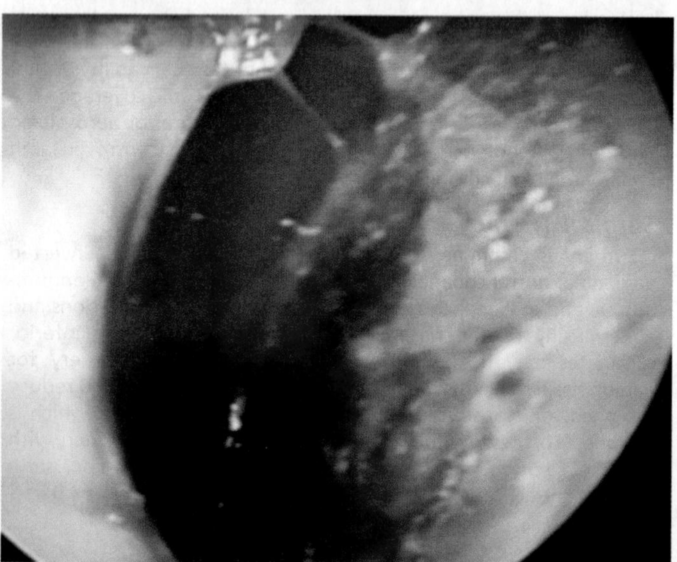

FIGURE 452–5 • Dilated nasal vessels and crusting typical of a patient with epistaxis.

Diagnosis

History

A patient with ear pain should be asked to reveal the location of the discomfort, the duration of the symptoms, and any activities related to the onset of the condition. As an example, recent swimming would make otitis externa more likely, whereas a recent upper respiratory infection with hearing loss would suggest otitis media. Questions should address possible hearing loss, vertigo, otorrhea, hoarseness, voice change, dysphagia, odynophagia, dyspnea, hemoptysis, hematemesis, and weight loss. A social history with specific concentration on tobacco and alcohol use should be obtained. A possible family history of upper aerodigestive tract and nasopharyngeal carcinoma should be sought. A past surgical history can reveal distant ear or throat surgery.

Physical Examination

A complete head and neck examination, including a general assessment for trauma and a basic eye examination, is required. The outer ear and pinna should be examined first. The ear canal should be first palpated, then inspected. An otoscope with a pneumatic bulb attachment is critical to establish the presence or absence of a middle ear effusion. Inspection of the tympanic membrane should be accomplished with notations made about patency and perforation, translucency of the eardrum, position and definition of the malleus, and the eardrum's mobility with the ear canal sealed and a puff of air delivered by the pneumatic bulb (Fig. 452–6). Abnormalities may be caused by infection (Fig. 452–7) or barotrauma (Fig. 452–8). A tuning fork examination with a 512-Hz tuning fork should be accomplished to determine lateralization of the sound (Weber examination) and should be used to determine whether air conduction is superior to bone conduction (Rinne examination). Facial nerve function should be assessed (Chapter 446) by determining whether the patient can close the eyes. The presence or absence of nystagmus should be recorded. Inspection of the nose, oral cavity, oropharynx, and neck should be accompanied by a cranial nerve examination (Chapter 418). Palpation of the tongue and tonsils is especially important if the ear pain is intense and persistent. A careful neck examination should look for masses. Oral cavity infections (Chapter 451) such as a peritonsillar abscess or severe tonsillitis may arise as ear pain, and the physical examination should reveal trismus, erythema, mass effect, and other common signs of pharyngitis.

Laboratory

An audiogram can assess hearing loss (Chapter 454). A tympanogram measures compliance of the middle ear system and is an accurate method

TABLE 452–2 CAUSES OF OTOLAGIA

Causes of Otalgia	External Ear	Middle Ear	Upper aerodigestive tract
Likely	Otitis externa Herpes zoster oticus Chondritis Foreign body	Acute otitis media Acute eardrum perforation Barotrauma Chronic otitis media with impending complication	Tonsillitis Tonsil abscess Deep neck abscess Tumor (especially tongue base, tonsil, hypopharynx, larynx, nasopharynx)
Unlikely	Malignant otitis externa Tumor	Tumor	

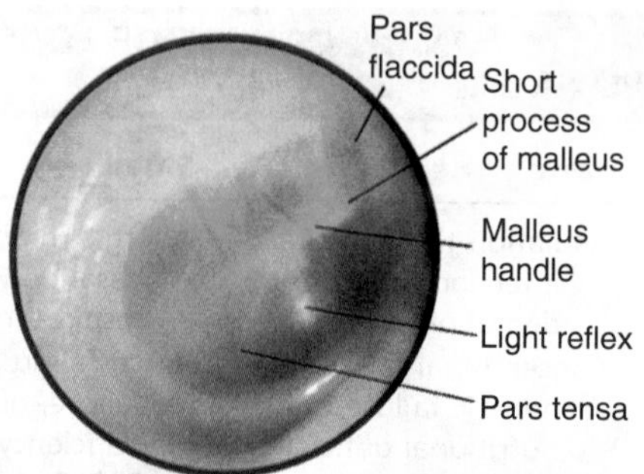

FIGURE 452–6 • A normal tympanic membrane. (From Dhillon RS, East CA [eds]: Ear, Nose and Throat and Head and Neck Surgery, 2nd ed. Edinburgh, Churchill Livingstone, 1994, p 2.)

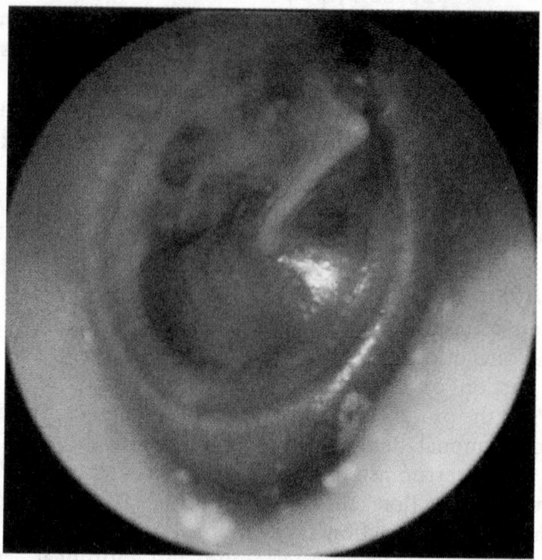

FIGURE 452–7 • Otoscopic appearance in otitis media with effusion. The handle and short process of the malleus are brought into relief by retraction of the eardrum. There is a slightly yellow appearance of the eardrum related to the middle ear effusion. (From Dhillon RS, East CA [eds]: Ear, Nose and Throat and Head and Neck Surgery, 2nd ed. Edinburgh, Churchill Livingstone, 1994, p 7.)

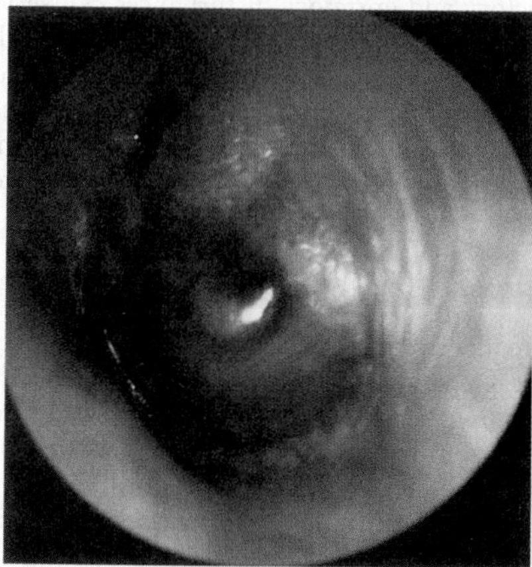

FIGURE 452–8 • Blood in the middle ear (hemotympanum). Causes include otitic barotraumas, secretory otitis media, and high jugular bulb. (From Dhillon RS, East CA [eds]: Ear, Nose and Throat and Head and Neck Surgery, 2nd ed. Edinburgh, Churchill Livingstone, 1994, p 26.)

used to diagnose otitis media. Cultures are rarely used because they require tympanocentesis, and cultures of the external ear can reveal a vast variety of organisms that are often treated empirically with antibiotics. If a fever and middle ear effusion are present and neck stiffness is part of the physical examination picture, a lumbar puncture may rarely be recommended (Chapter 437).

Imaging

In general, imaging is indicated if there are suspected complications of acute or chronic otitis media or to look for occult causes in the upper aerodigestive tract. If a patient is suspected to have meningitis, epidural or subdural abscess, brain abscess, or sagittal sinus thrombosis, imaging is mandatory. Imaging is also useful for operative planning in cases of chronic otitis media or (rarely) to evaluate tumors of the middle or external ear.

Differential Diagnosis

Otitis externa, which is an infection of the skin of the ear canal, is often due to manipulating the ear after swimming or trying to scratch an ear canal that itches because of skin irritation. Erythema of the canal skin and extreme pain on manipulating the ear canal are present. In the presence of concomitant cranial neuropathies, especially in diabetic or otherwise immunocompromised patients, malignant otitis externa with osteomyelitis should be suspected. Inspection of the tympanic membrane may reveal fluid (see Fig. 452–7), consistent with otitis media; the tuning fork examination should support the presence of a conductive hearing loss. Vesicles on the conchal portion of the pinna, especially when accompanied by a facial nerve paralysis, strongly suggest herpes zoster oticus with Ramsay Hunt syndrome (Chapter 454). A perforation of the eardrum suggests either acute or chronic otitis media, traumatic perforation, or possibly cholesteatoma (Chapter 454) if the perforation is in the posterior superior quadrant. Chronic draining otorrhea of long standing with a deep boring pain and a perforation of the tympanic membrane suggests a complication of otitis media.

If the ear and cranial nerve examination is negative but the patient's complaints of otalgia are persistent, special efforts need to be made to visualize the upper aerodigestive tract including the nasopharynx, oral cavity, oropharynx, larynx, and hypopharynx to be sure that infection or tumor is not present in these hard-to-examine areas. MRI can be very useful in these cases.

Treatment

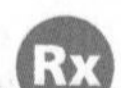

Otitis externa is often treated with office suctioning of debris using a microscope and the application of antibiotic drops (ciprofloxacin, tobramycin, neomycin, polymyxin B) with or without hydrocortisone in various combinations. Often, a small wick or sponge is placed into the ear canal to help maintain patency of the canal and to allow facile application of the medications. For otitis media, oral antibiotic treatment is directed at eradicating *H. influenzae, M. catarrhalis, S. pneumoniae,* and *S. aureus* with amoxicillin or erythromycin as for sinusitis (see earlier). The benefit is notable for children aged 2 years or younger with bilateral otitis and for older children with otitis plus otorrhea, whereas other patients can be observed without antibiotics. [3] Interestingly, the natural history of acute otitis media is acute perforation of the eardrum, which often results in otorrhea and a relief of pain. Most middle ear effusions clear spontaneously within 3 months whether or not they are treated. Most perforations of an eardrum caused by trauma heal without surgical intervention, but if an eardrum perforation persists for more than about 3 months, surgical closure utilizing tympanoplasty with or without mastoidectomy can be contemplated. Chronic draining perforations, especially if located in the posterior superior quadrant of the tympanic membrane, may require tympanomastoid surgery.

Patients with suspected herpes zoster can be started on acyclovir 800 mg by mouth every 4 hours for about 10 days with or without prednisone (Chapter 398). Intracranial complications of otitis media often need to be addressed surgically.

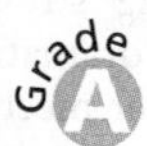

1. Folker RJ, Marple BF, Mabry RL, et al: Treatment of allergic fungal sinusitis: A comparison trial of postoperative immunotherapy with specific fungal antigens. Laryngoscope 1998;108:1623–1627.
2. Ponikau JU, Sherris DA, Weaver A, et al: Treatment of chronic rhinosinusitis with intranasal amphotericin B: A randomized, placebo-controlled, double-blind pilot trial. J Allergy Clin Immunol 2005;115:125–131.
3. Rovers MM, Glasziou P, Appelman CL, et al: Antibiotics for acute otitis media: A meta-analysis with individual patient data. Lancet 2006;368:1429–1435.

SUGGESTED READINGS

Osguthorpe JD, Nielsen DR: Otitis externa: Review and clinical update. Am Fam Physician 2006;74:1510–1516. *An excellent review of otitis externa.*

Piccirillo JF: Acute bacterial sinusitis. N Engl J Med 2004;351:902–910. *A case-based review.*

Prenner BM, Schenkel E: Allergic rhinitis: Treatment based on patient profiles. Am J Med 2006;119:230–237. *A comprehensive review.*

453 SMELL AND TASTE

Robert W. Baloh

Millions of people suffer from disorders of taste and smell, but these disorders are often neglected because they are not fatal and, unlike abnormalities of vision and hearing, are not considered serious handicaps. Chemosensory disorders, however, often reduce the enjoyment and quality of life and are important to patients who suffer from them.

Definition

The sensory receptor for taste, the taste bud, is made up of 50 to 150 cells arranged to form a pear-shaped organ. The lifespan of these cells is 10 to 14 days, and they are constantly being renewed from dividing epithelial cells surrounding the bud. Taste buds are located on the tongue, soft palate, pharynx, larynx, epiglottis, uvula, and the upper third of the esophagus. The taste buds located on the anterior two thirds of the tongue and on the palate are innervated by the chorda tympani branch of the seventh cranial nerve. The ninth cranial nerve innervates the posterior third of the tongue. The 9th and 10th nerves innervate taste buds in the pharynx and larynx. Afferent signals from the taste buds project to the nucleus of the solitary tract in the medulla and then via a series of relays to the thalamus and postcentral somatosensory cerebral cortex (primary ipsilateral). Free nerve endings of the fifth cranial nerve are found on the tongue and in the oral cavity, and lesions involving these pathways can also alter taste perception.

Olfactory receptors lie in a roughly dime-sized area of specialized pigmented epithelium that arches along the superior aspect of each side of the nasal mucosa. Specialized bipolar sensory cells in this region thrust short receptor hairs into the overlying mucosa to detect aromatic molecules as they dissolve. As with taste buds, the specialized receptor portion of the bipolar neuron undergoes continuous renewal, with turnover occurring approximately every 30 days. Thin axons of the bipolar neurons course through small holes in the cribriform plate of the ethmoid bone to form connections in the overlying olfactory bulb on the ventral surface of the frontal lobe. From here, second- and third-order neurons project directly and indirectly to the prepiriform cortex and parts of the amygdaloid complex of both sides of the brain, which represents the primary olfactory cortex.

Pathobiology

Pathology

Disorders of taste interfere with digestion because taste stimulants alter salivary and pancreatic flow, gastric contractions, and intestinal motility. Smell also contributes to the anticipation and ingestion of food because much of what is tasted derives from olfactory stimulation during ingestion and chewing. An inability to detect noxious tastes and odors can result in food or gas poisoning, particularly in elderly subjects. In the extreme, chemosensory disorders can lead to overwhelming stress, anorexia, and depression. Over the past few years there has been dramatic progress in modern understanding of the cellular and molecular mechanisms of chemoreception. Genes encoding for chemoreceptor proteins belonging to the G protein–coupled receptor superfamily account for up to 1% of mammalian genomes. Sequence diversity in these genes encodes unique structural motifs that bind to different ligands signaling different odors and tastes.

TABLE 453–1 COMMON CAUSES OF LOSS OF TASTE AND SMELL

	Taste	Smell
Local	Radiation therapy, oral infections, dentures, dental procedures	Allergic rhinitis, sinusitis, nasal polyposis, upper respiratory infection
Systemic	Cancer, renal failure, hepatic failure, nutritional deficiency (vitamin B_3, zinc), Cushing's syndrome, hypothyroidism, diabetes mellitus, infection (viral), drugs (antirheumatic and antiproliferative)	Renal failure, hepatic failure, nutritional deficiency (vitamin B_{12}), Cushing's syndrome, hypothyroidism, diabetes mellitus, infection (viral hepatitis, influenza), drugs (nasal sprays, antibiotics)
Neurologic	Bell's palsy, familial dysautonomia, multiple sclerosis	Head trauma, multiple sclerosis, Parkinson's disease, frontal tumor

Pathophysiology

Disorders of taste and smell can be divided into local, systemic, and neurologic categories (Table 453–1). The taste buds and the specialized receptor portion of the bipolar olfactory cells are constantly being renewed, and the process of renewal can be affected by nutritional, metabolic, and hormonal states, therapeutic radiation, drugs, and age. For example, with interruption of mitosis by antiproliferative agents, return of normal taste function takes a minimum of 10 days, whereas return to normal olfactory function takes more than 30 days. Diuretics can block apical ion channels on a taste bud, and antifungal drugs inhibit cytochrome P-450–dependent enzymes at the level of the receptors. Numerous local conditions such as colds and allergies, chronic sinusitis, and nasal polyposis can influence the sense of smell by restricting airway patency. Accidental blows to the head can shear the fine axons of the bipolar olfactory neurons and result in loss of smell. Lesions of the fifth, seventh (*chorda tympani*), and ninth nerves can lead to disordered taste sensation. Olfactory and gustatory disturbances can serve as important diagnostic signs for focal neurologic lesions (e.g., frontal lobe tumors). Hallucinations of smell and taste occur with epileptogenic lesions affecting the mesial temporal lobe and insular region, respectively. Finally, olfactory disturbances and hallucinations occur with a number of psychiatric illnesses (particularly depressive illness and schizophrenia).

Clinical Manifestations

The most frequently encountered causes of loss of smell are local obstructive disease, viral infections, head injuries, and normal aging. Patients can lose their sense of smell not only from chronic allergies and sinusitis but also from the nasal sprays and drops that they use to treat these conditions. The most common causes of loss of the sense of taste are viral infections and drug ingestion, particularly antirheumatic and antiproliferative drugs. Many of the systemic disorders listed in Table 453–1 probably produce their effect by decreasing the rate of turnover of sensory receptors on the tongue and olfactory epithelia. Disturbances of smell and taste in malnourished patients may be due to specific deficiencies in vitamins and minerals, such as zinc. Viral illnesses such as influenza and viral hepatitis produce disorders in both taste and smell. Multifocal neurologic disorders such as multiple sclerosis can affect the central olfactory and gustatory pathways at multiple levels; as a result, abnormalities of taste and smell are common in such patients.

Diagnosis

Olfaction can be tested grossly at the bedside with a few easily recognized odors such as coffee, chocolate, and the roselike aroma of the compound phenylethyl alcohol. (Nasal irritants should be avoided.) Each nostril is tested separately to determine whether the problem is unilateral or bilateral. Gustatory sensation is typically tested with weak solutions of sugar, salt, and acetic acid, or vinegar. The patient must keep the tongue protruded and respond to questions either by nodding the head or pointing to names of the tastes written on cards. The anterior two thirds and posterior third of the tongue should be tested separately.

Treatment

Treatment of olfactory dysfunction secondary to nasal disease is aimed at opening the air passageways while preserving the olfactory epithelium (Chapter 452). Intranasal steroids, antibiotics, and allergic therapies are useful in selected cases. Drugs known to affect taste or smell should be removed for a trial. Vitamin and mineral therapies are of unproven benefit.

SUGGESTED READINGS

Boyce JM, Shone GR: Effects of ageing on smell and taste. Postgrad Med J 2006;82:239–241. *Reviews the causes and treatment of smell and taste dysfunction in older people.*

Bramerson A, Nordin S, Bende M: Clinical experience with patients with olfactory complaints, and their quality of life. Acta Otolaryngol 2007;127:167–174. *A description of patients seeking medical attention for olfactory disorders and an overview of the etiologies and diagnosis.*

Doty RL, Bromley SM: Effects of drugs on olfaction and taste. Otolaryngol Clin North Am 2004;37:1229–1254. *Explains how and why so many drugs affect taste and smell.*

454 HEARING AND EQUILIBRIUM

Robert W. Baloh

Definition

The neural pathways subserving hearing and those most important for equilibrium and spatial orientation are anatomically proximate in much of their course from their end organs in the inner ear to their termination in the superior portion of the temporal lobe. Because of the close anatomic linkage, disorders that affect hearing often affect equilibrium and vice versa. For this reason, they are considered together here.

Pathobiology

Despite their anatomic propinquity, however, substantial pathophysiologic differences make clinical examination of the two systems quite different. The auditory system is physiologically relatively isolated, so that its function and dysfunction can be tested independently of other neural systems. The vestibular system, in contrast, has many close physiologic links with other neural systems (particularly the cerebellum, oculomotor system, and autonomic nervous system) and can be tested only indirectly by noting secondary effects on these systems.

Diagnosis

Abnormalities of the auditory system lead to only a few well-defined and unique symptoms (i.e., hearing loss or tinnitus). Abnormalities of the vestibular system can cause symptoms that mimic disorders of the other neural structures. Such symptoms include dizziness, visual distortion (oscillopsia), imbalance, nausea, vomiting, and even syncope.

DISORDERS OF THE AUDITORY SYSTEM

Definition

Anatomy and Physiology of Hearing

In normal hearing, sound waves are transmitted from the tympanic membrane through the three ossicles of the air-filled middle ear (air conduction) to the oval window and the basilar membrane of the fluid-sealed cochlea. The ossicles increase the gain from the tympanum to oval window about 18-fold, compensating for the loss that sound waves moving from air to fluid would otherwise suffer. In the absence of this system, sound may reach the cochlea by vibration of the temporal bone (bone conduction) but with much less efficiency (approximately 60-dB loss). Hair cells, tonotopically organized along the cochlear basilar membrane, detect the vibratory movement of that membrane and transduce vibration into nerve impulses. The nerve impulses are relayed by nerve cells that synapse at the base of hair cells and have their bodies in the spiral ganglion to the cochlear nucleus of the ipsilateral pontine tegmentum. The spiral cochlea mechanically analyzes the frequency content of sound. For high-frequency tones, only sensory cells in the basilar region are activated, whereas for low-frequency tones, all or nearly all sensory cells are activated. Therefore, with lesions of the cochlea and its afferent nerve, the hearing levels for different frequencies are usually unequal, typically resulting in better hearing sensitivity for low-frequency than for high-frequency tones. Within the brain stem, auditory signals ascend from the ventral and dorsal cochlear nuclei to reach the superior olivary nuclei of both sides. Thus, nervous system lesions central to the cochlear nucleus do not cause monaural hearing loss and, conversely, unilateral central lesions do not cause deafness. From these structures the pathway projects by way of the lateral lemnisci to the inferior colliculi. Each inferior colliculus transmits to the other and to its ipsilateral medial geniculate body, which in turn sends the final projection to the transverse auditory gyrus lying in the superior portion of the ipsilateral temporal lobe.

The normal ear can detect sound frequencies ranging between 20 and 20,000 Hz; the upper range drops off fairly rapidly with advancing age. The ear is most sensitive between 500 and 4000 Hz, which roughly corresponds to the frequency range most important for understanding speech. The hearing level in this range has several practical implications in terms of the degree of handicap and the potential for useful correction with amplification. A 30- to 40-dB hearing level in the speech range would impair normal conversation, whereas an 80-dB hearing level would make everyday auditory communication almost impossible (the social definition of deafness).

Pathobiology

Localization of Lesions within the Auditory Pathways

Conductive hearing loss results from lesions involving the external or middle ear. It is typically characterized by an approximately equal loss of hearing at all frequencies and by well-preserved speech discrimination once the threshold for hearing is exceeded. Patients with conductive hearing loss can hear speech in a noisy background better than in a quiet background because they can understand loud speech as well as anyone.

Sensorineural hearing loss results from lesions of the cochlea or auditory division, or both, of the eighth cranial nerve. With sensorineural hearing loss, the hearing levels for different frequencies are usually unequal, typically resulting in better hearing for low- than for high-frequency tones. Patients with sensorineural hearing loss often have difficulty hearing speech that is mixed with background noise and may be annoyed by loud speech. Three important manifestations of sensorineural lesions are diplacusis, recruitment, and tone decay. Diplacusis and recruitment are common with cochlear lesions; tone decay usually accompanies eighth nerve involvement.

Central hearing disorders result from lesions of the central auditory pathways. As a rule, patients with central lesions do not have impaired hearing for pure tones, and they can understand speech as long as it is clearly spoken in a quiet environment. If the listener's task is made more difficult with the introduction of background noise or competing messages, performance deteriorates more markedly in patients with central lesions than in normal subjects.

Diagnosis

Evaluation

Bedside Test

A quick test for hearing loss in the speech range is to observe the response to spoken commands at different intensities (whisper, conversation, shouting). Tuning fork tests permit a rough assessment of the hearing level for pure tones of known frequency. The clinician can use his or her own hearing level as a reference standard. In the Rinne test, nerve conduction is compared with bone conduction by holding a tuning fork (preferably 512 Hz) against the mastoid process until the sound can no longer be heard. It is then placed 1 inch from the ear and, in normal subjects, can be heard about twice as long by air as by bone. If bone conduction is better than air conduction, the hearing loss is conductive, but care must be taken to ensure that the bone conduction is not heard in the normal ear. In the Weber test, the tuning fork is placed on the patient's forehead or upper teeth. Normally, this sound is referred to the center of the head. If it is referred to the side of unilateral hearing loss, the hearing loss is conductive; if it is referred away from the side of unilateral hearing loss, the loss is sensorineural.

Audiometry

Pure tone testing is the cornerstone of most auditory examinations. Pure tones at selected frequencies are presented through either earphones (air conduction) or a vibrator pressed against the mastoid portion of the temporal bone (bone conduction), and the minimal level that the subject can hear (threshold) is determined for each frequency. Two speech tests are routinely used. The *speech reception threshold* (SRT) is the intensity at which the patient can correctly repeat 50% of the words presented. The SRT is a test of hearing sensitivity for speech and should reflect the hearing level for pure tones in the speech range. The *speech discrimination test* is a measure of the patient's ability to understand speech when it is presented at a level that is easily heard. In patients with eighth nerve lesions, speech discrimination scores can be severely reduced, even when pure tone thresholds are normal or nearly normal; by comparison, in patients with cochlear lesions, discrimination tends to be proportional to the magnitude of hearing loss.

Brain stem auditory-evoked responses can be recorded from scalp electrodes at 0 to 10 msec (early), 10 to 50 msec (middle), and 50 to 500 msec (late) following a click (a high-frequency stimulus). The early potentials reflect electrical activity at the cochlea, eighth cranial nerve, and brain stem; the later potentials reflect cortical activity. Computer averaging of the responses to 1000 to 2000 clicks separates the evoked potential from background noise. Early evoked responses may be used to estimate the magnitude of hearing loss and to differentiate among cochlea, eighth nerve, and brain stem lesions.

Hearing Loss

Pathobiology

Conductive Hearing Loss

The logic for identifying common causes of hearing loss is shown in Figure 454–1. The history, examination, and audiometry usually provide the key differential features. The most common cause of conductive hearing loss is *impacted cerumen* in the external canal. This benign condition is usually first noticed after bathing or swimming when a droplet of water closes the remaining tiny passageway. The most common serious cause of conductive hearing loss is inflammation of the middle ear, *otitis media,* either infective (suppurative; Fig. 452–7) or noninfective (serous). Fluid accumulates in the middle ear, impairing the conduction of airborne sound to the cochlea. Because the air cavity of the middle ear is in direct connection with the mastoid air cells, infection can spread through the mastoid bone and, occasionally, into the intracranial cavity. Chronic otitis media with perforation of the tympanic membrane can result in an invasion of the middle ear and other pneumatized areas of the temporal bone by keratinizing squamous epithelium (*cholesteatoma*). Cholesteatomas can produce erosion of the ossicles and bony labyrinth, resulting in a mixed conductive sensorineural hearing loss. Barotrauma to the middle ear arises with otalgia and hearing loss and can be associated with serous effusion or hematotympanum (Fig. 452–8). *Otosclerosis* commonly produces progressive conductive hearing loss by immobilizing the stapes with new bone growth in front of and below the oval window. The hearing loss is typically conductive, although in some persons the cochlea may be invaded by foci of otosclerotic bone, producing an additional sensorineural hearing loss. Otosclerosis usually stabilizes when the hearing level reaches 50 to 60 dB and rarely progresses to deafness. Other common causes of conductive hearing loss include trauma, congenital malformations of the external and middle ear, and glomus body tumors.

Sensorineural Hearing Loss

Hereditary Deafness

Genetically determined deafness, usually from hair cell aplasia or deterioration, may be present at birth or may develop in adulthood. The diagnosis of *hereditary deafness* rests on the finding of a positive family history. Mutations in connexin 26, a key component of gap junctions in the inner ear, account for the majority of cases of recessively inherited deafness. *Intrauterine factors* resulting in congenital hearing loss include infection (especially rubella); toxic, metabolic, and endocrine disorders; and anoxia associated with Rh incompatibility and difficult deliveries.

Cochlear Damage

Acute unilateral deafness usually has a cochlear basis. *Bacterial or viral infections* of the labyrinth, *head trauma* with fracture or hemorrhage into the cochlea, or *vascular occlusion* of a terminal branch of the anterior inferior cerebellar artery can extensively damage the cochlea and its hair cells. An acute idiopathic, often reversible, unilateral hearing loss strikes young adults and is presumed to reflect an isolated viral infection of the cochlea and auditory nerve terminals.

Sudden unilateral hearing loss often associated with vertigo and tinnitus can result from a *perilymphatic fistula.* Such fistulas may be congenital or may follow stapes surgery or head trauma.

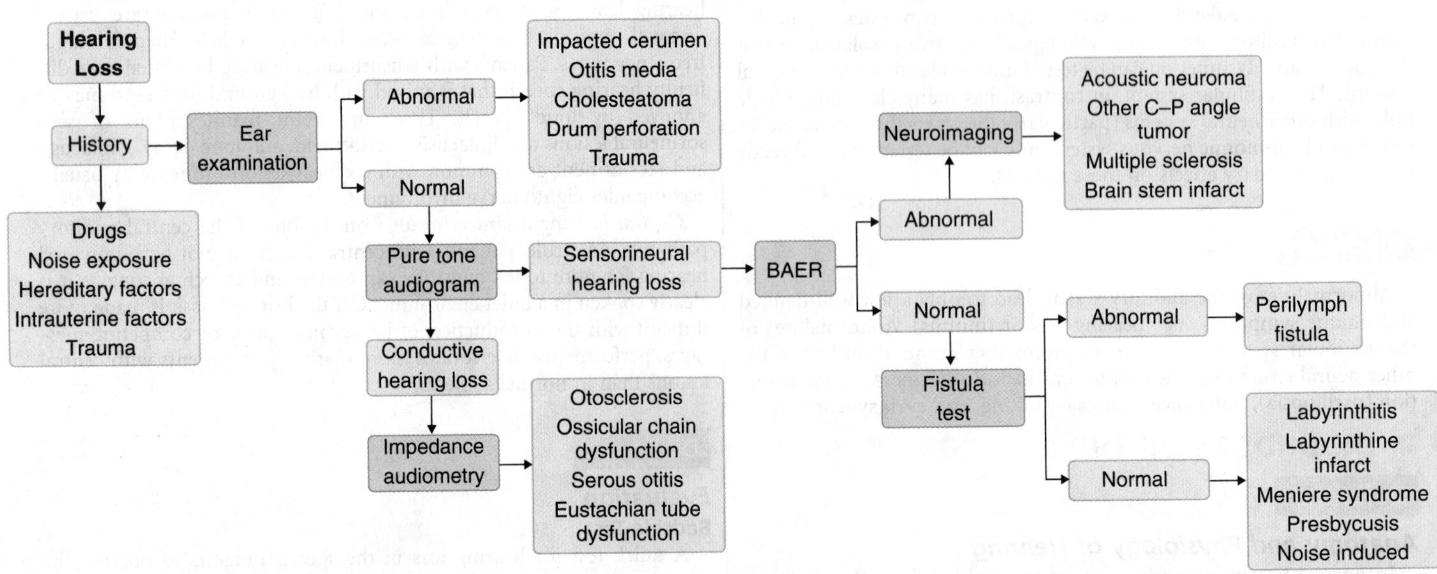

FIGURE 454–1 • Evaluation of hearing loss. BAER = brain stem auditory-evoked response; C–P = cerebellopontine.

Drugs

Drugs cause acute and subacute bilateral hearing impairment. Salicylates, furosemide, and ethacrynic acid have the potential to produce transient deafness when taken in high doses. More toxic to the cochlea are aminoglycoside antibiotics (gentamicin, tobramycin, amikacin, kanamycin, streptomycin, and neomycin). These agents can destroy cochlear hair cells in direct relation to their serum concentrations. Some antineoplastic chemotherapeutic agents, particularly cisplatin, cause severe ototoxicity.

Meniere's Syndrome

Subacute relapsing cochlear deafness occurs with *Meniere's syndrome,* a condition associated with fluctuating hearing loss and tinnitus, recurrent episodes of abrupt and often severe vertigo, and a sensation of fullness or pressure in the ear. Recurrent endolymphatic hypertension (hydrops) is believed to cause the episodes. Pathologically, the endolymphatic sac is dilated, and the hair cells become atrophic. The resulting deafness is subtle and reversible in the early stages but subsequently becomes permanent and is characterized by diplacusis and loudness recruitment. The disorder is usually unilateral, but in about 20 to 40% of patients, bilateral involvement occurs.

Presbycusis

The gradual, progressive, bilateral hearing loss commonly associated with advancing age is called *presbycusis.* Presbycusis is not a distinct disease entity but rather represents multiple effects of aging on the auditory system. It may include conductive and central dysfunction, although the most consistent effect of aging is on the sensory cells and neurons of the cochlea. The typical audiogram of presbycusis is a symmetrical high-frequency hearing loss gradually sloping downward with increasing frequency. The most consistent pathology associated with presbycusis is degeneration of sensory cells and nerve fibers at the base of the cochlea.

Noise-Induced Hearing Loss

The recurrent trauma of *noise-induced hearing loss* affects approximately the same cochlear region and is almost as common, particularly among those with exposure to loud explosive or industrial noises. Loud, blaring, modern music has become a recent offender. The loss almost always begins at 4000 Hz and does not affect speech discrimination until late in the disease process. With only brief exposure to loud noise (hours to days), there may be only a temporary threshold shift, but with continued exposure, permanent injury begins. The duration and intensity of exposure determine the degree of permanent injury.

Hearing loss from direct damage to the acoustic nerve in the petrous canal occasionally results from infection within or trauma to the surrounding bone; severe deafness of abrupt onset marks the event and is usually associated with acute vertigo related to concurrent vestibular nerve injury. Progressive unilateral hearing loss, which arises insidiously, initially in the high frequencies, and worsens by almost imperceptible degrees, is characteristic of benign neoplasms of the cerebellopontine angle, most commonly *acoustic neuromas.* In about 10% of cases, the hearing loss can be acute, apparently owing to either hemorrhage into the tumor or compression of the labyrinthine vasculature. Magnetic resonance imaging (MRI) with contrast reliably identifies small acoustic neuromas.

Central Hearing Loss

Central hearing loss is unilateral only if it results from damage to the pontine cochlear nuclei on one side of the brain stem from conditions such as *ischemic infarction* of the lateral brain stem (e.g., occlusion of the anterior inferior cerebellar artery [Chapter 431]), a plaque of *multiple sclerosis* (Chapter 436), or, rarely, invasion or compression of the lateral pons by a *neoplasm* or *hematoma* (Chapters 199 and 422). Bilateral *degeneration* of the cochlear nuclei accompanies some of the rare recessive inherited disorders of childhood. As noted, clinically important unilateral hearing loss never results from neurologic disease arising rostral to the cochlear nucleus. Although bilateral hearing loss could, in theory, result from bilateral destruction of central hearing pathways, in practice this is rare because involvement of neighboring structures in the brain stem or hemisphere would usually produce overwhelming neurologic disability.

Treatment

If an underlying disorder has not yet destroyed the auditory system and can be ameliorated medically or surgically, hearing may be improved or preserved. Most patients with otosclerosis respond to stapedectomy. Closure of a perilymph fistula may improve hearing. Antibiotic and decongestive treatment of otitis media (Chapter 452) should prevent permanent hearing loss. A low-salt diet and diuretics (see Table 454–2) are effective in selective cases of Meniere's syndrome. Folic acid supplementation can reduce the rate of hearing loss in the elderly. [1] Hearing aids amplify sound, usually with the goal of making speech intelligible. Patients with conductive hearing loss require simple amplification, but those with sensorineural hearing loss often need frequency-selective amplification to make hearing aids useful. Advances in acoustic technology have markedly improved the outlook for the latter. Serial audiograms in patients with noise or ototoxic drug exposure are critical for prevention of permanent hearing loss.

Tinnitus

Diagnosis

The evaluation of common causes of tinnitus (Fig. 454–2) begins with a careful history to identify common offending drugs.

Objective Tinnitus

With *objective tinnitus,* the patient hears a sound arising external to the auditory system, a sound that can usually be heard by the examiner with a stethoscope. Objective tinnitus usually has benign causes such as noise from temporomandibular joints, opening of eustachian tubes, or repetitive muscle contractions. Sometimes, in a quiet room, the patient can hear the pulsatile flow in the carotid artery or a continuous hum of normal venous outflow through the jugular vein. The latter can be obliterated by compression of the jugular vein or extreme lateral rotation of the neck. Pathologic objective tinnitus occurs when patients hear turbulent flow in vascular anomalies or tumors (e.g., glomus jugulare tumor). Objective tinnitus may also be an early sign of increased intracranial pressure. Such tinnitus, which probably arises from turbulent flow through compressed venous structures at the base of the brain, is usually overshadowed by other neurologic abnormalities.

Subjective Tinnitus

Subjective tinnitus can arise from sites anywhere in the auditory system. The sounds most frequently reported are metallic ringing, buzzing, blowing, roaring, or, less often, bizarre clanging, popping, or nonrhythmic beating. Tinnitus heard as a faint, moderately high-pitched, metallic ring can be observed by almost anyone who concentrates attention on auditory events in a quiet room. Sustained louder tinnitus accompanied by audiometric evidence of deafness occurs in association with both conductive and sensorineural hearing loss. Tinnitus observed with otosclerosis tends to have a roaring or hissing quality, and that associated with Meniere's syndrome often produces sounds that vary widely in intensity with time and quality, sometimes including roaring or clanging. Tinnitus with auditory nerve lesions tends to be higher pitched and ringing in quality. Audiometric and brain stem evoked response testing can help distinguish between lesions involving the conducting apparatus, the cochlea, and the auditory nerve. Tinnitus without observable deafness appears sporadically and for variable lengths of time in many persons without other evidence of an ongoing pathologic process.

Treatment

Most patients with tinnitus can be helped by detailed interview together with the relevant examination and laboratory investigations followed by reassurance when appropriate. Often, exacerbating factors such as chronic anxiety and depression can be treated. In patients with hearing loss and tinnitus, a hearing aid may improve tinnitus because the amplification of ambient sound may effectively mask the tinnitus. This mechanism probably explains the frequent

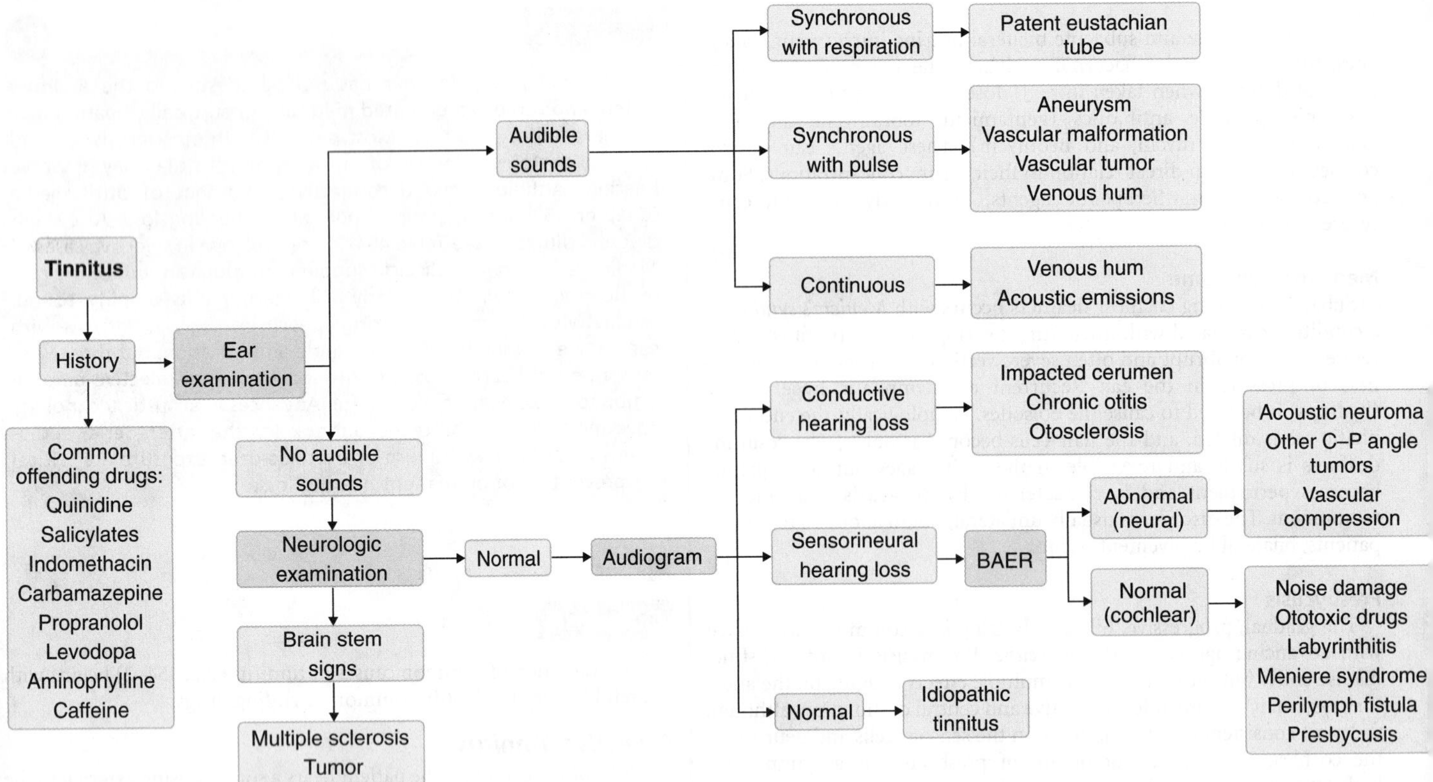

FIGURE 454–2 • Evaluation of tinnitus. BAER = brain stem auditory-evoked response; C–P = cerebellopontine.

Rx

observation that removal of cerumen from the external auditory canal to improve ambient hearing also improves tinnitus. Also, when cerumen is attached to the tympanic membrane, tinnitus may result from local mechanical effects on the conductive system. For patients who find their tinnitus most obtrusive when trying to sleep, a bedside frequency modulation (FM) clock radio tuned between stations can provide an effective masking sound; some such radios can be programmed to switch off after the patient falls asleep. A careful drug history should be taken, and a drug-free trial period should be considered when possible. Some patients who notice that caffeine, alcohol, or nicotine exacerbates their tinnitus experience significant relief when these drugs are discontinued. Benzodiazepines or tricyclic amines may provide temporary symptomatic relief of tinnitus, but cognitive behavioral therapy is a more effective long-term approach. 2

Equilibrium-Vestibular System

Pathobiology

Anatomy and Physiology of the Vestibular System

The paired vestibular end organs lie within the temporal bones next to the cochlea. Each organ consists of three semicircular canals that detect angular acceleration and two otolith structures, the utricle and saccule, that detect linear acceleration (including gravitational). Like the cochlea, these organs possess hair cells that act as force transducers, converting the forces associated with head acceleration into afferent nerve impulses. The hair cells of the three semicircular canals, each of which is oriented at right angles to the others, are located in the crista, where their cilia are embedded in a gelatinous mass called the cupula. Movement of the head causes the endolymph to flow either toward or away from the cupula, bending the cilia and, depending on the direction of endolymphatic movements, either exciting or inhibiting the afferent nerves at the base of the hair cells. Because the afferent nerves are tonically active, the baseline activity can be increased or decreased depending on the direction of hair cell bending. Furthermore, the two sets of semicircular canals are approximately mirror images of each other, so that rotational movement of the head that excites one canal inhibits the analogous canal on the opposite side. The hair cells of the utricle and saccule are located in an area called the *macule*. The macule of the utricle lies approximately in the plane of the horizontal canal, and the macule of the saccule is approximately in the plane of the anterior canal. The hair cell cilia are embedded in a membrane that contains calcium carbonate crystals or otoliths; the density of otoliths is considerably greater than that of the endolymph. Linear accelerations of the head combine with the linear acceleration of gravity to distort the otolith membrane, thereby bending the cilia of the hair cells and modulating the activity of the afferent nerve terminals at the base of the hair cells.

The afferent vestibular nerves have their cell bodies in Scarpa's ganglion. The nerve fibers travel in the vestibular portion of the eighth cranial nerve contiguous to the acoustic portion. Fibers from different receptor organs terminate in different vestibular nuclei at the pontomedullary junction. There are also direct connections with many portions of the cerebellum, the greatest representation being in the flocculonodular lobe, the so-called vestibular cerebellum. Efferent fibers from the brain stem travel through the vestibular nerve to reach hair cells of the semicircular canals and macules, where they modulate afferent activities. From the vestibular nuclei, second-order neurons make important connections to the vestibular nuclei of the other side, to the cerebellum, to motor neurons of the spinal cord, to autonomic nuclei in the brain stem, and, most important for the examining clinician, to the nuclei of the oculomotor system. Fibers from the vestibular nuclei also ascend through the brain stem and thalamus to reach the cerebral cortex bilaterally.

Diagnosis

Evaluation

History

Most vestibular problems presented to the physician are episodic, and often there are neither symptoms nor signs when the physician examines the patient. The history, therefore, can become paramount for identifying vestibular dysfunction. The history should attempt to distinguish vertigo (the illusion of movement in space) from lightheadedness (presyncope), ataxia (disequilibrium of the body without true movement in space), and psychogenic symptoms (the feeling of dissociation or, sometimes, disequilibrium).

Vertigo can be caused by either the peripheral or central vestibular apparatus. In general, peripheral vertigo is more severe, is more likely to be associated with hearing loss and tinnitus, and often leads to nausea and vomiting. Nystagmus associated with peripheral vertigo is usually inhibited by visual fixation. Central vertigo is generally less severe than peripheral vertigo and is often associated with other signs of central nervous system disease. The nystagmus of central vertigo is not inhibited by visual fixation and frequently is prominent when vertigo is mild or absent.

Common Causes of Vertigo (Fig. 454–3)

Physiologic Vertigo

Physiologic vertigo includes common disorders that occur in healthy people such as *motion sickness, space sickness,* and *height vertigo.* In these conditions, vertigo (defined as an illusion of movement) is minimal while autonomic symptoms predominate. With height vertigo, patients may experience acute anxiety and panic reaction. Individuals with motion sickness and space sickness typically develop perspiration, nausea, vomiting, increased salivation, yawning, and generalized malaise. Gastric motility is reduced and digestion impaired. Even the sight or smell of food is distressing. Hyperventilation is a common sign, and the resulting hypocapnia leads to changes in blood volume, with pooling in the lower parts of the body predisposing to postural hypotension and syncope. An unusual variant of motion-induced dizziness occurs when the subject returns to stationary conditions after prolonged exposure to motion (so-called *mal de débarquement syndrome*). Typically, affected patients report that they feel the persistent rocking sensation of a boat long after returning to solid ground. Rarely, the syndrome can last for months to years after exposure to motion and can even be incapacitating. The cause is unknown.

Physiologic vertigo can often be suppressed by supplying sensory cues that help to match the signals originating from different sensory systems. Thus, motion sickness, which is caused by a mismatch of visual and vestibular signals, is exacerbated by sitting in a closed space or reading (giving the visual system the miscue that the environment is stationary). It may be improved by looking out at the horizon. Height vertigo, caused by a mismatch between sensation of normal body sway and lack of its visual detection, can often be relieved either by sitting or by visually fixating a nearby stationary object.

Benign Positional Vertigo

Benign positional vertigo is by far the most common type of vertigo. Patients with this condition develop brief episodes of vertigo (less than 1 minute) with position change, typically when turning over in bed, getting in and out of bed, bending over and straightening up, or extending the neck to look up (so-called top shelf vertigo). Benign positional vertigo results when otolith debris inadvertently enters one of the semicircular canals. It can occur after head trauma or inner ear infection but most commonly occurs spontaneously in older people. The diagnosis rests on finding characteristic positional nystagmus in the plane of the affected canal (see later). It is important to recognize this syndrome because, in most patients, it can be cured by simple bedside maneuvers (see Table 454–2). If the history or findings are atypical, the condition must be distinguished from other causes of positional vertigo that may occur with tumors or infarcts of the posterior fossa.

Acute Peripheral Vestibulopathy ("Vestibular Neuritis")

One of the most common clinical neurologic syndromes at any age is the acute onset of vertigo, nausea, and vomiting lasting for several days and not associated with auditory or neurologic symptoms. Most affected patients gradually improve over 1 to 2 weeks, but residual dizziness and imbalance can persist for months. Many report an upper respiratory tract illness 1 to 2 weeks before the onset of vertigo. This syndrome occasionally occurs in epidemics (epidemic vertigo), may affect several members of the same family, and more often erupts in the spring and early summer. All of these factors suggest a viral origin, but attempts to isolate an agent have been unsuccessful, except for occasional findings of a herpes zoster infection. Pathologic studies showing atrophy of one or more vestibular nerve trunks, with or without atrophy of their associated sense organs, are evidence of a vestibular nerve site and, probably, viral cause for many patients with this syndrome In vestibular neuritis, high-dose steroids (see Table 454–2) given acutely improve symptoms and may decrease the amount of vestibular damage, [3] but patients typically compensate even if there is permanent damage.

Meniere's Syndrome

The typical clinical features of Meniere's syndrome are described earlier. This disorder accounts for about 10% of all patients with vertigo. The diagnosis is based on documenting episodic severe attacks accompanied by fluctuating hearing levels on audiometric testing beginning in the low frequencies.

Migraine

Vertigo is a common symptom with migraine (Chapter 421). It can occur with headaches or in separate isolated episodes, and it can predate the onset of headache. So-called benign paroxysmal vertigo of childhood is often the first symptom of migraine. The mechanism of vertigo with migraine is not clear, but damage to the inner ear occurs in about one fourth of patients. A few develop typical features of Meniere's syndrome.

Post-traumatic Vertigo

Vertigo, hearing loss, and tinnitus often follow a blow to the head (Chapter 422) that does not result in temporal bone fracture, the so-called *labyrinthine concussion.* Although they are protected by a bone capsule, the delicate labyrinthine membranes are susceptible to blunt trauma. Blows to the occipital or mastoid region are particularly likely to

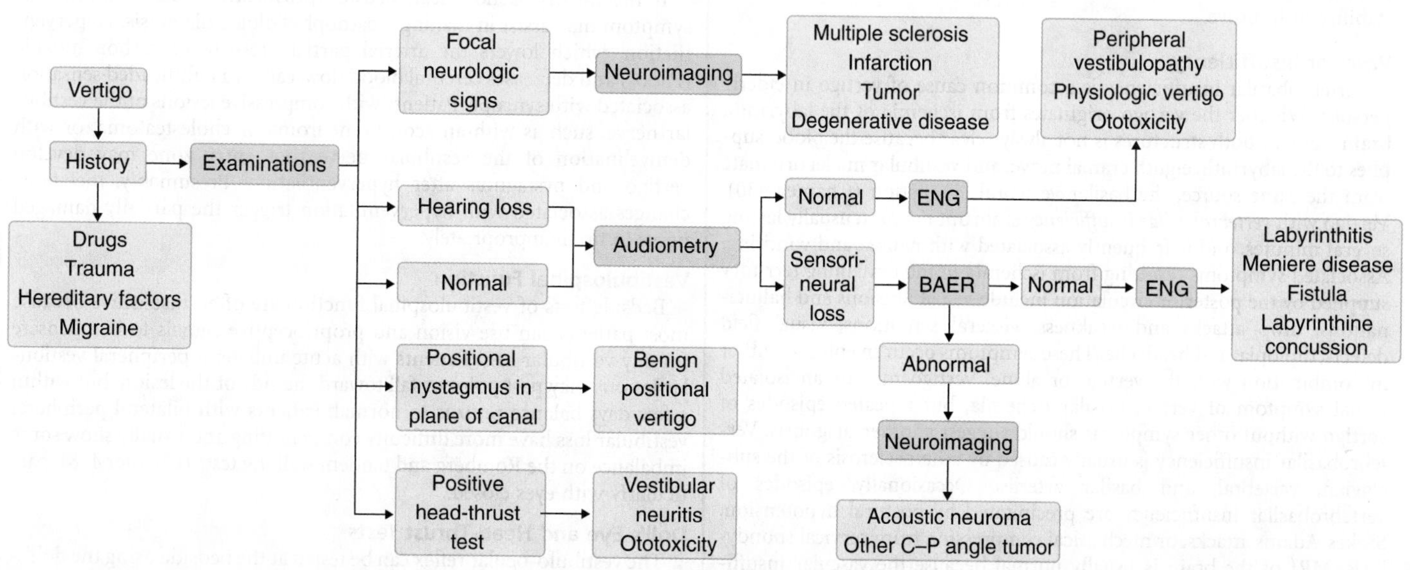

FIGURE 454–3 • Evaluation of vertigo. BAER = brain stem auditory-evoked response; C–P = cerebellopontine; ENG = electronystagmography.

produce labyrinthine damage. *Transverse fractures* of the temporal bone typically pass through the vestibule of the inner ear, tearing the membranous labyrinth and lacerating the vestibular and cochlear nerves. Complete loss of vestibular and cochlear function is the usual sequela, and the facial nerve is interrupted in approximately 50% of cases. Examination of the ear often reveals hemotympanum (see Fig. 452–8), but bleeding from the ear seldom occurs because the tympanic membrane usually remains intact. As noted earlier, *benign positional vertigo* is also a common sequela of head trauma. *Fistulas* of the oval and round windows can result from impact noise, deep-water diving, severe physical exertion, or blunt head injury without skull fracture. The mechanism of the rupture is a sudden negative or positive pressure change in the middle ear or a sudden increase in cerebrospinal fluid pressure transmitted to the inner ear through the cochlear aqueduct and internal auditory canal. Clinically, the rupture leads to the sudden onset of vertigo or hearing loss, or both. Surgical exploration of the middle ear is warranted when there is a clear relationship between the onset of vertigo or hearing loss, or both, and the onset of severe exertion, barometric change, head injury, or impact noise.

Postconcussion Syndrome

The so-called postconcussion syndrome refers to a vague dizziness (rarely vertigo) associated with anxiety, difficulty in concentrating, headache, and photophobia induced by a head injury resulting in concussion (Chapter 422). Occasionally, similar but less pronounced symptoms are associated with mild head injury judged to be trivial at the time. The cause is unknown, but animal studies indicate that small multifocal brain lesions (petechiae) commonly occur after concussive brain injury.

Other Peripheral Causes of Vertigo

Vertigo can be associated with *chronic bacterial otomastoiditis*, either from direct invasion of the inner ear by the bacteria or by erosion of the labyrinth by a cholesteatoma. Radiographic studies of the temporal bone readily identify these disorders. *Autoimmune inner ear disease* typically arises with episodic vertigo and fluctuating hearing levels similar to Meniere's syndrome, but it is more fulminant with early bilateral involvement. It can occur in isolation or with other systemic features of autoimmune disease. About two thirds of patients have antibodies directed against heat shock protein 70. The aminoglycosides streptomycin and gentamicin are remarkably selective for vestibular ototoxicity. The patient may suffer acute vertigo if the toxic effect is asymmetric. More often there is a progressive symmetrical loss of vestibular function leading to imbalance but not vertigo. Unfortunately, many patients being treated with ototoxic drugs are initially bedridden and unaware of the vestibular impairment until they recover from their acute illness and try to walk. Then they discover that they are unsteady on their feet and that the environment tends to jiggle in front of their eyes (*oscillopsia*). The diagnosis can be made at the bedside with a head-thrust test (bilateral corrective saccades; see later). Electronystagmography (ENG) can document the degree of vestibular loss. The best treatment is prevention. If the drug is discontinued early during the course of symptoms, the disorder may stabilize or improve.

Vascular Insufficiency

Vertebrobasilar insufficiency is a common cause of vertigo in elderly persons. Whether the vertigo originates from ischemia of the labyrinth, brain stem, or both structures is not always clear because the blood supplies to the labyrinth, eighth cranial nerve, and vestibular nuclei originate from the same source, the basilar vertebral circulation (Chapter 430). Vertigo with *vertebrobasilar insufficiency* is abrupt in onset, usually lasting several minutes, and is frequently associated with nausea and vomiting. Associated symptoms resulting from ischemia in the remaining territory supplied by the posterior circulation include visual illusions and hallucinations, drop attacks and weakness, visceral sensations, visual field defects, diplopia, and headache. These symptoms occur in episodes either in combination with the vertigo or alone. Vertigo may be an isolated initial symptom of vertebrobasilar ischemia, but repeated episodes of vertigo without other symptoms should suggest another diagnosis. Vertebrobasilar insufficiency is usually caused by atherosclerosis of the subclavian, vertebral, and basilar arteries. Occasionally, episodes of vertebrobasilar insufficiency are precipitated by postural hypotension, Stokes-Adams attacks, or mechanical compression from cervical spondylosis. MRI of the brain is usually normal because the vascular insufficiency is transient and function returns to normal between episodes. MR angiography can identify occlusive vascular disease most commonly involving the vertebral-basilar junction.

Vertigo is a common symptom with *infarction of the lateral brain stem* or *cerebellum* (Chapter 431), or both. The diagnosis is usually clear, based on the characteristic acute history and pattern of associated symptoms and neurologic findings. Occasionally, cerebellar infarction or hemorrhage arises with severe vertigo, vomiting, and ataxia without associated brain stem symptoms and signs that might suggest the erroneous diagnosis of an acute peripheral vestibular disorder. The key differential is the finding of clear cerebellar signs (extremity and gait ataxia) and of direction-changing, gaze-evoked nystagmus. Such patients must be watched carefully for several days because they may develop progressive brain stem dysfunction owing to compression by a swollen cerebellum.

Cerebellopontine-Angle Tumors

Most tumors growing in the cerebellopontine angle (e.g., *acoustic neuroma, meningioma, epidermal cyst*) grow slowly, allowing the vestibular system to accommodate so that they produce only a vague sensation of disequilibrium rather than acute vertigo (Chapter 199). Occasionally, however, episodic vertigo or positional vertigo heralds the presence of a cerebellopontine-angle tumor. In virtually all patients, retrocochlear hearing loss is present, best identified by an abnormal brain stem auditory evoked response. MRI with contrast is the most sensitive diagnostic study for identifying a cerebellopontine-angle tumor.

Other Central Causes of Vertigo

Acute vertigo may be the first symptom of *multiple sclerosis* (Chapter 436), although only a small percentage of young patients with acute vertigo eventually develop multiple sclerosis. Vertigo in multiple sclerosis is usually transient and often associated with other neurologic signs of brain stem disease, in particular, internuclear ophthalmoplegia or cerebellar dysfunction. Vertigo may also be a symptom of *parainfectious encephalomyelitis* or, rarely, *parainfectious cranial polyneuritis*. In this instance, the accompanying neurologic signs establish the diagnosis. The *Ramsay Hunt syndrome* (geniculate ganglion herpes) is characterized by vertigo and hearing loss associated with facial paralysis and, sometimes, pain in the ear. The typical lesions of herpes zoster (Chapter 398), which may follow the appearance of neurologic signs, are found in the external auditory canal and over the palate in some patients. Rarely is herpes zoster responsible for vertigo in the absence of the full-blown syndrome. *Granulomatous meningitis* (Chapter 437) or *leptomeningeal metastasis* and cerebral or systemic *vasculitis* (Chapter 291) may involve the eighth nerve, producing vertigo as an early symptom. In these disorders, cerebrospinal fluid analysis usually suggests the diagnosis (Chapter 418). Patients suffering from *temporal lobe epilepsy* (Chapter 426) occasionally experience vertigo as the aura. Vertigo in the absence of other neurologic signs or symptoms is never caused by epilepsy or other diseases of the cerebral hemispheres.

Bedside Tests

Hyperventilation

If the history is not clear, bedside provocative tests to mimic the symptom may assist in making a pathophysiologic diagnosis. Hyperventilation, which lowers the arterial partial pressure of carbon dioxide ($Paco_2$) and decreases cerebral blood flow, causes a lightheaded sensation associated with syncope. Patients with compressive lesions of the vestibular nerve, such as with an acoustic neuroma or cholesteatoma, or with demyelination of the vestibular nerve root entry zone may develop vertigo and nystagmus after hyperventilation. Presumably, metabolic changes associated with hyperventilation trigger the partially damaged nerve to fire inappropriately.

Vestibulospinal Function

Bedside tests of vestibulospinal function are often insensitive because most patients can use vision and proprioceptive signals to compensate for any vestibular loss. Patients with acute unilateral peripheral vestibular lesions may past point or fall toward the side of the lesion, but within a few days balance returns to normal. Patients with bilateral peripheral vestibular loss have more difficulty compensating and usually show some imbalance on the Romberg and tandem walking tests (Chapter 418), particularly with eyes closed.

Doll's-Eye and Head-Thrust Tests

The vestibulo-ocular reflex can be tested at the bedside using the doll's-eye and head-thrust tests. In an alert human, rotating the head back and forth in the horizontal plane induces compensatory horizontal eye movements that are dependent on both the visual and vestibular systems. The *doll's-eye test* is a test of vestibular function in a comatose patient (Chapter 428) because such patients cannot generate pursuit or corrective fast components. In this setting, conjugate compensatory eye movements indicate normally functioning vestibulo-ocular pathways. Because the vestibulo-ocular reflex has a much higher frequency range than the smooth pursuit system, a qualitative bedside test of vestibular function can be made with the *head-thrust test.* It is performed by grasping the patient's head and applying brief, small-amplitude, high-acceleration head thrusts first to one side and then the other. The patient fixates on the examiner's nose and the examiner watches for corrective saccades, which are a sign of an inappropriate compensatory slow phase.

Caloric Test

The caloric test induces endolymphatic flow in the horizontal semicircular canal and horizontal nystagmus by creating a temperature gradient from one side of the canal to the other. With a cold caloric stimulus, the column of endolymph nearest the middle ear falls because of its increased density. This causes the cupula to deviate away from the utricle (ampullofugal flow) and produces horizontal nystagmus with the fast phase directed away from the stimulated ear. A warm stimulus produces the opposite effect, causing ampullopedal endolymph flow and nystagmus directed toward the stimulated ear (a mnemonic is COWS, meaning cold opposite, warm same). Because of its ready availability, ice water (approximately 0° C) can be used for bedside caloric testing. To bring the horizontal canal into the vertical plane, the patient lies in the supine position with head tilted 30 degrees forward. Infusion of 1 to 3 mL of ice water induces a burst of nystagmus usually lasting about a minute. Greater than a 20% asymmetry in nystagmus duration suggests a lesion on the side of the decreased response. The ice water caloric test is a useful way to test the integrity of the oculomotor pathways in a comatose patient. In this case, ice water induces only a slow tonic deviation toward the side of stimulation.

Positional Tests

Examination for pathologic vestibular nystagmus should include a search for spontaneous and positional nystagmus (see Table 450–5). Because vestibular nystagmus secondary to peripheral vestibular lesions is inhibited with fixation, the yield is increased by impairing fixation with +30 lenses (Frenzel glasses) or infrared video recordings. Two types of positional testing are typically performed: moving the patient from the sitting to head-hanging right and head-hanging left positions (Dix-Hallpike test) and turning the head to the right and left while the patient lies supine. Induced positional nystagmus may be paroxysmal or persistent, and it may be in the same direction in all positions or change directions in different positions. The most common cause of positional nystagmus is otolith debris in the semicircular canals, either free floating (paroxysmal) or attached to the cupula (persistent). This type of nystagmus always occurs in the plane of the affected canal—vertical torsional for the vertical canals and horizontal torsional for the horizontal canal. By contrast, central positional nystagmus is often pure vertical or horizontal and cannot be explained by stimulating a single semicircular canal.

Electronystagmography

ENG tests oculomotor control by inducing and recording eye movements (with electro-oculography or video-oculography). A standard ENG test battery includes (1) tests of visual ocular control (saccades, smooth pursuit, and optokinetic nystagmus), (2) a careful search for pathologic nystagmus with fixation and with eyes open in darkness, and (3) measurement of induced vestibular nystagmus (caloric and rotational). ENG can be helpful in identifying a vestibular lesion and localizing it within the peripheral and central pathways.

Evaluating the "Dizzy" Patient

The history is key because it determines the type of dizziness (vertigo, near-faint, psychophysiologic disequilibrium), associated symptoms (neurologic, audiologic, cardiac, psychiatric), precipitating factors (position change, trauma, stress, drug ingestion), and predisposing illness (systemic viral infection, cardiac disease, cerebrovascular disease; Table 454–1). The history provides direction for both the examination and the diagnostic evaluation. When focal neurologic signs are found, neuroimaging usually leads to a specific diagnosis. When vertigo is present without focal neurologic symptoms or signs, head-thrust and positional testing are key to localizing the lesion to the labyrinth or eighth nerve. Audiometry and ENG are useful if the cause of vertigo is not clear after the history and examination. Patients with psychophysiologic dizziness should be identified early so that needless tests are not obtained. A detailed cardiac evaluation (including loop monitoring) often identifies the cause of episodic near fainting (Chapters 61, 65, and 427).

Treatment

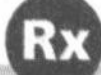

Treatment of vertigo can be divided into three general categories: specific, symptomatic, and rehabilitative. Specific therapies include particle repositioning maneuvers for benign positional vertigo, steroids for vestibular neuritis, and low-salt diet and diuretics for Meniere's syndrome (Table 454–2). When possible, treatment should be directed at the underlying disorder.

In many cases, however, symptomatic treatment is either combined with specific therapy or is the only treatment available. Many different classes of drugs have been found to have antivertiginous properties, and in most instances the exact mechanism of action is

TABLE 454–2 TREATMENT OF COMMON VERTIGO SYNDROMES

Syndrome	Treatment
Benign positional vertigo	
Posterior canal variant	Epley maneuver (Fig. 454–4)
Horizontal canal variant	Barbecue roll toward normal side (side with less nystagmus), sleep with normal ear down
Vestibular neuritis	Methylprednisolone 100 mg × 3 days, gradual taper over 22 days (must start within 3 days of onset)
Meniere's syndrome	
Medical	Low salt (1–2 g Na^+/day) + hydrochlorothiazide (25–50 mg/day)
Surgical	Intratympanic gentamicin, vestibular nerve section

TABLE 454–1 DESCRIPTION, MECHANISM, AND FOCUS OF DIAGNOSTIC WORKUP FOR COMMON TYPES OF DIZZINESS

Type of Dizziness	Description	Mechanism	Focus of Diagnostic Evaluation
Vertigo	Spinning (environment moves), tilt, drunkenness	Imbalance in tonic vestibular activity	Auditory and vestibular systems
Near faint	Lightheaded, swimming	Decreased blood flow to entire brain	Cardiovascular system
Psychophysiologic	Dissociated from body, spinning inside (environment still)	Impaired central integration of sensory signals	Psychiatric assessment
Disequilibrium	Off balance, unsteady on feet	Loss of vestibulospinal, proprioceptive, cerebellar, or motor function	Neurologic assessment

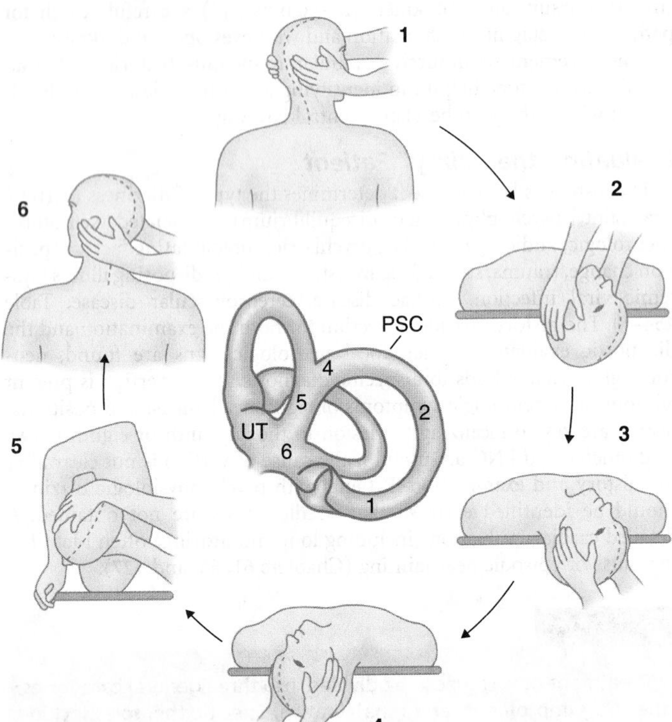

FIGURE 454–4 • Treatment maneuver for benign positional vertigo affecting the right posterior semicircular canal (PSC). The procedure is reversed for treating the left PSC. The numbers in the PSC correspond to the position of the otolith debris in each head position as it moves toward the utricle (UT). Positions 2 and 3 are the same except that the therapist has moved from the front to the back of the patient to continue the maneuver easily. The entire sequence should be repeated until no nystagmus is elicited. (Courtesy Carol A. Foster, MD.)

Rx

uncertain. All of these agents produce potentially unpleasant side effects, and the decision concerning which drug or combination to use is based on their known complications and on the severity and duration of the vertigo. An episode of prolonged, severe vertigo is one of the most distressing symptoms that a patient can experience. Affected patients prefer to lie still with eyes closed in a quiet, dark room. Antivertiginous drugs with sedation such as promethazine HCl (Phenergan; 25 mg) or diazepam (5 mg) may be helpful. Prochlorperazine suppositories (25 mg) may stop vomiting. In more chronic vertiginous disorders, when the patient is trying to carry on normal activity, less sedating antivertiginous medications such as meclizine (25 mg) or transdermal scopolamine (0.5 mg every 3 days) may provide relief. Chronic use of these drugs should be avoided.

Vestibular rehabilitation exercises are designed to help the patient compensate for permanent loss of vestibular function. [4] As the acute stage of nausea and vomiting subsides, the patient should attempt to focus the eyes and to move and hold them in the direction that provokes the most dizziness. A useful exercise involves staring at a visual target while oscillating the head from side to side or up and down, slow at first and then fast. The patient should try to stand and walk, at first in contact with a wall or with an assistant, and make slow supported turns. As improvement occurs, head movements should be added while standing and walking.

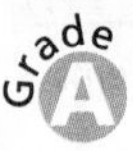

1. Durga J, Verhoef P, Anteunis LJ, et al: Effects of folic acid supplementation on hearing in older adults: A randomized, controlled trial. Lancet 2007;369:208–216.
2. Martinez Devesa P, Waddell A, Perera R, et al: Cognitive behavioural therapy for tinnitus. Cochrane Database Syst Rev 2007;24:1.
3. Strupp M, Zingler VC, Arbusow V, et al: Methylprednisolone, valacyclovir, or the combination for vestibular neuritis. N Engl J Med 2004;351:354–361.
4. Yardley L, Donovan-Hall M, Smith H, et al: Effectiveness of primary care-based vestibular rehabilitation for chronic dizziness. Ann Intern Med 2004;141:598–605.

SUGGESTED READINGS

Aw ST, Todd MJ, Aw GE, et al: Benign positional nystagmus: A study of its three-dimensional spatio-temporal characteristics. Neurology 2005;64:1897–1905. *How to diagnose and treat different types of benign positional vertigo.*

Bagai A, Thavendiranathan P, Detsky AS: Does this patient have hearing impairment? JAMA 2006;295:416–428. *A case-based review.*

Cook JA, Hawkins DB: Hearing loss and hearing aid treatment options. Mayo Clin Proc 2006;81:234–237. *A comprehensive review.*

Gates GA, Mills JH: Presbycusis. Lancet 2005;366:1111–1120. *Comprehensive overview.*

Neuhauser HK, Radtke A, von Brevern M, et al: Migrainous vertigo: Prevalence and impact on quality of life. Neurology 2006;67:1028–1033. *Migranous vertigo is common but underdiagnosed.*

455 THROAT DISORDERS

Thomas A. Tami

The functions of deglutition, respiration, voice, and alimentation are influenced by disorders of the throat. Because the anatomy in this area is characterized by indistinct boundaries, symptoms are often difficult to ascribe to a specific anatomic area without a careful physical examination.

Pathobiology

The pharynx is usually divided into three regions (Fig. 455–1). The *nasopharynx*, which is the region of the pharynx located above the soft palate and uvula, is usually very difficult to visualize directly unless the examiner is adept at using small nasopharyngeal mirrors or is able to use a fiberoptic endoscope introduced through the nose. Anatomic structures in the nasopharynx include the adenoids, the openings of the eustachian tubes, and the posterior tips of the inferior turbinates of the nasal cavity.

The *oropharynx* is anatomically defined as the region beginning at the level of the soft palate and extending inferiorly to the tip of the epiglottis. This anatomic area includes the faucial tonsils, the base of the tongue, the lingual tonsils, the soft palate, the uvula, and part of the posterior pharyngeal wall.

The *hypopharynx* is the lower part of pharynx extending from the tip of the epiglottis above to the introitus of the esophagus (the

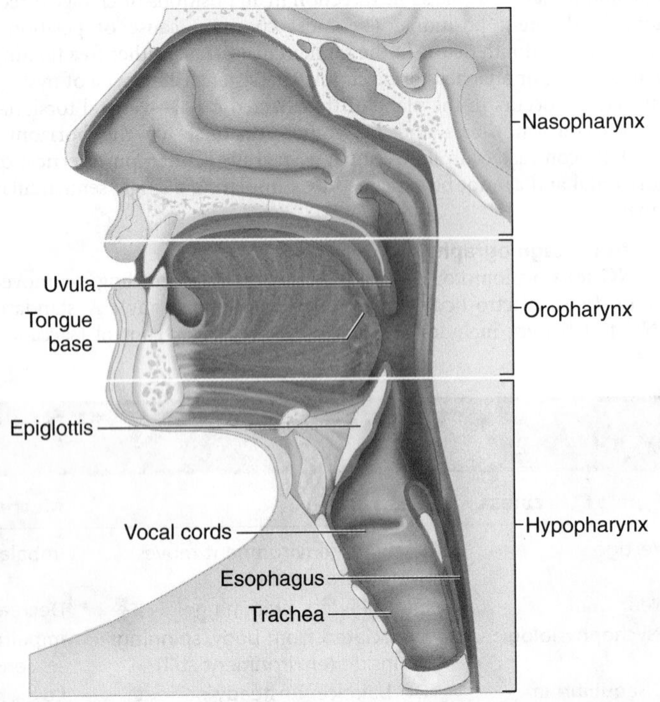

FIGURE 455–1 • The pharynx (throat) is typically divided into three distinct anatomic regions (nasopharynx, oropharynx, and hypopharynx).

cricopharyngeus muscle) below. This region includes the entire larynx (epiglottis, arytenoids, glottis or true vocal cords), the pyriform sinuses (pharyngeal folds lateral to the larynx), and the posterior pharyngeal wall. Although the tip of the epiglottis can occasionally be visualized by using a routine flashlight and tongue blade during a routine oral examination, this region can usually be clearly visualized only by using a laryngeal mirror or, more commonly, a fiber optic nasopharyngoscope.

DISEASE OF THE PHARYNX

Nasopharynx

Clinical Manifestations

Typically, diseases occurring in the nasopharynx produce few symptoms until the process is well advanced and produces nasal obstruction (Chapter 452), epistaxis (Chapter 452), ear pain (Chapter 452), headache (Chapter 421), or cranial nerve abnormalities owing to extension to the skull base. Symptoms of postnasal drainage, including cough and sore throat, can be caused by acute or chronic sinusitis or by allergic or non-allergic rhinitis. Treatment is for the underlying cause (Chapter 452). Examination using fiberoptic technology can often easily establish the appropriate diagnosis, but magnetic resonance imaging (MRI) or computed tomographic (CT) scanning can also be helpful (Chapter 452), especially when extension outside the nasopharynx is suspected (Chapter 200).

Nasopharyngeal carcinoma (Chapter 200), which is uncommon in Western populations but more common in Asian populations, particularly southern Chinese, is related to Epstein-Barr virus infection. Common presenting symptoms include nasal obstruction, unilateral or bilateral serous otitis media, epistaxis, cervical lymph node enlargement, or cranial nerve neuropathy that often arises as diplopia.

Oropharynx

Pharyngitis

In the oropharynx, sore throat (pharyngitis) is the most common presenting symptom (Fig. 455–2), and tonsillitis is the most important cause. Although the faucial tonsils are occasionally the only site of infection, the lingual tonsils and the adenoids are also usually involved. The clinical evaluation must differentiate among viral pharyngitis, bacterial causes (usually streptococcus (Chapter 313), tonsillitis, peritonsillar abscess, and (rarely) acute epiglottitis (Table 455–1).

Antibiotic treatment is recommended in patients at reasonable risk for bacterial infection (Chapter 313). [1] Penicillin (penicillin VK, 250 mg three times a day or 500 mg twice a day for 5 to 10 days) is usually chosen to treat acute bacterial pharyngitis, but cefuroxime axetil (250 mg twice a day for 5 to 10 days) is even more effective for primary treatment [2] and can be very effective for persistent infection. For patients who are allergic to penicillin, azithromycin (500 mg/day for 3 days) is an alternative. Infectious mononucleosis (Chapter 400) often produces disabling tonsillitis with impressive exudative tonsillar hypertrophy (Fig. 455–3). Corticosteroids are very effective during the acute phase of infectious mononucleosis, particularly for patients with potential airway obstruction related to tonsillar hypertrophy. Because this systemic viral disease can also produce other medical problems, such as hepatitis and thrombocytopenia, these possibilities should be considered during the clinical evaluation.

Peritonsillar abscess can usually be diagnosed by physical examination (Fig. 455–4). A peritonsillar abscess can usually be managed in an outpatient setting using surgical or needle drainage by an ear, nose, and throat specialist and oral antibiotics, such as amoxicillin plus metronidazole or clindamycin or amoxicillin clavulanate.

By comparison, a deep neck abscess is more serious condition because of its anatomic access to the fascial planes of the neck and chest. These patients usually present in a more toxic condition, often have swelling of the external neck, trismus or torticollis, and, occasionally, a compromised airway. These infections must be recognized immediately, often using imaging techniques, and managed aggressively, usually by external incision and drainage as well as with intravenous broad-spectrum antibiotic coverage of aerobic and anaerobic bacteria (e.g., clindamycin 600 mg intravenously every 8 hours, ampicillin-sulbactam 3 g every 6 hours, or penicillin G 2 million units every 4 hours plus metronidazole 500 mg every 6 hours).

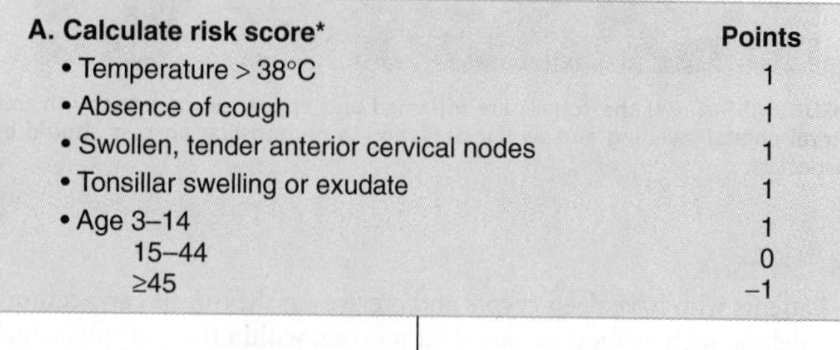

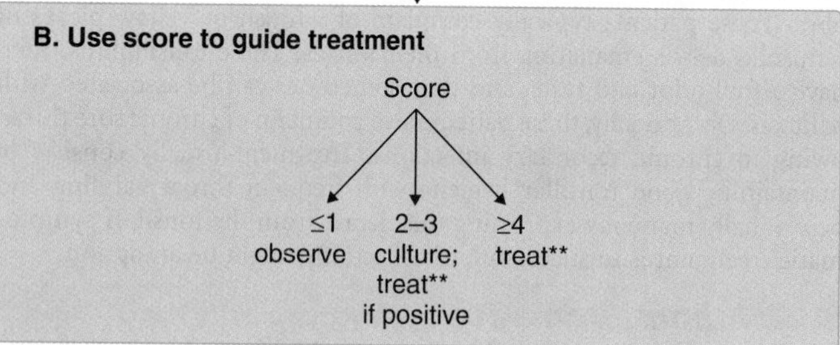

FIGURE 455–2 • Approach to diagnosis and treatment of the patient with a sore throat. *McIsaac WJ, Kellner JD, Aufricht P, et al: Empirical validation of guidelines for the management of pharyngitis in children and adults. JAMA 2004;291:1587–1595. **Treat for streptococcal infection; see text.

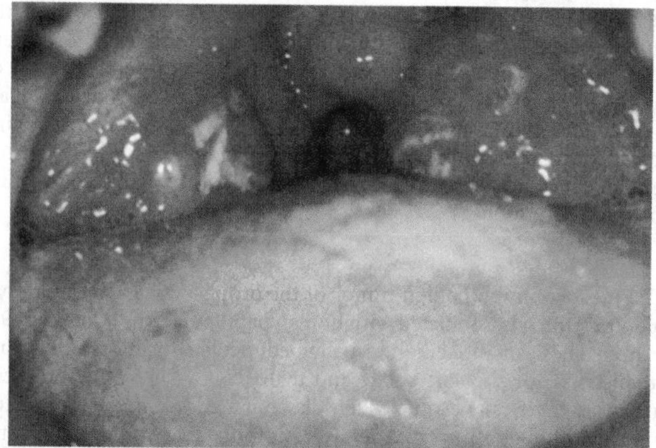

FIGURE 455–3 • Mononucleosis can produce impressive symmetrical exudative tonsillitis as shown in this patient.

TABLE 455–1 CLINICAL DIFFERENTIATION OF COMMON CONDITIONS ARISING AS SORE THROAT

Feature	Viral Pharyngitis	Bacterial Tonsillitis	Peritonsillar Abscess	Epiglottitis
Tonsillar enlargement	Usual	Rare	None	None
Tonsillar exudates	Occasional (mononucleosis)	Usual	Often	None
Tonsillar asymmetry	None	None	Usual	None
Trismus (inability to open jaw)	None	None	Usual	None
Cervical adenopathy	Occasional	Usual (tender)	Usual (tender)	None
Tender larynx	Rare	None	None	Usual

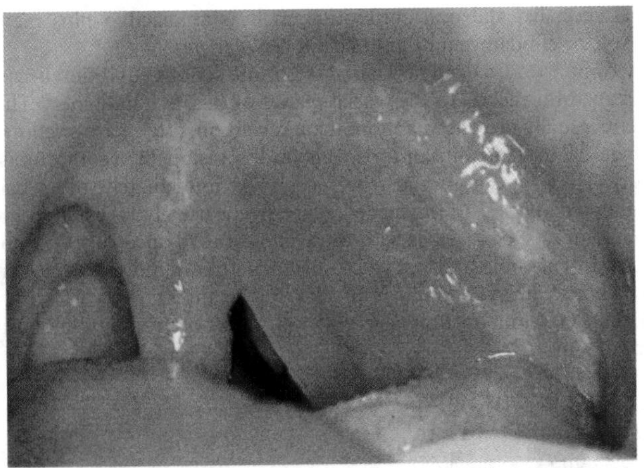

FIGURE 455–4 • If the tonsils are inflamed and appear asymmetric with unilateral palatal swelling and uvular deviation, a peritonsillar abscess should be suspected.

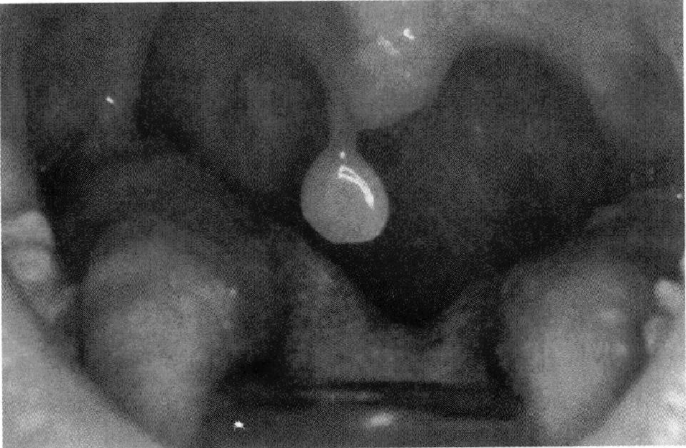

FIGURE 455–5 • Benign squamous papilloma. A benign squamous papilloma usually arises as a solitary lesion of the oropharynx, usually on the palate or uvula, but occasionally, especially in immunocompromised patients, the papillomatosis can become widespread on the oral and oropharyngeal mucosal surfaces.

Tonsils

Patients who have deep crypts and crevices in the tonsils can accumulate debris, such as food or sloughed mucosa, within these crypts, which provide an ideal environment for the growth of bacteria, especially anaerobes. These patients typically complain of whitish or yellow pieces of semisolid debris emanating from their tonsils. These tonsilloliths often have a foul odor and taste, and they sometimes can be associated with halitosis. Occasionally, these patients also complain of chronic sore throat owing to chronic secondary infections. Treatment usually consists of maintaining good tonsillar hygiene with frequent throat gargling and occasionally manually expressing this debris from the tonsil. If symptomatic treatment is unsuccessful, tonsillectomy might be an option.

Aphthous Stomatitis

Aphthous stomatitis, typically encountered in the oral cavity (Chapter 451), can also occur in the oropharynx. The spectrum of causes and their treatment are similar to those for oral stomatitis.

Thrush

Oral and pharyngeal candidiasis (thrush) is usually easily recognized by its typical "cottage cheese" exudative appearance. However, in the atrophic form of thrush, the inflammatory mucositis can be present without typical exudates. Treatment with either topical (clotrimazole or nystatin) or systemic (fluconazole) agents usually results in immediate and dramatic symptomatic improvement (Chapter 359). Underlying medical conditions commonly associated with thrush include diabetes, immune deficiency, malignancies, prolonged use of antibiotics, and xerostomia (dry mouth).

Tumors

The most common benign tumor of the oropharynx is the squamous papilloma, which is associated with human papillomavirus (Chapter 396) infection. These small, benign, usually pedunculated tumors often have a predilection for the soft palate and uvula (Fig. 455–5). In some circumstances, these can become widely disseminated within the mouth and pharynx. Although they are rarely symptomatic, removal is recommended when these produce undue concern on the part of the patient or the physician.

Hypopharynx

The hypopharynx is difficult to examine and assess. Nevertheless, when the presenting symptoms cannot be easily explained on the basis of the standard oral and oropharyngeal examination, conditions in the hypopharynx and larynx should be considered.

Epiglottitis

Epiglottitis (supraglottitis) is an uncommon problem but now is more common in adults than in children because of vaccination against *Haemophilus influenzae* in children (Chapter 323). The typical adult presenting with epiglottitis has a severe sore throat and odynophagia, often with fever and occasionally with a compromised airway, despite few or no findings on the oral or oropharyngeal examination. An examination of the larynx, preferably using a nasal fiberoptic endoscope, typically reveals swelling, erythema, and occasionally exudates of the epiglottis and other supraglottic structures. During the examination, palpation or manual movement of the larynx by external palpation produces significant pain. Patients with a confirmed diagnosis of epiglottitis require intravenous antibiotics (e.g., cefotaxime 2 g every 6 hours or ceftriaxone 1 to 2 g/day intravenously) and close observation because of the risk of developing a compromised airway. Although it is controversial, some otolaryngologists also recommend corticosteroids (e.g., dexamethasone 0.6 mg/kg given once) because of their benefit for croup in children. [3]

Hoarseness

The symptom of hoarseness invariably points to the larynx as the site of pathology. Benign lesions are most common, including vocal nodules (screamer's nodules), vocal cord cysts, vocal cord granulomas (usually resulting from intubation trauma or laryngopharyngeal reflux), and vocal cord papillomas. Malignancies must be suspected (Chapter 200), especially in patients with a strong smoking history.

Of the malignant tumors that can occur in the hypopharynx and larynx, squamous cell carcinoma is the most common and is usually associated with tobacco and ethanol use. Squamous cell carcinoma (Chapter 200) can occur on essentially any mucosal surface in the head and neck. Symptoms can range from mild sore throat to hoarseness, severe dysphagia, and odynophagia. Pain is often referred to the jaw or ear. Associated cervical lymph node enlargement is also common in advanced disease. Successful management depends on early detection by a careful examination of the entire upper aerodigestive tract, biopsy with histopathologic examination, and aggressive treatment based on the clinical stage and site of the lesion. Symptoms of hoarseness or of odynophagia (Chapter 140), hemoptysis (Chapters 83 and 89), aspiration (Chapter 94), enlarging neck nodes (Chapters 174 and 200), and otherwise unexplained ear pain (Chapter 452), especially when present for more than 4 to 6 weeks, should be investigated carefully with a thorough head and neck examination, which must include either indirect or a direct laryngoscopy.

Neurologic conditions affecting the larynx include unilateral vocal cord paralysis, which produces a "breathy" voice because the vocal cords cannot meet in the midline. The mobile cord often compensates over several months by moving across the midline to meet the paralyzed cord, thereby improving the voice. However, when compensation is inadequate or when aspiration occurs, vocal cord medialization procedures can be considered.

Bilateral vocal cord paralysis, either iatrogenic owing to thyroid surgery or thoracic surgery or, on occasion, owing to the Arnold-Chiari malformation (Chapter 444), may not produce severe impairment of voice because the cords are often positioned very close to one another in the midline; however, airway obstruction, especially with exertion, can be severe. In spasmodic dysphonia (Chapter 434), central nervous system–mediated dystonia of the vocal cord musculature causes a strained and tight-sounding voice that worsens with continued usage. Severely affected patients are often unable to maintain a voice beyond one or two words. Botulinum toxin injected directly into the vocalis muscle of the vocal cord can provide substantial symptomatic relief for up to 6 months.

Dysphagia and Esophageal Reflux

Dysphagia (Chapter 140) can have its origins in the hypopharynx, and the possibility of a mass lesion producing swallowing dysfunction must always be considered early in the diagnostic evaluation (see Hoarseness).

Symptoms of gastroesophageal reflux disease (GERD) may include intermittent hoarseness, chronic cough, postnasal drip, "globus" sensation, reactive airway disease, halitosis, and a brackish or acid taste in the back of the mouth and throat. Laryngoscopy typically reveals posterior laryngitis, with swollen and erythematous arytenoid cartilages, thickening of the vocal folds, interarytenoid edema, and thickening of the mucosa. When treatment aimed at nasal disorders (topical steroids, antihistamines, mucolytics, decongestants) fails to provide symptomatic relief, reflux disease should be suspected. Treatment is a therapeutic trial of a proton pump inhibitor (Chapter 140) for up to 3 months.

Spasm or thickening of the cricopharyngeus muscle, also know as the upper esophageal sphincter (Chapter 140), can cause poor pharyngeal emptying and occasionally cause spillage and penetration of secretions into the larynx with aspiration. This finding is common in patients with GERD and also seems to increase with age. Chronic cricopharyngeal spasm can result in the development of a diverticulum of the hypopharynx (Zenker's diverticulum; Fig. 140–8). These diverticula, which can slowly enlarge, can also serve as a reservoir for lodged food, medication, or other ingested materials for hours. The hallmark of Zenker's diverticulum is regurgitation of undigested food up to 4 hours following a meal; when large or symptomatic, these diverticula can usually be managed surgically.

Progressive neurologic conditions such as multiple sclerosis (Chapter 436) or amyotrophic lateral sclerosis (Chapter 435) can arise as slowly progressive dysphagia owing to loss of coordination of the swallowing musculature. Although these underlying neurologic conditions are not curable, attention to adequate alimentation and protection of the airway from aspiration are paramount. A careful evaluation by a swallowing therapist can provide invaluable management recommendations including alterations of swallowing techniques, changes in food consistency, and timing of other interventions, such as gastrostomy tube feedings or even tracheostomy for airway management.

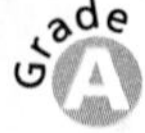

1. Del Mar CB, Glasziou PP, Spinks AB: Antibiotics for sore throat. Cochrane Database Syst Rev 2006;4:CD000023.
2. Casey JR, Pichichero ME: Meta-analysis of cephalosporins versus penicillin for treatment of group A streptococcal tonsillopharyngitis in adults. Clin Infect Dis 2004;38:1526–1534.
3. Bjornson CL, Klassen TP, Williamson J, et al: A randomized trial of a single dose of oral dexamethasone for mild croup. N Engl J Med 2004;351:1306–1313.

SUGGESTED READINGS

Ford CN: Evaluation and management of laryngopharyngeal reflux. JAMA 2005;294:1534–1540. *A practical review.*

Hopkins C, Yousaf U, Pedersen M: Acid reflux treatment for hoarseness. Cochrane Database Syst Rev 2006;1:CD005054. *It is unclear if antireflux therapy for patients with hoarseness, which may be due to laryngopharyngeal and gastro-esophageal reflux, is effective.*

Humair JP, Revaz SA, Bovier P, et al: Management of acute pharyngitis in adult: Reliability of rapid streptococcal tests and clinical findings. Arch Intern Med 2006;166:640–644. *RSAT had high sensitivity (91%) and specificity (95%) for streptococcal pharyngitis, leading to nearly optimal treatment (94%) and antibiotic prescription (37%), with minimal antibiotic overuse (3%) and underuse (3%).*

McIsaac WJ, Kellner JD, Aufricht P, et al: Empirical validation of guidelines for the management of pharyngitis in children and adults. JAMA 2004;291:1587–1595. *Recommends using guidelines to select patients for throat cultures but antibiotic treatment only in those with positive cultures or rapid strep tests.*

Merati AL, Heman-Ackah YD, Abaza M, et al: Common movement disorders affecting the larynx: A report from the neurolaryngology committee of the AAO-HNS. Otolaryngol Head Neck Surg 2005;133:654–665. *A detailed review.*

Scully C: Clinical practice. Aphthous ulceration. N Engl J Med 2006;355:165–172. *An excellent overview of aphthous ulceration.*

Section XXVII

Medical Consultation

Cecil Medicine 23

456 PRINCIPLES OF MEDICAL CONSULTATION

Gerald W. Smetana

APPROACH TO MEDICAL CONSULTATION

A general medical or subspecialty medical physician may be requested to perform a consultation for a variety of purposes. In some settings a single consultative encounter will be requested, or the consultant will determine that only one visit, either in the inpatient or in the outpatient setting, is necessary. In other circumstances the most appropriate consultative approach will include one or more follow-up visits to meet the goals of the consultation from the perspectives of the requesting physician, patient, and consultant. The consultant may become a co-manager who continues to care for a component of the patient's needs in an ongoing fashion while being careful to coordinate this co-management with the requesting physician. Finally, in some situations it may be most appropriate for the physician who initially requested the consultation no longer to play an active role in the care of the patient but rather to transfer ongoing care exclusively to the consultant.

From a practical perspective, consulting medical physicians, whether they are generalists or subspecialists, enter into the consultative mode in a relatively limited number of ways. Surgeons may request a preoperative medical consultation to assess operative risk and obtain recommendations regarding perioperative care (Chapter 457) or, postoperatively, to seek help in managing specific postoperative complications or help with the patient's long-term management. Both general medical physicians and medical subspecialists appropriately seek help from a subspecialist with particular knowledge in problems outside their own area of expertise. Sometimes these requests are directly related to procedures, but oftentimes requests seek cognitive guidance as well. Finally, noninternists may seek medical consultation in settings other than the preoperative or postoperative period. For example, medical physicians may often be called on to help determine whether the somatic symptoms of a psychiatric patient represent important medical conditions (Chapter 460). In the peripartum setting, specific complications of pregnancy may require sophisticated medical consultation (Chapter 259). In the United States, the transition from general practitioners to family physicians has created a group of primary care doctors whose longer training (3 years after medical school rather than 1) has resulted in far fewer consultative requests to general internists but a continued stream of consultations for medical subspecialists.

Each of these settings raises different challenges for the medical consultant. In all settings, however, a number of general principles apply and can improve the effectiveness of consultations. In addition to the universal need for sufficient content expertise to address the medical problem at hand, consultants must have a set of personal, interactive skills, which come naturally to some physicians but can and should be learned by others. These skills facilitate the ability to impart advice, to collaborate with the requesting physician, to interact effectively with the patient, and to improve outcomes in ways that reassure the patient, help but not threaten the requesting physician, and provide professional satisfaction for the consultant.

SETTING-SPECIFIC CONSULTATIVE ISSUES

An effective consultant must recognize the setting in which the consultation is requested and possess the required content knowledge. Distressingly, a number of studies have demonstrated that the requesting physician and the consultant often have different views on the reasons why a consultation was requested, and this initial disconnection, if present, will doom any medical consultation.

Preoperative Surgical Consultation

In the preoperative setting, the medical consultant should not "clear" a patient for surgery and must avoid the temptation to do so even if asked. Clearance may incorrectly imply that the procedure has no risk or that the medical consultant will take responsibility for having misled the patient and surgeon. Instead, the medical consultant should help determine the inherent risk associated with the proposed procedure for the particular patient, whether the patient is in the best possible condition for it, and whether any generic or patient-specific interventions would be beneficial (Chapter 457). Effective consultation also requires a substantial knowledge base, whether the consultation is focusing on a particular organ system or on overall perioperative risk (Chapter 457).

Postoperative Surgical Consultation

Surgeons typically request a postoperative medical consultation when a complication has developed that is beyond their area of expertise. These problems are commonly urgent, so the goal is expeditious consultation and prompt intervention. One postoperative model is the rapid response team, whereby a consultative team sees sick, hospitalized patients at the time that abnormalities develop that are thought to indicate impending serious complications. Two studies of this model of postoperative care have shown that care improves over baseline after the introduction of such a service.

Another reason for a postoperative consultation is to obtain assistance in post-hospitalization care. Consultants should aid in the transition to the outpatient or long-term care setting by taking primary or consultative roles as appropriate.

Medical-Medical Consultations

Cross-consultations between medical subspecialists or between a subspecialist and a generalist, in either direction, are quintessential examples of collaboration. For subspecialty consultations, the key is to provide requested expertise without overstepping into the domain of expertise of the requesting physician. Medical-medical consultations oftentimes result in ongoing co-management, thereby making collegiality especially important.

A growing example of medical-medical consultation is when a hospitalist assumes principal responsibility for an inpatient admission and then returns the patient to the primary care physician after hospital discharge. In this consultative interaction, close communication is critical because primary responsibility for the patient's care has shifted from the outpatient medical physician to the inpatient physician. This transfer of responsibility is not dissimilar to what occurs when a patient is submitted to the care of a subspecialist for a procedure such as cardiac catheterization or gastrointestinal endoscopy. Similar issues also arise when a critically ill patient with a condition such as a complicated myocardial infarction (Chapters 72 and 108) or shock (Chapters 107, 108, and 109) is managed principally by an inpatient-oriented medical specialist and is then expected to return to the care of the primary physician after hospital discharge. However, a key difference is that the inpatient hospitalist physician, unlike the consulting subspecialist, typically will not have any ongoing co-management role. Because of the higher risk of discontinuity, effective communication at the time of hospitalization, whenever key issues arise during hospitalization, and at the time of discharge is even more important in the inpatient hospitalist model than in the other settings in which subspecialists may take on more of a co-management role.

Consultations for Special Populations

When consulting for psychiatrists or in the peripartum period, the consultant requires special expertise to understand the oftentimes different expressions of signs and symptoms in specific populations, as well as how and when to modify typical medical recommendation because of special circumstances (Chapters 259 and 460). Although these consultations occasionally result in long-term co-management, more commonly they revolve around the resolution of an isolated problem.

Consultations for general practitioners or family physicians generally follow the same guidelines as those for general internists. However, because both the training and ongoing practices of such physicians may or may not include the same spectrum and complexity of disease encountered by typical general internists, the subspecialty consultant must use judgment regarding both the initial consultation and the advisability of ongoing co-management.

STRATEGIES FOR EFFECTIVE CONSULTATION

It is critical that requesting and consulting physicians agree about the reason for the consultative request. For example, the nature of a preoperative medical consultant's evaluation would differ substantially if the request were (1) routine, (2) for advice on perioperative insulin management in a patient with type 1 diabetes, or (3) to assist in determining the risks and benefits of proceeding to vascular surgery in a high-risk patient with coronary artery disease and a previous stroke. Effective communication at the time of the request will improve the value of the consultation and clarify the question. When there is doubt regarding the reason for the consultation, the consultant should speak directly to the referring physician before completing the evaluation of the patient.

Common reasons for medical consultations include assessment of perioperative risk; interpretation of a laboratory abnormality; help in obtaining a procedure, advice, or therapy; and aid in providing long-term care. Prophylactic strategies (venous thromboembolism, endocarditis, and surgical site infection) infrequently generate requests for medical consultation because they are commonly standardized to conform to practice guidelines at individual institutions.

Determining the question will also help narrow the scope of the consultant's advice and minimize the number of recommendations. This focus is especially important because evidence indicates that adherence by the requesting physician to any of the recommendations made by the consultant is higher for consultations with fewer recommendations. Another strategy to minimize the number of recommendations is to restrict advice to pertinent issues at the time, preferably in order of their importance. For example, a consultant who is asked to aid in the care of a critically ill pregnant patient with the HELLP syndrome (hemolysis, elevated liver enzymes, and low platelet count) (Chapters 164 and 259) should not also make recommendations regarding the value of cigarette cessation (Chapter 30), even though this issue will become very important after the mother and child have survived the acute event.

Requesting physicians are also more likely to adhere to recommendations when the patient is sicker, when the consultation is performed promptly, when advice is given to institute specific therapy rather than perform more diagnostic testing, and when the consultant writes frequent follow-up notes. When giving advice about medications, consultants should indicate specific doses and duration of treatment. When a recommendation is likely to be controversial (e.g., postpone surgery), it is always preferable to speak directly to the requesting physician before writing a consultation note in the hope that direct conversation will provide an opportunity to develop a consensus that may then be reflected in the formal consultation note.

Consultants should be careful to restrict their advice to their particular area of expertise. For example, unless a particular antipsychotic medication is contraindicated because of a medical issue (Chapter 460), it is wisest to defer decision making regarding psychiatric management to the psychiatrist. A strongly worded consultation note that advises against a particular strategy will put another physician in a difficult medicolegal position if it differs from the physician's usual or recommended practice.

SPECIAL CONSULTATIVE SITUATIONS

Curbside Consultation

Informal consultations are commonly termed "curbside" consultations. In the current era, ready access to online medical references may potentially reduce curbside requests. Consultants in "cognitive" specialties such as infectious diseases, rheumatology, and endocrinology provide a disproportionate amount of informal (as compared with formal) consultations. Informal consultations may occur by telephone, by e-mail, or in person. Curbside consultation is ingrained into the fabric of medical care.

Both generalists and specialists participate in an average of three to four curbside consultations per week. These consultations commonly involve questions about diagnostic tests, treatment plans, and the potential value of a formal consultation (which follows approximately a third of curbside consultations) in the future. To be effective, curbside consultations should be brief, involve a single question, and require no direct examination of the patient or medical records.

An important limitation of curbside consultations is that the consultant must rely on limited, secondhand information from the requesting physician rather than primary data from direct evaluation of the patient. Consultants report that such indirect information is often inaccurate on subsequent formal consultation. This reality, along with lack of financial compensation, leads to a greater degree of dissatisfaction with the curbside process by consultants than by requesting physicians. Salaried consultants may view a request for a curbside consultation more favorably than those whose livelihood depends on a fee-for-service model of care.

Although requesting physicians may perceive reduced medicolegal risk when they obtain and even document a curbside consultation, consultants may fear the risk of malpractice liability themselves when offering such advice. However, courts have consistently found that curbside consultants have no liability because no direct physician-patient relationship exists. Rather, the relationship is only between the requesting and consulting physicians.

Mandatory Consultations

In some situations, mandatory consultations may help enforce a standard of care. For example, mandatory inpatient infectious disease consultations can improve the use of antimicrobial agents in the hospital and after discharge. Similarly, instituting routine consultation for patients with certain sentinel conditions, such as diabetes, may improve outcomes.

Co-management

A consultation that begins with an initial encounter or a limited number of follow-up visits may evolve into ongoing co-management. In such an arrangement, the physician initially serving in a consultative role becomes at least coequal to the requesting physician in the provision of ongoing care. In some situations, the consultant may actually become the primary physician. This arrangement is obvious in situations in which the consultation was requested specifically for the provision of ongoing care. Other examples include situations in which an oncologist assumes principal care of a patient with a malignancy or a nephrologist assumes principal care of a patient with end-stage renal disease on dialysis. In some of these situations, a general internist who initially requested the consultation may now become the consultant and provide advice on preventive care and occasional help with intercurrent medical problems.

Co-management is also increasingly common in the hospital setting. Medical consultants may become co-managers of postoperative surgical patients, with a potential for improving outcomes. In one randomized trial of perioperative patients, formal co-management, in which a medical physician took responsibility for managing medical problems rather than acting in a consultative role, reduced postoperative complications; in addition, both nurses and surgeons preferred this model. [1] In some settings the outpatient primary care physician may retain a co-management role even as a cardiologist cares for a patient with an acute myocardial infarction, a pulmonologist cares for a patient in the intensive care unit, a hospitalist cares for a patient in the general medical setting, or a noninternist addresses a specific problem.

RESPONSIBILITIES OF THE CONSULTANT

The consultant is responsible to two parties: the patient and the referring physician. A paternalistic approach is not desirable. The consultant should not limit communication to just the referring physician and must not withhold discussion and recommendations from the patient. However, the consultant should not usurp the role of the referring physician, who remains responsible for assembling information and advice from varied sources, as well as for developing an integrated plan with the patient. For example, in the preoperative setting, the consultant should not express a final opinion regarding the suitability of proceeding to surgery without first discussing all relevant considerations with the referring surgeon.

In the trilateral deliberative model, the patient, referring physician, and consultant each have responsibilities and constraints inherent in their relationships (Table 456–1). Above all, the role of the consultant is to improve patient care and outcomes.

IMPACT OF CONSULTATIONS ON PATIENT OUTCOME

Few studies have investigated the impact of medical consultations on outcomes. One randomly assigned 355 patients whose surgeons had requested a preoperative consultation to either an outpatient medical

TABLE 456–1 THE TRILATERAL DELIBERATIVE MODEL

	Primary Physician-Patient Relationship	Consultant-Patient Relationship	Consultant–Primary Physician Relationship
Physician role	Friend or teacher	Friend or teacher	Both physicians as teacher-colleagues, consultant as counselor, primary physician as leader
Duties of physician	Giving information, interpreting the patient's values, deliberating with the patient to maximize autonomous choices Orchestration of care Ultimate responsibility, with the patient, for medical care	Giving information, interpreting the patient's values, deliberating with the patient to maximize autonomous choices	Giving information, interpreting options, deliberating to maximize quality of medical care
Constraints on the physician	Avoid undue dominance over consultant	Minimize unnecessary duplication of tests Minimize expression to the patient of insignificant differences in judgment with the primary physician Generally defer to the primary physician's ultimate judgment	Either physician should keep the patient's confidences from the other physician if the patient so desires and if the information is not relevant to immediate health care
Exceptions and negotiable areas between physicians		Direct discussion with the patient over a difference with the primary physician is permissible to avoid serious harm to the patient or in the event of malpractice by the primary physician	Primary responsibility during specific procedures or periods can be the consultant's, at which point the consultant temporarily assumes the primary physician's role

Adapted with permission from Emmanuel LL, Richter J: The consultant and the patient-physician relationship. A trilateral deliberative model. Arch Intern Med 1994;154:1785–1790.

consultation or usual care (inpatient consultation at the discretion of the surgeon). Length of stay did not differ between the two groups, but there were fewer unnecessary admissions (those that did not result in surgery) in the outpatient consultation group. [2] Other reports indicate that anywhere from 10 to 50% of preoperative medical consultations result in changes in patient management.

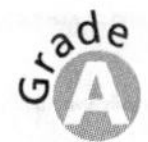

1. Huddleston JM, Long KL, Naessens JL, et al: Medical and surgical comanagement after elective hip and knee arthroplasty. A randomized, controlled trial. Ann Intern Med 2004;141:28–38.
2. Macpherson DS, Lofgren RP: Outpatient internal medicine preoperative evaluation: A randomized controlled trial. Med Care 1994;32:498–507.

SUGGESTED READINGS

Bellomo R, Goldsmith D, Uchino S, et al: Prospective controlled trial of effect of medical emergency team on postoperative morbidity and mortality rates. Crit Care Med 2004;32:916–921. *An ICU-based medical emergency team was associated with a reduced incidence of postoperative adverse outcomes.*

Linzer M, Myerburg RJ, Kutner JS, et al: Exploring the generalist-subspecialist interface in internal medicine. Am J Med 2006;119:528–537. *Recommendations on whether and when to refer for a variety of diseases.*

MERIT Study Investigators: Introduction of the medical emergency team (MET) system: A cluster-randomised controlled trial. Lancet 2005;365:2091–2097. *The MET system did not reduce adverse events, but both the intervention and control groups did significantly better than patients just before the trial began.*

Salerno SM, Hurst FP, Halvorson S, et al: Principles of effective consultation: An update for the 21st century consultant. Arch Intern Med 2007;167:271–275. *Emphasizes that different types of physicians and surgeons prefer different approaches to consultations.*

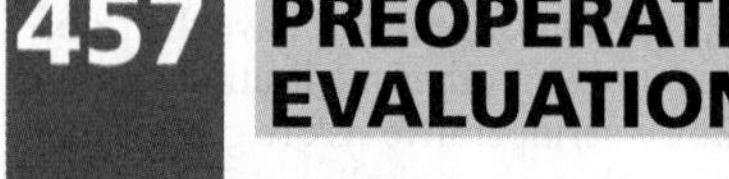

457 PREOPERATIVE EVALUATION

Steven L. Cohn

PREOPERATIVE EVALUATION

Each year in the United States, more than 25 million inpatient surgical procedures and an additional 25 million outpatient procedures are performed. Although over a third of these surgical patients are older than 65 years, overall morbidity and mortality are relatively low, in part because of modern anesthetic and surgical techniques. A crucial aspect of safety is careful preoperative evaluation of the patient, not only by the surgeon and anesthesiologist but also, in many instances, by a general medical consultant or medical subspecialist.

Operative Risk Assessment

The components of perioperative risk include those related to the patient, procedure, provider, and anesthesia. Anesthetic risk is low, with mortality less than 0.03% in a normal healthy patient—American Society of Anesthesiology (ASA) class 1—but increasing to 0.2% in ASA class 2 (mild systemic disease), 1.2% in class 3 (severe systemic disease), 8% in class 4 (severe systemic disease that is a constant threat to life), and 34% in class 5 (a moribund patient not expected to survive for 24 hours without surgery). Meta-analysis suggests that when feasible, neuraxial (spinal or epidural) anesthesia may reduce postoperative complications when compared with general anesthesia (Chapter 458), but decisions regarding the anesthetic technique should be the responsibility of the anesthesiologist and not be part of the preoperative medical consultation. With respect to the provider, data support a "learning curve," with better outcomes when procedures are performed by more experienced, higher-volume surgeons.

General Risk Assessment

History and Physical Examination

The medical history and physical examination are the most important components in assessing a patient's risk for surgery. The consultation should focus (Chapter 456) on pertinent medical problems, particularly cardiopulmonary symptoms and diseases that are associated with risk and are likely to influence perioperative management. The importance of the past surgical history is to determine whether the patient was able to undergo major surgery in the recent past or had any perioperative medical or anesthetic-related complications that could occur again. The social history should assess and quantify the amount, duration, and last use of tobacco, alcohol, or illicit substances. It is important to document allergies to medications, foods, and latex, as well as to obtain an accurate list of the patient's current prescription and over-the-counter medications, including doses and adherence. The family history is relevant primarily for any genetically associated complications such as malignant hyperthermia. The review of systems should include the presence or absence of chest pain and dyspnea, as well as the patient's exercise capacity. The physical examination must include the vital signs, assessment of the airway and respiratory status, cardiovascular examination, and documentation of any neurologic deficit.

Preoperative Tests

Screening preoperative test results in otherwise healthy individuals are usually normal and, even when abnormal, rarely affect management (generally <1%) (Table 457–1). Most significant abnormalities can be predicted from the clinical information obtained, which then guides selective testing based on the history, the physical findings, and the planned type of surgery and anesthesia. Most patients undergoing low-risk surgery with local anesthesia require no preoperative testing. Repeat testing should be avoided if recent (within 3 months) results were normal, unless the patient's condition or medications have changed.

Perioperative Medications

Decisions regarding whether to continue a medication perioperatively should consider the drug's pharmacokinetics (Chapter 27), as well as its effects on the primary disease and perioperative risk, including potential interactions with anesthetic agents. Some medications are essential to continue (e.g., cardiac medications and corticosteroids), whereas others must be discontinued (e.g., oral hypoglycemic agents) or have their dose altered (e.g., insulin and anticoagulants). Still other medications should be started prophylactically to minimize perioperative risk (e.g., anticoagulants for prophylaxis against venous thromboembolism [Chapter 81] and antibiotic prophylaxis for surgical site infection or endocarditis [Chapter 76]). Although data are often lacking or conflicting, Table 457–2 briefly summarizes "consensus" perioperative recommendations for the major classes of drugs.

Cardiac Risk Assessment

A significant proportion of patients who undergo surgery have either known coronary artery disease or risk factors for it, and postoperative cardiac complications are second only to direct surgical complications as a cause of perioperative mortality. The goal is to clinically risk-stratify patients and determine whether additional testing, new medications, or cardiac interventions will be beneficial.

History and Physical Examination

Important information includes any history of previous cardiac disease (myocardial infarction, angina, heart failure, arrhythmias, valvular disease), cardiac interventions (coronary artery bypass grafting, percutaneous coronary intervention), cardiac evaluation (noninvasive testing, angiography), risk factors (hypertension, diabetes mellitus, dyslipidemia, cigarette smoking), and associated diseases (peripheral arterial disease, stroke, chronic kidney disease, and chronic obstructive pulmonary disease [COPD]). Current status regarding chest pain or dyspnea, functional capacity, and medications should be assessed. The physical examination serves to confirm findings in the history, as well as to assess severity and control of the disease (e.g., heart failure, hypertension, valvar disease). The preoperative electrocardiogram rarely changes management unless it demonstrates evidence of a recent or silent myocardial infarction, but it is often useful as a baseline against which to compare postoperative tracings.

Cardiac Risk Indices

Over the years a number of risk indices have been proposed to assist in preoperative cardiac evaluation. The most current approach, developed during the evaluation of several thousand patients and validated in thousands more, is the revised cardiac risk index (Table 457–3). Consensus guidelines developed by the American College of Cardiology and the American Heart Association incorporate risk into a stepwise strategy and are updated periodically. Based on these approaches and on more recent randomized trials and meta-analyses, data support a systematic approach to perioperative testing and treatment in patients with suspected or known cardiac disease (Figs. 457–1 and 457–2).

Noninvasive Tests

A resting echocardiogram (Chapter 53) is indicated to evaluate valvar heart disease in patients with clinically suspicious murmurs and left ven-

TABLE 457–1 RECOMMENDATIONS FOR PREOPERATIVE LABORATORY TESTING

Test	% Abnormal	% Influencing Management	Indications
Hemoglobin	1.8	0.1	Expected major blood loss, symptoms of anemia, chronic kidney disease
White blood count	0.7	0.0	Suspected infection, myeloproliferative disorder, myelotoxic medications
Platelet count	0.9	0.02	Bleeding diathesis, myeloproliferative disorder, myelotoxic medications
Prothrombin time	0.3	0.0	Bleeding diathesis, liver disease, malnutrition, antibiotic use, anticoagulants
Partial thromboplastin time	6.5	0.1	Bleeding diathesis, anticoagulant use
Electrolytes	12.7	1.8	Renal disease, medications affecting electrolytes (e.g., diuretics, digoxin, ACE inhibitor, ARBs)
Glucose	9.3	0.5	Known DM, steroids, morbid obesity
Renal function	8.2	2.6	Renal disease, DM, HTN, major surgery, older age, medications affecting renal function
Liver function tests	0.4	0.1	Known liver disease, albumin level if at risk for needing postoperative parenteral nutrition
Urinalysis	19.1	1.4	No indication unless GU symptoms or instrumentation planned
Electrocardiogram (<50 years old)	29.6 (19.7)	2.6	Age >40 in men or >50 in women or symptoms/signs of or previous known diagnosis of cardiac disease, DM, or HTN
Chest radiograph (<50 years old)	21.2 (4.9)	3.0	Age >50 or symptoms/signs or previous known diagnosis of cardiac or pulmonary disease

ACE = angiotensin-converting enzyme; ARB = angiotensin receptor blocker; DM = diabetes mellitus; GU = genitourinary; HTN = hypertension.
Modified from Smetana GW, Macpherson DS: The case against routine preoperative laboratory testing. Med Clin North Am 2003;87:7–40.

TABLE 457–2 PERIOPERATIVE MANAGEMENT OF MEDICATIONS

Medication Class	Recommendation
Anticoagulants (heparins, warfarin)	Continue for minor surgery Discontinue at an appropriate interval before major surgery Consider bridging anticoagulation for patients at high risk for interim thrombosis (Table 35–2)
Antiplatelet drugs	Continue for minor surgery Discontinue clopidogrel at least 5 days before surgery If discontinuing aspirin, do so at least 5–7 days before surgery
Cardiovascular medications	Continue most agents Initiate β-blockers in patients at high risk for perioperative cardiac morbidity Withhold diuretics on the morning of surgery, especially if signs of volume depletion are present
Lipid-lowering agents	Continue "statins" Discontinue other agents
Pulmonary agents	Continue
Gastrointestinal agents	Continue
Diabetic agents (see text)	Withhold oral hypoglycemic agents on the morning of surgery; restart when the patient resumes eating For type 1 diabetics, continue some form of insulin (long acting or intravenous) at all times For type 2 diabetics, decrease the dose of morning intermediate insulin
Thyroid agents (hypothyroidism and hyperthyroidism) (see text)	Continue thyroid replacement Continue antithyroid medication and postpone surgery until the hyperthyroidism is controlled
Oral contraceptives, hormone replacement, and SERMs	May discontinue 3 weeks before surgery only in patients at high risk for perioperative venous thromboembolism; otherwise continue
Corticosteroids (see text)	Continue chronic corticosteroids; increase the dosage to account for surgical stress
Psychotropic agents	Continue SSRIs but consider withholding them several weeks before CNS surgery Continue tricyclic antidepressants, benzodiazepines, lithium, and antipsychotics Usually discontinue MAOs 10–14 days before surgery
Chronic opioids	Continue; substitute equianalgesic or higher doses for surgical pain
Rheumatologic agents	Continue methotrexate Discontinue other DMARDs and anticytokines Continue hypouricemic agents
Neurologic agents	Continue antiseizure medications Withold antiparkinsonian agents briefly Continue agents for myasthenia gravis
Herbal agents	Discontinue all agents

CNS = central nervous system; DMARD = disease-modifying antirheumatic drug; MAO = monoamine oxidase; SERM = selective estrogen receptor modulator; SSRI = selective serotonin reuptake inhibitor.
Adapted from Cohn SL, Macpherson DS: Perioperative medication management. *In* Cohn SL, Smetana GW, Weed HG, eds: Perioperative Medicine: Just the Facts. New York: McGraw-Hill, 2006.

TABLE 457–3 CLINICAL FACTORS IMPORTANT IN ASSESSING PERIOPERATIVE CARDIAC RISK

Revised cardiac risk index criteria*

Patients are at risk and are candidates for perioperative β-blockers if they have
- **Ischemic heart disease** or any two of the following:
- **Heart failure,†** defined as
  - S3 or bilateral rales on physical examination or pulmonary edema on chest radiograph
- **Cerebrovascular disease,** defined as
  - History of transient ischemic attack or history of cerebrovascular accident
- **Insulin-dependent diabetes mellitus**
- **Chronic renal insufficiency,** defined as
  - Baseline creatinine of 2.0 mg/dL or greater
- **High-risk surgery,** defined as
  - Intrathoracic, intra-abdominal, or suprainguinal vascular surgery

*Lee TH, Marcantonio ER, Mangione CM, et al: Derivation and prospective validation of a simple index for prediction of cardiac risk of major noncardiac surgery. Circulation 1999;100:1043–1049.
†Use of β-blockers must be individualized and used with caution in patients with heart failure.
Reproduced from Auerbach AD, Goldman L: Assessing and reducing the cardiac risk of non-cardiac surgery. Circulation 2006;113:1361–1376.

tricular function in patients with heart failure. Other than for the assessment of aortic stenosis (see later), it is not a reliable predictor of perioperative cardiac events. Exercise testing (with or without imaging) is preferred to pharmacologic stress testing because it assesses functional capacity (see Table 48–3), but its use is often limited by a patient's inability to achieve the target heart rate.

Pharmacologic Stress Testing

Pharmacologic stress testing (either dipyridamole or adenosine with nuclear imaging [Chapters 54 and 70] or dobutamine echocardiography [Chapters 53 and 70]) is indicated when a patient cannot perform adequate exercise (see Table 70–5 and Fig. 70–4). Both tests have equivalent sensitivity for predicting perioperative ischemic complications, whereas stress echocardiography has fewer false-positive results. Dipyridamole and adenosine can cause bronchospasm and are best avoided in patients with symptomatic or severe asthma or obstructive lung disease, but they are commonly preferred in patients with left bundle branch block, in whom exercise or stress echocardiography is more likely to give false-positive results. Quantitatively, the number and extent of reperfusion defects or wall motion abnormalities correlate with the severity of disease, likelihood of complications, and need for further evaluation by angiography.

Risk Reduction Strategies for Ischemic Heart Disease

Medical Therapy

Prophylactic β-blockers (e.g., atenolol or bisoprolol) have been shown to decrease perioperative cardiac risk in higher-risk patients, but a

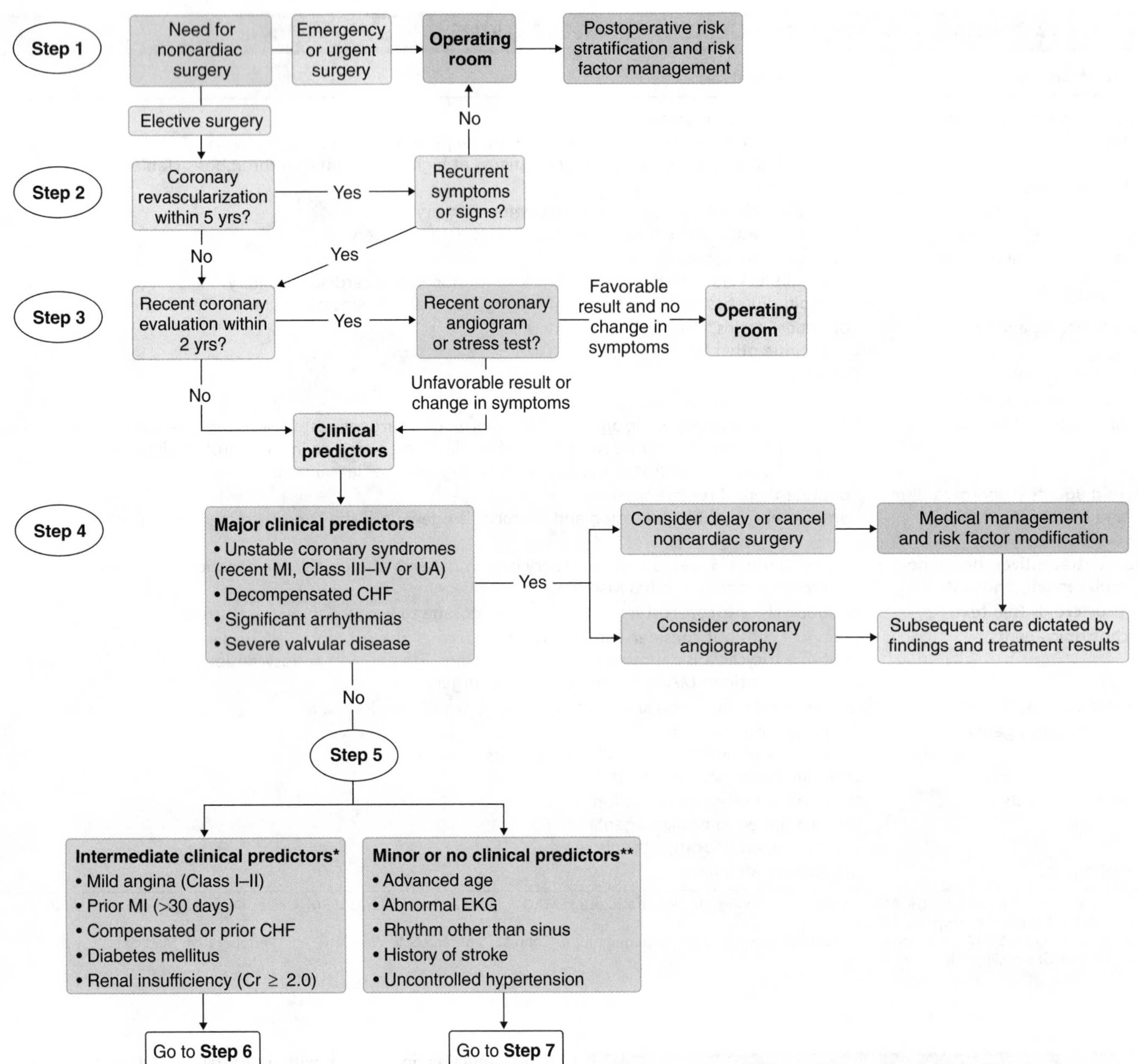

FIGURE 457–1 • Algorithm for patient selection for cardioprotective agents and cardiac testing before elective major noncardiac surgery (part 1). CHF = congestive heart failure; Cr = creatine; EKG = electrocardiogram; METS = metabolic equivalents; MI = myocardial infarction; UA = unstable angina. (From Cohn SL, Goldman L: Preoperative risk evaluation and perioperative management of patients with coronary artery disease. Med Clin North Am 2003;87:111–136. Adapted from Eagle KA, Berger PB, Clakins H, et al: ACC/AHA guideline update for perioperative cardiovascular evaluation for noncardiac surgery—executive summary: A report of the American College of Cardiology/American Heart Association Task Force on Practice Guidelines [Committee to Update the 1996 Guidelines on Perioperative Cardiovascular Evaluation for Noncardiac Surgery]. Published simultaneously in J Am Coll Cardiol 2002;39:542–553 and Circulation 2002;105:1257–1267.)

meta-analysis of all randomized trials has shown that the 50% or greater benefit found in all studies combined does not currently meet statistical significance. 1 β-Blockers probably benefit higher-risk patients (see Fig. 457–1) and are most likely to be used when incorporated into routine local guidelines and titrated to a heart rate of 55 to 65 beats per minute. Various recommended regimens are listed in Table 457–4.

If a patient has contraindications to β-blockers (bronchospasm, bradyarrhythmia, acute heart failure, advanced heart block), an α_2-adrenergic agonist (i.e., clonidine, 0.2 mg orally the night before and morning of surgery) may be an alternative choice based on data that such medications also reduce ischemia and possibly perioperative myocardial infarction and death, especially in patients undergoing major vascular surgery. 2 Limited data on prophylactic calcium antagonists or nitrates have not shown major benefits in preventing complications after noncardiac surgery.

Statins (Chapter 217) may be beneficial by stabilizing endothelial plaque. Although the manufacturers' package inserts currently recommend discontinuing statins before surgery, current data suggest that they should be continued perioperatively and be started prophylactically preoperatively in patients who meet criteria for their ongoing use (Chapter 217).

Invasive Therapies

Prophylactic coronary revascularization in patients who have stable cardiac symptoms and no aortic stenosis and do not meet standard criteria for the procedure (Chapter 70) does not reduce perioperative myocardial infarction, death within 30 days, or long-term mortality at an average of 2.7 years in patients who receive appropriate medical therapy. 3 Preoperative coronary revascularization is indicated only if the patient meets the criteria for coronary angiography or revascularization independent of the need for surgery.

For bare metal stents, limited data suggest that surgery should be delayed for at least 2 weeks and preferably for 6 weeks after stenting because of the risk for in-stent thrombosis when dual antiplatelet therapy

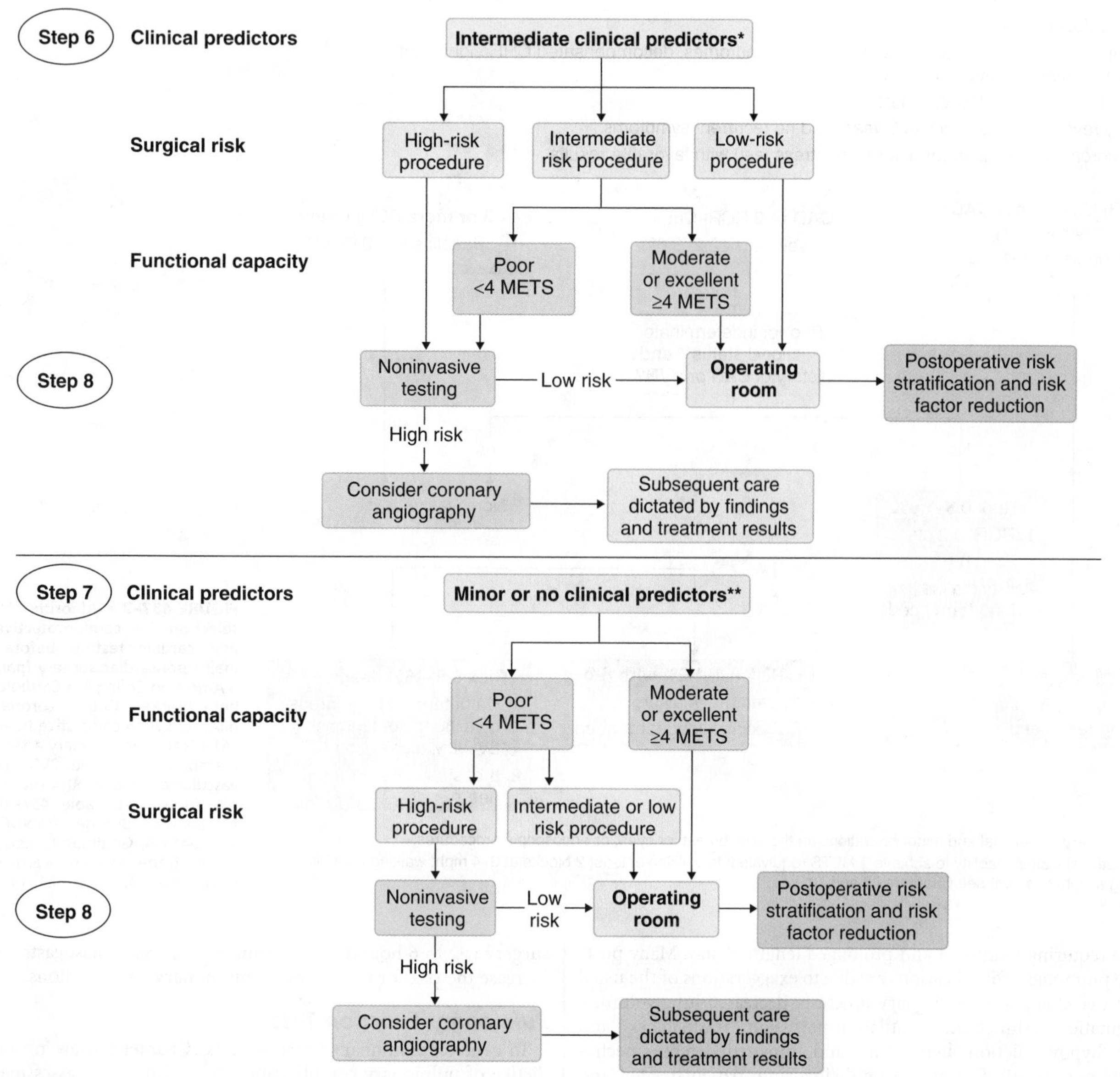

FIGURE 457–1, cont'd

with aspirin and clopidogrel is discontinued early or because of the alternative risk for bleeding if surgery is performed in patients receiving such antiplatelet therapy (Chapter 73). Similar concerns apply with drug-eluting stents for which dual antiplatelet therapy should be continued uninterrupted for a minimum of 12 months because of the risk of late in stent thrombosis. However, no studies have reported outcomes for noncardiac surgery after placement of these stents. The antiplatelet therapy is usually discontinued 5 to 7 days before the noncardiac procedure. For balloon angioplasty without stenting, a delay of at least 7 to 10 days is generally recommended.

Other Cardiovascular Diseases

Heart Failure

Heart failure, which is a major risk factor for surgery, requires treatment and optimization before surgery (Chapter 58). Routine use of *pulmonary artery catheters* does not reduce morbidity or mortality in patients undergoing elective noncardiac surgery. 4

Aortic Stenosis

Patients with symptomatic *aortic stenosis* who meet the criteria for valve replacement (Chapter 75) independent of their need for surgery should undergo the valvar surgery before the noncardiac surgery. However, patients usually survive surgery with intensified care if they refuse valve replacement or time does not permit it. Balloon aortic valvuloplasty may be an option in severe cases. An asymptomatic valvar gradient higher than 25 to 30 mm Hg also carries an increased risk for perioperative complications but is an indication for more careful monitoring rather than valve surgery. Endocarditis prophylaxis is appropriate for patients with valvar heart disease (Chapter 76).

Hypertension

Hypertension with diastolic blood pressure lower than 110 mm Hg and no significant target organ damage does not increase the risk for major perioperative cardiac complications. Even when the preoperative diastolic blood pressure is higher, limited data suggest that surgery is safe after additional antihypertensive therapy.

Arrhythmias

Although patients with arrhythmias have increased perioperative risk, the risk is increased because the arrhythmias are usually markers of more serious heart disease or cause hemodynamic problems and not because of the arrhythmias themselves. Patients with tachyarrhythmias and bradyarrhythmias should generally be treated as in the nonoperative setting (Chapters 63 and 64), except for the special circumstance of anticoagulation in the perioperative setting (Chapter 35).

Pulmonary Risk Assessment

Postoperative pulmonary complications are as common as cardiac complications and are associated with significant morbidity and mortality. Major complications include respiratory failure (e.g., reintubation, prolonged mechanical ventilation), pneumonia, atelectasis requiring bronchoscopy, and to a lesser degree, bronchospasm or an exacerbation

Exclude patients with:

- ACC major clinical predictors (unstable coronary syndromes, decompensated CHF, significant arrhythmias, severe valvular disease)
- Contraindications to β-blockers (β-b)
- Coronary revascularization within 5 years and no recurrent symptoms
- Recent coronary evaluation (angiogram or stress test) with favorable results

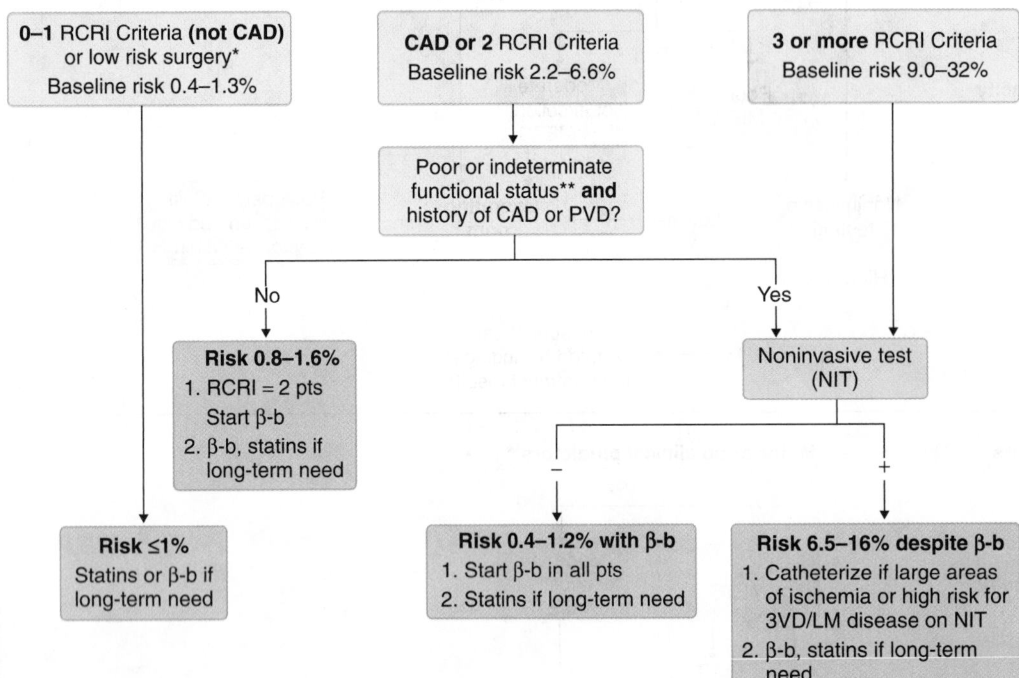

*Low risk surgery: superficial and minor operations on the skin, breast, or eyes, or endoscopic procedures.

**Poor functional status: inability to achieve 4 METS (equivalent to walking at least 2 blocks at 3–4 mph, walking up a hill, or climbing a flight of stairs) see Chapters 48 and 70.

FIGURE 457–2 • Algorithm for patient selection for cardioprotective agents and cardiac testing before elective major noncardiac surgery (part 2). ACC = American College of Cardiology; β-b = beta blocker; CAD = coronary artery disease; CHF = congestive heart failure; LM = left main coronary artery; METS = metabolic equivalents; PVD = peripheral vascular disease; RCRI = revised cardiac risk index (see Table 457–3); 3VD = three-vessel disease. (Modified from Auerbach A, Goldman L: Assessing and reducing the risk of noncardiac surgery. Circulation 2006;113:1361–1376.)

of COPD requiring treatment and prolonged length of stay. Many postoperative pulmonary complications are due to exaggerations of the usual postoperative changes in pulmonary function: decreased lung volumes, diaphragmatic dysfunction, ventilation-perfusion mismatches and shunting, hypoventilation, hypoxemia, and impaired defense mechanisms. Pulmonary risk factors can be divided into patient-related and procedure-related factors, the latter of which includes the type of surgery, anesthesia, and related factors.

Patient-Related Factors

COPD (Chapter 88) increases the risk for postoperative pulmonary complications approximately twofold, depending on its severity, whereas well-controlled *asthma* (Chapter 87) does not increase risk. Active cigarette smokers are at increased risk, mainly related to the number of pack years smoked; smoking cessation at least 8 weeks before surgery may reduce the risk, but stopping soon before surgery may increase the risk, possibly related to changes in cough and sputum production. *Obstructive sleep apnea* (Chapter 101), typically associated with obesity, confers an increased risk for hypercapnia and hypoxemia, and obese patients are at increased risk for atelectasis. Advanced age, poor functional status, an altered mental state, and suppressed immune status from chronic steroid use, alcohol use, or diabetes may also increase the risk for postoperative pulmonary complications.

Procedure-Related Factors

Pulmonary function decreases by approximately 50% after thoracic surgery, upper abdominal procedures, and abdominal aortic aneurysm repair and does not fully return to normal for several weeks. Lower abdominal surgery is associated with a 25% decrease in pulmonary function. Laparoscopic procedures are usually associated with lower rates of postoperative pulmonary complications and shorter hospital stays than open procedures are. Neuraxial anesthesia (epidural or spinal) may be associated with decreased risk when compared with general anesthesia, but the decision about which type of anesthesia to use is best left to the anesthesiologist. Emergency surgery, prolonged duration of anesthesia or surgery (>2 to 6 hours), and routine postoperative nasogastric tube use increase the risk for postoperative pulmonary complications.

Pulmonary Function Tests

In general, pulmonary function tests (Chapter 85) are no more predictive of pulmonary complications than clinical risk assessment alone is. Even a postoperative predicted forced expiratory volume in 1 second (FEV_1) of less than 800 mL for lung resection, which is thought to portend a very high risk for death or prolonged mechanical ventilation, is not an absolute contraindication to surgery (Chapter 102). Preoperative arterial blood gas evaluation is also of little benefit in predicting postoperative pulmonary complications.

Risk Reduction Strategies

Unfortunately, many of the risk factors for postoperative pulmonary complications cannot be modified. Inhaled bronchodilators (β-agonists and anticholinergics) and steroids can optimize the respiratory status of patients with COPD/asthma. Broad-spectrum antibiotics should be used to treat exacerbations caused by bacterial infection. Chest physiotherapy may be helpful. Smoking should be stopped at least 8 weeks before surgery, if possible.

Lung expansion maneuvers (either incentive spirometry or deep-breathing exercises) can significantly improve pulmonary function, minimize atelectasis, and reduce risk, especially for thoracic and upper abdominal surgery. Pain control (Chapter 28) improves pulmonary function by allowing deeper breathing. Epidural analgesia reduces postoperative pulmonary complications and, when possible, is preferable to parenteral narcotics.

Endocrine Conditions

Diabetes Mellitus

The major risks associated with surgery in diabetic patients are cardiac complications and wound infections. Complications are probably related more to associated diseases and end-organ involvement (coronary artery

TABLE 457–4 PROTOCOLS FOR PROPHYLACTIC PERIOPERATIVE β-BLOCKERS

GENERAL PRINCIPLES

Start β-blocker at least 1 week before surgery (if possible)
Titrate the dose to an ideal target heart rate of 55–65 beats per minute
Use half the dose if the heart rate is <65 beats per minute, if systolic blood pressure is <120 mm Hg, or in a small elderly or frail patient
Hold the dose if the heart rate is <55 beats per minute or systolic blood pressure is <100 mm Hg
Continue β-blocker postoperatively for at least 1–4 weeks (or indefinitely if independent criteria such as known coronary artery disease, peripheral arterial disease, or hypertension are present). Taper the dose if discontinuing

SPECIFIC DRUGS: ATENOLOL, BISOPROLOL, OR METOPROLOL

Preoperatively (recommended starting dose, then titrate to the target heart rate):
- Atenolol: start at 25 mg orally daily
- Bisoprolol: start at 5 mg orally daily at least 7 days before surgery
- Metoprolol: start at 25–50 mg orally twice daily up to 30 days preoperatively

Day of surgery—continue the usual dose or increase the oral dose to control the heart rate or give additional IV doses (atenolol or metoprolol, 5–10 mg) as needed if unable to take orally. Esmolol can also be used (500-μg/kg IV loading dose over a 1-min period; then infuse at 50–200 μg/kg/min and titrate to the target heart rate)

Postoperatively—continue the usual preoperative dose:
- Atenolol: 25–100 mg orally daily for at least 7 days
- Bisoprolol: 5–10 mg orally daily for at least 30 days
- Metoprolol: 25–100 mg orally twice daily for at least 14 days
- Substitute IV atenolol or metoprolol (5-mg doses) as needed if unable to take medication orally

disease, chronic kidney disease, and autonomic neuropathy) than to the glucose level itself. However, glucose levels higher than 300 mg/dL may impair wound healing and interfere with leukocyte defense mechanisms, and tighter control of the glucose level may improve outcomes in critically ill patients. [5]

Patients whose diabetes is controlled by diet require only perioperative glucose monitoring (finger sticks) with short-acting insulin coverage on an as-needed basis. Patients taking oral hypoglycemic agents (Chapter 248) should not take them on the morning of surgery (chlorpropamide should be stopped 2 to 3 days before and metformin preferably 1 day before) and should be monitored with sliding-scale insulin coverage as needed. Patients taking insulin are most often given half to two thirds of their usual intermediate-acting insulin on the morning of surgery and are then given short-acting insulin on a sliding scale based on finger stick monitoring (Chapter 247). Continuous intravenous insulin, which provides tighter glucose control but is associated with more episodes of hypoglycemia and requires a monitored setting, is typically used in patients undergoing cardiac surgery and in critically ill patients. There are no published guidelines regarding the management of patients taking long-acting basal insulin (glargine)—either it can be continued or the dose can be reduced on the morning of surgery. Regardless of the mode of treatment, frequent monitoring of the glucose level is critical.

Exogenous Corticosteroids and Adrenal Insufficiency

The stress of surgery activates the hypothalamic-pituitary-adrenal (HPA) axis, which in turn stimulates release of adrenocorticotropic hormone (ACTH) and subsequent secretion of cortisol (Chapter 245), but a patient who is taking exogenous corticosteroids may have suppression of the HPA axis and not be able to respond to this stress adequately. As a result, hypotension and shock may occur.

In general, a daily dose equivalent to 5 mg or less of prednisone (Chapter 245), alternate-day short-acting therapy, or corticosteroids given for less than 3 weeks do not cause clinically significant HPA suppression, so no supplemental therapy is indicated. Conversely, doses greater than 20 mg/day of prednisone for longer than 3 weeks usually suppress the HPA axis and warrant perioperative supplemental corticosteroids. In patients who are taking intermediate dosing regimens or who took large doses in the past year but are not taking corticosteroids or are taking lower doses now, the options are to perform an ACTH (cosyntropin) stimulation test, if time permits, and treat only patients with an inadequate response (Chapter 245) or to prescribe supplemental corticosteroids empirically.

When supplemental corticosteroids are appropriate, short-term therapy tailored to the level of expected stress can provide protection without adverse affects on wound healing and with only short-term problems with glucose intolerance and fluid retention. For minor procedures or local anesthesia, the recommended approach is to give the patient's usual dose before surgery without further supplementation. For moderate surgical stress (e.g., open cholecystectomy, lower extremity vascular surgery), a reasonable approach is 50 mg of hydrocortisone intravenously before surgery, followed by 25 mg every 8 hours for 1 to 2 days, and then the patient's usual dose. For major surgical stress, patients are typically given 100 mg of hydrocortisone intravenously before induction of anesthesia, followed by 50 mg every 8 hours for 2 to 3 days, and then their usual dose.

Thyroid Disease

An inadequately treated or undiagnosed hyperthyroid patient is potentially at risk for thyroid storm postoperatively. Elective surgery should be postponed in patients who are symptomatic or have resting tachycardia until they are euthyroid. Treatment of a thyrotoxic patient undergoing urgent or emergency surgery includes a combination of β-blockers, antithyroid agents, and iodine to control the resting heart rate to less than 90 beats per minute, as well as prophylactic corticosteroid supplementation, as used for thyroid storm (Chapter 244).

Conversely, patients with mild to moderate hypothyroidism tolerate surgery reasonably well. Patients with markedly symptomatic hypothyroidism should be treated with oral levothyroxine (T_4) for several weeks before elective surgery. For emergency surgery, intravenous liothyronine (T_3) or T_4 (200 to 300 μg intravenously, then 50 to 200 μg/day) and supplemental corticosteroids (hydrocortisone, 100 mg intravenously, then 25 to 50 mg every 6 hours; also correct fluid and electrolyte abnormalities) should be given. Myxedema coma is a rare complication of surgery.

Liver Disease

Routine preoperative testing of liver function is not recommended, but elective surgery should be avoided in patients with acute viral or alcoholic hepatitis. Patients with stable mild chronic hepatitis tolerate surgery well.

Patients with alcoholic liver disease or cirrhosis are at risk for postoperative complications, including bleeding, infection, poor wound healing, and delirium. The severity of disease as assessed by Turcotte-Pugh criteria and the MELD (Model for End-Stage Liver Disease) score (Chapter 158) can be used to estimate risk. Aggressive treatment of coagulopathy, ascites, and encephalopathy is indicated before surgery.

Hematologic Problems

Anemia increases the risk for postoperative complications only when it is severe, and operative patients generally tolerate hemoglobin levels as low as 7 g/dL. Preoperative transfusion should not be triggered solely by the hemoglobin level but should also consider the expected blood loss from the surgical procedure and the patient's comorbid conditions. For patients with cardiopulmonary disease, however, a goal of 10 g/dL is typically recommended.

Patients without a history of abnormal bleeding require no preoperative testing of coagulative function, but those with such a history should be evaluated. Ideally, the prothrombin time should be within 3 seconds of control (international normalized ratio <1.5), the partial thromboplastin time within 10 seconds of control, and the platelet count above a minimum of 50,000, depending on the type of surgery.

The approach to perioperative anticoagulation, both in terms of prevention of venous thromboembolism and for the management of a patient taking warfarin, aspirin, or other antithrombotic medications, is described elsewhere (Chapter 35).

Renal Disorders

Patients with chronic kidney disease typically have other comorbid diseases and may also have fluid and electrolyte abnormalities, anemia, and bleeding diatheses, which should be treated and optimized before surgery. Patients maintained on dialysis should ideally undergo dialysis the day before surgery to optimize their volume status, prevent hyperkalemia, and minimize acute shifts in acid-base balance.

Neurologic Problems

The risk for a postoperative stroke in unselected patients after general surgery is less than 0.5%, but patients with a history of stroke and those undergoing vascular surgery, especially carotid surgery, have higher risk. Patients with symptomatic carotid bruits require further investigation and possible intervention before elective surgery (Chapter 431). However, there is no evidence to support preoperative intervention in patients with asymptomatic bruits before noncardiac surgery. The general recommendation is to delay elective surgery for at least 2 to 4 weeks after a stroke.

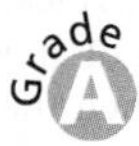

1. Devereaux PJ, Beattie WS, Choi PT, et al: How strong is the evidence for the use of perioperative beta blockers in non-cardiac surgery? Systematic review and meta-analysis of randomised controlled trials. BMJ 2005;331:313–321.
2. Wijeysundera DN, Naik JS, Beattie WS: Alpha-2 adrenergic agonists to prevent perioperative cardiovascular complications: A meta-analysis. Am J Med 2003;114:742–752.
3. McFalls EO, Ward HB, Moritz TE, et al: Coronary-artery revascularization before elective major vascular surgery. N Engl J Med 2004;351:2795–804.
4. Sandham JD, Hull RD, Brant RF, et al: A randomized, controlled trial of the use of pulmonary-artery catheters in high-risk surgical patients. N Engl J Med 2003;348:5–14.
5. van den Berghe G, Wouters P, Weekers F, et al: Intensive insulin therapy in the critically ill patients. N Engl J Med 2001;345: 1359–1367.

SUGGESTED READINGS

Auerbach AD, Goldman L: Assessing and reducing the cardiac risk of non-cardiac surgery. Circulation 2006;113:1361–1376. *An updated review.*

Cohn SL, Smetana GW, Weed HG (eds): Perioperative Medicine—Just the Facts. New York, McGraw Hill, 2006. *A concise text.*

Devereaux P, Goldman L, Yusuf S, et al: Surveillance and prevention of major perioperative ischemic cardiac events in patients undergoing noncardiac surgery: A review. CMAJ 2005;173:627–634.

Eagle KA, Berger PB, Clakins H, et al: ACC/AHA guideline update for perioperative cardiovascular evaluation for noncardiac surgery—executive summary: A report of the American College of Cardiology/American Heart Association Task Force on Practice Guidelines (Committee to Update the 1996 Guidelines on Perioperative Cardiovascular Evaluation for Noncardiac Surgery). Published simultaneously in J Am Coll Cardiol 2002;39:542–553 and Circulation 2002;105:1257–1267. Available at http://www.acc.org/clinical/guidelines/perio/index.html. *An extensive review with evidence and consensus-based recommendations.*

Smetana GW, Lawrence VA, Cornell JE; American College of Physicians: Preoperative pulmonary risk stratification for noncardiothoracic surgery: Systematic review for the American College of Physicians. Ann Intern Med 2006;144:581–595. *Systematic review of preoperative pulmonary risk factors.*

Section XXVII Consultation

458 OVERVIEW OF ANESTHESIA

Jeanine P. Wiener-Kronish

In the United States, more than 40 million procedures, including outpatient procedures, that require an anesthetic are performed annually. With modern techniques, anesthesia causes or contributes to mortality in about 1 per 200,000 healthy patients. Perioperative mortality is now more often related to the patient's underlying diseases (Chapter 457).

PREOPERATIVE ASSESSMENT

Important aspects of preoperative risk assessment include the type of surgery to be performed, the patient's underlying medical problems, and the particular demands for anesthesia (Chapter 457).

Airway Assessment

Assessment of the airway is always necessary even if regional anesthesia is planned because general anesthesia may be required if regional anesthesia cannot be accomplished. Patients with restrictive mouth openings cannot undergo routine laryngoscopy and cannot have specialized intubation devices inserted. Endotracheal intubation in patients with small mouth openings can be accomplished by placing the endotracheal tube using a fiberoptic bronchoscope through either the nose or mouth. If this approach is not successful, a surgical airway must be created. The prevalence of difficult intubation is about 6% for nonobese patients.

Malignant Hyperthermia

Malignant hyperthermia (MH) (Chapter 302) is characterized by acute hyperpyrexia developing during or immediately after general anesthesia. The channels that regulate the duration and amplitude of calcium efflux from the sarcoplasmic reticulum are the ryanodine receptors, which exist as three isoforms. Gain-of-function mutations affecting RyR1, the receptor expressed primarily in skeletal muscle, are present in 1 per 15,000 to 50,000 people and are associated with enhanced sensitivity to halothane and caffeine and with MH and central core disease. More than 80 distinct mutations have been detected, and mutation of the adult skeletal muscle sodium channel, SCN4A, may also cause the syndrome. Patients with mutations predisposing to MH function normally at resting conditions, but exposure to volatile anesthetics, including halothane, isoflurane, enflurane, desflurane, and sevoflurane, or exposure to a depolarizing muscle relaxant, succinylcholine, can precipitate life-threatening muscle contractures, increases in heart rate and body temperature, rhabdomyolysis, myoglobinuria, and metabolic acidosis. The mortality rate is 80% in untreated patients but about 5% with current treatment. Note that succinylcholine causes a release of myoglobin from muscle in small amounts even in normal patients.

Patients with MH do not predictably respond to triggering agents, and some patients with MH have had muted symptoms of MH after the administration of nontriggering agents. MH appears to occur now in muted forms, probably because of the decreased use of succinylcholine by anesthesiologists, the diagnostic awareness of MH by anesthesiologists, the routine use of carbon dioxide monitors so that increases in end-expiratory carbon dioxide are detected quickly, and the availability of dantrolene. If MH is suspected by obtaining a family history of adverse events with the administration of anesthesia or when a patient has a reaction suspicious for MH, a muscle biopsy is usually obtained for in vitro contracture testing, which tests the muscle contracture responses to caffeine or halothane. Genetic investigations are also recommended but MH cannot be excluded on the basis of genetic testing alone because of the diversity of mutations and genes that can be involved in this syndrome. The Malignant Hyperthermia Association of the United States (*www.mhaus.org*) is available for information to the public and all medical personnel can obtain information 24 hours every day on the MH hotline, 1-800-MHHYPER or 1-800-644-9737.

Dantrolene is the drug of choice to prevent and to reverse the symptoms of MH. Dantrolene decreases muscle sensitivity to caffeine, reduces the calcium release from the sarcoplasmic reticulum, and produces some muscle weakness. Dantrolene comes in 20-mg bottles and must be dissolved in sterile water; the recommended doses are 2 mg/kg every 5 minutes intravenously up to a total dose of 10 mg/kg, but doses of 29 mg/kg have been reported. Other treatments for MH include stopping volatile anesthetics, hyperventilating the patients and administering 100% oxygen, administering bicarbonate for severe acidosis, controlling fevers and maintaining temperature below 39° C (but not causing hypothermia) with iced fluids, surface cooling, and cooling of body cavities if necessary. Monitoring of temperature and vital signs, urinary outputs, muscle enzymes, glucose, coagulation studies, acid-base status, and gas exchange is recommended.

Two other diseases associated with mutations of RyR1 are central core disease and multiminicore disease, which are rare congenital myopathies. Patients with central core disease present with infantile hypotonia; a muscle biopsy is needed for definitive diagnosis. Multiminicore disease is a nonprogressive congenital myopathy with infants presenting with hypotonia, ophthalmoplegia, and arthrogryposis. These children develop scoliosis and eventually may require chronic ventilation. Avoidance of triggering agents is advised for these syndromes and for patients with other myopathies. Both MH and central core disease are thought to be inherited as autosomal dominant diseases, but extensive genetic analysis has revealed overlapping phenotypes.

Monamine Oxidase Inhibitors, Opioid Analgesics, and Serotonin Toxicity

Anesthesiologists routinely ask whether patients are taking monoamine oxidase inhibitors (MAOIs) because of the routine use of analgesics in perioperative patients and the problems with drug interactions these drugs cause (see later). Also, serotonin toxicity has features similar to those of MH and must be distinguished from it. Serotonin toxicity, characterized as a triad of neuromuscular hyperactivity (tremor, clonus, myoclonus, hyperreflexia, and pyramidal rigidity), autonomic hyperactivity (diaphoresis, fever, tachycardia, and tachypnea), and altered mental status (agitation, excitement, and confusion), can be precipitated by the administration of MAOIs and serotonin re-uptake inhibitors. Rigidity, decreasing arterial carbon dioxide levels, and a temperature of more than 38.5° C are associated with life-threatening toxicity. Ecstasy, 3,4-methylenedioxymethamphetamine, combined with MAOIs, including moclobemide, can lead to fatalities because they act as serotonin releasers. Tramadol, used for pain relief, and venlafaxine, an antidepressant, act as serotonin releasers and have been involved in the development of toxicity with the concurrent administration of MAOIs.

ANAPHYLAXIS IN THE PERIOPERATIVE PERIOD

The incidence of life-threatening hypersensitivity reactions during anesthesia is 1:4000 to 1:25,000. Anaphylaxis is caused by immunoglobulin E (IgE)-mediated reactions (Chapter 274), whereas anaphylactoid reactions produce the same clinical picture but are not IgE mediated. Anaphylaxis during anesthesia can arise as cardiovascular collapse, airway obstruction, flushing, or edema of the skin. Neuromuscular blocking agents, such as succinylcholine, and opioid analgesics can cause nonimmunologic release of histamine from mast cells and produce a similar clinical syndrome Antibiotics, protamine, and blood transfusions, all given routinely during operations (Chapter 183), can also elicit a variety of systemic reactions. About 75% of perioperative hypersensitivity reactions appear to be due to muscle relaxants, especially rocuronium and vecuronium, with a mortality of 3 to 6%. Skin tests (prick tests) for all the substances to which the patient was exposed are usually done, and IgE levels in the patients' blood are assessed to determine whether the patient had an allergic reaction that was IgE mediated.

Latex Allergies

For sensitized patients (Chapter 274), exposure to even low amounts of latex-containing particles is sufficient for induction of severe anaphylactic reactions. A latex-free operating environment, in which no latex gloves or latex accessories are used, is key for patients with known allergy. Skin prick tests with latex extracts should be considered in patients at high risk for latex allergy.

Nausea and Vomiting

Postoperative nausea and vomiting are more likely with volatile anesthetics but are also common when perioperative opioids are administered. Prophylactic ondansetron, dexamethasone, and droperidol each independently reduce postoperative nausea and vomiting by about 26%, [1] with the main predictor for efficacy being the patient's risk for postoperative nausea and vomiting. Note that droperidol has received a "black box" warning from the Food and Drug Administration and is no longer used often in the United States. Total intravenous anesthesia with propofol reduces postoperative nausea and vomiting only about one fifth, often because narcotics are still administered. The use of spinal or epidural anesthesia, or both, may decrease the incidence of nausea and vomiting.

Conscious Sedation versus General Anesthesia

General anesthesia can be achieved with a balanced drug regimen that induces a loss of consciousness, which can range from deep sedation requiring airway support to states requiring full ventilatory support because of weakness and loss of respiratory drive. In contrast, conscious sedation denotes a state in which patients can still control their airway, do not require ventilatory support, but are sleepy, have less pain, and are amnestic. The same drugs are often used for general anesthesia and conscious sedation; achievement of the two different conditions in the appropriate patients requires knowledge of the pharmacokinetics of the drugs (Table 458–1).

Propofol

Propofol, an alkyl phenol, is perhaps the most frequently used intravenous anesthetic. It is lipid soluble and quickly cleared from the central compartment so that it is rapidly eliminated even after long periods of continuous infusion. However, the clearance of propofol is changed by gender (men have lower clearance rates than women), size (children require higher doses), and age (elderly patients have decreased clearance rates and experience increased effects with the drug). Propofol also appears to inhibit the enzymatic degradation of narcotics. Because of its predilection for causing apnea, propofol is a dangerous drug for conscious sedation. Propofol also decreases arterial blood pressure, causes pain with injection, and can precipitate myoclonus. Large quantities of propofol can cause the propofol infusion syndrome, which is associated with cardiomyopathy, metabolic acidosis, skeletal myopathy, hyperkalemia, hepatomegaly, and lipemia. Despite these problems, propofol is frequently used because the recovery from propofol is within minutes, even after it is given as a prolonged continuous infusion, in contrast to the longer duration of drug effects seen after the administration of other intravenous sedatives.

Midazolam

Midazolam, a benzodiazepine that produces muscle relaxation through a central mechanism, is hypnotic, sedative, anxiolytic, amnesic, and anticonvulsant. Its amnesic and anticonvulsant effects are mediated through α_1 and $GABA_A$ receptors, and the anxiolytic and muscle relaxation effects are mediated through α_2 and $GABA_A$ receptors. Only 20% receptor occupancy is needed to produce anxiolysis, whereas unconsciousness requires 60%. Long-term administration of benzodiazepines produces tolerance, which appears to decrease receptor binding and function. Benzodiazepines cause dose-related respiratory system depression, with a peak

TABLE 458–1 COMMON ANESTHETIC APPROACHES FOR VARIOUS TYPES OF SURGERY

SURGERY ON INTRA-ABDOMINAL OR INTRATHORACIC ORGANS

Examples include cardiac surgery, lung resections, gastric bypass.

General anesthesia usually administered because mechanical ventilation is often required. Drugs include premedication for anxiety with midazolam, general anesthesia with volatile anesthetics (desflurane, sevoflurane, nitrous oxide), neuromuscular blockade, and opioid analgesics.

Epidural anesthesia and analgesia are also utilized. Drugs include ropivacaine or lidocaine with fentanyl.

SURGERY ON LIMBS

Examples include hip replacement, knee replacement, foot or arm surgeries.

Can perform with epidural or spinal anesthesia, depending on limb. Examples of medications are tetracaine, lidocaine, ropivacaine, and fentanyl or morphine.

Can perform axillary or scalene block. Examples of drugs are lidocaine and ropivacaine.

For postoperative pain control, can perform regional blocks that leave catheter in place, including femoral nerve block, axillary nerve blocks.

CATARACT SURGERY, LOCAL ANESTHESIA ON EYE WITH OR WITHOUT SEDATION

Examples of drugs used for sedation are midazolam and fentanyl.

effect at 3 minutes and significant depression persisting for 60 to 120 minutes. The rate of administration of the drug affects the onset of depression: the faster the drug is given, the quicker the respiratory depression. Benzodiazepines and opioids appear to produce additive respiratory depression, including apnea. Unlike propofol, benzodiazepines used alone decrease blood pressure only modestly. Other drugs, particularly drugs that affect the cytochrome P-450 3A4 enzyme (including azole antifungals, human immunodeficiency virus [HIV] protease inhibitors, and calcium-channel inhibitors), affect the clearance of midazolam and prolong its half-life significantly; there are several reports of prolonged amnesia in HIV patients who received midazolam for conscious sedation. Midazolam also has an active metabolite and is often associated with delirium in elderly persons (Chapter 26), perhaps because it impairs both implicit and relational memory.

Opioids

Opioids (Chapter 32) are classified as naturally occurring (morphine, codeine), semisynthetic (heroin), and synthetic (methadone, fentanyl, remifentanil). There are four opiate receptors—mu, kappa, delta, and nociceptin receptors—which are G protein–coupled receptors. Chronic exposure to agonists leads to cellular adaptation mechanisms that are probably involved in tolerance, dependence, and withdrawal. Clinically, mu agonists (morphine, fentanyl, and meperidine) are utilized almost exclusively for analgesia to relieve pain. However, these agents have other important effects, including respiratory depression, decreased gastric emptying, nausea, vomiting, sedation, constipation, pruritus, and dependence and tolerance, when given repeatedly. When opioids are given with propofol or benzodiazepines, or both, there is a synergistic depressive effect on respiration, hence the rational for monitoring patients who receive medications for conscious sedation.

Ketamine

Ketamine is unique among the intravenous agents because it has analgesic properties and decreases tolerance to opiates. Ketamine produces dose-related analgesia, which may be profound even when patients can keep their eyes open, breathe spontaneously, and protect their own airway with conserved swallowing and cough reflex. Side effects include increased lacrimation, salivation, and increased muscle tone. Ketamine increases cerebral blood flow, can increase seizure activity, and can produce undesirable psychological reactions; these side effects are dose related and may be minimized by concomitant use of benzodiazepines. Ketamine is also a bronchial smooth muscle relaxant and can prevent experimentally induced bronchospasm. Ketamine is usually associated with an increase in blood pressure, heart rate, and cardiac output. These features make ketamine a useful drug for sedating patients with hemodynamic instability or with difficult airways.

Volatile Anesthetics

Volatile (inhalational) anesthetics include desflurane, sevoflurane, isoflurane, halothane, and nitrous oxide. Inhaled anesthetics are absorbed through the respiratory epithelium and mucous membranes of the respiratory tract, and they are excreted mainly by exhalation. Access to the circulation is almost instantaneous owing to the large pulmonary surface area. The pharmacologic effects of inhaled anesthetics depend primarily on alveolar ventilation, the ventilation/perfusion ratio, coadministered gases, gas flow, and the physicochemical properties of the anesthetic gas rather than on the quantity of drug administered, the extent and rate of absorption, protein binding, excretion, secretion, or metabolism.

Severe hepatotoxicity, which led to the discontinuation of the use of chloroform, carbon tetrachloride, and trichloroethylene anesthetics, is seen as fatal hepatic necrosis with halothane in 1 in 10,000 anesthetics. This problem appears to occur much less frequently with isoflurane and desflurane exposures. Mild halothane hepatotoxicity is self-limited and can occur with a single exposure, whereas fulminant halothane hepatitis occurs only after multiple exposures to the drug, has a high mortality rate (50%), and is associated with antibodies to halothane-altered antigens.

Nitrous oxide, which is the only nonhalogenated agent still used, is not metabolized in human tissues. It irreversibly oxidizes the cobalt atom of vitamin B_{12}, thereby inhibiting the activity of the cobalamin-dependent enzyme methionine synthase. Individuals with vitamin B_{12} deficiency or with mutations of methionine synthase may be at risk for neurologic injury from nitrous oxide, and it should not be used in patients at risk. Exposure to high concentrations of over 10^3 ppm may be associated with an increased incidence of abortions and decreased fertility, and its use should be avoided in patients and personnel at risk. General anesthesia can be achieved only by giving combinations of drugs along with nitrous oxide to achieve the desired effects.

Neuromuscular Blockers

Neuromuscular blockers are used to paralyze muscles to facilitate endotracheal intubation and mechanical ventilation, to decrease shivering during induced hypothermia, or to improve conditions for optimal surgery. Succinylcholine causes prolonged depolarization of the neuromuscular junction, resulting in failure to generate an action potential. Within 9 to 13 minutes after 1 mg/kg of succinylcholine, 90% of muscle strength is restored. The rapid onset and rapid return of muscle function make succinylcholine a useful drug for difficult intubations. Side effects of succinylcholine include hyperkalemia, myalgia, masseter spasm, sinus bradycardia and nodal rhythms, and increased intraocular pressure.

Most of the other neuromuscular drugs utilized by anesthesiologists are nondepolarizing in that they compete with acetylcholine for the neuromuscular junction and can be reversed by increasing the quantity of acetylcholine. Clinically, a drug is often chosen for its duration of action: shorter acting agents include rapacuronium and mivacurium; intermediate agents, acting for 20 to 50 minutes, include vecuronium, rocuronium, atracurium, and cisatracurium.

These drugs were utilized routinely in critically ill ventilated patients until it was discovered that their chronic administration was associated with prolonged paralysis, particularly in patients given concomitant steroids. There are other notable interactions with nondepolarizing agents: antibiotics can increase neuromuscular blockade; magnesium sulfate potentiates neuromuscular blockade; lithium can potentiate neuromuscular blockade with succinylcholine and with pipecuronium; and antiepileptic drugs cause resistance to nondepolarizing muscle blockade so that larger doses must be administered for paralysis, and patients receiving anticonvulsants have accelerated recovery from neuromuscular blockade.

General versus Regional Anesthesia

The decision regarding the type of anesthesia to be administered often depends on the requirements of the surgery. For example, laparoscopic surgery requires general anesthesia because the insufflation of gases impairs the ability to breathe adequately. General anesthesia is also required for surgeries on the airway or thorax because mechanical ventilation is usually needed to sustain adequate respiration. Procedures that do not allow any movement (e.g., precise procedures in the brain) often require general anesthesia and paralysis.

Side effects of general anesthesia depend on the drugs utilized to achieve anesthesia, whether neuromuscular blockade is administered, and whether mechanical ventilation is utilized. Complications of endotracheal intubation include local pain, trauma to the airway, swelling, vocal cord paralysis, increased bronchospasm, and death related to improper placement. Volatile anesthetics are associated with postoperative atelectasis (Chapter 90); regional anesthesia helps preserve respiratory dynamics. Postoperative cognitive dysfunction (Chapter 26) does not seem to depend on the type of anesthesia administered.

Neuraxial (Spinal and Epidural) Anesthesia and Analgesia

Spinal anesthesia and epidural anesthesia were first thought of as an alternative to general anesthesia. Spinal anesthesia is the instillation of local anesthetics into the cerebrospinal fluid (CSF). Epidural anesthesia is the instillation of larger volumes of local anesthetics into the epidural space, or the potential space that exists just before the CSF. Data suggest that neuraxial anesthesia may be preferred over general anesthesia when either approach is feasible. 2 Because spinal anesthesia is associated with an increased incidence of headache in younger patients, epidural anesthesia is often used. The drugs used in spinal and epidural anesthesia are basically the same, but the doses are different, as less medication is required when it is instilled into the CSF. Complications of epidural and spinal anesthesia and analgesia include failed blocks, post–dural puncture headaches, and toxicity from the local anesthetics (see Regional Anesthesia). Epidural hematoma remains a rare event, occurring in fewer than 1 in 150,000 operations even in the presence of potent antithrombotic agents. Other more rare complications of epidural and spinal anesthetics include intracranial subdural hematoma, transverse myelitis, hypotension, and cardiac arrest.

With postoperative epidural analgesia, either local anesthetic or local anesthetic and narcotics are instilled into the epidural space for postoperative pain control. In randomized trials in high-risk patients, this approach provides superior pain relief, slightly decreased length of stay in the intensive care unit, and a slight decrease in the requirement for mechanical ventilation. [3, 4]

Regional Anesthesia

Regional anesthesia includes the deposition of local anesthetics near nerves, including local anesthetics in the epidural space and in the CSF. The local anesthetics bind to the nerves, permeate the nerve's axon, and reside in the axoplasm. The binding of the local anesthetic to the sodium channels prevents opening of the channels. The rates of onset and recovery from nerve blockade are controlled by the diffusion of the local anesthetic into and out of the whole nerve.

Examples of regional anesthesia include the deposition of local anesthetics near the brachial plexus to anesthetize the arms (axillary or intrascalene blocks), deposition near the femoral or sciatic nerves to anesthetize the legs, deposition near ulnar or radial nerves for lower arm blocks, and deposition near the pudendal nerves or caudal space for groin procedures. Dentists use this technique frequently when they inject local anesthetic near various nerves in the oral cavity. Surgeries that can be performed with regional anesthesia include carotid surgery and the placement of fistulas for dialysis.

The dangers of regional anesthesia include the injection of local anesthetic into the systemic circulation or a failed block, which requires the administration of either conscious sedation or general anesthesia. Systemic toxicity is manifested as convulsions and respiratory depression. Tinnitus, visual and auditory disturbances, and dizziness are signs of milder central nervous toxicity. Cardiac toxicity can be manifested by decreases in heart rate, prolonged conduction times, and negative inotropic effects. Bupivacaine toxicity is associated with ventricular fibrillation. Despite its appeal in appropriate patients, regional anesthesia is not obviously better than general anesthesia for cesarean section. [5]

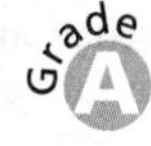

1. Apfel CC, Korttila K, Abdalla M, et al: A factorial trial of six interventions for the prevention of postoperative nausea and vomiting. N Engl J Med 2004;350:2441–2451.
2. Rigg JR, Jamrozik K, Myles PS, et al: Epidural anaesthesia and analgesia and outcome of major surgery: A randomised trial. Lancet 2002;359:1276–1282.
3. Park WY, JS Thompson, Lee KK: Effect of epidural anesthesia and analgesia on perioperative outcome: A randomized, controlled Veterans Affairs cooperative study. Ann Surg 2001;234:560–569.
4. Ballantyne JC, Kupelnick B, McPeek B, et al: Does the evidence support the use of spinal and epidural anesthesia for surgery? J Clin Anesth 2005;17:382–391.
5. Afolabi BB, Lesi FE, Merah NA: Regional versus general anaesthesia for caesarean section. Cochrane Database Syst Rev 2006;4: CD004350.

SUGGESTED READINGS

Campagna JA, Miller KW, Forman SA: Mechanisms of actions of inhaled anesthetics. N Engl J Med 2003;348:2110–2124. *A review of the mechanisms of the commonly used volatile anesthetics.*

Chassot PG, Bettex DA: Anesthesia and adult congenital heart disease. J Cardiothorac Vasc Anesth 2006;20:414–437. *Overview with specific recommendations.*

Gillman PK: Monoamine oxidase inhibitors, opioid analgesics and serotonin toxicity. Br J Anaesth 2005;95:434–441. *Opioids that are associated with a toxidrome that has some of the features of malignant hyperthermia.*

Litman RS, Rosenberg H: Malignant hyperthermia: Update on susceptibility testing. JAMA 2005;293:2918–2924. *A comprehensive review.*

Reich DL, Hossain S, Krol M, et al: Predictors of hypotension after induction of general anesthesia. Anesth Analg 2005;101:622–628. *A useful clinical review.*

Shiga T, Wajima Z, Inoue T, et al: Predicting difficult intubation in apparently normal patients: A meta-analysis of bedside screening test performance. Anesthesiology 2005;103:429–437. *Tests proposed to help practitioners identify difficult intubation have poor to moderate sensitivity.*

459 POSTOPERATIVE CARE AND COMPLICATIONS

Donald Redelmeier

POSTOPERATIVE CARE

Team Psychology

The medical consultant in the postoperative setting must have both a knowledge of medicine and an appreciation of team psychology (Chapter 456). In contrast to other settings, the internist is not the team leader, often does not maintain an ongoing relationship with the patient, and does not have the authority of the most responsible physician. Moreover, patients may be dispersed across diverse surgical services, each with their own orientation and culture. The challenges of coordination and communication are enormous, particularly given the multiple other health care professionals involved in complex surgical cases. Considerable tact is often needed to avoid antagonizing the surgeon, disrupting the team dynamics, or inducing a cascade of cumbersome inopportune testing.

Focusing on Recovery

Facilitating the patient's recovery from surgery differs somewhat from managing patients with acute exacerbations of chronic disease. In the postoperative setting, many therapies need to be discontinued at some point because the patient has recovered; for example, discontinuing a urinary catheter because the patient can now void spontaneously or discontinuing a major tranquilizer because the patient is now orientated and coherent. Discontinuing many other interventions requires substantial judgment, such as the decision when to discontinue intravenous access, supplemental oxygen, and intermittent laxatives. Much depends on experience and on reconsidering individual patients on a regular basis.

Reading Anesthesia Records

A careful but focused review of the anesthesia record for details about the surgery is essential because the consultant is rarely present during the operation. Perhaps the most basic information to identify is the date of surgery because the elapsed time helps in interpreting the patient's current state of recovery. Moreover, sometimes the date is not immediately evident if more than one surgery has been performed, a planned operation was cancelled, or misquotations arise over time. Data about the duration of surgery, type of anesthesia (e.g., regional, spinal, or general [Chapter 458]), and major intraoperative events help establish reasonable expectations about the future course, as well as the possibility of specific complications (e.g., epidural hematoma after spinal anesthesia). Sharing some of the basic data with the patient is often helpful because a surprising number either benefit from repetition or are not otherwise informed.

Patterns of Mistakes

Medical errors (Chapter 11) that arise in postoperative care often seem mundane in retrospect yet are lethal if undetected. Some patterns of mistakes have the feature of "double trouble," such as when a patient has both a potassium level of 2.0 and a prothrombin time of 2.0 but care focuses only on one of these abnormalities. Other mistakes arise because a single problem develops at an awkward moment, such as a patient in whom acute dyspnea develops when another patient is having a seizure. Still other mistakes relate to the fallibility of human memory and attention, such as when a normal blood sugar value in the morning leads clinicians to assume that the level is still normal in the afternoon. These errors can result in substantial harm, failures of clinicians to learn from past mistakes, and unprofessional reactions related to embarrassment. None of these patterns are unique to postoperative care, yet the fast and unfamiliar terrain of surgical settings can make even simple mistakes difficult to avoid.

Checking Orders

The first method to reduce errors after surgery is to check the postoperative orders already written for the patient. Such double checking is a tedious task, and clinicians often direct insufficient attention to this review in the mistaken belief that most of the work is already done. Ironically, checking orders written by another clinician sometimes requires more than customary attention because of the challenges of following someone else's legibility, sequencing, and preferences. The set of orders may need to be read twice: once for errors of commission (e.g., a calcium-channel blocker ordered at the wrong dose) and once for errors of omission (e.g., a β-blocker inadvertently not reordered after surgery). A classic mistake on postoperative orders is failure to follow-through on interventions initiated immediately before surgery (e.g., endocarditis prophylaxis). A particularly vexing issue is the need for repeated rechecking on subsequent days (e.g., new orders for sedative drugs).

Recommended Prophylaxis

Some complications are sufficiently frequent and serious that routine prophylaxis is merited in the postoperative setting. For example, antibiotics are indicated for patients at high risk for endocarditis (Chapter 76). Systemic anticoagulation with heparin is indicated for patients at high risk for postoperative deep vein thrombosis (Chapters 35 and 81). β-Blockers appear to be protective for patients at high risk for cardiac ischemia (Chapter 457). Gastric acid suppression (Chapter 142) is justified for patients at high risk for postoperative gastric bleeding. Parenteral antibiotics are indicated for patients undergoing prosthetic joint replacement. The optimal method to gauge whether a patient is at high risk for each complication is contentious and thereby leads to variation in practice patterns across different settings.

Future Prevention

A postoperative consultant who maintains communication, facilitates the patient's recovery, and avoids postoperative mistakes also has the chance to initiate unrelated medical interventions for general medical care. Such opportunities for prevention might include influenza vaccination, colon cancer screening, or cholesterol reduction. The main advantage of such comprehensive care is that it conforms to the ideal of providing all services possible to the individual. The main disadvantage of such comprehensive care is the potential for creating unintended chaos, confusion, or misquotation (Chapter 456). Such unintended consequences distract the surgical team from the primary goal and also carry some risk of complications from the comprehensive care at a time when the patient is trying to recover from surgery. Many effective postoperative consultants will defer such opportunities for prevention to the physicians who assume long-term responsibility for the patient's care.

COMPLICATIONS

Symptoms and Signs

Chest Pain

Chest pain is a common problem after surgery and has an extensive differential diagnosis (Chapter 48). In the postoperative setting, the immediate consideration is an acute ischemic myocardial event. The diagnosis of postoperative myocardial infarction (MI) differs somewhat from community-acquired MI (Table 459–1). Interpretation of a patient's symptoms, examination, and electrocardiogram is often problematic because of changes related to surgery and anesthesia. Instead, diagnosis is heavily dependent on specific biomarkers, such as an elevated troponin level, especially since a large proportion of postoperative MIs are painless. Management priorities include supplemental oxygen, heart rate control, and correction of hemoglobin. Thrombolysis is often contraindicated, but percutaneous coronary intervention may be considered. In the absence of data from randomized trials for acute MI in this setting, other beneficial therapies such as aspirin and angiotensin-converting enzyme inhibitors should be used on a case-by-case basis (Chapter 72).

TABLE 459–1 CRITERIA FOR DIAGNOSING POSTOPERATIVE MYOCARDIAL INFARCTION

The diagnosis of perioperative MI requires any one of the following criteria:

Criterion 1: A typical rise in the troponin level or a typical fall in an elevated troponin level detected at its peak after surgery in a patient without a documented alternative explanation for an elevated troponin level (e.g., pulmonary embolism) or a rapid rise and fall in CK-MB only if troponin measurement is unavailable.* This criterion requires that one of the following criteria be met:

- Ischemic signs or symptoms (e.g., chest, arm, or jaw discomfort; shortness of breath; pulmonary edema)
- Development of pathologic Q waves on an ECG
- ECG changes indicative of ischemia
- Coronary artery intervention
- New or presumed new cardiac wall motion abnormality on echocardiography or new or presumed new fixed defect on radionuclide imaging

Criterion 2: Pathologic findings of acute or healing MI

Criterion 3: Development of new pathologic Q waves on an ECG if troponin levels were not obtained or were obtained at times that could have missed the clinical event

*Because CK-MB is both less sensitive and less specific than troponin levels in the perioperative setting than in other settings, it should be used for diagnostic purposes only when troponin levels are not obtainable.

CK-MB = creatine kinase MB isoenzyme; ECG = electrocardiogram; MI = myocardial infarction.

Reproduced with permission from Devereaux PJ, Goldman L, Yusuf S, et al: Surveillance and prevention of major perioperative ischemic cardiac events in patients undergoing noncardiac surgery: A review. CMAJ 2005;173:779–788.

Dyspnea

Shortness of breath (Chapter 83) after surgery has an extensive differential diagnosis (Table 459–2). The three key considerations are fluid overload/heart failure (Chapter 57), pulmonary embolism (Chapter 99), and air space disease (a continuum encompassing atelectasis [Chapter 90], bronchitis [Chapter 96], aspiration [Chapter 94], mucous plugging, and pneumonia). Distinguishing among these three considerations requires focusing on the speed of onset, the timing relative to surgery, vital signs, oxymetry, and the physical examination (Chapter 83). Fluid overload is most commonly seen soon after the cessation of positive pressure ventilation or vasodilating neuraxial anesthesia or analgesia. It is also common 3 to 5 days postoperatively when fluid that has been "third spaced" is mobilized into the intravascular compartment. Interventions that are safe in most situations include oxygen and withholding sedation. The use of continuous positive airway pressure can reduce the rate of reintubation in hypoxemic postoperative patients. [1] Other interventions that will be helpful or harmful, depending on the specific situation, include diuretics, elaborate medical imaging, and physiotherapy.

Anorexia

Loss of appetite after surgery has an extensive differential diagnosis (Chapter 134) that can be narrowed substantially if the patient was eating properly before surgery. The immediate priority is to search for and correct underlying contributors. Oral, enteral, or parenteral support is not the priority initially, although such support may become necessary. Drug toxicity is a particularly common, easily detected when considered, and rapidly reversible contributor to postoperative anorexia. Anatomic abnormalities are usually evident by medical imaging studies. Other common metabolic contributors include abnormalities in electrolytes, calcium, phosphorus, and magnesium. Acalculous cholecystitis (Chapter 159) is an important postoperative complication that must be considered in a patient with right upper quadrant tenderness. Multiple antinausea medications are available for symptomatic relief (e.g., ondansetron, dexamethasone, droperidol) and act in an additive manner when used in combination. [2]

Vomiting

Vomiting is the extreme form of nausea in the postoperative setting, and the two symptoms share the same differential diagnosis. In most patients, vomiting is rare and unexpected and merits immediate care. Initial management is to ensure that the patient's airway is protected, discontinue oral medications (and find parenteral substitutes if necessary), and consider inserting a nasogastric tube. In patients after gastrointestinal surgery, the priorities are an anastomotic leak, peritoneal abscess, or

TABLE 459–2 DISTINGUISHING AMONG COMMON CAUSES OF ACUTE POSTOPERATIVE DYSPNEA

	Pulmonary Air Space	Fluid Overload/Heart Failure	Pulmonary Thromboembolism
CHARACTERISTICS OF TIMING			
Days since surgery	1–7 days	0–5 days	5–28 days
Speed of onset	1–3 days	1–24 hours	1–5 minutes
PREVIOUS HISTORY			
Previous lung disease	++		
Previous heart failure		++	
Previous venous thrombosis			++
ABNORMAL VITAL SIGNS			
Temperature			
Heart rate	+	+	+
Blood pressure	+	+	++
Respiratory rate	+	++	+
Oxymetry	++	+	+
PHYSICAL EXAMINATION			
Jugular venous distention		+	+
Pulmonary rales	+	++	
S_3 gallop		++	
RESPONSE TO TREATMENT			
Oxygen	+	+	+
Anticholinergic bronchodilators	+	+	+
Withdrawal of sedatives	+	+	+
Aggressive physiotherapy	++		
Diuretics/afterload reduction		++	

other anatomic abnormality. In patients after operations on more remote parts of the body, the priorities are emetogenic medications (such as postoperative chemotherapy), gastroparesis associated with an autonomic neuropathy, and fecal impaction. If no reversible contributor is identified, the default diagnosis is prolonged idiopathic ileus, and a therapeutic trial of intravenous neostigmine can be considered.

Diarrhea

Diarrhea (Chapter 143) is relatively rare after surgery and involves a limited number of possibilities if the patient's bowel movements were normal before surgery. In such cases the situation represents an acute-onset diarrhea that is usually secretory in nature. The immediate priority is to exclude toxic megacolon, which is caused by overgrowth of toxigenic *Clostridium difficile* and is a potential emergency. Clinical evaluation for toxic megacolon requires assessment for tachycardia, hypotension, delirium, and other signs of sepsis rather than waiting on initial stool studies for *C. difficile*. Risk factors for antibiotic-associated diarrhea include advanced age, use of broad-spectrum antibiotics (e.g., third-generation cephalosporins), and unknown host susceptibility factors (e.g., past episodes of pseudomembranous colitis). Oftentimes a definitive diagnosis is never established and treatment focuses on feeding the patient a lactose-free diet while avoiding intestinal paralytics. Complete resolution is typical, provided that adequate fluid and electrolyte levels are maintained.

Weakness

Weakness after surgery is almost inevitable, but focal weakness may reflect nerve damage caused by intraoperative positioning (e.g., fascial nerve damage after carotid endarterectomy) and rarely indicates a spontaneous new intracranial event (e.g., intracerebral bleeding [Chapter 432] secondary to anticoagulation). Such deficits are often overlooked during the initial postoperative interval and may become apparent only after the patient has regained strength elsewhere in the body. Conversely, new deficits that are evident early after surgery and resolve rapidly thereafter may reflect an old stroke that is fully compensated during less stressful circumstances. Medical imaging of the brain is worthwhile if no explanation is apparent on initial assessment. Nonfocal weakness commonly responds to physical therapy.

Delirium

Mental status changes after surgery are common, especially in elderly patients (Chapter 26), and can be remarkably difficult to diagnose and correct. The immediate priority is to determine whether the impairment is acute or chronic and to detect easily reversible contributors (such as infection, hypoglycemia, alkalosis). A complete assessment is often unnecessary if the patient had normal mental status before surgery because many dementia syndromes are thereby excluded (such as vitamin B_{12} deficiency, tertiary syphilis, Alzheimer's disease). Immediate treatment usually focuses on discontinuing medications, especially anticholinergics, narcotics, and tranquilizers. The patient may also benefit from the continuous presence of friends and family members, who can provide frequent orientation and constant attention. A sense of patience is necessary because delirium rarely resolves instantly. The benefit of low-dose neuroleptics (e.g., risperidone, 0.5 mg twice daily) remains uncertain.

Seizures

The development of uncontrolled seizures (Chapter 426) after surgery is rare. The immediate priority is to exclude status epilepticus, uncover any past history of a chronic seizure disorder, and identify provocative factors. Neurosurgical patients typically undergo a standardized treatment protocol, including steroids and imaging. Other conditions that can cause abnormal movement, such as septic rigors, delirium tremens, Parkinson's disease, major psychopathology, hypothermic shivering, and hypercapnic asterixis, must be excluded. Additional considerations include detecting and correcting any underlying metabolic abnormalities such as hypocalcemia, hypoxemia, hyponatremia, hypophosphatemia, and drug toxicity. Treatment primarily focuses on reversing the underlying precipitating cause and providing nonspecific care with benzodiazepines, phenytoin, and ongoing monitoring.

Hypertension

Hypertension may reflect a variety of disorders and must be treated in a manner that neither overreacts nor underreacts to the situation. Hypertension is particularly common after neurosurgical procedures or carotid endarterectomy. The initial assessment focuses on whether the patient has chronic hypertension based on the past history, current electrocardiogram, or findings on funduscopy. Special attention should also be directed toward excluding undertreated pain, agitated delirium, fluid overload, alcohol withdrawal, and inadvertent discontinuation of chronic antihypertensive medications. In uncertain cases, systemic analgesia is often helpful, along with nitrates (e.g., nitroglycerin, 0.4 mg/hr transdermally) and β-blockers (e.g., metoprolol, 5 mg intravenously). The major complication of treatment is the potential for overcorrection and inadvertent hypotension—such errors are particularly common in patients with no evidence of past hypertension.

Hypotension

Hypotension (Chapter 7) after surgery is generally an emergency, and the immediate concern is often internal bleeding, especially after intra-abdominal operations or when anticoagulation is used to prevent venous thrombosis. The initial stages of hypotension are frequently unrecognized because of biologic stress responses by patients, psychological denial by clinicians, and misattribution to the concurrent use of analgesia. Early hypotension is particularly easy to miss if the patient has coexisting chronic hypertension and the apparently "normal" blood pressure is dismissed as unremarkable. Treatment usually entails volume supplementation, serial assessment, vasopressors as needed (Chapters 108 and 109), and a search for underlying causes, especially possible sepsis. Sometimes an extensive differential diagnosis needs to be considered if no anatomic cause related to surgery is evident (Chapter 107). Routine use of pulmonary artery catheters for diagnosis or to guide therapy is not helpful. 3

Tachycardia

Tachycardia after surgery can be caused by a myriad of arrhythmias (Chapters 63 and 64) and may contribute to postoperative cardiac ischemia. Distinguishing between newly identified and newly incident tachycardia can sometimes be accomplished by determining whether the patient does or does not complain of palpitations. The initial assessment almost always requires review of the electrocardiogram to distinguish atrial fibrillation from other disorders. The goal of treatment is to identify and correct precipitating factors such as pain, blood loss, hypoxia, electrolyte abnormalities, fluid overload, hypotension, pulmonary embolism, and drug withdrawal. Most arrhythmias respond to correction of the underlying abnormality. Specific antiarrhythmic treatment, when needed, is generally similar to that used in the nonoperative setting (Chapters 63 and 64). For atrial fibrillation, anticoagulation is sometimes contraindicated; in such situations, cardioversion within 48 hours merits consideration.

Fever

Fever (Chapter 302) after surgery is common, frequently perplexing, and often multifactorial. Worrisome possibilities include transfusion reactions (Chapter 183), hospital-acquired pneumonia (Chapter 97), urinary tract infection (Chapter 306), line sepsis (Chapter 304), and wound infection. In many cases no definitive cause is found, the patient recovers spontaneously, and the default diagnosis is atelectasis. Detailed evaluation, when necessary, requires culture of blood, urine, and the wound to identify specific microbiologic organisms. Selection of empirical antibiotics is usually based on local practice patterns and hospital ecology, with the main disadvantage being the breeding of resistant organisms. Hydration, nutrition, and general supportive care are important, yet frequently neglected needs of patients with prolonged elevations in body temperature.

Edema

Peripheral edema (Chapter 48), which is often first noticed by nursing staff after surgery, is rarely life-threatening unless treated with excessive diuretics. The cause is often multifactorial and includes both increased hydrostatic pressure (including heart failure and gravity from intraoperative positioning), decreased oncotic pressure (related to hypoalbuminemia from decreased liver production or increased losses), and capillary leak (potentially caused by medications or tissue reactions). Treatment focuses on correcting any underlying abnormalities, maintaining nutrition, judicious use of diuretics, monitoring renal function, providing systemic anticoagulation against deep vein thrombosis, and efforts toward mobilizing the patient. Selected use of echocardiography, a low-salt diet, afterload reduction, and spironolactone may be helpful in patients in whom heart failure (Chapter 58) is the dominant mechanism.

Laboratory Test Results

Leukocytosis

An elevated white cell count (Chapter 173) can have many causes, but the immediate priority is to exclude a life-threatening septic process (Chapters 107 and 109). Direct microscopic examination of the peripheral blood smear (Chapter 161) can be helpful to check for toxic granulations (see Fig. 161–29), Döhle's bodies (Fig. 161–30), and a shift toward primitive band cells (Fig. 161–24). Many cases are caused by noninfectious causes, including infarcted tissue (brain, heart, intestinal tract), inflammatory conditions (renal insufficiency, diabetic ketoacidosis, lupus erythematosus), or demargination stress reactions (dehydration, systemic corticosteroids, ionotropes). In the absence of direct evidence, some clinicians may initiate empirical antibiotics, whereas others may elect waiting. Substantial controversy remains about the proper duration of empirical antibiotics when no cause is discovered and the patient is otherwise recovering.

Anemia

Anemia (Chapter 162) is common and sometimes underappreciated because coexisting volume depletion causes the blood hemoglobin concentration to underestimate the degree of blood loss. The initial priority is to differentiate bleeding at the surgical site from other causes. In many cases the exact cause is unclear and substantial uncertainty may arise over the need to initiate gastric acid suppression therapy or sacrifice systemic anticoagulation originally directed against venous thrombosis. Guidelines for transfusion therapy depend on the patient's cardiac reserve, as well as the available blood bank supply at the particular medical center. A reasonable goal is to maintain a hemoglobin level of 7 mg/dL or higher, except in patients with cardiovascular disease, in whom a hemoglobin goal of 10 mg/dL is reasonable. The immediate postoperative interval is not usually the appropriate time to initiate erythropoietin, oral iron replacement, or detailed evaluations for other hematologic abnormalities.

Platelet Count Abnormalities

Patients often have abnormal platelet counts after surgery yet rarely require further evaluation or treatment. In most cases the thrombocytopenia is mild, does not require transfusion therapy, resolves in a few weeks, and is not a sign of an ominous disorder (e.g., sepsis or heparin-induced thrombocytopenia). Platelet transfusions are indicated if the decrease in platelet count is extreme, accompanied by evidence of major blood loss, or related to recent surgery on the central nervous system (including the eye). Thrombocytosis is also common about a month after surgery and is sometimes extreme. However, even postoperative thrombocytosis exceeding 1,000,000/mL rarely necessitates treatment, does not predispose patients to unwanted clotting disorders, and typically resolves spontaneously after a few weeks.

Abnormal Sodium

Both hyponatremia and hypernatremia (Chapter 117) are frequent complications in the postoperative setting. The immediate priority is to assess the patient's intravascular volume status and correct possible volume depletion. Hyponatremia is often multifactorial, including excessive use of diuretics, excess intrinsic antidiuretic hormone (as a result of factors such as drugs, pain, or mechanical ventilation), and unmeasured osmoles (e.g., intravenous contrast agents). Hypernatremia is always due to free water deficiency, which may indicate severe cognitive impairment or other factors interfering with the ability to express thirst or ingest water. Correction is similar to that in the nonoperative setting. Abnormalities in sodium concentration require careful follow-up, can develop or recur at any point after an operation, yet are rarely the root cause of a patient's inability to recover from surgery.

Abnormal Serum Potassium

Hyperkalemia and hypokalemia (Chapter 117) are also frequent postoperative complications. The immediate priority is to assess and stabilize the patient's electrocardiogram. Hyperkalemia is usually due to cellular shifts, renal failure, and tissue destruction (including hemolysis). Hyperkalemia will generally correct with treatments that shift potassium into cells (e.g., intravenous glucose with or without insulin or β-agonists) and enhance excretion (e.g., gastrointestinal binding agents). Hypokalemia is usually due to inadequate intake, excessive loss, or cellular shifts. Hypokalemia will generally correct with replacement therapy and rarely requires aldosterone antagonism. Both abnormalities can usually be treated as in the nonoperative setting (Chapter 117). The prognosis is favorable if the patient's electrocardiogram shows no major abnormalities and renal function is preserved.

Alkalosis

Systemic alkalosis (Chapter 119) typically requires volume supplementation because the cause is generally intravascular volume depletion. Blood gas determinations may be necessary in some cases to exclude the possibility of concurrent carbon dioxide retention with compensatory metabolic alkalosis. Untreated, alkalosis can result in altered mentation, cardiac arrhythmias, and delayed mobilization. Most patients with postoperative alkalosis do not require carbonic anhydrase inhibitors or intravenous acid. The prognosis is usually favorable, with gradual correction over a period of several days. Rapid correction of alkalosis, unlike rapid correction of hyponatremia, is not known to cause neurologic injury.

Azotemia

The initial assessment of an elevated serum creatinine concentration (Chapter 115) focuses on reviewing previous values (to distinguish acute from chronic renal insufficiency) and identifying contributing factors (such as prerenal volume depletion, intrarenal nephrotoxins, or postrenal urethral obstruction). A trial of intravenous fluids may be useful on both a diagnostic and therapeutic basis. Treatment is the same as in the nonoperative setting. Subsequent monitoring is always necessary, with serum creatinine measurements obtained on a daily basis. Serial measurements of urinary volume and body weight and urine cultures are occasionally helpful in selected cases. Prognosis is dependent on the underlying factors and is less favorable after cardiac surgery.

Hyperbilirubinemia

Elevations in serum bilirubin (Chapter 150) are rare after surgery, even though abnormalities in liver enzymes are frequent with general anesthesia. The most benign explanation is Gilbert's syndrome, but the immediate priority is to assess for possible hepatic failure (especially in patients who have received halothane). As in the nonoperative setting, treatment involves withdrawing potential hepatoxins, supporting the patient, and allowing time for liver function to recover (Chapter 158). Treatment of hepatic encephalopathy is particularly important because of the constipation and generalized catabolic state that follow major surgery. Monitoring should include serial measurement of liver function on a daily basis because each component (e.g., bilirubin, albumen, prothrombin time) can be altered in postoperative patients by factors unrelated to the liver. The prognosis is unfavorable if the patient's liver function fails to recover quickly.

Blood Glucose Abnormalities

In patients with diabetes mellitus (Chapter 247), serum blood sugar concentrations often become erratic after surgery because of altered dietary intake, decreased physical activity, and release of counter-regulatory hormones. The priorities are to avoid hypoglycemia, severe hyperglycemia, diabetic ketoacidosis, cerebral damage, and repeated events. Rapid reversal of sepsis or focal infection can lead to a precipitous decrease in insulin requirements; in such cases, vigilance is required because unsuspected hypoglycemia may cause permanent damage or be fatal in a patient who may seem to be sleeping. Recent studies have suggested but not uniformly confirmed benefits of maintaining blood sugar tightly within the normal range in critically ill patients. Patients need to be forewarned that temporary doses of subcutaneous insulin may be required but do not commit the patient to chronic insulin therapy. Monitoring involves serial measurement of blood sugar until the patient is eating in a reliable manner.

Special Situations

Some postoperative complications are difficult to classify because no single dominant problem is apparent by symptoms, signs, or laboratory testing. Instead, the patient has two or more problems that need to be addressed simultaneously. The immediate goal is to set priorities and avoid the temptation to try to eliminate every possibility on the first day. The corollary is to continue to check progress over the many days that may be required for complete diagnosis and successful therapy. Because so many concerns require attention in the postoperative interval, the risk is that clinicians will lose track of a nonemergency issue and make an error that seems obvious in retrospect.

Postoperative complications sometimes generate multiple consultations with physicians who have overlapping abilities. An example might be a patient with a postoperative fever that prompts consultations from pulmonology, nephrology, dermatology, general medicine, and infectious diseases. In theory, gathering a critical mass of medical experts together should increase the likelihood of accurate diagnosis, timely treatment, and foolproof follow-up. In reality, however, the coordination and communication are never perfect. Personal rivalries, diffusion of responsibility, and many other psychological factors may impede interactions among consultants. Opportunities for miscommunication may be further accentuated if the patient has an exotic diagnosis that is a special draw on the consultant's attention (e.g., pheochromocytoma). Arguing in front of the patient, in view of other professionals, or in the medical record can be demoralizing. The priority is to communicate effectively with the surgical team responsible for the patient and encourage that team to make the final decision.

Another vexation occurs when an urgent request is not connected to a clear rationale (Chapter 456). Diplomacy is needed to establish whether the motivation reflects medicolegal concerns rather than a biologic change in the patient. Sometimes the stimulus that drives the consultation can best be addressed by providing reassurance and confirmation. Sometimes the stimulus is an obscure preexisting disorder (e.g., moyamoya disease), and the surgical team has neither the experience nor the time to investigate how this unrelated medical condition can influence recovery from surgery. Sometimes the stimulus is an unspoken political wish to transfer the care of a burdensome patient from one physician to another. A consultant should develop an understanding of how to interact with other clinicians under such ambiguous circumstances.

In many postoperative cases the original reason for consultation may resolve and no major issues may remain. The situation now provides an opportunity to review the patient, particularly for the appropriate use of unrelated medications. The consultant may often detect excessive medications that were appropriate early in the hospital course and that have ceased to be necessary, thereby justifying discontinuation (e.g., diuretics, antibiotics, bronchodilators). Discontinuing medications that have become superfluous requires initiative and wisdom, and the common mistake is to propagate unnecessary medications in stable patients under the rationale of "don't mess with success." The ability to watch the patient for several hours or for a day or two often presents an ideal opportunity for the safe withdrawal of medications. Ironically, discontinuing a treatment sometimes requires more skill, time, and initiative than starting it.

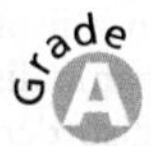

1. Squadrone V, Coha M, Cerutti E, et al: Continuous positive airway pressure for treatment of postoperative hypoxemia: A randomized controlled trial. JAMA 2005;293:589–595.
2. Apfel CC, Korttila K, Abdalla M, et al: A factorial trial of six interventions for the prevention of postoperative nausea and vomiting. N Engl J Med 2004;350:2441–2451.
3. Sandham JD, Jull RD, Brant RF, et al: A randomized, controlled trial of the use of pulmonary-artery catheters in high-risk surgical patients. N Engl J Med 2003;348:5–14.

SUGGESTED READINGS

Bergmann MA, Murphy KM, Kiely DK, et al: A model for management of delirious postacute care patients. J Am Geriatr Soc 2005;53:1817–1825. *Description of a multifactorial pragmatic model for the management of postoperative delirium.*

Devereaux PJ, Goldman L, Cook DJ, et al: Perioperative cardiac events in patients undergoing noncardiac surgery: A review of the magnitude of the problem, the pathophysiology of the events and methods to estimate and communicate risk. CMAJ 2005;173:627–634. *Review of the pathophysiology and epidemiology of postoperative cardiac events.*

Duggan M, Kavanagh BP: Pulmonary atelectasis: A pathogenic perioperative entity. Anesthesiology 2005;102:838–854. *Extensive summary on prevention, detection, and treatment of postoperative atelectasis.*

Selim M: Perioperative stroke. N Engl J Med 2007;356:706–713. *A clinical review.*

Van den Berghe G, Wilmer A, Hermans G, et al: Intensive insulin therapy in the medical ICU. N Engl J Med 2006;354:449–461. *Did not confirm benefits seen in a prior randomized trial of surgical ICU patients.*

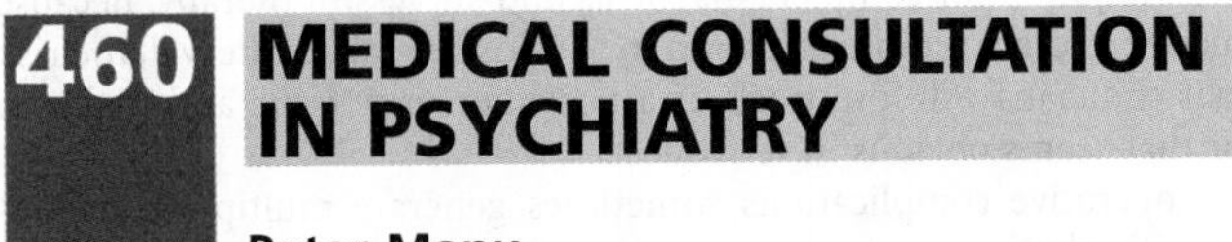

460 MEDICAL CONSULTATION IN PSYCHIATRY

Peter Manu

HEALTH STATUS IN PSYCHIATRIC PATIENTS

The physical health of psychiatric patients is poor, with a higher risk for death at an early age than in the mentally sane. The magnitude of the problem is greatest in patients with schizophrenia, who have a 50% increased risk for death and 20% shorter lifespan. Poverty, social neglect, substandard medical care, unhealthy life habits, and complications of psychiatric treatments are major contributors to this increased morbidity and mortality. The problem is actually worsening even in First-World countries; in Stockholm County, Sweden, the standardized mortality ratio (observed/expected deaths) of 9.4 in males and 3.6 in females with schizophrenia in 1991 to 1995 was two-fold higher than in the previous decade.

MEDICAL EVALUATION IN PSYCHIATRIC SETTINGS

Requirements for medical training in psychiatry vary. In the United States, psychiatric residents have up to 4 months of inpatient medical training. Data suggest that psychiatrists have limited skills in assessing nonpsychiatric problems in terms of history taking, a reluctance to perform physical examinations, and a tendency toward premature diagnostic closure. As a result, the need for medical consultation is enormous. In one study, 1001 consecutively admitted psychiatric patients generated 2120 initial consultations (Table 460–1) and 1800 follow-up visits. The highest rate of medical utilization was for patients with dementia, schizophrenia, substance abuse disorders, and mental retardation. About 10% of patients seen by a medical consultant required transfer to a medical or surgical unit. Medical consultation in psychiatry is not more difficult than in other clinical settings but must be informed by knowledge about the serious complications of psychiatric treatments (Table 460–2). This chapter provides details about some of the most important entities specific to the psychiatric setting.

EVALUATION OF CHIEF COMPLAINTS

Medical consultation for psychiatric patients creates unique challenges in evaluation of the chief complaint. Many patients with outpatient psychiatric disorders have somatic symptoms such as fatigue, weakness, dizziness, headache, insomnia, widespread pain, and constipation. In most of these patients, the underlying mental illnesses are mood disorders (unipolar depression and dysthymia), anxiety disorders (panic disorder and generalized anxiety disorder), somatoform disorders, substance use disorders (most often alcohol, opiates, cocaine, and benzodiazepine), and borderline personality disorder. As a group, these patients have many physical complaints and resist a psychological explanation for their symptoms even when the medical evaluation fails to identify objective abnormalities.

In contrast, patients admitted for inpatient psychiatric treatment often have psychotic disorders, developmental abnormalities, or dementia with behavioral disturbance; they are frequently vague or silent about physical suffering and only rarely voice somatic delusions. Such patients even may deny pain after bowel perforation or myocardial infarction.

A rigorous diagnostic evaluation is therefore required to avoid the errors of omission created by the weak correlation between complaints and pathology. This evaluation should include consideration of physical disorders, drug effects (adverse reaction, toxicity, or withdrawal), cognitive impairment (delirium), sensory impairment (loss of vision, hearing, speech, or postural balance), and situational maladjustment (isolation, overload, or loss of privacy). Attribution of symptoms to the patient's psychiatric condition should remain a diagnosis of exclusion.

TABLE 460–1 REASONS FOR INPATIENT MEDICAL CONSULTATION FOR 1001 CONSECUTIVE PSYCHIATRIC PATIENTS

SYMPTOMS	
Fall	6.4%
Rash	5.6%
Constipation	5.2%
Cough	5.1%
Abdominal pain	5.1%
Pain in the extremities	5.1%
Chest pain	5%
Nausea or vomiting	4.9%
Diarrhea	3.8%
Eye redness	3.7%
Sore throat	3.4%
Back pain	3.1%
PHYSICAL FINDINGS	
Hypertension	6.3%
Edema	5.8%
Hypotension	3.5%
Fever	3.4%
LABORATORY ABNORMALITIES	
Hyperglycemia	8.6%
Anemia	7.5%
Abnormal urinalysis	6.3%
Abnormal electrocardiogram	6.3%
Azotemia	4.6%
Abnormal potassium level	4.6%
Abnormal leukocyte count	3.3%
Abnormal thyroid function	3.1%
Hyponatremia	3.1%
RISK ASSESSMENT	
Medical clearance for electroconvulsive therapy	3.7%

MEDICAL COMPLICATIONS OF PSYCHIATRIC TREATMENTS

Antipsychotic-Induced Metabolic Syndrome

Metabolic syndrome is more prevalent (range, 29 to 63%) in schizophrenic and other psychiatric patients treated with atypical antipsychotic drugs such as clozapine, olanzapine, risperidone, and quetiapine than in the general population. Clozapine and olanzapine are the worst offenders because they induce substantial weight gain, thereby leading to insulin resistance (with or without fasting hyperglycemia) and atherogenic dyslipidemia. This gain in weight may be related to affinity for the histamine H_1-receptor and to neurobiologic mechanisms that regulate appetite and metabolism via the production and activity of serotonin, leptin, and tumor necrosis factor-α. Within 18 months, 30% of patients treated with olanzapine will increase their body weight by more than 7%, with an average increase of 43 mg/dL in triglycerides, 15 mg/dL in blood glucose, and 0.41% in glycosylated hemoglobin. Not surprisingly, these changes result in about a two-fold increased risk for diabetes and coronary heart disease events. Nonetheless, controlled trials have identified olanzapine and clozapine as the most effective drugs for patients with schizophrenia and other psychotic disorders, and the beneficial therapeutic response sometimes correlates with the amount of weight gained during treat-

TABLE 460–2 MAJOR MEDICAL COMPLICATIONS OF PSYCHOTROPIC DRUGS

CARDIOVASCULAR	
Cardiomyopathy	Clozapine
Hypertension	MAO inhibitors, venlafaxine
Myocarditis	Clozapine
Orthostatic hypotension	Tricyclics, trazodone, antipsychotics
QTc prolongation	Antipsychotics, tricyclics
Venous thromboembolism	Clozapine, risperidone, phenothiazines
RESPIRATORY	
Choking	Antipsychotics, tricyclics
Laryngospasm	Antipsychotics
Respiratory depression	Benzodiazepines, barbiturates, methadone, antidepressants, atypical antipsychotics
GASTROINTESTINAL	
Bowel obstruction	Tricyclics, antipsychotics
Dysphagia	Tricyclics, antipsychotics
Hepatic impairment	Carbamazepine, valproic acid, phenothiazines, mirtazapine, nefazodone, quetiapine, olanzapine, clozapine, MAO inhibitors, naltrexone
Pancreatitis	Carbamazepine, valproic acid, clozapine, olanzapine
KIDNEY AND URINARY TRACT	
Renal insufficiency	Lithium, clozapine
Urinary retention	Antipsychotics, tricyclics
ENDOCRINE	
Hyperprolactinemia	First-generation antipsychotics, risperidone
Hypothyroidism	Lithium, quetiapine
Inappropriate ADH secretion	Serotonin re-uptake inhibitors, methadone, tricyclics
Metabolic syndrome	Clozapine, olanzapine, risperidone, quetiapine
HEMATOLOGIC	
Leukocytosis	Lithium
Neutropenia	Clozapine, olanzapine, risperidone, carbamazepine, valproate, mirtazapine
Thrombocytopenia	Carbamazepine, valproate
MUSCULOSKELETAL	
Rhabdomyolysis*	Antipsychotics, serotonin re-uptake inhibitors, MAO inhibitors
SKIN	
Stevens-Johnson syndrome	Lamotrigine, carbamazepine, barbiturates
OTHER	
Fever*	Antipsychotics, serotonin re-uptake inhibitors, MAO inhibitors
Seizure	Bupropion, MAO inhibitors, tricyclics, phenothiazines

*Includes neuroleptic malignant syndrome and serotonin syndrome.
ADH = antidiuretic hormone; MAO = monoamine oxidase.

ment. 3-Hydroxy-3-methylglutaryl coenzyme A (HMG-CoA) reductase inhibitors (statins) must be used aggressively to achieve individualized low-density lipoprotein cholesterol targets (Chapter 217). Blood pressure control should be obtained with judicious use of diuretics, angiotensin-converting enzyme inhibitors, angiotension receptor blockers, or calcium-channel blockers (Chapter 66). β-Adrenergic blockers are problematic in patients with comorbid depressive disorders, and α-adrenergic blockers should be used cautiously in patients receiving neuroleptics because they increase the potential for orthostatic hypotension, syncope, and falls. The glucose intolerance often seen in patients treated with antipsychotic agents is due to insulin resistance and is best treated by weight reduction (Chapter 239), metformin, thiazolidinediones (pioglitazone or rosiglitazone; Chapter 239), or any combination of these measures. Smoking cessation programs combining transdermal or transmucosal nicotine replacement, bupropion, and cognitive-behavioral therapy should be strongly recommended despite the dismally high failure rates that have been reported in patients with chronic schizophrenia (Chapter 30).

Antipsychotic-Induced Myocarditis and Cardiomyopathy

Antipsychotic-induced myocarditis and cardiomyopathy (Chapter 59) are most common in patients treated with clozapine (0.9%) and fluphenazine (0.4%). In contrast, the risk for these complications is only 0.1% in patients receiving haloperidol, thioridazine, and risperidone.

The accepted pathophysiologic explanation for myocarditis is that of an IgE-mediated acute hypersensitivity reaction, similar to the allergic myocarditis produced by penicillins, sulfonamides, and methyldopa. In a small number of patients, a competing hypothesis proposes that clozapine induces hypereosinophilic myocarditis, colitis, hepatitis, pancreatitis, alveolitis, and interstitial nephritis. A direct cardiotoxic effect of drug metabolites cannot be excluded.

In patients in whom myocarditis develops, the mortality rate is as high as 50%, with almost half the deaths occurring suddenly and unexpectedly. The average duration of exposure to clozapine before diagnosis or death is 21 days, and the dosage range is 50 to 725 mg/day. Common symptoms are fever (48%), dyspnea (35%), "flulike illness" (30%), chest pain (22%), and fatigue (17%). Laboratory features include left ventricular hypokinesia or reduced ejection fraction (48%) or pericardial effusion (17%) on echocardiography, nonspecific repolarization abnormalities on electrocardiography (35%), peripheral eosinophilia (35%), elevated creatine kinase and troponin levels (22%), and radiographic evidence of heart failure (13%). The diagnosis can be confirmed by endomyocardial biopsy showing fraying of myocytes and perivascular infiltrates with degranulated eosinophils. Among survivors, symptoms resolve or substantially improve after discontinuation of clozapine and treatment with high-dose corticosteroids (e.g., prednisone, 1 mg/kg/day for 4 days, tapered to 0.33 mg/kg/day for the following 4 days).

Clozapine-induced dilated cardiomyopathy may be caused by an evolving myocarditis or by chronic injury mediated by free radicals, similar to the myocarditis produced by doxorubicin (Chapter 59). The demographic features are similar to those of myocarditis, but the mean duration of treatment before diagnosis is much longer (9 months vs. 3 weeks) and the mortality rate is lower (22 vs. 51%). Patients have clinical or echocardiographic evidence of left ventricular dysfunction without eosinophilia or enzymatic evidence of myocardial necrosis.

Prolonged QTc Interval and Sudden Death

Significant prolongation of the QTc interval (Chapter 64) leading to ventricular tachyarrhythmias and sudden cardiac death (Chapter 62) can occur after antipsychotic treatment with the usual doses of thioridazine, haloperidol, and sertindole. Abnormal myocardial repolarization has been observed during treatment with most antipsychotic medications and after intentional or accidental overdoses of tricyclic antidepressants, lithium, and methadone (Chapter 111). All antipsychotics affect the cardiac potassium channel by blocking the rapidly activating component of the rectifier potassium current (Chapter 60). This effect translates into a dose-dependent increase in the duration of phase 3 of the action potential. The drug concentration that produces 50% inhibition of rapid potassium outflow varies for each drug (e.g., 1 nmol/L for haloperidol and 6 nmol/L for olanzapine). For first-generation antipsychotics, the mean changes in QTc from baseline to the recommended steady-state drug dose range from 36 msec for thioridazine to 6 msec for quetiapine, 5 msec for haloperidol, and 0.2 msec for risperidone. In one study, QTc prolongation (to greater than 450 msec in males or 470 msec in females) was observed in 3% of patients treated with risperidone and quetiapine, 1% of patients receiving ziprasidone, but none of those treated with olanzapine. [1] All patients about to start antipsychotic drugs should be asked about a personal history of syncope and a family history of long QT syndrome or sudden death at a young age. A baseline electrocardiogram and serum electrolytes should be obtained before starting antipsychotic drug therapy, tricyclic antidepressants, and methadone. Interval electrocardiograms should be obtained after each increase in medication in older patients, patients with known heart disease, and those starting other drugs known to produce QTc prolongation or hypokalemia (Chapter 64) A QTc interval of 500 msec or greater requires the discontinuation of all drugs that affect membrane repolarization. QTc intervals greater than 450 msec in males and 470 msec in females, QTc dispersion (difference between the longest and shortest QTc on a 12-lead electrocardiogram) greater than 100 msec, and an increase in QTc duration of more than 60 msec in comparison to the baseline measurement should prompt a re-evaluation of the risks and benefits associated with the drugs in question.

Choking and Laryngeal Dystonia

Asphyxia deaths from choking occur at a rate of 0.8% per 1000 psychiatric patients each year, a frequency that is more than 100 times greater than in the general population. In addition, videofluoroscopy demonstrates silent aspiration in 38% of psychiatric patients who survive a choking incident. Choking and silent aspiration are manifestations of dysphagia (Chapter 140), which is common in the mentally ill. Half the psychiatric patients with dysphagia have a fast-eating syndrome seen in association with restlessness, poor chewing skills, food pocketing in the cheeks, and attention deficits that characterize psychotic disorders and mental retardation. Bradykinetic dysphagia, which is seen in 25% of psychiatric patients with choking episodes, is due to the antidopaminergic and anticholinergic effects of psychotropic medications. This condition, which features reduced lingual range of motion, increased oral transit time, decreased pharyngeal peristalsis, and delayed initiation of the swallowing reflex, is seen in patients with neurologic features of drug-induced parkinsonism (Chapter 433). Dyskinetic dysphagia (7% of choking cases), which generally occurs in patients maintained on long-term antipsychotic medication, is part of the clinical spectrum of tardive dyskinesia (Chapter 434). The examination reveals involuntary contractions of the tongue and perioral musculature, clumsiness of voluntary movements of the tongue, and discontinuous bolus propulsion in the oral stage. In the remaining patients, the dysphagia is due to cerebrovascular disease (11%) or to pharyngeal or esophageal pathology (7%).

Laryngeal dystonia, which is a life-threatening complication of antipsychotic drug therapy, primarily with haloperidol and phenothiazines, is produced by acute spasmodic contraction of the adductor laryngeal muscles. Symptoms include respiratory distress, dysphonia, and stridor. Neuroleptic-induced bronchospasm may precede the onset of stridor. Patients typically indicate extreme subjective distress by clutching their anterior cervical area. The majority of patients also have other dystonias involving the head and neck, including torticollis, retrocollis, trismus, tongue protrusion, and deviation of the eyes up, down, or sideward. In general, the symptoms and signs develop in the first week after starting or rapidly increasing the dose of neuroleptic medications. Similar dystonic phenomena have been described after treatment with the antiemetics promethazine, prochlorperazine, and metoclopramide. A reduction in the dose of anticholinergic or antiparkinsonian medication used to prevent or treat extrapyramidal symptoms can also precipitate laryngeal dystonia. The condition is more common in young males and must be distinguished from epiglottitis, allergic/anaphylactic laryngeal edema or laryngospasm, mechanical obstruction, and psychogenic stridor. Intravenous administration of diphenhydramine (initial dose, 25 mg; may repeat after 5 minutes if symptoms persist) is the treatment of choice, and endotracheal intubation is seldom required.

Drug-Induced Neutropenia and Agranulocytosis

Drug-induced neutropenia with absolute neutrophil counts of less than 1500/mL has been observed during treatment with most second-generation antipsychotics (clozapine, olanzapine, risperidone, and quetiapine) and mood stabilizers (carbamazepine, valproic acid, and lamotrigine), as well as some antidepressant drugs (tricyclic antidepressants and mirtazapine). Clozapine-induced neutropenia occurs in 4 to 5% of patients within 6 months after starting treatment and progresses to agranulocytosis in 10% or more of neutropenic patients if the drug is continued. In vitro, clozapine toxicity requires peroxide and peroxidase, and the defect in oxidation is related to abnormalities in the *NQO2* (quinone oxidoreductase) gene involved in drug detoxification. The cytotoxic effect can be blocked in vitro by exogenous glutathione, *N*-acetylcysteine, and ascorbic acid, but the therapeutic effect of these agents has not yet been studied. Treatment with clozapine should be started only if the baseline absolute neutrophil count is greater than 1500/μL. The concomitant use of carbamazepine, angiotensin-converting enzyme inhibitors, sulfonamides, and propylthiouracil should be avoided. Clozapine should be stopped and the patient evaluated immediately for fever, oral ulcerations, and symptoms or signs of infection. Complete blood counts should be obtained once a week for the first 26 weeks and every other week thereafter, and clozapine should be stopped and all medications reassessed if the absolute neutrophil count drops below 1500/μL. Clozapine-related agranulocytosis has been treated successfully with colony-stimulating factors (either granulocyte or granulocyte-macrophage colony-stimulating factor).

Neutropenia has also been associated with olanzapine, risperidone, and quetiapine in patients who have never received clozapine. Treatment with anticonvulsant mood stabilizers, particularly carbamazepine, is associated with a dose-dependent neutropenia and thrombocytopenia in approximately 10% of patients in the first 6 months of treatment and should be monitored with complete blood counts twice each month during this period.

Neuroleptic Malignant Syndrome

Neuroleptic malignant syndrome, which occurs in approximately 0.2% of patients receiving neuroleptics, must be part of the differential diagnosis of fever and rhabdomyolysis (Chapter 114) in a psychiatric patient (Table 460–3). The frequency is greater in young males and patients who are malnourished or dehydrated, have Parkinson's disease, or are treated parenterally with large doses of neuroleptics over short periods. The main diagnostic criteria are elevated temperature (higher than 104° F in 40% of patients) and diffuse muscle rigidity (ranging from mild hypertonicity to severe "lead pipe" stiffness). In addition, two or more of the following are required for a definitive diagnosis: (1) autonomic instability (tachycardia, elevated or labile blood pressure, postural hypotension, diaphoresis, sialorrhea, and urinary incontinence), (2) changes in mental status (ranging from confusion to mutism or coma), (3) leukocytosis (up to 20,000/mL), and (4) elevated creatine kinase (up to 100,000 IU/L). Other clinical manifestations include bradykinesia, chorea, dystonias, dysphagia, dysarthria or aphonia, seizures, and tremor. The severity of

TABLE 460–3 DIFFERENTIAL DIAGNOSIS OF NEUROLEPTIC MALIGNANT SYNDROME

Infection of the central nervous system
Infection in patients with drug-induced parkinsonism
Drug overdose (psychostimulants, antidepressants, lithium, anticholinergics)
Alcohol or drug withdrawal (benzodiazepines, barbiturates, antiparkinsonians)
Side effects of nonpsychotropic dopamine-depleting drugs (reserpine, metoclopramide, prochlorperazine, promethazine)
Cholinergic rebound
Serotonin syndrome
Thyrotoxicosis
Malignant hyperthermia

rhabdomyolysis correlates with the creatine kinase level and with the presence of myoglobinemia, myoglobinuria, metabolic acidosis, and azotemia. The electroencephalogram shows nonspecific slowing in slightly more than half of patients.

The time lag from starting the drug to the onset of neuroleptic malignant syndrome is generally short, with 30% of cases developing within 48 hours and 96% within the first month of treatment. The exception appears to be clozapine-associated neuroleptic malignant syndrome, which has an average time lag of 50 days. Neuroleptic syndrome is sometimes confused with severe catatonia (Chapter 420), but the catatonic signs in neuroleptic malignant syndrome are usually restricted to mutism and akinesia. Furthermore, hyperthermia, rigidity, tremor, and rhabdomyolysis are not present in patients with catatonia. Nonetheless, close medical follow-up of severely catatonic patients is warranted because they are at very high risk (22%) for neuroleptic malignant syndrome.

Untreated, neuroleptic malignant syndrome has a mortality of 10% as a result of acute renal failure, aspiration pneumonia, adult respiratory distress syndrome, disseminated intravascular coagulation, and cerebellar neuronal degeneration. Most fatalities are avoidable if the diagnosis is made early, the neuroleptic agent is discontinued rapidly, and the patient is immediately transferred to an intensive care setting for supportive and specific therapy. Bromocriptine (2.5 mg three times daily orally or through a nasogastric tube; may increase by 2.5 mg three times daily to a maximum daily dose of 40 mg) or amantidine (100 mg orally or through a nasogastric tube twice daily; may increase to 300 mg/day in divided doses) should be used in moderately severe cases and continued until the muscle rigidity and metabolic abnormalities have significantly improved. The skeletal muscle relaxant dantrolene (starting with a dose of 1 mg/kg intravenously and titrated to a maximum of 10 mg/kg/day divided into three intravenous or oral doses) should be added to bromocriptine or amantidine in patients with fulminant hypermetabolic features and those with persistent muscle rigidity despite treatment with dopamine agonists. Refractory neuroleptic malignant syndrome improves after electroconvulsive therapy (ECT).

Serotonin Syndrome

Serotonin syndrome (Chapters 7 and 458) is an adverse drug reaction primarily produced by excess serotonergic agonism of central nervous system and peripheral serotonin receptors. The complication is induced by selective serotonin re-uptake inhibitors (SSRIs; sertraline, fluoxetine, paroxetine, and citalopram), monoamine oxidase inhibitors (phenelzine, moclobemide clorgiline), heterocyclic antidepressants (trazodone and nefazodone), dual-uptake inhibitors (venlafaxine), psychostimulants (amphetamines and cocaine), and buspirone. Other causative drugs in psychiatric patients include mood stabilizers (lithium and valproic acid), analgesics (tramadol, meperidine, and fentanyl), antiemetics (metoclopramide), cough suppressants (dextromethorphan), and dietary supplements (tryptophan, St. John's wort, and ginseng). In postmarketing surveillance studies of the newer antidepressants, the syndrome has an incidence of four cases per 10,000 patient months in patients who start taking nefazodone and has been shown to occur in 15% of patients with intentional overdose of SSRIs. The etiology of serotonin syndrome is overstimulation of 5-HT1A and possibly also 5-HT2 receptors through excess of serotonin precursors or agonists, increased serotonin release, reduced serotonin uptake, and decreased serotonin metabolism. Severe cases of the syndrome have been more frequently reported in patients treated with monoamine oxidase inhibitors who took over-the-counter dextromethorphan or the illegal methylenedioxymethamphetamine (Ecstasy) or who started treatment with serotonin re-uptake inhibitors or meperidine.

Potentially life-threatening, the syndrome is characterized by changes in mental status (ranging from agitation to confusion and coma), autonomic instability (tachycardia, labile or high blood pressure, diaphoresis, and diarrhea), neuromuscular abnormalities (myoclonus, mydriasis, ocular clonus, rigidity, hyperreflexia, tremors, and shivering), and hyperthermia. Death may occur as a consequence of rhabdomyolysis with renal failure, hyperkalemia, disseminated intravascular coagulation, and acute respiratory distress syndrome. The symptoms occur within the first 24 hours and sometimes within minutes after the initial use of medication, a change in dose, addition of a new drug, or overdose attempt. The differential diagnosis includes neuroleptic malignant syndrome, viral or bacterial meningitis or encephalitis, heat stroke, anticholinergic "toxidrome," and drug or alcohol withdrawal.

General management includes immediate discontinuation of serotonergic drugs, comprehensive supportive therapy, and benzodiazepines for control of agitation and myoclonus. Specific therapy relies on the use of cyproheptadine (an H_1-receptor antagonist with antiserotonergic and anticholinergic properties) and chlorpromazine (a 5-HT1A and 5-HT2 receptor antagonist). Cyproheptadine should be started at a dose of 12 mg administered orally or through a nasogastric tube and additional 2-mg doses given every 2 hours until symptoms improve or the maximum dose of 32 mg has been reached. The usual maintenance dose of cyproheptadine is 8 mg three times daily. Chlorpromazine (50 mg intramuscularly; may repeat three or four times daily and increase gradually to 400 mg/day in divided doses) is indicated in patients with severe symptoms who must be treated parenterally. Rapid improvement has also been observed after single doses of olanzapine (10 mg administered sublingually). Chlorpromazine and olanzapine should be used only after the possibility of neuroleptic malignant syndrome has been excluded.

Antipsychotic-Induced Hyperprolactinemia

Drug-induced hyperprolactinemia is produced by first-generation antipsychotic medications and by risperidone, but it is quite rare with other atypical antipsychotics such as aripiprazole, olanzapine, and ziprasidone. In patients treated with prolactin-raising antipsychotic medications, hormone levels are above the normal limit in 60% of females and 40% of males. Symptomatic hyperprolactinemia (Chapter 242) occurs in about a third of these patients and is generally associated with a 10-fold increase above baseline levels. Excess prolactin leads to dysfunction of target tissues (galactorrhea, oligomenorrhea and amenorrhea, infertility, sexual impairment, and gynecomastia), as well as an increased risk for breast cancer, osteoporosis, and cardiovascular disease. The mechanism of antipsychotic-related hyperprolactinemia is suppression of dopamine inhibition of lactotroph cells in the hypothalamus. Brain imaging is required in symptomatic patients and those with significant elevated prolactin levels to exclude tumors of the pituitary and hypothalamus.

Psychogenic Polydipsia and Drug-Induced Hyponatremia

Hyponatremia is common in psychiatric patients and can lead to severe complications, including seizure, coma, brain stem herniation, and death (Chapter 117). The diagnosis is often delayed because traditional manifestations of hyponatremia such as lethargy, restlessness, weakness, and disorientation overlap with features of psychiatric disorders. The differential diagnosis in psychiatric settings must emphasize psychogenic polydipsia and the drug-induced syndrome of inappropriate secretion of antidiuretic hormone (SIADH) (Chapter 117).

Patients with psychogenic polydipsia typically have serum hypo-osmolality and a maximally dilute urine (urine osmolality less than 100 mOsm/L). The incidence of polydipsia is 20% and the incidence of water intoxication is 5% in inpatient psychiatric facilities. Urinary incontinence and nocturnal enuresis may be part of the clinical manifestation. The mechanism of increased thirst is poorly understood but may involve incomplete suppression of antidiuretic hormone (ADH) by the hypothalamus, as well as response to the mouth dryness produced by the anticholinergic effect of many psychotropic drugs. The differential diagnosis includes diuretic effect, renal insufficiency, glucocorticoid deficiency, and hypothyroidism. Stringent measures to restrict fluid intake are generally effective in patients with moderate hyponatremia, and clozapine limits polydipsia and improves water intoxication in refractory cases.

Drug-induced SIADH is predominantly related to SSRIs, and animal experiments have suggested that the excess serotonin stimulates release of ADH and will lead to hyponatremia, provided that water intake is sufficient. Other drugs commonly used by psychiatric patients that may produce SIADH include tricyclic antidepressants, monoamine oxidase inhibitors, carbamazepine, first-generation antipsychotic medications, benzodiazepines, methadone, and nicotine. Elderly patients, patients with a lower body mass index, and those with a baseline plasma sodium level less than 138 mEq/L are at higher risk. The median time to diagnosis after starting SSRIs is 9 days. Urinary excretion of sodium usually is greater than 20 mEq/L, and urine osmolality is higher than 300 mOsm/L. In patients with mild asymptomatic hyponatremia, SSRIs can be continued with careful monitoring while the patient is placed on supervised fluid restriction.

Risk Assessment before Electroconvulsive Therapy

ECT is highly effective for the treatment of drug-refractory major depression and other psychiatric disorders. The procedure requires a brief period of general anesthesia with sodium penthothal, etomidate, or propofol, as well as muscle paralysis with succinylcholine, during which the patient receives bag-valve-mask ventilation with supplemental oxygen and is monitored with continuous electrocardiography and pulse oximetry. Bronchospasm may follow induction of anesthesia, particularly in patients already at risk for respiratory compromise. During electrical stimulation of the brain, parasympathetic activation can lead to bradycardia or several seconds of asystole, which can be avoided by premedicating the patient with intravenous glycopyrrolate. The parasympathetic effect lasts until onset of the akinetic seizure, when sympathetic tone increases and produces tachycardia, an elevation in blood pressure, and increased myocardial demand for oxygen. These changes can be corrected with intravenous esmolol. At the same time, because of the enhanced neuronal metabolic rate, augmented blood flow to the brain increases intracranial pressure. This elevated sympathetic tone causes ECT-related myocardial ischemia, tachyarrhythmias, and potential rupture of aortic or intracranial aneurysms. The elevated intracranial pressure may lead to brain herniation in patients with a space-occupying lesion. Older patients have a high rate of prolonged confusion, arrhythmias, and falls after ECT. A structured medical evaluation before ECT can address risks and the potential for complications (Fig. 460–1). All effort must be made to optimize the patient's active medical conditions before ECT. For high-risk patients one must require that ECT be performed in a setting that allows immediate access to an intensive care unit rather than in the ECT suite of a self-standing psychiatric hospital. Essential medications should be administered with a small amount of fluid 6 hours before ECT. Drugs that can increase or decrease the seizure threshold, such as lidocaine, theophylline, phenothiazine, tricyclic antidepressants, and benzodiazepines, must be discontinued before ECT. Optimal pre-ECT risk assessment, careful anesthesia, and post-ECT monitoring result in a serious complication rate of only 0.9% and essentially no fatalities.

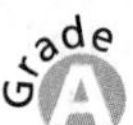

1. Lieberman JA, Stroup TS, McEvoy JP, et al: Effectiveness of antipsychotic drugs in patients with chronic schizophrenia. N Engl J Med 2005;353:1209–1223.

Section XXVII Consultation

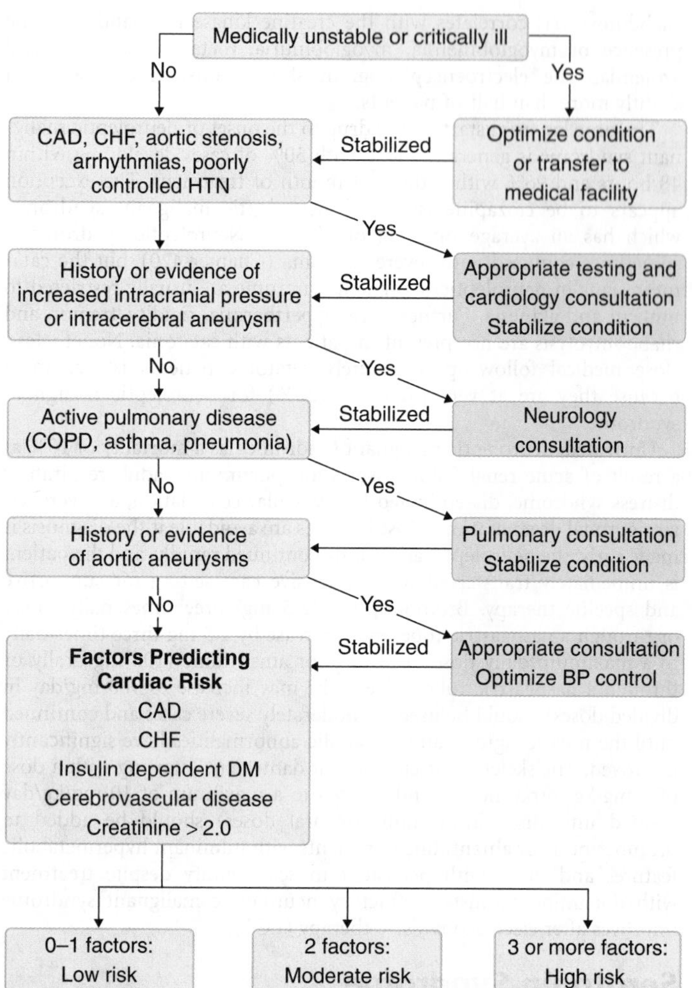

FIGURE 460–1 • Risk assessment before electroconvulsive therapy. BP = blood pressure; CAD = coronary artery disease; CHF = congestive heart failure; COPD = chronic obstructive pulmonary disease; DM = diabetes mellitus; HTN = hypertension. (Modified after Frederickson A, Manu P: Risk assessment prior to electroconvulsive therapy. *In* Manu P, Suarez RE, Barnett BJ [eds]: Handbook of Medicine in Psychiatry. Washington, DC, American Psychiatric Publishing, 2006, pp 687–700.)

SUGGESTED READINGS

Boyer EW, Shannon M: The serotonin syndrome. N Engl J Med 2005;352: 1112–1120. *Comprehensive review of the clinical manifestation, etiology, and management of serotonin syndrome.*

Brookes G, Ahmed AG: Pharmacological treatments for psychosis-related polydipsia. Cochrane Database Syst Rev 2006;4:CD003544. *Limited clinical trial data for two treatment modalities, demeclocycline and naloxone.*

Casey DE: Metabolic issues and cardiovascular disease in patients with psychiatric disorders. Am J Med 2005;118:15S–22S. *A clinical review.*

Manu P, Suarez RE, Barnett BJ: Medicine in psychiatry: What do we need to know? *In* Manu P, Suarez RE, Barnett BJ (eds): Handbook of Medicine in Psychiatry. Washington, DC, American Psychiatric Publishing, 2006, pp xxv–xxvii. *Systematic evaluation of the reasons for medical consultation in an inpatient psychiatric setting.*

Marder SR, Essock SM, Miller AL, et al: Physical health monitoring of patients with schizophrenia. Am J Psychiatry 2004;161:1334–1349. *Practical recommendations regarding the major medical complications of antipsychotic drug therapy.*

Merrill DB, Dec GW, Goff DC: Adverse cardiac effects associated with clozapine. J Clin Psychopharmacol 2005;25:32–41. *A meta-analysis of reported cases of clozapine-induced myocarditis and cardiomyopathy.*

Sachdev PS: Neuroleptic-induced movement disorders: An overview. Psychiatr Clin North Am 2005;28:255–274. *Updated information regarding neuroleptic malignant syndrome and drug-induced extrapyramidal syndromes.*

Section XXVIII

Skin Diseases

461 STRUCTURE AND FUNCTION OF THE SKIN

David A. Norris

KEY FUNCTIONS OF THE SKIN

The skin, which is the largest organ in the body, is a tough, resilient barrier that covers the body and shields the muscle compartment and internal structures. It is composed of an outer epidermis of ectodermal origin and an underlying dermis of mesenchymal origin. The structure of the skin varies considerably from one area of the body to another, including changes in the thickness of its components and in its specialized structures of epithelial origin (e.g., hair, nails, sweat glands, and sebaceous glands). The skin is commonly affected in systemic diseases, and it is also the location of many diseases limited to the skin. It is often damaged by external stimuli such as radiation, sunlight, toxins, irritants, allergens, and infectious agents.

The skin serves critical functions.

PROTECTION. Melanin pigment and antioxidant enzymes are positioned in the epidermis to protect the skin against radiation. The thick reticular dermis is a barrier to injury and trauma, as well as a cushion for underlying structures. The epidermis resists friction and tangential stress. The stratum corneum, which is an impenetrable barrier to external substances, is thickened on the palms and soles to provide padding and protection.

THERMOREGULATION. Evaporation from eccrine sweat glands is critical for thermoregulation. Vascular dilation and constriction help regulate the exchange of heat in the skin to preserve heat in cold climates and eliminate heat after exercise.

IMMUNOLOGIC RESPONSE. The skin is the outermost arm of the immune response and is designed to defend against infection, transformed cells, and toxins by means of highly developed innate and acquired local immune responses.

BARRIER TO WATER LOSS. The stratum corneum is the critical component of normal skin that prevents transepidermal water loss.

SECRETION OF WASTES. Eccrine and apocrine sweat glands transport wastes and also provide excretion of odiferous substances.

SENSATION. The skin is the largest sensory organ. The skin and mucous membranes are the principal sites of pleasurable sensation and also sites of unpleasant sensations.

STRUCTURE OF THE SKIN

The skin consists of two distinct layers: the *epidermis* and the *dermis* (Fig. 461–1). The skin is derived from two germinal cell lineages: the ectoderm, which gives rise to the epidermis, and the mesenchyme, which produces the dermis. These two layers are joined at a basement membrane zone termed the *basal lamina.*

The epidermis, which is a stratified squamous epithelial layer, contains several different levels of structure and function. It is held together by distinctive adhesion structures termed *desmosomes* (Fig. 461–2). The *stratum corneum*, which is the product of the dying epidermis, resists the penetration of external organisms and toxins and prevents water loss. The *basal lamina* is a very complex structure of epidermal and dermal-derived proteins that attach the epidermis to the dermis and resist shear stress.

The *papillary dermis* is a collagenous matrix containing the blood vessels that feed the epidermis. The *reticular dermis* is a tougher cushion protecting underlying tissue and containing the epidermal adnexal structures. The blood vessels and nerves are separated into a superficial plexus in the papillary dermis and a deeper plexus that serves the adnexal structures. The dermis is separated from the fascia and underlying muscle by a layer of subcutaneous adipose tissue that allows the skin to move freely relative to deeper internal structures.

The epidermally derived adnexal structures (eccrine sweat glands, apocrine sweat glands, sebaceous glands, and hair follicles) are anchored in the dermis but penetrate the epidermis and the barrier of the stratum corneum (see Fig. 461–1). The hair follicle is a cycling structure containing specialized populations of epithelial cells, pigment cells, and mesenchymal cells that control the hair cycle. Eccrine sweat glands discharge sweat directly through the stratum corneum. Apocrine sweat glands discharge their products into hair follicles. Sebaceous glands drain into sebaceous hair follicles on the scalp, face, chest, back, axilla, and groin. An extensive network of blood vessels and nerves serves the skin. The superficial vascular plexus feeds the epidermis through an extensive complex of capillary loops in the papillary dermis. The deep vascular and nerve plexus serve the adnexal structures in the dermis. The hair follicles, with their apocrine and sebaceous glands, and the eccrine sweat glands are potential avenues for transepidermal absorption of drugs because they penetrate the stratum corneum.

Cells of the Epidermis and Epidermal Differentiation

The epidermis is a stratified squamous epithelium composed mostly of keratinocytes, with other resident cells in distinct locations (melanocytes, Langerhans cells, and Merkel cells). In response to various stimuli, migrating cells such as lymphocytes, dermal macrophages, neutrophils, and eosinophils enter the epidermis. Keratinocytes are attached firmly to each other through desmosomes (see Fig. 461–2), which connect to the rigid keratin intermediate filament network and give the epidermis strength. The basal layer of the rigid epidermis connects to the basement membrane zone by means of hemidesmosomes, which are highly organized adhesion structures linked to the basal keratin network. Adherens junctions link surrounding keratinocytes and connect them to the actin microfilament network. These junctions provide more plastic adhesions that are also involved in actin-mediated movement. Junctions on melanocytes and Langerhans cells attach through E-cadherin–containing adherens junctions to keratinocytes to maintain their dendritic structure.

Keratinocytes and Epidermal Differentiation

Epidermal Differentiation

Epidermal differentiation is a genetically programmed process by which keratinocytes differentiate from proliferating cells in the germinative layer to form tightly attached "prickle" cells in the malpighian layer, dying cells in the granular layer, and corneocytes in the stratum. During this process, keratinocytes undergo tremendous changes reflecting their different functional characteristics. Keratinocytes are named for the intermediate filament protein keratin, which forms insoluble stiff filaments that give the epidermis its strength. The keratins are made of tetramers composed of two basic and two acidic keratins (K5/14 in the basal layer, K1/10 in the spinous layer, K6/16 in the hyperproliferative epidermis, K9/19 in the palms and soles). Keratin has versatile properties and is the major component of hair and nails in humans and of beaks, hooves, and feathers in other animals.

The attachments within the epidermis are formed by desmosomes and adherens junctions. The adherens junctions that form between keratinocytes are characterized by homophilic binding of cell surface cadherins and by binding of the adhesion structure to actin microfilaments within the cell by catenins (Fig. 461–3A). Desmosomes are composed of molecules called desmogleins and desmocollins, which are homologous to cadherins and form adhesion structures with keratins through numerous associated proteins such as plakoglobin and plakophilin (see Fig. 461–3B). The basal keratinocytes are attached to the basal lamina at the hemidesmosome, a specialized adhesion structure linked to the basal cell keratin filament network (see Fig. 461–3C). The progressive differentiation of the epidermis is associated with specific changes in protein expression and function.

Functions of the Epidermal Layers

The *germinative (basal) layer* of the epidermis is responsible for cell proliferation. This layer is resistant to apoptosis because of defenses maintained by receptors for growth factors and matrix molecules. The germinative layer can become a migrating epithelial tongue to aid in wound healing.

The *spinous layer* produces a dense keratin filament network (keratins 1/10) that interacts with desmosomes, and it synthesizes involucrin (which is involved in protein cross-linking with the plasma membrane in the granular layer), a protective antioxidant network (glutathione reductase, peroxidases, catalases), cytokines, chemokines, lamellar bodies, and keratohyaline granules.

Cells in the *granular layer* undergo programmed cell death (apoptosis). Keratohyaline granule profilaggrin is activated into filaggrin, thereby inducing keratin cross-linking. Lamellar body contents are secreted into

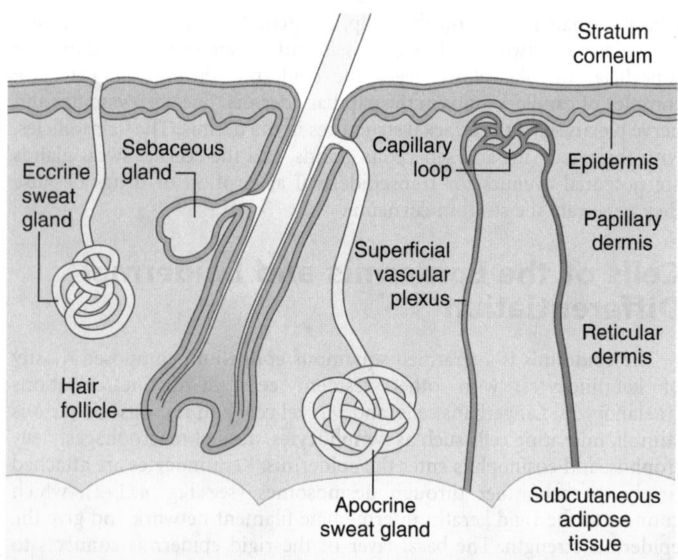

FIGURE 461–1 • The skin and adnexal structures. The relationship of the epidermis and its adnexal structures (sebaceous and sweat glands and hair follicles) to the dermis and subcutaneous adipose tissue is shown. Note how these structures are associated with breaks in the barrier of the stratum corneum.

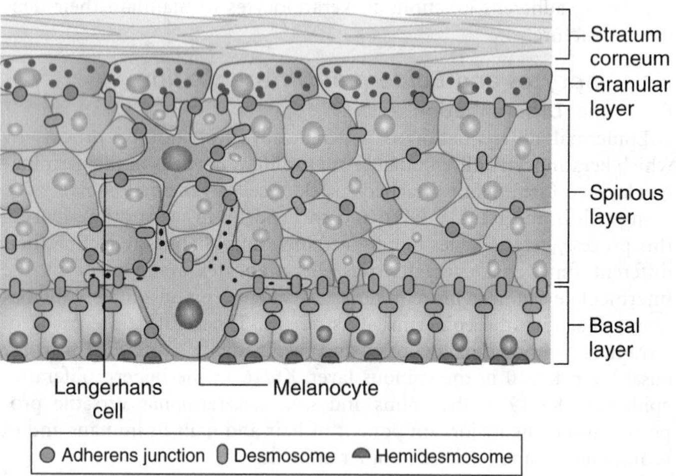

FIGURE 461–2 • Cell attachment in the epidermis. The epidermal keratinocytes, melanocytes, and Langerhans cells form a network of attachments crucial to normal epidermal function.

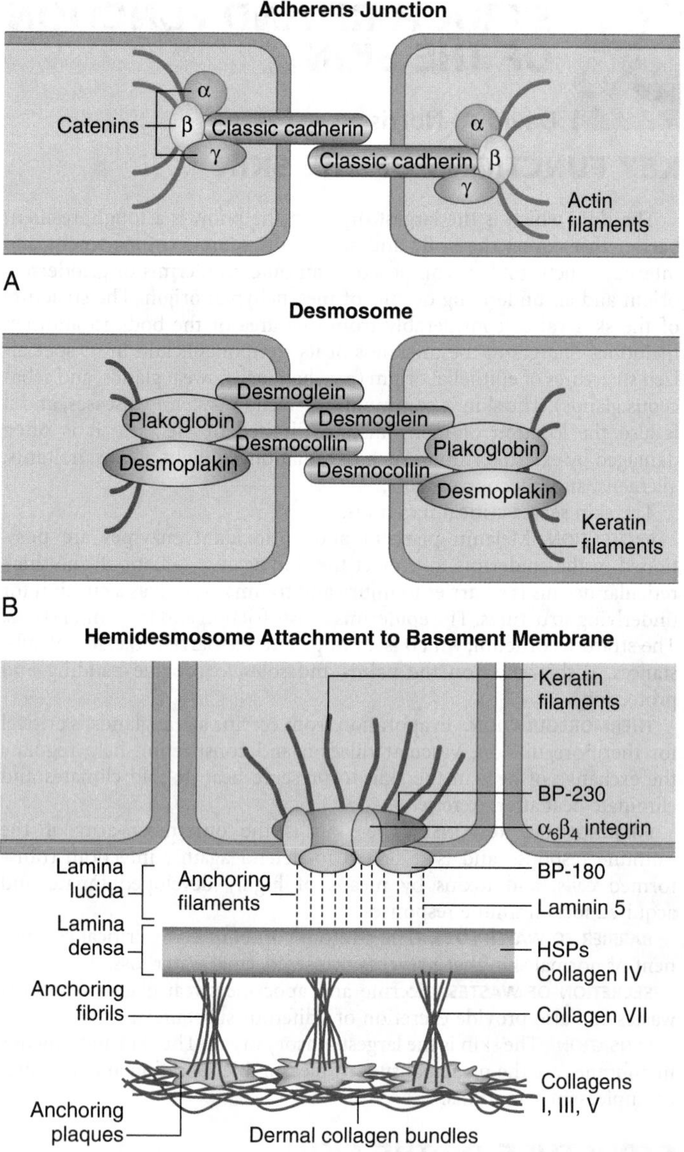

FIGURE 461–3 • Molecular aspects of key epidermal adhesion structures and connection of the epidermis to the dermis. A–C, These structures are crucial to the normal integrity of the skin. Mutations or autoimmune damage to these structures has devastating effects on skin function. HSP = heat shock protein.

the extracellular space by fusion of the lamellar body to the cell membrane. Cross-linking of involucrin and cornifin to the cell membrane by transglutaminase produces a thickened, cornified envelope. Protein synthesis ceases as cells die to form intact corneocytes, which contain cross-linked keratin filaments and a thick cornified envelope.

Flat corneocytes surrounded by phospholipid lamellae form the impervious *stratum corneum*. Although the cornified layer provides a thin, flexible barrier to protect sensitive cells from the external environment, molecules can diffuse through the cornified layer. Indeed, this transepidermal route is the major route of penetration of topical medications (Chapter 462). After a defined period, desquamation of superficial corneocytes occurs by enzymatic degradation of extracellular material.

Melanocytes

Melanocytes, which are dendritic cells that synthesize and secrete the pigment melanin, are derived embryonically from neural crest cells and typically migrate to the epidermal-dermal junction during development, although a few can be found in the dermis. Melanocytes are localized in the basal layer of the epidermis, with the ratio of melanocytes to keratinocytes ranging from about 1:4 to about 1:10 at different locations in the skin. The relative number of melanocytes is roughly the same for both sexes and for all races, approximately 1500 melanocytes per square millimeter of skin surface. A totally separate population of melanocytes resides in hair follicles that produce pigmented hairs. Differences in the coloration of skin are therefore determined by the relative activity of these cells, not their numbers. Epidermal melanocytes are attached to the basal lamina by integrin receptors, and they are attached to surrounding keratinocytes by E-cadherin–mediated attachments. Melanin pigment is synthesized in melanocyte-specific organelles termed *melanosomes*. Melanosome transfer is achieved when keratinocytes actively engulf the melanosome-containing cytoplasmic tips of the dendritic processes of the melanocytes. Exposure to ultraviolet (UV) light increases the rate of formation of melanosomes and enhances their rate of delivery to keratinocytes.

Melanin is a complex heteropolymer that absorbs light across the entire UV and visible spectrum; it is the principal protection of the skin against solar radiation. Melanization is a complex biochemical process controlled largely by three genes: tyrosinase (rate-limiting step), which oxidizes tyrosine to 3,4-dihydroxyphenylalanine (dopa); tyrosinase-related protein 1 (TyRP-1); and tyrosinase-related protein 2 (TyRP-2). Control of melanization is a complex genetic and environmental process. One important level of control is binding of melanocyte-stimulating hormone to the melanocortin-1 receptor (MC-1R) on melanocytes. The enzymes that control melanization are transported into the melanosome, where the biochemical processes occur in a protected organelle-bound environment. The whole organelle is then transported to keratinocytes, where it resides in a "helmet" location above the nucleus. Polymorphisms in MC-1R control the relative amounts of the three key enzymes. Decreases in TyRP-1 and TyRP-2 lead to the production of pheomelanin, a brown-red pigment with inferior photoprotective properties. This type of pigment is seen in red-haired individuals and is associated with decreased sun protection, increased photoaging, and a higher rate of melanoma and nonmelanoma skin cancer. UV light can transform melanocytes into malignant melanoma, the most deadly form of skin cancer (Chapter 214).

Melanocytes are terminally differentiated cells with no stem cell population to repopulate interfollicular melanocytes. A melanocyte precursor population in the outer root sheath of the hair follicle can be mobilized to repopulate lost interfollicular melanocytes—an approach to repigmentation that is used for vitiligo. However, melanocyte stem cell populations are believed to exist in the hair follicle, where they replenish the melanocytes of the hair bulb during each cycle of hair regeneration in the transition from telogen to anagen (see Hair).

Langerhans Cells

Dendritic Langerhans cells are an important subset of antigen-presenting cells located in the midportion of the epidermis. These cells become more abundant at sites of inflammatory skin disorders, including allergic reactions such as contact dermatitis (Chapter 464). Langerhans cells are migratory, and they contain characteristic striated, rodlike structures known as Birbeck granules. They also bear several important immunologic cell surface receptors (DC1, major histocompatibility complex [MHC] class II, IgG receptor, C3 receptor). In contact sensitization (contact dermatitis), Langerhans cells internalize and process antigen, migrate to regional lymph nodes, and present the antigen to naive lymphocytes. When the antigen is reapplied to skin (challenge), the Langerhans cells again process and present the antigen to sensitized lymphocytes in the skin or in lymph nodes.

Merkel Cells

Merkel cells are scattered among the basal keratinocytes and are more abundant in some areas than others. These cells are often found near or in contact with very fine, unmyelinated nerves, and they form synapses with peripheral nerve fiber endings. Merkel cells are present singly or in clusters called tactile corpuscles. They are attached to adjacent epidermal cells by numerous desmosome connections, but their tonofilaments, unlike those of keratinocytes, are not grouped into bundles. In the cytoplasm of Merkel cells are numerous membrane-bounded dense granules that contain catecholamines. It is believed that Merkel cells serve as adapting mechanoreceptors. Merkel cell tumors are uncommon but are among the most deadly of skin cancers.

The Dermal-Epidermal Junction

The dermal-epidermal junction is a transitional zone in which the basal layer of the epithelium is connected to penetrating deep collagenous anchors that originate in the papillary dermis. The connection is composed of collagenous rods, globular domains, and cruciate protein complexes that form a firm attachment that resists friction and tangential stress. This junction, which is the weakest structure point in the skin, is the site of blistering induced by cold, heat, and immunologically and genetically mediated blistering disorders.

Downgrowths of the epidermis form tiny ridges, called rete pegs, that add bonding surface area between the dermis and epidermis (Table 461–1). The sandwiched basal lamina follows the ridges, which are more pronounced in areas of high abrasion. The lamina has three zones: the lamina lucida, the lamina densa, and the fibroreticular lamina. Keratin filaments in the basal cells anchor in the hemidesmosomes, which connect to anchoring filaments of the lamina lucida and then to the dense collagen and heparan sulfate proteoglycan matrix of the lamina densa. Anchoring fibrils of type VII collagen form the fibroreticular lamina and end in the anchoring plaques that intercalate with type III and VI collagen in the papillary dermis.

TABLE 461–1 COMPONENTS OF THE DERMAL-EPIDERMAL JUNCTION

Location	Structure	Macromolecules
Basal keratinocytes Plasma membrane	Hemidesmosomes	BPAg 230 (BPAg1) BPAg 180 (BPAg2) Plectin Integrins $\alpha_6\beta_4$ and $\alpha_3\beta_1$
Lamina lucida	Anchoring filaments	Laminin isoforms Part of BPAg2
Lamina densa	Electron-dense band	Type IV collagen Entactin Heparan sulfate proteoglycan
Sublamina densa fibrillar zone	Anchoring fibrils Microfibrils Collagen fibers Microthread-like fibers	Type VII collagen Fibrillin 1 and 2 Collagen types I, III, and VI Linkin

The Dermis

The thickness of the dermis varies considerably in different parts of the body. For descriptive purposes, the dermis is divided into the papillary layer, which is the thinner inner layer next to the epidermis, and the reticular layer, which is composed of denser connective tissue and constitutes the bulk of the dermis. The papillary layer, which forms the dermal papillary ridges, is composed of collagen and reticular and elastic fibers that are woven into a loose network. The extracellular matrix consists of mucopolysaccharides. The dermis contains many different cell types, including fibroblasts, fibrocytes, macrophages, leukocytes, and plasma cells. The vascular supply to the skin is confined to the dermis, where small arteries enter from the subcutaneous tissue and form deep and superficial sheetlike plexus. Capillary loops ascend into the dermal papillae and return via venous plexus. The postcapillary venule portion of the vascular network, which is where leukocytes enter the tissue, is an important target of damage in allergic vasculitis. The nerve supply to the skin is very profuse and consists of both myelinated and nonmyelinated fibers. Specialized sensory structures such as pacinian and Meissner's corpuscles are located prominently in the hands and feet. Because up to 4 to 5% of the total blood volume can be stored in the dermis, it plays an important role in thermal regulation; sympathetic nerve fibers control blood flow to and from the skin.

Epidermal Appendages of the Skin

Sebaceous Glands

Sebaceous glands, or oil glands, are found throughout the dermis except for the palms of the hands and the soles of the feet. Most of these glands, which are greatly activated at the onset of puberty, discharge their contents via a single duct into the lumen of hair follicles. Where these glands occur independently of hairs (e.g., the glans penis, lips, labia minora, and eyelids), they open directly onto the surface of the skin. The sebaceous glands are holocrine in their secretion; that is, the entire cell is discharged as a secretory body. Mature cells filled with triglycerides, waxy esters, squalene, cholesterol, and fatty acids degenerate and disintegrate (necrosis); the entire debris is discharged as sebum. Contraction of the erector pili muscles aids in discharging the contents of these glands.

Eccrine Sweat Glands

Sweat glands are merocrine in secretion; that is, they discharge components of cytoplasm into the sweat duct. *Eccrine* sweat glands are positioned over the entire skin but are concentrated most densely in the palms, the soles, and the head. Eccrine sweat glands, which number about 3 million, are innervated by postganglionic, cholinergic sympathetic nerves. Excess heat causes sweating to begin on the forehead and to spread elsewhere over the body. Eccrine sweat glands secrete a watery solution that is high in sodium chloride but also contains urea, uric acid, potassium, and immunoglobulins. Histologically, these glands are simple tubular structures composed of a coiled glandular portion and a straight duct, which on entry into the epidermis is continuous with a spiral cleft opening to the surface of the skin. On the outside of the secretory epithelium are myoepithelial cells.

Apocrine Sweat Glands

Apocrine glands remain small until early puberty, when they enlarge and begin to secrete. Histologically, these glands consist of two portions: the coiled secretory gland, which is situated in the dermis and subcutaneous tissue, and a straight excretory duct, which is composed of two layers of epithelial cells. Apocrine release can be secretion or excretion. Secretion is a continuous process, but excretion is episodic. Excretion occurs when there is actual propulsion, presumably provided by the myoepithelial sheath, which is innervated by adrenergic sympathetic fibers. Apocrine glands are scent glands whose secretion is increased by fear, sexual excitement, and other forms of heightened tension. Apocrine glands are present in the axilla, the external genitalia, the areolar skin around nipples, and the perianal area. Specialized apocrine glands include Moll's glands on the eyelid and ceruminous (wax) glands in the auditory canal.

Nails

The nail is composed of a proximal germinative epithelium that is called the nail matrix, a keratinized product that is called the nail plate or body, an underlying specialized epithelium that is called the nail bed and is attached to the undersurface of the nail, and a protective loop of skin that is called the proximal nail fold. Underlying the proximal part of the body of the nail is a collection of germinal cells that form an opaque spot on the nail, the lunula. The lunula is white because the papillary dermis in this region is less vascular, and the stratum germinativum is thick and opaque; this is the site of the proliferating nail matrix that is responsible for growth of the nail. As these epidermal cells are formed, they become tightly packed and keratinized, but they do not desquamate. Nails grow at a rate of 0.5 to 1.5 mm/wk, with toenails growing much more slowly than fingernails.

Hair

There are three types of hair follicles: vellus hair follicles located over most of the body; terminal hair follicles located on the scalp, beard area, axilla, groin, and other hairy areas; and sebaceous hair follicles located on the scalp, face, beard, chest, back, axilla, and groin. Sebaceous hair follicles have a minimal hair shaft but hypertrophied sebaceous glands. Terminal hairs form the long hairs of the scalp and beard. The hair follicles of the eyelashes and eyebrows also have specialized characteristics determined by local mesenchymal factors. Hair follicle growth is determined by influences of the dermis and is strongly stimulated by androgens by means of the type II androgen receptor.

Hairs are dead shafts composed of fused plates of keratin that project from the surface of the epidermis. Hair does not grow continuously but rather passes through a cycle (Fig. 461–4). Anagen is the growth phase. Then comes a short catagen stage in which portions of the hair follicle involute and growth ceases. Next is the telogen, or resting, phase. Near the end of the telogen phase, the hair falls out or is easily pulled out. A shed hair is called a club hair because of the shape of the root. This overall cycle varies depending on the hair and the location on the body. For scalp hairs, the anagen phase can last 3 to 10 years, but it may be as short as 4 months in other areas of the body. The hair growth cycle can be synchronized during pregnancy so that a larger number of hair follicles will enter the telogen phase together and therefore be shed together after delivery of the fetus, thereby causing temporary thinning of the hair 3 to 4 months after pregnancy (telogen effluvium). Hair is pigmented by melanocytes situated in the hair bulb close to the papillae. Keratinocytes in the papillary region engulf the pigment granules, much as they do in the skin.

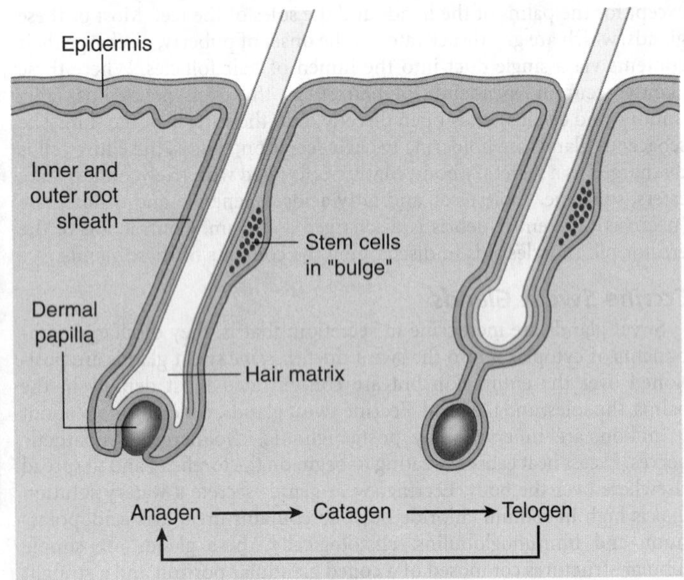

FIGURE 461–4 • Hair follicle cycle. Communications between the dermal papilla, the matrix, the follicle sheath, and the stem cells control the hair cycle through its anagen, catagen, and telogen phases.

The hair cycle depends on synchronized cooperation among four major components of the hair follicle: the dermal papilla, the hair matrix, the outer root sheaths, and the stem cells in the bulge region. During the actively growing anagen phase of the hair cycle, signals from the dermal papilla maintain the proliferating hair matrix. When these signals terminate, the follicle enters the catagen phase in which the matrix and root sheaths of the lower follicle die by apoptosis. The follicle then enters a resting telogen phase. When the follicle re-enters the anagen phase, signals from the dermal papilla stimulate stem cells in the bulge region of the follicle, and these cells migrate to form the new matrix, initiate a new hair shaft, and cause the old hair to fall out. In normal follicles in young healthy adults, the anagen phase is almost 3 years and the telogen phase is about 3 months. At any time, 10 to 15% of the hairs are in telogen on a healthy young scalp.

In "telogen effluvium," the shift to telogen is abrupt, and hairs fall from the scalp precipitously in 3 months when new anagen hairs are formed in the follicles. This pattern is commonly seen 3 to 4 months after a severe systemic illness or at the termination of pregnancy. A gradual shift to the telogen phase occurs with age and is even greater in androgenic alopecia.

SPECIALIZED ASPECTS OF SKIN STRUCTURE AND FUNCTION

Clinical Correlates

Genetic diseases that affect the function of the dermis and epidermis are listed in Table 461–2 and are described further in subsequent chapters.

Skin-Associated Immune System

The skin is the most external component of the immune response, with well-developed elements of both the innate and acquired immune systems (Chapter 42). The barrier of the stratum corneum is broken by adnexal structures such as hair and sweat glands, and infections in these sites are suppressed by a network of innate immune responses and defenses. The skin is also a principal site for invasion by bacteria, parasites, and viruses, and it is an important site of tumor induction; all these processes are influenced by a well-developed acquired immune response. The skin contains several populations of antigen-presenting cells, including the epidermal Langerhans cells. Trafficking of T cells to the skin occurs through skin-specific homing receptors such as the cutaneous lymphocyte antigen.

The skin's innate immune system includes macrophages, dendritic cells, and neutrophils, as well as a very extensive epidermal network of cytokines (e.g., interleukin-1 [IL-1] and tumor necrosis factor-α [TNF-α]) and chemokines. The skin has a number of receptors for foreign organisms (CD14, Toll-like receptors, mannose receptors), defensins and other antibacterial proteins, and networks that augment and inhibit complement in the papillary dermis.

The skin's acquired immune system includes an epidermal network of specialized dendritic cells (Langerhans cells) plus dermal dendritic cells. The cutaneous lymphocyte antigen stimulates the trafficking of lymphocytes to the skin. Both T_H1 and T_H2 responses are well developed in skin, but most inflammatory skin diseases have a T_H1 response. Hair follicles may be immunologically privileged sites because they lack MHC class I.

Control of Apoptosis in the Skin

Apoptosis is a normal part of the cycle of epidermal differentiation. In the granular cell layer, transglutaminase-mediated cross-linking of

TABLE 461–2 CLINICAL CORRELATES OF THE STRUCTURE AND FUNCTION OF THE SKIN: GENETIC DISEASES AFFECTING FUNCTION OF THE EPIDERMIS AND DERMIS

Disease	Cells Involved	Gene and/or Protein Affected
IMMUNOBULLOUS DISORDERS (Chapter 465)		
Pemphigus vulgaris	Keratinocytes	Antibody to desmoglein 3
Pemphigus foliaceous	Keratinocytes	Antibody to desmoglein 1
Bullous pemphigoid	Keratinocytes	Antibody to BP180 and/or BP230
Epidermolysis bullosa acquisita	Subepidermal blister	Antibody to CVII
Bullous systemic lupus erythematosus	Subepidermal blister	Antibody to CVII
MECHANOBULLOUS DISORDERS (Chapter 465)		
Epidermolytic hyperkeratosis	Suprabasal keratinocyte	K1, K10
Epidermolytic palmoplantar keratoderma	Suprabasal keratinocyte	K9
Epidermolysis bullosa simplex	Basal keratinocyte	K5, K14
Junctional epidermolysis bullosa	Subepidermal blister	Laminin V
Dystrophic epidermolysis bullosa	Subepidermal blister	CVII
DISORDERS OF CORNIFICATION		
Ichthyosis vulgaris	Granular, stratum corneum	Reduced/absent filaggrin
Harlequin ichthyosis	Stratum corneum	Reduced K1/K10, filaggrin
X-linked ichthyosis	Stratum corneum	Steroid sulfatase
Lamellar ichthyosis	Stratum corneum	*TGM1* (transglutaminase type 1)
DISORDERS OF KERATINOCYTE ATTACHMENT		
Darier's disease	Suprabasal keratinocytes	*ATP2A2* (*SERCA2*)
Hailey-Hailey disease	Suprabasal keratinocytes	*ATP2C1*
DISORDERS OF PIGMENTATION (Chapter 467)		
Piebaldism	Melanocytes	c-*kit* (stem cell factor receptor)
Hermansky-Pudlak syndrome	Melanocyte (melanosome)	HPS-1p
	Platelet (platelet dense bodies) lysosomes	β3A subunit of the AP-3 adaptor complex
Chédiak-Higashi syndrome	Melanocyte (melanosome) lysosomes	*LYST* gene
Albinism	Melanocyte/melanosomes	Tyrosinase, *TRP1*
Vitiligo	Melanocyte	Cytotoxic damage (immune, chemical)

involucrin initiates formation of the cornified envelope, which is a specialized apoptotic envelope. Unlike other apoptotic cells, the corneocyte is not phagocytized or fragmented. Epidermal stem cells, melanocytes, and proliferating transit-amplified cells of the basal and suprabasal epidermis are resistant to apoptosis, and these defenses against apoptosis are mediated by integrin and growth factor receptor ligation. Integrin and growth factor expression are lost in the differentiating epidermal compartment, and these cells are susceptible to apoptosis induced by chemotherapy, activation of death receptors such as Fas, and UV radiation (Fig. 461–5). In the granular cell layer, apoptosis initiates terminal changes in keratinocytes, thereby producing the dead corneocytes that are the "bricks" of the stratum corneum.

Endothelial cells are also resistant to apoptosis by virtue of their attachment to basement membrane proteins through integrin receptors and because of antiapoptotic proteins that are induced during inflammation to protect these cells. Conversely, during vessel remodeling, the antiapoptotic defenses decrease and endothelial cells die.

Activated lymphocytes, Langerhans cells, and granulocytes that enter the skin are all sensitive to apoptosis. Most phototherapy protocols to treat inflammatory skin diseases rely on UV light–induced apoptosis to destroy Langerhans cells and lymphocytes, whereas the relative resistance of keratinocytes and melanocytes to UV light protects the normal underlying skin cells.

Ultraviolet Radiation and the Skin

The skin is uniquely susceptible to damage induced by exposure to radiation from the sun. Visible and UV light penetrates into the skin and produces important biologic effects. Some effects, such as photoactivation of vitamin D, are beneficial, but most are damaging.

The skin has a number of natural defenses against UV light. First, melanin, a heteropolymer that is transferred from melanocytes to keratinocytes, protects the basal keratinocytes against UV radiation. Second, antioxidant enzymes (e.g., catalase, peroxidase, thioredoxin, and superoxide dismutase) protect skin cells against oxidant damage. Macrophages are induced by UV radiation to enter the epidermis to remove damaged cells. UV radiation also induces Langerhans cells to exit the epidermis and present antigens to T cells in regional lymph nodes. Finally, keratinocytes produce large amounts of IL-1 and TNF-α in response to UV radiation, and a complex system of antagonists and decoy receptors buffer the epidermis from cytokine-induced damage.

Despite these defenses, UV radiation damages keratinocytes and induces malignancy. UV radiation damage also induces both local and systemic immunosuppression, and it can induce autoimmunity when apoptotic keratinocytes and autoantigens are presented to lymphocytes in patients with diseases such as lupus erythematosus.

Itching

The sensations of both itch and pain are transmitted by unmyelinated C fibers. It is assumed that the receptors are the free nerve endings in the dermis and epidermis. Multiple compounds induce pruritus: amines (histamine and serotonin), proteases (papain, kallikrein, trypsin), neuropeptides (substance P, vasoactive intestinal peptide, calcitonin gene–related peptide), eicosanoids, opioids, cytokine growth factors, and

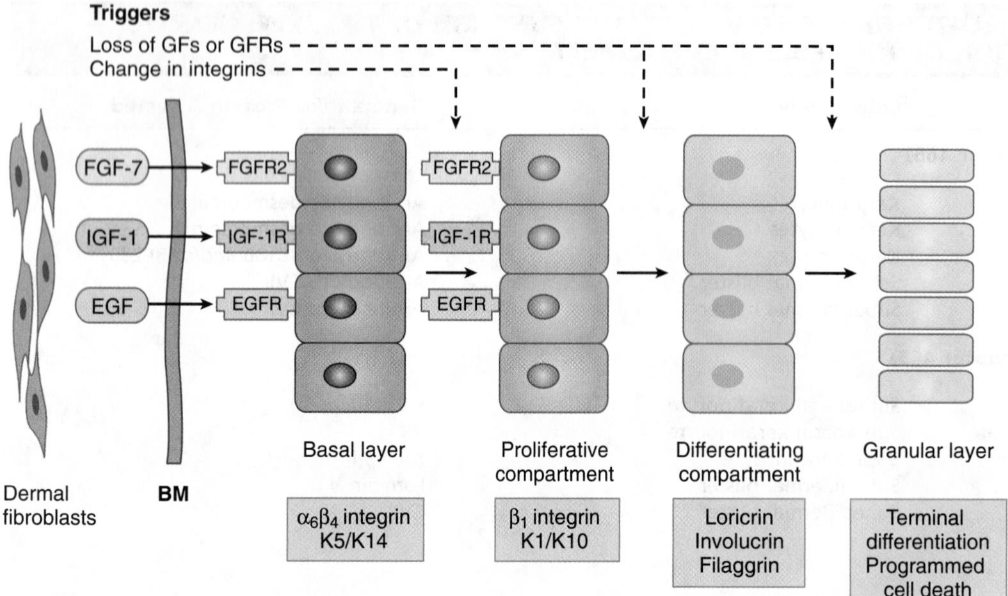

FIGURE 461–5 • Epidermal differentiation. Differentiation of the epidermis, controlled by growth factor receptors and integrin receptors, also modulates the susceptibility of the epidermis to apoptosis induced by external and internal triggers. BM = basal membrane; EGF = epidermal growth factor; EGFR = EGF receptor; FGF = fibroblast growth factor; FGFR = FGF receptor; IGF = insulin-like growth factor.

TABLE 461–3 CLINICAL ASSOCIATIONS WITH PRURITUS

SKIN DISEASES

Dermatitis, including contact dermatitis
Bullous disorders, especially dermatitis herpetiformis and bullous pemphigoid
Drug effects (opiates, aspirin, quinidine)
Urticaria and angioedema
Lichen planus
Sunburn
Seborrheic dermatitis
Infestations (e.g., scabies, pediculosis)
Xerosis (dry skin)
Irritant particles (e.g., fiberglass, "itching powder")

SYSTEMIC DISEASES

Uremia
Obstructive biliary disease (primary biliary cirrhosis, cholestatic hepatitis, cholestasis of pregnancy, extrahepatic biliary obstruction)
Hematologic and myeloproliferative disorders (lymphoma, polycythemia vera, iron deficiency anemia)
Endocrine disorders (thyrotoxicosis, hypothyroidism, diabetes, carcinoid)
Carcinomas (breast, stomach, or lung)
Psychiatric disorders (e.g., delusional states, stress, psychosis)
Neurologic disorders (e.g., multiple sclerosis, notalgia paresthetica, neuropathy)
Mastocytosis (urticaria pigmentosum, telangiectasia macularis eruptive perstans)

products of eosinophils and platelets. Many of these compounds act through their effects as mast cell degranulators. Histamine is the major itch-inducing product of mast cells, but other mediators may also be involved. Pruritus is a frequent component of many skin and systemic diseases (Table 461–3).

Pruritus is a common clinical problem whose treatment is often unsatisfactory. Treatment of any underlying skin or systemic disease is necessary for long-term success. Drugs that inhibit the effects of mast cell products (H_1 or H_2 blocking antihistamines, antileukotrienes) or that inhibit mast cell degranulation (phosphodiesterase inhibitors, β-agonists) are effective as oral agents. Neuropeptide-mediated itching can be inhibited by desensitization with capsaicin. Opiate antagonists block the central opiate receptors that induce the pruritus associated with opiate use. UV radiation treatment can effectively treat the intractable pruritus that occurs in patients with renal failure.

Wound Healing

The skin is the major target of wounding in most people and is the preeminent model used to study wound healing in animals and humans. Wound healing is a complex process with three sequential phases: inflammation, proliferation and tissue formation, and tissue remodeling. The phase of tissue remodeling extends for weeks and months after the closure of wounds, and the fibroblast is the cornerstone of remodeling of the dermis, vessels, and basement membrane.

Vascular abnormalities (arterial insufficiency, venous stasis, and microangiopathy) are commonly associated with poor wound healing. Poor wound healing is also a serious problem in patients with chronic infections or malnutrition. Patients with extensive skin disease, especially mechanobullous or immunobullous disorders such as epidermolysis bullosa or pemphigus, likewise demonstrate defects in wound healing. Efforts to promote wound healing in these situations focus on repair and reversal of vascular disease, reversal of tissue edema, application of growth factors to stimulate angiogenesis and keratinocyte migration, and the use of antibiotics to decrease local infection

SUGGESTED READINGS

Fuchs E: Scratching the surface of skin development. Nature 2007;445:834–842. *A comprehensive review of skin stem cells.*

Pulkkinen L, Ringpfeil F, Uitto J: Progress in heritable skin diseases: Molecular basis and clinical implications. J Am Acad Dermatol 2002;47:91–104. *Details on the clinical findings induced by specific mutations in genes that control the structure and function of the skin.*

Yosipovitch G, Greaves MW, Schmelz M: Itch. Lancet 2003;361:690–694. *Overview of pathophysiology, diagnosis, and therapy.*

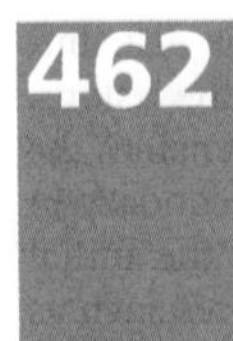

462 EXAMINATION OF THE SKIN AND APPROACH TO DIAGNOSING SKIN DISEASES

Cheryl A. Armstrong

EXAMINATION OF THE SKIN

The examination of the skin is a critical component of the comprehensive medical approach to the patient. By learning how to examine the skin and approach the diagnosis of skin diseases, the physician can focus on the lesions that warrant therapy or provide important information about the systemic health of the patient. Other lesions may be of cosmetic concern to the patient even though they have little or no medical significance.

As the organ system that is an interface with the environment, the skin has an extensive array of mechanical, biochemical, immunologic, and neurologic properties that both inform and protect each individual. The skin also has a vast ability to alter its cellular and acellular components in response to internal or external insults, a process that leads to changes that are subsequently defined as disorders or diseases. The physical examination of the skin can provide information about both cutaneous and systemic diseases, and the examination can sometimes diagnose serious medical conditions at an otherwise asymptomatic stage.

Skin disorders can usually be visualized directly by both the patient and the physician. For example, the patient not only feels the itch and discomfort of an allergic contact dermatitis reaction to poison ivy but also sees the vesicular and crusted skin lesions. The appearance of new lesions or a sudden change in existing lesions can elicit emotional reactions in patients or their family members. The physician must learn to see the same eruptions using a careful and systematic approach that leads to a specific and treatable diagnosis.

History and Physical Examination

Most dermatologists conduct the dermatologic history and examination simultaneously. The physician can best focus the history and full skin examination by first visualizing the lesion or lesions that constitute the patient's primary skin complaint. Because there are hundreds of described dermatoses, the systematic approach is based on pattern recognition.

Physical Examination

SETTING. A skin examination can be conducted in virtually any medical setting. It is most effectively performed in an office equipped with an examination table, adequate natural or artificial fluorescent lighting, examination gowns for patients to wear, and a sink for thorough handwashing before and after each examination. If natural light through a window is used, it is critical to ensure the patient's privacy inside the examination room. A movable focused artificial light beam and a lighted magnifying glass can be used to shine obliquely on the skin to assess the elevation of skin lesions. Many dermatologists prefer to examine all lesions at a 1:1 ratio without magnification, but others prefer magnifying certain types of lesions to ascertain morphologic features. For example, the follicular plugging of the lesions of discoid lupus erythematosus (Chapter 287) or the telangiectasias associated with a basal cell carcinoma (Chapters 214 and 466) may be better appreciated with magnification. Gowns that can be positioned to uncover parts of the skin surface while leaving other parts covered help ensure the patient's comfort during the examination.

PRECAUTIONS. Universal precautions against infectious diseases should be practiced during every skin examination or cutaneous procedure. Handwashing with soap and warm water ensures that the physician is taking appropriate steps to avoid spreading organisms from a previous patient. When examining intact skin, it is not necessary to wear gloves. For the protection of both the patient and physician, gloves should be worn when the physician touches nonintact skin surfaces. Because of the increasing incidence of allergies to latex in the health care setting, nonlatex gloves should be used for all patients. Gloves should be discarded after the examination is complete or after touching the mouth or the genital area.

TOTAL BODY EXAMINATION. A total body skin examination is usually recommended for each new patient to assess existing pigmented lesions and determine whether any are serious, although there are no data to document the yield of such an approach (Chapter 13). With the steady increase in squamous cell carcinoma, basal cell carcinoma, and cutaneous melanomas over the past several decades, the total body skin examination is an opportunity to diagnose lesions in an early treatable stage as well as to educate patients about their own risk factors for developing skin cancer. Subsequently, total body skin examinations can be scheduled at 3- to 12-month intervals for patients at high risk for developing new or recurrent malignant lesions (Chapter 214), whereas patients at low risk should be examined at less frequent intervals, such as every 1 to 3 years.

Many dermatologists approach this examination by using the following sequence: face (forehead, eyelids, lips, ears, nose, cheeks, chin), neck, scalp and hair, back, chest, abdomen, arms, hands (including palms and fingernails), legs, and feet (including soles and toenails). Having the patient change into a comfortable gown with undergarments removed facilitates the ease of the examination. Some dermatologists perform part of the examination with the patient in a sitting position and part of the examination with the patient lying back on the examination table. The goal is to ensure that the skin can be well visualized and that the patient is comfortable with the amount of skin being exposed at one time.

ASSESSING SKIN FEATURES. Basic skin features such as skin pigmentation, skin turgor, abnormal skin color (jaundice, pallor), and the degree of photodamage to sun-exposed skin surfaces should be assessed, and these findings guide the medical history and subsequent, detailed examination. For example, patients with lightly pigmented skin and evident photodamage to the hands and face warrant a careful history to inquire about prior skin cancers in themselves and their immediate family members as well as a full body skin examination to look for precancerous or potentially malignant lesions of which the patient may be unaware. Patients with abnormal skin color, such as a yellow hue (jaundice; Chapter 150) should be questioned about known medical conditions, examined for any other cutaneous signs associated with disease of that organ, and assessed with the appropriate laboratory studies.

It is often helpful to touch the lesion and the skin surrounding the lesion. Features such as firmness, movability from the underlying skin, fluctuance, and depressibility are helpful in characterizing the lesion. Darier's sign, which is the appearance of an urticarial wheal and flare reaction after rubbing a skin lesion, is observed in lesions that contain large numbers of mast cells (e.g., urticaria pigmentosa) and is the result of the mechanical degranulation of the mast cells and the resulting release of histamine. Nikolsky's sign is dislodgement of the epidermis with the appearance of a moist, glistening defect after pushing, rubbing, or rotating normal skin near bullous lesions; this sign is typical of disorders in which epidermal cells are not well adhered together (e.g., pemphigus and toxic epidermal necrolysis).

Obtaining the History

After seeing and palpating the lesion, the physician can obtain a more detailed history and continue with a more comprehensive examination of the skin as indicated. Pertinent questions should assess duration of the lesion or eruption, what the lesion looked like when it first began, how the lesion feels (e.g., itch, sting, tenderness, pain), and how the condition has changed since it was first noticed. It is also helpful to inquire about a history of prior similar lesions and how they progressed. A medication history is important because both systemic and topical medications can cause or exacerbate a number of skin conditions. It is also important to inquire specifically about how the patient may have tried to treat the lesion because many treatments can change the natural appearance of the lesion.

The past medical history should be targeted to obtain information about major illnesses, especially those that would lead to immunodeficiency states, as well as prior dermatologic diseases. The presence of known heritable dermatologic conditions in the family should be determined. In particular, patients should be specifically questioned about a personal or family history of atopic dermatitis, hay fever, or asthma (atopy). All patients should be asked about a personal or family history of malignant melanoma and nonmelanoma skin cancers. The social and work history can also provide critical clues to the diagnosis of a particular skin condition because many are related to occupational or recreational activities. A travel history to determine whether patients have encountered environmental stresses such as sun, heat, or cold or have been exposed to parasitic infestations can also be useful. Because psychological stress can exacerbate many dermatoses, it is useful to inquire about overall levels of anxiety and stress or recent stressful situations.

After visualizing the lesion of concern, it is often helpful to look systematically at all the skin again. It is also important to watch the patient's behavior in the examination room. Many patients think that they should not scratch lesions and they tell the physician that the lesions itch but that they do not scratch. However, direct observation shows the patient rubbing, tapping, scratching, or picking the lesion while engaged in conversation with the physician. These behaviors can change a primary lesion to a secondary lesion.

Melanoma

Patients at high risk for the development of melanoma require the most comprehensive skin examinations, commonly by a dermatologist. Photography (conventional or digital) as well as detailed "maps" of the nevi are used over time to assess changes in lesions or the presence of new lesions that warrant removal. A hair dryer at the low setting can be used to blow aside the hair to allow visualization of the entire scalp. The skin of the external and internal labia is examined for pigmented lesions in women. The comprehensive skin examination is also an ideal opportunity to educate the patient about performing self-examinations that include exposed and unexposed skin including the buttocks, posterior thighs, and calves.

DIAGNOSING SKIN DISEASES

Categorization of Skin Lesions

Four major features of skin lesions or eruptions allow the skin disease to be placed in diagnostic categories that facilitate specific diagnosis: (1) the morphologic appearance of the individual lesions, (2) the distribution of lesions over the body surface, (3) the arrangement of the lesions, and (4) the number of lesions present. This information also enables the physician to determine whether the lesions are primary or secondary in nature. Primary lesions are defined as those that represent the initial pathologic change; secondary lesions result from external forces such as scratching, picking, or infection of primary lesions. An experienced dermatologist can often make the diagnosis from this descriptive information before even seeing the patient.

Morphology of Lesions

The morphology of individual lesions can be described in the following ways (Table 462–1): (1) whether they are flat, raised above the surface of the skin, or depressed; (2) the range of their size; (3) whether they are solid or contain fluid; and (4) how their color compares with the patient's normal skin. Morphologic terms have been developed to assess alterations in the stratum corneum and dermal or subcutaneous tissue. For example, the stratum corneum in psoriatic plaques can be silvery in color with densely adherent layers so that it looks like the mineral mica; this pattern is called a *micaceous scale.* Another usual morphologic feature is whether the individual lesions are monomorphic or polymorphic: all monomorphic lesions are the same shape, size, color, and consistency. Certain diseases, such as eruptive xanthoma, almost always have monomorphic papules, whereas other diseases, such as acne, are more likely to have polymorphic lesions that may represent either changes over time or a basic variability.

Distribution of Lesions

Many skin diseases commonly affect particular parts of the body surface (Table 462–2). In certain cases, the pattern of distribution is consistent with our understanding of the pathogenesis of a disease. For

TABLE 462–1 TERMINOLOGY TO DESCRIBE THE MORPHOLOGY OF INDIVIDUAL SKIN LESIONS

Term	Definition	Example
PRIMARY SKIN LESIONS: INITIAL PATHOLOGIC CHANGE		
Macule	Circumscribed change in skin color that is flush with the surrounding skin. Lesion is <1 cm in diameter	Solar lentigo Traumatic purpura
Patch	Circumscribed change in skin color that is flush with the surrounding skin. Lesion is ≥1 cm in diameter	Cafe au lait spot Vitiligo
Papule	A solid or cystic elevation <1 cm in diameter	Acne Eruptive xanthoma
Nodule	A solid or cystic elevation >1 cm but <2 cm in diameter	Dermatofibroma
Tumor	A solid or cystic elevation >2 cm in diameter	Follicular cyst
Plaque	An elevated lesion that is >1 cm in diameter	Psoriasis
Scale	Desiccated, thin plates of cornified epidermal cells that form flakes on the skin surface	Ichthyosis
Wheal	Circumscribed, flat-topped, firm elevation of skin with a well-demarcated and palpable margin	Urticaria
Vesicle	Circumscribed, elevated lesion containing clear serous or hemorrhagic fluid that is <1 cm in diameter	Contact dermatitis Herpes simplex
Bulla	Circumscribed, elevated lesion containing clear serous or hemorrhagic fluid that is >2 cm in diameter	Bullous pemphigoid
Pustule	A vesicle containing purulent exudate	Folliculitis
Atrophy	A depression from the surface of the skin with underlying loss of epidermal or dermal substance	Lichen sclerosis et atrophicus
Erosion	A depression from the surface of the skin with a loss of all or part of the epidermis Can be a secondary lesion	Burn Ruptured bulla
Ulceration	A depression from the surface of the skin with a loss of the entire epidermis and at least some of the dermis Can be a secondary lesion	Ecthyma Excoriation of acne papule
SECONDARY SKIN LESIONS: RESULT FROM EXTERNAL FORCES SUCH AS SCRATCHING, PICKING, INFECTION, OR HEALING OF PRIMARY LESIONS		
Lichenification	Dry, leathery thickening of the skin with exaggerated skin markings	Chronic eczema
Scar	An elevated or depressed area of fibrosis of the dermis or subcutaneous tissue resulting from an antecedent destructive process	Healing wound
Fissure	A deep linear split in the skin extending through the epidermis	Traumatized eczema
Crust	Dried exudates of serum, blood, sebum, or purulent material on the surface of the skin	Acute and/or secondarily infected eczema

example, acne lesions are found on the parts of the skin that contain the highest concentration of sebaceous glands, which are known to be involved in the development of acne. Other skin diseases are precipitated or caused by sun exposure, and their lesions are present only in sun-exposed areas of the body (e.g., lupus erythematosus or phototoxic drug eruptions). Dermatologic disorders that are the direct result of the patient's manipulation of the skin are found only where the patient can reach (e.g., the posterior shoulders but not the middle of the back).

The pattern of distribution, although poorly understood from a pathogenetic perspective, is extremely helpful for diagnosis (Fig. 462–1). For example, psoriasis often symmetrically affects the scalp, extensor arms and legs (elbows, knees, and shins), umbilicus, intragluteal cleft, and fingernails (Fig. 462–2; Chapter 464). Psoriatic lesions can involve the entire body surface, but an awareness of its common distribution guides the physical examination and aids accurate diagnosis. Conversely, atopic dermatitis (Chapter 464) typically often involves the flexural arms and legs (antecubital fossae and popliteal fossae), wrists, nipples, and eyelids.

TABLE 462–2 PREFERENTIAL DISTRIBUTION OF SELECTED SKIN DISEASES

Distribution on the Skin	Skin Disease
Skin chronically exposed to sunlight (face, neck, hands, arms)	Actinic keratosis, basal cell carcinoma, squamous cell carcinoma
Central chest, shoulders, and earlobes	Keloids
Extensor arms and legs, intragluteal cleft, umbilicus	Psoriasis
Antecubital fossa, popliteal fossa	Atopic dermatitis
Anterior surface of lower legs	Palpable purpura, pretibial myxedema, necrobiosis lipoidica diabeticorum, erythema nodosum
Axilla and inguinal areas	Hidradenitis suppurativa
Posterior neck and back	Folliculitis
Web spaces of toes and sides of feet	Tinea pedis
Web spaces of fingers and wrists	Scabies
Palms and soles	Secondary syphilis, erythema multiforme

It is important to examine the mucous membranes of the mouth and the genital areas. Lichen planus (Chapter 464), a papulosquamous skin disease, often involves the volar wrists, shins, buccal mucosa, and shaft of the penis. In lichen planus, the oral and genital lesions may be asymptomatic and the medical history cannot substitute for a careful physical examination.

Arrangement of Lesions

The arrangement of several lesions in relation to each other can provide valuable diagnostic information. Terms that are commonly used to describe the relationship of lesions to each other include *clustered, grouped, linear, zosteriform, annular,* and *coalescing* (Table 462–3). *Clustered* lesions are arranged within a few millimeters of each other. When vesicular lesions are clustered on an erythematous base, the word *herpetiform* is used to describe their arrangement because this is the classical appearance of herpes simplex (Fig. 462–3; Chapters 397 and 465). *Grouped* lesions are arranged in the same body site, such as over a shoulder or elbow. A *linear* arrangement of lesions looks like a geometric line over any part of the body surface. One type of linear arrangement is called *Koebnerization* (or the Koebner phenomenon), which occurs in particular skin diseases, such as psoriasis, in which new lesions evolve after traumatic injury. Linear lesions are frequently seen in allergic contact dermatitis if the offending antigen brushed against the skin to create a

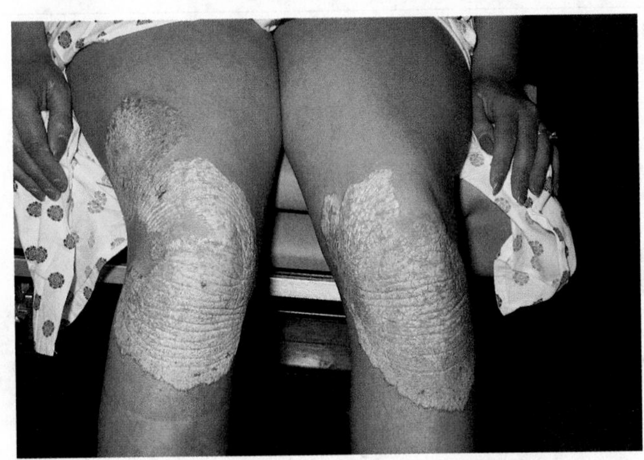

FIGURE 462–2 • The distribution of psoriatic lesions is often symmetrical over the extensor surfaces of the skin.

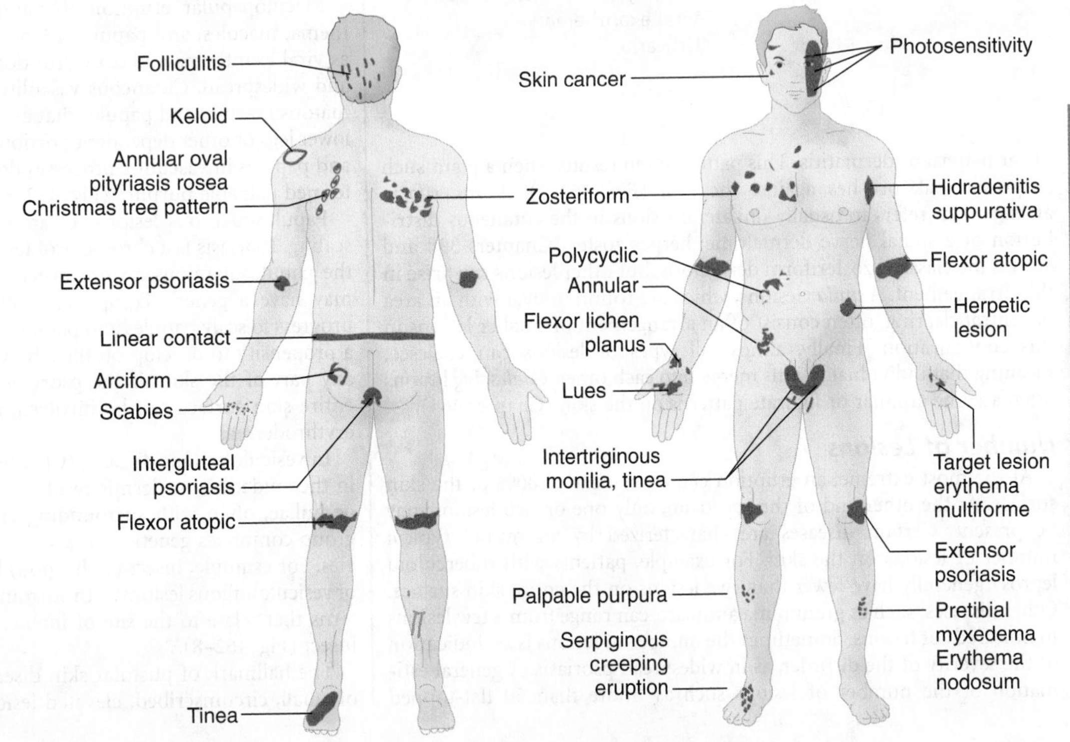

FIGURE 462–1 • Configurational and regional diagnostic aids for the diagnosis of primary and secondary skin lesions.

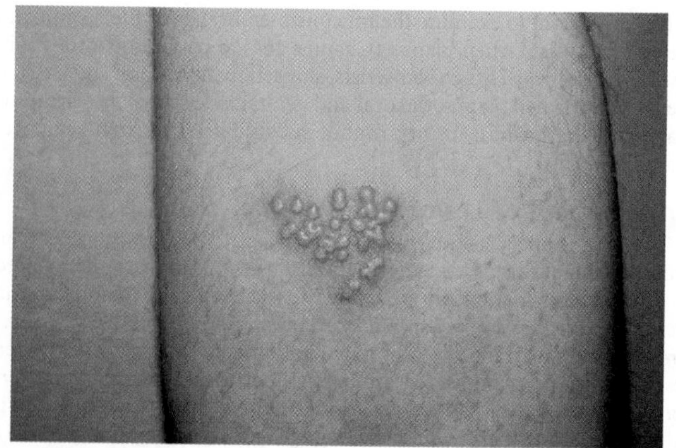

FIGURE 462–3 • This arrangement of vesicular lesions clustered on an erythematous base, seen here in a patient with herpes simplex, is termed *herpetiform*.

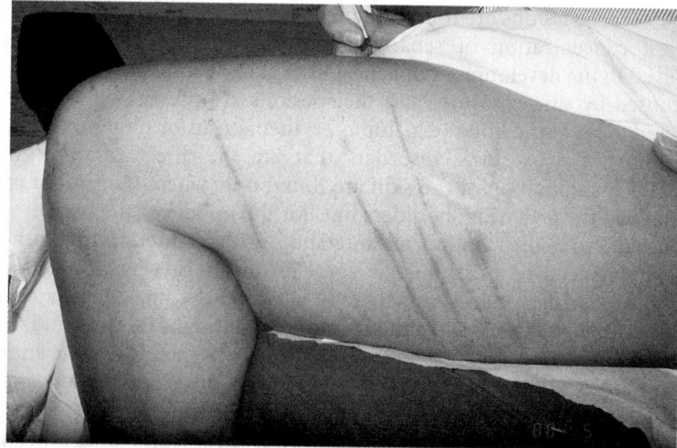

FIGURE 462–4 • Allergic contact dermatitis occurring in a linear arrangement when the offending antigen, such as poison oak, is brushed against the skin in this way.

TABLE 462–3 ARRANGEMENT OF SKIN LESIONS

Type of Arrangement	Example of Skin Disease
Clustered	Herpes simplex
Grouped	Lichen planus Granuloma annulare Dermatitis herpetiformis
Linear	Allergic contact dermatitis Epidermal nevus Morphea Koebnerized psoriasis
Zosteriform	Herpes zoster Metastatic breast carcinoma Hemangiomas of Sturge-Weber syndrome
Annular without scale	Secondary syphilis Lupus erythematosus Urticaria Hansen's disease (leprosy)
Annular with scale	Dermatophytosis Pityriasis rosea Erythema annulare centrifugum
Coalescing	Psoriasis Drug hypersensitivity eruption Viral exanthema Urticaria

linear pattern of dermatitis. This pattern often results when a plant such as poison oak brushes against the skin (Fig. 462–4). A *zosteriform* arrangement refers to usually unilateral lesions in the cutaneous distribution of a spinal nerve dermatome; herpes zoster (Chapters 398 and 465) is the classical zosteriform dermatosis, but other lesions can arise in this arrangement. *Annular* lesions, which are round to oval with an area of central clearing, often consist of an arrangement of smaller lesions in this configuration. Finally, almost all types of lesions can coalesce, meaning that individual lesions merge into each other. *Coalescing* lesions often assume annular or figurate patterns on the skin (Chapter 464).

Number of Lesions

At the most extreme, an eruption can cover nearly 100% of the skin surface. At the other end of the spectrum, only one or two lesions may be present. Certain diseases are characterized by an overall typical number of lesions on the skin. For example, patients with tuberculoid leprosy generally have fewer than five lesions on the entire skin surface. Other diseases, such as granuloma annulare, can range from a few lesions to hundreds of lesions. Sometimes the number of lesions is an indication of the severity of the disorder, as in widespread psoriasis. A general estimation of the number of lesions such as "more than 50 flat-topped papules distributed on the shins and wrists bilaterally" or "8 to 10 orange-colored papules on each elbow" can also assist in guiding the physician to the correct diagnosis.

Major Classifications

After carefully identifying the clinical features of skin lesions or eruptions, the physician can use the recognized patterns to classify the disease into a general category of skin disorders. The ability to identify the clinical features of a lesion's morphology allows cutaneous disorders to be placed in categories that narrow the differential diagnosis to a reasonable number of choices, which can then be further refined by considering the distribution, arrangement, and number of lesions (Table 462–4).

Eczematous dermatitis (Chapter 464) is a common superficial skin inflammation that is characterized by erythematous macules and papules in the early and mild stages. These changes can progress to vesiculation, oozing, fine scaling, and crusting. Because eczematous dermatitis is associated with pruritus (itching), the patient often excoriates the involved skin. In the chronic setting, lichenification caused by repeated rubbing is a typical secondary clinical feature of eczematous dermatitis. The localized distribution of an eczematous eruption at the site of allergen exposure helps distinguish allergic contact dermatitis (Fig. 462–5) from other types of eczematous dermatoses, such as atopic dermatitis and stasis dermatitis, that tend to be bilaterally symmetrical and involve particular areas of the skin.

Maculopapular eruptions (Chapter 465) are characterized by erythema, macules, and papules. Many of these cutaneous eruptions, such as viral exanthems and drug eruptions, are often symmetrical, bilateral, and widespread. Cutaneous vasculitis shows clinical features of erythematous macules and papules that are commonly most prominent on the lower legs or other dependent portions of the skin. When the red macules and papules in vasculitic processes do not blanch with pressure, they are termed palpable purpura (Fig. 462–6).

Papulosquamous lesions (Chapter 464) are defined as papules with scaling. Psoriasis is a chronic proliferative epidermal disease that typifies the papulosquamous skin disorders. This inflammatory disease, which may have a genetic component, often begins with red macules that progress to scaly papules and plaques (Fig. 462–7). Psoriatic plaques have a propensity to develop on the elbows, knees, and scalp but can involve any part of the skin. If the psoriatic process becomes widespread, the entire skin surface can be involved, and the syndrome is then termed erythroderma.

In vesiculobullous diseases (Chapter 465), cleavage at particular levels in the epidermis or dermis results in the clinical appearance of vesicles or bullae, often with surrounding erythema. This broad morphologic group comprises genetic and acquired diseases with a variety of etiologies. For example, insect (arthropod) bite reactions are a common cause of vesiculobullous lesions with surrounding erythema, distributed in patterns that relate to the site of interaction with the particular offending insect (Fig. 462–8).

The hallmark of pustular skin diseases (Chapter 465) is the presence of small, circumscribed, elevated lesions containing purulent exudates,

TABLE 462–4 MORPHOLOGY-BASED CLASSIFICATION OF MAJOR SKIN DISORDERS

Group	Clinical Morphology	Examples of Diseases in the Group
Eczematous dermatitis	Erythematous macules, papules, vesicles, lichenification, fine scaling, excoriations, crusting	Contact dermatitis, atopic dermatitis, stasis dermatitis, photodermatitis, exfoliative dermatitis
Maculopapular eruptions	Macules, erythema, papules	Viral exanthems, drug hypersensitivity reactions, Kawasaki's disease, vasculitic, purpuric eruptions
Papulosquamous dermatoses	Papules, plaques, and erythema with scales	Psoriasis, Reiter's syndrome, pityriasis rosea, lichen planus, seborrheic dermatitis, ichthyosis, secondary syphilis, mycosis fungoides
Vesiculobullous diseases	Vesicles, bullae, erythema	Herpes simplex and zoster, hand-foot-and-mouth disease, insect bites, bullous impetigo, scalded skin syndrome, pemphigus, bullous pemphigoid, dermatitis herpetiformis, porphyria cutanea tarda, erythema multiforme
Pustular diseases	Pustules, cysts, erythema	Acne vulgaris rosacea, pustular psoriasis, folliculitis
Urticaria and cellulitis	Wheals and figured, raised erythema, scaling	Urticaria, erythema annulare centrifugum and erysipelas
Nodular lesions	Nodules and tumors, some associated with erosions and ulceration	Benign and malignant tumors—basal cell cancer, squamous cell cancer, rheumatoid nodules, xanthomas
Telangiectasia, atrophic, scarring, ulcerative diseases	Atrophic, sclerotic telangiectasia, ulcerative changes	Connective tissue diseases, radiation dermatitis, lichen sclerosus et atrophicus, vascular insufficiency (arterial and venous), pyoderma gangrenosum
Hypermelanosis and hypomelanosis	Increased and decreased melanin deposition in skin	Acanthosis nigricans, cafe au lait spots, vitiligo, tuberous sclerosis, xeroderma pigmentosum, melasma, freckles

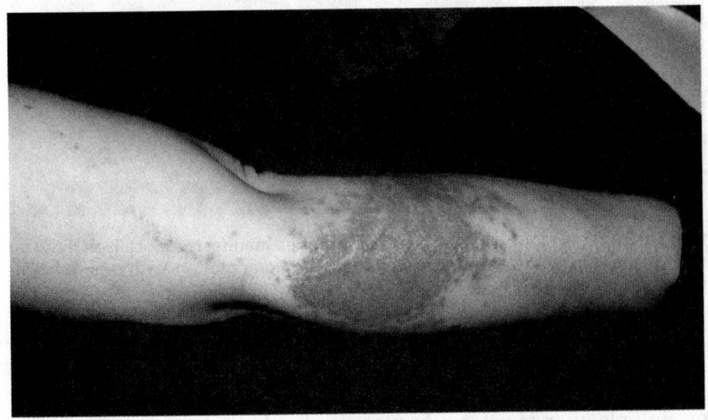

FIGURE 462–5 • Allergic contact dermatitis on the arm at the site of application of a topical antibacterial ointment to treat a burn wound. This cutaneous allergic response manifests as erythematous macules, papules, and vesicles where the allergen comes in contact with the skin.

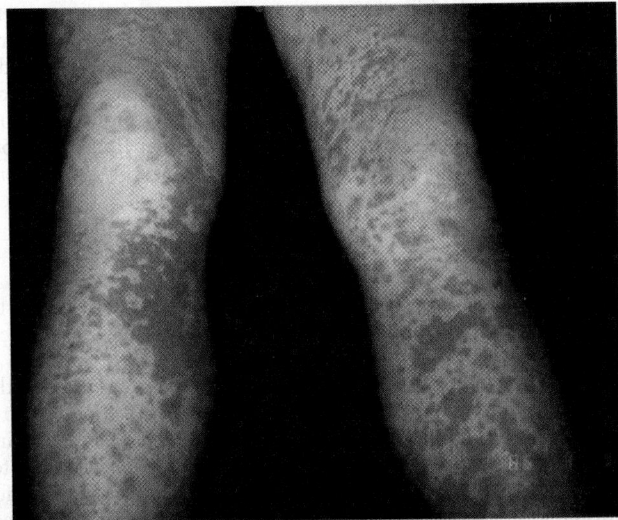

FIGURE 462–6 • Palpable purpura (nonblanching red macules and papules) on the lower legs is typical of many types of cutaneous vasculitis.

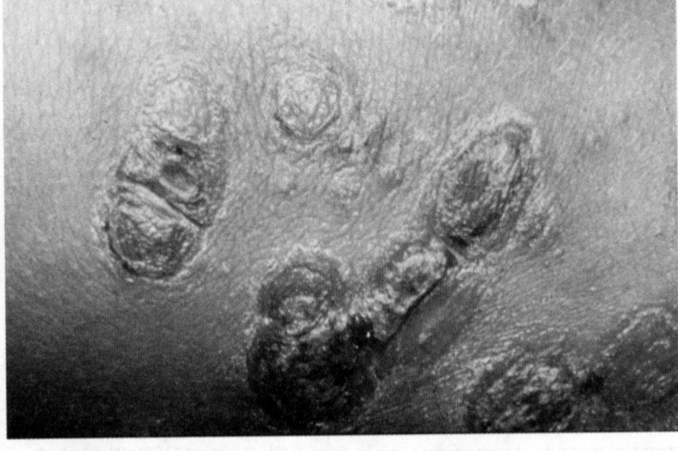

FIGURE 462–7 • Psoriasis is characterized by erythematous, scaling papules and plaques.

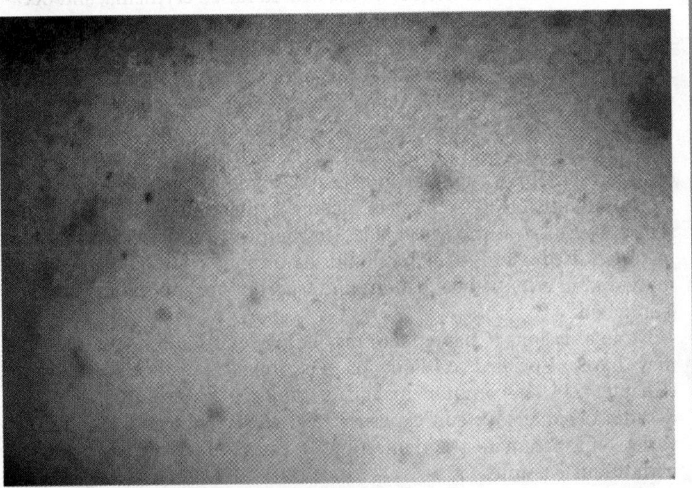

FIGURE 462–8 • Arthropod bite reactions on the skin of the back appear as multiple papulovesicles with surrounding erythema from assault by sand fleas while the patient was sleeping on the beach.

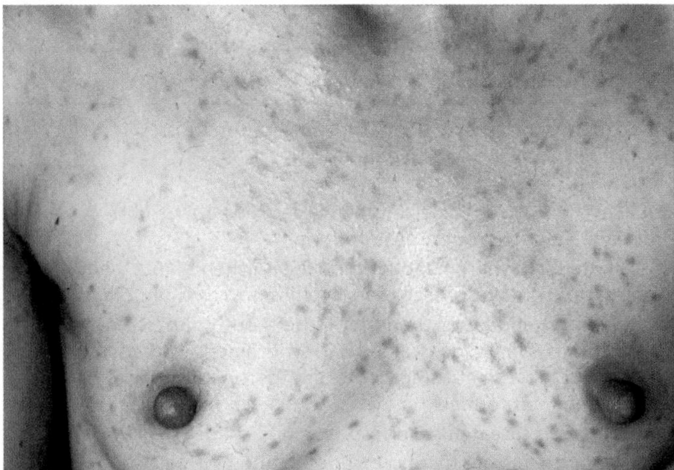

FIGURE 462–9 • Monomorphous follicularly oriented pustules on the chest are seen in pityrosporum folliculitis.

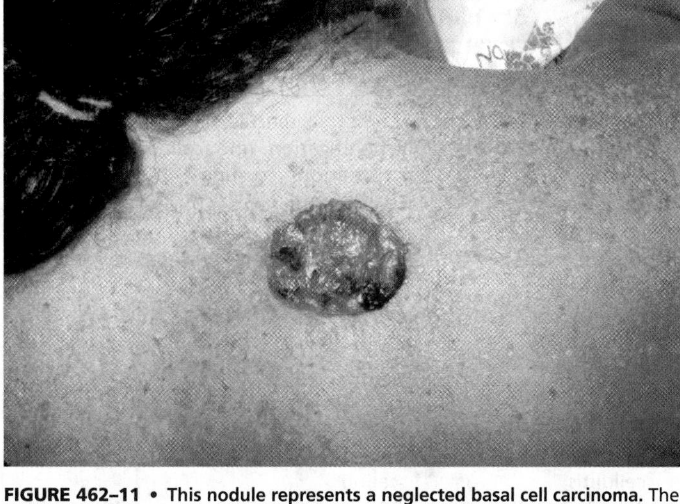

FIGURE 462–11 • This nodule represents a neglected basal cell carcinoma. The lesion is well defined and sharply demarcated from normal skin. The rolled smooth border with telangiectasias surrounds several crusted ulcerations.

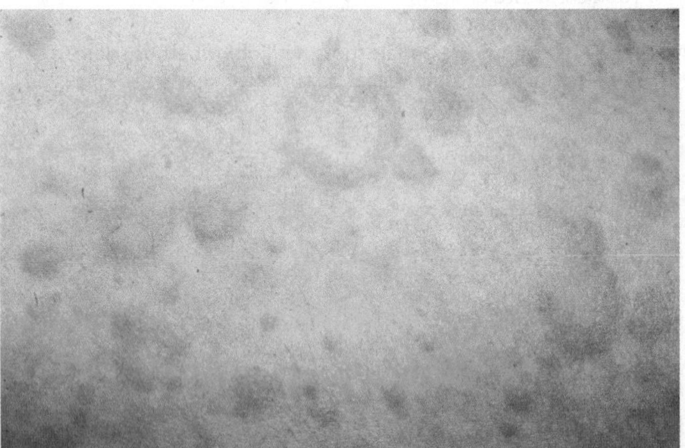

FIGURE 462–10 • This eruption consisting of evanescent, annular wheals is termed urticaria.

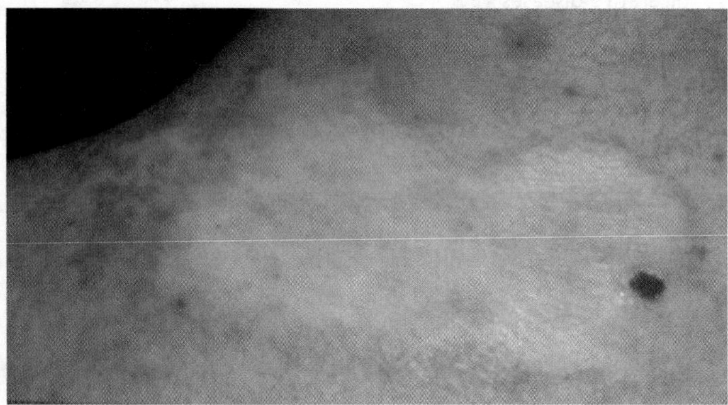

FIGURE 462–12 • This single plaque of morphea manifests as localized induration of the skin with central atrophy and hypopigmentation with a peripheral rim of erythema.

often with associated erythema. Cystic lesions are pustular lesions greater than 1 cm in size. Pustules may be sterile, as in pustular psoriasis, or may contain microbial organisms, as in acne (Chapter 465). Folliculitis is a pustular skin infection located within hair follicles and often surrounded by erythema (Fig. 462–9).

Skin disorders arising as urticaria (Chapter 466) or cellulitis (Chapter 467) share clinical features of wheals, figured raised erythema, and occasionally scaling. Urticaria is an inflammatory mast cell–mediated process that may have an allergic or nonallergic cause and is characterized by clinical lesions called wheals, which are evanescent, erythematous, rounded or flat-topped, elevated (edematous) lesions (Fig. 462–10). Although the borders of a wheal are sharply demarcated, they tend to be transient and may appear and disappear in a matter of hours. Wheals may be round, oval, serpiginous, or annular in appearance and can range in size from several millimeters to over 10 cm. Itching is often intense in the affected skin but resolves as the wheal fades. In contrast to urticaria, the erythematous, raised lesions seen in cellulitis have an infectious cause and tend to expand in a centrifugal pattern until appropriate antibiotic treatment is initiated.

Nodular lesions (Chapter 466) may be single or multiple nodules and may have associated erosions or ulcerations. Basal cell carcinoma (Chapter 214), a common malignant tumor of the skin, is linked to decades of cutaneous sun exposure (Fig. 462–11). In addition, a large variety of inflammatory and infectious diseases of the skin are associated with nodular lesions.

Skin diseases sharing the morphologic features of telangiectasia, atrophy, scarring, and ulceration can be classified together, although there is a wide range of causes, including connective tissue diseases, such as localized or systemic scleroderma. A localized type of cutaneous scleroderma, termed morphea (Chapter 288), is characterized by single or multiple discrete patches or plaques of indurated skin, often accompanied by cutaneous atrophy and pigmentary changes (Fig. 462–12).

Hypermelanosis and hypomelanosis (Chapter 467) occur in a wide range of cutaneous disorders in which there is increased or decreased melanin deposition in the skin. These skin lesions may appear dark (hyperpigmented), as seen with cafe au lait spots, or pale (hypopigmented), as seen with vitiligo. Xeroderma pigmentosum is a rare, genetic disease in which patients cannot repair DNA damage induced by ultraviolet irradiation and develop early freckling that progresses to widespread hypopigmented and hyperpigmented macules over time (Fig. 462–13). Most important, without meticulous protection from ultraviolet irradiation of the skin, these patients suffer from cutaneous neoplasms, including malignant melanoma (Chapter 214), in the early decades of life.

Diagnostic Tests

After a reasonable differential diagnosis has been created, diagnostic tests can narrow the differential or confirm the correct diagnosis (Table 462–5). The potassium hydroxide preparation of scale and pustules is used to look for microscopic hyphae or pseudohyphae that indicate the presence of a dermatophyte infection or yeast infection (Fig. 462–14; Chapter 464). The Gram stain of pustules or bullae is used to determine whether bacteria are present or whether the lesion is sterile (Chapter 465). The Tzanck preparation of the base of a vesicle is used to look for rounded, multinucleated keratinocytes that indicate a herpesvirus infection (Fig. 462–15; Chapter 465). The oil mount of skin scrapings from the base of a burrow or pruritic papule is used to look for the mites or eggs that indicate a scabies infestation (Fig. 462–16; Chapter 380).

Skin Biopsy

When an infection is suspected, it is often necessary to obtain specimens for culture by swabbing pustules, bullae, or abscesses. Any overlying crust should be removed before obtaining the culture specimen. Scale from the surface of the skin can also be sent for fungal culture to increase the detection of dermatophyte infections, especially those involving the nails. If bacterial cellulitis is suspected, tissue from the dermis can be cultured by obtaining a skin biopsy that is sent for culture or by injecting the site with sterile saline and aspirating material to send for culture. To diagnose deep fungal or mycobacterial infections, tissue usually must be obtained by biopsy and sent for culture under appropriate temperature conditions.

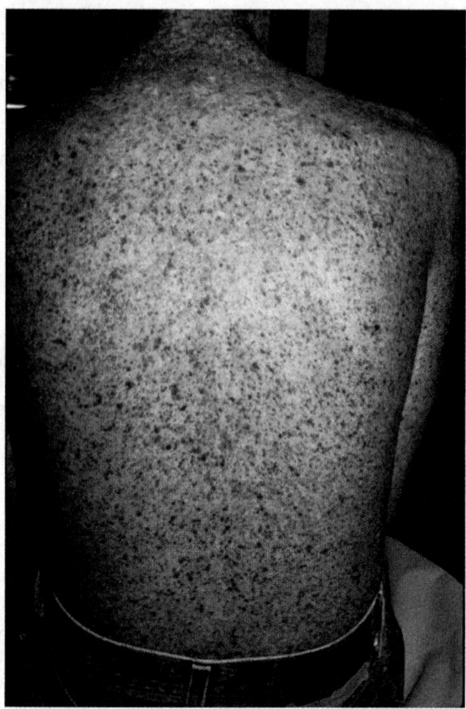

FIGURE 462–13 • Widespread hypopigmented and hyperpigmented macules on sun-exposed skin are a clinical feature of xeroderma pigmentosum after exposure to normal amounts of sunlight over time.

Skin biopsies, which can be performed on growths from inflammatory eruptions, are an essential tool when the diagnosis is not certain (Fig. 462–17). The term *biopsy* may also be applied to the surgical removal of benign skin lesions such as warts and skin tags. Many dermatologists follow the general practice of sending all excised skin tissue for histologic assessment.

Biopsy of Possible Malignancy

Any lesions that have features of basal cell carcinoma or squamous cell carcinoma should be biopsied (Chapters 214 and 466). Clinical indica-

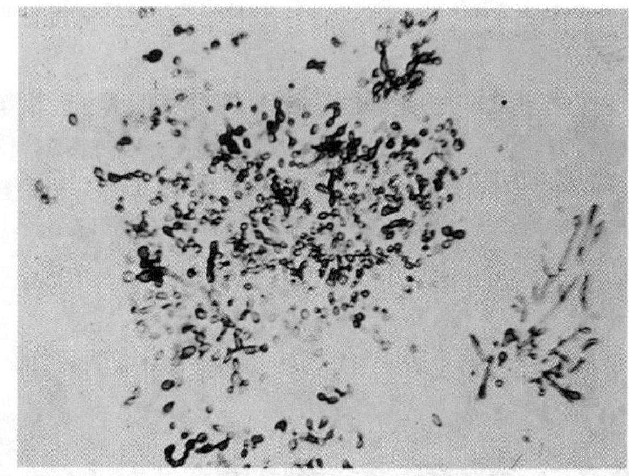

FIGURE 462–14 • *Candida albicans.* Potassium hydroxide examination of candidal skin lesion shows short, stubby hyphae and budding yeast elements.

TABLE 462–5 DIAGNOSTIC TESTING FOR SKIN DISEASES

Diagnostic Test	Material to Obtain	Indications	Findings
TESTS PROCESSED IN THE OFFICE			
Potassium hydroxide preparation and microscopic examination	Skin scraping from scale or pustules	Presence of scale or pustules	Hyphae or pseudohyphae indicating dermatophyte or yeast infection
Gram stain and microscopic examination	Skin scraping from pustules or bullae	Presence of pustules or bullae	Gram-positive or gram-negative bacteria
Tzanck stain and microscopic examination	Skin scraping from the base of a vesicle	Presence of vesicles	Rounded, multinucleated keratinocytes indicating a herpesvirus infection
Oil mount and microscopic examination	Skin scraping from the base of a burrow or nonexcoriated papule	Presence of burrows or pruritic papules	Mites or eggs indicating scabies infestation
TESTS PROCESSED IN AN OUTSIDE LABORATORY			
Punch biopsy	Core of anesthetized skin using a punch biopsy instrument	Lesions suspected to be malignant (such as BCC or SCC) or an undiagnosed inflammatory skin lesion	Microscopic alterations in the epidermis, dermis, and subcutaneous tissue
Shave or snip biopsy	All or part of an anesthetized skin lesion that protrudes from the surface of the skin	Raised lesions suspected to be malignant (such as BCC or SCC) or bothersome raised lesions	Microscopic alterations in the epidermis and the upper dermis
Excisional biopsy	An entire anesthetized skin lesion	Lesions suspected to be malignant (such as melanoma) or bothersome flat lesions	Microscopic alterations in the epidermis, dermis, and subcutaneous tissue with the entire architecture of the lesion in the specimen

BCC = basal cell carcinoma; SCC = squamous cell carcinoma.

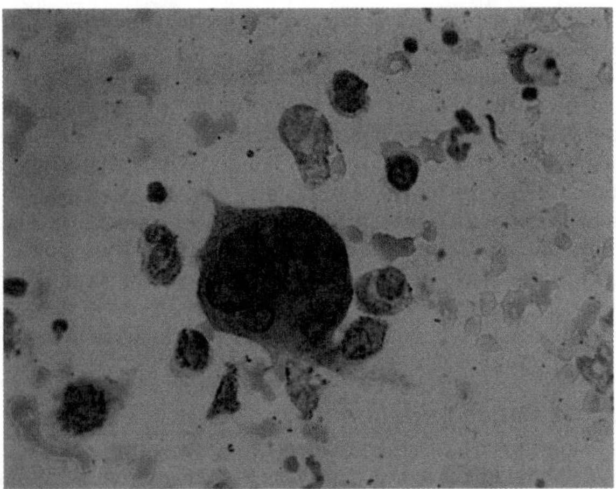

FIGURE 462–15 • Tzanck smear of herpes simplex. Positive Tzanck smear is seen as multinucleated giant cell.

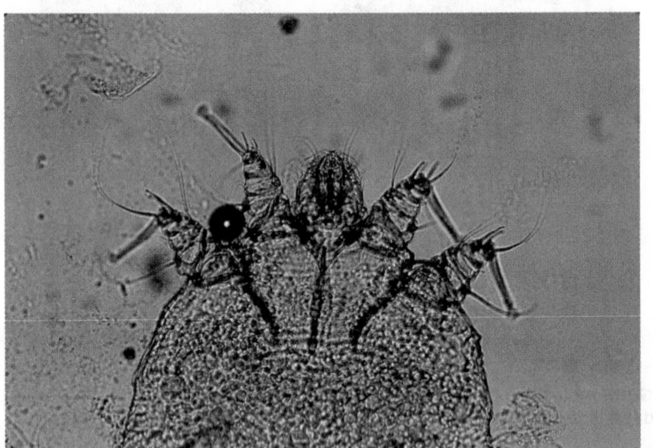

FIGURE 462–16 • A scabies mite is seen on this microscopic examination of an oil mount of a scraping taken from the end of a small burrow on the wrist.

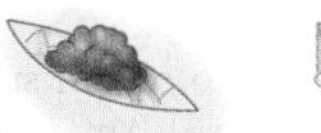
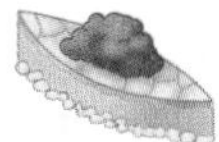

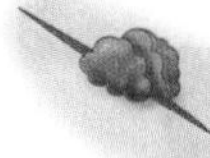
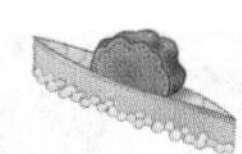

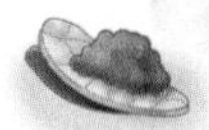
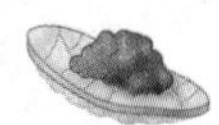

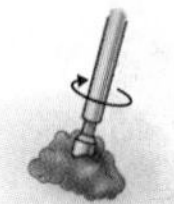
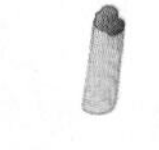

FIGURE 462–17 • Methods of skin biopsy.

tions for biopsy of lesions suspected to be malignant include lesions that fail to heal, increase in size, bleed easily, or ulcerate spontaneously. Actinic keratoses, which are considered to be precancerous lesions, are usually treated without preceding biopsy. The usual biopsy approach to non-melanotic lesions that protrude from the surface of the skin is to perform either a snip biopsy (with scissors) or a shave biopsy (with a blade). If the entire lesion is removed, it can be considered an excisional biopsy.

Punch Biopsy

For inflammatory skin lesions, it is usually necessary to obtain tissue down to subcutaneous fat for an accurate assessment of the inflammatory process. A punch biopsy using an instrument 3 to 8 mm in diameter to "core out" a piece of skin tissue is the preferred approach. If multiple lesions are present, it is prudent to select a lesion that is not in a cosmetically important area because a scar will occur at the punch biopsy site but to be sure to select a representative lesion that has not been altered by scratching, infection, or lichenification. The punch biopsy wound heals best when closed with one to two sutures, but it can be left to heal by granulation. Some inflammatory skin disorders, especially bullous disorders, have characteristic autoantibody deposition that can be assessed by direct immunofluorescence of biopsy tissue. This test is performed in specialized dermatopathology laboratories.

The approach to biopsying lesions that have clinical features of malignant melanoma is critical. First, there is only one opportunity to obtain tissue correctly to maximize the chance of accurate diagnosis. Second, an improperly obtained biopsy can make it impossible to assess the patient's risk of metastatic disease. When malignant melanoma is suspected, the lesion should be removed entirely with an elliptic excisional biopsy; margins of normal skin are not included in the biopsied tissue. A shave biopsy should be avoided because it does not allow the full depth of the lesions to be determined histologically. The thickness of the lesion remains the most accurate way to predict metastatic disease and is critical for planning adjuvant therapy (Chapters 214 and 466). A punch biopsy should be avoided because it does not provide the dermatopathologist with the full histologic architecture of the lesion. When clinical features of a pigmented lesion of the skin are highly suggestive of malignant melanoma, the patient should usually be referred to a dermatologist before performing the biopsy to ensure that the most accurate histologic information is obtained to guide clinical treatment.

SUGGESTED READINGS

Argenziano G, Puig S, Zalaudek I, et al: Dermoscopy improves accuracy of primary care physicians to triage lesions suggestive of skin cancer. J Clin Oncol 2006;24:1877–1882. *Dermoscopy improves diagnosis by primary care physicians.*

Losina E, Walensky RP, Geller A, et al: Visual screening for malignant melanoma: A cost-effectiveness analysis. Arch Dermatol 2007;143:21–28. *One-time screening for melanoma in persons older than 50 appears to be cost effective.*

Moore MM, Geller AC, Zhang Z, et al: Skin cancer examination teaching in US medical education. Arch Dermatol 2006;142:439–444. *Demonstrates need for better training.*

463 PRINCIPLES OF THERAPY

Victoria P. Werth

The goal of therapy is to improve a skin condition with the least toxic and most specific approach. Because many treatments or medications can be applied directly to the skin, the option for topical therapy is attractive for treating many dermatologic diseases. However, many diseases require systemic therapies, particularly when patients have widespread involvement of the skin or a disease that cannot be improved with topical therapy. Therapies work by improving barrier function, removing scale, altering inflammation in the skin, altering blood flow, providing antimicrobial effects, or affecting proliferating cells. Recent advances in the understanding of cutaneous biology have not been routinely accompanied by evidence-based documentation of the benefits of many specific therapies.

PRINCIPLES OF TOPICAL THERAPY

Soaks and Dressings

Water or saline applied by soaks and wet dressings can be beneficial for many skin conditions, including ulcers, by promoting healing of the

epidermis and débridement of crusts. Soaked gauze is applied to involved areas for 15 to 30 minutes several times a day, and care should be taken not to allow the gauze to dry and adhere. If adherence occurs, the gauze should be soaked before the dressing is removed. Use of strong antiseptic solutions, including hydrogen peroxide, is not recommended because of toxicity to cells. Whirlpool action can enhance débridement. When large areas of skin are involved, baths are a convenient way to treat the skin with medications that reduce itching and inflammation. The best time to apply moisturizers that help trap water in the upper layers of skin is immediately after a bath or shower.

Wet-to-dry dressings are rarely used, except when initial vigorous wound débridement is necessary. Continued use after wounds are débrided traumatizes wounds and delays healing. Moist wound healing, which is often ideal, can be accomplished using a topical antibiotic such as a combination of polymyxin B and bacitracin (Polysporin) or mupirocin (Bactroban), gauze impregnated with petrolatum (Vaseline), or an occlusive hydrocolloid dressing. Little evidence indicates that débriding enzymes are beneficial. Compression with an Unna or multilayered boot, which includes an elastic dressing such as COBAN, can decrease local edema and can facilitate wound healing. Polysporin/petrolatum gauze or occlusive dressings are placed underneath, an approach that is helpful for chronic venous, diabetic, and pressure ulcers, as well as for acute wounds. Closed wet dressings, in which gauze is soaked and is then covered with an impervious material, can help when maceration and heat retention are needed. Biologic dressings with skin substitutes or keratinocytes can be beneficial for wounds that are resistant to healing. Skin grafts can also facilitate healing of otherwise nonhealing wounds. Platelet-derived growth factor, which is approved for use in diabetic ulcers, can modestly improve wound healing.

Topical Medications

Topical medications mix an active drug with preservatives, emulsifying agents, and an appropriate base or vehicle. Systemic absorption varies among patients, sites, and vehicles. Topically applied drugs are absorbed more readily through inflamed, thin skin. The base can be any of the following: a *powder,* which promotes dryness and is used to reduce maceration in intertriginous area; a *lotion,* which is a suspension of oil in water; *solutions,* which include water, alcohol, and propylene glycol, but not oil; *gels,* which are solid at room temperature but melt on contact with the skin; a *cream,* which is an emulsion of oil in water that leaves a thin oil coating as the water evaporates; an *ointment,* which combines oils, such as petrolatum (Vaseline), with small amounts of water, and which is more occlusive and hence increases the absorption of medication but also results in a greasier appearance; a *paste,* which is a mixture of powder and ointment; or a *spray.* Lotions, solutions, and gels provide less penetration than ointments, but they are especially useful for treatment of hair-bearing areas such as the scalp, where greasiness is displeasing. Creams are less greasy than ointments and are useful for the face, groin, and intertriginous areas. Ointments are often more effective for dry, scaly conditions such as eczema and psoriasis and are helpful in areas such as the palms and soles that have thick skin, but they should be avoided in infected or intertriginous areas. The choice of base is determined by the skin condition and location. Impregnated tapes are another delivery method to provide occlusion and to protect the skin from manipulation.

ANTI-INFLAMMATORY AGENTS

Glucocorticoids

Topical glucocorticoids work because of their effects on vasoconstriction, proliferation, immunosuppression, and inflammation. Assays related to the ability to vasoconstrict and clinical trials of efficacy have allowed the division of glucocorticoids into various classes based on potency (Table 463–1). These medications are typically used twice a day. Side effects include atrophy of the skin, telangiectasias, purpura, striae, local skin infections (e.g., folliculitis, tinea, and candidiasis), hypopigmentation, hypertrichosis, systemic adrenal suppression when these agents are used on as little as 20% diseased skin surface area, and glaucoma when they are used around the eye. Side effects are especially prevalent when fluorinated steroids are used on thin skin (e.g., face, groin, or scrotum), and prolonged use on the face can result in facial dermatitis, acne, and an eruption resembling acne rosacea that often is exacerbated when use of the steroid is terminated. Certain conditions are more responsive to steroids, and the steroid's potency must be chosen based on the condition and location (Table 463–2). The superpotent class I agents should be restricted to patients with severe dermatoses, and their use should normally not exceed 2 weeks. Patients who receive these potent agents require frequent follow-up and must be carefully evaluated for the need to continue strong topical steroids. Use of any fluorinated steroid on the face requires an exact diagnosis and should be limited in the extent of application and duration of use. Intralesional glucocorticoids can be injected into individual lesions to improve delivery of the medication, and this method is commonly used to treat patients with acne cysts, hypertrophic scars, keloids, alopecia areata, granuloma annulare, discoid and panniculitic lupus erythematosus (Chapter 287), psoriasis, and lichen simplex chronicus. Triamcinolone acetonide is most frequently used, followed by the longer-acting triamcinolone hexacetonide. It is important to use proper dilutions, such as 2.5 mg/mL on the face and 5 mg/mL elsewhere, to avoid local skin atrophy.

Systemic glucocorticoids are used for acute and chronic conditions in dermatology, but they should be avoided, if possible, or minimized because of their well-known side effects (Chapter 33). Acute conditions that commonly require systemic steroids include severe contact dermatitis such as poison ivy, photodermatitis, severe atopic dermatitis, and acute urticaria. Many skin conditions such as psoriasis and eczema become exacerbated when steroids are tapered, so steroids should be avoided when possible in these conditions. The dose of steroid must be individualized to the condition and severity of the presentation. Steroid-sparing drugs, such as immunosuppressive agents, can be used to minimize the long-term use of steroids in selected conditions.

TABLE 463–1 RANKING OF SOME COMMONLY USED TOPICAL STEROIDS BY POTENCY

Super potency	Clobetasol propionate (Temovate ointment and cream), betamethasone dipropionate (Diprolene cream and ointment), diflorasone diacetate (Psorcon E ointment), halobetasol propionate (Ultravate ointment)
High potency	Amcinonide, mometasone furoate ointment, diflorasone diacetate (Florone ointment), halcinonide 0.1% cream, fluocinonide, desoximetasone, triamcinolone acetonide, diflorasone diacetate ointment and cream, betamethasone dipropionate (Diprosone), betamethasone benzoate and valerate
Medium potency	Fluticasone propionate, mometasone furoate cream, halcinonide 0.25% ointment, triamcinolone acetonide 0.1% cream and lotion, fluocinolone acetonide 0.2%, 0.25%, and 0.1% cream and 0.25% ointment and 0.5% solution, hydrocortisone valerate 0.2% ointment and cream, alclometasone dipropionate 0.5% ointment, betamethasone dipropionate 0.5% lotion, hydrocortisone butyrate 0.1% cream, betamethasone benzoate 0.25% cream, betamethasone valerate 0.1% cream and 0.5% lotion, flumethasone pivalate 0.3% cream, desonide 0.5% cream
Low potency	Hydrocortisone 1% cream

TABLE 463–2 CLINICAL APPLICATION OF TOPICAL GLUCOCORTICOIDS

Super potency and high potency	Plaque and palmoplantar psoriasis, lichen planus, dyshidrotic eczema, lichen simplex chronicus, granuloma annulare, sarcoidosis
Medium potency	Dermatitis: allergic contact, atopic, neurodermatitis
Low potency	Intertrigo, pruritus ani, seborrheic dermatitis

Nonsteroidal Anti-inflammatory Agents

PSORIASIS THERAPIES. Tars and anthralin are used for psoriasis (Chapter 464). Tars are most commonly used in conjunction with ultraviolet B (UVB) light, as part of the Goeckerman regimen. Tars are also used in shampoos and bath oils to treat seborrhea and psoriasis. Anthralin is a synthetic hydroxyanthrone that inhibits keratinocyte proliferation; it stains and can be irritating, but it can be effective therapy (Chapter 464).

CALCIPOTRIOL. Calcipotriol is a vitamin D derivative that has antiproliferative and immunomodulatory effects on skin. Hypercalcemia can occur if more than 100 g/week is used, so this agent cannot be used for widespread disease. It is applied twice daily, can be irritating on thin skin, and takes 6 to 8 weeks to be effective.

RETINOIDS. The retinoids are a group of compounds, including vitamin A and its derivatives. Their effects are mediated through several different classes of receptors, and the receptor-drug complex has effects on other regulatory proteins that affect growth factors, oncogenes, keratins, or transglutaminases. Retinoids affect cell growth, differentiation, and morphogenesis, inhibit tumor promotion and malignant cell growth, have immunomodulatory effects, and alter cell cohesion.

Topical retinoids include all-*trans* retinoic acid (tretinoin), which is approved for acne (Retin-A) and photoaging (Renova 0.05% cream) and which is also useful for hyperpigmentation, steroid-induced atrophy, and early stretch marks. Tretinoin is available as a cream (0.025%, 0.05%, 0.1%), a gel (0.01%, 0.025%), and a solution (0.05%). Adapalene (Differin, 0.1% gel) and tazarotene (Tazorac) are used for acne (Chapter 465). Tazarotene is also used for psoriasis, often in combination with topical steroids to minimize irritation. Topical retinoids can be irritating and frequently cause an exacerbation before improvement. However, they should be used regularly on lesion-prone skin to produce improvement. Moisturizers may be needed to minimize drying effects.

Systemic retinoids commonly used for the skin include isotretinoin, acitretin, and bexarotene (Targretin). They have many uses, but most frequently isotretinoin (Accutane) is used for cystic and conglobate acne, acitretin for severe psoriasis (especially erythrodermic and pustular forms), and bexarotene for cutaneous T-cell lymphoma. Isotretinoin and acitretin have also been used to treat several forms of ichthyosis and lupus erythematosus, and for the chemoprevention of skin cancers, particularly in immunosuppressed transplant recipients. The many side effects of systemic retinoids include teratogenicity, cheilitis, hair loss, headaches, hyperlipidemias, abnormal liver enzymes, vertebral hyperostosis, tendon and ligament calcification, osteoporosis, and central hypothyroidism with bexarotene. Pregnancy must be avoided, and the use of retinoids in women of childbearing age therefore requires careful monitoring. Treatment for acne is reserved for cases of cystic acne not responding to less toxic therapies; in this setting, a 4- to 5-month course of Accutane, at 0.5 to 1 mg/kg/day, is curative in 85 to 90% of patients.

ANTIMALARIAL DRUGS. Aminoquinolines include chloroquine, hydroxychloroquine, and quinacrine. These agents have inhibitory effects on proinflammatory cytokine production, DNA replication, and chemotaxis. They are useful in patients with connective tissue diseases, polymorphous light eruption, sarcoidosis (Chapter 95), porphyria cutanea tarda (Chapter 465), sclerosing conditions, and vasculitis. Side effects include diarrhea, headache, irritability, psychosis, skin dyspigmentation, and, rarely, retinopathy. Retinopathy is rare if doses of chloroquine are 3.5 mg/kg/day or less and hydroxychloroquine are 6.5 mg/kg/day or less. Combinations of hydroxychloroquine or chloroquine with quinacrine are frequently helpful when a solitary agent is inadequate. The combination of hydroxychloroquine and chloroquine should not be used because of the additive risk of retinopathy.

Dapsone

Dapsone is a sulfone that inhibits the response of neutrophils and possibly eosinophils to chemotactic stimuli. It is useful for dermatitis herpetiformis (Chapter 465), cutaneous vasculitis (Chapter 466), pyoderma gangrenosum (Chapter 144), bullous lupus erythematosus (Chapter 287), Behçet's disease (Chapter 291), and autoimmune bullous diseases (Chapter 465). Side effects include hemolysis, methemoglobinemia, peripheral neuropathy, agranulocytosis, and, rarely, a hypersensitivity syndrome with hepatitis, fevers, and rash. A glucose-6-dehydrogenase level should be checked before starting the drug, and it is common for patients with a normal glucose-6-dehydrogenase level to experience a 2 g/dL decrease in hemoglobin after achieving therapeutic doses of 100 to 200 mg/day.

THALIDOMIDE. Thalidomide has potent anti-inflammatory effects, likely resulting from inhibition of tumor necrosis factor-α. It also modifies adhesion molecules on circulating leukocytes. Thalidomide is a serious teratogen, and patients must comply with strict birth control and monitoring. It is effective at a dose of 50 to 100 mg/day, with improvement beginning at 2 weeks and a full clinical response seen at 2 to 3 months in patients with severe cutaneous lupus erythematosus (Chapter 287), erythema nodosum leprosum (Chapter 464), aphthae, Behçet's disease (Chapter 291), actinic prurigo, chronic graft-versus-host disease (Chapter 184), multiple myeloma (Chapter 198), and numerous other inflammatory dermatoses. Beside teratogenesis, the main side effects include peripheral neuropathy, constipation, sedation, and, rarely, amenorrhea.

GOLD. Intramuscular gold has been used to treat pemphigus vulgaris (Chapter 465), with success as a solitary agent. A total dose of 400 to 600 mg of gold is often required to stop the formation of blisters; after the initial test doses, gold is administered at 50 mg once a week.

COLCHICINE. Colchicine, usually at a dose of 0.6 mg twice a day, is used for leukocytoclastic vasculitis (Chapter 465) and Behçet's disease. The main side effect of this low oral dose is diarrhea.

ANTIMICROBIAL AGENTS

Antibacterials

Topical antibiotics are used to treat superficial skin diseases, such as acne and folliculitis that are related to infectious organisms, and skin wounds or ulcers. They may work by decreasing neutrophil chemotaxis and other anti-inflammatory mechanisms. Topical solutions, gels, pledgets, and ointments are available, depending on the agent, and antibiotics include erythromycin, clindamycin, tetracycline, and metronidazole. Benzoyl peroxide also has antibacterial properties and is quite effective for mild to moderate acne (Chapter 465). [1] Bacitracin and Polysporin ointments are typically used for wounds, but they can cause contact hypersensitivity; neomycin should be avoided because of the high incidence of allergic reactions. Mupirocin is particularly effective against *Staphylococcus* and *Streptococcus* species, and it can be used in the nose for carriers of staphylococci. Systemic antibiotics such as penicillins, cephalosporins, and erythromycin are used for patients with soft tissue infections such as impetigo, folliculitis, furuncles, carbuncles, cellulitis, ecthyma, erysipelas, postoperative wound infections, and necrotizing fasciitis. Tetracycline, doxycycline, and minocycline are used for acne, rosacea, and perioral dermatitis. Fluoroquinolones such as ciprofloxacin are useful for treatment of gram-negative soft tissue infections.

Antifungals

Topical antifungal agents are used for patients with limited superficial fungal infections of the skin (Chapter 464). The numerous topical antifungal drugs available include the azoles (clotrimazole, econazole, ketoconazole, oxiconazole, and miconazole), which are available as creams and lotions, applied once or twice a day. The creams tend to be more effective. Topical agents used for dermatophytes, but not *Candida,* are haloprogin and tolnaftate. The newer allylamine antifungals are naftifine and terbinafine, which have fungicidal effects. Ciclopirox 8% topical solution was recently approved for use in treating and preventing relapses of onychomycosis. Nystatin creams, oral suspensions, and vaginal tablets are effective for treatment of *Candida* infections. The combination of antifungals with potent topical steroids such as betamethasone dipropionate is not advised because of increased side effects from the steroid and decreased efficacy of the antifungal as a result of the concomitant steroid.

Systemic antifungal agents include griseofulvin, terbinafine (allylamine), ketoconazole (imidazole), itraconazole, and fluconazole. These agents are used for extensive or severe superficial skin fungal infections (Chapter 464) caused by dermatophytes, *Candida,* or *Malassezia furfur* or for local infections not responsive to topical drugs, such as those found in the nails and scalp. Itraconazole and terbinafine are the only oral antifungals approved in the United States for treatment of onychomycosis, and griseofulvin is the only oral agent approved for tinea capitis. Griseofulvin is best taken with a fatty meal to improve absorption and is the only antifungal drug not requiring regular monitoring of liver enzymes.

Griseofulvin shows weak affinity for keratin, and thus it must be used for 18 months for onychomycosis of the toenails and 6 months for the fingernails to achieve even relatively poor cure rates. Terbinafine is the only fungicidal drug, whereas the rest are fungistatic. The number of interactions with medications is lower with terbinafine than with the triazole antifungals and ketoconazole because terbinafine does not inhibit or induce hepatic isoenzyme CYP 3A4 (Chapter 27). However, terbinafine affects CYP 2D6, another hepatic isoenzyme, so it is relatively contraindicated in patients who are taking cyclosporine or rifampin. Itraconazole and fluconazole have been used in pulse-dosing regimens for treatment of onychomycosis. Fluconazole and terbinafine are not dependent on gastric acidity for optimal gastrointestinal absorption. Overall, the side effects of the systemic antifungal agents are similar and include headache and gastrointestinal symptoms (griseofulvin, terbinafine), nausea and vomiting (itraconazole, fluconazole, ketoconazole), hepatitis, and lupus-like syndromes (terbinafine).

Antivirals

Verrucae are treated with various destructive modalities, including 50 to 80% dichloroacetic acid and trichloroacetic acid solutions, podophyllin resin, and podofilox. Topical antiviral creams such as penciclovir and acyclovir do not significantly shorten the course of herpes simplex. Systemic antiviral drugs include acyclovir, valacyclovir, famciclovir, and foscarnet, which are used to treat primary and recurrent herpes simplex (Chapter 397) and herpes zoster (Chapter 398), although only acyclovir is approved for use in herpes zoster. These agents specifically block the function of herpesvirus DNA polymerase. Valacyclovir and famciclovir are only available orally in the United States, but the prolonged intracellular half-life allows for less frequent dosing than with acyclovir. Patients with herpes zoster require higher doses than do patients with herpes simplex. Side effects include nausea and headaches.

Antiparasitics

Topical antiparasitic medications are used to treat pediculosis capitis, pediculosis pubis, and scabies. In addition, topical metronidazole has anti-inflammatory properties used to treat rosacea. For pediculosis and scabies, clothing and bedding must be washed, and all family members must be treated. Effective treatment includes 1% γ-benzene hexachloride (lindane), a chlorinated hydrocarbon pesticide that should not be used in young children or in pregnant or lactating women. It is ineffective against nits and thus must be reapplied after 1 week. Permethrin 5% cream (Elimite) for scabies or 1% cream rinse is particularly effective for head lice and requires just one application; 10% crotamiton (Eurax) and 5% topical sulfur ointments are less effective. Malathion is a moderately toxic organophosphate insecticide, but it must be applied overnight to treat lice. Pyrethrins (RID, Nix) are best used twice, one week apart, to treat head lice and nits.

ANTIPRURITIC OR ANESTHETIC AGENTS

Topical Analgesics

Capsaicin is an active ingredient of cayenne peppers and other plants of the Capsicum family that is used for postherpetic neuralgia and other painful nerve-related conditions. It causes excitation of neural afferent C-fibers and reduces substance P. Capsaicin causes a burning sensation and is applied four to five times a day for 5 to 6 weeks. Eutectic mixture of local anesthetic (EMLA) is a mixture of lidocaine and prilocaine used under occlusion to induce cutaneous anesthesia before a procedure. Lidocaine can be used as a topical anesthetic, but benzocaine should be avoided because it is a sensitizer.

Antipruritic Agents

Doxepin 5% cream is used for localized pruritus. Menthol is a cyclic terpene plant alcohol used for non–histamine-related itching. Pramoxine hydrochloride is a topical anesthetic used for mild to moderate itching. Oral antihistamines play an important role in controlling pruritus for many skin conditions (Table 463–3), especially for those conditions mediated by histamine, such as urticaria, angioedema, and urticaria pigmentosa. The sedating and anticholinergic properties of many H_1-receptor antihistamines likely account for some of their efficacy. H_1-receptor antihistamines are cornerstones of routine therapy, and if an agent from one group of H_1-receptor antihistamines is ineffective, then an agent from a different class should be administered or combined. Second-generation H_1-receptor antihistamines are less sedating and are used if patients cannot tolerate or do not improve after taking first-generation agents. The combination of two different H_1-receptor antihistamines can be used when a solitary agent does not work; in particular, use of a sedating antihistamine at night and a second-generation antihistamine during the day can be helpful. Both H_1- and H_2-receptors are in skin, and occasionally combining H_1- and H_2-receptor antagonists can be beneficial. Usually, first-generation agents (e.g., hydroxyzine, 10 to 25 mg every 6 hours) are started at low doses and are increased as tolerated, and regular continuous dosing is recommended. The tricyclic antidepressant doxepin, normally started at 10 to 25 mg at bedtime, has both anti–H_1- and H_2-receptor activity, but it interacts with drugs metabolized by the cytochrome P-450 pathway. Side effects of commonly used first-generation antihistamines include sedation, dry mouth, blurred vision, constipation, and urinary retention, and lower doses may be required in elderly patients. The recommended dose for second-generation antihistamines (e.g., fexofenadine, 60 mg twice a day) should not be exceeded.

AGENTS THAT IMPROVE SURFACE FUNCTIONS (LUBRICATION, SCALE)

Moisturizers

Moisturizers improve skin by diminishing scale and increasing water content. They usually contain mixtures of water and fatty substances such as petrolatum, lanolin, lanolin derivatives, and fatty alcohols. Greasy moisturizers tend to function better, but they are less acceptable cosmetically.

Keratolytics

α-Hydroxy acids (lactic acid, glycolic acid, citric acid, glucuronic acid, pyruvic acid) are extremely effective keratolytics. They are helpful in treating disorders of keratinization and photoaging, as well as acne. Propylene glycol, used as 40 to 60% aqueous solutions, can decrease scaling. Salicylic acid, which works by decreasing keratinocyte adhesion and hydrating keratins, is used in a range of concentrations in many different bases to remove scale, to soften the stratum corneum, or as destructive therapy to remove warts and calluses. Urea is used in varying concentrations to treat scaling.

IMMUNE THERAPIES

Immunosuppressive Agents

Topical cytotoxic drugs include 5-fluorouracil, mechlorethamine (nitrogen mustard), carmustine (BCNU), bleomycin, and the calcineurin inhibitors tacrolimus and pimecrolimus. Topical 5-fluorouracil interferes with pyrimidine metabolism and action and blocks DNA synthesis. It is used to treat actinic keratoses, superficial basal cell cancers, and Bowen's disease, bowenoid papulosis, actinic cheilitis, and warts. Topical use does not cause systemic toxicity, but expected side effects include local irritation, erythema, and pain. Nitrogen mustard and BCNU, which have alkylating agents that inhibit DNA, RNA, and protein synthesis, are used to treat cutaneous T-cell lymphoma (Chapter 195); they can cause cutaneous reactions and myelosuppression, and nitrogen mustard commonly causes a cutaneous hypersensitivity reaction.

Intralesional bleomycin, which disrupts DNA synthesis, has been used to treat warts. Topical tacrolimus (Prograf) and pimecrolimus, immunosuppressive macrolides that act on T lymphocytes to inhibit interleukin-2 transcription, are used for atopic dermatitis, allergic contact dermatitis, psoriasis, and several other inflammatory skin conditions. They frequently cause a burning sensation in the skin; although systemic absorption is minimal, ongoing studies are assessing whether the risk of cancer is increased by their topical use. Systemic immunosuppressives such as methotrexate, azathioprine, thioguanine, hydroxyurea, mycophenolate (CellCept), cyclophosphamide, chlorambucil, and cyclosporine are used

TABLE 463–3 OVERVIEW ANTIHISTAMINES

Antihistamine Group	Generic Name	Average Oral Adult Doses
FIRST-GENERATION H_1-TYPE ANTIHISTAMINES		
Alkylamine	Brompheniramine (Dimetapp)	4 mg q4–6h
	Chorpheniramine (Chlor-Trimeton)	4 mg q4–6h (short acting); 8–12 mg q8–12h (long acting)
Amino alkyl ether (ethanolamine)	Clemastine fumarate	1.34 mg bid or 2.68 mg qd–tid
	Diphenhydramine (Benadryl)	25–50 mg q4–6h
Ethylenediamine	Pyrilamine (Triaminic)	30 mg bid
Phenothiazine	Promethazine (Phenergan)	10–12.5 mg qid
	Trimeprazine (Temaril)	2.5 mg q6h
Piperidine	Azatadine	1–2 mg q8–12h
	Cyproheptadine	4 mg q8h
	Diphenylpyraline	2 mg tid–qid
Piperazine	Hydroxyzine (Atarax)	25–100 mg tid–qid
SECOND-GENERATION H_1-TYPE ANTIHISTAMINES		
Alkylamine	Acrivastine (combined with pseudoephedrine in allergy medication)	8 mg qid
Piperidine	Astemizole (Hismanal)	10 mg qd
	Loratidine (Claritin)	10 mg qd
	Fexofenadine (Allegra)	60 mg bid or 180 mg qd
Piperazine	Cetirizine (Zyrtec)	5–10 mg/day
H_2-TYPE ANTIHISTAMINES		
	Cimetidine (Tagamet)	400 mg bid
	Ranitidine (Zantac)	150 mg bid
	Famotidine	10 mg bid
	Nizatidine	300 mg hs
H_1- AND H_2-TYPE ANTIHISTAMINES		
	Doxepin (Sinequan)	10–25 mg hs

bid = twice daily; hs = at bedtime; qd = once daily; qid = four times daily; tid = three times daily.

in numerous inflammatory or immunologically mediated skin conditions, particularly in widespread psoriasis (Chapter 464) and as glucocorticoid-sparing agents for autoimmune blistering diseases.

Immunomodulatory Therapies

Imiquimod, available as a 5% cream, is an imidazoquinolinamine that has antitumor and antiviral activity. It induces local production of γ-interferon, and it is used to treat warts and superficial skin cancers.

Many systemic immunomodulatory drugs are currently used in dermatology. These include interferons and tumor necrosis factor-α inhibitors such as etanercept and infliximab (Remicade). 2 Interferon-α2b is used both intralesionally and subcutaneously to treat genital warts, high-risk melanoma, Kaposi's sarcoma, hemangiomas, cutaneous T-cell lymphoma, keloids, Behçet's disease, cryoglobulinemia and vasculitis from hepatitis C (Chapter 152), and perhaps basal cell and squamous cell carcinomas. Total interferon doses are generally 3 million IU or less per session, and systemic doses are usually administered 3 days per week. Side effects include flulike symptoms, leukopenia, anemia, and hepatitis. Numerous drugs approved for treatment of psoriasis affect T cells, either by blockade of costimulatory signals, as with efalizumab, or of T-cell activation, as with alefacept. Intravenous immunoglobulin, which is used to treat certain autoimmune skin diseases including pemphigus vulgaris, cicatricial pemphigoid, and dermatomyositis, likely works through Fc receptor modulation and anti-idiotype interactions. Extracorporeal photochemotherapy (photopheresis), which combines 8-methoxypsoralen and ultraviolet A (UVA) irradiation of lymphocytes, is used for Sézary syndrome, the leukemic form of cutaneous T-cell lymphoma (Chapter 195). Plasmapheresis, used in combination with other immunosuppressive therapies, can remove autoantibodies and immune complexes in patients in whom autoimmune disease or cryoglobulinemia is resistant to other therapies.

OTHER THERAPIES

Phototherapy and Laser

UV treatments are given with different wavelengths, depending on the condition and the response to treatment. Currently, clinicians use broadband UVB (290 to 320 nm), narrow-band 311-nm UVB, PUVA (psoralen with UVA 320 to 400 nm), and UVA1 (340 to 400 nm). Both forms of UVB and PUVA are used for psoriasis and vitiligo, but other conditions such as nummular and atopic dermatitis, pruritus resulting from uremia, and cutaneous T-cell lymphoma are treated in this way. High-dose UVA1 is used, mainly in Europe, to treat atopic dermatitis, localized scleroderma, and mastocytosis. PUVA is associated with an increased risk of skin cancers, including melanoma. The risks of long-term UVA therapy are currently unknown, but photoaging is associated with UVA, and there have been reports of an increase of melanoma associated with use of suntanning beds, in which much of the exposure is to UVA. Laser therapy is used to treat vascular lesions such as port wine stains, tattoos, psoriasis, benign skin tumors, and photodamage, as well as to remove hair. Photodynamic therapy involves activation of a photosensitizer by illumination with visible light that leads to photochemical tissue destruction or immunomodulation. Photodynamic therapy can be used to treat actinic keratoses, Bowen's disease, and superficial basal cell carcinomas by causing selective tissue necrosis and tumor destruction.

Dermatologic Surgery

Although approaches such as dessication and curettage can be used for some skin tumors, others require excisional surgery or Mohs' microscopic controlled surgery to ensure complete lesion removal. If the tumors are recurrent, of a pathologic type that increases the likelihood of recurrence, or large and requiring clearance of the tumor before repair, the Mohs approach can provide rapid documentation of full removal while sparing as much normal tissue as possible. After the margins have been cleared of tumor, flaps and grafts can be immediately utilized for repair of the resultant defects.

Patients with extensive actinic damage resulting in either large numbers of actinic keratoses or photodamage can be treated with various ablative approaches that utilize either chemical peels or laser resurfacing with the carbon dioxide laser. Chemical peels can be performed at different depths and intensities, and agents can include glycolic acid, acetic acid, or even phenol. Lasers used to remove sun-induced lentigines include the q-switched lasers, such as the neodymium:yttrium-aluminum-garnet laser, the ruby, and the alexandrite. Many patients seek treatment for wrinkles with soft tissue augmentation that uses human-derived collagen and hyaluronic acid or with a muscle relaxer, botulinum type A exotoxin.

Hair transplants are a surgical approach to the problem of hair loss. The process includes harvesting hair grafts from the posterior scalp and placing the grafts in areas of alopecia.

Sunscreen

Transparent sunscreens absorb photons of light. They are rated by the sun protection factor (SPF), which is determined by the ratio of UV exposure needed to cause erythema in protected versus unprotected skin. Most sunscreens work in the UVB range or shorter UVA wavelengths. Examples of UVB-absorptive compounds include aminobenzoates, cinnamates, salicylates, and benzophenones. Short-wavelength UVA-absorptive compounds include benophenones and anthranilates. The best UVA blocking agent in the United States is avobenzone (Parsol 1789), which can be combined with UVB screens. Some sunscreens are water resistant or waterproof, as determined by the substantivity of the sunscreen, and these agents provide continued protection after sweating or swimming. Sunscreens can cause irritation and, rarely, contact allergic reactions. Physical sunscreens, such as zinc oxide and titanium dioxide, reflect light from the skin and include newer micronized reflecting powders that provide broad-spectrum (UVB and UVA) protection. Sunscreens decrease skin cancers and photodamage. UVB is partially reflected by clothing, and sun-protective clothing can provide substantial protection (Solumbra, SPF of 30).

Cosmetics: Camouflage, Bleaching, and Hair Loss

Patients with numerous skin conditions benefit from camouflage cosmetics, which can also cause contact hypersensitivity. Products such as Dermablend can be blended to match skin colors, are thicker, can cover disfiguring lesions, and can be fixed with powder. Hydroquinones, topical retinoic acid, and azelaic acid (inhibits tyrosinase) are used to treat hyperpigmented conditions such as melasma and lentigines; these agents can be irritating and cause dyspigmentation. Topical minoxidil 2% (available over the counter) and 5% solutions are used for androgenic alopecia and alopecia areata. Finasteride, a 5α-reductase inhibitor, is effective in men with androgenetic alopecia.

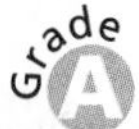

1. Ozolins M, Eady EA, Avery AJ, et al: Comparison of five antimicrobial regimens for treatment of mild to moderate inflammatory facial acne vulgaris in the community: Randomized controlled trial. Lancet 2004;364:2188–2195.
2. Leonardi CL, Powers JL, Matheson RT, et al: Etanercept as monotherapy in patients with psoriasis. N Engl J Med 2003;349:2014–2022.

SUGGESTED READINGS

Haider A, Shaw JC: Treatment of acne vulgaris. JAMA 2004;292:726–735. *Overview of topical and oral therapies.*

Kim EJ, Hess S, Richardson SK, et al: Immunopathogenesis and therapy of cutaneous T cell lymphoma. J Clin Invest 2005;115:798–812. *A scholarly review.*

Nickoloff BJ, Stevens SR: What have we learned in dermatology from the biologic therapies? J Am Acad Dermatol 2006;54:S143–S151. *A review of cell-based and cytokine-based therapies.*

Werth VP, Duvic M: Medical dermatology. Dermatol Clin 2002;19:603–772. *Review of treatment of many serious dermatologic illnesses.*

464 ECZEMAS, PHOTODERMATOSES, PAPULOSQUAMOUS (INCLUDING FUNGAL) DISEASES, AND FIGURATE ERYTHEMAS

Henry W. Lim

ECZEMA

The more commonly encountered eczemas (Table 464–1) share similar histologic characteristics. However, they have varying degrees of edema within the epidermis (spongiosis) and of infiltration with lymphocytes and macrophages in the superficial dermis.

Nummular Dermatitis

Nummular dermatitis occurs most frequently in patients who are in their 50s to 60s and is usually associated with significant dryness of the skin (xerosis). Both sexes are affected; in temperate climates, this condition is most frequently seen in the winter. The condition appears to be more frequent among Asians. The origin of nummular dermatitis is unclear, although xerosis plays a significant role in its pathogenesis.

Patients usually present with pruritic, coin-shaped, erythematous patches with some scales and occasionally with pinhead-sized vesicles (Fig. 464–1). Lesions may be excoriated and lichenified (i.e., thickened skin with accentuation of skin markings). Legs and arms are the commonly affected sites, although lesions can also occur on the trunk. All patients should be educated about the care of dry skin, such as the use of emollients and moisturizing soaps and avoidance of long, hot showers. Topical corticosteroid ointments (e.g., triamcinolone ointment, 0.1% twice daily for 1 to 2 weeks) are helpful for active lesions, and oral antihistamines (e.g., fexofenadine, 180 mg every morning, and hydroxyzine,

TABLE 464–1 ECZEMAS
Nummular dermatitis
Dyshidrosis
Atopic dermatitis
Seborrheic dermatitis
Allergic contact dermatitis
Irritant contact dermatitis

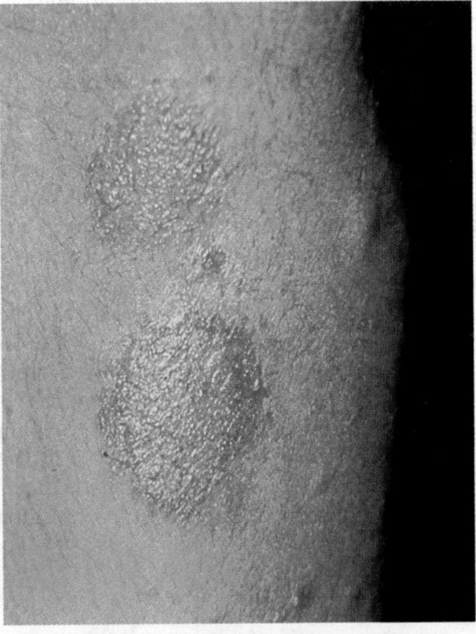

FIGURE 464–1 • Coin-shaped erythematous patches in a patient with nummular dermatitis.

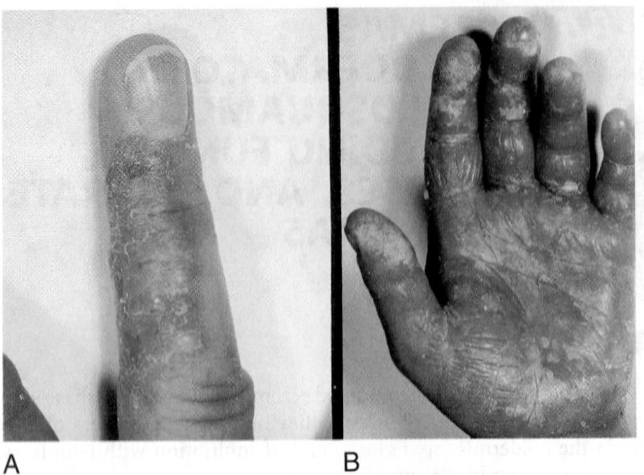

FIGURE 464–2 • Dyshidrosis. A, Scaly erythematous patch with erosions on the side of a finger. **B,** Erythema, scaliness, and peeling of the palm.

25 to 50 mg at bedtime, as needed) are useful for pruritus. In severe cases, narrow-band ultraviolet B (NB-UVB) phototherapy, psoralen combined with UVA (PUVA), or a short course of oral corticosteroids (prednisone, 0.5 to 1 mg/kg/day, with a maximum dose of 60 mg/day, for 1 to 2 weeks, then taper in 10 to 14 days) is beneficial.

Dyshidrosis

Dyshidrosis appears as deep-seated, pinhead-sized vesicles, most commonly along the sides of the fingers (Fig. 464–2). Occasionally, the palms and soles may also be involved. Lesions are usually pruritic, associated with xerosis of the surrounding skin. Fissuring of the tip and the side of the fingers frequently occurs. Dyshidrosis is seen in individuals who wash their hands frequently, such as health care and restaurant workers and mothers of young infants. Treatment follows a sequential order: (1) minimizing of hand washing, (2) liberal use of over-the-counter emollients, (3) topical corticosteroid ointments (e.g., fluocinonide ointment, 0.05% twice daily for 2 weeks), and (4) oral antihistamines (e.g., fexofenadine, 180 mg every morning, and hydroxyzine, 25 to 50 mg at bedtime, as needed).

Atopic Dermatitis

Atopic dermatitis is most commonly seen among young children, but severe cases persist into adulthood. In more than 80% of the patients, the disease starts before the age of 5 years. The prevalence has been estimated at between 15 and 23%. Patients usually present with xerosis, erythematous scaly patches, small vesicles, excoriations, crusting, and, not infrequently, impetiginization (Fig. 464–3). With chronic scratching and rubbing, hyperpigmentation and lichenification occur. Commonly affected sites include the periorbital area and flexor areas such as the neck, antecubital fossa, and popliteal fossa. In severe cases, the entire skin surface may be involved. Diagnosis is made by the typical morphologic features and by the distribution of the lesions, as well as by a family and personal history of atopy. The therapeutic ladder consists of the following: (1) over-the-counter emollients; (2) topical corticosteroid ointments (e.g., triamcinolone ointment, 0.1% twice daily for 1 to 2 weeks), or topical calcineurin inhibitors (tacrolimus ointment, 0.1% for 3 to 4 weeks, or pimecrolimus cream, 1% for 3 to 4 weeks). [1,2] The latter have been given a "black box warning" by the U.S. Food and Drug Administration for their potential association with the development of malignant disease; therefore, continuous prolonged use (i.e., >2 to 3 months) should be minimized; (3) oral antihistamines (e.g., fexofenadine, 180 mg every morning, and hydroxyzine, 25 to 50 mg at bedtime, as needed); (4) NB-UVB phototherapy [3]; and (5) PUVA. In patients with recalcitrant cases, oral prednisone (0.5 to 1 mg/kg/day), cyclosporine (3 to 5 mg/kg/day), and mycophenolate mofetil (1 to 2 g/day) have been successful.

Seborrheic Dermatitis

Seborrheic dermatitis is a common condition that occurs as erythematous patches with fine, greasy-appearing scales, most commonly on

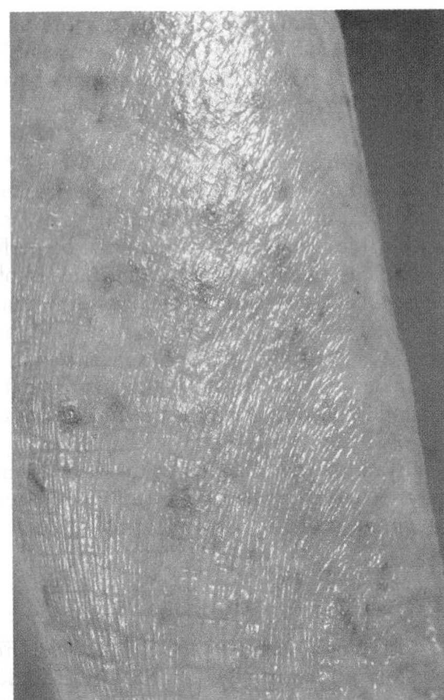

FIGURE 464–3 • Atopic dermatitis. Note the erythema, excoriation, and lichenification.

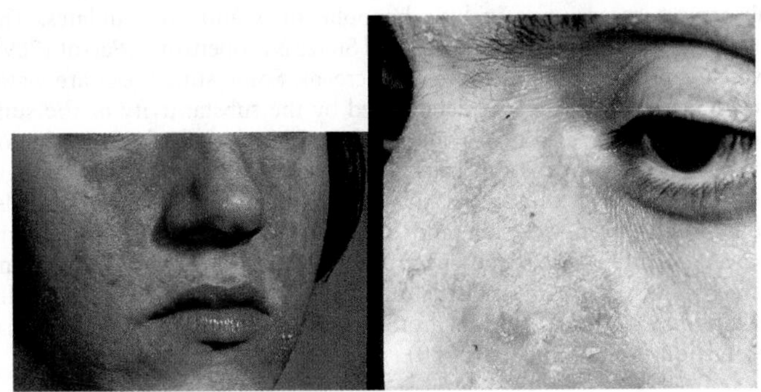

FIGURE 464–4 • Erythematous patches with greasy-appearing scales on the malar area of two patients with seborrheic dermatitis.

the malar area, midforehead, midchest, and scalp (Fig. 464–4). This condition is common in patients with human immunodeficiency virus (HIV) infection (Chapter 415). The pathogenesis is unknown, although *Pityrosporum ovale* is believed to play a role. The diagnosis can usually be made on clinical grounds alone. Topical corticosteroids (e.g., hydrocortisone cream 2.5%, twice daily for 1 to 2 weeks) can rapidly reduce the inflammation; then topical ketoconazole cream, 2% twice daily as needed (or shampoo 2% daily or every other day for the scalp), is safe for long-term treatment.

Allergic Contact Dermatitis and Irritant Contact Dermatitis

Allergic contact dermatitis and irritant contact dermatitis are induced by exogenous agents. Allergic contact dermatitis is a delayed hypersensitivity response to external allergens, whereas irritant contact dermatitis is a nonspecific toxic response to contact irritants. In both conditions, lesions occur in the exposed area, but in patients with severe cases, nonexposed areas may also have milder lesions. In allergic contact dermatitis, patients present with erythematous pruritic papules followed by vesicles. Lesions resolve with fine scales. Postinflammatory hyperpigmentation may be observed, especially in dark-skinned individuals. Histologically, epidermal edema and dermal histiocytic infiltrates are observed. Irritant contact dermatitis manifests with lesions morphologically similar to those of allergic contact dermatitis. However, irritant contact dermatitis is usually associated with a burning sensation rather than with pruritus. Postinflammatory hyperpigmentation is frequently observed. Histologic changes consist of necrotic keratinocytes, epidermal necrosis, and neurophilic infiltrates. Management includes identification and removal of the offending agent, as well as symptomatic treatments such as topical corticosteroids and oral antihistamines.

PHOTODERMATOSES

Photodermatoses indicate the development of cutaneous eruption secondary to exposure to UV or visible radiation (Table 464–2). By convention, electromagnetic radiation in the UV region is divided into UVC (200 to 290 nm), UVB (290 to 320 nm), UVA-2 (320 to 340 nm), and UVA-1 (340 to 400 nm). Visible light extends from 400 to 760 nm. Because UVC emitted by the sun is absorbed by ozone in the stratosphere, UVC does not reach the Earth's surface. UVB, UVA, and visible light are the relevant spectra in photodermatoses.

Polymorphous Light Eruption

Polymorphous light eruption, the most common idiopathic photodermatosis, occurs in 10 to 20% of the general population. It usually occurs in young adults, has a slight female predominance, and is seen worldwide. Affected individuals are less susceptible to cutaneous photoimmunosuppression and hence have an enhanced response to UV-induced neoantigens in the skin. Lesions usually occur in early spring within a few hours of exposure to sunlight. Lesions can manifest as pinhead papules, papules, papulovesicles, or, less commonly, vesicles (Fig. 464–5); they can also be minimally pruritic. Usually, lesions persist for several days and resolve spontaneously. The condition tends to improve as the sunny season progresses, a phenomenon known as "hardening."

The course is chronic; only 11% of patients have complete resolution of the disease in 16 years and 24% in 32 years. Diagnosis is based on the typical history and morphologic features of the lesion; the diagnosis can be confirmed by the induction of lesions with provocative phototesting. When lesions occur primarily on the face, a diagnosis of lupus must be excluded. Management consists of sun avoidance, the use of broad-spectrum sunscreens, topical corticosteroids, and oral antihistamines. In severe cases, desensitization treatment using NB-UVB or PUVA has been successful. Desensitization is usually performed in early spring by exposing patients to increasing doses of NB-UVB or PUVA.

TABLE 464–2 PHOTODERMATOSES

Polymorphous light eruption
Chronic actinic dermatitis
Solar urticaria
Phototoxicity and photoallergy
Porphyrias

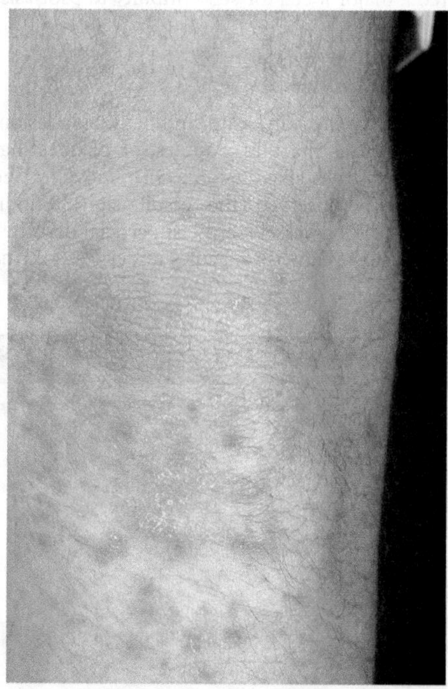

FIGURE 464–5 • Erythematous papules a few hours after exposure to the sun in a patient with polymorphous light eruption.

Chronic Actinic Dermatitis

Chronic actinic dermatitis is a chronic photodermatosis that occurs most commonly in men in their 60s and 70s. It has been seen in patients of all ethnic groups, but in the United States, it is more commonly seen in dark-skinned individuals. It occurs in 5 to 17% of patients referred for evaluation of photosensitivity. Chronic actinic dermatitis can evolve from photoallergic contact dermatitis, allergic contact dermatitis, or exposure to a known photosensitizing agent; however, it can also arise de novo. Investigators have postulated that this condition represents a delayed hypersensitivity response to an unidentified antigen.

Patients present with erythematous papules and plaques with superficial scaling and, frequently, with lichenification (Fig. 464–6). The distribution of lesions is primarily on sun-exposed areas, such as the forehead, nose, cheeks, "V" area of the neck, dorsum of the hands, and forearms. Typically, sun-protected areas, such as the postauricular area, the area underneath the chin, the area above the eyes, and the trunk, are spared. This chronic photosensitivity occurs in the absence of any continued exposure to known photosensitizers. Histologically, one sees a dermal lymphohistiocytic infiltrate; atypical mononuclear cells may be observed. On phototesting, patients have decreased sensitivity to UVA, UVB, and/or visible light. In a study of 178 cases, 10% resolved in 5 years and 50% in 15 years. An association with HIV infection (Chapter 415) has been reported.

The diagnosis is based on the patient's history and on the morphologic features and distribution of the lesions. It is confirmed by phototesting.

Management is challenging. During the sunny season, it is critical that patients practice maximal photoprotection, consisting of staying in the shade, using broad-spectrum sunscreens, clothing, and wearing a wide-brimmed hat. Other treatment modalities, in approximate sequential order, are topical tacrolimus ointment, oral mycophenolate mofetil (1 to 2 g/day), oral cyclosporine (3 to 5 mg/kg/day), and azathioprine (50 to 200 mg/day). In recalcitrant cases, the following may be used: PUVA in conjunction with oral corticosteroids or a combination of mycophenolate mofetil, PUVA, and oral corticosteroids.

Solar Urticaria

Solar urticaria occurs worldwide. In photodermatology referral centers, it accounts for 5 to 7% of patients. The mean age at onset is usually in the fourth decade, with a slight female predominance. In one study, the mean duration of disease at the time of diagnosis was 3.6 years. Patients develop urticaria that appears within minutes of sun exposure and persists for less than 24 hours. Lesions are most commonly induced by visible light, but they can also be induced by UVA or UVB. Similar to polymorphous light eruption, improvement may occur as the summer season progresses (hardening). The diagnosis is confirmed by induction

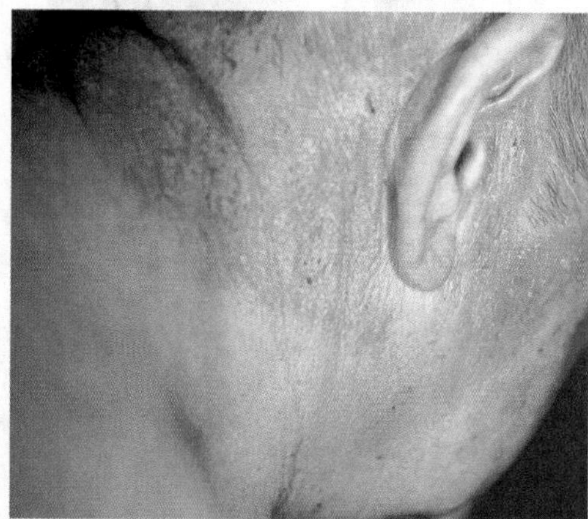

FIGURE 464–6 • Erythema and lichenification in a patient with chronic actinic dermatitis. Note sparing of the sun-protected areas of the neck, infra-auricular area, and lower cheeks.

of the lesion after controlled exposure to the appropriate light source. Management consists of photoprotection and the use of oral antihistamines (e.g., fexofenadine, 180 mg every morning, and hydroxyzine, 25 to 50 mg at bedtime). In severe cases, graduated exposure to UVA or PUVA is helpful.

Phototoxicity and Photoallergy

The terms *phototoxicity* and *photoallergy* refer to the development of skin lesions after combined exposure to an oral or topical photosensitizer and electromagnetic radiation. Phototoxicity is a nonspecific cutaneous toxic reaction, whereas photoallergy is a delayed hypersensitivity response. For most photosensitizers, the action spectrum for both lies in the UVA range. Most of the phototoxic agents are systemic medications, whereas the most common photoallergens are the various ultraviolet filters in sunscreen. In both conditions, patients present with erythematous papules and vesicles confined to sun-exposed areas. Vesicular eruption is distinctly more common in phototoxicity, whereas pruritic eczematous eruption is more common in photoallergy. Histologically, phototoxicity is characterized by necrotic keratinocytes and infiltrates consisting predominantly of neutrophils, whereas photoallergy is characterized by epidermal edema (spongiosis) and lymphohistiocytic dermal infiltrate. The diagnosis is based on a careful history for exposure to photosensitizers combined with the typical morphologic features. Management consists of identification and removal of photosensitizer and the use of topical corticosteroids (e.g., triamcinolone ointment, 0.1% twice daily for 2 weeks) and oral antihistamines (e.g., fexofenadine, 180 mg every morning, and hydroxyzine, 25 to 50 mg at bedtime as needed (Chapter 463).

Porphyrias

The most common cutaneous porphyria is porphyria cutanea tarda, in which patients present with skin fragility and blister formation on sun-exposed areas, most commonly the dorsum of the hands and the forearms (Fig. 464–7; Chapter 229). Erosion and crusting on the face can also be noted. Patients usually have periorbital hypertrichosis and, less frequently, periorbital mottled hyperpigmentation and hypopigmentation. Sclerodermoid skin changes can occur in both sun-exposed and sun-protected areas. The defective enzyme is uroporphyrinogen decarboxylase. Porphyria cutanea tarda is associated with excessive alcohol intake, exposure to estrogens, hepatitis C infection (Chapter 152), HIV infection (Chapter 415), and hemochromatosis (Chapter 231). Patients invariably have an elevated level of ferritin and frequently have elevated liver enzyme values.

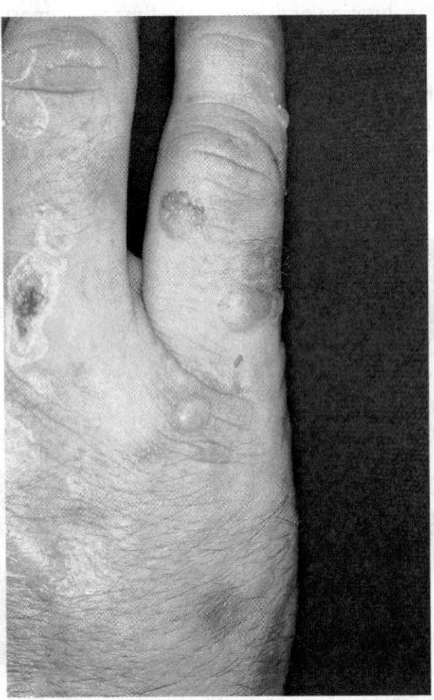

FIGURE 464–7 • Erosion, crusting, and vesicles on the dorsum of the hand of a patient with porphyria cutanea tarda.

The diagnosis is suggested by the typical clinical appearance and is confirmed by the characteristic porphyrin profile (elevated levels of 8-, 7-, 6-, 5-, and 4-carboxyl porphyrins in the urine and isocoproporphyrin in feces; Chapter 229). Management consists of avoidance of precipitating factors (alcohol, iron-containing vitamins, estrogen-containing birth control pills) and weekly phlebotomy. In patients who are anemic (e.g., those with HIV infection), low-dose hydroxychloroquine (200 mg/week) is beneficial. With appropriate treatment, remission can persist for years.

PAPULOSQUAMOUS (INCLUDING FUNGAL) DISEASES

Common papulosquamous diseases are listed in Table 464–3.

Psoriasis

Epidemiology

Psoriasis is the most commonly recognized papulosquamous disease. It occurs in 2 to 3% of the general population, with considerable variation in different parts of the world. It affects male and female patients equally. Approximately one third of the patients have a positive family history. Psoriasis has bimodal peak of onset, at age 22.5 years and again at age 55 years. The onset of psoriasis before the age of 15 years is associated with a higher prevalence of positive family history of psoriasis and with more severe disease.

Pathobiology

Psoriasis was initially thought to be purely a disease of keratinocyte hyperproliferation; however, it has now clear that it is an immunologically mediated disease. Factors playing a role in the pathogenesis include T cells, cytokines, chemokines, growth factors, dendritic cells, eicosanoids, neutrophils, and mast cells. Investigators have postulated that, in genetically susceptible individuals, exposure to precipitating factors such as infections (e.g., streptococcal or HIV infections), stress, or physical injury results in activation of T cells and generation of cytokines, followed by influx of neutrophils and subsequent release of inflammatory mediators, which lead to the development of cutaneous lesions.

A linkage disequilibrium (i.e., higher than expected association) occurs between psoriasis and human leukocyte antigens (HLAs), the most common being HLA-Cw6. However, HLA-Cw6 is unlikely to be the disease allele, because psoriasis develops in only about 10% of HLA-Cw6–positive individuals. PSORS1, mapped to chromosome 6p21.3, is now considered a major locus for susceptibility to psoriasis.

Clinical Manifestations

Psoriasis can involve the skin, scalp, and nails. Skin lesions are characterized by erythematous macules, papules, or plaques that are usually covered with silvery scales (Fig. 464–8). On removal of the scales, pinpoint bleeding may be observed (the Auspitz sign), a finding reflecting the proliferation of blood vessels in the superficial dermis. Nail involvement includes pittings, yellowish macules underneath the nail plate ("oil

TABLE 464–3 PAPULOSQUAMOUS DISEASES
Psoriasis
Pityriasis rubra pilaris
Pityriasis rosea
Lichen planus
Lichen nitidus
Secondary syphilis
Pityriasis lichenoides
Parapsoriasis
Mycosis fungoides
Dermatophytosis
Tinea versicolor

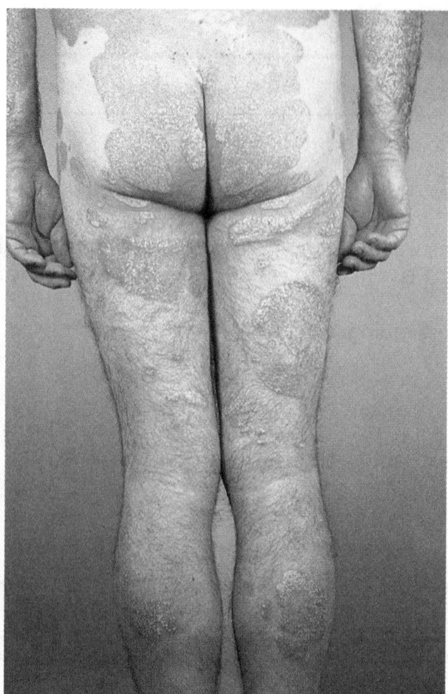

FIGURE 464–8 • Erythematous plaques with silvery scales in a patient with psoriasis.

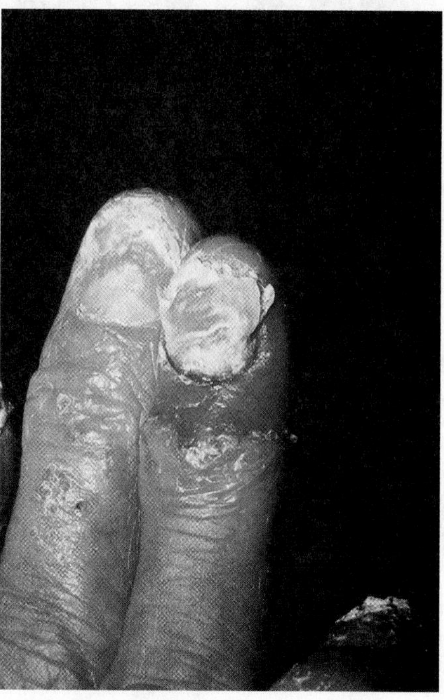

FIGURE 464–9 • Thickening and crumbling of the nail plate (onychodystrophy) in a patient with psoriasis. Note the erythematous patches with silvery scales in the periungual area.

drop" sign), and thickening of the nail (onychodystrophy) (Fig. 464–9). Minor injury to the skin can result in the development of psoriatic lesions (Koebner's phenomenon). The association of psoriasis with HIV infection (Chapter 415) has been well documented; HIV-associated psoriasis tends to be inflammatory and is usually more resistant to treatment compared with non–HIV-associated psoriasis.

Several distinct forms of psoriasis are recognized. *Psoriasis vulgaris,* the most common type, appears as a persistent erythematous scaly papule and plaque on elbows, knees, and scalp; however, it may also involve any part of the body. *Guttate psoriasis* usually occurs after viral or bacterial (most commonly streptococcal) infection; it appears as small, erythematous, scaly papules scattered over a large area of the body in a raindrop distribution (guttate = droplike). *Inverse psoriasis* refers to psoriasis that occurs in skinfold areas such as the groin, axilla, and inframammary folds. It appears as an erythematous, somewhat shiny patch; because of the constant friction in the involved areas, scales are usually absent. *Erythrodermic psoriasis* appears as widespread, sometimes generalized erythroderma with fine silvery scales, frequently associated with fissures. *Palmoplantar psoriasis* manifests as keratotic scaly patches and plaques on the palms and soles, very frequently with accompanying fissures, which can be painful. *Pustular psoriasis of von Zumbusch* is a rare variant of psoriasis occurring with generalized pustules that are 2 to 3 mm in diameter and associated with the onset of fever.

Five to 30% of patients with psoriasis may also have psoriatic arthritis, which may precede that appearance of cutaneous lesions (Chapter 286). Most of these patients present with peripheral asymmetrical oligoarthritis involving the interphalangeal joints of the hands and feet, the large joints of the legs, or combinations of both. Psoriatic arthritis has been associated with HLA-B57, although some studies have also reported HLA-Cw6 in more than 50% of all persons with this disease.

Diagnosis

In most cases, the diagnosis of psoriasis can be made based on the history and physical examination alone. However, in patients with erythrodermic psoriasis, other causes of generalized erythroderma (including pityriasis rubra pilaris, drug eruption, and cutaneous T-cell lymphoma) must be excluded.

Treatment

Therapy includes topical medications, UV-based treatment, and systemic drugs. For mild disease, topical therapy such as with topical corticosteroids (e.g., triamcinolone ointment, 0.1% twice daily for 1 to 2 weeks), anthralin, calcipotriene cream (0.005%, twice daily as needed), tazarotene (0.05% gel, once or twice daily as needed) or with tar preparations (crude coal tar, 2% daily for 2 weeks), used alone or in combination, is effective. In patients who have widespread lesions, NB-UVB is the best option, whereas PUVA should be considered for patients in whom NB-UVB therapy has failed. For patients with recalcitrant disease, oral medications such as methotrexate (7.5 to 15 mg/week), acitretin (25 to 50 mg/day), cyclosporine (3 to 5 mg/kg/day), hydroxyurea (1 g/day), and mycophenolate mofetil (1 to 2 g/day) have all been used with success.

The most recent advance in the treatment of psoriasis is the use of the biologic agents, which are most appropriately used in patients who have widespread disease and in whom UV-based therapy or treatment with one of the systemic medications has failed (Table 464–4). Tumor necrosis factor-α (TNF-α) inhibitors include the following: etanercept, a human TNF-receptor/immunoglobulin G1 fusion protein; infliximab, a chimeric mouse anti–TNF-α antibody; and adalimumab, a human immunoglobulin G1 anti–TNF-α antibody. A CD2 antagonist is alefacept, a protein that is fused to IgG and that contains the binding site of lymphocyte function–associated antigen-3, which binds to CD2 markers on the surface of memory T cells. An anti-CD11a is efalizumab, a humanized monoclonal antibody.

Pityriasis Rubra Pilaris

Epidemiology

Pityriasis rubra pilaris occurs equally in men and women; the incidence ranges from 1 in 5000 new dermatology patients in Great Britain to 1 in 50,000 in India. This disease most frequently occurs as the acquired form, although a familial form (autosomal dominant with variable expression) also occurs. Sixty percent of patients have adult-onset disease, with peak incidences in the first, second, and fifth to sixth decades. Abnormal vitamin A metabolism has been postulated as a possible cause.

TABLE 464–4 BIOLOGIC AGENTS FOR PSORIASIS

Biologic Agents	Dose/Duration	Monitoring	Side Effects
TNF-α INHIBITORS			
Etanercept (Enbrel)	50 mg SC twice a week for 12 weeks, then 50 mg SC weekly indefinitely	PPD, chest radiograph, CBC	Injection site reaction
Infliximab (Remicade)	5–10 mg/kg IV at week 0, 2, 6, then every 8 wk indefinitely	PPD, chest radiograph, CBC, LFTs	Infusion reaction, sepsis, lupus-like syndrome, aplastic anemia (rare)
Adalimumab (Humira)	40 mg SC every 2 wk indefinitely	PPD, chest radiograph, CBC	Infection
ANTI-CD2			
Alefacept (Amevive)	15 mg IM weekly for 12–16 wk; consider a second course after a 12-wk interval	PPD, chest radiograph, CD4	Infection
ANTI-CD11a			
Efalizumab (Raptiva)	0.7 mg/kg SC, then 1 mg/kg every wk indefinitely	PPD, chest radiograph, CBC, platelet count	Infection, flare of psoriasis

CBC = complete blood count; IM = intramuscularly; IV = intravenously; LFTs = liver function tests; PPD = purified protein derivative; SC = subcutaneously; TNF = tumor necrosis factor.

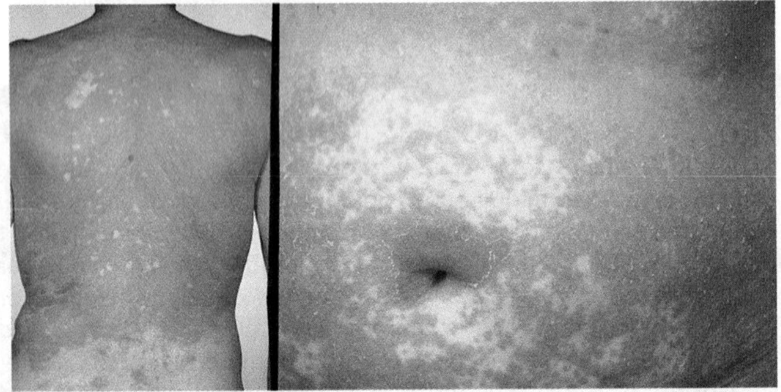

FIGURE 464–10 • Pityriasis rubra pilaris. Note the erythematous orange plaques with islands of sparing.

Clinical Manifestations

Clinically, patients present with erythematous to orange papules and plaques on all parts of the body (Fig. 464–10). Characteristically, skin appears normal between these lesions ("islands of sparing"). Erythema, hyperkeratosis, and fissures of the palms and soles are common; when severe, these lesions result in functional impairment. Many patients have follicular keratotic papules on the dorsa of the fingers and occasionally on the elbows as well as on the wrists. The nails are yellow and thickened, with distal splinter hemorrhages. In adult patients, the condition typically starts on the face and moves to the lower extremities; in the juvenile form, it usually starts in the lower half of the body. Ectropion may occur, and pruritus is observed in approximately 20% of patients. In contrast to psoriasis, arthritis is uncommon. Pityriasis rubra pilaris has been associated with HIV infection (Chapter 415).

Diagnosis

Definitive diagnosis can usually be made based on the clinical presentations and by the characteristic histologic findings of alternating vertical and horizontal parakeratosis in the stratum corneum.

Treatment

Rx

The most effective treatment is with oral retinoids (acitretin, 25 to 50 mg/day for 1 to 2 months). Methotrexate (7.5 to 15 mg/week), either as a monotherapy or in combination with oral acitretin (25 to 50 mg/day), is also beneficial. Other options include PUVA

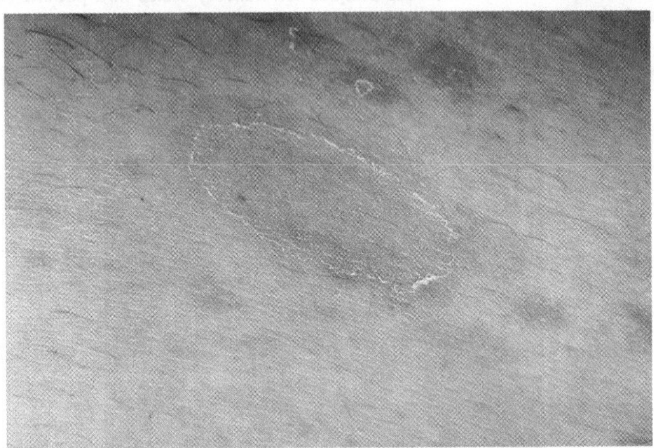

FIGURE 464–11 • Large erythematous oval patch (herald patch) of pityriasis rosea accompanied by smaller erythematous patches.

(8-methoxypsoralen, 0.4 to 0.6 mg/kg, with gradually increasing doses of UVA, three times weekly for 8 to 10 weeks), or cyclosporine (3 to 5 mg/kg/day). For all patients, topical over-the-counter emollients should be used as needed, and topical keratolytic agents, such as ammonium lactate lotion 12%, twice daily as needed, are helpful as adjunctive therapy.

Pityriasis Rosea

Epidemiology and Pathobiology

The incidence of pityriasis rosea has been reported as 3 to 30 per 1000 patients. It occurs in all ethnic groups, most commonly in the third and fourth decades of life, with a slight female predominance. The cause is not known, and a possible association with human herpesviruses 6 and 7 has been reported.

Clinical Manifestations

In 50 to 90% of patients, pityriasis rosea starts with a primary lesion (herald patch), which is an erythematous, scaly, oval patch a few centimeters in diameter. This lesion is usually followed within a few days by smaller erythematous scaly patches on the trunk, less commonly on the proximal extremities (Fig. 464–11). As a rule, the palms and soles are spared. The distribution of the eruption, especially on the back, tends to follow the lines of cleavage of the skin, with a resulting "Christmas tree" distribution. Lesions are most commonly asymptomatic, although they may be mildly pruritic. The eruption is self-limiting and resolves within 6 to 8 weeks. In rare instances, lesions may persist.

Diagnosis

The diagnosis can usually be made clinically. The most important differential diagnosis is secondary syphilis, which, in contrast to pityriasis rosea, usually involves the palms and soles. In many instances, a rapid plasma reagin test is advisable to exclude syphilis.

Treatment

Rx

Treatment is primarily symptomatic, including topical corticosteroids and oral antihistamines. NB-UVB phototherapy or PUVA should be reserved for patients with severe, recalcitrant cases.

Lichen Planus

Epidemiology

Lichen planus occurs most commonly in patients between 30 and 60 years of age. Women are affected more frequently than men and tend to be somewhat older at the onset of disease. The prevalence in the general population is about 1%.

Pathobiology

Histologically, lichen planus is characterized by dense lymphocytic infiltrate at the dermal-epidermal junction. The infiltrates consist of predominantly T cells, a finding suggesting the pathogenic role of cell-mediated immunity. Because lichen planus or lichen planus–like eruptions can occur after exposure to drugs or chemicals (e.g., color film developer), the role of drugs and chemicals in inducing a T-cell–mediated response against the epidermis has been postulated. Lichen planus may be associated with hepatitis C infection (Chapter 152).

Clinical Manifestations

Clinically, patients usually present with erythematous to violaceous flat-topped papules, often with white lacy lines (Wickham's striae) on the wrists, forearms, and genitalia (Fig. 464–12). *Oral lichen planus* occurs as white papules and plaques with a reticulated appearance, most commonly along the bite line on the buccal mucosa. Occasionally, erosion may occur. *Hypertrophic lichen planus* usually occurs on the lower extremities as lichenified, violaceous plaques, probably secondary to chronic rubbing and scratching of the lichen planus lesions. *Erosive lichen planus* occurs as erosion usually surrounded by violaceous discoloration at the periphery; this variant tends to occur more commonly on the feet. *Bullous lichen planus* occurs as vesicles or bullae arising from a preexisting lesion of lichen planus. *Lichen planopilaris* occurs as violaceous papules and plaques involving the scalp, most prominently surrounding the hair follicles; it progresses to scarring alopecia. *Lichen planus actinicus*, a variant of lichen planus occurring most commonly in the Middle East, tends to occur on the sun-exposed areas such as the forehead; it occurs as papules or plaques with minimally elevated rolled edges. *Atrophic lichen planus* resembles typical lichen planus lesion but with a central area of superficial atrophy. *Lichen planus of the nails* occurs as thinning of the nail with longitudinal ridges; it may progress to complete loss of the nail plate (pterygium formation).

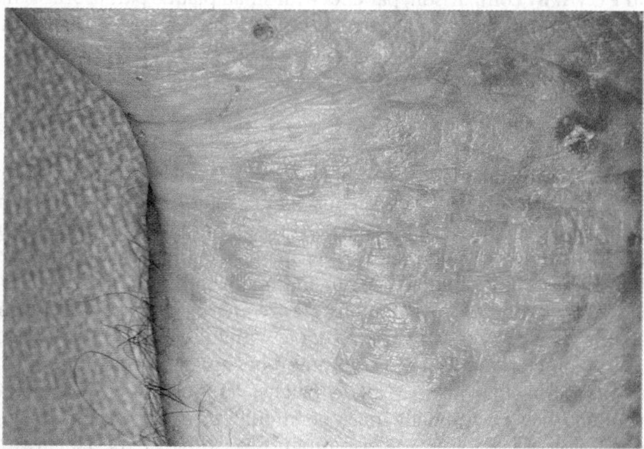

FIGURE 464–12 • Erythematous papules on the wrist of a patient with lichen planus.

Diagnosis

The diagnosis can be made by clinical appearance. It is confirmed by the characteristic histologic findings of infiltration by lymphocytes at the dermal-epidermal junction.

Treatment

Several treatment options are available. Topical corticosteroids (e.g., triamcinolone ointment, 0.1% twice daily for 1 to 2 weeks) are helpful in patients with limited disease. Hypertrophic lichen planus can be treated with topical corticosteroids (fluocinonide 0.05% ointment twice daily for 2 to 3 weeks), with occlusion at night, or with interlesional corticosteroid injections (triamcinolone suspension, 3 to 5 mg/mL). A 6- to 8-week course of oral corticosteroid is helpful in patients with widespread lichen planus. NB-UVB phototherapy or PUVA is helpful for widespread conditions. Oral acitretin (25 to 50 mg/day) or systemic cyclosporine (3 to 5 mg/kg/day) has been used with good success in some patients. Oral lesions can be treated with topical corticosteroids (triamcinolone 0.1% paste, twice daily for 2 to 3 weeks), topical retinoids (tretinoin gel 0.01% twice daily for 3 to 4 weeks), or cyclosporine solution (100 mg/mL, 1 mL, twice daily, swish and swallow). Without treatment, cutaneous lesions resolve in approximately 1 year, whereas oral and hypertrophic lesions tend to be much more chronic, persisting for 4.5 years and 8.5 years, respectively.

Lichen Nitidus

Lichen nitidus is a rather uncommon condition that usually occurs in children or young adults. The incidence has been estimated to be 3.4 cases per 10,000 population. It is more commonly observed in dark-skinned individuals. The cause is unclear, and no infectious agent has been identified.

The lesions are 1- to 2-mm, shiny, skin-colored discrete papules, sometimes with fine scales on their surface, occurring most commonly on the genitalia or forearms and occasionally on the trunk. A generalized form has rarely been reported. Lesions are usually asymptomatic. Histologically, one sees a dense lymphocytic infiltrate in the superficial dermis and at the dermal epidermal junction. In contrast to lichen planus, in which the infiltrate tends to involve the entire section of the skin, the infiltrate in lichen nitidus tends to be much more focal and localized.

The diagnosis usually can be confirmed from the typical clinical appearance and the characteristic histologic changes. The condition tends to remit spontaneously in a few years, so therapy, with topical corticosteroids (e.g., triamcinolone ointment, 0.1% twice daily for 2 weeks) and oral antihistamines (e.g., fexofenadine, 180 mg every morning, and hydroxyzine, 25 to 50 mg at bedtime, as needed) should be reserved for symptomatic cases only.

Secondary Syphilis

Lesions of secondary syphilis typically occur 1 to 2 months after the development of a primary chancre lesion (Chapter 340). However, up to 25% of patients may not remember having a chancre. Once the eruption occurs, it lasts for 1 to 3 months.

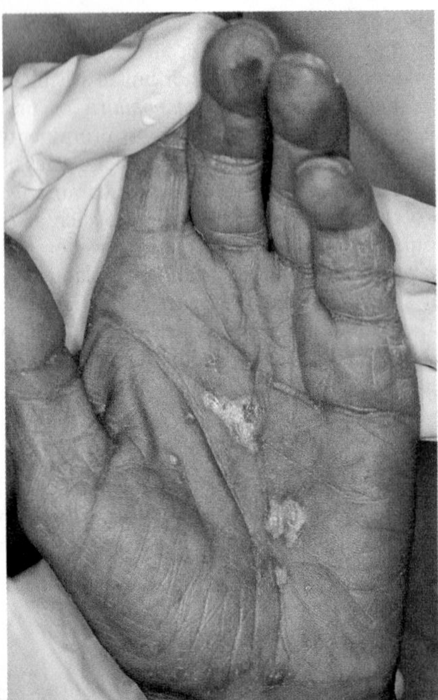

FIGURE 464–13 • Scaly papules and plaques on the palm of a patient with secondary syphilis.

Clinically, secondary syphilis may appear as erythematous macules ("roseola syphilitica"), erythematous to hyperpigmented oval or circular papules and plaques covered with scales, or a maculopapular eruption. Nodular eruption may also occur occasionally. The lesions tend to be widespread, and the palms and soles are very frequently involved (Fig. 464–13). The diagnosis is made based on the history, physical examination, and a positive rapid plasma reagin test. Skin biopsy shows the proliferation of endothelial cells in the dermis and a dense dermal infiltrate containing many plasma cells. Intramuscular penicillin is the treatment of choice.

Pityriasis Lichenoides

Pityriasis lichenoides occurs as erythematous papules that may be minimally pruritic and covered with scales, scattered on all parts of the body. In the acute form (pityriasis lichenoides et varioliformis acuta [PLEVA]), the central part of the lesions develops vesicles, pustules, and hemorrhages, with eventual crusting of the lesions. The patient may have mild constitutional symptoms of fever and malaise. The chronic form (pityriasis lichenoides chronica [PLC]) occurs as asymptomatic erythematous to hyperpigmented papules and plaques covered with fine scales; the trunk and extremities are common sites. Histologically, both PLEVA and PLC are characterized by dense lymphocytic infiltrates in the dermis, with CD8 lymphocytes predominating in PLEVA and CD4 lymphocytes in PLC.

PLEVA usually resolves in a few months, although it can persist. PLC usually lasts for a few years. PLEVA is less common than PLC, although both disorders affect patients of all ages, with a slight male predominance.

Treatment generally follows a sequential order: (1) topical corticosteroids (e.g., triamcinolone ointment, 0.1% twice daily for 1 to 2 weeks) and antihistamines, (2) tetracycline (1 to 2 g/day), or erythromycin (1 to 2 g/day), (3) NB-UVB phototherapy (three times weekly for 8 to 10 weeks with increasing doses of NB-UVB) or PUVA, and (4) methotrexate (7.5 to 15 mg/week).

Parapsoriasis

The two common variants of parapsoriasis are large plaque parapsoriasis and small plaque parapsoriasis. The peak incidence is in the fifth decade, although rare cases may begin in childhood. Large plaque parapsoriasis appears as oval to circular, erythematous to hyperpigmented macules and patches with fine scales and superficial atrophy (crinkling atrophy) scattered on all parts of the body (Fig. 464–14). These lesions are usually larger than 5 cm. Although lesions may be minimally pruritic, they are usually asymptomatic. Large plaque parapsoriasis is considered

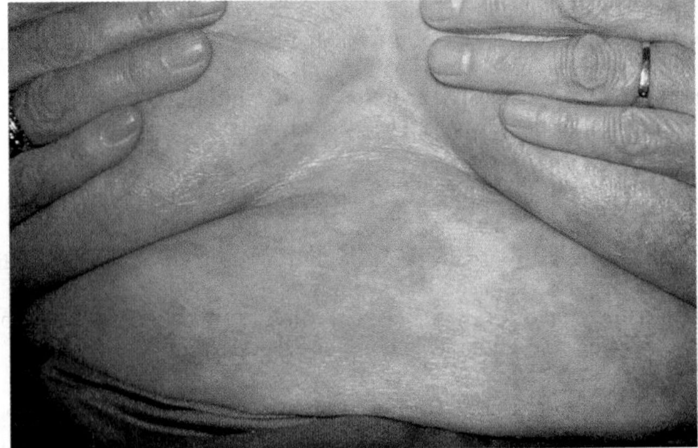

FIGURE 464–14 • Erythematous patches with fine scales in a patient with large plaque parapsoriasis.

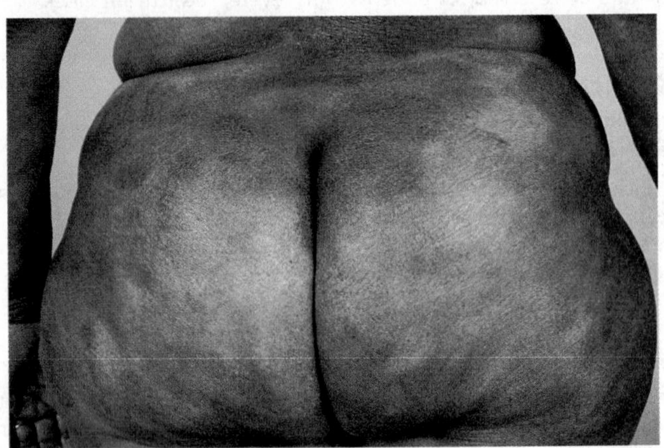

FIGURE 464–15 • Hyperpigmented patches in a patient with mycosis fungoides.

by some to be a less aggressive variant of mycosis fungoides (see later). Small plaque parapsoriasis appears as circular to oval erythematous to hyperpigmented patches or minimally elevated plaques, with lesions less than 5 cm in diameter and usually covered with fine scales. Digitate dermatosis is a distinct variant of small plaque parapsoriasis in which lesions appear along the line of cleavage, usually on the lateral aspect of the trunk in the shape of fingerprints. Histologically, large plaque parapsoriasis is characterized by a dermal lymphocytic infiltrate, which may extend into the epidermis, whereas small plaque parapsoriasis is characterized by spongiotic dermatitis, with a mild superficial lymphocytic infiltrate in the dermis. In up to one third of patients, large plaque parapsoriasis may evolve into mycosis fungoides. As a result, treatment of large plaque parapsoriasis is similar to that of early-stage mycosis fungoides: high-potency topical corticosteroids, topical nitrogen mustard, NB-UVB phototherapy, and PUVA. By comparison, patients with small plaque parapsoriasis have a benign course, and management of small plaque parapsoriasis should be symptomatic only, with emollients, topical corticosteroids, and NB-UVB phototherapy.

Mycosis Fungoides

Mycosis fungoides is a variant of cutaneous T-cell lymphoma (Chapter 196). The four types of cutaneous manifestations are patch, plaque, tumor, and erythrodermic. The patch stage of mycosis fungoides manifests as patches with fine "cigarette paper" wrinkling of the epidermis. The patches can be skin colored or minimally erythematous; hyperpigmented or hypopigmented lesions are frequently seen in dark-skinned patients. The patches can vary from a few millimeters to a few centimeters in diameter; they are more common on sun-protected areas such as the buttocks (Fig. 464–15). The patches are usually asymptomatic, although they occasionally may be mildly pruritic. Lesions may be present for years. As the disease progresses, some of the patches may become more indurated and may evolve into more elevated plaques. Nodular lesions may occur in patients without any patch or plaque lesions, although more commonly these lesions occur in conjunction with patches and plaques. Erythrodermic mycosis fungoides occurs as a generalized erythroderma with significant scaling and pruritus. Hyperkeratosis of the palms and soles, as well as fissuring of hands and feet, are quite common. In dark-skinned patients, mycosis fungoides may appear as hypopigmented patches.

The diagnosis is confirmed by histologic demonstration of atypical mononuclear cells both in the epidermis and in the dermis, as well as immunophenotypic markers showing predominance of CD4 cells in the infiltrate. Therapy for mycosis fungoides generally follows a sequential order: (1) topical nitrogen mustard (i.e., mechlorethamine, 10 mg in 60 mL of water, applied daily until lesions resolve, then taper), or NB-UVB, each of which can be combined with topical corticosteroids (e.g., triamcinolone ointment, 0.1% twice daily for 1 to 2 months); (2) PUVA; (3) topical retinoids (e.g., bexarotene gel, 1% once to four times daily, until lesions resolve); and (4) one of the following: oral bexarotene (300 mg/m^2/day for 2 to 4 months) or interferon-α (3 to 9 million U subcutaneously 3 times weekly for 2 to 4 months). Erythrodermic disease is most effectively treated with extracorporeal photopheresis.

Dermatophytoses

Fungal infections that occur as papulosquamous eruptions include tinea corporis, tinea manuum, tinea cruris, and tinea pedis. Tinea corporis causes a polycyclic erythematous scaly patch that has elevated borders and consists of papules and sometimes pustules. As the lesion progresses, the border advances centrifugally. The trunk is the most common site. Tinea cruris has similar morphologic features, except it is located in the inguinal folds and expands centrifugally from the folds. In men, the scrotum is usually spared. Tinea manuum presents as an erythematous scaly patch with an advancing active border, usually located on the dorsum of the hands, or it may occur as diffuse scaly patches with mild hyperkeratosis involving part or the entire surface of the palm and palmar aspect of the fingers. Tinea pedis also has two clinical manifestations: it can occur as scaly macerated lesions with erythema in the toe webs or as patchy or diffuse scaliness on the sole extending to the medial and lateral aspect of the foot (moccasin distribution). The latter presentation can be associated with diffuse scaliness of one but not both palms, a condition known as the "one-hand, two-feet syndrome." The diagnosis can be confirmed by examination of skin scrapings using 10% potassium hydroxide preparation and/or by fungal culture. Treatment consists of topical or oral antifungal medications (e.g., clotrimazole cream, 1%, twice daily for 2 to 4 weeks, or terbinafine, 250 mg for 2 to 12 weeks, depending on the site involved).

Tinea Versicolor

Tinea versicolor is a fungal infection of the skin caused by *Malassezia furfur.* It occurs in otherwise healthy young individuals, especially in warm and moist environments during the summer. Clinically, it appears as macules and patches with very fine scales; the color can be hypopigmented, skin colored, minimally erythematous, or light brown (Fig. 464–16). The patches start as perifollicular macules, with the midchest and midback the most common sites. As the lesions progress, hypopigmentation of the skin may also occur. The lesion usually is asymptomatic. The diagnosis is confirmed by the characteristic appearance of the fungal elements on a 10% potassium hydroxide preparation: grapelike clusters of yeast and short, septate branching hyphae ("spaghetti and meatballs" appearance). Treatment is with 2.5% selenium sulfide shampoo (applied for 10 minutes then wash off, 5 times weekly for 4 to 6 weeks), topical antifungal preparations (e.g., clotrimazole cream, 1% twice daily for 4 weeks), or a 1- to 3-day course of oral ketoconazole (200 mg/day) or itraconazole (200 mg/day).

FIGURATE ERYTHEMAS

These conditions appear as erythematous circular or polycyclic plaques with central clearing and, frequently, centrifugally migrating border (Table 464–5). Occasionally, fine scaling may also be observed. The extremities are the most common sites. The diagnosis can frequently be made by the typical history and morphologic features.

Erythema annulare centrifugum is most commonly idiopathic; however, it can also be a manifestation of a hypersensitivity response to medications. Management includes identification of a precipitating agent (if possible) and treatment with topical or systemic corticosteroids.

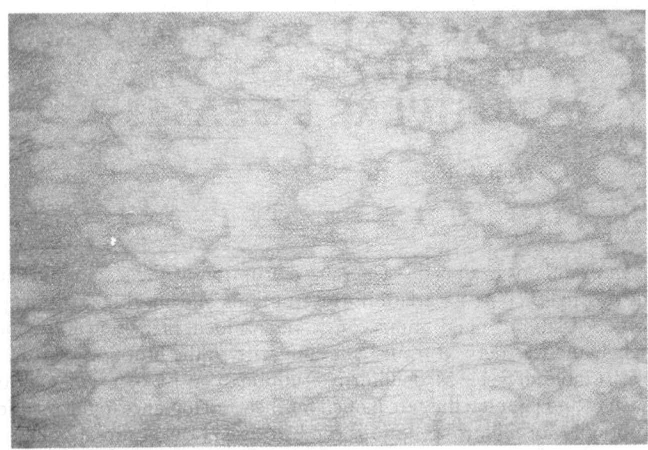

FIGURE 464–16 • Hypopigmented patches of tinea versicolor.

TABLE 464–5 FIGURATE ERYTHEMAS

Erythema annulare centrifugum
Erythema gyratum repens
Erythema chronicum migrans

Erythema gyratum repens occurs as concentric erythematous plaques with fine scales, resembling a "wood-grain" pattern. This unusual form of figurate erythema has been associated with malignant hematologic diseases and with carcinomas of the breast, lung, gastrointestinal tract, prostate, and cervix. Treatment of the underlying malignant disease results in the resolution of the skin lesion in a few months. *Erythema chronicum migrans*, which is a cutaneous manifestation of Lyme disease and is caused by the spirochete *Borrelia burgdorferi* (Chapter 342), appears as a concentric ring of erythema that progresses centrifugally from the site of a tick bite. Occasionally, it may appear as a circular erythematous patch. The diagnosis is made by a history of a tick bite, the characteristic cutaneous lesion, and/or elevated serum antibodies to *B. burgdorferi*. Management is the same as for Lyme disease.

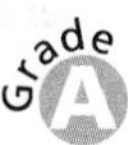

1. Ashcroft DM, Dimmock P, Garside R, et al: Efficacy and tolerability of topical pimecrolimus and tacrolimus in the treatment of atopic dermatitis: Meta-analysis of randomized controlled trials. BMJ 2005;330:516–521.
2. Paller AS, Lebwohl M, Fleischer AB Jr, et al, US/Canada Tacrolimus Ointment Study Group. Tacrolimus ointment is more effective than pimecrolimus cream with a similar safety profile in the treatment of atopic dermatitis: Results from 3 randomized, comparative studies. J Am Acad Dermatol 2005;52:810–822.
3. Reynolds NJ, Franklin V, Gray JC, et al: Narrow-band ultraviolet B and broad-band ultraviolet A phototherapy in adult atopic eczema: A randomised controlled trial. Lancet 2001;357: 2012–2016.

SUGGESTED READINGS

de Quatrebarbes J, Esteve E, Bagot M, et al: Treatment of early-stage mycosis fungoides with twice-weekly applications of mechlorethamine and topical corticosteroids: A prospective study. Arch Dermatol 2005;141:1117–1120. *The combination appeared to be beneficial.*

Liao WC, Mutasim DF: Infliximab for the treatment of adult-onset pityriasis rubra pilaris. Arch Dermatol 2005;141:423–425. *A biologic agent was useful.*

Lowes MA, Bowcock AM, Krueger JG: Pathogenesis and therapy of psoriasis. Nature 2007;445:866–873. *A molecular and pathophysiologic review.*

Morison WL: Photosensitivity. N Engl J Med 2004;350:1111–1117. *A case-based review.*

Schön MP, Boehncke W-H: Psoriasis. N Engl J Med 2005;352:1899–1912. *A comprehensive review.*

Warshaw EM, Wohlhuter RJ, Liu A, et al: Results of a randomized, double-blind, vehicle-controlled efficacy trial of pimecrolimus cream 1% for the treatment of moderate to severe facial seborrheic dermatitis. J Am Acad Dermatol 2006; [Epub ahead of print]. *Pimecrolimus may be effective.*

Watanabe T, Kawamura T, Jacob SE, et al: Pityriasis rosea is associated with systemic active infection with both human herpesvirus-7 and human herpesvirus-6. J Invest Dermatol 2002;119:779–780. *A carefully done study on the association of herpesviruses with pityriasis rosea.*

Williams HC: Atopic dermatitis. N Engl J Med 2005;352:2314–2324. *A comprehensive review.*

465 MACULAR, PAPULAR, VESICULOBULLOUS, AND PUSTULAR DISEASES

Neil J. Korman

MACULAR AND PAPULAR EXANTHEMS

An exanthem is an acute generalized eruption of the skin, and there are two major types: scarlatiniform eruptions and morbilliform eruptions. Scarlatiniform eruptions consist of confluent blanching erythema; their name was derived from their similarity to the eruption of scarlet fever (Table 465–1). Morbilliform eruptions consist of erythematous macules and papules; they are named for their resemblance to the measles eruption. Morbilliform eruptions can be caused by exposure to medications (Chapter 466) or viral infections.

Scarlatiniform Eruptions

Scarlet Fever

Scarlet fever is caused by infection of the ears, nose, throat, and skin with toxin-producing β-hemolytic streptococci (Chapter 312). It most commonly occurs in children after streptococcal wound infections, burns, and upper respiratory tract infections. Occasional cases of scarlet fever can also be caused by *Staphylococcus aureus* (Chapter 310), *Haemophilus influenzae* (Chapter 323), and *Clostridium* species (Chapter 319). The rash is due to a circulating toxin that induces local production of inflammatory mediators and alteration of cutaneous cytokines. Patients may have an abrupt onset of fever, headache, vomiting, malaise, chills, and sore throat. The mucous membranes are usually erythematous with petechiae, and the tongue commonly has a white membrane. Red, exudative tonsils are present with pharyngeal infections. The skin eruption appears after the fever and is characterized by fine erythematous papules, first on the upper part of the trunk and then in a more general distribution. The face is flushed, and circumoral pallor is seen. This eruption lasts for 4 to 5 days, followed by fine desquamation, the extent and duration of which are related to the severity of the eruption. Treatment is 1.2 million units of benzathine penicillin G given intramuscularly or oral penicillin VK, 1000 mg twice daily for 10 days. Most patients recover after 4 to 5 days, and the rash usually resolves completely over a period of several weeks.

Toxic Shock Syndrome

Definition

Toxic shock syndrome is an acute febrile illness caused by toxin-producing strains of *S. aureus* (Chapter 310) or, less commonly, *Streptococcus* (toxic shock–like syndrome [Chapter 311]).

TABLE 465–1 MACULAR AND PAPULAR ERUPTIONS

SCARLATINIFORM ERUPTIONS
Scarlet fever
Toxic shock syndrome
Kawasaki's disease
MORBILLIFORM ERUPTIONS
Measles
Rubella
Erythema infectiosum
Roseola
PAPULAR ERUPTIONS
Molluscum contagiosum
Warts

Pathobiology

Most cases of staphylococcal toxic shock syndrome or streptococcal toxic shock–like syndrome occur in young healthy persons aged 20 to 50 years. These toxins cause massive release of tumor necrosis factor-α and interleukin-1, cytokines that mediate fever, rash, hypotension, tissue injury, and shock.

Clinical Manifestations

The hallmarks of the disease are fever, rash, hypotension, and involvement of multiple organs, including the lungs, kidneys, liver, and gastrointestinal tract. Desquamation of the palms and soles follows onset of the illness by 1 to 2 weeks. There is diffuse macular erythema with flexural accentuation, mucous membrane erythema, and severe conjunctival involvement. Blood cultures are positive in 5 to 15% of patients with staphylococcal toxic shock syndrome and approximately 50% of those with streptococcal toxic shock–like syndrome.

Treatment

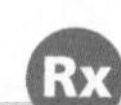

Treatment is supportive and includes hydration, vasopressors, appropriate antibiotics, and drainage of infected sites. Patients with staphylococcal toxic shock should be treated with intravenous vancomycin to cover methicillin-resistant staphylococci, 1 g every 12 hours for 10 to 15 days, with dose adjustment based on creatinine clearance. Patients with streptococcal toxic shock should be treated with both intravenous penicillin G, 3 to 4 million units every 4 hours, and intravenous clindamycin, 600 to 900 mg every 8 hours for 10 to 15 days, followed by oral therapy. Double antibiotic coverage is the standard of care for streptococcal toxic shock syndrome because this infection is characterized by extremely large numbers of stationary bacteria and penicillin alone is not effective in this scenario inasmuch as penicillin binding proteins are not expressed during the stationary group phase of streptococci. Silver sulfadiazine cream may lead to increased toxin production; therefore, mupirocin ointment should be used for infected sites.

Prognosis

The mortality rate in patients with staphylococcal toxic shock syndrome is 5 to 15%, whereas that for streptococcal toxic shock–like syndrome may be five times higher.

Kawasaki's Disease

Epidemiology

Kawasaki's disease, a systemic vasculitis of unknown etiology, occurs in children of all races but is most prevalent in Japan. Though primarily an illness of children younger than 5 years, Kawasaki's disease also occurs in adults. Its epidemiologic and clinical manifestations imply that an infection is the cause, but bacterial, viral, and serologic studies have yet to confirm such an etiology.

Clinical Manifestations

The clinical hallmarks are fever lasting up to 2 weeks, with spikes to 40° C (104° F), and a toxic-appearing patient. During the acute phase, the polymorphic eruption may be scarlatiniform, urticarial, morbilliform, or targetoid. Desquamation occurs in the perianal area 2 days after the onset of fever and on the extremities 2 to 3 weeks later. Patients often have hemorrhagic, dry fissured lips, conjunctival injection, a "strawberry tongue," and cervical lymphadenitis. Myocarditis and coronary artery aneurysms may develop in untreated patients, so prompt diagnosis is critical. Other findings include arthralgias and arthritis, urethritis, aseptic meningitis, pneumonitis, and diarrhea.

Diagnosis

Despite the lack of specific diagnostic tests for this syndrome, the typical skin eruption accompanied by myocarditis is characteristic.

Treatment Rx

Recommended therapy in the acute phase includes intravenous gamma globulin, 400 mg/kg/day for 4 days, and acetylsalicylic acid, 100 mg/kg, until the patient has been afebrile for several days. During the subacute and convalescent phase, acetylsalicylic acid is usually given at 3 to 8 mg/kg for 6 to 8 weeks. The optimal salicylate regimen for Kawasaki's disease remains uncertain, and there are no controlled trials to prove that aspirin reduces coronary artery aneurysms.

Morbilliform Eruptions

Measles

Measles is caused by a paramyxovirus (Chapter 390) that infects respiratory epithelium and is highly transmissible. The incubation period is 7 to 14 days. The prodrome consists of cough, coryza, and conjunctivitis. The enanthem, or Koplik's spots, predates the exanthem by 1 to 2 days and lasts 2 to 4 days. These blue-white spots surrounded by a red halo appear on the buccal mucosa and are pathognomonic for measles. The exanthem begins on the fourth or fifth day as papules on the face and behind the ears; it then spreads to the trunk and extremities. Measles is diagnosed on clinical grounds. Active immunization with live attenuated virus has dramatically reduced the incidence of measles infection (Chapter 16) and is the most important preventive measure. Treatment consists of supportive care, with attention to maintaining good hydration.

Rubella

Rubella is an RNA virus of the Togaviridae family (Chapter 391). Infection with this virus leads to an illness involving the skin, lymph nodes, and occasionally the joints, primarily in young children. The disease is spread by nasal droplet infection and has an incubation period of 14 to 21 days. Patients are most contagious when the rash is erupting. In children there may be no prodrome; in adults, however, fever, sore throat, and rhinitis may be present. The exanthem begins as pink macules and papules on the face that spread to the trunk and extremities; it lasts 1 to 3 days. Generalized tender lymphadenopathy, especially the suboccipital, postauricular, and cervical nodes, is the hallmark of rubella. In normal children and adolescents, the diagnosis is made clinically and laboratory work is unnecessary. If the diagnosis is questioned, a rising IgM antibody titer over a 2-week period indicates recent infection. No treatment exists, and the disease is usually self-limited. Rest and fluids are appropriate. The best protection is vaccination given with measles and mumps vaccine (i.e., MMR) at 12 to 15 months and again at 4 to 6 years (Chapter 16).

Erythema Infectiosum

Erythema infectiosum is an exanthem caused by human parvovirus B19 (Chapter 394). It has a 4- to 14-day incubation period and is spread by aerosolized respiratory droplets. Acute infection leads to the production of IgM antibodies and the formation of immune complexes, which are deposited in the skin and joints. Bright red erythema appears abruptly over the cheeks. Within 1 to 4 days, an erythematous morbilliform eruption occurs on the extremities; it fades within several days to a reticulate pattern (Fig. 465–1). There may also be malar erythema or a reticulate eruption on the extremities. Exposure of adults to parvovirus B19 leads to an acute polyarthropathy of the hands, wrists, knees, and ankles. Parvovirus B19 can interfere with erythropoiesis (Chapter 171) and can cause aplastic crisis in patients with sickle cell disease (Chapter 167). The diagnosis is clinical, and further testing is not generally necessary. Erythema infectiosum is usually a benign, self-limited disease.

Roseola

Roseola (exanthem subitum) is caused by human herpesvirus 6 (Chapter 397). Virus replication occurs in leukocytes and salivary glands. Early invasion of the central nervous system (CNS) may lead to seizures. The classic patient is a healthy 9- to 12-month-old with an abrupt onset of high fever (40° C [104° F]) lasting for 3 days. Febrile seizures occur in 15% of cases. Its rapid defervescence is striking, with the onset of a generalized pink morbilliform exanthem. The eruption lasts 2 days and

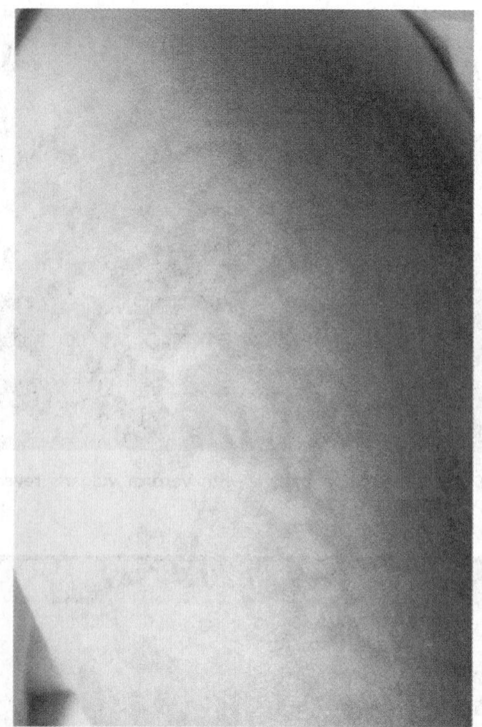

FIGURE 465–1 • Reticulate macular erythema on the thigh of a patient with erythema infectiosum.

consists of pink papules or blanchable macular erythema. The lack of symptoms during the febrile phase and appearance of the exanthem as the fever subsides help with the diagnosis, but rubella and measles must also be considered. In an immunocompromised child or adult, there is usually an abrupt onset of fever, malaise, and sometimes CNS involvement. Virus isolation, seroconversion (IgM), or detection of viral DNA sequences in peripheral blood mononuclear cells can confirm the diagnosis. No antiviral therapy is available for roseola, and treatment is supportive. Practically all immunocompetent patients recover from roseola without sequelae, but chronic infection with multisystem complications may develop in immunocompromised patients.

Papular Eruptions

Molluscum Contagiosum

Molluscum contagiosum is a cutaneous infection caused by a large DNA poxvirus that affects both children and adults. Firm, smooth, umbilicated papules, usually 2 to 6 mm in diameter, are present in groups or widely disseminated on the skin and mucosal surfaces. Patients infected with human immunodeficiency virus (HIV) may have hundreds of lesions, and some lesions can be larger than 15 mm (Chapter 415). The diagnosis is made on clinical grounds. Molluscum contagiosum is self-limited, with the goal of treatment being destruction of the lesions. Commonly used treatments are all topical and include cryotherapy with liquid nitrogen, curettage, cantharidin, podophyllin, and tretinoin.

Warts

Warts are benign proliferations of skin and mucosa caused by human papillomaviruses (HPVs) (Chapter 396). More than 150 types of HPV have been identified. Certain types of HPV occur at particular anatomic sites; however, warts of any HPV type may be found at any site. Variants include common warts, genital warts, flat warts, and deep palmoplantar warts. Common warts, known as verruca vulgaris, are hard papules that range in size from 1 mm to more than 1 cm with a rough scaly surface (Fig. 465–2) and can occur anywhere on the body. Warts are transmitted by direct contact, and disruption of the epithelial barrier is a predisposing factor. HPV subtypes 6, 11, 16, 18, 31, and 35 may be associated with malignancies (Chapter 396). Malignant transformation, though uncommon, can occur in patients with genital warts or in immunocompromised patients. Infection is confined to the epithelium and does not result in systemic viral dissemination. The diagnosis is made on clinical grounds. Viral DNA identification via Southern blot hybridization is used to iden-

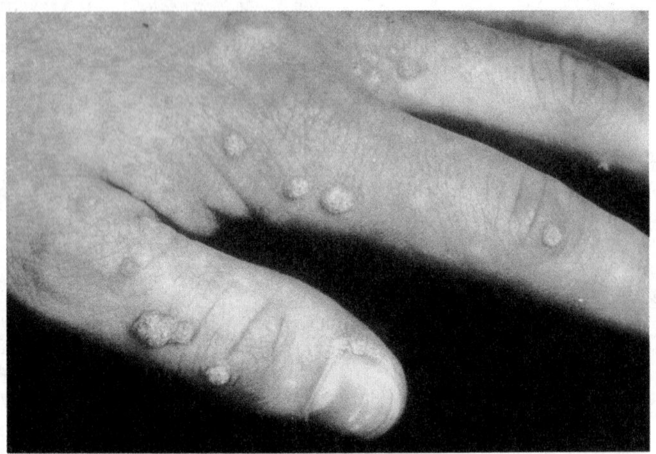

FIGURE 465–2 • Hand of a patient with verruca vulgaris revealing many verrucous papules.

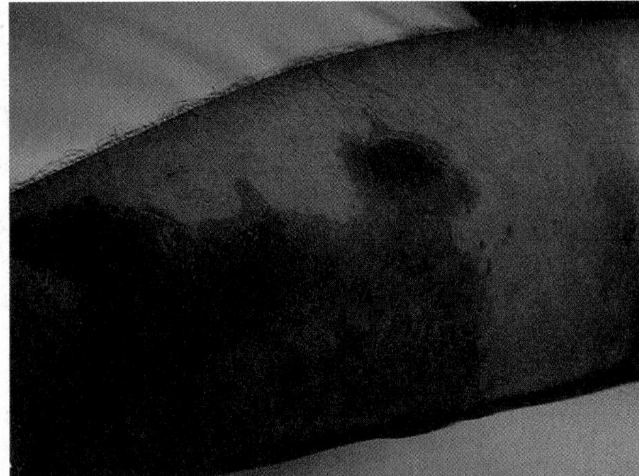

FIGURE 465–3 • Purpura fulminans. Purpura and hemorrhagic blisters are seen on the arm of this patient.

TABLE 465–2 PURPURIC ERUPTIONS

NONPALPABLE PURPURA
CUTANEOUS DISORDERS
Solar purpura
Steroid purpura
Pigmented purpuric dermatosis
SYSTEMIC DISORDERS
Idiopathic thrombocytopenic purpura
Abnormal platelet function in renal or hepatic disease
Thrombocytosis in myeloproliferative diseases
Clotting factor abnormalities
Ehlers-Danlos syndrome
Scurvy
Amyloidosis
Disseminated intravascular coagulation
Thrombotic thrombocytopenic purpura
Monoclonal cryoglobulinemia
Warfarin necrosis
Emboli
Cholesterol emboli
Fat emboli
Tumor emboli from atrial myxomas
Emboli from endocarditis
PALPABLE PURPURA
VASCULITIS
Leukocytoclastic vasculitis
Henoch-Schönlein purpura
Urticarial vasculitis
Polyarteritis nodosa
INFECTIOUS EMBOLI
Meningococcemia
Gonococcemia
Rocky Mountain spotted fever
Ecthyma gangrenosum

tify specific HPV subtypes. All therapies are methods of physical destruction of the skin where the virus is located because there are no specific antipapillomavirus medications. Common topical therapies include in-office treatment with liquid nitrogen, cantharidin, or podophyllin, as well as prescription-strength tretinoin or imiquimod. Over-the-counter liquid nitrogen is not as cold nor as effective as in-office treatment.

Purpuric Eruptions

Purpura occurs when red blood cell extravasation leads to visible hemorrhage in the skin (Table 465–2). Petechiae (<3 mm) and purpura (>3 mm) may be nonpalpable or palpable. When the condition is severe, petechiae and purpuric lesions may become confluent and form ecchymoses larger than 1 cm.

Nonpalpable Purpura

Dermal Causes

Frequent causes of nonpalpable purpura include solar purpura, steroid purpura, and Schamberg's disease. Solar purpura, caused by chronic sun exposure and aging, is usually found on the forearms. Steroid purpura, which is due to prolonged use of topical or systemic steroids, can occur in any location (Chapter 33). Both conditions are caused by changes in the dermal connective tissue surrounding blood vessels. Schamberg's disease, or pigmented purpuric dermatosis, is a capillaritis with yellow-brown macules and petechiae on the lower part of the legs. This capillaritis occurs as a result of red blood cell extravasation secondary to perivascular lymphocyte inflammation.

Systemic Causes

Systemic causes of nonpalpable purpura include idiopathic thrombocytopenia purpura (Chapter 179), abnormal platelet function as a result of renal or hepatic insufficiency (Chapters 131 and 158) or thrombocytosis as seen in myeloproliferative diseases (Chapter 177), and clotting factor abnormalities (Chapter 181). Fragility of the blood vessels, especially the capillaries, is found in Ehlers-Danlos syndrome (Chapter 281), scurvy (Chapter 232), and systemic amyloidosis (Chapter 296).

Thrombi

Thrombus formation within skin blood vessels also leads to purpura in patients with disseminated intravascular coagulation (Chapter 181), thrombotic thrombocytopenia purpura (Chapter 179), monoclonal cryoglobulinemia (Chapter 198), and drug reactions to warfarin (Chapter 35). Disseminated intravascular coagulation may be caused by infectious agents (bacterial, particularly meningococcemia, viral, or rickettsial) and by malignancies such as leukemia (Chapter 181). Purpura fulminans is a type of disseminated intravascular coagulation associated with fever and hypotension; it is usually found in children after a bacterial or viral infection. Widespread purpura and hemorrhagic bullae can be seen in disseminated intravascular coagulation and purpura fulminans (Fig. 465–3). Thrombotic thrombocytopenia purpura (Chapter 179) is manifested as fever, purpura, renal failure, microangiopathic hemolytic anemia, and neurologic disease. Monoclonal cryoglobulinemia may be associated with leukemia, lymphoma, multiple myeloma, and Waldenström's macroglobulinemia. Mixed cryoglobulinemia is frequently associated with hepatitis C infection (Chapter 152). Widespread purpura along with ulcerations limited to the lower extremities or fingers and toes can occur. Skin biopsy specimens may reveal intracapillary deposits of precipitated cryoglobulins. Disease can be worsened by exposure to cold. The vessels of the lungs, brain, and kidneys may be involved. Warfarin necrosis of the skin (Chapter 35) is an uncommon reaction that occurs between the third and tenth day of therapy and is characterized by painful erythematous to purpuric plaques in which hemorrhagic bullae develop. The most common sites include the breasts, thighs, and buttocks. The onset of disease is unrelated to the dose of warfarin, and continued warfarin therapy does not alter the course of the disease.

Emboli

Cholesterol emboli are found in the lower extremities of patients with severe atherosclerosis as a result of occlusion of small- and medium-caliber arteries by cholesterol crystals (Chapter 126). Cholesterol emboli are triggered by vascular procedures or thrombolytic therapy, but they can also occur spontaneously. Other sources of emboli that may cause petechiae or purpura include fat emboli occurring after major injury (Chapters 99 and 113), tumor emboli from atrial myxomas (Chapter 59), emboli from infective endocarditis (Chapter 76), or nonbacterial thrombotic endocarditis (Chapters 59 and 189).

Palpable Purpura

Vasculitis

Palpable purpura results from inflammatory damage to cutaneous blood vessels. Leukocytoclastic vasculitis, which is manifested as palpable purpura (Fig. 465–4), may be idiopathic or associated with sepsis, drug reactions, connective tissue diseases, cryoglobulinemia, hepatitis B or C infection, or underlying malignancies. Appropriate evaluation of patients with palpable purpura should always include histopathologic evaluation to confirm the diagnosis. Skin biopsy specimens from patients with leukocytoclastic vasculitis reveal angiocentric inflammation with endothelial cell swelling, fibrinoid necrosis of blood vessel walls, a neutrophilic cellular infiltrate with fragmentation of nuclei (karyorrhexis or leukocytoclasia) around and within blood vessel walls, and extravasated red blood cells (Fig. 465–5). Fresh skin biopsy specimens processed for direct immunofluorescence reveal deposits of immunoglobulins and complement in blood vessel walls. Once the diagnosis is confirmed, routine blood tests (including testing of renal and liver function) and urinalysis should be performed in all patients, whereas specialized tests should be targeted to specific patients with suggestive findings. If an etiologic agent can be identified and treated, the vasculitis will often resolve. Patients with idiopathic leukocytoclastic vasculitis can be treated with oral colchicine (0.6 mg twice daily), oral dapsone (100 mg once daily), or in the most severe cases, immunosuppressive agents such as azathioprine (up to 2.5 mg/kg for as long as the disease is active, as guided by the thiopurine methyltransferase level) or cyclophosphamide (up to 2 mg/kg for as long as the disease is active).

FIGURE 465–4 • Palpable purpura. Leukocytoclastic vasculitis commonly causes raised purpuric and ulcerated lesions on the legs.

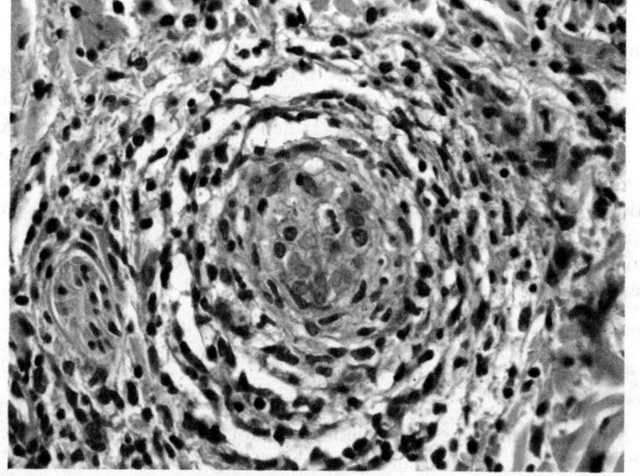

FIGURE 465–5 • Leukocytoclastic vasculitis. Histologic evaluation reveals a smudged blood vessel in the dermis with neutrophils, neutrophilic, dust, and red blood cells.

Henoch-Schönlein purpura is a leukocytoclastic vasculitis that affects children and young adults; it is often preceded by an upper respiratory infection with associated fever, arthralgias, abdominal pain, and renal vasculitis (Chapter 179). Direct immunofluorescence reveals IgA deposits in dermal blood vessels.

Urticarial or hypocomplementemic vasculitis (Chapter 291) is characterized by urticarial lesions that last longer than 24 hours; arthritis, facial, and laryngeal edema; and low serum complement levels. In some patients, systemic lupus erythematosus (Chapter 287) may develop. In polyarteritis nodosa (Chapter 291), vasculitis of the arterial blood vessels leads to ischemia of the skin. Skin lesions usually include ulcerated nodules and ecchymoses.

Cutaneous Emboli

In addition to vasculitis, cutaneous emboli can also lead to the development of palpable purpura. Infectious emboli (Chapter 76) can be caused by gram-negative cocci, gram-negative rods, *Rickettsia,* and in immunocompromised patients, *Candida* and opportunistic fungi. Acute meningococcemia (Chapter 311) occurs after an upper respiratory tract infection and is associated with headache, fever, meningitis, hypotension, and disseminated intravascular coagulation. The embolic lesions, which are found on the trunk and lower extremities, can range from 1 mm up to several centimeters. Disseminated gonococcal infection (Chapter 322) is accompanied by fever, arthralgias, tenosynovitis, and a small number of vesiculopustules with purpura or hemorrhagic necrosis over the distal ends of the extremities. Rocky Mountain spotted fever (Chapter 348) is a tick-borne disease characterized by headache, fever, chills, photophobia, and myalgias. The cutaneous eruption starts acrally and spreads centripetally as small, erythematous, blanchable macules that evolve into petechiae, palpable purpura, and ecchymoses. Ecthyma gangrenosum is manifested as erythematous papules and plaques in which central purpura and hemorrhagic necrosis develop; *Pseudomonas aeruginosa* (Chapter 328) is the most common organism, but *Klebsiella* (Chapter 309), *Escherichia coli* (Chapter 327), and *Serratia* (Chapter 309) have also been implicated. In immunocompromised patients, ecthyma gangrenosum may develop as a result of infection with *Candida* or opportunistic fungi.

VESICULOBULLOUS DISEASES

Vesicles are clear, fluid-filled lesions measuring less than 5 mm; bullae or blisters are clear, fluid-filled lesions larger than 5 mm. Vesiculobullous lesions in the skin may be caused by immunologically mediated mechanisms, hypersensitivity reactions, metabolic disorders, inherited genetic defects, and infections (Table 465–3).

Immunologically Mediated Blistering Diseases

Bullous Pemphigoid

Definition

Bullous pemphigoid is an autoimmune blistering disease of the elderly. Tense blisters and urticarial plaques occur on the flexor surfaces of the arms and legs, axilla, groin, and abdomen (Fig. 465–6).

Pathobiology

IgG autoantibodies bind to the epidermal basement membrane and activate complement, which attracts inflammatory cells. These inflammatory cells release proteases that degrade basement membrane proteins and lead to blister formation. Histology reveals a subepidermal blister with an eosinophilic infiltrate. Direct immunofluorescence shows linear deposits of IgG and C3 at the basement membrane. Indirect immunofluorescence studies using salt-split skin demonstrate circulating IgG antibodies that bind to the epidermal side.

TABLE 465–3 VESICULOBULLOUS DISEASES

IMMUNOLOGICALLY MEDIATED DISEASES
Bullous pemphigoid
Herpes gestationis
Mucous membrane pemphigoid
Epidermolysis bullosa acquisita
Dermatitis herpetiformis
Linear IgA bullous dermatosis
Pemphigus
Vulgaris
Foliaceus
Paraneoplastic
HYPERSENSITIVITY DISEASES
Erythema multiforme minor
Erythema multiforme major (Stevens-Johnson syndrome)
Toxic epidermal necrolysis
METABOLIC DISEASES
Porphyria cutanea tarda
Pseudoporphyria
Diabetic blisters
INHERITED GENETIC DISORDERS
Epidermolysis bullosa
Simplex
Junctional
Dystrophic
INFECTIOUS DISEASES
Impetigo
Staphylococcal scalded skin syndrome
Herpes simplex
Varicella
Herpes zoster

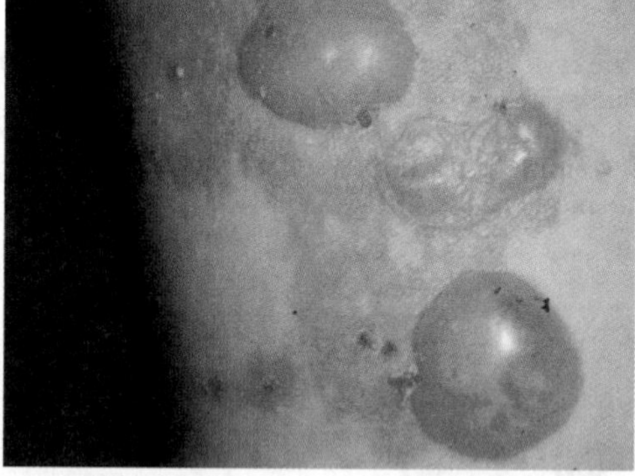

FIGURE 465–6 • Bullous pemphigoid. Tense subepidermal bullae are seen on an erythematous base.

Treatment

Rx

Treatment is dictated by the degree of involvement and the rate of progression of the disease. A randomized, multicenter trial demonstrated that 40 g of the ultrapotent topical steroid clobetasol, applied twice daily to the skin of patients with bullous pemphigoid until 15 days after disease control was obtained, was effective and superior to oral corticosteroid treatment in patients with both moderate and severe disease. [1] Nevertheless, the practicality of such potent topical steroids is controversial, and many experts use oral prednisone, 1 mg/kg in an early morning daily dose, as a foundation of therapy for patients with generalized bullous pemphigoid. Other treatments include tetracycline (500 mg four times daily), dapsone (up to 150 mg daily), azathioprine (up to 2.5 mg/kg as guided by the thiopurine methyltransferase level), methotrexate (up to 15 mg weekly), mycophenolate mofetil (35 to 45 mg/kg divided into two daily doses), and cyclophosphamide (up to about 2 mg/kg). The duration of therapy with all of these medications varies, depending on the activity of the disease. Left untreated, bullous pemphigoid generally persists for months to years. Spontaneous remissions and exacerbations occur. The mortality rate is relatively low, even without treatment.

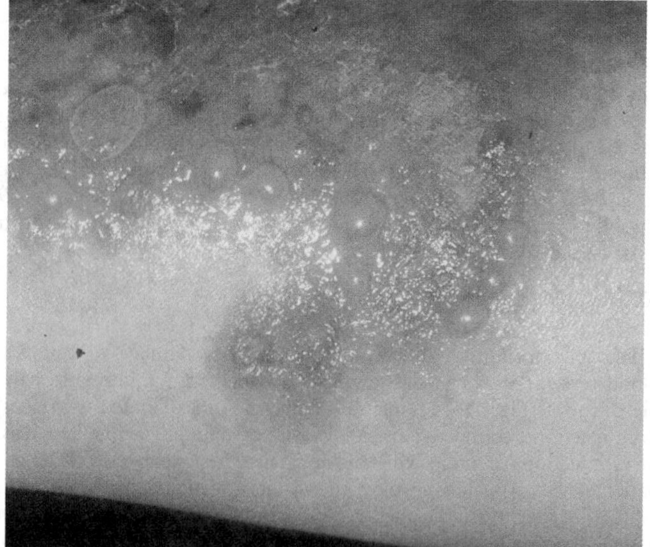

FIGURE 465–7 • Herpes gestationis. Multiple tense blisters and erosions on an erythematous base are present.

Herpes Gestationis

Herpes gestationis is a rare autoimmune dermatosis of pregnancy. Despite the name, herpes gestationis has no relationship to herpesvirus infection. Most patients have intense pruritus. Periumbilical urticarial plaques progress to vesicles and blisters. The eruption spreads peripherally (Fig. 465–7), typically sparing the face, palms, soles, and mucous membranes. IgG autoantibodies are produced against bullous pemphigoid antigen II, which is critical in epidermal-dermal adhesion. Antibody binding triggers an immune response leading to blister formation. Histology reveals a subepidermal blister, and direct immunofluorescence shows linear C3 deposits at the basement membrane.

Corticosteroids are the mainstay of therapy. Patients with mild disease are treated with moderate- to high-potency topical corticosteroids, such as 0.05% fluocinonide ointment applied twice daily to affected areas, whereas patients with extensive disease usually require systemic corticosteroids, such as prednisone, 1 mg/kg given once daily as an early morning dose. Disease clears within 1 to 2 weeks after initiation of treatment. There is an increased risk for premature delivery and birth of infants who are small for gestational age, thus suggesting that these women should be managed by obstetricians experienced in high-risk pregnancies.

Mucous Membrane Pemphigoid

Definition

Mucous membrane pemphigoid, previously called cicatricial pemphigoid, is a group of subepithelial blistering diseases that involve the mucosal surfaces. Patients have blisters of the oral, ocular, nasopharyngeal, laryngeal, anogenital, and esophageal mucosa that heal with scarring, which causes the major morbidity associated with the disease.

Pathobiology

There are several subgroups of mucous membrane pemphigoid. Some patients have circulating IgG autoantibodies that bind to the dermal side of salt-split skin and recognize laminin 5. A second subgroup includes patients who have pure ocular disease and IgG antibodies directed against β4 integrin. A third subgroup has mucosal disease and skin lesions. The fourth variant includes patients with oral disease but without skin disease. Histology reveals a subepidermal blister with an inflammatory cell infiltrate. Direct immunofluorescence shows linear IgG, IgA, and C3 deposits at the basement membrane. Indirect immunofluorescence reveals circulating IgG or IgA antibodies, or both.

Treatment

Rx

Treatment is dictated by the extent, severity, and location of disease; it ranges from topical corticosteroids, such as 0.05% fluocinonide ointment applied twice daily to affected areas under occlusion in patients with only oral disease, to prednisone, 1 mg/kg given once daily as an early morning dose, and cyclophosphamide, up to 2 mg/kg given as an early morning dose for up to 2 years, for severe ocular disease. Management teams should include ophthalmologists, otolaryngologists, dermatologists, and internists for patients with severe disease. Patients with both circulating IgG and IgA antibodies tend to have more severe disease.

Prognosis

Mucous membrane pemphigoid is a chronic disease. Untreated ocular disease can result in blindness.

Epidermolysis Bullosa Acquisita

Epidermolysis bullosa acquisita is an acquired autoimmune blistering disease that generally occurs in middle age. There are two types of skin lesions: noninflammatory acral blisters that heal with scarring and milia formation and widespread inflammatory vesiculobullous disease.

Pathobiology

Epidermolysis bullosa acquisita is characterized by IgG autoantibodies that target collagen VII, the major protein of anchoring fibrils. These autoantibodies alter dermal-epidermal adhesion and lead to blister formation. Histology reveals a subepidermal blister containing few inflammatory cells when mechanobullous lesions are sampled or a neutrophil-rich infiltrate when inflammatory blisters are sampled. Direct immunofluorescence reveals linear IgG deposits at the basement membrane. Indirect immunofluorescence shows circulating IgG autoantibodies that bind the dermal side of salt-split skin.

Treatment

Rx

Epidermolysis bullosa acquisita is a chronic disease that is very difficult to treat. Dapsone (at doses up to 150 mg daily), colchicine (0.6 mg twice daily), azathioprine (up to 2.5 mg/kg as guided by the thiopurine methyltransferase level), or cyclophosphamide (2 mg/kg given as an early morning dosage) alone or along with prednisone (60 mg given once daily as an early morning dose) is only occasionally successful. Cyclosporine at doses of up to 5 mg/kg or extracorporeal photopheresis has been used successfully in patients with severe disease. Because of nephrotoxicity, cyclosporine should be reserved for crisis management of patients who have severe disease and are experiencing a major flare.

Dermatitis Herpetiformis

Dermatitis herpetiformis is an immune-mediated vesicular disease that usually occurs in the young to middle aged. Skin lesions are extremely pruritic grouped vesicles and erosions located on the scalp, posterior of the neck, and extensor surfaces of the elbows, knees, and buttocks (Fig. 465–8). Most patients have a subclinical gluten-sensitive enteropathy (Chapter 143) that is reversible with a gluten-free diet. Diet alone can sometimes control the skin disease, with clearance of the cutaneous granular IgA deposits at the basement membrane. Biopsy specimens of skin lesions reveal dermal papillary neutrophilic microabscesses. Direct immunofluorescence shows dermal papillary granular IgA deposits in all patients. Dermatitis herpetiformis can be treated with dapsone, usually 100 mg daily given chronically. Dermatitis herpetiformis is a lifelong disease.

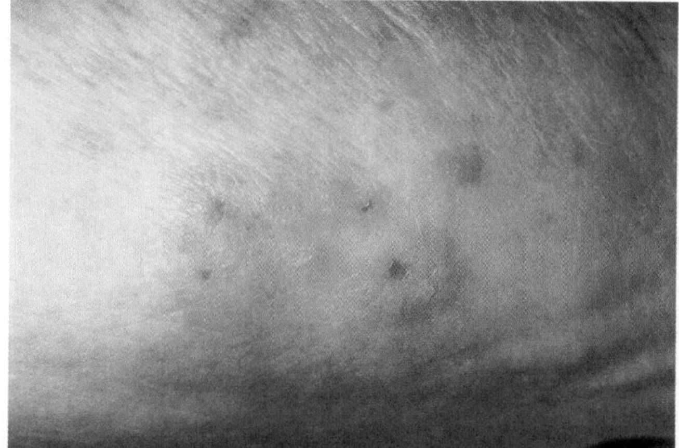

FIGURE 465–8 • Dermatitis herpetiformis. The elbow of a patient has eroded erythematous papules and papulovesicles.

Linear IgA Bullous Dermatosis

Linear IgA bullous dermatosis is an acquired autoimmune blistering disease of the skin. The primary lesions are papulovesicles, and involvement of the oral mucous membranes is common. The disease occurs throughout adulthood. Deposition of IgA antibody specific for a portion of bullous pemphigoid antigen II leads to complement activation and neutrophil chemotaxis. Proteolytic enzymes are released, destroy the dermal-epidermal junction, and cause blister formation. Histology reveals a subepidermal vesicle or cleft with neutrophil predominance. Direct immunofluorescence shows linear deposits of IgA at the basement membrane. Indirect immunofluorescence demonstrates circulating IgA antibodies. The majority of patients respond to dapsone, 100 mg daily, given chronically. Patients whose disease is not controlled with dapsone may benefit from the addition of oral prednisone, 1 mg/kg once daily as an early morning dose. The disease tends to be chronic in adults, but the childhood version (called chronic bullous disease of childhood) may run a several-year course and then remit.

Pemphigus

Definition

Pemphigus refers to a group of autoimmune blistering intraepidermal diseases of the skin and mucous membranes that are most common in middle age.

Clinical Manifestations

Patients with pemphigus vulgaris have flaccid blisters and erosions in the oropharynx (Fig. 465–9), trunk, head, neck, and intertriginous areas. Pemphigus foliaceus is accompanied by erythema, scaling, and crusting of the face, scalp, and upper part of the trunk. Patients with paraneoplastic pemphigus have ocular and oral blisters and erosions along with skin lesions resembling erythema multiforme and an associated underlying malignancy that is generally lymphoreticular in origin (Chapter 189).

Pathobiology

Autoantibodies in pemphigus vulgaris target desmoglein III, and autoantibodies in pemphigus foliaceus target desmoglein I. Circulating

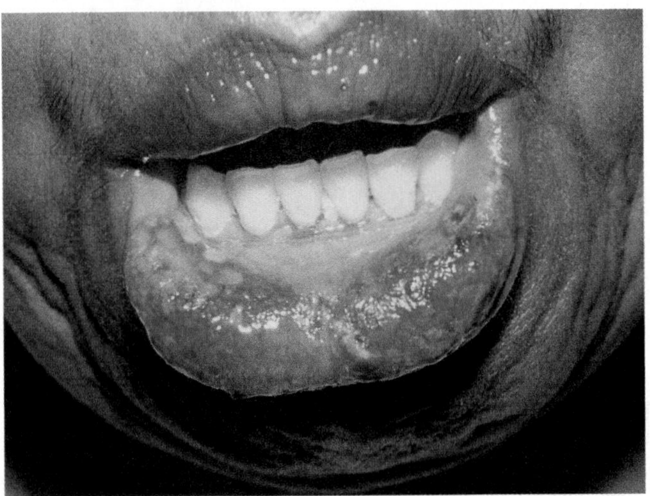

FIGURE 465–9 • Pemphigus vulgaris. The lower lip of a patient has confluent erosions with scattered crusting.

antibodies in paraneoplastic pemphigus recognize a complex of proteins, including desmoplakin I and II, bullous pemphigoid antigen I, envoplakin, periplakin, and desmoglein I and III.

Diagnosis

Skin biopsy specimens from patients with pemphigus vulgaris reveal suprabasilar acantholysis, whereas pemphigus foliaceus biopsy specimens demonstrate subcorneal acantholysis. Biopsy specimens of paraneoplastic pemphigus show suprabasilar acantholysis and dyskeratotic keratinocytes with basal cell vacuolization.

Direct immunofluorescence demonstrates cell surface deposits of IgG in patients with pemphigus vulgaris and foliaceus, whereas indirect immunofluorescence reveals circulating IgG antibodies. Patients with paraneoplastic pemphigus have circulating and tissue-bound IgG antibodies that are indistinguishable from those in pemphigus vulgaris and that also recognize the cell surface of simple epithelia, including the liver and heart.

Treatment

Rx

Treatment regimens depend on the patient's age, the degree of involvement, the rate of disease progression, and the subtype of pemphigus. Systemic corticosteroids (e.g., oral prednisone, 1 mg/kg once daily as an early morning dose) are required for pemphigus vulgaris, whereas topical corticosteroids (e.g., 0.05% fluocinonide ointment applied twice daily to affected areas) occasionally control pemphigus foliaceus. Steroid-sparing agents include dapsone (up to 150 mg daily), the combination of tetracycline (500 mg four times daily) and niacinamide (500 mg three times daily), hydroxychloroquine (administered at less than 6 mg/kg of lean body mass divided into two daily doses), mycophenolate mofetil (35 to 45 mg/kg/day divided into two daily doses), azathioprine (up to 2.5 mg/kg as guided by the thiopurine methyltransferase level), and cyclophosphamide (up to 2 mg/kg given as an early morning dose). The duration of therapy with each of these medications varies according to the level of disease activity. Although the use of steroid-sparing agents is supported by clinical experience, few controlled studies have demonstrated their benefit. For paraneoplastic pemphigus caused by benign tumors such as Castleman's disease (Chapter 196), tumor removal is curative. Patients with associated malignant tumors have recalcitrant disease, although there are occasional successes with pulse corticosteroids (methylprednisolone, 1000 mg given daily for 3 consecutive days), pulse cyclophosphamide (500 to 1000 mg given monthly for 6 months to 1 year, often along with varying doses of prednisone), immunoapheresis, and immunoablative high-dose cyclophosphamide (50 mg/kg/day for 4 days).

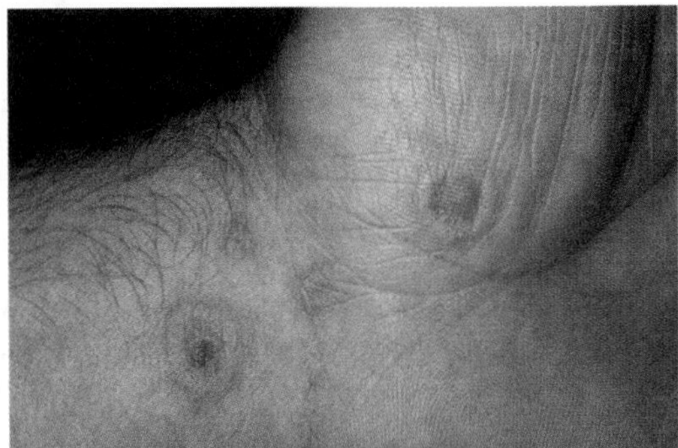

FIGURE 465–10 • Erythema multiforme. Target or "bull's-eye" annular lesions with central vesicles and bullae are characteristic of erythema multiforme.

Prognosis

Before the availability of corticosteroids, 60 to 90% of patients with pemphigus vulgaris died, whereas the mortality rate has now decreased to the 5 to 10% range. The prognosis of patients with paraneoplastic pemphigus is related to the type of associated neoplasm. Patients with benign tumors usually experience clearance of their lesions after tumor resection, whereas those with malignant tumors generally have a poor prognosis.

Hypersensitivity Reactions That Cause Blisters

Erythema Multiforme

Definition

Erythema multiforme is an acute blistering eruption that occurs in all age groups. Erythema multiforme minor is localized, with minimal or no mucosal involvement. Erythema multiforme major, also known as Stevens-Johnson syndrome, is a more severe mucosal and skin disease characterized by signs and symptoms reminiscent of serum sickness (Chapter 44).

Clinical Manifestations

Toxic epidermal necrolysis is at the most severe end of the erythema multiforme spectrum. The primary lesions of erythema multiforme minor are erythematous macules and edematous papules with vesicular centers that become dusky violet. Target or iris lesions are found on extensor surfaces of the extremities and spread centripetally (Fig. 465–10). The skin lesions of Stevens-Johnson syndrome resemble those of erythema multiforme minor but are likely to be generalized and show confluent erythema with urticarial and purpuric lesions. Erosions of two or more mucosal surfaces occur in Stevens-Johnson syndrome and may include hemorrhagic crusting of the lips, ulceration of the ocular mucosa, and genital involvement. Patients with erythema multiforme major have a 1- to 14-day prodrome that includes fever, cough, sore throat, vomiting, and diarrhea. Patients with toxic epidermal necrolysis may have a similar prodrome, rapidly followed by generalized macular erythema that progresses to confluent erythema with skin tenderness. Large blisters follow soon afterward, and then skin sloughing occurs as the large blisters break and leave denuded skin.

Pathobiology

Common etiologic associations of erythema multiforme include infections such as herpes simplex (Chapter 397) (especially recurrent erythema multiforme minor), *Mycoplasma pneumoniae* (Chapter 338), and drug reactions (Chapter 275). Sulfonamides, penicillins, barbiturates, carbamazepine, phenytoin, allopurinol, and nonsteroidal anti-inflammatory drugs (NSAIDs) are the most common drugs implicated in Stevens-Johnson syndrome and toxic epidermal necrolysis.

Diagnosis

The diagnosis of erythema multiforme is clinical.

Treatment

Rx

Chronic antiviral treatment with acyclovir (400 mg twice daily for 6 months) decreases outbreaks in a subset of patients with recurrent erythema multiforme minor. Treatment of erythema multiforme major is otherwise nonspecific, with attention to fluid and electrolyte balance and eye disease being critical. If a drug is suspected, it must be withdrawn. Systemic corticosteroid treatment is contraindicated in Stevens-Johnson syndrome. Treatment of toxic epidermal necrolysis is very difficult, but uncontrolled studies suggest that intravenous immunoglobulin (2 to 3 g/kg over a period of 2 to 5 days) may improve the prognosis.

Prognosis

Erythema multiforme minor usually subsides within 2 to 3 weeks. Erythema multiforme major takes 3 to 6 weeks to clear and has less than a 5% mortality rate. Toxic epidermal necrolysis has a mortality rate approaching 30%, and patients are best managed in an intensive care or burn unit.

Metabolic Disorders That Cause Blisters

Porphyria Cutanea Tarda

Porphyria cutanea tarda is caused by deficient activity of the heme synthetic enzyme uroporphyrinogen decarboxylase (Chapter 229). The fragility of sun-exposed skin leads to erosions and bullae, which are worst on the dorsal surface of the hands (Fig. 465–11), forearms, and face. Healing of crusted erosions and blisters leaves scars, milia, and hyperpigmented and hypopigmented atrophic patches. Hypertrichosis is common and most florid over the temporal and malar areas. Urinary porphyrin levels are abnormally high. Histology reveals a subepidermal blister with minimal dermal infiltrate, and direct immunofluorescence demonstrates immunoglobulin and complement deposition in dermal capillaries and at the basement membrane. Phlebotomy is the standard treatment, and the goal is to reduce serum ferritin to the lower limit of the normal range. Another treatment option is oral hydroxychloroquine at a dose (200 mg twice weekly until the disease is under control) that is much lower than that used for photoprotective indications. Alcohol and estrogen use should be discontinued because they can cause the disease to flare.

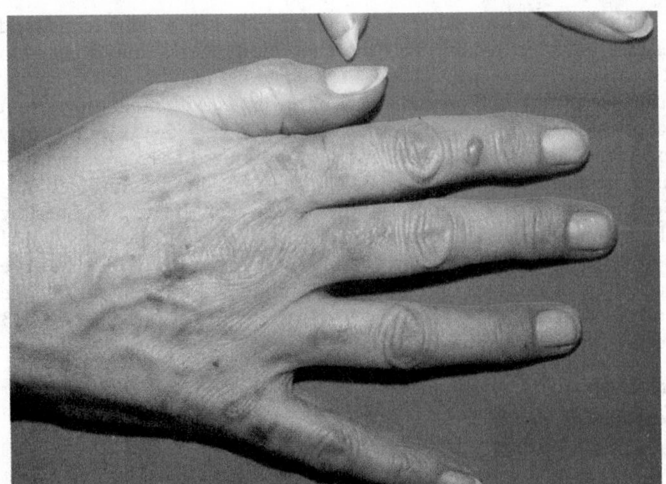

FIGURE 465–11 • Porphyria cutanea tarda. A blister and erosions are present on the dorsal surface of the hand.

Pseudoporphyria

Pseudoporphyria is a bullous eruption that mimics porphyria cutanea tarda clinically and histologically without porphyrin abnormalities. Many medications can cause pseudoporphyria, including propionic acid–derivative NSAIDs (e.g., naproxen, diflunisal, ketoprofen, nabumetone, oxaprozin, and mefenamic acid), furosemide, tetracycline, fluoroquinolones, amiodarone, cyclosporine, dapsone, etretinate, and flutamide. The prognosis is good for patients with pseudoporphyria after the offending agent has been discontinued. However, resolution of the disease may take several months. In patients with chronic renal failure treated by hemodialysis, true porphyria cutanea tarda or pseudoporphyria may develop and is very difficult to treat.

Diabetes Mellitus

Distal extremity blisters may occasionally develop in patients with diabetes mellitus (Chapter 247). There is no correlation between the development of blisters and the severity, duration, or complications of diabetes. The mechanism of blister formation is not understood.

Inherited Genetic Disorders That Cause Blisters

Epidermolysis bullosa is a group of inherited bullous disorders characterized by blister formation in response to mechanical trauma. Subtypes include epidermolysis bullosa simplex (intraepidermal skin separation) (Fig. 465–12), junctional epidermolysis bullosa (skin separation in the lamina lucida), and dystrophic epidermolysis bullosa (sublamina densa separation). Infancy is an especially difficult time, and epidermolysis bullosa may be accompanied by blistering that is complicated by infection and sepsis. Many patients with junctional epidermolysis bullosa have severe disease that can lead to death, usually secondary to infection, and metastatic squamous cell carcinoma may develop in some patients with recessive dystrophic epidermolysis bullosa and can also lead to death. In contrast, epidermolysis bullosa simplex, milder forms of junctional epidermolysis bullosa, and dominant dystrophic epidermolysis bullosa do not usually affect life expectancy. Epidermolysis bullosa simplex is caused by mutations of the genes coding for keratins 5 and 14. Junctional epidermolysis bullosa has a variable molecular etiology, and mutations in genes coding for laminin 5 subunits, bullous pemphigoid antigen I, $\alpha 6$ integrin, and $\beta 4$ integrin have been demonstrated. Dystrophic epidermolysis bullosa is caused by mutations of the type VII collagen gene. Epidermolysis bullosa is a lifelong disease. Some subtypes, especially the milder forms, improve with age. No medications are known to correct the underlying molecular defects, but gene therapy is being actively pursued.

Infectious Diseases That Cause Blisters

Impetigo

Impetigo is a bacterial infection of the superficial layers of the epidermis. Bullous impetigo is caused by *S. aureus* (Chapter 310), and nonbullous impetigo is caused by group A β-hemolytic streptococci (Chapter

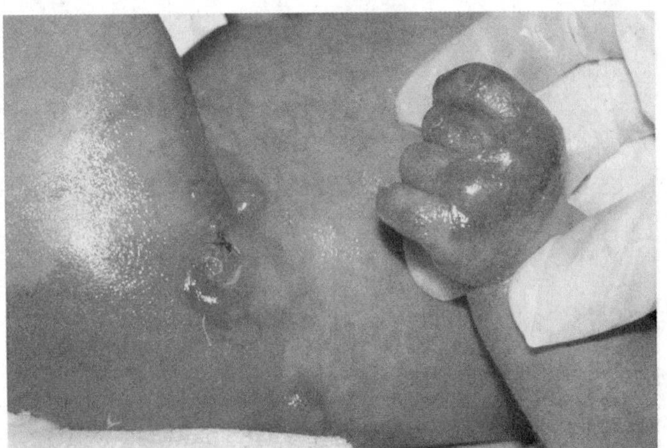

FIGURE 465–12 • Epidermolysis bullosa simplex. Tense blisters and erosions are present on the trunk and extremities of a newborn.

312). Bullous impetigo is manifested as vesicles and bulla (Fig. 465–13). Lesions are common on the face but may appear anywhere. Nonbullous impetigo is characterized by fragile vesicles or pustules that rupture and leave honey-colored crusted papules or plaques, especially near the nose and mouth and on the extremities. Lesions develop on normal or traumatized skin or are superimposed on preexisting conditions, including scabies, varicella, or atopic dermatitis. The causative agent of bullous impetigo is coagulase-positive *S. aureus*, which produces exfoliatins A and B. The toxins cause cleavage within or below the stratum granulosum. Impetigo is diagnosed clinically. Culture and sensitivity studies are recommended if topical or oral treatment is ineffective. Oral antibiotics, including dicloxacillin (500 mg four times daily for 7 days) or cephalexin (500 mg three times daily for 7 days), applied twice daily for 7 days, are used for extensive disease or in patients refractory to topical mupirocin. Gentle débridement of crusts is recommended. Lesions resolve after 7 to 10 days of treatment. Acute glomerulonephritis (Chapter 122) develops in 2 to 5% of young children with nonbullous impetigo, usually within 10 days after the skin lesions appear.

Staphylococcal Scalded Skin Syndrome

Staphylococcal scalded skin syndrome is a blistering disease caused by an exotoxin produced by *S. aureus* (Chapter 310). It is most common in young children but may occur in adults who have renal insufficiency or are immunocompromised. The site of the staphylococcal infection is usually extracutaneous. Staphylococcal scalded skin syndrome is manifested as a sudden onset of fever and tender, blanchable erythema. It starts on the central part of the face, neck, and intertriginous areas and rapidly generalizes. The palms, soles, and mucous membranes are spared. Flaccid blisters occur within 1 to 2 days and soon exfoliate in large sheets, with superficially denuded skin remaining (Fig. 465–14). The disease must be distinguished from toxic epidermal necrolysis by skin biopsy. In staphylococcal scalded skin syndrome there is an upper epidermal blister, whereas toxic epidermal necrolysis causes a dermal-epidermal blister. Patients with the most severe staphylococcal scalded skin syndrome should be treated with intravenous nafcillin or oxacillin, 2 g every 4 to 6 hours for 10 to 14 days. If the patient is found to have methicillin-resistant staphylococci, vancomycin, 1 g every 12 hours (with dose adjustment based on creatinine clearance), should be given for 10 to 14 days. Patients with mild disease may be treated with oral dicloxacillin, 500 mg four times daily for 10 to 14 days, unless the staphylococcal isolate is methicillin resistant, in which case the choice of antibiotics should be guided by the results of sensitivity testing.

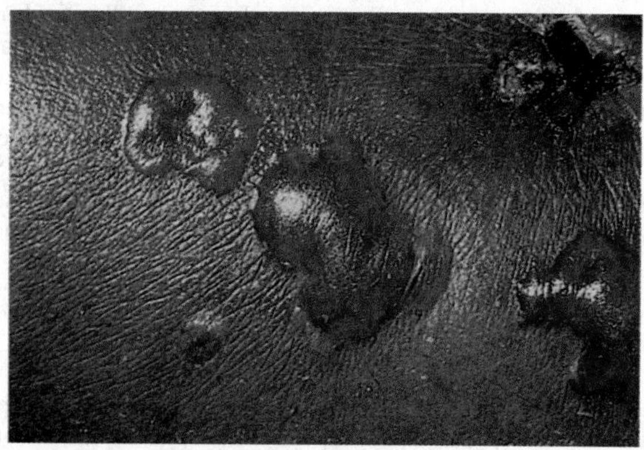

FIGURE 465–13 • Bullous impetigo. Multiple blisters are present on the trunk of this patient.

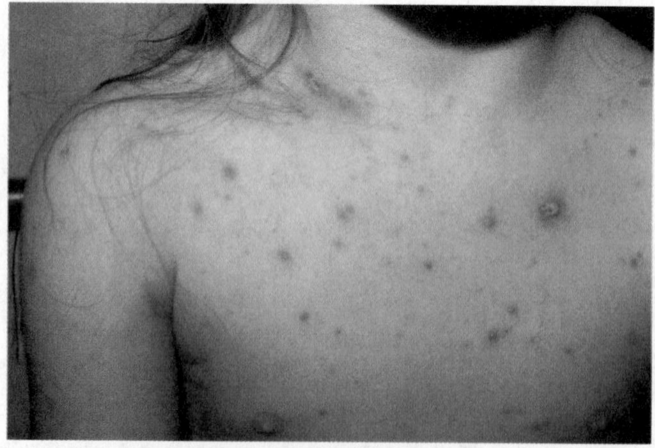

FIGURE 465–14 • Staphylococcal scalded skin syndrome. Confluent erythema with exfoliation of skin is seen on the trunk.

Herpes Simplex Virus Infection

Pathobiology

Herpes simplex virus (HSV) infection (Chapter 397) may be caused by type 1 or type 2 HSV. The hallmark of HSV infection is its ability to establish latent infection. Disease commonly occurs as a recurrent vesicular eruption of the oral, perioral (typically HSV-1), or genital (typically HSV-2) regions, although primary gingivostomatitis (typically in children and young adults and caused by HSV-1) and primary genital herpes (typically HSV-2) are less common.

Clinical Manifestations

Patients with primary gingivostomatitis have high fever, regional lymphadenopathy, and malaise. Patients with primary genital herpes have fever, flulike symptoms, tender inguinal adenopathy, and aseptic meningitis. These infections all reveal grouped vesicles on an erythematous base. Recurrent eruptions can be triggered by skin trauma, cold or heat, concurrent infection, and menstruation. Chronic erosive ulcers of the face and anogenital areas may develop in immunocompromised patients.

Diagnosis

Tzanck smear of fluid from the roof of a vesicle can be helpful in confirming the diagnosis (see Fig. 462–15), but viral culture is the diagnostic "gold standard." The direct fluorescent antibody test is an antigen-based technique that not only yields same-day results but can also distinguish HSV from varicella-zoster virus (VZV) and is becoming widely used.

Treatment

In healthy individuals, HSV infection is self-limited. The goal of treatment is to shorten the current attack and prevent recurrences. Acyclovir is effective in the treatment of HSV infections; valacyclovir and famciclovir are closely related, effective medications with improved oral bioavailability. The doses and duration of therapy vary depending on whether the infection is limited to the oral or genital mucous membranes or is disseminated and on whether it is primary or recurrent disease (Chapter 397).

Chickenpox

Chickenpox is caused by VZV (Chapter 398). It is usually a childhood disease, but affected adults have more morbidity. Skin lesions occur 10 to 21 days after exposure to VZV. Erythematous macules appear on the scalp, face, trunk, and proximal ends of the limbs, with rapid progression to papules, vesicles, pustules, and crusting (Fig. 465–15). Adults may experience a more widespread eruption, prolonged fever, and pneumonia. The diagnosis is usually made clinically, but direct fluorescent antibody or culture confirmation is sometimes needed. Treatment of healthy children is unnecessary because the disease is self-limited. Adults should be treated with oral acyclovir, 800 mg five times a day for 7 days. The varicella vaccine given once to healthy children 12 to 18 months of age and twice, in a 4- to 8-week interval, to susceptible persons older than 13 years (Chapter 16) is highly effective.

Herpes Zoster

Pathobiology

Herpes zoster is caused by reactivation of VZV from a previous chickenpox infection. The disease is more common in older or immunocompromised patients.

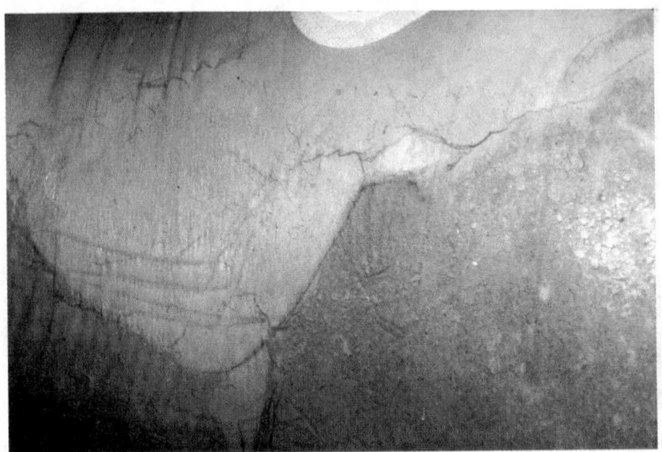

FIGURE 465–15 • Erythematous macules and vesicles with crusted erosions on the chest of a patient with varicella.

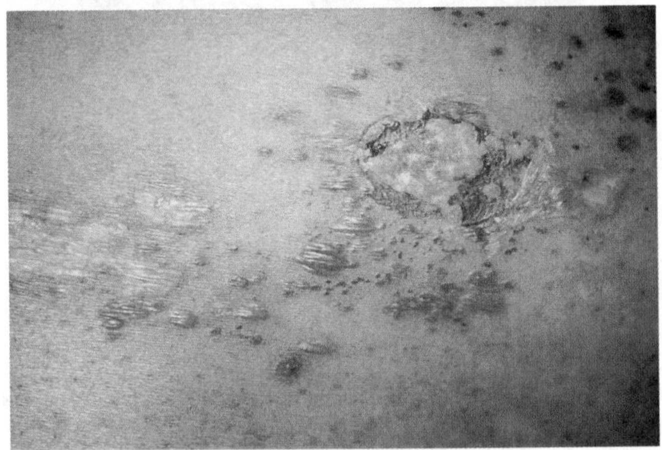

FIGURE 465–16 • Herpes zoster. Necrotic blisters and erosions in a dermatomal pattern are seen on the trunk of this patient.

Clinical Manifestations

The typical manifestation is painful grouped herpetiform vesicles on an erythematous base confined to cutaneous surfaces innervated by one sensory nerve and preceded by radicular pain (Fig. 465–16). The major morbidity, which is pain within the affected dermatome, can be severe and persist after the skin lesions have resolved (postherpetic neuralgia). Immunocompromised patients have an increased risk for cutaneous dissemination and visceral involvement of the bladder, lungs, and CNS.

Treatment

Rx

Acyclovir (800 mg orally five times daily for 7 days) and its derivatives valacyclovir (500 mg orally three times daily for 7 days) and famciclovir (500 mg orally three times daily for 7 days) are safe and effective in the treatment of active disease and prevention of postherpetic neuralgia. In an immunocompromised patient, acyclovir should be given intravenously (10 mg/kg every 8 hours for 7 to 10 days). The earlier antiviral medications are started, the more effective they are in shortening the duration of herpes zoster and in preventing or decreasing the severity of postherpetic neuralgia. Although older uncontrolled studies suggested that 3 weeks of oral prednisone may decrease the incidence of both acute pain and postherpetic neuralgia, more recent controlled studies have failed to demonstrate any beneficial effects of systemic corticosteroids. Patients with postherpetic neuralgia of more than 3 months' duration benefit from the use of gabapentin, 1600 or 2400 mg daily, with a significant reduction in pain. [2] VZV vaccine markedly reduces both the morbidity from herpes zoster and postherpetic neuralgia in healthy adults older than 60 years. [3]

PUSTULAR ERUPTIONS

Acne Vulgaris

Definition

Acne vulgaris is the most common pustular skin condition. Teenagers are usually affected, but the disease may persist into adulthood. The comedo, which is the primary lesion, can be either closed (whitehead) or open (blackhead).

Pathobiology

Androgen production after puberty stimulates the release of sebum by sebaceous glands. Sebum flow is impeded because of abnormal keratinization within the pilosebaceous canal, a process that leads to the formation of comedones. Bacterial (*Propionibacterium acnes*) proliferation within the comedo predisposes to rupture of the pilosebaceous unit with extravasation into the surrounding dermis, which results in papules, pustules, and cysts.

Treatment

Patients with mild disease are treated topically with benzoyl peroxide, tretinoin, adapalene, or tazarotene, which normalize follicular keratinization. In patients with mild to moderate disease, treatment with benzoyl peroxide is the most cost-effective therapy. [4] The addition of topical antibiotics helps control inflammatory papules and pustules. More significant disease is often treated with oral tetracycline (250 to 1000 mg/day), doxycycline (200 mg/day), or minocycline (200 mg/day). Dapsone gel (5%) is safe and effective. [5] Another approach is oral contraceptives containing ethinyl estradiol and norgestimate, which are superior to placebo in the treatment of acne in women. Isotretinoin (Accutane) (1 mg/kg given for 5 months), which decreases sebaceous gland size and sebum production, is reserved for severe cystic disease because of its teratogenicity, possible associated risk for depression, and other significant side effects. Acne may be exacerbated by the use of oil-based cosmetics or hair preparations. Androgenic hormones, systemic corticosteroids, lithium, phenytoin, phenobarbital, isoniazid, and endocrinologic conditions such as polycystic ovary disease and adrenal or ovarian tumors may produce acneiform eruptions or aggravate preexisting acne.

Rosacea

Rosacea, which is a chronic inflammatory disease of the face, affects the pilosebaceous units and blood vessels and generally occurs in middle age. Erythema, telangiectases, erythematous papules, and pustules occur on the central part of the face. Ocular rosacea can lead to keratitis, iritis, blepharitis, and recurrent chalazion; it should be managed by an ophthalmologist. In its most severe form, rosacea can cause sebaceous gland hyperplasia leading to a large red bulbous nose known as rhinophyma (Fig. 465–17). Rosacea is more likely to develop in patients with a tendency toward facial flushing. Flushing can be due to heat, spicy foods, hot drinks, alcohol, or emotional stimuli. With time, the flushing reaction lasts longer and longer until it persists. Topical antibiotics, including 1% metronidazole, are helpful in mild disease. Patients with more severe disease require oral tetracycline, 500 mg twice daily for 3 to 4 months and then slowly decreased as tolerated. Azelaic acid gel (15%) can significantly improve papulopustular rosacea. [6]

Perioral Dermatitis

Perioral dermatitis is characterized by erythematous papules and pustules, as well as scaling patches around the mouth and eyes (Fig. 465–18). Most patients have used potent topical corticosteroids inappropriately for long periods. The eruption generally clears after stopping the corticosteroid and using tetracycline, 250 mg orally twice daily for 6 weeks.

Acute Exanthematous Pustulosis

Acute exanthematous pustulosis is a generalized pustular eruption that is associated with fever and frequently caused by antibiotics. Pustules

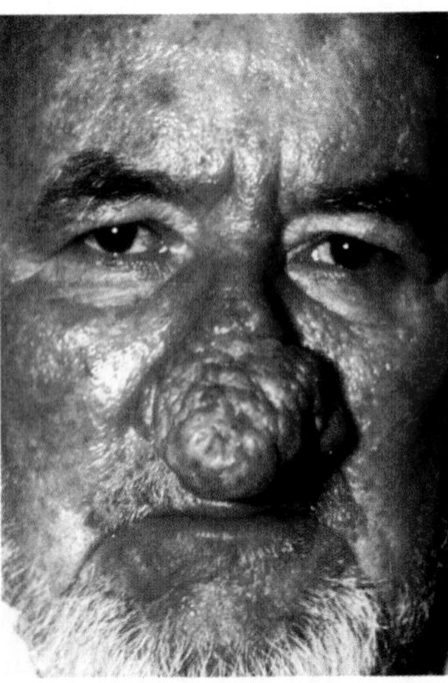

FIGURE 465–17 • Sebaceous gland hyperplasia. A large red bulbous nose known as rhinophyma is characteristic of late-stage rosacea.

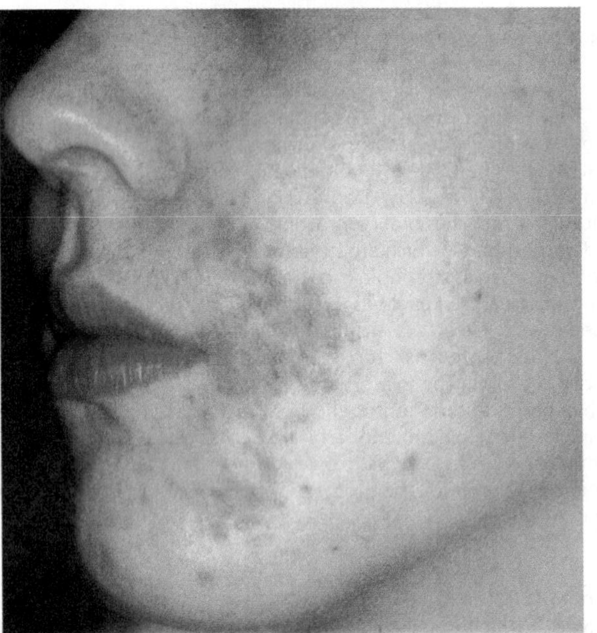

FIGURE 465–18 • Perioral dermatitis. Erythematous papules and pinpoint pustules are evident around the mouth.

develop within 2 days of drug administration, start on the face or in flexural areas, and rapidly disseminate (Fig. 465–19). Spontaneous resolution occurs in less than 2 weeks.

Pustular Psoriasis

Pustular psoriasis is a variant of psoriasis (Chapter 464) that localizes to the palms and soles or generalizes over the entire body. Patients with generalized disease have fever and leukocytosis and require systemic therapy. Pustules can also be seen in patients with septic emboli of bacterial or fungal origin, including gonococcemia and systemic candidiasis (see Purpuric Eruptions).

Folliculitis

Folliculitis is inflammation of the hair follicles caused by infection with staphylococci. It is due to obstruction of individual hair follicles and associated pilosebaceous units. Folliculitis is more common in patients with diabetes mellitus, obesity, or immunocompromised states. The primary lesion is a pustule with a central hair. Typical affected sites are the scalp, thighs, trunk, axilla, and inguinal area. Sometimes the infection can extend deeper into the dermis and form larger erythematous nodules from one (furuncle) or more (carbuncle) follicles. Treatment with oral antibiotics such as cephalexin, 500 mg twice daily for 14 days, clears

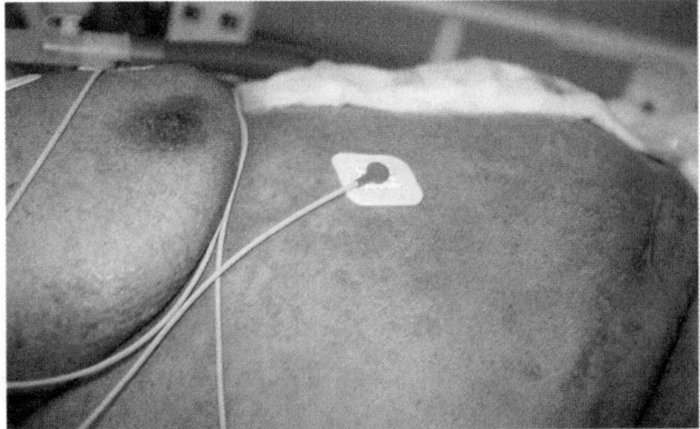

FIGURE 465–19 • Acute generalized exanthematous pustulosis. Erythematous macules and numerous superficial pustules are present on the trunk of this patient.

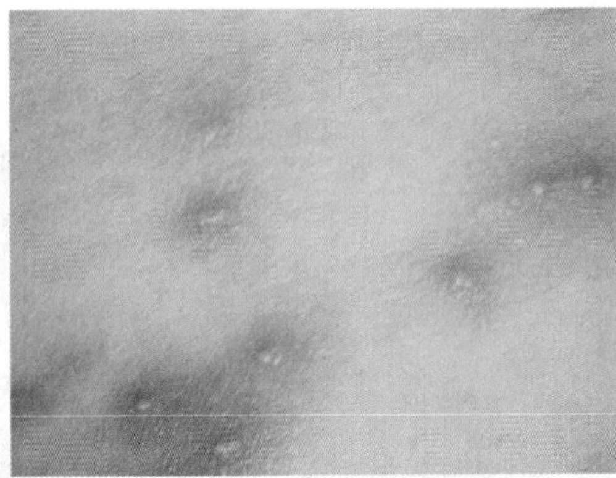

FIGURE 465–20 • *Pseudomonas* folliculitis. The trunk of this patient has numerous pustules on an erythematous base.

extensive infections, whereas topical antibiotics (e.g., clindamycin solution applied twice daily for 2 weeks or longer) and antibacterial soaps (e.g., Dial or Lever 2000) help in milder disease.

Pseudomonas Folliculitis

Pseudomonas folliculitis is acquired from hot tubs contaminated with *Pseudomonas aeruginosa* (Chapter 328). The typical finding is papules and pustules in areas of skin occluded by a bathing suit (Fig. 465–20). Treatment with ciprofloxacin at 500 mg twice daily for 10 to 14 days is usually curative.

Pityrosporum folliculitis is a pruritic, acne-like eruption that occurs on the upper part of the back and the chest, arms, and face and is caused by *Pityrosporum ovale.* Treatment is with oral ketoconazole, 200 mg/day for 2 weeks, and 2% ketoconazole shampoo applied to the affected area daily for 1 month.

Eosinophilic Pustular Folliculitis

Eosinophilic pustular folliculitis is a sterile, intensely pruritic folliculitis usually found on the face, chest, and back of patients who are positive for HIV (Chapter 415). Skin biopsy is needed to confirm the diagnosis. Treatment is difficult, but options include potent topical corticosteroids, such as 0.1% triamcinolone ointment applied twice daily for several months (although this class 4 steroid should not be used on the face); antihistamines, such as hydroxyzine, 25 mg every 8 hours as needed; and ultraviolet light therapy.

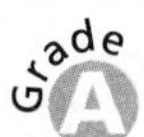

1. Joly P, Roujeau JC, Benichou J, et al: A comparison of oral and topical corticosteroids in patients with bullous pemphigoid. N Engl J Med 2002;346:321–327.
2. Rice AS, Maton S, Postherpetic Neuralgia Study Group: Gabapentin in post herpetic neuralgia: A randomized, double blind, placebo-controlled study. Pain 2001;94:215–224.
3. Oxman MN, Levin MJ, Johnson GR, et al: A vaccine to prevent herpes zoster and postherpetic neuralgia in older adults. N Engl J Med 2005;352:2271–2284.
4. Ozolins M, Eady EA, Avery AJ, et al: Comparison of five antimicrobial regimens for the treatment of mild to moderate inflammatory facial acne vulgaris in the community: Randomized controlled trial. Lancet 2004:364;2188–2195.

5. Draelos ZD, Carter E, Maloney JM, et al: Two randomized studies demonstrate the efficacy and safety of dapsone gel 5% for the treatment of acne vulgaris. J Am Acad Dermatol 2007;56:439.
6. Thiboutot D, Thieroff-Ekerdt R, Graupe K: Efficacy and safety of azelaic acid (15%) gel as a new treatment for papulopustular rosacea: Results from two vehicle-controlled, randomized phase III studies. J Am Acad Dermatol 2003;48:836–845.

SUGGESTED READINGS

Crowson AN, Mihm MC Jr, Magro CM: Cutaneous vasculitis: A review. J Cutan Pathol 2003;30:161–173. *An excellent review of the vasculitides of the skin.*
Fontaine J, Joly P, Roujeau JC: Treatment of bullous pemphigoid. J Dermatol 2003;30:83–90. *A comprehensive update.*
Gibbs S, Harvey I: Topical treatments for cutaneous warts. Cochrane Database Syst Rev 2006;3:CD001781. *An overview of the topical treatments for cutaneous warts.*
Gupta AK, Chaudhry MM: Rosacea and its management: An overview. J Eur Acad Dermatol Venereol 2005;19:273–285. *Review of rosacea and its variants.*
James WD: Acne. N Engl J Med 2005;352:1463–1472. *A comprehensive review.*
Letko E, Papaliodis DN, Papliodis GN, et al: Stevens-Johnson syndrome and toxic epidermal necrolysis: A review of the literature. Ann Allergy Asthma Immunol 2005;94:419–436. *A comprehensive update.*
Newburger JW, Takahashi M, Gerber MA, et al: Diagnosis, treatment, and long-term management of Kawasaki disease. Circulation 2004;110:2747–2771. *The American Academy of Pediatrics recommendations on diagnosis, treatment, and management.*
Stanley J, Amagai M: Pemphigus, bullous impetigo, and the staphylococcal scalded-skin syndrome. N Engl J Med 2006;355:1800–1810. *A review of these blistering diseases.*
Uitto J, Richard G: Progress in epidermolysis bullosa: From eponyms to molecular genetic classification. Clin Dermatol 2005;23:33–40. *A comprehensive review.*
van der Wouden JC, Menke J, Gajadin S, et al: Interventions for cutaneous molluscum contagiosum. Cochrane Database Syst Rev 2006;2:CD004767. *A review of the possible treatments for cutaneous molluscum contagiosum.*

466 URTICARIA, DRUG HYPERSENSITIVITY RASHES, NODULES AND TUMORS, AND ATROPHIC DISEASES

Madeleine Duvic

URTICARIA

Definition and Epidemiology

Urticaria, also known as hives, is one of the most common cutaneous reaction patterns (Fig. 466–1). It is triggered by a wide variety of antigens—internal or external—or by physical stimuli, including but not limited to cold, pressure, and sunlight (Chapter 273; Table 466–1).

Urticaria is typically transient and self-limited, without leakage of blood cells into the skin or damage to the blood vessels. Chronic urticaria, defined as urticaria that recurs over a period of 6 weeks or more, is often of unknown cause. Chronic urticaria can be related to the ingestion of aspirin or agents that cross-react with salicylates, such as sodium benzoate (a common food preservative) or tartrazine (yellow dye #5). The number of mast cells has been found to be increased in the gastrointestinal tract of individuals with chronic urticaria, even in absence of gastrointestinal symptoms.

Pathobiology

Urticaria can be due to allergic IgE-mediated type I hypersensitivity reactions or to non–immunologically mediated physical factors. Local degranulation of mast cells with the release of histamine and other factors, such as slow-reacting substance of anaphylaxis, precipitates urticaria. Injections of corticotropin-releasing hormone (CRH) and acute stress cause degranulation of mast cells and increased vascular permeability, mediated through activation of CRH receptor 1 and mast cell histidine decarboxylase, both of which are elevated in the skin of patients with chronic urticaria. As a result of transient leakage of plasma into the dermis from capillaries and small postcapillary venules, a demarcated, pink, raised lesion (hive) develops. Larger raised plaques or annular forms (giant urticaria) and deep tissue swelling (angioedema) are less frequent manifestations.

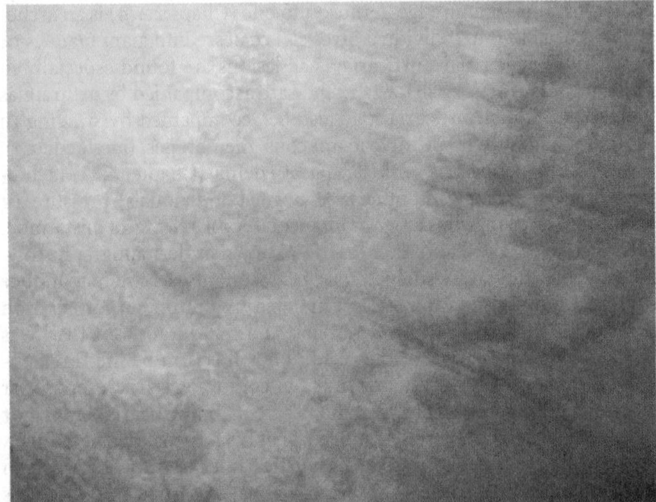

FIGURE 466–1 • Urticaria. (From dermnetnz.org/reactions/urticaria.html.)

TABLE 466–1 COMMON CAUSES OF URTICARIA

URTICARIA MAY BE ACCOMPANIED BY ANGIOEDEMA AND ANAPHYLAXIS
Blood products: red cells, platelets, gamma globulin
Drugs
Antibiotics: penicillins, cephalosporins, sulfonamides, isoniazid
Aspirin: salicylates, benzoates, phenylbutazone
Anticonvulsants: hydantoin
Chemotherapy: doxorubicin, daunorubicin, L-asparaginase, chlorambucil, cyclophosphamide, melphalan, methotrexate, nitrogen mustard, procarbazine
Dextran
Opiates
Quinidine
Radiocontrast dyes, iodine
Environmental: animal dander or proteins, formaldehyde, pollen, mold, plants, latex, plastic tubing, exercise, heat, cold, sunlight
Foods: berries, eggs, milk, nuts, tomatoes, shellfish, soy
Food additives: sodium benzoate, tartrazine (yellow dye #5)
Hormones
Infections: streptococcal, staphylococcal, sinusitis or abscesses, viral hepatitis, Epstein-Barr virus mononucleosis, *Candida*
Insect bites or venom: Hymenoptera, mosquitoes, mites, scabies
Vaccines
URTICARIAL-LIKE ERUPTIONS AND REACTIVE ERYTHEMAS
Erythema multiforme: herpes simplex, DNA viruses, *Mycoplasma pneumoniae*, drugs
Erythema marginatum: streptococcal rheumatic fever
Juvenile rheumatoid arthritis
Erythema chronicum migrans: *Borrelia* infections
Erythema annulare centrifugum: tinea, drugs
Figurate erythemas: erythema repens (often with underlying carcinoma)
Urticaria pigmentosa (mastocytosis)

Clinical Manifestations

Individual urticarial lesions are pink to light red, blanch with pressure, and are raised above the surface of the skin. The center of the lesions may be paler than the leading edge. A mosquito bite (Chapter 274) is an archetypal urticarial lesion. Individual hives can coalesce into giant plaques or annular rings called giant urticaria; such lesions are found especially in serum sickness (Chapter 44), where they are accompanied by arthralgias and fever. Confluent urticaria may also be accompanied by swelling of the underlying soft tissue or the mucous membranes (angioedema), as well as by anaphylaxis with laryngeal edema (Chapter 274), a life-threatening emergency. In otherwise normal individuals, pressure or writing on the skin will cause spontaneous local release of histamine, which induces a wheal and flare reaction known as dermatographism.

Other physical stimuli such as cold, heat, sun, or exercise may induce urticaria. Cold urticaria may be precipitated by putting an ice cube on the skin; the interval until hives develop and the duration of the hives correlate with the severity of the condition, which can be life-threatening if the patient is suddenly immersed in cold water. Heat, exercise, or exertion may be accompanied by small, 2- to 3-mm urticarial lesions or cholinergic urticaria. Exercise-induced anaphylaxis may be hereditary, but the defect is unknown. Cases of urticaria caused by exposure to the sun (solar urticaria) or to water (aquagenic urticaria) are less common forms of physically induced urticaria. By comparison, pruritus without detectible lesions represents the mildest expression of urticarial reactions.

Diagnosis

Urticaria typically results from exposure to antigen only minutes to a few hours before onset of the lesions. In many cases, pruritus may proceed onset of the rash or be the major feature. The most common triggers of IgE-mediated allergic urticarial reactions are drugs (especially penicillin, sulfa drugs, antibiotics, and contrast dye), foods (shellfish, salicylates in berries, tomatoes, yeast, and penicillin in blue cheese), food additives (sodium benzoate), nuts (especially peanuts), or insect bites (mosquitoes, bees, wasps, scabies, or animal mites). Nonimmunologic mediators of urticaria include aspirin and opiates, as well as physical agents that work through the prostaglandin pathway or degranulate mast cells.

Acute urticaria can also be triggered by skin contact with an antigen, such as latex, and can progress to anaphylaxis. In addition, urticaria can be a sign or prodrome of a latent infection, especially streptococcal pharyngitis in children or viral hepatitis in adults. The migratory urticarial rash accompanying rheumatic fever, erythema marginatum (Fig. 466–2), is characterized by evanescent, scalloped lesions that change location over the course of hours.

When urticarial lesions are present for more than 24 hours, underlying urticarial vasculitis should be suspected. Skin biopsy is required to distinguish urticarial vasculitis from urticaria in which no damage to the blood vessels is evident. Erythema multiforme (Chapter 465), most commonly precipitated by herpes simplex infections, other DNA viruses, or drugs, is characterized by lesions that are hybrids between urticaria and vasculitis. Erythema multiforme lesions are known as target or bull's-eye lesions and have deep red centers and pink urticarial rims (see Fig. 465–10). When vascular damage or purpura is present, the lesion is termed *leukocytoclastic vasculitis,* the most severe expression of hypersensitivity reactions involving cutaneous blood vessels (see Fig. 465–4).

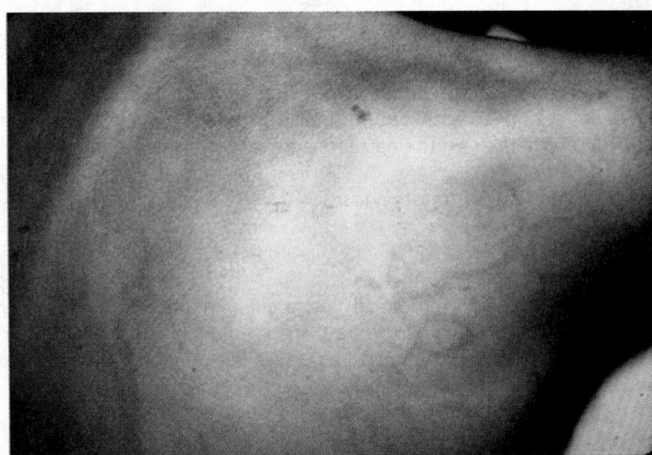

FIGURE 466–2 • Erythema marginatum. (From http://www.medscape.com/content/1998/00/41/73/417394/art-m5649.fig2.jpg.)

Chronic urticaria can be caused by occult infections (sinusitis, gallbladder disease, *Helicobacter pylori,* yeast infections, tooth abscesses, or silent hepatitis), as well as by collagen vascular diseases and tumors, especially Hodgkin's lymphoma. Deficiency of the C1 esterase inhibitor can be manifested as chronic urticaria with angioedema (Chapter 273). Although a thorough medical evaluation may aid in diagnosis, the cause of chronic urticaria may remain uncertain. In the absence of a known antigen, stress is often invoked as the underlying cause of chronic recurrent idiopathic urticaria.

Systemic mastocytosis (Chapter 276) may be accompanied by urticarial lesions, as well as gastrointestinal symptoms. In the form of mastocytosis known as *urticaria pigmentosa,* stroking the lesions produces urticaria, known as *Darier's sign.*

Treatment

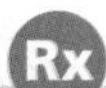

Management of urticaria depends on its severity and the duration of the problem (Chapter 273). For mild urticaria limited to the skin, traditional antihistamines (diphenhydramine [Benadryl], hydroxyzine) or the newer nonsedating agents (terfenadine [Seldane], cetirizine [Zyrtec], loratadine [Claritin]) can be administered by mouth intermittently as needed (Table 466–2). Acute urticaria is often treated with diphenhydramine, 25 to 50 mg orally; if the urticaria is severe, short-term corticosteroids, up to 1 mg/kg, can be used. For urticaria associated with wheezing or anaphylaxis, subcutaneous epinephrine and intravenous corticosteroids, as well as oxygen, should be administered immediately.

TABLE 466–2 TREATMENT OF URTICARIA

1. Avoid the inciting agent!
2. Medications based on severity
   - A. Mild to moderate, acute urticaria
     - Oral antihistamines, e.g., diphenhydramine (Benadryl), 10–50 mg PO q12h, or hydroxyzine, 10–25 mg PO q8h; nonsedating alternatives include cetirizine (Zyrtec), 5–10 mg, or loratadine (Claritin), 10 mg/day
   - B. Severe urticaria with or without angioedema
     - Antihistamines, e.g., diphenhydramine (Benadryl), 25–50 mg PO q6–8h or 10–50 mg IV q2–4h, not to exceed 400 mg/24 hr
     - Corticosteroids, e.g., prednisone, 10–60 mg PO every morning with tapering over a 2-wk period, triamcinolone (Kenalog), 40 mg IM for one dose, or dexamethasone, 0.6–0.75 mg/m^2/day IV in divided doses q6–12h, depending on severity
   - C. Anaphylaxis
     - A—Airway (intubation)
     - B—Breathing (oxygen)
     - C—Circulation: parenteral aqueous epinephrine, 1:1000 IV, saline or volume expanders
     - IV corticosteroids (e.g., methylprednisolone, 125 mg)
     - Histamine H_1- and H_2-antagonists (50 mg each of diphenhydramine and ranitidine)
   - D. Chronic idiopathic urticaria—combination therapy
     - Nonsedating antihistamine: cetirizine, 10 mg/day, or fexofenadine, 20–240 mg twice daily, alone or with montelukast, 10 mg/day, or H_1- and H_2-antagonists (50 mg each of diphenhydramine and ranitidine) and/or low-dose corticosteroids (if unavoidable)

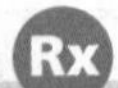

Finding the cause plus removing the antigen of chronic recurrent urticaria is highly preferable to recurrent or chronic administration of corticosteroids or antihistamines. The patient should avoid aspirin compounds and other drugs that could be the cause. The cyclooxygenase inhibitor montelukast (10 mg/day) may also help patients with aspirin-induced urticaria. Allergy testing is recommended if the history is unrevealing (Chapter 270). If lesions remain present for more than 24 hours, skin biopsy is indicated to determine whether vasculitis or mastocytosis is present. If infection, collagen vascular disease, or a tumor is suspected, a full serologic evaluation should be undertaken.

DRUG RASHES

Definition

Drugs have been associated with every type of cutaneous reaction pattern ranging from mild and self-limited to severe and life-threatening (see Table 27–5).

Pathobiology

Delayed hypersensitivity reactions are due to T-lymphocyte infiltrates, with or without eosinophils. Helper T cells are more abundant, but $CD8^+$ suppressor cells that express granzyme B and perforin are implicated in keratinocyte damage. Peripheral eosinophilia, which is induced by interleukin-5 and eotaxin, can also occur.

Clinical Manifestations and Diagnosis

A careful drug history is critical. Most drug rashes are either immediate (urticaria) or delayed hypersensitivity reactions (exanthems). Immediate reactions such as pruritus, hives, angioedema, and anaphylaxis occur within minutes to a few hours after the drug is taken (see earlier). The most common drug-related rash (Table 466–3) is a macular, bright pink to salmon-colored exanthem that appears as early as 7 to 10 days and as late as 14 days after a drug is first administered. Delayed hypersensitivity reactions can be macular or papular exanthems (or both), morbilliform eruptions, annular erythemas, or confluent erythema (Fig. 466–3). Once sensitization to a particular drug has occurred, readministration of the same drug may trigger an eruption within 24 to 72 hours. Drug hypersensitivity reactions are typically very symmetrical. They characteristically begin on the upper part of the trunk and face and progress to the lower extremities. The lesions may become purpuric on the lower extremities or dependent areas as a result of gravity. Exanthems secondary to drugs most often become confluent erythematous patches after several days.

Pruritus may or may not accompany drug rashes; when present, it is helpful for making the diagnosis. The differential diagnosis for drug rashes includes viral exanthems (Chapter 465), graft-versus-host disease or the leukocyte recovery rash after allogeneic bone marrow transplantation, erythematous exanthems that accompany streptococcal (scarlet fever; Chapter 311) or staphylococcal (toxic shock syndrome; Chapter 310) infections, and the acute manifestation of collagen vascular diseases. A similar exanthema occurs when ampicillin is administered to patients who have infectious mononucleosis (Chapter 400).

Treatment and Prognosis

If use of the drug is discontinued, delayed hypersensitivity reactions resolve in about a week. Corticosteroids, such as 0.01% triamcinolone cream applied several times per day to the affected area, and antihistamines given orally three to four times daily are helpful in reducing the itching and shortening the course if given for a few days.

TABLE 466–3 DELAYED HYPERSENSITIVITY DRUG RASHES BY CATEGORY

MACULOPAPULAR EXANTHEMS—ANY DRUG CAN PRODUCE A RASH 7–10 DAYS AFTER THE FIRST DOSE
Allopurinol Antibiotics: penicillin, sulfonamides Antiepileptics: phenytoin, phenobarbital Antihypertensives: captopril, thiazide diuretics Contrast dye: iodine Gold salts Hypoglycemic drugs Meprobamate Phenothiazines Quinine
DRUG RASH WITH EOSINOPHILIA AND SYSTEMIC SYMPTOMS (DRESS)
Anticonvulsants: phenytoin, phenobarbital Antibiotics: sulfonamides, minocycline, dapsone Allopurinol Phenothiazines
ERYTHEMA MULTIFORME/STEVENS-JOHNSON SYNDROME
Sulfonamides, phenytoin, barbiturates, carbamazepines, allopurinol, amikacin, phenothiazines Toxic epidermal necrolysis: same as for erythema multiforme but also acetazolamide, gold, nitrofurantoin, pentazocine, tetracycline, quinidine
ACUTE GENERALIZED EXANTHEMIC PUSTULOSIS
Antibiotics: penicillins, macrolides, cephalosporins, clindamycin, imipenem, fluoroquinolones, isoniazid, vancomycin, minocycline, doxycycline, linezolid Antimalarials: chloroquine, hydroxychloroquine Antifungals: terbinafine, nystatin Anticonvulsants: carbamazepine Calcium-channel blockers Furosemide Systemic corticosteroids Protease inhibitors
COLLAGEN VASCULAR OR LUPUS-LIKE REACTIONS
Procainamide, hydralazine, phenytoin, penicillamine, trimethadione, methyldopa, carbamazepine, griseofulvin, nalidixic acid, oral contraceptives, propranolol
ERYTHEMA NODOSUM
Oral contraceptives, penicillin, sulfonamides, diuretics, gold, clonidine, propranolol, opiates Fixed drug reactions: phenolphthalein, barbiturates, gold, sulfonamides, meprobamate, penicillin, tetracycline, analgesics

Specific Syndromes

Drug Rash with Eosinophilia and Systemic Symptoms

An especially severe hypersensitivity *drug rash with eosinophilia and systemic symptoms* (DRESS) is most frequently seen with phenytoin (Dilantin) or carbamazepine (Tegretol) or when allopurinol is coadministered with thiazide diuretics (Fig. 466–4). DRESS may be delayed in onset by 4 to 6 weeks, persists longer than classic drug-induced eruptions do, and becomes generalized and severe, even when use of the agent is discontinued. Continued administration of the drug can result in generalized exfoliative erythroderma, toxic necrolysis, and systemic hypersensitivity, including hepatitis (50%), nephritis (10%), or less commonly,

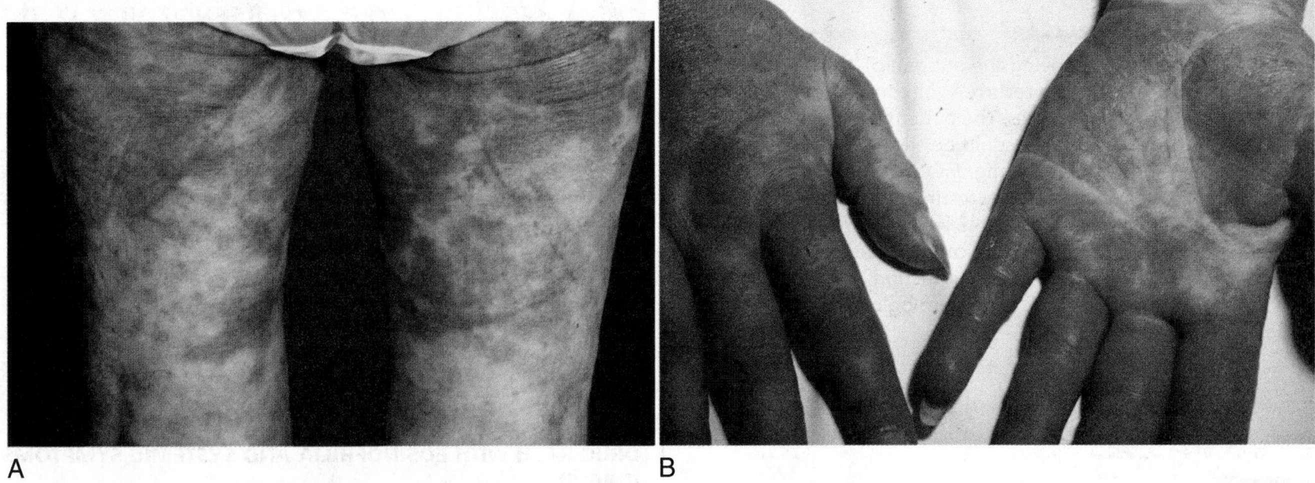

FIGURE 466–3 • Delayed hypersensitivity reaction. A, Drug reaction. **B,** acral erythema.

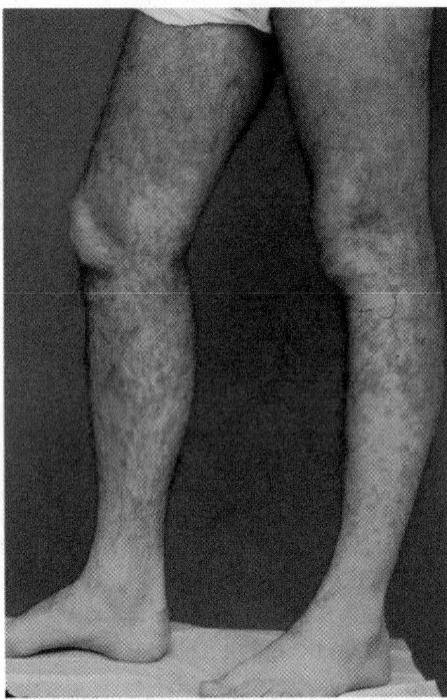

FIGURE 466–4 • Hypersensitivity drug rash caused by phenytoin.

pneumonitis, myocarditis, pericarditis, or atypical lymphocytosis and lymphadenopathy mimicking mononucleosis or T-cell lymphoma. With visceral involvement there is a 10% mortality rate, usually from liver failure.

Erythema Multiforme

Drugs are almost always implicated when blistering conditions known as *erythema multiforme* (see Fig. 465–10), *Stevens-Johnson syndrome,* or *toxic epidermal necrolysis* develop in adults (Fig. 466–5). Commonly implicated medications include allopurinol, phenytoin, and sulfa drugs (see Table 27–5).

Leukocytoclastic Vasculitis

Severe drug reactions can also be manifested as vasculitis, neutrophilic eruptions, and ulcerations. Vasculitis is further categorized by the size of the involved vessel and the nature of the cellular reaction and immune complexes. *Leukocytoclastic vasculitis* (Chapter 465), which is the most common form of vasculitis induced by drugs, is manifested as palpable purpura, usually on the extremities (see Fig. 465–4).

Neutrophilic Drug Reactions

Neutrophilic drug reactions include iododermas and bromodermas, as well as drug-induced Sweet's syndrome (see Inflammatory and Hematopoietic Papular and Tumors) and *acute generalized exanthemic pustulosis* (see Fig. 465–19), which is characterized by numerous (>100), small (<5 mm), nonfollicular subcorneal pustules that arise on erythematous skin, often beginning in skin creases or on the face. High fever and peripheral neutrophilia may proceed or accompany the eruption. The pustules are sterile, present for 5 to 10 days, and followed by desquamation. Ninety percent of cases are due to drugs and usually appear within 2 to 3 days after the administration of antibiotics or 1 to 2 weeks after other drugs; the pustules resolve within 15 days. This syndrome has also been called pustular drug rash, pustular psoriasis after corticosteroid withdrawal, and toxic pustuloderma. When severe, it may be confused with toxic epidermal necrolysis, but the mortality rate is only 1 to 2%. Skin patch testing is frequently positive.

Fixed Drug Eruptions

A fixed drug reaction is an eruption that occurs at the same location every time that the drug is ingested. The mucous membranes of the mouth or genital region are most commonly involved. The lesion may begin as erythema and then become gray or brown. Phenolphthalein-containing laxatives, barbiturates, and acetaminophen are common causes. If skin that is involved in a fixed drug reaction is grafted to another area, the eruption will be transferred to the new location, thereby suggesting that local antigens are important.

Photosensitivity and Withdrawal Reactions

Light may combine with drugs (Table 466–4) to produce photosensitivity reactions (Chapter 464) that can be quite severe. Thiazides, tetracyclines, sulfa drugs, antipsychotic agents, and hydralazine are often implicated in photosensitivity reactions.

Drugs can exacerbate existing cutaneous diseases. Examples are steroid withdrawal, β-blockers, and lithium, which worsen psoriasis. Photosensitizing drugs may exacerbate lupus erythematosus or porphyria cutanea tarda.

Contact Dermatitis

Allergic contact dermatitis, which is a T-cell–mediated delayed hypersensitivity reaction, can result from topical drug application. In clinical practice, contact dermatitis manifested by erythema and microvesiculation occurs in the area where the drug has been applied but may spread beyond the area (termed an *ID reaction*). Common contact sensitizers include Neosporin (polymyxin B/neomycin/bacitracin), bacitracin, diphenhydramine, doxepin, lidocaine, lanolin, mercury, and *p*-aminobenzoic acid.

BENIGN NODULES AND TUMORS

The skin is a heterogeneous organ composed of epidermis, dermis, subcutaneous compartments, and blood vessels. The skin hosts a number of migrating cells (Chapter 461), all of which can give rise to benign or malignant tumors. Lesions that arise from epidermal keratinocytes are usually papules (warts, sebaceous hyperplasia) or plaques (psoriasis, Bowen's disease; Chapter 465). Nodules are deep lesions that are best felt

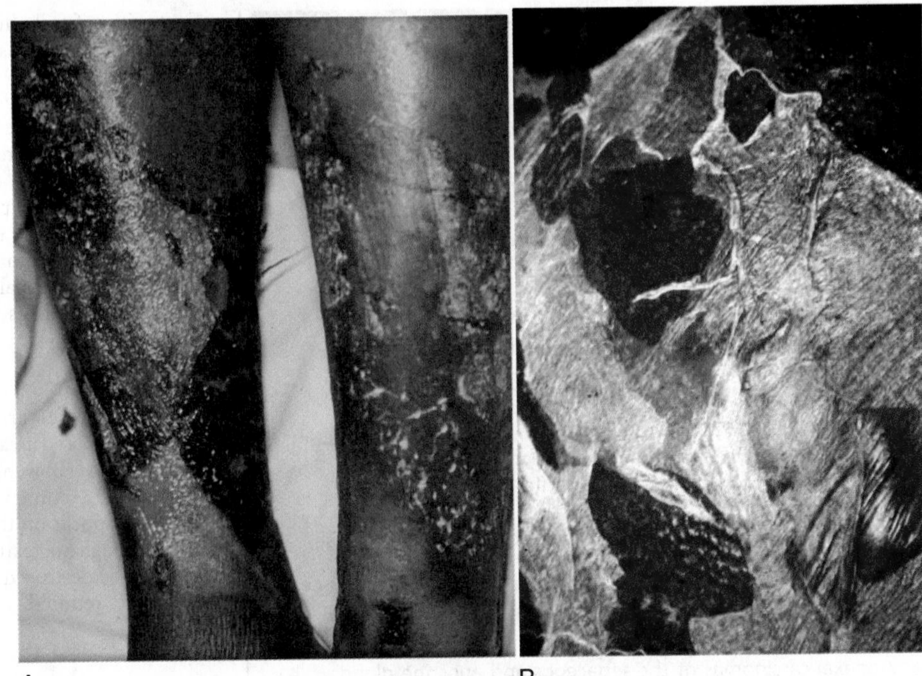

FIGURE 466–5 • Toxic epidermal necrolysis. A, Clinical appearance. B, Close-up appearance of epidermal sheets.

TABLE 466–4 DRUGS ASSOCIATED WITH SUN SENSITIVITY

PHOTOTOXIC
Chlorpromazine
Hydralazine
Levaquin
Procainamide
Psoralens
Porphyrins
Tetracyclines
Thiazide diuretics
Sulfonamides
PHOTOALLERGIC
Promethazine
Griseofulvin
Chlorothiazide
Hypoglycemic drugs

rather than seen because they arise in the dermis or in subcutaneous tissue. Nodules may arise from collections of cells around vessels or in fat, from foreign bodies, or from metabolic deposits. Nodules may induce no surface change or be accompanied by an overlying epidermal reaction such as hyperpigmentation, erythema, or scaling. Dermal invasion by a malignant basal or squamous cell carcinoma or invasive melanoma may also produce nodules (Chapter 214).

Nodules may be tender or asymptomatic and single or multiple. They can have a purple vascular component and may break down to form ulcers. Nodules are classified as inflammatory (granulomas, vasculitis, or panniculitis), infectious, or metabolic or as benign or malignant tumors arising from skin or invading cells (Table 466–5). Nodules that are smaller and symmetrical are more likely to be benign than lesions that grow rapidly, are larger, or invade surrounding tissue. Any rapidly changing skin nodule should be investigated with an excisional biopsy to the level of fat for correct histopathologic diagnosis. Culture of the lesion is also highly recommended because deep fungal infections and tuberculosis may be manifested as nodules.

Benign Epidermal Tumors

The top layer of skin is the avascular epidermis, which is composed of resident keratinocytes, as well as migratory melanocytes, Langerhans cells, and in disease states, inflammatory cells (Chapter 461). Epidermal stem cells arising near the hair follicle differentiate to form adnexal organs, including hair follicles and glands (sebaceous, eccrine, and apocrine), each of which can give rise to benign or malignant tumors.

Seborrheic Keratoses

The most common benign epidermal tumors are seborrheic keratoses, which are pleomorphic verrucous, oval lesions that have regular borders, are often raised, and appear to be stuck onto the skin (Fig. 466–6). Seborrheic keratoses arise from a keratinocyte clone and are often inherited in an autosomal dominant pattern. Their color can be white, flesh colored, pink, yellow, tan, brown, or black, and several different colors can be present in the same patient and in the same lesion. Seborrheic keratoses may be friable and peel off with scraping. The appearance of large numbers of eruptive seborrheic keratoses may also signal an internal carcinoma that is producing a growth factor such as epidermal growth factor. Seborrheic keratoses can be distinguished from melanocytic nevi, melanomas, and pigmented basal cell carcinoma by the presence of white to yellow horn cysts on their surface, which are best appreciated under magnification. Although seborrheic keratoses are benign, they must be differentiated from other pigmented lesions, especially superficial spreading melanoma (see Fig. 214–3).

Papules

Papules (Chapter 465) include *warts* (see Fig. 465–2), which are caused by the human papillomavirus (HPV). HPV can also be detected in squamous carcinomas arising on the digits and in keratoacanthoma, a low-grade, well-demarcated, dome-shaped squamous cell carcinoma that grows rapidly and spontaneously involutes in 6 to 8 weeks. In acrodermatitis verruciformis, multiple warts that have the appearance of seborrheic keratoses (see later) are found on the extremities and give rise to squamous carcinomas. *Tricholemmomas* are wartlike epidermal lesions found in association with Cowden's syndrome, which is associated with mutations in the *PTEN* gene; Cowden's syndrome is defined by warty papules on the gums, tricholemmomas (Fig. 466–7), fibrous papules, and multiple hamartomas involving the breast, thyroid, intestines, ovary, and cerebellum (Chapter 203). *Molluscum contagiosum* (Chapter 465) (Fig. 466–8), caused by a DNA virus, are small, shiny, domed-shaped, 1- to 5-mm papules with a central dell; they are common in children and immunocompromised patients. Epidermoid tumors on the scalp in a

TABLE 466–5 TUMORS AND NODULES OF THE SKIN

Benign, nonpigmented tumors and nodules
Epidermal: warts, acrochordons, tricholemmomas, sebaceous hyperplasia
Adnexal: epidermal cysts, syringomas, follicular cysts, pilomatricoma, apocrine or eccrine adenomas
Dermal and subcutaneous: lipomas, angiolipomas, neurofibromas, leiomyomas
Benign, pigmented tumors and nodules
Epidermal: seborrheic keratoses
Melanocytic compound nevi (junctional nevi are flat)
Spitz nevus
Blue nevus
Dermatofibromas
Malignant, nonpigmented tumors and nodules
Basal cell carcinoma (nodular, superficial, morpheaform, pigmented)
Squamous cell carcinoma (actinic keratoses, Bowen's disease, keratoacanthomas)
Cutaneous T- and B-cell lymphomas
Amelanotic melanomas
Merkel cell carcinomas
Adnexal carcinomas of the sebaceous and apocrine glands
Malignant, pigmented tumors and nodules
Pigmented basal cell carcinoma
Malignant melanoma: in situ, superficial spreading, nodular, acral lentiginous
Dermatofibrosarcoma protuberans
Inflammatory nodules over joints
Gottren's papules (dermatomyositis)
Gouty tophi
Heberden's nodes (osteoarthritis)
Multicentric reticulohistiocytosis (paraneoplastic syndrome)
Rheumatoid nodules
Granuloma annulare
Inflammatory nodules of the lower extremities
Panniculitis
Vasculitis: periarteritis nodosa
Metabolic nodules of the skin
Amyloidosis
Gouty tophi
Xanthomas, necrobiotic xanthogranuloma
Xanthelasma
Vascular lesions
Benign: nevus flammeus, angiokeratomas, spider hemangiomas, capillary hemangiomas, cavernous hemangiomas, blue rubber bleb nevi, pyogenic granulomas
Malignant: Kaposi's sarcoma, angiosarcoma

patient with a family history of colon cancer are helpful in making the diagnosis of Gardner's syndrome (Chapter 203).

Adnexal Tumors

Adnexal tumors arise from the hair follicles or from sebaceous or other glands and are commonly found on the face. *Trichoepitheliomas* have features similar to basal cell carcinoma, whereas sebaceous hyperplasia describes small yellow papules with a central depression. *Sebaceous carcinomas* occur around the upper part of the face or eyelids as solitary lesions or as markers for the Muir-Torre syndrome of familial breast and colon cancer. Epidermal or sebaceous cysts, which are found in acne or as single firm nodules with a central pore, are filled with sebum or keratin.

Actinic Keratoses

Actinic keratoses arise from sun-induced DNA damage to keratinocytes in exposed areas. They are precursor lesions of in situ squamous cell carcinoma (Bowen's disease) and invasive squamous carcinoma (Chapter 214). Actinic keratoses are scaly, 0.1- to 1.0-cm, white or pink lesions that appear on the forearms, hands, face, and scalp (Fig. 466–9). They are rough in texture and may have little induration. Individual lesions can be destroyed locally by cryotherapy or topical agents such as fluorouracil, retinoid, or imiquimod. Pink or red scaly lesions with

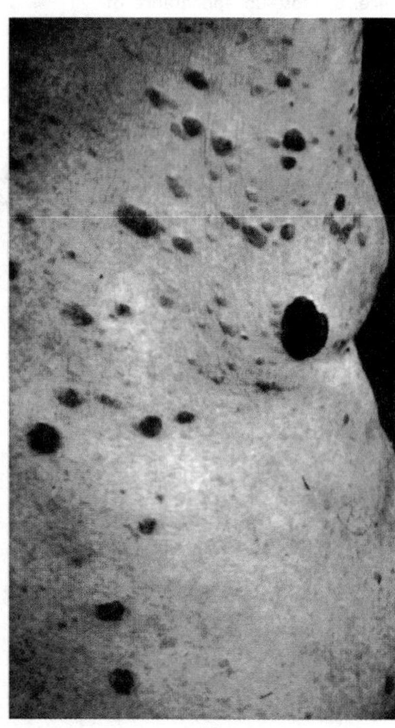

FIGURE 466–6 • Seborrheic keratoses.

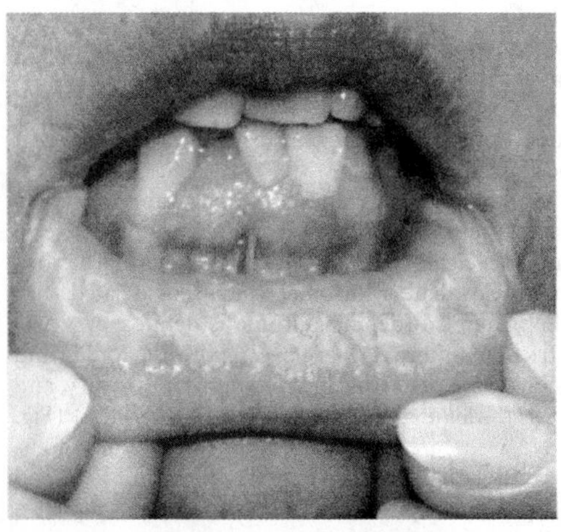

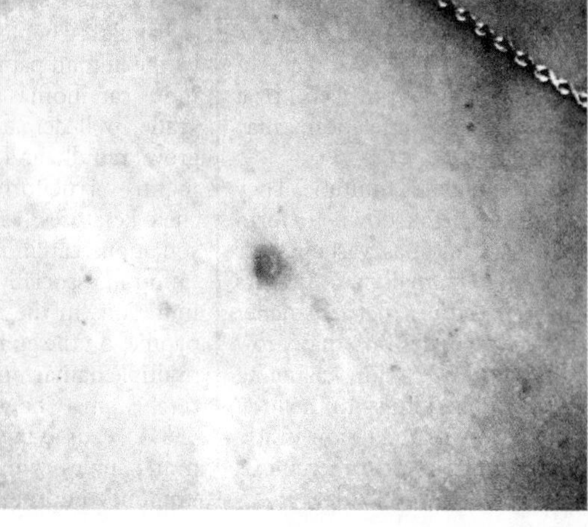

FIGURE 466–7 • Cowden's syndrome: cobblestone gums (left) and tricholemmoma (right).

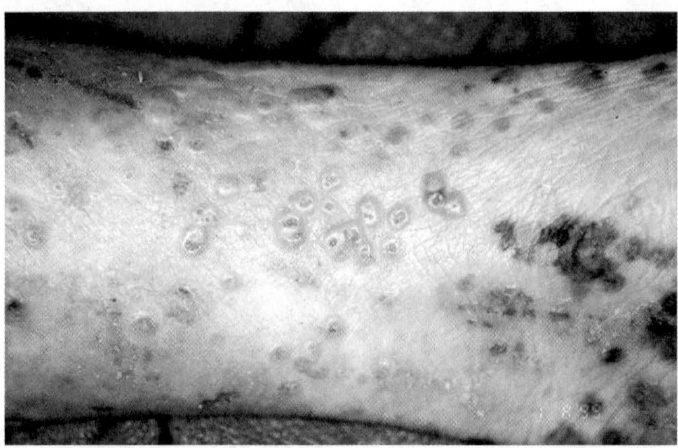

FIGURE 466–8 • Molluscum contagiosum in an immunocompromised patient.

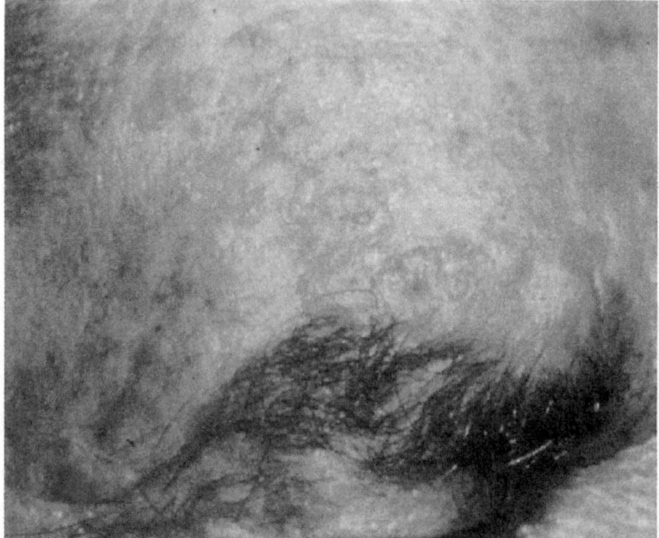

FIGURE 466–9 • Actinic keratoses.

induration, thick crusts, ulceration, or pain must be sampled to exclude invasive squamous cell carcinoma. Because the skin on which actinic keratoses arise is photodamaged and may carry mutations in *p53*, a more effective approach is to treat the entire area with 5-fluorouracil cream (5%) applied daily for 2 weeks or twice weekly for 8 weeks, with use of a topical antibiotic for a shorter period.

Benign Tumors of Cells That Migrate into Skin

Melanocytes

Benign melanocytic moles or nevi (new) are discrete nests of melanocytes acquired during childhood and young adulthood and stimulated by sun exposure. *Nevi* are benign lesions, in contrast to malignant melanomas, which also arise from melanocytes (Chapter 214). Nevi tend to regress with age and may change in color during pregnancy. Benign melanocytic nevi are formed by nests of melanocytes at the epidermal junction (junctional nevi), in the dermis (intradermal nevi), or in both compartments (compound nevi). The appearance of moles depends on the type and age of the lesion. *Junctional nevi* (Fig. 466–10) are small, flat, and light to dark brown. *Intradermal nevi* are soft, flesh-colored to pink papules with smooth regular borders and surface. *Compound nevi* are also papules but have brown pigmentation. *Blue nevi* (Fig. 466–11) are flat, grayish blue, and regular. Small congenital nevi are dark brown, whereas large (>20 cm) congenital nevi have variegated colors and are more likely to transform with melanoma (Fig. 466–12). Patients who have more than 10 large, atypical moles with irregular borders and colors that resemble melanoma have a very high risk for the development of melanoma, especially if there is a family history; such patients require regular surveillance examinations. Other recognized risk factors for melanoma include having more than 50 small nevi, red or blonde hair, or fair skin that burns and a history of blistering sunburns as a child.

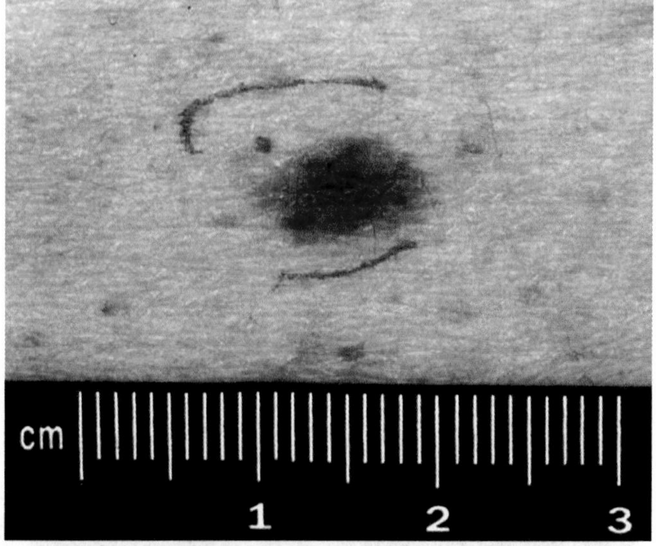

FIGURE 466–10 • Junctional nevus.

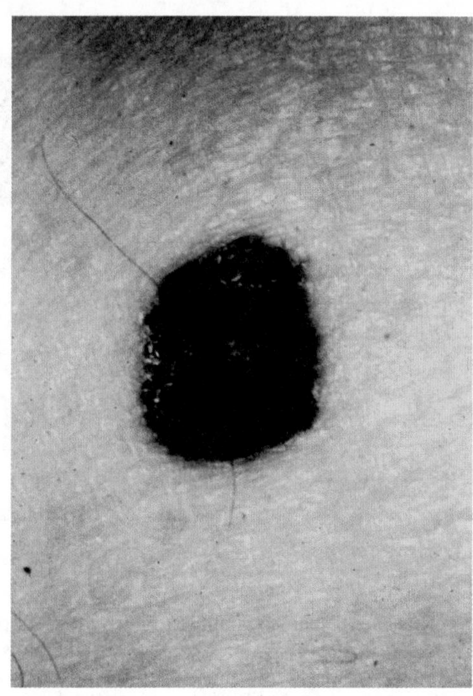

FIGURE 466–11 • Benign blue nevus.

Langerhans Cell Histiocytosis

The skin immune system includes surveillance mediated by antigen-presenting cells such as Langerhans cells and dermal dendritic cells, as well as skin-homing T lymphocytes. Langerhans cells migrate from lymph nodes, process antigen, and present peptides to T cells. Proliferation of Langerhans cells characterizes one form of histiocytosis. Childhood histiocytosis X is manifested as severe seborrheic dermatitis of the scalp and gluteal areas with underlying purpura and may result in the hemophagocytic syndrome. In adults, lesions appear in the intertriginous areas (Fig. 466–13). Patients with the non–Langerhans cell histiocytosis have lytic bone involvement (eosinophilic granulomas) or diabetes insipidus (Hand-Schüller-Christian syndrome).

Dermal Tumors

Dermatofibromas

Fibroblasts are the resident cells of the dermis and are responsible for producing collagen, elastin, and mucopolysaccharides. Accumulation of

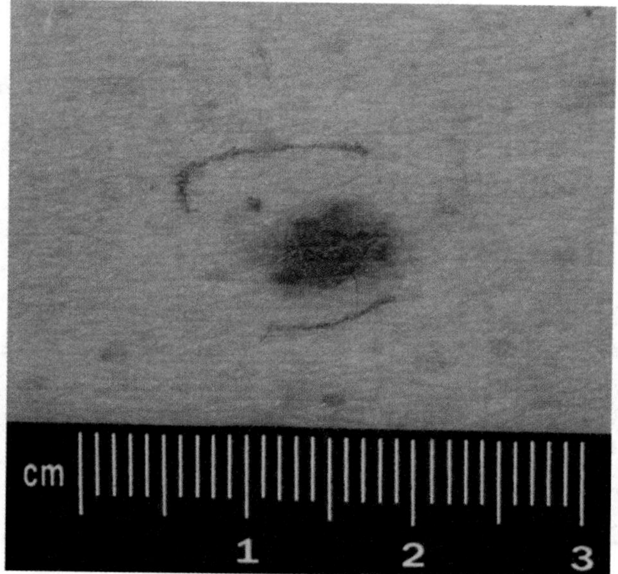

FIGURE 466–12 • Dysplastic nevus syndrome.

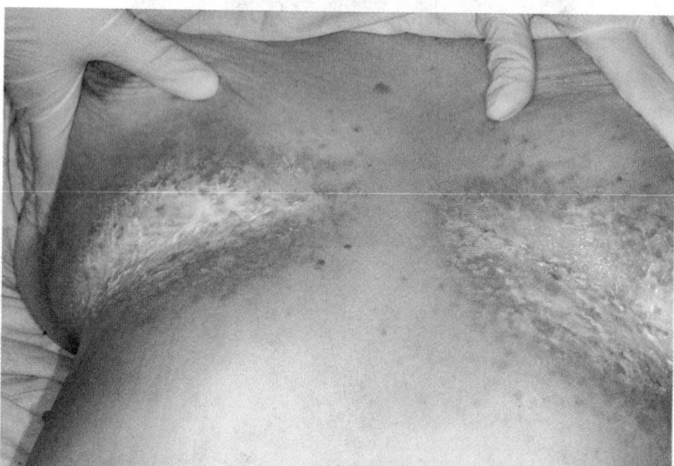

FIGURE 466–13 • Histiocytosis X.

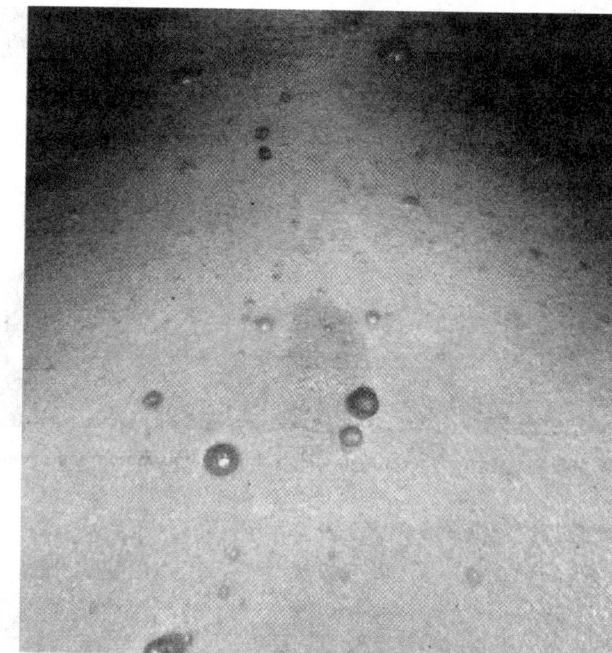

FIGURE 466–14 • Neurofibromatosis with cafe au lait spots and neurofibromas.

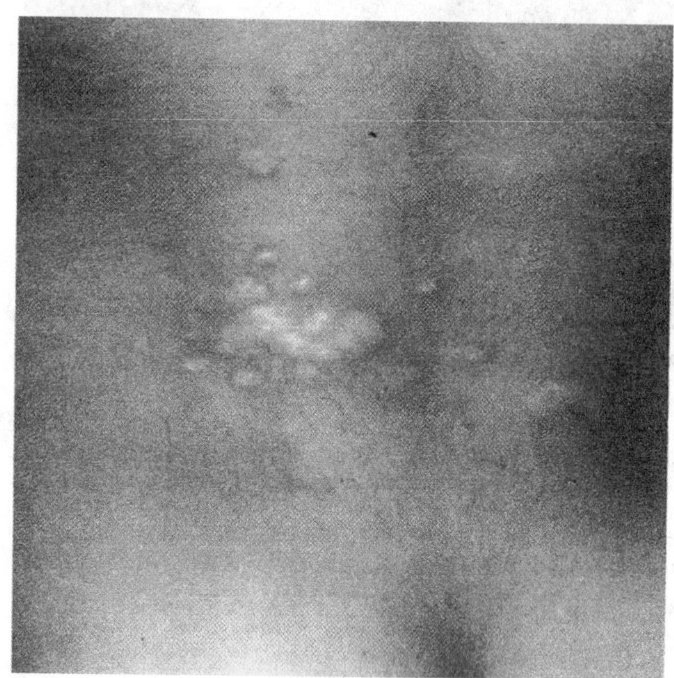

FIGURE 466–15 • Schwannoma.

these products results in sclerosis, papules, or nodules. Fibroblasts in small dense clusters form firm papules or nodules known as *dermatofibromas,* which are brown papules most commonly found on the extremities and form after insect bites or trauma. They are firm and well-demarcated papules with puckering around them when lateral pressure is applied. Dermatofibromas can be treated, but increased scarring may occur. The malignant counterpart is dermatofibroma sarcoma protuberans, which is a poorly defined, rapidly expanding, dermal malignant tumor. Overlying erythema or hyperpigmentation is often present.

Collagenomas

Collagenomas and elastic tumors with the appearance of small white to yellow papules are found in the skin and bone of patients with Buschke-Ollendorff syndrome. *Pseudoxanthoma elasticum* (Chapter 281), an autosomal recessive disorder, is typically manifested as cutaneous yellow plaques about the neck or antecubital fossa from damaged elastin tissue. *Mucin cysts* are gray, shiny, well-demarcated round nodules that generally arise on the mucosa or on the digits, where they may have an underlying connection to the joint space.

Benign tumors in the dermis can also arise from neural crest cells: *neurofibromas* (soft, flesh-colored papules; Fig. 466–14) and *schwannomas* (larger subcutaneous soft tumors or plaques; Fig. 466–15). Although solitary neurofibromas may occur, the presence of multiple lesions plus cafe au lait spots (tan macules) or axillary freckling (Crowe's sign) is diagnostic of neurofibromatosis type I, an autosomal dominant disorder caused by mutations in neurofibromin (Chapter 444). Schwannomas can become malignant and be manifested as dermal nodules.

Merkel Cell Carcinoma

Merkel cell carcinoma is a particularly aggressive small cell tumor arising from the cutaneous nerve endings or Meissner's corpuscles. Merkel cell tumors are accompanied by translucent or purple papules or plaques on sun-exposed areas (Fig. 466–16), but their appearance is not distinctive. Treatment requires full excision, radiation therapy, and often chemotherapy because the cancer tends to recur and metastasize. Glomus tumors are benign and blue or purple, with small, painful tumors arising from nerve endings. Soft, well-demarcated nodules of fatty tissue, called *lipomas,* are benign and may be multiple; they may have a vascular component or be painful.

Vascular Lesions

Hemangiomas

Benign capillary hemangiomas are bright cherry-red to purple raised papules less than 5 mm in diameter that appear on the trunk with aging and may be numerous (Fig. 466–17). *Pyogenic granulomas,* which are sterile collections of polymorphonuclear leukocytes, can resemble capillary hemangiomas, but they have a friable epidermal surface and bleed easily; they may be similar in appearance to amelanotic melanoma. In the presence of multiple pyogenic granuloma-like lesions, infectious bacillary angiomatosis should be considered (Chapter 336). Flat red macules found on the posterior of the neck are due to a benign capillary network and are referred to as nevus flammeus or stork bite. *Cavernous* or *strawberry hemangiomas* can also appear in the neonatal period as rapidly growing vascular tumors; they may obstruct the eye or the pharynx before regressing. Corticosteroids, interferon, or antiangiogenic factors can be used to treat these lesions successfully. Cavernous hemangiomas are deeper and less likely to resolve than smaller lesions. When associated with platelet consumption, the Kasabach-Merritt syndrome is present (Chapter 179).

Kaposi's Sarcoma

Kaposi's sarcoma (Chapter 415) is a disseminated angiomatosis that arises from viral interleukin-8 production by herpesvirus 8. The lesions are often symmetrical and can appear as purple patches; as raised purple, brown, or gray plaques; or as small papules, firm nodules, or ulcers (Fig. 466–18). Mucosal involvement is more common in advanced disease. Kaposi's sarcoma in young African adults and Kaposi's sarcoma associated with human immunodeficiency virus (HIV) infection often have a more aggressive course than Kaposi's sarcoma in elderly men of Mediterranean background, in whom the disease tends to be indolent and confined to the lower extremities. Treatment of HIV disease with highly active retroviral therapy has been associated with a decreased incidence and severity of HIV-associated Kaposi's sarcoma. *Angiosarcomas* are malignant purple to red vascular tumor nodules that are more common in elderly individuals or on the extremities of patients with chronic lymphedema.

Inflammatory and Hematopoietic Papules and Tumors

Inflammatory diseases of the skin often involve the vessels of the dermis or deeper subcutaneous tissue. The inflammatory infiltrates can be mixed or restricted in nature. Lymphocytes, polymorphonuclear leukocytes, histocytes, eosinophils, and plasma cells are the most common components of inflammatory reactions. Hematologic malignancies can be manifested in the skin as patches, nodules, papules, or vasculitic lesions. T cells that home to skin give rise to cutaneous T-cell lymphoma, a heterogeneous group of extranodal non-Hodgkin's lymphomas (Chapter 196). In mycosis fungoides, the lesions are usually pleomorphic pink, white, or brown patches or plaques; patches of alopecia can occur, and diffuse erythroderma is found with blood involvement (Sézary's syndrome) or with staphylococcal colonization. Tumors occur late in the disease or if the cells have transformed to a large phenotype,

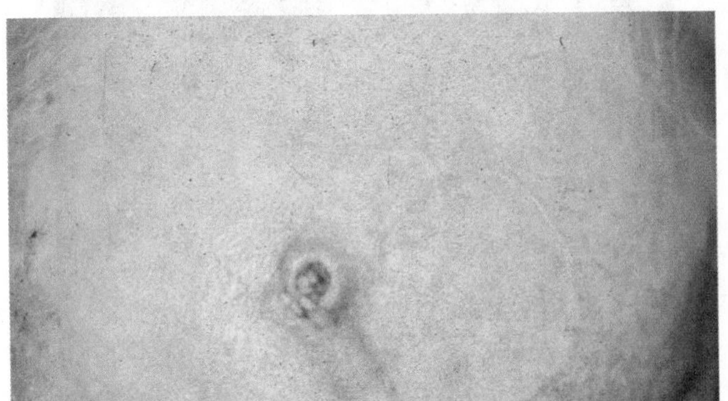

FIGURE 466–16 • Merkel cell tumor.

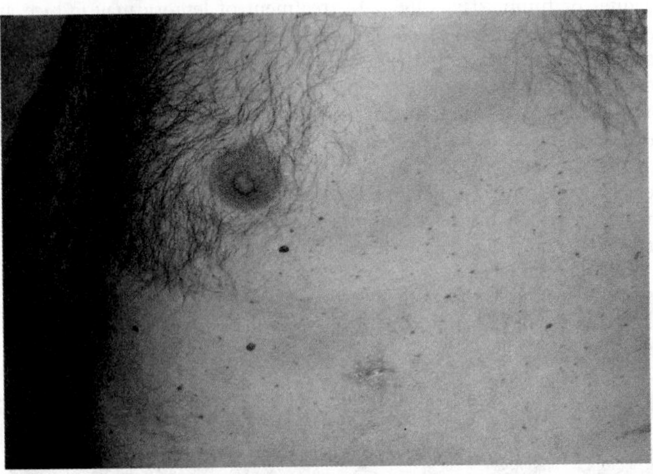

FIGURE 466–17 • Benign capillary hemangioma.

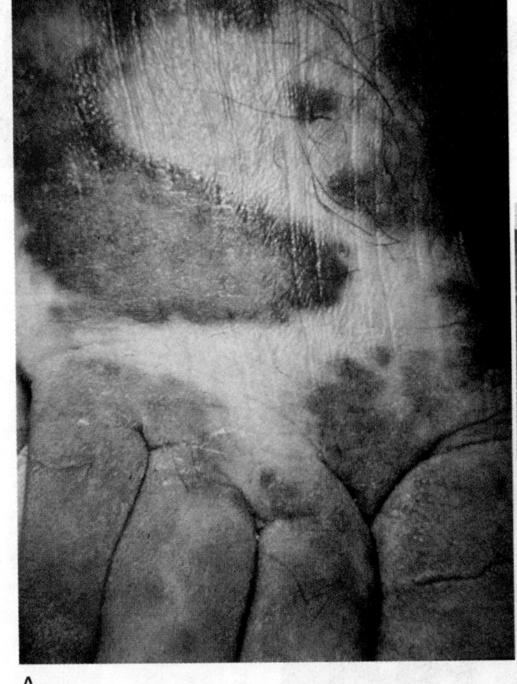

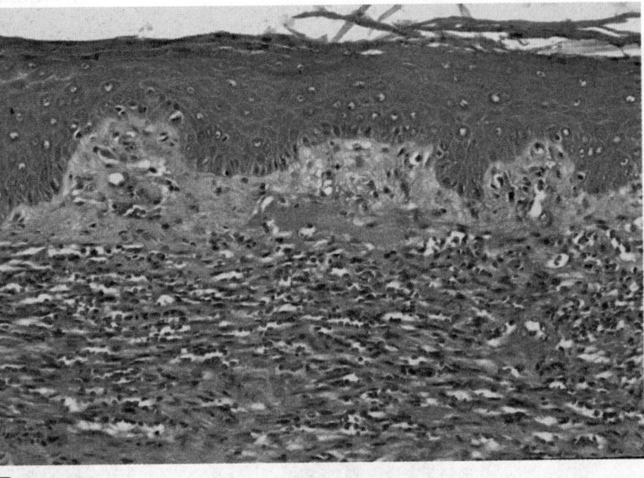

FIGURE 466–18 • Kaposi's sarcoma. **A,** Involvement of the lower extremity (Mediterranean Kaposi's sarcoma). **B,** Histology.

which may express CD30 (see Fig. 465–15). The early phase of mycosis fungoides is indistinguishable from chronic eczematous or psoriasiform dermatitis. Peripheral cutaneous T-cell lymphomas may also be found in subcutaneous tissue as panniculitic lesions. Lymphomatoid papulosis is characterized by crops of red to pink regressing papules with a histologic picture of anaplastic large cell lymphoma, including expression of the Ki-1 or CD30 antigen. The lesions are self-regressing and should be distinguished from $CD30^+$ lymphoma and transformed mycosis fungoides for the purpose of treatment. Natural killer T-cell lymphomas and immunoblastic lymphomas may be manifested in skin as brown dermal nodules.

B-cell lymphomas in skin are pink, infiltrated, dome-shaped shiny papules or tumors that are most commonly located on the face, scalp, or upper part of the back. With the exception of large cell lymphoma, many B-cell lymphomas of the skin are indolent and some are stimulated by *Borrelia* infection or chronic inflammation. Plasmacytomas can arise in the skin, as well as in bone, with multiple myeloma or independent of it. Extramedullary hematopoiesis or endometriosis can be associated with red or brown nodules in the dermis.

Sarcoidosis

Sarcoidosis (Chapter 95) is an inflammatory granulomatous process manifested as ichthyosis, papules, plaques, or tumors with an apple jelly color (Fig. 466–19). Patients with *lepromatous leprosy* have histiocytic plaques or tumors (Fig. 466–20); treatment of leprosy may induce an inflammatory reaction called erythema nodosum leprosum. Granulomatous inflammation within the dermis can result in damage to collagen, as seen in granuloma annulare (ringlike pink to red infiltrated lesions often on the hands or elbows), rheumatoid nodules that occur on the extensor surface of the arms, and necrobiosis lipoidica on the shins of diabetics. All three lesions typically include fibrin deposits within dermal blood vessels. Multicentric reticulohistiocytosis is a rare paraneoplastic syndrome in which histiocytic nodules form over joints with associated arthritis.

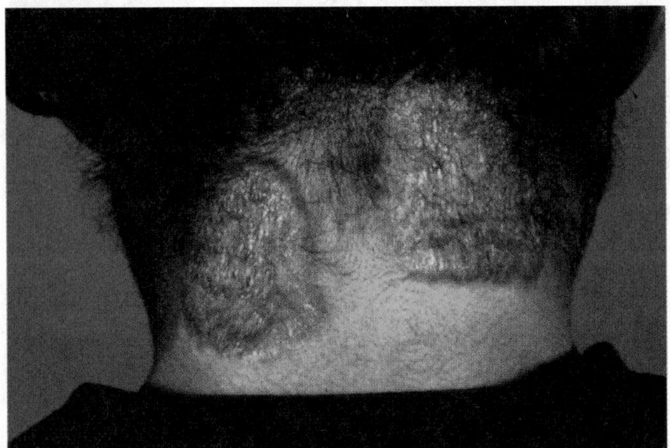

FIGURE 466–19 • Cutaneous sarcoidosis.

Inflammatory Skin Nodules

Inflammatory skin nodules arise from inflamed deeper structures, especially blood vessels (vasculitis) or adipose tissue (panniculitis); both can arise in response to underlying infection or antigen stimulation with influx of inflammatory cells. Vasculitis is further categorized by the size of the vessels and the type of circulating immune complexes. Damage to blood vessels results in leakage of red blood cells with the development of purpura (nonblanching red to purple lesions; Chapter 291). *Erythema elevatum diutinum* is manifested as multiple, infiltrated pink or yellow to red and violaceous nodules or papules that may be painful or asymptomatic. The lesions can coalesce to form gyrate lesions on the dorsum of the hands or extensor surfaces similar to granuloma annulare. Erythema elevatum diutinum is associated with upper respiratory infections (especially *Streptococcus*), HIV infection, and inflammatory bowel disease. The underlying histopathology is a necrotizing vasculitis with neutrophils and hyalinization of the vessels. Erythema elevatum diutinum must be distinguished from *Sweet's syndrome* (recurrent febrile, neutrophilic dermatosis of Sweet), which is characterized by similar lesions clinically (Fig. 466–21). Sweet's syndrome is accompanied by fever, and biopsy specimens show sheets of leukocytes filling the upper dermis in the absence of infection. It occurs in patients with leukemia, inflammatory bowel disease, or rheumatoid arthritis. Sweet's syndrome, but not erythema elevatum diutinum, is highly responsive to corticosteroids, whereas dapsone can improve both conditions.

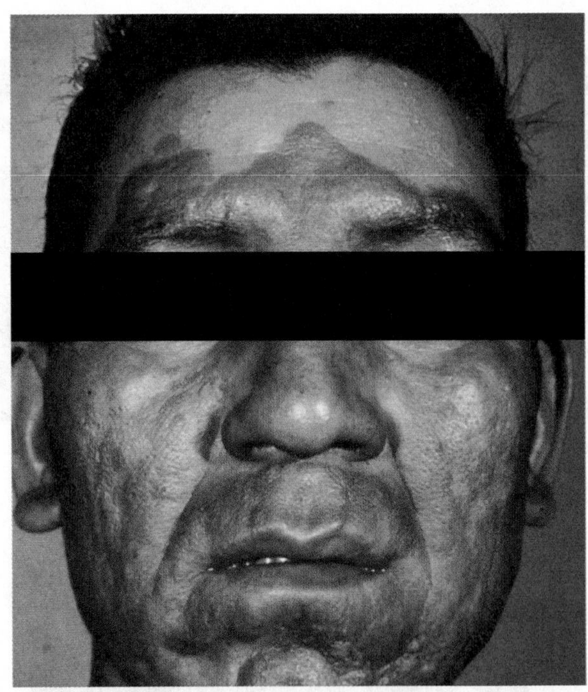

FIGURE 466–20 • Leonine facies associated with lepromatous leprosy.

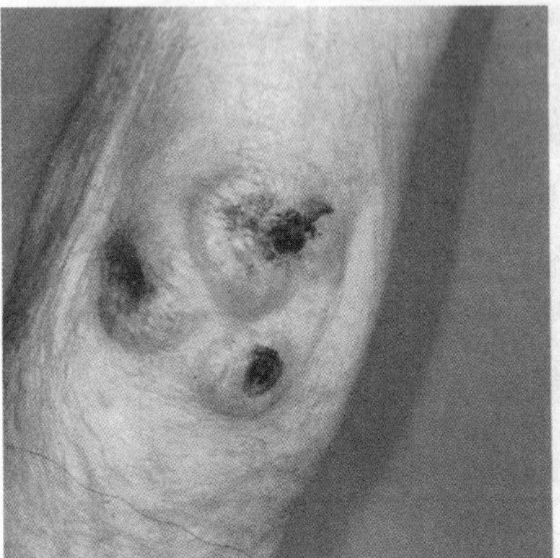

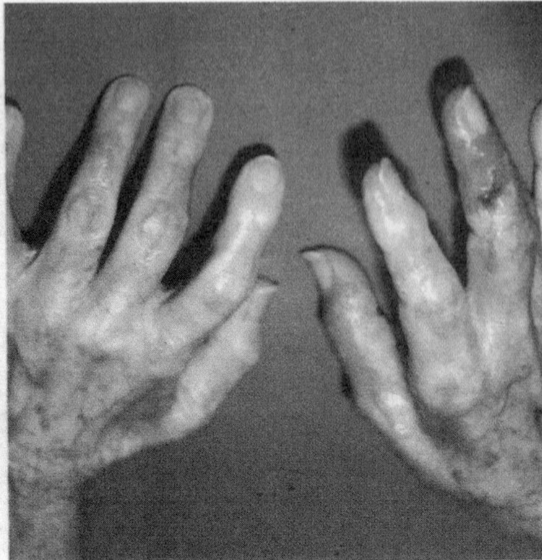

FIGURE 466–21 • Sweet's syndrome in patients with leukemia.

Polyarteritis Nodosa

Polyarteritis nodosa (Chapter 291) arises in larger arterioles and may be associated with hepatitis C infection, mesenteric aneurysms, cryoglobulinemia, cutaneous ulceration, and livedo reticularis. Polyarteritis nodosa is distinct from small vessel leukocytoclastic vasculitis, which is characterized by smaller areas (a few millimeters) of purpura.

In the clinical setting, *panniculitis* occurs more frequently than nodular vasculitis. The differential diagnosis of vasculitis versus septal or lobular panniculitis requires an excisional biopsy, including fat, with appropriate cultures and stains. Lobular panniculitis with necrosis and purpura is actually called nodular vasculitis or erythema induratum. Nodular vasculitis is characterized by painful, chronic recurrent nodules that develop on the shin or thighs and that become bluish, ulcerate, and heal with scarring. *Erythema induratum* (Fig. 466–22), which is exacerbated by cold exposure, is sometimes associated with infection with *Mycobacterium tuberculosis* (Chapter 345). True *lobular panniculitis,* with or without fat necrosis, occurs more often in males with underlying pancreatitis (Chapter 147) and may precede the detection of pancreatic cancer (Chapter 204). The lesions have a predilection for the anterior aspect of the shins and may be fluctuant as a result of fat necrosis. Lupus panniculitis or lupus profundus involves the fat and is diagnosed by overlying granular immune complex deposition of IgM along the dermal-epidermal junction. Lupus panniculitis of the breast can be mistaken for adenocarcinoma; it is treated with antimalarials or corticosteroids. Lobular panniculitis with calcification of the small arterioles, which occurs in the setting of renal failure with hyperparathyroidism, is called calciphylaxis (Chapter 131).

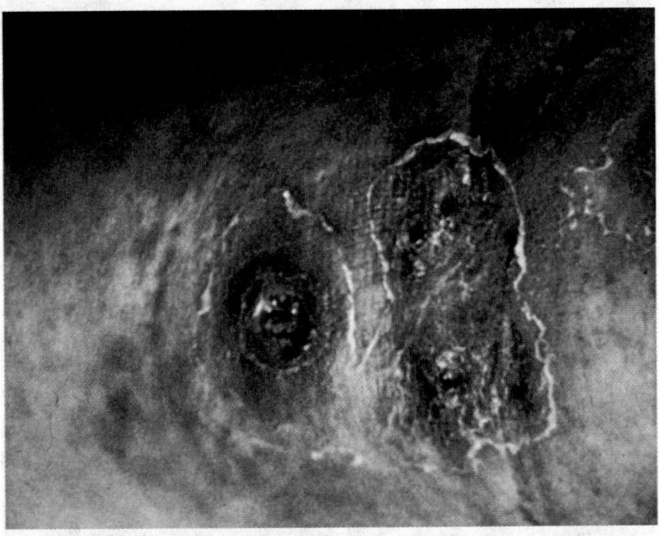

FIGURE 466–22 • Erythema induratum.

Fungal Infections

Especially in immunocompromised patients, necrotic or granulomatous lobular panniculitis can be caused by disseminated fungal infections with *Candida, Sporothrix schenckii, Cryptococcus, Histoplasma, Nocardia, Rhizopus, Aspergillus, Fusarium,* or chromomycosis. Fungal mycelia invade vessel walls, where they produce purpuric and painful lesions that may ulcerate. Osler's nodes, which are tender nodular vasculitic lesions on the extremities, occur in the setting of bacterial endocarditis (Chapter 76). Staphylococcal or streptococcal sepsis may be manifested as pustules, papules, or panniculitic lesions. *Klebsiella* and *Pseudomonas* are associated with hemorrhagic necrosis of vessels or ecthyma gangrenosa. Granulomatous lobular panniculitis may also arise in the setting of syphilis, atypical mycobacterial infection, tuberculosis, or leprosy.

Erythema Nodosum

Erythema nodosum (Fig. 466–23) is characterized by tender nodules, 1 to 2 cm in diameter, that have warm, pink, overlying epidermis and appear in crops on the extremities. A perivascular inflammatory infiltrate is present around small intralobular vessels without vasculitis. Erythema nodosum frequently arises in response to various infections, inflammatory bowel disease, or drug use, but often the underlying cause remains unknown (Table 466–6).

TABLE 466–6 TRIGGER FACTORS ASSOCIATED WITH ERYTHEMA NODOSUM

Infections Bacterial: *Streptococcus,* tuberculosis, leprosy, *Mycoplasma, Yersinia, Salmonella,* leptospirosis, tularemia Fungal: coccidioidomycosis, blastomycosis, histoplasmosis, dermatophytosis Viruses and *Chlamydia:* paravaccinia, Epstein-Barr virus, lymphogranuloma venereum, cat-scratch disease, psittacosis, hepatitis B
Drugs: sulfonamides, bromides, oral contraceptives
Malignancies: lymphoma, leukemia, carcinoma, post-tumor radiation
Inflammatory: ulcerative colitis, Crohn's disease, Whipple's disease, Behçet's syndrome, Sweet's syndrome, collagen vascular diseases
Pregnancy

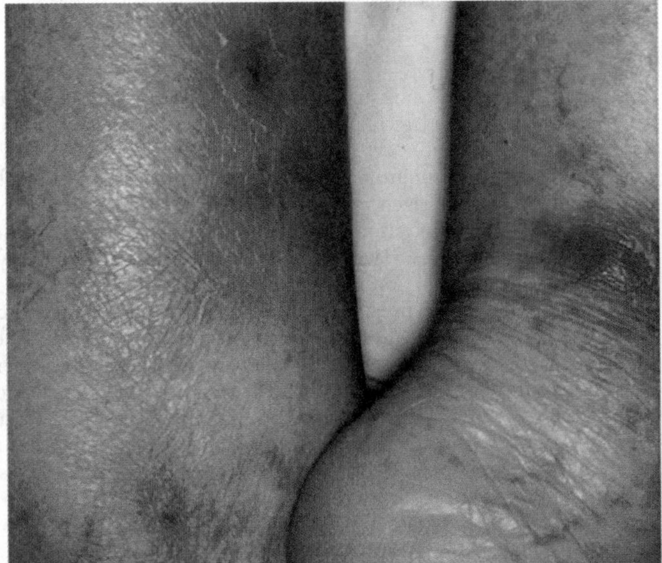

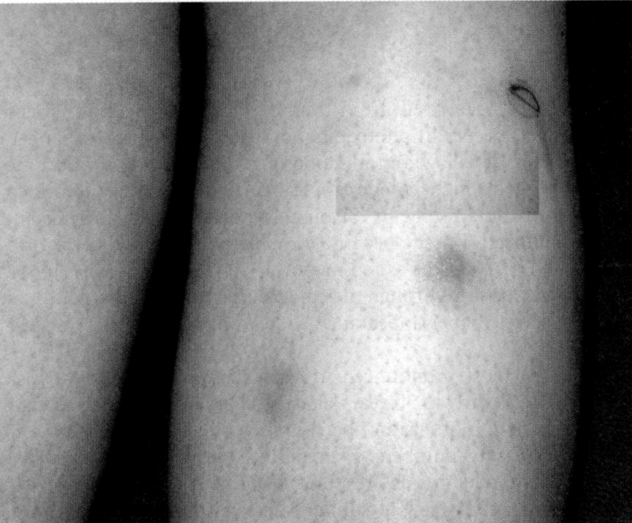

A B

FIGURE 466–23 • Erythema nodosum. A and B, Erythema nodosum and septal panniculitis of the lower extremities.

TABLE 466–7 ATROPHIC SKIN CONDITIONS WITH SCARRING, ULCERATIONS, AND/OR TELANGIECTASES

ATROPHY
Epidermal: chronic corticosteroid use, photoaging, mycosis fungoides
Dermal elastin: anetoderma, cutis laxa, intrinsic aging
Dermal collagen: Ehlers-Danlos syndrome, aging
Subcutaneous: granulomatous slack skin (a mycosis fungoides variant)
Lipodystrophy (loss of fat)
SCARRING OR ATROPHY WITH TELANGIECTASES
Discoid and subacute cutaneous lupus erythematosus
Dermatomyositis
Keloid formation
Large plaque parapsoriasis (poikiloderma vasculare atrophicans variant of mycosis fungoides)
Photoaging
Necrobiosis lipoidica diabeticorum
Radiation dermatitis
Porphyrias
Thermal burns (erythema ab igne)
SCLEROSIS OR INFILTRATIVE PROCESSES
Amyloidosis
Systemic sclerosis, scleroderma
Localized sclerosis, morphea
Lichen sclerosis et atrophicus
Lichen myxedematosus/papular mucinosis (mucopolysaccharide deposition with paraproteinemia)
Myxedema (mucin deposits with anti–thyroid-stimulating hormone receptor antibodies)
ULCERATIONS
Secondary breakdown of any blister or nodule: infectious, inflammatory, tumor, vasculitis
Decubitus or pressure ulcers
Genital ulcers: syphilis, herpes simplex, chancroid, lymphogranuloma venereum, Behçet's syndrome
Pyoderma gangrenosum, Sweet's syndrome

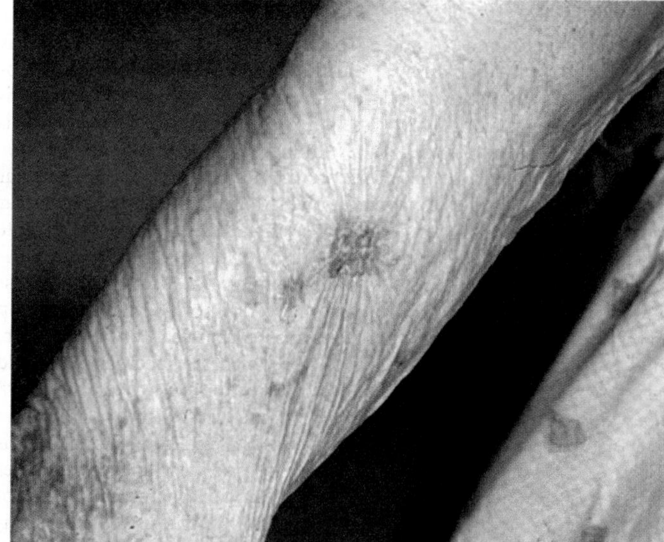

FIGURE 466–24 • Atrophic skin in Ehlers-Danlos syndrome type 2.

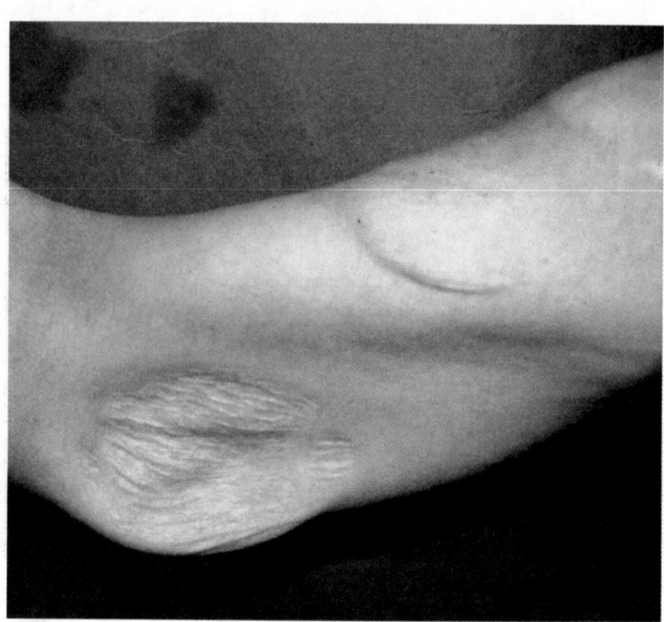

FIGURE 466–25 • Anetoderma.

ATROPHIC AND SCLEROTIC LESIONS

(Table 466–7)

Atrophic Lesions

Atrophic lesions can result from thinning or loss of the normal epidermal layers, as occurs in photoaging, in lupus erythematosus, and in genetic disorders of collagen production (e.g., Ehlers-Danlos syndrome; Fig. 466–24). Use of high-potency topical corticosteroids also produces loss of collagen and atrophy. In Cushing's syndrome, the epidermis and underlying connective tissue become atrophic and promote the formation of striae. Striae appear as red or purple streaks because the underlying dermis can be seen through the epidermis. Epidermal wrinkling can result in a cigarette paper appearance with prominence of the underlying blood vessels.

Aging skin is most pronounced in sun-exposed areas, but intrinsic aging beginning as early as 30 years of age is characterized by abnormalities in the formation of elastin fibers. Aging of the skin is also accompanied by decreasing numbers of epidermal-dermal involutions (rete ridges) and poor circulation as a result of changes in dermal blood vessels. Aging of the skin secondary to sunlight involves the induction or production of proteolytic enzymes that digest the underlying collagen and elastin (wrinkles). These changes can be partially prevented or restored with the use of topical vitamin A creams on a regular basis and with use of sun protection, including sunscreen. In addition, sun exposure induces pigment incontinence (freckling), increased junctional nevi, and proliferation of benign keratinocyte growths (seborrheic keratoses).

Atrophy can also result from ongoing inflammatory processes that lead to scarring, such as collagen vascular disease or mycosis fungoides. Anetodermas, which are localized sclerotic lesions (Fig. 466–25) with distinctive clinical features, have likewise been attributed to underlying inflammatory processes. Connective tissue diseases often produce sclerosis and atrophy after active inflammation. The cutaneous and discoid forms of *lupus erythematosus* (Chapter 287) are manifested as scaly plaques with atrophy or alopecia on sun-exposed areas; the systemic form is characterized by malar rash, urticaria, or vasculitic lesions. *Dermatomyositis* (Chapter 290) can be associated with collagen vascular disease or malignancy; periorbital suffusion, telangiectasia of the nail beds, and Gottron's papules or scaly lesions over the joints are the skin manifestations.

Eosinophilic fasciitis is accompanied by nodules or sclerosis of the lower extremities, myopathy, pulmonary disease, and eosinophilia. This syndrome, which follows the ingestion of L-tryptophan or its contaminants (Fig. 466–26), resembles the panniculitis seen in systemic sclerosis, in which fat lobules are replaced by new collagen formation. *Eosinophilic*

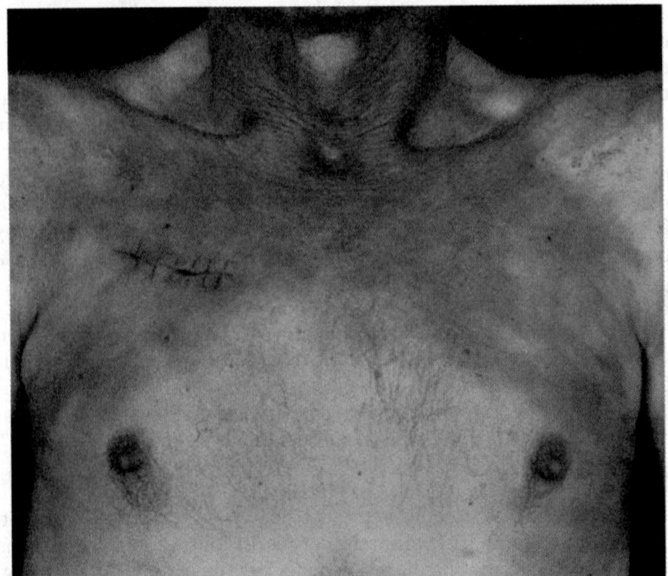

FIGURE 466–26 • Eosinophilic fasciitis secondary to tryptophan.

cellulitis, or *Wells' syndrome,* is manifested as nodules, papules, or ulcerative lesions, as well as red plaques; in this disorder, eosinophils infiltrate the area between collagen fibers.

Sclerotic Lesions

Sclerotic lesions are accompanied by more collagen production; the skin has a thicker or glossy appearance. Sclerosis may also result from the accumulation of mucopolysaccharides in scleromyxedema or lichen myxedematosus or from amyloid deposits. A new entity associated with renal failure—nephrogenic fibrosing dermopathy—is also characterized by acral fibrosis and deposition of hyaluronate in the skin. In *scleroderma* (Chapter 288), collagen deposition is associated with Raynaud's syndrome, calcinosis, and telangiectasia. A localized form of scleroderma, termed *morphea,* may occur down the center of the face (coup de sabre), in plaques on the extremities (Fig. 466–27), after radiation exposure, or with *Borrelia* infections. *Lichen sclerosis et atrophicus* is a superficial inflammatory morphea characterized by white atrophic patches, especially in the genital regions. Widespread systemic sclerosis may also follow bone marrow transplantation in the setting of chronic graft-versus-host disease.

Telangiectasia

Telangiectasia, or prominence of skin blood vessels, frequently accompanies atrophic as well as sclerotic processes and is common in photoaged skin. Telangiectasia of the mucous membranes is found in Osler-Weber-Rendu syndrome, and vascular spiders are found both in α_1-antitrypsinase deficiency and alcoholism. The presence of telangiectasia and hyperpigmentation and hypopigmentation (poikiloderma) in sun-shielded areas of the body should alert the clinician to the diagnosis of early mycosis fungoides.

Ulcers

Ulcers are secondary skin lesions that may arise from trauma, loss of proper blood supply, aging, vasculitis, blister formation, infection, or underlying neoplasia. Ulcers may be shallow erosions (loss of the epidermis) or be deeper and involve the dermis and underlying subcutaneous structures. Ulcers most commonly appear on the lower extremities, where they result from status dermatitis and venous insufficiency, arteriolar insufficiency, diabetic neuropathy, or vasculitis. For example, pyoderma gangrenosum is a trauma-induced ulcer that is part of the spectrum of Sweet's syndrome, accompanies other conditions, and may require immunosuppressive therapy. In contrast, decubitus ulcers require débridement, elimination of local pressure, and attention to nutrition (Chapter 232). In some cases, diagnosis may require skin biopsy, cultures, and serologic testing for other associated diseases.

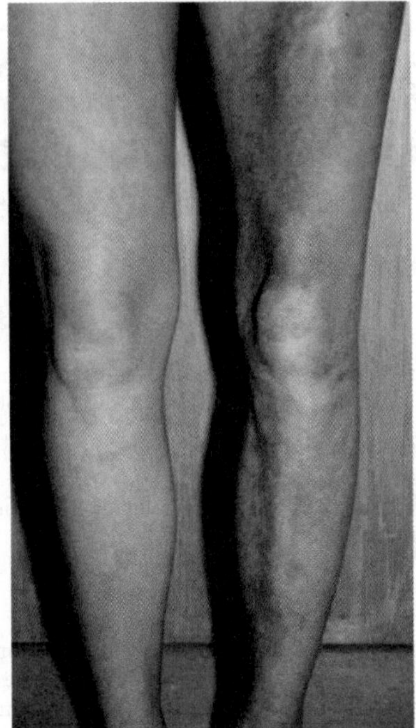

FIGURE 466–27 • Linear morphea.

After an inflammatory or ulcerated skin wound heals, scarring is common. Epidermal stem cells that reside in the bulge region of the hair follicle are capable of regenerating a normal epidermis. When a wound is deeper than the bulge region, scarring and loss of hair are likely to occur. Scarring alopecia (lichen planopilaris, discoid lupus, scarring folliculitis) results in permanent baldness and must be distinguished from the less severe, nonscarring conditions such as telogen effluvium or alopecia areata. Scarring also accompanies the most severe epidermolysis bullosa disorders caused by sub-basement membrane defects in proteins. Scarring accompanies third-degree burns, deep cryotherapy, or other trauma to the dermis. Scarring may also follow severe inflammation (discoid lupus) or infection (syphilis, leprosy).

Keloids

Some individuals have more pronounced and hypertrophic scar formation known as keloids, with an autosomal dominant inheritance pattern. Keloids are tumor-like in appearance and result from an overproduction of collagen. They are especially common on the anterior of the chest, neck, and earlobes and may require antineoplastic treatment after surgical removal.

SUGGESTED READINGS

Askari SK, Schram SE, Wenner RA, et al: Evaluation of prospectively collected presenting signs/symptoms of biopsy-proven melanoma, basal cell carcinoma, squamous cell carcinoma, and seborrheic keratosis in an elderly male population. J Am Acad Dermatol 2007. *Study that describes the common signs/symptoms of BCC, SCC, and seborrheic keratosis.*

Dibbern DA Jr: Urticaria: Selected highlights and recent advances. Med Clin North Am 2006;90:187–209. *Review.*

Gruchalla RS, Pirmohamed M: Clinical practice. Antibiotic allergy. N Engl J Med 2006;354:601–609. *A comprehensive overview of allergic reactions to antibiotics (including drug rash).*

Markel A: Allopurinol-induced DRESS syndrome. Isr Med Assoc J 2005;7:656–660. *Review of DRESS.*

O'donoghue M, Tharp MD: Antihistamines and their role as antipruritics. Dermatol Ther 2005;18:333–340. *A comprehensive overview.*

Pereira FA, Mudgil AV, Rosmarin DM: Toxic epidermal necrolysis. J Am Acad Dermatol 2007;56:181–200. *A comprehensive review of the classification, clinical presentation, etiology, pathophysiology, prognosis, and treatment of TEN.*

467 INFECTIONS, HYPER- AND HYPOPIGMENTATION, REGIONAL DERMATOLOGY, AND DISTINCTIVE LESIONS IN BLACK SKIN

Jean Bolognia

INFECTIONS, INCLUDING CELLULITIS

Cutaneous infections can be divided into four major categories: bacterial, fungal (Chapter 464), viral, and parasitic (Table 467–1).

Bacterial Infections

Of the bacterial infections, impetigo, folliculitis, furuncles, and cellulitis are most commonly encountered.

Impetigo

Impetigo, which is caused by *Staphylococcus aureus* or group A β-hemolytic streptococci, is usually seen as honey-colored crusts (Fig. 467–1); less often, subcorneal (superficial) bullae are present. This infection is most commonly found on the face in children, but it can develop at any site where the cutaneous barrier has been disrupted (e.g., areas of dermatitis, sites of trauma, or arthropod bites). A deeper, but less common bacterial infection of the skin is *ecthyma*, which is most frequently streptococcal in origin; it is characterized by thick hemorrhagic crusts overlying erosions or ulcerations, usually 0.5 to 1.5 cm in diameter. These lesions favor the extremities, especially in the setting of lymphedema. Ecthyma should not be confused with ecthyma gangrenosum, which represents an embolic phenomenon most often caused by bacteremia with gram-negative bacilli. Although mild cases of impetigo usually respond to topical mupirocin, oral antibiotics that cover *S. aureus* (e.g., dicloxacillin, 250 mg orally four times a day, or cephalexin, 250 mg orally four times a day) are needed to treat severe impetigo and ecthyma.

TABLE 467–1 SKIN INFECTIONS

BACTERIAL DISEASES
Impetigo
Ecthyma
Folliculitis
Furuncle/carbuncle
Cellulitis
Necrotizing fasciitis
Ecthyma gangrenosum
Other
Gram-negative cocci: meningococcemia, gonococcemia
Gram-positive bacilli: erythrasma, anaerobic cellulitis
Spirochetes: Lyme disease, syphilis, endemic treponematoses
Mycobacteria
VIRAL DISEASES
Herpes simplex virus: oral, genital
Human papillomavirus: common warts, condyloma acuminata
Pox virus: molluscum contagiosum
Varicella-zoster virus
Viral exanthems (e.g., enteroviruses, rubeola, rubella, parvovirus, human immunodeficiency virus)
FUNGAL DISEASES
Candidiasis
Tinea (dermatophytoses): pedis, corporis, cruris
Pityriasis (tinea) versicolor
Emboli (e.g., *Aspergillus, Mucor*)
ECTOPARASITES/PARASITES
Scabies
Lice: scalp, pubic, body
Leishmaniasis
Schistosomiasis, human and animal
Onchocerciasis
Strongyloidiasis
Amebiasis
Trypanosomiasis
Hookworm infections, human and animal

Folliculitis

The initial lesions of folliculitis are perifollicular pustules that are often surrounded by a rim of erythema (Chapter 465). *Pseudomonas* folliculitis, which favors the trunk, is usually associated with the use of hot tubs or whirlpools because their higher temperatures (vs. swimming pools) make eradication of *Pseudomonas* more difficult (see Fig. 465–20).

Furuncles

Furuncles, also called boils, represent an *S. aureus* cutaneous infection that is localized primarily within the dermis. In contrast to folliculitis, the lesions are larger and manifested as tender erythematous nodules (Fig. 467–2). A central follicular structure may be noted, as well as a central pustule ("pointing"). Because a furuncle is an abscess, the preferred treatment is incision and drainage followed by oral antistaphylococcal

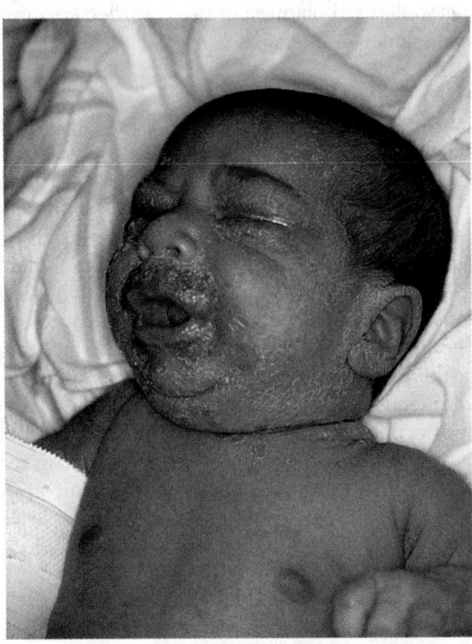

FIGURE 467–1 • Impetigo in an infant and marked involvement of the face with honey-colored crusts and superficial erosions. (Courtesy of Yale Dermatology Residents' Slide Collection.)

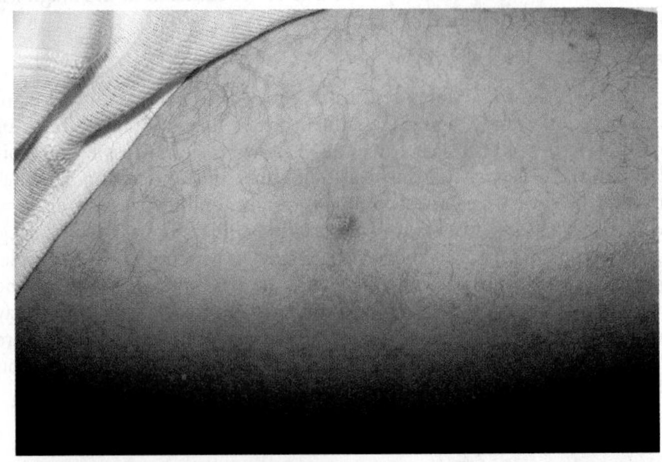

FIGURE 467–2 • Furuncle with surrounding cellulitis. (Courtesy of Yale Dermatology Residents' Slide Collection.)

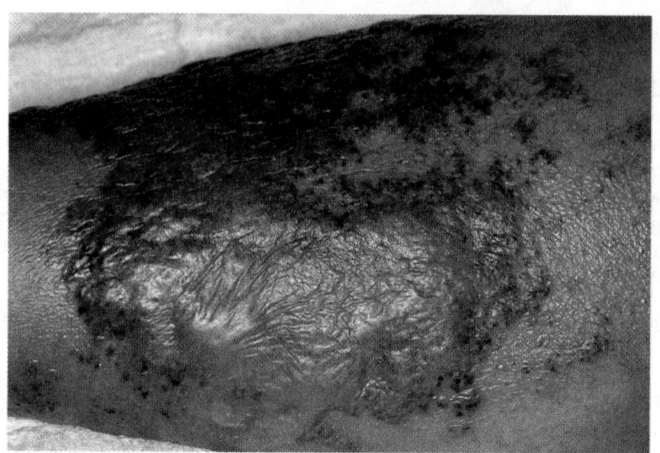

FIGURE 467–3 • Bullous and hemorrhagic cellulitis of the shin. (Courtesy of University of Southern California Dermatology Residents' Slide Collection.)

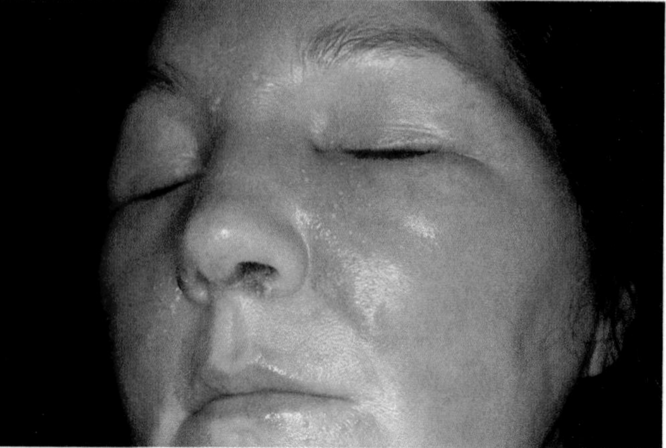

FIGURE 467–4 • Erysipelas of the face with well-demarcated erythematous plaques. (Courtesy of Yale Dermatology Residents' Slide Collection.)

antibiotics (e.g., dicloxacillin, 250 mg orally four times a day, or cephalexin, 250 mg orally four times a day); if methicillin-resistant *S. aureus* is likely (e.g., use of health care facilities such as dialysis units, participation in skin-to-skin contact sports), treatment should be changed to clindamycin, trimethoprim-sulfamethoxazole, or linezolid. *Carbuncles* are larger, more complex, and more extensive versions of furuncles; they may be accompanied by systemic symptoms such as fever and may require a more prolonged course of therapy.

Cellulitis

Cellulitis is a fairly common cutaneous infection that occurs most often on the lower extremities. Locally, it is manifested as erythema, edema, warmth, and tenderness; systemic findings can include fever, malaise, and leukocytosis. The vast majority of cases are bacterial in origin, but some are caused by fungal infections (e.g., *Cryptococcus*) or chemical reactions (e.g., extravasated oxacillin or calcium salts). Bacterial cellulitis is most commonly caused by group A β-hemolytic streptococci and *S. aureus,* with the former being associated with the more severe, necrotizing variant. In patients who have diabetes or who are immunocompromised, cellulitis can be caused by gram-negative bacilli or atypical mycobacteria. Risk factors include a preceding break in the skin barrier, edema secondary to venous hypertension, lymphedema, and previous bouts of cellulitis.

Although the diagnosis of cellulitis is usually fairly straightforward (Fig. 467–3), it can sometimes be difficult in patients with chronic lower extremity edema, especially those who are afebrile. One complication of chronic lower extremity edema is lipodermatosclerosis (i.e., inflammation followed by fibrosis of subcutaneous fat), which is seen acutely as erythema, warmth, and tenderness and is easily confused with cellulitis. The skin above the medial malleolus is often the initial site of involvement with lipodermatosclerosis, but the inflammation can extend onto the shin and calf. The chronic phase of lipodermatosclerosis is characterized by induration, a permanent brown-red to violet discoloration of the skin, and an "inverted wine bottle" appearance of the distal end of the lower extremity. It is important for the clinician to realize that in patients with chronic lipodermatosclerosis and superimposed cellulitis, the skin will never return to its normal color, even after adequate antibiotic therapy.

Unless there is an associated bacteremia, the diagnosis of cellulitis is primarily clinical. In immunocompromised hosts, a saline injection followed by aspiration and culture can be helpful. Histologically, cellulitis is characterized by an infiltrate of neutrophils within the dermis. Skin biopsy can exclude disorders that may be confused with cellulitis, such as contact dermatitis, erythema migrans, inflammatory carcinoma, and Wells' syndrome (an idiopathic disorder in which eosinophils infiltrate the dermis). Treatment of cellulitis varies from oral cephalexin to intravenous vancomycin plus intravenous ceftazidime, depending on the suspected pathogens, the host, and the severity of systemic toxicity.

Cellulitis resides in the middle of a spectrum of soft tissue infections that includes *erysipelas* (more superficial and more sharply demarcated; Fig. 467–4) at one end and *necrotizing fasciitis* (deeper, more necrotic, and undermining) at the other. In healthy adults, erysipelas can be treated with oral penicillin (200,000 units four times daily) or, if *S. aureus* is of concern, oral dicloxacillin (500 mg four times daily) for a 10-day course. Necrotizing fasciitis is usually caused by multiple organisms, including anaerobic streptococci; its diagnosis requires a high index of suspicion, and it must be considered when there are areas of violaceous induration or a foul-smelling discharge. Prompt surgical débridement and broad-spectrum systemic antibiotics (e.g., a β-lactam/β-lactamase inhibitor such as intravenous piperacillin/tazobactam, 4.5 g every 6 hours for a total of 18 g/day [16 g piperacillin/2 g tazobactam]), with or without ciprofloxacin (400 mg orally or intravenously every 12 hours), for at least 2 weeks are mandatory. Unless only a single organism is seen on Gram stain and isolated on culture, broad-spectrum antibiotic coverage should be continued because of the polymicrobial nature of necrotizing fasciitis and the difficulty of culturing anaerobes.

Although *Clostridium perfringens* can cause anaerobic cellulitis and gas gangrene, the most common cutaneous infection by gram-positive bacilli is *erythrasma,* which is manifested as interdigital toe web maceration with fissures, as well as shiny or scaly brown-red patches in the axillae and groin. The latter is often confused with tinea cruris (Chapter 464). A diagnostic finding is the presence of coral (orange-pink) fluorescence on Wood's lamp illumination (ultraviolet A). The responsible organism is *Corynebacterium minutissimum.* Treatment options include topical and oral erythromycin (e.g., 333 mg three times a day for 7 to 14 days).

Toxic Erythemas

Eruptions caused by the release of toxins (e.g., exfoliative toxins ET-A and ET-B) produced by *S. aureus* and streptococci include *staphylococcal scalded skin syndrome* (Chapters 310 and 465), *scarlet fever* (Chapter 311), and *toxic shock syndrome* (Chapter 465). Staphylococcal scalded skin syndrome (see Fig. 465–14) is characterized by large areas of tender erythema in which superficial desquamation (peeling) develops, often with scaling and crusting in a radial array around the mouth. The areas of erythema are sterile; the conjunctivae, nasopharynx, or a distant site on the skin is the usual site of the primary staphylococcal infection. A clue to the diagnosis of scarlet fever is the presence of a strawberry tongue with prominent red papillae. Management involves treatment of the systemic infection (Chapters 310 and 465).

Neisseria Infections

Both *gonococcemia* (Chapter 322) and *meningococcemia* (Chapter 321) can manifest as cutaneous lesions. The former gives rise to a small number of vesicopustules on an erythematous base, generally acral in location (Fig. 467–5); these lesions represent septic emboli and are accompanied by fever, arthritis, and tendonitis. The earliest lesions of *acute meningococcemia* may be subtle (macular areas of erythema), but central hemorrhage (petechiae and purpura) and necrosis (gun metal gray color) soon follow (Fig. 467–6). The lesions may become quite extensive; when accompanied by disseminated intravascular coagulation, severe peripheral ischemia may result. Cutaneous involvement in *chronic meningococcemia* is a reflection of lymphocytic or leukocytoclastic vasculitis rather than septic emboli. Management is systemic treatment (Chapters 321 and 322).

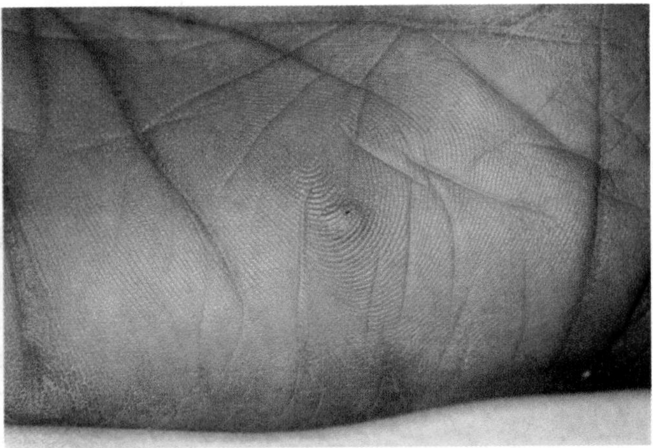

FIGURE 467–5 • Disseminated gonococcal infection with an acral pustule on a red-violet base. (Courtesy of Yale Dermatology Residents' Slide Collection.)

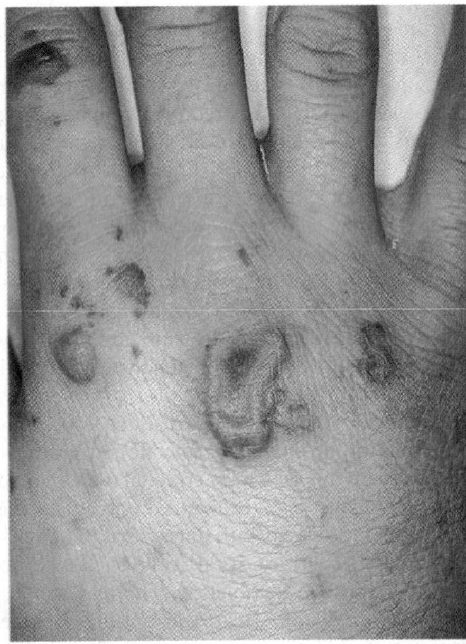

FIGURE 467–6 • Purpuric and necrotic embolic lesions of meningococcemia. (Courtesy of Yale Dermatology Residents' Slide Collection.)

Pseudomonas Infections

Pseudomonas infections of the skin vary from "hot tub" folliculitis (Chapter 465) to soft tissue infections of the external ear. Interdigital toe web infections that begin as simple tinea pedis can be complicated by superimposed *Pseudomonas* infection and result in erythema, swelling, tenderness, and drainage. Depending on its severity, treatment varies from topical antiseptics to oral or intravenous fluoroquinolones (e.g., ciprofloxacin, 500 mg orally every 12 hours for 7 to 14 days). In immunocompromised hosts, *Pseudomonas* and other gram-negative bacilli can produce cellulitis as well as secondary septic emboli in the skin. The latter begin as purpura or purpuric bullae in which central necrosis then develops. These lesions, which arise as a result of ischemic infarction of the skin, are termed *ecthyma gangrenosum*. Management is treatment of the systemic pseudomonal disease (Chapter 328).

Spirochetes

Spirochetal infections have a wide range of skin findings from erythema migrans secondary to *Borrelia burgdorferi* (Chapter 342), to endemic treponematoses such as *yaws* and *pinta* (Chapter 341), to the cutaneous manifestations of the three stages of *syphilis* (Chapter 340). Syphilitic lesions include a firm, generally nontender ulceration (chancre) in primary syphilis; a generalized papulosquamous eruption (Chapter 464) plus alopecia, oral ulcers, and condylomata lata in secondary syphilis; and thick plaques and ulcers in tertiary disease. Management involves treatment of the systemic disease.

Mycobacteria Infections

Infections with *Mycobacterium tuberculosis* and mycobacteria other than *M. tuberculosis* are associated with skin lesions such as verrucous papules, scarring granulomatous plaques, and draining ulcers. In immunocompetent hosts in developed countries, *Mycobacterium marinum* (Chapter 346) is most commonly associated with skin disease, which is usually manifested in a lymphocutaneous (i.e., sporotrichoid) pattern. Treatment of cutaneous mycobacterial disease (Chapters 345 and 346), including leprosy (Chapter 347), is the same as for systemic disease.

Viral Infections

The most common viral infections of the skin are verrucae (warts; see Fig. 465–2), recurrent oral and genital herpes simplex (Chapters 397 and 465), molluscum contagiosum (see Fig. 466–8 and Chapter 466), and exanthems (Chapter 465). Varicella and herpes zoster are seen less frequently (Chapter 398).

Fungal Infections

A variety of fungal infections involve the skin and nails and are most commonly due to dermatophytes (tinea), *Candida* species, and *Pityrosporum* (pityriasis versicolor) (Chapter 464; also see Table 467–1). Although both dermatophyte infections and pityriasis versicolor are associated with scaling, cutaneous candidiasis is characterized by erythema, a more erosive quality, and satellite pustules. Treatment is described in Chapter 464.

Septic emboli caused by *Candida* or other opportunistic fungi such as *Aspergillus* (Chapter 360) or *Fusarium* often have a clinical appearance similar to that of ecthyma gangrenosum secondary to gram-negative rods such as *Pseudomonas.* The responsible organisms can be detected histologically in biopsy specimens or by bedside examination of dermal scrapings; culture confirms the specific organism. Cutaneous plaques secondary to *Pneumocystis jiroveci* favor the internal ear. Treatment is for the underlying fungal infection.

Ectoparasites and Parasites

Ectoparasites: Scabies and Lice

The most common ectoparasitic cutaneous infestations are (1) scabies from the human variant of the *Sarcoptes* mite and (2) lice, of which there are three subtypes: head, body, and pubic. *Scabies* is characterized by pruritus in association with papules, papulovesicles, and linear burrows, as well as signs of scratching, such as excoriations and areas of dermatitis. Sites of predilection include the wrists, ankles, fingers, toes (including the web spaces), areolae, and genitalia (especially the penis). The number of mites living within the stratum corneum is limited in immunocompetent hosts; when scraped and examined microscopically, linear burrows provide the highest yield of mites and eggs. In elderly and immunosuppressed patients, a form of scabies known as crusted or Norwegian scabies presents as multiple areas of scaling and crusting that are teeming with mites.

Infestations with scalp *lice* are seen most commonly in children, who may be asymptomatic or have marked pruritus. In addition to the lice, multiple egg casings ("nits") are attached to the proximal portions of scalp hairs. In developed countries, body lice are seen primarily in homeless individuals; patients typically have multiple erythematous papules at the sites of "bites," as well as signs of scratching. The lice and their eggs are found in the patient's clothing. Pubic lice are sometimes called "crabs" because their bodies are shorter and broader than those of scalp or body lice and thus resemble the shape of a crab. As a result of their leg span, these lice reside on pubic hairs and less often on axillary hairs or eyelashes.

The most effective Food and Drug Administration–approved treatments of head lice, pubic lice, and routine scabies are topical 0.5% malathion, 5% permethrin cream, and 5% permethrin cream, respectively; each of these topical medications is applied for 8 to 12 hours on days 1 and 8. For crusted scabies, oral ivermectin (250 to 400 μg/kg; off-label use) is often required to eradicate the infestation. Treatment of body lice involves discarding egg- and lice-infested clothing; for head lice, potential sources of reinfection, such as hairbrushes, should be discarded. Sexual and household contacts of patients with pubic lice and scabies, respectively, must be treated similarly to the symptomatic patient.

Other Parasites

Cutaneous lesions are seen in leishmaniasis (Chapter 369), amebiasis (Chapter 373), schistosomiasis (Chapter 376), onchocerciasis (Chapter 379), strongyloidiasis (Chapter 378), and hookworm infections (Chapter 378). Exposure to water infested with the cercariae of animal schistosomes results in multiple erythematous papules, which occur most commonly on the feet and is termed "swimmer's itch." Dog and cat hookworm infections lead to *cutaneous larva migrans,* with serpiginous erythematous tracks that correspond to the path of migration of the hookworm larvae. Both these infections are self-limited because the parasite's life cycle cannot be completed in humans. In immunocompromised hosts, cutaneous plaques can occasionally develop from free-living amebae such as *Acanthamoeba.*

DISORDERS OF HYPOPIGMENTATION AND HYPERPIGMENTATION

Disorders of pigmentation can be divided into four major categories: diffuse, linear, circumscribed, and either reticulated (in the case of hyperpigmentation) or guttate (in the case of hypopigmentation) (Table 467–2).

Hypopigmentation

Albinism

The primary disorder of diffuse hypopigmentation is *oculocutaneous albinism,* an autosomal recessive disorder in which there is a pigmentary dilution of melanin-containing structures (i.e., the eyes, hair, and skin). The phenotype varies from total absence of melanin pigment to a subtle decrease whose recognition requires comparison with first-degree relatives; the density of melanocytes in skin is normal, but their ability to produce pigment is absent or decreased. Ninety percent of patients with oculocutaneous albinism have mutations in the genes that encode either tyrosinase (type I) or P protein (type II). Complications of oculocutaneous albinism include decreased visual acuity, nystagmus, photophobia, and an increase in cutaneous carcinomas, especially squamous cell carcinoma. These signs and symptoms are most severe in those who produce the least pigment. The differential diagnosis includes total vitiligo (absence of melanocytes histologically) and a few inborn errors of metabolism (e.g., phenylketonuria). Treatment consists of longitudinal ophthalmologic care and minimizing sun exposure.

Linear Hypopigmentation

Disorders of *linear hypopigmentation* consist primarily of nevoid conditions (e.g., hypomelanosis of Ito, systematized nevus depigmentosus) in which streaks of hypomelanosis follow Blaschko's lines (an embryonic development pattern that involves all layers of the skin and becomes clinically apparent in the setting of mosaicism). Some patients have associated central nervous system and musculoskeletal abnormalities.

Circumscribed (Patchy) Hypopigmentation

Vitiligo

Vitiligo (Fig. 467–7) is usually slowly progressive and occurs principally in periorificial areas (around the eyes, nose, lips, genitalia) and the hands, feet, flexor surface of the wrists, ankles, elbows, knees, and major body folds. Vitiligo, which is caused by a loss of melanocytes within the skin, is also associated with autoimmune endocrinopathies (Chapter 250) and alopecia areata (see later). T cells that recognize antigens on the surface of melanocytes (and melanoma cells) are found within the skin and in peripheral blood. Treatment includes topical corticosteroids, topical immunomodulators (e.g., tacrolimus), and phototherapy. The differential diagnosis is primarily chemical leukoderma secondary to compounds that are cytotoxic to melanocytes (e.g., catechols, phenols), the leukoderma of melanoma (often metastatic), and the leukoderma of scleroderma with retention of perifollicular pigmentation.

Guttate Hypopigmentation

Idiopathic guttate hypomelanosis, in which well-demarcated hypopigmented macules measure only 2 to 4 mm in diameter, is the most common cause of guttate ("raindrop") leukoderma (Fig. 467–8). The favored sites for this common age-related disorder, which may be related to chronic sun exposure, are the shins and the extensor surface of the forearms.

TABLE 467–2 DISORDERS OF PIGMENTATION

HYPOPIGMENTATION

DIFFUSE (PIGMENTARY DILUTION)
- Oculocutaneous albinism
- Generalized (total) vitiligo
- Inborn errors of metabolism (e.g., phenylketonuria)

CIRCUMSCRIBED
- Decrease in pigment
  - Acquired: postinflammatory hypopigmentation (e.g., atopic dermatitis, sarcoidosis, lupus erythematosus, mycosis fungoides), pityriasis (tinea) versicolor secondary to *Malassezia*
  - Congenital: nevus depigmentosus, ash-leaf spots of tuberous sclerosis
- Absence of pigment
  - Acquired: vitiligo, chemical leukoderma, leukoderma of scleroderma, leukoderma of melanoma
  - Congenital: piebaldism

LINEAR
- Nevoid hypopigmentation (e.g., hypomelanosis of Ito)

GUTTATE
- Idiopathic guttate hypomelanosis
- Confetti macules of tuberous sclerosis

HYPERPIGMENTATION

DIFFUSE
- Drug reactions (e.g., cyclophosphamide, zidovudine)
- Addison's disease
- Ectopic adrenocorticotropic hormone production (e.g., small cell lung cancer)
- Hemochromatosis
- Scleroderma
- Primary biliary cirrhosis
- Hyperthyroidism
- Vitamin B_{12} or folate deficiency
- Porphyria cutanea tarda
- Melanosis secondary to metastatic melanoma
- Argyria

CIRCUMSCRIBED
- Postinflammatory hyperpigmentation (e.g., acne vulgaris, arthropod bites, dermatitis, lichen planus)
- Melasma
- Pityriasis (tinea) versicolor
- Mastocytosis
- Fixed drug reactions
- Deposits of drugs and their metabolites

LINEAR
- Exposure to psoralen-containing plants (e.g., limes) plus ultraviolet A light
- Drug reactions (e.g., bleomycin)
- Nevoid hyperpigmentation
- Genodermatoses (e.g., incontinentia pigmenti)

RETICULATED
- Erythema ab igne
- Genodermatoses

Other Acquired Causes

Circumscribed hypomelanosis is seen in patients with pityriasis (tinea) versicolor (see Fig. 464–16) and *postinflammatory hypopigmentation.* Although postinflammatory hypopigmentation is most often associated with atopic dermatitis, it can also occur with sarcoidosis (Chapter 95), lupus erythematosus (Chapter 287), and mycosis fungoides (Chapter 464).

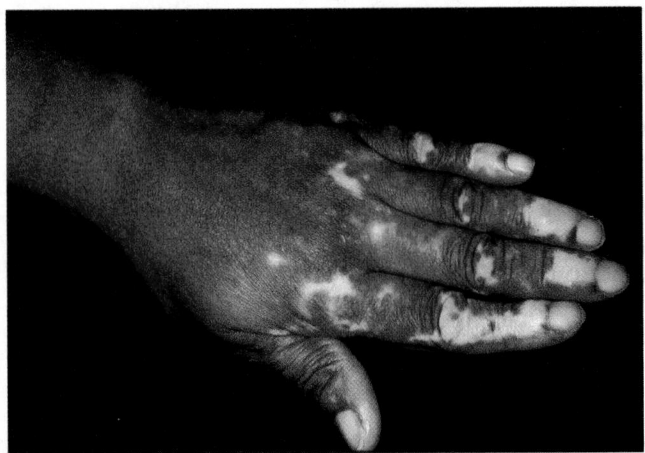

FIGURE 467–7 • Striking leukoderma of the hand in a patient with vitiligo.

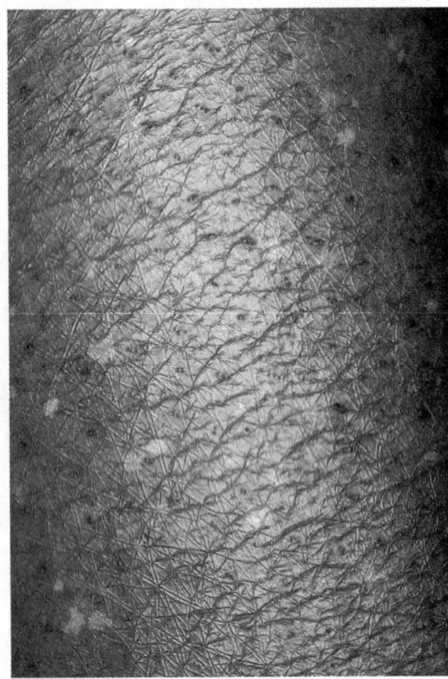

FIGURE 467–8 • Idiopathic guttate hypomelanosis with small, well-demarcated hypopigmented macules on the shin.

Congenital Causes

Congenital circumscribed areas of hypomelanosis include *nevus depigmentosus,* a common tan "birthmark" seen in 1 in 50 infants with a partial decrease in pigment; *piebaldism,* an unusual autosomal dominant disorder with areas of complete absence of pigment caused by mutations in the *KIT* gene; *nevus anemicus,* a localized area of vasoconstriction; and the *ash-leaf spots* of tuberous sclerosis (Chapter 444), with a partial decrease in pigment.

Hyperpigmentation

Diffuse Hyperpigmentation

Diffuse hyperpigmentation is most commonly due to drugs (e.g., cyclophosphamide, zidovudine) and endocrinopathies associated with increased circulating levels of adrenocorticotropic hormone (ACTH) (e.g., Addison's disease [Chapter 245], ectopic ACTH production by tumors such as small cell lung carcinoma [Chapter 201]). ACTH, as well as melanocyte-stimulating hormone, can bind and activate the melanocortin-1 receptors on melanocytes, thereby leading to increased melanin production. Additional causes include hemochromatosis (Chapter 231), scleroderma (Chapter 288), primary biliary cirrhosis (Chapter 159), and hyperthyroidism (Chapter 244). Systemic exposure to silver (argyria; Chapter 20) can lead to a slate-gray color.

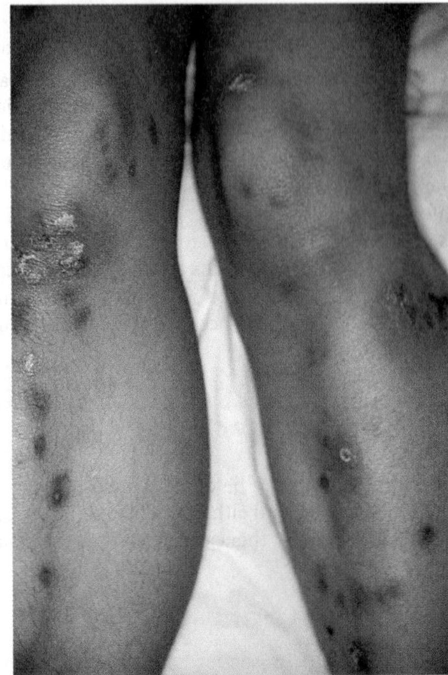

FIGURE 467–9 • Postinflammatory hyperpigmentation secondary to arthropod bites. (Courtesy of Yale Dermatology Residents' Slide Collection.)

Linear and Reticulated Hyperpigmentation

Linear streaks of hyperpigmentation can be due to nevoid (i.e., hamartomatous) conditions that reflect cutaneous mosaicism, as in linear hypopigmentation (see earlier) and genodermatoses (inherited disorders with cutaneous manifestations, e.g., incontinentia pigmenti secondary to mutations in the gene *NEMO*), as well as exposure to either plant-derived psoralens (e.g., from limes) plus ultraviolet A irradiation or systemic bleomycin (flagellate pigmentation). Reticulated hypermelanosis is also seen in several genodermatoses (e.g., dyskeratosis congenita) and after chronic exposure to heat (erythema ab igne). The latter corresponds to the cutaneous venous plexus and is seen most commonly in the lumbosacral region where heating pads have been applied.

Circumscribed (Patchy) Hyperpigmentation

The most common causes of circumscribed hypermelanosis are tinea versicolor (which can present as both hypopigmentation and hyperpigmentation, hence its name), postinflammatory hyperpigmentation, and melasma. *Postinflammatory hyperpigmentation* (Fig. 467–9) is observed more frequently in darkly pigmented individuals and often follows acne vulgaris, arthropod bites, chronic dermatitis, and lichen planus. Additional causes of circumscribed darkening of the skin are cutaneous mastocytosis (urticaria pigmentosa; Chapter 276), deposits of drugs such as antimalarials and minocycline (blue-gray discoloration), and medications that produce fixed drug reactions, most frequently trimethoprim-sulfamethoxazole and nonsteroidal anti-inflammatory drugs. In *melasma* (Fig. 467–10), symmetrical hyperpigmented patches are seen on the lateral aspect of the forehead, upper part of the cheek, and mandibular area. At least 90% of patients with melasma are women. The lesions are exacerbated by ultraviolet light and estrogen (oral contraceptives, pregnancy). Melasma is treated with daily broad-spectrum sunscreens and lightening agents such as hydroquinone (4% cream) and retinoic acid (0.025 to 0.10% cream) for 3 to 4 months; the creams are applied on alternate days or daily to limit irritation.

REGIONAL DERMATOSES

Several common dermatoses have a predilection for particular anatomic sites (Fig. 467–11 and Table 467–3). A classic example is the preference of plaques of psoriasis for the extensor surfaces (e.g., elbows and knees), in contrast to atopic dermatitis, which favors the antecubital and popliteal fossae.

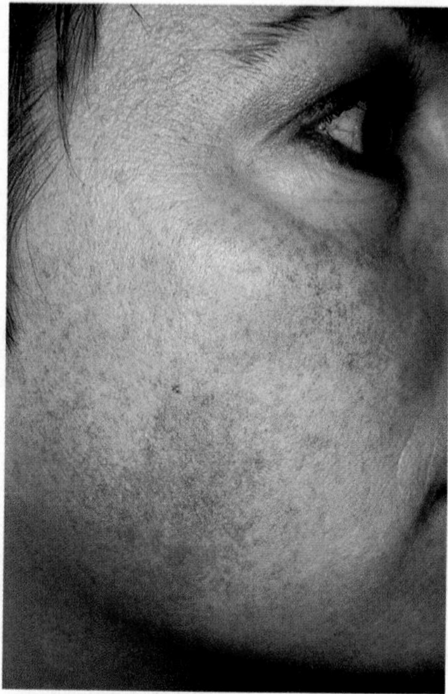

FIGURE 467–10 • Hyperpigmented patches on the cheek in a patient with melasma.

Diseases of Nails

Abnormalities of the nail apparatus are most commonly the result of infections or cutaneous inflammatory diseases but can also be seen in a number of systemic diseases (Table 467–4).

Infections

Infections are primarily caused by dermatophytes or *Candida* species. In tinea unguium (Chapter 464), there is yellow-brown discoloration and thickening of the nail plate, as well as subungual debris. Infections with *Candida* species lead either to chronic paronychia with loss of the cuticle plus swelling and slight erythema of the periungual region, which may result in ridging of the nail plate, or to onycholysis, which is lifting of the distal end of the nail plate from the nail bed. Onycholysis is usually related to chronic exposure to water and irritants; it may be complicated by *Pseudomonas* colonization, which leads to a green discoloration of the nail.

Inflammation

The major inflammatory disorder that causes nail changes is *psoriasis* (Chapter 464), which can result in onycholysis, subungual debris, and localized areas of yellow-brown discoloration (oil-drop changes). The characteristic pitting of the nails (see Fig. 464–9) is caused by involvement of the proximal nail matrix (the matrix is the site of proliferation) in which circumscribed collections of incompletely differentiated cells cover the surface of the "dead" nail plate; subsequent sloughing of these cells leads to the pits. Nail pits are also seen in alopecia areata, where their

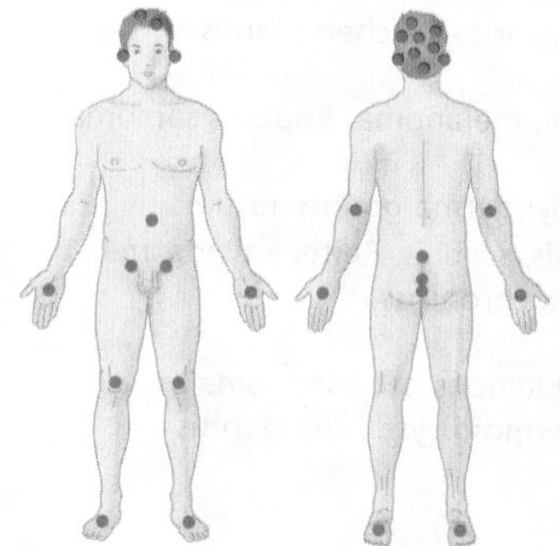

Psoriasis
Scalp, ears, scalpline
Palms, soles
Dorsal hands, feet
Elbows, knees/shins
Presacrum
Intergluteal fold
Nails

Inverse Psoriasis
Submammary
Inguinal fold
Umbilicus

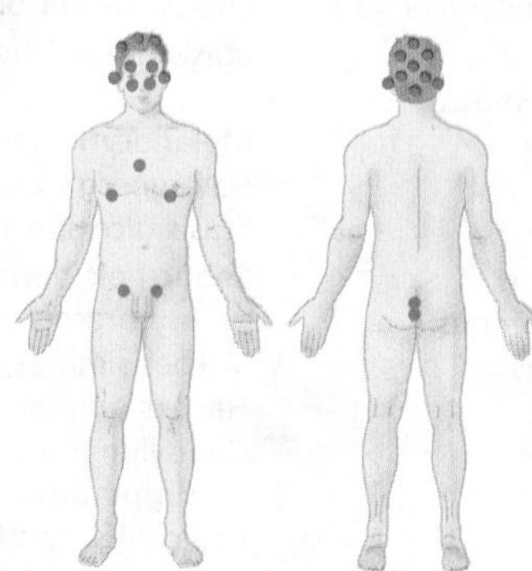

Seborrheic Dermatitis
Scalp, ears, postauricular
Eyebrows
Nasolabial folds
Central chest
Intergluteal fold
Submammary
Inguinal fold

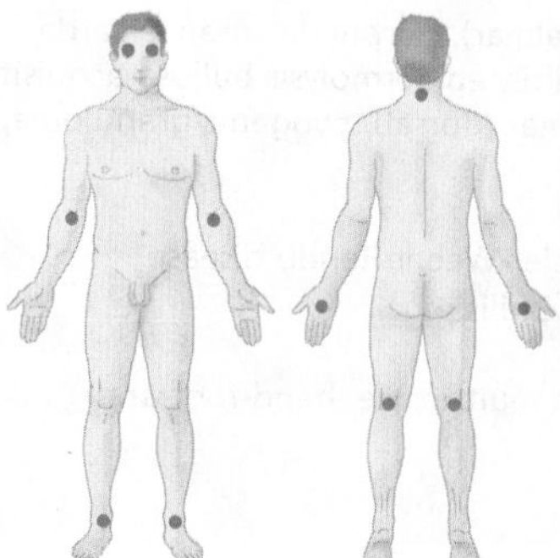

Atopic Dermatitis (adults)
Eyelids
Antecubital fossa
Popliteal fossa
Posterior neck
Ankles
Hands

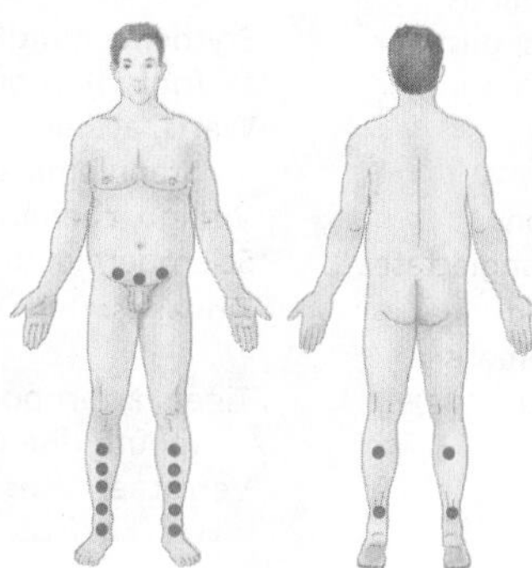

Stasis Dermatitis (adults)
Legs, below knees, but greater on shins than calves
Lower pannus

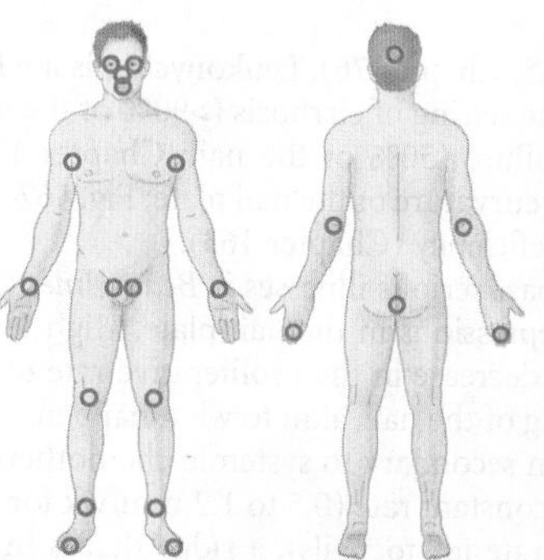

Vitiligo
Loss of color:
Around eyes
Around nose
Around mouth
Axillae, groin
Wrists (flexor)
Poliosis (streak of white hairs)
Elbows, knees, ankles
Backs of hands/feet (includes digits)
Perianal

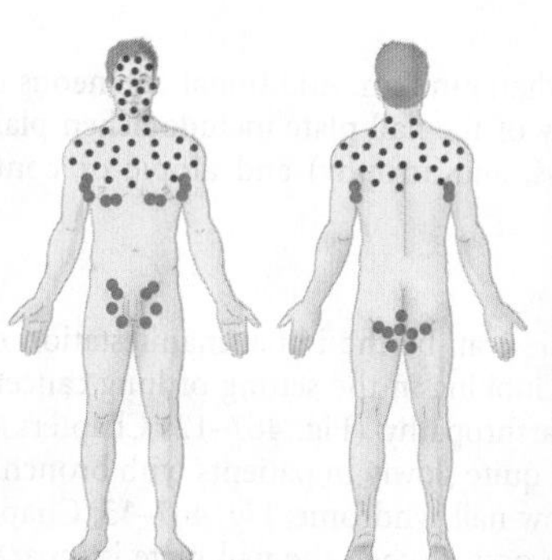

Acne Vulgaris/ Hidradenitis Suppurativa
∴ = papulopustules, blackheads or whiteheads Face/neck/upper trunk/shoulders
● = nodules of hidradenitis suppurativa

FIGURE 467–11 • Regional involvement of specific skin diseases.

TABLE 467–3 REGIONAL DERMATOLOGY

Region of Skin	Type of Skin Group	Disease Process
Scalp	Papulosquamous and eczematous	Seborrheic dermatitis, psoriasis, tinea capitis, eczema (atopic, contact)
	Pustular	Folliculitis, kerion
	Papulonodular	Melanocytic nevi, seborrheic keratoses, pilar cysts, verrucae
	Atrophic and telangiectatic	Discoid lupus erythematosus
Face	Pustular	Acne, rosacea, folliculitis (beard), tinea
	Papulosquamous and eczematous	Seborrheic dermatitis, psoriasis (hairline), contact dermatitis (e.g., cosmetics), atopic dermatitis, impetigo, lupus erythematosus, photodermatitis
	Vesicular	Herpes simplex, herpes zoster, bullous impetigo
	Papulonodular	Melanocytic nevi, actinic keratoses, seborrheic keratoses, basal cell carcinomas, squamous cell carcinomas, melanomas
Trunk	Papulosquamous and eczematous	Psoriasis, atopic dermatitis, contact dermatitis, tinea versicolor, pityriasis rosea, scabies, secondary syphilis
	Vesiculobullous	Bullous pemphigoid, pemphigus, erythema multiforme/Stevens-Johnson syndrome
	Maculopapular	Morbilliform drug reactions, viral exanthems
	Papulonodular	Melanocytic nevi, seborrheic keratoses, angiomas, lipomas, basal and squamous cell carcinomas, keloids, neurofibromas, melanoma
	Pustular	Acne, folliculitis
	Urticarial	Hives, drug reactions
Arms and forearms	Eczematous and papulosquamous	Contact dermatitis (e.g., plants), atopic dermatitis, psoriasis, lichen planus
	Papulonodular	Melanocytic nevi, verrucae, seborrheic keratoses, actinic keratoses
	Purpuric	Actinic (solar) purpura
	Atrophic and telangiectatic	Lupus, dermatomyositis
Legs	Eczematous and papulosquamous	Stasis dermatitis, contact dermatitis, atopic dermatitis, psoriasis, lichen planus
	Papulonodular	Melanocytic nevi, dermatofibromas, erythema nodosum, melanoma, Kaposi's sarcoma
	Purpuric	Schamberg's disease (capillaritis), vasculitis
	Ulcerative	Stasis ulcers, arterial insufficiency, neuropathic ulcers, pyoderma gangrenosum
Genitalia and groin	Eczematous and papulosquamous	Seborrheic dermatitis, tinea, psoriasis, contact dermatitis, scabies, Reiter's syndrome, erythrasma, candidiasis, lichen planus, lichen simplex chronicus
	Vesiculobullous	Herpes simplex, Stevens-Johnson syndrome
	Ulcerative	Herpes simplex, syphilis, chancroid, Behçet's disease, squamous cell carcinoma
	Papulonodular	Condyloma accuminata, molluscum contagiosum, epidermoid cyst, hidradenitis suppurativa, squamous cell carcinoma
	Pustular	Folliculitis, candidiasis, hidradenitis suppurativa
Hands	Eczematous and papulosquamous	Irritant and allergic contact dermatitis, atopic dermatitis, tinea, scabies, secondary syphilis
	Vesiculobullous, pustular	Erythema multiforme, hand-foot-and-mouth disease (palmar), porphyria cutanea tarda (dorsal), psoriasis, herpetic whitlow, blistering dactylitis, epidermolysis bullosa acquisita
	Papulonodular	Warts, actinic keratoses (dorsal), squamous cell carcinomas (dorsal), pyogenic granuloma, granuloma annulare, digital mucous cysts (dorsal)
	Depigmentation	Vitiligo, chemical leukoderma
	Periungual telangiectases	Scleroderma, dermatomyositis, lupus erythematosus, Osler-Weber-Rendu disease
Feet	Eczematous and papulosquamous	Tinea, psoriasis, contact dermatitis, atopic dermatitis, syphilis
	Vesiculobullous	Tinea, arthropod bites, epidermolysis bullosa, erythema multiforme, hand-foot-and-mouth disease, epidermolysis bullosa acquisita
	Papules	Verrucae, corns

configuration is gridlike rather than random. Additional cutaneous disorders associated with dystrophy of the nail plate include lichen planus (longitudinal ridging, roughness, and atrophy) and atopic or contact dermatitis (horizontal ridging).

Systemic Diseases

Occasionally, nail abnormalities can be the initial manifestation of a systemic disease. Examples are clubbing in the setting of lung cancer or hypertrophic pulmonary osteoarthropathy (Fig. 467–12; Chapters 189 and 201), yellow nails that grow quite slowly in patients with bronchiectasis and pleural effusions (yellow nail syndrome; Fig. 467–13; Chapters 90 and 100); onycholysis, which occurs when the nail plate is separated from the nail bed and is a sign of hyperthyroidism (Fig. 467–14; Chapter 244); and linear "splinter" hemorrhages in the nail bed secondary to bacterial endocarditis (Fig. 467–15; Chapter 76). Leukonychia is a white discoloration of the nail seen in the setting of cirrhosis (>90% of the nail; Chapter 157) or chronic renal failure (50% of the nail; Chapter 131). Spooning (koilonychia, a concave curvature of the nail plate; Fig. 467–16) can occur in patients with iron deficiency (Chapter 163).

A nail change that can "date" past serious illnesses is *Beau's lines* (Fig. 467–17), which are horizontal depressions in the nail plate. High fevers and severe illnesses can lead to a decrease in the proliferative rate of the nail matrix with resultant thinning of the nail, akin to what happens with the hair shaft in anagen effluvium secondary to systemic chemotherapy. Because the nail grows at a fairly constant rate (0.5 to 1.2 mm/wk for fingernails and half to a third that rate for toenails), a ridge that is in the midportion of all the fingernails reflects an insult 2.5 to 3 months previously. It is also important to examine the periungual region for *cuticular*

TABLE 467–4 NAIL DISEASES

INFLAMMATORY DISORDERS
Psoriasis, Reiter's disease (pitting of the nails)
Dermatitis (including atopic, contact)
Lichen planus
Alopecia areata
INFECTIOUS DISEASES
Dermatophytes
Candida spp
Saprophytes (toenails)
POSSIBLE SIGNS OF SYSTEMIC DISEASE
Splinter hemorrhages: bacterial endocarditis or vasculitis, but trauma is the most common cause
Transverse depressions in the nail plate (Beau's lines): chemotherapy, stressful event (e.g., high fever, severe illness)
Onycholysis: hyperthyroidism or porphyria, but psoriasis and chronic contact with irritants or water are more common causes
Clubbing: congenital heart disease, hypertrophic pulmonary osteoarthropathy, lung cancer, chronic pulmonary infections
Spooning (koilonychia): iron deficiency
White transverse bands: chronic hypoalbuminemia (Muehrcke's lines)* or arsenic exposure (Mees' lines)†, but trauma is the most common cause
Diffuse white discoloration (leukonychia): >90%—cirrhosis; 50%—chronic renal failure
Yellow and slow growing: yellow nail syndrome (pleural effusion, bronchiectasis)
Longitudinal streaks: lentigo, benign nevus, melanoma, but trauma (fair-skinned individuals) or physiologic (dark-skinned individuals) are the most common causes

*Disappear with pressure to the nail bed.
†Do not disappear with pressure to the nail bed.

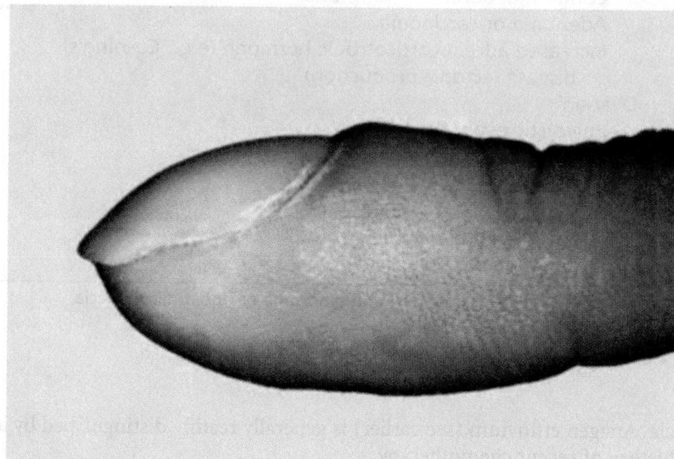

FIGURE 467–12 • Clubbing. Available at The Dermatologists' Image Resource: *http://www.dermnet.com/image.cfm?passedArrayIndex=3&moduleID=13&moduleGroupID=183.* Accessed May 24, 2006.

telangiectases, which are seen in dermatomyositis (Chapter 290), systemic lupus erythematosus (Chapter 287), scleroderma (Chapter 288), and hereditary hemorrhagic telangiectasia (Chapter 179).

Diseases of Hair

Alopecia

In the clinical examination of a patient with alopecia, the initial step is to determine the distribution: diffuse, patterned, or circumscribed.

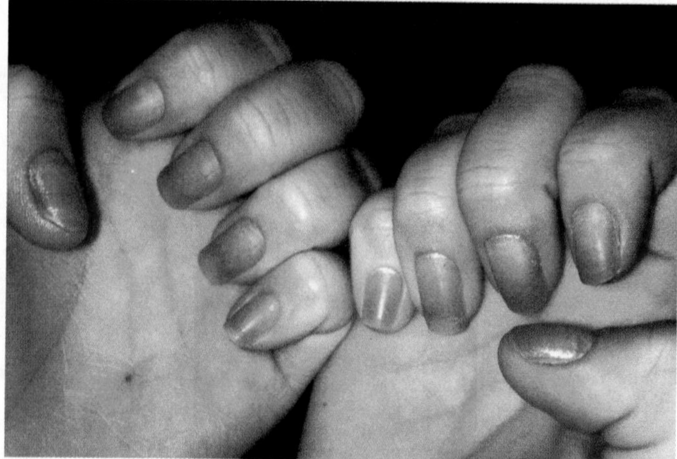

FIGURE 467–13 • Yellow nail. Available at DermAtlas: *http://dermatlas.med.jhmi.edu/derm/indexdisplay.cfm?ImageID=1047137097.* Accessed May 24, 2006.

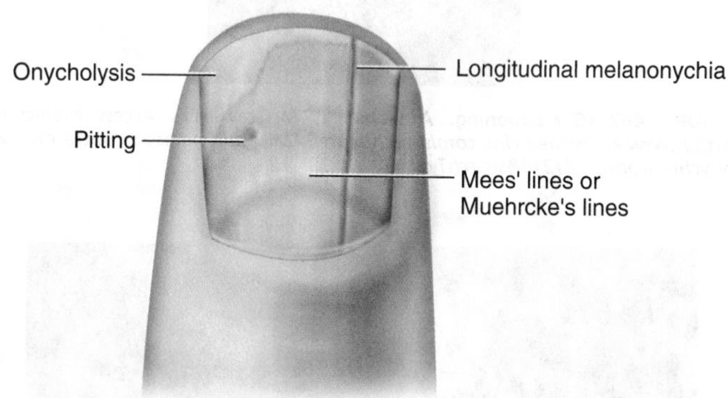

FIGURE 467–14 • Some pathologic findings in the nail.

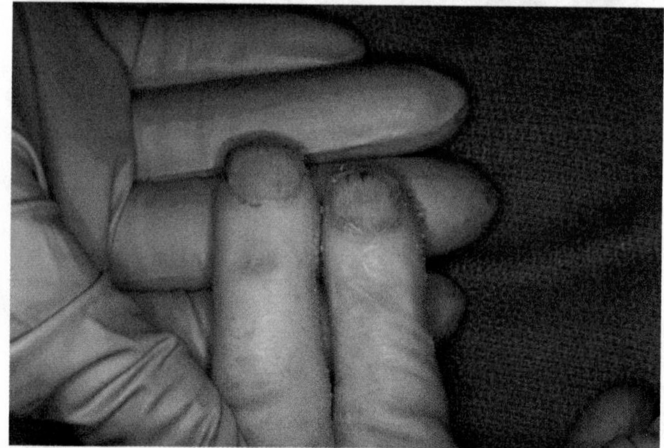

FIGURE 467–15 • Splinter hemorrhage. Available at *http://library.med.utah.edu/WebPath/CVHTML/CV105.html.*

Diffuse Alopecia

The major cause of diffuse alopecia is *telogen effluvium,* which is characterized by increased shedding with resultant diffuse thinning of the scalp hair (Table 467–5). Telogen effluvium is reversible and is caused by enhanced synchronization of the hair cycle so that more than the usual number of hairs are in telogen at one time (Chapter 461). The precipitating event has often occurred 2 to 3 months before the onset of shedding.

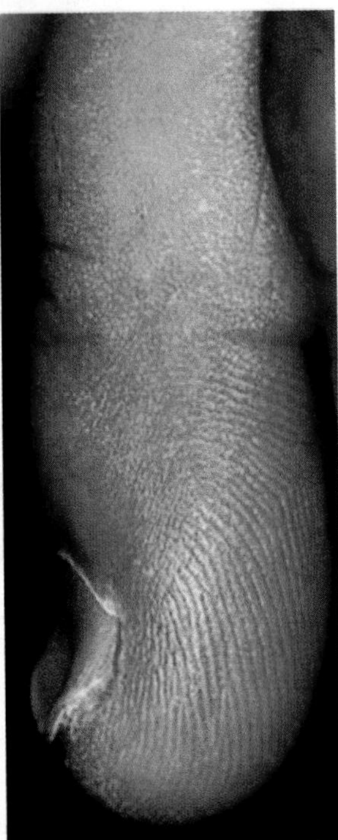

FIGURE 467–16 • Spooning. Available at McGraw-Hill's Access Medicine: *http://www.accessmedicine.com/search/searchAMResultImg.aspx?rootterm=koilonychia&rootID=41210&searchType=1.*

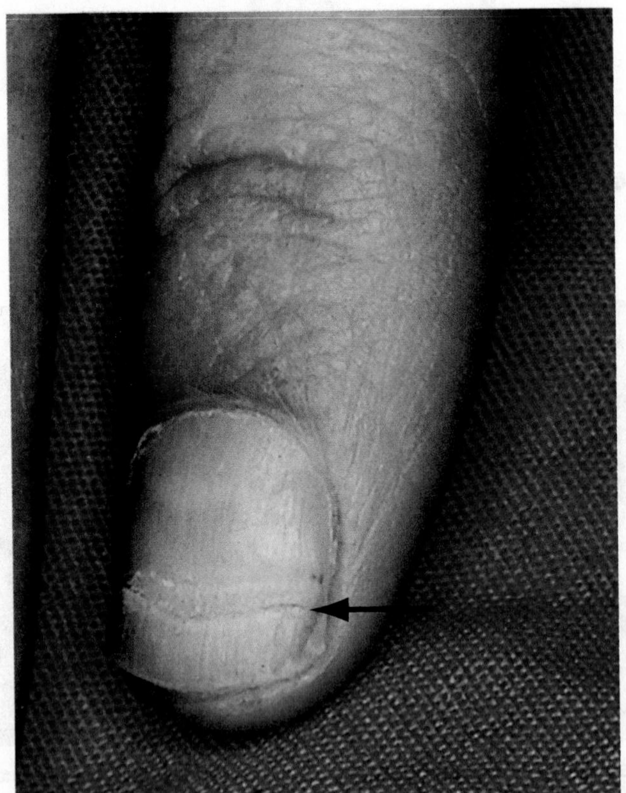

FIGURE 467–17 • Beau's lines. (From Fawcett RS, Linford S, Stulberg DL: Nail abnormalities: Clues to systemic disease. Am Fam Physician 2004;69:1421.)

Drugs that can lead to diffuse alopecia include lithium, warfarin, β-blockers, retinoids, and interferon. In patients with diffuse alopecia, it is important to exclude hyperthyroidism (Chapter 244), hypothyroidism (Chapter 244), and iron deficiency (Chapter 163) and to review all medications carefully, including over-the-counter, "natural," and illicit agents (e.g., amphetamines). Occasionally, systemic lupus erythematosus (Chapter 287) and genodermatoses can be accompanied by diffuse alopecia. Anagen effluvium (see earlier) is generally readily distinguished by a history of recent chemotherapy.

TABLE 467–5 CAUSES OF ALOPECIA AND HIRSUTISM

ALOPECIA
NONSCARRING
Primary cutaneous disorders
Androgenetic alopecia (male pattern and female pattern)
Telogen effluvium
Traction alopecia
Alopecia areata
Tinea capitis
Trichotillomania
Drugs (e.g., lithium, warfarin, β-blockers, retinoids, interferon)
Systemic diseases
Hyperthyroidism
Hypothyroidism
Deficiencies of protein, iron, biotin, and zinc
Human immunodeficiency virus infection
Systemic lupus erythematosus
Secondary syphilis
Hypopituitarism
SCARRING
Primary cutaneous disorders
Lichen planus
Discoid lupus erythematosus
Folliculitis decalvans
Central centrifugal cicatricial alopecia*
Linear scleroderma (morphea)
Systemic diseases
Systemic lupus erythematosus with cutaneous involvement (discoid lesions)
Sarcoidosis
Cutaneous metastases
HIRSUTISM
End-organ sensitivity (i.e., constitutional)
Hyperandrogenemia
Adrenal
Congenital adrenal hyperplasia
Adenoma or carcinoma
Increased adrenocorticotropic hormone (e.g., Cushing's disease, ectopic production)
Ovarian
Polycystic ovary syndrome
Hyperthecosis
Tumors
Pituitary
Hyperprolactinemia
Drugs (e.g., anabolic steroids)

*Also termed follicular degeneration syndrome or hot comb alopecia.

Patterned Alopecia

The most common form of patterned alopecia, also known as male pattern or female pattern alopecia, is *androgenetic* alopecia. In the male pattern, there is midline accentuation with recession of the frontal scalp line. The alopecia is the result of gradual miniaturization of the individual hair follicles/hair shafts because of the effects of dihydrotestosterone. Increased "end-organ sensitivity" is the usual explanation for androgenetic alopecia, but it can also be a reflection of hyperandrogenism (Chapter 261). Because hair follicles are not completely lost, the process is theoretically reversible. The follicles within a U-shaped band on the lower part of the scalp do not miniaturize (despite exposure to dihydrotestosterone) and therefore serve as a reservoir for hair transplantation. Androgenetic alopecia can first become apparent when there is a superimposed telogen effluvium, especially in women. The differential diagnosis includes traction alopecia from hairstyles that chronically pull on hair. Topical 2 to 5% minoxidil (men and women) and oral finasteride (men; 1 mg/day) are therapeutic options for androgenetic alopecia.

Circumscribed Alopecia

Circumscribed nonscarring alopecia can be a manifestation of *alopecia areata,* which is an autoimmune process in which T lymphocytes surround the hair bulb deep in the dermis. Discrete areas of hair loss with no clinical evidence of inflammation are seen, with initial lesions often being the size of a quarter. The natural history can vary from stabilization and spontaneous regrowth of hair to rapid spread and coalescence. In a minority of patients, involvement of the entire scalp (alopecia totalis) or the entire body (alopecia universalis) can be observed. Patients with alopecia areata have an increased incidence of vitiligo and autoimmune polyendocrinopathies. Treatment consists primarily of intralesional corticosteroids and topical irritants (e.g., anthralin) or allergens (e.g., squaric acid dibutyl ester). Additional causes of circumscribed nonscarring alopecia include tinea capitis (Chapter 464), syphilis (Chapter 340), and trichotillomania, in which people pull out their scalp hairs, usually because of anxiety.

The major causes of scarring alopecia are *lichen planus* (Chapter 464) and *discoid lupus erythematosus* (Chapter 287), in which there is permanent loss of hair follicles. In patients with active lesions, scalp inflammation is seen, especially at the periphery of the areas of alopecia. Sarcoidosis (Chapter 95), cutaneous metastases, and morphea (linear scleroderma; Chapter 288) are uncommon causes of scarring alopecia. A total body skin examination (including nails and oral mucosa) can provide clues to the diagnosis, especially in the case of lichen planus and discoid lupus erythematosus, but histologic evaluation is required to establish the diagnosis of scarring alopecia.

Hirsutism (Chapter 261)

Hirsutism is an increase in hair growth in particular anatomic sites that are androgen dependent (e.g., lateral aspect of the face, chin, neck, central part of the chest, lower part of the abdomen, and groin), whereas hypertrichosis is increased hair growth anywhere on the body. Because of the involvement of androgens, hirsutism is not normally seen before puberty. There can be either increased end-organ sensitivity (in this case the hair follicle) or hyperandrogenemia (see Table 467–5). The former is often familial, and the latter is often related to ovarian or adrenal dysfunction (the two sites of androgen production in women). Endocrinologic evaluation is recommended, including measurement of circulating levels of free testosterone, dehydroepiandrosterone sulfate, and prolactin (Chapter 261). Treatments include bleaches, chemical or wax depilatories, topical eflornithine, electrolysis, and laser therapy.

DISTINCTIVE LESIONS IN BLACK SKIN

Although some diseases are more common in patients of African ancestry (e.g., tinea capitis, pseudofolliculitis barbae, dissecting cellulitis), others are simply more noticeable (e.g., vitiligo and postinflammatory hypopigmentation) (Table 467–6). The explanation for the increased incidence is speculative in most instances, with the exception of curled hairs leading to pseudofolliculitis barbae. Tightly curled hairs, when shaved, are usually cut at an oblique angle, which results in a sharp tip at the distal end of the hair shaft that allows penetration of the skin adjacent to the hair follicle and subsequent inflammation. Some cutaneous disorders are seen less commonly in black skin (e.g., acne rosacea and scabies).

Another entity seen more commonly in individuals of African descent is keloids (Fig. 467–18). Keloids generally appear at sites of trauma (e.g., ear piercing) but can occasionally develop spontaneously, especially on the trunk. In the former situation, they are thought to represent an exaggerated response to wound healing, with increased formation of collagen not only at the site of the trauma (as in hypertrophic scars) but also in adjacent, previously uninvolved skin. Treatment options include intralesional corticosteroids and intralesional interferon or excision followed by radiation therapy.

TABLE 467–6 DISORDERS SEEN MORE COMMONLY IN PATIENTS OF AFRICAN ANCESTRY

HEAD AND NECK
Folliculitis decalvans/dissecting cellulitis
Tinea capitis
Traction alopecia
Central centrifugal cicatricial alopecia*
Acne keloidalis nuchae
Pseudofolliculitis barbae
Pomade acne
Dermatosis papulosa nigra
Inherited patterned lentiginosis
Melasma
Discoid lupus erythematosus
PALMAR
Keratosis punctata of the palmar creases
LOWER EXTREMITIES
Ulcers secondary to sickle cell anemia
GENERALIZED
Keloids
Cutaneous sarcoidosis
Papular eczema and follicular-based inflammation

*Also termed follicular degeneration syndrome or hot comb alopecia.

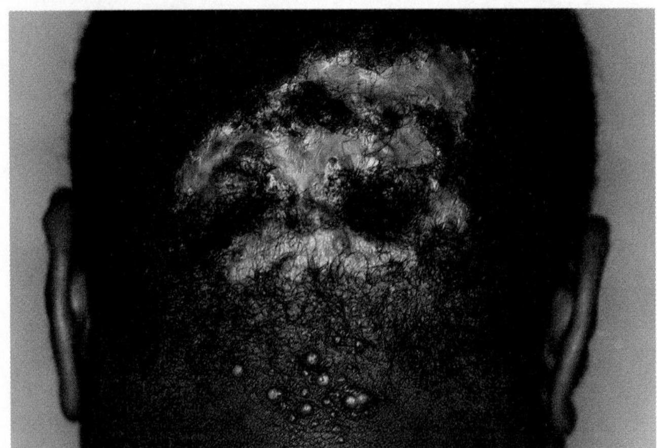

FIGURE 467–18 • Acne keloidalis in an African American man. (Courtesy of Kalman Watsky, MD.)

SUGGESTED READINGS

Falagas ME, Vergidis PI: Narrative review: Diseases that masquerade as infectious cellulitis. Ann Intern Med 2005;142:47–55. *Provides an extensive differential diagnosis.*

Grimes PE: New insights and new therapies in vitiligo. JAMA 2005;293:730–735. *A clinical review.*

Piraccini BM, Iorizzo M, Antonucci A, et al: Drug-induced nail abnormalities. Expert Opin Drug Saf 2004;3:57–65. *Side effects of medications as they pertain to the nail apparatus.*

Seghal VN, Srivastava G: Vitiligo treatment options: An evolving scenario. J Dermatolog Treat 2006;17:262–275. *A comprehensive review.*

Stough D, Stenn K, Haber R, et al: Psychological effect, pathophysiology, and management of androgenetic alopecia in men. Mayo Clin Proc 2005;80: 1316–1322. *A comprehensive review.*

Swartz MN: Clinical practice. Cellulitis. N Engl J Med 2004;350:904–912. *An excellent approach to diagnosis and treatment of this disorder.*

Appendix

REFERENCE INTERVALS AND LABORATORY VALUES*

Ronald J. Elin

Reference intervals are valuable guidelines for the clinician to assess health and disease, but they should not be used as absolute indicators of health and disease. For essentially every test, significant overlap exists between healthy and diseased populations. Many factors may influence the determination of the reference interval. The method and mode of standardization are variables for the reference interval, particularly for immunologic and enzymatic tests. The selection of the "normal" population is also important because factors such as age, gender, race, diet, personal habits (e.g., alcohol consumption, smoking), and exercise may influence the reference interval for a given analyte. Finally, the statistics chosen to define the reference interval are also a factor. These multiple variables for determining the reference interval indicate why differences exist among institutions for the same analyte.

The values in this chapter are primarily for adults in the fasting state. Values for other groups, when included, are clearly identified. Prefixes and abbreviations are listed in Table Appendix–1. For convenience, this chapter is divided into the following three sections: clinical chemistry, toxicology, and serology (Table Appendix–2); hematology and coagulation (Table Appendix–3); and drugs, therapeutic and toxic (Table Appendix–4). The list includes reference intervals for the most common tests used in the practice of internal medicine.

All laboratory values are given in conventional and international units. If the value and units for a reference interval are the same for conventional and international units, the interval is listed only in the column for international units. The temperature for all enzyme assays listed in the chapter is 37° C. The pertinent prefixes denoting the decimal factors and abbreviations are listed in Table Appendix–1.

TABLE APPENDIX–1 PREFIXES AND ABBREVIATIONS

PREFIXES DENOTING DECIMAL FACTORS

Prefix	Symbol	Factor
mega	M	10^6
kilo	k	10^3
hecto	h	10^2
deca	da	10^1
deci	d	10^{-1}
centi	c	10^{-2}
milli	m	10^{-3}
micro	μ	10^{-6}
nano	n	10^{-9}
pico	p	10^{-12}
femto	f	10^{-15}

ABBREVIATIONS

AU	Arbitrary units
CSF	Cerebrospinal fluid
EDTA	Ethylenediaminetetra-acetic acid
EU	Ehrlich unit
GD	General diagnostics
Hb	Hemoglobin
hpf	High-power field
IFA	Immunofluorescent assay
IU	International unit (of hormone activity)
Kat	Katal
Pa	Pascal
RBC	Red blood cell
RIA	Radioimmunoassay
RID	Radial immunodiffusion
S	Substrate
U	International unit (of enzyme activity)
WBC	White blood cell

SUGGESTED READINGS

Burtis CA, Ashwood ER, Bruns DE (eds): Tietz Textbook of Clinical Chemistry and Molecular Diagnosis, 4th ed. St. Louis, Elsevier Saunders, 2006. *A comprehensive text.*

Wu AHB (ed): Tietz Clinical Guide to Laboratory Tests, 4th ed. St. Louis, Elsevier Saunders, 2006. *A comprehensive text of reference intervals.*

*The material in this chapter was partially extracted from Tietz NW (ed): Clinical Guide to Laboratory Tests. Philadelphia, WB Saunders, 1995. The material for the section on therapeutic drug concentrations was partially extracted from Burtis CA, Ashwood ER (eds): Tietz Textbook of Clinical Chemistry, Philadelphia, WB Saunders, 1994. The main contributors to this section of the book are P. C. Painter, J. Y. Cope, and J. L. Smith. Other sources are listed under the suggested readings for this chapter.

TABLE APPENDIX–2 CLINICAL CHEMISTRY, TOXICOLOGY, AND SEROLOGY

Test	Specimen	Reference Interval (Conventional Units)	Reference Interval (International Units)
Acetoacetate Semiquantitative	Serum or plasma (fluoride/oxalate)	Negative (<1 mg/dL)	Negative (<0.1 mmol/L)
Acetone Semiquantitative	Urine Serum or plasma (fluoride or oxalate)	Negative Negative (<1 mg/dL)	Negative Negative (0.17 mmol/L)
Acid phosphatase (S:p-nitrophenylphosphate)	Serum		M: 2.5–11.7 U/L F: 0.3–9.2 U/L
Adrenocorticotropic hormone (ACTH)	Plasma (heparin)	0800 hr: <120 pg/mL 1600–2000 hr: <85 pg/mL	<26 pmol/L <19 pmol/L
Alanine aminotransferase (ALT, SGPT)	Serum	M: 10–40 U/L F: 7–35 U/L	0.17–0.68 μKat/L 0.12–0.60 μKat/L
Albumin Nephelometric, colorimetric Turbidimetric	Serum CSF Urine	3.4-4.8 g/dL <45 mg/dL <80 mg/day at rest <150 mg/day ambulatory	34-48 g/L <450 mg/L <80 mg/day <150 mg/day
Aldolase	Serum	1.0–7.5 U/L	0.2–0.13 μKat/L
Aldosterone	Plasma (heparin EDTA) or serum	Adult, average sodium diet Supine: 3–16 ng/dL Upright: 7–30 ng/dL	 0.8–0.44 nmol/L 0.19–0.83 nmol/L
Alkaline phosphatase (S:4-NPP)	Serum	Adult (>20 yr): 25–100 U/L	0.43–1.70 μKat/L
Aluminum	Serum	<5.41 μg/L	<0.2 μmol/L
δ-Aminolevulinic acid (δ-ALA)	Serum Urine	15-23 μg/dL 1.5–7.5 mg/day	1.1–8 μmol/L 11.4–57.2 μmol/day
Ammonia nitrogen Resin or enzymatic	Serum or plasma (Na-heparin) Urine, 24-hr	Adult: 15–45 μg N/dL 140–1500 mg/day	11-32 μmol/L 10–107 mmol/day
Amylase (S:Beckman, defined substrate)	Serum Urine, timed specimen	27–131 U/L	0.46–2.23 μKat/L 1–17 U/hr
Angiotensin I	Peripheral venous plasma (EDTA)	<25 pg/mL	<25 ng/L
Angiotensin II	Plasma (EDTA) Arterial blood	10–60 pg/mL	10–60 ng/L
α_1-Antitrypsin (nephelometry)	Serum	78–200 mg/dL	0.78–2 g/L
Anion gap [$Na^+ - (Cl^- + HCO_3^-)$]	Serum or plasma (heparin)	7–16 mEq/L	7–16 mmol/L
Arsenic	Whole blood (heparin)	0.2–2.3 μg/dL Chronic poisoning: 10–50 μg/dL Acute poisoning: 60–93 μg/dL	0.3–0.31 μmol/L 1.33–6.65 μmol/L 7.98–12.37 μmol/L
Ascorbic acid (see Vitamin C)			
Aspartate aminotransferase (AST, SGOT)	Serum	10–30 U/L	0.17–0.51 μKat/L
Base excess	Whole blood (heparin)	–2 to 3 mEq/L	–2–3 mmol/L
Bicarbonate	Serum	22–29 mEq/L	22–29 mmol/L
Bile acids, total	Serum, fasting Serum, 1-hr postprandial Feces	0.3–2.3 μg/mL 1.8–3.2 μg/mL 120–225 mg/day	0.74–5.64 μmol/L 4.41–7.84 μmol/L 294–551 μmol/day
Bilirubin, conjugated (direct)	Serum	0–0.2 mg/dL	0–3.4 μmol/L
Bilirubin, total	Serum Urine	0.3–1.2 mg/dL	5–21 μmol/L Negative
B-type natriuretic peptide (BNP)	Whole blood or plasma (EDTA)	<100 pg/mL	<28.8 pmol/L
Calcium, ionized (iCa)	Serum	4.65–5.28 mg/dL	1.16–1.32 mmol/L
Calcium, total	Serum Urine, 24-hr CSF	8.6–10.0 mg/dL 100–300 mg/d 4.2–5.4 mg/dL	2.15–2.50 mmol/L 2.5–7.5 mmol/day 1.5–1.35 mmol/L
Cancer antigen 125 (CA 125)	Serum	<35 U/mL	<35 kU/L
Cancer antigen 15-3 (CA 15-3)	Serum	<30 U/mL	<30 kU/L
Carbohydrate antigen 19-9 (CA 19-9)	Serum	<37 U/mL	<37 kU/L
Carbon dioxide, partial pressure (Pco_2)	Whole blood, arterial (heparin)	M: 35–48 mm Hg F: 32–45 mm Hg	4.66–6.38 kPa 4.26–5.99 kPa

TABLE APPENDIX–2 CLINICAL CHEMISTRY, TOXICOLOGY, AND SEROLOGY—cont'd

Test	Specimen	Reference Interval (Conventional Units)	Reference Interval (International Units)
Carbon dioxide, total (Tco_2)	Serum or plasma (heparin)	23–29 mEq/L	23–29 mmol/L
Carcinoembryonic antigen (CEA)	Serum	Nonsmokers: <2.5 ng/mL	<2.5 μg/L
β-Carotene	Serum	10–85 μg/dL	0.19–1.58 μmol/L
Catecholamines, total	Urine, 24-hr	<100 μg/day	<5.91 nmol/day
Ceruloplasmin	Serum	18–45 mg/dL	180–450 mg/L
Chloride	Serum or plasma (heparin)	98–106 mEq/L	98–106 mmol/L
	CSF	118–132 mEq/L	118–132 mmol/L
	Urine, 24-hr	110–250 mEq/day	110–250 mmol/day
Cholesterol, total	Serum or plasma (EDTA)	Recommended: <200 mg/dL Moderate risk: 200–239 mg/dL High risk: ≥240 mg/dL	<5.18 mmol/L 5.18–6.19 mmol/L 6.22 mmol/L
Chorionic gonadotropin, β-subunit (β-HCG)	Serum or plasma (EDTA)	M and nonpregnant F: <5.0 mIU/mL	<5.0 IU/L
Complement			
Total hemolytic Complement activity	Serum	75–160 U/mL	75–160 kU/L
Copper	Serum	M: 70–140 μg/dL F: 80–155 μg/dL	10.99–21.98 μmol/L 12.56–24.34 μmol/L
	Erythrocyte (heparin)	90–150 μg/dL	14.13–23.55 μmol/L
	Urine, 24-hr	3–35 μg/day	0.47–0.55 μmol/day
Coproporphyrin	Urine, 24-hr	34–234 μg/day	51–351 nmol/day
	Feces, 24-hr	<30 μg/g dry wt 400–1200 μg/day	<45 nmol/g dry wt 600–1800 nmol/day
Corticosterone	Serum	0800 hr: 130–820 ng/dL 1600 hr: 60–220 ng/dL	4–24 nmol/L 2–6 nmol/L
Cortisol	Serum or plasma (heparin)	0800 hr: 5–23 μg/dL 1600 hr: 3–15 μg/dL 2000 hr: ≤50% of 0800 hr	138–635 nmol/L 82–413 nmol/L Fraction of 0800 hr: ≤0.50
Cortisol, free	Urine, 24-hr	20–90 μg/day	55–248 nmol/day
C-peptide	Serum	0.78–1.89 ng/mL	0.26–0.62 nmol/L
C-reactive protein	Serum	68–8200 ng/mL	68–8200 μg/L
Creatine kinase (CK)	Serum		M: 38–174 U/L F: 26–140 U/L
Isoenzymes, fraction 2 (MB)	Serum	<4–6% of total (method-dependent)	Fraction of total: <0.4–0.6
Creatinine Jaffe, kinetic or enzymatic	Serum or plasma	M: 0.7–1.3 mg/dL F: 0.6–1.1 mg/dL	62–115 μmol/L 53–97 μmol/L
	Urine, 24-hr	M: 14–26 mg/kg/day F: 11–20 mg/kg/day	124–230 μmol/kg/day 97–177 μmol/kg/day
Creatinine clearance (endogenous)	Serum or plasma, and urine	M: 90–139 mL/min/1.73 m^2 F: 80–125 mL/min/1.73 m^2	0.87–1.34 mL/sec/m^2 0.77–1.20 mL/sec/m^2
Dehydroepiandrosterone (DHEA)	Serum	M: 1.8–12.5 ng/mL F: 1.3–9.8 ng/mL	6.2–43.3 nmol/L 4.5–34. nmol/L
11-Deoxycortisol (compound S)	Serum	12–158 ng/dL	0.3–4.6 nmol/L
Erythropoietin	Serum		5–36 U/L
Estrogens, total	Serum	M: 20–80 pg/mL F, cycle: Postmenopausal: ≤130 pg/mL Follicular phase: 60–200 pg/mL Luteal phase: 160–400 pg/mL	20–80 ng/L ≤130 ng/L 60–200 ng/L 160–400 ng/L
	Urine, 24-hr		M: 15–40 μg/day F: Preovulation: 4–25 μg/day Ovulation: 28–100 μg/day Luteal peak: 22–80 μg/day Pregnancy, term: <45,000 μg/day Postmenopausal: <20 μg/day
Fat, fecal	Feces, 72-hr		<7 g/day Fat-free diet: <4 g/day
Fatty acids, nonesterified (free)	Serum or plasma (heparin)	8–25 mg/dL	0.28–0.89 mmol/L
Ferritin	Serum	M: 20–250 ng/mL F: 10–120 ng/mL	20–250 μg/L 10–120 μg/L
$α_1$-Fetoprotein	Serum	<10 ng/mL	<10 μg/L
Fibrinogen (see Table Appendix–3)			

Continued

TABLE APPENDIX–2 CLINICAL CHEMISTRY, TOXICOLOGY, AND SEROLOGY—cont'd

Test	Specimen	Reference Interval (Conventional Units)	Reference Interval (International Units)
Folate	Serum	3–16 ng/mL	7–36 nmol/L
	Erythrocytes (EDTA)	140–628 ng/mL packed cells	317–1422 nmol/L packed cells
Follitropin (FSH)	Serum or plasma (heparin)	M: 4–25 mIU/mL	4–25 IU/L
		F: Follicular phase: 1–9 mIU/L	1–9 IU/L
		Ovulatory peak: 6–26 mIU/mL	6–26 IU/L
		Luteal phase: 1–9 mIU/mL	1–9 IU/L
		Postmenopausal: 30–118 mIU/mL	30–118 IU/L
	Urine, 24-hr		M: 3–11 IU/day
			F: 2–15 IU/day
Gastrin	Serum	25–90 pg/mL	25–90 ng/L
Glucose	Serum	Adult: 74–106 mg/dL	4.1–5.9 mmol/L
		>60 y: 80–115 mg/dL	4.4–6.4 mmol/L
	Whole blood (heparin)	65–95 mg/dL	3.6–5.3 mmol/L
	CSF	40–70 mg/dL	2.2–3.9 mmol/L
Quantitative, enzymatic	Urine	<0.5 g/day	<2.8 mmol/day
Qualitative	Urine		Negative
Glucose, 2-hr postprandial	Serum	<126 mg/dL	<7.0 mmol/L
Glucose, tolerance test (GTT), oral	Serum	mg/dL: Normal / Diabetic	mmol/L: Normal / Diabetic
		Fasting: 70–105 / >140	3.9–5.8 / >7.8
		60 min: 120–170 / ≥200	6.7–9.4 / ≥11
		90 min: 100–140 / ≥200	5.6–7.8 / ≥11
		120 min: 70–120 / ≥140	3.9–6.7 / ≥7.8
γ-Glutamyltransferase (GGT) (Szasz method)	Serum	M: 2–30 U/L	0.03–0.51 μKat/L
		F: 1–24 U/L	0.02–0.41 μKat/L
Glycerol, free	Plasma	0.29–1.72 mg/dL	0.03–0.19 mmol/L
Growth hormone (hGH, somatotropin)	Serum	Adult, M: 0–4 ng/mL	0–4 μg/L
		F: 0–18 ng/mL	0–18 μg/L
		>60 y, M: 1–9 ng/mL	1–9 μg/L
		F: 1–16 ng/mL	1–16 μg/L
Haptoglobin (see Hematology and Coagulation section)			
HDL cholesterol (HDLC) (5th percentile from Lipid Research Clinics)	Serum or plasma (EDTA)	M: >29 mg/dL	>0.75 mmol/L
		F: >35 mg/dL	>0.91 mmol/L
Hemoglobin A_{1c} (electrophoresis)	Whole blood (heparin, EDTA, or oxalate)	5.0–7.5% of total Hb	Fraction of Hb: 0.050–0.075
Homovanillic acid (HVA)	Urine, 24-hr	1.4–8.8 mg/day	8–48 μmol/day
17-Hydroxycorticosteroids (17-OHCS)	Urine, 24-hr	M: 3.0–10.0 mg/day	8.3–27.6 μmol/day
		F: 2.0–8.0 mg/day	5.5–22.1 μmol/day
5-Hydroxyindole acetic acid (5-HIAA)			
Qualitative	Fresh random urine		Negative
Quantitative	Urine, 24-hr	2–6 mg/day	10.4–31.2 μmol/day
17-Hydroxyprogesterone (17-OHP)	Serum	M: 0.5–2.5 ng/mL	1.5–7.5 nmol/L
		F: Follicular: 0.2–1.0 ng/mL	0.6–3.0 nmol/L
		Luteal: 1.–5.0 ng/mL	3.0–15.5 nmol/L
		Postmenopausal: ≤0.7 ng/mL	≤2.1 nmol/L
Immunoglobulin A (IgA)	Serum	40–350 mg/dL	400–3,500 mg/L
Immunoglobulin D (IgD)	Serum	0–8 mg/dL	0–80 mg/L
Immunoglobulin E (IgE)	Serum	0–380 IU/mL	0–380 kIU/L
Immunoglobulin G (IgG)	Serum	650–1,600 mg/dL	6.5–16 g/L
	CSF	0.5–5 mg/dL	5–50 mg/L
Immunoglobulin M (IgM)	Serum	55–300 mg/dL	550–3000 mg/L
Insulin (12-hr fasting), immunoreactive	Serum	0.7–9.0 μIU/mL	5–63 pmol/L
Intrinsic factor (see Vitamin B_{12})			
Iron	Serum	M: 65–175 μg/dL	11.6–31.3 μmol/L
		F: 50–170 μg/dL	9.0–30.4 μmol/L
Iron-binding capacity, total (TIBC)	Serum	250–450 μg/dL	44.8–80.6 μmol/L
Iron saturation	Serum		Fraction of iron saturation:
		M: 20–50	0.20–0.5
		F: 15–50	0.15–0.5

TABLE APPENDIX-2 CLINICAL CHEMISTRY, TOXICOLOGY, AND SEROLOGY—cont'd

Test	Specimen	Reference Interval (Conventional Units)	Reference Interval (International Units)
17-Ketogenic steroids (17-KGS)	Urine, 24-hr	M: 5–23 mg/day F: 3–15 mg/day	17–80 μmol/day 10–52 μmol/day
Ketone bodies Qualitative	Serum Urine, random	Negative (0.5–3 mg/dL)	Negative (5–30 mg/L) Negative
17-Ketosteroids, total (17-KS)	Urine, 24-hr	M: 10–25 mg/day F: 6–15 mg/day	37–87 μmol/day 21–52 μmol/day
L-Lactate	Whole blood (heparin)	Venous: 8.1–15.3 mg/dL Arterial: <11.3 mg/dL	0.9–1.7 mmol/L <1.3 mmol/L
Lactate dehydrogenase (LDH)	Serum		208–378 U/L
LDH isoenzymes (electrophoresis, agarose)	Serum	% Fraction 1: 18–33 Fraction 2: 28–40 Fraction 3: 18–30 Fraction 4: 6–16 Fraction 5: 2–13	Fraction of total: 0.18–0.33 0.28–0.40 0.18–0.30 0.06–0.16 0.02–0.13
Lead	Whole blood (heparin)	<25 μg/dL Toxic: ≥100 μg/dL	<1.21 μmol/L ≥4.83 μmol/L
	Urine	<80 μg/dL	<0.39 μmol/L
Lipase	Serum	31–186 U/L	0.5–3.2 μKat/L
Low-density lipoprotein cholesterol (LDLC)	Serum or plasma (EDTA)	Recommended: <130 mg/dL Moderate risk: 130–159 mg/dL High risk: ≥160 mg/dL	<3.37 mmol/L 3.37–4.12 mmol/L ≥4.14 mmol/L
Lutropin (LH)	Serum or plasma (heparin)	M: 1–8 mU/mL F: Follicular phase: 1–2 mU/mL Midcycle: 16–104 mU/mL Luteal: 1–12 mU/mL Postmenopausal: 16–66 mU/mL	1–8 U/L 1–12 U/L 16–104 U/L 1–12 U/L 16–66 U/L
	Urine		M: 9–23 U/day F: non-midcycle, 4–30 U/day
Lysozyme	Serum, plasma	0.4–1.3 mg/dL	4–13 mg/L
Magnesium	Serum Urine, 24-hr	1.3–2.1 mEq/L 6.0–10.0 mEq/day	0.65–1.05 mmol/L 3.00–5.00 mmol/day
Mercury	Whole blood (EDTA) Urine, 24-hr	<5.0 μg/dL <20 μg/L Toxic: >150 μg/L	<0.25 μmol/L <0.1 μmol/L <0.75 μmol/L
Metanephrine, total	Urine, 24-hr	0.05–1.20 μg/mg creatinine	0.03–0.69 mmol/mol creatinine
Myelin basic protein	CSF		<2.5 μg/L
Myoglobin	Serum		M: 19–92 μg/L F: 12–76 μg/L
	Urine, random		Negative
Osmolality	Serum Urine, random		275–295 mOsmol/kg 50–1,200 mOsmol/kg, depending on fluid intake After 12-hr fluid restriction: >850 mOsmol/kg
	Urine, 24-hr		~390–900 mOsmol/kg
Oxalate	Serum	1–2.4 μg/mL Ethylene glycol poisoning: >20 μg/mL	11-27 μmol/L Ethylene glycol poisoning: >228 μmol/L
Oxygen (Po_2)	Whole blood, arterial (heparin)	83–108 mm Hg	11–14.4 kPa
Oxygen saturation	Whole blood, arterial (heparin)	95–98%	Fraction saturated: 0.95–0.98
Parathyroid hormone	Serum	Varies with laboratory N-terminal: 8–24 pg/mL C-terminal: 50–330 pg/mL Intact: 10–65 pg/mL	 8–24 ng/L 50–330 ng/L 10–65 ng/L
pH (37° C)	Whole blood, arterial (heparin)		7.35–7.45
Phosphorus, inorganic	Serum	2.7–4.5 mg/dL >60 yr, M: 2.3–3.7 mg/dL F: 2.8–4.1 mg/dL	0.87–1.45 nmol/L 0.74–1.2 nmol/L 0.90–1.3 nmol/L
	Urine, 24-hr	0.4–1.3 g/day	13–42 mmol/day

Continued

TABLE APPENDIX–2 CLINICAL CHEMISTRY, TOXICOLOGY, AND SEROLOGY—cont'd

Test	Specimen	Reference Interval (Conventional Units)	Reference Interval (International Units)
Porphobilinogen (PBG)			
Quantitative	Urine, 24-hr	0–2.0 mg/day	0–8.8 μmol/day
Qualitative	Urine, fresh random		Negative
Potassium	Serum	3.5–5.1 mEq/L	3.5–5.1 mmol/L
	Plasma (heparin)	3.5–4.5 mEq/L	3.5–4.5 mmol/L
	Urine, 24-hr	25–125 mEq/day	25–125 mmol/day
Pregnanediol	Urine, 24-hr	M: 0–1.9 mg/day	0–5.9 μmol/day
		F: Follicular: <2.6 mg/day	<8 μmol/day
		Luteal: 2.6–10.6 mg/day	8–33 μmol/day
		Postmenopausal: 0.2–1.0 mg/day	0.6-3.1 μmol/day
Progesterone	Serum	M: 0.13–0.97 ng/mL	0.4–3.1 nmol/L
		F: Follicular: 0.15–0.70 ng/mL	0.5–2.2 nmol/L
		Luteal: 2.0–25 ng/mL	6.4–79.5 nmol/L
Prolactin (hPRL)	Serum	M: 3.0–14.7 ng/mL	3.0–14.7 μg/L
		F: 3.8–23.2 ng/mL	3.8–23.2 μg/L
Prostate-specific antigen (PSA)	Serum, freeze	M: <4 ng/mL	<4 μg/L
Protein			
Total	Serum	6.4–8.3 g/dL	64.0–83.0 g/L
Electrophoresis (cellulose acetate)	Serum	Albumin: 3.5–5.0 g/dL	35–50 g/L
		α_1-Globulin: 0.1–0.3 g/dL	1–3 g/L
		α_2-Globulin: 0.6–1.0 g/dL	6–10 g/L
		β-Globulin: 0.7–1.1 g/dL	7–11 g/L
		γ-Globulin: 0.8–1.6 g/dL	8–16 g/L
Total	Urine, 24-hr		50–80 mg/day at rest
Total	CSF	Lumbar: 15–45 mg/dL	150–450 mg/L
Pyruvic acid	Whole blood (heparin)	0.3–0.9 mg/dL	0.03–0.10 mmol/L
Renin (normal diet)	Plasma (EDTA)	Supine: 0.2–1.6 ng/mL/hr	0.2–1.6 μg/L/hr
		Standing: 0.7–3.3 ng/mL/hr	0.7–3.3 μg/L/hr
Riboflavin (see Vitamin B_2)			
Sediment	Urine, fresh, random		Hyaline: occasional (0–1) casts/hpf
Casts			RBC: not seen
			WBC: not seen
			Tubular epithelial: not seen
			Transitional and squamous epithelial: not seen
Cells			RBC: 0–2/hpf
			WBC: M: 0–3/hpf
			F: 0–5/hpf
			Epithelial: few
			Bacteria:
			Unspun: no organisms/oil immersion field
			Spun: <20 organisms/hpf
Sodium	Serum or plasma (heparin)	136–146 mEq/L	136–146 mmol/L
	Urine, 24-hr	40–220 mEq/day	40–220 mmol/day
Specific gravity	Urine, random		1.002–1.030
	Urine, 24-hr		1.015–1.025
Testosterone, free	Serum	M: 50–210 pg/mL	174–729 pmol/L
		F: 1.0–8.5 pg/mL	3.5–29.5 pmol/L
Testosterone, total	Serum	M: 280–1100 ng/dL	9.7–38.2 nmol/L
		F: 15-70 ng/dL	0.5–2.4 nmol/L
	Urine	20–50 yr,	
		M: 50–135 μg/day	173–470 nmol/day
		F: 2–12 μg/day	7–42 nmol/day
		>50 yr,	
		M: 40–60 μg/day	139–210 nmol/day
		F: 2–8 μg/day	7–28 nmol/day
Thiamine (see Vitamin B_1)	Serum	0.10–0.54 μg/dL	2.9–16.1 nmol/L
Thyroglobulin (Tg)	Serum	3–42 ng/mL	3–42 μg/L
Thyroglobulin antibodies	Serum		<1:10

TABLE APPENDIX–2 CLINICAL CHEMISTRY, TOXICOLOGY, AND SEROLOGY—cont'd

Test	Specimen	Reference Interval (Conventional Units)	Reference Interval (International Units)
Thyroid microsomal antibodies	Serum		Nondetectable (hemagglutination) or <1:10 (IFA)
Thyrotropin (hTSH)	Serum or plasma	0.4–4.2 μU/mL	0.4–4.2 mU/L
Thyrotropin-releasing hormone	Plasma	5–60 pg/mL	5–60 ng/L
Thyroxine, free (FT_4)	Serum	0.8–2.4 ng/dL	10–31 pmol/L
Thyroxine (T_4), total	Serum	M: 4.6–10.5 μg/dL F: 5.5–11.0 μg/dL	59–135 nmol/L 71–142 nmol/L
Thyroxine-binding globulin (TBG)	Serum	15.0–34.0 μg/mL	15.0–34.0 mg/L
Thyroxine index, free	Serum		4.2–13.0
Transcortin	Serum	M: 18.8–25.2 mg/L F: 14.9–22.9 mg/L	323–433 nmol/L 256–393 nmol/L
Transferrin	Serum	200–400 mg/dL >60 yr:180–380 mg/dL	2.0–4.0 g/L 1.80-3.80 g/L
Transthyretin (prealbumin)	Serum	10–40 mg/dL	100–400 mg/L
Triglycerides (TG)	Serum, after ≥12-hr fast	Recommended: <250 mg/dL	2.83 mmol/L
Tri-iodothyronine, free	Serum	260–480 pg/dL	4.0–7.4 pmol/L
Tri-iodothyronine, total (T_3)	Serum	100–200 ng/dL	1.54–3.08 mmol/L
Tri-iodothyronine resin uptake test (T_3RU)	Serum	24–34%	24–34 AU (arbitrary units)
Troponin-I	Serum		<10 μg/L
Troponin-T	Serum		0–0.1 μg/L
Urea nitrogen	Serum or plasma Urine	6–20 mg/dL 12–20 g/day	2.1–7.1 mmol/L 0.43–0.71 mol/day
Urea nitrogen/creatinine ratio	Serum		12/1–20/1
Uric acid (uricase)	Serum Urine, 24-hr	M: 3.5–7.2 mg/dL F: 2.6–6.0 mg/dL 250–750 mg/day	0.21–0.42 mmol/L 0.15–0.35 mmol/L 1.48–4.43 mmol/day
Urinary sediment (see Sediment)			
Uroporphyrin	Urine, 24-hr Feces, 24-hr specimen Erythrocytes (heparin or EDTA)	<50 μg/day 10–40 μg/day	<60 nmol/day 12-48 nmol/day Negative
Vanillylmandelic acid (VMA)	Urine, 24-hr	2–7 mg/day	10.1–35.4 μmol/day
Viscosity	Serum		1.10–1.22 centipoise
Vitamin A	Serum	30–80 μg/dL	1.05–2.8 μmol/L
Vitamin B_1 (Thiamine)	Serum	0–2 μg/dL	0–75 nmol/L
Vitamin B_2 (Riboflavin)	Serum	4–24 μg/dL	106–638 nmol/L
Vitamin B_6	Plasma (EDTA)	5–30 ng/mL	20–121 nmol/L
Vitamin B_{12}	Serum	200–835 pg/mL	148–616 pmol/L
Vitamin C	Plasma (oxalate, heparin, or EDTA)	0.5–1.5 mg/dL 5–50 μg/day	28–85 μmol/L 0.67–0.665 μmol/day
Vitamin D_3, 1,25-dihydroxy	Serum	25–45 pg/mL	60–108 pmol/L
Vitamin D_3, 25-hydroxy	Plasma (heparin)	Summer: 15–80 ng/mL Winter: 14–42 ng/mL	37.4–200 nmol/L 34.9–105 nmol/L
Vitamin E	Serum	5.0–18.0 μg/mL	12–42 μmol/L
Zinc	Serum	70–150 μg/dL	10.7–22.9 μmol/L

TABLE APPENDIX–3 HEMATOLOGY AND COAGULATION

Test	Specimen	Reference Interval (Conventional Units)	Reference Interval (International Units)
Activated partial thromboplastin time (APTT)	Plasma (Na citrate)		25–35 sec
Antithrombin III	Plasma (Na citrate)	85–115% of normal human plasma	0.85–1.15
Bleeding time (BT)	Blood from skin		
Ivy			Normal: 2–7 min Borderline: 7–11 min
Simplate (G-D)			2.75–8 min
Blood volume	Whole blood (heparin)		M: 52–83 mL/kg F: 50–75 mL/kg
Bone marrow	Bone marrow aspirate	% (mean)	Number fraction (mean)
Differential count			
Myeoblasts		0.3–5.0(2.0)	0.003–0.05 (0.02)
Promyelocytes		1.0–8.0 (5.0)	0.01–0.08 (0.05)
Myelocytes			
Neutrophilic		5.0–19.0 (12.0)	0.05–0.19 (0.12)
Eosinophilic		0.5–3.0 (1.5)	0.005–0.03 (0.015)
Basophilic		0.0–0.5 (0.3)	0.00–0.005 (0.003)
Metamyelocytes		13.0–32.0 (22.0)	0.13–0.32 (0.22)
Polymorphonuclear neutrophils		0.7–3.0 (2.0)	0.007–0.03 (0.02)
Polymorphonuclear eosinophils		0.5–4.0 (2.0)	0.005–0.04 (0.02)
Polymorphonuclear basophils		0.0–0.7 (0.2)	0.0–0.007 (0.002)
Lymphocytes		3.0–17.0 (10.0)	0.03–0.17 (0.10)
Plasma cells		0.0–2.0 (0.4)	0.00–0.02 (0.004)
Monocytes		0.5–5.0 (2.0)	0.005–0.05 (0.02)
Reticulum cells		0.1–2.0 (0.2)	0.001–0.02 (0.002)
Megakaryocytes		0.3–3.0 (1.0)	0.003–0.03 (0.01)
Pronormoblasts		1.0–8.0 (4.0)	0.01–0.08 (0.04)
Normoblasts		7.0–32.0 (18.0)	0.07–0.32 (0.18)
Clot lysis, 37° C	Whole clotted blood		47–72 hr
Clot retraction screen	Whole blood (no anticoagulant)		Retraction begins at 1 hr maximum at 24 hr
Clotting time, Lee-White, 37° C	Whole blood (no anticoagulant)		5–8 min
Differential count (see Bone Marrow Differential Count or Leukocyte Differential Count)			
Eosinophil count	Whole blood (EDTA); capillary blood	50–400 cells/μL (mm³)	50–400 × 10⁶ cells/L
Erythrocyte count (RBC count)	Whole blood (EDTA)	×10⁶ cells/μL M: 4.3–5.7 F: 3.8–5.1	×10¹² cells/L 4.3–5.7 3.8–5.1
Erythrocyte sedimentation rate (ESR), Wintrobe			M: 0–15 mm/hr F: 0–20 mm/hr
Ferritin (see Table Appendix–2)			
Fibrin degradation products (agglutination, Thrombo-Wellco test)	Whole blood: special tube containing thrombin and proteolytic inhibitor	<10 μg/mL <0.25 μg/mL	<10 mg/L <0.25 mg/L
Fibrinogen	Plasma (Na citrate)	200–400 mg/dL	2.00–4.00 g/L
Glucose-6-phosphate dehydrogenase (G6PD) in erythrocytes	Whole blood (ACD, EDTA, or heparin)	12.1 ± 2.09 U/g Hb (1 SD)	0.78 ± 0.13 MU/mol Hb (1 SD)
Haptoglobin (Hp)	Serum; avoid hemolysis	26–85 mg/dL	260–1850 mg/L
Hematocrit (HCT, Hct)	Whole blood (EDTA)		
Calculated from MCV and RBC (electronic displacement or laser)		M: 39–49% F: 35–45%	0.39–0.49 volume fraction 0.35–0.45 volume fraction*
Hemoglobin (Hb)	Whole blood (EDTA)	M: 13.5–17.5 g/dL F: 12.0–16.0 g/dL	2.09–2.71 mmol/L 1.86–2.48 mmol/L
	Plasma (heparin, ACD)	<3 mg/dL	<0.47 μmol/L
	Urine, fresh, random		Negative

TABLE APPENDIX–3 HEMATOLOGY AND COAGULATION—cont'd

Test	Specimen	Reference Interval (Conventional Units)		Reference Interval (International Units)	
Hemoglobin electrophoresis	Whole blood (EDTA, citrate, or heparin)			Mass function	
		HbA > 95%		HbA > 0.95	
		HbA_2 1.5–3.5%		HbA_2 0.15–0.35	
		HbF < 2%		HbF < 0.02	
Leukocyte count (WBC count)	Whole blood (EDTA)	4.5–11.0 × 10^3 cells/μL (mm^3)		4.5–11.0 × 10^9 cells/L	
	CSF	0.5 mononuclear cells/μL		0.5 × 10^6 cells/L	
Leukocyte	Whole blood (EDTA)	% Cells/μL (mm^3)		Number fraction cells × 10^6/L	
Differential count					
Myelocytes		0	0	0	0
Neutrophils—bands		3–5	150–400	0.03–0.05	150–400
Neutrophils—segmented		54–62	3000–5800	0.54–0.62	3000–5800
Lymphocytes		23–33	1500–3000	0.23–0.33	1500–3000
Monocytes		3–7	285–500	0.03–0.07	285–500
Eosinophils		1–3	50–250	0.01–0.03	50–250
Basophils		0–0.75	15–50	0–0.0075	15–50
Leukocyte	CSF	%		Number fraction	
Differential count					
Lymphocytes		62 ± 34		0.62 ± 0.34	
Monocytes (includes pia-arachnoid mesothelial cells)		36 ± 20		0.36 ± 0.20	
Neutrophils		2 ± 5		0.02 ± 0.05	
Histocytes				Rare	
Ependymal cells				Rare	
Eosinophils				Rare	
Mean corpuscular hemoglobin (MCH)	Whole blood (EDTA)	26–34 pg/cell		0.40–0.53 fmol/cell	
Mean corpuscular hemoglobin centration (MCHC)	Whole blood (EDTA)	31–37% Hb/cell or gHb/dL RBC		4.81–5.74 mmolHb/L RBC	
Mean corpuscular volume (MCV)	Whole blood (EDTA)			80–100 fL	
Methemoglobin (MetHb)	Whole blood (EDTA, heparin, or ACD)	0.06–0.24 g/dL		9.3–37.2 μmol/L	
Plasma volume	Plasma (heparin)	M: 25–43 mL/kg F: 28–45 mL/kg		0.025-0.043 L/kg 0.028–0.045 L/kg	
Platelet count (thrombocyte count)	Whole blood (EDTA)	150–450 × 10^3/μL (mm^3)		150–450 × 10^9/L	
Prothrombin consumption	Whole blood (no anticoagulant)			>30 sec	
Prothrombin time, one-stage	Plasma (Na citrate)	Reference values will vary with the type of thromboplastin		In general: 11–16 sec	
International normalized ratio (INR)		Relevant only in patients on warfarin (see Chapter 188, Antithrombotic Therapy Prevention): $INR = \left[\frac{\text{Patient PT}}{\text{Normal mean PT}}\right]^{ISI\dagger}$ ISI = International Sensitivity Index of thromboplastin		INR 2.0–3.0	
RBC count (see Erythrocyte Count)					
Red cell volume	Whole blood (heparin)	M: 20–36 mL/kg F: 19–31 mL/kg		M: 0.020–0.036 L/kg F: 0.019–0.031 L/kg	
Reticulocyte count	Whole blood (EDTA, heparin, or oxalate)	0.5–1.5% of erythrocytes		0.005–0.015 (number fraction)	
Sulfhemoglobin	Whole blood (EDTA, heparin, or EDTA)	≤1.0% of total Hb		<0.010 of total Hb (mass fraction)	
Thrombin time	Whole blood (Na citrate)			Time of control ±25 when control is 9–13 sec	
Thromboplastin time, activated (see Activated partial thromboplastin time [APTT])					

TABLE APPENDIX–4 DRUGS: THERAPEUTIC AND TOXIC

Drug	Specimen	Reference Interval (Conventional Units)		Reference Interval (International Units)
Acetaminophen	Serum or plasma (heparin or EDTA)	Therapeutic: Toxic:	10–30 μg/mL >200 μg/mL	66–199 μmol/L >1324 μmol/L
Amikacin	Serum or plasma (EDTA)	Therapeutic: Peak Trough (severe infection) Toxic: Peak Trough	 25–35 μg/mL 4–8 μg/mL >35 μg/mL >10 μg/mL	 43–60 μmol/L 6.8–13.7 μmol/L >60 μmol/L >17 μmol/L
ε-Aminocaproic acid	Serum or plasma (heparin or EDTA); trough	Therapeutic:	100–400 μg/mL	0.76–3.05 mmol/L
Amitriptyline	Serum or plasma (heparin or EDTA); trough (>12 hr after dose)	Therapeutic: Toxic:	120–250 ng/mL >500 ng/mL	433–903 nmol/L >1805 nmol/L
Amobarbital	Serum	Therapeutic: Toxic:	1–5 μg/mL >10 μg/mL	4-22 μmol/L >44 μmol/L
Amphetamine	Serum or plasma (heparin or EDTA)	Therapeutic: Toxic:	20–30 ng/mL >200 ng/mL	148–222 nmol/L >1480 nmol/L
Bromide	Serum	Toxic:	>1250 μg/mL	>15.6 mmol/L
Caffeine	Serum or plasma (heparin or EDTA)	Therapeutic: Toxic:	3–15 μg/mL >50 μg/mL	15–77 μmol/L >258 μmol/L
Carbamazepine	Serum or plasma (heparin or EDTA); trough	Therapeutic: Toxic:	4–12 μg/mL >15 μg/mL	17–51 μmol/L >63 μmol/L
Carbenicillin	Serum or plasma	Therapeutic: Toxic:	Dependent on minimum inhibitory concentration of specific organism >250 μg/mL	Same >660 μmol/L
Chloramphenicol	Serum or plasma (heparin or EDTA); trough	Therapeutic: Toxic:	10–25 μg/L >25 μg/mL	31–77 μmol/L >77 μmol/L
Chlordiazepoxide	Serum or plasma (heparin or EDTA); trough	Therapeutic: Toxic:	700–1000 ng/mL >5000 ng/mL	2.34–3.34 μmol/L >16.7 μmol/L
Chlorpromazine	Serum or plasma (heparin or EDTA); trough	Therapeutic: Toxic:	50–300 ng/mL >750 ng/mL	157–942 nmol/L >2355 nmol/L
Cimetidine	Serum or plasma (heparin or EDTA); trough	Therapeutic:	0.5–1.2 μg/mL	2–5 μmol/L
Clonazepam	Serum or plasma (heparin or EDTA); trough	Therapeutic: Toxic:	15–60 ng/mL >80 ng/mL	48–190 nmol/L >254 nmol/L
Clonidine	Serum or plasma (heparin or EDTA)	Therapeutic:	1.0–2.0 ng/mL	4.4–8.7 nmol/L
Clorazepate	Serum or plasma (heparin or EDTA)	As desmethyldiazepam: Therapeutic:	 0.12–1.0 μg/mL	 0.36–3.01 μmol/L
Cocaine	Serum or plasma (heparin or EDTA) on ice	Therapeutic: Toxic:	100–500 ng/mL >1000 ng/mL	330–1650 nmol/L >3300 nmol/L
Codeine	Serum	Therapeutic: Toxic:	10–100 ng/mL >200 ng/mL	33–334 nmol/L >668 nmol/L
Cyclosporine	Serum (12 hr after dose)	Therapeutic: Toxic:	100–400 ng/mL >400 ng/mL	83–333 nmol/L >333 nmol/L
Desipramine	Serum or plasma (heparin or EDTA); trough (≥12 hr after dose)	Therapeutic: Toxic:	75–300 ng/mL >400 ng/mL	281–1125 nmol/L >1500 nmol/L
Diazepam	Serum or plasma (heparin or EDTA); trough	Therapeutic: Toxic:	100–1000 ng/mL >5000 ng/mL	0.35–3.51 μmol/L >17.55 μmol/L
Digitoxin	Serum or plasma (heparin or EDTA) ≥6 hr after dose	Therapeutic: Toxic:	20–35 ng/mL >45 ng/mL	26–46 nmol/L >59 nmol/L
Digoxin	Serum or plasma (heparin or EDTA) trough (≥12 hr after dose)	Therapeutic: Congestive heart failure Arrhythmias: Toxic:	 0.8–1.5 ng/mL 1.5–20 ng/mL >2.5 ng/mL	 1.0–1.9 nmol/L 1.9–2.6 nmol/L >3.2 nmol/L
Diphenylhydantoin (see Phenytoin)				

Appendix

TABLE APPENDIX–4 DRUGS: THERAPEUTIC AND TOXIC—cont'd

Drug	Specimen	Reference Interval (Conventional Units)		Reference Interval (International Units)
Disopyramide	Serum or plasma (heparin or EDTA); trough	Therapeutic:		
		Arrhythmias:		
		Atrial	2.8–3.2 μg/mL	8.3–9.4 μmol/L
		Ventricular	3.3–7.5 μg/mL	9.7–22 μmol/L
		Toxic:	>7 μg/mL	>20.7 μmol/L
Doxepin	Serum or plasma (heparin or EDTA); trough (≥12 hr after dose)	Therapeutic:	30–150 ng/mL	107–537 nmol/L
		Toxic:	>500 ng/mL	>1790 nmol/L
Ephedrine	Serum	Therapeutic:	0.05–0.10 μg/mL	0.30–0.61 μmol/L
		Toxic:	>2 μg/mL	>12.1 μmol/L
Ethchlorvynol	Serum or plasma (heparin or EDTA)	Therapeutic:	2–8 μg/mL	14–55 μmol/L
		Toxic:	>20 μg/mL	>138 μmol/L
Ethosuximide	Serum or plasma (heparin or EDTA); trough	Therapeutic:	40–100 μg/mL	283–708 μmol/L
		Toxic:	>150 μg/mL	>1062 μmol/L
Fenoprofen	Plasma (EDTA)	Therapeutic:	20–65 μg/mL	82–268 μmol/L
Flecainide	Serum or plasma (heparin or EDTA); trough	Therapeutic:	0.2–1.0 μg/mL	0.5–2.4 μmol/L
		Toxic:	>1.0 μg/mL	>2.4 μmol/L
Flurazepam	Serum or plasma (EDTA)	Therapeutic:	Not well defined	
		Toxic:	>0.2 μg/mL	>0.5 μmol/L
Furosemide	Serum (30 min after dose)	Therapeutic:	1–2 μg/mL	3–6 μmol/L
Gentamicin	Serum or plasma (EDTA)	Therapeutic:		
		Peak (severe infection)	8–10 μg/mL	16.7–20.9 μmol/L
		Trough (severe infection)	<2–4 μg/mL	<4.2–8.4 μmol/L
		Toxic:		
		Peak	>10 μg/mL	>21 μmol/L
		Trough	>4 μg/mL	>8.4 μmol/L
Glutethimide	Serum	Therapeutic:	2–6 μg/mL	9–28 μmol/L
		Toxic:	>5 μg/mL	>23 μmol/L
Haloperidol	Serum or plasma (heparin or EDTA)	Therapeutic:	6–245 ng/mL	16–652 nmol/L
		Toxic:	Not defined	
Ibuprofen	Serum or plasma (heparin or EDTA)	Therapeutic:	10–50 μg/mL	49–243 μmol/L
		Toxic:	100–700 μg/mL	485–3395 μmol/L
Imipramine	Serum or plasma (heparin or EDTA); trough (≥12 hr after dose)	Therapeutic:	125–250 ng/mL	446–893 nmol/L
		Toxic:	>500 ng/mL	>1784 nmol/L
Isoniazid	Serum or plasma (heparin or EDTA)	Therapeutic:	1–7 μg/mL	7–51 μmol/L
		Toxic:	20–710 μg/mL	146–5176 μmol/L
Kanamycin	Serum or plasma (EDTA)	Therapeutic:		
		Peak	25–35 μg/mL	52–72 μmol/L
		Trough (severe infection)	4–8 μg/mL	8–16 μmol/L
		Toxic:		
		Peak	>35 μg/mL	>72 μmol/L
		Trough	>10 μg/mL	>21 μmol/L
Lidocaine	Serum or plasma (heparin or EDTA); ≥45 min following bolus dose	Therapeutic:	1.5–6.0 μg/mL	6.4–26 μmol/L
		Toxic:		
		Central nervous system or cardiovascular depression	6–8 μg/mL	26–34.2 μmol/L
		Seizures, obtundation, decreased cardiac output	>8 μg/mL	>34.2 μmol/L
Lithium	Serum or plasma (heparin or EDTA); (>12 hr after last dose)	Therapeutic:	0.6–1.2 mEq/L	0.6–1.2 nmol/L
		Toxic:	>2 mEq/L	>2 mmol/L
Lorazepam	Serum or plasma (heparin or EDTA)	Therapeutic:	50–240 ng/mL	156–746 nmol/L
Meperidine	Serum or plasma (heparin or EDTA)	Therapeutic:	400–700 ng/mL	1620–2830 nmol/L
		Toxic:	>1 μg/mL	>4043 nmol/L
Meprobamate	Serum	Therapeutic:	6–12 μg/mL	28–55 μmol/L
		Toxic:	>60 μg/mL	>275 μmol/L
Methadone	Serum or plasma (heparin or EDTA)	Therapeutic:	100–400 ng/mL	0.32–1.29 μmol/L
		Toxic:	>2000 ng/mL	>6.46 μmol/L

Continued

TABLE APPENDIX–4 DRUGS: THERAPEUTIC AND TOXIC—cont'd

Drug	Specimen	Reference Interval (Conventional Units)		Reference Interval (International Units)
Methamphetamine	Serum	Therapeutic: Toxic:	0.01–0.05 μg/mL >0.5 μg/mL	0.07–0.34 μmol/L >3.35 μmol/L
Methaqualone	Serum or plasma (heparin or EDTA)	Therapeutic: Toxic:	2–3 μg/mL >10 μg/mL	8–12 μmol/L >40 μmol/L
Methotrexate	Serum or plasma (heparin or EDTA)	Therapeutic: Toxic: Low-dose therapy (1–2 wk) High-dose therapy (48 hr)	variable >9.1 ng/mL >227 ng/mL	variable >20 nmol/L >0.5 μmol/L
Methsuximide (*N*-desmethyl methsuximide)	Serum	Therapeutic: Toxic:	10–40 μg/mL >40 μg/mL	53–212 μmol/L >212 μmol/L
Methyldopa	Plasma (EDTA)	Therapeutic: Toxic:	1–5 μg/mL >7 μg/mL	4.7–23.7 μmol/L >33 μmol/L
Methyprylon	Serum	Therapeutic: Toxic:	8–10 μg/mL >50 μg/mL	43–55 μmol/L >273 μmol/L
Morphine	Serum or plasma (heparin or EDTA)	Therapeutic: Toxic:	10–80 ng/mL >200 ng/mL	35–280 nmol/L >700 nmol/L
N-Acetylprocainamide	Serum or plasma (heparin or EDTA); trough	Therapeutic: Toxic:	5–30 μg/mL >40 μg/mL	18–108 μmol/L >144 μmol/L
Netilmicin	Serum or plasma (EDTA)	Therapeutic: Peak (severe infection) Trough (severe infection) Toxic: Peak Trough	 8–10 μg/mL <4 μg/mL >12 μg/mL >4 μg/mL	 17–21 μmol/L <8 μmol/L >25 μmol/L >8 μmol/L
Nitroprusside	Serum or plasma (EDTA)	As thiocyanate: Therapeutic:	 6–29 μg/mL	 103–499 μmol/L
Nortriptyline	Serum or plasma (heparin or EDTA); trough (≥12 hr after dose)	Therapeutic: Toxic:	50–150 ng/mL >500 ng/mL	190–570 nmol/L >1,900 nmol/L
Oxazepam	Serum or plasma (heparin or EDTA)	Therapeutic:	0.2-1.4 μg/mL	0.70-4.9 μmol/L
Oxycodone	Serum	Therapeutic: Toxic:	10–100 ng/mL >200 ng/mL	32–317 nmol/L >634 nmol/L
Pentazocine	Serum or plasma (EDTA)	Therapeutic: Toxic:	0.05–0.2 μg/mL >1 μg/mL	0.2–0.7 μmol/L >3.5 μmol/L
Pentobarbital	Serum or plasma (heparin or EDTA); trough	Therapeutic, hypnotic: Therapeutic coma: Toxic:	1–5 μg/mL 20–50 μg/mL >10 μg/mL	4–22 μmol/L 88–221 μmol/L >44 μmol/L
Phenacetin	Plasma (EDTA)	Therapeutic: Toxic:	1–30 μg/mL 50–250 μg/mL	6–167 μmol/L 279–1395 μmol/L
Phencyclidine	Serum or plasma (heparin or EDTA)	Toxic:	90–800 ng/mL	370–3288 nmol/L
Phenobarbital	Serum or plasma (heparin or EDTA); trough	Therapeutic: Toxic: Slowness, ataxia, nystagmus Coma with reflexes Coma without reflexes	15–40 μg/mL 35–80 μg/mL 65–117 μg/mL >100 μg/mL	65–172 μmol/L 151–345 μmol/L 280–504 μmol/L >430 μmol/L
Phensuximide (both parent and *N*-desmethyl metabolites)	Serum or plasma (heparin or EDTA)	Therapeutic:	40–60 μg/mL	228–324 μmol/L
Phenylbutazone	Plasma (EDTA)	Therapeutic: (not well defined) Toxic:	50–100 μg/mL >100 μg/mL	162–324 μmol/L >324 μmol/mL

TABLE APPENDIX–4 **DRUGS: THERAPEUTIC AND TOXIC—cont'd**

Drug	Specimen	Reference Interval (Conventional Units)		Reference Interval (International Units)
Phenylpropanolamine	Serum	Therapeutic: Toxic:	0.05–0.10 μg/mL >5 μg/mL	0.33–0.66 μmol/L >33.7 μmol/L
Phenytoin	Serum or plasma (heparin or EDTA); trough	Therapeutic: Toxic:	10–20 μg/mL >20 μg/mL	40–79 μmol/L >79 μmol/L
Primidone	Serum or plasma (heparin or EDTA) trough	Therapeutic: Toxic:	5–12 μg/mL >15 μg/mL	23–55 μmol/L >69 μmol/L
Procainamide	Serum or plasma (heparin or EDTA); trough	Therapeutic: Toxic: Also consider effect of metabolite, *N*-acetylprocainamide	4–10 μg/mL >10–12 μg/mL	17–42 μmol/L >42–51 μmol/L
Propoxyphene	Plasma (EDTA)	Therapeutic: Toxic:	0.1–0.4 μg/mL >0.5 μg/mL	0.3–1.2 μmol/L >1.5 μmol/L
Propranolol	Serum or plasma (heparin or EDTA); trough	Therapeutic:	50–100 ng/mL	193–386 nmol/L
Protriptyline	Serum or plasma (heparin or EDTA); trough (≥12 hr after dose)	Therapeutic: Toxic:	70–250 ng/mL >500 ng/mL	266–950 nmol/L >1900 nmol/L
Quinidine	Serum or plasma (heparin or EDTA); trough	Therapeutic: Toxic:	2–5 μg/mL >6 μg/mL	6–15 μmol/L >18 μmol/L
Salicylates	Serum or plasma (heparin or EDTA); trough	Therapeutic: Toxic:	150–300 μg/mL >300 μg/mL	1086–2172 μmol/L >2,172 μmol/L
Secobarbital	Serum	Therapeutic: Toxic:	1–2 μg/mL >5 μg/mL	4.2–8.4 μmol/L >21.0 μmol/L
Theophylline	Serum or plasma (heparin or EDTA)	Therapeutic: Toxic:	8–20 μg/mL >20 μg/mL	44–111 μmol/L >110 μmol/L
Thiocyanate	Serum or plasma (EDTA)	Nonsmoker: Smoker: Therapeutic, after nitroprusside infusion:	1–4 μg/mL 3–12 μg/mL 6–29 μg/mL	17–69 μmol/L 52–206 μmol/L 103–499 μmol/L
Thiopental	Serum or plasma (heparin or EDTA); trough	Hypnotic: Coma: Anesthesia: Toxic:	1–5 μg/mL 30–100 μg/mL 7–130 μg/mL >10 μg/mL	4.1–20.7 μmol/L 124–413 μmol/L 29–536 μmol/L >41 μmol/L
Thioridazine	Serum or plasma (heparin or EDTA)	Therapeutic: Toxic:	1.0–1.5 μg/mL >10 μg/mL	2.7–4.1 μmol/L >27 μmol/L
Tobramycin	Serum or plasma (heparin or EDTA)	Therapeutic: Peak (severe infection) Trough (severe infection) Toxic: Peak Trough	 8–10 μg/mL <4 μg/mL >10 μg/mL >4 μg/mL	 17–21 μmol/L <9 μmol/L >21 μmol/L >9 μmol/L
Tocainide	Serum or plasma (heparin or EDTA)	Therapeutic:	4–10 μg/mL	21–52 μmol/L
Tolbutamide	Serum	Therapeutic: Toxic:	80–240 μg/mL >640 μg/mL	299–888 μmol/L >2368 μmol/L
Valproic acid	Serum or plasma (heparin or EDTA); trough	Therapeutic: Toxic:	50–100 μg/mL >100 μg/mL	347–693 μmol/L >693 μmol/L
Vancomycin	Serum or plasma (heparin or EDTA); trough	Therapeutic: Toxic: (not well established)	5–10 μg/mL >80–100 μg/mL	3–7 μmol/L >55–69 μmol/L
Verapamil	Serum or plasma (heparin or EDTA)	Therapeutic:	100–500 ng/mL	220–1100 nmol/L
Warfarin	Serum or plasma (heparin or EDTA)	Therapeutic:	1–10 μg/mL	3–32 μmol/L

Index

Note: Page numbers followed by f refer to figures; page numbers followed by t refer to tables. **Boldface** numbers refer to main discussions.

I